STEDMAN'S® SUBENTRY LOCATOR

A unique dictionary-within-a-dictionary that serves as a master cross-reference index of subentry terms alphabetize ... words. For additional information see page S-1.

Use it:

- **To locate the governing main entry under which an elusive subentry term will be found**
- **For information related by the commonality of like words in multiple-word terms**
- **As a handy spelling checker for modifiers**

acral lentiginous: melanoma
acrid: poison
acrocentric: chromosome
acrodynic: erythema
acrofacial: dysostosis; syndrome
acromegalic: gigantism
acromial: angle; artery; extremity; network; process; reflex
acromial articular: facies; surface
acromioclavicular: disk; joint; ligament
acromion: presentation
acromiothoracic: artery
acroparesthesia: syndrome
acrosomal: cap; granule; vesicle
acrylic: resin
acrylic resin: base; tooth; tray

cap

acrosomal c., head c.; acrosome; a collapsed membranous vesicle that covers the anterior part of the nucleus of the spermatozoon, derived from the acrosomal granule; the carbohydrate-rich substance of the c. is associated with hydrolytic enzymes.

granule

acrosomal g., the single g. within an acrosomal vesicle which results from the coalescence of proacrosomal g.'s.

vesicle

acrosomal v., a v. derived from the Golgi apparatus during spermiogenesis whose limiting membrane adheres to the nuclear envelope; together with the acrosomal granule within, it spreads in a thin layer over the pole of the nucleus to form the acrosomal cap.

---

antemortem: clot; thrombus
anterior: asynclitism; choroiditis; component; curvature; embryotoxon; guide; megalophthalmus; nephrectomy; occlusion; rhinoscopy; rhizotomy; scleritis; sclerotomy; staphyloma; symblepharon; synechia; urethritis; uveitis; vitrectomy
anterior anatomical structures (specific anterior anatomical and histological structures are listed under the following): arch; area; artery; base; border, bundle; canal; cell; chamber, column; commissure; convolution; crest; cusp; division; epithelium; extremity; fissure; fontanel; foramen; fossa; funiculus; gland; groove; gyrus; horn; joint; layer; ligament; limb; line; lip; lobe; lobule; margin; membrane; muscle; naris; nerve; node; notch; part; pillar; pituitary; plexus; pole; portal; process; pyramid; recess; region; ring; root; segment; sinus; spine; substance; sulcus; surface; tract; triangle; tooth; tubercle; valve; vein; velum; wall
anterior chamber cleavage: syndrome
anterior facial: height
anterior focal: point
anterior myocardial: infarction
anterior pelvic: exenteration
anterior pituitary: gonadotropin

Stedman's
MEDICAL DICTIONARY

25th Edition

ILLUSTRATED

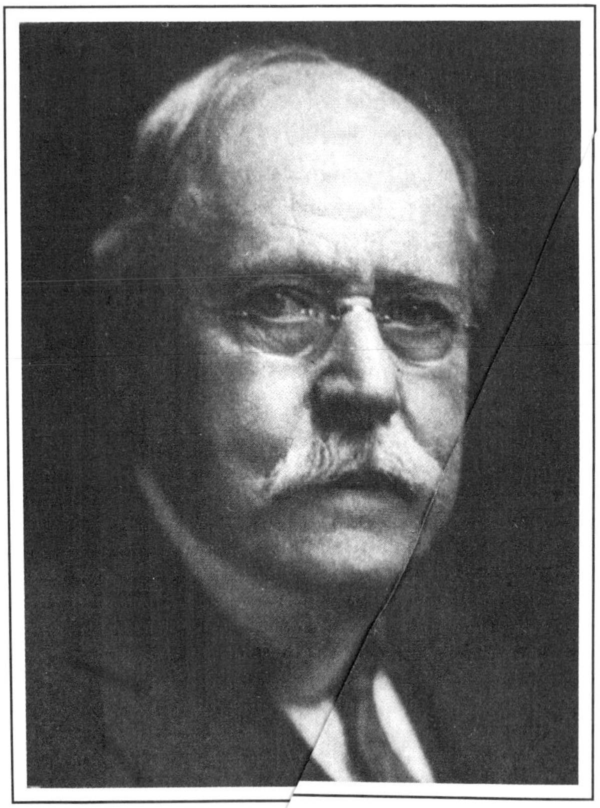

THOMAS LA HROP STEDMAN
853-1938)
Courtesy of the Library he New York Academy of Medicine

Stedman's
MEDICAL DICTIONARY

25th Edition

ILLUSTRATED

SANS TACHE

Williams & Wilkins

BALTIMORE • PHILADELPHIA • HONG KONG
LONDON • MUNICH • SYDNEY • TOKYO

A WAVERLY COMPANY

Editor: William R. Hensyl
Associate Editor: Harriet Felscher
Administrative Assistant: Julie Rodowsky
Administrative Aide: Gertrude A. Wilder
Project Editor: Bill Cady
Designers: Robert C. Och / Dan Pfisterer
Illustration Planner: Wayne J. Hubbel
Production Coordinator: Raymond E. Reter

Accurate indications, adverse reactions, and dosage schedules for drugs are provided in this book, but it is possible that they may change. The reader is urged to review the package information data of the manufacturers of the medications mentioned.

Printed in the United States of America

English Language Co-editions
Asian 1967, 1972, 1976
Indian 1967, 1973
Taiwan 1972, 1978

Translated Editions
Greek 1976
Indian 1977
Japanese 1977, 1985
Portuguese 1976
Spanish (in press)

Library of Congress Cataloging-in-Publication Data

Stedman, Thomas Lathrop, 1853–1938.
[Medical dictionary]
Stedman's medical dictionary.—25th ed.
p. cm.
ISBN 0-683-07916-6 REGULAR EDITION
ISBN 0-683-7925-5 DELUXE EDITION
1. Medicine—Dictionaries. I. Title. II. Title: Medical dictionary
[DNLM: 1. Dictionaries, Medical. W 13 S812m]
R121.S8 1989
610'.3—dc20
DNLM/DLC
for Library of Congress
89-16579
CIP

94
10

CONTENTS

LIST OF COLOR PLATES

(Between pages 824 and 825)

LIST OF TABLES

(According to Main Entry Title)

CONSULTANTS

William K. Beatty — **Etymology, Biography, and History**
Professor of Medical Bibliography, Northwestern University Medical School, Chicago, Illinois

Everett S. Beneke, Ph.D. — **Mycology**
Professor, Departments of Microbiology and Public Health and of Botany and Plant Pathology, Michigan State University, East Lansing, Michigan

Alfred Jay Bollet, M.D. — **Internal Medicine**
Clinical Professor of Medicine, Yale University School of Medicine, New Haven, Connecticut; Adjunct Professor of Medicine, New York Medical College, New York, New York; Chairman, Department of Medicine, Danbury Hospital, Danbury, Connecticut; Editor, *Resident and Staff Physician*

M. Desmond Burke, M.D. — **Clinical Pathology, Hematology, and Laboratory Medicine**
Professor of Pathology and Director of Clinical Laboratories, School of Medicine and University Hospital, State University of New York at Stony Brook, Stony Brook, New York

Michael J. Burridge, B.V.M.&S., M.P.V.M., Ph.D. — **Veterinary Medicine**
Chairman and Professor, Department of Infectious Diseases, College of Veterinary Medicine, University of Florida, Gainesville, Florida

Malcolm B. Carpenter, M.D. — **Neuroanatomy**
Professor of Anatomy, F. Edward Hébert School of Medicine, Uniformed Services University of the Health Sciences, Bethesda, Maryland

Waldo E. Cohn, Ph.D. — **Biochemistry and Chemistry**
Senior Biochemist, Retired, and Consultant, Biology Division, Oak Ridge National Laboratory, Oak Ridge, Tennessee; Director, Office of Biochemical Nomenclature; Editor, *Progress in Nucleic Acid Research and Molecular Biology*

Clark E. Corliss, Ph.D. — **Embryology**
Professor Emeritus of Anatomy, University of Tennessee, Memphis, Tennessee

Donald J. Ferguson, M.D., Ph.D. — **General Surgery**
Professor Emeritus of Surgery, University of Chicago, Chicago, Illinois

John P. Frazer, M.D. — **Otorhinolaryngology**
Professor of Otolaryngology, University of Rochester Medical Center, Rochester, New York

Robert M. Goldwyn, M.D. — **Plastic and Reconstructive Surgery**
Clinical Professor of Surgery, Harvard Medical School, Boston, Massachusetts; Editor, *Plastic and Reconstructive Surgery*

Nicholas M. Greene, M.D. **Anesthesiology**
Professor of Anesthesiology, Yale University School of Medicine, New Haven, Connecticut

Donald Heyneman, Ph.D. **Parasitology**
Professor of Parasitology, University of California, San Francisco, California; Associate Dean for Health and Medical Sciences, School of Public Health, University of California, Berkeley, California; Chairman, University of California, Berkeley/University of California, San Francisco, Joint Medical Progress

Frank Hinman, Jr., M.D. **Urology and Urologic Surgery**
Clinical Professor of Urology, University of California, San Francisco, California

Joseph L. Hirschmann, Pharm. D. **Pharmacology and Toxicology**
General Manager, First DataBank, San Bruno, California

Paul B. Hoffer, M.D. **Nuclear Medicine**
Professor of Diagnostic Radiology and Director, Section of Nuclear Medicine, Yale University School of Medicine, New Haven, Connecticut

Steven E. Hyler, M.D. **Psychiatry**
Associate Clinical Professor of Psychiatry, Columbia University, and Psychiatrist, New York State Psychiatric Institute, New York, New York

Naomi M. Kanof, M.D.† **Dermatology**
Clinical Professor Emeritus of Medicine (Dermatology), Georgetown University School of Medicine, and Dermatologist in Private Practice, Washington, D.C.

Frederick H. Kasten, Ph.D. **Stains and Staining Procedures**
Professor of Anatomy, Louisiana State University Medical Center, New Orleans, Louisiana

Ralph H. Kellogg, M.D., Ph.D. **Physiology**
Professor of Physiology, University of California, San Francisco, California

E. Frederick Lang, M.D. **Radiology**
Radiologist, Retired, Grosse Pointe, Michigan

Edwin H. Lennette, M.D., Ph.D. **Immunology and Virology**
California Public Health Foundation and Director Emeritus, Viral and Rickettsial Diseases Laboratory, California Department of Health Services, Berkeley, California

Erwin F. Lessel, Ph.D. **Bacteriology**
Chief Editor, Editorial Services Department, Lederle Laboratories, Pearl River, New York

Joseph D. Matarazzo, Ph.D. **Psychology**
Chairman, Department of Medical Psychology, School of Medicine, Oregon Health Sciences University, Portland, Oregon

†Deceased

David N. Menton, Ph.D. **Histology**
Associate Professor of Anatomy, Washington University School of Medicine, St. Louis, Missouri

Edmond A. Murphy, M.D., Sc.D. **Genetics**
Professor of Medicine, The Johns Hopkins University School of Medicine, Baltimore, Maryland

Frank W. Newell, M.D., M.Sc. **Ophthalmology**
Raymond Distinguished Professor of Ophthalmology, The University of Chicago, Chicago, Illinois; Editor-in-Chief, *American Journal of Ophthalmology*

Maxine Patrick, R.N., Dr.P.H. **Nursing**
Professor, Department of Physiological Nursing, University of Washington School of Nursing, Seattle, Washington

Leonard F. Peltier, M.D., Ph.D. **Orthopaedics**
Professor and Acting Head, Department of Surgery, University of Arizona Health Sciences Center, Tucson, Arizona

Roy R. Peterson, Ph.D. **Gross Anatomy**
Professor Emeritus and Lecturer in Anatomy, Washington University School of Medicine, St. Louis, Missouri

George S. Schuster, D.D.S., Ph.D. **Dentistry**
Ione and Arthur Merritt Professor, Coordinator of Oral Biology/Microbiology, School of Dentistry, Medical College of Georgia, Augusta, Georgia

Thomas W. Shields, M.D. **Thoracic Surgery**
Professor of Surgery, Northwestern University Medical School, Chicago, Illinois

E. Stewart Taylor, M.D. **Obstetrics and Gynecology**
Professor Emeritus of Obstetrics and Gynecology, University of Colorado School of Medicine, Denver, Colorado; Editor, *Obstetrical and Gynecological Survey*

A. Earl Walker, M.D. **Neurology, Neuropathology, and Neurosurgery**
Professor Emeritus of Neurological Surgery, The Johns Hopkins University School of Medicine, Baltimore, Maryland; Professor Emeritus of Neurology and Neurosurgery, The University of New Mexico School of Medicine, Albuquerque, New Mexico

William H. Wehrmacher, M.D. **Cardiology**
Clinical Professor of Medicine and Adjunct Professor of Physiology, Loyola University Stritch School of Medicine, Maywood, Illinois

Colin Wood, M.D. **Pathological Anatomy**
Professor of Pathology and Dermatology, University of Maryland School of Medicine, Baltimore, Maryland

CONTRIBUTORS

Mary L. Borysewicz, Managing Editor, *American Journal of Ophthalmology*

Show-Hong Duh, Ph.D., Department of Pathology, University of Maryland School of Medicine, Baltimore, Maryland

Thomas R. Koch, Ph.D., D.A.B.C.C., Department of Pathology, University of Maryland School of Medicine, Baltimore, Maryland

David L. Schaffner, D.D.S., M.D., Department of Pathology, Baylor College of Medicine, Houston, Texas

Jorge Sequeiros, M.D., Assistant Professor of Medical Genetics, Instituto de Ciências Biomédicas de Abel Salazar, Universidade do Porto, Portugal

ILLUSTRATORS

Diane Abeloff, Medical Illustrator, Baltimore, Maryland

Ranice W. Crosby, Associate Professor Emeritus and Director Emeritus, Department of Art as Applied to Medicine, The Johns Hopkins University School of Medicine, Baltimore, Maryland

A. Hooker Goodwin, Professor Emeritus of Medical and Dental Illustration, University of Illinois at the Medical Center, Chicago, Illinois

Lydia V. Kubiuk, Medical Illustrator, Baltimore, Maryland

Biagio J. Melloni, Ph.D., Medical Illustrator, Bethesda, Maryland

ILLUSTRATION CREDITS

Basmajian, J.V.: *Grant's Method of Anatomy,* 9th ed. Baltimore: Williams & Wilkins, 1975. Kidney

Basmajian, J.V.: *Primary Anatomy,* 7th ed. Baltimore: Williams & Wilkins, 1976. Anterior View of Normal Heart

Carpenter, M.B.: *Human Neuroanatomy,* 7th ed. Baltimore: Williams & Wilkins, 1976. Brodmann's Areas, Capsula Interna, Gamma Loop, Segments of Spinal Cord (Medulla Spinalis), Mesencephalon

Comroe, J.H., Jr.: *The Lung,* 2nd ed. Chicago: Year Book Medical Publishers, 1962. Subdivisions of Total Lung Capacity

Copenhaver, W.M., Kelley, D.E., and Wood, R.L.: *Bailey's Textbook of Histology,* 17th ed. Baltimore: Williams & Wilkins, 1978. Cell, Mature Human Spermatozoon

Corliss, C.B.: *Patten's Human Embryology.* New York: McGraw-Hill Book Co., 1976. Ovary

Davey, T.H.: *Guide to Human Parasitology.* London: H.K. Lewis & Co., Ltd., 1958. *Ascaris lumbricoides*

Gorin, G., and Posner, A.: *Slit-Lamp Gonioscopy,* 3rd ed. Baltimore: Williams & Wilkins, 1967. Optics of Goldmann Gonioscopic Mirror

Herndon, C.N., in Morehead, R.P.: *Human Pathology.* New York: McGraw-Hill Book Co., 1965. Chromosome Aberrations

Hobbins, J.C., and Winsberg, F.: *Ultrasonography in Obstetrics and Gynecology.* Baltimore: Williams & Wilkins, 1977. Ultrasonography

Langman, J.: *Medical Embryology,* 4th ed. Baltimore: Williams & Wilkins, 1981. Human Blastocyst, Coloboma Iridis, Neural Crest, Meckel's Diverticulum, Embryo, Epispadias and Ectopia of Bladder, Tracheoesophageal Fistula, Maturing Follicle, Fonticuli in Skull of Newborn, Congenital Diaphragmatic Hernia, Hypospadias, Karyotype of Normal Human Cell, Embryonic Germ Layers, Cleft Lip, Omphalocele, Cleft Palate, Full Term Placenta, Sclerotome, Scrotum, Spina Bifida

Najarian, H.H.: *Textbook of Medical Parasitology.* Baltimore: Williams & Wilkins, 1967. *Cimex lectularis, Demodex folliculorum, Entamoeba histolytica, Giardia lamblia, Ornithodoros moubata, Pediculus humanus, Pthirus pubis, Sarcoptes scabiei*

Patten, B.M.: *Human Embryology,* 3rd ed. New York: McGraw-Hill Book Co., 1968. Amnion

Patten, B.M., and Carlson, B.A.: *Foundations of Embryology.* New York: McGraw-Hill Book Co., 1974. Formation of Gastrocele

Proctor, D.F.: *Anesthesia and Otolaryngology.* Baltimore: Williams & Wilkins, 1957. Tracheotomy

Salter, R.B.: *Textbook of Disorders and Injuries of the Musculoskeletal System.* Baltimore: Williams & Wilkins, 1970. Herniated Disk, Epiphyses of Femur

Schultz, R.J.: *The Language of Fractures.* Baltimore: Williams & Wilkins, 1972. Pseudarthrosis, Subluxation

Spaltsholz, W.: *Hand Atlas of Human Anatomy.* Philadelphia: J.B. Lippincott Co., 1959. Auricle of Ear

Taylor, E.S.: *Beck's Obstetrical Practice and Fetal Medicine,* 10th ed. Baltimore: Williams & Wilkins, 1976. Deceleration, Extraction, Types of Female Pelvis

Youmans, W.B.: *Fundamentals of Human Physiology,* 2nd ed. Chicago: Year Book Medical Publishers, 1962. Nomenclature of Lung Volumes

PUBLISHER'S PREFACE

This 25th edition of *Stedman's Medical Dictionary* celebrates a tradition of over one and one-half centuries of American medical lexicography and an ongoing dedication of the dictionary to the needs of the medical and allied health professions.

The tradition began in 1833 with publication of the first American medical dictionary, Dr. Robley Dunglison's *A New Dictionary of Medical Science and Literature,* a work that continued through successive editions until the 23rd edition, which was edited by Thomas Lathrop Stedman, M.D., in 1903. Five years later, respect for an "institution" from which he had learned the language of medicine prompted Dr. Stedman to write a modernized version of the Dunglison dictionary. It was published in 1911 as *A Practical Medical Dictionary* and now is commonly known as *Stedman's*.

By the early 1970s, *Stedman's* led the way as the first American medical dictionary to use database publishing in the form of electronic storage, retrieval, updating, and composition. Another first followed with the adaptation of this innovation to incorporate terms in the 1982 edition into electronic software as a stand-alone medical spelling reference and as part of editorial processing systems. Existing and developing technologies appear to offer limitless possibilities for development and dissemination of "word information" products drawn from the *Stedman's* database and tailored to the needs of any segment of the health-care market.

"User-friendly" is a concept that has been universally applied to computer hardware and software to promote easy and efficient use by both novice and expert. It is a concept that is equally applicable to the print media. Making *Stedman's* easier to use and easier to read has been a major focus in the preparation of this edition, from design of its specifications through construction of its individual entries. First-time medical dictionary users as well as seasoned veterans will immediately appreciate the difference.

Our increased page trim size enhances readability by allowing more white space around the vocabulary entries, wider text columns, and a larger and more open typeface. The traditional main entry-subentry format has been revamped to facilitate scanning for the sought-after term. In multiple-definition entries, the definition numbers are in boldface to distinguish each definition further.

The phonetic spelling used for pronunciation of entry terms has been simplified to a broad transcription to avoid inclusion of esoteric phonetic symbols, the need to remember a variety of stylistic conventions, and frequent consultation of the pronunciation key. For the most part, the phonetic spelling incorporates commonly understood sounds that are encountered in everyday English words.

The "*Stedman's* Subentry Locator," which now conveniently precedes section *A* of the vocabulary, is unique among medical dictionaries. It functions as an index of the adjectival or descriptive words in subentry terms cross-referenced to the main entries under which the subentries are found. This feature is a particularly useful tool for the dictionary user who is unfamiliar with the main entry-subentry format common to many medical and specialty dictionaries and who would seek a multiple-word term at the strictly alphabetical location common to general language dictionaries.

Users of *Stedman's* are urged to read carefully the section, "How to Use This Dictionary," which follows this preface. There the organization, format, and style of the dictionary are clearly explained, and actual vocabulary entries serve as illustrative examples. An understanding of the principles of *Stedman's* organization, format, and style not only will save time through an efficient search for information but also will increase the amount of information obtained.

The "Medical Etymology" section has been rewritten to concentrate on the principles of word formation that underlie the creation of medical and scientific terms, with special consideration given to the needs of those users of the dictionary who approach its vocabulary without a background in Greek and Latin.

Each entry in the present vocabulary of approximately 100,000 entries has been reviewed by at least one of the 36 specialty consultants, frequently by three, and often by five or six. This ongoing multispecialty review resulted in the addition and substantial revision (often re-revision) of over 10,000 entries. Noteworthy updating occurred in the terminologies of molecular biology, immunology, infectious diseases, endocrinology, genetics, and psychiatry and psychology. Four appendices, "Comparative Temperature Scales," "Temperature Equivalents," "Weights and Measures," and "Laboratory Reference Range Values," have been revised and updated to include SI units and equivalents.

During this editing cycle we continued to strive for optimum clarity of definitions by rewriting to make them as readable as possible within the constraints of conciseness. As an aid to understanding, all major words in a definition that one would expect to find in a medical dictionary can be found as defined entries in the vocabulary. However, the terminology of many advanced, sophisticated subjects frequently contains terms that can be adequately and clearly defined only to users who have had at least some basic introduction to the material.

Stedman's Medical Dictionary is a working dictionary, a record of a living language. As such, its words are formed, spelled, pronounced, and defined as they are used rather than as they should be. Every dictionary contains numerous words that by philological standards are misformed, misspelled, mispronounced, and misused. A dictionary may suggest standards, as by choosing to place definitions with the terms of an official nomenclature, but it cannot enforce them. *Stedman's,* therefore, serves as a guide for those who wish to speak and write more precisely and to coin new words more accurately.

Acknowledgments

This edition of *Stedman's,* like previous editions, is a tribute to its consultants and contributors, who are listed on the pages immediately preceding this preface. Their generous assistance in the form of recommended new entries, revisions, and "words of wisdom" has been invaluable to the preparation of this edition and doubtlessly will benefit editions to come.

We regret that it is not possible to cite individually all of the nomenclatures, glossaries, compendia, references, textbooks, journals, and other literature sources from which our entries have been derived. Our sincere appreciation is extended to the authors, editors, and publishers of the anonymous publications for their indirect contributions.

Special credit is due the copy editors of Williams & Wilkins and of Waverly Press who, as a result of regularly consulting *Stedman's* during the course of their work on book and journal manuscripts, have provided us with many useful ideas to enhance the dictionary's content.

We thank the numerous *Stedman's* owners who have written us to suggest new entries and revisions and to correct the inevitable errors. We welcome your comments on this edition.

WILLIAMS & WILKINS

William R. Hensyl
Managing Editor

HOW TO USE THIS DICTIONARY

ORGANIZATION OF THE VOCABULARY

Main Entry-Subentry Format

Entries in the vocabulary generally adhere to the organization of multiple-word terms located as subentries under governing single-word *noun* main entries, in an index-like arrangement. Thus, "hemorrhagic fever," "Q fever," and "Rocky Mountain spotted fever" will be found under *fever*; "carcinoid tumor," "giant cell tumor of bone," and "Wilms' tumor" will be found under *tumor*:

fever (fē'ver) [A.S. *fefer*]. Pyrexia; febris. **1.** A bodily temperature above the normal of 98.6°F (37°C). **2.** A disease in which there is an

hemorrhagic f., a syndrome that occurs in perhaps 20 to 40% of infections by arboviruses of the hemorrhagic f. group: al-

Q f. [*Q,* for "query," so named because etiologic agent was unknown], a disease caused by *Coxiella burnetii,* which is propagated

Rocky Mountain spotted f., an acute infectious disease of high mortality, characterized by frontal and occipital headache, intense

tumor (tū'mŏr) [L. *tumor,* a swelling]. **1.** Any swelling or tumefaction. **2.** Neoplasm. **3.** One of the four signs of inflammation (t., ca-

carcinoid t., argentaffinoma; a usually small, slow-growing neoplasm composed of islands of rounded, oxyphilic, or spindle-

giant cell t. of bone, giant cell myeloma; osteoclastoma; a soft, reddish brown, sometimes malignant, osteolytic t. composed of

Wilms' t., adenomyosarcoma; embryoma of the kidney; mesoblastic nephroma; nephroblastoma; renal carcinosarcoma; a malig-

In a specialty dictionary, as contrasted with a general language dictionary, the advantages of such categorization in an index-like arrangement of entries are obvious.

Verbs, adjectives, adverbs, combining forms, prefixes, abbreviations, and symbols follow the general rules of indexing and thus are located as main entries.

Multiple-word Terms as Main Entries

Certain multiple-word terms, such as compound words or chemical and drug terms, may deviate from the standard main entry-subentry format.

Compound words that usually are written closed up as one word or that are hyphenated are located as main entries rather than as subentries under the portion of the term that would otherwise represent the main entry. For example, "aftercontraction" is located in the *A's* rather than under *contraction*; "self-hypnosis" is located in the *S's* rather than under *hypnosis*.

Multiple-word chemical and drug terms generally are located as main entries unless the term includes a general noun that would logically be considered a type or kind or when the term's location as a subentry would appear to be illogical or forced. For example, "adrenergic blocking agent" (a type of agent) is under *agent,* but "Agent Orange" (a specific compound) is a main entry; "bile acid" (a type of acid) is under *acid,* but "acid red" (a stain that is neither an acid nor red) and "ribonucleic acid" (a molecule rather than an acid) are main entries.

Users of the dictionary who initially may be unable to discern the appropriate location of such terms should look for them at the alphabetical locations of the specific words making up the term.

Multiple-word Terms as Subentries

An elusive multiple-word term may be located as a subentry under another main entry that is synonymous with the *noun* in the sought-after term. For example, a certain surgical "procedure" might be spoken of or written about as an "operation," "technique," or "method" and be found under one of those main entries; similarly, "disease" and "syndrome" frequently are used interchangeably. At such main entries, a cross-reference will refer the user to the alternative main entries under which the desired term may be located as a subentry:

> **operation** (op-er-ā'shŭn). **1.** Any surgical procedure. **2.** The act, manner, or process of functioning. See also entries under method, procedure, technique.
>
> **procedure** (prō-sē'jŭr). Act or conduct of diagnosis, treatment, or operation. See also entries under method, operation, technique.
>
> **disease** (di-zēz') [Eng. *dis-* priv. + ease]. **1.** Morbus; illness; sickness; an interruption, cessation, or disorder of body functions, systems, or organs. **2.** A morbid entity characterized usually by at least two of these criteria: recognized etiologic agent(s), identifiable group of signs and symptoms, or consistent anatomical alterations. See also syndrome.
>
> **syndrome** (sin'drōm) [G. *syndromē,* a running together, tumultuous concourse; (in med.) a concurrence of symptoms, fr. *syn,* together, + *dromos,* a running]. The aggregate of signs and symptoms associated with any morbid process, and constituting together the picture of the disease. See also disease.

Location of elusive subentries can be determined in the following ways:

- The **"*Stedman's* Subentry Locator,"** immediately preceding section *A* of the vocabulary, is an alphabetical index of the adjectival or descriptive words of subentry terms and the noun main entry words under which they are located.

- ***Cross-reference locators*** beginning with the word "see," within the vocabulary, are found as main entries and as subentries and as part of the definition of an entry. Examples and additional information concerning cross-referencing are given on page xxi.
- For ***eponymic terms,*** the biographical surname main entry has cross-references to all eponymic terms attributed to that person. Examples and additional information are given under "Eponyms" on page xxii.

Alphabetization

Main Entries

Main entries are alphabetized letter by letter as spelled, rather than word by word as in a telephone directory:

blood	cross
blood bank	crossbreed
bloodletting	cross-cylinder
blood purple	crossing-over of genes
bloodstream	cross-matching
blood vessel	crossway

Alphabetization exceptions are as follows:

- Prepositions, conjunctions, articles, and the apostrophe s of possessive eponyms are disregarded, as are spaces, punctuation, Greek letters (*e.g.*, α, β, γ), numbers, configurational characters (*e.g.*, D-, +, −), and italicized forms (*e.g.*, *p*-, *N*-, *cis*-), whether as prefixes or as interior components in compound chemical terms.
- Prepositional phrases, especially Latin expressions, include the preposition in alphabetization. Therefore, *ante cibum* is in the *A's; in vitro* is in the *I's.*
- Spelled-out Greek letters and configurational forms are considered in alphabetization. Thus, "α-naphthylurea" is located in the *N's,* but "alpha-blocker" is in the *A's;* "L-dopa" is located in the *D's,* but "levodopa" is in the *L's.*

Capitalized words (proper nouns) precede lower case words (common nouns). Thus, "*Streptococcus*" appears before "streptococcus," and "Down" appears before "down."

Subentries

Subentries are alphabetized letter by letter following the same rules given above for main entries, but with some additional significant differences.

In subentry terms (as well as throughout definitions of both main entries and subentries), the governing main entry noun is represented by its initial letter, if it is singular; by addition of apostrophe and *s,* if it is a regular plural; or by a spelled-out form, if it is an irregular plural or a plural Latin word. Regardless of its form, the main entry word is disregarded in alphabetization of subentries, as also are prepositions, conjunctions, articles, and possessive forms used in eponymic terms:

crest	**gyrus**
gluteal c.	angular g.
c. of greater tubercle	gyri breves insulae
inguinal c.	central gyri
c.'s of nail bed	g. dentales
nasal c.	short gyri of insula
c. of neck of rib	gyri temporales transversi

Spelling

For alphabetizing letter by letter (as previously described), spelling disregards spaces, punctuation, Greek letters, numbers, configurational characters, and italicized forms, whether as prefixes or as interior components of compound chemical terms.

Alternative spellings, especially those of prefixed combining forms, are given as main entries with cross-references to the various spellings:

chilitis (kī-lī'tis). Cheilitis.

hem-, hema- [G. *haima,* blood]. Combining forms meaning blood. See also hemat-, hemato-, hemo-.

kyto-. See cyto-.

Older or outmoded spellings that have been superseded are also given as main entries with cross-references to the currently used spellings:

oari-, oario- [G. *ōarion,* a small egg, dim. of *ōon,* egg]. Obsolete combining forms denoting ovary. See oo-, oophor-, ovario-.

pleio-. Rarely used alternative spelling for pleo-.

Differences in British and American spellings, particularly those at or near the beginning of a word, are handled by prefix main entries that are cross-referenced from the British spelling to the American spelling:

ae-. For words so beginning and not found here, see under e-.

oe-. For words so beginning and not found here, see e-.

British spellings within compound words may also change the alphabetical location of some entries:

	British	**American**
*ae** for *e*	*ae*tiology	*e*tiology
	f*ae*ces	f*e*ces
	orthop*ae*dic	orthop*e*dic
oe for *e*	c*oe*liac	c*e*liac
	*oe*dema	*e*dema
	diarrh*oe*a	diarrh*e*a
our for *or*	tum*our*	tum*or*
re for *er*	fib*re*	fib*er*

**Ae* in the combining form aero- is accepted spelling in both usages, as in *aero*sol, an*aero*be, and other words derived from G. *aer,* air; *aero*plane/*air*plane is a well known exception.

Surnames, used as biographical main entry cross-references to associated eponymic terms, are alphabetized by their most commonly used spellings. Users should keep in mind spelling variations such as ä versus ae, ö versus oe, ü versus ue, and Mac versus Mc. For names beginning with prefixes, such as Van, van der, von, de, and which may be used with or without the prefix, cross-reference main entries have been provided to direct the user to the proper entry location. Regardless of the form of a surname (*e.g.*, Crohn, Bence Jones, d'Herelle, von Willebrand, Loeffler or Löffler), the name is alphabetized letter by letter as spelled.

ORGANIZATION OF ENTRIES AND CROSS-REFERENCES

The definition is given at only one location for two or more synonymous terms. Entries for the other synonymous terms are cross-referenced to the term where the definition is to be found. This system is also used for obsolete or outmoded terms, for spelling variations, or when there is a definite preference dictated by usage. The practice of placing a definition at only one location primarily serves to focus all of the information concerning a term at a single place, rather than strictly as an indicator of preference. It also keeps the size of *Stedman's* manageable by avoiding duplication of definitions.

Main Entries

Defined main entries usually are constructed as follows: (1) boldface entry word followed by its abbreviation or symbol (if any) in parentheses, (2) pronunciation in parentheses, (3) derivation in brackets, and (4) the definition proper:

① ② ③

electrocardiogram (ECG, EKG) (ē-lek-trō-kar′dē-ō-gram) [electro- + G. *kardia,* heart, + *gramma,* a drawing]. Graphic record of the heart's action currents obtained with the electrocardiograph.

④

If the entry word is used in the definition, it is abbreviated to its first letter or to its accepted abbreviation, *e.g.*, b. for bone, DNA for deoxyribonucleic acid, Hb for hemoglobin.

When there is more than one definition, each definition is indicated by a boldface number; however, the numerical sequence of the definitions is not necessarily an indication of importance or of preference:

> **mesocardia** (mez′ō-kar′dē-ă) [meso- + G. *kardia,* heart]. **1.** Atypical position of the heart in a central position in the chest, as in early embryonic life. **2.** Plural of mesocardium.

Synonyms, separated by semicolons, generally are placed at the beginning of a definition; a lightface number in parentheses following a synonym indicates the particular definition of that term with which the boldface entry word is synonymous:

> **nephropathy** (ne-frop′ă-thē) [nephro- + G. *pathos,* suffering]. Nephrosis (1); renopathy; any disease of the kidney.

When the list of synonyms is lengthy or may otherwise confuse the user, the synonyms are located separately at the end of the definition following the phrase "also called."

Systematic names of defined trivial or generic chemical and drug terms are likewise placed at the beginning of the definition, along with the molecular formula:

> **acetone** (as′e-tōn). Dimethyl ketone; CH_3COCH_3; a colorless, volatile, inflammable liquid; extremely small amounts are found in nor-

> **aspirin** (as′pi-rin). Acetylsalicylic acid; $C_6H_4(OCOCH_3)COOH$; a widely used analgesic, antipyretic, and anti-inflammatory agent.

Subentries

Defined subentries are organized much like main entries, as previously described on page xix. Pronunciation and derivation are provided when the principal words making up the subentry term are not provided as main entries in the vocabulary, as in the following example:

> **folie**
> **f. à deux** (ă-du) [Fr. two], identical or similar mental disorders, such as a paranoid fixation, usually affecting two members of the same family living together.

Multiple definitions are distinguished by boldface numbers in parentheses, but their numerical sequence is not necessarily indicative of importance or preference:

age
developmental a. (DA), **(1)** fetal a.; a. estimated by anatomic development since implantation; **(2)** a. of an individual estimated from the degree of anatomic, physiologic, mental, and emotional maturation.

In the definition, the main entry word, whenever used, is abbreviated to its first letter or to its accepted abbreviation as a space-saving device:

age
anatomical a., physical a.; a. in terms of structure rather than of function or of passage of time.

deoxyribonucleic acid (DNA)
competitor DNA, DNA from a test organism that is denatured and then used in *in vitro* hybridization experiments in which it competes with DNA (homologous) from a reference organism;

Cross-referencing of Synonyms and of Related Terms

Cross-references may be main entries or subentries or may be part of a main entry or subentry definition. They may serve to direct the user to a defined entry or to an entry where additional or related information can be found.

A cross-reference from a synonym to the defined synonymous term consists solely of the latter term. In the following example, the relevent synonym is a main entry:

boil (boyl) [A.S. *byl,* a swelling]. Furuncle.

callus (kal'ŭs) [L. hard skin]. **1.** Callosity. **2.** A composite mass of tissue that forms at a fracture site to establish continuity between the bone ends; it is composed initially of uncalcified fibrous tissue and cartilage, and ultimately of bone.

dermatitis
trefoil d., trifoliosis.

When the relevent synonym is a multiple-word term located as a subentry, the governing main entry word under which it will be found is *italicized,* as in the following example:

candle-power (kan'dl-pow'er). Luminous *intensity.*

commissurotomy (kom'i-syūr-ot'ō-mē). **1.** Surgical division of any commissure, fibrous band, or ring. **2.** Midline *myelotomy.*

fever
tertian f., vivax *malaria.*

When the synonym cross-reference is from one subentry to another subentry under the same main entry, the main entry word is abbreviated, as in the following example:

calculus
arthritic c., gouty *tophus.*
biliary c., gallstone.
dendritic c., staghorn c.
nephritic c., obsolete term for renal c.

Other cross-references, such as those to the location of a defined term, to related information, from spelling variations, or from outmoded or obsolete terms, use the same format but are preceded by "see" or "see also" or by descriptive wording:

anulus, pl. **anuli** (an′yū-lŭs, -lī) [L.] [NA]. Official alternative term for annulus.

border (bōr′der). The part of a surface that forms its outer boundary. See also edge; margin; margo.

capsid (kap′sid). See virion.

factor
f. III, in the clotting of blood, tissue thromboplastin. See thromboplastin.

oarium (ō-ar′ē-ŭm) [G. *ōarion,* a small egg]. Obsolete term for ovary.

oe-. For words so beginning and not found here, see e-.

reaction
oxidation-reduction r., see oxidation-reduction.

red [A.S. *reád*]. One of the primary colors, occupying the lower extremity of the spectrum at the other end from violet. For individual red dyes, see specific name.

Cf. (L. *confer,* compare) and *q.v.* (L. *quod vide,* which see) are used in definitions to direct the user to entries where comparative or related information can be found. The same format as for synonym cross-references and for other cross-references is used for these cross-references.

Eponyms

The surnames of persons to whom eponymic terms are attributed are given as brief biographical main entries that serve as locator cross-references to the eponyms. These cross-references are not necessarily to the defined entry, since a synonymous descriptive term may be the defined term; if this is the case, a cross-reference to the defined term is provided:

Down, John Langdon H., British physician, 1828–1896. See D.'s *syndrome.*

Hoffmann, Johann, German neurologist, 1857–1919. See H.'s muscular *atrophy, phenomenon, reflex, sign;* Werdnig-H. *disease.*

Sylvius (Dubois, de le Boë), Franciscus (Francois), Dutch physician, anatomist, and physiologist, 1614–1672. See sylvian *angle, aqueduct, fissure, line, point, valve, ventricle; fossa* of S.; *vallecula* sylvii.

Wilms, Max, German surgeon, 1867–1918. See W.'s *tumor.*

Note that the abbreviated possessive form of the surname in the cross-reference is apostrophe and *s* regardless of whether the spelled-out possessive form is apostrophe and *s* or *s* and apostrophe.

Traditionally, the possessive form has been appended to the name of the discoverer or describer of, for example, a disease (Down's syndrome, Wilms' tumor) but not to the name of the person having the disease (Christmas disease, Job syndrome), a compound name (Bence Jones proteinuria, Niemann-Pick disease), or the name of the location where the disease was first found to occur (Lyme disease, Pontiac fever). In recent years, this rule of thumb has not been followed consistently (Legionnaires disease, Legionnaire's disease, Legionnaires' disease). The use of the possessive form is increasingly less common, particularly in certain specialties.

Abbreviations and Symbols

Abbreviations and symbols, as well as acronyms and other contractions, are included in the vocabulary if they are accepted usage as opposed to *ad hoc* creations. They are located as main entries, generally as cross-references to the spelled-out terms where they are cited parenthetically in boldface immediately after the boldface entry word(s):

Cyt Symbol for cytosine.

PET Abbreviation for positron emission *tomography.*

stat. Abbreviation for L. *statim,* at once, immediately.

cytosine (Cyt) (sī'tō-sēn). 4-Amino-2(1*H*)-pyrimidinone; a pyrimi-

tomography
positron emission t. (PET), tomographic imaging of local meta-

statim (stat.) (stā'tim) [L.]. At once; immediately.

Some abbreviations and symbols are self-explanatory or are more appropriately defined at their entries than at a contrived entry for the spelled-out terms:

APUD [*a*mine *p*recursor *u*ptake, *d*ecarboxylase] Proposed designation for a group of cells in different organs secreting polypeptide hormones. Cells in this group have certain biochemical characteris-

b.i.d. Abbreviation for L. *bis in die,* twice a day.

FUO Abbreviation for fever of unknown origin.

M.D. Abbreviation of *Medicinae Doctor,* Doctor of Medicine.

PUVA Abbreviation for oral administration of *p*soralen and subsequent exposure to long wavelength ultraviolet light (*uv-a*); used to treat psoriasis.

Q_{CO_2} Symbol for the microliters STPD of CO_2 given off per milligram of tissue per hour.

Abbreviations may appear with or without periods. Some nomenclature conventions have eliminated the period from certain types of abbreviations. General use of periods with most abbreviations is progressively declining, but in some instances periods are retained to avoid confusion.

PRONUNCIATION

Conventions Used

Phonetic spelling for pronunciation is given in parentheses immediately after the boldface entry word(s). Pronunciation is provided in main entries except where it would be redundant because the phonetic spelling is the same as the spelling of the boldface entry word(s). Pronunciation is not given for subentry words unless they are foreign words or they do not appear as pronounced main entries. For Latin boldface subentry words, a prime (′) is used to indicate the stressed syllable.

The phonetic system used is a basic one and has only a few conventions:

- Two diacritical marks are used: the macron (¯) for long vowels; and the breve (˘) for short vowels.
- Principal stressed syllables are followed by a prime (′); monosyllables do not have a stress mark.
- Other syllables are separated by hyphens.

The following pronunciation key provides examples of vowel and consonant sounds encountered in the phonetic system. No attempt has been made to accommodate the slurred sounds common in speech or regional variations in speech sounds. Note that a vowel with a breve (˘) is used for the indefinite vowel sound of the *schwa* (ə). Native pronunciation of foreign words is approximated as closely as possible.

Pronunciation Key

Vowels

ā d*ay*, m*a*te, c*a*re, d*ai*ry, *a*orta, *a*pe, *a*te, f*a*ce, w*ay*, s*ai*l, *ai*r, *ae*ro, beh*a*ve, g*au*ge, h*ei*r, b*ei*ge, *ei*ght, th*ei*r, th*ey*, s*ue*de

a m*a*t, h*a*t, pl*ai*d, *a*ct, p*a*ra, d*a*mage, ban*a*na

ă *a*bortion, medi*a*, b*a*nan*a*, *a*bout, *a*lone, aort*a*, par*a*, hep*a*titis, ceph*a*lo, dam*a*ge, mount*ai*n, eq*ua*l

ah f*a*ther, hurr*ah*, w*a*sp, w*a*nder, y*a*cht

ar f*ar*, *ar*tery, gu*a*rd, c*ar*t, he*ar*t

aw f*a*ll, c*au*se, t*au*ght, t*a*ll, t*a*lk, c*a*lm, r*aw*, th*aw*, l*aw*yer, s*aw*, *au*to

ē b*e*, b*ee*, m*ee*t, d*ee*r, bl*ee*d, *e*qual, k*ey*, f*e*tal, *e*ven, perin*e*o, prosth*e*sis, t*ea*m, *ea*r, b*ea*t, bacter*i*a, anter*i*or, pit*y*, bus*y*, -log*y*, merid*i*an, mach*i*ne

e m*e*t, m*e*ridian, b*e*t, l*e*g, *e*dge, *e*rror, duch*e*ss, p*e*rineo, h*ei*fer, fr*ie*nd, s*ai*d, *a*ny, *ae*sthetic, d*ea*th, b*u*ry, gu*e*st

ĕ tak*e*n, syst*e*m, synth*e*sis, gen*e*sis

er t*er*m, *err*, m*err*y, op*er*ation, fath*er*, *ear*n, l*ear*n, f*ir*m, th*ir*st, m*yr*tle

ī p*ie*, p*i*ne, f*i*re, h*igh*, s*i*de, *i*ce, b*i*te, h*ei*ght, bu*y*, h*y*per, den*y*, p*y*lon

i p*i*t, m*i*rror, t*i*p, f*i*t, d*i*ffer, hab*i*t, eas*i*ly, per*i*neo, -*i*sm, arch*i*-, s*ie*ve, b*ui*ld, p*y*ramid, ph*y*sical, wom*e*n, walk*i*ng

ĭ penc*i*l

ō n*o*, n*o*te, f*o*re, f*o*r, s*o*, t*oe*, *o*pen, b*o*ne, ph*o*ne, perine*o*, th*o*rus, r*oa*d, b*oa*t, *o*we, sn*ow*, s*ou*l, f*ou*r, s*ew*

o n*o*t, r*o*tten, b*o*x, b*o*ther, c*o*t, *o*n, *o*ncology, *ou*ght, f*ou*ght, br*oa*d

ŏ *o*ccult, lem*o*n, c*o*llect, l*o*ve, s*o*n, t*o*n, fl*oo*d, d*oe*s, r*ou*gh

ow c*ow*, br*ow*, p*ow*er, pl*ow*, n*ow*, *ou*t, b*ou*gh, h*ou*r, l*ou*d, th*ou*

oy b*oy*, tr*oy*, t*oy*, v*oi*d, mast*oi*d, *oi*l, c*oi*n, bu*oy*, Fr*eu*d ū food, *oo*ze, p*oo*l, t*o*, t*oo*, t*oo*l, pr*o*ve, m*o*ve, can*oe*, r*u*le, l*u*pus, J*u*ne, fr*ui*t, ac*ou*stic, d*ew*, n*ew*, gr*ew*

u w*oo*d, f*oo*t, w*oo*l, t*oo*k, w*o*lf, w*ou*ld, p*u*ll, p*u*t

ŭ b*u*t, s*u*n, b*u*d, c*u*p, *u*p, h*u*mdr*u*m, f*u*dge, lup*u*s, occ*u*lt, adj*u*st, *u*s, c*ou*ple,tract*io*n, adj*u*st, uter*u*s

yū disp*u*te, p*u*re, *u*nit, *u*nion, c*u*rable, f*u*ture, *u*terus, y*ou*th, b*eau*ty, c*ue*, f*eu*d, f*u*se, f*ew*, v*iew*

Consonants

b	*b*ad, ta*b*le, ta*b*	n	*n*o, su*n*set, o*n*
ch	*ch*ild, tea*ch*er, mu*ch*	ng	si*ng*le, ri*ng*
d	*d*og, la*dd*er, le*d*	p	*p*an, u*pp*er, to*p*
dh	*th*is, rhy*th*m, smoo*th*	r	*r*ot, hu*rr*y, nea*r*
f	*f*it, di*ff*er, i*f*, rou*gh*, *ph*one	s	*s*o, pa*ss*ing, mi*ss*, *c*ent, dan*c*ing
g	*g*ot, bi*gg*er, le*g*	sh	*sh*ould, ten*si*on, planta*ti*on
h	*h*it, be*h*ave	t	*t*en, bu*tt*on, ca*t*
j	*j*ade, ad*j*ust, *g*erm, ed*ge*	th	*th*in, e*th*er, wi*th*
k	*c*at, a*c*tion, *k*ept, wa*k*e, boo*k*, *ch*ronic	v	*v*ery, li*v*er, ga*v*e
ks	e*x*quisite, e*x*cellent, ta*x*	w	*w*e, a*w*ay
kw	ex*qu*isite, ac*qu*ire, *qu*it	y	*y*es, law*y*er
l	*l*aw, a*l*one, a*ll*	z	*z*ero, ma*z*e, tho*s*e, brace*s*, say*s*, brow*s*e
m	*m*e, si*m*ple, hi*m*	*zh*	a*z*ure, mea*s*ure

In some words the initial sound is not that of the initial letter(s), or the initial letter(s) is not sounded or has a different sound, as in the following examples:

*ae*robe (ār′ōb)	*ph*thalein (thal′ē-in)
*ei*meria (ī-mē′rē-ă)	*p*neumonia (nū-mō′nē-ă)
*g*nathic (nath′ik)	*p*sychology (sī-kol′ō-jē)
*k*nuckle (nŭk-l)	*p*tosis (tō′sis)
*oe*dipism (ed′i-pizm)	*x*anthoma (zan-thō′mă)

DERIVATIONS

Organization

The origin or etymology of a boldface entry term is given in square brackets [ ] after the pronunciation. Of necessity, derivations are brief and as simple as possible to facilitate memory and promote association with similar derivatives. The information provided has three basic components: (1) the abbreviation of the language to which the original word(s) belongs; (2) in *italics,* the original word(s) from which the term is derived; and (3) the English translation of the word(s). For Greek and Latin verbs, the first person singular present form, rather than the infinitive, is used because the root word is more readily recognized in the former form; however, the English translation is given in the infinitive:

① ② ③

diphtheria (dif-thēr′ē-ă) [G. *diphthera,* leather]. Diphtheritis; a spe-

① ② ③

graph (graf) [G. *graphō,* to write]. A line or tracing denoting varying

① ② ③

union (yūn′yŭn) [L. *unus,* one]. **1.** The joining or amalgamation of

① ② ③

duct (dŭkt) [L. *duco,* pp. *ductus,* to lead]. Ductus; a tubular struc-

When the boldface entry term has the same or approximately the same meaning and/or spelling as the word(s) from which it is derived, the redundant material is not included in the derivation, as in the following examples:

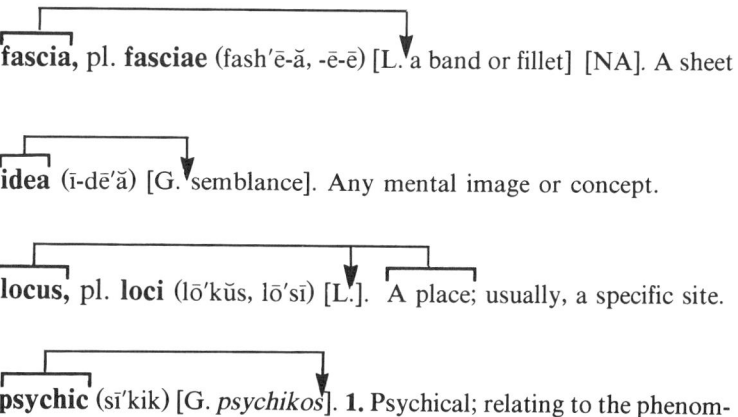

fascia, pl. **fasciae** (fash′ē-ă, -ē-ē) [L. a band or fillet] [NA]. A sheet

idea (ī-dē′ă) [G. semblance]. Any mental image or concept.

locus, pl. **loci** (lō′kŭs, lō′sī) [L.]. A place; usually, a specific site.

psychic (sī′kik) [G. *psychikos*]. **1.** Psychical; relating to the phenom-

Derivations frequently include additional components, especially when a derivation involves compound words or more than one word from one or more languages. A Greek or Latin verb may be hyphenated to indicate that the second part of the word exists as a simple verb with the same or approximately the same meaning, qualified by the addition of an adjectival or adverbial prefix; if the simple verb undergoes a change when forming part of a compound, that change is also shown:

apocrine (ap'ō-krin) [G. *apo-krinō,* to separate]. Denoting a mechanism of glandular secretion in which the apical portion of secretory cells is shed and incorporated into the secretion. See also a. *gland.*

component (kom-pō'nent) [L. *com-pono,* pp. *-positus,* to place together]. An element forming a part of the whole.

When words originating from more than one language are part of a derivation, the language of each word and the word's English translation are given; when the words are from the same language, the language is indicated only for the first word:

apicectomy (ap-i-sek'tō-mē) [L. *apex,* summit or tip, + G. *ektomē,* excision]. **1.** Opening and exenteration of air cells in the apex of the

gonarthrotomy (gon-ar-throt'ō-mē) [G. *gony,* knee, + *arthron,* joint, + *tomē,* incision]. Incision into the knee joint.

Prefixes and Suffixes

Combining forms used as prefixes or within compound words are listed in the vocabulary as boldface main entries with their own bracketed derivations and full definitions. When used in bracketed derivations of other boldface entry terms, which follow alphabetically in the vocabulary, their language of origin and English translation are not given:

neur-, neuri-, neuro- [G. *neuron,* nerve]. Combining forms denoting a nerve or relating to the nervous system.

neuralgia (nū-ral'jē-ă) [neur- + G. *algos,* pain]. Neurodynia; nerve pain; pain of a severe, throbbing, or stabbing character in the

neuritis, pl. **neuritides** (nū-rī'tis, nū-rit'i-dēz) [neuri- + G. *-itis,* inflammation]. Inflammation of a nerve, associated with neuralgia,

neurology (nū-rol'ō-jē) [neuro- + G. *logos,* study]. The branch of medical science concerned with the nervous system and its disor-

Combining forms used as suffixes and terminations are also listed in the vocabulary as boldface main entries with their own bracketed derivations and full definitions. When used in bracketed derivations of other boldface entry terms, the language of origin is indicated (only if different from the preceding word), and the English translation is given:

-osis, pl. **-oses** [G.]. Suffix, properly added only to words formed from G. roots, meaning a process, condition, or state, usually abnormal or diseased. It denotes primarily any production or in-

halitosis (hal-i-tō'sis) [L. *halitus,* breath, + G. *-ōsis,* condition]. Fetor oris; ozostomia; stomatodysodia; a foul odor from the mouth.

pneumoconiosis, pl. **pneumoconioses** (nū'mō-kō-nē-ō'sis, -sēz) [G. *pneumōn,* lung, + *konis,* dust, + *-ōsis,* condition]. Pneumonoconiosis; anthracotic tuberculosis; inflammation commonly

ABBREVIATIONS AND SYMBOLS USED IN THIS DICTIONARY

The abbreviations and symbols listed below are used in the derivations and definitions of entries in the dictionary. They should be distinguished from the abbreviations and symbols given as entries in the vocabulary or accompanying the spelled-out entry words that they represent, as discussed on page xxiii.

acc.	accusative
adj.	adjective
Am. Ind.	American Indian
Ar.	Arabic
A.S.	Anglo-Saxon
c., ca.	L. *circa,* about
cf.	L. *confer,* compare
Ch.	Chinese
char.	character
C.I.	Colour Index
D.	Dutch
dial.	dialect
dim.	diminutive
EC	Enzyme Commission
e.g.	L. *exempli gratia,* for example
Eng.	English
etym.	etymology
fem.	feminine
Fr.	French
fr.	from
fut.	future
G.	Greek
Gael.	Gaelic
gen.	genitive
Ger.	German
Hind.	Hindu
Ice.	Icelandic
i.e.	L. *id est,* that is
Ind.	Indian
It.	Italian
Jap.	Japanese
L.	Latin
L.L.	Late Latin
masc.	masculine
M.E.	Middle English
Med. L., Mediev. L.	Medieval Latin
Mod. L.	Modern Latin
myth.	mythological
NA	*Nomina Anatomica*
neut.	neuter
N.G.	New Guinea
ntr.	neuter
obs.	obsolete
O.E.	Old English
O. Fr.	Old French
O.H.G.	Old High German
O.N.	Old Norse
p.	participle
Pers.	Persian
Pg.	Portuguese
pl.	plural
pp.	past participle
priv.	privative, negative

pr. p.	present participle
q.v.	L. *quod vide,* which see
Sansk.	Sanskrit
Sc.	Scandinavian
sing.	singular
Sp.	Spanish
Sw.	Swedish
thr.	through
US	United States
W. Af.	West African
*	In biographical data, denotes year of birth when year of death is not given
†	In biographical data, denotes year of death when year of birth is not given

MEDICAL ETYMOLOGY

The vocabularies of the life sciences are straining to keep pace with the increasingly rapid growth of knowledge. Each new discovery, concept, or theory seems to require a new word or new grouping of words in order to be described or defined in speech and print. *Ad hoc* creations and counterfeit coinages often are produced in haste to satisfy the moment's need, without consideration of etymological standards or philological principles. Too often, such words become sufficiently established and cannot be ignored by any vocabulary that intends to be comprehensive and current.

One purpose of a dictionary is to show the sources of the words in its vocabulary. The origin and development of words is the subject of etymology. The derivation of individual words, an editorial feature of *Stedman's* since its first edition, helps to tell the history of a word, to show how it acquired its meaning, and as a result to make the understanding, remembering, and using of the word easier and more accurate. Spurious coinages only confound the process.

ORIGINS

Words were the first great tools of the mind and the beginning of knowledge. The growth of knowledge often can be traced by studying the history of words, and the development of modern medicine is no exception. Medical knowledge originally progressed orally from teacher to student; the students used the words of their mentors. As medicine developed and created new concepts, new words were required and were created. But where did these medical words originate? A frequently heard response is that most are derived from the "dead" classical languages of Greek and Latin. Only part of that statement is true. That these words are used daily in the classroom, in professional practice, and in the voluminous literature, and continue to be a source for new words and groups of words, attests to the continuing viability of both languages.

At the beginning of the Western medical tradition, Hippocrates spoke and wrote in his native language, Greek. He used such words, although not necessarily with their current meanings, as *adenoma, amblyopia, anthrax, borborygmus, bregma, cachexia, carcinoma, cholera, emphysema, erythema, exanthema, herpes, ileus, kyphosis, lordosis, meninges, nephritis, olecranon, paresis, phagedena, symphysis, thorax, typhus, ureter,* and *urethra*. By the time of Celsus, a Roman medical writer of the first century A.D., Greek was established as the language of medicine in the civilized world, although Latin words such as *abdomen, anus, cancer, delirium, fistula, hernia, maxilla, omentum, patella, pus, radius, scabies,* and *tibia* were in use.

In the middle of the next century, Galen, a Greek physician practicing in Rome, used in his extensive writings additional words such as *anthrax, ascites, chemosis, coccyx, diaphoresis, diastole, epididymis, gomphosis, hypophysis, hypospadias, iris, kerion, lysis, mydriasis, pemphigus, peritoneum, pityriasis, pylorus, sarcoma, skeleton, strabismus, syndrome, systole, tarsus, tenia, thymus,* and *trichiasis*. His surviving medical works passed through Latin and Arabic translations and became canonized as medical law until the emergence of scientific medicine nearly fifteen centuries later. During the

Middle Ages, Latin emerged as the language of the learned and literate and permanently imprinted its influence on the language of medicine.

Not all medical words have come to us from Greek and Latin. Arabic has provided words such as *alcohol, camphor, sugar,* and *syrup*. Occasionally, the Arabic definite article and a Greek stem have been combined to produce words, such as *alchemy* and *elixir*. Some of the other languages that have contributed words are Italian (*belladonna, malaria, scarlatina*), Spanish (*cascara, guaiac, marijuana*), German (*anlage, ester, gestalt*), Scandinavian (*ill, leg, skin*), and Japanese (*sodoku, tsutsugamushi, urushiol*). Anglo-Saxon origins are a source of many short words, especially anatomical words such as *arm, back, ear, foot, hand, neck, rib,* and *skull*; internal organs are represented by words such as *gut, heart, liver, lung, spleen,* and *tongue*.

French words are more numerous than those from any other modern language and appear in any of three basic forms: (1) unchanged or slightly modified forms, as represented by *bougie, chancre, malaise, tic douloureux,* and *tourniquet*; (2) Anglicized forms, such as *goiter, malinger, jaundice,* and *powder*; and (3) Gallicizations of Greek or Latin words, such as *diastase, migraine,* and *palsy*. A few, like *culdocentesis* and *culdoplasty,* are hybrids of French and Greek words.

WORD FORMATION

A reader who sees for the first time words such as "hemangioendothelioblastoma" or "acrocephalopolysyndactyly" may recoil in shock from what appears to be an unintelligible string of letters. However, when the individual components of these compound words are known, *i.e.,* when they are viewed as "hem-angio-endothelio-blast-oma" and "acro-cephalo-poly-syndactyly," the spelling, pronunciation, and understanding of such terms are relatively easy. Often a word's components provide its definition, *e.g., poly-chondr-itis,* many-cartilage-inflammation, a widespread inflammation of cartilage. An appreciation of the origins or derivations of words, particularly compound words, is difficult when one does not understand how they are formed. The fundamentals of compound word formation, especially from Greek and Latin words, involve some understanding of roots or bases, stems, inflections, and affixes.

Roots

The root or base of a word is that element that remains after any formative additions (inflections, affixes, etc.) are removed. For example, *gen* or *gn* is a root found in Greek, Latin, English, and other Indo-European languages with the sense of "beget" or "produce": Greek *genos* or Latin *genus,* birth; Latin *pregnans,* pregnant; English *king* or *kin*. A root, therefore, is the basic lexical unit in a language to which affixes or inflections are added to give it the form of a word. In English, a root often functions as an independent word (*e.g.,* do, love, help).

Stems

A stem is that part of a word consisting of a root or base (with any affixes) to which inflections are added or in which inflectional changes are made. For example, Latin *vox,* voice, become *voces,* voices, in the plural, *vocis,* of a voice, in the possessive (genitive), and *vocalis,* vocal, as an adjective; *voc-* is the root from which the derivatives are formed. In English, *do* is a root to which affixes (*un*do, do*er*) or inflections (do*ing*, do*es*) may be added to create new words or different meanings.

Inflections

An inflection is a change in the form of a word or an addition to a stem by which a certain grammatical relationship is expressed (*e.g.,* number, case, gender, mood, tense, adjectival comparison). Inflection is not as complex an element in English as it can be in Greek and Latin, especially since English has no declensions of nouns, noun genders, or gender and number agreements between noun and adjective. Some guidelines are given below concerning Greek and Latin inflections that should be remembered for derivations and word formation.

For **verbs,** the Greek future tense and the Latin passive past participle frequently provide a key for derivations. For example, the Greek verb *kinein,* to move, becomes *kinēso* (hence *kinēsis*) in the future and can be readily identified as a stem in *kinesi*ology and *kinesi*meter. The Latin verb, *solvere,* to loosen, becomes *solutus,* in the passive past participle; both forms are stems, respectively, in *solv*ent and *solut*ion.

The stem of a Greek or Latin **noun** may come from the nominative (subjective) case or from the genitive (possessive) case. For example, the Greek word for body is *sōma* in the nominative singular form and *sōmatos* in the genitive form; both forms are found as stems in such English medical words as chromo*som*e and *somat*otropic. The Latin word for eye, *oculus,* appears as *oculi* in both the genitive and plural forms; only one form needs to be remembered to recognize the stem in *ocul*ar, *ocul*ist, or *oculo*-motor.

Modifiers in Greek and Latin follow their nouns in number and gender. Most medical terms affected by this rule are Latin or are Greek assimilated into Latin. Familiarity and practice with the following guidelines for nouns and their modifiers may help to reduce the confusion often associated with plural nouns ending in *-a* that look like singular nouns, singulars ending in *-s* that look like plurals, and the correct forms of modifiers that accompany them.

Plurals are formed by adding inflections to a singular noun or its stem:

1. When the singular ending is *-e* or *-a,* the plural ending is *-ae.* EXAMPLE: G. *theke, thekae;* L. *theca, thecae;* L. *ala, alae.*

   However, if a Greek singular noun ends in *-a* preceded by *m,* the plural ends in *-ata.* EXAMPLE: *stigma, stigmata; papilloma, papillomata.*

2. When the singular ending is *-os* or *-us,* the plural ending is *-i.* EXAMPLE: G. *gyros, gyri;* L. *gyrus, gyri;* L. *sulcus, sulci.*

Some Latin nouns ending in *-us* change the *s* to *r*, often change the preceding vowel, and add *-a*. EXAMPLE: *corpus, corpora; viscus, viscera*. Others are the same in both singular and plural forms. EXAMPLE: *ductus, fetus, plexus*.

3. When the singular ending is *-on* or *-um*, the plural ending is *-a*. EXAMPLE: G. *kranion, krania;* L. *cranium, crania;* L. *ovum, ova*.

4. When the singular ending is *-is* or *-es*, the plural ending is *-es*. EXAMPLE: G. *paralysis, paralyses;* L. *pelvis, pelves;* L. *facies, facies*.

   Some of these nouns have a *d* or *t* inserted to form the plural. EXAMPLE: G. *arthritis, arthritides;* L. *paries, parietes*. Others, such as *biceps, herpes*, and *scabies*, are unchanged from singular to plural.

Adjectives usually encountered have one of the following endings, which can provide a clue to the number and gender of the nouns they modify:

-a	feminine singular	*-us*	masculine singular	*-um*	neuter singular
-ae	feminine plural	*-i*	masculine plural	*-a*	neuter plural

EXAMPLE: *theca externa, gyrus dentatus, cranium bifidum*.

Grammatically correct matching of nouns and adjectives is more than just their having the same endings that happen to rhyme. Thus, one sees such terms as *papilloma diffusum* (neuter singular), *corpus cavernosum* (neuter singular), and *ductus lactiferi* (masculine plural).

What may appear to be an adjective can be a noun in the genitive (possessive) case, *e.g., theca folliculi* (wall of a follicle), *gyri cerebri* (convolutions of the cerebral cortex), *stratum retinae* (layer of the retina). **Genitives** are often found in anatomical terms and, like adjectives, modify the noun in number and gender. As a general rule, a noun whose stem does not differ has a genitive singular ending that is the same as its plural when the noun is one following either of the first two guidelines above; *i.e.*, ending in *-ae* or *-i*. For a noun following the third guideline, the genitive singular ending is *-i*. When the stem differs, the genitive singular usually ends in *-is*. Genitive plurals usually end in *-arum* or *-orum*.

Compound Words

A compound word is a word formed from two or more stems joined by a connecting vowel. An ideally formed compound word would have all of its parts from one language, such as Greek or Latin. With the assimilation of Greek words into Latin, and later of classical Greek and Latin elements into English, hybridization became as common in words as in plants and as prolific as weeds. Native Latin compounds usually used *i* as the connecting vowel, as in *multiformis* (L. *multus* + *forma*). With the assimilation of Greek, *o* (widely used in that language) came to be commonly used as a connecting vowel between Latin elements and between Greek and Latin elements. Thus today one sees "dorsolateral" (L. *dorsus* + *laterus*) instead of "dorsilateral," hemodialysis" (G. *haima* + *dialysis*), and "psychosexual" (G. *psyche* + L. *sexus*).

Combining Forms

The formation of combining forms, those forms of the first word or stem in a compound word, has been and continues to be inconsistent. However, some general principles apply:

1. When the first stem ends in *-a* or *-e* and the second stem begins with a consonant, the vowel usually is replaced by *-o*. EXAMPLE: L. *lingua* + *versus* = linguo-version; G. *psyche* + *logos* = psychology.
2. When the first stem ends in a consonant and the second stem begins with a consonant, the consonant ending the first stem may be dropped and the remaining vowel may be left unchanged. EXAMPLE: G. *bradys* + *kardia* = bradycardia; G. *erythros* + *kytos* = erythrocyte.
3. When the first stem ends in a vowel and the second stem begins with a vowel, the vowel ending the first stem usually is dropped. EXAMPLE: L. *bursa* + G. *ektomē* = bursectomy; G. *plasma* + *aphairesis* = plasmapheresis.

Exceptions are abundant, as can be seen in *plasmacyte* and *archetype, neuroendocrine* and *psychoanalysis,* and *intra-abdominal* and *salpingo-oophorectomy*. Hundreds of combining forms, with their derivations and definitions, have been included in the *Stedman's* vocabulary as a guide to word formation and derivation.

Prefixes and Suffixes

Prefixes and suffixes are affixed (attached) to a word or stem, in contrast to the joining of two or more words or stems to form a compound word. Most of the prefixes and suffixes used in medical terminology have come almost unchanged from Greek and Latin prepositions, adverbs, and adjectives. They are included as entries in the *Stedman's* vocabulary, each with its own derivation and definition.

Prefixes

A prefix alters the meaning of the word to which it is attached, as in the negatives *a-* or *an-, in-* or *im-,* and *un-*. When a Greek or Latin preposition or adverb ending in a consonant is prefixed to a word beginning with a consonant, the final consonant of the prefix may change as a result of assimilation or for euphony, as in the following example:

n becomes *l* before words beginning with *l*. EXAMPLE: *in* + *lusus* = illusion.

n becomes *m* before words beginning with *b, m, p,* or *ph*. EXAMPLE: *in* + *bilanx* (*lanc-*) = imbalance; *in* + *muncus* = immune; *in* + *plusus* = impulse; *en* + *phasis* = emphasis.

n is dropped before words beginning with *s*. EXAMPLE: *syn* + *stello* = systole.

b and *d* change to the letter beginning the word. EXAMPLE: *ad* + *fero* = afferent; *ob* + *clusus* = occlusion; *sub* + *faux* (*faucis*) = suffocate.

Most Greek prefixes ending in a vowel retain it when the word to which it is attached begins with a consonant and drop it when the word begins with a vowel:

apo + *krinō* = apocrine; *apo* + *eidos* = apeidosis
dia + *gnōsis* = diagnosis; *dia* + *ourēsis* = diuresis

Suffixes

A suffix also can alter the function of a word by changing it from one part of speech to another, as from a noun to an adjective or from a verb to a noun. Most Latin and Greek suffixes that have been assimilated into English are familiar to its users.

One suffix worth noting is *-itis* (inflammation of), which is the feminine form of the Greek masculine *itēs* and agrees with the Greek feminine *nosos* (disease). Any qualifying adjective must therefore be feminine, *e.g.*, *dermatitis exfoliativa, retinitis pigmentosa*.

ALPHABETS AND PRONUNCIATION

Greek Alphabet

Although the Greek alphabet is the ancestor of the English alphabet, the order and shape of the English alphabet's letters are essentially the same as that of the Latin alphabet. Since most Greek has entered English via Latin, the latter has influenced the transliteration of Greek for use in English.

Classical Greek had no letters corresponding to our *c* or *h*. Kappa (κ) became a hard *c* in Latinized Greek words, as when the Greek *kranion* became *cranium*. An aspirate (‘), or rough breathing mark, over a beginning vowel or over rho (ρ) is transcribed as *h*. This sound is also part of theta (θ), phi (φ), and chi (χ), which are transcribed as *th, ph,* and *ch*.

Greek Alphabet

Letters: Capital	Small	Name of Letters	Sound	Transcription
Α	α	alpha	*fa*ther, *a*rt	A
Β	β	beta	*b*et	B
Γ	γ	gamma*	*g*et	G
Δ	δ	delta	*d*og	D
Ε	ε	epsilon	*e*nd	E
Ζ	ζ	zeta	*z*oo	Z
Η	η	eta	th*ey*	Ē
Θ	θ	theta	*th*in	TH
Ι	ι	iota	mach*i*ne	I
Κ	κ	kappa	*k*ey, *c*ar	K, C (Latin)
Λ	λ	lambda	*l*et	L
Μ	μ	mu	*m*at	M
Ν	ν	nu	*n*et	N
Ξ	ξ	xi	se*x*	X
Ο	ο	omikron	h*o*t	O
Π	π	pi	*p*at	P
Ρ	ρ	rho†	*r*at, *rh*eostat	R, RH
Σ	σ, ς	sigma‡	*s*it	S
Τ	τ	tau	*t*op	T
Υ	υ	upsilon	mo*o*n	Y or U
Φ	φ	phi	*ph*oto	PH
Χ	χ	chi	Ba*ch* (Ger.)	CH
Ψ	ψ	psi	ti*ps*	PS
Ω	ω	omega	*o*pen	Ō

* Before kappa (κ), gamma (γ), chi (χ), or xi (ξ), gamma has a nasal sound, as in si*n*ger.

† Rho (ρ) is doubled (ρρ) after a short vowel and is transcribed as *rrh*, as in dia*rrh*ea.

‡ ς is used at the end of a word; σ is used elsewhere.

Greek diphthongs are as follows:

Dipthong	Sound	Transcription
αι	*ai*sle	ae, e, ai
ει	r*ei*n	ei, i, e
οι	c*oi*n	oe, e, oi
υι	s*ui*te	ui
αυ	l*ou*d	au
ευ	met + t*oo*	eu
ου	gr*ou*p	u, ou

Diphthongs αι and οι were transcribed in Latin as *ae* and *oe*. These, plus *ei*, have been retained in British spellings. American spellings generally prefer the single vowels *e* and *i*.

Latin Alphabet

The order and the shape of letters in the Latin alphabet are essentially the same as those in the English alphabet, except that the former alphabet has no *j, k,* or *w*. English sounds associated with these consonants are generally handled in Latin by *i, c,* and *v*.

Consonant sounds are as in English, except for the following:

c	*c*at (not *c*ity)
ch	*ch*rome (not *ch*op)
g	*g*o (not *g*erm)
s	*s*at (not day*s*)
th	*th*in (not *th*en)
v	*w*ork

Vowel sounds are as follows:

a	f*a*ther (long), *a*lone (short)
e	th*ey* (long), b*e*t (short)
i	mach*ine* (long), s*i*t (short)
o	t*o*ne (long), h*o*t (short)
u	r*u*le (long), p*u*sh (short)
y	*ü*ber (German)

Diphthongs are pronounced as follows:

ae	*ai*sle	ui	su*i*te
oe	c*oi*n	eu	f*eu*d

Pronunciation

The original pronunciation of Greek and Latin words cannot be precisely determined. There are several methods of pronunciation, and the knowledgeable and experienced listener can often tell the speaker's educational background by the pronunciation used. *Stedman's* provides a general guide to pronunciation in the tables above as well as in the "Pronunciation Key" (p. xxv), which will enable users to pronounce the words in its vocabulary in a basic American manner.

Accentuation of Greek and Latin words transformed into English generally follows the same pattern. Words of two syllables are accented on the first syllable. Words of three syllables are accented on the next to the last syllable (penult) when it is *long* or on the syllable before that (antepenult) when the next to the last syllable is *short*.

Acknowledgments

Greek and Latin lexicons, as well as numerous textbooks of medical terminology, are available for anyone interested in pursuing medical etymology and word formation beyond the scope of this section. A particularly informative and enjoyable resource is *The Language of Medicine: Its Evolution, Structure, and Dynamics,* second edition, by John H. Dirckx (New York: Praeger Publishers, 1983).

William K. Beatty, our consultant for etymology, biography, and history, inspired the revision of this section and contributed significantly to its content.

STEDMAN'S SUBENTRY LOCATOR

The "*Stedman's* Subentry Locator" is a list of subentry terms from the *A* to *Z* vocabulary; these terms are arranged alphabetically letter by letter according to the first word(s) of the term. It functions as a master cross-referencing system for adjectival or descriptive terms contained in the vocabulary, in lieu of locator cross-references within the vocabulary. When used in conjunction with an understanding of the organization of the vocabulary, as explained on pages xiv–xxx of "How to Use This Dictionary," any subentry in *Stedman's* can readily be found. In addition, information related by the commonality of like word(s) used in multiple-word terms is brought into focus.

Each listing in the "*Stedman's* Subentry Locator" is made up of one or more boldface words, representing the adjectival or descriptive part of the subentry term, followed by one or more lightface words, each representing the noun that completes the subentry term and is the main entry under which the subentry is found in the vocabulary. For example:

acinous: carcinoma; cell; gland

carcinoma
  acinous c.
cell
  acinous c.
gland
  acinous g.

Special treatment has been given to *anatomical* terms that begin with words such as "anterior," "posterior," and "deep" by grouping them in listings such as **anterior anatomical structures,** instead of having a lengthy listing of each specific "anterior" anatomical structure. Note that there is a listing of **anterior** for nonanatomical terms.

For names of diseases and disorders, one should also check listings such as "acute," "congenital," "infectious," and "progressive," in addition to the specific name. For example, there are listings for **bulbar:** paralysis, **infectious bulbar:** paralysis, and **progressive bulbar:** paralysis.

Omitted from the listings are subentry terms that are easily located in the vocabulary because the first word of the subentry is the same as its noun main entry. These include:

- Latin nomenclature (**vena cava inferior** is under **vena; erythema multiforme** is under **erythema**).
- chemical and drug names (many of these are also main entries). See also the explanation in "How To Use This Dictionary," page xvi.
- prepositional terms (**angle of declination** is under **angle; law of denervation** is under **law**).

Eponyms derived from surnames are also omitted because the vocabulary contains biographical surname main entries that serve as locator cross-references to the attributed eponymic subentries. Note that adjectival forms (*e.g.*, addisonian, brownian, eustachian) and eponyms derived from places (*e.g.*, Lyme, Iceland, Rocky Mountain) are listed.

Significant adjectival words in subentry terms are defined as main entries in the vocabulary. Such defined entries often preclude the need for a subentry. For example: **chronic** as a defined main entry makes unnecessary "chronic disease" as a subentry under **disease.** However, in the "*Stedman's* Subentry Locator" there are 33 listings ranging from **chronic** to **chronic ulcerative** for specific entities whose names begin with "chronic" and are found as subentries in the vocabulary.

A

α: see alpha
A: band; bile; cell; chain; esotropia; exotropia; fiber; strabismus; wave
A_2: thalassemia
aaa: disease
abacterial thrombotic: endocarditis
abapical: pole
abarticular: gout
ABC, A.B.C.: lead; process
abdominal: angina; apoplexy; brain; canal; cavity; dropsy; fibromatosis; fissure; fistula; guarding; hernia; hysterectomy; hystereopexy; hysterotomy; migraine; myomectomy; nephrectomy; pad; part; pool; pregnancy; pressure; pulse; reflex; region; respiration; ring; sac; salpingectomy; salpingo-oophorectomy; salpingotomy; section; typhoid; zone
abdominal aortic: plexus
abdominal external oblique: muscle
abdominal internal oblique: muscle
abdominal muscle deficiency: syndrome
abdominocardiac: reflex
abdominojugular: reflux
abdominothoracic: arch
abdominovaginal: hysterectomy
abducens: nucleus
abducent: nerve
abductor: muscle
aberrant: artery; bundle; complex; duct; ductule; ganglion; goiter; hemoglobin
aberrant bile: duct
aberrant ventricular: conduction
ABLB: test
abnormal: cleavage; correspondence; occlusion
ABO: antigen; factor
ABO hemolytic: disease
aborted: systole
aborted ectopic: pregnancy
abortion: rate
abortive: neurofibromatosis; transduction
abortus: bacillus
abortus-Bang-ring: test
abraded: wound
abrasive: strip
abscopal: effect
absence: seizure
absent: state
absolute: agraphia; alcohol; dehydration; glaucoma; hemianopsia; humidity; hydration; hyperopia; leukocytosis; scale; scotoma; sterility; system; temperature; threshold; unit; viscosity; zero
absolute cell: increase
absolute intensity threshold: acuity
absolute refractory: period
absolute terminal innervation: ratio
absorbable gelatin: film; sponge
absorbable surgical: suture
absorbancy: index
absorbed: dose
absorbent: cotton; point; system; vessel
absorption: band; cell; chromatography; coefficient; collapse; fever; line; spectrum
absorptive: cell
abstinence: symptom
abstract: intelligence; thinking
acapnial: alkalosis
acarine: dermatosis
accelerated: conduction; eruption; reaction; rejection
accelerator: factor; fiber; globulin; nerve
access: opening
accessory: adrenal; atrium; auricle; breast; canal; cartilage; chromosome; cramp; flocculus; gland; ligament; nerve; organ; placenta; process; sign; spleen; symptom; thyroid; tubercle
accessory cephalic: vein
accessory cuneate: nucleus
accessory hemiazygos: vein
accessory lacrimal: gland
accessory nasal: cartilage
accessory nerve lymph: node
accessory obturator: artery
accessory olivary: nucleus
accessory pancreatic: duct
accessory parotid: gland
accessory phrenic: nerve
accessory plantar: ligament
accessory quadrate: cartilage
accessory saphenous: vein
accessory suprarenal: gland
accessory thyroid: gland
accessory vertebral: vein
accessory volar: ligament
accident: neurosis
accidental: abortion; hypothermia; image; murmur; symptom
acclimating: fever
accolé: form
accommodation: phosphene; reflex
accommodative: asthenopia; convergence; strabismus
accommodative convergence-accommodation: ratio
accompanying: vein
accordion: graft
accoucheur's: hand
accretion: line
accretionary: growth
acentric: chromosome
acetabular: artery; fossa; notch
acetate replacement: factor
acetic: fermentation; solution
acetone: body; chloroform; compound; fixative; test
acetone-insoluble: antigen
aceto-orcein: stain
acetosoluble: albumin
acetous: fermentation
acetyl: value
acetyl-activating: enzyme
achievement: age; motive; quotient; test
Achilles: bursa; reflex; tendon
achlorhydric: anemia
acholuric: jaundice
achondroplastic: dwarf
achrestic: anemia
achromatic: apparatus; lens; objective; threshold; vision
acid: agglutination; alcohol; cell; deoxyribonuclease; dyspepsia; fuchsin; gland; indigestion; intoxication; maltase; oxide; phospha-

tase; radical; reaction; rigor; salt; seromucoid; stain; sulfate; tartrate; tide; wave
acid-ash: diet
acid-base: balance; equilibrium
acid etch cemented: splint
acid-etched: restoration
acidic: dye
acidified serum: test
acidophil, acidophilic: adenoma; cell; granule; leukocyte
acidophilus: milk
acid perfusion: test
acid phosphatase: stain; test
acid reflux: test
acinar: carcinoma; cell
acinar cell: tumor
acinic cell: adenocarcinoma; carcinoma
acinose: carcinoma
acinotubular: gland
acinous: carcinoma; cell; gland
ackee: poisoning
acne: bacillus; keloid
acneform: syphilid
acorn-tipped: catheter
acoustic: agraphia; aphasia; area; cell; crest; lemniscus; nerve; neurilemoma; neurinoma; neuroma; papilla; radiation; schwannoma; spot; stria; tetanus; tolerance; tubercle; vesicle
acousticofacial: crest; ganglion
acousticopalpebral: reflex
acoustic reference: level
acoustic trauma: deafness
acquired: agammaglobulinemia; character; cuticle; distichia; drive; hyperlipoproteinemia; hypogammaglobulinemia; ichthyosis; immunity; leukodermia; leukopathia; methemoglobinemia; nevus; reflex; sensitivity; toxoplasmosis; trichoepithelioma
acquired centric: relation
acquired eccentric: relation
acquired enamel: cuticle
acquired epileptic: aphasia
acquired hemolytic: anemia; icterus
acquired immunodeficiency: syndrome
acral lentiginous: melanoma
acrid: poison
acridine: dye
acridine orange: stain
acrocentric: chromosome
acrodynic: erythema
acrofacial: dysostosis; syndrome
acromegalic: gigantism
acromelic: dwarfism
acromial: angle; artery; extremity; network; process; reflex
acromial articular: facies; surface
acromioclavicular: disk; joint; ligament
acromion: presentation
acromiothoracic: artery
acroparesthesia: syndrome
acrosomal: cap; granule; vesicle
acrylic: resin
acrylic resin: base; tooth; tray
ACTH-producing: adenoma
ACTH stimulation: test
actin: filament
actinic: cheilitis; conjunctivitis; dermatitis; granuloma; keratitis; keratosis; porokeratosis; ray; reticuloid
actinium: emanation
actinomycotic: appendicitis
action: current; potential; tremor
activated: atom; charcoal; epilepsy; hydrogen; resin; sludge; state
activated partial thromboplastin: time
activated sludge: method
activation: analysis
active: acetate; anaphylaxis; caries; congestion; electrode; formyl; hyperemia; immunity; immunization; methionine; methyl; movement; mutant; principle; prophylaxis; psychoanalysis; repressor; site; splint; sulfate; transport; vasoconstriction vasodilation
active chronic: hepatitis
active rosette: test
activity: coefficient
actual: cautery
acuminate papular: syphilid
acupuncture: anesthesia
acute: abdomen; abscess; alcoholism; angle; appendicitis; ataxia; chalazion; cholecystitis; delirium; glaucoma; glomerulonephritis; goiter; inflammation; malaria; nephritis; nephrosis; porphyria; pyelonephritis; rhinitis; rickets; trypanosomiasis; tuberculosis; urticaria
acute adrenocortical: insufficiency
acute African sleeping: sickness
acute anterior: poliomyelitis
acute ascending: paralysis
acute atrophic: paralysis
acute bacterial: endocarditis
acute brachial: radiculitis
acute bulbar: poliomyelitis
acute catarrhal: conjunctivitis
acute cellular: rejection
acute compression: triad
acute contagious: conjunctivitis
acute crescentic: glomerulonephritis
acute cutaneous: leishmaniasis
acute decubitus: ulcer
acute disseminated: encephalomyelitis; myositis
acute epidemic: conjunctivitis; leukoencephalitis
acute follicular: conjunctivitis
acute fulminating meningococcal: septicemia
acute hallucinatory: paranoia
acute hemorrhagic: conjunctivitis; encephalitis; glomerulonephritis; pancreatitis
acute idiopathic: polyneuritis
acute infectious: gastroenteritis
acute intermittent: porphyria
acute interstitial: nephritis; pneumonia
acute isolated: myocarditis
acute lymphonodular: pharyngitis
acute miliary: tuberculosis
acute necrotizing: encephalitis; gingivitis
acute neutrophilic: dermatosis
acute parenchymatous: hepatitis
acute phase: reactant
acute post-streptococcal: glomerulonephritis
acute primary hemorrhagic: meningoencephalitis
acute promyelocytic: leukemia
acute pulmonary: alveolitis
acute radiation: syndrome
acute recurrent: rhabdomyolysis
acute reflex bone: atrophy
acute rheumatic: arthritis
acute scalp: cellulitis
acute situational: reaction
acute splenic: tumor
acute transverse: myelitis
acute vascular: purpura
acute yellow: atrophy
acyclic: compound
acyl-activating: enzyme
acyl carrier: protein
acylmercaptan: bond
adamantine: membrane
adansonian: classification
adaptation: disease; syndrome

adaptive: behavior; enzyme; hypertrophy
adaptive behavior: scale
addisonian: anemia; crisis
addition: compound
addition-deletion: mutation
additive: effect
adductor: canal; muscle; reflex; tubercle
Aden: fever; ulcer
adeno-associated: virus
adenoid: disease; facies; tissue; tumor
adenoid cystic: carcinoma
adenoid squamous cell: carcinoma
adenoidal-pharyngeal-conjunctival: virus
adenomatoid: tumor
adenomatoid odontogenic: tumor
adenomatous: goiter; polyp
adenosatellite: virus
adequal: cleavage
adequate: stimulus
adherence: syndrome
adherent: leukoma; pericardium; placenta
adhesion: dyspepsia; phenomenon; test
adhesive: arachnoiditis; bandage; capsulitis; inflammation; pericarditis; peritonitis; phlebitis; pleurisy; tape; vaginitis
adhesive absorbent: dressing
adient: behavior
adipodermal: graft
adipokinetic: hormone
adipose: capsule; cell; degeneration; fold; fossa; infiltration; tissue; tumor
adiposogenital: degeneration; dystrophy; syndrome
adjacent: angle
adjustable: articulator
adjustable axis: face-bow
adjustable occlusal: pivot
adjustment: disorder
adjuvant: vaccine
adlerian: psychoanalysis; psychology
admaxillary: gland
adnexal: adenoma; carcinoma
adolescent: albuminuria; crisis; medicine; sterility
adolescent round: back
adoptive: immunity; immunotherapy
adrenal: androgen; apoplexy; body; capsule; cortex; crisis; gland; hermaphroditism; hypertension; rest; virilism
adrenal ascorbic acid depletion: test
adrenal cortical: carcinoma; syndrome
adrenaline: reversal
adrenal virilizing: syndrome
adrenal weight: factor
adrenergic: agent; amine; blockade; fiber; receptor
adrenergic blocking: agent
adrenergic neuronal blocking: agent
adrenocortical: adenoma; hormone; insufficiency
adrenocorticotropic: hormone; peptide
adrenogenital: syndrome
adrenotropic: hormone
adsorption: theory
adult: medulloepithelioma; rickets; tuberculosis
adult-onset: diabetes
adult pseudohypertrophic muscular: dystrophy
adult respiratory distress: syndrome
adult T-cell: leukemia; lymphoma
advancement: flap
adventitial: cell; neuritis
adventitious: albuminuria; bursa; cyst
adverse: reaction
adversive: movement
adynamic: ileus
A-E: amputation
aerial: mycelium
aerobic: dehydrogenase; respiration
aerosol: generator
aerospace: medicine
aestivoautumnal: fever
affect: displacement; hunger; memory; spasm
affective: disorder; psychosis; tone
afferent: fiber; lymphatic; nerve; vessel
afferent glomerular: arteriole
afferent loop: syndrome
affinity: chromatography; column
afibrillar: cementum
AFORMED: phenomenon
African: cachexia; histoplasmosis; trypanosomiasis
African furuncular: myiasis
African hemorrhagic: fever
African horse: sickness
African horse sickness: virus
African sleeping: sickness
African swine: fever
African swine fever: virus
afterloading: screw
afunctional: gingivitis; occlusion
A/G: ratio
Ag-AS: stain
agene: process
agglutinating: antibody
agglutinative: thrombus
aggregate: anaphylaxis; gland
aggregated lymphatic: follicle; nodule
aggressive: instinct
aggressive infantile: fibromatosis
agitated: depression
aglossia-adactylia: syndrome
agminate, agminated: gland
agnogenic myeloid: metaplasia
agonal: infection; leukocytosis; rhythm; thrombus
agony: clot
agranular: cortex; leukocyte
agranular cytoplasmic: reticulum
agranulocytic: angina
A-H: interval
A-H conduction: time
AIDS-related: complex; virus
air: bladder; cell; conduction; dose; embolus; pollution; sac; sickness; splint; syringe; thermometer; tube; vesicle
air-bone: gap
airbrasive: technique
air-conditioner: lung
airplane: splint
air-slaked: lime
airway: resistance
A-K: amputation
Akabane: virus
akamushi: disease
akinetic: epilepsy; mutism
Akureyri: disease
alactic oxygen: debt
alar: artery; chest; fold; lamina; ligament; part; plate; process; spine
alarm: reaction
albino: rat
albumin-globulin: ratio
albuminized: iron
albuminocytologic: dissociation
albuminoid: degeneration
albuminous: cell; degeneration; gland; swelling
albuminuric: retinitis
Alcian blue: stain
alcohol: diuresis
alcohol amnestic: syndrome
alcoholic: cardiomyopathy; cirrhosis; deterioration; extract; hyalin; psychosis; tincture

alcoholic hyaline: body
alcohol-soluble: eosin
aldehyde: base; fuchsin; reaction
aldehyde fuchsin: stain
alecithal: ovum
Aleppo: boil
aleukemic: leukemia; myelosis
Aleutian: disease
Aleutian disease of mink: virus
alexin: unit
algid: malaria; stage
algid pernicious: fever
algoid: cell
Alice in Wonderland: syndrome
alicyclic: compound
alignment: curve; mark
alimentary: apparatus; canal; diabetes; glycosuria; hyperinsulinism; lipemia; osteopathy; pentosuria; system; tract
alimentary tract: smear
aliphatic: compound
alisphenoid: cartilage
alizarin: indicator
alizarin red: stain
alkali: disease; metal; reserve; therapy
alkali denaturation: test
alkali-earth: metal
alkaline: earth; phosphatase; reaction; ribonuclease; tide; water; wave
alkaline-ash: diet
alkaline earth: element
alkaline milk: drip
alkaline phosphatase: stain
alkylating: agent
allantoenteric: diverticulum
allantoic: bladder; cavity; cyst; diverticulum; fluid; sac; stalk; vesicle
allantoid: membrane
allantoidoangiopagous: twin
allelic: additivity; exclusion; gene
allergenic: extract
allergic: angiitis; conjunctivitis; coryza; eczema; granulomatosis; inflammation; purpura; reaction; rhinitis
allergic granulomatous: angiitis
allied: reflex
alligator: forceps; skin
allogeneic: graft; inhibition
allomeric: function
allopathic: keratoplasty
all or none: law
allosteric: site
allotropic: personality
allotypic: determinant; marker
alloxan: diabetes
almond: nucleus
alpha (α-): angle; blocking; cell; fiber; granule; helix; hemolysin; hemolysis; particle; ray; rhythm; streptococcus; substance; thalassemia; unit; wave
alpha(α)-1-: antitrypsin
alpha (α)-adrenergic: receptor
alpha (α)-adrenergic blocking: agent
alphabetical: keratitis
alpha (α)-chymotrypsin-induced: glaucoma
alpha (α)-heavy-chain: disease
alpha (α_1)-trypsin: inhibitor
alphabetical: keratitis
Alpine: scurvy
ALT:AST: ratio
alterative: inflammation
altercursive: intubation
alternate: hemianesthesia
alternate binaural loudness balance: test
alternate cover: test
alternate day: strabismus
alternating: current; hemiplegia; mydriasis; pulse; strabismus; tremor
alternative: inheritance
altitude: chamber; erythremia; sickness
altitudinal: hemianopsia
alum: whey
aluminum: penicillin
alveolar: abscess; air; angle; arch; atrophy; body; bone; border; canal; cell; crest; duct; foramen; gas; gingiva; gland; index; macrophage; mucosa; osteitis; part; periosteum; point; process; ridge; sac; septum; ventilation; yoke
alveolar-arterial oxygen: difference
alveolar cell: carcinoma
alveolar dead: space
alveolar gas: equation
alveolar hydatid: cyst
alveolar soft part: sarcoma
alveolar supporting: bone
alveolobuccal: groove; sulcus
alveolodental: canal; ligament; membrane
alveololabial: groove; sulcus
alveololingual: groove; sulcus
alevolonasal: line
amacrine: cell
amalgam: carrier; matrix; strip; tattoo
amaurotic: mydriasis; nystagmus; pupil
amaurotic cat's: eye
amaurotic familial: idiocy
amber: mutation
ambient: behavior
ambiguous: nucleus
ambiguous external: genitalia
amboceptor: unit
Amboyna: button
Ambu: bag
ambulant: erysipelas; plague
ambulatory: automatism; plague; schizophrenia; surgery; typhoid
amebic: abscess; colitis; dysentery; granuloma; vaginitis
ameboid: astrocyte; cell; movement
amelanotic: melanoma
ameloblastic: fibroma; fibrosarcoma; layer; odontoma; sarcoma
ameloblastic adenomatoid: tumor
amelodental, amelodentinal: junction
amenorrhea-galactorrhea: syndrome
American: leishmaniasis; tarantula
American Law Institute: rule
amide: oxime
amino: sugar
***p*-aminohippuric acid:** clearance
ammonia: rash
ammoniacal: urine
ammoniated: mercuric chloride; mercury; tincture
amnemonic: agraphia
amnesic: aphasia
amnestic: aphasia; psychosis; syndrome
amniocardiac: vesicle
amnioembryonic: junction
amniogenic: cell
amnion: ring
amniotic: adhesion; band; cavity; corpuscle; duct; fluid; fold; raphe; sac
amniotic fluid: embolism; syndrome
amorphous: fraction; phosphorus
amorphous insulin zinc: suspension
amphibolic: fistula
amphibolous: fistula
amphiprotic: solvent
amphophil: granule
amphoric: rale; resonance; respiration; voice
amphoric voice: sound
amphoteric: electrolyte; element; reaction
amphotropic: virus

amplifier: host
amplifier type: electrocardiograph
amplitude of: accommodation; convergence
ampullar: abortion; pregnancy
ampullary: aneurysm; crest; limb; sulcus
amputating: ulcer
amputation: neuroma
Amsterdam: syndrome
amygdaloid: complex; fossa; nucleus; tubercle
amylaceous: corpuscle
amylase-creatinine clearance: ratio
amylic: fermentation
amylogenic: body
amyloid: body; corpuscle; degeneration; kidney; nephrosis; tumor
amyotrophic lateral: sclerosis
A-N: interval
anabiotic: cell
anaclitic: depression; psychotherapy
anacrotic: limb; pulse
anadicrotic: pulse
anaerobic: dehydrogenase; respiration
anal: atresia; canal; cleft; column; erotism; fascia; fissure; fistula; gland; membrane; orifice; pecten; phase; pit; plate; reflex; region; sac; sinus; triangle; valve; verge
analeptic: enema
analgesic: cuirass; nephritis; nephropathy
anal skin: tag
analytic: chemistry; psychiatry; psychology; therapy
analyzing: rod
anamnestic: reaction
anaphase: lag
anaphylactic: antibody; intoxication; shock
anaphylactoid: crisis; purpura; shock
anaplastic: carcinoma; cell
anarthritic rheumatoid: disease
anastomosed: graft
anastomosing: fiber
anastomotic: fiber; stricture; ulcer; vein
anatomic; anatomical: age; crown; element; neck; pathology; position; rigidity; root; sphincter; tooth; tubercle; wart
anatomical dead: space
anatrophic: nephrotomy
anchor: splint
anchoring: villus
anconal: fossa
anconeus: muscle
ancylostomiasis: dermatitis
androgen: unit
androgenic: alopecia; hormone; zone
android: pelvis
anechoic: chamber
anemic: anoxia; halo; hypoxia; infarct; murmur
anergic: leishmaniasis
aneroid: manometer
anesthesia: machine
anesthetic: record; circuit; depth; ether; gas; index; leprosy; shock; vapor
anestrous: ovulation
aneurysm: needle
aneurysmal: bruit; phthisis; sac; varix
aneurysmal bone: cyst
angel's: wing
anginose: scarlatina
angioblastic: cell
angiodysgenetic: myelomalacia
angiofollicular mediastinal lymph node: hyperplasia
angiogenesis: factor
angioid: streak
angioimmunoblastic: lymphadenopathy
angiolithic: degeneration; sarcoma
angiolymphoid: hyperplasia
angiomatoid: tumor
angioneurotic: edema; hematuria
angio-osteohypertrophy: syndrome
angioparalytic: neurasthenia
angiopathic: neurasthenia; retinopathy
angiopathic hemolytic: anemia
angioplastic: infantilism
angiotensin converting: enzyme
angiotensin converting enzyme: inhibitor
angle of: convergence
angle-closure: glaucoma
angular: acceleration; aldehyde; aperture; artery; cheilitis; conjunctivitis; convolution; curvature; gyrus; methyl; notch; stomatitis; vein
anhidrotic ectodermal: dysplasia
anhydrous: alcohol; chloral; lanolin
anicteric virus: hepatitis
aniline: fuchsin
aniline-water: solution
animal: charcoal; dextran; force; graft; lymph; model; pole; soap; starch; toxin; virus; wax
animal protein: factor
anion: gap
anion-exchange: resin
anionic: detergent
anisometropic: amblyopia
anisotropic: disk; lipoid
ankle: bone; clonus; jerk; joint; reflex; region
ankyloglossia superior: syndrome
ankylosed: tooth
ankylosing: hyperostosis; spondylitis
annealing: lamp; tray
annectant: gyrus
annihilation: radiation
annular: band; cartilage; cataract; ligament; pancreas; placenta; plexus; scleritis; scotoma; sphincter; staphyloma; stricture; synechia; syphilid
annulate: lamella
annulospiral: ending; organ
anococcygeal: body; ligament; nerve
anocutaneous: line
anodal: current
anodal closure: contraction; tetanus
anodal duration: tetanus
anodal opening: contraction; tetanus
anode: ray
anogenital: band; raphe
anomalous: complex; correspondence; trichromatism; uterus; viscosity
anomalous mitral: arcade
anomeric: carbon
anomic: aphasia
anonymous: artery; vein
anorectal: junction; spasm; syndrome
anorectal lymph: node
anosognosic: epilepsy; seizure
anospinal: center
anovular: menstruation
anovular ovarian: follicle
anovulational: menstruation
anovulatory: cycle
anoxemia: test
anoxic: anoxia
anserine: bursa; bursitis
ansiform: lobule
antagonistic: muscle; reflex
antalgic: gait
antebrachial: fascia
antebrachiocarpal: joint
antecedent: sign
antecubital: space
antegonial: notch

antegrade: cystography; pyelography; urography
antemortem: clot; thrombus
antenatal: diagnosis
anterior: asynclitism; choroiditis; component; curvature; embryotoxon; guide; megalophthalmus; nephrectomy; occlusion; rhinoscopy; rhizotomy; scleritis; sclerotomy; staphyloma; symblepharon; synechia; urethritis; uveitis; vitrectomy
anterior anatomical structures (specific anterior anatomical and histological structures are listed under the following): arch; area; artery; base; border, bundle; canal; cell; chamber, column; commissure; convolution; crest; cusp; division; epithelium; extremity; fissure; fontanel; foramen; fossa; funiculus; gland; groove; gyrus; horn; joint; layer; ligament; limb; line; lip; lobe; lobule; margin; membrane; muscle; naris; nerve; node; notch; part; pillar; pituitary; plexus; pole; portal; process; pyramid; recess; region; ring; root; segment; sinus; spine; substance; sulcus; surface; tract; triangle; tooth; tubercle; valve; vein; velum; wall
anterior chamber: trabecula
anterior chamber cleavage: syndrome
anterior facial: height
anterior focal: point
anterior myocardial: infarction
anterior ocular: segment
anterior pelvic: exenteration
anterior pituitary: gonadotropin
anterior pituitary-like: hormone
anterior spinal: paralysis
anterior tibial: bursa
anterior tibial compartment: syndrome
anterofacial: dysplasia
anterograde: amnesia; block; conduction; memory
anteroinferior myocardial: infarction
anterolateral: column; cordotomy; fontanel; groove; sulcus; surface; tractotomy
anterolateral central: artery
anterolateral myocardial: infarction
anterolateral striate: artery
anterolateral thalamostriate: artery
anteromedial: surface
anteromedial central: artery
anteromedial thalamostriate: artery
anteromedian: groove
anteroposterior: diameter; dysplasia
anteroposterior facial: dysplasia
anteroseptal myocardial: infarction
antevesical: hernia
anthracotic: tuberculosis
anthrax: pneumonia; septicemia; toxin
anthropoid: pelvis
anthroponotic cutaneous: leishmaniasis
antiacrodynia: factor
antialopecia: factor
antianemic: principle
antianxiety: agent
anti-basement membrane: antibody; glomerulonephritis; nephritis
antiberiberi: factor; vitamin
antibiotic: enterocolitis; sensitivity
antibiotic sensitivity: test
anti-black-tongue: factor
antibody: excess
antibody deficiency: disease; syndrome
anticoagulant: therapy
anticomplementary: factor; serum
anti-D: immunoglobulin
antidiuretic: hormone
antiepithelial: serum
antifoaming: agent
anti-G: suit
antigen: excess; interferon; unit
antigen-antibody: reaction
antigenic: competition; complex; determinant; drift; shift
antigen-responsive: cell
antigen-sensitive: cell
antiglobulin: test
antigravity: muscle
antihemophilic: factor; globulin; plasma
antihemorrhagic: factor; vitamin
antihuman: globulin
antihuman globulin: test
anti-idiotype: antibody; autoantibody
anti-kidney serum: nephritis
antilymphocyte: serum
antimicrobial: spectrum
anti-Monson: curve
antineuritic: factor; vitamin
antinuclear: antibody; factor
antipellagra: factor
antiperistaltic: anastomosis
antipernicious anemia: factor
antipodal: cone
anti-Pr cold: autoagglutinin
antipsychotic: agent
antirabies: serum
antirachitic: vitamin
antireflection: coating
antireticular cytotoxic: serum
antiscorbutic: vitamin
antisense: DNA
antiseptic: dressing
antiserum: anaphylaxis
antisocial: personality
antisocial personality: disorder
antisterility: factor; vitamin
antitoxic: serum
antitoxin: rash; unit
antitragohelicine: fissure
antitrypsin: deficiency
antitryptic: index
antivenene: unit
antiviral: immunity; protein
antral: pouch; sphincter
anvil: sound
anxiety: dream; hysteria; neurosis; reaction; state; syndrome
anxious: delirium
aortic: arch; area; atresia; body; bulb; dwarfism; facies; foramen; incompetence; insufficiency; murmur; nerve; notch; opening; ostium; plexus; reflex; regurgitation; sac; sinus; spindle; stenosis; sulcus; valve; vestibule; window
aortic arch: syndrome
aortic body: tumor
aortic septal: defect
aorticorenal: ganglion
aorticopulmonary septal: defect
aortocoronary: bypass
aortoiliac: bypass
aortoiliac occlusive: disease
aortopulmonary: septum
aortorenal: bypass
apallic: state; syndrome
apathetic: thyrotoxicosis
apatite: calculus
A-P-C: virus
ape: fissure; hand
aperiosteal: amputation
apex: beat; pneumonia
aphakic: eye; glaucoma
aphonic: pectoriloquy
aphthobullous: stomatitis
aphthous: fever; stomatitis
apical: abscess; angle; area; complex; cyst; dendrite; foramen; gland; granuloma; infection; ligament; periodontitis; process; segment; space
apical ectodermal: ridge
apical lymph: node

apical periodontal: abscess
apicoposterior: segment
aplanatic: lens
aplastic: anemia; lymph
apneic: oxygenation; pause
apneustic: breathing
apochromatic: lens; objective
apocrine: adenoma; carcinoma; chromhidrosis; gland; metaplasia; miliaria
apolar: cell
aponeurotic: fibroma; reflex
apophylactic: phase
apophysary: point
apophysial: fracture; point
apoplectic: cyst; retinitis
apparent: viscosity
appendiceal: abscess
appendicular: artery; colic; muscle; skeleton; vein
appendicular lymph: node
apperceptive: mass
appetite: juice
appetitive: behavior
applanation: tonometer
apple jelly: nodule
applied: anatomy; anthropology; chemistry
appliqué: form
apposition: suture
appositional: growth
approach-approach: conflict
approach-avoidance: conflict
approximation: suture
aptitude: test
APUD: cell
apyretic: tetanus; typhoid
aquagenic: pruritis
aqueduct: veil
aqueductal: intubation
aqueous: chamber; flare; humor; phase; vaccine; vein
aqueous influx: phenomenon
aquo-: ion
arachnoid, arachnoidal: cyst; foramen; granulation; membrane; villus
arborescent: cataract
arborization: block
arc: perimeter
arc-flash: conjunctivitis
arch: bar; form; length; wire
archaic-paralogical: thinking
arched: crest
archenteric: canal
arch length: deficiency
arch-loop-whorl: system
arciform: artery; vein
arcon: articulator
arcuate: artery; crest; eminence; fasciculus; fiber; line; nucleus; scotoma; uterus; vein; zone
arcuate popliteal: ligament
arcuate pubic: ligament
ardent: fever; spirit
areolar: choroiditis; choroidopathy; gland; tissue
argentaffin: cell; granule
Argentinian hemorrhagic: fever
arginine: oxytocin; vasopressin; vasotocin
argyrophilic: cell; fiber
aristotelian: method
arithmetic: mean
arm: phenomenon
armed: rostellum
armored: heart
aromatic: bitters; castor oil; compound; series; water
arousal: function; reaction
arrested: tuberculosis
arrested dental: caries
arrhenic: medication
arrow: poison
arrow point: tracing
arsenic, arsenical: keratosis; pigmentation; tremor
arseniureted: hydrogen
arterial: arch; blood; bulb; anal; capillary; circle; cone; duct; flap; forceps; groove; hemangioma; hyperemia; hypotension; ligament; line; murmur; nephrosclerosis; network; sclerosis; segment; spider; tension; transfusion; vein; wave
arteriocapillary: sclerosis
arteriococcygeal: gland
arteriolar: nephrosclerosis; sclerosis
arteriolosclerotic: kidney
arteriolovenular: anastomosis; bridge
arteriosclerotic: aneurysm; gangrene; kidney; psychosis; retinopathy
arteriovenous: anastomosis; aneurysm; fistula; nicking; shunt
arteriovenous carbon dioxide: difference
arteriovenous oxygen: difference
artery: needle
arthritic: atrophy; calculus
arthritic general: pseudoparalysis
arthrodial: cartilage; joint
articular: capsule; cartilage; chondrocalcinosis; circumference; corpuscle; crepitus; crescent; crest; disk; eminence; fossa; fracture; gout; lamella; leprosy; lip; margin; meniscus; muscle; nerve; network; pit; process; rheumatism; sensibility; surface; tubercle
articular vascular: circle
articulated: skeleton
articulating: paper
artificial: anatomy; ankylosis; anus; crown; dentition; eye; heart; hibernation; insemination; kidney; melanin; pacemaker; pneumothorax; pupil; radioactivity; respiration; selection; sphincter; stone; tear; ventilation
artificial active: immunity
artificial Carlsbad: salt
artificial Kissingen: salt
artificial passive: immunity
artificial Vichy: salt
artistic: anatomy
aryepiglottic: fold; muscle
arylated: alkyl
arytenoid: cartilage; gland; swelling
artenoidal articular: surface
asbestos: acne; body; corn; liner; wart
ascending: artery; colon; current; degeneration; myelitis; neuritis; paralysis; part; process; pyelonephritis
ascending cervical: artery
ascending frontal: convolution; gyrus
ascending lumbar: vein
ascending palatine: artery
ascending parietal: convolution; gyrus
ascending pharyngeal: artery; plexus
ascitic: agar
ascorbate-cyanide: test
aseptic: fever; necrosis; surgery
asexual: dwarfism; generation; reproduction
ashen: tuber; tubercle; wing
Asian: influenza
Asiatic: cholera; schistosomiasis
asiderotic: anemia
aspermatogenic: sterility
aspheric: lens
asphyxiating thoracic: chondrodystrophy; dysplsia
aspirating: needle
aspiration: biopsy; pneumonia
Assam: fever
assertive: conditioning; training
assident: sign; symptom
assimilation: pelvis; sacrum

assist-control: ventilation
assisted: respiration; ventilation
assisted cephalic: delivery
assistive: movement
associated: antagonist; movement
association: area; constant; cortex; fiber; mechanism; neurosis; system; test; time; tract
associative: aphasia; reaction; strength
assortative: mating
astacoid: rash
asteroid: body; hyalosis
asthma: crystal
asthmatic: bronchitis
asthmatoid: wheeze
astigmatic: dial; lens
astral: fiber
astroglia: cell
asymmetric motor: neuropathy
asymmetrical: chondrodystrophy
asymptomatic: coccidioidomycosis
asynchronous pulse: generator
atactic, ataxic: abasia; agraphia; aphasia; gait; nystagmus; paramyotonia; paraplegia
atavistic: epiphysis
atelectatic: rale
ateliotic: dwarfism
atheroma: embolism
atheromatous: degeneration; plaque
atherosclerotic: aneurysm
athlete's: foot
athletic: heart
atlantoaxial: articulation
atlantooccipital: articulation; joint; membrane
atmospheric: pressure
atom: meter
atomic: core; heat; number; theory; volume; weight
atomic absorption: spectrophotometry
atomic mass: unit
atomistic: psychology
atonic: absence; bladder; dyspepsia; ectropion; entropion; epilepsy; epiphora; impotence; ulcer
atopic: allergy; asthma; cataract; conjunctivitis; dermatitis; eczema; reagin
atrabiliary: capsule
atraumatic: needle; suture
atresic: teratosis
atretic: corpus
atretic ovarian: follicle
atrial: artery; auricle; auricula; bigeminy; capture; complex; dissociation; echo; extrasystole; fibrillation; flutter; gallop; kick; myxoma; sound; standstill; systole; tachycardia
atrial chaotic: tachycardia
atrial fusion: beat
atrial natriuretic: factor
atrial septal: defect
atrial synchronous pulse: generator
atrial transport: function
atrial triggered pulse: generator
atrial-well: technique
atriodigital: dysplasia
atriosystolic: murmur
atrioventricular (or A-V): band; block; bundle; canal; conduction; dissociation; extrasystole; gradient; groove; interval; nicking; node; rhythm; septum; sulcus; trunk; valve
atrioventricular canal: cushion
atrioventricular nodal: bigeminy; extrasystole; rhythm; tachycardia
atrophic: arthritis; excavation; gastritis; glossitis; heterochromia; inflammation; keratoconjunctivitis; kidney; pharyngitis; rhinitis; thrombosis; vaginitis
atropine: test
attached: craniotomy; gingiva
attached cranial: section
attachment: apparatus
attack: rate
attending: staff; surgeon
attention deficit: disorder
attentuated: tuberculous; virus
attitudinal: reflex
attraction: sphere
atypical: absence; achrocephalosyndactyly; achromatoposia; fibroxanthoma; insulin; lipoma; measles; pneumonia; pseudocholinesterase
atypical facial: neuralgia
atypical melanocytic: hyperplasia
atypical trigeminal: neuralgia
atypical verrucous: endocarditis
audiogenic: epilepsy
auditory: agnosia; alternans; aphasia; area; canal; capsule; cartilage; cortex; fatigue; field; ganglion; hair; hyperalgesia; hyperesthesia; lemniscus; localization; nerve; nucleus; ossicle; pathway; pit; placode; process; reflex; stria; string; synesthesia; threshold; tooth; tract; tube; vertigo; vesicle
auditory brainstem response: audiometry
auditory oculogyric: reflex
auditory receptor: cell
augmentation: graft; mammaplasty
augmented histamine: test
augmentor: fiber; nerve
aural: myiasis; vertigo
auramine O fluorescent: stain
auricular: appendage; appendectomy; appendix; arc; canaliculus; cartilge; complex; extrasystole; fibrillation; fissure; flutter; ganglion; index; ligament; notch; point; reflex; standstill; surface; systole; tachycardia; triangle; tubercle; vein
auriculo-infraorbital: plane
auriculopalpebral: reflex
auriculopressor: reflex
auriculotemporal: nerve
auriculotemporal nerve: syndrome
auriculoventricular: groove
auropalpebral: reflex
auscultatory: alternans; gap; percussion; sound
aussage: test
Australia: antigen
Australian X: disease; encephalitis
Australian X disease: virus
authoritarian: personality
authority: figure
autistic: parasite
autochthonous: idea; malaria; parasite
autocrine: hypothesis
autodermic: graft
autoerythrocyte: sensitization
autoerythrocyte sensitization: syndrome
autogenous: graft; keratoplasty; union; vaccine
autohemolysis: test
autoimmune: disease; thrombocytopenia; thyroiditis
autoimmune hemolytic: anemia
autokinetic: effect
autologous: protein
autolytic: enzyme
automated differential leukocyte: counter
automatic: absence; audiometer; audiometry; beat; chorea; condenser; contraction; epilepsy; plugger
autonomic: bladder; disorder; epilepsy; ganglion; imbalance; nerve; plexus

autonomic motor: neuron
autonomic nervous: system
autonomous: psychotherapy
autoparenchymatous: metaplasia
autophagic: vacuole
autopolymer, autopolymerizing: resin
autoscopic: phenomenon
autoserum: therapy
autosomal: gene
autumn: crocus; fever
autumnal: catarrh
auxanographic: method
auxetic: growth
auxiliary: abutment
auxotrophic: strain
A-V: see atrioventricular
A-V strabismus: syndrome
available arch: length
avalanche: conduction
avascular: necrosis
average pulse: magnitude
aversion: therapy
aversive: behavior; conditioning; training
avian: achondroplasia; diphtheria; erythroblastosis; influenza; leukosis; lymphomatosis; malaria; monocytosis; myeloblastosis; reticuloendotheliosis; sarcoma; spirochetosis; trichomoniasis
avian encephalomyelitis: virus
avian erhthroblastosis: virus
avian infectious: encephalomyelitis; laryngotracheitis
avian infectious laryngotracheitis: virus
avian influenza: virus
avian leukosis-sarcoma: complex; virus
avian lymphomatosis: virus
avian myeloblastosis: virus
avian neurolymphomatosis: virus
avian pneumoencephalitis: virus
avian sarcoma: virus
avian viral arthritis: virus
aviation: medicine; otitis
aviator's: disease; ear
avoidance: conditioning
avoidance-avoidance: conflict
avoidant: personality
avulsed: wound
avulsion: fracture
axial: amblyopia; ametropia; aneurysm; angle; cataract; current; filament; hyperopia; illumination; muscle; myopia; neuritis; plate; point; projection; skeleton; surface; view; wall
axial pattern: flap
axile: corpusle
axillary: anesthesia; arch; artery; cataract; cavity; fascia; fold; fossa; gland; line; nerve; plexus; region; space; triangle; vein
axillary lymph: node
axillary sweat: gland
axiolabiolingual: plane
axiomesiodistal: plane
axis: corpuscle; cylinder; deviation; ligament; shift; traction
axis-traction: forceps
axoaxonic: synapse
axodendritic: synapse
axon: hillock; reflex; terminal
axonal: process
axonal terminal: bouton
axoplasmic: transport
axosomatic: synapse
A.-Z.: test
azin: dye
azo: dye; itch
azocarmine: dye
azotemic: retinitis
azotobacter: nuclease
Aztec: ear
azure: lunula
azure A: stain
azurophil: granule
azygos: artery; vein
azygos vein: principle
azygos venous: line

B

β: see beta
B: bile; cell; chain; fiber; lymphocyte; virus; wave
B_T: factor
baby: tooth
bacillary: dysentery; layer; pyelonephritis
bacillus Calmette-Guérin: vaccine
back: cross; mutation; pressure; tooth
back-action: plugger
backboard: splint
background: radiation
back of foot: reflex
back vertex: power
backward: curvature
backward heart: failure
backwash: ileitis
bacterial: allergy; aneurysm; antagonism; capsule; endarteritis; endocarditis; hemolysin; interference; plaque; toxin; virus
bacteriocin: factor
bacteriocinogenic: plasmid
bacteriogenic: agglutination
bacteriolytic: serum
bacteriophage: immunity; resistance; typing
bacteriotropic: substance
Bagdad: boil
bag-gel: implant
bag of: waters
baked: tongue
baker's: eczema; itch
baking: soda
balance: theory
balanced: anesthesia; articulation; bite; occlusion; polymorphism; translocation
balancing: contact; side
balancing occlusal: surface
balanic: hypospadias
balantidial: dysentery
BALB: test
bald: tongue
Balkan: beam; frame; nephropathy; splint
ball: thrombus; valve; variance
ball-and-socket: joint
ballerina-foot: pattern
balloon: atrioseptostomy; cell
balloon cell: nevus
ballooning: colliquation; degeneration
balloon-tip: catheter
ball-valve: action; thrombus
bamboo: hair
bancroftian: filariasis
band: cell; neutrophil
bandage: sign
bandbox: reasonance
band-shaped: keratopathy
bar: clasp
Barbados: leg
barbed: broach
barber's: itch
barber's pilonidal: sinus
bar clasp: arm
bar clip: attachment
Barcoo: rot; vomit
bare: area
bare lymphocyte: syndrome
barium: enema
bar joint: denture
barometric: pressure
baroreceptor: nerve
barrel: chest
bar-sleeve: attachment
baryta: water
basal: age; anesthesia; body; bone; cell; corpuscle; diet; ganglion; granule; lamina; layer; metabolism; part; plate; ridge; rod; seat;

sphincter; striation; surface; tuberculosis; vein
basal cell: adenoma; carcinoma; epithelioma; hyperplasia; layer; nevus; papilloma
basal cell nevus: syndrome
basal joint: reflex
basal metabolic: rate
basaloid: carcinoma; cell
basal seat: area
basal skull: fracture
basal squamous cell: carcinoma
base: composition; deficit; excess; line; material; metal; pair; plate; projection; unit; view
baseball: finger
basedowian: insanity
baseline: tonus; variability
baseline fetal heart: rate
basement: lamina; membrane
baseplate: wax
basibregmatic: axis
basic: diet; dye; estropia; exotropia; fuchsin; metal; oxide; personality; salt; stain
basic fuchsin-methylene blue: stain
basic personality: type
basicranial: axis; flexure
basifacial: axis
basilar: angle; apophysis; artery; bone; cartilage; cell; crest; impression; index; invagination; lamina; leptomeningitis; membrane; meningitis; part; plexus; process; prognathism; sinus; sulcus; vertebra
basilic: vein
basinasal: line
basioccipital: bone
basipharyngeal: canal
basisphenoid: bone
basivertebral: vein
basket: cell
basophil: adenoma; cell; granule; substance
basophilic: degeneration; leukemia; leukocyte; leukocytosis; leukopenia
basophilocyte: leukemia
basosquamous: carcinoma
Bassora: gum
bath: itch; pruritus
bathing trunk: nevus
bathmic: evolution
battered child: syndrome
battle: fatigue; neurosis
battledore: placenta
bauxite: pneumoconiosis
bay: sore
bayonet: hair
BCG: vaccine
B-E: amputation
Be^a: antigen
beaded: hair
beaked: pelvis
beaker: cell
bearing-down: pain
beat-to-beat: variation
bed: sore
beechwood: sugar
beer: heart
beer-drinker's: cardiomyopathy
beet: sugar, tongue
behavior: chain; disorder; genetics; modification; reflex; therapy
behavioral: immunogen; manifestation; medicine; pathogen; psychology
BEI: test
Belgian Congo: anemia
bell: sound
bellmetal: resonance
bellows: murmur
bell-shaped: crown
belt: test
bending: fracture
benign: albuminuria; cementoblastoma; dyskeratosis; glycosuria; hypertension; lymphadenosis; lymphocytoma; lymphoma; mesothelioma; nephrosclerosis; stupor; tetanus; tumor
benign bone: aneurysm
benign bovine: theileriosis
benign chronic bullous: dermatosis
benign dry: pleurisy
benign essential: tremor
benign familial: icterus
benign inoculation: lymphoreticulosis; reticulosis
benign juvenile: melanoma
benign lymphoepithelial: lesion
benign mediastinal lymph node: hyperplasia
benign migratory: glossitis
benign mucosal: pemphigoid
benign myalgic: encephalomyelitis
benign paroxysmal: peritonitis
benign prostatic: hypertrophy
benign tertian: malaria
bentiromide: test
bentonite flocculation: test
benzene: nucleus; ring
benzidine: test
berlocque, berlock: dermatitis
berry: aneurysm; cell
beryllium: granuloma
beta (β-): angle; cell; corynebacteriophage; fiber; globulin; granule; hemolysin; hemolysis; leukocyte; oxidation; particle; phage; radiation; ray; rhythm; substance; thalassemia; wave
beta (β)-adrenergic: receptor
beta (β)-adrenergic receptor blocking: agent
beta (β)-adrenoreceptor: antagonist
beta (β)-carotene cleavage: enzyme
beta-delta (β-δ): thalassemia
beta (β)-hemolytic: streptococcus
beta-oxidation-condensation: theory
betel: cancer
bevelled: anastomosis
BH: interval
Bi: antigen
biauricular: axis
biaxial: joint
bi-bi: reaction
bicameral: abscess
bicanalicular: sphincter
biceps: muscle; reflex
biceps femoris: reflex
bicipital: aponeurosis; bursitis; fascia; groove; rib; ridge; tuberosity
bicipitoradial: bursa
biclonal: gammopathy
biconcave: lens
bicondylar: articulation; joint
biconvex: lens
bicoudate: catheter
bicuspid: tooth; valve
bidirectional ventricular: tachycardia
bidiscoidal: placenta
bifid: cranium; penis; rib; tongue; uterus; uvula
bifidus: factor
bifocal: lens; spectacles
bifoveal: fixation
bifurcated: ligament
bifurcation lymph: node
big: ACTH; head
bigeminal: body; pregnancy; pulse; rhythm
big liver: disease
bilaminar: blastoderm
bilateral: hemianopsia; hermaphroditism; left-sideness; lithotomy; synchrony
bile: acid; capillary; cyst; duct; papilla; peritonitis; pigment; thrombus
bile acid tolerance: test
bile pigment: hemoglobin

bile salt: agar
bilharzial: appendicitis; dysentry; granuloma
biliary: artesia; calculus; canaliculus; cirrhosis; colic; duct; ductule; dyskinesia; fever, fistula; steatorrhea; xanthomatosis
bilious: headache; typhoid
bilious remittent: fever; malaria
bilirubin: encephalopathy
bilobed: flap
bilocular: joint; stomach
bilocular femoral: hernia
bimanual: percussion; version
bimaxillary: protrusion
bimaxillary dentoalveolar: protrusion
bimaxillary protrusive: occlusion
Bimiti: virus
binangle: chisel
binary: combination; fission; nomenclature
binasal: hemianopsia
binaural: stethoscope
binaural alternate loudness balance: test
binauricular: arc
binding: energy
binocular: fixation; hemianopsia; heterochromia; loupe; microscope; ophthalmoscope; parallax; rivalry; vision
binomial: distribution; nomenclature
biochemical: genetics; metastasis; pharmacology; profile
bioelectric: potential
biogenetic: law
biologic; biological: chemistry; coefficient; control; evolution; half-life; hemolysis; time; vector
biological standard: unit
biomedical: engineering
biometrial: school
biopsy: needle
biorbital: angle
biotic: community; factor; potential
biparietal: diameter
bipartite: uterus
bipedicle: flap
bipennate: muscle
biphasic: insulin; response
bipolar: cautery; cell; lead; neuron; taxis; version
bird: face; unit
bird-breeder's: disease; lung
bird shot: retinochoroiditis
birth: amputation; canal; control; fracture; palsy; rate; trauma; weight
biscuit: bite
bisferious: pulse
Biskra: button
bismuth: line
bite: analysis; fork; gauge; plane; rim
bitemporal: hemianopsia
bitewing: film; radiograph
biting: louse; pressure; strength
bitter: almond oil; orange; tonic; water
bitterling: test
biundulant: meningoencephalitis
biuret: reaction; reagent; test
bivalent: antibody; chromosome
bivalent gas gangrene: antitoxin
bivalve: speculum
biventral: lobule
BK: virus
B-K: amputation
B-K mole: syndrome
black: cataract; death; disease; eye; fever; jaundice; lead; line; lung; measles; mustard; piedra; plague; sickness; spore; tarantula; tongue; urine; vomit; water
black currant: rash
black-dot: ringworm
black-legged: tick
black-tongue: disease
blackwater: fever
bladder: reflex; schistosomiasis
blade: bone
bland: diet; embolism; infarct
blanket: suture
blast: cell; chest; crisis; injury
blastodermic: disk; layer; vesicle
blastomycetic: dermitis
blastoporic: canal
bleached: wax
bleaching: powder
blear: eye
bleeding: polyp; time
blending; inheritance
blenorrheal: conjunctivitis
blighted: ovum
blind: boil; enema; fistula; foramen; gut; headache; spot; staggers; study; test
blinding: disease; glare
blind loop: syndrome
blind nasotracheal: intubation
blistering: collodion
block: anesthesia; vertebra
block design: test
blocked: aerogastria
blocking: activity; agent; antibody
blood: agar; albumin; bath; blister; calculus; capillary; cast; cell; circulation; clot; corpuscle; count; crisis; crystal; cyst; disk; dyscrasia; factor; gas; group; island; islet; lymph; mole; mote; plasma; plastid; plate; poisoning; pressure; quotient; relationship; serum; spavin; substitute; sugar; spot; tumor; type; typing; vessel
blood-air: barrier
blood-aqueous: barrier
blood-brain: barrier
blood-cerebrospinal fluid: barrier
blood gas: analysis
blood group: agglutinin; agglutinogen; antibody; antigen; antiserum; substance; system
blood group-specific: substance
bloodless: amputation; decerebration; operation; phlebotomy
blood plasma: fraction
blood urea: nitrogen
blood-vascular: system
blood volume: nomogram
blowing: wound
blow-out: fracture
blue: asphyxia; atrophy; baby; cataract; disease; edema; fever; line; nevus; pus; sclera; spot; vision; vitriol
blueberry muffin: baby
bluecomb: disease; virus
blue cone: monochromasy
blue dome: cyst
blue-green: algae; bacteria
blue pus: bacillus
blue rubber-bleb: nevus
bluetongue: virus
blunt duct: adenosis
boat: conformation; form
boat-shaped: abdomen
body: cavity; image; language; mechanics; plethysmography; schema; stalk
body mass: index
body righting: reflex
body-weight: ratio
bog: spavin
boilermaker's: deafness
boiling: point
Bolivian hemorrhagic: fever
bolster: finger
bolus: dressing
bomb: calorimeter
Bombay: phenomenon; trait
bone: abscess; ache; age; block; canaliculus; cell; charcoal; chips;

conduction; corpuscle; cyst; flap; forceps; graft; infarct; island; marrow; matrix; phosphate; plate; reflex; resorption; salt; sclerosis; sensibility; spavin; tissue; wax
bone marrow: transplantation
bony: ankylosis; crepitus; heart; labyrinth; palate; part
bony nasal: septum
bony semicircular: canal
booster: dose
Bordeaux: mixture
border: cell, molding; movement; seal
borderline: leprosy; personality; ray
borderline personality: disorder
border tissue: movement
Borna: disease
Borna disease: virus
Bornholm: disease
Bornholm disease: virus
bosch: yaws
Boston: exanthema; opium
bothropic, Bothrops: antitoxin
botryoid: sarcoma
botulinum: antitoxin
botulinus: toxin
botulism: antitoxin
bound: water
bounding: pupil
bouquet: fever
boutonneuse: fever
boutonnière: deformity
bovine: acetonemia; achondroplasia; adenovirus; antitoxin; babesiosis; borreliosis; brucellosis; colloid; hemoglobinuria; hyperkeratosis; ketosis; lymphosarcoma; mastitis; porphyria; rhinovirus; trichomoniasis
bovine cancer: eye
bovine congenital: ataxia
bovine ephemeral: fever
bovine granular: vaginitis
bovine herpes: mammillitis
bovine infectious: abortion
bovine leukemia: virus
bovine leukosis: virus
bovine papular: stomatitis
bovine papular stomatitis: virus
bovine serum: albumin
bovine sporadic: encephalomyelitis
bovine ulcerative: mammillitis
bovine vaccinia: mammillitis
bovine virus: diarrhea
bovine virus diarrhea: virus
bow-: leg
bowed: tendon
bowel: bypass; sound
bowel bypass: syndrome
bowenoid: papulosis
boxer's: ear; fracture
boxing: wax
brachial: anesthesia; artery; fascia; bland; muscle; neuritis; plexus; vein
brachial birth: palsy
brachial lymph: node
brachial plexus: neuropathy
brachiocephalic: muscle; trunk; vein
brachioradial: muscle; reflex
brachypellic: pelvis
bracken: poisoning; staggers
bradykinetic: analysis
bradykinin-potentiating: peptide
brain: cicatrix; concussion; congestion; contusion; death; edema; laceration; lipid; mantle; murmur; potential; sand; stem; sugar; swelling; wave
brain-heart infusion: agar
brain wave: complex; cycle
brainstem: hemorrhage
brainstem evoked response: audiometry
branched: calculus
branched chain: ketoaciduria; ketonuria
brancher deficiency: amylopectinosis
branchial: apparatus; arch; cartilage; cell; cleft; cyst; duct; fissure; fistula; groove; mesoderm; pouch
branchial cleft: cyst
branchial efferent: column
branching: enzyme; factor
branchiometric: muscle
branchiomotor: nucleus
brandy: nose
branny: desquamation; tetter
brassy: body; cough
brawny: arm; scleritis
Brazil: wax
Brazilian: ophthalmia; pemphigus
BrDu: banding
bread: pill
bread-and-butter: pericardium
break: shock
breakaway: phenomenon
breakbone: fever
breakoff: phenomenon
breast: bone; pang; pump
breath analysis: test
breath holding: test
breathing: bag; reserve
breech: delivery; extraction; presentation
bregmatic: fontanel
bregmatolambdoid: arc
bregmocardiac: reflex
brephoplastic: graft
brewers': yeast
brickdust: deposit
brickmaker's: anemia
bridge: corpuscle
bridging hepatic: necrosis
bridle: structure; suture
brightness difference: threshold
brilliant green bile salt: agar
brisket: disease
bristle: cell
British: gum
British thermal: unit
brittle: bone; diabetes
broad: fascia; ligament; spectrum
broadest: muscle
broad marginal confrontation: method
broad spectrum: antibiotic
bromide: acne
bromine: water
bromphenol: test
Brompton: cocktail
bromsulphalein: test
bronchial: adenoma; artery; asthma; breathing; bud; calculus; fremitus; gland; pneumonia; polyp; respiration; tube; vein; voice
bronchic: cell
bronchiolar: adenocarcinoma; carcinoma
bronchiolo-alveolar: carcinoma
bronchitic: asthma
bronchocentric: granulomatosis
bronchoesophageal: fistula; muscle
bronchogenic: carcinoma; cyst
bronchomediastinal: trunk
bronchopleural: fistula
bronchopulmonary: aspergillosis; dysplasia; segment; sequestration; spirochetosis
bronchopulmonary lymph: node
bronchoscopic: brush; smear; sponge
bronchovesicular: respiration
bronze: diabetes
bronzed: disease: skin
brood: capsule; cell
brother: complex
brow: presentation
brown: atrophy; edema; fat; induration; layer; pellicle; stria; tumor
brownian: motion; movement
brownian-Zsigmondy: movement
brucella strain 19: vaccine
brush: biopsy; border; burn; catheter

brush burn: abrasion
brush heap: structure
BSP: test
bubble gum: dermatitis
bubbling: rale
bubonic: plague
buccal: angle; artery; cavity; curve; embrasure; flange; gingiva; gland; nerve; occlusion; pit; region; smear; surface; tablet; vestibule
buccal lymph: node
buccinator: artery; crest; nerve
buccinator lymph: node
buccocervical: ridge
buccogingival: ridge
buccolingual: diameter, dimension; relation
bucconasal: membrane
bucconeural: duct
bucco-occlusal: angle
buccopharyngeal: fascia; membrane; part
buck: tooth
bucket-handle: incision; tear
buckled: aorta
buckthorn: polyneuropathy
bud: fission
buddeized: milk
buffalo: neck
buffer: capacity; index; pair; value
buffered crystalline: penicillin
buffy: coat
bulbar: apoplexy; conjunctiva; myelitis; palsy; paralysis; pulse; ridge; septum
bulbocavernosus: reflex
bulboid: corpuscle
bulbomimic: reflex
bulbosacral: system
bulbourethral: gland
bulbous: bougie
bulboventricular: loop; ridge
bulging eye: disease
bulk: modulus
bull: neck
bulldog: calf; forceps; head
bullet: bubo; forceps
bullous: edema; fever; impetigo; keratopathy; myringitis; pemphigoid; syphilid
bull's-eye: maculopathy
bundle: bone
bundle-branch: block
Bunyamwera: fever; virus
bunyavirus: encephalitis
bur: drill
Burdwan: fever
Burgundy: pitch
buried: flap; suture
burning drops: sign
burnt: alum
burr: cell
burrowing: hair
bursal: abscess; cyst; synovitis
Buruli: ulcer
Bush: sickness; yaws
Buss: disease
butanol-extractable: iodine
butanol-extractable iodine: test
butter: stool
butterfly: adrenal; eruption; fragment; lung; patch; rash; vertebra
button: suture
buttonhole: iridectomy; stenosis
buttress: foot; plate
buyo cheek: cancer
Bwamba: fever; virus
By: antigen
Byzantine arch: palate

C

C: banding; bile; cell; chain; factor; fiber; terminus; wave
C1: esterase
C1 esterase: inhibitor
C3: proactivator
c-a: interval
C-banding: stain
C carbohydrate: antigen
C group: virus
C-reactive: protein
"C" sliding: osteotomy
CA: virus
cabbage: goiter
cable: graft
cacao: butter
cachectic: edema; endocarditis; fever; pallor
cadaveric: rigidity; spasm
caddis: worm
cafe: coronary
café-au-lait: spot
Cagot: ear
Cain: complex
caisson: disease
cake: alum; kidney
caked: breast
Calabar: swelling
calcaneal: artery; bone; bursitis; gait; process; region; sulcus; tuber; tubercle; tuberosity
calcaneal articular: surface
calcanean: tendon
calcaneocuboid: joint; ligament
calcaneofibular: ligament
calcaneonavicular: ligament
calcaneotibial: ligament
calcareous: conjunctivitis; degeneration; infiltration; metastasis
calcarine: artery; fasciculus; fissure; sulcus
calcic: water
calcification: line
calcific nodular aortic: stenosis
calcified: cartilage
calcifying epithelial odontogenic: tumor
calcifying and keratinizing odontogenic: cyst
calcifying odontogenic: cyst
calcined: magnesia
calcinuric: diabetes
calcium: antagonist; gout; rigor; time
calcium channel-blocking: agent
calculated mean: organism
calculated serum: osmolality
calf: bone; diphtheria
caliciform, calyciform: cell; ending
California: encephalitis; virus
California psychological inventory: test
caliper: micrometer
callosal: convolution; gyrus; sulcus
callosomarginal: artery; fissure
calomel: electrode
caloric: nystagmus; test; value
calorigenic: action
calvarial: hook
cambium: layer
camel: pox
cameloid: anemia; cell
CAMP: factor; test
cAMP receptor: protein
camp: fever
camphorated: menthol; phenol
camptomelic: dwarfism
Canada: balsam; snakeroot; turpentine
canal: ray
canalicular: duct; sphincter
canarypox: virus
cancellous: bone; tissue
cancer: body; family; juice
cane: sugar
canefield: fever
canicola: fever
canine: amebiasis; babesiosis; borreliosis; carcinoma; ehrlichiosis; eminence; fossa; herpetovirus; hysteria; leishmaniasis; prominence; spasm; tooth
canine distemper: virus
canine hereditary: blindness

canine oral: papilloma
canine parvovirus: disease
canine venereal: granuloma
canker: sore
cannon: bone; sound; wave
cannonball: pulse
cantering: rhythm
canthal: hypertelorism
cantharidal: collodion
cantharis: camphor
canthomeatal: plane
cantilever: beam
caoutchouc: pelvis
cap: splint; stage
Cape: aloe; gum
capeline: bandage
capillary: angioma; arteriole; attraction; bed; circulation; drainage; fracture; hemangioma; lake; loop; nevus; pericyte; pulse; vein; vessel
capillary fragility: test
capillary permeability: factor
capillary resistance: test
Capim: virus
capital: operation
capitate: bone
capitular: joint
capon-comb-growth: test
capped: elbow; hock; knee; uterus
caprine: herpetovirus
capsular: advancement; antigen; cataract; cirrhosis; glaucoma; ligament; space
capsular flap: pyeloplasty
capsule: cell; forceps
capsulolenticular: cataract
capture: beat
car: sickness
Caraparu: virus
carbacrylamine: resin
carbamino: compound
carbocyclic: compound
carbohydrate: metabolism
carbohydrate-induced: hyperlipemia
carbohydrate utilization: test
carbol: fuchsin
carbol-fuchsin: paint
carbol-thionin: stain
carbon: cycle
carbonated: water
carbonate dehydrarase: inhibitor
carbon dioxide: acidosis; content; cycle; electrode; elimination
carbon dioxide-free: water
carbon dioxide withdrawal seizure: test
carbon disulfide: poisoning
carbonic: anhydrase; water
carbonic acid: gas
carbonic anhydrase: inhibitor
carbon monoxide: hemoglobin; poisoning
carboxymethyl: cellulose
carcinoembryonic: antigen
carcinoid: syndrome; tumor
carcinomatous: encephalomyelopathy; implant; myelopathy; myopathy; neuromyopathy
cardiac: accident; albuminuria; aneurysm; arrest; arrhythmia; asthma; calculus; catheter; cirrhosis; competence; cycle; decompression; diastole; diuretic; dysrhythmia; edema; failure; ganglion; gland; hemoptysis; heterotaxia; histiocyte; hormone; impression; impulse; incompetence; index; infarction; insufficiency; jelly; liver; lung; massage; monitor; murmur; muscle; neurosis; notch; opening; output; part; plexus; polyp; prominence; reserve; segment; skeleton; souffle; sound; standstill; symphysis; tamponade; telemetry; tube; vein
cardiac depressor: reflex
cardiac lymphatic: ring
cardiac muscle: tissue
cardiac valve: prosthesis
cardinal: ligament; point; symptom; vein
cardinal ocular: movement
cardioarterial: interval
cardioesophageal: relaxation
cardiogenic: plate; shock
cardiohepatic: angle; triangle
cardioid: condenser
cardiomuscular: bradycardia
cardiopulmonary: bypass; murmur; resuscitation
cardiorespiratory: murmur
ardiothoracic: index; ratio
cardiotoxic: myolysis
cardiovascular: system
carinate: abdomen
carnassial: tooth
carnauba: wax
carneous: degeneration; mole
caroticoclinoid: ligament
caroticotympanic: artery; nerve
carp: mouth
carrier: screening
carotid: artery; body; bruit; bulb; canal; duct; endarterectomy; foramen; ganglion; groove; sheath; shudder; sinus; sulcus; triangle; tubercle; wall
carotid body: tumor
carotid-cavernous: fistula
carotid sinus: nerve; reflex; syncope; syndrome
carpal: arch; artery; articulation; bone; canal; groove; joint; tunnel
carpal articular: surface
carpal tunnel: syndrome
carpometacarpal: joint; ligament
carpopedal: contraction; spasm
carrier: cell; state; strain
carrying: angle
cartesian: nomogram
cartilage: bone; capsule; cell; knife; lacuna; matrix; space
cartilage-hair: hypoplasia
cartilaginous: joint; neurocranium; part; septim; tissue; viscerocranium
cascade: stomach
caseation: necrosis
case-control: study
case fatality: rate
caseous: abscess; degeneration; lymphadenitis; necrosis; osteitis; pneumonia; tubercle
cassia: cinnamon
Castile: soap
casting: flask; ring; wax
castrate: cell
castration: anxiety; cell; complex
cat: unit
catabolite activator: protein
catabolite gene: activator
catacrotic: pulse
catadicrotic: pulse
catalactic: reaction
cataract: lens; needle; spoon
cataract-oligophrenia: syndrome
catarrhal: asthma; fever; gastritis; inflammation; jaundice; ophthalmia
catastrophic: reaction
catatonic: dementia; excitement; pupil; rigidity; schizophrenia; stupor
catatorulin: test
catatropic: image
cat-bite: disease; fever
cat-cry: syndrome
cat distemper: virus
categorical: trait
caterpillar: cell; dermatitis; flap; rash
caterpillar-hair: ophthalmia
catgut: suture

catheter: embolus; fever; gauge; guide
cathodal closure: contraction; tetanus
cathodal duration: tetanus
cathodal opening: clonus; contraction; tetanus
cathode: ray
cathode ray: oscilloscope; tube
cation-exchange: resin
cationic: detergent
cation-ion: difference
cat-scratch: disease; fever
cat's-eye: pupil; syndrome
cattle: plague; wart
cattle plague: virus
Catu: virus
cauda equina: syndrome
caudal: anesthesia; canal; flexure; ligament; neuropore; retinaculum; sheath; vertebra
caudal neurosecretory: system
caudal pancreatic: artery
caudal pharyngeal: complex
caudal transtentorial: herniation
caudal transverse: fissure
caudate: lobe; nucleus; process
caul: fat
cauliflower: ear
causal: additivity
caustic: alkali; potash; soda
cautery: conization; knife
caval: fold; valve
cavalry: bone
cavernous: angioma; artery; body; groove; hemangioma; lymphangiectasis; nerve; part; plexus; rale; resonance; respiration; rhonchus; sinus; tissue; voice
cavernous-carotid: aneurysm
cavernous sinus: syndrome
cavernous voice: sound
caviar: lesion
cavity: liner; margin; preparation; wall
cavity line: angle
cavity preparation: base; form
cavosurface: angle; bevel
CB: lead
CDE: antigen
ceasmic: teratosis
cecal: artery; fold; foramen; hernia; recess
cecocentral: scotoma
Celestin: tube
celiac: artery; axis; disease; ganglion; gland; plexus; rickets; trunk
celiac lymph: node
celiac plexus: reflex
celiotomy: incision
cell: body; bridge; center; culture; cycle; fusion; hybridization; inclusion; line; marker; matrix; membrane; nest; organelle; strain; transformation; wall
cell-bound: antibody
cell-mediated: reaction
cellular: biology; cartilage; embolism; immunity; immunodeficiency; infiltration; mosaicism; pathology; polyp; spill; tenacity; tumor
cellular blue: nevus
cellular immunity deficiency: syndrome
cellulitic: phlegmasia
cellulocutaneous: flap
celluloid: strip
CELO: virus
celomic: bay; pouch
celomic metaplasia: theory
cement: base; corpuscle; line
cemental: caries; dysplasia
cementodentinal: junction
cementoenamel: junction
cementum: hyperplasia
centigrade: scale
centimeter-gram-second: system; unit
central: amputation; apnea; apparatus; artery; bearing; body; bone; bradycardia; callus; canal; cataract; chromatolysis; deafness; ganglioneuroma; gyrus; illumination; implantation; incisor; inhibition; lacteal; lobule; necrosis; neuritis; nystagmus; osteitis; paralysis; pit; placenta; pneumonia; scotoma; spindle; sulcus; tendon; vein; vision
central angiospastic: retinitis; retinopathy
central areolar choroidal: atrophy; sclerosis
central-bearing: device; point
central-bearing tracing: device
central cementifying: fibroma
central cord: syndrome
central core: disease
Central European tick-borne: fever
Central European tick-borne encephalitis: virus
central excitatory: state
central gray: substance
central lymph: node
central nervous: system
central ossifying: fibroma
central pontine: myelinolysis
central serous: choroidopathy; retinopathy
central tegmental: fasciculus; tract
central terminal: electrode
central transactional: core
central venous: catheter; pressure
centrencephalic: epilepsy
centri-acinar: emphysema
centric: contact; fusion; occlusion; position; relation
centric jaw: relation
centrifugal: casting; current; nerve
centrifugal fast: analyzer
centrilobular: emphysema
centripetal: current; nerve
centroacinar: cell
centrodistal: joint
centrofacial: lentiginosis
centrolecithal: egg; ovum
centromedian: nucleus
centromere banding: stain
centromeric: index
centronuclear: myopathy
cephalic: angle; flexure; index; pole; presentation; reflex; tetanus; triangle; vein; version
cephalocaudal: axis
cephalomedullary: angle
cephalometric: analysis; roentgenogram; tracing
cephalo-oculocutaneous: telangiectasia
cephalo-orbital: index
cephalopalpebral: reflex
cephalorrhachidian: index
cephalotrigeminal: angiomatosis
ceramo-metal: casting
ceratocricoid: ligament
ceratopharyngeal: part
cerebellar: artery; ataxia; atrophy; cortex; cyst; fissure; gait; hemisphere; pyramid; rigidity; speech; syndrome; sulcus; tonsil
cerebellomedullary: cistern
cerebellomedullary malformation: syndrome
cerebellopontile: angle
cerebellopontine: angle; recess
cerebellopontine angle: syndrome; tumor
cerebellorubral: tract
cerebellothalamic: tract
cerebral: agraphia; angiography; anthrax; arteriography; artery; calculus; cladosporiosis; claudication; compression; cortex;

chorioptic: mange
choriovitelline: placenta
choroid: fissure; glomus; plexus; skein; tela; vein
choroidal: ring
choroidal vascular: atrophy
Chr^{a}: antigen
Christchurch (Ch^{1}): chromosome
Christmas: disease; factor
chromaffin: body; cell; reaction; system; tissue; tumor
chromate: stain
chromatic: aberration; apparatus; audition; fiber; granule; spectrum; vision
chromatin: body; network; nucleus; particle
chromatophorotropic: hormone
chrome: alum; ulcer
chrome alum hematoxylin-phloxine: stain
chrome-cobalt: alloy
chromic: catgut
chromidial: apparatus; net; substance
chromophil: adenoma; granule; substance
chromophobe: adenoma; cell; granule
chromosomal: deletion; gap; region; syndrome; trait
chromosomal breakage: syndrome
chromosomal instability: syndrome
chromosome: aberration; band; mosaicism; pair; satellite
chronic: abscess; alcoholism; anaphylaxis; appendicitis; bronchitis; cholecystitis; conjunctivitis; dysentery; eczema; glaucoma; glomerulonephritis; hepatitis; inflammation; malaria; nephritis; pyelonephritis; rejection; rheumatism; rhinitis; shock; soroche; trypanosomiasis; ulcer; urticaria; vertigo
chronic absorptive: arthritis
chronic acholuric: jaundice
chronic active liver: disease
chronic adrenocortical: insufficiency
chronic African sleeping: sickness
chronic allograft: rejection
chronic anterior: poliomyelitis
chronic atrophic: polychondritis; thyroiditis; vulvitis
chronic cicatrizing: enteritis
chronic constrictive: pericarditis
chronic cutaneous: leishmaniasis
chronic cystic: mastitis
chronic desquamative: gingivitis
chronic discoid: lupus (erythematosus)
chronic endemic: fluorosis
chronic familial: icterus; jaundice; polyneutritis
chronic follicular: conjunctivitis
chronic granulomatous: disease
chronic hemorrhagic villous: synovitis
chronic hypertensive: disease
chronic hypertrophic: vulvitis
chronic hyperventilation: syndrome
chronic idiopathic: jaundice
chronic interstitial: hepatitis; salpingitis
chronic mountain: sickness
chronic nonleukemic: myelosis
chronic obstructive pulmonary: disease
chronic progressive: chorea
chronic respiratory: disease
chronic rheumatic: arthritis
chronic subglottic: laryngitis
chronic ulcerative: proctitis
chronologic: age
chyle: cistern; corpuscle; cyst; peritonitis; vessel
chyliform: ascites
chylous: arthritis; ascites; hydrothorax; urine
cicatricial: alopecia; conjunctivitis; ectropion; entropion; horn; pemphigoid
cigarette: drain
cigarette-paper: scar
ciliary: blepharitis; body; canal; cartilage; crown; disk; fold; ganglion; gland; ligament; margin; movement; muscle; part; process; ring; staphyloma; vein; wreath; zone; zonule
ciliary ganglionic: plexus
ciliated: epithelium
ciliospinal: center; reflex
cincture: sensation
cinema: eye
cinematic: amputation
cineplastic: amputation
cingulate: convolution; gyrus; herniation
cingulum: rest
circadian: rhythm
circinate: retinitis; retinopathy
circle absorption: anesthesia
circling: disease
circular: amputation; anastomosis; bandage; dichroism; fiber; fold; layer; reaction; sinus; sulcus
circulation: time
circulatory: arrest; collapse; system
circumalveolar: fixation
circumanal: gland
circumferential: cartilage; clasp; fibrocartilage; implantation; lamella; wiring
circumferential clasp: arm
circumflex: nerve; vein
circumflex fibular: artery
circumflex scapular: artery
circummandibular: fixation
circumnevic: vitiligo
circumscribed: craniomalacia; edema; myxedema; peritonitis; pyocephalus; scleroderma
circumvallate: papilla
circumventricular: organ
circumzygomatic: fixation
circus: movement; rhythm
cirsoid: aneurysm; varix
cis: phase
cisternal: puncture
citrate: intoxication
citrated: calcium (carbimide)
citric acid: cycle
citrovorum: factor
CL: lead
clamp: band; forceps
clang: association
clasp: arm; bar; guideline
clasping: reflex
clasp-knife: effect; rigidity; spasticity
classic, classical: conditioning; migraine
classical cesarean: section
clastic: anatomy
clathrate: crystal
claustral: layer
clavate: papilla
clavicular: facet; notch; part; percussion
clavipectoral: fascia
claw: food; hand
clay pigeon: poisoning
cleansing: cream
clear: cell; layer
clear cell: acanthoma; adenocarcinoma; carcinoma; hidradenoma
clearing: factor; medium
clear liquid: diet
cleavage: cavity; cell; division; line; product; site; spindle
cleaved: cell
cleft: hand; lip; nose; palate; spine; tongue
cleidocranial: dysostosis; dysplasia
clenched fist: sign
clerical: spectacles

clicking: rale; tinnitus
clidocranial: dysostosis; dysplasia
client-centered: therapy
climacteric: psychosis; syndrome
climatic: bubo; keratopathy
climbing: fiber
clinical: chemistry; crown; diagnosis; eruption; fitness; genetics; lethal; medicine; nurse; pathology; pharmacologist; pharmacology; pharmacy; psychology; recording; root; spectrometry; spectroscopy; thermometer
clinoid: process
clip: forceps
clipped: speech
cloacal: membrane; plate; theory
clomiphene: test
clonal: aging
clonal selection: theory
clonic: convulsion; spasm
cloning: vector
clonogenic: cell
close: bite
closed: anesthesia; bite; circle; comedo; dislocation; drainage; fracture; hospital; reduction; surgery
closed-angle: glaucoma
closed chain: compound
closed chest: massage
closed circuit: method
closed head: injury
closed-loop: obstruction
closed skull: fracture
closing: contraction; membrane; snap; volume
clostridial: myonecrosis
closure: principle
clot retraction: time
clotting: factor; time
clouding of: consciousness
cloudy: swelling; urine
clover: disease
cloverleaf: skull
cloverleaf skull: syndrome
club: foot; hair; hand; moss
clubbed: digit; finger; penis
cluster: analysis; headache
CO_2: see carbon dioxide
coagulation: factor; necrosis; time
coal tar: naphtha
coaptation: splint; suture
coarctate: retina
coarse: dispersion; tremor
coast: erysipelas
coated: tongue
cobbler's: suture
cobra: hemotoxin
cobra venome: cofactor; factor
cocarde: reaction
coccidioidal: granuloma
coccidioidin: test
coccygeal: body; bone; dimple; fistula; foveola; ganglion; gland; horn; joint; muscle; nerve; part; plexus; sinus; vertebra; whorl
Cochin China: diarrhea
cochlear: aqueduct; area; canal; canaliculus; duct; implant; joint; labyrinth; nerve; nucleus; part; prosthesis; recess; root; window
cochlear hair: cell
cochleariform: process
cochleo-orbicular: reflex
cochleopalpebral: reflex
cochleopupillary: reflex
cochleostapedial: reflex
cockade: reaction
cockscomb: ulcer
cocoa: butter
coconut: sound
codfish: vertebra
coding: sequence
codominant: allele; gene; inheritance; trait
Coe: virus
coenzyme: factor
cofactor of: thromboplastin
coffee-ground: vomit
coffin: joint
cognitive: psychology; therapy
cognitive dissonance: theory
cognitive laterality: quotient
cogwheel: phenomenon; pupil; respiration; rigidity
cohesive: gold
cohort: study
coil: gland
coiled: artery
coin: lesion; test
coid: abscess; agglutination; agglutinin; allergy; autoagglutinin; autoantibody; cautery; conization; cream; gangrene; hemolysin; light; nodule; pack; snare; sore; stage; ulcer; urticaria; virus
cold bend: test
cold-blooded: animal
cold cure: resin
cold-curing: resin
cold hemagglutinin: disease
cold-rigor: point
coli: granuloma
colic: impression; intussusception; sphincter; surface; tenia; vein
collagen: disease; fiber; fibril
collagenous: colitis; fiber
collagen-vascular: disease
collapse: delirium; therapy
collapsing: pulse
collar: bone
collar-button: abscess
collared: flagellate
collar-stud: chalazion
collateral: artery; circulation; eminence; fissure; hyperemia; inheritance; ligament; sulcus; trigone; vessel
collateral digital: artery
collecting: tubule
collective: unconscious
collier's: lung
colliquative: albuminuria; degeneration; diarrhea; necrosis; sweat
collision: tumor
collodion: baby
colloid: acne; adenoma; body; cancer; carcinoma; corpuscle; cyst; degeneration; goiter; milium; system; theory
colloidal: dispersion; gel; metal; silicon dioxide; silver; solution
colloidal radioactive: gold
colocutaneous: fistula
coloileal: fistula
colon: bacillus
colonic: fistula; smear
color: aberration; blindness; chart; constancy; hearing; index; radical; scotoma; sense; spectrum; taste; vision
Colorado tick: fever
Colorado tick fever: virus
color-contrast: microscope
colorimetric: titration
colorimetric caries susceptibility: test
colostomy: bag
colostrum: corpuscle
colovaginal: fistula
colovesical: fistula
Columbia Mental Maturity: scale
Columbia S. K.: virus
column: cell; chromatography
columnar: epithelium; layer
coma: aberration; cast; scale; vigil
comb-growth: test
combination: beat; calculus; restoration
"combination" oral: contraceptive
combined: glaucoma; immunodeficiency; pregnancy; sclerosis; version
combined fat- and carbohydrate-induced: hyperlipemia
combined system: disease
combining: weight

comblike: septum
combustion: equivalent
comfort: zone
comma: bacillus; bundle; tract
commando: operation
commemorative: sign
commensal: parasite
comminuted: fracture
comminuted skull: fracture
commissural: cell; cheilitis; fiber; myelotomy
common: antigen; limb; migraine; opsonin; salt; wart
common basal: vein
common bile: duct
common cardinal: vein
common carotid: artery; plexus
common cold: virus
common facial: vein
common fibular: nerve
common hepatic: artery; duct
common iliac: artery; vein
common iliac lymph: node
common interosseous: artery
common palmar digital: artery; nerve
common peroneal: nerve
common plantar digital: artery; nerve
common synovial flexor: sheath
common tendinous: ring
common, variable: immunodeficiency
communicable: disease
communicating: artery; hydrocephalus
community: dentistry; psychiatry; psychology
community health: nurse
compact: bone; substance
companion: artery; vein
companion lymph: node
comparative: anatomy; pathology; physiology; psychology
comparator: microscope
compensated: acidosis; alkalosis; glaucoma
compensating: curve; emphysema; ocular
compensation: neurosis
compensatory: atrophy; circulation; emphysema; hypertrophy; pause; polycythemia
competitive: antagonist; inhibition
competitive binding: assay
competitor: deoxyribonucleic acid
complement: fixation; unit
complemental: air
complementary: air; color; deoxyribonucleic acid; hypertrophy; role; strand
complement binding: assay
complement chemotactic: factor
complement-fixation: reaction; test
complement-fixing: antibody
complete: abortion; achromatopsia; antibody; antigen; ascertainment; blood count; carcinogen; cataract; cleavage; denture; disinfectant; fistula; hemianopsia; hernia; iridoplegia; medium; metamorphosis; tetanus; transduction
complete atrioventricular (A-V): dissociation
complete denture: impression
complex: absence; odontoma
complex learning: process
complex partial: seizure
complex precipitated: epilepsy
complicated: cataract; fracture
composite: flap; graft; resin
composite dental: cement
compound: aneurysm; caries; character; cyst; dislocation; eye; fracture; gland; heterozygote; joint; lens; lipid; microscope; nevus; odontoma; pregnancy; protein; restoration
compound granule: cell
compound hyperopic: astigmatism
compound myopic: astigmatism
compound skull: fracture
comprehensive medical: care
compressed: sponge; tablet; yeast
compressible cavernous: body
compression: anesthesia; cyanosis; molding; paralysis; plating; retinopathy; syndrome; thrombosis
compressive: myelopathy; nystagmus; strength
compressor: muscle
compulsive: idea; neurosis; personality
computed: perimetry; tomography
computer: model; simulation
computerized axial: tomography
concave: lens; mirror
concavoconcave: lens
concavoconvex: lens
concealed: conduction; hemorrhage; hernia
concentrated human red blood: corpuscle
concentration: gradient
concentric: fibroma; hypertrophy; lamella
concept: formation
conchal: cartilage; crest
conchoidal: body
concomitant: immunity; strabismus; symptom
concordance: rate
concordant: alternans; alternation
concrete: operation; seborrhea; thinking
concurrent: validity
concussion: cataract; myelitis
condensation: compound
condensed: milk
condensing: enzyme; osteitis
conditionally lethal, conditional-lethal: mutant
conditioned: avitaminosis; hemolysis; reflex; response; stimulus
conduct: disorder
conducting: airway; system
conduction: analgesic; anesthesia; aphasia
conductive: deafness; heat
condylar: articulation; axis; canal; fossa; guidance; guide; joint; process
condylar emissary: vein
condylar guidance: inclination
condylar hinge: position
condyle: cord; path
condyloid: canal; process
cone: achromatopsia; cell; degeneration; disk; fiber; granule; vision
confluent: articulation; smallpox
confluent and reticulate: papillomatosis
confrontation: method
confusion: color
congelation: urticaria
congenic: strain
congenital: afibrinogenemia; agammaglobulinemia; alopecia; amputation; anemia; aplasia; baldness; cataract; conus dysphagocytosis; elephantiasis; epulis; glaucoma; hydrocele; hydrocephalus; hypophosphatasia; leukoderma; leukopathia; lymphedema; megacolon; methemoglobinemia; myxedema; nevus; nystagmus; pancytopenia; paramyotonia; pneumonia; stridor; syphilis; torticollis; toxoplasmosis; valve
congenital adrenal: hyperplasia
congenital aplastic: anemia
congenital aregenerative: anemia
congenital atonic: pseudoparalysis

congenital cerebral: aneurysm
congenital diaphragmatic: hernia
congenital dyserythropoietic: anemia
congenital dysplastic: angiectasia; angiomatosis; angiopathy
congenital ectodermal: defect; dysplasia
congenital erythropoietic: porphyria
congenital facial: diplegia
congenital generalized: fibromatosis
congenital hemolytic: anemia; icterus; jaundice
congenital hypoplastic: anemia
congenital ichthyosiform: erythroderma
congenital pyloric: stenosis
congenital sebaceous: hyperplasia
congenital spastic: paraplegia
congenital sutural: alopecia
congenital total: lipodystrophy
congestive: cirrhosis; failure; splenomegaly
Congo red: paper; stain
Congolian red: fever
congophilic: angiopathy
congruent: point
congruous: hemianopsia
conic: papilla
conical: catheter; cornea
conjoined: anastomosis; tendon; twins
conjoined equal or symmetrical: twins
conjoined unequal or asymmetrical: twins
conjoint: tendon; therapy
conjugal: cancer
conjugate: axis; deviation; diameter; disparity; division; focus; foramen; gaze; ligament; movement; nystagmus; paralysis; point
conjugate acid-base: pair
conjugated: antigen; bilirubin; compound; estrogen; hapten; protein
conjugated double: bond
conjugative: plasmid
conjunctival: artery; cul-de-sac; gland; layer; reflex; ring; sac; varix; vein
connecting: cartilage; stalk; tubule
connective: tissue; tumor
connective tissue: cell; disease; group
connector: bar
conoid: ligament; process; tubercle
conscious: perception
consecutive: amputation; aneurysm; angiitis; anophthalmus; esotropia
consensual: reaction; validation
consensual light: reflex
consistency: principle
consolidation: chemotherapy
consonating: rale
constancy: phenomenon
constant: coupling; region
constant field: equation
constant infusion: pump
constant positive pressure: breathing
constitutional: cause; disease; formula; hirsutism; psychology; reaction; symptom; thrombopathy; ulcer
constitutional hepatic: dysfunction
constitutive: heterochromatin
constriction: hyperemia; ring
constrictive: endocarditis
construct: validity
consulting: staff
consumption: coagulopathy
contact: allergy; area; catalysis; ceptor; cheilitis; dermatitis; illumination; inhibition; lens; point; splint; surface
contact-type: dermatitis
contagious: abortion; agalactia; aphthae; disease; ecthyma
contagious bovine: pleuropneumonia
contagious caprine: pleuropneumonia
contagious ecthyma: virus
contagious equine: metritis
contagious granular: conjunctivitis
contagious pustular: dermatitis
contagious pustular dermatitis: virus
contagious pustular stomatitis: virus
content: analysis; validity
continued: fever
continuous: beam; capillary; clasp; eruption; murmur; phase; spectrum; suture; tremor; variation
continuous bar: retainer
continuous epidural: anesthesia
continuous loop: wiring
continuous passive: motion
continuous positive airway: pressure
continuous positive pressure: ventilation
continuous spinal: anesthesia
contour: line
contraceptive: device; sponge
contracted: foot; heel; kidney; pelvis; tendon
contractile: stricture, vacuole
contraction: band
contractual: psychiatry; psychotherapy
contractural: diathesis
contracture: deformity
contralateral: hemiplegia; reflex; sign
contrary: sexual
contrast: bath; enema; enhancement; medium; sensitivity; stain
contrecoup: injury
control: animal; experiment; gene; group; syringe
controlled: hypotension; respiration; substance; ventilation
controlled mechanical: ventilation
contusion: pneumonia
convalescent: carrier; serum
convective: heat
convenience: form
conventional: animal; sign
convergence: excess; insufficiency; nucleus
convergent: evolution; squint; strabismus
converging: meniscus
conversion: disorder; electron; hysteria; reaction
conversion hysteria: neurosis
conversive: heat
convex: lens; mirror
convexoconcave: lens
convexoconvex: lens
convoluted: bone; gland; part; tubule
convoluted seminiferous: tubule
convulsant: threshold
convulsive: reflex; state; tic
cooled-knife: method
coolie: itch
coordinate: bond; convulsion
coordinated: reflex
copolymer: resin
copper: cataract; colic; nose
Copper Kettle: vaporizer
copper phosphate: cement
copper sulfate: method
copra: itch
coracoacromial: ligament
coracobrachial: bursa; muscle
coracoclavicular: ligament
coracohumeral: ligament
coracoid: process; tuberosity
coral: calculus
coralliform: cataract
cord: bladder; blood
cordate: pelvis
cordiform: pelvis; uterus
cordy: pulse
core: pneumonia

corn: ergot; sugar
corneal: astigmatism; corpuscle; decompensation; dystrophy; ectasia; facet; graft; layer; lens; margin; pannus; reflex; space; spot; staphyloma; transplantation; trepanation
corneoscleral: part
corniculate: cartilage; tubercle
corniculopharyngeal: ligament
cornified: layer
corn-meal, cornmeal: agar; disease
cornoid: lamella
cornual: pregnancy
coronal: plane; pulp; section; suture
coronary: artery; band; bypass; cataract; endarterectomy; failure; insufficiency; ligament; node; occlusion; plexus; sinus; sulcus; tendon; thrombosis; valve; vein
coronary care: unit
coronary nodal: rhythm
coronary ostial: stenosis
coronary sinus: rhythm
coronoid: fossa; process
corpuscular: lymph; radiation
corpus luteum: hematoma; hormone
corpus luteum deficiency: syndrome
corpus luteum hormone: unit
corrected: dextrocardia
corrective emotional: experience
correlation: coefficient
correlational: method
correlative: differentiation
corridor: disease
corrosion: preparation
corrosive: mercury; sublimate; ulcer
corrugator: muscle
cortical: apraxia; arch; artery; audiometry; blindness; bone; cataract; convexity; deafness; epilepsy; hormone; implantation; osteitis; part; sensibility; substance
corticobulbar: fiber; tract
corticonuclear: fiber
corticopontine: fiber; tract
corticopupillary: reflex
corticoreticular: fiber
corticospinal: fiber; tract
corticosteroid-binding: globulin; protein
corticosteroid-induced: glaucoma
corticotropic: hormone
corticotropin-releasing: factor; hormone
corymbose: syphilid
cosmetic: dermatitis; surgery
cosmic: ray
costal: angle; arch; cartilage; chondritis; fringe; groove; notch; part; pit; pleurisy; process; respiration; surface; tuberosity
costal arch: reflex
costoaxillary: vein
costocervical: artery, trunk
costochondral: joint; syndrome
costoclavicular: ligament; line; syndrome
costocolic: ligament
costodiaphragmatic: recess
costomediastinal: recess; sinus
costopectoral: reflex
costophrenic septal: line
costotransverse: foramen; joint; ligament
costovertebral: joint
costoxiphoid: ligament
cotton-fiber: embolism
cotton-mill: fever
cotton-wool: patch; spot
cotyledonary: placenta
cotyloid: cavity; joint; ligament; notch
couching: needle
cough: fracture; reflex
counseling: psychology
count: density
counter-: shock
countercurrent: distribution; mechanism
coup: injury
coupled: beat; pulse; rhythm
coupling: defect; factor; interval; phase
cover: glass; test
covert: sensitization
cover-uncover: test
cow: face; kidney
cowl: muscle
cowpox: virus
coxal: bone
coxitic: scoliosis
Coxsackie: encephalitis; virus
CR: lead
crab: hand; yaws
cracked: heel
cracked-pot: resonance; sound
crackling: jaw
cradle: cap
craft: palsy
cranial: arteritis; base; bone; capacity; cavity; flexure; fontanel; index; nerve; root; sinus; suture; synchondrosis; vertebra
craniocardiac: reflex
craniocarpotarsal: dysplasia; dystrophy
craniodiaphysial: dysplasia
craniofacial: angle; appliance; axis; dysostosis; fixation; notch; surgery
craniofacial dysfunction: fracture
craniofacial suspension: wiring
craniometaphysial: dysplasia
craniometric: point
craniopharyngeal: canal; duct
craniosacral: system
craniosinus: fistula
crater: arc
cravat: bandage
crazy chick: disease
cream of: tartar
crease: wound
creatinine: clearance; coefficient
creative: thinking
creep: recovery
creeping: eruption; myiasis; palsy; thrombosis; ulcer
cremaster: muscle
cremasteric: artery; fascia; reflex
crepitant: rale
crescendo: angina; murmur; sleep
crescent: cell
crescent cell: anemia
crescentic: lobule
CREST: syndrome
crevicular: epithelium; fluid
crib: death
cribriform: area; fascia; hymen; plate
cricoarytenoid: articulation; joint
cricoarytenoid articular: capsule
cricoesophageal: tendon
cricoid: cartilage
cricopharyngeal: ligament; part
cricosantorinian: ligament
cricothyroid: artery; articulation; joint; ligament; membrane; muscle
cricothyroid articular: capsule
cricotracheal: ligament; membrane
cricovocal: membrane
cri-du-chat: syndrome
Crimean-Congo hemorrhagic: fever
Crimean-Congo hemorrhagic fever: virus
criminal: abortion; anthropology; hygiene; insanity; irresponsibility; psychology
crisis: intervention
criterion-related: validity
critical: angle; illumination; organ; period; pH; point; pressure; rate; temperature
critical care: unit
critical flicker fusion: frequency
crocodile: tears
crocodile tears: syndrome

crop: gland; milk
cross: agglutination; birth; circulation; flap; hybridization; infection; mating; reaction; tolerance
cross-bite: tooth
cross-cut: bur
crossed: anesthesia; cylinder; diplopia; embolism; eye; fixation; hemianesthesia; hemianopsia; hemiplegia; immunoelectrophoresis; jerk; laterality; paralysis; reflex
crossed adductor; jerk; reflex
crossed extension: reflex
crossed knee: jerk; reflex
crossed phrenic: phenomenon
crossed pyramidal: tract
crossed spino-adductor: reflex
cross-linked: polymer; resin
cross-reacting: agglutinin; antibody; material
cross-sectional: echocardiography; method; study
crotalaria: poisoning
Crotalus: antitoxin
croup-associated: virus
croupous: bronchitis: conjunctivitis; inflammation; laryngitis; lymph; membrane; pharyngitis; rhinitis
crowing: inspiration
crown: bark; cavity; flask; glass; tubercle
crown-heel: length
crown-rump: length
CRST: syndrome
crucial: anastomosis; bandage; ligament
cruciate: anastomosis; eminence; ligament; muscle
cruciform: eminence; ligament; part
crude: drug; urine
crural: arch; artery; canal; fossa; hernia; ring; septum; sheath; triangle
crush: kidney; syndrome
crusted: ringworm; tetter
crutch: palsy; paralysis
Cruz: trypanosomiasis
cry: reflex
crypt: abscess
cryptogenic: cirrhosis; infection; pyemia; septicemia
cryptophthalamus: syndrome
cryptorchid: testis
crystal: cryoglobulinemia; rash; structure
crystalline: capsule; cataract; digitalin; interface; lens
crystalline insulin zinc: suspension
crystallized: trypsin
crystal violet: stain; vaccine
CT: number, unit
Cuban: itch
cubic: centimeter; niter
cubital: bone; fossa; joint; nerve
cubital lymph: node
cuboid: bone
cuboidal: epithelium
cuboidal articular: surface
cuboideonavicular: joint; ligament
cuboidodigital: reflex
cuirass: respirator
cul-de-sac: smear
cultivated: yeast
cultural: anthropology; shock
culture: medium
cumulative: action; dose; effect
cuneate: fasciculus; funiculus; nucleus
cuneiform: bone; cartilage; cataract; lobe; tubercle
cuneocerebellar: tract
cuneocuboid: joint; ligament
cuneometatarsal: joint
cuneonavicular: articulation; joint; ligament
cup biopsy: foceps
cupping: glass
cupular: part
cupular blind: sac
cupulate: part
cupuliform: cataract
curative: dose
curb: tenotomy
curby: hock
curd: soap
curdy: pus
curlicue: ureter
currant jelly: clot
curvature: aberration; hyperopia; myopia
curve: response
cushingoid: sign
cusp: angle; height
cuspal: interference
cuspid: tooth
cuspidate: tooth
cuspless: tooth
cutaneomandibular: polyoncosis
cutaneomeningospinal: angiomatosis
cutaneomucous: muscle
cutaneomucouveal: syndrome
cutaneous: absorption; albinism; ancylostomiasis; anthrax; apoplexy; diphtheria; emphysema; gangrene; habronemiasis; hemorrhoids; horn; larva migrans; layer; leishmaniasis; leprosy; muscle; nerve; reaction; reflex; test; tuberculosis; vasculitis; vein
cutaneous cervical: nerve
cutaneous pupil, cutaneous-pupillary: reflex
cutaneous systemic: angiitis
cutaneous tuberculin: test
cutireaction: test
cutis: graft; plate
cutting: edge; forceps; tooth
cuttlefish: disk
cuvette: oximeter
cyanide: poisoning
cyanide-nitroprusside: test
cyanotic: asphyxia; atrophy; induration
cyclic: adenylic acid; albuminuria; compound; estropia; neutropenia; phosphate; phosphoric acid; strabismus
cyclopean: eye
cyclothymic: disorder; personality
cylinder: retinoscopy
cylindric, cylindrical: bronchiectasis; epithelium; lens
cylindroid: aneurysm
cylindromatous: carcinoma
cynic: spasm
cystic: acne; artery; carcinoma; diathesis; disease; duct; fibrosis; goiter; hyperplasia; kidney; lymphangiectasis; maculopathy; mole; node; polyp; vein
cystic duct: cholangiography
cystic gall: duct
cystic medial: necrosis
cystic papillomatous: craniopharyngioma
cystine: calculus
cystine storage: disease
cystinotic: leukocyte
cystoduodenal: ligament
cystoid macular: degeneration; edema
cytoscopic: urography
cythemolytic: icterus
cytochrome: system
cytocrine: secretion
cytogenic: reproduction
cytoid: body
cytologic: examination; screening; smear; specimen
cytologic filter: preparation
cytomegalic: cell
cytomegalic inclusion: disease
cytomegalovirus: disease
cytopathic: effect

cytopathogenic: virus
cytophagic: panniculitis
cytophil: group
cytophilic: antibody
cytoplasmic: bridge; inheritance; matrix
cytoplasmic inclusion: body
cytoreductive: therapy
cytotonic: enterotoxin
cytotoxic: cell; reaction
cytotrophoblastic: shell
cytotropic: antibody
cytotropic antibody: test

D

δ: see delta
D: cell; enzyme; wave
daily: dose
Dakar: vaccine
dancing: chorea; disease; spasm
dandy: fever
Danubian endemic familial: nephropathy
DAPI: stain
DA pregnancy: test
dark: adaptation; cell; reaction
dark-adapted: eye
dark-field: condenser; illumination; microscope
dark-ground: illumination
dartoic: tissue
dartos: muscle
darwinian: ear; reflex; theory; tubercle
date: boil, fever
datum: plane
Datura: poisoning
daughter: cell; colony; cyst; star
dawn: phenomenon
day: blindness; hospital; residue; sight
dead: finger; nerve; pulp; space; tooth; tract
dead-end: host
dead fetus: syndrome
deadly: agaric; nightshade
deamidizing: enzyme
deaminating: enzyme
death: instinct; rate; trance
debrancher deficiency limit: dextrinosis
debranching: enzyme; factor
debulking: operation
decapitation: factor
decarboxylated: dopa
decay: constant; theory
decentered: lens
decerebrate: rigidity
decidual: cast; cell; endometritis; fissure; reaction
deciduate: placenta
deciduous: dentition; membrane; skin; tooth
decinormal: solution
declamping: phenomenon; shock
decomposition of: movement
decompression: chamber; disease; operation; sickness
decoy: cell
decremental: conduction
decubital: gangrene
decubitus: calculus; paralysis; ulcer
de-emetinized: ipecacuanha
deep: bite; percussion; reflex; scleritis; sensibility
deep abdominal: reflex
deep anatomical structures (specific deep anatomical or histological structures are listed under the following): arch; artery; bursa; cell; cortex; fascia; gyrus; head; layer; ligament; muscle; nerve; node; nucleus; part; plexus; ring; space; vein; vessel
deep punctate: keratitis
deer-fly: disease; fever
deer hemorrhagic: fever
deer hemorrhagic fever: virus
def: index
DEF caries: index
defective: bacteriophage; phage; probacteriophage; prophage; virus
defense: mechanism; reflex
defensive: circle; medicine
deferent: canal; duct
deferential: plexus
deferred: shock
defervescent: stage
deficiency: anemia; disease; symptom
definitive: callus; host; lysosome; method; prosthesis
deflective occlusal: contact
degenerative: arthritis; chorea; index; inflammation; myopia
degenerative joint: disease
degloving: injury
deglutition: apnea; pneumonia; reflex
dehydrated: alcohol
dehydration: fever
dehydrocholate: test
deiterospinal: tract
déjà vu: phenomenon
delayed: allergy; conduction; dentition; eruption; flap; graft; hypersensitivity; implantation; reaction; reflex; sensation; shock; suture
delayed reaction: experiment
Delhi: boil
delimiting: keratotomy
delirious: shock
delphian: node
delta: agent; alcoholism; antigen; cell; granule; hepatitis; rhythm; virus; wave
deltoid: crest; eminence; impression; ligament; muscle; region; tuberosity
deltoideopectoral: triangle; trigone
deltopectoral: flap
demand: pacemaker
demand pulse: generator
demarcation: current; line; potential
demigauntlet: bandage
demilune: body
demodectic: acariasis; blepharitis; mange
demonstration: ophthalmoscope
demyelinating: disease; encephalopathy
denaturation: temperature
denatured: alcohol; protein
dendriform: keratitis
dendritic: calculus; cataract; cell; depolarization; keratitis; process; spine; thorn
dendritic corneal: ulcer
dengue: fever, virus
dengue hemorrhagic: fever
dengue shock: syndrome
dense-deposit: disease
density: gradient
density gradient: centrifugation
dental: abscess; anatomy; anesthesia; ankylosis; apparatus; arch; articulation; biomechanics; biophysics; bulb; calculus; canal; cap; caries; cast; cement; cord; crest; crypt; curing; cuticle; drill; dysfunction; engineering; fiber; fistula; floss; follicle; forceps; formula; furnace; geriatrics; germ; granuloma; groove; hygienist; impaction; index; jurisprudence; lamina; ledge; lever; lymph; material; neck; nerve; orthopedics; osteoma; pathology; plaque; polyp; process; prophylaxis; prosthesis; prosthetics; pulp; pump; ridge; sac; senescence; shelf; sur-

geon; syringe; tubercle; tubule; ulcer; wedge
dentary: center
dentate: fascia; fissure; fracture; gyrus; line; nucleus; suture
dentatothalamic: tract
denticulate: hymen, ligament
dentigerous: cyst
dentin: globule
dentinal: canal; dysplasia; fiber; fluid; papilla; pulp; sheath; tubule
dentinal lamina: cyst
dentinocemental: junction
dentinoenamel: junction
dentoalveolar: joint
dentogingival: lamina
denture: base; border; brush; characterization; edge; esthetics; flange; flask; foundation; hyperplasia; packing; prognosis; retention; space; stability
denture basal: surface
denture-bearing: area
denture foundation: area; surface
denture impression: surface
denture occlusal: surface
denture polished: surface
denture sore: mouth
denture-supporting: area; structure
Denver: classification; shunt
deodorized: opium
deoxy: sugar
dependent: beat; drainage; edema; personality; variable
depletion: response
depolarizing: block; relaxant
depot: injection; reaction; therapy
depressed: fracture
depressed skull: fracture
depressive: stupor
depressor: fiber; muscle; nerve; reflex
deprivation: amblyopia
depth: compensation; dose; perception; psychology; recording
derby hat: fracture
derivative: chromosome
derived: protein
dermal: bone; graft; leishmanoid; papilla; sinus; system; tuberculosis
dermal duct: tumor
dermal-fat: graft
dermatogenic: torticollis
dermatologic: paste
dermatomic: area
dermatopathic: lymphadenitis; lymphadenopathy
dermoepidermal: interface
dermoepidermic: graft
dermoid: cyst; system; tumor
dermolytic bullous: dermatosis
dermotuberculin: reaction
descending: artery; colon; current; degeneration; neuritis; nucleus; part; tract
descending palatine: artery
descending scapular: artery
descriptive: anatomy; myology; statistics
desensitizing: paste
desert: fever; sore
desiccated: liver; pituitary
design: denture
desmoid: tumor
desmoplastic: fibroma; trichoepithelioma
despeciated: antitoxin
desquamative: pneumonia
desquamative inflammatory: vaginitis
desquamative interstitial: pneumonia
destructive: distillation
detached: craniotomy; retina
detached cranial: section
determinant: group
determinate: cleavage
detrusor: pressure
detrusor sphincter: dyssynergia
developmental: age; anatomy; anomaly; disability; groove; line; physiology; psychology
deviational: nystagmus
devil's: grip
devitalized: tooth
Devonshire: colic
dew: claw; itch; point
dexamethasone suppression: test
df, DF caries: index
dhobie: itch; mark
dhobie mark: dermatitis
Di: antigen
diabetic: acidosis; arthropathy; cataract; coma; dermopathy; diet; felopathy; gangrene; gingivitis; glomerulosclerosis; lipemia; myelopathy; neuropathy; puncture; retinitis; retinopathy
diabetogenic: factor
diachronic: study
diagnostic: anesthesia; audiometry; cast; sensitivity; specificity; ultrasound
diagnostic diphtheria: toxin
diagonal: conjugate
dial: manometer
dialysis: dementia; shunt
dialysis disequilibrium: syndrome
dialysis encephalopathy: syndrome
diamond: disk; fuchsin; skin
diamond cutting: instrument
diamond-shaped: murmur
diamond skin: disease
Diana: complex
diaper: dermatitis; rash
diaphragm: pessary; phenomenon
diaphragmatic: flutter; hernia; ligament; node; peritonitis; pleura; pleurisy; surface
diaphragmatic myocardial: infarction
diaphysial: aclasis; center; dysplasia
diaphysial juxtaepiphysial: exostosis
diarthrodial: cartilage; joint
diastatic skull: fracture
diastolic: afterpotential; murmur; pressure; shock; thrill
diastrophic: dwarfism
diathermic: therapy
diatomaceous: earth
diazo: reaction; reagent; stain
diazonium: salts
dibasic: acid; ammonium; calcium; potassium; sodium
dicarboxylic acid: cycle
dicentric: chromosome
dichorial: twins
dichorionic diamniotic: placenta
dicrotic: notch; pulse; wave
didactic: analysis
diencephalic: epilepsy; syndrome
diestrous: cycle
dietary: amenorrhea; fiber
dietetic: albuminuria
diethenoid: fatty acid
differential: diagnosis; growth; manometer; stain; stethoscope; thermometer; threshold
differential blood: pressure
differential renal function: test
differential spinal: anesthesia
differential ureteral catheterization: test
differential white: blood count
diffuse: abscess; aneurysm; choroiditis; emphysema; ganglion; glomerulonephritis; goiter; leishmaniasis; peritonitis; phlegmon; sclerosis
diffuse arterial: ectasia
diffuse cutaneous: leishmaniasis
diffused: reflex
diffuse deep: keratitis

diffuse idiopathic skeletal: hyperostosis
diffuse infantile familial: sclerosis
diffuse mesangial: proliferation
diffuse small cleaved cell: lymphoma
diffuse waxy: spleen
diffusible: stimulant
diffusing: capacity; factor
diffusion: anoxia; coefficient; constant; hypoxia; method; respiration; shell
digastric: fossa; groove; muscle; notch; triangle
digenetic: fluke
digestive: albuminuria; apparatus; fever; glycosuria; leukocytosis; system; tract; tube
digital: fossa; furrow; joint; pulp; reflex; vein; whorl
digital collateral: artery
digitalis: unit
digital subtraction: angiography
digitate: impression; wart
digitonin: reaction
dihydric: alcohol
dihydrogen: phosphate
dilated: cardiomyopathy; pore
dilating: laryngotome
dilation: thrombosis
dilator: muscle
dilute, diluted: acetic acid; alcohol; hydrochloric acid; phosphoric acid
dilution: anemia
dimensional: stability
dimidiate: hermaphroditism
dimorphic: anemia
dimorphous: leprosy
dimple: sign
dinitrophenylhydrazine: test
dinner: pad
dinoflagellate: toxin
Diogenes: cup
dioptric: aberration
diovular: twins
DIP: joint
dip: phenomenon
diphasic: complex
diphasic milk: fever
diphenylhydantoin: gingivitis
diphenylmethane: dye
diphtheria: antitoxin; toxin
diphtheria and tetanus toxoids and pertussis: vaccine
diphtheria antitoxin: unit
diphtheritic: conjunctivitis; enteritis; membrane; neuropathy; paralysis; ulcer
diphyllobothrium: anemia
diplobacillary: conjunctivitis
diploic: canal; vein
diploid: nucleus
dipolar: ion
dipole: theory
direct: astigmatism; auscultation; calorimetry; current; diplopia; diuretic; embolism; flap; fracture; illumination; image; lead; method; ophthalmoscope; ophthalmoscopy; oxidase; percussion; ray; retainer; retention; technique; transfusion; vision; zoonosis
direct acrylic: restoration
direct bone: impression
direct composite resin: restoration
direct Coombs': test
direct filling: resin
direct fluorescent antibody: test
directive: psychotherapy
direct lytic: factor
direct nuclear: division
direct pulp: capping
direct pyramidal: tract
direct reacting: bilirubin
direct resin: restoration
direct vision: spectroscope
disappearing bone: disease
disc (see also disk): electrophoresis; syndrome
discharging: tubule
disciform: degeneration; detachment
disclosing: solution
discoid: lupus (erythematosus)
discoidal: cleavage
disconnection: syndrome
discontinuation: test
discontinuous: phase; sterilization
discordant: alternans; alternation
discrete: smallpox
discriminant: function; stimulus
disease: determinant
dish: face
dish-pan: fracture
disintegration: constant
disjoined: pyeloplasty
disjugate: movement
disjunctive: absorption
disk (see also disc): kidney
disk sensitivity: method
disk-shaped: cataract
dislocation: fracture
disodium: phosphate
disorganized: schizophrenia
disparity: angle
dispensing: tablet
disperse: placenta
dispersed: phase
dispersing: electrode
dispersion: colloid; medium; phase
displacement: analysis; threshold
disproportionating: enzyme
dissecting: aneurysm; cellulitis
dissection: tubercle
disseminate, disseminated: aspergillosis; choroiditis; coccidioidomycosis; lipogranulomatosis; lupus (erythematosus); sclerosis; tuberculosis
disseminated cutaneous: gangrene; leishmaniasis
disseminated intravascular: coagulation
disseminated recurrent: infundibulofolliculitis
dissociated: anesthesia; nystagmus
dissociation: constant; sensibility
dissociative: anesthesia; reaction
distal: caries; centriole; end; ileitis; myopathy; occlusion; part; surface
distal interphalangeal: joint
distal radioulnar: articulation
distal splenorenal: shunt
distance: ceptor
distant: flap
distemper: virus
distention: cyst; ulcer
distilled: water
distortion: aberration
distraction: conus
distributed: effort
distributing: artery
distribution: coefficient; curve; leukocytosis; volume
distributive: analysis
disulfide: bond
diurnal: periodicity; rhythm
divergence: insufficiency
divergence excess: exotropia
divergence insufficiency: exotropia
divergent: squint; strabismus
diverging: meniscus
diver's, divers': paralysis; spectacles
divided: dose; spectacles
diving: goiter; reflex
divisional: nursing
dizygotic: twins
djenkol: poisoning
dmf, DMF caries: index
dmfs, DMFS caries: index
DNA: gap; helix; homology; hybridization; polymorphism; virus
dog: disease; nose; unit
dog distemper: virus
dogmatic: school
dolichoectatic: artery
dolichopellic: pelvis

E

emotional: age; amenorrhea; attitude; deprivation; disease; disorder; disturbance; leukocytosis; overlay; tone
empathic: index
emphysematous: cholecystitis; gangrene; phlegmon
empiric: risk
empirical: formula
empty: sella
empyema: tube
empyemic: scoliosis
emulsifying: wax
emulsion: colloid
enamel: cap; cell; cleavage; cleaver; crypt; cuticle; dysplasia; epithelium; fiber; fissure; germ; hypocalcification; hypoplasia; lamella; layer; ledge; membrane; niche; nodule; organ; pearl; projection; pulp; prism; rod; tuft; wall
enamel rod: inclination; sheath
enarthrodial: joint
encephalic: angioma; vesicle
encephalitis: virus
encephaloclastic: microcephaly
encephalocraniocutaneous: lipomatosis
encephaloid: cancer
encephalomyelonic: axis
encephalomyocarditis: virus
encephalo-ophthalmic: dysplasia
encephalotrigeminal: angiomatosis
encephalotrigeminal vascular: syndrome
encounter: group
encysted: calculus; pleurisy
end: artery; bud; bulb; organ; piece; plate; point; stage
endaural: incision
end-cutting: bur
end-diastolic: volume
endemic: deafmutism; funiculitis; goiter; hematuria; hemoptysis; hypertrophy; index; influenza; neuritis; stability; typhus
endemic nonbacterial infantile: gastroenteritis
endemic paralytic: vertigo
endobronchial: tube
endocardial: cushion; fibroelastosis; murmur; sclerosis
endocardial cushion: defect
endocervical: smear
endochondral: bone; ossification
endocrine: exophthalmos; gland; ophthalmopathy; system
endocrine polyglandular: syndrome
endodermal: cell; pouch
endodermal sinus: tumor
endodontic: stabilizer
endogenic: toxicosis
endogenomorphic: depression
endogenous: cycle; depression; fiber; hyperglyceridemia; infection
endogenous creatinine: clearance
endolymphatic: duct; hydrops; sac
endometrial: cyst; implant; smear
endometrial stromal: sarcoma
endometrioid: carcinoma; tumor
endomyocardial: fibroelastosis; fibrosis
end-on mattress: suture
endo-osseous: implant
endopelvic: fascia
endoplasmic: reticulum
endorectal pull-through: procedure
endoscopic: biopsy
endoscopic retrograde: cholangiopancreatography
endosteal: implant
endoteric: bacterium
endothelial: cell; cyst; dystrophy; leukocyte; myeloma
endotheliochorial: placenta
endothelio-endothelial: placenta
endothoracic: fascia
endotoxin: shock
endotracheal: anesthesia; intubation; stylet; tube
endovenous: septum
end-point: measurement
end-position: nystagmus
end-systolic: volume
end-tidal: sample
end-to-end: bite; occlusion
energy-rich: phosphate
engine: reamer
English: disease; position; rhinoplasty
ensheathing: callus
ensiform: cartilage; process
ensisternum: cartilage
enteric: fever; plexus; tuberculosis; virus
enteric coated: tablet
enteric cytopathogenic bovine orphan: virus
enteric cytopathogenic human orphan: virus
enteric cytopathogenic monkey orphan: virus
enteric cytopathogenic swine orphan: virus
entericoid: fever
enterochromaffin: cell
enterocutaneous: fistula
enteroendocrine: cell
enterogastric: reflex
enterogenous: cyanosis; cyst; methemoglobinemia
enterohepatic: circulation
enterokinetic: agent
enteropathic: arthritis
enterovaginal: fistula
enterovesical: fistula
entodermal: canal; cell; cloaca; pouch
entoptotic: pulse
entorhinal: area
entrance: block
entrapment: neuropathy
entry: zone
enuretic: absence
envelope: conformation; flap
environmental: psychology
enzootic: abortion; ataxia; encephalomyelitis; stability
enzootic bovine: leukosis
enzootic encephalomyelitis: virus
enzygotic: twins
enzymatic: synthesis
enzyme: antagonist
enzyme inhibition: theory
enzyme-linked immunosorbent: assay
enzyme-multiplied: immunoassay
eosin-methylene blue: agar
eosinopenic: reaction
eosinophil, eosinophilic: adenoma; granule; granuloma; leukemia; leukocyte; leukocytosis; leukopenia; meningitis; meningoencephalitis; pneumonia
eosinophil chemotactic: factor
eosinophilic: cellulitis
eosinophilic nonallergic: rhinitis
eosinophilic pustular: folliculitis
eosinophilocytic: leukemia
epactal: bone; ossicle
epamniotic: cavity
eparterial: bronchus
ependymal: cell; cyst; layer; zone
ephemeral: fever
ephemeral fever: virus
epibranchial: placode
epicranial: aponeurosis; muscle
epicritic: sensibility
epidemic: curve; dropsy; encephalitis; exanthema; hemoglobinuria; hepatitis; hiccup; hysteria; keratoconjunctivitis; myalgia; myositis; nausea; neuromyasthenia; parotiditis; pleurodynia; polyarthritis; roseola; tetany; tremor; typhus; vertigo; vomiting
epidemic benign dry: pleurisy

epidemic cerebrospinal: meningitis
epidemic diaphragmatic: pleurisy
epidemic gangrenous: proctitis
epidemic gastroenteritis: virus
epidemic hemorrhagic: fever
epidemic keratoconjunctivitis: virus
epidemic myalgia: virus
epidemic myalgic: encephalomyelitis; encephalomyelopathy
epidemic nonbacterial: gastroenteritis
epidemic parotitis: virus
epidemic pleurodynia: virus
epidemic transient diaphragmatic: spasm
epidemiological: distribution
epidermal: cyst; ridge
epidermal growth: factor
epidermal ridge: count
epidermic: cell; graft
epidermic-dermic: nevus
epidermoid: cancer; carcinoma; cyst
epidermolytic: hyperkeratosis
epidural: anesthesia; block; cavity; hematoma; meningitis; space
epigastric: angle; fold; fossa; hernia; reflex; region; vein; voice
epigastric lymph: node
epiglottic: cartilage; tubercle
epihyal: bone; ligament
epikeratophakic: keratoplasty
epilation: dose
epilemmal: ending
epileptic: absence; dementia
epileptiform: neuralgia
epileptogenic: zone
epimastical: fever
epinephrine: reversal
epiotic: center
epipapillary: membrane
epipericardial: ridge
epiphrenic: diverticulum
epiphysial: arrest; cartilage; eye; fracture; line; plate
epiphysial aseptic: necrosis
epiploic: appendage; foramen
epipteric: bone
epiretinal: membrane
episcleral: artery; lamina; space; vein
episternal: bone
epithelial: attachment; body; cancer; cast; cell; cyst; dysplasia; dystrophy; ectoderm; inlay; lamina; layer; migration; nest; pearl; plug; tissue
epithelial choroid: layer
epithelial reticular: cell
epitheliochorial: placenta
epithelioid: cell
epithelioid cell: nevus
epithermal: chemistry; neutron
epitrichial: layer
epitrochlear: node
epituberculous: infiltration
epitympanic: recess; space
epizoic: commensalism
epizootic: cellulitis; lymphangitis
epoxy: resin
epsilon: alcoholism
Epsom: salt
equal: cleavage
equation: division
equatorial: cleavage; plane; plate; staphyloma
equilibrium: constant; dialysis
equine: babeiosis; encephalitis; encephalomyelitis; gait; gonadotropin; influenza; rhinopneumonitis; rhinovirus; syphilis
equine abortion: virus
equine arteritis: virus
equine biliary: fever
equine coital exanthema: virus
equine gonadotropin: unit
equine infectious: anemia
equine infectious anemia: virus
equine influenza: virus
equine monocytic: ehrlichiosis
equine rhinopneumonitis: virus
equine serum: hepatitis
equine spinal: ataxia
equine swamp: fever
equine viral: arteritis
equine virus: abortion
equiphasic: complex
equivalence: zone
equivalent: extract; power; temperature; weight
equivalent form: reliability
equivocal: symptom
erect: illumination
erectile: tissue
erector: muscle
erector-spinal: reflex
erethistic: shock
erogenous: zone
E-rosette: test
erosive: adenomatosis
erotic: zoophilism
erotogenic: zone
erroneous: projection
eruptive: fever; phase; xanthoma
erythema: dose; threshold
erythematous: syphilid
erythredema: polyneuritis
erythremic: myelosis
erythroblastic: anemia
erythrocyte: index
erythrocyte adherence: phenomenon; test
erythrocyte fragility: test
erythrocyte maturation: factor
erythrocyte sedimentation: rate
erythrocytic: series
erythrodysesthesia: syndrome
erythrogenic: toxin
erythrohepatic: porphyria
erythroid: cell
erythrophore: reaction
erythropoietic: hormone; porphyria; protoporphyria
escape: beat; conditioning; impulse; interval phenomenon; rhythm
escape-capture: bigeminy
escaped: beat; contraction
escaped ventricular: contraction
Escherichia coli: enterotoxin; ribonuclease
esodic: nerve
esophageal: achalasia; artery; atresia; cardiogram; gland; impression; lead; manometry; opening; plexus; reflux; smear; speech; varix; vein; web
esophagogastric: junction; orifice; vestibule
esophagosalivery: reflex
essential: albuminuria; amino acid; bradycardia; dysmenorrhea; fever; fructosuria; hematuria; hypertension; oil; pentosuria; phthisis; pruritus; tachycardia; telangiectasia; thrombocytopenia
essential food: factor
essential progressive: atrophy
established cell: line
esterified: estrogen
esthesiodic: system
esthetic: surgery
estradiol benzoate: unit
estrogenic: hormone
estrone: unit
estrous: cycle
ether: cone; convulsion; test
ethereal: oil; solution; tincture
ethmoid: angle; bone; infundibulum
ethmoidal: bulla; cell; crest; foramen; groove; labyrinth; notch; process; sinus; vein
ethmoidal-lacrimal: fistula
ethmoidolacrimal: suture
ethmoidomaxillary: suture
ethmovomerine: plate
eucalyptus: gum
euglobulin clot lysin: test
eugnathic: anomaly
eunuchoid: gigantism; state; voice

euplastic: lymph
European: snakeroot; tarantula
euroxenous: parasite
eustachian: catheter; cushion; tonsil; tube; tuber; valve
eutectic: alloy; temperature
euthyroid: hypometabolism
evoked: potential; response
evoked response: audiometry
evolutionary: fitness
examining: table
exanthematous: disease; fever
excentric: amputation
excess: lactate
exchange: transfusion
excision: biopsy
excitable: area
excitation: spectrum; wave
excitatory postsynaptic: potential
excited: atom; catatonia; state
exciting: cause; electrode; eye
excitor: nerve
excitoreflex: nerve
exclamation point: hair
excretory: duct; ductule; gland; urography
exercise: bone; test
exertional: rhabdomyolysis
exfoliative: cytology; dermatitis; gastritis
exhaustion: atrophy; psychosis
existential: psychiatry; psychology; psychotherapy
exit: block; dose
exoccipital: bone
exocelomic: membrane
exocrine: gland
exodic: nerve
exoerythrocytic: cycle; stage
exogenic: toxicosis
exogenous: cycle; fiber; hemochromatosis; hyperglyceridemia; ochronosis; pigmentation
exogenous creatinine: clearance
exophthalmic: goiter; ophthalmoplegia
exophthalmos-producing: substance
exoteric: bacterium
expansion: arch
expansive: delusion
expectation: neurosis
experimental: group; medicine; method; neurosis; psychology
experimental allergic: encephalitis; encephalomyelitis
experimenter: effect
expiratory: center; resistance; stridor
expiratory reserve: volume
expired: gas
exploratory: drive
exploring: electrode; needle
explosive: decompression; speech
exponential: distribution
exposed: pulp
exposure: keratitis
expressed: mustard oil
expressed skull: fracture
expression: vector
expressive: aphasia
expulsive: pain
exsanguination: transfusion
exsiccated: alum; sodium
exsiccation: fever
extemporaneous: mixture
extended: clasp; pyelotomy
extended family: therapy
extended insulin zinc: suspension
extended radical: mastectomy
extension: form
extensor: aponeurosis; muscle; retinaculum; tetanus
external: absorption; defibrillator; fistula; fixation; hemorrhoids; hydrocephalus; medium; meningitis; ophthalmopathy; pacemaker; phase; pyocephalus; respiration; squint; strabismus; traction; urethrotomy; version
external anatomical structures (specific external anatomical and histological structures are listed under the following): artery; axis; canthus; capsule; cell; conjugate; crest; epithelium; fascia; fiber; fibrocartilage; foramen; genitalia; gland; ligament; lip; malleolus; meatus; muscle; nerve; node; nose; nucleus; plexus; pore; protuberance; ridge; ring; sulcus; surface; vein; wall
external cardiac: massage
external exudative: retinopathy
external malleolar: sign
external oblique: reflex
external pin: fixation
external urethral: opening
exterofective: system
extinction: coefficient
extra-: systole
extra-abdominal: desmoid
extraamniotic: pregnancy
extracapsular: ankylosis; fracture; ligament
extracardiac: murmur
extracellular: cholesterolosis; enzyme; fluid; toxin
extrachorial: pregnancy
extrachromosomal: element; inheritance
extracoronal: retainer
extracorporeal: circulation; dialysis
extracranial: pneumatocele; pneumocele
extracting: forceps
extraction: coefficient; ratio
extradural: anesthesia; hematorrhachis; hemorrhage
extraembryonic: blastoderm; celom; mesoderm
extraglomerular: mesangium
extramammary Paget: disease
extramembranous: pregnancy
extramural: practice
extranuclear: inheritance
extraoral: anchorage
extraoral fracture: appliance
extraperitoneal: fascia
extrapineal: pinealoma
extrapleural: pneumothorax
extrapyramidal: disease; dyskinesia; syndrome
extrapyramidal motor: system
extrasaccular: hernia
extrasensory: perception
extrasensory thought: transferase
extraskeletal: chondroma
extrauterine: pregnancy
extravasation: cyst
extravascular: fluid
extravital: ultraviolet
extreme: capsule
extreme somatosensory evoked: potential
extrinsic: asthma; color; factor; motivation; sphincter
extrinsic allergic: alveolitis
extrinsic incubation: period
extruded: tooth
exudation: cell; corpuscle; cyst
exudative: bronchiolitis; choroiditis; glomerulonephritis; inflammation; retinitis; vitreoretinopathy
exudative discoid and lichenoid: dermatitis
exudative retinal: detachment
eye: capsule; cup; drops; lens; ointment; reflex; socket; speculum; tooth
eye-closure: reflex
eye-ear: plane
eyelash: sign

F

F: actin; agent; duction; factor; gen-

F—*continued*
ote; pilus; plasmid; thalassemia; wave
F′: agent; factor; plasmid
f: wave
FA: virus
Fab: fragment; piece
face: form; presentation; validity
face-bow: fork; record
facet: rhizotomy
facial: angle; artery; axis; bone; canal; cleft; colliculus; diplegia; eczema; eminence; height; hemiatrophy; hemiplegia; hillock; index; muscle; nerve; neuralgia; palsy; paralysis; perception; plane; plexus; profile; reflex; root; spasm; surface; tic; triangle; trophoneurosis; vein; vision
facialis: phenomenon
facial lymph: node
faciodigitogenital: dysplasia
facioscapulohumeral: atrophy
facioscapulohumeral muscular: dystrophy
factitious: purpura; urticaria
factorial: experiment
facultative: anaerobe; heterochromatin; hyperopia; parasite; saprophyte
fading: time
faith: healing
falciform: cartilage; crest; ligament; lobe; margin; process
falciform retinal: fold
falciparum: fever; malaria
fallen: arch
falling: palate; sickness
falling of: womb
fallopian: aqueduct; arch; canal; hiatus; ligament; neuritis; pregnancy; tube
false: agglutination; albuminuria; anemia; aneurysm; angina; ankylosis; blepharoptosis; branching; cast; conjugate; coxa; cyanosis; cyst; dextrocardia; diphtheria; diverticulum; dominance; glottis; hematuria; hermaphroditism; hypertrophy; image; joint; knot; macula; masturbation; membrane; mole; negative; neuroma; nucleolus; pain; paracusis; pelvis; positive; pregnancy; projection; rib; ringbone; suture; thirst; vertebra; waters
false-negative: reaction
false-positive: reaction
false vocal: cord
familial: aggregation; amyloidosis; cancer; cystinuria; dysautonomia; emphysema; encephalopathy; glycinuria; goiter; hyperbetalipoproteinemia; hypercholesterolemia; hyperchylomicronemia; hyperlipoproteinemia; hyperprebetalipoproteinemia; hypertriglyceridemia; hypoparathyrodism; nephrosis; screening
familial amyloid: neuropathy
familial benign chronic: pemphigus
familial endocrine: adenomatosis
familial erythrobalstic: anemia
familial fat-induced: hyperlipemia
familial fibrous: dysplasia
familial high density lipoprotein: deficiency
familial hypercholesteremic: xanthomatosis
familial hypogonadotropic: hypogonadism
familial hypoplastic: anemia
familial intestinal: polyposis
familial juvenile: nephrophthisis
familial Mediterranean: fever
familial microcytic: anemia
familial nonhemolytic: jaundice
familial paroxysmal: polyserositis; rhabdomyolysis
familial periodic: paralysis
familial polyendocrine: adenomatosis
familial pseudoinflammatory: maculopathy
familial pseudoinflammatory macular: degeneration
familial pyridoxine-responsive: anemia
familial spinal muscular: atrophy
familial splenic: anemia
familial white folded: dysplasia
family: medicine; therapy
famine: fever
fan: sign
far: point; sight
far-and-near: suture
Far East Russian: encephalitis
farmer's: lung; skin
far point of: convergence
fascia: graft
fascial: hernia
fascicular: block; degeneration; graft; keratitis; ophthalmoplegia; sarcoma; ulcer
fasciculata: cell
fasciculate: bladder
fasciolar: gyrus
fast: rhythm; smear
fastidious: organism
fastigiobulbar: tract
fat: body; cell; embolism; graft; indigestion; metabolism; necrosis; pad; solvent; tide
fatality: rate
father: complex
fatigue: fever; fracture; strength
fat-soluble: vitamin
fat-storing: cell
fatty: alcohol; ascites; atrophy; cast; change; cirrhosis; degeneration; diarrhea; heart; hernia; infiltration; kidney; liver; metamorphosis; oil; phanerosis; series; tissue
fatty acid oxidation: cycle
faucial: paralysis; reflex; tonsil
faulty: union
faun tail: nevus
Fc: fragment; piece; receptor
feather: louse
featural: surgery
febrile: albuminuria; convulsion; crisis; psychosis; urine; urticaria
fecal: abscess; fistula; impaction; tumor; vomiting
feedback: inhibition; system
feeding: center; tube
feeling: tone
feigned: eruption
feline: agranulocytosis; leukemia; pneumonitis
feline infectious: enteritis; peritonitis
feline leukemia: virus
feline leukemia-sarcoma virus: complex
feline panleukopenia: virus
feline rhinotracheitis: virus
feline viral: rhinotracheitis
female: catheter; gonad; hermaphroditism; prostate; pseudohermaphroditism; sterility; urethra
femininity: complex
femoral: arch; artery; canal; fossa; hernia; muscle; nerve; opening; plexus; reflex; region; ring; septum; sheath; triangle; vein
femoroabdominal: reflex
femoropatellar: joint
femoropopliteal: bypass
femoropopliteal occlusive: disease
femorotibial: joint
fenestrated: capillary; membrane C; sheath
fenestration: operation
fermentation Lactobacillus casei: factor
fermentative: dyspepsia

fern: test
ferric: alum
ferric chloride: reaction; test
ferruginous: body
fertile: period
fertility: agent; factor; vitamin
fertilization: cone; membrane
fertilized: ovum
fescue: foot; poisoning
festinating: gait
fetal: adenoma; age; attitude; bradycardia; circulation; cortex; cotyledon; death; distress; dystocia; electrocardiography; erythroblastosis; fracture; habitus; hemoglobin; hydrops; inclusion; medicine; membrane; movement; ovoid; placenta; souffle; tachycardia; zone
fetal alcohol: syndrome
fetal aspiration: syndrome
fetal death: rate
fetal heart: rate
fetal hydantoin: syndrome
fetal warfarin: syndrome
fetoplacental: anasarca
fever: blister; therapy
feverish: urine
FF, ff: wave
FGT cytologic: smear
fibrillar: basket
fibrillary: chorea; contraction; myoclonia; neuroma; tremor; wave
fibrillation: threshold
fibrin: calculus; thrombus
fibrin/fibrinogen degradation: product
fibrinocartilaginous: ring
fibrinogen-fibrin conversion: syndrome
fibrinoid: degeneration; necrosis
fibrinolytic: purpura
fibrinopurulent: inflammation
fibrinous: adhesion; bronchitis; cast; cataract; degeneration; inflammation; iritis; lymph; pericarditis; pleurisy; polyp, rhinitis
fibrin-stabilizing: factor
fibroblast: interferon
fibrocaseous: peritonitis
fibrocystic: disease
fibroepithelial: papilloma
fibrohyaline: tissue
fibroid: adenoma; cataract; inflammation; lung; tumor
fibrolamellar liver cell: carcinoma
fibromatosis: virus
fibromuscular: dysplasia; hyperplasia
fibrosing: adenomatosis; adenosis
fibrositic: headache
fibrous: adhesion; ankylosis; appendix; astrocyte capsule; cavernitis; degeneration; dysplasia; goiter; hamartoma; histiocytoma; joint; layer; membrane; polyp; protein; ring; sheath; tissue; trigone; tubercle; tunic; union; xanthoma
fibrous articular: capsule
fibrous bacterial: virus
fibrous cortical: defect
fibular: artery; margin; node; notch; vein
fibular articular: surface
fibular collateral: ligament
Ficoll-Hypaque: technique
fictitious: feeding
field: block; fever; lens
field block: anesthesia
field of: consciousness; fixation; vision
fifth: disease; finger; ventricle
fifth cranial: nerve
fig: wart
figure-of-8 (eight): abnormality; bandage; suture
filamentary: keratopathy
filament-nonfilament: count
filamentous: bacteriophage; colony
filamentous bacterial: virus
filament polymorphonuclear: leukocyte
filar: mass; micrometer; substance
filarial: arthritis; dermatosis funiculitis; hydrocele; periodicity; synovitis
filariform: larva
filial: generation
filiform: bougie; papilla; pulse; wart
filler: graft
fillet: layer
filling: defect
filter: paper
filtering: cicatrix; operation
filtrable: virus
filtrate: factor; nitrogen
filtration: angle; coefficient; fraction; slit; space
fimbriated: fold
fimbriodentate: sulcus
final: host; impression
fine: structure; tremor
finger: agnosia; percussion; phenomenon
finger-nose: test
fingerprint: dystrophy
finger-thumb: reflex
finger-to-finger: test
finishing: bur
first: dentition; finger; messenger
first arch: syndrome
first cranial: nerve
first cuneiform: bone
first degree: burn
first duodenal: sphincter
first-order: reaction; receptor
first parallel pelvic: plane
first permanent: molar
first rank: symptom
first temporal: convolution
first visceral: cleft
fish: poison; skin; test
fish-mouth: meatus
fish-mouth mitral: stenosis
fish tapeworm: anemia
fission: fungus; product
fissural: cyst
fissure: bur; caries; sealant
fissured: fracture; tongue
fistula: knife; test
fistulous: withers
FIT: test
fixation: disparity; nystagmus; reaction
fixational ocular: movement
fixator: muscle
fixed: alkali; alkaloid; coupling; dressing; idea; macrophage; oil; pupil; torticollis; virus
fixed drug: eruption
fixed partial: denture
fixed-rate: pacemaker
fixed rate pulse: generator
fixing: eye
flaccid: ectropion; membrane; part
flag: flap; sign
flagellar: agglutinin; antigen
flail: chest; joint
flame: arc; figure; photometer; spot
flame emission: spectrophotometry
flammable: anesthetic
flange: contour
flank: bone; incision; position
flap: amputation; operation
flapless: amputation
flapping: tremor
flash: blindness; burn; dispersal; keratoconjunctivitis; method; point
flashing pain: syndrome
flask: closure
flat: affect; bone; chest; condyloma; electroencephalogram; flap; foot; hand; pelvis; plate; wart
flat papular: syphilid

flat top: wave
flatulent: dyspepsia
flatus: enema
flea-bitten: kidney
flea-borne: typhus
fleck, flecked: dystrophy; retina
flecked retina: syndrome
fleece: worm
fleshy: mole; polyp
flexible: collodion
flexion: crease
flexor: reflex; retinaculum; tetanus
flexural: eczema
flick: movement
flicker: fusion; perimetry; photometer
flicker fusion frequency: technique
flight: blindness
flight or fight: response
flint: disease; glass
flittering: scotoma
floating: cartilage; kidney; organ; patella; rib; spleen; villus
floccular: fossa
flocculation: reaction; test
flocculonodular: lobe
flood: fever
floor: cell; plate
floppy valve: syndrome
florid oral: papillomatosis
florid osseous: dysplasia
floriform: cataract
floss: silk
flotation: constant; method
floury: cornea
flow: cytophotometry
flower-spray: ending; organ
flowing: hyperostosis
flow-over: vaporizer
flow-volume: curve
fluid: extract; wave
fluorescein: angiography
fluorescein instillation: test
fluorescein string: test
fluorescence: microscopy; quenching; spectrum
fluorescence plus Giemsa: stain
fluorescent: antibody; microscope; screen; stain
fluorescent antibody: technique
fluorescent antinuclear antibody: test
fluorescent treponemal antibody-absorption: test
fluoridated: tooth
Flury strain: vaccine
Flury strain rabies: virus
flush: technique
flutter-fibrillation: wave
flux: density; ratio
fluxionary: hyperemia
fly: agaric; blister
flying: blister
flying spot: microscope
FMD: virus
foam: cell
foam stability: test
foamy: agent; virus
focal: amyloidosis; appendicitis; depth; distance; epilepsy; glomerulonephritis; illumination; infection; interval; necrosis; nephritis; point; reaction; sclerosis
focal dermal: hypoplasia
focal dermal hypoplasia: syndrome
focal embolic: glomerulonephritis
focal epithelial: hyperplasia
focal lymphocytic: thyroiditis
focal sclerosing: glomerulopathy
focal segmental: glomerulosclerosis
folded-lung: syndrome
folding: fracture
foliate: papilla
folic acid: antagonist; conjugate
folk: medicine
follian: process
follicle-stimulating: hormone; principle
follicle-stimulating hormone-releasing: factor; hormone
follicular: abscess; adenoma; antrum; carcinoma; conjunctivitis; cyst; cystitis; gland; goiter; hormone; impetigo; iritis; lymphoma; mange; mucinosis; papule; pharyngitis; stigma; syphilid; trachoma; urethritis; vulvitis
follicular epithelial: cell
follicular ovarian: cell
follicular predominantly large cell: lymphoma
follicular predominantly small cleaved cell: lymphoma
food: ball; fever; impaction; poisoning
foot: plate; plugger; presentation; process; rot; yaws
foot-and-mouth: disease
foot-and-mouth disease: virus
foot-and-mouth disease virus: vaccine
football: calf
footling: presentation
foot-pound-second: system; unit
foraminal: herniation; node
forced: alimentation; beat; cycle; duction; feeding; respiration
forced expiratory: flow; time; volume
forced grasping: reflex
forced vital: capacity
forceps: delivery
forcible: feeding
forebrain: eminence; prominence; vesicle
foreign: body; protein; serum
foreign body: granuloma; salpingitis; tumorigenesis
foreign body giant: cell
foreign protein: therapy
forensic: dentistry; medicine; odontology; psychiatry; psychology
forequarter: amputation
forest: yaws
formal: operation
formaldehyde: fixative
formalin: pigment
formative: cell
formed visual: hallucination
formol: titration
formol-calcium: fixative
formol-Müller: fixative
formol-saline: fixative
formol-Zenker: fixative
Fort Bragg: fever
fortification: figure; spectrum
fortified vitamin D: milk
forward: conduction
forward heart: failure
foudroyant: myelitis
founder: effect; principle
fountain: decussation; syringe
fourth: disease; finger; ventricle
fourth cranial: nerve
fourth lumbar: nerve
fourth parallel pelvic: plane
fourth turbinated: bone
foveated: chest
foveolar: cell
fowl: cholera; erythroblastosis; leukosis; lymphomatosis; myeloblastosis; paralysis; pest; plague; typhoid
fowl erythroblastosis: virus
fowl lymphomatosis: virus
fowl myeloblastosis: virus
fowl neurolymphomatosis: virus
fowl plague: virus
fowlpox: virus
fox: encephalitis
fox encephalitis: virus
FPS, fps: system; unit
fractional: distillation; dose; sterilization
fractional epidural: anesthesia

G

ganglioside: lipidosis
gangrenous: appendicitis; emphysema; pharyngitis; pneumonia; rhinitis; stomatitis
gap: arthroplasty; junction; phenomenon
Gap_1: period
Gap_2: period
garapata: disease
gargantuan: mastitis
gas: abscess; bacillus; cautery; chromatography; constant; cyst; embolism; gangrene; peritonitis; phlegmon; thermometer
gaseous: mediastinography; pulse
gas gangrene: antitoxin
gas-liquid: chromatography
gasping: disease
gasserian: ganglion
gastral: mesoderm
gastrea: theory
gastric: analysis; calculus; canal; colic; crisis; diastole; digestion; feeding; fistula; fold; follicle; freezing; gland; hemorrhage; impression; indigestion; juice; mucin; neurasthenia; pit; plexus; smear; stapling; surface; tetany; ulcer; vein; vertigo; volvulus
gastric inhibitory: polypeptide
gastric lymphatic: follicle
gastrocardiac: syndrome
gastrocnemius: muscle
gastrocolic: fistula; ligament; omentum; reflex
gastrocutaneous: fistula
gastrodiaphragmatic: ligament
gastroduodenal: artery; fistula; orifice
gastroduodenal lymph: node
gastroenteritis: virus
gastroepiploic: vein
gastroesophageal: hernia; reflux; vestibule
gastrogenous: diarrhea
gastrohepatic: omentum
gastroileac: reflex
gastrointestinal: fistula; hormone; tract
gastrojejunal loop obstruction: syndrome
gastrolienal: ligament
gastropancreatic: fold
gastrophrenic: ligament
gastrosplenic: ligament; omentum
gate-control: hypothesis; theory
gating: mechanism
gauntlet: bandage
gaussian: curve; distribution
gauze: bandage
gaze: nystagmus
G-banding: stain
GE: antigen
gel: diffusion; electrophoresis; filtration; structure
gelatin: sugar
gelatinous: ascites; infiltration; polyp; scleritis; substance; tissue; varix
gel diffusion: reaction
gel diffusion precipitin: test
gemästete: cell
geminated: tooth
gemistocytic: astrocyte; astrocytoma; cell; reaction
genal: gland
gender: identity; role
gene: deletion; flow; frequency; mosaicism; pool
gene dosage: compensation; effect
general: anatomy; anesthesia; anesthetic; bloodletting; hospital; immunity; peritonitis; physiology; sensation; stimulant; transduction; tuberculosis
general adaptation: reaction; syndrome
generalized: anaphylaxis; chondromalacia; emphysema; epilepsy; gangliosidosis; glycogenosis; lentiginosis; tetanus; vaccinia; xanthelasma
generalized anxiety: disorder
generalized cortical: hyperostosis
generalized eruptive: histiocytoma
generalized pustular: psoriasis
generalized Shwartzman: phenomenon
generalized tonic-clonic: seizure
general somatic afferent: column
general somatic efferent: column
general splanchnic afferent: column
general splanchnic efferent: column
general visceral afferent: column
general visceral efferent: column
generated occlusal: path
generative: empathy
generator: potential
genesial: cycle
genetic: amplification; anemia; association; carrier; code; colonization; compound; counseling; death; determinant; disequilibrium; dominant; drift; engineering; equilibrium; female; fitness; fixation; heterogeneity; homeostasis; immunity; isolate; lethal; linkage; load; locus; male; marker; polymorphism; psychology; recombination
genial: tubercle
genic: balance
geniculate: body; ganglion; neuralgia; otalgia
geniculocalcarine: radiation; tract
genioglossal: muscle
geniohyoid: muscle
genital: cord; corpuscle; duct; eminence; fold; furrow, gland; herpes; ligament; organ; phase; primacy; ridge; swelling; system; tract; tubercle; wart
genitocrural: nerve
genitofemoral: nerve
genitoinguinal: ligament
genitourinary: apparatus; fistula; system
gentian aniline: water
genucubital: position
genupectoral: position
geographic, geographical: choroidopathy; keratitis; stippling; tongue
geometric: isomerism; mean
geriatric: therapy
germ: cell; disk; layer; line; membrane; nucleus; theroy; tube
German: braxy; measles
German measles: virus
germinal: aplasia; area; cell; center; cord; disk; epithelium; localization; membrane; mosaicism; pole; rod; spot; vesicle
germinative: layer
germ layer: theory
germ tube: test
gestalt: phenomenon; psychology; theory; therapy
gestational: age; edema; proteinuria; psychosis
ghatti: gum
Gheel: colony
ghost: cell; corpuscle; tooth
ghost cell: glaucoma
ghoul: hand
giant: baby; cell; chromosome; colon; condyloma; drusen; fibroadenoma; hives; hypertrophy; melanosome
giant axonal: neuropathy
giant cell: aortitis; arteritis; carcinoma; epulis; fibroma; granuloma; hepatitis; myeloma; myocarditis; pneumonia; sarcoma; thyroiditis; tumor
giant follicular: lymphoblastoma
giant gastric: fold

H

head: botfly; cap; cavity; fold; kidney; mirror; nurse; presentation; process; tetanus; tremor
head-bobbing doll: syndrome
head-dropping: test
healed: tuberculosis; ulcer
health: care
hearing: level
heart: antigen; beat; block; failure; hormone; position; rate; reflex; sac; sound; stroke; transplantation
heart-failure: cell
heart-hand: syndrome
heart-lung: machine; preparation
heart-shaped: pelvis; uterus
heat: apoplexy; capacity; cramp; edema; exhaustion; hyperpyrexia; lamp; prostration; rash; rigor; stroke; treatment; urticaria
heat coagulation: test
heat-curing: resin
heat-instability: test
heat-rigor: point
heavy: chain; eye; hydrogen; nitrogen; oxygen; water
heavy chain: disease
α-heavy-chain: disease
γ-heavy-chain: disease
μ-heavy-chain: disease
heavy liquid: petrolatum
hebephrenic: dementia; schizophrenia
hebetic: cough
hectic: flush
hederiform: ending
heel: bone; fly; jar; tap; tendon
heel-tap: reaction; test
height: vertigo
height-length: index
height of: contour
HeLa: cell
helicine: artery
helicoid: choroidopathy; ginglymus
helicopod: gait
helium: speech
helmet: cell
helminthic: dysentery
helper: cell; virus
hemadsorption: virus
hemadsorption virus: test
hemagglutinating cold: autoantibody
hemaggluntination: inhibition
hemal: arch; gland; node; spine
hemangiectatic: hypertrophy
hemangioma-thrombocytopenia: syndrome
hematinic: principle
hematogenetic: calculus
hematogenous: abscess; embolism; jaundice; osteitis; pigment; theory
hematoidin: crystal
hematopoietic, hemopoietic: gland; system; tissue
hematoxylin: body
hematoxylin and eosin: stain
hematoxylin-malachite green-basic fuchsin: stain
hematoxyphil: body
hematuric bilious: fever
hemianopic: scotoma; spectacles
hemiazygos: vein
hemic: calculus; distomiasis; murmur
hemilateral: chorea
hemiopic: reaction
hemiopic pupillary: reaction
hemiplegic: amyotrophy; gait; migraine
hemisulfur: mustard
hemithoracic: duct
hemoccult: test
hemochorial: placenta
hemoclastic: reaction
hemoendothelial: placenta
hemoglobin C: disease
hemoglobin H: disease
hemoglobinuric: fever; nephrosis
hemohepatogenous: jaundice
hemolymph: gland; node
hemolysin: unit
hemolytic: anemia; chain; disease; gas; jaundice; splenomegaly; streptococcus; unit
hemolytic-uremic: syndrome
hemophilic: arthritis; joint
hemopoietic: see hematopoietic
hemorrhagic: anemia; ascites; bronchitis; colitis; cyst; dengue; diathesis; disease; endovasculitis; fever; gangrene; glaucoma; infarct; iritis; measles; nephritis; pachymeningitis; pain; plague; pleurisy; rickets; septicemia; shock; smallpox
hemorrhoidal: nerve; plexus; vein
hemostatic: collodion; forceps
hemotoxic: anemia
HEMPAS: cell
hen-cluck: stertor
HEP: vaccine
heparin: unit
hepatic: amebiasis; capsulitis; colic; coma; cord; cyst; duct; encephalopathy; fistula; flexure; infantilism; insufficiency; lamina; lobule; plexus; prominence; segment; steatosis; triad; vein
hepatic intermittent: fever
hepatic lymph: node
hepatic portal: vein
hepatic venous: segment
hepatitis A: virus
hepatitis B: vaccine; virus
hepatitis B core: antigen
hepatitis B e: antigen
hepatitis B surface: antigen
hepatitis delta: virus
hepatocellular: carcinoma; jaundice
hepatocolic: ligament
hepatocystic: duct
hepatoduodenal: ligament
hepatoenteric: recess
hepatoesophageal: ligament
hepatogastric: ligament
hepatogenous: jaundice; pigment
hepatojugular: reflex; reflux
hepatolenticular: degeneration; disease
hepatonephric: syndrome
hepatophosphorylase deficiency: glycogenosis
hepatopleural: fistula
hepatorenal: ligament; pouch; recess; syndrome
herald: patch
herd: immunity; instinct
hereditary: chorea; hemochromatosis; lymphedema; methemoglobinemia; myokymia; nephritis; photomyoclonus; spherocytosis
hereditary angioneurotic: edema
hereditary cerebellar: ataxia
hereditary deforming: chondrodysplasia; chondrodystrophy
hereditary fructose: intolerance
hereditary hemorrhagic: telangiectasis; thrombasthenia
hereditary methemoglobinemic: cyanosis
hereditary multiple: exostosis; trichoepithelioma
hereditary opalescent: dentin
hereditary progressive: arthro-ophthalmopathy
hereditary renal-retinal: dysplasia
hereditary sensory radicular: neuropathy
hereditary spinal: ataxia
heredofamilial: tremor
heredomacular: degeneration
hernia: knife

hernial: aneurysm; sac
herniated: disk
heroic: treatment
herpes: encephalitis; virus
herpes simplex: virus
herpes zoster: virus
herpetic: fever; keratitis; keratoconjunctivitis; meningoencephalitis; ulcer; whitlow
herpetiform: aphtha
herring-worm: disease
hertzian: experiment
herz: hormone
heterochromic: cyclitis; uveitis
heterocladic: anastomosis
heterocyclic: compound
heterocytotropic: antibody
heterodermic: graft
heterogametic: embryo
heterogeneous: nucleation; radiation; RNA; system
heterogenetic: antibody; antigen; parasite
heterogenic enterobacterial: antigen
heterogenous: keratoplasty; vaccine
heterologous: antiserum; desensitization; graft; insemination; protein; stimulus; tumor; twins
heteromeric: cell; peptide
heterometabolous: metamorphosis
heterometric: autoregulation
heteronomous: psychotherapy
heteronymous: diplopia; hemianopsia; image; parallax
heterophil: antibody; antigen; hemolysin; leukocyte
heteropycnotic: chromatin
heterotopic: bone; graft; pain; pregnancy
heterotropic: chromosome
heterotype: mitosis
heterotypic: cortex
heterotypical: chromosome
heterovaccine: therapy
heteroxenous: parasite
hexacanth: embryo
hexaxial reference: system
hexazonium: salts
hexokinase: method
hexon: antigen
hexone: base
hexose monophosphate: shunt
HFR, Hfr: strain
HG: factor
H-graft: anastomosis
hiatal, hiatus: hernia
hibernating: gland
hidden: part
hidebound: disease
hidrotic ectodermal: dysplasia
high: convex; enema; lithotomy; wine
high altitude: chamber
high calorie: diet
high-egg passage: vaccine
high endothelial postcapillary: venule
high energy: compound; phosphate
high energy phosphate: bond
higher order: conditioning
highest: concha
highest intercostal: artery; vein
highest nuchal: line
highest thoracic: artery
highest turbinated: bone
high fat: diet
high forceps: delivery
high frequency: currency; deafness; transduction
high lip: line
high output: failure
high pressure: oxygen
high resolution: banding
high spinal: anesthesia
high steppage: gait
hilar: dance
hilar cell: tumor
hilus: cell
hind: kidney
hindbrain: vesicle
hindquarter: amputation
hinge: axis; joint; movement; position; region
hinged: flap
hip: bone; joint; phenomenon
hip-flexion: phenomenon
hippocampal: commissure; convolution; fissure; gyrus; sclerosis
hippocratic: face; facies; finger; nail; school; succussion
hippocratic succussion: sound
Histalog: test
histamine: liberator; shock; test
histaminic: cephalagia; headache
histiocytic: leukemia
histiocytic medullary: reticulosis
histocompatibility: gene
histoid: leprosy; neoplasm; tumor
histologic: accommodation
histoplasmin-latex: test
histotoxic: anoxia
histrionic: personality; spasm
hitchhiker's: thumb
HL-A: antigen
HLA: complex
Ho: antigen
hobnail: cell; liver; tongue
hoe: excavator; scaler
hog: cholera
hog cholera: vaccine; virus
holandric: gene; inheritance
holiday: syndrome
holiday heart: syndrome
holistic: medicine; psychology
hollow: back; bone
holoblastic: cleavage
holocrine: gland
hologynic: inheritance
holometabolous: metamorphosis
holosystolic: murmur
homeometric: autoregulation
homeostatic: equilibrium
homigrade: scale
hominal: physiology
homing: valve
homochronous: inheritance
homocladic: anastomosis
homocyclic: compound
homocytotropic: antibody
homogametic: embryo
homogeneous: immersion; nucleation; radiation; system
homogenous: keratoplasty
homolecithal: egg
homologous: antiserum; chromosome; desensitizatoin; graft; insemination; series; stimulus; tumor
homologous serum: jaundice
homonymous: diplopia; hemianopsia; image; parallax
homosexual: panic
homotopic: pain
homotypic: cortex
homovanillic acid: test
homozygous: achondroplasia
honey: urine
honeycomb: lung; macula; ringworm; scall; tetter
Hong Kong: foot; influenza; toe
hoof-and-mouth: disease
hook: bundle
hookean: behavior
hooked: bone; fasiculus
hookless: tapeworm
hook-shaped: cataract
hookworm: anemia; disease
horizontal: atrophy; cell; fissure; fracture; heart; osteotomy; overlap; part; plane; plate; resorption; transmission; vertigo
hormonal: gingivitis
horny: layer
horsepox: virus
horseradish: peroxidase

horseshoe: fistula; kidney; placenta
hospital: fever; formulary; gangrene; record
hot: abscess; eye; flash; flush; gangrene; nodule; pack; snare; spot
hot salt: sterilizer
Hottentot: tea
hound-dog: facies
hourglass: contraction; head; murmur; pattern; stomach; vertebra
house: staff; surgeon
housemaid's: knee
H-R conduction: time
Hu (He): antigen
human: babesiosis; botfly; ecology; fibrinogen; genetics; insulin; serum; thrombin
human α_1 proteinase: inhibitor
human antihemophilic: factor; fraction
human botfly: myiasis
human chorionic: gonadotropin; somatomammotropin
human chorionic somatomammotropic: hormone
human diploid cell rabies: vaccine
human fibrin: foam
human gamma: globulin
human immunodeficiency: virus
humanistic: psychology
human leukemia-associated: antigen
human lymphocyte: antigen
human measles immune: serum
human menopausal: gonadotropin
human normal: immunoglobulin
human papilloma: virus
human pertussis immune: serum
human placental: lactogen
human scarlet fever immune: serum
human T-cell lymphoma/leukemia: virus
human T-cell lymphotropic: virus
humeral: artery; articulation; head
humeroradial: articulation; joint
humeroulnar: head; joint
humid: tetter
humoral: doctrine; immunity; pathology; theory
hunger: contraction; pain; swelling
hunting: phenomenon; reaction
hurloid: facies
H-V: interval
HVA: test
H-V conduction: time
H-Y: antigen
hyaline: body; cartilage; cast; degeneration; leukocyte; membrane; thrombus; tubercle
hyaline membrane: disease
hyaloid: artery; body; canal; fossa; membrane
hyaloideoretinal: degeneration
hybrid: prosthesis
hydatid: cyst; disease; fremitus; mole; polyp; pregnancy; rash; resonance; sand; thrill
hydatidiform: mole
hydralazine: syndrome
hydrated: alumina
hydrate microcrystal: theory
hydratic: crystal
hydraulic: conductivity
hydremic: edema
hydride: ion
hydroalcoholic: extract; tincture
hydrocephalic: idiocy
hydroelectric: bath
hydrogen: acceptor; bond; carrier; donor; electrode; ion; number; transport
hydrolytic: cleavage
hydrolyzing: enzyme
hydronium: ion
hydrophil, hydrophilic: colloid; petrolatum
hydrophobic: colloid; tetanus
hydropic: degeneration
hydrostatic: dilator; pressure
hydrous: wool fat
17-hydroxycorticosteroid: test
17-hydroxylase deficiency: syndrome
hygienic laboratory: coefficient
hygroscopic: expansion
hylic: tumor
hyobranchial: cleft
hyoepiglottic: ligament
hyoglossal: membrane; muscle
hyoid: apparatus; arch; bone
hyomandibular: cleft
hyparterial: bronchus
hyperabduction: syndrome
hyperacute: rejection
hyperbaric: anesthesia; chamber; oxygen; oxygenation
hyperbaric oxygen: therapy
hyperbaric spinal: anesthesia
hypercalcemic: sarcoidosis; uremia
hyperchromatic: anemia; macrocythemia
hyperchromic: anemia
hypercyanotic: angina
hyperemia: test
hypereosinophilic: syndrome
hyperergic: encephalitis
hyperextension-hyperflexion: injury
hyperfunctional: occlusion
hypergenic: teratosis
hyperglobulinemia: purpura
hyperglycemic-glycogenolytic: factor
hypergonadotropic: eunuchoidism
hyperimmunoglobulin E: syndrome
hyperkalemic periodic: paralysis
hyperkinetic: syndrome
hyperlucent: lung
hypermature: cataract
hypernatremic: encephalopathy
hyperopic: astigmatism
hyperosmolar hyperglycemic nonketonic: coma
hyperostotic: spondylosis
hyperplastic: arteriosclerosis; gingivitis; graft; inflammation; osteoarthritis; polyp; pulpitis
hyperprolactinemic: amenorrhea
hyperquantivalent: idea
hyperreactive malarious: splenomegaly
hypersecretion: glaucoma
hypersegmented: neutrophil
hypersensitive: dentin
hypersensitive xiphoid: syndrome
hypersensitivity: angiitis; pneumonitis; reaction
hypertensive: arteriopathy; arteriosclerosis; encephalopathy; iridocyclitis; retinopathy
hypertonic: absence
hypertrophic: arthritis; cardiomyopathy; gastritis; pulpitis; rhinitis; ringworm; rosacea; scar
hypertrophic cervical: pachymeningitis
hypertrophic hypersecretory: gastropathy
hypertrophic interstitial: neuropathy
hypertrophic pulmonary: osteoarthropathy
hypertrophic pyloric: stenosis
hypertrophied frenula: syndrome
hyperventilation: syndrome; test; tetany
hyperviscosity: syndrome
hypnagogic: hallucination; image
hypnogenic: spot
hypnopompic: image
hypnotic: psychotherapy; relationship; sleep; state
hypobaric spinal: anesthesia
hypobranchial: eminence
hypocalcemic: cataract
hypochondriac: region
hypochondriacal: melancholia

immune complex: disease; disorder; nephritis
immune electron: microscopy
immune fetal: hydrops
immune response: gene
immune serum: globulin
immune thrombocytopenic: purpura
immunity: deficiency
immunoblastic: lymphadenopathy; lymphoma; sarcoma
immunochemical: assay
immunodeficiency: syndrome
immunofluorescence: method; microscopy
immunofluorescent: stain
immunologic, immunological: competence; deficiency; enhancement; mechanism; paralysis; surveillance; tolerance
immunologic pregnancy: test
immunological deficiency: syndrome
immunologically activated: cell
immunologically competent: cell
immunoperoxidase: technique
immunoproliferative: disorder
immunoproliferative small intestinal: disease
immunoradiometric: assay
immunoreactive: insulin
impact: resistance
impacted: fetus; fracture; tooth
impedance: angle; method; plethysmography
imperative: conception
imperfect: fungus; stage; state
imperforate: anus; hymen
impetiginous: cheilitis; syphilid
implant: denture
implantation: cone; cyst; dermoid; graft; theory
implant denture: substructure; superstructure
implanted: suture
implosive: therapy
impression: area; compound; material; tray
impressive: aphasia
impulse control: disorder
impulsive: obsession
impure: flutter
inactivated poliovirus: vaccine
inactive: mutant; repressor; tuberculosis
inadequate: personality; stimulus
inanition: fever
inappropriate: affect; hormone
inborn: error
incarcerated: hernia; placenta
incarceration: symptom
incarial: bone
incasement: theory
incest: barrier
incident: angle; point; ray
incidental: color; image; learning; parasite
incipient: abortion; caries
incisal: edge; embrasure; guidance; guide; margin; path; point; rest; surface
incisal guide: angle
incised: wound
incision: biopsy
incisional: hernia
incisive: bone; canal; duct; foramen; fossa; papilla; suture
incisor: canal; crest; foramen; tooth
inclusion: blenorrhea; body; cell; compound; conjunctivitis; cyst; dermoid
inclusion body: disease; encephalitis
inclusion cell: disease
inclusion conjunctivitis: virus
incomitant: strabismus
incompatible blood transfusion: reaction
incompetent cervical: os
incomplete: abortion; achromatopsia; alexia; antibody; antigen; ascertainment; cleavage; disinfectant; fistula; fracture; hemianopsia; metamorphosis; neurofibromatosis; tetanus
incomplete atrioventricular (A-V): dissociation
incomplete conjoined: twins
incomplete foot: presentation
incongruent: nystagmus
incongruous: hemianopsia
incremental: line
incubation: period
incubative: stage
incubatory: carrier
incudal: fold; fossa
incudiform: uterus
incudomalleolar: joint
incudostapedial: articulation; joint
indentation: hardness
independent: assortment; variable
indeterminate: cleavage; leprosy
index: amblyopia; ametropia; case; finger; hypermetropia; myopia
index extensor: muscle
indexical: sign
India ink capsule: stain
Indian: ginger; gum; method; operation; podophyllum; rhinoplasty; sickness
Indian podophyllum: resin
indicator: system; yellow
indicator-dilution: curve
indifference to pain: syndrome
indifferent: cell; electrode; gonad; oxide; tissue; water
indigo: calculus
indirect: agglutination; assay; calorimetry; diuretic; fracture; lead; method (for inlay); ophthalmoscope; ophthalmoscopy; oxidase; placentography; ray; retainer; retention; technique; test; transfusion; vision
indirect Coombs': test
indirect fluorescent antibody: test
indirect hemagglutination: test
indirect inguinal: hernia
indirect nuclear: division
indirect pulp: capping
indirect pupillary: reaction
indirect reacting: bilirubin
individual: difference; psychology; therapy; tolerance
individuation: field
indolent: bubo; ulcer
indophenol: method
induced: abortion; apnea; enzyme; hypotension; malaria; mutation; phagocytosis; radioactivity; sensitivity; symptom; trance
inducer: cell
inducible: enzyme
induction: chemotherapy; period
inductive: resistance
indurative: myocarditis
industrial: deafness; disease; psychology
industrial methylated: spirit
indwelling: catheter
inert: gas
inertia: time
inevitable: abortion
infant: death
infantile: acropustulosis; autism; cataract; convulsion; diplegia; dwarfism; fibrosarcoma; gastroenteritis; hemiplegia; hernia; hypothyroidism; leishmaniasis; myxedema; osteomalacia; pellagra; scurvy; sexuality; spasm; tetany
infantile cortical: hyperostosis
infantile digital: fibromatosis
infantile gastroenteritis: virus
infantile muscular: atrophy

infantile neuroaxonal: dystrophy
infantile neuronal: degeneration
infantile progressive spinal muscular: atrophy
infantile purulent: conjunctivitis
infantile spastic: paraplegia
infant mortality: rate
infection: immunity
infection-exhaustion: psychosis
infectious: anemia; disease; endocarditis; enterohepatitis; granuloma; hepatitis; icterus; jaundice; mononucleosis; myositis; nucleic acid; ophthalmoplegia; papilloma; plasmid; polyneuritis; sinusitis; wart
infectious arteritis: virus
infectious avian: bronchitis
infectious bovine: keratitis; rhinotracheitis
infectious bovine rhinotracheitis: virus
infectious bronchitis: virus
infectious bulbar: paralysis
infectious bursal: disease
infectious canine: hepatitis
infectious canine hepatitis: virus
infectious ectromelia: virus
infectious eczematoid: dermatitis
infectious hepatitis: virus
infectious necrotic: hepatitis
infectious papilloma: virus
infectious porcine: encephalomyelitis
infectious porcine encephalomyelitis: virus
infective: disease; embolism; endocarditis; thrombus
inferential: statistics
inferior: laryngotomy; polioencephalitis
inferior anatomical structures (specific inferior structures are listed under the following): angle; aperture; arch; area; arteriole; artery; bone; border; brachium; bursa; canal; colliculus; concha; convolution; extremity; fascia; fasciculus; fissure; flexure; fold; foramen; fossa; ganglion; groove; gyrus; horn; joint; ligament; limb; line; lobe; lobule; margin; muscle; nerve; node; notch; nucleus; olive; part; peduncle; pit; plexus; pole; recess; retinaculum; root; segment; sinus; sulcus; surface; triangle; trunk; tubercle; vein; velum; vena; venule; wall
inferiority: complex
inferior myocardial: infarction
inferolateral: margin; surface
inferolateral myocardial: infarction
inferomedial: margin
infested: abortion
infiltrating: lipoma
infiltration: anesthesia
infinite: distance
inflamed: ulcer
inflammatory: carcinoma; corpuscle; edema; lymph; polyp; pseudotumor; rheumatism
inflammatory fibrous: hyperplasia
inflammatory papillary: hyperplasia
inflatable: implant; splint
influenza: bacillus; virus
influenzal: pneumonia
influenza virus: vaccine
information: theory
informational: ribonucleic acid
infra-auricular subfascial parotid lymph: node
infrabony: pocket
infracardiac: bursa
infraclavicular: fossa; infiltrate; part; triangle
infraclinoid: aneurysm
infracostal: line
infraduodenal: fossa
infraglenoid: tubercle; tuberosity
infraglottic: space
infragranular: layer
infrahyoid: bursa; muscle
infralobar: part
inframammary: region
infranatant: fluid
infranodal: extrasystole
infraorbital: artery; canal; foramen; groove; margin; nerve; region; suture
infraorbitomeatal: plane
infrapatellar: fold
infrapatellar fat: body
infrared: cataract; light; microscope; ray; spectroscopy; spectrum; thermography
infrascapular: artery; region
infrasegmental: part; vein
infraspinatus: bursa; fascia; muscle
infraspinous: fossa
infrasternal: angle
infratemporal: crest; fossa; surface
infratrochlear: nerve
infundibular: part; recess; stalk; stem; stenosis
infundibuliform: fascia; hymen; sheath
infundibulo-ovarian: ligament
infundibulopelvic: ligament
infusion: graft
infusion-aspiration: drainage
ingravescent: apoplexy
ingrowing: toenail
ingrown: hair; nail
inguinal: canal; crest; fold; fossa; gland; hernia; ligament; plexus; region; triangle; trigone
inguinal aponeurotic: fold
inguinocrural: hernia
inguinofemoral: hernia
inguinolabial: hernia
inguinoscrotal: hernia
inguinosuperficial: hernia
inhalation: analgesia; anesthesia; anesthetic; therapy
inherent: immunity
inherited: character
inherited albumin: variant
inhibiting: antibody
inhibition: factor
inhibitory: fiber; nerve; obsession
inhibitory postsynaptic: potential
initial: contact; dose; heat; hematuria
initiating: agent; codon
initiation: factor
injection: flask; mass; molding
injury: potential
inlay: graft; wax
innate: heat; immunity; reflex
inner: malleolus; table
inner cell: mass
inner dental: epithelium
inner enamel: epithelium
innermost intercostal: muscle
innervation: apraxia
innocent: murmur; tumor
innominate: artery; bone; cartilage; fossa; substance; vein
innominate cardiac: vein
inorganic: acid; catalyst; chemistry; compound; murmur; orthophosphate; pyrophosphatase
inorganic dental: cement
inquiline: parasite
insect: virus
insensible: perspiration; thirst
insertion: sequence
insertional: mutagenesis
insoluble: soap
inspiratory: capacity; center; stridor
inspiratory reserve: volume
inspired: gas
inspissated: cerumen
instantaneous: vector
instantaneous electrical: axis

instrumental: conditioning
insufflation: anesthesia
insular: area; artery; cortex; hypothesis; part; sclerosis; scotoma; vein
insulin: antagonist; injection; lipoatrophy; lipodystrophy; resistance; shock; unit
insulin-antagonizing: factor
insulin coma: therapy; treatment
insulin-dependent: diabetes
insulin hypoglycemia: test
insulin-like: activity
insulin-like growth: factor
insulinopenic: diabetes
insulin zinc: suspension
integumentary: system
intellectual: aura
intelligence: quotient; test
intensification: chemotherapy
intensive: care; psychotherapy
intensive care: unit
intention: spasm; tremor
intentional: replantation
interaction process: analysis
interalveolar: pore; septum; space
interannular: segment
interarch: distance
interarticular: fibrocartilage; joint
interarytenoid: notch
interatrial: foramen; septum
intercalary: neuron; staphyloma
intercalated: disk; duct; nucleus
intercapillary: cell
intercapital: ligament
intercapitular: vein
intercarotid: body
intercarpal: joint; ligament
intercartilaginous: part
intercavernous: sinus
intercellular: bridge; canaliculus; cement; digestion; junction; lymph
interceptive occlusal: contact
interchondral: articulation; joint
interclavicular: ligament; notch
interclinoid: ligament
intercolumnar: fascia; fiber
intercondylar: eminence; fossa; line; tubercle
intercondylic: fossa
intercondyloid: fossa; notch
intercornual: ligament
intercostal: anesthesia; figament; membrane; nerve; neuralgia; space; vein
intercostal lymph: node
intercostobrachial: nerve
intercostohumeral: nerve
intercrural: fiber; ganglion
intercuneiform: joint; ligament
intercuspal: position
interdental: canal; caries; papilla; septum; splint
interectopic: interval
interfacial: canal
interfacial surface: space
interfascial: space
interfascicular: fasciculus
interference: beat; dissociation; microscope
interfoveolar: ligament
intergenic: complementation
interglobular: space
interiliac lymph: node
interilioabdominal: amputation
interim: denture
interjudge: reliability
interlaminar: jelly
interlobar: artery; duct; surface; vein
interlobular: artery; duct; ductule; emphysema; pleurisy; vein
interlocal: additivity
interlocking: gyrus
intermaxillary: anchorage; bone; elastic; fixation; relation; segment; suture; traction
intermediary: movement; nerve; system
intermediate: abutment; amputation; body; bronchus; carcinoma; disk; ganglion; heart; hemorrhage; host; junction; lamella; layer; line; mesoderm; nerve; part; ray; trait; vein
intermediate antebrachial: vein
intermediate basilic: vein
intermediate cephalic: vein
intermediate cubital: vein
intermediate cuneiform: bone
intermediate dorsal cutaneous: nerve
intermediate great: muscle
intermediate lacunar: node
intermediate lumbar lymph: node
intermediate sacral: crest
intermediate supraclavicular: nerve
intermediate temporal: artery
intermediate vastus: muscle
intermediolateral: nucleus
intermediolateral cell: column
intermediomedial: nucleus
intermembranous: part
intermenstrual: pain
intermesenteric: plexus
intermetacarpal: joint; ligament
intermetatarsal: articulation; joint; ligament
intermittent: albuminuria; arthralgia; claudication; cramp; hydrarthrosis; hydrosalpinx; malaria; pulse; sterilization; tetanus; torticollis
intermittent acute: porphyria
intermittent explosive: disorder
intermittent malarial: fever
intermittent mandatory: ventilation
intermittent positive pressure: breathing; ventilation
intermuscular: septum
intermuscular gluteal: bursa
internal: antigen; attachment; base; decompression; fistula; fixation; hemorrhage; hemorrhoids; hydrocephalus; medicine; meningitis; ophthalmopathy; phase; pyocephalus; resorption; respiration; squint; strabismus; traction; urethotomy; version
internal anatomical structures (specific internal anatomical and histological structures are listed under the following): artery; axis; canthus; capsule; cell; conjugate; crest; fascia; fiber; fibrocartilage; foramen; gland; ligament; line; lip; malleolus; meatus; muscle; nerve; node; nostril; opening; plexus; pore; protuberance; ring; sulcus; surface; vein
internal adhesive: pericarditis
internal capsule: syndrome
internal conversion: electron
internal lacrimal: fistula
internasal: suture
international: unit
interneuromeric: cleft
internodal: segment
internuncial: neuron
interocclusal: clearance; distance; gap; record
interocclusal rest: space
interofective: system
interosseous: bursa; cartilage; crest; fascia; groove; margin; membrane; nerve
interosseous cuneocuboid: ligament
interosseous cuneometatarsal: ligament
interosseous metacarpal: ligament
interosseous metatarsal: ligament
interosseous sacroiliac: ligament
interosseous talocalcanean: ligament
interpalpebral: zone
interpapillary: ridge
interparietal: bone; sulcus; suture
interpectoral lymph: node

inverted: image; papilloma; pelvis; reflex; testis
inverted cone: bur
inverted follicular: keratosis
inverted radial: reflex
investigatory: reflex
investing: cartilage; tissue
investment: cast
invisible: differentiation; spectrum
in vitro: fertilization
in vivo: fertilization
involuntary: muscle
involuntary nervous: system
involution: cyst; form
involutional: melancholia; psychosis
iodate: reaction
iodide: acne
iodide transport: defect
iodinated: albumin; casein; glycerol
iodine: cyst; eruption; number; reaction; stain; valve
iodine-induced: hyperthyroidism
iodized: collodion
iodophil: granule
iodotyrosine deiodinase: defect
ion: channel
ion-exchange: resin
ionic: medication; strength
ionization: chamber
ionized: atom
ion-selective: electrode
ionizing: radiation
ipomea: resin
ipsilateral: reflex
Ir: gene
iridial: part
iridocorneal: angle
iridocorneal endothelial: syndrome
iridocorneal mesodermal: dysgenesis
IRI/G: ratio
iris: dehiscence; freckle; pit
Irish: moss
Irish moss: gelatin
iris-nevus: syndrome
iron: alum; hematoxylin; index; lung
iron-binding: capacity
iron deficiency: anemia
iron-dextran: complex
iron storage: disease
irradiated vitamin D: milk
irreducible: hernia
irregular: astigmatism; bone; dentin; nystagmus
irresistible: impulse
irreversible: colloid; hydrocolloid; pulpitis; reaction; shock
irritable: breast; colon; heart; testis
irritation: cell; dentin; fibroma
irruption: canal
ischemic: contracture; hypoxia; lumbago; necrosis
ischemic muscular: atrophy
ischemic optic: neuropathy
ischiadic: spine
ischial: bone; bursa; tuberosity
ischiatic: hernia; notch
ischiocapsular: ligament
ischiocavernous: muscle
ischiofemoral: ligament
ischiopubic: ramus
ischiorectal: abscess; fossa
island: disease; fever; flap
islet: cell; tissue
islet cell: adenoma
isoallotypic: determinant
isobaric spinal: anesthesia
isochromic: anemia
isocyclic: compound
isodiphasic: complex
isodynamic: law
isoelectric: line; period; point; zone
isoenzyme: electrophoresis
isogeneic: graft
isogenic: strain
isogenous: chondrocyte
isoimmune: thrombocytopenia
isionic: point
isolated: abutment, dextrocardia; dyskeratosis; hypoaldosteronism; protèinuria
isolated explosive: disorder
isolated parietal: endocarditis
isolecithal: egg; ovum
isologous: graft
isomeric: function; transition
isometric: exercise; interval; period; relaxation; ruler; traction
isomorphic: response
isomorphous: gliosis
isoniazid: neuropathy
isoperistaltic: anastomosis
isoplastic: graft
isoprene: rule
isopropanol precipitation: test
isorhythmic: dissociation
isosbestic: point
isoserum: treatment
isotonic: coefficient; traction
isotope: clearance
isotropic: disk; lipid
isovolume pressure-flow: curve
isovolumetric: relaxation
isovolumic: relaxation
Itai-Itai: disease
Italian: method; operation; rhinoplasty
^{131}I uptake: test
I-V: see intraventricular
ivory: exostosis; membrane

J

J: chain; point
jacket: crown
jacksonian: epilepsy
jail: fever
jake: paralysis
jalap: resin
Jamaican vomiting: sickness
Jamestown Canyon: virus
Japan: wax
Japanese B: encephalitis
Japanese B encephalitis: virus
Japanese river: fever
jargon: aphasia
jaw: bone; jerk; joint; movement; reflex; repositioning; separation; skeleton
jaw-winking: phenomenon; syndrome
jaw-working: reflex
JC: virus
jejunal: artery
jejunal and ileal: vein
jejunogastric: intussusception
jejunoileal: bypass; shunt
Jembrana: disease
Jericho: boil
jerk: finger
jerky: nystagmus; respiration
Jesuit: tea
jet: injection; injector; nebulizer
jet ejector: pump
jeweller's: forceps
j-g: complex
JH: virus
Jk: antigen
Job: syndrome
Jobbins: antigen
Jocasta: complex
jock: itch
jogger's: amenorrhea
joint: capsule; evil; gamete; ill; oil; sense
Js: antigen
J-sella: deformity
jugal: bone; ligament; point
jugular: duct; embryocardia; foramen; fossa; ganglion; gland; nerve; notch; process; pulse; sinus; trunk; tubercle; vein; wall
jugular foramen: syndrome
jugular venous: arch
jugulodigastric: node

K

L

lepromatous: leprosy
lepromin: reaction; test
leprosy: bacillus
leprous: neuropathy
leptomeningeal: carcinoma; carcinomatosis; fibrosis
leptospiral: jaundice
lesser: circulation
lesser anatomical structures (specific lesser structures are listed under the following): artery; bone; cartilage; cavity; circle; cul-de-sac; curvature; foramen; fossa; gland; horn; muscle; nerve; notch; omentum; pancreas; sac; spine; trochanter; tubercle; tuberosity; wing
lethal: coefficient; dose; dwarfism; equivalent; factor; gene; mutation
lethality: rate
lethal midline: granuloma
lethargic: hypnosis
letter: blindness
letter-shaped: keratitis
leucine: hypoglycemia
leukemic: leukemia; myelosis; reticuloendotheliosis, reticulosis; retinitis; retinopathy
leukemic hyperplastic: gingivitis
leukemoid: reaction
leukocyte: cream; inclusion
leukocyte bactericidal assay: test
leukocytic: sarcoma
leukocytoclastic: angiitis; vasculitis
leukocytosis-promoting: factor
leukoerythroblastic: anemia
leukopenic: factor; index; leukemia; myelosis
leukoplakic: vulvitis
levator: cushion; hernia; swelling
Levay: antigen
levoatrio-cardinal: vein
Lf, L_f: dose
libido: theory
licensed practical: nurse
lichen: amyloidosis
lichenoid: dermatosis; eczema; keratosis
lid: reflex
lid closure: reaction
lienal: artery
lienophrenic: ligament
lienorenal: ligament
lienteric: diarrhea
life: cycle; instinct; stress; table
life-belt: cataract
life-span: development
ligature: wire
light: adaptation; bath; cell; chain; difference; metal; reflex; sense; sleep; treatment
light-adapted: eye
light-differential: threshold
light-liquid: petrolatum
lightning: strip
lightning eye: movement
light-touch: palpation
light wire: appliance
ligneous: conjunctivitis; struma; thyroiditis
lilliputian: hallucination
limb: bud; lead
limb-girdle muscular: dystrophy
limbic: lobe; system
limb-kinetic: apraxia
liminal: stimulus; trait
limit: dextrin; dextrinase
limited range: audiometer
limiting: angle; layer; membrane; sulcus
limulus lysate: test
line: angle; test
linear: acceleration; accelerator; amputation; atrophy; craniectomy; fracture; phonocardiograph
linear absorption: coefficient
linear IgA bullous: disease
linear skull: fracture
lined: flap
lingual: aponeurosis; arch; artery; bar; bone; crypt; embrasure; flange; flap; follicle; gingiva; goiter; gyrus; lobe; nerve; occlusion; papilla; plate; plexus; quinsy; rest; splint; surface; tonsil; trophoneurosis; vein
lingual salivary gland: depression
linguocervical: ridge
linguogingival: fissure; groove; ridge
linin: network
lining: cell
linkage: analysis; disequilibrium; group; marker
linnaean: system
lion-jaw bone-holding: forceps
lip: reflex; sulcus
lip and leg: ulceration
lipedematous: alopecia
lipemic: retinopathy
lipid: granulomatosis; hystiocytosis; keratopathy; pneumonia; proteinosis
lipid-mobilizing: hormone
lipoatrophic: diabetes
lipoblastic: lipoma
lipogenous: diabetes
lipoid: dermatoarthritis; granuloma; granulomatosis; nephrosis; pneumonia; theory
lipomatous: hypertrophy; infiltration; polyp
lipomelanic: reticulosis
lipophagic: granuloma
lipophagic intestinal: granulomatosis
lipoprotein: electrophoresis; polymorphism
lipotropic: factor; hormone
lipotropic pituitary: hormone
liquefaction: degeneration
liquefactive: necrosis
liquefied: phenol
liquid: air; extract; glucose; paraffin; petrolatum; pitch
liquid crystal: thermography
liquid human: serum
liquid-liquid: chromatography
Listeria: meningitis
literal: agraphia
lithiasis: conjunctivitis
lithotomy: position
litigious: paranoia
litmus: paper
little: ACTH; finger; fossa
Little Leaguer's: elbow
littoral: cell
live: vaccine
liveborn: infant
livedo: vasculitis
livedoid: dermatitis
live oral poliovirus: vaccine
liver: acinus; bud; flap; palm; spot; starch
liver cell: carcinoma
liver filtrate: factor
liver Lactobacillus casei: factor
liver of: sulfur
living: anatomy
L-L: factor
Lo, L_0: dose
loading: dose
lobar: bronchus; pneumonia; sclerosis
lobster-claw: deformity; hand
lobular: carcinoma; glomerulonephritis; pneumonia
local: anaphylaxis; anemia; anesthesia; anesthetic; asphyxia; bloodletting; death; epilepsy; flap; glomerulonephritis; im-

munity; reaction; sign; stimulant; symptom; syncope; tetanus; tic
local anesthetic: reaction
local excitatory: state
localization: agnosia
localized: osteitis; peritonitis
localized nodular: tenosynovitis
localizing: electrode; symptom
lock: finger; jaw
locked: bite; facet; knee
locked-in: syndrome
locomotor: ataxia
locoweed: disease
loculated: empyema
loculation: syndrome
locust: gum
lod: method
logarithmic: phase; phonocardiograph
logistic: curve
logit: transformation
long: axis; bone; chain; muscle; process; pulse; root; sight; vinculum
long abductor: muscle
long-acting thyroid: stimulator
long adductor: muscle
long buccal: nerve
long central: artery
long ciliary: nerve
long cone: technique
long extensor: muscle
long fibular: muscle
long flexor: muscle
long incubation: hepatitis
longissimus capitis: muscle
longitudinal: aberration; arch; arc; canal; dissociation; duct; fissure; fold; fracture; layer; lie; ligament; method; sinus; study; sulcus
longitudinal oval: pelvis
longitudinal pontine: bundle
long-leg: arthropathy
long plantar: ligament
long posterior ciliary: artery
long radial extensor: muscle
long saphenous: nerve; vein
long subscapular: nerve
long-term: memory
long thoracic: artery; nerve; vein
loop: stoma
loose: body; cartilage; skin
lop: ear
lordosis: reflex
lordotic: albuminuria; pelvis
louping: ill
louping-ill: virus
louse: fly
louse-borne: typhus
low: convex; delirium; fever; wine
low-calorie: diet
low cervical cesarean: section
low-compliance: bladder
low-egg-passage: vaccine
lower: airway; extremity; eyelid; jaw; lip; lobe
lower abdominal periosteal: reflex
lower alveolar: point
lower lateral cutaneous: nerve
lower motor: neuron
lower nephron: nephrosis
lower nodal: extrasystole
lower respiratory tract: smear
lower ridge: slope
lower uterine: segment
lowest lumbar: artery
lowest splanchnic: nerve
lowest thyroid: artery
low fat: diet
low flow: principle
low forceps: delivery
low frequency: transduction
low lip: line
low output: failure
low salt: syndrome
low spinal: anesthesia
low tension: glaucoma
low tone: deafness
L-phase: variant
Lr, L_r: dose
L/S: ratio
Lu: antigen
lubricating: cream
lucid: interal
luetic: mask
lumbar: appendicitis; artery; enlargement; flexure; ganglion; hernia; nephrectomy; nerve; part; plexus; puncture; region; rheumatism; rib; triangle; trunk; vein; vertebra
lumbar iliocostal: muscle
lumbar lymph: node
lumbar puncture: needle
lumbar rotator: muscle
lumbar splanchnic: nerve
lumberman's: itch
lumbocostal: ligament
lumbocostoabdominal: triangle
lumbodorsal: fascia
lumboinguinal: nerve
lumbosacral: angle; joint; plexus; trunk
lumbrical: muscle
luminous: flux; intensity; retinoscope
lumpy: jaw
lumpy skin: disease
lumpy skin disease: virus
lunar: periodicity
lunate: bone; fissure; sulcus; surface
lung: bud; unit
Lunyo: virus
lupoid: hepatitis; leishmaniasis; sycosis; ulcer
lupus: nephritis
lupus band: test
lupus erythematosus (see also L.E.): cell
lupus erythematosus cell: test
luteal: cell; phase
luteal phase: defect; deficiency
lutein: cell
luteinizing: hormone; principle
luteinizing hormone/follicle-stimulating hormone-releasing: factor
luteinizing hormone-releasing: factor; hormone
luteoplacental: shift
luteotropic: hormone
luting: agent
luxus: heart
Lyme: arthritis; disease
lymph: capillary; cell; circulation; corpuscle; embolism; follicle; gland; node; nodule; sac; scrotum; sinus; space; varix; vessel
lymphadenoid: goiter
lymphadenopathy-associated: virus
lymphatic: angina; corpuscle; duct; edema; fistula; follicle; leukemia; plexus; ring; sarcoma; sinus; stroma; system; tissue; valve; vessel
lymphatic dissemination: theory
lymphedematous: keratoderma
lymph node permeability: factor
lymphoblastic: leukemia; lymphoma
lymphocyte: transformation
lymphocyte leukocyte: interferon
lymphocyte-mediated: cytotoxicity
lymphocytic: adenohypophysitis; choriomeningitis; leukemia; leukemoid reaction; leukocytosis; leukopenia; series
lymphocytic choriomeningitis: virus
lymphocytotoxic: antibody
lymphogenous: embolism
lymphogranuloma venereum: antigen; virus
lymphoid: cell; corpuscle; granulomatosis; hemoblast; hypophysi-

M

marginal ring: ulcer
marian: lithotomy
marine: pharmacology; soap
marital: counseling
marker: trait
marker X: chromosome
marmoset: virus
marriage: therapy
marrow: canal; cell
marrow-lymph: gland
Marseilles: fever
marsh: fever; gas
marsupial: notch
masculine: pelvis; uterus
masculinity-femininity: scale
masked: epilepsy; gout; virus
masklike: face
masochistic: personality
mason's: lung
mass: hysteria; infection; movement; number; peristalsis; reflex; spectrograph
mass action: theory
masseter: reflex
masseteric: artery; fascia; nerve; tuberosity; vein
massive: collapse
massive bowel resection: syndrome
mast: cell; leukocyte
mast cell: leukemia
master: cast; eye; gland
master-dominant: eye
mastery: motive
masticating: cycle; surface
masticator: nerve
masticatory: apparatus; diplegia; force; nucleus; spasm; surface; system
masticatory silent: period
mastoid: abscess; angle; antrum; artery; bone; canaliculus; cell; empyema; fontanel; foramen; fossa; groove; margin; notch; part; process; sinus; wall
mastoid emissary: vein
mastoid lymph: node
mat: burn; gold
matched: group
maternal: cotyledon; death; dystocia; inheritance; placenta
maternal death: rate
maternity: hospital
mathematical: genetics
mating: isolate; season
matrix: band; calculus; retainer
mattress: suture
maturation: arrest; factor; index; value
mature: bacteriophage; cataract; neutrophil
mature cell: leukemia
mature ovarian: follicle
maturity-onset: diabetes
matutinal: epilepsy
maxillary: angle; antrum; artery; dentition; eminence; gland; hiatus; nerve; plexus; process; protraction; sinus; surface; tuberosity; vein
maxillary sinus: roentgenogram
maxillofacial: prosthetics
maxillomandibular: fixation; record; registration; relation; traction
maximal: dose; stimulus
maximal Histalog: test
maximal permissible: dose
maximum: temperature; velocity
maximum breathing: capacity
maximum occipital: point
maximum urea: clearance
maximum voluntary: ventilation
Mayaro: virus
M:E: ratio
meadow: dermatitis; saffron
meadow grass: dermatitis
meal: worm
mean: caloric; temperature; vector
mean cell: hemoglobin; volume
mean cell hemoglobin: concentration
mean electrical: axis
mean foundation: plane
measles: immunoglobulin; virus
measles convalescent: serum
measles immune: globulin
measles, mumps, and rubella: vaccine
measles virus: vaccine
measured: intelligence
meatal: cartilage; spine
Mecca: balsam
mechanical: abrasion; alternation; antidote; dysmenorrhea; ileus; intelligence; jaundice; strabismus; vector; ventilation; vertigo
mechanically balanced: occlusion
mechanistic: school
meconial: colic
meconium: aspiration; ileus; peritonitis
meconium blockage: syndrome
medi: virus
medial: arteriosclerosis
medial anatomical structures (specific medial structures are listed under the following): angle; arch; arteriole; artery; body; bone; bundle; bursa; canthus; commissure; condyle; cord; crest; elevation; eminence; epicondyle; fasciculus; fillet; fold; fossa; groove; gyrus; lamina; layer; lemniscus; ligament; limb; line; lip; margin; meniscus; muscle; nerve; network; node; nucleus; part; plate; pole; process; retinaculum; ridge; root; rotator; segment; stria; surface; tubercle; tuberosity; vein; venule; wall
median: bar; laryngotomy; lithotomy; relation; rhinoscopy; strumectomy
median anatomical structures (specific median structures are listed under the following): aperture; artery; bud; crest; eminence; groove; joint; ligament; line; nerve; plane; point; raphe; sulcus; suture; vein
median retruded: relation
median rhomboid: glossitis
mediastinal: emphysema; fibrosis; part; pleura; space; vein
mediate: auscultation; contagion; percussion; transfusion
medical: anatomy; care; chemistry; diathermy; ethics; examiner; genetics; jurisprudence; model; mycology; pathology; psychology; record; selection; treatment
medical record: linkage
medicinal: charcoal; chemistry; eruption; soap; zinc
mediocolic: sphincter
mediodorsal: nucleus
mediopubic: reflex
mediotarsal: amputation
Mediterranean: anemia; fever; lymphoma; theileriosis
Mediterranean exanthematous: fever
Mediterranean-hemoglobin E: disease
medium: artery; vein
medullary: artery; bone; callus; carcinoma; cavity; center; chemoreceptor; cone; cord; groove; layer; membrane; plate; pyramid; pyramidotomy; ray; sarcoma; sheath; space; stria; substance; tenia; tube
medullary sponge: kidney
medullated nerve: fiber
Medusa: head

megacystic: syndrome
megakaryocytic: leukemia
megaloblastic: anemia
megalocytic: anemia
meibomian: blepharitis; conjunctivitis; cyst; gland; sty
meiotic: division; drive; phase
melamine: resin
melanocyte-stimulating: hormone
melanoflocculation: test
melanophore-expanding: principle
melanotic: carcinoma; freckle; pigment; progonoma; whitlow
melanotic neuroectodermal: tumor
melon-seed: body
melting: point; temperature
membrane: bone; potential
membrane attack: complex
membrane-coating: granule
membrane expansion: theory
membranoproliferative: glomerulonephritis
membranous: ampulla; cataract; cochlea; conjunctivitis; dysmenorrhea; glomerulonephritis; labyrinth; laryngitis; layer; lipodystrophy; neurocranium; ossification; part; pharyngitis; rhinitis; septum; urethra; viscerocranium; wall
memory: loop; span; trace
mendelian: character; genetics; inheritance; ratio
Mengo: encephalitis; virus
meningeal: carcinoma; carcinomatosis; hernia; leukemia; plexus; vein
meningitic: streak
meningocerebral: cicatrix
meningococcal: meningitis
meningotyphoid: fever
meningovascular: syphilis
meniscofemoral: ligament
meniscus: lens
menopausal: syndrome
menstrual: colic; cycle; edema; leukorrhea; molimina; period; sclerosis
menstrual extraction: abortion
mental: aberration; age; agraphia; apparatus; artery; canal; chronometry; deficiency; disease; disorder; foramen; health; hospital; hygiene; illness; image; impairment; impression; nerve; point; process; protuberance; region; retardation; scotoma; spine; structure; symphysis; tubercle
mentoanterior: position
mentolabial: furrow
mentoposterior: position
mentotransverse: position
mephitic: gas
mercurial: line; manometer; stomatitis; tremor
mercury: arc; poisoning
meridional: aberration; cleavage; fiber
meristic: variation
mermaid: deformity
meroblastic: cleavage
merocrine: gland
mesangial: cell; nephritis
mesangial proliferative: glomerulonephritis
mesangiocapillary: glomerulonephritis
mesatipellic: pelvis
mesencephalic: flexure; nucleus; tegmentum; tract; vein
mesenchymal: cell; epithelium; hyloma; tissue
mesenteric: gland; hernia; vein
mesenteric artery: occlusion
mesenteric lymph: node
mesentericoparietal: fossa; recess
mesethmoid: bone
mesh: graft
mesial: angle; caries; displacement; occlusion; surface
meso: compound
mesoblastic: nephroma; segment; sensibility
mesocaval: shunt
mesocolic lymph: node
mesoglia: cell
mesomelic: dwarfism
mesometanephric: carcinoma
mesometric: pregnancy
mesonephric: adenocarcinoma; duct; fold; rest; ridge; tissue; tubule
mesonephroid: tumor
mesopic: perimetry
mesothelial: cell; hyloma
mesovarian: margin
messenger: ribonucleic acid
metabisulfite: test
metabolic: acidosis; alkalosis; coma; craniopathy; encepatholopathy; equivalent; indican; pool
metabolized vitamin D: milk
metacarpal: index; ligament; vein
metacarpohypothenar: reflex
metacarpophalangeal: articulation; joint
metacarpothenar: reflex
metacentric: chromosome
metachromatic: body; granule; leukodystrophy; stain
metafacial: angle
metaherpetic: keratitis
metahypophysial: diabetes
metal: base; interface
metal fume: fever
metal insert: tooth
metallic: rale; tremor
metameric nervous: system
metanephric: bud; cap; diverticulum; duct; tubule
metanephrogenic: tissue
metaphysial: dysostosis; dysplasia
metaphysical fibrous cortical: defect
metaplastic: anemia; carcinoma; ossification; polyp
metastatic: abscess; calcification; carcinoma; choroiditis; mumps; ophthalmia; pneumonia; retinitis
metastatic carcinoid: syndrome
metatarsal: artery; ligament; reflex
metatarsophalangeal: articulation; joint
metatropic: dwarfism
metatypical: carcinoma
meter: angle
meter-kilogram-second: system; unit
methacrylate: resin
methanol: fixative
methionine-activating: enzyme
methionyl: dipeptidase
methodical: chorea
methonium: compound
3-methoxy-4-hydroxymandelic acid: test
methylated: spirit
methyl green-pyronin: stain
metopic: point; suture
metrial: gland
metric: system
metroperitoneal: fistula
metrotropic: test
Mexican: tea
Mexican hat: cell; corpuscle
Mexican spotted: fever
MHA-TP: test
Mi^2: antigen
mianeh: disease; fever
microangiopathic hemolytic: anemia
micro-Astrup: method
microbial: genetics; persistence; ribonuclease; vitamin
micrococcal: endonuclease; nuclease
microcrystalline: cellulose
microcystic: disease
microcystic epithelial: dystrophy

molluscum: body; conjunctivitis; corpuscle
molluscum contagiosum: virus
Monday morning: sickness
mongolian: fold; macula; spot
moniliasis: pneumonia
moniliform: hair
monkey: malaria
monkey B: virus
monkeypox: virus
monoamine oxidase: inhibitor
monoamniotic: twins
monobasic: acid; ammonium; potassium
monobromated: camphor
monochorial: twins
monochorionic diamniotic: placenta
monochorionic monoamniotic: placenta
monochromatic: aberration; ray
monoclonal: antibody; gammopathy; immunoglobulin; protein
monocrotic: pulse
monocular: diplopia; heterochromia; strabismus
monocytic: angina; leukemia; leukemoid reaction; leukocytosis; leukopenia
monocytoid: cell
monohydric: alcohol
monoleptic: fever
monomolecular: reaction
monomorphic: adenoma
mononuclear phagocytic: system
monophasic: complex
monophyletic: theory
monopolar: cautery
monorecidive: chancre
monostotic fibrous: dysplasia
monovalent: antiserum
monovular: twins
monozygotic: twins
moon: blindness; face
moral: ataxia; treatment
morbid: impulse; obesity; thirst
morbidity: rate
morgagnian: cyst
morning: diarrhea; sickness; vomiting
morning glory: anomaly; syndrome
morphogenetic: movement
morphologic: element
mortality: rate
mortar: kidney
mortise: joint
mosaic: fungus; inheritance; wart
mosquito: clamp; forceps
moss: starch
mossy: cell; fiber; foot
moth: patch
moth-eaten: alopecia
mother: cell; colony; cyst; liquor; star; surrogate; yaw
mother superior: complex
motile: leukocyte
motility test: medium
motion: sickness
motor: abreaction; agraphia; aphasia; apraxia; area; cell; cortex; decussation; endplate; fiber; image; impersistence; nerve; neuron; nucleus; paralysis; plate; point; root; unit; zone
motor dapsone: neuropathy
motor neuron: disease
motor speech: center
mottled: enamel; tooth
mountain: balm; sickness
mounting: medium
mouse: cancer; encephalomyelitis; hepatitis; leprosy; poliomyelitis; pox; unit
mouse antialopecia: factor
mouse encephalomyelitis: virus
mouse hepatitis: virus
mouse leukemia: virus
mouse mammary tumor: virus
mouse parotid tumor: virus
mouse poliomyelitis: virus
mousepox: virus
mousetail: pulse
mouse thymic: virus
mouse-tooth: forceps
mouth: breathing; mirror; rehabilitation
mouth-to-mouth: respiration; resuscitation
movable: heart; joint; kidney; pulse; spleen
moyamoya: disease
Mozart: ear
MP: joint
MSB trichrome: stain
MS-1: agent
MS-2: agent
Mu: antigen
mucilaginous: gland
mucin clot: test
mucinogen: granule
mucinoid: degeneration
mucinous: carcinoma; plaque
muciparous: gland
mucoalbuminous: cell
mucobuccal: fold
mucocutaneous: junction; leishmaniasis; muscle
mucocutaneous lymph node: syndrome
mucoepidermoid: carcinoma; tumor
mucoepithelial: dysplasia
mucoid: adenocarcinoma; colony; degeneration
mucoid medial: degeneration
mucomembranous: enteritis
mucoperichondrial: flap
mucoperiosteal: flap
mucopurulent: conjunctivitis
mucosal: disease; fold; graft; tunic
mucosal disease: virus
mucosal relief: roentgenography
mucoserous: cell
mucous: cast; cell; colic; cyst; diarrhea; gland; membrane; ophthalmia; patch; plaque; plug; polyp; rale; sheath
mucous connective: tissue
mucous neck: cell
mucus: impaction
mud: bed; fever
muffle: furnace
mu (μ)-heavy-chain: disease
mulberry: calculus; molar; ovary; spot
mule-spinner's: cancer
müllerian: adenosarcoma; duct
müllerian duct inhibitory: factor
müllerian regression: factor
multangular: bone
multiaxial: classification; joint
multicentric: reticulohistiocytosis
multicore: disease
multicuspid: tooth
multifactorial: inheritance
multifocal: choroiditis; lens; osteitis
multiform: layer
multi-infarct: dementia
multilamellar: body
multilocular: cyst; fat
multilocular adipose: tissue
multilocular hydatid: cyst
multimammate: mouse
multinodular: goiter
multinuclear: leukocyte
multipennate: muscle
multiphasic: screening
multiple: amputation; anchorage; embolism; endocrinoma; endocrinopathy; exostosis; fission; fracture; myeloma; myelomatosis; myositis; neuritis; parasitism; personality; pregnancy; sclerosis; serositis; stain; vision
multiple ego: state
multiple endocrine: neoplasia
multiple epiphysial: dysplasia
multiple hamartoma: syndrome
multiple idiopathic hemorrhagic: sarcoma

multiple intestinal: polyposis
multiple lentigines: syndrome
multiple mucosal neuroma: syndrome
multiple puncture tuberculin: test
multiple self-healing squamous: epithelioma
multiple symmetric: lipomatosis
multiplicative: division; growth
multipolar: cell; mitosis; neuron
multivalent: vaccine
multivariate: study
multivesicular: body
mummification: necrosis
mummified: pulp
mumps: meningoencephalitis; virus
mumps sensitivity: test
mumps skin test: antigen
mumps virus: vaccine
mumu: fever
mung bean: nuclease
municipal: hospital
mural: aneurysm; cell; endocarditis; pregnancy; thrombosis; thrombus
murine: hepatitis; leprosy; typhus
murine sarcoma: virus
Murray Valley: encephalitis; rash
Murray Valley encephalitis: virus
Murutucu: virus
muscle: bundle; curve; epithelium; fascicle; hemoglobin; plasma; plate; repositioning; resection; serum; sound; spasm; spindle
muscle-tendon: attachment; junction
muscular: anesthesia; artery; asthenopia; atrophy; dystrophy; fascia; fibril; hyperesthesia; incompetence; insufficiency; lacuna; layer; movement; murmur; process; pulley; reflex; relaxant; rheumatism; sense; substance; system; tissue; triangle; trophoneurosis; tunic
muscular subaortic: stenosis
musculocutaneous: amputation; flap; nerve
musculophrenic: artery; vein
musculospiral: groove; nerve; paralysis
musculotendinous: cuff
musculotubal: canal
mushroom: poisoning
mushroom-worker's: lung
music: blindness
musical: agraphia; alexia; murmur
musician's: cramp
muskeag: moss
mustard: gas
mutant: gene
mutation: rate
mutilating: keratoderma; leprosy
muttering: delirium
mutton-fat keratic: precipitate
mutual: resistance
MVE: virus
myasthenic: facies; reaction
mycoplasma, mycoplasmal: pneumonia
mycotic: abscess; aneurysm; keratitis
mydriatic: rigidity
myelin: body; figure; sheath
myelineated nerve: fiber
myelinic: degeneration
myeloblastic: leukemia; protein
myelocytic: crisis, leukemia; leukemoid reaction
myelogenic, myelogenous: leukemia; sarcoma
myeloid: cell; metaplasia; reticulosis; sarcoma; series; tissue
myelomonocytic: leukemia
myelopathic: anemia
myelophthisic: anemia
myeloproliferative: syndrome
myenteric: plexus; reflex
mylohyoid: fossa; groove; line; muscle; nerve; ridge
mylopharyngeal: part
myocardial: bridge; infarction; insufficiency; ischemia; rigor
myocardial depressant: factor
myoclonic: absence
myoclonic astatic: epilepsy
myoclonus: epilepsy
myocutaneous: flap
myodermal: flap
myoelastic: theory
myoepicardial: mantle
myoepithelial: cell
myofacial pain-dysfunction: syndrome
myofascial: syndrome
myofunctional: therapy
myogenic: paralysis; potential; theory
myoid: cell
myomatous: polyp
myometrial arcuate: artery
myometrial radial: artery
myoneural: blockade; junction
myopathic: atrophy; facies; scoliosis
myophosphorylase deficiency: glycogenosis
myopic: astigmatism; choroidopathy; conus; crescent; degeneration
myosin: filament
myotatic: contraction; irritability; reflex
myotonic: cataract; dystrophy
myotubular: myopathy
myovascular: sphincter
myovenous: sphincter
myxedema: heart; voice
myxedematous: infantilism
myxoid: cyst; degeneration
myxomatosis: virus
myxomatous: degeneration
myxomembranous: colitis
myxopapillary: ependymoma

N

nabothian: cyst; follicle
nacreous: ichthyosis
nail: bed; extension; fold; horn; matrix; pit; plate; pulse; skin
nail-patella: syndrome
Nairobi: disease
Nairobi sheep disease: virus
naked: virus
NAME: syndrome
NANB: hepatitis
nanoid: enamel
nanukayami: fever
nape: nevus
napkin: rash
narcoleptic: tetrad
narcotic: blockade; hunger; reversal
narrow angle: glaucoma
nasal: bone; calculus; capsule; catarrh; cavity; concha; crest; duct; feeding; foramen; ganglion; gland; glioma; height; hemorrhage; hydrorrhea; index; margin; muscle; myiasis; nerve; notch; part; pharynx; pit; placode; point; polyp; process; reflex; region; ridge; sac; septum; spine; surface; valve; venule
nasal venous: arch
Nasik: vibrio
nasion-pogonion: measurement
nasion-postcondylar: plane
nasion soft: tissue
nasobasilar: line
nasobregmatic: arc
nasociliary: nerve; root
nasofrontal: vein
nasogastric: tube
nasojugal: fold
nasolabial: groove; node

nasolacrimal: canal; duct
nasomandibular: fixation
nasomaxillary: suture
nasomental: reflex
naso-occipital: arc
nasopalatine: groove; nerve
nasopharyngeal: groove; leishmaniasis; passage
nasotracheal: intubation; tube
natal: cleft; tooth
native: albumin; protein
natural: antibody; dentition; dye; focus; hemolysin; immunity; mutation; selection
natural killer: cell
nature-nurture: issue
Nauheim: bath; treatment
navel: ill
navicular: abdomen; bone; disease; fossa
navicular articular: surface
NBT: test
ND: virus
near: point; reaction; reflex; sight
near point of: convergence
Nebraska calf diarrhea: virus
nebulous: urine
neck: reflex; sign
necrobiotic: xanthogranuloma
necrogenic: wart
necrogranulomatous: keratitis
necrolytic migratory: erythema
necrosis: bacillus
necrotic: angina; cirrhosis; cyst; inflammation; pulp; rhinitis
necrotic infectious: conjunctivitis
necrotizing: angiitis; arteriolitis; encephalitis; enterocolitis; encephalomyelopathy; fasciitis; papillitis; scleritis; sialometaplasia
necrotizing ulcerative: gingivitis
needle: bath; biopsy; culture; forceps
needle point: tracing
Neethling: virus
negative: accommodation; afterimage; anergy; catalyst; chronotropism; convergence; electrode; electrotaxis; feedback; meniscus; phase; politzerization; pressure; scotoma; stain; taxis; thermotaxis; transference; valence
negative base: excess
negative end-expiratory: pressure
negatively: bathmotropic; dromotropic; inotropic
negative strand: virus
Negishi: virus
negligible: glycosuria
nemaline: myopathy
neonatal: anemia; apoplexy; arthritis; diagnosis; hepatitis; herpes; hypoglycemia; isoerythrolysis; line; medicine; rate; ring; screening; tetany; tooth
neonatal calf diarrhea: virus
neoplastic: arachnoiditis; meningitis
neotype: culture; strain
neovascular: glaucoma
nephric: blastema; duct
nephritic: calculus; factor; syndrome
nephrogenic: adenoma; cord; diabetes; tissue
nephronic: loop
nephrotic: syndrome
nephrotomic: cavity
Neptune's: girdle
nerve: block; cell; conduction; deafness; decompression; ending; fascicle; fiber; field; force; ganglion; graft; implantation; pain; papilla; plexus; root; suture; tract; trunk
nerve block: anesthesia
nerve cell: body
nerve conduction: velocity
nerve growth: factor
nerve growth factor: antiserum
nerve-point: massage
nervous: asthenopia; asthma; bladder; dyspepsia; dysphagia; indigestion; lobe; system; tissue; tunic
net: flex; knot
nettle: rash
nettling: hair
neural: arch; axis; canal; crest; cyst; deafness; fold; ganglion; groove; layer; plate; segment; spine; tube
neural crest: syndrome
neuralgic: amyotrophy
neurasthenic: asthenopia
neurenteric: canal
neurilemma: cell
neuritic: atrophy; plaque
neurobiotactic: movement
neurocentral: joint; suture; synchondrosis
neurochronaxic: theory
neurocirculatory: asthenia
neurocutaneous: melanosis; syndrome
neuroectodermal: junction
neuroendocrine: cell
neuroendocrine transducer: cell
neuroepithelial: body; cell; layer
neurofibrillary: degeneration
neurogenic: atrophy; bladder; fracture; theory
neuroglia: cell
neurohumoral: secretion; transmission
neurolemma: cell
neuroleptic: agent
neuroleptic malignant: syndrome
neuromast: organ
neuromuscular: cell; junction; relaxant; spindle; system
neuromuscular blocking: agent
neuroparalytic: keratitis; ophthalmia
neuropathic: albuminuria; arthritis; arthropathy; joint
neuropsychologic: disorder
neurosecretory: cell; substance
neurosomatic: junction
neurotendinous: organ; spindle
neurotic: excoriation; manifestation
neurotonic: pupil; reaction
neurotrophic: atrophy
neurotropic: attraction; virus
neurovasclar: flap
neutral: axis; element; fat; mutation; occlusion; oxide; point; reaction; stain; zone
neutral buffered formalin: fixative
neutral lipid storage: disease
neutralization: plate; test
neutralizing: antibody
neutropenic: angina
neutrophil: granule
neutrophilic: leukemia; leukocyte; leukocytosis; leukopenia
nevoid: amentia; elephantiasis; hypertrichosis
nevus: cell
new: combination; growth; mutation
Newcastle: disease
Newcastle disease: virus
New Hampshire: rule
newtonian: aberration; constant; flow; fluid; viscosity
New World: leishmaniasis
new yellow: enzyme
New Zealand: mouse
niacin: test
nickel: dermatitis
nicotinic acid: maculopathy
nictitating: membrane; spasm
night: blindness; hospital; myopia; pain; palsy; sight; sweat; vision
nihilistic: delusion
nil: disease
ninhydrin: reaction
ninhydrin-Schiff: stain
ninth cranial: nerve
ninth-day: erythema

nipple: line; shield
nirvana: principle
nitrate: respiration
nitritoid: reaction
nitro: dye
nitro blue: tetrazolium
nitroblue tetrazolium: test
nitrogen: cycle; equivalent; mustard; narcosis
nitrogenous: equilibrium
nitroid: shock
nitroprusside: test
NK: cell
noble: cell; element; gas; metal
nociceptive: reflex
nocifensor: reflex
nocturnal: amblyopia; diarrhea; enuresis; epilepsy; myclonus; periodicity; vertigo
nodal: bigeminy; bradycardia; escape; extrasystole; fever; point; plane; rhythm; tachycardia; tissue
nodding: spasm
nodose: ganglion; rheumatism
nodular: amyloidosis; arteriosclerosis; body; disease; episcleritis; fasciitis; headache; hidradenoma; hyperplasia; iritis; leprosy; lymphoma; melanoma; mesoneuritis; panencephalitis; scleritis; sclerosis; syphilid; transformation; tuberculid; vasculitis
nodular histiocytic: lymphoma
nodular nonsuppurative: panniculitis
nodular non-X: histiocytosis
nodular regenerative: hyperplasia
nodular subepidermal: fibrosis
noetic: anxiety
noise: pollution
nomenclatural: type
nominal: aphasia
nomothetic: approach
non-A: hepatitis
nonabsorbable: ligature
nonabsorbable surgical: suture
nonaccommodative: esotropia
nonan: malaria
nonanatomic: tooth
non-arcon: articulator
non-B: hepatitis
nonbacterial thrombotic: endocarditis
nonbacterial verrucous: endocarditis
nonchromaffin: paraganglioma
nonclonogenic: cell
noncohesive: gold
noncommunicating: hydrocephalus
noncompetitive: inhibition
noncomplementary: role
nonconjugative: plasmid
nondeciduous: placenta
nondepolarizing: block; relaxant
nondepolarizing neuromuscular blocking: agent
nondirective: psychotherapy
nonessential: amino acid
nonfenestrated: forceps
nonfilament polymorphonuclear: leukocyte
nongonococcal: urethritis
nongranular: leukocyte
non-Hodgkin's: lymphoma
nonhomologous: chromosome
nonimmune: agglutination; serum
nonimmune fetal: hydrops
noninfiltrating lobular: carcinoma
noninflammatory: edema
non-insulin-dependent: diabetes
nonisolated: proteinuria
nonketotic: hyperglycemia
nonlamellar: bone
nonlipid: histiocytosis
nonmedullated: fiber
nonmotile: leukocyte
non-newtonian: fluid
nonobstructive: jaundice
nonoccluded: virus
nonossifying: fibroma
nonosteogenic: fibroma
nonovulational: menstruation
nonparticipant: observer
nonpedunculated: hydatid
nonpenetrant: trait
nonpenetrating: keratoplasty; wound
nonphasic sinus: arrhythmia
nonpolar: compound; solvent
nonprecipitating: antibody
nonprotein: nitrogen
non-rapid eye: movement
nonrebreathing: anesthesia; mask; valve
nonrefractive accommodative: esotropia
nonrenal: azotemia
nonsecretory: myeloma
nonsense: mutation; syndrome; triplet
nonseptate: mycelium
nonsexual: generation
nonspecific: anergy; cholinesterase; encephalomyeloneuropathy; immunity; protein; system; therapy; urethritis
nonthrombocytopenic: purpura
nontoxid: goiter
nontransmural myocardial: infarction
nontropical: sprue
nonvital: pulp; tooth
noogenic: neurosis
NOR: banding
Nordhausen: sulfuric acid
no reflow: phenomenon
normal: animal; antibody; antithrombin; antitoxin; axis; bite; concentration; distribution; dwarfism; hearing; occlusion; opsonin; ovariotomy; phosphate; serum; solution; tartrate; toxin; valve
normal cholesteremic: xanthomatosis
normal horse: serum
normal human: plasma; serum
normal human serum: albumin
normally posed: tooth
normal pressure: hydrocephalus
normochromic: anemia
normocytic: anemia
normoglycemic: glycosuria
normokalemic periodic: paralysis
normolipemic: xanthoma
normospermatogenic: sterility
North American: blastomycosis
Northern blot: analysis; technique
North Queensland tick: fever; typhus
Norwalk: agent
Norway: itch
Norwegian: scabies
nose-bridge-lid: reflex
nose-eye: reflex
nosocomial: gangrene
notched: tooth
note: blindness
notifiable: disease
notochordal: canal; plate; process; sheath; vertebrate
notoedric: mange
NPH: insulin
nuchal: fascia; ligament; plane; tubercle
nuclear: atom; bag; cataract; chemistry; energy; envelope; family; fusion; hyaloplasm; jaundice; layer; magneton; medicine; membrane; ophthalmoplegia; pacemaker; pore; reaction; ribonucleic acid; sap; sclerosis; spindle; stain
nuclear bag: fiber
nuclear chain: fiber
nuclear-cytoplasmic: ratio
nuclear inclusion: body

nuclear magnetic: resonance
nuclear magnetic resonance: imaging
nucleate: endonuclease
nucleic acid: base; probe
nucleinic: base
nucleolar: chromosome; organizer; satellite; zone
nucleoplasmic: index
nucleoside: pair; phosphorylases
nucleotide: deletion; pair
nude: mouse
null: cell; hypothesis
null-cell: adenoma
numerical: aperture; hypertrophy; taxonomy
nummular: sputum; syphilid
nun's: murmur
nurse: cell
nursemaid's: elbow
nutmeg: liver
nutrient: agar; artery; canal; enema; foramen; vessel
nutritional: amblyopia; anemia; cirrhosis; edema; encephalomalacia; energy; hemosiderosis; polyneuropathy
nutritional type cerebellar: atrophy
nutritive: equilibrium; ratio
nymphocaruncular: sulcus
nymphohymeneal: sulcus
nystagmus: test
nystagmus blockage: syndrome

O

O: agglutinin; antigen; colony
oasthouse urine: disease
oat: cell
oat cell: carcinoma
oatmeal-tomato paste: agar
OAV: syndrome
obeliar: area
obesity: index
object: blindness; constancy; glass; libido; relationship
objective: optometer; perimetry; psychology; sensation; sign; symptom; synonym
obligate: aerobe; anaerobe; parasite
oblique: amputation; bandage; bundle; cord; diameter; fiber; fissure; fracture; head; illumination; lie; ligament; line; muscle; part; ridge; sinus; vein
oblique arytenoid: muscle
oblique facial: cleft
oblique lateral jaw: roentgenogram
oblique popliteal: ligament
obliterating: endarteritis
obliterative: arachnoiditis; bronchitis
oblong: pit
obsessive: behavior
obsessive-compulsive: neurosis
obstacle: sense
obstetric, obstetrical: binder; conjugate; forceps; hand; paralysis; position
obstructed: testis
obstructive: apnea; appendicitis; dysmenorrhea; hydrocephalus; jaundice; murmur; thrombus
obturating: embolism
obturator: appliance; artery; canal; crest; fascia; foramen; groove; hernia; membrane; nerve; tubercle; vein
obturator lymph: node
occipital: anchorage; angle; artery; belly; bone; condyle; fontanel; groove; gyrus; horn; lobe; margin; neuralgia; neuritis; operculum; plane; plexus; point; pole; region; sinus; somite; triangle; vein
occipital emissary: vein
occipital lymph: node
occipitoanterior: position
occipitoaxial: ligament
occipitocollicular: tract
occipitofrontal: diameter; fasciculus; muscle
occipitomastoid: suture
occipitomental: diameter
occipitopontine: tract
occipitoposterior: position
occipitotectal: tract
occipitotemporal: sulcus
occipitothalamic: radiation
occipitotransverse: position
occluded: virus
occluding: frame; ligature; paper; relation
occluding centric relation: record
occlusal: adjustment; analysis; balance; caries; clearance; correction; curvature; disharmony; embrasure; force; form; harmony; imbalance; path; pattern; pivot; plane; position; pressure; radiograph; rest; rim; scheme; surface; system; table; trauma; wear
occlusal rest: bar
occlusal vertical: dimension
occlusion: rim
occlusive: dressing; ileus; meningitis
occult: bleeding; blood; border; carcinoma; fracture; hydrocephalus
occupation: neurosis; spasm
occupational: deafness; disease; therapy
occupational professional: spasm
ochre: mutation
ochronotic: arthritis
ocular: albinism; ataxia; bobbing; cone; crisis; cup; dysmetria; flutter; humor; hypertelorism; larva migrans; lens; lymphomatosis; micrometer; muscle; myiasis; myoclonus; myopathy; nystagmus; onchocerciasis; paralysis; pemphigoid; prosthesis; rigidity; sparganosis; scoliosis; tension; torticollis; vertigo; vesicle
ocular motor: apraxia
ocular-mucous membrane: syndrome
oculoauriculovertebral: dysplasia
oculobuccogenital: syndrome
oculocardiac: reflex
oculocephalic: reflex
oculocephalogyric: reflex
oculocerebrorenal: syndrome
oculocutaneous: albinism; syndrome
oculodentodigital: dysplasia; syndrome
oculodermal: melanosis
oculoencephalic: angiomatosis
oculogravic: illusion
oculogyral: illusion
oculogyric: crisis
oculomotor: nerve; response; system
oculopharyngeal: syndrome
oculovertebral: dysplasia; syndrome
oculovestibulo-auditory: syndrome
ODD: syndrome
odd: chromosome
odontoblastic: layer; process
odontogenic: cyst; dysplasia; myxoma
odontoid: ligament; process; vertebra
odoriferous: gland
oedipal: neurosis; period; phase
Oedipus: complex
OFD: syndrome
official: formula
17-OH-corticoids: test
oil: bath; cyst; embolism; gland; immersion; pneumonia; sugar; tumor; vaccine
oil red O: stain

oil retention: enema
oily: granuloma
OKT: cell
Old World: leishmaniasis
old yellow: enzyme
olecranon: bursitis; fossa; process; reflex
olefiant: gas
olfactory: anesthesia; angle; area; bulb; bundle; cortex; epithelium; foramen; gland; glomerulus; groove; hyperesthesia; hypesthesia; membrane; mucosa; nerve; neuroblastoma; organ; peduncle; pit; placode; pyramid; region; root; stria; sulcus; tract; trigone; tubercle
olfactory receptor: cell
oligemic: shock
oligodendroglia: cell
olivary: body; eminence
olive-tipped: catheter
olivocerebellar: tract
olivocochlear: bundle
olivopontocerebellar: atrophy; degeneration
olivospinal: tract
olympian: forehead
omega: oxidation
omega-oxidation: theory
omental: bursa; enterocleisis; graft; sac; tuber
OMM: syndrome
omnifocal: lens
omoclavicular: triangle
omohyoid: muscle
omotracheal: triangle
omphaloangiopagous: twins
omphalomesenteric: artery; duct
Omsk hemorrhagic: fever
Omsk hemorrhagic fever: virus
oncocytic hepatocellular: tumor
oncofetal: antigen; marker
oncogenic: virus
oncoplastic: carcinoma
oncosphere: embryo
oncotic: pressure
one-child: sterility
one-horned: uterus
onion: body
onion bulb: neuropathy
onlay: graft
on-off: phenomenon
ontogenic: homeostasis
O'nyong-nyong: fever; virus
oophoritic: cyst
opacifying: gallstone
opaline: patch
opaque: microscope
open: biopsy; bite; comedo; cordotomy; dislocation; drainage; flap; fracture; hospital; pneumothorax; reduction; tuberculosis; wound
open-angle: glaucoma
open chain: compound
open chest: massage
open circuit: method
open drop: anesthesia
open head: injury
open heart: surgery
opening: axis; contraction; movement; snap
open skull: fracture
opera-glass: hand
operant: behavior; conditioning
operating: microscope; table
operative: dentistry; myxedema
operator: gene
opercular: fold
ophryospinal: angle
ophthalmic: artery; hyperthyroidism; migraine; nerve; ointment; plexus; solution; vein; vertigo
ophthalmomandibulomelic: dysplasia
ophthalmoplegic: migraine
opiate: receptor
opossum: encephalitis
opponent: color
opportunistic: pathogen
opposer: muscle
oppositional: disorder
opsonic: index
optic: agnosia; axis; canal; capsule; chiasm; cup; decussation; disk; fissure; foramen; groove; keratoplasty; layer; nerve; neuritis; papilla; part; placode; radiation; recess; stalk; tract; vesicle
optical: aberration; activity; allachesthesia; antipode; density; illusion; image; iridectomy; maser; pachymeter; rotation
optical righting: reflex
optical rotatory: dispersion
optic nerve: drusen; hypoplasia
opticofacial: reflex
opticokinetic: nystagmus
optimum: dose; pH; temperature
optokinetic: nystagmus
O-R: system
oral: biology; cavity; contraceptive; fissure; hygiene; lichen; membrane; part; pathology; pharynx; phase; physiotherapy; plate; primacy; region; shield; smear; stereotypy; surgeon; surgery; tooth
oral epithelial: nevus
oral lactose tolerance: test
oral poliovirus: vaccine
orbicular: bone; ligament; muscle; process; zone
orbicularis: phenomenon
orbicularis oculi: reflex
orbicularis pupillary: reflex
orbital: abscess; apex; artery; axis; cavity; decompression; eminence; exenteration; fascia; gyrus; height; hernia; implant; index; lamina; layer; muscle; nerve; ophthalmoplegia; part; periostitis; plane; plate; process; region; sulcus; surface; syndrome; tubercle; width
orbitofrontal: artery; cortex
orbitonasal: index
orbitosphenoid: cartilage
orcein: stain
orcein elastic tissue: stain
orcinol: test
orf: virus
organ: culture
organic: acid; catalyst; chemistry; compound; contracture; deafness; disease; evolution; headache; murmur; pain; phosphate; principle; stricture; vertigo
organic brain: syndrome
organic dental: cement
organic mental: disorder; syndrome
organification: defect
organized: pneumonia
organoid: nevus; tumor
organ-specific: antigen
Oriboca: virus
Oriental: boil; button; ringworm; schistosomiasis; sore; ulcer
orienting: reflex; response
ornithine: cycle
ornithosis: virus
oroantral: fistula
orodigitofacial: dysostosis
orofacial: fistula
orofaciodigital: syndrome
oronasal: fistula; membrane
oropharyngeal: membrane
orotracheal: intubation; tube
Oroya: fever
orphan: drug; product; virus

orthodontic: appliance; band; therapy
orthogenic: evolution
orthognathic: surgery
orthograde: degeneration
orthomolecular: therapy
orthopaedic: surgery
orthopedic: surgery
orthoscopic: lens; spectacles
orthostatic: albuminuria; hypopiesis; hypotension; proteinuria
orthotopic: graft
oscillating: vision
oscillatory: potential
osmic acid: fixative
osmium tetroxide: stain
osmolal: clearance
osmotic: diuresis; nephrosis; pressure; shock
osseous: ampulla; cell; labyrinth; lacuna; part; polyp; tissue
osseous hydatid: cyst
osseous spiral: lamina
ossicular: chain
ossific: center
ossification: center
osteochondrogenic: cell
osteoclast activating: factor
osteocollagenous: fiber
osteogenetic: fiber; layer
osteogenic: cell; sarcoma; tissue
osteoid: osteoma; tissue
osteomalacic: pelvis
osteomyelofibrotic: syndrome
osteopathic: medicine; physician; scoliosis
osteoperiosteal: graft
osteoplastic: amputation; craniotomy; necrotomy
osteosclerotic: anemia
ostial: sphincter
Ot: antigen
Othello: syndrome
otic: abscess; barotrauma; capsule; ganglion; placode; vesicle
otitic: hydrocephalus; meningitis
otodectic: mange
otolithic: membrane
otomandibular: dysostosis; syndrome
otopalatodigital: syndrome
otopharyngeal: tube
outer: malleolus; table
outline: form
oval: amputation; corpuscle; fasciculus; foramen; fossa; window
ovale: malaria
ovale tertian: malaria
ovalocytic: anemia
ovarian: amenorrhea; artery; colic; cycle; cyst; dysmenorrhea; fimbria; follicle; fossa; ligament; plexus; pregnancy; varicocele; vein
ovarian ascorbic acid depletion: test
ovarian tubular: adenoma
ovarioabdominal: pregnancy
overanxious: disorder
overflow: wave
overhanging: restoration
overlay: denture
overproduction: theory
overriding: aorta
overripe: cataract
overt: homosexuality
ovine: acetonia; mastitis
ovular: membrane; transmigration
ovulational: sclerosis
ovulocyclic: porphyria
own: control
ox: bots
oxalate: calculus
oxazin: dye
Oxford: unit
oxidase: reaction
oxidation-reduction: electrode; indicator; potential; reaction; system
oxidative: phosphorylation
oxidized: cellulose
oxonium: ion
oxygen: capacity; consumption; debt; deficit; effect; electrode; poisoning; tent; therapy; toxocity
oxygen affinity: anoxia
oxygenated: hemoglobin
oxygen deprivation: theory
oxygen utilization: coefficient
oxyntic: cell; gland
oxyphil: adenoma; cell; chromatin; granule
oxyphilic: leukocyte
oxytalan fiber: stain

P

P: antigen; cell; enzyme; factor; wave
P-A: interval
P-A conduction: time
pacchonian: body; corpuscle; depression; gland; granulation
pacemaker: failure; output; sensitivity
Pacheco's parrot disease: virus
pachydermoperiostosis: syndrome
pacing: catheter
pacinian: corpuscle
packed cell: volume
packed human blood: cell
packing: process
pagetoid: cell; reticulosis
Pahvant Valley: fever; plague
pain: principle; reaction; threshold; tolerance
painful: anesthesia; hematuria; heel; paraplegia; point; toe
painful-bruising: syndrome
painless: hematuria; jaundice
pain-pleasure: principle
painter's: colic
paired: allosome; associate; beat; organelle
pajaroella: tick
palatal: abscess; bar; index; myoclonus; nystagmus; papillomatosis; plate; process; reflex; seal; shelf; triangle
palate: hook; myograph
palatine: aponeurosis; bone; gland; groove; index; papilla; process; raphe; reflex; ridge; spine; surface; tonsil; torus; vein
palatoethmoidal: suture
palatoglossal: arch
palatoglossus: muscle
palatomaxillary: index; suture
palatopharyngeal: arch; muscle
palatouvularis: muscle
palatovaginal: canal; groove
pale: globe; hypertension; infarct; thrombus
paleostriatal: syndrome
palindromic: DNA; encephalopathy; sequence
palisade: layer
pallesthetic: sensibility
palliative: treatment
pallidal: syndrome
palm: grasp; wax
palmar: aponeurosis; crease; fascia; fibromatosis; flexion; ligament; reflex; space; syphilid
palmar carpometacarpal: ligament
palmar digital: vein
palmar interosseous: artery; muscle
palmar metacarpal: artery; ligament; vein
palmar radiocarpal: ligament
palmar ulnocarpal: ligament
palmate: fold
palm-chin: reflex
palmin, palmitin: test

palmomental: reflex
palmoplantar: keratoderma
palpable: rale
palpatory: percussion
palpebral: artery; conjunctiva; fissure; gland; part; raphe
palpebronasal: fold
paludal: fever
pampiniform: body; plexus
panacinar: emphysema
pancake: kidney
pancervical: smear
pancreatic: cholera; colic; deoxyribonuclease; diabetes; digestion; diverticulum; dornase; duct; encephalopathy; infantilism; island; islet; juice; lithiasis; notch; plexus; ribonuclease; sphincter; steatorrhea; vein
pancreatic hyperglycemic: hormone
pancreaticoduodenal: transplantation; vein
pancreaticoduodenal lymph: node
pancreaticoenteric: recess
pancreaticosplenic lymph: node
pancreatogenous: diarrhea
pancreozymin-secretin: test
panic: attack; disorder
panleukopenia: virus
panlobular: emphysema
pannicular: hernia
panniculus carnosus: muscle
panoptic: stain
panoramic: roentgenogram
panoramic rotating: machine
panoramic x-ray: film
pansystolic: murmur
pantaloon: embolism
pantoate activating: enzyme
pantoscopic: spectacles
pantothenic acid: unit
pantropic: virus
PAP: technique
Pap: smear; test
paper: chromatography; plate
paper mill worker's: disease
papillary: adenocarcinoma; adenoma; carcinoma; duct; ectasia; foramen; hidradenoma; layer; muscle; process; stasis; tumor
papillary cystic: adenoma
papillary muscle: dysfunction; syndrome
papillotonic: pseudotabes
pappataci: fever
pappataci fever: virus
papular: acrodermatitis; dermatitis; fever; mucinosis; scrofuloderma; syphilid; tuberculid; urticaria
papular stomatitis: virus
papulonecrotic: tuberculid
papulosquamous: tuberculid
papyraceous: plate; scar
paraaortic: body
parabasal: body; filament
parabiotic: flap
paraboloid: condenser
parabrachial: nucleus
paracarcinomatous: encephalomyelopathy; myelopathy
paracarmine: stain
paracelsian: method
paracentral: artery; fissure; lobule; scotoma
paracentric: inversion
paracervical block: anesthesia
parachordal: cartilage; plate
parachute: deformity; reflex
parachute mitral: valve
paracoccidioidal: granuloma
paracolic: recess
paracolon: bacillus
paracyclic: ovulation
paracystic: pouch
paradoxical: contraction; embolism; incontinence; movement; pulse; pupil; reflex; respiration; sleep
paradoxical diaphragm: phenomenon
paradoxical extensor: reflex
paradoxical flexor: reflex
paradoxical patellar: reflex
paradoxical pupillary: phenomenon; reflex
paradoxical triceps: reflex
paraduodenal: fold; fossa; recess
paradysentery: bacillus
paraesophageal: hernia
paraffin: cancer; tumor; wax
parafollicular: cell
parafrenal: abscess
paraganglionic: cell
paragenital: tubule
paraglenoid: groove; sulcus
Paraguay: tea
parahippocampal: gyrus
parainfluenza: virus
parajejunal: fossa
parallax: method; test
parallel: attachment; ray
paraluteal: cell
paralytic: chorea; dementia; ectropion; ileus; miosis; mydriasis; myoglobinuria; rabies; scoliosis; strabismus
paralyzing: vertigo
paramammary lymph: node
paramastoid: process
paramedian: incision
paramesonephric: duct
parametric: abscess
parametritic: abscess
paranasal: sinus
paraneoplastic: acrokeratosis; syndrome
paranephric: abscess; body
paraneural: infiltration
paranoid: personality; schizophrenia
paranuclear: body
paraperitoneal: hernia; nephrectomy
parapharyngeal: space
paraphysial: cyst
pararectal: fossa; pouch
pararectal lymph: node
parasaccular: hernia
parasagittal: plane
paraseptal: cartilage; emphysema
parasinoidal: sinus
parasite-host: ecosystem
parasitic: cyst; disease; granuloma; hemoptysis; leiomyoma; melanoderma; otitis; thyroiditis; twin
parasitophorous: vacuole
parasol: insertion
parasternal: hernia; line
parasternal lymph: node
parastriate: area; cortex
parasympathetic: ganglion; nerve; part; root
parasympathetic nervous: system
parasystolic: beat
parataxic: distortion
paratenic: host
paraterminal: body; gyrus
parathyroid: gland; hormone; insufficiency: osteosis; tetany
parathyroprival: tetany
paratracheal: node
paratuberculous: lymphadenitis
paratyphoid: bacillus; fever
paraumbilical: vein
paraurethral: duct; gland
parauterine lymph: node
paravaccinia: virus
paravaginal: hysterectomy
paravaginal lymph: node
paraventricular: nucleus
paravertebral: anesthesia; ganglion; line; triangle

paravesical: fossa; pouch
paravesical lymph: node
paraxial: mesoderm; ray
parchment: heart; skin
parenchymal: cell
parenchymatous: cell; degeneration; goiter; hemorrhage; keratitis; mastitis; neuritis; tonsillitis
parent: cell; cyst
parental: generation; rejection
parenteral: absorption; alimentation; hyperalimentation; therapy
parenteric: fever
paretic: impotence
parietal: angle; bone; cell; eminence; eye; fistula; foramen; hernia; layer; lobe; margin; notch; plate; pleura; region; thrombus; tuber; vein; wall
parietal emissary: vein
parietomastoid: suture
parieto-occipital: artery; fissure; sulcus
parietopontine: tract
Paris: line
paroccipital: process
parolfactory: area
paroophoritic: cyst
parosteal: fasciitis
parotid: abscess; bubo; duct; fascia; gland; notch; papilla; plexus; recess; vein
paroxysmal: sleep; tachycardia
paroxysmal cerebral: dysrhythmia
paroxysmal nocturnal: dyspnea; hemoglobinuria
parrot: disease; fever; jaw; mouth; virus
parrot-beak: nail
parry: fracture
partial: agglutinin; anencephaly; aneuploidy; anodontia; antigen; cystectomy; denture; enterocele; epilepsy; group; lipoatrophy; pressure; sclerectasia; seizure; volume
partial adrenocortical: insufficiency
partial denture: impression; retention
partial ileal: bypass
partial-thickness: flap; graft
partial thromboplastin: time
participant: observer
partition: chromatography; coefficient
parturient: canal; paralysis; paresis
parvilocular: cyst
PAS: stain
passional: attitude
passive: agglutination; anaphylaxis; clot; congestion; duction; eruption; hemagglutination; hyperemia; immunity; immunization; incontinence; interval; learning; medium; movement; prophylaxis; transference; tremor; vasoconstriction; vasodilation
passive-aggressive: behavior; personality
passive cutaneous: anaphylaxis
passive cutaneous anaphylactic: reaction
pastil: radiometer
pastoral: counseling
patch: test
patellar: fossa; ligament; network; reflex; surface
patellar tendon: reflex
patello-adductor: reflex
patent: ductus; medicine
pathematic: aphasia
pathetic: nerve
pathogenic: occlusion
pathognomonic: symptom
pathologic: absorption; amenorrhea; amputation; anatomy; calcification; diagnosis; fracture; glycosuria; histology; myopia; physiology; rigidity; sphincter
pathologic retraction: ring
Patois: virus
patterned: alopecia
pattern sensitive: epilepsy
pavement: epithelium
pavlovian: conditioning
PBI: test
peak: magnitude
peak expiratory: flow
pearl: cyst; moss; tumor
pearl-worker's: disease
pear-shaped: area
peat: moss
peccant: humor
pecking: order
pecten: band
pectin: sugar
pectinate: fiber; line; muscle; zone
pectineal: ligament; line; muscle
pectiniform: septum
pectoral: fascia; gland; reflex; region; ridge; vein
pectoral lymph: node
pedal: system
pediatric: dentistry
pedicle: flap; graft
pediculous: blephoritis
pedigree: analysis
peduncular: ansa; loop; vein
pedunculated: hydatid; polyp
peg-and-socket: articulation; joint
pegged: tooth
pegtop: tooth
peliosis: hepatitis
pellagra-preventing: factor
pellet: implantation
pellucid: zone
pelvic: abscess; axis; brim; canal; cavity; cellulitis; diaphragm; exenteration; ganglion; girdle; hematocele; index; inlet; kidney; limb; outlet; part; peritonitis; plane; plexus; pole; presentation; promontory; surface; version
pelvic inflammatory: disease
pelvic splanchnic: nerve
pelvirectal: sphincter
pelvivertebral: angle
pelvofemoral muscular: dystrophy
pemphigoid: syphilid
pen: grasp
pencil: tenderness
pendular: movement; nystagmus
pendulous: abdomen; heart; palate
pendulum: rhythm
penetrant: gene
penetrating: keratoplasty; ulcer; wound
penile: fibromatosis; implant; raphe; urethra
penis: bone; envy; epine; thorn
pennate: muscle
penoscrotal: hypospadias
pension: neurosis
pentagastrin: test
pentavalent gas gangrene: antitoxin
penton: antigen
pentose phosphate: pathway
pep: pill
pepper and salt: fundus
peptic: cell; digestion; esophagitis; gland; ulcer
peptide: bond
peptonized: iron
peracute: mania
perambulating: ulcer
percept: analysis
perceptive: deafness
perceptual: expansion
percussion: sound; wave
percutaneous: cholangiography; stimulation
percutaneous radiofrequency: gangliolysis

percutaneous transluminal coronary: angioplasty
perfect: fungus; stage; state
perforated: layer; space; ulcer
perforating: abscess; artery; fiber; folliculitis; keratoplasty; ulcer; vein; wound
performance: test
performic acid: reaction
perfusion: cannula
perhydrase: milk
perialveolar: wiring
parianal odoriferous: gland
periapical: abscess; curettage; cyst; osteofibrosis; radiograph; roentgenogram; tissue
periapical cemental: dysplasia
periapical periodontal: granuloma
periappendiceal: abscess
periarterial: pad; plexus; sympathectomy
periarticular: abscess
pericallosal: artery
pericanalicular: fibroadenoma
pericapillary: cell
pericardiacophrenic: artery; vein
pericardial: cavity; decompression; fremitus; knock; murmur; poudrage; reflex; rub; vein; villus
pericardial friction: sound
pericardioperitoneal: canal
pericardiopleural: fold; membrane
pericemental: abscess; attachment
pericentral: fibrosis; scotoma
pericentric: inversion
perichondral: bone
perichoroid: space
periclaustral: lamina
pericolic membrane: syndrome
periconchal: sulcus
pericoronal: abscess; flap
pericorpuscular: synapse
pericytic: venule
peridental: ligament; membrane
peridontal: atrophy
peridural: anesthesia
peri-infarction: block
perilimbal suction: cup
perilymphatic: duct; space
perimuscular: fibrosis
perinatal: death; medicine
perinatal mortality: rate
perineal: artery; body; flexure; hernia; lithotomy; membrane; muscle; nerve; raphe; region; section; space; urethrostomy; urethrotomy
perineovaginal: fistula
perinephric: abscess
perineural: anesthesia; infiltration
perineuronal: satellite
perinuclear: cataract; space
periodic: arthralgia; catatonia; disease; edema; law; neutropenia; ophthalmia; paralysis; peritonitis; polyserositis; system
periodic acid-Schiff: stain
periodic migrainous: neuralgia
periodontal: abscess; anesthesia; atrophy; file; ligament; membrane; pocket; probe
peridontal ligament: fiber
perioplic: band
periorbital: membrane
periorificial: lentiginosis
periosteal: bone; bud; chondroma; elevator; ganglion; graft; implantation; reflex; sarcoma
periosteoplastic: amputation
periotic: bone; cartilage
peripharyngeal: space
peripheral: aneurysm; apnea; cataract; chemoreceptor; dysostosis; glare; iridectomy; resistance; scotoma; seal; tabes; vision
peripheral anterior: synechia
peripheral cementifying: fibroma
peripheral nervous: system
peripheral odontogenic: fibroma
peripheral ossifying: fibroma
peripolar: cell
periportal: space
perirectal: abscess
perirenal: fascia; insufflation
periscopic: lens; meniscus
perisinusoidal: space
peristatic: hyperemia
peristernal: perichondritis
peristriate: area; cortex
peritarsal: network
perithelial: cell
peritoneal: button; cavity; dialysis; fossa; transfusion; villus
peritoneovenous: shunt
peritonsillar: abscess
peritracheal: gland
peritubular: dentin; zone
peritubular contractile: cell
periungual: fibroma
periureteral: abscess
periurethral: abscess
perivascular fibrous: capsule
periventricular: fiber
perivisceral: cavity
perivitelline: space
permanent: callus; cartilage; restoration; stricture; tooth
permanent dominant: idea
permanent pedicle: flap
permeability: theory; vitamin
perna: disease
pernicious: anemia; malaria; vomiting
pernicious anemia type: metarubricyte; prorubricyte; rubriblast
peroneal: artery; bone; node; phenomenon; pulley; vein
peroneal communicating: nerve
peroneal muscular: atrophy
peroxidase: reaction; stain
perpendicular: fasciculus; plate
perpetually growing: tooth
persecution: complex
persecutory: delusion
Persian relapsing: fever
persistent: cloaca; tremor; truncus
persistent anterior hyperplastic primary: vitreous
persistent atrioventricular: canal
persistently growing: tooth
persistent posterior hyperplastic primary: vitreous
perivascular: cuff
personal: equation; motivation; space
personal growth: laboratory
personality: disorder; formation; integration; inventory; profile; test
perspiratory: gland
pertrochanteric: fracture
pertussis: immunoglobulin; vaccine
pertussis immune: globulin
Peruvian: tarantula; wart
pervasive developmental: disorder
pervenous: pacemaker
perverted: nystagmus
perverted ocular: movement
pessary: cell; corpuscle
petechial: angioma; fever; hemorrhage
petit: mal
petit mal: epilepsy
petro-occipital: fissure; joint
petrosal: bone; fossa; ganglion; impression; sinus; vein
petrosphenoidal: syndrome
petrosquamous: fissure; suture
petrotympanic: fissure
petrous: bone; ganglion; part; pyramid
PGSR: audiometry
pH: scale
phacoanaphylactic: uveitis

phacogenic: glaucoma; uveitis
phacolytic: glaucoma
phacomorphic: glaucoma
phaeomycotic: cyst
phagedenic: ulcer
phagocytic: index; pneumonocyte
phakic: eye
phalangeal: cell; joint
phallic: phase; tubercle
phantom: aneurysm; corpuscle; limb; pregnancy; tumor
phantom limb: pain
pharmaceutical: chemistry
pharmacologic: mediator
pharmacopeial: gel
pharyngeal: anesthesia; arch; bursa; calculus; canal; fistula; flap; gland; groove; hypophysis; isthmus; membrane; opening; pituitary; plexus; pouch; recess; reflex; space; tonsil; tubercle; vein
pharyngeal pouch: syndrome
pharyngobasilar: fascia
pharyngobranchial: duct
pharyngoconjunctival: fever
pharyngoconjunctival fever: virus
pharyngoepiglottic: fold
pharyngoesophageal: cushion; diverticulum; pad
pharyngomaxillary: space
pharyngonasal: cavity
pharyngopalatine: arch
pharyngotympanic: groove; tube
phase: microscope; rule
phase-contrast: microscope
phase I, phase II: block
phasic: reflex
phasic sinus: arrhythmia
PHC: syndrome
P-H conduction: time
phenanthrene: nucleus
phenol: coefficient
phenolsulfonphthalein: test
phenotypic: mixing; value
phentolamine: test
phenylalanyl: chain
phenylpyruvic: amentia
phenylthiocarbamoyl: peptide; protein
pheochrome: cell
phi: phenomenon
Phialophore-type: conidiophore
Philadelphia: chromosome; cocktail
philanthropic: hospital
philosopher's: stone
phlebotomus: fever
phlebotomus fever: virus
phlegmonous: abscess; cellulitis; enteritis; erysipelas; gastritis; mastitis; ulcer
phlogistone: theory
phlorizin; phloridzin: diabetes; glycosuria
phlyctenular: conjunctivitis; keratitis; ophthalmia; pannus
PhNCS: protein
phocomelic: dwarfism
phonemic: regression
phonic: spasm
phosphatase: unit
phosphate: diabetes; tetany
phosphogluconate: pathway
phosphohexose isomerase: deficiency
phosphoroclastic: cleavage; reaction
phosphorylase-rupturing: enzyme
phosphotungstic acid: hematoxylin; stain
phosphureted: hydrogen
photechic: effect
photic: driving; stimulation
photo: retinopathy
photoallergic: sensitivity
photochromic: lens; spectacles
photodynamic: sensitization
photoelectric: effect
photogenic: epilepsy
photomultiplier: tube
photon: density
photo-patch: test
photopic: adaptation; eye; vision
photoradiation: therapy
photoreactivating: enzyme
photoreceptor: cell
photosensor: oculography
photostress: test
phototoxic: sensitivity
phrenic: avulsion; ganglion; nerve; phenomenon; plexus; vein; wave
phrenicocolic: ligament
phrenicocostal: sinus
phrenicolienal: ligament
phrenicomediastinal: recess
phrenicopleural: fascia
phrenicosplenic: ligament
phrenic pressure: test
phrenogastric: ligament
phrenopericardial: angle
phrenosplenic: ligament
phrygian: cap
phthalein: test
phthinoid: chest
phyllodes: tumor
physaliphorous: cell
physical: age; allergy; anthropology; diagnosis; elasticity; examination; fitness; half-life; medicine; sign; therapy
physiologic, physiological: age; albuminuria; amenorrhea; anatomy; anemia; antidote; chemistry; congestion; cup; drive; dwarfism; elasticity; equilibrium; excavation; homeostasis; hypertrophy; icterus; incompatibility; jaundice; leukocytosis; occlusion; saline; sclerosis; scotoma; sphincter; unit
physiologically balanced: occlusion
physiologic dead: space
physiologic rest: position
physiologic retraction: ring
physiologic salt: solution
pi: monochromasy
pial: funnel
pial-glial: membrane
pianist's: cramp
pickwickian: syndrome
pi cone: monochromasy
picrocarmine: stain
picroformol: fixative
picronigrosin: stain
picture: element
piebald: eyelash; skin
piezogenic pedal: papule
pig: skin
pigeon: breast
pigeon-breeder's: disease
pigeon's: milk
pigment: cell; epitheliopathy; epithelium; induration
pigmentary: cirrhosis; glaucoma; retinopathy; syphilid
pigmented: ameloblastoma; dermatofibrosarcoma protuberans; epulis; layer
pigmented keratic: precipitate
pigmented purpuric lichenoid: dermatosis
pigmented villonodular: synovitis
pilar: cyst; tumor
piliferous: cyst
pillar: cell
piloid: astrocytoma; gliosis
pilomotor: fiber; reflex
pilon: fracture
pilonidal: cyst; fistula; sinus
pilous: gland
pilular: mass
pin: amalgam; implant
pincer: nail
pinch: graft
pineal: body; cell; cyst; eye; gland; habenula; recess; stalk
pineapple: test

ping-pong: bone; fracture; gaze; mechanism
pinhole: pupil
pink: disease; eye
pinocytotic: vesicle
pinworm: vaginitis
PIP: joint
pipe: bone
pipe-smoker's: cancer
pipestem: artery; fibrosis
piqure: diabetes
piriform, pyriform: area; cortex; fossa; muscle; opening; recess; sinus
pisciform: cataract
pisiform: bone
pisohamate: ligament
pisometacarpal: ligament
pisotriquetral: joint
pisounciform: ligament
pisouncinate: ligament
pistol-shot femoral: sound
piston: pulse
pit: caries
pit and fissure: caries
pitch: poisoning; wart
pitch-worker's: cancer
pithecoid: theory
pitted: keratolysis
pitting: edema
Pittsburgh: pneumonia
Pittsburgh pneumonia: agent
pituitary: adamantinoma; apoplexy; basophilia; cachexia; diverticulum; dwarfism; fossa; gigantism; gland; infantilism; membrane; myxedema; stalk
pituitary basophil: adenoma
pituitary gonadotropic: hormone
pituitary growth: hormone
pituitary stalk: section
pivot: joint
pivot shift: test
P-J: interval
place: theory
placenta: protein
placental: barrier; circulation; dystocia; lobe; membrane; plasmodium; polyp; presentation; septum; sign; souffle; thrombosis
placental dysfunction: syndrome
placental growth: hormone
placental parasitic: twin
placental sulfatase: deficiency
plague: bacillus; pneumonia; vaccine
plain: film
plane: joint; suture; wart
planoconcave: lens
planoconvex: lens
planographic: pelvimetry
plant: agglutinin; antitoxin; casein; dermatitis; indican; ribonuclease; toxin; virus
plantar: aponeurosis; arch; cushion; fascia; fibromatosis; flexion; ligament; muscle; reflex; space; syphilid; wart
plantar calcaneocuboid: ligament
plantar calcaneonavicular: ligament
plantar cuboideonavicular: ligament
plantar cuneocuboid: ligament
plantar cuneonavicular: ligament
plantar digital: vein
plantar interosseous: muscle
plantar metatarsal: artery; ligament; vein
plantar muscle: reflex
plantar quadrate: muscle
plantar venous: arch; network
plasma: cell; factor; fibronectin; layer; membrane; protein; scalpel; stain; substitute; therapy
plasma accelerator: globulin
plasma cell: balanitis; hepatitis; leukemia; mastitis; myeloma
plasmacrit: test
plasma iodoprotein: disorder
plasmal: reaction
plasma labile: factor
plasma protein: fraction
plasma renin: activity
plasma thromboplastin: antecedent; component; factor
plasmatic: stain
plasmic: stain
plasminogen: activator
plasmin prothrombins conversion: factor
plasmocytic: leukemoid reaction
plasmodial: trophoblast
plaster: bandage; splint
plaster of Paris: disease
plastic: anatomy; bronchitis; corpuscle; cyclitis; induration; iritis; lymph; motor; operation; pleurisy; surgery; tooth
plastic restoration: material
plastic section: stain
plate: thrombosis
plateau: iris; pulse
platelet: actomyosin; cofactor; factor; thrombosis
platelet-activating, -aggregating: factor
platelet aggregation: test
platelet-derived growth: factor
platelet tissue: factor
platypellic: pelvis
platypelloid: pelvis
play: therapy
pleasure: curve; principle
pleiotropic: gene
pleomorphic: adenoma; lipoma
plethysmographic: goggle
pleural: calculus; cavity; fluid; fremitus; poudrage; pressure; recess; sinus; space; villus
pleuritic: rub
pleuroesophageal: line; muscle
pleuropericardial: canal; hiatus; membrane; murmur
pleuroperitoneal: canal; cavity; fold; hiatus; membrane
pleuropneumonia-like: organism
plexiform: layer; neurofibroma; neuroma
plexogenic pulmonary: arteriopathy
plugging: instrument
plural: pregnancy
pluriglandular: adenomatosis
pluripotent: cell
plus: lens; strand
PM2: bacteriophage
PMA: index
pneocardiac: reflex
pneopneic: reflex
pneumatic: bone; cabinet; space; tonometer
pneumatic tire: injury
pneumatoenteric: recess
pneumococcal: polysaccharide; pneumonia; vaccine
pneumococcus: ulcer
pneumoenteric: recess
pneumogastric: nerve
pneumogenic: osteoarthropathy
pneumonia: virus
pneumonic: plague
pneumotaxic: localization
PNP: syndrome
P/O: ratio
pocketed: calculus
podalic: extraction; version
podiatric: medicine
podophyllum: resin
POEMS: syndrome
point: angle; deletion; epidemic; mutation
pointed: condyloma; wart
point system: test type
poker: back; spine
pokeweed: nitrogen
polar: anemia; body; cataract; cell; compound; globule; hypogenesis; plate; presentation; ring; solvent; star; zone

polarized: light
polarizing: microscope
pole: ligation
poliomyelitis: immunoglobulin; virus
poliomyelitis immune: globulin
poliovirus: vaccine
polishing: brush
polka: fever
poll: evil
pollen: antigen; extract
polyamine-methylene: resin
polyaxial: joint
polybasic: acid
polycarboxylate: cement
polychlorinated: biphenyl
polychromatic: cell
polychromatophil: cell
polycystic: disease; kidney; liver; ovary
polycystic liver: disease
polycystic ovary: syndrome
polydystrophic: dwarfism
polyendocrine deficiency: syndrome
polyester: resin
polygenic: inheritance
polyglandular deficiency: syndrome
polyleptic: fever
polymer fume: fever
polymorphic: reticulosis
polymorphic light: eruption
polymorphic superficial: keratitis
polymorphocytic: leukemia
polymorphonuclear: leukocyte
polymorphous: layer; perversion
polyneuritic: psychosis
polynuclear: leukocyte
polyoma: virus
polyostotic fibrous: dysplasia
polyovular ovarian: follicle
polyphenic: gene
polyphyletic: theory
polypoid: adenoma
polypous: endocarditis; gastritis
polysplenia: syndrome
polytene: chromosome
polyuria: test
polyvalent: allergy; antiserum; serum; vaccine
polyzygotic: twin
pomade: acne
pond: fracture
ponderal: index
pontile: apoplexy
pontine: angle; artery; cistern; flexure; hemorrhage; nucleus; vein
pontine angle: tumor
pontine gray: matter
pontocerebellar: cisternography; recess
pontomedullary: groove
pooled: serum
pooled blood: serum
poorly differentiated lymphocytic: lymphoma
popliteal: artery; fascia; fossa; groove; line; muscle; notch; plane; plexus; region; space; surface; vein
popliteal communicating: nerve
popliteal entrapment: syndrome
popliteal lymph: node
population: genetics
porcelain: inlay
porcine: adenovirus; amelia; graft; parakeratosis; valve
porcine encephalomyelitis: virus
porcupine: skin
portacaval: shunt
portal: canal; circulation; cirrhosis; fissure; hypertension; lobule; pyemia; system; vein
portal-systemic: encephalopathy
portasystemic vascular: shunt
Portuguese-Azorean: disease
port-wine: mark, stain
position: agnosia; effect; sense
positional: hypotension
position emission: tomography
positive: accommodation; afterimage; anergy; catalyst; chronotropism; convergence; electrode; electron; electrotaxis; feedback; meniscus; phase; ray; scotoma; stain; taxis; thermotaxis; transference; valence
positive end-expiratory: pressure
positively: bathmotropic, dromotropic, inotropic
positive-negative pressure: breathing
post: dam; implant
postadrenalectomy: syndrome
postage stamp: graft
postanal: gut
postaxilliary: line
postbasic: stare
postcapillary: venule
postcardiotomy: syndrome
postcentral: area; artery; fissure; gyrus; sulcus
postcholecystectomy: syndrome
postcloacal: gut
postcommissurotomy: syndrome
postcommunical: part
postconcussion: neurosis; syndrome
postcostal: anastomosis
post-dam: area
postdiphtheritic: paralysis
postdrive: depression
posterior: asynclitism; choroiditis; nephrectomy; occlusion; rhinoscopy; rhizotomy; rachischisis; scleritis; sclerosis; sclerotomy; staphyloma; symblepharon; synechia; urethritis; uveitis; vaginismus; vitrectomy
posterior anatomical structures (specific posterior structures are listed under the following): arch; area; artery; border; bundle; canal; cell; chamber; column; commissure; convolution; cord; crest; cusp; diameter; extremity; fauces; fissure; fontanel; foramen; fossa; funiculus; groove; gyrus; horn; joint; layer; ligament; limb; line; lip; lobe; lobule; margin; membrane; muscle; naris; nerve; node; notch; nucleus; part; pillar; pituitary; plexus; pole; process; pyramid; recess; region; root; segment; spine; substance; sulcus; surface; tooth; tract; triangle; tubercle; valve; vein; velum; wall
posterior column: cordotomy
posterior descending: embryotoxin
posterior focal: point
posterior inferior cerebellar artery: syndrome
posterior myocardial: infarction
posterior palatal: seal
posterior palatal seal: area
posterior pelvic: exenteration
posterior primary: division
posterior spinal: sclerosis
posterior tooth: form
posterior vaginal: hernia
posterolateral: fissure; fontanel; groove; sulcus
posterolateral central: artery
posteromedial central: artery
posteruption: cuticle
postextrasystolic: pause; wave
postganglionic motor: neuron
postgastrectomy: syndrome
postglenoid: foramen
posthemiplegic: athetosis; chorea
posthemorrhagic: anemia
posthepatic: cirrhosis
posthippocampal: fissure
posthypnotic: amnesia; psychosis; suggestion
posthypoglycemic: hyperglycemia
posticus: palsy; paralysis

postinfectious: bradycardia; psychosis
post-kala azar dermal: leishmanoid
postlaminar: part
postlingual: deafness; fissure
postlunate: fissure
postmaturity: syndrome
postmeiotic: phase
postmeningitic: hydrocephalus
postmenopausal: atrophy
postmortem: clot; delivery; examination; hypostasis; livedo; lividity; pustule; rigidity; suggillation; thrombus; tubercle; wart
postmyocardial infarction: syndrome
postnasal: drip
postnatal: life; pit
postnecrotic: cirrhosis
postnormal: occlusion
postoperative: parotiditis; pneumonia; tetany
postoperative pressure: alopecia
postoral: arch
postpalatal: seal
postpalatal seal: area
postpartum: alopecia; amenorrhea; cardiomyopathy; estrus; hemorrhage; hypertension; psychosis; tetanus
postpartum pituitary necrosis: syndrome
postparturient: hemoglobinuria
postperfusion: lung
postpericardiotomy: syndrome
postpharyngeal: space
postphlebitic: syndrome
postprandial: lipemia
postprimary: tuberculosis
postpyloric: sphincter
postpyramidal: fissure
postreduction: phase
postrenal: albuminuria
postrhinal: fissure
postrubella: syndrome
postsphenoid: bone
postsphygmic: interval
postsulcal: part
postsynaptic: membrane
post-term: infant
posttraumatic: amnesia; delirium; dementia; epilepsy; hydrocephalus; neurosis; osteoporosis; psychosis; syndrome
posttraumatic arterial or venous: thrombosis
posttraumatic leptomeningeal: cyst
posttraumatic neck: syndrome
posttraumatic stress: disorder; syndrome
posttussis suction: sound
posttussive: suction
postural: albuminuria; contraction; hypotension; ischemia; myoneuralgia; position; proteinuria; reflex; set; syncope; tremor; version; vertigo
posture: sense
postvaccinal: encephalitis
potable: water
potassium: inhibition
potato: nose; tumor
potato dextrose: agar
potential: energy
potentiometric: titration
Potomac horse: fever
poultry handler's: disease
poultryman's: itch
Powassan: encephalitis; virus
powdered: gold; ipecac; opium; stomach
power: failure; point
P-P: interval
P-Q: interval
P-R: interval; segment
PR: enzyme
practical: anatomy; unit
Prague: maneuver; pelvis
prairie: conjunctivitis; itch
preanesthetic: medication
preauricular: groove; point; sulcus
preauricular subfacial parotid lymph: node
preautomatic: pause
preaxillary: line
precancerous: lesion; melanosis
precapillary: anastomosis
prececal lymph: node
precentral: area; gyrus; sulcus
precentral cerebellar: vein
precervical: sinus
prechiasmatic: sulcus
prechordal: plate
precipitate: labor
precipitated: calcium; sulfur
precipitating: antibody
precipitation: test
precipitin: reaction; test
precision: attachment; rest
precocious: pseudopuberty; puberty
precollagenous: fiber
precommissural: bundle; septum
precommissural septal: area
precommunical: part
preconceptual: stage
precordial: lead
precordial catch: syndrome
precorneal: film
precostal: anastomosis
precuneal: artery
precursory: cartilage
predictive: validity; value
predisposing: cause
predorsal: bundle
preejection: period
preen: gland
preexcitation: syndrome
preextraction: record
preformation: theory
prefrontal: area; cortex, leukotomy; lobotomy; vein
preganglionic motor: neuron
pregenital: organization; phase
pregnancy: cell; diabetes; disease; luteoma; tumor
pregnant mare's serum: gonadotropin
pregranulosa: cell
prehyoid: gland
preinfarction: syndrome
preinterparietal: bone
prelaminar: part
prelaryngeal lymph: node
preliminary: impression
prelingual: deafness
prelogical: mind; thinking
premammary: abscess
premature: alopecia; beat; birth; contact; contraction; delivery; ejaculation; labor; systole
premature senility: syndrome
prematurity: myopia
premaxillary: bone; suture
premeiotic: phase
premenstrual: edema; syndrome; tension
premenstrual salivary: syndrome
premenstrual tension: syndrome
premolar: tooth
premotor: area; cortex; syndrome
prenatal: diagnosis; life; screening
prenodular: fissure
preoccipital: notch
pre-oedipal: phase
preoperative: record
preoptic: area; region
preoral: gut
prepapillary: sphincter
preparatory: iridectomy
prepared: chalk; ipecacuanha; suet
prepared mutton: tallow
prepatellar: bursa; bursitis
prepatient: period
prepericardiac lymph: node

prepiriform: gyrus
preputial: calculus; gland; ring; sac
prepyloric: sphincter; vein
prepyramidal: tract
prerectal: lithotomy
prereduction: phase
prerenal: albuminuria; azotemia
prerubral: field; nucleus
presacral: anesthesia; nerve; neurectomy; sympathectomy
presenile: dementia
presenile spontaneous: gangrene
presomite: embryo
presphenoid: bone
presphygmic: interval
presplenic: fold
pressor: amine; base; fiber; nerve; substance
pressorreceptive: mechanism
pressoreceptor: nerve; reflex; system
pressure: amaurosis; anesthesia; area; atrophy; collapse; dressing; epiphysis; gangrene; palsy; paralysis; plethysmograph; point; reversal; sense; sore; stasis
pressure-controlled: respirator
pressure-volume: index
presternal: notch; region
prestriate: area
presulcal: part
presumed ocular: histoplasmosis
presumptive: region
presynaptic: membrane
presystolic: gallop; murmur; thrill
pretectal: area; region
preterm: infant
pretibial: fever; myxedema
pretracheal: fascia; layer; node
preventive: dentistry; dose; medicine; treatment
prevertebral: fascia; ganglion; layer
prevertebral lymph: node
previllous: chorion; embryo
prickle: cell
prickle cell: layer
prickly: heat
primal: repression
primaquine: sensitivity
primary: adhesion; aerodontalgia; alcohol; aldosteronism; amenorrhea; amputation; amyloidosis; anesthetic; anophthalamus; atelectasis; bronchus; bubo; carcinoma; cardiomyopathy; caries; cementum; center; choana; coccidioidomycosis; color; complex; constriction; dementia; dentin; dentition; deviation; digestion; disease; dysmenorrhea; fissure; gain; hemochromatosis; hemorrhage; hydrocephalus; hyperoxaluria; hyperparathyroidism; hypertension; hyperthyroidism; hypogammaglobulinemia; hypogonadism; impression; irritant; lymphedema; lysosome; mesoderm; methemoglobinemia; metaplasia; narcissism; nodule; nondisjunction; oocyte; organizer; palate; pentosuria; point; process; proteose; pyodermia; ray; reaction; reinforcement; rejection; screwworm; sensation; sequestrum; shock; sodium; spermatocyte; syphilis; tooth; tuberculosis; union; villus; vitreous
primary adrenocortical: insufficiency
primary amebic: meningoencephalitis
primary atypical: pneumonia
primary biliary: cirrhosis
primary brain: vesicle
primary dental: lamina
primary dried: yeast
primary egg: membrane
primary embryonic: cell
primary erythroblastic: anemia
primary extrapulmonary: coccidioidomycosis
primary generalized: epilepsy
primary herpetic: stomatitis
primary idiopathic macular: atrophy
primary interatrial: foramen
primary irritant: dermatitis
primary labial: groove
primary macular: atrophy
primary medical: care
primary myeloid: metaplasia
primary neuronal: degeneration
primary ovarian: follicle
primary pigmentary: degeneration
primary progressive cerebellar: degeneration
primary pulmonary: lobule
primary refractory: anemia
primary renal: calculus
primary renal tubular: acidosis
primary sclerosing: cholangitis
primary senile: dementia
primary sex: character
primary skin: graft
primary visual: area; choana; cortex
primitive: aorta; chorion; furrow; groove; knot; node; palate; pit; ridge; streak
primitive costal: arch
primitive perivisceral: cavity
primitive reticular: cell
primordial: cartilage; cell; cyst; dwarfism; gigantism; kidney
primordial germ: cell
primordial ovarian: follicle
princeps cervicis: artery
principal: artery; focus; islet; piece; plane; point
principal optic: axis
prism: diopter
prism vergence: test
private: antigen, hospital
privet: cough
privileged: site
proacrosomal: granule
proactive: inhibition
probability: curve
probe: gorget; patency; syringe
problem-oriented: record
procaryotic: cell
procentriole: organizer
procerus: muscle
process: schizophrenia
prochordal: plate
procursive: chorea; epilepsy
prodromal: stage
prodromic: sign
productive: inflammation; peritonitis; pleurisy
product-moment: correlation
professional: neurosis; spasm
profile: record
profound: hypothermia
progestational: hormone
progesterone: unit
progressive: cataract; cleavage; hypocythemia; lipodystrophy; process; staining; vaccinia
progressive bacterial synergistic: gangrene
progressive bulbar: paralysis
progressive cerebellar: tremor
progressive cerebral: poliodystrophy
progressive choroidal: atrophy
progressive emphysematous: necrosis
progressive lingual: hemiatrophy
progressive multifocal: leukoencephalopathy
progressive muscular: atrophy; dystrophy
progressive pernicious: anemia
progressive pigmentary: dermatosis
progressive pneumonia: virus

psychogenic—*continued*
dipsia; purpura; torticollis; vomiting
psychogenic nocturnal: polydipsia
psychogenic nocturnal polydipsia: syndrome
psychogenic pain: disorder
psychographic: disturbance
psychological: test
psychomotor: epilepsy; retardation; seizure; test
psychopathic: personality
psychophysiologic: manifestation
psychosensory: aphasia
psychosexual: development; dysfunction
psychosomatic: disorder; medicine
psychotic: manifestation
PTA: stain
PTC: protein
pterygium: syndrome
pterygoid: canal; chest; depression; fissure; fossa; hamulus; lamina; nerve; notch; pit; plate; plexus; process; ridge; tubercle; tuberosity
pterygomandibular: ligament; raphe; space
pterygomaxillary: fissure; fossa; notch
pterygopalatine: canal; fossa; ganglion; groove; nerve
pterygopharyngeal: part
pterygospinal: ligament
pterygospinous: ligament; process
ptotic: organ
pubic: angle; arch; artery; baldness; body; bone; crest; ramus; region; spine; symphysis; tubercle
public: antigen; health; hospital
public health: dentistry; nurse
pubocapsular: ligament
pubococcygeal: muscle
pubofemoral: ligament
puboprostatic: ligament; muscle
puborectal: muscle
pubourethral: triangle
pubovaginal: muscle
pubovesical: ligament; muscle
pudding: opium
puddle: sign
pudendal: anesthesia; canal; cleavage; hernia; hematocele; nerve; sac; silt; ulcer; vein
pudic: nerve
puerile: respiration
puerperal: convulsion; eclampsia; fever; hemoglobinemia; hemoglobinuria; mastitis; morbidity; period; phlebitis; psychosis; sepsis; septicemia; tetanus
pullorum: disease
pulmonary: acariasis; acinus; adenomatosis; anthrax; arc; area; artery; aspergillosis; atresia; bella; circulation; collapse; cone; conus; distomiasis; edema; embolism; emphysema; fistula; glomangiosis; hamartoma; heart; hemosiderosis; hypertension; hypostasis; incompetence; insufficiency; ligament; murmur; opening; osteoarthropathy; pleurisy; plexus; pressure; pulse; ridge; salient; stenosis; sulcus; surface; transpiration; trunk; tuberculosis; valve; vein; ventilation
pulmonary alveolar: microlithiasis; proteinosis
pulmonary capillary wedge: pressure
pulmonary dismaturity: syndrome
pulmonary lymph: node
pulmonic: incompetence; murmur
pulmonocoronary: reflex
pulp: abscess; amputation; atrophy; calcification; calculus; canal; cavity; chamber; horn; nodule; polyp; pressure; stone; test
pulpal: well
pulpar: cell
pulpit: spectacles
pulpless: tooth
pulpy: testis
pulpy kidney: disease
pulsating: emphysema; metastasis, neurasthenia
pulse: curve; deficit; duration; generator; period; pressure; rate; therapy; wave
pulseless: disease
pulsion: diverticulum
pulsus: alternans
pumiced: foot
pump: failure; lung
punch: biopsy; graft
punchdrunk: syndrome
punctata albescens: retinopathy
punctate: basophilia; cataract; hemorrhage; hyalosis; keratitis; keratoderma; parotiditis; retinitis
puncture: diabetes; wound
pulpillary: athetosis; axis; distance; margin; membrane; reflex; zone
pupillary block: glaucoma
pupillary-skin: reflex
pure: absence; aphasia; color; culture; line
pure red cell: anemia; aplasia
pure tone: audiogram; audiometer; audiometry
purified: cotton; ozokerite; water
purified placental: protein
purified protein derivative of: tuberculin
purine: body
purine-restricted: diet
pursed lips: breathing
purse-string: instrument; suture
purulent: cyclitis; encephalitis; inflammation; ophthalmia; pleurisy; retinitis; synovitis
pus: basin; cell; corpuscle; tube
push-back: procedure
pustular: blepharitis; milaria; psoriasis; syphilid
putrescent: pulp
putrid: bronchitis; throat
putty: kidney
PVM: virus
pyelonephritic: kidney
pyemic: abscess; embolism
pyloric: antrum; artery; canal; cap; gland; incompetence; insufficiency; orifice; part; sphincter; stenosis; valve; vein
pyloric lymph: node
pyogenic: bacterium; fever; granuloma; infection; membrane; pachymeningitis; salpingitis
pyramid: sign
pyramidal: bone; cataract; cell; decussation; eminence; fiber; fracture; lobe; muscle; process; radiation; tract; tractotomy
pyramidal cell: layer
pyriform: (see piriform)
pyriform aperture: wiring
pyroligneous: alcohol; spirit; vinegar
pyroxylic: spirit
pyrrol, pyrrhol: cell
pyrrhole: nucleus
pyruvate kinase: deficiency
pyruvate oxidation: factor

Q

Q: angle; band; disk; enzyme; fever; wave
Q-banding: stain
Q-R: interval
Q-RB: interval
QRS: complex; interval
Q-S_2: interval
Q-T: interval
quack: medicine
quadrangular: cartilage; lobule; membrane; therapy

quadrantic: hemianopsia; scotoma
quadrate: ligament; lobe; lobule; muscle; part
quadrate pronator: muscle
quadriceps: artery; muscle; reflex
quadrigeminal: body; plate; pulse; rhythm
quadripedal extensor: reflex
quadruple: amputation; rhythm
quail bronchitis: virus
qualitative: alteration; analysis; trait
quality: control
quality control: chart
quantitative: alteration; analysis; genetics; hypertrophy; perimetry
quantum: limit; theory
Quaranfil: virus
quartan: fever; malaria; parasite
quarter: evil
quartz: glass
quaternary: ammonium; syphilis
quaternary carbon: atom
quellung: phenomenon; reaction; test
quick cure: resin
quiet: iritis; lung
quiet hip: disease
quilted: suture
quinacrine chromosome banding: stain
quinhydrone: electrode
quinine carbacrylic: resin
quinine carbacrylic resin: test
quotidian: fever; malaria

R

R: antigen; enzyme; factor; pilus; plasmid; wave
rabbit: fever; plague; snuffles
rabbit fibroma: virus
rabbit myxoma: virus
rabbitpox: virus
rabies: vaccine; virus
rabies immune: globulin
raccoon: eye
racemic: calcium
racemose: aneurysm; gland; hemangioma
rachitic: pelvis; rosary; scoliosis
racial: melanoderma
racket: amputation; nail
racquet: hypha
radial: acceleration; artery; border; bursa; eminence; fossa; head; immunodiffusion; keratotomy; nerve; notch; phenomenon; reflex; scar; vein
radial aplasia-thrombocytopenia: syndrome
radial collateral: artery; ligament
radial flexor: muscle
radial growth: phase
radial index: artery
radial recurrent: artery
radial sclerosing: lesion
radial styloid: tendovaginitis
radiant: energy; heat
radiate: crown; layer; ligament
radiate sternocostal: ligament
radiation: anemia; biology; burn; caries; cataract; chemistry; chimera; dermatosis; myelopathy; sickness; therapy
radical: cystectomy; hysterectomy; mastectomy; mastoidectomy; operation
radicular: abscess; artery; cyst; pulp; syndrome
radioactive: atom; constant; cyanocobalamin; equilibrium; iodine; isotope; probe; thyroxine
radioactive iodide uptake: test
radioallergosorbent: test
radiobicipital: reflex
radiocarpal: articulation: joint
radiochemical: purity
radioiodinated serum: albumin
radioisotopic: purity
radiological: anatomy; sphincter
radionuclide: angiography; cisternography; generator
radionuclidic: purity
radioperiosteal: reflex
radiopharmaceutical: purity
radioreceptor: assay
radiotelemetering: capsule
radioulnar: disk; syndesmosis
radium: emanation
radium beam: therapy
rag-sorter's: disease
RAI: test
railroad: nystagmus
rainbow: symptom
random: mating; sample; wave
random mating: equilibrium
random pattern: flap
range: paralysis
range of: accommodation; convergence
Ranikhet: disease
ranine: artery; tumor
rank-difference: correlation
raphe: nucleus
rapid: canities; decompression
rapid biplane: angiocardiography
rapid eye: movement
rapidly progressive: glomerulonephritis
rapid plasma reagin: test
rare: earth
rare-earth: element; metal
raspberry: tongue
rat: leprosy
rat-bite: fever
rate: constant; meter
ratio: scale
rational: formula; therapy
rat mite: dermatitis
raw: score
ray: fungus; therapeutics
R-banding: stain
reaction: center; formation; time
reactive: astrocyte; cell; depression; hyperemia; schizophrenia
reactive perforating: collagenosis
reading: frame
reading frame-shift: mutation
reaginic: antibody
real: focus; image
reality: adaptation; principle
real-time: ultrasound
reaper's: ophthalmia
rebound: phenomena; tenderness
rebreathing: anesthesia; technique
recapitulation: theory
receptive: aphasia
receptor: protein; site
recessive: character; gene; inheritance; trait
reciprocal: anchorage; arm; beat; bigeminy; force; inhibition; innervation; rhythm; transfusion; translocation
reciprocating: rhythm
reciprocity: law
reclotting: phenomenon
recognition: factor; time
recoil: atom; wave
recombinant: DNA; strain
recombination: fraction
reconstructive: mammaplasty; psychotherapy; surgery
record: base; rim
recovery: score
recreational: drug
recrudescent: typhus
recrudescent typhus: fever
recruiting: response
rectal: alimentation; anesthesia; column; fold; plexus; reflex; shelf; sinus; suppository; valve; valvotomy
rectal venous: plexus
rectangular: amputation
rectified: birch; spirit; tar; turpentine
rectocardiac: reflex

rectococcygeal: muscle
rectolabial: fistula
rectolaryngeal: reflex
rectosigmoid: sphincter
rectourethral: fistula; muscle
rectouterine: fold; pouch
rectovaginal: fistula; fold; septum
rectovesical: fascia; fistula; fold; muscle; pouch; septum
rectovestibular: fistula
rectovulvar: fistula
rectus: muscle
recurrence: risk
recurrent: albuminuria; artery; caries; encephalopathy; fever; hypopyon; nerve; stricture
recurrent aphthous: stomatitis; ulcer
recurrent central: retinitis
recurrent corneal: erosion
recurrent digital: fibroma
recurrent interosseous: artery
recurrent laryngeal: nerve
recurrent meningeal: nerve
recurrent scarring: aphtha
recurrent ulcerative: stomatitis
recurrent ulnar: artery
red: atrophy; corpuscle; degeneration; fever; gum; half-moon; hepatization; induration; infarct; lead; mange; muscle; neuralgia; nucleus; phosphorus; precipitate; pulp; reflex; sweat; test; thrombus; vision; wine
red blood: cell
red bone: marrow
red cell adherence: phenomenon, test
red pulp: cord
redox: electrode; indicator; potential; system
red oxide of: lead
reduced: eye; hematin; hemoglobin
reduced enamel: epithelium
reduced interarch: distance
reducible: hernia
reducing: diet; enzyme; sugar; valve
reduction: deformity; division; mammaplasty; nucleus; phase
reduplicated: cataract
redwater: fever
reed instrument: theory
reedy: nail
reel: foot
reentry: phenomenon; theory
reference: electrode; method; value
referred: pain; sensation
reflected: color; light; ray
reflecting: retinoscope
reflection: coefficient
reflex: angina; arc; asthma; control; cough; dyspepsia; epilepsy; headache; incontinence; inhibition; iridoplegia; ligament; movement; otalgia; sensation; symptom; therapy
reflex neurogenic: bladder
reflexogenic: pressosensitivity; zone
reflux: esophagitis; otitis
refracted: light
refracting: angle
refractive: amblyopia; index; keratotomy
refractive accommodative: esotropia
refractory: anemia; cast; flask; investment; period; state
refrigeration: anesthesia
regenerative: polyp
regional: anatomy; anesthesia; enteritis; enterocolitis; hyperthermia; perfusion
regional granulomatous: lymphadenitis
registered: nurse
regressing atypical: histiocytosis
regressive: staining
regressive-reconstructive: approach
regular: astigmatism
regular insulin: injection
regulator: gene
regulatory: albuminuria; sequence
regurgitant: fraction; murmur
regurgitation: jaundice
reinfection: tuberculosis
reinforced: anchorage
relapsing: fever; malaria; perichondritis; polychondritis
relational: threshold
relative: accommodation; amblyopia; dehydration; hemianopsia; humidity; immunity; incompetence; leukocytosis; polycythemia; scotoma; sensitivity; specificity; sterility; viscosity
relative refractory: period
relaxant: reversal
relaxation: factor; response; suture
release: phenomenon
released: substance
releasing: factor; hormone
reliability: coefficient
relief: area; chamber
REM: syndrome
reminiscent: aura; neuralgia
remittent: malaria
remittent malarial: fever
remote: memory
removable: bridge
removable partial: denture
renal: adenocarcinoma; agenesis; amyloidosis; artery; asthma; ballottement; calculus; capsulotomy; carcinosarcoma; cast; colic; collar; column; corpuscle; cortex; diabetes; epistaxis; fascia; ganglion; glycosuria; hematuria; hemophilia; hemorrhage; hypertension; hypoplasia; impression; infantilism; insufficiency; labyrinth; lobe; osteitis; osteodystrophy; papilla; pelvis; plexus; pyramid; reflex; retinopathy; rickets; segment; sinus; surface; threshold; transplantation; vein
renal cell: carcinoma
renal cortical: adenoma; lobule
renal fibrocystic: osteosis
renal papillary: necrosis
renal-splanchnic: steal
renal-splenic venous: shunt
renal tubular: acidosis
reniform: pelvis
renin-angiotensin: system
renovascular: hypertension
reovirus-like: agent
reparative: dentistry
reparative giant cell: granuloma
repeat action: tablet
repetition: rate
repetition-compulsion: principle
repetitive: DNA
replacement: bone; fibrosis; therapy
replicative: form
reportable: disease
repressible: enzyme
repressor: gene
reproductive: assimilation; cycle; nucleus; system
required arch: length
resectoscope: sheath
reserve: air; force
reserve tooth: germ
reservoir: bag; host
residual: abscess; affinity; body; capacity; cleft; inhibition; inhibitor; lumen; ridge; schizophrenia; urine; volume
residual ovary: syndrome
resistance: factor; form; plasmid; pyrometer; thermometer
resistance-inducing: factor
resistance-transfer: episone; factor
resistant ovary: syndrome
resistive: movement
resolution: acuity
resolving: power
resonance: theory
resorcinol-HCl: test
resorption: lacuna

respirable: aerosol
respiration: rate
respirator: brain
respiratory: acidosis; airway; alkalosis; apparatus; arrhythmia; bronchiole; burst; capacity; center; chain; coefficient; enzyme; epithelium; frequency; hippus; insufficiency; lobule; metabolism; metal; mucosa; murmur; pause; pigment; pulse; quotient; region; scleroma; sound; system; tract
respiratory dead: space
respiratory distress: syndrome
respiratory exchange: ratio
respiratory minute: volume
respiratory syncytial: virus
respondent: behavior; conditioning
response: hierarchy
response-produced: cue
rest: area; bite; body; nitrogen; pain; position; relation; seat
restiform: body; eminence
resting: cell; saliva; stage
resting tidal: volume
resting wandering: cell
rest jaw: relation
restless: legs
restless legs: syndrome
restorative: dentistry
restorative dental: material
restored: cycle
restrained: beam
restriction: endonuclease; enzyme; site
restriction (fragment) length: polymorphism
restriction-site: polymorphism
restructured: cell
rest vertical: dimension
retained: menstruation; placenta; testis
retarded: dentition
rete: cord; cyst; peg; ridge
retention: area; arm; cyst; form; groove; jaundice; point; polyp; suture; vomiting
retentive: arm
retentive circumferential clasp: arm
retentive fulcrum: line
rete ovarian: cyst
reticular: cartilage; cell; degeneration; dystrophy; formation; fiber; lamina; layer; membrane; substance; tissue
reticular activating: system
recticular erythematous: mucinosis
reticularis: cell
recticulated: bone; corpuscle
reticulating: colliquation
reticulin: stain
reticuloendothelial: cell; system
reticulohistiocytic: granuloma
reticulospinal: tract
reticulum cell: sarcoma
retiform: cartilage; tissue
retinal: adaptation; asthenopia; camera; cone; detachment; disparity; dysplasia; embolism; fold; image
retinal anlage: tumor
retinocerebral: angiomatosis
retractile: testis
retraction: nystagmus; syndrome
retroactive: inhibition
retroauricular lymph: node
retrobulbar: abscess; anesthesia; neuritis
retrocecal: abscess; recess
retroceccal lymph: node
retrocedent: gout
rectrocochlear: deafness
retrocolic: spasm
retrocursive: absence
retrocuspid: papilla
retroduodenal: artery; fossa; recess
retroflex: fasciculus
retrogasserian: neurectomy; neurotomy
retrograde: amnesia; aortography; beat; block; chromatolysis; conduction; degeneration; embolism; hernia; intussusception; memory; menstruation; metamorphosis; urography
retrograde P: wave
retrohyoid: bursa
retrolinguinal: space
retrolental: fibroplasia
retrolenticular: limb
retromammary: mastitis
retromandibular: fossa; vein
retromolar: fossa; pad
retromylohyoid: space
retroperitoneal: fibrosis; hernia; space
retropharyngeal: abscess; space
retropharyngeal lymph: node
retropubic: hernia; space
retrospective: falsification
retrosternal: hernia
retrotarsal: fold
retrusive: occlusion
return: extrasystole
returning: cycle
reverberating: circuit
reverse: banding; bevel; curve; mutation; osmosis; transcriptase
reversed: anaphylaxis; astigmatism; coarctation; peristalsis; shunt
reversed paradoxical: pulse
reversed passive: anaphylaxis
reversed Prausnitz-Küstner: reaction
reversed reciprocal: rhythm
reverse Eck: fistula
reverse Kingsley: splint
reversible: amblyopia; calcinosis; colloid; decortication; hydrocolloid; pulpitis; reaction; shock
Rh: antigen
rhagiocrine: cell
Rh blocking: test
rhegmatogenous retinal: detachment
rhesus: disease
rheumatic: arteritis; carditis; chorea; diesase; endocarditis; fever; pericarditis; pneumonia; tetany; torticollis; valvulitis
rheumatic heart: disease
rheumatoid: arteritis; arthritis; disease; factor; nodule; spondylitis
Rh_0 (D) immune: globulin
rhinal: fissure; sulcus
Rh null: syndrome
Rhodesian: trypanosomiasis
Rhodesian malignant: theileriosis
rhombencephalic: isthmus
rhombencephalic gustatory: nucleus
rhombic: groove; lip
rhomboid: fossa; impression; ligament
rhomboidal: sinus
rhonchal: fremitus
rhus: dermatitis
Rhus toxicodendron: antigen
Rhus venenata: antigen
rhythm: method
rhythmic: chorea
rib: spreader
ribbon: arch
ribbon arch: appliance
riboflavin: deficiency; unit
ribosomal: ribonucleic acid
ribosome-lamella: complex
rice: itch; body
ricefield: fever
rice-Tween: agar
rice-water: stool
rickettsia: vaccine
rickettsial: pox
Rida: virus
rider's: bone; bursa; leg; muscle
ridge: extension; relation; resorption
riding: embolism

Rift Valley: fever
Rift Valley fever: virus
right anatomical structures (specific right structures are listed under the following): appendage; artery; atrium; auricle; bronchus; crus; duct; fissure; flexure; heart; ligament; lobe; margin; node; part; plate; valve; vein; ventricle
right axis: deviation
right fibrous: trigone
righting: reflex
right ovarian vein: syndrome
right-to-left: shunt
right ventricular: failure; hypoplasia
rigid: pupil
rinderpest: virus
ring: abscess; chromosome; compound; finger; ligament; pessary; scotoma; syringe; test; ulcer
ringed: hair
ring-like corneal: dystrophy
ring precipitin: test
ring-wall: lesion
ringworm: yaws
ripe: cataract
rise: time
risk: factor
risorius: muscle
ritualistic: behavior
river: blindness
RNA: virus
RNA tumor: virus
robertsonian: translocation
Rochelle: salt
Rocio viral: encephalitis
rock: fever
rocket: immunoelectrophoresis
Rocky Montain spotted: fever
Rocky Mountain spotted fever: vaccine
rod: achromatopsia; cell; disk; fiber; granule; monochromasy; myopathy; vision
rodent: ulcer
rod nuclear: cell
roentgen: ray; unit
rolandic: epilepsy
role: conflict
roll: sulfur; tube
roller: bandage
roll-tube: culture
Roman: fever
R-on-T: phenomenon
roof: nucleus; plate
room: temperature
root: abscess; amputation; apex; canal; caries; dehiscence; filament; foramen; resection; resorption; sheath; tip
root canal: file; orifice; plugger; restoration; spreader; therapy; treatment
root caries: index
root end: cyst; granuloma
rooting: reflex
rope: burn; flap
rosacea-like: tuberculid
rosanilin: dye
rose: cold; spot
rose bengal radioactive (^{131}I): test
rosette-forming: cell
Ross River: fever; virus
rostral: lamina; neuropore
rostral transtentorial: herniation
rostrate: pelvis
rotary: joint; vertigo
rotation: center; flap
rotational: axis; nystagmus
rotator: cuff; muscle
rotatory: joint; nystagmus; spasm; tic
rote: learning
rough: colony
rough-surfaced cytoplasmic: reticulum
rouleaux: formation
round: atelectasis; bur; eminence; foramen; ligament; pelvis; window
round cell: sarcoma
round pronator: muscle
RPR: test
R-R: interval
Rs: virus
RS-T: segment
rubber: dam; pelvis; tissue
rubber-bulb: syringe
rubber dam: clamp
rubber dam clamp: forceps
rubbing: alcohol
rubeanic acid: stain
rubella: cataract; retinopathy; virus
rubella HI: test
rubella virus: vaccine
rubeola: virus
rubrobulbar: tract
rubroreticular: tract
rubrospinal: decussation; tract
ruby: spot
rufous: albinism
rum: nose
runt: disease
rupial: syphilid
ruptured: disk
rural cutaneous: leishmaniasis
Russian: fly
Russian autumn: encephalitis
Russian autumn encephalitis: virus
Russian spring-summer: encephalitis
Russian spring-summer encephalitis: virus
Russian tick-borne: encephalitis
rusty: sputum
Rye: classification

S

S: antigen; factor; peptide; phase; potential; protein; unit; wave
saber, sabre: shin; tibia
sabot: heart
saburral: amaurosis
saccadic: movement
sacciform: recess
saccular: aneurysm; bronchiectasis; gland; nerve; spot
sacculated: aneurysm; pleurisy
sacral: anesthesia; canal; crest; flexure; foramen; ganglion; hiatus; horn; index; nerve; part; plexus; region; triangle; tuberosity; vein; vertebra
sacral lymph: node
sacral splanchnic: nerve
sacral venous: plexus
sacred: bone
sacroanterior: position
sacrococcygeal: disk; joint; junction
sacrodural: ligament
sacrogenital: fold
sacroiliac: articulation; joint
sacropelvic: surface
sacroposterior: position
sacrosciatic: notch
sacrospinous: ligament
sacrotransverse: position
sacrotuberous: ligament
saddle: back; embolism; head; joint; nose
saddle block: anesthesia
sadomasochistic: relationship
safe: period
safety: lens; spectacles
sagittal: axis; border; crest; fontanel; groove; line; plane; section; sulcus; suture
sagittal split mandibular: osteotomy
sago: spleen
Saigon: cinnamon
sail: sound
sailor's: skin
Saint: see also St.
Saint Anthony's: dance

Saint Ignatius': itch
Saint John's: dance
Saint Vitus': dance
sakushu: fever
salaam: attack; convulsion; spasm
salicylic acid: collodion
saline: agglutin; purgative; solution; water
Salisbury common cold: virus
saliva: ejector; pump
salivary: calculus; colic; corpuscle; digestion; duct; fistula; gland; virus
salivary gland: hormone; virus
salivary gland virus: disease
salmon: disease; patch; poisoning
Salmonella food: poisoning
salpingopalatine: fold
salpingopharyngeal: fold; muscle
salt: action; depletion; dye; edema; fever; loading; poisoning; sensitivity; solution; wasting
saltatory: chorea; conduction; evolution; spasm
salt depletion: syndrome
salted: plasma; serum
salt-losing: nephritis
salt water: boil; soap
salvage: chemotherapy
sand: bath; body; tumor
sandal: foot
sandal strap: dermatitis
sandfly: fever
sandfly fever: virus
sandpaper: disk; gallbladder
sandworm: disease
sanguineous: cyst
sanious: pus
San Joaquin: fever
San Miguel sea lion: virus
Sao Paulo: fever
saphenous: nerve; opening; vein
saponification: number
sarcogenic: cell
sarcoidal: granuloma
sarcomatoid: carcinoma
sarcoplasmic: reticulum
sarcoptic: acariasis; mange
sartorius: bursa
satellite: abscess; cell; DNA; metastasis
satellite-rich: heterochromatin
satiety: center
saturated: color; fat; fatty acid; hydrocarbon; solution
saturation: analysis; index
saturnine: colic; encephalopathy; gout; tremor
saucer-shaped: cataract
sausage: finger
Savage: syndrome
S-BP: line
scabbard: trachea
scalded skin: syndrome
scalene: tubercle
scalenus-anticus: syndrome
scalp: contusion; infection; laceration; muscle
scalpriform: incisor
scaly: leg; ringworm; tetter
scamping: speech
scanning: speech
scanning electron: microscope
scaphoid: abdomen; bone; fossa; scapula; tuberosity
scapular: line; notch; reflex; region
scapulocostal: syndrome
scapulohumeral: atrophy; reflex
scapuloperiosteal: reflex
scar: cancer; carcinoma
scarf: bandage
scarification: test
scarlatinal: nephritis
scarlatiniform: erythema
scarlet: fever
scarlet fever: antitoxin
scarlet fever erythrogenic: toxin
scattered: radiation
scavenger: cell
scent: gland
schematic: eye
schindyletic: joint
schistosome: dermatitis; granuloma
schizencephalic: microcephaly
schizo-affective: psychosis
shizoid: personality
schizophreniform: disorder
schizotypical: personality
schneiderian: membrane
school: phobia
sciatic: foramen; hernia; nerve; neuralgia; neuritis; plexus; scoliosis; spine
scimitar: sign
scintillating: scotoma
scintillation: counter
scirrhous: carcinoma
scissor: gait
scleral: ectasia; resection; rigidity; ring; roll; spur; staphyloma; vein
scleral buckling: operation
sclerocorneal: junction
sclerocystic: disease
sclerosing: adenosis; agent; hamangioma; inflammation; keratitis; mastoiditis; osteitis; therapy
sclerotic: body; coat; dentin; gastritis; kidney; stomach, tooth
sclerotic cemental: mass
scoliotic: pelvis
scombroid: poisoning
scotopic: adaptation; eye; perimetry; vision
scout: roentgenogram
scratch: reflex; test
screen: defense; memory
screening: audiometry; test
screw: artery; elevator; joint
screwdriver: tooth
scrivener's: palsy
scrofulous: keratitis; ophthalmia; rhinitis
scroll: bone; ear
scrotal: artery; hernia; raphe; septum; swelling; tongue; vein
scrub: nurse; typhus
scurvy: rickets
sea: scurvy
sea-blue: histiocyte
sea-blue histiocyte: disease
sea gull: murmur
sealed jar: technique
seal-fin: deformity
seamstress's: cramp
sea urchin: granuloma
sebaceous: adenoma; cyst; epithelioma; follicle; gland; horn; tubercle
seborrheic: blepharitis; dermatitis; dermatosis; eczema; keratosis; verruca; wart
Sebright bantam: syndrome
second: finger; incisor; law; messenger; molar; sight; tooth
secondary: adhesion; aerodontalgia; agammaglobulinemia; alcohol; aldosteronism; amenorrhea; amputation; amyloidosis; anesthetic; anophthalmus; atelectasis; axis; buffer; calcium; carcinoma; cardiomyopathy; caries; cartilage; cataract; cementum; center; choana; coccidioidomyocosis; constriction; degeneration; dementia; dentin; dentition; deviation; dextrocardia; digestion; disease; drive; dysmenorrhea; elaboration; encephalitis; failure; fissure; follicle; gain; glaucoma; gout; hemochromatosis; hemorrhage; host; hydrocephalus; hyperparathyroidism; hyperthyroidism; hypogammaglobulinemia; hypogonadism; hypothyroidism; im-

secondary—*continued*
munodeficiency; infection; lysosome; mesoderm; metaplasia; methemoglobinemia; narcissism; nodule; nondisjunction; oocyte; palate; pellagra; point; process; proteose; pyoderma; ray; reinforcement; retinitis; saturation; screwworm; spermatocyte; suture; syphilid; syphilis; thrombus; tuberculosis; union; villus; vitreous
secondary abdominal: pregnancy
secondary adrenocortical: insufficiency
secondary antibody: deficiency
secondary egg: membrane
secondary generalized: epilepsy
secondary interatrial: foramen
secondary medical: care
secondary pulmonary: lobule
secondary refractory: anemia
secondary renal: calculus
secondary renal tubular: acidosis
secondary sensory: cortex; nucleus
secondary sex: character
secondary spiral: plate
secondary tympanic: membrane
secondary visual: area; cortex
secondary X: zone
second cranial: nerve
second cuneiform: bone
second degree: burn
second gas: effect
second-look: operation
second-order: conditioning
second parallel pelvic: plane
second signalling: system
second temporal: convolution
second tibial: muscle
secretin: test
secretor: factor
secretory: canaliculus; carcinoma; cyst; duct; granule; nerve; otitis
sectional: impression; roentgenography
sector: iridectomy
sedimentary: cataract
sedimentation: constant; rate
seed: corn
seesaw: murmur; nystagmus
segmental: anesthesia; artery; bronchus; fracture; glomerulonephritis; neuritis; neuropathy; plate; sphincter; zone
segmental alveolar: osteotomy
segmentation: cavity; nucleus
segmented: cell; leukocyte; neutrophil
segmenting: body
segregation: analysis; ratio
Seidlitz powder: test
selection: coefficient; pressure
selective: angiography; grinding; hypoaldosteronism; inattention; inhibition; medium; memory; stain
selenium: poisoning
self: concept
self-curing: resin
self-registering: thermometer
self-retaining: catheter
semantic: aphasia
semicircular: canal; duct
semiclosed: anesthesia; circle; line
semidirect: lead
semihorizontal: heart
semilente: insulin
semilunar: bone; cartilage; fascia; fasciculus; fibrocartilage; fold; ganglion; hiatus; line; notch; nucleus; valve
semilunar conjunctival: fold
semimembranosus: muscle
semimembranosus and semitendinosus: reflex
seminal: capsule; colliculus; duct; fluid; gland; granule; hillock; lake; vesicle
seminiferous: epithelium; tubercle
seminiferous tubule: dysgenesis
semi-open: anesthesia
semioval: center
semipermeable: membrane
semipolar: bond
semiprone: position
semispinal: muscle
semisulfur: mustard
semitendinous: muscle
semivertical: heart
Seneca: snakeroot
senegal: gum
senile: amyloidosis; arteriosclerosis; atrophoderma; atrophy; cataract; chorea; degeneration; delirium; dementia; deterioration; dwarfism; ectasia; elastosis; emphysema; fibroma; gangrene; halo; hemangioma; involution; keratoderma; keratoma; keratosis; lentigo; melanoderma; memory; nephrosclerosis; osteomalacia; paraplegia; plaque; psychosis; retinoschisis; tremor; vaginitis; wart
senile dental: caries
senile guttate: choroidopathy
senile hip: disease
senile lenticular: myopia
senile sebaceous: hyperplasia
senior: synonym
Sennetsu: fever
sensation: time
sense: organ
sense of: identity
sensible: heat; perspiration; temperature
sensitivity training: group
sensitized: antigen; cell; culture
sensitizing: dose; injection; substance
sensorial: area; idiocy
sensorimotor: area; theory
sensorineural: deafness
sensory: amblyopia; amusia; aphasia; area; cortex; crossway; decussation; deprivation; epilepsy; ganglion; image; inattention; nerve; neuronopathy; paralysis; receptor; root; tract; urgency
sensory precipitated: epilepsy
sensory speech: center
sentinel: animal; gland; pile; tag
sentinel spinous process: fracture
separating: medium; wire
separation: anxiety
septal: area; artery; bone; cartilage; cell; cusp; gingiva
septate: hymen; mycelium; uterus
septic: abortion; endocarditis; fever; infarct; intoxication; phlebitis; pneumonia; retinitis; shock
septicemic: abscess; plague
septic sore: throat
septomarginal: fasciculus; trabecula; tract
septo-optic: dysplasia
sequence: hypothesis
sequential multichannel: autoanalyzer
"sequential" oral: contraceptive
sequestration: cyst; dermoid
serial: extraction; roentgenography; section
serine: carboxypeptidase
serofibrinous: inflammation; pleurisy
seromucous: cell; gland
serous: apoplexy; atrophy; cell; coat; cyst; diarrhea; demilune; gland; hemorrhage; inflammation; iritis; ligament; membrane; meningitis; otitis; pleurisy; retinitis; synovitis; tunic
serpent: ulcer
serpentine: aneurysm
serpiginous: choroidopathy; keratitis; ulcer

serrate: suture
serum: accelerator; accident; agar; agglutinin; albumin; disease; eruption; hepatitis; nephritis; rash; reaction; shock; sickness; therapy
serum accelerator: globulin
serumal: calculus
serum hepatitis: virus
serum prothrombin conversion: accelerator
sesamoid: bone; cartilage
sessile: hydatid; polyp
seton: operation; wound
setting: expansion
seven-day: fever
seventh: sense
seventh-cranial: nerve
seven-year: itch
severe combined: immunodeficiency
sewer: gas
sewing: spasm
sex: cell; chromatin; chromosome; cord; determination; factor; hormone; linkage; object; ratio; reversal; role; skin
sex chromosome: imbalance
sex-influenced: inheritance
sex-limited: inheritance
sex-linked: character; gene; inheritance; locus
sexual: deviation; dimorphism; dwarfism; dysfunction; generation; gland; infantilism; instinct; intercourse; life; neurasthenia; perversion; potency; reproduction; selection
sexually transmitted: disease
shadow: cell; corpuscle; nucleus; test
shaggy: chorion; pericardium
shagreen: patch; skin
shake: culture; test
shaking: palsy
shallow: breathing
sham: feeding; rage
sham-movement: vertigo
shank: bone
sharp: spoon
shave: biopsy
shaving: cramp
shawl: muscle
shear: flow; rate; stress; thinning
shearing: edge
sheath: ligament; process
sheathed: artery
sheep: bots
sheep-pox: virus
shelf: procedure
shell: nail; shock
shellac: base
shell nail: syndrome
sherry: wine
shifting: dullness; pacemaker
shilling: scar
shimamushi: disease
shin: bone; splint
ship: fever
shipping: fever
shirt-stud: abscess
shock: antigen; index; lung; therapy; treatment
shocking: dose
shoe: boil
shoe dye: dermatitis
Shope: fibroma
Shope fibroma: virus
short: bone; chain; gyrus; head; process; root; sight; vinculum
short abductor: muscle
short adductor: muscle
short central: artery
short ciliary: nerve
shortening: reaction
short extensor: muscle
short fibular: muscle
short flexor: muscle
short gastric: artery; vein
short incubation: hepatitis
short palmar: muscle
short peroneal: muscle
short posterior ciliary: artery
short radial extensor: muscle
short saphenous: nerve; vein
short-term: memory
short-term exposure: limit
short-wave: diathermy
shotgun: prescription
shot-silk: phenomenon; reflex; retina
shotted: suture
shoulder: bursitis; girdle; joint; presentation
shoulder-girdle: syndrome
shoulder-hand: syndrome
shut-in: personality
SI: unit
Siamese: twins
sibilant: rale
sibling: rivalry
sicca: complex; syndrome
sick: headache; role
sickle: cell; flap; form; scotoma
sickle cell: anemia; crisis; dactylitis; disease; hemoglobin; retinopathy; test; trait
sickle cell-thalassemia: disease
sick sinus: syndrome
side: chain
side-: effect
side-chain: theory
sideratic: cataract
sideroachrestic: anemia
sideroblastic: anemia
sideropenic: dysphagia
siderotic: nodule
sieve: bone; graft; plate
sigma: effect; peptide
sigmoid: artery; colon; flexure; fossa; groove; notch; sinus; sulcus; vein
sigmoid lymph: node
sigmoidovesical: fistula
sign: blindness
signal: node
signet: ring
signet ring: cell
signet ring cell: carcinoma
silent: allele; area; electrode; gap; gallstone; ischemia; mutant; mutation; period
silent myocardial: infarction
silicate: cement; restoration
silicon: granuloma
siliculose, siliquose: cataract
silo-filler's: disease
silver: cell; cone; point; poisoning; stain
silver-ammoniacal silver: stain
silver fork: deformity; fracture
silverized: catgut
silver protein: stain
silver-tin: alloy
Simbu: virus
simian: crease; fissure; malaria; virus
simian vacuolating: virus
simple: absence; acne; anchorage; beam; color; conjunctivitis; diplopia; dislocation; epithelium; fission; fracture; glaucoma; goiter; heterochromia; hypertrophy; joint; lipid; lobule; lymphangiectasis; mastectomy; microscope; myopia; necrosis; obesity; protein; retinitis; schizophrenia; ulcer; urethritis
simple hyperopic: astigmatism
simple membranous: limb
simple myopic: astigmatism
simple pulmonary: eosinophilia
simple skull: fracture
simple squamous: epithelium
simulated: hypertrophy
simultaneous: contrast; perception
sincipital: presentation
Sindbis: fever; virus
singer's: node; nodule

single: ascertainment; bond; immunodiffusion; microscope
single (gel) diffusion precipitin: test
single photon emission computed: tomography
single-stranded nucleate: endonuclease
singlet: oxygen; state
sinoatrial: block; node
sinoatrial conduction: time
sinoatrial recovery: time
sinoauricular: block
sinuatrial: chamber
sinus: arrest; arrhythmia; barotrauma; block; bradycardia; histiocytosis; nerve; node; pause; phlebitis; reflex; rhythm; septum; standstill; tachycardia; tubercle
sinusoidal: capillary
sinuvertebral: nerve
SISI: text
sister chromatid: exchange
situation: anxiety
situational: psychosis; test
sitz: bath
sixth: disease; sense; ventricle
sixth cranial: nerve
sixth venereal: disease
sixth-year: molar
skein: cell
skeletal: extension; muscle; system; traction
skeletal muscle: fiber; tissue
skeleton: hand
skew: deviation; form
skim, skimmed: milk
skin: botfly; dose; flap; graft; groove; heart; reaction; reflex; ridge; stone; tag; test; traction
skinbound: disease
skin-muscle: reflex
skinnerian: conditioning
skin-puncture: test
skin-pupillary: reflex
skin-window: technique
skip: area
skipped: generation
skodiac: resonance
skull: fracture
slab-off: lens
slaked: lime
slant: culture
slaty: anemia
sleep: apnea; dissociation; drunkenness; epilepsy; paralysis; spindle
sleep-induced: apnea
sleeping: sickness
sleeve: graft
slender: fasciculus; lobule; process
slew: rate
slide: micrometer
sliding: flap; hernia; hook
sliding esophageal hiatal: hernia
sliding filament: hypothesis
sliding hiatal: hernia
sliding oblique: osteotomy
slime: fungus
sling: psychrometer
slipped: hernia; tendon
slipped tendon: disease
slipping: patella; rib
slipping rib: cartilage
slit: pore
slit ventricle: syndrome
slope: culture
slotted: attachment
sloughing: phagedena; ulcer
slow: combustion; fever; virus
slow channel-blocking: agent
slow-reacting: factor; substance
slow virus: disease
SLR: factor
sludged: blood
sluggish: layer
slurring: speech
Sm: antigen
small: artery; calorie; canal; intestine; pancreas; pelvis; trochanter; vein
small cardiac: vein
small cell: carcinoma
small cleaved: cell
small deep petrosal: nerve
smaller: muscle
smaller pectoral: muscle
smaller posterior straight: muscle
smaller psoas: muscle
smallest cardiac: vein
smallest scalene: muscle
smallest splanchnic: nerve
small increment sensitivity: index
small interarch: distance
small lymphocytic: lymphoma
smallpox: vaccine; virus
small pudendal: lip
small saphenous: vein
small sciatic: nerve
smear: culture
smell: blindness
smelling: salt
smoker's: patch; tongue
smoker's respiratory: syndrome
smooth: broach; chorion; colony; diet; leprosy; muscle
smooth muscle: relaxant; tissue
smooth muscular: sphincter
smooth surface: carrier
smooth-surfaced endoplasmic: reticulum
smudge: cell
S-N: line
S-N-A: angle
snail: fever
snap: finger
snapping: hip; reflex
S-N-B: angle
sneezing: gas
snout: reflex
snow: blindness; conjunctivitis
snowball: opacity
snowshoe hare: virus
snub-nose: dwarfism
soapsuds: enema
social: adaptation; control; disease; instinct; intelligence; maladjustment; psychiatry; therapy
socialized: medicine
social network: therapy
sociometric: distance
socket: joint
socotrine: aloe
sodium: pump
sodium-potassium: pump
sodium-responsive periodic: paralysis
soft: cataract; chancre; corn; diet; palate; papilloma; part; pulse; ray; soap; sore; sulfur; tubercle; ulcer; wart; water
solar: blindness; cheilitis; dermatitis; energy; fever; ganglion; keratosis; plexus; retinopathy; urticaria
soldier's: heart; patch
sole: nucleus; plate; reflex
soleal: line
sole-plate: ending
sole tap: reflex
soleus: muscle
solid: edema
solid phase: immunoassay
solitary: bundle; follicle; foramen; gland; nodule; tract
solitary bone: cyst
solitary osteocartilaginous: exostosis
solubility: test
soluble: antigen; glass; ligature; ribonucleic acid; soap; starch; tartar
soluble gun: cotton
soluble specific: substance
solution: pressure
solvent: drag; ether; inhalation
somatic: agglutinin; antigen; artery; cell; crossing-over; death; delu-

sion; layer; mesoderm; mitosis; mutation; nerve; nucleus; reproduction; swallow; teniasis
somatic cell: genetics; hybridization
somatic motor: neuron; nucleus
somatic mutation: theory
somatic sensory: cortex
somatization: disorder
somatoform: disorder
somatosensory: cortex
somatotropic: hormone
somatotropin release-inhibiting: factor
somatotropin-releasing: factor
somesthetic: area; system
somite: cavity
somitic: mesoderm
somnambulic: epilepsy
somnambulistic: trance
sonic: scaler; wave
sonomotor: response
sonorous: rale
soot: wart
sore: mouth; shin; throat
soremouth: virus
soul: pain
sound pressure: level
South African tick-bite: fever
South African type: porphyria
South American: blastomycosis; trypanosomiasis
Southern blot: analysis
space: maintainer; medicine; myopia; nerve; retainer; sense
spaced: teeth (see tooth)
spade: finger; hand
spallation: product
Spanish: fly
Spanish: influenza
sparing: action
spasmodic: apoplexy; asthma; diathesis; dysmenorrhea; laryngitis; mydriasis; stricture; tic; torticollis
spasmophilic: diathesis
spastic: abasia; anemia; aphonia; diplegia; ectropion; entropion; gait; hemiplegia; ileus; miosis; mydriasis; paraplegia; speech; syndrome
spastic flat: foot
spastic spinal: paralysis
spatial: acuity; formula; localization; vector; vectorcardiography
spatula: needle
special: anatomy; hospital; sensation; sense
specialized: transduction
special somatic afferent: column
special visceral efferent: column; nucleus
species: tolerance
specific: absorbance; action; activity; anergy; antiserum; antigen; bactericide; cause; cholinesterase; compliance; disease; epithet; extinction; gravity; heat; hemolysin; immunity; opsonin; parasite; reaction; rotation; serum; transduction; urethritis
specific absorption: coefficient
specific active: immunity
specific capsular: substance
specific dynamic: action
specific soluble: polysaccharide; sugar
spectacle: eye; plane
spectral: phonocardiograph; sensitivity
specular: glare; image; reflector
speculum: forceps
speech: audiogram; audiometer; audiometry; bulb; center; pathology
sperm: aster; cell; crystal; nucleus
spermacytic: seminoma
spermatic: cork; duct; filament; fistula; plexus; vein
sphagnum: moss
sphenoethmoidal: recess; suture; synchondrosis
sphenofrontal: suture
sphenoid: angle; bone; crest; process
sphenoidal: border; concha; fissure; fontanel; herniation; part; sinus; spine
sphenoidal sinus: aperture
sphenoidal turbinated: bone
sphenomandibular: ligament
sphenomaxillary: fissure; fossa; suture
sphenooccipital: joint; suture
sphenoorbital: suture
sphenopalatine: artery; foramen; ganglion; neuralgia; notch
sphenoparietal: sinus; suture
sphenopetrosal: fissure; synchondrosis
sphenosquamous: suture
sphenotic: center; foramen
sphenovomerine: suture
sphenozygomatic: suture
spherical: aberration; amalgam; lens; nucleus; recess
spherical form of: occlusion
spherocylindrical: lens
spherocytic: anemia; jaundice
spheroid: articulation; colony; joint
spherophakia-brachymorphia: syndrome
sphincter: muscle
sphincteroid: tract
sphingomyelin: lipidosis
sphygmic: interval
spica: bandage
spider: angioma; cancer; cell; finger; mole; nevus; pelvis; telangiectasia
spigelian: hernia
spike: potential
spike and wave: complex
spinach: stool
spinal: analgesia; anesthesia; anesthetic; angiography; apoplexy; arteriography; ataxia; atrophy; block; canal; column; concussion; cord; curvature; decompression; fusion; ganglion; headache; induction; marrow; muscle; nerve; nucleus; paralysis; part; point; puncture; pyramidotomy; quotient; reflex; root; shock; sign; stroke; tap; tract; tractotomy; vein
spinal accessory: nerve
spindle: cataract; cell; fiber
spindle cell: carcinoma; lipoma; nevus; sarcoma
spindle-celled: layer
spindle-shaped: muscle
spine: cell; sign
spinning disk: nebulizer
spino-adductor: reflex
spinocerebellar: tract
spinoglenoid: ligament
spinoolivary: tract
spinotectal: tract
spinothalamic: cordotomy; tract; tractotomy
spinous: layer; process
spiral: artery; bandage; crest; canal; fold; fracture; ganglion; groove; hypha; joint; ligament; line; membrane; organ; plate; prominence; septum; suture; tubule; valve; vein
spiral bulbar: septum
spiral foraminous: tract
spiral tip: catheter
spirillar: dysentery
spirillum: fever
spirit: lamp; thermometer
spirituous: liquor
spiro-: index
spironolactone: test
spiruroid: larva migrans
splanchnesthetic: sensibility

splanchnic: anesthesia; cavity; ganglion; layer; mesoderm; nerve; wall
spleen: deoxyribonuclease; endonuclease; phosphodiesterase
splenial: gyrus
splenic: anemia; apoplexy; artery; cell; cord; corpuscle; flexure; index; leukemia; plexus pulp; recess; sinus; vein; venography
splenic flexure: syndrome
splenic lymph: follicle; node; nodule
splenic portal: venography
splenius: muscle
splenorenal: ligament; shunt
splint: bone
splinted: abutment
splinter: hemorrhage
splintered: fracture
split: brain; fat; gene; hand; papule; pelvis; tolerance
split cast: method; mounting
split renal function: test
split-skin: graft
split-thickness: flap; graft
splitting: enzyme
Spondweni: virus
spondyloepiphysial: dysplasia
spondylolisthetic: pelvis
sponge: biopsy; tent
spongiform: encephalopathy; pustule
spongiose: part
spongy: body; bone; degeneration; iritis; spot; substance; urethra
spontaneous: abortion; agglutination; amputation; correction; combustion; evolution; fracture; gangrene; generation; mutation; phagocytosis; pneumothorax; recovery; remission; version
spontaneous cephalic: delivery
spontaneous intermittent mandatory: ventilation
spoon: nail
sporadic bovine: leukosis
sporotrichositic: chancre
sports: medicine
spot: test
spot-film: roentgenography
spotted: fever; sickness
spreading: depression; factor
spring: conjunctivitis; finger; lancet; ligament; ophthalmia
springing: mydriasis
spurious: ankylosis; cast; meningocele; pregnancy; torticollis
sputum: smear
squamocolumnar: junction
squamomastoid: suture
squamoparietal: suture
squamotympanic: fissure
squamous: cell; margin; metaplasia; pearl; suture
squamous cell: carcinoma
squamous odontogenic: tumor
square wave: stimulus
squint: hook
squinting: eye
squirrel: porphyria
squirrel plague: conjunctivitis
ST: junction; segment
St.: see also Saint
St. Louis encephalitis: virus
stab: cell; culture; drain; neutrophil; wound
stabilized: baseplate
stabilizing circumferential clasp: arm
stabilizing fulcrum: line
stable: colloid; equilibrium; factor; fracture; isotope
staccato: speech
staff: cell
stag-horn: calculus
stagnant: anoxia; hypoxia
stagnation: mastitis
staircase: phenomenon
stalked: hydatid
standard: atmosphere; bicarbonate; cell; deviation; lead; pressure; score; solution; temperature; volume
standard error of: difference; mean
standard serologic: test
standard urea: clearance
standby pulse: generator
standing: test
standing plasma: test
stapedial: artery; fold; membrane
stapedius: muscle
stapes: mobilization
stapes mobilization: operation
staphylococcal: enterotoxin; pneumonia
staphylococcal scalded skin: syndrome
staphylococcus: antitoxin; vaccine
staphylococcus food: poisoning
staphylo-opsonic: index
starch: equivalent; glycerite; gum; sugar
starch-iodine: test
starting: friction
startle: epilepsy; reaction; reflex
starvation: diabetes
stasis: cirrhosis; dermatitis; eczema; ulcer
state: hospital
state-dependent: learning
static: arthropathy; ataxia; compliance; convulsion; friction; gangrene; hysteresis; infantilism; medicine; perimetry; reflex; refraction; relation; scoliosis; sense; system; tremor
static bone: cyst
station: test
stationary: anchorage; cataract; phase
statistical: genetics
statoconial: membrane
statokinetic: reflex
statotonic: reflex
steady: state
steal: phenomenon
steam: cauterization; cautery
steam-fitter's: asthma
steeple: skull
stellate: abscess; block; cataract; cell; fracture; ganglion; hair; ligament; reticulum; retinopathy; vein; venule
stellate skull: fracture
stem: bronchus; cell
stem cell: leukemia
stenopeic, stenopaic: disk; iridectomy; spectacles
stenosal: murmur
stenoxous: parasite
steppage: gait
stepping: reflex
stercoraceous: vomiting
stercoral: abscess; appendicitis; fistula; ulcer
sterculia: gum
stereochemical: formula; isomerism
stereoscopic: acuity; microscope; parallax; pelvimetry; vision
stereotactic, stereotaxic: cordotomy; instrument; localization; surgery
sterile: abscess; cyst
sterile insect: technique
sternal: angle; artery; bar; cartilage; extremity; joint; line; membrane; muscle; notch; part; plane; puncture; synchondrosis
sternal articular: surface
sternobrachial: reflex
sternochondroscapular: muscle
sternoclavicular: angle; disk; joint; ligament; muscle
sternocleidomastoid: muscle; region; vein

sternocostal: articulation; joint; ligament; part; surface; triangle
sternohyoid: muscle
sternomastoid: artery; muscle
sternopericardial: ligament
sternothyroid: muscle
sternutatory; absence
steroid: acne; diabetes; fever; hormone; nucleus; ulcer
steroid metabolic clearance: rate
steroid production: rate
steroid secretory: rate
steroid withdrawal: syndrome
stethoscopic: phonocardiograph
stichochrome: cell
stiff: neck; toe
stiff lamb: disease
stiff-man: syndrome
stifle: bone; joint
still: layer
stillbirth: rate
stillborn: infant
stimulus: control; generalization; substitution; threshold
stimulus sensitive: myoclonus
stippled: epiphysis; tongue
stitch: abscess
stock: culture; strain; vaccine
Stockholm: syndrome
stocking: anesthesia
stoker's: cramp
stomach: ache; cough; drops; pump; reefing; tooth; tube; worm
stomal: ulcer
stomatognathic: system
stone: basket; heart
stone-manson's: disease
stop-: needle; speculum
storage: disease; oscilloscope
storiform: neurofibroma
strabismic: amblyopia; nystagmus
straddling: embolism
straight: gyrus; jacket; part; sinus; tubule; venule
straight back: syndrome
strain: fracture; gauge
strait: jacket
strangulated: hernia
strap: cell; muscle
stratified: epithelium; thrombus
stratified ciliated columnar: epithelium
stratified squamous: epithelium
stratiform: fibrocartilage
stratographic: analysis
straw: itch
straw-bed: itch
strawberry: birthmark; gallbladder; mark; nevus; tongue
strawberry-cream: blood
streak: culture; hyperostosis
streaked: gonad
streaming: movement
street: virus
strength-duration: curve
streptococcal: fibrinolysin; pneumonia
streptococcus erythrogenic: toxin
Streptococcus lactis R: factor
Streptococcus M: antigen
streptomycin: unit
stress: fracture; immunity; inoculation; reaction; ulcer
stress-bearing: area
stress-strain: curve
stretch: receptor; reflex
striate: area; body; cortex; keratopathy; vein
striated: border; duct; membrane; muscle
striated muscular: sphincter
string: test
stringed instrument: theory
stripped: atom
stripper's: asthma
stroboscopic: disk; microscope
stroke: output; volume
stroke work: index
stroma: plexus
stromal: hyperthecosis
strong silver: protein
structural: formula; gene; interface; isomerism
struvite: calculus
stuck: finger
stump: cancer; hallucination; neuralgia
stuporous: catatonia
stuttering: urination
Stuttgart: disease
styloauricular: muscle
styloglossus: muscle
stylohyoid: ligament; muscle
styloid: cornu; process; prominence
stylomandibular: ligament
stylomastoid: artery; foramen; vein
stylomaxillary: ligament
stylopharyngeal: muscle
styloradial: reflex
stylus: tracing
"s"-type: cholinesterase
stypic: collodion; colloid; cotton
subacromial: bursa; bursitis
subacute: abscess; glomerulonephritis; hepatitis; inflammation; nephritis; rheumatism
subacute bacterial: endocarditis
subacute combined: degeneration
subacute granulomatous: thyroiditis
subacute inclusion body: encephalitis
subacute migratory: panniculitis
subacute necrotizing: myelitis
subacute sclerosing: leukoencephalitis; panencephalitis
subacute spongiform: encephalopathy
subadventitial: fibrosis
subanconeus: muscle
subaortic: stenosis
subaortic lymph: node
subapical: segment
subarachnoid: anesthesia; cistern; cavity; hemorrhage; space
subarcuate: fossa
subareolar duct: papillomatosis
subastragalar: amputation
subcallosal: area; fasciculus; gyrus
subcapital: fracture
subcapsular: cataract
subcecal: fossa
subchorial: lake; space
subclavian: artery; duct; groove; loop; muscle; nerve; plexus; steal; sulcus; triangle; trunk; vein
subclavian steal: syndrome
subclinical: absence; diabetes
subcommissural: organ
subconscious: memory; mind
subcorneal pustular: dermatitis; dermatosis
subcortical arteriosclerotic: encephalopathy
subcostal: artery; groove; line; muscle; nerve; plane
subcrepitant: rale
subcrestal: pocket
subcrural: muscle
subcutaneous: bursa; emphysema; flap; implantation; mastectomy; myiasis; operation; part; ring; tenotomy; tissue; transfusion; vein
subcutaneous calcaneal: bursa
subcutaneous fat: necrosis
subcutaneous infrapatellar: bursa
subcuticular: suture
subdeltoid: bursa; bursitis
subdiaphragmatic: abscess; pyopneumothorax
subdigastric: node

subdural: cavity; hematoma; hemorrhage; hematorrachis; space
subendocardial: layer
subendocardial myocardial: infarction
subendothelial: layer
subepidermal: abscess
subfalcial: herniation
subfascial prepatellar: bursa
subgaleal: emphysema; hemorrhage
subgerminal: cavity
subgingival: calculus; curettage; space
subhepatic: recess
subhyoid: bursa
subinguinal: fossa; triangle
subjective; fremitus; psychology; sensation; sign; symptom; synonym; vision
sublenticular: limb
subleukemic: leukemia; myelosis
sublimed: sulfur
subliminal: self; stimulus; thirst
sublingual: artery; crescent; cyst; fold; fossa; ganglion; gland; nerve; pit; tablet; vein
submammary: mastitis
submandibular: duct; fossa; ganglion; gland; triangle
submandibular lymph: node
submaxillary: duct; fossa; ganglion; gland; triangle
submental: artery; triangle; vein
submental lymph: node
submental vertex: roentgenogram
submerged: tonsil
submetacentric: chromosome
submucosal: implant; plexus
subnasal: point
subneural: apparatus
suboccipital: decompression; muscle; nerve; neuralgia; neuritis; triangle
suboccipital venous: plexus
suboccipitobregmatic: diameter
suboccluding: ligature
subocclusal: surface
subpapillary: layer; network
subparietal: sulcus
subpellicular: fibril; mirotubule
subperiodic: periodicity
subperiosteal: abscess; amputation; fracture; implant
subperitoneal: appendicitis; fascia
subphrenic: abscess; pyopneumothorax; recess
subplasmalemmal dense: zone
subpopliteal: recess
subpubic: angle
subquadricipital: muscle
subsartorial: canal
subscapular: artery; bursa; fossa; muscle; nerve
subscapular lymph: node
subseptate: uterus
subserous: plexus
subsidiary atrial: pacemaker
substance: abuse
substance abuse: disorder
substernal: angle; goiter
substitution: product; therapy; transfusion
substitutive: therapy
subsuperior: segment
subsurface: cisterna
subtalar: joint
subtemporal: decompression
subtendinous: bursa
subtendinous iliac: bursa
subtendinous prepatellar: bursa
subthalamic: nucleus
subthreshold: stimulus
subtotal: hysterectomy
subungual: abscess; melanoma
subunit: vaccine
subvalvular: stenosis
subvocal: speech
succedaneous: dentition; tooth
succenturiate: placenta
successive: contrast
succinic acid: cycle
sucking: cushion; louse; pad; wound
suckling: reflex
sucrose hemolysis: test
suction: cup; drainage; ophthalmodynamometer; plate
suctorial: pad
sudanophobic: zone
sudden death: syndrome
sudden infant death: syndrome
sudomotor: fiber
sudoriferous: duct; gland
sudoriparous: abscess
suffocating: gas
suffocative: goiter
sugar: alcohol; cataract; tumor
sugar of: lead
sugar-coated: spleen
sugar-icing: liver
suggestive: psychotherapy; therapeutics
suicide: gesture
sulcal: artery
sulcomarginal: tract
sulcular: epithelium; fluid
sulcus: chancre
sulfate: respiration; water
sulfatide: lipidosis
sulfation: factor
sulfonium: ion
sulfosalicylic acid turbidity: test
sulfur: mustard; water
sulfurated: lime; potash
sulfureted: hydrogen
summation: beat; gallop
summer: asthma; disease; itch; prurigo; rash; sore
sump: drain; syndrome
sun: stroke
sun protection: factor
superciliary: arch; ridge
superfatted: soap
superficial: angioma; burn; cleavage; ectoderm; fascia; head; implantation; layer; part; reflex; tonsillitis; vein
superficial anatomical structures (specific superficial structures are listed under the following): arch; artery; ligament; muscle; nerve; node; plexus; ring; vein; vessel
superficial inguinal: pouch
superficial linear: keratitis
superficial punctate: keratitis
superficial pustular: perifolliculitis
superficial spreading: melanoma
superimposed: eclampsia; preeclampsia
superior: bursa; laryngotomy; paraplegia; polioencephalitis
superior anatomical structures (specific superior structures are listed under the following): angle; arch; area; arteriole; artery; articulation; border; brachium; colliculus; concha; convolution; extremity; fascia; fasciculus; fissure; fold; flexure; fossa; ganglion; gyrus; horn; joint; ligament; limb; line; lobe; lobule; margin; muscle; nerve; node; notch; nucleus; olive; part; peduncle; pit; plexus; pole; process; recess; retinaculum; root; segment; sinus; sulcus; surface; triangle; trunk; tubercle; vein; velum; vena; venule; wall
superior cerebellar artery: syndrome
superior hemorrhagic: polioencephalitis
superiority: complex
superior limbic: keratoconjunctivitis
superior mesenteric artery: syndrome
superior pulmonary sulcus: tumor
superior thoracic: aperture

superior vena caval: syndrome
supernatant: fluid
supernormal recovery: phase
supernumerary: kidney; mamma; organ; placenta
superolateral: surface
superomedial: margin
supersaturated: solution
supersonic: ray; wave
supersonic vibration: technique
supertemporal: fissure
supertraction: conus
supination: reflex
supinator: crest; jerk; muscle; reflex
supinator longus: reflex
supine: position
supine hypotensive: syndrome
supplemental: air; groove; lobe; ridge
supplementary: menstruation
supplementary motor: cortex
support: medium
supporting: area; cell; reaction; reflex
supportive: psychotherapy
suppressed: menstruation
suppressor: cell; gene; mutation
suppressor-sensitive: mutant
suppurating: gingivitis
suppurative: appendicitis; arthritis; cerebritis; chorioditis; encephalitis; hepatitis; hyalitis; mastitis; necrosis; nephritis; periodontitis; pleurisy; pneumonia; pulpitis; synovitis
supra-acetabular: groove; sulcus
supra-arytenoid: cartilage
supra-auricular: point
supracallosal: gyrus
supracervical: hysterectomy
suprachoroid: layer
supraclavicular: muscle; part
supraclavicular lymph: node
supraclinoid: aneurysm
supracondylar: fracture; process
supracrestal: line; plane
supraduodenal: artery
supraepicondylar: process
supragingival: calculus
supraglenoid: tubercle
suprahepatic: space
suprahisian: block
suprahyoid: gland; muscle
suprainterparietal: bone
supramarginal: convolution; gyrus
supramastoid: crest; fossa
supramaximal: stimulus
suprameatal: pit; spine; triangle
supranasal: point
supranormal: conduction; excitability
supranuclear: lesion; paralysis
supraoptic: commissure; nucleus
supraopticohypophysial: tract
supraorbital: arch; artery; foramen; margin; nerve; neuralgia; notch; point; reflex; ridge; vein
supraorbitomeatal: plane
suprapatellar: bursa; reflex
supraperiosteal: implant
suprapleural: membrane
suprapubic: cystotomy; lithotomy
suprarenal: body; capsule; cortex; gland; impression; plexus; vein
suprascapular: artery; ligament; nerve; notch; vein
suprasellar: cyst
supraspinatus: syndrome
supraspinous: fossa; ligament; muscle
suprasternal: bone; notch; plane; space
supratonsillar: fossa; recess
supratragic: tubercle
supratrochlear: artery; nerve; vein
supraumbilical: reflex
supravalvar: stenosis
supravalvar aortic stenosis: syndrome
supravalvar aortic stenosis-infantile hypercalcemia: syndrome
supraventricular: crest; extrasystole
supravesical: fossa
supravital: stain
supreme: concha
supreme intercostal: artery
supreme turbinated: bone
sural: artery; nerve; region
surdocardiac: syndrome
surface: analgesia; anatomy; catalysis; cell; epithelium; tension; thermometer
surface tension: theory
surface thalamic: vein
surgical: abdomen; anatomy; anesthesia; appliance; diathermy; emphysema; eruption; erysipelas; gut; ligation; maggot; microscope; neck; orthodontics; pathology; prosthesis; silk; splint; template
surging: faradism
surrogate: mother
survey: line
survival: time
suspended: animation; heart
suspension: colloid; laryngoscopy; stability
suspensory: bandage; ligament; muscle
sustained action: tablet
sustained release: tablet
sustentacular: cell; fiber
sutural: bone; cataract; ligament
suture: joint; ligature
SV40-adenovirus: hybrid
Sw^a: antigen
swallowing: reflex; threshold
swamp: fever; itch
swamp fever: virus
Swann: antigen
swan-neck: deformity
sweat: duct; gland; pore; test
sweat duct: adenoma
sweat gland: carcinoma
sweating: sickness; test
Swedish: gymnastics; movement
sweet: balm; precipitate
sweet clover: disease; poisoning
swelled: head
swim: bladder
swimmer's: itch
swimming: test
swimming pool: conjunctivitis; granuloma
swine: dysentery; erysipelas; fever; icteroanemia; influenza; pest; porphyria
swine edema: disease
swine encephalitis: virus
swine fever: virus
swineherd's: disease
swine influenza: virus
swinepox: virus
swine vesicular: disease
Swiss cheese: endometrium
Swiss mouse leukemia: virus
Swiss type: agammaglobulinemia
switching: site
swordfish: test
Sydney: crease; line
syllabic: speech
sylvatic: plague
sylvian: angle; aqueduct; fissure; line; point; valve; ventricle
symbiotic fermentation: phenomenon
symmetric, symmetrical: adenolipomatosis; asphyxia; gangrene
symmetric distal: neuropathy
sympathetic: agent; amine; blockade; ganglion; heterochromia; hormone; hypertonia; imbalance; iridoplegia; iritis; nerve; ophthal-

sympathetic—*continued*
mia; part; plexus; root; saliva; segment; symptom; trunk; uveitis
sympathetic formative: cell
sympathetic nervous: system
sympathetic reflex: dystophy
sympathicotropic: cell
sympathizing: eye
sympathochromaffin: cell
sympathomimetic: amine
symphysial: surface
symphysic: teratosis
symptom: complex; formation; group; substitution
symptomatic: anemia; epilepsy; erythema; fever; headache; impotence; leukemia; neuralgia; paramyotonia; porphyria; pruritus; reaction; torticollis; ulcer; varicocele
symptomatic myeloid: metaplasia
synaptic: bouton; cleft; conduction; ending; phase; resistance; terminal; trough; vesicle
synaptinemal: complex
synarthrodial: joint
synchondrodial: joint
synchronic: study
synchronized intermittent mandatory: ventilation
synchronous: reflex
synclonic: spasm
syncytial: bud; knot; sprout; trophoblast
syndermatotic: cataract
syndesmochorial: placenta
syndesmodial: joint
synergic: control
synergistic: muscle
syngeneic: graft
synovial: bursa; cell; chondromatosis; crypt; cyst; fluid; fold; frenulum; frenum; fringe; gland; hernia; joint; ligament; membrane; mesenchyme; osteochondromatosis; sarcoma; sheath; tuft; villus
synovial trochlear: bursa
syntactial: aphasia
synthesis: period
synthetic: chemistry; dye
syntonic: personality
syphilitic: abscess; aneurysm; aortitis; fever; leukoderma; meningoencephalitis; nephritis; osteochondritis; roseola; tooth; ulcer
Syriac: ulcer
Syrian: ulcer
syringomyelic: dissociation
systematic: anatomy; bacteriology; desensitization; vertigo
systematized: delusion; nevus
systemic: anaphylaxis; anatomy; chondromalacia; circulation; death; heart; hyalinosis; lupus; myelitis; poisoning
systemic autoimmune: disease
systemic febrile: disease
systemic vascular: resistance
systolic: click; gallop; gradient; honk; murmur; pressure; shock; thrill; whoop
systolic time: interval

T

T: agglutinogen; antigen; bandage; binder; cell; enzyme; group; lymphocyte; myelotomy; system; tube; tubule; wave
T-: bandage
T_3: toxicosis
***t*:** test
T.A.B.: vaccine
tabby-cat: striation
tabetic: arthropathy; crisis; cuirass; dissociation
table: salt
tablet: triturate
Tacaribe: complex; virus
tachycardia: window
tachycardia-bradycardia: syndrome
tactile: agnosia; anesthesia; cell; corpuscle; disk; elevation; fremitus; hair; hyperesthesia; image; meniscus; papilla; sense
tagged: atom
tagliacotian: operation
Tahyna: virus
tail: bone; bud; fold; sheath; vertebra
tailor's: cramp; muscle; spasm
talar: sulcus
talar articular: surface
talc: operation; pneumoconiosis
tallow: soap
talocalcaneal, talocalcanean: joint ligament
talocalcaneonavicular: joint
talocrural: articulation
talonavicular: ligament
tambour: sound
tamed: iodine
tangent: screen
tangential: wound
Tangier: disease
tank: respirator
tanned red: cell
tanner's: ulcer
tapered: bougie
tapetal light: reflex
tapetoretinal: degeneration; retinopathy
tapir: mouth
TAR: syndrome
tar: acne; camphor; keratosis
tarbagan: plague
tardive: cyanosis
tardive oral: dyskinesia
tardy: epilepsy
target: behavior; cell; gland; organ; patient; response
target cell: anemia
tarry: cyst
tarsal: arch; bone; canal; cartilage; cyst; fold; gland; joint; ligament; plate; sinus
tarsal tunnel: syndrome
tarsometatarsal: joint; ligament
tarsophalangeal: amputation
tarsotibial: amputation
tart: cell
tartrated: antimony
task-oriented: group
taste: blindness; bud; bulb; cell; corpuscle; deficiency; hair; pore; ridge
TATA: box
tautomeric: fiber
teacher's: node
teaching: hospital
tear: film; gas; sac; stone
teardrop: heart
tectobular: tact
tectonic: keratoplasty
tectopontine: tract
tectorial: membrane
tectospinal: decussation; tract
tegmental: decussation; field; syndrome; wall
telangiectatic: angioma; angiomatosis; cancer; fibroma; lipoma; wart
telangiectatic osteogenic: sarcoma
telencephalic: flexure; vesicle
telephone: theory
teleradium: therapy
telescopic: denture; spectacles
television: microscope
telocentric: chromosome
telogen: effluvium
telolecithal: egg; ovum
telomeric R-banding: stain
temperate: bacteriophage
temperature: coefficient; sense; spot
temperature-compensated: vaporizer

temperature-sensitive: mutant
template: ribonucleic acid
temporal: aponeurosis; apophysis; arteritis; bone; canal; cortex; dispersion; fascia; fossa; horn; line; lobe; muscle; plane; pole; process; region; ridge; surface; vein; venule
temporal lobe: epilepsy
temporary: base; callus; cartilage; denture; parasite; restoration; stricture; tooth
temporofrontal: tract
temporomandibular: arthrosis; articulation; joint; ligament; nerve; syndrome
temporomandibular articular: disk
temporomandibular joint: dysfunction
temporomandibular joint pain-dysfunction: syndrome
temporomaxillary: vein
temporoparietal: muscle
temporopontine: tract
temporozygomatic: suture
tenaculum: forceps
tender: line; point; zone
tendinous: arch; cord; inscription; intersection; opening; spot; synovitis
tendo achillis: reflex
tendon: advancement; bundle; cell; graft; recession; reflex; suture; transplantation
tendon sheath: syndrome
tennis: elbow; leg; thumb
tense: part; pulse
tensile: strength; stress
tension: cavity; curve; headache; pneumothorax; suture
tensor: muscle
tensor tarsi: muscle
tenth cranial: nerve
tentorial: angle; nerve; sinus
teratoid: tumor
teratomatous: cyst
teres major: muscle
teres minor: muscle
term: infant
terminal: artery; bar; bouton; bronchiole; cisterna; crest; deletion; endocarditis; filum; ganglion; hair; hematuria; ileitis; ileus; infection; leukocytosis; line; notch; nerve; nucleus; part; plate; pneumonia; sinus; stria; sulcus; thread; vein; ventricle; web
terminal addition: enzyme
terminal hinge: position
terminal jaw relation: record
terminal nerve: corpuscle
termination: codon; sequence
termino-terminal: anastomosis
ternary: complex
territorial: matrix
tertian: fever; malaria; parasite
tertiary: alcohol; amputation; cortex; dentin; syphilid; syphilis; villus; vitreous
tertiary egg: membrane
tertiary medical: care
Teschen: disease
Teschen disease: virus
tesselated: fundus
test: cross; meal; object; profile; solution; skein; tube; type
test handle: instrument
testicular: artery; cord; duct; dysgenesis; feminization; plexus; vein
testicular feminization: syndrome
testicular tubular: adenoma
testis: cord
testoid: hyperthecosis
test-retest: reliability
test-tube: baby
tetanic: contraction; convulsion
tetanoid: chorea; paraplegia
tetanus: antitoxin; immunoglobulin; toxin; vaccine
tetanus and gas gangrene: antitoxin
tetanus antitoxin: unit
tetanus immune: globulin
tetanus-perfringens: antitoxin
tetany: cataract
tethered cord: syndrome
tetracyclic: antidepressant
tetracyclic steroid: nucleus
tetraethyl: poisoning
tetrazonium: salts
Texas: fever; snakeroot
text: blindness
TG: virus
thalamic: syndrome; tenia
thalamic gustatory: nucleus
thalamostriate: vein
thallium: poisoning
thanatophoric: dwarfism
thebesian: foramen; valve; vein
theca: cell
theca cell: tumor
theca interna: cone
thecal: abscess; whitlow
theca-lutein: cell
thematic: paralogia; paraphasia
thematic apperception: test
thenar: eminence prominence; space
therapeutic: abortion; anesthesia; angiography; community; crisis; electrode; fever; group; incompatibility; index; iridectomy; malaria; nihilism; optimism; pessimism; pneumothorax; ratio
thermal: anesthesia; burn; capacity; sense; spectrum
thermic: anesthesia; fever; sense
thermo-: stromuhr
thermodynamic: potential; theory
thermoelectric: pile
thermogenic: action
thermolabile: opsonin
thermoluminescence: dosimetry
thermoprecipitin: reaction
thermostable: opsonin
thermostable opsonin: test
theta: rhythm; wave
thiamin chloride: unit
thiazide: diabetes
thiazin: dye
thigh: bone; joint
thin: section
thin-layer: chromatography; electrophoresis; immunoassay
thiochrome: method
thioclastic: cleavage
thiocyanogen: number; value
thioflavine T: stain
third: corpuscle; disease; eyelid; finger; molar; ovary; tonsil; trochanter; ventricle; ventriculostomy
third and fourth pharyngeal pouch: syndrome
third cranial: nerve
third cuneiform: bone
third degree: burn
third occipital: nerve
third parallel pelvic: plane
third peroneal: muscle
third temporal: convolution
thirst: fever
thixotropic: fluid
thoracic: axis; cage; cavity; choke; compliance; duct; fistula; ganglion; girdle; gland; goiter; index; limb; nerve; nucleus; part; respiration; spine; stomach; vertebra; vein; wall
thoracic aortic: plexus
thoracic cardiac: nerve
thoracic interspinal: muscle
thoracic intertransverse: muscle
thoracic longissimus: muscle
thoracic outlet: syndrome

thoracic-pelvic-phalangeal: dystrophy
thoracic rotator: muscle
thoracoacromial: artery; vein
thoracodorsal: artery; vein
thoracoepigastric: vein
thoracolumbar: aponeurosis; system
thoracolumbar venous: line
thorium: emanation
thorn apple: crystal
thought process: disorder
thready: pulse
threatened: abortion
three-cornered: bone
three-day: fever; measles
three-dimensional: record
three-glass: test
thresher's: lung
threshold: body; differential; percussion; shift; stimulus; substance
threshold limit: valve
thrombin: time
thrombocytic: series
thrombocytopenia-absent radius: syndrome
thrombocytopenic: purpura
thrombopathic: syndrome
thromboplastic plasma: component
thrombotic: apoplexy; gangrene; hydrocephalus; infarct; microangiopathy; phlegmasia
thrombotic thrombocytopenic: purpura
through: drainage
through-and-through myocardial: infarction
thrush: fungus
thumb: forceps; lancet; reflex
thunder: humor
thyme: camphor
thymic: abscess; agenesis; alymphoplasia; hypoplasia; vein
thymic lymphopoietic: factor
thymine: dimer
thymus: corpuscle; gland
thymus-dependent: zone
thyroarytenoid: muscle
thyrocardiac: disease
thyrocervical: trunk
thyroepiglottic: ligament; muscle
thyroglossal: duct
thyroglossal duct: cyst
thyrohyoid: membrane; muscle
thyrohypophysial: syndrome
thyroid: axis; body; bruit; cartilage; colloid; diverticulum; eminence; foramen; gland; storm; therapy; toxicosis; vein
thyroidal articular: surface
thyroid lymph: node
thyroid-stimulating: hormone
thyroid-stimulating hormone: test
thyroid-stimulating hormone-releasing: factor
thyroid-stimulating hormone stimulation: test
thyroid suppression: test
thyrolingual: duct
thyropharyngeal: part
thyrotoxic: coma; crisis; encephalopathy; myopathy; serum
thyrotoxic complement-fixation: factor
thyrotropic: hormone
thyrotropin-producing: adenoma
thyrotropin-releasing: factor; hormone
thyrotropin-releasing hormone stimulation: test
thyroxine-binding: globulin; prealbumin; protein
tibial: border; crest; nerve; phenomenon; tuberosity
tibial collateral: ligament
tibial communicating: nerve
tibial intertendinous: bursa
tibiocalcaneal: part
tibiofemoral: index
tibiofibular: articulation; joint; ligament; syndesmosis
tibionavicular: ligament; part
tick: fever; paralysis; typhus
tick-borne: encephalitis
tick-borne encephalitis: virus
tic-tac: rhythm; sound
tidal: air; drainage; volume; wave
tie-over: dressing
tiger: heart
tight: junction
tigroid: body; fundus; retina; striation; substance
tilt: table
time: constant; marker; sense
time compensation: gain
time-varied: gain
time-varied gain: control
Timothy hay: bacillus
tine: test
tinted denture: base
tissue: basophil; culture; displaceability; displacement; fluid; lymph; molding; registration; respiration; tension
tissue-bearing: area
tissue culture infectious: dose
tissue plasminogen: activator
tissue-specific: antigen
tissue thromboplastin inhibition: time
titratable acidity: test
Tj: antigen
TNM: staging
TO: virus
toad: skin
to-and-fro: anesthesia; murmur
toasted: shin
tobacco: heart
Tobruk: splint
toe: clonus; itch; phenomenon; reflex
toilet: training
tolbutamide: test
tolerance: dose
Tolu: balsam
toluidine blue O: stain
tone: color
tone decay: test
tongue: bone; depressor; flap; phenomenon
tonic: contraction; control; convulsion; epilepsy; pupil; reflex; spasm
tonoclonic: spasm
tonsil: position
tonsillar: calculus; crypt; fossa; fossulation; herniation; ring
tonsillolingual: sulcus
tooth: abrasion; avulsion; bud; cement; cough; form; germ; ligation; plane; polyp; pulp; sac; socket; spasm; transplantation
tooth-borne: base
toothed: vertebra
toper's: nose
tophaceous: gout
topical: anesthesia
topographic: anatomy
TORCH: syndrome
toric: lens
tornado: epilepsy
torsion: dystonia; fracture; neurosis; spasm
torsional: deformity
torsive: occlusion
torus: fracture
total: acidity; aphasia; cataract; cystectomy; elasticity; energy; hematuria; hyperopia; keratoplasty; mastectomy; necrosis; placenta (previa); sclerectasia; synechia; transfusion
total body: hypothermia
total catecholamine: test
total end-diastolic: diameter
total end-systolic: diameter
total joint: arthroplasty
total lung: capacity
total parenteral: nutrition
total pelvic: exenteration

total peripheral: resistance
total push: therapy
total refractory: period
total spinal: anesthesia
totipotent: cell
totipotential: protoplasm
touch: cell; corpuscle
tourniquet: poditis; test
tower: skull
toxemic: jaundice; retinopathy
toxic: amaurosis; amblyopia; anemia; cataract; cirrhosis; cyanosis; delirium; dementia; equivalent; goiter; hemoglobinuria; hydrocephalus; megacolon; nephrosis; neuritis; psychosis; retinopathy; shock; tetanus; unit
toxic epidermal: necrolysis
toxicogenic: conjunctivitis
toxic shock: syndrome
toxin: spectrum; unit
TPHA: test
TPI: test
Tr^a: antigen
trabecular: bone; carcinoma; meshwork; network; reticulum; zone
trace: conditioning; element
trace conditioned: reflex
tracheal: cartilage; fenestration; fistula; gland; pain; ring; triangle; tube; tugging; ulceration; vein
tracheal lymph: node
trachelobregmatic: diameter
tracheloclavicular: muscle
tracheobiliary: fistula
tracheobronchial: dyskinesia; groove
tracheoesophageal: fistula
tracheotomy: hook; tube
trachoma: body; gland; virus
trachomatous: conjunctivitis; keratitis; pannus
traction: alopecia; aneurysm; atrophy; diverticulum; epiphysis
trained: reflex
training: analysis; group
train-of-four: stimulus
trainwheel: rhythm
trance: coma
trans: phase
transactional: analysis; psychotherapy
transcellular: fluid
transcendental: anatomy
transcervical: fracture
transcondylar: fracture
transcortical: aphasia; apraxia
transcranial: roentgenogram
transducer: cell
transduodenal: sphincterotomy
transfer: coping; factor; gene; ribonucleic acid
transference: neurosis
transferred: ophthalmia; sensation
transferring: enzyme
transfixion: suture
transformed: lymphocyte
transforming: agent; factor; gene
transfusion: hepatitis; nephritis
transhiatal: esophagectomy
transient: agammaglobulinemia; albuminuria; hypogammaglobulinemia; myopia
transient acantholytic: dermatosis
transient ischemic: attack
transition: mutation; ray
transitional; cell; convolution; denture; epithelium; gyrus; leukocyte; zone
transitional cell: carcinoma; papilloma
translatory: movement
translocation: carrier; chromosome; mongolism
translumbar: aortography
transmembrane: potential
transmethylation: factor
transmissible: encephalopathy; enteritis; gastroenteritis; plasmid
transmissible gastroenteritis: virus
transmissible turkey enteritis: virus
transmissible venereal: tumor
transmitted: light
transmural: pressure
transmural myocardial: infarction
transneuronal: atrophy
transorbital: leukotomy: lobotomy
transosseous: venography
transovarial: transmission
transparent: dentin; septum; ulcer
transplantation: genetics
transplant lung: syndrome
transporionic: axis
transport: host; maximum; medium; number; tetany
transposable: element
transpulmonary: pressure
transpyloric: plane
transseptal: fiber; orchipexy
transsexual: surgery
transstadial: transmission
transsynaptic: chromatolysis; degeneration
transtentorial: herniation
transthoracic: esophagectomy; pressure
transureteroureteral: anastomosis
transurethral: resection
transverse: amputation; fracture; hermaphroditism; lie; myelitis; presentation
transverse anatomical structures (specific transverse structures are listed under the following): arch; artery; articulation; colon; convolution; crest; diameter; disk; ductule; fasciculus; fiber; fissure; flexure; fold; foramen; fornix; groove; gyrus; head; joint; ligament; line; muscle; nerve; part; pelvis; plane; process; ridge; septum; sinus; sulcus; suture; vein
transverse facial: fracture
transverse horizontal: axis
transversion: mutation
transversospinal: muscle
transversovertical: index
trapezium: bone
trapezius: muscle
trapezoid: body; bone; ligament; line; ridge
traumatic: alopecia; amenorrhea; amputation; anemia; anesthesia; aneurysm; asphyxia; cataract; dermatitis; encephalopathy; fever; gastritis; herpes; meningocele; myiasis; neurasthenia; neuritis; neuroma; neurosis; occlusion; orchitis; pneumonia; psychosis; retinopathy; tetanus
traumatic cervical: discopathy
traumatic progressive: encephalopathy
traumatogenic: occlusion
traumatopneic: wound
traveler's: diarrhea
treatment: denture
trefoil: dermatitis; tendon
trembling: palsy
tremulous: iris
trench: foot; hand; lung; mouth; nephritis
trephine: biopsy
treponema-immobilizing: antibody
treponemal: antibody
Treponema pallidum hemagglutination: test
Treponema pallidum immobilization: reaction; test
TRH stimulation: test
triad: syndrome
triadic: symbiosis
trial: base; case; denture; frame; lens
triangular: bandage; bone; cartilage; crest; disk; fascia; fold; fossa; lamella; ligament; muscle; pit; recess; ridge; uterus
triangularity of: tooth

triaxial reference: system
triazolopyridine: antidepressant
tribasilar: synostosis
TRIC: agent
tricarboxylic acid: cycle
triceps: bursa; muscle; reflex
triceps surae: reflex
trichilemmal: cyst
trichorhinophalangeal: syndrome
trichrome: stain
tricuspid: area; atresia; incompetence; insufficiency; murmur; orifice; stenosis; tooth; valve
tricyclic: antidepressant
trident: hands
trifacial: nerve; neuralgia
trifid: stomach
trifocal: lens
trigeminal: cavity; cough; crest; decompression; ganglion; impression; lemniscus; nerve; neuralgia; pulse; rhizotomy; rhythm; tractotomy
trigeminofacial: reflex
trigger: area; finger; point; zone
triggered: activity
trihydric: alcohol
triiodothyronine: toxicosis
triiodothyronine uptake: test
triketohydrindene: reaction
trilaminar: blastoderm
trimalleolar: fracture
triphammer: pulse
triphenylmethane: dye
triphyllomatous: teratoma
triplant: implant
triple: arthodesis; bond; phosphate; quartan; response; rhythm; vision
triple symptom: complex
triple X: syndrome
triplet: oxygen; state
triquetral: bone
triquetrous: cartilage
trisomy 8: syndrome
trisomy 13: syndrome
trisomy 18: syndrome
trisomy 20: syndrome
trisomy 21: syndrome
trisomy C: syndrome
trisomy D: syndrome
trisomy E: syndrome
tritiated: thymidine
triton: tumor
trochanter: reflex
trochanteric: bursa; bursitis; crest; fossa; syndrome
trochlear: fossa; nerve; notch; nucleus; process; spine
trochlear synovial: bursa
trochoid: articulation: joint
trophic: change; gangrene; nucleus; ulcer
trophoblastic: lacuna; operculum
trophoneurotic: atrophy; leprosy
trophotropic: zone
tropic: hormone
tropical: abscess; acne; anemia; boil; bubo; diarrhea; eczema; eosinophilia; lichen; mask; measles; medicine; myositis; pyomyositis; sore; splenomegaly; sprue; theileriosis; typhus; ulcer
tropical canine: pancytopenia
tropical splenomegaly: syndrome
true: albuminuria; aneurysm; ankylosis; apnea; cementoma; cholinesterase; conjugate; diverticulum; dwarfism; glottis; hermaphroditism; hypertrophy; knot; pelvis; rib; thirst; vertebra
true vocal: cord
truncate: ascertainment
truth: serum
trypanosome: fever; stage
trypsin: inhibitor
trypsin G-banding: stain
TSH stimulation: test
tsutsugamushi: disease; fever
tubal: abortion; cartilage; colic; dysmenorrhea; extremity; infantilism; insufflation; ligation; pregnancy; tonsil
tubal air: cell
tube: cast; tooth
tubed, tubed pedicle: flap
tuberal: nucleus
tubercle: bacillus
tuberculin: test
tuberculoid: leprosy
tuberculo-opsonic: index
tuberculosis: vaccine
tuberculous: abscess; bronchopneumonia; enteritis; lymphadenitis; meningitis; nephritis; peritonitis; rheumatism; scrofuloderma; spondylitis; wart
tuberoinfundibular: tract
tuberosity: reduction
tuberous: root; sclerosis
tuboabdominal: pregnancy
tubo-ovarian: abscess; pregnancy; variocele
tuboreticular: structure
tubotympanic: canal; recess
tubouterine: pregnancy
tubular: adenoma; aneurysm; carcinoma; cyst; forceps; gland; respiration; vision
tubular excretory: mass
tubuloacinar: gland
tubuloalveolar: gland
tubulointerstitial: nephritis
tufted: cell; phalanx
tularemic: chancre; conjunctivitis; pneumonia
tumbu dermal: myiasis
tumor: antigen; embolism; marker; stage; virus
tumoral: calcinosis
tumor angiogenic: factor
tumor lysis: syndrome
tumor necrosis: factor
tumor-specific transplantation: antigen
tuning: fork
tunnel: cell; disease; vision
T_3 uptake: test
turban: tumor
turbinal: varix
turbinated: body; bone; crest
turkey-meningoencephalitis: virus
Turkish: saddle
turnover: flap
turpentine: enema; poisoning
tussive: absence; fremitus
twelfth cranial: nerve
twelfth-year: molar
twenty-nail: dystrophy
twilight: sleep; state; vision
twin: cone; crystal; helix; placenta; pregnancy
twin-twin: transfusion
twist: form
twisted: hair
two-bellied: muscle
two-carbon: fragment
two-dimensional: chromatography; echocardiography; immunoelectrophoresis
two-glass: test
two-step exercise: test
two-sympathin: theory
two-way: catheter
tympanic: antrum; attic; body; bone; canal; cell; cavity; crest; ganglion; gland; groove; incisure; intumescence; lip; membrane; nerve; notch; opening; part; plate; plexus; promontory; ring; scute; sinus; vein; wall
tympanitic: resonance
tympanohyal: bone
tympanomastoid: fissure; suture
tympanosquamous: fissure
tympanostapedial: junction
type: culture; species; strain
type 1-4: dextrocardia

type 1-6: glycogenosis
type A: behavior; personality
type B: behavior; personality
type I-II: dip
trype I-III, V: acrocephalosyndactyly
type I-V familial: hyperlipoproteinemia
type I-VII: mucopolysaccharidosis
type II: cell; diabetes
type IS: mucopolysaccharidosis
typhoid: bacillus; bacteriophage; cholera; fever; pleurisy; pneumonia; septicemia; vaccine
typhoid-parathyroid: vaccine
typhus: vaccine
typical: absence; achromatopsia; acrocephalosyndactyly; pseudocholinesterase
typist's: cramp

U

U: wave
ulcerating: granuloma
ulcerative: colitis; dermatosis; pharyngitis; scrofuloderma; stomatitis
ulceromembranous: gingivitis; pharyngitis
ulnar: artery; bursa; eminence; head; margin; nerve; notch; reflex; vein
ulnar collateral: ligament
ulnar extensor: muscle
ulnar flexor: muscle
ultimate: principle; strength
ultimobranchial: body; pouch
ultra-: microscope
ultradian: rhythm
ultrafiltration: coefficient; hemodialyzer
ultralente: insulin
ultrasonic: cephalometry; cleaning; lithotresis; microscope; nebulizer; ray; therapy; wave
ultrasonic egg: recovery
ultrasound: cardiography
ultrastructural: anatomy
ultrathin: section
ultraviolet: keratoconjunctivitis; lamp; microscope; ray
ultropaque: method
Ulysses: syndrome
umbilical: artery; cord; cyst; fissure; fistula; fossa; fungus; hernia; notch; part; region; ring; souffle; vein; vesicle
umbilical prevesical: fascia
umbilicated: cataract
umbilicomammillary: triangle
umbilicovesical: fascia
Umbre: virus
unarmed: rostellum
unavoidable: hemorrhage
unbalanced: translocation
uncal: herniation
unciform: bone; fasciculus; pancreas; process
uncinate: attack; bundle; epilepsy; fasciculus; fit; gyrus; pancreas; process
uncompensated: acidosis; alkalosis
unconditioned: reflex; response; stimulus
unconjugated: bilirubin
unconscious: homosexuality
uncoupling: factor
uncovertebral: joint
uncus: band
undercut: gauge
undermining: ulcer
undescended: testis
undetermined: nitrogen
undifferentiated: cell
undifferentiated cell: adenoma
undifferentiated type: fever
undulant: fever
undulating: membrane; purse
unequal: cleavage; crossing-over
unequal retinal: image
unerupted: tooth
uneven: crossing-over
unformed visual: hallucination
ungual: phalanx; tuberosity
uniaxial: joint
unicameral: cyst
unicameral bone: cyst
unicanalicular: sphincter
unicellular: gland; sclerosis
unicorn: uterus
unidirectional: block; flux
unilateral: anesthesia; hemianopsia; hermaphroditism
unilocular: cyst; fat; joint
unilocular hydatid: cyst
unimolecular: reaction
uninhibited neurogenic: bladder
uninterrupted: suture
uniocular: hemianopsia
uniovular: twins
unipennate: muscle
unipolar: cell; electrocardiogram; lead; neuron
unit: character; fibril; membrane
uniting: canal; cartilage; duct
unit of: convergence
univalent: antibody
universal: appliance; donor; infantilism; solvent
unmyelinated: fiber
unpaired: allosome
unresolved: pneumonia
unsaturated: alcohol; fat; fatty acid
unstable: angina; colloid; equilibrium; fracture; hemoglobin
unstrained jaw: relation
unstriated: muscle
unsystematized: delusion
ununited: fracture
upbeat: nystagmus
upper: airway; extremity; eyelid; jaw; lip; lobe
upper abdominal periosteal: reflex
upper jaw: bone
upper lateral cutaneous: nerve
upper motor: neuron
upper motor neuron: lesion
upper nodal: extrasystole
upper uterine: segment
ur-: defense
urachal: cyst; fistula; fold; ligament
uracil: mustard
uranium: nephritis; unit
uranyl acetate: stain
urate crystals: stain
urban cutaneous: leishmaniasis
urea: clearance; concentration; cycle; frost; index; nitrogen
urea clearance: test
urease: test
uremic: breath; colitis; frost; lung; pericarditis; pneumonia; pneumonitis; polyneuropathy
ureteral: meatus; opening
ureteric: bud; dysmenorrhea; fold; plexus
ureterocutaneous: fistula
ureteroileal: anastomosis
ureteropelvic: obstruction
ureterorenal: reflux
ureterosigmoid: anastomosis
ureterotubal: anastomosis
ureteroureteral: anastomosis
ureterovaginal: fistula
ureterovesical: obstruction
urethral: artery; caruncle; crest; dilation; diverticulum; fever; gland; groove; hematuria; lacuna; opening; papilla; plate; sphincterotomy; surface; valve
urethral pressure: profile
urethrovaginal: fistula
urge: incontinence
uric acid: infarct
uricolytic: index
urinary: apparatus; bladder; cachexia; calculus; cast; cyst; fever; fistula; nitrogen; organ; reflex;

urinary—*continued*
sand; schistosomiasis; smear; stuttering; system; tract
urinary concentration: test
urinary exertional: incontinence
urinary stress: incontinence
uriniferous: tubule
urogenital: apparatus; canal; cleft; diaphragm; fistula; membrane; mesentery; region; ridge; septum; sinus; system; triangle
uropoietic: system
uropygial: gland
urorectal: fold; membrane; septum
urticarial: fever
USP: unit
uterine: appendage; artery; calculus; cavity; colic; contraction; dysmenorrhea; extremity; gland; inertia; insufficiency; milk; part; pregnancy; sinus; sinusoid; souffle; tetanus; tube; tympanities; vein
uterine venous: plexus
uteroabdominal: pregnancy
uteroepichorial: membrane
utero-ovarian: variocele
uteroperitoneal: fistula
uteroplacental: apoplexy; sinus
uterosacral: ligament
uterovaginal: canal; plexus
uterovesical: fold; pouch
utilization: time
utricular: nerve; reflex; spot
utriculoampullar: nerve
utriculosaccular: duct
uveal: part; staphyloma; tract
uveocutaneous: syndrome
uveo-encephalitic: syndrome
uveomeningitis: syndrome
uveoparotid: fever
uviol: lamp
Uzbekistan hemorrhagic: fever

V

V: antigen; esotropia; extropia; lead; wave
V-2: carcinoma
vaccine: body; lymph; virus
vaccinia: lymph; virus
vaccinoid: reaction
VACTERL: syndrome
vacuolar: degeneration; nephrosis
vacuolating: virus
vacuum: aspirator; casting; desiccator; extractor; flask; headache; investing; tube
vagabond's: disease
vagal: apnea; attack; part; trunk
vaginal: artery; atresia; celiotomy; column; dysmenorrhea; gland; hysterectomy; hysterotomy; laceration; lithotomy; myomectomy; nerve; opening; plug; pool; process; smear; synovitis
vaginal cornification: test
vaginal mucification: test
vaginal synovial: membrane
vaginal venous: plexus
vagovagal: reflex
vagrant's: disease
vagus: area; nerve; pulse
valence: electron
vallate: papilla
vallecular: dysphagia
valley: fever
valvotomy: knife
valvular: endocarditis; incompetence; insufficiency; pneumothorax; thrombus
vampire: bat
vanillylmandelic acid: test
vanishing: cream; lung
vanishing lung: syndrome
vapor: density; pressure
variable: coupling; deceleration; region
variant: angina; hemoglobin
varicella: encephalitis
varicella-zoster: virus
varicelloid: smallpox
varicose: aneurysm; eczema; ulcer; vein
variegate: porphyria
variola: virus
varioliform: syphilid
varioloid: varicella
vascular: bud; cataract; circle; cone; dementia; dentin; fold; gland; headache; hemophilia; keratitis; lacuna; layer; leiomyoma; murmur; nerve; papilla; plexus; polyp; ring; sclerosis; spur; stripe; system; zone
vasculocardiac: syndrome
vasoactive: amine
vasoactive intestinal: polypeptide
vasoformative: cell
vasogenic: shock
vasomotor: absence; ataxia; epilepsy; imbalance; nerve; paralysis; rhinitis; spasm
vasopressin-resistant: diabetes
vasopressor: reflex
vasovagal: attack; epilepsy; syncope; syndrome
VATER: complex
VCE: smear
VDRL: test
vector: loop
VEE: virus
vegetable: alkali; base; calomel; charcoal; gelatin; ophthalmia; sulfur; wax
vegetal: pole
vegetative: bacteriophage; endocarditis; life; pole; stage
vegetative nervous: system
veiled: puff
veiling: glare
vein: stone
Vel: antigen
velamentous: insertion
veldt: sore
vellus: hair
velocity: coefficient; constant
velopharyngeal: closure; insufficiency; seal
velvet: ant
Ven: antigen
venereal: bubo; disease; lymphogranuloma; sore; ulcer; wart
Venezuelan equine: encephalomyelitis
Venezuelan equine encephalomyelitis: virus
Venice: turpentine
venom: hemolysis
veno-occlusive: disease
venorespiratory: reflex
venous: angle; artery; blood; capillary; circle; congestion; embolism; gangrene; groove; heart; hum; hyperemia; insufficiency; lake; ligament; murmur; plexus; pulse; segment; sinus; star; valve
venous occlusion: plethysmography
venous-stasis: retinopathy
ventilation: meter
ventilation/perfusion: ratio
ventilation-perfusion: scan
ventilatory: compliance
ventral: hernia
ventral anatomical structures (specific ventral structures are listed under the following): aorta; artery; column; decussation; gland; horn; ligament; mesocardium; muscle; nucleus; pancreas; part; peduncle; plate; root; surface; tract
ventricular: aberration; afterload; aneurysm; artery; band; bigeminy; bradycardia; capture; complex; conduction; diverticulum; escape; extrasystole; fibrillation; fluid; flutter; fold; gradient; layer;

ligament; loop; plateau; preload; rhythm; septum; standstill; systole; tachycardia
ventricular filling: pressure
ventricular fusion: beat
ventricular inhibited pulse: generator
ventricular septal: defect
ventricular synchronous pulse: generator
ventricular triggered pulse: generator
ventriculoatrial: conduction
ventriculoradial: dysplasia
ventrobasal: nucleus
ventromedial: nucleus
verbal: agraphia
vermian: fossa
vermicular: colic; movement; pulse
vermiform: appendage; appendix; process
vermilion: border; zone
vermilion transitional: zone
verminous: abscess; aneurysm; appendicitis; bronchitis; ileus
vernal: catarrh; conjunctivitis; encephalitis; keratoconjunctivitis
Vernitrol: vaporizer
verrucous: carcinoma; endocarditis; hemangioma; hyperplasia; nevus; scrofuloderma; xanthoma
vertebra prominens: reflex
vertebral: arch; artery; canal; column; foramen; formula; fusion; ganglion; groove; nerve; notch; part; plexus; polyarthritis; pulp; region; rib; vein; venography
vertebral-basilar: system
vertebral cervical: instability
vertebral venous: plexus; system
vertebrated: catheter; probe
vertebroarterial: foramen
vertebrochondral: rib
vertebrocostal: trigone
vertebropelvic: ligament
vertebrosternal: rib
vertex: presentation
vertical: axis; dimension; elastic; heart; hymen; illumination; index; muscle; nystagmus; opening; osteotomy; overlap; parallax; plate; strabismus; transmission; vertigo
vertical banded: gastroplasty
vertical growth: phase
vertical retraction: syndrome
verticosubmental: view
vesical: calculus; diverticulum; fistula; gland; hematuria; lithotomy; plexus; reflex; surface; triangle
vesicating: gas
vesicle: hernia
vesicocolic: fistula
vesicocutaneous: fistula
vesicointestinal: fistula
vesicoumbilical: ligament
vesicoureteral: reflux; valve
vesicourethral: canal
vesicouterine: fistula; ligament; pouch
vesicovaginal: fistula
vesicovaginorectal: fistula
vesicular: appendage; exanthema; keratitis; keratopathy; mole; murmur; rale; resonance; respiration; rickettsiosis; stomatitis; transport
vesicular exanthema: virus
vesicular ovarian: follicle
vesicular stomatitis: virus
vesiculocavernous: respiration
vesiculotympanitic: resonance
vestibular: anus; area; canal; crest; fissure; fold; fossa; ganglion; gland; labyrinth; ligament; lip; membrane; nerve; nucleus; nystagmus; organ; part; root; screen; surface; vein; wall; window
vestibular blind: sac
vestibular hair: cell
vestibulocerebellar: ataxia
vestibulocochlear: nerve; organ
vestibulo-equilibratory: control
vestibulospinal: reflex; tract
vestigial: fold; muscle; organ
Veteran's Administration: hospital
veterinary: medicine
VI: antibody; antigen
vibrating: line
vibration: syndrome; tolerance
vibratory: massage; sensibility; urticaria
vibrionic: abortion
vicarious: hypertrophy; menstruation
vicious: cicatrix; circle; union
vidian: artery; canal; nerve; vein
villonodular pigmented: tenosynovitis
villous: adenoma; carcinoma; papilloma; placenta; tenosynovitis; tumor
vinous: liquor
violinist's: cramp
viral (see also virus): dysentery; envelope; gastroenteritis; hemagglutination; hepatitis; probe; strand; tropism; wart
viral hemorrhagic: fever
viral hemorrhagic fever: virus
virgin: generation; silk
virginal: membrane
Virginia: snakeroot
viridans: hemolysis
virile: member; reflex
virtual: focus; image
virulent: bacteriophage; bubo
virus (see also viral): blockade; encephalomyelitis; hepatitis; keratoconjunctivitis; pneumonia
virus A: hepatitis
virus-associated hemophagocytic: syndrome
virus B: hepatitis
virus-transformed: cell
virus X: disease
visceral: anesthesia; arch; brain; cavity; cleft; cranium; disorder; epilepsy; inversion; larva migrans; layer; leishmaniasis; lymphomatosis; mesoderm; node; plate; pleura; pleurisy; sense; skeleton; surface; swallow
visceral disease: virus
visceral motor: neuron
visceral nervous: system
visceral traction: reflex
viscerogenic: reflex
visceromotor: reflex
visceropannicular: reflex
viscerosensory: reflex
viscerotrophic: reflex
visible: spectrum
visibility: acuity
visiting: nurse
visna: virus
visual: acuity; allesthesia; angle; aphasia; area; axis; blackout; cortex; cycle; efficiency; extinction; field; image; inattention; pigment; projection; purple; threshold; violet; yellow
visual evoked: potential
visual orbicularis: reflex
visual receptor: cell
visual-spatial: agnosia
vita: glass
vital: capacity; center; force; index; knot; node; pulp; sign; spirit; stain; statistics; tooth; tripod; ultraviolet
vitality: test
vitamin A: unit
vitamin B_1 hydrochloride: unit
vitamin B_2, B_6: unit

vitamin B_{12}: neuropathy
vitamin C: test; unit
vitamin D: milk; unit
vitamin D-resistant: rickets
vitamin E: unit
vitamin K: unit
vitelliform: degeneration
vitelline: cord; duct; fistula; membrane; pole; reservoir; sac; vein; vessel
vitellointestinal: cyst; duct
vitiated: air
vitreoretinal choroidopathy: syndrome
vitreoretinal traction: syndrome
vitreo-tapetoretinal: dystrophy
vitreous: body; camera; cell; chamber; detachment; hernia; humor; lamella; membrane; table
vivax: fever; malaria
VMA: test
vocal: amusia; cord; fold; fremitus; ligament; muscle; nodule; process; resonance; shelf
voiding: cystogram
voiding flow: rate
volar carpal: ligament
volar interosseous: artery nerve
volatile: anesthetic; mustard; oil
volatile fatty acid: number
vole: bacillus
volitional: tremor
voltaic: taste; vertigo
volume: disease; element; index; substitute; unit
volume-controlled: respirator
volume-displacement: plethysmograph
volumetric: analysis; flask; solution
voluntary: dehydration; hospital; muscle; mutism; nystagmus
volutin: granule
vomeral: groove; sulcus
vomerine: canal; cartilage
vomerobasilar: canal
vomeronasal: organ
vomerorostral: canal
vomerovaginal: canal; groove
vomiting: gas; reflex
vortex: vein
vorticose: vein
VS: virus
vulnerable: period; phase
vulnerable child: syndrome
vulsella: forceps
vulvar: slit
vulvovaginal: anus; cystectomy; gland
Vw: antigen
V-Y: procedure

W

W: arch; chromosome; factor; procedure; ray
waddingtonian: homeostasis
waiter's: cramp
waking: numbness
walking: typhoid
walk-through: angina
wallerian: degeneration; law
wallet: stomach
waltzed: flap
wandering: abscess; cell; erysipelas; goiter; kidney; liver; organ; pacemaker; pneumonia
war: neurosis
warble: botfly; fly
warehouseman's: itch
warm: agglutinin; autoantibody
warm-blooded: animal
warm-cold: hemolysin
warty: dyskeratoma; horn; ulcer
wash-: bottle
washed: sulfur
washed field: technique
washerman's: mark
washerwoman's: itch
washing: soda
washout: cannula; test
wasserhelle: cell
wasted: ventilation
wasting: disease; palsy; paralysis
watchmaker's: cramp
water: aspirator; bath; bed; cancer; canker; depletion; diuresis; dressing; gas; glass; intoxication; itch; sore
water-clear: cell
water-hammer: pulse
watering-can: perineum; scrotum
watershed: infarction
water-soluble: chlorophyll (derivatives)
water-trap: stomach
water-whistle: sound
watery: eye
wattle: gum
wave: analyzer; form; number
wax: expansion; form; pattern
wax model: denture
wax-tipped: bougie
waxy: cast; degeneration; finger; kidney; liver; spleen
WDHA: syndrome
wear-and-tear: pigment
weaver's: cough
web: eye
Webb: antigen
webbed: finger; neck; penis; toe
weddellite: calculus
wedge: biopsy; bone; pressure; resection; spirometer
wedge-and-groove: joint; suture
wedge-shaped: fasciculus; tubercle
WEE: virus
weekend: hospital
weeping: eczema
welder's: conjunctivitis; lung
well differentiated lymphocytic: lymphoma
Wesselsbron: disease; fever
Wesselsbron disease: virus
West African: fever; trypanosomiasis
West African sleeping: sickness
Western blot: analysis; technique
western equine: encephalomyelitis
western equine encephalomyelitis: virus
West Indian: smallpox
West Nile: fever; virus
wet: beriberi; compress; cup; dream; gangrene; lung; nurse; pack; pleurisy; shock; tetter
wet and dry bulb: thermometer
wet cutaneous: leishmaniasis
wettable: sulfur
wheal-and-erythema: reaction
wheal-and-flare: reaction
wheat: gum
wheat pasture: poisoning
whetstone: crystal
whewellite: calculus
whey: alum; protein
whip: bougie
whiplash: injury
whispered: bronchophony; pectoriloquy
whispering: pectoriloquy
whistle-tip: catheter
whistling: deformity; rale
whistling face: syndrome
white: arsenic; beeswax; bile; commissure; corpuscle; diarrhea; fat; fiber; finger; gangrene; graft; infarct; lead; leg; line; matter; muscle; mustard; petrolatum; piedra; pine; pitch; pulp; spot; substance; thrombus; turpentine; wax; yolk
white blood: cell
white mercuric: precipitate
white muscle: disease
white-out: syndrome
white pupillary: reflex
white soft: paraffin
white sponge: nevus

white spot: disease
whole-body: counter
whole-body titration: curve
whole human: blood
whooping: cough
whooping-cough: vaccine
whorled: enamel
WI-38: cell
wide: plane; spectrum
wide field: ocular
wide-range: audiometer
wild: ginger; tobacco; type; yeast
wildfire: rash
wild-type: strain
willow: fracture
wind: contusion
Windigo, Wittigo: psychosis
window: level; width
wine: spirit
wing: cell; plate
winged: catheter; scapula
wink: reflex
winking: spasm
winter: dysentery; eczema; itch; sleep
wire: arch; splint
wire-loop: lesion
wiry: pulse
wisdom: tooth
Wistar: rat
witch's: milk
withdrawal: reflex; symptom
wolf: tooth
wolffian: body; cyst; duct; rest; ridge; tubule
wolffian duct: carcinoma
wood: charcoal; naphtha; spirit; sugar; vinegar
woodcutter's: encephalitis
wooden: resonance; tongue
wooden-shoe: heart
wool: ball; maggot
woolly: hair
woolly-hair: nevus
wool-sorter's: disease; pneumonia
word: blindness; deafness
working: bite; contact; occlusion; side
working occlusal: surface
working side: condyle
worm: abscess; aneurysm
wormian: bone
worsted: test
wound: clip; dehiscence; fever; myiasis
woven: bone
Wr^a: antigen
Wright: antigen
wrinkler: muscle
wrist: clonus; joint; sign
wrist clonus: reflex
writer's: cramp
writing: hand
wrought: wire
wry: neck

X

X: chromosome; disease; esotropia; exotropia; strabismus; zone
X-: body; ray
xanthene: dye
xanthogranulomatous: cholecystitis; pyelonephritis
X-chromosome-linked: achromatopsia
xeno-arc: photocoagulator
xenogeneic: graft
xenotropic: virus
xerotic: degeneration; keratitis
Xg: antigen
xiphisternal: joint
xiphisternal crunching: sound
xiphoid: cartilage; process
Xiphophorus: test
X-linked: agammaglobulinemia; gene; hypogammaglobulinemia; ichthyosis; inheritance; locus
X-linked hypophosphatemic: osteomalacia
X-linked infantile: hypogammaglobulinemia
XO: female; syndrome
x-ray: cap; dosimetry; microscope; therapy; tube
XX: male
XXX: female
XXY: male; syndrome
XYY: male; syndrome
xylose: test
xylostyptic: ether

Y

Y: axis; body; cartilage; chromosome; factor
y-: angle
Yaba: tumor
Yaba monkey: virus
Yangtze: edema
Yangtze Valley: fever
yeast: fungus; ribonuclease
yeast extract: agar
yellow: atrophy; blindness; body; cartilage; corallin; disease; fever; fiber; hepatization; ligament; mercury; precipitate; skin; spot; vision; wax; yolk
yellow bone: marrow
yellow fever: vaccine; virus
yellow soft: paraffin
yield: strength; stress
Y-linked: gene; inheritance; locus
yoke: bone
yolk: cell; cleavage; membrane; sac; stalk
yolk sac: tumor
Y-shaped: ligament
Yt^a: antigen

Z

Z: band; chromosome; disk; filament; line; procedure
Zambesi: ulcer
Zeisian: sty
zero-: gravity
zero degree: tooth
zero end-expiratory: pressure
zero-order: reaction
zeta: potential
zeta sedimentation: ratio
Zika: fever; virus
zinc: colic; gelatin
zinc-phosphate: cement
zinc sulfate flotation centrifugation: method
zirconium: granuloma
zonal: necrosis
zonary: placenta
zonular: band; cataract; fiber; layer; scotoma; space
zoonotic: infection; potential
zoonotic cutaneous: leishmaniasis
zooplastic: graft
zoster: encephalomyelitis
zoster immune: globulin
zwitter: hypothesis
zygal: fissure
zygapophysial: joint
zygomatic: arch; bone; diameter; fossa; margin; nerve; process; region
zygomatic: arch; bone; diameter; fossa; margin; nerve; process; region
zygomaticoauricular: index
zygomaticofacial: foramen
zygomaticomaxillary: suture
zygomatico-orbital: artery; foramen
zygomaticotemporal: foramen
zygomaxillary: point
zymatic: disease
zymogenic: cell
zymoplastic: substance
zymotic: papilloma

Stedman's
MEDICAL DICTIONARY

25th Edition
ILLUSTRATED

A

α **1.** First letter of the Greek alphabet, alpha; used as a classifier in the nomenclature of many sciences. **2.** Symbol for Bunsen's solubility *coefficient.* **3.** In chemistry, denotes the first in a series, a position immediately adjacent to a carboxyl group, the first of a series of closely related compounds, an aromatic substituent on an aliphatic chain, or the direction of a chemical bond away from the viewer. **4.** In chemistry, symbol for specific *rotation*. For terms beginning with this prefix, see the specific term.

A **1.** Abbreviation for ampere; adenine. **2.** Symbol for adenosine or adenylic acid in polynucleotides. **3.** Symbol (usually capitalized italic) for absorbance. **4.** As a subscript, refers to alveolar *gas.*

°A Symbol for degree absolute; replaced by K (kelvin).

Å Symbol for angstrom.

a **1.** Abbreviation for total *acidity;* area; asymmetric. **2.** Symbol for atto-. **3.** As a subscript, refers to systemic arterial blood.

a Symbol for specific absorption *coefficient.*

a-, an- [G. alpha, privative or negative, inseparable prefix, usually *an-* before a vowel or h]. Prefixes equivalent to the L. *in-* and E. *un-;* not, without, -less.

AA Abbreviation for amino acid; aminoacyl.

āā. Abbreviation for G. *ana,* of each; used in prescription writing following the name of two or more ingredients.

AAF Abbreviation for 2-acetylaminofluorene; 2-acetamidofluorene.

Aaron, Charles D., U.S. physician, 1866–1951. See A.'s *sign.*

Aarskog, Dagfinn J., 20th century Swedish pediatrician. See A.-Scott *syndrome.*

AAV Abbreviation for adeno-associated *virus.*

Ab Abbreviation for antibody.

ab-, abs- [L. *ab,* from, usually *abs-* before c, q, and t]. **1.** Prefix signifying from, away from, off. **2.** Prefix applied to electrical units in the CGS-electromagnetic system to distinguish them from units in the CGS-electrostatic system (prefix stat-) and those in the metric system or SI system (no prefix).

Abadie, Charles A., French ophthalmologist, 1842–1932. See A.'s *sign* of exophthalmic goiter.

Abadie, Joseph Louis Irénée Jean, French neurosurgeon, 1873–1946. See A.'s *sign* of tabes dorsalis.

abampere (ab-am'pēr). Electromagnetic unit of current equal to 10 absolute amperes; a current that exerts a force of 2π dynes on a unit magnetic pole at the center of a circle of wire (1 cm in radius).

abapical (ă-bap'i-kăl). Opposite the apex.

abarognosis (ab-ar-og-nō'sis) [G. *a-* priv. + *baros,* weight, + *gnōsis,* knowledge]. Loss of sense of weight estimation.

abasia (ă-bā'zē-ă) [G. *a-* priv. + *basis,* step]. Inability to walk.
atactic a., ataxic a., difficulty in walking due to ataxia of the legs.
choreic a., a. related to abnormal movements of the legs.
spastic a., a. due to a spastic contraction of the muscles when an attempt is made to walk.
a. trep'idans, a. due to trembling of the lower limbs.

abasia-astasia. See astasia-abasia.

abasic, abatic (ă-bā'sik, ă-bat'ik). Affected by, or associated with, abasia.

abaxial, abaxile (ab-ak'sē-ăl, -ak'sīl). **1.** Lying outside the axis of any body or part. **2.** Situated at the opposite extremity of the axis of a part.

abbau (ahb'bow) [Ger. *Abbau,* degradation, deterioration]. Those histologically demonstrable breakdown products noted in many degenerative diseases of the central nervous system.

Abbé, Ernst K., German physicist, 1840–1905. See A.'s *condenser;* A.-Zeiss *apparatus,* counting *chamber.*

Abbe, Robert, U.S. surgeon, 1851–1928. See A. *flap, operation.*

Abbott, Alexander C., U.S. bacteriologist, 1860–1935. See A.'s *stain* for spores.

Abbott, Edville G., U.S. orthopedic surgeon, 1871–1938. See A.'s *method.*

Abbott, W. Osler, U.S. physician, 1902–1943. See A.'s *tube,* Miller-A. *tube.*

abdomen (ab-dō'men; ab'dō-men) [L. *abdomen,* etym. uncertain] [NA]. Belly (1); venter (1); the part of the trunk that lies between the thorax and the pelvis. The a. does not include the vertebral region posteriorly but is considered by some anatomists to include the pelvis. It contains the greater part of the abdominal cavity, the cavum abdominis, and is divided by arbitrary planes into nine regions. See also *regiones* abdominis, under regio.
acute a., surgical a.; any serious acute intra-abdominal condition (such as appendicitis) attended by pain, tenderness, and muscular rigidity, and for which emergency surgery must be considered.
boat-shaped a., navicular a.
carinate a., a sloping of the sides with prominence of the central line of the a.
navicular a., boat-shaped or scaphoid a.; a condition in which the anterior abdominal wall is sunken and presents a concave rather than a convex contour.
a. obsti'pum, rarely used term for deformity of the a. due to congenitally short rectus muscles.
pendulous a., an a. with greatly relaxed walls that sag down over the pubic region.
protuberant a., unusual or prominent convexity of the a., due to excessive subcutaneous fat, poor muscle tone, or an increase in intra-abdominal content.
scaphoid a., navicular a.
surgical a., acute a.

abdominal (ab-dom'i-năl). Relating to the abdomen.

abdomino-, abdomin- [L. *abdomen*]. Combining forms denoting relationship to the abdomen.

abdominocentesis (ab-dom'i-nō-sen-tē'sis) [abdomino- + G. *kentēsis,* puncture]. Paracentesis of the abdomen.

abdominocyesis (ab-dom'i-nō-sī-ē'sis) [abdomino- + G. *kyēsis,* pregnancy]. **1.** Abdominal *pregnancy.* **2.** Secondary abdominal *pregnancy.*

abdominocystic (ab-dom-i-nō-sis'tik) [abdomino- + G. *kystis,* bladder]. Abdominovesical.

abdominogenital (ab-dom'i-nō-gen'i-tăl). Relating to the abdomen and the genital organs.

abdominohysterectomy (ab-dom'i-nō-his-ter-ek'tō-mē). Abdominal *hysterectomy.*

abdominohysterotomy (ab-dom'i-nō-his-ter-ot'ō-mē). Abdominal *hysterotomy.*

abdominoperineal (ab-dom'i-nō-păr-i-nē'ăl). Relating to both abdomen and parineum.

abdominoplasty (ab-dom'i-nō-plas-tē) [abdomino- + G. *plastos,* formed]. An operation performed on the abdominal wall for esthetic purposes.

abdominoscopy (ab-dom-i-nos'kō-pē) [abdomino- + G. *skopeō,* to examine]. Peritoneoscopy.

abdominoscrotal (ab-dom'i-nō-skrō'tăl). Relating to the abdomen and the scrotum.

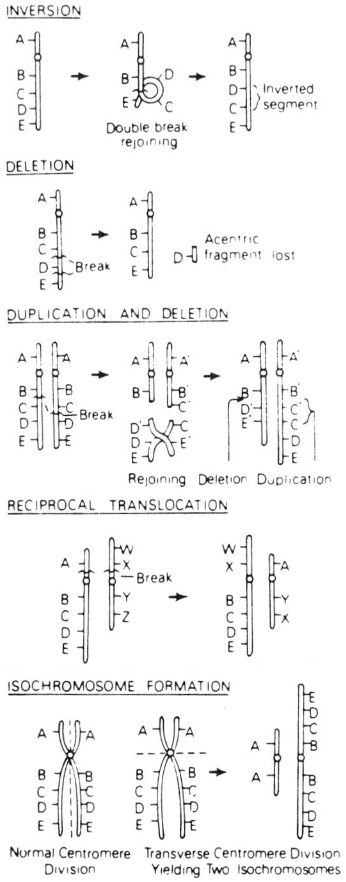

Chromosome Aberrations

abdominothoracic (ab-dom'i-nō-thō-ras'ik). Relating to both abdomen and thorax.

abdominovaginal (ab-dom'i-nō-vag'i-năl). Relating to both abdomen and vagina.

abdominovesical (ab-dom'i-nō-ves'i-kăl). Abdominocystic; relating to the abdomen and urinary bladder, or to the abdomen and gallbladder.

abduce (ab-dūs'). Abduct.

abducens (ab-dū'senz) [L.]. Abducent.
a. oc'uli, *musculus* rectus lateralis.

abducent (ab-dū'sent) [L. *abducens*]. Abducting; drawing away.

abduct (ab-dŭkt'). Abduce; to move away from the median plane.

abduction (ab-dŭk'shŭn) [L. *abductio*]. **1.** Movement of a body part away from the median plane (of the body, in the case of limbs; of the hand or foot, in the case of digits). **2.** Monocular rotation (duction) of the eye toward the temple. **3.** A position resulting from such movement. *Cf.* adduction.

abductor (ab-dŭk'ter, -tōr). A muscle that draws a part away from the median plane.

Abegg, Richard, Danish chemist, 1869–1910. See A.'s *rule.*

Abel, Rudolf, German bacteriologist, 1868–1942. See A.'s *bacillus.*

Abell-Kendall method. See under method.

Abelson, Herbert T., U.S. pediatrician, *1941. See A. murine leukemia *virus.*

abembryonic (ab'em-brē-on'ik) [L. *ab,* from, + embryonic]. Opposite the region at which the embryo is formed.

abenteric (ab-en-ter'ik) [L. *ab,* from, + G. *enteron,* intestine]. Apenteric.

Abernethy, John, British surgeon and anatomist, 1764–1831. See A.'s *fascia.*

aberrant (ab-er'ant) [L. *aberrans*]. **1.** Wandering off; said of certain ducts, vessels, or nerves taking an unusual course. **2.** Differing from the normal; in botany or zoology, said of certain atypical individuals in a species. **3.** Ectopic (1).

aberration (ab-er-ā'shŭn) [L. *aberratio*]. **1.** A straying from the normal situation. **2.** Deviant development or growth.
chromatic a., color a.; newtonian a.; chromatism (2); the difference in focus or magnification of an image arising because of a difference in the refraction of different wavelengths composing white light.
chromosome a., any deviation from the normal number or morphology of chromosomes.
color a., chromatic a.
coma a., the distortion of image formation created when a bundle of light rays enters an optical system not parallel to the optic axis.
curvature a., lack of spatial correspondence causing the image of a straight extended object to appear curved.
dioptric a., spherical a.
distortion a., the faulty formation of an image arising because the magnification of the peripheral part of an object is different from that of the central part when viewed through a lens.
lateral a., in spherical a., the distance between paraxial focus of central rays on the optic axis.
longitudinal a., in spherical a., the distance separating the focus of paraxial and peripheral rays on the optic axis.
mental a., an illogical and unreasonable thought or belief.
meridional a., an a. produced in the plane of a single meridian of a lens.
monochromatic a., a defect in an optical image arising because of the nature of lenses; the main types are spherical, coma, curvature, and distortion a., and astigmatism of oblique pencils.
newtonian a., chromatic a.
optical a., failure of rays from a point source to form a perfect image after traversing an optical system.
spherical a., dioptric or zonal a.; a monochromatic a. occurring in refraction at a spherical surface in which the paraxial and peripheral rays focus along the axis at different points.
ventricular a., aberrant ventricular *conduction.*

aberrometer (ab-er-rom'ē-ter) [L. *aberratio,* aberration, + G. *metron,* measure]. An instrument for measuring optical aberration or any error in experimentation.

abetalipoproteinemia (ā-bā'tă-lip'ō-prō'tēn-ē'mē-ă) [G. *a-,* priv., + *beta,* β, + lipoprotein + *-emia,* blood]. Bassen-Kornzweig syndrome; a disorder characterized by an absence from plasma of low density lipoproteins, presence of acanthocytes in blood, retinal pigmentary degeneration, malabsorption, engorgement of upper intestinal absorptive cells with dietary triglycerides, and neuromuscular abnormalities; autosomal recessive inheritance.

abeyance (ă-bā'ans) [fr. O. Fr.]. A state of temporary abolition of function.

abfarad (ab-far'ad). Electromagnetic unit of capacity equal to 10^9 farads.

ABG Abbreviation for arterial blood gas. See blood *gases.*

abhenry (ab-hen'rē). Electromagnetic unit of inductance equal to 10^{-9} henry.

abient (ab'ē-ent) [L. *abiens,* fr. *ab- eo,* to go from]. Having a tendency to move away from the source of a stimulus, as opposed to adient.

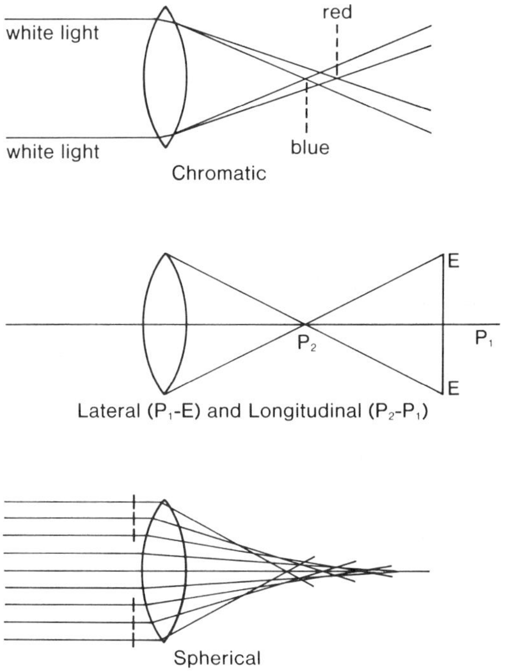

Optical Aberrations

ability (ă-bil'i-tē) [L. *habilitas,* aptitude]. The physical, mental, or legal competence to function.

abiogenesis (ab'ē-ō-jen'ĕ-sis) [G. *a-* priv. + *bios,* life, + *genesis,* production]. The origin of living matter without descent from other living matter; a theory of spontaneous generation.

abiogenetic (ab'ē-ō-jĕ-net'ik). Pertaining to abiogenesis.

abiosis (ab-ē-ō'sis) [G. *a-* priv. + *bios,* life]. **1.** Nonviability. **2.** Absence of life. **3.** Abiotrophy.

abiotic (ab-ē-ot'ik). Incompatible with life.

abiotrophy (ab-ē-ot'rō-fē) [G. *a-* priv. + *bios,* life, + *trophē,* nourishment]. Abiosis (3); an age-dependent manifestation of a genetically determined trait that has been latent from the time of conception.

abirritant (ab-ir'i-tănt). **1.** Abirritative; soothing, or relieving irritation. **2.** An agent possessing this property.

abirritation (ab-ir-i-tā'shŭn) [L. *ab,* from, + *irrito,* pp. *-atus,* to irritate]. Diminution or abolition of irritability in a part.

abirritative (ab-ir'i-tā-tiv). Abirritant (1).

abl. An oncogene found in the Abelson strain of mouse leukemia virus and involved in the Philadelphia chromosome translocation in chronic granulocytic leukemia.

ablactation (ab-lak-tā'shŭn) [L. *ab,* from, + lactation]. Weaning (1).

ablastemic (ā-blas-tem'ik) [G. *a-* priv. + *blastēma,* sprout]. Not germinal or blastemic.

ablastin (ă-blas'tin) [G. *a-* priv. + *blastos,* germ]. An antibody that seems to inhibit reproduction of trypanosomes; found in rats infected with *Trypanosoma lewisi.*

ablate (ab-lāt') [L. *au- fero,* pp. *ab- latus,* to take away]. To remove, or to destroy the function of.

ablation (ab-lā'shun) [L. see ablate]. Removal of a body part or the destruction of its function, as by a surgical procedure, morbid process, or noxious substance.

ablatio placentae (ab-lā'shē-ō pla-sen'tē). Abruptio placentae.

ablatio retinae (ab-lā'shē-ō ret'ĭ-nē). Obsolete term for retinal *detachment.*

ablepharia (ā-blef-ar'ē-ă) [G. *a-* priv. + *blepharon,* eyelid]. Congenital absence, partial or complete, of the eyelids.

ablepsia, ablepsy (ă-blep'sē-ă, ă-blep'sē) [G. *a-* priv. + *blepō,* to see]. Obsolete term for blindness.

abluent (ab'lū-ent) [L. *abluens,* fr. *ab-luo,* to wash off]. **1.** Cleansing. **2.** Anything with cleansing properties.

ablution (ab-lū'shŭn) [L. *ablutio,* washing off, cleansing]. An act of washing or bathing.

ablutomania (ab-lū-tō-mā'nē-ă) [L. *ablutio,* washing, + G. *mania,* insanity]. Rarely used term for a morbid preoccupation with thoughts about cleanliness, with frequent washing, as seen in obsessive-compulsive neurosis.

abnerval (ab-ner'văl). Abneural (1); away from a nerve; denoting specifically a current of electricity passing through a muscular fiber in a direction away from the point of entrance of the nerve fiber.

abneural (ab-nūr'ăl) [L. *ab,* away from, + G. *neuron,* nerve]. **1.** Abnerval. **2.** Away from the neural axis.

abnormal (ab-nōr'măl). Not normal; differing in any way from the usual state, structure, condition, or rule.

abnormality (ab-nōr-mal'i-tē). **1.** The state or quality of being abnormal. **2.** An anomaly, deformity, malformation, or dysfunction.
figure-of-eight a., a roentgenographic appearance produced by an anomalous drainage of the total pulmonary venous circulation into enlarged right and anomalous left venae cavae which produces a globular density above the heart; the silhouette suggests the figure eight.

ABO blood group. See Blood Groups appendix.

abohm (ab'ōm). Electromagnetic unit of resistance equal to 10^{-9} ohm.

aboiement (ah-bwah-mahn') [Fr. barking, yelping]. Rarely used term for the involuntary production of abnormal sounds, as seen in Gilles de la Tourette syndrome.

abomasitis (ab'ō-mas-ī'tis). Inflammation of the abomasum.

abomasum (ab-ō-mā'sŭm) [L. *ab,* from, + *omasum,* bullock's tripe]. The fourth compartment and the glandular portion of the stomach of a ruminant.

aborad, aboral (ab-ō'rad, -răl) [L. *ab,* from, + *os (or-),* mouth]. In a direction away from the mouth; opposite of orad.

abort (ă-bōrt') [L. *aborto,* to miscarry]. **1.** To give birth to an embryo or fetus before it is viable. **2.** To arrest a disease in its earliest stages. **3.** To arrest in growth or development; to cause to remain rudimentary. **4.** To remove products of conception before 20 weeks of gestation.

abortient (ă-bōr'shent). Abortifacient (1).

abortifacient (ă-bōr-ti-fā'shent) [L. *abortus,* abortion, + *facio,* to make]. **1.** Abortient; abortigenic; abortive (3); producing abortion. **2.** An agent that produces abortion.

abortigenic (ă-bōr-ti-jen'ik) [L. *abortus,* abortion, + *genesis,* production]. Abortifacient (1).

abortion (ă-bōr'shŭn). **1.** Giving birth to an embryo or fetus prior to the stage of viability at about 20 weeks of gestation (fetus weighs less than 500 g). A distinction is made between a. and premature birth: premature infants are those born after the stage of viability has been (occurring but before full term. A. may be either spontaneous (occurring from natural causes) or induced. **2.** The product of such nonviable birth. **3.** The arrest of any action or process before its normal completion.
accidental a., a. due to a fall, blow, or other injury.

ampullar a., a. resulting from pregnancy in tubal ampulla.
bovine infectious a., bovine *brucellosis.*
complete a., **(1)** the complete expulsion or extraction from its mother of a fetus or embryo. **(2)** complete expulsion of any other product of gestation. (*e.g.,* hydatidiform mole).
contagious a., bovine *brucellosis.*
criminal a., termination of pregnancy without medical or legal justification.
enzootic a. of ewes, a specific infectious a. of sheep caused by *Chlamydia psittaci.*
equine virus a., a highly contagious a. of mares, caused by equine rhinopneumonitis virus, sometimes associated with equine rhinopneumonitis.
habitual a., a condition in which a woman has had three or more consecutive, spontaneous a.'s.
imminent a., incipient a.
incipient a., imminent a.; impending a. characterized by copious vaginal bleeding, uterine contractions, and cervical dilation.
incomplete a., a. in which part of the products of conception have been passed but part (usually the placenta) remains in the uterus.
induced a., a. brought on purposefully by drugs or mechanical means.
inevitable a., a. characterized by rupture of the membranes in the presence of cervical dilation that has advanced beyond the possibility of preventing complete a.
infected a., a septic complication of an a.
justifiable a., therapeutic a.
menstrual extraction a., a technique for aspiration of early products of conception from the uterus a few days after the first missed menstrual period.
missed a., a. in which the fetus dies *in utero* but the product of conception is retained *in utero* for two months or longer.
septic a., an infectious a. complicated by fever, endometritis, and parametritis.
spontaneous a., a. that has not been artificially induced.
therapeutic a., justifiable a.; a. induced because of the mother's physical or mental health, or to prevent birth of a deformed child or a child resulting from rape.
threatened a., cramplike pains and slight show of blood that may or may not be followed by the expulsion of the fetus during the first 20 weeks of pregnancy.
tubal a., aborted ectopic pregnancy; rupture of an oviduct, the seat of ectopic pregnancy, or extrusion of the product of conception through the fimbriated end of the oviduct.
vibrionic a., a. of cattle or sheep caused by *Campylobacter fetus* (*Vibrio fetus*).

abortionist (ă-bōr'shŭn-ist). One who interrupts a pregnancy.

abortive (ă-bōr'tiv) [L. *abortivus*]. **1.** Not reaching completion; *e.g.,* said of an attack of a disease subsiding before it has fully developed or completed its course. **2.** Rudimentary. **3.** Abortifacient (1).

abortus (ă-bōr'tŭs) [L.]. Any product (or all products) of an abortion.

abouchement (ah-būsh-mahn') [Fr. *abouchement,* inosculation, anastomosis]. Junction of a small blood vessel with a large one.

aboulia (ă-bū'lē-ă). Abulia.

ABR Abbreviation for auditory brainstem response. See auditory brainstem response *audiometry.*

abrachia (ă-brā'kē-ă) [G. *a-* priv. + *brachiōn,* arm]. Congenital absence of arms.

abrachiocephaly, abrachiocephalia (ă-brā'kē-ō-sef'ă-lē, -se-fā'lē-ă) [G. *a-* priv. + *brachiōn,* arm, + *kephalē,* head]. Abrachiocephalia; acephalobrachia; congenital absence of arms and head.

abrade (ă-brād') [L. *ab-rado,* pp. *-rasus,* to scrape off]. **1.** To wear away by mechanical action. **2.** To scrape away the surface layer from a part.

Abrahams, Robert, U.S. physician, 1861–1935. See A.'s *sign.*

Abrams, Albert, U.S. physician, 1863–1924. See A.'s heart *reflex.*

abrasion (ă-brā'zhŭn) [see abrade]. **1.** Abraded wound; an excoriation, or circumscribed removal of the superficial layers of skin or mucous membrane. **2.** A scraping away of a portion of the surface. **3.** Grinding; in dentistry, the pathological grinding or wearing away of tooth substance by incorrect tooth-brushing methods, foreign objects, bruxism, or similar causes. *Cf.* attrition.
brush burn a., see brush *burn.*
gingival a., a lesion of the gingiva resulting from mechanical removal of a portion of the surface epithelium.
mechanical a., removal of the epidermis down to the tips of the papillae by rubbing with sandpaper, rotating wire brush, or other abrasive material; a method of removing or obliterating cutaneous scars or pits such as those produced by acne vulgaris.
tooth a., loss or wearing away of tooth structure caused by the abrasive characteristics of substances other than foods.

abrasive (a-brā'siv). **1.** Causing abrasion. **2.** Any material used to produce abrasions. **3.** A substance used in dentistry for abrading, grinding, or polishing.

abrasiveness (ă-brā'siv-nes). **1.** That property of a substance which causes surface wear by friction. **2.** The quality of being able to scratch or abrade another material.

abreact (ab-rē-akt'). **1.** To show strong emotion in reliving a previous traumatic experience. **2.** To discharge or release repressed emotion.

abreaction (ab-rē-ak'shŭn). In freudian psychoanalysis, an episode of emotional release or catharsis associated with the bringing into conscious recollection previously repressed unpleasant experiences.
motor a., the release of an unconscious thought, idea, or impulse through motor or muscular expression.

abruption (ab-rŭp'shŭ). A tearing away, separation, or detachment.

abruptio placentae (ab-rŭp'shē-ō pla-sen'tē). Ablatio or amotio placentae; premature detachment of a normally situated placenta.

Abrus (ā'brŭs) [more correctly *Habrus,* from G. *habros,* graceful]. A genus of leguminous plants. The root of *A. precatorius,* Indian liquorice, is sometimes used as a substitute for liquorice; the seeds are toxic and may cause vomiting, diarrhea, convulsions, and death if chewed.

abs. feb. Abbreviation for L. *absente febre,* when fever is absent.

ABSCESS

abscess (ab'ses) [L. *abscessus,* a going away]. **1.** A circumscribed collection of pus appearing in an acute or chronic localized infection, and associated with tissue destruction, and, frequently, swelling. **2.** A cavity formed by liquefactive necrosis within solid tissue.
acute a., hot a.; a recently formed a. with little or no fibrosis in the wall of the cavity.
alveolar a., dental, dentoalveolar, radicular, or root a.; an a. situated within the alveolar process of the jaws, most often caused by extension of infection from an adjacent nonvital tooth.
amebic a., tropical a.; an area of liquefaction necrosis of the liver or other organ containing amebae, often following amebic dysentery.
apical a., **(1)** periapical a.; **(2)** an a. in the apex of the lung.
apical periodontal a., periapical a.

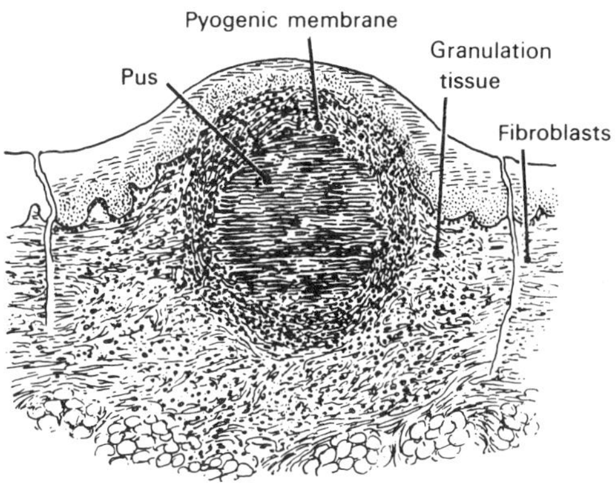

Abscess of Skin

appendiceal a., periappendiceal a.; an intraperitoneal a., usually in the right iliac fossa, resulting from extension of infection in acute appendicitis, especially with perforation of the appendix.
Bartholin's a., an a. of the vulvovaginal gland.
Bezold's a., an a. deep in the neck associated with suppuration in the mastoid tip cells.
bicameral a., an a. with two separate cavities or chambers.
bone a., suppuration within the medullary cavity (osteomyelitis), cortex, or periosteum of bone.
Brodie's a., a chronic a. of bone surrounded by dense fibrous tissue and sclerotic bone.
bursal a., suppuration within a bursa.
caseous a., an a. containing white solid or semisolid material of cheesy consistency; usually tuberculous.
chronic a., a long-standing collection of pus surrounded by fibrous tissue.
cold a., **(1)** an a. without heat or other usual signs of inflammation; **(2)** tuberculous a.
collar-button a., shirt-stud a.; an a. consisting of two cavities connected by a narrow isthmus, usually formed by rupture of an a. through a fascial layer in the hand or foot.
crypt a.'s, a.'s in crypts of Lieberkühn of the large intestinal mucosa; a characteristic feature of ulcerative colitis.
dental a., dentoalveolar a., alveolar a.
diffuse a., a collection of pus not circumscribed by a well defined capsule.
Douglas a., suppuration in Douglas pouch.
dry a., the remains of an a. after the pus is absorbed.
Dubois' a.'s, thymic a.'s; Dubois' disease; small cysts of the thymus containing polymorphonuclear leukocytes but lined by squamous epithelium; reported in congenital syphilis but also found in the absence of syphilis.
embolic a., an a. arising at the point of arrest of a septic embolus.
fecal a., stercoral a.
follicular a., an a. in a hair, tonsillar, or other follicle.
gas a., an a. containing gas caused by *Enterobacter aerogenes, Escherichia coli,* or other gas-forming microorganisms.
gingival a., gumboil; parulis; an a. confined to the gingival soft tissue.
gravitation a., perforating a.
gummatous a., syphilitic a.; an a. due to the softening and breaking down of a gumma, especially in bone.
hematogenous a., an a. caused by blood-borne organisms.
hot a., acute a.
hypostatic a., perforating a.
ischiorectal a., an a. involving the tissues in the ischiorectal fossa.
lacunar a., an a. involving the urethral lacunae.
lateral alveolar a., pericemental a.; an alveolar a. located along the lateral root surface of a tooth.
lateral periodontal a., an a. that forms at the depth of a periodontal pocket due to multiplication of pyogenic microorganisms or the presence of foreign material.
mastoid a., an a. of the mastoid air cells.
metastatic a., a secondary a. formed, at a distance from the primary focus, as a result of the transportation of pyogenic bacteria by the lymph or bloodstream.
migrating a., perforating a.
miliary a., one of a number of minute collections of pus, widely disseminated throughout an area or the whole body.
Munro's a., Munro's *microabscess.*
mycotic a., an a. caused by pathogenic fungi.
orbital a., retrobulbar a.; a circumscribed collection of pus within the orbit; frequently an extension of purulent infection of the paranasal sinuses, usually the ethmoids.
otic a., a cerebral a. secondary to suppuration of the middle ear.
palatal a., **(1)** a lateral periodontal a. associated with the lingual surface of a maxillary tooth; **(2)** an alveolar a. that has eroded the cortical plate, allowing extension into the palatal soft tissues.
parafrenal a., an a. that occurs on either side of the frenum of the penis.
parametric a., parametritic a., an a. in the connective tissue of the broad ligament of the uterus.
paranephric a., an a. in the region of the kidney, outside the renal fascia.
parotid a., rapidly progressive suppuration in parotid gland; a complication of parotitis.
Pautrier's a., Pautrier's *microabscess.*
pelvic a., an a. in the pelvic peritoneal cavity, developing as a complication of diffuse peritonitis or of localized peritonitis associated with abdominal or pelvic inflammatory disease, such as salpingitis; the pus frequently collects in the rectovesical or rectouterine pouch.
perforating a., an a. that breaks down tissue barriers to enter adjacent areas. Also called gravitation, hypostatic, migrating, or wandering a.
periapical a., apical a.; apical periodontal a.; an alveolar a. localized around the apex of a tooth root.
periappendiceal a., appendiceal a.
periarticular a., an a. surrounding a joint, not usually involving it.
pericemental a., lateral alveolar a.
pericoronal a., an a. developing in the inflamed dental follicular tissue overlaying the crown of a partially erupted tooth.
perinephric a., an a. surrounding or adjacent to the kidney.
periodontal a., an alveolar a. or a lateral periodontal a.
perirectal a., an a. in connective tissue adjacent to the rectum or anus.
peritonsillar a., quinsy; extension of tonsillar infection beyond the capsule with abscess formation usually above and behind the tonsil.
periureteral a., an a. surrounding the ureter.
periurethral a., an a. involving the tissues around the urethra.
phlegmonous a., circumscribed suppuration characterized by intense surrounding inflammatory reaction which produces induration and thickening of the affected area.
Pott's a., tuberculous a. of the spine.
premammary a., an a. in the subcutaneous tissue covering the mammary gland.
psoas a., an a., usually tuberculous, originating in tuberculous spondylitis and extending through the iliopsoas muscle to the inguinal region.
pulp a., an a. involving the soft tissue within the pulp chamber of a tooth, usually the sequella of caries or less frequently of trauma.
pyemic a., septicemic a.; a hematogenous a. resulting from pyemia, septicemia, or bacteremia.
radicular a., alveolar a.
residual a., an a. recurring at the site of a former a. resulting from

persistence of microbes and pus.
retrobulbar a., orbital a.
retrocecal a., an a. located posterior to the cecum, usually resulting from perforation of a retrocecal appendix.
retropharyngeal a., an a. arising, usually, in retropharyngeal lymph nodes, most commonly in infants.
ring a., an acute purulent inflammation of the corneal periphery in which a necrotic area is surrounded by an annular girdle of leukocytic infiltration.
root a., alveolar a.
satellite a., an a. closely associated with a primary a.
septicemic a., pyemic a.
shirt-stud a., collar-button a.
stellate a., a star-shaped necrotic area surrounded by epithelioid cells, seen within swollen inguinal lymph nodes in lymphogranuloma venereum.
stercoral a., fecal a.; a collection of pus and feces.
sterile a., an a. whose contents are not caused by pyogenic bacteria.
stitch a., an a. around a suture.
subacute a., an a. of several weeks' duration.
subdiaphragmatic a., subphrenic a.
subepidermal a., a microscopic a. located in the dermis just beneath the epidermis.
subperiosteal a., an a. between the periosteum and cortical plate of the bone.
subphrenic a., subdiaphragmatic a.; an a. directly beneath the diaphragm.
subungual a., suppuration beneath a fingernail or toenail.
sudoriparous a., a collection of pus in a sweat gland.
syphilitic a., gummatous a.
thecal a., suppuration in a tendon sheath.
thymic a.'s, Dubois' a.'s.
Tornwaldt's a., chronic infection of the pharyngeal bursa. See also Tornwaldt's *syndrome.*
tropical a., amebic a.
tuberculous a., cold a. (2); an a. caused by the tubercle bacillus.
tubo-ovarian a., a large a. involving a uterine tube and an adherent ovary, resulting from extension of purulent inflammation of the tube.
verminous a., worm a.
wandering a., perforating a.
worm a., verminous a.; a. due to parasitic worms or in which worms are found.

---

abscissa (ab-sis'ă) [L. *ab-scindo,* pp. *-scissus,* to cut away from]. In a plane cartesian coordinate system, the horizontal axis (*x*). *Cf.* ordinate.

abscission (ab-si'shŭn) [L. *ab-scindo,* pp. *-scissus,* to cut away from]. Cutting away.

absconsio (ab-skon'shē-ō) [Mod. L. fr. *abs-condo,* pp. *-conditus* or *-consus,* to hide]. A recess or cavity.

abscopal (ab-skō'păl, -skop'ăl). Denoting the remote effect that irradiation of a tissue has on nonirradiated tissue.

absence (ab'sens) [L. *absentia*]. Absence seizure; absentia epileptica; epileptic absence; petit mal; petit mal epilepsy; paroxysmal attacks of impaired consciousness, occasionally accompanied by spasm or twitching of cephalic muscles, which usually can be brought on by hyperventilation; depending on the type and severity of the a., the EEG may show an abrupt onset of a 3/sec spike and wave pattern as in simple a., or in atypical cases, a 4/sec spike and wave or faster spike complexes. The clinical states accompanying these EEG abnormalities may be classified as: 1) a. with no overt manifestations, *e.g.,* simple a.; epileptic a.; subclinical a.; 2) a. with clonic movements, *e.g.,* myoclonic a.; 3) a. with atonic states, *e.g.,* atonic a.; 4) a. with tonic contractions, *e.g.,* hypertonic muscular contraction; 5) a. with automatisms, *e.g.,* various stereotyped movements, usually of the face or hands; 6) a. with atypical features, *e.g.,* bizarre motor activity.
atonic a., a. with atonic states.
atypical a., a. with atypical features.
automatic a., a. with automatisms.
complex a., a. with automatisms.
enuretic a., a. with atypical features.
epileptic a., absence.
hypertonic a., a. with tonic contractions.
myoclonic a., a. with clonic components.
pure a., a. with no overt manifestations.
retrocursive a., a. with automatisms.
simple a., a. with no overt manifestations.
sternutatory a., a. with automatisms.
subclinical a., a. with no overt manifestations.
tussive a., a. with automatisms.
typical a., a. with no overt manifestations.
vasomotor a., a. with atypical features. *e.g.,* flushing.

absentia epileptica (ab-sen'shē-ă ep-i-lep'ti-kă). Absence.

Absidia (ab-sid'ē-ă). A genus of fungi (family Mucoraceae) commonly found in nature. Thermophilic species survive in compost piles at temperatures exceeding 45°C and may cause zygomycosis in humans.

absinthe (ab'sinth). A liqueur consisting of an alcoholic extract of absinthium and other bitter herbs.

absinthin (ab'sin-thin). A bitter principle, $C_{30}H_{40}O_8$, obtained from absinthium.

absinthium (ab-sin'thē-ŭm) [L., fr. G. *apsinthion*]. Wormwood; the dried leaves and tops of *Artemisia absinthium* (family Compositae). The infusion is now seldom used, but it has been used as a tonic; in large or frequently repeated doses it produces headache, trembling, and epileptiform convulsions.

absinthol (ab-sin'thawl). Thujone.

absolute (ab'sō-lūt) [L. *absolutus,* complete, pp. of *ab-solvo,* to loosen from]. Unconditional; unlimited; uncombined; certain.

absorb (ab-sōrb') [L. *ab-sorbeo,* pp. *-sorptus,* to suck in]. **1.** To take in by absorption. **2.** To reduce the intensity of transmitted light.

absorbance (*A*) (ab-sōr'bans). Absorbancy; absorbency; optical density; extinction (2); in spectrophotometry, equal to 2 minus the log of the percentage transmittance of light.
specific a., absorbance per unit of concentration. See specific absorption *coefficient.*

absorbancy (ab-sōr'ban-sē). Absorbance.

absorbefacient (ab-sōr-bē-fā'shŭnt) [L. *ab-sorbeo,* to suck in, + *facio,* to make]. **1.** Causing absorption. **2.** Any substance possessing such quality.

absorbency (ab-sōrb'en-sē). Absorbance.

absorbent (ab-sōr'bent). **1.** Bibulous; absorptive; having the power to absorb, soak up, or take into itself a gas, liquid, light rays, or heat. **2.** Any substance possessing such power. **3.** Material (usually caustic) for removal of carbon dioxide from circuits in which rebreathing occurs; *e.g.,* anesthesia and basal metabolism equipment.

absorber head (ab-sōr'ber hed). Portion of a rebreathing anesthesia circuit that contains carbon dioxide absorbent; often referred to as a canister.

absorption (ab-sōrp'shŭn). **1.** The taking in, incorporation, or reception of gases, liquids, light, or heat. *Cf.* adsorption. **2.** In radiology, the uptake of energy from radiation by the medium through which it passes.
cutaneous a., the percutaneous a. of drugs, allergens, atopens,

toxins, and other substances in contact with the intact epidermis.
disjunctive a., a. of living tissue in immediate relation with a necrosed part, producing the line of demarcation.
electron resonance a., see electron spin *resonance.*
external a., the a. of substances through skin, mucocutaneous surfaces, or mucous membranes.
interstitial a., the removal of water or of substances in the interstitial fluid by the lymphatics.
parenteral a., a. through the skin or subcutaneous tissues, or by any route other than the alimentary tract.
pathologic a., parenteral a. of any excremental or pathologic material into the bloodstream, *e.g.,* pus, urine, bile, etc.

absorptive (ab-sōrp'tiv). Absorbent (1).

absorptivity (ab-sōrp-tiv'i-tē). Specific absorption *coefficient.*
molar a., molar absorption *coefficient.*

abstinence (ab'sti-nens) [L. *abs-tineo,* to hold back, fr. *teneo,* to hold]. Specifically, refraining from the use of certain articles of diet, of alcoholic beverages, or from sexual intercourse.

abstract (ab'strakt) [L. *ab-straho,* pp. *-tractus,* to draw away]. **1.** A preparation made by evaporating a fluidextract to a powder and triturating with milk sugar. **2.** A condensation or summary of a scientific or literary article or address.

abstraction (ab-strak'shŭn) [L. *ab-straho,* pp. *-tractus,* to draw away]. **1.** Distillation or separation of the volatile constituents of a substance. **2.** Exclusive mental concentration. **3.** The making of an abstract from the crude drug. **4.** Malocclusion in which the teeth or associated structures are lower than their normal occlusal plane. See also odontoptosis. **5.** The process of selecting a certain aspect of a concept from the whole.

abstriction (ab-strik'shŭn) [L. *ab-,* from, + *strictura,* a contraction]. In fungi, the formation of asexual spores by cutting off portions of the sporophore through the growth of dividing partitions.

abterminal (ab-ter'mi-năl) [L. *ab,* from, + *terminus,* end]. In a direction away from the end and toward the center; denoting the course of an electrical current in a muscle.

abtropfung (ab-trop'fŭng) [Ger. *Abtropfung,* trickling down]. A theory that nevus cells are epidermal cells (melanocytes) that divide and drop off (migrate) into the dermis; or, in the presence of thinning of the basement membrane, reticulum and collagen encompass the nest of junctional cells forming the dermal component of the nevus.

abulia (ă-bū'lē-ă) [G. *a-* priv. + *boulē,* will]. Aboulia; loss or impairment of the ability to perform voluntary actions or to make decisions.

abulic (ă-bū'lik). Relating to, or suffering from, abulia.

abuse (ă-byūs'). **1.** Misuse, wrong use, especially excessive use, of anything. **2.** Injurious, harmful, or offensive treatment, as in child a.
drug a., habitual use of drugs solely to alter one's mood, affect, or state of consciousness.
substance a., excessive use of a substance, especially one that may modify body functions, such as caffeine-containing drinks, tobacco, and drugs.

abutment (ă-bŭt'ment). In dentistry, a natural tooth or implanted tooth substitute, used for the support or anchorage of a fixed or removable prosthesis.
auxiliary a., a tooth other than the one supporting the direct retainer, assisting in the overall support of a removable partial denture.
intermediate a., a natural tooth, or an implanted tooth substitute, without other natural teeth in proximal contact, used along with the mesial and distal a.'s to support a prosthesis; often called a "pier."
isolated a., a lone-standing tooth, or root, with edentulous areas mesial and distal to it.
splinted a., the joining of two or more teeth into a rigid unit by means of fixed restorations to form a single a. with multiple roots.

ABVD Abbreviation for a chemotherapy regimen of Adriamycin (doxorubicin), bleomycin, vinblastine, and dacarbazine; used to treat neoplastic diseases, such as Hodgkin's disease, shown to be resistant to MOPP therapy.

abvolt (ab'vōlt). Electromagnetic unit of difference of potential equal to 10^{-8} volt.

AC Abbreviation for alternating *current.*

Ac Symbol for actinium; acetyl.

aC Symbol for arabinosylcytosine.

a.c. Abbreviation for L. *ante cibum,* before a meal.

AC/A Abbreviation for accommodative convergence-accommodation *ratio.*

acacia (ă-kā'shē-ă) [G. *akakia*]. Gum arabic; the dried gummy exudation from *Acacia senegal* and other species of *A.* (family Leguminosae), prepared as a mucilage and syrup; used as an emollient, demulcent excipient, and suspending agent; formerly used as a transfusion fluid.

acalculia (ă-kal-kyū'lē-ă) [G. *a-* priv. + L. *calculo,* to reckon]. A form of aphasia characterized by inability to do simple mathematical problems; commonly seen in parietal lobe lesions.

acampsia (ă-kamp'sē-ă) [G. *a-* priv. + *kamptō,* to bend]. Stiffening or rigidity of a joint for any reason.

acamylophenine (ă-kam'ĕ-lō-fe-nēn). Camylofine.

acanth-. See acantho-.

acantha (ă-kan'thă) [G. *akantha,* a thorn]. A spine or spinous process.

acanthamebiasis (ă-kan'thă-mē-bī'ă-sis). Infection by free-living soil amebae of the genus *Acanthamoeba* that may result in a necrotizing dermal or tissue invasion, or a fulminating and usually fatal primary amebic meningoencephalitis.

Acanthamoeba (ă-kan-thă-mē'bă) [G. *akantha,* thorn, spine, + Mod. L. *amoeba,* fr. G. *amoibē,* change]. A genus of free-living ameba (family Acanthamoebidae, order Amoebida) found in and characterized by the presence of acanthopodia. Human infection includes invasion of skin or colonization following injury, corneal invasion and colonization, and possibly lung or genitourinary tract colonization; a few cases of brain or CNS invasion have occurred, but not solely by the olfactory epithelium route of entry as with the more virulent infections caused by *Naegleria fowleri.* Species responsible are chiefly *A. culbertsoni,* but cases have been reported involving *A. castellanii, A. polyphaga,* and *A. astronyxis,* though most cases have been chronic rather than fulminating and rapidly fatal as with *Naegleria fowleri* infection.

acanthella (ă-kan-thel'ă) [G. *akantha,* thorn, spine]. An intermediate larva stage of Acanthocephala, formed within the arthropod host; a preinfective, nonencysted stage leading to the infective cystacanth.

acanthesthesia (ă-kan-thes-thē'zē-ă) [G. *akantha,* thorn, + *aisthēsis,* sensation]. Paresthesia of a pinprick.

Acanthia lectularia (ă-kan'thē-ă lek-tyū-lār'ē-ă) [G. *akantha,* thorn, prickle; L. *lectus,* a bed]. Early name for *Cimex lectularius.*

acanthion (ă-kan'thē-on) [G. *akantha,* thorn]. Akanthion; the tip of the anterior nasal spine.

acantho- [G. *akantha,* thorn]. Combining form denoting relationship to a spinous process, or meaning spiny or thorny.

Acanthocephala (ă-kan-thō-sef'ă-lă) [acantho- + G. *kephalē,* head]. The thorny-headed worms, a phylum (formerly considered a class) of obligatory parasites without an alimentary canal, characterized by an anterior introvertible spiny proboscis. They superficially resemble nematodes but are cestode-like in other traits, and hence are grouped as a distinctive phylum of helminths. In the adult stage they are parasites of vertebrate animals, mostly fish and amphibians; the larval stage is passed in invertebrates, chiefly crustaceans and insects.

acanthocephaliasis (ă-kan'thō-sef-ă-lī'ă-sis). An illness caused by infection with a species of Acanthocephala.

Acanthocheilonema (ă-kan'thō-kī-lō-nē'mă) [acantho- + G. *cheilos,* lip, + *nēma,* thread]. A genus of filarial worms parasitic in man, now considered part of the genus *Mansonella.*

acanthocyte (ă-kan'thō-sīt) [acantho- + G. *kytos,* cell]. Acanthrocyte; an erythrocyte characterized by multiple spiny cytoplasmic projections, as in acanthocytosis.

acanthocytosis (ă-kan'thō-sī-tō'sis). Acanthrocytosis; a rare condition in which the majority of erythrocytes are acanthocytes; a regular feature of abetalipoproteinemia.

acanthoid (ă-kan'thoyd). Spine-shaped.

acantholysis (ak-an-thol'i-sis) [acantho- + G. *lysis,* loosening]. Separation or dissolution of individual prickle cells from their neighbor, as in conditions such as pemphigus vulgaris and keratosis follicularis.

acanthoma (ak-an-thō'mă) [acantho- + G. *-oma,* tumor]. Proliferation of epithelial squamous cells that may be malignant, benign, or even non-neoplastic. See also adenoacanthoma; keratoacanthoma.

a. adenoi'des cys'ticum, trichoepithelioma.

clear cell a., Degos' a.; a sharply demarcated epidermal lesion of a leg or arm with acanthosis and accumulation of glycogen in keratinocytes having pale staining cytoplasm.

Degos' a., clear cell a.

a. fissura'tum, a fissure bordered by acanthosis developing at a site of friction by spectacle frames, usually behind the ears.

intraepithelial a., Borst-Jadassohn type intraepidermal *epithelioma.*

acanthopodia (ă-kan-thō-pō'dē-ă) [acantho- + G. *pous, podos,* foot]. Toothlike pseudopodia observed in some amebae, typically in members of the genus *Acanthamoeba.*

acanthor (ă-kan'thōr) [G. *akantha,* thorn or spine]. The spindle-shaped embryo, with rostellar hooks and body spines, formed within the egg shell of Acanthocephala; this stage burrows into the body cavity of its first intermediate host, usually a crustacean in aquatic cycles, or insects in terrestrial cycles.

acanthorrhexis (ă-kan-thō-rek'sĭs) [acantho + G. *rhexis,* rupture]. Rupture of the intercellular bridges of the prickle cell layer of the epidermis, as in contact-type dermatitis.

acanthosis (ak-an-thō'sis) [acantho- + G. *-osis,* condition]. Hyperacanthosis; an increase in the thickness of the prickle cell layer of the epidermis.

glycogen a., elevated gray-white plaques of distal esophageal mucosa, with epithelium thickened by proliferation of large glycogen-filled squamous cells.

a. ni'gricans, keratosis nigricans; an eruption of velvet warty benign growths and hyperpigmentation occurring in the skin of the axillae, neck, anogenital area, and groins; in adults, may be associated with internal malignancy, endocrine disorders, or obesity; a benign (juvenile) type occurs in children. See also pseudoacanthosis nigricans.

acanthotic (ak-an-thot'ik). Pertaining to or characteristic of acanthosis.

acanthrocyte (a-kan'thrō-sīt). Acanthocyte.

acanthrocytosis (ă-kan'thrō-sī-tō'sis). Acanthocytosis.

acapnia (ă-kap'nē-ă) [G. *a-* priv. + *kapnos,* smoke]. Absence of carbon dioxide in the blood. Sometimes used synonymously with hypocapnia.

acarbia (ă-kar'bē-ă) [G. *a-* priv. + carbon]. Obsolete term denoting pronounced reduction in bicarbonate of the blood.

acardia (ā-kar'dē-ă) [G. *a-* priv. + *kardia,* heart]. Congenital absence of the heart; a condition sometimes occurring in the smaller parasitic member of conjoined twins when its partner monopolizes the placental blood supply.

acardiac (ā-car'dē-ak). Without a heart.

acardiotrophia (ă-kar'di-ō-trō'fē-ă) [G. *a-* priv. + *kardia,* heart, + *trophē,* nourishment]. Atrophy of the myocardium.

acardius (ă-kar'dē-ŭs). A conjoined twin without a heart, parasitic on, or utilizing the placental circulation of, its mate. *Cf.* holoacardius.

a. aceph'alus, acephalocardius; an acardiac fetus in which the head is absent.

a. amor'phus, a. anceps.

a. an'ceps, a. amorphus; an acardiac fetus with rudimentary head and extremities.

acariasis (ak-ar-ī'ă-sis). Acaridiasis; acarinosis; any disease caused by mites, usually a skin infestation. See mange.

demodectic a., infestation of the hair follicles with *Demodex folliculorum,* affecting man and many domestic animals.

psoroptic a., infestation of the skin with *Psoroptes* mites.

pulmonary a., infestation of the lungs of monkeys with the mite, *Pneumonyssus simicola.*

sarcoptic a., infestation of skin with *Sarcoptes scabiei.* See scabies (1).

acaricide (ă-kar'i-sīd) [Mod. L. *acarus,* a mite, fr. G. *akari* + L. *caedo,* to cut, kill]. An agent that kills acarines; commonly used to denote chemicals that kill ticks.

acarid (ak'ă-rid) [G. *akari,* mite]. Acaridan; acarus; a general term for a member of the family Acaridae or for a mite.

Acaridae (ă-kar'i-dē). A family of the order Acarina, a large group of exceptionally small mites, usually 0.5 mm or less, abundant in dried fruits and meats, grain, meal, and flour; frequently a cause of severe dermatitis among persons hypersensitized by frequent handling of infested products.

acaridan (ă-kar'i-dan). Acarid.

acaridiasis (ak'ar-i-dī'ă-sis). Acariasis.

Acarina (ak-ă-rī'nă) [G. *akari,* a mite]. An order of Arachnida that includes the mites and ticks.

acarine (ak'ă-rīn). A member of the order Acarina.

acarinosis (ak'ă-ri-nō'sis, ă-kar'i-). Acariasis.

acarodermatitis (ak'ă-rō-der-mă-tī'tis) [G. *akari,* mite, + *derma* (*dermat-*), skin]. A skin inflammation or eruption produced by a mite.

a. urticarioi'des, infestation with the grain itch mite, *Pediculoides ventricosis.*

acaroid (ak'ă-royd) [G. *akari,* mite, + *eidos,* resemblance]. Resembling a mite.

acarology (ak-ă-rol'ō-jē) [G. *akari,* mite, + *logos,* study]. The study of acarine parasites, the ticks and mites, and the diseases they transmit.

acarophobia (ak'ă-rō-fō'bē-ă) [G. *akari,* mite, + *phobos,* fear]. Morbid fear of small parasites, small particles, or of itching.

Acarus (ak'ă-rŭs) [G. *akari,* mite]. A genus of mites of the family Acaridae.

A. bala'tus, a tropical species of mite that causes a particularly severe type of scabies-like irritation.

A. folliculo'rum, *Demodex folliculorum.*

A. galli'nae, *Dermanyssus gallinae.*

A. horde'i, the barley mite, a species that penetrates beneath the skin.

A. rhizoglyp'ticus hyacin'thi, a species that develops in spoiled onions and may cause dermatitis.

A. scabie'i, *Sarcoptes scabiei.*

acarus (ak'ă-rŭs). Acarid.

acaryote (ă-kar'ē-ōt). Akaryocyte.

acatalasemia (ā-kat'ă-lā-sē'mē-ă). Acatalasia; anenzymia catalasia; Takahara's disease; absence of catalase from the blood, often manifest by recurrent infection or ulceration of the gums and related oral structures. Persons homozygous for the recessive gene may have complete absence (Japanese variety) or very low levels (Swiss variety) of catalase; persons heterozygous for the gene have reduced catalase levels (hypocatalasia) but with some overlap with the normal range.

acatalasia (ā-kat-ă-lā'zē-ă). Acatalasemia.

acatamathesia (ă-kat'ă-mă-thē'zē-ă) [G. *a-* priv. + *katamathēsis,* a thorough knowledge or understanding]. Obsolete term for the loss of the faculty of understanding, *e.g.,* in psychogenic deafness or disease.

acataphasia (ă-kat-ă-fā'zē-ă) [G. *a*-priv. + *kataphasis,* affirmation]. Inability to correctly formulate a statement.

acathectic (ak-ă-thek'tik). Relating to acathexia.

acathexia (ak-ă-thek'sē-ă) [G. *a-* priv. + *kathexis,* retention]. An abnormal release of secretions.

acathexis (ak-ă-thek'sis) [G. *a-* priv. + *kathexis,* retention]. A mental disorder in which certain objects or ideas fail to arouse an emotional response in the individual.

acathisia (ak-ă-thiz'ē-ă). Akathisia.

acaudal, acaudate (ā-kaw'dăl, ā-kaw'dāt) [G. *a-* priv. + L. *cauda,* tail]. Having no tail.

ACC Abbreviation for anodal closure *contraction.*

accelerans (ak-sel'er-anz) [L. accelerator]. **1.** Accelerating. **2.** Obsolete term for an accelerator nerve of the heart.

accelerant (ak-sel'er-ant). Accelerator.

acceleration (ak-sel-er-ā'shŭn) [see accelerator]. **1.** The act of accelerating. **2.** The rate of increase in velocity per unit of time; commonly expressed in *g* units; also expressed in centimeters or feet per second squared. **3.** The rate of increasing deviation from a rectilinear course. See radial a.

angular a., the rate of change of angular velocity; *e.g.,* when a centrifuge rotor is speeding up, or when there is a simultaneous change in velocity and direction, as in an aircraft in a tight spin.

linear a., the rate of change of velocity without a change in direction; *e.g.,* when the speed of an aircraft increases while flying a straight pathway.

radial a., the centripetal a. of a particle or vehicle moving along a curved path at a constant velocity; *e.g.,* turning a curve in an automobile, pulling out of a dive, or performing a loop maneuver in an aircraft. In aviation, a. varies directly with the square of the air speed and inversely with the radius of the turn ($a = V^2/r$, where V is air speed and r is radius of turn).

accelerator (ak-sel'er-ā-ter) [L. *accelerans,* pres. p. of *ac-celero,* to hasten, fr. *celer,* swift]. Accelerant. **1.** Anything that increases rapidity of action or function. **2.** In physiology, a nerve, muscle, or substance that quickens movement or response. **3.** A catalytic agent used to hasten a chemical reaction.

linear a., a device imparting high velocity and energy to atomic and subatomic particles; can be adapted for radiation therapy.

proserum prothrombin conversion a. (PPCA), *factor* VIII.

prothrombin a., *factor* V.

serum a., *factor* VII.

serum prothrombin conversion a. (SPCA), *factor* VII.

accelerin (ak-sel'er-in). Accelerator *globulin.*

accelerometer (ak-sel-er-om'ĕ-ter). An instrument for measuring the rate of change of velocity per unit of time.

accentuator (ak-sent'yū-ā-ter) [L. *accentus,* accent, fr. *cano,* to sing]. A substance, such as aniline, the presence of which allows a combination between a tissue or histologic element and a stain that might otherwise be impossible.

acceptor (ak-sep'ter) [L. *ac-cipio,* pp. *-ceptus,* to accept]. A compound that will take up a chemical group (*e.g.,* an amine group, a methyl group, a carbamoyl group) from another compound (the donor); under the action of transaminase, glutamic acid is an amine donor while pyruvic acid is an amine a.

hydrogen a., hydrogen *carrier.*

accés pernicieux (ak-sā' per-ni-syu') [Fr., pernicious attacks or symptoms]. A series of severe attacks of falciparum malaria, sometimes occurring in apparently mild cases; roughly classified as cerebral and algid.

access (ak'ses) [L. *accessus*]. A way or means of approach or admittance. In dentistry: **1.** The space required for visualization and for manipulation of instruments to remove decay and prepare a tooth for restoration. **2.** The opening in the crown of a tooth required to allow adequate admittance to the pulp space to clean, shape, and seal the root canal(s). Also called a. opening.

accessorius (ak-ses-ō'rē-ŭs) [L.]. Accessory.

a. willis'ii, *nervus* accessorius.

accessory (ak-ses'ō-rē) [L. *accessorius,* fr. *ac-cedo,* pp. *-cessus,* to move toward]. In anatomy, denoting certain muscles, nerves, glands, etc. that are auxiliary or supernumerary.

accident (ak'si-dent). A sudden unexpected event or injury occurring without omen or forewarning, or developing in the course of a disease.

cardiac a., sudden cardiac catastrophe, such as may result from coronary occlusion.

cerebrovascular a. (CVA), an obsolete and inappropriate term for stroke.

serum a., anaphylactic shock resulting from injection of foreign serum for therapeutic purposes. See also serum *sickness.*

accident-prone. 1. Having a greater number of accidents than would be expected of the average person in similar circumstances. **2.** Having personality characteristics predisposing one to accidents.

acclimation (ak-li-mā'shŭn). Acclimatization.

acclimatization (ă-klī'mă-ti-zā'shŭn). Acclimation; physiological adjustment of an individual to a different climate, especially to a change in environmental temperature or altitude.

accolé forms (ak-ō-lā'). See under form.

accommodation (ă-kom'ŏ-dā'shŭn) [L. *ac-commodo,* pp. *-atus,* to adapt, fr. *modus,* a measure]. **1.** The act or state of adjustment or adaptation. **2.** In sensorimotor theory, the alteration of schemata or cognitive expectations to conform with experience.

amplitude of a., the difference in refractivity of the eye at rest and when fully accommodated.

a. of eye, the increase in thickness and convexity of the eye's lens in order to focus an external object on the retina.

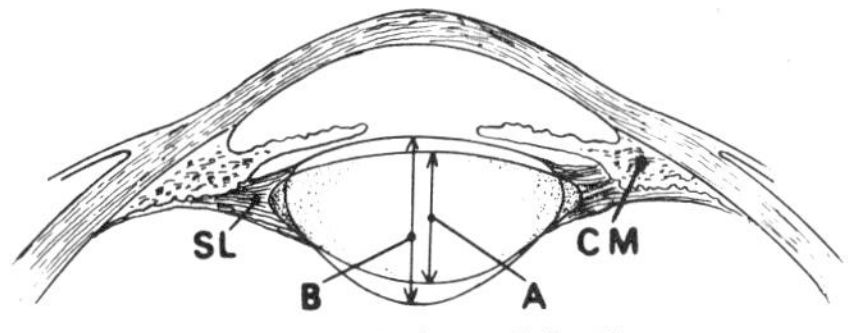

Accommodation of the Eye
A, shape of lens for far vision; *B,* shape of lens for near vision; *CM,* ciliary muscle; *SL,* suspensory ligament.

histologic a., pseudometaplasia; change in shape of cells to meet altered physical conditions, as the flattening of cuboidal cells in cysts as a result of pressure.

negative a., decreased a. for distance vision.

a. of nerve, the property of a nerve by which it adjusts to a slowly increasing strength of stimulus, so that the strength at which excitation occurs is greater than it would be were the strength to have risen more rapidly.

positive a., increased refractivity of the eye.

range of a., the distance between an object viewed with minimal refractivity of the eye and one viewed with maximal accommodation.

relative a., quantity of a. required for single binocular vision for any specified distance, or for any particular degree of convergence.

accommodative (ă-kom'ō-dā-tiv). Relating to accommodation.

accomplice (ă-kom'plis). A bacterium which accompanies the main infecting agent in a mixed infection and which influences the virulence of the main organism.

accouchement (a-kūsh-mawn') [Fr. from *coucher,* to lie down]. Childbirth, particularly parturition. See also birth.

a. forcé (fōr-sā'), forced, artificially hastened delivery, by means of forceps, version, etc.; originally applied to rapid dilation of the cervix with the hands, with version and forcible extraction of the fetus.

accoucheur (a-kū-sher'). Formerly used term for obstetrician.

accrementition (ak'rē-men-tish'ŭn) [L. *accresco,* pp. *-cretus,* to increase]. **1.** Reproduction by budding or germination. **2.** Accretion (1).

accretio cordis (ă-krē'shē-ō kōr'dis). Adhesion of the pericardium to adjacent extracardiac structures.

accretion (ă-krē'shŭn) [L. *accretio,* fr. *ad,* to, + *crescere,* to grow]. **1.** Accrementition (2); increase by addition to the periphery of material of the same nature as that already present; *e.g.,* the manner of growth of crystals. **2.** In dentistry, foreign material (usually plaque or calculus) collecting on the surface of a tooth or in a cavity. **3.** A growing together.

accrochage (ak-rō-shahj') [Fr. hooking, hitching]. Synchronization of two different rhythms of the heart or of other cellular elements as a result of contact, with each apparently influencing the behavior of the other but without either assuming dominance; seen in cases of isorhythmic dissociation.

acebutolol (as-ĕ-byū'tō-lol). *N*-[3-Acetyl-4-[2-hydroxy-3-[(1-methylethyl)amino]propoxy]phenyl]butanamide; a β-adrenergic blocking agent.

acecarbromal (as-ĕ-kar-brō'măl). Acetylcarbromal.

aceclidine (a-sek'li-dēn). 3-Quinuclidinol acetate ester; a cholinergic drug used for topical therapy of glaucoma.

acedapsone (as-ĕ-dap'sōn). Diacetyldiaminodiphenylsulfone; a derivative of dapsone with a longer duration of action; used to enhance the malaria chemoprophylaxis of quinine or of a combination of chloroquine-primaquine, and believed to act by interference with the utilization of folic acid.

acefylline piperazine (ă-sef'i-lēn). Piperazine theophylline-7-acetate; a diuretic and smooth muscle relaxant.

ACEI Abbreviation for angiotensin converting enzyme *inhibitor.*

acellular (ā-sel'yū-lăr) [G. *a-* priv. + L. *cellula,* a small chamber]. **1.** Noncellular (2); devoid of cells. **2.** A term applied to unicellular organisms that do not become multicellular and are complete within a single cell unit; frequently applied to protozoans to emphasize their complete organization within a single cell.

acelom (ā-sē'lom) [G. *a-* priv. + *koilōma,* hollow (celom)]. Absence of a true celom or body cavity lined with mesothelium; typically found in Platyhelminthes (flatworms), which have a syncytial mass of parenchymal cells instead of a true body cavity.

acelomate, acelomatous (ā-sē'lō-māt, ā-sē-lō'mă-tŭs). Not having a celom or body cavity.

acenesthesia (ă-sē-nes-thē'zē-ă, ă-sen-es-) [G. *a-* priv. + *koinos,* common, + *aisthēsis,* feeling]. Absence of the normal sensation of physical existence, or of the consciousness of visceral functioning.

acenocoumarin (ă-sē-nō-kū'mă-rin). Acenocoumarol.

acenocoumarol (ă-sē-nō-kū'mă-rol). Acenocoumarin; nicoumalone; 3-(α-acetonyl-*p*-nitrobenzyl)-4-hydroxycoumarin; an orally effective synthetic anticoagulant of the coumarin type, with similar actions.

acentric (ā-sen'trik) [G. *a-* priv. + *kentron,* center]. Without a center; in genetics, denoting a chromosome fragment without a centromere.

acephaline (ă-sef'ă-līn). Denoting members of the protozoan suborder Acephalina (order Eugregarinida), characterized by simple noncompartmentalized bodies, that parasitize invertebrates.

acephalia, acephalism (ă-se-fā'lē-ă, ă-sef'ă-lizm). Acephaly.

acephalobrachia (ă-sef'ă-lō-brā'kē-ă) [G. *a-* priv. + *kephalē,* head, + *brachiōn,* arm]. Abrachiocephaly.

acephalocardia (ă-sef'ă-lō-kar'dē-ă) [G. *a-* priv. + *kephalē,* head, + *kardia,* heart]. Absence of head and heart in a parasitic conjoined twin.

acephalocheiria, acephalochiria (ă-sef'ă-lō-kī'rē-ă) [G. *a-* priv. + *kephalē,* head, + *cheir,* hand]. Congenital absence of head and hands.

acephalocyst (ă-sef'ă-lō-sist) [G. *a-* priv. + *kephalē,* head, + *kystis,* bladder]. A hydatid cyst with no daughter cyst; a sterile hydatid, so called because it fails to develop scoleces or tapeworm heads.

acephalogaster (ă-sef'ă-lō-gas'ter) [G. *a-* priv. + *kephalē,* head, + *gastēr,* belly]. A parasitic conjoined twin consisting only of the pelvis and legs.

acephalogasteria (ă-sef'ă-lō-gas-tēr'ē-ă). Congenital absence of head, thorax, and abdomen in a parasitic twin with pelvis and legs only.

acephalopodia (ă-sef'ă-lō-pō'dē-ă) [G. *a-* priv. + *kephalē,* head, + *pous,* foot]. Congenital absence of head and feet.

acephalorrhachia (ă-sef'ă-lō-rak'ē-ă) [G. *a-* priv. + *kephalē,* head, + *rhachis,* spine]. Congenital absence of head and spinal column.

acephalostomia (ă-sef'ă-lō-stō'mē-ă) [G. *a-* priv. + *kephalē,* head, + *stoma,* mouth]. Congenital absence of the greater part of the head with, however, the presence of a mouthlike opening.

acephalothoracia (ă-sef'ă-lō-thōr-ā'sē-ă) [G. *a-* priv. + *kephalē,* head, + *thorax,* chest]. Congenital absence of head and thorax.

acephalous (ă-sef'ă-lŭs). Headless.

acephalus (ă-sef'ă-lŭs) [G. *a-* priv. + *kephalē,* head]. A malformed fetus in which the body lacks a head.

a. dibra'chius, a fetus lacking a head but having two recognizably developed arms.

a. di'pus, a fetus lacking a head but showing two recognizably developed feet.

a. monobra'chius, a fetus lacking a head and showing only one recognizable arm.

a. mon'opus, a fetus lacking a head and with fusion of the lower extremities so extreme that only a single foot is recognizable.

a. paraceph'alus, a malformed fetus with only partially developed skull and brain.

a. sym'pus, an a. showing fusion of all of the lower extremities.

acephaly (ă-sef'ă-lē) [G. *a-* priv. + *kephalē,* head]. Acephalia; acephalism; congenital absence of the head.

acervuline (ă-ser'vyū-līn) [Mod. L. *acervulus,* a little heap]. Occurring in clusters; aggregated.

acervulus (ă-ser'vyū-lŭs) [Mod. L. dim. of L. *acervus,* a heap]. *Corpora* arenacea.

acestoma (ă-ses-tō'mă) [G. *akestos,* curable, + *-ōma,* tumor]. Exuberant granulations that form a cicatrix.

acet-, aceto- Combining forms denoting the two-carbon fragment of acetic acid.

acetabula (as-ĕ-tab'yū-lă). Plural of acetabulum.

acetabular (as-ĕ-tab'yū-lăr). Relating to the acetabulum.

acetabulectomy (as'ĕ-tab-yū-lek'tō-mē) [acetabulum + G. *ektomē,* excision]. Excision of the acetabulum.

acetabuloplasty (as-ĕ-tab'yū-lō-plas-tē) [acetabulum + G. *plastos,* formed]. Any operation aimed at restoring the acetabulum to as near a normal state as possible.

acetabulum, pl. **acetabula** (as-ĕ-tab'yū-lŭm, -lă) [L. a shallow vinegar vessel or cup] [NA]. Cotyloid cavity; cotyle (2); a cup-shaped depression on the external surface of the hip bone, in which the head of the femur fits.

acetal (as'e-tal). Product of the addition of two moles of alcohol to one of an aldehyde, thus: $RCHO + 2R'OH \rightarrow RCH(OR')_2 + H_2O$; in mixed acetals (*e.g.,* glycosides), two different alcohols are bound to the original aldehyde group. See also hemiacetal.
a. phosphatid(at)e, older trivial name for alk-1-enylglycerophospholipid.

acetaldehyde (as-e-tal'dĕ-hīd). Acetic aldehyde; ethaldehyde; ethanal; CH_3CHO; an intermediate in yeast fermentation of carbohydrate and in alcohol metabolism.

acetamide (as-et-am'īd, ă-set'ă-mīd). Acetic amide; CH_3CONH_2; used in biomedical research.

acetamidine (as-e-tam'i-dēn). $CH_3C(NH)NH_2$; nitrogen analogue of acetic acid.

2-acetamidofluorene (AAF) (as'et-am'i-dō-flūr'ēn). 2-Acetylaminofluorene.

acetaminophen (as-et-ă-mē'nō-fen). Paracetamol; *N*-acetyl-*p*-aminophenol; *p*-acetamidophenol; an antipyretic and analgesic.

acetaminosalol (as-ĕ-tam'in-ō-sal'ol). Phenetsal; salicylic acid ester of acetyl-*p*- aminophenol; used as an analgesic, antipyretic, and intestinal antiseptic.

acetanilid (as-ĕ-tan'i-lid). *N*- Phenylacetamide; $C_6H_5NHCOCH_3$; an analgesic and antipyretic; continued use causes cyanosis.

acetarsol (as-ĕ-tar'sol). Acetarsone.

acetarsone (as-ĕ-tar'sōn). Acetarsol; acetylaminohydroxyphenylarsonic acid; *N*-acetyl-4-hydroxy-*m*-arsanilic acid; used in the treatment of amebiasis, and as a local application in Vincent's angina and in trichomoniasis vaginitis. The diethylamine salt is used as an antisyphilitic.

acetate (as'e-tāt). CH_3COO—; a salt or ester of acetic acid.
active a., acetyl-CoA.
a. kinase [EC 2.7.2.1], acetokinase; a phosphotransferase forming acetyl phosphate from ATP and acetate.
a. thiokinase, acetate-CoA ligase.

acetate-CoA ligase [EC 6.2.1.1]. Acetyl-CoA synthetase; acetyl-activating enzyme; acetate thiokinase; a ligase forming acetyl-CoA from acetate and CoA, at the expense of ATP.

acetazolamide (as'ĕ-tă-zol'ă-mīd). The heterocyclic sulfonamide, 5-acetylamido-1,3,4-thiadiazole-2-sulfonamide, which inhibits the action of carbonic anhydrase in the kidney, causing an increase in the urinary excretion of sodium, potassium, and bicarbonate, reduced excretion of ammonium, a rise in the pH of the urine, and a fall in the pH of the blood; used in respiratory acidosis for diuresis and control of fluid retention, in glaucoma to reduce intraocular pressure, and in epilepsy. A. sodium has the same actions and uses as a., but is more soluble and suitable for parenteral administration.

acetenyl (a-sē'ten-il). Ethynyl.

acetic (a-sē'tik, -set'ik) [L. *acetum,* vinegar]. **1.** Denoting the presence of the two-carbon fragment of acetic acid. **2.** Relating to vinegar; sour.

acetic acid. Ethanoic acid; CH_3COOH; a product of the oxidation of ethanol and of the destructive distillation of wood; used locally as a counterirritant and occasionally internally, and also as a reagent.
diluted a. a., contains 6% w/v of a. a.
glacial a. a., contains 99% absolute a. a.; a caustic for removal of corns and warts.

acetic aldehyde. Acetaldehyde.

acetic (acid) amide. Acetamide.

aceticoceptor (a-sē'ti-kō-sep'tōr) [L. *acetum,* vinegar, + *capio,* to take]. A side chain of molecules with a special affinity for the acetic acid radical.

acetic phosphoric anhydride. *Acetyl* phosphate.

acetify (ă-set'i-fī) [L. *acetum,* vinegar, + *facio,* to make; or *fieri,* to be made, to become]. To cause acetic fermentation; to make vinegar or become vinegar.

acetimeter (as-ĕ-tim'ĕ-ter) [L. *acetum,* vinegar, + G. *metron,* measure]. Acetometer; an apparatus for determining the content of acetic acid in vinegar or other fluid.

aceto- See acet-.

acetoacetate (as'e-tō-as'e-tāt). Diacetate (1); a salt or ion of acetoacetic acid.
a. decarboxylase [EC 4.1.1.4], a carboxy-lyase cleaving CO_2 from a. to form acetone.

acetoacetic acid (as'e-tō-a-sē'tik). Diacetic acid; CH_3COCH_2COOH; one of the ketone bodies, formed in excess and appearing in the urine in starvation or diabetes.

acetoacetyl-CoA (as'e-tō-a-sē'til). Acetoacetylcoenzyme A; intermediate in the oxidation of fatty acids; also formed from two molecules of acetyl-CoA; major role is condensation with acetyl-CoA to form the important *β*-hydroxy-*β*-methylglutaryl-CoA.

acetoacetyl-CoA reductase [EC 1.1.1.36]. An oxidoreductase catalyzing interconversion of a 3-oxoacyl-CoA, and the corresponding 3-hydroxyacyl-CoA, with NADP.

acetoacetyl-CoA thiolase. Acetyl-CoA acetyltransferase.

acetoacetylcoenzyme A (as'e-tō-as'e-til-kō-en'zīm). Acetoacetyl-CoA.

acetoacetyl-succinic thiophorase (as'e-tō-as'e-til-sŭk-sin'ik). 3-Oxo-CoA transferase.

acetohex'amide. (as-ĕ-tō-heks'ă-mīd). 1-[(*p*-Acetylphenyl)sulfonyl]-3-cyclohexylurea; an oral hypoglycemic agent that stimulates pancreatic insulin secretion; most useful therapeutically in mild cases of non-insulin dependent diabetes mellitus.

acetohydroxamic acid (as'e-tō-hī-drok'să-mik). *N*- Hydroxyacetamide; $C_2H_5NO_2$; an inhibitor of urease, used as adjunctive therapy in chronic urea-splitting urinary infections.

acetoin (as-et'-ō-in). 3-Hydroxy-2-butanone; $CH_3CH(OH)COCH_3$; a condensation product of two molecules of acetaldehyde.

acetokinase (as'e-tō-kī'nās). *Acetate* kinase.

acetol (as'e-tol). Obsolete term for 1-hydroxy-2-propanone, or hydroxyacetone, $CH_2OH\text{-}CO\text{-}CH_3$; also used as a proprietary name for certain commercial items.

α-acetolactic acid (as'e-tō-lak'tik). An intermediate in pyruvic acid catabolism and valine biosynthesis; $CH_3COC(OH)(CH_3)\text{-}COOH$.

acetolysis (as-e-tol'i-sis). Decomposition of an organic compound with the addition of the elements of acetic acid at the point of decomposition; analogous to hydrolysis and phosphorolysis.

acetomenaphthone (as'ĕ-tō-me-naf'thōn). Menadiol diacetate.

acetometer (as-ĕ-tom′ĕ-ter). Acetimeter.

acetone (as′e-tōn). Dimethyl ketone; CH_3COCH_3; a colorless, volatile, inflammable liquid; extremely small amounts are found in normal urine, but larger quantities occur in urine and blood of diabetic persons, sometimes imparting an ethereal odor to the urine and breath. The synthetic is used as a solvent in some pharmaceutical and commercial preparations.

acetonemia (as′ĕ-tō-nē′mē-ă) [acetone + G. *haima,* blood]. The presence of acetone or acetone bodies in relatively large amounts in the blood, manifested at first by erethism, and later by a progressive depression.
bovine a., a. found frequently in dairy cattle during the postparturient period.
ovine a., a. that occurs in ewes during the last weeks of pregnancy.

acetonemic (as′ĕ-tō-nē′mik). Relating to or caused by acetonemia.

acetonitrile (as′e-tō-nī′tril). Methyl cyanide; CH_3CN; a colorless fluid of aromatic odor, soluble in water and alcohol.

acetonuria (as′e-tō-nūr′ē-ă) [acetone + G. *ouron,* urine]. Excretion in the urine of large amounts of acetone, an indication of incomplete oxidation of large amounts of lipids; commonly occurs in diabetic acidosis.

acetophenazine maleate (as-ĕ-tō-fē′nă-zēn mal′ē-āt). 2-Acetyl-10{3-[4-(2-hydroxyethyl)piperazinyl]propyl}phenothiazine dimaleate; a phenothiazine tranquilizer.

acetophenetidin (as′ĕ-tō-fe-net′i-din). Phenacetin.

acetosulfone sodium (as′ĕ-tō-sŭl′fōn). 2-*N*-Acetylsulfamyl-4,4′-diaminodiphenylsulfone; a leprostatic administered orally.

acetous (as′e-tŭs). Relating to vinegar; sour-tasting.

acetphenolisatin (as′et-fē-nō-lī′să-tin). Oxyphenisatin acetate.

acetrizoate sodium (as-ĕ-trī-zō′āt). 3-Acetamido-2,4,6-triiodobenzoic acid sodium salt; a radiopaque medium.

acetum, pl. **aceta** (ă-sē′tŭm, -tă) [L. *vinum acetum,* soured wine, vinegar]. Vinegar.

aceturate (ă-set′yū-rāt). USAN-approved contraction for *N*-acetylglycinate, $CH_3CONHCH_2COO^-$

acetyl (Ac) (as′e-til). The radical, CH_3CO—; an acetic acid molecule from which the hydroxyl group has been removed.
a. chloride, CH_3COCl; a colorless liquid used as a reagent; also corrosive, causing severe burns because of hydrolysis to HCl.
a. phosphate, acetic phosphoric anhydride; $CH_3CO\text{-}OPO_3H_2$; a "high energy" phosphate that acts as an acetate donor in the metabolism of various bacteria.
a. transacylase, ACP-acetyltransferase.

acetyladenylate (as′e-til-ă-den′il-āt). Mixed anhydride between the carboxyl group of acetic acid and the phosphoric residue of adenosine 5′-phosphoric acid; Ado(5′)OP(O_2H)—$OCOCH_3$.

2-**acetylaminofluorene (AAF)** (as′e-til-am′i-nō-flūr′ēn). 2-Acetamidofluorene; *N*-2-fluorenylacetamide; a potent carcinogenic compound.

acetylase (a-set′il-ās). Any enzyme catalyzing acetylation or deacetylation, as in the formation of *N*-acetylglutamate from glutamate plus acetyl-CoA, or the reverse; a.'s are usually called acetyltransferases.

acetylation (a-set-i-lā′shŭn). Formation of an acetyl derivative.

acetylcarbromal (ă-sē′til-kar-brō′măl). Acecarbromal; *N*-acetyl-*N*′-(bromodiethylacetyl)urea; a sedative replaced by barbiturates and newer drugs.

acetylcholine (as-e-til-kō′lēn). (2-Acetoxyethyl)trimethylammonium ion; $CH_3CO\text{-}OCH_2CH_2\overset{+}{N}(CH_3)_3$; the acetic ester of choline, isolated from ergot, which causes cardiac inhibition, vasodilatation, gastrointestinal peristalsis, and other parasympathetic effects. It is liberated from preganglionic and postganglionic endings of parasympathetic fibers and from preganglionic fibers of the sympathetic as a result of nerve injuries, whereupon it acts as a transmitter on the effector organ; it is hydrolyzed into choline and acetic acid by acetylcholinesterase before a second impulse may be transmitted.
a. chloride, a miotic, administered subcutaneously for parasympathomimetic effect; used in cataract surgery.

acetylcholinesterase (as′e-til-kō-lin-es′ter-ās) [EC 3.1.1.7]. Choline esterase I; "e" -type, specific or true cholinesterase; the cholinesterases that hydrolyze acetylcholine within the central nervous system and at peripheral neuroeffector junctions (*e.g.,* motor endplates and autonomic ganglia).

acetyl-CoA. Acetylcoenzyme A; active acetate; condensation product of coenzyme A and acetic acid, symbolized as $CoAS{\sim}COCH_3$; intermediate in transfer of two-carbon fragment, notably in its entrance into the tricarboxylic acid cycle.

acetyl-CoA acetyltransferase [EC 2.3.1.9]. Acetoacetyl-CoA thiolase; acetyl-CoA thiolase; thiolase; an acetyltransferase forming acetoacetyl-CoA from two molecules of acetyl-CoA, releasing one CoA.

acetyl-CoA acylase. Acetyl-CoA hydrolase.

acetyl-CoA acyltransferase [EC 2.3.1.16]. β-Ketothiolase; 3-ketoacyl-CoA thiolase; an enzyme catalyzing the thioclastic cleavage of β-ketoacyl-CoA, forming an acyl-CoA with a carbon chain shorter by two atoms, the missing two atoms appearing as acetyl-CoA. See also acetyl-CoA acetyltransferase.

acetyl-CoA carboxylase [EC 6.4.1.2]. A ligase that catalyzes the reaction of acetyl-CoA, CO_2, and ATP, with Mn^{+2} as catalyst and covalently bound biotin, to form malonyl-CoA, ADP, and P_i, or the reverse decarboxylase); *N*- carboxybiotin is an intermediate.

acetyl-CoA deacylase. Acetyl-CoA hydrolase.

acetyl-CoA hydrolase [EC 3.1.2.1]. Acetyl-CoA acylase; acetyl-CoA deacylase; a hydrolase that cleaves acetate from acetyl-CoA.

acetyl-CoA synthetase. Acetate-CoA ligase.

acetyl-CoA thiolase. Acetyl-CoA acetyltransferase.

acetylcoenzyme A (as′e-til-kō-en′zīm). Acetyl-CoA.

acetylcysteine (as′ĕ-til-sis′tē-in). *N*- Acetyl-L-cysteine; a mucolytic agent that reduces the viscosity of mucous secretions; has been used to treat acetaminophen toxicity.

acetyldigitoxin (ă-sē′til-dij-i-tok′sin). The α-acetyl ester of digitoxin derived from lanatoside A, having the same actions and uses as digitoxin, but more rapid onset and shorter duration of action.

acetyldigoxin (ă-sē′til-dī-gok′sin). A digitalis glycoside with properties similar to those of digoxin; derived from digilanide C.

acetylene (a-set′i-lēn). HC≡CH; a colorless explosive gas, anesthetic in concentrations of 40 volumes percent.

***N*-acetylglutamate** (ă-sē′til-glū′tă-māt). An activator of carbamyl phosphate synthetase during urea synthesis; this amino acid causes a configurational change in the enzyme, increasing its affinity for adenosine triphosphate.

acetylornithinase (as′e-til-ōr′ni-thin-ās). Acetylornithine deacetylase.

acetylornithine deacetylase (as′e-til-ōr′ni-thēn) [EC 3.5.1.16]. Acetylornithinase; an enzyme catalyzing the hydrolysis of N^2-acetylornithine to ornithine.

3-**acetylpyridine** (as′e-til-pir′i-dēn). An antimetabolite of nicotinamide that produces symptoms of nicotinamide deficiency in mice.

acetylsalicylic acid (as′ĕ-til-sal-i-sil′ik). Aspirin.

***N*^{1}-acetylsulfanilamide.** Sulfacetamide.

***N*^{4}-acetylsulfanilamide** (as′e-til-sŭl-fă-nil′ă-mīd). *p*- Sulfamylacetanilide; an intermediate in the synthesis of sulfanilamide;

formed in animal bodies by acetylation of sulfanilamide.

acetyl sulfisoxazole. A derivative of sulfisoxazole with the same actions and uses.

acetyltannic acid (as′ĕ-til-tan′ik). Diacetyltannic acid; tannylacetate; an astringent used for treatment of diarrhea.

acetyltransferase (as′e-til-trans′fer-ās). Transacetylase; any enzyme transferring acetyl groups from one compound to another. See also acetyl-CoA, choline, and dihydrolipoamide acetyltransferases.

AcG, ac-g Abbreviation for accelerator *globulin.*

achalasia (ak-ă-lā′-zē-ă) [G. *a-* priv. + *chalasis,* a slackening]. Failure to relax; referring especially to visceral openings such as the pylorus, cardia, or any other sphincter muscles.
esophageal a., cardiospasm; phrenospasm; an obstruction which develops in the terminal esophagus just proximal to the cardioesophageal junction, the upper esophagus becoming dilated and filled with retained food; sometimes originates from a loss of motor innervation by fibers originating in the dorsal nucleus of the vagus nerve.

Achard, E. Charles, French physician, 1860–1941. See A. *syndrome,* A.-Thiers *syndrome.*

ache (āk). A pain of less than severe intensity that persists for a long time.
bone a., a dull pain in the bones, often severe; an extreme variety occurs in dengue.
stomach a., gastralgia; gastrodynia; pain in the abdomen, usually arising in the stomach or duodenum.

acheilia, achilia (ă-kī′lē-ă) [G. *a-* priv. + *cheilos,* lip]. Congenital absence of the lips.

acheilous, achilous (ă-kī′lŭs). Characterized by or relating to acheilia.

acheiria, achiria (ă-kī′rē-ă) [G. *a-* priv. + *cheir,* hand]. **1.** Congenital absence of the hands. **2.** Anesthesia in, with loss of the sense of possession of, one or both hands; a condition sometimes noted in hysteria. **3.** A form of dyscheiria in which the patient is unable to tell on which side of the body a stimulus has been applied.

acheiropody, achiropody (ă-kī-rop′ō-dē) [G. *a-* priv. + *cheir,* hand, + *podos,* foot]. Congenital absence of the hands and feet; autosomal recessive inheritance.

acheirous, achirous (ă-kī′rŭs). Characterized by or relating to acheiria (1).

Achenbach, Walter A., 20th century German internist. See A. *syndrome.*

achilia (ă-kī′lē-ă). Acheilia.

Achilles, Mythical Greek warrior, vulnerable only in the heel. See A. *bursa, reflex, tendon.*

achillobursitis (ă-kil′ō-ber-sī′tis). Retrocalcaneobursitis; inflammation of a bursa beneath the tendo calcaneus.

achillodynia (ă-kil-ō-din′ē-ă) [Achilles (tendon) + G. *odynē,* pain]. Pain due to inflammation of the bursa between the calcaneus and the tendo achillis (achillobursitis).

achillorrhaphy (ă-kil-ōr′ă-fē) [Achilles (tendon) + G. *rhaphē,* a sewing]. Suture of the tendo calcaneus.

achillotenotomy (ă-kil′ō-ten-ot′ō-mē) [Achilles (tendon) + G. *tenōn,* tendon, + *tomē,* a cutting]. Achillotomy.

achillotomy (ă-kil-ot′ō-mē) [Achilles (tendon) + G. *tomē,* incision]. Achillotenotomy; division of the tendo calcaneus.

achilous (a-kī-lŭs). Acheilous.

achiral (ā-kī′răl) [a- priv. + G. *cheir,* hand]. Not chiral; denoting an absence of chirality.

achiria (ă-kī′rē-ă). Acheiria.

achiropody (ă-kī-rop′ō-dē). Acheiropody.

achirous (ă-kī′rŭs). Acheirous.

achlorhydria (ā-klōr-hī′drē-ă) [G. *a-* priv. + chlorhydric (acid)]. Absence of hydrochloric acid from the gastric juice.

achlorophyllous (ā-klōr-ō-fī′lŭs). Without chlorophyll, as in fungi.

Acholeplasma, pl. **Acholeplasmata** (ă-kō-lē-plas′mă, mah-tă). A genus of bacteria (order Mycoplasmatales) that have characteristics identical to those of the species in the genus *Mycoplasma,* with the exception that the acholeplasmas do not require sterol for growth; saprophytic and parasitic species occur. The type species is *A. laidlawii.*
A. axan′thum, a species originally found in a murine leukemia cell line; ecology not determined.
A. granula′rum, *Mycoplasma granularum;* a species that occurs as a commensal in swine; pathogenicity not determined.
A. laidla′wii, *Mycoplasma laidlawii;* a species that occurs as a saprophyte in sewage, manure, humus, and soil; type species of the genus *A.*

acholia (ă-kō′lē-ă) [G. *a-* priv. + *cholē,* bile]. Suppressed or absent secretion of bile.

acholic (ă-kol′ik). Without bile, as in a. (pale) stools.

acholuria (ā-kō-lū′rē-ă) [G. *a-* priv. + *cholē,* bile, + *ouron,* urine]. Absence of bile pigments from the urine in certain cases of jaundice.

acholuric (ā-kō-lū′rik). Without bile in the urine.

achondrogenesis (ă-kon-drō-jen′ĕ-sis) [G. *a-* priv., + *chondros,* cartilage, + *genesis,* origin]. Dwarfism accompanied by various bone aplasias and hypoplasias of all four extremities, a normal or enlarged skull, and a short trunk with delayed ossification of the lower spine; autosomal recessive inheritance.

achondroplasia (ă-kon-drō-plā′zē-ă) [G. *a-* priv. + *chondros,* cartilage, + *plasis,* a molding]. Achondroplasty; osteosclerosis congenita; Parrot's disease (2); a type of chondrodystrophy characterized by an abnormality of conversion of cartilage into bone, predominantly affecting the epiphyses of long bones in which epiphysial growth is retarded and ceases early, resulting in dwarfism apparent at birth, with short extremities, but normal trunk; the head is frequently enlarged, with flattened nose, due to midfacial hypoplasia; autosomal dominant inheritance.

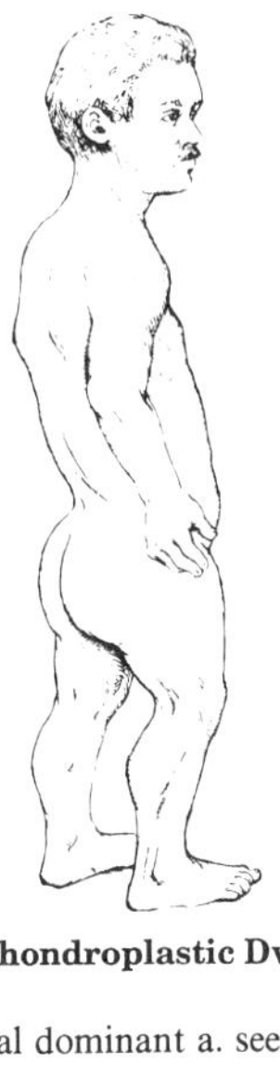

Achondroplastic Dwarf

avian a., an autosomal dominant a. seen in several breeds of domestic chickens.

bovine a., bull-dog *calf.*
homozygous a., severe a. affecting progeny whose parents are achondroplastic; usually fatal in the first year of life.

achondroplastic (ă-kon-drō-plas'tik). Relating to or characterized by achondroplasia.

achondroplasty (ă-kon'drō-plas-tē). Achondroplasia.

achordate, achordal (ā-kōr'dāt, ā-kōr'dăl). Referring to animal forms below the Chordata that do not develop a notochord or chorda.

achoresis (ă-kō-rē'sis) [G. *a-* priv. + *chōreō,* to make room, fr. *chōros,* space]. Permanent contraction of a hollow viscus, such as the stomach or bladder, whereby its capacity is reduced.

Achorion (ă-kō'rē-on) [G. *achōr,* dandruff]. Former name for *Trichophyton.*

achroacyte (ă-krō'ă-sīt) [G. *a-* priv. + *chroa,* color, + *kytos,* a hollow (cell)]. A colorless cell.

achroacytosis (ă-krō'ă-sī-tō'sis). Obsolete term for lymphocytosis.

achrodextrin (ak-rō-deks'trin) [G. a- priv. + *chrōma,* color, + dextrin]. Achroodextrin.

achroglobin (ak-rō-glō'bin) [G. a- priv. + *chrōma,* color, + globin]. A colorless respiratory protein compound present in certain invertebrates.

achromacyte (ă-krō'mă-sīt). Achromocyte.

achromasia (ak-rō-mā'sē-ă) [G. *achrōmos,* colorless]. **1.** Cachectic pallor; pallor associated with hippocratic facies, emaciation, and weakness, often heralding a moribund state. **2.** Achromia.

achromate (ă-krō'māt) [G. *a-* priv. + *chrōma,* color]. A person exhibiting achromatopsia.

achromatic (ā-krō-mat'ik) [G. *a-* priv. + *chrōma,* color]. **1.** Colorless. **2.** Not staining readily.

achromatin (ă-krō'mă-tin). The weakly staining components of the nucleus, such as the nuclear sap and euchromatin.

achromatinic (ă-krō-mă-tin'ik). Relating to or containing achromatin.

achromatism (ă-krō'mă-tizm). **1.** The quality of being achromatic. **2.** The annulment of chromatic aberration by combining glasses of different refractive indexes and different dispersion.

achromatocyte (ā-krō-mat'ō-sīt). Achromocyte.

achromatolysis (ă-krō-mă-tol'i-sis). Karyoplasmolysis; dissolution of the achromatin of a cell or of its nucleus.

achromatophil (ă-krō-mat'ō-fil) [G. *a-* priv. + *chrōma,* color, + *philos,* fond]. Achromophil. **1.** Achromophilic; achromophilous; not being colored by the histologic or bacteriologic stains. **2.** A cell or tissue that cannot be stained in the usual way.

achromatophilia (ă-krō'mat-ō-fil'ē-ă). A condition of being refractory to staining processes.

achromatopsia, achromatopsy (ă-krō-mă-top'sē-ă, ă-krō'mă-top-sē) [G. *a-* priv. + *chrōma,* color, + *opsis,* vision]. Achromatic vision; monochromasia; monochromasy; monochromatism (2); a severe congenital deficiency in color perception, often associated with nystagmus and reduced visual acuity.
atypical a., incomplete a. with normal visual acuity and no nystagmus.
complete a., typical a.; rod monochromasy; a. with absent color vision, nystagmus, reduced visual acuity, and light aversion.
cone a., a. previously believed due to a defect in neural transmission.
incomplete a., impaired, but not absent, color vision with less severely reduced visual acuity than in complete a.; inherited as an autosomal recessive or as an X-linked disorder (blue cone monochromasy; pi cone monochromasy).
rod a., a. previously believed due to a deficiency of normal cones.
typical a., complete a.
X-linked a., see incomplete a.

achromatosis (ă-krō-mă-tō'sis) [G. *a-* priv. + *chrōma,* color]. Achromia.

achromatous (ă-krō'mă-tŭs). Colorless.

achromaturia (ă-krō-mă-tū'rē-ă) [G. *a-* priv. + *chrōma,* color, + *ouron,* urine]. The passage of colorless or very pale urine.

achromia (ă-krō'mē-ă) [G. *a-* priv. + *chrōma,* color]. Achromasia (2); achromatosis. **1.** Absence or loss of natural pigmentation of the skin; may be congenital or acquired. **2.** Lack of capacity to accept stains in cells or tissue.
a. parasit'ica, a phase of lessening or absence of pigmentation in cutaneous lesions, caused by the fungus *Malassezia furfur.* See also *tinea* versicolor.
a. un'guium, leukonychia.

achromic (ā-krō'mik). Colorless.

achromocyte (ă-krō'mō-sīt) [G. *a-* priv. + *chrōma,* color, + *kytos,* hollow (cell)]. A hypochromic, crescent-shaped erythrocyte, probably resulting from artifactual rupture of a red cell with loss of hemoglobin. Also called achromatocyte; achromacyte; shadow (1); Ponfick's shadow; ghost, phantom, shadow, or Traube's corpuscle.

achromoderma (ă-krō-mō-der'mă). Leukoderma.

achromophil (ă-krō'mō-fil). Achromatophil.

achromophilic, achromophilous (ā-krō-mō-fil'ik, ā-krō-mof'i-lŭs). Achromatophil (1).

achromotrichia (ă-krō-mō-trik'ē-ă) [G. *a-* priv. + *chrōma,* color, + *thrix,* hair]. **1.** Absence or loss of pigment in the hair. See also canities. **2.** A graying of the hair of black rats in pantothenic acid deficiency.

achroodextrin (ak-rō'ō-deks'trin) [G. *achroos,* uncolored, + dextrin]. Achrodextrin; dextrin of low molecular weight, formed from starch in a stage of the digestion of the latter by amylase; it gives no color reaction with iodine.

achylia (ă-kī'lē-ă) [G. *a-* priv. + *chylos,* juice]. **1.** Absence of gastric juice or other digestive secretions. **2.** Absence of chyle.
a. gas'trica, diminished or abolished secretion of gastric juice associated with atrophy of the mucous membrane of the stomach.
a. pancreat'ica, deficiency or absence of pancreatic secretion, usually resulting in fatty stools, emaciation, and impaired nutrition.

achylous (ă-kī'lŭs) [G. *achylos,* without juice]. **1.** Lacking in gastric juice or other digestive secretions. **2.** Having no chyle.

acicular (ă-sik'yū-lar) [L. *acicular,* small pin]. Needle-shaped or needle-pointed; applied particularly to leaves and crystals.

acid (as'id) [L. *acidus,* sour]. **1.** A compound yielding a hydrogen ion in a polar solvent (*e.g.,* in water); a.'s form salts by replacing all or part of the ionizable hydrogen with an electropositive element or radical. An a. containing one ionizable atom of hydrogen in the molecule is called **monobasic**; one containing two such atoms, **dibasic**; and one containing more than two, **polybasic**. **2.** In popular language, any chemical compound that has a sour taste (given by the hydrogen ion). **3.** Sour; sharp to the taste. **4.** Relating to a.; giving an a. reaction. For individual acids, see specific names.
bile a.'s, taurocholic and glycocholic a.'s, used when bilary secretion is inadequate and for biliary colic.
dibasic a., see acid (1).
fatty a., see under F.
inorganic a., an a. made up of molecules not containing organic radicals; *e.g.,* HCl, H_2SO_4, H_3PO_4.
monobasic a., see acid (1).
organic a., an a. made up of molecules containing organic radicals; *e.g.,* acetic a., citric a., which contain the ionizable —COOH group.
polybasic a., see acid (1).

acidaminuria (as'id-am-i-nū'rē-ă). Obsolete term for aminoaciduria.

acidemia (as-i-dē'mē-ă) [acid + G. *haima,* blood]. An increase in the H-ion concentration of the blood or a fall below normal in pH, notwithstanding alterations in bicarbonate concentration. Individual types of a. are listed by specific name, *e.g.,* isovalericacidemia, aminoacidemia, etc.

acid-fast (as'id-fast). Denoting bacteria that are not decolorized by acid-alcohol after having been stained with dyes such as basic fuchsin; *e.g.,* the mycobacteria and a few nocardiae.

acidify (a-sid'i-fī). **1.** To render acid. **2.** To become acid.

acidity (a-sid'i-tē). **1.** The state of being acid. **2.** The acid content of a fluid.

total a. (a), an obsolete expression of gastric a., the a. being determined by titration with sodium hydroxide, using phenolphthalein as indicator.

acidocyte (ă-sid'ō-sīt) [acid + G. *kytos,* cell]. Obsolete term for eosinophilic *leukocyte.*

acidophil, acidophile (ă-sid'ō-fil, ă-sid'ō-fīl) [acid + G. *philos,* fond]. Acidophil *cell.*

acidophilic (as'i-dō-fil'ik, ă-sid'ō-fil-ik). Oxychromatic; having an affinity for acid dyes; denoting a cell or tissue element that stains with an acid dye, such as eosin.

acidosis (as-i-dō'sis) [acid + G. *-ōsis,* condition]. A state characterized by actual or relative decrease of alkali in body fluids in relation to the acid content; depending on the degree of compensation for the a., the pH of body fluids may be normal or decreased, an accumulation of acid metabolites often is present, and tissue function may be disturbed (most importantly that of the central nervous system), if compensation is inadequate.

carbon dioxide a., respiratory a.

compensated a., an a. in which the pH of body fluids is normal; compensation is achieved by respiratory or renal mechanisms.

diabetic a., decreased pH and bicarbonate concentration in the body fluids caused by accumulation of ketone bodies in diabetes mellitus.

lactic a., decreased pH and bicarbonate concentration in the body fluids caused by accumulation of lactic acid due to tissue hypoxia, drug reaction, or unknown etiology.

metabolic a., decreased pH and bicarbonate concentration in the body fluids caused either by the accumulation of acids or by abnormal losses of fixed base from the body, as in diarrhea or renal disease.

primary renal tubular a., a metabolic defect in the mechanism of urinary acidification that may either be the transient type, with onset in infancy, or the persistent type, with onset in childhood or adult years; both types are familial.

renal tubular a., a clinical syndrome characterized by inability to acidify urine, and by low plasma bicarbonate and high plasma chloride concentrations, often with hypokalemia; often complicated by osteomalacia, nephrocalcinosis, or renal calculi. See also primary and secondary renal tubular a.

respiratory a., carbon dioxide a.; a. caused by retention of carbon dioxide; due to inadequate pulmonary ventilation or hypoventilation, with decrease in blood pH unless compensated by renal retention of bicarbonate.

secondary renal tubular a., renal tubular a. that may occur as a complication of hypercalcemic states, hyperglobulinemic disorders, and in some other chronic renal conditions; a rather regular component of de Toni-Fanconi syndrome.

uncompensated a., an a. in which the pH of body fluids is subnormal, because restoration of normal acid-base balance is not possible or has not yet been achieved.

acidotic (as-i-dot'ik). Pertaining to or indicating acidosis.

acid red 87. *Eosin* Y.

acid red 91. *Eosin* B.

acidulate (a-sid'yū-lāt). To render more acid or sour.

acidulous (a-sid'yū-lŭs). Acid or sour.

aciduria (as-i-dū'rē-ă) [acid + G. *ouron,* urine]. **1.** Excretion of an acid urine. **2.** Excretion of an abnormal amount of any specified acid. Individual types of a. are prefixed by the specific acid; *e.g.,* aminoaciduria, ketoaciduria.

aciduric (as-i-dū'rik) [acid + L. *duro,* to endure]. Pertaining to bacteria that tolerate an acid environment.

acidyl (as'id-il). Obsolete term for acyl.

acinar (as'i-nar). Acinic; pertaining to the acinus.

Acinetobacter (as-i-nē'tō-bak'ter). *Lingelsheimia;* a genus of nonmotile, aerobic bacteria (family Neisseriaceae) containing Gram-negative or -variable coccoid or short rods, or cocci, often occurring in pairs. Spores are not produced. These bacteria grow on ordinary media without the addition of serum. They are oxidase-negative and catalase-positive; carbohydrates are oxidized or not attacked at all, and arginine dihydrolase is not produced. They occur frequently in clinical specimens. The type species is *A. calcoaceticus.*

A. calcoacet'icus, *Lingelsheimia anitrata;* a species of bacteria originally found in a quinate enrichment; strains of this organism which were identified as *Bacterium anitratum* were found in the genitourinary tract; it is the type species of the genus *A.*

acini (as'i-nī). Plural of acinus.

acinic (a-sin'ik). Acinar.

aciniform (a-sin'i-fōrm) [L. *acinus,* grape, + *forma,* shape]. Acinous.

acinitis (as-in-ī'tis). Inflammation of an acinus.

acinose (as'i-nōs). Acinous.

acinous (as'i-nŭs). Aciniform; acinose; resembling an acinus or grape-shaped structure.

acinus, gen. and pl. **acini** (as'i-nŭs, -nī) [L. berry, grape] [NA]. One of the minute grape-shaped secretory portions of an acinous gland. Some authorities use the terms a. and alveolus interchangeably, whereas others differentiate them by the constricted openings of the a. into the excretory duct.

liver a., the smallest functional unit of the liver, comprising all of the liver parenchyma supplied by a terminal branch of the portal vein and hepatic artery; typically involves segments of two lobules lying between two terminal hepatic venules.

pulmonary a., primary pulmonary lobule; respiratory lobule; that part of the airway consisting of a respiratory bronchiole and all of its branches.

aclasis (ak'lă-sis) [G. *a-* priv. + *klasis,* a breaking away, a fragment]. A state of continuity between normal and abnormal tissue.

diaphysial a., hereditary multiple *exostoses.*

aclastic (ă-klas'tik) [G. *a-* priv. + *klastos,* broken in pieces]. Nonrefractive; not refracting the rays of light.

acleistocardia (ă-klīs-tō-kar'dē-ă) [G. *a-* priv. + *kleistos,* closed, + *kardia,* heart]. Patency of the foramen ovale of the heart.

acme (ak'mē) [G. *akmē,* the highest point]. The period of greatest intensity of any symptom, sign, or process.

acmesthesia (ak-mes-thē'zē-ă) [G. *acmē,* point, + *aisthēsis,* sensation]. **1.** Sensitivity to pinprick. **2.** A cutaneous sensation of a sharp point.

acne (ak'nē) [probably a corruption (or copyist's error) of G. *akmē,* point of efflorescence]. An inflammatory follicular, papular, and pustular eruption involving the sebaceous apparatus.

a. agmina'ta, obsolete term for *lupus* miliaris disseminatus faciei.

a. al'bida, a. caused by milia.

a. artificia'lis, a. venenata; a. produced by external irritants, such

as tar (chloracne), or drugs internally administered, such as iodides or bromides.
asbestos a., acneform eruption resulting from occupational exposure to asbestos.
bromide a., follicular eruption on face, trunk, and extremities, due to bromide ingestion.
a. cachectico'rum, a. occurring in persons who have a debilitating constitutional disease; characterized by large, soft, purulent, ulcerative, cystic, and scarred lesions.
chlorine a., chloracne.
a. cilia'ris, follicular papules and pustules on the free edges of the eyelids.
colloid a., *elastosis* colloidalis conglomerata.
a. congloba'ta, severe cystic a., characterized by cystic lesions, abscesses, communicating sinuses, and thickened, nodular scars.
a. cosmet'ica, low-grade, non-inflammatory acne lesions from repeated application of comedogenic agents in cosmetics.
cystic a., a. in which the predominant lesions are cysts and deep-seated scars.
a. decal'vans, *folliculitis* decalvans.
a. erythemato'sa, rosacea.
a. fronta'lis, a. varioliformis.
a. genera'lis, a. lesions involving the face, chest, and back.
halogen a., an acneform eruption caused by bromides or iodides.
a. hypertroph'ica, a. vulgaris in which the lesions, on healing, leave hypertrophic scars.
a. indura'ta, deeply seated a., with large papules and pustules, large scars, and hypertrophic scars.
iodide a., a follicular eruption on the face, trunk, and extremities, due to injection or ingestion of iodide in a hypersensitive individual.
a. kerato'sa, an eruption of papules consisting of horny plugs projecting from the hair follicles, accompanied by inflammation.
a. lupoi'des, a. varioliformis.
a. medicamento'sa, acneform a. caused or exacerbated by several classes of drugs, *e.g.,* antiepileptic, halogens, steroids, tuberculostatic.
a. necrot'ica, a. varioliformis.
a. neonato'rum, a condition in newborn infants, characterized by papules and comedones on forehead and cheeks.
a. papulo'sa, a. vulgaris in which the papular lesions predominate.
pomade a., a. commonly found on the forehead and temples of black males after prolonged and repetitious application of hair creams.
a. puncta'ta, a condition that resembles chloracne in that black central comedones are present in all the lesions.
a. pustulo'sa, a. vulgaris in which the pustular lesions predominate.
a. ro'dens, a. varioliformis.
a. rosa'cea, rosacea.
a. scrofuloso'rum, papulonecrotic *tuberculid.*
a. seba'cea, *seborrhea* oleosa.
a. sim'plex, simple a., a. vulgaris.
steroid a., a. similar to a. vulgaris, but resulting from topical or oral administration of steroids.
a. syphilit'ica, pustular *syphilids.*
tar a., chloracne.
a. tar'si, follicular eruptions involving sebaceous glands of the eyelids.
a. telangiecto'des, rosacea-like *tuberculid.*
tropical a., a severe type of a. of the entire trunk, shoulders, upper arms, buttocks, and thighs; occurs in hot humid climates.
a. urtica'ta, an eruption of acne-like lesions, beginning as small urticarial wheals and followed by slight scarring.
a. variolifor'mis, a. frontalis, lupoides, necrotica, or rodens; a pyogenic infection involving follicles occurring chiefly on the forehead and temples; involution of the umbilicated and crusting lesions is followed by scar formation.
a. venena'ta, a. artificialis.
a. vulga'ris, a. simplex; simple a.; an eruption, predominantly of the face, upper back, and chest, comprised of comedones, cysts, papules, and pustules on an inflammatory base; the condition occurs primarily during puberty and adolescence, due to an overactive pilosebaceous apparatus, probably affected by hormonal activity.

acneform (ak'nē-fōrm). Acneiform; resembling acne.

acnegenic (ak-nē-jen'ik). Pertaining to substances thought to be responsible for causing or exacerbating lesions of acne.

acneiform (ak-nē'i-fōrm). Acneform.

acnemia (ak-nē'mē-ă) [G. *a-* priv. + *knēmē,* leg]. Congenital absence of legs.

acnitis (ak-nī'tis). Obsolete term for *lupus* miliaris disseminatus faciei.

acokanthera (ak-ō-kan'ther-ă) [G. *akōkē,* a point, + *anthēros,* blooming]. Juice from the leaves and stems of *Acokanthera ouabaio* (family Apocynaceae), a South African arrow poison containing ouabain.

acolasia (ak-ō-lā'sē-ă) [G. *akolasia,* licentiousness]. Morbid intemperance or lust.

acolous (ak'ō-lŭs) [G. *a-* priv. + *kōlon,* limb]. Without limbs.

acomia (ă-kō'mē-ă) [G. *a-* priv. + *komē,* hair of head]. Alopecia.

aconative (ă-kon'ă-tiv) [G. *a-* priv. + L. *conari,* to try]. Without the desire or wish to act.

aconitase (ă-kon'i-tās). Aconitate hydratase.

aconitate hydratase (ă-kon'i-tāt) [EC 4.2.1.3]. Aconitase; an enzyme catalyzing the dehydration of citric acid to *cis* -aconitic acid, a reaction of significance in the tricarboxylic acid cycle.

aconite (ak'ō-nīt). The dried root of *Aconitum napellus* (family Ranunculaceae), monkshood or wolfsbane; a powerful and rapid acting poison formerly used as an antipyretic, diuretic, diaphoretic, anodyne, cardiac and respiratory depressant, and externally as an analgesic.

***cis*-aconitic acid** (ak-ō-nit'ik). Dehydration product of citric acid; intermediate in the tricarboxylic acid cycle.

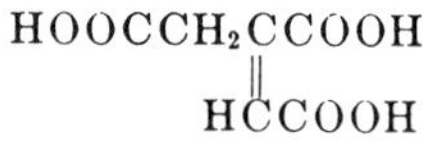

***cis*-Aconitic acid**

aconitine (a-kon'i-tēn). Acetylbenzoylaconine; the exceedingly poisonous active principle (alkaloid) of *Aconitum,* formerly used as a cardiac sedative and applied externally for neuralgia.

acorea (ă-kō'rē-ă) [G. *a-* priv. + *korē,* pupil]. Congenital absence of the ocular pupil.

acormus (ā-kōr'mŭs) [*a-* priv. + *kormos,* trunk of a tree]. A malformed fetus in which most of the trunk is absent.

Acosta, Joseph (José) de, Spanish Jesuit missionary, 1539–1600. See A.'s *disease.*

acouasm (ă-kū'ă-zm). Acousma.

acousma (ă-kūs'mă) [G. *akousma,* something heard]. Acouasm; rarely used term for an auditory hallucination in which indefinite sounds, such as ringing or hissing, are heard.

acousmatamnesia (ă-kūs'mă-tam-nē'zē-ă) [G. *akousma,* something heard, + *amnēsia,* forgetfulness]. A loss of memory for sounds.

acoustic (ă-kūs'tik). Relating to hearing or the perception of sound.

acousticophobia (ă-kūs'ti-kō-fō'bē-ă) [G. *akoustikos,* acoustic, + *phobos,* fear]. Morbid fear of sounds.

acoustics (ă-kūs'tiks) [G. *akoustikos*, relating to hearing]. The science concerned with sounds and of their perception.

ACP Abbreviation for acyl carrier *protein*.

ACP-acetyltransferase [EC 2.3.1.38]. Acetyl transacylase; enzyme transferring acetyl from acetyl-CoA to ACP to begin fatty acid snythesis.

ACP-malonyltransferase [EC 2.3.1.39]. Malonyl transacylase; an enzyme transferring malonyl from malonyl-CoA to ACP; a key step in fatty acid synthesis.

acquired (ă-kwīrd') [L. *ac-quiro (adq-)*, to obtain, fr. *quaero*, to seek]. Denoting a disease, predisposition, abnormality, etc., that is not inherited.

acquisition (ak-wi-zish'ŭn). In psychology, the empirical demonstration of an increase in the strength of the conditioned response in successive trials of pairing the conditioned and unconditioned stimulus.

acquisitus (ă-kwiz'i-tŭs). Acquired.

acral (ak'răl) [G. *akron*, extremity]. Relating to or affecting the peripheral parts, *e.g.*, limbs, fingers, ears, etc.

Acrania (ă-krā'nē-ă) [G. *a-* priv. + *kranion*, skull]. A group of the phylum Chordata whose members possess a notochord, gill slits, and nerve cord but no vertebrae, ribs, or skull; *e.g.*, *Amphioxus*, tunicates, and acorn worms.

acrania (ă-krā'nē-ă) [G. *a-* priv. + *kranion*, skull]. Complete or partial absence of a skull; associated with anencephaly.

acranial (ă-krā'nē-ăl). Having no cranium; relating to acrania or an acranius.

Acrel, Olof, Swedish surgeon, 1717–1806. See A.'s *ganglion*.

Acremonium (ak-rē-mō'nē-ŭm). A genus of fungi (family Moniliaceae, order Moniliales) that causes eumycotic mycetoma; three species, *A. falciforme*, *A. kiliense*, and *A. recifei*, produce whitish to yellow grains in the tissues.

acribometer (ak-ri-bom'ĕ-ter) [G. *akribēs*, exact, + *metron*, measure]. An instrument for measuring very minute objects.

acrid (ak'rid) [L. *acer (acr-)*, pungent]. Sharp, pungent, biting, or irritating.

acridine (ak'ri-dēn). Dibenzopyridine; 10-azaanthracene; a dye, dye intermediate, and antiseptic precursor (9-aminoacridine, acriflavine, proflavine hemisulfate) derived from coal tar and irritating to skin and mucous membranes.

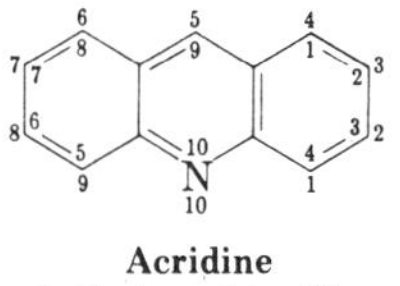

Acridine
Inner numbering is that used by *Chemical Abstracts* and *International Union of Pure and Applied Chemistry*.

tetramethyl a., a. orange.

acridine orange [C.I. 46005]. Tetramethyl a.; 3,6-bis(dimethylamino)acridine hydrochloride; a basic fluorescent dye useful as a metachromatic stain for nucleic acids; also used in screening cervical smears for abnormal and malignant cells, where unusual amounts of DNA and RNA occur during proliferation and in tumors (DNA fluoresces yellow to green; RNA fluoresces orange to red).

acridine yellow, 9- or 5-aminoacridine hydrochloride; a faintly yellow solution with strong bluish-violet fluorescence; used as a topical antiseptic and as a fluorescent stain in histology.

acriflavine (ak-ri-flā'vin) [C.I. 46000]. An acridine dye, a mixture of 3,6-diamino-10-methylacridinium chloride and 3,6-diaminoacridine; formerly used as a topical and urinary antiseptic, and used as one of Kasten's fluorescent Schiff reagents to reveal polysaccharides and DNA.

acrimonia (ak-ri-mō'nē-ă) [L. pungency]. In ancient humoral pathology, a sharp, pungent, disease-provoking humor.

acrimony (ak'rĭ-mō-nē) [L. *acrimonia*, pungency]. The quality of being intensely irritant, biting, or pungent.

acrinol (ak'ri-nol). Ethacridine lactate.

acrisorcin (ak-ri-sōr'sin). 9-Aminoacridine with 4-hexylresorcinol; a synthetic topical antifungal agent.

acritical (ă-krit'i-kăl, ā-) [G. *a-* priv. + *kritikos*, critical]. **1.** Not critical; marked by no crisis; denoting diseases terminating by lysis. **2.** Indeterminate, especially concerning prognosis.

acro- [G. *akron*, extremity; *akros*, extreme]. Combining form meaning: **1.** Extremity, tip, end, peak, topmost. **2.** Extreme.

acroagnosis (ak'rō-ag-nō'sis) [acro- + G. *agnōsia*, a not knowing]. Absence of acrognosis.

acroanesthesia (ak'rō-an-es-thē'zē-ă) [acro- + G. *an-* priv. + *aisthēsis* sensation]. Anesthesia of one or more of the extremities.

acroarthritis (ak-rō-arth-rī'tis) [acro- + G. *arthron*, joint, + *-itis*]. Inflammation of the joints of the hands or feet.

acroasphyxia (ak'rō-as-fik'sē-ă) [acro- + G. *asphyxia*, stoppage of the pulse]. Dead or waxy fingers; impaired digital circulation, possibly a mild form of Raynaud's disease, marked by a purplish or waxy white color of the fingers, with subnormal local temperature and paresthesia.

acroataxia (ak'rō-ă-tak'sē-ă) [acro- + ataxia]. Ataxia affecting the distal portion of the extremities, *i.e.*, hands and fingers, feet, and toes. *Cf.* proximoataxia.

acroblast (ak'rō-blast) [acro- + G. *blastos*, germ]. Component of the developing spermatid composed of numerous Golgi elements; it contains the proacrosomal granules.

acrobrachycephaly (ak'rō-brak-i-sef'ă-lē) [acro- + G. *brachys*, short, + *kephale*, head]. Type of craniosynostosis with premature closure of the coronal suture, resulting in abnormally short anteroposterior diameter of the skull.

acrobystitis (ak'rō-bis-tī'tis) [G. *akrobystia*, prepuce, + *-itis*, inflammation]. Obsolete term for posthitis.

acrocentric (ak-rō-sen'trik) [acro- + G. *kentron*, center]. Having the centromere close to the extremity, said of a chromosome.

acrocephalia (ak-rō-se-fā'lē-ă). Oxycephaly.

acrocephalic (ak-rō-se-fal'ik). Oxycephalic.

acrocephalopolysyndactyly (ak'rō-sef'ă-lō-pol'ē-sin-dak'ti-lē). Carpenter's syndrome; congenital malformation in which oxycephaly, brachysyndactyly of hand, and preaxial polydactyly of feet are associated with mental retardation.

acrocephalosyndactylia (ak'rō-sef'ă-lō-sin-dak-til'ē-ă). Acrocephalosyndactyly.

acrocephalosyndactylism (ak'rō-sef'ă-lō-sin-dak'til-izm). Acrocephalosyndactyly.

acrocephalosyndactyly (ak'rō-sef'ă-lō-sin-dak'ti-lē) [acrocephaly + G. *syn*, together, + *daktylos*, finger]. Acrocephalosyndactylia; acrocephalosyndactylism; acrosphenosyndactyly; acrodysplasia; a congenital syndrome characterized by peaked head, due to premature closure of skull sutures, associated with fusion or webbing of digits; autosomal dominant inheritance.

atypical a., see type II, III, and V a.

type I a., Apert's syndrome; typical a.; a. with the second through fifth digits fused into one mass with a common nail; often accompanied by moderately severe acne vulgaris of the forearms; autosomal dominant inheritance.

type II a., Apert-Crouzon syndrome; a. with facial characteristics

of Crouzon disease, with extremely hypoplastic maxilla; fusion of digits is less severe, with thumb and fifth finger usually separate; autosomal dominant inheritance.
type III a., Chotzen syndrome; mild acrocephaly, asymmetry of the skull, and soft tissue syndactyly of the second and third fingers and toes, often with other minor bony abnormalities; autosomal dominant inheritance.
type V a., Pfeiffer syndrome; a. with broad short thumbs and great toes, often with duplication (polydactyly) of the great toes and variable syndactyly of other digits; autosomal dominant inheritance.
typical a., type I a.

acrocephalous (ak-rō-sef'ă-lŭs). Oxycephalic.

acrocephaly (ak'rō-sef'ă-lē) [acro- + G. *kephalē,* head]. Oxycephaly.

acrochordon (ak-rō-kōr'don) [acro- + G. *chordē,* cord]. Skin *tag.*

acrocinesia, acrocinesis (ak'rō-sin-ē'zē-ă, -ē'sis) [acro- + G. *kinēsis,* movement]. Akrokinesia; excessive movement.

acrocontracture (ak'rō-kon-trak'chūr). Contracture of the joints of the hands or feet.

acrocyanosis (ak'rō-sī-an-ō'sis) [acro- + G. *kyanos,* blue, + *-osis,* condition]. Crocq's disease; a circulatory disorder in which the hands, and less commonly the feet, are persistently cold and blue; some forms are related to Raynaud's phenomenon.

acrocyanotic (ak'rō-sī-an-ot'ik). Characterized by acrocyanosis.

acrodermatitis (ak'rō-der-mă-tī'tis) [acro- + G. *derma,* skin, + *-itis,* inflammation]. Inflammation of the skin of the extremities.
a. chron'ica atroph'icans, a gradually progressive dermatitis appearing first on the feet, hands, elbows or knees, and comprised of indurated, erythematous plaques that become atrophic, giving a tissue-paper appearance of the involved sites.
a. contin'ua, *pustulosis* palmaris et plantaris.
a. enteropath'ica, an intermittently progressive defect of zinc metabolism defect in young children (3 weeks to 18 months), often first manifest as a blistering, oozing, and crusting eruption on an extremity or around one of the orifices of the body, followed by loss of hair and diarrhea or other gastrointestinal disturbances; autosomal recessive trait.
a. hiema'lis, a. occurring chiefly in winter.
papular a. of childhood, Gianotti-Crosti *syndrome.*
a. per'stans, *pustulosis* palmaris et plantaris.
a. vesiculos'a trop'ica, a form occurring in hot climates in which the skin of the extremities is glossy and shows numerous small vesicles.

acrodermatosis (ak'rō-der-mă-tō'sis) [acro- + G. *derma,* skin, + *-osis,* condition]. Any cutaneous affection involving the more distal portions of the extremities.

acrodolichomelia (ak'rō-dol'i-kō-mē'lē-ă) [acro- + G. *dolichos,* long, + *melos,* limb]. Congenital or acquired condition characterized by large size and disproportionate growth of the hands and feet.

acrodont (ak'rō-dont) [acro- + G. *odous,* tooth]. Tooth attachment in some lower vertebrates (mainly fish) in which the teeth rest on the edge of the jaw bone rather than in sockets or alveoli.

acrodynia (ak-rō-din'ē-ă) [acro- + G. *odynē,* pain]. **1.** Pain in peripheral or acral parts of the body. **2.** A syndrome caused almost exclusively by mercury poisoning: in children, characterized by erythema of the extremities, chest, and nose, polyneuritis, and gastrointestinal symptoms; in adults, by anorexia, photophobia, sweating, and tachycardia. Also known as erythredema; acrodynic erythema; pink or Swift's disease; dermatopolyneuritis. **3.** A condition caused in rats by a deficiency of pyridoxine, characterized by redness and swelling of the tips of the ears, nose, and paws, leading to necrosis of these parts.

acrodysesthesia (ak'rō-dis-es-thē'zē-ă) [acro- + dysesthesia]. Abnormal and unpleasant sensation in the peripheral portions of the extremities.

acrodysostosis (ak'rō-dis-os-tō'sis) [acro- + dysostosis]. A disorder, perhaps genetic, in which the hands and feet are abnormally small; facial changes and mental retardation are variable concomitants.

acrodysplasia (ak'rō-dis-plā'zē-ă) [acro- + dysplasia]. Acrocephalosyndactyly.

acroedema (ak'rō-ĕ-dē'mă). Edema of hand or foot, often permanent; occurs sometimes after an injury, and in certain neurological diseases.

acroesthesia (ak'ro-es-thē'zē-ă) [acro- + G. *aisthēsis,* sensation]. **1.** An extreme degree of hyperesthesia. **2.** Hyperesthesia of one or more of the extremities.

acrogenous (ak-roj'ĕ-nŭs) [acro- + G. *genos,* birth]. Denoting conida of fungi produced by the conidiogenous cell at the tip of a conidiophore.

acrogeria (ak-rō-jĕr'ē-ă) [acro- + G. *gerōn,* old]. Congenital reduction or loss of subcutaneous fat and collagen of the hands and feet, giving the appearance of senility.

acrognosis (ak-rog-nō'sis) [acro- + G. *gnōsis,* knowledge]. Cenesthesia, or sensory perception, of the extremities.

acrohyperhidrosis (ak'rō-hī'per-hī-drō'sis). Hyperhidrosis of the hands and feet.

acrokeratoelastoidosis (ak'rō-ker'ă-tō-ē-las-toy-dō'sis). A dominantly inherited papular keratosis of the palms and soles, with disorganization of dermal elastic fibers; sunlight and physical trauma are essential contributing factors.

acrokeratosis (ak'rō-ker-ă-tō'sis) [acro- + G. *keras,* horn, + *-osis,* condition]. Overgrowth of the horny layer of the skin, usually nodular configurations, of the dorsum of the fingers and toes, and occasionally on the rim of the ear and tip of the nose.
paraneoplastic a., Basex's *syndrome.*

acrokeratosis verruciformis (ak'rō-ker-ă-tō'sis vĕ-rū-si-fōrm'is) [acro- + keratosis; L. *verruca,* a wart, + *forma,* form]. A genodermatosis, probably related to Darier's disease, characterized by warty excrescences of the hands and feet.

acrokinesia (ak'rō-ki-nē'zē-ă). Acrocinesia.

acroleic acids (ak-rō'-lē-ik). Acrylic acids.

acroleukopathy (ak'rō-lū-kop'ă-thē). Depigmentation of the extremities.

acromegalia (ak'rō-mĕ-gā'lē-ă). Acromegaly.

acromegalic (ak'rō-mĕ-gal'ik). Pertaining to or characterized by acromegaly.

acromegalogigantism (ak'rō-meg'ă-lō-jī'gan-tizm) [acro- + G. *megas,* great, + *gigas,* giant]. Gigantism in which the facial features, disproportionate enlargement of the extremities, and other signs of acromegaly are prominent.

acromegaloidism (ak-rō-meg'ă-loyd-izm). A condition in which body proportions resemble those of acromegaly.

acromegaly (ak-rō-meg'ă-lē) [acro- + G. *megas,* large]. Acromegalia; a disorder marked by progressive enlargement of peripheral parts of the body, especially the head, face, hands, and feet, due to excessive secretion of somatotropin; organomegaly and other metabolic disorders occur, and diabetes mellitus may develop.

acromelalgia (ak-rō-mel-al'jē-ă) [acro- + G. *melos,* limb, + *algos,* pain]. A vasomotor neurosis marked by redness, pain, and swelling of the fingers and toes, headache, and vomiting; probably the same as erythromelalgia.

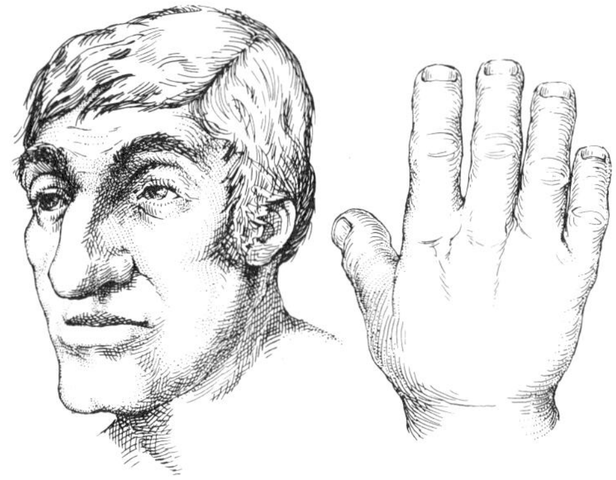

Acromegaly
Showing facial features and large, spadelike hand

acromelia (ak-rō-mē'lē-ă) [acro- + G. *melos,* limb, + *ia,* condition]. Acromelic dwarfism; a form of dwarfism in which shortening is most striking in the most distal segment of the limbs.

acromelic (ak-rō-mel'ik) [acro- + G. *melos,* limb]. Affecting the terminal part of a limb.

acrometagenesis (ak'rō-met-ă-jen'ĕ-sis) [acro- + G. *meta,* beyond, + *genesis,* origin]. Abnormal development of the extremities resulting in deformity.

acromial (ă-krō'mē-ăl). Relating to the acromion.

acromicria (ak-rō-mik'rē-ă, ak-rō-mī'krē-ă) [acro- + G. *mikros,* small]. The antithesis of acromegaly; a condition in which the bones of the face and extremities are small and delicate; possibly due to a deficiency of somatotropin.

acromioclavicular (ak-rō'mē-ō-kla-vik'yū-lăr). Scapuloclavicular (1); relating to the acromion and the clavicle; denoting the articulation between the clavicle and the scapula and its ligaments.

acromiocoracoid (ak-rō-mē-ō-kōr'ă-koyd). Coracoacromial.

acromiohumeral (ak-rō'mē-ō-hyū'mer-ăl). Relating to the acromion and the humerus.

acromion (ă-krō'mē-on) [G. *akrōmion,* fr. *akron,* tip, + *ōmos,* shoulder] [NA]. Acromial process; the lateral end of the spine of the scapula which projects as a broad flattened process overhanging the glenoid fossa; it articulates with the clavicle and gives attachment to part of the deltoid and of the trapezius muscles.

acromioscapular (ak-rō'mē-ō-skap'yū-lăr). Relating to both the acromion and body of the scapula.

acromiothoracic (ă-krō'mē-ō-thō-ras'ik). Thoracoacromial; thoracicoacromial; relating to the acromion and the thorax; denoting especially the arteria thoracoacromialis.

acromphalus (ak-rom'fal-ŭs) [acro- + G. *omphalos,* umbilicus]. Abnormal projection of the umbilicus.

acromyotonia (ak'rō-mī-ō-tō'nē-ă) [acro- + G. *mys,* muscle, + *tonos,* tension]. Acromyotonus; myotonia affecting the extremities only, resulting in spasmodic deformity of the hand or foot.

acromyotonus (ak-rō-mī-ot'ō-nŭs). Acromyotonia.

acroneurosis (ak'rō-nū-rō'sis). Any neurosis, usually vasomotor in nature, manifesting itself in the extremities.

acronine (ak'rō-nēn). 3,12-Dihydro-6-methoxy-3,3,12-trimethyl-7*H*-pyrano[2,3-*c*]acridin-7-one; an antineoplastic agent.

acronyx (ak'rō-niks) [acro- + G. *onyx,* nail]. An ingrowing nail.

acro-osteolysis (ak'rō-os-tē-ol'i-sis). Congenital condition manifested by palmar and plantar ulcerating lesions with osteolysis; acquired a. has been reported in workers exposed to vinyl chloride. See also Cheney *syndrome.*

acropachy (ak'rō-pak-ē, ă-krop'ă-kē) [acro- + G. *pachys,* thick]. Thickening of peripheral tissues; seen most often in hypothyroidism and hypertrophic pulmonary osteoarthropathy.

acropachyderma (ak'rō-pak-i-der'mă) [acro- + G. *pachys,* thick, + *derma,* skin]. Idiopathic Bamberger-Marie disease; Brugsch's or Uehlinger's syndrome; a disorder characterized by thickening of the skin of the face, scalp, and extremities together with clubbing of the fingers and deformities of the bones of the limb.

acroparesthesia (ak'rō-par-es-thē'zē-ă) [acro- + paresthesia]. **1.** Paresthesia of one or more of the extremities. **2.** An extreme degree of paresthesia.

acropathy (ă-krop'ă-thē) [acro- + G. *pathos,* disease]. Simple hereditary clubbing of the digits without associated pulmonary or other progressive disease, often more severe in males; autosomal dominant inheritance.

acropetal (ă-krop'ĕ-tăl) [acro- + L. *peto,* to seek]. **1.** In a direction toward the summit. **2.** Produced successively toward the apex, with the youngest conidium formed at the tip and the oldest at the base of a chain of conidia; pertaining to asexual spore production in fungi by successive budding of the distal spore in a spore chain.

acrophobia (ak-rō-fō'bē-ă) [acro- + G. *phobos,* fear]. Morbid fear of heights.

acropigmentation (ak'rō-pig-men-tā'shŭn). Hyperpigmentation of the dorsal surfaces of the fingers and toes beginning in early childhood and usually increasing with age; more common in persons of dark complexion.

acropleurogenous (ak'rō-plūr-oj'ĕ-nŭs). Denoting spores developing at the tip and along the sides of fungal hyphae.

acroposthitis (ak'rō-pos-thī'tis) [G. *akroposthia,* prepuce, + *-itis,* inflammation]. Posthitis.

acropustulosis (ak'rō-pŭs-tyū-lō'sis) [acro- + pustulosis]. Relapsing pustular eruptions of the hands and feet.
infantile a., a cyclically recurrent papulopustular and crusting eruption appearing soon after birth to 10 months; remission occurs at about 2 years of age.

acroscleroderma (ak'rō-sklēr-ō-der'mă) [acro- + G. *sklēros,* hard, + *derma,* skin]. Acrosclerosis.

acrosclerosis (ak'rō-sklĕ-rō'sis). Acroscleroderma; sclerodactyly; stiffness and tightness of the skin of the fingers, with atrophy of the soft tissue and osteoporosis of the distal phalanges of the hands and feet; a form of progressive systemic sclerosis occurring with Raynaud's phenomenon.

acrosin (ak'rō-sin) [EC 3.4.21.10]. A serine proteinase in spermatozoa.

acrosome (ak'rō-sōm) [acro- + G. *soma,* body]. Acrosomal *cap.*

acrosomin (ak-rō-sō'min). A lipoglycoprotein complex present in the acrosomal cap.

acrosphenosyndactyly (ak'rō-sfē'nō-sin-dak'ti-lē) [acro- + sphenoid + syndactyly]. Acrocephalosyndactyly.

acrospiroma (ak'rō-spī-rō'mă) [scro- + G. *speira,* coil, + -oma, tumor]. A tumor of the distal segment of a sweat gland.
eccrine a., clear cell or nodular hidradenoma; a tumor derived from the eccrine sweat ducts, often composed of glycogen-rich clear cells.

acrostealgia (ak-ros-tē-al'jē-ă). Painful inflammation of the bones of the hands and feet.

acroteric (ak-rō-ter'ik) [G. *akrōtērion,* the topmost point]. Relating to the extreme periphery, such as the tips of fingers and toes, the end of the nose.

Acrotheca (ak-rō-thē'kă) [see acrotheca]. Former name for *Rhinocladiella.*

acrotheca (ak-rō-thē'kă) [acro- + G. *thēkē,* box, case]. In fungi, a type of spore formation characteristic of the genus *Fonsecaea,* in which conidia are formed along the ends and sides of irregular club-shaped conidiophores.

acrotic (ă-krot'ik). **1** [G. *akrotēs,* extremity]. Relating to the surface of the body, especially the cutaneous glands. **2** [G. *a-* priv. + *krotos,* a striking]. Marked by great weakness or absence of the pulse; pulseless.

acrotism (ak'rō-tizm) [G. *a-* priv. + *krotos,* a striking]. Absence or imperceptibility of the pulse.

acrotrophodynia (ak'rō-trof-ō-din'ē-ă) [acro- + G. *trophē,* nourishment, + *odynē,* pain]. Neuritis of the extremities occurring as a sequel to trench foot.

acrotrophoneurosis (ak'rō-trof'ō-nū-rō'sis). Trophoneurosis of one or more of the extremities.

acrylate (ă-kril'āt). A salt or ester of acrylic acid.

acrylic (ă-kril'ik). Denoting certain synthetic plastic resins derived from a. acid. See also acrylic *resin.*

acrylic acids. Acroleic acids; a series of unsaturated aliphatic acids of the general formula R=CH—COOH; the prototype, acrylic acid (R=CH_2) or 2-propenoic acid, is derived from propionic acid by reduction or from glycerol by dehydration.

acrylonitrile (ak'ri-lō-nī'tril). Vinyl cyanide; $CH_2{=}CHCN$; a very toxic cyanide compound used in organic syntheses and in the manufacture of plastics and synthetic rubber.

ACTe Abbreviation for anodal closure *tetanus.*

ACTH Abbreviation for adrenocorticotropic *hormone.*

big ACTH, a form of ACTH, produced by certain tumors, which is a larger and more acidic peptide molecule than little ACTH, but is not immunochemically distinguishable from it and does not exert any of the biological effects characteristic of ACTH; tryptic digestion of big ACTH yields hormonally active little ACTH.

little ACTH, a term coined to denote the conventional ACTH molecule when contrasted with big ACTH.

acthiazidum (ak'thī-ă-zī'dŭm). Ethiazide.

actin (ak'tin). One of the protein components into which actomyosin can be split; it can exist in a fibrous form (F- actin) or a globular form (G-actin).

F-a., the association of G-a. subunits into a fibrous (F) protein caused by increase in salt concentration; the conversion of G-a. to F-actin is catalyzed by small concentrations of magnesium ion, is reversible, and is accompanied by the conversion of the bound ATP molecule to ADP and the conversion of one reactive —SH group to an unreactive form.

G-a., the globular (G) subunits of the a. molecule, having a molecular weight 57,000 and containing one molecule of ATP; it is soluble in dilute salt, polymerizing to F-a. when ionic strength is increased.

acting out. Overt expression of unconscious emotional feelings.

actinic (ak-tin'ik) [G. *aktis* (*aktin-*), a ray]. Relating to the chemically active rays of the electromagnetic spectrum.

actinides (ak'tin-ī-dēz) [*actinium,* first element of the series]. Actinide elements; those elements with atomic numbers 89 to 103, corresponding to the lanthanides in the Periodic Table.

actinism (ak'tin-izm). Archaic term for the effect of radiant energy, such as light, on chemicals or tissue.

actinium (ak-tin'ē-ŭm) [G. *aktis,* a ray]. An element, symbol Ac, atomic no. 89; it possesses no stable isotopes and exists in nature only as a disintegration product of uranium and thorium.

actino- [G. *aktis* (*aktin-*), a ray, beam]. Combining form meaning a ray, as of light; applied to any form of radiation or to any structure with radiating parts. See also radio-.

actinobacillosis (ak'tin-ō-bas-i-lō'sis). Wooden tongue of cattle; a disease of cattle and swine, occasionally reported in man, caused by *Actinobacillus lignieresii.* It affects the soft tissues, often the tongue and cervical lymph nodes, where granulomatous swellings are formed that eventually break down to form abscesses.

Actinobacillus (ak'tin-ō-bă-sil'lŭs) [actino- + L. *bacillus,* a little rod]. A genus of nonmotile, nonsporeforming, aerobic, facultatively anaerobic bacteria (family Brucellaceae) containing Gram-negative rods interspersed with coccal elements. The metabolism of these bacteria is fermentative. They are pathogenic to animals. The type species is *A. lignieresii.*

A. actinoi'des, a species of doubtful taxonomic position; it is nonpathogenic for laboratory animals but pathogenic for goats via the intratracheal route; isolated from calves with chronic pneumonia.

A. actinomyce'tem com'itans, a species of doubtful taxonomic position; not pathogenic for laboratory animals, and pathogenicity in man is questionable; occurs with actinomycetes in actinomycotic lesions.

A. equu'li, a species causing suppurative lesions, particularly in the kidneys and joints in foals and piglets, and endocarditis in pigs.

A. lignieres'ii, a species producing infections of the upper alimentary tract and mouth in cattle and swine (actinobacillosis) and suppurative lesions in the skin and lungs of sheep; it is the type species of its genus.

A. mal'lei, *Pseudomonas mallei.*

actinodermatitis (ak'ti-nō-der-mă-tī'tis) [actino- + G. *derma,* skin, + *-itis,* inflammation]. **1.** Inflammation of the skin produced by exposure to sunlight. **2.** Adverse reaction of skin to radiation therapy (ultraviolet, x-ray, or radium).

actinogen (ak-tin'ō-jen). Obsolete term for any radioactive element or, more generally, any substance that produces radiation.

actinogenesis (ak'ti-nō-jen'ĕ-sis) [actino- + G. *genesis,* origin]. Obsolete synonym for radiogenesis.

actinogenic (ak'ti-nō-jen'ik). Obsolete synonym for radiogenic.

actinogenics (ak'ti-nō-jen'iks). Obsolete synonym for radiogenics.

actinogram (ak-tin'ō-gram). Obsolete synonym for radiograph.

actinograph (ak-tin'ō-graf) [actino- + G. *graphō,* to write]. **1.** Obsolete term for radiograph. **2.** Obsolete apparatus for determining the proper exposure of a photographic plate according to the degree of light.

actinography (ak-ti-nog'ră-fē). Obsolete synonym for radiography.

actinohematin (ak'ti-nō-hē'mă-tin) [actino- + G. *haima,* blood]. A red respiratory pigment found in certain forms of *Actinia* (sea anemones).

actinolite (ak-tin'ō-līt). **1.** Any substance that undergoes a change when exposed to light. **2.** A greenish mineral, $Ca(Mg, Fe)_3(SiO_3)_4$.

actinolyte (ak-tin'ō-līt) [actino- + G. *lytos,* soluble, fr. *lyō,* to loose]. An obsolete apparatus formerly used in the application of the actinic rays.

Actinomadura (ak'ti-nō-mad'yū-ră) [actino- + *Madura,* India]. A genus of aerobic, Gram-positive, non-acid-fast fungi where filaments fragment into spores. *A. pelletieri* is an agent of mycetoma.

actinometry (ak-ti-nom'ĕ-trē) [actino- + G. *metron,* measure]. The determination of the photochemical action of light rays.

actinomycelial (ak'ti-nō-mī-sē'lē-ăl). Relating to the mycelium-like filaments of the Actinomycetales.

Actinomyces (ak'ti-nō-mī'sēz) [actino- + G. *mykēs,* fungus]. A genus of nonmotile, nonsporeforming, anaerobic to facultatively anaerobic bacteria (family Actinomycetaceae) containing Gram-positive, irregularly staining filaments; diphtheroid cells are predominant. Most of the species produce a filamentous microcolony. The metabolism of these chemoheterotrophs is fermentative; the products of glucose fermentation include acetic, formic, lactic and succinic acids but not propionic acid. These organisms are pathogenic for man and/or other animals. The type species is *A. bovis.*

A. bo'vis, a species of bacteria causing actinomycosis in cattle; infection in man is not established; it is the type species of its genus.
A. israe'lii, a species of bacteria causing human actinomycosis and, occasionally, infections in cattle.
A. naeslun'dii, a species whose natural habitat is the oral cavity; human infections have been reported, and it produces periodontal destruction in some species of animals.
A. odontoly'ticus, a species whose normal habitat is the human oral cavity; it has been isolated from deep dental caries.
A. visco'sus, a species that has been isolated from the oral cavity of humans and some species of other animals; it produces periodontal disease in animals and has been isolated from human dental calculus and root surface caries.

Actinomycetaceae (ak'ti-nō-mī'sē-tā'sē-ē). A family of nonsporeforming, nonmotile, ordinarily facultatively anaerobic (some species are aerobic and others are anaerobic) bacteria (order Actinomycetales) containing Gram-positive, non-acid fast, predominantly diphtheroid cells which tend to form branched filaments in tissue or in some stages of cultural development; the filaments readily fragment, producing diphtheroid or coccoid forms. The metabolism of these chemoheterotrophic bacteria is fermentative. This family contains the genera *Actinomyces* (type genus), *Arachnia, Bacterionema, Bifidobacterium,* and *Rothia.*

Actinomycetales (ak'ti-nō-mī'sē-tā'lēz). An order of bacteria consisting of moldlike, rod-shaped, clubbed or filamentous forms with decided tendency to true branching, without endospores, but sometimes developing conidia; it includes the families Mycobacteriaceae, Actinomycetaceae, Streptomycetaceae, and Nocardiaceae.

actinomycetes (ak'ti-nō-mī-sē'tēz). A term used to refer to members of the genus *Actinomyces;* sometimes improperly used to refer to any member of the family Actinomycetaceae or order Actinomycetales.

actinomycin (ak'tin-ō-mī'sin). A group of antibiotic agents, isolated from several species of *Streptomyces* (originally *Actinomycos*), that are active against gram-positive bacteria, fungi, and neoplasms. A.'s are chromopeptides, most containing the chromophore actinocin, and are derivatives of phenoxazine which differ in the amino acids and their sequence in the peptide chains; they form complexes with DNA and therefore inhibit RNA synthesis, primarily the ribosomal type.
a. A, the first of the a.'s isolated in crystalline form.
a. C, cactinomycin.
a. D, dactinomycin.
a. F_1, a. KS4; KS4; produced by actinomycin C-elaborating strains of *Streptomyces chrysomallus;* used as an antineoplastic agent.

actinomycoma (ak'ti-nō-mī-kō'mă) [actino- + G. *mykēs,* fungus, + *-oma,* tumor]. A swelling caused by an actinomycete.

actinomycosis (ak'ti-nō-mī-kō'sis) [actino- + G. *mykēs,* fungus, + *-osis,* condition]. Actinophytosis (1); lumpy jaw; a disease primarily of cattle and man caused by *Actinomyces bovis* in cattle and by *A. israelii* and *Arachnia propionica* in man. These actinomycetes are part of the normal bacterial flora of the mouth and pharynx, but when introduced into tissue they may produce chronic destructive abscesses or granulomas which eventually discharge a viscid pus containing minute yellowish granules (sulfur granules). In man, the disease commonly affects the cervicofacial area, abdomen, or thorax; in cattle, the lesion is commonly found in the mandible.

actinomycotic (ak'ti-nō-mī-kot'ik). Relating to actinomycosis.

Actinomyxidia (ak'ti-nō-mik-sid'ē-ă) [actino- + G. *myxa,* mucus]. A sporozoan order having a double cellular envelope, three polar capsules, and eight spores; parasitic chiefly in segmented worms, such as the common earthworm.

actinoneuritis (ak'ti-nō-nū-rī'tis). Obsolete term for radioneuritis.

actinophage (ak-tin'ō-fāj) [actino(myces) + G. *phagein,* to eat]. A virus specific for actinomycetes.

actinophytosis (ak'ti-nō-fī-tō'sis). **1.** Actinomycosis. **2.** Botryomycosis.

Actinopoda (ak-ti-nop'ō-dă) [actino- + G. *pous,* foot]. A class of Sarcodina having slender pseudopodia with a central axial filament.

actinosin (ak-tin'ō-sin). 2-Amino-4,6-dimethyl-3-oxo-3*H*-phenoxazine-1,9-dicarboxylic acid; a phenoxazone derivative that is the chromophore of the actinomycins.

actinotherapeutics (ak'ti-nō-thār-ă-pyū'tiks). Obsolete synonym for radiotherapeutics.

actinotherapy (ak'ti-nō-thār'ă-pē). **1.** In dermatology, ultraviolet light therapy. **2.** Obsolete term for radiotherapy.

actinotoxemia (ak'ti-nō-tok-sē'mē-ă). Obsolete synonym for radiotoxemia.

action (ak'shŭn) [L. *actio,* from *ago,* pp. *actus,* to do]. **1.** The performance of any of the vital functions, the manner of such performance, or the result of the same. **2.** The exertion of any force or power, physical, chemical, or mental. For the actions of some chemical substances, see under the substance.
ball valve a., intermittent blockage of a tube or outlet of a cavity by some object or material that permits passage in one direction but not in the other.
calorigenic a., thermogenic a.; increase of heat production of the body, as by the thyroid hormone.
cumulative a., cumulative *effect.*
salt a., any physicochemical effect produced by hypertonic concentrations of osmotically active electrolytes.
sparing a., the manner in which a nonessential nutritive component, by its presence in the diet, lowers the requirement for an essential component; thus nonessential cysteine spares essential methionine and nonessential tyrosine spares essential phenylalanine.
specific a., the a. of a drug or a method of treatment which has a direct and especially curative effect upon a disease, *e.g.,* the a. of vitamin B_{12} in pernicious anemia.
specific dynamic a. (SDA), increase of heat production caused by the ingestion of food, especially of protein.
thermogenic a., calorigenic a.

activate (ak'ti-vāt). **1.** To render active. **2.** To make radioactive.

activation (ak-ti-vā'shŭn). **1.** The act of rendering active. **2.** An increase in the energy content of an atom or molecule, through the raising of temperature, absorption of light photons, etc., which renders that atom or molecule more reactive. **3.** Techniques of stimulating the brain by light, sound, electricity, or chemical agents, in order to elicit hidden or latent abnormal activity in the electroencephalogram. **4.** Stimulation of cell division in an ovum by fertilization or by artificial means. **5.** The act of making radioactive.
EEG a., the low voltage, fast pattern of attentive wakefulness.

activator (ak'ti-vā-tōr). **1.** A substance that renders another substance, or catalyst, active, or that accelerates a process or reaction. **2.** The fragment, produced by chemical cleavage of a proactivator, that induces the enzymic activity of another substance. **3.** An apparatus for making substances radioactive; *e.g.,* neutron generator, cyclotron. **4.** A removable type of myofunctional orthodontic appliance that acts as a passive transmitter of force, produced by the function of the activated muscles, to the teeth and alveolar process, that are in contact with it.
catabolite gene a. (CGA), catabolite (gene) activator *protein.*
plasminogen a. [EC 3.4.21.31], urokinase; a proteinase converting plasminogen to plasmin by cleavage of a single (usually Arg-Val) bond in the former.
tissue plasminogen a. (TPA), a genetically engineered product which causes lysis of thrombi that are obstructing coronary arter-

ies; used in the management of acute myocardial infarction.

activity (ak-tiv'i-tē). **1.** In electroencephalography, the presence of neurogenic electrical energy. **2.** In physical chemistry, an ideal concentration for which the law of mass action will apply perfectly; the ratio of the a. to the true concentration is the a. coefficient, which becomes 1.00 · · · at infinite dilution.

blocking a., repression or elimination of electrical activity in the brain by the arrival of a sensory stimulus.

insulin-like a. (ILA), a measure of substances, usually in plasma, that exert biologic effects similar to those of insulin in various bioassays; sometimes used as a measure of plasma insulin concentrations; always gives higher values than immunochemical techniques for the measurement of insulin.

optical a., the ability of a compound in solution (one possessing no plane of symmetry, usually because of the presence of one or more asymmetric carbon atoms) to rotate the plane of polarized light either clockwise or counterclockwise.

plasma renin a. (PRA), estimation of renin in plasma by measuring the rate of formation of angiotensin I or II.

specific a., radioactivity per unit mass of the stated element or compound.

triggered a., one or a series of spontaneously generated heart beats originating from an action potential that produces an afterdepolarization which reaches activation threshold.

actomyosin (ak'-tō-mī'ō-sin). A protein complex composed of the actin and myosin; it is the essential contractile substance of muscle fiber, active with ATP.

platelet a., thrombosthenin; the contractile protein of platelets, responsible for clot retraction, platelet aggregation, and release of ADP and other biologic amines essential to platelet function.

Acuaria spiralis (ak-ū-ā'rē-ā spī-rā'lis) [L. *acus,* needle; Mod. L. *spiralis,* spiral]. A nematode parasite in the proventriculus and esophagus, and sometimes the intestine, of chickens, turkeys, pheasants, and other birds.

acuity (ā-kyū'i-tē) [thr. Fr., fr. L. *acuo,* pp. *acutus,* sharpen]. Sharpness, clearness, distinctness.

absolute intensity threshold a., the minimal light that can be seen.

resolution a., visual a.; detection of a target having two or more parts, often measured by using the Snellen test types; indicated by two numbers: the first represents the distance at which an individual sees the test types (usually 6 meters or 20 feet), and the second, the distance at which the test types subtend an angle of 5 minutes; *e.g.,* vision of 6/9 indicates a test distance of 6 meters and recognition of symbols which subtend an angle of 5 minutes at a distance of 9 meters.

spatial a., detection of the shape of a test object; *e.g.,* perceiving polygons of the same size but with different numbers of sides.

stereoscopic a., the detection of differences in distance by superimposition of slightly different retinal images into a single image to the brain.

Vernier a., detection of displacement of a portion of a line.

visibility a., recognition of an object on a background of different character.

visual a. (V), resolution a.

aculeate (ā-kyū'lē-āt) [L. *aculeātus,* pointed, fr. *acus,* needle]. Pointed; covered with sharp spines.

acuminate (ā-kyū'mi-nāt) [L. *acumino,* pp. *-atus,* to sharpen]. Pointed; tapering to a point.

acuology (ak-yū-ol'ō-jē) [L. *acus,* needle, + G. *logos,* study]. The study of the use of needles for therapeutic purposes, as in acupuncture.

acupuncture (ak-yū-punk'chūr) [L. *acus,* needle, + puncture]. Puncture with long, fine needles: **1.** An ancient Oriental system of therapy. **2.** More recently, acupuncture *anesthesia.*

acus (ā'kūs) [L.]. A needle.

acusection (ak'yū-sek-shŭn). Electrosurgery using a needle.

acusector (ak'yū-sek-ter) [L. *acus,* needle, + *secare,* to cut]. A needle used for electrosurgery.

acusis (ā-kyū'sis) [G. *akousis,* hearing]. Normal hearing; the ability to perceive sound normally.

acute (ā-kyūt') [L. *acutus,* sharp]. **1.** Of short and sharp course, not chronic; said of a disease. **2.** Sharp; pointed at the end.

acyanotic (ā-sī-ā-not'ik). Characterized by absence of cyanosis.

acyclic (ā-si'klik). Not cyclic; denoting especially an a. compound.

acycloguanosine (ā-sī-klō-gwan'ō-sēn). Acyclovir.

acyclovir (ā-sī'klō-vir). Acycloguanosine; a synthetic acyclic purine nucleoside analogue used as an antiviral agent in the treatment of genital herpes; the sodium salt is used for parenteral therapy.

acyl (as'il). An organic radical derived from an organic acid by the removal of the carboxylic hydroxyl group.

acyl-ACP dehydrogenase or **reductase.** Enoyl-ACP reductase (NADPH).

acyladenylate (as'il-ā-den'il-āt). A compound in which an acyl group is combined with AMP by elimination of H_2O between the OH's of a carboxyl group and of the phosphate residue of AMP, usually initially in the form of ATP and eliminating inorganic pyrophosphate in the condensation.

acylamidase (as-il-am'i-dās). Amidase.

***n*-acylamino acid** (as-il-am'i-nō). RCO-NH-CHR-COOH; an amino acid to the N of which an acyl group in attached, as in hippuric acid (*N*-benzoylglycine) or phenaceturic acid.

acylase (as'i-lās). Amidase.

acylation (as-i-lā'shŭn). Introduction of an acyl radical into an organic compound or formation of such a radical within an organic compound.

acyl-CoA. Acylcoenzyme A; $RCH_2CO{\sim}SCoA$; condensation product of a carboxylic acid and coenzyme A, and metabolic intermediate of importance, notably in the oxidation of fat.

acyl-CoA dehydrogenase ($NADP^+$) [EC 1.3.1.8]. 2-Enoyl-CoA reductase; enzyme catalyzing reduction of enoyl-CoA derivatives of chain length 4 to 16, with NADPH as the hydrogen donor.

acyl-CoA synthetase. 1. General term for enzymes (EC 6.2.1) that form acyl-CoA, now called ligases. **2.** Specifically, long-chain fatty acid–CoA ligase.

acylcoenzyme A (as'il-kō-en'zīm). Acyl-CoA.

acyl-malonyl-ACP synthase. 3-Oxoacyl-ACP synthase.

***N*-acylsphingol** (as-il-sfing'gol). Obsolete synonym for *N*-Acylsphingosine.

***N*-acylsphingosine** (as-il-sfing'gō-sēn). A condensation product of an organic acid with sphingosine at the amino group of the latter compound.

acyltransferases (as-il-trans'fer-ā-sez) [EC Class 2.3]. Transacylases; enzymes catalyzing the transfer of an acyl group from an acyl-CoA to various acceptors.

acystia (ā-sis'tē-ā) [G. *a-* priv. + *kystis,* bladder]. Congenital absence of the urinary bladder.

A.D. Abbreviation for *auris dexter* [L.], right ear.

ad- [L. *ad,* to]. Prefix denoting increase, adherence, or motion toward, and sometimes with an intensive meaning.

-ad [L. *ad,* to]. Suffix in anatomical nomenclature having the significance of the English -ward; denoting toward or in the direction of the part indicated by the main portion of the word.

adactylia, adactylism (ā-dak-til'ē-ā, -dak'til-izm). Adactyly.

adactylous (ā-dak'til-ŭs). Without fingers or toes.

adactyly (ā-dak'ti-lē) [G. *a-* priv. + *daktylos,* digit]. Adactylia;

adactylism; congenital condition characterized by the absence of digits (fingers or toes); autosomol recessive in Holstein cattle.

adamantine (ad-ă-man'tēn) G. *adamantinos,* very hard]. Exceedingly hard; formerly used in reference to the enamel of the teeth.

adamantinoma (ad-ă-man-ti-nō'mă). Obsolete term for ameloblastoma.
a. of long bones, a rare tumor of limb bones, usually the tibia, that microscopically resembles an ameloblastoma; the histogenesis is uncertain.
pituitary a., craniopharyngioma.

Adamkiewicz, Albert, Polish pathologist, 1850–1921. See *arteries* of A.

Adams, Robert, Irish physician, 1791–1875. See A.-Stokes or Stokes-A. *disease* or *syndrome,* Morgagni-A.-Stokes *syndrome.*

Adams, Sir William, British surgeon, 1760–1829. See A.'s *operation* for ectropion.

Adam's apple. *Prominentia* laryngea.

adaptation (ad-ap-tā'shŭn) [L. *ad-apto,* pp. *-atus,* to adjust]. **1.** Preferential survival of members of a species which have certain phenotypic features that give them an enhanced capacity to withstand a particular environment. **2.** An advantageous change in function or constitution of an organ or tissue to meet new conditions. **3.** Adjustment of the pupil and retina to varying degrees of illumination. **4.** A property of certain receptors through which they become less responsive or cease to respond to repeated or continued stimuli, the intensity of which is kept constant. **5.** The fitting, condensing, or contouring of a restorative material, foil, or shell to a tooth or cast so as to be in close contact. **6.** Adjustment (2); the dynamic process wherein the thoughts, feelings, behavior, and biophysiologic mechanisms of the individual continually change to adjust to a constantly changing environment.
dark a., scotopic a.; the visual adjustment occurring under reduced illumination in which the sensitivity to light is increased. See also dark-adapted *eye.*
light a., photopic a.; the visual adjustment occurring under increased illumination in which the sensitivity to light is reduced. See also light-adapted *eye.*
photopic a., light a.
reality a., the ability to adjust to the world as it exists.
retinal a., adjustment to degree of illumination.
scotopic a., dark a.
social a., adjustment to living in accordance with interpersonal, social, and cultural restrictions and demands.

adapter, adaptor (a-dap'ter, -tōr). **1.** A connecting part, joining two pieces of apparatus. **2.** A converter of electric current to a desired form.

adaptometer (ad-ap-tom'ĕ-ter). A device for determining the course of ocular dark adaptation and for measuring the minimum light threshold.

adaxial (ad-ak'sē-ăl). Toward an axis, or on one or other side of an axis.

add. Abbreviation for L. *adde,* add.

ad'der. Common name for many members of the family Viperidae (the vipers), applied to several genera, although true a.'s are of the genus *Vipera;* 11 species are known.

addict (ad'ikt). A person who is habituated to a substance or practice, especially one considered harmful.

addiction (ă-dik'shŭn) [L. *ad-dico,* pp. *-dictus,* consent, fr. *ad-* + *dico,* to say]. Habitual psychological and physiological dependence on a substance or practice which is beyond voluntary control.

Addis, Thomas, U.S. internist, 1881–1949. See A. *count.*

Addison, Christopher, British anatomist, 1869–1951. See A.'s clinical *planes.*

Addison, Thomas, British physician, 1793–1860. See A.'s *anemia, disease;* addisonian *anemia, crisis;* A.-Biermer *disease.*

addisonian (ad-i-sō'nē-an). Relating to or described by Thomas Addison.

additive (ad'i-tiv). **1.** A substance not naturally a part of a material (*e.g.,* food) but deliberately added to fulfill some specific purpose (*e.g.,* preservation). **2.** Tending to add or be added; cumulative; denoting addition.

additivity (ad-i-tiv'i-tē). The quality or state of being additive.
allelic a., the relationship between alleles such that the quantifiable phenotype of the heterozygote is at the midpoint between those for the two homozygotes; an absence of dominance.
causal a., the relationship between two or more causal components such that their combined effect is the algebraic sum of their combined effects.
interlocal a., the relationship among quantitative effects of different genetic loci such that their joint effect is equal to the sum of their individual effects; an absence of epistasis or interaction.

adducent (ă-dū'sent) [L. *adducens, pres. p. of ad-duco,* to bring]. Bringing to; adducting.

adduct (a-dŭkt') [L. *ad-duco,* pp. *-ductus,* to bring toward]. **1.** To draw toward the median plane. **2.** An addition product, or complex, or one part of the same.

adduction (ă-dŭk'shŭn). **1.** Movement of a body part toward the median plane, (of the body, in the case of limbs; of the hand or foot, in the case of digits). **2.** Monocular rotation (duction) of the eye toward the nose. **3.** A position resulting from such movement. *Cf.* abduction.

adductor (ă-dŭk'ter, tōr). A muscle that draws a part toward the median plane.

Ade Abbreviation for adenine.

adelomorphous (ă-del-ō-mōr'fŭs) [G. *adēlos,* uncertain, not clear, + *morphē,* shape]. Of not clearly defined form. In the past this term was applied to certain cells of the gastric glands.

aden-. See adeno-.

adenalgia (ad-ĕ-nal'jē-ă) [aden- + G. *algos,* pain]. Adenodynia; pain in a gland.

adendric (ā-den'drik). Adendritic.

adendritic (ā-den-drit'ik) [*G. a-* priv. + *dendron,* tree]. Adendric; without dendrites.

adenectomy (ad-ĕ-nek'tō-mē). [aden- + G. *ektomē,* excision]. Excision of a gland.

adenectopia (ad'ĕ-nek-tō'pē-ă) [aden- + G. *ek,* out of, + *topos,* place]. Presence of a gland other than in its normal anatomical position.

adenemphraxis (ad'ĕ-nem-frak'sis) [aden- + G. *emphraxis,* stoppage]. Rarely used term for an obstruction to the discharge of a glandular secretion.

adeniform (ă-den'i-fōrm). Adenoid (1).

adenine (ad'ĕ-nēn). 6-Aminopurine; one of the two major purines (the other being guanine) found in both RNA and DNA, and also in various free nucleotides of importance to the body, such as AMP (adenylic acid), ATP, NAD and NADP, and FAD; in all these compounds, a. is condensed with a sugar molecule at the nitrogen-9, forming adenosine. For structure, see adenylic acid.
a. arabinoside, misnomer for arabinosyladenine.
a. deoxyribonucleotide, deoxyadenylic acid.
a. nucleotide, adenylic acid.
a. sulfate, a. conjugated with sulfuric acid; used to stimulate leukocyte production in agranulocytosis.

adenitis (ad-ĕ-nī'tis) [aden- + G. *-itis,* inflammation]. Inflammation of a lymph node or of a gland.

adenization (ad-ĕ-nī-zā'shŭn). Conversion into glandlike structure.

adeno-, aden- [G. *adēn,* gland]. Combining forms denoting relation to a gland.

adenoacanthoma (ad'ĕ-nō-ak-an-thō'mă). Adenoid squamous cell carcinoma; a malignant neoplasm consisting chiefly of glandular epithelium (adenocarcinoma), usually well differentiated, with foci of metaplasia to squamous (or epidermoid) neoplastic cells.

adenoameloblastoma (ad'ĕ-nō-am'el-ō-blast-ō'mă). Adenomatoid odontogenic *tumor.*

adenoblast (ad'ĕ-nō-blast). [adeno- + G. *blastos,* germ]. A proliferating embryonic cell with the potential to form glandular parenchyma.

adenocarcinoma (ad'ĕ-nō-kar-si-nō'mă). Glandular cancer or carcinoma; a malignant neoplasm of epithelial cells in glandular or glandlike pattern.

acinic cell a., acinar, acinic cell, acinose, or acinous carcinoma; an a. arising from secreting cells of a racemose gland, particularly the salivary glands.

bronchiolar a., bronchiolar *carcinoma.*

clear cell a., **(1)** renal a.; **(2)** mesonephroma.

a. in si'tu, a noninvasive abnormal proliferation of glands believed to precede the appearance of invasive adenocarcinoma; reported in the endometrium and large intestine.

Lucké's a., Lucké's *carcinoma.*

mesonephric a., mesonephroma.

a. of Moll, a. arising from the ciliary (Moll's) glands.

mucoid a., sometimes applied to mucinous carcinoma, or a. containing mucin secreting neoplastic cells.

papillary a., an a. containing finger-like processes of vascular connective tissue covered by neoplastic epithelium, projecting into cysts or the cavity of glands or follicles; occurs most frequently in the ovary and thyroid gland.

renal a., clear cell a. (1); clear cell carcinoma of the kidney; renal cell carcinoma; hypernephroma; Grawitz' tumor; an a. arising in any part of the renal parenchyma, especially in middle-aged or older people of either sex (although more common in males); may form glands resembling renal tubules lined by cells with pale-staining cytoplasm, while in other cases the cytoplasm is more darkly staining; there may be a papillary or solid alveolar structure, or occasionally the tumor cells may be spindle-shaped.

adenocellulitis (ad'ĕ-nō-sel-yū-lī'tis). Inflammation of a gland, usually a lymph node, and of the adjacent connective tissue.

adenochondroma (ad'ĕ-nō-kon-drō'mă) [adeno- + G. *chondros,* cartilage, + *-oma,* tumor]. Pulmonary *hamartoma.*

adenocystoma (ad'ĕ-nō-sis-tō'mă). Adenoma in which the neoplastic glandular epithelium forms cysts.

adenocyte (ad'ĕ-nō-sīt) [adeno- + G. *kytos,* a hollow (cell)]. A secretory cell of a gland.

adenodiastasis (ad'ĕ-nō-dī-as'tă-sis) [adeno- + G. *diastasis,* a separation]. Separation or ectopia of glands or glandular tissue from their usual anatomical sites, *e.g.,* pancreatic glands in the wall of the small intestine, gastric glands in the wall of the esophagus.

adenodynia (ad'ĕ-nō-din'ē-ă) [adeno- + G. *odynē,* pain]. Adenalgia.

adenoepithelioma (ad'ĕ-nō-ep-i-thē-lē-ō'mă). Obsolete term for an epithelioma containing glandular elements.

adenofibroma (ad'ĕ-nō-fī-brō'mă). A benign neoplasm composed of glandular and fibrous tissues, with a relatively large proportion of glands.

adenofibromyoma (ad'ĕ-nō-fī'brō-mī-ō'mă). Adenomatoid *tumor.*

adenofibrosis (ad'ĕ-nō-fī-brō'sis). Sclerosing *adenosis.*

adenogenesis (ad'ĕ-nō-jen'ĕ-sis) [adeno- + G. *genesis,* production]. Development of a gland.

adenogenous (ad-ĕ-noj'en-ŭs). Having an origin in glandular tissue.

adenohypophysial (ad'ĕ-nō-hī-pō-fiz'ē-ăl). Relating to the adenohypophysis.

adenohypophysis (ad'ĕ-nō-hī-pof'i-sis) [NA]. Anterior lobe of the hypopysis; lobus anterior hypophyseos; lobus glandularis hypophyseos; it consists of the pars distalis, pars intermedia, and pars tuberalis (pars infundibularis). See also hypophysis.

adenohypophysitis (ad'ĕ-nō-hī-pof-ĭ-sī'tis). Inflammatory reaction or sepsis effecting the anterior pituitary gland, often related to pregnancy.

lymphocytic a., a diffuse lymphocytic infiltration of the adenohypophysis, often related to pregnancy; probably a disturbance in the immune system.

adenoid (ad'ĕ-noyd) [adeno- + G. *eidos,* appearance]. **1.** Adeniform; lymphoid (2); glandlike; of glandular appearance. **2.** See adenoids.

adenoidectomy (ad'ĕ-noy-dek'tō-mē) [adenoid + G. *ektomē,* excision]. An operation for the removal of adenoid growths in the nasopharynx.

adenoidism (ad'ĕ-noy-dizm). Symptoms and signs associated with enlarged nasopharyngeal lymphoid tissue.

adenoiditis (ad'ĕ-noy-dī'tis). Inflammation of nasopharyngeal lymphoid tissue.

adenoids (ad'ĕ-noydz). Adenoid disease (1); Meyer's disease; hypertrophy of the pharyngeal tonsil resulting from chronic inflammation.

adenoleiomyofibroma (ad'ĕ-nō-lī'ō-mī-ō-fī-brō'mă) [adeno- + G. *leios,* smooth, + *mys,* muscle, + fibroma]. Adenomatoid *tumor.*

adenolipoma (ad'ĕ-nō-li-pō'mă). A benign neoplasm composed of glandular and adipose tissues.

adenolipomatosis (ad'ĕ-nō-lip'ō-mă-tō'sis). A condition characterized by development of multiple adenolipomas.

symmetric a., multiple symmetric *lipomatosis.*

adenolymphocele (ad'ĕ-nō-lim'fō-sēl) [adeno- + L. *lympha,* spring water, + G. *kēlē,* tumor]. Cystic dilation of a lymph node following obstruction of the efferent lymphatic vessels.

adenolymphoma (ad'ĕ-nō-lim-fō'mă). Papillary cystadenoma lymphomatosum; Warthin's tumor; a benign glandular tumor usually arising in the parotid gland and composed of two rows of eosinophilic epithelial cells, which are often cystic and papillary, together with a lymphoid stroma.

adenolysis (ad-ĕ-nol'i-sis) [adeno- + G. *lysis,* destruction]. Obsolete term for enzymatic destruction or dissolution of glandular tissue.

adenoma (ad-ĕ-nō'mă) [adeno- + G. *-oma,* tumor]. An ordinarily benign neoplasm of epithelial tissue in which the tumor cells form glands or glandlike structures in the stroma; usually well circumscribed, tending to compress rather than infiltrate or invade adjacent tissue.

acidophil a., growth hormone-producing a.

ACTH-producing a., basophil a.; a pituitary tumor composed of corticotrophs that are densely granulated, basophilic, and PAS stain positive; it gives rise to Cushing's disease of Nelson's syndrome.

adnexal a., an a. arising in, or forming structures resembling, skin appendages.

adrenocortical a., a benign tumor of adrenal cortical cells; small unencapuslated nodules of adrenal cortex are probably localized areas of hyperplasia rather than a.'s; true a.'s are rare and may be symptomless or associated with Cushing's syndrome or primary aldosteronism.

apocrine a., papillary *hidradenoma.*

basal cell a., a benign encapsulated salivary gland a. of the parotid gland or upper lip, composed of small cells showing peripheral palisading.
basophil a., ACTH-producing a.
bronchial a., a slowly growing benign, or malignant but slowly progressing, polypoid epithelial tumor of bronchial mucosa, arising deep to the surface epithelium, possibly from mucous glands or their ducts; two histological types are recognized: carcinoid and cylindromatous.
chromophil a., any a. composed of cells that stain readily.
chromophobe a., null cell a.
colloid a., macrofollicular a.; a follicular a. of the thyroid, composed of large follicles containing colloid.
embryonal a., a benign neoplasm in which the glandular epithelial elements are not fully differentiated, resembling immature tissue observed in embryonic development.
eosinophil a., growth hormone-producing a.
fetal a., an a. occurring in the thyroid or anterior lobe of the pituitary, consisting of tall cylindrical cells arranged in tubular form, and resembling tissue observed in development of the fetus; epithelial elements are slightly more mature than those observed in embryonal a.
fibroid a., a. fibro'sum, fibroadenoma.
follicular a., an a. of the thyroid with a simple glandular pattern.
Fuchs' a., a benign epithelial tumor of the non-pigmented epithelium of the ciliary body, rarely exceeding 1 mm in diameter.
gonadotropin-producing a., a rare type of pituitary a. that produces FSH and LH; its cells can be identified only by immunochemical techniques.
growth hormone-producing a., acidophil or eosinophil a.; an a. that produces the clinical picture of gigantism or acromegaly, although a third of the cells have no granules or are a mixture of acidophils and chromophobes; some tumors may secrete both growth hormone and prolactin.
Hürthle cell a., a follicular a. of the thyroid in which the epithelium has undergone metaplasia into Hürthle cells. See also Hürthle cell *tumor*.
islet cell a., nesidioblastoma; a benign neoplasm of the pancreas composed of tissue similar in structure to that of the islets of Langerhans; it may contain functioning beta cells, and may cause hypoglycemia. See also insulinoma.
lactating a., an uncommon a. of the breast composed of tubuloacinar structures with pronounced secretory changes such as seen in pregnancy and lactation.
Leydig cell a., interstitial cell tumor of testis; small benign tumors of the testis that often produce testosterone, causing endocrine symptoms.
macrofollicular a., colloid a.
microfollicular a., a fetal a. of the thyroid composed of very small follicles and solid alveolar groups of thyroid epithelial cells.
monomorphic a., a benign ductal neoplasm of the salivary glands, with a uniform epithelial pattern and lacking the chondromyxoid stroma of a pleomorphic a.
nephrogenic a., a benign tumor of the urinary bladder mucosa, composed of glandular structures resembling renal tubules.
a. of nipple, subareolar duct *papillomatosis*.
null-cell a., undifferentiated cell a.; chromophobe or pituitary a.; an a. of the hypophysis composed of cells for which there is no overt evidence or hormone production, but which produce hypopituitarism and visual disturbances by compression of adjacent structures; approximately one third of these tumors have cells with abundant mitochondria (oncocytes) that are somewhat larger than the monocytic null cells.
ovarian tubular a., arrhenoblastoma.
oxyphil a., oncocytoma.
papillary cystic a., an a. in which the lumens of the acini are frequently distended by fluid, and the neoplastic epithelial elements tend to form irregular, fingerlike projections.
papillary a. of large intestine, villous a.
Pick's tubular a., androblastoma (1).
pituitary a., null-cell a.
pleomorphic a., mixed *tumor* of salivary gland.
polypoid a., adenomatous *polyp*.
prolactin-producing a., prolactinoma; a small, usually encapsulated, pituitary neoplasm composed of prolactin-producing cells; it gives rise to symptoms of nonpuerperal amenorrhea and galactorrhea (Forbes-Albright syndrome) in women and to impotence in men.
prostatic a., a term used for the growth in benign prostatic hyperplasia.
renal cortical a., one of the usually small a.'s sometimes found in the renal cortex and derived from renal tubular tissue.
sebaceous a., a benign tumor of sebaceous tissue, having a more progressive growth and less mature structure than in sebaceous gland hyperplasia. *Cf.* a. sebaceum.
a. seba'ceum, Pringle's disease; a hamartoma occurring on the face, composed of fibrovascular tissue and appearing as an aggregation of red or yellow papules which may be associated with tuberous sclerosis; sebaceous glands may be present but are not increased. *Cf.* sebaceous a.
sweat duct a., a benign tumor of the sweat duct, such as eccrine poroma.
testicular tubular a., androblastoma (1).
thyrotropin-producing a., a rare pituitary tumor usually associated with hypo- or hyperthyroidism.
tubular a., a benign neoplasm composed of epithelial tissue resembling a tubular gland.
undifferentiated cell a., null-cell a.
villous a., papillary a. of the large intestine; usually a solitary sessile, often large, tumor of colonic mucosa composed of mucinous epithelium covering delicate vascular projections; hypersecretion and malignant change occur frequently.

adenomatoid (ad-ĕ-nō'mă-toyd). Resembling an adenoma.

adenomatosis (ad'ĕ-nō-mă-tō'sis). A condition characterized by multiple glandular overgrowths.
erosive a. of nipple, subareolar duct *papillomatosis*.
familial endocrine a., type 1, multiple endocrine neoplasia, type 1; Wermer's syndrome; pluriglandular a.; multiple endocrinoma or endocrinopathy; endocrine polyglandular syndrome; presence of functioning tumors in more than one endocrine gland, commonly the pancreatic islets and parathyroid glands, which may be associated with Zollinger-Ellison syndrome; dominant inheritance.
familial endocrine a., type 2, multiple endocrine neoplasia, type 2; Sipple's syndrome; pheochromocytoma, medullary carcinoma of the thyroid, and neural tumors; autosomal dominant inheritance.
fibrosing a., sclerosing *adenosis*.
pluriglandular a., familial endocrine a., type 1.
pulmonary a., a neoplastic disease in which the alveoli and distal bronchi are filled with mucus and mucus-secreting columnar epithelial cells; characterized by abundant, extremely tenacious sputum, chills, fever, cough, dyspnea, and pleuritic pain.
pulmonary a. of sheep, jaagziekte; a chronic pulmonary disease of sheep, probably of viral origin, characterized by adenomatous proliferations in the alveoli and small bronchioles resembling neoplasia.

adenomatous (ad-ĕ-nō'mă-tŭs). Relating to an adenoma, and to some types of glandular hyperplasia.

adenomere (ad'ĕ-nō-mēr) [adeno- + G. *meros*, part]. Structural unit in the parenchyma of a developing gland.

adenomyoma (ad'ĕ-nō-mī-ō'mă). A benign neoplasm of muscle (usually smooth muscle) with glandular elements; occurs most frequently in uterus and uterine ligaments.

adenomyosarcoma (ad'ĕ-nō-mī'ō-sar-kō'mă). Wilms' *tumor.*

adenomyosis (ad'ĕ-nō-mī-ō'sis). The ectopic occurrence or diffuse implantation of adenomatous tissue in muscle (usually smooth muscle).
a. u'teri, a benign invasion of myometrium by endometrial tissue.

adenoneural (ad'ĕ-nō-nū'răl). Obsolete term relating to a gland and a nervous element. See neuroendocrine.

adenopathy (ad-ĕ-nop'ă-thē) [adeno- + G. *pathos,* suffering]. Swelling or morbid enlargement of the lymph nodes.

adenopharyngitis (ad'ĕ-nō-far-in-jī'tis). Inflammation of the adenoids and the pharyngeal lymphoid tissue.

adenophlegmon (ad'ĕ-nō-fleg'mon) [adeno- + G. *phlegmonē,* inflammation]. Acute inflammation of a gland and the adjacent connective tissue.

Adenophorasida (ad'ĕ-nō-fō-ras'i-dă) [G. *adēn,* gland, + *phōr,* thief]. Adenophorea; Aphasmidia; a class of nematodes lacking lateral canals opening into the excretory system and phasmids, with few or no caudal papillae, eggs unsegmented, and with polar plugs or hatching *in utero.* It includes the genera *Trichuris, Capillaria,* and *Trichinella* among important parasites of man and domestic animals. See also Secernentasida.

Adenophorea (ad'ĕ-nō-fō'rē-ă). Adenophorasida.

adenophyma (ad'ĕ-nō-fī'mă) [adeno- + G. *phyma,* tumor]. Rarely used term for any condition in which a gland or glandular organ is grossly enlarged as the result of inflammation.

adenosalpingitis (ad'ĕ-nō-sal-pin-jī'tis). *Salpingitis* isthmica nodosa.

adenosarcoma (ad'ĕ-nō-sar-kō'mă). A malignant neoplasm arising simultaneously or consecutively in mesodermal tissue and glandular epithelium of the same part.
müllerian a., a tumor of the uterus or ovaries, of low grade malignancy, characterized by benign appearing glands and a sarcomatous stroma.

adenose (ad'ĕ-nōs). Adenous; relating to a gland.

adenosinase (ad-ĕ-nō'sin-ās). *Adenosine* nucleosidase.

adenosine (A, Ado) (ă-den'ō-sēn). 9-β-D-Ribofuranosyladenine; a condensation product of adenine and D-ribose; a nucleoside found among the hydrolysis products of all nucleic acids and of the various adenine nucleotides. For structure, see adenylic acid.
a. cyclic phosphate, see adenosine 3',5'-cyclic phosphate.
a. deaminase [EC 3.5.4.4], an enzyme found in mammalian tissues, capable of catalyzing the deamination of adenosine, forming inosine.
a. diphosphate, see adenosine 5'-diphosphate.
a. kinase [EC 2.7.1.20], enzyme catalyzing the transfer of a phosphate group from ATP to adenosine, forming ADP and AMP.
a. monophosphate (AMP), adenylic acid; specifically, adenosine 5'-phosphate. See adenylic acid.
a. nucleosidase [EC 3.2.2.7], adenosinase; an enzyme cleaving adenosine to adenine and D-ribose.
a. phosphate, adenylic acid; specifically, adenosine 3'- or 5'-phosphate. See adenylic acid.
a. tetraphoshate, a condensation product of adenosine with tetraphosphoric acid at the 5' position.
a. triphosphate, adenosine 5'-triphosphate.

adenosine 3',5'-cyclic phosphate. An activator of phosphorylase kinase, formed in muscle from ATP by adenylate cyclase and broken down to 5'-AMP by a phosphodiesterase; sometimes referred to as the "second messenger." Also called cyclic adenylic acid, cyclic phosphate, cyclic AMP, although at least one other such compound (2',3') is known.

adenosine 5'-diphosphate (ADP). A condensation product of adenosine with pyrophosphoric acid, formed from ATP by the hydrolysis of the terminal phosphate group of the latter compound.

adenosine 3'-phosphate. 3'-Adenylic acid. See adenylic acid.

adenosine 5'-phosphate. 5'-Adenylic acid. See adenylic acid.

adenosine 3'-phosphate 5'-phosphosulfate (PAPS). Active sulfate; 3'-phosphoadenosine 5'-phosphosulfate; an intermediate in the formation of urinary ethereal sulfates, notable for containing a "high energy" sulfate bond; the 3'-OH of adenosine is replaced by $—OPO_3H_2$, the 5'-OH by $—OP(O_2H)\text{-}OS_3H$.

adenosine 5'-triphosphate (ATP). Adenosine triphosphate; adenosine (5)pyrophosphate; adenosine with triphosphoric acid esterfied at its 5' position; immediate precursors of adenine nucleotides in RNA.

adenosinetriphosphatase (ATPase) (a-den'ō-sēn-trī-fos'fă-tās) [EC 3.6.1.3]. Adenylpyrophosphatase; ATP-monophosphatase; triphosphatase; an enzyme in muscle (myosin) and elsewhere that catalyzes the release of the terminal phosphate group of adenosine 5'-triphosphate; visualized cytochemically in various cell membranes, mitochondria, and in the A band of striated muscle sarcomeres associated with myosin.

adenosis (ad-ĕ-nō'sis). A more or less generalized glandular disease.
blunt duct a., a. of the breast in which the ducts are enlarged but not increased in number.
fibrosing a., sclerosing a.
microglandular a., a. of the breast in which irregular clusters of small tubules are present in adipose or fibrous tissues, resembling tubular carcinoma but lacking stromal fibroblastic proliferation.
sclerosing a., fibrosing a. or adenomatosis; adenofibrosis; a nodular, benign breast lesion occurring most frequently in relatively young women and consisting of hyperplastic distorted lobules of acinar tissue with increased collagenous stroma; the changes may be difficult to distinguish microscopically from carcinoma.

adenosyl (a-den'ō-sil). The radical of adenosine minus an H or OH from one of the ribosyl OH groups, usually the 5', *e.g., S*-adenosylmethionine.

***S*-adenosylhomocysteine** (a-den'ō-sil-hō-mō-sis'te-ēn). *S*-(5'-Deoxy-5'-adenosyl)homocysteine; the compound formed by the demethylation of *S*-adenosylmethionine.

***S*-adenosylmethionine (AdoMet)** (a-den'ō-sil-me-thī'ō-nēn). Active methionine; *S*-(5'-deoxy-5'-adenosyl)methione; condensation product of adenosine and methionine involving replacement of the $—OPO_3H_2$ of adenylic acid by $—\overset{+}{S}(CH_3)CH_2CH_2CH(NH_2)CO_2H$ of methionine; a sulfonium compound bearing a methyl group that is transferred in transmethylation reactions. See also *methionine* adenosyltransferase.

adenotomy (ad-ĕ-not'ō-mē) [adeno- + G. *tomē,* a cutting]. Incision of a gland.

adenotonsillectomy (ad'ĕ-nō-ton-si-lek'tō-mē). Operative removal of tonsils and adenoids.

adenous (ad'ĕ-nŭs). Adenose.

Adenoviridae (ad'ĕ-nō-vir'i-dē). A family of double-stranded DNA viruses, commonly known as adenoviruses, that develop in the nuclei of infected cells in mammals and birds. The virion is 70 to 90 nm in diameter, naked, and ether-resistant; the capsids are icosahedral and composed of 252 capsomeres. The family includes two genera, *Mastadenovirus* and *Aviadenovirus,* and more than 80 antigenic types (species).

adenovirus (ad'ĕ-nō-vī'rŭs) [G. *adēn,* gland, + virus]. Adenoidal-pharyngeal-conjunctival or A-P-C virus; any virus of the family Adenoviridae.
bovine a.'s, viruses of the genus *Mastadenovirus,* with nine recognized serotypes, which can cause a mild upper respiratory tract disease in cattle.
porcine a.'s, viruses of the genus *Mastadenovirus,* with four rec-

ognized serotypes, which can cause a mild upper respiratory tract disease in swine.

adenyl (ad'e-nil). The radical or ion of adenine; often used for adenylyl, as in adenylosuccinic acid.
a. cyclase, former name for adenylate cyclase.

adenylate (a-den'i-lāt). Salt or ester of adenylic acid.
a. cyclase [EC 4.6.1.1], 3',5'-cyclic AMP synthetase; an enzyme acting on ATP to form 3',5'-cyclic AMP plus pyrophosphate.
a. kinase [EC 2.7.4.3], adenylic acid kinase; myokinase; a phosphotransferase that catalyzes the phosphorylation of one molecule of ADP by another, yielding ATP and AMP.

adenylic acid (ad-en-il'ik). Adenosine monophosphate or phosphate; adenine nucleotide; a condensation product of adenosine and phosphoric acid; a nucleotide found among the hydrolysis products of all nucleic acids. 3'-Adenylic acid (adenosine 3'-phosphate) and 5'-adenylic acid (adenosine 5'-phosphate) differ in the place of attachment of the phosphoric acid to the ribose; deoxyadenylic acid differs in having H instead of OH at the 2' position. See also entries under AMP.

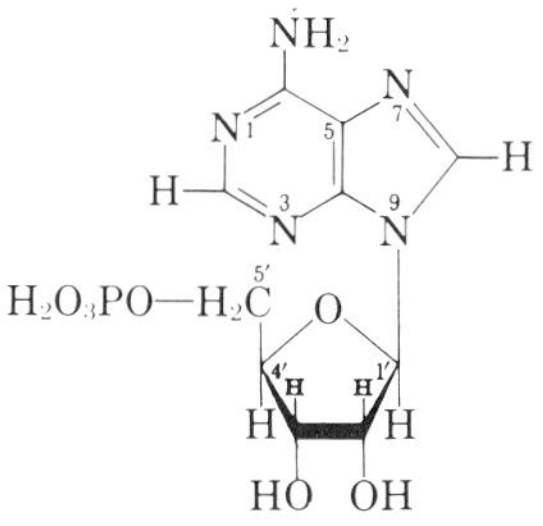

5'-Adenylic acid

cyclic a. a., adenosine 3',5'-cyclic phosphate.
a. a. deaminase, AMP deaminase.
a. a. kinase, *adenylate* kinase.

adenylosuccinase (ad'e-nil-ō-sŭk'sin-ās). Adenylosuccinate lyase.

adenylosuccinate lyase (ad'e-nil-ō-sŭk'sin-āt) [EC 4.3.2.2]. Adenylylsuccinate lyase; adenylosuccinase; an enzyme catalyzing the nonhydrolic cleavage of adenylosuccinic acid and also of 4-(*N*-succinocarboxamido)-5-aminoimidazole nucleotide to yield fumaric acid.

adenylosuccinate synthase [EC 6.3.4.4]. Adenylylosuccinate synthase; IMP-aspartate ligase; a ligase catalyzing the formation of adenylosuccinate from inosinic acid and aspartate, with concomitant hydrolysis of GTP to GDP.

adenylosuccinic acid (ad'e-nil-ō-sŭk'sin-ik). Adenylylosuccinic acid; a condensation product of aspartic acid and inosine phosphate; an intermediate in the biosynthesis of adenylic acid. Formally, it is adenylic acid with succinic acid replacing an H of the NH_2 group, forming a C-N bond.

adenylpyrophosphatase (ad'en-il-pī-rō-fos'fă-tās). Adenosinetriphosphatase.

adenylyl (a-den'i-lil). The radical of adenylic acid minus an OH from the phosphoric group; often shortened to adenyl in compound names, such as adenylosuccinic acid.
a. cyclase, former name for *adenylate* cyclase.
a. pyrophosphate, adenosine 5'-triphosphate.

adenylylosuccinate lyase (a-den'i-lil-ō-sŭk'sin-āt). Adenylosuccinate lyase.

adenylylosuccinate synthase. Adenylosuccinate synthase.

adenylylosuccinic acid (a-den'i-lil-ō-sŭk'sin-ik). Adenylosuccinic acid.

adeps, gen. **adipis, adipes** (ad'eps, ad'i-pis, -pēz) [L. lard, fat]. **1.** Denoting fat or adipose tissue. **2.** The rendered fat of swine, lard, used in the preparation of ointments. See also lanolin.
a. re'nis, the layer of adipose tissue surrounding the kidney.

adermia (ă-der'mē-ă) [G. *a-* priv. + *derma,* skin]. Congenital absence of skin.

adermine (ă-der'mēn). Obsolete term for pyridoxine.

adermogenesis (ă-der-mō-jen'ĕ-sis) [G. *a-* priv. + *derma,* skin, + *genesis,* origin]. Failure or imperfection in the regeneration of the skin, especially the imperfect repair of a cutaneous defect.

ADH Abbreviation for antidiuretic *hormone;* alcohol dehydrogenase.

adherence (ad-hēr'ens) [L. *adhero,* to stick to]. **1.** The act or quality of sticking to something. See also adhesion. **2.** The extent to which the patient continues the agreed-upon mode of treatment under limited supervision, in the face of conflicting demands. *Cf.* compliance (1); maintenance.

adhesins (ad-hē'zins) [L. *adhesio,* to stick to]. Microbial surface antigens that frequently exist in the form of filamentous projections (pili or fimbriae) and bind to specific receptors on epithelial cell membranes; usually classified according to their ability to induce agglutination of erythrocytes from various species, their differential attachment to epithelial cells of various origins, or their susceptibility to reversal of such binding activities in the presence of mannose.

adhesio, pl. **adhesiones** (ad-hē'zē-ō, ad-hē-zē-ō'nēz) [L.] [NA]. Adhesion.
a. interthalam'ica [NA], interthalamic adhesion; commissura cinerea or grisea; massa intermedia; the variable connection between the two thalamic masses across the third ventricle. It is absent in about 20% of human brains.

adhesion (ad-hē'zhŭn) [L. *adhesio,* to stick to]. **1.** Conglutination (1); the process of adhering or uniting of two surfaces or parts, especially the union of the opposing surfaces of a wound. **2.** In the plural, inflammatory bands that connect opposing serous surfaces. **3.** Physical attraction of unlike molecules for one another. **4.** Molecular attraction existing between the surfaces of bodies in contact.
amniotic a.'s, amniotic *bands.*
fibrinous a., an a. that consists of fine threads of fibrin resulting from an exudate of plasma or lymph, or an extravasation of blood.
fibrous a., fibrous strands resulting from the organization of fibrinous a.'s.
interthalamic a., *adhesio* interthalamica.
primary a., *healing* by first intention.
secondary a., *healing* by second intention.

adhesiotomy (ad-hē-sē-ot'ō-mē). Colliotomy; surgical section or lysis of adhesions.

adhesive (ad-hē'siv). **1.** Relating to, or having the characteristics of, an adhesion. **2.** Any material that adheres to a surface or causes adherence between surfaces.

adhib. Abbreviation for L. *adhibendus,* to be administered.

adiactinic (ā'dī-ak-tin'ik) [G. *a-* priv. + *dia,* through, + *aktis,* ray]. An obsolete term meaning opaque to photochemically active radiation.

adiadochocinesia, adiadochocinesis (ă-dī'ă-dō-kō-si-nē'sē-ă, -sis) [G. *a*-priv. + *diadochos,* successive, + *kinēsis,* movement]. Adiadochokinesis.

adiadochokinesis (ă-dī'ă-dō-kō-kin-ē'sis) [G. *a-* priv. + *diadochos,* successive, + *kinēsis,* movement]. Adiadochocinesia; adiadochocinesis; inability to perform rapid alternating movements. *Cf.* diadochokinesia. See also dysdiadochokinesia.

adiaphoresis (ā'dī-ă-fō-rē'sis) [G. *a*-priv. + *diaphorēsis,* perspiration]. Anhidrosis.

adiaphoretic (ā-dī′ă-fō-ret′ik). Anhidrotic.

adiaphoria (ă-dī-ă-fōr′ē-ă) [G. *a-* priv. + *dia,* through, + *phoros,* bearing]. Failure to respond to stimulation after a series of previously applied stimuli.

adiapneustia (ă-dī-ap-nū′stē-ă) [G. *a-* priv. + *diapneusis,* an exhaling]. Obsolete term for adiaphoresis.

adiaspiromycosis (ā′dē-ă-spī′rō-mī-kō′sis). A rare pulmonary mycosis of man and of rodents and other animals that dig in soil or are aquatic, caused by *Chrysosporium parvum.*

adiaspore (a′dē-ă-spōr) [G. *a-* priv. + *dia,* through, + *sporos,* seed]. A fungus spore which, when produced in the lungs of an animal or incubated *in vitro* at elevated temperatures, increases greatly in size without eventual reproduction or replication.

adiastole (ă-dī-as′tō-lē) [G. *a-* priv. + *diastolē,* dilation]. Absence or imperceptibility of the diastolic movement of the heart.

adiathermancy (ă-dī-ă-ther′man-sē) [G. *dia-thermainō,* to warm through, fr. *a-* priv. + *dia,* through, + *thermē,* heat]. Impermeability to heat.

Adie, William J., Australian physician, 1886–1935. See A.'s *pupil;* A. *syndrome;* Holmes-A. *pupil, syndrome.*

adiemorrhysis (ad′i-em-ōr′i-sis) [G. *a-* priv. + *dia,* through, + *haima,* blood, + *rhysis,* a flowing]. Arrest of the capillary circulation.

adient (ad′ē-ent) [L. *adiens,* pr. p. of *adeo,* to go toward]. Having a tendency to move toward the source of a stimulus, as opposed to abient.

Adinida (ă-din′i-dă) [G. *a-* priv. + *diēn,* a whirling]. A suborder of dinoflagellates, in which the flagella are free and do not lie in furrows.

adip-, adipo- [L. *adeps,* fat]. Combining forms relating to fat. See also lip-, lipo-.

adipectomy (ad-i-pek′tō-mē) [L. *adeps,* fat, + G. *ektomē,* excision]. Obsolete term for lipectomy.

adiphenine hydrochloride (ă-dif′ĕ-nen). α-Phenylbenzeneacetic acid 2-(diethylamino)ethyl ester hydrochloride; a spasmolytic agent used to decrease spasm of the biliary tract, gastrointestinal tract, uterus, and ureter.

adipic acid (ă-dip′ik). Hexanedioic acid; the dicarboxylic acid, $HOOC(CH_2)_4COOH$.

adipo-. See adip-.

adipocele (ad′i-pō-sēl) [adipo- + G. *kēlē,* tumor]. Lipocele.

adipocellular (ad′i-pō-sel′yū-lăr). Relating to both fatty and cellular tissues, or to connective tissue with many fat cells.

adipoceratous (ad-i-pō-ser′ă-tŭs). Relating to adipocere.

adipocere (ad′i-pō-sēr) [adipo- + L. *cera,* wax]. Grave wax; a fatty substance of waxy consistency into which dead animal tissues (as those of a corpse) are sometimes converted when kept from the air under certain favoring conditions of temperature.

adipocyte (ad′i-pō-sīt). Fat *cell.*

adipogenesis (ad′i-pō-jen′ĕ-sis). Lipogenesis.

adipogenic, adipogenous (ad′i-pō-jen′ik, ad-i-poj′ĕ-nŭs). Lipogenic.

adipoid (ad′i-poyd) [adipo- + G. *eidos,* resemblance]. Lipoid.

adipokinetic (ad′i-pō-ki-net′ik). Denoting a substance or factor that causes mobilization of stored lipid.

adipokinin (ad-i-pō-kī′nin). Adipokinetic hormone; an anterior pituitary hormone that causes mobilization of fat from adipose tissue.

adipometer (ad-i-pom′ĕ-ter) [adipo- + G. *metron,* measure]. An instrument for determining the thickness of the skin.

adiponecrosis (ad′i-pō-ne-krō′sis). Necrosis of fat, as in hemorrhagic pancreatitis.

adiposalgia (ad′i-pō-sal′jē-ă) [adipo- + G. *algos,* pain]. Painful areas of subcutaneous fat.

adipose (ad′i-pōs). Denoting fat.

adiposis (ad-i-pō′sis) [adipo- + G. *-osis,* condition]. Lipomatosis; liposis (1); pimelosis (1); steatosis (1); excessive local or general accumulation of fat in the body.
a. cardia′ca, fatty *heart* (2).
a. cerebra′lis, obesity resulting from intracranial disease, most commonly of the hypothalamus, resulting in hyperphagia.
a. doloro′sa, Anders' or Dercum's disease; lipomatosis neurotica; a condition characterized by a deposit of symmetrical nodular or pendulous masses of fat in various regions of the body, with discomfort or pain.
a. or′chica, *dystrophia* adiposogenitalis.
a. tubero′sa sim′plex, a condition resembling a. dolorosa in which the fat occurs in small nodular masses, which are sensitive to touch and may be spontaneously painful, on the abdomen or on the extremities.
a. universa′lis, excessive deposition of fat throughout all parts of the body, including the viscera.

adiposity (ad-i-pos′i-tē). **1.** Obesity. **2.** Excessive accumulation of lipids in a site or organ.

adiposuria (ad′i-pō-sū′rē-ă) [adipo- + G. *ouron,* urine]. Lipuria.

adipsia, adipsy (ă-dip′sē-ă, -dip′sē) [G. *a-* priv. + *dipsa,* thirst]. Absence of thirst or the lack of desire to drink.

aditus, pl. **aditus** (ad′i-tŭs) [L. access, fr. *ad-eo,* pp. *-itus,* go to] [NA]. An entrance to a cavity or channel.
a. ad an′trum [NA], the orifice leading from the epitympanic recess to the mastoid antrum.
a. ad aqueduc′tum cer′ebri, *anus* cerebri.
a. ad infundib′ulum, *recessus* infundibuli.
a. ad sac′cum peritonae′i mino′rum, *foramen* epiploicum.
a. glot′tidis infe′rior, *cavitas* infraglotticum.
a. glot′tidis supe′rior, the middle part of the laryngeal cavity, between the vestibular and vocal folds, with which the ventricles communicate.
a. laryn′gis [NA], the superior aperture of the larynx, bounded laterally by the aryepiglottic folds.
a. or′bitae [NA], the opening of the orbit, bounded by the supraorbital and infraorbital margins.
a. pel′vis, *apertura* pelvis superior.

adjustment (ă-jŭst′ment). **1.** In dentistry, any modification made upon a fixed or removable prosthesis during or after its insertion to perfect its adaptation and function. **2.** Adaptation (6).
occlusal a., modification of the occluding and incising surfaces of teeth to develop harmonious relationships between these surfaces.

adjuvant (ad′jū-vănt) [L. *ad-juvo,* pres. p. *-juvans,* to give aid to]. **1.** Adminiculum (2); a substance added to a drug product formulation which affects the action of the active ingredient in a predictable way. **2.** In immunology, a vehicle used to enhance antigenicity; *e.g.,* a suspension of minerals (alum, aluminum hydroxide or phosphate) on which antigen is adsorbed; or water-in-oil emulsion in which antigen solution is emulsified in mineral oil (Freund's incomplete a.), sometimes with the inclusion of killed mycobacteria (Freund's complete a.) to further enhance antigenicity.
Freund's complete a., water-in-oil emulsion of antigen, to which killed mycobacteria are added.
Freund's incomplete a., water-in-oil emulsion of antigen, without mycobacteria.

Adler, Alfred, Austrian psychiatrist, 1870–1937. See adlerian *psychology, psychoanalysis.*

Adler, Oscar, German physician, 1879–1932. See A.'s *test.*

adlerian (ad′ler-ē-an). Relating to or described by Alfred Adler.

ad lib. Abbreviation for L. *ad libitum,* freely, as desired.

admaxillary (ad-mak'si-lār-ē) [L. *ad,* to, + *maxilla,* jaw]. Near or connected to the maxilla.

admedial, admedian (ad-mē'dē-ăl, -dē-an). Toward or near the median plane.

adminiculum, pl. **adminicula** (ad-mi-nik'yū-lŭm, -yū-lă) [L. a hand-rest, prop, fr. *ad* + *manus,* hand] [NA]. That which gives support to a part.

a. lin'eae al'bae [NA], a triangular fibrous expansion, sometimes containing a few muscular fibers, passing from the superior pubic ligament to the posterior surface of the linea alba.

admov. Abbreviation for L. *admove,* apply.

adnerval (ad-ner'văl). Adneural. **1.** Lying near a nerve. **2.** In the direction of a nerve; said of an electric current passing through muscular tissue toward the point of entrance of the nerve.

adneural (ad-nūr'ăl). Adnerval.

adnexa, sing. **adnexum** (ad-nek'să, -sŭm) [L. connected parts]. Annexa; parts accessory to the main organ or structure. See also appendage.

a. o'culi, the eyelids, lacrimal glands, etc., associated with the eyeball.

a. u'teri, obsolete term for uterine appendages.

adnexal (ad-nek'săl). Annexal; relating to the adnexa.

adnexectomy (ad-nek-sek'tō-mē). Annexectomy. **1.** Excision of any adnexa. **2.** In gynecology, excision of the fallopian tube and ovary if unilateral and excision of both tubes and ovaries (adnexa uteri) if bilateral.

adnexitis (ad-neks-ī'tis) [L. *annexa,* adnexa, + *-itis,* inflammation]. Annexitis; inflammation of the adnexa uteri.

adnexopexy (ad-neks'ō-pek-sē) [L. *annexa,* adnexa, + G. *pēxis,* fixation]. Annexopexy; operation for suspension of the fallopian tube and ovary; usually, oophoropexy is accomplished without suspension of the tube.

adnexum (ad-nek'sŭm). Singular of adnexa.

Ado Symbol for adenosine.

adolescence (ad-ō-les'ens) [L. *adolescentia*]. The period of life beginning with puberty and ending with completed growth and maturity.

adolescent (ad-ō-les'ent). **1.** Pertaining to adolescence. **2.** An individual in that stage of development.

AdoMet Abbreviation for *S*-adenosylmethionine.

adonitol (ă-don'i-tol). Ribitol.

adoral (ad-ō'răl) [L. *ad,* to, + *os* (*or-*), mouth]. Near or directed toward the mouth.

ADP Abbreviation for adenosine 5′-diphosphate.

ADPase Apyrase.

adren-, adrenal-, adreno- [L. *ad,* toward, + *ren,* kidney]. Combining forms relating to the adrenal gland.

adrenal (ă-drē'năl) [L. *ad,* to, + *ren,* kidney]. **1.** Near or upon the kidney; denoting the glandula suprarenalis (adrenal gland). **2.** An adrenal gland or separate tissue thereof.

accessory a., adrenal rest; an island of cortical tissue separate from the adrenal gland, usually found in the retroperitoneal tissues, kidney, or genital organs.

butterfly a., *glandula* suprarenalis.

Marchand's a.'s, Marchand's rest; small collections of accessory a. tissue in the broad ligament of the uterus or in the testes.

adrenalectomy (ă-drē-năl-ek'tō-mē) [adrenal + G. *ektomē,* excision]. Suprarenalectomy; removal of one or both adrenal glands.

adrenaline (ă-dren'ă-lin, -lēn). Epinephrine.

a. oxidase, *amine* oxidase (flavin-containing).

adrenalitis (ă-drē-năl-ī'tis). Inflammation of the adrenal gland.

adrenalone (ă-dren'ă-lōn). 3′4′-Dihydroxy-2-(methylamino)acetophenone; 4-methylaminoacetopyrocatechol; precursor of epinephrine in some manufacturing processes; a topical adrenergic agent in ophthalmology.

adrenalopathy (ă-drē-nă-lop'ă-thē) [adrenal + G. *pathos,* suffering]. Adrenopathy; any pathologic condition of the adrenal glands.

adrenarche (ad'ren-ar-kē) [adren- + G. *archē,* beginning]. **1.** Menstruation and other signs of puberty induced by hyperactivity of the adrenal cortex. **2.** Physiologic change at puberty caused by adrenocortical secretion of androgenic hormones or precursors of them.

adrenergic (ad-rē-ner'jik) [adren- + G. *ergon,* work]. **1.** Relating to nerve cells or fibers of the autonomic nervous system that employ norepinephrine as their neurotransmitter. *Cf.* cholinergic. **2.** Relating to drugs that mimic the actions of the sympathetic nervous system. See α-adrenergic *receptor;* β-adrenergic *receptor.*

adrenic (ă-drē'nik). Relating to the adrenal gland.

adreno-. See adren-.

adrenoceptive (ă-dren-ō-sep'tiv). Referring to chemical sites in effectors with which the adrenergic mediator unites. *Cf.* cholinoceptive.

adrenocortical (ă-drē-nō-kōr'ti-kăl). Pertaining to adrenal cortex.

adrenocorticomimetic (ă-drē'nō-kōr'ti-kō-mi-met'ik). Mimicking or producing effects similar to adrenocortical function.

adrenocorticotropic, adrenocorticotrophic (ă-drē'nō-kōr'ti-kō-trō'pik, -trō'fik) [adrenal cortex + G. *trophē,* nurture; *tropē,* a turning]. Adrenotropic; adrenotrophic; stimulating growth or activity of the adrenal cortex.

adrenocorticotropin (ă-drē'nō-kōr-ti-kō-trō'pin). Adrenocorticotropic *hormone.*

adrenogenic, adrenogenous (ă-drē-nō-jen'ik, a-drē-noj'ē-nŭs) [adreno- + G. *-gen,* producing]. Of adrenal origin.

adrenoleukodystrophy (ALD) (ă-drē'nō-lū-kō-dis'trō-fē). Schaumberg's, Schilder's, Flatau-Schilder's, or Siemerling-Creutzfeld disease; encephalitis periaxialis diffusa; an X-linked recessive disorder affecting males, characterized by chronic adrenocortical insufficiency, skin hyperpigmentation, leukodystrophy, and progressive dementia, spastic paralysis, and other intellectual and neurological disturbances due to myelin degeneration in the white matter of the brain.

adrenolytic (ă-dren-ō-lit'ik) [adreno- + G. *lysis,* loosening, dissolution]. Denoting antagonism to or inhibition of the action of epinephrine, norepinephrine, and related sympathomimetics. See also adrenergic blocking *agent.*

adrenomegaly (ă-drē-nō-meg'ă-lē) [adreno- + G. *megas,* big]. Enlargement of the adrenal glands.

adrenomimetic (ă-drē'nō-mi-met'ik) [adreno- + G. *mimētikos,* imitative]. Having an action similar to that of the compounds epinephrine and norepinephrine, which are liberated from the adrenal medulla and adrenergic nerves; term proposed to replace the less accurate term, sympathomimetic. *Cf.* adrenergic; cholinomimetic.

adrenomyeloneuropathy (ă-drē'nō-mī'ĕ-lō-nū-rop'ă-thē) [adreno- + G. *myelos,* medulla, + *neuron,* nerve, + *pathos,* suffering]. A disorder pathologically similar to adrenoleukodystrophy but occurring in adults and predominantly involving the spinal cord.

adrenopathy (ă-drē-nop'ă-thē). Adrenalopathy.

adrenoprival (ă-drē-nō-prī'văl) [adreno- + L. *privo,* to deprive]. Indicating a loss of adrenal function, as a result of either disease or surgical excision.

adrenoreactive (ă-drē'nō-rē-ak'tiv). Responding to the catecholamines.

adrenoreceptors (ă-drē'nō-rē-sep'terz). Adrenergic *receptors.*

adrenosterone (a-drē-nos'ter-ōn). Andrenosterone; 4-androstene-3,11,17-trione; an androgen isolated from the adrenal cortex.

adrenotoxin (ă-drē-nō-tok'sin). A substance toxic for the adrenal glands.

adrenotropic, adrenotrophic (ă-drē-nō-trō'pik, -trō'fik). Adrenocorticotropic.

adrenotropin (ă-drē-nō-trō'pin). Adrenocorticotropic *hormone.*

adriamycin (ā'drē-ă-mī'sin). Doxorubicin.

adromia (ă-drō'mē-ă) [G. *a-* priv. + *dromos,* course]. Failure of muscle innervation.

ad sat. Abbreviation for L. *ad saturatum,* to saturation.

Adson, Alfred W., U.S. neurosurgeon, 1887–1951. See A.'s *procedure, test;* A. *forceps, maneuver;* Brown-A. *forceps.*

adsorb (ad-sōrb') [L. *ad,* to, + *sorbeo,* to suck in]. To take up by adsorption.

adsorbate (ad-sōr'bāt). Any substance adsorbed.

adsorbent (ad-sōr'bent). **1.** A substance that adsorbs, *i.e.,* a solid substance endowed with the property of attaching other substances to its surface without any covalent bonding. **2.** An antigen or antibody used in immune adsorption.

adsorption (ad-sōrp'shŭn) [L. *ad,* to, + *sorbeo,* to suck up]. The property of a solid substance to attract and hold to its surface a gas, liquid, or a substance in solution or in suspension. *Cf.* absorption.

immune a., **(1)** removal of antibody (agglutinin or precipitin) from antiserum by use of specific antigen; after aggregation has occurred, the antigen-antibody complex is separated either by centrifugation or by filtration; **(2)** removal of antigen by specific antiserum in a similar manner.

adsternal (ad-ster'năl). Near or upon the sternum.

adst. feb. Abbreviation for L. *adsente febre,* when fever is present.

ADTe Abbreviation for anodal duration *tetanus.*

adterminal (ad-ter'mi-năl). In a direction toward the nerve endings, muscular insertions, or the extremity of any structure.

adult (ă-dŭlt'). **1.** Fully grown and mature. **2.** A fully grown and mature individual.

adulterant (ă-dŭl'ter-ănt). An impurity; an additive that is considered to have an undesirable effect.

adulteration (ă-dŭl-ter-ā'shŭn). The alteration of any substance by the deliberate addition of a component not ordinarily part of that substance; usually used to imply that the substance is debased as a result.

adultomorphism (ă-dŭl-tō-mōr'fizm). Interpretation of children's behavior in adult terms.

ad us. ext. Abbreviation for L. *ad usum externum,* for external use.

adv. Abbreviation for L. *adversum,* against.

advance (ad-vans') [Fr. *avancer,* to set forward]. To move distally.

advanced life support. Definitive emergency medical care which includes defibrillation, airway management, and use of drugs and medications. *Cf.* basic life support.

advancement (ad-vans'ment). Surgical procedure in which a tendinous insertion or a skin flap is severed from its attachment and sutured to a more distal point.

capsular a., surgical reattachment of the anterior portion of Tenon's capsule.

tendon a., excision of the tendon of an eye muscle and attachment of it to a more anterior location on the globe.

adventitia (ad-ven-tish'ă) [L. *adventicius,* coming from abroad, foreign, fr. *ad,* to + *venio,* to come]. The outermost covering of any organ or structure which is properly derived from without and does not form an integral part of such organ or structure; specifically, the tunica adventitia.

adventitial (ad-ven-tish'ăl). Adventitious (3); relating to the outer coat or adventitia of a blood vessel or other structure.

adventitious (ad-ven-tish'ŭs). **1.** Arising from an external source or occurring in an unusual place or manner. See also extrinsic. **2.** Occurring accidentally or spontaneously, as opposed to natural or hereditary. **3.** Adventitial.

adynamia (ā-dī-nam'ē-ă, ad-i-nā'mē-ă) [G. *a-* priv. + *dynamis,* power]. **1.** Asthenia. **2.** Lack of motor activity or strength.

a. episod'ica heredita'ria, hyperkalemic periodic *paralysis.*

adynamic (ā-dī-nam'ik). Relating to adynamia.

ae-. For words so beginning and not found here, see under e-.

Aeby, Christopher T., Swiss anatomist, 1835–1885. See A.'s *muscle, plane.*

Aedes (ā-ē'dēz) [G. *aēdēs,* unpleasant, unfriendly]. A widespread genus of small mosquitoes frequently found in tropical and subtropical regions.

A. aegyp'ti, the yellow fever mosquito, a species that is also the vector of the pathogen of dengue; characterized by white lyre-shaped markings on the thorax.

A. albopic'tus, species that is an important vector of dengue viruses widespread in the Pacific basin.

A. cabal'lus, species that is an important vector of Rift Valley fever in South Africa.

A. leucocelae'nus, species that transmits yellow fever in South America.

A. polynesien'sis, species that is an important vector of filariasis and dengue in the Polynesian region.

A. scapular'is, species that is a vector of myxomatosis of rabbits.

A. sollic'itans, a common salt-marsh mosquito species and vector of eastern equine encephalomyelitis on the Atlantic and Gulf coasts of the United States.

A. variegat'us, a species that is a vector of filarial parasites in the Pacific Islands (Gilbert and Ellice group).

aelurophobia (ē-lū-rō-fō'bē-ă). Ailurophobia.

Aelurostrongylus (ē'lūr-ō-stron'ji-lŭs) [G. *ailuros,* cat, + Mod. L., fr. G. *strongylus,* round]. A common genus of lungworm in cats; land snails and slugs serve as intermediate hosts and snail-eating animals can serve as transport hosts.

aequorin (ē'kwō-rin). A bioluminescent protein isolated from the jellyfish *Aequorea* which emits blue light in the presence of even minute amounts of calcium ion; injected intramuscularly, it forms a useful calcium ion indicator in experiments on muscle tissue.

aer-, aero- [G. *aēr* (L. *aer*), air]. Combining forms denoting relationship to air or gas.

aerasthenia (ār-as-thē'nē-ă) [aer- + G. *asthenia,* weakness]. Aeroasthenia; aeroneurosis; a psychoneurotic condition occurring in pilots, characterized by worry, lack of self-confidence, mild depression, and varying constitutional disturbances.

aerated (ār'ā-ted). Charged with air or other gas.

aeration (ār-ā'shŭn). **1.** Airing. **2.** Saturating a fluid with air or other gas. **3.** The change of venous into arterial blood in the lungs.

aeremia (ār-ē'mē-ă) [aer- + G. *haima,* blood]. Air *embolism.*

aerendocardia (ār-en-dō-kar'dē-ă) [aer- + G. *endon,* within, + *kardia,* heart]. Presence of undissolved air in the blood within the heart.

aero-. See aer-.

aeroasthenia (ār'ō-as-thē'nē-ă). Aerasthenia.

aeroatelectasis (ār'ō-at-ē-lek'tă-sis). A partial, reversible, airless state of lung tissue most likely to occur in pilots exposed to high G forces, breathing 100% oxygen, and wearing an anti-G suit.

Aerobacter (ār-ō-bak'ter) [aero- + G. *baktērion,* a small staff]. An officially rejected generic name of bacteria. The type species is *A. aerogenes.* Motile organisms previously placed in this species are now placed in *Enterobacter aerogenes;* the nonmotile organisms have been transferred to *Klebsiella pneumoniae.* The species *A. cloacae* is now known as *Enterobacter cloacae.*

aerobe (ār'ōb) [aero- + G. *bios,* life]. **1.** An organism that can live and grow in the presence of oxygen. **2.** An organism that can use oxygen as a final electron acceptor in a respiratory chain.
obligate a., an organism which cannot live or grow in the absence of oxygen.

aerobic (ār-ō'bik). **1.** Aerophilic; aerophilous; living in air. **2.** Relating to an aerobe.

aerobiology (ār'ō-bī-ol'ō-jē). The study of atmospheric constituents, living and nonliving, of biological significance, *e.g.,* airborne spores, pathogenic bacteria, allergenic substances, pollutants.

aerobioscope (ār-ō-bī'ō-skōp) [aero- + G. *bios,* life, + *skopeō,* to view]. An apparatus for determining the bacterial content of the air.

aerobiosis (ār-ō-bī-ō'sis) [aero- + G. *biōsis,* mode of living]. Existence in an atmosphere containing oxygen.

aerobiotic (ār-ō-bī-ot'ik). Relating to aerobiosis.

aerocele (ār'ō-sēl) [aero- + G. *kēlē,* tumor]. Distention of a small natural cavity with gas.

Aerococcus (ār-ō-kok'ŭs) [aero- + G. *kokkus,* berry]. A genus of aerobic Gram-positive cocci that resemble enterococci but do not form chains. They are frequently isolated as airborne saphrophytes in hospitals and as a pathogen of lobsters; cause greening in blood agar and grow in the presence of 40% bile. The type and only species is *A. viridans.*

aerocolpos (ār-ō-kol'pos) [aero- + G. *kolpos,* lap, hollow]. Distention of the vagina with gas.

aerocystography (ār-ō-sis-tog'ră-fē) [aero- + G. *kystis,* bladder, + *graphō,* to write]. Obsolete synonym for pneumocystography.

aerocystoscope (ār-ō-sis'tō-skōp) [aero- + G. *kystis,* bladder, + *skōpeo,* to view]. An obsolete cystoscope for viewing the interior of the bladder distended with air or another gas.

aerocystoscopy (ār-ō-sis-tos'kō-pē). Obsolete procedure for inspection of the interior of the bladder with an aerocystoscope.

aerodermectasia (ār'ō-der-mek-tā'zē-ă) [aero- + G. *derma,* skin, + *ektasis,* a stretching out]. Subcutaneous *emphysema.*

aerodontalgia (ār'ō-don-tal'jē-ă) [aero- + G. *odous,* tooth, + *algos,* pain]. Aero-odontalgia; aero-odontodynia; dental pain caused by either increased or reduced atmospheric pressure.
primary a., dental pain associated with expansion of trapped gases within a tooth, as under a filling, an uncommon condition.
secondary a., pain referred to the dental area from an area of aerosinusitis; more commonly experienced than primary a.

aerodontia (ār-ō-don'shē-ă) [aero- + G. *odous,* tooth]. The science of the effect of either increased or reduced atmospheric pressure on the teeth.

aerodynamics (ār'ō-dī-nam'iks) [aero- + G. *dynamis,* force]. The study of air and other gases in motion, the forces that set them in motion, and the results of such motion.

aerodynamic size. In aerosols, the particle size with unit density which best represents the aerodynamic behavior of a particle.

aeroemphysema (ār'ō-em-fi-sē'mă). Obsolete term for decompression *sickness.*

aerogastria (ār-ō-gas'trē-ă). Distention of the stomach with gas.
blocked a., retention of gas in the stomach due to spasm of the sphincteric region of the lower esophagus which prevents belching.

aerogen (ār'ō-jen). A gas-forming microorganism.

aerogenesis (ār-ō-jen'ĕ-sis) [aero- + G. *genesis,* origin]. Production of gas, as by a microorganism.

aerogenic, aerogenous (ār-ō-jen'ik, -oj'ĕ-nŭs). Gas-forming.

aerohydrotherapy (ār'ō-hī-drō-thār'ă-pē) [aero- + G. *hydōr,* water, + *therapeia,* healing]. Treatment of disease by application, at different temperatures and by different methods, of both air and water.

aeromedicine (ār-ō-med'i-sin). Aviation *medicine.*

aeromonad (ār-ō-mō'nad). A vernacular term used to refer to any member of the genus *Aeromonas.*

Aeromonas (ār-ō-mō'nas). A genus of aerobic, facultatively anaerobic bacteria (family Pseudomonadaceae) containing Gram-negative, rod-shaped to coccoid cells which occur singly or in pairs or in clumps of chains; motile cells ordinarily possess a single, polar flagellum; some species are nonmotile. The metabolism of these organisms is both respiratory and fermentative. These bacteria are found in water and sewage; some are pathogenic to fresh water and marine animals. The type species is *A. hydrophila.*
A. hydroph'ila, a species causing red leg disease of frogs; it is the type species of *A.*

aeroneurosis (ār'-ō-nū-rō'sis). Aerasthenia.

aero-odontalgia (ār'ō-ō-don-tal'jē-ă). Aerodontalgia.

aero-odontodynia (ār'ō-ō-don-tō-din'ē-ă). Aerodontalgia.

aeropathy (ār-op'ă-thē) [aero- + G. *pathos,* suffering]. Any morbid state induced by a pronounced change in atmospheric pressure; *e.g.,* altitude sickness, decompression sickness.

aeropause (ār'ō-pawz). An upper region of the atmosphere, between the stratosphere and outer space, in which gas particles are so sparse as to provide almost no support for man's physiologic requirements or for vehicles that require air for burning fuel.

aerophagia, aerophagy (ār-ō-fā'jē-ă, -of'ă-jē) [aero- + G. *phagein,* to eat]. Pneumophagia; excessive swallowing of air.

aerophil, aerophile (ār'ō-fil, -fīl) [aero- + G. *philos,* fond]. **1.** Air-loving. **2.** An aerobic organism (aerobe), especially an obligate aerobe.

aerophilic, aerophilous (ār-ō-fil'ik, ār-of'i-lŭs). Aerobic.

aerophobia (ār-ō-fō'bē-ă) [aero- + G. *phobos,* fear]. Morbid dread of fresh air or of air in motion.

aeropiesotherapy (ār'ō-pī-ē'sō-thār'ă-pē) [aero- + G. *piesis,* pressure, + *therapeia,* medical treatment]. Treatment of disease by compressed (or rarified) air.

aeroplankton (ār-ō-plank'tōn) [aero- + G. *planktos,* ntr. *-on,* wandering]. An organism or a substance carried by air, *e.g.,* bacterium, pollen grain.

aeroplethysmograph (ār'ō-plē-thiz'mō-graf) [aero- + G. *plēthysmos,* enlargement, + *graphō,* to write]. Obsolete term for body *plethysmograph.*

aerosialophagy (ār'ō-sī-al-of'ă-jē). Sialoaerophagy.

aerosinusitis (ār-ō-sī-nū-sī'tis). Barosinusitis; inflammation of the paranasal sinuses caused by pressure difference within the sinus relative to ambient pressure, secondary to obstruction of the sinus orifice, sometimes due to high altitude flying or by descent from high altitude.

aerosis (ār-ō'sis) [aero- + G. *-osis,* condition]. Generation of gas in the tissues.

aerosol (ār'ō-sol). **1.** A liquid or solution dispersed in air in the form of a fine mist for therapeutic, insecticidal, or other purposes. **2.** A product that is packaged under pressure and contains therapeutically or chemically active ingredients intended for topical application, inhalation, or introduction into body orifices.
respirable a.'s, a.'s with an aerodynamic size under 10 μm.

aerosolization (ār-ō-sol-i-zā'shŭn). Dispersion in air of a liquid material or a solution in the form of a fine mist, usually for therapeutic purposes, especially to the respiratory passages.

aerotherapeutics, aerotherapy (ār'ō-thār-ă-pyū'tiks, -thār'ă-pē). Treatment of disease by fresh air, by air of different degrees of pressure or rarity, or by air medicated in various ways.

aerotitis media (ār-ō-tī'tis mē'dē-ă) [aero- + G. *ous*, ear, + *-itis*, inflammation]. Barotitis media; aviator's ear; aviation otitis; an acute or chronic inflammation of the middle ear caused by a reduction in pressure in the tympanic cavity relative to ambient pressure, secondary to eustachian tube obstruction; often occurs on descent from high altitude.

aerotonometer (ār'ō-ton-om'ĕ-ter) [aero- + G. *tonos*, tension, + *metron*, measure]. **1.** An instrument for estimating the tension or pressure of a gas. **2.** Tonometer (2).

aesculapian (es-kyū-lā'pē-an) [L. *Aesculapius*, G. *Asklēpios*, the god of medicine]. Esculapian; relating to Aesculapius, the art of medicine, or a medical practitioner.

aesculin (es'kyū-lin). Esculin.

aestival (es'ti-văl). Estival.

afebrile (ā-feb'ril). Apyretic.

afetal (ă-fē'tăl). Without relation to a fetus or intrauterine life.

affect (af'fekt) [L. *affectus*, state of mind, fr. *afficio*, to have influence on]. The emotional feeling, tone, and mood attached to a thought, including its external manifestations.
flat a., absence of or diminution in the amount of emotional tone or outward emotional reaction typically shown by others or oneself under similar circumstances.
inappropriate a., emotional tone or outward emotional reaction out of harmony with the idea, object, or thought accompanying it.
labile a., rapid shifts in outward emotional expresions; often associated with organic brain syndromes such as intoxication.

affect display. Facial expressions, postures, and gestures indicating emotional states.

affection (ă-fek'shŭn). **1.** A moderate feeling of tenderness, caring, or love. **2.** An abnormal condition of body or mind.

affective (af-fek'tiv). Pertaining to emotion, feeling, sensibility, or a mental state.

affectivity (af-fek-tiv'i-tē). Feeling *tone*.

affectomotor (af'fek-tō-mō'ter). Pertaining to muscular manifestations associated with affective tone.

afferent (af'er-ent) [L. *afferens*, fr. *af-fero*, to bring to]. Centripetal (1); eisodic; esodic; toward a center, denoting certain arteries, veins, lymphatics, and nerves.

affinity (ă-fin'i-tē) [L. *affinis*, neighboring, fr. *ad*, to, + *finis*, end, boundary]. **1.** In chemistry, the force that impels certain atoms to unite with certain others to form compounds. **2.** Selective staining of a tissue by a dye or the selective uptake of a dye, chemical, or other substance by a tissue.
residual a., secondary forces that enable apparently saturated atoms, ions, or molecules to attract other atoms or groups, causing such phenomena as complex formation, hydration, adsorption, etc.

affinous (af'i-nŭs). Pertaining to a marriage in which the partners are related, not by consanguinity, but through another marriage.

affirmation (af-fer-mā'shŭn). The stage in autosuggestion in which one exhibits a positive reactive tendency.

afflux, affluxion (af'lŭks, af-lŭk'shŭn) [L. *af-fluo*, pp. *-fluxus*, to flow toward]. A flowing toward; specifically, a flowing of blood toward any part. See congestion.

affusion (ă-fyū'zhŭn) [L. *af- fundo*, to pour into]. Pouring of water upon the body or any of its parts for therapeutic purposes.

AFH Abbreviation for anterior facial *height*.

afibrillar (ā-fī'bri-lăr). Denoting a biological structure that does not contain fibrils.

afibrinogenemia (ā-fī'brin-ō-jĕ-nē'mē-ă). The absence of fibrinogen in the plasma. See also hypofibrinogenemia.
congenital a., a rare disorder of blood coagulation in which little or no fibrinogen can be found in plasma; autosomal recessive inheritance.

aflatoxin (af'lă-tok'sin). Toxic metabolites of some strains of *Aspergillus flavus*, which play a role in the etiology of primary cancer of the liver in humans and produce disease in animals eating peanut meal and other feed contaminated by this fungus.

AFORMED See AFORMED *phenomenon*.

AFP Abbreviation for α-fetoprotein.

afterbirth (af'ter-berth). Secundina; secundinae; secundines; the placenta and membranes that are extruded from the uterus after birth.

aftercare (af'ter-kār). **1.** The care and treatment of a patient after an operation or during convalescence from an illness. **2.** Following psychiatric hospitalization, a continuing program of rehabilitation designed to reinforce the effects of the therapy.

aftercataract (af'ter-kat'ă-rakt). Secondary *cataract* (2).

afterchroming (af'ter-krōm'ing). Postchroming; additional treatment of a tissue specimen with chromate or a metal mordant to impart special staining properties.

aftercontraction (af'ter-kon-trak'shŭn). A muscular contraction persisting a noticeable time after the stimulus has ceased.

aftercurrent (af'ter-kŭr-ent). An electrical current induced in a muscle upon the termination of a constant current that has been passed through it.

afterdischarge (af-ter-dis'charj). Prolongation of response of neural elements after cessation of stimulation.

aftereffect (af'ter-ē-fekt'). A physical, physiologic, psychologic, or emotional phenomenon that continues after removal of the stimulus.

aftergilding (af'ter-gild'ing). The treatment of a fixed and hardened histologic specimen of nervous tissue with gold salts.

afterhearing (af-ter-hēr'ing). Aftersound.

afterimage (af'ter-im'ij). Persistence of the visual response after cessation of the stimulus.
negative a., a. in which the lightness relationship is reversed; if chromatic, it appears in complementary color.
positive a., a. in which the lightness relationship is the same as the original one; if chromatic, it appears in the same color.

afterimpression (af'ter-im-presh'ŭn). Aftersensation.

afterload (af'ter-lōd). **1.** The arrangement of a muscle so that, in shortening, it lifts a weight from an adjustable support or otherwise does work against a constant opposing force to which it is not exposed at rest. **2.** The load or force thus encountered in shortening.
ventricular a., formerly, the arterial pressure or some other measure of the force that a ventricle must overcome while it contracts during systolic ejection, contributed to by aortic or pulmonic artery impedance, peripheral vascular resistance, and mass and viscosity of blood; now, more rigorously expressed in terms of the wall stress, *i.e.*, the tension per unit cross-sectional area in the ventricular muscle fibers (calculated by Laplace's law from internal radius and wall thickness) that is required to produce the transmural pressure required for systolic ejection.

aftermovement (af'ter-mūv'ment). Kohnstamm's *phenomenon*.

afterpains (af'ter-pānz). Painful cramplike contractions of the uterus occurring after childbirth.

afterperception (af'ter-per-sep'shŭn). Appreciation of a stimulus only after it has ceased to act.

afterpotential (af'ter-pō-ten'shăl). The small changes in electrical potential in a stimulated nerve which follow the main, or spike, potential; they consist of an initial negative deflection followed by a positive deflection in the oscillograph record.

diastolic a., in the heart, a transmembrane potential change following repolarization, which may reach threshold magnitude and cause a rhythm disturbance; often recorded in poisoning, as by digitalis overdosage.

aftersensation (af'ter-sen-sā'shŭn). Afterimpression; a sensation persisting after its original cause has ceased to act.

aftersound (af'ter-sownd). Afterhearing; subjective sensation of a sound after the cause of the sound has ceased.

aftertaste (af'ter-tāst). A taste persisting after contact of the tongue with the sapid substance has ceased.

aftertouch (af'ter-tŭch). Persistence of touch sensation after removal of the stimulus.

aftosa (af-tō'să) [Sp. and It.]. Foot-and-mouth *disease.*

Ag 1. Symbol for silver (argentum). **2.** Abbreviation for antigen.

agalactia (ā-gal-ak'shē-ă) [G. *a-* priv. + *gala (galakt-),* milk]. Agalactosis; absence of milk in the breasts after childbirth.

contagious a., a generalized, debilitating disease of sheep and goats caused by *Mycoplasma agalactiae;* udder infection leads to a decrease in milk production.

agalactorrhea (ā-ga-lak-tō-rē'ă) [G. *a-* priv. + *gala,* milk, + *rhoia,* a flow]. Absence of the secretion or flow of breast milk.

agalactosis (ā-gal-ak-tō'sis). Agalactia.

agalactous (ă-gal-ak'tŭs). Relating to agalactia, or to the diminution or absence of breast milk.

agamete (ā-gam'ēt, ag'a-mēt) [G. *a-* priv. + *gametēs,* husband]. A protozoan organism produced by asexual multiple fission. See also schizogony.

agamic (ā-gam'ik). Agamous; denoting nonsexual reproduction, as by fission, budding, etc.

agammaglobulinemia (ā-gam'ă-glob'yū-li-nē'mē-ă). Absence of, or extremely low levels of, the gamma fraction of serum globulin; sometimes used loosely to denote absence of immunoglobulins in general. See also hypogammaglobulinemia.

acquired a., common variable *immunodeficiency.*

Bruton type a., X-linked *hypogammaglobulinemia.*

congenital a., primary a., X-linked *hypogammaglobulinemia.*

secondary a., secondary *immunodeficiency.*

Swiss type a., see severe combined *immunodeficiency.*

transient a., transient *hypogammaglobulinemia* of infancy.

X-linked a., X-linked *hypogammaglobulinemia.*

agamocytogeny (ā-gam'ō-sī-toj'ĕ-nē) [G. *agamos,* unmarried, + *kytos,* cell, + *genesis,* becoming]. Schizogony.

Agamofilaria (ā-gam'ō-fī-lā'rē-ă) [G. *agamos,* unmarried, + L. *filum,* thread]. A name given to immature filarial forms, the genera of the adult forms being undetermined.

agamogenesis (ag'ă-mō-jen'ĕ-sis, ā-gan-ō-) [G. *agamos,* unmarried, + *genesis,* production]. Asexual *reproduction.*

agamogenetic (ag'ă-mō-jĕ-net'ik, -ā-gam-ō-). Indicating asexual reproduction.

agamogony (ag-ă-mog'ō-nē) [G. *agamos,* unmarried, + *gonos,* offspring]. Asexual *reproduction.*

Agamomermis culicis (ag-ă-mō-mer'mis kyū'li-kis) [G. *agamos,* unmarried, + Mod. L., fr. G. *mermis,* cord; L. *culex,* gnat]. A species of nematode parasitic in the mosquito; a few cases have been recorded in humans, usually larval worms found emerging from body openings, presumably after ingestion of infected insects or application of moist earth bearing free-living larval stages.

agamont (ag'ă-mont) [G. *agamos,* unmarried, + *ōn (ont-),* being]. Schizont.

agamous (ag'ă-mŭs) [G. *agamos,* unmarried]. Agamic.

aganglionic (ā-gang-glē-on'ik). Without ganglia.

aganglionosis (ā-gang'glē-ō-nō'sis). The state of being without ganglia; *e.g.,* absence of ganglion cells from the myenteric plexus as a characteristic of congenital megacolon.

agapism (ah'gahp-ism) [G. *agapē,* brotherly love]. The doctrine that exalts nonsexual (brotherly) love.

agar (ah'gar, ā'gar) [Bengalese]. A polysaccharide (a sulfated galactan) derived from seaweed (various red algae); used as a solidifying agent in culture media.

ascitic a., a form of serum a.

bile salt a., an a. medium containing lactose, peptone, sodium taurocholate, and neutral red, for the growth and isolation of Gram-negative rods.

blood a., a mixture of blood and nutrient a., used for the cultivation of certain fastidious microorganisms.

Bordet-Gengou potato blood a., glycerine-potato a. with 25% of blood.

brain-heart infusion a., a medium used for the isolation of fastidious fungi.

brilliant green bile salt a., a culture medium consisting of a. with peptone, lactose, sodium taurocholate, brilliant green, and picric acid solution.

chocolate a., blood a. heated until the blood becomes brown or chocolate in color.

cholera a., an alkaline a. medium for cultivating *Vibrio cholerae.*

Conradi-Drigalski a., Drigalski-Conradi a.; a selective, nutrient medium for isolation of *Salmonella typhi* and other intestinal pathogens from fecal specimens; it contains the dye crystal violet, which generally inhibits growth of Gram-positive, but not Gram-negative, bacteria.

cornmeal a., a culture medium that is low in nutrients, used extensively in the study of yeastlike and filamentous fungi; it suppresses vegetative growth while stimulating sporulation of many species, and is widely used for producing the distinctive and rapidly diagnostic chlamydospores of *Candida albicans.*

Czapek's solution a., Czapek-Dox medium; a culture medium used for the cultivation of fungus species and for identification of *Aspergillus* and *Penicillium* species.

Drigalski-Conradi a., Conradi-Drigalski a.

EMB a., eosin-methylene blue a.

Endo a., Endo's medium; a medium containing peptone, lactose, dipotassium phosphate, a., sodium sulfite, basic fuchsin, and distilled water; originally developed for the isolation of *Salmonella typhi,* this medium is now most useful in the bacteriological examination of water; coliform organisms ferment the lactose, and their colonies become red and color the surrounding medium; non-lactose-fermenting organisms produce clear, colorless colonies against the faint pink background of the medium.

Endo's fuchsin a., fuchsin a.; nutrient a. containing lactose, alcoholic solution of fuchsin, sodium sulfite, and soda solution, used as a culture medium to differentiate *Salmonella typhi* from coliform bacteria.

eosin-methylene blue a., EMB a.; a lactose medium for isolation of coliform bacteria.

French proof a., Sabouraud's a.

fuchsin a., Endo's fuchsin a.

Guarnieri's gelatin a., a type of a., similar to Stoddart's gelatin a., used for the cultivation of *Streptococcus pneumoniae.*

lactose-litmus a., a. made by adding 2% lactose and litmus to acid-free nutrient a.; formerly used in the identification of *Salmonella typhi.*

MacConkey a., a primary isolation medium for recovery of aerobic and facultatively anaerobic Gram-negative bacteria.

Novy and MacNeal's blood a., a nutrient a. containing two volumes of defibrinated rabbit's blood; suitable for the cultivation of a

number of trypanosomes.
nutrient a., a simple solid medium containing beef extract, peptone, agar, and water; used for growing many common heterotrophic bacteria.
oatmeal-tomato paste a., a special culture medium for the production of ascospore formation in the dermatophytes.
Pfeiffer's blood a., solid a. with a few drops of human blood smeared on the surface.
potato dextrose a., a culture medium used extensively for the cultivation of fungi; especially good for development of conidia and other sporulating forms by which an organism is identified microscopically.
rice-Tween a., a useful medium for the development of the differential chlamydospores in *Candida albicans* and for preparation of slide cultures for other forms of sporulation in other fungal species.
Sabouraud's a., a culture medium for fungi containing neopeptone or polypeptone a. and glucose, with final pH 5.6; it is the standard, most universally used medium in mycology and is the international reference. Modified Sabouraud's a. (Emmons modification) with less glucose is better for pigment development in the colonies.
serum a., an enriched medium for cultivation of fastidious organisms; prepared by adding sterile serum to melted a.
yeast extract a., a medium used to induce sporulation and reduce vegetative growth in the cultivation of fungi.

agaric (ă-gar′ik) [G. *agarikon,* a kind of fungus]. Amadou; the dried fruit body of *Polyporus officinalis* (family Polyporaceae), occurring in the form of brownish or whitish light masses, which contains agaric acid.
deadly a., *Amanita phalloides.*
fly a., *Amanita muscaria.*

agaric, agaricic, or **agaricinic acid** (ă-gar′ik, ă-gar-ik′ik, ă-gar-i-sin′ik). α-Hexadecylcitric acid; 2-hydroxy-1,2,3-nonadecanetricarboxylic acid; obtained from agaric and responsible for the anhidrotic action of the mushroom; used as an anhidrotic agent.

Agaricus (ă-gar′i-kŭs) [L. *agaricum,* fr. G. *agarikon,* a tree fungus]. A large genus of mushrooms of which many are edible and others poisonous.

agarose (ag′ă-rōs). The neutral polysaccharide fraction found in agar preparations, generally comprised of galactose and altered anhydrogalactose residues; used in chromatography.

agastric (ă-gas′trik) [G. *a-* priv. + *gastēr,* belly]. Without stomach or digestive tract.

agastroneuria (ă-gas-trō-nūr′ē-ă) [G. *a-* priv. + *gastēr,* belly, + *neuron,* nerve]. Lessened nervous control of the stomach.

age (āj) [F. *âge,* L. *aetas*]. **1.** The period that has elapsed since birth. **2.** One of the periods into which human life is divided, distinguished by physical evolution, equilibrium, and involution; *e.g.,* the seven a.'s of man are: infancy, childhood, adolescence, maturity, middle life, senescence, and senility. **3.** To grow old; to gradually develop changes in structure which are not due to preventable disease or trauma and which are associated with decreased functional capacity and an increased probability of death. **4.** To cause artificially the appearance characteristic of one who has lived long or of a thing that has existed a long time. **5.** In dentistry, to heat an alloy for amalgam so as to make it set more slowly, increase strength, reduce flow, and have a stable shelf life; aging occurs by relieving internal strains.
achievement a., the relationship between the chronologic age and the age of achievement, as established by standard achievement tests.
anatomical a., physical a.; a. in terms of structure rather than of function or of passage of time.
basal a., highest mental a. level of the Stanford-Binet intelligence scale at which all items are passed.
Binet a., the a. of the normal child with whose intelligence (as measured by the Stanford-Binet scale) the intelligence of the abnormal child corresponds (of the profoundly retarded, 1 to 2 years; of the moderately to severely retarded, 3 to 7 years; of the borderline to mildly retarded, 8 to 12 years).
bone a., stage of development of bone as adjudged by x-ray, in contrast to chronologic age.
childbearing a., the period in a woman's life between puberty and menopause.
chronologic a. (CA), a. expressed in years and months; used as a measurement against which to evaluate a child's mental a. in computing his Stanford-Binet intelligence quotient.
developmental a. (DA), **(1)** fetal a.; age estimated by anatomic development since implantation; **(2)** age of an individual estimated from the degree of anatomic, physiologic, mental, and emotional maturation.
emotional a., a measure of emotional maturity by comparison with average emotional development.
fetal a., developmental a. (1).
gestational a., the duration of pregnancy as measured from the first day of the last normal menstrual period to the birth; expressed as the number of completed weeks and completed days.
mental a. (MA), a measure, expressed in years and months, of a child's relative intelligence as determined by the Stanford-Binet intelligence scale.
physical a., anatomical a.
physiologic a., a. estimated in terms of function.

agenesis (ă-jen′ĕ-sis) [G. *a-* priv. + *genesis,* production]. Absence, failure of formation, or imperfect development of any part.
gonadal a., gonadal *aplasia.*
renal a., absence of one or both kidneys, most commonly unilateral with absence of the ipsilateral müllerian duct and its derivatives; renal function is normal as long as the remaining kidney is intact; bilateral or complete renal a. is associated with Potter's facies and neonatal death.
thymic a., absence of the thymus, which may be associated with parathyroid a. in Di George syndrome.

agenitalism (ă-jen′i-tal-izm). Congenital absence of genitals.

agenosomia (ă-gen-ō-sō′mē-ă) [G. *a-* priv. + *genos,* sex, + *soma,* body]. Markedly defective formation or absence of the genitalia in a fetus; usually accompanied by protrusion of the abdominal viscera through an incomplete abdominal wall.

agent (ā′jent) [L. *ago,* pres. p. *agens* (*agent-*), to perform]. An active force or substance capable of producing an effect. For agents not listed here, see the specific name.
adrenergic blocking a., a compound that selectively blocks or inhibits responses to sympathetic adrenergic nerve activity (sympatholytic a.) and to epinephrine, norepinephrine, and other adrenergic amines (adrenolytic a.); two distinct classes exist, alpha- and beta-adrenergic receptor blocking a.'s.
α-adrenergic blocking a., alpha-blocker; an agent that competitively blocks α-adrenergic receptors; used in the treatment of hypertension.
β-adrenergic blocking a., beta-blocker; β-adrenergic receptor blocking a.; β-adrenoreceptor antagonist; a class of drugs that compete with β-adrenergic agonists for available receptor sites; some compete for both β_1 and β_2 receptors while others are primarily either β_1 or β_2 blockers; used in the treatment of a variety of cardiovascular diseases where β-adrenergic blockade is desirable.
adrenergic neuronal blocking a., a drug that prevents the responses evoked by sympathetic nerve impulses; it does not inhibit the responses of the adrenergic receptors to circulating epinephrine, norepinephrine, and other adrenergic amines.
β-adrenergic receptor blocking a., β-adrenergic blocking a.
alkylating a.'s, cytotoxic a.'s, such as nitrogen mustards, ethylenimines, and alkyl sulfonates, that cause alkylation of cellu-

lar constituents; their physiological action is thought to arise from such alterations, including cross-linking and cyclizing of portions of DNA, of DNA to protein, or of protein to protein.

antianxiety a., anxiolytic (1); minor tranquilizer; a functional category of drugs useful in the treatment of anxiety and able to reduce anxiety at doses which do not cause excessive sedation.

antifoaming a.'s, chemicals that lower surface tension (hence production of foam), used in laboratory evaporations, and also administered with oxygen to relieve the respiratory obstruction aggravated by the foam of edema fluid in pulmonary edema.

antipsychotic a., antipsychotic (1); major tranquilizer; a functional category of neuroleptic drugs that are helpful in the treatment of psychosis and have a capacity to ameliorate thought disorders.

Bittner a., mammary tumor *virus* of mice.

blocking a., a class of drugs that inhibit (block) a biologic activity or process, such as axonal conduction or transmission, or ions across a cell membrane; frequently called "blockers."

calcium channel-blocking a., slow channel-blocking a.; calcium antagonist; a class of drugs that have the ability to inhibit movement of calcium ions across the cell membrane; of particular value in the treatment of cardiovascular disorders because of pharmacologic effects such as depression of mechanical contraction of cardiac and smooth muscle and of both impulse formation and conduction velocity.

chimpanzee coryza a. (CCA), respiratory syncytial *virus.*

cholinergic a., an a. that mimics the action of the parasympathetic nervous system.

delta a., hepatitis delta *virus.*

Eaton a., *Mycoplasma pneumoniae.*

embedding a.'s, materials such as celloidin, paraffin, etc. in which specimens of tissue are set before being cut into sections for microscopic examination.

enterokinetic a., an a. used to relieve intestinal atony.

F a., F *plasmid.*

F' a., F' *plasmid.*

fertility a., F *plasmid.*

foamy a.'s, foamy *viruses.*

ganglionic blocking a., an a. that impairs the passage of impulses in autonomic ganglia.

initiating a., see initiation.

LDH a., lactate dehydrogenase *virus.*

luting a., a fastening material or cement; *e.g.*, plaster or wax to hold casts to an articulator, or cement to hold teeth on a metal base.

MS-1 a., a strain of hepatitis A virus.

MS-2 a., a strain of hepatitis B virus.

neuroleptic a., neuroleptic (1); any of a family of parenterally administered drugs producing analgesia, sedation, and tranquilization. See also antipsychotic a.

neuromuscular blocking a., a compound which, by virtue of its actions on the neuromuscular junction, inhibits the ability of motor nerve stimuli to produce skeletal muscle contraction (*e.g.*, curare, succinylcholine, gallamine, pancuronium).

nondepolarizing neuromuscular blocking a., a compound that paralyzes skeletal muscle primarily by inhibiting transmission of nerve impulses at the neuromuscular junction rather than by affecting the membrane potention of motor endplate or muscle fibers.

Norwalk a. [*Norwalk*, O, where first implicated in disease], a strain of epidemic gastroenteritis virus.

Pittsburgh pneumonia a., *Legionella micdadei.*

promoting a., see promotion.

reovirus-like a., rotavirus.

sclerosing a., a compound which acts by irritation of the veinous intimal epithelium; used in the treatment of varicose veins.

slow channel-blocking a., calcium channel-blocking a.

sympathetic a., see sympathomimetic *amine.*

transforming a., mitogen.

TRIC a.'s, strains of *Chlamydia trachomatis* that cause *tr*achoma and *i*nclusion *c*onjunctivitis a.'s. See *Chlamydia trachomatis.*

Agent Orange. An herbicide and defoliant, consisting of (2,4,5-trichlorophenoxy)acetic acid, (2,4-dichlorophenoxy)acetic acid, and dioxin, that was widely used in the Vietnam War; it has been shown to possess residual post-exposure carcinogenic and teratogenic properties in humans.

agerasia (ă-jer-ā'zē-ă) [G. *agērasia,* eternal youth, fr. *a-* priv. + *gēras,* old age]. An appearance of youth in old age.

ageusia (ă-gū'sē-ă) [G. *a-* priv. + *geusis,* taste]. Ageustia; gustatory anesthesia; loss of the sense of taste.

ageustia (ă-gūs'tē-ă). Ageusia.

agger, pl. **aggeres** (aj'er, ag'er, -ēz) [L. mound] [NA]. An eminence or projection.

a. na'si [NA], nasal ridge; an elevation on the lateral wall of the nasal cavity lying between the atrium of the middle meatus and the olfactory sulcus; it is formed by the mucous membrane covering the base of the ethmoidal crest of the maxilla.

a. perpendicula'ris, *eminentia* fossae triangularis.

a. val'vae ve'nae, a slight prominence on the wall of a vein corresponding to the location of a valve.

agglomerate, agglomerated (ă-glom'er-āt) [L. *ag-glomero,* to wind into a ball; from *ad,* to, + *glomus,* a ball]. Aggregated.

agglomeration (ă-glom-er-ā'shŭn). Aggregation.

agglutinant (ă-glū'ti-nant) [L. *ad,* to + *gluten,* glue]. A substance that holds parts together or causes agglutination.

agglutinate (ă-glū'ti-nāt). To accomplish, or be subjected to, agglutination.

agglutination (ă-glū-ti-nā'shŭn) [L. *ad,* to, + *gluten,* glue]. **1.** The process by which suspended bacteria, cells, or other particles of similar size are caused to adhere and form into clumps; similar to precipitation, but the particles are larger and are in suspension rather than being in solution. For specific a. reactions in the various blood groups, see Blood Groups appendix. **2.** Adhesion of the surfaces of a wound.

acid a., the clumping together of certain microorganisms at high hydrogen ion concentration.

bacteriogenic a., the clumping of erythrocytes as a result of effects of bacteria or their products.

cold a., a. of red blood cells by their own serum (see autoagglutination), or by any other serum when the blood is cooled below body temperature, but most pronounced below 25°C; the phenomenon results from cold agglutinins; although it is seen occasionally in the blood of apparently normal persons, it is more frequent in scarlet fever, staphylococcal infections, primary atypical pneumonia, certain hemolytic anemias, and trypanosomiasis.

cross a., group a.

false a., pseudoagglutination.

group a., cross a.; a. by antibodies specific for minor (group) antigens common to several microorganisms, each of which possesses its own major specific antigen.

immune a., a. caused by antibody (agglutinin) that is specific for the suspended microorganism, cell, or for an antigen that has been coated on a particle of suitable size.

indirect a., passive a.

mixed a., mixed agglutination *reaction.*

nonimmune a., **(1)** a. caused by a lectin having a degree of specificity, the mechanism of which is not understood; **(2)** a. that results from nonspecific factors, as in the case of acid a. or spontaneous a.

passive a., indirect a.; a. of particles that have been coated with soluble antigen, by antiserum specific for the adsorbed antigen.

spontaneous a., nonspecific clumping of organisms in saline related to lack of polar groups in electrolyte solution.

agglutinative (ă-glū'ti-nă-tiv). Causing, or able to cause, agglutination.

agglutinin (ă-glū'ti-nin). **1.** Immune a.; agglutinating antibody; an antibody that causes clumping or agglutination of the bacteria or other cells which either stimulated the formation of the a., or contain immunologically similar, reactive antigen. **2.** A substance, other than a specific agglutinating antibody, that causes organic particles to agglutinate, commonly qualified, *e.g.,* plant a.
blood group a.'s, see Blood Groups appendix.
chief a., major a.
cold a., an a. associated with cold agglutination.
cross-reacting a., group a.
flagellar a., H a. (1).
group a., cross-reacting a.; an immune a. specific for a group antigen.
H a., **(1)** flagellar a.; an a. that is formed as the result of stimulation by, and which reacts with, the thermolabile antigen(s) in the flagella of motile strains of microorganisms; **(2)** see ABO blood group, Blood Groups appendix.
immune a., agglutinin (1).
major a., chief a.; immune a. present in greatest quantity in an antiserum and evoked by the most dominant of a mosaic of antigens.
minor a., partial a.; immune a. present in an antiserum in lesser concentration than the major a.
O a., **(1)** somatic a.; an a. that is formed as the result of stimulation by, and that reacts with, the relatively thermostable antigen(s) in the cell bodies of microorganisms; **(2)** see ABO blood group, Blood Groups appendix.
partial a., minor a.
plant a., a lectin.
saline a., complete antibody; an anti-Rh antibody which causes agglutination of Rh+ erythrocytes when they are suspended either in saline or in a protein medium.
serum a., incomplete antibody (2); an anti-Rh antibody which coats Rh+ erythrocytes; the cells do not agglutinate when suspended in saline, but do agglutinate when suspended in serum or other protein media such as albumin.
somatic a., O a. (1).
warm a.'s, see autoantibody.

agglutinogen (ă-glū-tin'ō-jen) [agglutinin + G. *-gen,* production]. Agglutogen; an antigenic substance that stimulates the formation of specific agglutinin, which, under certain conditions, causes agglutination of cells that contain the antigen or particles coated with the antigen.
blood group a.'s, see Blood Groups appendix.
T a., an a. formed from a latent receptor on human red cells by the action of an enzyme in cultures of certain bacteria.

agglutinogenic (ă-glū'tin-ō-jen'ik). Agglutogenic; capable of causing the production of an agglutinin.

agglutinophilic (ă-glū'tin-ō-fil'ik) [agglutination + G. *phileō,* to love]. Readily undergoing pronounced agglutination.

agglutinophore (ă-glū'tin-ō-fōr) [agglutinin + G. *phoros,* bearing]. Obsolete term for an antibody-binding site, the portion of the antibody molecule that reacts with specific antigen.

agglutinoscope (ă-glū'tin-ō-skōp) [agglutination + G. *skopeō,* to view]. A magnifying glass or simple system of lenses used to observe agglutination *in vitro.*

agglutogen (ă-glū'tō-jen). Agglutinogen.

agglutogenic (ă-glū-tō-jen'ik). Agglutinogenic.

aggregate (ag'rē-gāt) [L. *ag-grego,* pp. *-atus,* to add to, fr. *grex* (greg-), a flock]. **1.** To unite or come together in a mass or cluster. **2.** The total of individual units making up a mass or cluster.

aggregated (ag'rē-gā-ted). Agglomerate; agglomerated; agminate; agminated; collected together, thereby forming a cluster, clump, or mass of individual units.

aggregation (ag-rē-gā'shŭn). Agglomeration; agmen; a crowded mass of independent but similar units; a cluster.
familial a., occurence of a trait in more members of a family than can be readily accounted for by chance; presumptive but not cogent evidence of the operation of genetic factors.

aggregometer (ag-rē-gom'ĕ-ter). An instrument for measuring platelet adhesiveness.

aggressin (ă-gres'in) [L. *agressor,* an assailant, fr. *ad-gredio,* pp. *-gressus,* to attack]. A substance postulated to inhibit the resistance mechanisms of the host.

aggression (ă-gresh'ŭn) [L. *agressus,* fr. *ad-gredio,* to accost, attack]. A domineering, forceful, or assaultive verbal or physical action toward another person as the motor component of the affects of anger, hostility, or rage.

aggressive (ă-gres'iv). **1.** Denoting aggression. **2.** Denoting a competitive forcefulness or invasiveness, as of a behavioral pattern, a pathogenic organism, or a disease process.

aging (ā'jing). **1.** The process of growing old, especially by failure of replacement of cells in sufficient number to maintain full functional capacity; particularly affects cells (*e.g.,* neurons) incapable of mitotic division. **2.** The gradual deterioration of a mature organism resulting from time-dependent, irreversible changes in structure that are intrinsic to the particular species, and which eventually lead to decreased ability to cope with the stresses of the environment, thereby increasing the probability of death.
clonal a., the deterioration in successive generations of a clone; thus paramecia and other simple forms, if allowed to reproduce asexually for a number of generations, invariably undergo deterioration, the characters of each group of descendants progressively departing from those of the original sexually produced ancestor.

agit. a. us. Abbreviation for L. *agita ante usum,* shake before using.

agit. bene Abbreviation for L. *agita bene,* shake well.

agitographia (aj'i-tō-graf'ē-ă) [L. *agito,* to hurry, + G. *graphō,* to write]. A condition in which one writes with great rapidity, leaving out words or parts of words.

agitolalia (aj'i-tō-lā'lē-ă). Agitophasia.

agitophasia (aj'i-tō-fā'zē-ă) [L. *agito,* to hurry, + G. *phāsis,* speech]. Agitolalia; abnormally rapid speech in which words are imperfectly spoken or dropped out of a sentence.

aglobulia (ā-glō-byū'lē-ă) [G. *a-* priv. + L. *globulus.* globule]. Obsolete term for anemia.

aglobuliosis (ā'glō-byū-lē-ō'sis). Obsolete term for a condition characterized by anemia.

aglobulism (ā-glob'yū-lizm). Obsolete term for anemia.

aglomerular (ā-glō-mer'yū-lăr). Having no glomeruli; said especially of a kidney in which the glomeruli have been destroyed, or kidneys of certain fish, *e.g.,* toad fish, that possess tubules but no glomeruli.

aglossia (ă-glos'ē-ă) [G. *a-* priv. + *glōssa,* tongue]. Congenital absence of the tongue.

aglossostomia (ă-glos-ō-stō'mē-ă) [G. *a-* priv. + *glōssa,* tongue, + *stoma,* mouth]. Congenital absence of the tongue, with a malformed (usually closed) mouth.

aglucon (ā-glū'kon). The portion of a glucoside other than the glucose.

aglutition (ā-glū-tish'ŭn). Dysphagia.

aglycon (ā-glī'kon). The noncarbohydrate portion of a glycoside.

aglycosuria (ā-glī-kō-sū'rē-ă). Absence of carbohydrate in the urine.

aglycosuric (ā-glī-kō-sū'rik). Relating to aglycosuria.

agmen, pl. **agmina** (ag'men, ag'min-ă) [L. a multitude]. Aggregation.
a. peyerian'um, *folliculi* lymphatici aggregati.
agminate, agminated (ag'mi-nāt, ag'mi-nā-ted) [L. *agmen,* a multitude]. Aggregated.
agnail (ag'nāl). Hangnail.
agnathia (ag-nā'thē-ă) [G. *a-* priv. + *gnathos,* jaw]. Congenital absence of the lower jaw, usually accompanied by approximation of the ears. See also otocephaly and synotia.
agnathous (ag'nā-thŭs). Relating to agnathia.
agnea (ag-nē'ă) [G. *agnoia,* want of perception]. Agnosia.
Agnew, Cornelius R., U.S. ophthalmologist, 1830–1888. See A.-Verhoeff *incision.*
agnogenic (ag-nō-jen'ik) [G. *a-* priv. + *gnosis,* knowledge, + *genesis,* origin]. Idiopathic (1).
agnosia (ag-nō'sē-ă) [G. ignorance; from *a-* priv. + *gnōsis,* knowledge]. Agnea; lack of sensory-perceptual ability to recognize objects.
auditory a., central auditory imperception of sound; inability to interpret the significance of sound perceived by the end organ.
finger a., inability to perceive a stimulus applied to the fingers.
ideational a., loss of conceptualization of objects.
localization a., inability to recognize the area where the skin is touched.
optic a., inability to interpret visual images.
position a., failure to recognize the posture of an extremity.
tactile a., inability to recognize objects by the touch.
visual-spatial a., disturbance in spatial orientation and in perception of the spatial relations of objects seen.
-agogue, -agog [G. *agōgos,* leading forth]. Suffixes indicating a promoter or stimulant of.
agomphosis, agomphiasis (ag-om-fō'sis, fī'ă-sis) [G. *a-* priv. + *gomphos,* peg, bolt]. Anodontia.
agonadal (ă-gon'ă-dăl). Denoting the absence of gonads.
agonal (ag'on-ăl). An obsolete term relating to the process of dying or the moment of death, so called because of the former erroneous notion that dying is a painful process.
agonist (ag'on-ist) [G. *agōn,* a contest]. **1.** Denoting a muscle in a state of contraction, with reference to its opposing muscle, or antagonist. **2.** A drug capable of combining with receptors to initiate drug actions; it possesses affinity and intrinsic activity.
agony (ag'ŏ-nē) [G. *agōn,* a struggle, trial]. Intense pain or anguish of body or mind.
agoraphobia (ag'ōr-ă-fō'bē-ă) [G. *agora,* marketplace, + *phobos,* fear]. An irrational fear of leaving the familiar setting of home, so pervasive that a large number of external life situations are entered into reluctantly or are avoided.
agoraphobic (ă-gōr-ă-fō'bik). Relating to or characteristic of agoraphobia.
agouti (ah-gu'tē) [Fr., fr. native Indian]. *Dasyprocta.*
-agra [G. *agra,* a seizure]. Suffix meaning sudden onslaught of acute pain.
agraffe (ă-graf') [Fr. *agrafe,* a hook, clasp]. An appliance for clamping together the edges of a wound, used in lieu of sutures.
agrammatica (ag-ră-mat'i-kă). Agrammatism.
agrammatism (ă-gram'ă-tizm) [G. *agrammatos,* unlearned]. Agrammatica; agrammatologia; a form of aphasia characterized by an inability to construct a grammatical or intelligible sentence; words are uttered, but not in proper sequence.
agrammatologia (ă-gram'mă-tō-lō'jē-ă). Agrammatism.
agranulocyte (ă-gran'yū-lō-sīt) [G. *a-* priv. + L. *granulum,* granule, + G. *kytos,* cell]. A nongranular leukocyte.
agranulocytosis (ă-gran'yū-lō-sī-tō'sis). Agranulocytic or neutropenic angina; angina lymphomatosa; an acute condition characterized by pronounced leukopenia with great reduction in the number of polymorphonuclear leukocytes (frequently less than 500 granulocytes per mm^3); infected ulcers are likely to develop in the throat, intestinal tract, and other mucous membranes, as well as in the skin.
feline a., panleukopenia.
agranuloplastic (ă-gran'yū-lō-plas'tik) [G. *a-* priv. + L. *granulum,* granule, + G. *plastikos,* formative]. Capable of forming nongranular cells, and incapable of forming granular cells.
agraphia (ă-graf'ē-ă) [G. *a-* priv. + *graphō,* to write]. Anorthography; logagraphia; impairment of the ability to write.
absolute a., atactic or literal a.; a. in which not even unconnected letters can be written.
acoustic a., acquired inability to write from dictation.
amnemonic a., a. in which letters and words can be written, but not connected sentences.
atactic a., absolute a.
cerebral a., graphic or graphomotor aphasia; mental a.; the inability to express ideas in writing.
literal a., absolute a.
mental a., cerebral a.
motor a., a. due to muscular incoordination.
musical a., loss of power to write musical notation.
verbal a., a. in which single letters can be written, but not words.
agraphic (ă-graf'ik). Relating to or marked by agraphia.
agriothymia (ag'rē-ō-thī'mē-ă) [G. *agriothymos,* wild of temper, fr. *agrios,* wild, + *thymos,* spirit]. Obsolete term for a wild, ferocious mania.
agromania (ag-rō-mā'nē-ă) [G. *agros,* field, + *mania,* frenzy]. Morbid impulse to live in the open country or in solitude.
agrypnia (ă-grip'nē-ă) [G. sleeplessness, fr. *agreō,* to hunt after, + *hypnos,* sleep]. Rarely used term for insomnia.
agrypnocoma (ă-grip'nō-kō'mă) [G. *agrypnos,* sleepless, + *kōma,* coma]. A wakeful, apathetic, or lethargic state.
ague (ā'gū) [Fr. *aigu,* acute]. **1.** Archaic term for malarial fever. **2.** A chill.
agyiophobia (aj'ē-ō-fō'bē-ă) [G. *agyia,* street, + *phobos,* fear]. A form of agoraphobia characterized by a morbid fear of being in the street.
agyria (ă-jī'rē-ă) [G. *a-* priv. + *gyros,* circle]. Lissencephalia; lissencephaly; congenital lack of convolutional pattern in the cerebral cortex due to defect of development.
AHF Abbreviation for antihemophilic *factor.*
AHG Abbreviation for antihemophilic *globulin.*
Ahumada, J.C., Argentinian physician. See A.-Del Castillo *syndrome.*
ahylognosia (ā-hī-log-nō'sē-ă) [G. *a-* priv. + *hyle,* matter, + *gnosis,* recognition]. Inability to recognize differences of density, weight, and roughness.
Aicardi, J. Dennis, 20th century French neurologist. See A.'s *syndrome.*
aichmophobia (īk-mō-fō'bē-ă) [G. *aichmē,* a point, + *phobos,* fear]. Morbid fear of being touched by the finger or any slender pointed object.
AID Abbreviation for donor of heterologous (artificial) insemination.
aidoi-, aidoio- [G. *aidoia,* genitals]. Archaic combining forms relating to the genitals.
AIDS Acquired immunodeficiency syndrome; a disease characterized by opportunistic infections (*e.g., Pneumocystis carinii* pneumonia, candidiasis, isosporiasis, cryptococcosis, toxoplasmosis)

and malignancies (*e.g.,* Kaposi's sarcoma, non-Hodgkin's lymphoma) in immunocompromised persons; caused by the human immunodeficiency virus transmitted by exchange of body fluids (*e.g.,* semen, blood, saliva) or transfused blood products; hallmark of the immunodeficiency is depletion of T4+ helper/inducer lymphocytes, primarily the result of selective tropism of the virus for these lymphocytes.

AIH Abbreviation for homologous (artificial) insemination.

aileron (ā'ler-on) [Fr. *aile,* wing]. A winglike extension of a fascia or sheath.

ailurophobia (ī'lū-rō-fō'bē-ă, ā'lu-). [G. *ailouros,* cat, + *phobos,* fear]. Aelurophobia; morbid fear of or aversion to cats.

ainhum (ī'yūm) [fr. Af. (Lagos), to saw]. Dactylolysis spontanea; an acquired slowly progressive fibrous constriction that develops in the digitoplantar fold, usually of the little toe, gradually resulting in loss of the toe; most commonly affects black males in the tropics.

air (ār) [G. *aēr;* L. *aer*]. Atmosphere (1); a mixture of gases in the following approximate percentages by volume after water vapor has been removed: oxygen, 20.94; nitrogen, 78.03; argon and other rare gases, 0.99; carbon dioxide, 0.04. Formerly used to mean any respiratory gas, regardless of its composition.
alveolar a., alveolar *gas.*
complemental a., inspiratory reserve *volume.*
complementary a., inspiratory *capacity.*
functional residual a., functional residual *capacity.*
liquid a., a. that by means of intense cold and pressure, has been liquefied.
minimal a., the volume of gas that remains in the lungs and cannot be expelled after they have been removed from the body, or after the chest has been opened.
reserve a., expiratory reserve *volume.*
residual a., residual *volume.*
supplemental a., expiratory reserve *volume.*
tidal a., tidal *volume.*
vitiated a., a. containing a reduced percentage of oxygen.

Aird, Robert B., U.S. neurologist, *1903. See Flynn-A. *syndrome.*

airsacculitis (ār'sak-yū-lī'tis). Inflammation of the mucous membrane of the air sacs of birds.

air'sickness. A condition resembling seasickness or other forms of motion sickness occurring in airplane flight as a result of vibration, deflections from linear flight, and gravitational forces.

airway (ār'wā). **1.** Any part of the respiratory tract through which air passes during breathing. **2.** In anesthesia or resuscitation, a device for correcting obstruction to breathing, especially an oropharyngeal and nasopharyngeal a., endotracheal a., or tracheotomy tube.
conducting a., the a. from the nasal cavity to a terminal bronchiole.
lower a., the portion of the respiratory tract that extends from the subglottis to and including the terminal bronchioles.
respiratory a., that part of the a. where interchange of gases occurs; it includes respiratory bronchioles, alveolar ducts, sacs, and alveoli.
upper a., the portion of the respiratory tract that extends from the nares or mouth to and including the larynx.

Ajellomyces capsulatum (ah-jĕ-lō-mī'sēz kap-sū-lā'tŭm). Emmonsiella capsulata; the ascomycetous (perfect, sexual) state of *Histoplasma capsulatum.*

Ajellomyces dermatitidis (ah-jĕ-lō-mī'sēz der-mă-tit'i-dis). The perfect state of the fungus *Blastomyces dermatitidis;* the (+) and (−) mating types cause disease with equal frequency. This sexual state is placed in the family Gymnoascaceae.

ajmaline (aj'mă-lēn). An indole alkaloid from the roots of *Rauwolfia serpentina,* related to reserpine, serpentine, and yohimbine; used for treatment of hypertension and as a tranquilizer or sedative.

ajowan oil (aj'ō-wan). Ptychotis oil; a volatile oil distilled from the fruit of *Carum copticum,* one of the sources of thymol; a carminative, aromatic, and expectorant.

akanthion (ă-kan'thē-on). Acanthion.

akaryocyte (ā-kar'ē-ō-sīt) [G. *a-* priv. + *karyon,* kernel, + *kytos,* a hollow (cell)]. Acaryote; akaryote; a cell without a nucleus (karyon), such as the erythrocyte.

akaryote (ā-kar'ē-ōt) [G. *a-* priv. + *karyon,* kernel]. Akaryocyte.

akatama (ah-kah-tah'mah) [W. Af]. An endemic peripheral neuritis affecting the adult native population of West Central Africa, characterized by burning, prickling, numbness, and erythema.

akatamathesia (ă-kat'ă-mă-thē'zē-ă). Acatamathesia.

akathisia (ak-ă-thiz'ē-ă) [G. *a-* priv. + *kathisis,* a sitting]. Acathisia; a syndrome characterized by an inability to remain in a sitting posture, with motor restlessness and a feeling of muscular quivering.

akembe (ă-kem'bē). Onyalai.

akeratosis (ă-ker-ă-tō'sis). Deficiency or absence of the horny tissue.

Åkerlund, A. Olof, Swedish radiologist, 1885–1958. See Å's *deformity.*

akinesia (ā-ki-nē'sē-ă, ā-kī-) [G. *a-* priv. + *kinēsis,* movement]. Akinesis. **1.** Absence or loss of the power of voluntary motion. **2.** The postsystolic interval of rest of the heart. **3.** A neurosis accompanied by paretic symptoms.
a. al'gera [G. *algos,* pain], a condition marked by severe neuralgic pain of indeterminate origin which is excited by any movement.
a. amnes'tica, loss of muscular power from disuse.

akinesic (ā-ki-nē'sik, ā-kī-). Akinetic.

akinesis (ā-ki-nē'sis, ā-kī-). Akinesia.

akinesthesia (ā-kin'es-thē'zē-ă) [G. *a-* priv. + *kinēsis,* motion, + *aisthēsis,* sensation]. Absence of the sense of perception of movement or of the muscular sense.

akinetic (ā-ki-net'ik, -kī-net'ik). Akinesic; relating to or suffering from akinesia.

akiyami (ah-kē-yah'mē). Hasamiyami.

aklomide (ak'lō-mīd). 2-Chloro-4-nitrobenzamide; a coccidiostat used in veterinary practice.

Al Symbol for aluminum.

ALA Abbreviation for δ-aminolevulinic acid.

Ala Symbol for alanine or its mono- or diradical.

ala, gen. and pl. **alae** (ā'lă, ā'lē) [L. wing]. **1** [NA]. Any winglike or expanded structure. **2.** *Fossa* axillaris.
a. au'ris, auricula (1).
a. cerebel'li, a. lobuli centralis.
a. cine'rea, *trigonum* nervi vagi.
a. cris'tae gal'li [NA], wing of crista galli; alar process; a small lateral expansion of the ethmoid bone from the front of the crista galli on each side that articulates with the frontal bone and forms the foramen cecum.
alae lin'gulae cerebel'li, *vincula* lingulae cerebelli.
a. lob'uli centra'lis [NA], a. cerebelli; the lateral winglike projection of the central lobule of the cerebellum.
a. ma'jor os'sis sphenoida'lis [NA], a. temporalis; greater wing of sphenoid bone.
a. mi'nor os'sis sphenoida'lis [NA], Ingrassia's apophysis or wing; a. orbitalis; lesser wing of sphenoid bone.
a. na'si [NA], pinna nasi; wing of nose; the outer more or less flaring wall of each nostril.
a. orbitalis, a. minor osis sphenoidalis.
a. os'sis il'ii [NA], wing of ilium; the upper flaring portion of the ilium.

a. sacra'lis [NA], wing of sacrum; the upper surface of the lateral part of the sacrum adjacent to the body.
a. tempora'lis, a. major ossis sphenoidalis.
a. vespertilio'nis [L. bat's wing], obsolete, but descriptive, term for broad ligament of the uterus.
a. vo'meris [NA], wing of vomer; an everted lip on either side of the upper border of the vomer, between which fits the rostrum of the sphenoid bone.

alacrima (ă-lak'rē-mă) [G. *a-* priv. + L. *lacrima,* tear]. Absence of tears.

Alajouanine, Théophile, French neurologist, 1890–1980. See A's. *syndrome;* Foix-A. *myelitis.*

alalia (ă-la'lē-ă) [G. *a-* priv. + *lalia,* talking]. Loss of the power of speech through impairment in the articulatory apparatus. See aphonia.

alalic (ă-lal'ik). Relating to alalia.

alanine (Ala) (al'ă-nēn). 2- or α-Aminopropionic acid; $CH_3CH(NH_2)COOH$; one of the amino acids occurring widely in proteins.

β-alanine. 3- or β-Aminopropionic acid; $NH_2CH_2CH_2COOH$; a decarboxylation production of aspartic acid.

alanine aminotransferase (ALT) [EC 2.6.1.2]. Alanine transaminase; (serum) glutamic-pyruvic transaminase; an enzyme transferring amino groups from L-alanine to 2-ketoglutarate, or the reverse (from L-glutamate to pyruvate); the D form (EC 2.6.1.21) effects the same reaction, but with D-alamine and D-glutamate.

alanine-oxomalonate aminotransferase [EC 2.6.1.47]. An enzyme that accomplishes the transfer of the amino groups of L-alanine to oxomalonate, an action similar to that of alanine aminotransferase.

alanine racemase [EC 5.1.1.1]. An enzyme, requiring pyridoxal phosphate as coenzyme, that catalyzes the racemization of L-alanine to D-alanine; found in various microorganisms, where it may play a role in the biosynthesis of the D-amino acids present in the capsular proteins.

alanine transaminase. Alanine aminotransferase.

alanosine (ă-lan'ō-sēn). An antibiotic substance produced by *Streptomyces alanosinicus;* possesses antineoplastic and antiviral activity.

Alanson, Edward, British surgeon, 1747–1823. See A.'s *amputation.*

alantin (ă-lan'tin). Inulin.

alantol (al'an-tol). Inulol; a yellowish liquid obtained by distillation from the root of *Inula helenium* or elecampane; used internally as an irritating tonic and externally as a mild rubefacient.

alant starch (ă-lant'). Inulin.

alanyl (al'ă-nil). The acyl radical of alanine.

alar (ā'lăr). **1.** Relating to a wing; winged. **2.** Axillary. **3.** Relating to the ala of such structures as the nose, sphenoid, sacrum, etc.

alastrim (ă-las'trim) [Pg. *alastrar,* to scatter over]. A mild form of smallpox caused by a less virulent strain of the virus. Also called Cuban itch; milkpox; pseudosmallpox; whitepox; West Indian smallpox; Kaffir pox; pseudovariola; variola minor.

alba (al'bă) [fem. of L. *albus,* white]. *Substantia* alba.

Albarran y Dominguez, Joaquin, Cuban urologist, 1860–1912. See A.'s *glands, test, tubules.*

albedo (al-bē'dō) [L. whiteness]. The light reflected by a surface.

Albers-Schönberg, Heinrich E., German radiologist, 1865–1921. See A.-S. *disease.*

Albert, Eduard, Austrian surgeon, 1841–1900. See A.'s *disease, suture.*

Albert, Henry, U.S. physician, 1878–1930. See A.'s *stain.*

albicans, pl. **albicantia** (al'bi-kanz, -kan'tē-ă) [L.]. **1.** White. **2.** *Corpus* albicans.

albiduria (al-bi-dū'rē-ă) [L. *albidus,* whitish, + G. *ouron,* urine]. Albinuria; the passing of pale or white urine of low specific gravity, as in chyluria.

albidus (al'bi-dŭs) [L.]. White, whitish.

Albini, Giuseppe, Italian physiologist, 1827–1911. See A.'s *nodules.*

albinism (al'bi-nizm) [L. *albus,* white]. Congenital leukoderma or leukopathia; an inherited (usually autosomal recessive) deficiency or absence of pigment in the skin, hair, and eyes, or eyes only, due to an abnormality in production of melanin.
cutaneous a., a heritable condition characterized by patterned loss of skin pigment on extremities and ventral thorax; a white forelock is often present, but no ocular findings.
ocular a., absence of pigment chiefly in the iris, choroid, and retinal pigment epithelium; X-linked inheritance.
oculocutaneous a., hereditary absence of pigment in skin, hair, and eyes; in the **tyrosinase negative type,** there is an absence of tyrosinase; in the **tyrosinase positive type,** there is normal tyrosinase which cannot enter pigment cells; it is transmitted by an autosomal recessive inheritance.
rufous a., xanthism.

albino (al-bī'nō) [L. *albus,* white]. An individual with albinism.

albinotic (al-bi-not'ik). Pertaining to albinism.

albinuria (al-bi-nū'rē-ă). Albiduria.

Albinus (Weiss), Bernhard S., German anatomist and surgeon, 1697–1770. See A.'s *muscle.*

albocinereous (al-bō-si-nē'rē-ŭs) [L. *albus,* white, + *cinereus,* ashen, fr. *cinis* (*ciner-*), ashes]. Relating to both the white and the gray matter of the brain or spinal cord.

Albrecht, Karl M.P., German anatomist, 1851–1894. See A.'s *bone.*

Albright, Fuller, U.S. physician, 1900–1969. See A.'s *disease, syndrome,* hereditary *osteodystrophy;* Forbes-A. *syndrome;* McCune-A. *syndrome.*

albuginea (al-byū-jin'ē-ă) [L. *albugineus,* fr. *albugo,* white spot]. A white fibrous tissue layer, such as the tunica albuginea. See tunica albuginea entries under tunica.

albugineotomy (al-byū-jin-ē-ot'ō-mē) [albuginea + G. *tomē,* cutting]. Incision into any tunica albuginea.

albugineous (al-byū-jin'ē-ŭs) [L. *albugineus,* fr. *albugo,* white spot]. **1.** Resembling boiled white of egg. **2.** Relating to any tunica albuginea.

albugo (al-bū'gō) [L. *albugo* (*-in-*), a white spot]. Leukoma.

albumen (al-byū'men) [L. the white of egg]. Ovalbumin.

albumin (al-byū'min) [L. *albumen* (*-min-*), the white of egg]. A type of simple protein, varieties of which are widely distributed throughout the tissues and fluids of plants and animals; a.'s are soluble in pure water, precipitable from solution by strong acids, and coagulable by heat in acid or neutral solution.
a. A, the normal or common type of human serum a.
acetosoluble a., Patein's a.
a. B, see inherited albumin *variants.*
Bence Jones a., see Bence Jones *protein.*
blood a., serum a.
bovine serum a. (BSA), a source of a. commonly used in *in vitro* biological studies.
dried human a., normal human serum a.
egg a., ovalbumin.
a. Ghent, see inherited albumin *variants.*
iodinated ^{125}I serum a., Radioiodinated serum a.; a sterile, buffered, isotonic solution prepared to contain not less than 10 mg of radioiodinated normal human serum albumin per ml, and adjusted

to provide not more than 1 mCi of radioactivity per ml; used as a diagnostic aid in determining blood volume and cardiac output.
iodinated ^{131}I human serum a., a sterile, buffered, isotonic solution prepared to contain not less than 10 mg of radioiodinated normal human serum a. per ml, and adjusted to provide not more than 1 mCi of radioactivity per ml; used as a diagnostic aid in the measurement of blood volume and cardiac output.
macroaggregated a. (MAA), conglomerates of human serum a. in a suspension; usually refers to particles 10 to 50 μm in size; used as a tagged agent for lung scanning.
a. Mexico, see inherited albumin *variants.*
a. Naskapi, see inherited albumin *variants.*
native a., a. existing in its natural state, the two principal forms being serum a. and egg a.; it is soluble in water and not precipitated by diluted acids.
normal human serum a., dried human a.; a sterile preparation of serum a. obtained by fractionating blood plasma proteins from healthy persons; used as a transfusion material and to treat edema due to hypoproteinemia.
Patein's a., acetosoluble a.; a substance resembling serum a., but soluble in acetic acid.
radioiodinated serum a. (RISA), iodinated ^{125}I serum a.
a. Reading, see inherited albumin *variants.*
serum a., blood a.; seralbumin; the principal protein in plasma, present in blood plasma and in serous fluids.
a. tannate, an astringent powder obtained by the action of tannic acid on a.; contains about 50% tannic acid; used as an astringent disinfectant in diarrhea and as a dusting powder.
a. X, an antithrombin in blood plasma; the normal antithrombin of blood.
a. X_1, heparin cofactor, required for the antithrombotic action of heparin.

albuminate (al-byū'min-āt). The product of the reaction between native albumin and dilute acids or dilute bases, thereby resulting in acid a.'s or alkali a.'s; both types are characterized by solubility in dilute acid or alkali, and relative insolubility in water, dilute solutions of salts, and alcohol.

albuminaturia (al-byū'mi-nă-tū'rē-ă) [albuminate + G. *ouron,* urine]. The presence of an abnormally large quantity of albuminates in the urine when voided.

albuminiferous (al-byū-min-if'er-ŭs) [albumin + L. *fero,* to bear]. Producing albumin.

albuminiparous (al-byū-min-ip'ăr-ŭs) [albumin + L. *pario,* to bring forth]. Forming albumin.

albuminocholia (al-byū'min-ō-kō'lē-ă) [albumin + G. *cholē,* bile]. Obsolete term for protein in the bile.

albuminogenous (al-byū-min-oj'en-ŭs). Producing or forming albumin.

albuminoid (al-byū'min-oyd). Albumoid. **1.** Resembling albumin. **2.** Any protein. **3.** Scleroprotein; glutinoid; a simple type of protein, insoluble in neutral solvents, present in horny and cartilaginous tissues and in the lens of the eye; *e.g.,* keratin, elastin, collagen.

albuminolysis (al-byū-min-ol'i-sis) [albumin + G. *lysis,* dissolution]. Proteolysis.

albuminoptysis (al-byū-mi-nop'ti-sis) [albumin + G. *ptysis,* a spitting]. Albuminous expectoration.

albuminorrhea (al-byū-min-ō-rē'ă) [albumin + G. *rhoia,* a flow]. Albuminuria.

albuminous (al-byū'min-ŭs). Relating to, containing, or consisting of albumin.

albuminuria (al-byū-mi-nū'rē-ă) [albumin + G. *ouron,* urine]. Albuminorrhea; proteinuria (2); presence of protein in urine, chiefly albumin but also globulin; usually indicative of disease, but sometimes resulting from a temporary or transient dysfunction.
adolescent a., functional a. occurring at about the time of puberty; it is usually cyclic or orthostatic a.
adventitious a., false a.; a. resulting from the presence of blood escaping somewhere in the urinary tract, of chyle, or of some other albuminous fluid, not caused by filtration of albumin from the blood through the kidneys.
a. of athletes, a form of functional a. following excessive muscular exertion.
Bamberger's a., obsolete term for hematogenous a. that is sometimes observed during the later phases of advanced anemia.
benign a., essential a.; a collective term for types that are not the result of pathologic changes in the kidneys.
cardiac a., a. caused by congestive heart failure.
colliquative a., an a. that is at first slight in degree, but unexpectedly becomes greatly increased during convalescence from highly febrile disease, *e.g.,* typhoid fever.
cyclic a., pseudalbuminuria; pseudoalbuminuria; recurrent a.; a functional a. sometimes observed intermittently in cycles of 12 to 36 hours' duration, chiefly in younger persons; the degree of a. is usually slight.
dietetic (digestive) a., the excretion of protein in the urine following the ingestion of certain foods.
essential a., benign a.
false a., adventitious a.
febrile a., a. associated with fever.
functional a., physiologic a. (2); a collective term denoting types of benign a. that are associated with physical exertion or other conditions in which there are physiologic changes such as during pregnancy or adolescence.
intermittent a., functional a. occurring at intervals, such as cyclic a. or a. of athletes.
lordotic a., orthostatic a.; so-called on the theory that the a. results from pressure due to lordosis in the lumbar spine.
neuropathic a., a. associated with epilepsy or other convulsive disorders, trauma to the brain, and cerebral hemorrhage.
orthostatic a., lordotic or postural a.; orthostatic or postural proteinuria; the appearance of albumin in the urine when the patient is erect and its disappearance when recumbent.
physiologic a., **(1)** presence of slight traces of protein in otherwise normal urine; **(2)** functional a.
postrenal a., a. caused by disease distal to the kidney.
postural a., orthostatic a.
prerenal a., a. caused by disease other than disease of the kidney or genitourinary tract.
recurrent a., cyclic a.
regulatory a., transitory a. occurring after unusual physical exertion.
transient a., a. of a temporary or short-lived nature.

albuminuric (al-byū-mi-nū'rik). Relating to or characterized by albuminuria.

albumoid (al-byū'moyd). Albuminoid.

albuterol (al-byū'ter-ol). Salbutamol; α'-[(*tert-* butylamino)-methyl]-4-hydroxy-*m-* xylene-α,α'-diol; a sympathomimetic bronchodilator with very selective effects on β_2 receptors, by inhalation.

Alcaligenes (al-kă-lij'en-ēz) [alkali + G. *-gen,* producing]. A genus of Gram-negative, rod-shaped bacteria (family Achromobacteraceae) which are either motile and peritrichous or nonmotile. They are strictly aerobic; some strains are capable of anaerobic respiration in the presence of nitrate or nitrite. Their metabolism is respiratory, never fermentative. They do not utilize carbohydrates. They are found mostly in the intestinal canal, decaying materials, dairy products, and soil. These organisms are placed by some authorities in the genus *Brucella.* The type species is *A. faecalis.*

alcapton (al-kap'tōn). Homogentisic acid.

alcaptonuria (al-kap-tō-nū'rē-ă). Alkaptonuria.

Alcian blue (al'sē-an) [C.I. 74240]. A complex phthalocyanin dye used as a stain to distinguish sulfomucins from sialomucins and uronic acid mucins, to demonstrate sulfated polysaccharides, and to detect glycoproteins in electrophoresis; often used in combination with PAS or aldehyde fuchsin.

alclofenac (al-klō'fē-nak). [4-(Allyloxy)-3-chlorophenyl]acetic acid; an anti-inflammatory agent.

alclometasone (al-klō-met'ă-sōn). 7-Chloro-11,17,21-trihydroxy-16-methylpregna-1,4-diene-3,20-dione; a potent corticosteroid used as the 17,21-dipropionate in topical therapy for psoriasis and other deep-seated dermatoses.

Alcock, Benjamin, Irish anatomist, *1801. See A.'s *canal.*

alcogel (al'kō-jel). A hydrogel, with alcohol instead of water as the dispersion medium.

alcohol (al'kō-hol) [Ar. *al,* the, + *kohl,* fine antimonial powder, the term being applied first to a fine powder, then, to anything impalpable (spirit)]. **1.** One of a series of organic chemical compounds in which a hydrogen (H) attached to carbon is replaced by a hydroxyl (OH); a.'s react with acids to form esters and with alkali metals to form alcoholates. For individual a.'s not listed here, see specific name. **2.** Ethanol; ethyl alcohol; grain alcohol; rectified or wine spirit; CH_3CH_2OH; a liquid containing 92.3% by weight, corresponding to 94.9% by volume, at 15.56°, of C_2H_50H; made from sugar, starch, and other carbohydrates by fermentation with yeast, and synthetically from ethylene or acetylene. It has been used in beverages and as a solvent, vehicle, and preservative; medicinally, it is used externally as a rubefacient, coolant, and disinfectant, and internally as an analgesic, stomachic, sedative, and antipyretic.

absolute a., **(1)** anhydrous a.; 100% a., water having been removed; **(2)** dehydrated a.; a. with a minimum admixture of water, at most 1%.

acid a., ethyl a. (70%) containing 1% hydrochloric acid.

anhydrous a., absolute a. (1).

dehydrated a., absolute a. (2).

denatured a., methylated or industrial methylated spirit; ethyl a. rendered unfit for consumption as a beverage by the addition of one or several chemicals for commercial purposes.

dihydric a., a. containing two OH groups in its molecule; *e.g.,* ethylene glycol.

dilute a., an a. in water mixtures of various concentrations, *e.g.,* 90, 80, 70, 60, 50, 45, 25, and 20% v/v of C_2H_5OH.

fatty a., a long chain a., analogous to the fatty acids, of which the fatty a. may be viewed as a reduction product; *e.g.,* octadecanol from stearic acid.

grain a., a. (2).

monohydric a., an a. containing one OH group.

primary a., an a. characterized by the univalent radical, $—CH_2OH$.

pyroligneous a., *methyl* alcohol.

rubbing a., an alcoholic mixture intended for external use; it usually contains 70% by volume of absolute a.; the remainder consists of water, denaturants (with and without coal tar colors), and perfume oils; used as a rubefacient.

secondary a., an a. characterized by the bivalent atom group, $>CHOH$.

sugar a., see sugar alcohol.

tertiary a., an a. characterized by the trivalent atom group, $\geqslant COH$.

trihydric a., an a. containing three OH groups; *e.g.,* glycerol.

unsaturated a.'s, those a.'s whose carbon chains contain one or more double or triple bonds.

alcohol acids. A group of compounds that contain both the carboxyl and hydroxy radicals; *e.g.,* glycolic acid.

alcoholate (al-kō-hol'āt). **1.** A tincture or other preparation containing alcohol. **2.** A chemical compound in which the hydrogen in the OH group of an alcohol is replaced by an alkali metal; *e.g.,* sodium methylate, CH_3ONa.

alcohol dehydrogenase (ADH) [EC 1.1.1.1]. Aldehyde reductase; DPNH → aldehyde transhydrogenase; an oxidoreductase converting an alcohol to an aldehyde (or ketone) with NAD^+ as the H acceptor. See also alcohol dehydrogenase (acceptor); alcohol dehydrogenase ($NADP^+$); alcohol dehydrogenase ($NAD(P)^+$).

alcohol dehydrogenase (acceptor) [EC 1.1.99.8]. An oxidoreductase converting primary alcohols to aldehydes with an H acceptor other than NAD^+.

alcohol dehydrogenase ($NADP^+$) [EC 1.1.1.2]. Retinaldehyde reductase; retinal reductase; an oxidoreductase converting alcohols to aldehydes (or ketones) with $NADP^+$ as H acceptor.

alcohol dehydrogenase ($NAD(P)^+$) [EC 1.1.1.71]. An oxidoreductase converting alcohols to aldehydes, or the reverse, with NAD^+ or $NADP^+$ as H acceptor; also reduces retinal to retinol.

alcoholic (al-kō-hol'ik). **1.** Relating to, containing, or produced by alcohol. **2.** One who suffers from alcoholism.

alcoholism (al'kō-hol-izm). Alcohol abuse, dependence, or addiction; chronic excessive drinking of alcoholic beverages resulting in impairment of health and social or occupational functioning, and increasing adaptation to the effects of alcohol requiring increasing doses to achieve and sustain a desired effect; specific signs and symptoms of withdrawal are usually shown upon sudden cessation of such drinking.

acute a., intoxication (2); a temporary deterioration in mental function, accompanied by muscular incoordination and paresis, induced by the ingestion of alcoholic beverages in toxic amounts.

alpha a., Jellinek's term for a still controllable and strictly psychological dependence on alcohol, as to relieve emotional or physical pain, with resulting interference with interpersonal relationships.

beta a., Jellinek's term for the physical complaints associated with excessive use of alcohol, such as polyneuropathy, gastritis, and liver cirrhosis.

chronic a., a pathologic condition, affecting chiefly the nervous and gastroenteric systems, caused by the habitual use of alcoholic beverages in toxic amounts.

delta a., Jellinek's term for an advanced form of gamma a. in which the individual has lost the ability to abstain from partaking of alcohol even for a brief period.

epsilon a., Jellinek's term for "spree-drinking," such as might occur during periods away from home.

gamma a., Jellinek's term for a severe stage of a. characterized by a progression from psychological to physiological dependence upon alcohol, including tissue dependence and withdrawal symptoms, with loss of control over alcohol intake and destructive effects on interpersonal relationships.

alcoholization (al'kō-hol-i-zā'shŭn). Permeation or saturation with alcohol.

alcoholophobia (al'kō-hol-ō-fō'bē-ă) [alcohol + G. *phobos,* fear]. Morbid fear of alcohol, or of becoming an alcoholic.

alcoholysis (al-kō-hol'i-sis) [alcohol + G. *lysis,* dissolution]. Splitting of a chemical bond with the addition of the elements of alcohol at the point of splitting.

alcuronium chloride (al-kyūr-ō'nē-ŭm). *N,N'*-Diallylnortoxiferinium dichloride; a skeletal muscle relaxant active as a non-depolarizing neuromuscular blocking agent.

ALD Abbreviation for adrenoleukodystrophy.

aldadiene (al-dă-dī'ēn). A metabolite of spironolactone that contains double bonds between C-4 and C-5 and between C-6 and C-7; formed upon removal of the 7α-acetylthiol side chain from spironolactone and as potent a diuretic as the parent compound.

aldaric acid (al'dar-ik). One of a group of sugar acids characterized by the formula HOOC—$(CHOH)_n$—COOH; *e.g.,* saccharic acid.

aldehol (al'dĕ-hol). An oxidation product of kerosene; used for denaturing ethyl alcohol.

aldehyde (al'dĕ-hīd). A compound containing the radical —CH=O, reducible to an alcohol (CH_2OH), oxidizable to an acid (COOH); *e.g.,* acetaldehyde.
angular a., the a. group attached to carbon 13 (between rings C and D) of the steroid nucleus in aldosterone.
a. reductase, alcohol dehydrogenase.

aldehyde base. Obsolete term for an imide.

aldehyde dehydrogenase (acylating) [EC 1.2.1.10]. An oxidoreductase converting an aldehyde and CoA to acyl-CoA with NAD^+ as H acceptor.

aldehyde dehydrogenase (NAD^+) [EC 1.2.1.3]. Aldehyde → DPN transhydrogenase; an oxidoreductase converting aldehydes to acids with NAD^+ as H acceptor.

aldehyde dehydrogenase ($NADP^+$) [EC 1.2.1.4]. Aldehyde → TPN transhydrogenase; an oxidoreductase converting aldehydes to acids with $NADP^+$ as H acceptor.

aldehyde dehydrogenase ($NAD(P)^+$) [EC 1.2.1.5]. An oxidoreductase converting aldehydes to acids with NAD^+ or $NADP^+$ as H acceptor.

aldehyde → DPN transhydrogenase. Aldehyde dehydrogenase (NAD^+).

aldehyde fuchsin. See Gomori's aldehyde fuchsin *stain.*

aldehyde-lyases [EC sub-subgroup 4.1.2]. Enzymes catalyzing the reversal of an aldol condensation.

aldehyde → TPN transhydrogenase. Aldehyde dehydrogenase ($NADP^+$).

Alder, Albert von. See A.'s *anomaly,* A. *bodies.*

alditol (al'di-tol). The alcohol derived by reduction of an aldose; *e.g.,* sorbitol. See also *aldose* reductase.

aldobiuronic acid (al'dō-bī-yū-ron'ik). Condensation products of an aldose and a uronic acid; such groupings occur among the components of various mucopolysaccharides, notably hyaluronic acid.

aldocortin (al'dō-kōr'tin). Aldosterone.

aldohexose (al-dō-heks'ōs). A 6-carbon sugar characterized by the (potential) presence of an aldehyde group in the molecule; *e.g.,* glucose, galactose.

aldoketomutase (al'dō-kē-tō-myū'tās). Lactoylglutathione lyase.

aldolase (al'dō-lās). **1.** Generic term for aldehyde-lyase. **2.** Name sometimes applied to fructose-bisphosphate aldolase.

aldonic acids (al-don'ik). Glyconic acids; monosaccharide derivatives in which the aldehyde group has been oxidized to a carboxyl group.

aldopentose (al-dō-pen'tōs). A monosaccharide with five carbon atoms, of which one is a (potential) aldehyde group; *e.g.,* ribose.

aldose (al'dōs). A monosaccharide potentially containing the characteristic group of the aldehydes, —CHO.
a. mutarotase, aldose 1-epimerase.
a. reductase [EC 1.1.1.21], polyol dehydrogenase ($NADP^+$); an oxidoreductase that converts aldoses to alditols (*e.g.,* glucose to sorbitol) with NADPH as hydrogen donor. See also sorbitol-6-phosphate dehydrogenase.

aldose 1-epimerase [EC 5.1.3.3]. Aldose mutarotase; mutarotase; an enzyme catalyzing interconversion of α- and β-D-glucose; also acts on L-arabinose, D-xylose, D-galactose, maltose, and lactose.

aldoside (al'dō-sīd). A glucoside in which the sugar moiety is an aldose.

aldosterone (al-dos'ter-ōn). Aldocortin; 11β,21-dihydroxy-3,30-dioxopregn-4-en-18-al(11→18 lactone); a steroid hormone produced by the zona glomerulosa of the adrenal cortex; its major action is to facilitate potassium exchange for sodium in the distal renal tubule, causing sodium reabsorption and potassium and hydrogen loss.

aldosteronism (al-dos'ter-on-izm). Hyperaldosteronism; a disorder caused by excessive secretion of aldosterone.
idiopathic a., primary a.
primary a., idiopathic a.; Conn's syndrome; an adrenocortical disorder caused by excessive secretion of aldosterone and characterized by headaches, nocturia, polyuria, fatigue, hypertension, hypokalemic alkalosis, potassium depletion, hypervolemia, and decreased plasma renin activity; may be associated with small benign adrenocortical adenomas.
secondary a., a. resulting not from a defect intrinsic to the adrenal cortex but from a stimulation of hormonal secretion caused by extra-adrenal disorders; associated with increased plasma renin activity and occurs in heart failure, nephrotic syndrome, cirrhosis, and hypoproteinemia.

aldotetrose (al-dō-tet'rōs). A four-carbon aldose; *e.g.,* threose, erythrose.

aldoxime (al-doks'ēm). A compound derived by the reaction of an aldose with hydroxylamine, thus containing the a. group —HC=NOH.

Aldrich, Robert Anderson, U.S. pediatrician, *1917. See A. *syndrome,* Wiskott-A. *syndrome.*

al'drin. A hexachlorohexahydrodimethanonaphthalene; a volatile chlorinated hydrocarbon used as an insecticide; if absorbed through the skin, it causes toxic symptoms consisting of irritability followed by depression.

alecithal (ă-les'i-thal) [G. *a-* priv. + *lekithos,* yolk]. Without yolk; denoting ova with little or no deutoplasm.

Alectorobius talaje (ă-lek-tōr-ō'bē-ŭs tă-lă'jē). An insect, commonly found in Mexico and South America, whose bites, like those of the bedbug, may suppurate.

alemmal (ă-lem'ăl) [G. *a-* priv. + *lemma,* husk]. Denoting a nerve fiber lacking a neurolemma.

alethia (ă-lē'thē-ă) [G. *a-* priv. + *lēthē,* forgetfulness]. Rarely used term for an incapacity to forget past events.

aletocyte (ă-lē'tō-sīt) [G. *alētēs,* a wanderer, + *kytos,* cell]. Obsolete term for a wandering cell of uncertain origin.

aleukemia (ă-lū-kē'mē-ă) [G. *a-* priv. + *leukos,* white, + *haima,* blood]. **1.** Literally, a lack of leukocytes in the blood. The term is generally used to indicate varieties of leukemic disease in which the white blood cell count in circulating blood is normal or even less than normal (*i.e.,* no leukocytosis), but a few young leukocytes are observed; sometimes used more restrictedly for unusual instances of leukemia with no leukocytosis and no young forms in the blood. **2.** Leukemic changes in bone marrow associated with a subnormal number of leukocytes in the blood. See also subleukemic *leukemia.*

aleukemic (ă-lū-kē'mik). Pertaining to aleukemia.

aleukemoid (ă-lū-kē'moyd). Resembling aleukemia symptomatically.

aleukia (ă-lū'kē-ă) [G. *a-* priv. + *leukos,* white]. **1.** Absence or extremely decreased number of leukocytes in the circulating blood; sometimes also termed aleukemic myelosis. **2.** Obsolete name for thrombocytopenia.

aleukocytic (ă-lū-kō-sit'ik). Manifesting absence or extremely reduced numbers of leukocytes in blood or lesions.

aleukocytosis (ă-lū-kō-sī-tō'sis) [G. *a-* priv. + *leukos,* white, + *kytos,* a hollow (cell)]. Absence or great reduction (relative or absolute) of the number of white blood cells in the circulating blood (*i.e.,* an advanced degree of leukopenia), or the lack of leukocytes in an anatomical lesion.

aleurioconidium (ă-lū'rē-ō-kō-nid'ē-ŭm) [G. *aleuron,* flour, + conidium]. Aleuriospore; a conidium developed from the blownout end of conidiogenous cells or hyphal branches, and released by rupture below the base of attachment.

aleuriospore (ă-lū'rē-ō-spōr). Aleurioconidium.

aleuron (al'ū-rōn) [G. flour]. Protein granules in the endosperm of seeds, supposed to contain the vitamins of edible seeds and grains.

aleuronate (ă-lū'rō-nāt). Protein from the aleuron layer (endosperm) of cereal grains; used to make bread for diabetics.

aleuronoid (ă-lū'rō-noyd). Resembling flour.

Alexander, W. Stewart, contemporary British pathologist. See A.'s *disease.*

Alexanders's deafness. See under deafness.

alexia (ă-lek'sē-ă) [G. *a-* priv. + *lexis,* a word or phrase]. Word or text blindness; visual aphasia (1); loss of the ability to grasp the meaning of written or printed words and sentences. Also called **optical, sensory,** or **visual a.,** in distinction to **motor a.** (anarthria), in which there is loss of the power to read aloud although the significance of what is written or printed is understood.
incomplete a., dyslexia.
musical a., music or note blindness; loss of the power to read musical notation.

alexic (ă-lek'sik). Pertaining to alexia.

alexin (ă-lek'sin) [G. *alexō,* to ward off]. Buchner's term for the bactericidal substances of cell-free serum, the activity of which is destroyed by heating at 56°C; applied by Bordet to the heat-labile substance normally present in serum and distinct from the sensitizing substance (antibody) produced by infection or immunization. In this sense it is synonymous with complement.

alexipharmac (ă-lek-si-far'mak) [G. *alexipharmakos,* preserving against poison]. **1.** Antidotal. **2.** An antidote.

alexithymia (ă-lek-si-thī'mē-ă) [G. *a-* priv. + *lexis,* word, + *-thymia,* feelings, passion]. Difficulty in recognizing and describing one's emotions, defining them in terms of somatic sensations or behavioral reactions.

aleydigism (ă-lī'dig-izm). Aplasia of Leydig cells, seen in hypogonadotrophic hypogonadism.

Alezzandrini, A.A., 20th century Argentinian ophthalmologist. See A.'s *syndrome.*

alfacalcidol (al-fă-kal'si-dol). 1-α-Hydroxycholecalciferol; a derivative of vitamin D used in the treatment of hypoparathyroidism, vitamin D dependent rickets, and rickets associated with malabsorption syndromes.

alfadolone acetate (al-fad'ō-lōn). Alphadolone acetate; 21-acetoxy-3α-hydroxy-5α-pregnane-11,20-dione; a weak anesthetic agent used primarily to enhance the solubility of alfaxalone.

alfaxalone (al-faks'ă-lōn). Alphaxalone; 3α-hydroxy-5α-pregnane-11,20-dione; a short-acting general anesthetic used with alfadolone acetate.

alfentanil hydrochloride (al-fen'tă-nil). $C_{21}H_{32}N_6O_3 \cdot HCl \cdot H_2O$; a narcotic agonist analgesic used as an anesthetic or as an adjunct in the maintenance of general anesthesia.

algae (al'jē) [pl. of L. *alga,* seaweed]. A division of eukaryotic, photosynthetic, nonflowering organisms that includes many seaweeds.
blue-green a., former name for the blue-green bacteria, now classified as Cyanobacteria.

algal (al'găl). Resembling or pertaining to algae.

algaroba (al-gă-rō'bă). Carob flour; locust gum; ground meal of the fruit of *Ceratonia siliqua;* used as an adsorbent-demulcent in the treatment of diarrhea.

alge-, algesi-, algio-, algo- [G. *algos,* pain]. Combining forms meaning pain.

algedonic (al-jē-don'ik) [G. *algos,* pain, + *hēdonē,* pleasure]. Relating to a mixed sensation or emotion of pleasure and pain.

algefacient (al-jē-fā'shent) [L. *algeo,* to be cold, + *facio,* pr. pl. *-iens,* to make]. An agent that has a cooling action.

algesi-. See alge-.

algesia (al-jē'zē-ă) [G. *algēsis,* a sense of pain]. Algesthesia.

algesic (al-jē'sik). Algetic.

algesichronometer (al-jē'zē-krō-nom'ĕ-ter) [G. *algēsis,* sense of pain, + *chronos,* time, + *metron,* measure]. An instrument for recording the time required for the perception of a painful stimulus.

algesidystrophy (al-jē-si-dis'trō-fē) [G. *algēsis,* sense of pain, + *dys-,* bad, + *trophē,* nourishment]. Algodystrophy.

algesimeter (al-jē-sim'ĕ-ter). Algesiometer.

algesiogenic (al-jē'zē-ō-jen'ik) [G. *algēsis,* sense of pain, + *-gen,* production]. Algogenic; pain-producing.

algesiometer (al-jē-zē-om'ĕ-ter) [G. *algēsis,* sense of pain, + *metron,* measure]. Algesimeter; algometer; odynometer; an instrument for measuring the degree of sensitivity to a painful stimulus.

algesthesia (al-jes-thē'zē-ă) [G. *algos,* pain, + *aisthēsis,* sensation]. Algesia; algesthesis. **1.** The appreciation of pain. **2.** Hypersensitivity to pain.

algesthesis (al-jes-thē'sis). Algesthesia.

algestone acetophenide (al-jes'tōn ă-sē-tō-fē'nīd). Alphasone acetophenide; 16α,17-dihydroxypregn-4-ene-3,20-dione cyclic acetal with acetophenone; a progestogen with contraceptive properties.

algetic (al-jet'ik). Algesic. **1.** Painful, or relating to or causing pain. **2.** Relating to hypersensitivity to pain.

-algia [G. *algos,* pain]. Suffix meaning pain or painful condition.

algicide (al'ji-sīd) [algae, + L. *caedo,* to kill]. An agent active against algae.

algid (al'jid) [L. *algidus,* cold]. Chilly, cold.

algin (al'jin). Sodium alginate; a carbohydrate product from a seaweed, *Macrocystis pyrifera;* used as a gel in pharmaceutical preparations.

alginate (al'ji-nāt). An irreversible hydrocolloid consisting of salts of alginic acid, a colloidal acid polysaccharide obtained from seaweed and composed of mannuronic acid residues; used in dental impression materials.

algio-. See alge-.

algiomotor (al-jē-ō-mō'tōr). Algiomuscular; causing painful muscular contractions.

algiomuscular (al'jē-ō-mŭs'kyū-lăr). Algiomotor.

algiovascular (al'jē-ō-vas'kyū-lăr). Algovascular.

algo-. See alge-.

algodystrophy (al-gō-dis'trō-fē) [algo- + G. *dys-,* bad, + *trophē,* nourishment]. Algesidystrophy; a painful local disturbance of growth, particularly due to focal aseptic necrosis of bone and cartilage.

algogenesis, algogenesia (al-gō-jen'ĕ-sis, -jē-nē'zē-ă) [algo- + G. *genesis,* origin]. The production or origin of pain.

algogenic (al-gō-jen'ik). Algesiogenic.

algolagnia (al-gō-lag'nē-ă) [algo- + G. *lagneia,* lust]. Algophilia (2); form of sexual perversion in which the infliction or the experiencing of pain increases the pleasure of the sexual act or causes sexual pleasure independent of the act; includes both sadism (active a.) and masochism (passive a.).

algometer (al-gom'ĕ-ter) [algo- + G. *metron,* measure]. Algesiometer.

algometry (al-gom'ĕ-trē). The process of measuring pain.

algophilia (al-gō-fil'ē-ă) [algo- + G. *phileō*, to love]. **1.** Pleasure experienced in the thought of pain in others or in oneself. **2.** Algolagnia.

algophobia (al-gō-fō'bē-ă) [algo- + G. *phobos*, fear]. Abnormal fear of or sensitiveness to pain.

algopsychalia (al-go-si-ka'lĭ-ah) [algo- + G. *psychē*, mind]. Psychalgia (1).

algorithm (al'gō-ridhm). A step-by-step written protocol for management of health care problems.

algoscopy (al-gos'kŏ-pē) [L. *algor*, cold, + G. *skopeō*, to view]. Cryoscopy.

algospasm (al'gō-spazm) [G. *algos*, pain, + *spasmos*, convulsion]. Spasm produced by pain.

algovascular (al-gō-vas'kyū-lăr) [G. *algos*, pain]. Algiovascular; relating to changes in the lumen of the blood vessels occurring under the influence of pain.

alible (al'i-bl) [L. *alibilis*, nutritive, fr. *alo*, to nourish]. Nutritive.

alicyclic (al-i-sik'lik). Denoting an alicyclic compound.

alienation (ā-lē-en-ā'shŭn) [L. *alieno*, pp. *-atus*, to make strange]. A condition characterized by lack of meaningful relationships to others, sometimes resulting in depersonalization and estrangement from others.

alienia (ā-li-ē'nē-ă) [G. *a-* priv. + L. *lien*, spleen]. Congenital absence of the spleen.

alienist (āl'yen-ist, ā-lē'en-ist). Obsolete term for one who treats mental diseases.

aliflurane (al-i-flū'rān). 1-Chloro-1,2,2,3-tetrafluoro-3-methoxycyclopropane; a synthetic compound with anesthetic properties.

aliform (al'i-fōrm) [L. *ala*, + *forma*, shape]. Wing-shaped.

alignment (ă-līn'ment). Alinement. **1.** The longitudinal position of a bone or limb. **2.** The act of bringing into line. **3.** In dentistry, the arrangement of the teeth in relation to the supporting structures and the adjacent and opposing dentitions.

aliment (al'i-ment) [L. *alo*, to nourish]. **1.** Food; nourishment. **2.** In sensorimotor theory, that which is assimilated to a schema; analogous to a stimulus.

alimentary (al-i-men'ter-ē) [L. *alimentarius*, fr. *alimentum*, nourishment]. Relating to food or nutrition.

alimentation (al-i-men-tā'shŭm). Providing nourishment. See also feeding.

forced a., forced *feeding*.

parenteral a., providing nourishment intravenously.

rectal a., nourishment provided by retention enemas.

alinasal (al'i-nā'săl) [L. *ala*, + *nasus*, nose]. Relating to the alae nasi, or flaring portions of the nostrils.

alinement (ă-līn'ment). Alignment.

alinjection (al'in-jek'shŭn). Injection of alcohol for hardening and preserving pathologic and histologic specimens.

aliphatic (al-i-fat'ik) [G. *aleiphar* (*aleiphat-*), fat, oil]. Denoting the acyclic carbon compounds, most of which belong to the fatty acid series.

aliphatic acids. The acids of nonaromatic hydrocarbons (*e.g.*, acetic, propionic, butyric acids); the so-called fatty acids of the formula R-COOH, where R is a nonaromatic (aliphatic) hydrocarbon.

alipoid (ā-lip'oyd) [G. *a-* priv. + *lipoidēs*, resembling fat]. Characterized by absence of lipoids.

alipotropic (ā'lip-ō-trōp'ik) [G. *a-* priv. + *lipos*, fat, + *tropos*, a turning]. Having no effect upon fat metabolism, or upon the movement of fat to the liver.

aliquant (al'ĭ-kwant). In chemistry and immunology, pertaining to a portion that results from dividing the whole in a manner that some is left after the a.'s (equal in volume or weight) have been apportioned.

aliquot (al'i-kwot). In chemistry and immunology, pertaining to a portion of the whole; loosely, any one of two or more samples of something, of the same volume or weight.

alisphenoid (al-i-sfē'noyd) [L. *ala*, + *sphēn*, wedge]. Relating to the greater wing of the sphenoid bone.

alizarin (ă-liz'ă-rin) [C.I. 58000]. 1,2-Dihydroxyanthraquinone; a red dye that occurs in the root of madder (***Rubia tinctorum***) in glucose combination (ruberythric acid) as orange needles, slightly soluble in water; used by the ancients as a dye. Now made synthetically from anthracene and used in the manufacture of dyes, *e.g.*, a. blue, a. orange, "Turkey red." As an indicator, it changes from yellow to red at pH 5.5 to 6.8; other modified a.'s have other colors and change color at other pH values.

a. cyanin [C.I. 58610], the disulfonate of hexahydroxyanthraquinone, $C_{14}H_6O_{14}S_2Na_2$; an acid dye used as a nuclear stain after mordanting and as a fluorochrome in ultraviolet microscopy.

a. purpurin, purpurin.

a. red S [C.I. 58005], sodium a. sulfonate; used as a stain for calcium in bone (calcium appears red-orange, magnesium, aluminum, and barium are varying shades of red), in the determination of fluorine; as a pH indicator it changes from yellow to purple between pH 3.7 and 5.2.

alkadiene (al-kă-dī'ēn). An acyclic hydrocarbon (alkane) containing two double bonds.

alkalemia (al-kă-lē'mē-ă) [alkali + G. *haima*, blood]. A decrease in H-ion concentration of the blood or a rise in pH, irrespective of alterations in the level of bicarbonate ion.

alkalescence (al-kal-es'ens). **1.** A slight alkalinity. **2.** The process of becoming alkaline.

alkalescent (al-kal-es'ent). **1.** Slightly alkaline. **2.** Becoming alkaline.

alkali, pl. alkalis, alkalies (al'kă-lī, -līz) [Ar., *al*, the, + *qalīy*, soda ash]. A strongly basic substance yielding hydroxide ions (OH^-) in solution; *e.g.*, sodium hydroxide, potassium hydroxide.

caustic a., a highly ionized (in solution) alkali; *e.g.*, NaOH.

fixed a., any a. other than a weakly ionized one, like ammonia.

vegetable a., a mixture of potassium hydroxide and carbonate.

alkaline (al'kă-līn). Relating to or having the reaction of an alkali.

alkalinity (al-kă-lin'i-tē). The state of being alkaline.

alkalinization (al'kă-lin-i-zā'shŭn). Alkalization.

alkalinuria (al'kă-li-nū'rē-ă) [alkaline + G. *ouron*, urine]. Alkaluria; the passage of alkaline urine.

alkalitherapy (al'kă-lī-thār'ă-pē). Therapeutic use of alkali for local or systemic effect.

alkalization (al'kal-i-zā'shŭn). Alkalinization; the process of rendering alkaline.

alkalizer (al'kă-līz-er). An agent that neutralizes acids or renders a solution alkaline.

alkaloid (al'kă-loyd). Vegetable base; originally, any one of hundreds of plant products distinguished by alkaline (basic) reactions, but now restricted to heterocyclic nitrogen-containing and often complex structures possessing pharmacological activity; their trivial names usually end in -ine. A.'s are synthesized by plants and are found in the leaf, bark, seed, or other parts, usually constituting the active principle of the crude drug; they are a loosely defined group, but may be classified according to the chemical structure of their main nucleus. For medicinal purposes, the salts of a.'s are usually used.

fixed a., a nonvolatile a.

alkalosis (al-kă-lō'sis). A pathophysiological disorder characterized by H-ion loss or base excess in body fluids (metabolic a.), or caused by CO_2 loss due to hyperventilation (respiratory a.).
acapnial a., respiratory a.
compensated a., a. in which there is a change in bicarbonate but the pH of body fluids approaches normal; respiratory a. may be compensated by increased production of metabolic acids or increased renal excretion of bicarbonate; metabolic a. is rarely compensated by hypoventilation.
metabolic a., an a. associated with an increased arterial plasma bicarbonate concentration, possibly resulting from an excessive intake of alkaline materials or an excessive loss of acid in the urine or through persistent vomiting; the base excess and standard bicarbonate are both elevated. See also compensated a.
respiratory a., acapnial a.; a. resulting from abnormal loss of CO_2 produced by hyperventilation, either active or passive, with concomitant reduction in arterial plasma bicarbonate concentration. See also compensated a.
uncompensated a., a. in which the pH of body fluids is elevated because of lack of the compensatory mechanisms of compensated a.

alkalotic (al-kă-lot'ik). Relating to alkalosis.

alkaluria (al-kă-lū'rē-ă). Alkalinuria.

alkane (al'kān). The general term for a saturated acyclic hydrocarbon; *e.g.,* propane, butane.

alkanet (al'kă-net) [C.I. 75530, 75520]. The root of a herb, *Alkanna,* or *Anchusa tinctoria* (family Boraginaceae), that yields red dyes alkannan and alkannin; used as a coloring agent; also used, combined with tannin, as an astringent.

alkannan (al'kă-nan) [C.I. 75520]. A minor red dye component derived from alkanet.

alkannin (al'kă-nin) [C.I. 75530]. Anchusin; (-)-5,8-dihydroxy-2-(1-hydroxy-4-methyl-3-pentenyl)-1,4-naphthoquinone; the major red dye derived from alkanet; used as an astringent, and in cosmetics and foods; can be used as an indicator: red at pH 6.8, changing to purple at pH 8.8 and blue at pH 10.0; also used as a fat stain.

alkapton (al-kap'tōn) [Boedeker's coinage fr. alkali + G. *kaptein,* to suck up greedily]. Homogentisic acid.

alkaptonuria (al-kap-tō-nū'rē-ă) [alkapton + G. *ouron,* urine]. Alcaptonuria; homogentisuria; excretion of homogentisic acid (alkapton) in the urine due to congenital lack of the enzyme homogentisate 1,2-dioxygenase, which mediates an essential step in the catabolism of phenylalanine and tyrosine; urine turns dark if allowed to stand or is alkalinized (a result of formation of polymerization products of homogentisic acid); frequently occurs throughout relatively long periods or may recur and subside at irregular intervals; arthritis and ochronosis are late complications; autosomal recessive inheritance.

alkatriene (al-kă-trī'ēn). An acyclic hydrocarbon containing three double bonds; *e.g.,* octatriene, CH_3—CH=CH—CH=CH—CH=CH—CH_3.

alkavervir (al-kă-ver'vir). A mixture of alkaloids obtained by the selective extraction of *Veratrum viride* with various organic solvents; used orally or parenterally as a hypotensive agent.

alkene (al'kēn). An acyclic hydrocarbon containing one double bond; *e.g.,* ethylene.

alkenyl (al'ken-il). The radical of an alkene.

alk-1-enyl. The radical of an alkene in which the double bond indicated by "en(e)" is between carbons 1 and 2 (carbon 1 being the radical or "yl" carbon), *i.e.,* R—CH=CH—; sometimes expressed as alk-1-en-1-yl.

alk-1-enylglycerophospholipid. A phosphatidate in which at least one of the radicals attached to the glycerol is an alk-1-enyl rather than the usual acyl radical (*i.e.,* is derived from an aldehyde rather than an acid, hence the older trivial names phosphatidal and acetal phosphatid(at)e); "plasmenic acid" has been proposed as a name for such phosphatidates.

alkide (al'kīd). Alkyl (2).

alkyl (al'kil). **1.** A hydrocarbon radical of the general formula C_nH_{2n+1}. **2.** Alkide; a compound, such as tetraethyl lead, in which a metal is combined with alkyl radicals.
arylated a., aralkyl.

alkylamine (al-kil'ă-mēn). An alkane containing an —NH_2 group in place of one H atom; *e.g.,* ethylamine.

alkylation (al'ki-lā'shŭn). Substitution of an alkyl radical for a hydrogen atom; *e.g.,* introduction of a side chain into an aromatic compound.

ALL Abbreviation for acute lymphocytic leukemia. See lymphocytic *leukemia.*

allachesthesia (al'ă-kes-thē'zē-ă) [G. *allachē,* elsewhere, + *aisthēsis,* sensation]. A condition in which a sensation is referred to a point other than that to which the stimulus is applied.
optical a., visual *allesthesia.*

allantiasis (al-an-tī'ă-sis) [G. *allas* (*allant-*), sausage]. Obsolete term for sausage poisoning due to botulism.

allanto-, allant- [G. *allas,* sausage]. Combining forms for allantois, allantoid.

allantochorion (ă-lan-tō-kōr'ē-on). Extraembryonic membrane formed by the fusion of the allantois and chorion.

allantogenesis (ă-lan-tō-jen'ĕ-sis) [allanto- + G. *genesis,* origin]. Development of the allantois.

allantoic (ă-lan-tō'ik). Relating to the allantois.

allantoid (ă-lan'toyd) [allanto- + G. *eidos,* appearance]. **1.** Sausage-shaped. **2.** Relating to, or resembling, the allantois.

allantoidoangiopagus (ă-lan-toyd'ō-an-jē-op'ă-gŭs) [allantoid + G. *angeion,* vessel, + *pagos,* fastened]. See allantoidoangiopagous *twins.*

allantoin (ă-lan'tō-in). Glyoxyldiureide; cordianine; 5-ureidohydantoin; a substance present in allantoic fluid, fetal urine, and elsewhere; also an oxidation product of uric acid and the end product of purine metabolism in animals other than man and the other primates.

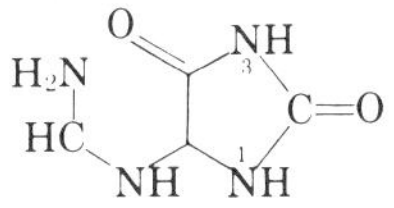

Allantoin

allantoinase (ă-lan-tō'i-nās) [EC 3.5.2.5]. An enzyme (an amidohydrolase) that catalyzes the hydrolysis of allantoin to allantoic acid.

allantoinuria (ă-lan'tō-in-yū'rē-ă) [allantoin + G. *ouron,* urine]. The urinary excretion of allantoin; normal in most mammals, abnormal in man.

allantois (ă-lan'tō-is) [allanto- + G. *eidos,* appearance]. Allantoid membrane; a fetal membrane developing from the hindgut (or yolk sac, in man). In man it is vestigial; externally, in mammals, it contributes to the formation of the umbilical cord and placenta; in birds and reptiles it lies close beneath the porous shell and serves as an organ of respiration.

allaxis (ă-laks'is) [G. *allattein,* to alter]. Metamorphosis.

allele (ă-lēl') [G. *allelōn,* reciprocally]. Allelomorph; any one of a series of two or more different genes that may occupy the same position or locus on a specific chromosome. As autosomal chromosomes are paired, each autosomal locus is represented twice in normal somatic cells. If the same a. occupies both loci, the individual or cell is homozygous for this a. If the a.'s at the two loci are different, the individual or cell is heterozygous for both a.'s. See also *dominance* of genes.

codominant a., see codominant.

silent a., amorph.

allelic (ă-lē'lik). Allelomorphic; relating to an allele.

allelism (al'ē-lizm). Allelomorphism; the state held in common by alleles.

allelocatalysis (ă-lē'lō-kă-tal'i-sis) [G. *allēlōn,* mutually, reciprocally, + *catalytikos,* able to dissolve]. Self-stimulation of growth in a bacterial culture by addition of similar cells.

allelocatalytic (ă-lē'lō-kat-ă-lit'ik). Mutually catalytic; denoting two substances each of which is decomposed in the presence of the other.

allelomorph (ă-lē'lō-mōrf) [G. *allēlōn,* reciprocally, + *morphē,* shape]. Allele.

allelomorphic (ă-lē-lō-mōr'fik). Allelic.

allelomorphism (ă-lē-lō-mōr'fizm). Allelism.

allelotaxis, allelotaxy (ă-lēl-ō-taks'is, -taks'ē) [G. *allēlōn,* reciprocally, + *taxis,* an arranging]. Development of an organ from a number of embryonal structures or tissues.

Allen, Alfred Henry, U.S. chemist, 1846–1904. See A.'s *test.*

Allen, Edgar, U.S. endocrinologist, 1892–1943. See A.-Doisy *test, unit.*

Allen, Edgar Van Nuys, U.S. physician, 1900–1961. See A. *test;* radial compression *test* of A.

Allen, Willard Myron, U.S. gynecologist, *1904. See Corner-A. *test, unit;* A.-Masters *syndrome.*

allergen (al'er-jen) [allergy + G. *-gen,* producing]. Antigen; von Pirquet's term for an incitant of altered reactivity (allergy).

allergenic (al-er-jen'ik). Antigenic.

allergic (ă-ler'jik). Relating to any response stimulated by an allergen.

allergic salute. A characteristic wiping or rubbing of the nose with a transverse or upward movement of the hand, as seen in children with allergic rhinitis.

allergin (al'er-jin). A seldom used term denoting the reactive substance in the passive transference of anaphylaxis.

allergist (al'er-jist). One who specializes in the treatment of allergies.

allergization (al'er-ji-zā'shŭn). Active sensitization as a result of allergens being naturally or artificially brought into contact with susceptible tissues; the procedure of being allergized.

allergized (al'er-jīzd). Specifically altered in reactivity; rendered capable of exhibiting one or another aspect of allergy.

allergodermia (al'er-gō-der'mē-ă). An allergic dermatitis.

allergosis (al'er-gō'sis) [allergy + G. *-osis,* condition]. Any abnormal condition characterized by allergy.

allergy (al'er-jē) [G. *allos,* other, + *ergon,* work]. **1.** Acquired or induced sensitivity; the immunologic state induced in a susceptible subject by an antigen (allergen), characterized by a marked change in the subject's reactivity; on initial contact with the antigen, no immunologic reaction occurs, but after a latent period of several days to two weeks or so, the subject becomes sensitive, even to antigen that persists from the initial inoculation (as in serum sickness); thereafter, the specific antigen evokes a reaction within minutes or hours, the severity of which depends upon quantitative relationships and route of entrance. The term "allergy" was coined by von Pirquet as an all-inclusive one for the various forms of changed reactivity which had been discovered by immunologists; "immune" was to be reserved for the state of complete freedom from reaction to substances which might be allergenic (antigenic) in some other subject. For a time, "allergy" was restricted in usage, in some areas to type I allergic reactions, but the present tendency is to return to the more general usage. See also allergic *reaction;* anaphylaxis. **2.** That branch of medicine concerned with the study, diagnosis, and treatment of allergic manifestations. **3.** An acquired hypersensitivity to certain drugs and biologic preparations.

atopic a., see atopy.

bacterial a., **(1)** the unproven concept that the atopic kind of type I allergic reactions may be caused by bacterial allergens; **(2)** the delayed type of skin test, so-called because of its early association with bacterial antigens (*e.g.,* the tuberculin test).

cold a., physical symptons produced by hypersensitivity to cold.

contact a., cutaneous reaction caused by direct contact with an allergen to which the individual is hypersensitive.

delayed a., a type IV allergic reaction; so called because in a sensitized subject the reaction becomes evident only several or more hours after contact with the allergen (antigen), reaches its peak after 36 to 48 hours, then recedes slowly. *Cf.* immediate a. See also delayed *reaction.*

drug a., sensitivity (hypersensitivity) to a drug or other chemical.

immediate a., a type I allergic reaction; so called because in a sensitized subject the reaction becomes evident usually within minutes after contact with the allergen (antigen), reaches its peak within an hour or so, then rapidly recedes. *Cf.* delayed a. See also immediate *reaction.*

latent a., a. that causes no signs or symptoms but can be revealed by means of certain immunologic tests with specific allergens.

physical a., excessive response to factors in the environment such as heat or cold.

polyvalent a., allergic response manifested simultaneously for several or numerous specific allergens.

Allescheria boydii (al-es-kē'rē-ă boy'dē-ī). *Pseudallescheria boydii.*

allesthesia (al-es-thē'zē-ă) [G. *allos,* other, + *aisthēsis,* sensation]. Allocheiria; allochiria; alloesthesia; Bamberger's sign (2); a form of allachesthesia in which the sensation of a stimulus in one limb is referred to the opposite limb.

visual a., optical allachesthesia; a disorder characterized by the transposition of images from one half of the visual field to the opposite.

allethrins (al'ĕ-thrinz). Allethrolone esters of chrysanthemum-monocarboxylic acids and synthetic analogs of pyrethrins, which are pyrethrolone esters of the same acids; viscous liquids, insoluble in water, that can be absorbed by lungs, skin, and mucous membranes and may cause liver and kidney injury, with lung congestion; used as an insecticide.

allethrolone (ă-leth'rō-lōn). 2-Methyl-4-oxo-3-(2-propenyl)-2-cyclopentenol; an analog of pyrethrolone (2-propenyl replacing the 2,4-pentadienyl group) used in allethrins.

alligation (al-i-gā'shŭn) [L. *alligatio,* fr. *al-ligo* (*adl-*), pp. *-atus,* to bind to]. A rule of mixtures whereby 1) the cost of a mixture may be determined, given the proportions and prices of the several ingredients; or 2) in pharmacy, the relative amounts of solutions of different percentages which must be taken to form a mixture of a given strength.

Allis, Oscar Huntington, U.S. surgeon, 1836–1921. See A.'s *forceps, sign.*

alliteration (ă-lit-er-ā'shŭn) [Fr. *allitération,* fr. L. *ad,* to, + *litteram,* letter of alphabet]. In psychiatry, a speech disturbance in which words commencing with the same sounds, usually consonants, are notably frequent.

allium (al'ē-ŭm). Garlic; *Allium sativum* (family Liliaceae), whose bulb contains up to 0.9% of volatile irritating oil with antiseptic action (see alliin); has been used as a diaphoretic, diuretic, and expectorant.

allo- [G. *allos,* other]. **1.** Prefix meaning "other" or differing from the normal or usual. **2.** Prefix formerly used with amino acids whenever their side chain contained an asymmetric carbon; now used only for the alloisoleucines and allothreonines.

alloalbuminemia (al'ō-al-byū'mi-nē'mē-ă). The condition of having serum albumin of a variant type that differs in mobility on electrophoresis from the usual type A; individuals are heterozygous or homozygous for one of the genes for variant albumin types, a genetic polymorphism without known clinical significance. See also inherited albumin *variants.*

alloantibody (al-ō-an'ti-bod-ē). An antibody specific for an alloantigen. Isoantibody is sometimes used in this sense.

alloantigen (al-ō-an'ti-jen). An antigen that occurs in some, but not in other members of the same species. Isoantigen is sometimes used in this sense.

alloarthroplasty (al-ō-arth'rō-plas-tē) [allo- + G. *arthron,* joint, + *plastos,* formed]. Formation of another or a new joint, using material not from the human body; *e.g.,* total joint replacement with prostheses.

allobarbital (al-ō-bar'bi-tal). 5,5-Diallylbarbituric acid; a hypnotic with intermediate duration of action.

allocentric (al-ō-sen'trik) [allo- + G. *kentron,* center]. Heterocentric; characterized by or denoting interest centered in other persons rather than in one's self. *Cf.* egocentric.

allocheiria, allochiria (al-ō-kī'rē-ă) [allo- + G. *cheir,* hand]. Allesthesia.

allochezia, allochetia (al-ō-kē'zē-ă, -kē'shē-ă) [allo- + G. *chezō,* to defecate]. Passage of feces through a fistula or other false passage.

allochiria (al'-ō-kī'rē-ă). Allocheiria.

allocholane (al-ō-kō'lān). See cholane.

allocholesterol (al-ō-kō-les'ter-ol). Coprostenol; cholest-4-en-3β-ol; an isomer of cholesterol, differing in the position of the one double bond.

allochroic (al-ō-krō'ik). Changed or changeable in color; relating to allochroism.

allochroism (al-ō-krō'izm) [allo- + G. *chrōa,* color]. A change or changeableness in color.

allochromasia (al-ō-krō-mā'zē-ă) [allo- + G. *chrōma,* color]. Change of color of the skin or hair.

allocortex (al'ō-kōr'teks) [allo- + L. *cortex,* bark (cortex)]. Heterotypic cortex; O. Vogt's term denoting several regions of the cerebral cortex, in particular the olfactory cortex and the hippocampus, characterized by fewer cell layers than the isocortex; see also *cortex* cerebri.

α-**allocortol** (al-ō-kōr'tol). 5α-Pregnane-3α,11β,17,20α,21-pentaol; the 5α enantiomer of α-cortol; a metabolite of hydroxycortisone found in the urine.

β-**allocortol.** 5α-Pregnane-3α,11β,17,20β,21-pentaol; the 20β isomer of α-allocortol and 5α enantiomer of β-cortol; a metabolite of hydrocortisone found in urine.

α-**allocortolone** (al-ō-kōr'tō-lōn). 3α,17,20α,21-Tetrahydroxy-5α-pregnane-11-one; the 5α enantiomer of α-cortolone; a metabolite of hydrocortisone found in urine.

β-**allocortolone.** 3α,17,20β,21-Tetrahydroxy-5α-pregnane-11-one; the 20β isomer of α-allocortolone and 5α enantiomer of β-cortolone; a metabolite of hydrocortisone found in urine.

allodiploid (al-ō-dip'loyd). See alloploid.

allodynia (al-ō-din'ē-ă) [allo- + G. *odynē,* pain]. The distress resulting from painful stimuli.

alloerotic (al'ō-ĕ-rot'ik). Heteroerotic; pertaining to or characterized by alloerotism.

alloeroticism (al'ō-ĕ-rot'i-sizm). Alloerotism.

alloerotism (al-ō-ār'ō-tizm) [allo- + G. *erōs,* love]. Alloeroticism; heteroerotism; sexual attraction toward another person. *Cf.* autoerotism.

alloesthesia (al-ō-es-thē'zē-ă). Allesthesia.

allogamy (al-og'ă-mē) [allo- + G. *gamos,* marriage]. Fertilization of the ova of one individual by the spermatozoa of another. *Cf.* autogamy.

allogenic, allogeneic (al-ō-jen'ik, -jĕ-nē'ik). **1.** Formerly, pertaining to a different species, or race. **2.** Pertaining to different gene constitutions within the same species.

allogotrophia (al'ō-gō-trō'fē-ă) [allo- + G. *trophē,* nourishment]. Growth or nourishment of one part or tissue at the expense of another part of the body.

allograft (al'ō-graft). Homograft; allogeneic, homologous, or homoplastic graft; a graft transplanted between genetically nonidentical individuals of the same species.

allogroup (al'ō-grūp). A term formerly used to denote a haplotype composed of closely linked allotypic markers.

allohexaploid (al-ō-heks'ă-ployd). See alloploid.

alloisomer (al-ō-ī'sōm-er). A geometric isomer.

allokeratoplasty (al-ō-ker'ă-tō-plas-tē). Replacement of opaque corneal tissue with a transparent prosthesis, usually plastic.

allokinesis (al-ō-ki-nē'sis, -kī-nē'sis) [allo- + G. *kinēsis,* movement]. **1.** Passive *movement.* **2.** Reflex *movement.*

allolalia (al-ō-lā'lē-ă) [allo- + G. *lalia,* talking]. Any speech defect, especially one due to disease affecting the speech center.

allomaleic acid (al-ō-mal'ē-ik). Fumaric acid.

allomerism (ă-lom'er-izm) [allo- + G. *meros,* part]. The state of differing in chemical composition but having the same crystalline form.

allometron (al-ō-me'tron) [allo- + G. *metron,* measure]. An evolutionary change in size or proportion of organic beings.

allomorphism (al-ō-mōr'fizm) [allo- + G. *morphē,* form]. **1.** Change of shape in cells due to mechanical causes, such as flattening from pressure, or to progressive metaplasia, such as the change of bile duct cells into liver cells. **2.** The state of being similar in chemical composition but differing in form (especially crystalline).

allongement (al-onzh'-maw) [Fr. elongation]. Lengthening of a structure during an operation by appropriate incisions.

allonomous (ă-lon'ō-mŭs) [allo- + G. *nomos,* law]. Governed by external stimuli.

allopath (al'ō-path). Allopathist. **1.** One who is a practitioner of allopathy. **2.** Erroneously, a traditional medical physician, as distinguished from eclectic or homeopathic practitioners.

allopathic (al-ō-path'ik). Relating to allopathy.

allopathist (al-op'ă-thist). Allopath.

allopathy (al-op'ă-thē) [allo- + G. *pathos,* suffering]. Substitutive therapy; a therapeutic system in which a disease is treated by producing a second condition that is incompatible with or antagonistic to the first. *Cf.* homeopathy.

allopentaploid (al-ō-pent'ă-ployd). See alloploid.

allophanamide (al'ō-fan-am'id). Biuret.

allophanic acid (al-ō-fan'ik). *N*-Carboxyurea; carbamoylcarbamic acid; urea carbonic acid, $NH_2CONHCOOH$; its amide is biuret (allophanamide).

allophasis (al-of'ă-sis) [allo- + G. *phasis,* speech]. Speech that is incoherent, disordered.

allophenic (al-ō-fē'nik). Pertaining to an animal with different cellular phenotypes produced by combining dividing fertilized eggs (blastomeres) of different genotypes (*i.e.*, from different pairs of parents).

allophore (al'ō-fōr). Erythrophore.

allophthalmia (al-of-thal'mē-ă). Heterophthalmus.

alloplasia (al-ō-plā'zē-ă) [allo- + G. *plasis*, a molding]. Heteroplasia.

alloplast (al'ō-plast) [allo- + G. *plastos*, formed]. **1.** A graft of an inert metal or plastic material. **2.** An inert foreign body used for implantation into tissues.

alloplasty (al'ō-plas-tē). Repair of defects by allotransplantation.

alloploid (al'ō-ployd) [allo- + -ploid]. Relating to a hybrid individual or cell with two or more sets of chromosomes derived from two different ancestral species; depending on the number of multiples of haploid sets, a.'s are referred to as allodiploids, allotriploids, allotetraploids, allopentaploids, allohexaploids, etc. See also heterokaryon.

alloploidy (al-ō-ploy'dē). The condition of being alloploid.

allopolyploid (al-ō-pol'i-ployd). An alloploid having two or more multiples of haploid sets of chromosomes.

allopolyploidy (al-ō-pol'i-ploy-dē). The condition of being allopolyploid.

allopregnane (al-ō-preg'nān). Original name for 5α-pregnane. See pregnane.

α-allopregnanediol (al'ō-preg-nān-dī'ol). 5α-Pregnane-3α,20α-diol; a metabolite of progesterone and adrenocortical hormones, found in urine.

β-allopregnanediol. The 5α-pregnane-3β,20α(and β)-diols; found in urine.

allopsychic (al-ō-sī'kik) [allo- + G. *psychē*, mind]. Denoting the mental processes in their relation to the outer world.

allopurinol (al-ō-pyū'ri-nol). 4-Hydroxypyrazolo-[3,4-*d*] pyrimidine; inhibitor of xanthine oxidase, used in the treatment of gout and to retard the rapid metabolic degradation of 6-mercaptopurine.

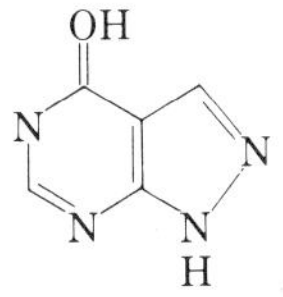

Allopurinol

allorhythmia (al-ō-rith'mē-ă) [allo- + G. *rhythmos*, rhythm]. An irregularity in the cardiac rhythm that repeats itself again and again.

allorhythmic (al-ō-rith'mik). Relating to or characterized by allorhythmia.

all or none. See Bowditch's *law*.

allose (al'ōs). $C_6H_{12}O_6$; a hexose sugar isomeric with glucose.

allosome (al'ō-sōm) [allo- + G. *sōma, body*]. Heterochromosome; heterotypical chromosome; one of the chromosomes differing in appearance or behavior from the autosomes and sometimes unequally distributed among the germ cells.
paired a., diplosome.
unpaired a., accessory *chromosome*.

allosteric (al-ō-stăr'ik). Pertaining to or characterized by allosterism.

allosterism, allostery (ă-los'ter-ism, -los'-ter-ē). The influencing of an enzyme activity by a change in the conformation of the enzyme, brought about by the noncompetitive binding of a nonsubstrate at a site (allosteric site) other than the active site of the enzyme.

allotetraploid (al-ō-tet'ră-ployd). See alloploid.

allotherm (al'ō-therm) [allo- + G. *thermē*, heat]. Poikilotherm.

allothreonines (al-o-thrē'ō-nēnz). Two of the four diastereoisomers of threonine, differing from the L and D threonines in the configuration of the hydroxyl group in the side chain.

allotopia (al-ō-tō'pē-ă) [allo- + G. *topos*, place]. Dystopia.

allotransplantation (al'ō-tranz-plan-ta'shŭn). Homotransplantation; transplantation of an allograft.

allotrichia circumscripta (al-ō-trik'ē-ă ser-kŭm-skrip'tă) [allo- + G. *thrix*, hair, + L. *circumscriptio*, a boundary]. Woolly-hair *nevus*.

allotriodontia (al-ot'rē-ō-don'shē-ă) [G. *allotrios*, foreign, + *odous* (*odont-*), tooth]. **1.** Growth of a tooth in some abnormal location. **2.** Transplantation of teeth.

allotriogeustia (al-ot'rē-ō-gū'stē-ă) [G. *allotrios*, foreign, + *geusis*, taste]. Perverted taste for innutritious or unusual substances.

allotriophagy (al-ot-rē-of'ă-jē) [G. *allotrios*, foreign, + *phagein*, to eat]. The habit of eating innutritious or unusual substances. See also pica.

allotriosmia (al-ot-rē-oz'mē-ă) [G. *allotrios*, foreign, + *osmē*, smell]. Incorrect recognition of odors.

allotriploid (al-ō-trip'loyd). See alloploid.

allotrope (al'ō-trōp) [allo- + G. *tropos*, a turning]. A substance in one of the allotropic forms that the element may assume.

allotrophic (al-o-trō'fik) [allo- + G. *trophē*, nourishment]. Having an altered nutritive value.

allotropic (al-ō-trop'ik). **1.** Relating to allotropism. **2.** Denoting a type of personality characterized by a preoccupation with the reactions of others.

allotropism, allotropy (ă-lot'rō-pizm, -lot'rō-pē). [allo- + G. *tropos*, a turning]. The existence of certain elements, in several forms differing in physical properties; *e.g.*, carbon black, graphite, and diamond are all pure carbon.

allotype (al'ō-tīp). Allotypic marker; any one of the genetically determined antigenic differences within a given class of immunoglobulin which occur among members of the same species. See also antibody.

allotypic (al-ō-tip'ik). Pertaining to an allotype.

alloxan (ă-loks'-an). An oxidation product of uric acid, 2,4,5,6-pyrimidinetetrone; administration to experimental animals causes hypoglycemia due to insulin liberation, followed by hyperglycemia due to destruction of the islets of Langerhans (alloxan diabetes).

alloxantin (ă-loks'an-tin). Uroxin; a condensation product of two molecules of alloxan, formed in the presence of reducing agents; a diabetogenic.

alloxazine (ă-loks'ă-zēn). Isomer of isoalloxazine.

alloxuremia (al-oks-yū-rē'mē-ă, al-ok-sū-rē'mē-ă) [alloxan + G. *haima*, blood]. The presence of purine bases in the blood.

alloxuria (al-oks-yū'rē-ă, al-ok-sū'rē-ă) [alloxan + G. *ouron*, urine]. The presence of purine bodies in the urine.

alloy (al'oy). A substance composed of a mixture of two or more metals.
chrome-cobalt a.'s, a.'s of cobalt and chromium containing molybdenum and/or tungsten plus trace elements; used in dentistry for denture bases and frameworks, and other structures.
eutectic a., an a., generally brittle and subject to tarnish and corrosion, with a fusion temperature lower than that of any of its components; used in dentistry mainly in solders.
gold a., an a. whose principal ingredient is gold, usually contains copper or platinum and silver; used in dentistry for restorations requiring considerable strength.
Raney a., an a. of Ni and Al in equal proportions, used in the

preparation of Raney Nickel.

silver-tin a., any a. of silver and tin; commonly 3 parts Ag and 1 part Sn, forming Ag_3Sn, the chief intermetallic compound in dental amalgam.

all-*trans*-retinal. *Trans*-retinal; visual yellow; the orange retinaldehyde resulting from the action of light on the rhodopsin of the retina, which converts the 11-*cis*-retinal component of the rhodopsin to all-*trans*-retinal plus opsin.

allspice oil (awl'spīs). Pimenta oil.

D-allulose (al'yū-lōs). D-Psicose.

allyl (al'il). 2-Propenyl; the monovalent radical, $CH_2{=}CHCH_2$—.

a. alcohol, vinyl carbinol; 2-propenol; $CH_2{=}CHCH_2OH$; a colorless liquid of pungent odor used in making resins and plasticizers; highly irritating to mucous membranes and readily absorbed, causing depression and coma.

a. cyanide, 3-butenenitrile; $CH_2{=}CHCH_2CN$; found in some mustard oils.

a. isothiocyanate, volatile mustard CH– allylisosulfocyanate; isothiocyanic allyl ester; $CH_2{=}CH{-}CH_2{-}NCS$; obtained from *Brassica nigra* or produced synthetically; a vesicant, used in 10% solution in 50% alcohol as a counterirritant in neuralgia. See also mustard oils.

a. sulfide, diallyl sulfide; thioallyl ether; "oil garlic"; $(CH_2{=}CHCH_2)S$; a constituent of garlic oil used in the manufacture of flavors.

allylamine (al-il-am'ēn). 3-Aminopropylene; $CH_2{=}CH{-}CH_2{-}NH_2$; a colorless liquid derived from crude oil of mustard and used in the pharmaceutical industry, *e.g.,* in the manufacture of mercurial diuretics.

allylbarbital (al-il-bar'bi-tal). Butalbital.

allylestrenol (al-il-es'trē-nol). 17-Allylestr-4-en-17β-ol; a progestational agent.

allylmercaptomethylpenicillin (al'il-mer-kap'tō-meth'il-pen-i-sil'in). *Penicillin* O.

***N*-allylnormorphine** (al'il-nor-mor'fēn). Nalorphine.

allysines (al'i-sēnz). Two or more six-carbon α-amino acids connected by a carbon-carbon bond; constituents of connective tissue and other structural elements. See also desmins.

Almeida, Floriano Paulo de, Brazilian physician. See A.'s *disease,* Lutz-Splendore-A. *disease.*

Almén, August Teodor, Swedish physiologist, 1833–1903. See A.'s *test* for blood.

almond oil (aw'mŭnd, awl'mŭnd). A fixed oil expressed from sweet almonds, the kernels of varieties of *Prunus amygdalus;* used in ointments.

bitter a. oil, a volatile oil from the dried ripe kernels of bitter a.'s and from other kernels containing amygdalin; it contains between 2 and 4% of hydrocyanic acid and 95% of benzaldehyde.

aloe (al'ō). **1.** The dried juice from the leaves of plants of the genus *Aloe* (family Liliaceae), from which are derived aloin, resin, emodin, and volatile oils. **2.** The dried juice from the leaves of *Aloe perryi* (socotrine a.'s), of *A. barbadensis* (Barbados and Curaçao a.'s), or of *A. capensis* (Cape a.'s); used as a purgative.

aloe-emodin (al'ō-em'ō-din). Rhabarberone; 1,8-dihydroxy-3-(hydroxymethyl)anthraquinone; 3-hydroxymethylchrysazin; the trimethyl ether of emodin; used as a laxative. See aloin; emodin.

aloetin (al-ō-ē'tin). Aloin.

alogia (ă-lō'jē-ă) [G. *a-* priv. + *logos,* speech]. **1.** Aphasia. **2.** Inability to speak due to mental deficiency or confusion.

aloin (al'ō-in). Barbaloin; aloetin; 1,8-dihydroxy-3-hydroxymethyl-10-(6-hydroxymethyl-3,4,5-trihydroxy-2-pyranyl)anthrone; 10-(1',5'-anhydroglucosyl)-aloe-emodin- 9-anthrone; a yellow crystalline principle made up of aloe-emodin and glucose, obtained from aloe; used as a laxative.

alopecia (al-ō-pē'shē-ă) [G. *alōpekia,* a disease like fox mange, fr. *alōpex,* a fox]. Acomia; calvities; pelade; baldness; loss of hair.

a. adna'ta, a. congenitalis.

androgenic a., male-type alopecia in females, associated with other evidence of excessive androgen activity, such as hirsutism.

a. area'ta, a condition of undetermined etiology characterized by circumscribed, noninflamed areas of baldness on the scalp, eyebrows, and bearded portion of the face. Also called a. circumscripta or celsi; Celsus' a. or area; Jonston's a. or area; porrigo decalvans; vitiligo capitis; Cazenave's or Celsus' vitiligo.

a. cap'itis tota'lis, a form of a. usually first noted as a. areata and progressing to involve the entire scalp, but occasionally occurring as an acute disease with total loss of scalp hair within a few days.

a. cel'si, Celsus' a., a. areata.

cicatricial a., a cicatrisa'ta, a. produced by scar formation in dermatoses such as folliculitis decalvans, pseudopelade, and lupus erythematosus.

a. circumscrip'ta, a. areata.

a. congenita'lis, congenital a., congenital baldness; a. adnata; hypotrichiasis (2); absence of all hair at birth.

congenital sutural a., *dyscephalia* mandibulo-oculofacialis.

a. dissemina'ta, loss of hair from all parts of the body.

a. dynam'ica, hair loss due to some destructive disease process affecting the hair follicles.

a. follicula'ris, *folliculitis* decalvans.

a. heredita'ria, male pattern a. or baldness; patterned a.; a resulting from sex-influenced dominant inheritance, with androgen stimulation required to produce hair loss in heterozygous individuals; homozygous females may have minor hair loss without androgen stimulation.

Jonston's a., a. areata.

a. leproti'ca, **(1)** a rare, moth-eaten, patchy type of a. seen in leprosy; **(2)** the more common lepromatous thinning or total loss of eyebrows and eyelashes.

a. limina'ris fronta'lis, a. marginalis; hair loss at the hair line, a condition most commonly seen in blacks; may be associated with seborrheic dermatitis but is commonly caused by friction or other trauma.

lipedematous a., a. with itching, soreness, or tenderness of the scalp in adult black women; the scalp is thickened and soft, subcutaneous fat is increased, and the hair is sparse and short.

male pattern a., a. hereditaria.

a. margina'lis, a. liminaris frontalis.

a. medicamento'sa, diffuse hair loss, most notably of the scalp, caused by administration of various types of drugs.

moth-eaten a., patchy hair loss of parietal and occipital regions of the scalp, characteristic of secondary syphilis.

a. mucino'sa, a relatively unusual condition of unknown origin that may develop as areas of erythema and edema in the bearded portion of the face or in the scalp.

a. neurot'ica, a. of trophoneurotic origin.

a. parvicula'ta, pseudopelade.

patterned a., a. hereditaria.

a. pityro'des, a loss of hair, of the body as well as of the scalp, accompanied by an abundant branlike desquamation.

postoperative pressure a., loss of hair over a circumscribed area on the posterior scalp, resulting from the necessarily continuous pressure on the occiput in a lengthy operative procedure.

postpartum a., temporary diffuse telogen loss of scalp hair at the termination of pregnancy.

premature a., a. prematu'ra, male pattern baldness appearing at an unusually early age.

a. preseni'lis, ordinary or common baldness occurring in early or middle life without any apparent disease of the scalp.

a. seni'lis, the normal loss of scalp hair in old age.

a. symptomat'ica, a. occurring in the course of various constitutional or local diseases, or following prolonged febrile illness.

a. syphilit'ica, moth-eaten a. of secondary syphilis.

a. tota'lis, total loss of hair of the scalp either at one time or within a very short period of time. *Cf.* universalis.

a. tox'ica, hair loss attributed to febrile illness.

traction a., traumatic a.

traumatic a., traction a.; circumscribed or diffuse loss of hair resulting from repetitive traction on the hair by pulling or twisting; also occurs after excessive application of hair "softeners" such as permanent wave solutions or hot combs.

a. triangula'ris congenita'lis, a congenital defect consisting of a triangular patch of baldness on the frontal or temporal region of the scalp.

a. universa'lis, total loss of hair from all parts of the body. *Cf.* a. totalis.

alopecic (al-ō-pē'sik). Relating to alopecia.

aloxiprin (ă-lok'si-prin). A condensation product of aluminum oxide and aspirin, used as an analgesic.

Alpers, Bernard J., U.S. neurologist, *1900. See A. *disease.*

alpha (al'fă). First letter of the Greek alphabet, α(*q.v.*).

alpha amylase. A starch-splitting enzyme obtained from a nonpathogenic bacterium of the *Bacillus subtilis* class, used in the treatment of inflammatory conditions and edema of soft tissues associated with traumatic injury; its therapeutic usefulness has not been fully established and its mode of action is not known.

alpha-blocker (al'fă-blok'er). α-Adrenergic blocking *agent.*

alphadione (al-fă-dī'ōn). An intravenous anesthetic containing two steroids, alfaxalone, and alfadolone acetate, dissolved in 20% polyoxyethylated castor oil.

alphadolone acetate (al-fad'ō-lōn). Alfadolone acetate.

alphaprodine (al-fă-prō'dēn). α-1,3-Dimethyl-4-phenyl-4-piperidinyl propionate; a narcotic analgesic related to meperidine; physical and psychic dependence may develop.

alphasone acetophenide (al'fă-sōn). Algestone acetophenide.

Alphavirus (al'fă-vī-rŭs). A genus of viruses (family Togaviridae) formerly classified as group A arboviruses.

alphaxalone (al-faks'ă-lōn). Alfaxalone.

alphodermia (al-fō-der'mē-ă) [G. *alphos,* leprosy, + *derma,* skin]. Leukoderma.

alphos (al'fos) [G. *alphos,* leprosy]. Psoriasis.

Alport, Arthur Cecil, South African physician, 1880–1959. See A.'s *syndrome.*

alprazolam (al-praz'ō-lam). A benzodiazepine minor tranquilizer used for management of anxiety disorders; abuse may lead to habituation or addiction.

alprenolol hydrochloride (al-pren'ō-lol). The hydrochloride salt of 1-(*o*-allylphenoxy)-3-(isopropylamino)propan-2-ol; a β-receptor blocking agent, used for the treatment of cardiac arrhythmias.

alprostadil (al-pros'tă-dil). Prostaglandin E_1; 11,15-dihydroxy-9-oxoprost-13-en-1-oic acid; a vasodilator used for palliative therapy to temporarily maintain patency of the ductus arteriosus in neonates with congenital heart defects.

ALS Abbreviation for amyotrophic lateral *sclerosis;* antilymphocyte *serum.*

alseroxylon (al'ser-ok'si-lon). A fat-soluble alkaloidal fraction extracted from the root of *Rauwolfia serpentina,* containing reserpine and other nonadrenolytic amorphous alkaloids; used as a sedative in psychoses, in mild hypertension, and as an adjunct to more potent hypotensive drugs.

Alström, Carl-Henry, Swedish geneticist, *1907. See A.'s *syndrome.*

ALT Abbreviation for alanine aminotransferase.

alter (awl'ter) [Mediev. L. *altero,* pp. *-atus,* to change, fr. L. *alter,* other]. To remove the gonads from an animal.

alteration (awl-ter-ā'shŭn). **1.** A change. **2.** A changing; a making different.

modal a., in electric irritability, a change in the mode of response of degenerated muscle to electric stimulation, the contraction being sluggish instead of quick.

qualitative a., in electric irritability, a change in which the muscle contracts as readily on application of the anode as on that of the cathode.

quantitative a., in electric irritability, a gradual loss of contractility in a muscle in response to static, faradic, and galvanic currents successively.

alteregoism (awl-ter-ē'gō-izm). Identification with people of similar personality to one's own.

alternans (awl-ter'nanz) [L.]. Alternating; often used substantively for alternation of the heart.

auditory a., auscultatory a.

auscultatory a., auditory a.; alternation in the intensity of heart sounds or murmurs in the presence of a regular cardiac rhythm as a result of alternation of the heart.

concordant a., simultaneous occurrence of right ventricular and pulmonary artery a. with peripheral pulsus a.

discordant a., presence of right ventricular and pulmonary artery a. with peripheral pulsus a., but with the strong beat of the right ventricle coinciding with the weak beat of the left and vice versa.

electrical a., electrical alternation of the heart.

pulsus a., see under pulsus.

Alternaria (al-ter-nā'rē-ă). A genus of fungi easily isolated from air and considered to be a common laboratory contaminant and an allergen; occasionally pathogenic in humans.

alternation (awl-ter-nā'shŭn). The occurrence of two things or phases in succession and recurrently.

concordant a., a. in either the mechanical or electrical activity of the heart, occurring in both systemic and pulmonary circuits.

discordant a., a. in cardiac activities of either the systemic or the pulmonic circuits, but not of both.

electrical a. of heart, a disorder in which the ventricular complexes are regular in time but of alternating pattern; a. of P waves occurs rarely.

a. of generations, metagenesis; a succession of generations of individuals like and unlike the original parents, or an a. of sexual and nonsexual generations.

a. of the heart, mechanical a.; disorder in which contractions of the heart are regular in time but are alternately stronger and weaker.

mechanical a., a. of the heart.

alternocular (awl-ter-nok'yū-lăr). Denoting the use of each eye separately instead of binocularly.

althea (al-thē'ă) [L., fr. G. *althaia,* marshmallow]. Marshmallow root; the root of *Althea officinalis* (family Malvaceae), used in the form of syrup or lozenge as a demulcent in irritation of the mouth and pharynx; dried leaves have also been used.

Altherr, Franz. See Meyenburg-A.-Uehlinger *syndrome.*

alt. hor. Abbreviation for L. *alternis horis,* every other hour.

altitudinal (al-ti-tū'di-năl). Relating to vertical relationships; *e.g.,* a. hemianopsia.

Altmann, Richard, German histologist, 1852–1900. See A.'s *fixative, granule,* anilin-acid fuchsin *stain, theory;* A.-Gersh *method.*

altrigendrism (al-trĭ-jen'drizm) [L. *altri,* fr. *alteri,* other, + Fr. *gendre,* fr. L. *genus,* sort]. Natural, wholesome, nonerotic activity between the sexes.

altrose (al'trōs). An aldohexose isomeric with glucose, tallose, allose, etc.

alum (al'ŭm). A double sulfate of aluminum and of an alkaline earth element or ammonium; chemically, an a. is any one of the markedly astringent double salts formed by a combination of a sulfate of aluminum, iron, manganese, chromium, or gallium with a sulfate of lithium, sodium, potassium, ammonium, cesium, or rubidium; used locally as styptics.

burnt a., dried a.

cake a., *aluminum* sulfate octadecahydrate.

chrome a., the sulfate of chromium and potassium; used as a mordant in histologic staining.

dried a., burnt a.; a. deprived of its water of crystallization by heat; an astringent dusting powder.

exsiccated a., a. heated to complete dryness; a local astringent.

ferric a., ferric ammonium sulfate.

iron a., ferric ammonium sulfate.

whey a., an astringent and styptic preparation made by boiling a. (1 oz.) in milk (10 oz.).

alum-hematoxylin (al'ŭm-hē-mă-tok'si-lin). A purple nuclear stain used in histology; a mixture of an aqueous solution of ammonium alum and an alcoholic solution of hematoxylin which is ripened or oxidized to hematein.

alumina (ă-lū'mi-nă). *Aluminum* oxide.

hydrated a., *aluminum* hydroxide.

aluminated (ă-lū'mi-nā-ted). Containing alum.

aluminon (ă-lū'min-on). The ammonium salt of aurintricarboxylic acid, so-called because of its usefulness in the detection of aluminum in biologic material, foods, etc.

aluminosis (ă-lū-min-ō'sis). A pneumoconiosis caused by inhalation of aluminum particles into the lungs.

aluminum (ă-lū'min-ŭm) [L. *alumen,* alum]. A white silvery metal of very light weight; symbol Al, atomic no. 13, atomic weight 26.98.

a. acetate, used as a disinfectant by embalmers; proposed as desiccant and deodorant powder for eczema and chronic skin ulcers.

a. acetotartrate, basic aluminum acetate (70%) and tartaric acid (30%); antiseptic.

a. acetylsalicylate, a. aspirin.

a. ammonium sulfate, $AlNH_4(SO_4)_2$; an astringent.

a. aspirin, a. acetylsalicylate; an analgesic and antipyretic.

a. bismuth oxide, *bismuth* aluminate.

a. carbonate, basic, $Al_2O_3CO_2$; an a. hydroxide-carbonate complex consisting of white lumps, insoluble in water; aqueous suspensions bind phosphorus in the intestine and lower serum inorganic phosphorus resulting in an increase in reabsorption of phosphorus by renal tubules and reduction of urinary excretion of phosphorus; it reduces formation of phosphatic urinary calculi and gastric acidity.

a. chlorate nonahydrate, mallebrin; $Al(ClO_3)_3 \cdot 9H_2O$; an antiseptic.

a. chloride hexahydrate, $AlCl_3 \cdot 6H_2O$; used as an astringent or antiseptic in solution.

a. diacetate, a. subacetate.

a. hydrate, a. hydroxide.

a. hydroxide, hydrated alumina; a. hydrate; $Al(OH)_3$; an astringent dusting powder; also used internally as a mild astringent antacid.

a. hydroxide gel, a suspension containing Al_2O_3, mainly in the form of a. hydroxide, used as an antacid; a dried form, with the same use, is obtained by drying the product of interaction in aqueous solution of an a. salt with ammonium or sodium carbonate.

a. hydroxychloride, an antiperspirant.

a. magnesium silicate, *magnesium* aluminum silicate.

a. monostearate, a compound of a. with a mixture of solid organic acids obtained from fats, and consisting chiefly of a. monostearate and a. monopalmitate; used as a suspending medium in pharmaceutical preparations.

a. nicotinate, tris(nicotinato)aluminum; a lipopenic agent with peripheral vasodilator action.

a. oleate, $Al(C_{18}H_{33}O_2)_3$; used as an ointment in certain cutaneous affections and in burns.

a. oxide, alumina; Al_2O_3; used as an abrasive, as a refractory, and in chromatography.

a. penicillin, see under penicillin.

a. phenolsulfonate, $Al(C_6H_4(OH)SO_3)_3$; antiseptic and astringent for local application, usually for cutaneous ulcers.

a. phosphate, $AlPO_4$; an infusible powder, insoluble in water but soluble in alkali hydroxides, used for dental cements with calcium sulfate and sodium silicate.

a. phosphate gel, an aqueous suspension of between 4.0 and 5.0% of a. phosphate; used as an antacid.

a. potassium sulfate, potassium alum; $AlK(SO_4)_2$; an astringent and styptic; also used in veterinary medicine for ulcerative stomatitis, leukorrhea, and conjunctivitis.

a. salicylate, basic, used in the treatment of ozena and pharyngitis.

a. salicylate, basic, soluble, ammoniated basic a. salicylate; used in solution as a spray for diseases of the upper air passages.

a. silicate, kaolin.

a. subacetate, a. diacetate; $Al(CH_3CO_2)_2OH$; used in solution as an astringent, as an ingredient in mouthwashes, and in embalming fluids.

a. sulfate octadecahydrate, cake alum; astringent detergent for skin ulcers.

aluminum group. Aluminum, boron, gallium, indium, and thallium.

alvei (al'vē-ī). Plural of alveus.

alveoalgia (al'vē-ō-al'jē-ă) [alveolus + G. *algos,* pain]. Dry socket; alveolalgia; alveolar osteitis; a postoperative complication of tooth extraction in which the blood clot in the socket disintegrates, resulting in an inflamed empty socket; pain usually begins on the second or third day after the extraction and may persist for days.

alveolalgia (al'vē-ō-lal'jē-ă). Alveoalgia.

alveolar (al-vē'ō-lăr). Relating to an alveolus.

alveolate (al-vē'ō-lāt) [L. *alveolus,* dim. of *alveus,* trough, hollow sac, cavity]. Pitted like a honeycomb.

alveolectomy (al'vē-ō-lek'tō-mē) [alveolus + G. *ektomē,* excision]. Surgical excision of a portion of the dentoalveolar process, for recontouring of the alveolar ridge at the time of tooth removal to facilitate a dental prosthesis.

alveoli (al-vē'ō-lī). Plural of alveolus.

alveolingual (al'vē-o-ling'gwăl). Alveololingual.

alveolitis (al'vē-ō-lī'tis). **1.** Inflamation of alveoli. **2.** Inflammation of a tooth socket.

acute pulmonary a., acute inflammation involving the pulmonary alveoli, with exudate into alveolar passages and impaired gas exchange; may result in necrosis with hemorrhage into the lungs and may occur in Goodpasture's syndrome, in association with glomerulonephritis.

extrinsic allergic a., hypersensitivity pneumonitis; pneumoconiosis resulting from hypersensitivity due to repeated inhalation of organic dust, usually specified according to occupational exposure; in the acute form, respiratory symptoms and fever start several hours after exposure to the dust; in the chronic form, there is eventual diffuse pulmonary fibrosis after exposure over several years. See also entries under disease, lung.

alveolo- [L. *alveolus*]. Combining form denoting relation to an alveolus or to the alveolar process.

alveoloclasia (al-vē'ō-lō-klā'zē-ă) [alveolo- + G. *klasis,* breaking]. Destruction of the alveolus.

alveolodental (al-vē'ō-lō-den'tăl). Relating to the alveoli and the teeth.

alveololabial (al-vē'ō-lō-lā'bē-ăl). Relating to the labial or outer surface of the alveolar processes.

alveololabialis (al-vē'ō-lō-lā-bē-ā'lis) [L.]. Relating to the alveololabial sulcus region.

alveololingual (al-vē'ō-lō-ling'gwăl). Alveolingual; relating to the lingual or inner surface of the alveolar process.

alveolopalatal (al-vē'ō-lō-pal'ă-tăl). Relating to the palatal surface of the alveolar process.

alveoloplasty (al-vē'ō-lō-plas-tē) [alveolo- + G. *plassō,* to form]. Alveoplasty; surgical preparation of the alveolar ridges for the reception of dentures; shaping and smoothing of socket margins after extraction of teeth with subsequent suturing to insure optimal healing.

interradicular a., intraseptal a., removal of the interradicular bone and collapsing of the cortical plates to a more desirable alveolar contour.

alveoloschisis (al-vē-ō-los'ki-sis) [alveolo- + G. *schisis,* cleaving]. Gnathoschisis; a cleft of the alveolar process.

alveolotomy (al-vē-ō-lot'ō-mē) [alveolo- + G. *tomē,* incision]. Surgical opening into a dental alveolus to allow drainage of pus from a periapical or other intraosseous abscess.

alveolus, gen. and pl. **alveoli** (al-vē'ō-lŭs, -ō-lī) [L. dim. of *alveus,* trough, hollow sac, cavity] [NA]. A small cell or cavity. **1.** A cell containing air; one of the terminal saclike dilations of the alveolar ducts in the lung. **2.** One of the terminal secretory portions of an alveolar or racemose gland. **3.** One of the honeycomb pits in the wall of the stomach. **4.** A. dentalis.

a. dentalis, pl. **alveoli dentales** [NA], alveolus (4); tooth socket; a socket in the alveolar process of the maxilla or mandible, into which each tooth fits and is attached by means of the periodontal ligament.

alveoli pulmo'nis [NA], air cells (1); bronchic cells; air vesicles; thin-walled saclike dilations of the respiratory bronchioles, alveolar ducts, and alveolar sacs across which gas exchange occurs between alveolar air and the pulmonary capillaries.

alveoplasty (al'vē-ō-plas-tē). Alveoloplasty.

alveus, pl. **alvei** (al'vē-ŭs, -vē-ī) [L. tray, trough, cavity, fr. *alvus,* belly]. A channel or trough.

a. hippocam'pi [NA], alveus of the hippocampus; a thin white band of fornix fibers covering the ventricular surface of the hippocampus.

a. urogenita'lis, *utriculus* prostaticus.

alvinolith (al-vin'ō-lith, al-vī'nō-lith) [L. *alvus,* belly, + G. *lithus,* stone]. Obsolete term for coprolith.

A.L.W. Abbreviation for arch-loop-whorl *system.*

alymphia (ă-lim'fē-ă). Absence or deficiency of lymph.

alymphocytosis (ă-lim'fō-sī-tō'sis). Absence or great reduction of lymphocytes.

alymphoplasia (ă-lim-fō-plā'zē-ă). Aplasia or hypoplasia of lymphoid tissue.

Nezelof type of thymic a., cellular *immunodeficiency* with abnormal immunoglobulin synthesis.

thymic a., lymphopenic thymic dysplasia; hypoplasia with absence of Hassall's corpuscles and deficiency of lymphocytes in the thymus and usually in lymph nodes, spleen, and gastrointestinal tract; there is peripheral lymphopenia and often hypogammaglobulinemia and absence of plasma cells; presents in early infancy with respiratory infections and leads to death within a few months. See also *immunodeficiency* with hypoparathyroidism.

Alzheimer, Alois, German neurologist, 1864–1915. See A.'s *dementia, disease, sclerosis.*

Am Symbol for americium.

amacrine (am'ă-krin) [G. *a-* priv. + *makros,* long, + *is* (*in-*), fiber]. **1.** A cell or structure lacking a long, fibrous process. **2.** Denoting such a cell or structure. See also amacrine *cell.*

amadou (ahm'ah-dū) [Fr.]. Agaric.

amalgam (ă-mal'gam) [G. *malagma,* a soft mass]. An alloy of an element or a metal with mercury. In dentistry, primarily of two types: silver-tin alloy, containing small amounts of copper and zinc, and a second type containing more copper (12 to 30% by weight); they are used for filling teeth and making dies.

pin a., an a. restoration held in place largely by small metal rods protruding from holes drilled into tooth structure.

spherical a., an alloy for dental a. composed of spherical particles instead of filings.

amalgamate (ă-mal'gă-māt). To make an amalgam.

amalgamation (ă-mal-gă-mā'shŭn). The process of combining mercury with a metal or an alloy to form a new alloy.

amalgamator (ă-mal'gă-mā-tŏr). A device for combining mercury with a metal or an alloy to form a new alloy.

Amanita (am-ă-nī'tă) [G. *amanitai,* fungi]. A genus of fungi, many members of which are highly poisonous.

A. musca'ria, fly agaric; a toxic species of mushroom with yellow to red pileus and white gills; it contains muscarine, which produces psychosis-like states and other symptoms.

A. phalloi'des, deadly agaric; a species containing poisonous principles, including phalloidin and amanitin, that cause gastroenteritis, hepatic necrosis, and renal necrosis.

α-amanitin (am-ă-nī'tin). A highly toxic, heat-stable cyclic polypeptide in *Amanita phalloides.*

amantadine hydrochloride (ă-man'tă-dēn). 1-Adamantanamine; an antiviral agent; also used to treat parkinsonism.

amara (ă-mah'ră) [neut. pl. of L. *amarus,* bitter]. Bitters (2).

amaranth, amaranthum (am'ă-ranth, am-ă-ran'thŭm) [G. *amaranthon,* a never-fading flower] [C.I. 16185]. An azo dye, 1-(4-sulfo-1-naphthylazo)-2-naphthol-3,6-disulfonate (trisodium salt); a soluble reddish brown powder, the color turning to magenta red in solution; used as a food and cosmetic coloring agent, and occasionally in histology.

amarine (am'ă-rin) [L. *amarus,* bitter]. A name applied to various bitter principles derived from plants, especially to a poisonous substance, 2,4,5-triphenylimidazoline, obtained from oil of bitter almond.

amaroid (am'ă-royd) [L. *amarus,* bitter, + G. *eidos,* like]. A bitter extractive that does not belong to the class of glycosides, alkaloids, or any of the known proximate principles of plants.

amaroidal (am-ă-roy'dăl). Resembling bitters; having a slightly bitter taste.

amarum (ă-mah'rŭm) [neut. of L. *amarus,* bitter]. One of a class of vegetable drugs of bitter taste, such as gentian and quassia, used as appetizers and tonics.

amastia (ă-mas'tē-ă) [G. *a-* priv. + *mastos,* breast]. Amazia; absence of the breasts.

amastigote (ă-mas'ti-gōt) [G. *a-* priv. + *mastix,* whip]. Leishman-Donovan *body.*

amathophobia (ă-math-ō-fō'bē-ă) [G. *amathos,* dust, + *phobos,* fear]. Morbid dread of dust or dirt.

amativeness (ahm'ă-tiv-nes) [L. *amo,* pp. *amatus,* to love]. Rarely used term for the propensity to love.

amaurosis (am-aw-rō'sis) [G. *amauros,* dark, obscure, + *-osis,* condition]. Gutta serena; blindness, especially that occurring without apparent change in the eye itself, as from a cortical lesion.

a. centra'lis, a. caused by a central nervous system abnormality.

a. congeni'ta of Leber, an autosomal recessive cone-rod abiotrophy causing blindness or severely reduced vision at birth.

a. fu'gax, a transient blindness that may result from a transient ischemia due to carotid artery insufficiency or to centrifugal force (visual blackout in flight).

pressure a., loss of vision occurring a few seconds after intraocular pressure exceeds systolic pressure of retinal arteries.

saburral a., a. associated with symptoms of acute gastric disturbance.

toxic a., blindness due to optic neuritis caused by methyl alcohol, lead, arsenic, quinine, or other poisons.

amaurotic (am-aw-rot'ik). Relating to or suffering from amaurosis.

amaxophobia (ă-mak-sō-fō'bē-ă) [G. *amaxa, hamaxa,* a carriage, + *phobos,* fear]. Hamaxophobia; morbid fear of, or of riding in, a vehicle.

amazia (ă-mā'zē-ă). Amastia.

ambageusia (am-bă-gū'sē-ă) [L. *ambo,* both, + G. *a-* priv. + *geusis,* taste]. Loss of taste from both sides of the tongue.

Ambard, Léon, French pharmacologist, 1876–1962. See A.'s *constant, laws.*

ambenonium chloride (am-bē-nō'nē-ŭm). *N,N'*-Bis-2-[(2-chlorobenzyl)diethylammonium chloride]ethyloxamide; a cholinesterase inhibitor similar to neostigmine in actions; used chiefly in the management of myasthenia gravis and occasionally for intestinal and urinary tract obstruction.

Amberg, Emil, U.S. otologist, 1868–1948. See A.'s lateral sinus *line.*

ambergris (am'ber-gris) [Mod. L. *ambra grisea,* gray amber]. A grayish pathologic secretion from the intestine of the sperm whale that occurs as a flammable waxy mass (melting point about 60°C), insoluble in water; contains cholesterol and benzoic acid, and is used as a base for perfume.

ambi- [L. *ambo,* both]. Prefix meaning round; all (both) sides. See also ambo-.

ambidexterity (am-bi-deks-ter'i-tē). Ambidextrism; the ability to use both hands with equal ease.

ambidextrism (am-bi-deks'trizm). Ambidexterity.

ambidextrous (am-bi-deks'trŭs). Having equal facility in the use of both hands.

ambient (am'bē-ent) [L. *ambiens,* going around]. Surrounding, encompassing; pertaining to the environment in which an organism or apparatus functions.

ambiguous (am-big'yū-ŭs) [L. *ambiguus,* fr. *ambigo,* to wander]. **1.** Having more than one interpretation. **2.** In anatomy, wandering; having more than one direction. **3.** In neuroanatomy, applied to a nucleus supplying special visceral efferent fibers to vagus and glossopharyngeal nerves.

ambilateral (am-bi-lat'er-ăl) [ambi- + L. *latus,* side]. Relating to both sides.

ambilevous (am-bi-lē'vŭs) [ambi- + L. *laevus,* left]. Ambisinister; ambisinistrous; awkward in the use of both hands.

ambisexual (am-bi-seks'yū-ăl). Bisexual.

ambisinister (am-bi-sin'is-ter) [ambi- + L. *sinister,* left]. Ambilevous.

ambisinistrous (am'bi-sin'is-trŭs). Ambilevous.

ambivalence (am-biv'ă-lens) [ambi- + L. *valentia,* strength]. The coexistence of antithetical attitudes or emotions toward a given person or thing, as in the simultaneous feeling and expression of love and hate toward the same person.

ambivalent (am-biv'ă-lent). Relating to or characterized by ambivalence.

ambivert (am'bi-vert). One who falls between the two extremes of introversion and extroversion, possessing some of the tendencies of each.

ambly- [G. *amblys,* dull]. Combining form denoting dullness, dimness.

amblyaphia (am-bli-ā'fē-ă) [ambly- + G. *haphē,* touch]. Diminution in tactile sensibility.

amblygeustia (am-bli-gūs'tē-ă) [ambly- + G. *geusis,* taste]. A blunted sense of taste.

Amblyomma (am-blē-om'ă) [ambly- + G. *omma,* eye, vision]. A genus of ornate, hard ticks (family Ixodidae) characterized by having eyes, festoons, and deeply imbedded ventral plates near the festoons in males.

A. america'num, the Lone-Star tick, a species that is an important pest and vector of Rocky Mountain spotted fever, found primarily in the southern United States and northern Mexico; it occurs on dogs and many other hosts, including domestic animals, birds, and man; it bites man in larval, nymphal, and adult stages.

A. cajennen'se, the Cayenne tick, a species that is an important pest in southern Texas, Central and South America, and the larger Caribbean islands, and a vector of Rocky Mountain spotted fever in Mexico and Central and South America; all stages attack man and many species of domestic and wild animals.

A. hebrae'um, the South African bont tick, an important vector of heartwater in southern Africa.

A. macula'tum, the Gulf Coast tick, a species that is a pest of livestock in the southeastern United States.

A. variega'tum, the tropical bont tick, a serious pest of domestic livestock and an important vector of heartwater in Africa and the Caribbean; it is closely associated with the development of severe clinical dermatophilosis in cattle in the Caribbean.

amblyopia (am-blē-ō'pē-ă) [G. *amblyōpia,* dimness of vision, fr. *amblys* dull, + *ōps,* eye]. Unilateral decreased visual acuity without detectable organic disease of the eye.

anisometropic a., cortical suppression of vision as a result of marked difference in refractive error of the two eyes.

axial a., a. resulting from a disproportion between the length of the eyeball and the refractivity of its optical surfaces.

deprivation a., sensory a.

eclipse a., solar or eclipse blindness; chorioretinitis affecting the fovea centralis due to the thermal action of infrared rays consequent to watching a solar eclipse with inadequate ocular protection. See also photoretinopathy.

a. ex anop'sia, obsolete term denoting cortical suppression of central vision due to disuse; now usually designated as anisometropic, sensory, or strabismic a.

functional a., reversible a.; that form of a. reversible with appropriate treatment.

hysterical a., a. occurring as a manifestation, usually, of a conversion reaction.

index a., an a. resulting from an alteration of the refractive index of the lens of the eye.

nocturnal a., nyctalopia.

nutritional a., a. resulting from lack of vitamin B-complex constituents.

refractive a., cortical inhibition of vision, caused by severe refractive error.

relative a., decreased visual acuity in which sensory a. is associated with functional a.

reversible a., functional a.

sensory a., deprivation a.; cortical suppression of central vision as a result of faulty ocular image formation secondary to corneal scars, cataract, or blepharoptosis.

strabismic a., cortical suppression of central vision as a result of crossing of the eyes.

toxic a., see toxic *amaurosis.*

amblyopic (am-blē-ō'pik). Relating to, or suffering from, amblyopia.

amblyoscope (am'blē-ō-skōp) [amblyopia + G. *skopeō,* to view]. A reflecting stereoscope used to evaluate or stimulate binocular vision. See also haploscope.

major a., an a. in which intensity of illumination as well as targets may be varied.

Worth's a., the original a.; a hand-held a. consisting of angled tubes that can be swiveled to any degree of convergence or divergence.

ambo- [L. *ambo,* both]. Prefix meaning round; all (both) sides. See also ambi-.

amboceptor (am'bō-sep-tōr) [ambo- + L. *capio,* to take]. Ehrlich's term for his concept, now obsolete, of the structure of complement-fixing antibody; now used chiefly to denote the anti-sheep erythrocyte antibody used in the hemolytic system of complement-fixation tests.

ambomalleal (am-bō-mal'ē-ăl). Relating to the ambos, or incus, and the malleus.

ambos (am'bōs) [Ger.]. Incus.

ambrosin (am-brō'sin). A principle in ragweed related to absinthin.

ambucetamide (am-byū-set'ă-mīd). α-Dibutylamino-α-(*p*-methoxyphenyl)acetamide; an intestinal antispasmodic.

ambulatory, ambulant (am'byū-lă-tōr-ē, am'byū-lant) [L. *ambulans,* walking]. Walking about or able to walk about; denoting a patient who is not confined to bed as a result of disease or surgery.

ambuphylline (am-byū'fi-lin). Theophylline aminoisobutanol; a diuretic and bronchodilator.

ambustion (am-bŭs'chŭn) [L. *amb-uro,* pp. *-ustus,* to burn around, scorch]. A burn or scald.

amcinonide (am-sin'ō-nid). A glucocorticoid used topically in the treatment of dermatoses.

amdinocillin (am'di-nō-sil'in). Mecillinam; $C_{15}H_{23}N_3O_3S$; a penicillin derivative of amidinopenicillamic acid which, unlike other penicillins, is very active against a wide range of Gram-negative bacteria.

ameba, pl. amebae, amebas (ă-mē'bă, -bē, -băz). Common name for *Amoeba* and similar naked, lobose, sarcodine protozoa.

amebacide (ă-mē'bă-sīd). Amebicide.

amebaism (ă-mē'bă-izm). **1.** Ameboidism (1). **2.** Ameboididity.

amebiasis (ă-mē-bī'ă-sis) [ameba + G. *-iasis,* condition]. Amebism; infection with *Entamoeba histolytica* or other pathogenic amebas.

canine a., infection of dogs with *Entamoeba histolytica* acquired from man; dogs are seldom cyst passers, and therefore are not a reservoir for human infection.

a. cu'tis, a serpiginous, ulcerating eruption with bloody, necrotic crust, appearing usually as an extension of underlying infection (*e.g.,* anus or site of surgical intervention of bowel or liver lesion), but occasionally at site of direct contact.

hepatic a., infection of the liver with *Entamoeba histolytica;* may occur with or without antecedent amebic dysentery.

amebic (ă-mē'bik). Relating to, resembling, or caused by amebas.

amebicidal (ă-mē-bi-sī'dăl). Destructive to amebas.

amebicide (ă-mē'bi-sīd) [ameba + L. *caedo,* to kill]. Amebacide; any agent that causes the destruction of amebas.

amebiform (ă-mē'bi-fōrm) [ameba + L. *forma,* shape]. Of the shape or appearance of an ameba.

amebiosis (ă-mē-bī-ō'sis). Obsolete term for amebiasis.

amebism (ă-mē'bizm). Amebiasis.

amebocyte (ă-mē'bō-sīt) [ameba, + *kytos,* cell]. **1.** A wandering cell found in invertebrates. **2.** Obsolete term for leukocyte. **3.** An *in vitro* tissue culture leukocyte.

ameboid (ă-mē'boyd) [ameba + G. *eidos,* appearance]. **1.** Resembling an ameba in appearance or characteristics. **2.** Of irregular outline with peripheral projections; denoting the outline of a form of colony in plate culture.

ameboididity (ă-mē-boy-did'i-tē). Amebaism (2); the power of locomotion after the manner of an ameboid cell.

ameboidism (ă-mē'boyd-izm). **1.** Amebaism (1); the performance of movements similar to those of an ameba. **2.** Denoting a condition sometimes seen in certain nerve cells.

ameboma (ă-mē-bō'mă) [ameba + G. *-oma,* tumor]. Amebic granuloma; a nodular, tumor-like focus of proliferative inflammation sometimes developing in chronic amebiasis, especially in the wall of the colon.

amebula, pl. amebulae (ă-mē'byū-lă, -lē) [fr. G. *amoibē,* a change, alteration]. Term applied to the excysted young amebas of *Entamoeba* species that emerge from the cyst in the human or vertebrate gut and their immediate progeny, usually totalling eight, prior to their localization in the large intestine.

amebule (ă-mē'byūl). A minute ameba.

ameburia (am-ē-byū'rē-ă) [ameba + G. *ouron,* urine]. The presence of amebas in the urine.

amelanotic (ā-mel-ă-not'ik) [G. *a-* priv. + *melas,* black]. Lacking in melanin.

amelia (ă-mē'lē-ă) [G. *a-* priv. + *melos,* a limb]. Congenital absence of a limb or limbs.

porcine a., autosomal recessive a. in piglets.

amelioration (ă-mēl-yō-rā'shŭn) [L. *ad,* to, + *melioro,* to make better]. Improvement; moderation in the severity of a disease or the intensity of its symptoms.

ameloblast (ă-mel'ō-blast, am-ĕ-lō'blast) [Early E. *amel,* enamel, + G. *blastos,* germ]. Adamantoblast; enamel cell; one of the columnar epithelial cells of the inner layer of the enamel organ of a developing tooth, concerned with the formation of enamel.

ameloblastoma (am'ĕ-lō-blas-tō'mă) [ameloblast + G. *-oma,* tumor]. A benign odontogenic epithelial neoplasm that histologically mimics the embryonal enamel organ but does not differentiate to the point of forming dental hard tissues; it behaves as a slowly growing expansile radiolucent tumor, occurs most commonly in the posterior regions of the mandible, and has a marked tendency to recur if inadequately excised.

pigmented a., melanotic neuroectodermal *tumor.*

amelodentinal (am'ĕ-lō-den'ti-năl). Dentinoenamel.

amelogenesis (am'ĕ-lō-jen'ĕ-sis). Enamelogenesis; the deposition and maturation of enamel.

a. imperfec'ta, enamelogenesis imperfecta; enamel dysplasia; a group of heriditary disorders in which the enamel is defective in structure or deficient in quantity. Two major groups are recognized: hypoplastic types, characterized by defective enamel matrix deposition but with normal mineralization; hypomineralization types, characterized by normal matrix but with defective mineralization.

amenia (ă-mē'nē-ă) [G. *a-* priv. + *mēn,* month]. Rarely used term for amenorrhea.

amenorrhea (ă-men-ō-rē'ă) [G. *a-* priv. + *mēn,* month, + *rhoia,* flow]. Absence or abnormal cessation of the menses.

dietary a., loss of menstrual function due to rapid weight loss or gain.

emotional a., a. caused by a strong emotional disturbance, *e.g.,* fright, grief.

hyperprolactinemic a., a. associated with abnormally high levels of serum prolactin; often accompanied by unphysiological lactation.

hypophysial a., a. due to inadequate gonadotrophic secretions by the anterior lobe of the hypophysis.

hypothalamic a., secondary a. arising from defective hypothalamic stimulation.

jogger's a., temporary cessation of menstrual function due to strenuous, daily exercise, as in jogging.

lactation a., physiological suppression of menses while nursing.
ovarian a., a. due to deficiency of estrogenic hormone.
pathologic a., a. due to organic disease, either uterine or other, *e.g.,* ovarian or pituitary failure, Simmonds' disease, anemic debility.
physiologic a., a. of pregnancy or the menopause, not associated with an organic disorder.
postpartum a., permanent a. following childbirth, sometimes due to pituitary failure resulting from postpartum hemorrhage and consequent necrosis of the pituitary.
primary a., a. in which the menses have never occurred.
secondary a., a. in which the menses appeared at puberty but subsequently ceased.
traumatic a., absence of menses because of endometrial scarring or cervical stenosis.

amenorrheal, amenorrheic (ă-men-ō-rē'ăl, -rē'ik). Relating to, accompanied by, or due to amenorrhea.

amentia (ă-men'shē-ă) [L. madness, fr. *ab,* from, + *mens,* mind]. **1.** Mental *retardation.* **2.** Dementia.
nevoid a., Brushfield-Wyatt *disease.*
phenylpyruvic a., a. accompanied by the appearance of phenylpyruvate in the urine.
Stearns alcoholic a., a temporary alcoholic mental disorder resembling delirium tremens but lasting for a longer time and showing a greater degree of amnesia and other mental defects.

amential (ă-men'shē-al). Pertaining to amentia.

American Law Institute rule. See under rule.

American Red Cross. The national Red Cross society of the United States, established by Congress to assist in caring for the sick and wounded, serving as a communications link between members of the U.S. armed forces and their families, conducting disaster relief and prevention programs, and furnishing other humanitarian services, the largest of which is a network of regional blood centers providing blood and blood products.

americium (am'ĕ-ris'ē-ŭm). An element obtained by the bombardment of uranium with neutrons or β decay of plutoniums 241 and 243; symbol Am, atomic no. 95.

amerism (am'er-izm) [G. *a-* priv. + *meros,* part]. The condition or quality of not dividing into parts, segments, or merozoites.

ameristic (am-ĕ-ris'tik). Endowed with amerism; not dividing into parts or segments.

Ames, B.N., U.S. molecular biologist, *1928 See A. *assay, test.*

amethopterin (ă-meth-ō-ter'in, am-ĕ-thop'tĕ-rin). Methotrexate.

ametria (ă-mē'trē-ă) [G. *a-* priv. + *mētra,* uterus]. Congenital absence of the uterus.

ametriodinic acid (ă'mĕ-trē-ō-din'ik). Iodamide.

ametrometer (am'ĕ-trom'ĕ-ter) [ametropia + G. *metron,* measure]. An appliance for measuring the degree of ametropia.

ametropia (am-ĕ-trō'pē-ă) [G. *ametros,* disproportionate, fr. *a-* priv. + *metron,* measure, + *ōps,* eye]. The optical condition in which there is an error of refraction so that with the eye at rest the retina is not in conjugate focus with light rays from distant objects, *i.e.,* only objects located a finite distance from the eye are focused on the retina.
axial a., that resulting from a shortening or lengthening of the eyeball on the optic axis, causing hyperopia or myopia, respectively.
index a., that resulting from alteration in the refractive index of the lens of the eye.

ametropic (am-ĕ-trō'pik). Relating to, or suffering from, ametropia.

amiantaceous (am'i-an-tā'shŭs) [G. *amiantus,* asbestos]. Asbestos-like; describing a type of crusting of a cutaneous lesion.

amianthoid (am-i-an'thoyd) [G. *amianthus,* asbestos]. Asbestoid; having a crystalline appearance like asbestos.

-amic. Suffix denoting the replacement of one COOH group of a dicarboxylic acid by a carboxamide group (—$CONH_2$); applied only to trivial names (*e.g.,* succinamic acid).

amicrobic (ā-mī-krō'bik). Not microbic; not related to or caused by microorganisms.

amicroscopic (ā'mī-krō-skop'ik). Submicroscopic.

amidase (am'i-dās) [EC 3.5.1.4]. Acylase; acylamidase; an enzyme that catalyzes the hydrolysis of monocarboxylic amides to free acid plus NH_3.

amidases. Amidohydrolases.

amide (am'īd, am'id). A substance formally derived from ammonia through the substitution of one or more of the hydrogen atoms by acyl groups, R—CO—NH_2, or from a carboxylic acid by replacement of a carboxylic OH by NH_2. Replacement of one hydrogen atom constitutes a **primary a.**; that of two hydrogen atoms, a **secondary a.**; and that of three atoms, a **tertiary a.**

amidine (am'i-din). The monovalent radical —C(NH)-NH_2.

amidinohydrolases (am'i-din-ō-hī'drō-lās-ez) [EC sub-subgroup 3.5.3]. Enzymes cleaving linear amidines; *e.g.,* arginase, creatinase.

amidinotransferases (am'i-din-ō-trans'fer-ās-ez) [EC sub-subclass 2.1.4]. Transamidinases; enzymes catalyzing a transamidination reaction (*e.g.,* glycine amidinotransferase).

amido-. Prefix denoting the amide radical, R-CO-NH- or R-SO_2-NH-, etc.

amido black 10B (am'i-dō) [C.I. 20470]. An acid diazo dye, $C_{12}H_{14}N_6O_9S_2Na_2$, used as a connective tissue stain, for staining protein in paper chromatography, and in electrophoresis.

amidogen (am'i-dō-jen). The amino group —(NH_2).

amidohydrolases (am'i-dō-hī'drō-lā-sez) [EC class 3.5.1 and 3.5.2]. Amidases; deamidases; deamidizing enzymes; enzymes hydrolyzing C-N bonds of amides; *e.g.,* asparaginase, barbiturase, urease, amidase.

amidonaphthol red (am'i-dō-naf'thol) [C.I. 18050]. Azophloxin; an azo dye, $C_{18}H_{13}N_3S_2Na_2$, used in light and fluorescence microscopy as a real acid counterstain.

amidopyrine (am-i-dō-pī'rēn). Aminopyrine.

Amidostomum anseris (am-i-dos'tō-mŭm an'ser-is) [amido- + G. *stoma,* mouth, + L. *anser,* goose]. A species of bloodsucking nematodes, similar to those of the genus *Trichostrongylus,* that parasitizes the gizzard and sometimes also the proventriculus and esophagus of domestic and wild ducks and geese; it causes heavy mortality in young birds.

amidoximes (am-i-doks'īmz, -dok'sēmz). Amide oximes; the oximes of amides with the general formula, R-C(NH_2)-NOH.

amidoxyl (am-i-dok'sil). The radical of an amide oxime (amidoxime), the terminal H (of the NOH) having been lost.

amikacin sulfate (am-i-kā'sin). An antibiotic agent with antimicrobial activity similar to that of kanamycin; also effective against *Pseudomonas aeruginosa.*

amiloride hydrochloride (ă-mil'ō-rīd). *N*-Amidino-3,5-diamino-6-chloropyrazinecarboxamide monohydrochloride dihydrate; a nonsteroidal compound exerting an effect similar to that of an aldosterone inhibitor, *i.e.,* urinary sodium excretion is enhanced and potassium excretion is reduced.

amimia (ă-mim'ē-ă) [G. *a-* priv. + *mimos,* a mimic]. Loss of the power to express ideas by gestures or signs.

aminacrine hydrochloride (am'i-nak'rin). 9-Aminoacridine hydrochloride; bactericidal agent for external use. See also aminocridine hydrochloride (acridine yellow).

aminate (am'i-nāt). To combine with ammonia.

amine (ă-mēn′, am′in). A substance formally derived from ammonia by the replacement of one or more of the hydrogen atoms by hydrocarbon or other radicals. The substitution of one hydrogen atom constitutes a **primary a.**, *e.g.*, NH_2CH_3; that of two atoms, a **secondary a.**, *e.g.*, $NH(CH_3)_2$; that of three atoms, a **tertiary a.**, *e.g.*, $N(CH_3)_3$; and that of four atoms, a **quaternary ammonium ion**, *e.g.*, $\overset{+}{N}(CH_3)_4$, a positively charged ion isolated only in association with a negative ion. The a.'s form salts with acids.

adrenergic a., adrenomimetic a., sympathomimetic a.

a. oxidase (copper-containing) [EC 1.4.3.6], a. oxidase (pyridoxal-containing); diamine oxidase; diamino oxyhydrase; histaminase; an oxidoreductase containing copper, and perhaps pyridoxal phosphate, and carrying out the same reaction as a. oxidase (flavin-containing).

a. oxidase (flavin-containing) [EC 1.4.3.4], monoamine oxidase; tyramine oxidase; tyraminase; diamine oxidase; adrenalin oxidase; an oxidoreductase containing flavin and oxidizing amines with the aid of O_2 to aldehydes or ketones with the release of NH_3 and H_2O_2.

a. oxidase (pyridoxal-containing), a. oxidase (copper-containing).

pressor a., pressor *base.*

sympathetic a., sympathomimetic a.

sympathomimetic a., adrenergic, adrenomimetic, or sympathetic a.; an agent that evokes responses similar to those produced by adrenergic nerve activity (*e.g.*, epinephrine, ephedrine, isoproterenol).

vasoactive a., a substance, such as histamine or serotonin, that contains amino groups and is pharmacologically characterized by its action on the blood vessels (altering vascular caliber or permeability).

amino-. Prefix denoting a compound containing the radical, $—NH_2$.

amino acid (AA) (ă-mē′nō). An organic acid in which one of the CH hydrogen atoms has been replaced by NH_2. See also α-amino acid.

a. a. dehydrogenases, enzymes catalyzing the oxidative deamination of amino acids to the corresponding oxo (keto) acids; two relatively nonspecific varieties exist, L and D (EC 1.4.1.5 and EC 1.4.99.1), for which L-amino acids and D-amino acids are the respective substrates; the products include NH_3 and a reduced hydrogen acceptor (NADH in the L case); a. a. dehydrogenases of greater specificity exit, (*e.g.*, glycine dehydrogenase). *Cf.* a. a. oxidases.

essential a. a.'s, α-amino acids required by an organism and which must be supplied in its diet (*i.e.*, cannot be synthesized by the organism either as free a. a.'s or in proteins.

nonessential a. acids, those a. a.'s that may be synthesized by an organism and are thus not required as such in its diet.

a. a. oxidases, enzymes (EC 1.4.3.2 and 1.4.3.3) oxidizing, with O_2, L- and D-amino acids respectively, to the corresponding keto acids, NH_3 and H_2O_2. *Cf.* a. a. dehydrogenases.

α-amino acid. An amino acid of the general formula $R\text{-}CHNH_2\text{-}COOH$ (*i.e.*, the NH_2 in the α position); the L forms of these are the hydrolysis products of proteins.

aminoacidemia (ă-mē′nō-as-i-dē′mē-ă, am′i-nō-) [amino acid + G. *haima*, blood]. The presence of excessive amounts of specific amino acids in the blood.

aminoacid-tRNA ligases. Recommended name for aminoacyl-tRNA synthetases (EC 6.1.1.1 - EC 6.1.1.22); *e.g.*, tyrosine-tRNA ligase for tyrosyl-tRNA synthetase (EC 6.1.1.1).

aminoaciduria (am′i-nō-as-i-dū′rē-ă) [amino acid + G. *ouron*, urine]. Acidaminuria; hyperaminoaciduria; excretion of amino acids in the urine, especially in excessive amounts.

9-aminoacridine (ă-mē-nō-ak′ri-dēn). 5-Aminoacridine; one of the acridine group of antiseptics (flavins); highly fluorescent in solution; used topically as an antiseptic.

5- or 9-**aminoacridine hydrochloride.** *Acridine* yellow.

aminoacyl (AA) (ă-mē′nō-as′il). The radical formed from an amino acid by removal of OH from a COOH group.

aminoacyladenylate (ă-mē′nō-as-il-ă-den′i-lāt). The product formed by the condensation of the acyl radical of an amino acid and adenosine 5′-phosphate (originally in the form of adenosine 5′-triphosphate, with elimination of a pyrophosphoric group).

aminoacylase (ă-mē′nō-as′i-lās) [EC 3.5.1.14]. An enzyme catalyzing hydrolysis of a wide variety of *N*-acyl amino acids to the amino acids. Also known as dehydropeptidase II and hippuricase (from substances on which it acts), benzamide, and histozyme.

α-aminoacyl-peptide hydrolases. Aminopeptidases.

aminoacyl-tRNA. Generic term for those compounds in which amino acids are esterfied through their COOH groups to the 3′ (or 2′) OH's of the terminal adenosine residues of transfer RNA's (*e.g.*, alanyl-tRNA, glycyl-tRNA); each compound involves one or a small number of tRNA's of specific chemical structure.

α-aminoadipic acid (ă-mē′nō-ă-dip′ik). 2-Amino-1,6-hexanedioic acid; an intermediate of lysine biosynthesis and degradation in higher fungi and bacteria, but not in algae and higher plants.

aminobenzene (ă-mē′nō-ben′zēn). Aniline.

***o*-aminobenzoic acid** (ă-mē′nō-ben-zō′ik). Anthranilic acid.

***p*-aminobenzoic acid (PABA).** Vitamin B_x; a factor in the vitamin B complex, a part of all folic acids and required for its formation; neutralizes the bacteriostatic effects of the sulfonamides since it furnishes an essential growth factor for bacteria, the utilization of which the sulfonamides interfere with.

D(−)-α-aminobenzylpenicillin (ă-mē-nō-ben′zil-pen-i-sil′in). Ampicillin.

γ-aminobutyric acid (GABA, γ-Abu) (ă-mē′nō-byū-tēr′ik). $NH_2(CH_2)_3COOH$; a constituent of the central nervous system; quantitatively the principal inhibitory neurotransmitter.

aminocaproic acid (ă-mē′nō-că-prō′ik). ε-Aminocaproic acid; 6-aminohexanoic acid; an antifibrinolytic agent, used to prevent bleeding in hemophilia, and after heart and prostate surgery when plasminogen or urokinase may be activated.

aminocarbonyl (am-i-nō-kar′bon-il). Carboxamide.

aminoglutethimide (ă-mē′nō-glū-teth′i-mīd). 2-(*p*-Aminophenyl)-2-ethylglutarimide; used, in conjunction with other anticonvulsant agents, in the management of mild convulsive disorders, but side effects are frequent; also has adrenal cortex inhibitory action and is used in the treatment of Cushing's syndrome and carcinomas.

aminoglycoside (am′i-nō-glī′kō-sīd). Any one of a group of bacteriocidal antibiotics derived from species of *Streptomyces* or *Micromonosporum* and characterized by two or more amino sugars joined by a glycoside linkage to a central hexose; a.'s act by causing misreading and inhibition of protein synthesis on bacterial ribosomes and are effective against aerobic Gram-negative bacilli and *Mycobacterium tuberculosis.* Some commonly used a.'s are streptomycin, neomycin, and gentamycin.

***p*-aminohippuric acid (PAH)** (ă-mē′nō-hi-pyūr′ik). *N*-(4-Aminobenzoyl) glycine; used in renal function tests.

***p*-aminohippuric acid synthase.** An enzyme in the liver that catalyzes the synthesis of *p*-aminohippuric acid from *p*-aminobenzoic acid and glycine.

5-aminoimidazole ribose 5′-phosphate (ă-mē′nō-im-id-az′ōl). 5-Amino-1-β-D-ribofuranosylimidazole 5′-phosphate; an intermediate in the biosynthesis of purines.

α-aminoisobutyric acid (ă-mē′nō-ī-sō-byū-tēr′ik). 2-Amino-2-methylpropionic acid; a synthetic amino acid useful in the study of amino acid transport across cell membranes; it is not metabolized by the cell.

β-aminoisobutyric acid. 3-Amino-2-methylpropionic acid; an end product of thymine catabolism; high urinary levels (200-300 mg/day) have been noted in some individuals, either from some disease process or following a genetic pattern.

aminoisometradine (ă-mē'nō-ī-sō-met'ră-dēn). Amisometradine.

α-amino-β-ketoadipic acid. 2-Amino-3-oxo-1,6-hexanedioic acid; an intermediate of porphobilinogen synthesis formed by δ-aminolevulinic acid synthase from succinyl-CoA and glycine; it rapidly decarboxylates to δ-aminolevulinic acid.

δ-aminolevulinic acid (ALA) (ă-mē'nō-lev-yū-lin'ik). $NH_2CH_2COCH_2CH_2COOH$; an acid formed by δ-aminolevulinate synthase (EC 2.3.1.37) from glycine and succinyl-coenzyme A; a precursor of porphobilinogen, hence an important intermediate in the biosynthesis of hematin.

δ-aminolevulinate dehydratase (ă-mē'nō-lev-yū-lin'āt). *Porphobilinogen* synthase.

aminolysis (am-i-nol'i-sis). Replacement of a halogen in an alkyl or aryl molecule by an amine radical, with elimination of hydrogen halide.

aminometradine (ă-mē'nō-met'ră-dēn). Aminometramide.

aminometramide (ă-mē'nō-met'ră-mīd). Aminometradine; 1-allyl-6-amino-3-ethyluracil; synthetic uracil derivative; an orally effective diuretic that is believed to act by inhibiting the reabsorption of sodium by the renal tubules; used in the treatment of edema due to congestive heart failure, liver disease, pregnancy, and certain drugs.

aminopeptidase (cytosol) [EC 3.4.11.1]. Leucine aminopeptidase; an enzyme of broad specificity, containing zinc, and catalyzing the hydrolysis of the N-terminal amino acid of a peptide.

aminopeptidase (microsomal) [EC 3.4.11.2 (formerly 3.4.1.2)]. An aminopeptidase of broad specificity, but preferring alanine and discriminating against proline.

aminopeptidases (ă-mē'nō-pep'ti-dās-ez) [EC sub-group 3.4.11]. α-aminoacyl-peptide hydrolases; enzymes catalyzing the breakdown of a peptide, removing the amino acid at the amino end of the chain; found in intestinal secretions.

aminophenazone (ă-mē-nō-fen'ă-zōn). Aminopyrine.

aminopherases (ă-mē'nō-fer-ās-ez). Aminotransferases.

aminophylline (ă-mē-nō-fil'in, am-i-nof'i-lin, -ēn). Theophylline ethylenediamine; $(C_7H_8N_4O_2)_2C_2H_4(NH_2)_22H_2O$; diuretic, vasodilator, and cardiac stimulant; also used in asthma that is resistant to epinephrine, and in veterinary medicine.

aminopromazine (ă-mē-nō-prō'mă-zēn). 10-[2,3-Bis(dimethylamino)propyl]phenothiazine; an intestinal antispasmodic.

***p*-aminopropiophenone (PAPP)** (ă-mē'nō-prō-pē-ō-fē'nōn). 1-(4-Aminophenyl)-1-propanone; an antidote for cyanide poisoning.

aminopterin (am-i-nop'ter-in). 4-Aminopteroylglutamic acid; 4-aminofolic acid; a folic acid antagonist used in the treatment of acute leukemia and other neoplastic diseases.

6-aminopurine (ă-mē'nō-pyūr'ēn). Alenine.

4-aminopyridine (am-i-nō-pir'i-dēn). An antagonist of nondepolarizing neuromuscular blockade; devoid of muscarinic side-effects but associated with central nervous system stimulation.

aminopyrine (am'i-nō-pī'rēn). Amidopyrine; aminophenazone; dipyrine; dimethylaminoantipyrine; 4-dimethylamino-2,3-dimethyl-1-phenyl-3-pyrazolin-5-one; used as an antipyretic and analgesic in rheumatism, neuritis, pulmonary tuberculosis, and common colds; may cause leukocytopenia.

aminorex (ă-min'ō-reks). 2-Amino-5-phenyl-2-oxazoline; a sympathomimetic appetite suppressant.

***p*-aminosalicylic acid (PAS, PASA)** (am'i-nō-sal-i-sil'ik). 4-Amino-2-hydroxybenzoic acid; a bacteriostatic agent against tubercle bacilli, used as an adjunct to streptomycin; the potassium, sodium, and calcium salts have the same use.

5-aminosalicyclic acid. Mesalamine.

α-aminosuccinic acid (ă-mē'nō-sŭk-sin'ik). Aspartic acid.

amino-terminal (ă-mē'nō-ter'min-ăl). N- or NH_2-terminal; the α-NH_2 group or the aminoacyl residue containing it at one end of a peptide or protein (usually at left as written).

aminotransferases (ă-mē'nō-trans'fer-ās-ez) [EC sub-group 2.6.1]. Aminopherases; transaminases; enzymes transferring amino groups between an α-amino acid to (usually) a 2-keto acid; *e.g.*, alanine and 2-ketoglutarate.

aminotriazole (am'i-nō-trī'ă-zol). Amitrole; 3-amino-1*H*-1,2,4-triazole; an effective weed killer that also possesses some antithyroid activity.

aminuria (am-i-nū'rē-ă) [amine + G. *ouron*, urine]. Excretion of amines in the urine.

amiodarone hydrochloride (ă-mē'ō-dă-rōn). (2-Butyl-3-benzofuranyl)[4-[2-(diethylamino)ethoxyl]-3,5-diiodophenyl]methanone; a coronary vasodilator used in the control of ventricular and supraventricular arrhythmias, and in the management of angina pectoris.

amisometradine (am'i-sō-met'ră-dēn). Aminoisometradine; 6-amino-3-methyl-1-(2-methylallyl)uracil; an oral diuretic.

amithiozone (am-i-thī'ō-zōn). Thiacetazone; 4'-formylacetanilide thiosemicarbazone; a leprostatic agent.

amitosis (am-i-tō'sis) [G. *a-* priv. + mitosis]. Remak's or direct nuclear division; direct division of the nucleus and cell, without the complicated changes in the nucleus that occur in the ordinary process of cell reproduction.

amitotic (am-i-tot'ik). Relating to or marked by amitosis.

amitriptyline hydrochloride (am-i-trip'ti-lēn). 10,11-Dihydro-*N,N*- dimethyl-5*H*- dibenzo[*a,d*]cycloheptene-$\Delta^{5,\gamma}$-propylamine hydrochloride; chemically and pharmacologically related to imipramine hydrochloride; an antidepressant agent with mild tranquilizing properties, used in the treatment of mental depression and in the depressive phase of manic-depressive states.

amitrole (am'i-trōl). Aminotriazole.

ammeter (am'mē-ter). An instrument for measuring strength of electric current in amperes.

Ammon, Friedrich A. von, German ophthalmologist and pathologist, 1799–1861. See A.'s *fissure, operation, prominence.*

ammonemia (am-ō-nē'mē-ă). Ammoniemia.

ammonia (ă-mō'nē-ă). A volatile gas, NH_3, very soluble in water, forming the weak base, NH_4OH, which combines with acids to form ammonium compounds.

ammoniac (ă-mō'nē-ak). A gum resin from a plant of western Asia, *Dorema ammoniacum* (family Umbelliferae); used internally as a stimulant and expectorant, and externally as a counterirritant plaster.

ammoniacal (ă-mō-nī'ă-kl). Relating to ammonia.

ammonia-lyases. Enzymes removing ammonia or an amino compound nonhydrolytically (hence lyases, EC class 4), by rupture of a C—N bond leaving a double bond (EC subgroup 4.3); *e.g.*, aspartate ammonia-lyase (aspartase) (EC 4.3.1.1).

ammoniated (ă-mō'nē-āt-ed). Containing or combined with ammonia.

ammoniemia (ă-mō-nē-ē'mē-ă) [ammonia + G. *haima*, blood]. Ammonemia; the presence of ammonia or some of its compounds in the blood, thought to be formed from the decomposition of urea; it usually results in subnormal temperature, weak pulse, gastroenteric symptoms, and coma.

ammonio-. Combining form indicating an ammonium group; *e.g.*, trimethylammonioethanol (choline).

ammonium (ă-mō'nē-ŭm). The ion, NH_4^+, formed by combination of NH_3 and H^+; behaves as a univalent metal in forming ammonium compounds.
a. benzoate, $C_6H_5COONH_4$; a stimulant diuretic, urinary antiseptic, and antirheumatic.
a. bromide, NH_4Br; a sedative.
a. carbonate, $(NH_4)_2CO_3$; a cardiac and respiratory stimulant and carminative expectorant.
a. chloride, muriate of ammonia; sal ammoniac; NH_4Cl; a stimulant expectorant and cholagogue; used to relieve alkalosis and to promote lead excretion.
dibasic a. phosphate, $(NH_4)_2HPO_4$; used for fireproofing, in baking powder, and as an antirheumatic.
a. ferric sulfate, ferric ammonium sulfate.
a. ichthosulfonate, ichthammol.
a. iodide, NH_4I; an expectorant.
a. mandelate, mandelic acid ammonium salt; a urinary antiseptic.
a. molybdate, $H_{24}Mo_7N_6O_{24}$; used in electron microscopy as a negative stain, and as a reagent for alkaloids and other substances.
monobasic a. phosphate, $(NH_4)H_2PO_4$; used in baking powder.
a. nitrate, NH_4NO_3; used in making nitrous oxide gas, in freezing mixtures, matches, and fertilizers; also used in veterinary medicine.

ammoniuria (ă-mō-nē-yū'rē-ă) [ammonia + G. *ouron,* urine]. Ammoniacal urine; excretion of urine that contains an excessive amount of ammonia.

ammonolysis (ă-mō-nol'i-sis) [ammonia + G. *lysis,* dissolution]. The breaking of a chemical bond with the addition of the elements of ammonia (NH_2 and H) at the point of breakage.

amnesia (am-nē'zē-ă) [G. *amnēsia,* forgetfulness]. A disturbance in the memory of information stored in long-term memory, in contrast to short-term memory, manifested by total or partial inability to recall past experiences.
anterograde a., a. in reference to events occurring after the trauma or disease that caused the condition.
lacunar a., localized a., a. in reference to isolated events.
posthypnotic a., selective forgetting, after a hypnotic state, of events occurring during hypnosis or of information stored in long-term memory, such as one's name, address, and names of relatives.
retrograde a., a. in reference to events that occurred before the trauma or disease that caused the condition.

amnesiac (am-nē'sē-ak). One suffering from amnesia.

amnesic (am-nē'sik). Amnestic (1); relating to or characterized by amnesia.

amnestic (am-nes'tik). **1.** Amnesic. **2.** An agent causing amnesia.

amnio- [G. *amnion*]. Combining form relating to the amnion.

amniocentesis (am'nē-ō-sen-tē'sis) [amnio- + G. *kentēsis,* puncture]. Transabdominal aspiration of fluid from the amniotic sac.

amniochorial, amniochorionic (am'nē-ō-kōr'ē-ăl, -kōr-ē-on'ik). Relating to both amnion and chorion.

amniogenesis (am'nē-ō-jen'ĕ-sis) [amnio- + G. *genesis,* production]. Formation of the amnion.

amniography (am-nē-og'ră-fē) [amnio- + G. *graphō,* to write]. Roentgenography of the amniotic sac after the injection of an opaque, water-soluble solution into the sac, by which it becomes possible to see the outline of the umbilical cord, the placenta, and the soft tissues of the fetal body. See also fetography.

amnioma (am-nē-ō'mă) [amnio- + G. *-oma,* tumor]. Broad flat tumor of the skin resulting from antenatal adhesion of the amnion.

amnion (am'nē-on) [G. the membrane around the fetus, fr. *amnios,* lamb]. Amniotic sac; indusium (2); innermost of the membranes enveloping the embryo *in utero* and containing the amniotic fluid; it consists of an internal embryonic layer with its ectodermal component, and an external somatic mesodermal component; in the later stages of pregnancy the amnion expands to come in contact with and partially fuse to the inner wall of the chorionic vesicle.

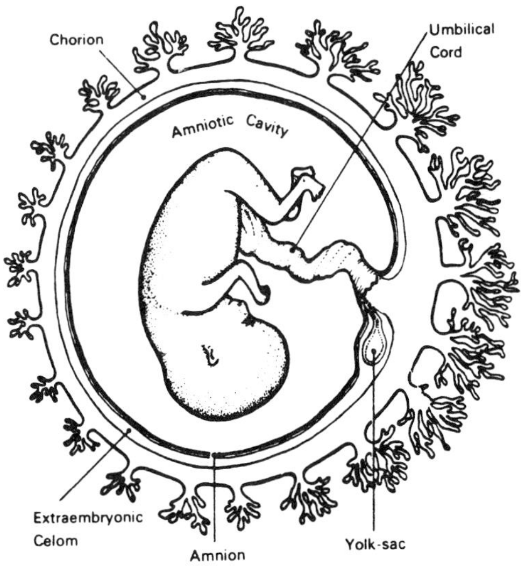

Amnion

a. nodo'sum, squamous metaplasia of amnion; nodules in the a. that consist of typical stratified squamous epithelium.

amnionic (am-nē-on'ik). Amniotic; relating to the amnion.

amnionitis (am'nē-ō-nī'tis) [amnion + G. *-itis,* inflammation]. Inflammation resulting from infection of the amniotic sac, which, in turn, usually results from premature rupture of the membranes (a condition often associated with neonatal infection).

amniorrhea (am-nē-ō-rē'ă) [amnio- + G. *rhoia,* flow]. Escape of amniotic fluid.

amniorrhexis (am-nē-ō-rek'sis) [amnio- + G. *rhēxis,* rupture]. Rupture of the amniotic membrane.

amnioscope (am'nē-ō-skōp). An endoscope for studying amniotic fluid through the intact amniotic sac.

amnioscopy (am-nē-os'kō-pē) [amnio- + G. *skopeō,* to view]. Examination of the amniotic fluid in the lowest part of the amniotic sac by means of an endoscope introduced through the cervical canal.

Amniota (am'nē-ō'tă). A group of vertebrates whose embryos are enclosed in an amnion; it includes all the reptiles, birds, and mammals.

amniotic (am-nē-ot'ik). Amnionic.

amniotome (am'nē-ō-tōm) [amnio- + G. *tomē,* cutting]. An instrument for puncturing the fetal membranes.

amniotomy (am-nē-ot'ō-mē). Artificial rupture of the fetal membranes as a means of inducing or expediting labor.

amobarbital (am-ō-bar'bi-tahl). 5-Ethyl-5-isoamylbarbituric acid; a central nervous system depressant with an intermediate duration of action; also used as the sodium salt.

A-mode. In diagnostic ultrasound, a one-dimensional presentation of a reflected sound wave in which echo amplitude (A) is displayed along the vertical axis and time of rebound (depth) along the horizontal axis; the echo information is presented from interfaces along a single line in the direction of the sound beam.

amodiaquine hydrochloride (am-ō-dī'ă-kwīn). 4-(7-Chloro-4-quinolylamino)-α-diethylamino-*o*-cresol dihydrochloride dihydrate; an antimalarial drug, also used in the treatment of amebic hepatitis; large doses may result in sialorrhea, nausea, vomiting, diarrhea, insomnia, palpitations, spasticity, and possibly convulsions.

amoeb-. See ameb-.

Amoeba (ă-mē'bă) [Mod. L. fr. G. *amoibē*change]. A genus of naked, lobose, pseudopod-forming protozoa of the class Sarcodina (or Rhizopoda), that are abundant soil-dwellers, especially in rich organic debris, and are also commonly found as parasites. The typical parasites of man are now placed in the genera *Entamoeba, Endolimax, Iodamoeba,* and *Dientamoeba*. See also *Naegleria.*

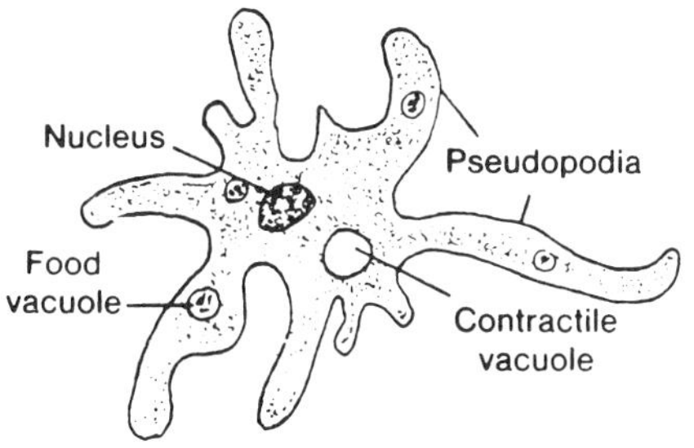

Amoeba

A. bucca'lis, *Entamoeba gingivalis.*
A. co'li, *Entamoeba coli.*
A. denta'lis, *Entamoeba gingivalis.*
A. dysenter'iae, *Entamoeba histolytica.*
A. histolyt'ica, *Entamoeba histolytica.*
A. meleag'ridis, *Histomonas meleagridis.*
A. pro'teus, an abundant, nonparasitic species, remarkable for the number and varied shapes of its pseudopodia.

Amoebotaenia (ă-mē'bō-tē'nē-ă) [amoeb- + L. fr. G. *tainia,* band, tape, a tapeworm]. A genus of small intestinal tapeworms of birds, seldom possessing more than 30 segments. *A. cuneata* (*A. sphenoides*) is a species common in domestic fowl; its cysticercoid is developed in earthworms.

amok (ă-mok') [native word]. **1.** A psychic disturbance originally observed in Malaya in which the subject becomes dangerously maniacal ("running amok"). **2.** Amuck; colloquialism denoting maniacal, wild, or uncontrolled behavior threatening injury to others.

amorph (ā'mōrf) [G. *a-* neg. + *morphē,* form, shape]. Silent allele; an allele that has no phenotypically recognizable product and therefore the existence of which can be inferred on negative evidence only, depending on the subtlety of the means of detection available.

amorphagnosia (ă-mōr-fag-nō'sē-ă) [G. *a-,* priv., + *morphē,* shape, + *gnosis,* recognition]. Inability to recognize the size and shape of objects.

amorphia, amorphism (ă-mōr'fē-ă, -fizm) [G. *a-* priv. + *morphē,* form]. Condition of being amorphous (1).

amorphosynthesis (ă-mōr'fō-sin'thĕ-sis) [G. *a*-priv. + *morphē,* form, + synthesis]. A disorder of awareness of space and of body schema.

amorphous (ă-mōr'fŭs). **1.** Without definite shape or visible differentiation in structure. **2.** Not crystallized.

amorphus (ă-mōr'fŭs). A malformed fetus with rudimentary head, limbs, and heart.

Amoss, Harold L., U. S. physician, 1886–1956. See A.'s *sign.*

amotio placentae (ă-mō'shē-ō plă-sen'tē). Abruptio placentae.

amotio retinae (ă-mō'shē-ō ret'ĭ-nē). Obsolete term for retinal *detachment.*

amoxapine (ă-mok'să-pēn). 2-Chloro-11-(1-piperazinyl)dibenz[*b,f*][1,4]oxazepine; a tricyclic antidepressant drug with uses similar to those of imipramine.

amoxicillin (ă-mok-si-sil'in). A semisynthetic penicillin antibiotic with an antimicrobial spectrum similar to that of ampicillin.

AMP Abbreviation for *adenosine* monophosphate (see adenylic acid); specifically, the 5'-phosphate unless modified by a numerical prefix.

AMP deaminase [EC 3.5.4.6]. Adenylic acid deaminase; an enzyme converting adenylic acid to inosinic acid and NH_3.

amperage (am'pĕr-ij). Strength of electric current. See ampere.

Ampère, André-Marie, French physicist, 1775–1836. See ampere; statampere; A.'s *postulate.*

ampere (A) (am-pēr) [A. *Ampère*]. The practical unit of electrical current; the absolute, practical a. originally was defined as having the value of 1/10 of the electromagnetic unit (see abampere and coulomb). Present definitions are: **1.** Legal: the current that, flowing for 1 second, will deposit 1.118 mg of silver from silver nitrate solution. **2.** Scientific (SI): the current that, if maintained in two straight parallel conductors of infinite length and of negligible circular cross-sections and placed 1 m apart in a vacuum, produces between them a force of 2×10^{-7} N/m.

amperometry (am-pĕr-om'ĕ-trē). Determination of any analyte concentration by measurement of the current generated in a suitable chemical reaction.

amph-. See amphi-, and ampho-.

ampheclexis (am-fĕ-klek'-sis) [G. *amphi,* two-sided, + *eklexis,* selection]. Reciprocal sexual selection, *i.e.,* by both male and female.

amphetamine (am-fet'ă-mēn). α-Methylphenethylamine; 1-phenyl-2-aminopropane; (phenylisopropyl)amine; $C_6H_5CH_2CH(NH_2)CH_3$; closely related in its structure and action to ephedrine and other sympathomimetic amines.
a. (4-chlorophenoxy)acetate, same actions and uses as a. sulfate.
a. phosphate, same actions and uses as a. sulfate.
a. sulfate, exerts less vasopressor, cardiac, and bronchial effect than ephedrine, but has a greater central nervous stimulating effect, decreasing the sensation of fatigue; used in the treatment of narcolepsy and certain types of paralysis agitans, and to reduce appetite in obesity.

***d*-amphetamine phosphate.** Dextroamphetamine phosphate.

***d*-amphetamine sulfate.** Dextroamphetamine sulfate.

amphi- [G. *amphi,* two-sided]. Combining form meaning on both sides, surrounding, double.

amphiarthrodial (am'fi-ar-thrō'dē-ăl). Relating to amphiarthrosis.

amphiarthrosis (am'fi-ar-thrō'sis) [amphi- + G. *arthrōsis,* joint]. Symphysis (1).

amphiaster (am-fi-as'ter) [amphi- + G. *astēr,* star]. Diaster; the double-star figure formed by the two asters and their connecting spindle fibers during mitosis.

amphibaric (am-fi-bar'ik) [amphi- + G. *baros,* pressure]. Denoting a pharmacologic material that may lower or elevate arterial blood pressure, depending on the dose.

amphiblestrodes (am'fi-bles-trō'dēz) [G. *amphiblēstroeidēs,* net-like]. Obsolete term for retina.

amphicelous (am-fi-sē'lŭs) [amphi- + G. *koilos,* hollow]. Concave at each end, as the body of a vertebra of a fish.

amphicentric (am-fi-sen'trik) [amphi- + G. *kentron,* center]. Centering at both ends, said of a rete mirabile that begins by the vessel breaking up into a number of branches and ends by the branches joining again to form the same vessel.

amphichroic (am-fi-krō'ik). Amphichromatic.

amphichromatic (am'fi-krō-mat'ik) [amphi- + G. *chrōma,* color]. Amphichroic; having the property of exhibiting either of two colors; *e.g.*, litmus, an a. pigment which is red in acids and blue in alkalis.

amphicrania (am-fi-krā'nē-ă) [amphi- + G. *kranion*, skull]. Neuralgic pain on both sides of the head.

amphicyte (am'fi-sīt) [amphi- + G. *kytos*, cell]. Capsule cell; one of the cells located around the bodies of the cerebrospinal and sympathetic ganglionic neurons.

amphigenetic (am'fi-jĕ-net'ik). Amphogenetic; produced by both sexes.

amphikaryon (am'fē-kar'ē-on) [amphi- + G. *karyon*, kernel]. A diploid nucleus containing two haploid groups of chromosomes.

amphileukemic (am'fi-lū-kē'mik). Denoting a leukemic condition that corresponds in degree to the changes in the organ or tissue.

Amphimerus (am-fim'er-ŭs) [amphi- + G. *meros*, segment]. A genus of opisthorchid trematodes found in the bile ducts of mammals, birds, and reptiles; probably transmitted by fish.

amphimicrobe (am'fi-mī'krōb). A microorganism that is either aerobic or anaerobic, according to the environment.

amphimixis (am-fi-mik'sis) [amphi- + G. *mixis*, mingling]. **1.** Union of the paternal and maternal chromatin after impregnation of the ovum. **2.** In psychoanalysis, a combination of genital and anal eroticism.

amphinucleolus (am'fi-nū-klē'ō-lŭs) [amphi- + L. *nucleolus*, dim. of *nucleus*, kernel]. A double nucleolus having both basophilic and oxyphilic components.

Amphioxus (am-fē-ok'sŭs) [amphi- + G. *oxys*, sharp]. A genus of small, translucent, fishlike chordates found in warm marine waters. Members are structurally similar to vertebrates in having a notochord, gills, digestive tract, and nerve cord, but they lack paired fins, vertebrae, ribs, or a skull.

amphipathic (am-fē-path'ik) [amphi- + G. *pathos*, feeling]. Amphiphilic; amphiphobic; denoting a molecule, such as comprises detergents or wetting agents, that contains groups with characteristically different properties, e.g., both hydrophilic and hydrophobic properties.

amphiphilic (am-fē-fil'ik) [amphi- + G. *philos*, fond]. Amphipathic.

amphiphobic (am-fē-fōb'ik) [amphi- + G. *phobos*, fear]. Amphipathic.

amphistome (am-fis'tōm) [amphi- + G. *stoma*, mouth]. A common name for any trematode of the genus *Paramphistomum*.

amphithymia (am-fi-thī'mē-ă) [amphi- + G. *thymos*, soul]. Obsolete term for a mental condition marked by periods of depression and elation.

amphitrichate, amphitrichous (am-fit'ri-kāt, am-fit'ri-kŭs) [amphi- + G. *thrix*, hair]. Having a flagellum or flagella at both extremities of a microbial cell; denoting certain microorganisms.

amphitypy (am-fit'i-pē). The property of being characteristic of two types.

amphixenosis (am-fiks-en-ō'sis) [amphi- + G. *xenos*, stranger, + G. *-osis*, condition]. A zoonosis maintained in nature by man and lower animals, *e.g.*, certain staphylococcoses. *Cf.* anthropozoonosis, zooanthroponosis.

ampho- [G. *amphō*, both]. Combining form meaning on both sides, surrounding, double.

amphochromatophil, amphochromatophile (am'fō-krō-mat'ō-fil, -ō-fīl). Amphophil.

amphochromophil, amphochromophile (am-fō-krō'mō-fil, -fīl) [ampho- + G. *chrōma*, color, + *philos*, fond]. Amphophil.

amphocyte (am'fō-sīt). Amphophil (2).

amphodiplopia (am'fō-di-plō'pē-ă) [ampho- + G. *diploos*, double, + *ōps*, vision]. Obsolete term for double vision in each eye.

amphogenetic (am'fō-jĕ-net'ik). Amphigenetic.

ampholyte (am'fō-līt). Amphoteric *electrolyte*.

amphomycin (am-fō-mī'sin). An antibiotic substance produced by *Streptomyces canus;* used topically for skin infections.

amphophil, amphophile (am'fō-fil, -fīl) [ampho- + G. *philos*, fond]. Amphochromatophil; amphochromatophile; amphochromophil; amphochromophile. **1.** Amphophilic; amphophilous; having an affinity for both acid and for basic dyes. **2.** Amphocyte; a cell that stains readily with either acid or basic dyes.

amphophilic, amphophilous (am-fō-fil'ik, am-fof'i-lŭs). Amphophil (1).

amphoric (am-fōr'ik) [G. *amphora*, a jar]. Denoting the sound heard in percussion and auscultation, resembling the noise made by blowing across the mouth of a bottle.

amphoriloquy (am-fō-ril'ō-kwē) [G. *amphora*, a jar, + *loquor*, to speak]. Presence of amphoric voice.

amphorophony (am-fōr-of'ō-nē) [G. *amphora*, a jar, + *phōnē*, voice]. Amphoric *voice*.

amphoteric (am-fō-tār'ik) [G. *amphoteroi* (pl.), both, fr. *amphō*, both]. Having two opposite characteristics, especially having the capacity of reacting as either an acid or a base; *e.g.*, $Al(OH)_3 \equiv$ - H_3AlO_3.

amphotericin, amphotericin B (am-fō-tār'i-sin). $C_{46}H_{73}NO_{20}$; an amphoteric polyene antibiotic prepared from *Streptomyces nodosus and* available as the sodium deoxycholate complex; also a nephrotoxic antifungal agent used extensively in the treatment of systemic mycoses.

amphotonia, amphotony (am-fō-tō'nē-ă, am-fot'ō-nē) [ampho- + G. *tonos*, tension]. Increased excitability of both the parasympathetic and sympathetic nervous systems.

ampicillin (am-pi-si'lin). D-(-)-α-Aminobenzylpenicillin; R– = $C_6H_5CH(NH_2)$– ; an acid-stable semisynthetic penicillin derived from 6-aminopenicillanic acid; it has a broader spectrum of antimicrobial action than penicillin G, inhibits the growth of Gram-positive and Gram-negative bacteria, and is not resistant to penicillinase; also available as a. sodium and a. trihydrate.

amplexus (am-plek'sŭs) [L. an embrace, fr. *amplector*, pp. *-plexus*, to wind around]. The pairing of male and female at the time that eggs and sperm are discharged simultaneously in those species, such as frogs, in which fertilization occurs externally.

amplification (am'pli-fi-kā'shŭn) [L. *amplificationis*, an enlarging]. The process of making larger, as in increasing an auditory or visual stimulus to enhance its perception.

genetic a., a process for producing an increase in pertinent genetic material, particularly for increasing the proportion of plasmid DNA to that of bacterial DNA.

amplitude (am'pli-tūd) [L. *amplitudo*, fr. *amplus*, large]. Largeness; extent; breadth or range.

a. of accommodation, a. of convergence, see under accommodation, convergence.

a. of pulse, see average pulse *magnitude;* peak *magnitude*.

ampoule (am'pul). Ampule.

amprotropine phosphate (am'prō-trō'pēn). 3-Diethylamino-2,2-dimethylpropyl tropate phosphate; an antispasmodic, similar in action to atropine.

ampule, ampul (am'pūl) [L. *ampulla*]. Ampoule; a hermetically sealed container, usually made of glass, containing a sterile medicinal solution, or powder to be made up in solution, to be used for subcutaneous, intramuscular, or intravenous injection.

ampulla, gen. and pl. **ampullae** (am-pul'lă, -ē) [L. a two-handled bottle] [NA]. A saccular dilation of a canal or duct.

Bryant's a., that portion of an artery on the proximal side of a ligature containing the clot, its upper boundary being marked by a

slight constriction.
a. canalic'uli lacrima'lis [NA], a. ductus lacrimalis; a slight dilation in the lacrimal duct just beyond the punctum lacrimalis.
a. chy'li, *cisterna* chyli.
a. duc'tus deferen'tis [NA], a. of vas deferens; Henle's a.; the dilation of the ductus deferens where it approaches its fellow just before it is joined by the duct of the seminal vesicle.
a. duc'tus lacrima'lis, a. canaliculi lacrimalis.
duodenal a., **(1)** a duodeni; **(2)** a. hepatopancreatica.
a. duode'ni [NA], duodenal a. (1); the dilated portion of the superior part of the duodenum. See also duodenal *cap.*
Henle's a., a. ductus deferentis.
a. hepat'opancreat'ica [NA], duodenal a. (2); Vater's a.; the dilation within the major duodenal papilla that normally receives both the common bile duct and the main pancreatic duct.
a. lactif'era, *sinus* lactiferi.
a. membrana'cea, pl. **ampullae membrana'ceae** [NA], membranous a.; a nearly spherical enlargement of one end of each of the three semicircular ducts, anterior, posterior, and lateral, where they connect with the utricle. Each contains a neuroepithelial crista.
membranous a., a. membranacea.
a. of milk duct, *sinus* lactiferi.
a. os'sea, pl. **ampullae os'seae** [NA], osseous a.; a circumscribed dilation of one extremity of each of the three bony semicircular canals, anterior, posterior, and lateral; each contains a membranous a.
osseous a., a. ossea.
a. rec'ti [NA], a. of rectum; a dilated portion of the rectum just above the anal canal.
a. of rectum, a. recti.
Thoma's a., a dilation of the arterial capillary beyond the sheathed artery of the spleen.
a. tu'bae uteri'nae [NA], a. of uterine tube; the wide portion of the uterine (fallopian) tube near the fimbriated extremity; it has a complexly folded mucosa with a columnar epithelium of mostly ciliated cells between which are secretory cells.
a. of uterine tube, a. tubae uterinae.
a. of vas deferens, a. ductus deferentis.
Vater's a., a. hepatopancreatica.

ampullar (am-pul'ăr). Relating in any sense to an ampulla.

ampullitis (am-pul-lī'tis). Inflammation of any ampulla, especially of the dilated extremity of the vas deferens or of the ampulla of Vater.

ampullula (am-pul'ū-lă) [Mod. L. dim. of L. *ampulla*]. A circumscribed dilation of any minute lymphatic or blood vessel or duct.

AMPUTATION

amputation (am-pyū-tā'shŭn) [L. *amputatio,* fr. *am-puto,* pp. *-atus,* to cut around, prune]. **1.** The cutting off of a limb or part of a limb, the breast, or other projecting part. **2.** In dentistry, removal of the root of a tooth, or of the pulp, or of a nerve root or ganglion; a modifying adjective is therefore used (pulp a.; root a.).
A-E a., abbreviation for *a*bove-the-*e*lbow a.
A-K a., abbreviation for *a*bove-the-*k*nee a.
Alanson's a., a circular a., the stump shaped like a cone.
aperiosteal a., a. with removal of periosteum from bone at the site of a.
B-E a., abbreviation for *b*elow-the-*e*lbow a.
Bier's a., osteoplastic a. of tibia and fibula.

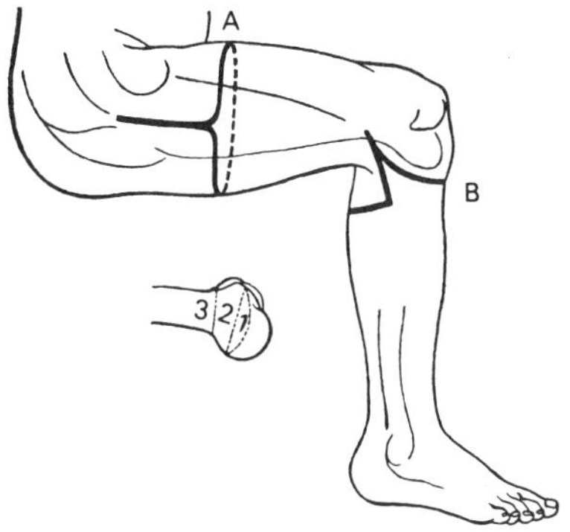

Amputation
A, racket incision for amputation of the hip; *B*, incision for Carden's, Gritti-Stokes, and Stokes' amputations. Inset shows the lines of section of the femur for (*1*) Carden's, (*2*) Gritti-Stokes, and (*3*) Stokes' amputations.

birth a., congenital a.
B-K a., abbreviation for *b*elow-the-*k*nee a.
bloodless a., dry a.; a. in which, by means of a tourniquet, the escape of blood from the cut surfaces is slight.
Callander's a., tenontoplastic a. through the femur at the knee.
Carden's a., transcondylar a. of the leg, the femur is sawed through the condyles just above the articular surface.
central a., a. in which the flaps are so united that the cicatrix runs across the end of the stump.
cervical a., a. of the uterine cervix.
Chopart's a., mediotarsal a.; a. through the midtarsal joint; *i.e.,* between the tarsal navicular and the calcaneocuboid joints.
cinematic a., cineplastic a.
cineplastic a., cinematic or kineplastic a.; cineplastics; kineplastics; cinematization; a method of a. of an extremity whereby the muscles and tendons are so arranged in the stump that they are able to execute independent movements and to communicate motion to a specially constructed prosthetic apparatus.
circular a., guillotine or linear a.; a. performed by a circular incision through the skin, the muscles being similarly divided higher up, and the bone higher still.
congenital a., intrauterine or birth a.; spontaneous a. (1); a. produced *in utero;* formerly attributed to the pressure of constricting bands; later regarded as the result of an intrinsic deficiency of embryonic tissue; recently again attributed to the pressure of constricting bands.
consecutive a., A revision or secondary succeeding amputation of a limb.
a. in continuity, a. through a segment of a limb, not at a joint.
double flap a., a. in which a flap is cut from the soft parts on either side of the limb.
dry a., bloodless a.
Dupuytren's a., a. of the arm at the shoulder joint.
eccentric a., a. with the scar of the stump off-center.
elliptical a., circular a. in which the sweep of the knife is not exactly vertical to the axis of the limb, the outline of the cut surface being therefore elliptical.
excentric a., a. in which the line of union of the flaps does not run across the end of the stump.
Farabeuf's a., **(1)** a. of the leg, the flap being large and on the outer side; **(2)** a. of the foot; disarticulation of the foot through the subtalar joint and the talo-navicular joint.
flap a., flap operation (1); an a. in which flaps of the muscular and cutaneous tissues are made to cover the end of the bone.
flapless a., an a. without any tissue to cover the stump

forequarter a., interscapulothoracic a.
Gritti-Stokes a., Gritti's operation; supracondylar a. of the femur, the patella being preserved and applied to the end of the bone, its articular cartilage being removed so as to obtain union.
guillotine a., circular a.
Guyon's a., a. above the malleoli, a modification of Syme's a.
Hancock's a., a. of the foot through the astragalus.
Hey's a., a. of the foot in front of the tarsometatarsal joint.
hindquarter a., hemipelvectomy.
immediate a., a. necessitated by irreparable injury to the limb, performed within twelve hours after the injury.
interilioabdominal a., hemipelvectomy.
intermediate a., intrapyretic or primary a.; an a. formerly performed during the period between trauma or incipient gangrene and suppuration.
interpelviabdominal a., hemipelvectomy.
interscapulothoracic a., forequarter a.; a. of the arm with removal of the scapula and a portion of the clavicle.
intrapyretic a., intermediate a.
intrauterine a., congenital a.
Jaboulay's a., hemipelvectomy.
kineplastic a., cineplastic a.
Kirk's a., a. at the lower end of the femur, using the tendon of the quadraceps extensor to cover the end of the bone.
Krukenberg's a., a cineplastic a. at the carpus with the distal end of the forearm used to create a fork-like stump; especially valuable in the blind because the stump has proprioception.
Larrey's a., a. at the shoulder joint.
Le Fort's a., a modification of Pirogoff's a.; the calcaneus is sawed through horizontally instead of vertically so that the patient steps on the same part of the heel as before.
linear a., circular a.
Lisfranc's a., Lisfranc's operation; a. of the foot at the tarsometatarsal joint, the sole being preserved to make the flap.
Mackenzie's a., a modification of Syme's a. at the ankle joint, the flap being taken from the inner side.
major a., a. of the lower or upper extremity above the ankle or the wrist, respectively.
Malgaigne's a., subastragalar a.
mediotarsal a., Chopart's a.
Mikulicz-Vladimiroff a., Vladimiroff-Mikulicz a.; an osteoplastic resection of the foot in which the talus and calcaneus are exsected, the anterior row of tarsal bones being united to the lower end of the tibia, the articular surfaces of both being removed; the lower end of the stump is therefore the anterior portion of the foot, the patient walking thereafter on tiptoe.
minor a., a. of a hand or foot or any parts of either.
multiple a., a. of two or more limbs or parts of limbs performed at the same operation.
musculocutaneous a., a. with a flap of muscle and skin.
oblique a., a. in which the line of section through an extremity is at other than a right angle; this yields an oval appearance to the cut surface (hence sometimes, though rarely, referred to as an oval a.).
osteoplastic a., an a., *e.g.,* through the tarsus, in which the cut surface of another bone is brought in apposition with the one primarily divided so that the two unite, thus giving a better stump.
oval a., **(1)** a. in which the flaps are obained by oval incisions through the skin and muscle; **(2)** rarely used term for oblique a.
pathologic a., a. necessitated by cancer or other disease of the limb and not by an injury.
periosteoplastic a., subperiosteal a.
Pirogoff's a., a. of the foot; the lower articular surfaces of the tibia and fibula are sawed through and the ends covered with a portion of the os calcis which has also been sawed through from above posteriorly downward and forward.
primary a., intermediate a.
pulp a., pulpotomy.
quadruple a., a. of both arms and both legs.
racket a., a circular or slightly oval a., in which a long incision is made in the axis of the limb.
rectangular a., a. in which the flaps are fashioned in the shape of a rectangle.
root a., radectomy; radiectomy; radisectomy; surgical removal of one or more roots of a multirooted tooth, the remaining root canal(s) usually being treated endodontically.
secondary a., a. performed some time after a previous a. that has failed to heal satisfactorily.
spontaneous a., **(1)** congenital a.; **(2)** a. as the result of a pathologic process rather than from external trauma.
Stokes a., a modification of the Gritti-Stokes a. in that the line of section of the femur is slightly higher.
subastragalar a., Malgaigne's a.; a. of the foot in which only the astragalus is retained.
subperiosteal a., periosteoplastic a.; a. in which the periosteum is stripped back from the bone and replaced afterward, forming a periosteal flap over the cut end.
Syme's a., Syme's operation; a. of the foot at the ankle joint, the malleoli being sawed off, and a flap being made with the soft parts of the heel.
tarsotibial a., a. through the ankle joint.

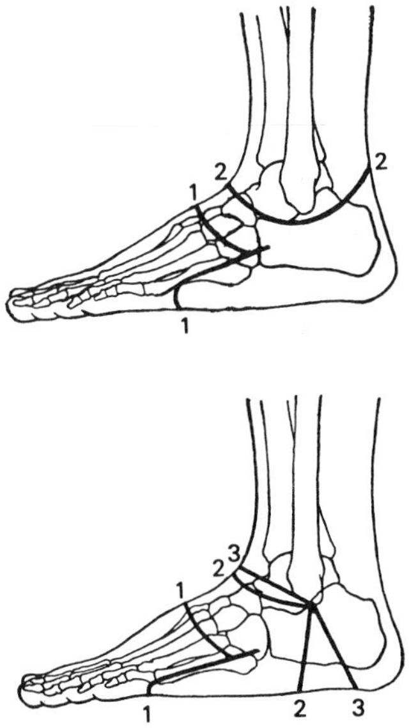

Tarsal Amputations
Above: 1, Chopart's; *2,* Mackenzie's. *Below:* Lines of incision for amputations: *1–1,* Lisfranc's; *2–2,* Pirogoff's; *3–3,* Syme's.

Teale's a., **(1)** a. of the forearm in its lower half, or of the thigh, with a long posterior rectangular flap and a short anterior one; **(2)** a. of the leg, with a long anterior rectangular flap and a short posterior one.
tertiary a., an a. formerly performed after infection had been controlled.
a. by transfixion, a. performed by transfixing the soft parts with a long knife and cutting the flap or flaps from within outward.
transverse a., a. in which the line of section through the extremity is at right angles to the long axis.
traumatic a., a. resulting from accidental or nonsurgical injury; may be complete or incomplete.
Tripier's a., a modification of Chopart's a., in that a part of the calcaneus is also removed.

Vladimiroff-Mikulicz a., Mikulicz-Vladimiroff a.

---

amputee (am'pyū-tē). A person with an amputated limb.

amrinone lactate (am'ri-nōn). 5-Amino-(3,4'-bipyridin)-6(1*H*)-one; an inotropic agent with vasodilator activity, used in management of congestive heart failure.

Amsler, Marc, Swiss ophthalmologist, 1891–1968. See A.'s *chart, marker;* A. *test.*

amu Abbreviation for atomic mass *unit.*

amuck (ă-mŭk'). Amok (2).

amusia (ă-myū'zē-ă) [G. *a-* priv. + *mousa,* music]. A form of aphasia characterized by loss of the faculty of musical expression or of the recognition of simple musical tones.
sensory a., failure to interpret or appreciate musical sounds.
vocal a., the inability to sing, although the individual is capable of other motor and speech performance.

Amussat, Jean Z., French surgeon, 1796–1856. See A.'s *valve, valvula.*

amychophobia (am'ī-kō-fō'bē-ă) [G. *amychē,* a scratch, + *phobos,* fear]. Morbid fear of being scratched.

amyctic (ă-mik'tik) [G. *amyssein,* to scratch, scarify]. Itchy or irritating.

amyelencephalia (ă-mī'el-en-sĕ-fā'lē-ă) [G. *a-* priv. + *myelos,* marrow, + *enkephalos,* brain]. Congenital absence of both brain and spinal cord.

amyelencephalic, amyelencephalous (ă-mī'el-en-se-fal'ik, -sef'ă-lŭs). Denoting or characteristic of amyelencephalia.

amyelia (ă-mī-ē'lē-ă) [G. *a-* priv. + *myelos,* marrow]. Congenital absence of the spinal cord, found only in association with anencephaly.

amyelic (ă-mī-ē'lik). Amyelous.

amyelinated (ă-mī'ĕ-li-nā'ted). Unmyelinated.

amyelination (ă-mī'ĕ-li-nā'shŭn). Absence of the myelin sheath of a nerve.

amyelinic (ă-mī'ĕ-lin'ik). Unmyelinated.

amyeloic, amyelonic (ă-mī-ĕ-lō'ik, ă-mī-ĕ-lon'ik) [G. *a-* priv. + *myelos,* marrow]. **1.** Amyelous. **2.** In hematology, sometimes used to indicate the absence of bone marrow or the lack of functional participation of bone marrow in hemopoiesis.

amyelous (ă-mī'ĕ-lŭs). Amyelic; amyeloic (1); amyelonic (1); without spinal cord.

amygdala, gen. and pl. **amygdalae** (ă-mig'dă-lă, -lē) [L. fr. G. *amygdalē,* almond; in Mediev. & Mod. L., a tonsil]. **1.** *Corpus* amygdaloideum. **2.** Tonsilla; denoting the cerebellar tonsil, as well as the lymphatic tonsils (pharyngeal, palatine, lingual, laryngeal, and tubal).
a. cerebel'li, *tonsilla* cerebelli.

amygdalase (ă-mig'dă-lās). β-D-Glucosidase.

amygdalin (ă-mig'dă-lin). Amygdaloside; mandelonitrile-β-gentiobioside; a glucoside present in almonds and seeds of other plants of the family Rosaceae; the principal component of laetrile. Emulsin splits a. into benzaldehyde, glucose, and hydrocyanic acid.

amygdaline (ă-mig'dă-līn). **1.** Relating to an almond. **2.** Relating to a tonsil, or to the brain structure called amygdala or amygdaloid nuclear complex. **3.** Tonsillar.

amygdaloid (ă-mig'dă-loyd) [amygdala + G. *eidos,* appearance]. Resembling an almond or a tonsil.

amygdaloside (ă-mig'dă-lō-sīd). Amygdalin.

amyl-. See amylo-.

amyl (ā'mil). Pentyl; the radical formed from a pentane, C_5H_{12}, by removal of one H. Several isomeric forms exist, the more important being $CH_3CH_2CH_2CH_2CH_2$— (amyl or pentyl); $(CH_3)_2CHCH_2CH_2$— (isoamyl or isopentyl); $CH_3CH_2CH_2CH(CH)_3$— and $(CH_3CH_2)_2CH$— (secondary amyl or pentyl); and $CH_3CH_2C(CH_3)_2$— (tertiary amyl or pentyl).
a. alcohol, 1-pentanol; used as a solvent for varnishes and oils; highly toxic, with irritating vapors. See also fusel oil.
a. hydrate, *amylene* hydrate.
a. nitrite, $C_5H_{11}NO_2$; a vasodilator used in angina pectoris and cyanide poisoning.
tertiary a. alcohol, *amylene* hydrate.
a. valerate, apple oil; isoamyl isovalerate; used as a sedative; formerly used in the treatment of gallstones because of its solvent action on cholesterol.

amylaceous (am'i-lā'shŭs). Starchy.

amylase (am'il-ās). One of a group of amylolytic enzymes that cleave starch, glycogen, and related α-1,4-glucans.

α-amylase [EC 3.2.1.1]. Ptyalin; glycogenase; a glucanohydrolase yielding α-glucose and maltose in a random manner from 1,4-α-glucans.

β-amylase [EC 3.2.1.2]. Saccharogen amylase; glycogenase; a glucanohydrolase yielding β -maltose units from the nonreducing ends of 1,4-α -glucans.

γ-amylase. Exo-1,4-α-D-glucosidase.

amylasuria (am-i-lā-sū'rē-ă). Diastasuria; the excretion of amylase (sometimes termed diastase) in the urine, especially increased amounts likely in acute pancreatitis.

amylemia (am-i-lē'mē-ă) [amylo- + G. *haima,* blood]. The hypothetical presence of starch in the circulating blood.

amylene (am'i-lēn). Trimethylethylene; 2-methyl-2-butene; $(CH_3)_2C{=}CHCH_3$; a flammable liquid hydrocarbon formed by the decomposition of amyl alcohol; has anesthetic properties but undesirable side actions.
a. chloral, dimethylethylcarbinolchloral; a hypnotic.
a. hydrate, tertiary amyl alcohol; amyl hydrate; dimethylethylcarbinol; *tert*-pentanol; a hypnotic used as a solvent for tribromoethanol.

amylin (am'i-lin). The cellulose of starch; the insoluble envelope of starch grains.

amylo-, amyl- [G. *amylon,* starch] Combining forms indicating starch, or polysaccharide nature or origin.

amylocaine hydrochloride (am'i-lō-kān). 1-(Dimethylaminomethyl)-1-methylpropyl benzoate hydrochloride; benzoylethyldimethylaminopropanol hydrochloride; an early local anesthetic once widely used but eventually abandoned because of side effects.

amyloclast (am'i-lō-klast) [amylo- + G. *klastos,* broken in pieces]. Obsolete term for amylase.

amylodextrin (am-i-lō-deks'trin). End product of hydrolysis of amylopectin by β-amylase; further hydrolysis requires amylo-1,6-glucosidase, which attacks the branch points.

amylogenesis (am-i-lō-jen'ĕ-sis) [amylo- + G. *genesis,* production]. Biosynthesis of starch.

amylogenic (am-i-lō-jen'ik). Relating to amylogenesis.

amyloglucosidase (am-i-lō-glū'kō-si-dās). Exo-1,4-α-D-glucosidase.

amylo-1,6-glucosidase [EC 3.2.1.33]. Dextrin 6-α-D-glucosidase; an enzyme hydrolyzing α-D-1,6 links (branch points) in chains of 1,4-linked α-D-glucose residues, hence the term debranching enzyme or factor; deficiency causes type 3 glycogenosis.

amyloid (am'i-loyd) [amylo- + G. *eidos,* resemblance]. Any of a group of chemically diverse proteins that appears microscopically homogeneous, but is composed of linear nonbranching aggregated fibrils arranged in sheets when seen under the electron microscope;

it stains dark brown with iodine, produces a characteristic green color in polarized light after staining with Congo red, is metachromatic with either methyl violet (pink-red) or crystal violet (purple-red), and fluoresces yellow after thioflavine T staining; a. occurs characteristically as pathologic extracellular deposits (amyloidosis), especially in association with reticuloendothelial tissue; the chemical nature of the proteinaceous fibrils is dependent upon the underlying disease process.

amyloidosis (am′i-loy-dō′sis) [amyloid + G. *-osis,* condition]. A disease characterized by extracellular accumulation of amyloid in various organs and tissues of the body; may be primary or secondary.

a. cu′tis, lichen a.; infiltration of the papillae of the epidermis by amyloid; the eruption consists of itching papules, small nodules, and plaques, most commonly on the lower legs, the extensors of the forearms, and the lumbar area.

familial a., familial amyloid *neuropathy.*

focal a., nodular a.

lichen a., a. cutis.

macular a., a form of a. cutis characterized by pruritic symmetrical brown reticulated macules; microscopically, amyloid is deposited as small subepidermal globules.

a. of multiple myeloma, foci of a. in mesenchymal tissues of some persons with multiple myeloma; no direct relation between amyloid and Bence Jones protein is conclusively known.

nodular a., focal a.; amyloid tumor; a form of a. in which amyloid occurs as small masses or nodules beneath the skin or mucous membranes, *e.g.,* in the larynx.

primary a., a form of a., sometimes familial and not associated with other recognized disease, which tends to involve diffusely the arterial walls and mesenchymal tissues in the tongue, lungs, intestinal tract, skin, skeletal muscle, and myocardium; the amyloid frequently does not manifest the usual affinity for Congo red, and sometimes provokes a foreign-body type of inflammatory reaction in the adjacent tissue.

renal a., amyloid nephrosis (1); renal deposits of amyloid, especially in glomerular capillary walls, which may cause albuminuria and the nephrotic syndrome.

secondary a., a. occurring in association with another chronic inflammatory disease; organs chiefly involved are the liver, spleen, and kidneys, and the adrenal glands less frequently.

senile a., a common form of a. in very old people, usually mild and limited to the heart.

amylolysis (am-i-lol′i-sis) [amylo- + G. *lysis,* dissolution]. Hydrolysis of starch into sugar.

amylolytic (am-i-lō-lit′ik). Relating to amylolysis.

amylomaltase (am-i-lō-mal′tās). 4-α-D-Glucanotransferase.

amylopectin (am-i-lō-pek′tin). A branched-chain polyglucose (glucan) in starch. *Cf.* amylose.

amylopectin 6-glucanohydrolase [EC 3.2.1.69]. Former name for α-dextrin endo-1,6-α-glucosidase.

amylopectin 1,6-glucosidase [EC 3.2.1.9]. Former name for an enzyme now known to be at least two enzymes, α-dextrin endoglucanohydrolase and isoamylase.

amylopectinosis (am′i-lō-pek-tin-ō′sis) [amylopectin + G. *-osis,* condition]. Glycogenosis due to deficiency of branching enzyme.

branching deficiency a., type 4 *glycogenosis.*

amylophagia (am′i-lō-fā′jē-ă) [amylo- + G. *phagein,* to eat]. Starch-eating; a morbid craving for starch.

amylophosphorylase (am′i-lō-fos-fōr′i-lās). Phosphorylase.

amyloplast (am′i-lō-plast) [amylo- + G. *plastos,* formed]. Amylogenic body; a granule in the protoplasm of a plant cell that is the center of a starch-forming process.

amylorrhea (am′i-lō-rē′ă) [amylo- + G. *rhoia,* flow]. Passage of undigested starch in the stools, implying a deficiency of amylase activity in the intestine.

amylose (am′i-lōs). An unbranched polyglucose (glucan) in starch, similar to cellulose. *Cf.* amylopectin.

amylosuria (am′i-lō-sū′rē-ă). Amyluria; excretion of starch in the urine.

amylo-(1,4→1,6)-transglucosidase or **-transglucosylase.** 1,4-α-D-Glucan branching enzyme.

amylum (am′i-lŭm). Starch.

amyluria (am-i-lū′rē-ă). Amylosuria.

amyocardia (ă-mī-ō-kar′dē-ă) [G. *a-* priv. + *mys,* muscle, + *kardia,* heart]. Myasthenia cordis; weakness of the heart muscle.

amyoesthesia, amyoesthesis (ă-mī′ō-es-thē′zē-ă, -thē′sis) [G. *a-* priv. + *mys,* muscle, + *aisthēsis,* perception]. Loss of muscle sensation.

amyoplasia (ă-mī-ō-plā′zē-ă) [G. *a-* priv. + *mys,* muscle, + *plasis,* a molding]. Deficient formation of muscle tissue.

a. congen′ita, *arthrogryposis* multiplex congenita.

amyostasia (ă-mī-ō-stā′zē-ă) [G. *a-* priv. + *mys,* muscle, + *stasis,* standing]. Difficulty in standing, due to muscular tremor or incoordination.

amyostatic (ă-mī-ō-stat′ik). Showing muscular tremors.

amyosthenia (ă-mī′os-thē′nē-ă) [G. *a-* priv. + *mys,* muscle, + *sthenos,* strength]. Muscular weakness.

amyosthenic (ă-mī-os-then′ik). Relating to or causing muscular weakness.

amyotaxy, amyotaxia (ă-mī′ō-tak-sē, ă-mī-ō-tak′sē-ă) [G. *a-* priv. + *mys,* muscle, + *taxis,* order]. Muscular ataxia.

amyotonia (ă-mī-ō-tō′nē-ă) [G. *a-* priv. + *mys,* muscle, + *tonos,* tone]. Myatonia.

a. congen′ita, Oppenheim's disease or syndrome; myatonia congenita; congenital atonic pseudoparalysis; atonic pseudoparalysis of congenital origin (neither familial nor hereditary), observed especially in infants and characterized by absences of muscular tone only in muscles innervated by the spinal nerves.

amyotrophia (ă-mī-ō-trō′fē-ă). Amyotrophy.

amyotrophic (ă-mī-ō-trō′fik). Relating to muscular atrophy.

amyotrophy (ă-mī-ot′rō-fē) [G. *a-* priv. + *mys,* muscle, + *trophē,* nourishment]. Amyotrophia; muscular wasting or atrophy.

hemiplegic a., muscular atrophy following hemiplegia.

neuralgic a., brachial plexus *neuropathy.*

progressive spinal a., progressive muscular *atrophy.*

amyous (am′ē-ŭs) [G. *a-* priv. + *mys,* muscle]. Lacking in muscular tissue, or in muscular strength.

amyxia (ă-mik′sē-ă) [G. *a-* priv. + *myxa,* mucus]. Obsolete term for absence of mucus.

amyxorrhea (ă-mik-sō-rē′ă) [G. *a-* priv. + *myxa,* mucus, + *rhoia,* flow]. Absence of the normal secretion of mucus.

an-. See a-.

ana- [G. *ana,* up]. Prefix meaning up, toward, apart; distinguished from *an-,* which is *a-* privative with *n* before a vowel.

Anabaena (an-ă-bē′nă). A genus of Cyanobacteria causing odors in water supplies.

anabiosis (an′ă-bī-ō′sis) [G. a reviving, fr. *ana,* again, + *biōsis,* life]. Resuscitation after apparent death.

anabiotic (an′ă-bī-ot′ik). **1.** Resuscitating or restorative. **2.** A revivifying remedy; a powerful stimulant.

anabolic (an-ă-bol′ik). Relating to or promoting anabolism.

anabolism (ă-nab′ō-lizm) [G. *anabolē,* a raising up]. The building up in the body of complex chemical compounds from smaller simpler compounds (*e.g.,* proteins from amino acids), usually with the use of energy. *Cf.* catabolism.

anabolite (ă-nab′ō-līt). Any substance formed as a result of anabolic processes.

anabrosis (an-ă-brō′sis) [G. fr. *ana,* up, + *bibrōskō,* to eat up]. Superficial erosion or ulceration.

anabrotic (an-ă-brot′ik). A substance that produces ulceration or erosion of the skin surface.

anacamptometer (an-ă-kamp-tom′ĕ-ter) [G. *anakampsis,* a bending back, reflection, + *metron,* measure]. Instrument for measuring the intensity of the deep reflexes.

anacardiol (an-ă-kar′dē-ol). 3-Ethoxy-*N,N*-diethyl-4-hydroxybenzamide; an analeptic.

anacatadidymus (an′ă-kat-ă-did′i-mŭs) [G. *ana,* up, + *kata,* down, + *didymos,* twin]. Conjoined twins united in the middle but separated above and below.

anacatesthesia (an′ă-kat′es-thē′zē-ă) [G. *ana,* up, + *kata,* down, + *aisthēsis,* sensation]. A hovering sensation.

anacidity (an-ă-sid′i-tē). Absence of acidity; used especially to denote absence of hydrochloric acid in the gastric juice.

anaclasis (ă-nak′lă-sis) [G. a bending back, reflection]. **1.** Reflection of light or sound. **2.** Refraction of the ocular media.

anaclitic (an-ă-klit′ik) [G. *ana,* toward, + *klinein,* to lean]. Leaning or depending upon; in psychoanalysis, relating to the dependence of the infant on the mother or mother substitute.

anacmesis (an-ak′mē-sis). Obsolete spelling for anakmesis.

anacrotic (an-ă-krot′ik). Anadicrotic; referring to the upstroke or ascending limb of the arterial pulse tracing; an abbreviated form for anadicrotic, twice beating on the upstroke.

anacrotism (ă-nak′rō-tizm) [G. *ana,* up, + *krotos,* a beat]. Peculiarity of the pulse wave. See anacrotic *pulse.*

anacusis (an′ă-kū′sis) [G. *an-* priv. + *akousis,* hearing]. Anakusis; total loss or absence of the ability to perceive sound as such.

anadenia (an-ă-dē′nē-ă) [G. *an-* priv. + *adēn,* gland]. Absence of glands or abeyance of glandular function.

a. ventric′uli, absence of glands from the stomach.

anadicrotic (an-ă-dī-krot′ik). Anacrotic.

anadicrotism (an-ă-dik′rō-tizm) [G. *ana,* up, + *di-krotos,* double beating]. Anacrotism.

anadidymus (an-ă-did′i-mŭs) [G. *ana,* up, + *didymos,* twin]. *Duplicitas* anterior.

anadipsia (an-ă-dip′sē-ă) [G. *ana,* intensive, + *dipsa,* thirst]. Extreme thirst. See also polydipsia.

anadrenalism (an-ă-drē′năl-izm). Complete lack of adrenal function.

anaerobe (an′ār-ōb, an-ār′ōb) [G. *an-* priv. + *aēr,* air, + *bios,* life]. A microorganism that can live and grow in the absence of oxygen.

facultative a., an a. able to grow in the presence or absence of free oxygen.

obligate a., an a. that will grow only in the absence of free oxygen.

anaerobic (an-ār-ō′bik). Relating to an anaerobe; living without oxygen.

anaerobiosis (an-ār-ō-bī-ō′sis) [G. *an-* priv. + *aēr,* air, + *biōsis,* way of living]. Existence in an oxygen-free atmosphere.

anaerogenic (an-ār-ō-jen′ik) [G. *an-* priv. + *aēr,* air, + *-gen,* producing]. Not producing gas.

anaerophyte (an-ār′ō-fīt) [G. *an-* priv. + *aēr,* air, + *phyton,* plant]. **1.** A plant that grows without air. **2.** An anaerobic bacterium.

anaeroplasty (an-ār′ō-plas-tē) [G. *an-*priv. + *aēr,* air, + *plastos,* formed]. Treatment of wounds by exclusion of air.

anagen (an′ă-jen) [G. *ana,* up, + *-gen,* producing]. Growth phase of the hair cycle.

anagenesis (an-ă-jen′ĕ-sis) [G. *ana,* up, + *genesis,* production]. **1.** Repair of tissue. **2.** Regeneration of lost parts.

anagenetic (an′ă-jĕ-net′ik). Pertaining to anagenesis.

anagestone acetate (an-ă-jes′tōn). 17-Hydroxy-6α-methylpregn-4-en-20-one acetate; a progestational agent.

Anagnostakis, Andrei, Cretan ophthalmologist, 1826–1897. See A.’s *operation.*

anagogy (an-ă-gō′jē) [G. *anagōgē,* fr. *an- ago,* to lead up]. Psychic content of an idealistic or spiritual nature.

anákhré (an-ah-krā′) [Fr. fr. Af. native term meaning “big nose”]. Goundou.

anakmesis (an-ak′mē-sis) [G. *an-* priv. + *akmēnos,* full grown, fr. *akmē,* highest point]. Arrest of maturation of leukocytes in their production centers, thereby resulting in greater numbers of young forms and progressively smaller proportions of mature granular cells in the bone marrow, as observed in agranulocytosis.

anakusis (an-ă-kū′sis). Anacusis.

anal (ā′năl). Relating to the anus.

analbuminemia (an′al-bū-mi-nē′mē-ă) [G. *an-* priv. + albumin + G. *haima,* blood]. Absence of albumin from the serum.

analeptic (an-ă-lep′tik) [G. *analēptikos,* restorative]. **1.** Strengthening, stimulating, or invigorating. **2.** A restorative remedy. **3.** A central nervous system stimulant, particularly used to denote agents that reverse depressed central nervous system function.

analgesia (an-ăl-jē′zē-ă) [G. insensibility, fr. *an-* priv. + *algēsis,* sensation of pain]. A condition in which nociceptive stimuli are perceived but are not interpreted as pain; usually accompanied by sedation without loss of consciousness.

a. al′gera, a. dolorosa; spontaneous pain in a part, associated with loss of sensibility.

conduction a., sensory denervation in a portion of the body (regional anesthesia), produced by pharmacological means.

a. doloro′sa, a. algera.

inhalation a., a. produced by inhalation of a central nervous system depressant gas (especially nitrous oxide) or vapor.

spinal a., euphemism for spinal *anesthesia.*

surface a., topical *anesthesia.*

analgesic (an-ăl-jē′zik). **1.** Analgetic (1); a compound capable of producing analgesia, *i.e.,* one that relieves pain by altering perception of nociceptive stimuli without producing anesthesia or loss of consciousness. **2.** Antalgic; characterized by reduced response to painful stimuli.

analgesimeter (an′ăl-jē-zim′i-ter) [analgesia + G. *metron,* measure]. A device for measuring pain under experimental conditions.

analgetic (an-ăl-jet′ik). **1.** Analgesic (1). **2.** Associated with decreased pain perception.

anality (ā-nal′i-tē). Referring to the psychic organization derived from, and characteristic of, the anal period of psychosexual development.

anallergic (an-ă-ler′jik). Not allergic.

analog (an′ă-log). [G. *analogos,* proportionate]. Analogue. **1.** One of two organs or parts in different species of animals or plants which differ in structure or development but are similar in function. **2.** A compound that resembles another in structure but is not necessarily an isomer (*e.g.,* 5-fluorouracil is an analog of thymine); a.’s are often used to block enzymatic reactions by combining with enzymes (*e.g.,* isopropyl thiogalactoside vs. lactose).

analogous (ă-nal′ō-gŭs). Possessing a functional resemblance, but having a different origin or structure.

analogue (an′ă-log). Analog.

analphalipoproteinemia (an-al′fă-lip′ō-prō′tēn-ē′mē-ă) [G. *an-,* priv., + *alpha*, α, + lipoprotein + *-emia*, blood]. Tangier *disease*.

analysand (ă-nal′i-sand). In psychoanalysis, the person being analyzed.

analysis, pl. analyses (ă-nal′i-sis, -sēz) [G. a breaking up, fr. *ana*, up, + *lysis*, a loosening]. **1.** The breaking up of a chemical compound or mixture into simpler elements; a process by which the composition of a substance is determined. **2.** The examination and study of a whole in terms of the parts composing it. **3.** See psychoanalysis.

activation a., the identification and quantification of unknown elements from their characteristic electromagnetic spectra and decay constants after they have been made radioactive by exposure to high levels of particulate radiation.

bite a., occlusal a.

blood gas a., the direct electrode measurement of the partial pressure of oxygen and carbon dioxide in the blood.

bradykinetic a., the a. of a movement by means of slow cinematography.

cephalometric a., a study of the skeletal and dental relationships used in orthodontic case a., as calculated from cephalograms.

character a., a. of the defenses and personality traits that characterize an individual.

cluster a., a statistical procedure, using correlation, by which the dynamic interaction of a number of factors can be studied simultaneously.

content a., any of a variety of techniques for classification and study of the verbal products of normal or of psychologically disabled individuals.

didactic a., training a.

displacement a., competitive binding *assay*.

distributive a., in psychobiology, the a. of information gained about the patient and its distribution by the physician, as indicated by the patient's complaint and symptoms.

Downs' a., a series of cephalometric criteria used as an aid in orthodontic diagnosis.

ego a., psychoanalytic study of the ways in which the ego deals with intrapsychic conflicts.

gastric a., measurement of pH and acid output of stomach contents; basal acid output can be determined by collecting the overnight gastric secretion or by a 1-hr collection; maximal acid output is determined following injection of histamine; output is measured by titration with a strong base.

interaction process a., in psychology, a. of small group behavior in terms of 12 specific categories, *e.g.*, solidarity, tension release, agreement.

linkage a., the estimation, from empirical phenotypic data on pedigrees, of the probability of genetic recombination of genes at two or more loci.

Northern blot a. [coined to distinguish it from eponymic Southern blot a.], a procedure similar to the Southern blot a., used mostly to separate and identify RNA fragments.

occlusal a., bite a.; a study of the relations of the occlusal surfaces of opposing teeth and their effect upon related structures.

pedigree a., the formal study of the pattern of a trait in a pedigree to determine such properties as its mode of inheritance, age of onset, and variability in phenotype.

percept a., psychologic survey of an individual's personality using Rorschach's series of inkblots.

qualitative a., determination of the nature, as opposed to the quantity, of each of the elements composing a substance.

quantitative a., determination of the amount, as well as the nature, of each of the elements composing a substance.

saturation a., competitive binding *assay*.

segregation a., in genetics, the enumeration of progeny according to distinct and mutually exclusive phenotypes; used as a test of a putative pattern of inheritance, *e.g.*, mendelian, dominant autosomal.

Southern blot a., a procedure to separate and identify DNA sequences; DNA fragments are separated by electrophoresis on an agarose gel, transferred (blotted) onto a nitrocellulose or nylon membrane, and hybridized with complementary (labeled) nucleic acid probes.

stratographic a., chromatography.

training a., didactic a.; psychoanalytic treatment of an analytic candidate carried out under the official auspices of a psychoanalytic training institute.

transactional a., a psychotherapy system, used in both individual and group treatment, involving a systematic understanding of the qualities of interpersonal interactions in the treatment sessions; includes four components: 1) structural analysis of intrapsychic phenomena; 2) transactional a. proper, determination of the currently dominant ego state (parent, child, or adult) of each participant; 3) game analysis, identification of the games played in their interactions and of the gratifications provided; 4) script analysis, uncovering of the causes of the patient's emotional problems.

volumetric a., quantitative a. by the addition of graduated amounts of a standard test solution to a solution of a known amount of the substance analyzed, until the reaction is just at an end; depends upon the stoichiometric nature of the reaction between the test solution and the unknown.

Western blot a. [coined to distinguish it from eponymic Southern blot a.], a procedure in which proteins separated by electrophoresis in polyacrylamide gels are transferred (blotted) onto nitrocellulose or nylon membranes and identified by specific complexing with antibodies that are either pre- or post-tagged with a labeled secondary protein.

analyst (an′ă-list). **1.** One who makes analytical determinations. **2.** Short term for psychoanalyst.

analyte (an′ă-līt). Any substance or chemical constituent of blood, urine, or other body fluid that is analyzed.

analytic, analytical (an-ă-lit′-ik, -i-kăl). **1.** Relating to analysis. **2.** Relating to psychoanalysis.

analyzer, analyzor (an′ă-līz-er, ŏr). **1.** The prism in a polariscope by means of which the polarized light is examined. **2.** The neural basis of the conditioned reflex; includes all of the sensory side of the reflex arc and its central connections. **3.** A device that electronically determines the frequency and amplitude of a particular channel of an electroencephalogram. **4.** Any instrument that performs an analysis.

centrifugal fast a., an automatic spectrophotometer that uses centrifugal force to mix samples and reagents, and propels the reactants at high speed about a detector that makes multiple absorbance readings.

kinetic a., an instrument that measures the rate of change in a chemical substance; used mainly for enzyme measurement.

wave a., an apparatus that can take a complex mixture of wave forms, separate out their component frequencies, and indicate their distribution on a record.

anamnesis (an-am-nē′sis) [G. *anamnēsis*, recollection]. **1.** The act of remembering. **2.** The medical history of a patient.

anamnestic (an-am-nes′tik). **1.** Mnemonic; assisting the memory. **2.** Relating to the medical history of a patient.

anamnionic, anamniotic (an-am-nē-on′ik, -ot′ik). Without an amnion.

Anamniota (an-am-nē-ō′tă). A group of vertebrates whose embryos are not enclosed in an amnion; it includes the cyclostomes, fish, and amphibians.

anamorphosis (an′ă-mōr-fō′sis) [G. *ana*, up, + *morphē*, form]. **1.** In phylogeny, a progressive series of changes in the evolution of a group of animals or plants. **2.** In optics, the process of correcting a distorted image with a curved mirror.

ananaphylaxis (an'an-ă-fī-lak'sis). Desensitization (1).

ananastasia (an'an-ă-stā'zē-ă) [G. *a-* priv. + *anastasis,* stand up]. Inability to stand up.

anancasm (an'an-kazm) [G. *anagkasma,* compulsion]. Any form of repetitious stereotyped behavior which, if prevented, results in anxiety.

anancastia (an-an-kas'tē-ă) [G. *anankastos,* compelled]. An obsession in which a person feels himself forced to act or think against his will.

anancastic (an-an-kas'tik). Pertaining to anancasm or anancastia.

anandria (an-an'drē-ă) [G. want of manhood, fr. *an-* priv. + *anēr-* (*andr-*), man]. Absence of masculinity.

anangioplasia (an-an'jē-ō-pla'zē-ă) [G. *an-*priv. + *angeion,* vessel, + *plassotos,* formed]. Imperfect vascularization of a part due to nonformation of vessels, or vessels with inadequate caliber.

anangioplastic (an-an'jē-ō-plas'tik). Relating to, characterized by, or due to anangioplasia.

anapeiratic (an'ă-pī-rat'ik) [G. *ana-peiraomai,* to try again, fr. *peiraō,* to try]. Resulting from overuse; denoting certain occupational neuroses.

anaphase (an'ă-fāz) [G. *ana,* up, + *phasis,* appearance]. The stage of mitosis or meiosis in which the chromosomes move from the equatorial plate toward the poles of the cell. In mitosis a full set of daughter chromosomes (46 in man) moves toward each pole. In the first division of meiosis one member of each homologous pair (23 in man), consisting of two chromatids united at the centromere, moves toward each pole. In the second division of meiosis the centromere divides, and the two chromatids separate with one moving to each pole.

anaphia (an-ā'fē-ă, an-af'ē-ă) [G. *an-* priv. + *haphē,* touch]. Anhaphia; absence of the sense of touch.

anaphoresis (an'ă-fō-rē'sis) [G. *ana,* up + *phorēsis,* a being borne]. Movement of negatively charged particles (anions) in a solution or suspension toward the anode in electrophoresis. *Cf.* cataphoresis.

anaphoretic (an'ă-fō-ret'ik). Relating to anaphoresis (1).

anaphoria (an-ă-fō'rē-ă) [G. *ana,* up, + *phoros,* bearing]. A tendency of the eyes, with fusion suspended, to turn upward.

anaphrodisia (an'af-rō-diz'ē-ă) [G. insensibility to love, from *an-* priv. + *Aphroditē,* the goddess of love]. Rarely used term denoting absence of sexual feeling.

anaphrodisiac (an'af-rō-diz'ē-ak). Antaphrodisiac; antaphroditic (1). **1.** Relating to anaphrodisia. **2.** Repressing or destroying sexual desire. **3.** An agent that lessens or abolishes sexual desire.

anaphylactic (an'ă-fī-lak'tik). Relating to anaphylaxis; manifesting extremely great sensitivity to foreign protein or other material.

anaphylactogen (an'ă-fī-lak'tō-jen). A substance (antigen) capable of rendering an individual susceptible to anaphylaxis; a substance (antigen) that will cause an anaphylactic reaction in such a sensitized individual.

anaphylactogenesis (an'ă-fī-lak-tō-jen'ĕ-sis). The production of anaphylaxis.

anaphylactogenic (an'ă-fī-lak-tō-jen'ik). Producing anaphylaxis; pertaining to substances (antigens) that result in an individual becoming susceptible to anaphylaxis.

anaphylactoid (an'ă-fī-lak'toyd) [anaphylaxis + G. *eidos,* resemblance]. Pseudoanaphylactic; resembling anaphylaxis.

anaphylatoxin (an'ă-fil-ă-tok'sin) [anaphylaxis + toxin]. Anaphylotoxin. **1.** A substance postulated to be the immediate cause of anaphylactic shock and that is assumed to result from the *in vivo* combination of specific antibody and the specific sensitizing material, when the latter is injected as a shock dose in a sensitized animal. **2.** The small fragment (C3a) split from the third component (C3) of complement by C3 convertase and that releases histamine from rat peritoneal mast cells, causes pig ileum to contract, and produces a local wheal following intracutaneous injection in man; also used with reference to a small fragment (C5a) split from the fifth component (C5) of complement by the EAC1243 complex which has chemotactic properties as well.

anaphylatoxin inactivator. An α-globulin (MW 300,000) which destroys the activity of the anaphylatoxic complement fragments. See anaphylatoxin (2).

anaphylaxis (an'ă-fī-lak'sis) [G. *ana,* away from, back from, + *phylaxis,* protection]. A term coined by Portier and Richet to indicate a lessened resistance to a toxin which results from a previous inoculation of the same material, and in this sense was synonymous with hypersensitivity in its original usage of a postulated increased sensitivity to a toxin; shortly thereafter, a. was used by Arthus to indicate an induced sensitivity; at times a. is used for anaphylactic shock. The term is commonly used to denote the immediate, transient kind of immunologic (allergic) reaction characterized by contraction of smooth muscle and dilation of capillaries due to release of pharmacologically active substances (histamine, bradykinin, serotonin, and slow-reacting substance), classically initiated by the combination of antigen (allergen) with mast cell-fixed, cytophilic antibody (chiefly IgE); the reaction can be initiated, also, by relatively large quantities of serum aggregates (antigen-antibody complexes, and others) that seemingly activate complement leading to production of anaphylatoxin, a reaction sometimes termed "aggregate a."

active a., reaction following inoculation of antigen in a subject previously sensitized to the specific antigen, in contrast to passive a.

aggregate a., see a.

antiserum a., passive a.

chronic a., *enteritis* anaphylactica.

generalized a., systemic a.; the immediate response, involving smooth muscles and capillaries throughout the body of a sensitized individual, that follows intravenous (and occasionally intracutaneous) injection of antigen (allergen). See also anaphylactic *shock.*

inverse a., anaphylactic shock in an animal (*e.g.,* guinea pig) whose tissues contain Forssman antigen, resulting from an intravenous injection of serum that contains Forssman's antibody.

local a., the immediate, transient kind of response that follows the injection of antigen (allergen) into the skin of a sensitized individual and is limited to the area surrounding the site of inoculation. See also skin *test.*

passive a., antiserum a.; a reaction resulting from inoculation of antigen in an animal previously inoculated intravenously with specific antiserum from another animal, a latent period being required between the two inoculations.

passive cutaneous a., a reaction that occurs in the guinea pig when antiserum is injected into the skin and, 6 to 24 hours later, specific antigen and a dye such as Pontamine blue or Evans blue are inoculated intravenously; the size of the blue areas at the sites of the antibody injections is a measure of the degree of altered permeability to dye-bound albumin.

reversed a., reversed passive a.

reversed passive a., reversed a.; an anaphylactic reaction induced in an animal injected with a specific antigen, which will bind to reactive tissue, and then, after a latent period, with serum from another animal previously sensitized to the identical antigen.

systemic a., generalized a.

anaphylotoxin (an'ă-fil-ō-tok'sin). Anaphylatoxin.

anaplasia (an-ă-plā'sē-ă) [G. *ana,* again, + *plasis,* a molding]. Dedifferentiation (2); loss of structural differentiation, especially as seen in most, but not all, malignant neoplasms.

Anaplasma (an-ă-plas'mă) [G. *an-* priv. + *plasma,* something formed or molded]. A genus of bacteria (family Anaplasmataceae) that parasitize red blood cells, where they appear as spherical chromatic granules; there is no demonstrable multiplication of these organisms in other tissues. These organisms are natural parasites of ruminants (families Bovidae and Camelidae) and are transmitted by arthropods. Initially regarded as protozoa, they are now placed in the order Rickettsiales. The type species is *A. marginale.*

A. centra'le, a species that causes benign anaplasmosis of cattle.

A. margina'le, a species that causes malignant anaplasmosis of cattle; it is the type species of the genus *A.*

A. o'vis, a species that is the agent of anaplasmosis in sheep and goats; cattle are refractory.

anaplasmosis (an'ă-plas-mō'sis). An infectious disease of ruminants, varying from peracute to chronic, caused by *Anaplasma* species and characterized by progressive anemia, icterus, and fever; it is transmitted by at least 20 species of ticks and mechanically by hepatophagous insects including horseflies (*Tabanus*), stable flies (*stomoxys*), deerflies (*Chrysops*), and mosquitoes.

anaplastic (an-ă-plas'tik). **1.** Relating to anaplasty. **2.** Characterized by or pertaining to anaplasia. **3.** Growing without form or structure.

anaplasty (an'ă-plas-tē) [G. *ana,* again, + *plastos,* formed]. Obsolete term for plastic *surgery.*

anapophysis (an-ă-pof'i-sis) [G. *ana,* back, + *apophysis,* offshoot]. An accessory spinal process of a vertebra, found especially in the thoracic or lumbar vertebrae.

anaptic (ă-nap'tik). Relating to anaphia.

anarithmia (an-ă-rith'mē-ă) [G. *an-* priv. + *arithmos,* number]. Aphasia characterized by an inability to count or use numbers.

anarthria (an-ar'thrē-ă) [G. fr. *an-arthos,* without joints; (of sound) inarticulate]. Loss of the power of articulate speech. See also aphasia and alexia.

anasarca (an-ă-sar'kă) [G. *ana,* through, + *sarx* (*sark-*), flesh]. Hydrosarca; a generalized infiltration of edema fluid into subcutaneous connective tissue.

fetoplacental a., edema of fetus and placenta as found in fetal hydrops.

anasarcous (an-ă-sar'kŭs). Characterized by anasarca.

anastigmatic (an'as-tig-mat'ik). Not astigmatic.

anastole (an-as'tō-lē) [G. *anastolē,* the laying bare of a wound]. Obsolete term for the gaping of a wound.

anastomose (ă-nas'tō-mōs). Inosculate. **1.** To open one structure into another directly or by connecting channels, said of blood vessels, lymphatics, and hollow viscera; also incorrectly applied to nerves. **2.** To unite by means of an anastomosis, or connection between formerly separate structures.

anastomosis, pl. **anastomoses** (ă-nas'tō-mō'sis, -sez) [G. *anastomōsis,* from *anastomoō,* to furnish with a mouth]. Inosculation. **1.** A natural communication, direct or indirect, between two blood vessels or other tubular structures. Also incorrectly applied to nerves. See communication. **2.** An operative union of two hollow or tubular structures. **3.** An opening created by surgery, trauma, or disease between two or more normally separate spaces or organs.

antiperistaltic a., an a. diverting the normal flow of contents.

arteriolovenular a., a. arteriovenosa.

a. arterioveno'sa [NA], arteriovenous or arteriolovenular a.; vessels through which blood is shunted from arterioles to venules without passing through the capillaries.

arteriovenous a., a. arteriovenosa.

Béclard's a., arcus raninus; an a. between the right and the left end-branch of the arteria profunda linguae.

bevelled a., a. performed after cutting each of the structures to be joined in an oblique fashion.

Billroth I and II a., Billroth's *operations* I and II.

Braun's a., after gastroenterostomy, a. between afferent and efferent loops of jejunum.

circular a., a. performed after cutting each structure to be joined in a plane vertical to the ultimate flow through the structures.

Clado's a., a. in the broad ligament between the appendicular and ovarian arteries.

conjoined a., the joining together of two small blood vessels by side-to-side elliptical a. to create a single larger stoma for subsequent end-to-end a.

cruciate a., crucial a., an a. between branches of the perforating, gluteal, and circumflex femoral arteries located behind the upper part of the femur.

elliptical a., a modification of direct a. whereby one or both tubular structures are spatulated beforehand, thus creating an ellipse of greater cross-sectional as well as circumferential dimension than would be possible with a bevelled or circular a.

Galen's a., Galen's nerve; a nerve at the posterior surface of the larynx connecting the superior and inferior laryngeal nerves, supplying sensory fibers to the latter.

heterocladic a., a. between branches of different arteries.

Hofmeister-Pólya a., see Hofmeister's *operation;* Pólya's *operation.*

homocladic a., a. between branches of same artery.

Hoyer's a.'s. Sucquet-Hoyer *canals.*

Hyrtl's a., Hyrtl's *loop.*

intestinal a., enteroenterostomy.

isoperistaltic a., an a. allowing flow of contents in the same and normal direction.

Jacobson's a., a portion of the tympanic plexus.

microneurovascular a., a. of very small blood vessels and nerves performed under a surgical microscope.

microvascular a., a. of very small blood vessels performed under a surgical microscope.

postcostal a., longitudinal a. of intersegmental arteries giving rise to the vertebral artery.

Potts' a., Potts' *operation.*

precapillary a., an a. between arterioles just before they become capillaries.

precostal a., longitudinal a. of intersegmental arteries giving rise to thyrocervical and costocervical trunks.

Riolan's a., Riolan's *arcade.*

Roux-en-Y a., Roux-en-Y operation; a. of the distal end of the divided jejunum to the stomach, bile duct, or another structure, with implantation of the proximal end into the side of the jejunum at a suitable distance below the first a., the bowel then forming a Y-shaped pattern.

Schmidel's anastomoses, abnormal channels of communication between the caval and portal venous systems.

Sucquet's a.'s, Sucquet-Hoyer a.'s, Sucquet-Hoyer *canals.*

termino-terminal a., an operation by which the central end of an artery is connected with the peripheral end of the corresponding vein, and the peripheral end of the artery with the central end of the vein.

transureteroureteral a., transureteroureterostomy.

uretero-ileal a., a. between the ureter and an isolated segment of ileum.

ureterosigmoid a., a. between the ureter and an isolated segment of the sigmoid colon.

ureterotubal a., obsolete procedure for a. between the ureter and the fallopian tube.

ureteroureteral a., a. from one part of a ureter to another part of the same ureter.

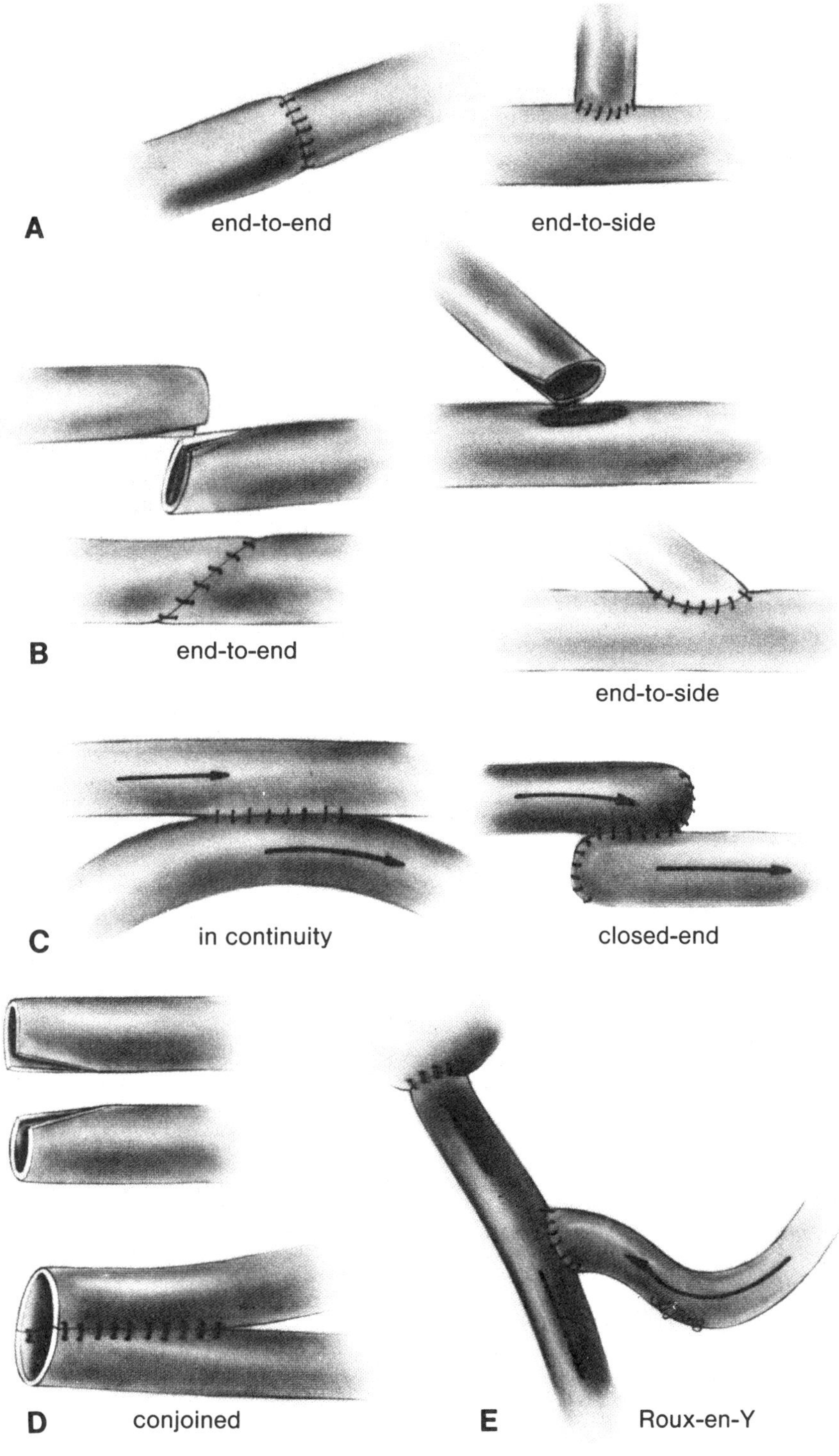

Anastomosis

Various methods applicable to vessels and other tubular structures: *A*, circular (end-to-end, end-to-side); *B*, spatulated elliptical (end-to-end, end-to-side); *C*, side-to-side (in continuity, closed-end); *D*, conjoined; *E*, Roux-en-Y. Arrows indicate direction of flow.

anastomotic (a-nas-tō-mot′ik). Pertaining to an anastomosis.

anastomotica magna (ă-nas-tō-mot′i-kă mag′nă). **1.** *Arteria* collateralis ulnaris inferior. **2.** *Arteria* genus descendens.

anastral (an-as′trăl). Lacking an aster.

anatomical (an′ă-tom′i-kăl). **1.** Relating to anatomy. **2.** Structural.

anatomical snuffbox (snŭf′boks). Tabatière anatomique; a hollow seen on the radial aspect of the wrist when the thumb is extended fully; it is bounded by the prominences of the tendon of the extensor pollicis longus posteriorly and of the tendons of the extensor pollicis brevis and abductor pollicis longus anteriorly. The radial artery crosses the floor which is formed by the scaphoid and the trapezium bones.

anatomicomedical (an-ă-tom′i-kō-med′i-kăl). Referring to both medicine and anatomy.

anatomicopathological (an-ă-tom′i-kō-path-ŏ-loj′i-kăl). Relating to anatomical pathology.

anatomicosurgical (an-ă-tom′i-kō-ser′ji-kăl). Relating to surgical anatomy.

anatomist (ă-nat′ŏ-mist). A specialist in the science of anatomy.

anatomy (ă-nat′ŏ-mē) [G. *anatomē*, dissection, from *ana*, apart, + *tomē*, a cutting]. **1.** The morphologic structure of an organism. **2.** The science of the morphology or structure of organisms. **3.** Dissection. **4.** A work describing the form and structure of an organism and its various parts.

applied a., the practical application of anatomical knowledge to diagnosis and treatment.

artificial a., the manufacture of models of anatomic structures, or the study of a. from such models.

artistic a., the study of a. for artistic purposes, as applied to painting, drawing, or sculpture.

clastic a., plastic a.; the construction or study of models in layers which can be removed one after the other to show the structure of the organism and/or organ.

comparative a., the comparative study of animal structure with regard to homologous organs or parts.

dental a., that branch of gross a. concerned with the morphology of teeth, their location, position, and relationships.

descriptive a., systematic a.; a description of, especially a treatise describing, physical structure, more particularly that of man.

developmental a., a. of the structural changes of an individual from fertilization to adulthood; includes embryology, fetology, and postnatal development.

functional a., physiological a.

general a., the study of gross and microscopic structures as well as of the composition of the body, its tissues and fliuds.

gross a., macroscopic a.; general a., so far as it can be studied without the use of the microscope.

living a., the study of a. in the living individual by inspection.

macroscopic a., gross a.

medical a., a. in its bearing upon the diagnosis and treatment of internal disorders.

microscopic a., the branch of a. in which the structure of cells, tissues, and organs is studied with the light microscope. See histology.

pathological a., anatomical *pathology.*

physiological a., functional a.; a. studied in its relation to function.

plastic a., clastic a.

practical a., a. studied by means of dissection.

radiological a., the study of the body through radiographs.

regional a., topographic a.; topology (1); a. of certain related parts or divisions of the body.

special a., the a. of certain definite organs or groups of organs involved in the performance of special functions; descriptive a. dealing with the separate systems.

surface a., the study of the configuration of the surface of the body, especially in its relation to deeper parts.

surgical a., applied a. in reference to surgical diagnosis and treatment.

systematic a., descriptive a.

systemic a., a. of the systems of the body.

topographic a., regional a.

transcendental a., the theories and deductions based upon the morphology of the organs and individual parts of the body.

ultrastructural a., the ultramicroscopic study of structures too small to be seen with a light microscope.

anatopism (ă-nat′ō-pizm) [G. *ana*, backward, + *topos*, place]. Failure to conform to the cultural pattern.

anatoxic (an-ă-tok′sik). Pertaining to the characteristic properties of anatoxin (toxoid).

anatoxin (an-ă-tok′sin). Toxoid.

anatricrotic (an′ă-trī-krot′ik). Characterized by anatricrotism; denoting a sphygmographic tracing with three waves on the ascending limb.

anatricrotism (an′ă-trik′rō-tizm) [G. *ana*, up, + *tri-*, thrice, *krotos*, beating]. A condition of the pulse manifested by a triple beat on the ascending limb of the sphygmographic tracing.

anatripsis (an-ă-trip′sis) [G. a rubbing, fr. *tribō*, fut. *tripsō*, to rub]. Therapeutic use of rubbing or friction with or without simultaneous application of a medicament.

anatriptic (an-ă-trip′tik). **1.** Pertaining to anatripsis. **2.** A remedy to be applied by friction or rubbing.

anatropia (an-ă-trō′pē-ă) [G. *ana*, up, + *tropē*, a turning]. Upward deviation of one eye.

anaudia (an-aw′dē-ă) [G. *an-* priv. + *audān*, to speak]. Aphonia.

anaxon, anaxone (an-aks′on, -aks′ōn) [G. *an-* priv. + *axōn*, axis]. Having no axon; denoting certain nerve cells first described by S. Ramón y Cajal as amacrine cells in the retina, and later discovered in several brain regions.

anazoturia (an′az-ō-tū′rē-ă) [G. *an-* priv. + azoturia]. A deficiency or lack of nitrogenous metabolic products excreted in the urine; pertains especially to unusually small quantities of urea in the urine.

AnCC Abbreviation for anodal closure *contraction.*

anchone (ang-kō′nē) [G. *agchonē*, a strangling]. Spasm of the throat muscles, often a conversion reaction.

anchorage (ang′kŏr-ij) [L. *ancora*, fr. G. *ankyra*, anchor]. **1.** Operative fixation of loose or prolapsed abdominal or pelvic organs. **2.** The part to which anything is fastened. In dentistry, a tooth or an implanted tooth substitute to which a fixed or removable partial denture, crown, or restorative material is retained. **3.** The nature and degree of resistance to displacement offered by an anatomical unit when used for the purpose of effecting tooth movement.

cervical a., a. in which the back of the neck is used for resistance by means of a cervical strap.

extraoral a., a. in which the resistance unit is outside the oral cavity; *e.g.*, cranial, occipital, or cervical a.

intermaxillary a., a. in which the units in one jaw are used to effect tooth movement in the other jaw.

intramaxillary a., a. in which the resistance units are all situated within the same jaw.

intraoral a., a. in which the resistance units are all located within the oral cavity.

multiple a., reinforced a.; a. in which more than one type of resistance unit is utilized.

occipital a., a. in which the top and back of the head are used for resistance by means of a headgear.

reciprocal a., a. in which the movement of one or more teeth is balanced against the movement of one or more opposing teeth.

reinforced a., multiple a.

simple a., a. in which the resistance to the movement of one or more teeth comes solely from resistance to tipping movement of the a. unit.

stationary a., a. in which the resistance to the movement of one or more teeth comes from the resistance to bodily movement of the a. unit; a questionable concept since the selected teeth remain only relatively stable.

anchusin (an'kū-sin). Alkannin.

ancillary (an'si-lār-ē) [L. *ancillaris,* relating to a maid servant]. Auxiliary, accessory, or secondary.

ancipital, ancipitate, ancipitous (an-sip'i-tăl, -i-tāt, -i-tŭs) [L. *anceps,* two- headed]. Two-headed; two-edged.

ancon (ang'kŏn) [G. *ankon,* elbow]. Elbow (1).

anconad (ang'kō-nad) [G. *ankōn,* elbow, + L. *ad,* to]. Toward the elbow.

anconal, anconeal (ang'kŏ-năl, ang-kō'nē-ăl). **1.** Relating to the elbow (ancon). **2.** Relating to the anconeus muscle.

anconeus (ang-kō'nē-ŭs) [L.]. *Musculus* anconeus.

anconitis (an-kō-nī'tis) [G. *ankōn,* elbow, + *-itis,* inflammation]. Inflammation of the elbow joint.

anconoid (ang'kō-noyd). Resembling the elbow.

ancrod (an'krod). A fraction obtained from the venom of the pit viper, *Angkistrodon rhodostoma,* which contains a fibrinogen-splitting enzyme; produces hypofibrinogenemia and diminution of both whole blood and plasma viscosity for improvement of the rheologic properties of blood, and is used in treatment of chronic peripheral vascular disease.

ancylo-. See ankylo-.

Ancylostoma (an-si-los'tō-mă, an-ki-) [G. *ankylos,* curved, hooked, + *stoma,* mouth]. *Ankylostoma;* a genus of Nematoda, the Old World hookworm, the members of which are parasitic in the duodenum. They attach themselves to villi in the mucous membrane, suck blood, and may cause a state of anemia, especially in cases of malnutrition. The eggs are passed with the feces, and the larvae develop in moist soil to become infectious third-stage (filariform) larvae that enter the body of man through the skin and possibly in drinking water; they migrate by the bloodstream to lung alveoli, are carried to bronchi and trachea, swallowed, and passed to the intestine where they mature. See also ancylostomiasis; *Necator americanus.*

A. brazilien'se, a species characterized by one pair of ventral buccal teeth, normally an intestinal parasite of dogs and cats but also found in man as a cause of human cutaneous larva migrans.

A. cani'num, a species possessing three pairs of ventral teeth in the oral cavity; common in dogs, but also occurring in human skin as a cause of cutaneous larva migrans.

A. ceylan'icum, species found in the civet cat of Ceylon; rarely reported from man as an intestinal parasite in Southeast Asia.

A. duodena'le, the Old World hookworm of man, a species widespread in temperate areas, in contrast to the more tropical distribution of the New World hookworm. See *Necator americanus.*

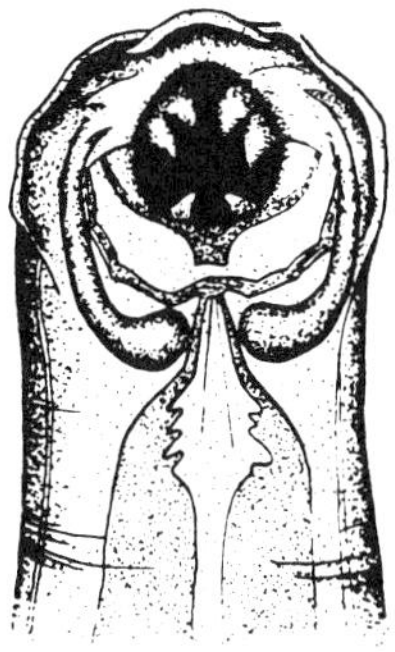

Ancylostoma duodenale
Mouth and buccal cavity.

ancylostomatic (an'si-lō-stō-mat'ik, an'ki-). Referring to hookworms of the genus *Ancylostoma.*

ancylostomiasis (an'si-lō-stō-mī'ă-sis, an'ki-). Ankylostomiasis; miner's disease (1); tunnel disease; intertropical or tropical hyphemia; uncinariasis; hookworm disease caused by *Ancylostoma duodenale* and characterized by eosinophilia, anemia, emaciation, dyspepsia, and, in children with severe long-continued infections, swelling of the abdomen with mental and physical maldevelopment.

cutaneous a., small vesicles and pustules on the skin at sites of penetration of larvae of *Ancylostoma;* these itching lesions, which begin most commonly on the feet and between the toes, frequently precede the onset of intestinal symptoms, particularly after sensitizing exposures. Also called a. cutis; ancylostomiasis dermatitis; coolie, dew, ground, toe, or swamp itch; swimmer's itch (1); water itch (1); water sore.

a. cu'tis, cutaneous a.

ancyroid (an'si-royd) [G. *ankyra,* anchor, + *eidos,* resemblance]. Ankyroid; shaped like the fluke of an anchor; denoting the cornua of the lateral ventricles of the brain and the coracoid process of the scapula.

Andernach, Johann W. (Guenther von Andernach), German physician, 1505–1574. See A.'s *ossicle.*

Anders, James Meschter, U.S. physician, 1854–1936. See A.'s *disease.*

Andersch, Carolus Samuel, German anatomist, 1732–1777. See A.'s *ganglion, nerve.*

Andersen, Dorothy Hansine, U.S. pediatrician, *1901. See A.'s *disease.*

Anderson, Evelyn, U.S. physician, *1899. See A. Collip *test.*

Anderson, James C., British urologist, *1899. See A.-Hynes *pyeloplasty.*

Anderson, Roger, U.S. surgeon, *1891. See A. *splint.*

Anderson-Collip test. See under test.

andira (an-dī'rā) [West Indian native name]. Worm bark; cabbage tree; the bark of *Andira inermis,* a leguminous tree of tropical America, used as an emetic, purgative, and anthelmintic.

andirine (an-dī'rin). *N*- Methyltyrosine; an alkaloid derived from Andira that has negligible stimulating action.

Andral, Gabriel, French physician, 1797–1876. See A.'s *decubitus.*

andrenosterone (an-drē-nos'ter-ōn). Adrenosterone.

Andrews, C.J., U.S. surgeon. See Brandt-A. *maneuver.*

andriatrics, andriatry (an-dri-at'riks, -drī'ă-trē) [G. *anēr,* a man, + *iatreia,* medical treatment]. Medical science relating to diseases of male genital organs and of men in general.

andro- [G. *anēr* (gen. andros), male]. Combining form meaning masculine; pertaining to the male of the species.

androblastoma (an'drō-blas-tō'mă). **1.** Pick's tubular or testicular tubular adenoma; Sertoli cell tumor; a testicular tumor microscopically resembling fetal testis, with varying proportions of tubular and stromal elements; the tubules contain Sertoli cells, which may cause feminization. **2.** Arrhenoblastoma.

androgen (an'drō-jen). Testoid (2); generic term for an agent, usually a hormone (*e.g.,* androsterone, testosterone), that stimulates activity of the accessory male sex organs, encourages development of male sex characteristics, or prevents changes in the latter that follow castration; natural a.'s are steroids, derivatives of androstane.

adrenal a., any androgenic hormone of adrenocortical origin; *e.g.,* dehydroepiandrosterone (and its sulfate), androstenedione, 11β-

hydroxyandrostenedione.

androgenesis (an-drō-jen'ĕ-sis) [andro- + G. *genesis*, production]. Egg development in the presence only of paternal chromosomes.

androgenic (an-drō-jen'ik). Testoid (1); relating to an androgen; having a masculinizing effect.

androgenous (an-droj'ĕ-nŭs). Giving birth predominantly to males.

androgynism (an-droj'i-nizm). Female *pseudohermaphroditism*.

androgynoid (an-droj'i-noyd) [andro- + G. *gynē*, woman, + *eidos*, resemblance]. A male resembling a female, or possessing hermaphroditic features.

androgynous (an-droj'i-nŭs). Pertaining to androgyny.

androgyny (an-droj'i-nē) [andro- + G. *gynē*, woman]. **1.** Female *pseudohermaphroditism*. **2.** Having both masculine and feminine characteristics, as in attitudes and behaviors that contain features of stereotyped, culturally sanctioned sexual roles of both male and female.

android (an'droyd) [andro- + G. *eidos*, resemblance]. Resembling a man in form and structure.

andrology (an-drol'ō-jē) [andro- + G. *logos*, treatise]. The branch of medicine concerned with diseases peculiar to the male sex, particularly infertility and sexual dysfunction.

andromania (an-drō-mā'nē-ă) [andro- + G. *mania*, frenzy]. Obsolete term for nymphomania.

andromedotoxin (an-drom'ĕ-dō-tok'sin). A strongly emetic active principle obtained from several species of *Andromeda* and *Rhododendron* (family Ericaceae); it is a cardiac poison, first stimulating and then paralyzing the vagus; it also paralyzes the motor nerve ends in striated muscle.

andromorphous (an-drō-mōr'fŭs) [andro- + G. *morphē*, form]. Having a male form or habitus.

andropathy (an-drop'ă-thē) [andro- + G. *pathos*, suffering]. Any disease, such as prostatitis, peculiar to the male sex.

androphobia (an-drō-fō'bē-ă) [andro- + G. *phobos*, fear]. Morbid fear of men, or of the male sex, resulting in avoidance of situations where men are present.

androstane (an'drō-stān). The parent hydrocarbon of the androgenic steroids. For structure, see steroids.

androstanediol (an-drō-stān'dī-ol). 5α-Androstane-$3\beta,17\beta$-diol; a steroid metabolite, of which 5β isomers are also known.

androstanedione (an-drō-stān'dī-ōn). 5α-Androstane-3,17-dione; a steroid metabolite, of which the 5β isomer is also known.

androstene (an'drō-stēn). Androstane with an unsaturated (*i.e.*, —CH=CH—) bond in the molecule.

androstenediol (an-drō-stēn'dī-ol). 5-Androsten-$3\beta,17\beta$-diol; a steroid metabolite differing from androstanediol by possessing a double bond between C-5 and C-6.

androstenedione (an-drō-stēn'dī-ōn). 4-Androstene-3,17-dione; androstanedione with a double bond between C-4 and C-5; an androgenic steroid, of weaker biological potency than testosterone; secreted by the testis, ovary, and adrenal cortex.

androstenolone (an-drō-stēn-ō-lōn). Dehydro-3-epiandrosterone.

androsterone (an-dros'ter-ōn). *cis*- Androsterone; 3α-hydroxy-5α-androstan-17-one; (3α-hydroxyetioallocholan-17-one; 3-epihydroxyetioallocholan-17-one); a steroid metabolite, found in male urine, having weak androgenic potency.

AnDTe Abbreviation for anodal duration *tetanus*.

anechoic (an-ĕ-kō'ik). Sonolucent.

anectasis (an-ek'tă-sis) [G. *an*- priv. + *ektasis*, dilation]. Primary *atelectasis*.

Anel, Dominique, French surgeon, 1679–1725. See A.'s *method*, *probe*.

anelectrode (an-ĕ-lek'trōd). Anode.

anelectrotonic (an-ē-lek-trō-ton'ik). Relating to anelectrotonus.

anelectrotonus (an'ē-lek-trot'ō-nŭs) [anelectrode + G. *tonos*, tension]. Changes in excitability and conductivity in a nerve or muscle cell in the neighborhood of the anode during the passage of a constant electric current.

ANEMIA

anemia (ă-nē'mē-ă) [G. *anaimia*, fr. *an*- priv. + *haima*, blood]. Any condition in which the number of red blood cells per cu mm, the amount of hemoglobin in 100 ml of blood, and the volume of packed red blood cells per 100 ml of blood are less than normal; clinically, generally pertaining to the concentration of oxygen-transporting material in a designated volume of blood, in contrast to total quantities as in oligocythemia, oligochromemia, and oligemia. A. is frequently manifested by pallor of the skin and mucous membranes, shortness of breath, palpitations of the heart, soft systolic murmurs, lethargy, and fatigability.

achlorhydric a., Faber's a. or syndrome; a form of chronic hypochromic microcytic a. associated with achlorhydria or achylia gastrica; observed most frequently in women in the third to fifth decades.

achrestic a. [G. *a*- priv. + *chrēsis*, a using], a form of chronic progressive macrocytic a., frequently fatal, in which the changes in bone marrow and circulating blood closely resemble those of pernicious a., but in which there is only transient or no response to therapy with vitamin B_{12}; glossitis, gastrointestinal disturbances, central nervous system disease, and pyrexia are not observed, and there is only little bleeding or hemolysis.

acquired hemolytic a., nonhereditary acute or chronic a. associated with or caused by extracorpuscular factors, *e.g.*, certain infectious agents, chemicals (including therapeutic agents), burns, toxic materials from higher plant and animal forms (including snake venoms), autoantibodies.

Addison's a., addisonian a., pernicious a.

angiopathic hemolytic a., a rare postpartum a. of unknown etiology with uremia and nephrosclerosis; may be a rare complication following use of contraceptive steroids.

aplastic a., Ehrlich's a.; a. gravis; a. characterized by a greatly decreased formation of erythrocytes and hemoglobin, usually associated with pronounced granulocytopenia and thrombocytopenia, as a result of hypoplastic or aplastic bone marrow.

asiderotic a., chlorosis.

autoallergic hemolytic a., autoimmune hemolytic a.

autoimmune hemolytic a., autoallergic hemolytic a.; **(1)** cold-antibody type, caused by hemagglutinating cold antibody and resulting from severe hemolysis in cold hemagglutinin disease; **(2)** warm-antibody type, acquired hemolytic a. due to serum autoantibodies (usually IgG class) that react with the patient's red blood cells; it varies in severity, occurs in all age groups of both sexes, and may be idiopathic or secondary to neoplastic, autoimmune, or other disease. The Coombs test is positive for IgG and complement, IgG alone, or complement alone.

Belgian Congo a., kasai.

Biermer's a., pernicious a.

brickmaker's a., a. associated with hookworm disease.

cameloid a., elliptocytic a.

chlorotic a., chlorosis.

congenital a., *erythroblastosis* fetalis.

congenital aplastic a., Fanconi's a.

congenital aregenerative a., congenital hypoplastic a.

congenital dyserythropoietic a., a group of a.'s characterized by ineffective erythropoiesis, bone marrow erythroblastic multinuclearity, and secondary hemochromatosis; probably autosomal recessive inheritance. Three types are described: **type I,** macrocytic, megaloblastic a. with erythroblastic internuclear chromatin bridges; **type II,** normoblastic a. with multinucleated erythroblasts; **type III,** macrocytic a. with erythroblastic multinuclearity and gigantoblasts.
congenital hemolytic a., accelerated destruction of red blood cells due to an inherited defect, such as a defect in the membrane which occurs in hereditary spherocytosis.
congenital hypoplastic a., congenital aregenerative, familial hypoplastic, or pure red cell a.; erythrogenesis imperfecta; Diamond-Blackfan a. or syndrome; normocytic normochromic a. resulting from congenital hypoplasia of the bone marrow, which is grossly deficient in erythroid precursors but other elements are normal; a. is progressive and severe, but leukocyte and platelet counts are normal or slightly reduced; survival of transfused erythrocytes is normal; minor congenital anomalies are found in some patients.
Cooley's a., *thalassemia* major.
crescent cell a., sickle cell a.
deficiency a., nutritional a.
Diamond-Blackfan a., congenital hypoplastic a.
dilution a., hydremia.
dimorphic a., a. in which two distinct forms of red cells are circulating.
diphyllobothrium a., fish tapeworm a.; a rare form of pernicious a. associated with *Diphyllobothrium latum* infection, especially in Finland.
dyshemopoietic a., any a. resulting from defective function of the bone marrow.
Ehrlich's a., aplastic a.
elliptocytic a., cameloid or ovalocytic a.; a. characterized by elliptical erythrocytes (ovalocytes) resembling those observed normally in camels; 1 to 15% of erythrocytes in nonanemic persons may be oval, but greater proportions are observed in certain patients with microcytic a. See also elliptocytosis.
equine infectious a., swamp fever (1); a worldwide infectious disease of horses and other equids, caused by equine infectious a. virus and marked by general debility, remittent fever, staggering gait, progressive a., and loss of flesh; it is transmitted by bloodsucking insects and by contact, oral infection, or the use of unsterilized syringes and needles.
erythroblastic a., an outmoded term for thalassemia major.
Faber's a., achlorhydric a.
false a., pseudoanemia.
familial erythroblastic a., an outmoded term for thalassemia major.
familial hypoplastic a., congenital hypoplastic a.
familial microcytic a., a rare type of hypochromic microcytic a. associated with a defect of iron metabolism characterized by high serum iron, hepatic iron deposits, and absence of stainable bone marrow iron stores.
familial pyridoxine-responsive a., a rare hereditary hypochromic a. that may be an X-linked or autosomal trait, and is responsive to pyridoxine.
familial splenic a., Gaucher's *disease.*
Fanconi's a., Fanconi's syndrome (1); Fanconi's or congenital pancytopenia; congenital aplastic a.; a type of idiopathic refractory a. characterized by pancytopenia, hypoplasia of the bone marrow, and congenital anomalies, occurring in members of the same family (probably resulting from a recessive gene); the a. is normocytic or slightly macrocytic, macrocytes and target cells may be found in the circulating blood, and the leukopenia usually is due to neutropenia; congenital anomalies include short stature, microcephaly, hypogenitalism, strabismus, anomalies of the thumbs, radii, and kidneys, mental retardation, and microphthalmia.
fish tapeworm a., diphyllobothrium a.
genetic a., any a. associated with an inherited defect in the structure or function of the erythrocytes and erythropoietic tissue.
globe cell a., hereditary *spherocytosis.*
goat's milk a., nutritional a. in infants maintained chiefly with goat's milk, which is relatively poor in iron content.
a. gra'vis, aplastic a.
ground itch a., a. associated with hookworm disease.
Hayem-Widal a., obsolete eponym for acquired hemolytic a.
hemolytic a., any a. resulting from an increased rate of erythrocytes destruction.
hemolytic a. of newborn, **(1)** *erythroblastosis* fetalis; **(2)** a disease similar to erythroblastosis fetalis, seen in foals, piglets, and puppies.
hemorrhagic a., a. resulting directly from loss of blood.
hemotoxic a., toxic a.
hookworm a., a. associated with heavy infections by *Ancylostoma duodenale* or *Necator americanus.*
hyperchromic a., hyperchromatic a., a. characterized by an increase in the ratio of the weight of hemoglobin to the volume of the erythrocyte, *i.e.,* the mean corpuscular hemoglobin concentration is greater than normal; although the weight of hemoglobin per cell may be greater in the macrocytes of pernicious a., the increase is proportional to the larger volume and such cells are not truly hyperchromic.
hypochromic a., a. characterized by a decrease in the ratio of the weight of hemoglobin to the volume of the erythrocyte, *i.e.,* the mean corpuscular hemoglobin concentration is less than normal; the individual cells contain less hemoglobin than they could have under optimal conditions.
hypochromic microcytic a., a. due to iron deficiency or thalassemia, and characterized by smaller than normal mean corpuscular volume, mean corpuscular hemoglobin, and mean corpuscular hemoglobin concentration.
hypoferric a., iron deficiency a.
hypoplastic a., progressive nonregenerative a. resulting from greatly depressed, inadequately functioning bone marrow; as the process persists, aplastic a. may occur.
icterohemolytic a., hereditary *spherocytosis.*
a. infan'tum pseudoleuke'mica, obsolete term for a syndrome observed in infants and young children, characterized by a deficiency of hemoglobin, anisocytosis and poikilocytosis, numerous erythroblasts, conspicuous leukocytosis with relative lymphocytosis, splenomegaly, hepatomegaly, and enlarged lymph nodes; now known to be associated with a variety of conditions, *e.g.,* malnutrition, gastrointestinal disorders, thalassemia, iron deficiency, tuberculosis.
infectious a., a. developing as a complication of infection, especially persistent suppurative disease and septicemia; probably results from depressed formation and short survival of erythrocytes.
intertropical a., a. occurring in hookworm disease, chiefly necatoriasis.
iron deficiency a., hypoferric a.; hypochromic microcytic a. characterized by low serum iron, increased serum iron-binding capacity, and decreased marrow iron stores.
isochromic a., normochromic a.
lead a., a. associated with poisoning from lead; thought to result from a defect in synthesis of hemoglobin based on the failure of iron being combined in the porphyrin ring.
Lederer's a., obsolete eponym for a form of acute acquired hemolytic a. associated with abnormal hemolysins and sometimes with hemoglobinuria.
leukoerythroblastic a., leukoerythroblastosis.
local a., a. resulting from a decreased supply of blood to a part, as in the occlusion of a vessel.
a. lymphat'ica, Hodgkin's *disease.*
macrocytic a., megalocytic a.; any a. in which the average size of

circulating erythrocytes is greater than normal, *i.e.,* the mean corpuscular volume is 94 cu μm or more (normal range, 82 to 92 cu μm), including such syndromes as pernicious a., sprue, celiac disease, macrocytic a. of pregnancy, a. of diphyllobothriasis, and others.
macrocytic achylic a., pernicious a.
macrocytic a. of pregnancy, an a. occurring in pregnancy, related to folate deficiency and characterized by a low level of hemoglobin and a reduced number of erythrocytes, which are larger than normal (macrocytes).
malignant a., pernicious a.
Marchiafava-Micheli a., paroxysmal nocturnal *hemoglobinuria.*
Mediterranean a., an outmoded collective term for thalassemia.
megaloblastic a., any a. in which there is a predominant number of megaloblasts, and relatively few normoblasts, among the hyperplastic erythroid cells in the bone marrow (as in pernicious a.).
megalocytic a., macrocytic a.
metaplastic a., pernicious a. in which the various formed elements in the blood are changed, *e.g.,* multisegmented, unusually large neutrophiles (macropolycytes), immature myeloid cells, bizarre platelets.
microangiopathic hemolytic a., hemolysis due to narrowing or obstruction of small blood vessels; causing fragmentation of red blood cells.
microcytic a., any a. in which the average size of circulating erythrocytes is smaller than normal, *i.e.,* the mean corpuscular volume is 80 cu μm or less (normal range, 82 to 92 cu μm).
microdrepanocytic a., sickle cell-thalassemia disease; a., clinically resembling sickle cell a., in which individuals are heterozygous for both the sickle cell gene and a thalassemia gene; about 60 to 80% of hemoglobin is Hb S, up to 20% Hb F, and the remainder Hb A.
milk a., a type of hypochromic microcytic a., resulting from deficiency of iron, sometimes occurring in infants maintained on a milk diet for too long a time.
molecular a., a. due to the presence in the blood of an abnormal hemoglobin; *e.g.,* sickle cell a., thalassemia.
myelophthisic a., myelopathic a., leukoerythroblastosis.
neonatal a., a. neonato'rum, *erythroblastosis* fetalis.
normochromic a., isochromic a.; any a. in which the concentration of hemoglobin in the erythrocytes is within the normal range, *i.e.,* the mean corpuscular hemoglobin concentration is from 32 to 36%.
normocytic a., any a. in which the erythrocytes are normal in size, *i.e.,* the mean corpuscular volume ranges from 82 to 92 cu μm.
nutritional a., deficiency a.; any a. resulting from a dietary deficiency of materials essential to red blood cell formation, *e.g.,* iron, vitamins, protein.
osteosclerotic a., a leukoerythroblastosis.
ovalocytic a., elliptocytic a.
pernicious a., Addison's, addisonian, Biermer's, or malignant a.; macrocytic achylic a.; Biermer's or Addison-Biermer disease; a chronic progressive a. of older adults (occurring more frequently during the fifth and later decades, rarely prior to 30 years of age), thought to result from a defect of the stomach accompanied by atrophy and associated with lack of an "intrinsic" factor; characterized by numbness and tingling, weakness, and a sore smooth tongue, as well as dyspnea after slight exertion, faintness, pallor of the skin and mucous membranes, anorexia, diarrhea, loss of weight, and fever; laboratory studies usually reveal greatly decreased red blood cell counts, low levels of hemoglobin, numerous characteristically oval shaped macrocytic erythrocytes (color index greater than normal, but not truly hyperchromic), and hypo- or achlorhydria, in association with a predominant number of megaloblasts and relatively few normoblasts in the bone marrow; the leukocyte count in peripheral blood may be less than normal, with relative lymphocytosis and hypersegmented neutrophils; a low level of vitamin B_{12} is found in peripheral red blood cells; administration of vitamin B_{12} results in a characteristic reticulocyte response, relief from symptoms, and an increase in erythrocytes, provided that pernicious a. is not complicated by another disease; the condition is not actually "pernicious," as it was prior to therapeutic use of liver and vitamin B_{12}.
physiologic a., apparent a. caused by increased fluid volume of the blood (overhydration).
polar a., a form of a. sometimes observed in natives of temperate climates when they migrate to the Arctic or Antarctic regions.
posthemorrhagic a., traumatic a.; an acute a. caused by fairly sudden and rapid loss of blood, as by traumatic laceration of a relatively large vessel, erosion of an artery in a duodenal ulcer, hemorrhage in an ectopic pregnancy, or the result of such diseases as hemophilia and acute leukemia.
primary erythroblastic a., *thalassemia* major.
primary refractory a., any of a group of anemic conditions in which there is persistent, frequently advanced a. that is not successfully treated by any means except blood transfusions, and that is not associated with another primary disease.
refractory a., see primary refractory a.; secondary refractory a.
pure red cell a., congenital hypoplastic a.
radiation a., hypoplastic a. sometimes occurring after high level acute or low level chronic exposure to ionizing radiation.
secondary refractory a., any persistent a. that is successfully treated only by blood transfusions, and that is associated with another condition.
sickle cell a., crescent cell a.; an inherited a. characterized by the presence of crescent- or sickle-shaped erythrocytes and by accelerated hemolysis, due to substitution of a single amino acid (valine for glutamic acid) in the sixth position of the beta chain of hemoglobin; affected homozygotes have 85-95% Hb S and severe anemia, while heterozygotes (said to have sickle cell trait) have 40-45% Hb S, the rest being normal Hb A; low oxygen tension causes polymerization of the abnormal beta chains, thus distorting the shape of the red blood cells. Homozygotes develop "crises" characterized by episodes of severe pain due to microvascular occlusions, bone infarcts, leg ulcers, and autoinfection of the spleen associated with increased susceptibility to bacterial infections.
sideroblastic a., sideroachrestic a., refractory a. characterized by the presence of sideroblasts in the bone marrow.
slaty a., an ash-gray pallor in poisoning from acetanelid or silver (argyria).
spastic a., local a. resulting from nontransitory contraction of the arterial vessels in the affected region.
spherocytic a., hereditary *spherocytosis.*
splenic a., Banti's *syndrome.*
target cell a., any a. with a conspicuous number of target cells in the peripheral blood; characteristic of thalassemia minor, and also found in several hemoglobinopathies.
toxic a., hemotoxic a.; any a. resulting from the destructive effects of a chemical, metabolic poison, bacterial toxin, venom, and similar materials.
traumatic a., posthemorrhagic a.
tropical a., various syndromes frequently observed in persons in tropical climates, usually resulting from nutritional deficiencies or hookworm or other parasitic diseases.

---

anemic (ă-nē'mik). Pertaining to or manifesting the various features of anemia.

anemometer (an-ĕ-mom'ĕ-ter) [G. *anemos,* wind, + *metron,* measure]. An instrument for measuring the velocity of air flow.

anemonol (ă-nem'ō-nol). A volatile oil, possessing markedly toxic properties, obtained from plants of the genus *Anemone.*

anemophobia (an'ĕ-mō-fō'bē-ă) [G. *anemos,* wind, + *phobos,* fear]. Morbid fear of wind.

anemotrophy (an-ĕ-mot'rō-fē) [G. *an-* priv. + *haima,* blood, + *trophē,* nourishment]. Lack of substances essential to the formation of blood, thereby resulting in hypoplastic anemia.

anencephalia (an'en-se-fā'lē-ă). Anencephaly.

anencephalic (an-en-se-fal'ik). Anencephalous; relating to anencephaly.

anencephalous (an-en-sef'ă-lŭs). Anencephalic.

anencephaly (an'en-sef'ă-lē) [G. *an-* priv. + *enkephalos,* brain]. Anencephalia; congenital defective development of the brain, with absence of the bones of the cranial vault, the cerebral and cerebellar hemispheres, a rudimentary brainstem, and traces of basal ganglia.
partial a., hemicephalia.

anenterous (an-en'ter-ŭs) [G. *an-* priv. + *entera,* intestines]. Having no intestine; denoting certain parasites, such as tapeworms.

anenzymia (an-en-zī'mē-ă). Congenital absence of a specific enzyme.
a. catala'sia, acatalasemia.

anephric (ā-nef'rik). Lacking kidneys.

anepia (ă-nep'ē-ă) [G. *an-* priv. + *epos,* word]. Aphasia.

anepiploic (an-ep-i-plō'ik). Lacking an omentum (epiploon).

anergasia (an-er-gā'zē-ă) [G. *an-* priv. + *ergasia,* work]. Absence of psychic activity as the result of organic brain disease.

anergastic (an-er-gas'tik). Pertaining to or characterized by anergasia.

anergia (an-er'jē-ă). Anergy (2).

anergic (an-er'jik). Relating to, or marked by, anergy.

anergy (an'er-jē) [G. *an-* priv. + *energeia,* energy, from *ergon,* work]. **1.** Absence of demonstrable sensitivity reaction in a subject to substances that would be antigenic (immunogenic, allergenic) in most other subjects. **2.** Anergia; lack of energy.
negative a., nonspecific a.; a reduction of the normal or usual immunologic responses because of unrelated intervening disease.
nonspecific a., negative a.
positive a., specific a.; a reduction of the normal or usual immunologic response resulting from a reaction to a specific allergen.
specific a., positive a.

aneroid (an'er-oyd) [G. *a-* priv. + *nēros,* wet, + *eidos,* form]. Without fluid; denoting a form of barometer without mercury, in which the varying air pressure is indicated by a pointer governed by the movement of the elastic wall of an evacuated chamber. Also used to denote a mercury-free pressure gauge used with some sphygmomanometers.

anerythroplasia (an'ĕ-rith-rō-plā'zē-ă) [G. *an-* priv. + erythro(cyte) + G. *plasis,* a molding]. A condition in which there is no formation of red blood cells.

anerythroplastic (an'ĕ-rith-rō-plas'tik). Pertaining to or characterized by anerythroplasia.

anerythroregenerative (an-ĕ-rith'thrō-rē-jen'er-ă-tiv). Pertaining to or characterized by lack of regeneration of red blood cells.

anesthecinesia (an-es'thē-si-nē'zē-ă). Anesthekinesia.

anesthekinesia (an-es'thē-ki-nē'zē-ă) [G. *an-* priv. + *aesthēsis,* sensation, + *kinēsis,* movement]. Anesthecinesia; combined sensory and motor paralysis.

ANESTHESIA

anesthesia (an'es-thē'zē-ă) [G. *anaisthēsia,* fr. *an-* priv. + *aisthēsis,* sensation]. **1.** A state characterized by loss of sensation, the result of pharmacologic depression of nerve function or of neurological disease. **2.** Broad term for anesthesiology as a clinical specialty.
acupuncture a., acupuncture (2); percutaneous insertion of, and stimulation by, needles placed in critical areas of the body to produce loss of sensation in another area.
axillary a., loss of sensation in the distal two-thirds of the upper extremity following injection of a local anesthetic solution about the nerve trunks in the axilla.
balanced a., a technique of general a. based on the concept that administration of a mixture of small amounts of several neuronal depressants summates the advantages, but not the disadvantages of, the individual components of the mixture.
basal a., parenteral administration of one or more sedatives to produce a state of depressed consciousness short of a general a.
block a., conduction a.
brachial a., anesthetization of an upper extremity by injection of local anesthetic solution about the brachial plexus.
caudal a., regional a. by injection of local anesthetic solution into the epidural space via the sacral hiatus.
cervical a., regional a. of the neck by injection of a local anesthetic solution about the cervical nerves.
circle absorption a., inhalation a. in which a circuit with carbon dioxide absorbent is used for complete (closed) or partial (semi-closed) rebreathing of exhaled gases.
closed a., inhalation a. in which there is total rebreathing of all exhaled gases, except carbon dioxide which is absorbed; gas flow into the anesthetic circuit consists only of oxygen, in amounts equal to the patient's metabolic consumption, plus small amounts of other gases (*e.g.,* nitrous oxide) which undergo continued uptake by and distribution in the patient.
compression a., pressure a.
conduction a., block a.; regional a. in which local anesthetic solution is injected about nerves to inhibit nerve transmission; includes spinal, epidural, nerve block, and field block a., but not local or topical a.
continuous epidural a., fractional epidural a.; insertion of a catheter into the lumbar or caudal epidural space for the repeated injection of local anesthetic solutions as a means of prolonging duration of anesthesia.
continuous spinal a., fractional spinal a.; insertion of a catheter into the spinal subarachnoid space and leaving it *in situ* to permit serial intermittent injection of local anesthetic solution for prolonged spinal a.
crossed a., a. of one side of the face and the other side of the body due to a brainstem lesion.
dental a., general, conduction, local, or topical a. for operations upon the teeth, gingivae, or associated structures.
diagnostic a., a. administered for evaluation of the mechanism responsible for a painful condition.
differential spinal a., a form of diagnostic spinal a. producing blockade of different types of nerves in the subarachnoid space, based upon their differences in sensitivity to local anesthetics; also observed during surgical spinal a.
dissociated a., loss of sensation for pain and temperature without loss of tactile sense.
dissociative a., a form of general a., but not necessarily complete unconsciousness, characterized by catalepsy, catatonia, and amnesia, especially that produced by phenylcyclohexylamine compounds, including ketamine.
a. doloro'sa, painful a.; severe spontaneous pain occurring in an anesthetic zone.
electric a., a., usually general a., produced by application of an electrical current.
endotracheal a., intratracheal a.; inhalation a. technique in which anesthetic and respiratory gases pass through a tube placed in the trachea via the mouth or nose.
epidural a., peridural a.; regional a. produced by injection of local

anesthetic solution into the peridural space.
extradural a., anesthetization, by local anesthetics, of nerves near the spinal canal external to the dura mater; often refers to epidural a., but may include paravertebral a.
field block a., conduction a. in which small nerves are not anesthetized individually, as in nerve block a., but instead are blocked *en masse* by local anesthetic solution injected to form a barrier proximal to the operative site.
fractional epidural a., continuous epidural a.
fractional spinal a., continuous spinal a.
general a., loss of ability to perceive pain associated with loss of consciousness produced by intravenous or inhalation anesthetic agents.
girdle a., a. distributed as a band encircling the abdomen.
glove a., loss of sensation in the distribution usually covered by a glove.
gustatory a., ageusia.
high spinal a., spinal a. in which the level of sensory denervation extends to the second or third thoracic dermatome.
hyperbaric a., inhalation of depressant gases or vapors at pressures greater than 1 atmosphere, especially as a means of producing general a. with agents too weak to produce a. at 1 atmosphere.
hyperbaric spinal a., spinal a. in which spread of local anesthetic solution in the subarachnoid space is controlled by adjusting the position of the patient after the specific gravity of local anesthetic solution has been made greater than that of cerebrospinal fluid by addition of glucose.
hypobaric spinal a., spinal a. in which spread of local anesthetic solution in the subarachnoid space is controlled by adjusting the position of the patient after the specific gravity of the local anesthetic solution has been made lower than that of cerebrospinal fluid by addition of distilled water.
hypotensive a., a. in which arterial hypotension is deliberately induced as a means of decreasing operative blood loss.
hypothermic a., general a. administered in conjunction with artificial lowering of body temperature.
hysterical a., a. as a manifestation of hysteria, usually involving half the body or isolated patches.
infiltration a., local a.
inhalation a., general a. resulting from breathing of anesthetic gases or vapors.
insufflation a., maintenance of inhalation a. by delivery of anesthetic gases or vapors directly to the airway of a patient spontaneously breathing room air.
intercostal a., regional a. produced by injection of local anesthetic solution about intercostal nerves.
intramedullary a., intraosseous a.; rarely used method of general a. by injection of intravenous anesthetic agent(s) into the medullary canal of long bones.
intranasal a., **(1)** insufflation a. in which an inhalation anesthetic is added to inhaled air passing through the nose or nasopharynx; **(2)** a. of nasal passages by infiltration and topical application of local anesthetic solution to nasal mucosa.
intraoral a., **(1)** insufflation a. in which an inhalation anesthetic is added to inhaled air passing through the mouth; **(2)** regional a. of the mouth and associated structures when local anesthetic solutions are used by topical application to oral mucosa, by local infiltration, or as nerve blocks.
intraosseous a., intramedullary a.
intraspinal a., injection of local anesthetic solution directly into the spinal cord; inaccurately used as a synonym for spinal a.
intratracheal a., endotracheal a.
intravenous a., general a. produced by injection of central nervous system depressants into the venous circulation.
intravenous regional a., Bier's method (1); regional a. by intravenous injection of local anesthetic solution distal to an occlusive tourniquet in an extremity previously exsanguinated by pressure or gravity.
isobaric spinal a., spinal a. in which spread of local anesthetic solution within the subarachnoid space is limited by making the specific gravity of the solution equal to that of cerebrospinal fluid.
local a., infiltration a.; regional a. produced by direct infiltration of local anesthetic solution into the operative site or, rarely, by freezing.
low spinal a., spinal a. in which the level of sensory denervation extends to the tenth or eleventh thoracic dermatome.
muscular a., loss of the muscle sense, or of the ability to determine the position of a limb or to recognize a difference in weights.
nerve block a., conduction a. in which local anesthetic solution is injected about peripheral nerves.
nonrebreathing a., a technique for inhalation a. in which valves exhaust all exhaled air from the circuit.
olfactory a., anosmia.
open drop a., inhalation a. by vaporization of a liquid anesthetic placed drop by drop on a gauze mask covering the mouth and nose.
painful a., a. dolorosa.
paracervical block a., regional a. of the cervix uteri by injection of local anesthetic solution into tissues adjacent to the cervix.
paravertebral a., **(1)** a. by injection of local anesthetic solution about nerves as they exit from the vertebral canal; **(2)** combined presynaptic, postsynaptic, and ganglionic sympathetic block by injection of local anesthetic solution about paravertebral sympathetic chains.
peridural a., epidural a.
perineural a., injection of an anesthetic agent about a nerve.
periodontal a., a. of the periodontal ligament, produced by injection of a local anesthetic drug.
pharyngeal a., a. of the pharynx occasionally complicating nervous disorders, most commonly in hysteria.
presacral a., injection of local anesthetic solution anterior to the sacrum, to block nerves as they exit from the sacral foramina.
pressure a., compression a.; loss of sensation produced by pressure applied to a peripheral nerve.
pudendal a., local a. produced by blocking the pudendal nerves near the spinal processes of the ischium; used in obstetrics.
rebreathing a., a technique for inhalation a. in which a portion or all of the gases that are exhaled are subsequently inhaled after carbon dioxide has been absorbed.
rectal a., general a. produced by instillation into the rectum of a solution containing a central nervous system depressant.
refrigeration a., cryoanesthesia.
regional a., use of local anesthetic solution(s) to produce circumscribed areas of loss of sensation; a generic term including conduction, nerve block, spinal, epidural, field block, infiltration, and topical a.
retrobulbar a., injection of a local anesthetic behind the eye to produce sensory denervation of the eye.
sacral a., regional a. limited to those areas innervated by sacral sensory nerves.
saddle block a., a form of spinal a. limited in area to the buttocks, perineum, and inner surfaces of the thighs.
segmental a., loss of sensation limited to an area supplied by one or more spinal nerve roots.
semi-closed a., inhalation a. using a circuit in which a portion of the exhaled air is exhausted from the circuit and a portion is rebreathed following absorption of carbon dioxide.
semi-open a., inhalation a. in which a portion of inhaled gases is derived from an anesthesia circuit while the remainder consists of room air.
spinal a., **(1)** subarachnoid a.; sensory denervation produced by injection of local anesthetic solution(s) into the spinal subarachnoid space; **(2)** loss of sensation produced by disease of the spinal cord.
splanchnic a., visceral a.; loss of sensation in those areas of the

visceral peritoneum innervated by the splanchnic nerves.
stocking a., loss of sensation in the area covered by a stocking.
subarachnoid a., spinal a. (1).
surgical a., **(1)** any a. administered for the purpose of permitting performance of an operative procedure, as differentiated from obstetrical, diagnostic, and therapeutic a.; **(2)** loss of sensation with muscle relaxation adequate for an operative procedure.
tactile a., loss or impairment of the sense of touch.
therapeutic a., administration of an anesthetic as a means of treatment.
thermal or **thermic a.,** loss of the ability to sense heat.
to-and-fro a., a. by means of a valveless closed a. circuit in which respired gases pass back and forth through a carbon dioxide absorbent interposed between patient and respiratory reservoir bag.
topical a., surface analgesia; superficial loss of sensation in mucous membranes or skin, produced by direct application of local anesthetic solutions, ointments, or jellies.
total spinal a., spinal a. extensive enough to produce loss of sensation in all extracranial sensory roots.
traumatic a., loss of sensation resulting from nerve injury.
unilateral a., hemianesthesia.
visceral a., splanchnic a.

anesthesiologist (an'es-thē-zē-ol'ō-jist). **1.** A physician specializing solely in anesthesiology and related areas. **2.** An individual with a doctorate degree who is board-certified and legally qualified to administer anesthetics and related techniques. *Cf.* anesthetist.

anesthesiology (an'es-thē-zē-ol'ō-jē) [anesthesia + G. *logos,* treatise]. The medical specialty concerned with the pharmacological, physiological, and clinical basis of anesthesia and related fields, including resuscitation, intensive respiratory care, and pain.

anesthesiophore (an-es-thē'zē-ō-fōr) [anesthesia + G. *phoros,* bearing]. The active group of a molecule that confers anesthetic or hypnotic effect.

anesthetic (an-es-thet'ik). **1.** A compound that reversibly depresses neuronal function, producing loss of ability to perceive pain and/or other sensations. **2.** Collective designation for anesthetizing agents administered to an individual at a particular time. **3.** Characterized by loss of sensation or capable of producing loss of sensation. **4.** Associated with or due to the state of anesthesia.
flammable a., an inhalation a. that supports combustion and forms explosive mixtures with oxidizing gases.
general a., a compound that produces loss of sensation associated with loss of consciousness.
inhalation a., a gas or a liquid with sufficient vapor pressure to produce general anesthesia when breathed.
intravenous a., a compound that produces anesthesia when injected intravenously.
local a., a compound that, when applied directly to mucous membranes or when injected about nerves, produces loss of sensation by inhibiting nerve excitation or conduction.
primary a., the compound that contributes most to loss of sensation when a mixture of anesthetics is administered.
secondary a., a compound that contributes to, but is not primarily responsible for, loss of sensation when two or more anesthetics are simultaneously administered.
spinal a., a local anesthetic agent capable of producing loss of sensation when injected into the subarachnoid space.
volatile a., a liquid a. that at room temperature volatilizes to a vapor which when inhaled is capable of producing general anesthesia. See also anesthetic *vapor.*

anesthetist (ă-nes'thĕ-tist). One who administers an anesthetic, whether an anesthesiologist, a physician who is not an anesthesiologist, a nurse a., or an anesthesia assistant.

anesthetization (ă-nes'thĕ-ti-zā'shun). The act of producing loss of sensation.

anesthetize (ă-nes'thĕ-tīz). To produce loss of sensation.

anestrous (an-es'trŭs). Relating to the anestrus.

anestrus (an-es'trŭs) [G. *a-* priv. + *oistros,* a gadfly, mad desire (estrus)]. The period of sexual quiescence between the estrus cycles of mammals; may be: 1) a prolonged period in monestrous animals (dogs) or seasonally polyestrous animals (sheep) or 2) a prolonged period of failure of estrus in mature nonpregnant, polyestrous animals.

anethopath (ă-nē'thō-path) [G. *an-* priv. + *ethos,* custom, + *pathos,* suffering]. A morally uninhibited person.

anetoderma (an-ĕ-tō-der'mă) [G. *anetos,* relaxed, + *derma,* skin]. Primary idiopathic macular atrophy; atrophia maculosa varioliformis cutis; an unusual form of atrophoderma characterized by circumscribed translucent lesions in which the skin becomes baglike and wrinkled.
Jadassohn-Pellizzari a., atrophy preceded by erythematous or urticarial lesions of the trunk and upper portions of the extremities, and enlarging to 2-3 cm before undergoing involution.
Schweninger-Buzzi a., sudden appearance of bluish-white balloon-like lesions, soft and readily indented, chiefly on the trunk and extremities of women.

aneuploid (an'yū-ployd) [G. *an-* priv. + euploid]. Having an abnormal number of chromosomes not an exact multiple of the haploid number, as contrasted with abnormal numbers of haploid sets of chromosomes, such as diploid, triploid, etc.

aneuploidy (an'yū-ploy-dē). State of being aneuploid.
partial a., a type of mosaicism in which some cells have a normal number of chromosomes and some have an abnormal number.

aneurine (an'yū-rēn). Thiamin.
a. hydrochloride, *thiamin* hydrochloride.

aneurolemmic (ă-nū-rō-lem'ik). Without a neurolemma.

aneurysm (an'yū-rizm) [G. *aneurysma* (-mat-), a dilation, fr. *eurys,* wide]. Circumscribed dilation of an artery, or a blood-containing tumor connecting directly with the lumen of an artery.

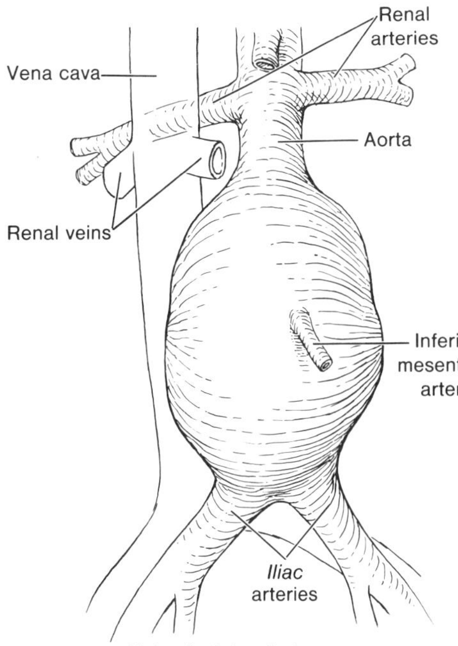

Abdominal Aortic Aneurysm

ampullary a., saccular a.
a. by anastomosis, a mass of dilated anastomosing vessels that produce a pulsating tumor usually in a superficial position.
arteriosclerotic a., atherosclerotic a.; the commonest type of a., occurring in the abdominal aorta and other large arteries, primarily in the elderly, and due to weakening of the tunica media by atherosclerosis.
arteriovenous a., a dilated arteriovenous shunt.
atherosclerotic a., arteriosclerotic a.
axial a., an a. involving the entire circumference of a blood vessel.
bacterial a., embolic a.
benign bone a., aneurysmal bone *cyst.*
Bérard's a., an arteriovenous a. in the tissues outside of the injured vein.
berry a., a small saccular a. of a cerebral artery that resembles a berry.
cardiac a., mural or ventricular a.; thinning, stretching, and bulging of a weakened ventricular wall, usually as a result of myocardial infarction.
cavernous-carotid a., a fistulous communication, of spontaneous or traumatic origin, between the cavernous sinus and the traversing internal carotid artery; a pulsating unilateral exophthalmos and a detectable cranial bruit are common accompaniments.
cirsoid a., racemose a. or hemangioma; cirsoid varix; dilation of a group of blood vessels due to congenital malformation with arteriovenous shunting.
compound a., an a. in which some of the coats of the artery are ruptured, others intact.
congenital cerebral a., localized dilation of a primitive vessel; often a berry a.
consecutive a., diffuse a.
cylindroid a., tubular a.
diffuse a., consecutive a; an a. that has enlarged and spread to the surrounding tissues in consequence of rupture of its walls.
dissecting a., splitting or dissection of an arterial wall by blood entering through an intimal tear or by interstitial hemorrhage; more common in the aorta, with an intimal tear near the aortic valve and distal dissection of the media for a variable distance, frequently rupturing through the outer wall; also a common aortic disease of turkeys.
ectatic a., an a. in which all the coats of the artery, though stretched, are unruptured.
embolic a., bacterial a.; an a. resulting from softening of the arterial wall at the site of lodgement of a septic embolus.
embolomycotic a., obsolete term for an a. caused by an embolism composed of an infected vegetation from a cardiac valve.
false a., **(1)** pulsating, encapsulated hematoma in communication with the lumen of the ruptured vessel; **(2)** pseudoaneurysm.
fusiform a., an elongated spindle-shaped dilation of an artery.
hernial a., the protrusion of the stretched inner coats of an artery through a wound in the adventitia.
infraclinoid a., an intracranial a. occurring within or below the cavernous sinus.
intracranial a., an a., either congenital, degenerative, posttraumatic, or mycotic, of the intracranial branches of the carotid or vertebral arterial systems.
miliary a., one of a number of minute sacculated or fusiform dilations of the smaller cerebral arteries.
mural a., cardiac a.
mycotic a., an a. caused by the growth of fungi within the vascular wall, usually following impaction of a septic embolus.
Park's a., an arteriovenous a. in which the brachial artery communicates with the brachial and median basilic veins.
peripheral a., **(1)** lateral a.; a saclike a. springing from one side of an artery; **(2)** an a. of one of the smaller branches of an artery.
phantom a., aortismus abdominalis; a palpable throbbing aorta, mistaken by novices for an a.
Pott's a., aneurysmal *varix.*
racemose a., cirsoid a.
Rasmussen's a., aneurysmal dilation of a branch of a pulmonary artery in a tuberculous cavity, rupture of which may cause serious hemoptysis.
saccular a., sacculated a., ampullary a.; a saclike bulging on one side of an artery.
serpentine a., dilation and tortuosity of an artery, sometimes affecting the temporal artery in the aged.
supraclinoid a., an intracranial a. of the internal carotid artery, occurring above the clinoid bone.
syphilitic a., an a., usually involving the thoracic aorta, resulting from tertiary syphilitic aortitis.
traction a., an aortic a. assumed to be due to the pull of a persistent ductus arteriosus.
traumatic a., an a. resulting from physical damage to the wall of an artery; usually a false a. or arteriovenous a.
true a., localized dilation of an artery with an expanded lumen lined by stretched remnants of the arterial wall.
tubular a., cylindroid a.; the uniform dilation of an artery along a considerable distance.
varicose a., a blood-containing sac, communicating with both an artery and a vein.
ventricular a., cardiac a.
verminous a., worm a., an a. in horses caused by ***Strongylus vulgaris*** larvae; usually involving the mesenteric arteries.

aneurysmal, aneurysmatic (an-yū-riz′măl, -riz-mat′ik). Relating to an aneurysm.

aneurysmectomy (an-yū-riz-mek′tō-mē) [aneurysm + G. *ektomē,* excision]. Excision of an aneurysm.

aneurysmogram (an′yū-riz′mō-gram). Demonstration of an aneurysm, usually by means of x-rays and a contrast medium.

aneurysmoplasty (an-yū-riz′mō-plas-tē) [aneurysm + G. *plastos,* formed]. Matas operation; endoaneurysmorrhaphy; endoaneurysmoplasty; repair of an aneurysm by opening the sac and suturing its walls to restore the normal dimension to the lumen of the artery. See also aneurysmorrhaphy.

aneurysmorrhaphy (an′yū-riz-mōr′ă-fē) [aneurysm + G. *raphē,* suture]. Closure by suture of the sac of an aneurysm to restore the normal lumen dimensions.

aneurysmotomy (an′yū-riz-mot′ō-mē) [aneurysm + G. *tomē,* incision]. Incision into the sac of an aneurysm.

ANF Abbreviation for antinuclear *factor.*

angei-. See angi-.

angelica root (an-jel′i-kă). The root of *Angelica archangelica* (family Umbelliferae); a tonic and stimulant that may cause nausea; used as a carminative, diuretic, and externally as a counterirritant.

Angelucci, Arnaldo, Italian ophthalmologist, 1854–1934. See A.'s *syndrome.*

Anger, Hal, U.S. electrical engineer, *1920. See A. *camera.*

Anghelescu, Constantin, Roumanian surgeon, 1869–1948. See A.'s *sign.*

angi-. See angio-.

angialgia (an-jē-al′jē-ă) [angio- + G. *algos,* pain]. Angiodynia; pain in blood vessel.

angiasthenia (an′jē-as-thē′nē-ă) [angio- + G. *astheneia,* weakness]. Vascular instability.

angiectasia, angiectasis (an-jē-ek-tā′zē-ă, -ek′tă-sis) [angio- + G. *ektasis,* a stretching]. Dilation of a lymphatic or blood vessel.
congenital dysplastic a., Klippel-Trenaunay-Weber *syndrome.*

angiectatic (an-jē-ek-tat′ik) [angio- + G. *ektatos,* capable of extension]. Marked by the presence of dilated blood vessels.

angiectomy (an-jē-ek'tō-mē) [angio- + G. *ektomē*, excision]. Excision of a section of a blood vessel.

angiectopia (an-jē-ek-tō'pē-ă) [angio- + G. *ektopos*, out of place]. Angioplany; abnormal location of a blood vessel.

angiitis, angitis (an-jē-ī'tis, an-jī'tis) [angio- + G. *-itis*, inflammation]. Vasculitis; inflammation of a blood vessel (arteritis, phlebitis) or of a lymphatic vessel (lymphangitis).
allergic a., cutaneous *vasculitis*.
allergic granulomatous a., Churg-Strauss *syndrome*.
consecutive a., a. caused by extension of the inflammatory process from the surrounding tissues.
cutaneous systemic a., cutaneous *vasculitis*.
hypersensitivity a., an inflammatory reaction in a blood vessel, the result of a specific reaction to an antigenic (allergic) substance or other agents to which the individual expresses unusual vascular sensitization.
leukocytoclastic a., cutaneous *vasculitis*.
a. live'do reticula'ris, *livedo* reticularis.
necrotizing a., inflammatory reaction of blood vessels resulting in fibrinoid necrosis of tissue, especially of the blood vessel wall.

angileucitis (an-jē-lū-sī'tis) [angio- + G. *leukos*, white, + *-itis*, inflammation]. Obsolete term for lymphangitis.

angina (an'ji-nă, an-jī'nă) [L. quinsy]. **1.** A severe constricting pain, usually referring to a. pectoris. **2.** Old term for a sore throat from any cause.
abdominal a., a. abdom'inis, intestinal a.; intermittent abdominal pain, frequently occurring at a fixed time after eating, caused by inadequacy of the mesenteric circulation from arteriosclerosis or other arterial disease.
agranulocytic a., agranulocytosis.
crescendo a., a. pectoris that occurs with increasing frequency, intensity, or duration.
a. cru'ris, intermittent claudication of the leg.
a. decu'bitus, a. pectoris decubitus.
a. diphtherit'ica, diphtheria involving the pharynx or larynx.
a. of effort, a. pectoris precipitated by physical exertion.
a. epiglottid'ea, inflammation of epiglottis.
false a., a. pectoris vasomotoria.
Heberden's a., a. pectoris.
hypercyanotic a., anginal pain in cyanotic patients with congenital heart disease or chronic pulmonary disease, the pain developing with intensification of the cyanosis during activity.
intestinal a., abdominal a.
a. inver'sa, Prinzmetal's a.
Ludwig's a., cellulitis, usually of odontogenic origin, involving the submandibular, sublingual, and submental spaces, resulting in painful swelling of the floor of the mouth, elevation of the tongue, dysphasia, dysphonia, and (at times) compromise of the airway.
lymphatic a., monocytic a.; an affection resembling Vincent's disease marked by an increase in the number of lymphocytes in the blood.
a. lymphomato'sa, agranulocytosis.
monocytic a., lymphatic a.
necrotic a., a form occurring usually as a complication of scarlet fever and more rarely of diphtheria, in which gangrenous patches are found in the mucous membrane of the air passages.
neutropenic a., agranulocytosis.
a. no'tha, a. pectoris vasomotoria.
a. pec'toris, breast pang; heart stroke (2); stenocardia; Heberden's a.; Rougnon-Heberden disease; severe constricting pain in the chest, often radiating from the precordium to the left shoulder and down the arm, due to ischemia of the heart muscle usually caused by coronary disease.
a. pec'toris decu'bitus, a. decubitus; anginal pain developing while the subject is recumbent.
a. pec'toris si'ne do'lore, Gairdner's *disease*.
a. pec'toris vasomoto'ria, reflex a.; vasomotor a.; a. notha; a. spuria; false a. pseudoangina; a. vasomotoria; a. pectoris in which the breast pain is comparatively slight, but pallor followed by cyanosis, and coldness and numbness of the extremities are marked.
Prinzmetal's a., a. inversa; variant a. pectoris; a form of a. pectoris, characterized by pain that is not precipitated by cardiac work, is of longer duration, is usually more severe, and is associated with unusual electrocardiographic manifestations including elevated ST segments in leads that are ordinarily depressed in typical a.
reflex a., a. pectoris vasomotoria.
a. scarlatino'sa, sore throat of scarlet fever.
a. si'ne do'lore, symptoms of coronary insufficiency occurring without pain.
a. spu'ria, a. pectoris vasomotoria.
unstable a., a. pectoris characterized by pain in the chest of coronary origin occurring in response to less exercise or other stimuli than ordinarily required to produce a.
variant a. pectoris, Prinzmetal's a.
vasomotor a.; a. vasomotor'ia, a. pectoris vasomotoria.
Vincent's a., an ulcerative infection of the tonsils and pharynx caused by fusiform and spirochetal organisms; it is usually associated with necrotizing ulcerative gingivitis and may cause suffocative attacks.
walk-through a., a circumstance in which continuing activity, such as walking, does not increase or prolong the pain of angina pectoris but brings about pain relief.

anginal (an'ji-năl, an-jī'). Relating to angina in any sense.

anginiform (an-jin'i-fōrm). Resembling angina.

anginoid (an'jin-oid). Resembling an angina, especially angina pectoris.

anginophobia (an'ji-nō-fō'bē-ă) [angina + G. *phobos*, fear]. Extreme fear of an attack of angina pectoris.

anginose, anginous (an'ji-nōs, -ji-nŭs). Relating to any angina.

angio-, angi- [G. *angeion*, vessel]. Combining forms relating to blood or lymph vessels.

angioarchitecture (an'jē-ō-ar'ki-tek-chūr). **1.** The arrangement and distribution of the blood vessels of any organ. **2.** The vascular framework of an organ or tissue.

angioblast (an'jē-ō-blast) [angio- + G. *blastos*, germ]. **1.** Vasoformative cell; a cell taking part in blood vessel formation. **2.** Primordial mesenchymal tissue from which embryonic blood cells and vascular endothelium are differentiated.

angioblastoma (an'jē-ō-blas-tō'mă). Hemangioblastoma.

angiocardiography (an'jē-ō-kar-dē-og'ră-fē) [angio- + G. *kardia*, heart, + *graphō*, to write]. Cardioangiography; x-ray imaging of the heart and great vessels made visible by injection of a radiopaque solution.
rapid biplane a., synchronous a. in two planes at right angles to each other.

angiocardiokinetic, angiocardiocinetic (an'jē-ō-kar'dē-ō-ki-net'ik, -dē-ō-si-net'ik) [angio- + G. *kardia*, heart, + *kinēsis*, movement]. Causing dilation or contraction in the heart and blood vessels.

angiocardiopathy (an'jē-ō-kar-dē-op'ă-thē) [angio- + G. *kardia*, heart, + *pathos*, disease]. Disease affecting both heart and blood vessels.

angiocarditis (an'jē-ō-kar-dī'tis) [angio- + G. *kardia*, heart, + *-itis*, inflammation]. Inflammation of the heart and blood vessels.

angiocholecystitis (an'jē-ō-kō'lē-sis-tī'tis) [angio- + G. *cholē*, bile, + *kystis*, bladder, + *-itis*, inflammation] Inflammation of the bile vessels and gallbladder.

angiocholitis (an'jē-ō-kō-lī'tis). Cholangitis.

angiocyst (an'jē-ō-sist). A small vesicular aggregation of embryonic mesodermal cells that may give rise to vascular endothelium and blood cells.

angiodermatitis (an′jē-ō-der-mă-tī′tis) [angio- + G. *derma*, skin, + *-itis*, inflammation]. Inflammation of the cutaneous blood vessels.

angiodiascopy (an′jē-ō-dī-as′kō-pē) [angio- + G. *dia*, through, + *skopeō*, to view]. Examination of the vessels in a part by transillumination.

angiodynia (an-jē-ō-din′ē-ă) [angio- + G. *odynē*, pain]. Angialgia.

angiodysplasia (an′jē-ō-dis-plā′zē-ă). Degenerative dilation of the normal vasculature.

angiodystrophy, angiodystrophia (an′jē-ō-dis′trō-fē, -dis-trō′fē-ă) [angio- + G. *dys-*, bad, + *trophē*, nourishment]. Defective formation or growth associated with marked vascular changes.

angioedema (an′jē-ō-ĕ-dē′mă). Angioneurotic *edema*.

angioelephantiasis (an′jē-ō-el′ĕ-fan-tī′ă-sis). Extensive increase in vascularity of the subcutaneous tissue, producing great thickening simulating large, diffuse angioma formation.

angioendotheliomatosis (an′jē-ō-en-dō-thē′lē-ō-mă-tō′sis). Proliferation of endothelial cells within blood vessels.

proliferating systematized a., a rare generalized cutaneous and visceral intracapillary proliferation of endothelial cells, with vascular thrombosis and obstruction. The condition has been divided into a benign reactive type and a rapidly fatal neoplastic type; however, some of the latter cases have been shown to be intravascular large-cell lymphomas.

angiofibrolipoma (an′jē-ō-fī′brō-li-pō′mă). A neoplasm composed of fibrocytes, capillaries, and adipose tissue.

angiofibroma (an′jē-ō-fī-brō′mă). Telangiectatic *fibroma*.

juvenile a., juvenile hemangiofibroma; a markedly vascular fibrous tumor occurring in the nasopharynx of males, usually in the second decade of life; epistaxis and local invasion may result, but spontaneous regression may occur after sexual maturity.

angiofibrosis (an′jē-ō-fī-brō′sis). Fibrosis of the walls of blood vessels.

angiogenesis (an′jē-ō-jen′ĕ-sis) [angio- + G. *genesis*, production]. Development of blood vessels.

angiogenic (an′jē-ō-jen′ik). **1.** Relating to angiogenesis. **2.** Of vascular origin.

angioglioma (an′jē-ō-glī-ō′mă). A mixed glioma and angioma.

angiogliomatosis (an′jē-ō-glī′ō-mă-tō′sis). Occurrence of multiple areas of proliferating capillaries and neuroglia.

angiogliosis (an′jē-ō-glī-ō′sis). Glial scarring about a blood vessel.

angiogram (an′jē-ō-gram) [angio- + G. *gramma*, a writing]. Radiograph obtained in angiography.

angiographic (an-jē-ō-graf′ik). Relating to or utilizing angiography.

angiography (an-jē-og′ră-fē) [angio- + G. *graphō*, to write]. Radiography of vessels after the injection of a radiopaque material.

cerebral a., cerebral arteriography; radiographic visualization of the blood vessels supplying the brain, including their extracranial portions; the injection of contrast media may be made by percutaneous puncture in **closed a.** or in **open a.** after exposure of the aortic arch, brachial artery by catheterization or retrograde injection, carotid artery, femoral artery with catheterization and serial selective visualization of carotid and vertebral systems, subclavian artery, and vertebral artery.

digital subtraction a., computer-assisted roentgenographic a. permitting visualization of the cardiovascular system without superimposed bone and soft tissue density; images made before and after intravenous injection allow subtraction (separation and removal) of images not delineated by the contrast medium.

fluorescein a., photographic visualization of the passage of fluorescein through intraocular vessels after intravenous injection.

radionuclide a., the display, by means of a stationary scintillation camera device, of the passage of a bolus of a rapidly injected radiopharmaceutical.

selective a., a. in which visualization is improved by concentrating the contrast medium in the region to be studied; with the aid of a pressure apparatus the medium is injected through a catheter into the area for study.

spinal a., spinal arteriography; radiographic visualization of the spinal cord vessels by controlled injection of a contrast medium into the aorta at the site of origin of appropriate vessels, performed by artery catheterization.

therapeutic a., use of diagnostic angiographic methods which have been improved or modified to serve as therapeutic measures; *e.g.*, for reduced or increased regional blood flow, vascular delivery of medicinal agents.

angiohemophilia (an′jē-ō-hē-mō-fil′ē-ă). von Willebrand's *disease*.

angiohyalinosis (an′jē-ō-hī′ă-li-nō′sis) [angio- + G. *hyalos*, glass, + *-osis*, condition]. Hyaline degeneration of the walls of the blood vessels.

angiohypertonia (an′jē-ō-hī-per-tō′nē-ă) [angio- + G. *hyper*, over, + *tonos*, tension]. Vasospasm.

angiohypotonia (an′jē-ō-hī-pō-tō′nē-ă) [angio- + G. *hypo*, under, + *tonos*, tension]. Vasoparalysis.

angioid (an′jē-oyd) [angio- + G. *eidos*, resemblance]. Resembling blood vessels.

angioinvasive (an′jē-ō-in-vā′siv). Denoting a neoplasm or other pathologic condition capable of entering the vascular bed.

angiokeratoma (an′jē-ō-ker-ă-tō′mă) [angio- + G. *keras*, horn, + *-ōma*, tumor]. Telangiectatic wart; telangiectasia verrucosa; keratoangioma; a superficial intradermal capillary hemangioma, over which there is a wartlike hyperkeratosis and acanthosis.

a. corpo′ris diffu′sum, Fabry's *disease*.

Fordyce's a., asymptomatic vascular papules of the scrotum, appearing in late adolescence; much less common in the vulva.

Mibelli's a.'s, telangiectatic small papules of the dorsa of the hands and feet, as well as on the elbows and knees, that enlarge to over 0.05 cm; familial incidence.

angiokeratosis (an′jē-ō-ker-ă-tō′sis). The occurrence of multiple angiokeratomas.

angiokinesis (an′jē-ō-ki-nē′sis) [angio- + G. *kinēsis*, movement]. Vasomotion.

angiokinetic (an′jē-ō-ki-net′ik). Vasomotor.

angioleiomyoma (an′jē-ō-lī′ō-mī-ō′mă). Vascular *leiomyoma*.

angiolipofibroma (an′jē-ō-lip′ō-fī-brō′mă). Angiofibrolipoma.

angiolipoma (an′jē-ō-li-pō′mă). Angiolipofibroma; lipoma cavernosum; telangiectatic lipoma; a lipoma that contains an unusually large number, or foci of proliferated, neoplastic-like, frequently dilated vascular channels.

angiolith (an′jē-ō-lith) [angio- + G. *lithos*, stone]. An arteriolith or a phlebolith.

angiolithic (an′jē-ō-lith′ik). Relating to an angiolith.

angiologia (an′jē-ō-lō′jē-ă) [angio- + G. *logos*, treatise, discourse] [NA]. Angiology.

angiology (an-jē-ol′ō-jē) [angio- + G. *logos*, treatise, discourse]. The science concerned with the blood vessels and lymphatics in all their relations.

angiolupoid (an′jē-ō-lū′poyd) [angio- + L. *lupus*, wolf, + G. *eidos*, resemblance]. A sarcoid-like eruption of the skin in which the granulomatous telangiectatic papules are distributed over the nose and cheeks.

angiolysis (an-jē-ol′i-sis) [angio- + G. *lysis*, destruction]. Obliteration of a blood vessel, such as occurs in the newborn infant after tying of the umbilical cord.

angioma (an-jē-ō'mă) [angio- + G. *-ōma,* tumor]. A swelling or tumor due to proliferation, with or without dilation, of the blood vessels (hemangioma) or lymphatics (lymphangioma).
capillary a., *nevus* vascularis.
cavernous a., cavernous *hemangioma.*
cherry a., senile *hemangioma.*
encephalic a., a collection of dilated arteries in the brain.
a. lymphat'icum, lymphangioma.
petechial a.'s, multiple lesions resembling petechiae but due to dilation of capillary walls; they are obliterated by pressure.
a. serpigino'sum, essential telangiectasia (2); the presence of rings of red dots on the skin, which tend to widen peripherally, due to proliferation, with subsequent atrophy, of the superficial capillaries.
spider a., arterial *spider.*
superficial a., *nevus* vascularis.
telangiectatic a., a. composed of dilated vessels.
a. veno'sum racemo'sum, tortuous swelling caused by varicosities of superficial veins.

angiomatoid (an-jē-ō'mă-toyd). Resembling a tumor of vascular origin.

angiomatosis (an'jē-ō-mă-tō'sis). A condition characterized by multiple angiomas.
cephalotrigeminal a., Sturge-Weber *syndrome.*
congenital dysplastic a., congenital dysplastic angiopathy; a. in which there is dysplasia of the underlying tissues, sometimes with overgrowth of bone (Klippel-Trenaunay-Weber syndrome), or encephalotrigeminal a. (Sturge-Weber syndrome) in which there is an angioma in the distribution of one or more branches of the trigeminal nerve, with vascular anomalies and calcification of the cerebral cortex.
cutaneomeningospinal a., Cobb *syndrome.*
encephalotrigeminal a., Sturge-Weber *syndrome.*
oculoencephalic a., an incomplete form of Sturge-Weber syndrome, consisting of angiomas only of the choroid and meninges.
retinocerebral a., Lindau's *disease.*
telangiectatic a., disseminated capillary and venous vascular malformations of the cerebral hemispheres and leptomeninges, occurring in Sturge-Weber syndrome.

angiomatous (an-jē-ō'mă-tŭs). Relating to or resembling an angioma.

angiomegaly (an'jē-ō-meg'ă-lē) [angio- + G. *megas,* large]. Enlargement of blood vessels or lymphatics.

angiometer (an-jē-om'ĕ-ter) [angio- + G. *metron,* measure]. Instrument for measuring the diameter of a blood vessel.

angiomyocardiac (an'jē-ō-mī'ō-kar'dē-ak) [angio- + G. *mys,* muscle, + *kardia,* heart]. Relating to the blood vessels and the cardiac muscle.

angiomyofibroma (an'jē-ō-mī'ō-fī-brō'mă). Vascular *leiomyoma.*

angiomyolipoma (an'jē-ō-mī'ō-li-pō'mă) [angio- + G. *mys,* muscle, + *lipos,* fat, + *-oma,* tumor]. A benign neoplasm of adipose tissue (lipoma) in which muscle cells and vascular structures are fairly conspicuous; most commonly a renal tumor containing smooth muscle, often associated with tuberous sclerosis.

angiomyoma (an'jē-ō-mī-ō'mă) [angio- + G. *mys,* muscle, + *-ōma,* tumor]. Vascular *leiomyoma.*

angiomyoneuroma (an'jē-ō-mī'ō-nū-rō'mă). Glomus *tumor.*

angiomyopathy (an'jē-ō-mī-op'ă-thē) [angio- + G. *mys,* muscle, + *pathos,* suffering]. Any disease of blood vessels involving the muscular layer.

angiomyosarcoma (an'jē-ō-mī'ō-sar-kō'mă). A myosarcoma that has an unusually large number of proliferated, frequently dilated, vascular channels.

angiomyxoma (an'jē-ō-miks-ō'mă). A myxoma in which there is an unusually large number of vascular structures.

angioneuralgia (an'jē-ō-nū-ral'jē-ă). Obsolete term for an affection, marked by a burning pain in an extremity, accompanied by redness and edema of the affected area, thought to be an early stage of Raynaud's disease.

angioneurectomy (an'jē-ō-nū-rek'tō-mē) [angio- + G. *neuron,* nerve, + *ektomē,* excision]. Exsection of the vessels and nerves of a part. **1** [angio- + G. *neuron,* nerve, + *ektomē,* excision]. Exsection of the vessels and nerves of a part. **2** [G. *neuron,* cord]. Exsection of a segment of the spermatic cord to produce sterility.

angioneuredema (an'jē-ō-nūr-ĕ-dē'mă) [angio- + G. *neuron,* nerve, + *oidēma,* a swelling]. Obsolete term for angioneurotic edema.

angioneuromyoma (an'jē-ō-nū'rō-mī-ō'mă). Glomus *tumor.*

angioneurosis (an'jē-ō-nū-rō'sis). Vasoneurosis; a disorder due to disease or injury of the vasomotor nerves or center.

angioneurotic (an'jē-ō-nū-rot'ik). Relating to an angioneurosis.

angioneurotomy (an'jē-ō-nū-rot'ō-mē) [angio- + G. *neuron,* nerve, + *tomē,* a cutting]. Division of both nerves and vessels of a part.

angioparalysis (an'jē-ō-pă-ral'i-sis). Vasoparalysis.

angioparesis (an'jē-ō-pă-rē'sis, -par'ĕ-sis). Vasoparesis.

angiopathic (an'jē-ō-path'ik). Relating to angiopathy.

angiopathy (an-jē-op'ă-thē) [angio- + G. *pathos,* suffering]. Angiosis; any disease of the blood vessels or lymphatics.
cerebral amyloid a., a pathological condition of small cerebral vessels characterized by deposits of amyloid in the vessel walls which may lead to infarcts or hemorrhage.
congenital dysplastic a., congenital dysplastic *angiomatosis.*
congophilic a., a condition of blood vessels characterized by deposits in the vessel walls of a substance, usually amyloid, that take a Congo red stain.

angiophacomatosis, angiophakomatosis (an'jē-ō-fak'ō-mă-tō'sis). The angiomatous phacomatoses: Lindau's disease and the Sturge-Weber syndrome.

angioplany (an'jē-ō-plā-nē) [angio- + G. *planē,* a wandering]. Angiectopia.

angioplasty (an'jē-ō-plas-tē) [angio- + G. *plastos,* formed]. Reconstruction of a blood vessel.
percutaneous transluminal a., an operation for enlarging a narrowed arterial lumen by peripheral introduction of a balloon-tip catheter and dilating the lumen on withdrawal of the inflated catheter tip.

angiopoiesis (an'jē-ō-poy-ē'sis) [angio- + G. *poiesis,* making]. Vasifaction; vasoformation; formation of blood or lymphatic vessels.

angiopoietic (an'jē-ō-poy-et'ik). Vasifactive; vasofactive; vasoformative; relating to angiopoiesis.

angiopressure (an'jē-ō-presh-er). Pressure on a vessel for the arrest of bleeding.

angiorrhaphy (an-jē-ōr'ă-fē) [angio- + G. *rhaphē,* a seam]. Suture repair of any vessel, especially of a blood vessel.

angiorrhexis (an'jē-ō-rek'sis) [angio- + G. *rhēxis,* rupture]. Rupture of any vessel, especially of a blood vessel.

angiosarcoma (an'jē-ō-sar-kō'mă). A rare malignant neoplasm occurring most often in the breast and skin, and believed to originate from the endothelial cells of blood vessels; microscopically composed of closely packed round or spindle-shaped cells, some of which line small spaces resembling vascular clefts.

angioscope (an'jē-ō-skōp) [angio- + G. *skopeō,* to view]. A modified microscope for studying the capillary vessels.

angioscopy (an-jē-os'kō-pē) [angio- + G. *skopeō,* to view]. Visualization with a microscope of the passage of substances (*e.g.,* contrast media, radiopaque agents) through capillaries after intravenous injection.

angioscotoma (an'jē-ō-skō-tō'mă) [angio- + G. *skotōma,* dizziness, vertigo]. Cecocentral scotoma (2); ribbon-shaped defect of the visual fields caused by the retinal vessels overlying photoreceptors.

angioscotometry (an'jē-ō-skō-tom'ĕ-trē) The measurement or projection of the angioscotoma pattern.

angiosis (an-jē-ō'sis). Angiopathy.

angiospasm (an'jē-ō-spazm). Vasospasm.
labyrinthine a., Lermoyez' *syndrome.*

angiospastic (an'jē-ō-spas'tik). Vasospastic.

angiostaxis (an'jē-ō-stak'sis) [angio- + G. *staxis,* a trickling, fr. *stazō,* to drip]. Rarely used term for: **1.** An oozing of blood. **2.** Hemophilia.

angiostenosis (an'jē-ō-stĕ-nō'sis) [angio- + G. *stenōsis,* a narrowing]. Narrowing of one or more blood vessels.

angiostomy (an-jē-os'tō-mē) [angio- + G. *stoma,* mouth]. Operative opening into a blood vessel and insertion of a cannula.

angiostrongylosis (an'jē-ō-stron-ji-lō'sis). Eosinophilic meningitis; infection of animals and man with nematodes of the genus *Angiostrongylus.*

Angiostrongylus (an'jē-ō-stron'jĭ-lŭs) [G. *angeion,* vessel, + *strongylos,* round]. A genus of metastrongyle nematodes parasitic in respiratory or circulatory systems of rodents, carnivores, and marsupials.
A. cantonen'sis, lungworm of rodents, a species transmitted by infected mollusks ingested by rodents; larvae develop in the brain and migrate to lungs, where the adult worms are found; thought to cause eosinophilic encephalomeningitis in man in the Pacific basin; larvae have been removed from cerebrospinal fluid and the anterior chamber of the eye from persons in Thailand who had eaten raw snails.
A. costaricen'sis, *Morerastrongylus costaricensis;* a nematode parasite of rats and other rodents in Central America, recently found to infect humans, where they localize in the mesenteric arteries; infective third-stage larvae have been found in the slug, *Vaginulus plebeius.*
A. malaysien'sis, species of *A.* found in Malaysia, a common rodent parasite similar to *A. cantonensis* and an actual or potential agent of eosinophilic meningitis in that region.
A. vaso'rum, *Haemostrongylos vasorum;* a species occurring in the pulmonary artery and, rarely, in the right ventricle of the dog and fox; thrombi may occur in the lungs, and hypertrophy of the heart and liver may result in ascites; affected animals suffer from dyspnea and occasionally may die from cardiac insufficiency.

angiostrophy (an-jē-os'trō-fē) [angio- + G. *strophē,* a twist]. Twisting the cut end of a blood vessel to arrest bleeding.

angiotelectasis, angiotelectasia (an'jē-ō-tē-lek'tă-sis, -tel'ek-tā'sē-ă) [angio- + G. *telos,* end, + *ektasis,* a stretching out]. Dilation of the terminal arterioles, venules, or capillaries.

angiotensin (an-jē-ō-ten'sin). A family of peptides of known and similar sequence, with vasoconstrictive activity, produced by enzymatic action of renin upon angiotensinogen. See a. I; a. II.

angiotensin I. A decapeptide of slightly variable sequence, depending on the animal source, formed from the tetradecapeptide angiotensinogen by the removal of four amino acid residues, a reaction catalyzed by renin; a peptidase cleaves two more residues to yield a. II, the physiologically active form.

angiotensin II. An octapeptide formed by the removal of two amino acid residues from a. I; a potent vasopressor agent and the most powerful stimulus for production and release of aldosterone from the adrenal gland.

angiotensin III. A heptapeptide derivative of a. II that has similar effects except for a relatively weaker effect on the adrenal cortex.

angiotensin amide. A synthetic substance closely related to the naturally occurring a. II; a potent vasopressor agent useful in the management of certain types of shock and circulatory collapse.

angiotensinase (an-jē-ō-ten'sin-ās) [EC 3.4.99.3]. Former name for the enzyme responsible for converting angiotensin I to II; now applied to the enzyme that degrades angiotensin II.

angiotensinogen (an'jē-ō-ten-sin'ō-jen). A tetradecapeptide formed by the liver (formerly considered to be a circulating α_2-globulin) that is converted by renin to angiotensin I.

angiotensinogenase (an'jē-ō-ten-sin'ō-jen-ās). Renin.

angiotensin precursor. Angiotensinogen.

angiotomy (an-jē-ot'ō-mē) [angio- + G. *tomē,* cutting]. Sectioning of a blood vessel, or the creation of an opening into a vessel prior to its repair.

angiotonia (an'jē-ō-tō'nē-ă). Vasotonia.

angiotonic (an'jē-ō-ton'ik). Vasotonic (1).

angiotribe (an'jē-ō-trīb) [angio- + G. *tribō,* to bruise]. Vasotribe; a crushing instrument, in the shape of strong forceps with screw attachment, used to crush the end of a blood vessel, together with the tissue in which it is embedded, to arrest hemorrhage.

angiotripsy (an'-jē-ō-trip'sē) [angio- + G. *tripsis,* friction, bruising]. Vasotripsy; the use of the angiotribe to arrest hemorrhage.

angiotrophic (an'jē-ō-trof'ik) [angio- + G. *trophē,* nourishment]. Rarely used term for vasotrophic.

angitis (an-jī'tis). Angiitis.

Angle, Edward Hartley, U.S. orthodontist, 1855–1930. See A.'s *classification of malocclusion.*

ANGLE

angle (ang'gl) [L. *angulus*]. The meeting point of two lines or planes; the figure formed by the junction of two lines or planes; the space bounded on two sides by lines or planes that meet. See also angulus. For a.'s not listed below, see the descriptive term; *e.g.,* axioincisal, distobuccal, labiogingival, linguogingival (2), mesiogingival, proximobuccal, etc.

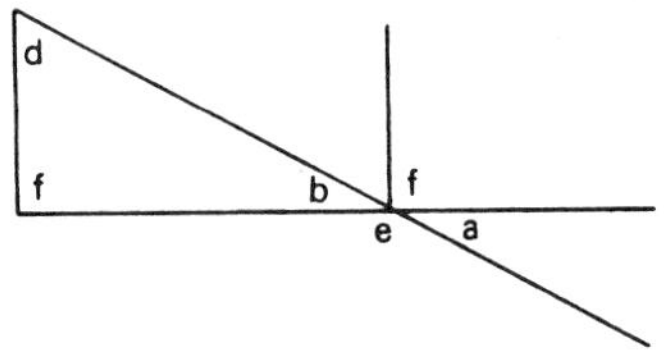

Geometric Angles
a, Acute angle; *b,* adjacent angle; *d,* oblique angle; *e,* obtuse angle; *f, f,* right angles.

acromial a., *angulus* acromialis.
acute a., any a. less than 90°.
adjacent a., an a. with a line in common with another a.
alpha a., **(1)** the a. between the visual and optic axes as they cross at the nodal point of the eye; **(2)** the a. between the visual line and the major axis of the corneal ellipse.
alveolar a., the a. between the horizontal plane and a line connecting the base of the nasal spine and the middle point of the projection of the alveolus of the maxilla.
a. of anomaly (abnormality), a. of deviation (3); a. of squint; in strabismus, the degree of deviation from parallelism in an eye.
a. of anteversion, a. of declination.
a. of aperture, the a. formed by lines drawn from the ends of the

diameter of a lens to its point of focus. See also angular *aperture.*
apical a., refracting a. of a prism; the a. between two plane surfaces of a prism.
axial a., an a. formed by two surfaces of a body, the line of union of which is parallel with its axis; the axial a.'s of a tooth are the distobuccal, distolabial, distolingual, mesiobuccal, mesiolabial, and mesiolingual.
basilar a., an a. formed by the intersection at the basion of lines coming from the nasal spine and the nasal point.
Bennett a., the a. formed by the sagittal plane and the path of the advancing condyle during lateral mandibular movement as viewed in the horizontal plane.
beta a., the a. formed by a line connecting the bregma and hormion meeting the radius fixus.
biorbital a., an a. formed by the meeting of the axes of the orbits.
Broca's a.'s, **(1)** Broca's basilar a.; **(2)** Broca's facial a.; **(3)** *angulus* occipitalis ossis parietalis.
Broca's basilar a., Broca's a. (1); the a. formed at the basion of lines drawn from the nasion and the alveolar point.
Broca's facial a., Broca's a. (2); the a. formed by the intersection at the biauricular axis of lines drawn from the supraorbital point and the alveolar point.
buccal a.'s, a.'s formed by the buccal surface of a tooth joining the other surfaces.
bucco-occlusal a., the line of junction of the buccal and occlusal surfaces of a tooth.
cardiohepatic a., cardiohepatic triangle; the a. formed by the upper border of the liver and the right border of the heart, especially as defined by percussion.
carrying a., the a. made by the arm and the forearm, with the elbow in full extension.
cavity line a., in dentistry, the a. formed by two walls of a cavity, *e.g.,* a tooth cavity, meeting along a line.
cavosurface a., the a. formed by the junction of a cavity wall and the surface of the tooth.
cephalic a., one of several a.'s formed by the intersection of two lines passing through certain points of the face or cranium.
cephalomedullary a., the a. made by the junction of the cerebrum and the brain stem.
cerebellopontile a., cerebellopontine a.
cerebellopontine a., cerebellopontile a.; pontine a.; the recess at the junction of the cerebellum, pons, and medulla.
a. of convergence, see under convergence.
costal a., *angulus* costae.
craniofacial a., the a. formed by the basifacial and basicranial axes at the midpoint of the sphenoethmoidal suture.
critical a., limiting a.; the a. of incidence of a ray of light in passing between two media changes from refraction to total reflection.
cusp a., **(1)** the a. made by the slopes of a cusp with the plane which passes through the tip of the cusp and which is perpendicular to a line bisecting the cusp, measured mesiodistally or buccolingually; **(2)** the a. made by the slopes of a cusp with a perpendicular line bisecting the cusp, measured mesiodistally or buccolingually; **(3)** one-half of the included a. between the buccal and lingual or mesial and distal cusp inclines.
Daubenton's a., occipital a. (2); an a. formed by the junction, at the opisthion, of lines coming from the basion and from the projection in the median plane of the lower border of the orbits. See also Daubenton's *line,* Daubenton's *plane.*
a. of declination, a. of anteversion; the a. formed by a line drawn through the center of the long axis of the neck of the femur meeting a line drawn in the transverse axis of the condyles, when the bone is viewed from above, looking straight down through the head of the femur; used to illustrate the normal degree of anteversion about 12° of the neck of the femur, which may be increased or decreased in some diseases.

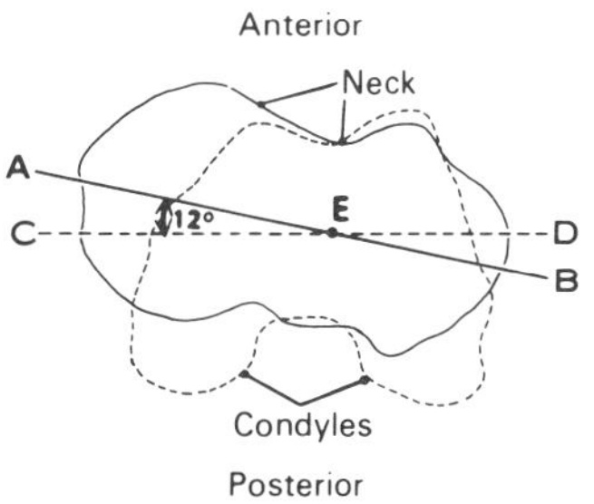

Angle of Declination of Femur

Superior view of right femur, showing angle of declination (*AEC*), with proximal end (*continuous line*) projected over distal end (*interrupted line*); *AB*, long axis of neck; *CD*, transverse axis of condyles.

a. of depression, a. of inclination.
a. of deviation, **(1)** in a prism, the sum of the a.'s of incidence and emergence minus the apical a. of a prism; **(2)** in optics, a. of refraction; **(3)** in strabismus, a. of anomaly.
disparity a., the difference in position of images on the retina, still permitting fusion.
duodenojejunal a., *flexura* duodenojejunalis.
a. of eccentricity, in strabismus, the a. between the line of fixation and the line of normal foveal fixation.
a. of emergence, the a. formed by a light ray emerging from the second surface of a prism and a line parallel to the incident ray.
epigastric a., the a. formed by the xiphoid process with the body of the sternum.
ethmoid a., the a. made by the plane of the cribriform plate of the ethmoid bone extended to meet the basicranial axis.
facial a., **(1)** any of several variously named and variously defined anatomical a.'s that have been used to quantify facial protrusion; **(2)** in dentistry, the a. formed by the intersection of the Frankfort plane with the nasion-pogonion line (inner lower a.), which establishes the anteroposterior relation of the mandible to the upper face at the Frankfort plane.
filtration a., *angulus* iridocornealis.
Frankfort-mandibular incisor a., the a. of procumbency of the mandibular incisor to the Frankfort plane.
frontal a. of parietal, *angulus* frontalis ossis parietalis.
a. of Fuchs, a crevice between the ciliary and pupillary zones of the iris formed by atrophy of superficial layers of the iris in the pupillary zone.
gamma a., the a. formed between a line joining the fixation point to the center of the eye and the optic axis.
hypsiloid a., y-a.
impedance a., a term expressing the ratio of electric resistance to electric capacitance (ohms to microfarads) in the tissues of the body or any other substance.
a. of incidence, incident a.; **(1)** the a. that a ray entering a refracting medium makes with a line drawn perpendicular to the surface of this medium; **(2)** the a. that a ray striking a reflecting surface makes with a line perpendicular to this surface.
incident a., a. of incidence.
incisal guide a., the a. formed with the horizontal plane by drawing a line in the sagittal plane between incisal edges of the maxillary and mandibular central incisors when the teeth are in centric occlusion.
a. of inclination, a. of depression; the a. formed by the meeting of a line drawn through the shaft of the femur with one passing through the long axis of the femoral neck; normally it is about 127°.
inferior a. of scapula, *angulus* inferior scapulae.
infrasternal a., *angulus* infrasternalis.

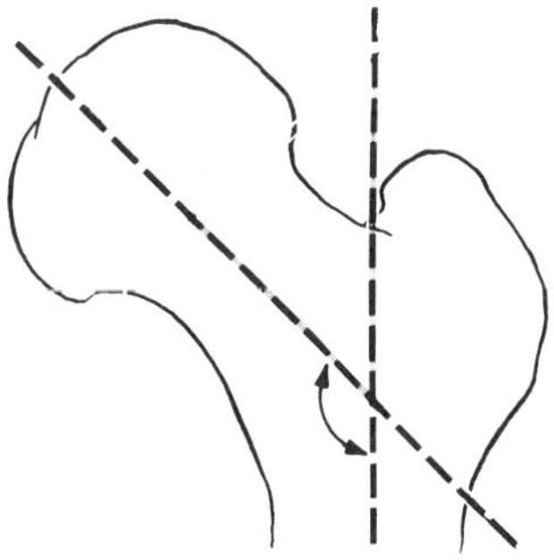

Angle of Inclination

iridocorneal a., *angulus* iridocornealis.
a. of iris, *angulus* iridocornealis.
Jacquart's facial a., a facial a. with the intersection always at the nasal spine point; additional variation uses the supraorbital point instead of the glabella, and this latter version is also known as ophryospinal facial a. or Topinard's facial a.
a. of jaw, *angulus* mandibulae.
kappa a., the a. between the pupillary axis and the visual axis; it is positive when the pupillary axis is nasal to the visual axis, and negative when the pupillary axis is temporal to the visual axis.
lateral a. of eye, *angulus* oculi lateralis.
lateral a. of scapula, *angulus* lateralis scapulae.
lateral a. of uterus, the upper part of the side of the uterus at the point of its junction with the uterine tube.
limiting a., critical a.
line a., in dentistry, the junction of two surfaces of the crown of a tooth, or of a tooth cavity (cavity line a.).
Louis' a., *angulus* sterni.
Lovibond's a., Lovibond's profile sign; the a. made at the meeting of the proximal nail fold and the nail plate when viewed from the radial aspect; normally, less than 180° but exceeding this in clubbing of the fingers.
Ludwig's a., *angulus* sterni.
lumbosacral a., the angle between the long axis of the lumbar part of the vertebral column and that of the sacrum.
a. of mandible, *angulus* mandibulae.
mastoid a. of parietal, *angulus* mastoideus ossis parietalis.
maxillary a., the a. formed by a line drawn from the ophryon and another from the point of the mandible and meeting at the contact between the upper and lower incisor teeth.
medial a. of eye, *angulus* oculi medialis.
mesial a., the a. formed by the meeting of the mesial with the labial (or buccal) or lingual surface of a tooth.
metafacial a., Serres' a.; the a. between the pterygoid processes and the base of the skull.
meter a., unit of ocular convergence; the amount of convergence required to view binocularly an object 1 meter distant and exerting 1 diopter of accommodation.
a. of mouth, *angulus* oris.
occipital a. of parietal, **(1)** *angulus* occipitalis ossis parietalis; **(2)** Daubenton's a.
olfactory a., the a. formed by the plane of the lamina cribrosa and the basicranial axis.
ophryospinal a., see Jacquart's facial a.
parietal a., Quatrefages' a.; an a. formed by the meeting of the prolongation of two lines tangential to the most prominent part of the zygomatic arch and to the parietofrontal suture on each side; when the lines remain parallel the a. is zero; when they diverge it is negative.
pelvivertebral a., the a. made by the pelvis with the general axis of the trunk or vertebral column.
phrenopericardial a., the a. made by the pericardium with the upper surface of the diaphragm.
Pirogoff's a., venous a. (1).
point a., the junction of three surfaces of the crown of a tooth, or of the walls of a cavity.
a. of polarization, the a. of incidence at which the reflected light is all polarized.
pontine a., cerebellopontine a.
pubic a., *angulus* subpubicus.
Q a., the a. formed when the resultant pull of the quadriceps muscle crosses the line of the patellar tendon.
Quatrefages' a., parietal a.
Ranke's a. [J. Ranke], the a. formed by the horizontal plane of the head and a line passing from the center of the margin of the alveolar arch of the maxilla, below the nasal spine to the center of the frontonasal suture.
a. of reflection, the a. that a ray reflected from a surface makes with a line drawn perpendicular to this surface; it is equal to the a. of incidence (2).
refracting a. of a prism, apical a.
a. of refraction, a. of deviation (2); the a. that a ray leaving a refracting medium makes with a line drawn perpendicular to the surface of this medium.
Rolando's a., the a. which the fissure of Rolando (central sulcus) makes with the midplane.
Serres' a., metafacial a.
S-N-A a. [sella-nasion-subspinale (or point *A*)], in cephalometrics, an a. measuring the anteroposterior relationship of the maxillary basal arch on the anterior cranial base; it shows the degree of maxillary prognathism. See also subspinale.
S-N-B a. [sella-nasion-supramentale (or point *B*)], an a. showing the anterior limit of the mandibular basal arch in relation to the anterior cranial base. See also supramentale.
sphenoid a., sphenoidal a., **(1)** a. formed by the intersection at the top of the sella turcica (dorsum sellae), of lines coming from the nasal point and from the tip of the rostrum of the sphenoid; **(2)** *angulus* sphenoidalis ossis parietalis.
a. of squint, a. of abnormality.
sternal a., *angulus* sterni.
sternoclavicular a., the a. formed by the junction of the clavicle with the sternum.
subpubic a., *angulus* subpubicus.
substernal a., *angulus* infrasternalis.
superior a. of scapula, *angulus* superior scapulae.
sylvian a., the a. formed by the sylvian line and a line perpendicular to the horizontal plane tangential to the highest point of the hemisphere.
tentorial a., the a. made by the plane of the tentorium and the basicranial axis.
Topinard's facial a., see Jacquart's facial a.
a. of torsion, the amount of rotation of a long bone along its axis or between two axes, measured in degrees.
venous a., **(1)** Pirogoff's a.; the junction of the internal jugular and subclavian veins, toward which converge the external and the anterior jugular and the vertebral veins, the thoracic duct in the left a. and the right lymphatic duct in the right a.; **(2)** in neuroradiology, the a. of union of the superior thalamostriate vein (vena terminalis) with the internal cerebral vein, usually closely behind the interventricular foramen of Monro.
Virchow's a., Virchow-Holder a.; an a. formed by the meeting of a line drawn from the middle of the nasofrontal suture to the base of the anterior nasal spine with a line drawn from this last point to the center of the external auditory meatus.
Virchow-Holder a., Virchow's a.
visual a., the a. formed at the retina by the meeting of lines drawn from the periphery of the object seen.
Vogt's a. [K. Vogt], a craniometric a. formed by the nasobasilar

and alveolonasal lines.

Weisbach's a., a craniometric a. formed by the junction, at the alveolar point, of lines passing from the basion and from the middle of the frontonasal suture.

Welcker's a., *angulus* sphenoidalis ossis parietalis.

y-a., hypsiloid a.; in craniometry, the a. at the inion formed by lines drawn from the hormion and the lambda.

---

angor (ang'gōr) [L. quinsy, anguish]. Rarely used term for extreme distress or mental anguish.

a. an'imi, a. pectoris (2); the sense of being in the act of dying, differing from the fear of death or the desire for death; a symptom that may occur with angina pectoris and occasionally in diseases of the medulla.

a. pec'toris, **(1)** Gairdner's *disease;* **(2)** a. animi.

angostura bark (an-gos-tū'ră). Cusparia bark; the bark of *Galipea officinalis;* formerly used as a bitter tonic and antipyretic.

Ångström, Anders J., Swedish physicist, 1814–1874. See angstrom; Å.'s *law, unit;* Å. *scale.*

angstrom (Å) (ang'strŏm) [A.J. Ångström]. A unit of wavelength, 10^{-10} m, roughly the diameter of an atom; equivalent to 0.1 nm.

Anguillula (ang-gwil'lū-lă) [Mod. L. dim. of L. *anguilla,* eel]. Old name for a genus of free-living nematodes. See *Turbatrix.*

angulation (ang'gū-lā'shŭn). Formation of an angle; an abnormal angle or bend in an organ.

angulus, gen. and pl. **anguli** (ang'gyū-lŭs, -lī) [L.] [NA]. An angle or corner. See angle.

a. acromia'lis [NA], acromial angle; the prominent angle at the junction of the posterior and lateral borders of the acromion.

a. cos'tae [NA], costal angle; the rather abrupt change in curvature of the body of a rib posteriorly, such that the neck and head of the rib are directed upward.

a. fronta'lis os'sis parieta'lis [NA], frontal angle of parietal; the anterior superior angle of the parietal bone.

a. infectio'sus, angular *stomatitis.*

a. infe'rior scap'ulae [NA], inferior angle of scapula; the acute angle formed by junction of the medial and lateral borders of the scapula.

a. infrasterna'lis [NA], infrasternal or substernal angle; the angle between the lower borders of the costal cartilages of the two sides as they approach the sternum.

a. ir'idis, a. iridocornealis.

a. iridocornea'lis [NA], a. iridis; angle of iris; iridocorneal or filtration angle; the acute angle between the iris and the cornea at the periphery of the anterior chamber of the eye.

a. latera'lis scap'ulae [NA], lateral angle of scapula; the blunt, concave head of the scapula forming the glenoid cavity at the junction of the superior and lateral borders of the bone.

a. mandib'ulae [NA], angle of mandible; angle of jaw; the angle formed by the lower margin of the body and the posterior margin of the ramus of the mandible.

a. mastoid'eus os'sis parieta'lis [NA], mastoid angle of parietal; the posteroinferior point of the parietal bone.

a. occipita'lis os'sis parieta'lis [NA], occipital angle of parietal (1); Broca's angle (3); the posterior superior angle of the parietal bone.

a. oc'uli latera'lis [NA], lateral angle of eye; a. oculi temporalis; lateral or external canthus; the angle formed by the junction of the lateral parts of the upper and lower eyelids.

a. oc'uli media'lis [NA], medial angle of eye; a. oculi nasalis; medial or internal canthus; the angle formed by the union of the upper and lower eyelids medially.

a. oc'uli nasa'lis, a. oculi medialis.

a. oc'uli temporalis, a. oculi lateralis.

a. o'ris [NA], angle of mouth; the lateral limit of the oral fissure.

a. sphenoida'lis os'sis parieta'lis [NA], sphenoid or sphenoidal angle (2); Welcker's angle; the anterior inferior angle of the parietal bone.

a. ster'ni [NA], sternal angle; Louis' or Ludwig's angle; the angle between the manubrium and the body of the sternum.

a. subpu'bicus [NA], subpubic or pubic a.; the a. formed by the inferior rami of the pubic bones.

a. supe'rior scap'ulae [NA], superior angle of scapula; formerly named the medial angle, it lies at the junction of the superior and medial borders of the bone.

anhalonidine (an-hă-lon'i-dēn). 1,2,3,4-Tetrahydro-6,7-dimethoxy-1-methyl-8-isoquinolinol; an alkaloid from *Lophophora williamsii.*

anhalonine (an-hal'ō-nēn). $C_{12}H_{15}NO_3$; an alkaloid from *Lophophora williamsii;* has been used in asthma and angina pectoris.

Anhalonium lewinii (an-hă-lō'nē-ŭm lū-win'ē-ī). *Lophophora williamsii.*

anhaphia (an-haf'ē-ă). Anaphia.

anhedonia (an-hē-dō'nē-ă) [G. *an-* priv. + *hedonē,* pleasure]. Absence of pleasure from the performance of acts that would ordinarily be pleasurable.

anhidrosis (an-hī-drō'sis) [G. *an-* priv. + *hidrōs,* sweat]. Anidrosis; adiaphoresis; ischidrosis; absence of sweating.

anhidrotic (an-hī-drot'ik). Anidrotic; adiaphoretic. **1.** Relating to, or characterized by, anhidrosis. **2.** An agent that reduces, prevents, or stops sweating. **3.** Denoting a reduction or absence of sweat glands, characteristic of congenital ectodermal defect and anhidrotic ectodermal dysplasia.

anhistic, anhistous (an-his'tik, -tŭs) [G. *an-* priv. + *histos,* web]. Without apparent structure.

anhydrase (an-hī'drās). An enzyme that catalyzes the removal of water from a compound; most such enzymes are now known as hydrases, hydro-lyases, or dehydratases.

carbonic a., *carbonate* dehydratase.

anhydration (an-hī-drā'shŭn). Dehydration (1).

anhydride (an-hī'drīd). An oxide that can combine with water to form an acid or that is derived from an acid by the abstraction of water.

anhydro- [G. *an*-priv., + *hydōr,* water]. Chemical prefix denoting the removal of water. *Cf.* pyro- (2).

anhydrogitalin (an-hī'drō-jit'ă-lin). Gitoxin.

anhydroleucovorin (an-hī'drō-lū-kō-vōr'in). 5,10-Methenyltetrahydrofolic acid; an intermediate formed in the folic acid-catalyzed glycine-serine interconversion.

anhydrosugars (an-hī'drō-shug-ărz). Dehydrosugars; sugars from which one or more molecules of water, other than water of crystallization, have been eliminated.

anhydrous (an-hī'drŭs). Containing no water, especially water of crystallization.

aniacinamidosis (ă-nī'ă-sin-am-i-dō'sis). Aniacinosis; deficiency of niacinamide which may be associated with pellagra.

aniacinosis (ă-nī'ă-sin-ō'sis). Aniacinamidosis.

anicteric (an-ik-ter'ik). Not icteric.

anidean (an-id'ē-an) [see anideus]. Anidous; shapeless; denoting a formless mass of tissue.

anideus (an-id'ē-ŭs) [G. *an-* priv. + *eidos,* shape]. Fetus anideus; a parasitic fetus consisting of a poorly differentiated mass of tissue with slight indications of parts.

embryonic a., a blastoderm without axial organization.

anidous (an-ī'dŭs). Anidean.

anidrosis (an-i-drō'sis). Anhidrosis.

anidrotic (an-i-drot'ik). Anhidrotic.

anile (ā'nīl, an'il) [L. *anilis,* fr. *anus,* an old woman]. In one's dotage.

anileridine (an-i-ler'i-dēn). Ethyl 1-(4-aminophenethyl)-4-phenylisonipecotate; related chemically and pharmacologically to meperidine hydrochloride; used for relief of moderate to severe pain; also mildly antihistaminic and spasmolytic; addiction liability is equivalent to that of morphine.

anilide (an'i-lid). An *N*-acyl aniline; *e.g.,* acetanilide.

anilinction, anilinctus (ā-ni-lingk'shŭn, -lingk'tŭs). Anilingus.

aniline (an'i-lin, -lēn) [Ar. *an-nil,* indigo]. Phenylamine; aminobenzene; benzeneamine; $C_6H_5(NH_2)$; an oily, colorless or brownish liquid, of aromatic odor and acrid taste, that is the parent substance of many synthetic dyes; formally derived from benzene by the substitution of the group $—NH_2$ for one of the hydrogen atoms.

aniline blue [C.I. 42755]. A mixture of sulfonated triphenylmethane dyes used widely as a connective tissue stain and counterstain.

anilingus (ā-ni-ling'gŭs) [L. *anus,* + *lingo,* to lick]. Analinction; anilinctus; sexual stimulation by licking or kissing the anus; a type of oral-genital sexual activity.

anilinism (an'il-in-izm). Anilism.

anilinophil, anilinophile (an-i-lin'ō-fil, -fīl) [aniline + G. *philos,* fond]. Anilinophilous; denoting a cell or histologic structure that stains readily with an aniline dye.

anilinophilous (an-i-li-nof'ĭ-lŭs). Anilinophil.

anilism (an'il-izm). Anilinism; chronic aniline poisoning characterized by gastric and cardiac weakness, vertigo, muscular depression, intermittent pulse, and cyanosis.

anility (ă-nil'i-tē) [L. *anilitas,* fr. *anus,* an old woman]. Dotage.

anima (an'i-mă) [L. breath, soul]. **1.** The soul or spirit. See animus (4). **2.** In jungian psychology, the inner self, in contrast to persona; a female archtype in a man. *Cf.* animus (5).

animal (an'i-măl) [L.]. **1.** A living, sentient organism that has membranous cell walls, requires oxygen and organic foods, and is capable of voluntary movement as distinguished from a plant or mineral. **2.** One of the lower a. organisms as distinguished from man.

cold-blooded a., poikilotherm.

control a., in research, an a. submitted to the same conditions as the others used for the experiment, but with the crucial factor (such as the injection of antitoxin, the administration of a drug, etc.) omitted. See also control; control *experiment.*

conventional a., an a. colonized by the burden of resident microorganisms normally associated with its particular species.

Houssay a., an a. that has been pancreatectomized and hypophysectomized. Named after the discoverer of the principle that a.'s are more sensitive to insulin after removal of the pituitary, and that after this operation the intensity of diabetes in depancreatized a.'s is diminished.

normal a., in research, an experimental a. that has neither suffered an attack of a particular disease nor received an injection of a specific microorganism or its toxin.

sentinel a., an a. deliberately placed in a particular environment to detect the presence of an infectious agent, such as a virus.

warm-blooded a., homeotherm.

animal black. Animal *charcoal.*

animalcule (an-i-mal'kyūl) [Mod. L. *animalculum,* dim. of L. *animal,* a living being]. **1.** Obsolete term for a microscopic animal organism or protozoan. **2.** Term used by believers in the preformation theory to designate the supposed miniature body contained in a gamete.

animation (an-i-mā'shŭn) [L. *animo,* pp. *-atus,* to make alive; *anima,* breath, soul]. **1.** The state of being alive. **2.** Liveliness; high spirits.

suspended a., a temporary state resembling death, with cessation of respiration; may also refer to certain forms of hibernation in animals or to endospore formation by some bacteria.

animatism (an'i-mă-tizm). Attribution of mental or spiritual qualities to both living beings and nonliving things. See also animism.

animism (an'i-mizm) [L. *anima,* soul]. The view that all things in nature, both animate and inanimate, contain a spirit or soul; held by primitive peoples and young children. See also animatism.

animus (an'i-mŭs) [L. *animus,* breath, rational soul in man, will]. **1.** An animating or energizing spirit. **2.** Intention to do something; disposition. **3.** In psychiatry, a spirit of active hostility or grudge. **4.** The ideal image toward which a person strives. **5.** In jungian psychology, a male archetype in a woman. *Cf.* anima (2).

anion (an'ī-on). An ion that carries a negative charge, going therefore to the positively charged anode; in salts, acid radicals are a.'s.

anion exchange. The process by which an anion in a mobile (liquid) phase exchanges with another anion previously bound to a solid, positively charged phase, the latter being an anion exchanger. It takes place when Cl^- is exchanged for OH^- in desalting. The reaction is Cl^- (in solution) + (OH^- on anion exchanger$^+$) → (Cl^- on anion exchanger) + OH^- (in solution); combined with cation exchange, NaCl is removed from solution. Anion exchange may also be used chromatographically, to separate anions, and medicinally, to remove an anion (*e.g.* Cl^-) from gastric contents or bile acids in the intestine.

anion exchanger. An insoluble solid, usually a polystyrene or a polysaccharide, with cation groups, (*e.g.,* $—NR_3^+$ or $—NR_2H^+$) which can attract and hold anions that pass by in a moving solution in exchange for anions previously held.

anionic (an-ī-on'ik). Referring to a negatively charged ion.

anionotropy (an'-ī-on-ot'rō-pē). The migration of a negative ion in tautomeric changes.

aniridia (an-i-rid'ē-ă) Absence of the iris; when congenital, a rudimentary iris root is usually present. *Cf.* irideremia.

anisakiasis (an'i-să-kī'ă-sis) [G. *anisos,* unequal, + *akis,* a point, + *-iasis,* condition]. Herring-worm disease; infection of the intestinal wall by larvae of *Anisakis marina* and other genera of anisakid nematodes (*Contracaecum, Phocanema*), characterized by intestinal eosinophilic granuloma and symptoms like those of peptic ulcer or tumor.

anisakid (an-i-să'kid). Common name for nematodes of the family Anisakidae.

Anisakidae (an-i-să'ki-dē). Family of large nematode worms (superfamily Heterocheilidae) found in the stomach and intestines of fish-eating birds and marine mammals, infection being acquired from marine fish; human cases of anisakiasis have been reported from Japan. See also *Anisakis.*

Anisakis (an-i-să'kis) [G. *anisos,* unequal, + *akis,* a point]. Genus of nematodes (family Anisakidae) that includes many common parasites of marine fish-eating birds and marine mammals.

anisate (an'ĭ-săt). A salt of anisic acid, usually possessing antiseptic properties.

anise (an'is). The fruit of *Pimpinellla anisum* (family Umbelliferae); an aromatic and carminative.

aniseikonia (an'ī-sī-kō'nē-ă) [G. *anisos,* unequal, + *eikōn,* an image]. An ocular condition in which the image of an object in one eye differs in size or shape from the image of the same object in the fellow eye.

anisic (an-is'ik). Relating to anise.

anisic acid (an-is'ik). 4-Methoxybenzoic acid; a crystalline volatile acid obtained from anise; its compounds are the antiseptic anisates.

anisindione (an'i-sin-dī'ōn). 2-*p*-Anisylindan-1,3-dione; an anticoagulant with pharmacologic actions similar to those of phenindone and bishydroxycoumarin.

aniso- [G. *anisos,* unequal]. Combining form meaning unequal or dissimilar.

anisoaccommodation (an-ī'sō-ă-kom-ō-dā'shŭn) [aniso- + L. *accommodare,* to adapt]. Variation between the two eyes in accommodation capacity.

anisochromasia (an-ī'sō-krō-mā'zē-ă) [aniso- + G. *chroma,* color]. The unequal distribution of hemoglobin in the red blood cells, such that the periphery is pigmented and the central region is virtually colorless, as observed in films of blood from persons with certain forms of anemia caused by deficiency of iron; normal red blood cells show mild a. because of their biconcave shape.

anisochromatic (an-ī'sō-krō-mat'ik). Not uniformly of one color.

anisocoria (an-ī-sō-kō'rē-ă) [aniso- + G. *korē,* pupil]. A condition in which the two pupils are not of equal size.

anisocytosis (an-ī'sō-sī-tō'sis) [aniso- + G. *kytos,* cell, + *-osis,* condition]. Considerable variation in the size of cells that are normally uniform, especially with reference to red blood cells.

anisodactylous (an-ī'sō-dak'ti-lŭs). Relating to anisodactyly.

anisodactyly (an-ī'sō-dak'ti-lē) [aniso- + G. *daktylon,* finger]. Unequal length in corresponding fingers.

anisogamy (an'-i-sog'ă-mē) [aniso- + G. *gamos,* marriage]. Fusion of two gametes unequal in size or form; fertilization as distinguished from isogamy or conjugation.

anisognathous (an-i-sog'nă-thŭs) [aniso- + G. *gnathos,* jaw]. Having jaws of unequal size, the upper being wider than the lower.

anisokaryosis (an-ī'sō-kar-ē-ō'sis) [aniso- + G. *karyon,* nut (nucleus), + *-osis,* condition]. Variation in size of nuclei, greater than the normal range for a tissue.

anisole (an'i-sōl). Methoxybenzene; $C_6H_5OCH_3$; obtained from anisic acid; used in perfumery.

anisomastia (an-i-sō-mas'tē-ă) [aniso- + G. *mastos,* breast]. Breasts of unequal size.

anisomelia (an-i-sō-mē'lē-ă) [aniso- + G. *melos,* limb]. A condition of inequality between two paired limbs.

anisometropia (an-ī'sō-me-trō'pē-ă) [aniso- + G. *metron,* measure, + *ōps,* sight]. A difference in the refractive power of the two eyes.

anisometropic (an-ī'sō-me-trop'ik). **1.** Relating to anisometropia. **2.** Having eyes of unequal refractive power.

anisophoria (an-ī-sō-fō'rē-ă) [aniso- + G. *phora,* a carrying]. Heterophoria in which the degree of phoria varies with the direction of gaze.

anisopiesis (an-ī-sō-pī-ē'sis) [aniso- + G. *piesis,* pressure]. Unequal arterial blood pressure on the two sides of the body.

anisorrhythmia (an-ī-sō-rith'mē-ă) [aniso- + G. *rhythmos,* rhythm]. Irregular action of the heart, or absence of synchronism in the rate of auricles and ventricles.

anisosphygmia (an-ī-sō-sfig'mē-ă) [aniso- + G. *sphygmos,* pulse]. Difference in volume, force, or time of the pulse in the corresponding arteries on two sides of the body, *e.g.,* the two radials, or femorals.

anisospore (an-ī'sō-spōr) [aniso- + G. *sporos,* seed]. A sexual cell capable of uniting with one of the opposite sex to form a new organism, as distinguished from the nonsexual cell, or isospore.

anisosthenic (an-ī-sos-then'ik) [aniso- + G. *sthenos,* strength]. Of unequal strength; denoting two muscles or groups of muscles that are either paired or are antagonists.

anisotonic (an-ī-sō-ton'ik) [aniso- + G. *tonus,* tension]. Not having equal tension; having unequal osmotic pressure.

anisotropic (an-ī-sō-trop'ik) [aniso- + G. *tropos,* a turning]. Not having properties that are the same in all directions.

anisotropine methylbromide (an'i-sō-trō'pēn). 8-Methyltropinium bromide 2-propylvalerate; an anticholinergic and intestinal antispasmodic.

Anitschkow, Nikolai, Russian pathologist, 1885–1964. See A. *cell, myocyte.*

ankle (ang'kl). **1.** *Articulatio* talocruralis. **2.** The region of the a. joint. **3.** Talus.

ankylo- [G. *ankylos,* bent, crooked; *ankylōsis,* stiffness or fixation of a joint]. Combining form meaning bent, crooked, stiff, or fixed. See also ancylo-.

ankyloblepharon (ang'ki-lō-blef'ă-ron) [ankylo- + G. *blepharon,* eyelid]. Blepharosynechia.

ankylocolpos (ang'ki-lō-kol'pos) [ankylo- + G. *kolpos,* womb (vagina)]. Vaginal *atresia.*

ankylodactyly, ankylodactylia (ang'ki-lō-dak'ti-lē, -dak-til'ē-ă) [ankylo- + G. *daktylos,* finger]. Adhesion between two or more fingers or toes. See also syndactyly.

ankyloglossia (ang'ki-lō-glos'ē-ă) [ankylo- + G. *glōssa,* tongue]. Tongue-tie.

ankylomele (ang'ki-lō-mē'lē) [ankylo- + G. *mēlē,* probe]. A curved or bent probe.

ankylopoietic (ang'ki-lō-poy-et'ik). Forming ankylosis.

ankyloproctia (ang'ki-lō-prok'shē-ă) [ankylo- + G. *prōktos,* anus]. Imperforation or stricture of the anus.

ankylosed (ang'ki-lōsd). Stiffened; bound by adhesions; denoting a joint in a state of ankylosis.

ankylosis (ang'ki-lō'sis) [G. *ankylōsis,* stiffening of a joint]. Stiffening or fixation of a joint as the result of a disease process, with fibrous or bony union across the joint.

artificial a., arthrodesis.

bony a., synostosis.

dental a., bony union of the radicular surface of a tooth to the surrounding alveolar bone in an area of previous partial root resorption.

extracapsular a., spurious a.; stiffness of a joint due to induration or heterotopic ossification of the surrounding tissues.

false a., fibrous a.

fibrous a., false a.; pseudankylosis; stiffening of a joint due to the presence of fibrous bands between and about the bones forming the joint.

intracapsular a., stiffness of a joint due to the presence of bony or fibrous adhesions between the articular surfaces of the joint.

spurious a., extracapsular a.

true a., synostosis.

Ankylostoma (ang-ki-los'tō-mă). *Ancylostoma.*

ankylostoma (ang-ki-los'tō-mă) [ankylo- + G. *stoma,* mouth]. Trismus.

ankylostomiasis (ang'ki-lō-stō-mī'ă-sis). Ancylostomiasis.

ankylotic (ang-ki-lot'ik). Characterized by or pertaining to ankylosis.

ankylurethria (ang-kil-yū-rē'thrē-ă) [ankylo- + G. *ourēthra,* urethra, + *-ia,* condition]. Obsolete term for imperforation or stricture of the urethra.

ankyroid (an'ki-royd). Ancyroid.

anlage, pl. **anlagen** (ahn'lah-ge, -gen) [Ger. hereditary factor]. **1.** Primordium. **2.** In psychoanalysis, genetic predisposition to a given trait or personality characteristic.

anneal (an-nēl') [A.S. *anaelan,* to burn]. **1.** To soften or temper a metal by controlled heating and cooling; the process makes a metal more easily adapted, bent, or swaged, and less brittle. **2.** In dentistry, to heat gold leaf preparatory to its insertion into a cavity, in order to remove adsorbed gases and other contaminants.

annectent (a-nek'tent) [L. *an-necto,* pres. p. *-nectnes,* pp. *-nexus,* to join to]. Connected with; joined.

Annelida (an'nĕ-lī'dă). A phylum that includes the segmented or true worms, such as the earthworm.

annelids (an'nĕ-lids). Common name for members of the phylum Annelida.

annellide (an'ĕ-līd) [Fr. *annelide,* fr. L. *anellus,* a ring]. A conidiogenous cell that produces conidia in succession, each leaving a ring-like collar on the cell wall when released.

annelloconidium (an'ĕ-lō-kō-nid'ē-um). A conidium produced by an annellide.

annexa (a-nek'să). Adnexa.

annexal (a-neks-ăl). Adnexal.

annexectomy (an-eks-ek'tō-mē). Adnexectomy.

annexitis (an-eks-ī'tis). Adnexitis.

annexopexy (an-eks'ō-pek-sē). Adnexopexy.

annotto (ă-not'ō). Coloring matter extracted from the seeds of *Bixa orellana;* contains bixin and several other yellow to orange-red pigments; used for coloring butter, margarine, cheese, and oils.

annular (an'yū-lăr) [L. *anulus,* ring]. Ring-shaped.

annuloplasty (an'yū-lō-plas-tē) [L. *anulus,* ring, + G. *plastos,* formed]. Reconstruction of an incompetent (usually mitral) cardiac valve.

annulorrhaphy (an-yū-lōr'ă-fē) [L. *anulus,* ring, + G. *raphē,* seam]. Closure of a hernial ring by suture.

annulus (an'yū-lŭs) [NA]. Anulus; ring; a ring-shaped or circular structure surrounding an opening or level area. See also entries under ring.

a. abdomina'lis, a. inguinalis profundus.

a. cilia'ris, orbiculus ciliaris.

a. conjuncti'vae [NA], anulus conjunctivae; conjunctival ring; a narrow ring at the junction of the periphery of the cornea with the conjunctiva.

a. femora'lis [NA], anulus femoralis; femoral ring; crural ring; the superior opening of the femoral canal, bounded anteriorly by the inguinal ligament, posteriorly by the pectineus muscle, medially by the lacunar ligament, and laterally by the femoral vein.

a. fibrocartilagin'eus [NA], anulus fibrocartilagineus; fibrocartilaginous ring; Gerlach's annular tendon; the thickened portion of the circumference of the tympanic membrane that is fixed in the tympanic sulcus.

a. fibro'sus [NA], anulus fibrosus; fibrous ring; **(1)** coronary tendon; Lower's ring; one of four fibrous rings that surround atrioventricular and arterial orifices of the heart; **(2)** the ring of fibrocartilage and fibrous tissue forming the circumference of the intervertebral disk.

a. of fibrous sheath, *pars* annularis vaginae fibrosae.

Haller's a., Haller's *insula.*

a. hemorrhoida'lis, *zona* hemorrhoidalis.

a. inguina'lis profun'dus [NA], anulus inguinalis profundis; deep inguinal ring; internal inguinal ring; a. abdominalis; abdominal ring; the opening in the transversalis fascia through which the ductus deferens (or round ligament in the female) and gonadal vessels enter the inguinal canal.

a. inguina'lis superficia'lis [NA], anulus inguinalis superficialis; superficial inguinal ring; subcutaneous ring; external inguinal ring; the slit-like opening in the aponeurosis of the external oblique muscle of the abdominal wall through which the spermatic cord (round ligament in the female) emerges from the inguinal canal.

a. ir'idis, ring of iris; either of two zones on the anterior surface of the iris, separated by a circular line concentric with the pupillary border; **a. iridis minor** [NA], the narrow inner zone of the iris; **a. iridis major** [NA], the outer, broader of the two zones of the iris.

a. lymphat'icus car'diae [NA], anulus lymphaticus cardiae; lymphatic ring of cardia; cardiac lymphatic ring; a group of lymph nodes surrounding the cardia of the stomach.

a. ova'lis, *limbus* fossae ovalis.

a. preputia'lis, preputial *ring.*

a. tendin'eus commu'nis [NA], anulus tendineus communis; common tendinous ring; Zinn's ligament, ring, or tendon; a fibrous ring that surrounds the optic canal and the medial part of the superior orbital fissure; it gives origin to the four rectus muscles of the eye and is partially fused with the sheath of the optic nerve.

a. tympan'icus [NA], anulus tympanicus; tympanic ring; tympanic bone; in the fetus, a more or less complete bony ring at the medial end of the cartilaginous external acoustic meatus, to which is attached the tympanic membrane.

a. umbilica'lis [NA], anulus umbilicalis; umbilical ring; canalis umbilicus; an opening in the linea alba through which pass the umbilical vessels in the fetus; in young embryos it is relatively nearer to the pubis, but gradually ascends to the center of the abdomen; it is closed in the adult, its site being indicated by the umbilicus or navel.

a. urethra'lis, *musculus* sphincter vesicae.

Vieussens' a., *limbus* fossae ovalis.

AnOC Abbreviation for anodal opening *contraction.*

anochlesia (an'ō-klē'zē-ă) [G. *an-* priv. + *ochlēsis,* disturbance]. **1.** Catalepsy. **2.** Quietude.

anochromasia (an'ō-krō-mā'zē-ă) [G. *anō,* upward, + *chrōma,* color]. **1.** Failure of cells or other elements of tissue to be colored in the usual manner when treated with a stain (or stains). **2.** Accumulation of hemoglobin in the peripheral zone of erythrocytes, thereby resulting in a pale, virtually colorless central portion.

anociassociation (ă-nō'sē-ă-sō-sē-ā'shŭn) [G. *a-,* priv. + L. *noceo,* to injure, + association]. Theory advanced by G. W. Crile that afferent stimuli, especially pain, contribute to the development of surgical shock, and, as a corollary, that nerve blocks protect against shock.

anococcygeal (a-nō-kok-sij'ē-ăl). Relating to both anus and coccyx.

anodal (an-ōd'ăl). Anodic; of, pertaining to, or emanating from an anode.

anode (an'ōd) [G. *anodos,* a way up, fr. *ana,* up, + *hodos,* a way]. Anelectrode; positive electrode; the positive pole of a galvanic battery or the electrode connected with it; an electrode toward which negatively charged ions (anions) migrate. *Cf.* cathode.

anodic (an-ōd'ik). Anodal.

anodontia (an-ō-don'shē-ă) [G. *an-* priv. + *odous,* tooth]. Agomphosis; agomphiasis; absence of the teeth.

partial a., hypodontia.

anodontism (an-ō-dont'izm). Congenital absence of tooth germ development.

anodyne (an'ō-dīn) [G. *an-* priv. + *odynē,* pain]. A compound less potent than an anesthetic or a narcotic but capable of relieving pain.

anoetic (an-ō-et'ik) [G. *anoēsia,* from *a-* priv. + *noos,* perception]. Lacking the power of comprehension, as in severe and profound levels of mental retardation.

anogenital (ā'nō-jen'ī-tăl). Relating in any way to both the anal and the genital regions.

anomalad (ă-nom'ă-lad) [see anomaly]. A malformation together with its subsequently derived structural changes.

anomaloscope (ă-nom'ă-lō-skōp) [G. *anōmalos,* irregular, + *skopeō,* to examine]. An instrument used to diagnose abnormalities of color perception in which one-half of a field of color is matched by mixing two other colors.

anomaly (ă-nom'ă-lē) [G. *anōmalia,* irregularity]. Deviation from the average or norm; anything structurally unusual or irregular or contrary to a general rule.

Alder's a., coarse azurophilic granulation of leukocytes, especcially granulocytes, which may be associated with gargoylism and Morquio's disease.

Aristotle's a., when a small object is held between the first and second fingers crossed in such a way that it touches or presses upon skin surfaces which ordinarily are not pressed upon simultaneously by a single object, it is perceived falsely as two.

Chédiak-Steinbrinck-Higashi a., Chédiak-Steinbrinck-Higashi *syndrome.*

developmental a., an a. established during intrauterine life; a congenital a.

Ebstein's a., Ebstein's disease; congenital downward displacement of the tricuspid valve into the right ventricle.

eugnathic a., eugnathia.

Freund's a., a narrowing of the upper aperture of the thorax by shortening of the first rib and its cartilage; formerly believed to predispose to tuberculosis because of defective expansion of the lung apex.

Hegglin's a., May-Hegglin a.; a disorder in which neutrophils and eosinophils contain basophilic structures known as Döhle or Amato bodies and in which there is faulty maturation of platelets, with thrombocytopenia.

May-Hegglin a., Hegglin's a.

morning glory a., congenital a. of the optic disk in which the nerve head is funnel-shaped, with a dot of white tissue at the end of the excavation, and is surrounded by an elevated pigmented annulus; the retinal vessels seen are multiple narrow bands at the edge of the disk.

Pelger-Huët nuclear a., congenital inhibition of lobulation of the nuclei of neutrophilic leukocytes; most cells present band or bilobulate appearance, and only an occasional cell has trilobed structure; it is not associated with disease, but may be confused with leukocyte "shift to left;" autosomal dominant inheritance.

Peters' a., anterior chamber cleavage *syndrome.*

Rieger's a., iridocorneal mesodermal *dysgenesis.*

Shone's a., coarctation of the aorta, subaortic stenosis, and stenosing ring of the left atrium found in association with a parachute mitral valve.

Uhl a., right ventricular myocardial aplasia, causing a dilated, thin-walled, and contracting right ventricle without murmurs; death results in early childhood.

anomer (an'ō-mer). One of two sugar molecules that are epimeric at the hemiacetal carbon atom (carbon-1 in aldoses, carbon-2 in ketoses); *e.g.,* α-D-glucose and β-D-glucose. *Cf.* epimer. See also sugars.

anomia (ă-nō'mē-ă) [G. *a-* priv. + *ōnoma,* name]. Nominal *aphasia.*

anomie (an'ō-mē) [Fr., fr. G. *anomia,* lawlessness]. **1.** Lawlessness; absence or weakening of social norms or values, with corresponding erosion of social cohesion. **2.** In psychiatry, absence or weakening of individual norms or values; characterized by anxiety, isolation, and personal disorientation.

anonychia, anonychosis (an-ō-nik'ē-ă, an-ō-nī-kō'sis) [G. *an-* priv. + *onyx* (*onych-*), nail]. Absence of the nails.

anonyma (ă-non'i-mă) [G. *an-* priv. + *onyma,* name]. Without name; a term formerly applied to the large vessels in the thorax, now called the truncus brachiocephalicus and the venae brachiocephalicae.

Anopheles (ă-nof'ĕ-lēz) [G. *anōphelēs,* useless, harmful, fr. *an-* priv. + *ōpheleō,* to be of use]. A genus of mosquitoes (family Culicidae, subfamily Anophelinae). The sporogenous cycle of the malarial parasite is passed in the body cavity of female mosquitoes of certain species of this genus; a few selected vectors (from among over 90 species) are listed below.

A. albima'nus, a species having white hind feet, a common carrier of the malaria parasite in the West Indies and Central America.

A. albitar'sus, a South American species that transmits malaria.

A. balabacen'sis, a vector species in Southeast Asia, Burma, and India.

A. culicifa'cies, a species that is a common malaria vector in India and Sri Lanka, China, and elsewhere in the Orient.

A. darling'i, a South American species, an important carrier of the malarial parasite.

A. fluviatil'is, a species that is an important vector in India and Pakistan.

A. freebor'ni, a species that is a vector in the western U.S. (although endemic cases are no longer present).

A. funes'tus, an important African species that transmits malaria.

A. gam'biae, an African species that is a most important vector of malaria.

A. labranch'iae, a species that is an important vector in southern Europe and the Mediterranean basin.

A. macula'tus, a species that is a vector in Malaysia and Indonesia.

A. maculipen'nis, the type species of this genus; its wings are marked by spots formed of collections of scales; one of the most widely spread species active in the dissemination of malaria (formerly an important vector in continental Europe).

A. min'imus, a species that is an important vector throughout the Orient.

A. pseudopunctipen'nis, a South American vector species.

A. quadrimacula'tus, a species that was formerly an important carrier of malaria in the southern United States.

A. stephen'si, a widespread species that is an important vector of malaria in Asia.

A. sundai'cus, a species that is an important vector in the Orient and Southeast Asia.

A. superpic'tus, a species that is an important vector in the Mediterranean region, Middle East, and southern Asia.

anophelicide (ă-nof'ĕ-li-sīd). An agent that destroys the *Anopheles* mosquito.

anophelifuge (ă-nof'ĕ-li-fūj). An agent that drives away or prevents the bite of *Anopheles* mosquitoes.

Anophelinae (an-of-ĕ-lī'nē). A subfamily of the mosquitoes (Culicidae) consisting of several genera, including *Anopheles.*

anopheline (ă-nof'ĕ-līn). Referring to the *Anopheles* mosquito.

Anophelini (ă-nof-ĕ-lī-nī) [G. *anōphelēs,* useless, troublesome]. The tribe of mosquitoes (family Culicidae) that includes the genus *Anopheles.*

anophelism (ă-nof'ĕ-lizm). The habitual presence in any region of *Anopheles* mosquitoes.

anophthalmia (an-of-thal'mē-ă) [G. *an-* priv. + *ophthalmos,* eye]. Congenital absence of all tissues of the eyes.

consecutive a., a. due to trophy or degeneration of optic vesicle.

primary a., failure of optic primordium to form.

secondary a., a. with abnormal development of the anterior part of the neural tube.

anoplasty (ā'nō-plas-tē) [L. *anus* + G. *plastos,* formed]. Plastic surgery of the anus.

Anoplocephala (an-op'lō-sef'ă-lă) [G. *anoplos,* unarmed, + *kephalē,* head]. A genus of large tapeworms (family Anoplocephalidae) with strong linear segmentation, numerous scattered testes, and eggs with a pyriform apparatus; they are parasitic in herbivores, with terrestrial mites serving as intermediate hosts.

A. perfolia'ta, *Taenia equina; Taenia quadrilobata;* a cosmopolitan species of the horse, donkey, mule, and zebra; cysticercoid larvae are found in arthropods.

Anoplura (an-ō-plū'ră) [G. *anoplos,* unarmed, + *oura,* tail]. The order of insects that includes the bloodsucking lice of mammals, with some 450 species arranged in 6 families, of which 4 contain species of medical or veterinary importance: *Haematopinus, Linognathus,* and *Solenopotes* of domestic mammals, and the human sucking lice *Pediculus humanus.*

anorchia (an-ōr'kē-ă). Anorchism.

anorchism (an-ōr'kizm) [G. *an-* priv. + *orchis,* testis]. Anorchia; congenital absence of the testes.

anorectal (ā'nō-rek'tăl). Relating to both anus and rectum.

anorectic, anoretic (an-ō-rek'tic, -ret'ik). Anorexic. **1.** Relating to, characteristic of, or suffering from anorexia, especially anorexia nervosa. **2.** An agent that causes anorexia.

anorexia (an-ō-rek'sē-ă) [G. fr. *an-* priv. + *orexis,* appetite]. Diminished appetite; aversion to food.
a. nervo'sa, a mental disorder manifested by extreme fear of becoming obese and an aversion to food, usually occurring in young women and often resulting in life-threatening weight loss, accompanied by a disturbance in body image.

anorexiant (an-ō-rek'sē-ănt). A drug, process, or event that leads to anorexia.

anorexic (an-ō-rek'sik). Anorectic.

anorexigenic (an'ō-rek-si-jen'ik). Promoting or causing anorexia.

anorgasmy, anorgasmia (an-ōr-gaz'mē, -gaz'mē-ă). Failure to experience an orgasm.

anorthography (an-ōr-thog'ră-fē) [G. *an-* priv. + *orthos,* straight, + *graphō,* to write]. Agraphia.

anoscope (ā'nō-skōp). A short speculum for examining the anal canal and lower rectum.
Bacon's a., an instrument resembling a rectal speculum, with a long slit on one side and an electric light opposite.

anosigmoidoscopy (ā'nō-sig-moy-dos'-kō-pē). Endoscopy of the anus, rectum and sigmoid colon.

anosmia an-oz'mē-ă) [G. *an-* priv. + *osmē,* sense of smell]. Olfactory anesthesia; smell blindness; loss of the sense of smell. It may be: **essential** or **true,** due to lesion of the olfactory nerve; **mechanical** or **respiratory,** due to obstruction of the nasal fossae; **reflex,** due to disease in some other part or organ; or **functional,** without any apparent causal lesion.

anosmic (an-oz'mik). Relating to anosmia.

anosodiaphoria (ă-nō'sō-dī-ă-fōr'ē-ă) [G. *a-* priv. + *nosos,* disease, + *diaphoria,* difference]. Indifference, real or assumed, regarding the presence of disease, specifically of paralysis.

anosognosia (ă-nō'sog-nō'sē-ă) [G. *a-* priv. + *nosos,* disease, + *gnōsis,* knowledge]. Ignorance, real or feigned, of the presence of disease, specifically of paralysis.

anosognosic (ă-nō-sog-nō'sik). Relating to anosognosia.

anospinal (ā'nō-spī'năl). Relating to the anus and the spinal cord.

anosteoplasia (an-os'tē-ō-plā'zē-ă) [G. *an-* priv. + *osteon,* bone, + *plassō,* to form]. Failure of bone formation.

anostosis (an-os-tō'sis) [G. *an-* priv. + *osteon,* bone]. Failure of ossification.

anotia (an-ō'shē-ă) [G. *an-* priv. + *ous,* ear]. Congenital absence of one or both ears.

anovesical (ā'nō-ves'i-kăl). Relating in any way to both anus and urinary bladder.

anovular (an-ov'yū-lăr). Anovulatory; absence of discharge of an ovum from the ovary during an ovarian cycle.

anovulation (an-ov-yū-lā'shŭn). Suspension or cessation of ovulation.

anovulatory (an-ov'yū-lă-tōr-ē). Anovular.

anoxemia (an-ok-sē'mē-ă) [G. *an-* priv. + oxygen + G. *haima,* blood]. Absence of oxygen in arterial blood; formerly often used to include moderate decrease in oxygen now properly distinguished as hypoxemia.

anoxia (an-ok'sē-ă) [G. *an-* priv. + oxygen]. Absence or almost complete absence of oxygen from inspired gases, arterial blood, or tissues; formerly often used to include moderate decrease in oxygen now properly distinguished as hypoxia.
anemic a., a term formerly considered synonymous with anemic hypoxia, but now reserved for extremely severe cases in which oxygen is almost completely lacking.
anoxic a., a term formerly considered synonymous with hypoxic hypoxia, but now reserved for extremely severe cases in which oxygen is almost completely lacking.
diffusion a., diffusion hypoxia severe enough to result in the absence of oxygen in alveolar gas.
histotoxic a., poisoning of the respiratory enzyme systems of the tissues, as in the inhibition of cytochrome oxidase by cyanides; owing to the inability of tissue cells to utilize oxygen, its tension in arterial and capillary blood is usually greater than normal.
a. neonator'um, any a. observed in newborn infants.
oxygen affinity a., a. due to inability of hemoglobin to release oxygen.
stagnant a., stagnant hypoxia severe enough to result in the absence of oxygen in tissues.

anoxic (an-ok'sik). Denoting or characteristic of anoxia.

Anrep, G.V., 20th century Lebanese physiologist in Britain. See A. *phenomenon.*

ansa, gen. and pl. **ansae** (an'să, -sē) [L. loop, handle] [NA]. Any anatomical structure in the form of a loop or an arc.
a. cervica'lis [NA], cervical loop; a loop in the cervical plexus consisting of fibers from the first three cervical nerves, some of which accompany the hypoglossal nerve for a short distance.
Haller's a., *ramus* communicans cum nervo glossopharyngeo (1).
Henle's a., nephronic *loop.*
a. hypoglos'si, former name for a. cervicalis.
lenticular a., a. lenticularis.
a. lenticula'ris [NA], lenticular a. or loop; the pallidal efferent fibers curving around the medial border of the internal capsule.
ansae nervo'rum spina'lium, loops of the spinal nerves, connecting ventral branches of the spinal nerves.
peduncular a., a. peduncularis.
a. peduncula'ris [NA], peduncular a. or loop; Reil's a.; a complex fiber bundle curving around the medial edge of the internal capsule and connecting the anterior part of the temporal lobe (temporal cortex), amygdala, and olfactory cortex with the mediodorsal nucleus of the thalamus; it enters the thalamus as a component of the inferior thalamic peduncle which also contains a major part of the fibers connecting the mediodorsal nucleus to the orbitofrontal cortex.
Reil's a., a. peduncularis.
a. sacra'lis, a nerve cord connecting the sympathetic nerve trunk and ganglion impar.
a. subcla'via [NA], subclavian loop; Vieussens' loop or a.; a nerve cord connecting the middle cervical and stellate sympathetic ganglia, forming a loop around the subclavian artery.
Vieussens' a., a. subclavia.

ansate (an'sāt). Ansiform.

anserine [L. *anserinus,* fr. *anser,* goose]. **1** (an'ser-īn). Resembling or characteristic of a goose. See *cutis* anserina and *pes* anserinus. **2** (an'ser-ēn). Methylcarnosine; N^{a}-(β-alanyl)-π-methyl-L-histidine; present in muscle.

ansiform (an'si-fōrm) [L. *ansa,* handle, + *forma,* shape]. Ansate; in the shape of a loop or arc.

ansotomy (an-sot'ō-mē) [L. *ansa,* handle + G. *tomē,* cutting]. **1.** Surgical division of a loop, usually a constricting loop. **2.** Section of the ansa lenticularis for treatment of striatal syndromes.

ant-. See anti-.

ant. One of the most numerous insects (order Hymenoptera), characterized by an extraordinary development of colonial dwelling and caste specialization.
harvester a., *Pogonomyrmex.*
velvet a., a wingless mutilid wasp (family Mutilidae, order Hymenoptera) known for its venomous sting.

antacid (ant-as'id). Antiacid. **1.** Neutralizing an acid. **2.** Any agent that reduces or neutralizes acidity, as of the gastric juice or any other secretion.

antagonism (an-tag'on-izm) [G. *antagōnisma,* from *anti,* against, + *agōnizomai,* to fight, fr. *agōn,* a contest]. Mutual resistance; denoting mutual opposition in action between structures, agents, diseases, or physiologic processes. *Cf.* synergism.
bacterial a., the killing, injury, or inhibition of one bacterium by products of another.

antagonist (an-tag'ō-nist). Something opposing or resisting the action of another; certain structures, agents, diseases, or physiologic processes that tend to neutralize or impede the action or effect of others. *Cf.* synergist.
β-adrenoreceptor a., β-adrenergic blocking *agent.*
associated a., one of two muscles or groups of muscles which pull in nearly opposite directions, but which, when acting together, move the part in a path between their diverging lines of action.
calcium a., calcium channel-blocking *agent.*
competitive a., an antimetabolite.
enzyme a., an antimetabolite or inhibitor of enzyme action.
folic acid a.'s, modified pterins, such as aminopterin and amethopterin, that interfere with the action of folic acid and thus produce the symptoms of folic acid deficiency; have been used in cancer chemotherapy.
insulin a., substances in the β- and γ-globulin or β_1-lipoprotein fractions of serum which may induce a functional insulin deficiency; may include nonprecipitating antibodies against nonhuman insulin.

antalgesia (ant-al-jē'zē-ă) [anti- + G. *algēsis,* sense of pain]. The lowering of a previous elevation in pain threshold.

antalgic (ant-al'jik). Analgesic (2).

antalkaline (ant-al'kă-līn). Reducing or neutralizing alkalinity.

antaphrodisiac (ant'af-rō-diz'ē-ak). Anaphrodisiac.

antaphroditic (ant'af-rō-dit'ik). **1.** Anaphrodisiac. **2.** Antivenereal.

antarthritic (ant'ar-thrit'ik). Antiarthritic. **1.** Relieving arthritis. **2.** A remedy for arthritis.

antasthenic (ant-as-then'ik) [anti- + G. *astheneia,* weakness]. **1.** Strengthening or invigorating. **2.** An agent possessing such qualities.

antasthmatic (ant-az-mat'ik). Antiasthmatic. **1.** Tending to relieve or prevent asthma. **2.** An agent that prevents or arrests an asthmatic attack.

antatrophic (ant-ă-trof'ik). **1.** Preventing or curing atrophy. **2.** An agent that promotes the restoration of atrophied structures.

antazoline hydrochloride (an-taz'ō-lēn). Phenazoline hydrochloride; 2-(*N*-benzylanilino- methyl)-2-imidazoline hydrochloride; a histamine-antagonizing agent used in treating allergy; also available as a. phosphate.

ante- [L. *ante,* before]. Prefix denoting before. See also pre-, pro-(1).

antebrachial (an'te-brā'kē-ăl). Relating to the forearm.

antebrachium (an-te-brā'kē-ŭm) [ante- + L. *brachium,* arm]. [NA]. Forearm.

antecardium (an-te-kar'dē-ŭm). Precordia.

antecedent (an-te-sē'dent) [L. *antecedo,* to go before]. A precursor.
plasma thromboplastin a. (PTA), *factor* XI.

ante cibum (a.c.) (an'tē sī'bŭm) [L.]. Before a meal.

antecubital (an-te-kyū'bi-tăl) [ante- + L. *cubitum,* elbow]. In front of the elbow.

antefebrile (an-te-feb'ril) [ante- + L. *febris,* fever]. Antepyretic.

anteflex (an'te-fleks) [ante- + L. *flecto,* pp. *flexus,* to bend]. To bend forward, or cause to bend forward.

anteflexion (an-te-flek'shŭn). A bending forward; a sharp forward curve or angulation; denoting especially a forward bend in the uterus at the junction of corpus and cervix uteri.

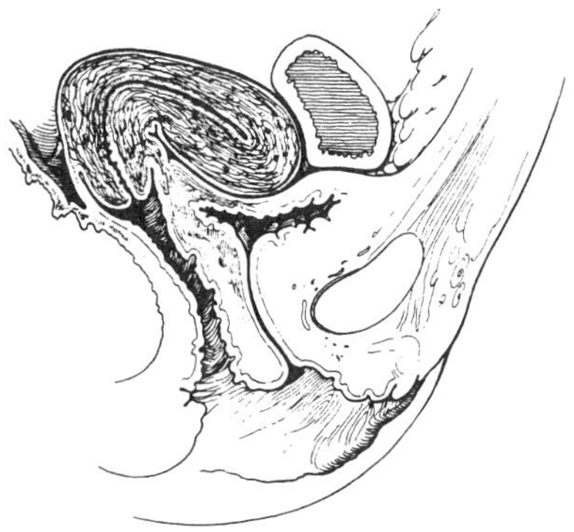

Anteflexion of the Uterus

a. of iris, the condition of the rotated iris after severe iridodialysis so that the pigmented layer faces forward.

antegrade (an'tē-grād). In radiology and urology, moving forward, as in peristalsis.

antemortem (an'te-mōr-tem) [ante- + L. acc. case of *mors* (*mort-*), death]. Before death. *Cf.* postmortem.

antenatal (an-te-nā'tăl) [ante- + L. *natus,* birth]. Prenatal.

antepartum (an'te-par-tŭm) [ante- + L. *pario,* pp. *partus,* to bring forth]. Before labor or childbirth. *Cf.* intrapartum; postpartum.

antephialtic (ant'ef-i-al'tik) [anti- + G. *ephialtēs,* nightmare]. Alleviating nightmares or distressing dreams.

anteposition (an'te-pō-si'shŭn). Forward or anterior position.

anteprostate (an-te-pros'tāt). *Glandula* bulbourethralis.

antepyretic (an'te-pī-ret'ik) [ante- + G. *pyretos,* fever]. Antefebrile; before the occurrence of fever; before the period of reaction following shock.

anterior (an-tēr'ē-ōr) [L.]. **1.** Before, in relation to time or space. **2** [NA]. Ventral (2); ventralis; in human anatomy, denoting the front surface of the body; often used to indicate the position of one structure relative to another, *i.e.,* situated nearer the front part of the body. **3.** Near the head or rostral end of certain embryos. **4.** Undesirable and confusing substitute for *cranial* in quadrupeds. In veterinary anatomy, a. is restricted to parts of the eye and inner ear.

antero-. Prefix denoting anterior.

anteroexternal (an'ter-ō-eks-ter'năl). In front and to the outer side.

anterograde (an'ter-ō-grād) [L. *gradior,* pp. *gressus,* to step, go]. **1.** Moving forward. *Cf.* antegrade. **2.** Extending forward from a particular point in time; used in reference to amnesia.

anteroinferior (an'ter-ō-in-fēr'ē-ōr). In front and below.

anterointernal (an'ter-ō-in-ter'năl). In front and to the inner side.

anterolateral (an'ter-ō-lat'er-ăl). In front and away from the middle line.

anteromedial (an'ter-ō-mē'dē-ăl). In front and toward the middle line.

anteromedian (an'ter-ō-mē'dē-an). In front and in the central line.

anteroposterior (an'ter-ō-pos-tēr-ē-er). **1.** Relating to both front and rear. **2.** In x-ray imaging, describing the direction of the beam through the patient from anterior to posterior, *e.g.*, an A-P view of the abdomen.

anterosuperior (an'ter-ō-sū-pē'rē-er). In front and above.

anterotic (ant-er-ot'ik) [anti- + G. *erōtikos*, pertaining to love]. Pertaining to an effort to avoid erotic feelings.

antesystole (an-te-sis'tō-lē). Premature activation of the ventricle responsible for the pre-excitation syndrome of the Wolff-Parkinson-White or Lown-Ganong-Levine types.

anteversion (an-te-ver'shŭn) [ante- + Mediev. L. *versio*, a turning]. Turning forward, inclining forward as a whole without bending.

anteverted (an-te-vert'ed). Tilted forward; in a position of anteversion.

anthelix (ant'hē-liks, an'thē-liks) [anti- + G. *helix*, coil] [NA]. Antihelix; an elevated ridge of cartilage anterior and roughly parallel to the posterior portion of the helix of the external ear.

anthelminthic (ant-hel-min'thik). Anthelmintic (1).

anthelmintic (ant-hel-min'tik, an-thel-) [anti- + G. *helmins*, worm]. **1.** Anthelminthic; helminthagogue; helminthic; helmintic; vermifuge; an agent that destroys or expels intestinal worms. **2.** Vermifugal; having the power to destroy or expel intestinal worms.

anthelone (an'thĕ-lōn). Urogastrone.

a. E, enterogastrone.

a. U, urogastrone.

anthelotic (ant-hē-lot'ik) [anti- + G. *hēlos*, nail, callus]. A remedy for corns.

anthema (an-thē'mă, an'thē) [G. *anthein*, to blossom]. Generalized eruption with sudden onset.

anthiolimine (an-thī-ō'li-mēn). Lithium antimony thiomalate; used in the treatment of filariasis and schistosomiasis.

anthocyanins (an-thō-sī'ă-ninz) [G. *anthos*, flower, + *kyanos*, a blue substance]. A group of floral pigments, existing as glycosides in combination with glucose or cellobiose molecules, that range from red to blue and are often pH dependent; soluble in water and alcohol but not in ether. A. are divided into derivatives of pelargonidin, cyanidins, and delphinidins. Some have been used as hematoxylin substitutes.

Anthomyia (an-thō-mī'yă) [G. *anthos*, flower, + *myia*, fly]. A genus of muscoid flies similar in appearance to the common housefly.

A. canicula'ris, a small black horsefly, the larvae of which have been reported as accidental parasites in the intestine of man, being hatched there from the ingested eggs; symptoms of gastroenteric irritation may be caused by it; adults may transport eggs of the tropical warble fly of man, *Dermatobia hominis*, a cause of myiasis.

anthoxanthins (an-thō-zan'thinz). Compounds responsible for the yellow and ivory shades of flowers; usually divided into flavones and flavonols.

anthracemia (an-thră-sē'mē-ă). Anthrax septicemia; the presence of *Bacillus anthracis* in the circulating blood, usually resulting from previously developed anthrax of the skin or lungs.

anthracene (an'thră-sēn) [G. *anthrax*, coal]. Anthracin; a hydrocarbon obtained from coal tar; it oxidizes to anthraquinone, which is converted to alizarin dyes.

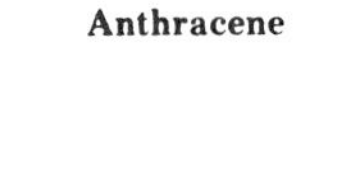

Anthracene

anthracia (an-thrā'sēă) [G. *anthrax*, carbuncle]. The occurrence of carbuncles.

anthracic (an-thras'ik). Relating to anthrax.

anthracin (an'thră-sin). Anthracene.

anthraco- (an'thră-kō-) [G. *anthrax*, coal, charcoal, carbuncle]. Combining form relating to coal or to carbuncle.

anthracoid (an'thră-koyd) [G. *anthrax*, carbuncle, + *eidos*, resemblance]. **1.** Resembling a carbuncle or cutaneous anthrax. **2.** Resembling anthrax.

anthracosilicosis (an'thră-kō-sil'i-kō'sis) [anthraco- + silicosis]. Pneumonoconiosis from accumulation of carbon and silica in the lungs from inhaled coal dust; the silica content produces fibrous nodules.

anthracosis (an-thră-kō'sis) [anthraco- + G. *-osis*, condition]. Collier's or miner's lung; melanedema; pneumonoconiosis from accumulation of carbon from inhaled smoke or coal dust in the lungs. See also pneumomelanosis.

anthracotic (an-thră-kot'ik). Characterized by anthracosis.

anthralin (an'thră-lin). Dithranol; 1,8,9-anthracenetriol; 1,8,9-anthratriol; 1,8,9-dihydroxyanthranol; used as a substitute for chrysarobin in ointment for treatment of psoriasis and ringworm infestation.

anthramucin (an-thră-myū'sin). A neutralizing material from the capsule of *Bacillus anthracis* that neutralizes serum and tissue antimicrobial action.

anthranilic acid (an-thră-nil'ik). *o*-Aminobenzoic acid; one of the products of tryptophan catabolism.

anthraniloyl (an-thră-nil'ō-il). The acyl radical of anthranilic acid.

anthrapurpurin (an'thră-pūr'pū-rin). 1,2,7-Trihydroxyanthraquinone; $C_{14}H_8O_5$; a purple dye used in histology as a reagent for calcium, although the specificity has been questioned.

9,10-**anthraquinone** (an'thră-kwi'nōn). 9,10-Dioxoanthracene; the basis of natural cathartic principles in plants; used as a reagent.

anthrax (an'thraks) [G. *anthrax* (*anthrak-*), charcoal, coal, a carbuncle]. **1.** Carbuncle (2); a disease in man caused by infection of subcutaneous tissues with *Bacillus anthracis;* marked by hemorrhage and serous effusions in various organs and body cavities and by symptoms of extreme prostration. **2.** Charbon; an infectious disease of animals, especially herbivores, due to presence in the blood of *Bacillus anthracis.*

cerebral a., a form of a., associated with pulmonary or intestinal a., in which the specific bacilli invade the capillaries of the brain; in addition to the symptoms of pulmonary or intestinal a., there is violent delirium; frequently associated with hemorrhagic meningitis.

cutaneous a., malignant pustule; a characteristic lesion that begins as a papule and soon becomes a vesicle and breaks, discharging a bloody serum; the seat of this vesicle, in about 36 hours, becomes a bluish black necrotic mass; constitutional symptoms are severe: high fever, vomiting, profuse sweating, and extreme prostration; the affection is often fatal.

intestinal a., a usually fatal form of a. marked by chill, high fever, pain in the head, back, and extremities, vomiting, bloody diarrhea, prostration, and frequently hemorrhages from the mucous membranes and in the skin (petechiae). See also *mycosis* intestinalis.

pulmonary a., a. pneumonia; wool-sorters' disease or pneumonia; rag-sorters' disease; a form of a. acquired by inhalation of dust containing *Bacillus anthracis;* there is an initial chill followed by pain in the back and legs, rapid respiration, dyspnea, cough, fever, rapid pulse, and extreme prostration.

anthrone (an'thrōn). 9,10-Dihydro-9-oxoanthracene; a reagent used in the detection of carbohydrates.

anthropo- [G. *anthrōpŏs*, man]. Combining form meaning human, or denoting some relationship to man.

anthropobiology (an'thrō-pō-bī-ol'ō-jē). The study of the biologic relationships of the human race.

anthropocentric (an'thrō-pō-sen'trik) [anthropo- + G. *kentron,* center]. With a human bias, under the assumption that man is the central fact of the universe.

anthropogenesis (an'thrō-pō-jen'ĕ-sis). Anthropogeny.

anthropogenic, anthropogenetic (an'thrō-pō-jen'ik, -jĕ-net'ik). Relating to anthropogeny.

anthropogeny (an-thrō-poj'ĕ-nē) [anthropo- + G. *genesis,* origin]. Anthropogenesis; anthropogony; the origin and development of man, both individual and racial.

anthropogony (an-thrō-poj'ō-nē). Anthropogeny.

anthropography (an-thrō-pog'ră-fē) [anthropo- + G. *graphō,* to write]. The geographical distribution of the varieties of mankind.

anthropoid (an'thrō-poyd) [G. *anthrōpo-eidēs,* man-like]. **1.** Resembling man in structure and form. **2.** One of the monkeys resembling man; an ape.

Anthropoidea (an'thrō-pō-id'ē-ă). A suborder of Primates, including man and the monkeys.

anthropology (an-thrō-pol'ō-jē) [anthropo- + G. *logos,* treatise]. The branch of science concerned with origin and development of humans in all their physical, social, and cultural relationships.
applied a., a fusion of modern cultural a. and some aspects of sociology in the study of literate peoples in their cultures and deriving applications therefrom.
criminal a., a. in relation to the physical and mental characteristics, heredity, and social relations of the criminal. See also criminology.
cultural a., study of all aspects of culture resulting from human behavior, including, among others, speech and language, systems of thought, social systems, and the artifacts produced by a culture.
physical a., the study of the physical attributes of human beings.

anthropometer (an-thrō-pom'ĕ-ter). An instrument for measuring various dimensions of the human body.

anthropometric (an-thrō-pō-met'rik). Relating to anthropometry.

anthropometry (an-thrō-pom'ĕ-trē) [anthropo- + G. *metron,* measure]. The branch of anthropology concerned with comparative measurements of the human body.

anthropomorphism (an'thrō-pō-mōr'fizm) [anthropo- + G. *morphē,* form]. Ascription of human shape or qualities to nonhuman creatures or inanimate objects. *Cf.* theriomorphism.

anthroponomy (an-thrō-pon'ō-mē) [anthropo- + G. *nomos,* law]. The study of the laws governing the development of the human race and the relation of man to his environment.

anthropopathy (an-thrō-pop'ă-thē) [anthropo- + G. *pathos,* suffering]. Attribution of human feelings to nonhumans, *e.g.,* to gods or lower animals.

anthropophilic (an'thrō-pō-fil'ik) [anthropo- + G. *phileō,* to love]. Man-seeking or man-preferring, especially with reference to: 1) bloodsucking arthropods, denoting the preference of a parasite for the human host as a source of blood or tissues over an animal host; and 2) dermatophytic fungi which grow preferentially on man rather than other animals.

anthropophobia (an'thrō-pō-fō'bē-ă) [anthropo- + G. *phobos,* fear]. Phobanthropy; morbid aversion to or dread of human companionship.

anthroposcopy (an'thrō-pos'kō-pē). [anthropo- + G. *skopeō,* to view]. Judging body type and build by inspection.

anthroposomatology (an'thrō-pō'sō-mă-tol'ō-jē) [anthropo- + G. *sōma,* body, + *logos,* study]. That part of anthropology concerned with the human body, *e.g.,* anatomy, physiology, or pathology.

anthropozoonosis (an'thrō-pō-zō'ō-nō'sis) [anthropo- + G. *zōon,* animal, + *nosis,* disease]. A zoonosis maintained in nature by animals and transmissible to man; *e.g.,* rabies, brucellosis. *Cf.* zooanthroponosis, amphixenosis.

anti- [G. *anti,* against]. **1.** Prefix signifying against, opposing, or, in relation to symptoms and diseases, curative. **2.** Prefix denoting an antibody (immunoglobulin) specific for the thing indicated; *e.g.,* antitoxin (antibody specific for a toxin).

antiacid (an-tē-as'id). Antacid.

antiadrenergic (an'tē-ad-rĕ-ner'jik). Antagonistic to the action of sympathetic or other adrenergic nerve fibers.

antiagglutinin (an'tē-ă-glū'ti-nin). A specific antibody that inhibits or destroys the action of an agglutinin.

antialexin (an'tē-ă-lek'sin). Anticomplement.

antiallergic (an'tē-ă-ler'jik). Relating to any agent or measure that prevents, inhibits, or alleviates an allergic reaction.

antianaphylaxis (an'tē-an'ă-fi-lak'sis). Desensitization (1).

antiandrogen (an-tē-an'drō-jen). Any substance capable of preventing full expression of the biological effects of androgenic hormones on responsive tissues, either by producing antagonistic effects on the target tissue, as estrogens do, or by merely inhibiting androgenic effects, as do agents like cyproterone.

antianemic (an'tē-ă-nē'mik). Pertaining to factors or substances that prevent or correct anemic conditions.

antiantibody (an'tē-an'tē-bod-ē). Antibody specific for another antibody.

antiantitoxin (an'tē-an-tē-tok'sin). An antiantibody that inhibits or counteracts the effects of an antitoxin.

antiarachnolysin (an-tē-ar-ak-nol'i-sin) [anti- + G. *arachnē,* spider, + lysin]. An antivenin counteracting the poison (lysin) of a spider.

antiarrhythmic (an'tē-ă-rith'mik). Antidysrhythmic; combating an arrhythmia.

antiarthritic (an'tē-ar-thrit'ik). Antarthritic.

antiasthmatic (an'tē-az-mat'ik). Antasthmatic.

antiautolysin (an'tē-aw-tol'i-sin). An antibody that inhibits or neutralizes the activity of an autolysin.

antibacterial (an'tē-bak-tēr'ē-ăl). Destructive to or preventing the growth of bacteria.

antibechic (an-tē-bek'ik) [anti- + G. *bēx* (*bēch-*), cough]. Antitussive.

antibiogram (an-tē-bī'ō-gram). A record of the resistance of microbes to various antibiotics.

antibiont (an-tē-bī'ont). A microorganism producing antimicrobial substance.

antibiosis (an'tē-bī-ō'sis) [anti- + G. *biōsis,* life]. **1.** An association of two organisms which is detrimental to one of them, in contrast to probiosis. **2.** Production of an antibiotic by bacteria or other organisms inhibitory to other living things, especially among soil microbes.

antibiotic (an'tē-bī-ot'ik). **1.** Relating to antibiosis. **2.** Prejudicial to life. **3.** A soluble substance derived from a mold or bacterium that inhibits the growth of other microorganisms. **4.** Relating to such an action.
broad spectrum a., an a. having a wide range of activity against both Gram-positive and Gram-negative organisms.

antibiotic-resistant. Indicating microorganisms that continue to multiply although exposed to antibiotic agents.

antibiotin (an-tē-bī'ō-tin). Avidin.

antiblennorrhagic (an'tē-blen-ō-raj'ik). Rarely used term for: **1.** Preventive or curative of a mucous discharge (blennorrhagia).

2. A remedy possessing such properties.

antibody (Ab) (an'tē-bod-i). Antisubstance; sensitizer (1); immune or protective protein; originally, a body or substance evoked in man or other animals by an antigen, and characterized by reacting specifically with the antigen in some demonstrable way, antibody and antigen each being defined in terms of the other. Now, it is supposed that antibodies may also exist naturally, without being present as a result of the stimulus provided by the introduction of an antigen: 1) in the broad sense any body or substance, soluble or cellular, which is evoked by the stimulus provided by the introduction of antigen and which reacts specifically with antigen in some demonstrable way; 2) one of the classes of globulins (immunoglobulins) present in the blood serum or body fluids of an animal as a result of antigenic stimulus or occurring "naturally." Different genetically inherited determinants, Gm (found on IgG H chains), Am (found on IgA H chains), and Km (found on K-type L chains and formerly called InV), control the antigenicity of the antibody molecule; subclasses are denoted either alphabetically or numerically (*e.g.,* G3mb1 or G3m5). The various classes differ widely in their ability to react in different kinds of serologic tests. See also immunoglobulin.

agglutinating a., agglutinin (1).

anaphylactic a., cytotropic a.

anti-basement membrane a., autoantibodies to renal glomerular basement membrane antigens.

anti-idiotype a., idiotype a.; an antiantibody, the activity of which is directed specifically against the idiotype of a particular immunoglobulin (antibody) molecule.

antinuclear a., an a. showing an affinity for cell nuclei, demonstrated by exposing a cell substrate to the serum to be tested, followed by exposure to an antihuman-globulin serum conjugated with fluorescein; development of specific nuclear fluorescence is a positive reaction; this a. is found in the serum of a high proportion of patients with systemic lupus erythematosus, rheumatoid arthritis, and certain collagen diseases, in some of their healthy relatives, and in about 1% of normal controls.

bivalent a., a. that causes a visible reaction with specific antigen as in agglutination, precipitation, and so on; so-called because according to the "lattice theory" aggregation occurs when the antibody molecule has two or more receptors which link across from one particle of antigen to another; probably a characteristic of the class of immunoglobulin.

blocking a., **(1)** a. which, in certain concentrations, does not cause precipitation after combining with specific antigen, and which, in this combined state, "blocks" activity of additional a. added to increase the concentration to a level at which precipitation would ordinarily occur; **(2)** the IgG class of immunoglobulin which combines specifically with an atopic allergen but does not elicit a type I allergic reaction, the combined IgG a. "blocking" available IgE class (reaginic) a. activity.

blood group a.'s, see Blood Groups appendix.

cell-bound a., a term sometimes used for supposed a. on the surface of cells that effects cell-mediated (delayed type) sensitivity.

CF a., complement-fixing a.

complement-fixing a., CF a.; sensitizing substance; a. that combines with and sensitizes antigen leading to the activation of complement, sometimes, but not always, resulting in lysis.

complete a., saline *agglutinin.*

cross-reacting a., **(1)** a. specific for group antigens, *i.e.,* those with identical functional groups; **(2)** a. for antigens that have functional groups of closely similar, but not identical, chemical structure.

cytophilic a., cytotropic a.

cytotropic a., cytophilic or anaphylactic a.; a. that has an affinity for certain kinds of cells, in addition to and unrelated to its specific affinity for the antigen that induced it, because of the properties of the Fc portion of the heavy chain. See also heterocytotropic a., homocytotropic a.; cytotropic antibody *test.*

fluorescent a., an immunoglobulin (antibody) to which a fluorescent dye has been attached.

Forssman a., heterophil a.; a heterogenetic a. specific for the Forssman group of heterogenetic antigens.

heterocytotropic a., a cytotropic a. (chiefly of the IgG class) similar in activity to homocytotropic a., but having an affinity for cells of a different species rather than for cells of the same or a closely related species.

heterogenetic a., an a. that reacts to a heterogenetic antigen.

heterophil a., heterophile a., Forssman a.

homocytotropic a., reaginic a.; a. of the IgE class which has an affinity for tissues (notably mast cells) of the same or a closely related species and that, upon combining with specific antigen, triggers the release of pharmacological mediators of anaphylaxis from the cells to which it is attached; the tropism seems to be dependent upon the Fc portion of the antibody molecule; the Prausnitz-Küstner a. (IgE class of immunoglobulins) is the prototype for this a., but in anaphylaxis in the guinea pig, the homocytotropic a. involved is of the γG class.

idiotype a., anti-idiotype a.

immobilizing a., treponema-immobilizing a.

incomplete a., **(1)** univalent a.; **(2)** serum *agglutinin.*

inhibiting a., univalent a.

lymphocytotoxic a.'s, a.'s specific for histocompatibility antigens of lymphocytes and which, upon combining with the antigens, induce cellular damage or death.

monoclonal a., an a. produced by a clone or genetically homogenous population of hybrid cells; hybrid cells are cloned to establish cell lines producing a specific a.

natural a., normal a.

neutralizing a., a form of a. that reacts with an infectious agent (usually a virus) and destroys or inhibits its infectivity and virulence; may be demonstrated by means of mixing serum with the suspension of infectious agent, and then injecting the mixture into animals that are susceptible to the agent in question.

nonprecipitating a., nonprecipitable a., a. that, under conditions normally employed in precipitin tests, is refractory to precipitation by specific a., demonstrable when antigen is added serially in small amounts; nonprecipitating a. will precipitate under special conditions such as addition of complement.

normal a., natural a.; a. demonstrable in the serum or plasma of various persons or animals not known to have been stimulated by specific antigen, either artificially or as the result of naturally occurring contact.

Prausnitz-Küstner a., atopic reagin; one of the IgE class of a.'s first demonstrated by Prausnitz and Küstner by passive transfer to the skin. See homocytotropic a.

precipitating a., precipitin.

reaginic a., homocytotropic a.

treponema-immobilizing a., immobilizing a.; treponemal a.; a., evoked during syphilitic infections, possessing specific affinity for *Treponema pallidum,* and which in the presence of complement immobilizes the organism.

treponemal a., treponema-immobilizing a.

univalent a., incomplete a. (1); inhibiting a.; an "incomplete" form of a. that may coat antigen, but which according to the "lattice theory" does not have a second receptor for attachment to another molecule of antigen; in the case of Rh+ erythrocytes, such an anti-Rh antibody may coat the cells but not cause them to agglutinate in saline; however, agglutination does occur when such coated cells are suspended in serum or other protein media, such as albumin, therefore called serum agglutinin.

Vi a., a form of a. that agglutinates highly virulent strains of *Salmonella typhosa, i.e.,* cells with Vi antigen; such bacteria are not agglutinable with O antiserum until the Vi antigen is destroyed. See Vi *antigen.*

Wassermann a., a., evoked during syphilitic infections, that combines with cardiolipin in the presence of lecithin and cholesterol; it is distinct from the treponema-immobilizing a.

antibrachial (an-tē-brā'kē-ăl). Incorrect spelling of antebrachial.

antibrachium (an-tē-brā'kē-ŭm). Incorrect spelling of antebrachium.

antibromic (an-tē-brō'mik) [anti- + G. *brōmos,* smell]. **1.** Deodorizing. **2.** A deodorizer.

anticalculous (an-tē-kal'kyū-lŭs). Antilithic.

anticarious (an'tē-kār'ē-ŭs). Preventing or inhibiting caries.

anticathexis (an'tē-kă-thek'sis). Counterinvestment; in psychoanalysis, the shifting of an emotional charge to an impulse or action of an opposite character; *e.g.,* unconscious hatred expressed as conscious love.

anticephalalgic (an'tē-sef-ă-lal'jik). Headache-relieving.

anticholagogue (an-tē-kol'ă-gog). An agent or process that reduces or suspends the flow of bile.

anticholinergic (an'tē-kol-i-ner'jik). Antagonistic to the action of parasympathetic or other cholinergic nerve fibers.

anticholinesterase (an'tē-kō-lin-es'ter-ās). One of the drugs that inhibit or inactivate acetylcholinesterase, either reversibly (*e.g.,* physostigmine) or irreversibly (*e.g.,* tetraethyl pyrophosphate).

anticipate (an-tis'i-pāt) [L. *anticipo,* pp. *-cipatus,* to anticipate, fr. *anti* (old form of *ante*), before, + *capio,* to take]. To come before the appointed time; said of a periodic symptom or disease, such as a malarial paroxysm, when it recurs at progressively shorter intervals.

anticipation (an-tis-i-pā'shŭn). **1.** Appearance before the appointed time of a periodic symptom or sign, such as a malarial paroxysm. **2.** Progressively earlier age of onset of a hereditary disease in successive generations; may be factitious (because of heightened awareness to early signs of the disease or because more conspicuous in the young) or authentic (because of progressive loss of epistatic and modifier genes by recombination and segregation).

anticlinal (an-tē-klī'năl) [anti- + G. *klinō,* to incline]. Inclined in opposite directions, as two sides of a pyramid.

anticnemion (an-tik-nē'mē-on) [G. *antiknēmion*]. Shin.

anticoagulant (an'tē-kō-ag'yū-lant). **1.** Preventing coagulation. **2.** An agent having such action.

anticodon (an-tē-kō'don). The trinucleotide sequence complementary to a codon; *e.g.,* if a codon is A-G-C, its anticodon is U (or T)-C-G. The complementarity principle arises from Watson-Crick base-pairing, in which A is complementary to U (or T), G is complementary to C. Sometimes called "nodoc."

anticomplement (an-tē-kom'plĕ-ment). Antialexin; a substance that combines with a complement and so neutralizes its action by preventing its union with the antibody.

anticomplementary (an'tē-kom-plĕ-men'tă-rē). Denoting a substance possessing the power of diminishing or abolishing the action of a complement.

anticontagious (an'tē-kon-tā'jŭs). Preventing contagion.

anticonvulsant (an'tē-kon-vŭl'sant). Anticonvulsive. **1.** Preventing or arresting convulsions. **2.** An agent having such action.

anticonvulsive (an'tē-kon-vŭl'siv). Anticonvulsant.

anticus (an-tī'kŭs) [L. in the very front, fr. *ante,* before]. A term in anatomical nomenclature to designate a muscle or other structure which of all similar structures is nearest the front or ventral surface. Nomina Anatomica uses "anterior" in place of this term.

anticytotoxin (an'tē-sī-tō-tok'sin). A specific antibody that inhibits or destroys the activity of a cytotoxin.

antidepressant (an'tē-dē-pres'ănt). **1.** Counteracting depression. **2.** An agent used in treating depression.

tetracyclic a., a class of a.'s similar to the tricyclic a.'s and also related to the phenothiazine antipsychotics; *e.g.,* maprotiline.

triazolopyridine a., a class of a.'s structurally and pharmacologically unrelated to other a.'s; clinical effectiveness appears to be equivalent to the tricyclic a.'s, but with less anticholinergic side effects; *e.g.,* trazodone.

tricyclic a., a class of a.'s structurally related to the phenothiazine antipsychotics; *e.g.,* amitriptyline, imipramine.

antidiabetic (an'tē-dī-ă-bet'ik). Counteracting diabetes; denoting an agent that lowers blood sugar.

antidiarrheal, antidiarrhetic (an'tē-dī-ă-re'ăl, -dī-ă-ret'ik). **1.** Having the property of opposing or correcting diarrhea. **2.** An agent having such action.

antidiuresis (an'tē-dī-yū-rē'sis). Reduction of urinary volume.

antidiuretic (an'tē-dī-yū-ret'ik). An agent that reduces the output of urine.

antidotal (an-tē-dō'tăl). Relating to or acting as an antidote.

antidote (an'tē-dōt) [G. *antidotos,* from *anti,* against, + *dotos,* what is given, fr. *didōmi,* to give]. An agent that neutralizes a poison or counteracts its effects.

chemical a., a substance that unites with a poison to form an innocuous chemical compound.

mechanical a., a substance that prevents the absorption of a poison.

physiologic a., an agent that produces systemic effects contrary to those of a given poison.

antidromic (an-tē-drom'ik) [anti- + G. *dromos,* a running]. Relating to propagation of an impulse along an axon in a direction the reverse of the normal; *Cf.* orthodromic.

antidysenteric (an'tē-dis-en-ter'ik). Relieving or preventing dysentery.

antidysrhythmic (an'tē-dis-rith'mik). Antiarrhythmic.

antidysuric (an'tē-dis-yū'rik). Preventing or relieving strangury or distress in urination.

antiemetic (an'tē-ĕ-met'ik) [anti- + G. *emetikos,* emetic]. **1.** Preventing or arresting vomiting. **2.** A remedy that tends to control nausea and vomiting.

antienergic (an'tē-en-er'jik) [anti- + G. *energos,* active]. Acting against or in opposition.

antienzyme (an-tē-en'zīm). An agent or principle that retards, inhibits, or destroys the activity of an enzyme; may be an inhibitory enzyme or an antibody to an enzyme.

antiepileptic (an'tē-ep-i-lep'tik). Indicating a drug or any measure that tends to prevent an epileptic seizure.

antiestrogen (an'tē-es'trō-jen). Any substance capable of preventing full expression of the biological effects of estrogenic hormones on responsive tissues, either by producing antagonistic effects on the target tissue, as androgens and progestogens do, or by competing with estrogens at estrogen receptors at the cellular level.

antifebrile (an-tē-fē'brīl, -feb'ril) [anti- + L. *febris,* fever]. Antipyretic (1).

antifibrinolysin (an'tē-fī-bri-nol'i-sin). Antiplasmin.

antifibrinolytic (an'tē-fī-brin-ō-lit'ik). Denoting a substance that decreases the breakdown of fibrin; *e.g.,* aminocaproic acid.

antifolic (an-tē-fō'lik). **1.** Antagonistic to the action of folic acid. **2.** Any agent with this effect. See also folic acid *antagonists.*

antifungal (an-tē-fŭng'ăl). Antimycotic.

anti-G In the strict sense, a term that means "antigravity" but, as commonly used, an adjectival term that implies protection against the effects of gravity (*e.g.,* anti-G *suit*).

antigalactagogue (an'tē-ga-lak'tă-gog). An agent for suppressing lactation.

antigalactic (an-tē-ga-lak′tik) [anti- + G. *gala,* milk]. Diminishing or arresting the secretion of milk.

ANTIGEN

antigen (Ag) (an′ti-jen) [anti(body) + G. *-gen,* producing]. Allergen; immunogen; any substance that, as a result of coming in contact with appropriate tissues of an animal body, induces a state of sensitivity and/or resistance to infection or toxic substances after a latent period (8 to 14 days) and which reacts in a demonstrable way with tissues and/or antibody of the sensitized subject *in vivo* or *in vitro.* Modern usage tends to retain the broad meaning of a., employing the terms "antigenic determinant" or "determinant group" for the particular chemical group of a molecule that confers antigenic specificity. See also hapten.

ABO a.'s. see ABO blood group, Blood Groups appendix.

acetone-insoluble a., cardiolipin.

Au a., (1) see Auberger blood group, Blood Groups appendix. **(2)** Australia a.

Australia a., Aus a., Au a., so-called because it was first recognized in an Australian aborigine, but now known to be an a. associated with hepatitis B virus.

Be^a a., Becker a., see low frequency blood groups, Blood Groups appendix.

Bi a., Bile's a., see low frequency blood groups, Blood Groups appendix.

blood group a., blood group substance; generic term for any inherited antigen found on the surface of erythrocytes that determines a blood grouping reaction with specific antiserum; a.'s of the ABO and Lewis blood groups may be found also in saliva and other body fluids; the genes controlling development of blood group a.'s vary in frequency in different population and ethnic groups. See also Blood Groups appendix.

By a., see low frequency blood groups, Blood Groups appendix.

capsular a., that found only in the capsules of certain microorganisms; *e.g.,* the specific polysaccharides of various types of pneumococci.

carcinoembryonic a. (CEA), a glycoprotein constituent of the glycocalyx of embryonic entodermal epithelium, generally absent from adult cells with the exception of some carcinomas in which it may also be detected in the patient's serum.

C carbohydrate a., see β-hemolytic *streptococci;* Lancefield *classification; Streptococcus pneumoniae.*

CDE a.'s, see Rh blood group, Blood Groups appendix.

cholesterinized a., cardiolipin to which cholesterol has been added.

Chr^a a., see low frequency blood groups, Blood Groups appendix.

common a., heterogenic enterobacterial a.; a common hapten that occurs in the bacterial cell wall and is shared by most Gram-negative bacteria; antibody to common a. is found in many patients with inflammatory bowel disease, and may be found (in low titer) in the serum of healthy blood donors and in commercial lots of gamma globulin.

complete a., any a. capable of stimulating the formation of antibody with which it reacts *in vivo* or *in vitro,* as distinguished from incomplete a. (hapten).

conjugated a., conjugated *hapten.*

delta a., hepatitis delta *virus.*

Dharmendra a., a chloroform-ether extracted suspension of *Mycobacterium leprae;* used to produce the Fernandez reaction in a lepromin test.

Di a., see Diego blood group, Blood Groups appendix.

Duffy a.'s., see Duffy blood group, Blood Groups appendix.

flagellar a., the heat-labile a.'s associated with bacterial flagella which, with specific antibody, are agglutinated into loose fluffy masses which are easily disintegrated by shaking, in contrast to somatic a.

Forssman a., a type of heterogenetic a. found in dogs, horses, sheep, cats, turtles, eggs of some fish, in certain bacteria (*e.g.,* some strains of enteric organisms and pneumococci), and varieties of corn; usually found in the tissues and organs (not in blood), but is present in sheep erythrocytes, though not in this animal's tissues; with the exception of guinea pigs and hamsters, Forssman a. is not found in rodents, or in frogs, hogs, and most primates; the antibody that develops in infectious mononucleosis of man reacts specifically with the Forssman. a.

Fy a.'s., see Duffy blood group, Blood Groups appendix.

G a. [Ger. *gebundenes,* bound], internal a.; an antigenic viral nucleoprotein.

Ge a., see high frequency blood groups, Blood Groups appendix.

Good a., see low frequency blood groups, Blood Groups appendix.

Gr a., Vw a.

group a.'s, a.'s that are shared by related genera of microorganisms.

H a., (1) the a. in the flagella of motile bacteria; so named because first identified in motile bacteria from a film (Ger. *Hauch*) of spreading growth on agar medium. See also O a. **(2)** the chemical precursor of a.'s of the ABO blood group locus.

He a.'s, Hu a.'s, see MNSs blood group, Blood Groups appendix.

heart a., cardiolipin.

hepatitis-associated a. (HAA), a term used for the surface a. of hepatitis B virus before its nature was established. See hepatitis B surface a.

hepatitis B core a. (HB_cAg), the a. found in the core (seemingly the nucleocapsid) of the Dane particle (seemingly the hepatitis B virus) and also in hepatocyte nuclei in hepatic B infections.

hepatitis B e a. (HBe, HB_eAg), an a., or group of a.'s, associated with hepatitis B infection and distinct from the surface a. (HB_sAg) and the core a. (HB_cAg); there is evidence that it is associated with the viral DNA polymerase; the a. and its antiserum (anti-e) seem to be associated with vertical transmission (or lack of transmission) of infection.

hepatitis B surface a. (HB_sAg), a. of the small (20 nm) spherical and filamentous forms of hepatitis B a., and a surface a. of the larger (42 nm) Dane particle (seemingly the hepatitis B virus). See also hepatitis B core a., hepatitis B e a.

heterogenetic a., heterophil a.; an a. which is possessed by a variety of different phylogenetically unrelated species; *e.g.,* the various organ- or tissue-specific a.'s, the alpha- and beta-crystalline protein of the lens of the eye, and Forssman a.

heterogenic enterobacterial a., common a. of Kunin.

heterophil a., heterogenetic a.

hexon a., see hexon.

HL-A a.'s, original designation for *h* uman *l* ymphocyte histocompatibility a.'s determined by alleles at locus *A* (the first recognized); "HLA" is now the system designation, locus A being designated HLA-A. See human lymphocyte a.'s.

Ho a., see low frequency blood groups, Blood Groups appendix.

human leukemia-associated a.'s, a.'s on the surface of leukemic cells which seem not to be present on the surfaces of the same type of normal cells; the myeloblast a. of acute myelogenous leukemia found in chronic myelogenous leukemia is thought to be associated with a "blastic" transformation.

human lymphocyte a.'s (HLA), system designation for the gene products of at least four linked loci (A, B, C, and D) on the sixth human chromosome which have been shown to have a strong influence on human allotransplantation, transfusions in refractory patients, and certain disease associations; more than 50 alleles are recognized, most of which are at loci HLA-A and HLA-B.

H-Y a., an a. factor, dependent on the Y chromosome, responsible for the differentiation of the human embryo into the male phenotype by inducing the initially bipotential embryonic gonad to develop into a testis; in the absence of this a., the indifferent gonad develops into an ovary.
I a.'s, i a.'s, see I blood group, Blood Groups appendix.
incomplete a., hapten.
internal a., G a.
Jk a.'s, see Kidd blood group, Blood Groups appendix.
Jobbins a., see low frequency blood groups, Blood Groups appendix.
Js a., see Sutter blood group, Blood Groups appendix.
K a.'s, k a.'s, see Kell blood group, Blood Groups appendix.
Kveim a., Kveim-Stilzbach a., a saline suspension of human sarcoid tissue prepared from the spleen of an individual with active sarcoidosis; used in the Kveim test.
Lan a., see high frequency blood groups, Blood Groups appendix.
Le a.'s, see Lewis blood group, Blood Groups appendix.
Levay a., see low frequency blood groups, Blood Groups appendix.
Lu a.'s, see Lutheran blood group, Blood Groups appendix.
lymphogranuloma venereum a., a sterile preparation of inactivated chlamydiae grown in the yolk sac of domestic fowl and used as an a. in the Frei *test.*
M a., see β-hemolytic *streptococci; Streptococcus pheumoniae;* blood group a.
M_1, M_2, M^c, M^g a.'s, see MNSs blood group, Blood Groups appendix.
Mi^2 a., see MNSs blood group, Blood Groups appendix.
Mitsuda a., an autoclaved suspension of human tissue naturally infected with *Mycobacterium leprae;* used to produce the Mitsuda reaction in a lepromin test.
MNSs a.'s, see MNSs blood group, Blood Groups appendix.
Mu a., see MNS blood group, Blood Groups appendix.
mumps skin test a., a sterile suspension of killed mumps virus in isotonic sodium chloride solution, used to determine susceptibility to mumps or to confirm a tentative diagnosis.
O a., (1) somatic a. of nonmotile bacteria that colonize on agar medium without forming a film (Ger. *ohne Hauch*). See also H a. (2) see ABO blood group, Blood Groups appendix.
oncofetal a.'s, tumor-associated a.'s present in fetal tissue but not in normal adult tissue, including α-fetoprotein and carcinoembryonic a.
organ-specific a., tissue-specific a.; a heterogenetic antigen with organ specificity; *e.g.,* in addition to species-specific a., kidney of one species contains a. that is identical to that in kidney of other species.
Ot a., see low frequency blood groups, Blood Groups appendix.
P a.'s, see P blood group, Blood Groups appendix.
partial a., hapten.
penton a., see penton.
pollen a., an extract of the antigenic protein from the pollen of plants; *i.e.,* pollen allergen, used in the diagnosis and prevention of hay fever.
private a.'s, see low frequency blood groups, Blood Groups appendix.
public a.'s, see high frequency blood groups, Blood Groups appendix.
R a., see β-hemolytic *streptococci.*
Rh a.'s, see Rh blood group, Blood Groups appendix.
Rhus toxicodendron a., an extract of fresh leaves of poison ivy, with 0.4% of procaine hydrochloride; used by intradermal injection to determine sensitiveness to the poison of *Rhus toxicodendron.*
Rhus venenata a., an extract of fresh leaves of poison sumac; used to determine sensitiveness to the plant or to relieve the dermatitis caused by contact with its leaves.
S a., soluble a.
sensitized a., the complex formed when a. combines with specific antibody; so called because the a., by the mediation of antibody, is rendered sensitive to the action of complement.
shock a., an a. capable of producing anaphylactic shock in an animal that has been sensitized to it.
Sm a., see high frequency blood groups, Blood Groups appendix.
soluble a., S a.; viral a. that remains in solution after the particles of virus have been removed by means of centrifugation; in the case of the influenza viruses, it is the internal helical structure, free of the external envelope.
somatic a., an a. located in the body of a bacterium in contrast to one in the flagella (flagellar a.) or in a capsule (capsular a.).
species-specific a., antigenic components in the tissues and fluids of members of a species of animal, by means of which various species may be immunologically distinguished; *e.g.,* serum albumin of horses is immunologically different from that of man, dogs, sheep, and so on.
specific a.'s, a.'s that characterize a single genus of microorganisms.
Stobo a., see low frequency blood groups, Blood Groups appendix.
Streptococcus M a., M protein (1); the somatic a. associated with virulence and type specificity of group A streptococci; removed from cell surface by trypsin digestion.
Sw^a a., see low frequency blood groups, Blood Groups appendix.
Swann a.'s, see low frequency blood groups, Blood Groups appendix.
T a.'s, tumor a.'s. See also β-hemolytic *streptococci.*
tissue-specific a., organ-specific a.
Tj a., see P blood group, Blood Groups appendix.
Tr^a a., see low frequency blood groups, Blood Groups appendix.
tumor a.'s, T a.'s; neo-antigens; a.'s present in tumors induced by certain types of adenoviruses and papovaviruses or in cells transformed *in vitro* by those viruses; tumor a.'s are unrelated to virus capsid a.'s but seem to be peculiar to the inducing virus and probably result from virus-specific messenger RNA present in the virion-free tumor cells; several kinds have been identified as proteins of various molecular weights.
tumor-specific transplantation a.'s (TSTA), surface a.'s of DNA tumor virus-transformed cells, which elicit an immune rejection of the virus-free cells when transplanted into an animal that has been immunized against the specific cell-transforming virus. Also called tumor-specific a.'s or tumor-associated transplantation a.'s.
V a., viral a. that is intimately associated with the virus particle, is protein in nature, has multiple antigenicities, and is strain-specific; antibody to such a. is demonstrable as protective or neutralizing antibody.
Vel a., see high frequency blood groups, Blood Groups appendix.
Ven a., see low frequency blood groups, Blood Groups appendix.
Vi a., "virulence a.," an external nonflagellar a. of enterobacteria formerly thought to be related to increased virulence.
Vw a., Gr a. See MNSs blood group, Blood Groups appendix.
Webb a., see low frequency blood groups, Blood Groups appendix.
Wr^a a., see low frequency blood groups, Blood Groups appendix.
Wright a.'s, see low frequency blood groups, Blood Groups appendix.
Xg a., see Xg blood group, Blood Groups appendix.
Yt^a a., see high frequency blood groups, Blood Groups appendix.

antigenemia (an'ti-jĕ-nē'mē-ă) [antigen + G. *haima,* blood]. Persistence of antigen in circulating blood; *e.g.,* HB_s-antigenemia (presence of hepatitis B virus surface antigen in blood serum).

antigenic (an-ti-jen'ik). Allergenic; immunogenic; having the properties of an antigen (allergen).

antigenicity (an'ti-jĕ-nis'i-tē). Immunogenicity; the state or property of being antigenic.

antigonorrheic (an′tē-gon-ō-rē′ik). Curative of gonorrhea.

antigravity (an-tē-grav′i-tē). See anti-G.

anti-HB_c (HB_cAb). Antibody to the hepatitis B core antigen (HB_cAg).

anti-HB e (HB_eAb). Antibody to the hepatitis B e antigen (HB_eAg).

anti-HB_s (HB_sAb). Antibody to the hepatitis B surface antigen (HB_sAg).

antihelix (an-tē-hē′liks). Anthelix.

antihemagglutinin (an′tē-hē-mă-glū′ti-nin, an′tē-hem-ă-). A substance (including antibody) that inhibits or prevents the effects of hemagglutinin.

antihemolysin (an′tē-hē-mol′i-sin, an′tē-hem-ol′-). A substance (including antibody) that inhibits or prevents the effects of hemolysin.

antihemolytic (an′tē-hē-mō-lit′ik, an′tē-hem-ō-). Preventing hemolysis.

antihemorrhagic (an′tē-hem-ō-răj′ik). Hemostatic (2); arresting hemorrhage.

antihidrotic (an′tē-hī-drot′ik, -hi-drot′ik). Antiperspirant.

antihistamines (an-tē-his′tă-mēnz). Drugs having an action antagonistic to that of histamine; used in the treatment of allergy symptoms.

antihistaminic (an′tē-his-tă-min′ik). **1.** Tending to neutralize or antagonize the action of histamine or to inhibit its production in the body. **2.** An agent having such an effect, used to relieve the symptoms of allergy.

antihormones (an-tē-hōr′mōnz). Substances demonstrable in serum that inhibit or prevent the usual effects of certain hormones, and which, in certain instances at least, are specific antibodies.

antihydriotic (an′tē-hī-drē-ot′ik). Antiperspirant.

antihydropic (an′tē-hī-drop′ik). **1.** Relieving edema (dropsy). **2.** An agent that mobilizes accumulated fluids.

antihypertensive (an′tē-hī-per-ten′siv). Indicating a drug or mode of treatment that reduces the blood pressure of hypertensive individuals.

antihypnotic (an′tē-hip-not′ik). **1.** Preventing or tending to prevent sleep. **2.** An arousing agent, or one antagonistic to sleep.

anti-icteric (an′tē-ik-ter′ik). Preventing or curing icterus (jaundice).

anti-inflammatory (an′tē-in-flam′ă-tō-rē). Reducing inflammation by acting on body mechanisms, without directly antagonizing the causative agent; denoting agents such as antihistamines and glucocorticoids.

antiketogenesis (an′tē-kē-tō-jen′ĕ-sis). Prevention or reduction of ketosis either by decreased production or increased utilization of ketone bodies.

antiketogenic (an′tē-kē-tō-jen′ik). Inhibiting the formation of ketone bodies, or accelerating their utilization.

antileukocidin (an′tē-lū-kos′i-din, lū-kō-sī′din). **1.** A substance that inhibits or prevents the effects of leukocidin. **2.** A leukocidin-specific antibody.

antileukotoxin (an′tē-lū-kō-tok′sin). A substance (including antibody) that inhibits or prevents the effects of leukocytoxin; frequently regarded as synonymous with antileukocidin.

antilewisite (an-tē-lū′i-sīt). Dimercaprol.

antilipotropic (an′tē-lip-ō-trop′ik). Pertaining to substances depressing choline synthesis (*e.g.,* by competing for methyl groups) and thus enhancing dietary fatty liver.

antilithic (an-tē-lith′ik) [anti- + G. *lithos,* stone]. **1.** Anticalculous; preventing the formation of calculi or promoting their dissolution. **2.** An agent so acting.

antilobium (an-tē-lō′bē-ŭm) [L., fr. G. *antilobion*]. Tragus (1).

antiluteogenic (an′tē-lū-tē-ō-jen′ik). Inhibiting the growth or hastening involution of the corpus luteum.

antilysin (an-tē-lī′sin). An antibody that inhibits or prevents the effects of lysin.

antimalarial (an′tē-mă-lā′rē-ăl). **1.** Preventing or curing malaria. **2.** A chemotherapeutic agent that inhibits or destroys malarial parasites.

antimer (an′ti-mer). Enantiomer.

antimere (an′ti-mēr) [anti- + G. *meros,* a part]. **1.** A segment of an animal body formed by planes cutting the axis of the body at right angles. **2.** One of the symmetrical parts of a bilateral organism. **3.** The right or left half of the body.

antimesenteric (an′tē-mez′en-ter′ik). Pertaining to the part of the intestine that lies opposite the mesenteric attachment.

antimetabolite (an′tē-me-tab′ō-līt). A substance that competes with, replaces, or antagonizes a particular metabolite; *e.g.,* ethionine is an a. of methionine.

antimetropia (an′tē-me-trō′pē-ă) [anti- + G. *metron,* measure, + *ōps,* eye]. A form of anisometropia in which one eye is myopic and the other hypermetropic.

antimicrobial (an′tē-mī-krō′bē-ăl). Tending to destroy microbes, to prevent their development, or to prevent their pathogenic action.

antimitotic (an′tē-mī-tot′ik). **1.** Having an arresting action upon mitosis. **2.** A drug having such an effect; *e.g.,* a folic acid antagonist that is used in leukemia to inhibit the multiplication of white cells.

antimongoloid (an-tē-mon′gō-loyd). The condition in which the lateral portion of the palpebral fissure is lower than the medial portion.

antimonid (an-tē-mō′nid). A chemical compound containing antimony in union with a more positive element; *e.g.,* sodium a., Na_3Sb.

antimonium (an-ti-mō′nē-ŭm). Antimony.

antimonous oxide (an-ti-mō′nŭs). *Antimony* trioxide.

antimony (an′-ti-mō-nē). Antimonium; stibium; a metallic element, symbol Sb, atomic no. 51, atomic weight 121.77, valences +3, +5; used in alloys; toxic and irritating to the skin and mucous membranes.

a. chloride, a. trichloride.

a. dimercaptosuccinate, stibocaptate; 2,3-dimercaptosuccinic acid cyclic thioantimonate; an antiparasitic effective against *Schistosoma mansoni* and *S. haematobium.*

a. oxide, a. trioxide.

a. potassium tartrate, tartar emetic; tartrated a.; potassium antimonyltartrate; a compound used as an expectorant and in the treatment of schistosomiasis japonicum, although it is extremely toxic and must be administered very slowly intravenously; common toxic manifestations are phlebitis, tachycardia, and hypotension; sudden deaths have been reported, chiefly from circulatory collapse.

a. sodium gluconate, stibogluconate sodium.

a. sodium tartrate, sodium antimonyl tartrate; $Na(SbO)C_4H_4O_6$; used in the treatment of schistosomiasis, and as an emetic.

a. sodium thioglycollate, a compound of a. trioxide and thioglycolic acid, used for tropical parasites.

tartrated a., a. potassium tartrate.

a. thioglycollamide, the triamide of a. thioglycolic acid; $Sb(SCH_2CONH_2)_3$; used in the treatment of trypanosomiasis, kala azar, and filariasis.

a. trichloride, a. chloride; butter of a.; $SbCl_3$; combines with vitamin A to form a blue compound and with β-carotene to form a green one, as a method for assay of these substances; also used externally as a caustic.

a. trioxide, a. oxide; antimonous oxide; flowers of antimony; Sb_2O_3; used technically in paints and flame-proofing; also used as an expectorant and emetic.

antimonyl (an-tim'ō-nil). The univalent radical, SbO–, of antimony.

antimuscarinic (an'tē-mŭs'kă-rin'ik). Inhibiting or preventing the actions of muscarine and muscarine-like agents, or the effects of parasympathetic stimulation at the neuroeffector junction (*e.g.,* atropine).

antimutagen (an-tē-myū'tă-jen). A factor that reduces or interferes with the mutagenic actions of effects of a substance.

antimutagenic (an'tē-myū-tă-jen'ik). Pertaining to or characteristic of an antimutagen.

antimyasthenic (an'tē-mī'as-then'ik). Tending toward the correction of the symptoms of myasthenia gravis, *e.g.,* as in the action of neostigmine.

antimycotic (an'-tē-mī-kot'ik) [anti- + G. *mykēs,* fungus]. Antifungal; antagonistic to fungi.

antinatriferic (an'tē-nā-trif'er-ik). Tending to inhibit sodium transport.

antinauseant (an-tē-naw'sē-ănt). Having an action to prevent nausea.

antineoplastic (an'tē-nē-ō-plas'tik). Preventing the development, maturation, or spread of neoplastic cells.

antinephritic (an'tē-nĕ-frit'ik). Preventing or relieving inflammation of the kidneys.

antineuralgic (an'tē-nū-ral'jik). Relieving the pain of neuralgia.

antineuritic (an'tē-nū-rit'ik). Relieving neuritis.

antineurotoxin (an'tē-nū-rō-tok'sin). An antibody to a neurotoxin.

antiniad (an-tin'ē-ad). Toward the antinion.

antinial (an-tin'ē-ăl). Relating to the antinion.

antinion (an-tin'ē-on) [anti- + G. *inion,* nape of the neck]. The space between the eyebrows; the point on the skull opposite the inion.

antinomy (an-tin'ō-mē) [anti- + G. *nomos,* law]. A contradiction between two principles, each of which is considered true.

antinuclear (an-tē-nū'klē-er). Having an affinity for or reacting with the cell nucleus.

antiodontalgic (an'tē-ō-don-tăl-jik) [anti- + G. *odous,* tooth, + *algos,* pain]. **1.** Relieving toothache. **2.** A toothache remedy.

antioncogene (an-tē-on'kō-jēn). A tumor-suppressing gene involved in controlling cellular growth; inactivation of this type of gene leads to deregulated cellular proliferation, as in cancer.

antioxidant (an-tē-oks'i-dănt). An agent that inhibits oxidation and thus prevents rancidity of oils or fats or the deterioration of other materials through oxidative processes.

antiparallel (an-tē-par'ă-lel). Denoting molecules that are parallel but point in opposite directions; *e.g.,* the two strands of a DNA double helix.

antiparasitic (an'tē-par-ă-sit'ik). Destructive to parasites.

antiparastata (an'tē-pa-ras'tă-tă) [anti- + G. *parastatēs,* a testicle]. *Glandula* bulbourethralis.

antipedicular (an'tē-pe-dik'yū-lăr). Destructive to lice.

antipediculotic (an'tē-pe-dik-yū-lot'ik). Effective in the treatment of pediculosis, especially denoting such an agent.

antiperiodic (an'tē-pēr-ē-od'ik). Preventing the regular recurrence of a disease (*e.g.,* malaria) or a symptom.

antiperistalsis (an'tē-per-i-stal'sis). Reversed *peristalsis.*

antiperistaltic (an'tē-per-i-stal'tik). **1.** Relating to antiperistalsis. **2.** Impeding or arresting peristalsis.

antiperspirant (an-tē-per'spi-rant). Antihidrotic; antihydriotic; antisudorific. **1.** Having an inhibitory action upon the secretion of sweat. **2.** An agent having such an action.

antiphagocytic (an'tē-fag-ō-sit'-ik). Impeding or preventing the action of the phagocytes.

antiphlogistic (an'tē-flō-jis'tik) [anti- + G. *phogistos,* burnt up]. Antipyrotic (1). **1.** Preventing or relieving inflammation. **2.** An agent that reduces inflammation.

antiphobic (an-tē-fō'bik). A mechanism or drug designed to control phobias.

antiplasmin (an-tē-plaz'min). Antifibrinolysin; a substance that inhibits or prevents the effects of plasmin; found in plasma and some tissues, especially the spleen and liver.

antiplatelet (an-tē-plāt'let). A substance that manifests a lytic or agglutinative action on the blood platelets, thereby inhibiting or destroying the effects of the latter.

antipneumococcic (an'tē-nū-mō-kok'sik). Destructive to, or repressing the growth of, the pneumococcus.

antipodal (an-tip'ō-dăl). Denoting opposite positions; positioned at opposite sides of a cell or other body.

antipode (an'ti-pōd) [G. *antipous,* with the feet opposite]. That which is diametrically opposite.

optical a., enantiomer.

antiport (an'tē-pōrt) [anti- + L. *porto,* to carry]. The coupled transport of two different molecules or ions through a membrane in opposite directions by a common carrier mechanism (antiporter). *Cf.* symport; uniport.

antiporter (an'tē-pōr-ter). A carrier mechanism that transports two different molecules or ions simultaneously in opposite directions through a membrane.

antiposic (an-tē-pō'sik). **1.** Inhibitory to the drinking of water and other beverages. **2.** An agent that has this effect.

antiprecipitin (an'tē-prē-sip'i-tin). A specific antibody that inhibits or prevents the effects of a precipitin.

antiprogestin (an'tē-prō-jes'tin). A substance that inhibits progesterone formation, that interferes with its carriage or stability in the blood, or that reduces its uptake by, or effects on, target organs.

antiprostate (an-tē-pros'tāt). *Glandula* bulbourethralis.

antiprothrombin (an'tē-prō-throm'bin). An anticoagulant that inhibits or prevents the conversion of prothrombin into thrombin; examples are heparin, which is present in various tissues (especially in liver), and dicoumarin, which is isolated from partially decomposed sweet clover.

antipruritic (an'tē-prū-rit'ik). **1.** Preventing or relieving itching. **2.** An agent that relieves itching.

antipsoric (an-tē-sō'rik) [anti- + G. *psōra,* itch]. Curative of scabies, or of itching.

antipsychotic (an'tē-sī-kot'ik). **1.** Antipsychotic *agent.* **2.** Denoting the actions of such an agent.

antipyogenic (an'tē-pī-ō-jen'ik) [anti- + G. *pyon,* pus, + *-gen,* production]. Preventing suppuration.

antipyresis (an'tē-pī-rē'sis). Symptomatic treatment of fever rather than of the underlying disease.

antipyretic (an'tē-pī-ret'ik) [anti- + G. *pyretos,* fever]. **1.** Antifebrile; febrifugal; reducing fever. **2.** Febrifuge; an agent that reduces fever.

antipyrine (an-tē-pī'rin, -pī'rēn). 2,3-Dimethyl-1-phenyl-3-pyrazoline-5-one; an analgesic and antipyretic.

a. acetylsalicylate, a compound of a. and aspirin; an antirheumatic and analgesic.

a. salicylacetate, an analgesic, antirheumatic, and antipyretic.

a. salicylate, an analgesic and antipyretic; used in dysmenorrhea, influenza, and acute rhinitis in the early stages.

antipyrotic (an'tē-pī-rot'ik) [anti- + G. *pyrōtikos,* burning, inflaming]. **1.** Antiphlogistic. **2.** Relieving the pain and promoting the healing of superficial burns. **3.** A topical application for burns.

antirachitic (an'tē-ră-kit'ik). Promoting the cure of rickets or preventing its development.

antirheumatic (an'tē-rū-mat'ik). **1.** Denoting an agent which suppresses manifestations of rheumatic disease; usually applied to anti-inflammatory agents or agents that are capable of delaying progression of the basic disease process in rheumatic arthritis. **2.** An agent possessing such properties.

antiricin (an-tē-rī'sin). An antibody or antitoxin that inhibits or prevents the effects of ricin.

antiruminant (an-tē-rū'mi-nănt). Denoting a method to 1) control regurgitation of food or 2) break a compulsive trend of thought.

anti-S See MNSs blood group, Blood Groups appendix.

antiscorbutic (an'tē-skōr-byū'tik). **1.** Preventive or curative of scurvy (scorbutus). **2.** A treatment for scurvy.

antiseborrheic (an'tē-seb-ō-rē'ik). **1.** Preventing or relieving excessive flow of sebum; preventing or relieving seborrheic dermatitis. **2.** An agent having such actions.

antisecretory (an'tē-sē-krē'tō-rī). Inhibitory to secretion, said of certain drugs that reduce or suppress gastric secretion.

antisepsis (an-tē-sep'sis) [anti- + G. *sēpsis,* putrefaction]. Prevention of infection by inhibiting the growth of infectious agents. See also disinfection.

antiseptic (an-tē-sep'tik). **1.** Relating to antisepsis. **2.** An agent or substance capable of effecting antisepsis.

antiserum (an-tē-sē'rŭm). Immune serum; serum that contains demonstrable antibody or antibodies specific for one (monovalent or specific a.) or more (polyvalent a.) antigens; may be prepared from the blood of animals inoculated parenterally (under certain conditions) with an antigenic material or from the blood of animals and persons that have been stimulated by natural contact with an antigen (as in those who recover from an attack of disease).

blood group a.'s, see Blood Groups appendix.

heterologous a., an a. that reacts with (*e.g.,* agglutinates) certain microorganisms or other complexes of antigens, even though the a. was produced by means of stimulation with a different microorganism or antigenic material. See also homologous a.

homologous a., an a. in which there is complete correspondence between the content of antibodies and the antigenic material used for producing the a.; *e.g.,* if Bacterium I (with antigens *a, b, c,* and *d*) is used to produce an a., the a. would contain antibodies *A, B, C,* and *D,* and would be homologous for Bacterium I but also *heterologous* for various bacteria that might contain any one, two, or three (but not all four) of the same antigens.

monovalent a., see a.

nerve growth factor (NGF) a., an a. containing antibodies against nerve growth factor; when injected into newborn animals the majority of sympathetic ganglion cells are permanently destroyed, resulting in hypoinnervation of peripheral tissues.

polyvalent a., see a.

specific a., see a.

antisialagogue (an-tē-sī-al'ă-gog) [anti- + G. *sialon,* saliva, + *agōgos,* drawing forth]. An agent that diminishes or arrests the flow of saliva.

antisialic (an-tē-sī-al'ik). Reducing the flow of saliva.

antisideric (an-tē-sid'er-ik) [anti- + G. *sideros,* iron]. Counteracting the physiological action of iron, probably by chelating or precipitation.

antisocial (an-tē-sō'shŭl). Behaving in violation of the social or legal norms of society; *e.g.,* the antisocial personality. *Cf.* asocial.

antispasmodic (an'tē-spaz-mod'ik). **1.** Preventive or curative of convulsions or spasmodic affections. **2.** An agent that quiets spasm.

antistaphylococcic (an'tē-staf'i-lō-kok'sik). Antagonistic to staphylococci or their toxins.

antistaphylolysin (an'tē-staf-i-lol'i-sin). A substance that antagonizes or neutralizes the action of staphylolysin.

antisteapsin (an'tē-stē-ap'sin). An antibody counteracting the action of triacylglycerol lipase (steapsin).

antistreptococcic (an'tē-strep-tō-kok'sik). Destructive to streptococci or antagonistic to their toxins.

antistreptokinase (an'tē-strep-tō-kī'nās). An antibody that inhibits or prevents the dissolution of fibrin by streptokinase.

antistreptolysin (an'tē-strep-tol'i-sin). An antibody that inhibits or prevents the effects of streptolysin O elaborated by group A streptococci; the amount of a. in the serum is frequently increased during and after streptococcal disease, and comparative titers may be a diagnostic and prognostic aid.

antisubstance (an-tē-sŭb'stans). Antibody.

antisudorific (an'tē-sū-dōr-if'ic). Antiperspirant.

antitetanic (an'tē-te-tan'ik). Tending to relax tetanic muscular contraction.

antithenar (an-tē-thē'nar). Hypothenar (1).

antithermic (an-tē-ther'mik) [anti- + G. *thermē,* heat]. Rarely used term for antipyretic (1).

antithrombin (an-tē-throm'bin). Any substance that inhibits or prevents the effects of thrombin in such a manner that blood does not coagulate.

normal a., an a. naturally occurring in blood and certain tissues under normal conditions in contrast to abnormal states or a. from other sources.

antithyroid (an-tē-thī'royd). Relating to an agent that suppresses thyroid function.

antitonic (an-tē-ton'ik). Diminishing muscular or vascular tonus.

antitoxic (an-tē-tok'sik). Neutralizing the action of a poison; specifically, relating to an antitoxin. See also antidotal.

antitoxigen (an-tē-toks'i-jen). Antitoxinogen.

antitoxin (an-tē-tok'sin) [anti- + G. *toxicon,* poison]. Antibody formed in response to antigenic poisonous substances of biologic origin, such as bacterial exotoxins (*e.g.,* those elaborated by *Clostridium tetani* or *Corynebacterium diphtheriae*), phytotoxins, and zootoxins; in general usage, a. refers to whole, or globulin fraction of, serum from animals (usually horses) immunized by injections of the specific toxoid. A. neutralizes the pharmacologic effects of its specific toxin *in vitro,* and also *in vivo* if the toxin is not already fixed in the tissue cells; the combination of a. with toxin does not necessarily result in destruction of either substance, and the union may frequently be dissociated by means of appropriate procedures.

bivalent gas gangrene a., a. specific for the toxins of *Clostridium perfringens* and *C. septicum.*

bothropic a., Bothrops a., a. specific for the venom of pit vipers of the genus *Bothrops* (*Bothrophora*) of the family Crotalidae.

botulism a., botulinum a., a. specific for a toxin of one or another strain of *Clostridium botulinum.*

bovine a., a. prepared from cattle instead of horses, used in the treatment of persons who are sensitive to horse serum; the cattle are immunized against the toxin for which specific a. is desired.

Crotalus a., a. specific for venom of rattlesnakes (*Crotalus* species).

despeciated a., an antitoxic serum treated in an appropriate manner to alter the species-specific protein, so that a person sensitized to the animal protein is not likely to have a serious reaction when the a. is administered.

diphtheria a., a. specific for the toxin of *Corynebacterium diphtheriae.*

dysentery a., a. specific for the neurotoxin of *Shigella dysenteriae.*
gas gangrene a., pentavalent gas gangrene a.; a. specific for the toxin of one or more species of *Clostridium* that cause gaseous gangrene and associated toxemia, especially *C. perfringens* (*C. welchii*), *C. novyi, C. septicum, C. histolyticum,* and *C. oedematiens;* commercially available preparations are usually polyvalent, *i.e.,* contain a. for two or more species.
normal a., serum that is capable of neutralizing an equivalent quantity of a normal toxin solution.
pentavalent gas gangrene a., gas gangrene a.
plant a., a. specific for a phytotoxin.
scarlet fever a., a. specific for the erythrogenic toxin of strains of group A β-hemolytic streptococci.
staphylococcus a., a preparation from native serum containing antitoxic globulins or their derivatives that specifically neutralize the lethal, skin-necrosing, and hemolytic properties of the α-toxin of *Staphylococcus aureus.*
tetanus a., a. specific for the toxin of *Clostridium tetani.*
tetanus and gas gangrene a.'s, a solution of antitoxic substances obtained from animals immunized against the toxins of *Clostridium tetani, C. perfringens,* and *C. septicum.*
tetanus-perfringens a., an a. prepared from animals immunized against the toxins of *Clostridium tetani* and *C. perfringens* (*C. welchii*).

antitoxinogen (an'tē-tok-sin'ō-jen) [antitoxin + G. *-gen,* producing]. Antitoxigen; any antigen that stimulates the formation of antitoxin in an animal or person, *i.e.,* a toxin or a toxoid.

antitragicus (an'tē-traj'i-kŭs). See *musculus* antitragicus.

antitragohelicine (an'tē-trā'gō-hel'i-sēn). See *fissura* antitragohelicina.

antitragus (an-tē-trā'gŭs) [G. *anti-tragos,* the eminence of the external ear, fr. *anti,* opposite, + *tragos,* a goat, the tragus] [NA]. A projection of the cartilage of the auricle, in front of the cauda helicis, just above the lobule, and posterior to the tragus from which it is separated by the intertragic notch.

antitreponemal (an'tē-trep-ō-nē'măl). Treponemicidal.

antitrismus (an-tē-triz'mŭs). A condition of tonic muscular spasm preventing closure of the mouth.

antitrope (an'ti-trōp) [anti- + G. *tropē,* a turn]. An organ or appendage that forms a symmetrically reversed pair with another of the same type, *e.g.,* the right and left legs of a vertebrate.

antitropic (an-tē-trō'pik). Similar, bilaterally symmetrical, but in an opposite location (as in a mirror image), *e.g.,* the right thumb in relation to the left thumb.

antitrypsic (an-tē-trip'sik). Antitryptic.

antitrypsin (an-tē-trip'sin). A substance that inhibits or prevents the action of trypsin.

α-1-antitrypsin. Human α_1-proteinase inhibitor; α_1-trypsin inhibitor; a glycoprotein that is the major protease inhibitor of human serum, is synthesized in the liver, and is genetically polymorphic due to the presence of over 20 alleles; individuals appropriately homozygous are deficient in α-1-trypsin and are predisposed to pulmonary emphysema and juvenile hepatic cirrhosis because of alterations in the amino acid and sialic acid components of the glycoprotein.

antitryptic (an-tē-trip'tik). Antitrypsic; possessing properties of antitrypsin.

antitumorigenesis (an'tē-tū-mōr-i-jen'ĕ-sis). Inhibition of the development of a neoplasm.

antitussive (an-tē-tŭs'iv) [anti- + L. *tussis,* cough]. Antibechic. **1.** Relieving cough. **2.** A cough remedy.

antityphoid (an-tē-tī'foyd). Preventive or curative of typhoid fever.

antivenene (an-tē-ven'ēn). Antivenin.

antivenereal (an'tē-ve-nē'rē-ăl). Preventive or curative of venereal diseases.

antivenin (an-tē-ven'in) [anti- + L. *venenum,* poison]. Antivenene; an antitoxin specific for an animal or insect venom.

antiviral (an-tē-vī'răl). Opposing a virus; weakening or abolishing its action.

antivitamin (an-tē-vī'tă-min). A substance that prevents a vitamin from exerting its typical biological effects. Most a.'s have chemical structures similar to vitamins (*e.g.,* pyridoxine and its a., deoxypyridoxine) and appear to function as competitive antagonists; some a.'s produce effects, in addition, that are unrelated to vitamin antagonism.

antivivisection (an'tē-viv-i-sek'shŭn). Opposition to the use of living animals for experimentation. See vivisection.

antixerophthalmic (an'tē-zē-rof-thal'mik) [anti- + G. *xēros,* dry, + *ophthalmos,* eye]. Denoting agents (vitamin A and retinoic acid) that inhibit pathologic drying of the conjunctiva (xerophthalmia).

antixerotic (an'tē-zē-rot'ik). Preventing xerosis.

Anton, Gabriel, German neuropsychiatrist, 1858–1933. See A.'s *syndrome.*

Antoni, Nils, Swedish neurologist, 1887–1968. See A. types A and B *neurilemoma.*

antra (an'tră). Plural of antrum.

antral (an'trăl). Relating to an antrum.

antrectomy (an-trek'tō-mē) [antrum + G. *ektomē,* excision]. **1.** Removal of the walls of an antrum. **2.** Removal of the antrum (distal half) of the stomach; often combined with bilateral excision of portions of vagus nerve trunks (vagectomy) in treatment of peptic ulcer.

antro- [L. *antrum,* from G. *antron,* a cave]. Combining form denoting relationship to any antrum.

antroduodenectomy (an'trō-dū-ō-dē-nek'tō-mē). Surgical removal of the antrum of the stomach and the ulcer-bearing part of the duodenum.

antronasal (an-trō-nā'săl). Relating to a maxillary sinus and the corresponding nasal cavity.

antrophose (an'trō-fōz) [antro- + G. *phos,* light]. A subjective sensation of light or color originating in the visual centers of the brain. See also phosphene.

antropyloric (an'trō-pī-lōr'ik). Related to or affecting the antrum pyloricum.

antroscope (an'trō-skōp) [antro- + G. *skopeō,* to view]. An instrument to aid in the ocular examination of any cavity, particularly the antrum of Highmore.

antroscopy (an-tros'cō-pē). Examination of any cavity, especially of the antrum of Highmore, by means of an antroscope.

antrostomy (an-tros'tō-mē) [antro- + G. *stoma,* mouth]. Formation of an opening into any antrum.
intraoral a., Caldwell-Luc *operation.*

antrotomy (an-trot'ō-mē) [antro- + G. *tomē,* incision]. Incision through the wall of any antrum.

antrotonia (an-trō-tō'nē-ă). Tonus of the muscular walls of an antrum, such as that of the stomach.

antrotympanic (an'trō-tim-pan'ik). Relating to the mastoid antrum and the tympanic cavity.

antrum, gen. **antri,** pl. **antra** (an'trŭm, -trī, -tră) [L. fr. G. *antron,* a cave]. **1** [NA]. Any nearly closed cavity, particularly one with bony walls. **2.** The pyloric end of the stomach, partially shut off, during digestion, from the cardiac end, or fundus, by the prepyloric sphincter.
a. au'ris, *meatus* acusticus externus.

a. cardi'acum, forestomach; a dilation that occasionally occurs in the esophagus near the stomach.
antra ethmoida'le, *sinus* ethmoidales.
follicular a., the cavity of an ovarian follicle filled with liquor folliculi.
a. of Highmore, *sinus* maxillaris.
mastoid a., a. mastoideum.
a. mastoid'eum [NA], mastoid or tympanic a.; Valsalva's a.; a cavity in the petrous portion of the temporal bone, communicating posteriorly with the mastoid cells and anteriorly with the epitympanic recess of the middle ear.
maxillary a., *sinus* maxillaris.
pyloric a., a. pyloricum.
a. pylor'icum [NA], pyloric a.; lesser cul-de-sac; a bulging of the pyloric end of the stomach wall along the greater curvature when the organ is distended. See antrum (2).
tympanic a., a. mastoideum.
Valsalva's a., a. mastoideum.

ANTU Abbreviation for α-naphthylthiourea.

Antyllus, Greek physician, *ca.* 150 A.D. See A.'s *method.*

ANUG Abbreviation for acute necrotizing ulcerative *gingivitis.*

anulus, pl. **anuli** (an'yū-lŭs, -lī) [L.] [NA]. Official alternative term for annulus.
a. conjuncti'vae [NA], official alternate term for *annulus* conjunctivae.
a. femora'lis [NA], official alternate term for *annulus* femoralis.
a. fibrocartilagin'eus [NA], official alternate term for *annulus* fibrocartilagineus.
a. fibro'sus [NA], official alternate term for *annulus* fibrosus.
a. inguina'lis profun'dus [NA], official alternate term for *annulus* inguinalis profundus.
a. inguina'lis superficia'lis [NA], official alternate term for *annulus* inguinalis superficialis.
a. lymphat'icus car'diae [NA], official alternate term for *annulus* lymphaticus cardiae.
a. tendin'eus commu'nis [NA], official alternate term for *annulus* tendineus communis.
a. tympan'icus [NA], official alternate term for *annulus* tympanicus.
a. umbilica'lis [NA], official alternate term for *annulus* umbilicalis.

anuresis (an-yū-rē'sis) [G. *an-* priv. + *ourēsis,* urination]. Inability to pass urine.

anuretic (an-yū-ret'ik). Relating to anuresis.

anuria (an-yū'rē-ă). Absence of urine formation.

anuric (an-yūr'ik). Relating to anuria.

anus, gen. **ani,** pl. **anus** (ā'nŭs, -nī, -nŭs) [L.] [NA]. Anal orifice; fundament (2); the lower opening of the digestive tract, lying in the fold between the nates, through which fecal matter is extruded.
artificial a., an opening into the bowel, usually in the right or left flank, as a result of a colostomy.
Bartholin's a., a. cerebri.
a. cer'ebri, Bartholin's a.; aditus ad aqueductum cerebri; entrance to the cerebral aqueduct (of Sylvius) from the caudal part of the third ventricle.
imperforate a., anal *atresia.*
a. vesica'lis, rectal emptying into the urinary bladder.
vestibular a., vulvovaginal a., a congenital malformation in which the a. is imperforate, but the rectum opens into the vagina just above the vulva.

an'vil. Incus.

anxiety (ang-zī'ĕ-tē) [L. *anxietas,* anxiety, fr. *anxius,* distressed, fr. *ango,* to press tight, to torment]. **1.** Apprehension of danger and dread accompanied by restlessness, tension, tachycardia, and dyspnea unattached to a clearly identifiable stimulus. **2.** In experimental psychology, a drive or motivational state learned from previously neutral cues.
castration a., castration *complex.*
free-floating a., in psychoanalysis, a pervasive unrealistic expectation unattached to a clearly formulated concept or object of fear; observed particularly in a. neurosis and may be seen in some cases of latent schizophrenia.
noetic a., in existential psychotherapy, a. caused by confusion or loss of meaning in life.
separation a., a child's apprehension or fear associated with removal from or loss of a parent or significant other.
situation a., a. related to current life problems.

anxiolytic (ang'zē-ō-lit'ik) [anxiety + G. *lysis,* a dissolution or loosening]. **1.** Antianxiety *agent.* **2.** Denoting the actions of such an agent.

AOC Abbreviation for anodal opening *contraction.*

aorta, gen. and pl. **aortae** (ā-ōr'tă, ā-ōr'tē) [Mod. L. fr. G. *aortē,* from *aeirō,* to lift up] [NA]. A large artery of the elastic type which is the main trunk of the systemic arterial system, arising from the base of the left ventricle and ending at the left side of the body of the fourth lumbar vertebra by dividing to form the right and left common iliac arteries. The a. is formed from: pars ascendens aortae; arcus aortae; and pars descendens aortae, which is divided into the pars thoracica aortae and the pars abdominalis aortae. See entries at pars and arcus.
a. abdomina'lis, *pars abdominalis* aortae. See under pars.
a. angus'ta, congenital narrowness of a.
a. ascen'dens, *pars ascendens* aortae. See under pars.
buckled a., pseudocoarctation.
a. descen'dens, *pars descendens* aortae. See under pars.
dynamic a., abnormally marked pulsations of abdominal a.
kinked a., pseudocoarctation.
overriding a., a congenitally malpositioned a. whose origin straddles the ventricular septum and so receives ejected blood from the right ventricle as well as from the left; it is found especially in tetralogy of Fallot.
primitive a., the paired aortic primordia in young embryos.
a. thorac'ica, *pars thoracica* aortae. See under pars.
ventral a.'s, the paired vessels ventral to the pharynx, which give rise to the aortic arches.

aortal (ā-ōr'tăl). Aortic.

aortalgia (ā-ōr-tal'jē-ă) [aorta + G. *algos,* pain]. Pain assumed to be due to aneurysm or other pathologic conditions of the aorta.

aortarctia (ā-ōr-tark'shē-ă) [aorta + L. *arcto,* properly *arto,* to narrow]. Aortostenosis.

aortartia (ā-ōr-tar'shē-ă). Aortostenosis.

aortectasis, aortectasia (ā-ōr-tek'tă-sis, -tek-tā'zē-ă) [aorta + G. *ektasis,* a stretching]. Dilation of aorta.

aortectomy (ā-ōr-tek'tō-mē) [aorta + G. *ektomē,* excision]. Excision of a portion of the aorta.

aortic (ā-ōr'tik). Aortal; relating to the aorta or the a. orifice of the left ventricle of the heart.

aorticorenal (ā-ōr'ti-kō-rē'năl). Related to the aorta and kidney, specifically the ganglion aorticorenale.

aortismus abdominalis (ā-ōr-tis'mŭs ab-dō-mi-nā'lis) [L.]. Phantom *aneurysm.*

aortitis (ā-ōr-tī'tis). Inflammation of the aorta.
giant cell a., giant cell arteritis involving the aorta.
syphilitic a., the commonest manifestation of tertiary syphilis, involving the thoracic aorta, where destruction of elastic tissue in the media results in dilation and aneurysm formation.

aortocoronary (ā-ōr'tō-kōr'ō-nār-ē). Relating to the aorta and the coronary arteries.

aortogram (ā-ōr′tō-gram). X-ray demonstration of the aorta after the injection of contrast medium (may be direct puncture or intravenous).

aortography (ā-ōr-tog′ră-fē) [aorta + G. *graphō,* to write]. Radiographic visualization of the aorta and its branches by injection of contrast medium using percutaneous puncture or catheterization technique.
retrograde a., a. by the injection of the contrast medium into the aorta through one of its branches; that is, in a direction against the blood stream; *e.g.,* the brachial branch.
translumbar a., a. by injection into the abdominal aorta through a needle just below the twelfth rib and four fingerbreadths to the left of the spinal processes of the vertebrae.

aortopathy (ā-ōr-top′ă-thē) [aorta + G. *pathos,* suffering]. Disease affecting the aorta.

aortoplasty (ā-ōr′tō-plas′tē). A procedure for surgical repair of the aorta.

aortoptosia, aortoptosis (ā-ōr-top-tō′zē-ă, -top-tō′sis) [aorta + G. *ptōsis,* a failing]. A sinking down of the abdominal aorta in splanchnoptosia.

aortorrhaphy (ā-ōr-tōr′ă-fē) [aorta + G. *rhaphē,* seam]. Suture of the aorta.

aortosclerosis (ā-ōr′tō-skler-ō′sis). Arteriosclerosis of the aorta.

aortostenosis (ā-ōr-tō-stĕ-nō′sis) [aorta + G. *stenōsis,* a narrowing]. Aortarctia; aortartia; narrowing of the aorta.

aortotomy (ā-ōr-tot′ō-mē) [aorta + G. *tomē,* a cutting]. Incision of the aorta.

APA Abbreviation for antipernicious anemia *factor.*

apallesthesia (ă-pal-es-thē′zē-ă) [G. *a-* priv. + *pallo,* to tremble, quiver, + *aisthēsis,* feeling]. Pallanesthesia.

apallic (ă-pal′ik) [G. *a-* priv. + L. *pallium,* brain mantle (cerebral cortex)]. Denoting a state of unresponsiveness due to diffuse cortical or brainstem damage, as in a persistent vegetative state. See also vegetative (1).

apancreatic (ă-pan-krē-at′ik). Without a pancreas.

aparalytic (ă-par′ă-lit′ik). Not paralyzed; without paralysis.

aparathyroidism (ă-par-ă-thī′royd-izm). Congenital absence of the parathyroid glands, with an extreme degree of hypoparathyroidism.

apareunia (ă-par-yū′nē-ă) [G. *a-* priv. + *para,* alongside, + *eunē,* bed]. Absence or impossibility of coitus.

apathetic (ap-ă-thet′ik). Exhibiting apathy; indifferent.

apathism (ap′ă-thizm). A sluggishness of reaction. *Cf.* erethism.

apathy (ap′ă-thē) [G. *apatheia,* fr. *a-* priv. + *pathos,* suffering]. Absence of emotion, with reduced activity; indifference; insensibility.

apatite (ap′ă-tīt). Generic name for a class of minerals with compositions that are variants of the formula D_5T_3M, where D is a divalent cation, T is a trivalent tetrahedral compound ion, and M is a monovalent anion; calcium phosphate a.'s are important mineral constituents of bones and teeth. See fluoroapatite, hydroxyapatite.

apazone (ap′ă-zōn). Azapropazone; 5-(dimethylamino)-9-methyl-2-propyl-1*H*-pyrazolo[1,2-*a*][1,2,4]benzotriazine-1,3(2*H*)-dione; an anti-inflammatory agent.

APC Abbreviation for *a*cetylsalicylic acid, *p*henacetin, and *c*affeine combined as an antipyretic and analgesic; antigen-presenting *cell.*

apeidosis (ap-ī-dō′sis) [G. *apo,* away, + *eidos,* form]. Departure from the normal histologic picture or the characteristic manifestations of a disease.

apellous (ă-pel′ŭs) [G. *a-* priv. + L. *pellis,* skin]. **1.** Without skin. **2.** Without foreskin; circumcised.

apenteric (ap-en-ter′ik) [G. *apo,* from, + *enteron,* intestine]. Abenteric; away from the intestine, said of a morbid process occurring elsewhere which would normally occur in the intestine.

apepsinia (ā-pep-sin′ē-ă). Rarely used term for lack of pepsin in the gastric juice.

aperiodic (ā-pēr-ē-od′ik). Not occurring periodically.

aperistalsis (ā′per-i-stal′sis). Absence of peristalsis.

aperitive (ă-per′i-tiv) [Fr. *apéritif,* from L. *aperio,* to open]. Stimulating the appetite.

Apert, Eugène, French pediatrician, 1868–1940. See A.'s *hirsutism, syndrome;* A.-Crouzon *syndrome.*

apertognathia (ă-per-tō-nath′ē-ă) [L. *apertus,* open, + G. *gnathos,* jaw]. Open bite (2); an open bite deformity, a type of malocclusion characterized by premature posterior occlusion and absence of anterior occlusion.

apertometer (ap-er-tom′ĕ-ter). Instrument for measuring the angular aperture of a microscope objective.

apertura, pl. aperturae (ap-er-tū′ră, -rē) [L. fr. *aperio,* pp. *apertus,* to open] [NA]. Aperture (1); opening; in anatomy, an open gap or hole.
a. exter′na aqueduc′tus vestib′uli [NA], the external opening of the vestibular aqueduct on the posterior surface of the petrous part of the temporal bone near the groove for the sigmoid sinus.
a. exter′na canalic′uli coch′leae [NA], the external opening of the cochlear aqueduct on the temporal bone medial to the jugular fossa.
a. latera′lis ventric′uli quar′ti [NA], lateral aperture of the fourth ventricle; foramen lateralis ventriculi quarti; foramen of Luschka, of Retzius, or of Key-Retzius; one of the two lateral openings of the fourth ventricle into the subarachnoid space.
a. media′na ventric′uli quar′ti [NA], median aperture of the fourth ventricle; arachnoid foramen; foramen of Magendie; metapore; the large midline opening in the posterior inferior part of the roof of the fourth ventricle, connecting the ventricle with the cerebellomedullary cistern.
a. pel′vis infe′rior [NA], a. pelvis minoris; pelvic outlet; pelvic plane of outlet; fourth parallel pelvic plane; inferior strait; plane of outlet; the lower opening of the true pelvis, bounded anteriorly by the pubic arch, laterally by the rami of the ischium and the sacrotuberous ligament on either side, and posteriorly by these ligaments and the tip of the coccyx.
a. pel′vis mino′ris, a. pelvis inferior.
a. pel′vis supe′rior [NA], pelvic plane of inlet; aditus pelvis; first parallel pelvic plane; superior strait; pelvic brim or inlet; plane of inlet; the upper opening of the true pelvis, bounded anteriorly by the pubic symphysis and the pubic crest on either side, laterally by the iliopectineal lines, and posteriorly by the promontory of the sacrum.
a. pirifor′mis [NA], piriform opening; the anterior nasal opening in the skull.
a. si′nus fronta′lis [NA], frontal sinus aperture; one of a pair of openings on the nasal part of the frontal bone through which the frontal sinuses communicate with the ethmoidal infundibulum.
a. si′nus sphenoidal′is [NA], sphenoidal sinus aperture; one of the pair of openings in the body of the sphenoid bone through which the sphenoid sinuses communicate with the sphenoethmoidal recess of the nasal cavity.
a. thora′cis infe′rior [NA], inferior thoracic aperture; the inferior boundary of the bony thorax composed of the twelfth thoracic vertebra and the lower margins of the rib cage and sternum.
a. thora′cis supe′rior [NA], superior thoracic aperture; the upper boundary of the bony thorax composed of the first thoracic vertebra and the upper margins of the first ribs and manubrium of the sternum.
a. tympan′ica canalic′uli chor′dae tym′pani [NA], tympanic

opening of canal for chorda tympani; the opening of the canal for the chorda tympani into the middle ear.

aperture (ap'er-chūr) [L. *apertura,* an opening]. **1.** Apertura. **2.** The diameter of the objective of a microscope.
angular a., the angle, in air, of light which passes from the object to the ends of the diameter of the front lens of the microscope objective.
frontal sinus a., *apertura* sinus frontalis.
inferior thoracic a., *apertura* thoracis inferior.
lateral a. of the fourth ventricle, *apertura* lateralis ventriculi quarti.
median a. of the fourth ventricle, *apertura* mediana ventriculi quarti.
numerical a. (N.A.), defined by the formula *n* sine *a,* where *n* is the refractive index of the medium between the object and objective lens and *a* is the angle between the central and the marginal ray entering the objective.
sphenoidal sinus a., *apertura* sinus sphenoidalis.
superior thoracic a., *apertura* thoracis superior.

apex, gen. **apicis,** pl. **apices** (ā'peks, ap'i-sis, ap'i-sēs) [L. summit or tip] [NA]. The extremity of a conical or pyramidal structure, such as the heart or the lung.
a. of arytenoid cartilage, a. cartilaginis arytenoideae.
a. auric'ulae [NA], tip of the auricle; a. satyri; a point projecting upward and posteriorly from the free outcurved margin of the helix a little posterior to its upper end.
a. cap'itis fib'ulae [NA], a. of head of fibula; styloid process of fibula; the pointed upper end of the fibular head to which is attached the arcuate popliteal ligament and part of the biceps femoris tendon.
a. cartila'ginis arytenoi'deae [NA], a. of arytenoid cartilage; the pointed upper end of the cartilage which supports the corniculate cartilage and the aryepiglottic fold.
a. cor'dis [NA], a. of heart; mucro cordis; vertex cordis; the blunt extremity of the heart formed by the left ventricle. See apex *beat.*
a. cor'nus posterio'ris [NA], tip of the posterior horn; caput cornus; the pointed extremity of each posterior gray column or cornu of the spinal cord.
a. cus'pidis den'tis [NA], a. of cusp of tooth.
a. of dens, a. dentis.
a. den'tis [NA], a. of dens; the tip of the dens of the axis to which is attached the apical ligament of the dens.
a. of head of fibula, a. capitis fibulae.
a. of heart, a. cordis.
a. lin'guae [NA], tip of tongue.
a. of lung, a. pulmonis.
a. na'si [NA], tip of nose.
orbital a., the posterior part of the orbit into which the optic canal opens.
a. os'sis sa'cri [NA], a. of sacrum; the tapering lower end of the sacrum that articulates with the coccyx.
a. par'tis petro'sae [NA], a. of petrous part of temporal bone; the blunt medial extremity of the petrous part on which the carotid canal opens.
a. of patella, a. patellae.
a. patel'lae [NA], a. of patella; the pointed lower end of the patella from which the ligamentum patellae passes to insert on the tibial tuberosity.
a. of petrous part of temporal bone, a. partis petrosae.
a. prosta'tae [NA], a. of prostate; the lowermost part of the prostate, situated above the urogenital diaphragm.
a. of prostate, a. prostatae.
a. pulmo'nis [NA], a. of lung; the rounded, upper extremity of each lung that extends into the cupula of the pleura.
a. rad'icis den'tis [NA], root a.; root tip; the tip of a tooth root, the part farthest from the incisal or occlusal side.
root a., a. radicis dentis.
a. of sacrum, a. ossis sacri.
a. sat'yri, a. auriculae.
a. of urinary bladder, a. vesicae.
a. vesi'cae [NA], a. of urinary bladder; the junction of the superior and anteroinferior surfaces of the bladder, continuous above with the median umbilical ligament.

apexcardiogram (ā-peks-kar'dē-ō-gram). Graphic recording of the movements of the chest wall produced by the apex beat of the heart.

apexification (ā-pek'si-fi-kā'shŭn). Induced tooth root development or closure of the root apex by hard tissue deposition.

apexigraph (ā-pek'si-graf) [apex + G. *graphō,* to write]. A device for determining the size and position of the apex of a tooth root.

APF Abbreviation for animal protein *factor.*

Apgar, Virginia, U.S. anesthesiologist, 1909–1974. See A. *score.*

aphagia (ă-fā'jē-ă) [G. *a-* priv. + *phagein,* to eat]. Dysphagia.
a. al'gera, failure to eat or swallow because it causes pain.

aphakia (ă-fā'kē-ă) [G. *a-* priv. + *phakos,* lentil, anything shaped like a lentil]. Absence of the lens of the eye.

aphakial, aphakic (ă-fā'kē-ăl, ă-fā'kik). Denoting aphakia.

aphalangia (ă-fă-lan'jē-ă) [G. *a-* priv. + phalanx]. Congenital absence of a digit, or more specifically, absence of one or more of the long bones (phalanges) of a finger or toe.

aphanisis (ă-fan'i-sis) [G. *aphaneia,* disappearance]. Loss of sexuality.

aphasia (ă-fā'zē-ă) [G. speechlessness, fr. *a-* priv. + *phasis,* speech]. Alogia (1); anepia; logagnosia; logamnesia; logasthenia; impaired or absent comprehension of or communication by speech, writing, or signs, due to dysfunction of brain centers in the dominant hemisphere.
acoustic a., auditory a.
acquired epileptic a., Landau-Kleffner *syndrome.*
amnestic a., amnesic a., inability to find or remember words.
anomic a., nominal a.
associative a., conduction a.
ataxic a., motor a.
auditory a., word deafness; acoustic a.; an impairment in comprehension of the auditory forms of language and communication in the presence of normal hearing.
Broca's a., motor a.
conduction a., associative a.; a form of a. in which the subject can speak and write, but skips or repeats words or substitutes one word for another, the lesion being in the association tracts connecting the various language centers.
expressive a., motor a.
functional a., a. related to conversion hysteria.
global a., total a.; loss of all forms of communication.
graphic a., graphomotor a., cerebral *agraphia.*
impressive a., sensory a.
jargon a., a. in which the patient talks in nonsense syllables or in which several words are run together as one.
Kussmaul's a., mutism in psychosis.
mixed a., a mixture of motor and sensory a.
motor a., ataxic, expressive, or Broca's a.; any of the varieties of a. in which the power of expression by writing, speaking, or signs is lost.
nominal a., anomic a.; anomia; a. in which the patient has difficulty in recalling or is unable to recall the names of persons and things.
pathematic a., mutism related to anger or strong emotions.
psychosensory a., inability to comprehend written or spoken words.
pure a.'s, rare a.'s affecting one type of communication, *e.g.,* read-

ing, while related communication forms such as writing, auditory comprehension, etc. remain intact.
receptive a., sensory a.
semantic a., a. in which objects are correctly named; there is little disturbance in the articulation of words; individual words are understood, but the broader meaning of what is heard cannot be grasped.
sensory a., impressive or receptive a.; loss of the ability to comprehend written, printed, or spoken words.
syntactical a., a. in which the words are fairly well pronounced but are spoken in short phrases or poorly constructed sentences without articles, prepositions, or conjunctions.
total a., global a.
transcortical a., a. caused by damage to association pathways.
visual a., **(1)** alexia; **(2)** improperly used as a synonym for anomia.
Wernicke's a., auditory a. and nominal a.

aphasiac, aphasic (ă-fā'zē-ak, ă-fā'sik). Relating to or suffering from aphasia.

aphasiologist (ă-fā'zē-ol'ō-gist). A specialist in speech disorders due to dysfunction of the dominant hemisphere.

aphasiology (ă-fā'zē-ol'ō-gē). The science of disorders of speech.

aphasmid (ā-faz'mid). **1.** Lacking phasmids, as seen in nematodes of the class Adenophorasida (Aphasmidia). **2.** Common name for a member of the class Aphasmidia, now Adenophorasida.

Aphasmidia (ā-faz-mid'ē-ă). Adenophorasida.

apheliotropism (ap-hē-lē-ot'rō-pizm) [G. *apo*, away, + *helios*, sun, + *tropein*, to turn]. Negative heliotaxis.

aphemesthesia (ă-fē-mes-thē'zē-ă) [G. *a-* priv. + *phēmē*, speech, + *aisthēsis*, sensation]. Loss of the sense of articulate speech; inability to recognize what oneself is saying.

aphemia (ă-fē'mē-ă) [a- priv. + G. *phēmē*, voice]. Obsolete term for a form of motor aphasia in which the ability to express ideas in spoken words is lost.

aphemic (ă-fē'mik). Relating to aphemia.

aphephobia (a-fē-fō'bē-ă) Haphephobia.

apheresis (ā-fer-ē'sis) [G. *aphairesis*, withdrawal]. Infusion of a patient's own blood from which certain cellular or fluid elements have been removed.

aphilopony (ā-fil-op'ō-nē) [G. *a-* priv. + *philō*, to like, + *ponos*, work]. Obsolete term for an aversion, or lack of desire, to work.

aphonia (ă-fō'nē-ă) [G. *a-* priv. + *phōnē*, voice]. Anaudia; loss of the voice as a result of disease or injury of the organ of speech.
hysterical a., loss of voice for psychogenic reasons, as in some varieties of hysteria.
a. paralyt'ica, a. due to paralysis of the vocal cords.
spastic a., a spasmodic contraction of the adductor muscles excited by an attempt at phonation.

aphonic (ă-fon'ik). Aphonous; relating to aphonia.

aphonogelia (ă-fon-ō-jē'lē-ă) [G. *a-* priv. + *phonē*, sound, + *gelān*, to laugh]. Inability to laugh out loud.

aphonous (af'ō-nŭs). Aphonic.

aphotesthesia (ă-fō-tes-thē'zē-ă) [G. *a-* priv. + *phōs*, light, + *aisthēsis*, perception]. Decreased sensitivity of the retina to light caused by excessive exposure to sunlight.

aphrasia (ă-frā'zē-ă) [G. *a-* priv. + *phrasis*, speaking]. Inability to speak, from any cause.

aphrodisia (af-rō-diz'ē-ă) [G. *aphrodisios*, relating to Aphrodite]. Sexual desire, especially when excessive.

aphrodisiac (af-rō-diz'ē-ak). **1.** Increasing sexual desire. **2.** Anything that arouses or increases sexual desire.

aphrodisiomania (af-rō-diz'ē-ō-mā'nē-ă) [G. *aphrodisia*, sexual pleasures, + *mania*, insanity]. Abnormal and excessive erotic interest.

aphtha, pl. aphthae (af'thă, af'thē) [G. ulceration]. **1.** In the singular, a small ulcer(s) on a mucous membrane. **2.** In the plural, stomatitis charactized by intermittent episodes of painful oral ulcers of unknown etiology that are covered by gray exudate, are surrounded by an erythematous halo, and range from several millimeters to 2 cm in diameter; they are limited to oral mucous membranes that are not bound to periosteum, occur as solitary or multiple lesions, and heal spontaneously in one to two weeks. Also called aphthae minor, recurrent aphthous stomatitis or ulcers; recurrent ulcerative stomatitis; aphthous or ulcerative stomatitis; canker sores.
Bednar's aphthae, traumatic ulcers located bilaterally on either side of the midpalatal raphe in infants.
contagious aphthae, foot-and-mouth *disease.*
herpetiform aphthae, a variant of oral aphthae, of unknown etiology, characterized by up to several dozen ulcers, 2-3 mm in diameter, organized in a clustered herpetiform distribution.
aphthae ma'jor, periadenitis mucosa necrotica recurrens; recurrent scarring aphthae, Sutton's disease; Mikulicz' aphthae; a severe form of aphthae characterized by unusually numerous, large, deep, and frequent ulcers; healing may take as long as six weeks and results in scarring.
Mikulicz' aphthae, *periadenitis* mucosa necroticae recurrens.
aphthae mi'nor, aphthae (2).
recurrent scarring aphthae, aphthae major.

aphthoid (af'thoyd). Resembling aphthae.

aphthongia (af-thon'jē-ă) [G. *a-* priv. + *phthongos*, voice]. A spasm of the muscles of speech sometimes affecting public speakers; a variety of occupational neurosis analogous to writer's cramp.

aphthosis (af-thō'sis). Any condition characterized by the presence of aphthae.

aphthous (af'thŭs). Characterized by or relating to aphthae or aphthosis.

aphylactic (ā-fī-lak'tik). Pertaining to or characterized by aphylaxis.

aphylaxis (ā-fī-lak'sis) [G. *a-* priv. + *phylaxis*, a guarding]. Nonimmunity; lack of protection against disease.

apical (ap'i-kăl). Apicalis. **1.** Relating to the apex of a pyramidal or pointed structure. **2.** Situated nearer to the apex of a structure in relation to a specific reference point; opposite of basal.

apicalis (ap-i-kā'lis) [L.] [NA]. Apical.

apicectomy (ap-i-sek'tō-mē) [L. *apex*, summit or tip, + G. *ektomē*, excision]. **1.** Opening and exenteration of air cells in the apex of the petrous part of the temporal bone. **2.** In dental surgery, an obsolete synonym for apicoectomy.

apiceotomy (ă-pis-ē-ot'ō-mē). Apicotomy.

apices (ap'i-sēs). Plural of apex.

apicitis (ap-i-sī'tis). Inflammation of the apex of a structure or organ.

apico- [L. *apex*, summit or tip]. Combining form relating to any apex.

apicoectomy (ap'i-kō-ek'tō-mē) [apico- + G. *ektomē*, excision]. Root resection; surgical removal of a dental root apex.

apicolocator (ap'i-kō-lō'kā-tōr). A device for locating the root apex of a tooth.

apicolysis (ap-i-kol'i-sis) [apico- + G. *lysis*, destruction]. Surgical collapse of the upper portion of the lung by the operative detachment of the parietal pleura allowing a medial displacement of the pulmonary apex.

Apicomplexa (ap-i-kom-plek'să) [L. *apex*, pl. *apicis*, tip, summit, + *complexus*, woven together]. A phylum of the subkingdom Protozoa, which includes the class Sporozoea and the subclasses Coccidia and Piroplasmia, and is characterized by the presence of an apical complex.

apicostome (ap'i-kō-stōm). The trocar and cannula used in apicostomy.

apicostomy (ap-i-kos'tō-mē) [apico- + G. *stoma,* mouth]. An operation in which the labial or buccal alveolar plate is perforated with a trocar and cannula; done to reach the root apex and to take cultures from this area.

apicotomy (ap-i-kot'ō-mē) [apico- + G. *tomē,* a cutting]. Apiceotomy; incision into an apical structure.

apiculate (ā-pik'yū-lāt) [L. *apiculus,* a tip or point]. Terminated abruptly by a small point.

apiculus (ă-pik'yū-lŭs) [L.]. A short, sharp projection on one end of a fungus spore at the point of attachment, or on the wall, of a hypha or condiophore.

apicurettage (ap-i-kyū'rĕ-tahzh). Apical curettage after removal of an infected tooth.

apinealism (ă-pin'ē-al-izm). Congenital or acquired absence of the pineal gland.

apiphobia (ā-pi-fō'bē-ă) [L. *apis,* bee, + G. *phobos,* fear]. Melissophobia; morbid fear of bees.

apituitarism (ā-pi-tū'i-tăr-izm). Total lack of functional pituitary tissue; may be iatrogenic (*e.g.,* as a consequence of hypophysectomy) or the result of a spontaneous disease process.

aplacental (ā-pla-sen'tăl). Without a placenta; denoting the monotremes (which lay eggs and have no placenta) and the marsupials (which have a transitory simple yolk-sac placenta).

aplanatic (ap-la-nat'ik). Pertaining to aplanatism, or to an aplanatic lens.

aplanatism (ă-plan'ă-tizm) [G. *a-* priv. + *planētos,* wandering]. Freedom from spherical aberration; said of a lens.

aplasia (ă-plā'zē-ă) [G. *a-* priv. + *plasis,* a molding]. **1.** Defective development or congenital absence of an organ or tissue. **2.** In hematology, incomplete, retarded, or defective development, or cessation of the usual regenerative process.

congenital a. of thymus, *immunodeficiency* with hypoparathyroidism.

a. cu'tis congen'ita, congenital absence or deficiency of a localized area of skin, with the base of the defect covered by a thin translucent membrane; most often a single area near the vertex of the scalp, but may occur in other areas; underlying structures may also be affected.

germinal a., seminiferous tubule *dysgenesis.*

gonadal a., gonadal agenesis; congenital absence of essentially all gonadal tissue; the external genitalia and genital ducts are female, but if interstitial cells of Leydig are present, the external genitalia are commonly ambiguous and the genital ducts are female.

a. pilo'rum pro'pia, monilethrix.

pure red cell a., a transitory arrest of red blood cell production which may occur in the course of a hemolytic anemia, often preceded by infection, or as a complication of certain drugs; if the arrest persists anemia may result. See also congenital hypoplastic *anemia.*

aplastic (ā-plas'tik, ă-). Pertaining to aplasia, or conditions characterized by defective regeneration, as in a. anemia.

apleuria (ă-plūr'ē-ă). Congenital absence of one or more ribs; usually associated with absent transverse process or processes.

apnea (ap'nē-ă) [G. *apnoia,* want of breath]. Absence of breathing.

central a., a. as the result of medullary depression which inhibits respiratory movement.

deglutition a., inhibition of breathing during swallowing.

induced a., intentional respiratory arrest during general anesthesia produced by hypocapnia, a muscle relaxant drug, respiratory center depression, or sudden cessation of controlled respiration.

obstructive a., peripheral a., a. either as the result of obstruction of the air passages or inadequate respiratory muscle activity.

sleep a., a. caused by upper airway obstruction during sleep, associated with frequent awakening and often with daytime sleepiness. *Cf.* sleep-induced a.

sleep-induced a., Ondine's curse; a. resulting from failure of the respiratory center to stimulate adequate respiration during sleep; divided into respiratory pause (cessation of air flow for less than 10 seconds) and apneic pause (cessation of air flow greater than 10 seconds).

true a., a. vera.

vagal a., cessation of respiration during general anesthesia following stimulation of the vagus nerve in the chest above the heart level or in the cervical and higher regions.

a. ve'ra, true a.; absence of respiratory movements, owing to hypocapnia and the consequent lack of stimulus by carbon dioxide to the respiratory centers.

apneic (ap'nē-ik). Related to or suffering from apnea.

apneumatosis (ap-nū-mă-tō'sis) [G. *a*-priv. + *pneumatoō,* to inflate, + *-osis,* condition]. Congenital atelectasis.

apneumia (ap-nū'mē-ă) [G. *a-* priv. + *pneumōn,* lung]. Congenital absence of the lungs.

apneusis (ap-nū'sis) [G. *a-* priv. + *pneusis,* a breathing, fr. *pneō,* to breathe]. An abnormal form of respiration following experimental section of the pons just behind its anterior border and consisting of prolonged inspirations alternating with short expiratory movements.

apneustic (ap-nū'stik). Pertaining to apneusis.

apo- [G. *apo,* away from, off]. Combining form meaning, usually, separated from or derived from.

apobiosis (ap-ō-bī-ō'sis) [G. death, fr. *apo,* from, + *biōsis,* life]. Death, especially local death of a part of the organism.

apocarteresis (ap'ō-kar-ter-ē'sis) [G. *apocarterein,* to starve oneself to death]. Suicide by starvation.

apocleisis (ap-ō-klī'sis) [G. *apo,* away, + *kleisis,* closure]. Aversion to food.

apocrine (ap'ō-krin) [G. *apo-krinō,* to separate]. Denoting a mechanism of glandular secretion in which the apical portion of secretory cells is shed and incorporated into the secretion. See also a. *gland.*

apocrustic (ap-ō-krŭs'tik) [G. *apokroustikos,* able to beat off, fr. *apo,* off, + *krouō,* to strike]. **1.** Astringent and repellent. **2.** An agent with such action.

apodal (ă-pō'dal) [G. *a-* priv. + *pous,* foot]. Apodous; relating to apodia.

apodemialgia (ap'ō-dē-mē-al'jē-ă) [G. *apodēmia,* being away from home, + *algos,* pain]. Wanderlust; longing to get away from home or to travel. *Cf.* nostalgia.

apodia (ă-pō'dē-ă) [G. *a-* priv. + *pous,* foot]. Apody; congenital absence of feet.

apodous (ap'ō-dŭs). Apodal.

apody (ap'ō-dē). Apodia.

apoenzyme (ap'ō-en-zīm). The protein portion of an enzyme as contrasted with the nonprotein portion, or coenzyme, or prosthetic portion (if present).

apoferritin (ap-ō-fer'i-tin). A protein in the intestinal wall that combines with a ferric hydroxide-phosphate compound to form ferritin, the first stage in the absorption of iron.

apogamia, apogamy (ap-ō-gam'ē-ă, ă-pog'ă-mē) [G. *apo,* away, + *gamein,* to wed]. Parthenogenesis.

apolar (ā-pō-'lăr). Without poles; denoting specifically embryonic nerve cells (neuroblasts) that have not yet begun to sprout processes.

apolipoprotein (ap'ō-lip-ō-prō'tēn). The protein component of lipoprotein complexes which is a normal constituent of plasma chylomicrons, HDL, LDL, and VLDL in man.

apomixia (ap-ō-mik'sē-ă) [G. *apo,* from, + *mixis,* a mingling]. Parthenogenesis.

apomorphine hydrochloride (ap-ō-mōr'fēn). $C_{17}H_{17}NO_2$- HC1; a derivative of morphine used as an expectorant, emetic, and hypnotic.

aponeurectomy (ap'ō-nū-rek'tō-mē). Excision of an aponeurosis.

aponeurology (ap'ō-nū-rol'ō-jē). The branch of anatomy concerned with aponeuroses and their relations.

aponeurorrhaphy (ap'ō-nū-rōr'ă-fē) [aponeurosis + G. *rhaphē,* suture]. Fasciorrhaphy.

aponeurosis, pl. **aponeuroses** (ap'ō-nū-rō'sis, -sēz) [G. the end of the muscle where it becomes tendon, fr. *apo,* from, + *neuron,* sinew] [NA]. A fibrous sheet or expanded tendon, giving attachment to muscular fibers and serving as the means of origin or insertion of a flat muscle; it sometimes also performs the office of a fascia for other muscles.

bicipital a., a. bicipita'lis, a. musculi bicipitis brachii.

Denonvilliers' a., *septum* rectovesicale.

epicranial a., a. epicranialis.

a. epicrania'lis [NA], epicranial a.; *galea* aponeurotica.

extensor a., a triangular tendinous expansion including the tendon of the extensor digitorum centrally, interosseus tendons on each side, and a lumbrical tendon laterally. It covers the dorsal aspect of the metacarpophalangeal joint and the proximal phalanx.

a. of insertion, a tendinous sheet serving for the insertion of a broad muscle.

a. of investment, a fibrous membrane covering and keeping in place a muscle or group of muscles.

a. lin'guae [NA], lingual a.; the thickened lamina propria of the tongue to which the lingual muscles attach.

lingual a., a. linguae.

a. mus'culi bicip'itis bra'chii [NA], bicipital a.; a. bicipitalis; lacertus fibrosus; bicipital or semilunar fascia; radiating fibers from the tendon of insertion of the biceps passing obliquely over the hollow of the elbow to the ulnar side and becoming merged into the deep fascia of the forearm.

a. of origin, a tendinous expansion serving as the attachment of origin of a broad muscle.

a. palat'ina [NA], palatine a.; the expanded tendons of the tensor veli palatini muscles in the anterior two-thirds of the soft palate to which the other palatine muscles attach.

palatine a., a. palatina.

palmar a., a. palmaris.

a. palma'ris [NA], palmar a.; palmar fascia; Dupuytren's fascia; the thickened, central portion of the fascia ensheathing the hand; it radiates toward the bases of the fingers from the tendon of the palmaris longus muscle.

Petit's a., [P. Petit]. the posterior layer of the broad ligament of the uterus.

a. pharynge'a, *fascia* pharyngobasilaris.

plantar a., a. plantaris.

a. planta'ris [NA], plantar a.; plantar fascia; the very thick, central portion of the fascia investing the plantar muscles; it radiates toward the toes from the medial process of the calcaneal tuberosity and gives attachment to the short flexor muscle of the toes.

Sibson's a., *membrana* suprapleuralis.

temporal a., *fascia* temporalis.

thoracolumbar a., *fascia* thoracolumbalis.

aponeurositis (ap'ō-nū-rō-sī'tis). Inflammation of an aponeurosis.

aponeurotic (ap'ō-nū-rot'ik). Relating to an aponeurosis.

aponeurotome (ap-ō-nū'rō-tōm). Instrument for dividing an aponeurosis.

aponeurotomy (ap'ō-nū-rot'ō-mē). Incision of an aponeurosis.

apopathetic (ap'ō-pă-thet'ik) [G. *apo,* away, + *pathētikos,* relating to the feelings]. Denoting a form of behavior in which one conspicuously alters his conduct in the presence of other people.

apophylaxis (ap'ō-fī-lak'sis). A diminution of the phylactic power of the body fluids, as sometimes observed in the negative phase of therapy with immunizing agents.

apophysary (ă-pof'i-sā-rē). Apophysial.

apophysial, apophyseal (ă-pō-fiz'ē-ăl). Apophysary; relating to or resembling an apophysis.

apophysis, pl. **apophyses** (ă-pof'i-sis, -sēz) [G. an offshoot]. An outgrowth or projection, especially one from a bone. A bony process or outgrowth that lacks an independent center of ossification.

basilar a., *pars* basilaris ossis occipitales.

a. con'chae, *eminentia* conchae.

a. hel'icis, *spina* helicis.

Ingrassia's a., *ala* minor ossis sphenoidalis.

lenticular a., *processus* lenticularis.

temporal a., *processus* mastoideus.

apophysitis (ă-pof-i-sī'tis). Inflammation of any apophysis.

a. tibia'lis adolescen'tium, Osgood-Schlatter *disease.*

apoplasmia (ap-ō-plaz'mē-ă). A decrease in the amount of blood plasma.

apoplectic (ap-ŏ-plek'tik). Relating to, suffering from, or predisposed to apoplexy.

apoplectiform (ap-ŏ-plek'ti-fōrm). Apoplectoid.

apoplectoid (ap-ŏ-plek'toyd). Apoplectiform; resembling apoplexy.

apoplexy (ap'ŏ-plek-sē) [G. *apoplēxia*]. **1.** A classical but obsolete term for stroke due to intracerebral hemorrhage, but sometimes used for stroke due to cerebral thrombosis. **2.** Encephalorrhagia (2); an effusion of blood into a tissue or organ.

abdominal a., mesenteric hemorrhage, thrombosis, or embolus involving the mesenteric or abdominal blood vessels.

adrenal a., hemorrhage into the adrenal glands or thrombosis of the adrenal veins, followed by acute adrenal insufficiency, occurring in the Waterhouse-Friderichsen syndrome.

bulbar a., pontile a.; a. due to vascular lesion in the brainstem.

cutaneous a., sudden rush of blood to skin and subcutaneous tissue.

embolic a., a. caused by the plugging of an artery of the brain by an embolus.

functional a., a condition simulating a. without any cerebral lesion; a form of conversion hysteria.

heat a., **(1)** heatstroke; **(2)** ardent *fever.*

ingravescent a., the slowly progressive onset of stroke.

neonatal a., intracranial hemorrhage in newborn children.

pituitary a., spontaneous hemorrhage into or ischemic necrosis of a normal or adenomatous pituitary gland.

pontile a., bulbar a.

Raymond type of a., a form of ingravescent a. in which there is paresthesia of the hand on the side to become paralyzed.

serous a., a. due to edema or local exudation of serum.

spasmodic a., the occurrence of apoplectic symptoms caused by a temporary spasm of a cerebral artery.

spinal a., hematorrhachis.

splenic a., peracute anthrax often seen in ruminants, in which death occurs very quickly after the appearance of the first signs of the disease; grossly enlarged spleen and capillary hemorrhages are often the only lesions.

thrombotic a., stroke caused by cerebral thrombosis.

uteroplacental a., Couvelaire *uterus.*

apoprotein (ap-ō-prō'tēn). A polypeptide chain (protein) not yet complexed with the prosthetic group that is necessary to form the active holoprotein.

apoptosis (ap-ō-tō'sis, ap'op-tō'sis) [G. a falling or dropping off, fr. *apo,* off, + *ptosis,* a falling]. Cell deletion by fragmentation into membrane-bound particles which are phagocytosed by other cells.

aporepressor (ap'ō-rē-pres'er). Inactive *repressor.*

aporia (ă-pōr'ē-ă) [G. *aporia,* difficulty, doubt]. Doubt, especially deriving from incompatible views on the same subject.

aporioneurosis (ă-pōr'ē-ō-nū-rō'sis) [G. *aporia,* difficulty, doubt, + neurosis]. Obsolete term for anxiety *neurosis.*

aposome (ap'ō-sōm) [G. *apo,* from, + *sōma,* body]. A cytoplasmic inclusion produced by the cell itself.

apostaxis (ap-ō-staks'is) [G. a trickling down]. Slight hemorrhage, or bleeding by drops.

aposthia (ă-pos'thē-ă) [G. *a-* priv. + *posthē,* foreskin]. Congenital absence of the prepuce.

apostilb (ap'ō-stilb) [G. *apo,* from + *stilbe,* lamp]. A unit of brightness equal to 0.1 millilambert.

apothanasia (ap'-ō-thă-nā'zē-ă) [G. *apo,* away, + *thanatos,* death]. Postponement of death; prolongation of life, as opposed to euthanasia.

apothecary (ă-poth'ĕ-kār-ē) [G. *apothēkē,* a barn, storehouse, fr. *apo,* from, + *thēkē,* a box]. Obsolescent term for pharmacist or druggist.

apothem, apotheme (ap'ō-them, ap'ō-thēm) [G. *apo,* from, + *thema,* something set down, fr. *tithēmi,* to place]. A precipitate caused by long boiling of a vegetable infusion or by its exposure to air.

apoxesis (ap-ok-sē'sis) [G. *apo,* away, + *xeein,* to scrape]. Subgingival *curettage.*

apozem, apozema (ap'ō-zem, ap-oz'ē-mă) [apo- + G. *zema,* something boiled]. Decoction.

apparatus, pl. **apparatus** (ap-ă-rā'tŭs, -rat'ŭs) [L. equipment. fr. *ap-paro,* pp. *-atus,* to prepare]. **1.** A collection of instruments adapted for a special purpose. **2.** An instrument made up of several parts. **3** [NA]. A group or system of glands, ducts, blood vessels, muscles, or other anatomical structures concerned in the performance of some function. See also system, systema.

Abbé-Zeiss a., Thoma-Zeiss *hemocytometer.*

achromatic a., the nonstaining asters and spindle fibers in a dividing cell.

alimentary a., a. digestorius.

attachment a., the tissues that attach the tooth to the alveolar process: cementum, periodontal membrane, and alveolar bone.

Barcroft-Warburg a., Warburg's a.

Beckmann's a., a. for the accurate measurement of melting points and boiling points in connection with molecular weight determinations.

Benedict-Roth a., a device employed to measure the amount of oxygen utilized in quiet breathing in the basal state for the estimation of the basal metabolic rate; the subject rebreathes oxygen through soda lime from a recording spirometer.

branchial a., the aggregate of the pharyngeal arches, pouches, clefts, and membranes seen in the developing embryo of vertebrates.

central a., the centrosome and centrosphere.

chromatic a., the deeply staining mass of chromosomes in a dividing cell.

chromidial a., the aggregate of extranuclear network, irregular strands, and masses of basophilic staining material permeating the protoplasm of the cell. See also ribosome; endoplasmic *reticulum.*

dental a., masticatory *system.*

digestive a., a. digestorius.

a. digesto'rius [NA], digestive a.; systema digestorium; alimentary a.; alimentary or digestive system; the digestive tract from the mouth to the anus with all its associated glands and organs.

genitourinary a., a. urogenitalis.

Golgi a., Golgi complex; Golgi internal reticulum; Holmgren-Golgi canals; a membranous system of cisternae and vesicles located between the nucleus and the secretory pole or surface of a cell; concerned with the investment and intracellular transport of membrane-bounded secretory proteins.

Haldane's a., a device used for the analysis of respiratory gases.

Heyns' abdominal decompression a., a vacuum chamber enclosing the abdomen of the pregnant woman, creating pressure during the first stage of labor.

hyoid a., a. hyoideus.

a. hyoi'deus, hyoid a.; veterinary anatomy term for hyoid bones, a modified portion of the ancestral branchial skeleton consisting of an articulated chain of bones extending from the mastoid region of the skull on each side to the base of the tongue; in humans, it is reduced to a single bone, os hyoideum; in a typical mammal (the dog), it consists of a tympanohyoid cartilage attached to the skull, followed by the stylohyoid, epihyoid, keratohyoid, basihyoid, and thyrohyoid bones.

juxtaglomerular a., juxtaglomerular *complex.*

Kirschner's a., Kirschner's *wire.*

Kjeldahl a., an a. for distilling ammonia arising from acid decomposition of an organic compound; used in nitrogen analysis.

a. lacrima'lis [NA], lacrimal a.; consisting of the lacrimal gland, the lacrimal lake, the lacrimal canaliculi, the lacrimal sac, and the nasolacrimal duct.

lacrimal a., a. lacrimalis.

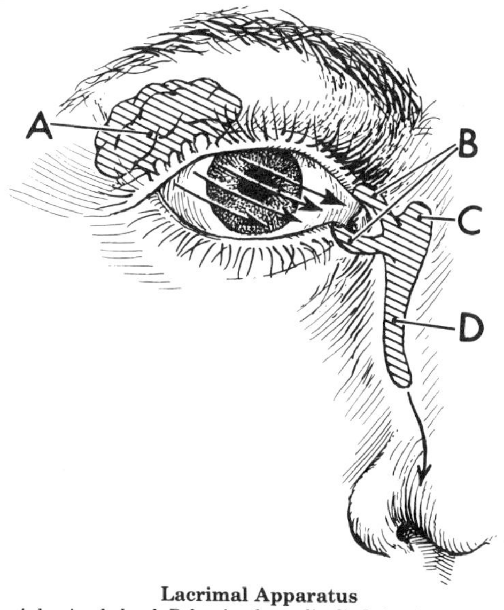

Lacrimal Apparatus
A, lacrimal gland; *B,* lacrimal canaliculi; *C,* fornix of lacrimal sac; *D,* nasolacrimal duct; *arrows* indicate the direction of flow of tears secreted by the lacrimal gland (*A*).

a. ligamento'sus col'li, *ligamentum* nuchae.

a. ligamento'sus weitbrecht'i, *membrana* tectoria.

masticatory a., **(1)** masticatory *system;* **(2)** stomatognathic *system.*

mental a., mental structure; in psychoanalysis, the topographic structure of the mind.

pyriform a., a pear-shaped structure within the eggshell of certain tapeworms (family Anoplocephalidae), of uncertain function.

a. respirato'rius [NA], respiratory apparatus or system; systema respiratorium; all the air passages from the nose to the pulmonary alveoli.

respiratory a., a. respiratorius.

Roughton-Scholander a., Roughton-Scholander syringe; a syringe-like device for analyzing the respiratory gases in a small sample of blood.
Sayre's suspension a., Sayre's suspension *traction.*
Scholander a., a device used for determining the oxygen and carbon dioxide percentage in 0.5 ml of a respiratory gas.
subneural a., modified sarcoplasm in a motor end-plate.
a. suspenso'rius len'tis, *zonula* ciliaris.
Taylor's a., Taylor's back *brace.*
Tiselius a., an a. for separating proteins in solution by electrophoresis and thus for determining the isoelectric point, molecular weight, and related physical properties; the direction and rate of migration of the protein and the characteristics of the boundary phase between the protein solution and the supernatant salt solution are recorded by photography of the changes in refractive index at the boundary.
urinary a., urinary *system.*
urogenital a., a. urogenitalis.
a. urogenita'lis [NA], systema urogenitale; urogenital a. or system; genitourinary a. or system; includes all the organs concerned in reproduction and in the formation and voidance of the urine.
Van Slyke a., an a. for determining the amounts of respiratory gases in the blood.
Warburg's a., Barcroft-Warburg a.; an a. for measuring the oxygen consumption of incubated tissue slices by manometric measurement of changes in gas pressure produced by oxygen absorption in an enclosed flask.

apparent (ă-păr'ent) [L. *apparens,* visible, fr. *appareo,* to come in sight]. **1.** Manifest; obvious; evident; *e.g.,* a clinically a. infection. **2.** Frequently used (confusingly) to mean "seeming to be," ostensible, pseudo-.

appendage (ă-pen'dij) [L. *appendix*]. Appendix; any part, subordinate in function or size, attached to a main structure. See also adnexa.
auricular a., **(1)** *auricula* atrialis; **(2)** a small congenital swelling usually located anterior to the auricle of the ear.
drumstick a., an a. of the nucleus that represents the XX chromosome seen in 3% of the neutrophil leukocytes of human females.
epiploic a., *appendix* epiploica.
a.'s of eye, the eyelids with their lashes, eyebrows, lacrimal apparatus, and conjunctiva.
a.'s of the fetus, amnion, yolk sac, and the fetal (chorionic) part of the placenta together with the umbilical cord.
left auricular a., *auricula* sinistra.
right auricular a., *auricula* dextra.
a.'s of skin, the hairs, nails, and sweat, sebaceous, and mammary glands.
uterine a.'s, the ovaries, uterine (fallopian) tubes, and ligaments.
vermiform a., *appendix* vermiformis.
vesicular a., *appendix* vesiculosa.

appendalgia (ap-pen-dal'jē-ă) [appendix + G. *algos,* pain]. Pain in the right lower quadrant of the abdomen in the region of the vermiform appendix.

appendectomy (ap-pen-dek'tō-mē) [appendix + G. *ektomē,* excision]. Appendicectomy; surgical removal of the vermiform appendix.
auricular a., excision of the heart's auricular appendix.

appendical (ă-pen'di-kăl). Appendiceal.

appendiceal (ă-pen-dis'ē-ăl). Appendical; relating to an appendix.

appendicectasis (ap-pen-di-sek'tă-sis). Ectasia of the appendix.

appendicectomy (ap-pen-di-sek'tō-mē). Appendectomy.

appendicism (ă-pen'di-sizm). Rarely used term for any chronic disease of the vermiform appendix, or a symptomatic uneasiness in that area.

appendicitis (ă-pen-di-sī'tis) [appendix + G. *-itis,* inflammation]. Inflammation of the vermiform appendix.
actinomycotic a., chronic suppurative a. due to infection by *Actinomyces israelii,* sometimes resulting in a fecal fistula following appendectomy.
acute a., acute inflammation of the appendix, usually due to bacterial infection, which may be precipitated by obstruction of the lumen by a fecalith; symptoms of periumbilical colicky pain and vomiting are followed by fever, leukocytosis, persistent pain, and signs of peritoneal inflammation in the right lower quadrant of the abdomen; perforation or abscess formation is a frequent complication.
bilharzial a., a. caused by the deposition of the eggs of the blood fluke, *Schistosoma mansoni,* in the vermiform appendix.
chronic a., fibrous adhesions, scarring, or deformity of the appendix following subsidence of acute a.; fibrous obliteration of the distal lumen is not abnormal in older persons.
focal a., acute a. involving only part of the appendix, sometimes at the site of, or distal to, an obstruction of the lumen.
gangrenous a., acute a. with necrosis of the wall of the appendix, most commonly developing in obstructive a. and frequently causing perforation and acute peritonitis.
lumbar a., a retrodisplaced appendix in the lumbar region.
obstructive a., acute a. due to infection of retained secretion behind an obstruction of the lumen by a fecalith or some other cause, including carcinoma of the cecum.
stercoral a., a. following a lodgment of fecal material in the appendix.
subperitoneal a., a. of a subperitoneally displaced appendix.
suppurative a., acute a. with purulent exudate in the lumen and wall of the appendix.
verminous a., a. caused by obstruction or response to the presence of parasitic worms such as *Ascaris lumbricoides, Strongyloides stercoralis,* or the pinworm *Enterobius vermicularis*

appendiclausis (ă-pen-di-klaw'sis) [appendix + L. *clausus,* closed]. Obsolete term for atrophy or obstruction of the appendix.

appendico- [L. *appendix,* appendage]. Combining form relating, usually, to the vermiform appendix.

appendicocele (ă-pen'di-kō-sēl) [appendico- + G. *kēlē,* hernia]. The vermiform appendix in a hernial sac.

appendicoenterostomy (ă-pen'di-kō-en-ter-os'tō-mē). [appendico- + G. *enteron,* intestine, + *stoma,* mouth]. **1.** The establishment of an artificial opening between the appendix and the small intestine. **2.** Appendicostomy.

appendicolithiasis (ă-pen'di-kō-li-thī'ă-sis) [appendico- + G. *lithos,* stone]. The presence of concretions in the vermiform appendix.

appendicolysis (ă-pen-di-kol'i-sis) [appendico- + G. *lysis,* a loosening]. An operation for freeing the appendix from adhesions.

appendicostomy (ă-pen-di-kos'tō-mē) [appendico- + G. *stoma,* mouth]. Appendicoenterostomy (2); an operation for opening into the intestine through the tip of the vermiform appendix, previously attached to the anterior abdominal wall.

appendicular (ap'en-dik'yū-lăr). **1.** Relating to an appendix or appendage. **2.** Relating to the limbs, as opposed to axial, which refers to the trunk and head.

appendix, gen. **appendicis,** pl. **appendices** (ă-pen'diks, -di-sis, -di-sēs) [L. appendage, fr. *ap- pendo,* to hang something on]. **1** [NA]. Appendage. **2.** Specifically, the appendix vermiformis.
auricular a., *auricula* atrialis.
a. ce'ci, a. vermiformis.
a. epididym'idis [NA], a. of epididymidis; pedunculated hydatid; a small pedunculated body attached to the head of the epididymis.
a. of epididymidis, a. epididymidis.
a. epiplo'ica, pl. **appen'dices epiplo'icae** [NA], epiploic appendage; one of a number of little processes or sacs of peritoneum pro-

jecting from the serous coat of the large intestine, except the rectum; they are generally distended with fat.
a. fibro'sa hep'atis [NA], fibrous a. of liver; a fibrous process, into which the tip of the left lobe of the liver may taper out, that passes with the left triangular ligament to be attached to the diaphragm.
fibrous a. of liver, a. fibrosa hepatis.
Morgagni's a., *lobus* pyramidalis glandulae thyroideae.
a. tes'tis [NA], ovarium masculinum; nonpedunculated or sessile hydatid; a vesicular nonpedunculated structure attached to the cephalic pole of the testis; a vestige of the cephalic end of the paramesonephric (müllerian) duct.
a. ventric'uli laryn'gis, *sacculus* laryngis.
vermiform a., a. vermiformis.
a. vermifor'mis [NA], vermiform a.; vermix; vermiform process; processus vermiformis; vermiform appendage; a. ceci; a wormlike intestinal diverticulum extending from the blind end of the cecum; it varies in length and ends in a blind extremity.
a. vesiculo'sa, pl. **appen'dices vesiculo'sae** [NA], vesicular appendage; Morgagni's or stalked hydatid; morgagnian cyst; a small fluid-filled cyst attached by a slender stalk to the fimbriated end of the uterine tube; a vestigial remnant of the embryonic mesonephric duct.

apperception (ap-er-sep'shŭn) [L. *ad,* to, + *per- cipio,* pp. *-ceptus,* to take wholly, perceive]. **1.** Comprehension; conscious perception; the full apprehension of any psychic content. **2.** The process of referring the perception of ideas to one's own personality.

apperceptive (ap-er-sep'tiv). Relating to, involved in, or capable of apperception.

appersonation, appersonification (ă-per'sŏ-nā'shŭn, ap-er-son'i-fi-kā'shŭn). A delusion in which one assumes the character of another person.

appestat (ap'e-stat) [appetite + G. *statos,* standing]. The mechanism in the brain (possibly in the hypothalamus) concerned with the appetite and control of food intake.

appetite (ap'ĕ-tīt) [L. *ad-peto,* pp. *-petitus,* to seek after, desire]. Orexia (2); a desire or longing to satisfy any conscious physical or mental need.

appetition (ap-ĕ-tish'ŭn) [L. *appetitio,* strong desire]. Desire directed toward a definite goal or object.

applanation (ap'lan-ā'shŭn) [L. *ad,* toward, + *planum,* plane]. In tonometry, the flattening of the cornea by pressure. Intraocular pressure is directly proportional to external pressure, and inversely proportional to the area flattened. See also applanation *tonometer.*

applanometry (ap-lan-om'ĕ-trē). Use of an applanation tonometer.

apple oil. *Amyl* valerate.

appliance (ă-plī'ans). A device used to provide function to a part, or for therapeutic purposes.
craniofacial a., a device used to immobilize and/or reduce mandibular or midfacial fractures. See also subentries under fixation.
edgewise a., a fixed, multibanded orthodontic a. using an attachment bracket the slot of which receives a rectangular archwire horizontally, which gives precise control in all three planes of space.
extraoral fracture a., a device used for extraoral reduction and fixation of maxillary or mandibular fractures, in which pins, clamps, or screws interjoined with metal or acrylic connectors are used to align the fractured segments. See also external pin *fixation.*
Hawley a., Hawley *retainer.*
intraoral fracture a., a metal or acrylic device attached to the teeth with wire or cement; used to immobilize fractures of the maxilla and mandible.
labiolingual a., an orthodontic a. that consists of a maxillary labial arch wire and a mandibular lingual arch wire.
light wire a., an orthodontic a. utilizing small gauge labial wires with expansion and contraction loops formed into it and attached to bands fitted to individual teeth; sometimes called Begg light wire differential force technique.
obturator a., an a. used to obliterate congenital or acquired defects of the jaws and surrounding structures, usually made of acrylic or rubber.
orthodontic a., a mechanism for the application of pressure to the teeth and their supporting tissues to produce changes in the relationship of the teeth and/or the related osseous structures.
ribbon arch a., an a. consisting of a rectangular wire inserted into a specially designed bracket attached to the labial and buccal surfaces of the teeth.
Roger-Anderson pin fixation a., an a. used in extraoral fixation of mandibular fractures and prognathic corrections in which pins placed in the bone segments are joined by metal connecting rods. See also external pin *fixation.*
surgical a., a metal or plastic a. constructed prior to surgery and used to immobilize or support mucosal, skin, bone, or bone marrow grafts during the postoperative phase.
universal a., a combination of the edgewise and ribbon arch a. techniques, affording precise control of individual teeth in all planes of space.

applicator (ap'li-kā-tōr) [L. *ap-plico,* to attach to]. A slender rod of wood, flexible metal, or synthetic material, at one end of which is attached a pledget of cotton or other substance for making local applications to any accessible surface.

apposition (ap-ō-zish'ŭn) [L. *ap-pono,* pp. *-positus,* to place at or to]. **1.** The placing in contact of two substances. **2.** The condition of being placed or fitted together. **3.** The relationship of fracture fragments to one another.

approach (ă-prōch'). In psychiatry, a term used to describe how interpersonal relationships are negotiated.
idiographic a., the comprehensive study of an individual as a basis for understanding human behavior in general.
nomothetic a., a frame of psychologic reference that attempts to provide norms and general principles of behavior by the study of groups.
regressive-reconstructive a., a form of psychotherapy in which regression, in order to resurrect some original psychic trauma, is an integral part of the treatment.

approximate (ă-prok'si-māt) [L. *ad,* to, + *proximus,* nearest]. To bring close together. In dentistry: **1.** Proximate, denoting the contact surfaces, either mesial or distal, of two adjacent teeth. **2.** Close together; denoting the teeth in the human jaw, as distinguished from the separated teeth in certain of the lower animals.

approximation (ă-prok-si-mā'shŭn). In surgery, bringing tissue edges into desired apposition for suturing.

apractagnosia (ā-prak-tag-nō'sē-ă) [G. *a-* priv. + *practa,* things to be done, + *gnosis,* recognition]. Inability to perform tasks involving spatial analysis; disorganization of construction and drawing.

apractic (ă-prak'tik). Apraxic.

apragmatism (ă-prag'mă-tizm) [G. *a-* priv. + pragmatism]. An interest in theory or dogmatism rather than in practical results.

apraxia (ă-prak'sē-ă) [G. *a-* priv. + *prattō,* to do]. Parectropia. **1.** A disorder of voluntary movement, consisting in partial or complete incapacity to execute purposeful movements, notwithstanding the preservation of muscular power, sensibility, and coordination in general. **2.** Object blindness; a psychomotor defect in which the proper use of an object can not be carried out although the object can be named and its uses described.
a. al'gera, a hysterical condition in which speaking, reading, writing, or consecutive thinking is impossible owing to the severe headache it causes.
cortical a., motor a.
ideational a., ideatory a., misuse of objects due to a disturbance of identification (agnosia).
ideokinetic a., ideomotor a., transcortical a.; a form of a. in which

simple but not complicated acts may be performed, presumably because the connections between the hypothetical ideational centers, which initiate such complex acts, and the motor cortex are interrupted.

innervation a., motor a.
limb-kinetic a., motor a.
motor a., cortical, innervation, or limb-kinetic a.; an inability to make movements or to use objects for the purpose intended.
ocular motor a., Balint's syndrome; inability to fixate objects in the peripheral visual field.
transcortical a., ideokinetic a.

apraxic (ă-prak'sik). Apractic; marked by or pertaining to apraxia.

apricot kernel oil (ā'pri-kot). See persic oil.

aprobarbital (ap-rō-bar'bi-tawl). 5-Allyl-5-isopropylbarbituric acid; allylisopropylmalonylurea; a hypnotic and sedative with intermediate action; available as a. sodium, with the same uses.

aproctia (ă-prok'shē-ă) [G. *a-* priv. + *prōktos,* anus]. Congenital absence or imperforation of the anus.

aprofen, aprofene, aprophen (ap'rō-fen, ap'rō-fēn, ap'rō-fen). 2-Diethylaminoethyl 2,2-diphenylpropionate; analgesic and antispasmodic.

aprophoria (ap'rō-fōr'ē-ă) [G. *a-* priv. + *prophora,* utterance]. Aphasia, including agraphia.

aprosexia (ap-rō-sek'sē-ă) [G. *a-* priv. + *prosexis,* attention, fr. *pros-echō,* to hold to]. Inattention, due to a sensorineural or mental defect.

aprosody (ă-pros'ō-dē) [G. *a-* priv. + *prosōdia,* voice modulation]. Absence, in speech, of the normal pitch, rhythm, and variations in stress.

aprosopia (ap-rō-sō'pē-ă) [G. *a-* priv. + *prosōpon,* face]. Congenital absence of the greater part or all of the face, usually associated with other malformations.

aprotinin (ā-prō'ti-nin). A protease and kallikrein inhibitor obtained from animal organs; a polypeptide with a molecular weight of about 6000. May be useful in the treatment of pancreatitis.

apsithyria (ap'si-thī'rē-ă) [G. *a-* priv. + *psithyrizō,* to whisper]. Loss of the ability to whisper.

aptyalia, aptyalism (ap-tī-ā'lē-ă, ap-tī'al-ism) [G. *a-* priv. + *ptyalon,* saliva]. Asialism.

APUD [*a*mine *p*recursor *u*ptake, *d*ecarboxylase] Proposed designation for a group of cells in different organs secreting polypeptide hormones. Cells in this group have certain biochemical characteristics in common, the first letters of which form the name: they contain amines, such as catecholamine and 5-hydroxytryptamine, take up precursors of these amines *in vivo,* and contain amino-acid decarboxylase.

apurinic acid (a-pyū-rin'ik). DNA from which the purine bases have been removed by mild acid treatment.

apyknomorphous (ā-pik-nō-mōr'fŭs) [G. *a-* priv. + *pyknos,* thick, + *morphē,* shape, form]. Denoting a cell or other structure that does not stain deeply because the stainable or chromophil material is not closely aggregated.

apyrase (ă-pī'rās) [EC 3.6.1.5.]. ADPase; ATP-diphosphatase; an enzyme catalyzing hydrolytic removal of two orthophosphate residues from adenosine triphosphate to yield adenosine monophosphate; *i.e.,* ATP + $H_2O \rightarrow$ AMP + $2P_i$.

apyretic (ā-pī-ret'ik). Afebrile, apyrexial; without fever, denoting apyrexia; having a normal body temperature.

apyrexia (ă-pī-rek'sē-ă) [G. *a-* priv. + *pyrexis,* fever]. Absence of fever.

apyrexial (ā-pī-rek'sē-ăl). Apyretic.

apyrimidinic acid (ă-pī'rim-i-din'ik). DNA from which the pyrimidine bases have been removed by chemical treatment.

aqua, gen. and pl. **aquae** (ak'wă, ah'kwah) [L.]. Water; H_2O. Pharmaceutical waters, aquae, are aqueous solutions of volatile substances. See water (3). Pharmaceutical solutions, liquors, are aqueous solutions of nonvolatile substances. See solution (3).

a. re'gia, a. rega'lis [L. royal water, so called from its power to dissolve gold], nitrohydrochloric acid.

aquacobalamin (ak'wă-kō-bal'ă-min). Aquocobalamin; vitamin B_{12a} (tautomeric with B_{12b}); a cobalamin derivative in which the sixth coordinate bond of the cobaltic ion is attached to a water molecule. See also vitamin B_{12}.

aquaphobia (ak-wă-fō'bē-ă) [L. *aqua,* water, + G. *phobos,* fear]. Morbid fear of water.

aquapuncture (ak-wă-pŭnk'chyūr) [L. *aqua,* water, + *punctura,* puncture]. Rarely used term for a hypodermic injection of water.

Aquaspirillum (ah-kwah-spī-ril'ŭm) [L. *aqua,* water, + *spirillum,* coil]. A genus of motile, nonsporeforming, aerobic bacteria (family Spirillaceae) containing Gram-negative, rigid, helical or helically curved cells which are 0.2 to 1.5 μm in diameter. Motile cells contain fascicles of flagella at one or both poles. Some species can grow anaerobically with nitrate instead of oxygen as the terminal electron acceptor. These organisms are chemoorganotrophic, possessing a strictly respiratory metabolism. They do not ferment carbohydrates; a few species can oxidize a limited variety of carbohydrates. The habitat of these organisms is fresh water. The type species is *A. serpens.*

aquatic (ă-kwat'ik). **1.** Of or pertaining to water. **2.** Denoting an organism that lives in water.

aqueduct (ak'we-dŭkt) [L. *aqueductus*]. Aqueductus.

a. of cerebrum, *aqueductus* cerebri.
cochlear a., *ductus* perilymphaticus.
Cotunnius' a., *aqueductus* vestibuli.
fallopian a., *canalis* facialis.
sylvian a., *aqueductus* cerebri.
a. of vestibule, *aqueductus* vestibuli.

aqueductus, pl. **aqueductus** (ak-we-dŭk'tŭs) [L. fr. *aqua,* water, + *ductus,* a leading, fr. *duco,* pp. *ductus,* to lead] [NA]. Aqueduct; a conduit or canal.

a. cer'ebri [NA], aqueduct of the cerebrum; a sylvii; iter a tertio ad quartum ventriculum; sylvian aqueduct; an ependymal-lined canal in the mesencephalon about $^3/_4$ inch long, connecting the third to the fourth ventricle.
a. coch'leae, *ductus* perilymphaticus.
a. cotun'nii, a. vestibuli.
a. fallo'pii, *canalis* facialis.
a. syl'vii, a. cerebri.
a. vestib'uli [NA], aqueduct of vestibule; a. cotunnii; Cotunnius' aqueduct or canal; **(1)** a bony canal running from the vestibule and opening on the posterior surface of the petrous portion of the temporal bone, giving passage to the endolymphatic duct and a small vein; **(2)** *ductus* endolymphaticus.

aqueous (ak'wē-ŭs, ā'kwē-ŭs). Watery; of, like, or containing water.

aquiparous (ă-kwip'er-ŭs) [L. *aqua,* water, + *pario,* to bring forth]. Secreting or excreting a watery fluid.

aquocobalamin (ak'wō-kō-bal'ă-min). Aquacobalamin.

aquo-ion (ak'wō-ī'on). A hydrated ion; an ion containing one or more water molecules; *e.g.,* $Cu(H_2O)_4{}^{2+}$.

aquosity (ă-kwos'i-tē). **1.** The state of being watery. **2.** Moisture.

Ar Symbol for argon.

Ara Symbol for arabinose, or its mono- or diradical.

ara-. Prefix for arabinose or arabinosyl.

arab- [G. *araps,* arab]. Combining form originally from gum arabic.

araban (a'ră-ban). A polysaccharide that yields arabinose on hydrolysis; a constituent of some pectins.

arabic (a'ră-bik). Relating to or derived from various species of *Acacia* having a gummy or resinous exudate.

arabic acid. Arabin.

arabin (a'ră-bin). Arabic acid; a carbohydrate gum, hydrolyzing to arabinose and hexoses, found naturally in union with calcium, potassium, and magnesium, when it is called gum arabic.

arabinoadenosine (a'ră-bin-ō-ah-den'ō-sēn). Arabinosyladenine.

arabinocytidine (a'ră-bin-ō-sī'ti-dēn). Arabinosylcytosine.

arabinofuranosylcytosine (a'ră-bin-ō-fūr'ă-nō-sil-sī'tō-sēn). Arabinosylcytosine.

arabinose (Ara) (ă-rab'i-nōs, a'ră-bin-ōs). Pectin sugar; a pentose widely distributed in plants, usually in complex polysaccharides; used in culture media. For structure, see sugars.

arabinosis (ă-rab-i-nō'sis). Disordered metabolism of arabinose.

arabinosuria (ă-rab'i-nō-sū'rē-ă). Excretion of arabinose in the urine.

arabinosyladenine (a'ră-bin-ō-sil-ă'den-ēn). Arabinoadenosine; 9-β-D-arabinofuranosyladenine; used for herpes simplex corneae and vaccinial keratitis.

arabinosylcytosine (araC,aC) (a'ră-bin-ō-sil-sī'tō-sēn). Arabinofuranosylcytosine; arabinocytidine; cytarabine; a compound of arabinose and cytosine, analogous to ribosylcytosine (cytidine), that inhibits the biosynthesis of DNA; used as a chemotherapeutic agent because of antiviral and tumor-growth inhibiting properties.

arabitol (ă-rab'i-tol). 1,2,3,4,5-pentanepentol; $C_5H_{12}O_5$; a sugar alcohol obtained from the reduction of arabinose.

araC Symbol for arabinosylcytosine.

arachic acid (ă-rak'ik). Arachidic acid.

arachidic acid (a-ră-kid'ik). Arachic acid; *n*-eicosanoic or *n*-icosanoic acid; $CH_3(CH_2)_{18}COOH$; a fatty acid contained in peanut oil, butter, and other fats.

arachidonic acid (ă-rak-i-don'ik). 5,8,11,14-Eicosatetraenoic (icosatetraenoic) acid; $CH_3(CH_2)_3(CH_2CH{=}CH)_4(CH_2)_3COOH$; an unsaturated fatty acid essential in nutrition; the biological precursor of the prostaglandins, the thromboxanes, and the leukotrienes collectively known as eicosanoids.

arachidonic acid cascade. Eicosanoids.

arachis oil (ar'ă-kis). Peanut oil.

arachnephobia (ă-rak-nē-fō'bē-ă) [G. *arachne*, spider, + *phobos*, fear]. Arachnophobia; morbid fear of spiders.

Arachnia (ă-rak'nē-ă). A genus of nonmotile, nonsporeforming, facultatively anaerobic bacteria (family Actinomycetaceae) containing Gram-positive, non-acid fast, branched, diphtheroid rods (0.2 to 0.3 by 3.0 to 5.0 μm and longer). These organisms produce filamentous microcolonies. Their metabolism is fermentative. Primarily propionic and acetic acids are produced from glucose. Catalase is not produced. The cell wall contains diaminopimelic acid but not arabinose. These organisms are pathogenic for man, causing lacrimal canaliculitis and typical actinomycosis. The type species is *A. propionica*.

A. propio'nica, a species causing lacrimal canaliculitis and typical actinomycosis; it is the type species of the genus *A*.

Arachnida (ă-rak'ni-dă) [G. *arachne*, spider]. A class of arthropods in the subphylum Chelicerata, consisting of spiders, scorpions, harvestmen, mites, ticks, and allies.

arachnidism (ă-rak'ni-dizm). Systemic poisoning following the bite of a spider (especially of the black widow spider).

arachnodactyly (ă-rak-nō-dak'ti-lē) [G. *arachnē*, spider, + *daktylos*, finger]. Dolichostenomelia; spider fingers; a condition in which the hands and fingers, and often the feet and toes, are abnormally long and slender; a characteristic of Marfan's syndrome and Achard syndrome.

arachnoid (ă-rak'noyd) [G. *arachnē*, spider, cobweb, + *eidos*, resemblance]. Ectodermal derivative resembling a cobweb; denoting specifically the arachnoidea covering the brain and spinal cord.

arachnoidal (ă-rak-noy'dăl). Relating to the arachnoid membrane, or arachnoidea.

arachnoidea, arachnoides (ă-rak-noyd'ē-ă, -dēz) [Mod. L. *arachnoideus* fr. G. *arachnē*, spider, + *eidos*, resemblance] [NA]. Arachnoid membrane; meninx serosa; a delicate fibrous membrane forming the middle of the three coverings of the brain (**a. enceph'ali**) and spinal cord (**a. spina'lis**); it is closely applied to the inner surface of the dura mater, from which it may be separated by the subdural cleft; between the arachnid and the pia mater lies the subarachnoid space.

arachnoiditis (ă-rak-noy-dī'tis). Inflammation of the arachnoid membrane and subjacent subarachnoid space. See also leptomeningitis.

adhesive a., obliterative a.; thickening of the leptomeninges, sometimes with obliteration of the subarachnoid space; commonly related to acute or chronic leptomeningitis of bacterial or chemical origin. See also leptomeningeal *fibrosis*.

neoplastic a., neoplastic *meningitis*.

obliterative a., adhesive a.

arachnolysin (ă-rak-nol'i-sin). A hemolytic substance in the venom of certain spiders.

arachnophobia (ă-rak-nō-fō'bē-ă). Arachnephobia.

aralkyl (ă-ral'kil). Arylated alkyl; a radical in which an aryl group is substituted for a hydrogen atom of an alkyl group; *e.g.*, $C_6H_5CH_2$—.

Aran, François A., French physician, 1817–1861. See A.-Duchenne *disease*, Duchenne-A. *disease*.

araneism (ă-ră'nē-izm). Rarely used term for arachnidism.

Arantius (Aranzio), Giulio C., Italian anatomist and physician, 1530–1589. See A.'s *ligament, nodule, ventricle; corpora* arantii; *ductus* venosus arantii.

araphia (ă-ră'fē-ă) [G. *a-* priv. + *rhaphe*, a seam]. Holorachischisis.

arbor, pl. **arbores** (ar'bōr, ar-bō'rēz) [L. tree]. In anatomy, a treelike structure with branchings.

a. vi'tae [NA], the arborescent appearance of gray and white matter in sagittal sections of the cerebellum.

a. vi'tae u'teri, *plicae* palmatae.

arborescent (ar-bō-res'ent). Dendriform.

arborization (ar'bōr-i-ză'shŭn). **1.** The terminal branching of nerve fibers or blood vessels in a branching treelike pattern. **2.** The branched pattern formed under certain conditions by a dried smear of cervical mucus.

arborize (ar'bōr-īz). To spread in a treelike branching pattern.

arboroid (ar'bōr-oyd) [L. *arbor*, tree, + G. *eidos*, resemblance]. Denoting a colony of protozoa, each of which remains attached to another cell or to the main stem at one point, forming a branching or dendritic figure.

arborvirus (ar'bōr-vī'rŭs). Arbovirus.

arbovirus (ar'bō-vī'rŭs) [*ar*, arthropod, + *bo*, borne, + virus]. Arborvirus; a large, heterogenous group of RNA viruses from 20 to 100 nm or more in diameter, and divisible into groups on the basis of characteristics of the virions. The 350 or so species, which are distributed among several families (Togaviridae, Bunyaviridae, Arenaviridae, Rhabdoviridae, Reoviridae) have been recovered from arthropods, bats, and rodents, and most, but not all, are arthropod-borne. Although about 75 species can infect man, only about 45 species produce disease, in most instances, of a very mild nature and difficult to distinguish from illnesses caused by viruses of other taxonomic groups. Apparent infections may be separated into three clinical syndromes: undifferentiated type fevers (systemic febrile disease), hemorrhagic fevers, and encephalitides.

ARC Abbreviation for AIDS-related *complex.*

arc (ark) [L. *arcus,* a bow]. **1.** A curved line or segment of a circle. **2.** Continuous luminous passage of an electric current in a gas or vacuum between two or more separated carbon or other electrodes.
auricular a., binauricular a., a line carried over the cranium from the center of one external auditory meatus to that of the other.
bregmatolambdoid a., the line running along the sagittal suture from the bregma to the apex of the lambdoid suture.
crater a., an a. of a direct current that forms a pitlike excavation at the positive pole.
flame a., an a. between two impregnated electrodes that causes volatilization of the core with resultant flame.
longitudinal a. of skull, the line carried over the skull from the nasion to the opisthion.
mercury a., an electric discharge through mercury vapor between electrodes one of which is usually mercury; provides a rich source of therapeutic ultraviolet rays; the containing tube is usually quartz; may also be glass with a fluorite window.
nasobregmatic a., a line running through the midline of the forehead from the nasion to the bregma.
naso-occipital a., the a. in the midline from the root of the nose to the inferior limit of the external occipital protuberance.
pulmonary a., pulmonary *salient.*
reflex a., the route followed by nerve impulses in the production of a reflex act, from the periphery through the afferent nerve to the nervous system and thence through the efferent nerve to the effector organ.

arcade (ar-kād) [L. *arcus,* arc, bow]. An anatomical structure resembling a series of arches.
anomalous mitral a., short chordae tendineae extending from both papillary muscles to the central portion of the anterior leaflet of the mitral valve and resulting in stenosis or incompetence of the valve.
Flint's a., a series of vascular arches at the bases of the pyramids of the kidney.
Riolan's a., Riolan's anastomosis; the anastomoses of the intestinal vessels in the mesentery.

arcate (ar'kāt). Arcuate.

arch-, arche-, archi-, archo- [G. *archē,* origin, beginning]. Combining forms meaning primitive, or ancestral; also first, or chief.

ARCH

arch [thru O. Fr. fr. L. *arcus,* bow]. In anatomy, any vaulted or archlike structure. See arcus.
abdominothoracic a., the line of the false ribs on either side with the lower end of the sternum, marking roughly the boundary line between the abdomen and thorax.
alveolar a. of mandible, *arcus* alveolaris mandibulae.
alveolar a. of maxilla, *arcus* alveolaris maxillae.
anterior a. of atlas, *arcus* anterior atlantis.
anterior palatine a., *arcus* palatoglossus.
aortic a., a. of the aorta, *arcus* aortae.
aortic a.'s, a series of arterial channels encircling the embryonic pharynx in the mesenchyme of the branchial a.'s. There are potentially six pairs, but in mammals the fifth pair is poorly developed or absent. The first and second pairs are functional only in very young embryos; the third pair is involved in the formation of the carotids; the fourth a. on the left is incorporated in the a. of the aorta; the sixth pair forms the proximal part of the pulmonary arteries.
arterial a.'s of colon, branches of the colic arteries that form a.'s in the mesocolon from which the walls of the colon are supplied.
arterial a.'s of ileum, a.'s formed by branches of the superior mesenteric artery from which vessels pass between the layers of the mesentery to the wall of the ileum.
arterial a.'s of jejunum, a.'s formed by branches of the superior mesenteric artery which supply the walls of the jejunum.
arterial a. of lower eyelid, *arcus* palpebralis inferior.
arterial a. of upper eyelid, *arcus* palpebralis superior.
axillary a., Langer's a. or muscle; an anomalous muscle or tendinous slip that passes across the axilla from the pectoralis major to insert with the latissimus dorsi onto the humerus.
branchial a.'s, visceral or pharyngeal a.'s; typically, 6 a.'s in vertebrates; in the lower vertebrates, they bear gills; in the higher vertebrates, they appear transiently and give rise to specialized structures in the head and neck.
carpal a.'s, two anastomotic arterial twigs running transversely across the wrist: the palmar or anterior lies in front of the carpus, being formed by palmar carpal branches of the radial and ulnar arteries; the dorsal or posterior lies on the dorsal surface of the carpus, being formed by the dorsal carpal branches of the radial and ulnar arteries.
Corti's a., the a. formed by the junction of the heads of Corti's inner and outer pillar cells.
cortical a.'s of kidney, the portions of renal substance (cortex) intervening between the bases of the pyramids and the capsule of the kidney.
costal a., *arcus* costalis.
a. of cricoid cartilage, *arcus* cartilaginis cricoideae.
crural a., *ligamentum* inguinale.
deep palmar a., *arcus* palmaris profundus.
deep palmar venous a., *arcus* venosus palmaris profundus.
dental a., the curved composite structure of the natural dentition and the residual ridge, or the remains thereof after the loss of some or all of the natural teeth.
dorsal venous a. of foot, *arcus* venosus dorsalis pedis.
expansion a., an orthodontic appliance that moves the dental structures distally, bucally, or labially, creating increased molar to molar width and arch length.
fallen a.'s, a breaking down of the a.'s of the foot, either longitudinal, transverse, or both; the resulting deformity is flat or spread foot, or both.
fallopian a., *ligamentum* inguinale.
femoral a., *ligamentum* inguinale.
a.'s of the foot, see *arcus* pedis longitudinalis; *arcus* pedis transversalis; *arcus* plantaris.
glossopalatine a., *arcus* palatoglossus.
Gothic a., needle point *tracing.*
Haller's a.'s, see *ligamentum* arcuatum laterale; *ligamentum* arcuatum mediale.
hemal a.'s, three or four V-shaped bones located ventral to the bodies of the third to sixth coccygeal vertebrae; they represent intercentra and usually enclose the ventral caudal artery and vein.
hyoid a., the second visceral, or branchial, a; the second postoral a. in the branchial a. series.
iliopectineal a., *arcus* iliopectineus.
inferior dental a., *arcus* dentalis inferior.
jugular venous a., *arcus* venosus juguli.
labial a., an orthodontic a. wire that approximates the labial surfaces of the teeth.
Langer's a., axillary a.
lateral longitudinal a., *arcus* pedis longitudinalis, pars lateralis.
lateral lumbocostal a., *ligamentum* arcuatum laterale.
lingual a., an orthodontic a. wire that approximates the lingual surfaces of the teeth.
longitudinal a. of foot, *arcus* pedis longitudinalis.

malar a., *arcus* zygomaticus.
mandibular a., mandibular process; the first postoral a. in the branchial a. series.
medial longitudinal a., *arcus* pedis longitudinalis, pars medialis.
medial lumbocostal a., *ligamentum* arcuatum mediale.
nasal venous a., an a. formed at the root of the nose by the two supratrochlear veins connected by a transverse vein.
neural a., *arcus* vertebrae.
a. of the palate, the vaulted roof of the mouth.
palatoglossal a., *arcus* palatoglossus.
palatopharyngeal a., *arcus* palatopharyngeus.
pharyngeal a.'s, branchial a.'s.
pharyngopalatine a., *arcus* palatopharyngeus.
plantar a., **(1)** *arcus* plantaris; **(2)** either of two bony a.'s of the foot, longitudinal a. or transverse a.
plantar venous a., *arcus* venosus plantaris.
posterior a. of atlas, *arcus* posterior atlantis.
posterior palatine a., *arcus* palatopharyngeus.
postoral a.'s, the series of branchial a.'s caudal to the mouth; the first is the mandibular, the second is the hyoid; caudal to the hyoid, the a.'s are unnamed, and designated only by their postoral number.
primitive costal a.'s, a.'s formed in the thoracic region of the vertebral column in the embryo from the costal processes or costal elements which give rise to the ribs.
pubic a., *arcus* pubis.
ribbon a., a thin, ribbon-shaped, rectangular orthodontic a. wire applied to the dental a.'s so that its widest dimension is parallel to the labial or buccal surfaces of the teeth.
superciliary a., *arcus* superciliaris.
superficial palmar a., *arcus* palmaris superficialis.
superficial palmar venous a., *arcus* venosus palmaris superficialis.
superior dental a., *arcus* dentalis superior.
supraorbital a., *margo* supraorbitalis.
tarsal a., see *arcus* palpebralis inferior and *arcus* palpebralis superior.
tendinous a., *arcus* tendineus; **t. a. of pelvic fascia,** *arcus* tendineus fasciae pelvis; **t. a. of levator ani muscle,** *arcus* tendineus musculi levatoris ani; **t. a. of soleus muscle,** *arcus* tendineus musculi solei.
a. of thoracic duct, see *ductus* thoracicus.
transverse a. of foot, *arcus* pedis transversalis.
Treitz' a., a fold of peritoneum arching between the left border of the ascending portion of the duodenum and the medial border of the left kidney; it contains the superior branch of the left colic artery and the inferior mesenteric vein.
vertebral a., *arcus* vertebrae.
visceral a.'s, branchial a.'s.
W-a., a fixed maxillary expansion device attached to the lingual part of the molars, with either bilateral or unilateral extension arms.
wire a., a wire conforming to the dental a.; used to restore the normal curve to the denture.
zygomatic a., *arcus* zygomaticus.

archaeus (ar-kē'ŭs) [L. fr. G. *archaios,* chief, leader]. Archeus; term first used by Valentine and later by Paracelsus and van Helmont to denote a spirit that presided over and governed bodily processes.

archaic (ar-kā'ik) [G. *archaikos,* ancient]. Ancient; old; in jungian psychology, denoting the ancestral past of mental processes.

Archambault, LaSalle, U.S. neurologist, 1879–1940. See Meyer-A. *loop.*

arche-. See arch-.

archenteron (ark-en'ter-on) [G. *archē,* beginning, + *enteron,* intestine]. Gastrocele (1).

archeocyte (ar'kē-ō-sīt) [G. *archaios,* ancient, + *kytos,* cell]. Obsolete term for ameboid cell (1).

archeokinetic (ar-kē-ō-ki-net'ik) [G. *archaios,* ancient, + *kinētikos,* relating to movement]. Denoting a low and primitive type of motor nerve mechanism, such as is found in the peripheral and the ganglionic nervous systems. *Cf.* neokinetic, paleokinetic.

archetype (ar'kē-tīp) [G. *archetypos,* first molded, fr. *archē,* origin, + *typiō,* to beat, stamp]. **1.** A primitive structural plan from which various modifications have evolved. **2.** Imago (2); in jungian psychology, structural manifestation of the collective unconscious.

archeus (ar-kē'ŭs). Archaeus.

archi-. See arch-.

archicerebellum (ar'ki-ser-ĕ-bel'ŭm) [archi- + L. *cerebellum*] [NA]. Vestibulocerebellum; the small phylogenetically oldest portion of the cerebellum, also called vestibulocerebellum because its afferents arise from the vestibular ganglion and nuclei; in mammals, it is represented by four subdivisions of the cerebellum: nodulus, uvula vermis, flocculus, and lingua cerebelli.

archicortex (ar'ki-kōr'teks) [archi- + L. *cortex*]. Archipallium. **1.** Typically, the phylogenetically older parts of the cerebral cortex. **2.** More specifically, the cortex forming the hippocampus. See also allocortex, and *cortex* cerebri.

archil (ar'kil). [old C.I. 1242]. Roccellin; orchella; orchil; a violet dye from the lichens *Rocella tinctoria* and *R. fuciformis.*

archin (ar'kin). Emodin.

archipallium (ar-ki-pal'ē-ŭm) [archi- + L. *pallium*]. Archicortex.

architectonics (ar-ki-tek-ton'iks). Cytoarchitecture.

archo-. **1** [G. *archē,* origin, beginning]. Variant of the combining form arch-. **2** [G. *archos,* rectum]. Obsolete combining form denoting the rectum. See procto- and recto-.

archwire (arch'wīr). A device consisting of a wire conforming to the alveolar or dental arch, used as an anchorage in correcting irregularities in the position of the teeth.

arciform (ar'ki-fōrm). Arcuate.

arctation (ark-tā'shŭn) [L. *arto* (improp. *arcto*), pp. *-atus,* to tighten]. A narrowing, contraction, stricture, or coarctation.

arcual (ar'kyū-ăl). Relating to an arch.

arcuate (ar'kyū-āt) [L. *arcuatus,* bowed]. Arcate; arciform; denoting a form that is arched or has the shape of a bow.

arcuation (ar-kyū-ā'shŭn). A bending or curvature.

ARCUS

arcus, gen. and pl. **arcus** (ar'kŭs) [L. a bow] [NA]. Any structure resembling a bent bow or an arch; an arc.
a. adipo'sus, a. cornealis.
a. alveola'ris mandib'ulae [NA], alveolar arch of mandible; limbus alveolaris (1); the free margin of the alveolar process of the mandible.
a. alveola'ris maxil'lae [NA], alveolar arch of maxilla; limbus alveolaris (2); the free border of the alveolar process of the maxilla.
a. ante'rior atlan'tis [NA], anterior arch of atlas; an arch that connects the lateral masses of the atlas anteriorly and articulates with the dens of the axis.
a. aor'tae [NA], aortic arch; arch of aorta; the curve between the ascending and descending portions of the aorta; it lies behind the manubrium sterni; it gives off the brachiocephalic trunk, the left common carotid, and the left subclavian arteries.
a. cartila'ginis cricoi'deae [NA], arch of cricoid cartilage; the

narrow part of the cartilage that encircles the air passage anterior to the lamina.

a. cornea'lis, a. adiposus, juvenilis, lipoides, or senilis; gerontoxon; an opaque, grayish ring at the periphery of the cornea just within the sclerocorneal junction, of frequent occurrence in the aged; it results from a deposit of fatty granules in, or hyaline degeneration of, the lamellae and cells of the cornea.

a. costa'lis [NA], costal arch; a. costarum; that portion of the inferior aperture of the thorax formed by the cartilages of the seventh to tenth ribs.

a. costa'rum, a. costalis.

a. denta'lis infe'rior [NA], inferior dental arch; mandibular dentition; the teeth supported by the alveolar part of the mandible, whether the 10 deciduous teeth or the 16 permanent teeth.

a. denta'lis supe'rior [NA], superior dental arch; maxillary dentition; the teeth supported by the alveolar process of the two maxillae, whether the 10 deciduous teeth or the 16 permanent teeth.

a. duc'tus thorac'ici [NA], arch of thoracic duct. See *ductus* thoracicus.

a. glossopalati'nus, a. palatoglossus.

a. iliopectin'eus [NA], iliopectineal arch; iliopectineal ligament; ligamentum iliopectineale; the fascial partition that separates the vascular and muscular lacunae deep to the inguinal ligament.

a. inguina'lis [NA], *ligamentum* inguinale.

a. juveni'lis, a. cornealis.

a. lipoi'des, a. cornealis.

a. lumbocosta'lis latera'lis, *ligamentum* arcuatum laterale.

a. lumbocosta'lis media'lis, *ligamentum* arcuatum mediale.

a. palati'ni, pillars of fauces; see a. palatoglossus and a. palatopharyngeus.

a. palatoglos'sus [NA], palatoglossal arch; glossopalatine arch or fold; anterior palatine arch; a. glossopalatinus; anterior pillar of fauces; one of a pair of ridges or folds of mucous membrane passing from the soft palate to the side of the tongue; it encloses the palatoglossus muscle.

a. palatopharyn'geus [NA], palatopharyngeal arch; pharyngopalatine arch; posterior palatine arch; posterior pillar of fauces; one of a pair of ridges or folds of mucous membrane which passes downward from the posterior margin of the soft palate to the lateral wall of the pharynx. It encloses the palatopharyngeus muscle.

a. palma'ris profun'dus [NA], deep palmar arch; a. volaris profundus; the arterial arch located deep to the long flexor tendons in the hand. It is formed by the radial artery in conjunction with the deep palmar branch of the ulnar artery.

a. palma'ris superficia'lis [NA], superficial palmar arch; a. volaris superficialis; the arterial arch in the hand located superficial to the long flexor tendons. It is formed principally by the ulnar artery and is usually completed by a communication with the superficial palmar branch of the radial artery.

a. palpebra'lis infe'rior [NA], arterial arch of lower eyelid; formed by the medial palpebral artery which communicates with a branch of the lacrimal artery along the tarsal margin.

a. palpebra'lis supe'rior [NA], arterial arch of upper eyelid; formed by communicating branches of the medial and lateral palpebral arteries. Often two arches are present, one located near the free border of the tarsal plate, the other along the upper border of the tarsus.

a. pe'dis longitudina'lis [NA], longitudinal arch of foot; it consists of the following: **a.p.l. pars medialis** medial longitudinal arch; formed by the calcaneus, talus, navicular, three cuneiform bones, and the three medial metatarsals; **a.p.l. pars lateralis** lateral longitudinal arch; formed by calcaneus, cuboid and two lateral metatarsals; the arch is supported normally by ligaments, intrinsic muscles, and the tendons of extrinsic muscles of the foot.

a. pe'dis transversa'lis [NA], transverse arch of foot; the arch formed by the proximal parts of the metatarsal bones, the three cuneiform bones, and the cuboid.

a. planta'ris [NA], plantar arch (1); the arterial arch formed by the lateral plantar artery running across the bases of the metatarsal bones and anastomosing with the dorsal artery of the foot.

a. poste'rior atlan'tis [NA], the posterior arch of the atlas that connects the lateral masses of the atlas posteriorly.

a. pu'bis [NA], pubic arch; the arch formed by the inferior rami of the pubic bones.

a. rani'nus, Béclard's *anastomosis.*

a. seni'lis, a. cornealis.

a. supercilia'ris [NA], superciliary arch or ridge; a fullness extending laterally from the glabella on either side, above the orbital margin of the frontal bone.

a. tar'seus, see a. palpebralis inferior and a. palpebralis superior.

a. tendin'eus [NA], tendinous arch; a fibrous band arching over a vessel or nerve as it passes through a muscle, and protecting it from injurious compression.

a. tendin'eus fas'ciae pel'vis [NA], tendinous arch of pelvic fascia; a linear thickening of the superior fascia of the pelvic diaphragm extending posteriorly from the body of the pubis alongside the bladder (and vagina in the female) and giving attachment to the supporting ligaments of the pelvic viscera.

a. tendin'eus mus'culi levato'ris ani [NA], tendinous arch of levator ani muscle; a thickened portion of the obturator fascia that extends in an arching line from the pubis posteriorly to the ischial spine and gives origin to part of the levator ani muscle.

a. tendin'eus mus'culi so'lei [NA], tendinous arch of soleus muscle; a tendinous arch stretching over the popliteal vessels between the tibia and fibula, that gives origin to the central portion of the soleus muscle.

a. un'guium, whitish area near the root of the nail.

a. veno'sus dorsa'lis pe'dis [NA], dorsal venous arch of foot; the arch in the subcutaneous tissue of the dorsum of the foot formed by the dorsal and digital veins; it unites medially with the dorsal vein of the great toe to form the great saphenous vein, and laterally with the dorsal vein of the little toe to form the small saphenous.

a. veno'sus jug'uli [NA], jugular venous arch; a connecting vein between the two anterior jugular veins in the suprasternal space.

a. veno'sus palma'ris profun'dus [NA], deep palmar venous arch; the venous arch that accompanies the deep palmar arterial arch; it usually consists of paired venae comitantes.

a. veno'sus palma'ris superficia'lis [NA], superficial palmar venous arch; the venous arch accompanying the superficial palmar arterial arch; it consists usually of paired venae comitantes.

a. veno'sus planta'ris [NA], plantar venous arch; the arch formed by the plantar digital veins from the toes.

a. ver'tebrae [NA], vertebral arch; neural arch; the posterior projection from the body of a vertebra that encloses the vertebral foramen; it consists of paired pedicles and laminae; the spinous, transverse, and articular processes arise from the arch. See also hemal *arches.*

a. vola'ris profun'dus, a. palmaris profundus.

a. vola'ris superficia'lis, a. palmaris superficialis.

a. zygomat'icus [NA], zygomatic arch; malar arch; zygoma (2); the arch formed by the temporal process of the zygomatic bone that joins the zygomatic process of the temporal bone.

---

ardanesthesia (ard'an-es-thē'zē-ă) [L. *ardor,* heat, + G. *an-* priv. + *aisthēsis,* sensation]. Thermoanesthesia.

ardor (ar'dōr) [L. fire, heat]. Old term for a hot or burning sensation.

ARDS Abbreviation for adult respiratory distress *syndrome.*

AREA

area, pl. **areae** (ār'ē-ă, -ēē) [L. a courtyard] **1** [NA]. Any circumscribed surface or space. **2.** All of the part supplied by a given artery or nerve. **3.** A part of an organ having a special function, as the motor a. of the brain. See also regio, region, space, spatium, zone, zona.

acoustic a., a. acustica.

a. acu'stica, acoustic a.; the floor of the lateral recess of the fourth ventricle, extending medially to the sulcus limitans and overlying the cochlear and vestibular nuclei of the rhombencephalon.

anterior intercondylar a., a. intercondylaris anterior.

aortic a., the region of the chest wall over the second right costal cartilage, where sounds produced at the aortic orifice are often best heard.

apical a., the a. about the root end of a tooth.

association a.'s, association *cortex.*

auditory a., auditory *cortex.*

bare a. of liver, a. nuda hepatis.

bare a. of stomach, the part of posterior surface of the fundus of the stomach between the two diverging layers of the gastrophrenic ligament, that is not covered by peritoneum.

basal seat a., that portion of the oral structures which is available to support a denture.

Broca's a., Broca's *center.*

Broca's parolfactory a., a. parolfactoria.

Brodmann's a.'s, a.'s of the cerebral cortex mapped out on the basis of the cortical cytoarchitectural patterns. See *cortex* cerebri.

a. of cardiac dullness, a triangular a. determined by percussion of the front of the chest; it corresponds to the part of the heart that is not covered by lung tissue.

Celsus' a., *alopecia* areata.

a. centra'lis, *macula* retinae.

a. coch'leae [NA], cochlear a.; the a. inferior to the transverse crest of the fundus of the internal acoustic meatus through which the filaments of the cochlear nerve pass to enter the cochlea.

cochlear a., a. cochleae.

Cohnheim's a., Cohnheim's field; a polygonal mosaic-like figure formed by a group of myofibrils, as seen in the cross-section of a skeletal muscle fiber examined under the microscope; a shrinkage artifact of fixation.

contact a., contact point; point of proximal contact; that part of the proximal surface of a tooth which touches the adjacent tooth mesially or distally.

cribriform a., a. cribrosa.

a. cribro'sa [NA], cribriform a.; the apex of a renal papilla pierced by 10 to 22 openings of the papillary ducts, the foramina papillaria.

denture-bearing a., denture foundation a.

denture foundation a., denture-bearing a.; that portion of the basal seat which supports the complete or partial denture base under occlusal load.

denture-supporting a., denture *foundation.*

dermatomic a., dermatome (3).

embryonal a., embryonic a., the a. of the blastoderm on either side of, and immediately cephalic to, the primitive streak where the component cell layers have become thickened.

entorhinal a., Brodmann's a. 28; a cytoarchitecturally well defined a. of multilaminate cerebral cortex on the medial aspect of the parahippocampal gyrus, immediately caudal to the olfactory cortex of the uncus; the a. is the origin of the major fiber system afferent to the hippocampus, the so-called perforant pathway.

excitable a., motor *cortex.*

a. of facial nerve, a. nervi facialis.

Flechsig's a.'s, three divisions (anterior, lateral, posterior) of each lateral half of the medulla as seen on transverse section, marked off by the root fibers of the hypoglossal and vagus nerves.

frontal a., frontal *cortex.*

fronto-orbital a., orbitofrontal *cortex.*

fusion a., Panum's a.

a. gas'trica [NA], one of a number of small polygonal a.'s, separated by linear depressions, on the surface of the mucous membrane of the stomach; they contain the gastric foveolae.

germinal a., a. germinati'va, a. germinativa; the place in the blastoderm where the embryo begins to be formed.

Head's a.'s, a.'s of skin exhibiting reflex hyperasthesia and hyperalgesia due to visceral disease.

impression a., in dentistry, that surface which is recorded in an impression.

inferior vestibular a., a. vestibularis inferior.

insular a., insula (1).

a. intercondyla'ris ante'rior [NA], anterior intercondylar a.; the broad depressed a. between the tibial condyles anteriorly to which attach the anterior ends of the menisci and the anterior cruciate ligament.

a. intercondyla'ris poste'rior [NA], posterior intercondylar a.; the deep notch between the tibial condyles posteriorly to which attaches the posterior cruciate ligament.

Jonston's a., *alopecia* areata.

Kiesselbach's a., Little's a.; an a. on the anterior portion of the nasal septum rich in capillaries and often the seat of epistaxis.

Little's a., Kiesselbach's a.

macular a., *macula* retinae.

Martegiani's a., Martegiani's *funnel.*

mitral a., the region of the chest over the apex of the heart, where the sounds, normal or pathologic, produced at the mitral valve are usually heard most distinctly.

motor a., motor *cortex.*

a. ner'vi facia'lis [NA], a. of facial nerve; the a. in the fundus of the internal acoustic meatus superior to the transverse crest through which the facial nerve passes to enter the facial canal.

a. nu'da hep'atis [NA], bare area of liver; the a. on the posterior surface of the liver which is fused with the diaphragm and therefore not covered by peritoneum.

obeliar a., the rhomboid region limited by lines uniting the parietal foramen of each side to the extremities of the straight portion of the sagittal suture.

olfactory a., *substantia* perforata anterior.

a. opa'ca, the peripheral a. of the blastoderm of birds and reptiles which is opaque because of adherent yolk.

oval a. of Flechsig, see *fasciculus* semilunaris.

Panum's a., fusion a.; the a. in and about the macula retinae in which stimulation of corresponding retinal points results in stereoscopic vision.

parastriate a., see visual *cortex.*

a. parolfacto'ria (Brocae) [NA], parolfactory a.; Broca's parolfactory a.; a small region of cerebral cortex on the medial surface of the frontal lobe, formed by the junction of the gyrus rectus with the gyrus cinguli, demarcated from the gyrus subcallosus by the sulcus parolfactorius posterior.

parolfactory a., a. parolfactoria.

pear-shaped a., retromolar *pad.*

a. pellu'cida, the translucent central part of the blastoderm of birds and reptiles.

peristriate a., see visual *cortex.*

piriform a., piriform *cortex.*

Pitres' a., prefrontal cortex of the cerebral hemisphere. See frontal *cortex.*

postcentral a., the cortex of the postcentral gyrus.

post dam a., posterior palatal seal a.

posterior intercondylar a., a. intercondylaris posterior.
posterior palatal seal a., post dam a.; postpalatal seal a.; the soft tissues along the junction of the hard and soft palates on which pressure within the physiologic limits of the tissues can be applied by a denture to aid in the retention of the denture.
postpalatal seal a., posterior palatal seal a.
a. postre'ma, a small, elevated a. in the lateral wall of the inferior recess of the fourth ventricle; one of the few loci in the brain where the blood-brain barrier is lacking; a chemoreceptor associated with vomiting.
precentral a., the cortex of the precentral gyrus.
precommissural septal a., a. subcallosa.
prefrontal a., prefrontal cortex. See frontal *cortex.*
premotor a., premotor *cortex.*
preoptic a., preoptic *region.*
prestriate a., secondary visual cortex; see visual *cortex.*
pretectal a., pretectal region; pretectum; a narrow, transversally oriented rostral zone of the mesencephalic tectum, bounded caudally by the superior colliculus, rostrally by the trigonum habenulae, and laterally by the pulvinar thalami; the a. contains several nuclei that receive fibers from the optic tract; it has bilateral efferent connections with the Edinger-Westphal nucleus of the oculomotor nuclear complex by way of which it mediates the pupillary light reflex.
primary visual a., see visual *cortex.*
pulmonary a., the region of the chest at the second left intercostal space, where sounds produced at the pulmonary orifice of the right ventricle are heard most distinctly.
relief a., in dentistry, the portion of the denture-bearing a. over which the denture base is altered to reduce functional pressure.
rest a., rest seat; the portion of a tooth structure or of a restoration in a tooth that is prepared to receive the positive seating of the metallic occlusal, incisal, lingual, or cingulum rest of a removable prosthesis.
retention a., an a. of a tooth provided during its preparation for restoration that will aid in holding the restoration in place. See also retention *groove,* retention *point.*
Rolando's a., motor *cortex.*
secondary visual a., see visual *cortex.*
sensorial or sensory a.'s, see *cortex* cerebri.
sensorimotor a., the precentral and postcentral gyri of the cerebral cortex.
septal a., the region of the cerebral hemisphere that stretches as a thin sheet of brain tissue between the fornix bundle and the ventral surface of the corpus callosum, forming the medial wall of the lateral ventricle's frontal horn; it extends ventrally through the narrow interval between the anterior commissure and the rostrum corporis callosi as the precommissural septum or gyrus subcallosus, which is continuous caudally with the preoptic a. and hypothalamus, as well as more laterally with the substantia innominata; it's major functional connections are with the hippocampus and hypothalamus.
silent a., any a. of the cerebral or cerebellar surface in which lesions cause no definite sensory or motor symptoms.
skip a.'s, subsidiary segments of diseased intestine in regional enteritis, separated from the region of major involvement.
somesthetic a., somatic sensory *cortex.*
stress-bearing a., **(1)** denture *foundation;* **(2)** surfaces of oral structures that resist forces, strains, or pressures brought upon them during function.
striate a., see visual *cortex.*
Stroud's pectinated a., the a. of the anal canal lying just below the rectal columns.
a. subcallo'sa [NA], *gyrus* subcallosus.
subcallosal a., *gyrus* subcallosus.
superior vestibular a., a. vestibularis superior.
supporting a., **(1)** those areas of the maxillary and mandibular edentulous ridges which are considered best suited to carry the forces of mastication when the dentures are in function; **(2)** denture *foundation.*
tissue-bearing a., denture *foundation.*
tricuspid a., the region of the chest wall over the lower part of the body of the sternum, where the sounds produced at the right atrioventricular orifice are heard most distinctly.
trigger a., trigger *point.*
vagus a., a portion of the floor of the fourth ventricle overlying the vagoglossopharyngeal nuclei.
a. vasculo'sa, the part of the a. opaca of the embryonic blastoderm of the chick, where the first blood vessels appear.
vestibular a., see a. vestibularis inferior and a. vestibularis superior.
a. vestibula'ris infe'rior [NA], inferior vestibular a.; the a. of the fundus of the internal acoustic meatus inferior to the transverse crest through which the saccular nerve passes.
a. vestibula'ris supe'rior [NA], superior vestibular a.; the a. in the fundus of the internal acoustic meatus superior to the transverse crest through which the superior part of the vestibular nerve passes to reach the macula utriculus and the ampullae of the anterior and lateral semicircular ducts.
visual a., visual *cortex.*
Wernicke's a., Wernicke's *center.*

---

areatus, areata (ă-rē-ā'tŭs, -tă) [L.]. Occurring in patches or circumscribed areas.

Areca (ar'ĕ-kă) [Malay]. A genus of palms of India and the Malay Archipelago. A species, *A. catechu,* furnishes a. nuts, or betel nuts, which contain arecoline and 15% red tannin, are chewed in the East Indies, and have an anthelmintic action. See also betel nut.

arecaidine (ă-rek'ā-dēn). Arecaine; 1,2,5,6-tetrahydro-1-methylnicotinic acid; a crystalline alkaloid resembling betaine, derived from the betel nut.

arecaine (ă-rek'ān). Arecaidine.

arecoline (ă-rek'ō-lēn). $C_8H_{13}NO_2$; a colorless oily alkaloid from the betel nut.

areflexia (ā-rē-flek'sē-ă). Absence of reflexes.

arenaceous (ar-ĕ-nā'shŭs) [L. *arena,* sand]. Sandy; of sand-like consistency.

Arenaviridae (ă-rē-nă-vir'i-dē) [L. *arēna* (*harēna*), sand]. A family of RNA viruses that includes lymphocytic choriomeningitis virus, Lassa virus, and the Tacaribe virus complex. The virions are 50 to 300 nm (average 100 nm) in diameter, enveloped, ether-sensitive, and contain single-stranded, segmented RNA (molecular weight 3 to 5 $\times$ 10^6); they also contain electron-dense, RNA-containing granules (20 to 30 nm in diameter) that resemble ribosomes, with an electron-microscopic appearance of sandiness.

Arenavirus (ă-rē'nă-vī'rŭs). The single genus of viruses in the family Arenaviridae.

areola, pl. **areolae** (ă-rē'ō-lă, -lē) [L. dim. of *area*]. **1** [NA]. Any small area. **2.** One of the spaces or interstices in areolar tissue. **3.** A mammae. **4.** Halo (3); a pigmented, depigmented, or erythematous zone surrounding a papule, pustule, wheal, or cutaneous neoplasm.
Chaussier's a., a ring of indurated tissue surrounding the lesion of cutaneous anthrax.
a. mam'mae [NA], a. papillaris; areola (3); a circular pigmented area surrounding the nipple or papilla mammae; its surface is dotted with little projections due to the presence of Montgomery's glands beneath.
a. papilla'ris, a. mammae.
a. umbilicus, a pigmented ring around the umbilicus in the pregnant woman.

areolar (ă-rē'ō-lăr). Relating to an areola.

areometer (ar-ē-om'ĕ-ter) [G. *araios,* thin, + G. *metron,* measure]. Hydrometer.

Arg Symbol for arginine or its mono- or diradical.

Ar'gas. A genus of soft ticks of the family Argasidae, some species of which usually infest birds but may attack man.
A. per'sicus, the abode, fowl, or Persian tick, a species that is a bloodsucking parasite of poultry; it may transmit fowl spirochetosis.
A. reflex'us, the pigeon tick, a species that may cause a cutaneous inflammatory lesion in man.

argasid (ar-gas'id). Common name for members of the family Argasidae.

Argasidae (ar-gas'i-dē). Family of ticks (superfamily Ixodoidea, order Acarina), the soft ticks, so called because of their wrinkled, leathery, tuberculated appearance that fills out when the tick is engorged with blood. A dorsal shield (scutum) is not present; the mouthparts (capitulum) are subterminal or ventral in a depression (camerostome) that extends above the capitulum to form the anterior margin of the cephalothorax (hood). A. contains about 85 species in 4 genera: *Argas, Ornithodoros, Otobius,* and *Antricola;* argasid ticks, chiefly species of *Ornithodoros,* harbor and transmit spirochetes of the genus *Borrelia* that cause relapsing fever in birds and mammals.

argentaffin, argentaffine (ar-jen'tă-fin, -fēn) [L. *argentum,* silver, + *affinitas,* affinity]. Pertaining to cells or tissue elements that reduce silver ions in solution, thereby becoming stained brown or black.

argentaffinoma (ar'jen-tă-fi-nō'mă, -taf-i-nō'mă). Carcinoid *tumor.*

argentation (ar-jen-tā'shŭn). Impregnation with a silver salt. See also argyria.

argentic (ar-jen'tik). **1.** Argyric (1); relating to silver. **2.** Denoting a chemical compound containing silver as the rare, doubly charged (Ag^{2+}) ion.

argentine (ar'jen-tēn). Relating to, resembling, or containing silver.

argentophil, argentophile (ar-jen'tō-fil, -fīl). Argyrophil.

argentous (ar-jen'tŭs). Denoting a chemical compound containing silver as a singly charged (Ag^{+}) ion. The vast majority of silver compounds contain the a. ion; where the ionic state of silver is not specifically stated, as in silver nitrate, the a. state is assumed.

argentum, gen. **argenti (Ag)** (ar-jen'tŭm, -jen'tī) [L.]. Silver.

arginase (ar'ji-nās) [EC 3.5.3.1]. Arginine amidase; canavanase; an enzyme of the liver that catalyzes the hydrolysis of arginine to ornithine and urea; a key enzyme of the urea cycle.

arginine (Arg) (ar'ji-nēn). 2-Amino-5-guanidinopentanoic acid; one of the amino acids occurring among the hydrolysis products of protein, particularly abundant in the basic proteins such as histones and protamines, and forming with lysine and histidine the group of basic amino acids called hexone bases or 6-carbon amino acids.
a. amidase, arginase.
a. deiminase [EC 3.5.3.6], a. dihydrolase or iminohydrolase; an enzyme catalyzing the hydrolytic deamination of a. to citrulline.
a. dihydrolase, a. deiminase.
a. glutamate, a compound composed of arginine and glutamic acid, given intravenously to detoxify ammonia; used in the treatment of ammoniemia resulting from liver dysfunction.
a. hydrochloride, a form of a. used for intravenous administration as an adjunct in the treatment of encephalopathies associated with liver diseases and ammoniacal azotemia.
a. iminohydrolase, a. deiminase.
a. phosphate, phosphoarginine.

argininosuccinase (ar'ji-ni-nō-sŭk'si-nās). Argininosuccinate lyase.

argininosuccinate lyase (ar'ji-ni-nō-sŭk'si-nāt) [EC 4.3.2.1]. Argininosuccinase; an enzyme cleaving L-argininosuccinate nonhydrolytically to L-arginine and fumarate.

argininosuccinic acid (ar'ji-ni-nō-sŭk-sin'ik). HOOC-$CH_2CH(COOH)$-NH-C(NH)-$NH(CH_2)_3CHNH_2$-COOH; formed as an intermediate in the conversion of citrulline to arginine in the urea cycle, in a reaction involving aspartic acid and adenosine triphosphate.

argininosuccinicaciduria (ar-ji-nin'ō-sŭk-sin'ik-as-i-dū'rē-ă). A possibly heritable disorder characterized by excessive urinary excretion of argininosuccinic acid, epilepsy, ataxia, mental retardation, liver disease, and friable, tufted hair; presumed to be the consequence of a deficiency of an enzyme responsible for splitting argininosuccinic acid to arginine and fumaric acid.

arginyl (ar'jin-il). The aminoacyl radical of arginine.

argipressin (ar-ji-pres'in). Arginine *vasopressin.*

argon (ar'gon) [G. ntr. of *argos,* lazy, inactive, fr. *a-* priv. + *ergon,* work]. A gaseous element, symbol Ar, atomic no. 18, atomic weight 39.95, present in the atmosphere in the proportion of about 1%; one of the noble gases.

Argonz, J., Argentinian physician. See A.-Del Castillo *syndrome.*

Argyll Robertson. See Robertson, Douglas Argyll.

argyria (ar-jir'ē-ă, -jī'rē-ă) [G. *argyros,* silver]. Argyriasis; argyrosis; argyrism; silver poisoning; a slate-gray or bluish discoloration of the skin and deep tissues, due to the deposit of insoluble albuminate of silver, occurring after the medicinal administration for a long period of a soluble silver salt; formerly fairly common from use of proprietary preparations of silver-containing materials in the nose and sinuses.

argyriasis (ar-ji-rī'ă-sis). Argyria.

argyric (ar-jir'ik). **1.** Argentic (1). **2.** Relating to argyria.

argyrism (ar'ji-rizm). Argyria.

argyrophil, argyrophile (ar-jī'rō-fil, -fīl) [G. *argyros,* silver, + *philos,* fond]. Argentophil, argentophile; pertaining to tissue elements that are capable of impregnation with silver ions and being made visible after an external reducing agent is used.

argyrosis (ar-ji-rō'sis). Argyria.

arhinia (ă-rin'ē-ă). Arrhinia.

Arias-Stella, Javier, Peruvian pathologist, *1924. See A.-S. *effect, phenomenon, reaction.*

ariboflavinosis (ă-rī'bō-flā-vi-nō'sis). Properly hyporiboflavinosis: a nutritional condition produced by a deficiency of riboflavin in the diet, characterized by cheilosis and magenta tongue.

aristogenics (ă-ris-tō-jen'iks) [G. *aristos,* best, + *genikos,* pertaining to race]. Eugenics.

aristolochic acid (ă-ris-tō-lō-kik). 8-Methoxy-6-nitrophenanthro[3,4-d]-1,3-dioxole-5-carboxylic acid; an aromatic bitter derived from plants of the genus *Aristolochia.*

aristotelian (ar'is-tō-tē'lē-ăn, ar'i-stō-tēl'yan). Attributed to or described by Aristotle.

Aristotle of Stagira, Greek philosopher and scientist, 384–322 B.C. See A.'s *anomaly,* aristotelian *method.*

arithmomania (ă-rith-mō-mā'nē-ă). A morbid impulse to count.

Arizona (ar'i-zō'nă). A genus of motile, peritrichous, nonsporeforming, aerobic to facultatively anaerobic bacteria (family Enterobacteriaceae) containing Gram-negative rods. These organisms do not produce urease and do not grow in media containing potassium cyanide. They decarboxylate lysine, arginine, and ornithine. Lactose is generally fermented. These organisms have been isolated from a wide variety of animals, including man; they may cause gastroenteritis in man and frequently are involved in localized lesions in man and lower animals. There is a single species, *A. hinshawii,* the type species.

Arlt, Carl Ferdinand von, Austrian ophthalmologist, 1812–1887. See A.'s *operation, sinus.*

arm [L. *armus,* forequarter of an animal; G. *harmos,* a shoulder joint]. **1.** brachium; the segment of the superior limb between the shoulder and the elbow; commonly used to mean the whole superior limb. **2.** A specifically shaped and positioned extension of a removable partial denture framework.

bar clasp a., a clasp a. which has its origin in the denture base or major connector; it consists of the a. which traverses but does not contact the gingival structures, and a terminal end which approaches its contact with the tooth in a gingivo-occlusal direction.

brawny a., a swollen arm caused by lymphedema, particularly after homolateral radical mastectomy.

circumferential clasp a., a clasp a. which has its origin in a minor connector and which follows the contour of the tooth approximately in a plane perpendicular to the path of insertion of the partial denture.

clasp a., a portion of a clasp of a removable partial denture which projects from the clasp body and helps retain the partial denture in position in the mouth. See clasp (2).

dynein a., a structure extending clockwise from one tubule of each of the 9 doublet microtubules toward the adjacent doublet seen in the axoneme of cilia or flagella (including human sperm tails); congenital absence of dynein, reflected structurally by absence of dynein a.'s, can account for symptoms seen in Kartagener's syndrome and in immotile cilia syndromes.

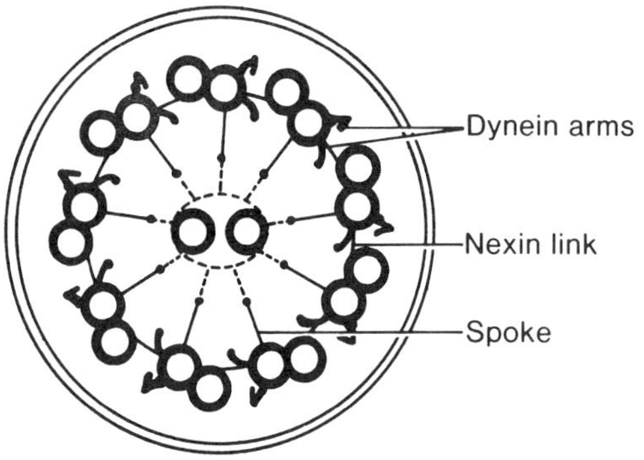

Dynein Arm
Cross-section of a cilium or central portion of a sperm tail; the exact attachment sites of the nexin links are tentative.

reciprocal a., a clasp a. or other extension used on a removable partial denture to oppose the action of some other part or parts of the appliance.

retentive a., retention a., a flexible segment of a removable partial denture that engages an undercut on an abutment and is designed to retain the denture.

retentive circumferential clasp a., an a. that is flexible and engages the infrabulge at the terminal end of the a.

stabilizing circumferential clasp a., an a. that is relatively rigid and embraces the height of contour of the tooth.

armamentarium (ar'mă-men-tār'ē-ŭm) [L. an arsenal, fr. *armamenta,* implements, tackle, fr. *arma,* armor, arms]. All the therapeutic means available to the health practitioner for the practice of his profession.

Armanni, Luciano, Italian pathologist, 1839–1903. See A.-Ebstein *kidney.*

armarium (ar-mar'ē-ŭm) [L. a closet, chest, fr. *arma,* armor]. Rarely used term for the physician's library, as part of his armamentarium.

Armillifer (ar-mil'i-fer) [O. Fr. *armille,* fr. L. *armilla,* a bracelet]. A genus of Pentastomida (order Porocephalida, family Porocephalidae); adults are found in the lungs of reptiles and the young in many mammals, including man.

A. armilla'tus, *Porocephalus armillatus;* species occurring in the python, the larva or nymph being occasionally found in man.

arm'pit. *Fossa* axillaris.

Armstrong, Arthur R., Canadian physician, *1904. See King-A. *unit.*

Armstrong, Henry E., British physician. See King-A. *unit.*

Arndt, G., German physician. See A.-Gottron *syndrome.*

Arndt, Rudolph, German psychiatrist, 1835–1900. See A.'s *law.*

Arneth, Joseph, German physician, 1873–1955. See A. *classification, count, formula, index, stages.*

arnica (ar'ni-kă) [Mod. L.]. Leopard's bane; mountain tobacco; the dried flower heads of *Arnica montana* (family Compositae); a cardiac sedative, but seldom given internally; used externally for sprains and bruises.

Arnold, Friedrich, German anatomist, 1803–1890. See A.'s *bundle, canal, ganglion, nerve, tract; foramen* of A.

Arnold, Julius, German pathologist, 1835–1915. See A.'s *bodies;* A.-Chiari *deformity, malformation, syndrome.*

aromatic (ar-ō-mat'ik) [G. *arōmatikos,* fr. *arōma,* spice, sweet herb]. **1.** Having an agreeable, somewhat pungent, spicy odor. **2.** One of a group of vegetable drugs having a fragrant odor and slightly stimulant properties. **3.** See aromatic *compound.*

aromatic L-amino-acid decarboxylase [EC 4.1.1.28]. Dopa decarboxylase; tryptophan decarboxylase; hydroxytryptophan decarboxylase; an enzyme that catalyzes the decarboxylation of dopa to dopamine, of tryptophan to tryptamine, and of hydroxytryptophan to serotonin; important in the biosynthetic pathway of catecholamines and melanin.

aroyl (a'rō-il). The radical of an aromatic acid (*e.g.,* benzoyl); analogous to acyl, the more general term.

arrack (a-rak') [Ar. sweet juice]. A strong alcoholic liquor distilled from dates, rice, sap of the coconut palm, and other substances.

arrector, pl. **arrectores** (ă-rek'tōr, ă-rek-tō'rēz) [L. that which raises, fr. *ar-rigo,* pp. *-rectus,* to raise up]. Erector.

arrecto'res pilo'rum, a bundle of smooth muscle between the connective sheath of the hair follicle and the papillary layer of the dermis; contraction of the muscle erects the hair and causes cutis anserina (goose flesh).

arrest (ă-rest') [O.Fr. *arester,* fr. LL. *adresto,* to stop behind]. **1.** To stop, check, or restrain. **2.** A stoppage; interference with, or checking of, the regular course of a disease, a symptom, or the performance of a function. **3.** Inhibition of a developmental process, usually at the ultimate stage of development; premature a. may lead to a congenital abnormality.

cardiac a. (CA), a loss of effective cardiac function, which results in cessation of circulation; may be due to asystole in which there is no observable myocardial activity or to ventricular fibrillation.

circulatory a., cessation of the circulation of blood as a result of ventricular standstill or fibrillation.

epiphysial a., early and premature fusion between epiphysis and diaphysis.

maturation a., cessation of complete differentiation of cells at an immature stage; in spermatogenic maturation a., the seminiferous tubules contain spermatocytes but no spermatozoa develop.

sinus a., cessation of sinus activity; the ventricles may continue to beat under A-V nodal or idioventricular control. See also sinus and atrial *standstill.*

arrhenic (ă-ren'ik). Relating to arsenic.

Arrhenius, Svante A., Swedish chemist, 1859–1927. See A. *doctrine, equation, law;* A.-Madsen *theory.*

arrhenoblastoma (ă-rē'nō-blas-tō'mă) [G. *arrhēn,* male, + *blastos,* germ, + *-ōma,* tumor]. Ovarian tubular adenoma; androblastoma (2); gynandroblastoma (1); a rare ovarian tumor that produces masculinization and often contains tubules and luteinized cells.

arrhenogenic (ă-rē-nō-jen'ik) [G. arrhēn, male, + *genesis,* production]. Productive of males only.

arrhenotocia (ă-rē-nō-tō'sē-ă) [G. *arrhēn,* male, + *tokos,* birth]. A form of parthenogenesis in which the virgin female gives birth to males only, as in the case of the queen bee.

arrhigosis (ă-ri-gō'sis) [G. *a-* priv. + *rigoun,* to shiver]. Lack of perception of cold.

arrhinencephaly, arrhinencephalia (ă-rin-en-sef'ă-lē, -se-fā'lē-ă) [G. *a-* priv. + *rhis (rhin-),* nose, + *enkephalos,* brain]. Congenital absence or rudimentary state of the rhinencephalon, or olfactory lobe of the brain, on one or both sides, with a corresponding lack of development of the external olfactory organs.

arrhinia (ă-rin'ē-ă) [G. *a-* priv. + *rhis (rhin-),* nose]. Arhinia; congenital absence of the nose.

arrhythmia (ă-ridh'mē-ă) [G. *a-* priv. + *rhythmos,* rhythm]. Loss of rhythm; denoting especially an irregularity of the heartbeat. *Cf.* dysrhythmia. See also entries under rhythm.
cardiac a., see cardiac *dysrhythmia.*
juvenile a., sinus a.
nonphasic sinus a., sinus a. in which variations in rhythm are not related to the phases of respiration.
phasic sinus a., respiratory a.; sinus a. in which the irregularity is related to the phases of respiration, the rate being faster in inspiration and slower in expiration.
respiratory a., phasic sinus a.
sinus a., juvenile a.; irregularity of the heartbeat, the heart being under the control of its normal pacemaker, the sinoatrial node.

arrhythmic (ă-ridh'mik, ā-). Marked by loss of rhythm; pertaining to arrhythmia.

arrhythmogenic (ă-ridh-mō-jen'ik) [G. *a-* priv. + *rhythmos,* rhythm, + *-gen,* production]. Capable of inducing cardiac arrhythmias.

arrhythmokinesis (ă-ridh'mō-ki-nē'sis) [G. *a-* priv. + *rhythmos,* rhythm, + *kinēsis,* movement]. Inability to preserve the rhythm of voluntary alternating movements.

arrowroot (ar'ō-rūt). The rhizome of *Maranta arundinacea,* a plant of tropical America, which is the source of a form of starch formerly used as a dietary supplement.

Arroyo, Carlos F., U.S. physician, 1892–1928. See A.'s *sign.*

Arruga, Count Hermenegildo, Spanish ophthalmologist, 1886–1972. See A.'s *forceps.*

arsacetin (ar-să-sē'tin). *p-* Acetamidobenzenearsonic acid; formerly used as an antisyphilitic agent.

arsenamide (ar-sen'ă-mīd). {[(*p-* Carbamoylphenyl)arsylene]dithio}diacetic acid; $H_2NCO\text{-}C_6H_4\text{-}As(SCH_2COOH)_2$; used in the treatment of filariasis.

arsenate (ar'sĕ-nāt). A salt of arsenic acid.

arseniasis (ar-sen-ī'ă-sis). Arsenicalism; chronic arsenical poisoning.

arsenic (ar'sĕ-nik) [Mod. L. fr. G. *arsenikon,* fr. *arsēn,* strong]. Arsenium; ratsbane; a metallic element, symbol As, atomic no. 33, atomic weight 74.9; forms a number of poisonous compounds, some of which are used in medicine.
a. trihydride, arsine.
a. trioxide, arsenous oxide; white a.; As_2O_3; dissolves in water to give arsenous acid, H_3AsO_3; used in the treatment of skin diseases and malaria, and as a tonic; also used externally as a caustic.
white a., a. trioxide.

arsenic (ar-sen'ik). Arsenical (2); arsenous (2); arsenious; denoting the element arsenic or one of its compounds, especially arsenic acid.

arsenic acid. $H_3AsO_4 \cdot {}^1/_2H_2O$; the hydrate of arsenic oxide or arsenic pentoxide which forms arsenates with certain bases.

arsenical (ar-sen'i-kăl). **1.** A drug or agent, the effect of which depends on its arsenic content. **2.** Denoting or containing arsenic.

arsenicalism (ar-sen'i-kăl-izm). Arseniasis.

arsenic-fast. Resistant to the poisonous action of arsenic; denoting especially spirochetes and other protozoan parasites, which acquire resistance after repeated administration of the drug.

arsenide (ar'sĕ-nīd). Arseniuret; a compound of arsenic with a metal or other positively charged atoms or groups in which the arsenic is not bound to any atoms of oxygen.

arsenious (ar-sen'ē-ŭs). Arsenic (adj.).

arsenium (ar-sē'nē-ŭm). Arsenic.

arseniuret (ar-se'nyū-ret). Arsenide.

arseniureted (ar-sē'nyū-ret-ed). Combined with arsenic so as to form an arsenide.

arsenotherapy (ar'sen-ō-thār'ă-pē). Therapeutic treatment with arsenic.

arsenous (ar'-sen-ŭs). **1.** Denoting a compound of arsenic with a valence of +3. **2.** Arsenic (adj.).

arsenous acid. See *arsenic* trioxide.

arsenous hydride. Arsine.

arsenous oxide. *Arsenic* trioxide.

arsenoxides (ar-sĕ-nok'i-dēs). Oxidation products in the body of arsphenamines; believed to be the agents active against spirochetes.

arsine (ar'sēn). Arsenic trihydride; arseniureted hydrogen; arsenous hydride; AsH_3; a cell and blood poison, many organic derivatives of which have been used in chemical warfare.

arsonic acid (ar-son'ik). A derivative of arsenic acid by replacement of a hydroxyl group by an organic radical.

arsonium (ar-son'ē-ŭm). The positively charged ion, AsH_4^+; analogous to the ammonium ion, NH_4^+.

arsphenamine (ars-fen'ă-min). Phenarsenamine; 3,3'-diamino-4,4'-dihydroxyarsenobenzene dihydrochloride; formerly used in the treatment of syphilis, yaws, and some other diseases of protozoan origin, after neutralization with NaOH. The synthesis of a. in 1907 and the demonstration of its usefulness as a therapeutic agent by Paul Ehrlich and co-workers (1909) marked the beginning of chemotherapy.

arsthinol (ars'thī-nol). Cyclic (hydroxymethyl)ethylene ester of 3-acetamido-4-hydroxydithiobenzenearsonous acid; an amebicide.

artefact (ar'tĕ-fakt). Artifact.

arteri-. See arterio-.

ARTERIA

arteria, gen. and pl. **arteriae** (ar-tēr'ē-ă, ar-tēr'ī-e) [L. from G. *artēria,* the windpipe, later an artery as distinct from a vein] [NA]. Artery; a blood vessel conveying blood in a direction away from the heart. With the exception of the pulmonary and umbilical arteries, the arteries convey red or aerated blood. At the major arteries, the arterial branches are listed separately following the designation *branches.* See also ramus for additional listings and definitions of arterial branches.
a. acetab'uli, *ramus* acetabularis.
a. alveola'ris infe'rior [NA], inferior alveolar artery; inferior den-

tal artery; *origin,* maxillary artery; *distribution,* through mandibular canal to lower teeth; *branches,* mylohyoid, mental, dental.
a. alveola'ris supe'rior ante'rior [NA], anterior superior alveolar artery; anterior superior dental artery; *origin,* infraorbital artery; *distribution,* upper incisors and canine teeth, maxillary sinus.
a. alveola'ris supe'rior poste'rior [NA], posterior superior alveolar or posterior alveolar artery; posterior dental artery; *origin,* maxillary artery; *distribution,* molar and premolar teeth, gingiva.
a. anastomot'ica auricula'ris mag'na, Kugel's *artery.*
a. anastomot'ica mag'na, **(1)** a. collateralis ulnaris inferior; **(2)** a. genus descendens.
a. angula'ris [NA], angular artery (1); the terminal branch of the facial artery; *distribution,* muscles and skin of side of nose; *anastomoses,* lateral nasal, and dorsal artery of nose and palpebrals from the ophthalmic.
a. anon'yma, *truncus* brachiocephalicus.
a. appendicula'ris [NA], appendicular artery; the branch of the ileocolic artery that supplies the vermiform appendix.
a. arcua'ta [NA], arcuate artery; a. metatarsalis; metatarsal artery; *origin,* dorsalis pedis; *branches,* deep plantar, dorsal metatarsals and dorsal digitals.
arte'riae arcua'tae renis, arcuate arteries of kidney; arciform arteries; branches of the interlobar arteries of the kidney which at the junction of the cortex and medulla turn and run at right angles to the parent stem and approximately parallel to the surface of the kidney.
a. articula'ris az'ygos, a. genus media.
a. ascen'dens [NA], ascending artery; the branch of the ileocolic artery that communicates with a branch of the right colic artery and supplies the ascending colon.
arteriae atria'les [NA], atrial arteries; branches of the right and left coronary arteries distributed to the muscle of the atria.
a. auditi'va inter'na, a. labyrinthi.
a. auricula'ris poste'rior [NA], posterior auricular artery; *origin,* external carotid; *branches,* muscular, posterior tympanic, auricular, occipital, and stylomastoid.
a. auricula'ris profun'da [NA], deep auricular artery; *origin,* maxillary; *distribution,* articulation of jaw, parotid gland, and external acoustic meatus; *anastomoses,* branches of superficial temporal and posterior auricular.
a. axilla'ris [NA], axillary artery; the continuation of the subclavian in the axilla, becoming the brachial in the arm; *branches,* superior thoracic, thoracoacromial, lateral thoracic, subscapular, posterior and anterior circumflex humeral.
a. basila'ris [NA], basilar artery; formed by union of the two vertebral arteries; runs from the lower to the upper border of the pons, where it bifurcates into the two posterior cerebral arteries; *branches,* anterior, inferior, cerebellar, labyrinthine, pontine, mesencephalic, and superior cerebellar.
a. brachia'lis [NA], brachial artery; humeral artery; *origin,* is a continuation of the axillary; *branches,* deep brachial, superior ulnar collateral, inferior ulnar collateral, muscular, and nutrient; bifurcates at the elbow into radial and ulnar.
a. brachia'lis superficia'lis [NA], superficial brachial artery; an occasional variation in which the brachial artery lies superficial to the median nerve in the arm.
a. bucca'lis [NA], buccal artery; buccinator artery; *origin,* maxillary; *distribution,* buccinator muscle, skin, and mucous membrane of cheek; *anastomoses,* buccal branch of facial.
a. bul'bi pe'nis [NA], artery of bulb of penis; a. bulbi urethrae; a branch of the internal pudendal artery which supplies the bulb of the penis.
a. bul'bi ure'thrae, a. bulbi penis.
a. bul'bi vestib'uli [NA], artery of bulb of vestibule; the branch of the internal pudendal artery in the female that supplies the bulb of the vestibule.
a. calcari'na, *ramus* calcarinus.
a. callo'somargina'lis [NA], callosomarginal artery; the second branch of the pericallosal artery running in the cingulate sulcus and sending branches to supply part of the medial and superolateral surfaces of the cerebral hemisphere.
a. cana'lis pterygoid'ei [NA], artery of pterygoid canal; vidian artery; a tiny artery running in the pterygoid canal connecting the maxillary and internal carotid arteries.
arte'riae carot'icotympan'ici [NA], caroticotympanic arteries; rami caroticotympanici; small branches from the petrous part of the internal carotid artery supplying the tympanic cavity.
a. carot'is commu'nis [NA], common carotid artery; *origin,* right from brachiocephalic, left from arch of aorta; runs upward in the neck and divides opposite upper border of thyroid cartilage into *terminal branches,* external and internal carotid.
a. carot'is exter'na [NA], external carotid artery; *origin,* common carotid; *branches,* superior thyroid, lingual, facial, occipital, posterior auricular, ascending pharyngeal, and *terminal branches,* maxillary and superficial temporal.
a. carot'is inter'na [NA], internal carotid artery; arises from the common carotid opposite upper border of thyroid cartilage, and terminates in the middle cranial fossa by dividing into the anterior and middle cerebral arteries; for descriptive purposes it is divided into four parts: pars cervicalis, pars petrosa, pars cavernosa, and pars cerebralis. See under pars.
a. cau'dae pancrea'tis [NA], caudal pancreatic artery; *origin,* splenic artery near the left gastroepiploic; *distribution,* the tail of the pancreas; *anastomoses,* with other pancreatic arteries.
a. ceca'lis ante'rior [NA], anterior cecal artery; *origin,* ileocolic artery; *distribution,* anterior region of cecum.
a. ceca'lis poste'rior [NA], posterior cecal artery; *origin,* ileocolic artery; *distribution,* posterior region of cecum.
a. celia'ca, *truncus* celiacus.
arte'riae centra'les anterolatera'les [NA], anterolateral central or striate arteries; arteriae thalamostriatae anterolaterales; anterolateral thalamostriate arteries; lateral striate arteries; lenticulostriate arteries (1); numerous small branches from the sphenoidal part of the middle cerebral arteries supplying the lateral and anterior parts of the corpus striatum.
arte'riae centra'les anteromedia'les [NA], anteromedial central arteries; arteriae thalamostriatae anteromediales; anteromedial thalamostriate arteries; several small branches of the precommunical part of the anterior cerebral artery; they are distributed to the anteromedial part of the corpus striatum part of the thalamus.
a. centra'lis brev'is [NA], short central artery; a branch of the precommunical part of the anterior cerebral artery.
a. centra'lis long'a [NA], long central artery; a. recurrens; recurrent artery; artery of Heubner; a branch of the precommunical part of the anterior cerebral artery supplying the anterior and inferior portions of the head of the caudate, putamen, and the anterior part of the internal capsule.
arte'riae centra'les posterolatera'les [NA], posterolateral central arteries; circumflex mesencephalic branches; several small branches of the postcommunical part of the posterior cerebral artery distributed to the lateral posterior part of the midbrain.
arte'riae centra'les posteromedia'les [NA], posteromedial central arteries; interpeduncular perforating branches; several small branches from the precommunical part of the posterior cerebral artery supplying the posterior medial part of the midbrain.
a. centra'lis ret'inae [NA], central artery of retina; a. retinae centralis; Zinn's artery; a branch of the ophthalmic artery which penetrates the optic nerve 1 cm behind the eye to enter the eye at the optic papilla in the retina; it divides into superior and inferior temporal and nasal branches.
a. cerebel'li infe'rior ante'rior [NA], anterior inferior cerebellar artery; *origin,* basilar; *distribution,* lower surface of lateral lobes of cerebellum; *anastomoses,* posterior inferior cerebellar.
a. cerebel'li infe'rior poste'rior [NA], posterior inferior cerebellar

artery; *origin,* vertebral; *distribution,* medulla, choroid plexus, and cerebellum; *anastomoses,* superior cerebellar and anterior inferior cerebellar.

a. cerebel'li supe'rior [NA], superior cerebellar artery; *origin,* basilar; *distribution,* upper surface of cerebellum and colliculi; *anastomoses,* posterior inferior cerebellar.

a. cer'ebri ante'rior [NA], anterior cerebral artery; one of the two terminal branches of the internal carotid; it passes posteriorly in the interhemispheric fissure along with its fellow of the opposite side, the two being joined by the anterior communicating artery; for descriptive purposes it is divided into two parts: the pars precommunicalis, supplying branches to the thalamus and corpus striatum, and the pars postcommunicalis, or a. pericallosa, supplying branches to the cortex of the medial parts of the frontal and parietal lobes.

a. cer'ebri me'dia [NA], middle cerebral artery; one of the two large terminal branches of the internal carotid artery; it passes laterally around the pole of the temporal lobe, then posteriorly in the depth of the lateral cerebral fissure; for descriptive purposes it is divided into three parts: 1) the pars sphenoidalis, supplying perforating branches to the internal capsule, thalamus, and corpus striatum; 2) the pars insularis, supplying branches to the insula and adjacent cortical areas; and 3) the pars terminalis or pars corticalis, supplying a large part of the central cortical convexity.

a. cer'ebri poste'rior [NA], posterior cerebral artery, formed by the bifurcation of the basilar artery; it passes around the cerebral peduncle to reach the medial aspect of the hemisphere; for descriptive purposes it is divided into three parts: 1) the pars precommunicalis, the part before the junction with the posterior communicating artery, supplying part of the thalamus and hypothalamus; 2) the pars postcommunicalis, supplying the thalamus, cerebral peduncles, and the choroid plexuses of the lateral and third ventricles; and 3) the pars terminalis or pars corticalis, supplying the cortex of the temporal and occipital lobes.

a. cervica'lis ascen'dens [NA], ascending cervical artery; cervicalis ascendens (2); *origin,* inferior thyroid, sometimes independently from the thyrocervical trunk; *distribution,* muscles of neck and spinal cord; *anastomoses,* branches of vertebral, occipital, ascending pharyngeal, and deep cervical.

a. cervica'lis profun'da [NA], deep cervical artery; *origin,* costocervical trunk; *distribution,* posterior deep muscles of neck; *anastomoses,* branches of occipital, ascending cervical, and vertebral.

a. cervica'lis superficia'lis [NA], superficial cervical artery. See *ramus* superficialis arteriae transversae colli.

a. cervicovagina'lis, cervicovaginal *artery.*

a. choroi'dea ante'rior [NA], anterior choroidal artery; *origin,* internal carotid or middle cerebral artery; *distribution,* optic tract, crus cerebri, uncus, hippocampus, globus pallidus, posterior part of internal capsule, geniculate bodies of the thalamus, and choroid plexus in the inferior horn of the lateral ventricle.

a. choroi'dea poste'rior, posterior choroidal artery; one of several choroidal rami of the posterior cerebral artery that supply the choroid plexus of the body of the lateral ventricle and of the third ventricle.

a. cilia'ris ante'rior [NA], anterior ciliary artery; one of several arteries derived from muscular branches of the ophthalmic which perforate the anterior part of the sclera and anastomose with posterior ciliary arteries.

a. cilia'ris poste'rior bre'vis [NA], short posterior ciliary artery; one of several ciliary branches of the ophthalmic distributed to the choroid coat of the eye.

a. cilia'ris poste'rior lon'ga [NA], long posterior ciliary artery; one of two branches of the ophthalmic running forward between the sclerotic and choroid coats to the iris, at the outer and inner margins of which they form by anastomosis two circles.

a. circumflex'a fem'oris latera'lis [NA], lateral circumflex a. of thigh; *origin,* profunda femoris; *distribution,* hip joint, thigh muscles; *anastomoses,* medial circumflex femoral, inferior gluteal, superior gluteal.

a. circumflex'a fem'oris media'lis [NA], medial circumflex artery of thigh; *origin,* profunda femoris; *distribution,* hip joint, muscles of thigh; *anastomoses,* inferior gluteal, superior gluteal, lateral circumflex femoral.

a. circumflex'a hu'meri ante'rior [NA], anterior circumflex humeral artery; *origin,* axillary; *distribution,* shoulder joint and biceps muscle; *anastomoses,* posterior circumflex humeral.

a. circumflex'a hu'meri poste'rior [NA], posterior circumflex humeral artery; *origin,* axillary; *distribution,* muscles and structures of shoulder joint; *anastomoses,* anterior circumflex humeral, suprascapular, thoracoacromial, and profunda brachii.

a. circumflex'a il'ium profun'da [NA], deep circumflex iliac artery; *origin,* external iliac; *distribution,* muscles and skin of lower abdomen, sartorius and tensor fasciae latae; *anastomoses,* lumbar, inferior epigastric, superior gluteal, iliolumbar, and superficial circumflex iliac.

a. circumflex'a il'ium superficia'lis [NA], superficial circumflex iliac artery; *origin,* femoral; *distribution,* inguinal lymph nodes and integument of that region; sartorius, and tensor fasciae latae muscles; *anastomoses,* deep circumflex iliac.

a. circumflex'a scap'ulae [NA], circumflex scapular artery; *origin,* subscapular; *distribution,* muscles of shoulder and scapular region; *anastomoses,* branches of suprascapular and transverse cervical.

a. col'ica dex'tra [NA], right colic artery; *origin,* superior mesenteric, sometimes by a common trunk with the ileocolic; *distribution,* ascending colon; *anastomoses,* middle colic, ileocolic.

a. col'ica me'dia [NA], middle colic artery; *origin,* superior mesenteric; *distribution,* transverse colon; *anastomoses,* right and left colic.

a. col'ica sin'istra [NA], left colic artery; *origin,* inferior mesenteric; *distribution,* descending colon and splenic flexure; *anastomoses,* middle colic, sigmoid.

a. collatera'lis me'dia [NA], middle collateral artery; the posterior terminal branch of the profunda brachii, anastomosing with the arteries which form the rete articulare cubiti.

a. collatera'lis radia'lis [NA], radial collateral artery; the anterior terminal branch of the profunda brachii, anastomosing with the radial recurrent.

a. collatera'lis ulna'ris infe'rior [NA], inferior ulnar collateral artery; great anastomotic artery (1); a. anastomotica magna (1); anastomotica magna (1); *origin,* brachial; *distribution,* arm muscles at back of elbow; *anastomoses,* anterior and posterior ulnar recurrent, superior ulnar collateral, profunda brachii, and recurrent interosseous.

a. collatera'lis ulna'ris supe'rior [NA], superior ulnar collateral artery; *origin,* brachial; *distribution,* elbow joint; *anastomoses,* posterior ulnar recurrent and inferior ulnar collateral.

a. co'mes ner'vi media'ni, a. mediana.

a. co'mes ner'vi phren'ici, a. pericardiacophrenica.

a. com'itans ner'vi ischiad'ici [NA], companion artery to sciatic nerve; *origin,* inferior gluteal; *distribution,* sciatic nerve; *anastomoses,* branches of profunda femoris.

a. commu'nicans ante'rior [NA], anterior communicating artery; a short vessel joining the two anterior cerebral arteries and completing the cerebral arterial circle (circle of Willis) anteriorly.

a. commu'nicans poste'rior [NA], posterior communicating artery; *origin,* internal carotid; *distribution,* optic tract, crus cerebri, interpeduncular region, and hippocampal gyrus; *anastomoses,* with posterior cerebral to form the cerebral arterial circle (circle of Willis).

a. conjunctiva'lis ante'rior [NA], anterior conjunctival artery; one of a number of small branches of the anterior ciliary arteries that supplies the conjunctiva.

a. conjunctiva'lis poste'rior [NA], posterior conjunctival artery; one of a series of branches from the tarsal arterial arches that supplies the conjunctiva.
a. corona'ria dex'tra [NA], right coronary artery; *origin,* right aortic sinus; *distribution,* it passes around the right side of the heart in the coronary sulcus, giving branches to the right atrium and ventricle, including the atrioventricular branches and the posterior interventricular branch.
a. corona'ria sin'istra [NA], left coronary artery; *origin,* left aortic sinus; *distribution,* it divides into two major branches, an anterior interventricular which descends in the anterior interventricular sulcus, and a circumflex branch which passes to the diaphragmatic surface of the left ventricle; gives atrial, ventricular, and atrioventricular branches.
a. cremaster'ica [NA], cremasteric artery; external spermatic artery; *origin,* inferior epigastric; *distribution,* coverings of spermatic cord; *anastomoses,* external pudendal, spermatic, and perineal a.
a. cys'tica [NA], cystic artery; *origin,* right branch of hepatic; *distribution,* gall bladder and visceral surface of the liver.
a. deferentia'lis, a. ductus deferentis.
a. digita'lis dorsa'lis [NA], dorsal digital artery; one of the collateral digital branches of the dorsal metatarsal arteries in the foot, and of the dorsal metacarpal arteries in the hand.
a. digita'lis palma'ris commu'nis [NA], common palmar digital artery; one of three arteries arising from the superficial palmar arch and running to the interdigital clefts where each divides into two proper palmar digital arteries.
a. digita'lis palma'ris pro'pria [NA], proper palmar digital artery; collateral digital or digital collateral artery; the artery that passes along the side of each finger.
a. digita'lis planta'ris commu'nis [NA], common plantar digital artery; one of four arteries arising from a superficial plantar arch, when present as a variation. They unite with the plantar metatarsal arteries.
a. digita'lis planta'ris pro'pria [NA], proper plantar digital artery; collateral digital artery; one of the digital branches of the plantar metatarsal arteries.
a. dorsa'lis clitori'dis [NA], dorsal artery of clitoris; one of the two terminal branches of the internal pudendal artery in the female, the other being the a. profunda clitoridis.
a. dorsa'lis na'si [NA], dorsal artery of nose; a. nasi externa; external artery of the nose; *origin,* ophthalmic; *distribution,* skin of side of nose; *anastomoses,* angular.
a. dorsa'lis pe'dis [NA], dorsal artery of foot; a continuation of the anterior tibial; *branches,* lateral tarsal, arcuate, dorsal metatarsal; *anastomoses,* with the lateral plantar to form the plantar arch.
a. dorsa'lis pe'nis [NA], dorsal artery of penis; the dorsal terminal branch of the internal pudendal artery in the male.
a. dorsa'lis scap'ulae [NA], dorsal scapular artery; a. scapularis dorsalis; descending scapular artery; a. scapularis descendens; ramus profundus arteriae transversae colli; ramus profundus arteriae scapularis descendens; *origin,* subclavian or transverse cervical; *distribution,* muscles and skin along the medial border of the scapula; *anastomoses,* suprascapular and scapular circumflex.
a. duc'tus deferen'tis [NA], artery of ductus deferens; a. deferentialis; *origin,* anterior division of internal iliac, or sometimes superior vesical; *distribution,* ductus deferens, seminal vesicles, testicle, ureter; *anastomoses,* testicular, cremasteric branch of inferior epigastric.
a. epigas'trica infe'rior [NA], inferior epigastric artery; deep epigastric a.; *origin,* external iliac; *branches,* cremasteric, muscular and pubic; *anastomoses,* superior epigastric, obturator.
a. epigas'trica superficia'lis [NA], superficial epigastric artery; *origin,* femoral; *distribution,* inguinal nodes and integument of lower abdomen; *anastomoses,* inferior epigastric, superficial circumflex iliac and external pudendal.
a. epigas'trica supe'rior [NA], superior epigastric artery; *origin,* the medial terminal branch of internal thoracic; *distribution,* abdominal muscles and integument, falciform ligament; *anastomoses,* inferior epigastric.
a. episclera'lis [NA], episcleral artery; one of many small branches of the anterior ciliary arteries that perforate the sclera behind the cornea to supply the iris and ciliary body.
a. ethmoida'lis ante'rior [NA], anterior ethmoidal artery; *origin,* ophthalmic; *distribution,* cerebral membranes in anterior cranial fossa, anterior ethmoidal cells, frontal sinus, anterior upper part of nasal mucous membrane, skin of dorsum of nose.
a. ethmoida'lis poste'rior [NA], posterior ethmoidal artery; *origin,* ophthalmic; *distribution,* posterior ethmoidal cells and upper posterior part of lateral wall of nasal cavity.
a. facia'lis [NA], facial artery; a. maxillaris externa; external maxillary artery; *origin,* external carotid; *branches,* ascending palatine, tonsillar and glandular branches, submental, inferior labial, superior labial, masseteric, buccal, lateral nasal branches, and angular.
a. femora'lis [NA], femoral artery; crural artery; *origin,* continuation of external iliac, beginning at inguinal ligament; *branches,* external pudendal, superficial epigastric, superficial circumflex iliac, profunda femoris, descending genicular, terminating in the popliteal at the upper part of the popliteal space.
a. fibula'ris [NA], official alternate term for a. peronea.
a. fronta'lis, a. supratrochlearis.
a. frontobasa'lis latera'lis [NA], lateral frontobasal artery; ramus orbitofrontalis lateralis; orbitofrontal artery; lateral orbitofrontal branch; a branch of the insular part of the middle cerebral artery distributed to the cortex of the lateral, inferior part of the frontal lobe.
a. frontobasa'lis media'lis [NA], medial frontobasal artery; orbital artery; ramus orbitofrontalis medialis; medial orbitofrontal branch; the first branch of the pericallosal artery; it supplies the medial half of the inferior surface of the frontal cortex.
arte'riae gas'tricae bre'ves [NA], short gastric arteries; vasa brevia; four or five small arteries given off from the splenic, passing to the greater curvature of the stomach, and anastomosing with the other arteries in that region.
a. gas'trica dex'tra [NA], right gastric artery; pyloric artery; *origin,* hepatic; *distribution,* pyloric portion of stomach on the lesser curvature; *anastomoses,* left gastric.
a. gas'trica sin'is'tra [NA], left gastric artery; coronary artery (1); *origin,* celiac; *distribution,* lesser curvature of stomach, abdominal part of the esophagus, and, frequently, a portion of the left lobe of the liver; *anastomoses,* esophageal, right gastric.
a. gastroduodena'lis [NA], gastroduodenal artery; *origin,* hepatic; terminal *branches,* right gastroepiploic, superior pancreaticoduodenal.
a. gastroepiplo'ica dex'tra, a. gastro-omentalis dextra.
a. gastroepiplo'ica sin'istra, a. gastro-omentalis sinistra.
a. gastro-omenta'lis dex'tra [NA], right gastro-omental artery; a. gastroepiploica dextra; right gastroepiploic artery; *origin,* gastroduodenal; *distribution,* greater curvature and walls of stomach and greater omentum; *anastomoses,* frequently unites with left gastroepiploic, and branches from this arch anastomose with branches of right and left gastric.
a. gastro-omenta'lis sin'istra [NA], left gastro-omental artery; a. gastroepiploica sinistra; left gastroepiploic artery; *origin,* splenic; *distribution,* greater curvature of stomach and greater omentum, frequently joining right gastroepiploic; *anastomoses,* see a. gastro-omentalis dextra.
a. ge'nus descen'dens [NA], descending artery of the knee; great anastomotic artery (2); a. anastomotica magna (2); anastomotica magna (2); *origin,* femoral; *distribution,* knee joint and adjacent parts; *anastomoses,* medial superior genicular, medial inferior genicular, lateral superior genicular, lateral inferior genicular and anterior tibial recurrent.
a. ge'nus infe'rior latera'lis [NA], lateral inferior genicular artery;

origin, popliteal; *distribution,* knee joint; *anastomoses,* lateral superior genicular and anterior tibial recurrent (and posterior).
a. ge'nus infe'rior media'lis [NA], medial inferior genicular artery; *origin,* popliteal; *distribution,* knee joint; *anastomoses,* anterior and posterior tibial recurrent and medial superior genicular.
a. ge'nus me'dia [NA], middle genicular artery; a. articularis azygos; *origin,* popliteal; *distribution,* synovial membrane and cruciate ligaments of knee joint.
a. ge'nus supe'rior latera'lis [NA], lateral superior genicular artery; *origin,* popliteal; *distribution,* knee joint; *anastomoses,* lateral circumflex femoral, third perforating, anterior tibial recurrent, lateral inferior genicular.
a. ge'nus supe'rior media'lis [NA], medial superior genicular artery; *origin,* popliteal; *distribution,* knee joint; *anastomoses,* descending genicular, lateral superior genicular.
a. glu'tea infe'rior [NA], inferior gluteal artery; a. ischiadica (ischiatica); *origin,* internal iliac; *distribution,* hip joint and gluteal region; *anastomoses,* branches of internal pudendal, lateral sacral, superior gluteal, obturator, medial and lateral circumflex femoral.
a. glu'tea supe'rior [NA], superior gluteal artery; *origin,* internal iliac; *distribution,* gluteal region; *anastomoses,* lateral sacral, inferior gluteal, internal pudendal, deep circumflex iliac, lateral circumflex femoral.
a. gy'ri angula'ris [NA], artery of angular gyrus; angular artery (2); the last branch of the terminal part of the middle cerebral artery distributed to parts of the temporal parietal and occipital lobes.
a. helici'na [NA], helicine artery; one of the coiled arteries in the erectile tissue of the penis.
a. hepat'ica commu'nis [NA], common hepatic artery; *origin,* celiac; *branches,* right gastric, gastroduodenal, and proper hepatic.
a. hepat'ica pro'pria [NA], proper hepatic artery; *origin,* common hepatic; *branches,* right and left hepatic.
a. hyaloi'dea [NA], hyaloid artery; the terminal branch of the primitive ophthalmic artery which forms in the embryo an extensive ramification in the primary vitreous and a vascular tunic around the lens; by $8^1/_2$ months, these vessels have atrophied almost completely, but a few persistent remnants are evident entoptically as muscae volitantes.
a. hypogas'trica, a. iliaca interna.
a. hypophysia'lis infe'rior [NA], inferior hypophysial artery; a small branch of the cavernous part of the internal carotid to the hypophysis.
a. hypophysia'lis supe'rior [NA], superior hypophysial artery; a small branch of the cerebral part of the internal carotid artery supplying the hypophysis.
arte'riae ilea'les [NA], ileal arteries; *origin,* superior mesenteric; *distribution,* ileum; *anastomoses,* other branches of superior mesenteric.
a. ileocol'ica [NA], ileocolic artery; *origin,* superior mesenteric, often by a common trunk with the right colic; *distribution,* terminal part of ileum, cecum, vermiform appendix, and ascending colon; *anastomoses,* right colic and ileal.
a. ili'aca commu'nis [NA], common iliac artery; one of the two terminal branches of the abdominal aorta; opposite the lumbosacral articulation, it bifurcates to form the internal iliac and the external iliac.
a. ili'aca exter'na [NA], external iliac artery; *origin,* common iliac; *branches,* inferior epigastric, deep circumflex iliac; becomes the femoral at the inguinal ligament.
a. ili'aca inter'na [NA], internal iliac artery; a. hypogastrica; hypogastric artery; *origin,* common iliac; *branches,* iliolumbar, lateral sacral, obturator, superior gluteal, inferior gluteal, umbilical, superior vesical, inferior vesical, middle rectal, and internal pudendal.
a. iliolumba'lis [NA], iliolumbar artery; *origin,* internal iliac; *distribution,* pelvic muscles and bones; *anastomoses,* deep circumflex iliac, lumbar.
a. infraorbita'lis [NA], infraorbital artery; *origin,* maxillary; *distribution,* upper canine and incisor teeth, inferior rectus and inferior oblique muscles, lower eyelid, lacrimal sac, and upper lip; *anastomoses,* branches of ophthalmic, facial, superior labial, transverse facial, and buccal.
arte'riae insula'res [NA], insular arteries; branches from the insular part of the middle cerebral artery distributed to the cortex of the insula.
a. intercosta'lis ante'rior [NA], anterior intercostal artery; a. intercostalis anterosuperior; a. intercostalis suprema; supreme or highest intercostal artery; *origin,* costocervical trunk; *distribution,* structures of first and second intercostal spaces; *anastomoses,* anterior intercostal branches of internal thoracic.
a. intercosta'lis anterosupe'rior, a. intercostalis anterior.
a. intercosta'lis poste'rior [NA], posterior intercostal artery; one of nine pairs of arteries arising from the thoracic aorta and distributed to the nine lower intercostal spaces, vertebral column, spinal cord, and muscles and integument of the back; they anastomose with branches of the musculophrenic, internal thoracic, superior epigastric, subcostal and lumbar.
a. intercosta'lis supre'ma, a. intercostalis anterior.
arte'riae interloba'res [NA], interlobar arteries; the branches of the segmental arteries of the kidney; they run between the renal lobes and give rise to the arcuate arteries.
arteriae interlobula'res [NA], interlobular arteries; arteries that pass between lobules of an organ; **a. i. hepatis,** the many terminal branches of the hepatic artery passing between hepatic lobules; **a. i. renis,** the branches of the interlobar arteries of the kidney passing outward through the cortex and supplying the glomeruli.
a. interos'sea ante'rior [NA], anterior interosseous artery; a. interossea volaris; volar interosseous artery; *origin,* common interosseous; *distribution,* deep parts of the forearm anteriorly; *anastomoses,* posterior interosseous.
a. interos'sea commu'nis [NA], common interosseous artery; *origin,* ulnar; *branches,* anterior and posterior interosseous.
a. interos'sea poste'rior [NA], posterior interosseous artery; dorsal interosseous artery (1); *origin,* common interosseous; *distribution,* deep parts of forearm posteriorly.
a. interos'sea recur'rens [NA], recurrent interosseous artery; *origin,* posterior interosseous; *distribution,* elbow joint; *anastomoses,* branches of profunda brachii and inferior ulnar collateral.
a. interos'sea vola'ris, a. interossea anterior.
arte'riae intestina'les, intestinal arteries; see arteriae ileales and arteriae jejunales.
a. ischiad'ica, a. ischiat'ica, a. glutea inferior.
arteriae jejuna'les [NA], jejunal arteries; *origin,* superior mesenteric; *distribution,* jejunum; *anastomoses,* by a series of arches with each other and with ileal arteries.
arte'riae labia'les anterio'res, *rami* labiales anteriores.
a. labia'lis infe'rior [NA], inferior labial artery; *origin,* facial; *distribution,* structures of lower lip; *anastomoses,* the artery from the opposite side, mental and sublabial.
a. labia'lis supe'rior [NA], superior labial artery; superior coronary artery; *origin,* facial; *distribution,* structures of upper lip and, by a septal branch, the anterior and lower part of the nasal septum; *anastomoses,* the artery of the opposite side and the sphenopalatine.
a. labyrin'thi [NA], artery of labyrinth; a. auditiva interna; internal auditory artery; a branch of the basilar artery that enters the labyrinth through the internal acoustic meatus.
a. lacrima'lis [NA], lacrimal artery; *origin,* ophthalmic; *distribution,* lacrimal gland, lateral and superior rectus muscles, superior eyelid, forehead, and temporal fossa.
a. laryn'gea infe'rior [NA], inferior laryngeal artery; *origin,* inferior thyroid; *distribution,* muscles and mucous membrane of larynx; *anastomoses,* superior laryngeal.

a. laryn'gea supe'rior [NA], superior laryngeal artery; *origin,* superior thyroid; *distribution,* muscles and mucous membrane of larynx; *anastomoses,* cricothyroid branch of superior thyroid and terminal branches of inferior laryngeal.
a. liena'lis [NA], a. splenica.
a. ligamen'ti tere'tis u'teri [NA], artery of round ligament of uterus; *origin,* inferior epigastric; *distribution,* round ligament.
a. lingua'lis [NA], lingual artery; *origin,* external carotid; *distribution,* runs along under surface of tongue, terminates as ranine artery, a. profunda linguae; *branches,* suprahyoid and dorsal lingual branches and sublingual artery.
a. lo'bi cauda'ti [NA], artery of caudate lobe; *origin,* left branch of proper hepatic; *distribution,* caudate lobe of the liver.
a. lumba'lis [NA], lumbar artery; one of four or five pairs; *origin,* abdominal aorta; *distribution,* lumbar vertebrae, muscles of back, abdominal wall; *anastomoses,* intercostal, subcostal, superior and inferior epigastric, deep circumflex iliac, and iliolumbar.
a. lumba'lis i'ma [NA], lowest lumbar artery; *origin,* middle sacral; *distribution,* sacrum and iliac muscle; *anastomosis,* deep circumflex iliac artery.
a. luso'ria, an aberrant right subclavian artery arising from the descending aorta; it passes posterior to the esophagus, often producing dysphagia.
a. malleola'ris ante'rior latera'lis [NA], anterior lateral malleolar artery; *origin,* anterior tibial; *distribution,* ankle joint; *anastomoses,* peroneal, lateral tarsal.
a. malleola'ris ante'rior media'lis [NA], anterior medial malleolar artery; *origin,* anterior tibial; *distribution,* ankle joint and neighboring integument; *anastomoses,* branches of posterior tibial.
arte'riae malleola'res posterio'res latera'les, *rami* malleolares laterales.
arte'riae malleola'res posterio'res media'les, *rami* malleolares mediales.
a. mamma'ria inter'na, a. thoracica interna.
a. masseter'ica [NA], masseteric artery; *origin,* maxillary; *distribution,* deep surface of masseter muscle; *anastomoses,* branches of transverse facial and masseteric branches of facial.
a. maxilla'ris [NA], maxillary artery; internal maxillary artery; *origin,* external carotid; *branches,* deep auricular, anterior tympanic, middle meningeal, inferior alveolar, masseteric, deep temporal, buccal, superior posterior alveolar, infraorbital, descending palatine, artery of pterygoid canal, sphenopalatine.
a. maxilla'ris exter'na, a. facialis.
a. media'na [NA], median artery; a. comes nervi mediani; *origin,* anterior interosseous; *distribution,* accompanies median nerve to palm; *anastomoses,* branches of superficial palmar arch.
arte'riae mediastina'les ante'riores, *rami* mediastinales (1).
a. menin'gea ante'rior [NA], anterior meningeal artery; *origin,* anterior ethmoidal; *distribution,* meninges in anterior cranial fossa; *anastomoses,* branches of middle meningeal and meningeal branches of internal carotid and lacrimal.
a. menin'gea me'dia [NA], middle meningeal artery; *origin,* maxillary; *branches,* petrosal, superior tympanic, frontal and parietal; *distribution,* to parts mentioned and through terminal branches to anterior and middle cranial fossae; *anastomoses,* meningeal branches of occipital, ascending pharyngeal, ophthalmic and lacrimal, stylomastoid, accessory meningeal branch of maxillary, and deep temporal.
a. menin'gea poste'rior [NA], posterior meningeal artery; *origin,* ascending pharyngeal; *distribution,* dura mater of posterior cranial fossa; *anastomoses,* branches of middle meningeal and vertebral.
a. menta'lis [NA], mental artery; the terminal branch of the inferior alveolar; *distribution,* chin; *anastomosis,* inferior labial artery.
a. mesenter'ica infe'rior [NA], inferior mesenteric artery; *origin,* aorta; *branches,* left colic, sigmoid, superior rectal; *anastomoses,* middle colic and middle rectal.
a. mesenter'ica supe'rior [NA], superior mesenteric artery; *origin,* aorta; *branches,* inferior pancreaticoduodenal, jejunal, ileal, ileocolic, appendicular, right colic, middle colic; *anastomoses,* superior pancreaticoduodenal and left colic.
a. metacar'pea dorsa'lis [NA], dorsal metacarpal artery; dorsal interosseous artery (2); one of four arteries running in the back of the interosseous muscles of the hand.
a. metacar'pea palma'ris [NA], palmar metacarpal artery; palmar interosseous artery; one of the three arteries springing from the deep palmar arch and running in the three medial interosseous spaces; they anastomose with the dorsal metacarpal arteries.
a. metatarsa'lis, a. arcuata.
a. metatar'sea dorsa'lis [NA], dorsal metatarsal artery; one of four arteries running in the back of the interosseous muscle of the foot. Lateral toes and the lateral side of the second toe through the collateral branches, the dorsal digital.
a. metatar'sea planta'ris [NA], plantar metatarsal artery; one of four branches of the plantar arch that divide into plantar digital arteries to supply the toes.
a. musculophren'ica [NA], musculophrenic artery; *origin,* the lateral terminal branch of internal thoracic; *distribution,* diaphragm and intercostal muscles; *anastomoses,* branches of pericardiacophrenic, inferior phrenic, and posterior intercostal arteries.
arte'riae nasa'les posterio'res latera'les [NA], posterior lateral nasal arteries; branches of the sphenopalatine artery that supply the posterior parts of the conchae and lateral nasal wall.
a. nasa'lis poste'rior sep'ti [NA], posterior septal artery of nose; a branch of the sphenopalatine artery that supplies the nasal septum and accompanies the nasopalatine nerve.
a. na'si exter'na [NA], official alternate term for a. dorsalis nasi.
a. nutri'cia [NA], nutrient artery; nutrient vessel; an artery of variable origin that supplies the medullary cavity of a long bone.
arte'riae nutri'ciae hu'meri [NA], nutrient arteries of humerus; *origin,* deep brachial; *distribution,* the medullary cavity of the humerus.
a. obturato'ria [NA], obturator artery; *origin,* anterior division of the internal iliac; *distribution,* ilium, pubis, obturator and adductor muscles; *anastomoses,* iliolumbar, inferior epigastric, medial circumflex femoral; *branches,* pubic, acetabular, anterior, and posterior.
a. obturato'ria accesso'ria [NA], accessory obturator artery; the term applied to the pubic branch of the inferior epigastric artery when it contributes a significant supply through the obturator canal.
a. occipita'lis [NA], occipital artery; *origin,* external carotid; *branches,* sternocleidomastoid, meningeal, auricular, occipital, mastoid, and descending.
a. occipita'lis latera'lis [NA], lateral occipital artery; one of the terminal branches of the posterior cerebral artery; it supplies, by several named branches, the lateral portions of the temporal lobe.
a. occipita'lis media'lis [NA], medial occipital artery; one of the terminal branches of the posterior cerebral artery; it is distributed, by several named branches, to the posterior corpus callosum and the medial and superolateral portions of the occipital lobe including the visual cortex.
a. ophthal'mica [NA], ophthalmic artery; *origin,* internal carotid; *branches,* ciliary, central artery of retina, anterior meningeal, lacrimal, conjunctival, episcleral, supraorbital, ethmoidal, palpebral, dorsal nasal, and supratrochlear.
a. ova'rica [NA], ovarian artery; *origin,* aorta; *distribution,* ureter, ovary, ovarian ligament and uterine tube; *anastomoses,* uterine.
a. palati'na ascen'dens [NA], ascending palatine artery; *origin,* facial; *distribution,* lateral walls of pharynx, tonsils, auditory tubes, and soft palate; *anastomoses,* tonsillar branch of facial, dorsal lingual, and descending palatine.
a. palati'na descen'dens [NA], descending palatine artery; *origin,* maxillary; *distribution,* soft palate, gums, and bones and mucous

membrane of hard palate; *anastomoses,* sphenopalatine, ascending palatine, ascending pharyngeal, and tonsillar branches of facial.
a. palati'na ma'jor [NA], greater palatine artery; anterior branch of descending palatine artery, supplying the gums and mucous membrane of the hard palate.
a. palati'na mi'nor [NA], lesser palatine artery; one of several posterior branches of the descending palatine in the greater palatine canal, distributed to the soft palate and tonsil.
arte'riae palpebra'les [NA], palpebral arteries; branches of the ophthalmic supplying the upper and lower eyelids, consisting of two sets, lateral and medial.
a. pancreat'ica dorsa'lis [NA], dorsal pancreatic artery; great superior pancreatic artery; *origin,* splenic; *distribution,* head and body of pancreas; *anastomoses,* superior pancreaticoduodenal.
a. pancreat'ica infe'rior [NA], inferior pancreatic artery; transverse pancreatic artery; *origin,* dorsal pancreatic; *distribution,* body and tail of pancreas; *anastomoses,* pancreatica magna.
a. pancreat'ica mag'na [NA], great pancreatic artery; *origin,* splenic; *distribution,* tail of pancreas; *anastomoses,* inferior and caudal pancreatic arteries.
a. pancreat'icoduodena'lis infe'rior [NA], inferior pancreaticoduodenal artery; one of two arteries, anterior and posterior; *origin,* superior mesenteric; *distribution,* head of pancreas, duodenum; *anastomoses,* superior pancreaticoduodenal.
a. pancreat'icoduodena'lis supe'rior [NA], superior pancreaticoduodenal artery; one of two arteries, anterior and superior; *origin,* gastroduodenal; *distribution,* head of pancreas, duodenum, common bile duct; *anastomoses,* inferior pancreaticoduodenal, splenic.
a. paracentra'lis [NA], paracentral artery; the third branch of the pericallosal artery supplying the cerebral cortex of the paracentral lobule and both sides of the medial part of the central sulcus.
arte'riae parieta'les [NA], parietal arteries; branches of the terminal part of the middle cerebral artery, divided into two branches. **a. p. anterior** [NA], anterior parietal artery; the branch distributed to the anterior part of the parietal lobe, and **a. p. posterior** [NA], posterior parietal artery; the branch distributed to the posterior part of the parietal lobe.
a. pari'eto-occipita'lis [NA], parieto-occipital artery; superior internal parietal artery; the largest cortical branch of the pericallosal artery supplying the medial and superolateral surface of the parietal lobe posterior to the paracentral lobule; rarely does it extend to supply part of the occipital lobe.
arte'riae perforan'tes [NA], perforating arteries; *origin,* a. profunda femoris; *distribution,* as three or four vessels that pass through the adductor magnus to the posterior and lateral parts of the thigh.
a. pericallo'sa [NA], pericallosal artery; the continuation of the anterior cerebral artery after the anterior communicating artery; it supplies branches to the cerebral cortex as it passes along the corpus callosum.
a. pericardiacophren'ica [NA], pericardiacophrenic artery; a. comes nervi phrenici; *origin,* internal thoracic; *distribution,* pericardium, diaphragm, and pleura; *anastomoses,* musculophrenic, inferior phrenic, mediastinal and pericardial branches of the internal thoracic.
a. perinea'lis [NA], perineal artery; *origin,* internal pudendal; *distribution,* superficial structures of the perineum; *anastomoses,* external pudendal arteries.
a. pero'nea [NA], peroneal artery; fibular artery; a. fibularis; *origin,* posterior tibial; *distribution,* soleus, tibialis posterior, flexor longus hallucis, peroneal muscles, inferior tibiofibular articulation, and ankle joint; *anastomoses,* anterior lateral malleolar, lateral tarsal, lateral plantar, dorsalis pedis.
a. pharyn'gea ascen'dens [NA], ascending pharyngeal artery; *origin,* external carotid; *distribution,* wall of pharynx and soft palate.
a. phren'ica infe'rior [NA], inferior phrenic artery; *origin,* the first paired branch from the abdominal aorta inferior to the diaphragm; *distribution,* diaphragm; *anastomoses,* superior phrenic, internal thoracic, and musculophrenic.
a. phren'ica supe'rior [NA], superior phrenic artery; one of a pair of small arteries given off from the thoracic aorta just superior to the diaphragm; *distribution,* diaphragm; *anastomoses,* musculophrenic, pericardiacophrenic, and inferior phrenic.
a. planta'ris latera'lis [NA], lateral plantar artery; larger of the two terminal branches of the posterior tibial; *distribution,* forms the plantar arch and through it supplies the sole of the foot and plantar surfaces of the toes; *anastomoses,* medial plantar, dorsalis pedis.
a. planta'ris media'lis [NA], medial plantar artery; one of the terminal branches of the posterior tibial; *distribution,* medial side of the sole of the foot; *anastomoses,* dorsalis pedis, lateral plantar.
arte'riae pon'tis [NA], pontine arteries; arteries of pons; rami ad pontem; several small branches of the basilar artery distributed to the pons.
a. poplit'ea [NA], popliteal artery; continuation of femoral in the popliteal space, bifurcating at the lower border of the popliteus muscle into the anterior and posterior tibial; *branches,* lateral and medial superior genicular, middle genicular, lateral and medial inferior genicular, and sural arteries.
a. precunea'lis [NA], precuneal artery; inferior internal parietal artery; the last cortical branch of the pericallosal artery; it supplies the inferior part of the precuneus.
a. prin'ceps pol'licis [NA], chief artery of thumb; principal artery of thumb; princeps pollicis; *origin,* radial; *distribution,* palmar surface and sides of thumb; *anastomoses,* arteries on dorsum of thumb.
a. profun'da bra'chii [NA], deep brachial artery; *origin,* brachial; *distribution,* humerus and muscles and integument of arm; *anastomoses,* radial recurrent, recurrent interosseous, ulnar collateral, posterior circumflex humeral.
a. profun'da clitori'dis [NA], deep artery of clitoris; the deep terminal branch of the internal pudendal artery in the female; it supplies the crus of the clitoris.
a. profun'da fem'oris [NA], deep artery of thigh; *origin,* femoral; *branches,* lateral circumflex femoral, medial circumflex femoral, terminating in three or four perforating branches.
a. profun'da lin'guae [NA], deep artery of tongue; a. ranina; ranine artery; termination of lingual; *distribution,* muscles and mucous membrane of under surface of tongue.
a. profun'da pe'nis [NA], deep artery of penis; *origin,* terminal branch of the internal pudendal artery; *distribution,* corpus cavernosum of the penis.
a. puden'da inter'na [NA], internal pudendal artery; *origin,* internal iliac; *branches,* inferior rectal, perineal, posterior scrotal (or labial), urethral, artery of bulb of penis (or of vestibule), deep artery of penis (or clitoris), dorsal artery of penis (or clitoris).
arte'riae puden'dae exter'nae [NA], external pudendal arteries; *origin,* femoral; *distribution,* skin over pubis, skin over penis, scrotum, or labium majus; *anastomoses,* dorsal artery of penis or clitoris, posterior scrotal or labial arteries.
a. pulmona'lis, *truncus* pulmonalis.
a. pulmona'lis dex'tra [NA], right pulmonary artery; one of two branches of the pulmonary trunk, it passes transversely across the mediastinum to enter the hilum of the right lung. Branches are distributed with the bronchi; frequent variations occur in which subsegmental bronchi receive independent branches. The NA lists the following branches; ramus apicalis, r. posterior descendens, r. anterior descendens, r. anterior ascendens, r. posterior ascendens, r. lobi medii (r. lateralis, r. medialis), r. apicalis [superior] lobi inferioris, pars basalis, from which arise r. subapicalis [subsuperior], r. basalis medialis [cardiacus], r. basalis anterior, r. basalis lateralis, and r. basalis posterior.
a. pulmona'lis sin'istra [NA], left pulmonary artery; it enters the hilum of the left lung. Its branches accompany the segmental and

subsegmental bronchi and are listed as follows in the NA: ramus apicalis, r. anterior descendens, r. posterior, r. anterior ascendens, r. lingularis (r. lingularis superior, r. lingularis inferior), r. apicalis [superior] lobi inferioris, pars basalis, from which arise r. subapicalis [subsuperior], r. basalis medialis, r. basalis anterior, r. basalis lateralis, and r. basalis posterior.

a. radia'lis [NA], radial artery; *origin,* brachial; *branches,* radial recurrent, dorsal metacarpal, dorsal digital, princeps pollicis, radial index, palmar metacarpal, and muscular, carpal, and perforating.

a. radia'lis in'dicis [NA], radial index artery; a. volaris indicis radialis; *origin,* radial; *distribution,* radial side of index finger.

a. rani'na, a. profunda linguae.

a. recta'lis infe'rior [NA], inferior rectal artery; inferior hemorrhoidal artery; *origin,* internal pudendal; *distribution,* anal canal, muscles and skin of the anal region, and skin of the buttock; *anastomoses,* middle rectal, perineal, and gluteal.

a. recta'lis me'dia [NA], middle rectal artery; middle hemorrhoidal artery; *origin,* internal iliac; *distribution,* middle portion of rectum; *anastomoses,* superior and inferior rectal.

a. recta'lis supe'rior [NA], superior rectal artery; superior hemorrhoidal artery; *origin,* inferior mesenteric; *distribution,* upper part of rectum; *anastomoses,* middle and inferior rectal.

a. recur'rens [NA], a. centralis longa.

a. recur'rens radia'lis [NA], radial recurrent artery; *origin,* radial; *distribution,* ascends around lateral side of elbow joint; *anastomoses,* radial collateral, interosseous recurrent.

a. recur'rens tibia'lis ante'rior [NA], anterior tibial recurrent artery; a branch of the anterior tibial artery which ascends to supply the front and sides of the knee joint.

a. recur'rens tibia'lis poste'rior [NA], posterior tibial recurrent artery; an inconstant branch of the posterior tibial artery which ascends anterior to the popliteus muscle, anastomoses with branches of the popliteal artery, and sends a twig to the tibiofibular joint.

a. recur'rens ulna'ris [NA], recurrent ulnar artery; *origin,* ulnar artery; *distribution,* two branches, anterior and posterior, pass medially in front of and behind the elbow joint; *anastomoses,* superior and inferior ulnar collateral.

a. rena'lis [NA], renal artery; *origin,* aorta; *branches,* segmental, ureteral, and inferior suprarenal; *distribution,* kidney.

arte'riae re'nis [NA], arteries of kidney; the branches of the renal artery that supply the kidney tissue. Usually five in number, they give off interlobar, arcuate and interlobular arteries in sequence. The latter send afferent arterioles to the glomeruli as well as branches to the kidney capsule.

a. ret'inae centra'lis, a. centralis retinae.

a. retroduodena'lis [NA], retroduodenal artery; posterior pancreaticoduodenal a.; *origin,* one of several small branches from the gastroduodenal artery posterior to the duodenum; *distribution,* first part of duodenum.

a. sacra'lis latera'lis [NA], lateral sacral artery; one of two arteries which arise from the internal iliac artery; they supply muscles and skin in the neighborhood and send branches into the sacral canal.

a. sacra'lis media'na [NA], median sacral artery; middle sacral artery; *origin,* back of abdominal aorta just above the bifurcation; *distribution,* lower lumbar vertebrae, sacrum, and coccyx; *anastomoses,* lateral sacral, superior and middle rectal.

a. scapula'ris descen'dens, a. scapularis dorsalis.

a. scapula'ris dorsa'lis [NA], alternative term for a. dorsalis scapulae.

a. segmen'ti [NA], segmental artery; one of five end arteries, each supplying an anatomical segment of the kidney. See subentries below.

a. segmen'ti anterio'ris inferio'ris re'nis [NA], artery of the anterior inferior segment of kidney; *origin,* anterior branch of renal.

a. segmen'ti anterio'ris superio'ris re'nis [NA], artery of anterior superior segment of kidney; *origin,* anterior branch of renal.

a. segmen'ti inferio'ris re'nis [NA], artery of inferior segment of kidney; *origin,* anterior branch of renal.

a. segmen'ti posterio'ris re'nis [NA], artery of posterior segment of kidney; *origin,* continuation of the posterior branch of renal.

a. segmen'ti superio'ris re'nis [NA], artery of superior segment of kidney; *origin,* anterior branch of renal.

arte'riae sigmoi'deae [NA], sigmoid arteries; *origin,* inferior mesenteric; *distribution,* descending colon and sigmoid flexure; *anastomoses,* left colic, superior rectal.

a. spermat'ica inter'na, a. testicularis.

a. sphe'nopalati'na [NA], sphenopalatine artery; *origin,* maxillary; *distribution,* posterior portion of lateral nasal wall and septum; *anastomoses,* branches of descending palatine, superior labial, and infraorbital.

a. spina'lis ante'rior [NA], anterior spinal artery; *origin,* vertebral; *distribution,* spinal cord and pia mater; *anastomoses,* spinal of intercostal and lumbar arteries.

a. spina'lis poste'rior [NA], posterior spinal artery; *origin,* vertebral; *distribution,* medulla, spinal cord, and pia mater; *anastomoses,* spinal branches of intercostal arteries.

a. sple'nica [NA], splenic artery; a. lienalis; lienal artery; *origin,* celiac trunk; *branches,* pancreatic, left gastroepiploic, short gastric, and splenic.

a. stylomastoi'dea [NA], stylomastoid artery; *origin,* posterior auricular; *distribution,* external acoustic meatus, mastoid cells, semicircular canals, stapedius muscle, and vestibule; *anastomoses,* tympanic branches of internal carotid and ascending pharyngeal, and labyrinthine branch of basilar.

a. subcla'via [NA], subclavian artery; *origin,* right from brachiocephalic, left from arch of aorta; *branches,* vertebral, thyrocervical trunk, internal thoracic; costocervical trunk, descending scapular; it is directly continuous with the axillary.

a. subcosta'lis [NA], subcostal artery; *origin,* thoracic aorta; *distribution,* inferior to twelfth rib in a manner similar to posterior intercostal arteries.

a. sublingua'lis [NA], sublingual artery; *origin,* lingual; *distribution,* extrinsic muscles of tongue, sublingual gland, mucosa of region; *anastomoses,* the artery of opposite side and submental.

a. submenta'lis [NA], submental artery; *origin,* facial; *distribution,* mylohyoid muscle, submandibular and sublingual glands, and structures of lower lip; *anastomoses,* inferior labial, mental branch of inferior dental and sublingual.

a. subscapula'ris [NA], subscapular artery; *origin,* axillary; *branches,* circumflex scapular, thoracodorsal; *distribution,* muscles of shoulder and scapular region; *anastomoses,* branches of transverse cervical, suprascapular, lateral thoracic, and intercostals.

a. sul'ci centra'lis [NA], artery of central sulcus; central artery; a branch of the terminal part of the middle cerebral artery distributed to the cortex on either side of the central sulcus.

a. sul'ci postcentra'lis [NA], artery of postcentral sulcus; postcentral artery; a branch of the terminal part of the middle cerebral artery distributing to the cortex on either side of the postcentral sulcus.

a. sul'ci precentra'lis [NA], artery of precentral sulcus; precentral artery; a branch of the terminal part of the middle cerebral artery distributed to the cortex on either side of the precentral sulcus.

a. supraduodena'lis [NA], supraduodenal artery; *origin,* gastroduodenal; *distribution,* first part of duodenum.

a. supraorbita'lis [NA], supraorbital artery; *origin,* ophthalmic; *distribution,* frontalis muscle and scalp; *anastomoses,* branches of the superficial temporal and supratrochlear.

a. suprarena'lis infe'rior [NA], inferior suprarenal artery; *origin,* renal; *distribution,* suprarenal gland.

a. suprarena'lis me'dia [NA], middle suprarenal artery; *origin,* aorta; *distribution,* suprarenal gland.

a. suprarena'lis supe'rior [NA], superior suprarenal artery; *origin,* inferior phrenic artery; *distribution,* suprarenal gland.

a. suprascapula'ris [NA], suprascapular artery; transverse scapular artery; *origin,* thyrocervical trunk; *distribution,* clavicle, scapula, muscles of shoulder, and shoulder joint; *anastomoses,* transverse cervical circumflex scapular.

a. supratrochlea'ris [NA], supratrochlear artery; a. frontalis; frontal artery; *origin,* ophthalmic; *distribution,* anterior portion of scalp; *anastomoses,* branches of supraorbital.

a. sura'lis [NA], sural artery; artery of calf; one of four or five arteries arising (sometimes by a common trunk) from the popliteal; *distribution,* muscles and integument of the calf; *anastomoses,* posterior tibial, medial, and lateral inferior genicular.

a. tar'sea latera'lis [NA], lateral tarsal artery; *origin,* dorsalis pedis; *distribution,* tarsal joints and extensor digitorum brevis muscle; *anastomoses,* arcuate, peroneal, lateral plantar, anterior lateral malleolar.

a. tar'sea media'lis [NA], medial tarsal artery; one of two small branches of the dorsalis pedis; *distribution.*

a. tempora'lis ante'rior [NA], anterior temporal artery; a branch of the insular part of the middle cerebral artery distributed to the cortex of the anterior part of the temporal lobe.

a. tempora'lis interme'dia [NA], intermediate temporal artery; a branch of the insular part of the middle cerebral artery supplying the cortex of the temporal lobe between the anterior and posterior temporal arteries.

a. tempora'lis media [NA], middle temporal artery; *origin,* superficial temporal; *distribution,* temporal fascia and muscle; *anastomoses,* branches of maxillary.

a. tempora'lis poste'rior [NA], posterior temporal artery; a branch of the insular part of the middle cerebral artery distributed to the cortex of the posterior part of the temporal lobe.

a. tempora'lis profun'da [NA], deep temporal artery, two in number, anterior and posterior; *origin,* maxillary; *distribution,* temporal muscle; *anastomoses,* branches of superficial temporal, lacrimal, and middle meningeal.

a. tempora'lis superficia'lis [NA], superficial temporal artery; *origin,* a terminal branch of the external carotid; *branches,* transverse facial, middle temporal, orbital, parotid, anterior auricular, frontal, and parietal.

a. testicula'ris [NA], testicular artery; a. spermatica interna; internal spermatic artery; *origin,* aorta; *branches,* ureteral, cremasteric, epididymal; *distribution,* testicle and parts designated by names of branches; *anastomoses,* branches of renal, inferior epigastric, deferential.

arte'riae thalamostria'tae anterolatera'les [NA], *arteriae* centrales anterolaterales.

arte'riae thalamostria'tae anteromedia'les [NA], official alternate term for *arteriae* centrales anteromediales.

a. thora'cica inter'na [NA], internal thoracic artery; a. mammaria interna; internal mammary artery; *origin,* subclavian; *branches,* pericardiacophrenic, anterior intercostal, sternal, mediastinal, thymic, bronchial, muscular, and perforating branches, and bifurcates into the musculophrenic and superior epigastric.

a. thora'cica latera'lis [NA], lateral thoracic artery; external mammary artery; long thoracic artery; *origin,* axillary; *distribution,* muscles of chest and mammary gland.

a. thora'cica supe'rior [NA], superior thoracic artery; *origin,* axillary; highest thoracic artery; *distribution,* muscles of chest; *anastomoses,* branches of suprascapular, internal thoracic, and thoracoacromial.

a. thoracoacromia'lis [NA], thoracoacromial artery; acromiothoracic artery; thoracic axis (1); *origin,* axillary; *distribution,* muscles and skin of shoulder and upper chest; *anastomoses,* branches of superior thoracic, internal thoracic, lateral thoracic, posterior and anterior circumflex humeral, and suprascapular.

a. thoracodorsa'lis [NA], thoracodorsal artery; dorsal thoracic artery; *origin,* subscapular; *distribution,* muscles of upper part of back; *anastomoses,* branches of lateral thoracic.

arte'riae thy'micae, *rami* thymici.

a. thyroi'dea i'ma [NA], lowest thyroid artery; Neubauer's artery; an inconstant artery; *origin,* arch of aorta or brachiocephalic artery; *distribution,* thyroid gland.

a. thyroi'dea infe'rior [NA], inferior thyroid artery; *origin,* thyrocervical trunk; *branches,* ascending cervical, inferior laryngeal, and muscular, esophageal, and tracheal.

a. thyroi'dea supe'rior [NA], superior thyroid artery; *origin,* external carotid; *branches,* infrahyoid, superior laryngeal, sternocleidomastoid, cricothyroid, and two terminal branches.

a. tibia'lis ante'rior [NA], anterior tibial artery; *origin,* popliteal; *branches,* posterior and anterior tibial recurrent, lateral and medial anterior malleolar, dorsalis pedis, lateral tarsal, medial tarsal, arcuate, dorsal metatarsal, and dorsal digital.

a. tibia'lis poste'rior [NA], posterior tibial artery; the larger and more directly continuous of the two terminal branches of the popliteal; *branches,* peroneal, nutrient of fibula, lateral and medial posterior malleolar, nutrient of tibia, medial and lateral plantar.

a. transver'sa cer'vicis [NA], a. transversa colli.

a. transver'sa col'li [NA], transverse artery of neck; transverse cervical artery; a. transversa cervicis; *origin,* thyrocervical trunk; *branches,* superficial (superficial cervical) and deep (descending scapular).

a. transver'sa facie'i [NA], transverse facial artery; *origin,* superficial temporal; *distribution,* parotid gland, parotid duct, masseter muscle, and overlying skin; *anastomoses,* infraorbital and buccal branches of maxillary, and buccal and masseteric branches of facial.

a. tympan'ica ante'rior [NA], anterior tympanic artery; glaserian artery; *origin,* maxillary; *distribution,* middle ear; *anastomoses,* tympanic branches of internal carotid and ascending pharyngeal and stylomastoid.

a. tympan'ica infe'rior [NA], inferior tympanic artery; *origin,* ascending pharyngeal; *distribution,* middle ear; *anastomoses,* tympanic branches of other arteries.

a. tympan'ica poste'rior [NA], posterior tympanic artery; *origin,* stylomastoid; *distribution,* middle ear; *anastomoses,* other tympanic arteries.

a. tympan'ica supe'rior [NA], superior tympanic artery; *origin,* middle meningeal; *distribution,* middle ear; *anastomoses,* other tympanic arteries.

a. ulna'ris [NA], ulnar artery; *origin,* brachial; *branches,* ulnar recurrent, common interosseous, dorsal and palmar carpal, deep palmar, and superficial palmar arch with its digital branches.

a. umbilica'lis [NA], umbilical artery; before birth the a. is a continuation of the internal iliac; after birth it is obliterated between the bladder and umbilicus, forming the medial umbilical ligament, the remaining portion, between the internal iliac artery and bladder, being reduced in size and giving off the superior vesical arteries.

a. urethra'lis [NA], urethral artery; *origin,* perineal artery; *distribution,* membranous urethra.

a. uteri'na [NA], uterine artery; *origin,* internal iliac; *distribution,* uterus, upper part of vagina, round ligament, and medial part of uterine (fallopian) tube; *anastomoses,* ovarian, vaginal, inferior epigastric.

a. vagina'lis [NA], vaginal artery; *origin,* internal iliac; *distribution,* vagina, base of bladder, rectum; *anastomoses,* uterine, internal pudendal.

arte'riae ventricula'res [NA], ventricular arteries; branches of the right and left coronary arteries distributed to the muscle of the ventricles.

a. vertebra'lis [NA], vertebral artery; the first branch of the subclavian artery; for descriptive purposes, divided into four parts:

1) pars prevertebralis, the portion before it enters the foramen of the transverse process of the sixth cervical vertebra; 2) pars transversaria, the portion in the transverse foramina of the first six cervical vertebrae; 3) pars atlantica, the portion running along the posterior arch of the atlas; and 4) pars intracranialis, the portion within the cranial cavity to its union with the artery from the other side to form the basilar artery.
a. vesica'lis infe'rior [NA], inferior vesical artery; *origin,* internal iliac; *distribution,* base of bladder, ureter, and (in the male) seminal vesicles, ductus deferens, and prostate; *anastomoses,* middle rectal, and other vesical branches.
a. vesica'lis supe'rior [NA], superior vesical artery; *origin,* umbilical; *distribution,* bladder, urachus, ureter; *anastomoses,* other vesical branches.
a. vitelli'na, vitelline artery; an artery carrying blood to the yolk sac from the embryo.
a. vola'ris ind'icis radia'lis, a. radialis indicis.
a. zygomat'ico-orbita'lis [NA], zygomatico-orbital artery; *origin,* superficial temporal, sometimes middle temporal; *distribution,* orbicularis oculi muscle and portions of the orbit; *anastomoses,* lacrimal and palpebral branches of ophthalmic.

arterial (ar-tē'rē-ăl). Relating to one or more arteries or to the entire system of arteries.

arterialization (ar-tē'rē-ăl-ī-zā'shŭn). **1.** Making or becoming arterial. **2.** Aeration or oxygenation of the blood whereby it is changed in character from venous to arterial. **3.** Vascularization. **4.** Conversion of a venous structure to function as an artery.

arteriarctia (ar-tēr-ē-ark'shē-ă) [L. *arteria,* artery, + *arcto,* to constrict]. Obsolete term for vasoconstriction of the arteries.

arteriectasis, arteriectasia (ar-tēr-ē-ek'tă-sis, -ek-tā'zē-ă) [L. *arteria,* artery, + G. *ektasis,* distention]. Obsolete term for vasodilation of the arteries.

arteriectomy (ar-tēr-ē-ek'tō-mē) [L. *arteria,* artery, + G. *ektomē,* excision]. Excision of part of an artery.

arterio-, arteri- [L. *arteria,* fr. G. *artēria,* artery]. Combining forms meaning artery.

arterioatony (ar-tēr'ē-ō-at'ō-nē) [arterio- + G. *atonia,* atony]. A relaxed state of the arterial walls.

arteriocapillary (ar-tēr'ē-ō-cap'i-lār-ē). Relating to both arteries and capillaries.

arteriogram (ar-tēr'ē-ō-gram) [arterio- + G. *gramma,* something written]. X-ray demonstration of an artery after injection of contrast medium into it.

arteriographic (ar-tēr'ē-ō-graf'ik). Relating to or utilizing arteriography.

arteriography (ar-tēr-ē-og'ră-fē) [arterio- + G. *graphō,* to write]. Visualization of an artery or arteries by x-ray imaging after injection of a radiopaque contrast medium.
cerebral a., cerebral *angiography.*
spinal a., spinal *angiography.*

arteriola, pl. **arteriolae** (ar-tēr-ē-ō'lă, -ō'lē) [Mod. L. dim. of *arteria,* artery] [NA]. Arteriole; a minute artery with a muscular wall; a terminal artery continuous with the capillary network.
a. macula'ris infe'rior [NA], inferior macular arteriole; *origin,* central artery of retina; *distribution,* inferior part of macula.
a. macula'ris supe'rior [NA], superior macular arteriole; *origin,* central artery of retina; *distribution,* upper part of macula.
a. media'lis ret'inae [NA], medial arteriole of retina; an arteriole supplying the part of the retina between the optic disk and the macula.
a. nasa'lis ret'inae infe'rior [NA], inferior nasal arteriole of retina; the branch of the central artery of the retina that supplies the lower medial, or nasal, part of the retina.
a. nasa'lis ret'inae supe'rior [NA], superior nasal arteriole of retina; the branch of the central artery of the retina that passes to the upper medial, or nasal, part of the retina.
arterio'lae rec'tae [NA], straight vessels into which the efferent arteriole of the juxtamedullary glomeruli breaks up; they form a leash of vessels which, arising at the bases of the pyramids, run through the renal medulla toward the apex of each pyramid, then reverse direction in a hairpin turn, and run straight back again toward the base of the pyramid as venae rectae.
a. tempora'lis ret'inae infe'rior [NA], inferior temporal arteriole of retina; the branch of the central artery of the retina that passes laterally below the macula to supply the lower lateral or temporal part of the retina.
a. tempora'lis ret'inae supe'rior [NA], superior temporal arteriole of retina; the branch of the central artery of the retina that passes laterally above the macula to supply the upper lateral or temporal part of the retina.

arteriolar (ar-ter-ē-ō'lăr). Of or pertaining to an arteriole or the arterioles collectively.

arteriole (ar-tēr'ē-ōl). Arteriola.
afferent glomerular a., a branch of an interlobular artery of the kidney that conveys blood to the glomerulus.
capillary a., a minute artery that terminates in a capillary.
efferent glomerular a., the vessel that carries blood from the glomerular capillary network to the capillary bed of the proximal convoluted tubule.
inferior macular a., *arteriola* macularis inferior.
inferior nasal a. of retina, *arteriola* nasalis retinae inferior.
inferior temporal a. of retina, *arteriola* temporalis retinae inferior.
medial a. of retina, *arteriola* medialis retinae.
superior macular a., *arteriola* macularis superior.
superior nasal a. of retina, *arteriola* nasalis retinae superior.
superior temporal a. of retina, *arteriola* temporalis retinae superior.

arteriolith (ar-tēr'ē-ō-lith) [L. *arteria,* artery, + G. *lithos,* a stone]. A calcareous deposit in an arterial wall or thrombus.

arteriolitis (ar-tēr'ē-ō-lī'tis) [L. *arteriola,* arteriole, + G.*-itis,* inflammation]. Inflammation of the wall of the arterioles.
necrotizing a., arteriolonecrosis; necrosis in the media of arterioles, characteristic of malignant hypertension.

arteriolo- [L. *arteriola,* arteriole]. Combining form relating to arterioles.

arteriology (ar-tēr'ē-ol'ō-jē) [L. *arteria,* artery, + G. *logos,* study]. The anatomy of the arteries: usually associated with the study of the other vessels under the name angiology.

arteriolonecrosis (ar-tēr-ē-ō'lō-nĕ-krō'sis) [L. *arteriola,* arteriole, + G. *nekrōsis,* a killing]. Necrotizing *arteriolitis.*

arteriolonephrosclerosis (ar-tēr-ē-ō'lō-nef'rō-skler-ō'sis). Arteriolar *nephrosclerosis.*

arteriolosclerosis (ar-tēr-ē-ō'lō-skler-ō'sis). Arteriolar sclerosis; arteriosclerosis affecting mainly the arterioles, seen especially in chronic hypertension.

arteriolovenous (ar-tērē-ō'lō-vē'nŭs). Involving both the arterioles and veins.

arteriolovenular (ar-tēr-ē-ō'lō-vē'nyū-lăr). Arteriolovenous.

arteriomalacia (ar-tēr'ē-ō-mă-lā'shē-ă) [arterio- + G. *malakia,* softness]. Softening of the arteries.

arteriometer (ar-tēr-ē-om'ĕ-ter) [arterio- + G. *metron,* measure]. An instrument for measuring the diameter of an artery, or its change in size during pulsation.

arteriomotor (ar-tēr'ē-ō-mō'ter). Causing changes in the caliber of an artery; vasomotor with special reference to the arteries.

arteriomyomatosis (ar-tēr'ē-ō-mī'ō-mă-tō'sis) [arterio- + G. *mys,* muscle, + *-oma,* tumor, + *-osis,* condition]. Thickening of the walls of an artery by an overgrowth of muscular fibers arranged irregularly, intersecting each other without any definite relation to the axis of the vessel.

arterionephrosclerosis (ar-tēr'ē-ō-nef'rō-skler-ō'sis). Arterial *nephrosclerosis.*

arteriopalmus (ar-tēr'ē-ō-pal'mŭs) [arterio- + G. *palmos,* throbbing]. Subjective sensation of throbbing of an artery.

arteriopathy (ar-tēr-ē-op'ă-thē) [arterio- + G. *pathos,* suffering]. Any disease of the arteries.
hypertensive a., arterial degeneration resulting from hypertension.
plexogenic pulmonary a., Ayerza's *disease.*

arterioplania (ar-tēr'ē-ō-plā'nē-ă) [arterio- + G. *planē,* a straying]. Presence of an anomaly in the course of an artery.

arterioplasty (ar-tēr'ē-ō-plas-tē) [arterio- + G. *plastos,* formed]. Any operation for the reconstruction of the wall of an artery.

arteriopressor (ar-tēr'ē-ō-pres'ser). Causing increased arterial blood pressure.

arteriorrhaphy (ar-tēr-ē-ōr'ă-fē) [arterio- + G. *rhaphē,* seam]. Suture of an artery.

arteriorrhexis (ar-tēr'ē-ō-rek'sis) [arterio- + G. *rhēxis,* rupture]. Rupture of an artery.

arteriosclerosis (ar-tēr'ē-ō-skler-ō'sis) [arterio- + G. *sklērōsis,* hardness]. Arterial or vascular sclerosis; sclerosis or hardening of the arteries; types generally recognized are: atherosclerosis, Mönckeberg's a., hypertensive a., and arteriolosclerosis.
hyperplastic a., hyperplasia of the intima and internal elastic layer and hypertrophy of the media independent of atheromatous lesions.
hypertensive a., progressive increase in muscle and elastic tissue of arterial walls, resulting from hypertension; in longstanding hypertension, elastic tissue forms numerous concentric layers in the intima and there is replacement of muscle by collagen fibers and hyaline thickening of the intima of arterioles; such changes can develop with increasing age in the absence of hypertension and may then be referred to as senile a.
medial a., Mönckeberg's a.
Mönckeberg's a., medial a.; Mönckeberg's degeneration, sclerosis, or calcification; arterial sclerosis involving the peripheral arteries, especially of the legs of older people, with deposition of calcium in the medial coat (pipestem arteries) but with little or no encroachment on the lumen.
nodular a., atheromas occurring in the arterial intima as discrete tumors.
a. oblit'erans, a. producing narrowing and occlusion of the arterial lumen.
senile a., a. similar to hypertensive a., but as a result of advanced age rather than hypertension.

arteriosclerotic (ar-tēr'ē-ō-skler-ot'ik). Relating to or affected by arteriosclerosis.

arteriospasm (ar-tēr'ē-ō-spazm). Spasm of an artery or arteries.

arteriostenosis (ar-tēr'ē-ō-stĕ-nō'sis) [arterio- + G. *stenōsis,* a narrowing]. Narrowing of the caliber of an artery, either temporary, through vasoconstriction, or permanent, through arteriosclerosis.

arteriostrepsis (ar-tēr'ē-ō-strep'sis) [arterio- + G. *strepsis,* a twisting]. Twisting the divided end of an artery to arrest bleeding.

arteriotome (ar-tēr'ē-ō-tōm). A lancet for performing arteriotomy.

arteriotomy (ar-tēr-ē-ot'ō-mē) [arterio- + G. *tomē,* incision]. Any surgical incision into the lumen of an artery, *e.g.,* to remove an embolus.

arteriotony (ar-tēr-ē-ot'ō-nē) [arterio- + G. *tonos,* tension]. Blood *pressure.*

arteriovenous (A-V) (ar-tēr'ē-ō-vē'nŭs). Arteriolovenular; relating to both an artery and a vein or to both arteries and veins in general; both arterial and venous.

arteritis (ar-ter-ī'tis) [L. *arteria,* artery, + G. *-itis,* inflammation]. Inflammation involving an artery or arteries.
cranial a., temporal a.
equine viral a., epizootic cellulitis; a highly contagious viral disease caused by equine arteritis virus and characterized by a high fever and respiratory and digestive tract signs; the essential lesions involve smaller arteries, with necrosis which may be followed by thrombosis, infarction, hemorrhages, and edema; abortion is a common result.
giant cell a., temporal a.
granulomatous a., temporal a.
Horton's a., temporal a.
a. nodo'sa, *polyarteritis* nodosa.
a. oblit'erans, obliterating a., *endarteritis* obliterans.
rheumatic a., a. due to rheumatic fever; Aschoff bodies are frequently found in the adventitia of small arteries, especially in the myocardium, and may lead to fibrosis and constriction of the lumens.
rheumatoid a., a. associated with rheumatoid arthritis, especially aortitis with aortic valve incompetence reported with ankylosing spondylitis.
temporal a., cranial, giant cell, granulomatous, or Horton's a.; panarteritis with medial necrosis and multinucleated giant cells in temporal, retinal, or intracerebral arteries; occurs in elderly persons and may be manifested by constitutional symptoms, severe bitemporal headache, and ocular symptoms including sudden loss of vision in one eye.

ARTERY

artery (ar'ter-ē) [L. *arteria,* fr. G. *artēria*]. Arteria.
aberrant a., a. having an unusual origin or course.
accessory obturator a., *arteria* obturatoria accessoria.
acetabular a., *ramus* acetabularis.
acromial a., *ramus* acromialis arteriae thoracoacromialis.
acromiothoracic a., *arteria* thoracoacromialis.
a.'s of Adamkiewicz, *rami* spinales (1c).
alar a. of nose, a branch of the angular a. that supplies the ala of the nose.
angular a., **(1)** *arteria* angularis; **(2)** *arteria* gyri angularis.
a. of angular gyrus, *arteria* gyri angularis.
anonymous a., *truncus* brachiocephalicus.
anterior cecal a., *arteria* cecalis anterior.
anterior cerebral a., *arteria* cerebri anterior.
anterior choroidal a., *arteria* choroidea anterior.
anterior ciliary a., *arteria* ciliaris anterior.
anterior circumflex humeral a., *arteria* circumflexa humeri anterior.
anterior communicating a., *arteria* communicans anterior.
anterior conjunctival a., *arteria* conjunctivalis anterior.
anterior descending a., *ramus* interventricularis anterior.
anterior ethmoidal a., *arteria* ethmoidalis anterior.
anterior inferior cerebellar a., *arteria* cerebelli inferior anterior.
a. to anterior inferior segment of kidney, *arteria* segmenti anterioris inferioris renis.
anterior intercostal a., *arteria* intercostalis anterior.
anterior interosseous a., *arteria* interossea anterior.
anterior interventricular a., *ramus* interventricularis anterior.
anterior labial a.'s, *rami* labiales anteriores.
anterior lateral malleolar a., *arteria* malleolaris anterior lateralis.

anterior medial malleolar a., *arteria* malleolaris anterior medialis.
anterior meningeal a., *arteria* meningea anterior.
anterior parietal a., *arteria* parietalis.
anterior peroneal a., *ramus* perforans.
anterior spinal a., *arteria* spinalis anterior.
anterior superior alveolar a., *arteria* alveolaris superior anterior.
anterior superior dental a., *arteria* alveolaris superior anterior.
a. to anterior superior segment of kidney, *arteria* segmenti anterioris superioris renis.
anterior temporal a., *arteria* temporalis anterior.
anterior tibial a., *arteria* tibialis anterior.
anterior tibial recurrent a., *arteria* recurrens tibialis anterior.
anterior tympanic a., *arteria* tympanica anterior.
anterolateral central a.'s, *arteriae* centrales anterolaterales.
anterolateral striate a.'s, *arteriae* centrales anterolaterales.
anterolateral thalamostriate a.'s, *arteriae* centrales anterolaterales.
anteromedial central a.'s, *arteriae* centrales anteromediales.
anteromedial thalamostriate a.'s, *arteriae* centrales anteromediales.
appendicular a., *arteria* appendicularis.
arciform a.'s., *arteriae* arcuatae renis.
arcuate a., *arteria* arcuata.
arcuate a.'s of kidney, *arteriae* arcuatae renis.
ascending a., *arteria* ascendens.
ascending cervical a., *arteria* cervicalis ascendens.
ascending palatine a., *arteria* palatina ascendens.
ascending pharyngeal a., *arteria* pharyngea ascendens.
atrial a.'s, *arteriae* atriales.
axillary a., *arteria* axillaris.
azygos a. of vagina, one of two a.'s that run longitudinally in the midline on the anterior and posterior aspects of the vagina; they take origin from the uterine a.
basilar a., *arteria* basilaris.
brachial a., *arteria* brachialis.
bronchial a.'s, *rami* bronchiales (1,2).
buccal a., buccinator a., *arteria* buccalis.
a. of bulb of penis, *arteria* bulbi penis.
a. of bulb of vestibule, *arteria* bulbi vestibuli.
calcaneal a.'s, *rami* calcanei.
calcarine a., *ramus* calcarinus.
a. of calf, *arteria* suralis.
callosomarginal a., *arteria* callosomarginalis.
caroticotympanic a.'s, *arteriae* caroticotympanici.
carotid a.'s, see *arteria* carotis communis; *arteria* carotis externa; *arteria* carotis interna.
carpal a., see *ramus* carpeus dorsalis arteriae radialis and ulnaris; *ramus* carpeus palmaris arteriae radialis and ulnaris.
caudal pancreatic a., *arteria* caudae pancreatis.
a. of caudate lobe, *arteria* lobi caudati.
cavernous a.'s, a number of small branches of the cavernous part of the internal carotid a.; see *ramus* tentorii basalis; *ramus* tentorii marginalis; *ramus* meningeus; ramus ganglionis trigemini; *rami* trigeminales et trocleares; and *ramus* sinus cavernosi.
cecal a.'s, see *arteria* cecalis anterior; *arteria* cecalis posterior.
celiac a., *truncus* celiacus.
central a., *arteria* sulci centralis.
central a. of retina, *arteria* centralis retinae.
a. of central sulcus, *arteria* sulci centralis.
cerebellar a.'s, see *arteria* cerebelli inferior anterior; *arteria* cerebelli inferior posterior; *arteria* cerebelli superior.
cerebral a.'s, see *arteria* cerebri anterior; arteria cerebri media; arteria cerebri posterior.
a. of cerebral hemorrhage, lenticulostriate a.
cervicovaginal a., arteria cervicovaginalis; an anastomotic communication between the uterine a. and the vaginal a.; it courses along the lateral aspect of the cervix and vagina.
Charcot's a., lenticulostriate a.'s (2).
chief a. of thumb, *arteria* princeps pollicis.
circumflex fibular a., *ramus* circumflexus fibulae.
circumflex scapular a., *arteria* circumflexa scapulae.
coiled a. of the uterus, spiral a.
collateral a., **(1)** one that runs parallel with a nerve or other structure; **(2)** one through which a collateral circulation is established.
collateral digital a., *arteria* digitalis palmaris propria.
common carotid a., *arteria* carotis communis.
common hepatic a., *arteria* hepatica communis.
common iliac a., *arteria* iliaca communis.
common interosseous a., *arteria* interossea communis.
common palmar digital a., *arteria* digitalis palmaris communis.
common plantar digital a., *arteria* digitalis plantaris communis.
communicating a., an a. that connects two larger a.'s.
companion a. to sciatic nerve, *arteria* comitans nervi ischiadici.
conjunctival a.'s, see *arteria* conjunctivalis anterior; *arteria* conjunctivalis posterior.
coronary a., **(1)** *arteria* gastrica sinistra; **(2)** see *arteria* coronaria dextra; *arteria* coronaria sinistra.
cortical a.'s, branches of the anterior, middle, and posterior cerebral a.'s that supply the cerebral cortex.
costocervical a., *truncus* costocervicalis.
cremasteric a., *arteria* cremasterica.
cricothyroid a., *ramus* cricothyroideus.
crural a., *arteria* femoralis.
cystic a., *arteria* cystica.
deep auricular a., *arteria* auricularis profunda.
deep brachial a., *arteria* profunda brachii.
deep cervical a., *arteria* cervicalis profunda.
deep circumflex iliac a., *arteria* circumflexa ilium profunda.
deep a. of clitoris, *arteria* profunda clitoridis.
deep epigastric a., *arteria* epigastrica inferior.
deep a. of penis, *arteria* profunda penis.
deep temporal a., *arteria* temporalis profunda.
deep a. of thigh, *arteria* profunda femoris.
deep a. of tongue, *arteria* profunda linguae.
descending a. of knee, *arteria* genus descendens.
descending palatine a., *arteria* palatina descendens.
descending scapular a., *arteria* scapularis dorsalis.
digital collateral a., *arteria* digitalis palmaris propria.
distributing a., muscular a.
dolichoectatic a., a distorted, dilated, and elongated artery commonly compressing a neural structure.
dorsal a. of clitoris, *arteria* dorsalis clitoridis.
dorsal digital a., *arteria* digitalis dorsalis.
dorsal a. of foot, *arteria* dorsalis pedis.
dorsal interosseous a., **(1)** *arteria* interossea posterior; **(2)** *arteria* metacarpea dorsalis.
dorsal metacarpal a., *arteria* metacarpea dorsalis.
dorsal metatarsal a., *arteria* metatarsea dorsalis.
dorsal a. of nose, *arteria* dorsalis nasi.
dorsal pancreatic a., *arteria* pancreatica dorsalis.
dorsal a. of penis, *arteria* dorsalis penis.
dorsal scapular a., *arteria* scapularis dorsalis.
dorsal thoracic a., *arteria* thoracodorsalis.
a. of ductus deferens, *arteria* ductus deferentis.
elastic a., a large a., such as the aorta or pulmonary a., which has many elastic lamella in its tunica media.
end a., terminal a.; an a. with insufficient anastomoses to maintain viability of the tissue supplied if occlusion of the a. occurs.
episcleral a., *arteria* episcleralis.
esophageal a.'s, *rami* esophageales.
external carotid a., *arteria* carotis externa.
external iliac a., *arteria* iliaca externa.
external mammary a., *arteria* thoracica lateralis.
external maxillary a., *arteria* facialis.

external a. of nose, *arteria* dorsalis nasi.
external pudendal a.'s, *arteriae* pudendae externae.
external spermatic a., *arteria* cremasterica.
facial a., *arteria* facialis.
femoral a., *arteria* femoralis.
fibular a., *arteria* peronea.
frontal a., *arteria* supratrochlearis.
gastroduodenal a., *arteria* gastroduodenalis.
glaserian a., *arteria* tympanica anterior.
great anastomotic a., (1) *arteria* collateralis ulnaris inferior; (2) *arteria genus descendens.*
great pancreatic a., *arteria* pancreatica magna.
great superior pancreatic a., *arteria* pancreatica dorsalis.
greater palatine a., *arteria* palatina major.
helicine a., *arteria* helicina.
a. of Heubner, *arteria* centralis longa.
highest intercostal a., *arteria* intercostalis anterior.
highest thoracic a., *arteria* thoracica superior.
humeral a., *arteria* brachialis.
hyaloid a., *arteria* hyaloidea.
hypogastric a., *arteria* iliaca interna.
ileal a.'s, *arteriae* ileales.
ileocolic a., *arteria* ileocolica.
iliolumbar a., *arteria* iliolumbalis.
inferior alveolar a., *arteria* alveolaris inferior.
inferior dental a., *arteria* alveolaris inferior.
inferior epigastric a., *arteria* epigastrica inferior.
inferior gluteal a., *arteria* glutea inferior.
inferior hemorrhoidal a., *arteria* rectalis inferior.
inferior hypophysial a., *arteria* hypophysialis inferior.
inferior internal parietal a., *arteria* precunealis.
inferior labial a., *arteria* labialis inferior.
inferior laryngeal a., *arteria* laryngea inferior.
inferior mesenteric a., *arteria* mesenterica inferior.
inferior pancreatic a., *arteria* pancreatica inferior.
inferior pancreaticoduodenal a., *arteria* pancreaticoduodenalis inferior.
inferior phrenic a., *arteria* phrenica inferior.
inferior rectal a., *arteria* rectalis inferior.
a. of inferior segment of kidney, *arteria* segmenti inferioris renis.
inferior suprarenal a., *arteria* suprarenalis inferior.
inferior thyroid a., *arteria* thyroidea inferior.
inferior tympanic a., *arteria* tympanica inferior.
inferior ulnar collateral a., *arteria* collateralis ulnaris inferior.
inferior vesical a., *arteria* vesicalis inferior.
infraorbital a., *arteria* infraorbitalis.
infrascapular a., a small branch of the arteria circumflexa scapulae.
innominate a., *truncus* brachiocephalicus.
insular a.'s, *arteriae* insulares.
interlobar a.'s, *arteriae* interlobares.
interlobular a.'s, *arteriae* interlobulares.
intermediate temporal a., *arteria* temporalis intermedia.
internal auditory a., *arteria* labyrinthi.
internal carotid a., *arteria* carotis interna.
internal iliac a., *arteria* iliaca interna.
internal mammary a., *arteria* thoracica interna.
internal maxillary a., *arteria* maxillaris.
internal pudendal a., *arteria* pudenda interna.
internal spermatic a., *arteria* testicularis.
internal thoracic a., *arteria* thoracica interna.
intestinal a.'s, arteriae intestinales; see *arteriae* ileales; *arteriae* jejunales.
jejunal a.'s, *arteriae* jejunales.
a.'s of kidney, *arteriae* renis.
Kugel's a., arteria anastomotica auricularis magna; a vessel of variable origin, most commonly a branch of the circumflex a., coursing posteriorly through the base of the interatrial septum toward the crux of the heart, anastomosing with coronary a. branches supplying the atrioventricular node, the atrioventricular bundle (bundle of His), and the upper posterior walls of the left ventricle.
a. of labyrinth, *arteria* labyrinthi.
lacrimal a., *arteria* lacrimalis.
lateral circumflex a. of thigh, *arteria* circumflexa femoris lateralis.
lateral frontobasal a., *arteria* frontobasalis lateralis.
lateral inferior genicular a., *arteria* genus inferior lateralis.
lateral nasal a., a branch of the facial a. which supplies the dorsum and ala of the nose.
lateral occipital a., *arteria* occipitalis lateralis.
lateral plantar a., *arteria* plantaris lateralis.
lateral sacral a., *arteria* sacralis lateralis.
lateral splanchnic a.'s, a.'s that arise in the embryo from the dorsal aorta to supply the mesonephros, testis (or ovary), and the adrenal gland.
lateral striate a.'s, *arteriae* centrales anterolaterales.
lateral superior genicular a., *arteria* genus superior lateralis.
lateral tarsal a., *arteria* tarsea lateralis.
lateral thoracic a., *arteria* thoracica lateralis.
left colic a., *arteria* colica sinistra.
left coronary a., *arteria* coronaria sinistra.
left gastric a., *arteria* gastrica sinistra.
left gastroepiploic a., *arteria* gastro-omentalis sinistra.
left gastro-omental a., *arteria* gastro-omentalis sinistra.
left pulmonary a., *arteria* pulmonalis sinistra.
lenticulostriate a.'s, (1) *arteriae* centrales anterolaterales; (2) Charcot's a.; a. of cerebral hemorrhage; any one of a variety of small a.'s entering the base of the brain through the substantia perforata anterior and supplying the striatum, globus pallidus, and internal capsule; most of these perforating a.'s are branches of the middle cerebral and anterior choroidal a.'s.
lesser palatine a., *arteria* palatina minor.
lienal a., *arteria* splenica.
lingual a., *arteria* lingualis.
long central a., *arteria* centralis longa.
long posterior ciliary a., *arteria* ciliaris posterior longa.
long thoracic a., *arteria* thoracica lateralis.
lowest lumbar a., *arteria* lumbalis ima.
lowest thyroid a., *arteria* thyroidea ima.
lumbar a., *arteria* lumbalis.
macular a.'s, see *arteriola* macularis inferior; *arteriola* macularis superior.
marginal a. of colon, a. formed by anastomoses between the right and left colic a.'s; it passes downward from the left colic flexure to the aboral end of the pelvic colon.
masseteric a., *arteria* masseterica.
mastoid a., *ramus* mastoideus.
maxillary a., *arteria* maxillaris.
medial circumflex a. of thigh, *arteria* circumflexa femoris medialis.
medial frontobasal a., *arteria* frontobasalis medialis.
medial inferior genicular a., *arteria* genus inferior medialis.
medial occipital a., *arteria* occipitalis medialis.
medial plantar a., *arteria* plantaris medialis.
medial striate a.'s, *rami* striati arteriae cerebri mediae.
medial superior genicular a., *arteria* genus superior medialis.
medial tarsal a., *arteria* tarsea medialis.
median a., *arteria* mediana.
median sacral a., *arteria* sacralis mediana.
medium a., muscular a.
medullary a.'s of brain, branches of the cortical a.'s which penetrate to and supply the white matter of the cerebrum.
mental a., *arteria* mentalis.

metatarsal a., *arteria* arcuata.
middle cerebral a., *arteria* cerebri media.
middle colic a., *arteria* colica media.
middle collateral a., *arteria* collateralis media.
middle genicular a., *arteria* genus media.
middle hemorrhoidal a., *arteria* rectalis media.
middle meningeal a., *arteria* meningea media.
middle rectal a., *arteria* rectalis media.
middle sacral a., *arteria* sacralis mediana.
middle suprarenal a., *arteria* suprarenalis media.
middle temporal a., *arteria* temporalis media. See also *arteria* temporalis intermedia; arteria temporalis posterior.
muscular a., medium or distributing a.; an a. with a tunica media composed principally of circularly arranged smooth muscle.
musculophrenic a., *arteria* musculophrenica.
myometrial arcuate a.'s, branches of the uterine and ovarian a.'s.
myometrial radial a.'s, continuations of the myometrial arcuate a.'s.
Neubauer's a., *arteria* thyroidea ima.
nutrient a., *arteria* nutricia.
nutrient a. of femur, one of two a.'s, superior and inferior, arising from the first and third perforating respectively (sometimes second and fourth).
nutrient a. of fibula, *origin,* peroneal (fibular); *distribution,* fibula.
nutrient a.'s of humerus, *arteriae* nutriciae humeri.
nutrient a. of the tibia, a. derived from the upper part of the posterior tibial a.; it enters through the nutrient foramen on the posterior surface of the tibia.
obturator a., *arteria* obturatoria.
occipital a., *arteria* occipitalis.
omphalomesenteric a., obsolete term for *arteria* vitellina.
ophthalmic a., *arteria* ophthalmica.
orbital a., *arteria* frontobasalis medialis.
orbitofrontal a., *arteria* frontobasalis lateralis.
ovarian a., *arteria* ovarica.
palmar interosseous a., *arteria* metacarpea palmaris.
palmar metacarpal a., *arteria* metacarpea palmaris.
palpebral a.'s, *arteriae* palpebrales.
paracentral a., *arteria* paracentralis.
parietal a.'s, *arteriae* parietales.
parieto-occipital a., *arteria* parieto-occipitalis.
a.'s of penis, see *arteria* dorsalis penis; *arteria* profunda penis.
perforating a.'s, *arteriae* perforantes.
perforating a.'s of foot, *rami perforantes* arteriae metatarsearum plantares. See under ramus.
perforating a.'s of hand, *rami perforantes* arteriae metacarpalium palmares. See under ramus.
perforating a.'s of internal mammary, *rami perforantes* arteriae thoracicae internae. See under ramus.
perforating a. of peroneal, *ramus* perforans.
pericallosal a., *arteria* pericallosa.
pericardiacophrenic a., *arteria* pericardiacophrenica.
perineal a., *arteria* perinealis.
peroneal a., *arteria* peronea.
pipestem a.'s, a.'s hardened by calcification as seen in Mönckeberg's arteriosclerosis; descriptive of the characteristic feeling to the finger of an examiner.
plantar metatarsal a., *arteria* metatarsea plantaris.
pontine a.'s, a.'s of pons, *arteriae* pontis.
popliteal a., *arteria* poplitea.
postcentral a., *arteria* sulci postcentralis.
a. of postcentral sulcus, *arteriae* sulci postcentralis.
posterior alveolar a., *arteria* alveolaris superior posterior.
posterior auricular a., *arteria* auricularis posterior.
posterior cecal a., *arteria* cecalis posterior.
posterior cerebral a., *arteria* cerebri posterior.
posterior choroidal a., *arteria* choroidea posterior.
posterior circumflex humeral a., *arteria* circumflexa humeri posterior.
posterior communicating a., *arteria* communicans posterior.
posterior conjunctival a., *arteria* conjunctivalis posterior.
posterior dental a., *arteria* alveolaris superior posterior.
posterior descending a., *ramus* interventricularis posterior.
posterior ethmoidal a., *arteria* ethmoidalis posterior.
posterior inferior cerebellar a., *arteria* cerebelli inferior posterior.
posterior intercostal a., *arteria* intercostalis posterior.
posterior interosseous a., *arteria* interossea posterior.
posterior interventricular a., *ramus* interventricularis posterior.
posterior labial a.'s, *rami* labiales posteriores.
posterior lateral nasal a.'s, *arteriae* nasales posteriores laterales.
posterior meningeal a., *arteria* meningea posterior.
posterior pancreaticoduodenal a., *arteria* retroduodenalis.
posterior parietal artery, arteria parietales anterior. See arteriae parietales under arteria.
posterior peroneal a.'s, *rami* malleolares laterales.
a. to posterior segment of kidney, *arteria* segmenti posterioris renis.
posterior septal a. of nose, *arteria* nasalis posterior septi.
posterior spinal a., *arteria* spinalis posterior.
posterior superior alveolar a., *arteria* alveolaris superior posterior.
posterior temporal a., *arteria* temporalis posterior.
posterior tibial a., *arteria* tibialis posterior.
posterior tibial recurrent a., *arteria* recurrens tibialis posterior.
posterior tympanic a., *arteria* tympanica posterior.
posterolateral central a.'s, *arteriae* centrales posterolaterales.
posteromedial central a.'s, *arteriae* centrales posteromediales.
precentral a., *arteria* sulci precentralis.
a. of precentral sulcus, *arteria* sulci precentralis.
precuneal a., *arteria* precunealis.
princeps cervicis a., *ramus* descendens (2).
principal a. of thumb, *arteria* princeps pollicis.
proper hepatic a., *arteria* hepatica propria.
proper palmar digital a., *arteria* digitalis palmaris propria.
proper plantar digital a., *arteria* digitalis plantaris propria.
a. of pterygoid canal, *arteria* canalis pterygoidei.
pubic a.'s, see *ramus* pubicus arteriae epigastricae inferioris; *ramus* pubicus arteriae obturatoriae.
pulmonary a., *truncus* pulmonalis. See also *arteria* pulmonalis dextra and *arteria* pulmonalis sinistra.
a. of pulp, the first section of a penicillus of the spleen.
pyloric a., *arteria* gastrica dextra.
quadriceps a. of femur, *ramus* descendens (1).
radial a., *arteria* radialis.
radial collateral a., *arteria* collateralis radialis.
radial index a., *arteria* radialis indicis.
radial recurrent a., *arteria* recurrens radialis.
radicular a.'s, *rami* spinales (1).
ranine a., *arteria* profunda linguae.
recurrent a., *arteria* centralis longa.
recurrent interosseous a., *arteria* interossea recurrens.
recurrent ulnar a., *arteria* recurrens ulnaris.
renal a., *arteria* renalis.
retroduodenal a., *arteria* retroduodenalis.
right colic a., *arteria* colica dextra.
right coronary a., *arteria* coronaria dextra.
right gastric a., *arteria* gastrica dextra.
right gastroepiploic a., *arteria* gastro-omentalis dextra.
right gastro-omental a., *arteria* gastro-omentalis dextra.
right pulmonary a., *arteria* pulmonalis dextra.
a. of round ligament of uterus, *arteria* ligamenti teretis uteri.
a. to sciatic nerve, *arteria* comitans nervi ischiadici.
screw a.'s, coiled a.'s into the uterine mucosa or in the macular

region of the retina.
scrotal a.'s, see *rami* scrotales anteriores; *rami* scrotales posteriores.
segmental a., *arteria* segmenti.
septal a., a branch of the superior labial a. that supplies the lower part of the nasal septum.
sheathed a., a subdivision of the penicillus of the spleen surrounded by macrophages and a reticular stroma.
short central a., *arteria* centralis brevis.
short gastric a.'s, *arteriae* gastricae breves.
short posterior ciliary a., *arteria* ciliaris posterior brevis.
sigmoid a.'s, *arteriae* sigmoideae.
small a.'s, unnamed muscular a.'s, usually with fewer than six or seven layers of muscle.
somatic a.'s, a.'s that arise in the embryo from the dorsal aorta and supply the body wall; they persist almost unchanged as the posterior intercostal, subcostal, and lumbar a.'s.
sphenopalatine a., *arteria* sphenopalatina.
spiral a., coiled a. of the uterus; one of the corkscrew-like a.'s in premenstrual or progestational endometrium.
splenic a., *arteria* splenica.
stapedial a., a small a. in the embryo that passes through the ring of the stapes, and is later obliterated; it is a second aortic arch derivative.
sternal a.'s, *rami* sternales.
sternomastoid a., see *rami* sternocleidomastoidei; *ramus* sternocleidomastoideus.
stylomastoid a., *arteria* stylomastoidea.
subclavian a., *arteria* subclavia.
subcostal a., *arteria* subcostalis.
sublingual a., *arteria* sublingualis.
submental a., *arteria* submentalis.
subscapular a., *arteria* subscapularis.
sulcal a., a small branch of the anterior spinal a. running in the anterior median fissure of the spinal cord.
superficial brachial a., *arteria* brachialis superficialis.
superficial cervical a., *arteria* cervicalis superficialis.
superficial circumflex iliac a., *arteria* circumflexa ilium superficialis.
superficial epigastric a., *arteria* epigastrica superficialis.
superficial palmar a., *ramus* palmaris superficialis arteriae radialis.
superficial temporal a., *arteria* temporalis superficialis.
superficial volar a., *ramus* palmaris superficialis arteriae radialis.
superior cerebellar a., *arteria* cerebelli superior.
superior coronary a., *arteria* labialis superior.
superior epigastric a., *arteria* epigastrica superior.
superior gluteal a., *arteria* glutea superior.
superior hemorrhoidal a., *arteria* rectalis superior.
superior hypophysial a., *arteria* hypophysialis superior.
superior internal parietal a., *arteria* parieto-occipitalis.
superior labial a., *arteria* labialis superior.
superior laryngeal a., *arteria* laryngea superior.
superior mesenteric a., *arteria* mesenterica superior.
superior pancreaticoduodenal a., *arteria* pancreaticoduodenalis superior.
superior phrenic a., *arteria* phrenica superior.
superior rectal a., *arteria* rectalis superior.
a. to superior segment of kidney, *arteria* segmenti superioris renis.
superior suprarenal a., *arteria* suprarenalis superior.
superior thoracic a., *arteria* thoracica superior.
superior thyroid a., *arteria* thyroidea superior.
superior tympanic a., *arteria* tympanica superior.
superior ulnar collateral a., *arteria* collateralis ulnaris superior.
superior vesical a., *arteria* vesicalis superior.
supraduodenal a., *arteria* supraduodenalis.
supraorbital a., *arteria* supraorbitalis.
suprascapular a., *arteria* suprascapularis.
supratrochlear a., *arteria* supratrochlearis.
supreme intercostal a., *arteria* intercostalis anterior.
sural a., *arteria* suralis.
terminal a., end a.
testicular a., *arteria* testicularis.
thoracoacromial a., *arteria* thoracoacromialis.
thoracodorsal a., *arteria* thoracodorsalis.
transverse cervical a., *arteria* transversa colli.
transverse facial a., *arteria* transversa faciei.
transverse a. of neck, *arteria* transversa colli.
transverse pancreatic a., *arteria* pancreatica inferior.
transverse scapular a., *arteria* suprascapularis.
ulnar a., *arteria* ulnaris.
umbilical a., *arteria* umbilicalis.
urethral a., *arteria* urethralis.
uterine a., *arteria* uterina.
vaginal a., *arteria* vaginalis.
venous a., *truncus* pulmonalis.
ventral splanchnic a.'s, a.'s that arise on the embryo from the dorsal aorta and are distributed to the digestive tube.
ventricular a.'s, *arteriae* ventriculares.
vertebral a., *arteria* vertebralis.
vidian a., *arteria* canalis pterygoidei.
vitelline a., *arteria* vitellina.
volar interosseous a., *arteria* interossea anterior.
Wilkie's a., the right colic a. when it occasionally crosses the duodenum.
Zinn's a., *arteria* centralis retinae.
zygomatico-orbital a., *arteria* zygomatico-orbitalis.

---

arthr-. See arthro-.
arthragra (arth-rag'rǎ) [G. *arthron,* joint, + *agra,* seizure]. Obsolete term for articular *gout.*
arthral (ar'thrǎl). Articular.
arthralgia (ar-thral'jē-ǎ) [G. *arthron,* joint, + *algos,* pain]. Arthrodynia; severe pain in a joint, especially one not inflammatory in character.
intermittent a., periodic a.
periodic a., intermittent a.; a condition in which pain and swelling of one or more joints, most commonly the knee, occurs at regular intervals; there is sometimes abdominal pain, purpura, or edema; the disease may show a familial tendency.
a. saturni'na, severe pain, chiefly on flexion of the joints of the lower extremities, in lead poisoning.
arthralgic (ar-thral'jik). Arthrodynic; relating to or affected with arthralgia.
arthrectomy (ar-threk'tō-mē) [G. *arthron,* joint, + *ektomē,* excision]. Exsection of a joint.
arthresthesia (ar-thres-thē'zē-ǎ) [G. *arthron,* joint, + *aisthesis,* sensation]. Articular *sensibility.*
arthrifuge (ar'thri-fūj) [arthritis + L. *fugo,* to chase away]. A gout remedy.
arthritic (ar-thrit'ik). Relating to arthritis.
arthritide (ar'thri-tēd) [Fr.]. A skin eruption of assumed gouty or rheumatic origin.
arthritides (ar-thrit'i-dēz). Plural of arthritis.
arthritis, pl. **arthritides** (ar-thrī'tis, ar-thrit'i-dēz) [G. fr. *arthron,* joint, + *-itis,* inflammation]. Articular rheumatism; inflammation of a joint or a state characterized by inflammation of joints.
acute rheumatic a., a. due to rheumatic fever.
atrophic a., obsolete term for a. without new bone formation, now usually called rheumatoid a.
chlamydial a., serous polyarthritis of cattle and sheep from

chlamydial infection.
chronic absorptive a., a. accompanied by pronounced resorption of bone with shortening and deformity, especially of the hands; when the deformity is extreme, the condition has also been termed a. mutilans.
chylous a., a. with a high lymph content in synovial fluid, usually due to filariasis.
a. defor'mans, rheumatoid a.
degenerative a., osteoarthritis.
enteropathic a., a form of a. sometimes resembling rheumatoid a. which may complicate the course of ulcerative colitis, Crohn's disease, or other intestinal disease.
filarial a., a. occurring in filariasis, probably due to extravasation of lipid-rich lymph resembling chyle into the joint space.
gouty a., inflammation of the joints (especially of the great toe) in gout.
hemophilic a., joint disease resulting from hemophilic bleeding into a joint.
hypertrophic a., osteoarthritis.
Jaccoud's a., Jaccoud's arthropathy; a rare form of chronic a., reported to occur after attacks of acute rheumatic fever, characterized by an unusual form of bone erosion of the metacarpal heads and by ulnar deviation of the fingers; it resembles rheumatoid a., but there is less overt inflammation, and rheumatoid factor is absent.
juvenile a., juvenile rheumatoid a., chronic a. beginning in childhood, most cases of which are pauciarticular, *i.e.,* affecting few joints. Several patterns of illness have been identified: in one subset, primarily affecting girls, iritis is common and antinuclear antibody is usually present; another subset, primarily affecting boys, frequently includes spinal a. resembling ankylosing spondylitis; some cases are true rheumatoid a. beginning in childhood and characterized by the presence of rheumatoid factor and destructive deforming joint changes, often undergoing remission at puberty. See also Still's *disease.*
Lyme a., the arthritic manifestation of Lyme disease.
a. mu'tilans, a form of chronic rheumatoid a. in which osteoporosis occurs with extensive destruction of the joint cartilages and pronounced deformities, chiefly of the hands and feet; similar changes can occur in some cases of psoriatic a.
neonatal a. of foals, bacterial polyarthritis caused by umbilical infections by several bacterial species.
neuropathic a., neuropathic *joint.*
a. nodo'sa, **(1)** rheumatoid a.; **(2)** gout.
ochronotic a., osteoarthritis occurring as a complication of ochronosis.
proliferative a., rarely used term for rheumatoid a., based on the characteristic proliferation of the synovial membrane seen in joints affected by the disease.
psoriatic a., the concurrence of psoriasis and a., resembling rheumatoid a. but thought to be a specific disease entity. See also a. mutilans.
rheumatoid a., a. deformans; a. nodosa (1); nodose rheumatism (1); a systemic disease, occurring more often in women, which affects connective tissue; a. is the dominant clinical manifestation, involving many joints, especially those of the hands and feet, accompanied by thickening of articular soft tissue, with extension of synovial tissue over articular cartilages, which become eroded; the course is variable but often is chronic and progressive, leading to deformities and disability.
suppurative a., pyarthrosis; purulent or suppurative synovitis; acute inflammation of synovial membranes, with purulent effusion into a joint, due to bacterial infection; the usual route of infection is hematogenic to the synovial tissue, causing destruction of the articular cartilage, and may become chronic, with sinus formation, deformity, and disability.
a. urat'ica, gout.

arthro-, arthr- [G. *arthron,* joint]. Combining forms denoting a joint or articulation.

Arthrobacter (ar-thrō-bak'ter) [G. *arthron,* joint, + *baktron,* staff or rod]. A genus of strictly aerobic, Gram-positive bacteria (family Corynebacteriaceae) whose cells undergo a change from a coccoid form to a rod shape following transfer to fresh complex growth medium. Although primarily found in soil, species identified as belonging to this genus have been found in the advancing front of lesions of dental caries. The type species is *A. globiformis.*

arthrocele (ar'thrō-sēl) [arthro- + G. *kēlē,* hernia, tumor]. **1.** Hernia of the synovial membrane through the capsule of a joint. **2.** Any swelling of a joint.

arthrocentesis (ar'thrō-sen-tē'sis) [arthro- + G. *kentēsis,* puncture]. Aspiration of fluid from a joint through a puncture needle.

arthrochondritis (ar'thrō-kon-drī'tis) [arthro- + G. *chondros,* cartilage, + *-itis,* inflammation]. Inflammation of an articular cartilage.

arthroclasia (ar-thrō-klā'zē-ă) [arthro- + G. *klasis,* a breaking]. The forcible breaking up of the adhesions in ankylosis.

arthrodesis (ar-throd'ĕ-sis, ar-thrō-dē'sis) [arthro- + G. *desis,* a binding together]. Artificial ankylosis; syndesis; the stiffening of a joint by operative means.
triple a., surgical fusion of the talonavicular, talocalcaneal, and calcaneocuboid joints.

arthroconidium (ar'thrō-kō-nid'ē-um) [G. *arthron,* joint, + conidium]. Arthrospore; a conidium released by fragmentation or separation at the septum of cells of the hypha.

arthrodia (ar-thrō'dē-ă) [G. *arthrōdia,* a gliding joint, fr. *arthron,* joint, + *eidos,* form]. *Articulatio* plana.

arthrodial (ar-thrō'dē-ăl). Relating to arthrodia.

arthrodynia (ar-thrō-din'ē-ă) [arthro- + G. *odynē,* pain]. Arthralgia.

arthrodynic (ar-thrō-din'ik). Arthralgic.

arthrodysplasia (ar'thrō-dis-plā'zē-ă) [arthro- + G. *dys,* bad, + *plasis,* a molding]. Congenital defect of joint development.

arthroendoscopy (ar'thrō-en-dos'kō-pē). Arthroscopy.

arthroereisis (ar-thrō-ĕ-rī'sis). Arthrorisis.

arthrogenous (ar-throj'ĕ-nŭs). **1.** Of articular origin; starting from a joint. **2.** Forming an articulation.

arthrogram (ar'thrō-gram). Roentgenogram of a joint; usually implies the introduction of a contrast agent into the joint capsule.

arthrography (ar-throg'ră-fē) [arthro- + G. *graphō,* to describe]. Roentgenography of a joint usually after injecting one or more contrast media into the joint.

arthrogryposis (ar'thrō-gri-pō'sis) [arthro- + G. *gryphōsis,* a crooking]. Congenital defect of the limbs characterized by contractures, flexion, and extension.
a. mul'tiplex congen'ita, amyoplasia congenita; limitation of range of joint motion and contractures present at birth, usually involving multiple joints; a syndrome probably of diverse etiology that may result from changes in spinal cord, muscle, or connective tissue.

arthrokatadysis (ar'thrō-kă-tad'i-sis) [arthro- + G. *katadysis,* a dipping under, a setting, fr. *dyō,* to make sink]. Otto's *disease.*

arthrolith (ar'thrō-lith) [arthro- + G. *lithos,* stone]. A loose body in a joint.

arthrolithiasis (ar'thrō-li-thī'ă-sis). Rarely used term for articular *gout.*

arthrologia (ar-thrō-lō'jē-ă) [NA]. Arthrology.

arthrology (ar-throl'ō-jē) [arthro- + G. *logos,* study]. Arthrologia; syndesmologia; syndesmology; synosteology; the branch of anatomy concerned with the joints.

arthrolysis (ar-throl'i-sis) [arthro- + G. *lysis,* a loosening]. Restoration of mobility in stiff and ankylosed joints.

arthrometer (ar-throm'ĕ-ter). Goniometer (3).

arthrometry (ar-throm'ĕ-trē) [arthro- + G. *metron,* measure]. Measurement of the range of movement in a joint.

arthronosos (ar-thrō-nō'sos) [arthro- + G. *nosos,* disease]. Rarely used term for any disease of the joints.

arthro-onychodysplasia (ar'thrō-on'i-kō-dis-plā'zē-ă). Nail-patella *syndrome.*

arthro-ophthalmopathy (ar'thrō-of'thal-mop'ă-thē) [arthro- + ophthalmo- + G. *pathos,* suffering]. Disease affecting joints and eyes.
hereditary progressive a., Stickler syndrome; autosomal dominant a. associated with progressive multiple dysplasia of the epiphyses, overtubulation of long bones, cleft lip and palate, hypermobility of joints, flattened vertebral bodies, pelvic bone deformities, and deafness.

arthropathia (ar-thrō-path'ē-ă) [L.]. Arthropathy.
a. psoriat'ica, inflammatory involvement of joints in persons suffering from psoriasis.

arthropathology (ar'thrō-pa-thol'ō-jē). The study of diseases of joints.

arthropathy (ar-throp'ă-thē) [arthro- + G. *pathos,* suffering]. Arthropathia; any disease affecting a joint.
diabetic a., a neuropathic a. occurring in diabetes.
Jaccoud's a., Jaccoud's *arthritis.*
long-leg a., a degenerative joint disease that develops after many years in the knee of the longer leg of a person with unequal leg lengths.
neuropathic a., neuropathic *joint.*
static a., secondary involvement of a joint following disease in a joint of the same extremity; *e.g.,* knee or ankle involvement in hip disease.
tabetic a., neuropathic *joint.*

arthrophlysis (ar-throf'li-sis) [arthro- + G. *phlysis,* eruption, fr. *phlyō,* to boil over]. An eczematous eruption in gouty or rheumatic persons.

arthrophyma (ar-thrō-fī'mă) [arthro- + G. *phyma,* swelling, tumor]. An articular tumor or swelling.

arthroplasty (ar'thrō-plas-tē) [arthro- + G. *plastos,* formed]. **1.** Creation of an artificial joint to correct ankylosis. **2.** An operation to restore as far as possible the integrity and functional power of a joint.
Charnley hip a., a form of total hip replacement consisting of the application of an acetabular cup and a femoral head prosthesis.
gap a., the surgical correction of ankylosis by creating a space between the ankylosed part of a joint and the portion for which movement is desired.
interposition a., surgical correction of ankylosis by separation of the immobile part of a joint from the mobilized part and interposition of a substance (*e.g.,* fascia, cartilage, metal, or plastic) between them.
intracapsular temporomandibular joint a., operative recontouring of the articular surface of the mandibular condyle without the removal of the articular disk.
total joint a., a. in which both joint surfaces are replaced with artificial materials, usually metal and high-density plastic.

arthropneumoroentgenography (ar'thrō-nū'mō-rant'gen-og'ră-fē). X-ray examination of a joint after it has been injected with air.

arthropod (ar'thrō-pod) [arthro- + G. *pous,* foot]. A member of the phylum Arthropoda.

Arthropoda (ar-throp'ō-dă) [arthro- + G. *pous,* foot]. A phylum of the Metazoa that includes the classes Crustacea (crabs, shrimps, crayfish, lobsters), Insecta, Arachnida (spiders, scorpions, mites, ticks), Chilopoda (centipedes), Diplopoda (millipedes), Merostomata (horseshoe crabs), and various other extinct or lesser known groups. A. forms the largest assemblage of living organisms, 75% insects, of which over a million species are known.

arthropodiasis (ar'thrō-pō-dī'ă-sis). Direct effects of arthropods upon vertebrates including acariasis, allergy, dermatosis, entomophobia, and actions of contact toxins.

arthropodic, arthropodous (ar-thrō-pō'dik, ar-throp'ō-dŭs). Pertaining to arthropods.

arthropyosis (ar'thrō-pī-ō'sis) [arthro- + G. *pyōsis,* suppuration]. Suppuration in a joint.

arthrorisis (ar'thrō-rī'sis) [arthro- + G. *ereisis,* a propping up]. Arthroerisis; an operation for limiting motion in a joint in cases of undue mobility from paralysis, usually by means of a bone block.

arthrosclerosis (ar'thrō-skler-ō'sis) [arthro- + G. *sklērōsis,* hardening]. Stiffness of the joints, especially in the aged.

arthroscope (ar'thrō-skōp). An endoscope for examining joint interiors.

arthroscopy (ar-thros'kō-pē) [arthro- + G. *skopeō,* to view]. Arthroendoscopy; endoscopic examination of the interior of a joint.

arthrosis (ar-thrō'sis). **1** [G. *arthrōsis,* a jointing]. Articulatio. **2** [arthro- + G. *-osis,* condition]. A degenerative affection of a joint.
temporomandibular a., a noninfectious degenerative dysfunction of the temporomandibular joint characterized by pain, cracking, and limited mandibular opening. See also myofacial pain-dysfunction *syndrome.*

arthrospore (ar'thrō-spōr) [arthro- + G. *sporos,* seed]. Arthroconidium.

arthrosteitis (ar-thros-tē-ī'tis) [arthro- + G. *osteon,* bone, + *-itis,* inflammation]. Inflammation of the osseous structures of a joint.

arthrostomy (ar-thros'tō-mē) [arthro- + G. *stoma,* mouth]. Establishment of a temporary opening into a joint cavity.

arthrosynovitis (ar'thrō-sin-ō-vī'tis). Inflammation of the synovial membrane of a joint.

arthrotome (ar'thrō-tōm). A large, strong scalpel used in cutting cartilaginous and other tough joint structures.

arthrotomy (ar-throt'ō-mē) [arthro- + G. *tomē,* a cutting]. Cutting into a joint.

arthrotropic (ar-thrō-trop'ik) [arthro- + G. *tropos,* a turning]. Tending to affect joints.

arthrotyphoid (ar-thrō-tī'foyd). Obsolete term for typhoid fever with joint involvement due to metastatic infection.

arthroxesis (ar-throk'sĕ-sis) [arthro- + G. *xesis,* a scraping]. Removal of diseased tissue from a joint by means of the sharp spoon or other scraping instrument.

Arthus, Nicolas Maurice, French bacteriologist, 1862–1945. See A. *phenomenon, reaction.*

artiad (ar'tē-ad) [G. *artios,* exact, (of numbers) even]. Obsolete term for an element of even valence.

articular (ar-tik'yū-lăr). Arthral; relating to a joint.

articulare (ar-tik-yū-lā'rē). In cephalometrics, the point of intersection of the external dorsal contour of the mandibular condyle and the temporal bone; the midpoint is used when a profile radiograph shows double projections of the rami.

articulate [L. *articulo,* pp. *-atus,* to articulate]. (ar-tik'yū-lit). **1.** Articulated. **2.** Capable of distinct and connected speech. (ar-tik'yū-lāt). **3.** To join or connect together loosely to allow motion between the parts. **4.** To speak distinctly and connectedly.

articulated (ar-tik'yū-lā-ted). Articulate (1); jointed.

ARTICULATIO

articulatio, pl. **articulationes** (ar-tik-yū-lā'shē-ō, -lā-shē-ō'nēz) [L. a forming of vines]. Articulation (1); arthrosis (1); junctura (1); joint; articulus; in anatomy, the place of union, usually more or less movable, between two or more bones. Joints between skeletal elements exhibit a great variety of form and function, and are classified into three general morphological types: articulationes fibrosae; articulationes cartilagineae; and articulationes synoviales.

a. acromioclavicula'ris [NA], acromioclavicular joint; a plane synovial joint between the acromial end of the clavicle and the medial margin of the acromion.

a. atlantoaxia'lis latera'lis [NA], lateral atlantoaxial joint; lateral atlantoepistrophic joint; a condylar synovial joint between the inferior articular pits of the atlas and the superior articular surfaces of the axis.

a. atlantoaxia'lis media'na [NA], median atlantoaxial joint; middle atlantoepistrophic joint; Cruveilhier's joint; a pivot synovial joint between the dens of the axis and the ring formed by the anterior arch and the transverse ligament of the atlas.

a. atlan'to-occipita'lis [NA], atlanto-occipital articulation or joint; a condylar synovial joint between the superior articular pits of the atlas and the condyles of the occipital bone.

a. bicondyla'ris [NA], bicondylar articulation or joint; a synovial joint in which two more or less distinct, rounded surfaces of one bone articulate with shallow depressions on another bone.

a. calca'neocuboi'dea [NA], calcaneocuboid joint; a somewhat saddle-shaped synovial joint between the anterior surface of the calcaneus and the posterior surface of the cuboid.

a. cap'itis cos'tae [NA], joint of head of rib; capitular joint; the synovial joint between a rib and bodies of two adjacent vertebrae; the joint cavity is divided by an intra-articular ligament which attaches to the intervertebral disk; the first, tenth, eleventh, and twelfth ribs articulate with only one vertebra.

articulatio'nes carpometacar'peae [NA], carpometacarpal joints; the synovial joints between the carpal and metacarpal bones; these are all plane joints except that of the thumb, which is saddle-shaped.

a. carpometacar'pea pol'licis [NA], carpometacarpal joint of thumb; the saddle-shaped synovial articulation between the trapezium and the base of the first metacarpal bone.

a. cartilag'inis [NA], cartilaginous joint; synarthrodial joint (2); junctura cartilaginea; a joint in which the apposed bony surfaces are united by cartilage; they are divided into synchondroses and symphyses; in synchondroses, the cartilage connecting the apposed surfaces is, as a rule, ultimately converted to bone, as between epiphyses and diaphyses of long bones; exceptions are the sternal synchondroses and the cartilaginous union of the first rib and the manubrium of the sternum; in symphyses the bones are connected by a flat disk of fibrocartilage which remains unossified throughout life; *e.g.,* the intervertebral disk and the symphysis pubis.

articulatio'nes cing'uli mem'bri inferio'ris [NA], joints of inferior limb girdle; juncturae cinguli membri inferioris; the joints that unite the sacrum and the two hip bones to form the pelvic girdle; these are the sacroiliac joints, the pubic symphysis, the sacrotuberal and sacrospinal ligaments, and the obturator membrane.

articulatio'nes cin'guli mem'bri superio'ris [NA], joints of superior limb girdle; juncturae cinguli membri superioris; the joints uniting the scapulae and clavicles to each other and the latter to the sternum forming the superior limb girdle; these are the acromioclavicular and the sternoclavicular joints.

a. compos'ita [NA], compound joint; a joint composed of three or more skeletal elements.

a. condyla'ris [NA], a. ellipsoidea.

a. costochondra'lis [NA], costochondral joint; the cartilaginous joint between the sternal end of a rib and the lateral end of a costal cartilage.

a. cos'totransversa'ria [NA], costotransverse joint; the synovial articulation between the neck and tubercle of a rib and the transverse process of a vertebra.

articulatio'nes costovertebra'les [NA], costovertebral joints; the synovial joints uniting ribs and vertebrae; they consist of the a. capitis costae and the a. costotransversaria.

a. cotyl'ica [NA], a. spheroidea.

a. cox'ae [NA], hip or thigh joint; the ball-and-socket synovial joint between the head of the femur and the acetabulum.

a. cricoarytenoid'ea [NA], cricoarytenoid articulation or joint; the synovial joint between the base of each arytenoid cartilage and the upper border of the lamina of the cricoid cartilage.

a. cricothyroid'ea [NA], cricothyroid articulation or joint; the synovial articulation between the inferior horn of the thyroid cartilage and the side of the cricoid cartilage.

a. cu'biti [NA], cubital or elbow joint; a compound hinge synovial joint between the humerus and the bones of the forearm; it consists of the a. humeroradialis and the a. humeroulnaris.

a. cuneonavicula'ris [NA], cuneonavicular articulation or joint; the synovial joint between the anterior surface of the navicular and the posterior surfaces of the three cuneiform bones.

a. dentoalveola'ris [NA], gomphosis.

a. ellipsoi'dea [NA], ellipsoidal joint; a. condylaris; condylar articulation or joint; a modified ball-and-socket synovial joint in which the joint surfaces are elongated or ellipsoidal; it is a biaxial joint, *i.e.,* two axes of motion at right angles to each other, the radiocarpal being an example.

a. fibro'sa [NA], fibrous joint; junctura fibrosa; synarthrodia; synarthrodial joint (1); immovable joint; a union of two bones by fibrous tissue such that there is no joint cavity and almost no motion possible; the types of fibrous joints are sutura, syndesmosis, and gomphosis.

a. ge'nus [NA], knee joint; a compound condylar synovial joint consisting of the joint between the condyles of the femur and the condyles of the tibia, the semilunar cartilages being interposed, and the articulation between femur and patella.

a. hu'meri [NA], humeral articulation; shoulder joint; a ball-and-socket synovial joint between the head of the humerus and the glenoid cavity of the scapula.

a. humeroradia'lis [NA], humeroradial articulation; humeroradial joint; the portion of the elbow joint between the capitulum of the humerus and the head of the radius.

a. humeroulna'ris [NA], humeroulnar joint; the portion of the elbow joint between the trochlea of the humerus and the trochlear notch of the ulna.

a. incudomallea'ris [NA], incudomalleolar joint; the saddle synovial joint between the incus and the malleus.

a. incudostape'dia [NA], incudostapedial articulation or joint; the synovial joint between the lenticular process on the long crus of the incus and the head of the stapes.

articulatio'nes intercar'peae [NA], intercarpal or carpal joints; the synovial joints between the carpal bones.

articulatio'nes interchondra'les [NA], interchondral articulations or joints; the synovial joints between the contiguous surfaces of the fifth, sixth, seventh, eighth, ninth, and tenth costal cartilages.

articulatio'nes intermetacar'peae [NA], intermetacarpal joints; the synovial joints between the bases of the second, third, fourth, and fifth metacarpal bones.

articulatio'nes intermetatar'seae [NA], intermetatarsal articulations or joints; the synovial joints between the bases of the five metatarsal bones.

articulatio'nes interphalan'geae [NA], interphalangeal articulations or joints; digital joints; or phalangeal joints; the hinge synovial joints between the phalanges of the fingers (articulationes interphalangeae manus) or toes (articulationes interphalangeae pedis).
articulatio'nes intertar'seae [NA], intertarsal articulations or joints; tarsal joints; the synovial joints which unite the tarsal bones.
a. lumbosacra'lis [NA], lumbosacral joint; junctura lumbosacralis; the articulation of the fifth lumbar vertebra with the sacrum.
a. mandibula'ris, a. temporomandibularis.
articulatio'nes ma'nus [NA], articulations of hand; these joints include the radiocarpal or wrist joint; intercarpal, carpometacarpal, intermetacarpal; metacarpophalangeal and interphalangeal joints.
a. mediocar'pea [NA], middle carpal joint; the synovial joint between the proximal and distal rows of carpal bones.
articulatio'nes mem'bri inferio'ris li'beri [NA], joints of free inferior limb; juncturae membri inferioris liberi; the joints uniting the bones of the free inferior limb to one another and to the pelvic girdle; they are the hip joint, knee joint, tibiofibular joints, and the joints of the foot.
articulatio'nes mem'bri superio'ris li'beri [NA], joints of free superior limb; juncturae membri superioris liberi; the joints uniting the bones of the free superior limb girdle; they are the shoulder joint, elbow joint, radioulnar joints, and joints of the hand.
articulatio'nes metacarpophalan'geae [NA], metacarpophalangeal articulations or joints; MP joints (1); the spheroid synovial joints between the heads of the metacarpals and the bases of the proximal phalanges.
articulationes metatarsophalan'geae [NA], metatarsophalangeal articulations or joints; MP joints (2); the spheroid synovial joints between the heads of the metatarsals and the bases of the proximal phalanges of the toes.
articulatio'nes ossiculo'rum audi'tus [NA], joints of ear bones; the joints of the ossicular chain consisting of a. incudomallearis, a. incudostapedia, and syndesmosis tympanostapedia.
a. os'sis pisifor'mis [NA], articulation of the pisiform bone; pisotriquetral joint; the synovial joint between the pisiform and triquetrum; it is separate from the other intercarpal joints.
a. ovoida'lis [NA], a. sellaris.
articulatio'nes pe'dis [NA], articulations of foot, joints including the talocrural, intertarsal, tarsometatarsal, intermetatarsal, metatarsophalangeal and interphalangeal joints.
a. pla'na [NA], plane joint; arthrodia; arthrodial or gliding joint; a synovial joint in which the opposing surfaces are nearly planes and in which there is only a slight, gliding motion, as in the intermetacarpal joints.
a. radiocar'pea [NA], radiocarpal articulation or joint; carpal articulation; wrist joint; the synovial joint between the distal end of the radius and its articular disk and the proximal row of carpal bones with the exception of the pisiform bone.
a. radioulna'ris dista'lis [NA], distal radioulnar articulation; inferior radioulnar joint; the pivot synovial joint between the head of the ulna and the ulnar notch on the radius; an articular disk passes across the distal part of the joint.
a. radioulna'ris proxima'lis [NA], proximal radioulnar articulation; superior radioulnar joint; the pivot synovial joint between the head of the radius and the ring formed by the radial notch of the ulna and the anular ligament.
a. sacrococcyge'a [NA], sacrococcygeal junction or joint; coccygeal joint; symphysis sacrococcygea; junctura sacrococcygea; the cartilaginous articulation of the coccyx with the sacrum.
a. sacroili'aca [NA], sacroiliac articulation or joint; the synovial joint on either side between the auricular surface of the sacrum and that of the ilium.
a. sellar'is [NA], saddle joint; a. ovoidalis; a biaxial synovial joint in which the double motion is effected by the opposition of two surfaces, each of which is concave in one direction and convex in the other; as in the carpometacarpal articulation of the thumb.

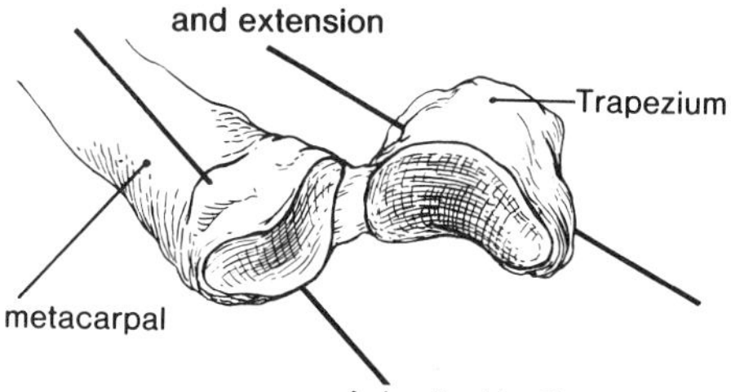

Articulatio Sellaris (Saddle Joint)

a. sim'plex [NA], simple joint; one composed of two bones only.
a. spheroi'dea [NA], spheroid articulation; a. cotylica; cotyloid, enarthrodial, or ball-and-socket joint; enarthrosis; socket or spheroid joint; a multiaxial synovial joint in which a more or less extensive sphere on the head of one bone fits into a rounded cavity in the other bone, as in the hip joint.
a. sternoclavicula'ris [NA], sternoclavicular joint; the synovial articulation between the medial end of the clavicle and the manubrium of the sternum and cartilage of the first rib; an articular disk subdivides the joint into two cavities.
articulatio'nes sternocosta'les [NA], sternocostal articulations or joints; the joints between the cartilages of the first seven ribs and the sternum; synovial cavities are variable in occurrence in these joints.
a. subtala'ris [NA], subtalar joint; talocalcaneal joint; a plane synovial joint between the inferior surface of the talus and the posterior articular surface of the calcaneus.
a. synovia'lis [NA], diarthrodial or synovial joint; movable joint; diarthrosis; perarticulation; junctura synovialis; a joint in which the opposing bony surfaces are covered with a layer of hyaline cartilage or fibrocartilage, there is a joint cavity containing synovial fluid, lined with synovial membrane and reinforced by a fibrous capsule and ligaments, and there is some degree of free movement possible.
a. tal'ocalca'neonavicula'ris [NA], talocalcaneonavicular joint; a ball-and-socket synovial joint, part of the transverse tarsal joint, formed by the head of the talus articulating with the navicular bone and the anterior part of the calcaneus.
a. talocrural'is [NA], talocrural articulation; ankle joint; mortise joint; ankle (1); a hinge synovial joint between the tibia and fibula above and the talus below.
a. tar'si transver'sa [NA], transverse tarsal articulation or joint; Chopart's joint; midtarsal joint; the synovial joint between the talus and calcaneus posteriorly and the navicular and cuboid bones anteriorly.
articulatio'nes tarsometatar'seae [NA], tarsometatarsal joints; cuneometatarsal joints; Lisfranc's joints; the three synovial joints between the tarsal and metatarsal bones, consisting of a medial joint between the first cuneiform and first metatarsal, an intermediate joint between the second and third cuneiforms and corresponding metatarsals, and a lateral joint between the cuboid and fourth and fifth metatarsals.
a. temporomandibula'ris [NA], temporomandibular articulation or joint; a. mandibularis; mandibular or jaw joint; the synovial articulation between the head of the mandible and the mandibular fossa and articular tubercle of the temporal bone; an articular disk divides the joint into two cavities.
a. tibiofibula'ris [NA], tibiofibular articulation; superior tibial

articulation; superior tibiofibular joint; the plane synovial joint between the lateral condyle of the tibia and the head of the fibula.

a. trochoid'ea [NA], trochoid articulation or joint; rotary, rotatory, or pivot joint; helicoid or lateral ginglymus; cyclarthrosis; a synovial joint in which a section of a cylinder of one bone fits into a corresponding cavity on the other, as in the proximal radioulnar articulation.

articulatio'nes zygapophysea'les [NA], zygapophysial joints; interarticular joints; juncturae zygopophyseales; the synovial joints between zygapophyses or articular processes of the vertebrae.

---

articulation (ar-tik-yū-lā'shŭn) [see articulatio]. **1.** Articulatio. **2.** A joining or connecting together loosely so as to allow motion between the parts. **3.** Distinct connected speech or enunciation. **4.** In dentistry, the contact relationship of the occlusal surfaces of the teeth during jaw movement.

atlanto-occipital a., *articulatio atlanto-occipitalis.*

balanced a., balanced *occlusion.*

bicondylar a., *articulatio* bicondylaris.

carpal a., *articulatio* radiocarpea.

condylar a., *articulatio* ellipsoidea.

confluent a., a tendency to run the syllables together in speech.

cricoarytenoid a., *articulatio* cricoarytenoidea.

cricothyroid a., *articulatio* cricothyroidea.

cuneonavicular a., *articulatio* cuneonavicularis.

dental a., gliding occlusion; the contact relationship of the occlusal surfaces of the upper and lower teeth when moving into and away from centric occlusion.

distal radioulnar a., *articulatio* radioulnaris distalis.

a.'s of foot, *articulationes* pedis.

a.'s of hand, *articulationes* manus.

humeral a., *articulatio* humeri.

humeroradial a., *articulatio* humeroradialis.

incudostapedial a., *articulatio* incudostapedia.

interchondral a.'s, *articulationes* interchondrales.

intermetatarsal a.'s, *articulationes* intermetatarseae.

interphalangeal a.'s, *articulationes* interphalangeae.

intertarsal a.'s, *articulationes* intertarseae.

metacarpophalangeal a.'s, *articulationes* metacarpophalangeae.

metatarsophalangeal a.'s, *articulationes* metatarsophalangeae.

peg-and-socket a., gomphosis.

a. of pisiform bone, *articulatio* ossis pisiformis.

proximal radioulnar a., *articulatio* radioulnaris proximalis.

radiocarpal a., *articulatio* radiocarpea.

sacroiliac a., *articulatio* sacroiliaca.

spheroid a., *articulatio* spheroidea.

sternocostal a.'s, *articulationes* sternocostales.

superior tibial a., *articulatio* tibiofibularis.

talocrural a., *articulatio* talocruralis.

temporomandibular a., *articulatio* temporomandibularis.

tibiofibular a., *articulatio* tibiofibularis.

transverse tarsal a., *articulatio* tarsi transversa.

trochoid a., *articulatio* trochoidea.

articulator (ar-tik'yū-lā-tŏr). Occluding frame; a mechanical device which represents the temporomandibular joints and jaw members to which maxillary and mandibular casts may be attached.

adjustable a., **(1)** an a. which may be adjusted to permit movement of the casts into recorded eccentric relationships; **(2)** an a. capable of adjustment to more than one eccentric position.

arcon a., **(1)** an a. with the equivalent condylar guides fixed to the upper member and the hinge axis to the lower member; **(2)** an instrument that maintains a constant relationship between the occlusal plane and the arcon guides at any position of the upper member, thereby making possible more accurate reproductions of mandibular movements.

non-arcon a., an a. with the equivalent condylar guides attached to the lower member and the hinge axis to the upper member.

articulatory (ar-tik'yū-lă-tō-rē). Relating to articulate speech.

articulostat (ar-tik'yū-lō-stat). A research instrument that will position dentures and the head of an x-ray machine in such a manner that films made at separate times may be accurately superimposed.

articulus (ar-tik'yū-lŭs) [L. joint]. Articulatio.

artifact (ar'ti-fakt) [L. *ars,* art, + *facio,* pp. *factus,* to make]. Artefact. **1.** Anything, especially in a histologic specimen or a graphic record, that is caused by the technique used or is not a natural occurrence, but is merely incidental. **2.** A skin lesion produced or perpetrated by self-inflicted action, as in dermatitis artefacta.

artifactitious (ar'ti-fak-tish'ŭs). Artifactual.

artifactual (ar-ti-fak'chyū-ăl). Artifactitious; produced or caused by an artifact.

Artiodactyla (ar'ti-ō-dak'ti-lă) [G. *artios,* even in number, + *daktylos,* finger]. An order of even-toed ungulates having either two or four digits, with the axis between the third and fourth; *e.g.,* pig and hippopotamus with four; camel, deer, giraffe, antelope, and cow with two.

ARV Abbreviation for AIDS-related *virus.*

aryepiglottic (ar'ē-ep-i-glot'ik). Arytenoepiglottidean; relating to the arytenoid cartilage and the epiglottis; denoting a fold of mucous membrane (plica aryepiglottica) and a muscle contained in it (musculus aryepiglotticus).

aryl (a'ril). An organic radical derived from an aromatic compound by removing a hydrogen atom.

a. acylamidase [EC 3.5.1.13], arylamidase; an amidohydrolase cleaving the acyl group from an anilide by hydrolysis.

arylamidase (ar-il-am'i-dās). *Aryl* acylamidase.

arylarsonic acid (ar'il-ar-son'ik). An arsonic acid containing an aryl radical; *e.g.,* arsenilic acid.

arylsulfatase (ar-il-sŭl'fă-tās) [EC 3.1.6.1]. Sulfatase (2); an enzyme that cleaves phenol sulfates, including cerebroside sulfates.

arytenoepiglottidean (a-rit'ĕ-nō-ep'i-glo-tid'ē-an). Aryepiglottic.

arytenoid (ar-i-tē'noyd) [see arytenoideus]. Denoting a cartilage (cartilago arytenoidea) and muscles (musculus arytenoideus obliquе and transversus) of the larynx.

arytenoidectomy (ar'ī-tē-noy-dek'tō-mē) [arytenoid + G. *ektomē,* excision]. Excision of an arytenoid cartilage.

arytenoideus (ar-ĭ-tē-noy'dē-ŭs) [G. *arytainoeides,* ladle-shaped, applied to cartilage of the larynx, fr. *arytaina,* a ladle, + *eidos,* resemblance]. *Musculus* arytenoideus obliquus and transversus.

arytenoiditis (ă-rit'ĕ-noy-dī'tis). Inflammation of an arytenoid cartilage.

arytenoidopexy (ar'ĭ-tē-noy'dō-pek'sē) [arytenoid + G. *pēxis,* fixation]. Fixation by surgery of cartilages or muscles of arytenoids.

A.S. Abbreviation for *auris sinister* [L.], left ear.

As Symbol for arsenic.

asafetida (as-ă-fet'ĭ-dă) [Pers. *aza,* mastic, + L. *fetidus,* fetid]. A gum resin, the inspissated exudate from the root of *Ferula foetida* (family Umbelliferae); used as a repellant against dogs, cats, and rabbits, and formerly used as an antispasmodic; in Asia, used as a condiment and flavoring agent.

asaphia (ă-saf'i-ă, ă-sā'fi-ă) [G. *asapheia,* obscurity, fr. *a-* priv. + *saphēs,* clear]. Indistinctness in speech.

Asarum (as'ar-ŭm) [L., fr. G. *asaron,* hazelwort]. A genus of plants of the family Aristolochiaceae.

A. canaden'se, wild ginger; Indian ginger; Canada snakeroot; an aromatic stimulant and diaphoretic.

A. europae'um, hazelwort; European snakeroot; an emetic and cathartic.

asbestoid (as-bes'toyd). Amianthoid.

asbestos (as-bes'tŏs) [G. unquenchable; so called in the erroneous belief that when heated, it could not be quenched]. The commercial product, after mining and processing, obtained from a family of fibrous hydrated silicates divided mineralogically into amphiboles (amosite, anthrophyllite, and crocidolite) and serpentines (chrysotile); it is virtually insoluble and is used to provide tensile strength and moldability, thermal insulation, and resistance to fire, heat, and corrosion; inhalation of a. particles can cause asbestosis.

asbestosis (as-bes-tō'sis). Pneumoconiosis due to inhalation of asbestos fibers suspended in the ambient air; sometimes complicated by pleural mesothelioma or bronchogenic carcinoma; ferruginous bodies are the histiologic hallmark of exposure to asbestos.

ascariasis (as-kă-rī'ă-sis) [G. *askaris,* an intestinal worm, + *-iasis,* condition]. Disease caused by infection with *Ascaris* or related ascarid nematodes.

ascaricide (as-kar'i-sīd) [ascarid + L. *caedo,* to kill]. **1.** Causing the death of ascarid nematodes. **2.** An agent having such properties.

ascarid (as'kă-rid). **1.** A general name for any nematode of the family Ascarididae. **2.** Pertaining to such nematodes.

Ascaridae (as-kar'i-dē). Former spelling for Ascarididae.

Ascaridata (as-kă-rid'ă-tă). Ascaridida.

Ascaridia (as-kă-rid'i-ă). A genus of relatively large nematodes (family Heterakidae) that inhabit the intestine of birds and cause ascaridiasis. Their life cycle is direct, without an intermediate host; their appearance and habits are much like those of members of the family Ascarididae.

A. colum'bae, a common species that occurs in domestic and wild pigeons.

A. gal'li, a species abundant in the small intestine of chickens, turkeys, geese, guinea fowl, and many wild birds in most parts of the world.

ascaridiasis (as'kă-ri-dī'ă-sis). Disease caused by infection with a species of *Ascaridia,* commonly occurring in the intestine of fowl.

Ascaridida (as-kă-rid'i-dă). Ascaridorida; Ascarididea; Ascaridata; an order of nematode worms that includes many important human, domestic animal, and fowl parasites such as *Ascaris, Ascaridia, Subuluris, Heterakis,* and *Anisakis.*

Ascarididae (as-kă-rid'i-dē) [G. *askaris,* an intestinal worm]. A family of large intestinal roundworms that includes the important nematode of man, *Ascaris lumbricoides,* the abundant roundworm of swine, *Ascaris suum,* and the common ascarids of dogs and cats, *Toxocara* and *Toxascaris* species.

Ascarididea (as-kar-i-did'ē-ă). Ascaridida.

Ascaridoidea (as-kă-ri-doy'dē-ă). Superfamily of stout, 3-lipped intestinal roundworms that includes the family Ascarididae.

ascaridole (as-kar'ĭ-dōl). 1,4-Peroxido-*p*- menth-2-ene; a major constituent of oil of chenopodium; an anthelmintic.

Ascaridorida (as-kări-dōr'i-dă). Ascaridida.

Ascaris (as'kă-ris) [G. *askaris,* an intestinal worm]. A genus of large, heavy-bodied roundworms parasitic in the small intestine; abundant in man and many other vertebrates.

A. equo'rum, *Parascaris equorum.*

A. lumbricoi'des, a large roundworm of man, one of the commonest human parasites (8 to 12 inches in length); various symptoms such as restlessness, fever, and sometimes diarrhea, are attributed to its presence, but usually it causes no definite symptoms; the similar species, *A. suum* (or *A. lumbricoides suum*) is very common in swine, but is not readily transmitted to man, and vice versa; the types are morphologically and immunologically similar but apparently are host-adapted types, considered distinct species or races.

Ascaroidea (as-kă-roy'dē-ă). Former spelling for Ascaridoidea.

ascaron (as-kă-ron) [G. *askaris,* an intestinal worm, + *hormōn,* pres. part. of *hormaō,* to excite]. A toxic peptone present in helminths, especially the ascaridids; symptoms of a. poisoning are similar to those of anaphylactic shock.

Ascarops strongylina (as'kă-rops stron-ji-lī'nă) [G. *askaris,* an intestinal worm; *strongylos,* round]. A small bloodsucking worm found in the stomach of pigs and wild boars in many parts of the world. Larvae of this species develop in coprophagous beetles; worms adhere to the gastric mucosa of the pig, and may cause inflammation and ulceration in heavy infections.

ascendens (as-sen'denz) [L.]. Ascending. Going upward, ascending, toward a higher position.

ascensus (ă-sen'sŭs) [L. ascent]. A moving upward; having an abnormally high position.

ascertainment (as-ser-tān'ment). In genetic research, the method by which a person, pedigree, or cluster is brought to the attention of an investigator.

complete a., method by which all families with at least one affected individual in a population are equally likely to be ascertained by survey or an appropriate random sampling technique.

incomplete a., truncate a.; method of locating affected individuals in which probability of locating any specific patient has a known value between 0 and 1.

single a., method of locating affected individuals by hospital or clinic admission or another way in which probability of encountering the same family twice approaches zero; also, the probability that a family will be ascertained is proportional to the number of affected members.

truncate a., incomplete a.

Aschelminthes (ask-hel-min'thēz). Nemathelminthes; a former phylum of the Metazoa which included the class Nematoda and a disparate assortment of other pseudocelomates, each now accorded separate phylum status; they are nonsegmented, bilaterally symmetric, and cylindric or filiform, with a pseudocele body cavity and rounded or pointed ends; they vary considerably in size, and the male is usually smaller than the female.

Ascher, Karl W., U.S. ophthalmologist, 1887–1971. See A.'s aqueous influx *phenomenon, syndrome.*

Aschheim, Selmar, German obstetrician and gynecologist, 1878–1965. See A.-Zondek *test.*

Aschner, Bernhard, Austrian gynecologist, 1883–1960. See A.'s *phenomenon, reflex;* A.-Dagnini *reflex.*

Aschoff, Karl A. Ludwig, German pathologist, 1866–1942. See A. *bodies, nodules; node* of A. and Tawara; Rokitansky-A. *sinus.*

ascites (ă-sī'tēz) [L. fr. G. *askos,* a bag, + *-ites*]. Hydroperitoneum; hydroperitonia; abdominal dropsy; accumulation of serous fluid in the peritoneal cavity.

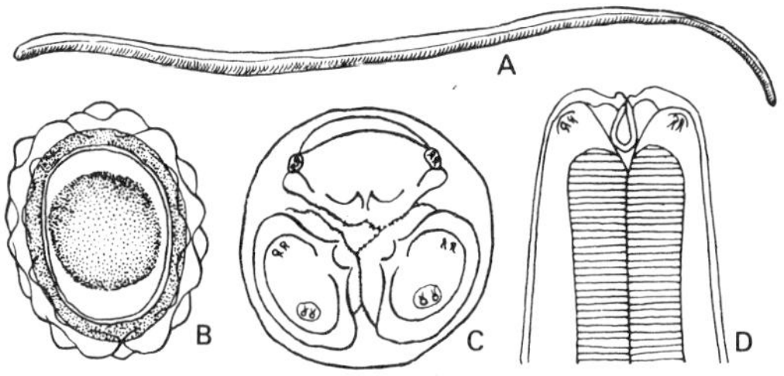

Ascaris lumbricoides

A, female; *B,* fertilized egg; *C,* head-on view of worm, showing lips and papillas; *D,* ventral view, showing anterior extremity of mature worm. Reduced from original magnifications of ×⅕ (*A*), ×500 (*B*), ×10 (*C*), ×5 (*D*).

a. adipo'sus, chylous a.
chyliform a., chylous a.
chylous a., a. chylo'sus, a. adiposus; chyliform, fatty, or milky a.; chyloperitoneum; presence in the peritoneal cavity of a milky fluid containing suspended fat, ordinarily caused by an obstruction or injury of the thoracic duct.
fatty a., chylous a.
gelatinous a., *pseudomyxoma* peritonei.
hemorrhagic a., bloody or blood-stained serous fluid, frequently resulting from metastatic carcinoma, in the peritoneal cavity.
milky a., chylous a.
a. pre'cox, a. appearing earlier than peripheral edema in cases of constrictive pericarditis.
pseudochylous a., presence in the peritoneum of an opalescent or cloudy fluid that does not contain fat.

ascitic (ă-sit'ik). Relating to ascites.

ascitogenous (as-i-toj'ĕ-nŭs). Producing ascites.

Asclepias (as-klē'pē-as) [G. *Asklēpios,* Aesculapius]. A genus of plants (family Asclepiadaceae), commonly called milkweeds; some species, *e.g., A. eriocarpa* and *A. galioides,* are toxic to herbivorous animals and fowl.

ascocarp (as'kō-karp) [G. *askos,* bag, + *karpos,* fruit]. A fungus structure, of varying complexity, which bears asci and ascospores.

ascogenous (as-koj'ĕ-nŭs). Denoting ascus-bearing fungus hypha or cell.

ascogonium (as-kō-gō'nē-ŭm). The female cell in an ascomycete which is fertilized by the male cell.

Ascoli, Alberto, Italian serologist, 1877–1957. See A. *reaction.*

Ascomycetes (as'kō-mī-sē'tēz) [G. *askos,* a bag, + *mykēs,* mushroom]. A class of fungi characterized by the presence of asci and ascospores. Such fungi have generally two distinct reproductive phases, the sexual or perfect stage and the asexual or imperfect stage. *Ajellomyces capsulatum* and *Ajellomyces dermatitidis* are pathogenic members of this class.

ascorbase (as-kōr'bās). *Ascorbate* oxidase.

ascorbate (as-kōr'bāt). A salt or ester of ascorbic acid.
a. oxidase [EC 1.10.3.3], ascorbase; a copper-containing enzyme that catalyzes the oxidation of ascorbic acid to dehydroascorbic acid.

ascorbic acid (as-kōr'bik). Vitamin C; antiscorbutic vitamin; cevitamic acid; 2,3-didehydro-L-*threo*-hexono-1,4-lactone; used in preventing scurvy, as a strong reducing agent, and as an antioxidant in foodstuffs.

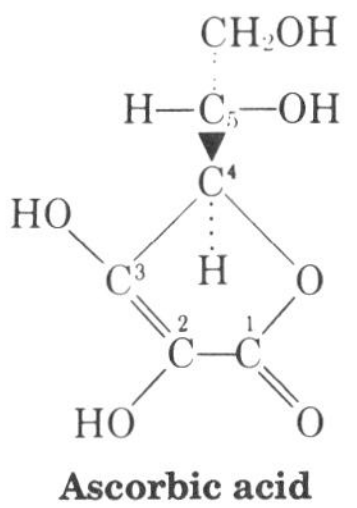

Ascorbic acid

ascorbyl palmitate (as-kōr'bil pal'mi-tāt). L-Ascorbic acid-6-palmitate; used as a preservative in pharmaceutical preparations.

ascospore (as'kō-spōr) [G. *askos,* bag, + *sporos,* seed]. A spore formed within an ascus; the sexual spore of Ascomycetes.

ascus, pl. **asci** (as'kŭs, as'ī) [G. *askos,* bag]. The saclike cell of Ascomycetes in which ascospores develop following nuclear fusion and meiosis.

-ase. A termination denoting an enzyme, suffixed to the name of the substance (substrate) upon which the enzyme acts; *e.g.,* phosphatase, lipase, proteinase. Enzymes named before the convention was established generally have an *-in* ending; *e.g.,* pepsin, ptyalin, trypsin.

asecretory (ā-sē-krē'tō-rē). Without secretion.

Aselli (Asellio, Asellius), Gasparo, Italian anatomist at Cremona, 1581–1626. See A.'s *gland, pancreas.*

asemasia, asemia (as-ĕ-mā'zē-ă, ă-sē'mē-ă) [G. *a-* priv. + *sēmasia,* the giving of a signal, fr. *sēma,* sign]. Asymbolia (2).

asepsis (ă-sep'sis, ā-) [G. *a-* priv. + *sēpsis,* putrefaction]. A condition in which living pathogenic organisms are absent; a state of sterility (2).

aseptate (ă-sep'tāt, ā-) [G. *a-* priv. + L. *saeptum,* a partition]. In fungi, a term describing absence of cross walls in a hyphal filament or a spore.

aseptic (ă-sep'tik, ā-). Marked by or relating to asepsis.

asepticism (ă-sep'ti-sizm, ā-). The practice of aseptic surgery.

asequence (ă-sē'kwens). Lack of normal sequence, specifically, between atrial and ventricular contractions.

asexual (ā-seks'yū-ăl). **1.** Without sex, as in a. reproduction. **2.** Having no sexual desire or interest.

ASF Abbreviation for African swine *fever.*

Asherman, Joseph G., Czechoslovakian gynecologist, *1889. See A.'s *syndrome.*

Ashley's phenomenon. See under phenomenon.

Ashman, R., 20th century U.S. physiologist. See A. *phenomenon.*

Ashman's phenomenon. See under phenomenon.

asialia (ā-sī-a'lē-ă). Asialism.

asialism (ă-sī'ă-lizm) [G. *a-* priv. + *sialon,* saliva]. Aptyalism; aptyalia; asialia; diminished or arrested secretion of saliva.

asitia (ă-sish'ē-ă) [G. *a-* priv. + *sitos,* food]. Disgust at the sight or thought of food.

Askanazy, Max, German pathologist, 1865–1940. See A. *cell.*

Ask-Upmark, E., 20th century Swedish pathologist. See A.-U. *kidney.*

Asn Symbol for asparagine or its mono- or diradical.

asocial (ā-sō'shŭl). Not social; indifferent to social rules or customs; withdrawn from society; *e.g.,* a recluse, a regressed schizophrenic person, a schizoid personality. *Cf.* antisocial.

asoma, pl. **asomata** (ā-sō'mă, -sō'mă-tă) [G. *a-* priv. + *sōma,* body]. A fetus with only a rudimentary body.

Asp Symbol for aspartic acid or its radical forms.

aspalasoma (as-pal-ă-sō'mă) [G. *aspalax,* a mole + *soma,* body]. Obsolete term for a malformed fetus with eventration at the lower part of the abdomen, presenting separate openings for intestine, bladder, and sexual organs.

asparaginase (as-par'ă-ji-nās). L-Asparaginase; asparaginase II. **1** [EC 3.5.1.1]. An enzyme catalyzing the hydrolysis of asparagine to aspartic acid and ammonia. **2.** The enzyme from *Escherichia coli,* used in the treatment of acute leukemia and other neoplastic diseases.

asparagine (Asn) (as-par'ă-jin). Asparamide; α-amino-β-succinamic acid; $NH_2COCH_2CH(NH_2)COOH$; the β-amide of aspartic acid, a nonessential amino acid occurring in proteins; a diuretic.
a. ligase [EC 6.3.1.1], a. synthetase; an acid: ammonia ligase (amide synthetase) forming asparagine from aspartate and NH_3, with cleavage of ATP to AMP.
a. synthetase, a. ligase.

asparaginic acid (as'par-ă-jin'ik). Aspartic acid.

asparaginyl (as-par'ă-jin-il). The aminoacyl radical of asparagine.

Asparagus (as-par'ă-gŭs) [L. fr. G. *asparagos*]. A genus of plants of the family Liliaceae. *A. officinalis* is an edible vegetable, the rhizome and roots of which, together with the young edible shoots, are used as a diuretic.

asparmide (as-par'ă-mīd). Asparagine.

aspartame (as'par-tām). *N*- L-α-Aspartyl-Lphenyalanine 1-methyl ester; a low-calorie sweetening agent about 200 times as sweet as sucrose.

aspartase (as-par'tās). *Aspartate* ammonia-lyase.

aspartate (as-par'tāt). A salt or ester of aspartic acid.
a. aminotransferase (AST) [EC 2.6.1.1], a. transaminase; glutamic-aspartic transaminase; (serum) glutamic-oxaloacetic transaminase; an enzyme catalyzing the transfer of an amine group from glutamic acid to oxaloacetic acid, forming α-ketoglutaric acid and aspartic acid, or vice versa.
a. ammonia-lyase [EC 4.3.1.1], aspartase; fumaric aminase; an enzyme catalyzing the conversion of aspartic acid to fumaric acid, splitting out ammonia.
a. carbamoyltransferase [EC 2.1.3.2], an enzyme catalyzing formation of ureidosuccinate (*N*-carbamoylaspartate) by the transfer of carbamoyl from carbamoylphosphate to the NH_2 of aspartate.
a. kinase [EC 2.7.2.4], an enzyme catalyzing the phosphorylation by ATP of aspartate to 4-phosphoaspartate (β-aspartyl phosphate).
a. transaminase, a. aminotransferase.

aspartate 1-decarboxylase [EC 4.1.1.11]. Glutamate decarboxylase.

aspartate 4-decarboxylase [EC 4.1.1.12]. Aspartate βdecarboxylase; a carboxy-lyase converting aspartate to alanine (releasing CO_2), decarboxylating aminomalonate, and (in bacteria) removing SO_2 from cysteinesulfinate. See also desulfinase.

aspartic acid (as-par'tik). α-Aminosuccinic acid; asparaginic acid; $HOOC–CH_2–CH(NH_2)–COOH$; one of the amino acids occurring in proteins.

aspartyl (as-par'til). The aminoacyl radical of aspartic acid.

β-aspartyl(acetylglucosamine) (as-par'til-as'e-til-glū'kō-să-mēn). Misnomer for 1-(β-asparagino)-*N*-acetylglucosamine or 1-(β-aspartamido)-*N*-acetylglucosamine, or, formally, 1-(β-L-aspartamido)-*N*-2-acetamido-1,2-dideoxy-β-D-glucose; a compound of *N*-acetylglucosamine and asparagine, linked via the amide nitrogen of the latter and carbon-1 of the former.

aspartylglycosamine (as-par'til-glī'kō-să-mēn). Generic term for compounds of asparagine and a 2-amino sugar; *e.g.*, β-aspartyl (acetylglucosamine).

aspartylglycosaminuria (as-par'til-glī'kō-să-mi-nūr'ē-ă). A disorder of glycoprotein catabolism characterized by the presence of an aspartylglycosamine in the urine, with coarse facies, mental retardation, and lens opacities resembling that in Hurler's syndrome and in hurloid facies; autosomal recessive inheritance.

aspect (as'pekt) [L. *aspectus*, fr. *a-spicio*, pp. *-spectus*, to look at]. **1.** The manner of appearance; looks. **2.** The side of an object that is directed in any designated direction.

aspergillic acid (as-per-jil'ik). 2-Hydroxy-3-isobutyl-6-(1-methylpropyl)pyrazine-1-oxide; produced by *Aspergillus flavus;* an antibiotic agent moderately active against Gram-positive and Gram-negative bacteria, but toxic to animal tissues.

aspergillin (as-per-jil'in). A black pigment obtained from various species of *Aspergillus;* improperly used to designate various antibiotics obtained from *Aspergillus.*

aspergilloma (as'per-ji-lō'mă). **1.** An infectious granuloma caused by *Aspergillus.* **2.** A variety of bronchopulmonary aspergillosis; a ball-like mass of *Aspergillis fumigatus* colonizing an existing cavity in the lung.

aspergillosis (as'per-ji-lō'sis). **1.** The presence of *Aspergillus* in the tissues or on a mucous surface of man and animals, and the symptoms produced thereby. **2.** Infection of the lungs and air sacs of birds, especially chickens and turkeys, with *Aspergillus fumigatus,* frequently introduced in spoiled, moldy feed.
bronchopulmonary a., pulmonary a.; an inflammatory and destructive disease of the bronchi and lungs due to the pressure and growth of *Aspergillus fumigatus.* There are four varieties: 1) a bronchial infection with allergic manifestations, in which the fungus grows in the mucus (evoked by the inflammation) which may be expectorated as yellow bronchial casts and may cause intermittent bronchial obstruction, with transient pulmonary shadows seen radiographically; asthma and blood eosinophilia are often present, and bronchial wall destruction may eventually result in a proximal form of bronchiectasis; 2) aspergilloma; 3) an infection with pulmonary necrosis as a pneumonic involvement of the lung in debilitated subjects; 4) disseminated a.
disseminated a., a variety of bronchopulmonary a. characterized by a generalized infection of the lung occurring usually in subjects with defective immune response.
invasive a., so-called because of the peculiar predilection of *Aspergillus fumigatus* to invade blood vessels and cause tissue infarction; it is second only to candidiasis as a cause of secondary fungal infection in patients whose immune mechanisms have been suppressed by chemotherapy.
pulmonary a., bronchopulmonary a.

Aspergillus (as-per-jil'ŭs) [Med. L. a sprinkler, fr. L. *aspergo,* to sprinkle]. A genus of fungi (class Ascomycetes) that contains many species, a number of them with black, brown, or green spores. A few species are pathogenic for man, other animals, and avians.

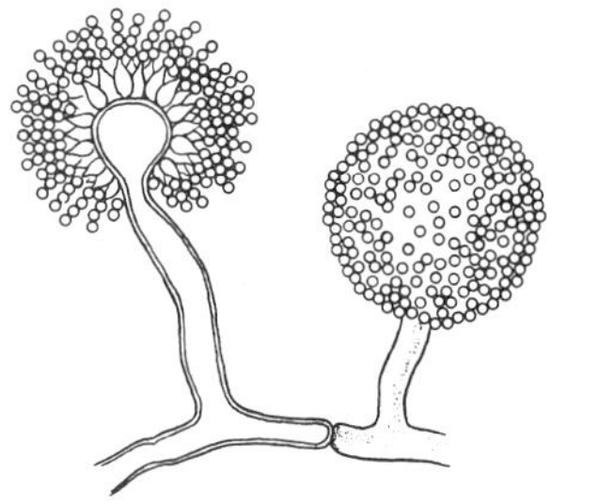

Aspergillus
Showing cross section (*left*).

A. clava'tus, a species isolated from soil and feces; it yields a carcinogenic mycotoxin known as patulin.
A. fla'vus, a species with yellow-green conidia that is found growing on grains; may produce aflatoxin, which is the cause of aflatoxicosis in poultry and cattle, and is carcinogenic for rats and man; occasionally causes aspergillosis in man and animals.
A. fumiga'tus, a species that yields the antibiotics fumigacin and fumigatin, and is the common cause of aspergillosis in man and birds.
A. nid'ulans, a species that causes one form of mycetoma, and occasionally causes aspergillosis in man.
A. ni'ger, a pathogenic species with black spores, often present in the external auditory meatus but not necessarily pathogenic; used in the commercial manufacturing of citric and gluconic acids.
A. ter'reus, a species that produces the antibiotic citrinin; it has been isolated from otomycosis, especially in Japan and Taiwan, and occasionally causes aspergillosis in man and animals.

aspermatism (ā-sper'mă-tizm, ă-sper') [G. *a-* priv. + *sperma,* seed]. Aspermia.

aspermatogenic (ā-sper'mă-tō-jen'ik, ă-sper') [G. *a-* priv. + *sperma,* seed, + *-gen,* production]. Failing in the production of spermatozoa.

aspermia (ā-sper'mē-ă, ă-sper') Aspermatism; lack of secretion or expulsion of semen following ejaculation.

aspersion (as-per'zhŭn) [L. *aspersio,* a sprinkling]. A form of hydrotherapy in which water of a given temperature is sprinkled on the body.

aspheric (ā-sfer'ik) [G. *a-* priv. + *sphaira,* sphere]. Denoting a paraboloidal surface, especially of a lens or mirror, that eliminates spherical aberration.

asphygmia (as-fig'mē-ă) [G. *a-* priv. + *sphygmos,* pulse]. Temporary absence of pulse.

asphyxia (as-fik'sē-ă) [G. *a-*priv. + *sphyzō,* to throb]. Impaired or absent exchange of oxygen and carbon dioxide on a ventilatory basis; combined hypercapnia and hypoxia or anoxia.
blue a., a. livida.
cyanotic a., traumatic a.
a. liv'ida, blue a.; a form of a. neonatorum in which the skin is cyanotic, but the heart is strong and the reflexes are preserved.
local a., stagnation of the circulation, sometimes resulting in local gangrene especially of the fingers; one of the symptoms usually associated with the local syncope of Raynaud's disease.
a. neonato'rum, a. occurring in the newborn.
a. pal'lida, a form of a. of the newborn, in which the skin is pale, the pulse weak and slow, and the reflexes absent.
symmetric a., Raynaud's *disease.*
traumatic a., cyanotic a.; pressure stasis; the extravasation of blood into the skin and conjunctivae, produced by a sudden mechanical increase in venous pressure, analogous to the Rumpel-Leede test; it is common in those who have been hanged, and is seen occasionally in crush injuries.

asphyxial (as-fik'sē-ăl). Relating to asphyxia.

asphyxiant (as-fik'sē-ănt). **1.** Asphyxiating; producing asphyxia. **2.** Anything, especially a gas, that produces asphyxia.

asphyxiate (as-fik'sē-āt). To induce asphyxia.

asphyxiating (as-fik'sē-āt-ing). Asphyxiant (1).

asphyxiation (as-fik-sē-ā'shŭn). The production of, or the state of, asphyxia.

Aspiculuris tetraptera (as-pik-yū-lū'ris tet-rap'ter-ă) [Pers. *espic,* fr. L. *spica,* ear, spike; *tetra-* + *pteron,* feather, wing]. The mouse pinworm, an abundant oxyurid nematode of the mouse cecum or large intestine, along with another common oxyurid pinworm of mice, *Syphacia obvelata;* it is also found in other rodents, including *Rattus.*

aspidin (as-pid'in). A toxic active principle, $C_{25}H_{32}O_8$, contained in aspidium.

aspidinol as-pid'i-nol). An alcohol, $C_{12}H_{16}O_4$, occurring in aspidium.

aspidium (as-pid'ē-ŭm) [G. *aspidion,* a little shield, dim. of *aspis,* shield]. The rhizomes and stipes of *Dryopteris filix-mas* (European a. or male fern), or of *Dryopteris marginalis* (American a. or marginal fern) (family Polypodiaceae); used in the treatment of tapeworm infestation, usually in the form of the oleoresin or extract, but because of its potential toxicity, its use is restricted to patients who do not respond to treatment with safer drugs such as dichlorophen, niclosamide, or quinacrine.

aspidosamine (as'pi-dō-sam'ēn). A strong base, $C_{22}H_{28}N_2O_2$, derived from quebracho; a toxic irritant.

aspidospermine (as'pi-dō-sper'mēn). An alkaloid, $C_{22}H_{30}N_2O_2$, obtained from quebracho, an irritant.

aspirate [L. *a-spiro,* pp. *-atus,* to breathe on, give the H sound]. **1** (as'pi-rāt). To remove by aspiration. **2** (as'pi-rit). The substance removed by aspiration.

aspiration (as-pi-rā'shŭn). **1.** Removal, by suction, of a gas or fluid from a body cavity, from unusual accumulations, or from a container. **2.** The inspiratory sucking into the airways of fluid or foreign body, as of vomitus. **3.** A surgical technique for cataract, requiring a small corneal incision, severance of the lens capsule, fragmentation of the lens material, and removal with a needle.
meconium a., intrauterine a. by the fetus of amniotic fluid contaminated by meconium resulting from fetal hypoxic distress.

aspirator (as'pi-rā-ter, -tōr). An apparatus for removing fluid by aspiration from any of the body cavities; it consists usually of a hollow needle or trocar and cannula, connected by tubing with a container vacuumized by a syringe or reversed air (suction) pump.
vacuum a., an instrument for removing the products of conception by suction after cervical dilation.
water a., a jet ejector pump operated by water and commonly used as a laboratory suction pump.

aspirin (as'pi-rin). Acetylsalicylic acid; $C_6H_4(OCOCH_3)COOH$; a widely used analgesic, antipyretic, and anti-inflammatory agent.

asplenia (ă-splē'nē-ă). Congenital absence of the spleen.

asplenic (ă-splen'ik). Having no spleen.

asporogenous (as-pō-roj'ĕ-nŭs) [G. *a-* priv. + *sporos,* seed, + *-gen,* production]. Not producing spores.

asporous (as-pōr'ŭs) [G. *a-* priv. + *sporos,* seed]. Incapable of producing spores.

asporulate (as-pōr'yū-lāt). Nonsporeforming.

assassin bug (ă-sas'in) [Fr., fr. It. *assassino,* fr. Ar. *hashshāshin,* those addicted to hashish]. An insect of the family Reduviidae (order Hemiptera) that inflicts irritating, painful bites in animals and man; related to the cone-nosed bugs (triatomines), a vector of South American trypanosomiasis.

assay (as'sā, ă-sā'). **1.** Analysis; test of purity; trial. **2.** To examine; to subject to analysis.
Ames a., Ames *test.*
clonogenic a., *in vitro* culturing of neoplastic cells to test their radiosensitivity or chemosensitivity, and probable clinical efficacy of a therapeutic agent.
competitive binding a., displacement or saturation analysis; general term for an a. in which a binder competes for labeled versus unlabeled ligand; following separation of free and bound ligand, the ligand (the analyte assayed) is quantitated by relating bound and unbound ratios to known standards. See also enzyme-linked immunosorbent a.; radioreceptor a.; immunoassay; enzyme-multiplied *immunoassay;* radioimmunoassay.
complement binding a., a test for the detection of immune complexes.
double antibody sandwich a., for antigen; an application of the ELISA method in which material being tested for antigen is added to wells coated with known antibody; the presence of antigen fixed to the antibody coat can be determined either directly, by adding human antibody linked to the enzyme of the indicator system, or indirectly, by first adding unlabeled known antibody, the attachment of which to the antigen can be demonstrated by addition of immunoglobulin-specific antibody linked to the enzyme.
enzyme-linked immunosorbent a. (ELISA), a sensitive method for serodiagnosis of specific infectious diseases; an *in vitro* competitive binding a. in which an enzyme and its substrate serve as the indicator system rather than a radioactive substance; in positive tests, the two yield a colored or other easily recognizable substance; tests are made in wells in polystyrene or other material to which immunoglobulins or antigenic (viral or other) preparations readily adsorb; the enzyme is linked to known immunoglobulin (or antigen) and in positive tests remains in the well as part of the antigen-antibody complex available to react with its substrate when added.
Grunstein-Hogness a., a procedure for identifying plasmid clones by colony hybridization.

immunochemical a., immunoassay.
immunoradiometric a., an a. that differs from conventional radioimmunoassay in that the compound to be measured combines directly with radioactively labeled antibodies.
indirect a., for antibody; an application of the ELISA method in which serum being tested for antibody is added to wells coated with known antigen; presence of antibody bound to the antigen coat can be determined by addition of immunoglobulin-specific antibody to which is linked the enzyme of the indicator system, followed by addition of substrate to the washed aggregate.
radioreceptor a., a competitive binding a. in which the binder is a membrane or tissue receptor rather than an antibody.
Raji cell radioimmune a., for immune complexes; a procedure by which immune complexes adsorbed from a test serum by a standard preparation of lymphoblastoid (Raji) cells are assayed by the capacity to bind ^{125}I-labeled antibody to immunoglobulin.

Assézat, Jules, French anthropologist, 1832–1876. See A.'s *triangle.*

assimilable (ă-sim′i-lă-bl). Capable of undergoing assimilation.

assimilation (ă-sim-i-lā′shŭ) [L. *as-similo,* pp. *-atus,* to make alike]. **1.** Incorporation of digested materials from food into the tissues. **2.** Amalgamation and modification of newly perceived information and experiences into the existing cognitive structure.
reproductive a., in sensorimotor theory, an active cognitive process by which past experience is applied to novel situations.

Assmann, Herbert, German internist, 1882–1950. See A.'s tuberculous *infiltrate.*

associate. 1 (ă-sō′shi-āt). Any item or individual grouped with others by some common factor. **2** (ă-sō′shē-āt). To accomplish association.
paired a.'s, words, syllables, digits, or other items learned in pairs, so that when one is given, its a. is to be recalled.

association (ă-sō-sē-ā′shŭn) [L. *as-socio,* pp. *-sociatus,* to join to; *ad* + *socius,* companion]. **1.** Union; a connection of persons, things, or ideas by some common factor. **2.** A functional connection of two ideas, events, or psychological phenomena established through learning or experience. See also conditioning.
clang a., psychic a.'s resulting from sounds; often encountered in the manic phase of manic-depressive psychosis.
dream a.'s, the memories and emotions mentioned by a patient trying to understand a dream at the request of a psychoanalyst.
free a., an investigative psychoanalytic technique in which the patient verbalizes, without reservation or censor, the passing contents of his mind; the verbalized conflicts that emerge constitute resistances that are the basis of the psychoanalyst's interpretations.
genetic a., the occurrence together in a population, more often than can be readily explained by chance, of two or more traits of which at least one is known to be genetic.

associationism (ă-sō-sē-ā′shŭn-izm). In psychology, the theory that man's understanding of the world occurs through ideas associated with sensory experience rather than through innate ideas.

assortment (ă-sōrt′ment). In genetics, the relationship between non-allelic genetic traits that are transmitted from parent to child more or less independently in accordance with the degree of linkage between the respective loci.
independent a., the pattern of transmission of unlinked loci.

AST Abbreviation for *aspartate* aminotransferase.

astasia (ă-stā′zē-ă) [G. unsteadiness, from *a*-priv. + *stasis,* standing]. Inability, through muscular incoordination, to stand.

astasia-abasia (ă-stā′zē-ă-ă-bā′zē′ă). Blocq's disease; the inability to either stand or walk in the normal manner; the person affected seems to collapse when attempting to walk, as if to prove that he cannot do so; a symptom of conversion hysteria.

astatic (ā-stat′ik). Pertaining to astasia.

astatine (as′tă-tēn) [G. *astatos,* unstable]. An artificial radioactive element of the halogen series; symbol At, atomic number 85.

asteatodes (ă-stē-ă-tō′dēz). Asteatosis.

asteatosis (ă-stē-ă-tō′sis) [G. *a-* priv. + *stear (steat-),* fat]. Asteatodes; diminished or arrested action of the sebaceous glands.
a. cu′tis, dry, scaly integument with decrease in sebaceous secretion.

aster (as′ter) [Mod. L. fr. G. *astēr,* a star]. Astrosphere.
sperm a., see sperm-aster.

astereognosis (ă-stēr′ē-og-nō′sis) [G. *a-* priv. + *stereos,* solid, + *gnōsis,* knowledge]. Stereoagnosis; stereoanesthesia; loss of the ability to judge the form of an object by touch.

asterion (ăstē′rē-on) [G. *asterios,* starry]. A craniometric point in the region of the posterolateral, or mastoid, fontanel, at the junction of the lambdoid, occipitomastoid and parietomastoid sutures.

asterixis (ă-ster-ik′sis) [G. *a-* priv. + *stērixis,* fixed position]. Flapping tremor; involuntary jerking movements, especially in the hands, best elicited by having the patient extend his arms, dorsiflex his wrists, and spread his fingers; commonly called a "liver flap" because of its frequent occurrence in patients with impending hepatic coma, although it may also be seen in other forms of metabolic encephalopathy.

asternal (ā-ster′năl) [G. *a-* priv. + *sternon,* chest]. **1.** Not related to or connected with the sternum, *e.g.,* a. rib. **2.** Without a sternum.

asternia (ă-ster′nē-ă). Congenital absence of the sternum.

Asterococcus (as′ter-ō-kok′kŭs) [Mod. L. fr. G. *astēr,* a star, + *kokkos,* a berry]. *Mycoplasma.*

asteroid (as′tē-royd) [G. *astēr,* star, + *eidos,* resemblance]. Resembling a star.

asthenia (as-thē′nē-ă) [G. *astheneia,* weakness, fr. *a-* priv. + *sthenos,* strength]. Adynamia (1); weakness or debility.
neurocirculatory a., Da Costa's or effort syndrome; irritable or soldier's heart; a syndrome of functional nervous and circulatory irregularities characterized by increased susceptibility to fatigue, palpitation, dyspnea, rapid pulse, precordial pain, and anxiety; observed especially in soldiers on active duty but also in civilians.

asthenic (as-then′ik). **1.** Relating to asthenia. **2.** Denoting a thin, delicate body habitus.

asthenopia (as-thē-nō′pē-ă) [G. *astheneia,* weakness, + *ōps,* eye]. Eyestrain; subjective symptoms of ocular fatigue, discomfort, lacrimation, and headaches arising from use of the eyes.
accommodative a., a. due to errors of refraction and excessive contraction of the ciliary muscle.
muscular a., a. due to imbalance of the extrinsic ocular muscles.
nervous a., a. due to functional or organic nervous disease.
neurasthenic a., retinal a.; a. due to neurasthenia, frequently after a debilitating disease.
retinal a., neurasthenic a.

asthenopic (as-thē-nop′ik). Relating to or suffering from asthenopia.

asthenospermia (as-thē-nō-sper′mē-ă) [G. *astheneia,* weakness, + *sperma,* seed, semen]. Loss or reduction of motility of the spermatozoa, frequently associated with infertility.

asthma (az′mă) [G.]. Originally, a term used to mean "difficult breathing"; now used to denote bronchial a.
atopic a., bronchial a. due to atopy.
bronchial a., a condition of the lungs in which there is widespread narrowing of airways, varying over short periods of time either spontaneously or as a result of treatment, due in varying degrees to contraction (spasm) of smooth muscle, edema of the mucosa, and mucus in the lumen of the bronchi and bronchioles; these changes are caused by the local release of spasmogens and vasoactive substances (*e.g.,* histamine, or certain leukotrienes or prostaglandins) in the course of an allergic process.

bronchitic a., catarrhal a.; a. precipitated by bronchitis.
cardiac a., an asthmatic attack, the bronchoconstriction being secondary to the pulmonary congestion and edema of left ventricular failure.
catarrhal a., bronchitic a.
extrinsic a., bronchial a. resulting from an allergic reaction to foreign substances, such as inhaled particles, vapors, or gases, or ingested foods, beverages, or drugs.
hay a., an asthmatic stage of hay fever.
intrinsic a., bronchial a. in which no extrinsic causes can be identified, and which is assumed to be due to an endogenous process, possibly allergic.
miller's a., a. caused by flour or grain allergens.
miner's a., the dyspnea of anthracosis or other pneumoconioses in miners.
nervous a., a. precipitated by psychic stress.
reflex a., a. occurring as a reflex in disease of the viscera, the nose, or other parts.
spasmodic a., a. due to spasm of the bronchioles.
steam-fitter's a., a. associated with asbestosis acquired by exposure to asbestos-insulated heating and plumbing components.
stripper's a., a. associated with byssinosis.
summer a., a. associated with hay fever or allergy to summer vegetation.

asthmatic (az-mat'ik). Relating to or suffering from asthma.

asthma-weed. 1. Lobelia. **2.** *Euphorbia pilulifera.*

asthmogenic (az'mō-jen'ik). Causing asthma.

astigmatic (as'tig-mat'ik). Relating to or suffering from astigmatism.

astigmatism (ă-stig'mă-tizm) [G. *a-* priv. + *stigma* (*stig- mat-*), a point]. Astigmia **1.** A lens or optical system having different refractivity in different meridians. **2.** A condition of unequal curvatures along the different meridians in one or more of the refractive surfaces (cornea, anterior or posterior surface of the lens) of the eye, in consequence of which the rays from a luminous point are not focused at a single point on the retina.

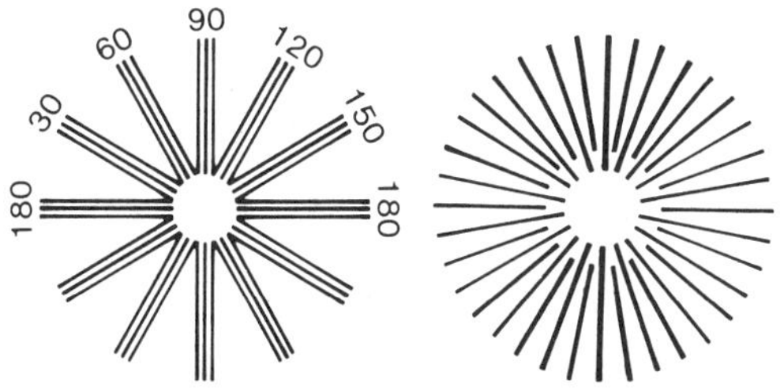

Astigmatism
Astigmatic dial (left) as seen by a person with astigmatism (right).

compound hyperopic a., a. in which all meridians are hyperopic but to different degrees.
compound myopic a. (M + Am), a. in which all meridians are myopic but to different degrees.
corneal a., a. due to a defect in the curvature of the corneal surface.
direct a., a. with the rule.
hyperopic a., simple hyperopic a.; that form of a. in which one meridian is hyperopic and the one at right angle to it is without a refractive error.
irregular a., a. in which different parts of the same meridian have different degrees of curvature.
lenticular a., a. due to defect in the curvature, position, or index of refraction of the lens.
mixed a., a. in which one meridian is hyperopic while the one at right angle to it is myopic.
myopic a., simple myopic a.; that form of a. in which one meridian is myopic and the one at right angle to it is without refractive error.
a. of oblique pencils, an aberration occurring when a bundle of light rays strikes a refracting medium in some other direction than parallel to the axis of the lens.
regular a., a. in which the curvature in each meridian is equal throughout its course, and the meridians of greatest and least curvature are at right angles to each other.
reversed a., a. against the rule.
a. against the rule, reversed a.; a. when the greater curvature or refractive power is in the horizontal meridian.
a. with the rule, direct a.; a. when the greater curvature or refractive power is in the vertical meridian.
simple hyperopic a., hyperopic a.
simple myopic a., myopic a.

astigmatometer, astigmometer (as-tig-mă-tom'ĕ-ter, as-tig-mom'ĕ-ter). Stigmatometer; an instrument for measuring the degree and determining the variety of astigmatism.

astigmatometry, astigmometry (ă-stig-mă-tom'ĕ-trē, as-tig-mom'ĕ-trē). Determination of the form and measurement of the degree of astigmatism.

astigmatoscope (as-tig-mat'ō-skōp). Astigmoscope; an instrument for detecting and measuring the degree of astigmatism.

astigmatoscopy (as-tig-mă-tos'kō-pē). Astigmoscopy; use of the astigmatoscope.

astigmia (ă-stig'mē-ă). Astigmatism.

astigmoscope (ă-stig'mō-skōp). Astigmatoscope.

astigmoscopy (as-tig-mos'kō-pē). Astigmatoscopy.

astomatous (ă-stō'mă-tŭs). Astomous; without a mouth.

astomia (ă-stō'mē-ă) [G. *a-* priv. + *stoma,* mouth]. Congenital absence of a mouth.

astomous (ă-stō'mŭs). Astomatous.

astragalar (as-trag'ă-lar). Relating to the astragalus or talus.

astragalectomy (as-trag-ă-lek'tō-mē) [astragalus, + G. *ektomē,* excision]. Removal of the astragalus, or talus.

astragalocalcanean (as-trag'ă-lō-kal-kā'nē-an). Relating to both the astragalus, or talus, and the calcaneus, or os calcis.

astragalofibular (as-trag'ă-lō-fib'yū-lar). Relating to both the astragalus, or talus, and the fibula.

astragaloscaphoid (as-trag'ă-lō-scaf'oyd). Talonavicular.

astragalotibial (as-trag'ă-lō-tib'ē-ăl). Relating to both the astragalus, or talus, and the tibia.

Astragalus (as-trag'ă-lŭs). A genus of plants (family Leguminosae), notably *A. mollissimus* (locoweed) on the range lands of western North America, capable of taking selenium from the soil and causing poisoning in sheep, cattle, and horses. *A. gummifer* is a source of tragacanth.

astragalus (as-trag'ă-lŭs) [G. *astragalos,* ball of the ankle joint]. Talus.

astral (as'tră). Relating to an astrosphere.

astrapophobia (as'tră-pō-fō'bē-ă) [G. *astrapē,* lightning, + *phobos,* fear]. Morbid fear of lightning.

astriction (as-trik'shŭn). **1.** Astringent action. **2.** Compression to arrest hemorrhage.

astringent (as-trin'jent) [L. *astringens*]. **1.** Causing contraction of the tissues, arrest of secretion, or control of bleeding. **2.** An agent having these effects.

astroblast (as'trō-blast) [G. *astron,* star, + *blastos,* germ]. A primitive cell developing into an astrocyte.

astroblastoma (as'trō-blas-tō'mă). Grade II or grade III astrocytoma; a relatively poorly differentiated glioma composed of young, immature, neoplastic cells of the astrocytic series, frequently arranged radially with short fibrils terminating in so-called "sucker feet" on small blood vessels.

astrocele (as'trō-sēl) [G. *astron*, star, + *koilia*, hollow]. Centrosphere.

astrocyte (as'trō-sīt) [G. *astron*, star, + *kytos*, hollow (cell)]. Astroglia; macroglia; astroglia or macroglia cell; spider cell (1); Cajal's cell (2); Deiters' cell (2); one of the large neuroglia cells of nervous tissue. See also neuroglia.
ameboid a., protoplasmic a. (1).
fibrous a., fibrillary a., stellate cell with long processes found in the white substance of the brain and spinal cord and characterized by having bundles of fine filaments in its cytoplasm.
gemistocytic a., protoplasmic a. (1).
protoplasmic a., **(1)** gemistocyte; gemästete cell; ameboid a.; ameboid cell (2); reactive a. or cell; gemistocytic a. or cell; a swollen neural cell possessing a well defined acidophilic cytoplasm; **(2)** one form of a., found in gray substance, having few fibrils and numerous branching processes.
reactive a., protoplasmic a. (1).

astrocytoma (as'trō-sī-tō'mă) [G. *astron*, star, + *kytos*, cell, + *-oma*, tumor]. A relatively well differentiated glioma composed of neoplastic cells that resemble one of the types of astrocytes, with varying amounts of fibrillary stroma; in children and persons less than 20 years of age, a.'s usually arise in a cerebellar hemisphere; in adults, a.'s usually occur in the cerebrum, sometimes growing rapidly and invading extensively.
gemistocytic a., protoplasmic a.
grade I a., solid or cystic a. of high differentiation.
grade II a., astroblastoma.
grade III a., astroblastoma.
grade IV a., glioblastoma.
piloid a., a slowing growing a. composed histologically of elongated fibrous astrocytes; often located in the optic chiasm or hypothalamus.
protoplasmic a., gemistocytoma; gemistocytic a.; a neoplasm composed of large, plump, swollen, acidophilic astrocytes.

astrocytosis (as'trō-sī-tō'sis). An increase in the number of astrocytes, frequently observed in an irregular, poorly or moderately well defined zone adjacent to degenerative lesions (*e.g.*, encephalomalacia), focal inflammations (*e.g.*, abscesses), or certain neoplasms in the brain; in some instances, a. may be diffuse in a relatively large region; a. represents a reparative defense mechanism.
a. cer'ebri, glioblastosis cerebri.

astroependymoma (as'trō-ē-pen'di-mō'mă). Mixed glioma; a glial neoplasm composed of a mixed population of astrocytic and ependymal cells.

astroglia (as-trog'lē-ă) [G. *astron*, star, + neuroglia]. Astrocyte.

astroid (as'troyd) [G. *astroeidēs*, fr. *astron*, star, + *eidos*, resemblance]. Star-shaped.

astrokinetic (as'trō-ki-net'ik). Relating to movement of the centrosome and astrosphere of a dividing cell.

astrosphere (as'trō-sfēr) [G. *astron*, star, + *sphaira*, ball]. Aster; paranuclear body; attraction sphere; Lavdovsky's nucleoid; a set of radiating microtubules extending outward from the cytocentrum and centrosphere of a dividing cell.

Astrup, Poul, Danish clinical chemist, *1915. See micro-Astrup *method.*

Astwood, Edwin B., U.S. endocrinologist, *1909. See A.'s *test.*

asverin (as'ver-in). 1-Methyl-3-piperidylidenedi(2-thienyl)methane; an antitussive.

Asx Symbol meaning "Asp or Asn."

asyllabia (ā-si-lā'bē-ă) [G. *a-* priv. + *syllabē*, syllable]. Form of alexia in which one recognizes individual letters, but cannot comprehend them when arranged collectively in syllables or words.

asylum (ă-sī'lŭm) [L. fr. G. *asylon*, a sanctuary, fr. *a-* priv. + *sylē*, right of seizure]. Old term for an institution for the housing and care of those who by reason of age or mental or bodily infirmities are unable to care for themselves.

asymbolia (ā-sim-bō'lē-ă) [G. *a-* priv. + *symbolon*, an outward sign]. **1.** Loss of the ability to appreciate by touch the form and nature of an object. **2.** Sign blindness; asemasia; asemia; a form of aphasia in which the significance of signs and symbols is not appreciated.

asymmetric (a) (ā-si-met'rik). Not symmetrical; denoting a lack of symmetry between two or more like parts.

asymmetry (ā-sim'ĕ-trē). **1.** Lack of symmetry; disproportion between two normally like parts. **2.** Significant difference in amplitude or frequency of two brain wave tracings taken simultaneously from the two sides of the brain under identical conditions of recording.

asymptomatic (ā'simp-tō-mat'ik). Without symptoms, or producing no symptoms.

asynclitism (ă-sin'kli-tizm) [G. *a-* priv. + *syn-klino*, to incline together]. Obliquity; absence of synclitism or parallelism between the axis of the presenting part of the child and the pelvic planes in childbirth.
anterior a., Nägele *obliquity*.
posterior a., Litzmann *obliquity*.

asyndesis (ă-sin'dĕ-sis) [G. *a-* priv. + *syn*, together, + *desis*, binding]. **1.** A mental defect in which separate ideas or thoughts cannot be joined into a coherent concept. **2.** A breaking up of the connecting links in language, said to be characteristic of language disturbance of schizophrenics.

asynechia (ă-si-nek'ē-ă) [G. *a-* priv. + *synecheia*, continuity]. Discontinuity of structure.

asynergia, asynergy (ă-sin-er'jē-ah, ă-sin'er-jē) [G. *a-* priv. + *syn*, with, + *ergon*, work]. Lack of cooperation or working together of parts that normally act in unison.

asynergic (ā'sin-er'jik). Characterized by asynergia.

asynesia, asynesis (ă-si-nē'zē-ă, -nē'sis) [G. *a-* priv. + *synesis*, union, understanding]. Lack of easy comprehension and practical intelligence.

asystematic (ā'sis-tĕ-mat'ik). Not systematic; not relating to one system or set of organs.

asystole (ă-sis'tō-lē) [G. *a-*priv, + *systolē*, a contracting]. Asystolia; cardiac standstill; absence of contractions of the heart.

asystolia (ă-sis-tō'lē-ă). Asystole.

asystolic (ă-sis-tol'ik). **1.** Relating to asystole. **2.** Not systolic.

At Symbol for astatine.

ata Abbreviation for *atmosphere* absolute.

atactilia (ā-tak-til'ē-ă) [G. *a-* priv. + L. *tactilis*, relating to touch, fr. *tango*, pp. *tactus*, to touch]. Loss of the sense of touch.

ataractic (at-ă-rak'tik) [G. *ataraktos*, calm]. Ataraxic. **1.** Having a calming or tranquilizing effect. **2.** A tranquilizer.

ataraxia (at-ă-rak'sē-ă) [G. *a-* priv. + *taraktos*, disturbed, + *-ia*]. Calmness and peace of mind; tranquility.

ataraxic (at-ă-rak'sik). Ataractic.

atavic (ă-tav'ik, at'ă-vik). Atavistic.

atavism (at'ă-vism) [L. *atavus*, a remote ancestor]. The appearance in an individual of characteristics presumed to have been present in some remote ancestor; reversion to an earlier biological type.

atavistic (at-ă-vis'tik). Atavic; relating to atavism.

atavus (at'ă-vŭs) [L. remote grandfather]. Throwback; a structure not commonly found in a contemporary organism that resembles a structure known to have existed in remote ancestral forms.

ataxia (ă-tak'sē-ă) [G. *a*-prov. + *taxis,* order]. Ataxy; dyssynergia; incoordination; an inability to coordinate the muscles in the execution of voluntary movement.
acute a., progressive a. of cerebellar type developing after severe infections.
bovine congenital a., an autosomal recessive a. seen in several European breeds of cattle.
Briquet's a., weakening of the muscle sense and increased sensibility of the skin, in hysteria.
Bruns a., difficulty in initiation of movements of the feet when they are in contact with the ground; a condition related to a frontal lobe lesion.
a. of calves, a specific cerebellar a. in the Jersey breed, probably a recessive genetic trait.
cerebellar a., loss of muscular coordination as a result of disease in the cerebellum.
a. cor'dis, atrial *fibrillation.*
enzootic a., swayback; a metabolic disease of lambs characterized clinically by progressive incoordination of the hind limbs and pathologically by disruption of neuron and myelin development in the central nervous system; caused by a deficiency of metabolizable copper in the ewe during the last half of her pregnancy.
equine spinal a., a disease of young horses characterized by progressive weakness and incoordination, most evident in the hind legs; it is associated with lesions in the cervical region of the spinal cord and is the result of compression of the spinal cord by malformed cervical vertebrae.
Friedreich's a., hereditary spinal a.
hereditary cerebellar a., Marie's a.; a disease of later childhood and early adult life, marked by ataxic gait, hesitating and explosive speech, nystagmus, and sometimes optic neuritis.
hereditary spinal a., Friedreich's a.; heredoataxia; sclerosis of the posterior and lateral columns of the spinal cord, occurring in children and marked by a. in the lower extremities, extending to the upper, followed by paralysis and contractures; autosomal recessive inheritance.
kinetic a., motor a.
a. of lambs, myelination failure seen in ewes on a copper-deficient diet.
Leyden's a., pseudotabes.
locomotor a. (1) motor a.; **(2)** *tabes* dorsalis.
Marie's a., hereditary cerebellar a.
moral a., inconstancy of ideas and of conscious intent, as a manifestation of hysteria.
motor a., kinetic a.; locomotor a. (1); a. developing upon attempting to perform coordinated muscular movements.
ocular a., nystagmus.
spinal a., a. due to spinal cord disease, as in tabes dorsalis.
static a., inability to preserve equilibrium while standing, due to loss of myesthesia.
a. telangiecta'sia, Louis-Bar syndrome; a familial single-gene autosomal recessive disease characterized by progressive cerebellar a., with oculocutaneous telangiectases and proneness to pulmonary infections; coarse nystagmoid oscillations appear, and there is immunodeficiency associated with both B- and T-type lymphocytes.
vasomotor a., a form of autonomic a. causing irregularity in the peripheral circulation, marked by alternations of pallor and suffusion, due to spasm of the smaller blood vessels.
vestibulocerebellar a., a. due to disease of the central vestibular system or its cerebellar components, manifested clinically by an unsteady gait, nystagmus, and incoordination of arm and leg movements.

ataxiadynamia (ă-tak'sē-ă-dī-nam'ē-ă). Muscular weakness combined with incoordination.

ataxiagram (ă-tak'sē-ă-gram). The recording made by an ataxiagraph.

ataxiagraph (ă-tak'sē-ă-graf). Ataxiameter; an instrument for measuring the degree and direction of the swaying of the body and head in static ataxia, with the individual's eyes closed.

ataxiameter (ă-tak'sē-ă-mē'ter). Ataxiagraph.

ataxiaphasia (ă-tak'sē-ă-fā'zē-ă) [G. *a*- priv. + *taxis,* order, + *phasis,* an affirmation, speech]. Inability to form connected sentences, although single words may perhaps be used intelligibly.

ataxic (ă-tak'sik). Relating to, marked by, or suffering from ataxia.

ataxiophemia (ă-tak-sē-ō-fē'mē-ă) [G. *a*- priv. + *taxis,* order, + *phēmē,* voice, speech]. Incoordination of the muscles concerned in speech production.

ataxiophobia (ă-tak'sē-ō-fō'bē-ă) [G. *a*- priv. + *taxis,* order, + *phobos,* fear]. Morbid dread of disorder or untidiness.

ataxy (ă-tak'sē). Ataxia.

-ate. Termination used as a replacement for "-ic acid" when the acid is neutralized (*e.g.,* sodium acetate) or esterfied (*e.g.,* ethyl acetate).

atelectasis (at-ē-lek'tă-sis) [G. *atelēs,* incomplete, + *ektasis,* extension]. Absence of gas from a part or the whole of the lungs, due to failure of expansion or resorption of gas from the alveoli. See also pulmonary *collapse.*
primary a., anectasis; nonexpansion of the lungs after birth, found in all stillborn infants and in liveborn infants who die before respiration is established.
round a., folded-lung *syndrome.*
secondary a., pulmonary collapse at any age, but particularly of infants, due to hyaline membrane disease or elastic recoil of the lungs while dying from other causes.

atelectatic (at-ē-lek-tat'ik). Relating to atelectasis.

atelia (ă-tē'lē-ă) Ateliosis.

ateliosis (ă-tē'lē-ō'sis) [G. *atelēs,* incomplete, + *-osis,* condition]. Atelia; incomplete development of the body or any of its parts, as in infantilism and dwarfism.

ateliotic (ă-tē-lē-ot'ik). Marked by ateliosis.

atelopidtoxin (ā-tel-op'id-tok'sin). A potent poison from the skin of the golden arrow frog (*Atelopus zeteki*) of Central and South America.

atenolol (ă-ten'ō-lol). 4-[2-Hydroxy-3[(1-methylethyl)amino]-propoxy]benzeneacetamide; a β-adrenergic blocking agent used primarily in the treatment of angina pectoris and hypertension.

athelia (ă-thē-lē-ă) [G. *a*- priv. + *thēlē,* nipple]. Congenital absence of the nipples.

athermancy (ă-ther'man-sē) [G. *athermantos,* not heated, fr. *a*- priv. + *thermaino,* to heat, fr. *thermē,* heat]. Impermeability to heat.

athermanous (ă-ther'mă-nŭs). Absorbing radiant heat; not permeable to heat rays.

athermosystaltic (ă-ther'mō-sis-tal'tik) [G. *a*- priv. + *thermos,* hot, + *systaltikos,* constringent]. Not contracted or constricted by ordinary variations of temperature; said of certain tissues.

athero- [G. *athērē,* gruel]. Combining form relating to the deposit of gruel-like, soft, pasty materials.

atheroembolism (ath'er-ō-em'bō-lizm). Cholesterol *embolism.*

atherogenesis (ath'er-ō-jen'ĕ-sis). Formation of atheroma, important in the pathogenesis of arteriosclerosis.

atherogenic (ath-er-ō-jen'ik). Having the capacity to initiate, increase, or accelerate the process of atherogenesis.

atheroma (ath-er-ō'mă) [G. *athērē,* gruel, + *-ōma,* tumor]. Atherosis; the lipid deposits in the intima of arteries, producing a yellow swelling on the endothelial surface; a characteristic of athero-sclero sis.

atheromatous (ath-er-ō'mă-tŭs). Relating to or affected by atheroma.

atherosclerosis (ath'er-ō-skler-ō'sis). Nodular sclerosis; arteriosclerosis characterized by irregularly distributed lipid deposits in the intima of large and medium-sized arteries; such deposits are associated with fibrosis and calcification. In lower animals, a. of swine and fowl mostly resemble a. of man.

atherosclerotic (ath'er-ō-skler-ot'ik). Relating to or characterized by atherosclerosis.

atherosis (ath-er-ō'sis). Atheroma.

atherothrombosis (ath'er-ō-throm-bō'sis).]. Clot formation in an atheromatous vessel.

atherothrombotic (ath'er-ō-throm-bot'ik). Denoting, characteristic of, or caused by atherothrombosis.

athetoid (ath'ĕ-toyd). Resembling athetosis.

athetosic, athetotic (ath-ĕ-tō'sik, -tot'ik). Pertaining to, or marked by, athetosis.

athetosis (ath-ĕ-tō'sis) [G. *athetos,* without position or place]. A condition in which there is a constant succession of slow, writhing, involuntary movements of flexion, extension, pronation, and supination of the fingers and hands, and sometimes of the toes and feet.
double a., Vogt *syndrome.*
double congenital a., congenital bilateral a., often associated with spastic paraplegia.
posthemiplegic a., posthemiplegic chorea; abnormal jerking or athetotic movements associated with hemiplegia.
pupillary a., rarely used term meaning hippus.

athrepsia, athrepsy (ă-threp'sē-ă, ath'rep-sē) [G. *a-* priv. + *threpsis,* nourishment]. **1.** Obsolete term for narasmus. **2.** Atrepsy; as used by Ehrlich, immunity to transplanted neoplastic cells due to a lack of nourishment in the sense of a deficiency of supposed substances required for the development of such cells.

athrocytosis (ath'rō-sī-tō'sis) [G. *athrō,* gathered together, + *kytos,* cell, + *-osis,* condition]. The capacity of cells to absorb and retain electronegative colloids, as shown by macrophages and at the apical surface of proximal convoluted tubule cells of the kidney.

athrombia (ă-throm'bē-ă) [G. *a-* priv. + thrombin]. A defect of blood clotting characterized by deficiency in formation of thrombin.

athymia (ă-thī'mē-ă) [G. *a-*priv. + *thymos,* mind, also thymus]. **1.** Absence of affect or emotivity; morbid impassivity. **2.** Athymism; congenital absence of the thymus gland, often with associated immunodeficiency.

athymism (ă-thī'mizm). Athymia (2).

athyrea (ă-thī'rē-ă). Athyroidism.

athyroidism (ă-thī'royd-izm). Athyrea; athyrosis; congenital absence of the thyroid gland or suppression of its secretion.

athyrosis (ă-thī-rō'sis). Athyroidism.

athyrotic (ă-thī-rot'ik). Relating to athyroidism.

ATL Abbreviation for adult T-cell *leukemia* or *lymphoma.*

atlantad (at-lan'tad). In a direction toward the atlas.

atlantal (at-lan'tăl). Atloid; relating to the atlas.

atlanto-, atlo- [G. *atlas*]. Combining forms relating to the atlas.

atlantoaxial (at-lan'tō-ak'sē-ăl). Atloaxoid; atlantoepistrophic; pertaining to the atlas and the axis; denoting the joint between the first two cervical vertebrae.

atlantodidymus (at-lan'tō-did'ĕ-mŭs) [atlanto- + G. *didymos,* twin]. Atlodidymus; conjoined twins with two heads on one neck and a single body.

atlantoepistrophic (at-lan'tō-ep'i-strof'ik). Atlantoaxial.

atlanto-occipital (at-lan'tō-ok-sip'i-tăl). Atlo-occipital; relating to the atlas and the occipital bone.

atlanto-odontoid (at-lan'tō-ō-don'toyd). Relating to the atlas and the dens of the axis.

atlas (at'las) [G. *Atlas,* in Greek mythology a Titan who supported the earth on his shoulders] [NA]. First cervical vertebra, articulating with the occipital bone and rotating around the dens of the axis.

atlo-. See atlanto-.

atloaxoid (at-lō-ak'soyd). Atlantoaxial.

atlodidymus (at-lō-did'ĕ-mŭs). Atlantodidymus.

atloid (at'loyd). Atlantal.

atlo-occipital (at'lō-ok-sip'i-tăl). Atlanto-occipital.

atm Symbol for standard *atmosphere.*

atmo- [G. *atmos,* vapor]. Prefix denoting steam or vapor, or derived by action of same.

atmolysis (at-mol'i-sis) [atmo- + G. *lysis,* dissolution]. Separation of mixed gases by passing them through a porous diaphragm, the lighter gases diffusing through at a faster rate.

atmometer (at-mom'ĕ-ter) [atmo- + G. *metron,* measure]. An instrument for measuring the rate of evaporation.

atmos [abbreviation of atmosphere] Obsolete abbreviation for a unit of pressure; replaced by atm.

atmosphere (at'mōs-fēr) [atmo- + G. *sphaira,* sphere]. **1.** Air. **2.** Any gas surrounding a given body; a gaseous medium. **3.** A unit of air pressure. See also standard a.; torr.
a. absolute (ata), a unit of absolute pressure (also known as barometric pressure) expressed in atm.
ICAO standard a., the standard a. adopted by the International Civil Aviation Organization, used for calibrating altimeters and for expressing hypobaric chamber pressures in terms of equivalent altitude; it ignores many deviations found in nature.
standard a. (atm), **(1)** the pressure of the a. at mean sea level, equivalent to 1,013,250 dynes/cm^2 or 101,325 pascals (newtons/m^2 in the SI system); **(2)** a standardized expression of the relation of barometric pressure, temperature, and other atmospheric variables as a function of altitude above sea level.

atmospherization (at'mō-sfēr-i-zā'shŭn). Conversion of venous into arterial blood.

Atmungsferment (aht'mungz-fer-ment) [Ger.]. Warburg's respiratory enzyme; a system of cytochromes and their oxidases that participate in respiratory processes.

atom (at'ŏm) [G. *atomos,* indivisible, uncut]. The once ultimate particle of an element, believed to be as indivisible as its name indicates. Discovery of radioactivity demonstrated the existence of subatomic particles, notably protons, neutrons and electrons, the first two comprising most of the mass of the atomic nucleus.
activated a., excited a.; an a. possessing more than normal energy as a result of input of energy. See also excited *state.*
Bohr's a., a concept or model of the a. in which the negatively charged electrons move in circular or elliptical orbits around the positively charged nucleus, energy being emitted or absorbed when electrons change from one orbit to another.
excited a., activated a.
ionized a., an a. that possesses an electrostatic charge as a result of loss or gain of electrons; *e.g.,* H^+, CA^{+2}, Cl^-, O^{-2}.
labeled a., tagged a.; a radioactive a., or a stable but rare one, which by its presence in a molecule helps identify that molecule.
nuclear a., a concept or model of the a. characterized by the presence of a small, massive nucleus at its center.
quaternary carbon a., an a. of carbon to which four other carbon a.'s are attached.

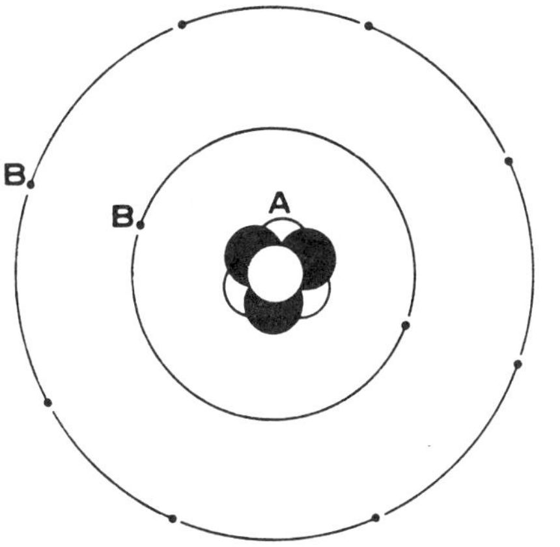

Structure of an Atom
A, nucleus, containing protons (*open circles*) and neutrons (*black circles*); *B,* electrons, traveling in orbits around nucleus.

radioactive a., an a. with an unstable nucleus, which emits particulate or electromagnetic radiation (radioactive emission) to achieve greater stability.
recoil a., the remainder of an a. from which a nuclear particle has been emitted or ejected; since this occurs with high velocity, the remainder recoils with a velocity inversely proportional to its mass.
stripped a., an a. minus all its electrons.
tagged a., labeled a.

atomic (ă-tom′ik). Relating to an atom.

atomism (at′ŏm-izm). The approach to the study of a psychological phenomenon through analysis of the elementary parts of which it is assumed to be composed. *Cf.* holism.

atomistic (at-ŏm-is′tik). Pertaining to atomism or a. psychology.

atomization (at-ŏm-i-zā′-shŭn). Spray production; reduction of a fluid to small droplets.

atomizer (at′ŏm-ī-zer). A device used to reduce liquid medication to fine particles in the form of a spray or aerosol; useful in delivering medication to the nose and throat. See also nebulizer; vaporizer.

atonia (ā-tō′nē-ă) [G. languor]. Atony.

atonic (ă-ton′ik). Relaxed; without normal tone or tension.

atonicity (at-ō-nis′i-tē). Atony.

atony (at′ŏ-nē) [G. *atonia,* languor]. Atonia; atonicity; relaxation, flaccidity, or lack of tone or tension.

atopen (at′ō-pen). The excitant causing any form of atopy.

atopic (ă-top′ik) [G. *atopos,* out of place; strange]. Relating to or marked by atopy.

atopognosia, atopognosis (ă-top-og-nō′zē-ă, -og-nō′sis) [G. *a-* priv. + *topos,* place, + *gnōsis,* knowledge]. Inability to locate a sensation properly.

atopy (at′ō-pē) [G. *atopia,* strangeness, fr. *a-* priv. + *topos,* a place]. Type I allergic reaction, specifically one with strong familial tendencies, caused by various allergens and associated with the Prausnitz-Küstner (IgE class) antibody.

atoxic (ā-tok′sik). Not toxic.

ATP Abbreviation for adenosine 5′-triphosphate.

ATPase Abbreviation for adenosinetriphosphatase.

ATPD Symbol indicating that a gas volume has been expressed as if it had been dried at the ambient temperature and pressure.

ATP-diphosphatase. Apyrase.

ATP-monophosphatase. Adenosinetriphosphatase.

ATPS Symbol indicating that a gas volume has been expressed as if it were saturated with water vapor at the ambient temperature and barometric pressure; the condition of an expired gas equilibrated in a spirometer.

atrabiliary (at-ră-bil′ē-ār-ē) [L. *atra bilis,* black bile]. Obsolete term for depressed melancholic.

atractosylidic acid (ă-trak′tō-sil-id′ik). Atractyligenin.

atractylic acid (ă-trak′til-ik). A highly poisonous steroid glycoside from *Atractylis gummifera L.* (*Compositae*), having a strychnine-like action that produces convulsions of a hypoglycemic nature; the aglycon, atractyliginin, is combined with glucose and isovaleric acid, and is the toxic principle. A. interferes with oxidative reactions, the citric acid cycle, and nerve conduction.

atractyligenin (ă-trak′til-i-jen′in). Atractosylidic acid; atractylin; the steroid aglycon and toxic principle of atractylic acid.

atractylin (ă-trak′til-in). Atractyligenin.

atracurium besylate (a-tră-kyūr′ē-ŭm). $C_{65}H_{82}N_2O_{18}S_2$; a non-depolarizing neuromuscular relaxant of intermediate duration of action; used as an adjunct to general anesthesia.

atrepsy (ă-trep′sē) [G. *a-* priv. + *trephō,* to nourish]. Athrepsia (2).

atresia (ă-trē′zē-ă) [G. *a-* priv. + *trēsis,* a hole]. Clausura; absence of a normal opening or normally patent lumen.
anal a., a. a′ni, imperforate anus; proctatresia; congenital absence of an anal opening due to the presence of a membranous septum (persistence of the cloacal membrane) or to complete absence of the anal canal.

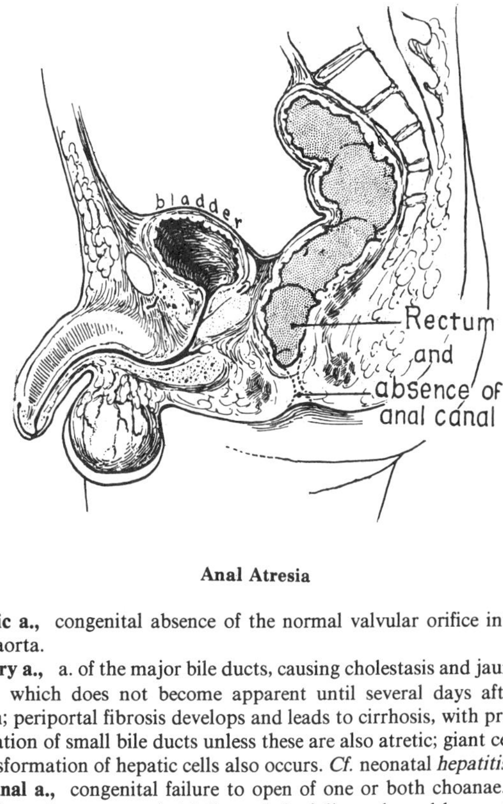

Anal Atresia

aortic a., congenital absence of the normal valvular orifice into the aorta.
biliary a., a. of the major bile ducts, causing cholestasis and jaundice, which does not become apparent until several days after birth; periportal fibrosis develops and leads to cirrhosis, with proliferation of small bile ducts unless these are also atretic; giant cell transformation of hepatic cells also occurs. *Cf.* neonatal *hepatitis.*
choanal a., congenital failure to open of one or both choanae.
esophageal a., congenital failure of the full esophageal lumen to develop.
a. follic′uli, a normal process affecting the primordial ovarian follicles in which death of the ovum results in cystic degeneration followed by cicatricial closure.

intestinal a., an obliteration of the lumen of the small intestine, with the ileum involved in 50% of cases and the jejunum and duodenum following in frequency; most frequent cause of intestinal obstruction in the newborn; etiology may be related to a failure of recanalization during early development or to some impairment of blood supply during intrauterine life.
a. i'ridis, atretopsia; congenital absence of pupillary opening.
laryngeal a., congenital failure of the laryngeal opening to develop, resulting in partial or total obstruction at or just above or below the glottis.
pulmonary a., congenital absence of the normal valvular orifice into the pulmonary artery.
tricuspid a., congenital lack of the tricuspid orifice.
vaginal a., ankylocolpos; colpatresia; congenital or acquired imperforation or occlusion of the vagina, or adhesion of the walls of the vagina.

atresic (ă-trē'zik). Atretic.

atretic (ă-tret'ik). Atresic; imperforate; relating to atresia.

atreto- [G. *atrētos,* imperforate] Prefix denoting lack of opening of the part named.

atretoblepharia (ă-trē'tō-ble-făr'ē-ă) [atreto- + G. *blepharon,* eyelid]. Symblepharia.

atretocystia (ă-trē'tō-sis'tē-ă) [atreto- + G. *kystis,* bladder]. Congenital or acquired absence of an opening of a bladder.

atretogastria (ă-trē'tōgas'trē-ă) [atreto- + G. *gastēr,* stomach]. Congenital absence of an opening of the stomach.

atretopsia (ă-trē-top'sē-ă) [atreto- + G. *ōps,* eye]. *Atresia* iridis.

atria (ā'trē-ă). Plural of atrium.

atrial (ā'trē-ăl). Relating to an atrium.

atrichia (ă-trik'ē-ă) [G. *a-* priv. + *thrix* (*trich-*), hair]. Atrichosis; absence of hair, congenital or acquired.

atrichosis (at-ri-kō'sis). Atrichia.

atrichous (at'ri-kŭs). Without hair.

atrio- [L. *atrium*]. Combining form relating to the atrium.

atriomegaly (ā'trē-ō-meg'ă-lē) [atrio- + G. *megas,* great]. Enlargement of the atrium.

atrionector (ā-trē-ō-nek'ter, -tōr) [atrio- + L. *necto,* to join]. *Nodus* sinuatrialis.

atriopeptin (ā'trē-ō-pep'tin). Atrial natriuretic *factor.*

atrioseptopexy (ā'trē-ō-sep'tō-pek-sē) [atrio- + L. *septum,* partition, + G. *pexis,* fixation]. A closed surgical technique for repairing atrial septal defects, in which a portion of the free wall of the right atrium is sutured so as to occlude the defect.

atrioseptoplasty (ā'trē-ō-sep'tō-plas-tē) [atrio- + L. *septum,* partition, + G. *plastos,* formed]. Surgical repair of an atrial septal defect.

atrioseptostomy (ā'trē-ō-sep-tos'tō-mē) [atrio- + L. *septum,* partition, + G. *stoma,* mouth]. Establishment of a communication between the two atria of the heart.
balloon a., tearing or enlarging the foramen ovale by pulling a balloon-bearing catheter across the atrial septum for the purpose of augmenting interatrial mixing of blood in the treatment of cyanotic congenital heart disease.

atriotome (ā'trē-ō-tōm). An instrument for opening an atrium.

atriotomy (ā-trē-ot'ō-mē) [atrio- + G. *tomē,* incision]. Surgical opening of an atrium.

atrioventricular (A-V) (ā'trē-ō-ven-trik'yū-lar). Relating to both the atria and the ventricles of the heart, especially to the ordinary, orthograde transmission of conduction or bloodflow.

atriplicism (ă-trip'li-sizm) [L. *atriplex* (*-plic-*), the orach, a vegetable]. An intoxication caused by the ingestion of certain species of *Atriplex,* eaten as greens in China; it is marked by pain and swelling of the fingers, spreading to the forearm; bullae and ulcers form, and the fingers may become gangrenous.

atrium, pl. **atria** (ā'trē-ŭm, ā'trē-ă) [L. entrance hall]. **1** [NA]. A chamber or cavity to which are connected several chambers or passageways. **2.** A. cordis. **3.** That part of the tympanic cavity that lies immediately deep to the eardrum. **4.** A. meatus medii. **5.** In the lung, a subdivision of the alveolar duct from which alveolar sacs open.
accessory a., *cor* triatriatum.
a. cor'dis [NA], a. of heart; atrium (2); the upper chamber of each half of the heart.
a. dex'trum [NA], right a., the a. of the right side of the heart which receives the blood from the venae cavae and coronary sinus.
a. glot'tidis, *vestibulum* laryngis.
a. of heart, a. cordis.
left a., a. sinistrum.
a. mea'tus me'dii [NA], atrium (4); the anterior expanded portion of the middle meatus of the nose, just above the vestibule.
a. pulmona'le, a. sinistrum.
right a., a. dextrum.
a. sinis'trum [NA], left a.; a. pulmonale; a. of the left side of the heart which receives the blood from the pulmonary veins.

Atropa (at'rō-pă) [G. *Atropos,* one of the Fates cutting the thread of life, because of the lethal effects of the plant]. A genus of plants (family Solanaceae) of which *A. belladonna* is typical. See belladonna.

atrophedema. (ă-trof'ĕ-dē'mă). Angioneurotic *edema.*

atrophia (ă-trō'fē-ă) [G. fr. *a-* priv. + *trophē,* nourishment]. Atrophy.
a. bulbo'rum hereditar'ria, Norrie's *disease.*
a. cu'tis, atrophoderma.
a. maculo'sa variolifor'mis cu'tis, anetoderma.
a. pilo'rum pro'pria, a general term that includes fragilitas crinium, trichorrhexis nodosa, monilethrix, and atrophy of the hair.

atrophic (ă-trof'ik). Denoting atrophy.

atrophie blanche (ă'trō-fi blahnsh') [Fr.]. Small smooth ivory-white areas with hyperpigmented borders and telangiectasis, developing into atrophic stellate scars; seen especially on the legs and ankles of middle-aged women, and associated with livedo reticularis and dermal hyalinizing vasculitis.

atrophied (at'rō-fēd). Characterized by atrophy.

atrophoderma (at'rō-fō-der'mă). Atrophia cutis; atrophy of the skin which may occur either in discrete localized areas or in widespread areas. See also anetoderma.
a. al'bidum, stocking-like type of atrophy affecting the extremities, probably congenital; first noted in early childhood on the lower limbs as a symmetric thinning that renders the parts sensitive.
a. biotrip'ticum, senile cutaneous atrophy.
a. diffu'sum, diffuse idiopathic cutaneous atrophy.
a. macula'tum, primary macular atrophy of the skin; a rare condition in which a macular lesion becomes involuted, leaving the area thin, soft, and slightly wrinkled.
a. neurit'icum, glossy *skin.*
a. of Pasini and Pierini, a form of slate-colored atrophy of the skin occurring in discrete, 2-cm or larger lesions, either singly or multiply, and occasionally confluent, increasing in number and size over a period of years and then remaining constant; thought by some to be of two types: one preceded by morphea, and the other appearing with no preceding identifiable pathology.
a. pigmento'sum, *xeroderma* pigmentosum.
a. reticula'tum symmet'ricum fa'ciei, a rarely used term for *folliculitis* ulerythematosa reticulata.
senile a., a. seni'lis, the loss of fat, increased pigmentation, and other changes of the skin associated with old age.

a. stria'tum, the condition marked by the presence of lineae albicantes.

a. vermicula'tum, *folliculitis* ulerythematosa reticulata.

atrophodermatosis (at'rō-fō-der-mă-tō'sis). Any cutaneous affection in which a prominent symptom is skin atrophy.

atrophy (at'rō-fē) [G. *atrophia,* fr. *a-* priv. + *trophē,* nourishment]. Atrophia; a wasting of tissues, organs, or the entire body, as from death and reabsorption of cells, diminished cellular proliferation, decreased cellular volume, pressure, ischemia, malnutrition, lessened function, or hormonal changes.

acute reflex bone a., Sudeck's a.

acute yellow a. of the liver, Rokitansky's disease (1); acute parenchymatous hepatitis; a lesion in which there is extensive and rapid death of parenchymal cells of the liver, sometimes with fatty degeneration; the necrosis may result from fulminant viral infection or chemical poisoning.

alveolar a., diminution in size of the supportive tissues of the teeth due to lack of function, reduced blood supply, or unknown causes.

arthritic a., a. of muscles rendered inactive by a chronically inflamed or fixed joint.

blue a., depressed blue atrophic scars due to injections in the skin of impure substances, as seen in narcotics addicts.

brown a., a. of the heart wall, especially in the elderly, in which the muscle is dark reddish brown and reduced in volume; the muscle fibers become pigmented especially about the nuclei, by lipochrome granules.

Buchwald's a., a progressive form of cutaneous a.

central areolar choroidal a., areolar *choroidopathy.*

cerebellar a., a degeneration of the cerebellum, particularly the Purkinje cells, as the result of abiotrophy or of toxic agents, as in alcoholism.

choroidal vascular a., a. affecting either all choroidal vessels or only the choriocapillaris, occurring either diffusely or confined to the posterior pole of the eye.

compensatory a., a. especially of an endocrine organ as a result of its function being assumed by a new source of hormone.

cyanotic a., red a.; a. due to destruction of the parenchymatous cells of an organ as a consequence of chronic venous congestion.

cyanotic a. of the liver, cardiac *cirrhosis.*

Erb's a., progressive muscular *dystrophy.*

essential progressive a. of iris, progressive a. of the iris without inflammatory signs, characterized by patchy loss of all layers of the iris with hole formation, migration of the pupil, degeneration of the corneal endothelium, peripheral anterior synechiae, and secondary glaucoma; usually unilateral, predominately affecting women in their middle years.

exhaustion a., a., especially of glandular cells, believed to result from excessive functional activity or overstimulation.

facioscapulohumeral a., facioscapulohumeral muscular *dystrophy.*

familial spinal muscular a., infantile muscular a.

fatty a., fatty infiltration secondary to an a. of the essential elements of an organ or tissue.

gingival a., gingival *recession.*

gray a., obsolete term for a degeneration of the optic disk in which it assumes a grayish or bluish gray color.

gyrate a. of choroid and retina, a slowly progressive a. of the choriocapillaris, pigmentary epithelium, and sensory retina, with irregular confluent atrophic areas and an associated ornithenuria; autosomal recessive inheritance.

Hoffmann's muscular a., infantile muscular a.

horizontal a., horizontal resorption; a progressive loss of alveolar and supporting bone surrounding the teeth, beginning at the most coronal level of the bone.

Hunt's a., neural a. of the small muscles of the hand without sensory disturbances; two types are recognized: *thenar,* from compression of the thenar branch of the median nerve; *hypothenar,* from compression of the deep palmar branch of the ulnar nerve.

idiopathic muscular a., progressive muscular *dystrophy.*

infantile muscular a., Hoffmann's muscular a.; Werdnig-Hoffmann disease; familial spinal muscular a.; infantile progressive spinal muscular a.; progressive muscular wasting due to degeneration of motor neurons in anterior horns of the spinal cord; onset is usually in the first year, with 80% mortality by the fourth year; autosomal recessive inheritance.

infantile progressive spinal muscular a., infantile muscular a.

ischemic muscular a., see Volkmann's *contracture.*

juvenile muscular a., Kugelberg-Welander or Wohlfart-Kugelberg-Welander disease; slowly progressive proximal muscular weakness with fasciculation and wasting, electromyographic and muscle biopsy findings of lower motor neuron disease, and onset usually between 2 and 17 years of age; autosomal recessive inheritance is usual.

Kienböck's a., acute a. of bone in an extremity following inflammation.

Leber's hereditary optic a., hereditary degeneration of the optic nerve and papillomacular bundle with resulting rapid loss of central vision, progressive for several weeks, then usually stationary with permanent central scotoma; age of onset is variable, most often in the third decade; males are predominantly affected and transmission is by normal females, but X-linkage is unlikely.

linear a., *striae* cutis distensae.

macular a., a rare condition of unknown cause, characterized by discrete, sharply defined areas of atrophy where the skin surface protrudes as small bladder-like tumors.

marantic a., marasmus.

muscular a., a wasting of muscular tissue, especially due to lack of use. *Cf.* myopathic a.

myopathic a., muscular a. due to disease of the muscle itself and not of paralytic or central nervous system origin.

neuritic a., neurotrophic a.

neurogenic a., fascicular *degeneration.*

neurotrophic a., neuritic a.; trophic change; a. of a muscle resulting from neuritis or degeneration of the motor nerves, usually beginning in the lower extremities, reaching the greatest extent in the legs, less in the upper extremities.

nutritional type cerebellar a., a moderately circumscribed cortical a. restricted largely to the anterior vermis and noted in cachetic patients, particularly those with chronic alcoholism.

olivopontocerebellar a., olivopontocerebellar degeneration; a progressive neurologic disease characterized by loss of neurons in the cerebellar cortex, basis pontis, and inferior olivary nuclei; results in ataxia, tremor, involuntary movement, and dysarthria; five clinical types (four with dominant, one with recessive inheritance) have been described, each type characterized by additional findings, such as sensory loss, retinal degeneration, ophthalmoplegia, and extrapyramidal signs.

periodontal a., decrease in size and/or cellular elements of the periodontium after it has reached normal maturity.

peroneal muscular a., Charcot-Marie-Tooth disease; fossicular degeneration characterized by slowly progressive wasting of distal muscles of the extremities, usually involving the legs before the arms; pes cavus is often the first sign; autosomal dominant, autosomal recessive, and X-linked recessive types exist, with severity related to genetic type.

Pick's a., Pick's disease (2); circumscribed a. of the cerebral cortex.

postmenopausal a., a. following menopause, as of the genital organs.

pressure a., the wasting of hard or soft tissue resulting from excessive pressure applied to tissue by a denture base.

primary idiopathic macular a., anetoderma.

primary macular a. of skin, *atrophoderma* maculatum.

progressive choroidal a., choroideremia (2).
progressive muscular a., progressive spinal amyotrophy; Duchenne-Aran, Aran-Duchenne, or Cruveilier's disease; muscular trophoneurosis; creeping palsy; wasting paralysis or palsy; a. of the cells of the anterior horns of the spinal cord, resulting in a slow progressive wasting and paralysis of the muscles of the extremities and of the trunk.
pseudohypertrophic muscular a., pseudohypertrophic muscular *dystrophy*.
pulp a., diminution in size and/or cellular elements of the dental pulp due to interference with the blood supply.
red a., cyanotic a.
scapulohumeral a., Vulpian's a.
senile a., geromarasmus; wasting of tissues and organs with advancing age from decreased catabolic or anabolic processes, at times due to endocrine changes, decreased use, or ischemia.
serous a., a degenerative change occurring in fat cells, the fat being absorbed and its place being taken by a serous fluid.
spinal a., *tabes* dorsalis.
striate a. of skin, linear pink striations occurring in the skin of debilitated, usually bedfast patients.
Sudeck's a., Sudeck's syndrome; posttraumatic osteoporosis; acute reflex bone a.; acute a. of bones, commonly of the carpal or tarsal bones, following a slight injury such as a sprain. See also causalgia, and sympathetic reflex *dystrophy*.
traction a., *striae* cutis distensae.
transneuronal a., transsynaptic *degeneration*.
trophoneurotic a., a. related to loss of innervation.
Vulpian's a., scapulohumeral a.; progressive spinal muscular a. beginning in the shoulder.
yellow a. of the liver, see acute yellow a. of the liver.
Zimmerlin's a., a variety of hereditary progressive muscular a. in which the a. begins in the upper half of the body.

atropine (at'rō-pēn). *dl*-Hyoscyamine; *dl*-tropyl tropate; tropine tropate; $C_{17}H_{23}NO_3$; an alkaloid obtained from *Atropa belladonna;* an antispasmodic, antisudorific, anticholinergic, and mydriatic.
a. methonitrate, the methylnitrate of a., with the same actions and uses as a.
a. methylbromide, methylatropine bromide.
a. sulfate, an anticholinergic.

atropinism (at'rō-pin-izm). Symptoms of poisoning by atropine or belladonna.

atropinization (at-rō'pin-i-zā'shŭn). Administration of atropine or belladonna to the point of achieving the pharmacologic effect.

atrotoxin (at-rō-toks'in). A component of diamondback rattlesnake (*Crotalus atrox*) venom that specifically and reversibly increases voltage-dependent calcium ion currents in isolated myocytes.

attachment (ă-tach'ment). **1.** A connection of one part with another. **2.** In dentistry, a mechanical device for the fixation and stabilization of a dental prosthesis.
bar-sleeve a.'s bar clip a.'s, fixed bar joints or rigid bar units used for splinting abutments with removable sleeves or clips within the partial denture for supporting and/or retaining the prosthesis.
epithelial a., junctional *epithelium*.
frictional a., precision a.
internal a., precision a.
key a., precision a.
keyway a., precision a.
muscle-tendon a., muscle-tendon junction; the union of a muscle and tendon fiber in which sarcolemma intervenes between the two; the end of the muscle fiber may be rounded, conical, or tapered.
parallel a., precision a.
pericemental a., the tissues surrounding the cementum of the tooth, *i.e.,* the periodontal ligament and alveolar bone.
precision a., frictional, internal, key, keyway, parallel, or slotted a.; **(1)** a frictional or mechanically retained unit used in fixed or removable prosthodontics, consisting of closely fitting male and female parts; **(2)** an a. that may be rigid in function or may incorporate a movable stress control unit to reduce the torque on the abutment.
slotted a., precision a.

attack (ă-tak'). The occurrence of some disease or episode, ordinarily with dramatic and sudden onset, such as an a. of shingles or heart a.
drop a., a. characterized by falling without warning, often upon movement of the head and probably due to cervical spondylosis compressing the vertebral arteries or to hyperirritable carotid sinus.
panic a., sudden onset of intense apprehension, fear, terror, or impending doom accompanied by various constitutional disturbances, depersonalization, and derealization.
salaam a., nodding *spasm*.
transient ischemic a. (TIA), a sudden loss of neurological function with complete recovery usually within 24 hours; the result of vascular impairment to the brain.
uncinate a., uncinate *epilepsy*.
vagal a., vasovagal a., syncope, or syndrome; Gowers' syndrome; a paroxysmal condition marked by a slow pulse, fall in blood pressure, and sometimes convulsions; thought to be due to sudden stimulation of the vagus nerve mediated through receptors in the carotid sinus, the aortic arch, or the heart.
vasovagal a., vagal a.

attar of rose (at'ăr) [Pers. *attara,* to smell sweet]. Rose oil.

attending (ă-tend'ing) [L. *attendo,* to bend to, notice]. In psychology, readiness to percieve, as in listening or looking; focusing of sense organs is sometimes involved.

attenuant (ă-ten'yū-ănt). **1.** Denoting that which attenuates. **2.** An agent, means, or method that attenuates.

attenuate (ă-ten'yū-āt) [L. *at-tenuo,* pp. *-tenuatus,* to make thin or weak, fr. *tenuis,* thin]. To dilute, thin, reduce, weaken, diminish.

attenuation (ă-ten-yū-ā'shŭn). **1.** The act of attenuating. **2.** Diminution of virulence in a strain of an organism, obtained through selection of variants which occur naturally or through experimental means. **3.** Loss of energy of a beam of radiant energy due to absorption, scattering, beam divergence, and other causes as the beam propagates through a medium.

attenuator (ă-ten'yū-ā-tŏr, -tōr). **1.** An electrical system of resistors and capacitors used to reduce the strength of the electrical signals in ultrasonography. **2.** Immunoglobulin(s) given during the incubation period to reduce or prevent clinical manifestations of infection.

attic (at'ik). *Recessus* epitympanicus.
tympanic a., *recessus* epitympanicus.

atticomastoid (at'i-kō-mas'toyd). Relating to the attic of the tympanic cavity and the mastoid antrum or cells.

atticotomy (at-i-kot'ō-mē) [attic + G. *tomē,* incision]. Operative opening into the tympanic attic.

attitude (at'i-tūd) [Mediev. L. *aptitudo,* fr. L. *aptus,* fit]. **1.** Posture; position of the body and limbs. **2.** Manner of acting. **3.** In social or clinical psychology, a relatively stable and enduring predisposition or set to behave or react in a certain way toward persons, objects, institutions, or issues.
emotional a.'s, passional a.'s.
fetal a., fetal *habitus*.
passional a.'s, emotional a.'s; a.'s expressive of any of the great passions; *e.g.,* anger, lust.

attitudinal (at-i-tū'di-năl). Relating to a posture of the body; *e.g.,* a. (statotonic) reflex.

atto- (a) [Danish *atten,* eighteen] Prefix used in the SI and metric systems to signify one quintillionth (10^{-18}).

attollens (ătol'ens) [L. *at- tollo,* pres. p. *-tollens,* to lift up]. Raising up; in anatomy, muscle action that lifts.
a. au'rem, a. auric'ulam, *musculus* auricularis superior.
a. oc'uli, *musculus* rectus superior.

attraction (ă-trak'shŭn) [L. *at-traho,* pp. *-tractus,* to draw toward]. The tendency of two bodies to approach each other.
capillary a., the force that causes fluids to rise up very fine tubes or through the pores of a loose material.
chemical a., the force impelling atoms of different elements or molecules to unite to form new substances or compounds.
magnetic a., the force that draws iron or steel toward a magnet.
neurotropic a., the pull of a regenerating axon toward the motor end-plate.

attrahens (at'ră-henz) [see attraction]. Drawing toward, denoting a muscle (attrahens aurem or auriculam) rudimentary in man, that tends to draw the pinna of the ear forward. See musculus auricularis anterior.

attrition (ă-trish'ŭn) [L. *at-tero,* pp. *-tritus,* to rub against, rub away]. **1.** Wearing away by friction or rubbing. **2.** In dentistry, physiological loss of tooth structure caused by the abrasive character of food or from bruxism. *Cf.* abrasion.

at wt Abbreviation for *atomic weight.*

atypia (ā-tip'ē-ă). Atypism; state of being not typical.

atypical (ā-tip'i-kal) [G. *a*-priv. + *typikos,* conformed to a type]. Not typical; not corresponding to the normal form or type.

atypism (ā-tip'izm). Atypia.

A.U. Abbreviation for *auris uterque* [L.], each ear or both ears.

Au Symbol for gold (aurum).

^{198}Au colloid. Radiogold colloid.

Aub, Joseph C., U.S. physician, 1890–1973. See A.-DuBois *table.*

Auberger (Au) blood group. See Blood Groups appendix.

Aubert, Hermann, German physiologist, 1826–1892. See A.'s *phenomenon.*

Auchmeromyia (awk'mer-ō-mī'yă) [G. *auchmeros,* without rain, hence unwashed, squalid, + *myia,* a fly]. A genus of bloodsucking botflies (family Calliphoridae, order Diptera).
A. luteo'la, the Congo floor maggot; the bloodsucking larva of this botfly species is found in Africa south of the Sahara, usually in or near human habitations; the resistant larvae or maggots crawl to sleeping humans and suck blood for 15 to 20 minutes, detach, and hide, repeating these nightly attacks during their developmental period; no disease transmission is known from this insect.

aucubin (aw'kū-bin). $C_{15}H_{24}O_9$; a glycoside contained in the seeds of *Acuba japonica* (family Cornaceae) and *Plantago ovata* (family Plantaginaceae); the seeds are used in the treatment of diarrhea.

audile (aw'dil). **1.** Relating to audition. **2.** Denoting the type of mental imagery in which one recalls most readily that which has been heard. *Cf.* motile; visile. **3.** Auditive.

audio- [L. *audio,* to hear]. Combining form relating to hearing.

audioanalgesia (aw'dē-ō-an-ăl-jē'zē-ă). Use of music or sound delivered through earphones to mask pain during dental or surgical procedures.

audiogenic (awd'ē-ō-jen'ik) [audio- + G. *genesis,* production]. **1.** Caused by sound, especially a loud noise. **2.** Sound-producing.

audiogram (aw'dē-ō-gram) [audio- + G. *gramma,* a drawing]. The graphic record drawn from the results of hearing tests with the audiometer, charts the threshold of hearing at various frequencies against sound intensity in decibels.
pure tone a., a chart of the threshold for hearing acuity at various frequencies usually expressed in decibels above normal threshold and usually covering frequencies from 128 to 8000 Hz.
speech a., the record of thresholds for spondaic word lists and scores for phonetically balanced word lists.

audiologist (aw-dē-ol'ōjist). A specialist in evaluation, habitation, and rehabilitation of those whose communication disorders center in whole or in part in the hearing function.

audiology (aw-dē-ol'ō-jē). The study of hearing disorders through the identification and measurement of hearing function loss as well as the rehabilitation of persons with hearing impairments.

audiometer (aw-dē-om'ĕ-ter) [audio- + G. *metron,* measure]. An electrical instrument for measuring the threshold of hearing for pure tones of frequencies generally varying from 200 to 8000 Hz (recorded in terms of decibels). It also records thresholds for lists of spoken words and discrimination percentage for phonetically balanced word lists.
automatic a., an a. that is operated by the patient, enabling him to control the intensity of the tone presented to him and thus track his own hearing thresholds.
Békésy a., an automatic a. in which the tone sweeps the audiometric scale while the patient controls intensity by pressing a button when he cannot hear the tone; may be operated either at a fixed frequency or at steadily changing frequencies.
group a., an a. designed to test the hearing of a group of people simultaneously, using more than one pair of headsets; used in screening procedures.
limited range a., a pure-tone a. designed to test restricted ranges of frequency and sound pressure.
pure-tone a., an electroacoustical generator which produces pure tones of selected frequencies and calibrated output.
speech a., an a. that provides spoken material at controlled sound pressure levels to obtain speech reception thresholds, tolerance for loud speech, and discrimination ability, utilizing either a live voice with a microphone or a recorded voice played over a turntable or tape recorder.
wide range a., a pure-tone a. which measures the major portion of the human auditory range in frequency and sound pressure level; used primarily for clinical and diagnostic purposes, and for determining hearing thresholds of children.

audiometric (aw'dē-ō-met'rik). Related to measurement of hearing levels.

audiometrician (aw'dē-ō-me-trish'ăn). A person specialized in the measurement of hearing levels.

audiometrist (aw-dē-om'ĕ-trist). A person trained in the use of the audiometer in testing hearing acuity.

audiometry (aw-dē-om'ĕ-trē). Use of the audiometer.
auditory brainstem response (ABR) a., brainstem evoked response a.; an electrophysiologic measure of auditory function utilizing responses produced by the auditory nerve and the brainstem.
automatic a., an audiometric technique using an automatic audiometer, which enables the patient to track his own hearing thresholds by controlling the intensity of the signal being presented to him, while the audiometer sweeps through the audible frequency range.
Békésy a., automatic a. utilizing the Békésy audiometer; the patient makes two threshold tracings, one in which the tone is rapidly turned on and off (interrupted tone) and one in which the tone is presented steadily (continuous tone); results may be suggestive of middle-ear, cochlear, or eighth nerve lesions.
brainstem evoked response (BSER) a., auditory brainstem response a.
cortical a., measurement of the potentials that arise in the auditory system above the level of the brainstem.
diagnostic a., measurement of hearing threshold levels to determine the nature and degree of hearing loss (*e.g.,* conductive, sensorineural, or mixed).
electrodermal a., a form of electrophysiologic a. used to deter-

mine hearing thresholds by measuring changes in skin resistance as a conditioned response to noise stimuli.

electrophysiologic a., measurement of a patient's response to a sound stimulus by using various types of objective audiometric equipment or techniques without necessarily having the patient's conscious cooperation.

evoked response a. (ERA), a type of electrophysiologic a. in which electrical potentials of neural impulses from the cochlear nerve and various levels in the brainstem are used to localize the site of a lesion causing a hearing loss.

group a., simultaneous testing of a group of people, using either pure tones or speech presented in such a way that each person may give reliable information regarding the test items heard.

pure-tone a., a. utilizing tones of various frequencies and intensities as auditory stimuli to measure hearing, including comparisons of results from testing air conduction and bone conduction.

screening a., rapid measurement of the hearing of an individual or a group against a predetermined limit of normalcy; auditory responses to different frequencies presented at a constant intensity level are tested.

speech a., measurement of overall performance in hearing, understanding, and responding to speech for a general assessment of hearing and an estimate of degree of practical handicap.

audiovisual (aw'dē-ō-vizh'yū-ăl). Pertaining to a communication or teaching technique that combines both audible and visible symbols.

audition (aw-dish'ŭn). Hearing.

chromatic a., color *hearing.*

gustatory a., a form of synesthesia in which a sensation of taste is noted when certain sounds are heard.

auditive (aw'di-tiv). Audile (3); one who recalls most readily that which has been heard.

auditory (aw'di-tōr-ē) [L. *audio,* pp. *auditus,* to hear]. Pertaining to the sense of hearing or to the organs of hearing.

Auenbrugger, Leopold, Austrian physician, 1722–1809. See A.'s *sign.*

Auer, John, U.S. physician, 1875–1948. See A. *bodies, rods.*

Auerbach, Leopold, German anatomist, 1828–1897. See A.'s *ganglion, plexus.*

Aufrecht, Emanuel, German physician, 1844–1933. See A.'s *sign.*

augnathus (awg-nath'ŭs) [G. *au,* again, + *gnathos,* jaw]. Dignathus.

Aujeszky, Aládar, Hungarian pathologist, 1869–1933. See A.'s *disease,* disease *virus.*

aura, pl. **au'rae** (aw'ră, -rē) [L. breeze, odor, gleam of light]. The beginning of a seizure as recognized by the patient, characterized by a peculiar sensation, often an epigastric feeling which may ascend to the head, or by sensory phenomena such as noises in the ears, flashes of light, vertigo, etc., or more complex experiences of a bizarre nature, called auditory, epigastric, vertiginous, etc., depending on its origin or characteristics.

intellectual a., reminiscent a.; a dreamy, detached, or reminiscent mental state preceding an epileptic seizure.

kinesthetic a., a feeling of movement of a part of the body when no movement occurs.

reminescent a., intellectual a.

aural (aw'răl). **1.** Relating to the ear (auris). **2.** Relating to an aura.

auramine O (aw'ră-mēn) [C.I. 41000]. A yellow fluorescent dye, $C_{17}H_{22}N_3Cl$, used as a stain for the tubercle bacillus and as a stain for DNA in Kasten's fluorescent Feulgen stain.

auranofin (aw-ran'ō-fin). $C_{20}H_{34}AuO_9PS$; a compound of radiogold colloid used to treat rheumatoid arthritis.

aurantiasis cutis (aw-ran-tī'ă-sis kyū'tis) [L. *aurantium,* orange, + G. *-iasis,* condition; *cutis,* skin]. Carotenosis cutis.

aureolic acid (aw-rē-ō'lik). Mithramycin.

auri- [L. *auris,* ear]. Combining form denoting the ear. See also ot-, oto-.

auriasis (aw-rī'ă-sis). Chrysiasis.

auric (aw'rik). Relating to gold (aurum).

auricle (aw'ri-kl). Auricula.

accessory a.'s, small, fleshy nodules or folds, sometimes with supporting cartilage, occasionally found along the margins of the embryonic branchial clefts.

atrial a., *auricula* atrialis.

cervical a., accessory a. on the neck.

left a., *auricula* sinistra.

right a., *auricula* dextra.

auricula, pl. **auriculae** (aw-rik'yū-lă, -lē) [L. the external ear, dim. of *auris,* ear]. Auricle. **1** [NA]. Pinna (1); ala auris; the projecting shell-like structure on the side of the head, constituting, with the external acoustic meatus, the external ear. **2.** A. atrialis.

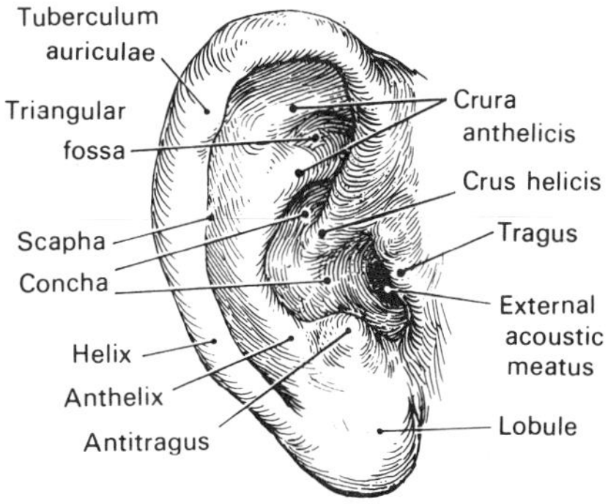

Auricle of the Ear

atrial a., a. atrialis.

a. a'tria'lis [NA], atrial a.; auricula (2); auricle; auricular appendage (1); auricular appendix; a small conical pouch projecting from the upper anterior portion of each atrium of the heart.

a. dex'tra [NA], right auricle; right auricular appendage; the small conical projection from the right atrium of the heart.

a. sinis'tra [NA], left auricle; left auricular appendage; the small conical projection from the left atrium of the heart.

auricular (aw-rik'yū-lăr). Relating to the ear, or to an auricle in any sense.

auriculare, pl. **auricularia** (aw-rik-yū-lā'rē, -rē-ă) [L. *auricularis,* pertaining to the ear]. Auricular point; a craniometric point at the center of the opening of the external acoustic meatus; or, in certain cases, the middle of the upper edge of this opening.

auriculocranial (aw-rik'yū-lō-krā'nē-ăl). Relating to the auricle or pinna of the ear and the cranium.

auriculotemporal (aw-rik'yū-lō-tem'pō-răl). Relating to the auricle or pinna of the ear and the temporal region.

auriculoventricular (aw-rik'yū-lō-ven-trik'yū-lăr). Obsolete synonym for atrioventricular.

aurid, pl. **aurides** (aw'rid, aw'ri-dēz) [L. *aurum,* gold, + *-id* (1)]. A skin lesion due to injection of gold salts.

auriform (aw'ri-fōrm). Ear-shaped.

aurin (aw'rin) [C.I. 43800]. Corallin; *p*- rosolic acid; a triphenylmethane derivative used as an indicator (changes from yellow to red at pH 6.8 to 8.2) and as a dye intermediate; also used to help differentiate tubercle bacilli from other acid-fast microorganisms.

aurintricarboxylic acid (aw'rin-trī'kar-boks-il'ik). Tris(3-carboxy-4-hydroxyphenyl)methane; a chelating agent that has a special affinity for beryllium and certain other materials, and may therefore be of use in combating beryllium poisoning; the ammonium salt is known as aluminon.

auris, pl. **aures** (aw'ris, aw'rēz) [L.] [NA]. Ear.
a. exte'rna [NA], external ear. See ear. See also auricula; external acoustic *meatus;* pinna.
a. inter'na [NA], internal ear. See ear. See also labyrinth; labyrinthus.
a. me'dia [NA], middle ear. See ear. See also *cavitas* tympanica.

auriscope (aw'ri-skōp) [L. *auris,* ear, + *skopeō,* to view]. Otoscope.

aurochromoderma (aw'rō-krō-mō-der'mă) [L. *aurum,* gold, + *chrōma,* color, + derma, skin]. Chrysiasis.

auromercaptoacetanilid (aw'rō-mer-kap'tō-as-ĕ-tan'i-lid). Aurothioglycanide; {[(phenylcarbamoyl)methyl]thio}gold; $AuSCH_2$-$CONH$–C_6H_5; an organic gold compound, insoluble in water; used in the treatment of rheumatoid arthritis, and administered by intramuscular injection; more slowly absorbed than the water-soluble gold salts.

aurone (aw'rōn). Benzalcoumaran-3-one; 2-benzylidene-3(2*H*)-benzofuranone; the parent compound of a series of plant pigments; they are substituted coumaranones, and may be formed from chalcones.

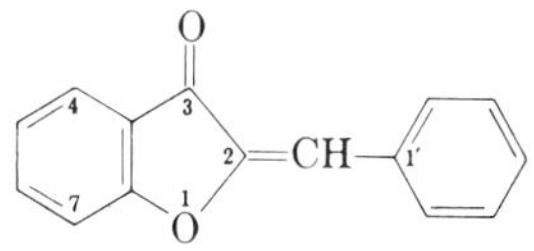

Aurone

aurotherapy (aw-rō-thăr'ă-pē) [L. *aurum,* gold]. Chrysotherapy.

aurothioglucose (aw'rō-thī-ō-glū'kōs). Gold thioglucose; organic gold preparation with –SAu group in place of 1-OH group of glucose; used in rheumatoid arthritis and nondisseminated lupus erythematosus.

aurothioglycanide (aw'-rō-thī-ō-glī'kă-nīd). Auromercaptoacetanilid.

aurum (aw'rŭm) [L.]. Gold.

auscultate, auscult (aws'kŭl-tāt, aws-kŭlt'). To perform auscultation.

auscultation (aws-kŭl-tā'shŭn) [L. *ausculto,* pp. *-atus,* to listen to]. Listening to the sounds made by the various body structures as a diagnostic method.
immediate a., direct a., a. by application of the ear to the surface of the body.
mediate a., a. performed with the use of a stethoscope.

auscultatory (aws-kŭl'tă-tō-rē). Relating to auscultation.

Austin Flint. See Flint, Austin.

aut-. See auto-.

autecic, autecious (aw-tē'sik, aw-tē'shŭs) [G. *autos,* same, + *oikion,* house]. Denoting a parasite that infects, throughout its entire existence, the same host.

autemesia (aw-tĕ-mē'zē-ă) [G. *autos,* self, + *emesis,* vomiting]. **1.** Idiopathic or functional vomiting. **2.** Vomiting induced by provoking the gag reflex.

authenticity (aw-then-tis'i-tē) [G. *authentikōs,* original, primary]. **1.** The quality of being authentic, genuine, and valid. **2.** In psychological functioning and personality, applied to the conscious feelings, perceptions, and thoughts that one expresses and communicates.

autism (aw'tizm) [G. *autos,* self]. A tendency to morbid self-absorption at the expense of regulation by outward reality.
infantile a., Kanner's syndrome; a severe emotional disturbance of childhood characterized by qualitative impairment in reciprocal social interaction and in communication, language, and symbolic development.

autistic (aw-tis'tik). Pertaining to or characterized by autism.

auto-, aut- [G. *autos,* self]. Prefixes meaning self, same.

autoactivation (aw'tō-ak-ti-vā'shŭn). Autocatalysis.

autoagglutination (aw'to-ă-glū-ti-nā'shŭn). **1.** Nonspecific agglutination or clumping together of cells (*e.g.,* bacteria, erythrocytes) due to physical-chemical factors. **2.** The agglutination of an individual's red blood cells in his own serum, as a consequence of specific autoantibody.

autoagglutinin (aw'tō-ă-glū'ti-nin). An agglutinating autoantibody.
anti-Pr cold a., a cold a. specific for the Pr (protease-sensitive) antigen of erythrocytes.
cold a., a heterogeneous group of autoantibodies that react at temperatures below 37°C, often most actively at 4°C; most are the IgM class of immunoglobulins with affinity for the Ii system of erythrocyte antigens, but some are anti-Pr cold a.'s; cold a.'s may be associated with infection (*e.g.,* primary atypical pneumonia, infectious mononucleosis and other virus infections, certain protozoan infections) and in such instances usually are not active *in vivo* (*i.e.,* they usually do not cause cold hemagglutinin disease); cold a.'s that are associated with cold hemagglutinin disease may be secondary to lymphoreticular neoplasms and may be monoclonal; positive direct antiglobulin tests are due to erythrocyte-fixed complement.

autoallergic (aw'tō-ă-ler'jik). Pertaining to autoallergy.

autoallergization (aw'tō-al'er-ji-zā'shŭn). Induction of autoallergy.

autoallergy (aw-tō-al'er-jē). An altered reactivity in which antibodies (autoantibodies) are produced against an individual's own tissues, causing a destructive rather than a protective effect.

autoanalysis (aw'tō-ă-nal'i-sis). Self-analysis; attempted analysis, or psychoanalysis, of one's self.

autoanalyzer (aw-tō-an'ă-līz-er). An instrument capable of conducting analyses automatically; commonly used in chemical analyses.
sequential multichannel a. (SMA), an automated instrument capable of performing multiple (usually chemical) analyses simultaneously by propelling samples and reagents in continuous flow fashion along tubes to the detector mechanisms.

autoanaphylaxis (aw'tō-an'ă-fī-lak'sis). Old term for certain kinds of autoallergy.

autoantibody (aw-tō-an'ti-bod-ē). Antibody occurring in response to antigenic constituents of the host's tissue, and which reacts with the inciting tissue component.
anti-idiotype a., idiotype a.; an a., the specificity of which is directed against one of one's own idiotypes. See also anti-idiotype *antibody.*
cold a., an a. that reacts at temperatures below 37°c.
Donath-Landsteiner cold a., cold hemolysin; an a. of the IgG class responsible for paroxysmal cold hemoglobinuria; it is adsorbed to red cells only at temperatures of 20°C or lower, causing the red cells to lyse in the presence of complement at higher temperatures; it has only slight agglutinating properties in spite of its marked lytic activity, and has a specificity within the blood group P; it is also occasionally present for short periods of time following measles and other infections, and formerly was frequently associated with syphilis.
hemagglutinating cold a., a cold autoagglutinin, with somewhat less affinity for complement than the Donath-Landsteiner type, that causes cold-hemagglutinin disease.

idiotype a., anti-idiotype a.

warm a., an a. that reacts optimally at 37°C.

autoanticomplement (aw'tō-an-ti-com'plĕ-ment). An anticomplement that is formed in the body of an animal and inhibits or destroys the complement of the same animal.

autoantigen (aw-to-an'ti-jen). A "self" antigen; any tissue constituent that evokes an immune response to the host's tissues.

autoassay (aw'tō-as-ā). Detection or estimation of the amount of a substance produced in an organism by means of a test object in that organism, as, for example, use of the denervated heart *in situ* of a cat to assay for epinephrine or sympathin liberated into its bloodstream.

autoblast (aw'tō-blast) [auto- + G. *blastos,* germ]. **1.** An independent cell. **2.** A single, independent microbe, protozoon, or single-celled (acellular) organism.

autocatalysis (aw'tō-kă-tal'i-sis). Autoactivation; a reaction in which one or more of the products formed acts to catalyze the reaction; beginning slowly, the rate of such a reaction rapidly increases. *Cf.* chain *reaction.*

autocatalytic (aw'tō-kat-ă-lit'ik). Relating to autocatalysis.

autocatheterization, autocatheterism (aw'tō-kath-ĕ-ter-i-zā'shŭn, -kath'ĕ-ter-izm). Passage of a catheter by the patient.

autochthonous (aw-tok'thon-ŭs) [auto- + G. *chthon,* land, ground, country]. **1.** Native to the place inhabited; aboriginal. **2.** Originating in the place where found; said of a disease originating in the part of the body where found, or of a disease acquired in the place where the patient is.

autoclasis, autoclasia (aw-tok'lă-sis, aw-tō-klā'zē-ă) [auto- + G. *klasis,* breaking]. **1.** A breaking up or rupturing from intrinsic or internal causes. **2.** Progressive immunologically induced tissue destruction.

autoclave (aw'tō-klāv) [auto- + L. *clavis,* a key, in the sense of self-locking]. **1.** An apparatus for sterilization by steam under pressure; it consists of a strong closed boiler containing a small quantity of water and, in a wire basket, the articles to be sterilized. **2.** To sterilize in an autoclave.

autocoid (aw'tō-koyd) [G. *autos,* self, + *eidos,* form]. A chemical substance functioning as produced by one type of cell which affects the function of different types of cells in the same region, thus functioning as a local hormone or messenger.

autocrine (aw'tō-krin) [auto- + G. *krinō,*to separate]. Denoting self-stimulation through cellular production of a factor and a specific receptor for it.

autocystoplasty (aw-tō-sis'tō-plas-tē) [auto- + G. *kystis,* bladder, + *plastos,* formed]. Autoplasty of the bladder.

autocytolysin (aw'tō-sī-tol'i-sin). Autolysin.

autocytolysis (aw'tō-sī-tol'i-sis). Autolysis.

autocytotoxin (aw'tō-sī-tō-toks'in). A cytotoxic autoantibody.

autodermic (aw-tō-der'mik) [auto- + G. *derma,* skin]. Relating to one's own skin; denoting especially an autodermic graft or dermatoautoplasty.

autodigestion (aw'tō-dī-jes'chŭn). Autolysis.

autodiploid (aw-tō-dip'loyd). See autoploid.

autodrainage (aw-tō-drān'ij). Drainage into contiguous tissues.

autoecholalia (aw'tō-ek-ō-lā'lē-ă) [auto- + echolalia]. Repetition of some or all the words in one's statements.

autoerotic (aw'tō-ĕ-rot'ik). Pertaining to autoerotism.

autoeroticism (aw'tō-ĕ-rot'i-sizm). Autoerotism.

autoerotism (aw-tō-ār'ō-tizm) [auto- + G. *erōtikos,* relating to love]. Autoeroticism; autosexualism(1). **1.** Sexual arousal or gratification using one's own body, as in masturbation. **2.** Sexual self-love. *Cf.* alloerotism. See also narcissism.

autofluoroscope (aw-tō-flūr'ō-skōp). A type of scintillation camera consisting of a matrix of individual sodium iodide crystals, each with their separate light pipe and photomultiplier tube; used for radioisotope scanning procedures.

autogamous (aw-tog'ă-mŭs). Relating to or characterized by autogamy.

autogamy (aw-tog'ă-mē) [auto- + G. *gamos,* marriage]. Automixis; a form of self-fertilization in which fission of the cell nucleus occurs without division of the cell, the two pronuclei so formed reuniting to form the synkaryon; in other cases, the cell body also divides, but the two daughter cells immediately conjugate.

autogenesis (aw-tō-jen'ĕ-sis) [auto- + G. *genesis,* production]. **1.** The origin of living matter within the organism itself. **2.** In bacteriology, the process by which vaccine is made from bacteria obtained from the patient's own body.

autogenetic, autogenic (aw'tō-jĕ-net'ik, jen'ik). Autogenous (1); relating to autogenesis.

autogenous (aw-toj'ĕ-nŭs) [G. *autogenēs,* self-produced]. **1.** Autogenetic. **2.** Originating within the body, applied to vaccines prepared from bacteria obtained from the affected person. *Cf.* endogenous.

autognosis (aw-tog-nō'sis) [auto- + G. *gnōsis,* knowledge]. Self-knowledge; recognition of one's own character, tendencies, and peculiarities.

autograft (aw'tō-graft) [auto- + A.S. *graef*]. Autoplast; autotransplant; autogeneic, autologous, or autoplastic graft; a tissue or an organ transferred by grafting into a new position in the body of the same individual.

autografting (aw-tō-graft'ing). Autotransplantation.

autogram (aw'tō-gram) [auto- + G. *gramma,* something written]. A wheal-like lesion on the skin following pressure by a blunt instrument or by stroking.

autographism (aw-tog'ră-fism). Dermatographism.

autohemagglutination (aw'tō-hē'mă-glū-ti-nā'shŭn). Autoagglutination of erythrocytes.

autohemolysin (aw'tō-hē-mol'i-sin). An autoantibody that in the presence of complement causes lysis of erythrocytes in the same individual in whose body the lysin is formed.

autohemolysis (aw'tō-hē-mol'i-sis). Hemolysis occurring in certain diseases as a result of an autohemolysin.

autohemotherapy (aw'tō-hē-mō-thār'ă-pē). Treatment of disease by the withdrawal and reinjection of the patient's own blood.

autohemotransfusion (aw'tō-hē-mō-tranz-fyū'zhŭn). Autotransfusion.

autohexaploid (aw-tō-heks'ă-ployd). See autoploid.

autohypnosis (aw'tō-hip-nō'sis). Autohypnotism; statuvolence; idiohypnotism; self-induced hypnosis, accomplished by concentrating on self-absorbing thought or on the idea of being hypnotized.

autohypnotic (aw'tō-hip-not'ik). Relating to autohypnosis.

autohypnotism (aw-tō-hip'nō-tizm). Autohypnosis.

autoimmune (aw-tō-i-myūn'). Arising from and directed against the individual's own tissues, as in autoimmune disease.

autoimmunity (aw'tō-i-myū'ni-tē). **1.** Literally, the condition in which "self" is exempt. **2.** In immunology, the condition in which one's own tissues are subject to deleterious effects of the immune system, as in autoallergy and in autoimmune disease.

autoimmunization (aw'tō-im'yū-ni-zā'shŭn). Induction of autoimmunity.

autoimmunocytopenia (aw-tō-im'yū-nō-sī-tō-pē'nē-ă). Anemia, thrombocytopenia, and leukopenia resulting from cytotoxic autoimmune reactions.

autoinfection (aw'tō-in-fek'shŭn). Autoreinfection; self-infection. **1.** Reinfection by microbes or parasitic organisms on or within the body that have already passed through an infective cycle, such as a succession of boils, or a new infective cycle with production of a new generation of larvae and adults, as by the nematode *Strongyloides stercoralis* or the cestode *Hymenolepsis nana.* **2.** Self-infection by direct contagion as with parasite eggs passed in the infectious state transmitted by fingernails (anal-oral route), as with the pinworm, *Enterobius vermicularis.*

autoinfusion (aw'tō-in-fyū'shŭn). Forcing the blood from the extremities, as by the application of a bandage or pressure device, to raise the blood pressure and fill the vessels in the vital centers; resorted to after excessive loss of blood or other body fluids. *Cf.* autotransfusion.

autoinoculable (aw'tō-in-ok'yū-lă-bl). Susceptible to autoinoculation.

autoinoculation (aw'tō-in-ok-yū-lā'shŭn). A secondary infection originating from a focus of infection already present in the body.

autointoxicant (aw'tō-in-toks'i-kant). Autotoxin; an endogenous toxic agent that causes autointoxication.

autointoxication (aw'tō-in-toks-i-kā'shŭn). Self-poisoning; autotoxicosis; enterotoxication; enterotoxism; endogenic toxicosis; intestinal intoxication; a disorder resulting from absorption of the waste products of metabolism, decomposed matter from the intestine, or the products of dead and infected tissue as in gangrene.

autoisolysin (aw'tō-ī-sol'i-sin). An antibody that in the presence of complement causes lysis of cells in the individual in whose body the lysin is formed, as well as in others of the same species.

autokeratoplasty (aw-tō-ker'ă-tō-plas-tē) [auto- + G. *keras,* horn, + *plassō,* formed]. Grafting of corneal tissue from one eye of a patient to the fellow eye.

autokinesia, autokinesis (aw-tō-ki-ne'sē-ă, aw-tō-ki-nē'sis) [auto- + G. *kinēsis,* movement]. Voluntary movement.

autokinetic (aw-tō-kĭ-net'ik). Relating to autokinesis.

autolesion (aw-tō-lē'zhŭn). A self-inflicted injury.

autologous (as-tol'ō-gŭs) [auto- + G. *logos,* relation]. **1.** Occurring naturally and normally in a certain type of tissue or in a specific structure of the body. **2.** Sometimes used to denote a neoplasm derived from cells that occur normally at that site, *e.g.,* a squamous cell carcinoma in the esophagus. **3.** In transplantation, referring to a graft in which the donor and recipient areas are in the same individual.

autolysate (aw-tol'i-sāt). The mixture of substances resulting from autolysis.

autolyse (aw'tō-līs). Autolyze.

autolysin (aw-tol'i-sin). Autocytolysin; an antibody that in the presence of complement causes lysis of the cells and tissues in the body of the individual in whom the lysin is formed.

autolysis (aw-tol'i-sis) [auto- + G. *lysis,* dissolution]. Autocytolysis, autodigestion; isophagy. **1.** Enzymatic digestion of cells (especially dead or degenerate) by enzymes present within them (autogenous). **2.** Destruction of cells as a result of a lysin formed in those cells or others in the same organism.

autolytic (aw-tō-lit'ik). Pertaining to or causing autolysis.

autolyze (aw'tō-līz). Autolyse; to undergo autolysis.

automallet (aw'tō-mal-et). Obsolete term for automatic *plugger.*

automatism (aw-tom'ă-tizm). Telergy. **1.** The state of being independent of the will or of central innervation, applicable, for example, to the heart's action. **2.** An epileptic attack consisting of stereotyped psychic, sensory, or motor phenomena carried out in a state of impaired consciousness and of which the individual usually has no knowledge. **3.** A condition in which an individual is consciously or unconsciously, but involuntarily, compelled to the performance of certain motor or verbal acts, often purposeless and sometimes foolish or harmful.

ambulatory a., a person's automatic performance of an action or series of actions without being consciously aware of the processes involved in the performance.

immediate posttraumatic a., a posttraumatic state in which the patient performs automatically without immediate or later memory of that behavior.

automatograph (aw-tō-mat'ō-graf). An instrument for recording automatic movements.

automixis (aw-tō-miks'is) [auto- + G. *mixis,* intercourse]. Autogamy.

automnesia (aw-tom-nē'zē-ă) [auto- + G. *mnēsis,* a remembering]. Spontaneous revival of memories of an earlier condition of life.

automysophobia (aw'tō-mis-ō-fō'bē-ă) [auto- + G. *mysos,* dirt, + *phobos,* fear]. Morbid dread of personal uncleanliness.

autonomic (aw-tō-nom'ik). **1.** Relating to the autonomic nervous system. **2.** Obsolete term for autonomous.

autonomotropic (aw'tō-nom-ō-trop'ik) [autonomic + G. *trepein,* to turn]. Acting on the autonomic nervous system.

autonomous (aw-ton'ō-mŭs). Having independence or freedom from control by external forces or, in a narrow sense, by the cerebrospinal nerve centers.

autonomy (aw-ton'ō-mē) [auto- + G. *nomos,* law]. The condition or state of being autonomous.

functional a., in social psychology, the tendency of a developed motive system (*e.g.,* motive of acquisition) to become independent of the primary or innate drive from which it originated (*e.g.,* need for food).

auto-oxidation (aw'tō-oks-i-dā'shŭn). Autoxidation; the direct combination of a substance with molecular oxygen at ordinary temperatures.

auto-oxidizable (aw'tō-oks-i-dīz'ă-bl). Denoting substances that react directly with oxygen (*e.g., b* hemochromogen in cytochrome) and do not require the action of dehydrogenases.

autopathic (aw-tō-path'ik). Rarely used synonym for idiopathic.

autopentaploid (aw-tō-pen'tă-ployd). See autoploid.

autopepsia (aw-tō-pep'sē-ă) [auto- + G. *pepsis,* digestion]. Self-digestion, said of ulceration of the gastric mucous membrane by its own secretion, or the digestion of the skin surrounding a gastrostomy or colostomy opening.

autophagia (aw-tō-fā'jē-ă) [auto- + G. *phagein,* to eat]. **1.** Biting one's own flesh; *e.g.,* as a symptom of Lesch-Nyhan syndrome. **2.** Maintenance of the nutrition of the whole body by metabolic consumption of some of the body tissues. **3.** Autophagy.

autophagic (aw-tō-fā'jik). Relating to or characterized by autophagia.

autophagolysosome (aw'tō-fā-gō-lī'sō-sōm). The digestive vacuole of autophagy which results from the fusion of a primary lysosome with an autophagic vacuole.

autophagy (aw-tof'ă-jē) [auto- + G. *phagein,* to eat]. Autophagia (3); segregation and disposal of damaged organelles within a cell.

autophilia (aw-tō-fil'ē-ă) [auto- + G. *phileō,* to love]. Narcissism (1).

autophobia (aw-tō-fō'bē-ă) [auto- + G. *phobos,* fear]. Morbid fear of solitude or of self.

autophony (aw-tof'ō-nē) [auto- + G. *phōnē,* sound]. Tympanophonia (2); increased resonance of one's own voice, breath sounds, arterial murmurs, etc., noted especially in disease of the middle ear or of the nasal fossae.

autoplast (aw'tō-plast) [auto- + G. *plastos,* formed]. Autograft.

autoplastic (aw'tō-plas-tik). Relating to autoplasty.

autoplasty (aw'tō-plas-tē). Repair of defects by autotransplantation.

autoploid (aw'tō-ployd) [auto- + -ploid]. Relating to an individual or cell with two or more sets of chromosomes derived from duplication of a single haploid set; depending on the number of multiples of the haploid set, a.'s are referred to as autodiploids, autotriploids, autotetraploids, autopentaploids, autohexaploids, etc.

autoploidy (aw'tō-ploy-dē). The condition of being autoploid.

autoplugger (aw'tō-plŭg-er). Obsolete term for automatic *plugger.*

autopod (aw'tō-pod). Autopodium.

autopodium, pl. **autopodia** (aw'tō-pō'dē-ŭm, dē-ă) [auto- + G. *pous (pod-),* foot]. Autopod; the distal major subdivision of a limb (hand or foot).

autopoisonous (aw-tō-poy'zŭn-ŭs). Autotoxic.

autopolymer (aw-tō-pol'i-mer). See autopolymer *resin.*

autopolymerization (aw-tō-pol'i-mer-i-zā'shŭn). Polymerization without the use of external heat, as a result of the addition of an activator and a catalyst.

autopolyploid (aw-tō-pol'i-ployd). An autoploid having two or more multiples of the haploid set of chromosomes.

autopolyploidy (aw-tō-pol'i-ploy-dē). The condition of being allopolyploid.

autopsy (aw'top-sē) [G. *autopsia,* seeing with one's own eyes]. **1.** Postmortem examination; necropsy; necroscopy; thanatopsy; an examination of the organs of a dead body to determine the cause of death or to study the pathologic changes present. **2.** In the terminology of the ancient Greek school of empirics, the intentional reproduction of an effect, event, or circumstance that occurred in the course of a disease and observation of its influence in ameliorating or aggravating the patient's symptoms.

autoradiogram (aw-tō-rā'dē-ō-gram). Autoradiograph.

autoradiograph (aw-tō-rā'dē-ō-graf). Autoradiogram; reproduction of the distribution and concentration of radioactivity in a tissue or other substance made by placing a photographic emulsion on the surface of, or in close proximity to, the substance.

autoradiography aw'tō-rā-dē-og'ră-fē). Radioautography; the process of producing an autoradiograph.

autoregulation (aw'tō-reg-yū-lā'shŭn). **1.** The tendency of the blood flow to an organ or part to remain at or return to the same level despite changes in the pressure in the artery which conveys blood to it. **2.** In general, any biologic system equipped with inhibitory feedback systems such that a given change tends to be largely or completely counteracted; *e.g.,* baroreceptor reflexes form a basis for autoregulation of the systemic arterial blood pressure.

heterometric a., the a. of the strength of contraction of the ventricle that occurs in direct relation to the end-diastolic fiber length in accordance with Starling's law of the heart.

homeometric a., the a. of strength of contraction of the ventricle by mechanisms or agents (*e.g.,* the staircase phenomenon or treppe, sympathetic nerves, norepinephrine) that do not depend upon change in the end-diastolic fiber length.

autoreinfection (aw'tō-rē-in-fek'shŭn). Autoinfection.

autoreproduction (aw'tō-rē-prō-duk'shŭn). Replication (2); the ability of a gene or virus, or nucleoprotein molecule generally, to bring about the synthesis of another molecule like itself from smaller molecules within the cell.

autorrhaphy (aw-tōr'ă-fē) [auto- + G. *raphē,* sewing]. Wound closure using strands of fascia from the edges of the wound.

autosensitize (aw-tō-sen'si-tīz). Isosensitize; to sensitize against one's own body cells.

autosepticemia (aw'tō-sep-ti-sē'mē-ă) [auto- + G. *sēpsis,* decay, + *haima,* blood]. Septicemia apparently originating from microorganisms existing within the individual and not introduced from without.

autoserotherapy (aw'tō-sē-rō-thār'ă-pē). Autotherapy (3); the treatment of certain conditions, such as dermatoses, by injection of the patient's own blood serum.

autoserum (aw-tō-sē'rŭm). Serum obtained from the patient's own blood and used in autoserotherapy.

autosexualism (aw-tō-sek'shū-ă-lizm). **1.** Autoerotism. **2.** Narcissism.

autosite (aw'tō-sīt) [auto- + G. *sitos,* food]. That member of abnormal, unequal conjoined twins that is able to live independently and nourish the other member (parasite) of the pair.

autosmia (aw-toz'mē-ă) [auto- + G. *osmē,* smell]. The smelling of one's own body odor.

autosomal (aw-tō-sō'măl). Pertaining to an autosome.

autosomatognosis (aw-tō-sō'mă-tog-nō'sis) [auto- + G. *sōma,* body, + *gnōsis,* recognition]. The sensation that an amputated portion of the body is still present. See phantom limb.

autosomatognostic (aw-to-sō'mă-tog-nos'tik). Pertaining to autosomatognosis.

autosome (aw'tō-sōm) [auto- + G. *sōma,* body]. Euchromosome; any chromosome other than a sex chromosome; a.'s normally occur in pairs in somatic cells and singly in gametes.

autosuggestibility (aw'tō-sŭg-jes-tĭ-bil'i-tē). A mental state in which autosuggestion (1) readily occurs.

autosuggestion (aw'tō-sŭg-jes'chŭn). **1.** Constant dwelling upon an idea or concept, thereby inducing some change in the mental or bodily functions. See also autohypnosis. **2.** Reproduction in the brain of impressions previously received which become then the starting point of new acts or ideas.

autosynnoia (aw'tō-sin-noy'ă) [auto- + G. *synnoia,* deep thought, fr. *syn,* with + *noeō,* to think]. Self-centeredness; a mental disorder in which one never has a thought not connected with himself.

autosynthesis (aw-tō-sin'thĕ-sis). Self-reproduction or -replication.

autotelic (aw-tō-tel'ik) [auto- + G. *telos,* end, completeness, purpose]. Denoting those traits closely associated with the central purposes of an individual.

autotemnous (aw-tō-tem'nŭs) [auto- + G. *temnō,* to cut]. Denoting a cell that propagates itself by fission without previous conjugation.

autotetraploid (aw-tō-tet'ră-ployd). See autoploid.

autotherapy (aw-tō-thār'ă-pē). **1.** Self-treatment. **2.** Spontaneous cure. **3.** Autoserotherapy. **4.** An obsolete method of treating disease by the administration of the patient's own pathologic excretions.

autotomy (aw-tot'ŏ-mē) [auto- + G. *tomē,* a cutting]. The act of casting off a body part as a means of escape; *e.g.,* the limb of a crab or the tail of a lizard.

autotopagnosia (aw'tō-top'ag-nō'zē-ă) [auto- + G. *topos,* place, + G. *a-* priv. + gnōsis]. Inability to recognize any part of one's own body; a condition resulting from a lesion of the dominant hemisphere. *Cf.* somatotopagnosis.

autotoxemia (aw'tō-tok-sē'mē-ă). Autointoxicants present in the blood, usually resulting in autointoxication.

autotoxic (aw-tō-toks'ik). Autopoisonous; relating to autointoxication.

autotoxicosis (aw'tō-tok-si-kō'sis). Autointoxication.

autotoxin (aw-tō-tok'sin). Autointoxicant.

autotransfusion (aw'tō-tranz-fyū'zhŭn). Autohemotransfusion; transfusing back into the body of blood removed. *Cf.* autoinfusion.

autotransplant (aw-tō-tranz'plant). Autograft.

autotransplantation (aw'tō-tranz-plan-tā'shŭn). Autografting; the performance of an autograft.

autotriploid (aw-tō-trip'loyd). See autoploid.

autotroph (aw'tō-trōf) [auto- + G. *trophē,* nourishment]. A microorganism which uses only inorganic materials as its source of nutrients; carbon dioxide serves as the sole carbon source.

autotrophic (aw-tō-trof'ik). Pertaining to an autotroph.

autovaccination (aw'tō-vak-si-nā'shŭn). A second vaccination with virus from a vaccine sore on the same individual.

autoxidation (aw-tok-si-dā'shŭn). Auto-oxidation.

autozygous (aw-tō-zī'gŭs) [auto- + G. *zygōtos,* yoked]. Denoting genes in a homozygote that are copies of the identical ancestral gene as a result of a consanguineous mating.

auxano-, aux-, auxo- [G. *auxanō,* to increase]. Prefix denoting relation to increase, *e.g.,* in size, intensity, speed.

auxanogram (awk-san'ō-gram) [auxano- + G. *gramma,* something written]. A plate culture of bacteria in which variable conditions are provided in order to determine the effect of these conditions on the growth of the bacteria.

auxanographic (awk'san-ō-graf'ik). Pertaining to auxanogram or auxanography.

auxanography (awk-san-og'ră-fē). The study, using auxanograms, of the effects of different conditions on the growth of bacteria.

auxanology (awk-san-ol'ō-jē) [auxano- + G. *logos,* study]. The study of growth.

auxesis (awk-sē'sis) [G. increase]. Increase in size, especially as in hypertrophy.

auxiliary (og-zil'yă-rē). **1.** Functioning in an augmenting capacity; supplementary. **2.** Functioning as a subordinate; secondary.

auxiliomotor (awg-zil'ē-ō-mō-tŏr). Aiding motion.

auxilytic (awk'si-lit'ik) [G. *auxō,* to increase, + *lysis,* dissolution]. Increasing the destructive power of a lysin, or favoring lysis.

auxo-. See auxano-.

auxocardia (awk-sō-kar'dē-ă) [auxo- + G. *kardia,* heart]. **1.** Enlargement of the heart, either hypertrophy or dilation. **2.** Cardiac *diastole.*

auxochrome (awk'sō-krōm) [auxo- + G. *chrōma,* color]. The chemical group within a dye molecule by which the dye is bound to reactive end groups in tissues.

auxodrome (awk'sō-drōm) [auxo- + G. *dromos,* course]. A course of growth as plotted on a Wetzel grid.

auxoflore (awk'sō-flōr). An atom or group of atoms that, by its presence in a molecule, shifts the latter's fluorescent radiation in the direction of the shorter wavelength, or increases the fluorescence. *Cf.* bathoflore.

auxogluc (awk'sō-gluk). An atomic grouping that, when present in a molecule, intensifies its sweetness.

auxometer (awks-om'ĕ-ter) [auxo- + G. *metron,* measure]. An instrument for measuring the magnifying power of a lens.

auxotonic (awk-sō-ton'ik). Denoting the condition in which a contracting muscle shortens against an increasing load. *Cf.* isometric (2); isotonic (3).

auxotox (awk'sō-toks). An atomic grouping that, when present in a molecule, intensifies its poisonous characteristics.

auxotroph (awk'sō-trōf) [auxo- + G. *trophē,* nourishment]. A mutant microorganism that requires some nutrient that is not required by the organism (prototroph) from which the mutant was derived.

auxotrophic (awk-sō-trof'ik, -trō'fik). Pertaining to an auxotroph.

A-V Abbreviation for arteriovenous; atrioventricular.

avalvular (ā-val'vyū-lăr). Nonvalvular; without valves.

avascular (ă-vas'kyū-ler, ā). Nonvascular; without blood or lymphatic vessels; may be a normal state as in certain forms of cartilage, or the result of disease.

avascularization (ă-vas'kyū-lar-ī-zā'shŭn, ā-). **1.** Expulsion of blood from a part, as by means of an Esmarch tourniquet or arterial compression. **2.** Loss of vascularity, as by scarring.

Avellis, Georg, German laryngologist, 1864–1916. See A.'s *syndrome.*

avenin (ă-vē'nin). Legumin; plant or vegetable casein; a prolamine, about 25% glutamic acid, found in oats (*Avena*) and in various legumes; considered highly nutritious.

Aviadenovirus (ā'vē-ad'ĕ-nō-vī'rŭs). A genus of viruses (family Adenoviridae) that includes types (species) of viruses found in birds.

avian (ā'vē-ăn) [L. *avis,* bird]. Pertaining to birds.

avidin (av'i-din). Antibiotin; a glycoprotein in nondenatured egg white that strongly binds biotin and prevents its absorption, thus leading to biotin deficiency; denaturation destroys the biotin-binding property.

Avipoxvirus (ā'vē-poks-vī'rŭs). The genus of viruses (family Poxviridae) that includes the poxviruses of birds, including canarypox and fowlpox viruses.

avirulent (ā-vir'yū-lent). Not virulent.

avitaminosis (ā-vī'tă-min-ō'sis). Properly, hypovitaminosis.
conditioned a., a. caused by any number of pathologic states or dysfunctions in which the supply of a vitamin absorbed by the body is inadequate for the needs under particular circumstances; *e.g.,* the reduced bacterial synthesis of the vitamins in the alimentary canal produced by antibiotic agents.

avivement (ah-vēv-maw') [Fr. *aviver,* to quicken, revive]. Excision of the edges of a wound to assist the healing process.

Avogadro, Amadeo, Italian physicist, 1776–1856. See A.'s *constant, hypothesis, law, number, postulate.*

avoirdupois (av'er-du-poyz') [Fr. to have weight, corrupted fr. O. Fr. *avoir,* property, + *de,* of, + *pois,* weight]. A system of weights in which 16 ounces make a pound, equivalent of 453.6 g. See Weights and Measures appendix.

AVP Abbreviation for antiviral *protein.*

avulsion (ă-vŭl'shŭn) [L. *a-vello,* pp. *-vulsus,* to tear away]. A tearing away or forcible separation. *Cf.* evulsion.
a. of caruncula lacrimalis, laceration of the inner one-sixth of the lower eyelid with rupture of the canaliculus lacrimalis.
nerve a., the pulling out of a portion of a nerve to produce a lasting paralysis, *e.g.,* a phrenic nerve a. to paralyze the diaphragm and collapse the lung.
tooth a., the traumatic separation of a tooth from its alveolus.

AW Abbreviation for atomic *weight.*

ax Abbreviation for axis.

Axenfeld, K. Theodor P.P., German ophthalmologist, 1867–1930. See A.'s *syndrome;* Morax-A. *conjunctivitis, diplobacillus.*

axenic (ā-zen'ik) [G. *a-* priv. + *xenos,* foreign]. Sterile, denoting especially a pure culture; *e.g.,* a protozoan culture free from bacteria. Also used to denote "germ-free" animals born and raised in a sterile environment. See also gnotobiote.

axes (ak'sēz). Plural of axis.

axial (ak'sē-ăl). **1.** Axile; relating to an axis. **2.** Relating to or situated in the central part of the body, in the head and trunk as distinguished from the limbs. **3.** In dentistry, relating to or parallel with the long axis of a tooth.

axifugal (ak-sif'yū-găl) [L. *axis* + *fugio,* to flee from]. Axofugal; extending away from an axis or axon.

axil (ak'sil). *Fossa* axillaris.

axile (ak'sīl). Axial (1).

axilla, gen. and pl. **axillae** (ak'sil'ă, ak-sil'ē) [L.]. *Fossa* axillaris.

axillary (ak'sil-ār-ē). Alar (2); relating to the axilla.

axio- [L. *axis*]. Combining form relating to an axis. See also axo-.

axiobuccal (ak'sē-ō-bŭk'ăl). Referring to the junction of the axial and buccal planes, usually a line.

axiobuccogingival (ak'sē-ō-bŭk-ō-jin'ji-văl). Referring to the junction of the axial, buccal and gingival planes; usually a point.

axioincisal (ak'sē-ō-in-sī'săl). Referring to the line angle formed by the junction of the incisal edge and axial walls of a tooth.

axiolabial (ak'sē-ō-lā'bē-ăl). Referring to the line angle of a cavity formed by the junction of the axial and the labial walls of a tooth.

axiolabiolingual (ak'sē-ō-lā'bē-ō-ling'qwăl). Referring to a section from labial to lingual along the longitudinal axis of a tooth.

axiolingual (ak'sē-ō-ling'qwăl). Referring to the line angle of a cavity formed by the junction of an axial and a lingual wall.

axiolinguocervical (ak'sē-ō-ling'gwō-ser'vi-kăl). Referring to the point angle formed by the junction of an axial, lingual, and cervical (gingival) wall of a cavity.

axiolinguoclusal (ak'sē-ō-ling'gwō-klū'săl). Referring to the point angle formed by the junction of an axial, lingual, and occlusal wall of a cavity.

axiolinguogingival (ak'sē-ō-ling'gwō-jin'ji-văl). Referring to the point angle formed by the junction of an axial, lingual, and gingival (cervical) wall of a cavity.

axiomesial (ak'sē-ō-mē'zē-ăl) Referring to the line angle of a cavity formed by the junction of an axial and a mesial wall.

axiomesiocervical (ak'sē-ō-mē'zē-ō-ser'vi-kăl). Referring to the point angle formed by the junction of an axial, mesial, and cervical (gingival) wall of a cavity.

axiomesiodistal (ak'sē-ō-mē'zē-ō-dis'tăl). See under plane.

axiomesiogingival (ak'sē-ō-mē'zē-ō-jin'ji-văl). Referring to the point angle formed by an axial, mesial, and gingival (cervical) wall of a cavity.

axiomesioincisal (ak'sē-ō-mē'zē-ō-in-sī'săl). Referring to the point angle formed by the junction of an axial, mesial, and incisal wall of a cavity.

axion (ak'sē-on). The brain and spinal cord (cerebrospinal axis).

axio-occlusal (ak'sē-ō-ŏklū'săl). Pertaining to the line angle formed by the junction of the axial and occlusal walls of a tooth.

axioplasm (ak'sē-ō-plazm). Axoplasm.

axiopodium, pl. **axiopodia** (ak'sē-ō-pō'dē-ŭm, -dē-ă). Axopodium.

axiopulpal (ak'sē-ō-pŭl'păl). Referring to the line angle formed by the junction of an axial and pulpal wall of a cavity.

axioversion (ak'sē-ō-ver'zhŭn). Abnormal inclination of the long axis of a tooth.

axipetal (ak-sip'ĕ-tăl) [L. *axis* + *peto,* to seek]. Centripetal (2).

axiramificate (ak'sē-ram-if'i-kāt). Denoting a nerve cell whose axon, usually short, breaks up into many branches, *e.g.,* Golgi's type II cells.

axis, pl. **axes (Ax)** (ak'sis, ak'sēz) [L. axle, axis]. **1.** A straight line passing through a spherical body between its two poles, and about which the body may revolve. **2.** The central line of the body or any of its parts. **3.** The vertebral column. **4.** The central nervous system. **5** [NA]. Epistropheus; toothed or odontoid vertebra; vertebra dentata; the second cervical vertebra. **6.** An artery that divides, immediately upon its origin, into a number of branches.

basibregmatic a., a line extending from the basion to the bregma.

basicranial a., a line drawn from the basion to the midpoint of the sphenoethmoidal suture.

basifacial a., facial a.; a line drawn from the subnasal point to the midpoint of the sphenoethmoidal suture.

biauricular a., a straight line joining the two auricularia. (*Cf.* auriculare).

a. bul'bi exter'nus [NA], external a. of eye; that part of the optic a. from the anterior surface of the cornea to the posterior surface of the sclera.

a. bul'bi inter'nus [NA], internal a. of eye; that part of the optic a. from the posterior surface of the cornea to the anterior surface of the retina.

celiac a., *truncus* celiacus.

cephalocaudal a., long a. of body.

cerebrospinal a., encephalomyelonic a.; neural a.; axion; the central nervous system; the brain and spinal cord.

condylar a., condyle cord; a line through the two mandibular condyles around which the mandible may rotate during a part of the opening movement.

conjugate a., conjugata.

craniofacial a., a straight line passing through the mesethmoid, presphenoid, basisphenoid, and basioccipital bones.

electrical a., the general direction of the electromotive force developed in the heart during its activation, usually represented in the frontal plane. See triaxial reference *system.*

embryonic a., the cephalocaudal a. established in the embryo by the primitive streak.

encephalomyelonic a., cerebrospinal a.

external a. of eye, a. bulbi externus.

facial a., basifacial a.

frontal a., the transverse a. of the eyeball, a line running transversely through the center of the globe of the eye.

hinge a., transverse horizontal a.

instantaneous electrical a., the resultant a. of the electromotive forces developing in the heart at any given moment.

internal a. of eye, a. bulbi internus.

a. of lens, a. lentis.

a. len'tis [NA], a. of the lens; a line connecting the anterior and posterior poles of the lens of the eye.

long a., a line parallel to an object lengthwise; in dentistry, the line extending inciso- (occluso-) cervically parallel to axial surfaces of a tooth.

long a. of body, cephalocaudal a.

mandibular a., tranverse horizontal a.

mean electrical a., the average magnitude and direction of all the electromotive forces developed during the cardiac event under consideration; *e.g.,* atrial or ventricular depolarization, or ventricular repolarization. See also axis *deviation.*

neural a., cerebrospinal a.

neutral a. of straight beam, the a. perpendicular to the plane of loading of a beam at stresses within the proportional limit; it lies at the gravity a. of the cross-section of the beam.

normal a., a mean electrical a. of the heart situated between $-30°$ and $+90°$. See hexaxial reference *system.*

opening a., an imaginary line around which the mandibular condyles may rotate during opening and closing movements. *Cf.* fulcrum *line.*

optic a., a. opticus.

a. op'ticus [NA], optic a.; the a. of the eye connecting the anterior and posterior poles; it usually diverges from the visual a. by five degrees or more.

orbital a., the line from the middle of the orbital opening to the center of the optic foramen.

pelvic a., a. pelvis.

a. pel'vis [NA], pelvic a.; plane of pelvic canal; a hypothetical curved line joining the center point of each of the four planes of the pelvis.

principal optic a., a line passing through the center of the lens of a refracting system at right angles to its surface.
pupillary a., a line perpendicular to the surface of the cornea, passing through the center of the pupil.
rotational a., fulcrum *line.*
sagittal a., **(1)** the anteroposterior a. of the eyeball; **(2)** in dentistry, the line in the frontal plane around which the working side condyle rotates during mandibular movement.
secondary a., any ray passing through the optical center of a lens.
a. of symmetry, an a. through a particle (*e.g.,* a virus) on such a plane that, if the particle is rotated on the a., there are two or more positions at which the particle appears identical.
thoracic a., **(1)** *arteria* thoracoacromialis; **(2)** *vena* thoracoacromialis.
thyroid a., *truncus* thyrocervicalis.
transporionic a., an imaginary line connecting the upper central points of the external auditory meatuses; used in roentgenographic cephalometry (see porion).
transverse horizontal a., hinge or mandibular a.; an imaginary line around which the mandible may rotate through the horizontal plane.
vertical a., **(1)** the vertical line passing through the center of the eyeball; **(2)** in dentistry, the line around which the working side condyle rotates in the horizontal plane during mandibular movement.
visual a., line of vision; the straight line extending from the object seen, through the center of the pupil, to the macula lutea of the retina.
Y-a., a cephalometric indicator of the vertical and horizontal coordinates of mandibular growth expressed in degrees of the inferior facial angle formed by the intersection of the sella-gnathion plane with the Frankfort horizontal plane.

axo- [G. *axōn,* axis]. Combining form meaning axis, usually relating to an axon.

axoaxonic (ak'sō-ak-son'ik). Relating to synaptic contact between the axon of one nerve cell and that of another. See synapse.

axodendritic (ak'sō-den-drit'ik). Pertaining to the synaptic relationship of an axon with a dendrite of another neuron. See synapse.

axofugal (ak-sof'yū-găl) [axo- + L. *fugio,* to flee]. Axifugal.

axograph (ak'sō-graf) [axo- + G. *graphō,* to write]. A device for recording scales or axes of predetermined magnitude on kymographic records.

axolemma (ak'sō-lem'ă) [axo- + G. *lemma,* husk]. Mauthner's sheath; the plasma membrane of the axon.

axolysis (ak-sol'i-sis) [axo- + G. *lysis,* dissolution]. Destruction or dissolution of a nerve axon.

axometer (ak-som'ĕ-ter). Axonometer; an instrument for determining the axis of a spectacle lens.

axon (ak'son) [G. *axōn,* axis]. The single process of a nerve cell that under normal conditions conducts nervous impulses away from the cell body and its remaining processes (dendrites). It is a relatively even filamentous process varying in thickness from about 0.25 to more than 10 μm. In contrast to dendrites, which rarely exceed 1.5 mm in length, a.'s can extend great distances from the parent cell body (some a.'s of the pyramidal tract are 40 to 50 cm long). A.'s 0.5 μm thick or over are generally enveloped by a segmented myelin sheath provided by oligodendroglia cells (in brain and spinal cord) or Schwann cells (in peripheral nerves). Like dendrites and nerve cell bodies, a.'s contain a large number of neurofibrils. With some exceptions, nerve cells synaptically transmit impulses to other nerve cells or to effector cells (muscle cells, gland cells) exclusively by way of the synaptic terminals of their a.

axonal (ak'sō-năl). Pertaining to an axon.

axoneme (ak'sō-nēm) [axo- + G. *nēma,* a thread]. **1.** The central thread running in the axis of the chromosome. **2.** Axial *filament.* **3.** The distinctive array of microtubules in the core of eukaryotic cilia and flagella comprising a central pair surrounded by a sheaf of nine doublet microtubules.

axonography (ak-son-og'ră-fē). Electroaxonography; the recording of electrical changes in axons.

axonometer (ak-sō-nom'ĕ-ter). Axometer.

axonopathy ak-sō-nop'ă-thē). Abnormal derangement of the axon of a neuron.

axonotmesis (ak'son-ot-mē'sis) [axon + G. *tmēsis,* a cutting]. Interruption of the axons of a nerve followed by complete degeneration of the peripheral segment, without severance of the supporting structure of the nerve; such a lesion may result from pinching, crushing, or prolonged pressure.

axopetal (ak-sop'ĕ-tăl) [axo- + L. *peto,* to seek]. Extending in a direction toward an axon.

axoplasm (ak'sō-plazm). Axioplasm; neuroplasm of the axon.

axopodium, pl. axopodia (ak-sō-pō'dē-ŭm, -ă) [Mod. L., fr. L. *axis* + G. *podion,* dim. of *pous* (*pod-*), foot]. Axiopodium; a permanent pseudopodium containing a stiff axial filament of differentiated protoplasm.

axosomatic (ak-sō-sō-mat'ik) [axo- + G. *sōma,* body]. Relating to the synaptic relationship of an axon with a nerve cell body. See synapse.

axostyle (ak'sō-stīl) [axo- + G. *stylos,* pillar]. An elongate supporting rod or tubule that runs the length of certain flagellate protozoans, frequently projecting out of the posterior end. Single or multiple, filamentous or rigid, they vary with the species but serve as an endoskeletal framework and may function in locomotion as well.

axotomy (ak-sot'ō-mē) [axo- + G. *tomē,* to cut]. Incision or cutting of an axon.

Ayala, A.G., Italian neurologist, 1878–1943. See A.'s *index, quotient.*

Ayerza, L., Argentinian physician, 1861–1918. See A.'s *disease, syndrome.*

Ayre, J. Ernest, U.S. gynecologist, *1910. See A. *brush.*

azacrine (ā'ză-krēn). 2-Methoxy-6-chloro-9-(5'-diethylamino-2'-pentyl)amino-3-azoacridine; an antimalarial; an effective schizontocide in acute falciparum infection.

azacyclonol hydrochloride (ā'ză-sī'klō-nol). γ-Pipradol hydrochloride; α,α-diphenyl-4-piperidine-methanol hydrochloride; a structural isomer of pipradol hydrochloride partially antagonistic to its actions, used with varying results in the treatment of hallucinations and confusion.

9-**azafluorene** (ā-ză-flūr'ēn). Carbazole.

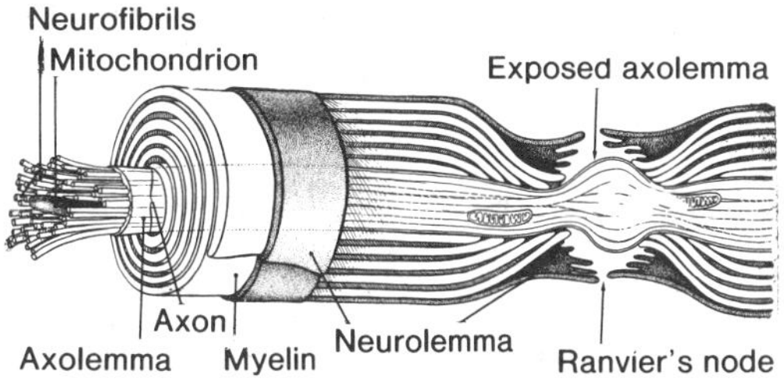

Detail of an Axon, Myelin Sheath, and Neurolemma

8-**azaguanine** (ā-ză-gwah'nēn). Guanazolo; triazologuanine; guanine with N for C in position 8; a guanine antagonist that has been used in the treatment of acute leukemia.

azamethonium bromide (ā'ză-me-thō'nē-ŭm). [(Methylimino)-

diethylene]bis-[ethyldimethylammonium bromide]: a ganglionic blocking agent.

azaperone (ā'za-per-ōn). 4'-Fluoro-4-[4-(2-pyridyl)-1-piperazinyl]butyrophenone; a tranquilizing agent.

azapetine phosphate (ā-zap'ĕ-tēn). 6-Allyl-6,7-dihydro-5*H*-dibenz[*c.e*]azepine phosphate; a potent adrenergic (α-receptor) blocking agent similar in action and uses to those of tolazoline; used in the treatment of peripheral vascular diseases.

azapropazone (ā-ză-prō'pă-zōn). Apazone.

azaribine (ā-zar'i-bēn). 2',3',5'-Triacetyl derivative of 6-azauridine; an antipsoriatic agent no longer used because of a high incidence of severe adverse reactions.

azaserine (ā-ză-sēr'ēn). Serine diazoacetate; *O*- O-diazoacetyl-L-serine; $N_2CH\text{-}CO\text{-}O\text{-}CH_2CH(NH_2)COOH$; an antibiotic inhibitor of purine synthesis.

azaspirodecanedione (ā-ză-spī'rō-dek-ān-dī'ōn). A class of anti-anxiety agents not chemically or pharmacologically related to other classes of sedative and anxiolytic drugs; *e.g.,* buspirone hydrochloride.

azatadine maleate (ă-zat'ă-dēn). 6,11-Dihydro-11-(1-methyl-4-piperidylidene)-5*H*- benzo[5,6]cyclohepta[1,2-b]pyridine dimaleate; an antihistamine with anticholinergic and antiserotonin properties.

azathioprine (ā-ză-thī'ō-prēn). 6-(1-Methyl-4-nitro-5-imidazolyl)-thiopurine; a derivative of 6-mercaptopurine, used as a cytotoxic and immunosuppressive agent in organ transplantation and in the treatment of autoimmune hemolytic anemias, systemic lupus erythematosus, leukemias, and rheumatoid arthritis.

6-azathymine (ā-ză-thī'mēn). Thymine with N for C in position 6; an antimetabolite of thymine.

6-azauridine (AzUR) (az-aw'ri-dēn). Uridine with N for C in position 6; a triazine analogue of uridine and an antimetabolite with selectivity for human neoplastic leukocytes; produces partial remissions in certain acute leukemias of adults.

azeotrope (ā-zē'ō-trōp) [G. *a-* priv.+ *zeein,* to boil,+ *tropos,* a turning]. A mixture of two liquids that boils without change in proportion of the two liquids, either in the liquid or the vapor phase; *e.g.,* 95% ethanol.
halothane-ether a., an azeotropic mixture in the proportions halothane 68 to diethyl ether 32, by volume, that combines the advantages of each anesthetic yet is non-flammable.

azeotropic (ā-zē-ō-trop'ik). Denoting or characteristic of an azeotrope.

azide (az'id). A compound that contains the monovalent $-N_3$ group.

azidothymidine (AZT) (az'i-dō-thī'mi-dēn). Zidovudine.

azlocillin sodium (az-lō-sil'in). Sodium (6R)-6-[D-2-(2-oxoimidazolidine-1-carboxamido)-2-phenylacetamido]penicillanate; an extended spectrum penicillin used in treatment of infections caused by *Pseudomonas aeruginosa, Escherichia coli,* and *Haemophilus influenzae.*

azo- [Fr. *azote,* name for nitrogen proposed by Lavoisier]. Prefix denoting the presence in a molecule of the group $\equiv C\text{-}N=N\text{-}C\equiv$. *Cf.* diazo-.

azobilirubin (az'ō-bil-i-rū'bin). The red-violet pigment formed by the condensation of diazotized sulfanilic acid with bilirubin in the van den Bergh reaction.

azocarmine B, azocarmine G (az-ō-kar'min) [C.I. 50090, C.I. 50085]. Red acid dyes, the former more soluble in water, useful in Heidenhain's azan stain.

azoic (ă-zō'ik, ā-) [G. *a-* priv. + *zōikos,* relating to an animal]. Containing no living things; without organic life.

azole (az'ōl). Pyrrole.

azolitmin (az-ō-lit'min) [old C.I. 1242]. A purplish red coloring matter obtained from natural litmus or synthesized by oxidizing orcinol in the presence of ammonia, lime, and potash; used as a broad indicator of pH (red at 4.5, blue at 8.3).

azoospermia (ā-zō-ō-sper'mē-ă) [G. *a-* priv. + *zōon,* animal, + *sperma,* seed]. Absence of living spermatozoa in the semen; failure of spermatogenesis. See also aspermia.

azophloxin (az-ō-flok'sin). Amidonaphthol red.

azoprotein (az-ō-prō'tēn). Any of the modified proteins produced by treatment with diazonium derivatives of various aromatic amines; used to elicit antibody formation and demonstrate antibody specificity.

azosulfamide (az-ō-sŭl'fă-mīd). 2-(4'-Sulfamylphenylazo)-7-acetamido-1-hydroxynaphthalene-3,6-disulfonate; a reddish derivative, soluble in water, less toxic but less effective than sulfanilamide; it owes its antibacterial activity to the sulfanilamide released.

azotemia (az-ō-tē'mē-ă) [azo- (azote) + G. *haima,* blood]. Uremia.
nonrenal a., prerenal a., nitrogen retention resulting from something other than primary renal disease.

azotemic (az-ō-tēm'ik). Relating to azotemia.

azothermia (az-ō-ther'mē-ă) [azote + G. *therme,* heat]. Fever resulting from uremia.

azoturia (az-ō-tūr'ē-ă) [azo- (azote) + G. *ouron,* urine]. An increased elimination of urea in the urine.
a. of horses, paralytic myoglobinuria; Monday morning sickness; hemoglobinemia paralytica; black water; an afebrile disease of horses, characterized by massive muscle degeneration, a rapidly developing paralysis of the hind legs, and myoglobinuria; onset is sudden, usually appearing shortly after the horse has returned to work after a few days' rest.

azovan blue (az'ō-van). Evans blue.

AZT Abbreviation for azidothymidine.

aztreonam (az-trē'ō-nam). 2-[[[1-(2-Amino-4-thiazolyl)-2-[2-methyl-4-oxo-1-sulf-3-azetidinyl)amino]-2-oxoethylidene]amino]oxy]-2-methylpropanoic acid; a synthetic bactericidal monobactam antibiotic with a wide spectrum of activity against Gram-negative aerobic pathogens.

azul (azh'yūl). Pinta.

AZUR Abbreviation for 6-azauridine.

azure (azh'yūr). A term for a group of basic blue methylthionine or phenothiazine dyes; used as biological stains, especially in blood and nuclear stains.
a. A [C.I. 52005], asymmetrical dimethylthionine chloride; $C_{14}H_{14}N_3SCl$; a blue dye used as a component of MacNeal's tetrachrome blood stain and of Romanowsky-type blood stains; also used as a stain for mucins, nucleic acids, and mast cell granules; gives a metachromatic violet to red color to highly acidic substances in tissues.
a. B [C.I. 52010], trimethylthionine chloride; $C_{15}H_{16}N_3SCl$; a blue dye used like a. A; also as a. B bromide to give metachromatic staining of RNA and DNA.
a. C [C.I. 52002], monomethylthione chloride; $C_{13}H_{12}N_3SCl$; a blue-violet thiazin dye used in the metachromatic staining of mucins and cartilage.
a. I, methylene a.; a mixture of a. A and B.
a. II, a mixture of a. I and methylene blue; the eosinate, a. II-eosin, is the principal ingredient of Giemsa stain.

azuresin (azh'yū-res'in). Quinine carbacrylic resin; a complex of azure A and carbacrylic resin; used as an indicator for the detection of gastric achlorhydria without intubation.

azurophil, azurophile (azh'yū-rō-fil, -fīl) [azure + G. *philos,* fond]. Staining readily with an azure dye, denoting especially the hyperchromatin and reddish purple granules of certain blood cells.

azygogram (az′i-gō-gram). Radiographic demonstration of the azygos venous system after injection of contrast medium.

azygography (az′i-gog′ră-fē). Radiography of the azygos venous system after injection of contrast medium.

azygos (az′ī-gos) [G. *a-* priv. + *zygon,* a yoke]. An unpaired (azygous) anatomical structure.

azygous (az′ī-gŭs, ă-zī′gŭs) [L. *azygos*]. Unpaired; single.

B

β **1.** Second letter of the Greek alphabet, beta. **2.** In chemistry denotes the second in a series, the second carbon from a functional (*e.g.*, carboxylic) group, or the direction of a chemical bond toward the viewer. For terms having this prefix, see the specific term.

B **1.** Symbol for boron. **2.** As a subscript, refers to barometric *pressure.*

b As a subscript, refers to blood.

Ba Symbol for barium.

Babbitt, Isaac, U.S. inventor, 1799–1862. See B. *metal.*

Babcock, Stephen M., U.S. chemist, 1843–1931. See B. *tube.*

Babès, Victor, Roumanian bacteriologist, 1854–1926. See *Babesia;* B.'s *nodes;* B.-Ernst *bodies.*

Babesia (bă-bē'zē-ă) [V. *Babès*]. The economically most important genus of the family Babesiidae; characterized by multiplication in host red blood cells to form pairs and tetrads; it causes babesiosis (piroplasmosis) in most types of domestic animals, and several species cause disease in splenectomized or normal people; known vectors are ixodid or argasid ticks. Sometimes divided into the genera *Piroplasma, Nuttallia, Babesiella,* and *Microbabesia,* but the single generic name is usually employed.

B. argenti'na, *B. bovis.*

B. ber'bera, *B. bovis.*

B. bigem'ina, species that is an etiologic agent of bovine babesiosis, transmitted by *Boophilus* ticks, especially *B. annulatus.*

B. bo'vis, *B. argentina* or *berbera;* a species that is a cause of bovine babesiosis; this parasite is smaller than *B. bigemina,* is transmitted by ticks of the genera *Boophilus, Rhipicephalus,* and *Ixodes,* and has caused fatal babesiosis in splenectomized people in Yugoslavia and the U.S.S.R.

B. cabal'li, species that is a cause of equine babesiosis in many parts of the world, including the southeastern U.S.; vector ticks are species of *Dermacentor, Hyalomma,* and *Rhipicephalus;* human cases also have been reported.

B. ca'nis, species found in dogs, wolves, and jackals in many tropical and subtropical areas of the Americas, Europe, Asia, and Africa; it is most pathogenic in dogs, causing mild to severe canine babesiosis, the severest disease occurring in dogs imported into areas where the disease is enzootic; the most important vector is *Rhipicephalus sanguineus.*

B. diver'gens, commonest species of *Babesia* in western and central Europe, causing a disease of cattle similar to that produced by *B. bovis;* vector tick is *Ixodes ricinus;* it has caused human babesiosis in splenectomized individuals in France, Ireland, Scotland, and Yugoslavia; also found in reindeer.

B. e'qui, species that occurs in horses, mules, donkeys, and zebras; it has a geographic distribution similar to that of *B. caballi,* but is smaller and more pathogenic, causing equine babesiosis; human cases also have been reported.

B. fe'lis, species found in domestic and wild members of the cat family, chiefly in Africa and India, causing babesiosis less severe than that caused by *B. canis.*

B. gibso'ni, species that infects dogs, wolves, and jackals, chiefly in India, Sri Lanka, and China, and is smaller than *B. canis;* only slightly pathogenic for the natural host, the jackal, but highly pathogenic in the dog.

B. micro'ti, a species naturally parasitizing certain rodents (*Peromyscus* and *Microtus* spp.) in North America; a number of human cases have been reported from Nantucket and Martha's Vineyard islands and nearby coastal New England. The local tick vector is *Ixodes dammini.*

B. mota'si, species that causes acute or chronic disease of sheep and goats in southern Europe, Africa, the Middle East, the U.S.S.R., and other areas; transmitted by ticks of the genera *Rhipicephalus, Haemaphysalis,* and *Dermacentor.*

B. o'vis, species described from sheep and goats in many tropical and subtropical areas of the eastern hemisphere as a cause of icterohematuria; it is smaller and less pathogenic than *B. motasi,* and immunologically distinct.

B. trautman'ni, species that causes mild or fatal babesiosis in pigs in southern Europe, the U.S.S.R., and Africa; the vector is *Rhipicephalus sanguineus.*

Babesiella (bă-bē-zē-el'ă). See *Babesia.*

Babesiidae (ba'bē-zī'i-dē, -zē'i-dē) A family of protozoan parasites (class Sporozoea, order Piroplasmida) occurring in the red blood cells of various mammals. The organisms are piriform, round, or oval in shape and reproduce by schizogony to form tetrads or by binary fission to form pairs in the red blood cells; transmission is effected by ticks. The family includes the genera *Babesia, Echinozoon,* and *Entopolypoides; Aegyptianella,* formerly included, is now thought to be a rickettsia. See also Theileriidae.

babesiosis (bă-bē'zē-ō'sis). Piroplasmosis; a disease caused by infection with a species of *Babesia,* the infection being transmitted by ticks. In animals, the disease is characterized by fever, malaise, listlessness, severe anemia, and hemoglobulinuria; the death rate frequently is higher in adult than in young animals.

bovine b., bovine hemoglobinuria; redwater fever (1); Texas fever; tick fever (3); an infectious disease of cattle caused by *Babesia species and transmitted by ticks.*

canine b., malignant fever in dogs caused by *Babesia* species.

equine b., equine biliary fever; biliary fever of horses; a disease of horses caused by species of *Babesia* and characterized by high fever, icterus, and enlargement of the spleen and lymph nodes.

human b., a rare human disease caused by infection with *Babesia* species (most frequently *B. divergens* in Europe and *B. microti* in the U.S.) that has been fatal in some splenectomized individuals.

Babinski, Joseph F., French neurologist, 1857–1932. See B.'s *phenomenon, sign;* B. *reflex.*

baby (bā'bē). An infant; a newborn child.

blue b., a child born cyanotic because of a congenital cardiac or pulmonary defect causing incomplete oxygenation of the blood.

blueberry muffin b., jaundice and purpura, especially of the face in the newborn, which may result from intrauterine viral infection.

collodion b., a newborn child with lamellar ichthyosis; at birth, the skin is bright red, shiny, translucent, and drawn tight, giving a distorted appearance (as if having been painted with collodion) of immobilization of the face; contraction of the skin causes ectropion, a pressed down appearance of the nose, and a gaping of the mouth and the labia.

giant b., macrosomia in the newborn, which may result from maternal diabetes.

test-tube b., popular term for a b. born after uterine implantation of a maternal ovum fertilized *in vitro.*

bacampicillin hydrochloride (bak'am-pi-sil'in). 1-(Ethoxycarbonyloxy)ethyl(6R)-6-(α-D-phenylglycylamino)- penicillanate hydrochloride; a semisynthetic penicillin with the same activity and uses as ampicillin, but better absorbed on oral administration.

baccate (bak'āt) [L. *bacca,* berry]. Berry-like.

Baccelli, Guido, Italian physician, 1832–1916. See B.'s *sign.*

bacciform (bak'sĭ-fōrm) [L. *bacca,* berry]. Berry-shaped.

Bachman, George W., U.S. parasitologist, *1890. See B. and Pettit *test.*

Bachmann. See Rivinus.

Bachmann, Jean George, U.S. physiologist, 1877–1959. See B.'s *bundle.*

Bacillaceae (bă-si-lā'sē-ē). A family of aerobic or facultatively anaerobic, sporeforming, ordinarily motile bacteria (order Eubacteriales) containing Gram-positive rods. These organisms are chemoheterotrophic. Some species are pathogenic. Ordinarily two genera, *Bacillus* and *Clostridium,* are included. The type genus is *Bacillus.*

bacillar, bacillary (bas'i-lar, bas'i-lā-rē). Shaped like a rod; consisting of rods or rodlike elements.

Bacille bilié de Calmette-Guérin (BCG) (bah-sēl' bi-lē-ā) [Fr.]. Calmette-Guérin bacillus; an attenuated strain of *Mycobacterium bovis* used in the preparation of BCG vaccine.

bacillemia (bas-i-lē'mē-ă) [bacillus + G. *haima,* blood]. The presence of rod-shaped bacteria in the circulating blood.

bacilli (bă-sil'ī). Plural of bacillus.

bacilliform (ba-sil'i-fōrm) [L. *bacillus,* a rod, + *forma,* form]. Rod-shaped.

bacillin (ba-sil'in). An antibiotic substance produced by *Bacillus subtilis.*

bacillomyxin (ba-sil-ō-mik'sin). An antibiotic active against certain pathogenic fungi obtained from cultures of *Bacillus subtilis.*

bacillosis (bas-i-lō'sis). A general infection with bacilli.

bacilluria (bas-i-lū'rē-ă) [bacillus + G. *ouron,* urine]. The presence of bacilli in the urine.

Bacillus (ba-sil'ŭs) [L. dim. of *baculus,* rod, staff]. A genus of aerobic or facultatively anaerobic, sporeforming, ordinarily motile bacteria (family Bacillaceae) containing Gram-positive rods. Motile cells are peritrichous. These organisms are chemoheterotrophic. They are found primarily in soil. A few species are animal pathogens; some species produce antibodies. The type species is *B. subtilis.*

B. amyloliquefa'ciens, a highly amylolytic species of soil bacteria that produces subtilisin.

B. an'thracis, a species that causes anthrax in man, cattle, swine, sheep, rabbits, guinea pigs, and mice.

B. bre'vis, a species found in soil, air, dust, milk, and cheese; some strains produce the antibiotic gramicidin or tyrocidin.

B. ce'reus, a species that causes an emetic type and a diarrheal type of food poisoning in humans, and can cause infections in humans and other mammals.

B. hemoly'ticus, former name for *Clostridium haemolyticum.*

B. histoly'ticus, former name for *Clostridium histolyticum.*

B. megate'rium, a saprophytic species of experimental interest; strains produce bacteriocins (megacins).

B. polymyx'a, a species found in soil, water, milk, feces, and decaying vegetables; some strains produce the antibiotic polymyxin.

B. pseudodiphthe'riae, *Corynebacterium bovis.*

B. sphae'ricus, a species that is an insect pathogen and that has been associated with human and other mammalian infections, especially in compromised hosts.

B. sub'tilis, grass or hay bacillus; a species found in soil and decomposing organic matter; some strains produce the antibiotic subtilin, subtenolin, or bacillomycin; it is the type species of the genus *B.*

B. thuringien'sis, a species that is an insect pathogen and that has been implicated in human and mammalian infections.

bacillus, pl. **bacilli** (ba-sil'ŭs, -ī) [L. dim. of *baculus,* a rod, staff]. **1.** A vernacular term used to refer to any member of the genus *Bacillus.* **2.** Term formerly used to refer to any rod-shaped bacterium.

Abel's b., *Klebsiella ozaenae.*

abortus b., *Brucella abortus.*

acne b., *Propionibacterium acnes.*

Bang's b., *Brucella abortus.*

Battey b. [Battey hospital in Rome, Ga], *Mycobacterium intracellulare.*

blue pus b., *Pseudomonas aeruginosa.*

Bordet-Gengou b., *Bordetella pertussis.*

Calmette-Guérin b., Bacille bilié de Calmette-Guérin.

cholera b., *Vibrio cholerae.*

colon b., see *Escherichia coli.*

comma b., *Vibrio cholerae.*

Döderlein's b., a large, Gram-positive bacterium occurring in normal vaginal secretions; although thought by some to be identical with *Lactobacillus acidophilus,* the identity of Döderlein's b. is still doubtful.

Ducrey's b., *Haemophilus ducreyi.*

dysentery b., an organism of the genus *Shigella* which causes dysentery.

Eberth's b., *Salmonella typhi.*

Flexner's b., *Shigella flexneri.*

Friedländer's b., *Klebsiella pneumoniae.*

Gärtner's b., *Salmonella enteritidis.*

gas b., *Clostridium perfringens.*

Ghon-Sachs b., *Clostridium septicum.*

glanders b., *Pseudomonas mallei.*

grass b., *Bacillus subtilis.*

Hansen's b., *Mycobacterium leprae.*

hay b., *Bacillus subtilis.*

Hofmann's b., *Corynebacterium pseudodiphtheriticum.*

influenza b., *Haemophilus influenzae.*

Johne's b., *Mycobacterium paratuberculosis.*

Kitasato's b., *Yersinia pestis.*

Klebs-Loeffler b., *Corynebacterium diphtheriae.*

Koch's b., **(1)** *Mycobacterium tuberculosis,* **(2)** *Vibrio cholerae.*

Koch-Weeks b., *Haemophilus influenzae.*

lactic acid b., a member of the genus *Lactobacillus.*

leprosy b., *Mycobacterium leprae.*

Loeffler's b., *Corynebacterium diphtheriae.*

mist b., *Mycobacterium smegmatis* (formerly *M. lacticola*).

Moeller's grass b., *Mycobacterium phlei.*

Morgan's b., *Proteus morganii.*

Much's b., an alleged non-acid fast granular form of the tubercle b.; not demonstrable by the Ziehl stain, but takes a modified Gram stain; it is said to be the form present in the tuberculous skin lesion.

necrosis b., *Fusobacterium necrophorum.*

paracolon b., any one of a number of diverse enteric bacteria which fail to ferment lactose promptly.

paradysentery b., *Shigella flexneri.*

paratyphoid b., one of the three organisms causing the three forms, A, B, and C, of paratyphoid fever. See also paratyphoid fever.

Park-Williams b., a special strain of *Corynebacterium diphtheriae* used for toxin production.

Pfeiffer's b., *Haemophilus influenzae.*

plague b., *Yersinia pestis.*

Plaut's b., probably *Fusobacterium nucleatum,* differentiated by some from Vincent's b.; the former is motile and nonpathogenic, the latter is nonmotile and pathogenic.

Plotz b., a small, Gram-positive bacterium suggested as the pathogenic agent of typhus fever.

Preisz-Nocard b., *Corynebacterium pseudotuberculosis.*

Sachs' b., *Clostridium septicum.*

Schmorl's b., *Fusobacterium necrophorum.*

Schottmüller's b., *Salmonella schottmülleri.*

Shiga b., *Shigella dysenteriae.*

Shiga-Kruse b., *Shigella dysenteriae.*

Sonne b., *Shigella sonnei.*

timothy hay b., *Mycobacterium phlei.*

tubercle b., **(1)** *Mycobacterium tuberculosis* (human); **(2)** *M. bovis* (bovine); **(3)** *M. avium* (avian).
typhoid b., *Salmonella typhi.*
Vincent's b., probably *Fusobacterium nucleatum.*
vole b., an acid-fast b. isolated from voles and used in the production of a vaccine against human and bovine tuberculosis.
Weeks' b., *Haemophilus influenzae.*
Welch's b., *Clostridium perfringens.*
Whitmore's b., *Pseudomonas pseudomallei.*

bacitracin (bas-i-trā'sin). An antibacterial polypeptide of known chemical structure isolated from cultures of an aerobic, Gram-positive, spore-bearing bacillus (member of the *Bacillus subtilis* group); active against hemolytic streptococci, staphylococci, and several types of Gram-positive, aerobic, rod-shaped organisms; usually applied locally. Zinc b. is also available.

back (bak). See dorsum.
adolescent round b., Scheuermann's *disease.*
hollow b., lordosis.
poker b., *spondylitis* deformans.
saddle b., lordosis.

backache (bak'āk). Nonspecific term used to describe back pain; generally refers to pain below the cervical level.

backbone (bak'bōn). *Columna* vertebralis.

backcross (bak'kros). Mating of an individual heterozygous for one or more gene pairs to an individual homozygous for the same gene pairs.

backing (bak'ing). In dentistry, a metal support which serves to attach a facing to a prosthesis.

back-knee (bak'nē'). *Genu* recurvatum.

backscatter (bak'skat-er). Induced radiation deflected more than 90° from the primary beam. See scattered *radiation.*

baclofen (bak'lō-fen). *β*-(Aminomethyl)-*p*- chlorohydrocinnamic acid; a muscle relaxant used in the symptomatic treatment of spinal cord injuries and multiple sclerosis.

Bacon, Harry E., U.S. proctologist, *1900. See B.'s *anoscope.*

bacteremia (bak-tēr-ē'mē-ă) [bacteria + G. *haima,* blood]. Bacteriemia; the presence of viable bacteria in the circulating blood.

bacteri-. See bacterio-.

bacteria (bak-tēr'ē-ă). Plural of bacterium.

bacterial (bak-tēr'ē-ăl). Relating to bacteria.

bactericholia (bak'tēr-i-kō'lē-ă). Bacteria in bile.

bactericidal (bak-tēr'i-sī'dăl). Bacteriocidal; causing the death of bacteria.

bactericide (bak-tēr'i-sīd) [bacteria + L. *caedo,* to kill]. Bacteriocide; an agent that destroys bacteria.
specific b., a bacteriolytic immune serum destructive to one bacterial species or genus only.

bacterid (bak'ter-id) [bacteria + *-id* (1)]. **1.** A recurrent or persistent eruption of discrete sterile pustules of the palms and soles, thought to be an allergic response to infection at a remote site. **2.** A dissemination of a previously localized bacterial skin infection.

bacteriemia (bak-tēr-ē-ē'mē-ă). Bacteremia.

bacterio-, bacteri- [see bacterium]. Combining forms relating to bacteria.

bacterioagglutinin (bak-tēr'ē-ō-ă-glū'ti-nin). An antibody that agglutinates bacteria.

bacteriochlorin (bak-tēr'-ē-ō-klōr'in). 7,8,17,18-Tetrahydroporphyrin; the basic structure of the bacteriochlorophylls.

bacteriochlorophyll (bak-tēr-ē-ō-klōr'ō-fil). Magnesium bacteriopheophytinate; either of two forms of chlorophyll: 1) *α*, $-CH{=}CH_2$ replaced by $-CO{-}CH_3$ in the chlorophyll *α* structure, two hydrogens also being added; 2) *β*, $-CH{=}CH_2$ replaced by $-CO{-}CH_3$ and $-CH_2{-}CH_3$ replaced by $-C{\equiv}CH$ in the chlorophyll *β* structure, two hydrogens also being added.

bacteriocidal (bak-tēr'ē-ō-sī'dăl). Bactericidal.

bacteriocide (bak-tēr'ē-ō-sīd). Bactericide.

bacteriocidin (bak-tēr'ē-ō-sī'din). Antibody having bactericidal activity.

bacteriocinogens (bak-tēr'ē-ō-sin'ō-jenz). Bacteriocinogenic *plasmids.*

bacteriocins (bak-tē'ē-ō-sinz). Proteins that are produced by certain bacteria possessing bacteriocinogenic plasmids and that exert a lethal effect on closely related bacteria; in general, b.'s have a narrower range of activity than antibiotics do and are more potent.

bacterioclasis (bak-tēr-ē-ok'lă-sis) [bacterio- + G. *klasis,* a breaking]. Fragmentation of bacteria, as in the Twort phenomenon.

bacteriofluorescin (bak-tēr'ē-ō-flūr-es'in). A fluorescent material produced by bacteria.

bacteriogenic (bak-tēr'ē-ō-jen'ik). Caused by bacteria.

bacteriogenous (bak-tēr-ē-oj'e-nŭs). **1.** Producing bacteria. **2.** Of bacterial origin or causation.

bacterioid (bak-tēr'ē-oyd) [bacterio- + G. *eidos,* resemblance]. Resembling bacteria.

bacteriologic, bacteriological (bak'tēr-ē-ō-loj'ik, -i-kăl). Relating to bacteria or to bacteriology.

bacteriologist (bak'ter-ē-ol'ō-jist). One who primarily studies or works with bacteria.

bacteriology (bak-tēr-ē-ol'ō-jē) [bacterio- + G. *logos,* study]. The branch of science concerned with the study of bacteria.
systematic b., that branch of b. concerned with nomenclature and classification (taxonomy).

bacteriolysin (bak-tēr-ē-ol'i-sin). Specific antibody that combines with bacterial cells (*i.e.,* antigen) and, when adequate complement is available, causes lysis or dissolution of the cells.

bacteriolysis (bak-tēr-ē-ol'i-sis) [bacterio- + G. *lysis,* dissolution]. The dissolution of bacteria, *e.g.,* by means of hypotonic solutions or by specific antibody and complement.

bacteriolytic (bak-tēr-ē-ō-lit'ik). Pertaining to lytic destruction of bacteria; manifesting the ability to cause dissolution of bacterial cells.

bacteriolyze (bak-tēr'ē-ō-līz). To cause the digestion or solution of bacterial cells.

bacteriopexy (bak-tēr'ē-ō-pek-sē) [bacterio- + G. *pēxis,* fixation]. Immobilization of bacteria by phagocytic cells.

bacteriophage (bak-tēr'ē-ō-fāj) [bacterio- + G. *phagein,* to eat]. Phage; a virus with specific affinity for bacteria, and the active agent in d'Herelle's phenomenon. B.'s have been found in association with essentially all groups of bacteria, including the Cyanobacteria; like other viruses they contain either (but never both) RNA or DNA and vary in structure from the seemingly simple filamentous bacterial virus to relatively complex forms with contractile "tails"; their relationships to the host bacteria are rather specific and, as in the case of temperate b., may be genetically intimate. B.'s are named after the bacterial species, group, or strain for which they are specific, *e.g.,* corynebacteriophage, coliphage; eight families are recognized and have been assigned provisional names: Corticoviridae, Cystoviridae, Inoviridae, Leviviridae, Microviridae, Myoviridae, Pedoviridae, and Styloviridae. See also coliphage.
defective b., defective phage; a temperate b. mutant whose genome does not contain all of the normal components and cannot become fully infectious virus, yet can replicate indefinitely in the bacterial genome as defective probacteriophage; many defective b.'s are mediators of transduction.
filamentous b., a b. that is rod-shaped and lacks the head-and-tail

structure characteristic of most b.'s.

mature b., the complete, infective form of b.

temperate b., b. whose genome incorporates with, and replicates with, that of the host bacterium; dissociation (and resultant development of vegetative b.) occurs at a slow rate resulting occasionally in lysis of a bacterium and release of mature b., thus rendering the bacterial culture capable of inducing general lysis if transferred to a culture of a susceptible bacterial strain.

typhoid b., b. specific for *Salmonella typhosa.*

vegetative b., the form of b. in which the b. nucleic acid (lacking its coat) multiplies freely within the host bacterium, independently of bacterial multiplication.

virulent b., a b. that regularly causes lysis of the bacteria that it infects; it may exist in one or the other of only two forms, vegetative or mature; it does not have a probacteriophage form (*i.e.,* its genome does not incorporate with that of the host bacterium), therefore it does not effect lysogenization.

bacteriophagia (bak-tēr'ē-ō-fā'jē-ă). Twort-d'Herelle *phenomenon.*

bacteriophagology (bak-tēr'ē-ō-fă-gol'ō-jē). Protobiology; the study of bacteriophages.

bacteriopheophorbide (bak-tēr'ē-ō-fē-ō-fōr'bīd). Bacteriophorbin with the side-chains found in bacteriochlorophyll, but lacking the phytyl group.

bacteriopheophorbin (bak-tēr'ē-ō-fē-ō-fōr'bin). De-esterfied bacteriopheophorbide, derived from bacteriochlorin.

bacteriopheophytin (bak-tēr'ē-ō-fē-ō-fī'tin). Bacteriopheophorbide with a phytyl ester on the C-17 propionic residue; bacteriochlorophyll less its magnesium residue.

bacteriophorbin (bak-tēr'ē-ō-fōr'bin). Phorbin further saturated by addition of two hydrogens to C-7 and C-8.

bacteriophytoma (bak-tēr'ē-ō-fī-tō'mă) [bacterio- + G. *phytos,* plant, + *-oma,* growth]. A growth in plant tissues produced by bacteria.

bacterioprotein (bak-tēr'ē-ō-prō'tēn). One of the albuminous substances, or proteins, within the cells of bacteria; these substances vary in their character and properties.

bacteriopsonin (bak-tēr-ē-op'sō-nin). An opsonin acting upon bacteria, as distinguished from a hemopsonin which affects red blood corpuscles.

bacteriosis (bak-tēr-ē-ō'sis). A localized or generalized bacterial infection.

bacteriostasis (bak-tēr-ē-os'tă-sis) [bacterio- + G. *stasis,* a standing still]. An arrest or retardation of growth of bacteria.

bacteriostat (bak-tēr'ē-ō-stat). Any agent that inhibits or retards bacterial growth.

bacteriostatic (bak-tēr'ē-ō-stat'ik). Inhibiting or retarding the growth of bacteria.

bacteriotoxic (bak-tēr'ē-ō-tok'sik). Poisonous or toxic to bacteria.

bacteriotropic (bak-tēr'ē-ō-trop'ik) [bacterio- + G. *tropē,* a turning]. Turning toward or moving in the direction of bacteria; having an affinity for bacteria.

bacteriotropin (bak-tēr-ē-ot'rō-pin). A constituent of the blood, usually a specific antibody, *i.e.,* opsonin, that combines with bacterial cells and renders them more susceptible to phagocytes.

bacteriotrypsin (bak-tēr'ē-ō-trip'sin). A trypsin-like enzyme produced by bacteria, particularly *Vibrio cholerae.*

Bacterium (bak-tēr'ē-ŭm) [Mod. L. fr. G. *baktērion,* dim. of *baktron,* a staff or club]. A bacterial generic name placed on the list of rejected names by the Judicial Commission and the International Committee on Systematic Bacteriology of the International Association of Microbiological Societies. As a consequence, *B.* is no longer used in bacteriology. Identifiable organisms formerly placed in the genus *B.* have all been transferred to other genera. Specifically, *B. anitratum* is now known as *Acinetobacter calcoaceticus; B. coli* is now called *Escherichia coli.*

bacterium, pl. **bacteria** (bak-tēr'ē-ŭm, -ă) [Mod. L. fr. G. *baktērion,* dim. of *baktron,* a staff]. A unicellular prokaryotic microorganism that usually multiplies by cell division and has a cell wall that provides a constancy of form; they may be aerobic or anaerobic, motile or nonmotile, and free-living, saprophytic, parasitic, or pathogenic. See also Cyanobacteria.

Binn's b., a type of the typhoid-paratyphoid subgroups of the nonlactose-fermenting bacteria.

blue-green b., see Cyanobacteria.

Chauveau's b., former name for *Clostridium chauvoei.*

endoteric b., a b. that forms an endotoxin.

exoteric b., a b. that secretes an exotoxin.

lysogenic b., **(1)** a b. in the symbiotic condition in which its genome includes the genome (probacteriophage) of a temperate bacteriophage; in occasional instances the probacteriophage dissociates from the bacterial genome, develops into vegetative bacteriophage, and then matures, causing lysis of the respective host b. and release into the culture medium of infective temperate bacteriophage; **(2)** formerly, a pseudolysogenic bacterial strain, *i.e.,* a "carrier" strain of bacteriophage of low infectivity.

pyogenic b., a b. that causes a pyogenic infection, such as the pyogenic cocci (staphylococci, streptococci, pneumococci, meningococci) and *Haemophilus influenzae.*

bacteriuria (bak-tēr-ē-ū'rē-ă). The presence of bacteria in the urine.

bacteroid (bak'ter-oyd). Resembling bacteria.

Bacteroidaceae (bak'ter-oy-dā'sē-ē). A family of obligately anaerobic (microaerophilic species may occur), nonsporeforming bacteria (order Eubacteriales) containing Gram-negative rods which vary in size from minute, filterable forms to long, filamentous, branching forms; pronounced pleomorphism may occur. Motile and nonmotile species occur; motile cells are peritrichous. Body fluids are frequently required for growth. Carbohydrates are usually fermented with the production of acid; gas may be produced in glucose or peptone media. These organisms occur primarily in the intestinal tracts and mucous membranes of warm-blooded animals. They may be pathogenic. The type genus is *Bacteroides.*

Bacteroides (bak-ter-oy'dēz) [G. *bakterion* + *eidos,* form]. A genus of obligately anaerobic, nonsporeforming bacteria (family Bacteroidaceae) containing Gram-negative rods. Both motile and nonmotile species occur; motile cells are peritrichous. Some species ferment carbohydrates and produce combinations of succinic, lactic, acetic, formic, or propionic acids, sometimes with short-chained alcohols; butyric acid is not a major product. Those species which do not ferment carbohydrates produce from peptone either trace to moderate amounts of succinic, formic, acetic, and lactic acids or major amounts of acetic and butyric acids with moderate amounts of alcohols and isovaleric, propionic, and isobutyric acids. They are part of the normal flora of the oral, respiratory, intestinal, and urogenital cavities of humans and animals; some species are pathogenic. The type species is *B. fragilis.*

B. bi'vivus, a species usually isolated from urogenital and abdominal infections.

B. capillo'sus, 16 a species isolated from human cysts and wounds, the mouth, and feces, and from the intestinal tracts of some animals.

B. corro'dens, a species now assigned in part to *B. urolyticus.*

B. di'siens, a species isolated from abdominal and urogenital infections, and from the mouth.

B. frag'ilis, a species that is one of the predominant organisms in the lower intestinal tract of man and other animals; also found in specimens from appendicitis, peritonitis, rectal abscesses, pilonidal cysts, surgical wounds, and lesions of the urogenital tract; it is the type species of the genus *B.*

B. furco'sus, a species found in an infected appendix, in lung and

abdominal abscesses, and in feces.
B. melaninogen'icus, a species found in the mouth, feces, infections of the mouth, soft tissue, respiratory tract, urogenital tract, and the intestinal tract.
B. nodo'sus, a species involved in the causation of foot rot in sheep and goats.
B. o'ris, a species isloated from the gingival crevice, systemic infections, face, neck, and chest abscesses, wound drainages, and blood and various bodily fluids.
B. ora'lis, a species found in the gingival crevice area of man and in infections of the oral cavity and upper respiratory and genital tracts.
B. pneumosin'tes, a species found in the nasopharynx, gingival crevice and periodontal pockets, blood, respiratory tract, brain abscesses, and head and neck infections.
B. praeacu'tus, a species isolated from the intestinal tracts of infants and adults, gangrenous lesions, lung abscesses, and blood.
B. putredi'nis, a species isolated from feces, cases of acute appendicitis, and abdominal and rectal abscesses; also from foot rot of sheep and from farm soil.
B. urolyt'icus, a species isolated from infections of the respiratory and intestinal tracts, and from the buccal cavity, intestinal tract, urogenital tract, and blood after a dental extraction.

bacteroidosis (bak'ter-oy-dō'sis). Infection with *Bacteroides.*

baculiform (bă-kyū'li-fōrm) [L. *baculum,* a rod, + *forma,* form]. Rod-shaped.

Baculoviridae (bak-yū-lō-vir'i-dē) [L. *baculum,* rod]. A family of viruses that multiply only in invertebrates; Virions are rod-shaped and measure 40 to 70 nm by 250 to 400 nm; genomes are of double-stranded, supercoiled DNA (MW 80 to 100 × 10^6). Genera of viruses that multiply only in invertebrates are also included in other families: *Iridovirus* (Iridoviridae), *Entomopoxvirus* (Poxviridae), *Densovirus* (Parvoviridae), cytoplasmic polyhedral virus group (Reoviridae), and *Sigmavirus* (Rhabdoviridae).

baculum (bak'yū-lŭm) [L. a rod]. *Os* penis.

Baehr, George, U.S. physician, *1887. See B.-Lohlein *lesion.*

Baelz, Erwin B., German physician in Tokyo, 1849–1913. See B.'s *disease.*

Baer, Karl E. von, Russian embryologist, 1792–1876. See B.'s *law.*

BAER Abbreviation for brainstem evoked response. See under evoked *response.*

Baeyer, Johann F.W.A. von, German chemist, 1835–1917. See B.'s *theory.*

bag [A.S. *baelg*]. A pouch, sac, or receptacle.
Ambu b., proprietary name for a self-reinflating b. used with positive pressure respiration during resuscitation, foam rubber being built into the walls of the b. so that its shape is automatically restored after compression with air or oxygen drawn into the b.
breathing b., reservoir b.; a collapsible reservoir from which gases are inhaled and into which gases may be exhaled during general anesthesia or artificial ventilation.
colostomy b., a bag worn over an artifical anus to collect feces.
Douglas b., a large b. in which expired gas is collected for several minutes to determine oxygen consumption in man under conditions of actual work.
nuclear b., the aggregation of nuclei occurring in the nonstriated center of an intrafusal muscle fiber of a neuromuscular spindle.
Petersen's b., an obsolete device consisting of a rubber b. introduced into the rectum and inflated to push up the bladder to facilitate performance of a suprapubic cystotomy.
Plummer's b., Plummer's *dilator.*
Politzer b., a pear-shaped rubber b. used for forcing air through the eustachian tube by the Politzer method.
reservoir b., breathing b.
b. of waters, colloquialism for the amniotic sac and contained amniotic fluid.

bagassosis (bag-ă-sō'sis). Extrinsic allergic alveolitis following exposure to sugar cane fiber (bagasse); variously attributed to inhalation of spores of soil fungi and, particularly, thermophilic actinomycetes.

Baggenstoss, Archie H., U.S. pathologist, *1908. See B. *change.*

Bagolini, B., 20th century Italian ophthalmologist, See B. *test.*

bahnung (bah'nŭng) [Ger. *Bahnung,* the making of a pathway]. Increased ease of transmission of a nerve impulse in a nerve tract as a result of prior stimulation.

Baillarger, Jules G.F., French neurologist, 1809–1890. See B.'s *band, lines.*

Bailliart, Paul, French ophthalmologist, 1877–1969. See B.'s *ophthalmodynamometer.*

Bainbridge, Francis A., British physiologist, 1874–1921. See B. *reflex.*

Baker, James Porter, U.S. physician, *1902. See Charcot-Weiss-B. *syndrome.*

Baker, John Randal, British zoologist, *1900. See B.'s pyridine *extraction,* acid *hematein.*

Baker, William M., British surgeon, 1839–1896. See B.'s *cyst.*

BAL Abbreviation for British anti-Lewisite.

balan-. See balano-.

balance (bal'ans) [L. *bi-,* twice, + *lanx,* dish, scale]. **1.** An apparatus for weighing; *e.g.,* scales. **2.** The normal state of action and reaction between two or more parts or organs of the body. **3.** Quantities, concentrations, and proportionate amounts of bodily constituents. **4.** The difference between intake and utilization, storage, or excretion of a substance by the body. See also equilibrium.
acid-base b., acid-base equilibrium; the normal b. between acid and base in the blood plasma, expressed in the hydrogen ion concentration or pH, resulting from the relative amounts of acidic and basic materials ingested and produced by body metabolism, compared to the relative amounts of acidic and basic materials excreted from the body and consumed by body metabolism; the normal state of acid-base b. is not one of neutrality, with equal concentrations of hydrogen and hydroxyl ions, but a more alkaline state with a certain excess of hydroxyl ions.
genic b., see balance *theory* of sex.
occlusal b., a condition in which there are simultaneous contacts of the occluding units of the opposing dental arches in centric and eccentric positions within the functional range.
Wilhelmy b., a device for measuring surface tension in terms of the pull exerted on a thin plate of platinum or other material suspended vertically through the surface; used in a Langmuir trough to study pulmonary surfactant.

balanic (ba-lan'ik) [G. *balanos,* acorn, glans]. Relating to the glans penis or glans clitoridis.

Balanites aegyptiaca (bal-ă-nī'tēz ē-jip-tī'ă-kă) [L. *balanos,* acorn]. A genus of trees growing in the Near East, whose berries contain an active principle that is deadly to mollusks, miracidia, cercariae, tadpoles, and fish and that is used as a prophylactic against schistosomiasis by adding it to drinking water.

balanitis (bal-ă-nī'tis) [G. *balanos,* acorn, glans, + *-itis,* inflammation]. Inflammation of the glans penis or glans clitoridis.
b. circina'ta, a form thought to be due to the presence of *Spirochaeta balanitidis.*
b. circumscrip'ta plasmacellula'ris, b. of Zoon.
b. diabet'ica, a form in diabetics resulting from irritation by the saccharine urine or urine contaminated with bacteria.
plasma cell b., b. of Zoon.
b. xerot'ica oblit'erans, atrophy and shrinking of the skin of the glans penis, which may result in urethral stenosis; the cause is un-

known, but the condition is believed to be lichen sclerosus et atrophicus of the glans penis.

b. of Zoon, Zoon's erythroplasia; b. circumscripta plasmacellularis; plasma cell b.; benign chronic circumscribed b. characterized histologically by subepithelial plasma cell infiltration and clinically by small erythematous papular lesions.

balano-, balan- [G. *balanos,* acorn, glans]. Combining forms relating to the glans penis.

balanoblennorrhea (bal'an-ō-blen-ōr-ē'ă) [balano- + G. *blennos,* mucus, + *rhoia,* flow]. Obsolete term for gonorrheal inflammation of the external surface of the glans penis.

balanocele (bal'an-ō-sēl) [balano- + G. *kēlē,* hernia]. Obsolete term for protrusion of the glans penis through a gangrenous opening in the prepuce.

balanoplasty (bal'an-ō-plas-tē) [balano- + G. *plastos,* formed]. Plastic surgery of the glans penis.

balanoposthitis (bal'an-ō-pos-thī'tis) [balano- + G. *posthē,* prepuce, + *-itis,* inflammation]. Inflammation of the glans penis and overlying prepuce.

balanopreputial (bal'an-ō-prē-pyū'shē-ăl). Relating to the glans penis and the prepuce.

balanorrhagia (bal'an-ō-rā'jē-ă) [balano- + G. *rhēgnymi,* to burst forth]. Obsolete term for running discharge from the glans penis.

balanorrhea (bal'an-ō-rē'ă) [balano- + G. *rhoia,* flow]. Obsolete term for balanitis with a purulent discharge.

balantidiasis (bal'an-ti-dī'ă-sis). Balantidosis; a disease caused by the presence of *Balantidium coli* in the large intestine; characterized by diarrhea, dysentery, and occasionally ulceration.

Balantidium (bal-an-tid'ē-ŭm) [G. *balantidion,* dim of *ballantion,* a bag]. A genus of ciliates (family Balantidiidae) found in the digestive tract of vertebrates and invertebrates.

B. co'li, a very large parasitic ciliate species, usually 50 to 80 μm in length, reaching up to 200 μm in pigs, found in the cecum or large intestine, swimming actively in the lumen; usually harmless in man but may invade and ulcerate the intestinal wall, producing a colitis resembling amebic dysentery.

B. su'is, a species originally considered distinct from the ciliate parasite of man, *B. coli,* but now considered synonymous with it; nonpathogenic in swine.

balantidosis (bal'an-ti-dō'sis). Balantidiasis.

balanus (bal'ă-nŭs) [G. *balanos,* acorn, glans penis]. *Glans* penis.

bald (bawld) [M.E. *balled*]. Having no hair, or a decrease in the amount of hair of the scalp.

baldness (bawld'nes). Alopecia.

congenital b., *alopecia* congenitalis.

male pattern b., *alopecia* hereditaria.

pubic b., pubomadesis.

Baldy, John M., U.S. gynecologist, 1860–1934. See B.'s *operation.*

Balint, Rudolph, Hungarian neurologist and psychiatrist, 1874–1929. See B.'s *syndrome.*

Ball, Sir Charles B., Irish surgeon, 1851–1916. See B.'s *operation.*

ball. 1. A round mass. See bezoar. **2.** In veterinary medicine, a large pill or bolus.

chondrin b., one of the globular masses formed by a group of cells inclosed in a capsule, in hyaline cartilage.

dust b., a mass sometimes found in the stomach or intestine of an animal fed on mill cleanings.

food b., phytobezoar.

b. of the foot, the padded portion of the sole, at the anterior extremity of the heads of the metatarsals, upon which the weight rests when the heel is raised.

fungus b., a compact mass of fungal mycelium and cellular debris, 1 to 5 cm in diameter, residing within a lung cavity; such cavities may be produced by bacterial as well as mycotic infectious agents, but they are usually produced by *Aspergillus fumigatus* or, more rarely, by *A. niger.* See also aspergilloma (2).

hair b., trichobezoar.

wool b., a trichophytobezoar formed chiefly of wool and vegetable matter in the stomach of sheep.

Ballance, Sir Charles A., British surgeon, 1856–1936. See B.'s *sign,* Koerte-B. *operation.*

Ballet, Gilbert, French neurologist, 1853–1916. See B.'s *disease, sign.*

balling gun, balling iron. An instrument used for administering boluses or capsules to animals.

ballism (bal'izm). Ballismus.

ballismus (bal-iz'mŭs) [G. *ballismos,* a jumping about]. Ballism; the occurrence of lively jerking or shaking movements, especially as observed in chorea.

ballistocardiogram (bal-is-tō-kar'dē-ō-gram) [G. *ballō,* to throw, + *kardia,* heart, + *gramma,* something written]. A record of the body's recoil caused by cardiac contraction and the ejection of blood into the aorta; may be used as a basis for calculating the cardiac output in man.

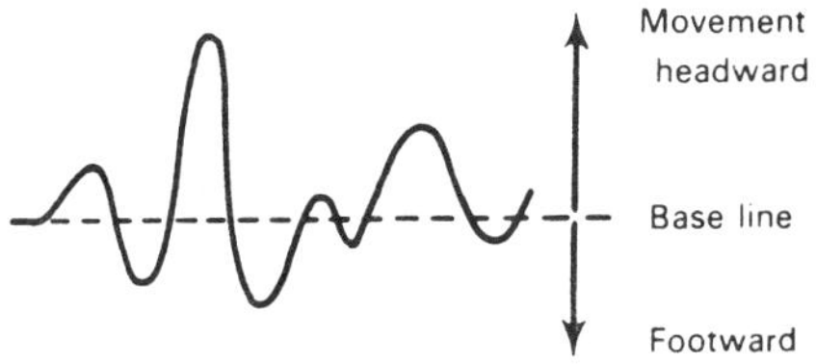

Ballistocardiogram

ballistocardiograph (BCG) (bal-is-tō-kar'dē-ō-graf). Instrument for taking a ballistocardiogram, consisting either of a moving table suspended from the ceiling, or of an apparatus that rests upon the patient's body, usually on the shins, together with a graphic recording system.

ballistocardiography (bal-is-tō-kar-dē-og'ră-fē). **1.** The graphic recording of movements of the body imparted by ballistic forces (cardiac contraction and ejection of blood, deceleration of blood flow through the great vessels; these minute movements are amplified and recorded on moving chart paper after being translated into an electrical potential by a pickup device. **2.** The study and interpretation of ballistocardiograms.

ballistophobia (bal-is-tō-fō'bē-ă) [G. *ballo,* to throw, + *phobos,* fear]. Morbid fear of a projectile or missile.

balloon (bă-lūn). **1.** An inflatable spherical or ovoid device used to retain tubes or catheters in, or provide support to, various body structures. **2.** To distend a body cavity with a gas or fluid to facilitate its examination.

balloonseptostomy (bă-lūn'sep-tos'tō-mē). Creation of an artificial interatrial septal defect by cardiac catheterization during which an inflated balloon is pulled across the interatrial septum through the foramen ovale; used in cases of transposition of the great vessels and tricuspid atresia.

ballottable (bal-ot'ăbl). Capable of exhibiting the phenomenon of ballottement.

ballottement (bal-ot-maw') [Fr. *balloter,* to toss up]. **1.** Maneuver used in physical examination to estimate the size of an organ not near the surface, particularly when there is ascites, by a flicking motion of the hand or fingers similar to that of dribbling a basketball. **2.** An infrequently used method of diagnosis of pregnancy: with the tip of the forefinger in the vagina, a sharp tap is made against the lower segment of the uterus; the fetus, if present, is tossed upward and (if the finger is retained in place) will be felt to strike against the wall of the uterus as it falls back.

renal b., a maneuver in which the kidney is moved by pressure from behind, allowing it to be felt between the hands and its size, shape, and mobility determined.

balm (bawlm) [L. *balsanum*, fr. G. *balsamon*, the balsam tree]. **1.** Balsam. **2.** An ointment, especially a fragrant one. **3.** A soothing application.

b. of Gilead, Mecca balsam; opobalsamum; an oleoresin from *Commiphora opobalsamum* (family Burseraceae), probably the myrrh of the Bible; used in perfumery.

mountain b., eriodictyon.

sweet b., melissa.

balneotherapeutics, balneotherapy (bal'nē-ō-thār-ă-pyū'tiks, -thār'ă-pē) [L. *balneum*, bath]. Immersion of part or all of the body in a mineral water bath as a form of therapy.

Baló, Jozsef, Hungarian physician, *1896. See B.'s *disease*.

balsam (bawl'sam) [G. *balsamon;* L. *balsamum*]. Balm (1); a fragrant, resinous or thick, oily exudate from various trees and plants.

Canada b., Canada turpentine; a yellowish liquid resin from the b. fir, *Abies balsamea* (family Pinaceae); contains kinene and bornyl acetate; used for mounting histologic specimens and as a cement for lenses.

b. of copaiba, copaiba.

Mecca b., *balm* of Gilead.

b. of Peru, a thick, dark brown liquid b. obtained from *Toluifera pereirae* (family Leguminosae), containing 60% cinnamein; used as a healing application to wounds.

Tolu b., a yellowish brown soft mass obtained from *Toluifera balsamum* (family Leguminosae), containing cinnamic and benzoic acids and esters; used as a stimulant expectorant.

balsamic (bawl-sam'ik). **1.** Relating to balsam. **2.** Fragrant.

Bamberger, Eugen B., Austrian physician, 1858–1921. See B.-Marie *disease, syndrome*.

Bamberger, Heinrich von, Vienna physician, 1822–1888. See B.'s *albuminuria, disease, sign*.

bamethan sulfate (bā'meth-an) α-[(Butylamino)methyl]-*p*-hydroxybenzyl alcohol sulfate; a sympathomimetic amine used as a peripheral vasodilator.

bamifylline hydrochloride (bă-mif'i-lin). 8-Benzyl-7-{2-[ethyl(2-hydroxyethyl)amino] ethyl}theophylline hydrochloride; a vasodilator and smooth muscle relaxant.

bamipine (bam-i-pēn). 4-*N*- Benzylanilino-1-methylpiperidine; an antihistaminic.

bancroftiasis, bancroftosis (ban-krof-tī'ă-sis, -tō'sis). Infection with *Wuchereria bancrofti*.

band. **1.** Any appliance or part of an apparatus that encircles or binds a part of the body. **2.** Any ribbon-shaped or cordlike anatomical structure that encircles or binds another structure or that connects two or more parts. See fascia, line, linea, stripe, stria, tenia.

A b.'s, Q b.'s or disks; A or anisotropic disks; the dark-staining anisotropic cross striations in the myofibrils of muscle fibers, comprising regions of overlapping thick (myosin) and thin (actin) filaments.

absorption b., the range of wavelengths or frequencies in the electromagnetic spectrum where radiant energy is absorbed by passage through a gaseous, liquid, or dissolved substance; it is exploited for analytical purposes in colorimetry or spectrophotometry, and is usually described in terms of the wavelength where maximum absorbance occurs (*i.e.*, λ_{max}).

amniotic b.'s, amniotic adhesions; annular b.; Streeter's b.'s; Simonart's b.'s (1); Simonart's ligaments or threads; constriction ring (2); strands of amniotic tissue adherent to the embryo or fetus; they may cause constriction of embryonic limbs. See also congenital *amputation*.

annular b., amniotic b.'s.

anogenital b., the first indication of the perineum in the embryo.

atrioventricular b., *truncus* atrioventricularis.

Baillarger's b.'s, Baillarger's *lines*.

Bechterew's b., *band* of Kaes-Bechterew.

Broca's diagonal b., a white fiber bundle descending in the precommissural septum toward the base of the forebrain, immediately rostral to the lamina terminalis; at the base, the bundle turns in the caudolateral direction; traveling through a ventral stratum of the substantia innominata alongside the optic tract, it fades before reaching the amygdala.

chromosome b., an area of darker or contrasting staining across the width of a chromosome; the pattern of b.'s is characteristic for most chromosomes. See banding.

Clado's b., the suspensory ligament of the ovary covered with peritoneum.

b.'s of colon, *teniae* coli.

contraction b., a microscopic change in myocardial cells in which excessive contraction, associated with elevated intracellular calcium and serum norepinephrine, causes the formation of transverse amorphous b.'s in the fibers which are then incapable of contracting again.

coronary b., corium coronae; a region of the pododerm; a prominent ridge of corium and underlying tela subcutanea at the top of the hoof from which most of the wall of the hoof grows.

Essick's cell b.'s, groups of cells in the developing rhombencephalon which migrate in two b.'s, one of which eventually forms the inferior olivary nucleus and the arcuate nucleus, and the other the pontine nuclei.

Gennari's b., *line* of Gennari.

b of Giacomini, uncus b. of Giacomini.

H b., Hensen's disk or line; H disk; the paler area in the center of the A b. of a striated muscle fiber, comprising the central portion of thick (myosin) filaments which are not overlapped by thin (actin) filaments.

His' b., *truncus* atrioventricularis.

Hunter-Schreger b.'s, Hunter-Schreger or Schreger's lines; alternating light and dark lines seen in dental enamel that begin at the dentoenamel junction and end before they reach the enamel surface; they represent areas of enamel rods cut in cross-sections dispersed between areas of rods cut longitudinally.

I b., I or isotropic disk; a light b. on each side of the Z line of striated muscle fibers, comprising a region of the sarcomere where thin (actin) filaments are not overlapped by thick (myosin) filaments.

iliotibial b., *tractus* iliotibialis.

b. of Kaes-Bechterew, band, layer of Bechterew, line of Kaes; line of Kaes-Bechterew; b. of horizontal myelinated fibers in the most superficial part of the third layer of the isocortex.

Ladd's b., a peritoneal attachment of an incompletely rotated cecum, causing obstruction of the duodenum, found in malrotation of the intestine.

Lane's b., Lane's kink; a congenital b. on the distal ileum causing stasis.

M b., M *line*.

Mach's b., a relatively bright or dark b. perceived in a zone where the luminance increases or decreases rapidly.

Maissiat's b., *tractus* iliotibialis.

matrix b., a metal or plastic b. secured around the crown of a tooth to confine restorative material to be adapted into a prepared cavity.

Meckel's b., Meckel's ligament; the portion of the anterior ligament of the malleus that extends from the base of the anterior process through the petrotympanic fissure, to attach to the spine of the sphenoid.

moderator b., *trabecula* septomarginalis.

orthodontic b., a thin strip of metal closely adapted to the crown of a tooth.
pecten b., a fibrous induration of the anal pecten resulting from passive congestion or a chronic form of inflammation in this region.
perioplic b., a narrow b. of corium and underlying tela subcutanea proximal to the coronary b. at the top of the hoof; the periople develops from it.
Q b.'s, A b.'s.
Reil's b., **(1)** *trabecula* septomarginalis; **(2)** *lemniscus* medialis.
Simonart's b.'s, **(1)** amniotic b.'s; **(2)** weblike band of tissue partially filling the gap between the medial and lateral portions of a cleft lip.
Soret b., the absorption b. of all porphyrins at about 400 nm.
Streeter's b.'s, amniotic b.'s.
uncus b. of Giacomini, frenulum or b. of Giacomini; tail of the dentate gyrus; cauda fasciae dentatae; a slender whitish b., the attenuated anterior continuation of the dentate gyrus (fascia dentata), crossing transversally the surface of the recurved part of the uncus gyri parahippocampalis.
ventricular b. of larynx, *plica* vestibularis.
Z b., Z *line.*
zonular b., *zona* orbicularis.

bandage (ban'dij). **1.** A piece of cloth or other material, of varying shape and size, applied to a body part to make compression, absorb drainage, prevent motion, retain surgical dressings. **2.** To cover a body part by application of a b.

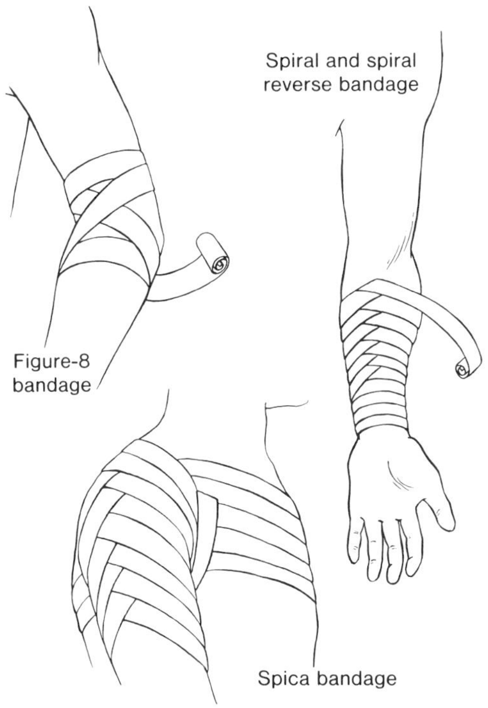

Bandage

adhesive b., a dressing of plain absorbent gauze affixed to plastic or fabric coated with a pressure-sensitive adhesive.
Barton's b., a figure-of-8 b. supporting the mandible below and anteriorly; used in mandibular fracture.
capeline b. [L. *capella,* a cap], a b. covering the head or an amputation stump like a cap.
circular b., one encircling an extremity, or a portion of it, or the trunk.
cravat b., a b. made by bringing the point of a triangular b. to the middle of the base and then folding lengthwise to the desired width.
crucial b., a b. in the shape of a cross; *e.g.,* a T-b.
demigauntlet b., a gauntlet b. that covers only the hand, leaving the fingers exposed.
Desault's b., a b. for fracture of the clavicle; the elbow is bound to the side, with a pad placed in the axilla.
elastic b., a b. containing stretchable material; used to make local pressure.
figure-of-8 b., a b. applied alternately to two parts, usually two segments of a limb above and below the joint, in such a way that the turns describe the figure 8; used primarily for the treatment of fractures of the clavicle.
four-tailed b., a strip of cloth split in two except for a central portion placed under the chin, with four tails tied over the head; used to limit motion of the mandible.
gauntlet b., a figure-of-8 b. covering the hand and fingers.
gauze b., see gauze.
Gibney's fixation b., herring-bone strapping of the foot and leg for sprain of the ankle.
Gibson's b., a b., resembling Barton's b., for stabilizing a fracture of the mandible.
hammock b., a b. for retaining dressings on the head: the dressings are covered by a wide gauze strip, the ends of which are brought down over the ears and held while a narrow circular b. is passed around the head; the ends of the gauze strip are then turned up over the circular b. and other turns are made securing them firmly.
immovable b., a b. of cloth impregnated with plaster of Paris, liquid glass, or the like, which hardens soon after its application.
many-tailed b., Scultetus b..
Martin's b., a roller b. of soft rubber used to make compression on a limb in the treatment of varicose veins or ulcers.
oblique b., a b. in which the successive turns proceed obliquely up or down the limb.
plaster b., a roller b. impregnated with plaster of Paris and applied moist; used to make a rigid dressing for a fracture or diseased joint.
roller b., a strip of material, of variable width, rolled into a compact cylinder to facilitate its application.
scarf b., triangular b.
Scultetus' b., many-tailed b.; a large oblong cloth, the ends of which are cut into narrow strips, which is applied to the thorax or abdomen, the strips being tied or overlapped and pinned.
spica b., [L. *spica,* ear of grain]. successive strips of material applied to the body and the first part of a limb, or to the hand and a finger, which overlap slightly in a V to resemble an ear of grain.
spiral b., an oblique b. encircling a limb, the successive turns overlapping those preceding.
suspensory b., suspensory; a bag of expansile fabric for supporting the scrotum and its contents.
T-b., T-*binder.*
triangular b., scarf b.; a piece of cloth cut in the shape of a right-angled triangle, used as a sling.
Velpeau's b., a b. which serves to immobilize arm to chest wall, with the forearm positioned obliquely across and upward on front of chest.

band'ing. The process of differential staining of metaphase chromosomes of cells to reveal the characteristic patterns of bands that permit identification of individual chromosomes; each of the 22 pairs of human chromosomes and the X and Y chromosomes has an identifying b. pattern.
BrDu-b., labeling of chromosomes in proliferating tissue by adding an excess of bromodeoxyuridine, which replaces the uridine incorporated in RNA and which fluoresces in ultraviolet light; the

bands result from sister chromatid exchanges.

C-b., a means of preferentially staining the regions of *c* onstitutive heterochromatin in the karyotype by denaturation with heat, acid, or alkali.

G-b., a process similar to C-b. in which *G* iemsa stain is used.

high-resolution b., b., especially in prophase, which increases the clarity and number of discernible chromosome bands.

NOR-b., a procedure which utilizes a silver stain that preferentially accumulates in the *n* ucleoli-*o* rganizing *r* egions, *i.e.,* the satellite regions of the acrocentric chromosomes.

prometaphase b., b. done in the stage of mitosis intermediate between prophase and metaphase.

Q-b., a process similar to C-b. in which *g* uinacrine and ultraviolet light are used.

R-b., a means of staining chromosomes utilizing a technique that is the *r* everse of that used for G-b., which results in a "photographic negative" of them; acridine orange and ultraviolet light are used.

reverse b., see R-b.

Bandl, Ludwig, German obstetrician, 1842–1892. See B.'s *ring.*

bandy-leg (ban'dē-leg). *Genu* varum.

bane (bān). A poison or blight.

Bang, Bernhard L.F., Danish veterinarian and physician, 1848–1932. See B.'s *bacillus, disease;* abortus-B.-ring *test.*

Bangerter, Alfred P.D., Swiss ophthalmologist, *1909. See B.'s *method.*

banisterine (ba-nis'tĕ-rēn). Harmine.

Bannister, Henry M., U.S. physician, 1844–1920. See B.'s *disease.*

Banti, Guido, Italian physician, 1852–1925. See B.'s *disease, syndrome.*

bar. 1. A unit of pressure equal to 1 megadyne (10^6 dyne) per cm^2 in the CGS system, 0.987 atmosphere, or $10^5 N/m^2$ in the SI system. **2.** Connector b. (1); one of the two convergent ridges on the ground surface of the hoof of a horse, united by the frog, and fused with the sole in front. **3.** A metal segment of greater length than width which serves to connect two or more parts of a removable partial denture. See also major *connector.* **4.** A segment of tissue or bone that unites two or more similar structures.

arch b., any one of several types of wires, b.'s, or splints conforming to the arch of the teeth, extending from one side of the arch to the other and located labially, or lingually; used for the treatment of jaw fractures and/or stabilization of injured teeth.

b. of bladder, *plica* interureterica.

clasp b., see clasp.

connector b., (1) bar (2); **(2)** see major or minor *connector.*

labial b., a major connector located labial to the dental arch joining two or more bilateral parts of a mandibular removable partial denture.

lingual b., a major connector located lingual to the dental arch joining two or more bilateral parts of a mandibular removable partial denture.

median b. of Mercier, a prominent band of fibromuscular tissue involving the interureteric ridge or neck of the urinary bladder, occasionally resulting in significant urinary obstruction.

Mercier's b., *plica* interureterica.

occlusal rest b., a minor connector used to attach an occlusal rest to a major part of a removable partial denture.

palatal b., a major connector which crosses the palate and unites two or more parts of a maxillary removable partial denture.

Passavant's b., Passavant's *cushion.*

sternal b., one of the transverse units of the developing sternum formed by the union of paired primordia.

terminal b., dark spots or b.'s (depending on the plane of section) in the lateral boundary between the apical ends of columnar epithelial cells; this region corresponds with the junctional complex and the thin filaments that anchor on the zonula adherans.

baragnosis (bar-ag-nō'sis) [G. *baros,* weight + *a-* priv., + *gnōsis,* a knowing]. Failure to appreciate the weight of objects held in the hand.

Bárány, Robert, Austrian otologist and Nobel laureate, 1876–1936. See B.'s *sign,* caloric *test.*

barba (bar'bă) [L.]. **1** [NA]. The beard. **2.** A hair of the beard.

barbaloin (bar-bal'ō-in). Aloin.

Barber. See Blount-B. *disease.*

barbiero (bar-bē-ā'rō) [Pg. the barber]. Brazilian term for the blood-sucking hemipteran triatomid bug, *Panstrongylus megistus,* an important vector of Chagas' disease, caused by *Trypanosoma cruzi.*

barbital (bar'bi-tawl). 5,5-Diethylbarbituric acid; diethylmalonylurea; a hypnotic and sedative; available as b. sodium (soluble b.), with the same uses.

barbiturate (bar-bich'yūr-āt). A derivative of barbituric acid, including phenobarbital and others, that act as CNS depressants and are used for their tranquilizing, hypnotic, and anti-seizure effects; some b.'s have the potential for abuse.

barbituric acid (bar-bi-chyūr'ik). Malonylurea; 2,4,6-trioxohexahydropyrimidine; 2,4,6-(1*H*,3*H*,5*H*) pyrimidinetrione; a crystalline dibasic acid from which barbital and other barbiturates are derived; has no sedative action.

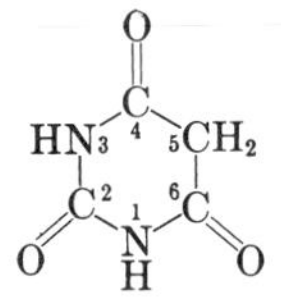

Barbituric acid

barbiturism (bar'bi-chyūr-izm). Chronic poisoning by any of the derivatives of barbituric acid; symptoms, which are not very distinctive, include cutaneous eruption accompanied by chills, fever, and headache.

barbotage (bar-bō-tahzh') [Fr. *barboter,* to dabble]. A method of spinal anesthesia in which a portion of the anesthetic solution is injected into the cerebral spinal fluid, which is then aspirated into the syringe and a second portion of the contents of the syringe is injected; the process is repeated until the entire contents of the syringe are injected.

barbula hirci (bar'byū-lă hir'sī) [L. dim. of *barba,* beard, + gen. sing. of *hircus,* goat]. The hairs growing from the tragus, antitragus, and incisura intertragica at the opening of the external acoustic meatus.

Barclay, Alfred E., British physician, 1877–1949. See B.-Baron *disease.*

Barcroft, Sir Joseph F., British physiologist, 1872–1947. See B.-Warburg *apparatus, technique.*

Bard, Louis, French physician, 1857–1930. See B.'s *sign.*

Bard, Philip, U.S. physiologist, *1898. See Cannon-B. *theory.*

Bardet, Georges, French physician, *1885. See B.-Biedl *syndrome;* Laurence-Moon-B.-Biedl *syndrome.*

Bardinet, Barthélemy A., French physician, 1809–1874. See B.'s *ligament.*

baresthesia (bar-es-thē'zē-ă) [G. *baros,* weight, + *aisthēsis,* sensation]. Pressure *sense.*

baresthesiometer (bar'es-thē'zē-om'ĕ-ter) [G. *baros,* weight, + *aisthēsis,* sensation, + *metron,* measure]. An instrument for measuring the pressure sense.

bariatric (bar-ē-at'rik). Relating to bariatrics.

bariatrics (bar-ē-at'riks) [G. *baros,* weight, + *iatreia,* medical treatment]. That branch of medicine concerned with the management (prevention or control) of obesity and allied diseases.

baric (ba'rik). Relating to barometric pressure (as in isobar) or to weight generally.

baricity (ba-ris'i-tē) [G. *baros,* weight]. The weight of one substance compared to the weight of an equal volume of another substance at the same temperature.

barilla (ba-ril'ā). Commercial, usually impure, sodium carbonate and sulfate.

baritosis (bar-i-tō'sis). A form of pneumoconiosis caused by barite or barium dust.

barium (ba'rē-ŭm, bā'rē-ŭm) [G. *barys,* heavy]. A metallic, alkaline, divalent earth element; symbol Ba, atomic weight 137.36, atomic no. 56.
b. chloride, formerly used as a heart tonic and for varicose veins; extremely toxic.
b. hydroxide, $Ba(OH)_2$; a caustic compound combined with calcium hydroxide in a carbon dioxide absorbent; used in anesthetic circuits. See also absorbent (3).
b. oxide, b. monoxide, baryta; BaO; it is caustic, forming the strong base, $Ba(OH)_2$, in water; used as a dehydrating agent.
b. sulfate, $BaSO_4$; given orally or rectally as a suspension for x-ray visualization of the gastrointestinal tract.
b. sulfide, a poisonous grayish yellow powder, used as a depilatory.

bark. 1. The envelope or covering of the roots, trunk, and branches of plants. B.'s of pharmacological significance not listed below are alphabetized under specific names. **2.** Cinchona.
cinchona, Jesuits', or Peruvian b., cinchona.

Barkan, Otto, U.S. ophthalmologist, 1887–1958. See B.'s *operation.*

Barkman, Åke, 20th century Swedish internist. See B.'s *reflex.*

Barkow, Hans K.L., German anatomist, 1798–1873. See B.'s *ligament.*

Barlow, John B., 20th century South African cardiologist. See B. *syndrome.*

Barlow, Sir Thomas, British physician, 1845–1945. See B.'s *disease.*

barn [fr. "big as the side of a barn" by humorous comparison with much smaller areas]. A unit of area for effective cross-section of atomic nuclei with respect to atomic projectiles; equal to 10^{-24} cm^2.

Barnes, Robert, British obstetrician, 1817–1907. See B.'s *curve, zone.*

Barnes' dystrophy. See under dystrophy.

baro- [G. *baros,* weight]. Combining form relating to weight or pressure.

baroceptor (bar'ō-sep-ter, -tōr). Baroreceptor.

barograph (bar'ō-graf). Barometrograph; a device that gives a continuous record of barometric pressure.

barometrograph (bar-ō-met'rō-graf). Barograph.

Baron. See Barclay-Baron *disease.*

barophilic (bar'ō-fil'ik) [G. *baros,* weight, + *phileō,* to love]. Thriving under high environmental pressure; applied to microorganisms.

baroreceptor (bar'ō-rē-sep'ter, -tōr). Baroceptor; pressoreceptor; sensory nerve ending in the wall of the auricles of the heart, vena cava, aortic arch, and carotid sinus, sensitive to stretching of the wall resulting from increased pressure from within, and functioning as the receptor of central reflex mechanisms that tend to reduce that pressure.

baroreflex (bar-ō-rē'fleks). A reflex triggered by stimulation of a baroreceptor.

baroscope (bar'ō-skōp). An instrument measuring changes in atmospheric pressure.

barosinusitis (bar'ō-sī-nus-ī'tis) [G. *baros,* weight, pressure, + sinusitis]. Aerosinusitis.

barostat (bar'ō-stat). A pressure-regulating device or structure, such as the baroreceptors of the carotid sinus and aortic arch, when connected to effectors providing negative feedback.

barotaxis (bar-ō-tak'sis) [G. *baros,* weight, + *taxis,* order]. Barotropism; reaction of living tissue to changes in pressure.

barotitis media (bar-ō-tī'tis mē'dē-ā). Aerotitis media.

barotrauma (băr'ō-traw'mă) [G. *baros,* weight, + trauma]. Injury, generally to the middle ear or paranasal sinuses, resulting from imbalance between ambient pressure and that within the affected cavity.
otic b., injury caused to the ear by imbalance in pressure between ambient air and the air in the middle ear.
sinus b., injury to air sinuses, resulting from imbalance in pressure between ambient air and air in the paranasal sinuses. See also aerosinusitis.

barotropism (bar-ot'rō-pizm) [G. *baros,* weight, + *tropē,* a turning]. Barotaxis.

Barr, Murray L., Canadian microanatomist, *1908. See B. chromatin *body.*

Barr, Yvonne M. See Epstein-B. *virus.*

Barraquer, Ignacio, Spanish ophthalmologist, 1884–1965. See B.'s *method.*

Barraquer Roviralta, Luis, Spanish physician, 1855–1928. See B.'s *disease.*

Barré, Jean A., French neurologist, *1880. See B.'s *sign;* Guillain-B. *reflex, syndrome;* Landry-Guillain-Barré *syndrome.*

barren (bar'en) [M.E. *bareyne*]. Unable to produce a pregnancy.

Barrett, Norma R., British physician, *1903. See B. *esophagus, syndrome;* B.'s *epithelium.*

barrier (bar'ē-er). **1.** An obstacle or impediment. **2.** In psychiatry, a conflictual agent that blocks resolving behavior.
blood-air b., the material intervening between alveolar air and the blood; it consists of a nonstructural film or surfactant, alveolar epithelium, basement lamina, and endothelium.
blood-aqueous b., a selectively permeable b. between the capillary bed in the processes of the ciliary body and the aqueous humor in the anterior chamber of the eye; consists of two layers of simple cuboidal epithelium joined at their apical surfaces with junctional complexes.
blood-brain b. (BBB), a selective mechanism opposing the passage of most ions and large-molecular compounds from the blood to brain tissue located in a continuous layer of endothelial cells connected by tight junctions; similar capillaries are found in the retina, iris, inner ear, and within the endoneurium of peripheral nerves.
blood-cerebrospinal fluid b., blood-CSF b., a b. located at the tight junctions which surround and connect the cuboidal epithelial cells on the surface of the choroid plexus; capillaries and connective tissue stroma of the choroid do not represent a b. to protein tracers or dyes.
incest b., in psychoanalysis, the learning or internalization of parental and social prohibitions against incest.
placental b., placental *membrane.*

Bart. Surname of the individual in whom *hemoglobin* Bart's was first reported.

Bart's syndrome. See under syndrome.

Bartels, Peter H., U.S. scientist, *1929. See B.'s *spectacles.*

Barth, Jean B., Strasburg physician, 1806–1877. See B.'s *hernia.*

Bartholin, Casper, Danish anatomist, 1655–1738. See B.'s *abscess, cyst, cystectomy, duct, gland.*

Bartholin, Thomas, Danish anatomist, 1616–1680. See B.'s *anus.*

bartholinitis (bar-tō-lin-ī'tis). Inflammation of a vulvovaginal (Bartholin's) gland.

Bartholomew, Rudolph A., U.S. obstetrician-gynecologist, 1886–1969. See B.'s *rule* of fourths.

Bartley, Samuel H., U.S. psychologist, *1901. See Brücke-B. *phenomenon.*

Barton, John Rhea, U.S. surgeon, 1794–1871. See B.'s *bandage, forceps, fracture.*

Bartonella (bar-tō-nel'ă) [A. L. *Barton*]. A genus of bacteria (family Bartonellaceae) placed in the order Rickettsiales; these organisms multiply in fixed-tissue cells and in erythrocytes and reproduce by binary fission; they are found in man and in arthropod vectors.
B. bacillifor'mis, a species found in the blood and epithelial cells of lymph nodes, spleen, and liver in Oroya fever and in blood and eruptive elements in verruga peruana; probably also found in sandflies (*Phlebotomus verrucarum*); known to be established only on the South American continent and perhaps in Central America; it is the type species of the genus *B.*

bartonellosis (bar-tō-nel-ō'sis). A disease, endemic in certain valleys of the Andes in Peru, Chile, Ecuador, Bolivia, and Colombia, caused by *Bartonella bacilliformis which is* transmitted by the bite of the nocturnally biting sandfly, *Phlebotomus verrucarum;* occurs in three forms: 1) Oroya *fever;* 2) *verruga* peruana; 3) a combination or sequence of these.

Bartter, Frederic C., U.S. physician, 1914–1983. See B.'s *syndrome.*

Baruch, Simon, U.S. physician, 1840–1921. See B.'s *law.*

baruria (bar-yū'rē-ă) [G. *barys,* heavy, + *ouron,* urine]. Rarely used term for excretion of urine that has an unusually high specific gravity, *e.g.,* greater than 1.025 to 1.030.

bary- [G. *barys,* heavy]. Combining form meaning heavy.

barye (ba'rē) [G. *barys,* heavy]. The CGS unit of pressure, equal to 1 $dyne/cm^2$. See bar (1).

baryglossia (bar-i-glos'ē-ă) [bary- + G. *glōssa,* tongue]. Baryphonia.

barylalia (bar-i-lā'lē-ă) [bary- + G. *lalia,* speech]. Baryphonia.

barymazia (bar-i-mā'zē-ă). [bary- + G. *mazos,* breast]. Rarely used term for hypertrophy of the breast.

baryphonia (bar-i-fō'nē-ă) [bary- + G. *phōnē,* voice]. Baryglossia; barylalia; a deep voice.

baryta (ba-rī'tă) [G. *barytēs,* weight]. *Barium* oxide.

baryto- Prefix indicating the presence of barium in a mineral.

basad (bā'sad). In a direction toward the base of any object or structure.

basal (bā'săl). **1.** Basalis; basialis (1); situated nearer the base of a pyramid-shaped organ in relation to a specific reference point; opposite of apical. **2.** In dentistry, denoting the floor of a cavity in the grinding surface of a tooth. **3.** Denoting a standard or reference state of a function, as a basis for comparison. More specifically, denoting the exact conditions for measurement of basal metabolic *rate* (*q.v.*); b. conditions do not always denote a minimum value, *e.g.,* metabolic rate in sleep is usually less than the b. rate, but is inconvenient for standard measurement.

basalioma (bā-sal-ē-ō'mă). Basal cell *carcinoma.*

basalis (bā-sā'lis) [L.] [NA]. Basal (1).

basaloid (bā'să-loyd). Resembling that which is basal, but not necessarily basal in origin or position.

basaloma (bā-să-lō'mă). Basal cell *carcinoma.*

Basan's syndrome. See under syndrome.

base (bās) [L. and G. *basis*]. **1.** Basement (1); basis; the lower part or bottom; the part opposite the apex; the foundation. **2.** In pharmacy, the chief ingredient of a mixture. **3.** In chemistry, an electropositive element (cation) that unites with an anion to form a salt; a compound ionizing to yield hydroxyl ion. See also Brønsted b. **4.** Nitrogen-containing organic compounds (*e.g.,* purines, pyrimidines, amines, alkaloids, ptomaines) that act as Brønsted b.'s. **5.** Cations, or substances forming cations. **6.** An element or radical containing an unshared pair of electrons (Lewis concept).

$$\begin{matrix} H \\ :\ddot{N}:H \\ \ddot{H} \end{matrix} + H^+ \rightarrow \left[\begin{matrix} H \\ H:\ddot{N}:H \\ \ddot{H} \end{matrix}\right]^+$$

acrylic resin b., a form made of acrylic resin molded to conform to the tissues of the alveolar process and used to support the teeth of a prothesis.
aldehyde b., obsolete term for an imide.
anterior cranial b., *fossa* cranii anterior.
b. of arytenoid cartilage, *basis* cartilaginis arytenoideae.
b. of bladder, *fundus* vesicae urinariae.
b. of brain, *facies* inferior cerebri.
Brønsted b., any molecule or ion that combines with a hydrogen ion; *e.g.,* OH^-, CN^-, NH_3; this definition replaces the older and more limited concepts of base (3).
cavity preparation b., cement b.
cement b., cavity preparation b.; in dentistry, a layer of dental cement, sometimes medicated, that is placed in the deep portion of a cavity preparation to protect the pulp, reduce the bulk of a metallic restoration, or eliminate undercuts.
b. of cochlea, *basis* cochleae.
cranial b., *basis* cranii interna.
denture b., saddle (2); **(1)** that part of a denture which rests on the oral mucosa and to which teeth are attached; **(2)** that part of a complete or partial denture which rests upon the basal seat and to which teeth are attached.
b. of heart, *basis* cordis.
hexone b.'s, histone b.'s, the α-amino acids arginine, histidine, and lysine, which are basic by virtue of the presence in the side chains of a guanidine, imidazole, and amine group, respectively; called "hexone" because each is a six-carbon compound.
internal b. of skull, *basis* cranii interna.
b. of lung, *basis* pulmonis.
b. of mandible, *basis* mandibulae.
b. of metacarpal bone, *basis* ossis metacarpalis.
metal b., a metallic portion of a denture b. forming a part of the wall of the basal surface of the denture; it serves as a b. for the attachment of the plastic (resin) part of the denture and the teeth.
b. of metatarsal bone, *basis* ossis metatarsalis.
b. of modiolus, *basis* modioli.
nucleic acid b., a purine or pyrimidine.
nucleinic b., obsolete term for purine.
b. of patella, *basis* patellae.
b. of phalanx, *basis* phalangis.
pressor b., pressor amine or substance; **(1)** one of several products of intestinal putrefaction believed to cause functional hypertension when absorbed; **(2)** any alkaline substance that raises blood pressure.
b. of prostate, *basis* prostatae.
record b., baseplate.
b. of renal pyramid, *basis* pyramidis renis.
b. of sacrum, *basis* ossis sacri.
Schiff b., a condensation (dehydration) product of a primary amine and an aldehyde with production of an N=C link, such as the intermediates formed by pyridoxal phosphate in transaminations and amino acid decarboxylations.

shellac b., a resinous wafer adapted to maxillary or mandibular casts to form baseplates.
b. of skull, *basis* cranii.
b. of stapes, *basis* stapedis.
temporary b., baseplate.
tinted denture b., a denture b. that simulates the coloring and shading of natural oral tissues.
b. of tongue, *radix* linguae.
tooth-borne b., the denture b. restoring an edentulous area which has abutment teeth at each end for support; the tissue which it covers is not used for support.
trial b., baseplate.
vegetable b., alkaloid.

basedoid (bahz'ĕ-doyd). Denoting a condition resembling Graves' disease (Basedow's disease), but without toxic symptoms.

Basedow, Karl A. von, German physician, 1799–1854. See B.'s *disease, pseudoparaplegia;* Jod-B. *phenomenon;* basedowian *insanity.*

basedowian (bahz-ĕ-dō'ē-an). Described by or attributed to K. Basedow.

basement (bās'ment). **1.** Base (1). **2.** A cavity or space partly or completely separated from a larger space above it.

baseplate (bās'plāt). Record, temporary, or trial base; a temporary form representing the base of a denture; used for making maxillomandibular (jaw) relation records and for the arrangement of teeth.
stabilized b., a b. lined with plastic material to improve its fit and stability.

Basex syndrome. See under syndrome.

bas-fond (bah-fawn'). Fundus.

basi-, basio-, baso- [G. and L. *basis,* base]. Combining forms meaning base, or basis.

basialis (bā-sē-ā'lis). Basal; relating to a basis or the basion.

basialveolar (bā'sē-al-vē'ō-lăr). Relating to both basion and alveolar points; denoting especially the b. length, or the shortest distance between these two points.

basic (bā'sik). Relating to a base.

basicity (bā-sis'i-tē). **1.** The valence or combining power of an acid, or the number of replaceable atoms of hydrogen in its molecule. **2.** The characteristic(s) of being a chemical base.

basic life support. Emergency cardiopulmonary resuscitation, control of bleeding, treatment of shock and poisoning, stabilization of injuries and wounds, and basic first aid.

basicranial (bā'si-krā'nē-ăl). Relating to the base of the skull.

Basidiobolus (ba-sid'ē-ō-bō'lŭs) [Mod. L. *basidium,* dim. of G. *basis,* base, + L. *bolus,* fr. G. *bolos,* lump or clod]. A genus of fungi belonging to the class Zygomycetes (Phycomycetes). *B. haptosporus* has been isolated from cases of entomophthoramycosis basidiobolae in man, especially in Indonesia, tropical Africa, and Southeast Asia.

Basidiomycetes (ba-sid'ē-ō-mī-sēt'ez) [Mod. L. *basidium,* dim. of G. *basis,* base, + *mykēs* (*mykēt*), fungus]. One of the four major classes of fungi, characterized by a spore-bearing organ (basidium), usually a single clavate cell, which bears basidiospores after karyogamy and meiosis. The class comprises the smuts, rusts, mushrooms, and puffballs. Excluding mycotoxins, there is only one human pathogen, the basidiomycetous stage of *Cryptococcus neoformans.*

basidiospore (ba-sid'ē-ō-spōr) [G. *basidon,* small base, + *sporos,* seed]. A fungal spore borne on a basidium, characteristic of the class Basidiomycetes.

basidium, pl. **basidia** (ba-sid'ē-ŭm, -ă) [L., fr G. *basis,* base]. A spore-bearing organ or conidiophore, the spore mother cell characteristic of Basidiomycetes. It bears a fixed number of asexual spores (basidiospores or conidia) externally after karyogamy and meiosis. It is composed of a swollen terminal cell situated on a slender stalk, and gives rise to slender filaments (sterigmata), usually four in number, from the ends of which the spores are developed.

basifacial (bā'si-fā'shăl). Relating to the lower portion of the face.

basihyal, basihyoid (bā'si-hī'ăl, bā-si-hī'oyd). The base or body of the hyoid bone.

basilar, basilaris (bas'i-lăr, bas-i-lā'ris). Relating to the base of a pyramidal or broad structure.

basilateral (bā'si-lat'er-ăl). Relating to the base and one or more sides of any part.

basilemma (bā-si-lem'ă) [basi- + G. *lemma,* rind]. Basement *membrane.*

basilicus (ba-sil'i-kŭs) [L. fr. G. *basilikos,* royal]. Denoting a prominent or important part or structure.

basin (bā'sin). A receptacle for fluids.
emesis b., kidney b., a shallow b. of curved, kidney-shaped design, used to collect body fluids or as a container for various other liquids.
pus b., a receptacle curved so as to fit closely the surface to which it is applied, used to receive the pus from a wound during its cleansing and redressing.

basinasal (bā'si-nā'săl). Relating to the basion and the nasion; denoting especially the b. length, or the shortest distance between the two points.

basio-. See basi-.

basioccipital (bā'sē-ok-sip'i-tăl). Relating to the basilar process of the occipital bone.

basioglossus (bā-sē-ō-glos'ŭs). The portion of the hyoglossus muscle that originates from the body of the hyoid bone.

basion (bā'sē-on) [G. *basis,* a base] [NA]. The middle point on the anterior margin of the foramen magnum, opposite the opisthion.

basipetal (bā-sip'ĕ-tăl) [basi- + L. *peto,* to seek]. **1.** In a direction toward the base. **2.** Pertaining to asexual conidial production in fungi, in which successive budding of the basal conidium forms in an unbranched chain with the youngest at the base.

basiphobia (bās-i-fō'bē-ă) [G. *basis,* a stepping, + *phobos,* fear]. Morbid fear of walking.

basis (bā'sis) [L. and G.] [NA]. Base (1).
b. cartilag'inis arytenoi'deae [NA], base of arytenoid cartilage; the part of the arytenoid cartilage that articulates with the cricoid cartilage and from which the muscular process extends laterally and the vocal process projects anteriorly.
b. cer'ebri, *facies* inferior cerebri.
b. coch'leae [NA], base of cochlea; the enlarged part of the cochlea that is directed posteriorly and medially and lies close to the internal acoustic meatus.
b. cor'dis [NA], base of the heart; that part of the heart formed mainly by the left atrium but to a small extent by the posterior part of the right atrium; it is directed backward and to the right and is separated from the vertebral column by the esophagus and aorta.
b. cranii externa [NA], official alternate term for *norma* basilaris.
b. cra'nii inter'na [NA], internal base of skull; cranial base; the interior aspect of the skull on which the brain rests.
b. mandib'ulae [NA], base of mandible; the rounded inferior border of the body of the mandible.
b. modi'oli [NA], base of modiolus; the part of the modiolus enclosed by the basal turn of the cochlea; it faces the lateral end of the internal acoustic meatus.
b. os'sis metacarpa'lis [NA], base of metacarpal bone; the expanded proximal extremity of each metacarpal that articulates with one or more of the distal row of carpal bones.
b. os'sis metatarsa'lis [NA], base of metatarsal bone; the ex-

panded proximal extremity of each metatarsal bone; it articulates with one or more of the distal row of tarsal bones.

b. os'sis sa'cri [NA], base of sacrum; the upper end of the sacrum that articulates with the body of the fifth lumbar vertebra in the midline and the alae on either side.

b. patel'lae [NA], base of patella; the superior border of the patella to which the tendon of the rectus femoris attaches.

b. pedun'culi, *crus* cerebri.

b. phalan'gis [NA], base of phalanx; the expanded proximal end of each phalanx in the hand or foot that articulates with the head of the next proximal bone in the digit.

b. prosta'tae [NA], base of prostate; the broad upper surface of the prostate contiguous with the bladder wall.

b. pulmo'nis [NA], base of lung; the lower concave part of the lung that rests upon the convexity of the diaphragm.

b. pyram'idis re'nis [NA], base of renal pyramid; the outer broad part of a renal pyramid that lies next to the cortex.

b. stape'dis [NA], base of stapes; footplate (1); the flat portion of the stapes that fits in the oval window.

basisphenoid (bā'si-sfē'noyd). Relating to the base or body of the sphenoid bone; denoting the independent center of ossification in the embryo that forms the posterior portion of the body of the sphenoid bone.

basitemporal (bā'si-tem'pō-răl). Relating to the lower part of the temporal region.

basivertebral (bā'si-ver'tĕ-brăl). Relating to the body of a vertebra.

bas'ket. 1. A basket-like arborization of the axon of cells in the cerebellar cortex, surrounding the cell body of Purkinje cells. **2.** Any basket-like device or structure.

fibrillar b.'s, the scleral end of neuroglia fibers of Müller which as fine, tapering, needlelike fibrillae ascend the proximal parts of rods and cones, giving them a fibrillar appearance.

stone b., an instrument passed through an endoscope to capture and extract urinary calculi.

Basle Nomina Anatomica (BNA). Basel anatomical nomenclature; the name adopted in 1895 in Basel, Switzerland (French spelling, Basle) by members of the German Anatomical Society which met to compile a Latin nomenclature of anatomical terms. Revisions of the resulting nomenclature were published at intervals until, in 1955 in Paris, France, the international membership of the Congress of Anatomists adopted a modification of the Basle Nomina Anatomica terminology. That modification dropped the reference to the original meeting place. See *Nomina Anatomica.*

baso-. See basi-.

basocyte (bā'sō-sīt) [G. *basis,* base, + *kytos,* cell]. Basophilic *leukocyte.*

basocytopenia (bā'sō-sī-tō-pē'nē-ă). Basophilic *leukopenia.*

basocytosis (bā'sō-sī-to'sis). Basophilic *leukocytosis.*

basoerythrocyte (bā'sō-e-rith'rō-sīt). A red blood cell that manifests changes of basophilic degeneration, such as basophilic stippling, punctate basophilia, or basophilic granules.

basoerythrocytosis (bā'sō-ĕ-rith'rō-sī-tō'sis). An increase of red blood cells with basophilic degenerative changes, frequently observed in diseases characterized by prolonged hypochromic anemia.

basograph (bā'sō-graf) [baso- + G. *graphō,* to write]. An instrument that makes graphic records of abnormalities of gait.

basolateral (bā-sō-lat'er-ăl). Basal and lateral; specifically used to refer to one of the two major cytological divisions of the amygdaloid complex. See *corpus* amygdaloideum.

basometachromophil, basometachromophile (bā'sō-met-ă-krō'mō-fil, -fīl). Staining metachromatically with a basic dye. See metachromasia.

basopenia (bā-sō-pē'nē-ă) [baso- + G. *penia,* poverty]. Basophilic *leukopenia.*

basophil, basophile (bā'sō-fil, -fīl) [baso- + G. *phileō,* to love]. **1.** A cell with granules that stain specifically with basic dyes. **2.** Basophilic. **3.** A phagocytic leukocyte of the blood characterized by numerous basophilic granules containing heparin and histamine; except for its segmented nucleus, it is morphologically and physiologically similar to the mast cell.

tissue b., mast *cell.*

basophilia (bā-sō-fil'ē-ă). Basophilism. **1.** A condition in which there is more than the usual number of basophilic leukocytes in the circulating blood (basophilic leukocytosis) or an increase in the proportion of parenchymatous basophilic cells in an organ (in the bone marrow, basophilic hyperplasia). **2.** Grawitz' b.; a condition in which basophilic erythrocytes are found in circulating blood, as in certain instances of leukemia, advanced anemia, malaria, and plumbism.

Grawitz' b., basophilia (2).

pituitary b., obsolete name for pituitary basophil *adenoma.*

punctate b., stippling (1).

basophilic (bā'sō-fil'ik). Basophil (2); denoting tissue components having an affinity for basic dyes under specific pH conditions.

basophilism (bā-sof'i-lizm). Basophilia.

Cushing's b., pituitary b., Cushing's *syndrome.*

basophilocyte (bā-sō-fil'ō-sīt). Basophilic *leukocyte.*

basoplasm (bā'sō-plazm). That part of the cytoplasm which stains readily with basic dyes.

Bassen, Frank A. See B.-Kornzweig *syndrome.*

Bassini, Edoardo, Italian surgeon, 1844–1924. See B.'s *operation.*

Bassler, Anthony U.S. physician, 1874–1959. See B.'s *sign.*

bassorin (bas'ōr-in). The insoluble portion (60 to 70%) of tragacanth that swells to form a gel; it contains complex methoxylated acids, particularly bassoric acid.

Bastedo, Walter A., U.S. physician, 1873–1952. See B.'s *sign.*

bat [M.E. *bakke*]. A member of the mammalian order Chiroptera.

vampire b., a member of the genus *Desmodus;* an important reservoir host of rabies virus in Central and South America.

bath [A.S. *baeth*]. **1.** Immersion of the body or any of its parts in water or any other yielding or fluid medium, or application of such medium in any form to the body or any of its parts. **2.** Apparatus used in giving a b. of any form, qualified according to the medium used, the temperature of the medium, the form in which the medium is applied, the medicament added to the medium, or according to the part bathed.

colloid b., a b. prepared by adding soothing agents such as sodium bicarbonate or oatmeal to the b. water to relieve skin irritation and pruritus.

contrast b., a b. in which a part is immersed in hot water for a period of a few minutes and then in cold, the hot and cold periods alternated regularly at half-hour intervals; used to increase the blood flow to the part.

douche b., the local application of water in the form of a large jet or stream.

dousing b., a luminous electric hot air b. given at a very high temperature.

electric b., electrotherapeutic b., (1) hydroelectric b.; a b. in which the medium is charged with electricity; **(2)** therapeutic application of static electricity, with the patient placed on an insulated platform.

Greville b., an obsolete treatment with nonluminous electric hot air given at a very high temperature.

hafussi b. [Ger. *hand,* hand, + *fuss,* foot], a modification of the Nauheim treatment, only the hands and feet of the patient being immersed in hot water through which carbon dioxide gas is made to pass.

hydroelectric b., electric b. (1).
light b., therapeutic exposure of the skin to radiant light.
Nauheim b., Nauheim *treatment.*
needle b., a b. in which water is projected forcibly against the body in many very fine jets.
oil b., in chemistry, a vessel containing oil, in which a container holding a substance to be heated or evaporated can be immersed.
sand b., in chemistry, an arrangement whereby a substance to be treated is in a vessel protected from the direct action of fire by a layer of sand.
sitz b. [Ger. *sitzen,* to sit], immersion of only the perineum and buttocks, with the legs being outside of the tub.
water b., in chemistry, a vessel containing water, in which a container holding a substance to be heated or evaporated can be immersed.

bathmotropic (bath-mō-trō'pik) [G. *bathmos,* threshold, + *tropē,* a turning]. Influencing nervous and muscular irritability in response to stimuli.
negatively b., lessening nervous or muscular irritability.
positively b., increasing nervous or muscular irritability.

batho- [G. *bathos,* depth]. Combining form relating to depth. See also bathy-.

bathochromic (bath-ō-krō'mik) [batho- + G. *chrōma,* color]. Denoting the shift of an absorption spectrum maximum to a longer wavelength.

bathoflore (bath'ō-flōr). An atom or group of atoms that, by its presence in a molecule, shifts the latter's fluorescent radiation in the direction of longer wavelength, or reduces the fluorescence. *Cf.* auxoflore.

bathophobia (bath-ō-fō'bē-ă) [G. *bathos,* depth, + *phobos,* fear]. Morbid fear of deep places or of looking into them.

bathy- [G. *bathys,* deep]. Combining form relating to depth. See also batho-.

bathyanesthesia (bath'ē-an-es-thē'zē-ă) [G. *bathys,* deep, + *an-* priv. + *aisthēsis,* sensation]. Loss of deep or mesoblastic sensibility.

bathycardia (bath-ē-kar'dē-ă) [G. *bathys,* deep, + *kardia,* heart]. A condition in which the heart occupies a lower position than normal but is fixed there, as distinguished from cardioptosia.

bathyesthesia (bath'ē-es-thē'zē-ă) [G. *bathys,* deep, + *aisthēsis,* sensation]. General term for all subcutaneous sensation; *i.e.,* sensation in the tissues beneath the skin. See also myesthesia.

bathygastry (bath-ē-gas'trē) [G. *bathys,* deep, + *gastēr,* stomach]. Gastroptosis.

bathyhyperesthesia (bath-ē-hī'per-es-thē'zē-ă) [G. *bathys,* deep, + *hyper,* above, + *aisthēsis,* sensation]. Exaggerated sensitiveness of the muscular tissues and other deep structures.

bathyhypesthesia (bath-ē-hip'es-thē'zē-ă) [G. *bathys,* deep, + *hypo,* under, + *aisthēsis,* sensation]. Impairment of sensation in the deeper parts; partial loss of the muscle sense.

Batson, Oscar V., U.S. otolaryngologist, 1894–1979. See B.'s *plexus,* Carmody-B. *operation.*

Batten, Frederick E., British ophthalmologist, 1865–1918. See B.-Mayou *disease.*

battery (bat'er-ē). A group or series of tests administered for analytic or diagnostic purposes.
Halstead-Reitan B., a b. of neuropsychological tests (category test, tactual performance test, Seashore test, speech sounds perception test, finger oscillation test, trail-making test, dynamometer strength of grip) used to determine the effects of brain damage on behavior.

Battle, William H., British surgeon, 1855–1936. See B.'s *incision, sign.*

Baudelocque, Jean L., French obstetrician, 1746–1810. See B.'s *diameter,* uterine *circle.*

Baudelocque, Louis A., French obstetrician, 1800–1864. See B.'s *operation.*

Bauer, Hans, 20th century German anatomist. See B.'s chromic acid leucofuchsin *stain.*

Bauer, Walter, U.S. internist, *1898. See B.'s *syndrome.*

Bauhin, Gaspard, Swiss anatomist, 1560–1624. See B.'s *gland, valve.*

Baumé, Antoine, French chemist and pharmacist, 1728–1805. See B.'s *scale.*

Baumès, Jean B.T., French physician, 1756–1828. See B.'s *symptom.*

Baumgarten, P. Clemens von, German pathologist, 1848–1928. See B.'s *veins;* Cruveilhier-B. *disease, murmur, sign, syndrome.*

bay (bā). **1.** In anatomy, a recess containing fluid. **2.** Especially, the lacrimal b.
celomic b.'s, medial and lateral recesses at either side of the urogenital mesentery of the embryo.
lacrimal b., *lacus* lacrimalis.

bayberry bark (bā'ber-ē). Myrica.

Bayes, Thomas, British mathematician, 1702–1761. See B. *theorem.*

Bayle, Antoine L.J., French physician, 1799-1858. See B.'s *disease.*

Bayley, Nancy, U.S. psychologist, *1899. See B. *Scales* of Infant Development.

bayonet (bā-ō-net') [Fr. *bayonette,* fr. *Bayonne,* France, where first made]. An instrument having a blade or nib that is offset and parallel to the shaft.

Bazett's formula. See under formula.

Bazin, Antoine P.E., French dermatologist, 1807–1878. See B.'s *disease.*

BBB Abbreviation for blood-brain *barrier.*

BBOT Abbreviation for 2,5-bis(5-*t*-butylbenzoxazol-2-yl) thiophene.

BCG Abbreviation for Bacille bilié de Calmette-Guérin; ballistocardiograph.

BCNU Carmustine.

B.D.S. Abbreviation for Bachelor of Dental Surgery.

B.D.Sc. Abbreviation for Bachelor of Dental Science.

Be Symbol for beryllium.

beaded (bēd'ed). **1.** Marked by numerous small rounded projections, often arranged in a row like a string of beads. **2.** Applied to a series of noncontinuous bacterial colonies along the line of inoculation in a stab culture. **3.** Denoting stained bacteria in which more deeply stained granules occur at regular intervals in the organism.

beading (bē'ding). **1.** Numerous small rounded projections, often in a row like a string of beads. **2.** The rounded elevation along the border of the tissue surface of the major connectors of a maxillary dental prosthesis. **3.** Protection of the formed borders of final impressions by the careful placement of wax sticks or a plaster-pumice combination adjacent to the borders prior to forming the master cast.
b. of the ribs, rachitic *rosary.*

beak (bēk) [L. *beccus*]. **1.** The nose of pliers used in dentistry for contouring and adjusting wrought or cast metal dental appliances. **2.** Sometimes used to describe a beak-shaped anatomical structure. See rostrum.

beaker (bē'ker). A thin glass vessel, with a lip (beak) for pouring, used as containers for liquids.

Béal's conjunctivitis. See under conjunctivitis.

Beale, Lionel S., British physician, 1828–1906. See B.'s *cell.*

beam (bēm) [O.H.G. *Boum*]. Any bar whose curvature changes under load; in dentistry, frequently used instead of "bar."

Balkan b., Balkan *frame.*

cantilever b., in dentistry, a b. that is supported by only one fixed support at only one of its ends.

continuous b., in dentistry, a b. that continues over three or more supports, those supports not at the b. ends being equally free supports.

restrained b., in dentistry, a b. that has two or more supports, at least one of which permits some freedom of rotation to the point of support but not as much as if the support were a free support.

simple b., in dentistry, a straight b. that has two, and only two, supports, one at either end.

bean (bēn). The flattened seed, contained in a pod, of various leguminous plants. B.'s of pharmacological significance are alphabetized by specific name.

bearing (bār'ing). A supporting point or surface.

central b., in dentistry, application of forces between the maxillae and mandible at a single point located as near as possible to the center of the supporting areas of the upper and lower jaws; used for the purpose of distributing closing forces evenly throughout the areas of the supporting structures during the recording of maxillomandibular (jaw) relations and during the correction of occlusal errors.

bearing down. Expulsive effort of a parturient woman in the second stage of labor.

beat (bēt) [A.S. *beatan*]. **1.** To strike; to throb or pulsate. **2.** A stroke, impulse, or pulsation, as of the heart or pulse. **3.** Activity of a cardiac chamber produced by catching a stimulus generated elsewhere in the heart.

apex b., the visible and/or palpable pulsation made by the apex of the left ventricle as it strikes the chest wall in systole; normally in the fifth intercostal space, about 10 cm to the left of the median line.

atrial fusion b., a b. that occurs when the atria are activated in part by the sinus impulse and in part by a retrograde impulse from A-V node or ventricle.

automatic b., automatic contraction; in contrast to forced b., an ectopic b. that arises *de novo* and is not precipitated by the preceding b.; thus escaped and parasystolic b.'s are automatic.

capture b., ventricular capture; the cardiac cycle resulting when, after a period of A-V dissociation, the atria regain control of the ventricles.

combination b., fusion b.

coupled b.'s, bigeminal *pulse.*

dependent b., forced b.

Dressler b., fusion b. interrupting a ventricular tachycardia and producing a normally narrow QRS complex as a result of the fusion of two impulses, one impulse from the ventricular tachycardia and the other from a supraventricular focus; Dressler b.'s prove the presence of ventricular tachycardia by interruption of it.

dropped b., a heart b. that fails to appear owing to A-V block.

echo b., extrasystole produced by the return of an impulse in the heart retrograde to a focus near its origin which then returns antegradely to produce a second contraction of the heart.

ectopic b., a cardiac b. originating elsewhere than at the sinoatrial node.

escape b., escaped b., escaped contraction; an automatic b., usually arising from the A-V node or ventricle, occurring after the next expected normal b. has defaulted; it is therefore always a late b., terminating a longer cycle than the normal.

forced b., dependent b.; **(1)** an extrasystole supposedly precipitated in some way by the preceding normal b. to which it is coupled; **(2)** an extrasystole caused by artificial stimulation of the heart.

fusion b., combination, mixed, summation b.; a cardiac contraction triggered by more than a single impulse, when the wave fronts coincide to act together on a single focus of activity; in the electrocardiogram, the atrial or ventricular complex when either atria or ventricles are activated by two simultaneously invading impulses.

heart b., ictus cordis; a complete cardiac cycle, including spread of the electrical impulse and the consequent mechanical contraction.

interference b., ventricular capture in A-V dissociation.

mixed b., fusion b.

paired b.'s, see bigeminy.

parasystolic b., parasystole.

premature b., extrasystole.

pseudofusion b., an electrocardiographic representation of a cardiac depolarization produced by superimposition of an ineffectual electronic pacemaker spike upon a QRS-complex originating from a spontaneous focus within the heart; the pacemaker spike is ineffectual because the electronic discharge, which it represents graphically, occurred within the absolute refractory period of the spontaneous beat and is therefore not indicative of pacemaker malfunction.

reciprocal b., see reciprocal *rhythm.*

retrograde b., a b. occurring as a contraction of a portion of a heart chamber cephalad to the chamber of origin, *e.g.,* an atrial b. triggered by an impulse originating in the ventricle.

summation b., fusion b.

ventricular fusion b., a fusion b. that occurs when the ventricles are activated partly by the descending sinus or A-V nodal impulse and partly by an ectopic ventricular impulse.

Beau, Joseph H.S., French physician, 1806–1865. See B.'s *lines.*

Beauvaria (bō-vā'rē-ă). A genus of fungi (class Hyphomycetes). *B. bassiana* is pathogenic for insects and holds promise in the biologic control of insects.

becanthone hydrochloride (be-can'thōn). 1-{[2- [Ethyl(2-hydroxy-2-methylpropyl)amino]ethyl]amino}- 4-methylthioxanthen-9-one; a schistosomicide.

Bechterew, Vladimir M. von, Russian neurologist, 1857–1927. See B.'s *band, disease, layer, nucleus, sign; line* of B.; *band* of Kaes-B.; B.-Mendel or Mendel-B. *reflex.*

Beck, Claude S., U.S. surgeon, *1894. See B.'s *triad.*

Beck, Emil G., U.S. surgeon, 1866–1932. See B.'s *method.*

Beck, E.V. See Bek, E.V.

Becker, B.J.P. See B.'s *disease.*

Becker, P.E. See B. type tardive muscular *dystrophy.*

Becker, Samuel W., U.S. dermatologist, 1894–1964. See B.'s *nevus.*

Becker's stain for spirochetes. See under stain.

Beckmann, Ernst O., German chemist, 1853–1923. See B.'s *apparatus.*

Beckwith, John Bruce, U.S. pathologist, *1933. See B.-Wiedemann *syndrome.*

Béclard, Pierre A., French anatomist, 1785–1825. See B.'s *anastomosis, hernia, triangle.*

beclomethasone dipropionate (be-klō-meth'ă-sōn). Dipropionate salt of 9-chloro-11β,17,21-trihydroxy-16β-methylpregna-1,4-diene-3,20-dione; a topical anti-inflammatory agent.

Becquerel, Antoine H., French physicist and Nobel laureate, 1852–1908. See becquerel; B. *rays.*

becquerel (Bq) (bek'rel) [A.H. *Becquerel*]. The SI unit of measurement of radioactivity, equal to 1 disintegration per second; 1 Bq = 3.70×10^{10} Ci.

bed. 1. In anatomy, a base or structure that supports another structure. **2.** A piece of furniture used for rest, recuperation, or treatment.

capillary b., the capillaries considered collectively and their volume capacity for blood.
fracture b., a narrow extra firm b. for treatment of fractures; usually incorporates an overhead frame for traction apparatus.
Gatch b., a b. with divided sections for independent elevation of a patient's head and knees.
mud b., a b. in which the mattress consists of semiliquid mud made from special clays, covered with a sheet of plastic material; used to widely distribute the pressure of the body weight over the dependent surface, for patients with burns or large anesthetic areas.
nail b., *matrix* unguis.
water b., a mattress in the form of a closed rubber bag filled with water; used to prevent or treat pressure sores by equalizing the distribution of the patient's weight against the support.

bed'bug. *Cimex lectularius.*

bedlam (bed'lăm) [corruption or contraction of St. Mary of *Bethlehem* Hospital in London]. **1.** Colloquialism for a mental hospital or institution. **2.** A place or scene of wild or riotous behavior. **3.** A disturbing uproar.

Bednar, Alois, Austrian physician, 1816–1888. See B.'s *aphthae.*

Bednar, Blahoslav, 20th century Czech pathologist. See B. *tumor.*

Bedsonia (bed-sō'nē-ă). A generic name formerly used for organisms now placed in the genus *Chlamydia.*

bedsore (bed'sōr). Decubitus *ulcer.*

bed-wet'ting. Nocturnal *enuresis.*

bee [A.S. *beó, bī*]. An insect of the genus *Apis;* the honeybee, *A. mellifica,* is the source of honey and wax.

beech oil. Beechwood tar.

beechwood tar (bēch'wud). Beech oil; a thick, oily, dark brown liquid with the odor of creosote; largely used as a source of creosote.

Beer, August, German physicist, 1825–1863. See B.'s *law.*

Beer, Georg J., Austrian ophthalmologist, 1763–1821. See B.'s *knife, operation.*

beeswax (bēz'waks). Wax (1).
white b., white *wax.*

beeturia (bē-tū'rē-ă). Betacyaninuria; urinary excretion of betacyanin after ingestion of beets, found in most iron-deficient individuals and in some normal persons.

Beevor, Charles E., British neurologist, 1854–1908. See B.'s *sign.*

Begbie, James, Scottish physician, 1798–1869. See B.'s *disease.*

Begg, P. Raymond, Australian orthodontist, *1898. See B. light wire differential force *technique.*

Béguez César, Antonio, Cuban pediatrician. See B. C. *disease.*

behavior (bē-hāv'yer). **1.** Any response emitted by or elicited from an organism. **2.** Any mental or motor act or activity. **3.** Specifically, parts of a total response pattern.
adaptive b., any b. that enables an organism to adjust to a particular situation or environment.
adient b., appetitive b.
ambient b., aversive b.
appetitive b., adient b.; movement of an organism toward a certain type of stimulus, such as food. *Cf.* aversive b.
aversive b., ambient b.; movement of an organism away from a certain type of stimulus, such as electric shock. *Cf.* appetitive b.
hookean b., the b. of a perfectly elastic body; *i.e.,* the strain is directly proportional to the stress. See also Hooke's *law.*
molar b., in psychology, b. described in large response units rather than smaller ones. *Cf.* molecular b.
molecular b., in psychology, b. described in small response units rather than larger ones; a specific response. *Cf.* molar b.
obsessive b., the repetitive stylized b. seen in obsessive-compulsive neurosis.
operant b., response (2).
passive-aggressive b., apparently compliant b., with intrinsic obstructive or stubborn qualities, to cover deeply felt aggressive feelings.
respondent b., b. in response to a specific stimulus; usually associated with classical conditioning.
ritualistic b., automatic b. of psychogenic or cultural origin.
target b., **(1)** operant; **(2)** in behavior modification therapy, the prescribed goal performance.
type A b., a b. pattern characterized by aggressiveness, ambitiousness, restlessness, and a strong sense of time urgency; associated with increased risk for coronary heart disease.
type B b., a b. pattern characterized by the absence or obverse of type A b. characteristics.

behavioral (bē-hāv'yer-ăl). Pertaining to behavior.

behaviorism (bē-hāv'yer-izm). Behavioral psychology; a branch of psychology that attempts to formulate, through systematic observation and experimentation, the laws and principles which underlie the behavior of man and animals; its major contributions have been made in the areas of conditioning and learning.

behaviorist (bē-hāv'yer-ist). An adherent of behaviorism.

Behçet, Hulusi, Turkish dermatologist, 1889–1948. See B.'s *disease, syndrome.*

behenic acid (bĕ-hen'ik). Docosanoic acid; $CH_3(CH_2)_{20}COOH$; a constituent of most fats and fish oils; large amounts are found in jamba, mustard seed, and rapeseed oils.

Behr, Carl, German ophthalmologist, 1874–1943. See B.'s *disease, syndrome.*

Behring, Emil A. von, German bacteriologist and Nobel laureate, 1854–1917. See B.'s *law.*

BEI Abbreviation for butanol-extractable *iodine.*

bej'el. Nonvenereal endemic syphilis found chiefly among Arab children; apparently due to *Treponema pallidum.*

Bek (or Beck), E.V. See Kashin-B. *disease.*

Békésy, Georg von, Hungarian biophysicist in U.S. and Nobel laureate, 1899–1972. See B. *audiometer; audiometry.*

bel [A.G. *Bell*]. Unit expressing the relative intensity of a sound. The intensity in bels is the logarithm (to the base 10) of the ratio of the power of the sound to that of a reference sound. Ordinarily, the reference sound is assumed to be one with a power of 10^{-16} watts per sq cm, approximately the threshold of a normal human ear at 1000 Hz.

belch'ing [A.S. *baelcian*]. Eructation.

belemnoid (be-lem'noyd) [G. *belemnon,* a dart, + *eidos,* resemblance]. Dart-shaped.

Bell, Sir Charles, Scottish surgeon, anatomist, and physiologist, 1774–1842. See B.'s *law,* respiratory *nerve, palsy, phenomenon, spasm;* external respiratory *nerve* of B.

Bell, John, Scottish surgeon and anatomist, 1763–1820. See B.'s *muscle.*

belladonna (bel-ă-don'ă) [It. *bella,* beautiful, + *donna,* lady]. Deadly nightshade; *Atropa belladonna* (family Solanaceae); a perennial herb with dark purple flowers and shining purplish black berries; the leaves (0.3% b. alkaloids) and root (0.5% b. alkaloids) contain atropine and related alkaloids which are anticholinergic. B. is used as a powder (0.3% b. alkaloids, calculated as hyoscyamine) and tincture in asthma, colic, and hyperacidity.

belladonnine (bel-ă-don'ēn). An artificial alkaloid derived from atropine by warming with hydrochloric acid.

bell-crowned (bel'krownd). Denoting a tooth the crown of which has a cross-sectional diameter much greater than that of the neck.

belle indifference. See la belle indifference.

Bellini, Lorenzo, Italian physician and anatomist, 1643–1704. See B.'s *ducts, ligament.*

belly (bel'ē) [O.E. *belig,* bag]. **1.** The abdomen. **2.** Venter (2). **3.** Popularly, the stomach or womb.
b.'s of digastric muscle, see *venter* anterior musculi digastrici; *venter* posterior musculi digastrici.
frontal b., *venter* frontalis.
occipital b., *venter* occipitalis.
b.'s of omohyoid muscle, see *venter* inferior musculi omohyoidei; *venter* superior musculi omohyoidei.
prune b., see abdominal muscle deficiency *syndrome.*

bellyache (bel'ē-āk). Colloquialism for abdominal pain, usually colicky.

belly button (bel'ē bŭt'ŏn). Umbilicus.

belonephobia (bel'ō-nē-fō'bē-ă) [G. *belonē,* needle, + *phobos,* fear]. Morbid fear of needles, pins, and other sharp-pointed objects.

Belsey, Ronald, contemporary British surgeon. See B. *operation.*

bemegride (bem'ĕ-grīd). 3-Ethyl-3-methylglutarimide; a central nervous system stimulant used as an analeptic in intoxications due to barbiturates and other central nervous system depressant drugs.

benactyzine hydrochloride (ben-ak'ti-zēn). 2-Diethylaminoethyl benzilate hydrochloride; an anticholinergic drug with the same actions but with approximately only one-fifth the activity of atropine; it is thought to raise the threshold of emotional reaction to external stimuli. Used as a psychotherapeutic and tranquilizing agent.

Bence Jones, Henry, British physician, 1814–1873. See B.J. *albumin, cylinders, myeloma, protein, reaction.*

bendazac (ben'dă-zak). [(1-Benzyl-1*H*- indazol-3-yl)oxy]-acetic acid; a topical anti-inflammatory agent.

Bender, Lauretta, U.S. psychiatrist, *1897. See B. gestalt *test.*

bendrofluazide (ben-drō-flū'ă-zīd). Bendroflumethiazide.

bendroflumethiazide (ben'drō-flū'mĕ-thī'ă-zīd). Bendrofluazide; 3-benzyl-3,4-dihydro-6-(trifluoromethyl)-2*H*-1,2,4-benzothiadiazine-7-sulfonamide-1,1-dioxide; a diuretic and antihypertensive agent.

bends (bendz) [fr. convulsive posture of those so afflicted]. Decompression *sickness.*

beneceptor (ben'ē-sep'ter, tōr) [L. *bene,* well, + *capio,* to take]. A nerve organ or mechanism (ceptor) for the appreciation and transmission of stimuli of a beneficial character. *Cf.* nociceptor.

Benedek, Ladislaus (László), Austrian neurologist, 1887–1945. See B.'s *reflex.*

Benedict, Francis G., U.S. metabolist, 1870–1957. See B.-Roth *apparatus, calorimeter.*

Benedict, Stanley R., U.S. chemist, 1884–1936. See B.'s *solution, test;* B.-Hopkins-Cole *reagent.*

Benedikt, Moritz, Austrian physician, 1835–1920. See B.'s *syndrome.*

benign (bē-nīn') [thru O. Fr., fr. L. *benignus,* kind]. Denoting the mild character of an illness or the nonmalignant character of a neoplasm.

Béniqué, Pierre Jules, French physician, 1806–1851. See B.'s *sound.*

benne oil (ben'nē). Sesame oil.

Bennett, Edward H., Irish surgeon, 1837–1907. See B.'s *fracture.*

Bennett, John H., British physician, 1812–1875. See B.'s *disease.*

Bennett, Norman G., British dentist, 1870–1947. See B. *angle, movement.*

Bennhold, H., German physician, *1893. See B.'s Congo red *stain.*

Benois, Louis, French physicist, *1856. See B. *scale.*

benoxaprofen (ben-oks-ă-prō'fen). (±)-2-(*p*- Chlorophenyl)-α-methyl-5-benzoxazoleacetic acid; a nonsteroidal anti-inflammatory and analgesic agent.

benoxinate hydrochloride (ben-oks'in-āt). Oxylonprocaine hydrochloride; 2-diethylaminoethyl-4-amino-3-*n*- butoxybenzoate hydrochloride; a soluble benzoic acid ester related to procaine, used as a surface anesthetic with bacteriostatic action.

benperidol (ben-per'i-dol). Benzperidol; 1-{1-[3-(*p*-Fluorobenzoyl)propyl]-4-piperidyl}-2-benzimidazolin-one; a tranquilizer.

Bensley, Robert R., U.S.-Canadian anatomist, 1867–1956. See B.'s specific *granules.*

Benson, Arthur H., British ophthalmologist, 1852–1912. See B.'s *disease.*

bentiromide (ben-tir'ō-mīd). 4-[[(2-Benzoylamino)-3-(4-hydroxyphenyl)-1-oxopropyl]amino]benzoic acid; a peptide used as a screening test for exocrine pancreatic insufficiency and to monitor the adequacy of supplemental pancreatic therapy.

bentonite (ben'ton-īt). Native colloidal hydrated aluminum silicate; an absorbent clay found in the western U.S.; it is sometimes used in the treatment of diarrhea and skin disorders.

benz-. Combining form denoting association with benzene.

benzalacetophenone (ben'zal-as-e-tō-fē'nōn). Chalcone.

benzalcoumaran-3-one (ben-zal-kū'mar-an-thrē'ōn). Aurone.

benzaldehyde (ben-zal'dĕ-hīd). C_6H_5CHO; benzoic aldehyde; an aldehyde produced artificially or obtained from oil of bitter almond, containing not less than 80% of b.; a flavoring agent used in orally administered medicines.

benzalkonium chloride (ben-zal-kō'nē-ŭm). A mixture of alkylbenzyldimethylammonium chlorides in which the alkyls are long-chain compounds (C_8 to C_{18}); a surface-active germicide for many pathogenic nonsporulating bacteria and fungi. Aqueous solutions of this agent have a low surface tension, and possess detergent, keratolytic, and emulsifying properties that aid the penetration and wetting of tissue surfaces.

benzamide (ben'ză-mīd). Aminoacylase.

benz[*a*]anthracene (ben-zan'thră-sēn). 1,2-Benzanthracene; benzanthrene; a carcinogenic hydrocarbon.

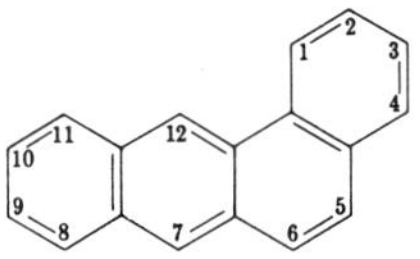

Benz [a] anthracene

benzanthrene (ben-zan'thrēn). Benz[*a*]anthracene.

benzene (ben'zēn). Benzol; cyclohexatriene; coal tar naphtha; $(CH)_6$ the basic structure in the aromatic compounds; a highly toxic hydrocarbon from light coal tar oil; used as a solvent.

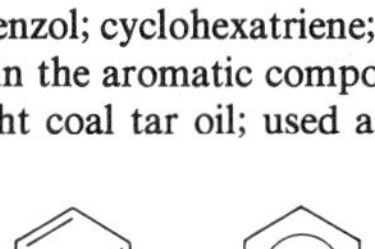

Benzene

b. bromide, a lacrimator or tear gas.

benzeneamine (ben-zēn'ă-mēn). Aniline.

(γ)-benzene hexachloride. Incorrect name for 1,2,3,4,5,6-hexachlorocyclohexane (lindane).

benzestrol (ben-zes'trol). 3-Ethyl-2,4-bis(*p*-hydroxyphenyl)acetate; a synthetic estrogenic substance.

benzethonium chloride (benz-ĕ-thō'nē-ŭm). A synthetic quaternary ammonium compound, one of the cationic class of detergents; germicidal and bacteriostatic.

benzidine (ben'zi-dēn). *p*-Diaminodiphenyl; $NH_2C_6H_4C_6H_4NH_2$; used to detect sulfates in water analysis, or for the identification of blood.

benzimidazole (ben-zim-i-dā'zōl). A ring system comprised of a benzene ring fused with an imidazole ring; occurs in nature as part of the vitamin B_{12} molecule.

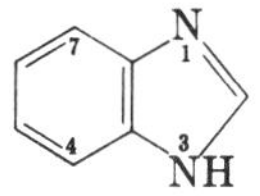

Benzimidazole

benzin, benzine (ben'zin, ben-zēn). *Petroleum* benzin.

benzindamine hydrochloride (ben-zin'dă-mēn). Benzydamine hydrochloride.

benziodarone (ben-zē'ō-dă-rōn). 2-Ethyl-3-benzofuranyl 4-hydroxy-3,5-diiodophenyl ketone; a coronary vasodilator.

benzoate (ben'zō-āt). A salt or ester of benzoic acid.

benzoated (ben'zō-āt-ed). Containing benzoic acid or a benzoate, usually sodium benzoate.

benzocaine (ben'zō-kān). Ethyl aminobenzoate; $NH_2C_6H_4$–$COO(C_2H_5)$; the ethyl ester of *p*- aminobenzoic acid; a topical anesthetic agent.

benzoctamine hydrochloride (ben'zok'tă-mēn). *N*- Methyl-9,10-ethanoanthracene-9(10*H*)-methylamine hydrochloride; a sedative with a muscle-relaxing agent.

benzodiazepine (ben'zō-dī-az'ĕ-pēn). Parent compound for the synthesis of a number of psychoactive compounds (*e.g.*, diazepam, chlordiazepoxide), with a common molecular configuration:

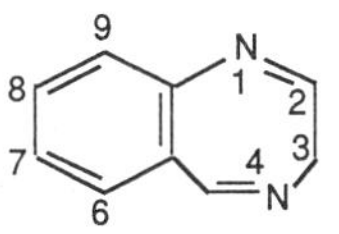

Benzodiazepine

benzoic (ben-zō'ik). Relating to or derived from benzoin.

benzoic acid. Benzoyl hydrate; flowers of benzoin; C_6H_5COOH; occurs naturally in gum benzoin; it is used as a food preservative, locally as a fungistatic, and orally as an antiseptic, diuretic, and expectorant. It is excreted rapidly as hippuric acid.

benzoic aldehyde. Benzaldehyde.

benzoin (ben'zō-in, ben'zoyn). Gum benzoin; gum benjamin; a balsamic resin obtained from *Styrax benzoin* (family Styracaceae), used as a stimulant expectorant, but usually by inhalation in laryngitis and bronchitis; it retards rancidification of fats and is used for this purpose in the official benzoinated lard.

benzol (ben'zol). Benzene.

benzomorphan (ben-zō-mōr'fan). 6,7-Benzomorphan; 1,2,3,4,5,6-hexahydro-2,6-methano-3-benzazocine; the parent compound of a series of analgesics including pentazocine and phenazocine; it does not possess analgesic properties itself.

benzonatate (ben-zō'nă-tāt). Nonaethyleneglycol monomethyl ether *p-n*-butylaminobenzoate; an antitussive agent related chemically to tetracaine.

benzopurpurin 4B (ben-zō-per'pūrin) [C.I. 23500]. A red acid dye, $C_{34}H_{26}N_6O_6S_2Na_2$, formerly used as a plasma stain and as an indicator (changes from violet to red in the pH range 1.2 to 4.0).

1,4-benzoquinone (ben-zō-kwin'ōn). Quinone (2); 2,5,-cyclohexadiene-1,4,-dione; an essential part of coenzyme Q and vitamin E, reducible to hydroquinone.

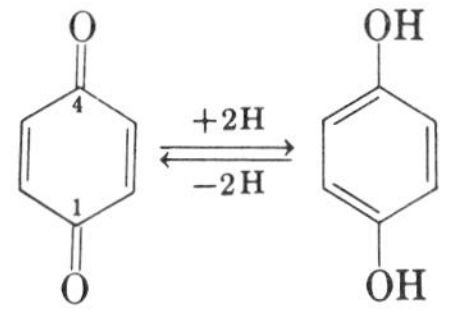

1,4-Benzoquinone

benzoquinonium chloride (ben'zō-kwī-nō'nē-ŭm). A skeletal muscle relaxant.

benzoresinol (ben-zō-res'i-nol). A resinous constituent of benzoin.

benzosulfimide (ben-zō-sŭl'fi-mīd). Saccharin.

benzothiadiazides (ben'zō-thī-ă-dī'ă-zīdz). A class of diuretics that increase the excretion of sodium and chloride and an accompanying volume of water, independent of alterations in acid-base balance; most of the compounds in this group are analogues of 1,2,4-benzothiadiazine-1,1-dioxide. See also benzthiazide.

benzoxiquine (ben-zoks'i-kwin). Benzoxyline; 8-quinolinol benzoate ester; a disinfectant.

benzoxyline (ben-zoks'i-lēn). Benzoxiquine.

benzoyl (ben'zō-il). The benzoic acid radical, C_6H_5CO—, forming benzoyl compounds.

b. chloride, C_6H_5COCl; a colorless liquid of pungent odor; a reagent.

b. hydrate, benzoic acid.

b. peroxide, C_6H_5CO–O–O–COC_6H_5; made by the interaction of sodium peroxide and b. chloride; used in oil as an application to ulcers and to burns and scalds, in promoting the polymerization of denture base resins, and as a keratolytic in the treatment of acne.

benzoylcholinesterase (ben'zō-il-kō-lin-es'ter-ās). Obsolete term for cholinesterase.

benzoylpas calcium (ben-zō'il-pas). 4-Benzamidosalicylic acid calcium salt; an antituberculous agent.

benzperidol (benz-per'i-dol). Benperidol.

benzphetamine hydrochloride (benz-fet'ă-mēn). *N*- Benzyl-*N*, α-dimethylphenethylamine hydrochloride; a sympathomimetic agent used as an anorexiant.

benzpyrinium bromide (benz-pī-rin'ē-ŭm). Benzstigminum bromidum; 1-benzyl-3-hydroxypyridinium bromide diethylcarbamate; a cholinergic drug with action and uses similar to those of neostigmine.

benzquinamide (benz-kwin'ă-mīd). A benzoquinoline amide used as an antiemetic agent.

benzstigminum bromidum (benz-stig'mi-nŭm). Benzpyrinium bromide.

benzthiazide (benz-thī'ă-zīd). 3-[(Benzylthio)methyl]-6-chloro-2*H*-1,2,4-benzothiadiazine-7-sulfonamide 1,1-dioxide; a diuretic and antihypertensive agent.

benztropine mesylate (benz-trō'pēn). 3-Diphenylmethoxytropane methanesulfonate; a parasympatholytic agent with atropine-like and antihistaminic actions.

benzydamine hydrochloride (ben-zid'ă-mēn). Benzindamine hydrochloride; 1-benzyl-3-[3-dimethylamino)propoxy]-1*H*-indazole; an analgesic and antipyretic.

benzyl (ben'zil). The hydrocarbon radical, $C_6H_5CH_2$–.

b. alcohol, phenmethylol; phenylcarbinol; $C_6H_5CH_2OH$; possesses local anesthetic and bacteriostatic properties.

b. benzoate, C_6H_5CO–$OCH_2C_6H_5$; an agent that reduces the contractility of unstriated muscular tissue, possessing marked antispasmodic properties; used now as a pediculicide and scabicide.

b. benzoate-chlorophenothane-ethyl aminobenzoate, a mixture of three components used in emulsions or ointments.

b. carbinol, phenylethyl alcohol.

b. cinnamate, cinnamein; *trans*-cinnamic benzyl ester; a constituent of balsams of Peru, Tolu, and styrax.

b. fumarate, dibenzyl fumarate; $(C_6H_5CH_2)$ OOCCHCH-COO$(CH_2C_6H_5$; used for the same purposes as b. benzoate.

b. mandelate, the b. ester of mandelic acid, having an antispasmodic action similar to that of b. benzoate.

b. succinate, dibenzyl succinate; $(C_6H_5CH_2)_2(CH_2CO_2)_2$; action and dosage are the same as those of b. benzoate.

benzylic (ben-zil'ik). Relating to or containing benzyl.

benzylidene (ben-zil'i-dēn). The hydrocarbon radical, $C_6H_5CH=$.

benzyloxycarbonyl (Cbz, Z) (ben'zil-kar'bon-il). Carbobenzoxy; amino-protecting radical used (as the chloride) in peptide synthesis, yielding $PhCH_2OCO$—NHR.

benzylpenicillin (ben'zil-pen-i-sil'in). *Penicillin* G.

bephenium hydroxynaphthoate (be-fen'ē-ŭm hī-droks'ē-naf'thō-āt). Benzyldimethyl-(2-phenoxyethyl)ammonium 3-hydroxy-2-naphthoate; a drug used against *Ancylostoma duodenale* and *Necator americanus* (hookworms of man); now largely replaced by mebendazole.

Beradinelli, Waldemar, Argentinian physician, 1903–1956. See B.'s *syndrome.*

Bérard, Auguste, French surgeon, 1802–1846. See B.'s *aneurysm.*

Béraud, Bruno J., French surgeon, 1825–1865. See B.'s *valve.*

berberine (ber'ber-ēn). Umbellatine; $C_{20}H_{19}NO_5$; an alkaloid from *Hydrastis canadensis* (family Berberidaceae); has been used as an antimalarial, antipyretic, and carminative, and externally for indolent ulcers.

Berg's stain. See under stain.

Berger, Emil, Austrian ophthalmologist, 1855–1926. See B.'s *space.*

Berger, Hans, German neurologist, 1873–1941. See B. *rhythm.*

Berger, Jean, 20th century French nephrologist. See B.'s focal *glomerulonephritis.*

Berger, Oskar, German physician, 1844–1885. See B.'s *paresthesia.*

Bergmann, Ernst von, German surgeon, 1836–1907. See B.'s *incision.*

Bergmann, Gottlieb H., German neurologist and anatomist, 1781–1861. See B.'s *cords, fibers.*

Bergmeister, O., Austrian ophthalmologist, 1845–1918. See B.'s *papilla.*

Bergonié, Jean A., French physician, 1857–1925. See B. *method.*

beriberi (ber'ē-ber'ē) [Singhalese, extreme weakness]. Kakké; endemic neuritis; panneuritis endemica; a specific polyneuritis, occurring in endemic form in eastern and southern Asia, sporadically in other parts of the world without reference to climate, and sometimes in alcoholics, resulting mainly from a dietary deficiency of thiamin; sensory nerves are more likely to be affected than motor nerves, with symptoms beginning in the feet and working upward with the hands affected late in the course of the disease. See also nutritional *polyneuropathy.*

dry b., paraplegic b., affecting chiefly the peripheral nerves; its clinical pattern is predominantly that of a neuropathy without congestive failure.

wet b., edematous b., in which congestive heart failure occurs in addition to peripheral neuropathy.

berkelium (berk'lē-um) [*Berkeley,* Calif., city where first prepared]. An artificial transuranium radioactive element; symbol Bk, atomic no. 97.

Berlin, Rudolf, German ophthalmologist, 1833–1897. See B.'s *edema.*

Berlin blue [C.I. 77510]. Prussian blue; ferric ferrocyanide; $Fe_4(Fe(CN)_6)_3$; a dye used to color injection masses for blood vessels and lymphatics, and in staining of siderocytes.

Bernard, Claude, French physiologist, 1813–1878. See B.'s *canal, duct, puncture;* B.-Cannon *homeostasis;* B.-Horner *syndrome;* B.-Sergent *syndrome.*

Bernard, Jean, 20th century French physician. See B.-Soulier *syndrome.*

Bernays, Augustus C., U.S. surgeon, 1854–1907. See B.'s *sponge.*

Bernhardt, Martin, German neurologist, 1844–1915. See B.'s *disease,* Roth-B. *disease,* B.-Roth *syndrome.*

Bernhardt's formula. See under formula.

Bernheim's syndrome. See under syndrome.

Bernoulli, Daniel, Swiss mathematician, 1700–1782. See B. *effect;* B.'s *law, principle, theorem.*

Bernstein, Lionel M., U.S. internist, *1923. See B. *test.*

Berry, Sir James, Canadian surgeon, 1860–1946. See B.'s *ligament.*

Berson, Solomon A., U.S. internist, *1918. See B. *test.*

Berthelot, Pierre Eugene Marcellin, French chemist, 1827–1907. See B. *reaction.*

Berthollet, Claude L., French chemist, 1748–1822. See B.'s *law.*

bertiellosis (ber'tē-ĕ-lō'sis). Infection of primates including man with cestodes of the genus *Bertiella.*

Bertin, Exupère J., French anatomist, 1712–1781. See B.'s *bone, column, ligament, ossicle.*

berylliosis (be-ril-ē-ō'sis). Beryllium poisoning characterized by the occurrence of granulomatous fibrosis, especially of the lungs, from chronic inhalation of beryllium.

beryllium (be-ril'ē-ŭm). A white metal element belonging to the alkaline earths; symbol Be, atomic weight 9.013, atomic no. 4.

Besnier, Ernest, French dermatologist, 1831–1909. See B.'s *prurigo;* B.-Boeck-Schauman *syndrome.*

Besnoitia (bes-noy'tē-ă). A genus of protozoan parasites (family Besnoitiidae, class Sporozoea), closely related to *Toxoplasma,* that localize in subcutaneous, connective, serous, and other tissues and are surrounded by a heavy, nucleated wall of host tissue, forming a cyst; hosts include domestic ruminants, reindeer, caribou, rodents, opossums, and reptiles.

B. bennet'ti, species occurring in horses and asses in North America and Africa, and causing a chronic disease with scabbing, scarring, and thickening of the skin.

B. besno'iti, species causing besnoitiasis of cattle, goats, and larger antelopes in Europe, Africa, the Middle East, South America, and Asia; it primarily causes a chronic low-grade infection; mechanical transmission is by bloodsucking tabanid horseflies.

B. taran'di, a species occurring in reindeer and caribou, giving rise to a condition called "corn-meal disease" because of the granular nature of the lesions on the skin.

besnoitiasis (bes-noy-tē-ā'sis). Besnoitiosis; a disease of cattle primarily caused by *Besnoitia besnoiti.* Cysts occur chiefly in the connective tissue of the skin, nasal mucous membranes, and serous membranes. Following a febrile stage, depilatory and seborrheic changes occur in the skin.

Besnoitiidae (bes-noy'tē-i-dē). A family of protozoan parasites, similar to those of the family Toxoplasmatidae, to which the genus Besnoitia belong.

besnoitiosis (bes'noy-tē-ō'sis). Besnoitiasis.

Best, Franz, German pathologist, 1878–1920. See B.'s *disease,* carmine *stain.*

bestiality (bes-tē-al'i-tē). Zooerastia; sexual relations with an animal.

beta (bā'tă) [G.]. Second letter of the Greek alphabet, β(*q.v.*).

beta-blocker (bā'tă-blok'er). β-Adrenergic blocking *agent.*

betacism (bā'tă-sizm) [G. *bēta,* the second letter of the alphabet]. A defect in speech in which the sound of *b* is given to other consonants.

betacyaninuria (bā-tă-sī'ă-ni-nū'rē-ă) [betacyanin + G. *ouron,* urine]. Beeturia.

betahistine hydrochloride (bā-tă-his'tēn). 2-[2-(Methylamino)ethyl]pyridine dihydrochloride; an inhibitor of diamine oxidase used as a histamine-like agent for treatment of Ménière's disease.

betaine (bē'tă-ēn). Trimethylglycocoll anhydride; oxyneurine; glycine or glycyl betaine; $(CH_3)_3\overset{+}{N}—CH_2COO^-$; an oxidation product of choline and a transmethylating intermediate in metabolism.

b. aldehyde, $(CH_3)_3\overset{+}{N}\text{-}CH_2CHO$; an intermediate in the interconversion of betaine and choline.

b. hydrochloride, trimethylglycine hydrochloride; $C_5H_{12}ClNO_2$; an acidifying agent used in the treatment of achlorhydria and hypochlorhydria.

betaine-aldehyde dehydrogenase [EC 1.2.1.8]. An oxidizing enzyme that catalyzes the oxidation of betaine aldehyde to betaine; part of the choline oxidase system.

betamethasone (bā-tă-meth'ă-sōn). Betadexamethasone; 9-fluoro-11β,17,21-trihydroxy-16β-methyl-a,4-pregnadiene-3,20- dione; 9α-fluoro-16β-methylprednisolone; a semisynthetic glucocorticoid with anti-inflammatory effects and toxicity similar to those of cortisol; not useful in the treatment of adrenal insufficiency because it causes little sodium retention. For systemic and topical therapy, its actions are similar to those of prednisone, but more potent. Also available as b. sodium phosphate, b. acetate, and b. valerate.

betanidine sulfate (be-tan'i-dēn). Bethanidine sulfate.

betatron (bā'tă-tron). A circular electron accelerator that is a source of either high energy electrons or x-rays.

betaxolol hydrochloride (be-taks'ō-lol). 1-[4-[2-(cyclopropylmethoxy) ethyl] phenoxy] - 3 - isopropylaminopropan - 2 - ol hydrochloride; a β-adrenergic blocking agent used primarily in the treatment of ocular hypertension and chronic open-angle glaucoma.

betazole hydrochloride (bā'tă-zōl). An analogue of histamine that stimulates gastric secretion with less tendency to produce the side effects seen with histamine; used, in place of histamine, to measure the gastric secretory response.

betel (bē'tl) [Pg. *betel, betle,* fr. Malayalam or Tamil *vetilla*]. The dried leaves of *Piper betle* (family Piperaceae), a climbing East Indian plant; used as a stimulant and narcotic.

betel nut. Areca nut, the nut of the areca palm, *Areca catechu* (family Palmae), of the East Indies, chewed by the natives.

bethanechol chloride (be-than'ĕ-kol). Carbamoylmethylcholine chloride; (2-hydroxypropyl)trimethylammonium chloride carbamate; a parasympathomimetic agent, used to relieve constipation, paralytic ileus, and urinary retention.

bethanidine sulfate (be-than'i-dēn). Betanidine sulfate; 1-benzyl-2,3-dimethylguanidine; an adrenergic blocking agent used for palliative treatment of hypertension.

Bethesda-Ballerup Group. A group of citrate-utilizing, slow lactose-fermenting bacteria (family Enterobacteriaceae) which share a similar series of antigens with the lactose-fermenting citrobacters; these organisms are now included in the genus *Citrobacter* without a distinction between prompt and slow lactose fermentation.

Betke-Kleihauer test. See under test.

Bettendorff, Anton J., German chemist, 1839–1902. See B.'s *test.*

betula oil (bet'yū-lă). Oil of sweet birch, a volatile oil obtained by distillation from the bark of *Betula lenta* (sweet birch). See also *methyl* salicylate.

Betz, Vladimir A., Russian anatomist, 1834–1894. See B. *cells.*

Beuren, A.J. See B. *syndrome.*

Bevan, Arthur D., U.S. surgeon, 1861–1943. See B.'s *incision.*

Bevan-Lewis, William, British physician and physiologist, 1847–1929. See B.-L. *cells.*

bevel (bev'ĕl). **1.** A surface having a sloped or slanting edge. **2.** The incline that one surface or line makes with another when not at right angles. **3.** The edge of a cutting instrument. **4.** To create a slanting edge on a body structure.

cavosurface b., the incline of the cavosurface angle of a prepared cavity wall in relation to the plane of the enamel wall.

reverse b., the sloping edge of a cutting instrument.

bevonium methyl sulfate (be-vō'nē-ŭm). Pyribenzyl methyl sulfate; 2-(hydroxymethyl)-1,1-dimethylpiperidinium methyl sulfate benzylate; an anticholinergic agent.

bezoar (bē'zōr) [Pers. *padzahr,* antidote]. A concretion formed in the alimentary canal of animals, and occasionally man; formerly considered to be a useful medicine with magical properties and apparently still used for this purpose in some places; according to the substance forming the ball, may be termed trichobezoar (hairball), trichophytobezoar (hair and vegetable fiber mixed), or phytobezoar (foodball).

Bezold, Albert von, German physiologist, 1836–1868. See B.'s *ganglion,* B.-Jarisch *reflex.*

Bezold, Friedrich, German otologist, 1842–1908. See B.'s *abscess, mastoiditis, perforation, sign, symptom, triad.*

bhang (bang) [Hind.]. Name given in the East to powdered preparation of *Cannabis sativa* which is chewed or smoked by the local residents. See also cannabis.

BHN Abbreviation for Brinell hardness *number.*

Bi Symbol for bismuth.

bi- [L.] **1.** Prefix meaning twice or double, referring to double structures, dual actions, etc. **2.** In chemistry, used to denote a partially neutralized acid (an acid salt); *e.g.,* bisulfate. *Cf.* bis-; di-.

Bial, Manfred, German physician, 1869–1908. See B.'s *test.*

bialamicol hydrochloride (bī-ă-lam'i-kol). Biallylamicol hydrochloride; 3,3'-bis[(diethylamino)methyl]-5,5'-bis(2 propenyl)-1,1'-biphenyl 4,4'diol hydrochloride; an amebicide.

Bianchi, Giovanni B., Italian anatomist, 1681–1761. See B.'s *nodule, valve.*

biarticular (bī'ar-tik'yū-lăr). Diarthric.

biasterionic (bī-as-ter-ē-on'ik). Relating to both asterions, especially the b. diameter, or b. width, the shortest distance from one asterion to the other.

biauricular (bī-aw-rik'yū-lăr). Relating to both auricles, in any sense.

bib. Abbreviation for L. *bibe,* drink.

bibasic (bī'bās-ik). Dibasic.

bibenzonium bromide (bī-ben-zō'nē-ŭm). [2-(1,2-Diphenylethoxy)ethyl]trimethylammonium bromide; an antitussive.

bibliomania (bib'lē-ō-mā'nē-ă) [G. *biblion,* book, + *mania,* frenzy]. Morbidly intense desire to collect and possess books, especially rare books.

bibulous (bib'yū-lŭs) [L. *bibulus,* drinking freely, absorbent]. Absorbent (1).

bicameral (bī-kam'er-ăl) [bi- + L. *camera,* chamber]. Having two chambers; denoting especially an abscess divided by a more or less complete septum.

bicapsular (bī-kap'sū-lăr). Having a double capsule.

bicarbonate (bī-kar'bon-āt). HCO_3^-; the ion remaining after the first dissociation of carbonic acid.

standard b., the plasma b. concentration of a sample of whole blood that has been equilibrated at 37°C with a carbon dioxide pressure of 40 mm Hg and an oxygen pressure greater than 100 mm Hg; abnormally high or low values indicate metabolic alkalosis or acidosis, respectively.

bicardiogram (bī-kar'dē-ō-gram). The composite curve of an electrocardiogram representing the combined effects of the right and left ventricles.

bicellular (bī-sel'yū-lăr). Having two cells or subdivisions.

bicephalus (bī-sef'ă-lŭs). Dicephalus.

biceps (bī'seps) [bi- + L. *caput,* head]. A muscle with two origins or heads.

Bichat, Marie F.X., French anatomist, physician, and biologist, 1771–1802. See B.'s *canal, fat-pad, fissure, foramen, fossa, ligament, membrane, protuberance, tunic.*

bichloride (bī-klōr'īd). Dichloride.

bicho (bē'cho). Epidemic gangrenous *proctitis.*

bichromate (bī-krō'māt). Dichromate.

biciliate (bī-sil'ē-āt). Having two cilia.

bicipital (bī-sip'i-tăl) [bi- + L. *caput,* head]. **1.** Two-headed. **2.** Relating to a biceps muscle.

Bickel, Gustav, 19th century German physician. See B.'s *ring.*

biclonal (bī-klō'năl). Pertaining to or characterized by biclonality.

biclonality (bī-klōn-al'i-tē). A condition in which some cells have markers of one cell line and other cells have markers of another cell line, as in biclonal leukemias.

biclonal peak. Two narrow electrophoretic bands thought to represent immunoglobulin of two cell lines.

biconcave (bī-kon'kāv). Concavoconcave; concave on two sides; denoting especially a form of lens.

biconvex (bī-kon'veks). Convexoconvex; convex on two sides; denoting especially a form of lens.

bicornous, bicornuate, bicornate (bī-kōr'nŭs, -nū-āt, -nāt) [bi- + L. *cornu,* horn]. Two-horned; having two processes or projections.

bicro-. Pico- (2).

bicron (bī'kron). Picometer.

bicuspid (bī-kŭs'pid) [bi- + L. *cuspis,* point]. Having two points, prongs, or cusps.

bicuspidization (bī-kŭs'pi-di-zā'shŭn). Surgical change of a normally tricuspid aortic valve into a functioning bicuspid valve; performed in correction of aortic valvar disease.

b.i.d. Abbreviation for L. *bis in die,* twice a day.

bidactyly (bī-dak'ti-lē) [bi- + G. *daktylos,* finger]. Abnormality in which the medial digits are lacking with only the first and fifth represented. See also lobster-claw *deformity.*

bidet (bē-dā') [Fr. a small horse]. A tub for a sitz bath, having also an attachment for giving vaginal or rectal infusions.

bidiscoidal (bī'dis-koy'dăl). Resembling, or consisting of, two disks.

BIDS Acronym for *b* rittle hair, *i* mpaired intelligence, *d* ecreased fertility, and *s* hort stature; usually manifested as an inherited deficiency of a high-sulfur protein.

biduous (bid'yū-ŭs) [L. *biduus,* lasting two days, fr. *bi-* + *dies,* day]. Of two days' duration.

Biebl, M. See B. *loop.*

Biebrich scarlet red [*Biebrich,* Germany] [C.I. 26905]. Scarlet red.

Biederman, Joseph B., U.S. physician, *1907. See B.'s *sign.*

Biedl, Artur, Austrian physician, 1869–1933. See Bardet-B., Laurence-B., Laurence-Moon-Bardet-B. *syndrome.*

Bielschowsky, Alfred, German ophthalmologist, 1871–1940. See B.'s *sign.*

Bielschowsky, Max, German neuropathologist, 1869–1940. See B.'s *disease, stain;* Jansky-B. *disease.*

Biemond, A., 20th century French neurologist. See B. *syndrome.*

Bier, August K.G., German surgeon, 1861–1949. See B.'s *amputation, hyperemia, method.*

Biermer, Anton, German physician, 1827–1892. See B.'s *anemia, disease, sign;* Addison-B. *disease.*

Biernacki, Edmund A., Polish pathologist, 1866–1912. See B.'s *sign.*

Biesiadecki, Alfred von, Polish physician, 1839–1888. See B.'s *fossa.*

bifascicular (bī'fă-sik'yū-lăr). Involving two of the three fascicles of the ventricular conduction system of the heart.

bifid (bī'fid) [L. *bifidus,* cleft in two parts]. Split or cleft; separated into two parts.

Bifidobacterium (bī'fī-dō-bak-tēr'ē-ŭm) [L. *bifidus,* cleft in two parts, + bacterium]. A genus of anaerobic bacteria (family Actinomycetaceae) containing Gram-positive rods of highly variable appearance; freshly isolated strains characteristically show bifurcated V and Y forms, uniform or branched, and club or spatulate forms. They frequently stain irregularly; two or more granules may stain with methylene blue, while the remainder of the cell is unstained. They are not acid-fast, are nonmotile, and do not produce spores; acetic and lactic acids are produced from glucose. Pathogenicity for man or other animals has not been reported, although they have been found in the feces and alimentary tract of infants, older people, and other animals. The type species is *B. bifidum.*

B. bi'fidum, *Lactobacillus bifidus;* type species of the genus *Bifidobacterium;* it is found in the feces and alimentary tract of breast- and bottle-fed infants and of older persons, rats, turkeys, and chickens; also found in the rumen of cattle; pathogenicity for man and other animals has not been reported. See also *Lactobacillus bifidus* subsp. *pennsylvanicus.*

bifocal (bī-fō'kăl). Having two foci.

biforate (bī-fō'rāt) [bi- + L. *foro,* pp. *-atus,* to bore, pierce]. Having two openings.

bifur'cate, bifur'cated (bī-fer'kāt, -kā-ted) [bi- + L. *furca,* fork]. Forked; two-pronged; having two branches.

bifurcatio (bī'fer-kā'shē-ō). Bifurcation.

b. aor'tae [NA], bifurcation of aorta; the division of the aorta into right and left common iliac arteries; it occurs at the level of the fourth and fifth lumbar vertebral body.

b. tra'cheae [NA], bifurcation of trachea; the division of the trachea into the right and left main bronchi; it occurs at the level of the fifth or sixth thoracic vertebral body and is marked internally by the presence of a carina or keel-like ridge between the diverging bronchi.

b. trun'ci pulmona'lis [NA], bifurcation of pulmonary trunk; the division of the pulmonary trunk into right and left pulmonary arteries.

bifurcation (bī-fer-kā'shŭn). Bifurcatio; a forking; a division into two branches.

b. of aorta, *bifurcatio* aortae.

b. of pulmonary trunk, *bifurcatio* trunci pulmonalis.

b. of trachea, *bifurcatio* tracheae.

Bigelow, Henry J., U.S. surgeon, 1818–1890. See B.'s *ligament, septum.*

bigemina (bī-jem'i-nă). Bigeminal *pulse.*

bigeminal (bī-jem′i-năl). Paired; double; twin.

bigemini (bī-jem′i-nī). Bigeminy.

bigeminum (bī-jem′i-nŭm) [L. ntr. of *bigeminus,* doubled]. One of the corpora bigemina.

bigeminy (bī-jem′i-nē) [bi- + L. *geminus,* twin]. Bigemini; twinning; pairing; especially, the occurrence of heart beats in pairs.
atrial b., pairing of atrial beats, as when an atrial extrasystole is coupled to each sinus beat.
atrioventricular (A-V) nodal b., nodal b.; paired beats, each pair consisting of an A-V nodal extrasystole coupled to a beat of the dominant, usually sinus, rhythm.
escape-capture b., paired beats, each couplet consisting of an escape beat followed by a conducted sinus beat.
nodal b., atrioventricular nodal b.
reciprocal b., paired beats, each pair consisting of an A-V nodal beat followed by a reciprocal beat.
ventricular b., paired ventricular beats, the common form consisting of ventricular extrasystoles coupled to sinus beats.

bigerminal (bī-jer′min-ăl). Relating to two germs or ova.

big-head. 1. In horses, usually denotes osteodystrophia fibrosa. **2.** Gas gangrene infection of tissues of the head, caused by *Clostridium novyi* in sheep, usually young rams with head wounds. **3.** Photosensitization in sheep.

bigitalin (bī-jit′ă-lin). Gitoxin.

Bignami, Amico, Italian physician, 1862–1929. See Marchiafava-B. *disease.*

bilabe (bī′lāb) [bi- + L. *labium,* lip]. An obsolete forceps for seizing and removing urethral or small vesical calculi.

bilateral (bī-lat′er-ăl) [bi- + L. *latus,* side]. Relating to, or having, two sides.

bilateralism (bī-lat′er-ăl-izm). A condition in which the two sides are symmetrical.

bile (bīl) [L. *bilis*]. Gall (1); fel; the yellowish brown or green fluid secreted by the liver and discharged into the duodenum where it aids in the emulsification of fats, increases peristalsis, and retards putrefaction; contains sodium glycocholate and sodium taurocholate, cholesterol, biliverdin and bilirubin, mucus, fat, lecithin, and cells and cellular debris.
A b., b. from the common duct.
B b., b. from the gallbladder.
C b., b. from the hepatic duct.
white b., see leukobilin.

Bilharzia (bil-har′zē-ă) [T. *Bilharz*]. An early name for *Schistosoma.*

bilharziasis (bil-har-zī′ă-sis). Schistosomiasis.

bilharzioma (bil-har-zē-ō′mă). A tumor-like swelling of the skin, due to schistosomiasis.

bilharziosis (bil-har-zē-ō′sis). Schistosomiasis.

bili- [L. *bilis,* bile]. Combining form relating to bile.

biliary (bil′ē-ār-ē). Bilious (1); relating to bile.

bilifaction, bilification (bil-i-fak′shŭn, -fi-kā′shŭn) [bili- + L. *facio,* pp. *factus,* to make]. Rarely used terms for bile formation.

biliferous (bil-if′er-ŭs). Rarely used term for containing or carrying bile.

biligenesis (bil-i-jen′ĕ-sis) [bili- + G. *genesis,* production]. Bile production.

biligenic (bil-i-jen′ik). Bile-producing.

bilin, biline (bī′lin). The chain of four pyrrole residues resulting from the cleavage of one bond of one of the four methylidene residues of the porphin part of a porphyrin; specifically, the unsubstituted tetrapyrrole; bilirubin and biliverdin are bilins. Sometimes called porphobilin.

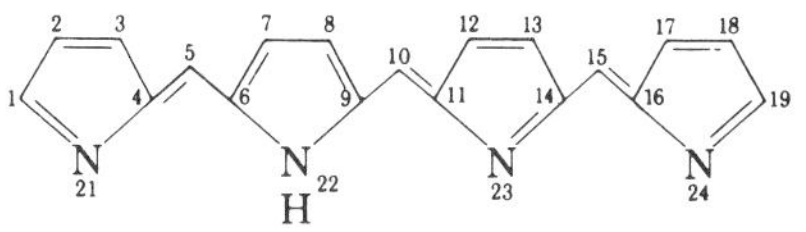

Bilin(e)
Numbering corresponds to porphyrin, from which it is derived.

bilious (bil′yŭs). **1.** Biliary. **2.** Relating to or characteristic of biliousness. **3.** Choleric; formerly, denoting a temperament characterized by a superficial dark complexion, high blood pressure, slow pulse, strong appetites, tenacity of purpose, and a quick, irritable temper.

biliousness (bil′yŭs-nes). An imprecisely delineated congestive disturbance with anorexia, coated tongue, constipation, headache, dizziness, pasty complexion, and, rarely, slight jaundice; assumed to result from hepatic dysfunction.

biliptysis (bil-ip′ti-sis) [bili- + G. *pytalon,* saliva]. Occurrence of bile in the sputum.

bilirachia (bil-i-rā′kē-ă) [bili- + G. *rachis,* spine]. Occurrence of bile pigments in the spinal fluid.

bilirubin (bil-i-rū′bin) [bili- + L. *ruber,* red]. A red bile pigment found as sodium bilirubinate (soluble), or as an insoluble calcium salt in gallstones, formed from hemoglobin during normal and abnormal destruction of erythrocytes by the reticuloendothelial system; a bilin with substituents on the 2, 3, 7, 8, 12, 13, 17, and 18 carbon atoms and with oxygens on carbons 1 and 19.
conjugated b., direct reacting b.
direct reacting b., conjugated b.; the fraction of serum b. which has been conjugated with glucuronic acid in the liver cell to form b. diglucuronide; so called because it reacts directly with the Erlich diazo reagent; increased levels are found in hepatobiliary diseases, especially of the obstructive variety.
indirect reacting b., unconjugated b.; the fraction of serum b. which has not been conjugated with glucuronic acid in the liver cell; so called because it reacts with the Erlich diazo reagent only when alcohol is added; increased levels are found in hepatic disease and hemolytic conditions.
unconjugated b., indirect reacting b.

bilirubinemia (bil′i-rū-bin-ē′mē-ă) [bilirubin + G. *haima,* blood]. The presence of bilirubin in the blood, where it is normally present in relatively small amounts; the term is usually used in relation to increased concentrations observed in various pathologic conditions where there is excessive destruction of erythrocytes or interference with the mechanism of excretion in the bile. Determination of the quantity of bilirubin in the blood serum reveals two fractions, namely direct reacting (conjugated) and indirect reacting (nonconjugated) bilirubin; determination of conjugated and total bilirubin in serum is an important and frequently used clinical laboratory test.

bilirubinglobulin (bil-i-rū′bin-glob′yū-lin). A bilirubin-globulin complex; a transport form of bilirubin to the liver where bilirubin is converted to a diglucuronic acid derivative and passes into the bile.

bilirubin-glucuronoside glucuronosyltransferase [EC 2.4.1.95]. Bilirubin monoglucuronide transglucuronidase; a transferase that transfers a glucuronoside from one molecule of bilirubin glucuronoside to another, forming bilirubin bisglucuronoside.

bilirubinoids (bil-i-rū′bin-oydz). Generic term denoting intermediates in the conversion of bilirubin to stercobilin by reductive enzymes in intestinal bacteria. Included are mesobilirubin, mesobilane mesobilene-b, urobilinogen, urobilin, reduction products of mesobilane (stercobilinogen) and mesobilene (stercobilin), and mesobiliviolin; most are found in normal urine and feces. Products related to these intermediates and found in pathological conditions (*e.g.,* jaundice, liver disease) are the structurally indefinite probilifuscins and propentdyopents found in gallstones.

bilirubinuria (bil'i-rū-bi-nū'rē-ă) [bilirubin + G. *ouron,* urine]. The presence of bilirubin in the urine.

bilitherapy (bil-i-thār'ă-pē). Treatment with bile or bile salts.

biliuria (bil-ē-yū'rē-ă) [bili- + G. *ouron,* urine]. Choluria; choleuria; the presence of various bile salts, or bile, in the urine.

biliverdin, biliverdine (bil-i-ver'din). Uteroverdine; verdine; dehydrobilirubin; choleverdin; a green bile pigment formed from the oxidation of bilirubin; a bilin with a structure almost identical to that of bilirubin.

biliverdinglobin (bil-i-ver'din-glō'bin). Choleglobin.

Bill, Arthur H., U.S. obstetrician, 1877–1961. See B.'s *maneuver.*

Billroth, C.A. Theodor, Austrian surgeon, 1829–1894. See B.'s *cords, operations* I and II, *venae* cavernosae; B. I and II *anastomosis.*

bilobate, bilobed (bī-lō'bāt, bī'lōbd). Having two lobes.

bilobular (bī-lob'yū-lăr). Having two lobules.

bilocular, biloculate (bī-lok'yū-lăr, -yū-lāt) [bi- + L. *loculus,* dim. of *locus,* a place]. Having two compartments or spaces.

bilophodont (bī-lof'ō-dont) [bi- + G. *lophos,* ridge, + *odous,* tooth]. Having two longitudinal ridges on the premolar and molar teeth; designating certain animals, such as the kangaroo.

bimanual (bī-man'yū-ăl) [bi- + L. *manus,* hand]. Relating to, or performed by, both hands.

bimastoid (bī-mas'toyd). Relating to both mastoid processes.

bimaxillary (bī-mak'si-lār-e). Relating to both the right and left maxillae; sometimes used when describing something affecting both upper jaws.

bimodal (bī-mō'dăl). Denoting a frequency curve characterized by two peaks.

bimolecular (bī-mō-lek'yū-lăr). Involving two molecules, as in a b. reaction.

binangle (bin-ang'-ūl) [L. *bini,* pair, + *angulus,* angle]. **1.** The second angle given the shank of an angled instrument to bring its working end close to the axis of the handle in order to prevent it from turning about the axis. **2.** A dental instrument possessing the above characteristics.

binary (bī'nār-ē) [L. *binarius,* consisting of two, fr. *bini,* double]. Denoting or comprised of two components, elements, molecules, etc.

binaural (bin-aw'răl) [L. *bini,* a pair, + *auris,* ear]. Binotic; relating to both ears.

bind (bīnd) [A.S. *bindan*]. **1.** To confine or encircle with a band or bandage. **2.** To join together with a band or ligature. **3.** To combine or unite molecules by means of reactive groups, either in the molecules *per se* or in a chemical added for that purpose; frequently used in relation to chemical bonds that may be fairly easily broken (*i.e.,* noncovalent), as in the binding of a toxin with antitoxin, or a heavy metal with a chelating agent, etc. **4.** A close interpersonal relationship in which one person feels compelled to act in a certain way to obtain the approval of the other person.

double b., a type of personal interaction in which one receives two mutually conflicting verbal or nonverbal instructions or demands from the same person or different individuals, resulting in a situation in which either compliance or noncompliance with either alternative threatens a needed relationship.

binder (bīnd'er). **1.** A broad bandage, especially one encircling the abdomen. **2.** Anything that binds. See bind (3).

obstetrical b., a supporting garment covering the abdomen from the ribs to the trochanters, tightly pinned at the back, affording support after childbirth or, rarely, during childbirth.

T-binder, T-bandage; two strips of cloth at right angles; used for retaining dressing, as on the perineum.

Binet, Alfred, French psychologist, 1857–1911. See B. *age, scale, test;* B.-Simon *scale, test;* Stanford-B. intelligence *scale.*

Bing, Paul Robert, German neurologist, 1878–1956. See B.'s *reflex.*

Bing, Richard J., U.S. physician, *1909. See Taussig-B. *disease, syndrome.*

Bingham, E.C., U.S. chemist, 1878–1945. See B. *flow, model, plastic.*

Binn's bacterium. See under bacterium.

binocular (bin-ok'yū-lăr) [L. *bini,* paired, + *oculus,* eye]. Adapted to the use of both eyes; said of an optical instrument.

binomial (bī-nō'mē-ăl) [bi- + G. *nomos,* name]. Consisting of two terms or names. See also binary *combination.*

binotic (bin-ot'ik) [L. *bini,* a pair, + G. *ous* (*ōt-*), ear]. Binaural.

binovular (bin-ov'yū-lar) [L. *bini,* pair, + Mod. L. *ovulum,* dim. of L. *ovum,* egg]. Diovular.

Binswanger, Otto Ludwig, German neurologist, 1852–1929. See B.'s *disease, encephalopathy.*

binuclear, binucleate (bī-nū'klē-ăr, -klē-āt). Having two nuclei.

binucleolate (bī-nū'klē-ō-lāt). Having two nucleoli.

Binz, Carl, German pharmacologist, 1832–1913. See B.'s *test.*

bio- [G. *bios,* life]. Combining form denoting life.

bioacoustics (bī'ō-ă-kūs'tiks). The science dealing with the effects of sound fields or mechanical vibrations in living organisms.

bioassay (bī-ō-as'ā). Determination of the potency or concentration of a compound by its effect upon animals, isolated tissues, or microorganisms, as compared with an analysis of its chemical or physical properties.

bioastronautics (bī'ō-as-trō-naw'tiks). The study of the effects of space travel and space habitation on living organisms.

bioavailability (bī'ō-ă-vāl'ă-bil'i-tē). The physiological availability of a given amount of a drug, as distinct from its chemical potency.

biocenosis (bī-ō-se-nō'sis) [bio- + G. *koinos,* common]. Biotic community; an assemblage of species living in a particular biotope.

biochemical (bī-ō-kem'i-kăl). Relating to biochemistry.

biochemistry (bī-ō-kem'is-trē). Biological or physiological chemistry; the chemistry of living organisms and of the chemical changes occurring thcrcin.

biochemorphic (bī'ō-kem-ōr'fik). Denoting the relation between biologic action and chemical structure, as of foods and drugs.

biochemorphology (bī'ō-kem-ōr-fol'ō-jē) [bio- + chemistry + G. *morphē,* shape, + *logos,* study]. **1.** The study of the relationship between biologic action and chemical structure. **2.** Macroscopic or gross morphology as revealed by biochemical techniques; *e.g.,* selective staining of enzymes, antibodies.

biocidal (bī-ō-sī'dăl) [bio- + L. *caedo,* to kill]. Destructive of life; particularly pertaining to microorganisms.

bioclimatology (bī'ō-klī-mă-tol'ō-jē). The science of the relationship of climatic factors to the distribution, numbers, and types of living organisms; an aspect of ecology.

biocytin (bī-ō-sī'tin). Biotinyllysine; ε-*N*-biotinyl-L-lysine; biotin condensed through its carboxyl group with the ε-amino group of a lysine in the apoenzymes to which biotin is the coenzyme; the predominant form in which biotin occurs.

biocytinase (bī-ō-sī'tin-ās). An enzyme in blood that catalyzes the hydrolysis of biocytin to biotin and lysine; probably biotinidase.

biodegradable (bī'ō-dē-grād'ă-bl). Denoting a substance that can be chemically degraded or decomposed by natural effectors (*e.g.,* weather, soil bacteria, plants, animals).

biodegradation (bī'ō-deg-rā-dā'shŭn). Biotransformation.

biodynamic (bī'ō-dī-nam'ik). Relating to biodynamics.

biodynamics (bī'ō-dī-nam'iks) [bio- + G. *dynamis,* force]. The science dealing with the force or energy of living matter.

bioecology (bī-ō-ē-kol'ō-jē). Ecology.

bioenergetics (bī'ō-en-er-jet'iks). The study of energy changes involved in the chemical reactions within living tissue.

bioengineering (bī'ō-en-jin-ēr'ing). See biomedical *engineering.*

biofeedback (bī-ō-fēd'bak). A training technique that enables an individual to gain some element of voluntary control over autonomic body functions; based on the learning principle that a desired response is learned when received information (feedback) indicates that a specific thought complex or action has produced the desired response.

bioflavonoids (bī-ō-flāv'on-oydz). Naturally occurring flavone or coumarin derivatives having the activity of the so-called vitamin P, notably rutin and esculin.

biogenesis (bī-ō-jen'ĕ-sis) [bio- + G. *genesis,* origin]. Term given by Huxley to the now generally accepted view that life originates only from preexisting life and never from nonliving material. See spontaneous *generation;* recapitulation *theory.*

biogenetic (bī'ō-jĕ-net'ik). Relating to biogenesis.

biogeochemistry (bī'ō-jē-ō-kem'is-trē). The study of the influence of living organisms and life processes on the chemical structure and history of the earth.

biogravics (bī-ō-grav'iks) [bio- + L. *gravis,* weight]. That field of study dealing with the effect on living organisms (particularly man) of abnormal gravitational effects produced, *e.g.,* by acceleration or by free fall; in the former case, heavier than normal weight is induced, and in the latter weightlessness.

bioinstrument (bī'ō-in'strū-ment). A sensor or device usually attached to or embedded in the human body or other living animal to record and to transmit physiologic data to a receiving and monitoring station.

biokinetics (bī'ō-ki-net'iks) [bio- + G. *kinēsis,* motion]. The study of the growth changes and movements that developing organisms undergo.

biologic, biological (bī'ō-loj'ik, -loj'i-kăl). Relating to biology.

biologist (bī-ol'ō-jist). A specialist or expert in biology.

biology (bī-ol'ō-jē) [bio- + G. *logos,* study]. The science concerned with the phenomena of life and living organisms.
cellular b., cytology.
molecular b., a field of b. concerned with biological phenomena in terms of molecular (or chemical) interactions; it differs from biochemistry in that the latter is concerned primarily with the chemical behavior of biologically important substances and analogues thereof, and differs from other fields of biology in its emphasis on chemical interactions, especially those involved in the replication of DNA, its "transcription" into RNA, and its "translation" into or expression in protein, *i.e.,* in the chemical reactions connecting genotype and phenotype.
oral b., that aspect of b. devoted to the study of biological phenomena associated with the oral cavity in health and disease (*e.g.,* dental caries, mastication, periodontal disease).
radiation b., that field of science which studies the biological effects of ionizing radiation on living systems.

bioluminescence (bī'ō-lū-min-es'ens) [bio- + L. *lumen* (*-inis*), light]. Cold light (1); light produced by certain organisms from the oxidation of luciferins through the action of luciferases and with negligible production of heat, chemical energy being converted directly into light energy.

biolysis (bī-ol'i-sis) [bio- + G. *lysis,* dissolution]. Disintegration of organic matter through the chemical action of living organisms.

biolytic (bī-ō-lit'ik). **1.** Relating to biolysis. **2.** Capable of destroying life.

biomass (bī'ō-mas). The total weight of all living things in a given area, biotic community, species population, or habitat; a measure of total biotic productivity.

biome (bī'ōm). The total complex of biotic communities occupying and characterizing a particular geographic area or zone.

biomechanics (bī-ō-me-kan'iks). The science concerned with the action of forces, internal or external, on the living body.
dental b., dental *biophysics.*

biomedical (bī-ō-med'i-kăl). **1.** Pertaining to those aspects of the natural sciences, especially the biologic and physiologic sciences, that relate to or underlie medicine. **2.** Biological and medical, *i.e.,* encompassing both the science(s) and the art of medicine.

biometer (bī-om'ĕ-ter) [bio- + G. *metron,* measure]. A device for measuring carbon dioxide given off by organisms and, hence, for determining the quantity of living matter present.

biometrician (bī-ō-me-trish'ăn). One who specializes in the science of biometry.

biometry (bī-om'ĕ-trē). The statistical analysis of biological data.

biomicroscope (bī-ō-mī'krō-skōp). Slitlamp; in ophthalmology, an instrument consisting of a microscope combined with a rectangular light source.

biomicroscopy (bī'ō-mī-kros'kŏ-pē). **1.** Microscopic examination of living tissue in the body. **2.** Examination of the cornea, aqueous humor, lens, vitreous humor, and retina by use of a slitlamp combined with a binocular microscope.

Biomphalaria (bī-om-fă-lā'rē-ă). An important genus of freshwater snails (family Planorbidae, subfamily Planorbinae), several species of which serve as intermediate hosts of *Schistosoma mansoni* in Africa, Saudi Arabia and Yemen, South America, and the Caribbean. Host snails formerly were placed in the genera *Australorbis, Tropicorbis,* and *Taphius* but are no longer considered generically distinct.

bion (bī'on) [G. pres. p. ntr. of *bioō,* to live]. A living thing.

Biondi, Aldolpho, Italian pathologist, 1846–1917. See B.-Heidenhain *stain.*

bionecrosis (bī-ō-ne-krō'sis). Necrobiosis.

bionic (bī-on'ik). Relating to or developed from bionics.

bionics (bī-on'iks) [bio- + electronics]. The science of biologic functions and mechanisms as applied to electronic chemistry; such as computers, employing various aspects of physics, mathematics, and chemistry; *e.g.,* improving cybernetic engineering by reference to the organization of the vertebrate nervous system.

bionomics (bī-ō-nom'iks). **1.** Bionomy. **2.** Ecology.

bionomy (bī-on'ō-mē) [bio- + G. *nomos,* law]. Bionomics (1); the laws of life; the science concerned with the laws regulating the vital functions.

biophage (bī'ō-fāj). An organism that derives the nourishment for its existence from another living organism.

biophagism (bī-of'ă-jizm) [bio- + G. *phagein,* to eat]. Biophagy; the deriving of nourishment from living organisms.

biophagous (bī-of'ă-gŭs). Feeding on living organisms; denoting certain parasites.

biophagy (bī-of'ă-jē). Biophagism.

biopharmaceutics (bī'ō-far-mă-sū'tiks). The study of the physical and chemical properties of a drug, and its dosage form, as related to the onset, duration, and intensity of drug action.

biophilia (bī-ō-fil'ē-ă) [bio- + G. *philia,* love, fondness for]. The instinct of self-preservation.

biophotometer (bī-ō-fō-tom'ĕ-ter). An instrument used for measuring the rate and degree of dark adaptation.

biophylactic (bī'ō-fī-lak'tik). Relating to biophylaxis.

biophylaxis (bī'ō-fī-lak'sis) [bio- + G. *phylaxis,* protection]. Nonspecific defense reactions of the body, *e.g.,* phagocytosis, vascular and other reactions of inflammatory processes.

biophysics (bī-ō-phyz'iks). **1.** The study of biological processes and materials by means of the theories and tools of physics. **2.** The study of physical processes (*e.g.,* electricity, luminescence) occurring in organisms.
dental b., dental biomechanics; the relationship between the biologic behavior of oral structures and the physical influence of a dental restoration.

bioplasm (bī'ō-plazm) [bio- + G. *plasma,* thing formed]. Protoplasm, especially in its relation to living processes and development.

bioplasmic (bī-ō-plas'mik). Relating to bioplasm.

biopsy (bī'op-sē) [bio- + G. *opsis,* vision]. **1.** Process of removing tissue from living patients for diagnostic examination. **2.** A specimen obtained by b.
aspiration b., needle b.
brush b., b. obtained by passing a bristled catheter into the ureter or pyelocalyceal system to remove cells from suspected areas of disease by entrapping them in the bristles.
endoscopic b., b. obtained by instruments passed through an endoscope or obtained by a needle introduced under endoscopic guidance.
excision b., excision of tissue for gross and microscopic examination in such a manner that the entire lesion is removed.
incision b., removal of only a part of a lesion by incising into it.
needle b., aspiration b.; any method in which the specimen for b. is removed by aspirating it through an appropriate needle or trocar that pierces the skin, or the external surface of an organ, and into the underlying tissue to be examined.
open b., surgical incision or excision of the region from which the b. is taken.
punch b., trephine b.; any method that removes a small cylindrical specimen for b. by means of a special instrument that pierces the organ directly or through the skin or a small incision in the skin.
shave b., a b. technique performed with a surgical blade or a razor blade; used for lesions that are elevated above the skin level or confined to the epidermis and upper dermis.
sponge b., abrasion of a lesion with a suitable sponge.
trephine b., punch b.
wedge b., excision of a cuneiform specimen.

biopsychology (bī'ō-sī-kol'ō-jē). An interdisciplinary area of study involving psychology, biology, physiology, biochemistry, the neural sciences, and related fields.

biopterin (bī-op'ter-in). 6-(1,2-Dihydroxypropyl)pterin; a pterin found in yeast, the fruit fly, and in normal human urine.

biopyoculture (bī-ō-pī'ō-kŭl-chūr) [bio- + G. *pyon,* pus, + culture]. A culture made from purulent exudate in which various cells, including the phagocytes, are still viable.

biorbital (bī-ōr'bī-tăl) [bi- + G. *orbita,* orbit]. Relating to both orbits.

biorheology (bī'ō-rē-ol'ō-jē) [bio- + G. *rheō,* to flow, + *logos,* study]. The science concerned with deformation and flow in biological systems.

biorhythm (bī'ō-rith-m) [bio- + G. *rhythmos,* rhythm]. A biologically inherent cyclic variation or recurrence of an event or state, such as the sleep cycle, circadian rhythms, or periodic diseases.

bioroentgenography (bī'ō-rent-jen-og'ră-fē). The making of x-ray pictures of subjects in motion.

biose (bī'ōs). Glycolaldehyde.

bioside (bī'ō-sīd). Disaccharide.

biosis (bī-ō'sis) [G. *biōsis,* way of living]. Life, in a general sense.

biosocial (bī-ō-sō'shŭl). Involving the interplay of biological and social influences.

biospectrometry (bī'ō-spek-trom'ĕ-trē) [bio- + L. *spectrum,* an image, + G. *metron,* measure]. Clinical spectrometry; spectroscopic determination of the types and amounts of various substances in living tissue or fluid from a living body.

biospectroscopy (bī'ō-spek-tros'kō-pē) [bio- + L. *spectrum,* image, + G. *skopeō,* to examine]. Clinical spectroscopy; spectroscopic examination of specimens of living tissue, including fluids removed therefrom.

biospeleology (bī'ō-spē'lē-ol'ō-jē) [bio- + G. *spēliaion,* cave]. The study of organisms whose natural habitat is wholly or partly subterranean.

biosphere (bī'ō-sfēr) [bio- + G. *sphaira,* sphere]. All the regions in the world where living organisms are found.

biostatics (bī-ō-stat'iks) [bio- + G. *statikos,* causing to stand]. The science of the relation between structure and function in organisms.

biostatistics (bī'ō-stă-tis'tiks). The science of statistics applied to biological or medical data.

biosynthesis (bī-ō-sin'thĕ-sis). Formation of a chemical compound by enzymes, either in the organism (*in vivo*) or by fragments or extracts of cells (*in vitro*).

biosynthetic (bī'ō-sin-thet'ik). Relating to or produced by biosynthesis.

biosystem (bī'ō-sis-tem). A living organism or any complete system of living things that can, directly or indirectly, interact with others.

Biot, Camille, 19th century French physician. See B.'s *breathing.*

biota (bī-ō'tă) [Mod. L., fr. G. *bios,* life]. The collective flora and fauna of a region.

biotaxis (bī-ō-tak'sis) [bio- + G. *taxis,* arrangement]. **1.** The classification of living beings according to their anatomical characteristics. **2.** Cytoclesis.

biotelemetry (bī-ō-tel-em'ĕ-trē). The technique of monitoring vital processes and transmitting data without wires to a point remote from the subject.

biotic (bī-ot'ik). Pertaining to life.

biotics (bī-ot'iks) [G. *biōtikos,* relating to life]. The science concerned with the functions of life, or vital activity and force.

biotin (bī'ō-tin). W factor; *cis-* hexahydro-2-oxo-1*H*- thieno[3,4-*d*] imidazoline-4-valeric acid; a component of the vitamin B_2 complex occurring in or required by most organisms and inactivated by avidin.

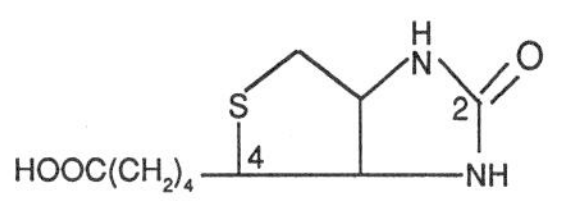

Biotin

b. oxidase, an enzyme (probably nonspecific) catalyzing the beta-oxidation of the b. side chain.

biotinidase (bī-ō-tin'i-dās) [EC 3.5.1.12]. An enzyme catalyzing the hydrolysis of biotin amide, biocytin, and other biotinides to biotin.

biotinides (bī-ot'i-nīdz). Compounds of biotin; *e.g.,* biocytin.

biotinyllysine (bī'ō-tin-il-lī'sin). Biocytin.

biotope (bī'ō-tōp) [G. *bios,* life, + *topos,* place]. The smallest geographical area providing uniform conditions for life; the physical part of an ecosystem.

biotoxicology (bī'ō-tok-si-kol'ō-jē). The study of poisons produced by living organisms.

biotoxin (bī-ō-tok'sin). Any toxic substance formed in an animal body, and demonstrable in its tissues or body fluids, or both.

biotransformation (bī'ō-trans-fōr-mā'shŭn). Biodegradation; the conversion of molecules from one form to another within an organism, often associated with change in pharmacologic activity; refers especially to drugs and other xenobiotics.

biotropism (bī-ō-trō'pizm) [bio- + G. *tropē,* a turning]. A theory that a drug eruption may be due to activation of a latent infection by the drug.

biotype (bī'ō-tīp). **1.** A population or group of individuals composed of the same genotype. **2.** In bacteriology, former name for biovar.

biovar (bī'ō-var). A group (infrasubspecific) of bacterial strains distinguishable from other strains of the same species on the basis of physiological characters. Formerly called biotype.

biovular (bī'ov-yū-lar). Diovular.

bipalatinoid (bī-pal'ă-ti-noyd). A capsule with two compartments, used for making remedies in nascent form; the reaction between the two substances takes place as the capsule dissolves in the stomach, thus activating the remedy.

biparasitism (bī-par'ă-sit-izm). Hyperparasitism.

biparental (bī-pa-ren'tăl). Having two parents, male and female.

biparietal (bī-pa-rī'ĕ-tăl) [bi- + L. *paries,* wall]. Relating to both parietal bones of the skull.

biparous (bip'ă-rŭs) [bi- + L. *pario,* to give birth]. Bearing two young.

bipartite (bī-par'tīt). Consisting of two parts of divisions.

biped (bī'ped) [bi- + L. *pes,* foot]. **1.** Two-footed. **2.** Any animal with only two feet.

bipedal (bī'ped-ăl). **1.** Relating to a biped. **2.** Capable of locomotion on two feet; *e.g.,* an iguana and some other lizards have this capability.

bipennate, bipenniform (bī-pen'āt, pen'i-fōrm) [bi- + L. *penna,* feather]. Pertaining to a muscle with a central tendon toward which the fibers converge on either side like the barbs of a feather.

biperforate (bī-per'fō-rāt). Having two foramina or perforations.

biperiden (bī-per'i-den). α-5-Norbornen-2-yl-α-phenyl-1-piperidinepropanol; an anticholinergic agent with sedative and central effects on the basal ganglia; used in the symptomatic treatment of parkinsonism and drug-induced parkinsonism. Also available as b. hydrochloride.

biphenamine hydrochloride (bī-fen'ă-mēn). Xenysalate hydrochloride; 2-diethylaminoethyl 2-hydroxy-3-phenylbenzoate hydrochloride; an antiseborrheic agent.

biphenotypic (bī'fē-nō-tip'ik). Pertaining to or characterized by biphenotypy.

biphenotypy (bī-fē'nō-tī'pē). The expression of markers more than one cell type by the same cell, as in certain leukemias.

biphenyl (bī-fen'il). Phenylbenzene; C_6H_5-C_6H_5; an aromatic hydrocarbon.

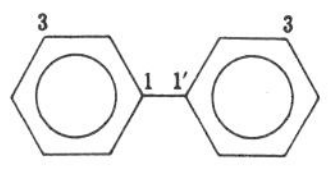

Biphenyl

polychlorinated b. (PCB), b. in which some or all of the hydrogen atoms attached to ring carbons are replaced by chlorine atoms; an industrial carcinogen.

bipolar (bī-pō'ler). Having two poles, ends, or extremes.

bipotentiality (bī'pō-ten-shē-al'i-tē). Capability of differentiating along two developmental pathways.

biramous (bī-rā'mŭs) [bi- + L. *ramus,* branch]. Having two branches.

Birbeck, Michael S., contemporary British cancer researcher. See B.'s *granule.*

Birch-Hirschfeld, Felix V., German pathologist, 1842–1899. See B.-H.'s *stain.*

birch tar (berch). Birch tar oil.

birch tar oil. B. tar; pyroligneous oil obtained by the dry distillation of the wood of *Betula alba* and rectified by steam distillation; used externally in the treatment of skin diseases.

Bird, Samuel D., Australian physician, 1833–1904. See B.'s *sign.*

birefringence (bī-rē-frin'jens). Double *refraction.*

birefringent (bī-rē-frin'-jent). Refracting twice; splitting a ray of light in two.

birotation (bī-rō-tā'shŭn). Mutarotation.

birth (berth). **1.** Passage of the offspring from the uterus to the outside world; the act of being born. **2.** Specifically, in the human, complete expulsion or extraction from its mother of a fetus irrespective of gestational age, and regardless of whether or not the umbilical cord has been cut or whether or not the placenta is attached.

cross b., obsolete term for: **(1)** transverse *lie;* **(2)** transverse *presentation.*

premature b., b. of an infant after viability has been achieved with gestation of at least 20 weeks or birth weight of at least 500 gr, but before full term.

birthmark (berth'mark). Nevus (1).

strawberry b., strawberry *nevus.*

bis- [L.] **1.** Prefix signifying two or twice. **2.** In chemistry, used to denote the presence of two identical but separated complex groups in one molecule. *Cf.* bi-; di-. See also bi-.

bisacodyl (bis-ak'ō-dil). 4,4'-(2-Pyridylmethylene)diphenol diacetate; bis(*p*-acetoxyphenyl)-2-pyridylmethane; a laxative used orally or rectally for constipation.

bisacromial (bis'ă-krō'mē-ăl). Relating to both acromion processes.

bisalbuminemia (bis'al-byū'mi-nē'mē-ă). The condition of having two kinds of serum albumin that differ in mobility on electrophoresis: normal albumin (albumin A) and any one of several variant types that migrate slower or faster than albumin A; individuals are heterozygous for the gene for albumin A and the gene for the variant albumin type. See also inherited albumin *variants.*

bisalt (bī'sawlt). Acid *salt.*

bisaxillary (bis-ak'si-lār-ē). Relating to both axillae.

2,5-bis(5-*t*-butylbenzoxazol-2-yl)thiophene (BBOT). A scintillator used in radioactivity measurements by scintillation counting.

bis(2-chloroethyl)sulfide. Mustard *gas.*

Bischof, W., 20th century German neurosurgeon. See B.'s *myelotomy.*

biscuit (bis'kit). A term associated with the firing of porcelain, and applied to the fired article before glazing. May be any stage after the fluxes have flowed enough to provide rigidity to the structure up to the stage where shrinkage is complete. Referred to as low, medium or high b., depending on the completeness of vitrification, also as hard or soft b.

biscuit-bake. Biscuit-firing; the initial bake(s) given fusing porcelain at lower than glazing temperature to control shrinkage during the process of building up the dental restoration.

biscuit-firing. Biscuit-bake.

bisdequalinium chloride (bis'de-kwă-lin'ē-ŭm). 1,1'-Decamethylene-4,4'-(1,10-decamethylenediimino)bis[quinaldinium chloride]; an antiseptic.

bisexual (bī-seks'yū-ăl). Ambisexual. **1.** Having gonads of both sexes. See also hermaphroditism and subentries. **2.** Denoting an individual who engages in both heterosexual and homosexual relations.

bisferious (bis-fĕr'ē-ŭs) [L. *bis,* twice, + *ferio,* to strike]. Striking twice; said of the pulse.

Bishop, Louis F., U.S. physician, 1864–1941. See B.'s *sphygmoscope.*

bishydroxycoumarin (bis-hī-drox'ē-kū'mă-rin). Dicumarol.

bisiliac (bis-il'ē-ak). Relating to any two corresponding iliac parts or structures, as the iliac bones or iliac fossae.

bis in die (b.i.d.) (bis in dē'ā) [L.]. Twice a day.

Bismarck brown R [C.I. 21010]. A diazo dye similar to Bismarck brown Y.

Bismarck brown Y [Ger. *bismarckbraun,* after Otto von *Bismarck,* Ger. chancellor] [C.I. 21000]. Vesuvin; a diazo dye used for staining mucin and cartilage in histologic sections, in the Papanicolaou technique for vaginal smears, and as one of Kasten's Schiff-type reagents in the PAS and Feulgen stains.

bismuth (biz'mŭth) [Ger. *Wismut*]. A trivalent metallic element; symbol Bi, atomic no. 83, atomic weight 209. Several of its salts are used in medicine; some contain BiO^+, rather than Bi^{3+}, and are called subsalts.

b. aluminate, aluminum b. oxide; a gastric antacid.

b. ammonium citrate, ammoniocitrate of b.; an intestinal astringent.

b. carbonate, b. subcarbonate.

b. chloride oxide, b. oxychloride.

b. citrate, used in the making of b. and ammonium citrate.

b. iodide, b. triiodide; BiI_3; used in electron microscopy to reveal synapses.

b. oxide, Bi_2O_3; used for the same purposes as the subnitrate.

b. oxycarbonate, b. subcarbonate.

b. oxychloride, bismuthyl chloride; b. chloride oxide; BiOCl; basic b. chloride, used for the same purposes as the subnitrate.

b. oxynitrate, b. subnitrate.

b. salicylate, see b. subsalicylate.

b. sodium tartrate, a basic sodium b. tartrate; an antisyphilitic agent.

b. sodium triglycollamate, sodium b. complex of nitrilotriacetic acid.

b. subcarbonate, b. oxycarbonate; b. carbonate; bismuthyl carbonate; $(BiO)_2CO_3$; used for the same purposes as b. subnitrate, but has lower toxicity.

b. subgallate, used internally in diarrhea and externally as an astringent and protective dusting powder.

b. subnitrate, b. oxynitrate; a basic salt, the composition of which varies with the conditions of preparation; used internally as an intestinal astringent and externally as a mild astringent and antiseptic; the metal is used as an electron microscope stain for nucleic acids.

b. subsalicylate, used as an intestinal antiseptic.

b. tribromophenate, b. tribromophenol, used externally as an antiseptic.

b. trichloride, butter of bismuth; $BiCl_3$; addition of water results in formation of b. oxychloride.

b. triiodide, b. iodide.

bismuthosis (bis-mŭ-thō'sis). Chronic bismuth poisoning.

bismuthyl (biz'mŭ-thil). The group, BiO^+, that behaves chemically as the ion of a univalent metal; its salts are subsalts of bismuth.

b. carbonate, *bismuth* subcarbonate.

b. chloride, *bismuth* oxychloride.

bisoxatin acetate (bis-ok'să-tin). 2,2-Bis(*p*-hydroxyphenyl)-2*H*-1,4-benzoxazin-3(4*H*)-one diacetate; a laxative.

1,4-bis(5-phenyloxazol-2-yl)benzene (POPOP). A liquid scintillation agent used in radioisotope measurement.

bistephanic (bī'stĕ-fan'ik). Relating to both stephanions; denoting particularly the b. width of the cranium, or b. diameter, the shortest distance from one stephanion to the other.

bisteroid (bī-stĕr'oyd). A molecule composed of two molecules of a given steroid joined together by a carbon-to-carbon bond.

bistoury (bis'tū-rē) [Fr. *bistouri,* fr. *bisorit,* dagger]. A long, narrow-bladed knife, with a straight or curved edge and sharp or blunt point (probe-point); used for opening or slitting cavities or hollow structures.

bistratal (bī-strā'tăl). Having two strata or layers.

bisulfate (bī-sŭl'fāt). Acid sulfate; a salt containing HSO_4^-.

bisulfide (bī-sŭl'fīd). A compound of the anion HS^-; an acid sulfide.

bisulfite (bī-sŭl'fīt). A salt or ion of HSO_3^-.

bit. The smallest unit of digital information expressed in the binary system of notation (either 0 or 1).

bitartrate (bī-tar'trāt). A salt or anion resulting from the neutralization of one of tartaric acid's two acid groups.

bitch [O.E. *bicche*]. A female dog of breeding age.

bite (bīt) [A.S. *bītan*]. **1.** To incise or seize with the teeth. **2.** The act of incision or seizure with the teeth. **3.** A morsel of food held between the teeth. **4.** Term used to denote the amount of pressure developed in closing the jaws. **5.** Undesirable jargon for terms such as interocclusal record, maxillomandibular registration, denture space, and interarch distance. **6.** A wound or puncture of the skin made by animal or insect. See bites.

balanced b., balanced *occlusion.*

biscuit b., maxillomandibular *record.*

close b., small interarch *distance.*

closed b., reduced vertical interarch distance with excessive vertical overlap of the anterior teeth.

deep b., an abnormally large vertical overlap of anterior teeth in centric occlusion.

edge-to-edge b., edge-to-edge *occlusion.*

end-to-end b., edge-to-edge *occlusion.*

jumping the b., an orthodontic technique for correcting a crossbite, usually anterior.

locked b., an occlusion in which the cusp arrangement restricts lateral excursions.

normal b., normal *occlusion* (1).

open b., **(1)** large interarch *distance;* **(2)** apertognathia.

rest b., a misnomer for physiologic rest *position.*

working b., working *contacts.*

bitemporal (bī-tem'pŏ-răl). Relating to both temples or temporal bones.

biteplate, biteplane (bīt'plāt, bīt'plān). A removable appliance that incorporates a plane of acrylic designed to occlude with the opposing teeth.

bites (bītz) [see bite]. Penetration of the skin (puncture or laceration) causing reactions that result from 1) mechanical injury; 2) injection of toxic material such as snake or scorpion venom; 3) injection of antigenic substance capable of inducing and eliciting allergic sensitization; 4) introduction of otherwise saprophytic flora such as *Staphylococcus pyogenes* in the instance of human bites; 5) invasion of the tissue as in myiasis; 6) transmission of disease such as typhus and rabies. Depending on the nature of the material propelled into the puncture of the skin and, in the case of antigenic material, on the previous exposure and immunity of the host, the local reaction will be immediate or delayed, accompanied by varying degrees of pain, itching and burning, and systemic manifestations specific for the offending agent.

bitewing (bīt'wing). See bitewing *radiograph.*

bithionol (bī-thī'ō-nol). 2,2'-Thiobis[4,6-dichlorophenol]; an antiparasitic agent used for treatment of the human lungworm, *Paragonimus westermani,* and the Oriental liver fluke, *Clonorchis sinensis;* also used as a bacteriostat in soaps and detergents; sodium bithionate is used as a topical bactericide and fungicide.

bitolterol mesylate (bī-tol'ter-ol). 4-[2-(*tert*- Butylamino)-1-hydroxyethyl]-o-phenylenedi(*p*- toluate)methanesulfonate; a sympathomimetic bronchodilator used in the prophylaxis and treatment of bronchial asthma and reversible bronchospasm.

Bitot, Pierre A., French physician, 1822–1888. See B.'s *spots.*

bitrochanteric (bī-trō-kan-ter'ik). Relating to two trochanters, either to the two trochanters of one femur or to both great trochanters.

bitropic (bī-trop'ik) [bi- + G. *tropē,* a turning]. Having a dual affinity, as in tissues or organisms.

bitter apple. Colocynth.

bit'ters. **1.** An alcoholic liquor in which bitter vegetable substances (*e.g.,* quinine, gentian) have been steeped. **2.** Amara; bitter vegetable drugs (*e.g.,* quassia, gentian, cinchona), usually used as tonics.
aromatic b., b. with a pleasant aromatic flavor.

Bittner, John J., U.S. oncologist, *1904. See B.'s *agent,* B. milk *factor.*

Bittorf, Alexander, German physician, 1876–1949. See B.'s *reaction.*

biuret (bī-ū-ret'). Allophanamide; carbamoylurea; $NH(CONH_2)_2$; a derivative of urea obtained by heating, eliminating NH_3 between two ureas.

bivalence, bivalency (bī-vā'lens, bī-vā'len-sē). Divalence; divalency; a combining power (valence) of two.

bivalent (bī-vā'lent, biv'ă-lent). **1.** Divalent; having a combining power (valence) of two. **2.** In cytology, a structure consisting of two paired homologous chromosomes, each split into two sister chromatids, as seen during the pachytene stage of prophase in meiosis.

biventer (bī-ven'ter) [bi- + L. *venter,* belly]. Two-bellied; denoting two-bellied muscles.
b. cer'vicis, *musculus* spinalis capitis.
b. mandib'ulae, *musculus* digastricus.

biventral (bī-ven'tral). Digastric (1).

bixin (bik'sin). A carotenoid (a carotene-dioic acid); the orange-red coloring matter from seeds of *Bixa orellana;* the ethyl ester is used as a food and drug colorant. See also annotto.

bizygomatic (bī'zī-gō-mat'ik). Relating to both zygomatic bones or arches.

Bizzozero, Giulio, Italian physician, 1846–1901. See B.'s red *cells,* B.'s *corpuscle.*

Bjerrum, Jannik P., Danish ophthalmologist, 1851–1920. See B.'s *scotoma, screen, sign.*

Bjornstad, R., 20th century Scandinavian dermatologist. See B.'s *syndrome.*

Bk Symbol for berkelium.

Black, Douglas A.K., Scottish physician, *1909. See B.'s *formula.*

Black, Greene V., U.S. dentist, 1836–1915. See B.'s *classification.*

Blackfan, Kenneth D., U.S. physician, 1883–1941. See Diamond-B. *anemia, syndrome.*

blackhead (blak'hed). **1.** Open *comedo.* **2.** Histomoniasis.

blackleg (blak'leg). Quarter evil; a highly fatal, specific, essentially gas-gangrenous infection caused by *Clostridium chavoei* (*feseri*) and affecting the muscular upper parts of the legs of young cattle and sheep.

blackout (blak'owt). **1.** Temporary loss of consciousness due to decreased blood flow to the brain. **2.** Momentary loss of consciousness as an absence.
visual b., see *amaurosis* fugax.

bladder (blad'er) [A.S. *blaedre*]. Vesica (1).
air b., swim b.; a two-chambered gas-filled sac that is present in most fish and functions as a hydrostatic organ; it is located beneath the vertebral column, and is connected with the esophagus in some fish.
allantoic b., a type of b. formed as an outgrowth of the cloaca.
atonic b., a large, dilated, and nonemptying b.; usually due to disturbance of innervation or to chronic obstruction.
autonomic neurogenic b., neuropathic b.; malfunctioning b., secondary to low spinal cord lesions. See cord bladder.
cord b., a b. after interruption of its nerve supply, marked by abnormal detrusor and sphincter function, generally with incomplete emptying, reduced or increased b. capacity, and deranged control of micturition.
fasciculate b., a b. with hypertrophied walls, the muscular bundles standing out like interlacing cords on the inner surface of the viscus.
gall b., see gallbladder; *vesica* biliaris.
ileal b., ideal *conduit.*
low-compliance b., a b. that has high pressure at low volumes in the absence of detrusor activity.
nervous b., a b. condition in which there is a neurotic wish to urinate frequently but sometimes with failure to empty the b. completely.
neurogenic b., any defective functioning of bladder due to impaired innervation, *e.g.,* cord b., neuropathic b.
pseudoneurogenic b., Hinman *syndrome.*
reflex neurogenic b., an abnormal condition of b. function whereby the b. is cut off from upper motor neuron control, but where the lower motor neuron arc is still intact.
swim b., air b.
uninhibited neurogenic b., a condition, either congenital or acquired, of abnormal b. function whereby normal inhibitory control of detrusor function by the central nervous system is impaired or underdeveloped, resulting in precipitant or uncontrolled micturition and/or anuresis.
urinary b., *vesica* urinaria.

bladderworm (blad'er-werm). Cysticercus.

bladevent (blăd'vent). A thin, wedge-shaped endo-osseous implant of metal that is inserted into a surgically prepared groove in the maxilla or mandible.

Blagden, Sir Charles, British physician, 1748–1820. See B.'s *law.*

blain (blān) [A.S. *blegen*]. A lesion on the skin.

Blainville, Henri M.D. de, French zoologist and anthropologist, 1777–1850. See B. *ears.*

Blair, Vilray P., U.S. surgeon, 1871–1955. See B.-Brown *graft.*

Blakemore, Arthur H., U.S. surgeon, *1897. See Sengstaken-B. *tube.*

Blalock, Alfred, U.S. surgeon, 1899–1965. See B.-Hanlon *operation;* B.-Taussig *operation.*

Blandin, Philippe F., French surgeon, 1798–1849. See B.'s *gland.*

blas [a Middle E. variant of *blast*]. Term invented by van Helmont to denote a mystical spirit or vital force which presided over and governed the various processes of the body. Each bodily function was supposed to have its own special b.; b. appears to be the counterpart of the archaeus of Paracelsus.

Blasius, Gerardus, 17th century Dutch anatomist. See B.'s *duct.*

Blaskovics, Laszlo, Hungarian ophthalmologist, 1869–1938. See B.'s *operation.*

-blast [G. *blastos,* germ]. Suffix indicating an immature precursor cell of the type indicated by the preceding word.

blastema (blas-tē'mă) [G. a sprout]. **1.** The primordial cellular mass from which an organ or part is formed. **2.** A cluster of cells competent to initiate the regeneration of a damaged or ablated structure.
nephric b., nephroblastema; the extension of nephrogenic cord tissue, caudal to the mesonephros, into which the ureteric buds grow to initiate development of the definitive mammalian kidney.

blastemic (blas-tem'ik). Relating to the blastema.

blasto- [G. *blastos,* germ]. Combining form used in terms pertaining to the process of budding (and the formation of buds) by cells or tissue.

blastocele (blas'tō-sēl) [blasto- + G. *koilos,* hollow]. Blastocoele; cleavage or segmentation cavity; the cavity in the blastula of a developing embryo.

blastocelic (blas-tō-sē'lik). Blastocoelic; relating to the blastocele.

blastocoele (blas'tō-sēl). Blastocele.

blastocoelic (blas'tō-sē'lik). Blastocelic.

Blastoconidium (blas'tō-cō-nid'ē-ŭm) [blasto- + conidium]. Blastospore; a holoblastic conidium that is produced singly or in chains, and detached at maturity leaving a bud scar, as in the budding in a yeast cell.

blastocyst (blas'tō-sist) [blasto- + G. *kystis,* bladder]. Blastodermic vesicle; the modified blastula stage of mammalian embryos, consisting of the inner cell mass and a thin trophoblast layer enclosing the blastocele.

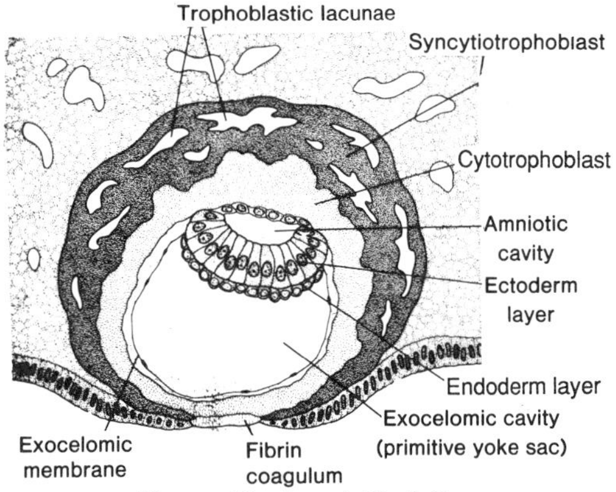

Human Blastocyst, Ninth Day

blastocyte (blas'tō-sīt) [blasto- + G. *kytos,* cell]. An undifferentiated blastomere of the morula or blastula stage of an embryo.

blastocytoma (blas'tō-sī-tō'mă). Blastoma.

blastoderm, blastoderma (blas'tō-derm, -tō-der'ma) [blasto- + G. *derma,* skin]. Membrana germinativa; germ or germinal membrane; the thin disk-shaped cell mass of a young embryo and its extraembryonic extensions over the surface of the yolk; when fully formed, all three primary germ layers (ectoderm, endoderm, and mesoderm) are present.
bilaminar b., the b. of a young embryo when it consists of only two of the three primary germ layers it will ultimately have.
embryonic b., that part of the b. that takes part in the formation of the embryonic body.
extraembryonic b., that part of the b. which is not incorporated in the embryo but forms membranes concerned in its nourishment and protection.
trilaminar b., the b. after all three of the primary germ layers have been established.

blastodermal, blastodermic (blas-tō-der'măl, -der'mik). Relating to the blastoderm.

blastodisk (blas'tō-disk). **1.** The disk of active cytoplasm at the animal pole of a telolecithal egg. **2.** The blastoderm, especially in very young stages when its extent is small.

blastogenesis (blas-tō-jen'ĕ-sis) [blasto- + G. *genesis,* origin]. **1.** Reproduction of unicellular organisms by budding. **2.** Development of an embryo during cleavage and germ layer formation. **3.** Transformation of small lymphocytes of human peripheral blood in tissue culture into large, morphologically primitive blastlike cells capable of undergoing mitosis; can be induced by a variety of agents including phytohemagglutinin, certain antigens to which the cell donor has been previously immunized, and leukocytes from an unrelated individual.

blastogenetic, blastogenic (blas'tō-je-net'ik, -tō-jen'ik). Relating to blastogenesis.

blastolysis (blas-tol'i-sis) [blasto- + G. *lysis,* loosening]. Dissolution of the blastocyst and subsequent death.

blastolytic (blas-tō-lit'ik). Relating to blastolysis.

blastoma (blas-tō'mă) [blasto- + G. *-oma,* tumor]. Blastocytoma; embryonal carcinosarcoma; a neoplasm composed chiefly or entirely of immature undifferentiated cells (*i.e.,* blast forms), with little or virtually no stroma.

blastomere (blas'tō-mēr) [blasto- + G. *meros,* part]. Cleavage cell; one of the cells into which the egg divides after its fertilization.

blastomerotomy (blas'tō-mēr-ot'ō-mē) [blastomere + G. *tomē,* incision]. Blastotomy.

blastomogenic (blas'tō-mō-jen'ik). Causing or producing a blastoma.

Blastomyces dermatitidis (blas-tō-mī'sēz der-mă-tit'i-dis) [blasto- + G. *mykēs,* fungus]. A dimorphic soil fungus that causes blastomycosis. It grows in mammalian tissues as budding cells and in culture as a white to buff-colored filamentous fungus bearing spherical or ovoid conidia on terminal or lateral short, slender conidiophores. In its perfect state it is known as *Ajellomyces dermatitidis.*

blastomycin (blas-tō-mī'sin). An antigen for intradermal testing prepared from sterile filtrates of cultures of the filamentous form of *Blastomyces dermatitidis.*

blastomycosis (blas'tō-mī-kō'sis). Gilchrist's disease; a chronic granulomatous and suppurative disease caused by Blastomyces dermatitidis; originates as a respiratory infection and disseminates, usually with pulmonary, osseous, and cutaneous involvement predominating. Formerly called North American b., the disease has now been found in African states as well as in Canada and the U.S.
North American b., see blastomycosis.
South American b., paracoccidioidomycosis.

blastoneuropore (blas'tō-nū'rō-pōr) [blasto- + neuropore]. A temporary opening formed in some embryos by the union of the blastopore and neuropore.

blastophore (blas'tō-fōr) [blasto- + G. *phorōs,* bearing]. An early stage of division of a coccidial schizont in which spheroid or ellipsoid structures are formed with a single peripheral layer of nuclei; merozoites form at the surface of the b. over each nucleus, grow out radially, and separate from the residual body (remnant of the b.); in a first-generation schizont such as *Eimeria bovis,* about 120,000 merozoites are produced.

blastopore (blas'tō-pōr) [blasto- + G. *poros,* opening]. The opening into the archenteron formed by invagination of the blastula to form a gastrula.

blastospore (blas'tō-spōr) [blasto- + G. *sporos,* seed]. Blastoconidium.

blastotomy (blas-tot'ō-mē) [blasto- + G. *tomē,* incision]. Blastomerotomy; experimental destruction of one or more blastomeres.

blastula (blas'tyū-lă) [G. *blastos,* germ]. An early stage of an embryo formed by the rearrangement of the blastomeres of the morula to form a hollow sphere.

blastular (blas'tyū-lar). Pertaining to the blastula.

blastulation (blas-tyū-lā'shŭn). Formation of the blastula or blastocyst.

Blatin, Marc, French physician, *1878. See B.'s *syndrome.*

Blatta (blat'ă) [L. cockroach]. A genus of insects (family Blattidae) that includes the abundant oriental cockroach, *B. orientalis.* The dried insect yields antihydropin, a diuretic principle.

Blattella (bla-tel'ă) [L. *blatta,* cockroach]. A genus of cockroaches, (family Blattidae) that includes *B. germanica,* the German cockroach or croton bug, probably the most familiar and widespread of the cockroaches.

Blattidae (blat'i-dē) [L. *blatta,* cockroach]. A family of insects (order Blattaria) consisting of over 4,000 species of cockroaches, largely tropical but worldwide in distribution, including a number of abundant pests of households, kitchens, and institutions or facilities, wherever food is present; noxious wherever found, yet not positively incriminated in natural transmission of pathogenic organisms to man. Common household pests include the German cockroach, *Blattella germanica,* the American cockroach, *Periplaneta americana,* and the oriental cockroach, *Blatta orientalis.*

bleb. A large flaccid vesicle.

bleed (blēd). To lose blood as a result of rupture or severance of blood vessels.

bleeder (blēd'er). Colloquialism for one suffering from hemophilia, Christmas disease, Osler's disease, or other bleeding disorders.

bleeding (blēd'ing). Losing blood as a result of the rupture or severance of blood vessels.

dysfunctional uterine b., uterine b. due to a benign endocrine imbalance rather than to any organic disease.

occult b., see occult *blood.*

blem'ish. **1.** A small circumscribed alteration of the skin considered to be unesthetic but insignificant. **2.** To alter the skin, rendering an unesthetic appearance.

blennadenitis (blen-ad-ĕ-nī'tis) [G. *blennos,* mucus, + *adēn,* gland, + *-itis,* inflammation]. Inflammation of the mucous glands.

blennemesis (blen-em'ĕ-sis) [G. *blennos,* mucus, + *emesis,* vomiting]. Vomiting of mucus.

blenno-, blenn- [G. *blenna, blennos,* mucus]. Combining forms relating to mucus.

blennogenic (blen-ō-jen'ik) [blenno- + G. *-gen,* to produce]. Muciparous.

blennogenous (ble-noj'ĕ-nŭs). Muciparous.

blennoid (blen'oyd) [blenno- + G. *eidos,* resemblance]. Muciform.

blennophthalmia (blen-of-thal'mē-ă). **1.** Conjunctivitis. **2.** Gonorrheal *ophthalmia.*

blennorrhagia (blen-ō-rā'jē-ă) [blenno- + G. *rhēgnymi,* to burst forth]. Blennorrhea.

blennorrhagic (blen-ō-raj'ik). Blennorheal.

blennorrhea (blen-ō-rē'ă) [blenno- + G. *rhoia,* a flow]. Blennorrhagia; myxorrhea; any mucous discharge, especially from the urethra or vagina.

b. conjunctiva'lis, gonorrheal *ophthalmia.*

inclusion b., inclusion *conjunctivitis.*

b. neonato'rum, *ophthalmia* neonatorum.

Stoerk's b., chronic, first purulent then dry, catarrh of the upper air passages with hypertrophy of the mucous membrane and submucosa, in many cases the same as scleroma.

blennorrheal (blen-ō-rē'ăl). Blennorrhagic; relating to blennorrhea.

blennostasis (blen-os'tă-sis) [blenno- + G. *stasis,* standing]. Rarely used term for diminution or suppression of secretion from the mucous membranes.

blennostatic (blen-ō-stat'ik). Diminishing mucous secretion.

blennuria (ble-nū'rē-ă) [blenno- + G. *ouron,* urine]. The excretion of an excess of mucus in the urine.

bleomycin sulfate (blē-ō-mī'sin). An antineoplastic antibiotic obtained from *Streptomyces verticillus.*

blephar-. See blepharo-.

blepharadenitis (blef'ar-ad-ĕ-nī'tis) [blephar- + G. *adēn,* gland, + *-itis,* inflammation]. Blepharoadenitis; inflammation of the meibomian glands or the marginal glands of Moll or Zeis.

blepharal (blef'ă-răl). Referring to the eyelids.

blepharectomy (blef'a-rek'tō-mē) [blepharo- + G. *ektomē,* excision]. Excision of all or part of an eyelid.

blepharedema (blef'ar-ĕ-dē'mă). Edema of the eyelids, causing swelling and often a baggy appearance.

blepharitis (blef'ă-rī'tis) [blepharo- + G. *-itis,* inflammation]. Inflammation of the eyelids.

b. acar'ica, demodectic b.

b. angula'ris, inflammation of the lid margins at the angles of the commissure.

ciliary b., b. marginalis.

demodectic b., b. acarica; inflammation of the eyelid associated with *Demodex folliculorum.*

b. follicula'ris, pustular b.; folliculitis interna or externa; a deep-seated suppurative inflammation of ciliary follicles and the glands of Zeis and Moll of the eyelid.

marginal b., b. marginalis.

b. margina'lis, psorophthalmia; ciliary or marginal b.; inflammation of the margins of the eyelids.

meibomian b., inflammation of the eyelid margin and the meibomian glands.

b. oleo'sa, seborrheic b.

b. parasit'ica, pediculous b.; b. phthiriatica; marginal b. due to the presence of lice.

pediculous b., b. parasitica.

b. phthiriat'ica, b. parasitica.

pustular b., b. follicularis.

b. rosa'cea, inflammation of the margins of the eyelids in association with acne rosacea.

seborrheic b., b. oleosa or squamosa; a common type of chronic inflammation of the margins of the eyelids with adherence of dry scales; often with an associated seborrheic dermatitis of scalp and face.

b. sic'ca, inflammation of the margins of the eyelids in which the lashes are powdered with dry scales.

b. squamo'sa, seborrheic b.

b. ulcero'sa, marginal b. with ulceration.

blepharo-, blephar- [G. *blepharon,* eyelid]. Combining forms meaning eyelid.

blepharoadenitis (blef'ă-rō-ad-ĕ-nī'tis). Blepharadenitis.

blepharoadenoma (blef'ă-rō-ad-ĕ-nō'mă) [blepharo- + G. *adēn,* gland, + *-oma,* tumor]. A tumor or adenoma of a gland of the eyelid.

blepharochalasis (blef'ă-rō-kal'ă-sis) [blepharo- + G. *chalasis,* a slackening]. Ptosis adiposa; dermatolysis palpebrarum; a condition in which there is a redundancy of the skin of the upper eyelids so that a fold of skin hangs down, often concealing the tarsal margin when the eye is open.

blepharochromidrosis (blef'ă-rō-krō-mi-drō'sis) [blepharo- + G. *chrōma,* color, + *hidrōsis,* sweat]. Chromidrosis of the eyelids.

blepharoclonus (blef-ar-ok'lō-nŭs) [blepharo- + G. *klonos,* a tumult]. Clonic spasm of the eyelids.

blepharocoloboma (blef'ă-rō-kol-ō-bō'mă) [blepharo- + coloboma]. A defect of the eyelid; may be congenital or acquired.

blepharoconjunctivitis (blef'ă-rō-kon-jŭnk-ti-vī'tis). Inflammation of the palpebral conjunctiva.

blepharodiastasis (blef'ă-rō-dī-as'tă-sis) [blepharo- + G. *diastasis,* separation]. Abnormal separation or inability to completely close the eyelids.

blepharokeratoconjunctivitis (blef'ă-rō-ker'ă-tō-kon-jŭnk'ti-vī'tis). An inflammation involving the eyelids, cornea, and conjunctiva.

blepharomelasma (blef'ă-rō-mē-laz'mă) [blepharo- + melasma]. A dark discoloration of the skin of the eyelid.

blepharon (blef'ă-ron) [G. *blepharon,* eyelid]. Palpebra.

blepharopachynsis (blef'ă-rō-pă-kin'sis) [blepharo- + G. *pachynsis,* a thickening]. A pathological thickening of an eyelid.

blepharophimosis (blef'ă-rō-fi-mō'sis) [blepharo- + G. *phimōsis,* an obstruction]. Blepharostenosis; decrease in the size of the palpebral aperture without fusion of lid margins.

blepharophyma (blef'ă-rō-fī'mă) [blepharo- + G. *phyma,* a tumor]. A tumor of the skin of the eyelid.

blepharoplast (blef'ă-rō-plast) [blepharo- + G. *plastos,* formed]. Basal *body.*

blepharoplastic (blef'ă-rō-plas'tik). Relating to blepharoplasty.

blepharoplasty (blef'ă-ro-plast-tē) [blepharo- + G. *plassō,* to form]. Any operation for the correction of a defect in the eyelids.

blepharoplegia (blef'ă-rō-plē'jē-ă) [blepharo- + G. *plēgē,* stroke]. Paralysis of an eyelid.

blepharoptosis, blepharoptosia (blef'ă-rop'tō-sis, -op-tō'sē-ă) [blepharo- + G. *ptōsis, a falling*]. Ptosis (2); drooping of the upper eyelid.

b. adipo'sa, excessive elasticity of skin so that it hangs over the free border of the eyelid.

false b., pseudoptosis.

blepharorrhaphy (blef-ar-ōr'ă-fē) [blepharo- + G. *rhaphē,* seam]. Tarsorrhaphy.

blepharospasm, blepharospasmus (blef'ă-rō-spazm, -spaz'mŭs). Spasmodic winking, or contraction of the orbicularis oculi muscle; may be associated with other dystonic contractions of facial, jaw, or neck muscles; usually initiated or aggravated by emotion, fatigue, or psychedelic drugs.

blepharostat (blef'ă-rō-stat) [blepharo- + G. *statos,* fixed]. Eye *speculum.*

blepharostenosis (blef'ă-rō-ste-nō'sis) [blepharo- + G. *stenōsis,* a narrowing]. Blepharophimosis.

blepharosynechia (blef'ă-rō-sin-ek'ē-ă) [blepharo- + G. *synecheia,* continuity, fr. *syn- echō,* to hold together]. Ankyloblepharon; pantankyloblepharon; adhesion of the eyelids to each other or to the eyeball.

blepharotomy (blef-ă-rot'ō-mē) [blepharo- + G. *tomē,* incision]. A cutting operation on an eyelid.

Blessig, Robert, Russian physician, 1830–1878. See B.'s *cysts.*

blind (blīnd). Unable to see; without useful sight. See blindness.

blindness (blīnd'nes). **1.** Typhlosis; loss of the sense of sight; absolute b. connotes no light perception. See also amblyopia; amaurosis. **2.** Loss of visual appreciation of objects although visual acuity is normal. **3.** Absence of the appreciation of sensation, *e.g.,* taste b.

canine hereditary b., an autosomal dominant condition seen in dogs of the collie and several other breeds.

color b., misleading term for anomalous or deficient color vision; complete color b. is the absence of one of the primary cone pigments of the retina. See protanopia, deuteranopia, tritanopia.

cortical b., loss of sight due to an organic lesion in the visual cortex.

day b., hemeralopia.

eclipse b., eclipse *amblyopia.*

flash b., a temporary loss of vision produced when retinal light-sensitive pigments are bleached by light more intense than that to which the retina is physiologically adapted at that moment.

flight b., visual blackout in aviators. See also *amaurosis* fugax.

functional b., loss of vision related to conversion reaction.

legal b., generally, visual acuity of less than 6/60 or 20/200 using Snellen test types, or visual field restriction to 20 degrees or less; the criteria used to define legal b. vary among different groups.

letter b., a form of aphasia in which one is unable to recognize the significance of letters.

mind b., psychanopsia; a type of aphasia in which the person no longer understands what he sees.

moon b., periodic *ophthalmia.*

music b., musical *alexia.*

night b., nyctalopia.

note b., musical *alexia.*

object b., apraxia (2).

river b., ocular *onchocerciasis.*

sign b., asymbolia (2).

smell b., anosmia.

snow b., severe photophobia secondary to ultraviolet keratoconjunctivitis.

solar b., eclipse *amblyopia.*

taste b., the lack of ability to appreciate a substance by taste.

text b., word b., alexia.

blis'ter. **1.** A fluid-filled thin-walled structure under the epidermis or within the epidermis (subepidermal or intradermal). **2.** To form a b. with heat or some other vesiculating agent.

blood b., a b. containing blood; resulting from a minor pinch or crushing injury.

fever b., colloquialism for herpes simplex of the lips.

fly b., a cantharidal b. caused by discharge of a vesicating body fluid by certain beetles, particularly members of the family Meloidae which produce cantharidin, *e.g., Lytta* (*Cantharis*) *vesicatoria,* the notorious "Spanish fly;" non-cantharidin vesicating fluid is produced by other beetles, such as rove beetles (family Staphylinidae), especially the genus *Paederus,* whose fluid, on contact with the skin, produces an intensely painful b.

flying b., a misnomer for a vesicator agent applied successively to different skin areas and kept in one place just long enough to cause redness but not long enough to cause a b.

blis'tering. Vesiculation (1).

bloat, bloating (blōt, blōt'ing). **1.** Abdominal distention from swallowed air or intestinal gas from fermentation. **2.** Distention of the rumen of cattle, caused by the accumulation of gases of fermentation, particularly likely to occur when the animals are pastured on rich legume grasses; if unrelieved, the condition may quickly lead to death.

Bloch, Bruno, Swiss dermatologist, 1878–1933. See B.-Sulzberger *disease, syndrome.*

Bloch, Marcel, French physician, 1885–1925. See B.'s *reaction.*

block [Fr. *bloquer*]. **1.** To obstruct; to arrest passage through. **2.** A condition in which the passage of a nervous impulse is arrested, wholly or in part, temporarily or permanently. **3.** Atrioventricular b.

anterograde b., conduction b. of an impulse traveling anywhere in its ordinary direction, from the sinoatrial node toward the ventricular myocardium.

arborization b., intraventricular b. supposedly due to widespread blockage in the Purkinje ramifications and manifested in the electrocardiogram by a pattern similar to bundle-branch b. but with complexes of low amplitude.

atrioventricular (A-V) b., block (3); heart b.; impairment of the normal conduction between atria and ventricles; in **first degree A-V b.**, there is prolongation of A-V conduction time (P-R interval); in **second degree A-V b.**, some but not all atrial impulses fail to reach the ventricles, thus some ventricular beats are dropped; in **complete A-V b.**, complete atrioventricular dissociation (2); no impulses can reach the ventricles despite a slow ventricular rate (under 45 per minute); atria and ventricles beat independently.

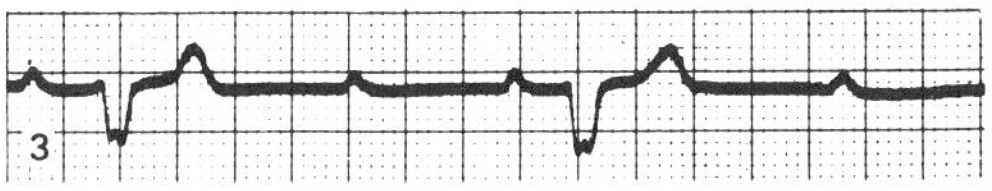

Complete Atrioventricular Block

bone b., a surgical procedure in which the bone adjacent to the joint is modified to limit the motion of the joint mechanically; *e.g.*, at the ankle joint to correct foot-drop by preventing extension below 90°, but allowing flexion within 90°.
bundle-branch b., intraventricular b. due to interruption of conduction in one of the two main branches of the bundle of His and manifested in the electrocardiogram by marked prolongation of the QRS complex.

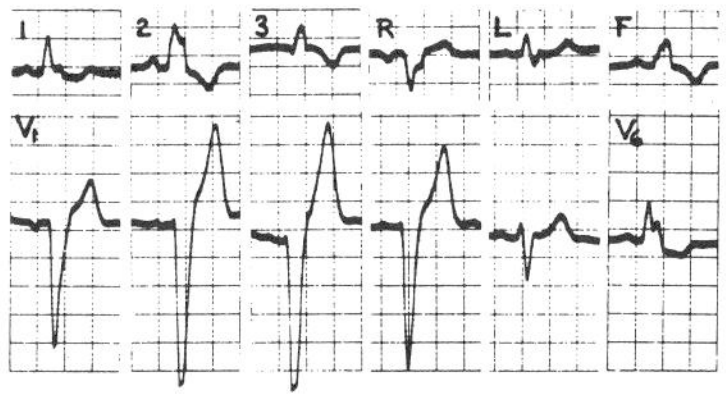

Left Bundle-Branch Block

depolarizing b., skeletal muscle paralysis associated with loss of polarity of the motor endplate, as occurs following administration of succinylcholine.
entrance b., protective b.
epidural b., obstruction of the epidural space by compression, hematoma, scar tissue, etc.; used inaccurately to refer to epidural anesthesia.
exit b., inability of an impulse to leave its point of origin, the mechanism for which is conceived as an encircling zone of refractory tissue denying passage to the emerging impulse.
fascicular b., a condition based on the concept that two fascicles in the left branch of the bundle of His provide three fascicles of a system of conduction, of which the right bundle branch constitutes the third, for the transmission of the cardiac impulse from the atrium above to the ventricle below the A-V node; block may occur in any or all fascicles, all three together producing complete A-V block. See also hemiblock.
field b., regional anesthesia produced by infiltration of local anesthetic solution into tissues surrounding an operative field.
heart b., atrioventricular b.
intra-atrial b., impaired conduction through the atria, manifested by widened and often notched P waves in the electrocardiogram.
intraventricular (I-V) b., delayed conduction within the ventricular conducting system or myocardium, including bundle-branch and peri-infarction b.'s., and the hemiblocks.
Mobitz types of atrioventricular b., type I, the dropped beat of the Wenckebach phenomenon; type II, a dropped cardiac cycle that occurs without alteration in the conduction of the preceding intervals.
nerve b., interruption of conduction of impulses in peripheral nerves or nerve trunks by injection of local anesthetic solution.
nondepolarizing b., skeletal mucle paralysis unaccompanied by changes in polarity of the motor endplate, as occurs following administration of tubocurarine.
peri-infarction b., an electrocardiographic abnormality associated with an old myocardial infarct and caused by delayed activation of the myocardium in the region of the infarct; characterized by an initial vector directed away from the infarcted region with the terminal vector directed toward it.
phase I b., inhibition of nerve impulse transmission across the myoneural junction associated with depolarization of the motor endplate, as in the muscle paralysis produced by succinylcholine.
phase II b., inhibition of nerve impulse transmission across the myoneural junction unaccompanied by depolarization of the motor endplate, as in the muscle paralysis produced by tubocurarine.
protective b., entrance b.; protection; an unexplained mechanism whereby a pacemaker is protected from being discharged by the impulse from another center; the mechanism, usually conceived as an encircling zone of unidirectionally refractory tissue permitting egress of impulses from the center but preventing access to the center, is seen in operation in ventricular parasystole where the parasystolic center is protected from discharge by the sinus pacemaker and so is able to maintain its intrinsic rhythm undisturbed.
retrograde b., impaired conduction backward from the ventricles or A-V node into the atria.
sinoatrial (S-A), sinoauricular, sinus b., failure of the impulse to leave the sinus node.
spinal b., obstruction of the flow of cerebrospinal fluid in the spinal subarachnoid space by a tumor, inflammation, scar tissue, etc.; used inaccurately to refer to spinal anesthesia.
stellate b., injection of local anesthetic solution in the vicinity of the stellate ganglion.
suprahisian b., atrioventricular conduction delay occurring above, or cephalad to, the bundle of His.
unidirectional b., b. that prevents passage of an impulse when it approaches from one direction but not from the other, as when b. in the A-V node prevents anterograde conduction to the ventricles while retrograde conduction to the atria remains intact.
Wilson b., the commonest form of right bundle-branch b., characterized in lead I by a tall slender R wave followed by a wider S wave of lower voltage.
Wolff-Chaikoff b., Wolff-Chaikoff effect; blocking of the organic binding of iodine and its incorporation into hormone caused by large doses of iodine; usually a transient effect, but in large doses in susceptible individuals it can be prolonged and cause iodine myxedema.

blockade (blok'ād). **1.** Intravenous injection of large amounts of colloidal dyes or other substances whereby the reaction of the reticuloendothelial cells to other influences (*e.g.*, by phagocytosis) is temporarily prevented. **2.** Arrest of peripheral nerve conduction or transmission at autonomic synaptic junctions, autonomic receptor sites, or myoneural junctions by a drug.
adrenergic b., selective inhibition by a drug of the responses of effector cells to adrenergic sympathetic nerve impulses (sympatholytic) and to epinephrine and related amines (adrenolytic).
cholinergic b., **(1)** inhibition by a drug of nerve impulse transmission at autonomic ganglionic synapses (ganglionic b.), at postganglionic parasympathetic effector cells (*e.g.*, by atropine), and at myoneural junctions (myoneural b.); **(2)** the inhibition of a cholinergic agent.
ganglionic b., inhibition of nerve impulse transmission at autonomic ganglionic synapses by drugs such as nicotine or hexamethonium.
myoneural b., inhibition of nerve impulse transmission at myoneural junctions by a drug such as curare.
narcotic b., the use of drugs to inhibit the effects of narcotic substances.
sympathetic b., interruption of transmission in sympathetic ganglia or conduction of impulses in pre- or postganglionic sympathetic nerve fibers.

virus b., the interference of one virus by another, either attenuated or unrelated.

blocker (blok'er). **1.** An instrument used to obstruct a passage. **2.** See blocking *agent.*

Macintosh b.'s, a system of tubes used during thoracic operations to block one lung, or lobe, from the other.

blocking (blok'ing). **1.** Obstructing; arresting of passage, conduction, or transmission. **2.** In psychoanalysis, a sudden break in free association occurring when a painful subject or repressed complex is touched. **3.** Sudden cessation of thoughts and speech, which may indicate the presence of a severe thought disorder or a psychosis.

alpha b., the desynchronization of the brain waves as seen on an electroencephalogram, produced by opening the eyes or by intense thought or emotion.

block-out (blok'owt). Elimination of undercuts by filling such areas with a medium such as wax or wet pumice.

Blocq, Paul O., French physician, 1860–1896. See B.'s *disease.*

blood (blŭd) [A.S. blōd]. Sanguis; the "circulating tissue" of the body; the fluid and its suspended formed elements that are circulated through the heart, arteries, capillaries, and veins; b. is the means by which 1) oxygen and nutritive materials are transported to the tissues, and 2) carbon dioxide and various metabolic products are removed for excretion. The b. consists of a pale yellow or gray-yellow fluid, plasma, in which are suspended red b. cells (erythrocytes), white b. cells (leukocytes), and platelets. See also arterial b.; venous b.

arterial b., b. that is oxygenated in the lungs, found in the left chambers of the heart and in the arteries, and relatively bright red.

cord b., b. present in the umbilical vessels at the time of delivery.

laky b., b. that is undergoing or has undergone laking. See lake (2); laky.

occult b., b. in the feces in amounts too small to be seen but detectable by chemical tests.

sludged b., b. in which the corpuscles, as a result of some general abnormal state, *e.g.,* burns, traumatic shock, and similar stresses, become massed together in the capillaries, and thereby block the vessels or move slowly through them.

strawberry-cream b., the appearance of the b. in advanced degrees of lipemia.

venous b., b. which has passed through the capillaries of various tissues, except the lungs, and is found in the veins, the right chambers of the heart, and the pulmonary arteries; it is usually dark red as a result of a lower content of oxygen.

whole b., b. drawn from a selected donor under rigid aseptic precautions; contains citrate ion or heparin as an anticoagulant; used as a b. replenisher.

blood bank. A place, usually a separate part or division of a hospital laboratory, in which blood is collected from donors, typed, and often separated into several components for transfusion to recipients.

blood count. Calculation of the number of red (RBC) or white (WBC) blood cells in a cubic millimeter of blood, by means of counting the cells in an accurate volume of diluted blood; also, the determination of the percentages of various types of leukocytes, *i.e.,* a differential count, as observed in a stained film of blood.

complete b. c. (CBC), a combination of the following determinations: red blood cell count, white blood cell count, erythrocyte indices, hematocrit, and differential blood count.

differential white b. c., an estimate of the percentage of white blood cell types which make up the total white blood cell count.

Schilling's b. c., Schilling's index; a method of counting blood in which the polymorphonuclear neutrophils are separated into four groups according to the number and arrangement of the nuclear masses in these cells.

blood dust. Hemoconia.

blood group. A system of genetically determined antigens or agglutinogens located on the surface of the erythrocyte. Each group is determined by a series of closely linked loci. Because of the antigen differences existing between individuals, b.g.'s are significant in blood transfusions, maternal-fetal incompatibilities (erythroblastosis fetalis), tissue and organ transplantation, disputed paternity cases, and in genetic and anthropologic studies; certain b.g.'s have been supposed to be related to susceptibility or resistance to certain diseases. Often used as synonymous with blood type. See Blood Groups appendix for individual groups: ABO, Auberger, Diego, Duffy, I, Kell, Kidd, Lewis, Lutheran, MNSs, P, Rh, Sutter, Xg, and the low frequency and high frequency b.g.'s.

blood grouping. Blood typing; the classification of blood samples by means of appropriate laboratory tests according to their agglutination reactions with respect to one or more blood groups. In general, a suspension of erythrocytes to be tested is exposed to a known specific antiserum; agglutination of the erythrocytes indicates that they possess the antigen for which the antiserum is specific, while absence of agglutination indicates absence of the antigen. Certain antisera require special testing conditions.

bloodless (blŭd'les). Without blood.

bloodletting (blŭd'let-ing). Removing blood, usually from a vein; formerly used as a general remedial measure, but used now in congestive heart failure and polycythemia.

general b., removing blood by arteriotomy or phlebotomy.

local b., removing blood from the smaller vessels, formerly by a cupping glass or by leeching.

blood puzzles. Foreign bodies or deformed blood cells that may be misinterpreted as infectious agents (*e.g.,* bacteria, fungi) in stained films as a result of similarities in morphology and staining properties.

bloodshot (blŭd'shot). Denoting locally congested smaller blood vessels of a part (*e.g.,* the conjunctiva) which are dilated and visible.

bloodstream (blŭd'strēm). The flowing blood as it is encountered in the circulatory system as distinguished from blood which has been removed from the circulatory system or sequestered in a part; thus, something added to the b. may be expected to become distributed to all parts of the body through which blood is flowing.

blood type. The specific reaction pattern of erythrocytes of an individual to the antisera of one blood group; *e.g.,* the ABO blood group consists of four major b.t.'s: O, A, B, and AB, depending on agglutination of erythrocytes by neither, one, the other, or both anti-A and anti-B testing sera. The b.t. is the genetic phenotype of the individual for one blood group system and may vary in detail with the number of different antisera available for testing. See also Blood Groups appendix.

blood typing. Blood grouping.

blood vessel. A tube (artery, capillary, vein, or sinus) conveying blood.

bloodworm (blŭd'werm). **1.** The filarial parasite of sheep, *Elaeophora schneideri.* **2.** Red aquatic larvae of certain dipterous gnats and midges. **3.** Marine annelids in the family Terebellidae with soft bodies and red blood. **4.** Blood-inhabiting worms, such as the blood flukes of man in the genus *Schistosoma.*

Bloom, David, U.S. dermatologist, *1892. See B.'s *syndrome.*

blot. See Northern, Southern, and Western blot *analysis.*

blotch. Commonly used term to denote a pigmented or erythematous lesion.

Blount, Walter P., U.S. orthopedist, *1900. See B.'s *disease,* B.-Barber *disease.*

blowfly (blō'flī). See *Calliphora, Lucilia, Phormia.*

blue (blū). A color between green and violet on the spectrum. For individual blue dyes, see the specific name.

blue'bag. Ovine *mastitis.*

bluetongue (blū'tŭng). Soremuzzle; an infectious disease of sheep, possibly of cattle, caused by bluetongue virus and transmitted by bloodsucking midges of the genus *Culicoides;* manifested by catarrhal inflammation of the mucosae of the mouth, nose, and intestinal tract, accompanied frequently by foot involvement and lameness; infection or vaccination with attenuated virus during early pregnancy causes brain and heart anomalies in lambs.

Blum, Paul, French physician, 1878–1933. See Gougerot and B. *disease.*

Blumberg, Jacob M., German surgeon and gynecologist, 1873–1955. See B.'s *sign.*

Blumenau, Leonid W., Russian neurologist, 1862–1932. See B.'s *nucleus.*

Blumenbach, Johann F., German physiologist, 1752–1840. See B.'s *clivus.*

Blumer, George, U.S. physician, 1858–1940. See B.'s *shelf.*

blush (blŭsh). **1.** A sudden and brief redness of the face and neck due to emotion. **2.** In angiography used metaphorically to describe neovascularity or, in some cases, extravasation.

BLV Abbreviation for bovine leukemia *virus.*

B-mode. A two-dimensional diagnostic ultrasound presentation of echo-producing interfaces in a single plane; the intensity of the echo is represented by modulation of the brightness (B) of the spot, and the position of the echo is determined from the position of the transducer and the transit time of the acoustical pulse.

BMR Abbreviation for basal metabolic *rate.*

BNA Abbreviation for *Basle Nomina Anatomica.*

bob'bing. An up-and-down movement.
inverse ocular b., slow downward eye movement followed by delayed quick upward return.
ocular b., sudden conjugate downward deviation of the eyes with a slow return to the normal position.

BOC, *t*-BOC Abbreviations formerly used for *t*-butoxycarbonyl; current usage is Boc.

Boc Abbreviation for *t*- butoxycarbonyl.

Bochdalek, Vincent A., Prague anatomist, 1801–1883. See B.'s *foramen, ganglion, gap, hernia, muscle, valve;* flower basket of B.

Bock, August C., German anatomist, 1782–1833. See B.'s *ganglion, nerve.*

Bockhart, Max, German physician, 1883–1921. See B.'s *impetigo.*

Bodansky, Aaron, U.S. biochemist, 1887–1961. See B. *unit.*

Bödecker, Charles F., U.S. oral histologist, embryologist, and pathologist, *1880. See B. *index.*

Bodian, David, U.S. anatomist, *1910. See B.'s copper Protargol *stain.*

Bodo (bō'dō). A genus of free-living, ovoid or slightly pyriform protozoa with two flagella, one projecting anteriorly and the other posteriorly; may be ingested as encysted forms in food or drink, or possibly deposited in feces or urine after excretion; in either instance, cysts frequently develop into trophozoites if the specimen is permitted to remain at room temperature for a few hours prior to examination; the organisms are not pathogenic in man.
B. cauda'tus, a species that is found in specimens of human feces (especially in tropical regions); the organisms are frequently termed coprozoic flagellates.
B. sal'tans, a species of the intestinal tract sometimes observed in ulcers.
B. urina'rius, a species found occasionally in the urine.

BODY

body (bod'ē) [A.S. *bodig*]. **1.** The head, neck, trunk, and extremities. **2.** The material part of man, as distinguished from the mind and spirit. **3.** The principal mass of any structure. **4.** A thing; a substance. See also corpus, soma.
acetone b., ketone b.
adrenal b., *glandula* suprarenalis.
alcoholic hyaline b.'s, Mallory b.'s.
Alder b.'s, granular inclusions in polymorphonuclear leukocytes; they take on a dark color with Giemsa-Wright stain and react metachromatically with toluidine blue. See also Alder's *anomaly.*
alveolar b., *processus* alveolaris.
amylogenic b., amyloplast.
amyloid b.'s of the prostate, small masses of colloid material often present in the tubules of the gland. See also *corpus* amylaceum.
anococcygeal b., *ligamentum* anococcygeum.
aortic b., *glomus* aorticum.
Arnold's b.'s, small portions or minute fragments of erythrocytes (sometimes mistaken for blood platelets), or small "ghosts" of erythrocytes.
asbestos b.'s, ferruginous b.'s with asbestos fibers as a core; a histiologic hallmark of exposure to asbestos.
Aschoff b.'s, Aschoff nodules; a form of granulomatous inflammation characteristically observed in acute rheumatic carditis; fully developed Aschoff b.'s consist of fibrinoid change in connective tissue, lymphocytes, occasional plasma cells, and abnormal characteristic histiocytes.
asteroid b., (1) an eosinophilic inclusion resembling a star with delicate radiating lines, occurring in a vacuolated area of cytoplasm of a multinucleated giant cell; especially frequent in sarcoidosis, but occurs also in other granulomas; (2) a structure that is characteristic of sporotrichosis when found in the skin or secondary lesions of this mycosis; in tissue, it surrounds the 3- to 5-μm in diameter ovoid yeast of *Sporothrix schenkii.*
Auer b.'s, Auer rods; rod-shaped structures of uncertain nature in the cytoplasm of immature myeloid cells, especially myeloblasts, in acute myelocytic leukemia; may be an abnormal form of lysosomes; they contain peroxidase and acid phosphatase, and stain red by azure-eosin stains.
Babès-Ernst b.'s, intracellular granules, present in many species of bacteria, which possess a strong affinity for nuclear stains. Also called volutin or metachromatic granules.
Barr chromatin b., sex *chromatin.*
basal b., basal corpuscle or granule; blepharoplast; kinetosome; an elongated centriolar structure situated at the base of each cilium at the apical margin of a cell; it has nine peripheral triplomicrotubules continuous with the peripheral diplomicrotubules of each cilium or flagellum.
bigeminal b.'s, *corpora* bigemina.
Bollinger b.'s, relatively large, spheroid or ovoid, usually somewhat granular, acidophilic, intracytoplasmic inclusion b.'s observed in the infected tissues of birds with fowlpox; when b.'s are ruptured large numbers of fowlpox virus particles are released.
Borrel b.'s, particles of fowlpox virus; aggregates of Borrel b.'s in infected cells result in the formation of Bollinger b.'s.
brassy b., a dark-colored, usually shrunken erythrocyte in which there is a malarial parasite.
Cabot's ring b.'s, ring-shaped or figure-of-eight structures that stain red with Wright's stain, found in red blood cells in severe anemias, possibly a remnant of the nuclear membrane; a form of basophilic degenerative process.

Call-Exner b.'s, small fluid-filled spaces between granulosal cells in ovarian follicles and in ovarian tumors of granulosal origin; they may form a rosette-like structure.
cancer b.'s, Plimmer's b.'s; discrete, acidophilic or amphophilic, hyaline b.'s of various shapes and sizes, occurring in the cytoplasm of some of the neoplastic cells and also extracellularly in the stroma of various carcinomas and sarcomas; formerly regarded by some observers as parasitic causal agents, but now thought to be products of cell necrosis (apoptosis).
carotid b., *glomus* caroticum.
cavernous b. of clitoris, *corpus* cavernosum clitoridis.
cavernous b. of penis, *corpus* cavernosum penis.
cell b., the part of the cell containing the nucleus.
central b., cytocentrum.
chromaffin b., paraganglion.
chromatin b., the genetic apparatus of bacteria. See nucleus (2).
ciliary b., *corpus* ciliare.
Civatte b.'s, colloid b.'s; eosinophilic hyaline b.'s seen in or just beneath the epidermis, particularly in lichen planus, and formed by necrosis of individual basal cells.
b. of clavicle, *corpus* claviculae.
b. of clitoris, *corpus* clitoridis.
coccygeal b., *corpus* coccygeum.
colloid b.'s, Civatte b.'s.
compressible cavernous b.'s, submucous venous plexuses found at the level of the pharyngoesophageal junction and anal canal, which assist in reducing or obliterating the lumen.
conchoidal b.'s, Schaumann b.'s.
Councilman (hyaline) b., Councilman's lesion; an eosinophilic globule, seen in the liver in yellow fever, derived from necrosis of a single hepatic cell.
Cowdry's type A inclusion b.'s, droplet-like masses of acidophilic material surrounded by clear halos within nuclei, with margination of chromatin on the nuclear membrane.
Cowdry's type B inclusion b.'s, droplet-like masses of acidophilic material surrounded by clear halos within nuclei, without other nuclear changes during early stages of development of the inclusion.
creola b.'s, large compact clusters of ciliated columnar cells found in the sputum of some asthmatic patients.
cytoid b.'s, swollen retinal nerve fibers which look like cells when cut transversely; found in cotton-wool patches.
cytoplasmic inclusion b.'s, see inclusion b.'s.
Deetjen's b.'s, platelet.
demilune b., a circular b. of extreme transparency except for a crescentic punctate substance on one edge which contains hemoglobin. The b. is much larger than a red blood cell, but is thought possibly to be a degenerated red blood cell swollen by imbibition; it has been found in malaria and in convalescence from typhoid fever; the transparent portion is called the glass b.
Döhle b.'s, Döhle or leukocyte inclusions; discrete round or oval b.'s ranging in diameter from just visible to 2 μm, which stain sky blue to gray blue with Romanowsky stains, found in neutrophils of patients with infections, burns, trauma, pregnancy, or cancer.
Donovan b., *Calymmatobacterium inguinale.*
Ehrlich's inner b., Heinz-Ehrlich b., a round oxyphil b. found in the red blood cell in case of hemocytolysis due to a specific blood poison.
elementary b.'s, **(1) (E.B.)** old term for virions, especially the largest virus particles, visible by light microscopy when stained; **(2)** platelets.
b. of epididymis, *corpus* epididymidis.
epithelial b., *glandula* parathyroidea.
fat b. of cheek, *corpus* adiposum buccae.
fat b. of ischiorectal fossa, *corpus* adiposum fossae ischiorectalis.
fat b. of orbit, *corpus* adiposum orbitae.
ferruginous b.'s, in the lungs, foreign inorganic or organic fibers coated by complexes of hemosiderin and glycoproteins, and believed to be formed by macrophages that have phagocytized the fibers. See also asbestos b.'s.
foreign b., anything in the tissues or cavities of the b. that has been introduced there from without, and that is not rapidly absorbable.
b. of fornix, *corpus* fornicis.
fuchsin b.'s, **(1)** Russell b.'s; **(2)** hyaline b.'s.
b. of gallbladder, *corpus* vesicae felleae.
Gamna-Favre b.'s, characteristic, relatively large, intracytoplasmic basophilic inclusion b.'s observed in endothelial cells in lymphogranuloma venereum; probably composed of degenerated nuclear material. See also Miyagawa b.'s.
Gamna-Gandy b.'s, Gandy-Gamna b.'s, Gamna-Gandy or siderotic nodules; small firm spheroidal or irregular foci that are yellow-brown, brown, or rustlike in color, occurring chiefly in the spleen in such conditions as congestive splenomegaly and sickle cell disease, and consisting of relatively dense fibrous tissue or collagenous fibers impregnated with iron pigment and calcium salts; probably result from organization and scarring of sites where small perivascular hemorrhages occurred.
geniculate b., see *corpus* geniculatum laterale, *corpus* geniculatum mediale.
glass b., see demilune b.
glomus b., glomus (2).
Guarnieri b.'s, intracytoplasmic acidophilic inclusion b.'s observed in epithelial cells in variola (smallpox) and vaccinia infections, and which include aggregations of Paschen b.'s or virus particles.
Halberstaedter-Prowazek b.'s, trachoma b.'s.
Hassall's b.'s, thymic *corpuscles.*
Hassall-Henle b.'s, Henle's warts; hyaline b.'s on the posterior surface of Descemet's membrane at the periphery of the cornea.
Heinz b.'s, beta substance; substantia metachromaticogranularis; minute b.'s sometimes seen in erythrocytes by the dark ground illumination method, after staining with azur I; regarded by Heinz as particles of dead cytoplasm, by others as composed of cholesterinolein.
Heinz-Ehrlich b., Ehrlich's inner b.
hematoxylin b.'s, hematoxyphil b.'s, poorly defined, homogeneous basophilic remnants of whole nuclei, an occasional finding in the fixed tissues of patients with systemic lupus erythematosus, but observed more frequently in the renal glomeruli and the walls of blood vessels, and probably are related to the L.E. phenomenon; so named because of their affinity for hematoxylin stain.
Herring b.'s, hyaline b.'s of pituitary.
Highmore's b., *mediastinum* testis.
Howell-Jolly b.'s, Jolly b.'s; spherical or ovoid eccentrically located granules, approximately 1 μm in diameter, occasionally observed in the stroma of circulating erythrocytes, especially in stained preparations (as compared with wet unstained films); probably represent nuclear remnants, inasmuch as they can be stained with dyes that are rather specific for chromatin; the significance of the b.'s is not exactly known, but they occur more frequently and in greater numbers after splenectomy.
hyaline b.'s, fuchsin b.'s (2); homogeneous eosinophilic inclusions in the cytoplasm of epithelial cells; in renal tubules, hyaline b.'s represent droplets of protein reabsorbed from the lumen. See also Mallory b.'s.; drusen.
hyaline b.'s of pituitary, Herring b.'s; accumulations of a gelatinous neurosecretory substance in the axons of the hypothalamohypophyseal tract in the posterior lobe of the hypophysis.
hyaloid b., *corpus* vitreum.
b. of hyoid bone, *corpus* ossis hyoidei.
b. of ilium, *corpus* ossis ilii.
immune b., an early term for antibody.
inclusion b.'s, distinctive structures frequently formed in the nu-

cleus or cytoplasm (occasionally in both locations) in cells infected with certain filtrable viruses, observed especially in nerve, epithelial, or endothelial cells; may be demonstrated by means of various stains, especially Mann's eosin methylene blue or Giemsa's techniques. **Nuclear i. b.'s** are usually acidophilic and are of two morphologic types: 1) granular, hyaline, or amorphous b.'s of various sizes, *i.e.,* Cowdry's type A i. b.'s, occurring in such diseases as herpes simplex infection or yellow fever; 2) more circumscribed b.'s, frequently with several in the same nucleus (and no reaction in adjacent tissue), *i.e.,* the type B b.'s, occurring in such diseases as Rift Valley fever and poliomyelitis. **Cytoplasmic i. b.'s** may be: 1) acidophilic, relatively large, spherical or ovoid, and somewhat granular, as in variola or vaccinia, rabies, and molluscum contagiosum; 2) basophilic, relatively large, complex combinations of viral and cellular material, as in trachoma, psittacosis, and lymphopathia venereum. In some instances, inclusion b.'s are known to be infective and probably represent aggregates of virus particles in combination with cellular material, whereas others are apparently not infective and may represent only abnormal products formed by the cell in response to the virus. Inclusion b.'s that resemble some of those known to be related to viral infections are occasionally observed in degenerative diseases and in lead poisoning.

b. of incus, *corpus* incudis.

infrapatellar fat b., *corpus* adiposum infrapatellare.

intercarotid b., *glomus* caroticum.

intermediate b. of Flemming, midbody.

interrenal b.'s, interrenal glands; distinct paired or unpaired structures in all fishes, which lie in close proximity to the kidney, homologous to the cortical tissue of the mammalian adrenal gland.

b. of ischium, *corpus* ossis ischii.

Jaworski's b.'s, mucous shreds in the gastric contents in hyperchlorhydria.

Joest b.'s, intranuclear inclusion b.'s (Cowdry's type B) produced in certain nerve cells by Borna disease virus.

Jolly b.'s, Howell-Jolly b.'s.

juxtaglomerular b., periarterial pad; a collection of cells around the renal glomerular arterioles which contain cytoplasmic granules, probably composed of renin.

juxtarestiform b., a medial subdivision of the inferior cerebellar peduncle (corpus restiforme) composed of fibers reciprocally connecting the vestibular nuclei with the cerebellum, in particular the latter's nodulus, flocculus, and uvula vermis. It also carries primary sensory fibers from the vestibular ganglia to the cerebellum, as well as cerebellar projections to the rhombencephalic reticular formation.

ketone b., acetone b.; one of a group of ketones that includes acetoacetic acid, its reduction product, β-hydrobutyric acid, and its decarboxylation product, acetone; high levels are found in tissues and body fluids in ketosis.

Koch's blue b.'s, schizonts of *Theileria parva,* the causative agent of East Coast fever; found principally within endothelial cells of the spleen and lymph nodes.

Kurloff's b.'s, palely basophilic, granular inclusions sometimes observed in the cytoplasm of the large mononuclear leukocytes (probably lymphocytes) of guinea pigs and certain other animals; thought by some observers to be an intracellular phase in the life cycle of the protozoan parasite *Leucocytozoon cobayae,* whereas others regard the b.'s as a stage in the development of leukocytic granules.

Lafora b., an intraneural inclusion b. composed of acid mucopolysaccharides, seen in familial myoclonus epilepsy.

Lallemand's b.'s, Trousseau-Lallemand b.'s; **(1)** old term for small gelatinoid concretions sometimes observed in seminal fluid; **(2)** old term for Bence Jones *cylinders.*

Landolt's b.'s, bipolar nerve cells lying between the retinal rods and cones in amphibia, reptiles, and birds.

lateral geniculate b., *corpus* geniculatum laterale.

L-D b., Leishman-Donovan b.

L.E. b., the amorphous round b. in the cytoplasm of an L.E. cell.

Leishman-Donovan b., amastigote; L-D b.; the intracytoplasmic, nonflagellated leishmanial form of certain intracellular parasites, such as species of *Leishmania* or the intracellular form of *Trypanosoma cruzi;* originally used for *Leishmania donovani* parasites in infected spleen or liver cells in kala azar.

Lewy b.'s, intracytoplasmic inclusion b.'s especially noted in pigmented brainstem neurons and seen in Parkinson's disease.

Lieutaud's b., *trigonum* vesicae.

Lindner's b.'s, initial b.'s resembling inclusion b.'s found in epithelial cells in scrapings in trachoma.

loose b., a solid tissue fragment lying free in a body cavity, especially in a joint or the peritoneal cavity; *e.g.,* joint mice, melon-seed b., rice b.

Luse b.'s, collagen fibers with abnormally long spacing (exceeding 1000 Å) between electron-dense bands.

Luys' b., *nucleus* subthalamicus.

Mallory b.'s, alcoholic hyalin; alcoholic hyaline b.'s; large, poorly defined accumulations of eosinophilic material in the cytoplasm of damaged hepatic cells in certain forms of cirrhosis and marked fatty change especially due to alcoholism.

malpighian b.'s, *folliculi* lymphatici lienales.

mamillary b., *corpus* mamillare.

b. of mammary gland, *corpus* mammae.

b. of mandible, *corpus* mandibulae.

b. of maxilla, *corpus* maxillae.

medial geniculate b., *corpus* geniculatum mediale.

melon-seed b., a small fibrous loose b. in the joints or tendon sheaths.

metachromatic b.'s, concentrated deposits consisting primarily of polymetaphosphate and occurring in many bacteria as well as in algae, fungi, and protozoa; m. b.'s differ in staining properties from the surrounding protoplasm. See metachromasia.

Michaelis-Gutmann b., a rounded homogenous or concentrically laminated b., 1 to 10 μ in diameter, containing calcium and iron; found within macrophages in the bladder wall in malakoplakia.

Miyagawa b.'s, a term used to refer to *Chlamydia trachomatis* (*Miyagawanella lymphogranulomatosis*), the elementary b.'s that develop in the intracytoplasmic microcolonies of lymphogranuloma venereum.

molluscum b., molluscum corpuscle; the central gelatinous mass contained in the lesions of molluscum contagiosum; it consists of degenerated cells and the inclusion b.'s (virus).

Mooser b.'s, a term used to refer to the rickettsiae found in the exudate (and in tissue) from the tunica vaginalis in endemic typhus fever (caused by *Rickettsia typhi*).

multilamellar b., cytosome (2).

multivesicular b.'s, membrane-bound b.'s, 0.5 to 1.0 μm wide, that occur in the cytoplasm of cells and contain a number of small vesicles; hydrolases (especially acid phosphatase) occur in the matrix.

myelin b., myelin *figure.*

b. of nail, *corpus* unguis.

Negri b.'s, Negri corpuscles; eosinophilic, sharply outlined, pathognomonic inclusion b.'s (2 to 10 μm in diameter) found in the cytoplasm of certain nerve cells containing the virus of rabies, especially in Ammon's horn of the hippocampus.

nerve cell b., the part of the neuron that includes the nucleus but excludes the processes.

neuroepithelial b., a corpuscular aggregate of nonciliated cells containing neurosecretory substance found in normal bronchial epithelium.

Nissl b.'s, Nissl *substance.*

nodular b., in fungi, a compact, roughly spherical or squarish structure formed by coiling and twisting of the end of a hypha; considered to be abortive growths toward sexual reproduction.

nuclear inclusion b.'s, see inclusion b.'s.
Odland b., keratinosome.
olivary b., oliva.
onion b.'s, obsolete term for epithelial *nests.*
pacchionian b.'s, *granulationes* arachnoideales.
pampiniform b., epoophoron.
b. of pancreas, *corpus* pancreatis.
Pappenheimer b.'s, phagosomes, containing ferruginous granules, found in red blood cells in diseases such as sideroblastic anemia, hemolytic anemia, and sickle cell disease; may contribute to spurious platelet counts by electro-optical counters.
para-aortic b.'s, *corpora* para-aortica.
parabasal b., a term formerly equivalent to the DNA kinetoplast, part of the giant mitochondrion of certain parasitic flagellates (see also kinetoplast). The parabasal b. plus the basal b. were previously thought to comprise a kinetoplast, or locomotory apparatus, but kinetoplast is now restricted to part of the DNA giant mitochondrion and parabasal b. is a distinct structure near the nucleus, probably equivalent to the metazoan Golgi apparatus.
paranephric b., a mass of fat lying behind the renal fascia.
paranuclear b., astrosphere.
paraterminal b., *gyrus* subcallosus.
Paschen b.'s, particles of virus observed in relatively large numbers in squamous cells of the skin (or the cornea of experimental animals) in variola (smallpox) or vaccinia.
b. of penis, *corpus* penis.
perineal b., *centrum* tendineum perinei.
b. of phalanx, *corpus* phalangis.
Pick's b.'s, intracytoplasmic argentophilic inclusion b.'s seen in neurons in Pick's disease.
pineal b., *corpus* pineale.
Plimmer's b.'s, cancer b.'s.
polar b., polar cell or globule; polocyte; one of two small cells formed by the ovum during its maturation; the first is usually released just prior to ovulation, the second not until discharge of the ovum from the ovary; in mammals, the second polar b. may fail to form unless the ovum has been penetrated by a sperm cell.
Prowazek b.'s, historic term for either of two types of inclusion b.'s associated with diseases caused by filtrable viruses: 1) trachoma b.'s; 2) tiny, ovoid, granular forms, frequently in pairs, observed in the cytoplasm and in Guarnieri b.'s in the cutaneous squamous cells of man and animals infected with variola (smallpox) or vaccinia virus; probably the same as Paschen b.'s.
Prowazek-Greeff b.'s, trachoma b.'s.
psammoma b.'s, **(1)** sand b.'s; mineralized b.'s occurring in the meninges, choroid plexus, and in certain meningiomas, composed usually of a central capillary surrounded by concentric whorls of meningocytes in various stages of hyaline change and mineralization; **(2)** *corpora* arenacea; **(3)** calcospherite.
psittacosis inclusion b.'s, intracytoplasmic chlamydial microcolonies observed in bronchial epithelial cells infected with *Chlamydia psittaci.*
pubic b., b. of pubic bone, *corpus* ossis pubis.
purine b.'s, any purine.
quadrigeminal b.'s, *corpora* quadrigemina.
residual b., a cytoplasmic vacuole (lysosome) containing accumulated particulate products of metabolism, *e.g.,* lipofuscin.
residual b. of Regaud, the excess cytoplasm that separates from the spermatozoon during spermiogenesis.
rest b., a small mass of cytoplasm remaining after the nucleus and cytoplasm of the schizont of certain sporozoan protozoa have divided into asexual spores or merozoites.
restiform b., *pedunculus* cerebellaris inferior.
b. of rib, *corpus* costae.
rice b., one of the small loose b.'s found in hygromas, tendon sheaths, and joints.
Russell b.'s, fuchsin b.'s; small, discrete, variably sized, spherical, intracytoplasmic, acidophilic, hyaline b.'s that stain deeply with fuchsin; they occur frequently in plasma cells in chronic inflammation, where they are believed to consist of γ-globulin.
sand b.'s, psammoma b.'s (1).
Sandström's b.'s, see *glandula* parathyroidea.
Savage's perineal b., *centrum* tendineum perinei.
Schaumann b.'s, conchoidal b.'s; concentrically laminated calcified b.'s found in granulomas, particularly in sarcoidosis.
sclerotic b.'s, copper pennies; vegetative rounded muriform cells of dematiaceous fungi, characteristic of the causal agents of chromomycosis in tissue.
segmenting b., schizont.
b. of sphenoid bone, *corpus* ossis sphenoidalis.
spongy b. of penis, *corpus* spongiosum penis.
b. of sternum, *corpus* sterni.
b. of stomach, *corpus* ventriculi.
striate b., *corpus* striatum.
suprarenal b., *glandula* suprarenalis.
b. of sweat gland, *corpus* glandulae sudoriferae.
Symington's anococcygeal b., *ligamentum* anococcygeum.
b. of talus, *corpus* tali.
b. of thigh bone, *corpus* ossis femoris.
threshold b., threshold *substance.*
thyroid b., *glandula* thyroidea.
b. of tibia, *corpus* tibiae.
tigroid b.'s, Nissl *substance.*
b. of tongue, *corpus* linguae.
trachoma b.'s., Prowazek-Greeff b.'s; Halberstaedter-Prowazek b.'s; Prowazek b.'s (1); distinctive, complex, intracytoplasmic forms found in the conjunctival epithelial cells of persons in the acute phase of trachoma, less frequently in later stages, varying from 1) discrete acidophilic granules (approximately 250 nm in diameter), to 2) irregular clumps of such material embedded in a basophilic matrix, to 3) relatively large basophilic b.'s (approximately 700 to 1000 nm in diameter), to 4) large basophilic b.'s that include discrete, tiny, acidophilic granules.
trapezoid b., *corpus* trapezoideum.
Trousseau-Lallemand b.'s, Lallemand's b.'s.
tuffstone b., membrane-bound electron-dense granules, measuring about 0.5 μm in diameter, found primarily in Schwann cells of patients suffering from metachromatic leukodystrophy; the name alludes to their resemblance to volcanic limestone.
turbinated b., **(1)** turbinal; a concha with its covering of mucous membrane and other soft parts; **(2)** *concha* nasalis inferior, media, superior, and suprema.
tympanic b., tympanic *gland.*
b. of ulna, *corpus* ulnae.
ultimobranchial b., a diverticulum from the fourth pharyngeal pouch of an embryo, regarded by some as a rudimentary fifth pharyngeal pouch and by others as a lateral thyroid primordium; the ultimobranchial b.'s of lower vertebrates contain large amounts of calcitonin; in mammals, the b.'s fuse with the thyroid gland and are thought to develop into the parafollicular cells.
b. of urinary bladder, *corpus* vesicae urinariae.
b. of uterus, *corpus* uteri.
vaccine b.'s, old term pertaining to intracellular b.'s that were erroneously thought to be forms in the life cycle of a protozoan organism, *Cytorrhyctes vaccinae,* postulated to be the causal agent of vaccinia.
Verocay b.'s, "clear" spaces outlined by opposing rows of parallel nuclei seen microscopically in neurilemomas.
b. of vertebra, *corpus* vertebrae.
Virchow-Hassall b.'s, thymic *corpuscles.*
vitreous b., *corpus* vitreum.
Weibel-Palade b.'s, rod-shaped bundles of microtubules seen by electron microscopy in vascular endothelial cells.
wolffian b., mesonephros.

Wolf-Orton b.'s, intranuclear inclusion b.'s seen in cells of malignant neoplasms, especially those of glial cell origin.
X b., Langerhans' *granule.*
Y b., a single fluorescent spot originating in the long arm of the Y chromosome and visible in somatic nuclei of buccal smears.
yellow b., *corpus* luteum.
zebra b., metachromaticly staining membrane-bound granules, measuring 0.5-1 μm in diameter and containing lamellae with a 5.8 nm spacing, reported in Schwann cells and macrophages of patients suffering from metachromatic leukodystrophy.
Zuckerkandl's b.'s, *corpora* paraaortica.

---

body burden. Activity of a radiopharmaceutical retained by the body at a specified time following administration.

Boeck, Caesar P.M., Norwegian dermatologist, 1845–1917. See B.'s *disease, sarcoid,* Besnier-B.-Schaumann *disease, syndrome.*

Boeck, Carl W., Norwegian physician, 1808–1875. See Danielssen-B. *disease.*

Boehmer, F. See B.'s *hematoxylin.*

Boerhaave, Hermann, Dutch physician, 1668–1738. See B.'s *glands, syndrome.*

Bogaert, Ludo van. See van Bogaert, Ludo.

bogbean (bog'bēn). Buckbean.

Bogros, Annet J., French anatomist, 1786–1823. See B.'s *space.*

Bogros, Antoine, 19th century French anatomist. See B.'s serous *membrane.*

Bohn, Heinrich, German physician, 1832–1888. See B.'s nodules.

Bohn's nodules. See Epstein's *pearls.*

Bohr, Christian, Danish physiologist, 1855–1911. See B. *effect;* B.'s *equation.*

Bohr, Niels H.D., Danish physicist, 1885–1962. See B.'s *atom, magneton, theory.*

boil (boyl) [A.S. *byl,* a swelling]. Furuncle.
Aleppo b., Bagdad b., the lesion occurring in cutaneous leishmaniasis.
blind b., a furuncle that does not have a fluctuant central point; it appears as a dull red painful papule.
date b., Delhi b., Jericho b., the lesion occurring in cutaneous leishmaniasis.
Madura b., mycetoma (1).
Oriental b., the lesion occurring in cutaneous leishmaniasis.
salt water b.'s, furuncles on hands and forearms of fishermen.
shoe b., capped elbow; olecranoid bursitis in the horse; so called because it may be caused by trauma from the shoe in the recumbent animal.
tropical b., the lesion occurring in cutaneous leishmaniasis.

boldenone (bōl'dĕ-nōn). Dehydrotestosterone; 17β-hydroxyandrosta-1,4-dien-3-one; an anabolic and androgenic agent used in veterinary medicine.

boldin (bol'din). Boldoglucin; a glycoside from boldus; a cholagogue and diuretic.

boldine (bol'dēn). A bitter alkaloid obtained from boldus.

boldo (bol'dō). Boldus.

boldoglucin (bol-dō-glū'sin). Boldin.

boldus (bol'dŭs) [Chilean]. Boldo; the leaves of *Boldu boldus* or *Peumus boldus* (family Monimiaceae), an evergreen shrub of Chile; used in various disturbances of liver function.

boletic acid (bol-et'ik). Fumaric acid.

Boley gauge. See under gauge.

Boll, Franz C., German histologist and physiologist, 1849–1879. See B.'s *cells.*

Bollinger, Otto, German pathologist, 1843–1909. See B. *bodies, granules.*

Bollman, Jesse L., U.S. physiologist, *1896. See Mann-B. *fistula.*

Bolognini's symptom. See under symptom.

bolometer (bō-lom'ĕ-ter) [G. *bolē,* a throw, a sunbeam, + *metron,* measure]. **1.** An instrument for determining minute degrees of radiant heat. **2.** An obsolete instrument for measuring the force of the heartbeat as distinguished from the blood pressure.

Bolton, Joseph S., British neurologist, 1867–1946. See B., B.-Broadbent, B.-nasion *plane;* B. *point;* B.-nasion *line.*

bolus (bō'lŭs) [L. fr. G. *bōlos,* lump, clod]. **1.** A single, relatively large quantity of a substance, usually one intended for therapeutic use, such as a b. dose of a drug. **2.** A masticated morsel of food or another substance ready to be swallowed, such as a b. of barium for x-ray studies.
intravenous b., a relatively large volume of fluid or dose of a drug or test substance given intravenously and rapidly to hasten or magnify a response.

bombard'. To expose a substance to particulate or electromagnetic radiations for the purpose of making it radioactive.

bombesin (bom'bĕ-sin). A peptide found in vagal nerve endings in the gastrointestinal mucosa and believed to be a neurotransmitter stimulating gastrin secretion.

bond. In chemistry, the force holding two neighboring atoms in place and resisting their separation; a b. is electrovalent if it consists of the attraction between oppositely charged groups, or covalent if it results from the sharing of one, two, or three pairs of electrons by the bonded atoms.
acylmercaptan b., —CO—S—; a "high energy" b. formed by the condensation of a carboxyl group (—COOH) and a mercaptan (or thiol) group (—SH); widely formed in the course of intermediary metabolism, notably in the oxidation of fats, where the —SH is part of coenzyme A and the —COOH is part of the fatty acid being oxidized.
conjugated double b.'s, two double b.'s separated by one single b.
coordinate b., semipolar b.
disulfide b., the —S—S— link binding two peptide chains (or different parts of one peptide chain); occurs as part of the molecule of the amino acid, cystine, and is important as a structural determinant in many protein molecules, notably keratin, insulin, and oxytocin.
double b., a covalent b. resulting from the sharing of two pairs of electrons; *e.g.,* $CH_2{=}CH_2$ (ethylene).
high energy phosphate b., see high energy *phosphates.*
hydrogen b., a b. arising from the sharing of a hydrogen atom, covalently bound to N or O, with another N or O. In substances of biological importance, the most common hydrogen b.'s are those in which H links N to O or N; such b.'s link purines on one strand to pyrimidines in the other strand of nucleic acids, thus maintaining double-stranded structures as in the Watson-Crick helix.

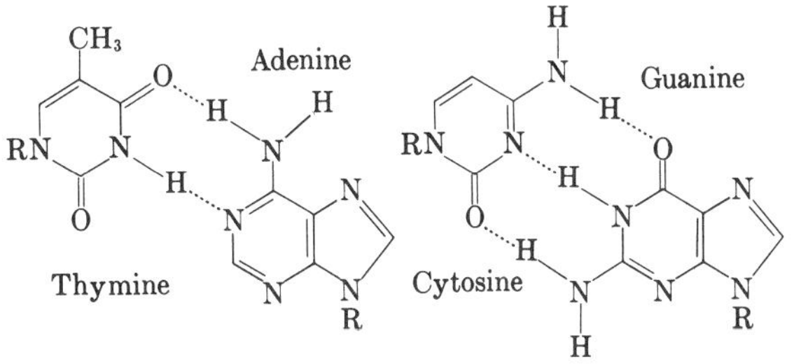

Hydrogen bonding between purines and pyrimidines

In these structures, hydrogen bonds are indicated by dotted lines; *R* = deoxyribose in chains.

peptide b., the common link (—CO—NH—) between amino acids in proteins, actually a form of amide linkage, formed by elimination of H_2O between the —CO—OH of one amno acid and the H_2N— of another.

semipolar b., coordinate b.; a b. in which the two electrons shared by a pair of atoms belonged originally to only one of the atoms; often represented by a small arrow pointing toward the electron receiver; *e.g.,* nitric acid, O(OH)N→O; phosphoric acid, $(OH)_3P \rightarrow O$.

single b., a covalent b. resulting from the sharing of one pair of electrons; *e.g.,* $CH_3—CH_3$ (ethane).

triple b., a covalent b. resulting from the sharing of three pairs of electrons; *e.g.,* CH≡CH (acetylene).

BONE

bone (bōn) [A.S. *bān*]. **1.** A hard connective tissue consisting of cells embedded in a matrix of mineralized ground substance and collagen fibers. The fibers are impregnated with a form of calcium phosphate similar to hydroxyapatite as well as with substantial quantities of carbonate, citrate sodium, and magnesium; by weight, b. is composed of 75% inorganic material and 25% organic material. **2.** For definitions of bones as part of the animal skeleton, see os.

Albrecht's b., a small b. between the basioccipital and basisphenoid.

alveolar b., **(1)** *processus* alveolaris; **(2)** alveolar supporting bone; in dentistry, the specialized bony structure which supports the teeth; it consists of the cortical b. that comprises the tooth socket into which the roots of the tooth fit, and is supported by the trabecular b.

alveolar supporting b., alveolar b. (2).

ankle b., talus.

basal b., the osseus tissue of the mandible and maxillae except the alveolar processes.

basilar b., os basilare; basioccipital b.; the basilar process of the occipital b. which unites with the condylar portions in about the fourth or fifth year.

basioccipital b., basilar b.

basisphenoid b., in comparative anatomy, the b. in the floor of the braincase in the region of the pituitary.

Bertin's b.'s, *conchae* sphenoidales.

blade b., scapula.

breast b., sternum.

Breschet's b.'s, *os* suprasternale.

brittle b.'s, *osteogenesis* imperfecta.

bundle b., immature b. containing thick bundles of collagen fibers arranged nearly parallel to one another with osteocytes in between; a similar type of b. is found in regions penetrated by fibers of Sharpey, as at ligament and tendon attachments.

calcaneal b., calcaneus.

calf b. [O.N. *kalfi,* fibula], fibula.

cancellous b., *substantia* spongiosa.

cannon b., shank b. (1); the middle metacarpal (or metatarsal b.) in the horse.

capitate b., *os* capitatum.

carpal b.'s, *ossa* carpi. See carpus (2).

cartilage b., endochondral b.

cavalry b., rider's b.

central b., *os* centrale.

central b. of ankle, *os* naviculare.

cheek b., *os* zygomaticum.

coccygeal b., *os* coccygis.

collar b., clavicula.

compact b., *substantia* compacta.

convoluted b., see entries under *concha* nasalis.

cortical b., *substantia* corticalis.

coxal b., *os* coxae.

cranial b.'s, *ossa* cranii.

cubital b., *os* triquetrum.

cuboid b., *os* cuboideum.

cuneiform b., see os triquetrum and entries for os cuneiforme under os.

dermal b., a b. formed by ossification of the cutis.

b.'s of digits, *ossa* digitorum.

dorsal talonavicular b., Pirie's b.

ear b.'s, *ossicula* auditus.

elbow b., ulna.

endochondral b., cartilage or replacement b.; a b. that develops in a cartilage environment after the latter is partially or entirely destroyed by calcification and subsequent resorption.

epactal b.'s, *ossa* suturarum.

epihyal b., an ossified stylomastoid ligament.

epipteric b., Flower's b.; a sutural b. occasionally present at the pterion or junction of the parietal, frontal, greater wing of the sphenoid, and squamous portion of the temporal b.'s.

episternal b., *os* suprasternale.

ethmoid b., *os* ethmoidale.

exercise b., rider's b.

exoccipital b. (eks-ok-sip′i-tăl). *pars lateralis* ossis occipitalis. See under pars.

facial b.'s, ossa faciei; bones of visceral cranium; the bones surrounding the mouth and nose and contributing to the orbits; they are the paired maxilla, zygomatic, nasal, lacrimal, palatine, inferior nasal concha; and the unpaired ethmoid, vomer, mandible, and hyoid.

first cuneiform b., *os* cuneiforme mediale.

flank b., *os* ilium.

flat b., *os* planum.

Flower's b., epipteric b.

fourth turbinated b., *concha* nasalis suprema.

frontal b., *os* frontale.

Goethe's b., **(1)** preinterparietal b.; **(2)** *os* incisivum.

greater multangular b., *os* trapezium.

hamate b., *os* hamatum.

heel b., calcaneus.

heterotopic b.'s, b.'s that do not belong to the main skeleton but that regularly develop in certain organs, *e.g.,* the heart, penis, clitoris, and snout of some animals.

highest turbinated b., *concha* nasalis suprema.

hip b., *os* coxae.

hollow b., *os* pneumaticum.

hooked b., *os* hamatum.

hyoid b., **(1)** *os* hyoideum; **(2)** see *apparatus* hyoideus.

iliac b., *os* ilium.

incarial b., *os* interparietale.

incisive b., *os* incisivum.

b.'s of inferior limb, *ossa* membri inferioris.

inferior turbinated b., *concha* nasalis inferior.

innominate b., *os* coxae.

intermaxillary b., *os* incisivum.

intermediate cuneiform b., *os* cuneiforme intermedium.

interparietal b., *os* interparietale.

irregular b., *os* irregulare.

ischial b., *os* ischii.

jaw b., mandibula.

jugal b., *os* zygomaticum.

Krause's b., small b. (secondary ossification center) in the triradiate cartilage between the ilium, the ischium, and the pubic b. in the

growing acetabulum.
lacrimal b., *os* lacrimale.
lamellar b., the normal type of adult mammalian b., whether cancellous or compact, composed of parallel lamellae in the former and concentric lamellae in the latter; lamellar organization reflects a repeating pattern of collagen fibroarchitecture.
lateral cuneiform b., *os* cuneiforme laterale.
lenticular b., *processus* lenticularis.
lentiform b., *os* pisiforme.
lesser multangular b., *os* trapezoideum.
lingual b., *os* hyoideum.
long b., *os* longum.
lunate b., *os* lunatum.
malar b., *os* zygomaticum.
marble b.'s, osteopetrosis.
mastoid b., *processus* mastoideus.
medial cuneiform b., *os* cuneiforme mediale.
medullary b., areas of b. formation present in the marrow spaces of the long b.'s of birds, which serve as a readily mobilized source of calcium for shell formation.
membrane b., a b. which develops embryologically within a membrane of vascularized primitive mesenchymal tissue without prior formation of cartilage.
mesethmoid b., in comparative anatomy, the b. present in some species as the most anterior b. of the floor of the braincase.
middle cuneiform b., *os* cuneiforme intermedium.
middle turbinated b., *concha* nasalis media.
multangular b., see *os* trapezium; *os* trapezoideum.
nasal b., *os* nasale.
navicular b., *os* naviculare.
navicular b. of hand, *os* scaphoideum.
nonlamellar b., woven b.
occipital b., *os* occipitale.
orbicular b., *processus* lenticularis.
palatine b., *os* palatinum.
parietal b., *os* parietale.
penis b., *os* penis.
perichondral b., periosteal b.; in the development of a long b. a collar or cuff of osseous tissue forms in the perichondrium of the cartilage model; the connective tissue membrane of this perichondral b. then becomes periosteum.
periosteal b., perichondral b.
periotic b., *pars petrosa* ossis temporalis. See under pars.
peroneal b., fibula.
petrosal b., petrous b., *pars* petrosa ossis temporalis.
ping-pong b., the thin shell of osseous tissue at the periphery of a giant cell tumor in a b.
pipe b., *os* longum.
Pirie's b., dorsal talonavicular b.; an anomalous b. of the foot located near the head of the talus.
pisiform b., *os* pisiforme.
pneumatic b., *os* pneumaticum.
postsphenoid b., the posterior portion of the body of the sphenoid b.
preinterparietal b., Goethe's b. (1); a large sutural b. occasionally found detached from the anterior portion of the interparietal b.
premaxillary b., *os* incisivum.
presphenoid b., in comparative anatomy, the b. in the floor of the braincase anterior to the basisphenoid b.
pubic b., *os* pubis.
pyramidal b., *os* triquetrum.
replacement b., endochondral b.
reticulated b., woven b.
rider's b., cavalry or exercise b.; heterotopic bone ossification of the tendon of the adductor longus muscle from strain in horseback riding.
Riolan's b.'s, several small sutural b.'s sometimes present in the petro-occipital suture.
sacred b. [so called from belief in indestructibility of the bone as the basis for resurrection], *os* sacrum.
scaphoid b., *os* scaphoideum.
scroll b.'s, see *concha* nasalis inferior, media, superior, and suprema.
second cuneiform b., *os* cuneiforme intermedium.
semilunar b., *os* lunatum.
septal b., (1) *septum* interalveolare; (2) *septum* interradicularia.
sesamoid b., *os* sesamoideum.
shank b., (1) cannon b.; (2) tibia.
shin b., tibia.
short b., *os* breve.
sieve b., *lamina* cribrosa ossis ethmoidalis.
sphenoid b., *os* sphenoidale.
sphenoidal turbinated b.'s, *conchae* sphenoidales.
splint b., (1) the second or fourth, or internal or external small metacarpal b.'s in the horse; these are splinter-like in shape and lie on either side of the metacarpal or cannon b.; (2) fibula.
spongy b., (1) *substantia* spongiosa; (2) turbinated b.'s.
stifle b., the patella of the stifle joint of a horse.
b.'s of superior limb, *ossa* membri superioris.
superior turbinated b., *concha* nasalis superior.
suprainterparietal b., a sutural b. at the posterior portion of the sagittal suture.
suprasternal b., *os* suprasternale.
supreme turbinated b., *concha* nasalis suprema.
sutural b.'s, *ossa* suturarum.
tail b., *os* coccygis.
tarsal b.'s, ossa tarsi. See tarsus (1).
temporal b., *os* temporale.
thigh b., *os* femoris.
third cuneiform b., *os* cuneiforme laterale.
three-cornered b., *os* triquetrum.
tongue b., *os* hyoideum.
trabecular b., *substantia* spongiosa.
trapezium b., *os* trapezium.
trapezoid b., *os* trapezoideum.
triangular b., *os* trigonum.
triquetral b., *os* triquetrum.
turbinated b.'s, see *concha* nasalis inferior, media, superior, and suprema.
tympanic b., *annulus* tympanicus.
tympanohyal b., a small nodule of b. forming the base of the cartilaginous styloid process of the temporal b. at birth.
unciform b., *os* hamatum.
upper jaw b., maxilla.
Vesalius' b., *os* vesalianum.
b.'s of visceral cranium, facial b.'s.
wedge b., *os* cuneiforme intermedium, laterale, and mediale.
wormian b.'s, *ossa* suturarum.
woven b., nonlamellar or reticulated b.; bony tissue characteristic of the embryonal skeleton in which the collagen fibers of the matrix are arranged irregularly in the form of interlacing networks.
yoke b., *os* zygomaticum.
zygomatic b., *os* zygomaticum.

---

bone architecture. The pattern of trabeculae and associated structures. See also Wolff's *law.*

bone ash. Tribasic *calcium* phosphate.

bone black. Animal *charcoal.*

bonelet (bōn'let). Ossiculum.

bone-salt. The main chemical compound in bone, deposited as minute crystals in a netlike matrix of collagenous fibers containing collagen; it closely resembles the naturally occurring fluorapatite

$3Ca_3(PO_4)_2 \cdot CaF_2$, but is probably a hydroxyapatite in which F is replaced by OH.

Bonhoeffer, Karl, German psychiatrist, 1868–1948. See B.'s *sign.*

Bonnet, Amédée, French surgeon, 1809–1858. See B.'s *capsule, operation, position.*

Bonnevie, Kristine, German physician, 1872–1950. See B.-Ullrich *syndrome.*

Bonnier, Pierre, French clinician, 1861–1918. See B.'s *syndrome.*

Bonwill, William G.A., U.S. dentist, 1833–1899. See B. *triangle.*

Böök, Jan A., Swedish geneticist, *1915. See B.'s *syndrome.*

Boophilus (bō-of'i-lŭs) [G. *bous,* ox, + *philos,* fond]. A genus of hard ticks (family Ixodidae) infesting cattle; members are important vectors of bovine babesiosis and anaplasmosis in various parts of the world. Previously thought to be synonymous with *Margaropus,* but now considered distinct; *B.* is distinguished by the presence of eyes, palpi and hypostome characteristics, and by lack of festoons.

B. annula'tus, species that formerly was the vector of bovine babesiosis in the southern United States, but is still an important species in Mexico and certain other countries.

B. decolora'tus, species that is a vector of bovine babesiosis and anaplasmosis in sub-Saharan Africa.

B. mi'cropus, the tropical cattle tick, a species that is an important vector of bovine babesiosis and anaplasmosis in Mexico, Central and South America, Africa, Australia, and oriental countries, and of relapsing fever by *Borrelia theileri* in South Africa and Australia.

booster (būs'ter). See under dose.

boot (būt). A boot-shaped appliance.

Junod's b., an airtight case into which the arm or leg is inserted and the air is then exhausted; used to divert a portion of the blood temporarily from the general circulation.

boracic acid (bō-ras'ik). Boric acid.

borate (bōr'āt). A salt of boric acid.

borated (bōr'āt-ed). Mixed or impregnated with borax or boric acid.

borax (bō'raks). *Sodium* borate.

borborygmus, pl. **borborygmi** (bōr-bō-rig'mŭs, -rig'mī) [G. *borborygmos,* rumbling in the bowels]. Rumbling or gurgling noises produced by movement of gas in the alimentary canal, and audible at a distance.

Bordeau (Bordeu), Théophile de, French physician, 1722–1776. See de B. *theory.*

border (bōr'der). The part of a surface that forms its outer boundary. See also edge; margin; margo.

alveolar b., **(1)** the most occlusal edge of the alveolar bone; **(2)** *processus* alveolaris.

anterior b., *margo* anterior.

brush b., limbus penicillatus; the apical epithelial surface bearing closely packed microvilli about 2 μm long, such as occur on the cells of the proximal tubule of the nephron.

denture b., denture edge; periphery (2); **(1)** the limit or boundary or circumferential margin of a denture base; **(2)** the margin of the denture base at the junction of the polished surface with the impression (tissue) surface; **(3)** the extreme edges of a denture base at the buccolabial, lingual, and posterior limits.

b.'s of eyelids, *limbi* palpebrales.

inferior b., *margo* inferior.

occult b. of nail, *margo* occultus unguis.

posterior b. of petrous part of temporal bone, *margo posterior* partis petrosae ossis temporalis. See under margo.

radial b., *margo lateralis* antebrachii. See under margo.

sagittal b., *margo* sagittalis.

sphenoidal b., *margo* sphenoidalis.

striated b., limbus striatus; the free surface of the columnar absorptive cells of the intestine formed by closely packed microvilli about 1 μm long, giving the appearance of parallel striations.

superior b. of petrous part of temporal bone, *margo superior* partis petrosae ossis temporalis. See under margo.

tibial b., *margo medialis* pedis. See under margo.

b. of uterus, *margo* uteri.

vermilion b., vermilion zone; vermilion transitional zone; the red margin of the upper and lower lip that commences at the exterior edge of the intraoral labial mucosa ("moist line") and extends outward, terminating at the extraoral labial cutaneous junction; a thinly keratinized type of stratified squamous epithelium deeply penetrated by well vascularized dermal papillae which show through the translucent epidermis to impart the typical red appearance of the lips.

Bordet, Jules, Belgian bacteriologist and Nobel laureate, 1870–1961. See Bordetella; B.-Gengou potato blood *agar, bacillus, phenomenon.*

Bordetella (bōr-dĕ-tel'ă) [J. *Bordet*]. A genus of strictly aerobic bacteria (family Brucellaceae) containing minute, Gram-negative coccobacilli. Motile and nonmotile species occur; motile cells are peritrichous. The metabolism of these organisms is respiratory. They require nicotinic acid, cysteine, and methionine; hemin (X factor) and coenzyme I (V factor) are not required. They are parasites and pathogens of the mammalian respiratory tract. The type species is *B. pertussis.*

B. bronchisep'tica, a species causing atrophic rhinitis of swine, bronchopneumonia in rodents, and bronchopneumonia secondary to distemper in dogs.

B. parapertus'sis, a species that causes a whooping cough-like disease.

B. pertus'sis, *Haemophilus pertussis;* Bordet-Gengou bacillus; a species that causes whooping cough; the type species of the genus *B.*

boric acid (bō'rik). Boracic acid; H_3BO_3; a very weak acid, used as an antiseptic dusting powder, in saturated solution as a collyrium, and with glycerin in aphthae and stomatitis.

borism (bōr'izm). Symptoms caused by the ingestion of borax or any compound of boron.

Börjeson, Mats, Swedish physician, *1922. See B.-Forssman-Lehmann *syndrome.*

Born, Gustav Jacob, German embryologist, 1851–1900. See B. *method* (of wax plate reconstruction).

bornane (bōr'nān). Camphane; 1,7,7-trimethylnorbornane; parent of borneols, camphene, and similar essential oils (terpenes).

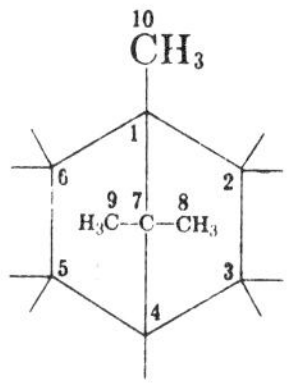

Bornane

boroglycerin (bō-rō-glis'er-in). Glyceryl borate; boroglycerol; a soft mass obtained by heating glycerin and boric acid; an antiseptic, usually used mixed with equal parts of glycerin, constituting glycerite.

boroglycerol (bō-rō-glis'er-ol). Boroglycerin.

boron (bōr'on). A nonmetallic trivalent element, symbol B, atomic weight 10.81, atomic no. 5; occurs as a hard crystalline mass or as a brown powder, and forms borates and boric acid.

Borrel, Amédée, French bacteriologist, 1867–1936. See B. *bodies,* blue *stain.*

Borrelia (bō-rē′lē-ă, bo-rel′ē-ă) [A. *Borrell*]. A genus of bacteria (family Treponemataceae) containing cells 8 to 16 μm in length, with coarse, shallow, irregular spirals and tapered, finely filamented ends. These organisms are parasitic on many forms of animal life, are generally hematophytic, or are found on mucous membranes. Some borreliae are transmitted by the bites of arthropods. The type species is *B. anserina.*

B. anseri′na, a species that causes spirochetosis of fowls; found in the blood of infected geese, ducks, other fowls, and vector ticks; it is the type species of the genus *B.*

B. burgdor′feri, a species causing Lyme disease in humans and borreliosis in dogs, cattle, and possibly horses.

B. cauca′sica, a species found as a cause of relapsing fever in the Caucasus; transmitted by *Ornithodoros verrucosus.*

B. crocidu′rae, a species that causes relapsing fever in Africa, Near East, and central Asia, and is transmitted by the small variety of the tick *Ornithodoros erraticus.*

B. dutto′nii, a species causing Central and South African relapsing fever; transmitted by a tick, *Ornithodoros moubata.*

B. herm′sii, a species found as a cause of relapsing fever in British Columbia, California, Colorado, Idaho, Nevada, Oregon, and Washington; transmitted by a tick, *Ornithodoros hermsi.*

B. hispan′ica, a species causing relapsing fever in Spain, Portugal, and northwest Africa, transmitted by the large variety of the tick *Ornithodorus erratica.*

B. koch′ii, a species causing African relapsing fever and transmitted by *Ornithodoros savigni.*

B. latysche′wii, a species that causes relapsing fever in Iran and central Asia; transmitted by the tick *Ornithodoros tartakovskyi* from rodents and reptiles.

B. mazzot′tii, a species that causes relapsing fever in Mexico and Central and South America; transmitted by the tick *Ornithodoros talajé.*

B. par′keri, a species found as a cause of relapsing fever in the western United States; transmitted by a tick, *Ornithodoros parkeri.*

B. per′sica, a species that causes relapsing fever in the Middle East and central Asia; the vector is the tick *Ornithodoros tholozani.*

B. recurren′tis, *Spirochaeta obermeieri;* Obermeier's spirillum; a species causing relapsing fever in South America, Europe, Africa, and Asia; transmitted by the bedbug, *Cimex lectularius,* and the louse, *Pediculus humanus* subsp. *humanus.*

B. thei′leri, a species that causes borreliosis in cattle and other mammals in South Africa and Australia; transmitted by the ticks *Boophilus micropus* and *Rhipicephalus evertsi.*

B. turica′tae, a species found as a cause of relapsing fever in Mexico, New Mexico, Texas, Oklahoma, and Kansas; transmitted by *Ornithodoros turicata.*

B. venezuelen′sis, a species causing spirochetal relapsing fever in Central and South America; transmitted by *Ornithodoros rudis* and *O. venezuelensis.*

borreliosis (bō-rē-lē-ō′sis). Disease caused by bacteria of the genus *Borrelia.*

bovine b., a disease of cattle caused by *Borrelia burgdorferi* and characterized by laminitis, arthritis, and synovitis.

canine b., a disease of dogs caused by *Borrelia burgdorferi* and characterized by lameness due to a migratory, intermittent, oligoarticular arthritis.

Borst, Maximilian, German pathologist, 1869–1946. See B.-Jadassohn type intraepidermal *epithelioma.*

boss (baws). **1.** A protuberance; a circumscribed rounded swelling. **2.** The prominence of a kyphosis.

bosselated (baws′ĕ-lā-ted) [Fr. *bosseler,* to emboss]. Marked by numerous bosses or rounded protuberances.

bosselation (baws-ĕ-lā′shŭn). **1.** A boss. **2.** A condition in which one or more bosses, or rounded protuberances are present.

Boston, Leonard N., U.S. physician, 1871–1931. See B.'s *sign.*

Botallo (Botallus), Leonardo, Italian physician in Paris, 1530–1600(?). See B.'s *duct, foramen, ligament.*

botfly (bot′flī). Robust, hairy fly of the order Diptera, often strikingly marked in black and yellow or gray, whose larvae produce a variety of myiasis conditions in man and various domestic animals, especially herbivores. See also *Gasterophilus.*

head b.'s, flesh flies of the dipterous families Oestridae and Cuterebridae; robust, hairy, black, yellow, or gray flies that, while flying, deposit newly hatched larvae or, in some cases, eggs, on or near the nostrils of sheep, goats, deer, horses, camels, and, rarely, man.

human b., *Dermatobia hominis.*

skin b.'s, *Dermatobia hominis.* See also *Cuterebra* species.

warble b., *Dermatobia hominis.* See also *Hypoderma.*

bothria (both′rē-ă). Plural of bothrium.

bothriocephaliasis (both′rē-ō-sef-ă-lī′ă-sis). Diphyllobothriasis.

Bothriocephalus (both′rē-ō-sef′ă-lŭs) [G. *bothrion,* dim. of *bothros,* pit or trench, + *kephalē,* head]. A genus of pseudophyllid tapeworms with both plerocercoid and adult stages in fishes; sometimes historically confused with *Diphyllobothrium.*

B. corda′tus, a species common in dogs and man in Greenland.

B. la′tus, former name for *Diphyllobothrium latum.*

B. manso′ni, former name for *Spirometra mansoni.*

B. mansonoi′des, former name for *Spirometra mansonoides.*

bothrium, pl. **bothria** (both′rē-ŭm, -rē-ă) [G. *bothros,* pit or trench]. One of the slitlike sucking grooves found on the scolex of pseudophyllidean tapeworms, such as the broad fish tapeworm of man, *Diphyllobothrium latum.*

botryoid (bot′rē-oyd) [G. *botryoeidēs,* like a bunch of grapes (*botrys*)]. Staphyline; uviform; having numerous rounded protuberances resembling a bunch of grapes.

Botryomyces (bot′rē-ō-mī′sēz) [G. *botrys,* a bunch of grapes, + *mykēs,* fungus]. A generic name applied to a supposed fungus causing botryomycosis. Since this disease is now known to be caused by several kinds of bacteria, staphylococci most commonly, the name is invalid and rarely used. The name of the disease has been retained, nevertheless, to indicate a peculiar type of tissue reaction.

botryomycosis (bot′rē-ō-mī-kō′sis) [fr. *Botryomyces*]. Actinophytosis (2); a chronic granulomatous condition of horses, cattle, swine, and man, usually involving the skin but occasionally also the viscera, and characterized by granules in the pus, consisting of masses of bacteria, generally staphylococci but sometimes other types, surrounded by a hyaline capsule which sometimes exhibits clublike bodies around its periphery; the anatomic structure of the lesion resembles that of actinomycosis and mycetoma.

botryomycotic (bot′rē-ō-mī-kot′ik). Relating to or affected by botryomycosis.

bots [Gael. *boiteag,* maggot]. The larvae of several species of botflies.

ox b., cattle grub; the larvae of the warble flies, *Hypoderma bovis* and *H. lineatum.*

sheep b., *Oestrus ovis* larvae.

Böttcher, Arthur, Estonian anatomist, 1831–1889. See B.'s *canal, cells, crystals, ganglion, space;* Charcot-B. *crystalloids.*

bottle (bot′tl). A container for liquids.

Mariotte b., a stoppered b. with bottom outlet, used as a reservoir for constant infusions; air enters only by bubbling through a tube extending down through the stopper almost to the bottom; a partial vacuum thus supports the variable height of liquid above the air inlet, providing a constant gravity head for outflow.

wash-b., **(1)** a bottle with a tube passing to the bottom, through which gases are forced into water to purify them; **(2)** a stoppered bottle with two tubes, one ending above and the other below a fluid, so that air blowing through the short tube forces liquid in a small stream from the free end of the long one; used for washing chemical apparatus.

Woulfe's b., a b. with two or three necks, used in a series, connected with tubes, for working with gases (washing, drying, absorbing, etc.).

botulin (bot'yū-lin). Botulinus *toxin.*

botulinogenic (bot'yū-lin-ō-jen'ik). Botulogenic.

botulism (bot'yū-lizm) [L. *botulus,* sausage]. An intoxication due to the ingestion of *Clostridium botulinum* toxin in improperly canned or preserved food; mainly affects man, chickens, water fowl, cattle, sheep, and horses, and is characterized by paralysis in all species; swine, dogs, and cats are somewhat resistant. See also *Clostridium botulinum.*

botulismotoxin (bot'yū-liz-mō-tok'sin). Botulinus *toxin.*

botulogenic (bot'yū-lō-jen'ik). Botulinogenic; botulism-producing.

boubas (bū'bahs) [native Brazilian]. Yaws.

Bouchard, Charles Jacques, French physician, 1837–1915. See B.'s *disease.*

bouche de tapir (būsh-dĕ-tă'pir) [Fr.]. Tapir *mouth.*

Bouchut, Jean A.E., French physician, 1818–1891. See B.'s *method, tube.*

Bouffardi's mycetomas. See under mycetoma.

bougie (bū-zhē') [Fr. candle]. A cylindrical instrument, usually somewhat flexible and yielding, used for calibrating or dilating constricted areas in tubular organs, such as the urethra or rectum; sometimes containing a medication for local application.

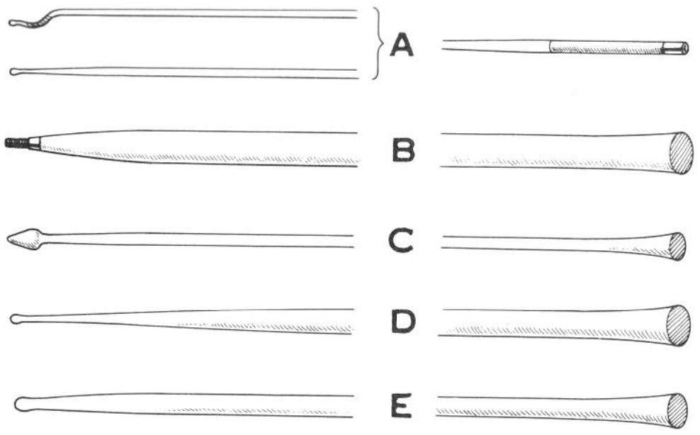

Bougies

A, filiform bougie with spiral or straight tip and threaded trailing end designed to accept following dilators; *B,* following bougie with threaded tip for insertion into filiform bougie; *C,* cone-tipped bougie; *D* and *E,* tapering olive-tipped bougies.

b. à boule (bū-zhē'ă-būl'), a ball-tipped b.

bulbous b., b. à boule; a b. with a bulb-shaped tip, some of which are shaped like an acorn or an olive.

elastic b., a b. made of rubber, latex, or other similarly flexible material.

elbowed b., a b. with a sharply angulated bend near its tip.

filiform b., a very slender b. usually used for gentle exploration of strictures or sinus tracts of small diameter where false passages can be encountered or created; the entering end can consist of either a straight or spiral tip, and the trailing end usually consists of a threaded cylinder into which the screw tip of a following b. can be inserted.

following b., a flexible tapered b. with a screw tip which is attached to the trailing end of a filiform b., to allow progressive dilation without danger of creating false passages.

Hurst b.'s, a series of mercury-filled tubes of graded diameter for dilating the cardioesophageal region.

Maloney b.'s, a series of b.'s similar to Hurst b.'s but having cone-shaped tips.

tapered b., a b. with gradually increasing caliber, used to dilate structures.

wax-tipped b., a long slender flexible b. with a wax tip, used for endoscopic passage into the ureter to confirm the presence of a calculus by scratching the surface of the tip with the sharp edges of the stone.

whip b., a b. tapered to a threadlike tip at the end.

bougienage (bū-zhē-nahzh'). Examination or treatment of the interior of any canal by the passage of a bougie or cannula.

Bouillaud, Jean B., French physician, 1796–1881. See B.'s *disease.*

bouillon (bū-yawṅ') [Fr. broth, fr. *bouillir,* to boil]. A clear beef tea.

Bouin, Paul, French histologist, 1870–1962. See B.'s *fixative.*

boulimia (bū-lim'ē-ă). *Bulimia* nervosa.

bound (bownd). **1.** Limited, circumscribed; enclosed. **2.** Denoting a substance, such as iodine, phosphorus, calcium, morphine, that is not in readily soluble form but exists in combination with a colloid, especially protein. **3.** Fixed to a receptor, such as on a cell wall.

bouquet (bū-ka') [Fr.]. A cluster or bunch of structures, especially of blood vessels, suggesting a b.

Riolan's b., the muscles and ligaments, "les fleurs rouges et les fleurs blanches" (the red and white flowers), arising from the styloid process.

Bourdon, Eugène, French engineer and inventor, 1808–1884. See B. *tube.*

Bourgery, Marc-Jean, French anatomist and surgeon, 1797–1849. See B.'s *ligament.*

Bourneville, Désiré-Magloire, French physician, 1840–1909. See B.'s *disease,* B.-Pringle *disease.*

Bourquin, Anne, U.S. chemist, *1897. See Sherman-B. *unit* of vitamin B_2.

bouton (bū-ton') [Fr. button]. A button, pustule, or knoblike swelling.

axonal terminal b.'s, axon *terminals.*

b. de Bagdad, b. de Biskra, or **d'Orient,** the lesion occurring in cutaneous leishmaniasis.

b. en chemise, small abscess of the intestinal mucosa, occurring in amebic dysentery.

b.'s en passage, consecutive synapses along the course of an axon.

synaptic b.'s, axon terminals. See under terminal.

terminal b.'s, b. terminaux, axon *terminals.*

boutonnière (bū-tŏn-nēr', -năr') [Fr. buttonhole]. A traumatically produced slit or buttonhole-like opening.

Bouveret, Leon, French physician, 1850–1929. See B.'s *sign.*

Bovicola (bō-vik'ō-lă). A genus of biting lice that is considered by some to be a subgenus of *Damalinia;* includes the species *B. bovis* (*Trichodectes scalaris*), the common red or biting ox louse of cattle; *B. caprae* (*Trichodectes climax*), found on sheep and goats; *B. equi* (*Trichodectes parumpilosus*), the common biting louse of horses; *B. ovis* (*Trichodectes sphaerocephalus*), the common biting louse of sheep. See also *Trichodectes.*

bovine (bō'vīn, -vin) [L. *bos* (*bov-*), ox]. Relating to cattle.

bow (bō). Any device bent in a simple curve or semicircle and possessing flexibility.

Logan's b., heavy stainless steel wire bent in an arc and taped to both cheeks to protect the incision and to relieve tension on a freshly repaired cleft lip.

Bowditch, Henry P., U.S. physiologist, 1840–1911. See B.'s *law.*

bow'el [through the Fr. from L. *botulus,* sausage]. Intestinum (1).

Bowen, John T., U.S. dermatologist, 1857–1941. See B.'s *disease,* precancerous *dermatosis;* bowenoid *papulosis.*

Bowie's stain. See under stain.

bowleg (bō'leg). *Genu* varum.

Bowles type stethoscope. See under stethoscope.

Bowman, Sir William, British ophthalmologist, anatomist, and physiologist, 1816–1892. See B.'s *capsule, disks, gland, membrane, muscle, operation, probe, space, theory.*

box (boks). Container; receptacle.

fracture b., an obsolete means of supporting a fractured leg, consisting of a container with only bottom and sides.

Hogness b., see TATA b.

Pribnow b., see TATA b.

Skinner b., an experimental apparatus in which an animal presses a lever to obtain a reward.

TATA b. [*box,* fr. enclosure of nucleotide letters in a rectangle], in molecular biology, a sequence of nucleotides rich in thymidylate (T) and deoxyadenylate (A) arranged in conventional 5′- to -3′ orientation which occurs in the promoter region of the DNA of many (if not all) genomes, just "upstream" (5′ direction) from the starting point of transcription by RNA polymerase. Sometimes called Hogness b. or Pribnow b. after the investigators who first noted the ubiquitous occurrence of the sequence in eukaryotes and prokaryotes respectively.

boxing (boks'ing). In dentistry, the building up of vertical walls, usually in wax, around a dental impression after beading, to produce the desired size and form of the dental cast, and to preserve certain landmarks of the impression.

Boyce, William H., U.S. urologist, *1918. See B.'s *operation.*

Boyden, Edward A., U.S. anatomist, 1886–1977. See B. *meal,* B.'s *sphincter.*

Boyer, Baron Alexis de, French surgeon, 1757–1833. See B.'s *bursa, cyst.*

Boyle, Hon. Robert, British physicist and chemist, 1627–1691. See B.'s *law.*

Bozeman, Nathan, U.S. surgeon, 1825–1905. See B.'s *operation, position;* B.-Fritsch *catheter.*

Bozzolo, Camillo, Italian physician, 1845–1920. See B.'s *sign.*

BP Abbreviation for blood *pressure; British Pharmacopoeia.*

b.p. Abbreviation for boiling *point.*

Br Symbol for bromine.

Braasch, William F., U.S. urologist, 1878–1975. See B. *catheter.*

brace (brās). An orthosis or orthopedic appliance that supports or holds in correct position any movable part of the body and that allows motion of the part, in contrast to a splint, which prevents motion of the part.

Taylor's back b., a steel spinal support.

bracelet (brās'let). An appliance for the wrist.

Nussbaum's b., an appliance designed for use with writer's cramp.

braces (brā'sez). Colloquialism for orthodontic appliances.

brachia (brā'kē-ă). Plural of brachium.

brachial (brā'kē-ăl). Relating to the arm.

brachialgia (brā-kē-al'jē-ă) [L. *brachium,* arm, + *algos,* pain]. Pain in the arm.

b. stat'ica paresthet'ica, pain in the arm and transient paresthesia occurring only at night.

brachio- [L. *brachium,* arm]. Combining form meaning: **1.** Arm. **2.** Radial.

brachiocephalic (brā'kē-ō-se-fal'ik). Relating to both arm and head.

brachiocrural (brā'kē-ō-krū'răl). Relating to both arm and thigh.

brachiocubital (brā'kē-ō-kyū'bi-tăl). Relating to both arm and elbow or to both arm and forearm.

brachiogram (brā'kē-ō-gram). Tracing of the brachial artery pulse.

brachium, pl. **brachia** (brā'kē-ŭm, -ă, brak') [L. arm, prob. akin to G. *brachiōn*] [NA]. **1.** Arm, specifically the segment of the upper limb between the shoulder and the elbow. **2.** An anatomical structure resembling an arm.

b. collic'uli inferio'ris [NA], b. of the inferior colliculus; b. quadrigeminum inferius; inferior quadrigeminal b.; a fiber bundle passing from the inferior colliculus on either side of the brainstem along the lateral border of the superior colliculus to the posterior part of the thalamus where it enters the medial geniculate body. It forms part of the major ascending auditory pathway.

b. collic'uli superio'ris [NA], b. of the superior colliculus; superior quadrigeminal b.; b. quadrigeminum superius; a band of fibers of the optic tract bypassing the lateral geniculate body to terminate in the superior colliculus and pretectal region.

b. conjuncti'vum cerebel'li, *pedunculus* cerebellaris superior.

b. of the inferior colliculus, b. colliculi superioris.

inferior quadrigeminal b., b. colliculi inferioris.

b. pon'tis, *pedunculus* cerebellaris medius.

b. quadrigem'inum infe'rius, b. colliculi inferioris.

b. quadrigem'inum supe'rius, b. colliculi superioris.

b. of superior colliculus, b. colliculi superioris.

superior quadrigeminal b., b. colliculi superioris.

Bracht, E., 20th century German pathologist. See B.-Wachter *lesion.*

Bracht, Erich Franz, German obstetrician and gynecologist, *1882. See B. *maneuver.*

brachy- [G. *brachys,* short]. Combining form meaning short.

brachybasia (brak-ē-bā'sē-ă) [brachy- + G. *basis,* a stepping]. The shuffling gait characteristic of pyramidal tract disease.

brachybasocamptodactyly (brak-ē-bā'sō-kamp-tō-dak'ti-lē) [brachy- + G. *basis,* base, + *campylos,* curved, + *daktylos,* finger]. Combined disproportionate shortness and crookedness of the fingers.

brachybasophalangia (brak-ē-bā'sō-fă-lan'jē-ă) [brachy- + G. *basis,* base, + phalanx]. Abnormal shortness of the phalanges.

brachycardia (brak-ē-kar'dē-ă). Bradycardia.

brachycephalia (brak-ē-sĕ-fā'lē-ă). Brachycephaly.

brachycephalic (brak-ē-se-fal'ik). Brachycephalous; relating to or characterized by brachycephaly.

brachycephalism (brak-ē-sef'ă-lizm) [brachy- + G. *kephalē,* head]. Brachycephaly.

brachycephalous (brak-ē-sef'ă-lŭs). Brachycephalic.

brachycephaly (brak-ē-sef'ă-lē) [brachy- + G. *kephalē,* head]. Brachycephalia; brachycephalism; disproportionate shortness of head, the skull having a cephalic index of over 80; among the brachycephalic races are the American Indians, Malayans, and Burmese.

brachycheilia, brachychilia (brak'ē-kī'lē-ă) [brachy- + G. *cheilos,* lip]. Abnormal shortness of the lips.

brachycnemic (brak-ē-nē'mik) [brachy- + G. *knēmē,* leg]. Having short legs; specifically, relating to a tibiofemoral index of less than 82 with a shank disproportionately shorter than the thigh.

brachycranic (brak-ē-krā'nik) [brachy- + G. *kranion,* skull]. Brachycephalic with a cephalic index of 80.0 to 84.9.

brachydactylia (brak-ē-dak-til'ē-ă) [brachy- + G. *daktylos,* finger]. Brachydactyly.

brachydactylic (brak-ē-dak-til'ik). Denoting brachydactyly.

brachydactyly (brak-ē-dak'ti-lē) [brachy- + G. *daktylos,* finger]. Brachydactylia; abnormal shortness of the fingers.

brachyesophagus (brak'ē-e-sof'ă-gŭs) [brachy- + esophagus]. An abnormally short esophagus.

brachyfacial (brak-ē-fā'shăl). Brachyprosopic.

brachyglossal (brak-ē-glos'ăl) [brachy- + G. *glōssa,* tongue]. Denoting an abnormally short tongue.

brachygnathia (brak-ig-nā'thē-ă) [brachy- + G. *gnathos,* jaw]. Bird face; abnormal shortness or recession of the mandible.

brachygnathous (brak-ig'nā-thŭs). Having a receding underjaw.

brachykerkic (brak-ē-ker'kik) [brachy- + G. *kerkis,* radius]. Relating to a radiohumeral index of less than 75, with a forearm relatively shorter than the upper arm.

brachymelia (brak-ē-mē'lē-ă) [brachy- + G. *melos,* limb]. Disproportionate shortness of the limbs.

brachymesophalangia (brak-ē-mes'ō-fă-lan'jē-ă) [brachy- + G. *mesos,* middle, + phalanx]. Abnormal shortness of the middle phalanges.

brachymetacarpalia, brachymetacarpalism (brak'ē-met-ă-kar-pā'lē-ă, -met-ă-kar'pă-lizm). Brachymetacarpia.

brachymetacarpia (brak'ē-met-ă-car'pē-ă). Brachymetacarpalia; brachymetacarpalism; abnormal shortening of the metacarpals, especially the fourth and fifth.

brachymetapody (brak'ē-me-tap'ō-dē) [brachy- + G. *meta-* (tarsal) + *pous (pod-),* foot]. Apparent shortness of toes or fingers resulting from shortness or hypoplasia of the metacarpals or metatarsals.

brachymetatarsia (brak'ē-met-ă-tar'sē-ă). Abnormal shortness of the metatarsals.

brachymorphic (brak'ē-mōr'fik) [brachy- + G. *morphē,* form]. Having, or denoting, a shorter form than that of the usually accepted norm.

brachyodont (brak'ē-ō-dont) [brachy- + G. *odous,* tooth]. Having abnormally short teeth.

brachypellic (brak-ē-pel'ik) [brachy- + pelvis]. Brachypelvic; denoting a transverse oval pelvis. See brachypellic *pelvis.*

brachypelvic (brak-ē-pel'vik). Brachypellic.

brachyphalangia (brak'ē-fă-lan'jē-ă) [brachy- + phalanx]. Abnormal shortness of the phalanges.

brachypodous (bra-kip'ō-dŭs) [brachy- + G. *pous,* foot]. Having abnormally short feet.

brachyprosopic (brak-ē-prō-sop'ik) [brachy- + G. *prosōpikos,* facial]. Brachyfacial; having a disproportionately short face.

brachyrhinia (brak-ē-rī'nē-ă) [brachy- + G. *rhis,* nose]. Abnormal shortness of the nose.

brachyrhynchus (brak-ē-ring'kŭs) [brachy- + G. *rhynchos,* snout]. Abnormal shortness of the nose and maxilla, often associated with cyclopia.

brachyskelic (brak-ē-skel'ik) [brachy- + G. *skelos,* leg]. Relating to abnormally short legs.

brachystaphyline (brak-ē-staf'i-lin) [brachy- + G. *staphylē,* uvula]. Having a short palate; having a palatomaxillary index above 85.

brachysyndactyly (brak'ē-sin-dak'i-lē) [brachy- + syndactyly]. Abnormal shortness of fingers or toes combined with a webbing between the adjacent digits.

brachytelephalangia (brak-ē-tel'ē-fă-lan'jē-ă) [brachy- + G. *telos,* end, + phalanx]. Abnormal shortness of the distal phalanges.

brachytherapy (brak-ē-thār'ă-pē). Radiotherapy in which the source of irradiation is placed close to the surface of the body or within a body cavity; *e.g.,* application of radium to the cervix.

brachytype (brak'ē-tīp). Endomorph.

brachyuranic (brak-ē-yū-ran'ik) [brachy- + G. *ouranos,* the sky, roof of the mouth]. Having a palatomaxillary index above 115.

bracing (brās'ing). In dentistry, resistance to horizontal components of masticatory force. See *component* of force.

bracket (brak'et). In dentistry, a small metal attachment that is soldered or welded to an orthodontic band or bonded directly to the teeth, serving to fasten the arch wire to the band or tooth.

Bradford, Edward H., U.S. orthopedist, 1848–1926. See B. *frame.*

brady- [G. *bradys,* slow]. Combining form meaning slow.

bradyarrhythmia (brad'ē-ă-rith'mē-ă) [brady- + G. *a-* priv. + *rhythmos,* rhythm]. Any disturbance of the heart's rhythm resulting in a rate under 60 beats per minute.

bradyarthria (brad-ē-arth'rē-ă) [brady- + G. *arthroō,* to utter distinctly, fr. *arthron,* a joint]. Bradyglossia (2); bradylalia; bradylogia; a form of dysarthria characterized by an abnormal slowness or deliberation in speech.

bradycardia (brad-ē-kar'dē-ă) [brady- + G. *kardia,* heart]. Brachycardia; bradyrhythmia; slowness of the heartbeat, usually defined as a rate under 60 beats per minute.
- **cardiomuscular b.,** b. due to disease of the cardiac musculature.
- **central b.,** b. due to disease of the central nervous system, usually with increased intracranial pressure.
- **essential b.,** idiopathic b.; a slow pulse for which no cause can be discovered.
- **fetal b.,** a fetal heart rate of less than 100 beats per minute.
- **idiopathic b.,** essential b.
- **nodal b.,** atrioventricular nodal *rhythm.*
- **postinfectious b.,** a toxic b. occurring during convalescence from various infectious diseases, such as influenza.
- **sinus b.,** b. originating in the normal sinus pacemaker.
- **ventricular b.,** slowness of ventricular rate, usually implying the presence of atrioventricular block.

bradycardiac (brad-ē-kar'dē-ak). Relating to or characterized by bradycardia.

bradycardic (brad-ē-kar'dik). Bradycardiac.

bradycinesia (brad-ē-si-nē'sē-ă). Bradykinesia.

bradycrotic (brad-ē-krot'ik) [*brady-* + G. *krotos,* a striking]. Relating to or characterized by a slow pulse.

bradydiastole (brad-ē-dī-as'tō-lē). Prolongation of the diastole of the heart.

bradyesthesia (brad-ē-es-thē'zē-ă) [brady- + G. *aisthēsis,* sensation]. Retardation in the rate of transmission of sensory impressions.

bradyglossia (brad-ē-glos'ē-ă) [brady- + G. *glōssa,* tongue]. **1.** Slow or difficult tongue movement. **2.** Bradyarthria.

bradykinesia (brad-ē-kin-ē'zē-ă) [brady- + G. *kinēsis,* movement]. Bradycinesia; extreme slowness in movement.

bradykinetic (brad-ē-ki-net'ik). Characterized by or pertaining to slow movement.

bradykinin (brad-ē-kī'nin) [brady- + G. *kinein,* to move]. Kallidin I; kallidin 9; the nonapeptide Arg-Pro-Pro-Gly-Phe-Ser-Pro-Phe-Arg, produced from the decapeptide kallidin (bradyininogen) that is produced from α_2-globulin by kallikrein, normally present in blood in an inactive form and similar to trypsin in action; b. is one of a number of the plasma kinins, is a potent vasodilator, and is one of the physiologic mediators of anaphylaxis released from cytotroic antibody-coated mast cells following reaction with antigen (allergen) specific for the antibody.

bradykininogen (brad'ē-ki-nin'ō-jen). Kallidin.

bradykinin potentiator B. 5-OxoPro-Gly-Leu-Pro-Pro-Arg-Pro-Lys-Ile-Pro-Pro; the undecapeptide precursor of bradykinin and the angiotensins.

bradylalia (brad-ē-lā'lē-ă) [brady- + G. *lalia,* speech]. Bradyarthria.

bradylexia (brad-ē-lek'sē-ă) [brady- + G. *lexis,* word]. Abnormal slowness in reading.

bradylogia (brad-ē-lō'jē-ă) [brady- + G. *logos,* word]. Bradyarthria.

bradymenorrhea (brad'ē-men-ō-rē'ă) [brady- + G. *mēn,* month, + *rhoia,* flow]. Slow menstrual flow or prolonged menstrual bleeding.

bradypepsia (brad-ē-pep'sē-ă) [brady- + G. *pepsis,* digestion]. Slowness of digestion.

bradyphagia (brad-ē-fā'jē-ă) [brady- + G. *phagein,* to eat]. Extreme slowness in eating.

bradyphasia (brad-ē-fā'zē-ă) [brady- + G. *phasis,* speaking]. Bradyphemia; a form of aphasia characterized by abnormal slowness of speech.

bradyphemia (brad-ē-fē'mē-ă) [brady- + G. *phēmē,* speech]. Bradyphasia.

bradypnea (brad-ip-nē'ă, brad-ē-nē-ă) [brady- + G. *pnoē,* breathing]. Abnormal slowness of respiration, specifically a low respiratory frequency.

bradypragia (brad-ē-prā'jē-ă) [brady- + G. *prassō,* to do, act]. Sluggish action; slow movement.

bradypsychia (brad-ē-sī'kē-ă) [brady- + G. *psychē,* soul]. Slowness of mental reactions.

bradyrhythmia (brad-ē-rith'mē-ă). Bradycardia.

bradyspermatism (brad-ē-sper'mă-tizm). Absence of ejaculatory force, so that the semen trickles away slowly.

bradysphygmia (brad-ē-sfig'mē-ă) [brady-+ G. *sphygmos,* pulse]. Slowness of the pulse; can occur without bradycardia, as in ventricular bigeminy when every alternate beat may fail to produce a peripheral pulse.

bradystalsis (brad-ē-stahl'sis) [G. *bradys,* slow, + (*peri*) *stalsis,* contracting around]. Slow bowel motion.

bradyteleocinesia (brad'ē-tel-ē-ō-sin-ē'sē-ă) [brady- + G. *teleos,* complete, + *kinēsis,* movement]. Bradytelokinesis; sudden arrest of a movement just before its intended termination, then after a pause it is completed slowly or by jerks; a symptom of cerebellar disease.

bradyteleokinesis (brad'ē-tel-ē-ō-ki-nē'sis). Bradyteleocinesia.

bradytocia (brad-ē-tō'sē-ă) [brady- + G. *tokos,* childbirth]. Tedious labor; slow delivery.

bradyuria (brad-ē-yū'rē-ă) [brady- + G. *ouron,* urine]. Slow micturition.

bradyzoite (brad-ē-zō'īt) [brady- + G. *zōē,* life]. A slowly multiplying encysted form of sporozoan parasite typical of chronic infection with *Toxoplasma gondii.* It has also been called a merozoite or zoite; the complex of b.'s within an enclosing membrane has also been called a pseudocyst, though it is now regarded as a true cyst.

braille (brāl) [Louis *Braille,* French teacher of blind, 1809–1852]. A system of writing and printing by means of raised dots corresponding to letters, numbers, and punctuation to enable the blind to read by touch.

Brailsford, James Frederick, British radiologist, 1888–1961. See B.-Morquio *disease.*

Brain, W. Russell, Lord, British physician, 1895–1966. See B.'s *reflex.*

brain (brān) [A.S. *braegen*]. Encephalon; that part of the central nervous system contained within the cranium. See also encephalon. *Cf.* cerebrum; cerebellum.

abdominal b., *plexus* celiacus.

respirator b., a swollen and congested b. with necrotic and autolytic changes seen in patients who have been on a respirator for a day or longer.

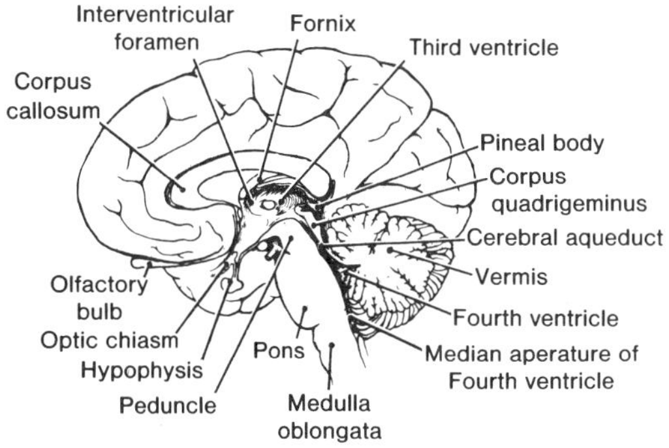

Parts of the Brain

Diagram of a brain which has been divided by a sagittal section between the hemispheres.

split b., a b. in which the corpus callosum and usually the anterior and posterior commissures have been sectioned.

visceral b., limbic *system.*

braincase (brān'kās). The cranium in its restricted sense, the part of the skull that encloses the brain; the neurocranium derived from membranous bone.

brainstem, brain stem (brān'stem). Originally, the entire unpaired subdivision of the brain, composed of (in anterior sequence) the rhombencephalon, mesencephalon, and diecephalon as distinguished from the brain's only paired subdivision, the telencephalon. More recently, the term's connotation has undergone several arbitrary modifications: some use it to denote no more than rhombencephalon plus mesencephalon, distinguishing that complex from the prosencephalon (diencephalon plus telencephalon); others restrict it even further to refer exclusively to the rhombencephalon. From both developmental and architectural viewpoints, the original interpretation seems preferable.

brainwashing (brān'wash'ing). Inducing a person to modify his attitudes and behavior in certain directions through various forms of pressure or torture.

bran. A by-product of the milling of wheat, containing approximately 20% of indigestible cellulose; a bulk cathartic, usually taken in the form of cereal or special bran products.

branch. Ramus; an offshoot; in anatomy, one of the primary divisions of a nerve or blood vessel. See ramus and subentries under arteria, nervus, and vena.

branchia, pl. **branchiae** (brang'kē-ă, -ē) [G. gill] [NA]. The gills, or organs of respiration, in water-living animals.

branchial (brang'kē-ăl). **1.** Relating to branchiae or gills. **2.** In embryology, denoting the various structures constituting the branchial *apparatus, q.v.*

branch'ing [Fr. *branche,* related to L. *branchium,* arm]. Dividing into parts; sending out offshoots; bifurcating.

false b., in bacteriology, the appearance of b. produced when a cell is pushed out of the general line of growth and develops a new line of growth while the remaining cells continue to develop along the original line of growth.

branchiogenic, branchiogenous (brang'kē-ō-jen'ik, -kē-oj'en-ŭs) [G. *branchia,* gill, *-gen,* to produce]. Originating from the branchial arches.

branchioma (brang-kē-ō'mă). A rare form of carcinoma that originates in remnants of epithelium in the branchial structures; most of the lesions occurring in this site are likely to be metastases from a primary neoplasm in another location.

branchiomere (brang'kē-ō-mēr) [G. *branchia,* gill, + *meros,* part].

An embryonic segment corresponding to one of the branchial arches.

branchiomerism (brang-kē-om'er-izm). Arrangement into branchiomeres.

branchiomotor (brang'kē-ō-mō'tōr). Relating to or controlling the movement of muscles derived from the branchial arches.

Brandt, M.L., U.S. obstetrician, *1894. See B.-Andrews *maneuver.*

bran'dy. Spiritus vini vitis; an alcoholic liquid obtained by the distillation of the fermented juice of sound ripe grapes and usually containing 48 to 54% ethyl alcohol.

Branham, H.H., 19th century U.S. surgeon. See B.'s *sign.*

Branhamella (bran-hă-mel'ă) [Sara *Branham*]. A subgenus of aerobic, nonmotile, nonsporeforming bacteria (family Neisseriaceae) containing Gram-negative cocci that occur in pairs with adjacent sides flattened; these organisms differ from those of the genus *Moraxella* and of other genera in the family by their DNA base content and composition. They occur in the mucous membranes of the upper respiratory tract. The type species is *B. catarrhalis.*

B. catarrha'lis, a species found in the mucous membranes of the respiratory tract of humans, occasionally causing disease; it is the type species of the genus *B.*

branny (bran'ē) [M.E. *bran,* broken coat of cereal grain]. Denoting desquamation of small husk-like scales.

Brasdor, Pierre, French surgeon, 1721–1798. See B.'s *method.*

Braun, Christopher Heinrich, German surgeon, 1847–1911. See B.'s *anastomosis.*

Braune, Christian W., German anatomist, 1831–1892. See B.'s *canal, muscle, valve.*

brawny (brahw'nē) [M.E. fleshy]. Thickening (lichenified) and dusky (a darkened hue), as of a swelling.

Braxton Hicks, John. See Hicks, John Braxton.

braxy (brak'sē) [Nor. *brad sot,* quick plague]. A fatal disease of sheep caused by *Clostridium septicum* and marked by inflammation of the abomasum and duodenum; symptoms preceding death in the less acute form are weakness, coma, and dyspnea.

German b., infectious necrotic *hepatitis* of sheep.

Bray, Charles William, U.S. otologist, *1904. See Wever-B. *phenomenon.*

brazilein (bră-zil'ē-in). $C_6H_{12}O_5$; a red oxidation product of brazilin.

brazilin (bră-zil'in) [C.I. 75280]. A red natural dye, $C_{16}H_{14}O_5$, obtained from the bark of several species of tropical trees and oxidized to the active red dye brazilein; resembles hematoxylin in origin, chemistry, and usage; used as a nuclear stain and as an indicator (red in alkalies, yellow in acids).

brazing (brā'zing). In dentistry, soldering.

BrDu Abbreviation for bromodeoxyuridine.

breakoff (brāk'awf). A feeling of physical separation from the earth when piloting an aircraft at high altitude.

breakthrough (brāk'thrū). A sudden manifestation of new and more constructive attitudes following a period of resistance during psychotherapy.

breast (brest) [A.S. *breōst*]. **1.** The anterior surface of the thorax. **2.** Mamma.

accessory b., *mamma* accessoria.

caked b., stagnation *mastitis.*

chicken b., *pectus* carinatum.

funnel b., *pectus* excavatum.

irritable b., swelling and induration of the b., not due to a neoplasm, and usually of comparatively brief duration.

male b., *mamma* masculina.

pigeon b., *pectus* carinatum.

breath (breth) [A.S. *braeth*]. **1.** The respired air. **2.** An inspiration.

uremic b., characteristic odor of the b. in patients with chronic renal failure, variously described as "fishy," "ammoniacal," and "fetid," which is indicative of the systemic accumulation of volatile metabolites, usually excreted by the kidneys; dimethylamine and trimethylamine have been identified and correlated with the classic fishy odor.

breath-holding (breth'hōld-ing). Voluntary or involuntary cessation of breathing, usually in the inspiratory position and in young children as a psychogenic effect.

breathing (brēdh'ing). Pneusis; inhalation and exhalation of air or gaseous mixtures.

apneustic b., a series of slow, deep inspirations, each one held for 30 to 90 seconds, after which the air is suddenly expelled by the elastic recoil of the lung.

Biot's b., Biot's *respiration.*

bronchial b., breath sounds of a harsh or blowing quality, heard on auscultation of the chest, made by air moving in the large bronchi and barely if at all modified by the intervening lung; duration of the expiratory sound is as long as or longer than that of the inspiratory sound, and its pitch as high as or higher than that of the inspiratory sound; may be heard over a consolidated lung, over a pulmonary cavity, and, rarely, above a pleural effusion due to an underlying compressed lung. Whispered pectoriloquy is another manifestation that usually can be elicited when bronchial b. is present.

continuous positive pressure b. (CPPB), controlled mechanical *ventilation.*

glossopharyngeal b., respiration unaided by the usual primary muscles of respiration; the air is forced into the lungs by use of the tongue and muscles of the pharynx.

intermittent positive pressure b. (IPPB), controlled mechanical *ventilation.*

mouth b., habitual respiration through the mouth instead of the nose, usually due to obstruction of the nasal airways; believed to be a contributing factor in malocclusion and gingival irritation.

positive-negative pressure b. (PNPB), inflation of the lungs with positive pressure and deflation with negative pressure by an automatic ventilator.

pursed lips b., a technique in which air is inhaled slowly through the nose and mouth and exhaled slowly through pursed lips; used by patients with chronic obstructive pulmonary disease to improve their breathing by controlling the rate and depth of respiration.

shallow b., a type of b. with abnormally low tidal volume.

Breda, Achille, Italian dermatologist, 1850–1933. See B.'s *disease.*

bredouillement (brā-dwē-mahn') [Fr.]. Omission of parts of words related to extremely rapid speech.

breech (brēch) [A.S. *brēc*]. Nates.

breeding (brēd'ing). Selected mating of individuals to produce a desired strain. See also hybridization; linebreeding; inbreeding.

bregma (breg'mă) [G. the forepart of the head] [NA]. The point on the skull corresponding to the junction of the coronal and sagittal sutures.

bregmatic (breg-mat'ik). Relating to the bregma.

brei (brī) [Ger. pulp]. A fine mince or mush of tissue in which the cells are for the most part intact. *Cf.* homogenate.

bremsstrahlung (bremz'strah-lŭng) [Ger. *Bremsstrahlung,* braking radiation]. Continuous spectrum radiation produced by the interaction of a beam of electrons and the nuclei which scatter them.

Brenn, Lena, 20th century U.S. researcher. See Brown-B. *stain.*

Brenner, Fritz, German pathologist, *1877. See B. *tumor.*

brepho- [G. *brephos,* embryo or newborn infant]. Rarely used prefix denoting a primitive stage of development.

Breschet (Brechet), Gilbert, French anatomist, 1784–1845. See

B.'s *bones, canals, hiatus, sinus, veins.*

Brescia, Michael J., U.S. nephrologist, *1933. See B.-Cimino *fistula.*

Breslow, Alexander, U.S. pathologist, 1928–1980. See B.'s *thickness.*

bretylium tosylate (bre-til'ē-ŭm). (*o*-Bromobenzyl)ethyldimethylammonium *p*-toluenesulfonate; a sympatholytic agent that prevents the release of norepinephrine from the nerve ending; used in the treatment of essential hypertension.

Breuer, Josef, Austrian internist 1842–1925. See Hering-B. *reflex.*

Breus, Carl, Austrian obstetrician, 1852–1914. See B. *mole.*

brevicollis (brev-ē-kol'is) [L. *brevis,* short, + *collum,* neck]. Abnormal shortness of the neck.

Brewer, George E., U.S. surgeon, 1861–1939. See B.'s infarct.

Bricker, Eugene M., U.S. urologist, *1908. See B. *operation.*

Brickner, Walter M., U.S. surgeon, 1876–1930. See B.'s *position.*

bridge (bridj). **1.** The upper part of the ridge of the nose formed by the nasal bones. **2.** One of the threads of protoplasm that appears to pass from one cell to another. **3.** Fixed partial *denture.*

arteriolovenular b., the largest capillary connecting arteriole to venule.

cell b.'s, intercellular b.'s.

cytoplasmic b.'s, intercellular b.'s.

Gaskell's b., *truncus* atrioventricularis.

intercellular b.'s, cell or cytoplasmic b.'s; slender cytoplasmic strands connecting adjacent cells; in histological sections of the epidermis and other stratified squamous epithelia, the b.'s are processes attached by a desmosome and are shrinkage artifacts of fixation; true b.'s with cytoplasmic confluence exist between incompletely divided germ cells.

myocardial b., a b. of cardiac muscle fibers extending over the epicardial aspect of a coronary artery; this finding, in cases of sudden unexpected death, has led to speculation that cardiac contraction during exertion could constrict the coronary artery.

removable b., removable partial *denture.*

Wheatstone's b., an apparatus for measuring electrical resistance; four resistors are connected to form the four sides or "arms" of a square; a voltage is applied to one diagonal pair of connections, while the voltage between the other diagonal pair is measured, *e.g.,* by a galvanometer; the bridge is "balanced" when the measured voltage is zero; then, the ratios of the two pairs of adjoining resistances must be identical.

bridgework (bridj'wŏrk). Partial *denture.*

bridle (brī'dl). **1.** Frenum. **2.** A band of fibrous material stretching across the surface of an ulcer or other lesion or forming adhesions between opposing serous or mucous surfaces.

b. of clitoris, *frenulum* clitoridis.

Bright, Richard, British internist and pathologist, 1789–1858. See B.'s *disease.*

Brill, Nathan E., U.S. physician, 1860–1925. See B.'s *disease,* B.-Symmers *disease,* B.-Zinsser *disease.*

bril'liant cres'yl blue. See cresyl blue.

bril'liant green [C.I. 42040]. Ethyl green; the sulfate of di-(*p*-diethylamino)-triphenyl carbinolanhydride. An indicator dye that changes from yellow to green at pH 0.0 to 2.6; also used as a topical antiseptic and as a selective bacteriostatic agent in culture media.

bril'liant vi'tal red. Vital red.

bril'liant yel'low [C.I. 13085]. An indicator dye that changes from yellow to orange or red at pH 6.4 to 8.0.

brim. The upper edge or rim of a hollow structure.

pelvic b., *apertura* pelvis superior.

brimstone (brim'stōn) [A.S. *brinnan,* to burn]. Sulfur.

brindle (brin'dl) [diminutive of O.E. *brinded*]. A hair coat color in which there is a uniform mixture of gray or tawny hairs with others of white or black; a composite color.

Brinell, Johan A., Swedish metallurgist, 1849–1925. See B. hardness *number.*

Briquet, Paul, French physician, 1796–1881. See B.'s *ataxia, syndrome.*

brisement forcé (briz-mon'fōr-sā') [Fr. forcible breaking]. Forcible manipulation, usually under anesthesia, in which the position of a deformed limb is corrected by tearing the soft tissue and crushing the bone, as in a once popular but no longer used correction for club foot deformities.

bris'ket [O.E. *brusket*]. The part of a beef animal (sometimes used of other species) that constitutes the caudoventral part of the neck and lies cranially to and between the forelimbs of the animal.

Brissaud, Edouard, French physician, 1852–1909. See B.'s *disease, infantilism, reflex;* B.-Marie *syndrome.*

British anti-Lewisite (BAL) (brit'ish an-tē-lū'is-īt). Dimercaprol.

British Pharmacopoeia (BP). See Pharmacopeia.

broach (brōch). A dental instrument for removing the pulp of a tooth or exploring the canal.

barbed b., a root canal instrument set with barbs; used for removing a dental pulp, pulp tissue remnants, or dentinal debris.

smooth b., an exploring instrument used in endodontic practice; a root canal tine.

Broadbent, Sir William H., British physician, 1835– 1907. See B.'s *law, sign;* Bolton-B. *plane.*

broad-spectrum. See under spectrum.

Broca, Pierre P., French surgeon, neurologist, and anthropologist, 1824–1880. See B.'s *angles, aphasia, area,* parolfactory *area,* diagonal *band, center, field, fissure, formula,* visual *plane, pouch.*

Brock, Sir Russell C., British surgeon, *1903. See B.'s *knife, syndrome;* B. *operation.*

Brockenbrough, E.C., U.S. surgeon, *1930. See B. *sign.*

Brocq, Louis A.J. French dermatologist, 1856–1928. See B.'s *disease.*

brocresine (brō-krē'sēn). α-(Aminooxy)-6-bromo-*m*-cresol; a histidine decarboxylase inhibitor.

Brödel, Max, German medical artist in the U. S., 1870–1941. See B.'s bloodless *line.*

Brodie, Sir Benjamin C., British surgeon, 1783–1862. See B.'s *abscess, bursa, disease, knee.*

Brodie, Charles Gordon, Scottish anatomist and surgeon, 1860–1933. See B.'s *ligament.*

Brodie, Thomas Gregor, British physiologist, 1866–1916. See B. *fluid.*

Brodmann, Korbinian, German neurologist, 1868–1918. See B.'s *areas.*

Broesike, Gustav, German anatomist, *1853. See B.'s *fossa.*

brom-, bromo- [G. *brōmos,* a stench]. Prefixes most commonly indicating the presence of bromine in a compound.

bromate (brō'māt). Salt or anion of bromic acid.

bromated (brō'māt-ĕd). Brominated; combined or saturated with bromine or any of its compounds.

bromazepam (brō-mā'zĕ-pam). 7-Bromo-1,3-dihydro-5-(2-pyridinyl)-2*H*-1,4-benzodiazepin-2-one; an antianxiety agent.

bromazine hydrochloride (brō-mă-zēn). Bromodiphenhydramine hydrochloride.

bromcresol green (brom-krē'sol). A substituted triphenylmethane dye (MW 698, pK 4.7), sparingly soluble in water but readily soluble in alcohol, ether, and ethyl acetate; used as an indicator of pH (yellow at pH 3.8, blue-green at pH 5.4).

bromcresol purple. A substituted triphenylmethane dye (MW 540, pK 6.3), practically insoluble in water but soluble in alcohol and dilute alkalies; used as an indicator of pH (yellow at pH 5.2, purple at pH 6.8).

bromelain, bromelin (brō'mĕ-lān, -lin) [C. *Bromelius (Bromel),* Swedish botanist, 1639–1705] [EC 3.4.22.4]. One of a group of peptide hydrolases, a cysteine proteinase, obtained from pineapple; used in tenderizing meats and in producing hydrolysates of proteins; orally administered in the treatment of inflammation and edema of soft tissues associated with traumatic injury.

bromhexine hydrochloride (brom-hek'sēn). 3,5-Dibromo-N^{α}-cyclohexyl-N^{α}-methyltoluene-α,2-diamine hydrochloride; an expectorant with mucolytic, antitussive, and bronchodilator properties.

bromhidrosis (brom-hi-drō'sis). Bromidrosis.

bromic (brō'mik). Relating to bromine; denoting especially bromic acid, $HBrO_3$.

bromide (brō'mīd). The anion Br^-; salt of hydrogen bromide (HBr).

bromidrosiphobia (brō'mi-drō-si-fō'bē-ă) [bromidrosis + G. *phobos,* fear]. Morbid fear of giving forth a bad odor from the body, sometimes with the belief that such an odor is present.

bromidrosis (brōm-i-drō'sis) [G. *brōmos,* a stench, + *hidrōs,* perspiration]. Bromhidrosis; osmidrosis; ozochrotia; fetid or foul smelling perspiration.

brominated (brō'min-āt-ĕd). Bromated.

bromindione (brō-min-dī'ōn). 2-(*p*-Bromophenyl)-1,3-indandione; an oral anticoagulant.

bromine (brō'mēn, -min) [Fr. *brome,* bromine, fr. G. *bromos,* stench]. Bromum; a nonmetallic, reddish, volatile, liquid element; symbol Br, atomic no. 35, atomic weight, 79.9; valences 1 to 7 inclusive; it unites with hydrogen to form hydrobromic acid, and this reacts with many metals to form bromides, some of which are used in medicine.

bromism, brominism (brō'mizm, -min-izm). Chronic bromide intoxication, characterized by headache, drowsiness, confusion and occasionally violent delirium, muscular weakness, cardiac depression, an acneform eruption, foul breath, anorexia, and gastric distress.

bromisovalum (brōm-i-sō-val'ŭm). A nonbarbiturate sedative and hypnotic.

bromo-. See brom-.

bromocresol green (brō-mō-krē'sol). Tetrabromo-m-cresolsulfonphthalein; an indicator dye changing from yellow to blue at pH 4.7; used to track DNA in agarose electrophoresis, and in a dye-binding method for analysis of serum albumin.

bromocriptine (brō-mō-krip'tēn). 2-Bromo-α-ergocryptine; an ergot derivative which slows dopamine turnover, inhibits prolactin secretion and release of prolactin by thyrotropin-releasing hormone, and retards tumor growth and hence is used in the treatment of hyperprolactinemia associated with various pituitary tumors.

bromodeoxyuridine (BrDu) (brō'mō-dē-ok'sē-yūr'i-dēn). A compound that competes with uridine for incorporation in RNA and fluoresces in ultraviolet light; used in BrDu-banding.

bromoderma (brō-mō-der'mă) [bromide + G. *derma,* skin]. An acneform or granulomatous eruption due to hypersensitivity to bromide.

bromodiphenhydramine hydrochloride (brō'mō-dī-fen-hī'dră-mēn). Bromazine hydrochloride; 2-(*p*-bromo-α-phenylbenzyloxy)-*N,N*-dimethylethylamine hydrochloride; an antihistamine that may cause drowsiness and xerostomia.

bromohyperhidrosis, bro'mohy'peridro'sis (brō'mō-hī'per-hi-drō'sis, -hī'per-i-drō'sis) [G. *brōmos,* a stench, + *hyper,* over, + *hidrōsis,* sweating]. Excessive secretion of sweat having a fetid odor.

bromophenol blue (brō-mō-fē'nol). Bromphenol blue.

bromopnea (brō-mop-nē'ă) [G. *brōmos,* a stench, + *pnoē,* breath]. Obsolete term for halitosis.

bromosulfophthalein (brō'mō-sŭl'fō-thal'ē-in). Sulfobromophthalein sodium.

5-bromouracil (brō-mō-yū'ră-sil). Synthetic analogue (antimetabolite) of thymine, in which a bromine atom takes the place of the methyl group in thymine.

brompheniramine maleate (brōm-fen-ir'ă-mēn). 2-[*p*-Bromo-α-(2-dimethylaminoethyl)benzyl]pyridine maleate; a potent antihistaminic agent.

bromphenol blue (brom-fē-nol). Bromophenol blue; a substituted triphenylmethane dye (MW 670, pK 4.0), used as an acid-base indicator (yellow at pH less than 3.1, blue at pH more than 4.7); also used for histochemical and electrophoretic demonstration of proteins.

bromsulfophthalein (brom-sŭl'fō-thal'ē-in). Sulfobromophthalein sodium.

bromthymol blue (brom-thī'mol). A substituted triphenylmethane dye (MW 624, pK 7.0), used primarily as a hydrogen ion indicator (yellow at pH 6.0, blue at pH 7.6); also a weak but toxic vital stain.

bromum (brō'mŭm). Bromine.

broncatar (bron'kă-tar). Camphoric acid compound (neutralized) with 2-amino-2-thiazoline (1:2); an antitussive and respiratory stimulant.

bronch-, bronchi-. See broncho-.

bronchi (brong'kī). Plural of bronchus.

bronchi-. See broncho-.

bronchia (brong'kē-ă) [G. pl. of *bronchion,* dim. of *bronchos,* trachea]. Bronchial *tubes;* the smaller divisions of the bronchi. See also bronchus; bronchiolus.

bronchial (brong'kē-ăl). Relating to the bronchi.

bronchiectasia (brong'kē-ek-tā'zē-ă). Bronchiectasis.
b. sicca, dry *bronchiectasis.*

bronchiectasic (brong-kē-ek-tā'zik). Bronchiectatic.

bronchiectasis (brong-kē-ek'tă-sis) [bronchi- + G. *ektasis,* a stretching]. Bronchiectasia; chronic dilation of bronchi or bronchioles as a sequel of inflammatory disease or obstruction.
cylindrical b., b. resulting in dilated bronchi of cylindrical shape; *i.e.,* of uniform caliber.
dry b., bronchiectasia sicca; b. characterized by lack of productive cough and by occasional hemoptysis.
saccular b., b. resulting in dilated bronchi of saccular or irregular shape.

bronchiectatic (brong-kē-ek-tat'ik). Bronchiectasic; relating to bronchiectasis.

bronchiloquy (brong-kil'ō-kwē) [bronchi- + L. *loquor,* to speak]. Bronchophony.

bronchiocele (brong'kē-ō-sēl). Bronchocele.

bronchiogenic (brong-kē-ō-jen'ik). Bronchogenic; of bronchial origin; emanating from the bronchi.

bronchiole (brong'kē-ōl). Bronchiolus.
respiratory b.'s, *bronchioli* respiratorii.
terminal b., bronchiolus terminalis; the end of the conducting airway; the lining is simple columnar or cuboidal epithelium without mucous goblet cells; most of the cells are ciliated, but a few nonciliated serious secreting cells occur.

bronchiolectasia (brong'kē-ō-lek-tā'zē-ă). Bronchiolectasis.

bronchiolectasis (brong'kē-ō-lek'tă-sis) [bronchiole + G. *ektasis,* a stretching]. Bronchiolectasia; bronchiectasis involving the bronchioles.

bronchioli (brong-kē'ō-lī). Plural of bronchiolus.

bronchiolitis (brong-kē-ō-lī'tis) [bronchiole + *-itis,* inflammation]. Inflammation of the bronchioles, often associated with bronchopneumonia.
exudative b., inflammation of the bronchioles, with fibrinous exudation.
b. fibro'sa oblit'erans, obstruction of bronchioles, especially terminal bronchioles, by fibrous granulation tissue arising from ulcerated mucosa; the condition may follow inhalation of irritant gases, or may complicate pneumonia.
proliferative b., b. with obliteration of bronchiolar lumen and alveoli by epithelial proliferation, which may follow influenza and giant-cell pneumonia.

bronchiolo- [L. *bronchiolus*]. Combining form relating to the bronchiole.

bronchiolopulmonary (brong'kē-ōlō-pul'mō-nār-ē). Relating to the bronchioles and the lungs.

bronchiolus, pl. bronchioli (brong-kē'ō-lŭs, -ō-lī) [Mod. L. dim. of *bronchus*] [NA]. Bronchiole; one of the finer subdivisions of the bronchi, less than 1 mm in diameter, and having no cartilage in its wall, but relatively abundant smooth muscle and elastic fibers.
bronchi'oli respirato'rii [NA], respiratory bronchioles; the smallest bronchioles (0.5 mm in diameter) that connect the terminal bronchioles to alveolar ducts; alveoli rise from part of the wall.
b. termina'lis, terminal *bronchiole.*

bronchiostenosis (brong'kē-ō-sten-ō'sis). Narrowing of the lumen of a bronchial tube.

bronchitic (brong-kit'ik). Relating to bronchitis.

bronchitis (brong-kī'tis). Inflammation of the mucous membrane of the bronchial tubes.
asthmatic b., b. which causes or aggravates bronchospasm.
Castellani's b., hemorrhagic b.
chronic b., a condition of the bronchial tree characterized by cough, hypersecretion of mucus, and expectoration of sputum over a long period of time, associated with frequent bronchial infection; usually due to inhalation, over a prolonged period, of air contaminated by dust or by noxious gases of combustion.
croupous b., fibrinous b.
fibrinous b., pseudomembranous, croupous, or plastic b.; inflammation of the bronchial mucous membrane, accompanied by a fibrinous exudation which often forms a cast of the bronchial tree with severe obstruction of air flow.
hemorrhagic b., Castellani's b.; bronchopulmonary spirochetosis; bronchospirochetosis; chronic b. due to infection with spirochetes (though other bacteria are usually present and contribute to the infection) and characterized by cough and bloody sputum.
infectious avian b., gasping disease; a specific infectious disease of young birds, caused by infectious bronchitis virus and associated with blocking of respiratory passages by exudate; it is highly transmissible, and often causes heavy losses of young chicks and heavy production losses among older laying birds.
obliterative b., b. oblit'erans, fibrinous b. in which the exudate is not expectorated but becomes organized, obliterating the affected portion of the bronchial tubes with consequent permanent collapse of affected portions of the lung.
plastic b., fibrinous b.
pseudomembranous b., fibrinous b.
putrid b., b. accompanied by an expectoration of foul-smelling sputum.
verminous b., hoose; b. and bronchopneumonia caused by invasion of the bronchi by lungworms; occurs commonly in cattle, swine, and sheep, but rarely in other species.

bronchium, pl. **bronchia** (brong'kē-ŭm, brong'kē-ă) [Mod. L. fr. G. *bronchion*]. Bronchus.

broncho-, bronch-, bronchi- [G. *bronchos,* windpipe]. Combining form denoting bronchus, and, in ancient usage, the trachea.

bronchoalveolar (brong'kō-al-vē'ō-lăr). Bronchovesicular.

bronchocavernous (brong-kō-kav'er-nŭs). Relating to a bronchus or bronchial tube and a pulmonary pathologic cavity.

bronchocele (brong'kō-sēl) [broncho- + G. *kēlē,* hernia]. Bronchiocele; a circumscribed dilation of a bronchus.

bronchoconstriction (brong-kō-kon-strik'shŭn). Reduction in the caliber of a bronchus or bronchi.

bronchoconstrictor (brong-kō-kon-strik'ter, -tōr). **1.** Causing a reduction in caliber of a bronchus or bronchial tube. **2.** An agent that possesses this action.

bronchodilatation (brong'kō-dil-ă-tā'shŭn). Increase in caliber of the bronchi and bronchioles in response to pharmacologically active substances or autonomic nervous activity.

bronchodilation (brong'kō-dīlā'shŭn). **1.** Alternative spelling for bronchodilatation. **2.** Rarely used term for bronchiectasis.

bronchodilator (brong-kō-dī-lā'ter, -tōr). **1.** Causing an increase in caliber of a bronchus or bronchial tube. **2.** An agent that possesses this power.

bronchoedema (brong'kō-ĕ-dē'mă). Swelling of the mucosa of the bronchi.

bronchoesophagology (brong'kō-ē-sof-ă-gol'ō-jē) [broncho- + G. *oisophagos,* esophagus, + *logos,* study]. The specialty concerned with the diagnosis and treatment of diseases of the tracheobronchial tree and esophagus by endoscope and other means.

bronchoesophagoscopy (brong'kō-ē-sof-ă-gos'kō-pē). Examination of the tracheobronchial tree or esophagus through appropriate endoscopes.

bronchofiberscope (brong-kō-fī'ber-skōp). A fiberoptic endoscope particularly adapted for visualization of the trachea and bronchi.

bronchogenic (brong-kō-jen'ik). Bronchiogenic.

bronchogram (brong'kō-gram). The radiograph obtained at bronchography.

bronchography (brong-kog'ră-fē) [broncho- + G. *graphē,* a drawing]. Radiographic examination of the tracheobronchial tree following the injection of one of several radiopaque materials.

broncholith (brong'kō-lith) [broncho- + G. *lithos,* stone]. Bronchial calculus; a hard concretion in a bronchus or bronchial tube.

broncholithiasis (brong'kō-li-thī'ă-sis). Bronchial inflammation or obstruction caused by broncholiths.

bronchomalacia (brong'kō-mă-lā'shē-ă) [broncho- + G. *malakia,* a softening]. Degeneration of elastic and connective tissue of bronchi and trachea.

bronchomotor (brong-kō-mō'ter). **1.** Causing a change in caliber, dilation, or contraction of a bronchus or bronchiole. **2.** An agent possessing this action.

bronchomycosis (brong'kō-mī-kō'sis) [broncho- + G. *mykēs,* fungus]. Any fungus disease of the bronchial tubes or bronchi.

bronchophony (brong-kof'ō-nē) [broncho- + G. *phōnē,* voice]. Bronchiloquy; bronchial voice; increased intensity and clarity of voice sounds heard over a bronchus surrounded by consolidated lung tissue. See also tracheophony.
whispered b., whispering *pectoriloquy.*

bronchoplasty (brong'kō-plas-tē) [broncho- + G. *plastos,* formed]. Surgical alteration of the configuration of a bronchus.

bronchopneumonia (brong'ko-nu-mo'nī-ah). Bronchial pneumonia; acute inflammation of the walls of the smaller bronchial tubes, with varying amounts of pulmonary consolidation due to spread of the inflammation into peribronchiolar alveoli and the alveolar ducts; may become confluent or may be hemorrhagic.

tuberculous b., an acute form of pulmonary tuberculosis characterized by widespread patchy consolidations.

bronchopulmonary (brong-kō-pul'mō-nār-ē). Relating to the bronchi tubes and the lungs.

bronchorrhaphy (brong-kōr'ă-fē) [broncho- + G. *raphē,* a seam]. Suture of a wound of the bronchus.

bronchorrhea (brong'kō-rē'ă) [broncho- + G. *rhoia,* a flow]. Excessive secretion of mucus from the bronchial mucous membrane.

bronchoscope (brong'kō-skōp) [broncho- + G. *skopeō,* to view]. An endoscope for inspecting the interior of the tracheobronchial tree, either for diagnostic purposes (including biopsy) or for the removal of foreign bodies.

bronchoscopy (brong-kos'kō-pē). Inspection of the interior of the tracheobronchial tree through a bronchoscope.

bronchospasm (brong'kō-spazm). Contraction of smooth muscle in the walls of the bronchi and bronchioles, causing narrowing of the lumen.

bronchospirochetosis (brong'kō-spī'rō-kē-tō'sis). Hemorrhagic *bronchitis.*

bronchospirography (brong'kō-spī-rog'ră-fē) [broncho- + L. *spiro,* to breathe, + G. *graphō,* to write]. Use of a single lumen endobronchial tube for measurement of ventilatory function of one lung.

bronchospirometer (brong'kō-spī-rom'ĕ-ter) [broncho- + L. *spiro,* to breathe, + G. *metron,* measure]. A device for measurement of rates and volumes of air flow into each lung separately, using a double lumen endobronchial tube.

bronchospirometry (brong'kō-spī-rom'ĕ-trē). Use of a bronchospirometer to measure ventilatory function of each lung separately.

bronchostaxis (brong'kō-stak'sis) [broncho- + G. *staxis,* a dripping]. Hemorrhage from the bronchi.

bronchostenosis (brong-kō-sten-ō'sis). Chronic narrowing of a bronchus.

bronchostomy (brong-kos'tō-mē) [broncho- + G. *stoma,* mouth]. Surgical formation of a new opening into a bronchus.

bronchotome (brong'kō-tōm) [broncho- + G. *tomē,* a cutting]. An instrument for incising a bronchus.

bronchotomy (brong-kot'ō-mē). Incision of a bronchus.

bronchotracheal (brong-kō-trā'kē-ăl). Relating to the trachea and bronchi.

bronchovesicular (brong'kō-vĕ-sik'yū-lăr). Bronchoalveolar; relating to the bronchioles and alveoli in the lungs.

bronchus, pl. bronchi (brong'kŭs, brong'kī) [Mod. L., fr. G. *bronchos,* windpipe] [NA]. One of the subdivisions of the trachea serving to convey air to and from the lungs. The trachea divides into right and left main bronchi which in turn form lobar, segmental, and subsegmental bronchi. In structure, the intrapulmonary bronchi have a lining of pseudostratified ciliated columnar epithelium, and a lamina propria with abundant longitudinal networks of elastic fibers; there are spirally arranged bundles of smooth muscle, abundant mucoserous glands, and in the outer part of the wall irregular plates of hyaline cartilage.

eparterial b., obsolete term for the right superior lobe b. which passes above the right pulmonary artery.

hyparterial bronchi, obsolete term for those bronchi which pass below the pulmonary arteries, *i.e.,* right middle and inferior lobar bronchi and left superior and inferior lobar bronchi.

intermediate b., b. intermedius, the portion of the right main b. between the upper lobe b. and the origin of the middle and inferior lobe bronchi.

left main b., b. principalis sinister.

lobar bronchi, bronchi lobares.

bronchi loba'res [NA], lobar bronchi; the divisions of the main bronchi that supply the lobes of the lungs; **b. lobaris superior, b. lobaris medius,** and **b. lobaris inferior** are the three lobar bronchi on the right; **b. lobaris superior** and **b. lobaris inferior** are the two on the left. The lobar bronchi divide into segmental bronchi.

primary b., the main b. arising at the tracheal bifurcation and extending into the developing lung of the embryo.

b. principa'lis dex'ter [NA], right main b.; it arises at the bifurcation of the trachea and enters the hilum of the right lung, giving off the superior lobe b. and continuing downward to give off the middle and inferior lobe bronchi.

b. principa'lis sinis'ter [NA], left main b.; it arises at the bifurcation of the trachea, passes in front of the esophagus and enters the hilum of the left lung where it divides into a superior lobe b. and an inferior lobe b.

right main b., b. principalis dexter.

segmental b., b. segmentalis.

b. segmenta'lis [NA], segmental b.; one of the divisions of a lobar b. that supplies a bronchopulmonary segment. In the right lung there are commonly ten: *in the superior lobe,* b. segmentalis apicalis, b. segmentalis posterior, b. segmentalis anterior; *in the middle lobe,* b. segmentalis lateralis, b. segmentalis medialis; *in the inferior lobe,* b. segmentalis apicalis or superior, b. segmentalis basalis medialis or cardiacus, b. segmentalis basalis anterior, b. segmentalis basalis lateralis, b. segmentalis basalis posterior. In the left lung there are commonly nine: *in the superior lobe,* b. segmentalis apicoposterior, b. segmentalis anterior, b. lingularis superior, b. lingularis inferior; *in the inferior lobe,* b. segmentalis apicalis or superior, b. segmentalis basalis medialis or cardiacus, b. segmentalis basalis anterior, b. segmentalis basalis lateralis, b. segmentalis basalis posterior.

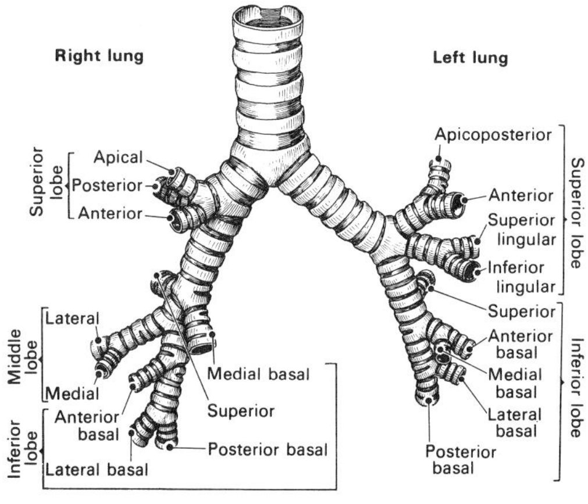

Segmental Bronchi

stem b., the main b. from which the branches of the bronchial tree arise.

Brønsted, Johannes N., Danish physical chemist, 1879–1947. See B. *base, theory.*

brontophobia (bront-ō-fō'bē-ă) [G. *brontē,* thunder, + *phobos,* fear]. Tonitrophobia; morbid fear of thunder.

brood (brūd). **1.** Litter (2). **2.** To ponder anxiously; to meditate morbidly.

Brooke, Bryan N., British surgeon, *1915. See B. *ileostomy.*

Brooke, Henry A.G., British dermatologist, 1854–1919. See B.'s *disease, tumor.*

broom (brūm). Scoparius.

brow [A.S. *brū*]. **1.** The eyebrow. See supercilium. **2.** Frons.

brow'lift. Operation to elevate the eyebrows and thereby remove excess skin folds or fullness in the upper eyelids.

Brown, Harold W., U.S. ophthalmologist, *1898. See B.'s *syndrome.*

Brown, James B., U.S. plastic surgeon, 1899–1971. See Blair-B. *graft;* B.-Adson *forceps.*

Brown, James H., U.S. microbiologist, *1884. See B.-Brenn *stain.*

Brown, Robert, British botanist, 1773–1858. See brownian *motion; movement;* brownian-Zsigmondy *movement.*

Browne, Sir Denis John, British surgeon, *1892. See Denis B. *pouch, splint.*

brownian (brown'ē-ăn). Relating to or described by Robert Brown.

Browning, William, U.S. anatomist and neurologist, 1855–1941. See B.'s *vein.*

Brown-Séquard, Charles E., French physiologist and neurologist, 1817–1894. See B.-S.'s *paralysis, syndrome.*

Brucella (brū-sel'lă) [Sir David *Bruce,* British surgeon, 1855–1931]. A genus of encapsulated, nonmotile bacteria (family Brucellaceae) containing short, rod-shaped to coccoid, Gram-negative cells. These organisms do not produce gas from carbohydrates, are parasitic, invading all animal tissues and causing infection of the genital organs, the mammary gland, and the respiratory and intestinal tracts, and are pathogenic for man and various species of domestic animals. The type species is *B. melitensis.*

B. abor'tus, Bang's bacillus; abortus bacillus; a species that causes abortion in cows (bovine brucellosis), mares, and sheep, undulant fever in man, and a wasting disease in chickens.

B. ca'nis, a species causing epididymitis, brucellosis, and abortion in dogs; occasionally causes mild human disease.

B. meliten'sis, a species that causes brucellosis in man, abortion in goats, and a wasting disease in chickens; it may infect cows and hogs and be excreted in their milk; it is the type species of the genus *B.*

B. su'is, a species causing abortion in swine, brucellosis in man, and a wasting disease in chickens; may also infect horses, dogs, cows, monkeys, goats, and laboratory animals.

Brucellaceae (brū-sel-ā'sē-ē). A family of bacteria (order Eubacteriales) containing small, coccoid to rod-shaped, Gram-negative cells which occur singly, in pairs, in short chains, or in groups. The cells may or may not show bipolar staining. Motile and nonmotile species occur; motile cells are peritrichous. V (phosphopyridine nucleotide) and/or X (hemin) factors are sometimes required for growth. Blood serum may be required or may enhance growth. Increased carbon dioxide tension may also favor growth, especially on primary isolation. These organisms are parasites and pathogens which affect warm-blooded animals, including man, rarely cold-blooded animals. It was formerly called Parvobacteriaceae. The type genus is *Brucella.*

brucellergin (brū-sel'er-jin). A fat-free nucleoprotein antigen derived from brucella; used in skin tests for brucellosis.

brucellin (brū-sel'in). A vaccine prepared from several species of *Brucella;* formerly thought to prevent or cure brucellosis.

brucellosis (brū-sel-ō'sis). Malta or undulant fever; Mediterranean fever (1); an infectious disease caused by *Brucella,* characterized by fever, sweating, weakness, aches, and pains, and transmitted to man by direct contact with diseased animals or through ingestion of infested meat, milk, or cheese, and particularly hazardous to veterinarians, farmers, and slaughterhouse workers; although some crossing over by species may occur, *Brucella melitensis, B. abortus, B. canis,* and *B. suis* characteristically affect goats, cattle, dogs, and swine, respectively.

bovine b., bovine infectious abortion; contagious abortion; Bang's disease; a disease in cattle caused by *Brucella abortus;* in pregnant cows, characterized by abortion late in pregnancy, followed by retained placenta and metritis; in bulls, orchitis and epididymitis may occur; the organism may localize in the udder and thus appear in milk from infected cows.

Bruch, Carl W.L., German anatomist, 1819–1884. See B.'s *glands, membrane.*

brucine (brū-sēn, -in) [J. *Bruce*]. Dimethoxystrychnine; an alkaloid from *Strychnos nux-vomica* and *S. ignatii* (family Loganiaceae), that produces paralysis of sensory nerves and peripheral motor nerves; the convulsive action which is characteristic of strychnine is almost entirely absent; used as a local anodyne and tonic.

Bruck, Alfred, German physician, *1865. See B.'s *disease.*

Brücke, Ernst W. von, Austrian physiologist, 1819–1892. See B.'s *muscle, tunic;* B.-Bartley *phenomenon.*

Brudzinski, Josef von, Polish physician, 1874–1917. See B.'s *sign.*

Brugia (brū'jē-ă). A genus of filarial worms transmitted by mosquitoes to man, primates, felid carnivores, and a number of other mammals.

B. mala'yi, the Malayan filaria species, an important agent of human filariasis and elephantiasis in Southeast Asia and Indonesia, transmitted to man by species of *Mansonia* and *Anopheles* mosquitoes; adult parasites cause lymphangitis and lymphadenitis, but there is less involvement of the genital region and lower extremities, and a relatively greater incidence of disease in the upper extremities than with *Wuchereria bancrofti* infection. Formerly called *Wuchereria malayi.*

Brugsch, K.L. Theodor, German internist, *1878. See B.'s *syndrome.*

bruise (brūz). An injury usually producing a hematoma without rupture of the skin.

bruissement (brwēs-mawhn') [Fr.]. A purring auscultatory sound.

bruit (brū-ē') [Fr.]. A harsh or musical, intermittent auscultatory sound, especially an abnormal one.

aneurysmal b., blowing murmur heard over an aneurysm.

carotid b., a systolic murmur heard at the root of the neck but not at the aortic area; any b. produced by blood flow in a carotid artery.

b. de canon, cannon sound; the loud first heart sound heard intermittently in complete atrioventricular block when the ventricles happen to contract shortly after the atria.

b. de diable [Fr. humming-top], venous *hum.*

b. de galop [Fr.], gallop.

b. de lime [Fr. file], introduced by R. Laënnec to describe a rough rasping murmur.

b. de moulin [Fr. mill], gurgling or splashing mill-wheel sounds heard when both fluid and air are present in the pericardial sac.

b. de rappel [Fr. drum-beat], double-shock sound; applied by J. B. Bouillaud to describe the cadence of a split-second heart sound, or of the second sound followed by an opening snap.

b. de Roger, Roger's *murmur.*

b. de scie ou de rape [Fr. saw, rasp], introduced by R. Laënnec to describe harsh, rasping murmurs.

b. de soufflet [Fr. bellows], introduced by R. Laënnec to describe a blowing murmur.

b. de tabourka [Fr. tambour], a loud tambour-like or bell-like second heart sound heard at the aortic area in syphilitic aortitis.

b. de triolet [Fr. a little trio], introduced by L. Gallavardin to describe the triple cadence produced by a systolic click.

thyroid b., vascular murmur heard over hyperactive thyroid gland, due to increased blood flow.

Traube's b., gallop.

Brumpt, Emile, French parasitologist, 1877–1951. See B.'s white *mycetoma.*

Brunn, Albert von, German anatomist, 1849–1895. See B.'s *membrane, nests.*

Brunn, Fritz, 20th century Czechoslovakian physician. See B. *reaction.*

Brunner, Johann C., Swiss anatomist, 1653–1727. See B.'s *glands.*

brunneroma (brūn-er-ō'mă). An adenoma of Brunner's glands; a rare solitary tumor.

brunnerosis (brūn-er-ō'sis). Benign nodular hyperplasia of Brunner's glands.

Bruns, Ludwig, German neurologist, 1858–1916. See B. *ataxia.*

Brunschwig, Alexander, U.S. surgeon, 1901–1969. See B.'s *operation.*

brush (brŭsh) [A.S. *byrst,* bristle]. An instrument made of some flexible material, such as bristles, attached to a handle or to the tip of a catheter.

Ayre b., a device, consisting of a long flexible tube with a b. at the distal end, for collecting gastric mucosal cells in cancer detection studies; after positioning in the stomach the b. is rotated and "sweeps" cells from the mucosa.

bronchoscopic b., a small b. for insertion through a bronchoscope to wipe off cells for microscopic identification in suspected bronchial carcinoma.

denture b., a b. used to clean removable dentures.

Haidinger's b.'s, the perception of two dark yellowish b.'s or sheaves radiating about 5 degrees from the point of fixation when an evenly illuminated surface, such as the blue sky, is viewed through a polarizing lens.

Kruse's b., a bunch of fine platinum wires attached to a holder; used in bacteriological work to spread material over the surface of a culture medium.

polishing b., a b. usually mounted in a rotating instrument, used to polish teeth or artificial replacements.

Brushfield, Thomas, British physician, 1858–1937. See B.'s *spots,* B.-Wyatt *disease.*

brushite (brŭsh'īt). $CaHPO_4.2H_2O$; a naturally occurring acid calcium phosphate occasionally found in dental calculus.

Bruton, Ogden C., U.S. pediatrician, *1908. See B.'s *disease,* B. type *agammaglobulinemia.*

bruxism (brŭk'sizm) [G. *brucho,* to grind the teeth]. A clenching of the teeth, associated with forceful lateral or protrusive jaw movements, resulting in rubbing, gritting, or grinding together of the teeth, usually during sleep; sometimes a pathologic condition.

Bryant, Sir Thomas, British surgeon, 1828–1914. See B.'s *ampulla, sign, traction, triangle.*

BSA Abbreviation for bovine serum *albumin.*

BSER Abbreviation for brainstem evoked response. See brainstem evoked response *audiometry.*

Bt_2cAMP $N^6,O^{2'}$-dibutyryladenosine 3':5'-cyclic phosphate, a dibutyryl derivative of cAMP.

BTPS Symbol indicating that a gas volume has been expressed as if it were saturated with water vapor at body temperature (37°C) and at the ambient barometric pressure; used for measurements of lung volumes.

BTU Abbreviation for British thermal *unit.*

buaki (bū-ak'ē). A nutritional (protein deficiency) disease observed in natives of the Congo and characterized by edema, skin lesions, and anemia; possibly related to kwashiorkor.

buba madre (bū'bă mah'dre). Mother *yaw.*

bubas (bū'bahs). Yaws.

b. brazilia'na, espundia.

bubo (bū'bō) [G. *boubōn,* the groin, a swelling in the groin]. Inflammatory swelling of one or more lymph nodes in the groin; the confluent mass of nodes usually suppurates and drains pus.

bullet b., a hard, painless swelling of a gland in the groin, accompanying a chancre.

chancroidal b., virulent b.; an ulcerating b., due to *Haemophilus ducreyi.*

climatic b., venereal *lymphogranuloma.*

indolent b., an indurated enlargement of an inguinal node.

malignant b., the b. associated with bubonic plague.

parotid b., a swelling of the parotid gland due to secondary septic infection.

primary b., a b. occurring as the first sign of venereal infection.

tropical b., venereal *lymphogranuloma.*

venereal b., an enlarged gland in the groin associated with any venereal disease, especially chancroid.

virulent b., chancroidal b.

bubonalgia (bū'bon-al'jē-ă) [G. *boubōn,* groin, + *algos,* pain]. Pain in the groin.

bubonic (bū-bon'ik). Relating in any way to a bubo.

bubonulus (bū-bon'yū-lŭs) [Mod. L. dim. of *bubo*]. **1.** An abscess occurring along the course of a lymphatic vessel. **2.** One of a number of hard nodules, often breaking down into ulcers, which form along the course of acutely inflamed lymphatic vessels of the dorsum of the penis.

bucardia (byū-kar'dē-ă) [G. *bous,* ox, + *kardia,* heart]. Cor bovinum; extreme hypertrophy of the heart.

bucca, gen. and pl. **buccae** (bŭk'ă, bŭk'ē) [L.] [NA]. Cheek.

buccal (bŭk'ăl). Pertaining to, adjacent to, or in the direction of the cheek.

buccinator (bŭk'si-nā'ter, -tōr) [L. *buccinator,* trumpeter]. See *musculus* buccinator.

bucco- [L. *bucca,* cheek]. Combining form relating to the cheek.

buccoaxial (bŭk-ō-ak'sē-ăl). Referring to the line angle formed by the buccal and axial walls of a cavity.

buccoaxiocervical (bŭk'ō-ak'sē-ō-ser'vi-kăl). Referring to the point angle formed by the junction of the buccal, axial, and cervical (gingival) walls of a cavity.

buccoaxiogingival (bŭk'ō-ak'sē-ō-jin'ji-văl). Referring to the point angle formed by the junction of a buccal, axial, and gingival (cervical) wall.

buccocervical (bŭk-ō-ser'vi-kăl). **1.** Relating to the cheek and the neck. **2.** In dental anatomy, referring to that portion of the buccal surface of a bicuspid or molar tooth adjacent to its cemento-enamel junction.

buccoclusal (bŭk-ō-klū'săl). Incorrect term referring to the line angle formed by the junction of a buccal and pulpal wall. See buccopulpal.

buccodistal (buk-ō-dis'tăl). Referring to the line angle formed by the junction of a buccal and distal wall of a cavity.

buccogingival (bŭk-ō-jin'ji-văl). Relating to the cheek and the gum.

buccolabial (bŭk-ō-lā'bē-ăl). **1.** Relating to both cheek and lip. **2.** In dentistry, referring to that aspect of the dental arch or those surfaces of the teeth in contact with the mucosa of lip and cheek.

buccolingual (bŭk-ō-ling'wăl). **1.** Pertaining to the cheek and the tongue. **2.** In dentistry, referring to that aspect of the dental arch or those surfaces of the teeth in contact with the mucosa of the lip or cheek and the tongue.

buccomesial (bŭk-ō-mē'zē-ăl). Referring to the line angle formed by the junction of a buccal and mesial wall of a cavity.

buccopharyngeal (bŭk'ō-fă-rin'jē-ăl). Relating to both cheek or mouth and pharynx.

buccopulpal (buk-ō-pŭl'păl). Referring to the line angle formed by the junction of a buccal and pulpal wall of a cavity.

buccoversion (bŭk'ō-ver-zhŭn). Malposition of a posterior tooth from the normal line of occlusion toward the cheek.

buccula (bŭk'yū-lă) [L. dim. of *bucca,* cheek]. Double chin; a fatty puffing under the chin.

Buchner, Eduard, German chemist, 1860–1917. See B. *extract, funnel.*

Buchner, Hans, German bacteriologist, 1850–1902. See B. *extract.*

buchu (bū'kū) [native]. Hottentot tea; the dried leaves of *Barosma betulina, B. crenulata,* or *B. serratifolia* (family Rutaceae), a shrub growing in South Africa; used as a carminative, diuretic, and urinary antiseptic.

Buchwald, Hermann Edmund. German physician, *1903. See B.'s *atrophy.*

Buck, Gurdon, U.S. surgeon, 1807–1877. See B.'s *extension, fascia, traction.*

buck'bean. Bogbean; menyanthes; water shamrock; marsh trefoil; the leaves of *Menyanthes trifoliata* (family Gentianaceae); credited with emmenagogue, antiscorbutic, and simple bitter properties.

buckthorn (bŭk'thōrn). *Rhamnus.*

Bucky, Gustav, U.S. radiologist, 1880–1963. See B. *diaphragm,* B.'s *rays.*

buclizine hydrochloride (bu'kli-zēn). 1-(*p-tert*-Butylbenzyl)-4-(*p*-phenylbenzyl)piperazine dihydrochloride; a mild sedative used for motion sickness, vertigo, and anxiety accompanying psychosomatic disorders.

buclosamide (buk-lō'să-mīd). *N*-Butyl-4-chlorosalicylamide; a topical antifungal agent.

bucrylate (byū'kri-lāt). Isobutyl 2-cyanoacrylate; a tissue adhesive used in surgery.

Bucy, Paul C., U.S. neurosurgeon, *1904. See Klüver-B. *syndrome.*

bud (bŭd). **1.** An outgrowth that resembles the b. of a plant, usually pluripotential, and capable of differentiating and growing into a definitive structure. **2.** To give rise to such an outgrowth. See also gemmation.

bronchial b., one of the outgrowths from the primordial endodermal bronchus, giving rise to pulmonary epithelium.

end b., tail b.

gustatory b., *caliculus* gustatorius.

limb b., an ectodermally covered mesenchymal outgrowth on the embryonic flank giving rise to either the forelimb or hindlimb.

liver b., the primordial cellular diverticulum from foregut endoderm of the embryo that gives rise to the parenchyma of the liver.

lung b., the endodermal lung primordium which will give rise to the epithelial lining of the respiratory tract.

median tongue b., *tuberculum* impar.

metanephric b., ureteric b.; the primordial cellular outgrowth from the mesonephric duct that gives rise to the epithelial lining of the ureter, pelvis, and calyces of the kidney, and the straight collecting tubules.

periosteal b., a vascular connective tissue bud from the perichondrium that invades the ossification center of the cartilaginous model of a developing long bone.

syncytial b., syncytial *knot.*

tail b., end b.; the rapidly proliferating mass of cells at the caudal extremity of the embryo.

taste b., *caliculus* gustatorius.

tooth b., the primordial structures from which a tooth is formed; the enamel organ, dental papilla, and the dental sac enclosing them.

ureteric b., metanephric b.

vascular b., an endothelial sprout arising from a blood vessel.

Budd, George, London physician, 1808–1882. See B.'s *cirrhosis, syndrome;* B.-Chiari *syndrome.*

Budde, E., Danish sanitary engineer, *1871. See B. *process.*

budding (bŭd'ing). Gemmation.

Budge, Julius L., German physiologist, 1811– 1888. See B.'s *center.*

Budin, Pierre C., French gynecologist, 1846–1907. See B.'s obstetrical *joint.*

Buerger, Leo, U.S. physician, 1879–1943. See Winiwarter-B. *disease.*

bufa-, bufo-. Combining forms denoting origin from toads; used in the systematic and trivial names of toxic substances (genins) isolated from plants and animals containing the bufanolide structure; prefixes denoting species origin are often attached.

bufadienolide (bū-fă-dī-en'ō-līd). See bufanolide.

bufagenins (bū'fă-jen-inz). Bufagins.

bufagins (bū'fă-jinz). Bufagenins; a group of steroids (bufanolides) in the venom of a family of toads (Bufonidae) having a digitalis-like action upon the heart. See also bufotoxins.

bufanolide (bū-fan'ō-līd). The fundamental steroid lactone of several squill-toad (family Bufonidae) venoms or toxins; also found in the form of glycosides in plants (*e.g.,* digitalis). The steroid is essentially a 5*β*-androstane, with a 14*β* H. The lactone at C-17 is structurally related to the $-CH(CH_3)CH_2CH_2CH_3$ radical attached to C-17 in the cholanes, and is in the same configuration as that of cholesterol (*i.e.,* 20*R*); in some species, b. is formed from cholesterol. Various b. derivatives having unsaturation in the lactone ring (20,22) or elsewhere (4) are known as **bufenolides** (one double bond), **bufadienolides** (two double bonds), **bufatrienolides** (three double bonds), etc; they have varying numbers of hydroxyl groups at positions 3, 5, 14, and 16, and these may be further substituted. For structure, see steroids.

bufatrienolide (bū-fă-trī-en'ō-līd). See bufanolide.

bufenolide (bū-fen'ō-līd). See bufanolide.

buffer (bŭf'er). **1.** A mixture of an acid and its conjugate base (salt), such as H_2CO_3/HCO_3^-; $H_2PO_4^-/HPO_4^{2-}$, that, when present in a solution, reduces any changes in pH that would otherwise occur in the solution when acid or alkali is added to it; thus, the pH of the blood and body fluids is maintained virtually constant (pH 7.45) although acid metabolites are continually being formed in the tissues and CO_2 (H_2CO_3) is lost in the lungs. See also conjugate acid-base *pair.* **2.** To add a b. to a solution and thus give it the property of resisting a change in pH when it receives a limited amount of acid or alkali.

secondary b., see Hamburger's *law.*

bufo-. See bufa-.

Bufonidae (bū-fon'ĭ-dē) [L. *bufo,* toad]. A family of toads whose dermal glands secrete several kinds of pharmacologically active substances having a cardiac action similar to that of digitalis.

buformin (bū-fōr'min). 1-Butylbiguanide; an oral hypoglycemic agent.

bufotenine (bū-fō-ten'ēn). Mappine; 3-(2-dimethylaminoethyl)indol-5-ol; *N,N*-dimethylserotonin; a psychotomimetic agent isolated from the venom of certain toads (family Bufonidae) and also present in several plants and one of the active principles of cohoba; raises the blood pressure by a vasoconstrictor action and produces psychic effects including hallucinations.

bufotoxins (bū-fō-toks'inz). A group of steroid lactones (conjugates of bufagins and suberylarginine at C-3) of digitalis present in the venoms of toads (family Bufonidae); their effects are similar to but weaker than those of the bufagins.

bug. An insect belonging to the suborder Heteroptera. For organisms so called, see the specific term.

buggery (bŭg'ger-ē) [O.F. *bougre,* heretic, fr. Med. L. *Bulgaris,* a Bulgar (hence a heretic)]. Sodomy.

bulb (bŭlb) [L. *bulbus,* a bulbous root]. **1.** Bulbus; any globular or fusiform structure. **2.** A short vertical underground stem of plants, as of the onion and garlic.

aortic b., *bulbus* aortae.
arterial b., *bulbus* aortae.
carotid b., *sinus* caroticus.
b. of corpus spongiosum, *bulbus* penis.
dental b., the papilla, derived from mesoderm, that forms the part of the primordium of a tooth which is situated within the cup-shaped enamel organ.
duodenal b., duodenal *cap.*
end b., one of the oval or rounded bodies in which the sensory nerve fibers terminate in mucous membrane.
b. of eye, *bulbus* oculi.
hair b., *bulbus* pili.
b. of jugular vein, *bulbus* venae jugularis.
Krause's end b.'s, *corpuscula* bulboidea.
b. of lateral ventricle, a rounded elevation in the dorsal part of the medial wall of the posterior horn of the lateral ventricle, produced by the forceps major.
olfactory b., *bulbus* olfactorius.
b. of penis, *bulbus* penis.
b. of posterior horn of lateral ventricle of brain, *bulbus* cornus posterioris.
Rouget's b., a venous plexus on the surface of the ovary.
speech b., a prosthetic speech aid; a restoration used to close a cleft or other opening in the hard or soft palate, or to replace absent tissue necessary for the production of good speech.
taste b., *caliculus* gustatorius.
b. of urethra, *bulbus* penis.
b. of vestibule, *bulbus* vestibuli.

bulbar (bŭl'bar). **1.** Relating to a bulb. **2.** Relating to the rhombencephalon (hindbrain). **3.** Bulb-shaped; resembling a bulb.

bulbi (bŭl'bī). Plural of bulbus.

bulbitis (bŭl-bī'tis). Inflammation of the bulbous portion of the urethra.

bulbo- [L. *bulbus,* bulb]. Combining form relating to a bulb, or bulbus.

bulbocavernosus (bŭl'bō-kav-er-nō'sŭs). See under musculus.

bulboid (bŭl'boyd) [bulbo- + G. *eidos,* resemblance]. Bulb-shaped.

bulbonuclear (bŭl-bō-nū'klē-ar). Relating to the nuclei in the medulla oblongata.

bulbopontine (bŭl-bō-pon'tēn). Relating to the rostral part of the rhombencephalon composed of the pons and overlying tegmentum.

bulbosacral (bŭl'bō-sā'krăl). See bulbosacral *system.*

bulbospinal (bŭl-bō-spī'năl). Spinobulbar; relating to the medulla oblongata and spinal cord, particularly to nerve fibers interconnecting the two.

bulbourethral (bŭl'bō-yū-rē'thrăl). Urethrobulbar; relating to the bulbus penis and the urethra.

bulbus, gen. and pl. **bulbi** (bŭl'bŭs, -bī) [L. a plant bulb] [NA]. Bulb (1).
b. aor'tae [NA], aortic bulb; arterial bulb; the dilated first part of the aorta containing the aortic semilunar valves and the aortic sinuses.
b. cor'dis, a transitory dilation in the embryonic heart where the arterial trunk joins the ventral roots of the aortic arches.
b. cor'nus posterior'is [NA], bulb of posterior horn of lateral ventricle of the brain; a curved elevation on the inner wall of the posterior horn produced by the fibers of the forceps major of the corpus callosum as they bend backward into the occipital lobe.
b. oc'uli [NA], bulb of eye; eyeball; globe of eye; the eye proper without the appendages.
b. olfacto'rius [NA], olfactory bulb; the grayish expanded rostral extremity of the olfactory tract, lying on the cribriform plate of the ethmoid and receiving the olfactory filaments.

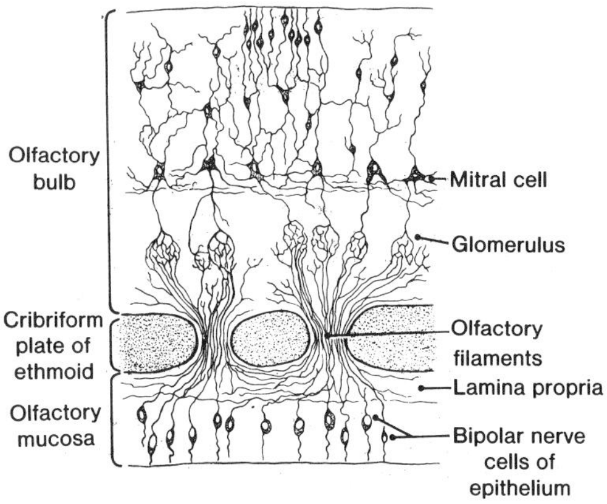

Bulbus Olfactorius

Diagram of olfactory mucosa and olfactory bulb (Ramón y Cajal), showing neuronal relations.

b. pe'nis [NA], bulb of corpus spongiosum, penis, or urethra; b. urethrae; the expanded posterior part of the corpus spongiosum penis lying in the interval between the crura of the penis.
b. pi'li [NA], hair bulb, the lower expanded extremity of the hair follicle that fits like a cap over the papilla pili.
b. ure'thrae, b. penis.
b. ve'nae jugula'ris [NA], bulb of jugular vein; one of two dilated parts of the internal jugular vein; the superior bulb (Heister's diverticulum) is a dilation at the beginning of the internal jugular vein in the jugular fossa of the temporal bone; the inferior bulb is a dilated portion of the vein just before it reaches the brachiocephalic vein.
b. vestib'uli [NA], bulb of vestibule; a mass of erectile tissue on either side of the vagina united anterior to the urethra by the commissura bulborum.

bulesis (bū-lē'sis) [G. *boulēsis,* a willing]. The will; a willing.

bulimia (bū-lim'ē-ă) [G. *bous,* ox, + *limos,* hunger]. B. nervosa.
b. nervo'sa, bulimia; boulimia, hyperorexia; a chronic morbid disorder involving repeated and secretive episodic bouts of eating characterized by uncontrolled rapid ingestion of large quantities of food over a short period of time, followed by self-induced vomiting, purging, and anorexia; accompanied by feelings of guilt, depression, or self-disgust.

bulimic (bū-lim'ik). Relating to, or suffering from, bulimia nervosa.

Bulinus (byū-lī'nŭs). A genus and subgenus of freshwater snails in the family Planorbidae (subfamily Bulininae), which includes many species that are intermediate hosts of the human blood fluke, *Schistosoma haematobium,* in Africa and the Middle East; divided into two subgenera, *Physopsis* and *Bulinus,* the former being responsible for transmission of *S. haematobium* south of the Sahara, the latter responsible for transmission of this bladder blood fluke in north Africa and the Middle East. Important species include *B. truncatus* and *B. forskalii,* hosts for human and animal schistosomes and several domestic animal amphistome flukes.

bulkage (bŭlk'ij). Anything, such as agar, that increases the bulk of material in the intestine, thereby stimulating peristalsis.

bulla, gen. and pl. **bullae** (bul'ă, -ē) [L. bubble]. **1.** A large vesicle appearing as a circumscribed area of separation of the epidermis from the subepidermal structure **(subepidermic b.)** or as a circumscribed area of separation of epidermal cells **(intraepidermic b.)** caused by the presence of serum, sometimes mixed with blood, and occasionally caused by a substance injected intra- or subepidermally. **2** [NA]. A bubble-like structure.
ethmoidal b., b. ethmoidalis.

b. ethmoida'lis [NA], ethmoidal b.; a bulging of the inner wall of the ethmoidal labyrinth in the middle meatus of the nose, just below the middle nasal concha; it is regarded as a rudimentary concha.
pulmonary b., **(1)** an air-filled blister on the surface of the lung; **(2)** a similar abnormality within the lung presenting as a thin-walled cavity.
b. tympan'ica, the bony capsule enclosing the middle ear of the cat and dog.

bullnose (bul'nōz). Necrotic *rhinitis* of pigs.

bullous (bul'ŭs). Relating to, of the nature of, or marked by, bullae.

bumetanide (byū-met'ă-nīd). 3-Butylamino-4-phenoxy-5-sulfamoylbenzoic acid; a diuretic used in the treatment of edema associated with congestive heart failure, hepatic cirrhosis, and renal disease.

Bumke, Oswald C.E., German neurologist, 1877–1950. See B.'s *pupil.*

BUN Abbreviation for blood urea *nitrogen.*

bunamidine hydrochloride (bŭn-am'i-dēn). *N,N*-Dibutyl-4-hexyloxynaphthamidine monohydrochloride; an anthelmintic.

bundle (bŭn'dl). A structure composed of a group of fibers, muscular or nervous; a fasciculus.
aberrant b.'s, a group, or groups, of fibers from the corticobulbar or corticonuclear tract, directed to each of the motor nuclei of cranial nerves.
anterior ground b., fasciculus anterior proprius. See *fasciculi* proprii.
Arnold's b., *tractus* temporopontinus.
atrioventricular (A-V) b., *truncus* atrioventricularis.
Bachmann's b., division of the anterior internodal tract which continues into the left atrium providing a specialized path for interatrial conduction.
comma b. of Schultze, *fasciculus* semilunaris.
Flechsig's ground b.'s, fasciculus anterior proprius and fasciculus lateralis proprius. See *fasciculi* proprii.
Gantzer's accessory b., see Gantzer's *muscle.*
Gierke's respiratory b., *tractus* solitarius.
ground b.'s, *fasciculi* proprii.
Held's b., *tractus* tectospinalis.
Helie's b., a vertically arched b. of fibers in the superficial layer of the myometrium.
Helweg's b., olivospinal *tract.*
His' b., b. of His, *truncus* atrioventricularis.
Hoche's b., see *fasciculus* semilunaris.
hooked b. of Russell, uncinate b. of Russell.
Keith's b., *truncus* atrioventricularis.
Kent's b., **(1)** *truncus* atrioventricularis; **(2)** a muscle fiber b. in the mammalian heart below the nodus atrioventricularis; may also occur in man.
Kent-His b., *truncus* atrioventricularis.
Killian's b., *pars* cricopharyngea.
Krause's respiratory b., *tractus* solitarius.
lateral ground b., fasciculus lateralis proprius. See *fasciculi* proprii.
Lissauer's b., *fasciculus* dorsolateralis.
Loewenthal's b., *tractus* tectospinalis.
longitudinal pontine b.'s, *fasciculi* longitudinalis pontis.
medial forebrain b., a fiber system coursing longitudinally through the lateral zone of the hypothalamus, connecting the latter reciprocally with the midbrain tegmentum and with various components of the limbic system; it also carries fibers from norepinephrine-containing and serotonin-containing cell groups in the brainstem to the hypothalamus and cerebral cortex, as well as dopamine-carrying fibers from the substantia nigra to the caudate nucleus and putamen.
medial longitudinal b., *fasciculus* longitudinalis medialis.
Meynert's retroflex b., *fasciculus* retroflexus.
Monakow's b., *tractus* rubrospinalis.
muscle b., a group of muscle fibers ensheathed by connective tissue (perimysium).
oblique b. of pons, *fasciculus* obliquus pontis.
olfactory b., a fiber system, described by E. Zuckerkandl as "Reichbündel," descending from the septum pellucidum in front of the anterior commissure toward the base of the forebrain; it contains precommissural fibers of the fornix, fibers from the septum to the hypothalamus and substantia innominata, as well as fibers ascending to the septum and hippocampus from the hypothalamus and midbrain; it bears no special relation to the sense of smell.
olivocochlear b., a group of fibers originating from small cell groups surrounding the superior olive (nucleus dorsalis corporis trapezoidei), passing peripherally with the contralateral vestibular nerve, then bridging over into the cochlear nerve, and terminating synaptically on the hair cells of Corti's organ. A smaller uncrossed bundle follows a similar course. This efferent system in the cochlear nerve modulates the responsiveness of the auditory receptor cells.
Pick's b., a b. of nerve fibers recurving rostralward from the pyramidal tract in the medulla oblongata, and believed to consist of corticonuclear fibers.
posterior longitudinal b., *fasciculus* longitudinalis medialis.
precommissural b., see olfactory b.
predorsal b., *tractus* tectospinalis.
Rathke's b.'s, *trabeculae* carneae.
Schütz' b., *fasciculus* longitudinalis dorsalis.
solitary b., *tractus* solitarius.
tendon b., a group of tendon fibers surrounded by a sheath of irregular connective tissue (peritendineum).
Türck's b., *tractus* pyramidalis anterior.
uncinate b. of Russell, hooked b. of Russell; uncinate fasciculus of Russell; fastigial efferent fibers that cross with the cerebellum and descend over the lateral surface of the superior cerebellar peduncle; these fibers largely terminate in the vestibular nuclei and the reticular formation of the pons and medulla.
Vicq d'Azyr's b., *fasciculus* mamillothalamicus.

bungpagga (bŭng-pag'ă). *Myositis* purulenta tropica.

bunion (bŭn'yŭn) [O.F. *buigne,* bump on the head]. A localized swelling at either the medial or dorsal aspect of the first metatarsophalangeal joint, caused by an inflammatory bursa; a medial b. is usually associated with hallux valgus.

bunionectomy (bŭn-yŭn-ek'tō-mē). Excision of a bunion.
Keller b., excision of the proximal portion of the proximal phalanx of the first toe.
Mayo b., excision of the head of the first metatarsal.

Bunnell, Sterling, U.S. surgeon, 1882–1957. See B.'s *suture.*

bunodont (bū'nō-dont) [G. *bounos,* mound, + *odous* (*odont-*), tooth]. Having molar teeth with rounded or low conical cusps, in contrast to lophodont.

bunolol hydrochloride (byū'nō-lol). DL-5-[3-*tert*- (Butylamino)-2-hydroxypropoxy]-3,4-dihydro-1(2*H*)-naphthalenone hydrochloride; a *β*-adrenergic blocking agent for treatment of cardiac arrhythmias.

bunolophodont (bū-nō-lof'ō-dont) [G. bunos, mound, + *lophos,* ridge, + *odous,* tooth]. Having molar teeth with transverse ridges and rounded cusps on the occlusal surface.

bunoselenodont (bū'nō-sĕ-len'ō-dont) [*bunos,* + *selēnē,* moon, + *odous,* tooth]. Having molar teeth with crescentic ridges and rounded cusps on the occlusal surface.

Bunostomum (byū-nō-stō'mŭm) [G. *bounos,* hill, mound, + *stoma,* mouth]. A genus of hookworms (family Ancylostomatidae, subfamily Necatorinae) found in cattle and other herbivores; similar to *Necator.*

B. phlebot'omum, a species that occurs in cattle, sheep, and some wild ruminants in many parts of the world.

B. trigonoceph'alum, a cosmopolitan hookworm species in the small intestines of sheep and goats.

Bunsen, Robert W., German chemist and physicist, 1811–1899. See B. burner, B.'s solubility *coefficient,* B.-Roscoe *law.*

Bunsen burner [R. W. Bunsen]. A gas lamp supplied with lateral openings admitting sufficient air so that the carbon is completely burned, thus giving a very hot but only slightly luminous flame.

Bunyaviridae (bŭn-yă-vir'i-dē) [*Bunyamwere,* Uganda]. A family of arboviruses composed of four genera: *Bunyvirus, Phlebovirus, Nairovirus,* and *Uukuvirus.* Virions are 90–100 nm in diameter, sensitive to lipid solvents and detergents, and enveloped with glycopolypeptide surface projections; the nucleocapsid is of helical symmetry containing single-stranded segmented RNA (MW 7×10^6).

Bunyavirus (bŭn'yă-vī'rŭs). A genus of the family Bunyaviridae which contains at least 145 viruses divided into 16 serological groups.

buphthalmia, buphthalmos, buphthalmus (būf-thal'mē-ă, -thal'-mos, -thal'mŭs) [G. *bous,* ox, + *ophthalmos,* eye]. Congenital glaucoma; hydrophthalmia; hydrophthalmos; hydrophthalmus; an affection of infancy, marked by an increase of intraocular pressure with enlargement of the eyeball.

bupivacaine (byū-piv'ă-kān). *dl*-1-Butylpipecoloxylidide; a potent, long-acting local anesthetic used in regional anesthesia.

buprenorphine hydrochloride (bū-pre-nōr'fēn). $C_{29}H_{41}NO_4{\cdot}HCl$; a semisynthetic opioid analgesic used for relief of moderate to severe pain.

bupropion hydrochloride (bū-prō'pē-on). 1-Propanone,1-(3-chlorophenyl)-2-[1,1-dimethylethyl)amino]-hydrochloride; an antidepressant.

bur (bŭr). A rotary cutting instrument, used in dentistry, consisting of a small metal shaft and a head designed in various shapes; used at various rotational velocities for excavating decay, shaping cavity forms, and for reduction of tooth structure. See also burr.

cross-cut b., a b. with blades located at right angles to its long axis.

end-cutting b., a b. with blades only on its end.

finishing b., a b. with numerous fine cutting blades placed close together; used to contour metallic restorations.

fissure b., a cylindrical or tapered rotary cutting tool intended for extending or widening fissures in a tooth, as for general surface reduction of tooth substance.

inverted cone b., a rotary cutting instrument in the shape of a truncated cone with the smaller end attached to the shaft; generally used for entering carious pits or creating undercuts in cavity preparations.

round b., a dental b. with the cutting blades spherically arranged.

Burchard, H., 19th century German chemist. See B.-Liebermann *reaction;* Liebermann-B. *test.*

Burchard-Liebermann reaction, Liebermann-Burchard test. See under reaction, test.

Burdach, Karl F., German anatomist and physiologist, 1776–1847. See B.'s *column, fasciculus, nucleus, tract.*

burden (ber'den). See body burden.

buret, burette (bū-ret') [Fr.]. A graduated glass tube with a tap as its lower end; used for measuring liquids in volumetric chemical analyses.

Bürger, Max. See B.-Grütz *syndrome.*

Burk, Dean, U.S. scientist, *1904. See Lineweaver-B. *equation.*

Burkitt, Denis P., 20th century Ugandan physician. See B.'s *lymphoma.*

Burlew disk. See under disk.

Burn, J.H. See B. and Rand *theory.*

burn (bern) [A.S. *baernan*] **1.** To cause a lesion by heat or any other agent, similar to that caused by heat. **2.** To suffer pain caused by excessive heat, or similar pain from any cause. **3.** A lesion caused by heat or any cauterizing agent, including friction, electricity, and electromagnetic energy; types of b.'s resulting from different agents are relatively specific and diagnostic. The division of b.'s into three degrees is recognized for geographical designation: **first degree b.,** involving only the epidermis and causing erythema and edema without vesiculation; **second degree b.,** involving the epidermis and dermis and usually forming blisters that may be superficial or deep dermal necrosis, but with epithelial regeneration extending from the skin appendages; **third degree b.,** destruction of the entire skin; deep third-degree b.'s extend into subcutaneous fat, muscle, or bone and often cause much scarring.

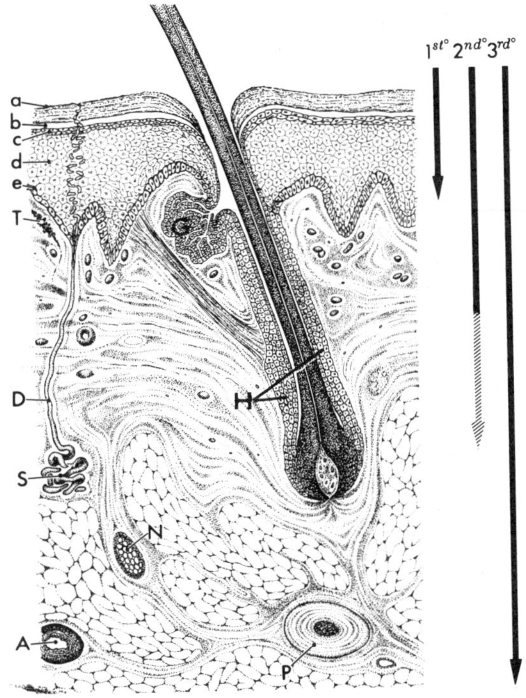

Burns

The five layers of epidermis, showing (*vertical arrows*) 1st, 2nd, and 3rd degree burns. *a,* Stratum corneum; *b,* stratum lucidum; *c,* stratum granulosum; *d,* stratum spinosum; *e,* stratum basale; *A,* artery; *D,* duct of sudoriferous gland; *G,* sebaceous gland; *H,* hair follicle; *N,* nerve; *P,* Pacinian corpuscle; *S,* sudoriferous gland; *T,* tactile corpuscle.

brush b., a b. caused by friction of a rapidly moving object against the skin or ground into the skin.

chemical b., a b. due to a caustic chemical.

first degree b., see burn (3).

flash b., a b. due to very brief exposure to intense radiant heat; the typical b. produced by atomic explosion.

full-thickness b., third degree b. See burn (3).

mat b., see brush b.

partial-thickness b., second degree b. See burn (3).

radiation b., a b. caused by planned or unplanned exposure to

radium, x-rays, atomic energy in any form, ultraviolet rays, etc.
rope b., see brush b.
second degree b., see burn (3).
superficial b., first degree b. See burn (3).
thermal b., a b. caused by heat.
third degree b., see burn (3).

Burnett, Charles H., U.S. physician, *1901. See B.'s *syndrome.*

burnisher (bŭr'nish-er) [O. F. *burnir,* to polish]. An instrument for smoothing and polishing the surface or edge of a dental restoration.

burnout (bern'owt). **1.** In dentistry, the elimination, by heat, of an invested pattern from a set investment in order to prepare the mold to receive casting metal. **2.** Colloquialism for a condition characterized by physical and emotional exhaustion resulting from chronic unrelieved job-related stress.

Burns, Allan, Scottish anatomist, 1781–1813. See B.'s *ligament,* falciform *process, space.*

Burow, Karl A. von, German surgeon, 1809–1874. See B.'s *operation, solution, triangle, vein.*

burr (bŭr). A drilling tool for enlarging a trephine hole in the cranium. See also bur.

burrow (ber'ō). **1.** A subcutaneous tunnel or tract made by a parasite, such as the itch mite. **2.** A sinus or fistula. **3.** To undermine or create a tunnel or tract through or beneath various tissue planes.

BURSA

bursa, pl. **bursae** (ber'să, ber'sē) [Mediev. L., a purse] [NA]. A closed sac or envelope lined with synovial membrane and containing fluid, usually found or formed in areas subject to friction; *e.g.,* over an exposed or prominent part or where a tendon passes over a bone.
Achil'les b., b. tendinis calcanei.
b. achil'lis [NA], official alternate term for b. tendinis calcanei.
b. of acromion, b. subcutanea acromialis.
adventitious b., a b.-like cyst formed between two parts as a result of friction.
b. anseri'na [NA], anserine b.; tibial intertendinous b.; the b. between the tibial collateral ligament of the knee joint and the tendons of the sartorius, gracilis, and semitendinosus muscles.
anserine b., b. anserina.
anterior tibial b., b. subtendinea musculi tibialis anterioris.
bicipitoradial b., b. bicipitoradialis.
b. bicip'itoradia'lis [NA], bicipitoradial b.; the b. between the tendon of the biceps brachii muscle and the anterior part of the tuberosity of the radius.
Boyer's b., b. retrohyoidea.
Brodie's b., **(1)** b. subtendinea musculi gastrocnemii medialis; **(2)** b. musculi semimembranosi.
Calori's b., a b. between the arch of the aorta and the trachea.
coracobrachial b., b. musculi coracobrachialis.
b. cubita'lis interos'sea [NA], interosseous b. of elbow; an inconstant b. located between the tendon of the biceps and the ulna or the oblique cord.
deep infrapatellar b., b. infrapatellaris profunda.
b. of extensor carpi radialis brevis, b. musculi extensoris carpi radialis brevis.
b. fabric'ii, the b. of Fabricius in poultry, a blind saclike structure located on the posterodorsal wall of the cloaca; it performs a thymus-like function.
Fleischmann's b., b. sublingualis; an inconstant serous b. at the level of the frenulum linguae, between the surface of the genioglossus muscle and the mucous membrane of the floor of the mouth.
b. of gastrocnemius, b. subtendinea musculi gastrocnemii.
gluteofemoral b., b. intermusculares musculorum gluteorum.
gluteus medius b.'s, bursae trochantericae musculi glutei medii.
gluteus minimus b., b. trochanterica musculi glutei minimi.
b. of great toe, the b. between the lateral side of the base of the first metatarsal bone and the medial side of the shaft of the second metatarsal.
b. of hyoid, b. retrohyoidea.
iliac b., b. subtendinea iliaca.
b. iliopectinea [NA], iliopectineal b.; a large b. between the iliopsoas tendon and the iliopubic eminence.
iliopectineal b., b. iliopectinea.
inferior b. of biceps femoris, b. subtendinea musculi bicipitis femoris inferior.
infracardiac b., a small serous sac sometimes present on the medial side of the base of the right lung in the embryo. See also pneumatoenteric *recess.*
infrahyoid b., b. infrahyoidea.
b. infrahyoi'dea [NA], infrahyoid b.; a b. sometimes found below the inferior margin of the body of the hyoid bone between the sternothyroid muscle and the median thyrohyoid membrane.
b. infrapatella'ris profun'da [NA], deep infrapatellar b.; the b. between the upper part of the tibia and the patellar ligament.
infraspinatus b., b. subtendinea musculi infraspinati.
intermuscular gluteal b., b. intermusculares musculorum gluteorum.
b. intermuscula'res mus'culorum gluteor'um [NA], intermuscular gluteal b.; gluteofemoral b.; two or three small bursae between the tendon of the gluteus maximus and the linea aspera.
interosseous b. of elbow, b. cubitalis interossea.
b. intratendin'ea olec'rani [NA], intratendinous b. of elbow; b. of Monro; a b. sometimes present within the tendon of insertion of the triceps brachii.
intratendinous b. of elbow, b. intratendinea olecrani.
b. ischiad'ica mus'culi glu'tei max'imi [NA], ischial b.; the b. between the gluteus maximus muscle and the tuberosity of the ischium.
b. ischiad'ica mus'culi obturato'ris inter'ni [NA], b. of obturator internus (1); the large, constant b. between the obturator internus tendon and the lesser sciatic notch.
ischial b., b. ischiadica musculi glutei maximi.
laryngeal b., b. subcutanea prominentiae laryngeae.
lateral malleolus b., b. subcutanea malleoli lateralis.
b. of latiss'imus dor'si, b. subtendinea musculi latissimus dorsi.
Luschka's b., b. pharyngea.
medial malleolar b., b. subcutanea malleoli medialis.
b. of Monro, b. intratendinea olecrani.
b. muco'sa, b. synovialis.
b. mus'culi bicip'itis femo'ris supe'rior [NA], superior b. of biceps femoris; a b. frequently found between the tendon of the long head of the biceps femoris and the ischial tuberosity and the tendon of the semimembranosus.
b. mus'culi coracobrachia'lis [NA], coracobrachial b.; a b. frequently present between the tendon of the coracobrachialis and the subscapularis muscle.
b. mus'culi extenso'ris car'pi radia'lis bre'vis [NA], b. of extensor carpi radialis brevis; the b. between the tendon of the extensor carpi radialis brevis and the base of the third metacarpal.
b. mus'culi pirifor'mis [NA], b. of the piriformis; a small b. located between the tendons of the piriformis and superior gemellus and the femur.
b. mus'culi semimembrano'si [NA], b. of semimembranosus; Brodie's b. (2); it lies between the muscle, the head of the gastrocnemius, and the knee joint.
b. mus'culi tenso'ris ve'li palati'ni [NA], b. of tensor veli palatini

muscle; a small b. located where the tendon of the tensor passes around the pterygoid hamulus.
b. of ob'turator inter'nus, **(1)** b. ischiadica musculi obturatoris interni; **(2)** b. subtendinea musculi obturatoris interni.
b. of olecranon, b. subcutanea olecrani.
omental b., b. omentalis.
b. omenta'lis [NA], omental b.; omental sac; lesser peritoneal sac or cavity; an isolated portion of the peritoneal cavity lying dorsal to the stomach and extending craniad to the liver and diaphragm and caudad into the greater omentum; it opens into the general peritoneal cavity at the epiploic foramen.
b. ovar'ica, the peritoneal recess between the medial aspect of the ovary and the mesosalpinx.
b. pharynge'a [NA], pharyngeal b.; Luschka's b.; Tornwaldt's cyst; a cystic notochordal remnant found inconstantly in the posterior wall of the nasopharynx at the lower end of the pharyngeal tonsil.
pharyngeal b., b. pharyngea.
b. of the piriformis, b. musculi piriformis.
b. of popliteus, *recessus* subpopliteus.
prepatellar b., b. subcutanea prepatellaris.
b. quadra'tus fem'oris, quadratus femoris b., between the front of the quadratus femoris muscle and the lesser trochanter of the femur.
radial b., *vagina* tendinis musculi flexoris pollicis longi.
retrohyoid b., b. retrohyoidea.
b. retrohyoi'dea [NA], retrohyoid b.; Boyer's b.; b. of hyoid; subhyoid b.; a b. between the posterior surface of the body of the hyoid bone and the thyrohyoid membrane.
rider's b., an adventitious b. on the inner side of the knee caused by horseback riding.
sartorius b.'s, bursae subtendineae musculi sartorii.
b. of semimembranosus, b. musculi semimembranosi.
subacromial b., b. subacromialis.
b. subacromia'lis [NA], subacromial b.; between the acromion and the capsule of the shoulder joint.
b. subcuta'nea acromia'lis [NA], b. of acromion; the b. between the acromion and the skin.
b. subcuta'nea calca'nea [NA], subcutaneous calcaneal b.; a b. between the skin and the posterior surface of the calcaneus.
b. subcuta'nea infrapatella'ris [NA], subcutaneous infrapatellar b.; a b. between the patellar ligament and the skin.
b. subcuta'nea malle'oli latera'lis [NA], lateral malleolar b., the b. between the lateral malleolus and the skin.
b. subcuta'nea malle'oli media'lis [NA], medial malleolar b.; the b. between the medial malleolus and the skin.
b. subcuta'nea olecra'ni [NA], b. of olecranon; b. between the olecranon process of the ulna and the skin.
b. subcuta'nea prepatella'ris [NA], prepatellar b.; a b. between the skin and the lower part of the patella.
b. subcuta'nea prominen'tiae laryn'geae [NA], laryngeal b.; the b. located between the junction of the laminae of the thyroid cartilage and the skin.
b. subcuta'nea trochanter'ica [NA], trochanteric b. (1); the b. between the greater trochanter of the femur and the skin.
b. subcuta'nea tuberos'itas tib'iae [NA], subcutaneous b. of tibial tuberosity; the b. located superficial to the tibial tuberosity, either subcutaneous or subfascial.
subcutaneous calcaneal b., b. subcutanea calcanea.
subcutaneous infrapatellar b., b. subcutanea infrapatellaris.
subcutaneous b. of tibial tuberosity, b. subcutanea tuberositas tibiae.
subdeltoid b., b. subdeltoidea.
b. subdeltoid'ea [NA], subdeltoid b.; the b. between the deltoid muscle and the capsule of the shoulder joint. It may be combined with the subacromial b.
subfascial prepatellar b., b. subfascialis prepatellaris.
b. subfascia'lis prepatella'ris [NA], subfascial prepatellar b.; a b. between the fascia lata and the quadriceps tendon anterior to the patella.
subhyoid b., b. retrohyoidea.
b. sublingua'lis, Fleischmann's b.
subscapular b., b. subtendinea musculi subscapularis.
b. subtendin'ea ilia'ca [NA], subtendinous iliac b.; iliac b.; the b. at the attachment of the iliopsoas muscle into the lesser trochanter.
b. subtendin'ea mus'culi bicip'itis femo'ris infe'rior [NA], inferior b. of biceps femoris; the b. between the tendon of the biceps femoris and the fibular collateral ligament of the knee joint.
b. subtendin'eae mus'culi gastrocne'mii [NA], b. of gastrocnemius; subtendinous b. of gastrocnemius, consisting of a lateral and a medial (Brodie's b. (1)) b. between the heads of the gastrocnemius and capsule of the knee joint.
b. subtendin'ea mus'culi infraspinat'i [NA], infraspinatus b.; the b. located between the tendon of the infraspinatus and the capsule of the shoulder joint.
b. subtendin'ea mus'culi latis'simus dor'si [NA], b. of latissimus dorsi; a constant b. between the tendons of the teres major and the latissimus dorsi near their intersections.
b. subtendin'ea mus'culi obturatōris inter'ni [NA], b. of obturator internus (2); the b. between the tendon of the obturator internus muscle and the capsule of the hip joint.
bursae subtendin'eae mus'culi sarto'rii [NA], sartorius b.'s; bursae, sometimes separate from the b. anserina, located between the tendons of the sartorius, semitendinosus, and gracilis muscles.
b. subtendin'ea mus'culi subscapula'ris [NA], subscapular b.; b. between the tendon of the subscapularis muscle and the neck of the scapula; it communicates with the shoulder joint.
b. subtendin'ea mus'culi tere'tis majo'ris [NA], b. of teres major; b. under the tendon of the teres major near its attachment.
b. subtendin'ea mus'culi tibia'lis anterio'ris [NA], anterior tibial b.; the small b. between the medial surface of the medial cuneiform bone and the tendon of the tibialis anterior.
b. subtendin'ea mus'culi trape'zii [NA], b. of trapezius; a b. between the tendon of the trapezius muscle and the medial end of the scapular spine.
b. subtendin'ea mus'culi tricip'itus bra'chii [NA], triceps b.; the b. located deep to the tendon of the triceps brachii near its insertion on the olecranon.
b. subtendin'ea prepatella'ris [NA], subtendinous prepatellar b.; a b. between the tendon of the quadriceps and the patella.
subtendinous b. of gastrocnemius, b. subtendineae musculi gastrocnemii.
subtendinous iliac b., b. subtendinea iliaca.
subtendinous prepatellar b., b. subtendinea prepatellaris.
superior b. of biceps femoris, b. musculi bicipitis femoris superior.
suprapatellar b., b. suprapatellaris.
b. suprapatella'ris [NA], suprapatellar b.; a large b. between the lower part of the femur and the tendon of the quadriceps femoris muscle. It usually communicates with the cavity of the knee joint.
synovial b., b. synovialis.
synovial trochlear b., *vagina* synovialis musculorum obliqui superioris.
b. synovia'lis [NA], synovial b.; b. mucosa; a sac containing synovial fluid which occurs at sites of friction, as between a tendon and a bone over which it plays, or subcutaneously over a bony prominence. The NA lists the following types: b. synovialis subcutanea, b. synovialis submuscularis, b. synovialis subfascialis, and b. synovialis subtendinea.
b. ten'dinis calca'nei [NA], bursa achillis; b. of tendo calcaneus; Achilles b.; b. between the tendo calcaneus and the upper part of the posterior surface of the calcaneum.
b. of tendo calca'neus, b. tendinis calcanei.
b. of tensor veli palatini muscle, b. musculi tensoris veli palatini.

b. of teres major, b. subtendinea musculi teretis majoris.
tibial intertendinous b., b. anserina.
b. of trapezius, b. subtendinea musculi trapezii.
triceps b., b. subtendinea musculi tricipitus brachii.
trochanteric b., **(1)** b. subcutanea trochanterica. **(2)** b. trochanterica musculi glutei maximi.
b. trochanter'ica mus'culi glu'tei max'imi [NA], trochanteric b. (2); a multilocular b. between the gluteus maximus muscle and the greater trochanter of the femur.
bur'sae trochanter'icae mus'culi glu'tei me'dii [NA], gluteus medius b.; the b. between the tendon of the gluteus medius and the greater trochanter and the b. between the piriformis and gluteus medius.
b. trochanter'ica mus'culi glu'tei min'imi [NA], gluteus minimus b.; a fairly large b. usually located between the gluteus minimus and the greater trochanter.
trochlear synovial b., *vagina* synovialis musculorum obliqui superioris.
ulnar b., *vagina* synovialis communis musculorum flexorum.

---

bursal (ber'săl). Relating to a bursa.

bursectomy (ber-sek'tō-mē) [bursa + G. *ektomē,* excision]. Surgical removal of a bursa.

bursitis (ber-sī'tis). Bursal synovitis; inflammation of a bursa.
anserine b., inflammation of the anserine bursa lying between the pes anserinus and the upper medial surface of the tibia.
bicipital b., intertubercular b.
calcaneal b., capped hock; inflammation of one of the bursae related to the tuber calcanei, usually a result of trauma to the subcutaneous bursa; occurs most frequently in the horse.
intertubercular b., bicipital or shoulder b.; inflammation of the intertubercular bursa of the biceps brachii muscle of the shoulder of the horse, usually the result of trauma.
olecranon b., inflammation of the olecranon bursa.
prepatellar b., housemaid's *knee.*
shoulder b., intertubercular b.
subacromial b., subdeltoid b.; Duplay's disease; calcification of the subacromial bursa.
subdeltoid b., subacromial b.
trochanteric b., inflammation of one of the trochanteric bursae of the horse, and a common cause of hip lameness.

bursolith (ber'sō-lith) [bursa + G. *lithos,* stone]. A calculus formed in a bursa.

bursopathy (ber-sop'ă-thē). Any disease of a bursa.

bursotomy (ber-sot'ō-mē) [bursa + G. *tomē,* a cutting]. Incision through the wall of a bursa.

burst (berst). A sudden increase in activity.
respiratory b., the marked metabolic increase that occurs in a phagocyte following ingestion of particles.

bursula (ber'sū-lă) [Mod. L. dim. of Mediev. L. *bursa,* purse]. A small pouch or bag.
b. tes'tium, scrotum.

Burton, Henry, British physician, 1799–1849. See B.'s *line.*

Bury, Judson S., British dermatologist, 1852–1944. See B.'s *disease.*

Buschke, Abraham, German dermatologist, 1868–1943. See B.'s *disease,* Busse-B. *disease,* B.-Löwenstein *tumor,* B.-Ollendorf *syndrome.*

buspirone hydrochloride (byū-spī'rōn). *N*- [4-[4-(2-Pyrimidinyl)-1-piperazinyl]butyl]-hydrochloride; an antianxiety agent used in the management of anxiety disorders or for short-term relief of the symptoms of anxiety.

Busquet, G. Paul, French physician, *1866. See B.'s *disease.*

Buss. Surname of the man on whose farm the disease was first diagnosed. See B. *disease.*

Busse, Otto, German physician, 1867–1922. See B.-Buschke *disease.*

busulfan, busulphan (byū-sŭl'fan). 1,4-Butanediol dimethanesulfonate; tetramethylene *bis* (methanesulfonate); $CH_3O_2SO(CH_2)_4OSO_2CH_3$; an antineoplastic alkylating agent used in the treatment of chronic myelocytic leukemia; known to be teratogenic in humans.

butabarbital (byū-tă-bar'bi-tawl). 5-*sec*- Butyl-5-ethylbarbituric acid; a sedative and hypnotic with intermediate duration of action; available as b. sodium, with same usages.

butacaine sulfate (byū'tă-kān). 3-(Dibutylamino)-1-propanol *p*-aminobenzoate sulfate; a local anesthetic.

butalbital (byū-tal'bi-tawl). Allylbarbital; 5-allyl-5-isobutylbarbituric acid; a barbiturate of intermediate duration of action; a sedative and hypnotic.

butamben (byū-tam'ben). *Butyl* aminobenzoate.

butane (byū'tān). C_4H_{10}; a gaseous hydrocarbon present in natural gas; various isomers are known, many of which are anesthetically active, as is b.

butanilicaine (byū-tă-nil'i-kān). 2-(Butylamino)-6'-chloro-*o*-acetotoluidide; an aminoacyl anilide formerly used as a local anesthetic.

butanoic acid (byū-tă-nō'ik). Systematic name for normal *butyric acid.*

butanol (byū'tă-nol). Preferred chemical name for butyl alcohol.

butanoyl (byū'tan-ō-il). Butyryl; C_3H_7COO—; the radical of butanoic acid.

butaperazine (byū-tă-per'ă-zēn). 1-{10-[3-(4-Methyl-1-piperazinyl)propyl]-phenothiazin-2-yl}-1-butanone; an antipsychotic.

butaverine (byū-tav'er-ēn). Butyl ester of β-phenyl-1-piperidinepropionic acid; an antispasmodic (as hydrochloride).

butethal (byū'tē-thawl). 5-Butyl-5-ethylbarbituric acid; a sedative and hypnotic.

butethamate (byū-teth'ă-māt). 2-Phenylbutyric acid 2-(diethylamino)ethyl ester; an intestinal antispasmodic agent.

butethamine hydrochloride (byū-teth'ă-mēn). 2-(Isobutylamino)ethyl-*p*- amino benzoate; a local anesthetic.

buthalital (byū-thal'i-tawl). 5-Allyl-5-isobutyl-2-thiobarbituric acid; formerly used for intravenous anesthesia.

buthiazide (byū-thī'ă-zīd). Thiabutazide; 6-chloro-3,4-dihydro-3-isobutyl-2*H*-1,2,4-benzothiadiazine-7-sulfonamide 1,1-dioxide; has diuretic and antihypertensive actions.

butoconazole nitrate (byū-tō-kō'nă-zōl). $C_{19}H_{17}Cl_3N_2S{\cdot}HNO_3$; an antifungal agent used primarily in the treatment of vulvovaginal candidiasis.

butopyronoxyl (byū'tō-pī-rō-nok'sil). Butyl mesityl oxide oxalate; an insect repellent, effective against the biting stable fly (*Stomoxys calcitrans*).

butorphanol tartrate (byū-tōr'fă-nōl). (−)-17- (Cyclobutylmethyl)morphinan-3,14-diol tartrate; a potent nonnarcotic analgesic agent.

butoxamine hydrochloride (byū-tok'să-mēn). α-[1-(*tert*-Butylamino)ethyl]-2,5-dimethoxybenzyl alcohol hydrochloride; an antilipemic agent.

***t*-butoxycarbonyl (Boc)** (byū-toks-ē-kar'bŏn-il). *tert*-Butyloxycarbonyl; $(CH_3)_3C$-O-CO-; an amino-protecting group used in peptide synthesis.

butriptyline hydrochloride (byū-trip'tĭ-lēn). *dl*-10,11-Dihydro-*N,N,β*-trimethyl-5*H*-dibenzo[*a,d*]cycloheptene-5-propylamine; an antidepressant.

butt (bŭt). **1.** To bring any two square-ended surfaces in contact so as to form a joint. **2.** In dentistry, to place a restoration directly against the tissues covering the alveolar ridge.

butter (bŭt'er) [L. *butyrum,* G. *boutyron,* prob. fr. *bous,* cow, + *tyron,* cheese]. **1.** A coherent mass of milk fat, obtained by churning or shaking cream until the separate fat globules run together, leaving a liquid residue, buttermilk. **2.** A soft solid having more or less the consistency of b.

b. of antimony, *antimony* trichloride.

b. of bismuth, *bismuth* trichloride.

cacao b., cocoa b., *theobroma* oil. See also cacao.

b. of tin, stannic chloride pentahydrate, $SnCl_4 \cdot 5H_2O$.

b. of zinc, *zinc* chloride.

Butter's cancer. See under cancer.

butterfly (bŭt'er-flī). **1.** Any structure or apparatus resembling in shape a butterfly with outstretched wings. **2.** Butterfly eruption, patch, or rash; a scaling lesion on each cheek, joined by a narrow band across the nose; seen in lupus erythematosus and seborrheic dermatitis.

but'termilk. The fluid containing casein and lactic acid, left after the process of making butter.

butter yellow [C.I. 11160]. Methyl yellow; dimethylaminoazobenzene; $C_6H_5N{:}NC_6H_4N(CH_3)_2$; a fat-soluble yellow dye (MW 225) that has hepatic carcinogenic action in experimental animals; used as an indicator of pH (red, at pH 2.9, yellow at pH 4.0).

buttocks (bŭt'oks). Nates.

button (bŭt'ŏn) [Middle Fr. *boton,* a bud, probably fr. L. *bottere,* to thrust]. A structure, lesion, or device of knob shape.

Amboyna b. [*Amboyna,* one of the Spice Islands in the Malay Archipelago], yaws.

Biskra b., the lesion occurring in cutaneous leishmaniasis.

Murphy's b., an obsolete appliance formerly used for intestinal anastomosis; it consists of two hollow cylinders, one of which is sutured into each open end of the intestine; the two are then joined and fasten automatically, maintaining the two ends of intestine in apposition by their serous surfaces; after firm union has occurred the cylinders slough away and are passed in the stools.

Oriental b., the lesion occurring in cutaneous leishmaniasis.

peritoneal b., a device used to drain ascitic fluid to subcutaneous space.

buttonhole (bŭt'ŏn-hōl). **1.** A short straight cut made through the wall of a cavity or canal. **2.** The contraction of an orifice down to a narrow slit; *i.e.,* the so-called mitral b. in extreme mitral stenosis. See buttonhole *stenosis.*

butyl (byū'til). C_4H_9—; a radical of butane.

b. alcohol, C_4H_9OH; several isomeric forms are known: **primary b. a.,** propylcarbinol, $CH_3CH_2CH_2CH_2OH$, the butyl alcohol of fermentation; **isobutyl alcohol,** isopropylcarbinol, 2-methylpropanol, $(CH_3)_2CHCH_2OH$; **secondary b. a.,** ethylmethylcarbinol, 1-methylpropanol, $CH_3CH_2CH(CH_3)OH$; and **tertiary b. a.,** trimethylcarbinol, 1,1-dimethylethanol, $(CH_3)_3COH$.

b. aminobenzoate, butamben; *n*-butyl *p*-aminobenzoate; a local anesthetic, very insoluble and only slightly absorbed.

***tert*-butyloxycarbonyl** (byū'til-oks'ē-kar'bŏn-il). *t*-Butoxycarbonyl.

butylparaben (byū-til-par'ă-ben). Butyl *p*-hydroxybenzoate; an antifungal preservative.

butyraceous (byū-tir-ā'shĭ-us). Buttery in consistency.

butyrate (byū'ti-rāt). A salt or ester of butyric acid.

butyrate-CoA ligase [EC 6.2.1.2]. Butyryl-CoA synthetase; fatty acid thiokinase (medium chain); acyl-activating enzyme (2); a ligase forming acyl-CoA's from medium-chain fatty acids and CoA at the expense of ATP.

butyric (byū-tir'ik). Relating to butter.

butyric acid (byū-tir'ik). An acid of unpleasant odor occurring in butter, cod liver oil, sweat, and many other substances. It exists in two forms: **normal b. a.,** butanoic acid, $CH_3CH_2CH_2COOH$, which occurs in combination with glycerol in cow's butter; and **isobutyric acid,** 2-methylpropanoic acid, $(CH_3)_2CHCOOH$, one of the intermediates in valine catabolism, found in combination with glycerol in croton oil and elsewhere.

γ-butyrobetaine (byū-tir'ō-be-tān). γ-(Trimethylammonium) butyric acid; a betaine of γ-aminobutyric acid; a precursor of carnitine by hydroxylation of the β-carbon.

butyrocholinesterase (byū'tir-ō-kō-lin-es'ter-ās). Cholinesterase.

butyroid (byū'ti-royd). **1.** Buttery. **2.** Resembling butter.

butyrometer (byū-ti-rom'ĕ-ter) [G. *boutyron,* butter, + *metron,* measure]. An instrument for determining the amount of butterfat in milk.

butyrophenone (byū'tir-ō-fē'nōn). One of a group of derivatives of 4-phenylbutylamine that have neuroleptic activity; *e.g.,* haloperidol.

butyrous (byū'ti-rŭs). Denoting a tissue or bacterial growth of butter-like consistency.

butyryl (byū'ti-ril). Butanoyl.

butyrylcholine esterase (byū'ti-ril-kō'lēn es'ter-ās). Cholinesterase.

butyryl-CoA synthetase. Butyrate-CoA ligase.

Buzzard, Thomas, British physician, 1831–1919. See B.'s *maneuver.*

Buzzi, Fausto, coworker of Ernst Schweninger. See Schweninger-B. *anetoderma.*

bypass (bī'pas). **1.** A shunt or auxiliary flow. **2.** To create new flow from one structure to another through a diversionary channel. See also shunt.

aortocoronary b., coronary b.

aortoiliac b., an operation in which a vascular prosthesis is united with the aorta and iliac artery to relieve obstruction of the lower abdominal aorta, its bifurcation, and the proximal iliac branches.

aortorenal b., insertion of a graft of autogenous artery, saphenous vein, or synthetic material between the aorta and the distal renal artery, to circumvent an obstruction of the renal artery.

bowel b., jejunoileal b.

cardiopulmonary b., diversion of the blood flow returning to the heart through a pump oxygenator (heart-lung machine) and then returning it to the arterial side of the circulation; used in operations upon the heart to maintain extracorporeal circulation.

coronary b., aortocoronary b.; vein grafts or other conduits shunting blood from the aorta to branches of the coronary arteries, in order to increase the flow beyond the local obstruction.

extraintracranial b., a shunt of extracranial to intracranial vessels, commonly, the superficial temporal to middle cerebral arteries.

femoropopliteal b., a vascular prosthesis that bypasses an obstruction in the femoral artery; may be synthetic material, autologous tissue, or heterologous tissue.

gastric b., Mason operation; high division of the stomach, anastomosis of the small upper pouch of the stomach to the jejunum, and closure of the distal part of the stomach that is retained; used for treatment of morbid obesity.

jejunoileal b., jejunoileal shunt; anastomosis of the upper jejunum to the terminal ileum for treatment of morbid obesity.

partial ileal b., division of the small intestine approximately at the junction of the middle and lower one-third, closure of the distal end, and anastomosis of the proximal end to the cecum.

byssinosis (bis-i-nō'sis) [G. *byssos,* flax, + *-osis,* condition]. Cotton-mill or mill fever; an occupational respiratory disease of cotton, flax, and hemp workers (usually allergic), characterized by symptoms (especially wheezing) most severe at the beginning of each work week (since lack of exposure over the weekend allows buildup of large quantities of mediators of allergy, such as histamine).

C

C **1.** Abbreviation or symbol for large *calorie;* carbon; cathodal; cathode; Celsius; centigrade; cervical vertebra (C1 to C7); closure (of an electrical circuit); congius (gallon); contraction; cylinder; cylindrical *lens;* cytidine. **2.** When followed by a subscript, indicates renal clearance of a substance (*e.g.,* C_{In}, inulin clearance); compliance (*e.g.,* C_L, compliance of the lungs); concentration (3).

c **1.** Symbol for centi-; small *calorie.* **2.** As a subscript, refers to blood *capillary.*

c̄ Abbreviation for L. *cum,* with.

CA Abbreviation for carcinoma; cardiac *arrest;* cancer; chronologic *age; cytosine* arabinoside; *Chemical Abstracts* Service.

Ca **1.** Abbreviation for cathode. **2.** Symbol for calcium.

ca. Abbreviation for L. *circa* (about, approximately).

caapi (ka'pē). Aya huasca; wild rue; a hallucinogenic preparation obtained from *Banisteria caapi* (family Malpighaceae), a South American jungle vine; contains harmine and other psychotomimetic principles.

cabbage tree (kab'ij trē). Andira.

cabinet (kab'i-net). A box or small chamber.

pneumatic c., an airtight chamber with plate glass front, large enough to accommodate a sitting person, in which the air may be compressed or rarified at will.

Sauerbruch's c., an airtight chamber permitting operation on the thorax under negative air pressure, the patient lying within the c. with his head outside.

Cabot, Richard C., U.S. physician, 1868–1939, See C.'s ring *bodies.*

Cabot-Locke murmur. See under murmur.

cac-, caci-. See caco-.

cacao (kă-ka'ō) [native Mexican origin]. Theobroma; prepared c., or cocoa, a powder prepared from the roasted cured kernels of the ripe seed of *Theobroma cacao Linné* (family Sterculiaceae); the tree yields a fat, theobroma oil.

c. oil, *theobroma* oil.

CaCC Abbreviation for cathodal closure *contraction.*

Cacchione, Aldo. See De Sanctis-C. *syndrome.*

caché (kah-shā') [Fr. hidden, covered]. A lead cone covered with several layers of paper, having a mica window at the bottom, used as an applicator in radiotherapy, the radium or other radioactive substance being at the apex of the cone and filters being placed below as required.

cachectic (kă-kek'tik). Relating to or suffering from cachexia.

cachectin (kak-hek'tin) [G. *kakos,* bad, + *hexis,* condition of body]. Tumor necrosis factor; a polypeptide hormone produced by endotoxin-activated macrophages which has the ability to modulate adipocyte metabolism, lyse tumor cells *in vitro,* and induce hemorrhagic necrosis of certain transplantable tumors *in vivo.*

cachet (kă-shā') [Fr. a seal]. A seal-shaped capsule or wafer for enclosing powders of disagreeable taste.

cachexia (kă-kek'sē-ă) [G. *kakos,* bad, + *hexis,* condition of body]. A general weight loss and wasting occurring in the course of a chronic disease or emotional disturbance.

c. aphtho'sa, sprue (1).

c. aquo'sa, an edematous form of ancylostomiasis.

c. hypophys'eopri'va, a condition following total removal of the hypophysis cerebri, marked by a fall of body temperature, electrolyte imbalance, and hypoglycemia, followed by coma and death.

hypophysial c., Simmonds *disease.*

malarial c., chronic *malaria.*

pituitary c., Simmonds' *disease.*

c. strumipri'va, c. thyropriva.

c. thyroid'ea, c. thyropriva.

c. thyropri'va, c. thyroidea; c. strumipriva; signs and symptoms of hypothyroidism (with or without myxedema) resulting from the loss of thyroid tissue, either from surgery or radiotherapy.

cachinnation (kak-i-nā'shŭn) [L. *cachinnare,* to laugh immoderately and loudly]. Laughter without apparent cause, often observed in schizophrenia.

caco-, caci-, cac- [G. *kakos,* bad]. Combining forms meaning bad or ill.

cacocholia (kak-ō-kō'lē-ă) [caco- + G. *cholē,* bile]. An abnormal state of the bile.

cacodemonomania (kak-ō-dē'mon-ō-mā'nē-ă) [caco- + G. *daimōn,* spirit, + *mania,* frenzy]. A mental condition in which the patient believes himself to be inhabited by or possessed by an evil spirit.

cacodyl (kak'ō-dil). Tetramethyldiarsine; dicacodyl; $(CH_3)_2As$-$As(CH_3)_2$; an oil resulting from the distillation together of arsenous acid and potassium acetate.

cacodylate (kak'ō-dil-āt). A salt or ester of cacodylic acid. See cacodylic acid.

cacodylic (kak-ō-dil'ik). Relating to cacodyl; denoting especially c. acid.

cacodylic acid. Dimethylarsinic acid; $(CH_3)_2AsOOH$; prepared by treating cacodyl and cacodyl oxide with mercuric oxide, and forms cacodylates with various bases which were used in skin diseases, tuberculosis, malaria, and other affections in which arsenic was considered of value.

cacogenesis (kak-ō-jen'ĕ-sis) [caco- + G. *genesis,* origin]. Abnormal growth or development.

cacogenic (kak-ō-jen'ik). Relating to cacogenesis.

cacogenics (kak-ō-jen'iks). Obsolete term for practices and policies that tend to result in deterioration of a stock by adverse sexual selection.

cacogeusia (kak-ō-gū'sē-ă) [caco- + G. *geusis,* taste]. A bad taste.

cacomelia (kak-ō-mē'lē-ă) [caco- + G. *melos,* limb]. Congenital deformity of one or more limbs.

cacoplastic (kak-ō-plas'tik) [caco- + G. *plastikos,* formed]. **1.** Relating to or causing abnormal growth. **2.** Incapable of normal or perfect formation.

cacosmia (kă-koz'mē-ă) [G. *kakosmia,* a bad smell, fr. *kakos,* bad, + *osmē,* the sense of smell]. A subjective perception of nonexistent disagreeable odors; a variety of parosmia.

cactinomycin (kak'ti-nō-mī'sin). Actinomycin C; produced by *Streptomyces chrysomallus.* A mixture of actinomycins C_1 (dactinomycin), C_2, and C_3 used as an antineoplastic, immunosuppressive agent. See also actinomycins.

cacumen, pl. **cacumina** (kak-yū'men, -mi-nă) [L. summit]. The top or apex of a plant or an anatomical structure.

cacuminal (kak-yū'mi-năl). Relating to a top or apex, particularly of a plant or anatomical structure.

cadaver (kă-dav'er) [L. fr. *cado,* to fall]. Corpse; a dead body.

cadaveric (kă-dav'er-ik). Relating to a dead body.

cadaverine (kă-dav'er-in). 1,5-Pentanediamine; $H_2N(CH_2)_5NH_2$; a foul-smelling diamine formed by bacterial decarboxylation of lysine; poisonous and irritating to the skin.

cadaverous (kă-dav'er-ŭs). Having the pallor and appearance resembling a corpse.

cade oil (kād). *Juniper* tar.

cadmium (kad'mē-ŭm) [L. *cadmia,* fr. G. *kadmeia* or *kadmia,* an ore of zinc, calamine]. A metallic element, symbol Cd, atomic no. 48, atomic weight 112.40; its salts are poisonous and little used in medicine. Various compounds of c. are used commercially in metallurgy, photography, electrochemistry, etc.; a few have been used as ascaricides, antiseptics, and fungicides.

CaDTe Abbreviation for cathodal duration *tetanus.*

caduca (kă-dū'kă) [L. fem. of *caducus,* fallen, falling]. *Membrana* decidua.

caduceus (kă-dū'sē-ŭs) [L. the staff of Mercury]. A staff with two oppositely twined serpents and surmounted by two wings; emblem of the U.S. Army Medical Corps. For veterinary medicine the double serpent was changed in 1972 to its present form with a single serpent. See also staff of Aesculapius.

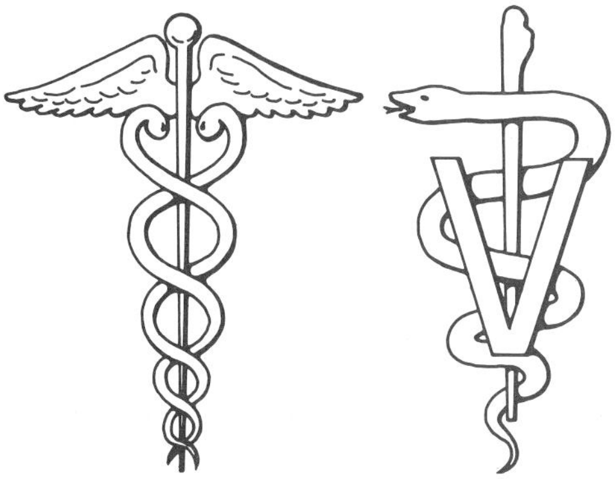

Caduceus
Left, insignia of the United States Army Medical Corps; *right,* insignia approved by the American Veterinary Medicine Association.

cae-. For words so beginning, see under ce-.

caffearine (kaf'ē-ă-rin). Trigonelline.

caffeine (kaf'ēn). Guaranine; thein; 1,3,7-trimethylxanthine; an alkaloid obtained from the dried leaves of *Thea sinensis,* tea, or the dried seeds of *Coffea arabica,* coffee; used as a diuretic and circulatory and respiratory stimulant, and in the treatment of headaches.
c. citrate, citrated c., a mixture of equal parts of c. and citric acid.
c. hydrate, monohydrate of c., a central nervous system stimulant.
c. and sodium benzoate, a mixture of equal parts of sodium benzoate and c., used to meet the indication of c.
c. and sodium salicylate, a mixture of sodium salicylate and c. used for the relief of headache and neuralgia.

caffeinism (kaf'ēn-izm). Caffeine intoxication characterized by restlessness, nervousness, excitement, insomnia, flushed face, diuresis, and gastrointestinal complaints, brought on by the ingestion of substances containing caffeine.

Caffey, John, U.S. pediatrician, 1895–1966. See C.'s *disease, syndrome;* C.-Silverman *syndrome.*

cage (kāj). **1.** An enclosure made partly or completely of open work and commonly used to house animals. **2.** A structure resembling such an enclosure.
thoracic c., compages thoracis.

Cajal (Ramón y Cajal), Santiago, Spanish histologist and Nobel laureate, 1852–1934. See C.'s *cell,* astrocyte *stain;* interstitial *nucleus* of C.

cajeput oil, cajuput oil (kaj'ĕ-pŭt, -yū-pŭt). A volatile oil distilled from the fresh leaves of *Cajuputi viridiflora,* a tree of tropical Asia and Australia; a stimulant, counterirritant, and expectorant.

cajeputol, cajuputol (kaj'ĕ-pyū-tol, -ŭ-pyū-tol). Cineole.

Cal Abbreviation for large *calorie.*

cal Abbreviation for small *calorie.*

Calabar bean (kal'ă-bar bēn). Physostigma.

calamine (kal'ă-mīn). Zinc oxide with a small amount of ferric oxide or basic zinc carbonate suitably colored with ferric oxide; used in dusting powders, lotions, and ointments, as a mild astringent and protective agent for skin disorders.

calamus (kal'ă-mŭs) [L. reed, a pen]. **1.** The dried, unpeeled rhizome of *Acorus calamus* (family Araceae), cultivated in Burma and Sri Lanka, a carminative and anthelminthic. **2.** A reed-shaped structure.
c. scripto'rius [L. writing pen], Arantius' ventricle; inferior part of the rhomboid fossa; the narrow lower end of the fourth ventricle between the two clavae.

calcaneal, calcanean (kal-kā'nē-al, kal-kā'nē-an). Relating to the calcaneus or heel bone.

calcaneo- [L. *calcaneum* heel]. Combining form relating to the calcaneus.

calcaneoapophysitis (kal-kā'nē-ō-ă-pof-i-sī'tis). Inflammation at the posterior part of the os calcis, at the insertion of the Achilles tendon.

calcaneoastragaloid (kal-kā'nē-ō-as-trag'ă-loyd). Relating to the calcaneus, or os calcis, and the talus, or astragalus.

calcaneocuboid (kal-kā'nē-ō-kyū'boyd). Relating to the calcaneus and the cuboid bone.

calcaneodynia (kal-kā'nē-ō-din'ē-ă) [calcaneo- + G. *odynē,* pain]. Painful *heel.*

calcaneonavicular (kal-kā'nē-ō-na-vik'yū-lăr). Calcaneoscaphoid; relating to the calcaneus and the navicular bone.

calcaneoscaphoid (kal-kā'nē-ō-skaf'oyd). Calcaneonavicular.

calcaneotibial (kal-kā'nē-ō-tib'ē-ăl). Relating to the calcaneus and the tibia.

calcaneovalgus (kal-kā'nē-ō-val'gŭs). See *talipes* calcaneovalgus.

calcaneovarus (kal-kā'nē-ō-vā'rŭs). See *talipes* calcaneovarus.

calcaneum (kal-kā'nē-ŭm) [L. the heel]. Calcaneus.

calcaneus, gen. and pl. **calcanei** (kal-kā'nē-ŭs, -kā'nē-ī) [L. the heel (another form of *calcaneum*)]. **1** [NA]. Calcaneum; calcaneal or heel bone; os calcis; the largest of the tarsal bones; it forms the heel and articulates with the cuboid anteriorly and the talus above. **2.** *Talipes* calcaneus.

calcar (kal'kar) [L. spur, cock's spur]. **1.** A small projection from any structure; internal spurs (septa) at the level of division of arteries and confluence of veins when branches or roots form an acute angle. **2.** A dull spine or projection from a bone. **3.** A horny outgrowth from the skin. See also subentries under spur.
c. a'vis [NA], hippocampus minor; Morand's spur; Haller's unguis; unguis avis; the lower of two elevations on the medial wall of the posterior horn of the lateral ventricle of the brain, caused by the depth of of the calcarine sulcus.
c. femora'le, Bigelow's septum; a bony spur springing from the underside of the neck of the femur above and anterior to the lesser trochanter, adding to the strength of this part of the bone.
c. pedis, calx (2).

calcareous (kal-kā'rē-ŭs) [L. *calcarius,* pertaining to lime, fr. *calx,* lime]. Chalky; relating to or containing lime or calcium, or calcific material.

calcarine (kal'kă-rēn). **1.** Relating to a calcar. **2.** Spur-shaped.

calcariuria (kal-kar-ē-yū'rē-ă) [L. *calcarius,* of lime, + G. *ouron,* urine]. Excretion of calcium (lime) salts in the urine.

calcergy (kal'ser-jē) [L. *calx,* chalk, calcium, + G. *ergon,* work, production]. Local calcification of soft tissue occurring at the site of injection of certain chemical compounds, such as lead acetate or cerium chloride; hydroxyapatite deposits are found in the calcified areas.

calces (kal'sēz). Plural of calx.

calcic (kal'sik). Relating to lime.

calcicosis (kal-si-kō'sis). Pneumoconiosis from the inhalation of limestone dust. Sometimes called marble cutter's phthisis.

calcidiol (kal-sĭ-dī'ol). Calcifediol; 25-hydroxycholecalciferol (a 3,25-diol); the first step in the biological conversion of vitamin D_3 to the more active form, calcitriol; it is more potent than vitamin D_3.

calcifediol (kal-sĭ-fĕ-dī'ol). Calcidiol.

calciferol (kal-sif'er-ol). Ergocalciferol.

calciferous (kal-sif'er-ŭs). Calcophorous. **1.** Containing lime. **2.** Producing any of the salts of calcium.

calcification (kal'si-fi-kā'shŭn) [L. *calx,* lime, + *facio,* to make]. Calcareous infiltration. **1.** Deposition of lime or other insoluble calcium salts. **2.** A process in which tissue or noncellular material in the body becomes hardened as the result of precipitates or larger deposits of insoluble salts of calcium (and also magnesium), especially calcium carbonate and phosphate (hydroxyapatite) normally occurring only in the formation of bone and teeth.
dystrophic c., c. occurring in degenerated or necrotic tissue, as in hyalinized scars, degenerated foci in leiomyomas, and caseous nodules.
metastatic c., c. occurring in nonosseous, viable tissue (*i.e.,* tissue that is not degenerated or necrotic), as in the stomach, lungs, and kidneys (and rarely in other sites); the cells of these organs secrete acid materials, and, under certain conditions in instances of hypercalcemia, the alteration in pH seems to cause precipitation of calcium salts in these sites.
Mönckeberg's c., Mönckeberg's *arteriosclerosis.*
pathologic c., c. occurring in excretory or secretory passages as calculi, and in tissues other than bone and teeth.
pulp c., endolith.

calcify (kal'si-fī). To deposit or lay down calcium salts, as in the formation of bone.

calcination (kal-si-nā'shŭn). The process of calcining.

calcine (kal'sēn). To expel water and volatile matter by heat.

calcinosis (kal-si-nō'sis) [calcium + *-osis,* condition]. A condition characterized by the deposition of calcium salts in nodular foci in various tissues other than the parenchymatous viscera; the two well-known forms, c. circumscripta and c. universalis, are not associated with tissue damage or demonstrable metabolic disease; other forms are the result of abnormal calcium and/or phosporous metabolism.
c. circumscrip'ta, localized deposits of calcium salts in the skin and subcutaneous tissues, usually surrounded by a zone of granulomatous inflammation; clinically, the lesions resemble the tophi of gout.
c. cu'tis, dystrophic c.; skin stones; a deposit of calcium in the skin; usually occurs secondary to a preexisting inflammatory, degenerative, or neoplastic dermatosis, and is frequently seen in scleroderma.
dystrophic c., c. cutis.
c. intervertebra'lis, calcium deposit in vertebral disk.
reversible c., a form of c. sometimes observed in patients who constantly ingest large quantities of milk and alkaline medicines, as in the treatment of peptic ulcer.
tumoral c., calcification of collagen, chiefly at the site of large joints, in South African blacks; probably genetic.
c. universa'lis, diffuse deposits of calcium salts in the skin and subcutaneous tissues, connective tissue, and other sites; may be associated with dermatomyositis, occurs more frequently in young persons, and is often fatal; serum levels of calcium and phosphorus are generally within normal limits.

calciol (kal'sē-ol). Cholecalciferol.

calciostat (kal'sē-ō-stat) [calcium + G. *statos,* standing]. Rarely used term denoting a postulated mechanism by which the parathyroid hormone production is increased when serum calcium is low and decreased when it is high.

calciotraumatic (kal'sē-ō-traw-mat'ik). Relating to the line of disturbed calcification that appears in the dentin of the incisor teeth of young rats placed on a rachitogenic diet: high in calcium and low in phosphorus, with no vitamin D.

calcipenia (kal-si-pē'nē-ă) [calcium + G. *penia,* poverty]. A condition in which there is an insufficient amount of calcium in the tissues and fluids of the body.

calcipenic (kal-si-pē'nik). Pertaining to calcipenia.

calcipexic (kal-si-pek'sik). Related or pertaining to calcipexis.

calcipexis, calcipexy (kal-si-pek'sis, kal'si-pek-sē) [calcium + G. *pēxis,* a fixing]. Fixation of calcium in the tissues, an occasional cause of tetany in infants.

calciphilia (cal-si-fil'ē-ă) [calcium + G. *phileō,* to love]. A condition in which the tissues manifest an unusual affinity for, and fixation of, calcium salts circulating in the blood.

calciphylaxis (kal'si-fī-lak'sis). A condition of induced systemic hypersensitivity in which tissues respond to appropriate challenging agents with a sudden, but sometimes evanescent, local calcification.

calciprivia (kal-si-priv'ē-ă). Absence or deprivation of calcium in diet.

calciprivic (kal-si-priv'ik). Deprived of calcium.

calcite (kal'sīt). Calcspar; $CaCO_3$; a naturally occurring mineral found in several forms, *e.g.,* chalk, Iceland spar, limestone, marble. See also calcium carbonate.

calcitetrol (kal-si-tet'rol). The 1,24,25-triol (a 1,3,24,24-tetrol) of cholecalciferol.

calcitonin (kal-si-tō'nin). Thyrocalcitonin; a peptide hormone, of which eight forms in five species are known; composed of 32 amino acids and produced by the parathyroid, thyroid, and thymus glands; its action is opposite to that of parathyroid hormone in that c. increases deposition of calcium and phosphate in bone; its level in the blood is increased by glucagon and by Ca^{2+}, and thus opposes postprandial hypercalcemia.

calcitriol (kal-si-trī'ol). 1α, 25-Dihydroxycholecalciferol (a 1,3,25-triol); the second step in the biological conversion of vitamin D_3 to its active form; it is more potent than calcidiol.

calcitroic acid (kal-si-trō'ik). A metabolite of calcitriol, involving the loss of carbons 24, 25, 26, and 27 and the oxidation of carbon 23 to a carboxylic acid; its function is unknown.

CALCIUM

calcium, gen. **cal'cii** (kal'sē-ŭm, -sē-ī) [Mod. L. fr. L. *calx,* lime]. A metallic dyad element; symbol Ca, atomic no. 20, atomic weight 40.09, density 1.54, melting point 810°. The oxide of c. is an alkaline earth, CaO, quicklime, which on the addition of water becomes c. hydrate, $Ca(OH)_2$, slaked lime. For some organic c. salts not listed below, see the name of the organic acid portion.
c. alginate, a topical hemostatic.

c. aminosalicylate, the c. salt of *p*-aminosalicylic acid, with the same uses.
c. benzoylpas, calcium 4-benzamidosalicylate; an antituberculous agent.
c. bromide, used to meet the same indications as potassium bromide.
c. carbaspirin, calcium salt of acetylsalicyclic acid compounded with urea (1:1 complex); an analgesic.
c. carbide, CaC_2; blackish crystalline lumps which when in contact with water yield acetylene gas.
c. carbimide, c. cyanamide; Ca=N—C≡N; a fertilizer and weed seed killer that also exhibits antithyroid activity; like disulfiram, it impairs ethanol metabolism; workers in cyanamide-producing plants exhibit systemic symptoms ("Monday-morning illness") after ingestion of alcohol.
c. carbonate, chalk; creta; $CaCO_3$; an astringent and antacid. See also calcite.
c. caseinate, the form of casein present in cow's milk; used in dietetic preparations; has been used for diarrhea in infants.
c. chloride, used to correct calcium deficiencies and in the treatment of magnesium intoxication and cardiac failure.
citrated c. carbimide, a mixture of two parts citric acid to one part c. carbimide; in the metabolism of ethanol, it slows the conversion of acetaldehyde to acetate; used in the treatment of alcoholism.
crude c. sulfide, sulfurated lime; used externally in the treatment of acne, scabies, and ringworm.
c. cyanamide, c. carbimide.
dibasic c. phosphate, c. monohydrogen phosphate; secondary c. phosphate; $CaHPO_4 \cdot 2H_2O$; used as a c. and phosphorus dietary supplement.
c. disodium edetate, *edetate* calcium disodium.
c. disodium ethylenediaminetetraacetate, *edetate* calcium disodium.
c. folinate, *leucovorin* calcium.
c. glubionate, calcium D-gluconate lactobionate monohydrate; a calcium replenisher.
c. gluceptate, c. glucoheptonate; used as a nutrient.
c. glucoheptonate, c. gluceptate.
c. gluconate, a salt of c. more palatable than the chloride.
c. glycerophosphate, a c. and phosphorus dietary supplement.
c. hippurate, said to be a solvent of uratic gravel and calculi.
c. hydroxide, $Ca(OH)_2$; used as a carbon dioxide absorbent.
c. hypophosphite, has been used for rickets and impaired nutrition.
c. iodate, used as a dusting powder and, in lotion and ointment, as an antiseptic and deodorant.
c. iodobehenate, a c. salt, $(C_{21}H_{42}ICOO)_2Ca$, used to meet the indications of the ordinary iodides.
c. ipodate, calcium salt of 3-[(dimethylaminomethylene)amino]-2,4,6-triiodohydrocinnamic acid; a radiopaque medium used in cholangiography and cholecystography.
c. lactate, used as a calcium replenisher.
c. lactophosphate, a mixture of c. lactate, c. acid lactate, and c. acid phosphate; used as a c. and phosphorus dietary supplement.
c. leucovorin, see under leucovorin.
c. levulinate, a hydrated c. salt of levulinic acid; it has the usual effects of c. administered orally or intravenously.
c. mandelate, c. salt of mandelic acid; a urinary anti-infective agent.
c. monohydrogen phosphate, dibasic c. phosphate.
c. oxalate, CaC_2O_4; found as sediment in the urine and in urinary calculi.
c. oxide, lime (1).
c. pantothenate, the c. salt of pantothenic acid; a vitamin B filtrate factor.
precipitated c. carbonate, $CaCO_3$; used as an antacid in the management of peptic ulcers and other conditions of gastric hyperacidity.
c. propionate, the c. salt of propionic acid; an antifungal agent.
racemic c. pantothenate, a mixture of the c. salts of the dextrorotatory and levorotatory isomers of pantothenic acid; same uses as c. pantothenate.
c. saccharate, c. D-saccharate; used as an antacid in dyspepsia and flatulence, as an antidote in carbolic acid poisoning, and as a stabilizer for c. gluconate solution for parenteral administration.
secondary c. phosphate, dibasic c. phosphate.
c. stearate, used in the preparation of tablets.
c. sulfate, CaO_4S; used in exsiccated form to make plaster of Paris. See also gypsum.
c. sulfite, used as an intestinal antiseptic, and locally in the treatment of parasitic skin diseases.
tertiary c. phosphate, tribasic c. phosphate.
tribasic c. phosphate, tricalcium phosphate; tertiary c. phosphate; bone phosphate; bone ash; $Ca_3(PO_4)_2$; used as an antacid.
c. trisodium pentetate, pentetate trisodium calcium.

---

calcium-45 (**^{45}Ca**). Most easily available of the radioactive c. isotopes; beta-emitter with a half-life of 164 days; used as a tracer.

calcium group. The metals of the alkaline earths: beryllium, magnesium, calcium, strontium, barium, and radium.

calciuria (kal-sē-yū'rē-ă). The urinary excretion of calcium; sometimes used as a synonym for hypercalciuria.

calcodynia (kal-kō-din'ē-ă) [L. *calx*, heel, + G. *odynē*, pain]. Painful *heel.*

calcophorous (kal-kof'er-ŭs) [L. *calx*, lime, + G. *phoros*, bearing]. Calciferous.

calcospherite (kal-kō-sfēr'īt) [L. *calx*, lime, + G. *sphaira*, sphere]. Psammoma bodies (3); a tiny, spheroidal, concentrically laminated body containing accretive deposits of calcium salts; found most frequently in papillary carcinomas of the thyroid and ovary, probably as the result of degenerative changes in the fibrovascular stroma.

calcspar (kalk'spar). Calcite.

calculi (kal'kyū-lī). Plural of calculus.

calculosis (kal-kyū-lō'sis) [L. *calculus*, small stone, + G. *-osis*, condition]. The tendency or disposition to form calculi or stones.

calculus, gen. and pl. **calculi** (kal'kyū-lŭs, -lī) [L. a pebble, a calculus]. Stone (1); a concretion formed in any part of the body, most commonly in the passages of the biliary and urinary tracts; usually composed of salts of inorganic or organic acids, or of other material such as cholesterol.
apatite c., a c. in which the crystalloid component consists of calcium fluophosphate.
arthritic c., gouty *tophus.*
biliary c., gallstone.
blood c., hemic c.; an angiolith or concretion of coagulated blood.
branched c., staghorn c.
bronchial c., broncholith.
cardiac c., cardiolith.
cerebral c., encephalolith.
combination c., alternating c.
coral c., staghorn c.
cystine c., a c. composed of cystine, soft and faintly radiopaque.
decubitus c., a c. formed in the urinary tract, as a result of long immobilization.
dendritic c., staghorn c.
dental c., **(1)** calcified deposits formed around the teeth; may appear as subgingival or supragingival c.; **(2)** tartar (2).
encysted c., pocketed c.; a urinary c. enclosed in a sac developed from the wall of the bladder.
fibrin c., a urinary c. formed largely from fibrinogen in blood.

fusible c., obsolete term for a c. formed from a mixture of calcium phosphate and triple phosphates which fuses to a black enamel-like mass when tested under a blowpipe.
gastric c., gastrolith.
hematogenetic c., serumal c.
hemic c., blood c.
indigo c., a c. formed by oxidation of indican in the urine.
intestinal c., a concretion in the bowel, either a coprolith or an enterolith.
lacrimal c., dacryolith.
mammary c., a concretion in one of the ducts of the breast.
matrix c., a yellowish-white to light tan urinary c. containing calcium salts, with the consistency of putty; composed chiefly of an organic matrix consisting of a mucoprotein and a sulfated mucopolysaccharide, and usually associated with chronic infection.
mulberry c., a hard smooth urinary c. composed of calcium oxalate, so-called because of its resemblance to a mulberry.
nasal c., rhinolith.
nephritic c., obsolete term for renal c.
oxalate c., a hard urinary c. of calcium oxalate; some are covered with minute sharp spines that can abrade the renal pelvic epithelium, whereas others are smooth.
pancreatic c., pancreatolith; pancreolith; a concretion, usually multiple, in the pancreatic duct, associated with chronic pancreatitis.
pharyngeal c., pharyngolith.
pleural c., pleurolith.
pocketed c., encysted c.
preputial c., postholith; a c. occuring beneath the foreskin.
primary renal c., a c. formed in an apparently healthy urinary tract, usually composed of oxalates, urates, or cystine.
prostatic c., prostatolith; a concretion formed in the prostate gland, composed chiefly of calcium carbonate and phosphate (corpora amylacea).
pulp c., endolith.
renal c., nephrolith; a c. occurring within the kidney collecting system.
salivary c., **(1)** a c. in a salivary duct or gland; **(2)** supragingival c.
secondary renal c., a c. associated with infection and/or obstruction, usually composed of struvite (magnesium ammonium phosphate).
serumal c., **(1)** hematogenetic c.; a greenish or dark brown calcareous deposit on the tooth, usually apical to the gingival margin; **(2)** subgingival c.
staghorn c., branched, coral, or dendritic c.; a c. occurring in the renal pelvis, with branches extending into the infundibula and calices.
struvite c., a c. in which the crystalloid component consists of magnesium ammonium phosphate.
subgingival c., serumal c. (2); calcareous deposit found on the tooth apical to the gingival margin.
supragingival c., salivary c. (2); calcified plaques adherent to tooth surfaces coronal to the free gingival margin.
tonsillar c., tonsillolith.
urinary c., urolith; a c. in the kidney, ureter, bladder, or urethra.
uterine c., uterolith; hysterolith; a calcified myoma of the uterus.
vesical c., cystolith; a urinary c. formed or retained in the bladder.
weddellite c., a c. in which the crystalloid component consists of calcium oxalate dihydrate.
whewellite c., a c. in which the crystalloid component consists of calcium oxalate monohydrate.

Calculus Surface Index (CSI). An index that measures only dental calculus, used for evaluating new calculus formation within a large group of test subjects.

Caldani, Leopoldo M.A., Italian anatomist, 1725–1813. See C.'s *ligament.*

Caldwell, George W., U.S. physician, 1834–1918. See C.-Luc *operation.*

Caldwell, William E., U.S. obstetrician, 1880–1943. See C.-Moloy *classification.*

Caldwell projection, Caldwell view. See under projection, view.

calefacient (kal-ĕ-fā'shent) [L. *calefacio,* fr. *caleo,* to be warm, + *facio,* to make]. **1.** Making warm or hot. **2.** An agent causing a sense of warmth in the part to which it is applied.

calf, pl. **calves** (kaf, kavz) [Gael. *kalpa*]. **1.** Sura. **2.** A young bovine animal, male or female.
bull-dog c., bovine achondroplasia; a c. with a short muzzle and brachycephalic skull, usually resulting from chondrodystrophy; associated with this condition are shortened limbs and anomalies of the vertebral centra; it often results in respiratory and feeding difficulties, and is sometimes fatal.
football c., an obsolete term used to describe the doughy sensation elicited on palpation of the c. when muscle necrosis has developed as a consequence of acute ischemia produced by acute arterial embolism.
gnome's c., an obsolete term denoting the very full rounded c. occurring in pseudohypertrophic muscular dystrophy affecting the gastrocnemius muscles.

calf-bone. Fibula.

caliber (kal'i-ber) [Fr. *calibre,* of uncert. etym.]. The diameter of a hollow tubular structure.

calibrate (kal'i-brāt). **1.** To graduate or standardize any measuring instrument. **2.** To measure the diameter of a tubular structure.

calibration (kal-i-brā'shŭn). The act of standardizing or calibrating an instrument or laboratory procedure.

calibrator (kal'ĭ-brā-ter, -tōr). A standard or reference material or substance used to standardize or calibrate an instrument or laboratory procedure.

caliceal (kal'i-se'al). Calyceal; relating to the calix.

calicectasis (kal-i-sek'tă-sis) [calix, + G. *ektasis,* dilation]. Caliectasis.

calicectomy (kal-i-sek'tō-mē) [calix, + G. *ektomē,* excision]. Caliectomy; calycectomy; excision of a calix.

calices (kal'i-sēz). Plural of calix.

caliciform (kă-lis'i-fōrm) [L. *calix* + *forma,* form]. Calyciform; shaped like a cup or goblet.

calicine (kal'i-sēn). Calycine; of the nature of, or resembling a calix.

Calicivirus (kă-lis'i-vī'rŭs) [G. *kalyx,* cup, + virus]. The sole genus of the family Caliciviridae; species include the vesicular exanthema virus of swine and related viruses of cats and sea lions.

calicoplasty (kă'lĭ-sō-plas-tē) [calix, + G. *plastos,* formed]. Calycoplasty; calioplasty; calyoplasty; plastic surgery of a calix, usually designed to increase its lumen at the infundibulum.

calicotomy (kal-ĭ-sot'ō-mē) [calix, + G. *tomē,* a cutting]. Calycotomy; caliotomy; calyotomy; incision into a calix, usually for removal of a calculus.

caliculus, pl. **caliculi** (kă-lik'yū-lŭs, lī) [L. dim. from G. *kalyx,* the cup of a flower]. Calycle; calyculus; a bud-shaped or cup-shaped structure, resembling the closed calyx of a flower.
c. gustato'rius [NA], taste or gustatory bud; taste bulb or corpuscle; Schwalbe's corpuscle; one of a number of flask-shaped cell nests located in the epithelium of vallate, fungiform, and foliate papillae of the tongue and also in the soft palate, epiglottis, and posterior wall of the pharynx; it consists of sustentacular, gustatory, and basal cells between which the intragemmal sensory nerve fibers terminate.
c. ophthal'micus, optic *cup.*

caliectasis (kă-lē-ek'tă-sis). Calicectasis; calyectasis; calycectasis;

pyelocaliectasis; dilation of the calices, usually due to obstruction or infection.

caliectomy (kā-lē-ek'tō-mē). Calicectomy.

californium (kal-i-fōr'nē-ŭm) [*California*, state and university where first prepared]. An artificial transuranium element, symbol Cf, atomic no. 98; half-life of ^{251}Cf (the most stable known isotope) is 900 years.

caligation (kal-i-gā'shŭn). Caligo.

caligo (kă-lī'gō) [L. fog, darkness]. Caligation; dimness of vision.

calioplasty (kā'lē-ō-plas-tē). Calicoplasty.

caliorrhaphy (kā'lē-ōr-a-fē) [calix, + G. *raphē*, suture, seam]. Calyorrhaphy. **1.** Suturing of a calix. **2.** Plastic surgery of a dilated or obstructed calix to improve urinary drainage, often requiring combination of two or more calices or the massive movement of pelvic mucosa to rebuild the caliceal drainage system.

caliotomy (kā-lē-ot'ō-mē). Calicotomy.

calipers (kal'i-perz) [a corruption of *caliber*]. An instrument used for measuring diameters; *e.g.*, in obstetrics, the pelvic diameters.

calisthenics (kal-is-then'iks) [G. *kalos*, beautiful, + *sthenos*, strength]. Systematic practice of various exercises with the object of preserving health and increasing physical strength.

calix, pl. **calices** (kā'liks, kal'i-sēz) [L. fr. G. *kalyx*, the cup of a flower] [NA]. Calyx; a flower-shaped or funnel-shaped structure; specifically one of the branches or recesses of the pelvis of the kidney into which the orifices of the malpighian renal pyramids project.
major calices, calices renales majores.
minor calices, calices renales minores.
calices rena'les majo'res [NA], major calices; the primary subdivisions of the renal pelvis, usually two or three in number.
calices rena'les mino'res [NA], minor calices; the subdivisions of the major calices, varying in number from 7 to 13, which receive the renal papillae.

Calkins, Leroy Adelbert, U.S. obstetrician-gynecologist, 1894–1960. See C. *sign*.

Call, Friedrich von, Vienna physician, 1844–1917. See C.-Exner *bodies*.

Callahan, John R., U.S. endodontist, 1853–1918. See C.'s *method*.

Callander, C. Latimer, San Francisco surgeon, 1892–1947. See C.'s *amputation*.

Calleja (Calleja y Sanchez), Camilo, Madrid anatomist, †1913. See *islands* of C.

Calliphora (kă-lif'ō-ră) [G. *kalli*, beauty, + *phoros*, bearing]. A genus of blowflies (family Calliphoridae, order Diptera), the bluebottle flies, the larvae of which feed on dead flesh. *C. vomitoria* and *C. vicina* are common species in the U.S.

Callison, James S., U.S. physician, *1873. See C.'s *fluid*.

Callitroga (kal-i-trō'gă). Former name for *Cochliomyia*.

callosal (ka-lō'săl). Relating to the corpus callosum.

callose (kal'ōs). A 1,3-β-D-glucan formed by certain enzymes from UDP-glucose, differing from cellulose (a β-1,4-glucan formed from GDP-glucose) and starch amylose (an α-1,4-glucan formed from ADP-glucose).

callositas (ka-los'i-tas). Callosity.

callosity (ka-los'i-tē) [L. fr. *callosus*, thick-skinned]. Callositas; callus (1); keratoma (1); poroma (1); tyle; tyloma; a circumscribed thickening of the keratin layer of the epidermis as a result of friction or intermittent pressure.

callosomarginal (ka-lō'sō-mar'jin-ăl). Relating to the corpus callosum and the gyrus cinguli; denoting the sulcus between them.

callous (kal'ŭs). Relating to a callus or callosity.

callus (kal'ŭs) [L. hard skin]. **1.** Callosity. **2.** A composite mass of tissue that forms at a fracture site to establish continuity between the bone ends; it is composed initially of uncalicifed fibrous tissue and cartilage, and ultimately of bone.
central c., medullary c.; the c. within the medullary cavity of a fractured bone.
definitive c., permanent c.; the c. which has become converted into osseous tissue.
ensheathing c., the mass of c. around the outside of the fractured bone.
medullary c., central c.
permanent c., definitive c.
provisional c., temporary c.; the c. that develops to keep the ends of the fractured bone in apposition; it is absorbed after union is complete.
temporary c., provisional c.

calmative (kahl'mă-tiv). Calming, quieting; allaying excitement; denoting such an agent.

Calmette, Leon C. A., French bacteriologist, 1863–1933. See *bacille* bilié de C.-Guérin, C. *test*, C.-Guérin *vaccine*.

calmodulin (kal-mod'yū-lin) [calcium + modulate]. A ubiquitous eukaryotic protein that binds calcium ions, thereby becoming the agent for many, if not most or all, of the cellular effects long ascribed to calcium ions. This calcium-protein complex binds to the apoenzyme, to form the holoenzyme, of certain phosphodiesterases; through these, or other as yet unknown mechanisms, the complex regulates adenylate and guanylate cyclases, many kinases, phospholipase A_2 activity, microtubule assembly, and other basic cellular functions.

calomel (kal'ō-mel). Mercurous chloride; mild mercury chloride; mercury monochloride, protochloride, or subchloride; sweet precipitate; HgCl; has been used as an intestinal antiseptic and laxative.
vegetable c., podophyllum.

calor (kā'lōr) [L.]. Heat, as one of the four signs of inflammation (c., rubor, tumor, dolor) enunciated by Celsus.

Calori, Luigi, Italian anatomist, 1807–1896. See C.'s *bursa*.

caloric (kă-lōr'ik) [L. *calor*, heat]. **1.** Relating to a calorie. **2.** Relating to heat.

calorie, calory (kal'ō-rē) [L. *calor*, heat]. A unit of heat content or energy. Calorie is being replaced by joule, the SI unit equal to 0.24 calorie. See also British Thermal *Unit*.
gram c., small c.
kilogram c. (kcal), large c.
large c. (C, Cal), kilogram c.; kilocalorie; the quantity of energy required to raise the temperature of 1 kg of water 1°C, more precisely from 15° to 16°C; it is 1000 times the value of the small c.; used in measurements of the heat production of chemical reactions, including those involved in biology.
mean c., one hundredth of the energy required to raise the temperature of 1 g of water from 0°C. to 100°C.
small c. (c, cal), gram c.; the quantity of energy required to raise the temperature of 1 g of water 1°C, or from 15° to 16° C in the case of normal or standard c.

calorific (cal-ō-rif'ik) [L. *calor*, heat]. Producing heat.

calorigenic (kă-lōr-i-jen'ik). [L. *calor*, heat, + G. *genesis*, production]. **1.** Capable of generating heat. **2.** Thermogenetic (2); stimulating metabolic production of heat.

calorimeter (kal-ō-rim'ĕ-ter) [L. *calor*, heat, + G. *metron*, measure]. An apparatus for measuring the amount of heat liberated in a chemical reaction.
Benedict-Roth c., see Benedict-Roth *apparatus*.
bomb c., an instrument for determining the potential energy of organic substances, including those in foods. It consists of a hollow

steel container, lined with platinum and filled with pure oxygen, into which a weighed quantity of food is placed and ignited with an electric fuse; the heat produced is absorbed by water surrounding the bomb and, from the rise in temperature, the calories liberated are calculated.

calorimetric (kă'lōr-i-met'rik). Relating to calorimetry.

calorimetry (kal-ō-rim'ĕ-trē). Measurement of the amount of heat given off by a reaction or group of reactions (as by an organism).
direct c., measurement of the heat produced by a reaction, as distinguished from indirect methods, which involve measurement of something other than heat production itself.
indirect c., determination of heat production of an oxidation reaction by measuring uptake of oxygen and/or liberation of carbon dioxide and nitrogen excretion, and then calculating the amount of heat produced.

caloritropic (kă-lōr'i-trop'ik). Relating to thermotropism.

calory (kal'ō-rē). Calorie.

Calot, Jean-François, French surgeon, 1861–1944. See C.'s *triangle.*

calumba (kă-lŭm'bă). Columbo; colomba; the dried root of *Jateorrhiza palmata* (family Menispermaceae), a tall climbing vine of east Africa; used as a bitter tonic.

calumbin (kal'ŭm-bin). Columbin; $C_{21}H_{24}O_7$; an amaroid from calumba that accounts for the bitterness of the crude drug.

calusterone (kal-yū'stĕ-rōn). 17β,17α-dimethyltestosterone; an antineoplastic agent.

calvaria, pl. **calvariae** (kal-vā'rē-ă, -vā'rē-ē) [L. a skull] [NA]. Skullcap; cranium cerebrale; cerebral cranium; roof of skull; the upper domelike portion of the skull.

calvarial (kal-vār'ē-ăl). Relating to the skullcap.

calvarium (kal-vār'ē-ŭm). Incorrectly used for calvaria.

Calvé, Jacques, French orthopedic surgeon, 1875–1954. See C.-Perthes *disease,* Legg-C.-Perthes *disease.*

calvities (kal-vish'e-ēz) [L. fr. *calvus,* bald]. Alopecia.

calx, gen. **calcis,** pl. **calces** (kalks, kal'sis, kal-sēs). **1** [L. limestone]. Lime (1). **2** [L. heel]. Heel (1); calcar pedis; the posterior rounded extremity of the foot.

calyceal (kal'i-se'ăl). Caliceal.

calycectasis (kal-i-sek'tă-sis). Caliectasis.

calycectomy (kal-i-sek'tō-mē). Caliectomy.

calyces (kal'i-sēz). Plural of calyx.

calyciform (kă-lis'i-fōrm). Caliciform.

calycine (kal'i-sēn). Calicine.

calycle, calyculus (kal'i-kl, kă-lik'yū-lŭs). Caliculus.

calycoplasty (kā'lē-sō-plas-tē). Calicoplasty.

calycotomy (kal-ē-sot-ō-mē). Calicotomy.

calyectasis (kā-lē-ek'tă-sis). Caliectasis.

Calymmatobacterium (kă-lim'mă-tō-bak-tēr'ē-ŭm) [G. *kalymma,* hood, veil, + *bakterion,* rod]. A genus of nonmotile bacteria (of uncertain taxonomic classification) containing Gram-negative, pleomorphic rods with single or bipolar condensations of chromatin; cells occur singly and in clusters. Outside of the human body, growth occurs only in the yolk sac or amniotic fluid of a developing chick embryo or in a medium containing embryonic yolk; the organisms are pathogenic only for man. The type species is *C. granulomatis.*
C. granulo'matis, Donovan body; a species causing granulomatous lesions (donovanosis) in man, particularly in the inguinal region (granuloma inguinale); the type species of the genus *C.*

calyoplasty (kā'lē-ō-plas-tē). Calicoplasty.

calyorrhaphy (kā'lē-ōr-a-fē). Caliorrhaphy.

calyotomy (kā-lē-ot'ō-mē). Calicotomy.

calyx, pl. **calyces** (kā'liks, kal'i-sēz) [G. cup of a flower]. Calix.

cambendazole (kam-ben'dah-zōl). Isopropyl 2-(4-triazolyl)-5-benzimidazolecarbamate; an anthelmintic.

cambium (kam'bē-ŭm) [L. exchange]. **1.** The inner layer of the periosteum. **2.** A layer between the wood and bark in plants.

camelpox (kam'el-poks). A disease of camels that may produce local lesions in man from contact; little information is available with respect to etiological agent.

camera, pl. (L.) **camerae,** (Eng.) **cameras** (kam'er-ă, -ē) [L. a vault]. **1.** A closed box; especially one containing a lens, shutter, and light-sensitive film or plates for photography. **2** [NA]. In anatomy, any chamber or cavity, such as one of the chambers of the heart, or eye.
Anger c., a nuclear medical radiation detecting system, employing a single thin crystal and multiple photodetecting circuits, that views the entire field at once and is most effective in the 100- to 511-keV energy range.
c. ante'rior bul'bi [NA], c. oculi anterior; c. oculi major; anterior chamber of eye; the space between the cornea and the iris, filled with a watery fluid (aqueous humor) and communicating through the pupil with the posterior chamber.
gamma c., any one of several nuclear medical scanners that records simultaneously counts from the entire operative field of view.
c. oc'uli ante'rior, c. anterior bulbi.
c. oc'uli ma'jor, c. anterior bulbi.
c. oc'uli mi'nor, c. posterior bulbi.
c. oc'uli poste'rior, c. posterior bulbi.
c. poste'rior bul'bi [NA], c. oculi posterior; c. oculi minor; posterior chamber of eye; the ringlike space, filled with aqueous humor, between the iris, the lens, and the ciliary body.
retinal c., an instrument for photographing the ocular fundus.
c. vi'trea bul'bi [NA], vitreous c.; vitreous chamber of eye; the large space between the lens and the retina; it is filled with the vitreous body.
vitreous c., c. vitrea bulbi.

camerostome (kam'er-ō-stōm) [L. *camera,* a vault, + G. *stoma,* mouth]. Ventral depression of the anterior cephalothorax of soft ticks (family Argasidae) in which the mouthparts (capitulum) lie.

camisole (kam'i-sōl). Straitjacket.

camomile (kam'ō-mil). Chamomile.

cAMP Abbreviation for adenosine 3′,5′-cyclic phosphate (cyclic AMP).

Campbell, Meredith F., 20th century U.S. pediatric urologist. See C. *sound.*

Campbell, William F., U.S. surgeon, 1867–1926. See C.'s *ligament.*

Camper, Pieter, Dutch physician and anatomist, 1722–1789. See C.'s facial *angle, chiasm, fascia, ligament, line, plane.*

camphane (kam'fān). Bornane.

camphene (kam'fēn). 2,2-Dimethyl-3-methylenenorbornane; a terpenoid occurring in many essential oils, *e.g.,* turpentine, camphor, citronella.

camphetamide (kam-fet'ă-mīd). Camphotamide.

camphor (kam'fōr) [mediev. L., fr. Ar. *kāfure*]. 1,7,7-Trimethylbicyclo[2.2.1]heptan-2-one; a ketone distilled from the bark and wood of *Cinnamonum camphora,* an evergreen tree of Southeast Asia and the adjoining islands, and also prepared synthetically from oil of turpentine; used in a variety of commercial products and as a topical anti-infective and antipruritic agent.
cantharis c., cantharidin.
c. liniment, camphorated oil; a mixture of camphor and cottonseed oil, or camphor and arachis oil; a mild counterirritant.
monobromated c., an antispasmodic, soporific, and sedative.
peppermint c., menthol.

tar c., naphthalene.
thyme c., thymol.

camphoraceous (kam-fō-rā'shŭs). Resembling camphor in appearance or odor.

camphorated (kam'fō-rā-ted). Containing camphor.

camphorated oil. *Camphor* liniment.

camphotamide (kam-fō'tă-mīd). Camphetamide; camphramine; 3-Diethylcarbamoyl-1-methylpyridinium camphorsulfonate; an analeptic and antianginal agent.

camphramine (kam'fră-mēn). Camphotamide.

campi foreli (kam'pē fōr-el'ē) [L. pl. of *campus,* field]. *Fields* of Forel.

campimeter (kam-pim'ĕ-ter) [L. *campus,* field, + G. *metron,* measure]. A portable, hand-held type of tangent screen used to measure central visual field.

camptocormia (kamp-tō-kōr'mē-ă) [G. *kamptos,* bent, + *kormos,* trunk of a tree]. Prosternation; a conversion reaction or hysterical condition in which the patient is bent completely forward and is unable to straighten up.

camptodactyly, camptodactylia (kamp-tō-dak'ti-lē, -dak-til'ē-ă) [G. *kamptos,* bent, + *daktylos,* finger]. Campylodactyly.

camptomelia (kamp-tō-mē'lē-ă) [G. *kamptos,* bent, + *melos,* limb]. A skeletal dysplasia characterized by a bending of the long bones of the extremities, resulting in a permanent bowing or curvature of the affected part.

camptomelic (kamp-tō-mel'ik). Denoting or characteristic of camptomelia.

camptospasm (kamp'tō-spazm). A nervous or hysterical forward bending of the trunk. See also nodding *spasm.*

Campylobacter (kam'pi-lō-bak'ter) [G. *campylos,* curved, + *baktron,* staff or rod]. A genus of bacteria containing Gram-negative, nonspore-forming, spirally curved rods with a single polar flagellum at one or both ends of the cell; they are motile with a characteristic corkscrew-like motion. The type species is *C. fetus.*
C. fe'tus, *Vibrio fetus;* a species that contains various subspecies which can cause human infections as well as abortion in sheep and cattle; it is the type species of the genus *C.*
C. fetus subsp. **jeju'ni,** a species that causes in man an acute gastroenteritis of sudden onset with constitutional symptoms (malaise, myalgia, arthralgia, and headache) and cramping abdominal pain; potential sources of human infection include poultry, cattle, sheep, pigs, and dogs.
C. sputo'rum, *Vibrio sputorum;* a species found in the genital tract of sheep and cattle and in the gingival crevice of man.

campylobacteriosis (kam'pi-lō-bak'ter-ē-ō'sis). Infection caused by microaerophilic bacteria of the genus *Campylobacter.*

campylodactyly (kam'pē-lō-dak'ti-lē) [G. *campylos,* curved, + *daktylos,* finger]. Camptodactylia; camptodactyly; streblodactyly; permanent flexion of one or both interphalangeal joints of one or more fingers, usually the little finger; often congenital in origin.

camylofine (kă-mil'ō-fin). Acamylophenine; *N*-[2-(diethylamino)ethyl]-2-phenylglycine isopentyl ester; an anticholinergic agent.

Canada, Wilma J., U.S. radiologist. See Cronkhite-C. *syndrome.*

canadine (kan'ă-dēn). Xanthopuccine; tetrahydroberberine; $C_{20}H_{21}NO_4$; an alkaloid present in *Hydrastis canadensis* (family Ranunculaceae) and in *Corydalis cava* (family Fumaraceae) with sedative and muscle relaxant properties.

CANAL

canal (kă-nal') [L. *canalis*] A duct or channel; a tubular structure. See also canalis and duct.
abdominal c., *canalis* inguinalis.
accessory c., lateral c.; a channel leading from the root pulp laterally through the dentin to the periodontal tissue; may be found anywhere in the tooth root, but is more common in the apical third of the root.
adductor c., *canalis* adductorius.
Alcock's c., *canalis* pudendalis.
alimentary c., digestive *tract.*
alveolar c.'s, *canales* alveolares.
alveolodental c.'s, *canales* alveolares.
anal c., *canalis* analis.
anterior condyloid c. of occipital bone, *canalis* hypoglossalis.
anterior semicircular c.'s, see *canales* semicirculares ossei.
archenteric c., notochordal c.; invagination of the blastopore into the notochordal process to form a cavity.
Arnold's c., *hiatus* canalis nervi petrosi minoris.
arterial c., *ductus* arteriosus.
atrioventricular c., the c. in the embryonic heart leading from the common sinuatrial chamber to the ventricle.
auditory c., *meatus* acusticus externus.
basipharyngeal c., *canalis* vomerovaginalis.
Bernard's c., *ductus* pancreaticus accessorius.
Bichat's c., *cisterna* venae magnae cerebri.
birth c., parturient c.; cavity of the uterus and vagina through which the fetus passes.
blastoporic c., an opening marking the remains of the neurenteric c.
bony semicircular c.'s, *canales* semicirculares ossei.
Böttcher's c., *ductus* utriculosaccularis.
Braune's c., the parturient c. formed by the uterine cavity, dilated cervix, vagina, and vulva.
Breschet's c.'s, *canale* diploici.
carotid c., *canalis* caroticus.
carpal c., **(1)** *canalis* carpi; **(2)** *sulcus* carpi.
caudal c., the space occupied by the sacral extension of the epidural space.
central c., *canalis* centralis.
central c.'s of cochlea, *canales* longitudinales modioli.
cervical c., *canalis* cervicis uteri.
ciliary c.'s, *spatia* anguli iridocornealis.
Civinini's c., *iter* chordae anterius.
Cloquet's c., *canalis* hyaloideus.
cochlear c., *canalis* spiralis cochleae.
condylar c., condyloid c., *canalis* condylaris.
Corti's c., Corti's *tunnel.*
Cotunnius' c., *aqueductus* vestibuli.
craniopharyngeal c., pituitary *diverticulum.*
crural c., *canalis* femoralis.
deferent c., *ductus* deferens.
dental c.'s, *canales* alveolares.
dentinal c.'s, *canaliculi* dentales.
diploic c.'s, *canales* diploici.
Dorello's c., a bony c. sometimes found at the tip of the temporal bone enclosing the abducens nerve and inferior petrosal sinus as these two structures enter the cavernous sinus.
Dupuytren's c., *vena* diploica.
endodermal c., the gut tube of young embryos.
facial c., *canalis* facialis.

fallopian c., *canalis* facialis.
femoral c., *canalis* femoralis.
Ferrein's c., *rivus* lacrimalis.
Fontana's c., *sinus* venosus sclerae.
galactophorous c.'s, *ductus* lactiferi.
Gartner's c., *ductus* epoophori longitudinalis.
gastric c., *canalis* ventriculi.
greater palatine c., *canalis* palatinus major.
gubernacular c., a small c. located between the permanent tooth germ and the apex of the deciduous tooth, containing remnants of dental lamina and connective tissue.
gynecophoric c., a ventral groove running the length of male schistosome flukes, into which the threadlike female worm fits.
Hannover's c., the space between the ciliary zonule and the vitreous body.
haversian c.'s, Leeuwenhoek's c.'s; vascular c.'s that run longitudinally in the center of haversian systems of compact osseous tissue.
Hensen's c., *ductus* reuniens.
c. of Hering, cholangiole.
Hirschfeld's c.'s, interdental c.'s.
Holmgrén-Golgi c.'s, Golgi *apparatus.*
c. of Hovius, an anastomotic circle between the anterior twigs of the venae vorticosae in the eyes of some animals, but not in normal human eyes.
Hoyer's c.'s, Sucquet-Hoyer c.'s.
Huguier's c., *iter* chordae anterius.
Hunter's c., *canalis* adductorius.
hyaloid c., *canalis* hyaloideus.
hypoglossal c., *canalis* hypoglossalis.
incisive c., incisor c., *canalis* incisivus.
inferior dental c., *canalis* mandibulae.
infraorbital c., *canalis* infraorbitalis.
inguinal c., *canalis* inguinalis.
interdental c.'s, Hirschfeld's c.'s; c.'s that extend vertically through alveolar bone between roots of mandibular and maxillary incisor and maxillary bicuspid teeth.
interfacial c.'s, intercellular spaces occurring in relation to intercellular attachments by desmosomes in stratified squamous epithelium, generally resulting from an artifact of fixation.
irruption c., the channel along which the periosteal vascular bud invades the cartilaginous matrix of growing bone.
Jacobson's c., *canaliculus* tympanicus.
Kürsteiner's (Kuersteiner's) c.'s, a fetal complex of vesicular, canalicular, and glandlike structures derived from parathyroid, thymus, or thymic cord; they are rudimentary and functionless unless persistent postnatally, when they may occur as cystic structures in the vicinity of parathyroid III and thymus III. Kursteiner described three types, type II c.'s being associated with thyroaplasia.
lateral c., accessory c.
lateral semicircular c.'s, see *canales* semicirculares ossei.
Laurer's c., a tube originating on the surface of the ootype of trematodes, directed dorsally to or near the surface; it may have originally served as a vagina or possibly as a reservoir of excess shell material.
Lauth's c., *sinus* venosus sclerae.
Leeuwenhoek's c.'s, haversian c.'s.
c.'s for lesser palatine nerves, *canales* palatini minores.
longitudinal c.'s of modiolus, *canales* longitudinales modioli.
Löwenberg's c., *ductus* cochlearis.
mandibular c., *canalis* mandibulae.
marrow c., *canalis* radicis dentis.
mental c., *foramen* mentale.
musculotubal c., *canalis* musculotubarius.
nasolacrimal c., *canalis* nasolacrimalis.
neural c., the c. within the embryonic neural tube; the primordium of the canalis centralis.
neurenteric c., a transitory communication between the neural tube and the gut in vertebrate embryos, including man.
notochordal c., archenteric c.
canal of Nuck, see *processus* vaginalis peritonei.
nutrient c., *canalis* nutricius.
obturator c., *canalis* obturatorius.
optic c., *canalis* opticus.
palatovaginal c., *canalis* palatovaginalis.
parturient c., birth c.
pelvic c., the passage from the superior to the inferior aperture of the pelvis.
pericardioperitoneal c., the constricted portion of the embryonic celom that joins the pericardial cavity to the peritoneal cavity, developing into the pleural cavities.
persistent atrioventricular c., endocardial cushion defect; the atrial and ventricular septa fail to meet, as in normal development, which results in a low atrial and high ventricular septal defect or a common atrioventricular c.
Petit's c.'s, *spatia* zonularia.
pharyngeal c., *canalis* palatovaginalis.
pleuropericardial c.'s, in the embryo, spaces or channels, one on each side, connecting the pericardial and pleural cavities.
pleuroperitoneal c., the communication between the embryonic pleural and peritoneal cavities.
portal c.'s, connective tissue spaces in the substance of the liver which are occupied by preterminal ramifications of the bile ducts, portal vein, and hepatic artery, as well as nerves and lymphatics.
posterior semicircular c.'s, see *canales* semicirculares ossei.
pterygoid c., *canalis* pterygoideus.
pterygopalatine c., *canalis* palatinus major.
pudendal c., *canalis* pudendalis.
pulp c., *canalis* radicis dentis.
pyloric c., *canalis* pyloricus.
Rivinus' c.'s, see *ductus* sublingualis major; *ductus* sublinguales minores.
root c. of tooth, *canalis* radicis dentis.
Rosenthal's c., *canalis* spiralis cochleae.
sacral c., *canalis* sacralis.
Santorini's c., *ductus* pancreaticus accessorius.
Schlemm's c., *sinus* venosus sclerae.
semicircular c.'s, see *canales* semicirculares ossei.
small c. of chorda tympani, *canaliculus* chordae tympani.
Sondermann's c., a blind outpouching of Schlemm's c., extending toward, but not communicating with, the anterior chamber of the eye.
spinal c., *canalis* vertebralis.
spiral c. of cochlea, *canalis* spiralis cochleae.
spiral c. of modiolus, *canalis* spiralis modioli.
Stilling's c., *canalis* hyaloideus.
subsartorial c., *canalis* adductorius.
Sucquet-Hoyer c.'s, Sucquet's c.'s, Sucquet-Hoyer anastomoses; Hoyer's c.'s or anastomoses; arteriovenous anastomoses controlling blood flow in the glomus bodies in the digits.
tarsal c., *sinus* tarsi.
temporal c., a c. in the zygomatic bone transmitting the zygomaticofacial and zygomaticotemporal nerves and vessels.
Theile's c., *sinus* transversus pericardii.
tubotympanic c., see tubotympanic *recess.*
tympanic c., *canaliculus* tympanicus.
uniting c., *ductus* reuniens.
urogenital c., urethra.
uterovaginal c., a median tubular structure produced in the embryo from the fusion of the caudal parts of the paramesonephric ducts.
van Horne's c., *ductus* thoracicus.
Velpeau's c., *canalis* inguinalis.
vertebral c., *canalis* vertebralis.

vesicourethral c., the cranial portion of the primitive urogenital sinus from which develop the bladder and part of the urethra.
vestibular c., *scala* vestibuli.
vidian c., *canalis* pterygoideus.
Volkmann's c.'s, vascular c.'s in bone which, unlike those of the haversian system, are not surrounded by concentric lamellae of bone; they run for the most part transversely, perforating the lamellae of the haversian system, and communicate with the c.'s of that system.
vomerine c., *canalis* vomerovaginalis.
vomerobasilar c., *canalis* vomerorostralis.
vomerorostral c., *canalis* vomerorostralis.
vomerovaginal c., *canalis* vomerovaginalis.
Walther's c.'s, *ductus* sublinguales minores.
Wirsung's c., *ductus* pancreaticus.

---

canales (kă-nā-lēz). Plural of canalis.

canalicular (kan-ă-lik'yū-lăr). Relating to a canaliculus.

canaliculi (kan-ă-lik'yū-lī). Plural of canaliculus.

canaliculitis (kan'ă-lik-yū-lī'tis) [canaliculus + G. *-itis,* inflammation]. Inflammation of the lacrimal canaliculus.

canaliculization (kan-ă-lik'yū-lī-zā'shŭn). The formation of canaliculi, or small canals, in any tissue.

canaliculus, pl. canaliculi (kan-ă-lik'yū-lŭs, -lī) [L. dim. fr. *canalis,* canal] [NA]. A small canal or channel.
auricular c., c. mastoideus.
biliary c., bile capillary; one of the intercellular channels, about 1 μm or less in diameter, that occurs between liver cells.
bone c., the c. interconnecting bone lacunae with one another or with a haversian canal; contains the interconnecting cytoplasmic processes of osteocytes.
canaliculi caroticotympan'ici [NA], small openings within the carotid canal that afford passage to the tympanic cavity of branches of the internal carotid artery and carotid sympathetic plexus.
c. chor'dae tym'pani [NA], small canal of chorda tympani; iter chordae posterius; a canal leading from the facial canal to the tympanic cavity through which the chorda tympani nerve enters this cavity.
c. coch'leae [NA], cochlear canaliculus; a minute canal in the temporal bone that passes from the cochlea inferiorly to open in front of the medial side of the jugular fossa. It contains the perilymphatic duct.
cochlear c., c. cochleae.
canalic'uli denta'les [NA], dental or dentinal tubules; tubuli dentales; dentinal canals; minute, wavy, branching tubes or canals in the dentin; they contain the long cytoplasmic processes of odontoblasts and extend radially from the pulp to the dentoenamel junction.
c. innomina'tus, foramen petrosum.
intercellular c., one of the fine channels between adjoining secretory cells, such as those between serous cells in salivary glands.
intracellular c., a fine canal formed by invagination of the cell membrane into the cytoplasm of a cell, such as those of the parietal cells of the stomach.
lacrimal c., c. lacrimalis.
c. lacrima'lis [NA], lacrimal c.; lacrimal duct; a curved canal beginning at the punctum lacrimale in the margin of each eyelid near the medial commissure and running transversely medially to empty with its fellow into the lacrimal sac.
mastoid c., c. mastoideus.
c. mastoid'eus [NA], mastoid c.; auricular c.; the canal that extends from the jugular fossa laterally through the mastoid process. It transmits the auricular branch of the vagus.
c. reu'niens, *ductus* reuniens.
secretory c., see intercellular or intracellular c.
Thiersch's canaliculi, minute channels in newly formed reparative tissue, permitting the circulation of nutritive fluids, precursors of new vascularization.
c. tympan'icus [NA], tympanic c.; Jacobson's canal; a minute canal passing from the inferior surface of the petrous portion of the temporal bone between the jugular fossa and carotid canal to the floor of the tympanic cavity. It transmits the tympanic branch of the glossopharyngeal nerve.

canalis, pl. canales (ka-nā'lis, -lēz) [L.] [NA]. A canal or channel.
c. adductor'ius [NA], adductor canal; Hunter's canal; subsartorial canal; the space in the thigh between the vastus medialis and adductor muscles, converted into a canal by the overlying sartorius muscle. It gives passage to the femoral vessels.
cana'les alveola'res [NA], alveolar canals; alveolodental or dental canals; canals in the body of the maxilla that transmit nerves and vessels from the alveolar foramina to the maxillary teeth.
c. ana'lis [NA], anal canal; the terminal portion of the alimentary canal; it extends from the pelvic diaphragm to the anal orifice.
c. carot'icus [NA], carotid canal; a passage through the petrous part of the temporal bone from its inferior surface upward, medially, and forward to the apex where it opens into the foramen lacerum. It transmits the internal carotid artery and plexuses of veins and autonomic nerves.
c. car'pi [NA], carpal canal (1); carpal tunnel; the space deep to the flexor retinaculum of the wrist through which the median nerve and the flexor tendons of the fingers and thumb pass; compression of the median nerve may occur here.
c. centra'lis [NA], central canal; syringocele (1); tubus medullaris; the ependyma-lined lumen (cavity) of the neural tube, the cerebral part of which remains patent to form the ventricles of the brain, while the spinal part in the adult often is reduced to a solid strand of modified ependyma.
c. cerv'icis u'teri [NA], cervical canal; a fusiform canal extending from the isthmus of the uterus to the opening of the uterus into the vagina.
c. condyla'ris [NA], condylar canal; condyloid canal; posterior condyloid foramen; the opening through the occipital bone posterior to the condyle on each side that transmits the occipital emissary vein.
cana'les diplo'ici [NA], diploic canals; Breschet's canals; channels in the diploë that accommodate the diploic veins.
c. facia'lis [NA], facial canal; fallopian aqueduct or canal; aqueductus fallopii; the bony passage in the temporal bone through which the facial nerve passes; it commences in the internal auditory meatus, passes at first anteriorly, then turns posteriorly to pass medial to the tympanic cavity; finally, it turns downward to reach the stylomastoid foramen.
c. femora'lis [NA], femoral canal; crural canal; the medial compartment of the femoral sheath.
c. hyaloid'eus [NA], hyaloid canal; Stilling's or Cloquet's canal; a minute canal running through the vitreous from the discus nervi optici to the lens, containing in fetal life a prolongation of the central artery of the retina, the hyaloid artery.
c. hypoglossa'lis [NA], hypoglossal canal; anterior condyloid canal of occipital bone; anterior condyloid foramen; the canal through which the hypoglossal nerve emerges from the skull.
c. incisi'vus [NA], incisive or incisor canal; one of several bony canals leading from the floor of the nasal cavity into the incisive fossa on the palatal surface of the maxilla; they convey the nasopalatine nerves and branches of the greater palatine arteries which anastomose with the septal branch of the sphenopalatine artery.
c. infraorbita'lis [NA], infraorbital canal; a canal running beneath the orbital margin of the maxilla from the infraorbital groove, in the floor of the orbit, to the infraorbital foramen; it transmits the infraorbital artery and nerve.
c. inguina'lis [NA], inguinal canal; abdominal canal; Velpeau's

canal; the obliquely directed passage through the layers of the lower abdominal wall that transmits the spermatic cord in the male and the round ligament in the female.

cana'les longitudina'les modio'li [NA], longitudinal canals of modiolus; central canals of the cochlea; centrally placed channels that convey vessels and nerves to the apical turns of the cochlea.

c. mandib'ulae [NA], mandibular canal; inferior dental canal; the canal within the mandible that transmits the inferior alveolar nerve and vessels. Its posterior opening is the mandibular foramen.

c. musculotuba'rius [NA], musculotubal canal; a canal beginning at the anterior border of the petrous portion of the temporal bone near its junction with the squamous portion, and passing to the tympanic cavity; it is divided by the cochleariform process into two canals: one for the auditory (eustachian) tube, the other for the tensor tympani muscle.

c. nasolacrima'lis [NA], nasolacrimal canal; the bony canal formed by the maxilla, lacrimal bone, and inferior concha that transmits the nasolacrimal duct from the orbit to the inferior meatus of the nose.

c. ner'vi petro'si superficial'is minor'ris, *hiatus* canalis nervi petrosi minoris.

c. nutri'cius [NA], nutrient canal; a canal in the shaft of a long bone or in other locations in irregular bones through which the nutrient artery enters a bone.

c. obturato'rius [NA], obturator canal; the opening in the superior part of the obturator membrane through which the obturator nerve and vessels pass from the pelvic cavity into the thigh.

c. op'ticus [NA], optic canal; optic foramen; foramen opticum; the short canal through the lesser wing of the sphenoid bone at the apex of the orbit that gives passage to the optic nerve and the ophthalmic artery.

c. palati'nus ma'jor [NA], greater palatine canal; pterygopalatine canal; the c. formed between the maxilla and palatine bones; it transmits the descending palatine artery and the greater palatine nerve.

cana'les palati'ni mino'res [NA], canals for lesser palatine nerves; c.'s located in the posterior part of the palatine bone.

c. palatovagina'lis [NA], palatovaginal canal; on the undersurface of the vaginal process of the sphenoid bone, a furrow that is converted into a canal by the sphenoidal process of the palatine bone; it transmits the pharyngeal branch of the maxillary artery and the pharyngeal nerve from the pterygopalatine ganglion.

c. pterygoi'deus [NA], pterygoid canal; vidian canal; an opening through the pterygoid process of the sphenoid bone through which pass the artery, vein, and nerve of the pterygoid canal.

c. pudenda'lis [NA], pudendal canal; Alcock's canal; the space within the obturator fascia lining the lateral wall of the ischiorectal fossa that transmits the pudendal vessels and nerves.

c. pylor'icus [NA], pyloric canal; the aboral segment (about 2 to 3 cm long) of the stomach; it succeeds the antrum and ends at the gastroduodenal junction.

c. rad'icis den'tis [NA], root canal of a tooth; marrow or pulp canal; the chamber of the dental pulp lying within the root portion of a tooth.

c. reu'niens, *ductus* reuniens.

c. sacra'lis [NA], sacral canal; the continuation of the vertebral canal in the sacrum.

cana'les semicircula'res os'sei [NA], bony semicircular canals; the three bony tubes in the labyrinth of the ear within which the membranous semicircular ducts are located; they lie in planes at right angles to each other and are known as **canales semicirculares anterior, posterior,** and **lateralis.**

c. spira'lis coch'leae [NA], spiral canal of cochlea; cochlear canal; Rosenthal's canal; the winding tube of the bony labyrinth which makes two and a half turns about the modiolus of the cochlea; it is divided incompletely into two compartments by a winding shelf of bone, the lamina spiralis ossea.

c. spira'lis modio'li [NA], spiral canal of modiolus; the space in the modiolus in which the spiral ganglion of the cochlear nerve lies.

c. umbil'icus, *annulus* umbilicalis.

c. ventric'uli [NA], gastric canal; the part of the body of the stomach that follows the lesser curvature; it is characterized by longitudinal mucosal folds.

c. vertebra'lis [NA], vertebral canal; spinal canal; tubus vertebralis; the canal that contains the spinal cord, spinal meninges, and related structures. It is formed by the vertebral foramina of successive vertebrae of the articulated vertebral column.

c. vomerorostra'lis [NA], vomerorostral canal; vomerobasilar canal; a small canal between the superior border of the vomer and the rostrum of the sphenoidal bone.

c. vomerovagina'lis [NA], vomerovaginal canal; basipharyngeal canal; vomerine canal; an opening between the vaginal process of the sphenoid and the ala of the vomer on either side. It conveys a branch of the sphenopalatine artery.

canalization (kan-ăl-ī-zā'shŭn). The formation of canals or channels in a tissue.

Canavan, Myrtelle M., U.S. pathologist, 1879–1953. See C.'s *disease, sclerosis.*

canavanase (kan-av'ă-nās). Arginase.

cancellated (kan'sĕ-lā-ted) [L. *cancello,* to make a lattice work]. Cancellous.

cancellous (kan'sĕ-lŭs). Cancellated; denoting bone that has a lattice-like or spongy structure.

cancellus, pl. **cancelli** (kan-sel'ŭs, -lī) [L. a grating, lattice]. A lattice-like structure, as in spongy bone.

cancer (CA) (kan'ser) [L. a crab, a cancer]. General term frequently used to indicate any of various types of malignant neoplasms, most of which invade surrounding tissues, may metastasize to several sites, and are likely to recur after attempted removal and to cause death of the patient unless adequately treated; especially, any such carcinoma or sarcoma, but, in ordinary usage, especially the former.

c. à deux [Fr. *deux,* two], carcinomas occurring at approximately the same time, or in fairly close succession, in two persons who live together.

betel c., buyo cheek c.; carcinoma of the mucous membrane of the cheek, observed in certain East Indian natives, probably as a result of irritation from chewing a preparation of betel nut and lime rolled within a betel leaf.

buyo cheek c. [Philippine *buyo,* betel], betel c.

chimney sweep's c., a carcinoma of the skin of the scrotum, occurring as an occupational disease in chimney sweeps.

colloid c., mucinous *carcinoma.*

conjugal c., c. à deux occurring in man and wife.

encephaloid c., medullary *carcinoma.*

c. en cuirasse (on-kwē-rahs') [Fr. breastplate], a carcinoma that involves a considerable portion of the skin of one or both sides of the thorax.

epidermoid c., epidermoid *carcinoma.*

epithelial c., any malignant neoplasm originating from epithelium, *i.e.*, a carcinoma.

familial c., c. occurring in blood relatives; the mode of inheritance may be either dominant, as in retinoblastoma, basal cell nevus syndrome, neurofibromatosis, and intestinal polyposis, or recessive, as in xeroderma pigmentosum. See also cancer *family.*

glandular c., adenocarcinoma.

green c., chloroma.

kang c., kangri c., kangri burn carcinoma; a carcinoma of the skin of the thigh or abdomen in certain Indian or Chinese workers; thought to result from irritation by heat from a hot brick oven (kang) or fire basket (kangri).

mouse c., any of various types of malignant neoplasms that occur naturally in mice, especially in certain inbred "c. strains" used for research studies.

mule-spinner's c., carcinoma of the scrotum or adjacent skin exposed to oil, observed in some workers in cotton-spinning mills.

paraffin c., carcinoma of the skin occurring as an occupational disease in paraffin workers.

pipe-smoker's c., squamous cell carcinoma of the lips occurring in pipe smokers.

pitch-worker's c., carcinoma of the skin of the face or neck, arms and hands, or the scrotum, resulting from exposure to carcinogens in pitch, which occurs naturally as asphalt, or as a residue in the distillation of tar.

scar c., scar *carcinoma.*

spider c., obsolete term for a malignant neoplasm with a rhizoid or filamentous edge of thin, threadlike, red lines that represent dilated vascular channels associated with the neoplasm; a form of telangiectatic c.

stump c., carcinoma of the stomach developing after gastroenterostomy or gastric resection for benign disease.

telangiectatic c., a c. with numerous dilated capillaries and "lakes" of blood within relatively large endothelium-lined channels.

water c., obsolete term for noma.

canceration (kan-ser-ā'shŭn). A change that results in properties and features usually associated with malignant neoplasms, *e.g.*, as in the development of a carcinoma in a site previously involved by a benign condition.

cancericidal (kan'ser-i-sī'dăl) [cancer + L. *caedo,* to kill]. Carcinolytic.

cancerigenic (kan'ser-i-jen'ik). Carcinogenic.

cancerocidal (kan'ser-ō-sī'dăl). Carcinolytic.

cancerophobia (kan'ser-ō-fō'bē-ă) [cancer + G. *phobos,* fear]. Carcinophobia; a morbid fear of acquiring a malignant growth.

cancerous (kan'ser-ŭs). Relating to or pertaining to a malignant neoplasm, or being afflicted with such a process.

cancra (kang'kră). Plural of cancrum.

cancriform (kang'kri-fōrm). Cancroid (1); resembling cancer.

cancroid (kang'kroyd) [cancer + G. *eidos,* resemblance]. **1.** Cancriform. **2.** Obsolete term for a malignant neoplasm that manifests a lesser degree of malignancy than that frequently observed with carcinoma or sarcoma.

cancrum, pl. **cancra** (kang'krŭm, -kră) [Mod. L., fr. L. *cancer,* crab]. A gangrenous, ulcerative, inflammatory lesion.

c. na'si, gangrenous, necrotizing, and ulcerative rhinitis, especially in children.

c. o'ris, noma.

candela (cd) (kan'de-lă) [L.]. Candle; the SI unit of luminous intensity, 1 lumen per m^2; the luminous flux emitted per unit of solid angle (steradian) by a full radiator having a temperature of the freezing point of platinum and an area of $^1/_{60}$ cm^2.

candicans (kan'di-kanz) [L. *candico,* pres. p. *-ans,* to be whitish]. One of the corpora albicantia.

candicidin (kan-di-sī'din). A fungistatic and fungicidal polyene antibiotic agent derived from a soil actinomycete similar to *Streptomyces griseus;* used in the treatment of vaginal candidiasis.

Candida (kan'did-ă) [L. *candidus,* dazzling white]. A genus of yeastlike fungi commonly found in nature; a few species are isolated from the skin, feces, and vaginal and pharyngeal tissue, but the gastrointestinal tract is the source of the single most important species, *C. albicans.*

C. al'bicans, thrush fungus; a species which is ordinarily a part of man's normal gastrointestinal flora, but which becomes pathogenic when there is a disturbance in the balance of flora or in debilitation of the host from other causes; resulting disease states may vary from limited to generalized cutaneous or mucocutaneous infections, to severe and fatal systemic disease including endocarditis, septicemia, and meningitis.

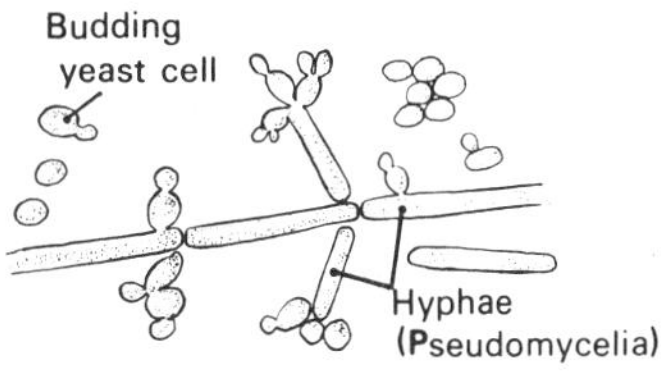

Candida albicans
(Original magnification, ×1000)

candidemia (kan-di-dē'mē-ă) [*Candida* + G. *haima,* blood]. Presence of cells of *Candida* species in the peripheral blood.

candidiasis (kan-di-dī'ă-sis). Candidosis; moniliasis; infection with, or disease caused by, *Candida,* especially *C. albicans.*

candidosis (kan-di-dō'sis). Candidiasis.

candle (kan'dl). Candela.

candle-meter (kan'dl-mē'ter). Lux.

candle-power (kan'dl-pow'er). Luminous *intensity.*

Canidae (kan'i-dē) [L. *canis,* dog]. A family of the *Carnivora* including the dogs, coyotes, wolves, and foxes.

canine (kā'nīn) [L. *caninus*]. **1.** Relating to a dog. **2.** Relating to the c. teeth. **3.** Dens caninus. **4.** Referring to the cuspid tooth.

caniniform (kā-nī'ni-fōrm). Resembling a canine tooth.

canister (kan'is-ter). A box or container; in anesthesiology, the container for carbon dioxide absorbent.

canities (kă-nish'ē-ēz) [L., fr. *canus,* hoary, gray]. A gradual dilution of pigment in hairs, producing a range of colors from normal to white, and perceived as gray. See also poliosis.

c. circumscrip'ta, piebald *eyelash.*

rapid c., whitening of hair overnight or over a few days; in the latter case, may be seen in alopecia areata, when surviving pigmented hairs are preferentially shed from gray hair.

c. un'guium, leukonychia.

canker (kang'ker) [L. *cancer*]. **1.** In cats and dogs, acute inflammation of the external ear and auditory canal. **2.** In the horse, a process similar to but more advanced than thrush; the horny frog is generally under-run with a whitish, cheeselike exudate, and the entire sole and even the wall of the hoof may be undermined.

water c., noma.

cannabidiol (kan-ă-bi-dī'ol). $C_{21}H_{30}O_2$; a constituent of *Cannabis,* related to cannabinol.

cannabinoids (ka-nab'i-noydz). Organic substances present in *Cannabis sativa,* having a variety of pharmacologic properties.

cannabinol (ka-nab'i-nol). 6,6,9-Trimethyl-3-pentyl-6*H*-dibenzo[*b,d*]-pyran-i-ol; a constituent of the resinous exudate of the pistillate flowers of *Cannabis sativa;* it has no psychotomimetic action as do the tetrahydro derivatives isolated from marijuana.

cannabis (kan'ă-bis) [L., fr. G. *kannabis,* hemp]. The dried flowering tops of the pistillate plants of *Cannabis sativa* (family Moraceae) containing isomeric tetrahydrocannabinols, cannabinol, and cannabidiol. Preparations of c. are smoked or ingested by members of various cultures and subcultures to induce psychotomimetic effects such as euphoria, hallucinations, drowsiness, and other mental changes. C. was formerly used as a sedative and analgesic; now available for restricted use in management of iatrogenic anorexia, especially that associated with oncologic chemotherapy and radiation therapy. Known by many colloquial or slang terms such as marijuana; marihuana; bhang; charas; ganja; hashish.

cannabism (kan'ă-bizm). Poisoning by preparations of cannabis.

Cannizzaro, Stanislao, chemist in Rome, 1826–1910. See C.'s *reaction.*

Cannon, Walter B., U.S. physiologist, 1871–1945. See C.'s *ring, theory;* C.-Bard *theory;* Bernard-C. *homeostasis.*

cannula (kan'yū-lă) [L. dim. of *canna,* reed]. A tube which can be inserted into a cavity, usually by means of a trocar filling its lumen; after insertion of the c., the trocar is withdrawn and the c. remains as a channel for the transport of fluid.
Karmen c., a c. used in performing early (menstrual extraction) abortion.
Lindemann's c., a c. used in blood transfusion.
perfusion c., a double-barreled c. used for irrigation of a cavity, the wash fluid passing into the cavity through one tube and out through the other.
washout c., a c. that can be irrigated without removal from the artery.

cannulation, cannulization (kan-yū-lā'shŭn, -yū-lī-zā'shŭn). Insertion of a cannula.

canrenone (kan-ren'ōn). 17-Hydroxy-3-oxo-17α-pregna-4,6-diene-21-carboxylic acid γ-lactone; an aldosterone antagonist and diuretic.

Cantelli's sign. See under sign.

canthal (kan'thăl). Relating to a canthus.

cantharidal (kan-thar'i-dăl). Relating to or containing cantharides.

cantharidate (kan-thar'i-dāt). A salt of cantharidic acid.

cantharides (kan-thar'i-dēz). Plural of cantharis.

cantharidic acid (kan-thar'i-dik). $C_{10}H_{14}O_5$; an acid, derived from cantharis, that forms salts (cantharidates) with alkalis.

cantharidin (kan-thar'i-din). Cantharis camphor; $C_{10}H_{12}O_4$; hexahydro-3α,7α-dimethyl-4,7-epoxyisobenzofuran-1,3-dione; the active principle of cantharis; the anhydride of cantharic acid.

cantharis, gen. **cantharidis,** pl. **cantharides** (kan'thar-is, kan-thar'i-dis, -dēz) [L., fr. G. *kantharis,* a beetle]. Spanish fly; Russian fly; a dried beetle, *Lytta (Cantharis) vesicatoria,* used as a counter-irritant and vesicant.

canthectomy (kan-thek'tō-mē) [G. *kanthos,* canthus, + *ektomē,* excision]. Excision of a palpebral canthus.

canthi (kan'thī). Plural of canthus.

canthitis (kan-thī'tis). Inflammation of a canthus.

cantholysis (kan-thol'i-sis) [G. *kanthos,* canthus, + *lysis,* loosening]. Canthoplasty (1).

canthoplasty (kan'thō-plas-tē) [G. *kanthos,* canthus, + *plassō,* to form]. **1.** Cantholysis; an operation for lengthening the palpebral fissure by incision through the lateral canthus. **2.** An operation for restoration of the canthus.

canthorrhaphy (kan-thōr'ă-fē) [G. *kanthos,* canthus, + *rhaphē,* suture]. Suture of the eyelids at either canthus.

canthotomy (kan-thot'ō-mē) [G. *kanthos,* canthus, + *tomē,* incision]. Slitting of the canthus.

canthus, pl. **can'thi** (kan'thŭs, -thī) [G. *kanthos,* corner of the eye]. The angle of the eye.
external c., *angulus* oculi lateralis.
internal c., *angulus* oculi medialis.
lateral c., *angulus* oculi lateralis.
medial c., *angulus* oculi medialis.

Cantor, Meyer O., Detroit physician, *1907. See C. *tube.*

CaOC Abbreviation for cathodal opening *contraction.*

CaOCl Abbreviation for cathodal opening *clonus.*

caoutchouc (kow'chuk) [S. A. Indian, *cahuchu*]. Rubber.

CAP Abbreviation for catabolite (gene) activator *protein.*

cap. Abbreviation for L. *capiat,* let him take.

cap (kap). **1.** Any anatomical structure that resembles a c. or cover. **2.** A protective covering for an incomplete tooth. **3.** Colloquialism for restoration of the coronal part of a natural tooth by means of an artificial crown. **4.** The nucleotide structure found at the 5′ terminus of many eukaryotic messenger RNAs, consisting of a 7-methylguanosine connected, via its 5′-hydroxyl group, by a triphosphate group to the 5′-hydroxyl group of the first nucleoside encoded by the DNA; usually symbolized as m^7 G(5′)ppp-(5′)N, where N is nucleoside number 1 in the transcribed mRNA and is often itself methylated; it is added posttranscriptionally.
acrosomal c., head c.; acrosome; a collapsed membranous vesicle that covers the anterior part of the nucleus of the spermatozoon, derived from the acrosomal granule; the carbohydrate-rich substance of the c. is associated with hydrolytic enzymes.
c. of the ampullary crest, *cupula* cristae ampullaris.
chin c., an extraoral appliance designed to exert an upward and backward force on the mandible by applying pressure to the chin, thereby preventing forward growth.
cradle c., colloquialism for seborrheic dermatitis of the scalp of the newborn.
dental c.'s, deciduous cheek teeth in the horse which remain attached to erupting permanent teeth.
duodenal c., duodenal bulb; pyloric c.; the first portion of the duodenum, as seen in a roentgenogram or by fluoroscopy.
Dutch c., a contraceptive vaginal diaphragm.
enamel c., the enamel covering the crown of a tooth.
head c., acrosomal c.
metanephric c., the concentrated mass of mesodermal cells about the metanephric bud in a young embryo; the cells of the cap form the uriniferous tubules of the permanent kidney.
phrygian c., on cholecystography, an incomplete septum, or a fold in the gallbladder, whose shape suggests the liberty cap of the French Revolution.
pyloric c., duodenal c.
x-ray c. of Zinn, prominence of the pulmonary arc in the cardiac silhouette in cases of patent ductus arteriosus.

capacitance (kă-pas'i-tans). The quantity of electric charge that may be stored upon a body per unit electric potential; expressed in farads, abfarads, or statfarads.

capacitation (kă-pas'i-tā'shŭn) [L. *capacitas,* fr. *capax,* capable of]. The physiologic process whereby ejaculated spermatozoa in the female genital tract acquire the ability to fertilize ova; characterized by rupture of the acrosomal cap which releases enzymes that facilitate penetration; c. has also been accomplished *in vitro.*

capacitor (kă-pas'i-ter, -tōr). Condenser (4); a device for holding a charge of electricity.

capacity (kă-pas'i-tē) [L. *capax,* able to contain; fr. *capio,* to take]. **1.** The potential cubic contents of a cavity or receptacle. **2.** Ability; power to do. See also volume.
buffer c., the amount of hydrogen ion (or hydroxyl ion) required to bring about a specific pH change in a specified volume of a buffer. See also buffer *value.*
cranial c., the cubic content of the skull obtained by determining the cubage of small shot, seeds, or beads required to fill the skull.
diffusing c. (symbol, D, followed by subscripts indicating location and chemical species), the amount of oxygen taken up by pulmonary capillary blood per minute per unit average oxygen pressure gradient between alveolar gas and pulmonary capillary blood; units are: ml/min/mm Hg; also applied to other gases such as carbon monoxide.
forced vital c. (FVC), vital c. measured with the subject exhaling as rapidly as possible; data relating volume, expiratory flow, and time form the basis for other pulmonary function tests, *e.g.,* flow-volume curve, forced expiratory volume, forced expiratory time, forced expiratory flow.

functional residual c. (FRC), functional residual air; the volume of gas remaining in the lungs at the end of a normal expiration; it is the sum of expiratory reserve volume and residual volume.
heat c., thermal c.; the quantity of heat required to raise the temperature of a system 1°C.
inspiratory c., complementary air; the volume of air that can be inspired after a normal expiration; it is the sum of the tidal volume and the inspiratory reserve volume.
iron-binding c. (IBC), the c. of iron-binding protein in serum (transferrin) to bind serum iron.
maximum breathing c. (MBC), maximum voluntary *ventilation.*
oxygen c., the maximum quantity of oxygen that will combine chemically with the hemoglobin in a unit volume of blood; normally it amounts to 1.34 ml of O_2 per gm of Hb or 20 ml of O_2 per 100 ml of blood.
residual c., residual *volume.*
respiratory c., vital c.
thermal c., heat c.
total lung c. (TLC), the inspiratory c. plus the functional residual c.; *i.e.,* the volume of air contained in the lungs at the end of a maximal inspiration; also equals vital c. plus residual volume.

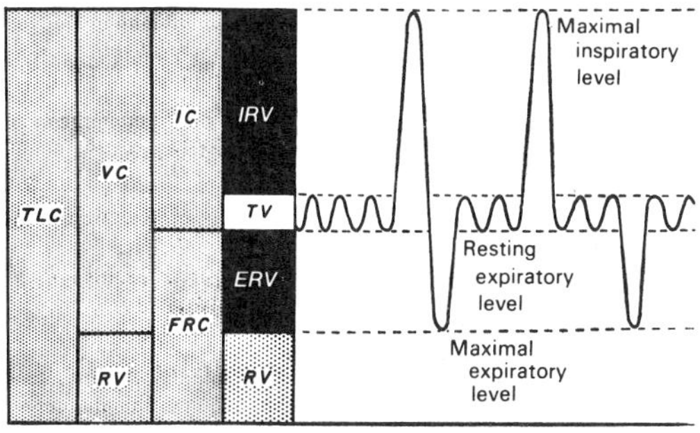

Subdivisions of the Total Lung Capacity

TLC, total lung capacity; *VC,* vital capacity; *RV,* residual volume; *IC,* inspiratory capacity; *FRC,* functional residual capacity; *IRV,* inspiratory reserve volume; *TV,* tidal volume; *ERV,* expiratory reserve volume.

vital c. (VC), respiratory c.; the greatest volume of air that can be exhaled from the lungs after a maximum inspiration.

capactins (kap-ak'tinz). A class of proteins capping the ends of actin filaments.

Capgras, Jean Marie Joseph, French psychiatrist, 1873–1950. See C.'s *syndrome.*

capillarectasia (kap'i-lar-ek-tā'zē-ă) [capillary + G. *ektasis,* extension]. Dilation of the capillary blood vessels.

Capillaria (kap-i-lā'rē-ă) [L. *capillaris,* fr. *capillus,* hair]. A genus of aphasmid nematode worms, characterized by threadlike appearance; related to *Trichuris.*
C. aeroph'ila, species occurring in the bronchi, bronchioles, and nasal sinuses of dogs, cats, and foxes; it causes rhinotracheitis, bronchitis, and nasal discharge in young animals.
C. bo'vis, species occurring in the small intestine of cattle, sheep, and goats.
C. brev'ipes, species found in the small intestine of cattle, sheep, and goats.
C. hepat'ica, species of threadworm that infects the liver in rodents; occasionally reported from man.
C. philippinen'sis, a species of threadworm that has been implicated as a cause of intestinal capillariasis among northern Philippine fishermen.
C. pli'ca, a fine threadworm species occurring in the urinary bladder and sometimes the kidney pelvis of the dog and cat; it apparently causes little damage in many instances.

capillariasis (kap'i-lăr-ī'ă-sis). A parasitic disease caused by infection with species of *Capillaria,* generally *C. philippinensis.*
intestinal c., a sprue-like diarrheal disease caused by infection with *Capillaria philippinensis,* large populations of which are built up by internal autoinfection in the intestinal mucosa; characterized by abdominal pain, edema, diarrhea, cachexia, hypoproteinemia, hypotension, cardiac failure, and hyporeflexia; severe infection is often manifested as a fulminating disorder that may be fatal.

capillariomotor (kap-i-lăr'ē-ō-mō'tōr). Vasomotor, with special reference to the capillaries.

capillarioscopy (kap'i-lar-ē-os'kō-pē). Microangioscopy; capillaroscopy; viewing the cutaneous capillaries at the base of the fingernail through the low power of the microscope.

capillaritis (kap'i-lar-ī'tis). Inflammation of a capillary or capillaries.

capillarity (kap-i-lar'i-tē). The rise of liquids in narrow tubes or through the pores of a loose material, as a result of capillary action.

capillaron (kap'i-lă-ron). An anatomical module composed of parenchymal cells together with their blood capillaries and extracapillary fluid in a compliant capsule; functions as a hydraulic unit which provides a theoretical basis for proposing that blood flow is regulated at the capillary.

capillaropathy (kap'i-lă-rop'ă-thē). Microangiopathy; any disease of the capillaries, often applied to vascular changes in diabetes mellitus.

capillaroscopy (kap'i-lar-os'kō-pē). Capillarioscopy.

capillary (kap'i-lār-ē) [L. *capillaris,* relating to hair]. **1.** Resembling a hair; fine; minute. **2.** A capillary vessel; *e.g.,* blood c., lymph c. **3.** Relating to a blood or lymphatic c. vessel.
arterial c., a c. opening from an arteriole or metarteriole.
bile c., biliary *canaliculus.*
blood c. (symbol c, as a subscript), a vessel whose wall consists of endothelium and its basement membrane; its diameter, when the c. is open, is about 8 μm; with the electron microscope, fenestrated c.'s and continuous c.'s are distinguished.
continuous c., a c. in which small vesicles (caveolae) are numerous and pores are absent.
fenestrated c., a c., found in renal glomeruli, intestinal villi, and some glands, in which ultramicroscopic pores of variable size occur; usually these are closed by a delicate diaphragm, although diaphragms are lacking in at least some renal glomerular c.'s.
lymph c., the beginning of the lymphatic system of vessels; it is lined with a highly attenuated endothelium with poorly developed basement membrane and a lumen of variable caliber. See lacteal (2).
sinusoidal c., a type of blood c. with caliber of from 10 to 20 μm or more; it is lined with a nonphagocytic fenestrated type of endothelium with a discontinuous basement membrane such as occurs in the liver.
venous c., a c. opening into a venule.

capillus, gen. and pl. **capilli** (ka-pil'ŭs, -lī) [L. hair] [NA]. A hair of the head.

capistration (kap-i-strā'shŭn) [L. *capistrum,* muzzle]. Obsolete term for paraphimosis (1).

capita (kap'i-tă). Plural of caput.

capitate (kap'i-tāt) [L. *caput (capit-),* head]. **1.** Head-shaped; having a rounded extremity. **2.** *Os* capitatum.

capitellum (kap-i-tel'ŭm) [L. dim. of *caput,* head]. **1.** Capitulum (1). **2.** *Capitulum* humeri.

capitium (kă-pit'ē-ŭm) [L. *caput,* head]. A bandage for the head.

capitonnage (kap'i-tō-nahzh) [Fr. upholstering]. Closure of a cyst cavity by use of sutures.

capitopedal (kap-i-tō-ped'ăl) [L. *caput,* head, + *pes* (*ped-*), foot]. Relating to the head and the feet.

capitula (kă-pit'yū-lă). Plural of capitulum.

capitular (kă-pit'yū-lăr). Relating to a capitulum.

capitulum, pl. **capitula** (kă-pit'yū-lŭm, -lă) [L. dim. of *caput,* head]. **1** [NA]. Capitellum (1); a small head or rounded articular extremity of a bone. See also caput. **2.** The bloodsucking, probing, sensing, and holdfast mouthparts of a tick, including the basal supporting structure; relative size and shape of mouthparts forming the c. are characteristic for the genera of hard ticks.

c. hu'meri [NA], capitellum; little head of humerus; the small rounded eminence on the lateral half of the distal end of the humerus for articulation with the radius.

Caplan, Anthony, British physician, 1907–1976. See C.'s *nodules, syndrome.*

capnogram (kap'nō-gram) [G. *kapnos,* smoke, + *gramma,* something written]. A continuous record of the carbon dioxide content of expired air.

capnograph (kap'nō-graf). Instrument by which a continuous graph of the carbon dioxide content of expired air is obtained.

cap'ping. A covering.

direct pulp c., a procedure for covering and protecting an exposed vital pulp.

indirect pulp c., the application of a suspension of calcium hydroxide to a thin layer of dentin overlying the pulp (near exposure) in order to stimulate secondary dentin formation and protect the pulp.

Capps, Joseph A., U.S. physician, 1872–1964. See C.'s *reflex.*

Capra (kap'ră) [L. a she-goat]. A genus of ruminants (family Bovidae) that includes the goat, ibex, and related animals; *C. hircus* is the domestic goat.

caprate (kap'rāt). A salt or ester of capric acid.

capreomycin sulfate (kap'rē-ō-mī'sin). Sulfate salt of the cyclic peptide antibiotic obtained from *Streptomyces capreolus,* used in the treatment of tuberculosis.

n-**capric acid** (kap'rik). Decanoic acid, $CH_3(CH_2)_8COOH$; a fatty acid found among the hydrolysis products of fat in goat's milk, cow's milk, and other substances. *Cf.* *n*-caproic acid; caprylic acid.

capriloquism (kă-pril'ō-kwizm) [L. *caper,* goat, + *loquor,* to speak]. Egophony.

caprin (kap'rin). Decanoin; glyceryl tricaprate; tridecanoylglycerol; one of the substances found in butter upon which its flavor depends.

caprine (kap'rēn). Norleucine.

caprine (kă'prīn) [L. *caprinus,* of goats]. Relating to goats; goatlike.

Capripoxvirus (kap'ri-poks-vī'rŭs) [L. *capra,* she-goat, + virus]. The genus of Poxviridae that includes the viruses of sheep-pox and goatpox.

caprizant (kap'ri-zant). Bounding; leaping; denoting a form of pulse beat.

caproate (kap'rō-āt). **1.** A salt or ester of *n* -caproic acid. **2.** USAN-approved contraction for hexanoate, $CH_3(CH_2)_4COO^-$.

n-**caproic acid** (kap-rō'ik). Hexanoic acid; $CH_3(CH_2)_4COOH$; a fatty acid found among the hydrolysis products of fat in butter and some other substances.

caproyl (kap'rō-il). Hexanoyl; the acyl radical of caproic acid.

caproylate (kap'rō-i-lāt). Hexanoate; a salt or ester of caproic acid.

caprylate (kap'ri-lāt). Octanoate; a salt or ester of caprylic acid.

caprylic acid (kap-ril'ik). Octanoic acid; $CH_3(CH_2)_6COOH$; a fatty acid found among the hydrolysis products of fat in butter and other substances.

capsaicin (cap-sā'i-sin). *trans* -8-Methyl-*N*- vanillyl-6-nonenamide; alkaloidal principle in the fruits of various species of *Capsicum,* with the same uses as capsicum.

capsicin (kap'sī-sin). A yellowish red oleoresin containing the active principle of capsicum.

capsicum (kap'si-kŭm). Cayenne, African, or red pepper, the dried ripe fruit of *Capsicum frutescens* (family Solanaceae); used as a carminative, gastrointestinal stimulant, and externally as a rubefacient.

capsid (kap'sid). See virion.

capsomer, capsomere (kap'sō-mēr). A subunit of the protein coat or capsid of a virus particle. See also hexon, penton, virion.

capsula, gen. and pl. **capsulae** (kap'sū-lă, -lē) [L. dim. of *capsa,* a chest or box] [NA]. Capsule (1). **1.** A membranous structure, usually dense collagenous connective tissue, that envelops an organ, a joint, or any other part. **2.** An anatomical structure resembling a capsule or envelope.

c. adipo'sa re'nis [NA], adipose capsule; the perirenal fat.

c. articula'ris [NA], articular or joint capsule; a sac enclosing a joint, formed by an outer fibrous membrane and an inner synovial membrane.

c. articula'ris cricoarytenoi'dea [NA], cricoarytenoid articular capsule; the capsule enclosing the joint between the arytenoid and cricoid cartilages.

c. articula'ris cricothyroi'dea [NA], cricothyroid articular capsule; the capsule enclosing the cricothyroid joint.

c. bul'bi, *vagina* bulbi.

c. cor'dis, pericardium.

c. exter'na [NA], external capsule; periclaustral lamina; a thin lamina of white substance separating the claustrum from the putamen or lateral portion of the lenticular nucleus. It joins the internal capsule at either extremity of the putamen, forming a capsule of white matter external to the lenticular nucleus.

c. extre'ma, extreme capsule; the layer of white matter separating the claustrum from the cortex of the insula, probably representing largely corticopetal and corticofugal fibers of the insular cortex.

c. fibro'sa [NA], the fibrous capsule of an organ; **c. f. glan'dulae thyroi'deae,** the fibrous sheath of the thyroid gland; **c. f. re'nis,** fibrous capsule of kidney; tunica fibrosa renis; a fibrous membrane ensheathing the kidney.

c. fibro'sa per'ivascula'ris [NA], perivascular fibrous capsule; Glisson's capsule; a layer of connective tissue ensheathing the hepatic artery, portal vein, and bile ducts as these ramify within the liver.

c. glomer'uli [NA], Bowman's or Müller's capsule; malpighian capsule (1); the expanded beginning of a nephron composed of an inner and outer layer: the visceral layer consists of podocytes which surround a tuft of capillaries (glomerulus); the parietal layer is simple squamous flat epithelium which becomes cuboidal at the tubular pole.

c. inter'na [NA], internal capsule; a massive layer (8 to 10 mm thick) of white matter separating the caudate nucleus and thalamus (medial) from the more laterally situated lentiform nucleus (globus pallidus and putamen). It consists of 1) fibers ascending from the thalamus to the cerebral cortex that compose, among others, the visual, auditory, and somatic sensory radiations, and 2) fibers descending from the cerebral cortex to the thalamus, subthalamic region, midbrain, hindbrain, and spinal cord. The internal capsule is the major route by which the cerebral cortex is connected with the brainstem and spinal cord. Laterally and superiorly it is directly continuous with the corona radiata which forms a major part of the cerebral hemisphere's white matter; caudally and medially it continues, much reduced in size, as the crus cerebri which contains, among others, the pyramidal tract. On horizontal section it appears in the form of a V opening out laterally; the V's obtuse angle is called genu (knee); its anterior and posterior limbs, respectively, the crus anterior and crus posterior.

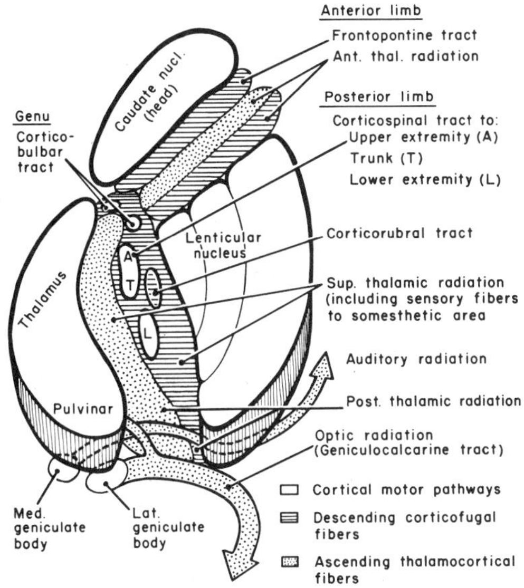

Capsula Interna
Right internal capsule and neighboring structures.

c. len'tis [NA], lenticular capsule; crystalline capsule; phacocyst; the capsule enclosing the lens of the eye.
c. li'enis, *tunica* fibrosa splenis.
c. vasculo'sa len'tis, in the embryo, the vascular mesenchymal capsule which invests the lens of the eye; the vessels of the dorsal part of the capsule are branches of the hyaloid artery, those of the ventral part are derived from the anterior ciliary arteries; normally all the vessels are atrophied by the end of the eighth month of intrauterine life.

capsular (kap'sū-lăr). Relating to any capsule.

capsulation (kap-sū-lā'shŭn). Enclosure in a capsule.

capsule (kap'sūl). **1.** Capsula. **2.** A fibrous tissue layer enveloping a tumor, especially if benign. **3.** A solid dosage form in which the drug is enclosed in either a hard or soft soluble container or "shell" of a suitable form of gelatin. **4.** A hyaline glycosaminoglycan sheath on the wall of a fungus cell, blastoconidium, or spore.
adipose c., *capsula* adiposa renis.
adrenal c., *glandula* suprarenalis.
articular c., *capsula* articularis.
atrabiliary c., *glandula* suprarenalis.
auditory c., auditory cartilage; the cartilage that, in the embryo, surrounds the developing auditory vesicle.
bacterial c., a layer of slime of variable composition which covers the surface of some bacteria; capsulated cells of pathogenic bacteria are usually more virulent than cells without capsules because the former are more resistant to phagocytic action.
Bonnet's c., the anterior part of the vagina bulbi.
Bowman's c., *capsula* glomeruli.
brood c.'s, small hollow projections from the lining membrane of a hydatid cyst from which the scoleces arise.
cartilage c., territorial matrix; the more intensely basophilic matrix in hyaline cartilage surrounding the lacunae in which lie the cartilage cells.
cricoarytenoid articular c., *capsula* articularis cricoarytenoidea.
cricothyroid articular c., *capsula* articularis cricothyroidea.
Crosby c., an attachment to the end of a flexible tube, used for peroral biopsy of the small intestine, by which a piece of mucosa is sucked into an opening in the c. and cut off.
crystalline c., *capsula* lentis.
external c., *capsula* externa.
extreme c., *capsula* extrema.
eye c., *vagina* bulbi.
fibrous c., *capsula* fibrosa.
fibrous articular c., *membrana* fibrosa.
fibrous c. of kidney, *capsula* fibrosa renis.
Gerota's c., *fascia* renalis.
Glisson's c., *capsula* fibrosa perivascularis.
internal c., *capsula* interna.
joint c., *capsula* articularis.
lenticular c., *capsula* lentis.
malpighian c., **(1)** *capsula* glomeruli; **(2)** a thin fibrous membrane enveloping the spleen and continued over the vessels entering at the hilus.
Müller's c., *capsula* glomeruli.
nasal c., the cartilage around the developing nasal cavity of the embryo.
optic c., the concentrated zone of mesenchyme around the developing optic cup; the primordium of the sclera of the eye.
otic c., the cartilage c. surrounding the inner ear mechanism; in elasmobranchs, it remains cartilaginous in the adult; in the embryos of higher vertebrates, it is cartilaginous at first but later becomes bony.
perivascular fibrous c., *capsula* fibrosa perivascularis.
radiotelemetering c., radiopill; an instrument that transmits measurements by radio impulses, from within the body; *e.g.,* measurements of pressure from within the small bowel.
seminal c., *vesicula* seminalis.
suprarenal c., *glandula* suprarenalis.
Tenon's c., *vagina* bulbi.

capsulitis (kap'sū-lī'tis). Inflammation of the capsule of an organ or part, as of the liver or the lens of the eye.
adhesive c., a condition in which there is limitation of motion in a joint due to inflammatory thickening of the capsule, a common cause of stiffness in the shoulder.
hepatic c., perihepatitis.

capsulolenticular (kap'sū-lō-len-tik'yū-lăr). Referring to the lens of the eye and its capsule.

capsuloplasty (kap'sū-lō-plas-tē) [L. *capsula,* capsule, + G. *plastos,* formed]. Plastic surgery of a capsule; more specifically, the capsule of a joint.

capsulorrhaphy (kap-sū-lōr'ă-fē) [L. *capsula,* capsule, + *raphē,* suture]. Suture of a tear in any capsule; specifically, suture of a joint capsule to prevent recurring dislocation of the articulation.

capsulotome (kap'sū-lō-tōm). Cystotome (2).

capsulotomy (kap-sū-lot'ō-mē) [L. *capsula,* capsule, + G. *tomē,* a cutting]. **1.** Creation of an opening through a capsule; *e.g.,* of a scar that might form around a foreign body. **2.** Specifically, incision of the capsule of the lens in the extracapsular cataract operation.
renal c., incision of the capsule of the kidney.

captodiamine (kap-tō-dī'ă-mēn). Captodiam; captodramin; 2-[*p*-(butylthio)-α-phenylbenzylthio]-*N,N*-dimethylethylamine; sedative and antianxiety agent.

captodramin (kap'tō-dră-mēn). Captodiamine.

captopril (kap'tō-pril). 1-(3-Mercapto-2-methyl-1-oxopropyl)-L-proline; an angiotensin converting enzyme inhibitor used in the treatment of hypertension.

capture (kap'chūr) [L. *capio,* pp. *-tus,* to take, seize]. Catching and holding a particle or impulse originating elsewhere.
atrial c., control of the atria after a period of independent beating, as in complete A-V block, by the retrograde impulse.
electron c., a mode of x-rays, of radioactive substances wherein an orbital electron (usually in the K shell) is captured by the nucleus, with the emission of a neutrino, characteristic K_α x-rays, and often

gamma rays.
ventricular c., c. *beat.*

capuride (kap'yū-rīd). (2-Ethyl-3-methylvaleryl)urea; formerly used as a hypnotic.

Capuron, Joseph, French physician, 1767–1850. See C.'s *points.*

caput, gen. **capitis,** pl. **capita** (kap'ut, ka'put; kap'i-tis, kap'ĭ-tă) [L.]. Head. **1** [NA]. The upper or anterior extremity of the animal body, containing the brain and the organs of sight, hearing, taste, and smell. **2** [NA]. The upper, anterior, or larger extremity, expanded or rounded, of any body, organ, or other anatomical structure. **3.** The rounded extremity of a bone. **4.** That end of a muscle which is attached to the less movable part of the skeleton.
c. angula're quadra'ti la'bii superio'ris, *musculus* levator labii superioris alaeque nasi.
c. bre've [NA], short head; in biceps brachii and biceps femoris, the head that has the more distal origin.
c. cor'nus, *apex* cornus posterioris.
c. cos'tae [NA], head of rib; the rounded medial extremity of a rib which, except for ribs 1, 10, 11, and 12, articulates by two facets with the bodies of two contiguous vertebrae.
c. epididymid'is [NA], head of epididymis; globus major; the upper and larger extremity of the epididymis.
c. fem'oris, c. ossis femoris.
c. fib'ulae [NA], head of fibula; the superior extremity of the fibula, which articulates by a facet with the undersurface of the lateral condyle of the tibia.
c. gallinaginis (gal-i-naj'i-nis) [Mod. L. snipe's head]. *colliculus* seminalis.
c. humera'le [NA], humeral head; the name applied to the heads of some of the muscles of the forearm that attach to the humerus.
c. hu'meri [NA], head of humerus; the upper rounded extremity fitting into the glenoid cavity of the scapula.
c. humeroulna're [NA], humeroulnar head; the head of the superficial flexor of the digits that attaches to both the humerus and the ulna.
c. infraorbita'le quadra'ti la'bii superio'ris, *musculus* levator labii superioris.
c. latera'le [NA], lateral head; one of the heads of origin of the triceps brachii and of the gastrocnemius.
c. long'um [NA], long head; the head that has the more proximal origin in the biceps and triceps brachii and the biceps femoris.
c. mal'lei [NA], head of malleus; the rounded portion of the malleus articulating with the body of the incus.
c. mandib'ulae [NA], head of mandible; the expanded articular portion of the condylar process of the mandible.
c. media'le [NA], medial head; one of the heads of origin of the triceps brachii and of the gastrocnemius.
c. medu'sae [*Medusa,* G. myth. char.], cirsomphalos; Medusa head; **(1)** varicose veins radiating from the umbilicus, seen in the Cruveilhier-Baumgarten syndrome; **(2)** dilated ciliary arteries girdling the corneoscleral limbus in rubeosis iridis.
c. nu'clei cauda'ti [NA], the head or anterior extremity of the caudate nucleus projecting into the anterior horn of the lateral ventricle.
c. obli'quum [NA], oblique head; one of the heads of origin of the adductor of the thumb and of the adductor of the great toe.
c. os'sis fem'oris [NA], head of thigh bone; head of femur; c. femoris; the hemispheric articular surface at the upper extremity of the thigh bone.
c. os'sis metacarpa'lis [NA], head of metacarpal bone; the expanded distal end of a metacarpal that articulates with the proximal phalanx of the same digit.
c. os'sis metatarsa'lis [NA], head of metatarsal bone; the expanded distal end of a metatarsal bone that articulates with the proximal phalanx of the same digit.
c. pancre'atis [NA], head of pancreas; that portion of the pancreas lying in the concavity of the duodenum.
c. phalan'gis [NA], head of phalanx; trochlea phalangis; the rounded articular surface at the distal end of the proximal and middle phalanx of each finger and toe.
c. profun'dum [NA], deep head; the head of short flexor of the thumb that arises from the trapezoid and capitate bones.
c. quadra'tum, a head of large size and square shape, owing to thickened parietal and frontal eminences, seen in rachitic children.
c. radia'le [NA], radial head; the name applied to one of the heads of origin of several forearm muscles that arise from the radius.
c. ra'dii [NA], head of radius; the disk-shaped upper extremity articulating with the capitulum of the humerus.
c. sta'pedis [NA], head of stapes; the portion of the stapes that articulates with the lenticular process of the incus.
c. succeda'neum, an edematous swelling formed on the presenting portion of the scalp of an infant during birth; the effusion overlies the periosteum and consists of serum; contrasted with cephalhematoma, in which condition the effusion lies under the periosteum and consists of blood.
c. superficia'le [NA], superficial head; the head of the short flexor of the thumb that arises from the flexor retinaculum and the trapezium.
c. ta'li [NA], head of talus; the rounded anterior portion of the talus articulating with the navicular bone.
c. transver'sum [NA], transverse head; one of the heads of origin of the adductor of the thumb and of the great toe.
c. ul'nae [NA], head of ulna; the small rounded distal extremity of the ulna articulating with the ulnar notch of the radius and the articular disk.
c. ulna're [NA], ulnar head; the name applied to one of the heads of several muscles of the forearm that arise from the ulna.
c. zygomat'icum quadra'ti la'bii superio'ris, *musculus* zygomaticus minor.

Carabelli, Georg C. (Edler von Lunkaszprie), Austrian dentist, 1787–1842. See *cusp* of C., C. *tubercle.*

caramel (kar'ă-mel). Burnt sugar; a concentrated solution of the substance obtained by heating sugar with an alkali; a thick, dark brown liquid used as a coloring and flavoring agent in pharmaceutical preparations.

caramiphen ethanedisulfonate (ka-ram'i-fen eth'ān-dī-sŭl'fō-nāt). Diethylaminoethyl 1-phenylcyclopentanecarboxylate ethanedisulfonate; an antitussive.

caramiphen hydrochloride. Diethylaminoethyl-1-phenylcyclopentane-1-carboxylate hydrochloride; a synthetic spasmolytic drug; used in the treatment of diseases of the basal ganglia, *e.g.,* parkinsonism and hepatolenticular degeneration.

carate (kă-rah'tē). Pinta.

carb-, carbo-. Prefixes indicating the attachment of a group containing a carbon atom.

carbachol (kar'bă-kol). A parasympathetic stimulant used locally in the eye for the treatment of glaucoma.

carbadox (kar'bă-doks). Methyl 3-(2-quinoxalinylmethylene)carbazate N^1,N^4-dioxide; an antibacterial agent.

carbamate (kar'bă-māt). Carbamoate; a salt or ester of carbamic acid; it forms the basis of urethane hypnotics.
c. kinase [EC 2.7.2.21], a phosphotransferase catalyzing the reaction of carbamoyl phosphate and ADP to form ATP, NH_3, and CO_2 (the reverse of the reaction catalyzed by carbamoyl-phosphate synthase).

carbamazepine (kar-bam-az'ĕ-pēn). 5-*H*-Dibenz[*b,f*]azepine-5-carboxamide; an anticonvulsant and also an analgesic especially useful in trigeminal neuralgia.

carbamic acid (kar-bam'ik). A hypothetical acid, NH_2-COOH, forming carbamates; the acyl radical is carbamoyl.

carbamide (kar'bă-mīd). Urea.

carbaminohemoglobin (kar-bam'i-nō-hē-mō-glō'bin). Carbhemoglobin; carbohemoglobin; carbon dioxide bound to hemoglobin by means of a reactive amino group on the latter, *i.e.*, Hb-NHCOOH; approximately 20% of the total content of carbon dioxide in blood is combined with hemoglobin in this manner.

carbamoate (kar'bă-mō-āt). Carbamate.

carbamoyl (kar'bă-mō-il). The acyl radical, NH_2-CO-, the transfer of which plays an important role in certain biochemical reactions; *e.g.*, in the urea cycle, carbamoyl phosphate.

carbamoylaspartate dehydrase (kar'bă-mō-il-as-par'tāt). Dihydro-orotase.

***N*-carbamoylaspartic** (kar'bă-mō-il-as-par'tik). Ureidosuccinic acid.

carbamoylation (kar-bă-mō-il-ā'shŭn). Transfer of the carbamoyl of carbamoyl phosphate to an amino group with elimination of inorganic phosphate.

carbamoylcarbamic acid (kar'bă-mō-il-kar-bam'ik). Allophanic acid.

carbamoylglutamic acid (kar'bă-mō-il-glū-tam'ik). $HOOC(CH_2)_2CH(NHCONH_2)COOH$; an intermediate in the carbamoylation of ornithine to citrulline in the urea cycle.

carbamoyl phosphate. H_2NCO-OPO_3H_2; a reactive intermediate capable of transferring its carbamoyl group (H_2NCO-) to an acceptor molecule, forming citrulline from ornithine in the urea cycle, and ureidosuccinic acid from aspartic acid in pyrimidine ring formation.

carbamoyl-phosphate synthase [EC 2.7.2.5]. A phosphotransferase catalyzing condensation of 2 ATP, NH_3, CO_2, and H_2O to yield 2 ADP + P_i + carbamoyl phosphate (the reverse of the reaction catalyzed by carbamate kinase).

carbamoyltransferases (kar'bă-mō-il-trans'fer-ās-ēz) [EC group 2.1.3]. Transcarbamoylases; enzymes transferring carbamoyl groups from one compound to another (*e.g.*, aspartate carbamoyltransferase, ornithine carbamoyltransferase).

carbamoylurea (kar'bă-mō-il-yū-rē'ă). Biuret.

carbamyl (kar'bă-mil). Former spelling of carbamoyl.

carbamylation (kar'bă-mil-ā'shŭn). Former spelling of carbamoylation.

carbanion (karb-an'ī-on). An organic anion in which the negative charge is on a carbon atom; the specific names are formed by adding -ide, -diide, etc. to the name of the parent compound; *e.g.*, methanide, $(CH_3)^-$.

carbarsone (kar-bar'sōn). 4-Ureidobenzenearsonic acid; *N*-carbamoylarsanilic acid; an amebicide.

carbazides (kar'bă-zīdz). Carbohydrazides; 1,3-diaminoureas; RNH-NHCONH-NHR'.

carbazochrome salicylate (kar-baz'ō-krōm). Adrenochrome monosemicarbazone-sodium salicylate complex; an oxidation product of epinephrine used for the systemic control of capillary bleeding associated with increased capillary permeability.

carbazole (kar'bă-zōl). Diphenylenimine; 9-azafluorene; reacts with carbohydrates (including uronates and deoxypentoses) giving colors characteristic of the sugar type; used for assay and analysis of carbohydrates and formaldehyde, and as a dye intermediate; sensitive to ultraviolet light.

carbazotic acid (kar-bă-zot'ik). Picric acid.

carbenicillin disodium (kar-ben-i-sil'in). Disodium salt of 6-(α-carboxy-α-phenylacetamido)penicillanic acid (α-carboxybenzylpenicillin); a semisynthetic extended spectrum penicillin active against a wide variety of Gram-positive and Gram-negative bacteria.

carbenium (kar-ben'ē-ŭm). See carbonium.

carbenoxolone disodium (kar-ben-oks'ō-lōn dī-sō'dē-ŭm). 3β-Hydroxy-11-oxoolean-12-en-30-oic hydrogen succinate disodium salt; a glucocorticoid used as an anti-inflammatory agent for the treatment of peptic ulcer.

carbetapentane citrate (kar'be-tă-pen'tān). 2-(Diethylaminoethoxy)ethyl 1-phenylcyclopentyl-1-carboxylate citrate; it has atropine-like and local anesthetic actions and effectively suppresses acute cough due to common upper respiratory infections.

carbhemoglobin (karb'hē-mō-glō'bin). Carbaminohemoglobin.

carbide (kar'bīd). A compound of carbon with an element more electropositive than itself; *e.g.*, CaC_2, calcium carbide.

carbidopa (kar-bi-dō'pă). α-Methyldopahydrazine; (−)-L-α-hydrazino-3,4-dihydroxy-α-methylhydrocinnamic monohydrate; a decarboxylation inhibitor, used in conjunction with levodopa in the treatment of Parkinson's disease.

carbimazole (kar-bī'mă-zōl). 1-Methyl-2-imidazolethiol ethyl carbonate; used in the treatment of hyperthyroidism.

carbinol (kar'bi-nol). *Methyl* alcohol.

carbinoxamine maleate (kar-bi-nok'să-mēn). Paracarbinoxamine maleate; 2-[*p*- chloro-α-(2-dimethylaminoethoxy)benzyl]pyridine maleate; an antihistaminic agent.

carbo [L. coal]. Charcoal.

carbo-. See carb-.

carbobenzoxy (Cbz, Z) (kar'bō-ben-zok'sē). Benzyloxycarbonyl.

carbocation (kar-bō-kat'ī-on). See carbonium.

carbochromene hydrochloride (kar-bō-krō'mēn hī-drō-klōr'īd). Chromonar hydrochloride.

carbohemoglobin (kar'bō-hē-mō-glō'bin). Carbaminohemoglobin.

carbohydrases (kar-bō-hī'drā-sez). Rarely used term for enzymes that hydrolyze carbohydrates.

carbohydrates (kar-bō-hī'drāts). Saccharides; class name for the aldehydic or ketonic derivative of polyhydric alcohols, the name being derived from the fact that the most common examples of such compounds have formulas that may be written $C_n(H_2O)_n$(*e.g.*, glucose, $C_6(H_2O)_6$; sucrose, $C_{12}(H_2O)_{11}$), although they are not true hydrates and the name is in that sense a misnomer. The group includes compounds with relatively small molecules, such as the simple sugars (monosaccharides, disaccharides, etc.), as well as macromolecular (polymeric) substances such as starch, glycogen, and cellulose polysaccharides. The c.'s most typical of the class contain carbon, hydrogen, and oxygen only, but carbohydrate metabolic intermediates in tissue contain phosphorus.

carbohydraturia (kar'bō-hī-dră-tū'rē-ă). General term denoting the excretion of one or more carbohydrates in the urine (*e.g.*, glucose, galactose, lactose, pentose), thus including such conditions as glycosuria (melituria), galactosuria, lactosuria, pentosuria, etc.

carbohydrazides (kar-bō-hī'dră-zīdz). Carbazides.

carbolate (kar'bō-lāt). **1.** Phenate. **2.** To carbolize.

carbolated (kar'bō-lā-ted). Phenolated.

carbol-fuchsin (kar'bol-fuk'sin). **1.** See Ziehl's *stain.* **2.** See carbol-fuchsin *paint.*

carbolic acid (kar-bol'ik). Phenol.

carbolize (kar'bō-līz). To mix with or add carbolic acid (phenol).

carboluria (kar-bō-lū'rē-ă) [carbolic acid + G. *ouron,* urine]. The presence of phenol (carbolic acid) in the urine.

carbomer (kar'bō-mer). A polymer of acrylic acid cross-linked with a polyfunctional compound, hence, a poly (acrylic acid) or polyacrylate; a suspending agent for pharmaceuticals.

carbometry (kar-bom'ĕ-trē). Carbonometry.

carbon (kar'bŏn) [L. *carbo,* coal]. A nonmetallic tetravalent element, symbol C, atomic no. 6, atomic weight 12.01. It has two natural isotopes, ^{12}C and ^{13}C (the former, set at 12.00000, being the standard for all molecular weights), and two artificial, radioactive isotopes of interest, ^{11}C and ^{14}C. The element occurs in two pure forms, diamond and graphite; in impure form in charcoal, coke, and soot; and in the atmosphere as CO_2. Its compounds are found in all living tissues, and the study of its vast number of compounds constitutes most of organic chemistry.

active c. dioxide, a complex of *N*-carboxybiotin (biotin + CO_2) and an enzyme; the form in which c. dioxide is added to methylcrotonyl-CoA to form β-methylglutaconyl in the catabolism of leucine, and to acetyl-CoA to form malonyl-CoA. See also acetyl-CoA carboxylase.

anomeric c., the reducing c. of a sugar; C-1 of an aldose, C-2 of a 2-ketose.

c. bisulfide, c. disulfide.

c. dichloride, tetrachlorethylene.

c. dioxide, carbonic anhydride; carbonic acid gas; CO_2; the product of the combustion of c. with an excess of air; in concentrations not less than 99.0% by volume of CO_2, used as a respiratory stimulant.

c. dioxide snow, dry ice; solid c. dioxide used in the treatment of warts, lupus, nevi, and other skin affections, and as a refrigerant.

c. disulfide, carbon bisulfide; CS_2; an extremely flammable (flashpoint -30°C), colorless, toxic liquid with a characteristic ethereal odor (fetid when impure); it is a parasiticide, but is seldom used other than as an industrial solvent.

c. monoxide, CO; a colorless, odorless, and poisonous gas formed by the incomplete combustion of c.; its toxic action is due to its strong affinity for hemoglobin and cytochrome, reducing oxygen transport and blocking oxygen utilization.

c. tetrachloride, tetrachloromethane; CCl_4; a colorless, mobile liquid having a characteristic ethereal odor resembling that of chloroform; it is used as a cleansing fluid and as a fire extinguisher, and has been used as an anthelmintic, especially against hookworm.

carbon-11 (^{11}C). A cyclotron-produced, positron-emitting radioisotope of carbon with a half-life of 20 minutes.

carbon-12 (^{12}C). The standard of atomic mass, 98.89% of natural carbon.

carbon-13 (^{13}C). A natural isotope, 1.11% of natural carbon.

carbon-14 (^{14}C). A beta-emitter with a half-life of 5730 years, widely used as a tracer in studying various aspects of metabolism; naturally occurring ^{14}C, arising from cosmic rays, is used to date relics containing natural carbonaceous materials.

carbonate (kar'bŏn-āt). **1.** A salt of carbonic acid. **2.** The ion $CO_3^{=}$.

c. dehydratase [EC 4.2.1.1], c. hydro-lyase; carbonic anhydrase; a zinc-containing enzyme in red blood cells that catalyzes the conversion of carbon dioxide (CO_2) entering the blood from the tissues into carbonic acid (H_2CO_3); the reverse reaction occurs when the blood reaches the lungs and carbon dioxide is liberated.

c. hydro-lyase, c. dehydratase.

carbonic (kar-bon'ik). Relating to carbon.

carbonic acid. H_2CO_3, formed from H_2O and CO_2.

carbonic anhydrase. *Carbonate* dehydratase.

carbonic anhydride. *Carbon* dioxide (1).

carbonium. (kar-bŏn'ē-ŭm). An organic cation in which the positive charge is on a carbon atom; *e.g.,* $(CH_3)^+$. It is now recommended that carbocation be used as the class name and carbenium be used for specific compound names.

carbonometer (kar-bō-nom'ĕ-ter) [L. *carbo (carbon-),* coal, + G. *metron,* measure]. An obsolete device used in carbonometry.

carbonometry (kar-bō-nom'ĕ-trē). Carbometry; an obsolete method for the determination of the presence and the proportion of carbon dioxide in the air or expired breath by the precipitation of calcium carbonate from lime water.

carbonuria (kar-bo-nū'rē-ă). Rarely used term denoting the excretion of carbon dioxide or other carbon compounds in the urine.

carbonyl (kar'bŏn-il). The characteristic group, —CO—, of the ketones, aldehydes, and organic acids.

carboprost tromethamine (kar'bō-prost trō-meth'ă-mēn). $C_{25}H_{38}O_5$; a prostaglandin used as an abortifacient and in the treatment of refractory postpartum bleeding.

carboxamide (kar-boks'am-īd). Aminocarbonyl; a molecular configuration (–$CONH_2$) that, together with the related carboximides (iminocarbonyls) (–CONH–), is a constituent of many hypnotics, including barbiturates, hydantoins, and thiazines.

carboximide (kar-boks'im-īd). See carboxamide.

carboxy-. Combining form indicating addition of CO or CO_2.

***N*-carboxyanhydrides** (kar-bok'sē-an-hī'drīdz). Heterocyclic derivatives of amino acids from which polypeptides may be synthesized.

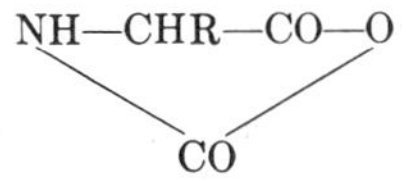

***N*-Carboxyanhydride**

carboxycathepsin (kar-bok'sē-kă-thep'sin). Peptidyl dipeptidase A.

carboxydismutase (kar-bok-sē-dis'mū-tās). Ribulose-bisphosphate carboxylase.

carboxyhemoglobin (HbCO) (kar-bok'sē-hē-mō-glō'bin). Carbon monoxide hemoglobin; a fairly stable union of carbon monoxide with hemoglobin. The formation of c. prevents the normal transfer of carbon dioxide and oxygen during the circulation of blood; thus, increasing levels of c. result in various degrees of asphyxiation, including death.

carboxyhemoglobinemia (kar-bok'sē-hē'mō-glō-bi-nē'mē-ă). Presence of carboxyhemoglobin in the blood, as in carbon monoxide poisoning.

carboxyl (kar-bok'sil). The characterizing group (—COOH) of certain organic acids; *e.g.,* HCOOH (formic acid), CH_3COOH (acetic acid), etc.

carboxylase (kar-bok'sil-ās). One of several carboxy-lyases, trivially named carboxylases or decarboxylases (EC subclass 4.1.1), catalyzing the addition of CO_2 to all or part of another molecule to create an additional —COOH group (*e.g.,* ribulose-bisphosphate carboxylase, EC 4.1.1.39).

carboxylation (kar-bok-si-lā'shŭn). Addition of CO_2 to an organic acceptor, as in photosynthesis, to yield a —COOH group; catalyzed by carboxylases.

carboxyltransferases (kar-bok-sil-trans'fer-ās-ez) [EC group 2.1.3]. Transcarboxylases; enzymes transferring carboxyl groups from one compound to another.

carboxypeptidase (kar-bok-sē-pep'ti-dās). A hydrolase that removes the amino acid at the free carboxyl end of a polypeptide chain.

acid c., serine c.

serine c. [EC 3.4.16.1], carboxypeptidase C; acid c.; a c. of broad specificity for terminal amino acid residues of peptides; the optimum pH is 4.5 to 6.0; sensitive to diisopropyl fluorophosphate.

carboxypeptidase A [EC 3.4.17.1]. Carboxypolypeptidase; a hydrolase that releases C-terminal amino acids, with exception of arginine, lysine, and proline.

carboxypeptidase B [EC 3.4.17.2]. Protaminase; a hydrolase that releases C-terminal lysine or arginine preferentially.

carboxypeptidase C [EC 3.4.12.1]. Serine c.

carboxypeptidase G. γ-Glutamyl hydrolase.

carboxypolypeptidase (kar-bok'sē-pol-ē-pep'ti-dās). Carboxypeptidase A.

***N*-carboxyurea** (kar-bok'sē-yū-rē'ă). Allophanic acid.

carbuncle (kar'bŭng-kl) [L. *carbunculus,* dim. of *carbo,* a live coal, a carbuncle]. **1.** Deep-seated pyogenic infection of the skin and subcutaneous tissues, usually arising in several contiguous hair follicles, with formation of connecting sinuses; often preceded or accompanied by fever, malaise, and prostration. **2.** Anthrax (1).

kidney c., renal c., formerly used term for coalescent multiple intrarenal abscesses.

carbuncular (kar-bŭng'kyū-lăr). Relating to a carbuncle.

carbunculosis (kar-bŭng-kyū-lō'sis). A condition marked by the occurrence of several carbuncles simultaneously or within a short period of time.

carburet (kar'bū-ret). **1.** Archaic term for carbide. **2.** To combine with carbon. **3.** To enrich a gas with volatile hydrocarbons, as in a carburetor.

carbutamide (kar-bū'tă-mīd). Aminophenurobutane; 1-butyl-3-sulfanilylurea; an oral hypoglycemic agent.

carbuterol hydrochloride (kar-bū'tĕ-rol). [5-[2-(*tert*- Butylamino)-1-hydroxyethyl]-2-hydroxyphenyl]urea monohydrochloride; a sympathomimetic drug with bronchodilatory activity.

carcass (kar'kăs) [F. *carcasse,* fr. It. *carcassa*]. The body of a dead animal; in reference to animals used for human food, the body after the hide, head, tail, extremities, and viscera have been removed.

carcino-, carcin- [G. *karkinos,* crab, cancer]. Combining forms relating to cancer.

carcinoembryonic (kar'si-nō-em-brē-on'ik). Relating to a carcinoma-associated substance present in embryonic tissue, as a c. antigen.

carcinogen (kar-sin'ō-jen, kar'si-nō-jen). Any cancer-producing substance, such as polycyclic aromatic hydrocarbons, or agents such as in certain types of irradiation.

complete c., a chemical c. that is able to induce cancer without provocation by a tumor-promoting agent introduced during therapy.

carcinogenesis (kar'si-nō-jen'ĕ-sis) [carcino- + G. *genesis,* generation]. The origin or production of cancer, including carcinomas and other malignant neoplasms.

carcinogenic (kar'si-nō-jen'ik). Cancerigenic; causing cancer.

carcinoid (kar'si-noyd). See carcinoid *tumor;* carcinoid *syndrome.*

carcinolytic (kar'si-nō-lit'ik) [carcino- + G. *lytikos,* causing a solution]. Cancericidal; cancerocidal; destructive to the cells of carcinoma.

CARCINOMA

carcinoma, pl. **carcinomas, carcinomata (CA)** (kar-si-nō'mă, -măz, -nō'mă-tă) [G. *karkinōma,* fr. *karkinos,* cancer, + *-oma,* tumor]. Any of the various types of malignant neoplasm derived from epithelial tissue in several sites, occurring more frequently in the skin and large intestine in both sexes, the bronchi and prostate gland in men, and the breast and cervix in women. C.'s are identified histologically on the basis of invasiveness and the changes that indicate anaplasia, *i.e.,* loss of polarity of nuclei, loss of orderly maturation of cells (especially in squamous cell type), variation in the size and shape of cells, hyperchromatism of nuclei (with clumping of chromatin), and increase in the nuclear-cytoplasmic ratio. C.'s may be undifferentiated, or the neoplastic tissue may resemble (to varying degree) one of the types of normal epithelium.

acinar c., acinic cell *adenocarcinoma.*

acinic cell c., acinic cell *adenocarcinoma.*

acinose c., acinous c., acinic cell *adenocarcinoma.*

adenoid cystic c., cylindromatous c.; a histologic type of c. characterized by large epithelial masses containing round, glandlike spaces or cysts which frequently contain mucus and are bordered by a few or many layers of epithelial cells without intervening stroma, forming a cribriform pattern like a slice of Swiss cheese; perineural invasion and hematogenous metastasis are common; occurs most commonly in salivary glands.

adenoid squamous cell c., adenoacanthoma.

adnexal c., a c. arising in, or forming structures resembling, skin appendages.

adrenal cortical c.'s, large invasive and metastasizing tumors which may cause virilism or Cushing's syndrome.

alveolar cell c., bronchiolar c.

anaplastic c., c. with absence of epithelial structural differentiation.

apocrine c., **(1)** a c. composed predominantly of cells with abundant eosinophilic granular cytoplasm, occurring in the breast; **(2)** a c. of the apocrine glands.

basal cell c., basal cell epithelioma; basaloma; basalioma; a slow-growing, locally invasive, but rarely metastasizing neoplasm derived from basal cells of the epidermis or hair follicles.

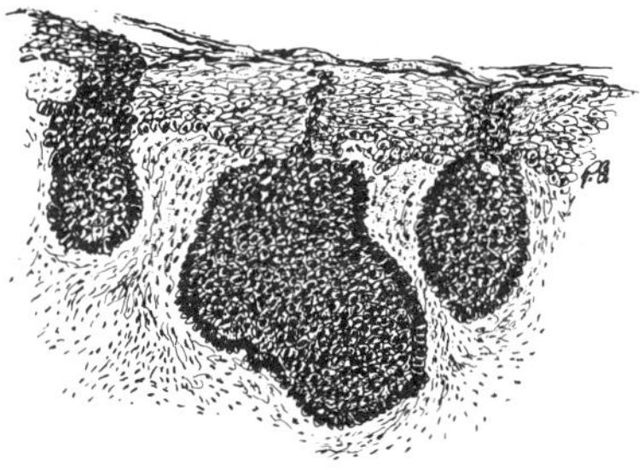

Basal Cell Carcinoma of the Skin

basaloid c., a poorly differentiated squamous cell c. of the anus that has some microscopic resemblance to basal cell c. of the skin, but which frequently metastasizes.

basal squamous cell c., basosquamous c.

basosquamous c., basisquamous c., basal squamous cell c.; intermediate or metatypical c.; a c. of the skin which in structure and behavior is considered transitional between basal cell and squamous cell c. The term should not be used for the much more common keratotic variety of basal cell c., in which the tumor cells are of basal type but which contains small foci of abrupt keratinization.

bronchiolar c., alveolar cell c.; bronchiolo-alveolar c.; bronchiolar adenocarcinoma; a c., thought to be derived from epithelium of terminal bronchioles, in which the neoplastic tissue extends along the alveolar walls and grows in small masses within the alveoli; involvement may be uniformly diffuse and massive, or nodular, or lobular; microscopically, the neoplastic cells are cuboidal or columnar and form papillary structures; mucin may be demonstrated in some of the cells and in the material in the alveoli, which also includes denuded cells; metastases in regional lymph nodes, and even in more distant sites, are known to occur, but are infrequent.

bronchiolo-alveolar c., bronchiolar c.

bronchogenic c., squamous cell or oat cell c. which arises in the

mucosa of the large bronchi and produces a persistent productive cough or hemoptysis; local growth causes bronchial obstruction and is observed radiologically as an enlarging lung mass; malignant tumor cells can be detected in the sputum, and they metastasize early to the thoracic lymph nodes and to the brain, adrenal glands, and other organs via the bloodstream.
canine c. 1, one of the few transplantable tumors of large animals; identified in 1954 at the School of Veterinary Medicine, University of Pennsylvania.
clear cell c. of kidney, renal *adenocarcinoma.*
colloid c., mucinous c.
c. cuta'neum, obsolete term for squamous or basal cell c. of the skin.
cylindromatous c., adenoid cystic c.
cystic c., a c. in which true epithelium-lined cysts are formed, or degenerative changes may result in cystlike spaces.
duct c., ductal c., a c. derived from epithelium of ducts, *e.g.,* in the breast or pancreas.
embryonal c., a malignant neoplasm of the testis, composed of large anaplastic cells with indistinct cellular borders, amphophilic cytoplasm, and ovoid, round, or bean-shaped nuclei that may have multiple large nucleoli; in some instances, the neoplastic cells may form tubular structures; embryonal c.'s may be malignant teratomas without differentiated elements.
endometrioid c., adenocarcinoma of the ovary resembling endometrial adenocarcinoma, possibly arising from ovarian foci of endometriosis.
epidermoid c., epidermoid cancer; a squamous cell c. of the skin.
fibrolamellar liver cell c., oncocytic hepatocellular tumor; primary hepatic c. in which malignant hepatocytes are intersected by fibrous lamellated bands.
follicular c.'s, c.'s of the thyroid composed of well or poorly differentiated epithelial follicles without papillary formation, which are difficult to distinguish from adenomas; the criteria include blood vessel invasion and the finding of metastases of follicular thyroid tissue in other structures such as cervical lymph nodes and bone; follicular c.'s may take up radioactive iodine.
giant cell c., a malignant epithelial neoplasm characterized by unusually large anaplastic cells.
giant cell c. of thyroid gland, a rapidly progressive undifferentiated c. observed in the thyroid gland, characterized by numerous, unusually large, anaplastic cells derived from glandular epithelium of the thyroid gland.
glandular c., adenocarcinoma.
hepatocellular c., malignant *hepatoma.*
Hürthle cell c., see Hürthle cell *tumor.*
inflammatory c., 52 c. of the breast presenting with edema, hyperemia, tenderness, and rapid enlargment of the breast; microscopically, there is extensive invasion of dermal lymphatics by the c.
c. in si'tu, intraepithelial c.; a lesion observed most commonly in stratified squamous epithelium and characterized by cytologic changes of the type associated with invasive c., but with the pathologic process limited to the lining epithelium and without histologic evidence of extension to adjacent structures; the distinctive changes are more apparent in the nucleus, *i.e.,* variation in size and shape, increase in chromatin, and numerous mitoses (including some that are atypical) in all layers of the epithelium, with loss of orderly maturation. The lesion is presumed to be the histologically recognizable precursor of invasive squamous cell c., *i.e.,* a localized and curable phase of c.; a similar process is also observed in glandular epithelium, but may be more difficult to identify.
intermediate c., basosquamous c.
intraductal c., a form of c. derived from the epithelial lining of ducts, especially in the breast, where most c.'s arise from ductal epithelium; the neoplastic cells proliferate in irregular papillary projections or masses, filling the lumens, that are solid, cribriform, or centrally necrotic; intraductal c. may be contained by the ductal basement membrane (intraductal c. in situ), but frequently invades surrounding stroma and may then metastasize.
intraepidermal c., c. in situ of the skin; *e.g.,* Bowen's disease.
intraepithelial c., c. in situ.
invasive c., a neoplasm in which collections of epithelial cells infiltrate or destroy the surrounding tissue.
juvenile c., secretory c.
kangri burn c., kangri *cancer.*
large cell c., an anaplastic c., particularly bronchogenic, composed of cells which are much larger than those in oat cell c. of the lung.
latent c., an epithelial neoplasm showing microscopic features of malignancy believed to have remained localized and asymptomatic for a long period; *e.g.,* small c.'s of the prostate in old men, often found incidentally at autopsy.
lateral aberrant thyroid c., a cervical nodule of thyroid c. situated outside the thyroid gland, formerly thought to arise from ectopic thyroid tissue but now believed to be metastatic from an occult c. within the gland.
leptomeningeal c., meningeal c.
liver cell c., malignant *hepatoma.*
lobular c., a form of acinic cell adenocarcinoma, especially of the breast, where lobular c. is less common than ductal c. and usually is composed of small cells.
lobular c. in situ, noninfiltrating lobular c.
Lucké c., Lucké's adenocarcinoma; a virus-associated adenocarcinoma of the kidney in adult frogs.
medullary c., encephaloid cancer; a malignant neoplasm, comparatively soft and branlike in consistency, that consists chiefly of neoplastic epithelial cells, with only a scant amount of fibrous stroma.
melanotic c., melanoma.
meningeal c., leptomeningeal c.; leptomeningeal carcinomatosis; meningeal carcinomatosis; an infiltration of c. cells in the arachnoid and subarachnoid space; may be primary or secondary.
mesometanephric c., mesonephroma.
metaplastic c., a c. in which some of the tumor cells are spindle shaped, suggesting a sarcoma, or in which the stroma shows foci of bone or cartilage; such c.'s occur in the upper respiratory or alimentary tract or in the breast.
metastatic c., secondary c.; a c. that has appeared in a region remote from its site of origin, as in metastasis (2).
metatypical c., basosquamous c.
microinvasive c., a variety of c. seen most frequently in the uterine cervix, in which c. in situ of squamous epithelium, on the surface or replacing the lining of glands, is accompanied by small collections of abnormal epithelial cells that infiltrate a very short distance into the stroma; this may represent the earliest stage of invasion, in which the neoplastic cells are capable of intrusion but not of sustained growth in connective tissue.
mucinous c., colloid c. or cancer; a variety of adenocarcinoma in which the neoplastic cells secrete conspicuous quantities of mucin, and, as a result, the neoplasms are likely to be glistening, sticky, and gelatinoid in consistency.
mucoepidermoid c., mucoepidermoid tumor; a salivary gland c. of low grade malignancy in children, but with variable malignancy in adults; composed of mucous, epidermoid, and intermediate cells, with mucous cells abundant only in low grade c.'s; recurrence is frequent, and high grade c.'s metastasize to cervical nodes.
c. myxomato'des, obsolete term for a form of colloid cancer in which there is myxomatous metaplasia of the cellular fibrous stroma.
noninfiltrating lobular c., lobular c. in situ; c. of the breast in which small tumor cells fill preexisting acini within lobules, without invading the surrounding stroma.
oat cell c., small cell c. (2); an anaplastic, highly malignant, and usually bronchogenic c. composed of small ovoid cells with very scanty cytoplasm; this c. and small round cell c.'s comprise over

one-third of c.'s of the lung.
occult c., a small c., either asymptomatic or giving rise to metastases without symptoms due to the primary c.
oncoplastic c., an undifferentiated c. showing no evidence by light microscopy of origin from a specific epithelial tissue, *e.g.,* squamous or glandular epithelium.
papillary c., a malignant neoplasm characterized by the formation of numerous, irregular, finger-like projections of fibrous stroma that is covered with a surface layer of neoplastic epithelial cells.
primary c., c. at the site of origin, with local invasion in that organ.
renal cell c., renal *adenocarcinoma.*
sarcomatoid c., spindle cell c.
scar c., scar cancer; adenocarcinoma of the lung arising from a peripheral lung scar or associated with interstitial fibrosis in a honeycomb lung.
scirrhous c., fibrocarcinoma; a hard c., fibrous in nature, resulting from a desmoplastic reaction by the stromal tissue to the presence of the neoplastic epithelium.
secondary c., metastatic c.
secretory c., juvenile c.; c. of the breast with pale-staining cells showing prominent secretory activity, as seen in pregnancy and lactation, but found mostly in children.
signet ring cell c., a poorly differentiated adenocarcinoma composed of cells with a cytoplasmic droplet of mucus that compresses the nucleus to one side along the cell membrane; arises most frequently in the stomach, occasionally in the large bowel or elsewhere.
c. sim'plex, **(1)** any form of c. in which the relative proportions of stroma and neoplastic epithelial cells are not unusual, *i.e.,* stromal elements are not comparatively abundant, nor are they reduced in amount or lacking; **(2)** a c. lacking any identifiable microscopic pattern, such as glandular structure.
small cell c., **(1)** an anaplastic c. composed of small cells; **(2)** oat cell c.
spindle cell c., sarcomatoid c.; a c. composed of elongated cells, frequently a poorly differentiated squamous cell c. which may be difficult to distinguish from a sarcoma.
squamous cell c., a malignant neoplasm derived from stratified squamous epithelium, but which may also occur in sites, such as bronchial mucosa, where glandular or columnar epithelium is normally present; variable amounts of keratin are formed, in relation to the degree of differentiation, and, if the keratin is not on the surface, it accumulates in the neoplasm as a keratin pearl; in instances in which the cells are well differentiated, intercellular bridges may be observed between adjacent cells; a common example in lower animals is ocular squamous cell c. of Hereford cattle.
sweat gland c., usually a solitary tumor, nodular and fixed to the skin and underlying structure, having slow growth for long periods followed by rapid spurts of growth and rapid dissemination.
trabecular c., Merkel cell *tumor.*
transitional cell c., a malignant neoplasm derived from transitional epithelium, occurring chiefly in the urinary bladder, ureters, or renal pelves (especially if well differentiated) frequently papillary; these c.'s are graded 1 to 3 or 4 according to the degree of anaplasia, grade 1 appearing histologically benign but being liable to recurrence. So-called transitional cell c. of the upper respiratory tract is more properly classified as squamous cell c.
tubular c., a well-differentiated form of breast c. with invasion of the stroma by small epithelial tubules.
V-2 c., a transplantable, highly malignant c. of experimental animals, that developed as a result of malignant change in a virus-induced papilloma of a domestic rabbit.
verrucous c., a well differentiated papillary squamous cell c., especially of the oral cavity or penis, that may invade locally but rarely metastasizes; the usual cytologic features of malignancy are absent.
villous c., a form of c. in which there are numerous, closely packed, papillary projections of neoplastic epithelial tissue.
Walker c., Walker *carcinosarcoma.*
wolffian duct c., mesonephroma.

carcinoma ex pleomorphic adenoma. Carcinoma arising in a benign mixed tumor of a salivary gland, characterized by rapid enlargement and pain.

carcinomata (kar-si-nō'mă-tă). Alternative plural of carcinoma.

carcinomatosis (kar'si-nō-mă-tō'sis). Carcinosis; a condition resulting from widespread dissemination of carcinoma in multiple sites in various organs or tissues of the body; sometimes also used in relation to involvement of a relatively large region of the body.
leptomeningeal c., meningeal *carcinoma.*
meningeal c., meningeal *carcinoma.*

carcinomatous (kar-si-nom'ă-tŭs). Pertaining to or manifesting the characteristic properties of carcinoma.

carcinophobia (kar'sin-ō-fō'bē-ă). Cancerophobia.

carcinosarcoma (kar'si-nō-sar-kō'mă). A malignant neoplasm that contains elements of carcinoma and sarcoma so extensively intermixed as to indicate neoplasia of epithelial and mesenchymal tissue. See also collision *tumor.*
embryonal c., blastoma.
renal c., Wilm's *tumor.*
Walker c., Walker carcinoma; a transplantable c. of the rat that originally appeared spontaneously in the mammary gland of a pregnant albino rat, and which now resembles a carcinoma in young transplants and a sarcoma in older transplants.

carcinosis (kar-si-nō'sis). Carcinomatosis.

carcinostatic (kar'si-nō-stat'ik). **1.** Pertaining to an arresting or inhibitory effect on the development or progression of a carcinoma. **2.** An agent that manifests such an effect.

carcoma (kar-kō'mă) [Sp. wood dust under the bark of a tree, caused by the wood louse]. Dark red-brown or mahogany-colored granular material that occurs in human feces in tropical regions; it yields a chemical reaction similar to that of urobilinogen and is composed of calcium oxide, iron, phosphoric and carbonic acids, urobilinogen, cholerythrogen, and other organic matter in varying proportions.

Carden, Henry D., British surgeon, †1872. See C.'s *amputation.*

cardi-. See cardio-.

cardia (kar'dē-ă) [G. *kardia,* heart]. *Pars* cardiaca ventriculi.

cardiac (kar'dē-ak) [L. *cardiacus*]. **1.** Pertaining to the heart. **2.** Pertaining to the esophageal opening of the stomach. **3.** A remedy for heart disease.

cardiac ballet (kar'dē-ak bal-ā'). Short runs of cardiac dysrhythmia consisting of uniform sequences of repetitive multiform extrasystoles.

cardialgia (kar-dē-al'jē-ă). [cardi- + G. *algos,* pain]. **1.** Obsolete term for pyrosis. **2.** Cardiodynia.

cardiataxia (kar'dē-ă-tak'sē-ă) [cardi- + G. *ataxia,* disorder]. Extreme irregularity in the action of the heart.

cardiatelia (kar'dē-ă-tē'lē-ă) [cardi- + G. *atelēs,* incomplete]. Incomplete development of the heart.

cardiectasia (kar'dē-ek-tā'zē-ă) [cardi- + G. *ektasis,* a stretching]. Dilation of the heart.

cardiectomy (kar-dē-ek'tō-mē) [cardi-(2) + G. *ektomē,* excision]. Excision of the cardiac part of the stomach.

cardiectopia (kar-dē-ek-tō'pē-ă) [cardi- + G. *ektopos,* out of place]. Abnormal placement of the heart.

cardinal (kar'di-năl) [L. *cardinalis,* principal]. Chief or principal; in embryology, relating to the main venous drainage.

card′ing. The procedure of placing individual sets of anterior or posterior teeth in trays lined with a wax strip.

cardio-, cardi- [G. *kardia,* heart]. Combining forms denoting: **1.** The heart. **2.** The cardia (ostium cardiacum).

cardioaccelerator (kar′dē-ō-ak-sel′er-ā-ter). Accelerator of the heart beat.

cardioactive (kar′dē-ō-ak′tiv). Influencing the heart.

cardioangiography (kar′dē-ō-an-jē-og′ră-fē). Angiocardiography.

cardioaortic (kar′dē-ō-ā-ōr′tik). Relating to the heart and the aorta.

cardioarterial (kar′dē-ō-ar-tēr′ē-ăl). Relating to the heart and the arteries.

cardiocairograph (kar-dē-ō-kī′rō-graf) [cardio- + G. *kairos,* the right point of time, + *graphō,* to write]. An instrument that synchronizes roentgen exposures of the thorax with selected phases of the cardiac cycle.

cardiocele (kar′dē-ō-sēl) [cardio- + G. *kēlē,* hernia]. A herniation or protrusion of the heart through an opening in the diaphragm, or through a wound.

cardiocentesis (kar′dē-ō-sen-tē′sis) [cardio- + G. *kentēsis,* puncture]. Paracentesis of the heart.

cardiochalasia (kar′dē-ō-kă-lā′zē-ă). Achalasia of the cardia.

cardioclasia (kar′dē-ō-klā′zē-ă). Cardiorrhexis.

cardiodiosis (kar′dē-ō-dē-ō′sis) [cardio- (2) + G. *diōsis,* a spreading open]. Maneuver to dilate the gastric cardia.

cardiodynamics (kar′dē-ō-dī-nam′iks). The mechanics of the heart's action, including its movement and the forces generated thereby.

cardiodynia (kar′dē-ō-din′ē-ă) [cardio- + G. *odynē,* pain]. Cardialgia (2); pain in the heart.

cardioesophageal (kar′dē-ō-ē-sof-ă-jē′ăl). Denoting the area at the junction of the esophagus and cardiac part of the stomach.

cardiogenesis (kar-dē-ō-gen′ĕ-sis) [cardio + G. *genesis,* origin]. Formation of the heart in the embryo.

cardiogenic (kar′dē-ō-jen′ik). Of cardiac origin.

cardiogram (kar′dē-ō-gram) [cardio- + G. *gramma,* a diagram]. **1.** The graphic tracing made by the stylet of a cardiograph. **2.** Generally used for any recording derived from the heart, with such prefixes as apex-, echo-, electro-, phono-, or vector- being understood.

esophageal c., tracing of left atrial contractions made by recording displacements of the column of air in an esophageal tube.

cardiograph (kar′dē-ō-graf) [cardio- + G. *graphō,* to write]. An instrument for recording graphically the movements of the heart, constructed on the principle of the sphygmograph.

cardiography (kar-dē-og′ră-fē). The use of the cardiograph.

ultrasound c., echocardiography.

cardiohemothrombus (kar′dē-ō-hē-mō-throm′bŭs). Cardiothrombus.

cardiohepatic (kar′dē-ō-hĕ-pat′ik). Relating to the heart and the liver.

cardiohepatomegaly (kar′dē-ō-hep′ă-tō-meg′ă-lē). Enlargement of both heart and liver.

cardioid (kar′dē-oyd) [cardi- + G. *eidos,* resemblance]. Resembling a heart.

cardioinhibitory (kar′dē-ō-in-hib′ĭ-tō-rē). Arresting or slowing the action of the heart.

cardiokinetic (kar′dē-ō-kĭ-net′ik) [cardio- + G. *kinēsis,* movement]. Influencing the action of the heart.

cardiokymogram (kar′dē-ō-kī′mō-gram). Record made by a cardiokymograph.

cardiokymograph (kar′dē-ō-kī′mō-graf). Noninvasive device, placed on the chest, capable of recording anterior left ventricle segmental wall motion; consists of a 5 cm diameter capacitive plate transducer as part of a high frequency, low-power oscillator with recording probe; changes in wall motion affect the magnetic field and thus the oscillatory frequency which is then recorded on a multichannel analog waveform polygraph.

cardiokymography (kar′dē-ō-kī-mog′ră-fē). Use of a cardiokymograph.

cardiolipin (kar′dē-ō-lip′in). Acetone-insoluble antigen; heart antigen; a 1,3-bis(phosphatidyl)glycerol with immunological properties; used in serological diagnosis of syphilis. When mixed with lecithin and cholesterol c. will combine with the Wassermann antibody but not with the treponema-immobilizing antibody.

cardiolith (kar′dē-ō-lith) [cardio- + G. *lithos,* stone]. Cardiac calculus; a concretion in the heart, or an area of calcareous degeneration in its walls or valves.

cardiologist (kar-dē-ol′ō-jist). Physician specializing in cardiology.

cardiology (kar-dē-ol′ō-jē) [cardio- + G. *logos,* study]. The medical specialty concerned with the diagnosis and treatment of heart disease.

cardiolysis (kar-dē-ol′i-sis) [cardio- + G. *lysis,* loosening]. An operation for breaking up the adhesions in chronic mediastinopericarditis; access is gained by resection of a portion of the sternum and the corresponding costal cartilages.

cardiomalacia (kar′dē-ō-mă-lā′shē-ă) [cardio- + G. *malakia,* softness]. Softening of the walls of the heart.

cardiomegaly (kar-dē-ō-meg′ă-lē) [cardio- + G. *megas,* large]. Macrocardia; megacardia; megalocardia; enlargement of the heart.

glycogen c., a form of glycogenosis due to abnormal storage of glycogen within the heart muscle cells.

cardiometry (kar-dē-om′ĕ-trē) [cardio- + G. *metron,* measure]. Measurement of the dimensions of the heart or the force of its action.

cardiomotility (kar′dē-ō-mō-til′ĭ-tē). Movements of the heart.

cardiomuscular (kar′dē-ō-mŭs′kyū-lăr). Pertaining to the cardiac musculature.

cardiomyoliposis (kar′dē-ō-mī′ō-li-pō′sis) [cardio- + G. *mys,* muscle, + *lipos,* fat, + *-osis,* condition]. Fatty degeneration of the myocardium.

cardiomyopathy (kar′dē-ō-mī-op′ă-thē) [cardio- + G. *mys,* muscle, + *pathos,* disease]. Myocardiopathy; disease of the myocardium. As a disease classification, the term is used in several different senses, but is limited by the World Health Organization to: "Primary disease process of heart muscle in absence of a known underlying etiology."

alcoholic c., myocardial disease occurring in some chronic alcoholics; may result either from thiamin deficiency or be of unknown pathogenesis.

beer-drinker's c., beer heart; myocardial degeneration with pericardial effusion, reported in heavy beer-drinkers.

dilated c., decreased systolic function of the left ventricle associated with its dilatation; most patients have global hypokinesia, although discrete regional wall movement abnormalities may occur; usually manifested by signs of overall cardiac failure, with congestive findings, as well as by fatigue indicative of a low output state.

hypertrophic c., thickening of the ventricular septum and walls of the left ventricle with marked myofibril disarray; often associated with greater thickening of the septum than of the free wall resulting in narrowing of the left ventricular outflow tract and dynamic outflow gradient; diastolic compliance is greatly impaired.

idiopathic c., primary c. (1).

postpartum c., cardiomegaly and congestive heart failure developing in the puerperium in the absence of any of the known causes of heart disease.

primary c., (1) idiopathic c.; c. of unknown or obscure cause; (2) a disease that affects mainly the heart muscle, sparing other cardiac structures and usually resulting in fibrosis or hypertrophy.

restrictive c., diverse group of conditions characterized by restriction of diastolic filling, a diagnosis limited by the World Health Organization to the hypereosinophilic type; often confused with constrictive pericarditis and the infiltrative cardiomyopathies; left ventricular size and systolic function are usually preserved but dyspnea results from increase in left ventricular diastolic filling pressure and signs of right ventricular failure may be prominent.

secondary c., disease that affects the myocardium secondarily to systemic disease, infection, or metabolic disease.

cardiomyotomy (kar'dē-ō-mī-ot'ō-mē) [cardio- (2) + G. *mys,* muscle, + *tomē,* cutting]. Esophagomyotomy.

cardionecrosis (kar'dē-ō-nĕ-krō'sis). Necrosis of the myocardium.

cardionector (kar'dē-ō-nek'tŏr, -tōr) [cardio- + L. *necto,* to join]. Term sometimes used for conducting *system* of the heart.

cardionephric (kar'dē-ō-nef'rik). Cardiorenal.

cardioneural (kar'dē-ō-nūr'ăl) [cardio- + G. *neuron,* nerve]. Relating to the nervous control of the heart.

cardioneurosis (kar'dē-ō-nū-rō'sis). Cardiac *neurosis.*

cardio-omentopexy (kar'dē-ō-ō-men'tō-pek-sē) [cardio- + omentum, + G. *pēxis,* fixation]. Operation for the attachment of omentum to the heart with the object of improving its blood supply.

cardiopaludism (kar'dē-ō-pal'ū-dizm) [cardio- + paludism, malaria, fr. L. *palus,* marsh]. Irregularity in the heart's action due to malaria.

cardiopath (kar'dē-ō-path). A sufferer from heart disease.

cardiopathia nigra (kar-dē-ō-path'ē-ă nī'gra). Ayerza's *syndrome.*

cardiopathy (kar-dē-op'ă-thē) [cardio- + G. *pathos,* disease]. Any disease of the heart.

cardiopericardiopexy (kar'dē-ō-pār-i-kar'dē-ō-pek-sē) [cardio- + pericardium, + G. *pēxis,* fixation]. An operation to increase the blood supply to the myocardium; sterile magnesium silicate (a form of talc) is spread within the pericardial sac to cause an adhesive pericarditis and an increase in blood supply to develop through the stimulation of interarterial coronary anastomoses and pericardial collaterals.

cardiophobia (kar'dē-ō-fō'bē-ă). Morbid fear of heart disease.

cardiophone (kar'dē-ō-fōn) [cardio- + G. *phōnē,* sound]. A stethoscope specially designed to aid in listening to the sounds of the heart.

cardiophony (kar'dē-of'ō-nē). A rarely used term for phonocardiography (1).

cardiophrenia (kar'dē-ō-frē'nē-ă). Phrenocardia.

cardioplasty (kar'dē-ō-plas-tē) [cardio- (2) + G. *plastos,* formed]. Esophagogastroplasty; an operation on the cardia of the stomach.

cardioplegia (kar'dē-ō-plē'jē-ă) [cardio- + G. *plēgē,* stroke]. **1.** Paralysis of the heart. **2.** An elective stopping of cardiac activity temporarily by injection of chemicals, selective hypothermia, or electrical stimuli.

cardioplegic (kar-dē-ō-plē'jik). Relating to cardioplegia.

cardioptosia (kar'dē-op-tō'sē-ă) [cardio- + G. *ptōsis,* a falling]. Drop heart; a condition in which the heart is unduly movable and displaced downward, as distinguished from bathycardia. See also *cor* mobile; *cor* pendulum.

cardiopulmonary (kar'dē-ō-pŭl'mo-nār-ē). Pneumocardial; relating to the heart and lungs.

cardiopyloric (kar'dē-ō-pī-lōr'ik, -pi-lōr'ik). Relating to the cardiac and pyloric extremities of the stomach.

cardiorenal (kar'dē-ō-rē'năl). Cardionephric; nephrocardiac; renicardiac; relating to the heart and the kidney.

cardiorrhaphy (kar-dē-ōr'ă-fē) [cardio- + G. *rhaphē,* suture]. Suture of the heart wall.

cardiorrhexis (kar-dē-ō-rek'sis) [cardio- + G. *rhēxis,* rupture]. Cardioclasia; rupture of the heart wall.

cardioschisis (kar-dē-os'ki-sis) [cardio- + G. *schisis,* a division]. Division of adhesions between the heart and the pericardium or the chest wall.

cardioscope (kar'dē-ō-skōp) [cardio- + G. *skopeō,* to view]. An instrument for inspecting the interior of the living heart.

cardioselective (kar'dē-ō-sē-lek'tiv). Denoting or having the properties of cardioselectivity.

cardioselectivity (kar'dē-ō-sē-lek-tiv'i-tē). The relatively predominant cardiovascular pharmacologic effect of a drug with multipharmacologic effects; used especially when describing beta-blocking agents.

cardiospasm (kar'dē-ō-spazm). Esophageal *achalasia.*

cardiosphygmograph (kar'dē-ō-sfig'mō-graf) [cardio- + G. *sphygmos,* pulse, + *graphō,* to write]. An instrument for recording graphically the movements of the heart and the radial pulse.

cardiotachometer (kar'dē-ō-tă-kom'ĕ-ter) [cardio- + G. *tachos,* rapidity, + *metron,* measure]. An instrument for measuring the rapidity of the heart beat.

cardiothrombus (kar'dē-ō-throm'bŭs). Cardiohemothrombus; a clot of blood within one of the heart's chambers.

cardiothyrotoxicosis (kar'dē-ō-thī-rō-tok-si-kō'sis). Hyperthyroidism with cardiac complications.

cardiotomy (kar-dē-ot'ō-mē) [cardio- + G. *tomē,* incision]. **1.** Incision of the heart wall. **2.** Incision of the cardiac part of the stomach.

cardiotonic (kar'dē-ō-ton'ik) [cardio- + G. *tonos,* tension]. Exerting a favorable, so-called tonic, effect upon the action of the heart.

cardiotoxic (kar'dē-ō-tok'sik) [cardio- + G. *toxikon,* poison]. Having a deleterious effect upon the action of the heart, due to poisoning of the cardiac muscle or of its conducting system.

cardiovalvotomy (kar'dē-ō-val-vot'ō-mē). Cardiovalvulotomy.

cardiovalvulitis (kar'dē-ō-val-vyū-lī'tis). Inflammation of the heart valves.

cardiovalvulotomy (kar'dē-ō-val-vyū-lot'ō-mē) [cardio- + Mod. L. *valvula,* a little valve + *tomē,* a cutting]. Cardiovalvotomy; an operation for the correction of valvular stenosis by cutting or excising a part of a heart valve.

cardiovascular (CV) (kar'dē-ō-vas'kyū-lăr) [cardio- + L. *vasculum,* vessel]. Relating to the heart and the blood vessels or the circulation.

cardiovasculorenal (kar'dē-ō-vas'kyū-lō-rē'năl). Relating to the heart, arteries, and kidneys, especially as to function or disease.

cardioversion (kar'dē-ō-ver'zhŭn). Restoration of the heart's rhythm to normal by electrical countershock.

cardioverter (kar'dē-ō-ver'ter). A machine used to perform cardioversion.

carditis (kar-dī'tis). Inflammation of the heart.

rheumatic c., pancarditis occurring in rheumatic fever, characterized by formation of Aschoff bodies in the cardiac interstitial tissue; may be associated with acute cardiac failure, endocarditis with small fibrin vegetations on the margins of closure of valve cusps (especially the mitral), and fibrinous pericarditis; it is frequently followed by scarring of the valves.

care (kār). In medicine and public health, a general term for the application of knowledge to the benefit of a community or individual.

comprehensive medical c., a concept that includes not only the traditional c. of the acutely or chronically ill patient, but also the

prevention and early detection of disease and the rehabilitation of the disabled.
health c., c. that encompasses the social, economic, and environmental influences, in addition to medical c.
intensive c., management and c. of critically ill patients. See also intensive c. *unit.*
medical c., the portion of c. under a physician's direction.
primary medical c., c. of a patient by a member of the health c. system who has initial contact with the patient.
secondary medical c., medical c. by a physician who acts as a consultant at the request of the primary physician.
tertiary medical c., specialized consultative c., usually on referral from primary or secondary medical c. personnel, by specialists working in a center that has personnel and facilities for special investigation and treatment.

carebaria (kar-ĕ-bā'rē-ă) [G. *karā,* head, + *barutēs,* heaviness]. Pressure or heaviness in the head.

caribi (kă-rē'bē). Epidemic gangrenous *proctitis.*

carica (kar'i-kă). Papaya.

caries (kār'ēz) [L. dry rot]. **1.** Destruction or necrosis of teeth. **2.** Obsolete term for tuberculosis of bones or joints.
active c., presence of lesions in teeth that prolapse toward pulp.
arrested dental c., carious lesions that have become inactive and may exhibit changes in color and/or consistency.
buccal c., c. beginning with decay on the buccal surface of a tooth.
cemental c., c. of the cementum of a tooth.
compound c., **(1)** c. involving more than one surface of a tooth; **(2)** two or more carious lesions joined to form one cavity.
dental c., saprodontia; a localized, progressively destructive disease of the teeth which starts at the external surface (usually the enamel) with the apparent dissolution of the inorganic components by organic acids that are produced in immediate proximity to the tooth by the enzymatic action of masses of microorganisms (in the bacterial plaque) on carbohydrates; the initial demineralization is followed by an enzymatic destruction of the protein matrix with subsequent cavitation and direct bacterial invasion; in the dentin, demineralization of the walls of the tubules is followed by bacterial invasion and destruction of the organic matrix.
distal c., loss of structure on the tooth surface that is directed away from the median plane of the dental arch.
fissure c., c. beginning in a fissure on the occlusal surfaces of posterior teeth.
incipient c., beginning c. or decay.
interdental c., c. between the teeth.
mesial c., c. on the tooth surface that is directed toward the median plane of the dental arch.
occlusal c., c. starting from the occlusal surface of a tooth.
pit c., a carious lesion, usually small, beginning in a pit on the labial, buccal, lingual, or occlusal surface of a tooth.
pit and fissure c., c. initiated in the areas where developmental pits and fissures are located on the tooth surface.
primary c., initial lesions produced by direct extension from an external surface.
proximal c., c. occurring in the proximal surface, either distal or mesial, of a tooth.
radiation c., c. of the cervical regions of the teeth, incisal edges, and cusp tips secondary to xerostomia induced by radiation therapy to the head and neck.
recurrent c., c. recurring in an area due to inadequate removal of the initial decay, usually beneath a restoration.
root c., c. of the root surface of a tooth, usually appearing as a broad shallow defect in the area of the cemento-enamel junction.
secondary c., c. of enamel beginning at the dento-enamel junction due to a rapid lateral spread of decay from the original decay.
senile dental c., c. occurring in old age, usually interproximally and in the cementum.
smooth surface c., c. initiated on the smooth surfaces of teeth.

carina, pl. **carinae** (kă-rī'nă, -rī'nē) [L. the keel of a boat]. **1.** In man, a term applied or applicable to several anatomical structures forming a projecting central ridge. **2.** That portion of the sternum in a bird, bat, or mole that serves as the origin of the pectoral muscles; it is not found in flightless birds and most mammals.
c. for'nicis, a ridge running along the undersurface of the fornix of the brain.
c. tra'cheae [NA], the ridge separating the openings of the right and left main bronchi at their junction with the trachea.
c. urethra'lis vagi'nae [NA], c. vaginae; the lower part of the anterior column of the vagina, in relation with the urethra.
c. vagi'nae, c. urethralis vaginae.

carinate (kar'i-nāt). Shaped like a keel; relating to or resembling a carina.

cario-. Combining form relating to caries.

cariogenesis (ka'rē-ō-jen'ĕ-sis). The process of producing caries; the mechanism of caries production.

cariogenic (ka'rē-ō-jen'ik). Producing caries; usually said of diets.

cariogenicity (ka'rē-ō-jĕ-nis'i-tē). Potential for caries production.

cariology (ka-rē-ol'ō-jē). The study of dental caries and cariogenesis.

cariostatic (kār-ē-ō-stat'ik). Exerting an inhibitory action upon the progress of dental caries.

carious (kār'ē-ŭs). Relating to or affected with caries.

carisoprodate (kar'i-sō-prō'dāt). Carisoprodol.

carisoprodol (kar'i-sō-prō'dol). Carisoprodate; isobamate; isopropyl meprobamate; *N*-isopropyl-2-methyl-2-propyl-1,2-propanediol dicarbamate; a skeletal muscle relaxant, chemically related to meprobamate.

carissin (ka-ris'sin). A glucoside obtained from *Carissa ovata stolonifera* of Australia; a powerful cardiac poison.

Carlen's tube. See under tube.

carmalum (kar-mal'ŭm). A 1% solution of carmine in 10% alum water, used as a stain in histology.

Carmichael, John P., U.S. dentist, 1856–1946. See C. *crown.*

carminate (kar'mi-nāt). A red salt of carminic acid.

carminative (kar-min'ă-tiv) [L. *carmino,* pp. *-atus,* to card wool; special Mod. L. usage, to expel wind]. **1.** Preventing the formation or causing the expulsion of flatus. **2.** An agent that relieves flatulence.

carmine (kar'min, kar'mēn) [Mediev. L. *carminus,* contr. fr. *carmisinus,* fr. Ar. *qirmizē,* the cochineal insect] [C.I. 75470]. Red coloring matter produced from coccinellin derived from cochineal; treatment of coccinellin with alum forms an aluminum lake of carminic acid, the essential constituent of c.
Schneider's c., a stain consisting of a 10% solution of c. in 45% acetic acid, used for fresh chromosome preparations.

carminic acid (kar-min'ik). A glucoside of an anthracenequinone carboxylic acid; the essential constituent of carmine.

carminophil, carminophile, carminophilous (kar-min'ō-fil, -fīl, kar-mi-nof'i-lŭs) [G. *phileō,* to love]. Staining readily with carmine dyes.

Carmody, Thomas Edward, U.S. oral surgeon, *1875. See C.-Batson *operation.*

carmustine (kar-mŭs'tēn). 1,3-Bis(2-chloroethyl)-1-nitrosourea; BCNU; an antineoplastic agent.

carnassial (kar-nas'ē-ăl). Adapted for shearing flesh; denoting those teeth designed to cut flesh.

carneous (kar'nē-ŭs) [L. *carneus*]. Fleshy.

carnes (kar'nēz) [L.]. Plural of caro.

Carnett's sign. See under sign.

carnification (kar′ni-fi-kā′shŭn) [L. *caro (carn-),* flesh, + *facio,* to make]. A change in tissues, whereby they become fleshy, resembling muscular tissue.

carnitine (kar′ni-tēn). Vitamin B_T; B_T factor; L-3-hydroxy-4-(trimethylammonium)butyrate; a trimethylammonium (betaine) derivative of γ-amino-β-hydroxybutyric acid, formed from N^{ϵ}-trimethyllysine and from γ-butyrobetaine; a thyroid inhibitor found in muscle, liver, and meat extracts; c. is an acyl carrier with respect to the mitochondrial membrane; it thus stimulates fatty acid oxidation and synthesis.

Carnivora (kar-niv′ō-ră) [L. *carnivorus,* fr. *caro (carn-),* flesh, + *voro,* to devour]. An order of chiefly flesh-eating mammals that includes the cats, dogs, bears, civets, minks, and hyenas, as well as the raccoon and panda; some species are omnivorous or herbivorous.

carnivore (kar′ni-vōr). One of the *Carnivora.*

carnivorous (kar-niv′ō-rŭs). Zoophagous; flesh-eating; subsisting on animals as food.

carnosine (kar′nō-sēn). Inhibitine; ignotine; *N*- β-alanyl-L-histidine; the dominant nonprotein nitrogenous component of brain tissue, first found in muscle.

carnosity (kar-nos′i-tē). **1.** Fleshiness. **2.** A fleshy protuberance.

Carnoy, Jean Baptiste, French biologist, 1836–1899. See C.'s *fixative.*

caro, gen. **carnis,** pl. **carnes** (kā′rō, kar′nis, -nes) [L.]. The fleshy parts of the body; muscular and fatty tissues.
c. quadra′ta syl′vii, *musculus* quadratus plantae.

carob flour (kar′ob). Algaroba.

Caroli, J., 20th century French physician. See C.'s *disease.*

carotenase (kar′-ō-ten-ās). β-Carotene 15,15′-dioxygenase.

carotene (kar′ō-tēn). Carotin; a class of carotenoids, yellow-red pigments (lipochromes) widely distributed in plants and animals, notably in carrots, and closely related in structure to the xanthophylls and lycopenes and to the open chain squalene; of particular interest in that they include precursors of the vitamins A (provitamin A carotenoids). Chemically, they consist of 8 isoprene units in a symmetrical chain with the 2 isoprenes at each end cyclized into α-carotene and β-carotene (γ-carotene has only one end cyclized). The cyclic ends of β-carotene are identical β-ionine-like structures; thus, on oxidative fission, β-carotene yields 2 molecules of vitamin A. The cyclic ends of α-carotene differ: one is an α-ionone, the other a β-ionone; on fission, α-carotene, like γ-carotene, yields 1 molecule of vitamin A (β-ionone derivative).

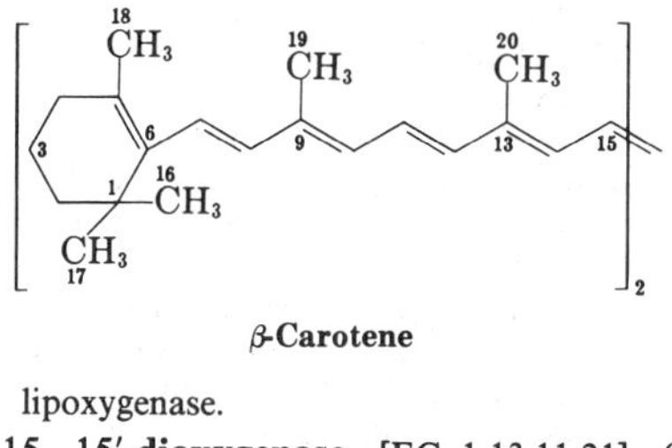

β-Carotene

c. oxidase, lipoxygenase.

β-carotene 15, 15′-dioxygenase [EC 1.13.11.21]. β-Carotene cleavage enzyme; carotenase; carotinase; an enzyme converting β-carotene to retinaldehyde, adding O_2.

carotenemia (kar′ō-te-nē′mē-ă). Carotinemia; xanthemia; carotene in the blood, especially pertaining to increased quantities, which sometimes cause a pale yellow-red pigmentation of the skin that may resemble icterus.

carotenoid (ka-rot′e-noyd). Carotinoid. **1.** Resembling carotene; having a yellow color. **2.** One of the carotenoids.

carotenoids (ka-rot′e-noydz). Generic term for a class of carotenes and their oxygenated derivates (xanthophylls) consisting of 8 isoprenoid units joined so that the orientation of these units is reversed at the center, placing the two central methyl groups in a 1,6 relationship in contrast to the 1,5 of the others. All c. may be formally derived from the acyclic $C_{40}H_{56}$ structure (part *IA* of the accompanying group of structures) with its long central chain of conjugated double bonds by hydrogenation, dehydrogenation, oxidation, cyclization, or combinations of these. Included as c. are some compounds arising from certain rearrangements or degradations of the carbon skeleton (structure *IB*), but not retinol and related C_{20} compounds. The nine-carbon end-groups may be acyclic with 1,2 and 5,6 double bonds (as in structure I*A*) or cyclohexanes with a single double bond at 5,6 or 5,4, or cyclopentanes or aryl groups; these are now designated by Greek letter prefixes (illustrated in part II of the accompanying group of structures) preceding "carotene" (α and δ, which are used in the trivial names α-carotene and δ-carotene, are not used for that reason). Suffixes (-oic acid, -oate, -al, -one, -ol) indicate certain oxygen-containing groups (acid, ester, aldehyde, ketone, alcohol); all other substitutions appear as prefixes (alkoxy-, epoxy-, hydro-, etc.). The configuration about all double bonds is *trans* unless *cis* and locant numbers appear. The prefix *retro-* is used to indicate a shift of one position of all single and double bonds; *apo-* indicates shortening of the molecule. See fig. on p. 252.

carotenosis cutis (kar-ō-te-nō′sis kyū′tis). Aurantiasis or carotinosis cutis; yellow coloration of the skin caused by an increase in carotene content.

carotic (kă-rot′ik) [G. *karōtikos,* stupefying]. **1.** Carotid. **2.** Stuporous.

caroticotympanic (ka-rot′i-kō-tim-pan′ik). Relating to the carotid canal and the tympanum.

carotid (ka-rot′id) [G. *karōtides,* the carotid arteries, fr. *karoō,* to put to sleep (because compression of the c. artery results in unconsciousness)]. Carotic (1); pertaining to any c. structure.

carotidynia (kă-rot′i-din′ē-ă). Carotodynia.

carotin (kar′ō-tin). Carotene.

carotinase (kar′ō-ti-nās). β-Carotene 15,15′-dioxygenase.

carotinemia (kar′ō-ti-nē′mē-ă). Carotenemia.

carotinoid (ka-rot′i-noyd). Carotenoid.

carotinosis cutis (ka-rot-i-nō′sis kyū′tis). *Carotenosis* cutis.

carotodynia (kă-rot′ō-din′ē-ă) [G. *odynē,* pain]. Carotidynia; pain caused by pressure on the carotid artery.

carpal (kar′păl). Relating to the carpus.

carpectomy (kar-pek′tō-mē) [G. *karpos,* wrist, + *ektomē,* excision]. Exsection of a portion or all of the carpus.

Carpenter, Charles C.J., U.S. immunologist, *1931. See C.'s *syndrome.*

Carpenter, George, British physician, 1859–1910. See C.'s *syndrome.*

carphenazine maleate (kar-fen′ă-zēn). 1{10-(3-[4-(2-Hydroxyethyl)-1-piperazinyl]propyl)phenothiazine-2-yl}-1-propanone bis-(hydrogen maleate); a phenothiazine tranquilizer of the piperazine group. Functionally classified as an antipsychotic agent, it is used in the treatment of chronic and acute schizophrenia; also possesses antiemetic, adrenolytic, anticholinergic, and dopamine-blocking actions.

carphologia, carphology (kar-fō-lō′jē-ă, -fol′ō-jē) [G. *karphologein*]. Floccillation.

carpitis (kar-pī′tis). Carpal arthritis in the horse and other animals.

carpocarpal (kar-pō-kar′păl). Mediocarpal (2).

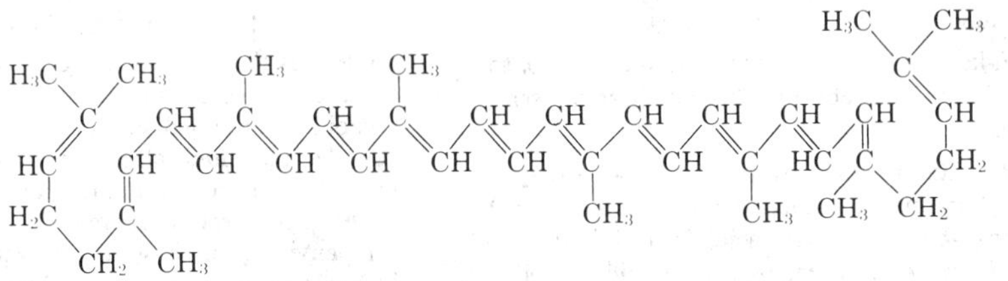

IA. Acyclic structures from which carotenoids are derived.

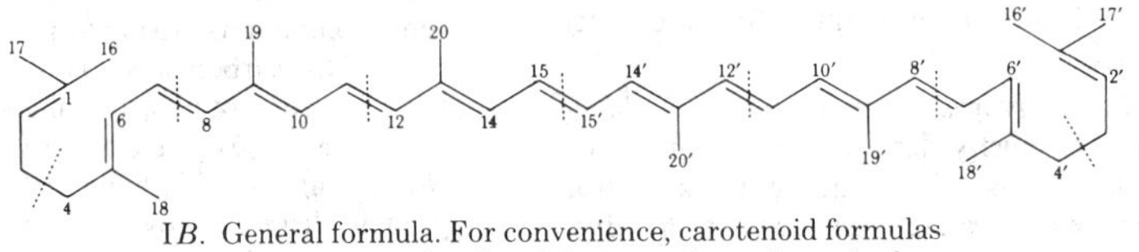

IB. General formula. For convenience, carotenoid formulas are often written in shorthand form as shown here; broken lines indicate formal division into isoprenoid units; numbering system is shown.

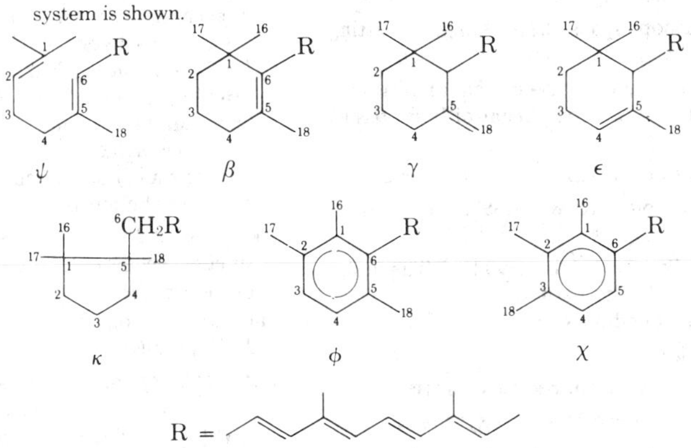

II. Designations of Greek letter prefixes

Carotenoids

Carpoglyptus (kar-pō-glip'tŭs) [G. *karpos,* fruit, + *glyphō,* , to carve]. A genus of mites including *C. passularum,* the fruit mite, which causes a dermatitis among handlers of dried fruit.

carpometacarpal (kar'pō-met-ă-kar'păl). Relating to both carpus and metacarpus.

carpopedal (kar'pō-ped'ăl) [G. *karpos,* wrist, + L. *pes (ped-),* foot]. Relating to the wrist and the foot, or the hands and feet; denoting especially c. spasm.

carpoptosis, carpoptosia (kar-pop-tō'sis, -tō'zē-ă) [G. *karpos,* wrist, + *ptōsis,* a falling]. Wrist-drop.

Carpue, Joseph C., British surgeon, 1764–1846. See C.'s *method.*

carpus, gen. and pl. **carpi** (kar'pŭs, kar'pī) [Mod. L. fr. Gr. *karpos*] [NA]. **1.** Wrist; the proximal segment of the hand consisting of the carpal bones and the associated soft parts. **2.** The ossa carpi, which articulate proximally with the radius and indirectly with the ulna, and distally with the five metacarpal bones; in domestic mammals, the bones of the proximal row are called radial, intermediate, ulnar, and accessory, while those of the distal row are termed first, second, third, and fourth carpal bones.
c. cur'vus, Madelung's *deformity.*

Carr, Francis H., British chemist, *1874. See C.-Price *reaction.*

carrageen, carragheen (kar'ă-jēn, -gēn). Chondrus (2).

carrageenan, carrageenin (kar-ă-gē'nan, -nin). A polysaccharide obtained from Irish moss; a galactosan sulfate resembling agar in molecular structure.

carre-four sensitif (kar-fūr'son-sē-tēf') [Fr. sensory crossroads]. A term given by Charcot to the posterior portion of the caudal limb of the internal capsule.

Carrel, Alexis, French-American surgeon in the U.S. and Nobel laureate, 1873–1944. See C.'s *treatment;* C.-Lindbergh *pump;* Dakin-C. *treatment.*

carrier (ka'rē-er). **1.** An individual with an asymptomatic infection that can be transmitted to other susceptible individuals. **2.** Any chemical capable of accepting an atom, radical, or subatomic particle from one compound, then passing it to another; *e.g.,* cytochromes are electron c.'s, homocysteine is a methyl c. **3.** A substance which, by having chemical properties closely related to or indistinguishable from those of a radioactive tracer, is thus able to carry the tracer through a precipitation or similar chemical procedure; the best c.'s are the nonradioactive isotopes of the tracer in question. See also tag.
amalgam c., an instrument used to transport triturated amalgam to a cavity preparation and to deposit it therein.
convalescent c., an individual who is clinically recovered from an infectious disease but is still capable of transmitting the infectious agent to others.
genetic c., an unaffected heterozygote bearing a usually harmful recessive gene.
hydrogen c., hydrogen acceptor; a molecule that, in conjunction with a tissue enzyme system, carries hydrogen from one metabolite (oxidant) to another (reductant) or to molecular oxygen to form H_2O.
incubatory c., an individual capable of transmitting an infectious

agent to others during the incubation period of the disease.
manifesting c., manifesting *heterozygote.*
translocation c., a person with balanced translocation.

Carrión, Daniel A., Peruvian medical student, 1859–1885, who inoculated himself with a disease later designated as C.'s *disease,* and died thereof.

Carswell, Sir Robert, British physician, 1793–1857. See C.'s *grapes.*

Carteaud, Alexandre, French physician, *1897. See Gougerot-C. *syndrome.*

Carter, Henry V., Anglo-Indian physician, 1831–1897. See C.'s *fever,* black *mycetoma.*

cartesian (kar-tē'zhŭn). Relating to Cartesius, Latinized form of Descartes.

carthamus (kar'tha-mŭs) [Ar. *qurtum,* fr. *qartama,* paint; the plant yields a dye]. Safflower; the dried florets of *Carthamus tinctorius* (family Compositae). See also safflower oil.

CARTILAGE

cartilage (kar'ti-lij) [L. *cartilago (cartilagin-),* gristle]. Gristle; chondrus (1); a connective tissue characterized by its nonvascularity and firm consistency; consists of cells (chondrocytes), an interstitial matrix of fibers (collagen), and a ground substance (proteoglycans). There are three kinds of c.: hyaline c., elastic c., and fibrocartilage. For a gross anatomical description, see cartilago and subentries.
accessory c., a sesamoid c.
accessory nasal c.'s, *cartilagines* nasales accessoriae.
accessory quadrate c., *cartilagines* alares minores.
c. of acoustic meatus, *cartilago* meatus acustici.
alisphenoid c., the c. in the embryo from which the greater wing of the sphenoid bone is developed.
annular c., *cartilago* cricoidea.
arthrodial c., *cartilago* articularis.
articular c., *cartilago* articularis.
arytenoid c., *cartilago* arytenoidea.
auditory c., auditory *capsule.*
c. of auditory tube, *cartilago* tubae auditivae.
auricular c., *cartilago* auriculae.
basilar c., fibrocartilago basalis; the c. filling the foramen lacerum.
branchial c.'s, c.'s developing within the vertebrate or embryonic branchial arches; they form the viscerocranium.
calcified c., c. in which calcium salts are deposited in the matrix; it occurs prior to replacement by osseous tissue and sometimes in aging c.
cellular c., an embryonic or immature stage of c. in which it consists chiefly of cells with very little matrix.
ciliary c., incorrect term sometimes applied to the tarsus inferior and tarsus superior. See tarsus (2).
circumferential c., **(1)** *labrum* acetabulare; **(2)** *labrum* glenoidale.
conchal c., *cartilago* auriculae.
connecting c., interosseous or uniting c.; the c. in a cartilaginous joint such as the symphysis pubis.
corniculate c., *cartilago* corniculata.
costal c., *cartilago* costalis.
cricoid c., *cartilago* cricoidea.
cuneiform c., *cartilago* cuneiformis.
diarthrodial c., *cartilago* articularis.
c. of ear, *cartilago* auriculae.
elastic c., yellow c.; a c. in which the cells are surrounded by a territorial capsular matrix outside of which is an interterritorial matrix containing elastic fiber networks in addition to the collagen fibers and ground substance.
ensiform c., ensisternum c., *processus* xiphoideus.
epiglottic c., *cartilago* epiglottica.
epiphysial c., *cartilago* epiphysialis.
falciform c., *meniscus* medialis.
floating c., loose c.; a loose piece of c. within a joint cavity, detached from the articular c. or from a meniscus.
greater alar c., *cartilago* alaris major.
Huschke's c.'s, two horizontal cartilaginous rods at the edge of the cartilaginous septum of the nose.
hyaline c., c. having a frosted glass appearance, with interstitial substance containing fine collagenous fibers obscured by the ground substance; in adult c., the cells are present in isogenous groups.
hypsiloid c., Y c.
innominate c., *cartilago* cricoidea.
interosseous c., connecting c.
intervertebral c., *discus* intervertebralis.
intra-articular c., *discus* articularis.
intrathyroid c., a narrow slip of c. sometimes found joining the laminae of the thyroid c. of the larynx in infancy.
investing c., *cartilago* articularis.
Jacobson's c., *cartilago* vomeronasalis.
c.'s of larynx, *cartilagines* laryngis.
lateral c., cartilaginous plates that extend above the hoof from the caudal angles of the distal phalanx of the horse; they are readily palpated under the skin of the sides of the hoof and assist in distributing the animal's weight during locomotion.
lateral c. of nose, *cartilago* nasi lateralis.
lesser alar c.'s, *cartilagines* alares minores.
loose c., floating c.
Luschka's c., a small cartilaginous nodule sometimes found in the anterior portion of the vocal cord.
mandibular c., Meckel's c.; a c. bar in the mandibular arch that forms a temporary supporting structure in the embryonic mandible; the cartilaginous primordium of the malleus and incus develop from its proximal end.
meatal c., *cartilago* meatus acustici.
Meckel's c., mandibular c.
Meyer's c.'s, the anterior sesamoid c.'s at the anterior attachments of the vocal ligaments.
Morgagni's c., *cartilago* cuneiformis.
c. of nasal septum, *cartilago* septi nasi.
orbitosphenoid c., the embryonic c. that develops on the side of the cartilaginous neurocranium into the lesser wing of the sphenoid bone.
parachordal c., c. primordia adjacent on either side to the cephalic portion of the notochord in young embryos; they represent an initial step in the formation of the chondrocranium.
paraseptal c., *cartilago* vomeronasalis.
periotic c., a cartilaginous mass on either side of the chondrocranium surrounding the developing auditory vesicle in the fetus; the otic capsule in its early cartilaginous stage.
permanent c., c. that is not replaced by bone.
c. of pharyngotympanic tube, *cartilago* tubae auditivae.
precursory c., temporary c.
primordial c., c. in an early stage in its development.
quadrangular c., *cartilago* septi nasi.
Reichert's c., a c. in the mesenchyme of the second branchial arch in the embryo, from which develop the stapes, the styloid processes, the stylohyoid ligaments, and the lesser cornua of the hyoid bone.
reticular c., retiform c., rarely used terms for fibrocartilage.
Santorini's c., *cartilago* corniculata.
secondary c., c., such as that in certain joints, which undergoes a

direct transformation into bone.
Seiler's c., a small rod of c. attached to the vocal process of the arytenoid c.
semilunar c., one of the articular menisci of the knee joint. See *meniscus* lateralis; *meniscus* medialis.
septal c., *cartilago* septi nasi.
sesamoid c. of larynx, *cartilago* sesamoidea laryngis.
sesamoid c.'s of nose, *cartilagines* nasales accessoriae.
slipping rib c., subluxation of rib c., at the costo-chondral junction, causing pain and audible click.
sternal c., a costal c. of one of the true ribs.
supra-arytenoid c., *cartilago* corniculata.
tarsal c., incorrect term sometimes applied to the tarsus inferior and tarsus superior. See tarsus (2).
temporary c., precursory c.; a c. that is normally replaced by bone, to form a part of the skeleton.
thyroid c., *cartilago* thyroidea.
tracheal c.'s, *cartilagines* tracheales.
triangular c., *discus* articularis radioulnaris.
triquetrous c., **(1)** *discus* articularis radioulnaris; **(2)** *cartilago* arytenoidea.
tubal c., *cartilago* tubae auditivae.
uniting c., connecting c.
vomerine c., vomeronasal c., *cartilago* vomeronasalis.
Weitbrecht's c., *discus* articularis acromioclavicularis.
Wrisberg's c., *cartilago* cuneiformis.
xiphoid c., *processus* xiphoideus.
Y c., Y-shaped c., hypsiloid c.; the connecting c. for the ilium, ischium, and pubis; it extends through the acetabulum.
yellow c., elastic c.

---

cartilagines (kar-ti-laj'i-nēz). Plural of cartilago.

cartilaginoid (kar-ti-laj'i-noyd). Chondroid (1).

cartilaginous (kar-ti-laj'i-nŭs). Chondral; relating to or consisting of cartilage.

cartilago, pl. **cartilagines** (kar-ti-lā'gō, -laj'i-nēs) [L. gristle] [NA]. Nonvascular, resiliant, elastic connective tissue found primarily in joints, the walls of the thorax, and tubular structures such as the larynx, air passages, and ears; comprises most of the skeleton in early fetal life, but is slowly replaced by bone. For a histological description, see cartilage.
c. ala'ris ma'jor [NA], greater alar cartilage; one of a pair of cartilages that form the tip of the nose. It consists of a medial crus that extends into the nasal septum with its fellow of the opposite side, and a lateral crus that forms the anterior part of the wing of the nose.
cartila'gines ala'res mino'res [NA], lesser alar cartilages; accessory quadrate cartilage; the two to four cartilaginous plates of the wing of the nose posterior to the greater alar cartilage.
c. articula'ris [NA], articular cartilage; arthrodial, diarthrodial, or investing cartilage; the cartilage covering the articular surfaces of the bones forming a synovial joint.
c. arytenoi'dea [NA], arytenoid cartilage; triquetrous cartilage (2); one of a pair of small pyramidal laryngeal cartilages that articulate with the lamina of the cricoid cartilage. It gives attachment to the posterior part of the corresponding vocal ligament and to several muscles. The base of the cartilage is hyaline but the apex is elastic.
c. auric'ulae [NA], cartilage of ear; auricular or conchal cartilage; the cartilage of the auricle.
c. cornicula'ta [NA], corniculate cartilage; supra-arytenoid cartilage; corniculum laryngis; Santorini's cartilage; a conical nodule of elastic cartilage surmounting the apex of each arytenoid cartilage.
c. costa'lis [NA], costal cartilage; costicartilage; the cartilage forming the anterior continuation of a rib.
c. cricoi'dea [NA], cricoid, annular, or innominate cartilage; the lowermost of the laryngeal cartilages; it is shaped like a seal-ring, being expanded into a nearly quadrilateral plate (lamina) posteriorly; the anterior portion is called the arch (arcus).
c. cuneifor'mis [NA], cuneiform cartilage; Morgagni's cartilage or tubercle; Wrisberg's cartilage; a small rod of elastic cartilage in the aryepiglottic fold above the corniculate cartilage.
c. epiglot'tica [NA], epiglottic cartilage; a thin lamina of elastic cartilage forming the central portion of the epiglottis.
c. epiphysia'lis [NA], epiphysial cartilage or plate; the disk of cartilage between the shaft and the epiphysis of a long bone during its growth.
cartila'gines laryn'gis [NA], cartilages of larynx. See specifically c. thyroidea, cricoidea, arytenoidea, cuneiformis, triticea, corniculata, sesamoidea laryngis, and epiglottis.
c. mea'tus acus'tici [NA], cartilage of acoustic meatus; meatal cartilage; the cartilage that forms the wall of the lateral part of the external acoustic meatus. It is incomplete above and is firmly attached to the margins of the bony part of the external meatus.
cartila'gines nasa'les accessor'iae [NA], accessory nasal cartilages; sesamoid cartilages of nose; variable small plates of cartilage located in the interval between the greater alar and lateral nasal cartilages.
cartila'gines na'si [NA], the cartilages of nose. See specifically c. nasi lateralis, alaris major, septi nasi, vomeronasalis; cartilagines alares minores, nasales accessoriae.
c. na'si latera'lis [NA], lateral cartilage of nose; the cartilage located in the lateral wall of the nose above the alar cartilage.
c. sep'ti na'si [NA], cartilage of nasal septum; quadrangular or septal cartilage; pars cartilaginea septi nasi; cartilaginous septum; a thin cartilaginous plate located between vomer, perpendicular plate of the ethmoid, and nasal bones, and completing the nasal septum anteriorly.
c. sesamoi'dea laryn'gis [NA], sesamoid cartilage of larynx; a small nodule of elastic cartilage sometimes present on the lateral border of the arytenoid cartilage.
c. thyroid'ea [NA], thyroid cartilage; the largest of the cartilages of the larynx; it is formed of two approximately quadrilateral plates (*laminae*) joined anteriorly at an angle of from 90° to 120°, the prominence so formed constituting the laryngeal prominence (Adam's apple).
cartila'gines trachea'les [NA], tracheal cartilages; tracheal ring; the 16 to 20 incomplete rings of hyaline cartilage forming the skeleton of the trachea; the rings are deficient posteriorly for from one-fifth to one-third of their circumference.
c. tritic'ea [L. *triticum*, wheat] [NA], corpus triticeum; triticeum; a rounded nodule of cartilage, the size of a grain of wheat, occasionally present in the posterior margin of the lateral hyothyroid ligament.
c. tu'bae auditi'vae [NA], cartilage of auditory tube or of pharyngotympanic tube; tubal cartilage; the trough-shaped cartilage that forms the medial wall, roof, and part of the lateral wall of the auditory tube.
c. vomeronasa'lis [NA], vomeronasal, vomerine, paraseptal, or Jacobson's cartilage; vomer cartilagineus; a narrow strip of cartilage located between the lower edge of the cartilage of the nasal septum and the vomer.

carubinose (kă-rū'bin-ōs). Mannose.

caruncle (kar'ŭng-kl). Caruncula.
Morgagni's c., *lobus* medius prostatae.
Santorini's major c., *papilla* duodeni major.
Santorini's minor c., *papilla* duodeni minor.
urethral c., a small, fleshy, sometimes painful protrusion of the mucous membrane, usually occurring at the meatus of the female urethra; it may be telangiectatic, papillomatous, or composed of granulation tissue.

caruncula, pl. **carunculae** (kă-rŭng'kyū-lă, -lē) [L. a small fleshy mass, fr. *caro,* flesh]. Caruncle. **1** [NA]. A small, fleshy protuberance, or any structure suggesting such a shape. **2.** In ungulates, one of about 200 specific disklike areas of the uterine endometrium that, in conjunction with the fetal cotyledon, forms a placentome of the placenta; as a site of fetal-maternal contact, the c. remains constant in position but enlarges greatly in size during pregnancy.

c. hymena'lis, pl. **carun'culae hymena'les** [NA], c. myrtiformis; one of the numerous tabs or projections surrounding the orifice of the vagina after rupture of the hymen.

c. lacrima'lis [NA], a small reddish body at the medial angle of the eye, containing modified sebaceous and sweat glands.

c. myrtifor'mis, pl. **carun'culae myrtifor'mes,** c. hymenalis.

c. saliva'ris, c. sublingualis.

c. sublingua'lis [NA], c. salivaris; a papilla on each side of the frenulum linguae marking the opening of the submandibular (Wharton's) duct.

Carus, Karl G., German anatomist and zoologist, 1789–1869. See C.'s *circle, curve.*

carvacrol (kar'vă-krol). 2-*p*-Cymenol; an isomer of thymol that occurs in several volatile oils (marjoram, origanum, savory, and thyme), with properties and activity that closely resemble those of thymol; has antiseptic properties, but is used chiefly as a perfume.

Carvallo's sign. See under sign.

carver (kar'ver). A dental hand instrument, available in a wide variety of end shapes, used for forming and contouring wax, filling materials, etc.

caryo- [G. *karyon,* nut, kernel]. For words beginning thus and not found here, see karyo-.

caryophyllus, caryophyllum (kar'ē-ō-fĭ'lŭs, -ŭm) [G. *karyophyllon,* clove tree, fr. *karyon,* nut, + *phyllon,* leaf]. Clove.

caryotheca (kar'ē-ō-thē'kă) [caryo- + G. *thēkē,* sheath, box]. Nuclear *envelope.*

Casal, Gasper, Spanish physician, 1691–1759. See C.'s *necklace.*

casamino acids (kās'ă-mē'nō). Trivial term for the mixture of amino acids derived by hydrolysis of casein; used in bacterial and similar growth media.

cascade (kas-kād') [Fr., fr. It. *cascare,* to fall]. **1.** A series of sequential interactions, as of a physiological process, which once initiated continues to the final one; each interaction is activated by the preceding one, sometimes with cumulative effect. **2.** To spill over, especially rapidly.

cascara (kas-kar'ă). C. sagrada.

c. amara, Honduras bark; the dried bark of a species of *Picramnia* (family Simarubaceae); used as a bitter tonic.

c. sagrada, cascara; the dried bark of *Rhamnus purshiana* (family Rhamnaceae); used as a laxative.

case (kās) [L. *casus,* an occurrence]. **1.** An instance of disease with its attendant circumstances. *Cf.* patient. **2.** A box or container.

index c., proband.

trial c., in refraction, a box containing lenses for testing.

caseation (kā-sē-ā'shŭn) [L. *caseus,* cheese]. Tyrosis (2); a form of coagulation necrosis in which the necrotic tissue resembles cheese and contains a mixture of protein and fat that is absorbed very slowly; occurs particularly in tuberculosis. See also caseous *necrosis.*

casein (cā'sē-in, kā'sēn). The principal protein of cow's milk and the chief constituent of cheese. It is insoluble in water, soluble in dilute alkaline and salt solutions, forms a hard insoluble plastic with formaldehyde, and is used as a constituent of some glues; various components are designated α-, β-, and κ-caseins.

c. iodine, iodinated c., caseo-iodine; a compound of c. with iodine formed by incubating the protein with the element, which becomes attached to tyrosine groups in the protein.

plant c., avenin.

caseinate (kā'sē-in-āt). A salt of casein.

caseinogen (kā-sē-in'ō-jen). "Soluble" or κ-casein which, when acted upon by rennin, is converted into paracasein.

caseo-iodine (kā'sē-ō-i'ō-dīn). *Casein* iodine.

caseose (kā'sē-ōs). Nondescript term for product resulting from the hydrolysis or digestion of casein.

caseous (kā'sē-ŭs). Pertaining to or manifesting the gross and microscopic features of tissue affected by caseation.

Caslick, Edward, 20th century U.S. veterinarian. See C.'s *operation.*

Casoni, Tommaro, Italian physician, 1880–1933. See C. intradermal *test,* skin *test.*

cassava starch (kă-sah'vah). Tapioca.

Casselberry, William E., U.S. laryngologist, 1858–1916. See C. *position.*

Casser (Casserio), Giulio, Italian anatomist, 1556–1616. See C.'s *fontanelle,* perforated *muscle.*

casserian (ka-sē'rē-an). Relating to or described by Casser.

cassette (kă-set') [Fr., dim. of *casse,* box]. **1.** A plate or film holder for use in photography and roentgenography. **2.** A perforated holder in which tissue blocks are placed for paraffin embedding.

cassia bark (kash'yă). Cinnamon.

cassia fistula. Purging c.; the dried ripe fruit of *Cassia fistula,* used as a laxative.

cassia oil. Cinnamon oil.

cast (kast). **1.** An object formed by the solidification of a liquid poured into a mold. **2.** Rigid encasement of a part, as with plaster or a plastic, for purposes of immobilization. **3.** An elongated or cylindrical mold formed in a tubular structure (*e.g.,* renal tubule, bronchiole) that may be observed in histologic sections or in material such as urine or sputum; results from inspissation of fluid material secreted or excreted in the tubular structures. **4.** Restraint of a large animal, usually a horse, with ropes and harnesses in a recumbent position. **5.** In dentistry, a positive reproduction of the form of the tissues of the upper or lower jaw, which is made by the solidification of plaster, metal, etc., poured into an impression, and over which denture bases or other dental restorations may be fabricated.

blood c., a c. usually formed in renal tubules, but may occur in bronchioles; consists of inspissated material that includes various elements of blood (*i.e.,* erythrocytes, leukocytes, fibrin, and so on), resulting from bleeding into the glomerulus or tubule, or into the alveolus or bronchiole.

coma c., Külz's cylinder; a renal c. of strongly refracting granules said to be indicative of imminent coma in diabetes.

decidual c., a mold of the interior of the uterus formed of the exfoliated mucous membrane in cases of extrauterine gestation.

dental c., a positive likeness of a part or parts of the oral cavity.

diagnostic c., a positive replica of the form of the teeth and tissues made from an impression.

epithelial c., a c. that contains epithelial cells and their remnants; occurs most frequently in renal tubules and urine.

false c., mucous or spurious c.; cylindroid; pseudocast; an elongated, ribbon-like mucous thread with poorly defined edges and pointed or split ends, often confused with a true urinary c.

fatty c., a renal or urinary c. consisting largely of fat globules; those containing doubly refractile bodies (composed of cholesterol) are found in the nephrotic syndrome.

fibrinous c., a yellow c. that somewhat resembles a waxy c.; more likely to occur in the urine of certain patients with acute nephritis.

granular c., a relatively dark, dense c. of coarsely or finely particulate cellular debris and other proteinaceous material. See also waxy c.

hair c., pseudonit; a c. composed of parakeratotic scales attached to scalp hair but freely movable up and down the hair shaft; found in scaling dermatitis of the scalp, including pityriasis capitis, psoriasis, and seborrheic dermatitis.

halo c., a c. applied to the shoulders in which metal bars are set that extend over the head to a halo, from which traction may be applied to the head by means of tongs or a halter.

hyaline c., a relatively transparent renal c. composed of proteinaceous material derived from disintegration of cells. See also waxy c.

investment c., refractory c.

master c., a replica of the prepared tooth surfaces, residual ridge areas, and/or other parts of the dental arch as reproduced from an impression.

mucous c., false c.

refractory c., investment c.; a c. made of material that will withstand the high temperatures of casting or soldering without disintegrating.

renal c., tube c.; any type of c. formed in a renal tubule, and found in the urine consisting of various materials, *e.g.*, albumin, cells, blood.

spurious c., false c.

tube c., renal c.

urinary c.'s, c.'s discharged in the urine.

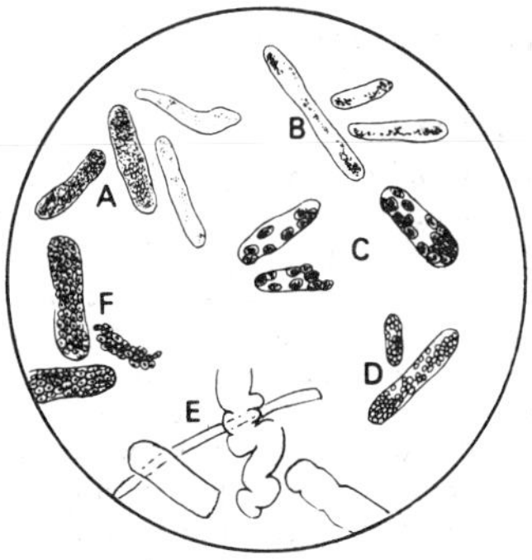

Urinary Casts

A, coarsely and finely granular casts; *B*, hyaline casts; *C*, leukocyte casts; *D*, erythrocyte casts; *E*, waxy casts; *F*, epithelial casts.

waxy c., a form of renal c. consisting of homogeneous proteinaceous material that has a high refractive index, in contrast to the low refractive index of hyaline c.'s; waxy c.'s probably represent an advanced stage of the disintegrative process that results in coarsely and finely granular c.'s, and are usually indicative of oliguria or anuria.

cast brace (kast brās). A specially designed plaster cast incorporating hinges and other brace components; used in the treatment of fractures to promote early activity and early joint motion.

Castellani, Sir Aldo, Italian physician, 1878–1971. See C.'s *bronchitis, paint;* C.-Low *sign.*

casting (kas'ting). **1.** A metallic object formed in a mold. **2.** The act of forming a c. in a mold.

centrifugal c., c. molten metal into a mold by spinning the metal from a crucible at the end of a revolving arm.

ceramo-metal c., a c. made of alloys containing or excluding precious metals, to which dental porcelain can be fused.

gold c., a c. made of gold, usually formed to represent and replace lost tooth structure.

vacuum c., the c. of a metal in the presence of a vacuum.

Castle, William B., U.S. physician, *1897. See C.'s intrinsic *factor.*

Castleman, Benjamin, U.S. pathologist, 1906–1982. See C.'s *disease.*

castor bean (kas'ter bēn). *Ricinus.*

castor oil. A fixed oil expressed from the seeds of *Ricinus communis* (family Euphorbiaceae); a purgative.

aromatic c. oil, contains cinnamon oil 3, clove oil 1, vanillin 1, saccharin 0.5, alcohol 30, in c. oil to make 1000; a cathartic.

castrate (kas'trāt) [L. *castro,* pp. *-atus,* to deprive of generative power (male or female)]. To remove the testicles or the ovaries.

castration (kas-trā'shŭn) [see castrate]. **1.** Sterilization (1); removal of the testicles or ovaries. **2.** See castration *complex.*

functional c., gonadal atrophy produced by prolonged treatment with sex hormones.

casualty (kazh'ū-ăl-tē). An injury, or the victim of an accident.

CAT Abbreviation for computerized axial *tomography.*

cata- [G. *kata,* down]. Combining form meaning down. See also kata-.

catabasial (kat-ă-bā'sē-ăl) [cata- + Mod. L. *basion*]. Denoting a skull in which the basion is lower than the opisthion.

catabiotic (kat'ă-bī-ot'ik) [cata- + G. *biōtikos,* relating to life]. Used up in the carrying on of the vital processes other than growth, or in the performance of function, referring to the energy derived from food.

catabolic (kat-ă-bol'ik). Relating to or promoting catabolism.

catabolism (kă-tab'ō-lizm) [G. *katabolē,* a casting down]. The breaking down in the body of complex chemical compounds into simpler ones (*e.g.*, glycogen to CO_2 and H_2O), often accompanied by the liberation of energy. *Cf.* anabolism.

catabolite (kă-tab'ō-līt). Any product of catabolism.

catachronobiology (kat'ă-kron'ō-bī-ol'ō-jē) [cata- + G. *chronos,* time, + biology]. The study of the deleterious effects of time on a living system.

catacrotic (kat-ă-krot'ik). Denoting a pulse tracing in which the downstroke is interrupted by one or more upward waves.

catacrotism (kă-tak'rō-tizm) [cata- + G. *krotos,* beat]. A condition of the pulse in which there are one or more secondary expansions of the artery following the main beat, producing secondary upward waves on the downstroke of the pulse tracing.

catadicrotic (kat'ă-dī-krot'ik). Denoting a pulse tracing in which there are two minor elevations interrupting the downtake.

catadicrotism (kat-ă-dī'krō-tizm) [cata + G. *di-,* two, + *krotos,* beat]. A condition of the pulse marked by two minor expansions of the artery following the main beat, producing two secondary upward waves on the downstroke of the pulse tracing.

catadidymus (kat-ă-did'i-mŭs) [cata- + G. *didymus,* twin]. *Duplicitas* posterior.

catadioptric (kat-ă-dī-op'trik). Employing both reflecting and refractive optical systems.

catagen (kat'ă-jen). A regressing phase of the hair growth cycle during which cell proliferation ceases, the hair follicle shortens, and an anchored club hair is produced.

catagenesis (kat-ă-jen'ĕ-sis) [cata- + G. *genesis,* origin]. Involution.

catalase (kat'ă-lās) [EC 1.11.1.6]. A hemoprotein catalyzing the decomposition of hydrogen peroxide to water and oxygen.

catalepsy (kat'ă-lep-sē) [G. *katalēpsis,* a seizing, catalepsy, fr. *kata,* down, + *lēpsis,* a seizure]. Anochlesia (1); a morbid condition characterized by waxy rigidity of the limbs, which may be placed in various positions that are maintained for a time, lack of response to stimuli, slow pulse and respiration, and pale skin.

cataleptic (kat-ă-lep'tik). Relating to, or suffering from, catalepsy.

cataleptoid (kat-ă-lep'toyd). Simulating or resembling catalepsy.

catalogia (kat-ă-lō'jē-ă) [cata- + G. *logion,* declaration]. Verbigeration.

catalysis (kă-tal'i-sis) [G. *katalysis,* dissolution]. The effect that a catalyst exerts upon a chemical reaction.

contact c., a process wherein the catalyst is a solid and the catalyzed reaction is produced in gases making contact with the solid.

surface c., c. at the surface of a solid particle or a macromolecule.

catalyst (kat'ă-list). Catalyzer; a substance that accelerates a chemical reaction but is not consumed or changed permanently thereby.

inorganic c., a c. such as a finely divided metal (Pt, Rh), carbon, etc.

negative c., a c. that retards a reaction.

organic c., enzyme.

positive c., see c.

Raney c., Raney Nickel.

catalytic (kat-ă-lit'ik). Relating to or effecting catalysis.

catalyze (kat'ă-līz). To act as a catalyst.

catalyzer (kat'ă-līz-er). Catalyst.

catamenia (kat-ă-mē'nē-ă) [G. the menses, ntr. pl. of *katamēnios,* monthly, fr. *mēn,* month]. Menses.

catamenial (kat-ă-mē'nē-ăl). Menstrual.

catamenogenic (kat'ă-men-ō-jen'ik). Causing menstruation.

catamnesis (kat-am-nē'sis) [cata- + G *mnēmē,* memory]. The medical history of a patient after an illness; the follow-up history.

catamnestic (kat-am-nes'tik). Related to catamnesis.

catapasm (kat'ă-pazm) [G. *katapasma,* a powder; *katapassō,* to sprinkle over]. A dusting powder applied to raw surfaces or ulcers.

cataphasia (kat-ă-fā'zē-ă) [cata- + G. *phasis,* a saying]. A disorder of speech in which there is an involuntary repetition several times of the same word. See also echolalia.

cataphora (kă-taf'ō-ră) [G. a falling down]. Semicoma or somnolence interrupted by intervals of partial consciousness.

cataphoresis (kat'ă-fō-rē'sis) [cata- + G. *phorēsis,* a being carried]. Movement of positively charged particles (cations) in a solution or suspension toward the cathode in electrophoresis. *Cf.* anaphoresis.

cataphoretic (kat'ă-fō-ret'ik). Relating to cataphoresis.

cataphylaxis (kat'ă-fī-lak'sis) [cata- + G. *phylaxis,* protection]. Seldom used term designating a deterioration in the natural defense mechanisms by which the body resists infectious disease.

cataplasia, cataplasis (kat-ă-plā'sē-ă, plā'sis) [cata- + G. *plasis,* a molding]. Retrograde metamorphosis; retrogression; retromorphosis; a degenerative change in cells or tissues that is the reverse of the constructive or developmental change; a return to an earlier or embryonic stage.

cataplasm (kat'ă-plazm) [G. *kataplasma,* poultice, fr. *kataplassō,* to spread over]. Poultice.

cataplectic (kat-ă-plek'tik). **1.** Developing suddenly. **2.** Pertaining to cataplexy.

cataplexy (kat'ă-plek-sē) [cata- + G. *plēxis,* a blow, stroke]. A transient attack of extreme generalized muscular weakness, often precipitated by an emotional state such as laughing heartily.

CATARACT

cataract (kat'ă-rakt) [L. *cataracta,* fr. G. *katarrhakiēs,* a downrushing, a waterfall, fr. *kata- rrhēgnymi,* to break down, rush down]. Cataracta; loss of transparency of the lens of the eye, or of its capsule.

annular c., disk-shaped, life-belt, or umbilicated c.; congenital c. in which a central white membrane replaces the nucleus.

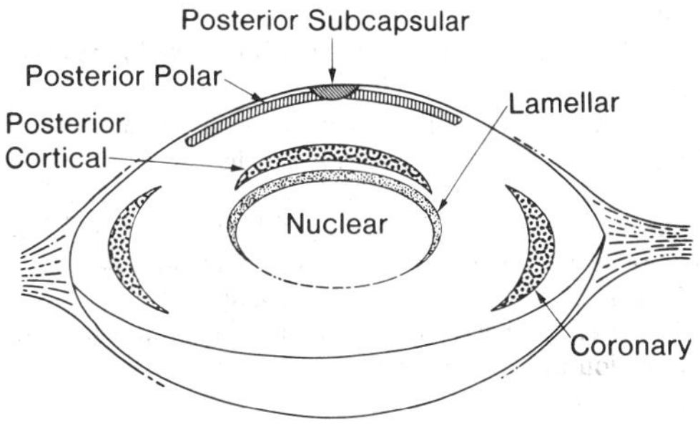

Cataracts

arborescent c., dendritic c.

atopic c., a c. associated with atopic dermatitis.

axial c., a lenticular opacity in the sagittal axis of the lens.

axillary c., a type of hereditary c. with opacities deep and central.

black c., cataracta brunescens; cataracta nigra; a c. in which the lens is hardened and of a dark brown color.

blue c., cataracta cerulea; coronary c. of bluish color.

capsular c., a c. in which the opacity affects the capsule only.

capsulolenticular c., a c. in which both the lens and its capsule are involved. See also membranous c.

central c., congenital c. limited to the embryonic nucleus.

complete c., mature c.

complicated c., secondary c. (1).

concussion c., traumatic c. occurring with or without a hole in the lens capsule.

congenital c., a c. present at birth; also seen as an autosomal recessive condition in calves of the Jersey breed.

copper c., *chalcosis* lentis.

coralliform c., congenital c. with round or elongated processes radiating from the center of the lens.

coronary c., peripheral cortical developmental c. occurring just after puberty; transmitted as a hereditary dominant characteristic.

cortical c., peripheral c.; a c. in which the opacity affects the cortex of the lens.

crystalline c., a hereditary c. with a coralliform or needle-shaped accumulation of crystals in the axial region of an otherwise clear lens.

cuneiform c., cortical c. in which the opacities radiate from the periphery like spokes of a wheel.

cupuliform c., saucer-shaped c.; a common form of senile c. often confined to a region just within the posterior capsule.

dendritic c., arborescent c.; a congenital sutural c. with complicated branching.

diabetic c., c. occurring in insulin-dependent diabetes mellitus.

disk-shaped c., annular c.

electric c., cataracta electrica; a c. caused by contact with a high-power electric current, or a lightning bolt.

embryonic c., a congenital c. situated near the anterior Y suture of the fetal lens nucleus.

fibroid c., fibrinous c., a sclerotic hardening of the capsule of the lens, following exudative iridocyclitis.

floriform c., a congenital c. with opacities arranged like the petals of a flower.

furnacemen's c., infrared c.

fusiform c., spindle c.

galactose c., a neonatal c. associated with intralenticular accumulation of galactose alcohol. See galactosemia.

glassworker's c., infrared c.

glaucomatous c., a nuclear opacity usually seen in absolute glaucoma.

gray c., a c. of gray color, usually seen in senile, mature, or cortical c.

hard c., nuclear c.
hook-shaped c., congenital c. with hook-like figures between the fetal and embryonic nuclei.
hypermature c., overripe c.; a c. in which the lens cortex becomes liquid, with the nucleus gravitating within the capsule (Morgagni's c.).
hypocalcemic c., a c. occurring with low serum calcium.
immature c., a stage of partial lens opacification.
infantile c., a c. affecting a very young child.
infrared c., furnacemen's or glassworker's c.; a c. secondary to absorption of heat by the lens, or by transmission from the adjacent iris.
intumescent c., a c. swollen because of fluid absorption.
juvenile c., a soft c. occurring in a child or young adult.
lamellar c., zonular c.; a c. in which the opacity is limited to the cortex.
life-belt c., annular c.
mature c., complete or ripe c.; a c. in which both the nucleus and cortex are opaque.
membranous c., a secondary c. composed of the remains of the thickened capsule and degenerated lens fibers.
Morgagni's c., sedimentary c.; a hypermature c. in which the nucleus gravitates within the capsule.
myotonic c., c. occurring in myotonic dystrophy.
nuclear c., hard c.; a c. involving the nucleus.
overripe c., hypermature c.
perinuclear c., a lamellar c. in which the nucleus is clear but is surrounded by a ring of opacity.
peripheral c., cortical c.
pisciform c., a hereditary c. with bilateral fish-shaped opacities in the axial region of the fetal nucleus.
polar c., a capsular c. limited to an area of the anterior or posterior pole of the lens.
posterior subcapsular c., a c. involving the cortex at the posterior pole of the lens.
progressive c., a c. in which the opacification process progresses to involve the entire lens.
punctate c., an incomplete c. in which there are opaque dots scattered through the lens.
pyramidal c., a cone-shaped, anterior polar c.
radiation c., a c. caused by excessive or prolonged exposure to x-rays, radium, beta rays, heat, or radioactive isotopes.
reduplicated c., a type of congenital c. with opacities situated at various levels in the lens.
ripe c., mature c.
rubella c., embryopathic c. secondary to intrauterine rubella infection.
saucer-shaped c., cupuliform c.
secondary c., **(1)** complicated c.; a c. that accompanies or follows some other eye disease such as uveitis; **(2)** aftercataract; a c. occurring in the retained lens or capsule after a c. extraction.
sedimentary c., Morgagni's c.
senile c., a c. occurring spontaneously in the elderly; mainly a cuneiform c., nuclear c., or posterior subcapsular c., alone or in combination.
sideratic c., a c. resulting from deposition of iron from an iron-containing intraocular foreign body.
siliculose c., siliquose c., calcareous degeneration of the capsule of the lens.
soft c., an advanced or mature c. in which the nucleus is not well developed.
spindle c., fusiform c.; a c. in which the opacity is fusiform, extending from one pole to the other.
stationary c., a c. that does not progress.
stellate c., congenital c. with lens opacities radiating toward the periphery, with subcapsular and cortical changes.
subcapsular c., a c. in which the opacities are concentrated beneath the capsule.
sugar c., any c. associated with intralenticular accumulation of pentose or hexose alcohols.
sutural c., a congenital type of c. with opacities along the Y sutures of the fetal lens nucleus.
syndermatotic c., a c. associated with skin disease.
tetany c., a c. that develops in hypocalcemia.
total c., a c. involving the entire lens.
toxic c., a c. caused by drugs or chemicals.
traumatic c., a c. caused by contusion, rupture, or a foreign body.
umbilicated c., annular c.
vascular c., cataracta adiposa, fibrosa, or ossea; congenital c. in which the degenerated lens is replaced with mesodermal tissue.
zonular c., lamellar c.

---

cataracta (kat-ă-rak'tă) [L.]. Cataract.
c. adipo'sa, vascular *cataract.*
c. brunes'cens, black *cataract.*
c. ceru'lea, blue *cataract.*
c. dermatog'enes, a cataract associated with skin disease.
c. elec'trica, electric *cataract.*
c. fibro'sa, vascular *cataract.*
c. membrana'cea accre'ta, adhesions between the lens capsule and the iris.
c. neurodermat'ica, cataract associated with atopic dermatitis.
c. ni'gra, black *cataract.*
c. nodifor'mis, an anterior dense, round concussion cataract.
c. os'sea, vascular *cataract.*

cataractogenesis (kat'ă-rak-tō-jen'ĕ-sis) [cataract + G. *genesis,* production]. The state of cataract formation.

cataractogenic (kat'ă-rak-tō-jen'ik). Cataract-producing.

cataractous (kat-ă-rak'tŭs). Relating to a cataract.

cataria (ka-tā'rē-ă) [L. *cattus,* male cat (post-class)]. Catnep; catnip; catmint; the dried flowering tops of *Nepeta cataria* (family Labiatae); an emmenagogue and antispasmodic; also reported to produce psychic effects.

catarrh (kă-tahr') [G. *katarrheō,* to flow down]. Simple inflammation of a mucous membrane.
autumnal c., hay *fever.*
malignant c. of cattle, malignant catarrhal *fever.*
nasal c., rhinitis.
vernal c., vernal *conjunctivitis.*

catarrhal (kă-tah'răl). Relating to or affected with catarrh.

Catarrhina (kat-ă-rī'nă) [kata- + G. *rhis* (*rhin-*), nose]. A genus of Old World monkeys in the superfamily Cercopithecoidea.

catarrhine (kat'ă-rīn). Relating to the *Catarrhina.*

catastalsis (kat-ă-stal'sis) [G. *kata-stellō,* to put in order, check]. A contraction wave resembling ordinary peristalsis but not preceded by a zone of inhibition.

catastaltic (kat-ă-stal'tik). **1.** Inhibitory, restricting, or restraining. **2.** An inhibitory or checking agent, such as an astringent or antispasmodic.

catastasis (kă-tas'tă-sis) [G.]. **1.** A condition or state. **2.** Restoration to a normal condition or a normal place.

catatonia (kat-ă-tō'nē-ă) [G. *katatonos,* stretching down, depressed, fr. *kata,* down, + *tonos,* tone]. A syndrome of psychomotor disturbances characterized by periods of physical rigidity, negativism, excitement, and stupor.
excited c., c. in which the patient is excited, impulsive, hyperactive, and combative.
periodic c., regularly reappearing phases of catatonic excitement.
stuporous c., c. in which the patient is subdued, mute, and negativistic, accompanied by varying combinations of staring, rigidity, and cataplexy.

catatonic, catatoniac (kat-ă-ton′ik, -tō′nē-ak). Relating to, or characterized by, catatonia.

catatrichy (kat′ă-tri-kē) [cata- + G. *thrix,* hair]. Presence of a forelock of hair that is separate or different in appearance; may be inherited.

catatricrotic (kat′ă-trī-krot′ik). Denoting a pulse tracing with three minor elevations interrupting the downstroke.

catatricrotism (kat-ă-trī′krō-tizm) [cata- + G. *tri-,* three, + *krotos,* beat]. A condition of the pulse marked by three minor expansions of the artery following the main beat, producing three secondary upward waves on the downstroke of the pulse tracing.

catechase (kat′ĕ-kās). Catechol 1,2-dioxygenase.

catechin (kat′ĕ-kin). Catechuic acid; catechinic acid; cyanidol; 3,3′,4′,5,7-flavanpentol; derived from catechu, and used as an astringent in diarrhea and as a stain.

catechinic acid (kat-ĕ-kin′ik). Catechin.

catechol (kat′ĕ-kol). **1.** Pyrocatechol. **2.** Term loosely used for catechin, which contains a pyrocatechol moiety, and as the root of catecholamines, which are pyrocatechol derivatives.
c. methyltransferase [EC 2.1.1.6], a transferase that catalyzes the methylation of the hydroxyl group at the 3 position of the aromatic ring of c.'s, including the catecholamines norepinephrine and epinephrine, the methyl group coming from *S*-adenosylmethionine.
c. oxidase [EC 1.10.3.1], *o*-diphenolase; diphenol oxidase; an enzyme oxidizing c.'s to 1,2-benzoquinones, with O_2. See also monophenol monooxygenase.
c. oxidase (dimerizing) [EC 1.1.3.14], an enzyme oxidizing c., with O_2, to a diphenylenedioxide quinone.

catecholamines (kat-ĕ-kol′ă-mēnz). Pyrocatechols with an alkylamine side chain; examples of biochemical interest are epinephrine, norepinephrine, and dopa.

catechol 1,2-dioxygenase [EC 1.13.11.1]. Catechase; pyrocatechase; an oxidoreductase catalyzing oxidation of pyrocatechol, with O_2, to *cis-cis-* muconate.

catechol 2,3-dioxygenase [EC 1.13.11.2]. Metapyrocatechase; an oxidoreductase oxidizing catechol, with O_2, to 2-hydroxymuconate semialdehyde.

catechu (kat′ĕ-chū, -kū) [East Indian name]. Gambir.
c. nigrum, cutch; black c., an extract of the heart wood of *Acacia catechu* (family Leguminosae), used as an astringent in diarrhea.

catechuic acid (kat-ĕ-chū′ik, -kū′ik). Catechin.

catelectrotonus (kat′ē-lek-trot′ō-nŭs) [cathode + electrotonus]. The changes in excitability and conductivity in a nerve or muscle in the neighborhood of the cathode during the passage of a constant electric current.

Catenabacterium (kat′ĕ-nă-bak-tēr′ē-ŭm) [L. *catena,* chain, + bacterium]. An obsolete genus of nonmotile, anaerobic bacteria containing Gram-positive, straight or curved rods which ordinarily occur in long chains or filaments. These organisms may be pathogenic. The type species is *C. helminthoides.* This genus is no longer recognized, and most of its species have been transferred to *Eubacterium* or *Lactobacillus.*
C. catenafor′me, *Lactobacillus catenaforme.*
C. contor′tum, *Eubacterium contortum.*
C. filamento′sum, *Eubacterium filamentosum.*
C. helminthoi′des, type species of the genus; this organism may be slightly pathogenic; it causes minor abscesses in rabbits.

catenating (kat′en-āt-ing) [L. *catenatus,* chained]. Occurring in a chain or series.

catenoid (kat′ĕ-noyd) [L. *catena,* chain, + G. *eidos,* resemblance]. **1.** Catenulate; like a chain, such as a chain of fungus spores or a colony of protozoa in which the individuals are joined end to end. **2.** Surface of net zero curvature generated by the rotation of a catenary (curve of repose of a suspended chain); the interventricular septum of the heart in idiopathic hypertrophic subaortic stenosis resembles a c., which makes it ineffective in increasing intracavity pressure or in reducing its volume as defined in Laplace's law.

catenulate (ka-ten′yū-lāt). Catenoid (1).

catgut (kat′gŭt) [probably from *kit,* a small violin, through confusion with kit, a small cat]. An absorbable surgical suture material made from the collagenous fibers of the submucosa of certain animals.
chromic c., c. impregnated with chromium salts to prolong its tensil strength and retard its absorption.
IKI c., c. sterilized in a solution of 1 part of iodine in 100 parts potassium iodide.
silverized c., c. prepared by immersion in a 2% solution of colloidal silver for 1 week and then in 95% alcohol for 15 to 30 minutes.

Catha edulis (kath′ă ed′yū-lis) [Ar. *khat*]. Flower of paradise; a plant of Abyssinia and Arabia (family Celastraceae), cultivated for use as a stimulant; khat (the fresh leaves and twigs) is chewed or used in the preparation of a beverage; the active principle is pharmacologically related to the amphetamines, probably *d*-norisoephedrine.

catharsis (kă-thar′sis) [G. *katharisis,* purification, fr. *katharos,* pure]. **1.** Purgation. **2.** Psychocatharsis; the release or discharge of emotional tension or anxiety by psychoanalytically guided emotional reliving of past, especially repressed, events.

cathartic (kă-thar′tik). **1.** Relating to catharsis. **2.** An agent having purgative action.

cathectic (kă-thek′tik). Pertaining to cathexis.

cathemoglobin (ka-thēm-ō-glō′bin). An artificial derivative of hemoglobin in which the globin is denatured and the iron oxidized.

cathepsin (kă-thep′sin). One of a number of proteinases and peptidases (peptide hydrolases) of animal tissues of varying specificities.

catheter (kath′ĕ-ter) [G. *kathetēr,* fr. *kathiēmi,* to send down]. **1.** A tubular instrument to allow passage of fluid from or into a body cavity. See also line (4). **2.** Especially a c. designed to be passed through the urethra into the bladder to drain it of retained urine.
acorn-tipped c., a c. used in ureteropyelography to occlude the ureteral orifice and prevent backflow from the ureter during and following the injection of an opaque medium.
c. à demeure (ă-dem-ĕr′) [Fr. *demeurer,* to dwell], an obsolete term for a c. that is retained for a considerable period in the urethra.
balloon-tip c., a tube with a balloon at its tip that can be inflated or deflated without removal after installation; the balloon may be inflated to facilitate passage of the tube through a blood vessel (propelled by the bloodstream) or to occlude the vessel in which the tube alone would allow free flow; such c.'s are used to enter the pulmonary artery to facilitate hemodynamic measurements.
bicoudate c., c. bicoudé (bī-kū-dā′) [bi + Fr. *coudé,* bent], an elbowed c. with a double bend.
Bozeman-Fritsch c., a slightly curved double-channel uterine c. with several openings at the tip.
Braasch c., a bulb-tipped c. used for dilation and calibration.
brush c., a ureteral c. with a finely bristled brush tip which is endoscopically passed into the ureter or renal pelvis and which by gentle to-and-fro movement brushes cells from the surface of suspected tumors.
cardiac c., intracardiac c.
central venous c., a c. passed through a peripheral vein, ending in the thoracic vena cava, for measurement of venous pressure or for infusion of concentrated solutions; the peripheral end may connect to a subcutaneous chamber for percutaneous injections given over periods of months or may exit from the skin at a distance from the vein.

conical c., a c. with a cone-shaped tip designed to dilate the ureter.
c. coudé (kū-da') [Fr. *coudé,* bent], elbowed c.
de Pezzer c., a self-retaining c. with a bulbous extremity.
double-channel c., two-way c.; a c. with two lumens, allowing irrigation and aspiration.
Drew-Smythe c., an instrument used for rupture of the amnion at a level several centimeters above the cervix for the purpose of inducing labor; it is passed through the cervix between the amnion and the endometrium.
elbowed c., c. coudé; prostatic c.; a c. with an angular bend near the beak; used to rise over prostatic obstruction.
eustachian c., a c. used for catheterization of the middle ear through the eustachian tube.
female c., a short, nearly straight c. for passage into the female bladder.
Fogarty c., a c. with an inflatable balloon near its tip; used to remove arterial emboli and thrombi from major veins (*e.g.,* iliofemoral) and to remove stones from the biliary ducts.
Foley c., a c. with a retaining balloon.
Gouley's c., a solid curved steel instrument grooved on its inferior surface so that it can be passed over a guide through a urethral stricture.
indwelling c., a c. left in place in the bladder, usually a balloon c.
intracardiac c., cardiac c.; a c. that can be passed into the heart through a vein or artery, to withdraw samples of blood, measure pressures within the heart's chambers or great vessels, and inject contrast media; used mainly in the diagnosis and evaluation of congenital, rheumatic, and coronary artery lesions.
Malecot c., a two- or four-winged c.
Nélaton's c., a flexible c. of red rubber.
olive-tipped c., a ureteral c. with an olive-shaped tip, used to dilate a constricted ureteral orifice; larger sizes are also used for dilating or calibrating urethral strictures.
pacing c., a cardiac c. with one or two electrodes at its tip which, when connected to a pulse generator and properly positioned in the right atrium or ventricle, will artificially pace the heart.
Pezzer c., see de Pezzer c.
Phillips' c., a c. with a filiform guide for the urethra.
prostatic c., elbowed c.
Robinson c., a straight urethral c. with two to six holes to facilitate drainage, especially in the presence of blood clots which may occlude one or more openings.
self-retaining c., a c. so constructed that it remains in urethra and bladder until removed, *e.g.,* indwelling c.; Foley c.
spiral tip c., a c. with an off-center filiform tip.
Swan-Ganz c., a thin (5 Fr), flexible, flow-directed c. using a balloon to carry it through the heart to a pulmonary artery; when it is positioned in a small arterial branch, pulmonary wedge pressure is measured in front of the temporarily inflated and wedged balloon.
two-way c., double-channel c.
vertebrated c., a c. made of several segments moving on each other like the links of a chain.
whistle-tip c., a c. with an opening at the end and side.
winged c., a soft rubber c. with little flaps at each side of the beak to retain it in the bladder.

catheterization (kath'ĕ-ter-ĭ-zā'shŭn). Passage of a catheter.

catheterize (kath'ĕ-ter-īz). To pass a catheter.

catheterostat (kath'ĕ-ter-ō-stat) [catheter + G. *statos,* standing]. A stand for holding catheters.

cathexis (kă-thek'sis) [G. *kathexis,* a holding in, retention]. Attachment of libido to a specific idea or object.

cathodal (kath'ō-dăl). Cathodic; of, pertaining to, or emanating from a cathode.

cathode (C, Ca) (kath'ōd) [G. *kathodos,* a way down, fr. *kata,* down, + *hodos,* a way]. Negative electrode; the negative pole of a galvanic battery or the electrode connected with it; the electrode toward which positively charged ions (cations) migrate and are reduced, and into which electrons are fed from their source (anode or generator). *Cf.* anode.

cathodic (kă-thod'ik). Cathodal.

catholysis (kath-ol'ĕ-sis). Electrolysis with a cathode needle.

cation (kat'ī-on) [G. *katiōn,* going down]. An ion carrying a charge of positive electricity, therefore going to the negatively charged cathode.

cation exchange. The process by which a cation in a liquid phase exchanges with another cation present as the counter-ion of a negatively charged solid polymer (cation exchanger). A cation-exchange reaction in removal of the Na^+ of a sodium chloride solution is $RSO_3^-H^+ + Na^+ \rightarrow RSO_3^-Na^+ + H^+$ (R is the polymer, RSO_3^- the cation exchanger); if this is combined with the anion-exchange reaction (see anion exchange), NaCl is removed from the solution (desalting). Cation exchange may also be used chromatographically, to separate cations, and medicinally, to remove a cation; *e.g.,* H^+, from gastric contents, or Na^+ and K^+ in the intestine.

cation exchanger. An insoluble solid (usually a polystyrene or a polysaccharide) that has negatively charged radicals attached to it (*e.g.,* $-COO^-$, $-SO_3^-$), which can attract and hold cations that pass by in a moving solution if these are more attracted to the acid groups than the counter ion present.

cationic (kat-ī-on'ik). Referring to positively charged ions and their properties.

cationogen (kat-ī-on'ō-jen). A substance that gives rise to positively charged ions.

catlin, catling (kat'lin, -ling). A long, sharp-pointed, double-edged knife used in amputations.

catmint (kat'mint). Cataria.

catnep, catnip (kat'nep, kat'nip). Cataria.

catochus (kat'ō-kŭs) [G. *katochē,* epilepsy (Galen), fr. *katechō,* to hold fast]. The trancelike phase of catalepsy in which the patient is conscious but cannot move or speak.

catoptric (ka-top'trik) [G. *katoptron,* mirror]. Relating to reflected light.

cauda, pl. caudae (kaw'dă, kaw'dē) [L. a tail]. Tail. **1** [NA]. Any tail, or tail-like structure, or tapering or elongated extremity of an organ or other part. **2.** In veterinary anatomy, a free appendage representing the caudal end of the vertebral column; covered by skin and hair, feathers, or scales.
c. epididym'idis [NA], tail of the epididymis; globus minor; the inferior part of the epididymis that leads into the ductus deferens; part of the reservoir of spermatozoa.
c. equi'na [L. horse tail] [NA], the bundle of spinal nerve roots arising from the lumbar enlargement and conus medullaris and running through the lower part of the subarachnoid space within the vertebral canal below the first lumbar vertebra; it comprises the roots of all the spinal nerves below the first lumbar.
c. fas'ciae denta'tae, uncus *band* of Giacomini.
c. hel'icis [NA], tail of helix; a flattened process terminating the cartilage of the helix of the ear, posteriorly and inferiorly.
c. nu'clei cauda'ti [NA], cauda striati; tail of the caudate nucleus; the elongated posterior extension of the caudate nucleus that parallels the body and inferior horn of the lateral ventricle.
c. pancre'atis [NA], tail of pancreas; the left extremity of the pancreas within the lienorenal ligament.
c. stria'ti, c. nuclei caudati.

caudad (kaw'dad). **1.** In a direction toward the tail. **2.** Situated nearer the tail in relation to a specific reference point; opposite of craniad. See also inferior.

caudal (kaw'dăl) [Mod. L. *caudalis*]. Caudalis; pertaining to the tail.

caudalis (kaw-dā'lis) [NA]. Caudal.

caudate (kaw'dāt). **1.** Tailed; possessing a tail. **2.** *Nucleus* caudatus.

caudatolenticular (kaw-dā'tō-len-tik'yū-lăr). Caudolenticular; relating to the nuclei caudatus and lenticularis.

caudatum (kaw-dā'tŭm). *Nucleus* caudatus.

caudocephalad (kaw-dō-sef'ăl-ad). In a direction from the tail toward the head.

caudolenticular (kaw'dō-len-tik'yū-lăr). Caudatolenticular.

caul (kawl) [Gaelic, *call*, a veil]. **1.** Galea (4); velum (2); veil (2); the amnion, either as a piece of membrane capping the baby's head at birth or the whole membrane when delivered unruptured with the baby. **2.** *Omentum* majus.

caumesthesia (kaw-mes-thē'zē-ă) [G. *kauma*, heat, + *aisthēsis*, sensation]. A sense of heat irrespective of the temperature of the air.

causalgia (kaw-zal'jē-ă) [G. *kausis*, burning, + *algos*, pain]. Persistent severe burning sensation of the skin, usually following direct or indirect (vascular) partial injury of a sensory nerve, accompanied by cutaneous changes (temperature and sweating).

cause (kawz) [L. *causa*]. That which produces an effect or condition; that by which a morbid change or disease is brought about.

constitutional c., a c. acting from within or through some systemic process or inborn error.

exciting c., procatarxis (1); the direct provoking c. of a condition.

predisposing c., anything that produces a susceptibility or disposition to a condition without actually causing it.

proximate c., the immediate c. that precipitates a condition.

specific c., a c. the action of which produces only one definite condition.

caustic (kaws'tik) [G. *kaustikos*, fr. *kaiō*, to burn]. Pyrotic (2). **1.** Exerting an effect resembling a burn. **2.** An agent producing this effect. **3.** Denoting a solution of a strong alkali; *e.g.*, caustic soda, NaOH.

cauterant (kaw'ter-ant). **1.** Cauterizing. **2.** A cauterizing agent.

cauterization (kaw-ter-ī-zā'shŭn). The act of cauterizing. See also subentries under cautery.

cauterize (kaw'ter-īz). To apply a cautery; to burn with a cautery.

cautery (kaw'ter-ē) [G. *kautērion*, a branding iron]. **1.** An agent or device used for scarring, burning, or cutting the skin or other tissues by means of heat, cold, electric current, or caustic chemicals. **2.** Use of a cautery.

actual c., technocausis; a c., such as electrocautery, acting directly through heat and not by chemical means.

bipolar c., electrocautery by high frequency electrical current passed through tissue from an active to a passive electrode; used for hemostasis.

chemical c., chemocautery.

cold c., cryocautery.

electric c., electrocautery.

galvanic c., obsolete term for electrocautery.

gas c., c. by means of a measured amount of a lighted gas jet.

monopolar c., electrocautery by high frequency electrical current passed from a single electrode, where the cauterization occurs, the patient's body serving as a ground.

cava (kā'vă). See *vena* cava inferior and superior.

cavagram (kā'vă-gram). Cavogram.

caval (kā'văl). Relating to a vena cava.

cavascope (kav'ă-skōp) [L. *cavum*, hole, + G. *skopeō*, to view]. Celoscope.

cave (kāv). A hollow or enclosed space or cavity. See cavum, cavitas, cavity, cavern, caverna.

caveola, pl. **caveolae** (kav-ē-ō'lă, -lē) [L.]. A small pocket, vesicle, cave or recess communicating with the outside of a cell and extending inward, indenting the cytoplasm and the cell membrane. Such caveolae may be pinched off to form free vesicles within the cytoplasm. They are considered to be sites of uptake of materials into the cell, expulsion of materials from the cell, or sites of addition or removal of cell (unit) membrane to or from the cell surface.

cavern (kav'ern). Caverna.

caverna, pl. **cavernae** (kă-ver'nă, -nē) [L. a grotto, fr. *cavus*, hollow]. [NA]. Cavern; an anatomical cavity with many interconnecting chambers.

cavernae corpo'ris spongio'si [NA], cavities of corpus spongiosum; the vascular spaces forming the erectile tissue of the corpus spongiosum penis in the male and the bulb of the vestibule in the female.

cavernae corpo'rum cavernoso'rum [NA], cavities of corpora cavernosa; the vascular spaces of the corpora cavernosa that, together with the intervening fibrous trabeculae, form the erectile tissue of the penis or clitoris.

caverniloquy (kav-er-nil'ō-kwē) [L. *caverna*, cavern, + *loqui*, to talk]. Low pitched resonant pectoriloquy heard over a lung cavity.

cavernitis (kav-er-nī'tis). Cavernositis; inflammation of the corpus cavernosum penis.

fibrous c., c. occasionally associated with Peyronie's disease.

cavernoscope (kav'er-nō-skōp). Celoscope.

cavernoscopy (kav-er-nos'kō-pē) [L. *caverna*, cavern, + G. *skopeō*, to view]. Celoscopy.

cavernositis (kav'er-nō-sī'tis). Cavernitis.

cavernostomy (kav-er-nos'tō-mē) [L. *caverna*, cavern, + G. *stoma*, mouth]. Speleostomy; opening of any cavity to establish drainage.

cavernous (kav'er-nŭs). Relating to a cavern or a cavity; containing many cavities.

Cavia (kā'vē-ă) [Mod. L., fr. native Indian]. A genus of the family Caviidae that includes the guinea pigs.

C. porcel'lus, guinea pig; a 1- to 2-pound rodent with a very short tail that is not visible externally; native to South America, where it is raised for food; used widely as a laboratory animal in bacteriologic, pathologic, and pharmacologic research.

cavitary (kav'i-tā-rē). **1.** Relating to a cavity or having a cavity or cavities. **2.** Denoting any animal parasite that has an enteric canal or body cavity and that lives within the host's body.

cavitas, pl. **cavitates** (kav'i-tas, -tā'tēs) [Mod. L.]. Cavity.

c. abdomina'lis [NA], abdominal cavity; cavum abdominis; enterocele (2); the space bounded by the abdominal walls, the diaphragm, and the pelvis; it usually is arbitrarily separated from the pelvic cavity by a plane across the superior aperture of the pelvis; however, it may include the pelvis with the abdomen; within the c. lie the greater part of the organs of digestion, the spleen, the kidneys, and the suprarenal glands.

c. articula're [NA], cavum articulare; a joint cavity.

c. corona'lis [NA], crown cavity; cavum coronale; the space within the crown of a tooth continuous with the root canal.

c. den'tis [NA], cavity of tooth; pulp cavity; cavum dentis; the central hollow of a tooth consisting of the crown cavity and the root canal; it contains the fibrovascular dental pulp and is lined throughout by odontoblasts.

c. glenoida'lis [NA], glenoid cavity or surface; glenoid fossa (1); the hollow in the head of the scapula that receives the head of the humerus to make the shoulder joint.

c. infraglot'ticum [NA], infraglottic space; aditus glottidis inferior; cavum infraglotticum; the part of the cavity of the larynx immediately below the glottis.

c. laryn'gis [NA], cavity of larynx; cavum laryngis; a cavity that is continuous above with the pharynx at the level of the aryepiglottic folds and extends downward through the rima glottidis to the infraglottic space.

c. medulla'ris [NA], medullary cavity; cavum medullare; the marrow cavity in the shaft of a long bone.

c. na'si [NA], nasal cavity; cavum nasi; the cavity on either side of the nasal septum, lined with ciliated respiratory mucosa, extending from the naris anteriorly to the choana posteriorly, and communicating with the paranasal sinuses through their orifices in the lateral wall, from which also project the three conchae; the cribriform plate, through which the olfactory nerves are transmitted, forms the roof; the floor is formed by the hard palate.

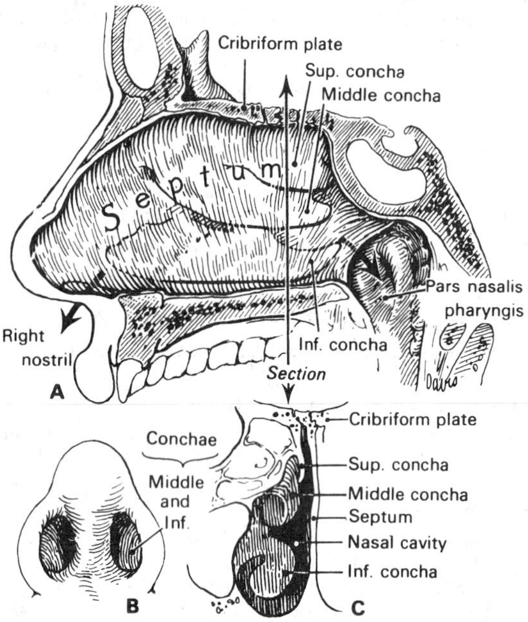

Cavitas Nasi

A, sagittal section showing right nasal cavity as seen through septum; *B,* nares viewed from below; *C,* coronal section at level indicated showing relationship between air passages and mucosal surfaces.

c. o'ris [NA], oral cavity; cavum oris; mouth (1); the region consisting of the vestibulum oris, the narrow cleft between the lips and cheeks, and the teeth and gums, and the c. oris propria.

c. o'ris pro'pria, oral cavity proper; the space between the dental arches, limited posteriorly by the isthmus of the fauces.

c. pel'vis [NA], pelvic cavity; cavum pelvis; the space bounded at the sides by the bones of the pelvis, above by the superior aperture of the pelvis, and below by the pelvic diaphragm; it contains the pelvic viscera.

c. pericardia'lis [NA], pericardial cavity (1); cavum pericardii; the potential space between the parietal and the visceral layers of the serous pericardium.

c. peritonea'lis [NA], peritoneal cavity; greater peritoneal cavity; cavum peritonei; the interior of the peritoneal sac, normally only a potential space between the parietal and visceral layers of the peritoneum.

c. pharyn'gis [NA], cavity of pharynx; cavum pharyngis; it consists of a nasal part continuous anteriorly with the nasal cavity and receiving the openings of the auditory tubes, an oral part opening through the fauces into the oral cavity, and a laryngeal part leading into the vestibule of the larynx and to the esophagus.

c. pleura'lis [NA], pleural cavity or space; cavum pleurae; the potential space between the parietal and visceral layers of the pleura.

c. thora'cis [NA], thoracic cavity; cavum thoracis; the space within the thoracic walls, bounded below by the diaphragm and above by the neck.

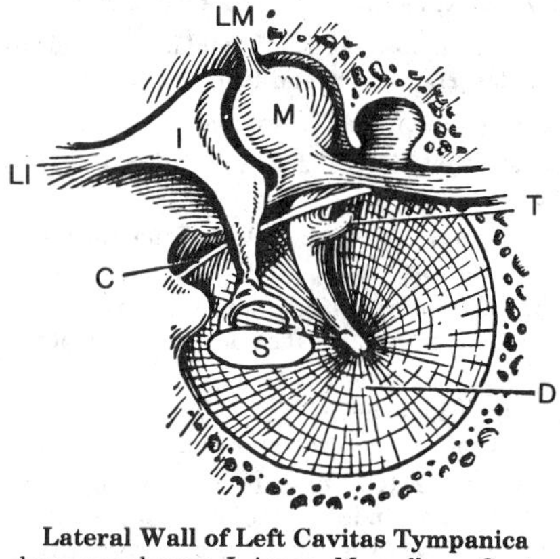

Lateral Wall of Left Cavitas Tympanica

D, drum membrane; *I,* incus; *M,* malleus; *S,* stapes; *C,* chorda tympani nerve; *LM,* ligament of malleus; *LI,* ligament of incus; *T,* tendon of tensor tympani muscle.

c. tympan'ica [NA], tympanic cavity; cavity of middle ear; cavum tympani; tympanum; an air chamber in the temporal bone containing the ossicles; it is lined with mucous membrane and is continuous with the auditory tube anteriorly and the tympanic antrum and mastoid air cells posteriorly.

c. u'teri [NA], cavity of uterus; cavum uteri; uterine cavity; the space within the uterus extending from the cervical canal to the openings of the uterine tubes.

cavitation (kav-i-tā'shŭn). Formation of a cavity, as in the lung in tuberculosis.

cavitis (kā-vī'tis). Celophlebitis.

cavity (kav'i-tē) [L. *cavus,* hollow]. **1.** A hollow space. See cave, cavum, cavitas, cavern, caverna. **2.** Lay term for the loss of tooth structure due to dental caries.

abdominal c., *cavitas* abdominalis.

allantoic c., the lumen of the allantois.

amniotic c., the fluid-filled c. inside the amnion which contains the developing embryo.

axillary c., fossa axillaris.

body c., see celom (2).

buccal c., *vestibulum* oris.

cleavage c., blastocele.

c. of concha, *cavum* conchae.

c.'s of corpora cavernosa, *cavernae* corporum cavernosorum.

c.'s of corpus spongiosum, *cavernae* corporis spongiosi.

cotyloid c., acetabulum.

cranial c., intracranial c.

crown c., *cavitas* coronalis.

ectoplacental c., epamniotic c.

ectotrophoblastic c., a developmental c. appearing between the trophoblast and the embryonic disk ectoderm in some mammals.

epamniotic c., ectoplacental c.; a developmental c. derived by division of the proamniotic space; it is further removed from the embryo than the amniotic c.

epidural c., *cavum* epidurale.

glenoid c., *cavitas* glenoidalis.

greater peritoneal c., *cavitas* peritonealis.

head c., the cephalic region in the embryos of vertebrates containing the modified somites that give rise to the eye muscles.

intracranial c., cranial c.; the space within the skull.

c. of larynx, *cavitas* laryngis.

lesser peritoneal c., *bursa* omentalis.

Meckel's c., *cavum* trigeminale.

medullary c., *cavitas* medullaris.
c. of middle ear, *cavitas* tympanica.
nasal c., *cavitas* nasi.
nephrotomic c., nephrocele (2).
oral c., *cavitas* oris.
oral c. proper, *cavitas* oris propria.
orbital c., orbita.
pelvic c., *cavitas* pelvis.
pericardial c., **(1)** *cavitas* pericardialis; **(2)** in the embryo, that part of the primary celom containing the heart; originally it is in open communication with the pleural c.'s and indirectly, through them, with the peritoneal part of the celom.
peritoneal c., *cavitas* peritonealis.
perivisceral c., primitive perivisceral c.; the space between the ectoderm and endoderm in the gastrula.
pharyngonasal c., *pars* nasalis pharyngis.
c. of pharynx, *cavitas* pharyngis.
pleural c., *cavitas* pleuralis.
pleuroperitoneal c., that part of the embryonic celom later partitioned to give rise to the pleural and peritoneal c.'s.
primitive perivisceral c., perivisceral c.
pulp c., *cavitas* dentis.
Retzius' c., *spatium* retropubicum.
segmentation c., blastocele.
c. of septum pellucidum, *cavum* septi pellucidi.
somite c., myocele (2).
splanchnic c., visceral c.; the celom or one of the body c.'s derived from it.
subarachnoid c., *cavum* subarachnoideale.
subdural c., *spatium* subdurale.
subgerminal c., gastrocele (1).
tension c., an expanding lung abscess.
thoracic c., *cavitas* thoracis.
c. of tooth, *cavitas* dentis.
trigeminal c., *cavum* trigeminale.
tympanic c., *cavitas* tympanica.
uterine c., c. of uterus, *cavitas* uteri.
visceral c., splanchnic c.

cavogram (kā'vō-gram). Cavagram; an angiogram of a vena cava.

cavography (kā-vog'ră-fē). Venacavography.

cavosurface (kā-vō-sŭr'făs). Relating to a cavity and the surface of a tooth.

cavum, pl. cava (ka'vŭm, -vă) [L. ntr. of adj. *cavus,* hollow] [NA]. A hollow, hole, or cavity.
c. abdom'inis, *cavitas* abdominalis.
c. articula're, *cavitas* articulare.
c. con'chae [NA], cavity of concha; the lower, larger portion of the concha below the crus helicis; it forms the vestibule to the external acoustic meatus.
c. corona'le, *cavitas* coronalis.
c. den'tis, *cavitas* dentis.
c. doug'lasi, *excavatio* rectouterina.
c. epidura'le [NA], epidural space or cavity; the space between the walls of the vertebral canal and the dura mater of the spinal cord.
c. infraglot'ticum, *cavitas* infraglotticum.
c. laryn'gis, *cavitas* laryngis.
c. mediastina'le, an inappropriate name sometimes applied to the mediastinum.
c. medulla're, *cavitas* medullaris.
c. na'si, *cavitas* nasi.
c. o'ris, *cavitas* oris.
c. pel'vis, *cavitas* pelvis.
c. pericar'dii, *cavitas* pericardialis.
c. perito'nei, *cavitas* peritonealis.
c. pharyn'gis, *cavitas* pharyngis.
c. pleu'rae, *cavitas* pleuralis.
c. psalte'rii, Verga's *ventricle.*
c. ret'zii, *spatium* retropubicum.
c. sep'ti pellu'cidi [NA], cavity of the septum pellucidum; fifth or sylvian ventricle; Duncan's, Vieussens, or Wenzel's ventricle; ventriculus quintus; pseudocele; pseudoventricle; a slitlike, fluid-filled space of variable width between the left and right septum pellucidum, which occurs in less than 10% of human brains and may communicate with the third ventricle.
c. subarachnoid'ea [NA], subarachnoid space or cavity; the space between the arachnoidea and pia mater, traversed by delicate fibrous trabeculae and filled with cerebrospinal fluid. Since the pia mater immediately adheres to the surface of the brain and spinal cord, the space is greatly widened wherever the brain surface exhibits a deep depression (for example, the deep sulci of the cerebral cortex); such widenings are called cisternae. All of the large blood vessels supplying the brain and spinal cord lie suspended in the subarachnoid space.
c. subdura'le, *spatium* subdurale.
c. thora'cis, *cavitas* thoracis.
c. trigemina'le [NA], trigeminal cavity; Meckel's cavity or space; the cleft in the meningeal layer of dura of the middle cranial fossa near the tip of the petrous part of the temporal bone; it encloses the roots of the trigeminal nerve and the trigeminal ganglion.
c. tym'pani, *cavitas* tympanica.
c. u'teri, *cavitas* uteri.
c. ver'gae, Verga's *ventricle.*
c. vesicouteri'num, *excavatio* vesicouterina.

cavy (kā'vē). Common name for *Cavia porcellus.*

Cazenave, Pierre L. Alphée, French dermatologist, 1795–1877. See C.'s *vitiligo.*

Cb Symbol for columbium.

C-banding. See C-banding *stain.*

CBC Abbreviation for complete *blood count.*

CBG Abbreviation for corticosteroid-binding *globulin.*

CBPP Abbreviation for contagious bovine *pleuropneumonia.*

Cbz Abbreviation for carbobenzoxy (benzyloxycarbonyl).

C.C. Abbreviation for chief complaint, as recorded on a patient's medical history.

cc, c.c. Abbreviation for cubic *centimeter.*

CCA Abbreviation for chimpanzee coryza *agent.*

CCC Abbreviation for cathodal closure *contraction.*

CCNU Lomustine.

CCTe Abbreviation for cathodal closure *tetanus.*

CCU Abbreviation for coronary care *unit;* critical care *unit.*

Cd Symbol for cadmium.

cd Symbol for candela.

CDC Abbreviation for Centers for Disease Control.

CDE blood group. See Rh blood group, Blood Groups appendix.

cDNA Abbreviation for complementary *deoxyribonucleic acid.*

CDP Abbreviation for cytidine 5′-diphosphate.

Ce Symbol for cerium.

CEA Abbreviation for carcinoembryonic *antigen.*

cebocephaly (sē-bō-sef'ă-lē) [G. *kēbos,* monkey, + *kephalē,* head]. Malformation in which the features are suggestive of a monkey; there is usually a tendency toward cyclopia, with defective or absent nose and closely set eyes.

cec-. See ceco-.

ceca (sē'kă). Plural of cecum.

cecal (sē'kăl). **1.** Relating to the cecum. **2.** Ending blindly or in a cul-de-sac.

cecectomy (sē-sek'tō-mē) [ceco- + G. *ektomē*, excision]. Typhlectomy; excision of the cecum.

cecitis (sē-sī'tis). Typhlenteritis; typhlitis; typhloenteritis; inflammation of the cecum.

ceco-, cec- [L. *caecum*, cecum]. Combining forms denoting the cecum. See also typhlo- (1).

cecocolostomy (sē'kō-kō-los'tō-mē). Formation of an anastomosis between cecum and colon.

cecofixation (sē'kō-fik-sā'shŭn). Cecopexy.

cecoileostomy (sē'kō-il-ē-os'tō-mē). Ileocecostomy.

cecopexy (sē'kō-pek-sē) [ceco- + G. *pexis*, fixation]. Typhlopexy; cecofixation; operative anchoring of a movable cecum.

cecoplication (sē'kō-pli-kā'shŭn) [ceco- + L. *plico*, pp. *-atus*, to fold]. Operative reduction in size of a dilated cecum by the formation of folds or tucks in its wall.

cecorrhaphy (sē-kōr'ă-fē) [ceco- + G. *rhaphē*, suture]. Typhlorrhaphy; suture of the cecum.

cecosigmoidostomy (sē'kō-sig-moy-dos'tō-mē). Formation of a communication between the cecum and the sigmoid colon.

cecostomy (sē-kos'tō-mē) [ceco- + G. *stoma*, mouth]. Typhlostomy; operative formation of a cecal fistula.

cecotomy (sē-kot'ō-mē) [ceco- + G. *tome*, incision]. Typhlotomy; incision into the cecum.

cecum, pl. **ceca** (sē'kŭm, sē'kă) [L. ntr. of *caecus*, blind] [NA]. **1.** Typhlon; blind gut; the cul-de-sac, about 6 cm in depth, lying below the terminal ileum forming the first part of the large intestine. **2.** Any similar structure ending in a cul-de-sac.
c. cupula're [NA], cupular blind sac; the upper blind extremity of the cochlear duct.
c. vestibula're [NA], vestibular blind sac; the lower extremity of the cochlear duct, occupying the cochlear recess in the vestibule.

cedar leaf oil (sē'der). Thuja oil; oil obtained by steam distillation from the fresh leaves of *Thuja occidentalis;* used as an insect repellent and counterirritant, and in perfumery.

cedar wood oil. Volatile oil obtained from the wood of *Juniperus virginiana* (family Pinaceae); used as an insect repellent, in perfumery, and as a clearing agent in microscopy.

Ceelen, W., 1884–1964. See C.-Gellerstedt *syndrome.*

cefaclor (sef'ă-klōr). A semisynthetic broad spectrum antibiotic derived from cephalosporin C; used orally.

cefadroxil (sef-ă-drok'sil). A semisynthetic broad spectrum antibiotic derived from cephalosporin C; used orally.

cefamandole nafate (sef-ă-man'dōl naf'āt). A semisynthetic broad spectrum antibiotic derived from cephalosporin C; used by injection.

cefazolin (se-faz'ō-lin). A broad spectrum cephalosporin antibiotic used to treat a wide variety of serious infections; available as the sodium salt for intramuscular or intravenous administration.

cefonicid disodium (se-fon'ĭ-sid). $C_{18}H_{16}N_6Na_2O_8S_3$; a broad spectrum long acting cephalosporin antibiotic structurally related to cefamandole.

cefoperazone sodium (se-fō-per'ă-zōn). $C_{25}H_{26}N_9NaO_8S_2$; a semisynthetic piperazine-cephalosporin antibiotic.

ceforanide (se-fōr'ă-nīd). $C_{20}H_{21}N_7O_6S_2$; a broad spectrum long lasting cephalosporin antibiotic.

cefotaxime sodium (se-fō-taks'ēm). $C_{16}H_{16}N_5NaO_7S_2$; a broad spectrum cephalosporin antibiotic.

cefotetan disodium (sef'ō-te-tan). $C_{17}H_{15}N_7Na_2O_8S_4$; a broad spectrum cephalosporin antibiotic.

cefoxitin sodium (se-fok'si-tin). A semisynthetic antibiotic derived from cephamycin C but structurally and pharmacologically similar to the cephalosporins; used by injection.

ceftazidime sodium (sef-taz'i-dēm). $C_{22}H_{21}N_6NaO_7S_2$; a cephalosporin antibiotic especially effective against enterobacteria and species of *Pseudomonas.*

ceftizoxime sodium (sef-ti-zoks'ēm). $C_{13}H_{12}N_5NaO_5S_2$; a broad spectrum cephalosporin antibiotic similar to cefotaxime sodium.

ceftriaxone disodium (sef-trī-aks'ōn). $C_{18}H_{16}N_8Na_2O_7S_3$; a semisynthetic parenteral cephalosporin antibiotic.

cel (sel) [L. *celer*, swift]. A unit of velocity; 1 cm per second.

-cele [G. *kēlē*, tumor, hernia]. Suffix denoting a swelling or hernia.

celectome (sē'lek-tōm) [G. *kēlē*, tumor, + *ektomē*, excision]. Obsolete term for an instrument, such as the harpoon, for obtaining a bit of tissue from the interior of a tumor for examination.

celenteron (sē-len'ter-on) [G. *koilos*, hollow, + *enteron*, intestine]. Gastrocele (1).

celery seed (sel'er-ē). The dried ripe fruit of *Apium graveolens* (family Umbelliferae); has been used in dysmenorrhea and as a sedative.

Celestin, Felix, French physician, *1900. See C. *tube.*

celestine blue B (sĕ-les'tēn) [C.I. 51050]. A dye recommended as a substitute for hematoxylin when it is unavailable.

celiac (sē'lē-ak) [G. *koilia*, belly]. Relating to the abdominal cavity.

celiagra (sē-lē-ag'ră) [G. *koilia*, belly, + *agra*, seizure]. Rarely used term for sudden painful affection of the stomach or other abdominal organs.

celiectomy (sē-lē-ek'tō-mē) [G. *koilia*, belly, + *ektomē*, excision]. Excision of any abdominal organ, or part of one.

celio- [G. *koilia*, belly]. Combining form denoting relationship to the abdomen. See also celo- (3).

celiocentesis (sē'lē-ō-sen-tē'sis) [celio- + G. *kentēsis*, puncture]. Rarely used term for paracentesis of the abdomen.

celioenterotomy (sē'lē-ō-en-ter-ot'ō-mē) [celio- + G. *enteron*, intestine, + *tomē*, incision]. Opening into the intestine through an incision in the abdominal wall.

celiogastrostomy (sē'lē-ō-gas-tros'tō-mē) [celio- + G. *gastēr*, stomach, + *stoma*, mouth]. Establishment of a gastric fistula through an incision in the abdominal wall.

celiogastrotomy (sē'lē-ō-gas-trot'ō-mē) [celio- + G. *gastēr*, stomach, + *tomē*, incision]. Abdominal section with incision of the stomach.

celiohysterectomy (sē'lē-ō-his-ter-ek'tō-mē) [celio- + G. *hystera*, womb, + *ektomē*, excision]. Abdominal *hysterectomy.*

celiohysterotomy (sē'lē-ō-his-ter-ot'ō-mē) [celio- + G. *hystera*, womb, + *tomē*, incision]. Abdominal *hysterotomy.*

celiomyalgia (sē'lē-ō-mī-al'jē-ă) [celio- + G. *mys*, muscle, + *algos*, pain]. Rarely used term for pain in the abdominal muscles.

celiomyomectomy (sē'lē-ō-mī-ō-mek'tō-mē) [celio- + myoma, + G. *ektomē*, excision]. Abdominal *myomectomy.*

celiomyomotomy (sē'lē-ō-mī-ō-mot'ō-mē) [celio- + myoma, + G. *tomē*, incision]. Incision into a myoma after abdominal incision.

celiomyositis (sē'lē-ō-mī-ō-sī'tis) [celio- + G. *mys*, muscle, + *-itis*, inflammation]. Inflammation of the abdominal muscles.

celioparacentesis (sē'lē-ō-par-ă-sen-tē'sis) [celio- + G. *parakentēsis*, a puncture for dropsy]. Rarely used term for paracentesis of the abdomen.

celiopathy (sē-lē-op'ă-thē) [celio- + G. *pathos*, disease]. Rarely used term for any abdominal disease.

celiorrhaphy (sē-lē-ōr'ă-fē) [celio- + G. *rhaphē*, seam]. Laparorrhaphy; suture of a wound in the abdominal wall.

celiosalpingectomy (sē'lē-ō-sal-pin-jek'tō-mē) [celio- + G. *salpinx*, trumpet + *ektomē*, excision]. Abdominal *salpingectomy.*

celiosalpingotomy (sē′lē-ō-sal-pin-got′ō-mē) [celio- + G. *salpinx,* trumpet, + *tomē,* incision]. Abdominal *salpingotomy.*

celioscopy (sē-lē-os′kŏ-pē) [celio- + G. *skopeō,* to view]. Peritoneoscopy.

celiotomy (sē-lē-ot′ō-mē) [celio- + G. *tomē,* incision]. Laparotomy (2); abdominal section; ventrotomy; transabdominal incision into the peritoneal cavity.

vaginal c., opening the peritoneal cavity through the vagina.

celitis (sē-lī′tis) [G. *koilia,* belly, + *-itis,* inflammation]. Any inflammation of the abdomen.

CELL

cell (sel) [L. *cella,* a storeroom, a chamber]. **1.** The smallest unit of living structure capable of independent existence, composed of a membrane-enclosed mass of protoplasm and containing a nucleus or nucleoid. C.'s are highly variable and specialized in both structure and function, though all must at some stage replicate proteins and nucleic acids, utilize energy, and reproduce themselves. **2.** A small closed or partly closed cavity; a compartment or hollow receptacle. **3.** A container of glass, ceramic, or other solid material within which chemical reactions generating electricity take place.

A c.'s, alpha c.'s of pancreas or of anterior lobe of hypophysis.

absorption c., a small glass chamber with parallel sides, in which absorption spectra of solutions can be obtained.

absorptive c.'s of intestine, c.'s on the surface of villi of the small intestine and the luminal surface of the large intestine which are characterized by having microvilli on their free surface.

acid c., parietal c.

acidophil c., acidophil; acidophile; a c. whose cytoplasm or its granules stain with acid dyes.

acinar c., acinous c.; any secreting c. lining an acinus, especially applied to the c.'s of the pancreas which furnish pancreatic juice, to distinguish them from the c.'s of the islets of Langerhans.

acinous c., acinar c.

acoustic c., a hair c. of the organ of Corti.

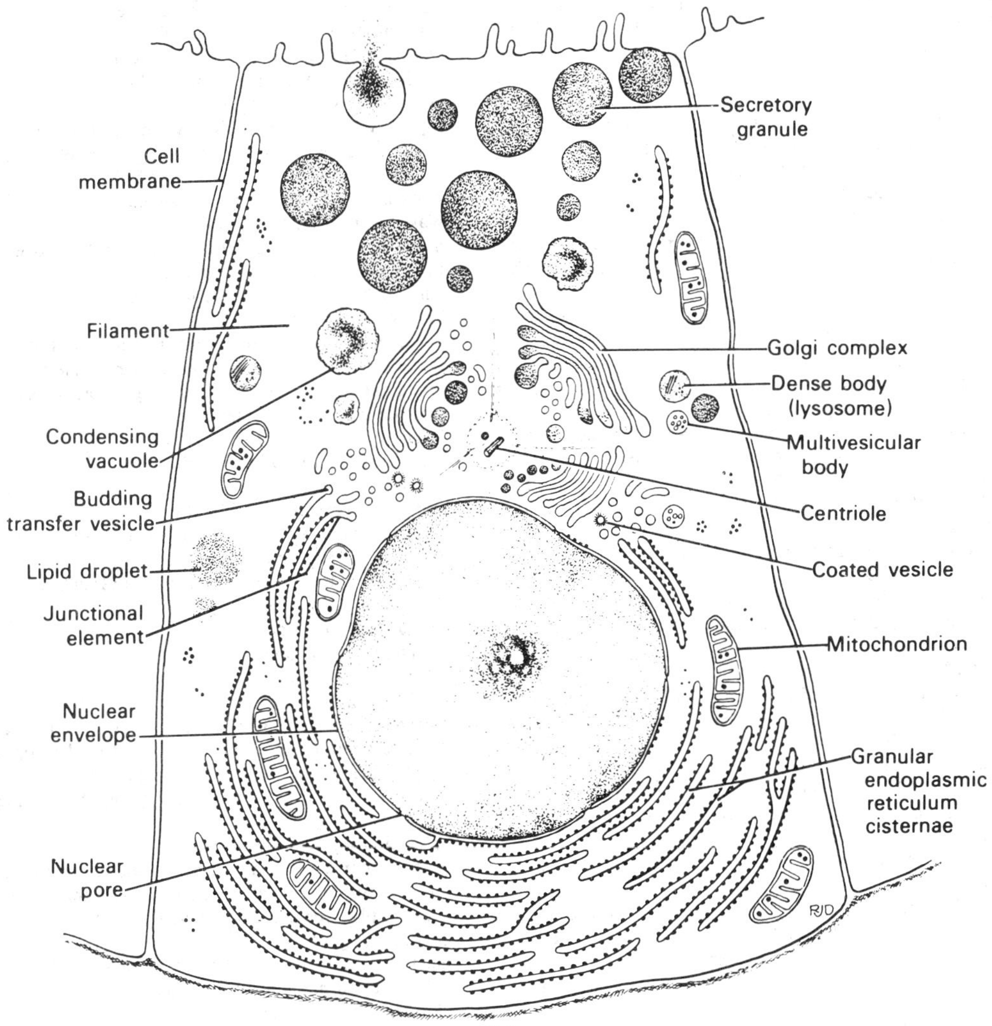

Cell

Diagram of a secretory cell as it would appear in a thin section viewed in an electron microscope.

adipose c., fat c.
adventitial c., pericyte.
air c.'s, (1) *alveoli* pulmonis; (2) air-containing spaces in the skull.
albuminous c., (1) serous c.; (2) zymogenic c.
algoid c., a c. appearing like c.'s of algae, sometimes found in chronic diarrhea.
alpha c.'s of anterior lobe of hypophysis, A c.'s; acidophil c.'s that constitute about 35% of the c.'s of the anterior lobe. There are two varieties: one that elaborates somatotropin; another that elaborates prolactin.
alpha c.'s of pancreas, A c.'s; c.'s of the islets of Langerhans that secrete glucagon.
alveolar c., pneumocyte; any of the c.'s lining the alveoli of the lung, including the squamous alveolar c.'s, the great alveolar c.'s, and the alveolar macrophages.
amacrine c., a nerve c. with short branching dendrites but believed to lack an axon; Cajal described and named such cells in the retina.
ameboid c., (1) wandering c.; a c. such as a leukocyte, having ameboid movements, with a power of locomotion; (2) protoplasmic *astrocyte* (1).
amniogenic c.'s, c.'s from which the amnion develops.
anabiotic c.'s, c.'s that are capable of resuscitation after apparent death; the existence of anabiotic tumor c.'s is postulated to explain the recurrence of a cancer after a very long symptomless period following operation.
anaplastic c., (1) a c. that has reverted to an embryonal state; (2) an undifferentiated c., characteristic of malignant neoplasms.
angioblastic c.'s, those c.'s in the early embryo from which primitive blood c.'s and endothelium develop.
Anitschkow c., cardiac *histiocyte.*
anterior c.'s, *sinus* anteriores.
antigen-presenting c. (APC), a c. originating in the bone marrow and subsequently found as a dendritic c. in various locations such as the skin (Langerhans' c.), the cortex of lymph nodes, the white pulp of the spleen, the thymus, and circulating in the blood and lymph (veil c.); it appears to facilitate the immune response by capturing antigen for presentation to lymphocytes in the regional lymph nodes or in the spleen.
antigen-responsive c., antigen-sensitive c.
antigen-sensitive c., antigen-responsive c.; a small lymphocyte that, although not itself an immunologically activated c., responds to antigenic (immunogenic) stimulus by a process of division and differentiation that results in the production of immunologically activated cells.
apolar c., a neuron without processes.
APUD c.'s, see APUD.
argentaffin c.'s, c.'s that contain granules which precipitate silver from an ammoniacal silver nitrate solution. See also enteroendocrine c.'s.
argyrophilic c.'s, c.'s that contain granules which precipitate silver only in the presence of a reducing agent. See also enteroendocrine c.'s.
Askanazy c., Hürthle c.
astroglia c., astrocyte.
auditory receptor c.'s, columnar c.'s in the epithelium of the organ of Corti, having hairs (stereocilia) on their apical ends. See Corti's c.'s.
B c., (1) beta c. of pancreas or of anterior lobe of hypophysis; (2) B *lymphocyte.*
balloon c., (1) an unusually large degenerated c. with pale-staining vacuolated or reticulated cytoplasm, as in viral hepatitis or in degenerated epidermal c.'s in herpes zoster; (2) a large form of nevus c. with abundant nonstaining cytoplasm, formed by vacular degeneration of melanosomes.
band c., band or stab neutrophil; rod nuclear c.; Schilling's band c.; stab or staff c.; any c. of the granulocytic (leukocytic) series that has a nucleus which could be described as a curved or coiled band, no matter how marked the indentation, if it does not completely segment the nucleus into lobes connected by a filament.
basal c., basilar c.; a c. of the deepest layer of stratified epithelium.
basaloid c., a c., usually of the epidermis, resembling a basal c.
basilar c., basal c.
basket c., (1) a neuron enmeshing the cell body of another neuron with its terminal axon ramifications; (2) smudge c.; (3) myoepithelial c.'s with branching processes which occur basal to the secretory c.'s of certain salivary gland and lacrimal gland alveoli.
basophil c. of anterior lobe of hypophysis, beta c. of anterior lobe of hypophysis.
beaker c., goblet c.
Beale's c., a bipolar ganglion c. of the heart with one spiral and one straight prolongation.
Berger c.'s, hilus c.'s.
berry c., a crenated red blood c. with surface spicules.
beta c. of anterior lobe of hypophysis, B c. (1); basophil c. of anterior lobe of hypophysis; one of a population of functionally diverse c.'s that contains basophilic granules and secrete hormones such as ACTH, lipotropin, thyrotropin, and the gonadotropins.
beta c. of pancreas, B c. (1); the predominant c. of the islets of Langerhans which secretes insulin.
Betz c.'s, Bevan-Lewis c.'s; large pyramidal c.'s in the motor area of the precentral gyrus of the cerebral cortex.
Bevan-Lewis c.'s, Betz c.'s.
bipolar c., a neuron having two processes, such as those of the retina or the spiral and vestibular ganglia of the eighth nerve.
Bizzozero's red c.'s, nucleated red blood c.'s in human blood.
blast c., an immature precursor c.; *e.g.,* erythroblast, lymphoblast, neuroblast. See also -blast.
blood c., blood corpuscle; one of the formed elements of the blood, a leukocyte or erythrocyte.
Boll's c.'s, basal c.'s in the lacrimal gland.
bone c., osteocyte.
border c.'s, c.'s forming the inner boundary of the organ of Corti.
Böttcher's c.'s, c.'s of the basilar membrane of the cochlea.
branchial c.'s, cartilage c.'s forming the branchial apparatus; possibly derived from the neural crest.
bristle c., hair c. of the inner ear.
bronchic c.'s, *alveoli* pulmonis.
brood c., mother c.
burr c., a crenated red blood c.
C c., (1) gamma c. of pancreas; a c. of the pancreatic islets of the guinea pig; (2) parafollicular c.
Cajal's c., (1) horizontal c. of Cajal; (2) astrocyte.
caliciform c., goblet c.
cameloid c., elliptocyte.
capsule c., amphicyte.
carrier c., phagocyte.
cartilage c., chondrocyte.
castration c.'s, castrate c.'s, signet ring c.'s (1); altered basophilic c.'s of the anterior lobe of the pituitary that develop following castration; the body of the c. is occupied by a large vacuole that displaces the nucleus to the periphery, giving the c. a resemblance to a signet ring.
caterpillar c., cardiac *histiocyte.*
centroacinar c., a c. of the pancreatic ductule that occupies the lumen of an acinus; it secretes bicarbonate and water, providing an alkaline pH necessary for enzyme activity in the intestine.
chalice c., goblet c.
chief c., the predominant cell type of a gland.
chief c. of corpus pineale, pinealocyte.
chief c. of parathyroid gland, a round clear c. with a centrally located nucleus; believed to secrete parathyroid hormone.
chief c. of stomach, zymogenic c.

chromaffin c., a c. that stains with chromic salts, in adrenal medulla and paraganglia of sympathetic nervous system.
chromophobe c.'s of anterior lobe of hypophysis, c.'s of the adenohypophysis that are devoid of specific acidophilic or basophilic granules when stained with common differential stains.
Clara c., a rounded, club-shaped, nonciliated c. protruding between ciliated c.'s in bronchiolar epithelium; believed to be secretory in function.
Claudius' c.'s, columnar c.'s on the floor of the ductus cochlearis external to the organ of Corti.
clear c., **(1)** a c. in which the cytoplasm appears empty with the light microscope, as occur in eccrine sweat glands and in the parathyroid glands when the glycogen is unstained; **(2)** any c., particularly a neoplastic one, containing abundant glycogen or other material which is not stained by hematoxylin or eosin, so that the c. cytoplasm is very pale in routinely stained sections.
cleavage c., blastomere.
cleaved c., a c. with single or multiple clefts in the nuclear membrane.
clonogenic c., a c. that has the potential to proliferate and give rise to a colony of c.'s; some daughter c.'s from each generation retain this potential to proliferate.
cochlear hair c.'s, Corti's c.'s; sensory c.'s in the organ of Corti in synaptic contact with sensory as well as efferent fibers of the cochlear (auditory) nerve; from the apical end of each c. about 100 stereocilia extend from the surface and make contact with the tectorial membrane.
column c.'s, neurons in the gray matter of the spinal cord whose axons are confined within the central nervous system.
commissural c., heteromeric c.; a neuron whose axon passes to the opposite side of the neuraxis.
compound granule c., gitter c.; gitterzelle; a microglial c. distended with phagocytosed debris.
cone c. of retina, cone (2).
connective tissue c., any of the c.'s of varied form occurring in connective tissue.
Corti's c.'s, cochlear hair c.'s.
crescent c., sickle c.
cytomegalic c.'s, c.'s containing large intranuclear and intracytoplasmic cytomegalic inclusion bodies.
cytotoxic c., suppressor c.
cytotrophoblastic c.'s, Langerhans' c.'s (2); stem c.'s that fuse to form the overlying syncytiotrophoblast of placental villi.
D c., delta c. of pancreas.
dark c.'s, c.'s in eccrine sweat glands having many ribosomes and mucoid secretory granules.
daughter c., one of the two or more c.'s resulting from the division of a parent c.
Davidoff's c.'s, Paneth's granular c.'s.
decidual c., an enlarged, ovoid connective tissue c. appearing in the endometrium of pregnancy.
decoy c.'s, benign exfoliated epithelial c.'s with pyknotic nuclei seen in urinary infections; may be mistaken for malignant c.'s.
deep c., mesangial c.
Deiters' c.'s, **(1)** phalangeal c.'s; **(2)** astrocytes.
delta c. of anterior lobe of hypophysis, a variety of c. having basophilic granules.
delta c. of pancreas, D c.; a c. of the islets having fine granules and containing somatostatin.
dendritic c.'s, in embryonic ectoderm, c.'s of neural crest origin with extensive processes; they early develop melanin.
Dogiel's c.'s, the different cell types in cerebrospinal ganglia.
dome c., one of the rounded surface c.'s of the periderm layer of the fetal epidermis.
Downey c., the atypical lymphocyte of infectious mononucleosis.
dust c., alveolar *macrophage.*
effector c., see effector.
egg c., the unfertilized ovum.
enamel c., ameloblast.
endodermal c.'s, entodermal c.'s; embryonic c.'s forming the yolk sac and giving rise to the epithelium of the alimentary tract and the parenchyma of associated glands.
endothelial c., one of the squamous c.'s forming the lining of blood and lymph vessels and the inner layer of the endocardium.
enterochromaffin c.'s, enteroendocrine c.'s.
enteroendocrine c.'s, enterochromaffin c.'s; Kulchitsky c.'s; c.'s with granules which may be either argentaffinic or argyrophilic; the c.'s, scattered throughout the digestive tract, are of several varieties and are believed to produce at least 20 different gastrointestinal hormones and neurotransmitters.
entodermal c.'s, endodermal c.'s.
ependymal c., a c. lining the central canal of the spinal cord (those of pyramidal shape) or one of the brain ventricles (those of cuboidal shape).
epidermic c., one of the c.'s of the epidermis.
epithelial c., one of the many varieties of c.'s that form epithelium.
epithelial reticular c., one of the many-branched epithelial c.'s that collectively form the supporting stroma for lymphocytes in the thymus; believed to produce thymosin and other factors that control thymic function.
epithelioid c., **(1)** a nonepithelial c. having certain characteristics of epithelium; **(2)** large mononuclear histiocytes having certain epithelial characteristics, particularly in tubercles where they are polygonal and have eosinophilic cytoplasm.
erythroid c., a c. of the erythrocytic series.
ethmoidal c.'s, *cellulae* ethmoidales.
external pillar c.'s, see pillar c.'s.
exudation c., exudation *corpuscle.*
Fañanás c., a specialized astrocyte found in the cerebellar cortex.
fasciculata c., a c. of the zona fasciculata of the adrenal cortex that contains numerous lipid droplets due to the presence of corticosteroids.
fat c., adipose c.; adipocyte; a connective tissue c. distended with one or more fat globules, the cytoplasm usually being compressed into a thin envelope, with the nucleus at one point in the periphery.
fat-storing c., lipocyte; a fat-filled c. present in the perisinusoidal space in the liver.
floor c., an obsolete term for the cell body of pillar c.'s in the floor of the arch of Corti.
foam c.'s, c.'s with abundant, pale-staining, finely vacuolated cytoplasm, usually histiocytes which have ingested or accumulated material that dissolves during tissue preparation, especially lipids. See also lipophage.
follicular epithelial c., a c. lining a follicle such as that of the thyroid gland.
follicular ovarian c.'s, c.'s of an ovarian follicle that surround the developing ovum; they form the stratum granulosum ovarii and cumulus oophorus.
foreign body giant c., a multinucleate "cell" or syncytium formed around particulate matter in chronic inflammatory reactions.
formative c.'s, inner cell mass c.'s of the blastocyst.
foveolar c.'s of stomach, theca c.'s of the foveolae of the stomach.
fuchsinophil c., a c. with a special affinity for fuchsin.
fusiform c.'s of cerebral cortex, spindle-shaped c.'s in the sixth layer of the cortex cerebri.
G c.'s, enteroendocrine c.'s that secrete gastrin, found primarily in the mucosa of the pyloric antrum of the stomach.
gamma c. of pancreas, C c. (1).
ganglion c., gangliocyte; originally, any nerve c. (neuron); in current usage, a neuron the c. body of which is located outside the limits of the brain and spinal cord, hence forming part of the peripheral nervous system; ganglion c.'s are either 1) the pseudounipolar c.'s of the sensory spinal and cranial nerves (sensory ganglia), or 2)

the peripheral multipolar motor neurons innervating the viscera (visceral or autonomic ganglia).
ganglion c.'s of dorsal spinal root, pseudounipolar nerve c. bodies in the ganglia of the dorsal spinal nerve roots; the sensory spinal nerves are composed of the peripheral axon branches of these sensory ganglion c.'s, whereas the central axon branch of each such c. enters the spinal cord as a component of the dorsal root.
ganglion c.'s of retina, the nerve c.'s of the retina whose central processes (fibers) form the optic nerve; their peripheral processes synapse with the bipolar c.'s and through them with the rod and cone c.'s; these c. bodies are round or flask-shaped and vary considerably in size.
Gaucher c.'s, large, finely and uniformly vacuolated c.'s derived from the reticuloendothelial system, and found especially in the spleen, lymph nodes, liver, and bone marrow of patients with Gaucher's disease; Gaucher c.'s contain kerasin (a cerebroside), which accumulates as a result of a genetically determined metabolic abnormality.
gemästete c., protoplasmic *astrocyte* (1).
gemistocytic c., protoplasmic *astrocyte* (1).
germ c., sex c.
germinal c., a c. from which other c.'s are proliferated.
ghost c., **(1)** a dead c. in which the outline remains visible, but without other cytoplasmic structures or stainable nucleus; **(2)** an erythrocyte after loss of its hemoglobin.
Giannuzzi's c.'s, serous *demilunes.*
giant c., a c. of large size, often with many nuclei.
gitter c. [Ger. *Gitterzelle,* fr. *Gitter,* lattice, wire-net], compound granule c.
glia c.'s, see neuroglia.
glitter c.'s, polymorphonuclear leukocytes that stain pale blue with gentian violet and contain cytoplasmic granules that exhibit brownian movement; observed in urine sediment and characteristic of pyelonephritis.
globoid c., a large c. of mesodermal origin that is found clustered in the intracranial tissues in globoid cell leukodystrophy.
glomerulosa c., a c. of the zona glomerulosa of the adrenal cortex that is the source of aldosterone; the c.'s are arranged in spherical or oval groups.
goblet c., beaker, caliciform, or chalice c.; an epithelial c. that becomes distended with a large accumulation of mucous secretory granules at its apical end, giving it the appearance of a goblet.
Golgi's c.'s, see Golgi type I *neuron;* Golgi type II *neuron.*
Golgi epithelial c., a glial cell found in the cerebellar cortex. See Bergman's *fibers.*
Goormaghtigh's c.'s, juxtaglomerular c.'s.
granule c.'s, **(1)** small nerve cell bodies in the external and internal granular layers of the cerebral cortex; **(2)** nerve cell bodies, of which only the nuclei are usually seen, in the granular layer of the cerebellar cortex.
granule c. of connective tissue, mast c.
granulosa c., a c. of the membrana granulosa lining the vesicular ovarian follicle which becomes a luteal c. of the corpus luteum after ovulation.
granulosa lutein c.'s, c.'s derived from the membrana granulosa of a mature ovarian follicle which secrete both estrogen and progesterone, and form the major component of the corpus luteum.
great alveolar c.'s, type II c.'s; granular pneumonocytes; cuboidal c.'s connected with the squamous pulmonary alveolar c.'s and having in their cytoplasm lamellated bodies (cytosomes) which represent the source of the surfactant that coats the alveoli.
guanine c., a c. whose cytoplasm contains glistening crystals of guanine.
gustatory c.'s, taste c.'s.
gyrochrome c., see gyrochrome.
hair c.'s, sensory epithelial c.'s present in the organ of Corti, in the maculae and cristae of the membranous labyrinth of the ear, and in taste buds; they are characterized by having long stereocilia or kinocilia (or both) which, with the light microscope, appear as fine hairs. See also vestibular hair c.'s; cochlear hair c.'s; taste c.'s.
hairy c.'s, medium sized leukocytes which have features of reticuloendothelial c.'s and multiple cytoplasmic projections (hairs) on the c. surface, but which may be a variety of B lymphocyte; they are found in hairy cell leukemia.
heart failure c., siderophore.
HeLa c.'s, the first continuously cultured human malignant c.'s, derived from a cervical carcinoma of a patient, Henrietta Lacks; used in the cultivation of viruses.
helmet c., a schistocyte shaped like a military helmet.
helper c., inducer c.; a subset of T lymphocytes that acts in cooperation with B lymphocytes to permit antibody formation.
HEMPAS c.'s, the abnormal erythrocytes of type II congenital dyserythropoietic anemia.
Hensen's c., one of the supporting c.'s in the organ of Corti, immediately to the outer side of the c.'s of Deiters.
heteromeric c., commissural c.
hilus c.'s, c.'s; in the hilus of the ovary which produce androgens; they are thought to be the ovarian counterpart of the interstitial c.'s of the testis.
hobnail c.'s, c.'s characteristic of a mesonephroma; a round expansion of clear cytoplasm projects into the lumen of neoplastic tubules, but the basal part of the c. containing the nucleus is narrow.
Hofbauer c., a large c. in the connective tissue of the chorionic villi; it appears to be a type of phagocyte.
horizontal c. of Cajal, Cajal's c. (1); a small fusiform c. found in the superficial layer of the cerebral cortex with its long axis placed horizontally.
horizontal c.'s of retina, c.'s in the outer part of the inner nuclear layer of the retina which lie with their axes more or less parallel with the surface. They are thought to connect the rods of one part of the retina with cones of another part.
Hortega c.'s, microglia.
Hürthle c., Askanazy c.; a large, granular eosinophilic c. derived from thyroid follicular epithelium by accumulation of mitochondria, *e.g.,* in Hashimoto's disease.
I c., inclusion c.; a cultured skin fibroblast containing membrane-bound inclusions.
immunologically activated c., an immunocyte that carries out an immune response, in contradistinction to an immunologically competent c.
immunologically competent c., a small lymphocyte capable of being immunologically activated by exposure to a substance that is antigenic (immunogenic) for the respective c.; activation involves either the capacity to produce antibody or the capacity to participate in the delayed type of sensitivity.
inclusion c., I c.
indifferent c., an undifferentiated, nonspecialized c.
inducer c., helper c.
intercapillary c., mesangial c.
internal pillar c.'s, see pillar c.'s.
interstitial c.'s, **(1)** Leydig's c.'s; c.'s between the seminiferous tubules of the testis which secrete testosterone; **(2)** c.'s derived from the theca interna of atretic follicles of the ovary; they resemble luteal c.'s and are an important source of estrogens; **(3)** pineal c.'s similar to glial c.'s with long processes.
irritation c., Türk's c.
islet c., one of the c.'s of the pancreatic islets.
Ito c.'s, fat-containing c.'s lining hepatic sinusoids.
juvenile c., metamyelocyte.
juxtaglomerular c.'s, Goormaghtigh's c.'s; c.'s, located at the vascular pole of the renal corpuscle which secrete renin and form a component of the juxtaglomerular complex; they are modified smooth muscle c.'s primarily of the afferent arteriole of the renal

glomerulus.
karyochrome c., see karyochrome.
killer c.'s, K c.'s, null c.'s (1); cytotoxic c.'s involved in c.-mediated immune responses; they appear to be T lymphocytes of the suppressor subset with receptors for the Fc portion of IgG molecules, and lyse or damage IgG coated target c.'s without mediation of complement.
Kulchitsky c.'s, enteroendocrine c.'s.
Kupffer c.'s, stellate c.'s of liver; reticuloendothelial c.'s lining the hepatic sinusoids.
lacis c. (lah-sē′) [Fr. *lacis,* meshwork], one of the c.'s of the juxtaglomerular apparatus found at the vascular pole of the renal corpuscle.
Langerhans' c.'s, (1) dendritic clear c.'s in the epidermis, containing distinctive granules which appear rod- or racket-shaped in section, but lacking tonofilaments, melanosomes, and desmosomes; they carry surface receptors for immunoglobulin (Fc) and complement (C3), and are believed to be antigen fixing and processing c.'s of monocytic origin; active participants in cutaneous delayed hypersensitivity. **(2)** centroacinar c.'s.
Langhans' c.'s, (1) Langhans'-type giant c.'s; multinucleated giant c.'s seen in tuberculosis and other granulomas; the nuclei are arranged in an arciform manner at the periphery of the c.'s; **(2)** cytotrophoblastic c.'s.
Langhans'-type giant c.'s, Langhans' c.'s (1).
LE c., lupus erythematosus c.; a polymorphonuclear leukocyte containing an amorphous round body which is a phagocytosed nucleus from another cell plus serum antinuclear globulin (IgG) and complement; formed *in vitro* in the blood of patients with systemic lupus erythematosus, or by the action of the patient's serum on normal leukocytes.
Leishman's chrome c.'s, basophilic granular leukocytes (basophils) observed in the circulating blood of some persons with blackwater fever.
lepra c.'s, distinctive, large, mononuclear phagocytes (macrophages) with a foamlike cytoplasm, and also poorly staining saclike structures resulting from degeneration of such c.'s, observed characteristically in leprous inflammatory reactions; indistinct staining results from numerous, fairly closely packed leprosy bacilli, which are acid-fast and resistant to staining by ordinary methods but may be vividly demonstrated by acid-fast staining procedures.
Leydig's c.'s, interstitial c.'s (1).
light c.'s of thyroid, parafollicular c.'s.
lining c., littoral c.
Lipschütz c., centrocyte (1).
littoral c. [L. *littoralis,* the seashore], lining c.; the c.'s lining the lymphatic sinuses of lymph nodes and the blood sinuses of bone marrow.
Loevit's c.'s, erythroblasts.
lupus erythematosus c., LE c.
luteal c., lutein c., a c. of the corpus luteum of the ovary which is derived from the granulosa cells of the preovulatory follicle; it secretes progesterone and estrogen.
lymph c., lymphocyte.
lymphoid c., a parenchymal c. of lymphatic tissue.
macroglia c., astrocyte.
malpighian c., a c. of the stratum spinosum of the epidermis.
Marchand's wandering c., a c. of the reticuloendothelial system.
marrow c., any c. of bone marrow, especially hemopoietic c.'s.
Martinotti's c., a small multipolar nerve c. with short branching dendrites scattered through various layers of the cerebral cortex; its axon ascends toward the surface of the cortex.
mast c., labrocyte; mastocyte; granule c. of connective tissue; tissue basophil; a connective tissue c. that contains coarse, basophilic, metachromatic granules; the c. is believed to contain heparin and histamine.
mastoid c.'s, *cellulae* mastoideae.
Mauthner's c., a large neuron of the spinal cord with its c. body located in the metencephalon of fish and amphibia.
Merkel's tactile c., *meniscus* tactus.
mesangial c., deep or intercapillary c.; a phagocytic c. in the capillary tuft of the renal glomerulus, interposed between endothelial c.'s and the basement membrane in the central or stalk region of the tuft.
mesenchymal c.'s, fusiform or stellate c.'s found between the ectoderm and endoderm of young embryos; the shape of the c.'s in fixed material is indicative of the fact that in life they were moving from their place of origin to areas where they would become reaggregated and specialized; most mesenchymal c.'s are derived from established mesodermal layers, but in the cephalic region they also develop from neural crest or neural tube ectoderm; they are the most strikingly pluripotential c.'s in the embryonic body, developing at different locations into any of the types of connective or supporting tissues, to smooth muscle, to vascular endothelium, or to blood cells.
mesoglial c.'s, mesoglia.
mesothelial c., one of the flat c.'s of mesothelium lining serous membranes.
Mexican hat c., target c. (1).
Meynert's c.'s., solitary pyramidal c.'s found in the cortex in the region of the calcarine fissure.
microglia c.'s, microglial c.'s, microglia.
middle c.'s, *sinus* mediae.
midget bipolar c.'s, bipolar c.'s in the inner nuclear layer of the retina that synapse with individual cone c.'s in the outer plexiform layer; other larger bipolar c.'s in the inner nuclear layer synapse with both rod and cone c.'s; the axons of both types synapse in the inner plexiform layer with the dendrites of the ganglion c.'s.
Mikulicz' c.'s, foamy macrophages containing *Klebsiella rhinoscleromatis;* found in the mucosal nodules in rhinoscleroma.
mirror-image c., (1) a c. whose nuclei have identical features and are placed in the cytoplasm in similar fashion; **(2)** a binucleate form of Reed-Sternberg c. often found in Hodgkin's disease; the twin nuclei are disposed in relation to an imaginary plane between them like a single nucleus together with its image in a mirror.

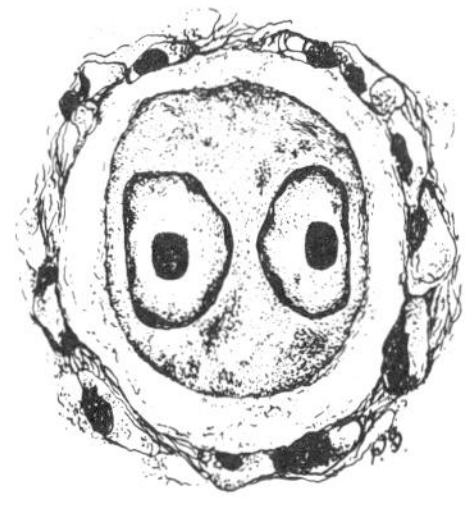

Mirror-Image Cell

mitral c.'s, large nerve c.'s in the olfactory lobe of the brain whose dendrites synapse (in glomeruli) with axons of the olfactory receptor c.'s of the nasal mucous membrane, and whose axons pass centrally in the olfactory tract to the olfactory cortex.
monocytoid c., a c. having morphological characteristics of a monocyte but which is nonphagocytic.
mossy c., one of the two types of neuroglia c.'s, consisting of a rather large body with numerous short branching processes.
mother c., brood or parent c.; metrocyte; a c. which, by division, gives rise to two or more daughter c.'s.
motor c., a neuron whose axon innervates peripheral effector c.'s such as muscle fibers or gland c.'s.
mucoalbuminous c.'s, mucoserous c.'s.
mucoserous c.'s, mucoalbuminous c.'s; seromucous c.'s; glandu-

lar c.'s intermediate in histologic characteristics between serous and mucous c.'s.
mucous c., a c. secreting mucus; *e.g.,* a goblet c.
mucous neck c., one of the mucin-secreting c.'s in the neck of a gastric gland.
Müller's radial c.'s, Müller's *fibers* (2).
multipolar c., a nerve c. with a number of dendrites arising from the c. body.
mural c., a nonendothelial c. enclosed within the basement membrane of retinal capillaries.
myeloid c., specifically, any young c. that develops into a mature granulocyte of blood, but frequently used as a synonym for marrow c.
myoepithelial c., a smooth muscle c. of ectodermal origin, found in a number of organs such as mammary, sweat, and lacrimal glands.
myoid c.'s, peritubular contractile c.'s; flattened smooth muscle-like c.'s of mesodermal origin which lie just outside the basal lamina of the seminiferous tubule.
Nageotte c.'s, c.'s found in the cerebrospinal fluid, one or two per cubic millimeter in health, but in greater numbers in various diseases.
natural killer c.'s, NK c.'s; spleen c.'s from normal (*i.e.,* nonimmunized) mice or blood lymphocytes from humans which lyse 'target' c.'s (tumor or virus-infected c.'s) without involvement of antibody or complement; the c.'s seem to be pre-T lymphocytes, but the mechanism involved in their killing activity is not clear; some, but not all, have surface Fc receptors, and interferon seems to play an as yet unexplained role.
nerve c., neuron (1).
Neumann's c.'s, nucleated c.'s in the bone marrow developing into red blood c.'s.
neurilemma c.'s, Schwann c.'s.
neuroendocrine c., **(1)** see neuroendocrine (2); **(2)** paraneurone.
neuroendocrine transducer c., an endocrine c. that releases its hormonal product into the bloodstream only upon receipt of a nervous impulse.
neuroepithelial c.'s, neuroepithelium.
neuroglia c.'s, see neuroglia.
neurolemma c.'s, Schwann c.'s.
neuromuscular c., a c. of a lower metazoan organism that is both sensitive and contractile.
neurosecretory c.'s, nerve c.'s, such as those of the hypothalamus, that elaborate a chemical substance (such as a releasing factor, neuropeptide, or, more rarely, a true hormone) that influences the activity of another structure (*e.g.,* anterior lobe of the hypophysis). See also neurosecretion.
nevus c., nevocyte; the c. of a pigmented cutaneous nevus which differs from a normal melanocyte in that it lacks dendrites.
Niemann-Pick c., Pick c.
NK c.'s, natural killer c.'s.
noble c.'s, obsolete term for the c.'s of the organs, nerves, and muscles, *i.e.,* the differentiated c.'s of the body as distinguished from the fixed or connective tissue and wandering c.'s having phagocytic properties.
nonclonogenic c., a c. that does not give rise to a colony of c.'s (large numbers of c.'s that are genetically identical); may undergo two or more c. divisions, but all daughter c.'s are destined to die or differentiate (lose all potential to divide).
null c.'s, **(1)** killer c.'s.; **(2)** c.'s of the adenohypophysis or lymphocytes which fail to be labeled with specific antibody markers for the major hormones produced by the adenohypophysis or for certain membrane-associated proteins of lymphocytes.
nurse c.'s, Sertoli c.'s.
oat c., a short, bluntly spindle-shaped c. that contains a relatively large, hyperchromatic nucleus, frequently observed in some forms of undifferentiated bronchogenic carcinoma.
OKT c.'s [*Ortho-Kung T* cell], monoclonal antibodies to T lymphocyte substrates: OKT-3 c.'s are T lymphocytes as a class, since all share a common leukocyte differentiation antigen; OKT-4 c.'s are helper c.'s; OKT-8 c.'s are suppressor c.'s. OKT-4/OKT-8 expresses the ratio of helper to suppressor c.'s, sometimes used as a measure of the functional status of the immune system and thus a basis for clinical diagnosis and prognosis.
olfactory receptor c.'s, Schultze's c.'s; very slender nerve c.'s, with large nuclei and surmounted by six to eight long, sensitive cilia in the olfactory epithelium at the roof of the nose; they are the receptors for smell.
oligodendroglia c.'s, see oligodendroglia.
Opalski c., a characteristically altered glial c. in the basal ganglia and thalamus in hepatolenticular degeneration.
osseous c., osteocyte.
osteochondrogenic c., one of the undifferentiated c.'s in the inner layer of the periosteum of an endochondrally developing bone capable of developing into an osteoblast or a chondroblast.
osteogenic c., one of the c.'s in the inner layer of the periosteum which forms osseous tissue.
osteoprogenitor c., preosteoblast; a mesenchymal c. that differentiates into an osteoblast.
oxyntic c., parietal c.
oxyphil c.'s, oxyphil (1); c.'s of the parathyroid gland which increase in number with age; the cytoplasm contains numerous mitochondria and stains with eosin. Similar c.'s, and tumors composed of them, are found in salivary glands and the thyroid; in the latter, also called Hürthle c.'s.
P c., a characteristic specialized c., with probable pacemaker function, found in the S-A node and A-V junction.
packed human blood c.'s, whole blood from which plasma has been removed; may be prepared any time during the dating period of the whole blood from which it is derived, but not later than six days after the blood has been drawn if separation of plasma and c.'s is achieved by centrifugation.
Paget's c.'s, pagetoid c.'s, relatively large, neoplastic epithelial c.'s (carcinoma c.'s) with hyperchromatic nuclei and palely staining cytoplasm; in Paget's disease of the breast, such c.'s occur in neoplastic epithelium in the ducts and in the epidermis of the nipple, areola, and adjacent skin.
Paneth's granular c.'s, Davidoff's c.'s; c.'s, located at the base of intestinal glands of the small intestine, which contain large acidophilic refractile granules and may produce lysozyme.
parafollicular c.'s, C c.'s (2); light c.'s of thyroid; c.'s present between follicles or interspersed among follicular c.'s; they are rich in mitochondria and are believed to be the source of thyrocalcitonin.
paraganglionic c.'s, c.'s of the embryonic sympathetic nervous system that become chromaffin c.'s.
paraluteal c., theca luteum c.
parenchymal c., see parenchyma.
parenchymatous c. of corpus pineale, pinealocyte.
parent c., mother c.
parietal c., acid or oxyntic c.; one of the c.'s of the gastric glands; it lies upon the basement membrane, covered by the chief c.'s, and secretes hydrochloric acid which reaches the lumen of the gland through fine intracellular and intercellular canals (canaliculi).
peptic c., zymogenic c.
pericapillary c., pericyte.
peripolar c., a granular c. located where the parietal and visceral capsules of the renal corpuscle meet; part of the c. faces the filtration space of Bowman.
perithelial c., pericyte.
peritubular contractile c.'s, myoid c.'s.
pessary c., a red blood c. in which the hemoglobin has disappeared from the center, leaving only the periphery visible.
phalangeal c.'s, Deiters' c.'s (1); the supporting c.'s of the organ of Corti, attached to the basement membrane and receiving between

their free extremities the hair c.'s. See also phalanx (2).
pheochrome c., (1) former term for enteroendocrine c.; (2) pheochromocyte.
photoreceptor c.'s., rod and cone c.'s of the retina.
physaliphorous c., c.'s containing a bubbly or vacuolated cytoplasm, *e.g.,* as characteristically seen in chordoma.
Pick c., Niemann-Pick c.; a relatively large, rounded or polygonal, mononuclear c., with indistinctly or palely staining, foamlike cytoplasm that contains numerous droplets of a phosphatide, sphingomyelin; such c.'s are widely distributed in the spleen and other tissues, especially those rich in reticuloendothelial components, in patients with Niemann-Pick disease.
pigment c., a c. containing pigment granules.
pigment c.'s of iris, c.'s of the stromal layer of the iris; in dark eyes (but not in blue) they contain granules of pigment.
pigment c.'s of retina, c.'s in the outermost layer of the retina that contain pigment granules.
pigment c. of skin, melanocyte.
pillar c.'s, pillar c.'s of Corti; Corti's pillars or rods; tunnel c.'s; c.'s forming the outer and inner walls of the tunnel in the organ of Corti.
pillar c.'s of Corti, pillar c.'s.
pineal c.'s, c.'s of the corpus pineale or pinealocyte.
plasma c., plasmacyte; an ovoid c. with an eccentric nucleus having chromatin arranged like a clock face or spokes of a wheel; the cytoplasm is strongly basophilic because of the abundant RNA in its endoplasmic reticulum; plasma c.'s are derived from B type lymphocytes and are active in the formation of antibodies.
pluripotent c.'s, primordial c.'s which may still differentiate into various specialized types of tissue elements; *e.g.,* mesenchymal c.'s.
polar c., polar *body.*
polychromatic c., polychromatophil c.; a primitive erythrocyte in bone marrow, with basophilic material as well as hemoglobin (acidophilic) in the cytoplasm.
polychromatophil c., polychromatic c.
posterior c.'s, *sinus* posteriores.
pregnancy c.'s, hypophysial chromophobe c.'s that increase in number and accumulate eosinophil granules during pregnancy.
pregranulosa c.'s, capsular c.'s surrounding the primordial ova in the embryonic ovary; they are derived from celomic epithelium.
prickle c., spine c.; one of the c.'s of the stratum spinosum of the epidermis; so called because of atypical shrinkage artifacts that occur in histological preparations, resulting in intercellular bridges at points of desmosomal adhesion.
primary embryonic c., in a very young embryo, a c. still capable of differentiation.
primitive reticular c., a c. with processes making contact with those of other similar c.'s to form a cellular network; along with the network of reticular fibers, the reticular c.'s form the stroma of bone marrow and lymphatic tissues.
primordial c., a c. from a group that constitutes the primordium of an organ or part of the embryo.
primordial germ c., gonocyte; the most primitive undifferentiated sex cell, found initially outside the gonad.
prolactin c., mammotroph.
pseudo-Gaucher c., a plasma c., microscopically resembling a Gaucher c., found in the bone marrow in some cases of multiple myeloma.
pseudounipolar c., unipolar *neuron.*
pseudoxanthoma c., relatively large phagocytic c.'s (macrophages) that contain numerous small lipid vacuoles or hemosiderin (or both), in organizing hemorrhagic or inflammatory lesions.
pulpar c., the specific macrophagic c. of the spleen substance.
Purkinje's c.'s, Purkinje's corpuscles; large nerve c.'s of the cerebellar cortex with a piriform cell body and dendrites arranged in a plane transverse to the folium.
pus c., pus *corpuscle.*
pyramidal c.'s, neurons of the cerebral cortex which, in sections perpendicular to the cortical surface, exhibit a triangular shape with a long apical dendrite directed toward the surface of the cortex; there are also lateral dendrites, and a basal axon which descends to deeper layers.
pyrrol c., pyrrhol c., a reticuloendothelial element that has a special affinity for pyrrol blue, taking up the dye by a process of pinocytosis.
Raji c., a c. of a cultured line of lymphoblastoid c.'s derived from a Burkitt's lymphoma; it possesses numerous receptors for certain complement components and is thus suitable for use in detection of immune complexes.
reactive c., protoplasmic *astrocyte* (1).
red blood c. (rbc, RBC), erythrocyte.
Reed-Sternberg c.'s, Reed c.'s, Sternberg, or Sternberg-Reed c.'s; large transformed lymphocytes generally regarded as pathognomonic of Hodgkin's disease; a typical c. has a pale-staining acidophilic cytoplasm and one or two large nuclei showing marginal clumping of chromatin and unusually conspicuous deeply acidophilic nucleoli; binucleate Reed-Sternberg c.'s frequently show a mirror-image form (mirror-image c.).
Renshaw c.'s, inhibitory interneurons that are innervated by collaterals from motoneurons and in turn form synapses with the same and adjacent motoneurons to exert inhibition; identified physiologically but not by Golgi technic.
resting c., a quiescent c.; one not undergoing mitosis.
resting wandering c., fixed macrophage.
restructured c., the viable c. produced by fusion of a karyoplast with a cytoplast.
reticular c., see primitive reticular c.
reticularis c., a c. of the zona reticularis of the innermost part of the adrenal cortex.
reticuloendothelial c., a c. of the reticuloendothelial system.
rhagiocrine c., macrophage.
Rieder c.'s, abnormal myeloblasts (12 to 20 μm in diameter) in which the nucleus may be widely and deeply indented (*i.e.,* suggestive of lobulation), or may actually be a bi- or multi-lobate structure; such c.'s are frequently observed in acute leukemia, and probably represent a more rapid maturation of the nucleus than that of the cytoplasm.
Rindfleisch's c.'s, obsolete eponym for eosinophilic *leukocytes.*
rod nuclear c., band c.
rod c. of retina, rod (2).
Rolando's c.'s, the nerve c.'s in Rolando's gelatinous substance of the spinal cord.
rosette-forming c.'s, T lymphocytes with an affinity for sheep erythrocytes and which, when suspended in serum, bind the uncoated, nonsensitized erythrocytes in a rosette formation.
Rouget c., spider c. (2); capillary pericyte; a c. with several slender processes that embraces the capillary wall in amphibia.
sarcogenic c., myoblast.
satellite c.'s, c.'s surrounding the c. body of a ganglion c. and continuous with the neurolemma of the processes.
satellite c. of skeletal muscle, sarcoplast; an elongated spindle-shaped c. occupying depressions in the sarcolemma and between it and the basal lamina; believed to play a role in muscle repair and regeneration by fusing with adjacent myofiber.
scavenger c., phagocyte.
Schilling's band c., band c.
Schultze's c.'s, olfactory receptor c.'s.
Schwann c.'s, neurolemma or neurilemma c.'s; c.'s of ectodermal (neural crest) origin that compose a continuous envelope around each nerve fiber of peripheral nerves; such c.'s are comparable to the oligodendroglia c.'s of brain and spinal cord; like the latter, they may form membranous expansions that wind around axons and thus form the axon's myelin sheath.
segmented c., a polymorphonuclear leukocyte matured beyond

the band c. so that two or more lobes of the nucleus occur.
sensitized c., **(1)** a c., including a bacterial c., that has combined with specific antibody to form a complex capable of reacting with complement components; **(2)** a small, "committed," c. derived, by division and differentiation, from a transformed lymphocyte.
septal c., a round pale c. of the lungs in the septa between the pulmonary alveoli.
seromucous c.'s, mucoserous c.'s.
serous c., albuminous c. (1); a c., especially of the salivary gland, that secretes a watery or thin albuminous fluid, as opposed to a mucous c.
Sertoli's c.'s, nurse c.'s; elongated c.'s in the seminiferous tubules to which spermatids are attached during spermiogenesis; they secrete androgen-binding protein and establish the blood-testis barrier by forming tight junctions with adjacent Sertoli's c.'s.
sex c., germ c.; a spermatozoon or an ovum.
Sézary c., an atypical T-lymphocyte seen in the peripheral blood in the Sézary syndrome; it has a large convoluted nucleus and scanty cytoplasm containing PAS -positive vacuoles.
shadow c.'s, smudge c.'s.
sickle c., crescent c.; drepanocyte; meniscocyte; an abnormal, crescentic erythrocyte that is characteristic of sickle c. anemia, resulting from an inherited abnormality of hemoglobin (hemoglobin S) causing decreased solubility at low oxygen tension.
signet ring c.'s, **(1)** castration c.'s; **(2)** c.'s containing a cytoplasmic droplet of mucus that compresses the nucleus to one side of the c.; found in certain adenocarcinomas.
silver c., one of a number of c.'s seen in plaques of multiple sclerosis, having round or oval nuclei, the body of the c. containing many yellow or light brown particles; the c.'s are characteristic of multiple sclerosis, but are found in other conditions, including syphilis.
skein c., reticulocyte.
small cleaved c., a lymphoid c. of follicular center c. origin which has an irregularly shaped nucleus with clumped chromatin, absent nucleoli, and one or more clefts in the nuclear membrane.
smudge c.'s, basket c.'s (2); shadow c.'s; Gumprecht's shadows; immature leukocytes of any type that have undergone partial breakdown during preparation of a stained smear or tissue section, because of their greater fragility; smudge c.'s are seen in largest numbers in acute leukemia.
somatic c.'s, the c.'s of an organism, other than the germ c.'s.
sperm c., spermatozoon.
spider c., **(1)** astrocyte; **(2)** Rouget c.; **(3)** a c. in a rhabdomyoma of the heart, with central nucleus and cytoplasmic mass connected to the cell wall by strands of cytoplasm separated by clear glycogen-filled areas.
spindle c., a fusiform c., such as those in the deeper layers of the cerebral cortex.
spine c., prickle c.
splenic c.'s, large round ameboid c.'s (macrophages) in the splenic pulp.
squamous c., a flat scalelike epithelial c.
squamous alveolar c.'s, type I c.'s; highly attentuated squamous c.'s that form the gas-permeable epithelium lining the alveoli of the lungs.
stab c., band c.
staff c., band c.
standard c., an electrical c. having a definite known voltage; used to calibrate other electric c.'s.
stellate c.'s of cerebral cortex, small star-shaped c.'s in the second and fourth layers of the cortex, and large stellate c.'s in the deeper part of the third layer in the visual cortex.
stellate c.'s of liver, Kupffer c.'s.
stem c., a c. whose daughter c.'s may differentiate into other c. types.
Sternberg-Reed c.'s, Sternberg c.'s, Reed-Sternberg c.'s.
stichochrome c., see stichochrome.
strap c., an elongated tumor c. of uniform width which may show cross-striations; found in rhabdomyosarcoma.
supporting c., sustentacular c.
suppressor c., cytotoxic c.; a subset of T lymphocytes that inhibits antibody formation by B lymphocytes and is involved in immune tolerance and in autoimmunity.
surface mucous c.'s of stomach, theca c.'s of stomach; c.'s lining the gastric surface and foveolae; a glycoprotein product at the apical end of each c. is secreted and forms a mucous protective film.
sustentacular c., supporting c.; one of the ordinary elongated c.'s resting on the basement membrane which surround and serve as a support to the shorter specialized c.'s in certain organs, such as the labyrinth of the inner ear or olfactory epithelium.
sympathetic formative c., a neuroblast of the embryonic autonomic nervous system.
sympathicotropic c.'s, c.'s in the hilum of the ovary associated with unmyelinated nerve fibers.
sympathochromaffin c., one of the c.'s in the embryo from which both sympathetic ganglion c.'s and chromaffin c.'s are developed.
synovial c., a c. in the synovial membrane of joints lying between the collagenous fibers.
T c., T *lymphocyte.*
tactile c., touch c.; one of the epithelioid c.'s of a corpusculum tactus.
tanned red c.'s, erythrocytes subjected to mild treatment with chemicals such as tannic acid so that they adsorb onto their surface soluble antigens; used in hemagglutination tests.
target c., **(1)** Mexican hat c.; an erythrocyte in target c. anemia, with a dark center surrounded by a light band which again is encircled by a darker ring; it thus resembles a shooting target; such c.'s also appear after splenectomy; **(2)** a c. lysed by cytotoxic T lymphocytes, as in graft rejection.
tart c., a monocyte with an engulfed nucleus in which the structure is still well preserved.
taste c.'s, gustatory c.'s; darkly staining c.'s in a taste bud that appear to have extending into the gustatory pore long hairlike microvilli containing a number of closely packed microtubules; the taste c.'s stand in synaptic contact with sensory nerve fibers of the facial, glossopharyngeal, or vagus nerves.
tendon c.'s, elongated fibroblastic c.'s arranged in rows between the collagenous tendon fibers.
theca lutein c., paraluteal c.; a steroid secretory c. of the corpus luteum that comes from the theca interna of the ovarian follicle at the time of ovulation.
theca c.'s of stomach, surface mucous c.'s of stomach.
Tiselius electrophoresis c., the special container in a Tiselius apparatus containing the solution to be analyzed electrophoretically.
totipotent c., an undifferentiated c. capable of developing into any type of c.; *e.g.,* the fertilized ovum.
touch c., tactile c.
Touton giant c., a xanthoma c. in which the multiple nuclei are grouped around a small island of nonfoamy cytoplasm.
transducer c., any c. responding to a mechanical, thermal, photic, or chemical stimulus by generating an electrical impulse synaptically transmitted to a sensory neuron in contact with the c.
transitional c., any c. thought to represent a phase of development from one form to another.
tubal air c.'s, *cellulae* pneumaticae tubae auditivae.
tufted c., a particular type of c. in the olfactory bulb comparable to the bulb's mitral c. with respect to afferent and efferent relationships, but smaller and more superficially located.
tunnel c.'s, pillar c.'s.
Türk c., irritation c.; Türk's leukocyte; a relatively large, immature c. with certain morphologic features resembling those of a plasma c., although the nuclear pattern is similar to that of a myeloblast; found in circulating blood only in pathologic conditions.
tympanic c.'s, *cellulae* tympanicae.

type II c.'s, great alveolar c.'s.
Tzanck c.'s, acantholytic c.'s seen in the Tzanck test.
undifferentiated c., a primitive c. that has not assumed the morphologic and functional characteristics which it will later acquire.
unipolar c., unipolar *neuron.*
vasoformative c., angioblast (1).
veil c., an antigen-presenting c. that has veil-like cytoplasmic processes and circulates in the blood and lymph.
vestibular hair c.'s, c.'s in the sensory epithelium of the maculae and cristae of the membranous labyrinth of the inner ear; afferent and efferent nerve fibers of the vestibular nerve end synaptically upon them; from the apical end of each c. a bundle of stereocilia and a kinocilium extend into the membrana statoconiorum of the maculae and the cupula of the cristae.
Virchow's c.'s, (1) the lacunae in osseous tissue containing the bone c.'s; also the bone c.'s themselves; **(2)** corneal *corpuscles.*
virus-transformed c., a c. that has been genetically changed to a tumor c., the change being hereditarily transmitted to daughter c.'s; c.'s transformed by oncornaviruses continue to produce virus in high concentration without being killed; DNA tumor virus-transformed c.'s develop (along with other changes) tumor-specific transplantation antigens and do not produce virus.
visual receptor c.'s, the rod and cone c.'s of the retina.
vitreous c., hyalocyte; a c. occurring in the peripheral part of the vitreous body which may be responsible for production of hyaluronic acid and possibly of collagen.
wandering c., ameboid c. (1).
Warthin-Finkeldey c.'s, giant c.'s with multiple overlapping nuclei, found in lymphoid tissue in measles, especially during the prodromal stage.
wasserhelle c., water-clear c. of parathyroid.
water-clear c. of parathyroid, wasserhelle c.; a variety of chief c., so-called because the cytoplasm contains much glycogen that is not preserved or stained in the usual preparation.
white blood c. (WBC), leukocyte.
WI-38 c.'s [*W*istar *I*nstitute], the first normal human cells, derived from fetal lung tissue, continuously cultivated.
wing c., one of the polyhedral c.'s in the corneal epithelium beneath the surface layer.
yolk c.'s, primitive embryonic c.'s lying between the endoderm and mesoderm; they probably give rise to the endothelium of vitelline vessels.
zymogenic c., albuminous c. (2); chief c. of stomach; peptic c.; a c. that secretes an enzyme; specifically a chief c. of a gastric gland or an acinar c. of the pancreas.

cella, gen. and pl. **cellae** (sel'ă, sel'ē) [L. storeroom, or compartment]. A room or cell.
c. me'dia, *pars* centralis ventriculi lateralis.

cellicolous (se-lik'ō-lŭs) [L. *cella,* cells, + *colere,* to abide in]. Living within cells.

cellobiase (sel-ō-bī'ās). β-D-Glucosidase.

cellobiose (sel-ō-bī'ōs). Cellose; a disaccharide obtained from cellulose; a glucose-(β1-4)-glucoside, differing only in the nature of the glycoside bond from maltose, which is α-linked.

cellohexose (sel-ō-heks'ōs). Glucose.

celloidin (se-loy'din). A solution of pyroxylin in ether and alcohol, used for embedding histologic specimens.

cellon (sel'on). Tetrachloroethane.

cellona (sel-ō'nă). A cellulose bandage impregnated with plaster of Paris.

cellose (sel'ōs). Cellobiose.

cellula, gen. and pl. **cellulae** (sel'yū-lă, -lē) [L. a small chamber, dim. of *cella*]. **1** [NA]. Cellule; in gross anatomy, a small but macroscopic compartment. **2.** In histology, a cell.
cel'lulae anterio'res, *sinus* anteriores.
cel'lulae co'li, *haustra* coli.
cel'lulae ethmoida'les [NA], ethmoidal cells; the numerous small air-filled cells in the ethmoidal labyrinth. See also *sinus* anteriores, *sinus* mediae, and *sinus* posteriores.
cel'lulae mastoid'eae [NA], mastoid cells; mastoid sinuses; numerous small intercommunicating cavities in the mastoid process of the temporal bone that empty into the mastoid or tympanic antrum.
cel'lulae me'diae, *sinus* mediae.
cel'lulae pneumat'icae tu'bae auditi'vae [NA], tubal air cells; occasional small air cells in the inferior wall of the auditory tube, near the tympanic orifice, communicating with the tympanic cavity.
cel'lulae posterio'res, *sinus* posteriores.
cel'lulae tympan'icae [NA], tympanic cells; numerous groovelike depressions in the walls of the tympanic cavity, communicating with the tubal air cells.

cellular (sel'yū-lăr) [L. *cellula,* dim. of *cella,* storeroom]. **1.** Relating to, derived from, or composed of cells. **2.** Having numerous compartments or interstices.

cellularity (sel-yū-lar'i-tē). The degree, quality, or condition of cells which are present.

cellulase (sel'yū-lās) [EC 3.2.1.4]. Endo-1,4-β-glucase; an enzyme catalyzing the hydrolysis of 1,4-β-glucoside links in cellulose and other β-D-glucans; found in a variety of microorganisms in soil and in the digestive tracts of herbivores.

cellule (sel'yūl). Cellula (1).

cellulicidal (sel'yū-li-sī'dăl) [cellula + L. *caedo,* to kill]. Destructive to cells.

cellulifugal (sel-yū-lif'yū-găl) [cellula + L. *fugio,* to flee]. Moving from, or extending in a direction away from, a cell or cell body; denoting certain cells repelled by other cells, or processes extending from the body of a cell.

cellulin (sel'yū-lin). Cellulose.

cellulipetal (sel-yū-lip'ĕ-tăl) [cellula + L. *peto,* to seek]. Moving toward, or extending in a direction toward, a cell or cell body.

cellulite (sel'yū-līt). **1.** Colloquial term for deposits of fat and other material believed to be trapped in pockets beneath the skin. **2.** Lipoedema.

cellulitis (sel-yū-lī'tis). Inflammation of cellular or connective tissue.
acute scalp c., nonlocalized inflammation of the scalp without suppuration.
dissecting c., *perifolliculitis* abscedens et suffodiens.
eosinophilic c., Wells' *syndrome.*
epizootic c., equine viral *arteritis.*
pelvic c., parametritis.
phlegmonous c., obsolete term for diffuse *phlegmon.*

cellulosan (sel'yū-lō-san). Hemicellulose.

cellulose (sel'yū-lōs). Cellulin; a polysaccharide comprised of cellobiose residues, differing in this respect from starch, which is comprised of maltose residues; it forms the basis of vegetable fiber and is the most abundant organic compound.
c. acetate, a polymer commonly used as a support medium for electrophoresis.
c. acetate phthalate, a reaction product of phthalic anhydride and a partial acetate ester of c.; used as a tablet-coating agent.
carboxymethyl c., CM-cellulose; c. in which some of the OH groups are modified to contain $—CH_2—COOH$ groups; used in column chromatography.
diethylaminoethyl c., DEAE-cellulose; c. to which diethylaminoethyl groups have been attached; used in anion-exchange chromatography.
microcrystalline c., purified, partially depolymerized c., pre-

pared by treating α-cellulose, obtained as a pulp from fibrous plant material, with mineral acids; used as a tablet diluent.
oxidized c., **(1)** cellulosic acid in the form of an absorbable gauze; used as a hemostatic in operations where ligation is not feasible (capillary or venous bleeding from small vessels) because cellulosic acid has a pronounced affinity for hemoglobin and produces an artificial clot; **(2)** a sterile absorbable substance prepared by the oxidation of cotton containing not less than 16% and not more than 22% of carboxyl. See also oxycellulose.

cellulosic acid (sel-yū-los'ik). See oxidized *cellulose.*

celo-. **1** [G. *koilōma,* hollow (celom)]. Combining form relating to the celom. **2** [G. *kēlē,* hernia]. Combining form meaning hernia. **3** [G. *koilia,* belly]. Combining form relating to abdomen. See also celio-.

celom, celoma (sē'lom, sēlō'mă) [G. *koilōma,* a hollow]. Coelom. **1.** The cavity between the splanchnic and somatic mesoderm in the embryo. **2.** The general body cavity in the adult.
extraembryonic c., that portion of the c. that extends beyond the confines of the embryonic body.

celomic (sē-lom'ik). Relating to the celom, or body cavity.

celonychia (sē-lō-nik'ē-ă) [G. *koilos,* hollowed, + *onyx* (*onych-*), nail]. Koilonychia.

celophlebitis (sē-lō-flĕ-bī'tis) [G. *koilos,* hollow, + phlebitis]. Cavitis; inflammation of a vena cava.

celoschisis (sē-los'ki-sis) [G. *koilia,* belly, + *schisis,* a fissure]. Obsolete term for gastroschisis.

celoscope (sē'lō-skōp) [G. *koilos,* hollow, + *skopeō,* to view]. Cavascope; cavernoscope; an optical device for examining the interior of a body cavity.

celoscopy (sē-los'kŏ-pē). Cavernoscopy; examination of any body cavity with an optical instrument.

celosomia (sē-lō-sō'mē-ă) [G. *kēlē,* hernia, + *sōma,* body]. Congenital protrusion of the abdominal or thoracic viscera, usually with defect of the sternum and ribs as well as of the abdominal walls.

celothelium (sē-lō-thē'lē-ŭm). Obsolete term for mesothelium.

celotomy (sē-lot'ō-mē) [G. *kēlē,* hernia, + *tomē,* incision]. Herniotomy.

celozoic (sē-lō-zō'ik) [G. *koilos,* hollow, + *zoikos,* pertaining to animals]. Inhabiting any of the cavities of the body; applied to certain parasitic protozoa, chiefly gregarines.

Celsius, Anders, Swedish astronomer, 1701–1744. See C. *scale.*

Celsus, Aulus (Aurelius) Cornelius, Roman physician and medical writer, *ca.* 30 B.C.–45 A.D. See C.'s *alopecia, area, kerion, papules, vitiligo.*

cement (se-ment') [see cementum]. **1.** Cementum. **2.** In dentistry, a nonmetallic material used for luting, filling, or permanent or temporary restorative purposes, made by mixing components into a plastic mass which sets, or as an adherent sealer in attaching various dental restorations in or on the tooth.
composite dental c., an organic dental c. modified by the inclusion of inorganic materials treated with a coupling agent to bond them to the polymers.
copper phosphate c., a dental preparation, the combination of a solution of orthophosphoric acid with a c. powder (usually zinc oxide, pretreated) modified with varying proportions of copper oxide.
dental c., see cement (2).
inorganic dental c., a dental c. consisting usually of metallic salts or oxides which, when mixed with a specific liquid, form a plastic mass that sets.
intercellular c., a hypothetical adhesive substance formerly believed to occur between some epithelial cells.
modified zinc oxide-eugenol c., dental c. obtained by mixing zinc oxide and eugenol with one or more additives.
organic dental c., a dental c. consisting mainly of synthetic polymers.
polycarboxylate c., a powder containing primarily zinc oxide mixed with a liquid containing polyacrylic acid which reacts to form a hard crystalline mass upon standing; when used to lute metal castings to teeth, it has the potential of bonding to the calcium contained in tooth structure as well as to any base metals contained in the casting.
silicate c., a dental filling material prepared by mixing a modified phosphoric acid solution with a powdered silica alumina fluoride glass.
tooth c., **(1)** cementum; **(2)** see cement (2).
unmodified zinc oxide-eugenol c., a dental c. obtained by mixing zinc oxide and eugenol without modifiers.
zinc phosphate c., a powder, containing primarily zinc oxide mixed with a liquid containing orthophosphoric acid to form a hard crystalline mass on standing, used in dentistry as a luting agent for cast metal restorations and orthodontic bands, and as a temporary restorative material, or a base under restorations, particularly in deep cavities.

cementation (sē-men-tā'shŭn). **1.** The process of attaching parts by means of a cement. **2.** In dentistry, attaching a restoration to natural teeth by means of a cement.

cementicle (se-men'ti-kl). A calcified spherical body, composed of cementum lying free within the periodontal membrane, attached to the cementum or imbedded within it.

cementification (se-men'ti-fi-kā'shŭn). Metaplastic production of cementum or cementoid within a less differentiated connective tissue, *e.g.,* c. of a fibroma.

cementoblast (se-men'tō-blast) [L. *cementum,* cement, + G. *blastos,* germ]. One of the cells concerned with the formation of the layer of cementum on the roots of teeth.

cementoblastoma (se-men'tō-blas-tō'mă). Benign c.; true cementoma; a benign odontogenic tumor of functional cementoblasts; it appears as a mixed radiolucent-radiopaque lesion attached to a tooth root and may cause expansion of the bone cortex or be associated with pain.
benign c., cementoblastoma.

cementoclasia (se-men-tō-klā'zē-ă) [L. *cementum,* cement, + G. *klasis,* fracture]. Destruction of cementum by cementoclasts.

cementoclast (se-men'tō-klast) [L. *cementum,* cement, + G. *klastos,* broken]. One of the multinucleated giant cells, identical with osteoclasts, that are associated with the destruction of cementum.

cementocyte (se-men'tō-sīt) [L. *cementum,* cement, + G. *kytos,* cell]. An osteocyte-like cell with numerous processes, trapped in a lacuna in the secondary cementum of the tooth.

cementodentinal (se-men'tō-den'ti-năl). Dentinocemental.

cementoma (se-men-tō'mă) [L. *cementum,* cement, + G. *-ōma,* tumor]. Nonspecific term referring to any benign cementum-producing tumor; four types are recognized: 1) periapical cemental dysplasia, 2) central ossifying fibroma, 3) cementoblastoma, 4) sclerotic cemental mass. When the type is not specified, c. usually refers to periapical cemental dysplasia.
gigantiform c., sclerotic cemental *mass.*
true c., cementoblastoma.

cementum (se-men'tŭm) [L. *caementum,* rough quarry stone, fr. *caedo,* to cut] [NA]. Cement (1); tooth cement (1); substantia ossea dentis; a layer of bonelike mineralized tissue covering the dentin of the root and neck of a tooth which blends with the fibers of the periodontal ligament.
afibrillar c., c. which, with the electron microscope, appears as laminated, electron-dense reticular material that sometimes overlies the enamel of the tooth.

primary c., c. that has no cementocytes; may cover the entire root of the tooth, but often is missing on the apical third of the root.
secondary c., c. that forms on the root surface after eruption; it contains cementocytes.

cenesthesia (sē-nes-thē′zē-ă) [G. *koinos,* common, + *aisthēsis,* sensation]. Coenesthesia; sixth sense; the general sense of bodily existence; the sensation caused by the functioning of the internal organs.

cenesthesic, cenesthetic (sē-nes-thē′zik, -sik; -thet′ik). Relating to cenesthesia.

cenesthopathy (sē-nes-thop′ă-thē) [G. *koinos,* common, + *aisthēsis,* sensation, + *pathos,* suffering]. A feeling or sense of general ill-being not related to any particular organ or part of the body.

ceno-. **1** [G. *koinos,* common]. Combining form meaning shared in common. **2** [G. *kainos,* new]. Combining form meaning new or fresh. **3** [G. *kenos,* empty]. Rarely used combining form denoting emptiness. See also coeno-.

cenocyte (sē′nō-sīt) [G. *koinos,* common, + *kytos,* cell]. Coenocyte; a multinucleate cell or hypha without cross walls, characteristic of the hyphae of Zygomycetes (Phycomycetes). See also nonseptate *mycelium.*

cenocytic (sē-nō-sit′ik). Coenocytic; pertaining to or having characteristics of a cenocyte.

cenogenesis (sē-nō-jen′ĕ-sis) [G. *kainos,* new, + *genesis,* a producing]. Production of characters differing from those of one's ancestors. *Cf.* palingenesis.

cenosite (sē′nō-sīt) [G. *koinos,* common, + *sitos,* food]. Coinosite; a facultative commensal organism; one that can sustain itself apart from its usual host.

cenotrope (sē′nō-trōp) [G. *koinos,* common, + *tropē,* a turning]. The behavior pattern shown by all members of a large group having the same biologic equipment and same experience.

censor (sen′sōr) [L. a judge, critic, fr. *censeo,* to value, judge]. In psychoanalytic theory, the psychic barrier that prevents certain unconscious thoughts and wishes from coming to consciousness unless they are so cloaked or disguised as to be unrecognizable.

center (sen′ter) [L. *centrum;* G. *kentron*]. **1.** The middle point of a body; loosely, the interior of a body. **2.** A group of nerve cells governing a specific function.
anospinal c., the c. in the spinal cord that controls the contraction of the anal sphincter.
Broca's c., Broca's field or area; motor speech c.; the posterior part of the inferior frontal gyrus of the left, or dominant, hemisphere, corresponding approximately to Brodmann's area 44; Broca identified this region as an essential component of the motor mechanisms governing articulated speech.
Budge's c., ciliospinal c.
cell c., cytocentrum.
chondrification c., a site of earliest cartilage formation in the body.
ciliospinal c., Budge's c.; the preganglionic motor neurons in the first thoracic segment of the spinal cord which give rise to the sympathetic innervation of the dilator muscle of the eye's pupil.
dentary c., a specific ossification c. of the mandible that gives rise to the lower border of its outer plate.
diaphysial c., primary c. of ossification in the shaft of a long bone.
epiotic c., the c. of ossification of the petrous part of the temporal bone that appears posterior to the posterior semicircular canal.
expiratory c., the region of the medulla oblongata that is electrically active during expiration and where electrical stimulation produces sustained expiration.
feeding c., colloquial and somewhat provisional term indicating a region of the lateral zone of the hypothalamus, electrical stimulation of which in the rat elicits uninterrupted eating; destruction of the region causes long-lasting anorexia.
germinal c. of Flemming, reaction c.; the lightly staining c. in a lymphatic nodule in which the predominant cells are large lymphocytes and macrophages.
inspiratory c., the region of the medulla oblongata that is electrically active during inspiration and where electrical stimulation produces sustained inspiration.
Kerckring's c., Kerckring's ossicle; an occasional independent ossification c. in the occipital bone; it appears in the posterior margin of the foramen magnum at about the sixteenth week of gestation.
medullary c., *centrum* semiovale.
motor speech c., Broca's c.
ossific c., the area of earliest destruction of cartilage prior to onset of ossification.
c. of ossification, *punctum* ossificationis.
primary c. of ossification, *punctum* ossificationis primarium.
reaction c., germinal c. of Flemming.
respiratory c., the region in the medulla oblongata concerned with integrating afferent information to determine the signals to the respiratory muscles; the inspiratory and expiratory c.'s considered together.
c. of ridge, the buccolingual midline of the residual ridge.
rotation c., a point or line around which all other points in a body move. See axis.
satiety c., colloquial term referring to the region of the ventromedial nucleus in the hypothalamus; destruction of this small region in the rat leads to continuous eating and extreme obesity.
secondary c. of ossification, *punctum* ossificationis secondarium.
semioval c., *centrum* semiovale.
sensory speech c., Wernicke's c.
speech c.'s, areas of the cerebral cortex centrally involved in speech function; one is in the left inferior frontal gyrus, a second one in the supramarginal, angular, and first and second temporal gyri. See also Broca's c. and Wernicke's c.
sphenotic c., one of the paired c.'s of ossification of the sphenoid bone.
vital c., c. essential to life, usually refers to the centers located in the medulla oblongata which are necessary for the maintenance of respiration and circulation.
Wernicke's c., Wernicke's area, field, region, or zone; sensory speech c.; the region of the cerebral cortex thought to be essential for understanding and formulating coherent, propositional speech; it encompasses a large region of the parietal and temporal lobes near the lateral sulcus of the left cerebral hemisphere; corresponding approximately to Brodmann's areas 40, 39, and 22.

Centers for Disease Control (CDC). The federal facility for disease eradication, epidemiology, and education headquartered in Atlanta, Georgia, which encompasses the Center for Infectious Diseases, Center for Environmental Health, Center for Health Promotion and Education, Center for Prevention Services, Center for Professional Development and Training, and Center for Occupational Safety and Health. Formerly named Center for Disease Control (1970), Communicable Disease Center (1946).

centesis (sen-tē′sis) [G. *kentēsis,* puncture, fr. *kenteō,* to prick, pierce]. Puncture, especially when used as a suffix, as in paracentesis.

centi- (c) [L. *centum,* one hundred]. Prefix used in the SI and metric systems to signify one hundredth (10^{-2}).

centibar (sen′ti-bar). One hundredth of a bar.

centigrade (C) (sen′ti-grād) [L. *centum,* one hundred, + *gradus,* step, degree]. **1.** Consisting of 100 degrees. See centigrade *scale.* **2.** One hundredth of a circle, equal to 3.6° of the astronomical circle.

centigram (sen′ti-gram). One hundredth of a gram; 0.1543 grain.

centiliter (sen'ti-lē-ter). One hundredth of a liter; 10 milliliters; 162.3 minims.

centimeter (cm) (sen'ti-mē-ter). One hundredth of a meter; 0.3937 inch.

cubic c. (cc, c.c.), one thousandth of a liter; 1 milliliter.

centimorgan (cM) (sen'ti-mōr-găn). See morgan.

centinormal (sen-ti-nōr'măl). One hundredth normal; denoting the concentration of a solution.

centipede (sen'ti-pēd) [L. *centum,* hundred, + *pes (ped-),* foot]. A venomous predatory arthropod of the order Chilopoda, characterized by one pair of legs per leg-bearing segment. The venom is injected through the first pair of leg-like appendages, modified into piercing claws; the bites may be painful and locally necrotic, but seldom are dangerous, except to very young children. Genera found in the U.S. include *Scutigera, Lithobius, Scolopendra,* and *Geophilus.*

centipoise (sen'ti-poyz). One hundredth of a poise.

centra (sen'tră). Plural of centrum.

centrad (sen'trad). **1.** Toward the center. **2.** A unit of measurement of the refracting strength of a prism; it corresponds to the deviation of a ray of light, the arc of which is $^{1}/_{100}$ of the radius of the circle, or 0.57°; it is expressed by the symbol ∇.

centrage (sen'trāj). The condition in which the optical centers of all the reflecting and refracting surfaces of an optical system are on the same axis.

centralis (sen-trā'lis) [L.] [NA]. Central; in the center.

centre médian de Luys (sen'tr mā-dē-an) [Fr.]. *Nucleus* centromedianus.

centrencephalic (sen'tren-se-fal'ik). Relating to the center of the encephalon.

-centric [G. *kentron,* center]. Combining form, in suffix position, denoting having a center (of a specific kind or number) or having a specific thing as its center (of interest, focus, etc.).

centric (sen'trik). Pertaining to a center.

centriciput (sen-tris'i-put) [L. *centrum,* center, + *caput,* head]. The central portion of the upper surface of the skull, between the occiput and the sinciput.

centrifugal (sen-trif'yū-găl) [L. *centrum,* center, + *fugio,* to flee]. **1.** Denoting the direction of the force pulling an object outward (away) from an axis of rotation. **2.** Sometimes, by analogy, extended to describe any movement away from a center. *Cf.* eccentric (2).

centrifugalization (sen-trif'yū-găl-i-zā'shŭn). Centrifugation.

centrifugalize (sen-trif'yū-găl-īz). Centrifuge (2).

centrifugation (sen-trif-yū-gā'shŭn). Centrifugalization; subjection to sedimentation, by means of a centrifuge, of solids suspended in a fluid.

density gradient c., ultracentrifugation of substances in concentrated solutions of cesium salts or of sucrose; at equilibrium, the medium exhibits a concentration (hence density) gradient increasing in the direction of centrifugal force and the substances of interest collect in layers at the levels of their densities.

centrifuge (sen'tri-fūj). **1.** An apparatus by means of which particles in suspension in a fluid are separated by spinning the fluid, the centrifugal force throwing the particles to the periphery of the rotated vessel. **2.** Centrifugalize; to submit to rapid rotary action, as in a c.

centrilobular (sen-tri-lob'yū-lăr). At or near the center of a lobule, *e.g.,* of the liver.

centriole (sen'trē-ōl) [G. *kentron,* a point, center]. Tubular structures, 150 nm by 300 to 500 nm, with a wall having 9 triple microtubules, usually seen as paired organelles lying in the cytocentrum; c.'s may be multiple and numerous in some cells, such as the giant cells of bone marrow.

distal c., the c. in the developing spermatozoon from which the flagellum develops.

proximal c., the c. that lies next to the head of the developing spermatozoon.

centripetal (sen-trip'ĕ-tăl) [L. *centrum,* center, + *peto,* to seek]. **1.** Afferent. **2.** Axipetal; denoting the direction of the force pulling an object toward an axis of rotation.

centro- [G. *kentron,* center]. Combining form relating to a center.

centroblast (sen'trō-blast) [centro- + G. *blastos,* germ]. A lymphocyte with a large non-cleaved nucleus.

Centrocestus (sen-trō-ses'tŭs) [G. *kentron,* point, center, + *kestos,* belt, both words fr. *kenteo,* to pierce]. A genus of extremely small fish-borne flukes (family Heterophyidae) that may produce intestinal lesions similar to those caused by *Heterophyes heterophyes. C. formosana* has been reported from man in Taiwan.

centrocyte (sen'trō-sīt) [centro- + G. *kytos,* cell]. **1.** Lipschütz cell; a cell whose protoplasm contains single and double granules of varying size stainable with hematoxylin; seen in lesions of lichen planus. **2.** A lymphocyte with a small cleaved nuclei.

centrokinesia (sen'trō-ki-nē'sē-ă) [centro- + G. *kinēsis,* movement]. Movement excited by a stimulus of central origin.

centrokinetic (sen'trō-ki-net'ik). **1.** Relating to centrokinesia. **2.** Excitomotor.

centrolecithal (sen-trō-les'i-thăl) [centro- + G. *lekithos,* yolk]. Denoting an ovum in which the deutoplasm accumulates centrally.

centromere (sen'trō-mēr) [centro- + G. *meros,* part]. **1.** Kinetochore; the nonstaining primary constriction of a chromosome which is the point of attachment of the spindle fiber and to provide the mechanism of chromosome movement during cell division; the c. divides the chromosome into two arms, and its position is constant for a specific chromosome: near one end (acrocentric), near the center (metacentric), or between (submetacentric). **2.** Obsolete term for the neck of the spermatozoon.

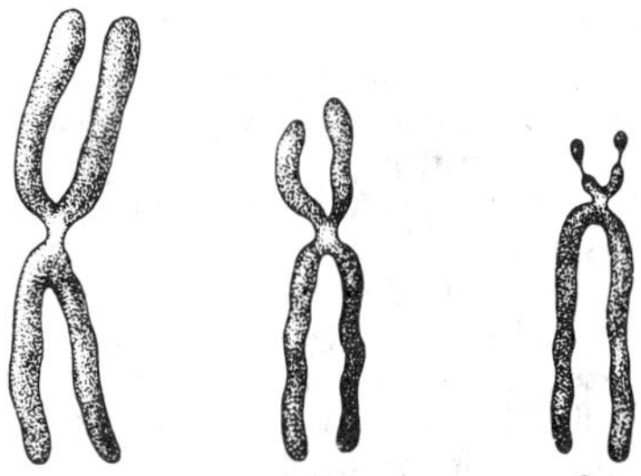

Normal Positions of the Centromere
A, metacentric; *B,* submetacentric; *C,* acrocentric, with satellites.

centroplasm (sen'trō-plazm) [centro- + G. *plasma,* thing formed]. The substance of the cytocentrum.

centrosome (sen'trō-sōm) [centro- + G. *sōma,* body]. Cytocentrum.

centrosphere (sen'trō-sfēr) [centro- + G. *sphaira,* a ball, sphere]. Astrocele; statosphere; the specialized, often gelated cytoplasm of the cytocentrum from which the astral fibers (microtubules) extend during mitosis.

centrostaltic (sen-trō-stal'tik) [centro- + G. *stallein,* set forth, fetch]. Relating to the center of motion.

centrum, pl. centra (sen'trŭm, sen'tră) [L. fr. G. *kentron*] [NA]. A center of any kind, especially an anatomical center.

c. media'num, *nucleus* centromedianus.

c. medulla're, c. semiovale.
c. ova'le, c. semiovale.
c. semiova'le, semioval center, medullary center; c. medullare; c. ovale; Vicq d'Azyr's c. semiovale; Vieussens' c.; the great mass of white matter composing the interior of the cerebral hemisphere; the name refers to the general shape of this white core in horizontal sections of the hemisphere.
c. tendin'eum diaphrag'mae [NA], central tendon of diaphragm; trefoil tendon; a three-lobed fibrous sheet occupying the center of the diaphragm.
c. tendin'eum peri'nei [NA], central tendon of perineum; perineal body; Savage's perineal body; the fibromuscular mass between the anal canal and the urogenital diaphragm in the median plane.
c. of a vertebra, **(1)** the ossification center of the central mass of the body of a vertebra; **(2)** the body of a vertebra as distinct from the arches.
Vicq d'Azyr's c. semiova'le, c. semiovale.
Vieussens' c., c. semiovale.
Willis' c. nervo'sum, *ganglia* celiaca.

Centruroides (sen-tru-roy'dēz), A genus of North American scorpions, the commonest species of which are *C. gracilis,* the margarite scorpion; *C. vittatus,* the stripe-back scorpion; and *C. sculpturatus,* the deadly sculptured scorpion. See also Scorpionida.

cenuris (se-nyū'ris) [G. *konos,* empty, + G. *uris,* tail]. A tapeworm bladderworm with multiple inverted scoleces attached to the inner germinative layer; produced by taeniid cestodes of the genus *Multiceps,* typically found in the brain or tissues of herbivores and the adult worm in the intestine of wolves, dogs, or other canids; rare cases of c. infections in man have been reported.

cenurosis, cenuriasis (sen-yū-rō'sis, sen-yū-rī'ă-sis). Coenurosis; disease produced by the presence of a cenuris cyst that, in sheep, causes a brain infection known as "gid" for the giddy gait induced in the infected animal; human c. has been reported but is extremely unusual, in contrast with hydatid disease.

CEP Abbreviation for congenital erythropoietic *porphyria.*

cephaeline (sef-a'ē-lēn). Desmethylemetine; dihydropsychotrine; $C_{28}H_{38}N_2O_2$; an alkaloid of ipecac; an emetic and amebicide.

Cephaelis (sef-ă-ē'lis) [G. *kephalē,* head, + *eilō,* to roll up, pack close]. *Uragoga.*

cephal-. See cephalo-.

cephalad (sef'ă-lad). Craniad; in a direction toward the head.

cephalalgia (sef'al-al'jē-ă) [cephal- + G. *algos,* pain]. Headache.
histaminic c., cluster *headache.*
Horton's c., cluster *headache.*

cephalea (sef-ă-lē'ă). Headache.
c. agita'ta, c. atton'ita, violent headache sometimes occurring in influenza and in the early stages of other infectious diseases.

cephaledema (sef'al-ē-dē'mă). Edema of the head.

cephalemia (sef-ă-lē'-mē-ă) [cephal- + G. *haima,* blood]. Congestion, active or passive, of the brain.

cephalexin (sef-ă-lek'sin). A broad spectrum antibiotic derived from cephalosporin C.

cephalhematocele (sef'ăl-hē-mat'ō-sēl) [cephal- + G. *haima,* blood, + *kēlē,* tumor]. Cephalohematocele; a cephalhematoma communicating with the cerebral sinuses.

cephalhematoma (sef'ăl-hē-mă-tō'mă) [cephal- + G. *haima,* blood, + *-ōma,* tumor]. Cephalohematoma; a blood cyst of the scalp in a newborn infant, due to an effusion of blood beneath the pericranium; contrasted with caput succedaneum, in which the effusion overlies the periosteum and consists of serum.

cephalhydrocele (sef-ăl-hī'drō-sēl) [cephal- + G. *hydōr,* water, + *kēlē,* tumor]. An extracranial serous cyst.

cephalic (se-fal'ik). Cranial (1).

cephalin (sef'ă-lin). Kephalin; a term formerly applied to a group of phosphatidic esters resembling lecithin but containing ethanolamine or serine in the place of choline; these are now known as phosphatidylethanolamine and phosphatidylserine. It is widely distributed in the body, especially in the brain and spinal cord, and is used as a local hemostatic and as a reagent in liver function test.

cephaline (sef'ă-līn). Denoting members of the protozoan suborder Cephalina (order Eugregarinida), characterized by bodies divided into chambers (anterior protomerite and posterior deutomerite, or anterior epimerite, protomerite, and terminal deutomerite); all are parasites of invertebrates.

cephalitis (sef-ă-lī'tis). Encephalitis.

cephalization (sef'ăl-ĭ-zā'shŭn). **1.** Evolutionary tendency for important functions of the nervous system to move forward in the brain. **2.** Initiation and concentration of the growth tendency at the anterior end of the embryo.

cephalo-, cephal- [G. *kephalē,* head]. Combining forms denoting the head.

cephalocaudal (sef'ă-lō-kaw'dăl) [cephalo- + L. *cauda,* tail]. Cephalocercal; relating to both head and tail, *i.e.,* to the long axis of the body.

cephalocele (sef'ă-lō-sēl). Encephalocele.

cephalocentesis (sef'ă-lō-sen-tē'sis) [cephalo- + G. *kentēsis,* puncture]. Passage of a hollow needle or trocar and cannula into the brain to drain or aspirate an abscess or the fluid of a hydrocephalus.

cephalocercal (sef'ă-lō-ser'kăl) [cephalo- + G. *kerkos,* tail]. Cephalocaudal.

cephalochord (sef'ă-lō-kōrd). Intracranial portion of the notochord in the embryo.

cephalodidymus (sef'ă-lō-did'i-mŭs) [cephalo- + G. *didymos,* twin]. Conjoined twins fused except in the cephalic region; a variety of duplicitas anterior.

cephalodiprosopus (sef'ă-lō-dī-pros'ō-pŭs) [cephalo- + G. *di-,* two, + *prosōpon,* face]. Asymmetrical conjoined twins with the head of the autosite carrying a reduced parasitic head. See also *diprosopus* parasiticus.

cephalodynia (sef'ă-lō-din'ē-ă) [cephalo- + G. *odynē,* pain]. Headache, specifically due to rheumatism of the fibrous structure of the scalp muscle.

cephalogenesis (sef'ă-lō-jen'ē-sis) [cephalo- + G. *genesis,* production]. Formation of the head in the embryonic period.

cephaloglycin (sef'a-lō-glī'sin). A semisynthetic broad spectrum antibiotic produced from cephalosporin C.

cephalogram (sef'ă-lō-gram). cephalometric *roentgenogram.*

cephalogyric (sef'ă-lō-jī'rik) [cephalo- + G. *gyros,* a circle]. Relating to circular movements of the head.

cephalohematocele (sef'ă-lō-hē-mat'ō-sēl). Cephalhematocele.

cephalohematoma (sef'ă-lō-hē-mă-tō'mă). Cephalhematoma.

cephalohemometer (sef'ă-lō-hē-mom'ē-ter) [cephalo- + G. *haima,* blood, + *metron,* measure]. An instrument showing the degree of intracranial blood pressure.

cephalomegaly (sef'ă-lō-meg'ă-lē) [cephalo- + G. *megas,* great]. Enlargement of the head.

cephalomelus (sef-ă-lom'ē-lŭs) [cephalo- + G. *melos,* a limb]. Malformed individual with an excrescence resembling a leg or arm, growing from the head.

cephalomeningitis (sef'ă-lō-men-in-jī'tis) [cephalo- + G. *mēninx* [*mening-*], membrane]. Inflammation of the membranes of the brain.

cephalometer (sef-ă-lom'ē-ter) [cephalo- + G. *metron,* measure]. Cephalostat; an instrument used to position the head to produce oriented, reproducible lateral and posterior-anterior headfilms.

cephalometrics (sef-ă-lō-met′riks) [cephalo- + G. *metron,* measure]. In oral surgery and orthodontics: **1.** The scientific measurement of the bones of the cranium and face, utilizing a fixed, reproducible position for lateral radiographic exposure of skull and facial bones. **2.** A scientific study of the measurements of the head with relation to specific reference points; used for evaluation of facial growth and development, including soft tissue profile.

cephalometry (sef-ă-lom′ĕ-trē) [cephalo- + G. *metron,* measure]. Measurements on the living head, or head without removal of the soft parts. See also cephalometrics.

ultrasonic c., Measurement of the fetal head by ultrasound.

cephalomotor (sef′ă-lō-mō′ter). Relating to movements of the head.

Cephalomyia (sef′ă-lō-mī′yă) [cephalo- + G. *myia,* fly]. Former name for *Oestrus.*

cephalont (sef′ă-lont) [cephalo- + G. *ōn (ont-),* being]. Adult stage of a cephaline gregarine, a sporozoan parasite commonly found in arthropods and other invertebrate hosts. The body is usually divided by a septum into an anterior epimerite and protomerite and a posterior deutomerite; acephaline gregarines lack a dividing septum.

cephalopagus (sef-ă-lop′ă-gŭs) [cephalo- + G. *pagos,* something fixed]. Conjoined twins with heads fused but the remainder of the bodies separate. See also craniopagus; *duplicitas* posterior.

cephalopathy (sef-ă-lop′ă-thē) [cephalo- + G. *pathos,* suffering]. Encephalopathy.

cephalopelvic (sef′ă-lō-pel′vik). Pertaining to the size of the fetal head in relation to the maternal pelvis.

cephalopelvimetry (sef′ă-lō-pel-vim′ĕ-trē). Pelvicephalography; pelvocephalography; roentgenographic measurement of the dimensions of the pelvis and the fetal head.

cephalopharyngeus (sef′ă-lō-fă-rin′jē-ŭs). See *musculus* constrictor pharyngis superior.

cephaloridine (sef-ă-lōr′i-dēn). A broad spectrum antimicrobial derived from cephalosporin C.

cephalorrhachidian (sef′ă-lō-ra-kid′ē-an) [cephalo- + G. *rhachis,* spine]. Relating to the head and the spine.

cephalosporanic acid (sef′ă-lō-spōr-an′ik). The basic chemical nucleus upon which cephalosporin antibiotic derivatives are based.

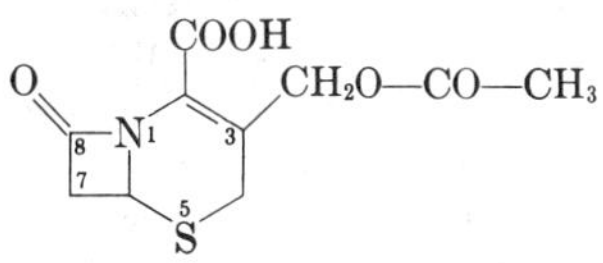

Cephalosporanic acid

cephalosporin (sef′ă-lō-spōr′in). One of several antibiotic substances obtained from *Cephalosporium acremonium, C. salmosynnematum,* and other fungi.

c. C, an antibiotic whose activity is due to the 7-aminocephalosporanic acid portion of the cephalosporanic acid molecule; it is effective against Gram-positive and Gram-negative bacteria, but is less potent than c. N. Addition of side chains produced semisynthetic broad spectrum antibiotics with greater antibacterial activity than that of c. C; the antibiotic activity is due to interference with bacterial cell-wall synthesis.

c. N, synnematin B; penicillin N; D-4-amino-4-carboxybutyl penicillinic acid; an antibiotic active against Gram-positive and Gram-negative bacteria, but inactivated by penicillinase; on hydrolysis it yields penicillamine.

c. P, a steroid antibiotic produced by *Cephalosporium,* chemically related to fusidic and helvolic acids, that is active only against Gram-positive bacteria.

cephalosporinase (sef′ă-lō-spōr′i-nās). *β*-Lactamase.

Cephalosporium (sef′ă-lō-spō′rē-ŭm). A genus of true fungi, usually a contaminant of laboratory media, but a few species have caused maduromycosis (mycetoma).

cephalostat (sef′ă-lō-stat) [cephalo- + G. *statos,* stationary]. Cephalometer.

cephalothin (sef-ă-lō′thin). 7-(Thiophene-2-acetamido)cephalosporanic acid; chemically modified cephalosporin C, a broad spectrum antibiotic.

cephalothoracic (sef′ă-lō-thō-ras′ik). Relating to the head and the chest.

cephalothoracoiliopagus (sef′ă-lō-thōr′ă-kō-il-i-op′ă-gŭs). Synadelphus.

cephalothoracopagus (sef′ă-lō-thōr-ă-kop′ă-gŭs) [cephalo- + G. *thorax,* chest, + *pagos,* something fixed]. Conjoined twins with the bodies fused in the cephalic and thoracic regions.

c. asym′metros, c. monosymmetros.

c. disym′metros, a form of c. with the fused head showing equally developed faces directed laterally.

c. monosym′metros, c. asymmetros; a form of c. in which only one of the faces is well developed.

cephalotome (sef′ă-lō-tōm) [cephalo- + G. *tomē,* a cutting]. Instrument formerly used for cutting into the fetal head to permit its compression in cases of dystocia.

cephalotomy (sef-ă-lot′ō-mē). Formerly used operation of cutting into the head of the fetus.

cephalotoxin (sef′ă-lōtok′sin). A poison, believed to be a protein, found in the salivary glands of cephalopods (octopus). See also eledoisin.

cephalotribe (sef′ă-lō-trīb) [G. *tribō,* to rub, bruise]. Forceps-like instrument, with strong blades and a screw handle, formerly used to crush the fetal head in cases of dystocia.

cephapirin sodium (sef-ă-pī′rin). A semisynthetic broad spectrum antibiotic derived from cephalosporin C; it is used by injection.

cephradine (sef′ră-dēn). A semisynthetic broad spectrum antibiotic derived from cephalosporin C; used orally and by injection.

-ceptor [L. *capio,* pp. *captus,* to take]. Suffix meaning taker or receiver.

ceptor (sep′ter, tōr) [L. *capio,* pp. *ceptus,* to take]. Receptor (2).

chemical c., c. that initiates chemical reactions in response to the appropriate stimuli.

contact c., a nerve c. in the surface layer of skin or mucous membrane by means of which impulses contributed by direct physical impact are received.

distance c., a nerve mechanism of one of the organs of special sense whereby the being is brought into relation with his distant environment.

cera (sē′ră) [L.]. Wax (1).

ceraceous (se-rā′shŭs) [L. *cera,* wax]. Waxen.

ceramidase (ser-am′i-dās). An enzyme that cleaves ceramides into sphingosine and fatty acids.

ceramide (ser′ă-mīd). Generic term for a class of sphingolipid, *N*-acyl (fatty acid) derivatives of a long chain base or sphingoid such as sphinganine or sphingosine; *e.g.,* $CH_3(CH_2)_{12}CH{=}CH$-CHOH-CH(CH_2OH)-NH-CO-*R,* where *R* is the fatty-acid residue, attached in this example to 4-sphingenine (sphingosine) in amide linkage.

c. dihexoside, the accumulated glycolipid noted in glycolipid lipidosis.

c. saccharide, glycosphingolipid.

cerasin (ser′ă-sin). Kerasin.

cerat-. For words beginning thus and not found here, see kerat-.

cerate (sē'rāt) [L. *cera,* wax]. A rarely used unctuous solid preparation, harder than an ointment, containing sufficient wax to prevent it from melting when applied to the skin.

ceratin (ser'a-tin). Keratin.

cerato-. For words beginning thus and not found here, see kerato-.

ceratocricoid (ser'ă-tō-krī'koyd). Keratocricoid; relating to the inferior cornua of the thyroid cartilage and to the cricoid cartilage, or the cricothyroid articulation.

ceratoglossus (ser'ă-tō-glos'ŭs) [L.]. *Musculus* chondroglossus.

ceratohyal (ser'ă-tō-hī'ăl). Keratohyal; relating to one of the cornua of the hyoid bone.

Ceratophyllidae (ser'ă-tō-fil'i-dē) [G. *keras,* horn, + *phyllodes,* like leaves]. A family of mammal and bird fleas, many of which have a wide host range and serve as important vectors of plague, sustaining the infection among wild and domestic rodent hosts. Important genera include *Nosopsyllus* and *Ceratophyllus.*

Ceratophyllus (ser-ă-tof'-lŭs) [cerat- (kerat-) + G. *phyllos,* leaved]. A genus of fleas (family Ceratophyllidae) found in temperate climates; includes important fleas of poultry such as *C. niger,* the western chicken flea, and *C. gallinae,* the European chicken flea, though these fleas have a wide range of hosts, including man.

C. punjaten'sis, a species abundant on wild and domestic rodents in India; may serve as a liaison agent between wild rodents and man in the transmission of plague.

cercaria, pl. **cerca'riae** (ser-kā'rē-ă, -rē-ē) [G. *kerkos,* tail]. The free-swimming trematode larva that emerges from its host snail; it may penetrate the skin of a final host (as in *Schistosoma* of man), encyst on vegetation (as in *Fasciola*), in or on fish (as in *Clonorchis*), or penetrate and encyst in various arthropod hosts. Body and tail are greatly varied in form, and specialized function is adapted to the particular life cycle demands of each species. See also sporocyst (1); redia.

cerci (ser'sī). Plural of cercus.

cerclage (sair-klazh') [Fr. an encircling, hooping, banding]. **1.** Tiring; bringing into close opposition and binding together the ends of an obliquely fractured bone or the fragments of a broken patella by a ring or by an encircling, tightly drawn wire loop. **2.** Operation for retinal detachment in which the choroid and retinal pigment epithelium are brought in contact with the detached sensory retina by a band encircling the sclera posterior to the insertion of the ocular rectus muscles. **3.** The placing of a nonabsorbable suture around an incompetent cervical os.

cercocystis (ser-kō-sis'tis) [G. *kerkos,* tail, + *kystis,* bladder]. A specialized form of tapeworm cysticercoid larva that develops within the vertebrate host villus rather than in an invertebrate host; *e.g.,* the c. of *Hymenolepis nana* in its direct or egg-borne cycle in man. See also Cysticercus, cysticercoid.

cercomer (ser'kō-mer) [G. *kerkos,* tail]. The caudal appendage of a larval cestode, the procercoid stage of pseudophyllid cestodes; it may also be found on the cysticercoid larvae of taenioid cestodes, as well as in many of the hymenolepidids (*e.g., Hymenolepis nana*). This appendage frequently bears the hooks originally used by the hexacanth in clawing its way into the intermediate host in which the procercoid or other larval stage develops.

cercomonad (ser-kō-mō'nad). Common name for members of the genus *Cercomonas.*

Cercomonas (ser-kō-mō'nas) [G. *kerkos,* tail + *monas* (*monad-*), unit, monad]. A genus of freshwater and coprophilic protozoan flagellates in which members have one anterior and one posterior flagellum. Species have been described from the intestine or feces of man and several types of domestic livestock, but have usually proved to be other genera such as *Trichomonas* or *Chilomastix.*

Cercopithecoidea (ser'kō-pith-ē-koy'dē-ă) [G. *kerkos,* tail, + *pithēkos,* monkey]. One of the three superfamilies of the suborder Anthropoidea; includes apes, Old World monkeys, and man.

Cercopithecus (ser-kō-pith-ē'kŭs). A genus of the family Cercopithecidae, represented by guenons and common African monkeys.

cercus, gen. and pl. **cerci** (ser'kŭs, -sē; ker'kŭs, -kē) [Mod. L., fr. G. *kerkos,* tail]. **1.** A stiff hairlike structure. **2.** A pair of specialized sensory appendages on the 11th abdominal segment of most insects.

cerea flexibilitas (sē'rē-ă flek-si-bil'i-tas) [L.]. "Waxy flexibility," in which the limb remains where placed; often seen in catatonia.

cerebellar (ser-e-bel'ar). Relating to the cerebellum.

cerebellin (ser-ĕ-bel'in). A cerebellum-specific hexadecapeptide localized in the perikarya and dendrites of cerebellar Purkinje cells; used as a marker for Purkinje cell maturation studies of neural development.

cerebellitis (ser-ĕ-bel-ī'tis). Inflammation of the cerebellum.

cerebello- [L. *cerebellum*]. Combining form relating to the cerebellum.

cerebellolental (ser-e-bel'ō-len'tăl). Relating to the cerebellum and the lens of the eye.

cerebellomedullary (ser-e-bel'ō-med'yū-lār-ē). Relating to the cerebellum and the medulla oblongata.

cerebello-olivary (ser-e-bel'ō-ol'i-vār-ē). Relating to the connection of the cerebellum with the inferior olive.

cerebellopontine (ser-e-bel'ō-pon'tēn). Relating to the cerebellum and the pons; denoting especially the c. recess or angle between these two structures.

cerebellorubral (ser-e-bel'ō-rū'brăl) [cerebello- + L. *ruber,* red]. Relating to the connection of the cerebellum with the red nucleus.

cerebellum, pl. **cerebella** (ser-e-bel'ŭm, -bel'ă) [L. dim. of *cerebrum,* brain] [NA]. The large posterior brain mass lying above the pons and medulla and beneath the posterior portion of the cerebrum; it consists of two lateral hemispheres united by a narrow middle portion, the vermis.

cerebr-. See cerebro-.

cerebra (sĕ-rē'bră). Plural of cerebrum.

cerebral (ser'ĕ-brăl, sĕ-rē'brăl). Relating to the cerebrum.

cerebralgia (ser-ĕ-bral'jē-ă) [cerebrum + G. *algos,* pain]. Headache.

cerebration (ser-ĕ-brā'shŭn). Activity of the mental processes, conscious or unconscious. See also mentation.

cerebri-. See cerebro-.

cerebriform (se-rē'bri-fōrm) [cerebri- + L. *forma,* shape, appearance, nature]. Resembling the external fissures and convolutions of the brain.

cerebritis (ser-ĕ-brī'tis). Nonlocalized inflammation of the brain without suppuration.

suppurative c., nonlocalized inflammation (phlegmon) of the brain with suppuration.

cerebro-, cerebr-, cerebri- [L. *cerebrum,* brain]. Combining forms relating to the cerebrum.

cerebrocuprein (ser'ĕ-brō-kū'prē-in). Cytocuprein.

cerebrogalactose (ser'ĕ-brō-gă-lak'tōs). D-Galactose.

cerebrogalactoside (ser'ĕ-brō-gă-lak'tō-sīd). Cerebroside.

cerebroma (ser-ĕ-brō'mă). Encephaloma.

cerebromalacia (ser'ĕ-brō-mă-lā'shē-ă). Encephalomalacia.

cerebromeningitis (ser'ĕ-brō-men-in-jī'tis). Meningoencephalitis.

cerebron (ser'ĕ-bron). Phrenosin.

cerebronic acid (ser-ĕ-bron'ik). Phrenosinic acid; 2-hydroxylignoceric acid, CH_3-$(CH_2)_{21}$-CHOH-COOH. A constituent of phrenosin (cerebron).

cerebropathia (ser'ĕ-brō-path'ē-ă). Encephalopathy.

cerebropathy (ser-ĕ-brop'ă-thē). Encephalopathy.

cerebrophysiology (ser'ĕ-brō-fiz-ē-ol'ō-jē). The physiology of the cerebrum.

cerebrosclerosis (ser'ĕ-brō-sklĕr-ō'sis) [cerebro- + G. *sklērōsis,* hardening]. Encephalosclerosis, specifically of the cerebral hemispheres.

cerebrose (ser'ĕ-brōs). D-Galactose.

cerebroside (ser'ĕ-brō-sīd). Cerebrogalactoside; galactolipid; galactolipin; a class of glycosphingolipid; specifically, a monoglycosylceramide (ceramide monosaccharide), the sugar being attached to the –CHOH– of the sphingoid. c's are found in the myelin sheath of nerve tissue; *e.g.,* kerasin, nervon, oxynervon, phrenosin, these names also being used for the fatty acid involved. C. is sometimes prefixed by gluco-, galacto-, etc., in place of the correct glucosylceramide, etc. The sulfate esters of c.'s are sulfatidates.

c.-sulfatase, c. sulfatidase [EC 3.1.6.8.], an enzyme that cleaves sulfate from a cerebroside 3-sulfate.

cerebrosidosis (ser'ĕ-brō-sī-dō'sis). Gaucher's *disease.*

cerebrosis (ser-ĕ-brō'sis). Encephalosis.

cerebrospinal (ser'ĕ-brō-spī-năl, sĕ-rē'brō-). Encephalorrhachidian; encephalospinal; relating to the brain and the spinal cord.

cerebrospinant (ser'ĕ-brō-spī'nant). **1.** Acting upon the cerebral nervous system, the brain and spinal cord. **2.** An agent affecting the cerebrospinal system.

cerebrosterol (ser'ē-brō-stēr'ol). 24β-Hydroxycholesterol; a hydroxylated cholesterol found in the brain and spinal cord.

cerebrotomy (ser-ĕ-brot'ō-mē) [cerebro- + G. *tomē,* incision]. Incision of the brain substance.

cerebrotonia (ser'ĕ-brō-tō'nē-ă) [cerebro- + G. *tonos,* tone]. A personality pattern associated with ectomorphic bodily type and with predominance of intellective processes; characterized by traits of inhibition, restraint, and concealment.

cerebrovascular (ser'ĕ-brō-vas'kyū-lăr). Relating to the blood supply to the brain, particularly with reference to pathologic changes.

cerebrum, pl. cerebra, cerebrums (ser'ĕ-brŭm, sĕ-rē'brŭm; -bră, -brŭmz) [L. *brain*] [NA]. Originally referred to the largest portion of the brain, including practically all parts within the skull except the medulla, pons, and cerebellum; it now usually refers only to the parts derived from the telencephalon and includes mainly the cerebral hemispheres (cerebral cortex and basal ganglia).

c. abdomina'le, *plexus* celiacus.

cerecloth (sēr'kloth) [L. *cera,* wax]. Gauze or cheese cloth impregnated with wax containing an antiseptic; used in surgical dressings.

Cerenkov, P.A., Russian physicist. See C. *radiation.*

ceresin (ser'ĕ-sin). Purified ozokerite; cerin; cerosin; earth wax; mineral wax (2); a natural mixture of hydrocarbons of high molecular weight; a substitute for beeswax, also used in dentistry for impressions.

cerin (se'rin). Ceresin.

Cerithidea (ser-i-thid'ē-ă). A genus of marine and brackish water operculate (prosobranch) snails that serve as first intermediate hosts of a number of trematodes. *C. cingulata* serves as host for *Heterophyes heterophyes* in Japan and Southeast Asia; *C. scalariformis* for cercariae that induce swimmer's itch in the southeastern U.S. from Florida to Texas.

cerium (sēr'ē-ŭm) [fr. *Ceres,* the planetoid]. A metallic element, symbol Ce, atomic no. 58, atomic weight 140.12.

c. oxalate, a mixture of the oxalates of c., lanthanum, and other rare earths; has been used in the treatment of vomiting.

cero- [L. *cera,* wax]. Combining form relating to wax.

ceroid (sē'royd). A waxlike, golden or yellow-brown pigment first found in fibrotic livers of choline-deficient rats, and also known to be present in some of the cirrhotic livers (and certain other tissues) of human beings. C. is acid-fast, insoluble in fat solvents, and probably a type of lipofuscin, although differing from true lipofuscins by failing to stain with Schmorl's ferric-ferricyanide reduction stain; it also exhibits autofluorescence.

ceroplasty (sē'rō-plas-tē) [G. *kēros,* wax, + *plassō,* to mold]. The manufacture of wax models of anatomical and pathologic specimens or of skin lesions.

cerosin (ser'ō-sin). Ceresin.

certifiable (ser-ti-fī'ă-bl). **1.** That which can or must be certified; said of infectious, industrial, and other diseases that are required by law to be reported to health authorities. **2.** Denoting a person showing disordered behavior of sufficient gravity to justify involuntary mental hospitalization.

certification (ser'ti-fi-kā'shŭn). **1.** The reporting to health authorities of notifiable disease. **2.** The attainment of board certification in a specialty. **3.** The court procedure by which a patient is committed to a mental institution. **4.** Involuntary mental hospitalization.

certify (ser'ti-fī) [L. *certus,* certain, + *facio,* to make]. **1.** To report to the health authorities the occurrence of a contagious or other reportable disease. **2.** To commit a patient to a mental hospital in accordance with the laws of the state.

cerulean (se-rū'lē-ăn) [L. *caeruleus,* blue, fr. *caelum,* sky]. Blue.

cerulein (se-rū'lē-in) [fr. *Hyla caerulea,* from which isolated]. A decapeptide with hypotensive activity; stimulates smooth muscle and increases digestive secretions; it is similar in structure to cholecystokinin and the gastrins, but much more potent as a stimulant to gallbladder contraction; also stimulates release of insulin.

ceruloplasmin (sĕ-rū'lō-plaz-min) [L. *caeruleus,* dark blue]. A blue copper-containing α-globulin of blood plasma, with a molecular weight of 150,000 and 8 atoms of copper per molecule; involved in copper transport and regulation, and can reduce O_2 directly without known intermediates; also has ferroxidase and polyamine oxidase properties of unknown significance.

cerumen (sĕ-rū'men) [L. *cera,* wax]. Earwax; the soft, brownish yellow, waxy secretion (a modified sebum) of the ceruminous glands of the external auditory meatus.

c. inspissa'tum, inspissated c., dried earwax plugging the external auditory canal.

ceruminal (se-rū'mi-năl). Relating to cerumen.

ceruminolytic (sĕ-rū'mi-nō-lit'ik) [cerumen, + G. *lysis,* a loosening]. One of several substances instilled into the external auditory canal to soften wax.

ceruminoma (sĕ-rū-mi-nō'mă). A usually benign adenomatous tumor of ceruminous glands of the external auditory canal.

ceruminosis (se-rū-mi-nō'sis). Excessive formation of cerumen.

ceruminous (sĕ-rū'mi-nŭs). Relating to cerumen.

ceruse (sē'rūs) [L. *cerussa*]. *Lead* carbonate.

cerveau isolé (ser-vō' ē-sō-lā') [Fr. detached brain]. An animal with its mesencephalon transected; it breathes spontaneously but is unresponsive, with abnormal pupils (usually dilated) and a continuous sleep pattern in the electroencephalogram. *Cf.* encephale isolé.

cervical (ser'vĭ-kal) [L. *cervix* (*cervic-*), neck]. Trachelian; relating to a neck, or cervix, in any sense.

cervicalis (ser-vi-kā'lis). Cervical.

c. ascen'dens, **(1)** *musculus* iliocostalis cervicis; **(2)** *arteria* cervicalis ascendens.

cervicectomy (ser-vi-sek'tō-mē) [cervix + G. *ektomē,* excision]. Trachelectomy; excision of the cervix uteri.

cervices (ser'vi-sēz). Plural of cervix.

cervicitis (ser-vi-sī'tis). Trachelitis; inflammation of the mucous membrane, frequently involving also the deeper structures, of the cervix uteri.

cervico- [L. *cervix,* neck]. Combining form relating to a cervix, or neck, in any sense.

cervicobrachial (ser'vi-kō-brā'kē-ăl). Relating to the neck and the arm.

cervicobuccal (ser'vi-kō-bŭk'ăl). Relating to the buccal region of the neck of a premolar or molar tooth.

cervicodynia (ser'vi-kō-din'ē-ă) [cervico- + G. *odynē,* pain]. Trachelodynia; neck pain.

cervicofacial (ser'vi-kō-fā'shăl). Relating to the neck and the face.

cervicography (ser-vi-kog'ră-fē) [cervix + G. *graphō,* to write]. Technique, equivalent to colposcopy, for photographing part or all of the uterine cervix.

cervicolabial (ser'vi-kō-lā'bē-ăl). Relating to the labial region of the neck of an incisor or canine tooth.

cervicolingual (ser'vi-kō-ling'gwăl). Relating to the lingual region of the cervix of a tooth.

cervicolinguoaxial (ser'vi-kō-ling'gwō-ak'sē-ăl). Referring to the point angle formed by the junction of the cervical (gingival), lingual, and axial walls of a cavity.

cervico-occipital (ser'vi-kō-ok-sip'i-tăl). Relating to the neck and the occiput.

cervicoplasty (ser'vi-kō-plas-tē). Plastic surgery on the cervix uteri or on the neck.

cervicothoracic (ser'vi-kō-thōr-as'ik). Relating to: **1.** the neck and thorax; **2.** the transition between the neck and thorax; **3.** the disk between the seventh cervical vertebra and first thoracic vertebra; **4.** the fusion of these vertebrae.

cervicotomy (ser-vi-kot'ō-mē) [cervico- + G. *tomē,* incision]. Trachelotomy; incision into the cervix uteri.

cervicovesical (ser'vi-kō-ves'i-kăl). Relating to the cervix of the uterus and the bladder.

cervix, gen. **cervicis,** pl. **cervices** (ser'viks, ser'vi-sis, -sēz) [L. neck] [NA]. **1.** Collum. **2.** Any necklike structure. **3.** Cervix uteri.
c. of the axon, the constricted portion of the axon just before the myelin sheath begins.
c. colum'nae posterio'ris, a slight constriction of the posterior gray column of the spinal cord, seen on cross-section just behind the gray commissure.
c. den'tis [NA], collum dentis; neck of tooth; dental neck; cervical zone of tooth; the slightly constricted part of a tooth, between the crown and the root.
c. u'teri [NA], cervix; neck of uterus or womb; the lower part of the uterus extending from the isthmus of the uterus into the vagina. It is divided into supravaginal and vaginal parts by its passage through the vaginal wall.
c. ves'icae urina'riae [NA], neck of urinary bladder; the lowest part of the bladder formed by the junction of the fundus and the inferolateral surfaces.

ceryl (sēr'il). Hexacosyl; the hydrocarbon radical, $C_{26}H_{53}$—, of ceryl alcohol (hexacosanol).

cesarean (se-zā'rē-ăn). Denoting a c. section, which was included under *lex cesarea,* Roman law (715 B.C.); not because performed at the birth of Julius Caesar (100 B.C.).

cesium (sē'zē-ŭm) [L. *caesius,* bluish gray]. A metallic element, symbol Cs, atomic no. 55, atomic weight 132.91; a member of the alkali metal group.

Cestan, Raymond, French neurologist, 1872–1934. See C.-Chenais *syndrome.*

Cestoda (ses-tō'dă) [G. *kestos,* girdle]. Eucestoda; a subclass of tapeworms (class Cestoidea), containing the typical members of this group, including the segmented tapeworms that parasitize man and domestic animals.

Cestodaria (ses-tō-dā'rē-ă). A subclass of the class Cestoidea, containing tapeworms that lack a scolex and are unsegmented (monozoic), in contrast to the typical tapeworms in the subclass Cestoda; larvae of c. (called lycophora) characteristically have 10 hooklets rather than six. C. are believed to be primitive tapeworms, parasitizing the intestine and celomic cavities of certain fish and a few reptiles.

cestode, cestoid (ses'tōd, -toyd). Common name for tapeworms of the class Cestoidea or its subclasses, Cestoda and Cestodaria.

cestodiasis (ses-tō-dī'ă-sis). Disease caused by infection with a cestode.

Cestoidea (ses-toy'dē-ă) [G. *kestos,* girdle, + *eidos,* form]. The tapeworms, a class of platyhelminth flatworms characterized by lack of an alimentary canal and, in typical forms (subclass Cestoda), by a segmented body with a scolex or holdfast organ at one end; adult worms are vertebrate parasites, usually found in the small intestine.

cetaceum (sē-tā'shē-ŭm) [G. *kētos,* a whale]. Spermaceti.

cetalkonium chloride (set'al-kō'nē-ŭm). Benzylhexadecyldimethylammonium chloride; an antibacterial agent.

cethexonium bromide (set-heks-ō'nē-ŭm). Hexadecyl(2-hydroxycyclohexyl)dimethylammonium bromide; an antiseptic.

cetostearyl alcohol (se-tō-stē'ă-ril). A component of the hydrophilic ointment ingredient known as emulsifying wax; a mixture of solid aliphatic alcohols consisting chiefly of stearyl and cetyl alcohols.

cetraria (sē-trā'rē-ă) [L. *caetra,* a short Spanish shield (from shape of the apothecia)]. Iceland moss; the dried plant, *Cetraria islandica* (family Parmeliaceae), a lichen, not a moss, used as a demulcent and as a folk remedy for bronchitis.

cetrimonium bromide (se-trī-mō'nē-ŭm). Hexadecyltrimethylammonium bromide; an antiseptic.

cetyl (sē'til). The univalent radical $C_{16}H_{33}$— of cetyl alcohol.
c. alcohol, 1-hexadecanol; palmityl alcohol; the 16-carbon alcohol corresponding to palmitic acid, so called because it is isolated from among the hydrolysis products of spermaceti; it is used as an emulsifying aid and in the preparation of "washable" ointment bases.
c. palmitate, $C_{15}H_{31}CO–OC_{16}H_{31}$; the chief constituent of spermaceti.

cetylpyridinium chloride (sē'til-pī-ri-din'ē-ŭm). The monohydrate of the quaternary salt of pyridine and cetyl chloride; a cationic detergent with antiseptic action against nonsporulating bacteria.

cetyltrimethylammonium bromide (sē'til-trī-me'thil-ă-mō'nē-ŭm). Cetrimide; a mixture of dodecyl-, tetradecyl-, and hexadecyltrimethylammonium bromides; an odorless surface-active agent, readily soluble in water; a disinfectant with a strong bacteriostatic action, used for the sterilization of instruments and utensils.

cevadilla (se-vă-dil'ă) [Sp. dim. of *cebada,* barley]. Sabadilla.

cevadine (sev'ă-dēn). $C_{32}H_{49}NO_9$; an alkaloid occurring in the seeds of *Schoenocaulon officinale (Sabadilla officinarum),* family Liliaceae; highly irritating to skin and mucous membranes. See also veratrine.

cevitamic acid (sev-i-tam'ik). Ascorbic acid.

CF Abbreviation for citrovorum *factor; coupling factor.*

Cf Symbol for californium.

CG Abbreviation for chorionic *gonadotropin.*

CGA Abbreviation for catabolite gene *activator.*

CGS, cgs Abbreviation for centimeter-gram-second. See under system, unit.

Chabertia (chă-ber'tē-ă). A genus of strongyle nematodes parasitic in animals. The species *C. ovina,* the bowel worm, is found in the digestive tract of sheep, goats, cattle, and some wild animals; it is not a bloodsucker ordinarily, but feeds on the mucosa of the gut, where in large numbers it can produce considerable damage.

Chaddock, Charles G., St. U.S. neurologist, 1861–1936. See C.'s *reflex, sign.*

Chadwick, James R., U.S. gynecologist, 1844–1905. See C.'s *sign.*

chaeta (kē'tă) [Mod. L. fr. G. *chaitē,* stiff hair]. Seta.

chafe (chāf) [Fr. *chauffer,* to heat, fr. L. *calefacio,* to make warm]. To cause irritation of the skin by friction.

Chagas, Carlos, Brazilian physician, 1879–1934. See C.'s *disease,* C.-Cruz *disease.*

chagoma (sha-gō'mă). The skin lesion in acute Chagas' disease.

chain (chān) [L. *catena*]. **1.** In chemistry, a series of atoms held together by one or more covalent bonds. **2.** In bacteriology, a linear arrangement of living cells that have divided in one plane and remain attached to each other.

A c., glycyl c.; a polypeptide component of insulin containing 21 amino acids, beginning with glycine (NH_2 terminus); insulin is formed by the linkage of an A c. to a B c. by two disulfide bonds; the amino-acid composition of the A c. is a function of species.

B c., phenylalanyl c.; a polypeptide component of insulin containing 30 amino acids, beginning with phenylalanine (NH_2 terminus); insulin is formed by the linkage of a B c. to an A c. by two disulfide bonds; the amino-acid composition of the B c. is a function of species.

behavior c., related behaviors in a series in which each response serves as a stimulus for the next response.

C c., C-peptide.

glycyl c., A c.

H c., heavy c.

heavy c., H c.; a polypeptide c. of high molecular weight, as the γ, α, μ, Δ, or ϵ c.'s in immunoglobulin.

hemolytic c., the hemolysis that occurs when complement is activated by the previously formed union of erythrocytes and specific antibody.

J c., a glycopeptide disulfide that is bonded to polymeric IgA and IgM; its function is to ensure correct polymerization of the subunits of IgA and IgM.

L c., light c.

light c., L c.; a polypeptide c. with low molecular weight, as the κ or λ c.'s in immunoglobulin.

long c., in bacteriology, a continuous line of more than eight cells.

ossicular c., *ossicula* auditus.

phenylalanyl c., B c.

respiratory c., cytochrome or electron-transport system; a sequence of energy-liberating oxidation-reduction reactions whereby electrons are accepted from reduced compounds and eventually transferred to oxygen with the formation of water.

short c., in bacteriology, a string of two to eight cells.

side c., a c. of noncyclic atoms linked to a benzene ring, or to any cyclic c. compound.

chaining (chān'ing). Learning related behaviors in a series in which each response serves as a stimulus for the next response.

chalasia, chalasis (kă-lā'zē-ă, -lā'sis) [G. *chalaō,* to loosen]. Inhibition and relaxation of any previously sustained contraction of muscle, usually of a synergic group of muscles.

chalaza (kă-lā'ză) [G. hail; a small tubercle, a sty (Galen)]. **1.** Chalazion. **2.** Suspensory ligament of the yolk in a bird's egg.

chalazion, pl. **chalazia** (ka-lā'zē-on, -zē-ă) [G. dim. of *chalaza,* a sty]. Chalaza (1); meibomian or tarsal cyst; a chronic inflammatory granuloma of a meibomian gland.

acute c., *hordeolum* internum.

collar-stud c., a c. that extends through the tarsal plate anteriorly (c. externum) and toward the conjunctiva.

chalcone (kal'kōn). Benzalacetophenone; 1,3-diphenyl-2-propen-1-one; $C_6H_5CH{=}CH\text{-}CO\text{-}C_6H_5$; the parent compound of a series of plant pigments.

chalcosis (kal-kō'sis) [G. *chalkos,* copper, brass]. Chalkitis; chronic copper poisoning.

c. len'tis, copper cataract; a cataract caused by excessive intraocular copper.

chalicosis (kal-i-kō'sis) [G. *chalix,* gravel]. Flint disease; pneumoconiosis caused by the inhalation of dust incident to the occupation of stone cutting.

chalinoplasty (kal'in-ō-plas-tē) [G. *chalinos,* bridle, corner of the mouth, + *plastos,* formed]. Rarely used term for the correction of defects of the mouth and lips, especially of the corners of the mouth.

chalk (chawk) [L. *calx*]. *Calcium* carbonate.

French c., talc.

prepared c., purified native calcium carbonate, usually molded into cones; used as a mild astringent and antacid.

chalkitis (kal-kī'tis) [G. *chalkos,* copper, brass]. Chalcosis.

chalone (kā'lōn). Originally, a hormone (*e.g.,* enterogastrone) that inhibits rather than stimulates; now, any one of a number of mitotic inhibitors elaborated by a tissue and active only on that type of tissue, regardless of species; a reversible tissue-specific mitotic inhibitor.

chalybeate (kal-ib'ē-āt) [G. *chalyps* (*chalyb-*), steel]. **1.** Impregnated with or containing iron salts. **2.** A therapeutic agent containing iron.

chamazulene (chă-maz'yū-lēn). 1,4-Dimethyl-7-ethylazulene; an anti-inflammatory agent.

chamber (chām'ber) [L. *camera*]. A compartment or enclosed space. See also camera.

Abbé-Zeiss counting c., Thoma-Zeiss *hemocytometer.*

altitude c., high altitude c.; a decompression c. for simulating a high altitude environment, particularly its low barometric pressure.

anechoic c., a room designed to absorb all sound so as to eliminate all echoes; used for isolation and sound research on human subjects.

anterior c. of eye, *camera* anterior bulbi.

aqueous c.'s, the anterior and posterior c.'s of the eye containing the aqueous humor. See *camera* anterior bulbi and *camera* posterior bulbi.

decompression c., a c. for exposing organisms to pressures below that of the atmosphere.

Haldane c., an obsolete c. for metabolic studies on animals.

high altitude c., altitude c.

hyperbaric c., a c. providing pressures greater than atmospheric, commonly used to treat decompression sickness and to provide hyperbaric oxygenation.

ionization c., a c. for detecting ionization of the enclosed gas; used for determining intensity of ionizing radiation.

posterior c. of eye, *camera* posterior bulbi.

pulp c., that portion of the pulp cavity which is contained in the crown or body of the tooth.

relief c., a recess in the impression surface of a denture to reduce or eliminate pressure from that specific area of the mouth.

Sandison-Clark c., a c. which can be fitted over a hole punched in a rabbit's ear, so that tissue will grow to fill the defect between two transparent plates; if the distance between the plates is small the living tissue can be studied microscopically.

sinuatrial c., the common c. formed by the single embryonic

atrium and the right and left horns of the sinus venosus.
Thoma's counting c., Thoma-Zeiss *hemocytometer*.
vitreous c. of eye, *camera* vitrea bulbi.
Zappert counting c., a special, standardized glass slide used for counting cells (especially erythrocytes and leukocytes) and other particulate material in a measured volume of fluid; the central portion is precisely ground in such a manner that the uniformly flat surface is exactly 0.1 mm lower than that of two parallel ridges on which a special, uniformly flat coverslip may be placed; accurately etched lines on the flat central portion form the boundaries of groups of squares of known areas, thereby providing the basis for determining the volume of fluid in which the cells are counted. Glass slides of this type are frequently known as hemocytometers.

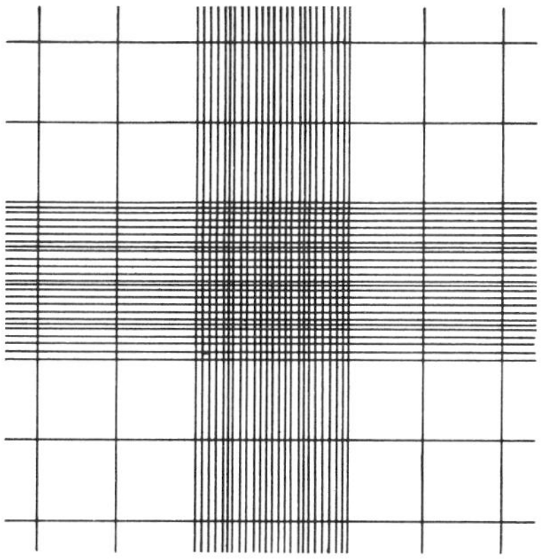

Diagram of Ruled Portion of Zappert Counting Chamber

Chamberlain, W.E., U.S. radiologist, 1891–1947. See C.'s *line*.

Chamberlen, Peter, British obstetrician, 1560–1631. See C. *forceps*.

chamecephalic (kam-ĕ-se-fal'ik) [G. *chamai*, on the ground (low, stunted), + *kephalē*, head]. Chamecephalous; having a flat head; denoting a skull with a vertical index of 70 or less; similar to tapinocephalic.

chamecephalous (kam-ĕ-sef'ă-lus). Chamecephalic.

chameprosopic (kam'ē-prō-sop'ik) [G. *chamai* (adv.), on the ground (low, spread out), + *prosōpikos*, facial]. Having a broad face.

chamfer (sham'fer) [fr. O.Fr. *chanfrein* (*t*), beveled edge]. A marginal finish on an extracoronal cavity preparation of a tooth which describes a curve from an axial wall to the cavosurface.

chamomile (kam'ō-mīl) [G. *chamaimēlon*, chamomile, fr. *chamai*, on the ground, + *mēlon*, apple]. Camomile; the flowering heads of *Anthemis nobilis* (family Compositae); a stomachic.

Champy, Christian, French physician, *1885. See C.'s *fixative*.

Chanarin, I., 20th century hematologist. See Dorfman-C. *syndrome*.

Chance, G.Q., 20th century British radiologist. See C. *fracture*.

chancre (shang'ker) [Fr. indirectly from L. *cancer*]. Hard c., sore or ulcer; syphilitic ulcer (1); ulcus venereum (1); the primary lesion of syphilis, which begins at the site of infection after an interval of 10 to 30 days as a papule or area of infiltration, of dull red color, hard, and insensitive; the center usually becomes eroded or breaks down into an ulcer that heals slowly after 4 to 6 weeks.
hard c., chancre.
mixed c., a sore resulting from simultaneous inoculation of a site with syphilis and chancroid.
monorecidive c., a c. that recurs at the site of a previously healed lesion.
c. re'dux, a second c. occurring in a syphilitic subject, possibly an allergic reaction without the presence of the specific spirochete.
soft c., chancroid.
sporotrichositic c., the initial lesion at the site of infection in sporotrichosis.
tularemic c., primary lesion, usually of finger, thumb, or hand, in tularemia.

chancriform (shang'kri-fōrm). Resembling chancre.

chancroid (shang'kroyd) [chancre + G. *eidos*, resemblance]. Soft chancre, sore, or ulcer; venereal sore or ulcer; ulcus venereum (2); an infectious venereal ulcer at the site of infection by *Haemophilus ducreyi*, beginning after an incubation period of 3 to 5 days.

chancroidal (shang-kroy'dăl). Relating to or of the nature of chancroid.

chancrous (shang'krŭs). Characterized by having a chancre.

Chandler, Paul, U.S. opthalmologist, *1896. See C. *syndrome*.

change (chanj). An alteration; in pathology, structural alteration of which the cause and significance is uncertain.
Armanni-Ebstein c., Armanni-Ebstein *kidney*.
Baggenstoss c., distention of pancreatic acini by proteinaceous secretion, seen in dehydration.
Crooke's hyaline c., Crooke's hyaline degeneration; replacement of cytoplasmic granules of basophil cells of the anterior pituitary by homogenous hyaline material; a characteristic finding in Cushing's syndrome, but usually not present in the cells of a basophil adenoma.
fatty c., fatty *metamorphosis*.
c. of life, colloquialism for **(1)** menopause; **(2)** climacteric.
trophic c., neurotrophic *atrophy*.

channel (chan'ĕl) [L. *canalis*]. A furrow, gutter, or groovelike passageway. See also canal; canalis.
ion c., a specific macromolecular protein pathway, with an aqueous "pore," that traverses the lipid bilayer of a cell's plasma membrane and maintains or modulates the electrical potential across this barrier by allowing controlled influx or exit of small inorganic ions such as Na^+, K^+, Cl^-, and Ca^{2+}. It plays an important role in propagation of the action potential in neurons, but also may control transduction of extracellular signals and contraction in muscle cells. In general, ion c.'s are characterized by their selectivity for certain ions, their specific regulation or gating of these ions, and their specific sensitivity to toxins.
ligand-gated c., a class of ion c.'s whose ionic permeability is regulated by cell membrane receptors that respond to specific extracellular chemical signals.
transnexus c., a hexagonal 15-20Å hydrophilic c. capable of transporting small ions between cardiac muscle cells.
voltage-gated c., a class of ion c.'s that open and close in response to change in the electrical potential across the plasma membrane of the cell; voltage-gated Na^+ c.'s are important for conducting action potential along nerve cell processes.

Chantemesse, André, French bacteriologist, 1851–1919. See C. *reaction*.

chaotropic (kā-ō-trōp'ik). Pertaining to chaotropism.

chaotropism (kā-ō-trōp'izm) [G. *chaos*, disorder, confusion, + *tropē*, a turning]. The property of certain substances, usually ions (*e.g.*, SCN^-, ClO_4^-, guanidinium), to distrupt the structure of water and thereby promote the solubility of nonpolar substances in polar solvents (*e.g.*, water), the unfolding of proteins, the elution from or movement through a chromatographic medium of an otherwise tightly bound substance, etc.

CHAP Acronym for cyclophosphamide, hexamethylmelamine, doxorubicin, and cisplatin, a chemotherapy regimen used in the treatment of ovarian cancer.

chappa (chap'pă) [W. Af.]. A disease marked by subcutaneous nodules, the size of a pigeon's egg, which break down, release a fatty looking material, and form ulcers; the eruption is preceded by severe muscular and articular pains.

chapped (chapt) [M.E. *chap,* to chop, split]. Having or pertaining to skin that is dry, scaly, and fissured, owing to the action of cold or to the excess rate of evaporation of moisture from the skin surface.

character (kar'ak-ter). Characteristic (1); an attribute, trait, or definite and distinct structural feature.
acquired c., a c. developed in a plant or animal as a result of environmental influences during the individual's life.
compound c., an inherited c. dependent upon two or more distinct genes.
dominant c., an inherited c. determined by a dominant gene. See *dominance* of genes.
inherited c., mendelian or unit c.; a single attribute of an animal or plant that is transmitted from generation to generation in accordance with genetic principles. See gene.
mendelian c., inherited c.
primary sex c.'s, the sex glands, testes or ovaries, and the accessory sex organs.
recessive c., an inherited c. determined by a recessive gene. See *dominance* of genes.
secondary sex c.'s, those c.'s peculiar to the male or female, *e.g.,* the beard of men and the breasts of women, which develop at puberty.
sex-linked c., an inherited c. determined by sex-linked gene. See gene.
unit c., inherited c.

character armor. A habitual pattern of organized defenses against anxiety.

characteristic (kar'ak-ter-is'tik). **1.** Character. **2.** Pertaining to a character.

characterization (kar'ak-ter-i-zā'shŭn). The description or attributing of distinguishing traits.
denture c., modification of the form and color of the denture base and/or teeth to produce a more lifelike appearance.

charas (char'as). A resin obtained from mature leaves of selected varieties of *Cannabis sativa;* used for smoking.

charbon (shar-bawn') [Fr. coal]. Anthrax (2).

charcoal (char'kōl). Carbo; carbon obtained by heating or burning wood with restricted access of air.
activated c., medicinal c.; the residue from the destructive distillation of various organic materials, treated to increase its adsorptive power; used in diarrhea, as an antidote in various forms of poisoning, and in purification processes in industry and research.
animal c., animal or bone black; bone c.; c. produced by incomplete combustion of animal tissues, especially bone.
bone c., animal c.
medicinal c., activated c.
vegetable c., wood c.; c. obtained by charring vegetable tissues, especially the wood of willow, beech, birch, or oak.
wood c., vegetable c.

Charcot, Jean M., French neurologist, 1825–1893. See C.'s *artery, disease,* intermittent *fever, gait, joint, syndrome, triad, vertigo;* C.-Leyden, C.-Neumann, C.-Robin *crystals;* C.-Böttcher *crystalloids;* C.-Marie-Tooth *disease;* C.-Weiss-Baker *syndrome;* Erb-C. *disease.*

charge transfer. See charge transfer *complex.*

charlatan (shar'lă-tan). Quack; a medical fraud claiming to cure disease by useless procedures, secret remedies, and worthless diagnostic and therapeutic machines.

charlatanism (shar'lă-tan-izm). Quackery; a fraudulent claim to medical knowledge; treating the sick without knowledge of medicine or authority to practice medicine.

Charles, Jacques C., French physicist, 1746–1823. See C.'s *law.*

charley horse (char'lē hōrs) [slang]. Localized pain or muscle stiffness following a contusion of a muscle.

Charlin (Correa), Carlos, Chilean ophthalmologist, 1886–1945. See C.'s *syndrome.*

Charlouis, M., 19th century Dutch army surgeon in Java. See C. *disease.*

Charlton, Willy, German physician, *1889. See Schultz-C. *phenomenon, reaction.*

Charnley, Sir John, 20th century British physician. See C. hip *arthroplasty.*

Charrière, Joseph F.B., French instrument maker, 1803–1876. See C. *scale.*

chart. 1. A recording of clinical data relating to a patient's case. **2.** Curve (2). **3.** In optics, symbols of graduated size for measuring visual acuity, or test types for determining far or near vision. See Snellen's *test types.*
Amsler's c., a 20-cm square divided into 5-mm squares upon which an individual may project a defect in the central visual field.
color c., an assembly of chromatic samples used in checking color vision.
quality control c., a c. illustrating the allowable limits of error in laboratory test performance, the limits being 2 SD about the mean of a control serum. See also quality *control.*
Tanner growth c., a series of c.'s showing distribution of parameters of physical development, such as stature, growth curves, and skinfold thickness, for children by sex, age, and stages of puberty.
Walker's c., a system of plotting the relative fetal and placental sizes.

Charters, W.J., U.S. dentist. See C. *method.*

charting. Clinical recording; making a record in tabular or graph form of the progress of a patient's condition.

Chassaignac, Edouard P.M., French surgeon, 1804–1879. See C.'s *space, tubercle.*

Chastek. Surname of the owner of a farm on which the disease later known as C. *paralysis* was first reported.

Chaudhry, Anand P. See Gorlin-C.-Moss *syndrome.*

Chauffard, Anatole M.E., French physician, 1855–1932. See C.'s *syndrome,* Still-C. *syndrome.*

chaulmoogra oil (chawl-mū'gră). Hydnocarpus oil; gynocardia oil; the fixed oil expressed from seeds of *Taraktogenos kurzii* (family Bixaceae) and *Hydnocarpus wightiana* (family Flacourtiaceae); formerly used in the treatment of leprosy.

Chaussier, François, French physician, 1746–1828. See C.'s *areola, line, sign.*

Chauveau, J.-B. Auguste, French veterinarian, physiologist, and microbiologist, 1827–1917. See C.'s *bacterium.*

Chayes, Herman E.S., U.S. prosthodontist, 1880–1933. See C.'s *method.*

Ch.B. Abbreviation for *Chirurgiae Baccalaureus,* Bachelor of Surgery.

Ch.D. Abbreviation for *Chirurgiae Doctor,* Doctor of Surgery.

Cheadle, Walter B., British pediatrician, 1835–1910. See C.'s *disease.*

Cheatle, Sir George L., British surgeon, 1865–1951. See C. *slit.*

checkbite (chek'bīt). Interocclusal *record.*

checkerberry oil (chek'er-bār'ē). Gaultheria oil.

Chédiak, Moisés. See C.-Higashi *disease,* C.-Steinbrinck-Higashi *anomaly* or *syndrome.*

cheek (chēk) [A. S. *ceáce*] Bucca; mala (1); gena; the side of the face forming the lateral wall of the mouth.

cheil-. See cheilo-.

cheilalgia, chilalgia (kī-lal'jē-ă) [cheil- + G. *algos,* pain]. Pain in the lip.

cheilectomy, chilectomy (kī-lek'tō-mē) [cheil- + G. *ektomē,* excision]. **1.** Excision of a portion of the lip. **2.** Chiseling away bony irregularities on the lips of a joint cavity that interfere with movements of the joint.

cheilectropion, chilectropion (kī-lek-trō'pē-on) [cheil- + G. *ektropos,* a turning out]. Eversion of the lips or a lip.

cheilion (kī'lē-on) [G. *cheilos,* lips]. A cephalometric point located at the angle (corner) of the mouth.

cheilitis, chilitis (kī-lī'tis) [cheil- + G. *-itis,* inflammation]. Inflammation of the lips or of a lip. See also cheilosis.

actinic c., solar c.

angular c., commissural c.; perlèche; inflammation and fissuring radiating from the commissures of the mouth secondary to predisposing factors such as lost vertical dimension in denture wearers, nutritional deficiencies, atopic dermatitis, or *Candida albicans* infection.

commissural c., angular c.

contact c., inflammation of the lips resulting from contact with a specific allergen.

c. exfoliati'va, an exfoliative dermatitis; it may be related to atopic dermatitis or to contact sensitivity.

c. glandula'ris, myxadenitis labialis; Volkmann's c.; Baelz' disease; an acquired disorder, of unknown etiology, of the lower lip characterized by swelling, ulceration, crusting, mucous gland hyperplasia, abscesses, and sinus tracts.

c. granulomato'sa, chronic, diffuse, soft swelling of the lips, of unknown etiology, microscopically characterized by granulomatous inflammation. See also Melkersson-Rosenthal *syndrome.*

impetiginous c., pyoderma of the lips.

solar c., actinic c.; mucosal atrophy, crusting, and fissuring of the vermillion border of the lips in older individuals, resulting from chronic exposure to sunlight; dysplastic (premalignant) changes are noted microscopically, analogous to solar keratosis.

c. venena'ta, allergic contact dermatitis of the lips, as in contact c.

Volkmann's c., c. glandularis.

cheilo-, cheil- [G. cheilos, lip]. Combining forms denoting relationship to the lips. See also chilo-, labio-.

cheiloalveoloschisis, chiloalveoloschisis (kī'lō-al-vē-ō-los'ki-sis) [cheilo- + alveolus, + G. *schisis,* cleft]. Cleft of the prepalate.

cheilognathoglossoschisis, chilognathoglossoschisis (kī'lō-nath'ō-glos-os'ki-sis, kī-log'nă-thō-) [cheilo- + G. *gnathos,* jaw, + *glōssa,* tongue, + *schisis,* cleft]. Associated condition of cleft mandible and lower lip, and bifid tongue.

cheilognathopalatoschisis, chilognathopalatoschisis (kī'lō-nath'ō-pal-ă-tos'ki-sis, kī-log'nă-thō-). Cheilognathouranoschisis.

cheilognathoprosoposchisis, chilognathoprosoposchisis (kī'lō-nath'ō-pros-ō-pos'ki-sis, kī-log'nă-thō-) [cheilo- + G. *gnathos,* jaw, + *prosōpon,* face, + *schisis,* cleft]. Oblique facial cleft, with cleft of lip and jaw.

cheilognathoschisis, chilognathoschisis (kī'lō-na-thos'ki-sis, kī-log'nă-) [cheilo- + G. *gnathos,* jaw, + *schisis,* cleft]. Cleft lip with a cleft in the jaw.

cheilognathouranoschisis, chilognathouranoschisis (kī-lō-nath'ō-yū-ră-nos'ki-sis, kī-log'nă-thō-) [cheilo- + G. *gnathos,* jaw, + *ouranos,* sky (roof of mouth), + *schisis,* cleft]. Cheilognathopalatoschisis; cleft lip with cleft jaw and palate.

cheilophagia, chilophagia (kī-lō-fā'jē-ă) [cheilo- + G. *phagein,* to eat]. Biting of the lips.

cheiloplasty, chiloplasty (kī'lō-plas-tē) [cheilo- + G. *plastos,* formed]. Plastic surgery of the lips.

cheilorrhaphy, chilorrhaphy (kī-lōr'ă-fē) [cheilo- + G. *raphē,* suture]. Suturing of the lip.

cheiloschisis, chiloschisis (kī-los'ki-sis) [cheilo- + G. *schisis,* cleft]. Cleft *lip.*

cheilosis, chilosis (kī-lō'sis) [cheil- + G. *-osis,* condition]. A condition characterized by dry scaling and fissuring of the lips; attributed by some to riboflavin and other nutritional deficiencies. See also cheilitis.

cheilostomatoplasty, chilostomatoplasty (kī-lō-stō'mă-tō-plas-tē) [cheilo- + G. *stoma,* mouth, + *plastos,* formed]. Plastic surgery of the lips and mouth.

cheilotomy, chilotomy (kī-lot'ō-mē) [cheilo- + G. *tomē,* incision]. Incision into the lip.

cheir-. See cheiro-.

cheirarthritis, chirarthritis (kī'rar-thrī'tis) [cheir- + arthritis]. Obsolete term for inflammation of the joints of the hand.

cheiro-, cheir- [G. *cheir,* hand]. Combining forms meaning hand. See also chiro-.

cheirobrachialgia, chirobrachialgia (kī'rō-brā'kē-al'jē-ă) [cheiro- + G. *brachiōn,* arm, + algos, pain]. Obsolete term for pain and paresthesia in the hand and arm.

cheirocinesthesia (kī'rō-sin-es-thē'zē-ă). Cheirokinesthesia.

cheirognostic, chirognostic (kī'rog-nos'tik) [cheiro- + G. *gnostikos,* perceptive]. Able to distinguish between right and left, as of the hands or of which side of the body is touched.

cheirokinesthesia, chirokinesthesia (kī'rō-kin-es-thē'zē-ă) [cheiro- + G. *kinēsis,* movement, + *aisthēsis,* sensation]. Cheirocinesthesia; chirocinesthesia; the subjective sensation of movement of the hands.

cheirokinesthetic (kī'rō-kin-es-thet'ik). Relating to cheirokinesthesia.

cheirology, chirology (kī-rol'ō-jē) [cheiro- + G. *logos,* word]. Dactylology.

cheiromegaly, chiromegaly (kī'rō-meg'ă-lē) [cheiro- + G. *megas,* large]. Macrocheiria.

cheiroplasty, chiroplasty (kī'rō-plas-tē) [cheiro- + G. *plastos,* formed]. Rarely used term for plastic surgery of the hand.

cheiropodalgia, chiropodalgia (kī'rō-pō-dal'jē-ă) [cheiro- + G. *pous,* foot, + *algos,* pain]. Pain in the hands and in the feet.

cheiropompholyx, chiropompholyx (kī-rō-pom'fō-liks) [cheiro- + G. *pompholyx,* a bubble, fr. *pomphos,* a blister]. Dyshidrosis.

cheirospasm, chirospasm (kī'rō-spazm) [cheiro- + G. *spasmos,* spasm]. Spasm of the muscles of the hand, as in writers' cramp.

chelate (kē'lāt). **1.** To effect chelation. **2.** Pertaining to chelation. **3.** A complex formed through chelation.

chelation (kē-lā'shŭn) [G. *chēlē,* claw]. Complex formation involving a metal ion and two or more polar groupings of a single molecule; thus, in heme, the Fe^{2+} ion is chelated by the porphyrin ring. C. can be used to remove an ion from participation in biological reactions, as in the c. of Ca^{2+} of blood by EDTA, which thus acts as an anticoagulant.

chelicera, pl. **cheli'cerae** (ke-lis'ĭ-ră, -ĭ-rē) [G. *chēlē,* claw, + *keras,* horn]. One of the two anterior appendages of arachnids; in ticks and parasitic mites, the chelicerae are piercing and cutting structures, and constitute important feeding organs.

chelidon (kel'ĕ-don) [G. *chelidōn,* a swallow, because of fancied resemblance to the shape of a swallow's tail]. *Fossa* cubitalis.

cheloid (kē'loyd). Keloid.

Chelonia (kē-lō'nē-ă) [G. *chelōnē,* a tortoise]. An order of reptiles, embracing the turtles, tortoises, and terrapins, whose bodies are enclosed in a bony shell covered with epidermal scutes and formed dorsally by expanded ribs and ventrally by a sternal plastron.

chelonian (kē-lō'nē-an). Resembling or relating to a turtle, tortoise, or terrapin.

chem-. See chemo-.

chemexfoliation (kem'eks-fō-lē-ā'shŭn). A chemosurgical technique designed to remove acne scars or treat chronic skin defects caused by exposure to sunlight.

chemiatry (kem'i-ă-trē). Iatrochemistry.

chemical (kem'i-kăl). Relating to chemistry.

chemicocautery (kem'i-kō-kaw'ter-ē). Chemocautery.

chemiotaxis (kem'ē-ō-taks'is). Chemotaxis.

chemise (shem-ēz') [Fr. shirt]. A square of gauze fastened to a catheter passed through its center; used to retain a tampon packed around the catheter inserted into a wound, such as that resulting from a perineal section. See also *catheter* en chemise.

chemist (kem'ist). A specialist or expert in chemistry.

chemistry (kem'is-trē) [G. *chēmeia,* alchemy]. The science concerned with the atomic composition of substances, the elements and their interreactions, and the formation, decomposition and properties of molecules.

analytic c., the application of c. to the determination of composition.

applied c., the application of the theories and principles of chemistry to practical purposes.

biological c., biochemistry.

clinical c., **(1)** the c. of human health and disease; **(2)** c. in connection with the management of patients, as in a hospital laboratory.

epithermal c., so-called "hot atom" c.; the science concerned with the chemical reactions of recoil atoms and free radicals produced in low energy nuclear processes.

inorganic c., the science concerned with compounds not involving covalent bonds.

macromolecular c., the c. of macromolecules (*e.g.,* proteins, nucleic acids) and polymers (nylon, polyethylene, etc.).

medical c., c. in its relation to pharmacy, physiology, or any science connected with medicine.

medicinal c., pharmaceutical c.

nuclear c., the science concerned with the c. of nuclear reactions and processes.

organic c., that branch of c. concerned with covalently linked atoms, centering around carbon compounds of this type; originally, and still including, the c. of natural products.

pharmaceutical c., pharmacochemistry; medicinal c. in its application to the analysis and the manufacture of drugs.

physiological c., biochemistry.

radiation c., the science concerned with the effects of ionizing or nuclear radiation on chemical reactions or materials.

synthetic c., the formation or building up of complex compounds by uniting the more simple ones.

chemo-, chem- [G. *chēmeia,* alchemy]. Combining forms relating to chemistry.

chemoautotroph (kem'ō-aw'tō-trōf, kē'mō) [chemo- + G. *autos,* self, + *trophikos,* nourishing]. Chemolithotroph; an organism that depends on chemicals for its energy and principally on carbon dioxide for its carbon.

chemoautotrophic (kem'ō-aw-tō-trof'ik, kē'mo-). Chemolithotrophic; pertaining to a chemoautotroph.

chemobiodynamics (kem'ō-bī-ō-dī-nam'iks, kē'mō-) [chemo- + G. *bios,* life, + *dynamis,* power]. Study devoted to elucidation of correlations between the chemical constitution of various materials and their ability to modify the function and morphology of biological systems.

chemobiotic (kem'ō-bī-ot'ik, kē-mō-). A combination of an antibiotic with a chemotherapeutic agent; *e.g.,* penicillin plus sulfanilamide.

chemocautery (kem'ō-kaw-ter-ē, kē'mō-). Chemical cautery; chemicocautery; any substance that destroys tissue upon application.

chemoceptor (kem'ō-sep-tōr, kē'mō-). Chemoreceptor.

chemodectoma (kem'ō-dek-tō'mă, kē'mō-). Aortic body, carotid body, chemoreceptor, or glomus jugulare tumor; nonchromaffin paraganglioma; receptoma; a relatively rare, usually benign neoplasm originating in the chemoreceptor tissue of the carotid body, glomus jugulare, and aortic bodies; consisting histologically of rounded or ovoid hyperchromatic cells that tend to be grouped in an alveolus-like pattern within a scant to moderate amount of fibrous stroma and a few large thin-walled vascular channels. *Cf.* paraganglioma.

chemodectomatosis (kem'ō-dek-tō-mă-to'sis, kē'mō-). Multiple tumors of perivascular tissue of carotid body or presumed chemoreceptor type, which have been reported in the lungs as minute neoplasms.

chemodifferentiation (kem'ō-dif-er-en-shē-ā'shŭn, kē'mō-). Invisible differentiation; differentiation of the cellular chemical constituents in the embryo prior to cytodifferentiation; sometimes recognizable histochemically.

chemoheterotroph (kem'ō-het'er-ō-trōf, kē'mō-) [chem- + G. *heteros,* other, + *trophē,* nourishment]. Chemoorganotroph.

chemoheterotrophic (kem'ō-het-er-ō-trof'ik, kē'mō-). Chemoorganotrophic.

chemoimmunology (kem'ō-im-yū-nol'ō-jē, kē'mō-). Immunochemistry.

chemokinesis (kem'ō-ki-nē'sis, kē'mō-) [chemo- + G. *kinēsis,* movement]. Stimulation of an organism by a chemical.

chemokinetic (kem'-ō-ki-net'ik, kē'mo-). Referring to chemokinesis.

chemolithotroph (kem'ō-lith'ō-trōf, kē'mō-). Chemoautotroph.

chemolithotrophic (kem'ō-lith-ō-trof'ik, kē'mō-). Chemoautotrophic.

chemoluminescence (kem'ō-lū-min-es'ens, kē'mō-). Light produced by chemical action.

chemolysis (kem-ol'i-sis) [chemo- + G. *lysis,* dissolution]. Chemical decomposition.

chemonucleolysis (kem'ō-nū-klē-ol'i-sis, kē'mō-). A change in the chemical structure of the nucleus pulposis of the vertebral disc caused by the injection of an emzyme; *e.g.,* a theraputic intervention for the treatment of a herniated nucleus pulposis, *i.e.,* "slipped disk."

chemoorganotroph (kem'ō-ōr'gă-nō-trōf, kē'mō-) [chemo- + G. *organon,* organ, + *trophē,* nourishment]. Chemoheterotroph; an organism that depends on organic chemicals for its energy and carbon.

chemoorganotrophic (kem'ō-ōr-gă-nō-trof'ik, kē'mō-). Chemoheterotrophic; pertaining to a chemoorganotroph.

chemopallidectomy (kem'ō-pal-i-dek'tō-mē, kē'mō-) [chemo- + globus pallidus + G. *ektomē,* excision]. Destruction of the globus pallidus by injection of a chemical agent.

chemopallidothalamectomy (kem'ō-pal'i-dō-thal-ă-mek'tō-mē, kē'mō-) [chemo- + globus pallidus + thalamus + G. *ektomē,* excision]. Destruction of portions of the globus pallidus and thalamus by injection of a chemical substance.

chemopallidotomy (kēm'ō-pal-i-dot'ō-mē, kē'mō-) [chemo- + globus pallidus + G. *tomē,* incision]. Injection of a chemical (usually necrotizing) into the globus pallidus.

chemoprophylaxis (kem'ō-pro'-fi-lak'sis, kē'mō-). Prevention of disease by the use of chemicals or drugs.

chemoreceptor (kem'ō-rē-sep'tŏr, kē'mō-). Chemoceptor; any cell that is activated by a change in its chemical milieu and thereby originates a flow of nervous impulses. Such cells can be either 1) "transducer" cells innervated by sensory nerve fibers (*e.g.*, the gustatory receptor cells of the taste buds; cells in the carotid body that are sensitive to changes in the oxygen and carbon dioxide content of the blood); or 2) nerve cells proper, such as the olfactory receptor cells of the olfactory mucosa, and certain cells in the brainstem that are sensitive to changes in the composition of the blood or cerebrospinal fluid.

medullary c., the c.'s in or near the ventrolateral surface of the medulla that are stimulated by local acidity.

peripheral c., the c.'s in the carotid and aortic bodies that are stimulated by chemical changes in the composition of the blood such as hypoxia.

chemoreflex (kem-ō-rē'fleks, kē-mō-). A reflex initiated by the stimulation of chemoreceptors, *e.g.*, of a carotid body.

chemoresistance (kem'ō-rē-zis'tans, kē'mō-). The resistance of bacteria or malignant cells to the inhibiting action of certain chemical substances used in treatment.

chemosensitive (kem-ō-sen'si-tiv, kē-mō-). Capable of perceiving changes in the chemical composition of the environment, *e.g.*, changes in the oxygen and carbon dioxide content of the blood.

chemoserotherapy (kem'ō-sēr'ō-thār-ă-pē, kē'mō-). An obsolete treatment of disease with a combination of drugs and serum.

chemosis (kē-mō'sis) [G. *chēmē*, a yawning, the cockle (from its gaping shell)]. Edema of the bulbar conjunctiva, forming a swelling around the cornea.

chemosmosis (kem-os-mō'sis) [chem- + G. *ōsmos*, a thrusting, an impulsion]. Chemical reaction between substances initially separated by a membrane.

chemosurgery (kem'ō-ser-jer-ē, kē'mō-). Excision of diseased tissue after it has been fixed *in situ* by chemical means.

chemotactic (kem-ō-tak'tik, kē-mō-). Relating to chemotaxis.

chemotaxis (kem-ō-tak'sis, kē-mo-) [chemo- + G. *taxis*, orderly arrangement]. Chemiotaxis; chemotropism; movement of cells or organisms in response to chemicals, whereby the cells are attracted (**positive c.**) or repelled (**negative c.**) by substances exhibiting chemical properties.

chemothalamectomy (kem'ō-thal-ă-mek'tō-mē, kē'mō-) [chemo- + thalamus, + G. *ektomē*, excision]. Chemothalamotomy; chemical destruction of a part of the thalamus, usually for relief of pain or dyskinesia.

chemothalamotomy (kem'ō-thal-ă-mot'ō-mē, kē'mō-). Chemothalamectomy.

chemotherapeutic (kem'ō-thār-ă-pyū'tik, kē'mō-). Relating to chemotherapy.

chemotherapeutics (kem'ō-thār-ă-pyū'tiks, kē'mō). The branch of therapeutics concerned with chemotherapy.

chemotherapy (kem'ō-thār-ă-pē, kē'mō-). Treatment of disease by means of chemical substances or drugs; usually used in reference to neoplastic disease. See also pharmacotherapy.

consolidation c., intensification c.; repetitive cycles of treatment during the immediate post-remission period, used especially for leukemia.

induction c., use of c. as initial treatment before surgery or radiotherapy of a malignancy.

intensification c., consolidation c.

salvage c., use of c. in a patient with recurrence of a malignancy following initial treatment, in hope of a cure or prolongation of life.

chemotic (kē-mot'ic). Relating to chemosis.

chemotransmitter (kem-ō-trans'mit-er, kē-mō-). A chemical substance produced to diffuse and cause responses of neurons or effector cells.

chemotropism (kem-ō-trōp'izm, kē-mō-) [chemo- + G. *tropos*, direction, turn]. Chemotaxis.

Chenais, Louis J., French physician, 1872–1950. See Cestan-C. *syndrome.*

Cheney, William D., U.S. radiologist, *1918. See C. *syndrome.*

chenodeoxycholic acid (kē'nō-dē-oks-ē-kō'lik). Chenodiol; 3α,7α-dihydroxy -5β-cholan-24-oic acid; a major bile acid in many vertebrates, usually conjugated with glycine or taurine, which facilitates cholesterol excretion and fat absorption; administered to dissolve cholesterol gallstones.

chenodiol (kē-nō-dī'ol). Chenodeoxycholic acid.

chenopodium (kē-nō-pō'dē-ŭm) [G. *chēn*, goose, + *pous* (*pod-*), foot]. Wormseed (2); Mexican or Jesuit tea; the dried ripe fruit of *Chenopodium ambrosoides* (family Chenopodiaceae), American wormwood, from which a volatile oil is distilled and used as an anthelmintic.

cherry juice (chār'ē). The juice expressed from the fresh ripe fruit of *Prunus cerasus*, containing not less than 1.0% of malic acid; used as a flavoring agent, and as a vehicle for cough syrups and other preparations for oral administrations.

cherubism (chār'ŭb-izm) [Hebr. *kerubh*, cherub]. Familial fibrous dysplasia of the jaws; a familial multilocular fibro-osseous disease, with enlargement of the jaw bones in young children (producing the characteristic facies) that tends to regress in adult life; bone formation is by osteoblasts (unlike fibrous dysplasia of bone).

Chervin, Claudius, French pedagogue, 1824–1896. See C.'s *method.*

chest [A.S. *cest*, a box]. Thorax.

alar c., phthinoid c.

barrel c., a c. permanently in the shape of a barrel, *i.e.*, with increased anteroposterior diameter, usually with some degree of kyphosis; seen in cases of emphysema.

blast c., trauma to c. and lungs by shock wave.

flail c., flapping chest wall; loss of stability of thoracic cage following fracture of sternum, ribs, or both.

flat c., a c. in which the anteroposterior diameter is shorter than the average.

foveated or **funnel c.,** *pectus* excavatum.

keeled c., *pectus* carinatum.

phthinoid c., alar or pterygoid c.; a long narrow c., the lower ribs being more oblique than usual and sometimes reaching almost to the crest of the ilium, with the scapulae projecting backward, the manubrium sterni depressed, and Louis' angle sharper than normal; such a c. was once considered indicative of pulmonary tuberculosis.

pterygoid c., phthinoid c.

chestnut (chest'nŭt). A small oval or round horny structure in the skin on the inner side of the legs of the horse. Since the architecture of c.'s varies in every individual, they may be used, like fingerprints of man, for positive identification of individuals.

Cheyne, John, Scottish physician, 1777–1836. See C.'s *nystagmus;* C.-Stokes *psychosis, respiration.*

Chiari, Hans, German pathologist, 1851–1916. See Arnold-C. *deformity, malformation, syndrome;* C.'s *disease, net, syndrome;* C.-Budd *syndrome.*

Chiari, Johann B., German obstetrician, 1817–1854. See C.-Frommel *syndrome.*

chiasm (kī'azm) [G. *chiasma*]. **1.** Chiasma. **2.** The crossing of intertwined chromosomes during prophase.

Camper's c., *chiasma* tendinum.

optic c., *chiasma* opticum.

chiasma, pl. **chiasmata** (kī-az'mă, kī-az'mă-tă) [G. *chiasma*, two crossing lines, fr. the letter *chi,* X] [NA]. Chiasm (1); a decussation or crossing of two tracts, such as tendons or nerves.

c. op'ticum [NA], optic chiasm; optic decussation; a flattened quadrangular body in front of the tuber cinereum and infundibulum, the point of crossing or decussation of the fibers of the optic nerves; most of the fibers cross to the opposite side, some run directly forward on each side without crossing, some pass transversely on the posterior surface between the two optic tracts and others pass transversely on the anterior surface between the two optic nerves.

c. ten'dinum [NA], crossing of the tendons; Camper's chiasm; the passage of the tendons of the flexor digitorum profundus (flexor digitorum longus in the foot) through the interval left by the decussation of the fibers of the tendons of the flexor digitorum superficialis (flexor digitorum brevis in the foot).

chiasmapexy (kī-as'mă-pek-sē) [G. *chiasma,* decussation, + *pexis,* fixation]. Surgical fixation of the optic chiasma.

chiasmatic (kī-az-mat'ik). Relating to a chiasm.

chiasmometer (kī-az-mom'ĕ-ter) [G. *chiasma,* decussation, + *metron,* measure]. An obsolete instrument used to measure the distance between the centers of rotation of the eyes.

chickenpox (chik'en-poks). Varicella.

Chick-Martin test. See under test.

Chievitz, Johan H., Danish anatomist, 1850–1901. See C.'s *layer, organ.*

chigger (chig'er). The six-legged larva of *Trombicula* species and other members of the family Trombiculidae; a bloodsucking stage of mites that includes the vectors of scrub typhus.

chigoe (chig'ō). Common name for *Tunga penetrans.*

chil-. See chilo-.

Chilaiditi, Demetrius. See C.'s *syndrome.*

chilalgia (kī-lal'jē-ă). Cheilalgia.

chilblain (chil'blān) [chill + A.S. *blegen,* a blain]. Erythema pernio; perniosis; erythema, itching, and burning, especially of the dorsa of the fingers and toes, and of the heels, nose, and ears on exposure to extreme cold (usually associated with high humidity); lesions can be single or multiple, and can become blistered and ulcerated.

CHILD See CHILD *syndrome.*

childbearing (chīld'bār-ing). Pregnancy and parturition.

childbirth (chīld'berth). Parturition; the process of labor and delivery in the birth of a child. See also birth, accouchement.

childhood (chīld'hud). The period of life between infancy and puberty.

chilectomy (kī-lek'tō-mē). Cheilectomy.

chilectropion (kī-lek-trō'pē-on). Cheilectropion.

chilitis (kī-lī'tis). Cheilitis.

chill [A.S. *cele,* cold]. **1.** A sensation of cold. **2.** Rigor (2); a feeling of cold with shivering and pallor, accompanied by an elevation of temperature in the interior of the body; usually a prodromal symptom of an infectious disease due to the invasion of the blood by toxins.

chilo-, chil- [G. *cheilos,* lip]. Combining forms denoting relationship to the lips. See also cheilo-, cheil-.

chiloalveoloschisis (kī'lō-al-vē-ō-los'ki-sis). Cheiloalveoloschisis.

chilognathoglossoschisis (kī'lō-nath'ō-glos-os'ki-sis). Cheilognathoglossoschisis.

chilognathopalatoschisis (kī'lō-nath'ō-pal-ă-tos'ki-sis). Cheilognathopalatoschisis.

chilognathoprosoposchisis (kī'lō-nath'ō-pros-ō-pos'ki-sis). Cheilognathoprosoposchisis.

chilognathoschisis (kī'-lō-nath-os'ki-sis). Cheilognathoschisis.

chilognathouranoschisis (kī'lō-nath'ō-yū-rā-nos'ki-sis). Cheilognathouranoschisis.

chilomastigiasis (kī'lō-mas-ti-gī'ă-sis). Chilomastosis; infection with *Chilomastix* flagellates, such as *C. mesnili* of the human cecum.

Chilomastix (kī-lō-mas'tiks) [chilo- + G. *mastix,* whip]. A genus of protozoan flagellates parasitic in the large intestine of man and other primates, and in many other mammals, birds, amphibia, and reptiles; it is ordinarily nonpathogenic, but one species, *C. mesnili,* may be an occasional cause of diarrhea in children.

chilomastosis (kī'lō-mas-tō'sis). Chilomastigiasis.

chilophagia (kī-lō-fā'jē-ă). Cheilophagia.

chiloplasty (kī'lō-plas-tē). Cheiloplasty.

Chilopoda (kī-lop'ō-dă) [chilo- + G. *pous,* foot]. A class of centipedes (phylum Arthropoda).

chilopodiasis (kī'lō-pō-dī'ă-sis). Invasion of one of the cavities, especially the nasal cavity, by a species of Chilopoda.

chilorrhaphy (kī-lōr'ă-fē). Cheilorrhaphy.

chiloschisis (kī-los'ki-sis) [chilo- + G. *schisis,* fissure]. Cleft *lip.*

chilosis (kī-lō'sis). Cheilosis.

chilostomatoplasty (kī-lō-stō'ma-tō-plas-tē). Cheilostomatoplasty.

chilotomy (kī-lot'ō-mē). Cheilotomy.

chimera (kī-mēr'ă, ki-) [L. *chimoera,* fr. G. *chimaira* (lit. a she-goat), a monster: the front a lion, the rear a dragon]. **1.** In experimental embryology, the individual produced by grafting an embryonic part of one animal on to the embryo of another, either of the same or of another species. **2.** An individual who has received a transplant of genetically and immunologically different tissue, such as bone marrow. **3.** Twins with two immunologically different types of erythrocytes. **4.** Sometimes used as a synonym for mosaic.

radiation c., an individual with mosaicism induced by exposure to ionizing radiation. See mosaic.

chimeric (kī-mēr'ik). **1.** Relating to a chimera. **2.** Composed of parts of different origin, or seemingly incompatible.

chimerism (kī-mēr'izm). The state of being a chimera.

chimpanzee (chim-pan'zē, chim'pan-zē') [African dial.]. Generic name for *Pan panisus* and *P. troglodytes.*

chin [A.S. *cin*] Mentum; the prominence formed by the anterior projection of the mandible, or lower jaw.

double c., buccula.

galoche c. (ga-lōsh), an abnormally narrow, protruding c.

chinic acid (chin'ik). Quinic acid.

chiniofon (kin'ē-ō-fon). A mixture of 7-iodo-8-hydroxyquinoline-5-sulfonic acid and sodium bicarbonate, used in the treatment of amebic dysentery.

chinoleine (chin'ō-lē-in). Quinoline.

chip. A small fragment resulting from breakage, cutting, or avulsion.

bone c.'s, small pieces of cancellous bone generally used to fill in bony defects and to promote reossification.

chip-blower. An instrument for blowing the debris out of, or drying, a tooth cavity that is being excavated for a filling; it consists of a rubber bulb with a metal nozzle.

chiral (kī'răl). Denoting an object, such as a molecule in a given configuration or conformation, that possesses chirality.

chirality (kī-ral'i-tē) [G. *cheir,* hand]. The property of nonidentity of an object with its mirror image; used in chemistry with respect to stereochemical isomers.

chirarthritis (kī-rar-thrī'tis). Cheirarthritis.

chiro-, chir- [G. *cheir,* hand]. Combining forms denoting the hand. See also cheiro-, cheir-.

chirobrachialgia (kī'rō-brā-kē-al'jē-ă). Cheirobrachialgia.

chirocinesthesia (kī-rō-sin-es-thē'zē-ă). Cheirokinesthesia.

chirognostic (kī-rog-nos'tik). Cheirognostic.

chirokinesthesia (kī-rō-kin-es-thē'-zē-ă). Cheirokinesthesia.

chirology (kī-rol'ō-jē). Dactylology.

chiromegaly (kī-rō-meg'ă-lē). Macrocheiria.

chiroplasty (kī'rō-plas-tē). Cheiroplasty.

chiropodalgia (kī'rō-pō-dal'jē-ă). Cheiropodalgia.

chiropodist (kī-rop'ō-dist) [chiro- + G. *pous,* foot]. Podiatrist.

chiropody (kī-rop'ō-dē). Podiatry.

chiropompholyx (kī-rō-pom'fō-liks). Dyshidrosis.

chiropractic (kī-rō-prak'tik) [chiro- + G. *praktikos,* efficient]. The system which utilizes the recuperative powers of the body and the relationship between the musculoskeletal structures and functions of the body, particularly of the spinal column and the nervous system, in the restoration and maintenance of health.

chiropractor (kī-rō-prak'tōr). One who is licensed and certified to practice chiropractic.

Chiroptera (kī-rop'ter-ă) [chiro- + G. *pteron,* wing]. The bats, an order of placental mammals of worldwide distribution, characterized by a modification of the forelimbs that enables them to fly. They are capable of emitting ultrasonic sounds that enable them to echolocate, find flying insect prey, and avoid objects in the dark. Though mostly insectivorous, some species feed on nectar, fruit, fish, and blood; the blood-feeding and insectivorous species are important reservoir hosts of rabies, in which the infection is thought to be frequently maintained without apparent pathology.

chiroscope (kī'rō-skōp) [chiro- + G. *skopeō,* to view]. A haploscopic instrument used for coordinating hand and eye as the patient draws while looking through it.

chirospasm (kī'rō-spazm). Cheirospasm.

chirurgeon (kī-rer'jon) [G. *cheirourgus,* fr. *cheir,* hand, + *ergon,* work]. Obsolete term for surgeon.

chirurgery (kī-rer'jer-ē) [G. *cheirourgia*] Obsolete term for surgery.

chirurgical (kī-rer'ji-kăl). Obsolete term for surgical.

chisel (chiz'l). A single beveled end-cutting blade with a straight or angled shank used with a thrust along the axis of the handle for cutting or splitting dentin and enamel.

binangle c., a c. with an angled shank to which a second angle is added in order to bring the cutting edge nearly in line with the axis of the handle so as to restore balance and to prevent it from turning about the axis; used when a c. must be angled for access.

chi-square (kī' skwār). A statistical technique whereby variables are categorized to determine whether a distribution of scores is due to chance or experimental factors.

chitin (kī'tin). A polymer of *N*-acetyl-D-glucosamine, similar in structure to cellulose and the second most abundant polysaccharide in nature, comprising the horny substance in the exoskeleton of beetles, crabs, certain microorganisms.

chitinase (kī'ti-nās) [EC 3.2.1.14]. Chitodextrinase; poly-β-glucosaminidase; an enzyme catalyzing the hydrolysis of chitin to *N*- acetylglucosamine; some enzymes of this type display lysozyme activity.

chitinous (kī'tin-ŭs). Of or relating to chitin.

chitobiose (kī-tō-bī'ōs). The disaccharide repeating unit in chitin; differs from cellobiose only in the presence of an *N*-acetylamino group on carbon-2 in place of the hydroxyl group.

chitodextrinase (kī-tō-deks'tri-nās). Chitinase.

chitoneure (kī'tō-nūr) [G. *chiton,* tunic, + *neuron,* sinew, nerve]. A rarely used collective term for the sheaths of nerves, nerve bundles, and nerve fibrils.

chitosamine (kī-tō'să-mēn). Glucosamine.

chiufa (chē-ū'fă). Kanyemba; an acute gangrenous proctitis and colitis with high fever, seen in southern Africa and South America at high altitudes; in women, the vulva and vagina may be affected.

Chlamydia (kla-mid'ē-ă) [G. *chlamys,* cloak]. *Chlamydozoon; Miyagawanella;* the single genus of the family Chlamydiaceae, including all the agents of the psittacosis-lymphogranuloma-trachoma disease groups. Two species are recognized, *C. psittaci* and *C. trachomatis;* the latter is differentiated from the former by its intracytoplasmic production of glycogen and its susceptibility to sulfadiazine. The type species is *C. trachomatis.* Formerly called *Bedsonia.*

C. oculogenita'lis, former name for *C. trachomatis.*

C. psitta'ci, *Rickettsia psittaci;* organisms that resemble *C. trachomatis,* but which form loosely bound intracytoplasmic microcolonies up to 12 μm in diameter, do not produce glycogen in sufficient quantity to be detected by iodine stains, and are not susceptible to sulfadiazine. Various strains of this species cause psittacosis in man and ornithosis in nonpsittacine birds; pneumonitis in cattle, sheep, swine, cats, goats, and horses; enzootic abortion of ewes; bovine sporadic encephalomyelitis; enteritis of calves; epizootic chlamydiosis of muskrats and hares; encephalitis of opossum; and conjunctivitis of cattle, sheep, and guinea pigs.

C. tracho'matis, spherical nonmotile organisms that form compact intracytoplasmic microcolonies up to 10 μm in diameter which (by division) give rise to infectious spherules 0.3 μm or more in diameter, accumulate glycogen for a limited period in sufficient quantity to be detected by iodine stain, and are susceptible to sulfadiazine and tetracycline; various strains of this species cause trachoma, inclusion and neonatal conjunctivitis, lymphogranuloma venereum, mouse pneumonitis, nonspecific urethritis, epididymitis, cervicitis, salpingitis, proctitis, and pneumonia; it is the type species of the genus *C.*

chlamydia, pl. **chlamydiae** (kla-mid'ē-ă, -mid'ē-ē). A vernacular term used to refer to any member of the genus *Chlamydia.*

Chlamydiaceae (kla-mid'ē-ā'sē-ē). Chlamydozoaceae; a family of the order Chlamydiales (formerly included in the order Rickettsiales) that includes the agents of the psittacosis-lymphogranuloma-trachoma group. The family contains small, coccoid, Gram-negative bacteria that resemble rickettsiae but which differ from them significantly by possessing a unique, obligately intracellular developmental cycle; intracytoplasmic microcolonies give rise to infectious forms by division. The classification of these organisms previously was in a state of flux, but they are now placed in a single genus, *Chlamydia,* the type genus of the family.

chlamydial (kla-mid'ē-ăl). Relating to or caused by any bacterium of the genus *Chlamydia.*

chlamydiosis (klă-mid-ē-ō'sis). General term for diseases caused by *Chlamydia psittaci* and *C. trachomatis.* See also ornithosis, psittacosis.

Chlamydoconidium (klam'i-dō-kō-nid'ē-um) [G. *chlamys,* cloak, + conidium]. A thallic conidium formed by modification of a preexisting hyphal cell which is usually enlarged, with a thicker wall and denser protoplasm; release is by separation from adjacent hyphal cells.

Chlamydophrys (kla-mid'ō-fris) [G. *chlamys,* cloak, + *ophrys,* brow]. A genus of shelled amebas, commonly found as fecal protozoans.

Chlamydozoaceae (kla-mid'ō-zō-ā'sē-ē, klam'i-dō-). Chlamydiaceae.

Chalmydozoon (klam'i-dō-zō'on). Chlamydia.

chloasma (klō-az'mă) [G. *chloazō,* to become green]. Moth patch; melanoderma or melasma characterized by the occurrence of extensive brown patches of irregular shape and size on the skin of the face and elsewhere; the pigmented patches are also called the mask of pregnancy, and are associated most commonly with pregnancy, menopause, and use of oral contraceptives.

c. bronzi'num, tropical mask; a bronze-colored pigmentation, probably produced by hormone imbalance, occurring in gradually increasing areas on the face, neck, and chest in persons exposed continuously to the tropical sun; similar to c. of the temperate zone, but intensified because of intense sunlight.

chlophedianol hydrochloride (klō-fē-dī'ă-nol). 2-Chloro-α-(2-dimethylaminoethyl)benzhydrol hydrochloride; an antitussive agent related chemically to the antihistamines.

chlor-, chloro- [G. *chloros,* green] Combining form denoting green; association with chlorine.

chloracetic acid (klōr-ă-sē'tik). Chloroacetic acid.

chloracne (klōr-ak'nē). Chlorine or tar acne; an acne-like eruption due to prolonged contact with certain chlorinated compounds (naphthalenes and diphenyls); keratinous plugs (comedones) form in the pilosebaceous orifices, and variously sized small papules (2 to 4 mm) develop.

chloral (klōr'ăl). Anhydrous chloral; trichloroacetaldehyde; CCl_3-CHO; a thin oily liquid with a pungent odor, formed by the action of chlorine gas on alcohol.

anhydrous c., chloral.

c. betaine, the adduct formed by chloral hydrate and betaine; it is slowly hydrolyzed in the alimentary tract to chloral hydrate; used as a hypnotic and sedative.

c. hydrate, $CCl_3CH(OH)_2$; a hypnotic, sedative, and anticonvulsant; it is also used externally as a rubefacient, anesthetic, and antiseptic.

***m*-chloral.** *p*-Chloral; metachloral; trichloral; a polymer of chloral obtained by prolonged contact with sulfuric acid; it has properties similar to those of chloral hydrate.

***p*-chloral.** *m*-Chloral.

chloralism (klōr'ăl-izm). Habitual use of chloral compounds as an intoxicant, or the symptoms caused thereby.

chlorambucil (klōr-am'byū-sil). Chloraminophene; chloroambucil; 4-{*p*-[bis(2-chloroethyl)amino]phenyl}butyric acid; a nitrogen mustard derivative that depresses lymphocytic proliferation and maturation.

chloramine B (klōr'ă-mēn). Sodium *N*-chlorobenzenesulfonamide; a nontoxic antiseptic substance used in wound irrigation as a substitute for c. T.

chloramine T. Chlorazene; sodium *N*-chloro-*p*-toluenesulfonamide; a nontoxic but strong antiseptic used in the irrigation of wounds and infected cavities.

chloraminophene (klōr-am'i-nō-fēn). Chlorambucil.

chloramiphene (klōr-am'i-fēn). Clomiphene citrate.

chloramphenicol (klōr-am-fen'i-kol). D-(−)-*threo*- 2,2-Dichloro-*N*- [β-hydroxy-α-(hydroxymethyl)-*p*- nitrophenethyl]acetamide; an antibiotic originally obtained from *Streptomyces Venezuelae.* It is effective against a number of pathogenic microorganisms including *Staphylococcus aureus, Brucella abortus,* Friedländer's bacillus, and the organisms of typhoid, typhus, and Rocky Mountain spotted fever; active by mouth. A serious reaction resulting in marrow damage with agranulocytosis or aplastic anemia may occur.

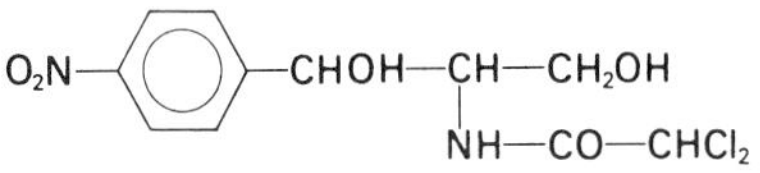

Chloramphenicol

c. palmitate, same action and use as c.

c. sodium succinate, chloramphenicol-α-(sodium succinate); the water-soluble sodium succinate derivative of c., suitable for parenteral administration; antibacterial activity, uses, and side effects are similar to those of the parent compound.

chlorate (klōr'āt). A salt of chloric acid.

chlorazanil (klō-raz'ă-nil). 2-Amino-4-(*p*-chloroanilino)-*s*-triazine; a diuretic.

chlorazene (klōr'ă-zēn). Chloramine T.

chlorazol black E (klor'ă-zol) [C.I. 30235]. An acid dye, $C_{34}H_{25}N_9O_7S_2Na_2$, used as a fat and general tissue stain, and to stain protozoa in fecal smears or in tissues.

chlorbenzoxamine (klōr-ben-zok'să-mēn). Chlorbenzoxyethamine; 1-[2-(*o*- chloro-α- phenylbenzyloxy)ethyl]-4-*o* methylbenzylpiperazine; an anticholinergic agent.

chlorbenzoxyethamine (klōr'ben-zok-sē-eth'ă-mēn). Chlorbenzoxamine.

chlorbetamide (klōr-bet'ă-mīd). 2,2-Dichloro-*N*-(2,4-dichlorobenzyl)-*N*-(2-hydroxyethyl)acetamide; an amebicide.

chlorbutol (klōr-byū'tol). Chlorobutanol.

chlorcyclizine hydrochloride (klōr-sik'li-zēn). 1-(*p*-Chlorobenzhydryl)-4-methylpiperazine hydrochloride; an antihistaminic agent.

chlordane (klōr'dān). A chlorinated hydrocarbon used as an insecticide; it may be absorbed through the skin with resultant severe toxic effects: hyperexcitability of central nervous system, tremors, lack of muscular coordination, convulsions, and death; also causes damage to the liver, kidneys, and spleen. It is only mildly toxic to animals.

chlordantoin (klōr-dan'tō-in). 5-(1-Ethylpentyl)-3-(trichloromethylthio)hydantoin; a topical antifungal agent.

chlordiazepoxide hydrochloride (klōr'dī-az-ē-pok'sīd). The hydrochloride of 7-chloro-2-methylamino-5-phenyl-3*H*- 1,4-benzodiazepine-4-oxide; an antianxiety agent.

chloremia (klō-rē'mē-ă). **1.** Chlorosis. **2.** Hyperchloremia.

chlorethene homopolymer (klōr'eth-ēn). Polyvinyl chloride.

chlorethyl (klōr-eth'il). *Ethyl* chloride.

chlorguanide hydrochloride (klōr-gwah'nīd). Chloroguanide hydrochloride.

chlorhexadol (klōr-heks'ă-dol). 2-Methyl-4-(2,2,2-trichloro-1-hydroxy-ethoxy)-2-pentanol; a hypnotic.

chlorhexidine hydrochloride (klōr-hek'si-dēn). 1,1'-Hexamethylenebis-[5- (*p*-chlorophenyl) biguanide] dihydrochloride; a topical antiseptic.

chlorhydria (klōr-hī'drē-ă). Hyperchlorhydria.

chloric acid (klōr'ik). An acid of pentavalent chlorine, $HClO_3$, existing only in solution and as chlorates.

chloride (klōr'īd). A compound containing chlorine, at a valence of −1, as in the salts of hydrochloric acid.

chloridimetry (klōr-ĭ-dim'ĕ-trē). The process of determining the amount of chlorides in the blood or urine, or in other fluids.

chloridometer (klōr-i-dom'ĕ-ter). An apparatus for determining the amount of chlorides in blood or urine, or other fluids.

chloriduria (klōr-i-dū'rē-ă). Chloruresis.

chlorin (klōr'in). 2,3-Dihydroporphin(e); 2,3-dihydroporphyrin; the root structure of the chlorophylls (for structure, see porphyrin). Addition of the two-carbon bridge (see structure of chlorophyll) to c. yields phorbin(e); addition of side-chains yields the phorbides, distinguished by a number of arbitrary prefixes (those found in the chlorophylls are pheo- and bacteriopheophorbide); esterification of the propionic group by phytyl yields the respective phytins, and the addition of magnesium yields the chlorophylls (magnesium phytinates).

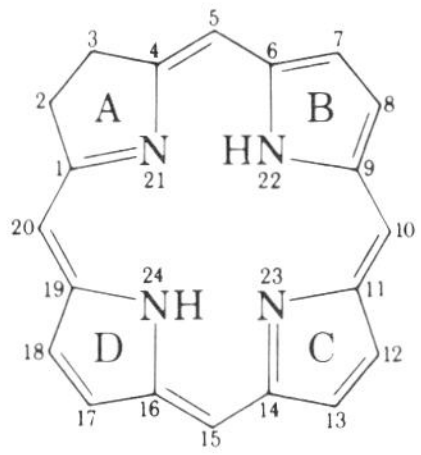

Chlorin

chlorinated (klōr'in-āt-ĕd). Having been treated with chlorine.

chlorindanol (klōr-in'dă-nol). 7-Chloro-4-indanol; a spermicide.

chlorine (klōr'ēn). A greenish, toxic, gaseous element; symbol Cl, atomic no. 17, atomic weight 35.46; a halogen used as a disinfectant and bleaching agent in the form of hypochlorite or of c. water, because of its oxidizing power.

chlorine group. The halogens.

chloriodized (klōr-ī'ō-dīzd). Containing both chlorine and iodine.

chloriodized oil. Iodochlorol; chlorinated and iodized peanut oil formed by the chemical addition of iodine monochloride; contains chlorine 7.5 and iodine 27.0%; used for roentgenography of sinus and bronchial tract.

chloriodoquin (klōr'ē-ō-dō'kwin). Iodochlorhydroxyguin.

chlorisondamine chloride (klōr-i-son'dă-mēn). 4,5,6,7-Tetrachloro-2-(2-dimethylaminoethyl)-2-methylisoindolinium chloride; a quaternary ammonium compound with ganglionic blocking action similar to, but more potent than, hexamethonium and pentolinium; used in the management of severe hypertension, including the malignant phase.

chlorite (klōr'īt). A salt of chlorous acid; the radical ClO_2^-.

chlormadinone acetate (klōr-mad'i-nōn). 6-chloro-17-hydroxy-4,6-pregnadiene-3,20-dione acetate; 6-chloro-6-dehydro-17α-acetoxyprogesterone; a progesterone derivative used in conjunction with estrogen as an oral contraceptive.

chlormerodrin (klōr-mer'od-rin). 1-[3-(Chloromercuri)-2-methoxypropyl]urea; a mercurial diuretic chemically related to meralluride.

chlormezanone (klōr-mez'ă-nōn). 2-(4-Chlorophenyl)-3-methyl-4-metathiazanone-1,1-dioxide; a muscle relaxant and tranquilizing agent with pharmacologic actions and uses similar to those of meprobamate.

chloro-. See chlor-.

chloroacetic acid (klōr'ō-ă-sē'tik). Chloracetic acid; an acetic acid in which one or more of the hydrogen atoms are replaced by chlorine. According to the number of atoms so displaced the acid is called monochloroacetic (chloroacetic), dichloroacetic, or trichloroacetic.

chloroacetophenone (klōr'ō-as'ĕ-tō-fē'nōn). $C_6H_5COCH_2Cl$; a lacrimatory gas.

chloroambucil (klōr-ō-am'byū-sil). Chlorambucil.

chloroanemia (klōr'ō-ă-nē'mē-ă). Chlorosis.

chloroazodin (klōr-ō-az'ō-din). α,α'-Azo-bis(chloroformamidine); a bactericidal agent used as a surgical antiseptic.

chlorobutanol (klōr-ō-byū'tă-nol). Acetone chloroform; chlorbutol; trichloro-*tert*-butyl alcohol; $Cl_3CC(CH_3)_2OH$; a hypnotic sedative and local anesthetic; used chiefly as a preservative in multiple-dose vials for parenteral use.

chlorocresol (klōr-ō-krē'sol). *p*-Chloro-*m*-cresol; used as an antiseptic and disinfectant; it is more active in acid than in alkaline solutions.

chlorocruorin (klōr-ō-krū'ōr-in). A greenish hemoglobin-like pigment found in certain worms; contains a porphyrin differing from protoporphyrin by a formyl group in place of the 2-vinyl group.

chloroethane (klōr-ō-eth'ān). *Ethyl* chloride.

chloroethylene (klōr-ō-eth'i-lēn). *Vinyl* chloride.

chloroform (klōr'ō-fōrm) [chlor(ine) + form(yl)]. Trichloromethane; methylene trichloride; $CHCl_3$; formerly used by inhalation to produce general anesthesia; also used as a solvent.
acetone c., chlorobutanol.

chloroformism (klōr'ō-fōrm-izm). Habitual chloroform inhalation, or the symptoms caused thereby.

chloroguanide hydrochloride (klōr-ō-gwah'nīd). Proguanil hydrochloride; chlorguanide hydrochloride; 1-(*p*-chlorophenyl)-5-isopropylbiguanide monohydrochloride; an antimalarial drug.

chlorohemin (klōr-ō-hē'min). Hemin.

chloroleukemia (klōr'ō-lū-kē'mē-ă) [chloro- + G. *leukos,* white, + *haima,* blood]. Chloroma.

chloroma (klō-rō'mă) [chloro- + G. *-ōma,* tumor]. Chloroleukemia; chloromyeloma; green cancer; a condition characterized by the development of multiple localized green masses of abnormal cells (in most instances, myeloblasts), especially in relation to the periosteum of the skull, spine, and ribs; the clinical course is similar to that of acute myeloid leukemia, although the tumors may precede the findings in blood and bone marrow; observed more frequently in children and young adults.

p-**chloromercuribenzoate (PCMB, *p* CMB)** (klōr'ō-mer'cyūr-ē-ben'zō-āt). Organic mercury compound ($ClHgC_6H_4COO^-$, $ClHgBzO^-$) that reacts with —SH groups of proteins; an inhibitor of action of those proteins (enzymes) that depend on —SH reactivity. See also *p* -mercuribenzoate.

chloromethane (klōr-ō-meth'ān). Methyl chloride; a refrigerant with anesthetic properties when inhaled; it hydrolyzes to methanol.

chlorometry (klo-rom'ĕ-trē). The measurement of chlorine content, or the use of analytical techniques involving the release or titration of chlorine.

chloromyeloma (klōr'ō-mī-ĕ-lō'mă) [chloro- + G. *myelos,* marrow, + *-ōma,* tumor]. Chloroma.

chloropenia (klōr-ō-pē'nē-ă) [chloro- + G. *penia,* poverty]. A deficiency in chloride.

chloropercha (klōr-ō-per'chă). A solution of gutta-percha in chloroform, used in dentistry as an agent to lute gutta-percha filling material to the wall of a prepared root canal.

chlorophenol (klōr-ō-fē'nol). One of several substitution products obtained by the action of chlorine on phenol; used as antiseptics.

o-**chlorophenol.** An antiseptic liquid, used in the treatment of lupus.

p-**chlorophenol.** Parachlorophenol.

chlorophenothane (klōr-ō-fen'ō-thān). Dichlorodiphenyltrichloroethane.

chlorophyll (klōr'ō-fil). The phorbin derivative found in photosynthetic organisms; light-absorbing green plant pigments that, in living plants, convert light energy into oxidizing and reducing power, thus fixing CO_2 and evolving O_2; the naturally occurring forms are c. *a, b, c,* and *d.* See also phorbin.

c. *a,* magnesium(II) pheophytinate *a* [(pheophytinato *a*)magnesium(II)]; the major pigment found in all oxygen-evolving photosynthetic organisms (higher plants, and red and green algae).
c. *b* (CH_3 at 7 replaced by CHO in the c. structure), magnesium(II) pheophytinate *b* [(pheophytinato *b*)magnesium(II)] ; the c. generally characteristic of higher plants (including the *Chlorophyta, Euglenaphyta,* and green algae).

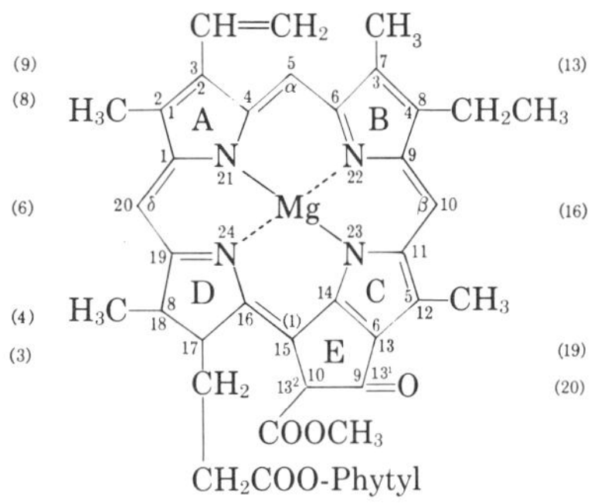

Chlorophyll *a*
Inner numbers: old system (Fischer), based on porphyrin.
Outer numbers: modern system, based on porphyrin.
Numbers in parentheses: Chemical Abstracts system, based on phorbin.

c. *c*, the c. present in brown algae, diatoms, and flagellates. Two variants are known: c_1, in which two hydrogens are lost from C-17 and C-18, thus resembling phytoporphyrin, and the side chain at C-17 becomes an acrylic residue, —CH=CH_2COOH; c_2, in which the same changes are noted, but two more hydrogens are lost from the ethyl group at C-8, making this a vinyl residue like that at C-3. The two compounds can thus be named in terms of phytoporphyrin: magnesium $3^1,3^2,17^1,17^2$-tetradehydro-13^2-(methoxycarbonyl)phytoporphyrinate and magnesium $3^1,3^2,8^1,8^2,17^1,17^2$-hexadehydro-$13^2$-(methoxycarbonyl)phytoporphyrinate.

c. *d* (—CH=CH_2 replaced by —CO—CH_3 in the c. structure), the c. found in red algae, together with c. *a*.

c. esterase, chlorophyllase.

water-soluble c. derivatives, the copper complex of sodium and/or potassium salts of saponified c., used topically for deodorization of chronic lesions and to promote wound repair.

chlorophyllase (klōr-ō-fil-ās) [EC 3.1.1.14]. Chlorophyll esterase; a hydrolyzing enzyme catalyzing the removal of the phytyl group from a chlorophyll, leaving a chlorophyllide.

chlorophyllide, chlorophyllid (klōr'ō-fil-id). That which remains of a chlorophyll molecule when the phytyl group is removed.

chloropicrin (klōr-ō-pik'rin). Nitrochloroform; trichloronitromethane; CCl_3NO_2; a toxic lung irritant and lacrimatory gas; it also causes vomiting, colic, and diarrhea, and therefore is called vomiting gas.

chloroplast (klōr'ō-plast) [chloro- + G. *plastos,* formed]. A plant cell inclusion body containing chlorophyll; occurs in cells of leaves and young stems.

chloroprednisone (klōr-ō-pred'ni-sōn). 6α-Chloro-17,21-dihydroxypregna-1,4-diene-3,11,20-trione; a topical anti-inflammatory agent.

chloroprocaine hydrochloride (klōr-ō-prō'kān). β-Diethylaminoethyl-2-chloro-4-aminobenzoate hydrochloride; a local anesthetic similar in action and use to procaine hydrochloride.

chloropsia (klo-rop'sē-ă) [chloro- + G. *opsis,* eyesight]. Green vision; a condition in which objects appear to be colored green, as may occur in digitalis intoxication.

chloropyramine (klōr-ō-pir'ă-mēn). 2-[*p*-Chlorobenzyl-(2-dimethylaminoethyl)amino]pyridine; an antihistaminic agent.

chloroquine (klōr'ō-kwīn). 7-Chloro-4-(4-diethylamino-1-methylbutylamino)quinoline; an antimalarial agent used for the treatment and suppression of *Plasmodium vivax, P. malariae,* and *P. falciparum;* available as the phosphate and sulfate. It does not produce a radical cure because it has no effect on the exoerythrocytic stages; c.-resistant strains of *P. falciparum* have developed in Southeast Asia, Africa, and South America. It is also used for hepatic amebiasis and for certain skin diseases, *e.g.,* lupus erythematosus and lichen planus.

chlorosis (klōr-ō'sis) [chloro- + G. *-osis,* condition]. Rarely used term for a form of chronic hypochromic microcytic (iron deficiency) anemia, characterized by a great reduction in hemoglobin out of proportion to the decreased number of red blood cells; observed chiefly in females from puberty to the third decade and usually associated with diets deficient in iron and protein. Also called chlorotic or asiderotic anemia; chloremia (1); chloroanemia; green sickness.

chlorothen citrate (klōr'ō-then). Chloromethapyrilene citrate; *N,N*- dimethyl-*N'*-(2-pyridyl)-*N'*-(5-chloro-2-thenyl)ethylenediamine citrate; an antihistaminic agent.

chlorothiazide (klōr-ō-thī'ă-zīd). 6-Chloro-7-sulfamyl-1,2,4-benzothiadiazine-1,1-dioxide; an orally effective diuretic inhibiting renal tubular reabsorption of sodium; used in the treatment of edema due to congestive heart failure, liver disease, pregnancy, premenstrual tension, and drugs; also used as an adjunct in the management of hypertension.

c. sodium, c. suitable for parenteral administration.

chlorothymol (klōr-ō-thī'mol). Monochlorothymol; chlorthymol; $C_{10}H_{13}OCl$; an antibacterial for topical use.

chlorotic (klō-rot'ik). Pertaining to or having the characteristic features of chlorosis.

chlorotrianisene (klōr'ō-trī-an'i-sēn). Chlorotris(*p*-methoxyphenyl)ethylene; a synthetic estrogen derived from stilbene, active by mouth.

chlorous (klōr'ŭs). **1.** Relating to chlorine. **2.** Denoting compounds of chlorine in which its valence is +3; *e.g.,* c. acid.

chlorous acid. $HClO_2$; an acid forming chlorites with bases.

β-chlorovinyldichloroarsine (klōr'ō-vī'nil-dī-klōr'ō-ar'sēn). Lewisite.

chlorphenesin (klōr-fen'ĕ-sin). 3-(*p*-Chlorophenoxy)-1,2-propenediol; a topical antifungal agent.

c. carbamate, carbamic acid 3-(4-chlorophenoxy)-2-hydroxypropyl ester; a skeletal muscle relaxant.

chlorphenindione (klōr-fen-in-dī'ōn). An anticoagulant related chemically to phenindione.

chlorpheniramine maleate (klōr-fen-ir'ă-mēn). (±)-2-[*p*-Chloro-α-[2-(dimethylamino)ethyl]benzyl]pyridine maleate; an antihistamine.

chlorphenol red (klōr-fē'nol). An acid-base indicator (MW 423, pK 6.0): yellow at pH values below 5.1, red above 6.7.

chlorphenoxamine (klōr-fen-ok'să-mēn). 2-(*p*-Chloro-α-methyl-α-phenylbenzyloxy)-*N,N*-dimethylethylamine hydrochloride; used in the management of idiopathic, arteriosclerotic, and postencephalitic parkinsonism, usually with concomitant administration of other anti-parkinsonian agents.

chlorphentermine hydrochloride (klōr-fen'ter-mēn). 4-Chloro-α,α-dimethylphenethylamine hydrochloride; a sympathomimetic amine used as an anorexiant.

chlorproethazine hydrochloride (klōr-prō-eth'ă-zēn). 2-Chloro-10-(3-diethylaminopropyl)phenothiazine; a skeletal muscle relaxant.

chlorproguanil hydrochloride (klōr-prō'gwah-nil). The 3,4-dichloro homologue of chloroguanide; used for causal prophylaxis and suppression of falciparum malaria.

chlorpromazine (klōr-prō'mă-zēn). 10-(3-Dimethylaminopropyl)-2-chlorophenothiazine; a phenothiazine antipsychotic agent with antiemetic, antiadrenergic, and anticholinergic actions. Although chemically related to promethazine, it has no antihistamine action, depresses conditioned reflexes and the hypothalamic centers, and has a hypotensive action of central origin.

c. hydrochloride, c. suitable for oral, intramuscular, and intravenous administration.

chlorpropamide (klōr-prō'pă-mīd). 1-(*p*-Chlorophenylsulfonyl)-3-propylurea; an orally effective hypoglycemic agent related chemically and pharmacologically to tolbutamide; used in controlling hyperglycemia in selected patients with diabetes mellitus.

chlorprothixene (klōr-prō-thik'sēn). 2-Chloro-9-(3-dimethylaminopropylidene)thiaxanthene; an antipsychotic of the thioxanthene group; it also possesses antiemetic, adrenolytic, spasmolytic, and antihistaminic actions.

chlorquinaldol (klōr-kwin'al-dol). 5,7-Dichloro-8-hydroxyquinaldine; a keratoplastic, antibacterial, and antifungal agent used in the treatment of cutaneous bacterial and mycotic infections.

chlortetracycline (klōr'tet-ră-sī'klēn). An antibiotic agent; a naphthacene derivative, obtained from *Streptomyces aureofaciens;* active against a wide range of pathogenic microorganisms including hemolytic streptococci, staphylococci, typhoid bacilli, and brucellae, as well as against certain viruses. Also available as c. calcium and c. hydrochloride.

chlorthalidone (klōr-thal'i-dōn). 2-Chloro-5-(1-hydroxy-3-oxo-1-isoindolinyl)benzenesulfonamide; an orally effective diuretic and antihypertensive agent, used in steroid therapy and the treatment of edema associated with congestive heart failure, renal disease, hepatic cirrhosis, pregnancy, obesity, and premenstrual tension; it produces an increase in the excretion of sodium, chloride, potassium, and water.

chlorthenoxazin (klōr-then-ok'să-zin). 2-(2-Chloroethyl)-2,3-dihydro-4*H*-1,3-benzoxazin-4-one; an antipyretic and analgesic.

chlorthymol (klōr-thī'mol). Chlorothymol.

chloruresis (klōr-yū-rē'sis). Chloruria; chloriduria; the excretion of chloride in the urine.

chloruretic (klōr-yū-ret'ik). Relating to an agent that increases the excretion of chloride in the urine, or to such an effect.

chloruria (klōr-yū'rē-ă). Chloruresis.

chlorzoxazone (klōr-zok'să-zōn). 5-Chloro-2-benzoxazolol; a skeletal muscle relaxant used in the treatment of painful muscle spasm due to musculoskeletal disorder of non-neurologic origin.

choana, pl. **choanae** (kō'an-ă, kō-ă'nē) [Mod. L. fr. G. *choanē,* a funnel] [NA]. Posterior naris; postnaris; isthmus pharyngonasalis; pharyngeal isthmus; the opening into the nasopharynx of the nasal cavity on either side.

primary or **primitive c.,** initial opening of the nasal pits of the embryo into the rostral part of the primordial oronasal cavity, before the formation of the secondary palate.

secondary c., internal nostril; the definitive c. opening into the nasopharynx, after the nasal chambers have been lengthened by the formation of the secondary palate.

choanal (kō'ă-năl). Pertaining to a choana.

choanate (kō'an-āt). Having a funnel, *i.e.,* with a ring or collar.

choanoflagellate (kō'an-ō-flaj'ĕ-lāt). Choanomastigote.

choanoid (kō'ă-noyd) [G. *choanē,* funnel, + *eidos,* resemblance]. Infundibuliform; funnel-shaped.

choanomastigote (kō'an-ō-mas'tī-gōt) [G. *choanē,* a funnel, + *mastix,* whip]. Choanoflagellate; collared flagellate; a term, in the series used to describe developmental stages of the parasitic flagellates, denoting the "barleycorn" form of the flagellate in the genus *Crithidia* characterized by a collarlike extension surrounding the anterior and through which the single flagellum emerges. See also amastigote; epimastigote; promastigote; trypomastigote.

Choanotaenia infundibulum (kō-ă-nō-tē'nē-ă) [G. *choanē,* a funnel, + L., fr. G. *tainia,* tapeworm]. An important species of cosmopolitan tapeworm of fowls, occurring in the small intestine and transmitted by houseflies and stableflies; related to *Dipylidium,* the double-pored dog tapeworm.

Chodzko's reflex. See under reflex.

choke (chōk). **1.** To prevent respiration by compression or obstruction of the larynx or trachea. **2.** Any obstruction of the esophagus in herbivorous animals by a partly swallowed foreign body.

thoracic c., obstruction by a foreign body in the thoracic portion of the esophagus of an animal.

chokes (chōks). A manifestation of decompression sickness or altitude sickness characterized by dyspnea, coughing, and choking.

chol-. See chole-.

cholagogic (kō-lă-goj'ik). Cholagogue (2).

cholagogue (kō'lă-gog) [chol- + G. *agōgos,* drawing forth]. **1.** An agent that promotes the flow of bile into the intestine, especially as a result of contraction of the gallbladder. **2.** Cholagogic; relating to such an agent or effect.

cholaic acid (kō-lā'ik). Taurocholic acid.

cholalic acid (kō-lal'ik). Cholic acid.

cholane, 5β-cholane (kō'lān). Parent hydrocarbon of the cholanic acids (cholic acids); androstane with a $—CH(CH_3)CH_2CH_2CH_3$ group in the 17 position. 5α-cholane is sometimes called allocholane. For structures, see steroids.

cholaneresis (kō-lă-ner'ĕ-sis). Increase in output of cholic acid or its conjugates.

cholangeitis (kō'lan-jē-ī'tis). Cholangitis.

cholangiectasis (kō-lan-jē-ek'tă-sis) [chol- + G. *angeion,* vessel, + *ektasis,* a stretching]. Dilation of the bile ducts, usually a sequel to obstruction.

cholangiocarcinoma (kō-lan'jē-ō-kar-si-nō'mă). An adenocarcinoma, primarily in intrahepatic bile ducts, composed of ducts lined by cuboidal or columnar cells that do not contain bile, with abundant fibrous stroma; cirrhosis is usually absent.

cholangioenterostomy (kō-lan'jē-ō-en-ter-os'tō-mē). Surgical anastomosis of bile duct to intestine.

cholangiofibrosis (kō-lan'jē-ō-fī-brō'sis) [chol- + G. *angeion,* vessel, + fibrosis]. Fibrosis of the bile ducts.

cholangiogastrostomy (kō-lan'jē-ō-gas-tros'tō-mē) [chol- + G. *angeion,* vessel, + *gastēr,* belly, + *stoma,* mouth]. Formation of a communication between a bile duct and the stomach.

cholangiogram (kō-lan'jē-ō-gram). The roentgenographic record of the bile ducts obtained by cholangiography.

cholangiography (kō-lan-jē-og'ră-fē) [chol- + G. *angeion,* vessel, + *graphō,* to write]. Roentgenographic examination of the bile ducts.

cystic duct c., roentgenography of the biliary system after introduction of contrast medium through the cystic duct.

percutaneous c., roentgenography of the biliary system after introduction of contrast medium by introducing a needle through the skin inferior to the right costal margin, and inserting it into the substance of the liver or into the gallbladder.

cholangiole (kō-lan'jē-ōl) [chol- + G. *angeion,* vessel, + *-ole,* small]. Canal of Hering; a ductule occurring between a bile canaliculus and an interlobular bile duct.

cholangiolitis (kō-lan'jē-ō-lī'tis). Inflammation of the small bile radicles or cholangioles.

cholangioma (kō-lan'jē-ō'mă) [chol- + G. *angeion,* vessel, + *-oma,* tumor]. A neoplasm of bile duct origin, especially within the liver; may be either benign or malignant (cholangiocarcinoma).

cholangiopancreatography (kō-lan'jē-ō-pan-krē-ă-tog'ră-fē). Roentgenographic examination of the bile ducts and pancreas.

endoscopic retrograde c. (ERCP), a method of c. using an endoscope as a cannula to inspect the pancreatic duct and common bile duct; it may also involve biopsy or introduction of contrast material for radiographic examination through a catheter.

cholangioscopy (kō-lan-jē-os'kō-pē) [chol- + G. *angeion,* vessel, + *skopeō,* to examine]. Choloscopy; visual examination of bile ducts utilizing a fiberoptic endoscope.

cholangiostomy (kō-lan-jē-os'tō-mē) [chol- + G. *angeion,* vessel, + *stoma,* mouth]. Formation of a fistula into a bile duct.

cholangiotomy (ko-lan-jī-ot'o-mī) [chol- + G. *angeion,* vessel, + *tomē,* incision]. Incision into a bile duct.

cholangitis (kō-lan-jī'tis) [chol- + G. *angeion,* vessel, + *-itis,* inflammation]. Cholangeitis; angiocholitis; inflammation of a bile duct or the entire biliary tree.

primary sclerosing c., recurrent or persistent obstructive jaundice, frequently with ulcerative colitis, due to extensive obliterative fibrosis of the extrahepatic or intrahepatic bile ducts; generally progresses to cirrhosis, portal hypertension, and liver failure; seen most commonly in young men.

cholanic acid (kō-lan'ik). Cholic acid.

cholanopoiesis (kō'lan-ō-poy-ē'sis) [chol- + G. *anō,* upward, + *poiēsis,* making]. Synthesis by the liver of cholic acid or its conjugates, or of natural bile salts.

cholanopoietic (kō'lan-ō-poy-et'ik). Pertaining to or promoting cholanopoiesis.

cholanthrene (kō-lan'thrēn). A polycyclic, somewhat carcinogenic hydrocarbon, structural parent of the highly carcinogenic 3 (or 20)-methylcholanthrene.

cholascos (kō-las'kos) [chol- + G. *askos,* bag]. Escape of bile into the free peritoneal cavity.

cholate (kō'lāt). A salt or ester of a cholic acid.

c. ligase [EC 6.2.1.7], c. synthetase or thiokinase; an enzyme that converts c. to choloylcoenzyme A, with cleavage of ATP to AMP.

c. synthetase, c. thiokinase, cholate-CoA ligase.

chole-, chol-, cholo- [G. *cholē,* bile]. Combining forms relating to bile. See also cholo-.

cholecalciferol (kō'lē-kal-sif'er-ol). Calciol; vitamin D_3; (5*Z*,7*E*)-(3*S*)-9,10-secocholesta-5,7,10(19)-trien-3-ol; formed by breakage of 9,10 bond in 7-dehydrocholesterol by ultraviolet irradiation, yielding a double bond between C-10 and C-19; probably the vitamin D of animal origin found in the skin, fur, and feathers of animals and birds exposed to sunlight, and also in butter, brain, fish oils, and egg yolk.

cholechromopoiesis (kō'lē-krō-mō-poy-ē'sis) [chole- + G. *chrōma,* color, + *poiesis,* making]. Synthesis of bile pigments by the liver.

cholecyst (kō'le-sist). *Vesica* biliaris.

cholecystagogic (kō'lē-sis-tă-goj'ik). Stimulating activity of the gallbladder.

cholecystagogue (kō-lē-sis'tă-gog) [chole- + G. *kystis,* bladder, + *agōgos,* leader]. A substance that stimulates activity of the gallbladder.

cholecystatony (kō'lē-sis-tat'ō-nē) [chole- + G. *kystis,* bladder, + *atonia,* atony]. Atonia, weakness, or failure of function of the gallbladder.

cholecystectasia (kō'lē-sis-tek-tā'zē-ă) [chole- + G. *kystis,* bladder, + *ektasis,* extension]. Dilation of the gallbladder.

cholecystectomy (kō'lē-sis-tek'tō-mē) [chole- + G. *kystis,* bladder, + *ektomē,* excision]. Surgical removal of the gallbladder.

cholecystendysis (kō'lē-sis-ten'dī-sis) [chole- + G. *kystis,* bladder, + *endysis,* an entering in]. Cholecystotomy.

cholecystenterostomy (kō'lē-sist-en-ter-os'tō-mē) [chole- + G. *kystis,* bladder, + *enteron,* intestine, + *stoma,* mouth]. Enterocholecystostomy; formation of a direct communication between the gallbladder and the intestine.

cholecystenterotomy (kō'lē-sist-en-ter-ot'ō-mē) [chole- + G. *kystis,* bladder, + enteron, intestine, + *tomē,* a cutting]. Enterocholecystotomy; incision of both intestine and gallbladder.

cholecystic (kō-lē-sis'tik). Relating to the cholecyst, or gallbladder.

cholecystis (kō-lē-sis'tis) [chole- + G. *kystis,* bladder]. *Vesica* biliaris.

cholecystitis (kō'lē-sis-tī'tis) [chole- + G. *kystis,* bladder, + *-itis,* inflammation]. Inflammation of the gallbladder.

acute c., congestion and or hemorrhagic necrosis, with variable infection, ulceration, and neutrophilic infiltration of the gallbladder wall; usually due to impaction of a stone in the cystic duct.

chronic c., chronic inflammation of the gallbladder, usually secondary to lithiasis, with lymphocytic infiltration and fibrosis that may produce marked thickening of the wall.

emphysematous c., c. due to infection with gas-producing bacteria, giving rise to gas in the gallbladder.

xanthogranulomatous c., chronic c. with conspicuous nodular infiltration by lipid macrophages; may be associated with biliary obstruction by calculi.

cholecystocolostomy (kō'-lē-sis'tō-kō-los'tō-mē) [chole- + G. *kystis,* bladder, + *kolon,* colon, + *stoma,* mouth]. Colocholecystostomy; cystocolostomy; establishment of a communication between the gallbladder and the colon.

cholecystoduodenostomy (kō-lē-sis'tō-dū-ō-dē-nos'tō-mē) [chole- + G. *kystis,* bladder, + L. *duodenum* + G. *stoma,* mouth]. Duodenocholecystostomy (1); establishment of a direct communication between the gallbladder and the duodenum.

cholecystogastrostomy (kō-lē-sis'tō-gas-tros'tō-mē) [chole- + G. *kystis,* bladder, + *gastēr,* stomach, + *stoma,* mouth]. Establishment of a communication between the gallbladder and the stomach.

cholecystogram (kō-lē-sis'tō-gram). The roentgenographic record of the gallbladder obtained by cholecystography.

cholecystography (kō-lē-sis-tog'ră-fē). [chole- + G. *kystis,* bladder, + *grapho,* to write]. Visualization of the gallbladder by roentgen rays after the administration of a radiopaque substance, such as sodium tetraiodophenolphthalein, or a radiopharmaceutical, such as technetium-99m, with a suitable detector.

cholecystoileostomy (kō-lē-sis'tō-il-ē-os'tō-mē) [chole- + G. *kystis,* bladder, + ileum + G. *stoma,* mouth]. Establishment of a communication between the gallbladder and the ileum.

cholecystojejunostomy (kō-lē-sis'tō-jē-jū-nos'tō-mē) [chole- + G. *kystis,* bladder, + jejunum, + G. *stoma,* mouth]. Establishment of a communication between the gallbladder and the jejunum.

cholecystokinase (kō-lē-sis-tō-kī'nās). An enzyme catalyzing the hydrolysis of cholecystokinin.

cholecystokinetic (kō'lē-sis'tō-ki-net'ik). Promoting emptying of the gallbladder.

cholecystokinin (kō'lē-sis-tō-kī'nin). Pancreozymin; a polypeptide (of 33 residues) hormone liberated by the upper intestinal mucosa on contact with gastric contents; stimulates contraction of the gallbladder. See also sincalide.

cholecystolithiasis (kō-lē-sis'tō-li-thī'ă-sis) [chole- + G. *kystis,* bladder, + *lithos,* stone]. Presence of one or more gallstones in the gallbladder.

cholecystolithotripsy (kō-lē-sis'tō-lith'ō-trip-sē) [chole- + G. *kystis,* bladder, + *lithos,* stone, + *tripsis,* a rubbing]. Crushing of a gallstone by manipulation of the unopened gallbladder.

cholecystomy (kō-lē-sis'tō-mē). Cholecystotomy.

cholecystopathy (kō'lē-sis-top'ă-thē). Disease of the gallbladder.

cholecystopexy (kō-lē-sis'tō-pek-sē) [chole- + G. *kystis*, bladder, + *pēxis*, fixation]. Suture of the gallbladder to the abdominal wall.

cholecystorrhaphy (kō'lē-sis-tōr'ă-fē) [chole- + G. *kystis*, bladder, + *rhaphē*, sewing]. Suture of an incised or ruptured gallbladder.

cholecystosonography (kō-lē-sis'tō-sō-nog'răfē). Ultrasonic examination of the gallbladder.

cholecystostomy (kō'lē-sis-tos'tō-mē) [chole- + G. *kystis*, bladder, + *stoma*, mouth]. Establishment of a fistula into the gallbladder.

cholecystotomy (kō'lē-sis-tot'ō-mē) [chole- + G. *kystis*, bladder, + *tomē*, incision]. Cholecystomy; cystifelleotomy; cholecystendysis; incision into the gallbladder.

choledoch-. See choledocho-.

choledoch (kō'lē-dok) [G. *cholēdochos*, containing bile, fr. *cholē*, bile, + *dechomai*, to receive]. *Ductus* choledochus.

choledochal (kō-lē-dok'ăl, kō-led'ō-kal). Relating to the common bile duct.

choledochectomy (kō-led-ō-kek'tō-mē) [choledoch- + G. *ektomē*, excision]. Surgical removal of a portion of the common bile duct.

choledochendysis (kō'led-ō-ken'dī-sis) [choledoch- + G. *endysis*, an entering in]. Choledochotomy.

choledochiarctia (kō'led-ō-ki-ark'tē-ă) [choledoch- + L. *artus* (improperly *arctus*), narrow]. Stenosis of the gall duct.

choledochitis (kō-led-ō-kī'tis) [choledoch- + G. *-itis*, inflammation]. Inflammation of the common bile duct.

choledocho-, choledoch- [G. *cholēdochos*, containing bile, fr. *cholē*, bile, + *dechomai*, to receive]. Combining forms relating to the ductus choledochus (the common bile duct).

choledochocholedochostomy (kō-led'ō-kō-kō-led'ō-kos'tō-mē) [choledocho- + choledocho- + G. *stoma*, mouth]. Operative joining of divided portions of common bile duct.

choledochoduodenostomy (kō-led'ō-kō-dū'ō-dē-nos'tō-mē) [choledocho- + duodenum + G. *stoma*, mouth]. Formation of a communication, other than the natural one, between the common bile duct and the duodenum.

choledochoenterostomy (kō-led'ō-kō-en-ter-os'tō-mē) [choledocho- + G. *enteron*, intestine, + *stoma*, mouth]. Establishment of a communication, other than the natural one, between the common bile duct and any part of the intestine.

choledochography (kō-led'ō-kog'ră-fē). Roentgenographic examination of the bile duct after the administration of a radiopaque substance.

choledochojejunostomy (kō-led'ō-kō-jĕ-jū-nos'tō-mē) [choledocho- + jejuno- + G. *stoma*, mouth]. Anastomosis between the common bile duct and the jejunum.

choledocholith (kō-led'ō-kō-lith) [choledocho- + G. *lithos*, stone]. Stone in the common bile duct.

choledocholithiasis (kō-led'ō-kō-lith-ī'ă-sis). Presence of a gallstone in the common bile duct.

choledocholithotomy (kō-led'ō-kō-li-thot'ō-mē) [choledocho- + G. *lithos*, stone, + *tomē*, incision]. Incision of the common bile duct for the extraction of an impacted gallstone.

choledocholithotripsy (kō-led'ō-kō-lith'ō-trip-sē) [choledocho- + G. *lithos*, stone, + *tripsis*, rubbing]. Choledocholithotrity; crushing of a gallstone in the common bile duct by manipulation without opening of the duct.

choledocholithotrity (kō-led'ō-kō-li-thot'ri-tē). Choledocholithotripsy.

choledochoplasty (kō-led'ō-kō-plas-tē). Plastic surgery of the common bile duct.

choledochorrhaphy (kō-led-ō-kōr'ră-fē) [choledocho- + G. *rhaphē*, suture]. Suturing together the divided ends of the common bile duct.

choledochostomy (kō-led-ō-kos'tō-mē) [choledocho- + G. *stoma*, mouth]. Establishment of a fistula into the common bile duct.

choledochotomy (kō-led-ō-kot'ō-mē) [choledocho- + G. *tomē*, incision]. Choledochendysis; incision into the common bile duct.

choledochous (kō-led'ō-kŭs). Containing or conveying bile.

choledochus (kō-led'ō-kŭs) [see choledoch]. *Ductus* choledochus.

choleglobin (kō-lē-glō'bin). Bile pigment hemoglobin; biliverdinglobin; green hemoglobin; verdoglobin; verdohemoglobin; a pigmented compound of globin and iron porphyrin (with an open ring due to cleavage of the α-methene bridge by α-methyl oxygenase); the first intermediate in the degradation of hemoglobin, further degraded successively to verdohemochrome, biliverdin, and bilirubin.

cholehematin (kō-lē-hē'mă-tin). A red pigment in the bile of herbivorous animals; derived from chlorophyll and a product of hematin oxidation.

cholehemia (kō-lē-hē'mē-ă) [chole- + G. *haima*, blood]. Cholemia.

choleic (kō-lē'ik). Cholic.

choleic acids. Compounds of bile acids and sterols.

cholelith (kō'lē-lith) [chole- + G. *lithos*, stone]. Gallstone.

cholelithiasis (kō'lē-li-thī'ă-sis). Chololithiasis; presence of concretions in the gallbladder or bile ducts.

cholelithotomy (kō'lē-li-thot'ō-mē) [chole- + G. *lithos*, stone, + *tomē*, incision]. Operative removal of a gallstone.

cholelithotripsy (kō-lē-lith'ō-trip-sē) [chole- + G. *lithos*, stone, + *tripsis*, a rubbing]. Cholelithotrity; the crushing of a gallstone.

cholelithotrity (kō-lē-li-thot'ri-tē) [chole- + G. *lithos*, stone, + L. *tero*, pp. *tritus*, to rub]. Cholelithotripsy.

cholemesis (kō-lem'ĕ-sis) [chole- + G. *emesis*, vomiting]. Vomiting of bile.

cholemia (kō-lē'mē-ă) [chole- + G. *haima*, blood]. Cholehemia; the presence of bile salts in the circulating blood.

cholemic (kō-lē'mik). Relating to cholemia.

cholepathia (kō-lē-path'ē-ă). **1.** Disease of bile ducts. **2.** Irregularity in contractions of the bile ducts.
c. spas'tica, spastic contraction of the bile ducts.

choleperitoneum (kō'lē-pār-i-tō-nē'ŭm). Bile in the peritoneum, which may lead to bile peritonitis.

choleperitonitis (kō'le-per-i-tō-nī'tis). Bile *peritonitis.*

cholepoiesis (kō'lē-poy-ē'sis) [chole- + G. *poiēsis*, making]. Cholopoiesis; formation of bile.

cholepoietic (kō'lē-poy-et'ik). Relating to the formation of bile.

cholera (kol'er-ă) [L. a bilious disease, fr. G. *cholē*, bile]. **1.** Formerly, a nonspecific term for a variety of gastrointestinal disturbances. **2.** Asiatic c.; an acute epidemic infectious disease caused by *Vibrio cholerae*, now occurring primarily in Asia. A soluble toxin elaborated in the intestinal tract by the vibrio alters the permeability of the mucosa, causing a profuse watery diarrhea, extreme loss of fluid and electrolytes, and a state of dehydration and collapse, but no gross morphologic change in the intestinal mucosa.
Asiatic c., c. (2).
fowl c., a destructive disease of domestic fowls caused by *Pasteurella multocida.*
hog c., swine fever or pest; an acute, highly contagious, and fatal disease of swine caused by the hog cholera virus and characterized by a sudden onset, high fever, depression, diarrhea, cutaneous hemorrhages, and frequently encephalomyelitic symptoms; pigs may die of the virus infection alone, or from complications of sec-

ondary bacterial infections; transmission is by direct contact or ingestion of contaminated food, particularly garbage.

c. infan'tum, old term for a disease of infants, characterized by vomiting, profuse watery diarrhea, fever, prostration, and collapse.

c. mor'bus, old term for acute severe gastroenteritis of unknown etiology, marked by severe colic, vomiting, and watery stools; formerly common during hot weather.

pancreatic c., obsolete term for Verner-Morrison *syndrome.*

c. sic'ca, an old term for a malignant form of disease seen during epidemics of Asiatic c. in which death occurs without diarrhea.

typhoid c., old term for c.(2) with predominantly cerebral manifestations such as confusion or dementia.

choleragen (kol'er-ă-jen) [cholera + G. *-gen,* producing]. A term suggested for a factor(s) produced during growth *in vitro* of the cholera vibrio and causes diarrhea.

choleraic (kol'er-ā'ik). Relating to cholera.

choleraphage (kol'er-ă-fāj) [cholera + G. *phagein,* to eat]. Bacteriophage of *Vibrio cholerae.*

choleresis (kō-ler-ē'sis). The secretion of bile as opposed to the expulsion of bile by the gallbladder.

choleretic (kol-er-et'ik). **1.** Relating to choleresis. **2.** An agent, usually a drug, that stimulates the liver to increase output of bile.

cholerheic (kol-ĕ-rē'ik). Denoting diarrhea produced secondary to unabsorbed bile salts.

choleric (kol'er-ik). Bilious (3).

choleriform (kol'er-i-fōrm). Choleroid; resembling cholera.

cholerigenic, cholerigenous (kol'er-i-jen'ik, -ij'en-ŭs). Causing or engendering cholera.

cholerine (kol'er-ēn). A mild form of diarrhea seen during epidemics of Asiatic cholera.

choleroid (kol'er-oyd). Choleriform.

cholerrhagia (kō-lē-rā'jē-ă) [chole- + G. *rhegnymi,* to burst forth]. Extensive flow of bile.

cholerrhagic (kō-lē-raj'ik). Referring to the flow of bile.

cholestane (kō'les-tān). The parent hydrocarbon of cholesterol. For structure, see steroids.

cholestanol (kō-les'tan-ol). Dihydrocholesterol; 3β-hydroxycholestane; differing from cholesterol in the absence of the double bond.

cholestanone (kō-les'tan-ōn). An oxidation product of cholestanol, differing from it in the presence of a ketone oxygen in place of the 3-hydroxyl group; an isomer of coprostanone.

cholestasia, cholestasis (kō-les-tā'sē-ă, -les'tă-sis) [chole- + G. *stasis,* a standing still]. An arrest in the flow of bile; c. due to obstruction of bile ducts is accompanied by formation of plugs of inspissated bile in the small ducts, canaliculi in the liver, and elevation of serum direct bilirubin and some enzymes.

cholestatic (kō-les-tat'ik). Tending to diminish or stop the flow of bile.

cholesteatoma (kō-les-tē-ă-tō'mă) [cholesterol + G. *stear (steat-),* tallow, + *-ōma,* tumor]. **1.** A tumor-like mass of keratinizing squamous epithelium and cholesterol in the middle ear, usually resulting from chronic otitis media, with squamous metaplasia or extension of squamous epithelium inward to line an expanding cystic cavity that may involve the mastoid and erode surrounding bone. **2.** An epidermoid cyst arising in the central nervous system in man or animals, commonly in the lateral ventricle of old horses.

cholestenone (kō-les'ten-ōn). A dehydrocholestanone, differing from cholestanone in the presence of a double bond between carbons 4 and 5.

cholesteremia (kō-les-ter-ē'mē-ă) [cholesterol + G. *haima,* blood]. Cholesterinemia; cholesterolemia; the presence of enhanced quantities of cholesterol in the blood.

cholesteride (kō-les'ter-īd). Obsolete term for a cholesteryl ester of a fatty acid.

cholesterin (kō-les'ter-in). Cholesterol.

cholesterinemia (kō-les'ter-in-ē'mē-ă) Cholesteremia.

cholesterinosis (kō-les'ter-in-ō'sis). Cholesterolosis.

cerebrotendinous c., cerebrotendinous *xanthomatosis.*

cholesterinuria (kō-les'ter-i-nū'rē-ă) [cholesterin + G. *ouron,* urine]. Cholesteroluria.

cholesteroderma (kō-les'ter-ō-der'mă). Xanthochromia.

cholesterol (kō-les'ter-ol). Cholesterin; 5-cholesten-3β-ol (cholestane with a 5,6 double bond and a 3β hydroxyl group); the most abundant steroid in animal tissues, especially in bile and gallstones, and present in food, especially that rich in animal fats; circulates in the plasma complexed to proteins of various densities and plays an important role in the pathogenesis of atheroma formation in arteries.

cholesterolemia (kō-les'ter-ol-ē'mē-ă) [cholesterol + G. *haima,* blood]. Cholesteremia.

cholesterologenesis (kō-les'ter-ol-ō-jen'ĕ-sis). The biosynthesis of cholesterol.

cholesterolosis (kō-les'ter-ol-ō'sis). Cholesterinosis; cholesterosis. **1.** A condition resulting from a disturbance in metabolism of lipids, characterized by deposits of cholesterol in tissue, as in Tangier disease. **2.** Cholesterol crystals in the anterior chamber of the eye, as in aphakia with associated retinal separation.

extracellular c., obsolete term for erythema elevatum diutinum characterized by lipid deposits in vessel walls.

cholesteroluria (kō-les'ter-ol-ū'rē-ă). Cholesterinuria; the excretion of cholesterol in the urine.

cholesterosis (kō'les-ter-ō'sis). Cholesterolosis.

c. cu'tis, xanthomatosis.

choleuria (kō-lē-yū'rē-ă). Biliuria.

choleverdin (kō-lē-ver'din). Biliverdin.

cholic (kō'lik). Choleic; relating to the bile.

cholic acid. Cholalic or cholanic acid; a family of steroids comprising the bile acids (or salts), generally in conjugated form (*e.g.,* glycocholic and taurocholic acids). Chemically, c.a.'s are cholan-24-oic (cholanic) acids (the terminal C_{24} of cholane becoming a —COOH group); biologically, c.a.'s are derived from cholesterol (a cholestane derivative) and display varying degrees of oxidation (OH groups) and orientation at positions 3, 7, and 12. It is these oxidations and orientations that distinguish the several c.a.'s; *e.g.,* c.a. is 3α,7α,12α-trihydroxy-5β-cholan-24-oic acid, deoxycholic acid is 3α,12α-di-hydroxy-5β-cholanic acid.

cholicele (kō'li-sēl) [G. *cholē,* bile, + *kēlē,* tumor]. Enlargement of the gallbladder due to retained fluids.

choline (kō'lēn). Lipotropic or transmethylation factor; (2-hydroxyethyl)trimethylammonium ion; $HOCH_2CH_2N(CH_3)_3{}^+$; found in most animal tissues either free or in combination as lecithin (phosphatidylcholine) or acetate (acetylcholine) or cytidine diphosphate (cytidinediphosphocholine). It is included in the vitamin B complex; as acetylcholine, it is essential for synaptic transmission. Several salts of choline are used in medicine.

c. acetylase, c. acetyltransferase.

c. acetyltransferase [EC 2.3.1.6], c. acetylase; an enzyme catalyzing the condensation of choline and acetyl-coenzyme A, forming acetylcholine.

c. chloride, a lipotropic agent.

c. dihydrogen citrate, (2-hydroxyethyl)trimethylammonium citrate; a lipotropic agent.

c. esterase I, acetylcholinesterase.

c. esterase II, cholinesterase.

c. kinase [EC 2.7.1.32], c. phosphokinase; an enzyme that cata-

lyzes the formation of phosphocholine from choline and ATP.
c. phosphatase, *phospholipase* D.
c. phosphokinase, c. kinase.
c. salicylate, c. salt of salicyclic acid; an analgesic and antipyretic (because of the salicylate moiety).
c. theophyllinate, oxtriphylline.

cholinephosphotransferase (kō'lēn-fos-fō-trans'fer-ās) [EC 2.7.8.2]. An enzyme catalyzing the reaction between CDP-choline and 1,2-diacylglycerol to form phosphatidylcholine.

cholinergic (kol-in-er'jik) [choline + G. *ergon,* work]. Relating to nerve cells or fibers that employ acetylcholine as their neurotransmitter. *Cf.* adrenergic.

cholinester (kō'lin-es-ter). An ester of choline; *e.g.,* acetylcholine.

cholinesterase (kō-lin-es'ter-ās) [EC 3.1.1.8]. Pseudocholinesterase; butyrylcholine esterase; butyrocholinesterase; choline esterase II; nonspecific or "s"-type c.; one of a family of enzymes capable of catalyzing the hydrolysis of acetylcholines and a few other compounds. See also acetylcholinesterase.
"e"-type c. ["e" in erythrocyte], acetylcholinesterase.
nonspecific c., cholinesterase.
specific c., acetylcholinesterase.
"s"-type c. ["s" in serum], cholinesterase.
true c., acetylcholinesterase.

cholinesterase reactivator. A drug that reacts directly with the alkylphosphorylated enzyme to free the active unit; the drugs used therapeutically to reactivate phosphorylated forms of acetylcholinesterase are oximes, *e.g.,* diacetylmonoxime, monoisonitrosoacetone.

cholinoceptive (kō'lin-ō-sep'tiv). Referring to chemical sites in effector cells with which acetylcholine unites to exert its actions. *Cf.* adrenoceptive.

cholinolytic (kō'lin-ō-lit'ik). Preventing the action of acetylcholine.

cholinomimetic (kol'i-nō-mi-met'ik). Having an action similar to that of acetylcholine, the substance liberated by cholinergic nerves; term proposed to replace the less accurate term, parasympathomimetic. *Cf.* adrenomimetic.

cholinoreactive (kō'lin-ō-rē-ak'tiv). Responding to acetylcholine and related compounds.

cholinoreceptors (kol'i-nō-rē-sep'terz, -tōrz). See cholinergic *receptors.*

cholistine sulphomethate sodium (kō-lis'tēn sul-fō-meth'āt). Colistimethate sodium.

cholo-. See chole-.

chololith (kol'ō-lith). Gallstone.

chololithiasis (kol-ō-li-thī'ă-sis). Cholelithiasis.

chololithic (kol-ō-lith'ik). Relating in any way to gallstones.

choloplania (kol-ō-plā'nē-ă) [cholo- + G. *planē,* a wandering]. The presence of bile salts in the blood or tissues.

cholopoiesis (kō-lō-poy-ē'sis). Cholepoiesis.

cholorrhea (kol-ō-rē'ă) [cholo- + G. *rhoia,* a flow]. An excessive secretion of bile.

choloscopy (kō-los'kŏ-pē). [cholo- + G. *skopeō,* to view]. Cholangioscopy.

cholothorax (kō-lō-thōr'aks). Bile in the pleural cavity.

choloyl (kō'lō-il). The radical of cholic acid or cholate.

choluria (kō-lū'rē-ă) [G. *cholē,* bile, + *ouron,* urine]. Biliuria.

cholylcoenzyme A (kō'lil-kō-en'zīm). A condensation product of cholic acid and coenzyme A; an intermediate in the formation of bile salts from bile acids, as taurocholic acid from cholic acid.

chondral (kon'drăl) [G. *chondros,* cartilage]. Cartilaginous.

chondralgia (kon-dral'jē-ă) [G. *chondros,* cartilage, + *algos,* pain]. Chondrodynia.

chondralloplasia (kon'dral-ō-plā'zē-ă) [G. *chondros,* cartilage, + *allos,* other, + *plasia,* formed]. Occurrence of cartilage in abnormal situations in the bony skeleton.

chondrectomy (kon-drek'tō-mē) [G. *chondros,* cartilage, + *ektomē,* excision]. Excision of cartilage.

Chondrichthyes (kon-drik'thi-ēz) [G. *chondros,* cartilage, + *ichthys,* a fish]. Class of cartilaginous fishes, including the sharks, rays, and chimeras.

chondrification (kon'dri-fi-kā'shŭn) [G. *chondros,* cartilage, + L. *facio,* to make]. Conversion into cartilage.

chondrify (kon'dri-fī). To become cartilaginous.

chondrin (kon'drin). Obsolete term for a gelatin-like substance obtained from cartilage by boiling. See collagen.

chondrio-. See chondro-.

chondritis (kon-drī'tis) [G. *chondros,* cartilage, + *-itis,* inflammation]. Inflammation of cartilage.
costal c., costochondritis.

chondro-, chondrio- [G. *chondrion,* dim. of *chondros,* groats (coarsely ground grain), grit, gristle, cartilage]. Combining forms denoting: **1.** Cartilage or cartilaginous. **2.** Granular or gritty substance.

chondroblast (kon'drō-blast) [chondro- + G. *blastos,* germ]. Chondroplast; a dividing cell of growing cartilage tissue.

chondroblastoma (kon'drō-blas-tō'mă). A benign tumor arising in the epiphyses of long bones, consisting of highly cellular tissue resembling fetal cartilage.

chondrocalcinosis (kon'drō-kal-si-nō'sis) [chondro- + calcium + G. *-osis,* condition]. Calcification of cartilage.
articular c., a disease characterized by calcified deposits, free from urate and consisting of calcium pyrophosphate crystals, in synovial fluid, articular cartilage, and adjacent soft tissue (pseudogout); causes various forms of arthritis commonly characterized by goutlike attacks of pain, swelling of the involved joints, and radiologic evidence of calcification in articular cartilage; seems to be inherited in some families and associated with certain diseases in others.

chondroclast (kon'drō-klast) [chondro- + G. *klastos,* broken in pieces]. A multinucleated cell involved in the reabsorption of calcified cartilage.

chondrocostal (kon-drō-kos'tăl) [chondro- + L. *costa,* rib]. Relating to the costal cartilages.

chondrocranium (kon-drō-krā'nē-ŭm) [chondro- + G. *kranion,* skull]. A cartilaginous skull; the cartilaginous parts of the developing skull.

chondrocyte (kon'drō-sīt) [chondro- + G. *kytos,* a hollow (cell)]. Cartilage cell; a cell that occupies a lacuna within the cartilage matrix.
isogenous c.'s, a group derived from one cell by division.

chondrodermatitis nodularis, chronica helicis (kon-drō-der-ma-tī'tis nod-yū-lar'is kron'i-kă hel'i-sis). Winkler's disease; a benign, chronic, small, painful nodule (or nodules) on the helix of the ear, which may occasionally become ulcerated.

chondrodynia (kon-drō-din'ē-ă) [chondro- + G. *odyne,* pain]. Chondralgia; pain in cartilage.

chondrodysplasia (kon'drō-dis-plā'zē-ă) [chondro- + G. *dys,* bad, + *plasis,* a molding]. Chondrodystrophy.
hereditary deforming c., obsolete term for hereditary multiple *exostoses.*
c. puncta'ta, *dysplasia* epiphysialis punctata.

chondrodystrophia (kon'drō-dis-trō'fē-ă). Chondrodystrophy.
c. calcif'icans congen'ita, *dysplasia* epiphysialis punctata.

c. congen'ita puncta'ta, Conradi's *disease.*

chondrodystrophy (kon-drō-dis'trō-fē) [chondro- + G. *dys,* bad, + *trophe,* nourishment]. Chondrodysplasia; chondrodystrophia; a disturbance in the development of the cartilage primordia of the long bones, especially the region of the epiphysial plates, resulting in arrested growth of the long bones and dwarfism in which the extremities are abnormally short, but the head and trunk are essentially normal.

asphyxiating thoracic c., asphyxiating thoracic *dysplasia.*

asymmetrical c., enchondromatosis.

hereditary deforming c., hereditary multiple *exostoses.*

chondroectodermal (kon'drō-ek-tō-der'măl). Relating to ectodermally derived cartilage; *e.g.,* branchial cartilages that may have developed from the neural crest.

chondrofibroma (kon'drō-fī-brō'mă). Chondromyxoid *fibroma.*

chondrogenesis (kon-drō-jen'ĕ-sis) [chondro- + G. *genesis,* origin]. Chondrosis (1); formation of cartilage.

chondroglossus (kon-drō-glos'ŭs) [chondro- + G. *glossa,* tongue]. See *musculus* chondroglossus.

chondrohypoplasia (kon'drō-hī-pō-plā'zē-ă). A mild form of achondroplasia; affected individuals survive into adult life.

chondroid (kon'droyd) [chondro- + G. *eidos,* resemblance]. **1.** Cartilaginoid; resembling cartilage. **2.** Uncharacteristically developed cartilage, primarily cellular with a basophilic matrix and thin or nonexistent capsules.

chondroitin (kon-drō'i-tin). A (muco)polysaccharide (proteoglycan) composed of alternating residues of β-D-glucuronic acid and *N*-acetylgalactosamine sulfate in alternating β1-3 and β1-4 linkages; present among the ground substance materials in the extracellular matrix of connective tissue.

c. sulfate A, c. with sulfuric residues esterifying the 4-hydroxyl groups of the galactosamine residues; found in connective tissue.

c. sulfate B, dermatan sulfate.

c. sulfate C, c. with sulfuric residues esterifying the 6-hydroxyl groups of the galactosamine residues.

chondrology (kon-drol'ō-jē) [chondro- + G. *logos,* treatise]. The study of cartilage.

chondrolysis (kon-drol'i-sis). Disappearance of articular cartilage as the result of lysis or dissolution of the cartilage matrix and cells.

chondroma (kon-drō'mă) [chondro- + G. *-ōma,* tumor]. A benign neoplasm derived from mesodermal cells that form cartilage.

extraskeletal c., a c. located in soft tissues, usually of the fingers, hands, and feet, not connected to underlying bone or periosteum.

juxtacortical c., periosteal c.

periosteal c., juxtacortical c.; a c. that develops from periosteum or periosteal connective tissue.

chondromalacia (kon'drō-mă-lā'shē-ă) [chondro- + G. *malakia,* softness]. Softening of any cartilage.

c. feta'lis, an intrauterine form of c. in which the fetus is born dead with soft pliable limbs.

generalized c., relapsing *polychondritis.*

c. of larynx, laryngomalacia; the presence of soft laryngeal cartilage, most often seen in relapsing polychondritis.

systemic c., relapsing *polychondritis.*

chondromatosis (kon'drō-mă-tō'sis). Presence of multiple tumor-like foci of cartilage.

synovial c., synovial osteochondromatosis; c. or osteocartilaginous nodules occurring in the synovial membrane of a joint.

chondromatous (kon-drō'mă-tŭs). Pertaining to or manifesting the features of a chondroma.

chondromere (kon'drō-mēr) [chondro- + G. *meros,* part]. A cartilage unit of the fetal axial skeleton developing within a single metamere of the body; a primordial cartilaginous vertebra together with its costal component.

chondromucin (kon-drō-myū'sin). Chondromucoid.

chondromucoid (kon-drō-myū'koyd). Chondromucin; chondroprotein; obsolete terms for a mucoprotein from cartilage; probably chondroitin sulfate, plus other materials.

chondromyxoma (kon'drō-mik-sō'mă). Chondromyxoid *fibroma.*

chondro-osseous (kon-drō-os'ē-ŭs). Relating to cartilage and bone, either as a mixture of the two tissues or as a junction between the two, such as the union of a rib and its costal cartilage.

chondro-osteodystrophy (kon'drō-os'tē-ō-dis'trō-fē). Osteochondrodystrophy; osteochondrodystrophia deformans; term used for a group of disorders of bone and cartilage which includes Morquio syndrome and similar conditions.

chondropathy (kon-drop'ă-thē) [chondro- + G. *pathos,* suffering]. Any disease of cartilage.

chondropharyngeus (kon'drō-făr-in-jē'ŭs). See *musculus* constrictor pharyngis medius.

chondrophyte (kon'drō-fīt) [chondro- + G. *phytos,* a growth]. An abnormal cartilaginous mass that develops at the articular surface of a bone.

chondroplast (kon'drō-plast) [chondro- + G. *plastos,* formed]. Chondroblast.

chondroplasty (kon'drō-plas-tē) [chondro- + G. *plastos,* formed]. Reparative or plastic surgery of cartilage.

chondroporosis (kon'drō-pōr-ō'sis) [chondro- + L. *porosus,* porous]. Condition of cartilage in which spaces appear, either normal (in the process of ossification) or pathologic.

chondroprotein (kon-drō-prō'tēn). Chondromucoid.

chondrosamine (kon-drō'să-mēn). Galactosamine.

chondrosarcoma (kon'drō-sar-kō'mă). A slowly growing malignant neoplasm derived from cartilage cells, occurring most frequently in pelvic bones or near the ends of long bones, in middle-aged and old people; most c.'s arise *de novo,* but some may develop in a preexisting benign cartilaginous lesion or in patients with enchondromatosis.

chondrosin, chondrosine (kon'drō-sin). A disaccharide composed of one molecule of D-glucuronic acid and one of galactosamine (chondrosamine); a component of the chondroitins.

chondrosis (kon-drō'sis). **1.** Chondrogenesis. **2.** Obsolete term for a cartilaginous tumor.

chondroskeleton (kon'drō-skel'ĕ-tŏn). A skeleton formed of hyaline cartilage; *e.g.,* that of the human embryo or of certain adult fishes such as the shark or ray.

chondrosome (kon'drō-sōm) [chondro- + G. + *sōma,* body]. Obsolete term for mitochondrion.

chondrosternal (kon-drō-ster'năl). **1.** Relating to a sternal cartilage. **2.** Relating to the costal cartilages and the sternum.

chondrosternoplasty (kon-drō-ster'nō-plas-tē). Surgical correction of malformations of the sternum.

chondrotome (kon'drō-tōm) [chondro- + G. *tomē,* cutting]. Cartilage knife; ecchondrotome; a very strong scalpel-shaped knife used in cutting cartilage.

chondrotomy (kon-drot'ō-mē) [chondro- + G. *tomē,* a cutting]. Division of cartilage.

chondrotrophic (kon-drō-trof'ik) [chondro- + G. *trophē,* nourishment]. Influencing the nutrition and thereby the development and growth of cartilage.

chondroxiphoid (kon-drō-zif'oyd) [chondro- + G. *xiphos,* sword, + *eidos,* appearance]. Relating to the xiphoid or ensiform cartilage.

chondrus (kon'drŭs) [G. *chondros,* gristle]. **1.** Cartilage. **2.** Irish or pearl moss; carrageen; carragheen; the plant *Chondrus crispus, Fucus crispus,* or *Gigartina mamillosa* (family Gigartinaceae); a demulcent in chronic and intestinal disorders.

chonechondrosternon (kō'nē-kon-drō-ster'non) [G.*choanē* (*chonē*), funnel, + *chondros,* cartilage, + *sternon,* sternum]. *Pectus* excavatum.

CHOP Acronym for cyclophosphamide, doxorubicin, vincristine, and prednisone, a chemotherapy regimen for treatment of lymphomas.

Chopart, François, French surgeon, 1743–1795. See C.'s *amputation, joint.*

chord- [G. *chordē,* cord]. Combining form meaning cord. See also cord-.

chorda, pl. **chordae** (kōr'dă, -dē) [L., cord] [NA]. A tendinous or a cordlike structure. See also cord.

c. dorsa'lis, notochord (2).

c. mag'na, *tendo* calcaneus.

c. obli'qua [NA], oblique cord; Weitbrecht's cord or ligament; Cooper's ligament (3); oblique or round ligament of elbow joint; a slender band extending from the lateral part of the coronoid process of the ulna distad and laterad to the radius immediately distal to the bicipital tuberosity.

c. spermat'ica, *funiculus* spermaticus.

chor'dae tendin'eae [NA], tendinous cords; the tendinous strands running from the papillary muscles to the atrioventricular valves (mitral and tricuspid).

c. tym'pani [NA], tympanichord; cord of tympanum, a nerve given off from the facial nerve in the facial canal which passes through the canaliculus of the c. tympani into the tympanic cavity, crosses over the tympanic membrane and handle of the malleus, and passes out through the petrotympanic fissure to join the lingual branch of the mandibular nerve; it conveys taste sensation from the anterior two-thirds of the tongue and carries parasympathetic preganglionic fibers to the submandibular and sublingual salivary glands.

c. umbilica'lis, *funiculus* umbilicalis.

c. vertebra'lis, notochord (2).

c. voca'lis, pl. **chor'dae voca'les,** *plica* vocalis.

chor'dae willis'ii, Willis' *cords.*

chordal (kōr'dăl). Relating to any chorda or cord, especially to the notochord.

chorda-mesoderm (kōr-dă-mes'ō-derm). That part of the protoderm of a young embryo which has the potentiality of forming notochord and mesoderm.

Chordata (kor-dā'tă) [L. *chorda,* fr. G. *chordē,* a string]. The phylum that includes the vertebrates, defined by possession of: 1) a single dorsal nerve cord (the brain and spinal cord of mammals); 2) a cartilaginous rod, the notochord, which forms dorsal to the primitive gut in the early embryo, and is surrounded and replaced by the vertebral column in the subphylum vertebrata; 3) by presence at some stage in development of gill slits in the pharynx or throat.

chordate (kōr'dāt). An animal of the phylum *Chordata.*

chordee (kōr-dē') [Fr. corded]. **1.** Penis lunatus; painful erection of the penis in gonorrhea or Peyronie's disease, with curvature resulting from lack of distensibility of the corpus cavernosum urethrae. **2.** Ventral curvature of the penis, most apparent on erection, as seen in hypospadias due to congenital shortness of the ventral skin and, on rare occasions, in patients with a normally situated meatus.

chorditis (kōr-dī'tis) [G. *chordē,* cord, + *-itis,* inflammation]. Inflammation of a cord; usually a vocal cord.

c. fibrino'sa, inflammation of the vocal cords with fibrinous exudation.

c. nodo'sa, c. tubero'sa, vocal cord *nodules.*

c. voca'lis, inflammation of the vocal cords.

c. voca'lis infe'rior, chronic subglottic laryngitis; an inflammation limited mainly to the undersurface of the vocal cords and adjacent parts.

chordoma (kōr-dō'mă) [(noto)chord + G. *-oma,* tumor]. A rare solitary slowly growing neoplasm of skeletal tissue in adults, derived from persistent portions of the notochord; composed of cells arranged in lobules, with abundant quantities of extracellular mucus; some cells contain vacuoles of mucus that resemble soap bubbles (physaliphorous cells).

chordoskeleton (kōr-dō-skel'ĕ-tŏn). The part of the embryonic skeleton that develops in conjunction with the notochord.

chordotomy (kōr-dot'ō-mē). Cordotomy.

chorea (kōr-ē'ă) [L. fr. G. *choreia,* a choral dance, fr. *choros,* a dance]. **1.** Irregular, spasmodic, involuntary movements of the limbs or facial muscles. **2.** Sydenham's c.

automatic c., uncontrollable abnormal movements.

chronic progressive c., hereditary c.

c. cor'dis, cardiac irregularity related to c.

dancing c., procursive c.;

degenerative c., hereditary c.

c. dimidia'ta, hemichorea.

electric c., **(1)** Dubini's disease; progressively fatal spasmodic disorder, possibly of malarial origin, occurring chiefly in Italy; **(2)** a severe form of Sydenham's c., in which the spasms are rapid and of a specially jerky character.

c. festi'nans, procursive c.

fibrillary c., Morvan's c.; fasciculations of the muscles of the legs and trunk.

c. gravida'rum, c. occurring in pregnancy.

habit c., tic.

hemilateral c., hemichorea.

Henoch's c., spasmodic *tic.*

hereditary c., Huntington's, disease or c.; chronic progressive or degenerative c.; a chronic disorder, beginning usually between the ages of 30 and 50 years, characterized by choreic movements in the face and extremities, accompanied by a gradual loss of the mental faculties ending in dementia; autosomal dominant inheritance.

Huntington's c., hereditary c.

hysterical c., conversion hysteria in which choreiform movements constitute the chief feature.

juvenile c., Sydenham's c.

laryngeal c., a spasmodic tic involving the muscles, resulting in an explosive manner of talking.

c. ma'jor, a spasmodic attack occurring in patients with conversion hysteria.

methodical c., c. in which the movements recur at definite intervals.

mimetic c., imitation of the c. movements of another person.

c. mi'nor, Sydenham's c.

Morvan's c., fibrillary c.

c. nu'tans, a functional manifestation characterized by rhythmic nodding.

paralytic c., weakness or paresis of an extremity or portion of the body associated with slight jerking movements.

posthemiplegic c., posthemiplegic *athetosis.*

procursive c., c. festinans; dancing c. or disease; a form in which the patient whirls around, runs forward, or exercises a sort of rhythmic dancing movement.

rheumatic c., Sydenham's c.

rhythmic c., patterned movement in conversion hysteria.

c. rotato'ria, a form in which the head is rotated or oscillates rapidly.

saltatory c., rhythmic dancing movements, as in procursive c.

senile c., a disorder resembling Sydenham's c., not associated with rheumatism or cardiac disease, occurring in the aged.

Sydenham's c., c. (2); c. minor; juvenile or rheumatic c.; Syden-

ham's disease; an acute toxic or infective disorder of the nervous system, usually associated with acute rheumatic fever, occurring in young persons and characterized by involuntary, irregular, jerky movement of the muscles of the face, neck, and limbs; they are intensified by voluntary effort but disappear in sleep.
tetanoid c., c. due to lenticular degeneration.

chorea-acanthocytosis (kōr-ē'ă-ă-kan'thō-sī-tō'sis). Familial degeneration of basal ganglia with acanthocytosis characterized by involuntary movements, acanthocytosis, and decreased or absent deep tendon reflexes.

choreal (kōr-ē'ăl). Relating to chorea.

choreic (kōr-ē'ik). Relating to or of the nature of chorea.

choreiform (kōr-ē'i-fōrm). Choreoid.

choreo-. Combining form relating to chorea.

choreoathetoid (kōr'ē-ō-ath'ĕ-toyd). Pertaining to or characterized by choreoathetosis.

choreoathetosis (kōr'ē-ō-ath-ĕ-tō'sis) [choreo- + G. *athētos,* unfixed, + *-ōsis,* condition]. Abnormal movements of body of combined choreic and athetoid pattern.

choreoid (kōr'ē-oyd). Choreiform; resembling chorea.

choreophrasia (kōr'ē-ō-frā'zē-ă) [choreo- + G. *phrasis,* speaking]. Continual repetition of meaningless phrases.

chorio- [G. *chorion,* membrane]. Combining form relating to any membrane, especially that which encloses the fetus.

chorioadenoma (kō'rē-ō-ad-ĕ-nō'mă). A benign neoplasm of chorion, especially with hydatidiform mole formation.
c. destru'ens, invasive mole; hydatidiform mole in which there is an unusual degree of invasion of the myometrium or its blood vessels, causing hemorrhage, necrosis, and occasionally rupture of the uterus or embolism of molar tissue to the lungs; there is marked proliferation of the trophoblast, but avascular villi may also be found.

chorioallantoic (kō'rē-ō-al-an-tō'ik). Pertaining to the chorioallantois.

chorioallantois (kō'rē-ō-ă-lan'tō-is). Extraembryonic membrane formed by the fusion of the allantois with the serosa or false chorion, especially in avian embryos.

chorioamnionitis (kō'rē-ō-am'nē-ō-nī'tis). Infection involving the chorion, amnion, and amniotic fluid; usually the placental villi and decidua are also involved.

chorioangioma (kō'rē-ō-an-jē-ō'mă) [chorion + angioma]. Benign tumor of placental blood vessels (hemangioma), usually of no clinical significance; large tumors may be associated with placental insufficiency; in some instances, the stroma is edematous and may resemble myxomatous tissue. See also chorioangiosis.

chorioangiomatosis (kō'rē-ō-an'jē-ō-mă-tō'sis). Chorioangiosis.

chorioangiosis (kō'rē-ō-an-jē-ō'sis) [chorio- + G. *angeion,* vessel, + *-osis,* condition]. Chorioangiomatosis; an abnormal increase in the number of vascular channels in placental villi; severe c. is associated with a high incidence of neonatal death and major congenital malformations.

choriocapillaris (kō'rē-ō-kap-i-lā'ris). *Lamina* choroidocapillaris.

choriocarcinoma (kō'rē-ō-kar-si-nō'mă). Chorionic epithelioma; chorioepithelioma; trophoblastoma; a highly malignant neoplasm derived from placental syncytial trophoblasts and cytotrophoblasts which forms irregular sheets and cords, which are surrounded by irregular "lakes" of blood; villi are not formed; neoplastic cells invade the myometrium and blood vessels. Hemorrhagic metastases develop relatively early in the course of the illness, and are frequently found in the lungs, liver, brain, and vagina and various other pelvic organs; c. may follow any type of pregnancy, especially hydatiform mole, and occasionally originates in teratoid neoplasms of the ovaries or testes.

choriocele (kō'rē-ō-sēl) [chorio- + G. *kēlē,* hernia]. A hernia of the choroid coat of the eye through a defect in the sclera.

chorioepithelioma (kō'rē-ō-ep-i-thē-lē-ō'mă). Choriocarcinoma.

choriogonadotropin (kō'rē-ō-gon'ă-dō-trō-pin). Chorionic *gonadotropin.*

chorioid-, chorioido-. For words beginning thus and not found here, see choroid-, choroido-.

chorioma (kō-rē-ō'mă). Rarely used term for a benign or malignant tumor of chorionic tissue.

choriomammotropin (kō'rē-ō-mam'ō-trō-pin). Human placental *lactogen.*

choriomeningitis (kō-rē-ō-men-in-jī'tis). A cerebral meningitis in which there is a more or less marked cellular infiltration of the meninges, often with a lymphocytic infiltration of the choroid plexuses, particularly of the third and fourth ventricles.
lymphocytic c., infection of mice and other animals, including man, with Arenaviridae; it often appears in animals used for experimental work, as a result of provocation by the injection of foreign materials into the nervous system.

chorion (kō'rē-on) [G. *chorion,* membrane enclosing the fetus]. Chorionic sac; the multilayered, outermost fetal membrane consisting of extraembryonic somatic mesoderm, trophoblast, and, on the maternal surface, villi bathed by maternal blood; as pregnancy progresses part of the c. becomes the definitive fetal placenta.
c. frondo'sum, shaggy c.; the part of the c. where the villi persist, forming the fetal part of the placenta.
c. lae've, smooth c.; the portion of the c. from which the villi disappear in the later stages of pregnancy.
previllous c., primitive c.
primitive c., previllous c.; the c. before its villi are well formed.
shaggy c., c. frondosum.
smooth c., c. laeve.

chorionic (kō-rē-on'ik). Relating to the chorion.

Chorioptes (kō-rē-op'tēz) [G. *chorion,* membrane, + *optos,* visible]. A genus of cosmopolitan and very common mange mites (family Psoroptidae) that cause chorioptic or symbiotic domestic animal mange, characterized by restriction of the mange to certain parts of the animal's body. Various species described, *i.e., C. equi* of horses, *C. caprae* of goats, *C. ovis* of sheep, *C. cunniculi* of rabbits, are now thought to be physiologic strains of one species, *C. bovis* of cattle.

chorioretinal (kō-rē-ō-ret'i-năl). Retinochoroid; relating to the choroid coat of the eye and the retina.

chorioretinitis (kō'rē-ō-ret-i-nī'tis). Retinochoroiditis.
c. sclopeta'ria [L. *sclopetum,* 14th century Italian handgun], proliferation of fibrous tissue in the choroid and retina as the result of contusion of the sclera by a high velocity missile.

chorioretinopathy (kō'rē-ō-ret-i-nop'ă-thē). A primary abnormality of the choroid with extension to the retina. See also choidopathy.

chorista (kō-ris'tă) [G. *chōristos,* separated]. A focus of tissue that is histologically normal per se, but is not normally found in the organ or structure in which it is located; *e.g.,* tissue displaced, during development, from its normal site. *Cf.* choristoma.

choristoblastoma (kō-ris'tō-blas-tō'mă) [choristoma + blastoma]. An autonomous neoplasm composed of relatively undifferentiated cells of a choristoma.

choristoma (kō-ris-tō'mă) [G. *chōristos,* separated, + *-ōma*]. A mass formed by maldevelopment of tissue of a type not normally found at that site.

choroid (ko'royd) [G. *choroeidēs,* a false reading for *chorioeidēs,* like a membrane]. Choroidea.

choroidal (kō-roy'dăl). Relating to the choroid (choroidea).

choroidea (kō-royd'ē-ă) [see choroid] [NA]. Choroid; the middle vascular tunic of the eye lying between the retina and the sclera.

choroideremia (kō-roy-der-ē'mē-ă) [choroid + G. *erēmia,* absence]. Progressive tapetochoroidal dystrophy; progressive choroidal atrophy; progressive degeneration of the choroid in males, beginning with peripheral pigmentary retinopathy, followed by atrophy of the retinal pigment epithelium and of the choriocapillaris, night blindness, progressive constriction of visual fields, and finally complete blindness; X-linked inheritance; heterozygous females show a pigmentary retinopathy but without visual defect and peripheral progression.

choroiditis (kō-roy-dī'tis). Posterior uveitis; inflammation of the choroid. *Cf.* choroidopathy, chorioretinopathy.
anterior c., disseminated c. restricted to peripheral choroid.
areolar c., inflammation of the choroid, with prominent pigment proliferation occurring first in the macular region and then more peripherally.
diffuse c., a widespread exudative inflammation of the choroid, with progressive resolution of older lesions as new ones occur.
disseminated c., chronic inflammation of the choroid, with multiple isolated foci.
exudative c., a circumscribed inflammation of the choroid, often with multiple lesions.
juxtapupillary c., c. adjacent to the optic disk.
metastatic c., inflammation of the choroid arising from microbial emboli.
multifocal c., macular, peripapillary, and peripheral c., often designated presumed ocular histoplasmosis.
posterior c., disseminated c. restricted to the central choroid.
proliferative c., the dense scar tissue produced by severe choroiditis.
suppurative c., purulent inflammation of the choroid.

choroido-. Combining form relating to the choroid.

choroidocyclitis (kō-roy'dō-si-klī'tis) [choroido- + G. *kyklos,* circle]. Inflammation of the choroid coat and the ciliary body.

choroidopathy (kō-roy-dop'ă-thē). Choroidosis; noninflammatory degeneration of the choroid.
areolar c., central areolar choroidal atrophy or sclerosis; a slowly progressive pigmentary degeneration in young persons; characterized by black foci closely set together and coalescent at the posterior pole and macular region.
central serous c., central angiospastic retinitis or retinopathy; central serous retinopathy. Detachment of the sensory retina induced by decreased adhesion between cells of the retinal pigment epithelium which permits plasma from the choriocapillaris to enter subretinal space.
Doyne's honeycomb c., drusen.
geographic c., helicoid or serpiginous c.; bilateral acquired abnormality of retinal pigment epithelium and choroid in which irregular multiple progressive swelling is followed by atropic scars in linear patterns.
guttate c., drusen.
helicoid c., geographic c.
myopic c., chronic degeneration of the sclera and choroid with posterior staphyloma, accompanying high myopia.
senile guttate c., drusen.
serpiginous c., geographic c.

choroidoretinitis (kō-roy'dō-ret-i-nī'tis). Retinochoroiditis.

choroidosis (ko'-roy-dō'sis). Choroidopathy.

Chotzen, F., 20th century German physician. See C. *syndrome.*

Christ, J., German dermatologist. See C.-Siemens *syndrome.*

Christensen, Erna, Danish pathologist. See C.-Krabbe *disease.*

Christian, Henry A., U.S. internist, 1876–1951. See C.'s *disease, syndrome;* Hand-Schüller-C. *disease;* Weber-C. *disease.*

Christison, Sir Robert, Scottish physician, 1797–1882. See C.'s *formula.*

Christmas. Surname of a child with the disease subsequently called Christmas *disease;* first case studied in detail. See also Christmas *factor, hemophilia* B.

chrom-, chromat-, chromato-, chromo- [G. *chrōma,* color]. Combining forms meaning color.

chromaffin (krō'maf-in) [chrom- + L. *affinis,* affinity]. Chromophil (3); chromaphil; pheochrome (1); giving a brownish yellow reaction with chromic salts; denoting certain cells in the medulla of the adrenal glands and in paraganglia.

chromaffinoma (krō-maf-in-ō'mă). Chromaffin tumor; a neoplasm composed of chromaffin cells derived from primitive sympathogonia, and occurring in the medullae of adrenal glands, the organs of Zuckerkandl, or the paraganglia of the thoracolumbar sympathetic chain; some c.'s secrete catecholamines. See also pheochromocytoma.

chromaffinopathy (krō'maf-in-op'ă-thē) [chromaffin + G. *pathos,* suffering]. Any pathologic condition of chromaffin tissue, as in the medullae of adrenal glands or the organs of Zuckerkandl.

chroman, chromane (krō'man, -mān). 3,4-Dihydro-2*H*-1-benzopyran; fundamental unit of the tocopherols (vitamin E). See also chromanol; chromene; chromenol.

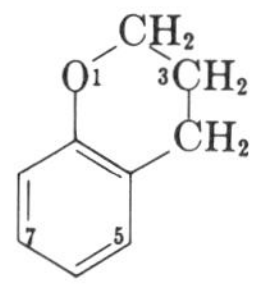

Chroman (Chromane)

chromanol (krō'man-ol). Hydroxychroman; 6-hydroxychroman (6-chromanol) is the fundamental unit of the tocopherols (vitamin E), tocols, and tocotrienols, as well as of ubi-, toco-, and phyllochromanol. See also chroman; chromene; chromenol.

chromaphil (krō'mă-fil). Chromaffin.

chromat-. See chrom-.

chromate (krō'māt). A salt of chromic acid.

chromatic (krō-mat'ik). Of or pertaining to color or colors; produced by, or made in, a color or colors.

chromatid (krō'mă-tid) [G. *chrōma,* color, + *-id* (2), *q.v.*]. Each of the two strands formed by longitudinal duplication of a chromosome that becomes visible during prophase of mitosis or meiosis; the two c.'s are joined by the still undivided centromere; after the centromere has divided at metaphase and the two c.'s have separated, each c. becomes a chromosome.

chromatin (krō'ma-tin) [G. *chrōma,* color]. The genetic material of the nucleus, consisting of deoxyribonucleoprotein, which occurs in two forms during the phase between mitotic divisions: 1) as heterochromatin, seen as condensed, readily stainable clumps; 2) as euchromatin, dispersed lightly staining or nonstaining material. During mitotic division the c. condenses and is seen as chromosomes.
heteropyknotic c., heterochromatin.
oxyphil c., oxychromatin.
sex c., Barr c. body; a small condensed mass of c. representing an inactivated X-chromosome usually located at the periphery of the interphase nucleus just inside the nuclear membrane; the number of sex c. bodies per nucleus is one less than the number of X-chromosomes, hence normal males and females with Turner's syndrome (XO) have none (sex c. negative), normal females and males with Klinefelter's syndrome (XXY) have one, and (XXX) females have two c. masses. For technical reasons only about half the cells in a preparation show typical masses. See also Lyon *hypothesis.*

chromatinolysis (krō′mă-ti-nol′i-sis). Chromatolysis.

chromatinorrhexis (krō-mat′i-nō-rek′sis) [chromatin + G. *rhēxis,* rupture]. Fragmentation of the chromatin.

chromatism (krō′mă-tizm) [G. *chrōma,* color]. **1.** Abnormal pigmentation. **2.** Chromatic *aberration.*

chromato-. See chrom-.

chromatogenous (krō-mă-toj′ĕ-nŭs) [chromato- + *-gen,* producing]. Producing color; causing pigmentation.

chromatogram (krō-mat′ō-gram). The graphic record produced by chromatography.

chromatograph (krō-mat′ō-graf). To perform chromatography.

chromatographic (krō′mat-ō-graf′ik). Pertaining to chromatography.

chromatography (krō-mă-tog′ră-fē) [chromato- + G. *graphō,* to write]. Stratographic analysis, absorption c.; the separation of chemical substances and particles (originally plant pigments and other highly colored compounds) by differential movement through a two-phase system. The mixture of materials to be separated is percolated through a column or sheet of some suitable chosen absorbent (*e.g.,* an ion-exchange material); the substances least absorbed are least retarded and emerge the soonest; those more strongly absorbed emerge later.
absorption c., chromatography.
affinity c., affinity column; c. where the absorbent has a unique chemical affinity for a particular component of the passing solution.
column c., a form of partition c. in which one phase is liquid (aqueous) flowing down a column packed with the second phase, a solid; the dissolved substances form a partition between the solid and liquid phases depending on the chemical and physical conditions of each phase; the more strongly adsorbed solutes reach the bottom of the column later than the less strongly adsorbed ones.
gas c., a chromatographic procedure in which the moving phase is a mixture of gases or vapors, which are separated in the process by their differential adsorption on a stationary phase.
gas-liquid c. (GLC), gas c., with the stationary phase being liquid rather than solid.
liquid-liquid c., c. in which both the moving phase and the stationary (or reverse-moving) phase are liquids, as in countercurrent distribution.
paper c., partition c. in which the moving phase is a liquid and the stationary phase is paper.
partition c., the separation of similar substances by repeated divisions between two immiscible liquids, so that the substances, in effect, cross the partition between the liquids in opposite directions; where one of the liquids is bound as a film on filter paper, the process is termed paper partition c. or paper c.
thin-layer c. (TLC), c. through a thin layer of cellulose or similar inert material supported on a glass or plastic plate.
two-dimensional c., paper c. in which a spot, located originally in one corner of a sheet, is developed in one direction along one side of the sheet, after which the sheet is rotated 90° and developed, with another solvent, in the new direction; the resultant spots are thus spread over the entire paper, giving a "map" or "fingerprint." Also generalized to include c. followed by electrophoresis (or vice versa), column c. followed by paper c., etc.

chromatoid (krō′mă-toyd) [chromato- + G. *eidos,* form]. A refractile substance composed of chromatin, thought to be a non-glycogen food reserve contained within the cytoplasm of certain protozoa; seen in cysts of *Entamoeba histolytica* as rounded bars or chromatoidal bodies in contrast to the splintery form of c. bodies in cysts of *Entamoeba coli.*

chromatokinesis (krō′mă-tō-ki-nē′sis) [chromato- + G. *kinēsis,* movement]. Rearrangement of the chromatin into various forms.

chromatolysis (krō-mă-tol′i-sis) [chromato- + G. *lysis,* dissolution]. Chromatinolysis; chromolysis; hypochromatosis; tigrolysis; the disintegration of the granules of chromophil substance (Nissl bodies) in a nerve cell body which may occur after exhaustion of the cell or damage to its peripheral process; other changes considered part of c. include swelling of the perikaryon and shifting of the nucleus from its central position to the periphery.
central c., retrograde c.; c. associated with significant axonal injury.
retrograde c., central c.
transsynaptic c., transsynaptic *degeneration.*

chromatolytic (krō-mă-tō-lit′ik). Relating to chromatolysis.

chromatometer (krō-mă-tom′ĕ-ter) [chromato- + G. *metron,* measure]. Colorimeter.

chromatopectic (krō′mă-tō-pek′tik). Chromopectic; relating to or causing chromatopexis.

chromatopexis (krō′mă-tō-pek′sis) [chromato- + G. *pēxis,* fixation]. Chromopexis; the fixation of color or staining fluid.

chromatophil, chromatophile (krō-mat′ō-fil, -fīl). Chromophil.

chromatophilia (krō′mă-tō-fil′ē-ă). Chromophilia.

chromatophilic, chromatophilous (krō-mă-tō-fil′ik, -tof′i-lŭs). Chromophilic.

chromatophobia (krō′mă-tō-fō′bē-ă). Chromophobia.

chromatophore (krō-mat′ō-fōr) [chromato- + G. *phoros,* bearing]. **1.** A colored plastid, due to the presence of chlorophyll or other pigments, found in certain forms of protozoa. **2.** A pigment-bearing phagocyte found chiefly in the skin, mucous membrane, and choroid coat of the eye, and also in melanomas. **3.** Chromophore.

chromatophorotropic (krō′mă-tō-fōr′ō-trop′ik) [chromatophore + G. *tropos,* a turning]. Denoting the attraction of chromatophores to the skin or other organs.

chromatoplasm (krō′mă-tō-plazm). The part of the cytoplasm containing pigment.

chromatopsia (krō-mă-top′sē-ă) [chromato- + G. *opsis,* vision]. A condition in which objects appear to be abnormally colored or tinged with color; designated according to the color seen: xanthopsia, yellow vision; erythropsia, red vision; chloropsia, green vision; cyanopsia, blue vision.

chromatotropism (krō-mă-tot′rō-pizm) [chromato- + G. *tropē,* turn]. **1.** A change of color. **2.** The phenomenon of orientation in response to color.

chromaturia (krō-mă-tū′rē-ă) [chromato- + G. *ouron,* urine]. Abnormal coloration of the urine.

chrome (krōm). Chromium, especially as a source of pigment.

chromene (krō′mēn). *2H*-1-Benzopyran; fundamental unit of the tocopherolquinones. See also chroman; chromanol; chromenol.

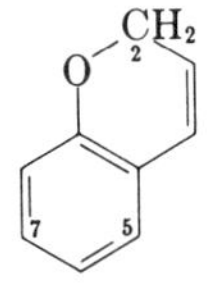

Chromene

chromenol (krō′men-ol). Hydroxychromene; 6-hydroxychromene (6-chromenol) is the fundamental unit of the tocopherolquinones (oxidized tocopherol) and plastochromenol-8. See also chroman; chromanol; chromene.

chrome red. Basic lead chromate, $PbCrO_4PbO$.

chromesthesia (krō-mes-thē′zē-ă) [G. *chrōma,* color, + *aisthēsis,* sensation]. **1.** The color sense. **2.** A condition in which another sensation, such as taste or smell, is excited by the perception of color.

chrome yellow [C.I. 77600]. Leipzig, lemon, or Paris yellow; lead chromate; a fine yellow powder used in paints and dyes.

chromhidrosis (krōm-hī-drō'sis) [chrom- + G. *hidros,* sweat]. Chromidrosis; a rare condition characterized by the excretion of sweat containing pigment; caused by ingestion of drugs or dyes.
apocrine c., excretion of colored sweat, usually black, from apocrine glands of the face; due to an abnormal lipochrome content of the secretion.

chromic acid (krō'mik). H_2CrO_4 or $H_2Cr_2O_7$; a strong oxidizing agent formed by dissolving chromium trioxide (CrO_3) in water.

chromidia (krō-mid'ē-ă). Plural of chromidium.

chromidiation (krō-mid-ē-ā'shŭn). Chromidiosis.

chromidiosis (krō-mid-ē-ō'sis). Chromidiation; an outpouring of nuclear substance and chromatin into the cell protoplasm.

chromidium, pl. **chromidia** (krō-mid'ē-ŭm, -ē-ă) [G. *chrōma,* color, + *-idion,* a diminutive termination]. A basophilic particle or structure in the cell cytoplasm, rich in RNA, often found in specialized cells.

chromidrosis (krō-mi-drō'sis). Chromhidrosis.

chromium (krō'mē-ŭm). A metallic element, symbol Cr, atomic no. 24, atomic weight 52.01.
c. trioxide, CrO_3; chromic acid, used as a caustic in the removal of warts and other small growths from the skin and genitals; the hydrated acid, H_2CrO_4, forms variously colored salts with potassium, lead, and other bases.

chromo-. See chrom-.

Chromobacterium (krō-mō-bak-tēr'ē-ŭm). A genus of bacteria (family Rhizobiaceae) containing Gram-negative, motile rods. These microorganisms produce a violet pigment (violacein) and are occasionally pathogenic to man and other animals. The type species is *C. violaceum.*
C. janthi'num, a species believed to cause a fatal septicemia in man and other animals.
C. viola'ceum, type species of the genus *C.;* it is found in soil and water.

chromoblast (krō'mō-blast). [chromo- + G. *blastos,* germ]. An embryonic cell with the potentiality of developing into a pigment cell.

chromoblastomycosis (krō'mō-blas'tō-mī-kō'sis) [chromo- + G. *blastos,* germ, + *mykē,* fungus, + *-osis,* condition]. Chromomycosis; a localized chronic mycosis of the skin and subcutaneous tissues characterized by skin lesions so rough and irregular as to present a cauliflower-like appearance; caused by dematiaceous fungi such as *Phialophora verrucosa, P. dermatitidis, Fonsecaea pedrosoi, F. compacta,* and *Cladosporuium carrionii;* fungal cells form rounded sclerotic bodies in tissue, with epidermal hyperplasia and intradermal microabscesses.

chromocenter (krō'mō-sen-ter). Karyosome.

chromocystoscopy (krō'mō-sis-tos'kō-pē) [chromo- + G. *kystis,* bladder, + *skopeō,* to view]. Cystochromoscopy.

chromocyte (krō'mō-sīt) [chromo- + G. *kytos,* cell]. Any pigmented cell, such as a red blood corpuscle.

chromogen (krō'mō-jen). **1.** A substance, itself without definite color, that may be transformed into a pigment; denoting especially benzene and its homologues toluene, xylene, quinone, naphthalene, and anthracene, from which the aniline dyes are manufactured. **2.** A microorganism that produces pigment.
Porter-Silber c.'s, yellow phenylhydrazones formed by the reaction of 17,21-dihydroxy-20-oxosteroids with a phenylhydrazine-ethanol-sulfuric acid reagent; used chiefly to determine plasma cortisol concentrations and the urinary output of 17-hydroxycorticoids.

chromogenesis (krō-mō-jen'ĕ-sis) [chromo- + G. *genesis,* production]. Production of coloring matter or pigment.

chromogenic (krō-mō-jen'ik). **1.** Denoting a chromogen. **2.** Relating to chromogenesis.

chromogranins (krō'mō-gran-inz). Soluble proteins of chromaffin granules; c. A, an acidic glycoprotein, accounts for approximately half of the total protein of the granule matrix.

chromoisomerism (krō'mō-ī-som'er-izm). Isomerism in which the isomers display different colors.

chromolipid (krō-mō-lip'id). Lipochrome (1).

chromolysis (krō-mol'i-sis). Chromatolysis.

chromomere (krō'mō-mēr) [chromo- + G. *meros,* a part]. **1.** A condensed segment of a chromonema. **2.** Granulomere.

chromometer (krō-mom'ĕ-ter). Colorimeter.

chromomycosis (krō'mō-mī-kō'sis) [chromo- + G. *mykēs,* fungus, + *-osis,* condition]. Chromoblastomycosis.

chromonar hydrochloride (krō'mō-nar). Carbochromene hydrochloride; [{3-[2-(diethylamino)ethyl]-4-methyl-2-oxo-2*H*-1-benzopyran-7-yl}oxy] acetic acid ethyl ester hydrochloride; used as a coronary vasodilator for treatment of angina pectoris.

chromone (krō'mōn). 4*H*- 1-Benzopyran-4-one; fundamental unit of various plant pigments and other substances. See also flavone; chromene; chromane.

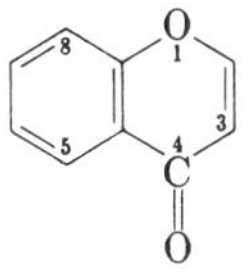

Chromone

chromonema, pl. **chromonemata** (krō-mō-nē'mă, -ma-tă) [chromo- + G. *nema,* thread]. Chromatic fiber; the coiled filament on which the genes are located, which extends the entire length of a chromosome and exhibits an intensely positive Feulgen test for DNA.

chromonychia (krō-mō-nik'ē-ă) [chromo- + G. *onyx* (*onych-*), nail]. Abnormality in the color of the nails.

chromopectic (krō-mō-pek'tik). Chromatopectic.

chromopexis (krō-mō-pek'sis). Chromatopexis.

chromophage (krō'mō-fāj) [chromo- + G. *phagein,* to eat]. A phagocyte that destroys pigment; term applied by Metchnikoff to the cells believed by him to be active in the reduction of pigment of the hair.

chromophanes (krō'mō-phānz) [chromo- + G. *phaino,* to show]. The colored oil globules in the retinal cones of some animal species.

chromophil, chromophile (krō'mō-fil, krō'mō-fīl) [chromo- + G. *phileō,* to love]. Chromatophil; chromatophile. **1.** Chromophilic. **2.** A cell or any histologic element that stains readily. **3.** Chromaffin.

chromophilia (krō-mō-fil'ē-ă) [chromo- + G. *phileō,* to love]. Chromatophilia; the property possessed by most cells of staining readily with appropriate dyes.

chromophilic, chromophilous (krō-mō-fil'ik, -mof'i-lŭs). Chromatophilic; chromatophilous; chromophil (1); staining readily; denoting certain cells and histologic structures.

chromophobe (krō'mō-fōb) [chromo- + G. *phobos,* fear]. Chromophobic; resistant to stains, staining with difficulty or not at all; denoting certain degranulated cells in the anterior lobe of the pituitary gland.

chromophobia (krō-mō-fō'bē-ă) [chromo- + G. *phobos,* fear]. Chromatophobia. **1.** Resistance to stains on the part of cells and tissues. **2.** A morbid dislike of colors.

chromophobic (krō-mō-fō'bik) [chromo- + *phobos,* fear]. Chromophobe.

chromophore (krō'mō-fōr) [chromo- + G. *phoros,* bearing]. Chromatophore (3); color radical; the atomic grouping upon which the color of a substance depends.

chromophoric, chromophorous (krō-mō-fōr'ik, -mof'ŏr-ŭs). **1.** Relating to a chromophore. **2.** Producing or carrying color; denoting certain microorganisms.

chromophototherapy (krō'mō-phō'tō-thār'ă-pē). Chromotherapy.

chromoplastid (krō-mō-plas'tid) [chromo- + G. *plastos,* formed, + *-id* (2)]. A pigmented plastid, containing chlorophyll, formed in certain protozoans.

chromoprotein (krō-mō-prō'tēn). One of a group of conjugated proteins, consisting of a combination of pigment with a protein; *e.g.,* hemoglobin.

chromosomal (krō'mō-sō'măl). Pertaining to chromosomes.

chromosomal map. A representation of the karyotype and of the positioning and ordering on it of those loci that have been localized by any of several mapping methods.

chromosome (krō'mō-sōm) [chromo- + G. *sōma,* body]. One of the bodies (normally 46 in man) in the cell nucleus that is the bearer of genes, has the form of a delicate chromatin filament during interphase, contracts to form a compact cylinder segmented into two arms by the centromere during metaphase and anaphase stages of cell divison, and is capable of reproducing its physical and chemical structure through successive cell divisons. In the case of microbes, the c. is procaryotic, not being enclosed within a nuclear membrane and not being subject to a mitotic mechanism.

accessory c., monosome; heterotropic or odd c.; unpaired allosome or c.; a c. existing without its normal homologous c.; at the reduction division of gametogenesis an accessory c. is likely to be included in one daughter cell and not in the other, but may be lost completely by lagging behind on the equatorial plate.

acentric c., a fragment of a c. lacking a centromere and which cannot attach to the mitotic spindle, therefore being unable to take part in the division of a nucleus and randomly distributed in daughter cells.

acrocentric c., a c. with the centromere placed very close to one end so that the shorter arm is very small, often with a satellite.

bivalent c., a pair of c.'s temporarily united.

Christchurch (Ch[1]) c., an abnormal small acrocentric c. (no. 21 or 22) with complete or almost complete deletion of the short arm, resulting in horseshoe or dumbbell shape; found in cultured leukocytes in some cases of chronic lymphocytic leukemia, also in some normal relatives of patients.

derivative c., translocation c.; an anomalous c. generated by translocation.

dicentric c., a c. with two centromeres, an abnormality that may result from reciprocal translocation.

fragile X c., an X c. with a fragile site near the end of the long arm, resulting in the appearance of an almost detached fragment; demonstrated only under special culture conditions; frequently associated with X-linked mental retardation (Renpenning's syndrome).

giant c., **(1)** polytene c.; **(2)** lampbrush c.

heterotropic c., accessory c.

heterotypical c., allosome.

homologous c.'s, members of a single pair of c.'s.

lampbrush c., giant c. (2); a large c. found in oocytes of certain animals characterized by many fine lateral projections giving the appearance of a test tube brush or lampbrush.

late replicating c., a c. (often anomalous) that is shown, *e.g.,* by incorporation of a labeled nucleotide, to undergo delayed duplication preliminary to mitosis; formerly used as a means of distinguishing members of a group of c.'s.

marker X c., a c. with cytologically distinctive characteristics.

metacentric c., a c. with a centrally placed centromere that divides the c. into two arms of approximately equal length.

nonhomologous c.'s, c.'s that are not members of the same pair.

nucleolar c., a c. regularly associated with a nucleolus.

odd c., accessory c.

Philadelphia (Ph[1]) c., an abnormal minute c. formed by a rearrangement of c.'s 9 and 22; found in cultured leukocytes of many patients with chronic granulocytic leukemia.

polytene c., giant c. (1); a stage of c. division that forms the giant c. found in the salivary gland of dipterous insects; the great width is the result of repeated divisions of the chromonema without subsequent separation of the filaments.

ring c., a c. with ends joined to form a circular structure; the normal form of the c. in certain bacteria.

sex c.'s, idiochromosome; gonosome; the pair of c.'s responsible for sex determination. In man and most animals, the sex c.'s are designated X and Y; females have two X c.'s, males have one X and one Y c. In certain birds, insects, and fishes the sex c.'s are designated Z and W; males have two Z c.'s, females may have one Z and one W c., or one Z and no W c.

submetacentric c., a c. with the centromere so placed that it divides the c. into two arms of unequal length.

telocentric c., a c. with a terminal centromere; such c.'s are unstable and arise by misdivision or breakage within the centromere region, and are usually eliminated within a few cell divisions or transformed into isochromosomes.

translocation c., derivative c.

unpaired c., accessory c.

W, X, Y, and Z c.'s, see sex c.'s.

chromosome map. A systematic semiabstract representation of the physical location of loci on a karyotype. *Cf.* genetic map.

chromosome mapping. The process of determining the position of specific genes on specific chromosomes and constructing a diagram of each chromosome showing the relative positions of genes; techniques include family studies with statistical analysis, somatic cell hybridization, and chromosome deletion mapping.

chromosome pairing. The process in synapsis whereby members of the chromosome pairs are aligned opposite each other before disjoining in the formation of the daughter cell; the apposition permits exchange of genetic material in crossing-over.

chromotherapy (krō-mō-thār'ă-pē). Chromophototherapy; treatment of disease by colored light.

chromotoxic (krō-mō-tok'sik). Caused by a toxic action on the hemoglobin, as in chromotoxic hyperchromemia, or resulting from the destruction of hemoglobin.

chromotrichia (krō-mō-trik'ē-ă) [chromo- + G. *thrix* (*trich-*), hair]. Colored or pigmented hair.

chromotrichial (krō-mō-trik'ē-ăl). Pertaining to the coloring of hair.

chromotrope (krō'mō-trōp). Any of several dyes containing chromotropic acid and which have the property of changing from red to blue on afterchroming.

chromotrope 2R [C.I. 16570]. A red acid dye, $C_{16}H_{10}N_2O_8S_2Na_2$, used as a counterstain and for staining red blood cells in sections.

chromotropic acid (krō'mō-trōp-ik). 4,5-Dihydroxynaphthalene-2,7-disulfonic acid; used as a reagent and in chromotropes.

chronaxia (krō-nak'sē-ă). Chronaxie.

chronaxie (krō'nak-sē) [G. *chronos,* time, + *axia,* value]. Chronaxia; chronaxis; chronaxy; a measurement of excitability of nervous or muscular tissue; the shortest duration of an effective electrical stimulus having a strength equal to twice the minimum strength required for excitation.

chronaximeter (krō-nak-sim'ĕ-ter). An instrument for measuring chronaxie.

chronaximetry (krō-nak-sim'ĕ-trē) [G. *chronos,* time, + *axia,* value, + *metrein,* to measure]. The measurement of chronaxie.

chronaxis (krō-nak'sis). Chronaxie.

chronaxy (krō'nak-sē). Chronaxie.

chronic (kron'ik) [G. *chronos,* time]. Of long duration; denoting a disease of slow progress and long continuance.

chronicity (kron-is'i-tē). The state of being chronic.

chrono- [G. *chronos,* time]. Combining form relating to time.

chronobiology (kron'ō-bī-ol'ō-jē) [chrono- + G. *bios,* life, + *logos,* study]. That aspect of biology concerned with the timing of biological events, especially repetitive or cyclic phenomena in individual organisms.

chronognosis (kron-og-nō'sis) [chrono- + G. *gnōsis,* knowledge]. Perception of the passage of time.

chronograph (kron'ō-graf) [chrono- + G. *graphō,* to record]. An instrument for graphic measurement and recording brief periods of time.

chronometry (krō-nom'ĕ-tre) [chrono- + G. *metron,* measure]. Measurement of intervals of time.
mental c., study of the duration of mental and behavorial processes.

chrono-oncology (kron'ō-on-kol'ō-jē) [G. *chronos,* time, + oncology]. The study of the influence of biological rhythms on neoplastic growth; also used to describe anti-cancer treatment based on the timing of drug administration.

chronopharmacology (kron'ō-far-mă-kol'ō-jē). A branch of chronobiology concerned with the effects of drugs upon the timing of biological events and rhythms, and the relation of biological timing to the effects of drugs.

chronophobia (kron'ō-fō'bē-ă). Morbid fear of the duration or immensity of time.

chronophotograph (kron-ō-fō'tō-graf). A photograph taken as one of a series for the purpose of showing successive phases of a motion.

chronotaraxis (kron'ō-tă-rak'sis) [chrono- + G. *taraxis,* confusion]. Distortion or confusion of the sense of time.

chronotropic (kron'ō-trop'ik). Affecting the rate of rhythmic movements such as the heartbeat.

chronotropism (kron-ot'rō-pizm) [chrono- + G. *tropē,* turn, change]. Modification of the rate of a periodic movement, *e.g.,* the heartbeat, through some external influence.
negative c., retardation of movement, especially of the heart rate.
positive c., acceleration of movement, especially of the heart rate.

chrys-, chryso- [G. *chrysos,* gold]. Combining forms meaning gold. See also auro-.

chrysanthemum-carboxylic acids (kri-san'thĕ-mŭm-kar-bok'si-lik). Cyclopropane carboxylic acids substituted in one position by two methyl groups, the other by 2-methyl-1-propenyl (chrysanthemum monocarboxylic acid) or by 3-methoxy-2-methyl-3-oxo-1-propenyl (chrysanthemum dicarboxylic acid methyl ester); these acids, esterfied with allethrolone or pyrethrolone, are the allethrins and pyrethrins, respectively.

chrysarobin (kris-ă-rō'bin) [G. *chrysos,* gold, + Brazil Ind. *araroba,* bark]. An extract of Goa powder; a complex mixure of reduction products of chrysophanic acid, emodin, and emodin monomethyl ether; used locally in ringworm, psoriasis, and eczema.

chrysazine (kris'ă-zin). Danthron.

chrysiasis (kri-sī'ă-sis) [G. *chrysos,* gold]. Chrysoderma; auriasis; aurochromoderma; a permanent slate-gray discoloration of the skin and sclera resulting from deposition of gold in the connective tissue of the skin and eye after administration of gold.

chrysocyanosis (kris'ō-sī-ă-nō'sis). Pigmentation of skin due to reaction to therapeutic use of gold salts.

chrysoderma (kris-ō-der'mă) [G. *chrysos,* gold, + *derma,* skin]. Chrysiasis.

chrysoidin (kris'oy-din) [C.I. 11270]. 2,4-Diaminoazobenzene hydrochloride; a dye (MW 249) made from aniline, used in histology and as an indicator (changing from orange to yellow at pH 4.0 to 7.0); also employed as a substitute for Bismark brown. C. citrate and c. thiocyanate are used as antiseptics.

Chrysomyia (kris-ō-mī'yă) [G. *chrysos,* gold, + *myia,* fly]. A genus of myiasis-producing fleshflies (family Calliphoridae) with medium-sized metallic-colored adults; includes the Old World screw worm, *C. bezziana* (sometimes called *Cochliomyia bezziana*), which is a primary invader, comparable to *Cochliomyia hominivorax,* the New World screw worm fly, whereas *C. megacephala* is an Old World equivalent to *Cochliomyia macellaria,* both being secondary or saprophytic invaders.

Chrysops (kris'ops) [G. *chrysos,* gold, + *ōpos,* eye]. The deer fly, a genus of biting flies with about 80 North American species, characterized by a splotched wing pattern; *C. discalis* is a vector of *Francisella tularensis* in the U.S.; *C. dimidiatus* and *C. silaceus* are the principal vectors of *Loa loa* in west Africa.

Chrysosporium parvum (kris-ō-spōr'ē-ŭm par'vŭm). A species of soil fungus that is the causative agent of adiaspiromycosis.

chrysotherapy (kris-ō-thār'ă-pē) [G. *chrysos,* gold]. Aurotherapy; treatment of disease by the administration of gold salts.

chthonophagia, chthonophagy (thon-ō-fā'jē-ă, -of'ă-jē) [G. *chthōn,* earth, + *phagein,* to eat]. Rarely used terms for geophagia.

chunking (chŭnk'ing). The process within short-term memory of combining disparate items of information so that they take up as little as possible of the limited space in short-term memory; *e.g.,* combining into one percept the three individual letters making up the word "cat."

Churg, Jacob, U.S. pathologist, *1910. See C.-Strauss *syndrome.*

chutta (chŭt'ă). Cancer of the roof of the mouth developing in Asians who smoke cigars with the lighted end inside the mouth. A similar association has been reported from South America and Sardinia.

Chvostek, Franz, Austrian surgeon, 1834–1884. See C.'s *sign.*

chyl-. See chylo-.

chylangioma (kī-lan-jē-ō'mă) [chyl- + G. *angeion,* vessel, + *-ōma,* tumor]. A mass of prominent, dilated lacteals and larger intestinal lymphatic vessels.

chylaqueous (kī-lā'kwē-ŭs) [chyl- + L. *aqua,* water]. Referring to watery chyle.

chyle (kīl) [G. *chylos,* juice]. A turbid white or pale yellow fluid taken up by the lacteals from the intestine during digestion and carried by the lymphatic system via the thoracic duct into the circulation. The milky appearance is due to chylomicrons in the lymph.

chylemia (kī-lē'mē-ă) [chyl- + G. *haima,* blood]. The presence of chyle in the circulating blood.

chylidrosis (kī-li-drō'sis) [chyl- + G. *hidrōs,* sweat]. Sweating of a milky fluid such as chyle.

chylifaction (kī-li-fak'shŭn) [chyl- + L. *facio,* to make]. Chylopoiesis.

chylifactive (kī-li-fak'tiv). Chylopoietic.

chyliferous (kī-lif'er-ŭs) [chyl- + L. *fero,* to carry]. Chylophoric; conveying chyle.

chylification (kī'li-fi-kā'shŭn). Chylopoiesis.

chyliform (kī'-li-fōrm). Resembling chyle.

chylo-, chyl- [G. *chylos,* juice, chyle]. Combining forms relating to chyle.

chylocele (kī'lō-sēl) [chylo- + G. *kēlē*, tumor]. A cystlike lesion resulting from the effusion of chyle into the tunica vaginalis propria and cavity of the tunica vaginalis testis.
parasitic c., *elephantiasis* scroti.

chylocyst (kī'lō-sist) [chylo- + G. *kystis*, bladder]. *Cisterna* chyli.

chyloderma (kī-lō-der'mă) [chylo- + G. *derma*, skin]. *Elephantiasis* scroti.

chylomediastinum (kī'lō-mē-dē-as-tī'nŭm). Abnormal presence of chyle in the mediastinum.

chylomicron, pl. **chylomicra, chylomicrons** (kī-lō-mi'kron, -mī'kră, -mi'kronz) [chylo- + G. *micros*, small]. A lipid droplet (about 1 nm diameter) of reprocessed lipid synthesized in epithelial cells of the small intestine, partially covered by β-lipoprotein and containing triglyceride and cholesterol ester; the least dense (0.93) of the plasma lipids which functions as a transport vehicle.

chylomicronemia (kī'lō-mī-krō-nē'mē-ă). The presence of chylomicrons, especially an increased number, in the circulating blood, as in type I familial hyperlipoproteinemia.

chylopericarditis (kī'lō-pār-i-kar-dī'tis). Chylopericardium.

chylopericardium (kī'lō-pār-i-kar'dē-ŭm). A milky pericardial effusion resulting from obstruction of the thoracic duct or from trauma.

chyloperitoneum (kī'lō-pār-i-tō-nē'ŭm). Chylous *ascites*.

chylophoric (kī-lō-fōr'ik) [chylo- + G. *phoros*, bearing]. Chyliferous.

chylopleura (kī-lō-plūr'ă). Chylothorax.

chylopneumothorax (kī'lō-nū-mō-thōr'aks). Free chyle and air in the pleural space.

chylopoiesis (kī'lō-poy-ē'sis) [chylo- + G. *poiesis*, a making]. Chylifaction; chylification; formation of chyle in the intestine and its absorption by the lacteals.

chylopoietic (kī'lō-poy-et'ik). Chylifactive; relating to chylopoiesis.

chylorrhea (kī-lō-rē'ă) [chylo- + G. *rhoia*, flow]. The flow or discharge of chyle.

chylosis (kī-lō'sis). The formation of chyle from the food in the intestine, its absorption by the lacteals, and its mixture with the blood and conveyance to the tissues.

chylothorax (kī-lō-thōr'aks). Chylopleura; chylous hydrothorax; an accumulation of milky chylous fluid in the pleural space, usually on the left.

chylous (kī'lŭs). Relating to chyle.

chyluria (kī-lū'rē-ă) [chyl- + G. *ouron*, urine]. The passage of chyle in the urine; a form of albiduria.

chymase (kī'mās). Chymosin.

chyme (kīm) [G. *chymos*, juice]. Pulp (3); the semifluid mass of partly digested food passed from the stomach into the duodenum.

chymification (kī-mi-fi-kā'shŭn) [G. *chymos*, juice, + L. *facio*, to make]. Chymopoiesis.

chymopapain (kī'mō-pap-ā'in) [EC 3.4.22.6]. A cysteine proteinase similar to papain; used to shrink slipped disks as an alternative to surgery, and as a meat tenderizer.

chymopoiesis (kī'mō-poy-ē'sis) [G. *chymos*, juice, chyme, + *poiesis*, a making]. Chymification; the production of chyme; the physical state of food (semifluid) brought about by digestion in the stomach.

chymorrhea (kī-mō-rē'ă) [G. *chymos*, juice, + *rhoia*, flow]. The flow of chyme.

chymosin (kī'mō-sin) [EC 3.4.23.4]. Chymase; pexin; rennase; rennet; rennin; a proteinase structurally homologous with pepsin, formed from prochymosin; the milk-curdling enzyme obtained from the glandular layer of the stomach of the calf.

chymosinogen (kī-mō-sin'ō-jen). Prochymosin.

chymotrypsin (kī-mō-trip'sin) [EC 3.4.21.1]. Chymotrypsin A or B; a serine proteinase of the gastrointestinal tract that preferentially cleaves carboxyl links of hydrophobic amino acids; synthesized in the pancreas as chymotrypsinogen, and subsequently converted to π-, δ-, and finally α-chymotrypsin by successive trypsin cleavages; proposed for use in the treatment of inflammation and edema associated with trauma and to facilitate intracapsular cataract extraction. Chymotrypsin C (EC 3.4.21.2) is similar to chymotrypsin but with broader specificity.

chymotrypsinogen (kī'mō-trip-sin'ō-jen). The precursor of chymotrypsin.

chymous (kī'mŭs). Relating to chyme.

C.I. **1.** Abbreviation for color *index*. **2.** Abbreviation for Colour Index.

Ci Abbreviation for curie.

Ciaccio, Carmelo, Italian pathologist, *1877. See C.'s *stain*.

Ciaccio, Giuseppe V., Italian anatomist, 1824–1901. See C.'s *glands*.

cib. Abbreviation for L. *cibus*, food.

cibophobia (sī-bō-fō'bē-ă) [L. *cibus*, food, + G. *phobos*, fear]. Fear of eating, or loathing for, food.

cicatrectomy (sik-ă-trek'tō-mē) [L. *cicatrix*, scar, + G. *ektomē*, excision]. Excision of a scar.

cicatrices (sik-ă-trī'sēz) Plural of cicatrix.

cicatricial (sik-ă-trish'ăl). Relating to a scar.

cicatricotomy, cicatrisotomy (sik'ă-trī-kot'ō-mē, -sot'ō-mē) [L. *cicatrix*, scar, + G. *tomē*, cutting]. Cutting a scar.

cicatrix, pl. **cicatrices** (sik'ă-triks, si-kā'triks; sik-ă-trī'sēz) [L.]. Scar.
brain c., a scarring of the brain resulting from injury (reactive gliosis), characterized by proliferation of mesodermal (vascular) and ectodermal (glial) elements. See also isomorphous *gliosis*.
filtering c., a c. through which fluid may seep; denoting especially a form of c. produced by an operation for glaucoma, through which there is subconjunctival drainage of aqueous humor.
meningocerebral c., scarring and adhesions involving contiguous brain and meninges; typically caused by head injury.
vicious c., a c. that by its contraction causes a deformity.

cicatrizant (sik-at'ri-zant). **1.** Causing or favoring cicatrization. **2.** An agent with such action.

cicatrization (sik'ă-tri-zā'shŭn). **1.** The process of scar formation. **2.** The healing of a wound otherwise than by first intention.

ciclopirox olamine (sī-klō-pir'oks ōl'ă-mēn). $C_{14}H_{24}N_2O_3$; a broad spectrum antifungal agent used to treat a variety of fungus and yeast skin infections.

cicutoxin (sik-yū-tok'sin). (−)-Heptadeca-*trans*-8,10,12-triene-4,6-diyne-1,4-diol; a toxic principle present in water hemlock, *Cicuta virosa* (family Umbelliferae); pharmacologic action is similar to that of picrotoxin.

ciguatera (sēg-wah-tār'ă) [Sp., prob. *cigua*, sea snail]. Poisoning due to the ingestion of the flesh or viscera of various marine fish of the tropical Caribbean and Pacific, such as barracuda, grouper, red snapper, amberjack, and dolphin, which contain ciguatoxin acquired through their food chain and unaffected by preservation or preparation procedures; characterized by varying combinations of vomiting and diarrhea, myalgia, dysesthesia and paresthesia of the extremities and perioral region, pruritis, headache, weakness, and diaphoresis.

ciguatoxin (sēg-wă-tok'sin). A marine saponin of unknown structure but with the empirical formula $C_{35}H_{65}NO_8$; the toxic substance causing ciguatera.

cili-. See cilio-.

cilia (sil'ē-ă). Plural of cilium.

ciliarotomy (sil'ē-ă-rot'ō-mē). Surgical division of the zona ciliaris.

ciliary (sil'ē-ar-ē) [Mod. L. *ciliaris,* relating to or resembling an eyelid, or eyelash, fr. L. *cilium,* eyelid]. **1.** Relating to any cilia or hairlike processes, specifically, the eyelashes. **2.** Relating to certain of the structures of the eyeball.

ciliastatic (sil-ē-ă-stat'ik). Denoting a drug or condition that slows or stops the beating of cilia (generally used with reference to respiratory mucosal cilia).

cilastatin sodium (sī-lă-stat'in). $C_{16}H_{25}N_2NaO_5S$; an inhibitor of the renal dipeptidase, dehydropeptidase 1, used, in conjunction with antibiotics subject to metabolism in the kidneys, to increase therapeutic response to the antibiotic.

Ciliata (sil-ē-ā'tă) [L. *cilium,* eyelid]. Formerly considered a class of Protozoa whose members bear cilia or structures derived from them, such as cirri or membranelles, but now placed within the phylum Ciliophora. Typical members, such as *Paramecium* or *Balantidium coli* (a parasite of man) possess two distinctive nuclei, a macronucleus and a micronucleus; only the latter bears the hereditary material exchanged in conjugation, a form of sexual reproduction found only in the C.

ciliated (sil'ē-ā-ted). Having cilia.

ciliates (sil'ē-āts). Common name for members of the Ciliata.

ciliectomy (sil-ē-ek'tō-mē). Cyclectomy.

cilio-, cili- [L. *cilium,* eyelid (eyelash)]. Combining forms relating to cilia or meaning ciliary, in any sense.

ciliogenesis (sil'ē-ō-jen'ē-sis). The formation of cilia.

Ciliophora (sil'ē-of'ō-ră) [cilio- + G. *phoros,* bearing]. A phylum of protozoa that includes the abundant free-living ciliates and the sessile suctorians; formerly classified as a subphylum of the phylum Protozoa.

cilioretinal (sil'ē-ō-ret'i -năl). Pertaining to the ciliary body and the retina.

cilioscleral (sil'ē-ō-sklē'răl). Relating to the ciliary body and the sclera.

ciliospinal (sil'ē-ō-spī'nal). Relating to the ciliary body and the spinal cord; denoting in particular the c. *center.*

ciliotomy (sil'ē-ot'ō-mē) [cilio- + G. *tomē,* incision]. Surgical section of the ciliary nerves.

ciliotoxicity (sil'ē-ō-tok-sis'i-tē). The characteristic of a drug or condition which impairs ciliary activity (generally refers to respiratory mucosal cilia).

cilium, pl. cilia (sil'ē-ŭm, -ă) [L. an eyelid]. **1** [NA]. Eyelash; one of the stiff hairs projecting from the margin of the eyelid. **2.** A motile extension of a cell surface, *e.g.,* of certain epithelial cells, containing nine longitudinal double microtubules arranged in a peripheral ring, together with a central pair.

cillo (sil'ō). Cillosis.

Cillobacterium (sil'ō-bak-tēr'ē-ŭm). An obsolete genus of motile, anaerobic bacteria containing Gram-positive, straight or curved rods. Motile cells are peritrichous. These organisms may be pathogenic. The type species is *C. moniliforme.* This genus is no longer recognized, and most of its species have been transferred to *Eubacterium: C. combesi* is now *Eubacterium combesi, C. moniliforme* is now *Eubacterium moniliforme, C. multiforme* is now *Eubacterium multiforme,* and *C. tenue* is now *Eubacterium tenue.*

cillosis (sil-ō'sis) [Mod. L., spelling influenced by Fr. *ciller,* to wink]. Cillo; spasmodic twitching of an eyelid.

cimetidine (si-met'i-dēn). *N*-Cyano-*N*′-methyl-*N*″-{2-[[(5-methyl-1*H*-imidazol-4-yl)methyl]thiol]ethyl}guanidine; a histamine analogue and antagonist used to treat peptic ulcer and hypersecretory conditions by blocking histamine receptor sites, thus inhibiting gastric acid secretion.

Cimex lectularius (sī'meks lek-tyū-lār-ē-ŭs) [L. *cimex,* bug, L. *lectulus,* a bed]. Bedbug; member of the family Cimicidae, with a flat, reddish-brown wingless body, prominent lateral eyes, and a three-jointed beak; it produces a characteristic pungent odor from thoracic stink glands and is an abundant pest in human abodes, especially in the tropics under poor sanitary conditions. Although the bedbug's bite produces an urticarial wheal, no important human disease has been proved to be routinely transmitted by it.

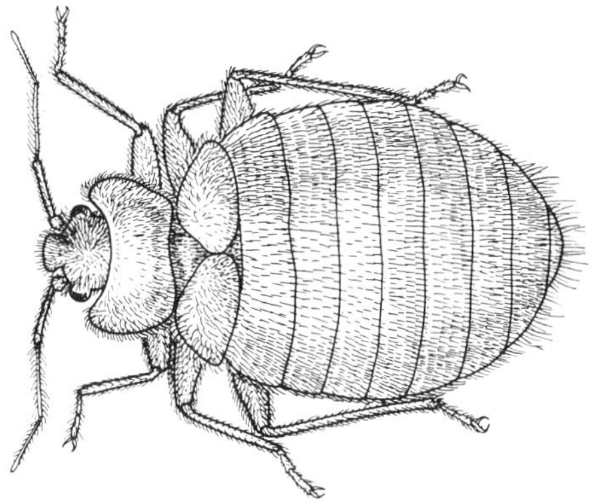

Cimex lectularius

cimicosis (sim-i-kō'sis). Lesions produced by bedbug bites of *Cimex lectularius.*

Cimino, James E., U.S. nephrologist, *1928. See Brescia-C. *fistula.*

cin-. See cine-.

cinanesthesia (sin'an-es-thē'zē-ă). Kinanesthesia.

cinanserin hydrochloride (si-nan'ser-in). 2′-[[3-(Dimethylamino)propyl]thio]cinnamanilide monohydrochloride; a serotonin inhibitor.

cinchol (sin'kol). β-Sitosterol.

cinchona (sin-kō'nă). Bark (2); cinchona, Jesuits', or Peruvian bark; quina; quinaquina; quinquina; the dried bark of the root and stem of various species of *Cinchona,* a genus of evergreen trees (family Rubiaceae), native of South America but cultivated in various tropical regions. The cultivated bark contains 7 to 10% of total alkaloids; about 70% is quinine. C. contains more than 20 alkaloids, of which two pairs of isomers are most important: quinine and quinidine, and cinchonidine and cinchonine.

cinchonic (sin-kon'ik). Relating to cinchona.

cinchonine (sin'-kō-nēn). A quinoline alkaloid prepared from the bark of several species of *Cinchona;* a tonic and antimalarial agent. Several c. salts are available.

cinchonism (sin'kō-nizm). Quininism; poisoning by cinchona, quinine, or quinidine; characterized by tinnitus, headache, deafness, and occasionally, anaphylactoid shock.

cinchophen (sin'kō-fen). 2-Phenylquinoline-4-carboxylic acid; 2-phenylcinchoninic acid; C_6H_5–(C_9H_5N)–COOH; an analgesic, antipyretic, and uricosuric agent that may produce liver damage and gastric lesions; used in experimental animals to produce gastric ulcer.

cinclisis (sing'-kli-sis) [G. *kinglizein,* to wag the tail, change constantly]. Rapid repetition of a movement, *e.g.,* rapidly repeated winking.

cine-, cin- [G. *kineō,* fut. *kinēsō,* to move]. Combining forms denoting movement, usually relating to motion pictures. See also kin-, kine-.

cineangiocardiography (sin'ē-an'jē-ō-kar-dē-og'ră-fē). Motion pictures of the passage of a contrast medium through chambers of the heart and great vessels.

cineangiography (sin'ē-an-jē-og'ră-fē). Motion pictures of the passage of a contrast medium through blood vessels.

cinefluorography (sin'ē-flūr-og'ră-fē). Cineradiography.

cinefluoroscopy (sin'ē-flūr-os'kō-pē). Cineradiography.

cinegastroscopy (sin'ē-gas-tros'kō-pē). Motion pictures of gastroscopic observations.

cinematics (sin-ē-mat'iks). Kinematics.

cinematization (sin'ē-mat-i-zā'shŭn). Cineplastic *amputation.*

cineole, cineol (sin'ē-ōl, -ol). Eucalyptol; cajeputol; cajuputol; 1,8-epoxy-*p*-menthane; a stimulant expectorant obtained from the volatile oil of *Eucalyptus globulus* and other species of *Eucalyptus.*

cinephotomicrography (sin'ē-fō'tō-mī-krog'ră-fē). The making of a motion picture of microscopic objects; time lapse photography is often used.

cineplastics (sin-ē-plas'tiks). Cineplastic *amputation.*

cineradiography (sin'ē-rā-dē-og'ră-fē). Cinefluorography; cinefluroroscopy; cineroentgenography; radiography of an organ in motion, *e.g.,* the heart, the gastrointestinal tract.

cinerea (si-nē'rē-ă) [L. fem. of *cinereus,* ashy, fr. *cinis,* ashes]. **1.** The gray matter of the brain and other parts of the nervous system. **2.** Obsolete term for mantle *layer.*

cinereal (si-nē'rē-ăl). Relating to the gray matter of the nervous system.

cineritious (si-ner-ish'ŭs). Ashen; denoting the gray matter of the brain, spinal cord, and ganglia.

cineroentgenography (sin'ē-rent-gen-og'ră-fē). Cineradiography.

cineseismography (sin'ē-sīz-mog'ră-fē). A technique for measuring movements of the body by continuous photographic recording of shaking or vibration.

cinetoplasm, cinetoplasma (sin-et'ō-plazm, sin-et-ō-plaz'mă). Kinetoplasm.

cineurography (sin'ē-yū-rog'ră-fē). Motion picture urography.

cingulate (sin'gyū-lāt). Relating to a cingulum.

cingulectomy (sin-gyū-lek'tō-mē) [cingulum + G. *ektomē,* excision]. Cingulotomy.

cingulotomy (sin-gyū-lot'ō-mē) [cingulum + G. *tomē,* a cutting]. Cingulectomy; formerly, a unilateral or bilateral surgical excision of the anterior half of the cingulate gyrus, but now accomplished by electrolytic destruction of the cortex and white matter of the cingulate gyrus and the anterior corpus callosum; performed for certain intractable psychoses, severe chronic pain, or addiction.

cingulum, gen. **cin'guli,** pl. **cingula** (sin'gyū-lŭm, -lă) [L. girdle, fr. *cingo,* to surround] [NA]. **1.** A structure that has the form of a belt or girdle. **2.** A well-marked fiber bundle passing longitudinally in the white matter of the gyrus cinguli (collateral gyrus); the bundle extends from the region of the anterior perforated substance back over the dorsal surface of the corpus callosum; behind the latter's splenium it curves down and then forward in the white matter of the parahippocampal gyrus; composed largely of fibers from the anterior thalamic nucleus to the cingulate and parahippocampal gyri, it also contains association fibers connecting these gyri with the frontal cortex, and their various subdivisions with each other.

c. den'tis [NA], c. of tooth; lingual lobe; basal ridge (2); a U- or W-shaped ridge at the base of the lingual surface of the crown of the upper incisors and cuspid teeth, the lateral limbs running for a short distance along the linguoproximal line angles, the central portion just above the gingiva.

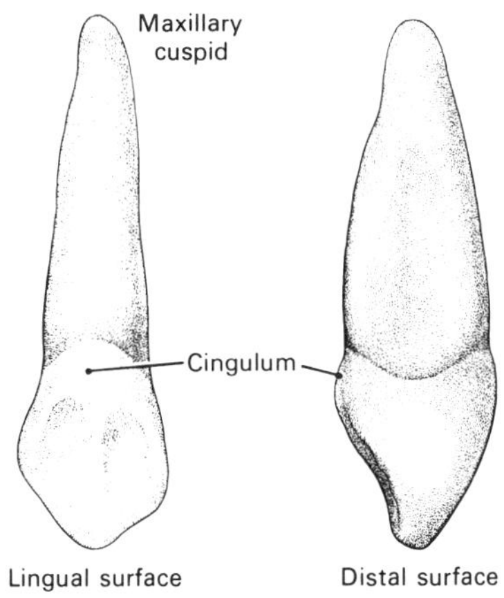

Cingulum Dentis

c. mem'bri inferior'is [NA], pelvic girdle; the bony ring formed by the hip bones and the sacrum, to which the inferior limbs are attached.

c. mem'bri superior'is [NA], shoulder or thoracic girdle; the bony ring, incomplete behind, that serves for the attachment and support of the upper limbs. It is formed by the manubrium sterni, the clavicles, and the scapulae.

c. of tooth, c. dentis.

cinnabar (sin'ă-bar) [G. *kinnabari*] Mercuric sulfide, red.

cinnamaldehyde (sin-ă-mal'de-hīd). Cinnamic aldehyde; 3-phenylpropenal; chief constituent of cinnamon oil.

cinnamate (sin'ă-māt). A salt or ester of cinnamic acid.

cinnamedrine (sin-am'ē-drēn). α-[1-(Cinnamylmethylamino)ethyl]benzyl alcohol; a smooth muscle relaxant used in the treatment of menstrual cramping.

cinnamein (sin'am-ē-in). *Benzyl* cinnamate.

cinnamene (sin'ă-mēn). Styrene.

cinnamic (si-nam'ik). Relating to cinnamon.

cinnamic acid. Phenylacrylic acid; 3-phenylpropenoic acid; cinnamylic acid; $C_6H_5CH{=}CHCOOH$; obtained from cinnamon oil, Peruvian and tolu balsams, or storax. It has been used in lupus as paint and in infectious diseases to promote leukocytosis.

cinnamic alcohol. Styrone.

cinnamic aldehyde. Cinnamaldehyde.

cinnamon (sin'ă-mon) [L. fr. G. *kinnamōmon,* cinnamon]. Cassia bark. **1.** Saigon c.; the dried bark of *Cinnamomum loureirii* Nees (family Lauraceae), an aromatic bark used as a spice and, in medicine, as an adjuvant, carminative, and aromatic stomachic. **2.** Ceylon c.; the dried inner bark of the shoots of *Cinnamomum zeylanicum.*

cassia c., Chinese c.; *Cinnamomum cassia* Nees (family Lauraceae); the unofficial source of most of the cinnamon in the shops; the source of c. oil.

Ceylon c., cinnamon (2).

Chinese c., cassia c.

Saigon c., cinnamon (1).

cinnamon oil. Cassia oil; the volatile oil distilled with steam from the leaves and twigs of *Cinnamomum cassia;* it contains not less than 80% by volume of the total aldehydes of cinnamon oil.

cinnamylic acid (sin-ă-mil'ik). Cinnamic acid.

cinnarizine (si-nar'i-zēn). Cinnipirine; 1-cinnamyl-4-(diphenylmethyl)piperazine; an antihistaminic.

cinnipirine (si-nip'i-rēn). Cinnarizine.

cinocentrum (sin-ō-sen'trŭm). Cytocentrum.

cinoxacin (si-noks'ă-sin). [1,3]Dioxolo[4,5-*g*]cinnoline-3-carboxylic acid, 1-ethyl-1,4-dihydro-4-oxo-; a synthetic organic acid, chemically related to nalidixic acid, used as an antibacterial to treat urinary tract infections.

cinoxate (si-nok'sāt). 2-Ethoxyethyl *p*-methoxycinnamate; an ultraviolet screen for topical application on the skin.

cion (sī'on) [G. *kiōn*, pillar, the uvula]. Archaic term for uvula.

ciprofloxacin hydrochloride (sip-rō-floks'ă-sin). $C_{17}H_{18}FN_3$-O_3·HCl·H_2O; a synthetic fluoroquinolone broad spectrum, antibacterial with activity against a wide range of Gram-negative and Gram-positive organisms.

cirantin (sir-an'tin). Hesperidin.

circadian (ser-kā'dē-ăn) [L. *circa*, about, + *dies*, day]. Relating to biologic variations or rhythms with a cycle of about 24 hours. *Cf.* infradian; ultradian.

circellus (sir-sel'ŭs) [L.]. Circle.

c. veno'sus hypoglos'si, *plexus* venosus canalis hypoglossi.

circhoral (ser-kō'răl). Occurring cyclically about once an hour.

circinate (ser'si-nāt) [L. *circinatus*, made round, pp. of *circino*, to make round, fr. *circinus*, a pair of compasses]. Circular; ring-shaped.

circle (ser'kl) [L. *circulus*] **1.** A ring-shaped structure or group of structures. **2.** A line or process with every point equidistant from the center.

arterial c. of cerebrum, *circulus* arteriosus cerebri.

articular vascular c., *circulus* articularis vasculosus.

Baudelocque's uterine c., pathologic retraction *ring.*

Carus' c., Carus' *curve.*

closed c., a circuit for administration of an inhalation anesthetic in which there is complete rebreathing with carbon dioxide absorption.

defensive c., obsolete term for the addition of a secondary affection which limits or arrests the progress of the primary affection, as thought to occur when pneumothorax supervenes on pulmonary tuberculosis, the two affections exerting a reciprocally antagonistic action.

greater arterial c. of iris, *circulus* arteriosus iridis major.

Haller's c., **(1)** *circulus* vasculosus nervi optici; **(2)** *plexus* venosus areolaris.

Huguier's c., anastomosis around the isthmus of the uterus (junction of the cervix with the body) between the right and left uterine arteries.

least diffusion c., in the configuration of rays emerging from a spherocylindrical lens system, the place where diverging rays of the lens first forming a line image are balanced by converging rays of the second lens.

lesser arterial c. of iris, *circulus* arteriosus iridis minor.

Pagenstecher's c., in the case of a freely movable abdominal tumor, the mass is moved throughout its entire range, its position at intervals being marked on the abdominal wall; when these points are joined, a c. is formed, the center of which marks the point of attachment of the tumor.

Ridley's c., *sinus* intercavernosi.

semi-closed c., a circuit for administration of an inhalation anesthetic in which partial rebreathing with carbon dioxide absorption is combined with loss from the circuit of a portion of respired gases through valves.

vascular c., **(1)** the c. around the mouth formed by the inferior and superior labial arteries; **(2)** *plexus* venosus areolaris.

vascular c. of optic nerve, *circulus* vasculosus nervi optici.

venous c. of mammary gland, *plexus* venosus areolaris.

vicious c., **(1)** the mutually accelerating action of two independent diseases, or of a primary and secondary affection; **(2)** the passage of food, after a gastroenterostomy, from the artificial opening through the intestinal loop by antiperistaltic action and back into the stomach again by the pyloric orifice, or the reverse.

c. of Willis, *circulus* arteriosus cerebri.

Zinn's vascular c., *circulus* vasculosus nervi optici.

circuit (ser'kit) [L. *circuitus*, a going round, fr. *circum*, around, + *eo*, pp. *itus*, to go]. The path or course of flow of cases or electric or other currents.

anesthetic c., equipment used during inhalation anesthesia to regulate concentrations of inhaled gases; includes a reservoir bag and usually directional valves, breathing tubes, and a carbon dioxide absorber.

Papez c., a long circuitous conduction chain in the mammalian forebrain, leading from the hippocampus by way of the fornix to the mammillary body and thence returning to the hippocampus by way of, sequentially, the anterior thalamic nuclei, gyrus cinguli, and gyrus parahippocampalis.

reverberating c., a theory of periodic conduction through the cerebral cortex of trains of impulses traveling in c.'s of neurons.

circulation (ser-kyū-lā'shŭn) [L. *circulatio*]. Movements in a circle, or through a circular course, or through a course which leads back to the same point; usually referring to blood c. unless otherwise specified.

blood c., the course of the blood from the heart through the arteries, capillaries, and veins back again to the heart.

capillary c., the course of the blood through the capillaries.

collateral c., c. maintained in small anastomosing vessels when the main vessel is obstructed.

compensatory c., c. established in dilated collateral vessels when the main vessel of the part is obstructed.

cross c., c. to an animal or one of its parts from the c. of another animal.

embryonic c., the basic plan of the c. of a young mammalian embryo, at first similar to that in aquatic forms, with an unpartitioned heart and conspicuous aortic arches in the branchial region; as gestation progresses, the arrangement of the major blood vessels gradually approaches that of an adult, but the routing of blood through the heart, characteristic of an adult, cannot be attained until lung breathing begins at birth.

enterohepatic c., c. of substances such as bile salts which are absorbed from the intestine and carried to the liver, where they are secreted into the bile and again enter the intestine.

extracorporeal c., the c. of blood outside of the body through a machine that temporarily assumes an organ's functions, *e.g.*, through a heart-lung machine or artificial kidney.

fetal c., the c. which serves the fetus *in utero*, with the placental circuit responsible for supplying oxygen and nutritive material and for eliminating CO_2 and nitrogenous wastes. See also embryonic c.

greater c., systemic c.

lesser c., pulmonary c.

lymph c., the slow passage of lymph through the lymphatic vessels and glands.

placental c., the c. of blood through the placenta during intrauterine life, serving the needs of the fetus for aeration, absorption, and excretion.

portal c., **(1)** c. of blood to the liver from the small intestine, the right half of the colon, and the spleen via the portal vein; sometimes specified as the hepatic portal c.; **(2)** more generally, any part of the systemic circulation in which blood draining from the capillary bed of one structure flows through a larger vessel(s) to supply the capillary bed of another structure before returning to the heart; *e.g.*, the hypothalamohypophyseal portal system.

pulmonary c., lesser c.; the passage of blood from the right ventricle through the pulmonary artery to the lungs and back through the pulmonary veins to the left atrium.

Servetus' c., obsolete eponym for the pulmonary c.

systemic c., greater c.; the c. of blood through the arteries, capillaries, and veins of the general system, from the left ventricle to the right atrium.

circulatory (ser'kyū-lă-tō-rē). **1.** Relating to the circulation. **2.** Sanguiferous.

circulus, gen. and pl. **circuli** (ser'kyū-lŭs, -lī) [L. dim. of *circus,* circle]. **1** [NA]. Any ringlike structure. **2.** A circle formed by connecting arteries, veins, or nerves.

c. arterio'sus cere'bri [NA], arterial circle of the cerebrum; circle of Willis; an anastomotic "circle" of arteries (roughly pentagonal in outline) at the base of the brain, formed, sequentially and in anterior to posterior direction, by the anterior communicating artery, the two anterior cerebral, the two internal carotid, the two posterior communicating, and the two posterior cerebral arteries.

c. arterio'sus hal'leri, c. vasculosus nervi optici.

c. arterio'sus ir'idis ma'jor [NA], greater arterial circle of iris; an arterial circle at the ciliary border of the iris.

c. arterio'sus ir'idis mi'nor [NA], lesser arterial circle of iris; an arterial circle near the pupillary margin of the iris.

c. articula'ris vasculo'sus [NA], articular vascular circle; an anastomosis of vessels encircling a joint.

c. vasculo'sus ner'vi op'tici [NA], c. arteriosus halleri; c. zinnii; vascular circle of the optic nerve; Zinn's vascular circle; Zinn's corona; Haller's circle (1); a network of branches of the short ciliary arteries on the sclera around the point of entrance of the optic nerve.

c. veno'sus hal'leri, *plexus* venosus areolaris.

c. veno'sus rid'leyi, *sinus* intercavernosi.

c. zin'nii, c. vasculosus nervi optici.

circum- [L. around]. Prefix denoting a circular movement, or a position surrounding the part indicated by the word to which it is joined. See also peri-.

circumanal (ser-kŭm-ā'năl). Perianal; periproctic; surrounding the anus.

circumarticular (ser'kŭm-ar-tik'yū-lăr) [circum- + L. *articulus,* joint]. Periarthric; periarticular; surrounding a joint.

circumaxillary (ser-kŭm-mak'si-lăr-ē). Periaxillary; around the axilla.

circumbulbar (ser-kŭm-bŭl'bar). Peribulbar.

circumcise (ser'kŭm-sīz). To perform circumcision, especially of the prepuce.

circumcision (ser-kŭm-sizh'ŭn) [L. *circumcido,* to cut around, fr. *circum,* around, + *caedo,* to cut]. **1.** Peritomy (2); posthetomy; operation to remove part or all of the prepuce. **2.** Cutting around an anatomical part (*e.g.,* the areola of the breast).

circumcorneal (ser-kŭm-kōr'nē-ăl). Pericorneal.

circumduction (ser-kŭm-dŭk'shŭn) [circum- + L. *duco,* pp. *ductus,* to draw]. **1.** Movement of a part, *e.g.,* an extremity, in a circular direction. **2.** Cycloduction.

circumference (ser-kŭm'fer-ens) [L. *circumferentia, a bearing around*]. Circumferentia; the outer boundary, especially of a circular area.

articular c. of radius, *circumferentia* articularis radii.

articular c. of ulna, *circumferentia* articularis ulnae.

circumferentia (ser-kŭm-fer-en'shē-ă) [L. a bearing around] [NA]. Circumference.

c. articula'ris ra'dii [NA], articular circumference of radius; the portion of the head of the radius that articulates with the radial notch of the ulna.

c. articula'ris ul'nae [NA], articular circumference of ulna; the portion of the head of the ulna that articulates with the ulnar notch of the radius.

circumflex (ser'kŭm-fleks) [circum- + L. *flexus,* to bend]. Describing an arc of a circle; denoting several anatomical structures: arteries, veins, nerves, and muscles.

circumgemmal (ser-kŭm-jem'ăl) [circum- + L. *gemma,* a bud]. Perigemmal; surrounding a budlike or bulblike body; denoting a mode of nerve termination by fibrils surrounding an end bulb.

circumintestinal (ser'kŭm-in-tes'ti-năl). Perienteric.

circumlental (ser-kŭm-len'tăl). Perilenticular.

circummandibular (ser'kŭm-man-dib'yū-lăr). Around or about the mandible.

circumnuclear (ser-kŭm-nū'klē-ăr). Perinuclear.

circumocular (ser-kŭm-ok'yū-lăr) [circum- + L. *oculus,* eye]. Periocular; periophthalmic; around the eye.

circumoral (ser-kŭm-ōr'ăl) [circum- + L. *os* (*oris*), mouth]. Perioral.

circumorbital (ser-kŭm-ōr'bi-tăl). Periorbital (2); around the orbit.

circumrenal (ser-kŭm-rē'năl) [circum- + L. *ren,* kidney]. Perinephric.

circumscribed (ser'kŭm-skrībd) [circum- + L. *scribo,* to write]. Bounded by a line; limited or confined.

circumscriptus (ser-kŭm-skrip'tŭs) [L.]. Circumscribed.

circumstantiality (ser'kŭm-stan-shē-al'i-tē) [L. *circum-sto,* pr. p. *-stans,* to stand around]. A disturbance in the thought process, either voluntary or involuntary, in which one gives an excessive amount of detail (circumstances) that is often tangential, elaborate, and irrelevant, to avoid making a direct statement or answer to a question; observed in schizophrenia and in obsessional disorders. *Cf.* tangentiality.

circumvallate (ser-kŭm-val'āt) [circum- + L. *vallum,* wall]. Denoting a structure surrounded by a wall, as the c. papillae of the tongue.

circumvascular (ser-kŭm-vas'kyū-lăr) [circum- + L. *vasculum,* vessel]. Perivascular.

circumventricular (ser'kŭm-ven-trik'yū-lăr). Around or in the area of a ventricle, as are the c. organs.

circumvolute (ser-kŭm-vol'ūt) [L. *circum-volvo,* pp. *-volutus,* to roll around]. Twisted around; rolled about.

cirrhogenous, cirrhogenic (sir-roj'ĕ-nŭs, -nō-jen'ik) [G. *kirrhos,* yellow (liver), + *-gen,* producing]. Tending to the development of cirrhosis.

cirrhonosus (sir-ron'ō-sŭs) [G. *kirrhos,* yellow (liver), + *nosos,* disease]. A disease of the fetus marked anatomically by a yellow staining of the peritoneum and pleura.

cirrhosis (sir-rō'sis) [G. *kirrgos,* yellow (liver), + *-osis,* condition]. Progressive disease of the liver characterized by diffuse damage to hepatic parenchymal cells, with nodular regeneration, fibrosis, and disturbance of normal architecture; associated with failure in the function of hepatic cells and interference with blood flow in the liver, frequently resulting in jaundice, portal hypertension, ascites, and ultimately hepatic failure.

alcoholic c., c. that frequently develops in chronic alcoholism, characterized in an early stage by enlargement of the liver due to fatty change with mild fibrosis, and later by Laënnec's c. with contraction of the liver.

biliary c., c. due to biliary obstruction, which may be a primary intrahepatic disease or secondary to obstruction of extrahepatic bile ducts; the latter may lead to cholestasis and proliferation in small bile ducts with fibrosis, but marked disturbance of the lobular pattern is infrequent. See also primary biliary c.

Budd's c., chronic enlargement of the liver without jaundice, formerly thought to be of intestinal origin.

capsular c. of liver, Glisson's c.

cardiac c., cardiac liver; cyanotic atrophy of the liver; pseudocirrhosis; congestive or stasis c.; an extensive fibrotic reaction within the liver as a result of prolonged congestive heart failure; true c. with fibrous bridging of lobules is unusual.

cholangiolitic c., a form of c. in which there is diffuse inflammation of the cholangioles, with inflammation, fibrosis, and regeneration; characterized by chronicity, relapses, and febrile episodes.
congestive c., cardiac c.
cryptogenic c., c. of unknown etiology, with no history of alcoholism or previous acute hepatitis.
fatty c., early nutritional c., especially in alcoholics, in which the liver is enlarged by fatty change, with mild fibrosis.
Glisson's c., capsular c. of the liver; chronic perihepatitis with thickening and subsequent contraction, resulting in atrophy and deformity of the liver.
Hanot's c., primary biliary c.
juvenile c., active chronic *hepatitis.*
Laënnec's c., portal c.; c. in which normal liver lobules are replaced by small regeneration nodules, sometimes containing fat, separated by a fairly regular framework of fine fibrous tissue strands (hobnail liver); usually due to chronic alcoholism.
necrotic c., postnecrotic c.
nutritional c., c. occurring in persons or animals with general or specific dietary deficiencies; methionine and cystine deficiency may produce changes of c. in animals, but it is uncertain whether malnutrition in humans leads to c. or only to reversible fatty infiltration of the liver.
pigmentary c., c. resulting from excessive deposits of iron in the liver, usually seen in hemochromatosis.
portal c., Laënnec's c.,
posthepatitic c., active chronic *hepatitis.*
postnecrotic c., necrotic c.; c. characterized by necrosis involving whole hepatic lobules, with collapse of the reticular framework to form large scars; regeneration nodules are also large; may follow viral or toxic necrosis, or develop as a result of ischemic necrosis in the course of nutritional c.
primary biliary c., Hanot's c.; a rare condition occurring mainly in middle-aged women, characterized by obstructive jaundice with hyperlipemia, pruritis, and hyperpigmentation of the skin; no obstruction of large bile ducts or proliferation of small bile ducts is found; the liver shows c. with marked portal infiltration by lymphocytes and plasma cells, and frequently by epithelioid cell granulomas; serum antimitochondrial antibodies are present in 85 to 90% of patients.
stasis c., cardiac c.
toxic c., c. of the liver resulting from chronic poisoning, as by lead or carbon tetrachloride.

cirrhotic (sir-rot'ik). Relating to or affected with cirrhosis.

cirri (sir'ī). Plural of cirrus.

cirrose, cirrous (sir'ōs, sir'ŭs). Relating to or having cirri.

cirrus, pl. **cirri** (sir'rŭs, -rī) [L. a curl]. A structure formed from a cluster or tuft of fused cilia, constituting one of the sensory or locomotor organs of certain ciliate protozoa.

cirsectomy (ser-sek'tō-mē) [G. *kirsos,* varix, + *ektomē,* excision]. Excision of a section of a varicose vein.

cirsocele (ser'sō-sēl) [G. *kirsos,* varix, + *kēlē,* tumor]. Varicocele.

cirsodesis (ser-sod'ĕ-sis) [G. *kirsos,* varix, + *desis,* a binding, fr. *deō,* to bind]. Ligation of varicose veins.

cirsoid (ser'soyd) [G. *kirsos,* varix, + *eidos,* appearance]. Varicoid.

cirsomphalos (ser-som'fă-los) [G. *kirsos,* varix, + *omphalos,* umbilicus]. *Caput* medusae.

cirsophthalmia (ser-sof-thal'mē-ă) [G. *kirsos,* varix, + *ophthalmos,* eye]. Varicose dilation of the conjunctival blood vessels.

cirsotome (ser'sō-tōm). A cutting instrument used in operating upon varicose veins.

cirsotomy (ser-sot'ō-mē) [G. *kirsos,* varix, + *tomē,* incision]. Treatment of varicose veins by multiple incisions.

cis- [L.] **1.** Prefix meaning on this side, on the near side; opposite of trans-. **2.** In genetics, a prefix denoting the location of two or more genes on the same chromosome of a homologous pair. **3.** In organic chemistry, a form of isomerism in which similar functional groups are attached on the same side of the plane that includes two adjacent, fixed carbon atoms (*e.g.,* the 2- and 3-OH groups of ribofuranose).

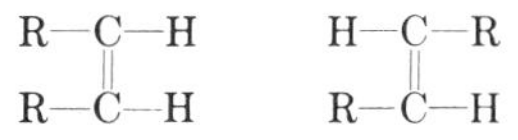

cis- *trans-*

cisplatin (sis'pla-tin). *cis*-Diamminedichloroplatinum; a chemotherapeutic agent with antitumor activity; c. binds DNA and interferes with DNA synthesis.

cissa (sis'ă) [G. *kissa, kitta,* longing for strange food by pregnant women]. Citta; cittosis; craving for unusual or unwholesome foods during pregnancy. See also pica.

cistern (sis'tern) [L. *cisterna*] Cisterna.
cerebellomedullary c., *cisterna* cerebellomedullaris.
c. of chiasm, *cisterna* chiasmatis.
chyle c., *cisterna* chyli.
c. of cytoplasmic reticulum, see cisterna (2).
c. of great vein of cerebrum, *cisterna* venae magnae cerebri.
interpeduncular c., *cisterna* interpeduncularis.
c. of lateral fossa of cerebrum, *cisterna* fossae lateralis cerebri.
c. of nuclear envelope, *cisterna* caryothecae.
Pecquet's c., *cisterna* chyli.
pontine c., *cisterna* pontis.
subarachnoidal c.'s, *cisternae* subarachnoideales.

cisterna, gen. and pl. **cister'nae** (sis-ter'nă, -ter'nē) [L. an underground cistern for water, fr. *cista,* a box]. Cistern. **1** [NA]. Any cavity or enclosed space serving as a reservoir, especially for chyle, lymph, or cerebrospinal fluid. **2.** An ultramicroscopic space occurring between the membranes of the flattened sacs of the endoplasmic reticulum, the Golgi complex, or the two membranes of the nuclear envelope.
c. am'biens, ambient c., c. venae magnae cerebri.
c. basa'lis, c. interpeduncularis.
c. caryothe'cae, cistern of the nuclear envelope; perinuclear space; the space between the internal and external membranes of the nuclear envelope; may be continuous in places with cisterns of the endoplasmic reticulum.
c. cerebellomedulla'ris [NA], cerebellomedullary cistern; c. magna; the largest of the subarachnoid cisterns between the undersurface of the cerebellum and the dorsal surface of the medulla oblongata.
c. chias'matis [NA], cistern of the chiasm; a dilation of the subarachnoid space below and anterior to the optic chiasm.
c. chy'li [NA], chyle cistern; receptaculum chyli; receptaculum pecqueti; ampulla chyli; Pecquet's cistern or reservoir; chylocyst; a dilated sac at the lower end of the thoracic duct into which the intestinal trunk and two lumbar lymphatic trunks open; it occurs inconstantly and when present is located behind the aorta opposite the first and second lumbar vertebrae.
c. crura'lis, c. interpeduncularis.
c. fos'sae latera'lis cer'ebri [NA], cistern of the lateral fossa of the cerebrum; an elongated expansion of the subarachnoid space where the arachnoid bridges over the opening of the Sylvian fissure.
c. interpeduncula'ris [NA], interpeduncular cistern; c. basalis; c. cruralis; Tarin's space; a dilation of the subarachnoid space in front of the pons, where the arachnoid membrane stretches across between the two temporal lobes over the base of the diencephalon.
c. mag'na, c. cerebellomedullaris.
c. perilymphat'ica, *spatium* perilymphaticum.
c. pon'tis, pontine cistern; an upward continuation of the subarachnoid space of the spinal cord, continuous about the medulla

with the c. cerebellomedullaris.

cister'nae subarachnoidea'les [NA], subarachnoidal cisterns; widening portions of the subarachnoid space within the cranium where the arachnoid bridges over a depression on the surface of the brain.

subsurface c., a cistern of the endoplasmic reticulum that lies close to the plasma membrane; such cisternae occur especially in the cell bodies of neurons.

c. superior'is, c. venae magnae cerebri.

terminal cisternae, pairs of transversely oriented tubules of the sarcoplasmic reticulum occurring at regular intervals in skeletal muscle fibers; together with an intermediate T tubule they make up a triad.

c. ve'nae mag'nae cer'ebri, cistern of the great vein of the cerebrum; c. ambiens; ambient c.; c. superioris; Bichat's canal or foramen; an expansion of the subarachnoid space extending forward between the corpus callosum and the thalamus; it encloses the internal cerebral veins which caudally join to form the vena magna cerebri (Galen's vein).

cisternal (sis-ter'năl). Relating to a cisterna.

cisternography (sis'tern-og'ră-fē). The roentgenographic study of the basal cisterns of the brain after the subarachnoid introduction of an opaque or other contrast medium, or a radiopharmaceutical with a suitable detector.

cerebellopontine c., the roentgenographic study of the cerebellopontine angle and contiguous structures after the introduction of a radiopaque contrast medium into the subarachnoid space.

radionuclide c., the demonstration of the cisterns at the base of the brain by a gamma-emitting substance.

cistron (sis'tron). The smallest functional unit of heredity; a length of chromosomal DNA associated with a single biochemical function. Under classical concepts, a gene might consist of more than one c.; in modern molecular biology, the c. is essentially equivalent to the gene.

cisvestism, cisvestitism (sis-ves'tizm, -ves'ti-tizm) [L. *cis,* on the near side of, + *vestio,* to dress]. The practice of dressing in clothes inappropriate to one's position or status. *Cf.* transvestism.

Citellus (si-tel'ŭs) [Mod. L.]. A genus of ground squirrel. *C. beecheyi, C. grammurus, C. pygmaeus, Yersinia C. townsendi,* and several other species act as an important reservoir of *Yersinia pestis.*

citral (sit'răl). An aldehyde from oils of lemon, orange, verbena, and lemon grass.

citrase, citratase (sit'rās, -ră-tās). *Citrate* lyase.

citrate (sit'rāt, sī'trāt). A salt or ester of citric acid; used as anticoagulants because they bind calcium ions.

c. aldolase, c. lyase.

c. lyase [EC 4.1.3.6], c. (*pro-* 3*S*)-lyase; citratase; citrase; citridesmolase; c. aldolase; an enzyme that catalyzes the cleavage of citric acid to oxaloacetic acid and acetic acid, in the absence of coenzyme A.

c. synthase [EC 4.1.3.7], c. (*si*)-synthase; citrogenase; condensing enzyme; oxaloacetate transacetase; an enzyme catalyzing the condensation of oxaloacetic acid and acetyl-CoA, forming citric acid and coenzyme A.

citrated (sit'rā-ted). Containing a citrate; specifically denoting blood serum or milk to which has been added a solution of potassium or sodium citrate, or both.

citric acid (sit'rik). 2-Hydroxypropane-1,2,3-tricarboxylic acid; the acid of citrus fruits, widely distributed in nature and a key intermediate in intermediary metabolism.

citridesmolase (sit-ri-des'mō-lās). *Citrate* lyase.

citrin (sit'rin). Vitamin P.

Citrobacter (sit'rō-bak-ter). A genus of motile bacteria (family Enterobacteriaceae) containing Gram-negative rods which utilize citrate as a sole source of carbon; the motile cells are peritrichous. Fermentation of lactose by these organisms is delayed or absent; they produce trimethylene glycol from glycerol. The type species is *C. freundii.*

C. amalona'tica, *Levinea amalonatica;* a species found in feces, soil, water, and sewage; isolated from clinical specimens as an opportunistic pathogen.

C. diver'sus, *C. koseri; Levinea malonatica;* a species found in feces, soil, water, sewage, and food; isolated from urine, throat, nose, sputum, and wounds; reported in cases of neonatal meningitis.

C. freun'dii *Escherichia freundii;* a species found in water, feces, and urine; it appears to be an inhabitant of the normal intestine, but it may occur in alimentary infections and in infections of the urinary tract, gallbladder, middle ear, and meninges; it is the type species of the genus *C.*

C. ko'seri, *C. diversus.*

citrogenase (si-troj'en-ās). *Citrate* synthase.

citronella (sit-rō-nel'ă). *Cymbopogon (Andropogon) nardus* (family Gramineae); a fragrant grass of Ceylon, from which is distilled a volatile oil (c. oil) used as a perfume and insect repellent.

citrulline (sit'rul-ēn). N^5-(Aminocarbonyl)-L-ornithine; α-amino-δ-ureidovaleric -ureidovaleric acid; 5-ureidonorvaline; an amino acid formed from ornithine in the course of the urea cycle; also found in watermelon (*Citrullus vulgaris*) and in casein.

citrullinemia (sit'rul-i-nē'mē-ă). A disease of amino acid metabolism (usually classed as a type of aminoaciduria) in which citrulline concentrations in blood, urine, and cerebrospinal fluid are elevated; manifested clinically by vomiting, ammonia intoxication, and mental retardation beginning in infancy; autosomal recessive inheritance.

citrullinuria (sit'rŭl-i-nū'rē-ă). Enhanced urinary excretion of citrulline; a manifestation of citrullinemia.

citta, cittosis (si'tă, si-tō'sis). Cissa.

Civatte, Achille, French dermatologist, 1877-1956. See C. *bodies, disease, poikiloderma.*

Civinini, Filippo, Italian anatomist, 1805–1844. See C.'s *canal, ligament, process.*

CK Abbreviation for *creatine* kinase.

Cl Symbol for chlorine.

cladiosis (klad-ē-ō'sis) [G. *klados,* branch or root, + *-osis,* condition]. A dermatophytosis resembling sporotrichosis, characterized by verrucous lesions and ascending lymphangitis; caused by *Scopulariopsis blochii.*

Clado, Spiro, French gynecologist, 1856–1905. See C.'s *anastomosis, band, ligament, point.*

Cladorchis watsoni (kla-dōr'kis wat-sō'nī). Incorrect term for *Watsonius watsoni.*

cladosporiosis (klad'ō-spō-rē-ō'sis). Infection with a fungus of the genus *Cladosporium.*

cerebral c., cerebral chromomycosis; a mycotic brain abscess due to *Cladosporium bantianum;* found especially in India.

Cladosporium (klad-ō-spōr'i-ŭm) [G. *klados,* a branch, + *sporos,* seed]. A genus of fungi having dematiaceous or dark-colored conidiophores with oval or round spores, commonly isolated in soil or plant residues.

C. bantia'num, a species that causes cerebral cladosporiosis.

C. carrion'ii, a species that is a cause of chromoblastomycosis in man.

C. wernec'kii, *Exophiala werneckii.*

clairvoyance (klār-voy'ans) [Fr.]. Perception of objective events (past, present, or future) not ordinarily discernible except by the senses; a type of extrasensory perception.

clamoxyquin hydrochloride (klam-ok'si-kwin). 5-Chloro-7-{[(3-diethylaminopropyl) amino]methyl}8-quinolinol dihydrochloride; an amebicide.

clamp (klamp). An instrument for compression of a structure. *Cf.* forceps.
Cope's c., a c. used in excision of colon and rectum.
Crafoord c., a c. used in heart and lung operations.
Crile's c., a rubber-covered c. for temporary stoppage of blood flow.
Fogarty c., a c. with rubber-shod blades having serrated surfaces, to provide an atraumatic grip on tissues.
Gant's c., a right-angled c. used in hemorrhoidectomy.
Gaskell's c., an instrument for crushing the atrioventricular bundle in experimental animals and thus producing heart block.
gingival c., a springlike metal piece encircling or grasping the cervix of a tooth and shaped so as to retract the gingival tissue.
Goldblatt's c., a c. applied experimentally to the renal artery to damp pulse pressure and thereby produce chronic hypertension by activation of the renin-angiotensin system.
Kelly c., a curved hemostat without teeth, introduced for gynecological surgery.
Kocher c., a heavy straight hemostat with interlocking teeth on the tip.
Mikulicz c., a c. used to crush walls between proximal and distal colon in two-stage colectomy.
mogen c. [Hebrew star], a circumcision instrument.
mosquito c., mosquito forceps; a small hemostat, straight or curved, with or without teeth; used to hold delicate tissue or for hemostasis.
Ochsner c., a straight hemostat with teeth.
Payr's c., a c. used in gastrectomy or enterectomy.
Potts' c., a fine-toothed, multiple-point, vascular fixation c. that imparts limited trauma to the vessel while securely holding it.
Rankin's c., a three-bladed c. used in resection of colon.
rubber dam c., a springlike metal piece encircling or grasping the cervix of a tooth and so shaped as to prevent a rubber dam from coming off the tooth.
Willett's c., Willett's *forceps.*

clamp connection. In fungi, a short hypha which bypasses a hyphal septum and is attached to the two cells adjacent to the septum; characteristic of some members of the class Basidiomycetes, especially certain mushrooms.

clapotage, clapotement (kla-pō-tahz', kla-pōt-mawn') [Fr.]. The splashing sound heard on succussion of a dilated stomach.

Clapton, Edward, British physician, 1830–1909. See C.'s *line.*

Clara, Max, Austrian anatomist, *1899. See C. *cell.*

clarificant (kla-rif'i-kant) [L. *clarus,* clear, + *facio,* to make]. An agent that makes a turbid liquid clear.

clarification (klar'i-fi-kā'shŭn). The process of making a turbid liquid clear.

Clark, A., 20th century U.S pharmacologist. See C.'s weight *rule.*

Clark, Eliot R., U.S. anatomist, 1881–1963, See Sandison-C. *chamber.*

Clark, Leland C., Jr., U.S. biochemist, *1918. See C. *electrode.*

Clark, Wallace H., Jr., U.S. dermatopathologist, *1924.

Clarke, Cecil. See C.-Hadfield *syndrome.*

Clarke, Sir Charles M., British physician, 1782–1857. See C.'s *ulcer.*

Clarke, Jacob A.L., British anatomist, 1817–1880. See C.'s *column, nucleus.*

clasmatocyte (klaz-mat'ō-sīt) [G. *klasma,* a fragment, + *kytos,* a hollow (cell)]. Macrophage.

clasmatosis (klaz-mă-tō'sis) [G. *klasma,* a fragment, + *-osis,* condition]. The extension of pseudopodia-like processes in unicellular organisms and blood cells by plasmolysis rather than by a true formation of pseudopodia.

clasp. 1. A part of a removable partial denture that acts as a direct retainer and/or stabilizer for the denture by partially surrounding or contacting an abutment tooth. **2.** A direct retainer of a removable partial denture, usually consisting of two arms joined by a body which connects with an occlusal rest; at least one arm of a clasp usually terminates in the infrabulge (gingival convergence) area of the tooth enclosed.
bar c., Roach c.; **(1)** a c. whose arms are bar-type extensions from major connectors or from within the denture base; the arms pass adjacent to the soft tissues and approach the point of contact on the tooth in a gingivo-occlusal direction; **(2)** a c. consisting of two or more separate arms located opposite to each other on the tooth; the bar arms arise from the framework or from a connector and may traverse the soft tissue; one arm (bar), the retentive arm, usually terminates in the infrabulge (gingival convergence) area of the tooth; the other, the reciprocal arm, usually terminates on the suprabulge (occlusal convergence) area.
circumferential c., **(1)** a c. that encircles more than 180° of a tooth, including opposite angles, and which usually contacts the tooth throughout the extent of the c., at least one terminal being in the infrabulge (gingival convergence) area; **(2)** a c. consisting of two circumferential c. arms, both of which originate from the same minor connector and are located on opposite surfaces of the abutment tooth.
continuous c., continuous bar *retainer.*
extended c., a c. that extends from its minor connector along the lingual and/or facial surface of two or more teeth.
Roach c., bar c.

class (klas) [L. *classis,* a class, division]. In biologic classification, the next division below the phylum (or subphylum) and above the order.

classification (klas'i-fi-kā'shŭn). A systematic arrangement into classes or groups.
adansonian c. [*Adanson,* Michel, French naturalist, 1727–1806], the c. of organisms based on giving equal weight to every character of the organism; this principle has its greatest application in numerical taxonomy.
Angle's c. of malocclusion, a c. of different types of malocclusion, based on the mesiodistal relationship of the permanent molars upon their eruption and locking, and comprised of three classes; *Class I:* normal relationship of the jaws, wherein the mesiobuccal cusp of the maxillary first molar occludes in the buccal groove of the mandibular first permanent molar; *Class II:* distal relationship of the mandible, wherein the distobuccal cusp of the maxillary first permanent molar occludes in the buccal groove of the mandibular first molar, and further classified as Division 1, labioversion of maxillary incisor teeth, and Division 2, linguoversion of maxillary central incisors, both of which may be unilateral conditions; *Class III:* mesial relationship of the mandible, wherein the mesiobuccal cusp of the maxillary first molar occludes in the embrasure between the mandibular first and second permanent molars, further classified as a unilateral condition.
Arneth c., a c. of the polymorphonuclear neutrophils according to the number of their nuclear lobes. See Arneth *stages.*
Black's c., a c. of cavities of the teeth based upon the tooth surface(s) involved.
Caldwell-Moloy c., a c. of the variations in the female pelvis; namely gynecoid, android, anthropoid, and platypelloid pelvis, based on the type of the posterior and anterior segments of the inlet.
Cummer's c., a listing of several types of removable partial dentures in accordance with the distribution of direct retainers.
Denver c., a system of nomenclature for human mitotic chromo-

somes, classifying them on the basis of length and position of the centromere.

Dukes c., a c. of the extent of operable adenocarcinoma of the colon or rectum commonly modified as follows: A (Dukes A), confined to the mucosa; B_1, into the muscularis mucosae; B_2, through the muscularis mucosae; C_1, limited to the bowel wall, with nodal metastases; C_2, through the bowel wall, with nodal metastases.

Galton's system of c. of fingerprints, see under fingerprint.

Jansky's c., the c. of the blood groups of the human race into I, II, III, and IV, now designated, respectively, as O, A, B, and AB.

Kennedy c., a listing of several forms of partially edentulous jaws in accordance with the distribution of the missing teeth.

Kiel c., Lennert c.; c. of non-Hodgkin's lymphoma into low-grade malignancy (lymphocytic, lymphoplasmacytoid, centrocytic, and centroblastic-centrocytic types) and high-grade malignancy (centroblastic, lymphoblastic of Burkitt's or convoluted cell, and immunoblastic types).

Lancefield c., a serologic c. dividing hemolytic streptococci into groups (A to O) which bear a definite relationship to their sources, based upon precipitation tests depending upon group-specific substances that are carbohydrate in nature; *e.g., Group A* contains strains pathogenic for man; *B,* strains from mastitis in cows and from normal milk, including a few strains from the human throat and vagina; *C,* strains from various lower animals, including a number from cattle; *D,* strains from cheese; *E,* strains from certified milk; *F,* strains mainly from the human throat, associated with tonsillitis; *G,* strains from man, a few from monkeys and dogs; and *H, K,* and *O,* nonpathogenic strains from normal human respiratory tracts.

Lennert c., Kiel c.

Lukes-Collins c., a c. of lymphomas according to the immunologic nature of the cell of origin, based on histologic and clinical data.

multiaxial c., a procedure used in DSM-III for diagnosing patients on five axes: 1) psychiatric syndrome present; 2) patient's history of personality and developmental disorders; 3) possible nonmental medical disorders; 4) severity of psychosocial stressors; 5) highest level of adaptive functioning in the past year.

Rappaport c., a histologic c. of lymphomas in use before the availability of recent methods for identification of B- and T-type lymphocytes.

Rye c. [*Rye,* NY, 1965], c. of Hodgkin's disease according to lymphocyte predominance, nodular sclerosing, mixed cellularity, and lymphocyte depletion types.

Salter-Harris c. of epiphysial fractures, the c. of epiphysial fractures into five groups (I to V), according to different prognoses regarding the effects of the injury on subsequent growth and subsequent deformity of the epiphysis.

clastic (klas'tik) [G. *klastos,* broken]. Breaking up into pieces, or exhibiting a tendency so to break or divide.

clastogen (klas'tō-jen) [G. *klastos,* broken, + *genos,* birth]. An agent (*e.g.,* certain chemicals, x-rays, ultraviolet light) capable of causing breakage of chromosomes.

clastogenic (klas-tō-jen'ik). Relating to the action of a clastogen.

clastothrix (klas'tō-thriks) [G. *klastos,* broken, + *thrix,* hair]. *Trichorrhexis* nodosa.

clathrate (klath'rāt) [L. *clathrare,* pp. *-atus,* to furnish with a lattice]. A type of inclusion compound in which small molecules are trapped in the cage-like lattice of macromolecules.

clathrin (klath'rin) [L. *clathri,* lattice]. The principal constituent of a polyhedral protein lattice that coats eukaryotic cell membranes (vesicles) and appears to be involved in protein secretion.

Clauberg, Karl W., German bacteriologist, *1893. See C. *test, unit.*

Claude, Henri, French psychiatrist, 1869–1945. See C.'s *syndrome.*

claudication (klaw-di-kā'shŭn) [L. *claudicatio,* fr. *claudico,* to limp]. Limping, usually referring to intermittent c.

cerebral c., intermittent cerebral symptoms due to insufficient blood supply to the brain related to narrowing of the arteries.

intermittent c., Charcot's syndrome; myasthenia angiosclerotica; a condition caused by ischemia of the muscles due to sclerosis with narrowing of the arteries; characterized by attacks of lameness and pain, brought on by walking, chiefly in the calf muscles; however, the condition may occur in other muscle groups.

claudicatory (klaw'di-kă-tōr-ē). Relating to claudication, especially intermittent claudication.

Claudius, Friedrich M., German anatomist, 1822–1869. See C.'s *cells, fossa.*

Clausen. See Dyggve-Melchior-C. *syndrome.*

claustra (klaws'tră). Plural of claustrum.

claustral (klaws'trăl). Relating to the claustrum.

claustrophobia (klaw-strō-fō'bē-ă) [L. *claustrum,* an enclosed space, + G. *phobos,* fear]. A morbid fear of being in a confined place.

claustrophobic (klaw-strō-fō'bik). Relating to or suffering from claustrophobia.

claustrum, pl. **claustra** (klaws'trŭm, klaws'tră) [L. barrier]. **1.** One of several anatomical structures bearing a resemblance to a barrier. **2** [NA]. A thin, vertically placed lamina of gray matter lying close to the outer portion (putamen) of the lenticular nucleus, from which it is separated by the external capsule. C. consists of two parts: 1) an insular part and 2) a temporal part between putamen and the temporal lobe. Cells of the c. have reciprocal connections with sensory areas of the cerebral cortex.

c. gut'turis, c. o'ris, *palatum* molle.

c. virgina'le, a rare term for hymen.

clausura (klaw-sū'ră) [L. a lock, bolt, fr. *claudo,* to close]. Atresia.

clava (klā'vă) [L. a club]. *Tuberculum* nuclei gracilis.

claval (klā'văl). Relating to the clava.

clavate (klā'vāt) [L. *clava,* a club]. Club-shaped.

clavi (klā'vi). Plural of clavus.

Claviceps purpurea (klav'i-seps pŭr-pū'rē-ă) [L. *clava,* club, + *caput,* head]. See ergot.

clavicle (klav'i-kl). Clavicula.

clavicotomy (klav-i-kot'ō-mē) [clavicle + G. *tomē,* incision]. Surgical division of the clavicle.

clavicula, pl. **clavic'ulae** (klă-vik'yū-lă) [L. *clavicula,* a small key, fr. *clavis,* key] [NA]. Clavicle; collar bone; a doubly curved long bone that forms part of the shoulder girdle. Its medial end articulates with the manubrium sterni, its lateral end with the acromion of the scapula.

clavicular (kla-vik'yū-lăr). Relating to the clavicle.

claviculus, pl. **claviculi** (kla-vik'yū-lŭs, -lī) [Mod. L. dim. of L. *clavus,* a nail]. One of the perforating collagen fibers of bone.

clavulanic acid (klav-yū-lan'ik). 3-(2-Hydroxyethylidene)-7-oxo-4-oxa-1-azabicyclo[3.2.0]heptane-2-carboxylic acid; a beta-lactam antibiotic structurally related to the penicillins that inactivate β-lactamase enzymes in penicillin-resistant organisms; usually used in combination with penicillins to enhance and broaden the spectrum of the penicillins.

clavus, pl. **clavi** (klā'vŭs, -vī) [L. a nail, wart, corn]. **1.** Corn (1); heloma; a small conical callosity caused by pressure over a bony prominence, usually on a toe. **2.** A condition resulting from healing of a granuloma of the foot in yaws, in which a core falls out, leaving an erosion.

claw (klaw) [L. *clavus,* a nail]. A sharp, slender, usually curved nail on the paw of an animal.

dew c., a rudimentary digit, not reaching the ground, on the feet

of many quadrupeds.
griffin c., clawhand.

clawfoot (klaw'fut). A condition of the foot characterized by hyperextension at the metatarsophalangeal joint and flexion at the interphalangeal joints, as a fixed contracture.

clawhand (klaw'hand). Griffin claw; main en griffe; atrophy of the interosseous muscles of the hand with hyperextension of the metacarpophalangeal joints and flexion of the interphalangeal joints.

Claybrook, Edwin B., U.S. surgeon, 1871–1931. See C.'s *sign.*

cleaning (klēn'ing). In dentistry, a procedure whereby accretions are removed from the teeth or from a dental prosthesis. See also dental *prophylaxis.*
ultrasonic c., in dentistry, the use of a high-frequency vibrating point to remove deposits from tooth structure; also the process of cleaning dentures by placing them in a special liquid in a container that generates high-frequency vibrations.

clearance (klēr'ans). **1** (C with a subscript indicating the substance removed). Removal of a substance from the blood, *e.g.,* by renal excretion, expressed in terms of the volume flow of arterial blood or plasma that would contain the amount of substance removed per unit time; measured in ml/min. Renal c. of any substance except urea or free water is calculated as the urine flow in ml/min multiplied by the urinary concentration of the substance divided by the arterial plasma concentration of the substance; normal human values are commonly expressed per 1.73 m^2 body surface area. **2.** A condition in which bodies may pass each other without hindrance, or the distance between bodies. **3.** Removal of something from some place; *e.g.,* "esophageal acid c." refers to removal from the esophagus of some acid that has refluxed into it from the stomach, evaluated by the time taken for restoration of a normal pH in the esophagus.
p- **aminohippurate c.,** a good measure of renal plasma flow, which it slightly underestimates; when a low plasma concentration of *p*-aminohippurate (PAH) is maintained by intravenous infusion, the kidney extracts and excretes almost all of the PAH from the plasma before it reaches the renal vein.
creatinine c., an accurate measure of glomerular filtration rate (GFR) in the dog; creatinine c. may overestimate GFR in man because of slight tubular secretion of creatinine.
endogenous creatinine c., a term distinguishing measurements based on the creatinine normally present in plasma; since no infusion is necessary, an average value may be obtained by collecting urine for a long period, *e.g.,* 24 hours.
exogenous creatinine c., a term distinguishing measurements based on infusing creatinine intravenously to raise its plasma concentration and facilitate its accurate chemical determination.
free water c., the amount of water excreted in the urine beyond that which would accompany the excreted solutes if the urine were isosmotic with plasma; it represents the loss of body water in excess of solute tending to raise body osmolality and making urine hyposmotic. Unlike other c.'s, it is calculated by subtracting the osmolal c. from the actual volume of urine excreted per minute. A negative value for free water c. represents the amount of water that the body has reclaimed from isosmotic tubule fluid to make the urine hyperosmotic and to lower body osmolality.
interocclusal c., freeway *space.*
inulin c., an accurate measure of the rate of filtration through the renal glomeruli, because inulin filters freely with water and is neither excreted nor reabsorbed through tubule walls. Inulin is not a normal constituent of plasma and must be infused continously to maintain a steady plasma concentration and a steady rate of urinary excretion during the measurement. Inulin c. in a normal adult person is about 120 ml/min (range 100–150) per 1.73 m^2 body surface area.
isotope c., the rate at which an isotope is removed (usually by blood flow) from a tissue or organ such as the brain.
maximum urea c., the urea c. when the urine flow exceeds 2 ml/min; normal value is about 75 ml blood/min per 1.73 m^2 body surface area.
occlusal c., a condition in which the opposing occlusal surfaces may glide over one another without any interfering projection.
osmolal c., the volume of urine that would be excreted per minute if the urinary solutes were accompanied by just enough water to make the urine isosmotic with plasma, *i.e.,* so that the solute excretion did not change the osmolality of body fluids. To calculate it, the volume of urine excreted per minute is multiplied by the urinary osmolality (usually measured by freezing point depression) and divided by the plasma osmolality. Osmolal c. is less than actual urine flow when urine is hyposmotic and exceeds it when urine is hyperosmotic.
standard urea c., Van Slyke's formula; the value obtained when the square root of the urine flow (when below 2 ml/min) is multiplied by the urine urea concentration and divided by the whole blood urea concentration; represents an old empirical adjustment for the effect of low urine flow on urea excretion; sometimes corrected for body size by dividing by some function of body weight or surface area. Later, plasma concentration was substituted for blood concentration in the calculation. The normal value is about 54 ml/min per 1.73 m^2 in an adult person.
urea c., the volume of plasma (or blood) that would be completely cleared of urea by one minute's excretion of urine; originally calculated as urine flow multiplied by urine urea concentration divided by concentration of urea in whole blood rather than plasma, representing blood urea c. rather than plasma urea c.

clearer (klēr'er). An agent, used in histological preparations, which is miscible in both the dehydrating or fixing fluid and the embedding substance.

cleavage (klēv'ij). **1.** Segmentation (2); series of cell divisions occurring in the ovum immediately following its fertilization. See also cleavage *division.* **2.** Scission (2); splitting of a complex molecule into two or more simpler molecules. **3.** Linear clefts in the skin indicating the direction of the fibers in the dermis. See also cleavage *lines.*

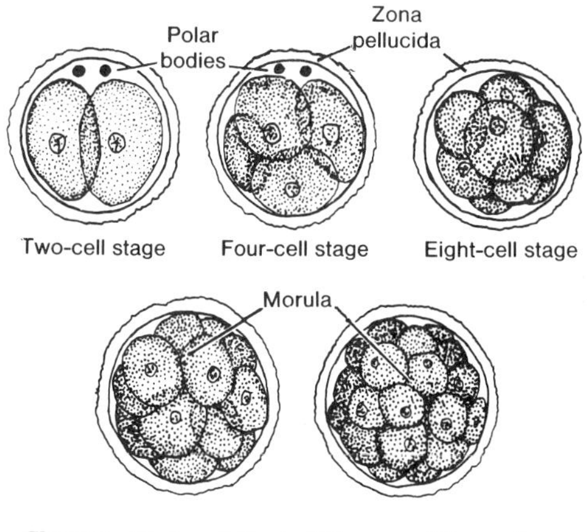

Cleavage (Segmentation) of Ovum and Formation of Morula

abnormal c. of cardiac valve, congenital malformation of a valve leaflet with a defect extending from the free margin.
adequal c., c. resulting in the formation of blastomeres of approximately equal size.
complete c., holoblastic c.
determinate c., c. resulting in blastomeres each capable of developing into a particular embryonic structure.
discoidal c., meroblastic c. limited to the small cap of protoplasm

of large-yolked eggs, such as the telolecithal eggs of birds.
enamel c., the splitting of enamel in a plane parallel to the direction of the enamel rods.
equal c., c. producing blastomeres of like size.
equatorial c., c. in which the plane of cytoplasmic division is at right angles to the axis of the ovum.
holoblastic c., complete c.; c. in which the blastomeres are completely separated.
hydrolytic c., hydrolysis.
incomplete c., meroblastic c.
indeterminate c., c. resulting in blastomeres of similar developmental potencies, each capable, when isolated, of producing an entire embryonic body.
meridional c., c. in a plane through the axis of the zygote.
meroblastic c., incomplete c.; incomplete separation of the blastomeres, with the divisions being limited to the nonyolked portion of the egg.
phosphoroclastic c., phosphorolysis.
progressive c., in fungi, a type of sporulation in which c. planes in the cytoplasm first produce protospores and then sporangiospores in a sporangium.
pudendal c., *rima* pudendi.
superficial c., meroblastic c. with the divisions limited to the peripheral cytoplasm of a centrolecithal egg.
thioclastic c., the splitting of a bond in fashion analogous to hydrolysis or phosphorolysis except that the elements of a substituted hydrogen sulfide (usually coenzyme A) are added across the break.
unequal c., c. producing blastomeres of different sizes.
yolk c., segmentation of the vitellus.

cleaver (klē'ver). A heavy knife for cutting or chopping.
enamel c., an instrument with a heavy shank and a very short blade at about 90° to the axis of the handle; used with a hoeing motion to strip enamel from the axial surfaces of a tooth in preparation for a crown.

Cleemann, Richard Alsop, U.S. physician, 1840–1912. See C.'s *sign.*

cleft (kleft). A fissure.
anal c., *crena* ani.
branchial c.'s, gill c.'s; a bilateral series of slitlike openings into the pharynx through which water is drawn by aquatic animals; in the walls of the c.'s are the vascular gill filaments that take up oxygen from the water passing through the c.'s; sometimes loosely applied to the branchial ectodermal grooves of mammalian embryos which are their imperforate, rudimentary homologues.
cholesterol c., a space caused by the dissolving out of cholesterol crystals in sections of tissue embedded in paraffin.
facial c., prosopoanoschisis; a c. resulting from incomplete merging or fusion of embryonic processes normally uniting in the formation of the face, *e.g.,* c. lip, or cleft palate.
first visceral c., hyomandibular c.
gill c.'s, branchial c.'s.
gingival c., a fissure associated with pocket formation and lined by mixed gingival and pocket epithelium.
gluteal c., *crena* ani.
hyobranchial c., the c. caudal to the hyoid arch of the embryo.
hyomandibular c., first visceral c.; the c. between the hyoid and mandibular arches of the embryo; the external auditory meatus is developed from its dorsal portion.
interneuromeric c.'s, c.'s between the neuromeric or segmental elevations in the primitive rhombencephalon.
Larrey's c., *trigonum* sternocostale.
Maurer's c.'s, Maurer's *dots.*
natal c., *crena* ani.
oblique facial c., prosoposchisis.
residual c., residual lumen; the remnants of the pituitary diverticulum which occurs between the pars distalis and pars intermedia; a distinct lumen is present in some animals, but, in man, is present only during prenatal development and sometimes in young children.
Schmidt-Lanterman c.'s, Schmidt-Lanterman *incisures.*
synaptic c., the space about 20 nm wide between the axolemma and the postsynaptic surface. See also synapse.
urogenital c., *rima* pudendi.
visceral c., any c. between two branchial (visceral) arches in the embryo.

cleid-. See cleido-.

cleidagra, clidagra (klī-dag'ră) [cleid- + G. *agra,* seizure]. Rarely used term for a sudden severe pain in the clavicle, resembling gout.

cleidal (klī'dăl). Clidal; relating to the clavicle.

cleido-, cleid- [G. *kleis,* clavicle]. Combining forms relating to the clavicle; also spelled clido-, clid-.

cleidocostal (klī-dō-kos'tăl) [cleido- + L. *costa,* rib]. Clidocostal; relating to the clavicle and a rib.

cleidocranial (klī'dō-krā'nē-ăl) [G. *kleis,* clavicle, + *kranion,* cranium]. Clidocranial; relating to the clavicle and the cranium.

-cleisis [G. *kleisis,* a closing]. Suffix meaning closure.

cleistothecium (klīs-tō-thē'sē-ŭm) [G. *kleistos,* enclosed, + *thēkē,* box]. In fungi, an ascocarp that is closed, with randomly dispersed asci.

Cleland, W. Wallace. See C.'s *reagent.*

clemastine (klem'as-tēn). Meclastine; D-2-[2-[(*p*-chloro-α-methyl-α-phenylbenzyl)oxy]ethyl]-1-methylpyrrolidine; an antihistaminic.

clemizole (klem'i-zōl). 1-Chlorobenzyl-2-(1-pyrrolidinylmethyl)-benzimidazole; an antihistaminic.

cleoid (klē'oyd) [A. S. *cle,* claw + G. *eidos,* resemblance]. A dental instrument with a pointed elliptical cutting end, used in excavating cavities or carving fillings and waxes.

cleptoparasite (klep-tō-par'ă-sīt) [G. *kleptō,* to steal, + parasite]. A parasite that develops on the prey of the parasite's host.

Cléret, M., French physician. See Launois-C. *syndrome.*

Clevenger, Shobal V., U.S. neurologist, 1843–1920. See C.'s *fissure.*

click (klik). A slight sharp sound.
ejection c., a clicking ejection sound. See under sound.
mitral c., the opening snap of the mitral valve.
systolic c., a sharp, clicking sound heard during cardiac systole; when heard in early systole it is usually an ejection sound; in late systole the c. usually signifies mitral insufficiency, as in the dysfunction of the mitral valvular apparatus when it prolapses into the left atrium during systole (see Barlow syndrome); may also be due to pleuropericardial adhesions or other extracardiac mechanisms.

clicking (klik'ing). A snapping, crepitant noise noted on excursions of the temporomandibular articulation, due to an asynchronous movement of the disk and condyle.

clid-. See clido-.

clidagra (klī-dag'ră). Cleidagra.

clidal (klī'dăl). Cleidal.

clidinium bromide (klī-din'ē-ŭm). 3-Hydroxy-1-methylquinuclidinium bromide benzilate; an anticholinergic.

clido-, clid- [G. *kleis,* clavicle]. Combining forms relating to the clavicle. See also cleido-.

clidocostal (klī-dō-kos'tăl). Cleidocostal.

clidocranial (klī-dō-krā'nē-ăl). Cleidocranial.

clidoic (klī-dō'ik). Cleidoic.

climacophobia (klī'mă-kō-fō'bē-ă) [G. *klimax,* ladder, + *phobos,* fear]. Morbid fear of stairs or of climbing.

climacteric (klī-mak'ter-ik, klī-mak-ter'ik) [G. *klimaktēr,* the rung of a ladder]. **1.** Climacterium; the period of endocrinal, somatic, and transitory psychologic changes occurring in the transition to menopause. **2.** A critical period of life.

grand c., the sixty-third year; the ninth of the seven-year periods, each of which from the third (twenty-first year) was formerly regarded as a critical time of life.

climacterium (klī-mak-tēr'ē-ŭm). Climacteric.

climatology (klī-mă-tol'ō-jē). The study of climate and its relation to disease.

climatotherapy (klī'mă-tō-thār'ă-pē). Treatment of disease by removal of the patient to a region having a climate more favorable for recovery.

climax (klī'maks) [G. *klimax,* staircase]. **1.** The height or acme of a disease; its stage of greatest severity. **2.** Orgasm.

climograph (klī'mō-graf) [G. *klima,* climate, + *graphō,* to record]. A diagram showing the effect of climate on health.

clindamycin (klin-dă-mī'sin). 7(*S*)-Chloro-7-deoxylincomycin; an antibacterial and antibiotic.

cline (klīn) [G. *klinein,* to slope]. A systematic relation between spatial distances and the frequencies of alleles; lines connecting points of equal frequency are termed isoclines, and the direction of the c. at any point is at right angles to an isocline.

clinic (klin'ik) [G. *klinē,* bed]. **1.** An institution, building, or part of a building where ambulatory patients are cared for. **2.** An institution, building, or part of a building in which medical instruction is given to students by means of demonstrations in the presence of the sick. **3.** A lecture or symposium on a subject relating to disease.

clinical (klin'i-kl). **1.** Relating to the bedside of a patient or to the course of his disease. **2.** Denoting the symptoms and course of a disease, as distinguished from the laboratory findings of anatomical changes. **3.** Relating to a clinic.

clinician (klin-ish'ŭn). A health professional engaged in the care of patients, as distinguished from one working in other areas.

clinicopathologic (klin'i-kō-path-ō-loj'ik). Pertaining to the signs and symptoms manifested by a patient, and also the results of laboratory studies, as they relate to the findings in the gross and histologic examination of tissue by means of biopsy or autopsy, or both.

clino- [G. *klinō,* to slope, incline, or bend]. Combining form denoting a slope (inclination or declination) or bend.

clinocephalic, clinocephalous (klī-nō-se-fal'ik, -sef'ă-lŭs). Relating to clinocephaly.

clinocephaly (klī'nō-sef'ă-lē) [clino- + G. *kephalē,* head]. Saddle head; craniosynostosis in which the upper surface of the skull is concave, presenting a saddle-shaped appearance in profile.

clinodactyly (klī'nō-dak'ti-lē) [clino- + G. *daktylos,* finger]. Permanent deflection of one or more fingers.

clinography (klin-og'ră-fē) [G. *klinē,* bed, + *graphō,* to write]. Graphic representation of the signs and symptoms exhibited by a patient.

clinoid (klī'noyd) [G. *klinē,* bed, + *eidos,* resemblance]. **1.** Resembling a bed. **2.** *Processus* clinoideus.

clinoscope (klī'nō-skōp) [clino- + G. *skopeō,* to view]. An instrument for measuring cyclophoria.

exogenous creatinine c., a term distinguishing measurements based on infusing creatinine intravenously to raise its plasma concentration and facilitate its accurate chemical determination.

clioquinol (klī-ō-kwin'ol). Iodochlorhydroxyquin.

clioxanide (klī-ok'să-nīd). 4'-Chloro-3,5-diiodosalicylanilide acetate; an anthelmintic.

clip (klip'). A fastener used to hold a part or thing together with another.

wound c. a metal clasp or device for surgical approximation of skin incisions.

clithrophobia (klīth-rō-fō'bē-ă) [G. *kleithron,* a bolt, + *phobos,* fear]. Morbid fear of being locked in.

clition (klit'ē-on) [G. *klitos,* a declivity]. A craniometric point in the middle of the highest part of the clivus on the sphenoid bone.

clitoridean (klit'ō-ri-dē'an). Relating to the clitoris.

clitoridectomy (klit'ō-ri-dek'tō-mē) [clitoris + G. *ektomē,* excision]. Removal of the clitoris.

clitoriditis (klit'ō-ri-dī'tis) [clitoris + G. *-itis,* inflammation]. Clitoritis; inflammation of the clitoris.

clitoris, pl. **clitorides** (klit'ō-ris, klī'tō-ris, -tōr'i-dēz) [G. *kleitoris*] [NA]. Membrum muliebre; penis femineus; penis muliebris; a cylindric, erectile body, rarely exceeding 2 cm in length, situated at the most anterior portion of the vulva and projecting between the branched extremities of the labia minora, which form its prepuce and frenulum. It consists of a glans, a corpus, and two crura, and is the homologue of the penis in the male, except that it is not perforated by the urethra and does not possess a corpus spongiosum.

clitorism (klit'ō-rizm). Prolonged and usually painful erection of the clitoris; the analogue of priapism.

clitoritis (klit-ō-rī'tis). Clitoriditis.

clitoromegaly (klit'ōr-ō-meg'ă-lē) [clitoris + G. *megas,* great]. An enlarged clitoris.

clival (klī'văl). Pertaining to the clivus.

clivus, pl. **clivi** (klī'vŭs, -vē) [L. slope] [NA]. **1.** A downward sloping surface. **2.** Blumenbach's c.; the sloping surface from the dorsum sellae to the foramen magnum composed of part of the body of the sphenoid and part of the pars basilaris of the occipital bone.

Blumenbach's c., clivus (2).

c. ocula'ris, the sloping walls of the fovea leading to the foveola.

cloaca (klō-ā'kă) [L. sewer]. **1.** In early embryos, the endodermally lined chamber into which the hindgut and allantois empty. **2.** In birds and monotremes, the common chamber into which open the hindgut, bladder, and genital ducts.

ectodermal c., the proctodeum of the embryo.

endodermal c., terminal portion of the hindgut internal to the cloacal membrane of the embryo.

persistent c., sinus urogenitalis (2); a condition in which the urorectal fold has failed to divide the c. of the embryo into rectal and urogenital portions.

cloacal (klō-ā'kăl). Pertaining to the cloaca.

cloacitis (klō-ă-sī'tis). An inflammation of the cloacal mucosa of fowls, with ulceration and chronic discharge.

clobetasol propionate (klō-bā'tă-sōl). Pregna-1,4-diene-3,20-dione, 21-chloro-9-fluoro-11-hydroxy-16-methyl-17-(1-oxopropoxy)-, (11β,16β)-; an anti-inflammatory corticosteroid usually used in topical preparations.

clocortolone (klō-kōr'tō-lōn). 9-Chloro-6α-fluoro-11β,21-dihydroxy-16α-methylpregna-1,4-diene-3,20-dione; an anti-inflammatory corticosteroid usually used in topical preparations; available as the acetate and the pivalate.

clofazimine (klō-faz'ĭ-mēn). 3-(*p*-Chloroanilino)-10-(*p*-chlorophenyl)-2,10-dihydro-2-(isopropylimino)phenazine; a tuberculostatic and leprostatic agent.

clofenamide (klō-fen'ă-mid). Monochlorphenamide; 4-chloro-*m*-benzenedisulfonamide; a diuretic.

clofibrate (klō'fi-brāt). Ethyl chlorophenoxyisobutyrate; an antilipemic agent that reduces plasma levels of cholesterol, triglycerides, and uric acid; used in the treatment of hypercholesterolemia and atherosclerosis.

clogestone acetate (klō-jes'tōn). 6-Chloro-3β,17-dihydroxypregna-4,6-dien-20-one diacetate; a progestational agent.

clomacran phosphate (klō'mă-kran). 2-Chloro-9-[3-(dimethylamino)propyl]acridan phosphate; a tranquilizer.

clomegestone acetate (klō-me-jes'tōn). 6-Chloro-17-hydroxy-16α-methylpregna-4,6-diene-3,20-dione acetate; a progestational drug.

clomiphene citrate (klō'mi-fēn). Chloramiphene; 2-[*p*-(2-chloro-1,2-diphenylvinyl)phenoxy]triethylamine dihydrogen citrate; an analogue of the nonsteroid estrogen, chlorotrianisene; a pituitary gonadotropin stimulant used therapeutically to induce ovulation; it competes with estrogen at the hypothalamic level, interrupting the negative feedback system and resulting in increased gonadotropin secretion.

clomipramine hydrochloride (klō-mip'ră-mēn). Chlorimipramine hydrochloride; 3-chloro-5-[3-(dimethylamino)propyl]-10,11-dihydro-5*H*- dibenz[*b,f*]azepine monohydrochloride; an antidepressant.

clonal (klō'năl). Pertaining to a clone.

clonazepam (klō-nā'zē-pam). 5-(*o*-Chlorophenyl)-1,3-dihydro-7-nitro-2*H*-1,4-benzodiazepin-2-one; an anticonvulsant drug.

clone (klōn) [G. *klōn*, slip, cutting used for propagation]. **1.** A colony or group of organisms (or an individual organism), or a colony of cells derived from a single organism or cell by asexual reproduction, all having identical genetic constitution. **2.** To produce such a colony or individual.

clonic (klon'ik). Relating to or characterized by clonus; marked by alternate contraction and relaxation of muscle.

clonicity (klon-is'i-tē). The state of being clonic.

clonicotonic (klon'i-kō-ton'ik). Both clonic and tonic; said of certain forms of muscular spasm.

clonidine hydrochloride (klō'ni-dēn). 2-(2,6-Dichloroanilino)-2-imidazoline hydrochloride; an antihypertensive agent with central and peripheral actions.

cloning (klōn'ing). Transplantation of a nucleus from a somatic cell to an ovum, which then develops into an embryo; many identical embryos can thus be reproduced by asexual reproduction.

clonism (klon'izm). A long continued state of clonic spasms.

clonixin (klō-niks'in). 2-(3-Chloro-*o*- toluidino)nicotinic acid; an analgesic.

clonogenic (klō-nō-jen'ik). Arising from or consisting of a clone.

clonograph (klon'ō-graf) [G. *klonos*, tumult, + *graphō*, to write]. An instrument for registering the movements in clonic spasm.

clonorchiasis (klō-nōr-kī'ă-sis). Clonorchiosis; a disease caused by *Clonorchis sinensis*, affecting the distal bile ducts of man and other fish-eating animals after ingestion of raw, smoked, or undercooked fish or raw crayfish; initial infection may be benign, but repeated or chronic infection induces an intense proliferative and granulomatous condition.

clonorchiosis (klō-nōr-kē-ō'sis). Chlonorchiasis.

Clonorchis sinensis (klō-nōr'kis sī-nen'sis). *Opisthorchis sinensis;* the Oriental Chinese liver fluke, a species of trematodes (family Opisthorchiidae) which in the Far East infects the bile passages of man and other fish-eating animals; cyprinoid fish serve as chief second intermediate hosts and various operculate snails serve as the first intermediate hosts.

clonospasm (klon'ō-spazm). Clonus.

clonus (klō'nŭs) [G. *klonos*, a tumult]. Clonospasm; a form of movement marked by contractions and relaxations of a muscle, occurring in rapid succession. See also contraction.
ankle c., a rhythmical contraction of the calf muscles following a sudden passive dorsal flexion of the foot, the leg being semiflexed.
cathodal opening c. (COCl, CaOCl), obsolete term for a c. produced near a cathode when the flow of current is stopped.
toe c., toe reflex (2); alternating movements of flexion and extension of the great toe following forcible extension at the metatarsophalangeal joint.
wrist c., rhythmical contractions and relaxations of the muscles of the forearm excited by a forcible passive extension of the hand.

clopamide (klō-pam'īd). 1-(4-Chloro-3-sulfamoylbenzamido)-2,6-dimethylpiperidine; a diuretic and antihypertensive agent.

Cloquet, Hippolyte, French anatomist, 1787–1840. See C.'s *space.*

Cloquet, Jules G., French anatomist, 1790–1883. See C.'s *canal, hernia, septum; node* of C.

clorazepate (klōr-az'ĕ-pāt). 7-Chloro-2,3-dihydro-2-oxo-5-phenyl-1*H*-1,4-benzodiazepine-3-carboxylate; the mono- or dipotassium salt is used as an anti-anxiety agent.

clorprenaline hydrochloride (klōr-pren'ă-lēn). Isoprophenamine hydrochloride; *o*-chloro-α-(isopropylaminomethyl)benzyl alcohol hydrochloride; a bronchodilator.

closiramine aceturate (klō-sir'ă-mēn). 8-Chloro-11-[2-(dimethylamino)ethyl]-6,11-dihydro-5*H*-benzo[5,6]cyclohepta[1,2-*b*] pyridine compound with *N*-acetylglycine; an antihistaminic.

clostridia (klos-trid'ē-ă). Plural of clostridium.

clostridial (klos-trid'ē-ăl). Relating to any bacterium of the genus *Clostridium.*

clostridiopeptidase A (klos-trid'ē-ō-pep'ti-dās). *Clostridium histolyticum* collagenase.

clostridiopeptidase B. Clostripain.

CLOSTRIDIUM

Clostridium (klos-trid'ē-ŭm) [G. *klōstēr*, a spindle]. A genus of anaerobic (or anaerobic, aerotolerant), sporeforming, motile (occasionally nonmotile) bacteria (family Bacillaceae) containing Gram-positive rods; motile cells are peritrichous. Many of the species are saccharolytic and fermentative, producing various acids and gases and variable amounts of neutral products; other species are proteolytic, some attacking proteins with putrefaction or more complete proteolysis. Some species fix free nitrogen. Exotoxins are sometimes produced by these organisms. They may cause disease in man and other animals. They are generally found in soil and in the intestinal tract of man and other animals. The type species is *C. butyricum.*

C. aerofoeti'dum, a species found in a case of gaseous gangrene and in feces.

C. bifermen'tans, a species found in putrid meat and gaseous gangrene; also commonly found in soil, feces, and sewage. Its pathogenicity varies from strain to strain.

C. botuli'num, a species which occurs widely in nature and which is a frequent cause of food poisoning (botulism) from preserved meats, fruits, or vegetables which have not been properly sterilized before canning. Including *C. parabotulinum* strains, there are six main types, A to F, characterized by antigenically distinct but pharmacologically similar, very potent neurotoxins, each of which can be neutralized only by the specific antitoxin; group C toxin contains at least two components; the recorded cases of human botulism have been due mainly to types A, B, E, and F; type Cα causes botulism in domestic and wild water fowl; Cβ and D are associated with intoxications in cattle.

C. butyr'icum, a species which occurs in naturally soured milk, in naturally fermented starchy plant substances, and in soil; it is not pathogenic. It is the type species of the genus *C.*

C. cadav'eris, a species found in a human cadaver and in the peritoneum of a rabbit; it is not pathogenic for guinea pigs or rabbits.

C. capitova'le, a species found in the pleural fluid of a sheep dead of gas gangrene, in cases of septicemia in humans, and in the feces of normal infants.
C. car'nis, a species found in a rabbit inoculated with soil; it is pathogenic for laboratory animals, in which an exotoxin produces edema, necrosis, and death.
C. chauvoe'i, *C. feseri;* a species which causes blackleg, black quarter, or symptomatic anthrax in cattle and other animals and which produces an exotoxin.
c. chromog'enes, a species found in pus from a perinephritic abscess in a human; weakly pathogenic for laboratory animals.
C. cochlear'ium, a species found in human war wounds and septic infections; it is not pathogenic for guinea pigs.
C. difficile (di-fi-sēl') [Fr. difficult], a species found in the feces of newborn infants; pathogenic for guinea pigs and rabbits.
C. fal'lax, a species found in war wounds, appendicitis, and black leg of sheep; it produces a weak exotoxin.
C. fese'ri, *C. chauvoei.*
C. gummo'sum, a species found in gaseous gangrene and in normal human (adult and infant) feces.
C. haemoly'ticum, a species found in cattle dying of icterohemoglobinuria; it is pathogenic and toxic for guinea pigs and rabbits and produces an unstable, hemolytic toxin.
C. histoly'ticum, a species found in war wounds, where it induces necrosis of tissue; it produces a cytolytic exotoxin which causes local necrosis and sloughing on injection; it is not toxic on feeding; it is pathogenic for small laboratory animals.
C. innomina'tum, a species found in septic and gangrenous war wounds.
C. microspo'rum, a species found in the abdominal contents of a fatal case of peritonitis.
C. multifermen'tans, a species found in a human muscle infected with gas gangrene; also found in fermented olives and spoiled chocolate candy.
C. nigri'ficans, a species found in canned corn showing "sulfur stinker spoilage." It is not pathogenic.
C. no'vyi, *C. oedematiens;* a species consisting of three types, A, B, and C; type A, from a case of gaseous gangrene and from human necrotic hepatitis, produces γ-toxin (a hemolytic lecithinase); B, from black disease (infectious necrotic hepatitis) of sheep, produces β-toxin (a hemolytic lecithinase); and C, found in bacillary osteomyelitis of water buffaloes, does not produce toxin.
C. oedema'tiens, *C. novyi.*
C. parabotuli'num, a species containing organisms formerly referred to as *C. botulinum* types A and B; the types are identified by protection tests with known type antitoxin; it produces a powerful exotoxin and is pathogenic for man and other animals.
C. paraputri'ficum, a species found in feces, especially those of infants, gaseous gangrene, and postmortem fluid and tissue cultures; it is not pathogenic for rabbits or guinea pigs.
C. perfrin'gens, *C. welchii;* gas bacillus; Welch's bacillus; a species which is the chief causative agent of gas gangrene in man and a cause of gas gangrene in other animals, especially sheep; it may also be involved in causing enteritis, appendicitis, food poisoning, and puerperal fever; this organism is found in soil, water, milk, dust, sewage, and the intestinal tract of man and other animals.
C. ramo'sum, *Ramibacterium ramosum;* a species found in the natural cavities of man and other animals as well as in sea water; it is also found in association with mastoiditis, otitis, pulmonary gangrene, putrid pleurisy, appendicitis, intestinal infections, balanitis, liver abscess, osteomyelitis, septicemia, and urinary infections, as well as in the vagina and in feces. It was formerly the type species of the obsolete genus *Ramibacterium.*
C. sep'ticum, Ghon-Sachs or Sachs' bacillus; vibrion septique; a species found in malignant edema of animals, in human war wounds, and in cases of appendicitis; it is pathogenic for guinea pigs, rabbits, mice, and pigeons and produces an exotoxin that is lethal and hemolytic.
C. sphenoi'des, a species found in gangrenous war wounds; it is not pathogenic for guinea pigs or rabbits.
C. sporo'genes, a species found in intestinal contents, gaseous gangrene, and soil; it is not pathogenic for guinea pigs or rabbits, but does produce a slight, temporary, local tumefaction.
C. ta'le, a species found in a case of acute appendicitis and in canned fish; pathogenicity for laboratory animals is variable.
C. ter'tium, a species found in wounds, but that is nonpathogenic for laboratory animals.
C. tet'ani, a species that causes tetanus; it produces a potent exotoxin (neurotoxin) that is intensely toxic for man and other animals when formed in tissues or injected, but not when ingested.
C. tetanoi'des, a species found in war wounds, postmortem blood cultures, and garden soil.
C. tetanomor'phum, a species found in war wounds and soil; it is not pathogenic for rabbits or guinea pigs.
C. thermosaccharoly'ticum, a species of thermophilic bacteria found in "hard swell" of canned goods; it is not pathogenic to laboratory animals.
C. welch'ii, *C. perfringens.*

---

clostridium, pl. **clostridia** (klos-trid'ē-ŭm, -ă). A vernacular term used to refer to any member of the genus *Clostridium.*

Clostridium histolyticum collagenase [EC 3.4.24.3]. Clostridiopeptidase A; collagenase A or I; an enzyme that catalyzes the hydrolysis of collagen.

Clostridium histolyticum proteinase B. Clostripain.

clostripain (klos'tri-pān) [EC 3.4.22.8]. *Clostridium histolyticum* proteinase B; clostridiopeptidase B; a cysteine proteinase cleaving preferentially at arginine CO—bonds.

closure (klō'zhŭr). **1.** The completion of a reflex pathway. **2.** The place of coupling between stimuli in the establishment of conditioned learning. **3.** To achieve or experience a sense of completion in a mental task.
flask c., in dentistry, the procedure of bringing the two halves or parts of a flask together; trial flask c.'s are preliminary c.'s made to eliminate excess denture-base material and to ensure that the mold is completely filled; the final flask c. is the last c. of a flask before curing, following trial packing of the mold with denture-base material.
velopharyngeal c., the apposition of the palate to the upper posterior pharyngeal wall as in deglutition and in some speech sounds.

closylate (klō'si-lāt). USAN-approved contraction for *p*-chlorobenzenesulfonate.

clot (klot). **1.** To coagulate, said especially of blood. **2.** A soft, nonrigid, insoluble mass formed when a liquid (*e.g.,* blood or lymph) gels.
agony c., a c. formed in the heart during the act of dying.
antemortem c., a blood c., found at autopsy, formed in any of the heart cavities or the great vessels before death.
blood c., crassamentum (1); the coagulated phase of blood; the soft, coherent, jelly-like red mass resulting from the conversion of fibrinogen to fibrin, thereby entrapping the red blood cells (and other formed elements) within the coagulated plasma.
chicken fat c., c. formed *in vitro* or postmortem from leukocytes and plasma of sedimented blood.
currant jelly c., a jelly-like mass of red blood cells and fibrin formed by the *in vitro* or postmortem clotting of whole or sedimented blood.
laminated c., a c. formed in a succession of layers such as occurs in the natural course of an aneurysm.
passive c., a c. formed in an aneurysmal sac consequent to the cessation of circulation through the aneurysm.
postmortem c., a c. formed in the heart or great vessels after death.

Schede's c., see Schede's *method.*

clotrimazole (klō-trim'ă-zōl). 1-(*o*-Chloro-α,α-diphenylbenzyl)imidazole; an antifungal agent used topically to treat a variety of fungal and yeast infections.

clottage (klot'ij). Blocking of any canal or duct by a blood clot.

Cloudman, Arthur M., 20th century U.S. pathologist. See C. *melanoma.*

clove oil (klōv). The volatile oil distilled with steam from cloves, *Eugenia caryophyllata* (family Myrtaceae); it contains not less than 85% by volume of total phenolic substances, chiefly eugenol; used as a dental analgesic.

cloxacillin sodium (klok-să-sil'in). [5-Methyl-3-(*o*-chlorophenyl)-4-isoxazolyl]penicillin sodium; a penicillinase-resistant penicillin.

clozapine (klō'ză-pēn). 8-Chloro-11-(4-methyl-1-piperazinyl)-5*H*-dibenzo[*b,e*][1,4]diazepine; a sedative.

CLQ Abbreviation for cognitive laterality *quotient.*

clubbing (klŭb'ing). A condition affecting the fingers and toes in which proliferation of distal tissues, especially the nail-beds, results in broadening of the extremities of the digits; the nails are abnormally curved and shiny.

clubfoot (klŭb'fut). *Talipes* equinovarus.

clubhand (klŭb'hand). Talipomanus.

clump (klŭmp) [A.S. *clympre,* a lump]. To form into clusters, small aggregations, or groups.

clumping (klŭmp-ing). The massing together of bacteria or other cells suspended in a fluid.

cluneal (klū'nē-ăl). Pertaining to the clunes.

clunes (klū'nēz) [pl. of L. *clunis,* buttock] [NA]. Nates.

cluttering (klŭt'er-ing). The dropping of letters or syllables by a hurried or nervous speaker.

Clutton, Henry H., British surgeon, 1850–1909. See C.'s *joints.*

-clysis [G. *klysis,* a drenching by a clyster]. Combining form, used as a suffix, denoting injection.

clysis (klī'sis) [G. *klysis,* a drenching by a clyster]. **1.** An infusion of fluid, usually subcutaneously, for therapeutic purposes. **2.** Formerly, a fluid enema; later, the washing out of material from any body space or cavity by fluids.

clyster (klis'ter) [G. *klystēr,* fr. *klyzō,* fut. *klysō,* to wash out]. An old term for enema.

C.M. Abbreviation for *Chirurgiae Magister,* Master in Surgery.

CM- Symbol for carboxymethyl radical.

Cm Symbol for curium.

cM Abbreviation for centimorgan.

cm Abbreviation for centimeter.

CMA Abbreviation for Certified Medical Assistant.

***p*-CMB** Abbreviation for *p*-chloromercuribenzoate.

CM-cellulose. Carboxymethyl *cellulose.*

CMI Abbreviation for cell-mediated *immunity.*

CMO Abbreviation for calculated mean *organism.*

CMP Symbol for cytidine 5′-phosphate (secondarily, for any cytidine monophosphate).

CMT Abbreviation for Certified Medical Transcriptionist. See medical transcriptionist.

CMV Abbreviation for controlled mechanical *ventilation;* cytomegalovirus.

cnemial (ne'mē-ăl) [G. *knēmē,* leg]. Relating to the leg, especially to the shin.

cnemis (nē'mis) [G. *knēmis* (*knēmid-*), a legging]. The shin.

cnida, pl. **cnidae** (nī'dă, nī'dē) [G. *knidē,* nettle]. Nematocyst.

cnidocyst (nī'dō-sist). Nematocyst.

cnidosis (nī-dō'sis) [G. *knidōsis,* nettle-rash, fr. *knidē,* a nettle]. Urticaria.

Cnidospora (nī-dō-spōr'ă) [G. *knidē,* nettle, sea nettle, + *sporos,* seed]. Microspora.

Cnidosporidia (nī'dō-spō-rid'ēă) [G. *knidē,* nettle, sea nettle, + Mod. L., fr. G. *sporos,* seed]. Microsporida.

C.N.M. Abbreviation for Certified Nurse Midwife.

CNS **1.** Abbreviation for central nervous *system.* **2.** Symbol for the thiocyanate radical, CNS^- or —CNS.

Co Symbol for cobalt.

co-. See con-.

CoA Abbreviation for coenzyme A.

coacervate (kō-as'er-vāt) [L. *coacervare,* pp. *-atus,* to collect in a mass]. An aggregate of colloidal particles separated out of an emulsion (coacervation) by the addition of some third component (coacervating agent).

coacervation (kō-as-er-vā'shŭn). Formation of a coacervate.

coadaptation (kō'ad-ap-tā'shŭn). The operation of selection jointly on two or more (usually linked) loci.

coagglutinin (kō-ă-glū'ti-nin). A substance that per se does not agglutinate an antigen, but does result in agglutination of antigen that is appropriately coated with univalent antibody. See also conglutination.

coagula (kō-ag'yū-lă). Plural of coagulum.

coagulable (kō-ag'yū-ă-bl). Capable of being coagulated or clotted.

coagulant (kō-ag'yū-lant). **1.** An agent that causes, stimulates, or accelerates coagulation, especially with reference to blood. **2.** Coagulative.

coagulate (kō-ag'yū-lāt) [L. *coagulo,* pp. *-atus,* to curdle]. **1.** To convert a fluid or a substance in solution into a solid or gel. **2.** To clot; to curdle; to change from a liquid to a solid or gel.

coagulation (kō-ag-yū-lā'shŭn). **1.** Clotting; the process of changing from a liquid to a solid, said especially of blood. **2.** A clot or coagulum. **3.** Transformation of a sol into a gel or semisolid mass; *e.g.,* the c. of the white of an egg by means of boiling. In any colloidal suspension, the dispersion of the disperse phase from the continuous phase is greatly reduced, thereby leading to a complete or partial separation of the latter; usually an irreversible phenomenon unless the basic nature of the substance is chemically altered.

disseminated intravascular c. (DIC), a hemorrhagic syndrome which occurs following the uncontrolled activation of clotting factors and fibrinolytic enzymes throughout small blood vessels; fibrin is deposited, platelets and clotting factors are consumed, and fibrin degradation products inhibit fibrin polymerization, resulting in tissue necrosis and bleeding. See also consumption *coagulopathy.*

coagulative (kō-ag'yū-lă-tiv). Coagulant (2); causing coagulation.

coagulopathy (kō-ag-yū-lop'ă-thē). A disease affecting the coagulability of the blood.

consumption c., a disorder in which marked reductions develop in blood concentrations of platelets with exhaustion of the coagulation factors in the peripheral blood as a result of disseminated intravascular coagulation.

coagulum, pl. **coagula** (kō-ag'yū-lŭm, -lă) [L. a means of coagulating, rennet]. Crassamentum (2); a clot or a curd; a soft, nonrigid, insoluble mass formed when a sol undergoes coagulation.

coal oil (kōl). Petroleum.

coal tar. A by-product obtained during the destructive distillation of bituminous coal; a very dark semisolid of characteristic naphthalene-like odor and a sharp, burning taste; used in the treatment of skin diseases.

coalescence (kō-ă-les′ens). Concrescence (1); fusion of originally separate parts.

coapt (kō′apt). To join or fit together.

coaptation (kō-ap-tā′shŭn) [L. *co-apto*, pp. *-aptatus*, to fit together]. Joining or fitting together of two surfaces; *e.g.*, the lips of a wound or the ends of a broken bone.

coarct (kō-arkt′) [L. *co-arcto*, pp. *-arctatus*, to press together]. Coarctate (1); to restrict or press together.

coarctate (kō-ark′tāt). **1.** Coarct. **2.** Pressed together.

coarctation (kō-ark-tā′shŭn). A constriction, stricture, or stenosis.
reversed c., aortic arch syndrome in which blood pressure in the arms is lower than in the legs.

coarctotomy (kō-ark-tot′ō-mē) [coarct + G. *tomē*, cutting]. Division of a stricture.

CoAS-, CoASH Symbols for the coenzyme A radical, reduced coenzyme A.

coat (kōt). **1.** The outer covering or envelope of an organ or part. **2.** One of the layers of membranous or other tissues forming the wall of a canal or hollow organ. See tunica.
buffy c., crusta inflammatoria or phlogistica; leukocyte cream; the upper, lighter portion of the blood clot (coagulated plasma and white blood cells), occurring when coagulation is delayed so that the red blood cells have had time to settle; the portion of centrifuged, anticoagulated blood which contains leukocytes and platelets.
sclerotic c., sclera.
serous c., *tunica* serosa.

coating (kōt′ing). A covering; a layer of some substance spread over a surface.
antireflection c., a film of magnesium fluoride spread on a lens to minimize reflections.

CoA transferases. See under coenzyme A.

Coats, George, British ophthalmologist, 1876–1915. See C.'s *disease.*

cobalamin (kō-bal′ă-min). General term for compounds containing the dimethylbenzimidazolylcobamide nucleus of vitamin B_{12}.
c. concentrate, the dried, partially purified product resulting from the growth of selected *Streptomyces* cultures or other cobalamin-producing microorganisms; contains at least 500 μg of c. in each gram.

cobalt (kō′bawlt) [Ger. *kobalt*]. A steel-gray metallic element, symbol Co, atomic no. 27, atomic weight 58.93; a constituent of vitamin B_{12}; certain of its compounds afford pigments, *e.g.*, c. blue.

cobalt-57 (**^{57}Co**). Half-life, 272 days; decays by electron capture with emission of a medium energy (123 keV) gamma ray.

cobalt-58 (**^{58}Co**). Positron emitter with half-life of 72 days.

cobalt-60 (**^{60}Co**). Half-life, 5.26 years; emits beta particles and energetic gamma rays, for which reason it is used in radiation therapy and diagnosis in place of radium (radon) and x-rays.

cobaltous chloride (kō-bawl′tŭs). $CoCl_2 \cdot 6H_20$; used in the treatment of various types of refractory anemia to improve the hematocrit, hemoglobin, and erythrocyte count.

cobamic acid (kō-bam′ik). Cobinic acid with a ribofuranose phosphate attached to the aminopropanol unit; a part of the vitamin B_{12} structure.

cobamide (kō-bam′īd). The hexa-amide of cobamic acid.

Cobb, Stanley, U.S. neuropathologist, *1887. See C. *syndrome.*

cobinamide (kō-bin′am-īd). The hexa-amide of cobinic acid; a part of the B_{12} vitamins (the cobalamins).

cobinic acid (kō-bin′ik). Cobyrinic acid with a 1-aminopropan-2-ol side chain attached to the $—CH_2CH_2COOH$ group on carbon-17 (side chain *f*); a part of the vitamin B_{12} structure.

cobra (kō′bră) [Port. snake, from L. *coluber*, snake]. Members of the highly venomous snake genus, *Naja* (family Elapidae); six species are recognized, all African except for the Asiatic c.; typical behavior includes spreading of the neck (hood), rearing one-third of the body off of the ground, and, in some species, the spitting of venom, which is primarily neurotoxic.

cobrotoxin (kō′brō-tok-sin). Direct lytic factor of cobra venom; a polypeptide of 62 residues; action on cells is similar to that of melittin in that it promotes disruption of membranes; used as an investigational antirheumatic agent.

cobyric acid (kō-bir′ik). Cobyrinamide; factor V_{1a}; the hexa-amide of cobyrinic acid; a part of the vitamins B_{12} structure.

cobyrinamide (kō-bir-in′ă-mīd). Cobyric acid.

cobyrinic acid (kō-bir-in′ik). Cobyrinic hexa-amide; corrin with 8 methyl groups at positions 1, 2, 5, 7, 12 (2), 15, 17; $—CH_2COOH$ groups at positions 2, 7, 18; $—CH_2CH_2COOH$ groups at positions 3, 8, 13, 17; and divalent cobalt centered among the four nitrogens. The acid side-chains are designated, in numerical order, *a, b, c, d, e, f, g.* It is a part of the vitamin B_{12} structure.

cobyrinic hexa-amide. Cobyric acid.

COC Abbreviation for cathodal opening *contraction.*

coca (kō′kă) [S. Am.]. The dried leaves of *Erythroxylon coca,* yielding not less than 0.5% of ether-soluble alkaloids; the source of cocaine and several other alkaloids.

cocaine (kō-kān). Benzoylmethylecgonine; an alkaloid obtained from the leaves of *Erythroxylon coca* (family Erythroxylaceae) and other species of *Erythroxylon,* or by synthesis from ecgonine or its derivatives; it has moderate vasoconstrictor activity and pronounced psychotropic effects; its salts are used as a topical anesthetic.

cocainization (kō′kān-i-zā′shŭn). Production of topical anesthesia of mucous membranes by the application of cocaine.

cocarboxylase (kō-kar-boks′i-lās). *Thiamin* pyrophosphate.

cocarcinogen (kō-kar′si-nō-jen). A substance that works symbiotically with a carcinogen in the production of cancer.

Coccaceae (kok-kā′sē-ē) [G. *kokkos,* a berry]. An obsolete term for a family of Eubacteriales which included all the spherical cells dividing in one (*Streptococcus*), two (*Micrococcus*), or three (*Sarcina*) planes, then forming cells, pairs, tetrads, cubes or larger packets, or chains.

coccal (kok′ăl). Relating to cocci.

cocci (kok′sī). Plural of coccus.

Coccidia (kok-sid′ē-ă) [Mod. L., fr. G. *kokkos,* berry]. Coccidiasina; a subclass of important protozoa (class Sporozoea, phylum Apicomplexa) in which the mature trophozoites are small and typically intracellular; schizogony and sporogony can occur in the same host, in contrast to the gregarines (subclass Gregarinia of class Sporozoea), which have large extracellular trophozoites in various invertebrates and do not reproduce by schizogony.

coccidia (kok-sid′ē-ă). Plural of coccidium.

coccidial (kok-sid′ē-ăl). Relating to coccidia.

Coccidiasina (kok-sid′ē-ă-sī′nă). Coccidia.

coccidioidal (kok-sid-ē-oy′dăl). Referring to the disease or to the infecting organism of coccidioidomycosis.

Coccidioides (kok-sid-ē-oy′dēz) [coccidium + G. *eidos,* resemblance]. A genus of fungi found in the soil of the semi-arid areas of the Southwestern U.S. and smaller areas throughout Central and South America, but has not been found elsewhere. The only pathogenic species, *C. immitis,* causes coccidioidomycosis.

coccidioidin (kok-sid-ē-oy′din). A sterile solution containing the by-products of growth of *Coccidioides immitis;* used as an intracutaneous skin test, diagnostically more valuable in non-endemic areas.

coccidioidoma (kok-sid′ē-oy-dō′mă). A benign localized residual granulomatous lesion or scar in a lung following primary coccidioidomycosis.

coccidioidomycosis (kok-sid-ē-oy′dō-mī-kō′sis) [coccidioides + G. *mykēs,* fungus, + *-osis,* condition]. Posadas' disease; an inapparent, benign, severe, or fatal systemic mycosis due to inhalation of dust particles containing arthrospores of *Coccidioides immitis.* In benign forms of the infection, the lesions are limited to the upper respiratory tract and lungs; in a low percentage of cases the disease disseminates to other visceral organs, bones, joints, and skin and subcutaneous tissues.
asymptomatic c., latent c.
disseminate c., a severe, chronic, and progressive form of c. resulting from rapid dissemination of endospores from the primary site of infection, or from reinfection in a previously sensitized patient, with widespread involvement of the central nervous system, bones, skin, and viscera.
latent c., asymptomatic c.; a form of c. not differentiated clinically from upper respiratory infections of viral or bacterial etiology; positive skin tests are useful in demonstrating past and present infections; tests for circulating serum antibodies are prognostic as well as diagnostic in some cases.
primary c., desert, valley, or San Joaquin fever; a disease common in the San Joaquin Valley of California and certain additional areas in the southwestern U.S. as well as the Chaco region of Argentina, caused by inhalation of the arthroconidia of *Coccidioides immitis;* acute onset of symptoms resemble pneumonia or pulmonary tuberculosis, productive of sputum usually containing spores of the fungus, and accompanied by aches, malaise, severe headache, and occasionally an early erythematous or papular eruption; erythema multiforme or erythema nodosum may appear later; the coccidioidin test is positive.
primary extrapulmonary c., a rare form of c. presenting near the site of local trauma with painless firm nodules occurring at one to two weeks, accompanied by regional adenopathy, with spontaneous healing in a few weeks.
secondary c., coccidiodal granuloma; progressive or disseminated extrapulmonary granulomatous lesions following primary c.

coccidiosis (kok-sid-ē-ō′sis). Group name for diseases due to any species of coccidia; a common and serious disease of many species of domestic animals and birds (not often serious in dogs and cats) and many wild animals kept in captivity; man and horses do not often suffer from c., but intestinal and pulmonary c. have been reported in individuals with AIDS.

coccidiostat (kok-sid′ē-ō-stat). A chemical agent generally added to animal feed to partially inhibit or delay the development of coccidiosis.

coccidium, pl. **coccidia** (kok-sid′ē-ŭm, -ē-ă) [Mod. L. dim. of G. *kokkos,* berry]. Common name given to protozoan parasites (order Eucoccidiida) in which schizogony occurs within epithelial cells, generally in the intestine, but in some species in the bile ducts and kidney; the final product of sexual fusion and differentiation that occurs within the host, the oocyst, generally passes to the soil in the feces, undergoes sporulation, and then acts as the infective form for another host. Coccidia are parasitic in most domestic and wild birds and mammals, occasionally in man, and are highly host-specific; the majority are nonpathogenic, but certain species rank among the most serious and economically important pathogens, causing coccidiosis in birds and mammals. See *Eimeria; Isospora.*

coccinella (kok-sin-el′ă). Cochineal.

coccinellin (kok-si-nel′in). The coloring principle derived from cochineal.

coccobacillary (kok′ō-bas′i-lār-ē). Relating to a coccobacillus.

coccobacillus (kok′ō-bă-sil′ŭs) [G. *kokkos,* berry]. A short, thick bacterial rod of the shape of an oval or slightly elongated coccus.

coccoid (kok′oyd) [G. *kokkos,* berry, + *eidos,* resemblance]. Resembling a coccus.

cocculin (kok′yū-lin). Picrotoxin.

coccus, pl. **cocci** (kok′ŭs, kok′sī) [G. *kokkos,* berry]. **1.** A bacterium of round, spheroidal, or ovoid form. **2.** Cochineal.
Neisser's c. *Neisseria gonorrhoeae.*
Weichselbaum's c., *Neisseria meningitidis.*

coccyalgia (kok-sē-al′jē-ă) [coccyx + G. *algos,* pain]. Coccygodynia.

coccycephaly (kok′si-sef′ă-lē) [G. *kokkyx,* cuckoo, + kephalē, head]. A malformation in which the cephalic profile suggests a beak.

coccydynia (kok-sē-din′ē-ă) [coccyx + G. *ōdyne, pain*]. Coccygodynia.

coccygalgia (kok-sē-gal′jē-ă) [coccyx + G. *algos,* pain]. Coccygodynia.

coccygeal (kok-sij′ē-ăl). Relating to the coccyx.

coccygectomy (kok-sē-jek′tō-mē) [coccyx + G. *ektomē,* excision]. Removal of the coccyx.

coccygeus (kok-si-jē′ŭs). See under musculus.

coccygodynia (kok′si-gō-din′ē-ă) [coccyx + G. *odynē,* pain]. Coccyalgia; coccydynia; coccygalgia; coccyodynia pain in the coccygeal region.

coccygotomy (kok-sē-got′ō-mē) [coccyx + G. *tomē,* a cutting]. Operation for freeing the coccyx from its attachments.

coccyodynia (kok′sē-ō-din′ē-ă). Coccygodynia.

coccyx, gen. **coccygis,** pl. **coccyges** (kok′siks, -si-jis, -si-jēs) [G. *kokkyx,* a cuckoo, the coccyx]. *Os* coccygis.

cochineal (kotch′i-nēl) [L. *coceineus,* scarlet] [C.I. 75470]. Coccinella; coccus (2); the dried female insects, *Coccus cacti,* enclosing the young larvae, or the dried female insect, *Dactylopius coccus,* containing eggs and larvae, from which coccinellin is obtained; used as a coloring agent and a stain. See carmine.

cochlea, pl. **cochleae** (kok′lē-ă, lē-ē) [L. snail shell] [NA]. A cone-shaped cavity in the petrous portion of the temporal bone, forming one of the divisions of the labyrinth or internal ear. It consists of a spiral canal making two and a half turns around a central core of spongy bone, the modiolus; this spiral canal of the cochlea contains the membranous cochlea, or ductus cochlearis, in which is the spiral organ (Corti).
membranous c., *ductus* cochlearis.

cochlear (kok′lē-ăr). Relating to the cochlea.

cochleare (kō-klē′ă, kok-lē-ā′rē) [L.]. A spoon.

cochleariform (kok-lē-ar′i-fōrm) [L. *cochleare,* spoon, + *forma,* form]. Spoon-shaped.

cochleate (kok′lē-āt) [L. *cochlea,* a snail shell]. **1.** Resembling a snail shell. **2.** Denoting the appearance of a form of plate culture.

cochleitis (kok-lē-ī′tis). Cochlitis.

cochleosacculotomy (kok′lē-ō-sac-yū-lot′ō-mē). An operation for Ménière's disease performed through the round window to create a shunt between the cochlear duct and the saccule.

cochleovestibular (kok′lē-ō-ves-tib′yū-lăr). Relating to the cochlea and the vestibule of the ear.

Cochliomyia (kok′lē-ō-mī′yă). A genus of fleshflies (family Calliphoridae) whose larvae develop in decaying flesh or carrion or in wounds or sores.
C. american'a, incorrect name for *C. hominivorax.*

C. hominivo'rax, the screw-worm fly, a species that is a serious pest of livestock from Mexico to Argentina and is the primary cause of myiasis in the western hemisphere; attracted by fresh blood, it deposits eggs on wounds, tick bites, or intact moist areas of the body, and the larvae invade living tissues, causing severe myiasis and often death; it is known to attack man, especially in the nose, although wounds, eyes, and other body openings have also been attacked.

C. macella'ria, the secondary screw-worm fly, a species attracted to decaying flesh (formerly used as surgical maggots); primarily a scavenger, but not implicated in primary myiasis as is *C. hominivorax,* though it may be a secondary wound invader in domestic animals in the Americas and has frequently been confused with the latter and improperly held responsible for primary myiasis; larvae may develop in neglected wounds.

cochlitis (kok-lī'tis). Cochleitis; inflammation of the cochlea.

cocillana (ko'sĕ-lah'nă). The dried bark of *Guarea rusbyi,* a Bolivia tree, used as an expectorant in bronchitis.

Cockayne, Edward A., British physician, 1880–1956. See C.'s *disease, syndrome;* Weber-C. *syndrome.*

cocks comb (koks kōm). *Crista* galli.

cocktail (kok'tāl). A drink that includes several ingredients or drugs.

Brompton c., [*Brompton* Chest Hospital, London, England, where developed], a c. of morphine and cocaine usually used for analgesia in terminal cancer patients; the formulations vary, but typically it contains 15 mg of morphine hydrochoride and 10 mg of cocaine hydrochloride per 10 ml of the c.

lytic c., a primarily European term for a mixture of drugs injected intravenously to produce sedation, analgesia, amnesia, hypotension, hypothermia, and blockade of sympathetic and parasympathetic nervous systems during surgical anesthesia.

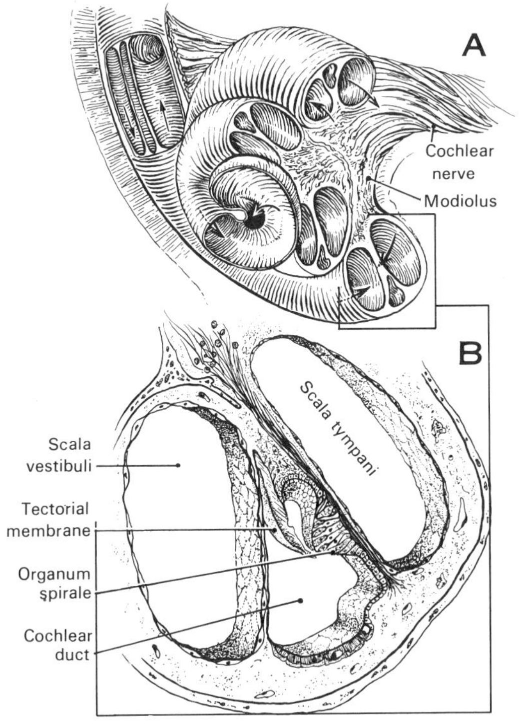

Cochlea

A, frontal view of right cochlea, with sections of spiral canal removed to show internal structure; *B,* section across spiral canal.

Philadelphia c., Rivers' c.

Rivers' c., Philadelphia c.; an intravenous slow injection of from 1000 to 2000 ml of 10% dextrose in isotonic saline to which thiamine hydrochloride and 25 units of insulin are added; used in acute alcoholism.

COCl Abbreviation for cathodal opening *clonus.*

cocoa (kō'kō). A powder prepared from the roasted kernels of the ripe seed of *Theobroma cacao* (family Sterculiaceae); used in the preparation of c. syrup, a flavoring agent. See also cacao.

coconsciousness (kō-kon'shŭs-nes). A splitting of consciousness into two streams.

cocto- [L. *coctus,* boiled] Prefix indicating boiled or modified by heat.

coctolabile (kok-tō-lā'bil, -bīl). Subject to alteration or destruction when exposed to the temperature of boiling water.

coctostabile, coctostable (kok-tō-stā'bil, -bīl; -stā'bl). Resisting the temperature of boiling water without alteration or destruction.

cod (kod). **1.** The fat-filled scrotum of a castrated bovine animal. **2.** A common marine fish (family Gadidae) related to the haddock and pollack.

code (kōd). **1.** A set of rules, principles, or ethics. **2.** Any system devised to convey information or facilitate communication. **3.** Term used in hospitals to describe an emergency situation requiring trained members of the staff, such as a cardiopulmonary resuscitation team, or the signal to summon such a team.

genetic c., the genetic information carried by the specific DNA molecules of the chromosomes; specifically, the system whereby particular combinations of three adjacent nucleotides in a DNA molecule control the insertion of particular amino acids in equivalent places in a protein molecule.

codecarboxylase (kō'dē-kar-boks'i-lās). Pyridoxal 5'-phosphate.

codehydrogenase I and II (kō'dē-hī-droj'ĕ-nās). Obsolete names for nicotinamide adenine dinucleotide and nicotinamide adenine dinucleotide phosphate, respectively.

codeine (kō'dēn) [G. *kōdeia,* head, poppy head]. Methylmorphine; morphine monomethyl morphine 3-methyl ether; obtained from opium, which contains 0.7 to 2.5%, but usually made from morphine. Used as an analgesic and antitussive; drug dependence (physical and psychic) may develop, but c. is less liable to produce addiction than is morphine.

Codex medicamentarius (kō'deks med'i-kă-men-tār'ē-ŭs) [L. a book pertaining to drugs]. The official title of the French Pharmacopeia.

cod liver oil. The partially destearinated fixed oil extracted from the fresh livers of *Gadus morrhuae* and other species of the family Gadidae, containing vitamins A and D; used as a supplementary source of vitamins A and D.

Codman, Ernest Amory, U.S. surgeon, 1869–1940. See C.'s *sign, triangle, tumor.*

codominant (kō-dom'i-nant). In genetics, denoting an equal degree of dominance of two genes, both being expressed in the phenotype of the individual; *e.g.,* genes A and B of the ABO blood group are codominant; individuals with both are type AB.

codon (kō'don). Triplet (3); a sequence of three nucleotides in a strand of DNA or RNA that provides the genetic information to incorporate a specific amino acid into a protein chain.

initiating c., the trinucleotide AUG (or sometimes GUG) that codes for the first amino acid in protein sequences, formylmethionine; the latter is often removed post-transcriptionally.

termination c., termination sequence; trinucleotide sequence (UAA, UGA, or UAG) that specifies the end of translation or transcription.

coe-. For words so beginning, and not found here, see ce-.

coefficient (kō-ĕ-fish'ĕnt) [L. *co-* + *efficio (exfacio)*, to accomplish]. **1.** The expression of the amount or degree of any quality possessed by a substance, or of the degree of physical or chemical change normally occurring in that substance under stated conditions. **2.** The ratio or factor that relates a quantity observed under one set of conditions to that observed under standard conditions, usually when all variables are either 1 or a simple power of 10.

absorption c., **(1)** the milliliters of a gas at standard temperature and pressure that will saturate 100 ml of liquid; **(2)** the amount of light absorbed in passing through 1 cm of a 1 molar solution of a given substance, expressed as a constant in Beer's law. *Cf.* specific absorption c. **(3)** in x-ray, a measure of the rate of decrease of intensity of a beam in its passage through a substance, resulting from a combination of scattering and conversion to other forms of energy.

activity c., see activity (2).

biological c., rarely used term denoting the energy expended by the body at rest.

Bunsen's solubility c. (α), the milliliters of gas STPD dissolved per milliliter of liquid and per atmosphere (760 mm Hg) partial pressure of the gas at any given temperature.

c. of consanguinity, c. of inbreeding.

correlation c.'s, a statistical term referring to the degree of relationship between two sets of paired measurements, but not indicative of one variable causing the other; may be positive, negative, or curvilinear, depending on whether the variations are in the same, opposite, or both directions.

creatinine c., the number of milligrams of creatinine excreted daily per kilogram of body weight.

diffusion c., diffusion constant; the mass of material diffusing across a unit area in unit time under a concentration gradient of unity.

distribution c., partition c.; the ratio of concentrations of a substance in two immiscible phases at equilibrium; the basis of many chromatographic separation procedures.

extinction c., specific absorption c.

extraction c., the percentage of a substance removed from the blood or plasma in a single passage through a tissue; *e.g.,* the extraction c. for *p*-aminohippuric acid (PAH) in the kidney is the difference between arterial and renal venous plasma PAH concentrations, divided by the arterial plasma PAH concentration.

filtration c., a measure of a membrane's permeability to water; specifically, the volume of fluid filtered in unit time through a unit area of membrane per unit pressure difference, taking into account both hydraulic and osmotic pressures.

hygienic laboratory c., Rideal-Walker c.

c. of inbreeding, c. of consanguinity; the probability that the individual concerned is homozygous by descent at an autosomal locus picked at random; equal to the c. of kinship of the parents.

isotonic c., the amount of salts in the blood plasma, or the amount that should be added to distilled water in order to prepare an isotonic solution.

c. of kinship, the probability that two genes at the same locus, picked at random from each of two individuals, are identical by descent.

lethal c., that concentration of disinfectant that kills bacteria at 20–25°C in the shortest period of time.

linear absorption c., that fraction of radiation absorbed in a material of unit thickness. See also absorption c.(3).

Long's c., Long's *formula.*

molar absorption c. (ϵ), molar absorbancy index; molar extinction c.; molar absorptivity; absorbance (of light) per unit path length (usually the centimeter) and per unit of concentration (moles per liter); a fundamental unit in spectrophotometry.

molar extinction c., molar absorption c.

Ostwald's solubility c., (λ), the milliliters of gas dissolved per milliliter of liquid and per atmosphere (760 mm of Hg) partial pressure of the gas at any given temperature. This differs from Bunsen's solubility c. (α) in that the amount of dissolved gas is expressed in terms of its volume at the temperature of the experiment, instead of STPD. Thus, $\lambda = \alpha\,(1 + 0.00367t)$, where t = temperature in degrees Celsius.

oxygen utilization c., the extraction c. for oxygen in any given tissue.

partition c., distribution c.

phenol c., Rideal-Walker c.

Poiseuille's viscosity c., an expression of the viscosity as determined by the capillary tube method; the coefficient $\eta = (\pi P r^4 t / 8 vl)$, where P is the pressure difference between the inlet and outlet of the tube, r the radius of the tube, l its length, and v the quantity of liquid delivered in the time t.

reflection c. (σ), a measure of the relative permeability of a particular membrane to a particular solute; calculated as the ratio of observed osmotic pressure to that calculated from van't Hoff's law; also equal to 1 minus the ratio of the effective pore areas available to solute and to solvent.

c. of relationship, the probability that a gene present in one mate is also present in the other and is derived from the same source.

reliability c., an index of the consistency of measurement often based on the correlation between scores obtained on the initial test and a retest (test-retest reliability) or between scores on two similar forms of the same test (equivalent-form reliability).

respiratory c., respiratory *quotient.*

Rideal-Walker c., phenol c.; hygienic laboratory c.; a figure expressing the disinfecting power of any substance; it is obtained by dividing the figure indicating the degree of dilution of the disinfectant that kills a microorganism in a given time by that indicating the degree of dilution of phenol which kills the organism in the same space of time under similar conditions.

selection c. (s), the proportion of progeny or potential progeny not surviving to sexual maturity; usually defined artificially by expressing the fitness of a phenotype as a fraction of the mean or optimal fitness to give the relative fitness, and subtracting this quantity from unity.

specific absorption c. (*a*), absorptivity; absorbancy index; specific extinction; extinction c.; absorbance (of light) per unit path length (usually the centimeter) and per unit of mass concentration. *Cf.* molar absorption c. (2).

temperature c., the fractional change in any physical property per degree rise in temperature.

ultrafiltration c., the filtration c. of a semipermeable membrane.

c. of variation (CV), standard deviation expressed as a percentage of a mean value.

velocity c., the rate of transformation of a unit mass of substance in a chemical reaction.

c. of viscosity, the value of the force per unit area required to maintain a unit relative velocity between two parallel planes a unit distance apart.

Coelenterata (sē-len-tē-rā'tă). One of the major phyla of invertebrates, to which such forms as jellyfish belong.

coelenterate (sē-len'ter-at). Common name for members of the Coelenterata.

coelom (sē'lom). Celom.

coenesthesia (kō-en-es-thē'zē-ă). Cenesthesia.

coeno- [G. *koinos,* common]. Combining form meaning shared in common. See also ceno-.

coenocyte (sē'nō-sīt). Cenocyte.

coenocytic (sē-nō-sit'ik). Cenocytic.

coenurosis (sē-nū-rō'sis). Cenurosis.

Coenurus (sē-nū'rŭs) [G. *koinos,* common, + *oura,* tail]. Former generic name, now used to designate larval forms of taenioid cestodes in which a bladder is formed with a number of invaginated scoleces developing within; distinguished from a hydatid cyst by the absence of free-floating daughter cyst colonies budded off within the bladder; C. larvae are found in members of the genus *Multiceps.*

C. cerebra'lis, the coenurus larvae of the tapeworm *Multiceps multiceps,* found in the brain and spinal cord of sheep, goats, and other ruminants (a few have been recorded in man); adults are found in the intestine of dogs, foxes, coyotes, and jackals.

C. seria'lis, the coenurus larvae of the tapeworm *Multiceps serialis,* found in subcutaneous and intramuscular tissues of rabbits and hares (a few have been recorded in man); adult worms are found in the intestine of dogs, foxes, and jackals.

coenzyme. (kō-en'zīm). Cofactor (1); a substance that enhances or is necessary for the action of enzymes; c.'s are of smaller molecular size than the enzymes themselves, are dialyzable and relatively heat-stable, and are usually easily dissociable from the protein portion of the enzyme; several vitamins are c.'s (*e.g.,* thiamin, pyridoxal, nicotinamide, riboflavin).

coenzyme I and II. Obsolete names for nicotinamide adenine dinucleotide and nicotinamide adenine dinucleotide phosphate respectively.

coenzyme A (CoA). A coenzyme containing pantothenic acid, adenosine 3'-phosphate 5'-pyrophosphate, and cysteamine; involved in the transfer of acyl groups, notably in transacetylations.

CoA transferases [EC Class 2.8.3], thiaphorases; thiophorases; enzymes transferring CoA from acetyl-CoA or succinyl-CoA to other acyl radicals.

coenzyme Q (CoQ). Quinones with isoprenoid side chains (specifically, ubiquinones) that mediate electron transfer between cytochrome *b* and cytochrome *c;* chemically similar to vitamins E and K, and to other tocopherols, quinones, and tocols.

coenzyme R. Biotin.

coeur (kūr) [Fr.]. Heart.

c. en sabot (awn sah-bo'), sabot heart; wooden-shoe heart; the roentgenographic configuration of the heart in the tetralogy of Fallot; the elevated apex combined with a transverse rectangular enlargement is likened to a wooden shoe.

cofactor (kō'fak'ter, tōr). **1.** Coenzyme. **2.** An atom or molecule essential for the action of a large molecule; *e.g.,* heme in hemoglobin, magnesium in chlorophyll.

c. V, *factor* VII.

cobra venom c., properdin *factor* B.

platelet c., *factor* VIII.

platelet c. II, *factor* IX.

c. of thromboplastin, *factor* V.

coferment (kō'fer-ment). Obsolete term for coenzyme.

Coffey, Robert C., U.S. surgeon, 1869–1933. See C. *suspension.*

Coffin, Grange S., U.S. pediatrician, *1923. See C.-Lowry *syndrome;* C.-Siris *syndrome.*

Cogan, David G., U.S. ophthalmologist, *1908. See C.'s *syndrome;* C.-Reese *syndrome.*

cognition (kog-ni'shŭn) [L. *cognitio*]. **1.** Generic term embracing the quality of knowing, which includes perceiving, recognizing, conceiving, judging, sensing, reasoning, and imagining. **2.** Any process whereby one acquires knowledge.

cognitive (kog'ni-tiv). Pertaining to cognition.

cohesion (kō-hē'zhŭn) [L. *co-haereo,* pp. *-haesus,* to stick together]. The attraction between molecules or masses that holds them together.

Cohnheim, Julius F., German histologist, pathologist, and physiologist, 1839–1884. See C.'s *area, field, theory.*

cohoba (kō-hō'bă). A psychotomimetic hallucinogenic substance obtained from *Acacia niopo* (family Leguminosae), a Central American plant, *Piptadenia peregrina,* and other plants; among its constituents are bufotenine and dimethyltryptamine; used in native localities as snuff or enema.

cohort (kō'hōrt). A defined population group followed prospectively in an epidemiological study.

coin-counting (koyn'kownt'ing). A sliding movement of the tips of the thumb and index finger, occurring in paralysis agitans.

coinosite (koyn'ō-sīt). Cenosite.

coital (ko'i-tăl). Pertaining to coitus.

Coiter (Koyter), Volcher, Dutch surgeon and anatomist, 1534–1600. See C.'s *muscle.*

coition (kō-ish'ŭn) [L. *co-eo,* pp. *-itus,* to come together]. Coitus.

coitophobia (kō'i-tō-fō'bē-ă) [L. *coitus,* sexual intercourse, + G. *phobos,* fear]. Morbid fear of sexual intercourse.

coitus (kō'i-tŭs) [L.]. Copulation (1); coition; pareunia; sexual intercourse; sexual union between male and female.

c. interrup'tus, onanism (1).

c. reserva'tus, c. in which ejaculation is postponed or suppressed.

col (kol). A crater-like area of the interproximal oral mucosa joining the lingual and buccal interdental papillae.

col-. See con-.

cola (kō'lă). Kola.

colchicine (kol'chi-sin) (USP, BP). $C_{22}H_{25}NO_6$; an alkaloid obtained from *Colchicum autumnale* (family Liliaceae); used for gout.

cold (kōld). **1.** A low temperature; the sensation produced by a temperature notably below an accustomed norm or a comfortable level. **2.** A virus infection involving the upper respiratory tract and characterized by congestion of the mucosa, watery nasal discharge, and general malaise, with a duration of 3 to 5 days. See also rhinitis.

c. in the head, acute rhinitis.

rose c., allergic rhinitis occurring in the spring and early summer.

cold-blooded (kōld-blŭd'ed). Poikilothermic.

Cole, Laurent, French pathologist, *1903. See Benedict-Hopkins-C. *reagent.*

Cole-Cecil murmur. See under murmur.

colectasia (kō-lek-tā'zē-ă) [G. *kolon,* colon, + *ektasis,* a stretching]. Ectacolia; distention of the colon.

colectomy (kō-lek'tō-mē) [G. *kolon,* colon, + *ektomē,* excision]. Excision of a segment or all of the colon.

coleitis (kol-ē-ī'tis) [G. *koleos,* sheath, + *-itis,* inflammation]. Obsolete term for vaginitis.

coleo- [G. *koleos,* sheath]. Combining form meaning sheath or, specifically, the vagina.

coleocele (kol'ē-ō-sēl) [G. *koleos,* sheath, + *kēlē,* tumor]. Colpocele (1).

Coleoptera (kō-lē-op'ter-ă) [G. *koleos,* sheath + *pteron,* wing]. An order of insects, the beetles, characterized by the possession of a pair of hard, horny wing covers overlying a pair of delicate membranous flying wings; it is the largest of the insect orders with the largest number of species of any animal or plant order.

coleoptosis (kō-lē-op'tō-sis). Coloptosis.

coleotomy (kol-ē-ot'ō-mē) [G. *koleos,* sheath, + *tomē,* incision]. **1.** Pericardiotomy. **2.** Vaginotomy.

coles (kō'lēz) [G. *kōlēs*]. Penis.

colestipol (kō-les'ti-pol). Tetraethylenepentamine polymer with 1-chloro-2,3-epoxypropane; an antilipemic drug.

colibacillosis (kō'li-bas-i-lō'sis). Diarrheal disease caused by *Escherichia coli.* Often called enteric c.

colibacillus, pl. colibacilli (kō'li-bă-sil'ŭs). Colon bacillus. See *Escherichia coli.*

colic (kol'ik) [G. *kōlikos,* relating to the colon]. **1.** Relating to the colon. **2.** Spasmodic pains in the abdomen. **3.** In young infants, paroxysms of gastrointestinal pain, with crying and irritability, due to a variety of causes, such as swallowing of air, emotional upset, or overfeeding.
appendicular c., vermicular c.; colicky pain occurring early in acute appendicitis.
biliary c., gallstone or hepatic c.; intense pain felt in the right upper quadrant of the abdomen from impaction of a gallstone in the cystic or hepatic duct or the ampulla of Vater.
copper c., an affection similar to lead c. occurring in chronic poisoning by copper.
Devonshire c., lead c.
gallstone c., biliary c.
gastric c., colicky pain associated with gastritis or peptic ulcer.
hepatic c., biliary c.
lead c., Devonshire, painter's, or saturnine c.; severe abdominal pain, with constipation, symptomatic of lead poisoning.
meconial c., abdominal pain of newborn infants.
menstrual c., intermittent cramp-like lower abdominal pains associated with menstruation.
milk c., enterotoxemia.
ovarian c., lower abdominal pain due to torsion or twisting of an ovary, as with an ovarian cyst.
painter's c., lead c.
pancreatic c., severe abdominal pain, resembling that of biliary c., caused by the passage of a pancreatic calculus.
renal c., severe pain caused by the impaction or passage of a calculus in the ureter or renal pelvis.
salivary c., periodic attacks of pain in the region of a salivary duct or gland, accompanied by an acute swelling of the gland, occurring in cases of salivary calculus.
saturnine c., lead c.
tubal c., lower abdominal pain due to spasmodic contraction of the oviduct excited by a blood clot, other irritant, or the injection of gas or oil.
uterine c., painful cramps of the uterine muscle sometimes occurring at the menstrual period, or in association with uterine disease.
vermicular c., appendicular c.
zinc c., c. resulting from chronic zinc poisoning.

colica (kol'i-kă). A colic artery. See entries under arteria.

colicin (kol'i-sin). Bacteriocin produced by strains of *Escherichia coli* and by other enterobacteria (*Shigella* and *Salmonella*) which carry the necessary plasmids.

colicinogeny (kol'i-si-noj'ĕ-nē). The bacterial property of producing a colicin.

colicky (kol'i-kē). Denoting or resembling the pain of colic.

colicoplegia (kol'i-kō-plē'jē-ă) [G. *kolikos,* suffering from colic, + *plēgē,* stroke]. Lead poisoning marked by both colic and palsy.

coliform (kō'li-fōrm, kol'i-fōrm). A general, ill-defined term used to denote Gram-negative, fermentative rods that inhabit the intestinal tract of man and other animals. Sometimes used to refer to all enteric bacteria, or used to refer only to lactose-fermenting enteric bacteria.

colimycin (kō-li-mī'sin). Colistin.

colipase (kō'lip-ās) [co- + lipase]. A small protein in pancreatic juice that is essential for the efficient action of pancreatic lipase.

coliphage (kō'li-fāj, kol'i-). A bacteriophage with an affinity for one or another strain of *Escherichia coli.* In general, c.'s, like other bacteriophages, are known by symbols that have significance only as a means of laboratory identification; additional notations, however, specifically identify variant characteristics, *e.g.,* λdgal denotes the deficient prophage (coliphage) λ, which carries the bacterial gene *gal* (galactose).

coliplication (kō'li-pli-kā'shŭn). Coloplication.

colipuncture (kō'li-pŭnk-chūr). Colocentesis.

colistimethate sodium (kō-lis-ti-meth'āte). Colistin (or cholistin) sulfomethate sodium; pentasodium colistinmethanesulfonate; contains the pentasodium salt of the penta(methanesulfonic acid) derivative of colistin A as the major component, with a small proportion of the pentasodium salt of the same derivative of colistin B; an effective antibiotic against most Gram-negative bacilli (except *Proteus*), given intramuscularly. See also *colistin* sulfate; polymyxin.

colistin (kō-lis'tin). Colimycin; a mixture of cyclic polypeptide antibiotics from a strain of *Bacillus polymyxa;* separable into polymyxins.
c. sulfate, the sulfate salt of an antibacterial substance produced by the growth of a strain of *Bacillus polymyxa,* consisting primarily of colistin A with small amounts of colistin B; it is effective against most Gram-negative bacteria (except *Proteus*); given orally for intestinal antibacterial action. See also colistimethate sodium; polymyxin.
c. sulfomethate sodium, colistimethate sodium.

colitis (kō-lī'tis) [G. *kolon,* colon, + *-itis,* inflammation]. Inflammation of the colon.
amebic c., inflammation of the colon in amebiasis.
collagenous c., c. occurring mostly in middle-aged women and characterized by persistent watery diarrhea and a deposit of a band of collagen beneath the basement membrane of colon surface epithelium.
c. cys'tica profun'da, intramural mucus-containing cysts of the large bowel; the condition may be mistaken for mucinous carcinoma but is not neoplastic.
c. cys'tica superficia'lis, a form of c. in which there is superficial cyst formation in the colon.
granulomatous c., changes, identical to those of regional enteritis, involving the colon.
c. gra'vis, obsolete term for ulcerative c.
hemorrhagic c., abdominal cramps and bloody diarrhea, without fever, attributed to a self-limited infection by a strain of *Escherichia coli.*
mucous c., myxomembranous c.; mucocolitis; an affection of the mucous membrane of the colon characterized by colicky pain, constipation or diarrhea (sometimes alternating), and passage of mucous or slimy pseudomembranous shreds and patches.
myxomembranous c., mucous c.
pseudomembranous c., pseudomembranous *enterocolitis.*
ulcerative c., a chronic disease of unknown cause characterized by ulceration of the colon and rectum, with rectal bleeding, mucosal crypt abscesses, inflammatory pseudopolyps, abdominal pain, and diarrhea; frequently causes anemia, hypoproteinemia, and electrolyte imbalance, and is less frequently complicated by peritonitis, toxic megacolon, or carcinoma of the colon.
uremic c., c. characterized by hemorrhages in the mucosa, occurring in renal failure, possibly owing to the irritant effect of ammonia formed by breakdown of increased urea in the intestinal secretions.

colitose (kol'ĭ-tōs). A polysaccharide somatic antigen of *Salmonella* species.

colla (kol'ă). Plural of collum.

collacin (kol'ă-sin). Collastin; degenerated collagen.

collagen (kol'lă-jen) [G *koila,* glue, + *-gen,* producing]. Ossein; osseine; ostein; osteine; the major protein (comprising over half of that in mammals) of the white fibers of connective tissue, cartilage, and bone which is insoluble in water, but can be altered to easily digestible, soluble gelatins by boiling in water, dilute acids, or alkalies. It is high in glycine, alanine, proline, hydroxyproline, but is low in sulfur and has no tryptophan. C. comprises a family of genetically distinct molecules all of which have a unique triple helix configuration of three polypeptide subunits known as α-chains; six types of c. have been identified, each with a different polypeptide chain. See also c. *fiber.*

type I c., the most abundant c., which forms large well-organized fibrils having high tensile strength.

type II c., c. unique to cartilage, nucleus pulposis, notochord, and vitreous body; it forms as thin highly glycosylated fibrils.

type III c., c. characteristic of reticular fibers.

type IV c., a less distinctly fibrillar form of c. characteristic of basement membranes.

collagenase A or **I** (kol'ă-jĕ-nās). *Clostridium histolyticum* collagenase.

collagenation (kol'ă-jĕ-nā'shŭn). Collagenization.

collagenic (kol-ă-jen'ik). Collagenous.

collagenization (ko-laj'ĕ-ni-zā'shŭn). Collagenation. **1.** Replacement of tissues or fibrin by collagen. **2.** Synthesis of collagen by fibroblasts.

collagenolytic (ko-laj'ĕ-nō-lit'ik). Causing the lysis of collagen, gelatin, and other proteins containing proline.

collagenosis (ko-laj-i-nō'sis). Collagen *disease.*

reactive perforating c., a rare skin disorder characterized by extrusion of collagen fibers through the epidermis; usually begins in infancy or childhood and appears clinically as recurrent umbilicated papules that resolve spontaneously.

collagenous (ko-laj'ĕ-nŭs). Collagenic; producing or containing collagen.

collapse (kō-laps') [L. *col-labor,* pp. *-lapsus,* to fall together]. **1.** A condition of extreme prostration, similar to hypovolemic shock and due to the same causes. **2.** A state of profound physical depression. **3.** A falling together of the walls of a structure or the failure of a physiological system.

absorption c., pulmonary c. due to rapid complete obstruction of a large bronchus.

circulatory c., failure of the circulation, either cardiac or peripheral.

c. of dental arch, movement of teeth to fill a space which would normally be filled by another, missing tooth, creating a malpositioning of adjacent and opposing teeth.

massive c., relatively sudden atelectasis of an entire lung or of a lobe.

pressure c., pulmonary c. due to external compression of the lung, as by a pleural effusion or pneumothorax.

pulmonary c., secondary atelectasis due to bronchial obstruction, pleural effusion or pneumothorax, cardiac hypertrophy, or enlargement of other structures adjacent to the lungs.

collar (kol'ăr). A band, usually denoting one encircling the neck.

renal c., in the embryo, a ring of veins around the aorta below the origin of the superior mesenteric artery.

c. of Venus, obsolete term for syphilitic *leukoderma.*

collarette (kol'er-et'). Iris frill; the sinuous, scalloped line in the iris that divides the central pupillary zone from the peripheral ciliary zone and marks the embryonic site of the atrophied minor vascular circle of the iris.

collastin (kol-as'tin). Collacin.

collateral (ko-lat'er-ăl). **1.** Indirect, subsidiary, or accessory to the main thing; side by side. **2.** A side branch of a nerve axon or blood vessel.

Colles, Abraham, Irish surgeon, 1773–1843. See C.'s *fascia, fracture, ligament, space.*

colliculectomy (ko-lik-yū-lek'tō-mē). Excision of the colliculus seminalis.

colliculitis (ko-lik-yū-lī'tis). Verumontanitis; inflammation of the urethra in the region of the colliculus seminalis.

colliculus, pl. **colliculi** (ko-lik'yū-lŭs, -lī) [L. mound, dim. of *collis,* hill] [NA]. A small elevation above the surrounding parts.

c. cartila'ginis arytenoi'deae [NA], the elevation on the anterolateral surface of the arytenoid cartilage above the triangular fovea.

facial c., c. facialis.

c. facia'lis, [NA], facial c. eminence, or hillock; eminentia abducentis or facialis; a prominent portion of the eminentia medialis, just above the striae medullares in the rhomboidal fossa; it is caused by the curve of the genu of the facial nerve around the nucleus of the abducens nerve.

inferior c., c. inferior.

c. infe'rior [NA], inferior c.; corpus quadrigeminum posterius; the ovoid, paired, inferior eminence of the lamina tecti mesencephali; it receives the lateral lemniscus and projects by way of the brachium colliculi inferioris to the medial geniculate body of the thalamus, and is thus an essential way-station in the central auditory pathway.

seminal c., c. seminalis.

c. semina'lis [NA], seminal c.; c. urethralis; seminal hillock; verumontanum; caput gallinaginis; an elevated portion of the urethral crest upon which open the two ejaculatory ducts and the prostatic utricle.

superior c., c. superior.

c. supe'rior [NA], superior c.; corpus quadrigeminum anterius; the paired, larger, rounded anterior eminence of the lamina tecti mesencephali; major afferent connections of the superficial layers are the retina and striate cortex; input to deep layers of the c.s. are polymodal. Its efferent connections are with the lower brainstem and spinal cord (tractus tectobulbaris and tectospinalis) and with the pulvinar and other cell groups in the caudal part of the thalamus; participates in extrageniculate visual pathway.

c. urethra'lis, c. seminalis.

Collier, James S., British physician, 1870–1935. See C.'s *tract.*

colligation (kol-i-gā'shŭn) [L. *cum,* together, + *ligāre,* to bind]. **1.** A combination in which the components are distinguishable from one another. **2.** The bringing of isolated events into a unified experience.

colligative (ko-lig'ă-tiv). Referring to properties of solutions that depend only on the concentration of dissolved substances and not on their nature (*e.g.,* osmotic pressure, elevation of boiling point).

collimation (kol-i-mā'shŭn). [L. *collineo,* to direct in a straight line]. The process, in x-ray, of restricting and confining the x-ray beam to a given area and, in nuclear medicine, of restricting the detection of emitted radiations from a given area of interest.

collimator (kol'i-mā-ter). A device of high absorption coefficient material used in collimation.

collinearity (kol'in-ē-ar'i-tē) [L. *collineo,* to direct in a straight line]. Identity in the orderings of the corresponding elements of DNA, the RNA transcribed from it, and the amino acid translated from the RNA.

Collins. See Lukes-Collins *classification.*

Collins, Edward Treacher, British ophthalmologist, 1862–1919. See Treacher Collins *syndrome.*

colliotomy (kol-ē-ot'ō-mē) [G. *kolla,* glue, + G. *tomē,* incision]. Adhesiotomy.

Collip, James B., Canadian endocrinologist, 1892–1965. See Noble-C. *procedure,* Anderson-C. *test.*

colliquation (kol-i-kwā'shŭn) [L. *col-,* together, + *liquo,* pp. *liquatus,* to cause to melt]. **1.** Excessive discharge of fluid. **2.** Liquidification in the process of necrosis.

ballooning c., obsolete term for ballooning *degeneration.*

reticulating c., obsolete term for reticular *degeneration.*

colliquative (ko-lik'wă-tiv). Denoting or characteristic of colliquation.

Collis, John Leighton, British thoracic surgeon, *1911. See C. *gastroplasty.*

collodion (ko-lō'dē-on). Collodium; a liquid made by dissolving pyroxylin or gun cotton in ether and alcohol; on evaporation it leaves a glossy contractile film; used as a protective for cuts or as a vehicle for the local application of medicinal substances.
blistering c., cantharidal c.
cantharidal c., c. vesicans; blistering c.; a powdered chloroform extract of cantharides in flexible c.; a vesicant.
flexible c., a mixture of camphor, castor oil, and c., or a mixture of castor oil, Canada turpentine, and c., used for the same purposes as c., but its film possesses the advantage, for certain conditions, of not contracting.
hemostatic c., styptic c.
iodized c., a 5% solution of iodine in flexible c.; a counterirritant.
salicylic acid c., salicylic acid and flexible c.; a keratolytic agent used in the treatment of corns and verrucae.
styptic c., styptic colloid; hemostatic c.; xylostyptic ether; tannic acid in flexible c.; an astringent and local hemostatic.
c. vesicans, cantharidal c.

collodium (ko-lō'dē-ŭm) [G. *kolla,* glue, + *eidos,* appearance]. Collodion.

colloid (kol'oyd) [G. *kolla,* glue, + *eidos,* appearance]. **1.** Aggregates of atoms or molecules in a finely divided state (submicroscopic), dispersed in a gaseous, liquid, or solid medium, and resisting sedimentation, diffusion, and filtration, thus differing from precipitates. See also hydrocolloid. **2.** Gluelike. **3.** Colloidin; a translucent, yellowish, homogeneous material of the consistency of glue, less fluid than mucoid or mucinoid, found in the cells and tissues in a state of c. degeneration. **4.** The stored secretion within follicles of the thyroid gland. For individual c.'s not listed below, see the specific name.
bovine c., conglutinin.
dispersion c., dispersoid.
emulsion c., emulsoid.
hydrophil c., hydrophilic c., emulsoid.
hydrophobic c., suspensoid.
irreversible c., unstable c.; a c. that is not again soluble in water after having been dried at ordinary temperature.
lyophilic c., emulsoid.
lyophobic c., suspensoid.
protective c., a c. that has the power of preventing the precipitation of suspensoids under the influence of an electrolyte.
reversible c., stable c.; a c. that is again soluble in water after having been dried at ordinary temperature.
stable c., reversible c.
styptic c., styptic *collodion.*
suspension c., suspensoid.
thyroid c., the semifluid material that occupies the lumen of thyroid follicles; it contains thyroglobulin mainly.
unstable c., irreversible c.

colloidal (ko-loyd'ăl). Denoting or characteristic of a colloid.

colloidin (ko-loy'din). Colloid (3).

colloidoclasia, colloidoclasis (ko-loy-dō-klā'sē-ă, -sis) [colloid + G. *klasis,* fracture]. Obsolete term for a rupture of the colloid equilibrium in the body.

colloidoclastic (ko-loy-dō-klas'tik). Obsolete term denoting colloidoclasia.

colloidogen (ko-loy'dō-jen). A substance capable of giving rise to a colloidal solution or suspension.

colloxylin (ko-lok'si-lin) [G. *kolla,* glue, + *xylinos,* woody, fr. *xylon,* wood]. Pyroxylin.

collum, pl. **colla** (kol'ŭm, kol'ă) [L.]. **1** [NA]. Neck (1); cervix (1); trachelos; the part between the shoulders or thorax and the head. **2.** A constricted or necklike portion of any organ or other anatomical structure.
c. anatom'icum hu'meri [NA], anatomical neck of humerus; a groove separating the head of the humerus from the tuberosities, giving attachment to the articular capsule.
c. chirur'gicum hu'meri [NA], surgical neck of humerus; the narrow portion below the head and tuberosities.
c. cos'tae [NA], neck of rib; the flattened portion of a rib between the head and the tuberosity.
c. den'tis, *cervix* dentis.
c. distor'tum, torticollis.
c. fem'oris, c. ossis femoris.
c. fib'ulae [NA], neck of fibula; the slightly constricted region between the head and body of the fibula.
c. folli'culi pi'li, neck of hair follicle; the narrowed part of the hair follicle between the hair bulb and the surface of the skin.
c. glan'dis pe'nis [NA], neck of glans penis; a constriction behind the corona glandis of the penis.
c. hu'meri, neck of humerus. See c. anatomicum humeri, c. chirurgicum humeri.
c. mal'lei [NA], neck of malleus; the constricted portion of the malleus between the head and the manubrium.
c. mandib'ulae [NA], neck of mandible; the constricted portion of the condylar process below the head of the mandible.
c. os'sis fem'oris [NA], neck of thigh bone; neck of femur; c. femoris; a short, constricted, strong bar projecting at an obtuse angle (about 125°) from the upper end of the shaft of the thigh bone and supporting its head.
c. ra'dii [NA], neck of radius; the narrow part of the shaft just below the head.
c. scap'ulae [NA], neck of scapula; a slight constriction marking the separation of that portion bearing the glenoid cavity and coracoid process from the remainder of the scapula.
c. ta'li [NA], neck of talus; a constriction separating the head, or anterior portion, from the body of the talus.
c. vesicae biliaris, c. vesicae felleae; neck of gallbladder; the narrow portion between the body of the gallbladder and beginning of the cystic duct.
c. ves'icae fel'leae [NA], c. vesicae biliaris.

collunarium (kol'yū-nā'rē-ŭm) [L. *col-luo* (*conl-*), to wash thoroughly, + *nares,* nostrils]. A nose wash; a nasal douche.

collutorium (kol-yū-tō'rē-ŭm) [Mod. L. fr. *col-luo,* pp. *-lutus,* to wash thoroughly]. Mouthwash.

collutory (kol'yū-tōr-ē) [L. *colluere,* to rinse]. Mouthwash.

Collyriclum (kol-ē-rik'lŭm). A genus of trematodes. *C. faba* causes the formation of subcutaneous cysts (cutaneous monostomiasis) in chickens, turkeys, and other birds.

collyrium (ko-lir'ē-ŭm) [G. *kollyrion,* poultice, eye salve]. Originally, any preparation for the eye; now, an eyewash.

colo- [G. *kolon,* colon]. Combining form relating to the colon.

coloboma (kol-ō-bō'mă) [G. *kolobōma,* lit., the part taken away in mutilation, fr. *koloboō,* to dock, mutilate]. Any defect, congenital, pathologic, or artificial, especially of the eye.
c. of choroid, a congenital defect of the choroid and retinal pigment epithelium exposing the sclera, which is usually situated below the optic disk in the region of fetal fissure.
Fuchs' c., congenital conus; a congenital crescent in the optic nerve not associated with myopia.
c. i'ridis, a congenital cleft of the iris, often associated with c. of the choroid, or the defect resulting from iridectomy. See fig. on p. 329.
c. len'tis, a segment of the lens equator devoid of zonular fibers, giving the appearance of a notch.
c. lo'buli, congenital fissure of the lobule of the ear.
macular c., a defect of the central retina as a result of arrested development or intrauterine retinal inflammation.
c. of optic nerve, a congenital notch in the formation of the optic

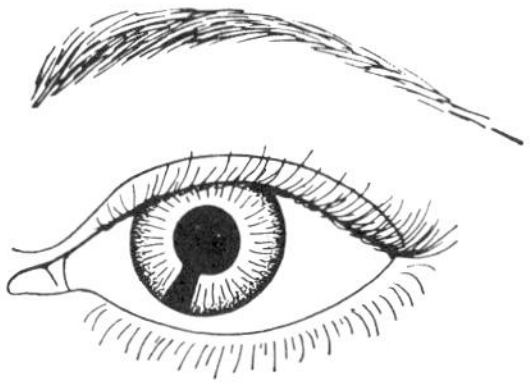

Coloboma Iridis

nerve, appearing as a craterlike excavation at the optic disk.

c. palpebra'le, a congenital notch in the eyelid margin.

c. of vitreous, a congenital indentation of the vitreous body by mesoderm; associated with severe myopia.

colocentesis (kō'lō-sen-tē'sis) [colo- + G. *kentēsis,* a puncture]. Colipuncture; colopuncture; puncture of the colon with a trochar or scalpel to relieve distention.

colocholecystostomy (kō'lō-kō-lē-sis-tos'tō-mē). Cholecystocolostomy.

colocolic (kō-lō-kol'ik). From colon to colon; said of a spontaneous or induced anastomosis between two parts of the colon.

colocolostomy (kō'lō-kō-los'tō-mē) [colo- + colo- + G. *stoma,* mouth]. Establishment of a communication between two noncontinuous segments of the colon.

colocynth (kol'ō-sinth) [G. *kolokynthē,* the round gourd or pumpkin]. Bitter apple; the peeled dried fruit of *Citrullus colcynthis* (family Cucurbitaceae), an herb of the sandy shores of the Mediterranean, resembling somewhat the watermelon plant; a hydrogogue cathartic.

colocystoplasty (kō-lō-sis'tō-plas-tē). Enlargement of the urinary bladder by attaching a segment of colon to it.

coloenteritis (kō'lō-en-ter-ī'tis). Enterocolitis.

colohepatopexy (kō-lō-hep'ă-tō-pek'sē) [colo- + G. *hēpar (hēpat-),* liver, + *pēxis,* fixation]. Attachment of the colon to the liver by adhesions.

cololysis (kō-lol'i-sis) [colo- + G. *lysis,* loosening]. Procedure of freeing the colon from adhesions.

colomba (kō-lom'bă). Calumba.

colominic acid (kol-ō-min'ik). Polymer of (α1,5)-*N*-acetylneuraminic acid; found in *Escherichia coli.*

colon (kō'lon) [G. *kolon*] [NA]. The division of the large intestine extending from the cecum to the rectum.

c. ascen'dens [NA], ascending c.; the portion of the c. between the ileocecal orifice and the right colic flexure.

ascending c., c. ascendens.

c. descen'dens [NA], descending c.; the part of the c. extending from the left colic flexure to the pelvic brim.

descending c., c. descendens.

giant c., megacolon.

iliac c., that portion of the descending c. which lies in the left iliac fossa, between the crest of the left ilium and the pelvic brim.

irritable c., tendency to colonic hyperperistalsis, sometimes with colicky pains and diarrhea.

lead-pipe c., the scarred rigid c. of advanced ulcerative colitis.

c. pelvi'num, c. sigmoideum.

sigmoid c., c. sigmoideum.

c. sigmoi'deum [NA], sigmoid c.; c. pelvinum; flexura sigmoidea; sigmoid flexure; S romanum; the part of the c. describing an S-shaped curve between the pelvic brim and the third sacral segment; it is continuous with the rectum.

transverse c., c. transversum.

c. transver'sum [NA], transverse c.; the part of the c. between the right and left colic flexures. It extends more or less transversely across the abdomen.

colonalgia (ko-lon-al'jē-ă) [colon + G. *algos,* pain]. Pain in the colon.

colonic (ko-lon'ik). Relating to the colon.

colonization (kol'on-i-zā'shŭn). **1.** Innidiation. **2.** The formation of compact population groups of the same type of microorganism, as the colonies that develop when a bacterial cell begins reproducing. **3.** The care of certain persons, *e.g.,* lepers, mental patients, in community groups.

genetic c., propagation of a gene by a host into which the gene has been introduced, naturally or artificially.

colonogram (ko-lon'ō-gram). Graphic recording of movements of the colon.

colonometer (kō'lō-nom'ĕ-ter). A device for counting bacterial colonies.

colonopathy (kō-lon-ap'ă-thē). Colopathy; any disordered condition of the colon.

colonorrhagia (kō-lon-ō-rā'jē-ă). Colorrhagia.

colonorrhea (kō'lon-ō-rē'ă). Colorrhea.

colonoscope (kō-lon'ō-skōp). An elongated endoscope, usually fiberoptic.

colonoscopy (kō-lon-os'kō-pē) [colon + G. *skopeō,* to view]. Coloscopy; visual examination of the inner surface of the colon by means of a colonoscope.

colony (kol'ō-nē) [L. *colonia,* a colony]. **1.** A group of cells growing on a solid nutrient surface, each arising from the multiplication of an individual cell; a clone. **2.** A group of people with similar interests, living in a particular location or area.

daughter c., a secondary c. growing on the surface of an older c.; it is smaller and may have characteristics different from those of the mother c.

filamentous c., in bacteriology, a c. composed of long, interwoven, irregularly disposed threads.

Gheel c., a c. in Gheel, Belgium, originating in the 13th century, for the informal communal care, in private homes, of severely mentally disordered persons.

H c. [Ger. *Hauch,* breath], a c. of motile organisms forming a thin film of growth. *Cf.* O c.

lenticular c., a bacterial c. shaped like a lentil or a double-convex lens.

mother c., a c. which gives rise to a secondary c. (a daughter c.), the latter growing on the surface of the former; the mother c. is larger than the daughter c., and the characteristics of the c.'s may differ.

mucoid c., a c. showing viscous or sticky growth typical of an organism producing large quantities of a carbohydrate capsule.

O c. [Ger. *ohne Hauch,* without breath], growth of a nonmotile bacterium in discrete, compact c.'s in contrast to a film of growth produced by some motile bacteria. *Cf.* H c.

rough c., a bacterial c. with a granular, flattened surface; this type of c. is usually associated with loss of virulence with respect to that of smooth c.'s.

smooth c., a bacterial c. with a glistening, rounded surface; this type of c. is usually associated with increased virulence with respect to that of rough c.'s.

spheroid c., a c. of protozoa in which the individual cells are held together in a coherent spherical mass by a gelatinoid material.

colopathy (kō-lop'ă-thē). Colonopathy.

colopexostomy (kō'lō-peks-os'tō-mē) [colo- + G. *pēxis,* fixation, + *stoma,* mouth]. Establishment of an artificial anus by creation of an opening into the colon after its fixation to the abdominal wall.

colopexotomy (kō'lō-pek-sot'ō-mē) [colo- + G. *pēxis,* fixation, + *tomē,* incision]. Incision into the colon after its fixation to the abdominal wall.

colopexy (kol'ō-pek-sē) [colo- + G. *pēxis,* fixation]. Obsolete term for attachment of a portion of the colon to the abdominal wall.

colophony (kō-lof'ō-nē) [*Colophōn,* Summit, a town in Ionia]. Rosin.

coloplication (kō'lō-pli-kā'shŭn) [colo- + Mod. L. *plica,* fold]. Reduction of the lumen of a dilated colon by making folds or tucks in its walls.

coloproctia (kō-lō-prok'shē-ă). Colostomy.

coloproctitis (kō'lō-prok-tī'tis) [colo- + G. *prōktos,* anus (rectum), + *-itis,* inflammation]. Colorectitis; proctocolitis; rectocolitis; inflammation of both colon and rectum.

coloproctostomy (kō'lō-prok-tos'tō-mē) [colo- + G. *prōktos,* anus (rectum), + *stoma,* mouth]. Colorectostomy; establishment of a communication between the rectum and a discontinuous segment of the colon.

coloptosis, coloptosia (kō-lop-tō'sis, -tō'sē-ă) [colo- + G. *ptōsis,* a falling]. Coleoptosis; downward displacement, or prolapse, of the colon, especially of the transverse portion.

colopuncture (kō-lō-pŭnk'chūr). Colocentesis.

color (kŭl'ŏr) [L.]. **1.** That aspect of the appearance of objects and light sources that may be specified as to hue, lightness (brightness), and saturation. **2.** That portion of the visible (370-760 nm) electromagnetic spectrum specified as to wavelength, luminosity, and purity.

complementary c.'s, pairs of different colors of light that produce white light when combined.

confusion c.'s, a set of c.'s (usually of colored wools), cream, buff, pale blue, gray, brown, green, violet, etc., used in tests for c. blindness.

extrinsic c., c. applied to the external surface of a dental prosthesis.

incidental c., a c. the impression of which remains after removal of the source. See also afterimage.

intrinsic c., the addition of c. pigment within the material of a dental prosthesis.

opponent c., pairs of c. that share c. channels in the retina (red-green, blue-yellow, black-white).

primary c., simple c.; the three c.'s of the retinal cone pigments (red, green, blue) that may be combined to match any hue.

pure c., a visual sensation produced by light of a specific wavelength.

reflected c.'s, those c.'s seen in light falling upon a pigmented surface.

saturated c., a c. containing a minimum amount of whiteness.

simple c., primary c.

tone c., timbre.

colorectal (kol'ō-rek'tăl). Relating to the colon and rectum, or to the entire large bowel.

colorectitis (kō'lō-rek-tī'tis). Coloproctitis.

colorectostomy (kō'lō-rek-tos'tō-mē). Coloproctostomy.

colorimeter (kŏl-er-im'ĕ-ter). Chromatometer; chromometer; an optical device for determining the color and/or intensity of the color of a liquid.

Duboscq's c., an apparatus for measuring the depth of tint in a fluid by comparing it with a standard fluid; glass cylinders are immersed in each of two cups containing, one the standard fluid, the other the fluid to be tested; on looking through the cylinders the tints are equalized by raising or lowering the cylinder in one cup, and the extent of this raising or lowering is indicated on a scale and gives the exact difference in tint.

colorimetric (kŏl-er-i-met'rik). Relating to colorimetry.

colorimetry (kol-er-im'ĕ-trē). A procedure for quantitative chemical analysis, based on comparison of the color developed in a solution of the test material with that in a standard solution; the two solutions are observed simultaneously in a colorimeter, and quantitated on the basis of the absorption of light.

color match. The result of adjusting color mixtures until all visually apparent differences are minimal.

colorrhagia (kō-lō-rā'jē-ă) [colo- + G. *rhēgnymi,* to burst forth]. Colonorrhagia; an abnormal discharge from the colon.

colorrhaphy (kō-lōr'ă-fē) [colo- + G. *rhaphē,* suture]. Suture of the colon.

colorrhea (kō-lō-rē'ă) [colo- + G. *rhoia,* a flow]. Colonorrhea; diarrhea thought to originate from a condition confined to or affecting chiefly the colon.

color solid. A schematic arrangement of color in space, the attributes of hue, saturation, and brightness being represented by cylindrical coordinates.

coloscopy (kō-los'kŏ-pē) [colo- + G. *skopeō,* to view]. Colonoscopy.

colosigmoidostomy (kō'lō-sig-moy-dos'kŏ-pē). Establishment of an anastomosis between any other part of the colon and the sigmoid colon.

colostomy (kō-los'tō-mē) [colo- + G. *stoma,* mouth]. Colopractia; establishment of an artificial cutaneous opening into the colon.

colostration (kō-los-trā'shŭn). Infantile diarrhea attributed to the action of the colostrum.

colostric (kō-los'trik). Relating to the colostrum.

colostrorrhea (kō-los-trōr-rē'ă) [colostrum, + G. *rhoia,* flow]. Abnormally profuse secretion of colostrum.

colostrous (kō-los'trŭs). Containing colostrum.

colostrum (kō-los'trŭm) [L.]. Foremilk; a thin white opalescent fluid, the first milk secreted at the termination of pregnancy; it differs from the milk secreted later by containing more lactalbumin and lactoprotein; c. is also rich in antibodies which confer passive immunity to the newborn.

colotomy (kō-lot'ō-mē) [colo- + G. *tomē,* incision]. Laparocolotomy; incision into the colon.

Colour Index (C.I.). A publication concerned with the chemistry of dyes, with each listed dye identified by a five-digit C.I. number, *e.g.,* methylene blue is C.I. 52015.

colp-. See colpo-.

colpatresia (kol-pa-trē'zēă) [colp- + G. *atrētos,* imperforate]. Vaginal *atresia.*

colpectasis, colpectasia (kol-pek'tă-sis, -pek-tā'sis) [colp- + G. *aktasis,* stretching]. Distention of the vagina.

colpectomy (kol-pek'tō-mē) [colp- + G. *ektomē,* excision]. Vaginectomy.

colpitis (kol-pī'tis) [colp- + G. *-itis,* inflammation]. Obsolete term for vaginitis.

c. mycot'ica, vaginomycosis.

colpo-, colp- [G. *kolpos,* any fold or hollow; specifically, the vagina]. Combining forms denoting the vagina. See also vagino-, vagin-.

colpocele (kol'pō-sēl) [colpo- + G. *kēlē,* hernia]. **1.** Vaginocele; coleocele; a hernia projecting into the vagina. **2.** Colpoptosis.

colpocleisis (kol-pō-klī'sis) [colpo- + G. *kleisis,* closure]. Operation for obliterating the lumen of the vagina.

colpocystitis (kol'pō-sis-tī'tis) [colpo- + G. *kystis,* bladder, + *-itis,* inflammation]. Obsolete term for inflammation of both vagina and bladder.

colpocystocele (kol-pō-sis'tō-sēl) [colpo- + G. *kystis,* bladder, + *kēlē,* hernia]. Cystocele.

colpocystoplasty (kol-pō-sis'tō-plas-tē) [colpo- + G. *kystis,* bladder, + *plastos,* formed]. Plastic surgery to repair the vesicovaginal wall.

colpocystotomy (kol'pō-sis-tot'ō-mē) [colpo- + G. *kystis,* bladder, + *tomē,* incision]. Incision into the bladder through the vagina.

colpocystoureterotomy (kol'pō-sis'tō-yū-rē-ter-ot'ō-mē) [colpo- + G. *kystis,* bladder, + *ourēter,* ureter, + *tomē,* incision]. Incision into the ureter by way of the vagina and the bladder.

colpodynia (kol-pō-din'ē-ă) [colpo- + G. *odynē,* pain]. Vaginodynia.

colpohyperplasia (kol'pō-hī-per-plā'zē-ă) [colpo- + hyperplasia]. Obsolete term for a condition marked by thickening of the vaginal mucous membrane.
c. cys'tica, c. emphysemato'sa, obsolete terms for *vaginitis* emphysematosa.

colpohysterectomy (kol'pō-his-ter-ek'tō-mē) [colpo- + G. *hystera,* uterus, + *ektomē,* excision]. Vaginal *hysterectomy.*

colpohysteropexy (kol-pō-his'ter-ō-pek-sē) [colpo- + G. *hystera,* uterus, + *pēxis,* fixation]. Operation for fixation of the uterus performed through the vagina.

colpohysterotomy (kol'pō-his-ter-ot'ō-mē) [colpo- + G. *hystera,* uterus, + *tomē,* incision]. Vaginal *hysterotomy.*

colpomicroscope (kol-pō-mī'krō-skōp). Special microscope for direct visual examination of the cervical tissue.

colpomicroscopy (kol'pō-mī-kros'kō-pē). Direct observation and study of cells in the vagina and cervix magnified *in vivo,* in the undisturbed tissue, by means of a colpomicroscope.

colpomycosis (kol'pō-mī-kō'sis). Vaginomycosis.

colpomyomectomy (kol'pō-mī-ō-mek'tō-mē) [colpo- + myoma + G. *ektomē,* excision]. Vaginal *myomectomy.*

colpopathy (kol-pop'ă-thē) [colpo- + G. *pathos,* suffering]. Vaginopathy.

colpoperineoplasty (kol'pō-pār-i-nē'ō-plas-tē) [colpo- + perineum, + G. *plastos,* formed]. Vaginoperineoplasty.

colpoperineorrhaphy (kol'pō-pār-i-nē-ōr'ă-fē) [colpo- + perineum, + G. *rhaphē,* sewing]. Vaginoperineorrhaphy.

colpopexy (kol'pō-pek-sē) [colpo- + G. *pēxis,* fixation]. Vaginofixation.

colpoplasty (kol'pō-plas-tē) [colpo- + G. *plastos,* formed]. Vaginoplasty.

colpopoiesis (kol'pō-poy-ē'sis) [colpo- + G. *poiēsis,* a making]. Surgical construction of a vagina.

colpoptosis, colpoptosia (kol-pō-tō'sis, kol-pop-tō'sis, -tō'sē-ă) [colpo- + G. *ptōsis,* a falling]. Colpocele (2); prolapse of the vaginal walls.

colporectopexy (kol-pō-rek'tō-pek-sē) [colpo- + rectum + G. *pēxis,* fixation]. Repair of a prolapsed rectum by suturing it to the wall of the vagina.

colporrhagia (kol-pō-rā'jē-ă) [colpo-+ G. *rhēgnymi,* to burst forth]. A vaginal hemorrhage.

colporrhaphy (kol-pōr'ă-fē) [colpo- + G. *rhaphē,* suture]. Repair of a rupture of the vagina by excision and suturing of the edges of the tear.

colporrhexis (kol-pō-rek'sis) [colpo- + G. *rhēxis,* rupture]. Vaginal laceration; tearing of the vaginal wall.

colposcope (kol'pō-skōp). Endoscopic instrument that magnifies cells of the vagina and cervix *in vivo* to allow direct observation and study of these tissues.

colposcopy (kol-pos'kō-pē) [colpo- + G. *skopeō,* to view]. Examination of vagina and cervix by means of an endoscope.

colpospasm (kol'pō-spazm). Spasmodic contraction of the vagina.

colpostat (kol'pō-stat) [colpo- + G. *statos,* standing]. Appliance for use in the vagina, such as a radium applicator, for treatment of cancer of the cervix.

colpostenosis (kol'pō-sten-ō'sis) [colpo- + G. *stenōsis,* narrowing]. Narrowing of the lumen of the vagina.

colpostenotomy (kol'pō-sten-ot'ō-mē) [colpo- + G. *stenōsis,* narrowing, + *tomē,* incision]. Surgical correction of a colpostenosis.

colpot'omy (kol-pot'ō-mē) [colpo- + G. *tomē,* incision]. Vaginotomy.

colpoureterotomy (kol'pō-yū-rē-ter-ot'ō-mē) [colpo- + G. *tomē,* incision]. Incision into a ureter through the vagina.

colpoxerosis (kol-pō-zē-rō'sis) [colpo- + G. *xērōsis,* dryness]. Abnormal dryness of the vaginal mucous membrane.

Colubridae (kol-yū'bri-dē) [L. *coluber,* serpent]. A family of largely nonpoisonous or mildly poisonous snakes comprising over 1000 species, found in North and South America, Asia, and Africa; some have small grooved fangs in the rear of the jaws.

columbin (ko-lŭm'bin). Calumbin.

columbium (Cb) (kol-ŭm'bē-ŭm) [*Columbia*]. Former name for niobium.

columbo (ko-lŭm'bō). Calumba.

columella, pl. **columellae** (kol-ū-mel'ă, -mel'ē) [L. dim. of *columna,* column]. **1.** Columnella; a column, or a small column. **2.** In fungi, a sterile invagination of a sporangium, as in Zygomycetes (Phycomycetes).
c. au'ris, the middle ear ossicle of amphibians, reptiles, and birds; homologous with the stapes of mammals.
c. coch'leae, modiolus.
c. na'si, the lower margin of the septum nasi.

column (kol'ŭm) [L. *columna*]. Columna. **1.** An anatomical part or structure in the form of a pillar or cylindric funiculus. See also fasciculus. **2.** A vertical object (usually cylindrical), mass, or formation.
affinity c., affinity *chromatography.*
anal c.'s, *columnae* anales.
anterior c. of medulla oblongata, *pyramis* medullae oblongatae.
anterior c. of spinal cord, *columna* anterior.
anterolateral c. of spinal cord, *funiculus* lateralis.
Bertin's c.'s, *columnae* renales.
branchial efferent c., special visceral or splanchnic efferent c.; a c. of gray matter in the brainstem of the embryo, represented in the adult by the nucleus ambiguus and the motor nuclei of the trigeminal and facial nerves.
Burdach's c., *fasciculus* cuneatus.
Clarke's c., *nucleus* thoracicus.
dorsal c. of spinal cord, *columna* posterior.
c. of fornix, *columna* fornicis.
general somatic afferent c., in the embryo, a c. of gray matter in the hindbrain and upper segments of the spinal cord, represented in the adult by the sensory nuclei of the trigeminal nerve.
general somatic efferent c., a c. of gray matter in the embryo, represented in the adult by the nuclei of oculomotor, trochlear, abducens, and hypoglossal nerves.
general visceral or **splanchnic afferent c.,** a c. of gray matter in the hindbrain of the embryo, developing into the nucleus of the solitary tract.
general visceral or **splanchnic efferent c.,** a c. of gray matter in the hindbrain of the embryo, represented in the adult by the dorsal nucleus of the vagus, the superior and inferior salivatory nuclei, and the Edinger-Westphal nucleus.
Goll's c., *fasciculus* gracilis.
Gowers' c., *tractus* spinocerebellaris anterior.
gray c.'s, *columnae* griseae.
intermediolateral cell c. of spinal cord, *nucleus* intermediolateralis.
lateral c. of spinal cord, *columna* lateralis.

Morgagni's c.'s, *columnae* anales.
posterior c. of spinal cord, **(1)** *columna* posterior; **(2)** in clinical parlance, the term often refers to the funiculus posterior of the spinal cord's white matter.
rectal c.'s, *columnae* anales.
renal c.'s, *columnae* renales.
Rolando's c., a slight ridge on either side of the medulla oblongata related to the descending trigeminal tract and nucleus.
Sertoli's c.'s, see Sertoli's *cells.*
special somatic afferent c., a c. of gray matter in the hindbrain of the embryo, represented in the adult by the nuclei of the auditory and vestibular nerves.
special visceral or **splanchnic efferent c.,** branchial efferent c.
spinal c., *columna* vertebralis.
Stilling's c., *nucleus* thoracicus.
Türck's c., *tractus* pyramidalis anterior.
vaginal c.'s, *columnae* rugarum.
ventral c. of spinal cord, *columna* anterior.
vertebral c., *columna* vertebralis.

columna, gen. and pl. **columnae** (ko-lŭm'nă, -nē) [L.] [NA]. Column.
colum'nae ana'les [NA], anal or rectal columns; Morgagni's columns; a number of vertical ridges in the mucous membrane of the upper half of the anal canal.
c. ante'rior [NA], anterior or ventral column of the spinal cord; the pronounced, ventrally oriented ridge of gray matter in each half of the spinal cord; it corresponds to the anterior or ventral horn appearing in transverse sections of the cord, and contains the motor neurons innervating the skeletal musculature of the trunk, neck, and extremities. See also columnae griseae.
colum'nae car'neae, *trabeculae* carneae.
c. for'nicis [NA], column of the fornix; anterior pillar of the fornix; that part of the fornix that curves down in front of the thalamus and the interventricular foramen of Monro, then continues through the gray matter of the hypothalamus to the mamillary body; consisting primarily of fibers originating in the hippocampus and subiculum, the c. fornicis is the direct continuation of the corpus fornicis.
columnae gris'eae [NA], gray columns; the three somewhat ridge-shaped masses of gray matter (c. anterior, posterior, and lateralis) that extend longitudinally through the center of each lateral half of the spinal cord; in transverse sections these columns appear as gray horns and are therefore commonly called ventral or anterior, dorsal or posterior, and lateral horn, respectively.
c. latera'lis [NA], lateral column of spinal cord; a slight protrusion of the gray matter of the spinal cord into the lateral funiculus of either side, especially marked in the thoracic region where it encloses preganglionic motor neurons of the sympathetic division of the autonomic nervous system; it corresponds to the lateral horn appearing in transverse sections of the spinal cord. See also columnae griseae.
c. na'si, the fleshy termination of the septum nasi.
c. poste'rior [NA], posterior or dorsal column of the spinal cord; the pronounced, dorsolaterally oriented ridge of gray matter in each lateral half of the spinal cord, corresponding to the posterior or dorsal horn appearing in transverse sections of the cord. See also *columnae* griseae.
colum'nae rena'les [NA], renal columns; Bertin's columns; the prolongations of cortical substance separating the pyramids of the kidney.
colum'nae ruga'rum [NA], vaginal columns; two slight longitudinal ridges, anterior and posterior, in the vaginal mucous membrane, each marked by a number of transverse mucosal folds.
c. vertebra'lis [NA], vertebral or spinal column; spina or spine (2); backbone; rachis; vertebrarium; spina dorsalis; dorsal spine; the series of vertebrae that extend from the cranium to the coccyx, providing support and forming a flexible bony case for the spinal cord.

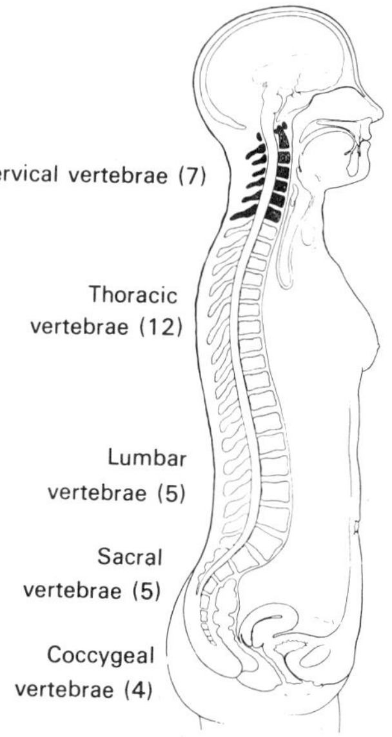

Columna Vertebralis
Adult vertebral column, shown in relation to the body.

columnella, pl. **columnellae** (ko-lŭm-nel'ă, -nel'ē) [L. dim. of *columna,* a column; another form of *columella*]. Columella (1).

colypeptic (kō-lē-pep'tik) [G. *kōlyō,* to hinder, + *pepsis,* digestion]. Rarely used term for retarding digestion.

com-. See con-.

coma (kō'mă) [G. *kōma,* deep sleep]. A state of profound unconsciousness from which one cannot be roused; may be due to the action of an ingested toxic substance or of one formed in the body, to trauma, or to disease.
c. carcinomato'sum, c. occurring in the final stage of cancerous cachexia.
diabetic c., Kussmaul's c.; c. that develops in severe and inadequately treated cases of diabetes mellitus and is commonly fatal, unless appropriate therapy is instituted promptly; results from reduced oxidative metabolism of the central nervous system that, in turn, stems from severe ketoacidosis and possibly also from the histotoxic action of the ketone bodies and disturbances in water and electrolyte balance.
hepatic c., c. occurring in advanced cirrhosis, hepatitis, poisoning, or other severe liver disease; may be preceded by neurologic abnormalities such as flapping tremor, mental confusion, or delirium; severe jaundice and acute disorders of ammonia, nitrogen, and amino acid metabolism may be present.
hyperosmolar hyperglycemic nonketonic c., c. in which blood glucose concentration is increased but without the presence of ketone bodies in plasma, largely as a result of dehydration of brain tissues due to high serum plasma osmolality caused by the high blood glucose concentration.
Kussmaul's c., diabetic c.
metabolic c., c. as the result of disorders of the neuronal mechanisms of energy transfer or of impairment or deprivation of the energy sources.
thyrotoxic c., c. preceding death in severe hyperthyroidism, as in thyroid storm or thyrotoxic crisis.
trance c., lethargic *hypnosis.*

comatose (kō'mă-tōs). In a state of coma.

combination (kom-bi-nā'shŭn). **1.** The act of combining (*i.e.,* by joining, uniting, or otherwise bringing into close association) separate entities. **2.** The state of being so combined.
binary c., the name of a species of bacteria consisting of two parts: a generic name and a specific epithet.
new c. (comb. nov.), the new name that results from the transfer of a microorganism from one genus to another; the generic name changes but, in most cases, the specific epithet remains the same.

combustible (kom-bus'ti-bl). Capable of combustion.

combustion (kom-bŭs'chŭn) [L. *comburo,* pp. *-bustus,* to burn up]. Burning, the rapid oxidation of any substance accompanied by the production of heat and light.
slow c., see decay.
spontaneous c., the ignition of a mass of material by heat developed within it by the oxidation of the substances composing it without external ignition.

Comby, Jules, Paris pediatrician, 1853–1947. See C.'s *sign.*

comedo, pl. **comedos, comedones** (kom'ē-dō, kō-mē'dō; kom'ē-dōz, kom -ē-dō'nēz) [L. a glutton, fr. *com-edo,* to eat up]. A dilated hair follicle infundibulum filled with keratin, squamae, and sebum; the primary lesion of acne vulgaris.
closed c., whitehead (2); a c. with a narrow or obstructed opening on the skin surface; closed c.'s may rupture, producing a low-grade dermal inflammatory reaction.
open c., blackhead (1); a c. with a wide opening on the skin surface capped with a blackened mass of epithelial debris.

comedocarcinoma (kō-mē'dō-kar-si-nō'mă). Form of carcinoma of the breast in which plugs of necrotic malignant cells may be expressed from the ducts.

comedogenic (kom'ē-dō-jen'ik) [comedo + G. *genesis,* production]. Tending to promote the formation of comedones.

comes, pl. **comites** (kō'mēz, kom'i-tēz) [L. a companion, fr. *com-,* together, + *eo,* pp. *itus,* to go]. A blood vessel accompanying another vessel or a nerve; the veins accompanying an artery, often two in number, are called venae comitantes or venae comites.

comitance (kom'i-tăns). Concomitance.

commensal (kŏ-men'săl). **1.** Pertaining to or characterized by commensalism. **2.** An organism participating in commensalism.

commensalism (kŏ-men'săl-izm). [L. *con-,* with, together, + *mensa,* table]. A symbiotic relationship in which one species derives benefit and the other is unharmed; *e.g., Entamoeba coli* in the human large intestine. *Cf.* metabiosis, mutualism, parasitism.
epizoic c., phoresis (2).

comminuted (kom'i-nū-ted) [L. *com-minuo,* pp. *-minutus,* to make smaller, break into pieces, fr. *minor,* less]. Broken into several pieces; denoting especially a fractured bone.

comminution (kom-i-nū'shŭn). A breaking into several pieces.

commissura, gen, and pl. **commissurae** (kom-i-syūr'ă, -yūr'ē) [L. a joining together, seam, fr. *com- mitto,* to send together, combine] [NA]. Commissure. **1.** Angle or corner of the eye, lips, or labia. **2.** A bundle of nerve fibers passing from one side to the other in the brain or spinal cord.
c. al'ba [NA], white or anterior white commissure; c. ventralis alba; a narrow band of white substance bordering on the anterior median fissure of the spinal cord in front of the anterior gray commissure, and consisting of nerve fibers crossing over from one half of the spinal cord to the other.
c. ante'rior [NA], anterior commissure; a round bundle of nerve fibers that crosses the midline of the brain near the anterior limit of the third ventricle. It consists of a smaller pars anterior, the fibers of which pass in part to the olfactory bulbs, and a larger pars posterior, which interconnects the left and right temporal lobes.
c. ante'rior gris'ea, see *substantia* intermedia centralis et lateralis.
c. bulbor'um, commissura of bulb; pars intermedia bulborum; a narrow median band that connects the two masses of erectile tissue (the bulbus vestibuli) on either side of the vaginal orifice.
c. cine'rea, *adhesio* interthalamica.
c. for'nicis [NA], commissure of the fornix; hippocampal commissure; commissura hippocampi; transverse fornix; delta fornicis; psalterium (1); the triangular subcallosal plate of commissural fibers resulting from the converging of the right and left fornix bundles which exchange numerous fibers and which curve back in the contralateral fornix to end in the hippocampus of the opposite side.
c. gris'ea, **(1)** *adhesio* interthalamica; **(2)** see *substantia* intermedia centralis et lateralis.
c. habenula'rum [NA], commissure of the habenulae; habenular commissure; the connection between the right and left habenular nuclei; the decussation of fibers of the two striae medullares, forming the dorsal portion of the peduncle of the pineal body.
c. hippocam'pi, c. fornicis.
c. labio'rum [NA], commissure or junction of lips; the junction of the lips lateral to the angle of the mouth.
c. labio'rum ante'rior [NA], anterior labial commissure; the junction of the labia majora anteriorly at the mons pubis.
c. labio'rum poste'rior [NA], posterior labial commissure; a slight fold uniting the labia majora posteriorly in front of the anus.
c. palpebra'rum latera'lis [NA], lateral palpebral commissure; the union of the upper and lower eyelids adjacent to the lateral angle.
c. palpebra'rum media'lis [NA], medial palpebral commissure; the union of the upper and lower eyelids adjacent to the medial angle.
c. poste'rior cer'ebri [NA], posterior cerebral commissure; a thin band of white matter, crossing from side to side beneath the habenula of the pineal body and over the aditus ad aqueductum cerebri; it is largely composed of fibers interconnecting the left and right pretectal region and related cell groups of the midbrain; dorsally, it marks the junction of the diencephalon and mesencephalon.
c. poste'rior gris'ea, see *substantia* intermedia centralis et lateralis.
commissu'rae supraop'ticae [NA], supraoptic commissures; commissures of Ganser, Gudden, and Meynert; the commissural fibers that lie above and behind the optic chiasm.
c. ventra'lis al'ba, c. alba.

commissural (kom-i-syūr'ăl). Relating to a commissure.

commissure (kom'i-syūr). Commissura.
anterior c., *commissura* anterior.
anterior labial c., *commissura* labiorum anterior.
anterior white c., *commissura* alba.
c. of bulb., *commissura* bulborum.
c. of cerebral hemispheres, *corpus* callosum.
c. of fornix, *commissura* fornicis.
Ganser's c.'s, *commissurae* supraopticae.
Gudden's c.'s, *commissurae* supraopticae.
c. of habenulae, *commissura* habenularum.
habenular c., *commissura* habenularum.
hippocampal c., *commissura* fornicis.
lateral palpebral c., *commissura* palpebrarum lateralis.
c. of lips, *commissura* labiorum.
medial palpebral c., *commissura* palpebrarum medialis.
Meynert's c.'s, *commissurae* supraopticae.
posterior cerebral c., *commissura* posterior cerebri.
posterior labial c., *commissura* labiorum posterior.
supraoptic c.'s, *commissurae* supraopticae.
Wernekinck's c., the decussation of the brachia conjunctiva before their entrance into the red nucleus of the tegmentum.
white c., *commissura* alba.

commissurotomy (kom'i-syūr-ot'ō-mē). **1.** Surgical division of any commissure, fibrous band, or ring. **2.** Midline *myelotomy.*
mitral c., opening the narrowed mitral orifice for the relief of mitral stenosis.

commitment (kŏ-mit′ment) [L. *com-mitto,* to deliver, consign]. Legal consignment, by certification, of an individual to a mental hospital or institution.

commotio (kō-mō′shē-ō) [L. a moving, commotion, fr. *com-moveo,* pp. *-motus,* to set in motion, agitate]. Concussion (2).
c. cer′ebri, brain *concussion.*
c. spina′lis, spinal *concussion.*

communicable (kŏ-myūn′i-kă-bl). Capable of being communicated or transmitted; said especially of disease.

communicans, pl. **communicantes** (kŏ-myū′ni-kans, kŏ-myū-ni-kan′tēz) [L. pres. p. of *communico,* pp. *-atus,* to share with some-one, make common]. Communicating; connecting or joining.

communication (kŏ-myū-ni-kā′shŭn) [L. *communicatio*]. **1.** An opening or connecting passage between two structures. **2.** In anatomy, a joining or connecting, said of fibrous, solid structures, *e.g.,* tendons and nerves. Anastomosis is incorrectly used as a synonym.

community (kŏ-myū′ni-tē). A given segment of a society or a population.
biotic c., biocenosis.
therapeutic c., a specially structured mental hospital or community health center milieu that provides an effective environment for behavioral changes in patients through resocialization and rehabilitation.

Comolli, Antonio, Italian pathologist, *1879. See C.'s *sign.*

comorbidity (kō-mōr-bid′i-tē). A concomitant but unrelated pathologic or disease process; usually used in epidemiology to indicate the coexistence of two or more disease processes.

compacta (kom-pak′tă). *Stratum* compactum.

compages thoracis (kom-pā′jēz thō-rā′sis) [NA]. Thoracic cage; the skeleton of the thorax consisting of the thoracic vertebrae, ribs, costal cartilages, and sternum.

comparascope (kom-par′ă-skōp) [L. *comparo,* to compare, + G. *skopeō,* to view]. A microscope accessory by means of which an observer may directly compare simultaneously the findings in two microscopic preparations.

compatibility (kom-pat-ĭ-bil′i-tē). The condition of being compatible.

compatible (kom-pat′ĭ-bl) [L. *con-,* with, + *patior,* to suffer]. **1.** Capable of being mixed without undergoing destructive chemical change or exhibiting mutual antagonism; said of the elements in a properly constructed pharmaceutical mixture. **2.** Denoting the ability of two biologic entities to exist together without nullification of, or deleterious effects on, the function of either; *e.g.,* blood, tissues, or organs that cause no reaction when transfused or no rejection when transplanted. **3.** Denoting satisfactory relationships in marriage or in sexual activities.

compensation (kom-pen-sā′shŭn) [L. *com-penso,* pp. *-atus,* to weigh together, counterbalance]. **1.** A process in which a tendency for a change in a given direction is counteracted by another change so that the original change is not evident. **2.** An unconscious mechanism by which one tries to make up for fancied or real deficiencies.
depth c., in echocardiography, control in the gain of the amplifier, to alter echo amplitude from varying depths. See time-varied gain *control.*
gene dosage c., the putative mechanism that adjusts the X-linked phenotypes of males and females to compensate for the haploid state in males and the diploid state in females.

compensatory (kom-pen′să-tōr-ē). Providing compensation; making up for a deficiency or loss.

competence (kom′pĕ-tens). **1.** The quality of being competent or capable of performing an allotted function. **2.** Integrity; especially the normal tight closure of a cardiac valve. **3.** The ability of a group of embryonic cells to respond to an organizer. **4.** The ability of a (bacterial) cell to take up free DNA, which may lead to transformation. **5.** In psychiatry, the mental ability to distinguish right from wrong and to manage one's own affairs.
cardiac c., ability of the ventricles to pump the blood returning to the atria, so that atrial pressure does not rise abnormally.
immunological c., immunocompetence.

competition (kom-pĕ-tish′ŭn). The process by which the activity or presence of one substance interferes with, or suppresses, the activity of another substance with similar affinities.
antigenic c., c. that occurs when two different antigens, each of which can evoke an immunological response when inoculated alone, are mixed in equal quantities and inoculated together; the response may be to only one, that to the other being largely or entirely suppressed.

complaint (kom-plānt′). A disorder, disease, or symptom, or the description of it.

complement (kom′plĕ-ment) [L. *complementum,* that which completes, fr. *com-pleo,* to fill up]. Ehrlich's term for the thermolabile substance, normally present in serum, that is destructive to certain bacteria and other cells sensitized by a specific complement-fixing antibody. C. is a serum protein complex, the activity of which is effected by a series of interactions resulting in enzymatic cleavages and which can follow one or the other of at least two pathways. In the case of immune hemolysis, the complex comprises nine components (designated C1 through C9) which react in a definite sequence and the activation of which is effected by the antigen-antibody complex; only the first seven components are involved in chemotaxis, and only the first four are involved in immune adherence or phagocytosis or are fixed by conglutinins. An alternative pathway (see properdin *system*) is activated by factors other than antigen-antibody complexes and involves components other than C1, C4, and C2 in the activation of C3. See also *component* of c.

complementarity (kom-plĕ-men-tār′i-tē). **1.** The degree of base-pairing (A opposite U or T, G opposite C) between two sequences of DNA and/or RNA molecules. **2.** The degree of affinity, or fit, of antigen and antibody combining sites.

complementation (kom′plĕ-men-tā′shŭn). **1.** Functional interaction between two defective viruses permitting replication under conditions inhibitory to the single virus. **2.** Interaction between two genetic units, one or both of which are defective, permitting the organism containing these units to function normally, whereas it could not do so if one unit were absent.
intergenic c., c. between pieces of genetic material which regulate the same function, such as a multienzyme pathway, but which have defects in regions of separate genetic function; such c. permits synthesis of normal end-product.
intragenic c., c. between pieces of genetic material, each of which has a different defect within the same gene; the resultant product of each is defective and nonfunctional, but the defective products may associate to produce a product which has some activity.

complex (kom′pleks) [L. *complexus,* woven together]. **1.** An organized constellation of feelings, thoughts, perceptions, and memories which may be in part unconscious and may strongly influence associations and attitudes. **2.** In chemistry, the relatively stable combination of two or more compounds into a larger molecule without covalent binding. **3.** A composite of chemical or immunological structures. **4.** A structural anatomical entity made up of three or more interrelated parts. **5.** An informal term used to denote a group of individual structures known or believed to be anatomically, embryologically, or physiologically related.
aberrant c., an anomalous c., more specifically an abnormal ventricular c. caused by abnormal intraventricular conduction of a supraventricular impulse.
AIDS-related c. (ARC), manifestations of AIDS in individuals who have not developed impaired immune systems, opportunistic

infections (*e.g., Pneumocystis carinii* pneumonia), or associated malignancies (*e.g.,* Kaposi's sarcoma).
amygdaloid c., *corpus* amygdaloideum.
anomalous c., a c. in the electrocardiogram differing significantly from the physiologic type in the same heart and lead.
antigenic c., a composite of different antigenic structures, such as a cell or a bacterium, or, by extension, a molecule containing two or more determinant groups of different antigenic specificities.
apical c., a set of anterior structures that characterize one or several developmental stages of members of the protozoan phylum Apicomplexa; includes the following structures, visible by electron microscopy: polar ring, conoid, rhoptries, micronemes, and subpellicular tubules.

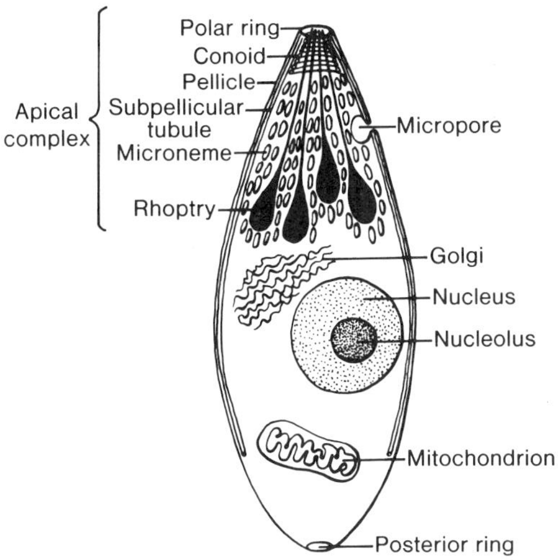

Apical Complex

atrial c., auricular c.; P wave in the electrocardiogram.
auricular c., atrial c.
avian leukosis-sarcoma (leukemia-sarcoma) c., **(1)** a term applied to avian sarcoma, myeloblastosis, erythroblastosis, leukosis, osteopetrosis, and lymphomatosis in the belief that these may all be manifestations of a single disease caused either by an ubiquitous virus or by a group of very closely related viruses (avian leukosis-sarcoma virus); **(2)** a division of the RNA tumor viruses (subfamily Oncovirinae) causing the avian leukosis-sarcoma c. of diseases; the viruses are subgrouped according to antigenic characteristics and growth in defined types of tissue culture cells. Also called avian leukosis-sarcoma virus; avian or fowl erythroblastosis virus; fowl lymphomatosis virus; avian or fowl myeloblastosis virus; avian sarcoma virus; avian lymphomatosis virus (1).
brain wave c., a specific combination of fast and slow electroencephalogram activity that recurs frequently enough to be identified as a discrete phenomenon.
brother c., Cain c.
Cain c. [*Cain,* biblical personage], brother c.; extreme envy or jealousy of a brother, leading to hatred.
castration c., castration anxiety; **(1)** a child's fear of injury to the genitals by the parent of the same sex as punishment for unconcious guilt over oedipal feelings; **(2)** fantasied loss of the penis by a female or fear of its actual loss by a male. **(3)** unconscious fear of injury from those in authority.
caudal pharyngeal c., the ultimobranchial body associated with the embryonic fourth and transitory fifth pharyngeal pouches.
charge transfer c., a c. between two organic molecules in which an electron from one (the donor) is transferred to the other (the acceptor), becoming generally distributed throughout the latter; subsequent transfer of a hydrogen atom completes the reduction of the acceptor; such c.'s are generally highly colored and may be so observed.
Diana c. [*Diana,* L. myth. char.], ideas leading to the adoption of masculine traits and behavior in a female.
diphasic c., a c. consisting of both positive and negative deflections.
Eisenmenger's c., Eisenmenger's tetralogy or disease; the combination of ventricular septal defect with pulmonary hypertension and consequent right-to-left shunt through the defect, with or without an associated overriding aorta.
Electra c. [*Electra,* G. myth. char.], father c.; female counterpart of the Oedipus c.
electrocardiographic c., a deflection or group of deflections in the electrocardiogram.
equiphasic c., isodiphasic c.
father c., Electra c.
feline leukemia-sarcoma virus c., viruses from cats that induce transmissible leukemia or transmissible fibrosarcoma in kittens.
femininity c., in psychoanalysis, the unconscious fear, in boys and men, of castration at the hands of the mother with resultant identification with the aggressor and envious desire for breasts and vagina.
Golgi c., Golgi *apparatus.*
HLA c., the major histocompatibility c. in humans. See also human lymphocyte *antigen.*
immune c., antigen combined with specific antibody, to which complement may also be fixed, and which may precipitate or remain in solution.
inferiority c., a sense of inadequacy which is expressed in extreme shyness, diffidence, or timidity, or as a compensatory reaction in exhibitionism or aggressiveness.
iron-dextran c., a colloidal solution of ferric hydroxide in c. with partially hydrolyzed dextran; used in the treatment of iron deficiency anemias by intramuscular injection.
isodiphasic c., equiphasic c.; a diphasic c. whose positive and negative deflections are approximately equal.
j-g c., juxtaglomerular c.
Jocasta c. [*Jocasta,* G. myth. char.], a mother's libidinous fixation on a son.
junctional c., the attachment zone between epithelial cells, typically consisting of the zonula occludens, the zonula adherens, and the macula adherens (desmosome).
juxtaglomerular c., j-g c.; juxtaglomerular apparatus; a c. consisting of the juxtaglomerular cells, which are modified smooth muscle cells in the wall of the afferent glomerular arteriole and sometimes also the efferent arteriole; extraglomerular mesangium lacis cells, which are located in the angle between the afferent and efferent glomerular arterioles; the macula densa of the distal convoluted tubule; and granular epithelial peripolar cells located at the angle of reflection of the parietal to the visceral capsule of the renal corpuscle; believed to provide some feedback control of extracellular fluid volume and glomerular filtration rate.
K c., slow waves in the electroencephalogram related to arousal from sleep by a sound.
Lear c. [*Lear,* Shakespearean character], a father's libidinous fixation on a daughter.
major histocompatibility c. (MHC), a group of linked loci, collectively termed H-2 c. in the mouse and HLA c. in humans, which codes for cell-surface histocompatibility antigens and is the principal determinant of tissue type and transplant compatibility. See also human lymphocyte *antigen.*
membrane attack c., complement components C5b, C6, C7, C8, and C9 assembled at sites of complement activation which attach to and may damage membranes of cells or bacteria.
Meyenburg's c., clusters of small bile ducts occurring in polycystic livers, separate from the portal areas.

monophasic c., a c. in the electrocardiogram that is entirely negative or entirely positive.
mother superior c., the tendency of a psychotherapist to play a mothering role to the detriment of the therapeutic process.
Oedipus c. [*Oedipus,* G. myth. char.], a developmentally distinct group of associated ideas, aims, instinctual drives, and fears generally observed in male children 3 to 6 years old: coinciding with the peak of the phallic phase of psychosexual development, the child's sexual interest is attached primarily to the parent of the opposite sex and is accompanied by aggressive feelings toward the parent of the same sex; in psychoanalytic theory, it is replaced by the castration c.
persecution c., a feeling that others have evil designs against one's well-being.
primary c., the typical lesions of primary pulmonary tuberculosis, consisting of a small peripheral focus of infection, with hilar or paratracheal lymph node involvement.
QRS c., the principal deflection in the electrocardiogram, representing ventricular depolarization.
ribosome-lamella c., a cylindrical cytoplasmic inclusion composed of concentrically arranged sheets of membranes alternating with rows of ribosomes; characteristic of the hairy cell in leukemic reticuloendotheliosis.
sicca c., dryness of the mucous membranes, as of the eyes and mouth, in the absence of a connective tissue disease such as rheumatoid arthritis.
spike and wave c., a c. of a slow wave and a fast one usually seen in the electroencephalogram in petit mal seizures.
Steidele's c., rarely used term for congenital absence of the aortic arch.
superiority c., term sometimes given to the compensatory behavior, *e.g.*, aggressiveness, self-assertion, associated with inferiority c.
symptom c., **(1)** see syndrome; **(2)** see complex (1).
synaptinemal c., a submicroscopic structure interposed between the homologous chromosome pairs during synapsis.
Tacaribe c. of viruses, a group of arenaviruses that includes the antigenically interrelated arboviruses Amapari, Junin, Latino, Machupo, Parana, Pichinde, Tacaribe, and Tamiami.
ternary c., term used to describe the tripartite combination of, for example, enzyme-cofactor-substrate, the active form involved in many enzyme reactions.
triple symptom c., Behçet's *syndrome.*
VATER c., a constellation of *v*ertebral defects, *a*nal atresia, *t*racheoesophageal fistula with *e*sophageal atresia, and *r*enal and *r*adial anomalies; associated with Fanconi's anemia.
ventricular c., the QRST wave in the electrocardiogram.

complexion (kom-plek'shŭn) [L. *complexio,* a combination, (later) physical condition]. The color, texture, and general appearance of the skin of the face.

complexus (kom-plek'sŭs) [L. an embracing, encircling]. Obsolete term for *musculus* semispinalis capitis.

compliance (kom-plī'ans). **1.** The consistency and accuracy with which a patient follows the regimen prescribed by a physician or other health professional. *Cf.* adherence (2); maintenance. **2 (C).** A measure of the ease with which a structure or substance may be deformed. In medicine and physiology, usually a measure of the ease with which a hollow viscus (*e.g.*, lung, urinary bladder, gallbladder) may be distended, *i.e.*, the volume change resulting from the application of a unit pressure differential between the inside and outside of the viscus; the reciprocal of elastance.
dynamic c. of lung, the value obtained when lung c. is estimated during breathing by dividing the tidal volume by the difference in instantaneous transpulmonary pressures at the ends of the respiratory excursions, when flow in the airway is momentarily zero; this value deviates markedly from static c. in patients in whom resistances and compliances are not uniform throughout the lung (*i.e.*, uneven time constants).
c. of heart, the passive or diastolic stiffness of the ventricle of the heart, most commonly of the left ventricle; one may distinguish between c. of the muscle and c. of the supportive structures, although ordinarily, both are considered together; a hypertrophied or scarred heart will manifest a stiff wall, *i.e.*, decreased c.
specific c., **(1)** the c. of a structure divided by its initial volume; **(2)** more specifically for the lungs, the c. divided by the functional residual capacity.
static c., the value obtained when c. is measured at true equilibrium, *i.e.*, in the absence of any motion.
thoracic c., that portion of total ventilatory c. ascribable to c. of the thoracic cage.
ventilatory c., the sum of dynamic c. of the lung and thoracic c.

complicated (kom'pli-kā-ted) [L. *com-plico,* pp. *-atus,* to fold together]. Made complex; denoting a disease upon which a morbid process or event has been superimposed, altering symptoms and modifying its course for the worse.

complication (kom-pli-kā'shŭn). A morbid process or event occurring during a disease which is not an essential part of the disease, although it may result from it or from independent causes.

component (kom-pō'nent) [L. *com-pono,* pp. *-positus,* to place together]. An element forming a part of the whole.
c. A of prothrombin, *factor* V.
anterior c. of force, a force operating to move teeth anteriorly.
c. of complement, any one of the nine distinct protein units (designated C1 through C9 and distributed in the α, β, and γ electrophoretic partitions of normal serum) that effect the immunological activities long associated with complement (*q.v.*). C1 is a complex of three subunits: C1q, C1r, and C1s. $C\overline{1q}$ (overbar indicates "active form") activates proenzyme C1r to $C\overline{1r}$ which activates C1s to $C\overline{1s}$(also known as C1 esterase), which converts proenzyme C2 to C2b and produces C4b from C4. C2b combines with C4b to form "classical-complement-pathway C3/C5 convertase" (also known as C3 convertase, C5 convertase, and $C\overline{42}$). This enzyme cleaves C3 to C3a and C3b, and C5 to yield C5a and C5b, as does "alternative-complement-pathway C3/C5 convertase" (also known as proenzyme factor B, properdin factor B, C3 proactivator, and heat-labile factor). Complement factor I (also known as C3b or C3b/C4b inactivator) inactivates C3b and C4b by a different proteolytic cleavage.
c. of force, **(1)** one of the factors from which a resultant force may be compounded or into which it may be resolved; **(2)** one of the vectors into which a force may be resolved.
c.'s of mastication, the various jaw movements that are made during the act of mastication, as determined by the neuromuscular system, the temporomandibular articulations, the teeth, and the food being chewed; divided, for purposes of analysis or description, into opening, closing, left lateral, right lateral, and anteroposterior c.'s.
c.'s of occlusion, the various factors involved in occlusion, such as the temporomandibular joint, the associated neuromusculature, the teeth, and the denture-supporting structures.
plasma thromboplastin c. (PTC), *factor* IX.
thromboplastic plasma c. (TPC), *factor* VIII.

composition (kom-pō-zish'ŭn) [L. *compono,* to arrange]. In chemistry, the kinds and numbers of atoms constituting a molecule.
base c., the proportions of the four bases (adenine, cytosine, guanine, and thymine present in DNA or RNA; usually expressed as the percentage (mol %) of G plus C.
modeling c., modeling *plastic.*

compos mentis (kom'pos men'tis) [L. possessed of one's mind; *compos,* having control, + *mens* (*ment-*), mind]. Of sound mind; sane; usually used in its opposite form, *non compos mentis.*

compound (kom'pownd) [thru O. Fr., fr. L. *compono*] **1.** In chemis-

try, a substance formed by the covalent or electrostatic union of two or more elements, generally differing entirely in physical characteristics from any of its components. **2.** In pharmacy, denoting a preparation containing several ingredients. For c.'s not listed here, see the specific chemical or pharmaceutical names.
acetone c., ketone *body.*
acyclic c., open chain or aliphatic c.; an organic c. in which the chain does not form a ring.
addition c., **(1)** strictly, a complex of two or more complete molecules in which each preserves its fundamental structure and no covalent bonds are made or broken (*e.g.,* hydrates of salts, adducts); **(2)** loosely, association of acids with basic organic c.'s (*e.g.,* amines with HCl); **(3)** more loosely, addition of two molecules without loss of any atom, but forming new covalent bonds (*e.g.,* $CH_2{=}CH_2 + Br_2 \rightarrow BrCH_2{-}CH_2Br$).
alicyclic c.'s, see cyclic c.
aliphatic c., acyclic c.
aromatic c., see cyclic c.
carbamino c., any carbamic acid derivative formed by the combination of carbon dioxide with a free amino group to form an *N*-carboxy group, -NH-COOH, as in hemoglobin forming carbaminohemoglobin.
carbocyclic c., see cyclic c.
closed chain c., cyclic c.
condensation c., a c. resulting from the combination of two or more simple substances, with the splitting off of some other substance, such as alcohol or water; *e.g.,* a peptide. *Cf.* conjugated c.
conjugated c., a c. formed by the union of two c.'s (as by the elimination of water between an alcohol and an organic acid to form an ester) and easily converted to the original c.'s (hydrolysis). *Cf.* condensation c. See also conjugation (4).
cyclic c., ring or closed chain c.; any c. in which the constituent atoms, or any part of them, form a ring. Used mainly in organic chemistry where: 1) numerous c.'s contain rings of carbon atoms (carbocyclic c.'s) or carbon atoms plus one or more atoms of other types (heterocyclic c.'s), usually nitrogen, oxygen, or sulfur; 2) where the atoms are all of the same element (homocyclic or isocyclic c.); 3) where the ring is saturated or contains nonconjugated double bonds (alicyclic c.), the c. is similar in properties to the corresponding acyclic c. (*e.g.,* cyclohexane resembles hexane); 4) where the ring contains conjugated double bonds (aromatic c.; *e.g.,* benzene, pyridine), it is more stable than the corresponding saturated ring and exhibits unusual chemical properties characteristic of itself and not of other types of rings or of acyclic c.'s.
genetic., compound *heterozygote.*
glycosyl c., the c. formed between a sugar and another organic substance in which the OH of the reducing (hemiacetal) group of the former is removed; *e.g.,* the natural nucleosides, in which a heterocyclic N becomes linked directly to the C-1 of ribose (or deoxyribose) to yield ribosyl compounds. *Cf.* glycoside.
heterocyclic c., see cyclic c.
high energy c.'s, classically, a group of phosphoric esters whose hydrolysis takes place with a free energy change of $-5{,}000$ to $-11{,}000$ calories per mole (in contrast to $-1{,}000$ to $-4{,}000$ for simple phosphoric esters like glucose 6-phosphate or α-glycerophosphates), thus being capable of driving energy-consuming reactions in living cells or reconstituted cell-free systems; adenosine 5′-triphosphate, with respect to the β and γ phosphates, is the best known and is regarded as the immediate energy source for most metabolic syntheses. The general types are acid anhydrides, phosphoric esters of enols, phosphamic acid ($R{-}NH{-}PO_3H_2$) derivatives, acyl thioesters (*e.g.,* of coenzyme A), sulfonium c.'s ($R_3\_\ S^+$), and aminoacyl esters of ribosyl moieties. See also high energy *phosphates.*
homocyclic c., see cyclic c.
impression c., modeling *plastic.*
inclusion c., the mechanical trapping of small molecules within spaces between other molecules; *e.g.,* the inclusion of iodine molecules by starch molecules to form the well-known red-to-black "addition c."
inorganic c., a c. in which the atoms or radicals are held together by electrostatic forces rather than by covalent bonds; capable of dissociation into ions in polar solvents (*e.g.,* H_2O). *Cf.* organic c.
isocyclic c., see cyclic c.
meso c.'s, c.'s containing more than one asymmetric carbon atom, with configurations about them so balanced that the molecule as a whole possesses a plane of symmetry, although the individual carbon atoms do not; such compounds are not optically active; *e.g.,* ribitol, mucic acid, meso-inositol.
methonium c.'s, agents that block impulses in ganglia (*e.g.,* hexamethonium) and are used in arterial hypertension.
modeling c., modeling *plastic.*
nonpolar c., a c. composed of molecules that possess a symmetrical distribution of charge, so that no positive or negative poles exist, and that are not ionizable in solution; *e.g.,* hydrocarbons. See also organic c.
open chain c., acyclic c.
organic c., a c. composed of atoms held together by covalent (shared electron) bonds. *Cf.* inorganic c.
polar c., a c. in which the electric charge is not symmetrically distributed, so that there is a separation of charge and formation of definite positive and negative pole; *e.g.,* H_2O. See also inorganic c.
ring c., cyclic c.

comprehension (kom-prē-hen′shŭn). Apperception (1).

compress (kom′pres) [L. *com-primo,* pp. *-pressus,* to press together]. A pad of gauze or other material applied for local pressure.
graduated c., layers of cloth thickest in the center, becoming thinner toward the periphery.
wet c., gauze moistened with saline or antiseptic solution.

compression (kom-presh′ŭn). A squeezing together; the exertion of pressure on a body in such a way as to tend to increase its density; the decrease in a dimension of a body under the action of two external forces directed toward one another in the same straight line.
c. of brain, cerebral c.
cerebral c., c. of the brain; pressure upon the intracranial tissues by an effusion of blood or cerebrospinal fluid, an abscess, a neoplasm, a depressed fracture of the skull, or an edema of the brain.
c. of tissue, tissue *displaceability.*

compressor (kom-pres′er, -ōr). **1.** A muscle, contraction of which causes compression of any structure. **2.** Compressorium; an instrument for making pressure on a part, especially on an artery to prevent loss of blood.
c. ve′nae dorsa′lis pe′nis, Houston's muscle; a variation of the ischiocavernosus muscle in which some fibers pass dorsal to the dorsal vein of the penis; thought at one time to be an important component in the mechanism of erection.

compressorium (kom-pres-ōr′ē-ŭm). Compressor (2).

Compton, Arthur H., U.S. physicist 1892–1962. See C. *effect.*

compulsion (kom-pŭl′shŭn) [L. *com-pello* pp. *-pulsus,* to drive together, compel]. Uncontrollable thoughts or impulses to perform an act, often repetitively, as an unconscious mechanism to avoid unacceptable ideas and desires which, by themselves, arouse anxiety; the anxiety becomes fully manifest if performance of the compulsive act is prevented.

compulsive (kom-pŭl′siv). Influenced by compulsion; of a compelling and irresistible nature.

con- [L. *cum,* with, together]. Prefix, to words of L. derivation, denoting with, together, in association; appears as com- before p, b, or m, as col- before l, and as co- before a vowel; corresponds to G. *syn-*.

conA, con A Abbreviation for concanavalin A.

conalbumin (kon-al-byū'min). Ovotransferrin; a glycoprotein containing mannose and galactose, constituting about 14% of egg white.

conanine (kon'ă-nēn). A steroid alkaloid; pregnane with a methylimino group bridging C-18 and C-20 (in α-configuration). See also conenine, conessine.

conarium (kō-nā'rē-ŭm) [G. *kōnarion* (dim. of *kōnos,* cone), the pineal body]. *Corpus* pineale.

conation (kō-nā'shŭn) [L. *conātio,* an undertaking, effort]. The conscious tendency to act, usually an aspect of mental process; historically aligned with cognition and affection, but more recently used in the wider sense of impulse, desire, purposeful striving.

conative (kon'ă-tiv). Pertaining to, or characterized by, conation.

conatus (kō-nah'tŭs, -nā'tŭs) [L. attempt]. A striving toward self-preservation and self-affirmation.

concameration (kon-kam-er-ā'shŭn) [L. *concameratio,* a vault; fr. *concamero,* pp. *-atus,* to vault over, fr. *camera,* a vault]. A system of interconnecting cavities.

concanavalin A (conA, con A) (kon-kă-nav'ă-lin). A phytomitogen, extracted from the jack bean, that agglutinates the blood of mammals and reacts with glucosans; like other phytohemagglutinins, conA stimulates T lymphocytes more vigorously than it does B lymphocytes.

concatenate (kon-kat'ĕ-nāt) [L. *con-cateno,* pp. *-atus,* to link together, fr. *catena,* a chain]. Denoting the arrangement of a number of structures, *e.g.,* enlarged lymph glands, in a row like the links of a chain.

Concato, Luigi M., Italian physician, 1825–1882. See C.'s *disease.*

concave (kon'kāv) [L. *concavus,* arched or vaulted]. Having a depressed or hollowed surface.

concavity (kon-kav'i-tē). A hollow or depression, with more or less evenly curved sides, on any surface.

concavoconcave (kon-kā'vō-kon'kāv). Biconcave.

concavoconvex (kon-kā'vō-kon'veks). Concave on one surface and convex on the opposite surface.

concentration (kon-sen-trā'shŭn) [L. *con-,* together, + *centrum,* center]. **1.** A preparation made by extracting a crude drug, precipitating from the solution, and drying. **2.** Increasing the amount of solute in a given volume of solution by evaporation of the solvent. **3.** The quantity of a substance per unit volume or weight. In renal physiology, symbol U for urinary c., P for plasma c.; in respiratory physiology, symbol C for amount per unit volume in blood, F for fractional c. (mole fraction or volume per volume) in dried gas; subscripts indicate location and chemical species.
M c., the maximum number of bacterial cells which can be produced in a unit volume of growth medium.
mean cell hemoglobin c. (MCHC), the average hemoglobin c. in a given volume of packed red cells, calculated from the hemoglobin therein and the hematocrit, in erythrocyte indices.
minimal alveolar (anesthetic) c., (MAC), the end-alveolar c. of an inhalation anesthetic which prevents somatic response to a painful stimulus in 50% of individuals; an index of relative potency of inhalation anesthetics.
minimal inhibitory c. (MIC), the lowest concentration of antibiotic sufficient to inhibit bacterial growth when tested *in vitro.*
molar c., see molar (4).
normal c., see normal (3).

concentric (kon-sen'trik). Having a common center, such that two or more spheres, circles, or segments of circles are within one another.

concept (kon'sept) [L. *conceptum,* something understood, pp. ntr. of *concipio,* to receive, apprehend]. Conception (1). **1.** An abstract idea or notion. **2.** An explanatory variable or principle in a scientific system.
no-threshold c., that the biologic effect of radiation is proportional to dose, even for minutely small doses.
self c., an individual's assessment of his or her status on a single trait or on many human dimensions using societal or personal norms as criteria.

concepti (kon-sep'tī). Plural of conceptus.

conception (kon-sep'shŭn) [L. *conceptio;* see concept]. **1.** Concept. **2.** Act of forming a general idea or notion. **3.** Act of conceiving, or becoming pregnant; fertilization of the oocyte (ovum) by a spermatozoon.
imperative c., a concept that does not arise from association but appears spontaneously and refuses to be banished.

conceptual (kon-sep'chū-ăl). Relating to the formation of ideas, to mental conceptions.

conceptus, pl. **concepti** (kon-sep'tŭs, -sep'tī). The product of conception, *i.e.,* embryo and membranes.

concha, pl. **conchae** (kon'kă, kon'kē) [L. a shell] [NA]. In anatomy, a structure comparable to a shell in shape, as the auricle or pinna of the ear or a turbinated bone in the nose.
c. auric'ulae [NA], concha of ear; the large hollow, or floor of the auricle, between the anterior portion of the helix and the antihelix; it is divided by the crus of the helix into the cymba above and the cavum below.
c. of ear, c. auriculae.
highest c., c. nasalis suprema.
inferior c., c. nasalis inferior.
middle c., c. nasalis media.
Morgagni's c., c. nasalis superior.
nasal c., *crista* ethmoidalis.
c. nasa'lis infe'rior [NA], inferior c.; inferior turbinated bone; **(1)** a thin, spongy, bony plate with curved margins, on the lateral wall of the nasal cavity, separating the middle from the inferior meatus; it articulates with the ethmoid, lacrimal, maxilla, and palate bones; **(2)** the above bony plate and its thick mucoperiosteum containing an extensive cavernous vascular bed for heat exchange.
c. nasa'lis me'dia [NA], middle c.; middle turbinated bone; **(1)** the middle thin, spongy, bony plate with curved margins, part of the ethmoidal labyrinth, projecting from the lateral wall of the nasal cavity and separating the superior meatus from the middle meatus; **(2)** the above bony plate and its thick mucoperiosteum containing a cavernous vascular bed for heat exchange.
c. nasa'lis supe'rior [NA], superior c.; superior turbinated bone; Morgagni's c.; **(1)** the upper thin, spongy, bony plate with curved margins, part of the ethmoidal labyrinth, projecting from the lateral wall of the nasal cavity and separating the superior meatus from the sphenoethmoidal recess; **(2)** the above bony plate and its thick mucoperiosteum, which is less vascular than that of the middle and inferior conchae.
c. nasa'lis supre'ma [NA], supreme c.; highest c.; supreme, highest, or fourth turbinated bone; c. santorini; Santorini's c.; supraturbinal; a small c. frequently present on the posterosuperior part of the lateral nasal wall; it overlies the supreme nasal meatus.
Santorini's c., c. santori'ni, c. nasalis suprema.
sphenoidal conchae, conchae sphenoidales.
con'chae sphenoida'les [NA], sphenoidal conchae; Bertin's bones or ossicles; sphenoidal turbinals; sphenoidal turbinated bones; paired ossicles of pyramidal shape, the spines of which are in contact with the medial pterygoid lamina, the bases forming the roof of the nasal cavity.
superior c., c. nasalis superior.
supreme c., c. nasalis suprema.

conchitis (kon-kī'tis). Inflammation of any concha.

conchoidal (kon-koy'dăl) [concha + G. *eidos,* appearance]. Shaped like a shell; having alternate convexities and concavities on the surface.

conchoscope (kon'kō-skōp) [concha + G. *skopeō,* to view]. A form of nasal speculum.

concomitance (kon-kom'i-tăns) [con- + L. *comito-,* pp. *-atus,* to accompany]. Comitance; in esotropia, one eye accompanying the other in all excursions, as in concomitant strabismus.

concordance (kon-kōr'dans) [L. *concordia,* agreeing, harmony]. Agreement in the type of two characteristics, either in the same individual or in two individuals (*e.g.,* twins or sibs) who are by hypothesis not independent; c. within the individual is usually termed genetic association and used as evidence of dependence.

concordant (kon-kōr'dant). Denoting or exhibiting concordance.

concrement (kon'krē-ment) [L. *con- cresco,* to grow together]. A concretion; a deposit of calcareous material in a part.

concrescence (kon-kres'ens) [see concrement]. **1.** Coalescence. **2.** In dentistry, the union of the roots of two adjacent teeth by cementum.

concretio cordis (kon-krē'shē-ō kōr'dis). Internal adhesive pericarditis; synechia pericardii; extensive adhesion between parietal and visceral layers of the pericardium with partial or complete obliteration of the pericardial cavity.

concretion (kon-krē'shŭn) [L. *cum,* together, + *crescere,* to grow]. The aggregation or formation of solid material.

concretization (kon'krēt-i-zā'shŭn). Inability to abstract with an overemphasis on specific details; seen in mental disorders, such as dementia and schizophrenia, and also normally in children.

concussion (kon-kŭsh'ŭn) [L. *concussio,* fr. *con- cutio,* pp. *-cussus,* to shake violently]. **1.** A violent shaking or jarring. **2.** Commotio; an injury of a soft structure, as the brain, resulting from a blow or violent shaking.
brain c., commotio cerebri; a clinical syndrome due to mechanical, usually traumatic, forces; characterized by immediate and transient impairment of neural function, such as alteration of consciousness, disturbance of vision and equilibrium, etc.
spinal c., commotio spinalis; a sudden, transient loss of function of the spinal cord, caused by injury but without permanent gross damage.

concussor (kon-kŭs-er, -sōr). A hammer-like instrument for tapping the parts as a form of massage.

condensation (kon-den-sā'shŭn) [L. *con- denso,* pp. *-atus,* to make thick, condense]. **1.** Making more solid or dense. **2.** The change of a gas to a liquid, or of a liquid to a solid. **3.** In psychoanalysis, an unconscious mental process in which one symbol stands for a number of others. **4.** In dentistry, the process of packing a filling material into a cavity, using such force and direction that no voids result.

condense (kon-dens'). To pack; to increase the density of; applied particularly to insertion of gold foil or silver amalgam in a cavity prepared in a tooth.

condenser (kon-den'ser). **1.** An apparatus for cooling a gas to a liquid, or a liquid to a solid. **2.** In dentistry, a manual or powered instrument used for packing a plastic or unset material into a cavity of a tooth; variation in sizes and shapes allows conformation of the mass to the cavity outline. **3.** The simple or compound lens on a microscope that is used to supply the illumination necessary for visibility of the specimen under observation. **4.** Capacitor.
Abbé's c., a system of two or three wide-angle, achromatic, convex and planoconvex lenses that may be moved upward or downward beneath the stage of a microscope, thereby regulating the concentration of light (directly from a bulb or reflected from a mirror) that passes through the material to be examined on the stage.
automatic c., automatic *plugger.*
cardioid c., a type of dark-field c.
dark-field c., an apparatus for throwing reflected light through the microscope field, so that only the object to be examined is illuminated, the field itself being dark.
paraboloid c., a type of dark-field c.

condition (kon-dish'ŭn). **1.** To train; to undergo conditioning. **2.** A certain response elicited by a specifiable stimulus or emitted in the presence of certain stimuli with reward of the response during prior occurrence. **3.** Referring to several classes of learning in the behavioristic branch of psychology.

conditioning (kon-dish'ŭn-ing). The process of acquiring, developing, educating, establishing, learning, or training new responses in an individual. Used to describe both respondent and operant behavior; in both usages, refers to a change in the frequency or form of behavior as a result of the influence of the environment.
assertive c., assertive *training.*
aversive c., aversive *training.*
avoidance c., the technique whereby an organism learns to avoid unpleasant or punishing stimuli by learning the appropriate anticipatory response to protect it from further such stimuli. *Cf.* escape c.
classical c., a form of learning, as in Pavlov's experiments, in which a previously neutral stimulus becomes a conditioned stimulus when presented together with an unconditioned stimulus. Also called stimulus substitution because the new stimulus evokes the response in question. See also respondent c.
escape c., the technique whereby an organism learns to terminate unpleasant or punishing stimuli by making the appropriate new response which ceases the delivery of such stimuli. *Cf.* avoidance c.
higher order c., the use of a previously conditioned stimulus to condition further responses, in much the same way unconditioned stimuli are used.
instrumental c., c. in which the response is a prerequisite to achieving some goal; often used as a synonym for operant c., but some psychologists make distinctions in the usages of these two terms.
operant c., skinnerian c.; a type of c. developed by Skinner in which an experimenter waits for the response to be conditioned to occur spontaneously, immediately after which the organism is given a reinforcer reward; after this procedure is repeated many times, the frequency of target response emission will have significantly increased over its pre-experiment base rate. See also *schedules* of reinforcement.
pavlovian c., respondent c.
respondent c., pavlovian c.; a type of c., first studied by I. P. Pavlov, in which a previously neutral stimulus (bell sound) elicits a response (salivation) as a result of pairing it (associating it contiguously in time) a number of times with an unconditioned or natural stimulus for that response (food shown to a hungry dog).
second-order c., the use of a previously successfully used stimulus as the unconditioned stimulus for further c.
skinnerian c., operant c.
trace c., c. when there is no temporal overlap between the c. stimulus and the unconditioned stimulus.

condom (kon'dom). Sheath or cover for the penis, for use in the prevention of conception or infection during coitus.

conductance (kon-dŭk'tans). **1.** A measure of conductivity; the ratio of the current flowing through a conductor to the difference in potential between the ends of the conductor; the c. of a circuit is the reciprocal of its resistance. **2.** The ease with which a fluid or gas enters and flows through a conduit, air passage, or respiratory tract; the flow per unit pressure difference.

conduction (kon-dŭk'shŭn) [L. *con- duco,* pp. *ductus,* to lead, conduct]. **1.** The act of transmitting or conveying certain forms of energy, such as heat, sound, or electricity, from one point to another, without evident movement in the conducting body. **2.** The transmission of stimuli of various sorts by living protoplasm.

aberrant ventricular c., ventricular aberration; abnormal intraventricular c. of a supraventricular beat, especially where surrounding beats are normally conducted.
accelerated c., pathologically increased speed of c. between the atrium and ventricles in the Wolff-Parkinson-White and Lown-Ganong-Levine syndromes; such accelerated pathways provide one of the bases for reentry tachycardia.
air c., in relation to hearing, the transmission of sound to the inner ear through the external auditory canal and the structures of the middle ear.
anterograde c., forward c.; c. from sinus node to ventricular myocardium.
atrioventricular (A-V) c., forward c. of the cardiac impulse from atria to ventricles via the A-V node, represented in the electrocardiogram by the P-R interval. P-H c. time is from the onset of the P wave to the first high frequency component of the His bundle electrogram (normally 119 $\pm$ 38 msec); A-H c. time is from the onset of the first high frequency component of the atrial electrogram to the first high frequency component of the His bundle electrogram (normally 92 $\pm$ 38 msec); P-A conduction time is from the onset of the P wave to the onset of the atrial electrogram (normally 27 $\pm$ 18 msec).
avalanche c., the discharge of an impulse from a neuron into a large number of neurons of the same physiologic system, thus producing the liberation of a very large amount of nervous energy by a given stimulus.
bone c., osteophony; in relation to hearing, the transmission of sound to the inner ear through vibrations applied to the bones of the skull.
concealed c., c. of an impulse through a part of the heart without direct evidence of its presence in the electrocardiogram; c. is inferred only because of its influence on the subsequent cardiac cycle.
decremental c., impaired c. in a portion of a fiber because of progressively lessening response of the unexcited portion of the fiber to the action potential coming toward it; it is manifested by decreasing speed of c., amplitude of action potential, and extent of spread of the impulse.
delayed c., first-degree A-V block. See atrioventricular *block.*
forward c., anterograde c.
intra-atrial c., c. of the cardiac impulse through the atrial myocardium, represented by the P wave in the electrocardiogram.
intraventricular c., ventricular c.; c. of the cardiac impulse through the ventricular myocardium, represented by the QRS complex in the electrocardiogram. H-R c. time is from the onset of the first high frequency component of the His bundle electrogram to the onset of the QRS complex of the surface electrocardiogram (normally 43 $\pm$ 12 msec); H-V c. time is from the onset of the first high frequency component of the His bundle electrogram to the onset of the ventricular electrogram (normally approximates the H-R interval but may be a little shorter).
nerve c., the transmission of an impulse along a nerve fiber.
Purkinje c., c. of the cardiac impulse through the Purkinje system.
retrograde c., retroconduction; ventriculoatrial c.; c. backward from the ventricles or from the A-V node into and through the atria.
saltatory c., c. in which the nerve impulse jumps from one node of Ranvier to the next.
supranormal c., transmission of an impulse during the brief period of the cardiac cycle when it would be expected to fail if it occurred outside this time interval; c. is, in fact, not supranormal, but only relatively improved in an abnormally depressed state of c. *Cf.* supranormal *excitability.*
synaptic c., the c. of a nerve impulse across a synapse.
ventricular c., intraventricular c.
ventriculoatrial (V-A) c., retrograde c.

conductivity (kon-dŭk-tiv'i-tē). **1.** The power of transmission or conveyance of certain forms of energy, as heat, sound, and electricity, without perceptible motion in the conducting body. **2.** The property, inherent in living protoplasm, of transmitting a state of excitation; *e.g.,* in muscle or nerve.
hydraulic c., ease of pressure filtration of a liquid through a membrane; specifically, $Kf = \eta(\dot{Q}/A)\ (\delta x/\delta P)$, where Kf = hydraulic c., η = viscosity of the liquid being filtered, $\dot{Q}/A$ = volume of liquid filtered per unit time and unit area, and $\delta x/\delta P$ = reciprocal of the pressure gradient through the membrane; solute concentrations should be identical on both sides of the membrane. Also applied more loosely to measurements on a total membrane of unknown area and thickness with unmeasured fluid viscosity ($K = \dot{Q}/\delta P$).

conductor (kon-dŭk'ter, -tōr). **1.** A probe or sound with a groove along which a knife is passed in slitting open a sinus or fistula; a grooved director. **2.** Any substance possessing conductivity.

conduit (kon'dū-it). A channel.
ileal c., an isolated segment of ileum serving as a replacement for another tubular organ; specifically, the use as a urinary conduit into which ureters can be implanted following total cystectomy or other loss of normal bladder function requiring supravesical diversion.

conduplicate (kon-dū'pli-kāt) [L. *con-,* with, + *duplico,* pp. *-atus*]. Folded upon itself lengthwise.

conduplicato corpore (kon-dū-pli-kā'tō kōr'pōr-ē). Condition in which the fetus is doubled up on itself in shoulder presentation.

condurango (kon-dū-rang'gō) [Peruv.]. The bark of *Gonolobus condurango, Marsdenia condurango* (family Asclepiadaceae), a shrub of Ecuador and Peru; an aromatic bitter and astringent.

condylar (kon'di-lăr). Relating to a condyle.

condylarthrosis (kon'di-lar-thrō'sis) [G. *kondylos,* condyle, + *arthrōsis,* a jointing]. A joint, like that of the knee, formed by condylar surfaces.

condyle (kon'dīl). Condylus.
c. of humerus, *condylus* humeri.
lateral c., *condylus* lateralis.
lateral c. of femur, *condylus* lateralis femoris.
lateral c. of tibia, *condylus* lateralis tibiae.
mandibular c., *processus* condylaris.
medial c., *condylus* medialis.
medial c. of femur, *condylus* medialis femoris.
medial c. of tibia, *condylus* medialis tibiae.
occipital c., *condylus* occipitalis.
working side c., in dentistry, the mandibular c. on the side toward which the mandible moves in a lateral excursion.

condylectomy (kon-di-lek'tō-mē) [G. *kondylos,* condyle, + *ektomē,* excision]. Excision of a condyle.

condylion (kon-dil'ē-on) [G. *kondylion,* dim. of *kondylos,* condyle]. A point on the lateral outer or medial inner surface of the condyle of the mandible.

condyloid (kon'di-loyd) [G. *kondylōdēs,* like a knuckle, fr. *kondylos,* condyle, + *eidos,* resemblance]. Relating to or resembling a condyle.

condyloma, pl. **condylomata** (kon-di-lō'mă, -mah'tă) [G. *kondylōma,* a knob]. Verruca mollusciformis; a wartlike excrescence at the anus or vulva, or on the glans penis.
c. acumina'tum, a projecting warty growth on the external genitals or at the anus, consisting of fibrous overgrowths covered by thickened epithelium showing koilocytosis, due to infection by human papilloma virus; it is almost always benign, although malignant change has been reported. Also called pointed c.; papilloma acuminatum or venereum; verruca acuminata; fig, genital, moist, pointed, or venereal wart.
flat c., **(1)** c. latum; **(2)** a c. of the uterine cervix caused by human

papilloma virus infection and characterized histologically by koilocytosis without papillomatosis.

giant c., Buschke-Löwenstein tumor; a large type of c. acuminatum found in the preputial sac of the penis of middle-aged, uncircumcised men; it tends to extend deeply and recur.

c. la'tum, flat c. (1); moist or mucous papule; a secondary syphilitic eruption of flat-topped papules, occurring in groups covered by a necrotic layer of epithelial detritus, and secreting a seropurulent fluid; they are found at the anus and wherever contiguous folds of skin produce heat and moisture.

pointed c., c. acuminatum.

condylomatous (kon-di-lō'mă-tŭs). Relating to a condyloma.

condylotomy (kon-di-lot'ō-mē) [G. *kondylos,* condyle, + *tomē,* incision]. Division, without removal, of a condyle.

condylus (kon'di-lŭs) [L. fr. G. *kondylos,* knuckle, the knuckle of any joint] [NA]. Condyle; a rounded articular surface at the extremity of a bone.

c. hu'meri [NA], condyle of humerus; the distal end of the humerus, including the trochlea, capitulum and the olecranon, coronoid and radial fossae.

c. latera'lis [NA], lateral condyle; **c. l. femoris,** lateral condyle of the femur; **c. l. tibiae,** lateral condyle of the tibia.

c. media'lis [NA], medial condyle; **c. m. femoris,** medial condyle of the femur; **c. m. tibiae,** medial condyle of the tibia.

c. occipita'lis [NA], occipital condyle; one of two elongated oval facets on the undersurface of the occipital bone, one on each side of the foramen magnum, which articulate with the atlas.

-cone. Suffix denoting the cusp of a tooth in the upper jaw.

cone (kōn) [G. *kōnos,* cone]. **1.** Conus (1); a figure having a circular base with sides inclined so as to meet at a point above. **2.** Cone cell of retina; the photosensitive, outward-directed, conical process of a c. cell essential for sharp vision and color vision; c.'s are the only photoreceptor in the fovea centralis and become interspersed with increasing numbers of rods toward the periphery of the retina.

antipodal c., the set of astral rays of a dividing cell extending from the centriole in a direction opposite to the equatorial plate.

arterial c., *conus* arteriosus.

elastic c., *conus* elasticus.

ether c., apparatus employed in the administration of ether by the open-drop technique.

fertilization c., a protuberance of the cytoplasm of the ovum at the point where the effective spermatozoon is attached.

gutta-percha c., a c.-shaped, semirigid root canal filling material composed of gutta-percha and zinc oxide.

Haller's c.'s, *lobuli* epididymidis.

implantation c., axon *hillock.*

keratosic c.'s, horny pointed or rounded elevations on the hands and feet, occasionally observed in cases of gonorrheal rheumatism.

c. of light, *pyramid* of light.

medullary c., *conus* medullaris.

ocular c., the c. of light in the interior of the eyeball with the base formed by the rays entering through the pupil and the apex focused on the retina.

Politzer's luminous c., *pyramid* of light.

pulmonary c., *conus* arteriosus.

retinal c.'s, see cone (2).

silver c., pure silver with standard conical shape, used with cement to obturate dental root canals.

theca interna c., the conical thickening of thecal cells of an ovarian follicle with its apex pointed toward the surface.

twin c., two retinal c.'s fused together.

vascular c.'s, *lobuli* epididymidis.

l-cone. Long wavelength sensitive c. (red c.).

m-cone. Middle wavelength sensitive c. (green c.).

s-cone. Short wavelength sensitive c. (blue c.).

conenine (kon'ĕ-nēn). Con-5-enine; conanine with a 5-6 double bond; precursor of conessine.

conessi (ko-nes'e) [E. Ind.]. Kurchi bark; the bark of *Holarrhena antidysenterica* (family Apocynaceae), an Indian tree; used as an astringent and in the treatment of dysentery and amebiasis.

conessine (kon'ĕ-sēn). Wrightine; neriine; roquessine; 3β-(dimethylamino)con-5-enine; 3β-dimethylamino-18α:20α-methylimino-5-pregnene; a steroid alkaloid derived from *Holarrhena antidysenterica* (conessi); a yellow astringent, used in the treatment of amebic dysentery and vaginal trichomoniasis.

conexus, pl. **conexus** (ko-nek'sŭs) [L.] [NA]. Official alternate term for connexus.

c. intertendin'eus [NA], official alternate term for *connexus* intertendineus.

confabulation (kon'fab-yū-lā'shŭn) [L. *con-fabular,* pp. *-fabulatus,* to talk together, fr. *fabula,* narrative]. The making of bizarre and incorrect responses, and a readiness to give a fluent answer, with no regard whatever to facts, to any question put; seen in amnesia, presbyophrenia, and Wernicke-Korsakoff syndrome.

confectio, gen. **confectionis,** pl. **confectiones** (kon-fek'shē-ō, -ō'nis, -ō'nēz) [L. fr. *conficio,* pp. *-fectus,* to make ready, prepare]. Confection.

confection (kon-fek'shŭn) [L. *confectio*]. Confectio; conserve; electuary; a pharmaceutical preparation consisting of a drug mixed with honey or syrup; a soft solid, sometimes used as an excipient for pill masses.

confertus (kon-fer'tŭs) [L. *confercio,* pp. *-fertus,* to cram together, fr. *farcio,* to fill full, cram]. Arranged closely together; confluent; coalescing.

confidentiality (kon'fi-den-shē-al'i-tē) [L. *con-fido,* to trust, be assured]. The statutorily protected right afforded specifically designated health professionals to nondisclosure of information discerned during consultation with a patient.

configuration (kon-fig-yū-rā'shŭn). **1.** The general form of a body and its parts. **2.** In chemistry, the spatial arrangement of atoms in a molecule. The c. of a compound (*e.g.,* a sugar) is the unique spatial arrangement of its atoms such that no other arrangement of these atoms is superimposable thereon with complete correspondence, regardless of changes in conformation (*i.e.,* twisting or rotation about single bonds); change of c. requires breaking and rejoining of bonds, as in going from D to L c.'s of sugars. *Cf.* conformation.

confinement (kon-fīn'ment) [L. *confine* (ntr.), a boundary, confine, fr. *con-* + *finis,* boundary]. Lying-in; giving birth to a child.

conflict (kon'flikt). Tension or stress experienced by an organism when satisfaction of a need, drive, or motive is thwarted by the presence of other attractive or unattractive needs, drives, or motives.

approach-approach c., a situation of indecision and vacillation in which an individual is confronted with two equally attractive alternatives.

approach-avoidance c., a situation of indecision and vacillation in which the individual is confronted with a single object or event which has both attractive and unattractive qualities.

avoidance-avoidance c., a situation of indecision and vacillation in which the individual is confronted with two equally unattractive alternatives.

role c., the stress on an individual required to play two different parts that cannot be harmonized.

confluence (kon'flū-ĕns) [L. *confluens*]. Confluens; a flowing together; a joining of two or more streams.

c. of sinuses, *confluens* sinuum.

confluens (kon-flū'enz) [L.] [NA]. Confluence.

c. si'nuum [NA], confluence of sinuses; torcular herophili; a meeting place, at the internal occipital protuberance, of the superior sagittal, straight, occipital, and two transverse sinuses of the dura mater.

confluent (kon'flū-ent) [L. *con-fluo,* to flow together]. **1.** Joining; running together; denoting certain skin lesions which become merged, forming a patch; denoting a disease characterized by lesions which are not discrete, or distinct one from the other. **2.** Denoting a bone formed by the blending together of two originally distinct bones.

conformation (kon-fōr-mā'shŭn). The spatial arrangement of a molecule achieved by rotation of groups about single covalent bonds, without breaking any covalent bonds; the latter restriction differentiates c. from configuration (as in anomers and related stereoisomers) where a bond or bonds must be broken in going from one form (configuration) to another. C. is one of the most important aspects of sugar chemistry and is basic to an understanding of the chemical properties of sugars.
boat c., see Haworth conformational formulas of cyclic *sugars.*
envelope c., see Haworth conformational formulas of cyclic *sugars.*

conformer (kon-fōr'mer) [L. *conformo,* to fashion]. A mold, usually of plastic material, used in plastic surgical repair to maintain space in a cavity or to prevent closing by healing of an artificial or natural opening affected by neighboring surgical repair.

confrontation (kon-frŏn-tā'shŭn). The act by the therapist, or another patient in a therapy group, of openly interpreting a patient's resistances, attitudes, feelings, or effects upon either the therapist, the group, or its member(s).

confusion (kon-fyū'zhŭn) [L. *confusio,* a confounding]. A mental state in which reactions to environmental stimuli are inappropriate because the person is bewildered, perplexed, or unable to orientate himself.

confusional (kon-fyū'zhŭn-ăl). Characterized by, or pertaining to, confusion.

congelation (kon-jĕ-lā'shŭn) [L. *con-gelo,* pp. *-atus,* to freeze]. **1.** Freezing. **2.** Frostbite.

congener (kon'jĕ-ner) [L. *con-,* with, + *genus,* race]. **1.** One of two or more things of the same kind, as of animal or plant with respect to classification. **2.** One of two or more muscles with the same function.

congenerous (kon-jen'er-ŭs) [see congener]. **1.** Having the same function; denoting certain muscles that are synergistic. **2.** Derived from the same source, or of a similar nature.

congenic (kon-jen'ik). Relating to an inbred strain of animals produced by repeated crossing of one gene line onto another inbred (isogenic) line.

congenital (kon-jen'i-tăl) [L. *congenitus,* born with]. Existing at birth, referring to certain mental or physical traits, anomalies, malformations, diseases, etc. which may be either hereditary or due to an influence occurring during gestation up to the moment of birth.

congenitus (kon-jen'i-tŭs) [L.]. Congenital.

congested (kon-jes'ted). Containing an abnormal amount of blood; in a state of congestion.

congestion (kon-jes'chŭn) [L. *congestio,* a bringing together, a heap, fr. *con-gero,* pp. *-gestus,* to bring together]. Presence of an abnormal amount of fluid in the vessels or passages of a part or organ; especially, of blood due either to increased afflux or to an obstruction to the return flow. See also hyperemia.
active c., c. due to an increased flow of arterial blood to a part.
brain c., encephalemia; increased volume of the intravascular compartment of the brain; often associated with brain swelling.
functional c., physiologic c.; hyperemia occurring during functional activity of an organ.
hypostatic c., hypostasis (2); c. due to pooling of venous blood in a dependent part.
passive c., c. caused by obstruction or slowing of the venous drainage, resulting in partial stagnation of blood in the capillaries and venules.
physiologic c., functional c.
venous c., overfilling and distention of the veins with blood as a result of mechanical obstruction or right ventricular failure.

congestive (kon-jes'tiv). Relating to congestion.

conglobate (kon-glō'bāt) [L. *con-globo,* pp. *-atus,* to gather into a *globus,* ball]. Formed in a single rounded mass.

conglobation (kon-glō-bā'shŭn). An aggregation of numerous particles into one rounded mass.

conglomerate (kon-glom'ĕ-rāt) [L. *con- glomero,* pp. *-atus,* to roll together, fr. *glomus,* a ball]. Composed of several parts aggregated into one mass.

conglutinant (kon-glū'ti-nant) [L. *con-glutino,* pp. *-atus,* to glue together, fr. *gluten,* glue]. Adhesive, promoting the union of a wound.

conglutination (kon-glū-ti-nā'shŭn). **1.** Adhesion (1). **2.** Agglutination of antigen(erythrocyte)-antibody-complement complex by normal bovine serum (and certain other colloidal materials); the procedure provides a means of detecting the presence of nonagglutinating antibody.

conglutinin (kon-glū'ti-nin). Bovine colloid; bovine serum protein that, when absorbed by erythrocyte-antibody-complement complexes, causes them to agglutinate; it is comparatively thermostable and apparently dissociates when diluted with physiologic saline solution.

congophilic (kon-gō-fil'ik). Denoting any substance that takes a Congo red stain.

Congo red (kong'gō) [C.I. 22120]. An acid direct cotton dye, sodium diphenyldiazo-bis-α-naphthylaminesulfonate; used as an indicator (pH 3.0, blue-violet, to pH 5.0, red) in testing for free hydrochloric acid in gastric contents; the dye is absorbed by amyloid and induces green fluorescence to amyloid in polarized light; used as a laboratory aid in the diagnosis of amyloidosis and as a histologic stain; see Bennhold's Congo red *stain.*

coni (kō'nī). Plural of conus.

conic, conical (kon'ik; kon'i-kăl). Resembling a cone.

-conid. Suffix denoting the cusp of a tooth in the lower jaw.

conidia (ko-nid'ē-ă). Plural of conidium.

conidial (ko-nid'ē-ăl). Relating to a conidium.

Conidiobolus (ko-nid'ē-ăl). A genus of fungi containing two species, *C. Coronatus* and *C. incongruus,* that cause entomophthoramycosis.

conidiogenous (ko-nid-ē-oj'ĕ-nŭs). Denoting a cell that gives rise to a conidium, *e.g.,* a phialide.

conidiophore (ko-nid'ē-ō-fōr) [conidium + G. *phoros,* bearing]. A specialized hypha which bears conidia in fungi.
Phialophore-type c., a type of spore formation, characteristic of the genus *Phialophora,* in which conidia are formed endogenously in flask-like c.'s called phialids.

conidium, pl. conidia (ko-nid'ē-ŭm, -ē-ă) [Mod. L. dim. fr. G. *konis,* dust]. An asexual spore of fungi borne externally in various ways.

coniine (kō'nē-ēn). Cicutine; conicine; 2-propylpiperidine; the toxic active alkaloid of conium; the hydrobromide and hydrochloride salts have been used as an antispasmodic.

coniofibrosis (kō'nē-ō-fī-brō'sis) [G. *konis,* dust, + fibrosis]. Fibrosis produced by dust, especially of the lungs by inhaled dust.

coniolymphstasis (kō'nē-ō-limf'stă-sis). Stasis of lymph caused by dust, presumably through the intervention of fibrosis.

coniometer (kō-nē-om'ĕ-ter) [G. *konis,* dust, + *metron,* measure].

A device for estimating the amount of dust in the air.

coniophage (kō'nē-ō-fāj) [G. *konis,* dust, + *phagein,* to eat]. Alveolar *macrophage.*

coniosis (kō-nē-ō'sis) [G. *konis,* dust]. Any disease or morbid condition caused by dust.

coniotomy (kō-nē-ot'ō-mē). Cricothyrotomy.

conium (kō-nē'ŭm) [L. fr. G. *kōneion,* hemlock]. Hemlock (poison hemlock); the dried unripe fruit of *Conium maculatum* (family Umbelliferae), also known as spotted cowbane or spotted parsley; it has been used as a sedative, antispasmodic, and anodyne.

conization (kō-nī-zā'shŭn). Excision of a cone of tissue, *e.g.,* mucosa of the cervix uteri.
cautery c., removal of a cone shape of endocervical tissue with electrocautery.
cold c., obtaining a cone of endocervical tissue with a cold knife blade so as to preserve histological characteristics and avoid desiccating tissue.

conjugant (kon'jū-gant) [L. *con-jugo,* to join]. A member of a mating pair of organisms or gametes undergoing conjugation. See also exconjugant.

conjugase (kon'jŭ-gās). γ-Glutamyl hydrolase.

conjugata (kon-jŭ-gā'tă) [L. fem. of *conjugatus,* pp. of *con-jugo,* to join together] [NA]. Distance from the promontory of the sacrum to the upper edge of the pubic symphysis. Also called conjugate or anteroposterior diameter of the pelvic inlet; conjugate axis; internal or true conjugate: conjugate of the inlet; conjugate (2); diameter medianus.
c. diagonal'is, diagonal *conjugate.*

conjugate (kon'jŭ-gāt) [L. *conjugatus,* joined together. See conjugata]. **1.** Conjugated; joined or paired. **2.** Conjugata.
diagonal c., false c. (1); conjugata diagonalis; the anteroposterior dimension of the inlet that measures the clinical distance from the promontory of the sacrum to the lower margin of the symphysis pubica.
effective c., false c. (2); the internal c. measured from the nearest lumbar vertebra to the symphysis, in spondylolisthesis.
external c., Baudelocque's diameter; the distance in a straight line between the depression under the last spinous process of the lumbar vertebrae and the upper edge of the symphysis pubica.
false c., (1) diagonal c.; **(2)** effective c.
folic acid c., a folate with three molecules of glutamic acid (pteropterin) instead of one, or with seven (pteroylheptaglutamic acid or vitamin B_c conjugate).
c. of inlet, conjugata.
internal c., conjugata.
obstetric c., the diameter that represents the shortest diameter through which the head must pass in descending into the superior strait and measures, by means of x-ray, the distance from the promontory of the sacrum to a point on the inner surface of the symphysis a few millimeters below its upper margin.
obstetric c. of outlet, the c. of the outlet lengthened by the backward displacement of the coccyx.
c. of outlet, the distance from the tip of the coccyx to the lower edge of the symphysis pubica. See also obstetric c. of outlet.
true c., conjugata.

conjugated (kon'jū-gāt-ed). Conjugate (1).

conjugation (kon-jŭ-gā'shŭn) [L. *con-jugo,* pp. *-jugatus,* to join together]. **1.** The union of two unicellular organisms or of the male and female gametes of multicellular forms followed by partition of the chromatin and the production of two new cells. **2.** Bacterial c., effected by simple contact, usually by means of specialized pili through which transfer genes and other genes of the plasmid are transferred to recipient bacteria. **3.** Sexual reproduction among protozoan ciliates, during which two individuals of appropriate mating types fuse along part of their lengths; their macronuclei degenerate and the micronuclei in each macronucleus divide several times (including a meiotic division); one of the resulting haploid pronuclei passes from each conjugant into the other and fuses with the remaining haploid nucleus in each conjugant; the organisms then separate (becoming exconjugants), undergo nuclear reorganization, and subsequently divide by asexual mitosis. **4.** The combination, especially in the liver, of certain toxic substances formed in the intestine, drugs, or steroid hormones with glucuronic or sulfuric acid; a means by which the biological activity of certain chemical substances is terminated and the substances made ready for excretion.

conjunctiva, pl. **conjunctivae** (kon-jŭnk-tī'vă, -vē) [L. fem. of *conjunctivus,* from *conjungo,* pp. *-junctus,* to bind together]. *Tunica* conjunctiva.
bulbar c., *tunica* conjunctiva bulbi.
palpebral c., *tunica* conjunctiva palpebrarum.

conjunctival (kon-jŭnk-tī'văl). Relating to the conjunctiva.

conjunctive (kon-jŭnk'tiv). Joining; connecting; connective.

conjunctiviplasty (kon-jŭnk-tī'vi-plas-tē). Conjunctivoplasty.

conjunctivitis (kon-jŭnk-ti-vī'tis). Blennophthalmia (1); inflammation of the conjunctiva.
actinic c., ultraviolet *keratoconjunctivitis.*
acute catarrhal c., simple c.; mucopurulent c.; c. with marked hyperemia and mucopurulent discharge, with a tendency toward spontaneous recovery.
acute contagious c., acute epidemic c., pinkeye (1); Koch-Weeks c.; an acute c. marked by intense hyperemia and profuse mucopurulent discharge; caused by *Haemophilus influenzae* (Koch-Weeks bacillus).
acute follicular c., an epidemic mucopurulent inflammation of the conjunctiva marked by follicles, especially in the lower fornix; may be caused by *Chlamydia,* adenoviruses, herpesvirus, and Newcastle disease virus.
acute hemorrhagic c., specific acute endemic c. with eyelid swelling, tearing, conjunctival hemorrhages, and follicles; usually caused by *Enterovirus* type 70.
allergic c., atopic c.; a conjuctival reaction to a substance producing a hypersensitivity response, either humoral or cellular.
angular c., Morax-Axenfeld c.; diplobacillary c.; a subacute bilateral conjunctival inflammation caused by the Morax-Axenfeld diplobacillus, marked by redness of the lateral canthi and scanty, stringy discharge that adheres to the lashes.
arc-flash c., ultraviolet *keratoconjunctivitis.*
c. ar'ida, xerophthalmia.
atopic c., allergic c.
Béal's c., acute inflammation of the conjunctiva with rapid onset, mild symptoms, and preauricular adenopathy.
blennorrheal c., gonococcal c.
calcareous c., c. petrificans; lithiasis c.; a condition in which the palpebral conjunctiva contains minute yellow concretions due to products of cellular degeneration in Henle's glands.
chemical c., conjunctival inflammation due to chemical irritants.
chronic c., a persistent, bilateral, conjunctival hyperemia with scanty exudation; there is a tendency toward remission and exacerbation.
chronic follicular c., catarrhal inflammation of the conjunctiva, with discrete follicles in fornices that may be infective, toxic, or irritant in nature.
cicatricial c., a chronic progressive ocular affection that produces scarring of the conjunctiva primarily and of the cornea sequentially, transient small vesicles, a viscid ropy discharge, symblepharon, xerosis, and trichiasis, eventually becoming bilateral; sometimes called ocular pemphigoid.
contagious granular c., trachoma.
croupous c., acute c. with membranous exudation, without infil-

tration of the underlying conjunctiva.
diphtheritic c., membranous c.; a severe conjunctival inflammation caused by *Corynebacterium diphtheriae* and characterized by an infiltrating membrane which on removal leaves a raw surface.
diplobacillary c., angular c.
follicular c., c. associated with hypertrophic lymphoid tissue in the lower fornices.
gonococcal c., blenorrheal c.; a purulent c. caused by *Neisseria gonorrhea* and marked by swollen congested conjunctiva, edematous eyelids, and a purulent discharge.
granular c., trachomatous c.
inclusion c., inclusion blenorrhea; swimming pool c.; a benign follicular c. caused by *Chlamydia trachomatis.*
infantile purulent c., *ophthalmia* neonatorum.
Koch-Weeks c., acute contagious c.
lacrimal c., a chronic c. associated with lacrimal passage obstruction and infection.
larval c., c. due to imbedding of larvae in the eye.
ligneous c., c. characterized typically by ligneous induration of the upper tarsal conjunctiva, whitish pseudomembrane, and, in severe cases, corneal opacity; usually bilateral.
lithiasis c., calcareous c.
c. medicamento'sa, a c. caused by medicine instilled into the conjunctival sac.
meibomian c., a c. associated with chronic inflammation of the meibomian glands, with swollen tarsal plates and frothy seborrheic secretion.
membranous c., diphtheritic c.
molluscum c., c. associated with lesions of molluscum contagiosum of the eyelid.
Morax-Axenfeld c., angular c.
mucopurulent c., acute catarrhal c.
necrotic infectious c., Pascheff's c.; a unilateral, suppurative, necrotic inflammation of the conjunctiva characterized by scattered, elevated white spots in the fornices and palpebral conjunctiva, and ipsilateral swelling of preauricular, parotid, and submaxillary lymph glands.
Parinaud's c., a chronic necrotic inflammation of the conjunctiva characterized by large, irregular, reddish follicles and regional lymphadenopathy.
Pascheff's c., necrotic infectious c.
c. petrif'icans, calcareous c.
phlyctenular c., phlyctenular or scrofulous ophthalmia; ophthalmia eczematosa; a circumscribed c. accompanied by the formation of small red nodules of lymphoid tissue (phlyctenulae) on the conjunctiva.
prairie c., a chronic c., characterized by the presence of small white spots on the palpebral conjunctiva, especially of the lower lid.
pseudomembranous c., a nonspecific inflammatory reaction characterized by the appearance on the conjunctiva of a coagulated fibrinous plaque that may be peeled off from intact epithelium.
purulent c., a violently acute inflammation of the conjunctiva, with copious pus and a marked tendency for corneal involvement.
simple c., acute catarrhal c.
snow c., ultraviolet *keratoconjunctivitis.*
spring c., vernal c.
squirrel plague c., tularemic c.
swimming pool c., inclusion c.
toxicogenic c., c. produced by topical application of a microbial toxin.
trachomatous c., granular c.; a chronic infection of the conjunctiva due to *Chlamydia trachomatis,* characterized by conjunctival follicles and subsequent cicatrization. See also trachoma.
tularemic c., c. tularen'sis, squirrel plague c.; c. due to *Francisella tularensis,* transmitted to man from rabbits and other rodents; characterized by chemosis, small necrotic ulcers, and regional adenopathy.
vernal c., vernal catarrh or keratoconjunctivitis; spring c. or ophthalmia; a chronic, bilateral conjunctival inflammation with photophobia and intense itching that recurs seasonally during warm weather; characterized in the palpebral form by cobblestone papillae in the upper palpebral conjunctiva and in the bulbar form by gelatinous nodules adjacent to the corneoscleral limbus.
welder's c., ultraviolet *keratoconjunctivitis.*

conjunctivodacryocystorhinostomy (kon-jŭnk'ti-vō-dak'rē-ō-sis'tō-rī-nos'tō-mē) [conjunctiva + G. *dakryon,* tear, + *kystis,* cyst, + *ris* (*rhin-*), nose, + *stoma,* mouth]. A procedure for providing lacrimal drainage when the canaliculi are closed; plastic tubes are inserted that extend from the conjunctival sac to the nose.

conjunctivodacryocystostomy (kon-jŭnk'ti-vō-dak'rē-ō-sis-tos'tō-mē) [conjunctiva + G. *dakryon,* tear, + *kystis,* sac, + *stoma,* mouth]. **1.** A surgical procedure through the conjunctiva, which provides an opening into the lacrimal sac. **2.** The opening so produced.

conjunctivoma (kon-jŭnk-ti-vō'mă). A homeoplastic tumor of the conjunctiva.

conjunctivoplasty (kon-jŭnk-tī'vō-plas-tē, kon-jŭngk'ti-vō-). Conjunctiviplasty; plastic surgery on the conjunctiva.

conjunctivorhinostomy (kon-jŭnk'ti-vō-rī-nos'tō-mē) [conjunctiva + G. *ris* (*rhin*), nose, + *stoma,* mouth]. **1.** A surgical procedure to construct a passageway through the conjunctiva into the nasal cavity. **2.** The opening so produced.

Conn, Harold J., U.S. microbiologist, 1886–1975. See Hucker-C. *stain.*

Conn, Jerome, U.S. physician, *1907. See C.'s *syndrome.*

connectins (kon-nek'tinz). Collective term for the protein components of the cytoskeleton (connective tissue); originally described in muscle, but later observed in erythrocyte and other cell membranes.

connection (kō-nek'shŭn). A union of elements or things.
intertendineus c.'s, *connexus* intertendineus.

connector (kō-nek'tōr, -tōr). In dentistry, a part of a partial denture which unites its components.
major c., a plate or bar (lingual bar, palatal bar) used for the purpose of uniting partial denture bases.
minor c., the connecting link (tang) between the major c. or base of a partial denture and other units of the prosthesis, such as clasps, indirect retainers, and occlusal rests.

Connell, F. Gregory, U.S. surgeon, 1875–1968. See C.'s *suture.*

connexon (kon-neks'on). A complex protein assembly that traverses the lipid bilayer of the plasma membrane and forms a continuous channel with a pore diameter of approximately 1.5 nm; a pair of c.'s from two adjacent cells join to form a gap junction which bridges the 2-4 nm gap between the cells, resulting in both electrical and metabolic couplings.

connexus (ko-nek'sŭs) [L.] [NA]. Conexus; a connecting structure.
c. intertendin'eus [NA], conexus intertendineus; juncturae tendinum; fibrous bands passing obliquely between the diverging tendons of the extensor digitorum on the dorsum of the hand.

conoid (kō'noyd) [G. *kōnoeidēs,* cone-shaped]. **1.** A cone-shaped structure. **2.** Part of the apical complex characteristic of the protozoan subphylum, Apicomplexa; seen in sporozoites, merozoites, or other developmental stages of sporozoans, less well developed in the piroplasms (families Babesiidae and Theileriidae). The function of the c. is unknown, but it is thought to be an organelle of penetration into the host cell, possibly aided by a protrusible form of the c.
Sturm's c., in optics, the pattern of rays formed after passage through a spherocylindrical combination.

conomyoidin (kō-nō-mī′oy-din) [G. *kōnos,* cone, + *mys,* muscle, + *eidos,* resemblance]. Contractile protoplasm at the inner end of the inner segment of retinal cones; motility is most evident in fishes and amphibians, and slight or absent in mammals.

conquinine (kon′kwi-nēn). Quinidine.

Conradi, Andrew C., Norwegian physician, 1809–1869. See C.'s *line.*

Conradi, Erich, German physician. See C.'s *disease.*

Conradi, Heinrich, German bacteriologist, *1876. See C.-Drigalski *agar,* Drigalski-C. *agar.*

consanguineous (kon-sang-gwin′ē-ŭs) [L. *cum,* with, + *sanguis,* blood: *consanguineus*]. Denoting consanguinity.

consanguinity (kon-sang-gwin′i-tē) [L. *consanguinitas,* blood relationship]. Blood relationship; kinship because of common ancestry.

conscious (con′shŭs) [L. *conscius,* knowing]. **1.** Aware; having present knowledge or perception of oneself, one's acts and surroundings. **2.** Denoting something occurring with the perceptive attention of the individual, as a c. act or idea, distinguished from automatic or instinctive.

consciousness (con′shŭs-nes) [L. *con-scio,* to know, to be aware of]. The state of being aware, or perceiving physical facts or mental concepts; a state of general wakefulness and responsiveness to environment.

clouding of c., a state in which the patient is not in contact with the environment.

double c., a condition in which one lives in two seemingly unrelated mental states, being, while in one, unaware of the other or of the acts performed in the other. See also dual *personality.*

field of c., the material of awareness at any given moment.

consensual (kon-sen′shū-ăl) [L. *con-,* with, + *sensus,* sensation]. Reflex (3); denoting what is done in response to a stimulus without cooperation of the will.

conservation (kon-ser-vā′shŭn) [L. *conservatio,* a preserving, keeping]. **1.** Preservation from loss, injury, or decay. **2.** In sensorimotor theory, the mental operation by which an individual retains the idea of an object after its removal in time or space.

c. of energy, the principle that the total amount of energy in a closed system remains always the same, none being lost or created in any chemical or physical process or in the conversion of one kind of energy into another, within that system.

conservative (kon-ser′vă-tiv). Denoting treatment by gradual, limited, or well-established procedures, as opposed to radical.

conserve (kon′serv). Confection.

consolidant (kon-sol′i-dant). A substance that promotes healing or union.

consolidation (kon-sol-i-dā′shŭn) [L. *consolido,* to make thick, condense, fr. *solidus,* solid]. Solidification into a firm dense mass; applied especially to inflammatory induration of a normally aerated lung due to the presence of cellular exudate in the pulmonary alveoli.

conspecific (kon-spe-sif′ik) [L. *con-,* with, + specific]. Of the same species.

constancy (kon′stan-sē). The quality of being constant.

color c., unchanging perception of the color of an object despite changes in lighting or viewing conditions.

object c., the tendency for objects to be perceived as unchanging despite variations in the positions in and conditions under which the objects are observed.

constant (kon′stănt). A quantity that, under stated conditions, does not vary with changes in the environment.

Ambard's c., see Ambard's *laws.*

association c., in experimental immunology, a mathematical expression of hapten-antibody interaction: average association c., K = [hapten-bound antibody]/[free antibody][free hapten].

Avogadro's c., Avogadro's *number.*

decay c., disintegration or radioactive c.; the c. in the mathematical expression for the number of atoms of a radionuclide decaying in a unit of time; λ in the equation $N/N_o = e^{-\lambda t}$.

diffusion c., diffusion *coefficient.*

disintegration c., decay c.

dissociation c. (K), the equilibrium c. involved in the dissociation of a compound into two or more ions.

dissociation c. of an acid (K_a), expressed by general equation $(H^+)(A^-)/(HA) = K_a$, where HA is the undissociated acid.

dissociation c. of a base (K_b), expressed by the general equation $(B^+)(OH^-)/(BOH) = K_b$, where BOH is the undissociated base.

dissociation c. of water (K_w), expressed by the equation $(H^+)(OH^-) = K_w = 10^{-14}$ at 25°C.

equilibrium c., in the reaction $A + B \rightleftarrows C + D$ at equilibrium (*i.e.,* no net change in *A, B, C,* or *D*), the concentrations of the four components are related by the equation $K = [C][D]/[A][B]$; K is the equilibrium c. If any component in the reaction has a multiplier (*e.g.,* $H_2 \rightleftarrows 2H$), that multiplier appears as an exponent in the calculation of $K = ([H]^2/[H_2])$. When this equation is applied to the ionization of a substance in solution, K is called the dissociation c. and its negative logarithm (base 10) is the pK. See also Henderson-Hasselbalch *equation.*

Faraday's c., see faraday.

flotation c. (S_f), negative S; Svedberg of flotation; characteristic sedimentation behavior of a lipoprotein fraction of plasma in a centrifugal field in a medium of appropriate density, achieved by adding a salt or D_2O to the plasma.

gas c., R (symbol for the constant) = 8.314 × 10^7 ergs per degree Celsius per mole = 8.314 J K^{-1} mol^{-1} (joule per kelvin mole).

Michaelis c., Michaelis-Menten c. (K_m), the concentration of the substrate at which half the maximum velocity of a reaction is achieved; the ratio of the rate c.'s $(k_2 + k_3)/k_1$ in the reaction Enzyme + Substrate $\underset{k_2}{\overset{k_1}{\rightleftarrows}}$ ES complex $\overset{k_3}{\rightarrow}$ Products + Enzyme. It is equal to substrate concentration × $[(V_{max} - V_{obs})/V_{obs}]$, the Michaelis-Menton equation. See also Lineweaver-Burk *equation.*

newtonian c. of gravitation (G), a universal c. relating the gravitational force, *f.,* attracting two masses, m_1 and m_2, toward each other when they are separated by a distance, *r,* in the equation: $f = G(m_1 m_2/r^2)$; it has the value of 6.6720 × 10^{-8} dyne $cm^2 gm^{-2}$ = 6.67 × $10^{-11} m^3 kg^{-1} s^{-2}$ in SI units.

Planck's c. (h), a c., 6.6256 × 10^{-34} J s (joule-seconds) or 6.6262 × 10^{-27} erg-seconds = 6.6262 × $10^{-34} JH_z{}^{-1}$(joule per hertz).

radioactive c. (λ), decay c.

rate c.'s, velocity c.'s.

sedimentation c., the c. *s* in Svedberg's equation for estimating the molecular weight of a protein from the rate of movement in a centrifugal field:

$$M = s\frac{RT}{D(1 - \bar{V}\rho)}$$

where M is the molecular weight, R the gas constant, T the absolute temperature, D the diffusion constant (in square centimeters per second), $\bar{V}$ the partial specific volume of the protein, ρ the density of the solvent. The constant *s,* with dimensions of time per unit of field force, is usually between 1 × 10^{-13} and 200 × 10^{-13} second. The Svedberg unit (S) is arbitrarily set at 1 × 10^{-13} second and is very often used to describe the sedimentation rate of macromolecules; *e.g.,* 4 S RNA.

time c., that part of the rate meter circuit that determines the time interval over which the rate of incoming events will be averaged.

velocity c.'s, rate c.'s; in enzymic reactions, k_1, k_2, and k_3 in the Michaelis-Menten c.

constellation (kon-stel-ā′shŭn). In psychiatry, all the factors that determine a particular action.

constipate (kon'sti-pāt). To cause constipation.

constipated (kon'sti-pāt-ed). Suffering from constipation.

constipation (kon-sti-pā'shŭn) [L. *con-stipo,* pp. *-atus,* to press together]. Costiveness; a condition in which bowel movements are infrequent or incomplete.

constitution (kon-sti-tū'shŭn) [L. *constitutio,* constitution, disposition, fr. *constituo,* pp. *-stitutus,* to establish, fr. *statuo,* to set up]. **1.** The physical makeup of a body, including the mode of performance of its functions, the activity of its metabolic processes, the manner and degree of its reactions to stimuli, and its power of resistance to the attack of pathogenic organisms. **2.** In chemistry, the number and kind of atoms in the molecule and the relation they bear to each other.

constitutional (kon-sti-tū'shŭn-ăl). **1.** Relating to a body's constitution. **2.** General; relating to the system as a whole; not local.

constriction (kon-strik'shŭn) [L. *con-stringo,* pp. *-strictus,* to draw together]. **1.** Binding or contraction of a part. See also stricture; stenosis. **2.** A subjective sensation as if the body or any part were tightly bound or squeezed.

primary c., the narrowing between the two arms of the chromosome represented by the centromere.

secondary c., a subsidiary narrowing of the chromosome associated in some cases with satellites.

constrictor (kon-strik'ter, -tōr) [L. fr. *constringo,* to draw together]. **1.** Anything that binds or squeezes a part. **2.** A muscle, the action of which is to narrow a canal; a sphincter.

consultand (kon-sŭl'tand) [see consultant]. In genetics, a person about whose future offspring the genetic counselor is to make predictions.

dummy c., a person in the line of descent from the last ancestor known to be affected by a genetic trait to the c. proper; for logical simplicity, the dummy c. is analyzed as if the c. proper.

consultant (kon-sŭl'tant) [L. *consulto,* pp. *-atus,* to deliberate, ask advice]. **1.** A physician or surgeon who does not take full responsibility for a patient, but acts in an advisory capacity, deliberating with and counseling the attending physician or surgeon. **2.** A member of a hospital staff who has no active service but stands ready to advise in any case, at the request of the attending physician or surgeon.

consultation (kon-sŭl-tā'shŭn). Meeting of two or more physicians or surgeons to evaluate the nature and progress of disease in a particular patient and to establish diagnosis, prognosis, and therapy.

consumption (kon-sŭmp'shŭn) [L. *con-sumo,* pp. *-sumptus,* to take up wholly, use up, waste]. **1.** The using up of something, especially the rate at which it is used. **2.** Obsolete term for a wasting of the tissues of the body, usually tuberculous.

oxygen c., **(1)** (Q_O or Q_{O_2}), the rate at which oxygen is used by a tissue; units: microliters of oxygen STPD used per milligram of tissue per hour; **(2)** ($\dot{V}_{O_2}$), the rate at which oxygen enters the blood from alveolar gas, equal in the steady state to the consumption of oxygen by tissue metabolism throughout the body; units: milliliters of oxygen STPD used per minute or mmol/min.

consumptive (kon-sŭmp'tiv). Relating to, or suffering from, consumption.

contact (kon'takt) [L. *con- tingo,* pp. *-tactus,* to touch, seize, fr. *tango,* to touch]. **1.** The touching or apposition of two bodies. **2.** A person who has been exposed to a contagious disease.

balancing c., balancing occlusal surface; **(1)** the c.'s between upper and lower dentures on the balancing or mediotrusive side for the purpose of stabilizing the dentures; **(2)** the c.'s between upper and lower dentures at the opposite side from the working or laterotrusive side (anteroposteriorly or laterally) for the purpose of stabilizing the dentures; **(3)** the c.'s between upper and lower natural or artificial teeth at the opposite side from the working or laterotrusive side.

centric c., centric *occlusion.*

deflective occlusal c., cuspal interference; interceptive occlusal c.; premature c.; a condition of tooth c.'s which diverts the mandible from a normal path of closure to centric jaw relation.

initial c., **(1)** the first meeting of opposing teeth upon elevation of the mandible toward the maxillae; **(2)** the initial occlusal c. of opposing teeth when the jaw is closed.

interceptive occlusal c., deflective occlusal c.

premature c., deflective occlusal c.

proximal c., proximate c., the area of touching of the surfaces of two adjacent teeth in the same arch.

c. with reality, correctly interpreting external phenomena in relation to the norms of one's social or cultural milieu.

working c.'s, working or occlusion; c.'s of teeth made on the side of the occlusion toward which the mandible has been moved.

contactant (kon-tak'tănt). Any of a heterogeneous group of allergens that elicit manifestations of induced sensitivity (hypersensitivity) by direct contact with skin or mucosa.

contagion (kon-tā'jŭn) [L. *contagio;* fr. *contingo,* to touch closely]. **1.** Contagium. **2.** Transmission of disease by contact with the sick. The term originated long before development of modern ideas of infectious disease and has since lost much of its significance, being included under the more inclusive term "communicable disease." **3.** Production of a neurosis or psychosis through imitation or autosuggestion.

immediate c., direct c. occurring as the result of actual contact with the sick.

mediate c., indirect c. effected through the medium of persons or objects that have been in contact with the sick.

psychic c., communication of a nervous disorder by imitation, as in mass hysteria.

contagious (kon-tā'jŭs). Relating to contagion; communicable or transmissible by contact with the sick or their fresh secretions or excretions.

contagiousness (kon-tā'jŭs-nes). The quality of being contagious.

contagium (kon-tā'jē-ŭm) [L. a touching]. Contagion (1); the agent of an infectious disease.

contaminant (kon-tam'i-nant). An impurity; any material of an extraneous nature associated with a chemical, a pharmaceutical preparation, a physiologic principle, or an infectious agent.

contaminate (kon-tam'i-nāt). To cause or result in contamination.

contamination (kon-tam-i-nā'shŭn) [L. *contamino,* pp. *-atus,* to stain, defile]. **1.** The act or process of rendering inferior, impure, unsuitable, or unhealthy by association, contact, mixture, or introduction of an unwholesome or undesirable element. **2.** The element involved. **3.** Freudian term for a fusion and condensation of words.

content (kon'tent) [L. *contentus,* fr. *con- tineo,* pp. *-tentus,* to hold together, contain]. **1.** That which is contained within something else, usually in this sense in the plural form, contents. **2.** In psychology, the form of a dream as presented to consciousness. **3.** Ambiguous usage for concentration (3); *e.g.,* blood hemoglobin c. could mean either its concentration or the product of its concentration and the blood volume.

carbon dioxide c., the total carbon dioxide available from serum or plasma following addition of acid; measured routinely in hospital laboratories as a component of electrolyte profiles.

latent c., the hidden, unconscious meaning of thoughts or actions, especially in dreams or fantasies.

manifest c., those elements of fantasy and dreams which are consciously available and reportable.

contiguity (kon-ti-gyū'i-tē) [L. *contiguus,* touching, fr. *contingo,* to touch]. **1.** Contact without actual continuity, *e.g.,* the contact of the bones entering into the formation of a cranial suture. *Cf.* continuity. **2.** Occurrence of two or more objects, events, or mental impressions together in space (**spatial c.**) or time (**temporal c.**).

contiguous (kon-tig'ū-ŭs). Adjacent or in actual contact.

continence (kon'ti-nens) [L. *continentia,* fr. *con- tineo,* to hold back]. **1.** Moderation, temperance, or self-restraint in respect to the appetites, especially to sexual intercourse. **2.** The ability to retain urine and/or feces until a proper time for their discharge.

continent (kon'ti-nent). Denoting continence.

continued (kon-tin'yūd) [L. *continuo,* to join together, make continuous]. Continuous; without intermission; said especially of protracted fever without apyretic intervals, such as typhoid fever, compared with the paroxysms of fever in malaria.

continuity (kon-ti-nu'i-tē) [L. *continuus,* continued]. Absence of interruption, a succession of parts intimately united, *e.g.,* the unbroken conjunction of cells and structures that make up a single bone of the skull. *Cf.* contiguity.

contour (kon'tūr) [L. *con-* (intens.), + *torno,* to turn (in a lathe), fr. *tornus,* a lathe]. **1.** The outline of a part; the surface configuration. **2.** In dentistry, to restore the normal outlines of a broken or otherwise misshapen tooth, or to create the external shape or form of a prosthesis.

flange c., the design of the flange of a denture.

gingival c., gum c.; the shape or form of the gingiva, either natural or artificial, around the necks of the teeth.

gum c., gingival c.

height of c., see under height.

contra- [L.]. Prefix signifying opposed, against. See also counter-.

contra-angle (kon'tră-ang'gl). **1.** One of the double or triple angles in the shank of an instrument by means of which the cutting edge or point is brought into the axis of the handle. **2.** An extension piece added to the end of a dental handpiece which, through a set of bevel gears, changes the angle of the axis of rotation of the bur in relation to the axis of the handpiece.

contra-aperture (kon'tră-ap'er-chūr). Counteropening.

contrabevel (kon'tră-bev'ĕl). A bevel located on the side opposite the customary side.

contraception (kon-tră-sep'shŭn). Prevention of conception or impregnation.

contraceptive (kon-tră-sep'tiv) [L. *contra,* against, + conceptive]. **1.** An agent for the prevention of conception. **2.** Relating to any measure or agent designed to prevent conception.

"combination" oral c., a mixture of a steroid having progestational activity and an estrogen; one such pill is taken daily for approximately 21 days of each menstrual cycle.

intrauterine c. device, see under device.

oral c., any orally effective preparation designed to prevent conception.

"sequential" oral c., a preparation providing two types of medication; the first type, containing only an estrogen, is taken daily from day 5 to approximately day 19 of the menstrual cycle; the second, containing an estrogen and a semisynthetic progestational steroid, is taken daily from day 20 to day 24 of the cycle.

contract [L. *con-traho,* pp. *-tractus,* to draw together]. **1** (kon-trakt'). To shorten; to become reduced in size; in the case of muscle, either to shorten or to undergo an increase in tension. **2** (kon-trakt'). To acquire by contagion or infection. **3** (kon'trakt). An explicit bilateral commitment by psychotherapist and patient to a defined course of action to attain the goal of the psychotherapy.

contractile (kon-trak'tĭl). Having the property of contracting.

contractility (kon-trak-til'i-tē). The ability or property of a substance, especially of muscle, of shortening, or becoming reduced in size, or developing increased tension.

contraction (C) (kon-trak'shŭn) [L. *contractio,* to draw together]. **1.** A shortening or increase in tension; denoting the normal function of muscular tissue. **2.** A shrinkage or reduction in size. **3.** Heart beat, as in premature c. See also subentries under beat.

after-c., see aftercontraction.

anodal closure c. (ACC, AnCC), obsolete term for the momentary c. of a muscle under the influence of the positive pole when the electrical circuit is established.

anodal opening c. (AOC, AnOC), obsolete term for the momentary c. of a muscle under the influence of the positive pole when the circuit is broken.

automatic c., automatic *beat.*

Braxton Hicks c., rhythmic myometrial activity occurring during the course of a pregnancy which causes no pain for the patient.

carpopedal c., carpopedal *spasm.*

cathodal closure c. (CCC, CaCC), obsolete term for the momentary c. of a muscle under the influence of the negative pole when an electrical circuit is established.

cathodal opening c. (COC, CaOC), obsolete term for the momentary c. of a muscle under the influence of the negative pole when the circuit is broken.

closing c., c. produced at the time of closing of the circuit when using direct current to stimulate the muscle.

escaped c., escaped *beat.*

escaped ventricular c., an escaped beat arising in the ventricle.

fibrillary c.'s, c.'s occurring spontaneously in individual muscle fibers; they are seen commonly a few days after damage to the motor nerves supplying the muscle, and this type of activity is distinguished from fasciculation, which is related to activation of motor units.

front-tap c., Gowers' c.; c. of the calf muscles when the anterior surface of the leg is struck.

Gowers' c., front-tap c.

hourglass c., constriction of the middle portion of a hollow organ, such as the stomach or the gravid uterus.

hunger c.'s, strong c.'s of the stomach associated with hunger pains.

idiomuscular c., myoedema.

myotatic c., a reflex c. of a skeletal muscle that occurs as a result of stimulation of the stretch receptors in the muscle, *i.e.,* as part of a myotatic reflex.

opening c., a c. produced at the time of opening the circuit when using direct current to stimulate the muscle or a motor nerve.

paradoxical c., a tonic c. of the anterior tibial muscles when a sudden passive dorsal flexion of the foot is made.

postural c., maintenance of muscular tension (usually isometric) sufficient to maintain posture.

premature c., see extrasystole.

tetanic c., see tetanus (2).

tonic c., sustained contraction of a muscle, as employed in the maintenance of posture.

uterine c., rhythmic activity of the myometrium associated with menstruation, pregnancy, or labor.

contracture (kon-trak'chūr) [L. *contractura,* fr. *con-traho,* to draw together]. A permanent muscular contraction due to tonic spasm or fibrosis, or to loss of muscular balance, the antagonists being paralyzed.

Dupuytren's c., a disease of the palmar fascia resulting in thickening and c. of fibrous bands on the palmar surface of the hand and fingers. See fig. on p. 348.

functional c., a muscular shortening that ceases during sleep or general anesthesia.

ischemic c. of the left ventricle, stone heart; myocardial rigor mortis; irreversible contraction of the left ventricle of the heart as a complication of cardiopulmonary bypass.

organic c., c., usually due to fibrosis within the muscle that persists whether the subject is conscious or unconscious.

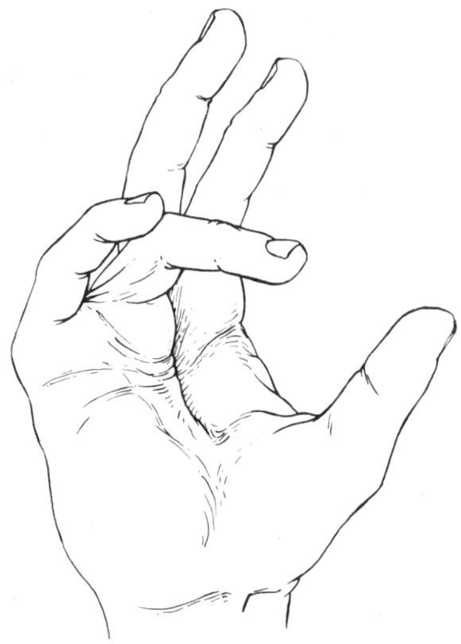

Dupuytren's Contracture

Volkmann's c., tissue degeneration produced by ischemia leading to a late c. involving muscles, tendons, fascia, and other soft tissues; caused by interference with blood flow, thus by direct vessel compression or prolonged spasm.

contrafissura (kon'tră-fi-shūr'ă) [L. *contra,* against, counter, + *fissura,* fissure]. Fracture by contrecoup; fracture of a bone, as in the skull, at a point opposite that where the blow was received.

contraindicant (kon-tră-in'di-kant). Indicating the contrary, *i.e.,* showing that a method of treatment which would otherwise be proper is inadvisable by special circumstances in the individual case.

contraindication (kon-tră-in-di-kā'shŭn). Any special symptom or circumstance that renders the use of a remedy or the carrying out of a procedure inadvisable, usually because of risk.

contralateral (kon-tră-lat'er-ăl) [L. *contra,* opposite, + *latus,* side]. Heterolateral; relating to the opposite side, as when pain is felt or paralysis occurs on the side opposite to that of the lesion.

contrast (kon'trast) [L. *contra,* against, + *sto,* pp. *status,* to stand]. A comparison in which differences are demonstrated or enhanced.
simultaneous c., the enhancement of the visual sensation of white when a white object is viewed adjacent to a black object; the black object also appears blacker as a result of the contiguity of white. Adjacent complementary colors also appear brighter; *e.g.,* green appears a brighter green and red a brighter red if these two colors are viewed side by side.
successive c., the visual effect caused by viewing a brightly colored object and then a gray surface; the latter appears tinged with the complementary color of the object. Viewing a surface colored in the complementary color of the object rather than in gray enhances the color intensity of the surface.

contrastimulant (kon-tră-stim'yū-lant). **1.** Annulling the effect of a stimulant. **2.** An agent whose action opposes that of a stimulant.

contrecoup (kawn-tr-kū') [Fr. counter-blow]. Denoting the manner of a contrafissura, as in the skull, at a point opposite that at which the blow was received. See also contrecoup *injury* of the brain.

contrectation (kon-trek-tā'shŭn) [L. *con- trecto,* pp. *-trectatus,* to handle]. **1.** Sexual foreplay prior to coition. **2.** The impulse to caress or embrace one of the opposite sex.

cont. rem. Abbreviation for L. *continuenter remedia,* continue the medicines.

control (kon-trōl') [Mediev. L. *contrarotulum,* a counterroll for checking accounts, fr. L. *rotula,* dim. of *rota,* a wheel]. **1.** To verify an experiment by means of another with the crucial variable omitted. **2.** A control animal or experiment. **3.** The regulation of maintenance of a function, action, reflex, etc.
biological c., c. of living organisms, including vectors and reservoirs of disease, by using their natural enemies (predators, parasites, competitors).
birth c., **(1)** restriction of the number of offspring by means of contraceptive measures; **(2)** projects, programs, or methods to control reproduction, by either improving or diminishing fertility.
idiodynamic c., nervous impulses from the medulla that preserve the normal trophic condition of the muscles.
own c.'s, a method of experimental c. in which the same subjects are used in both experimental and c. conditions.
quality c., the c. of laboratory analytical error by monitoring analytical performance with control sera and maintaining error within ± 2 SD of mean control values.
reflex c., nerve impulses transmitted to the muscles to maintain normal reflex action.
social c., the influence on the behavior of a person exerted by other persons or by society as a whole; *e.g.,* through social ostracism or the criminal law.
stimulus c., the use of conditioning techniques to bring the target behavior of an individual under environmental c.
synergic c., impulses transmitted from the cerebellum regulating the muscular activity of the synergic units of the body.
time-varied gain c. (TGC), time compensation gain; time-varied gain; change in gain at different depths with time, to compensate for the decrease in echo amplitude from greater depths in ultrasonic applications.
tonic c., nerve impulses that maintain a normal tonus or level of activity in muscle or other effector organs.
vestibulo-equilibratory c., nerve impulses transmitted from the semicircular canals, saccule, and utricle that serve to maintain the equilibrium of the body.

contusion (kon-tū'shŭn) [L. *contusio,* a bruising]. Any injury (usually caused by a blow) in which the skin is not broken. See also bruise, livedo.
brain c., a bruising, usually of the surface, of the brain with extravasation of blood but without rupture of the pia-arachnoid; healing results in a superficial depressed sclerotic area, possibly with incorporated meninges. See also brain *cicatrix.*
scalp c., intracutaneous or subcutaneous extravasation of blood without gross disruption of skin.
wind c., windage.

conular (kon'yū-lăr). Cone-shaped.

Conus (kō'nŭs). A genus of shellfish that inhabits the shores of some South Pacific islands. Several species, *C. geographus, C. textilis, C. aulicus, C. tulipa,* and *C. marmoreus* are poisonous, their sting or spine causing acute pain, edema, numbness, spreading paralysis, and sometimes coma and death.

conus, pl. **coni** (kō'nŭs, -nī) [L. fr. G. *kōnos,* cone]. **1** [NA]. Cone. **2.** Posterior staphyloma in myopic choroidopathy.
c. arterio'sus [NA], arterial cone; infundibulum (4); pulmonary c. or cone; the left or anterior portion of the cavity of the right ventricle of the heart, which terminates in the pulmonary artery.
congenital c., Fuchs' *coloboma.*
distraction c., a c. in which the optic nerve passes through the scleral canal in a markedly oblique direction.
c. elas'ticus [NA], elastic cone; membrana cricothyroidea; cricothyroid or cricovocal membrane; the thicker lower portion of the elastic membrane of the larynx.
co'ni epididym'idis [NA], official alternative term for *lobuli* epididymidis.
c. medulla'ris [NA], medullary cone; the tapering lower extremity

of the spinal cord.
myopic c., myopic *crescent.*
pulmonary c., c. arteriosus.
supertraction c., a reddish yellow c. or ring at the nasal margin of the optic disk, produced by displacement of the retinal pigment epithelium and lamina vitrea of the choroid; occurs in high myopia.
co'ni vasculo'si, *lobuli* epididymidis.

convalescence (kon-vă-les'ens) [L. *con-valesco,* to grow strong, fr. *valeo,* to be strong]. A period between the end of a disease and the patient's restoration to complete health.

convalescent (kon-vă-les'ent). **1.** Getting well or one who is getting well. **2.** Denoting the period of convalescence.

convallaria (kon-va-lăr'ē-ă) [L. *convallis,* an enclosed valley]. The flower, rhizome, and roots of *Convallaria majalis* (family Liliaceae), lily of the valley; they contain glycosides with digitalis-like action.

convection (kon-vek'shŭn) [L. *con-veho,* pp. *-vectus,* to carry or bring together]. Conveyance of heat in liquids or gases by movement of the heated particles, as when the layer of water at the bottom of a heated pot rises or the warm air of a room ascends to the ceiling.

convergence (kon-ver'jens) [L. *con-vergo,* to incline together]. **1.** The tending of two or more objects toward a common point. **2.** The direction of the visual lines to a near point.
accommodative c., the meter angle of c. expressed in diopters; equal to the product of the meter angles of c. times the interpupillary distance measured in centimeters.
amplitude of c., range of c.; the distance between the near point and far point of c.
angle of c., the angle that the visual axis makes with the median line when a near object is viewed.
far point of c., the point to which the visual lines are directed when c. is at rest.
near point of c., the point to which the visual lines are directed when c. is at its maximum.
negative c., the slight divergence of the visual axes when c. is at rest, as when observing the far point or during sleep.
positive c., inward deviation of the visual axes even when c. is at rest, as in cases of convergent squint.
range of c., amplitude of c.
unit of c., see meter *angle.*

convergent (kon-ver'jent). Tending toward a common point.

conversion (kon-ver'zhŭn) [L. *con-verto,* pp. *-versus,* to turn around, to change]. **1.** Change; transmutation. **2.** Transformation of an emotion into a physical manifestation, as in c. hysteria. **3.** In virology, the acquisition by bacteria of a new property associated with presence of a prophage. See also lysogeny.

convertase (kon'ver-tās). See *component* of complement.

convertin (kon-ver'tin). *Factor* VII.

convex (kon'veks, kŏn-veks') [L. *convexus,* vaulted, arched, convex, fr. *con-veho,* to bring together]. Applied to a surface that is evenly curved outward, the segment of a sphere.
high c., the segment of a sphere of short radius.
low c., the segment of a sphere of long radius.

convexity (kon-veks'i-tē). **1.** The state of being convex. **2.** A convex structure.
cortical c., *facies* superolateralis cerebri.

convexobasia (kon-vek-sō-bā'sē-ă) [L. *convexus,* outwardly curved, + *basis,* foundation]. Forward bending of the occipital bone.

convexoconcave. (kon-vek'sō-kon'kāv). Convex on one surface and concave on the opposite surface.

convexoconvex (kon-vek'sō-kon'veks). Biconvex.

convolute (kon'vō-lūt) [L. *con-volvo,* pp. *-volutus,* to roll together]. Convoluted; rolled together with one part over the other; in the shape of a roll or scroll.

convoluted (kon'vō-lū-ted). Convolute.

convolution (kon-vō-lū'shŭn) [L. *convolutio*] **1.** A coiling or rolling of an organ. **2.** Specifically, a gyrus of the cerebral or cerebellar cortex.
angular c., *gyrus* angularis.
anterior central c., *gyrus* precentralis.
ascending frontal c., *gyrus* precentralis.
ascending parietal c., *gyrus* postcentralis.
callosal c., *gyrus* cinguli.
cingulate c., *gyrus* cinguli.
first temporal c., *gyrus* temporalis superior.
hippocampal c., *gyrus* parahippocampalis.
inferior frontal c., *gyrus* frontalis inferior.
inferior temporal c., *gyrus* temporalis inferior.
middle frontal c., *gyrus* frontalis medius.
middle temporal c., *gyrus* temporalis medius.
posterior central c., *gyrus* postcentralis.
second temporal c., *gyrus* temporalis medius.
superior frontal c., *gyrus* frontalis superior.
superior temporal c., *gyrus* temporalis superior.
supramarginal c., *gyrus* supramarginalis.
third temporal c., *gyrus* temporalis inferior.
transitional c., transitional *gyrus.*
transverse temporal c.'s, *gyri* temporales transversi.
Zuckerkandl's c., *gyrus* subcallosus.

convulsant (kon-vŭl'sant). Causing convulsions. See also eclamptogenic; epileptogenic.

convulsion (kon-vŭl'shŭn) [L. *convulsio,* fr. *con-vello,* pp. *-vulsus,* to tear up]. **1.** A violent spasm or series of jerkings of the face, trunk, or extremities. **2.** Seizure (2).
clonic c., a c. in which the contractions are intermittent, the muscles alternately contracting and relaxing.
coordinate c., a clonic c. in which the movements are seemingly purposeful, being exaggerations of those that may occur naturally.
ether c., a c. occasionally associated with induction of ether anesthesia.
febrile c., a c. in infancy or early childhood, associated with fever.
hysterical c., hysteroid c., see hysteria.
immediate posttraumatic c., a c. beginning within seconds after injury.
infantile c., any c. occurring in infancy (0 to 2 years of age); may be associated with teething (tooth spasm), fever, etc.
mimic c., facial *tic.*
puerperal c.'s, puerperal *eclampsia.*
salaam c.'s, nodding *spasm.*
static c., saltatory *spasm.*
tetanic c., tonic c.
tonic c., tetanic c.; a c. in which muscle contraction is sustained.

convulsive (kon-vŭl'siv). Relating to convulsions; marked by or producing convulsions.

Cooke, A. Bennett, U.S. physician, *1869. See C.'s *speculum.*

Cooley, Thomas B., U.S. pediatrician, 1871–1945. See C.'s *anemia.*

Coolidge, William D., U.S. physicist, *1873. See C. *tube.*

Coomassie brilliant blue R-250 [C.I. 42660]. A general protein stain used in electrophoresis because of its unusual sensitivity.

Coombs, Carey F., British physician, 1879–1932. See C. *murmur.*

Coombs, Robin R.A., British veterinarian and immunologist, *1921. See Gell and C. *reactions;* C.'s *serum, test;* direct C. *test;* indirect C. *test.*

Cooper, Sir Astley Paston, British anatomist and surgeon, 1768–1841. See C.'s *fascia, hernia, herniotome, ligaments;* suspensory *ligaments* of C.

Cooperia (kū-pē'rē-ă). A genus of small, slender nematodes (family Trichostrongylidae) inhabiting the small intestine, rarely the abomasum, of ruminants; when fresh they are a bright pink color; they produce serious effects only when present in large numbers. In partly immune animals, these worms become enclosed in nodules in the wall of the intestine; they are less pathogenic in sheep and goats than the trichostrongyles *Haemonchus, Ostertagia,* and *Trichostrongylus.*

C. biso'nis, species that occurs in cattle, sheep, bison, and pronghorn antelopes.

C. curti'cei, species that occurs in sheep, goats, and wild deer in Europe, although cosmopolitan in distribution.

C. fiel'dingi, *C. punctata.*

C. oncoph'ora, *Strongylus radiatus; S. ventricosus;* species that occurs in cattle and domestic and wild sheep, but rarely in the horse; although worldwide in distribution, it is most common in the northern U.S. and Canada.

C. pectina'ta, species that occurs in cattle, sheep, water buffalo, dromedary camels, and various wild ruminants; it is common in the southern U.S.

C. puncta'ta, *C. fieldingi; Strongyloides bovis;* species that occurs mainly in cattle, less commonly in sheep, water buffalo, and several wild ruminants; although worldwide in distribution, it is especially widespread in North America and common in Hawaii.

C. spatula'ta, a species that occurs in cattle and sheep in the southern U.S., Kenya, Australia, and Malaysia.

Coopernail, George P., U.S. surgeon, *1876. See C.'s *sign.*

coordinate [see coordination]. **1** (kō-ōr'di-nit). Any of the scales or magnitudes that serve to define the position of a point. **2** (kō-ōr'di-nāt). To perform the act of coordination.

coordination (kō-ōr'di-nā'shun) [L. *co-,* together, + *ordino,* pp. *-atus,* to arrange, fr. *ordo (ordin-),* arrangement, order]. The harmonious working together; especially of several muscles or muscle groups in the execution of complicated movements.

Coors filter. See under filter.

co-ossification (kō-os'i-fi-kā'shŭn). State of being joined by bone formation.

co-ossify (kō-os'i-fī) [L. *co-,* together, + *os,* bone, + *facio,* to make]. To unite into one bone.

copaiba (kō-pī'bă) [Sp.]. Balsam of c.; the oleoresin of *Copaifera officinalis* and other species of *Copaifera* (family Leguminosae), a South American plant; c. oil is used as an expectorant, diuretic, and stimulant.

coparaffinate (kō-par'af-i-nāt). A mixture of water-insoluble isoparaffinic acids partially neutralized with isooctyl hydroxybenzyl-dialkyl amines; used as an antifungal agent for external application.

COPD Abbreviation for chronic obstructive pulmonary *disease.*

Cope, Sir Vincent Z., British surgeon, 1881–1974. See C.'s *clamp.*

cope (kōp). **1.** The upper half of a flask in the casting art; hence applicable to the upper or cavity side of a denture flask. **2.** To perform an act of coping.

copepod (kō'pē-pod). Any member of the order Copepoda.

Copepoda (kō-pep'ō-dă) [G. *kōpē,* an oar, + *pous (pod-),* a foot]. An order of abundant, free-living, freshwater and marine crustaceans of basic importance in the aquatic food chain in both the marine and freshwater environments; some species are commonly called water fleas. Some are ectoparasites of both cold-blooded and warm-blooded aquatic vertebrates; the parasitic copepods of fish and whales are often highly modified for deep penetration of the skin or for adherence by suckers and hooks (*e.g.,* the fish lice, *Argulus*). Certain copepods (*Cyclops, Diaptomus*) are important as intermediate hosts of *Diphyllobothrium latum* and of *Dracunculus medinensis.*

coping (kōp'ing). **1.** A thin metal covering or cap. **2.** An adaptive or otherwise successful method of dealing with individual or environmental situations that involve psychologic or physiologic stress or threat.

transfer c., in dentistry, a metallic, acrylic resin or other covering or cap used to position a die in an impression.

copolymer (kō'pol-i-mer). A polymer in which two or more monomers or base units are combined.

copper (kop'er) [L. *cuprum,* orig. *Cyprium, Cyprus,* where it was mined]. A metallic element, symbol Cu, atomic no. 29, atomic weight 63.55; several of its salts are used in medicine.

c. arsenite, cupric arsenite.

c. bichloride, chloride, or **dichloride,** cupric chloride.

c. citrate, cupric citrate.

c. sulfate, c. sulphate, cupric sulfate.

copper-64 (^{64}Cu). Beta and positron emitter with a half-life of 12.82 hr.

copper-67 (^{67}Cu). Beta and gamma emitter with a half-life of 59 hr.

copperas (kop'er-as). The impure commercial variety of ferrous sulfate.

copperhead (kop'er-hed). A poisonous snake of the genus *Denisonia* in Australia and *Agkistrodon* in the U.S.

copper pennies. Sclerotic *bodies.*

Coppet, Louis C. de, French physicist, 1841–1911. See C.'s *law.*

coprecipitation (kō'prē-sip-i-tā'shŭn). Precipitation of unbound antigen along with an antigen-antibody complex; may occur particularly when a soluble complex is precipitated by a second antibody specific for the Fc fragment of the immunoglobulin of the complex.

copremesis (kop-rem'ĕ-sis) [G. *kopros,* dung, + emesis]. Fecal *vomiting.*

copro- [G. *kopros,* dung]. Combining form denoting filth or dung, usually used in referring to feces. See also scato-, sterco-.

coproantibodies (kop'rō-an'ti-bod-ēz). Antibodies occurring in the intestinal content; they probably are formed by plasma cells in the intestinal mucosa and consist chiefly of the IgA class.

coprolagnia (kop-rō-lag'nē-ă) [copro- + G. *lagneia,* lust]. A form of sexual perversion in which the thought or sight of excrement causes pleasurable sensation.

coprolalia (kop-rō-lā'lē-ă) [copro- + G. *lalia,* talk]. Coprophrasia; involuntary utterances of vulgar or obscene words; seen in Gilles de la Tourette's syndrome.

coprolith (kop'rō-lith) [copro- + G. *lithos,* stone]. Fecalith; stercolith; a hard mass consisting of inspissated feces.

coprology (kop-rol'ō-jē) [copro- + G. *logos,* study]. Scatology (1).

coproma (kop-rō'mă) [copro- + G. *-ōma,* tumor]. Scatoma; fecaloma; stercoroma; fecal tumor; an accumulation of inspissated feces in the colon or rectum giving the appearance of an abdominal tumor.

coprophagous (kō-prof'ă-gŭs). Feeding on excrement.

coprophagy (kō-prof'ă-jē) [copro- + G. *phagein,* to eat]. Scatophagy.

coprophil, coprophilic (kop'rō-fil, -fil'ik) [see coprophilia]. **1.** Denoting microorganisms occurring in fecal matter. **2.** Relating to coprophilia.

coprophilia (kop-rō-fil'ē-ă) [copro- + G. *philos,* fond]. **1.** Attraction of microorganisms to fecal matter. **2.** In psychiatry, a morbid attraction to, and interest in (with a sexual element), fecal matter.

coprophobia (kop-rō-fō'bē-ă) [copro- + G. *phobos,* fear]. Morbid fear of defecation and feces.

coprophrasia (kop-rō-frā'zē-ă). Coprolalia.

coproplanesia (kop-rō-plan-ē'zē-ă) [copro- + G. *planesis*, a wandering]. Passage of feces through a fistula or artificial anus.

coproporphyria (kop'rō-pōr-fir'ē-ă). Presence of coproporphyrins in the urine, as in variegate porphyria.

coproporphyrin (kop-rō-pōr'fi-rin). One of two porphyrin compounds found normally in feces as a decomposition product of bilirubin (hence, from hemoglobin). See also porphyrinogens.

coproporphyrinogen (kop'rō-pōr-fi-rin'ō-jen). See porphyrinogens.

coprostane (kop-ros'tān). The parent hydrocarbon of coprosterol.

3β-coprostanol (kop-ros'tan-ol). Coprosterol.

***epi*-coprostanol,** *epi*-coprosterol; 5β-cholestan-3α-ol. (For structure of cholestane, see steroids.)

coprostanone (kop-ros'tan-ōn). 5β-Cholestan-3-one, an oxidation product of coprosterol.

coprostasis (kop-rō-stā'sis) [copro- + G. *stasis*, a standing]. Fecal *impaction.*

coprostenol (kop-ros'ten-ol). Allocholesterol.

coprosterin (kop-ros'ter-in). Coprosterol.

coprosterol (kop-ros'ter-ol). 3β-Coprostanol; coprosterin; stercorin; 5β-cholastan-3β-ol; a sterol of the feces produced by the reduction of cholesterol. For structure of coprostane and cholestane, see steroids.

***epi*-coprosterol,** *epi*-coprostenol.

coprostigmastane (kop-rō-stig·mas'tān). The 5β isomer of stigmastane.

coprozoa (kop-rō-zō'ă) [copro- + G. *zōon*, animal]. Protozoa that can be cultivated in fecal matter, although not necessarily living in feces within the intestine.

coprozoic (kop-rō-zō'ik). Relating to coprozoa.

coptosis (kop-tō'sis) [G. *kopto*, to tire, + *osis*, condition]. A state of perpetual fatigue.

copula (kop'yū-lă) [L. a bond, tie]. **1.** In anatomy, a narrow part connecting two structures, *e.g.*, the body of the hyoid bone; the hypobranchial eminence. **2.** Obsolete term for zygote.
His' c., hypobranchial *eminence.*
c. linguae, hypobranchial *eminence.*

copulation (kop-yū-lā'shŭn) [L. *copulatio*, a joining]. **1.** Coitus. **2.** In protozoology, conjugation between two cells that do not fuse but separate after mutual fertilization; observed in the ciliophora, as in *Paramecium.*

CoQ Abbreviation for coenzyme Q.

coquille (kō-kēl') [Fr.]. A spherical curved lens of uniform thickness.

cor, gen. **cordis** (kōr, kōr'dis) [L.] [NA]. Heart.
c. adipo'sum, fatty heart (2).
c. bilocula're, a heart in which the interatrial and interventricular septa are absent or incomplete.
c. bovi'num, bucardia.
c. mo'bile, movable heart; a heart that moves unduly on change of bodily position.
c. pen'dulum, pendulous heart; an extreme form of c. mobile in which the heart appears to be suspended by the great vessels.
c. pulmona'le, chronic c. p. is characterized by hypertrophy of the right ventricle resulting from disease of the lungs, except for lung changes in diseases that primarily affect the left side of the heart and excluding congenital heart disease; acute c. p. is characterized by dilation and failure of the right side of the heart due to pulmonary embolism. In both types, characteristic electrocardiogram changes occur, and in later stages there is usually right-sided cardiac failure.
c. triatria'tum, accessory atrium; a heart with three atrial chambers, the left atrium being subdivided by a transverse septum with a single small opening which separates the openings of the pulmonary veins from the mitral valve.
c. trilocula're, three-chmabered heart due to absence of the interatrial or of the interventricular septum; **c. t. biatriatum,** absence of the interventricular septum; **c. t. biventriculare,** absence of the interatrial septum.

coracidium (kō-ră-sid'ē-ŭm). The ciliated first-stage aquatic embryo of pseudophyllid and other cestodes with aquatic cycles; within the ciliated embryophore is a hooked larva, the hexacanth, that develops in the intermediate host, usually an aquatic crustacean, into the next larval stage, the procercoid.

coracoacromial (kōr'ă-kō-ă-krō'mē-ăl). Acromiocoracoid; relating to the coracoid and acromial processes.

coracobrachialis (kōr'ă-kō-brā-kē-ā'lis). Relating to the coracoid process of the scapula and the arm. See also *musculus* coracobrachialis.

coracoclavicular (kōr'ă-kō-kla-vik'yū-lăr). Scapuloclavicular (2); relating to the coracoid process and the clavicle.

coracohumeral (kōr'ă-kō-hyū'mer-ăl). Relating to the coracoid process and the humerus.

coracoid (kōr'ă-koyd) [G. *korakōdēs*, like a crow's beak, fr. *korax*, raven, + *eidos*, appearance]. Shaped like a crow's beak; denoting a process of the scapula.

corallin (kōr'ă-lin). Aurin.
yellow c., a sodium salt of aurin.

cord-. See chord-.

cord (kōrd) [L. *chorda*, a string]. **1.** In anatomy, any long ropelike structure. See also chorda. **2.** To become corded or stringlike, or having the appearance of a cord. **3.** In histopathology, a line of tumor cells only one cell in width.
Bergmann's c.'s, *striae* medullares ventriculi quarti.
Billroth's c.'s, splenic c.'s.
condyle c., condylar *axis.*
dental c., an aggregation of epithelial cells forming the rudimentary enamel organ.
false vocal c., *plica* vestibularis.
Ferrein's c.'s, see *plica* vocalis.
gangliated c., *truncus* sympathicus.
genital c., one of a pair of mesenchymal ridges bulging into the caudal part of the celom of a young embryo and containing the mesonephric and paramesonephric duct.
germinal c.'s, sex c.'s; the gonadal c.'s of the embryonic ovary or testis.
gonadal c.'s, columns of germinal and follicle cells penetrating centripetally into the embryonic ovarian cortex.
gubernacular c., the content of the gubernacular canal, usually composed of remnants of dental lamina and connective tissue.
hepatic c.'s, liver laminae as seen in sections.
lateral c. of brachial plexus, *fasciculus* lateralis plexus brachialis.
medial c. of brachial plexus, *fasciculus* medialis plexus brachialis.
medullary c.'s, **(1)** c.'s of dense lymphoid tissue between the sinuses in the medulla of a lymph node; **(2)** primordial cell c.'s in the medulla of the embryonic gonad from which the rete testis is formed in the male and the rete ovarii in the female.
nephrogenic c., a longitudinal dorsolateral tract of mesoderm derived from intermediate mesoderm; the primordium for both mesonephric and metanephric tubules.
oblique c., *chorda* obliqua.
posterior c. of brachial plexus, *fasciculus* posterior plexus brachialis.
psalterial c., *stria* vascularis ductus cochlearis.
red pulp c.'s, splenic c.'s.
rete c.'s, primordial cell c.'s in the embryonic gonads that become the rete testis of the male and the rete ovarii of the female.
sex c.'s, germinal c.'s.
spermatic c., *funiculus* spermaticus.

spinal c., *medulla* spinalis.
splenic c.'s, red pulp c.'s; Billroth's c.'s; the tissue occurring between the venous sinuses in the spleen.
tendinous c.'s, *chordae* tendineae.
testicular c., *funiculus* spermaticus.
testis c.'s, the germinal c.'s of the embryonic testis.
true vocal c., *plica* vocalis.
umbilical c., *funiculus* umbilicalis.
vitelline c., a persistent yolk stalk in the form of a solid cord of tissue connecting ileum to umbilicus.
vocal c., *plica* vocalis.
Weitbrecht's c., *chorda* obliqua.
Wilde's c.'s, transverse markings on the corpus callosum.
Willis' c.'s, chordae willisii; several fibrous c.'s crossing the superior sagittal sinus.

cordabrasion (kōrd'ă-brā-zhŭn). Abrasion of vocal cords to remove lesions.

cordate (kōr'dāt). Heart-shaped.

cordectomy (kōr-dek'tō-mē) [G. *chordē*, cord, + *ektomē*, excision]. Excision of a part or whole of a cord.

cordial (kōr'jŭl). A sweet aromatic liquor.

cordianine (kor-dī'ă-nēn). Allantoin.

cordiform (kōr'di-fōrm) [L. *cor* (*cord-*), heart, + *forma*, shape]. Heart-shaped.

cordis (kōr'dis) [gen. of L. *cor*, heart]. Of the heart.

cordopexy (kōr'dō-pek-sē) [G. *chordē*, cord, + *pēxis*, fixation]. **1.** Operative fixation of any displaced anatomical cord. **2.** Lateral fixation of one or both vocal cords to correct laryngeal stenosis.

cordotomy (kōr-dot'ō-mē) [G. *chordē*, cord, + *tomē*, a cutting]. Chordotomy. **1.** Any operation on the spinal cord. **2.** Division of tracts of the spinal cord, which may be performed percutaneously (stereotactic c.) or after laminectomy (open c.) by various techniques such as incision or radio frequency coagulation.
anterolateral c., spinothalamic c.; anterolateral or spinal tractotomy; division of the anterolateral quadrant of the spinal cord to section the spinothalamic tract.
open c., see c. (2).
posterior column c., division of the posterior column of the spinal cord.
spinothalamic c., anterolateral c.
stereotactic c., see c. (2).

Cordylobia (kōr-di-lō'bē-ă) [G. *kordylē*, a cudgel, swelling, or tumor]. A genus of calliphorid fleshflies.
C. anthropoph'aga, Tumbu fly of Africa south of the Sahara; a species that causes a boil-like furuncular myiasis; many animals besides man are attacked, especially domestic dogs, though rats are probably the chief reservoir of human infection.

cordylobiasis (kōr'di-lō-bī'ă-sis). African furuncular myiasis; tumbu dermal myiasis; infection of man and animals with larvae of flies of the genus *Cordylobia*.

core (kōr) [L. *cor*, heart]. **1.** The central mass of necrotic tissue in a boil. **2.** A metal casting, usually with a post in the canal of a root, designed to retain an artificial crown. **3.** A sectional record, usually of plaster of Paris or one of its derivatives, of the relationships of parts, such as teeth, metallic restorations, or copings.
atomic c., the nucleus plus the nonvalence electrons.
central transactional c., the reticular activating system of the brain.

core-, coreo-, coro- [G. *korē*, pupil]. Combining forms relating to the pupil.

corecleisis, coreclisis (kōr-ē-klī'sis) [G. *korē*, pupil, + *kleisis*, a closing]. Occlusion of the pupil.

corectasia, corectasis (kōr-ek-tā'zē-ă, kōr-ek'tă-sis) [G. *korē*, pupil, + *ektasis*, a stretching out]. Pathologic dilation of the pupil.

corectomedialysis (kōr-ek'tō-mē-dī-al'i-sis) [G. *korē*, pupil, + *ektomē*, excision, + *dialysis*, a loosening]. A peripheral iridectomy to form an artificial pupil.

corectopia (kōr-ek-tō'pē-ă) [G. *korē*, pupil, + *ektopos*, out of place]. Eccentric location of the pupil so that it is not in the center of the iris.

corediastasis (kōr'ē-dī-as'tă-sis) [G. *korē*, pupil, + *diastasis*, a separation]. A dilated state of the pupil.

corelysis (kō-rē-lī'sis) [G. *korē*, pupil, + *lysis*, a loosening]. The freeing of adhesions between the lens capsule and the iris.

coremium (kō-rē'mē-ŭm) [G. *korēma*, filth, refuse]. A sheaf-like tuft of conidiophores.

coreo-. See core-.

coreoplasty (kōr'ē-ō-plas-tē) [G. *korē*, pupil, + *plassō*, to form]. Coroplasty; the procedure to correct a deformed or occluded pupil.

corepexy (kōr-e-pek'sē) [G. *korē*, pupil, + *pēxis*, a fixing in place]. Corepraxy.

corepraxy (kōr-e-prak'sē) [G. *korē*, pupil, + *praxis*, action]. Corepexy; an operation to provide a central pupillary opening.

corepressor (kō-rē-pres'ŏr). A molecule, usually a product of a specific enzyme pathway, that combines with inactive repressor (produced by a regulator gene) to form active repressor, which then attaches to an operator gene site and inhibits activity of the structural genes controlled by the operator; a homeostatic mechanism for regulating enzyme production in repressible enzyme systems.

corestenoma (kōr-e-stĕ-nō'mă) [G. *korē*, pupil, + *stenōma*, a narrow pass]. A constriction of the pupil.
c. congen'itum, a partial occlusion of the pupil by congenital outgrowths from the sphincter margin.

Corey, R.B., U.S. chemist, 1897–1971. See Pauling-C. *helix*.

Cori, Carl F., U.S. biochemist and Nobel laureate, *1896. See C. *cycle, ester*.

Cori, Gerty Theresa, U.S. biochemist and Nobel laureate, 1896–1957. See C.'s *disease*.

coria (kō'rē-ă). Plural of corium.

coriander (kō-rē-an'der). The dried ripe fruit of *Coriandrum sativum* (family Umbelliferae); a mild stimulant aromatic and a flavoring agent.

corium, pl. coria (kō'rē-ŭm, -rē-ă) [L. skin, hide, leather] [NA]. Dermis; cutis vera; enderon; a layer of skin composed of a superficial thin layer that interdigitates with the epidermis, the stratum papillare, and the stratum reticulare; it contains blood and lymphatic vessels, nerves and nerve endings, glands, and, except for glabrous skin, hair follicles.
c. coro'nae, coronary *band*.
c. lim'bi, periople.
c. pari'etis, the wall of the pododerm.
c. so'leae, the sole of the pododerm.
c. un'gulae, pododerm.

Corlett, William T., U.S. dermatologist, 1854–1948. See C.'s *pyosis*.

corn (kōrn) [L. *cornu*, horn, hoof]. **1.** Clavus (1). **2.** A small inflammatory focus under the sole of the hoof of the horse; forefeet are most often affected, usually between the bar and the wall; sometimes seen in other hoofed animals.
asbestos c., asbestos wart; a granulomatous or hyperkeratotic lesion of the skin at the site of deposit of asbestos particles.
hard c., heloma durum; the usual form of c. over a toe joint.
seed c., a papilloma or wart on the sole of the foot.
soft c., heloma molle; a c. formed by pressure between two toes, the surface being macerated and yellowish in color.

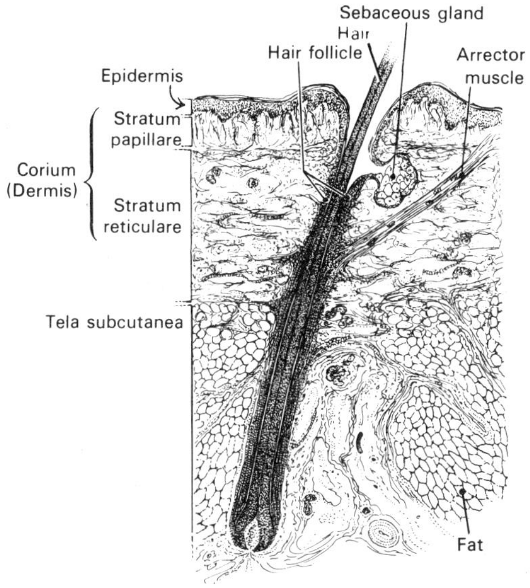

Corium

Section of thin skin, with portion of tela subcutanea

cornea (kōr'nē-ă) [L. fem. of *corneus,* horny] [NA]. The transparent tissue constituting the anterior sixth of the outer wall of the eye, with a 7.7 mm radius of curvature as contrasted with the 13.5 mm of the sclera; it consists of stratified squamous epithelium continuous with that of the conjunctiva, a substantia propria, substantially regularly arranged collagen imbedded in mucopolysaccharide, and an inner layer of endothelium.

conical c., keratoconus.

c. farina'ta, floury c.; bilateral speckling of the posterior part of the corneal stroma.

floury c., c. farinata.

c. pla'na congen'ita familia'res, a form of c. that is flatter than normal.

c. uri'ca, bilateral deposition of crystalline deposits of urea and sodium urate within corneal stroma.

c. verticilla'ta, congenital whorl-like opacities in the c.

corneal (kōr'nē-ăl). Relating to the cornea.

corneoblepharon (kōr'nē-ō-blef'ă-ron) [cornea + G. *blepharon,* eyelid]. Adhesion of the eyelid margin to the cornea.

corneocyte (kōr'nē-ō-sīt) [*cornea,* L. fem. of *corneus,* horny, + G. *kytos,* cell]. The dead keratin-filled squamous cell of the stratum corneum.

corneosclera (kōr'nē-ō-sklēr'ă). The combined cornea and sclera when considered as forming the external coat of the eyeball.

corneoscleral (kōr'nē-ō-sklēr'ăl). Pertaining to the cornea and sclera.

corneous (kōr'nē-ŭs) [L. corneus, fr. *cornu,* horn]. Horny.

Corner, Edred M., British surgeon, 1873–1950. See C.'s *tampon.*

Corner, George W., U.S. anatomist, 1889–1981. See C.-Allen *test, unit.*

corneum (kōr'nē-ŭm) [L., ntr. of *corneus,* horny, fr. *cornu,* horn]. See *stratum* corneum epidermidis; *stratum* corneum unguis.

corniculate (kōr-nik'yū-lāt) [L. *corniculatus,* horned]. **1.** Resembling a horn. **2.** Having horns or horn-shaped appendages.

corniculum (kōr-nik'yū-lŭm) [L. dim. of *cornu,* horn]. A cornu of small size.

c. laryn'gis, *cartilago* corniculata.

cornification (kōr-ni-fi-kā'shŭn) [L. *cornu,* horn, + *facio,* to make]. Keratinization.

cornified (kōr'ni-fīd). Keratinized.

corn oil. Maise or maize oil; the refined fixed oil expressed from the embryo of *Zea mays* (family Gramineae); a solvent.

cornsilk (kōrn'silk). Zea.

corn-smut (kōrn'smŭt). *Ustilago* maydis.

cornu, gen. **cornus,** pl. **cornua** (kōr'nū, -nūs, -nū-ă) [L. horn]. Horn. **1** [NA]. Any structure resembling a horn in shape. **2.** Any structure composed of horny substance. **3.** One of the coronal extensions of the dental pulp underlying a cusp or lobe. **4.** The major subdivisions of the lateral ventricle in the cerebral hemisphere (the frontal horn, occipital horn, and temporal horn). See also *ventriculus* lateralis.

c. ammo'nis, Ammon's *horn.*

c. ante'rius [NA], anterior or ventral horn; **(1)** frontal horn; the anterior or frontal division of the lateral ventricle of the brain, extending forward from Monro's interventricular foramen (see *ventriculus* lateralis); **(2)** the anterior or ventral gray column of the spinal cord as appearing in cross section. See also *columna* anterior; *columnae* griseae.

c. coccy'geum [NA], coccygeal horn; coccygeal c.; one of two processes that project upward from the dorsum of the base of the coccyx.

c. cuta'neum, cutaneous *horn.*

cornua of hyoid bone, see c. majus; c. minus.

c. infe'rius [NA], inferior horn; underhorn; a lower or downward prolongation of a part or structure of the body; **c. i. cartila'ginis thyroi'deae** [NA], inferior horn of thyroid cartilage; one of the pair of downward prolongations at the back of the thyroid cartilage; it articulates on each side with the cricoid cartilage; **c. i. hia'tus saph'enus** [NA], inferior horn of saphenous opening; the lower part of the falciform margin of the opening in the fascia lata through which the greater saphenous vein passes; **c. i. ventric'uli latera'lis** [NA], inferior horn of lateral ventricle; temporal horn; the part of the lateral ventricle extending downward and forward into the medial part of the temporal lobe (see *ventriculus* lateralis).

cornua of lateral ventricle, see c. anterius (1), c. inferius ventriculi lateralis, c. posterius (1).

c. latera'le [NA], lateral horn; the small lateral gray column of the spinal cord as appearing in transverse section. See also *columna* lateralis; *columnae* griseae.

c. ma'jus [NA], greater horn; the larger and more lateral of the two processes on either side of the hyoid bone.

c. mi'nus [NA], lesser horn; styloid c.; the shorter and more medial of the two processes on either side of the hyoid bone.

c. poste'rius [NA], posterior or dorsal horn; **c. p. ventriculi lateralis,** occipital horn; the posterior or occipital division of the lateral ventricle of the brain, extending backward into the occipital lobe (see *ventriculus* lateralis); the posterior gray column of the spinal cord as appearing in cross section (see also *columna* posterior; *columnae* griseae).

c. sacra'le [NA], sacral horn; the most caudal part of the intermediate sacral crest. On each side it forms the lateral margin of the sacral hiatus and articulates with the coccygeal c.

cornua of saphenous opening, c. inferius and c. superius hiatus saphenus.

cornua of spinal cord, see c. anterius (2), c. laterale, c. posterius (2).

styloid c., c. minus.

c. supe'rius [NA], superior horn; **c. s. cartilaginis thyroideae** [NA], superior horn of the thyroid cartilage; one of the pair of upward prolongations from the thyroid cartilage to which the lateral hyothyroid ligament attaches; **c. s. hiatus saphenus** [NA], superior horn of the saphenous opening; Burns' falciform process; Burns' or Hey's ligament; the upper part of the falciform margin of the opening in the fascia lata through which the greater saphenous vein passes.

cornua of thyroid cartilage, see c. inferius cartilaginis thyroideae; c. superius cartilaginis thyroideae.

c. uteri [NA], horn of uterus; uterine horn; the portion of the uterus to which the uterine tube attaches on either right or left.

cornua (kōr'nū-ă). Plural of cornu.

cornual (kōr'nū-ăl). Relating to a cornu.

coro-. See core-.

corona, pl. **coronae** (kō-rō'nă, -nē) [L. garland, crown, fr. G. *korōnē*] [NA]. Crown (1); any structure, normal or pathologic, resembling or suggesting a crown or a wreath.

c. cap'itis, crown of head; the topmost part of the head.

c. cilia'ris [NA], ciliary crown or wreath; the circular figure on the inner surface of the ciliary body, formed by the processes and folds (plicae) taken together.

c. clin'ica [NA], clinical crown; that part of the crown of a tooth visible in the oral cavity.

c. den'tis [NA], crown of a tooth; anatomical crown; the portion of a tooth covered with enamel.

c. glan'dis [NA], the prominent posterior border of the glans penis.

c. radia'ta, radiate crown; **(1)** [NA], a fan-shaped fiber mass on the white matter of the cerebral cortex, composed of the widely radiating fibers of the internal capsule; **(2)** a single layer of columnar cells derived from the cumulus oophorus which anchor on the zona pelucida of the oocyte in a secondary follicle.

c. seborrhe'ica, a red band at the hair line along the upper border of the forehead and temples occasionally observed in seborrheic dermatitis of the scalp.

c. vene'ris, papular syphilitic lesions (secondary eruption) along the anterior margin of the scalp or on the back of the neck.

Zinn's c., *circulus* vasculosus nervi optici.

coronad (kōr'ō-nad). In a direction toward any corona.

coronal (kōr'ō-năl). Coronalis; relating to a corona or the coronal plane.

coronale (kōr-ō-nā'lē) [L. neuter of *coronalis,* pertaining to a *corona,* crown]. **1.** *Os* frontale. **2.** One of the two most widely separated points on the coronal suture at the poles of the greatest frontal diameter.

coronalis (kōr-ō-nā'lis) [NA]. Coronal.

coronaria (kōr-ō-nā'rē-ă). A coronary artery, of the heart.

coronarism (kōr'ō-năr-izm) [coronary (artery) + *-ism*]. **1.** Coronary insufficiency. **2.** *Angina* pectoris.

coronaritis (kōr'ō-nă-rī'tis). Inflammation of coronary artery or arteries.

coronary (kōr'o-năr-ē) [L. *coronarius;* fr. *corona,* a crown]. **1.** Relating to or resembling a crown. **2.** Encircling; denoting various anatomical structures, *e.g.,* nerves, blood vessels, ligaments. **3.** Specifically, denoting the c. blood vessels of the heart and, colloquially, c. thrombosis.

cafe c., sudden collapse while eating that results from food impaction closing the glottis; often erroneously thought to stem from coronary artery disease.

Coronaviridae (kō-rō'nă-vir'i-dē) [L. *corona,* garland, crown]. A family of single-stranded RNA-containing viruses of medium size, some of which cause upper respiratory tract infections in man; others cause animal infections (infectious avian bronchitis, swine encephalitis, mouse hepatitis, neonatal calf diarrhea, and others). The viruses resemble myxoviruses except for the petal-shaped projections which give an impression of the solar corona. Virions are 80 to 130 nm in diameter, enveloped, and ether-sensitive. Nucleocapsids are thought to be of helical symmetry; they develop in cytoplasm and are enveloped by budding into cytoplasmic vesicles. *Coronavirus* is the only recognized genus.

coronavirus (kō-rō'nă-vī'rŭs). The single recognized genus in the family Coronaviridae, comprising the following species: avian infectious bronchitis virus (type species), neonatal calf diarrhea virus, human coronavirus (several serotypes), mouse (murine) hepatitis virus, porcine transmissible gastroenteritis virus, rat coronavirus, rat sialodacryoadenitis virus, and turkey bluecomb disease virus.

coronavirus (kō-rō'nă-vī'rŭs). Any virus of the family Coronaviridae.

coroner (kōr'on-er) [L. *corona,* a crown]. An official whose duty it is to investigate sudden, suspicious, or violent death to determine the cause; in some communities, the office has been replaced by that of medical examiner.

coronet (kōr'ō-net) [Fr. *coronette;* L. *corona,* crown]. The line of junction between the skin and the hoof or claw.

coronion (kŏ-rō'nē-on) [G. *korōnē,* crow]. Koronion; the tip of the coronoid process of the mandible; a craniometric point.

coronitis (kōr-ō-nī'tis). Inflammation of the coronary band of the horse's hoof, resulting in imperfect horn formation.

coronoid (kōr'ō-noyd) [G. *korōnē,* a crow, + *eidos,* resembling]. Shaped like a crow's beak; denoting certain processes and other parts of bones.

coronoidectomy (kōr'ō-noy-dek'tō-mē) [coronoid + G. *ektomē,* excision]. Surgical removal of the coronoid process of the mandible.

coroparelcysis (kō'rō-par-el'sī-sis) [G. *korē,* pupil, + *parelkō,* to draw aside]. An operation for displacing the pupil to one side in cases of central corneal opacity.

coroplasty (kōr'ō-plas-tē). Coreoplasty.

corotomy (kō-rot'ō-mē). Iridotomy.

corpora (kōr'pōr-ă). Plural of corpus.

corporeal (kōr-pō'rē-ăl). Pertaining to the body, or to a corpus.

corporin (kōr'pō-rin). Obsolete term for corpus luteum hormone.

corpse (kōrps) [L. *corpus,* body]. Cadaver.

corps ronds (kōr-ron') [Fr. round bodies]. Dyskeratotic round cells occurring in the epidermis, with a central round basophilic mass surrounded by a clear halo; characteristically found in keratosis follicularis.

corpulence, corpulency (kōr'pyū-lens, -len-sē) [L. *corpulentia,* magnification of *corpus,* body]. Obesity.

corpulent (kōr'pyū-lent). Obese.

CORPUS

corpus, gen. **corporis,** pl. **corpora** (kōr'pŭs, -pōr-is, -pōr-ă) [L. body] [NA]. **1.** The human body, consisting of head (caput), neck (collum), trunk (truncus), and limbs (membra). **2.** Any body or mass. **3.** The main part of an organ or other anatomical structure, as distinguished from the caput (head) or cauda (tail). See also body and soma.

c. adipo'sum buc'cae [NA], fat body of cheek; sucking cushion; sucking or suctorial pad; Bichat's fat-pad or protuberance; an encapsuled mass of fat in the cheek on the outer side of the buccinator muscle, especially marked in the infant; supposed to strengthen and support the cheek during the act of sucking.

c. adipo'sum fos'sae ischiorecta'lis [NA], fat body of ischiorectal fossa; the fat within the ischiorectal fossa.

c. adipo'sum infrapatella're [NA], infrapatellar fat body; the fatty mass that occupies the area between the patellar ligament and the

infrapatellar synovial fold of the knee joint.
c. adipo'sum or'bitae [NA], fat body of orbit; the mass of fat contained in the orbit that contributes to the support of the eyeball.
c. al'bicans [NA], atretic c. luteum; c. candicans; albicans (2); a retrogressed c. luteum characterized by increasing cicatrization and shrinkage of the cicatricial core with an amorphous, convoluted, completely hyalinized lutein zone surrounding the central plug of scar tissue.
cor'pora alla'ta, a pair of juvenile hormone-producing endocrine glands located near the brain in insects; action of the juvenile hormone is interrelated with that of brain hormone and ecdysone; a high concentration of the hormone at the time of molting will cause production of an additional larval instar; removal at an early larval stage causes precocious pupation, resulting in the formation of a midget adult; implantation at late larval stages can cause development of an oversized adult.
c. amygdaloi'deum [NA], amygdala (1); amygdaloid complex or nucleus; nucleus amygdalae; almond nucleus; a rounded mass of gray matter in the temporal lobe underneath the olfactory cortex of the uncus and immediately anterior to the inferior horn of the lateral ventricle; its major afferents are olfactory and its efferent connections are with the hypothalamus and mediodorsal nucleus of the thalamus and it is also reciprocally associated with the cortex of the temporal lobe; it is subdivided into two major nuclear groups; basolateral and corticomedial.
c. amyla'ceum, pl. **cor'pora amyla'cea,** one of a number of small ovoid or rounded, sometimes laminated, bodies resembling a grain of starch and found in nervous tissue, in the prostate, and in pulmonary alveoli; of little pathological significance, and apparently derived from degenerated cells or proteinaceous secretions. Also called amniotic, amylaceous, amyloid, or colloid corpuscle.
c. aor'ticum, *glomus* aorticum.
c. aran'tii, *nodulus* valvulae semilunaris.
cor'pora arena'cea, brain sand; psammoma bodies (2); acervulus; small calcareous concretions in the stroma of the pineal and other central nervous system tissues.
atretic c. luteum, c. albicans.
c. atret'icum, atretic ovarian *follicle.*
corpora bigem'ina, bigeminal bodies; a bilateral single swelling of the roofplate of the embryonic midbrain that later in development becomes subdivided into a superior and an inferior colliculus.
c. callo'sum [NA], commissure of the cerebral hemispheres; the great commissural plate of nerve fibers interconnecting the cortical hemispheres (with the exception of most of the temporal lobes which are interconnected by the anterior commissure). Lying at the floor of the longitudinal fissure, and covered on each side by the gyrus cinguli, it is arched from behind forward and is thick at each extremity (splenium and genu) but thinner in its long central portion (truncus); it curves back underneath itself at the genu to form the rostrum of the c. callosum.
c. can'dicans, c. albicans.
c. caverno'sum clitor'idis [NA], cavernous body of clitoris; one of the two parallel columns of erectile tissue forming the body of the clitoris; they diverge at the root to form the crura of the clitoris.
c. caverno'sum con'chae, *plexus* cavernosi concharum.
c. caverno'sum pe'nis [NA], cavernous body of penis; one of two parallel columns of erectile tissue forming the dorsal part of the body of the penis; they are separated posteriorly, forming the crura of the penis.
c. caverno'sum ure'thrae, c. spongiosum penis.
c. cilia're [NA], ciliary body; a thickened portion of the tunica vasculosa of the eye between the choroid and the iris; it consists of three parts or zones; orbiculus ciliaris, corona ciliaris, and musculus ciliaris.
c. clavic'ulae [NA], body of clavicle; the sinuous portion of the clavicle between the sternal and acromial extremities.
c. clitor'idis [NA], the body of the clitoris.
c. coccy'geum [NA], coccygeal body or gland; glomus coccygeum; arteriococcygeal gland; an arteriovenous (arteriolovenular) anastomosis supplied by the middle sacral artery and located on the pelvic surface of the coccyx. It was formerly called a gland (of Luschka) or a glomus and included with the paraganglia.
c. cos'tae [NA], the body of a rib.
c. denta'tum, *nucleus* dentatus cerebelli.
c. epididym'idis [NA], body of epididymis; the middle part that extends downward from the head to the tail of the epididymis on the posterior surface of the testis.
c. fem'oris, c. ossis femoris.
c. fibro'sum, the small fibrous cicatricial mass in the ovary formed following the atresia of an ovarian follicle; similar to a corpus albicans but smaller.
c. fib'ulae [NA], the shaft of the fibula.
c. fimbria'tum, (1) *fimbria* hippocampi; **(2)** the outer ovarian extremity of the oviduct.
c. for'nicis [NA], body of the fornix; the middle part of the fornix situated beneath the corpus callosum.
c. genicula'tum exter'num, c. geniculatum laterale.
c. genicula'tum inter'num, c. geniculatum mediale.
c. genicula'tum latera'le [NA], lateral geniculate body; c. geniculatum externum; the lateral one of a pair of small oval masses that protrude slightly from the posteroinferior aspects of the thalamus; its main (dorsal) subdivision serves as a processing station in the major pathway from the retina to the cerebral cortex, receiving fibers from the optic tract and giving rise to the geniculocalcarine radiation to the visual cortex in the occipital lobe.
c. genicula'tum media'le [NA], c. geniculatum internum; medial geniculate body; the medial one of a pair of prominent cell groups in the posteroinferior parts of the thalamus; it functions as the last of a series of processing stations along the auditory conduction pathway to the cerebral cortex, receiving the brachium of the inferior colliculus and giving rise to the auditory radiation to the auditory cortex in the superior temporal gyrus.
c. glan'dulae sudorif'erae, body of sweat gland; the coiled tubular secretory portion of a sweat gland located in the subcutaneous tissue or deep in the corium and connected to the surface of the skin by a long duct.
c. hemorrhag'icum, c. luteum hematoma; a hematoma with a lining formed by the thinned-out bright yellow lutein zone; gradual resorption of the blood elements leaves a cavity filled with a clear fluid, *i.e.,* a. c. luteum cyst.
c. high'mori, c. highmoria'num, *mediastinum* testis.
c. hu'meri [NA], shaft of humerus.
c. in'cudis [NA], body of incus; the main part of the incus that articulates with the malleus and from which the short and long limbs arise.
c. lin'guae [NA], body of tongue; the oral part of the tongue anterior to the terminal sulcus.
c. lu'teum [NA], yellow body; the yellow endocrine body, 1 to 1.5 cm in diameter, formed in the ovary at the site of a ruptured ovarian follicle immediately after ovulation; there is an early stage of proliferation or hyperemia, and vascularization before full maturity; later, there is a festooned and bright yellowish lutein zone traversed by trabeculae of theca interna containing numerous blood vessels; although the c. luteum secretes an estrogenic hormone, it elaborates a second hormone known as progesterone which is much more characteristic of it. If pregnancy does not occur, it is called a **c. luteum spurium,** which undergoes progressive retrogression to a c. albicans. If pregnancy does occur, it is called a **c. luteum verum,** which increases in size, persisting to the fifth or sixth month of pregnancy before retrogression.
c. luy'sii, *nucleus* subthalamicus.
c. mamilla're [NA], mamillary body; mamillary tubercle of hypothalamus; a small, round, paired cell group that protrudes into the interpeduncular fossa from the inferior aspect of the hypothala-

mus. It receives a major bundle of hippocampal fibers from the fornix and projects fibers to the anterior thalamic nuclei and into the brainstem tegmentum.
c. mam'mae [NA], body of mammary gland; the principal part of the breast, consisting of glandular tissue and its supporting fibrous tissue. It forms a conical mass converging toward the nipple and is surrounded by adipose tissue.
c. mandib'ulae [NA], body of mandible; the heavy, U-shaped, horizontal portion of the mandible extending posteriorly to the angle where it is continuous with the ramus; it supports the lower teeth.
c. maxil'lae [NA], body of maxilla; the central portion of the maxilla hollowed out by the maxillary sinus; it presents orbital, nasal, anterior, and infratemporal surfaces and supports four processes, frontal, zygomatic, palatine, and alveolar.
c. medulla're cerebel'li [NA], the interior white substance of the cerebellum.
c. nu'clei cauda'ti [NA], the suprathalamic part of the caudate nucleus lying in the floor of the central part of the lateral ventricle.
c. oliva're, oliva.
c. os'sis fem'oris [NA], body of thigh bone; shaft of femur; c. femoris; the cylindrical shaft of the thigh bone.
c. os'sis hyoi'dei [NA], the body of the hyoid bone.
c. os'sis il'ii [NA], body of ilium; it forms the upper two-fifths of the acetabulum and joins the pubis and ischium in the acetabulum. It continues above into the ala or wing of the ilium.
c. os'sis isch'ii [NA], body of ischium; the entire ischium with the exception of the ramus.
c. os'sis metacarpa'lis [NA], the shaft of one of the metacarpal bones.
c. os'sis pu'bis [NA], body of pubic bone; pubic body; the flattened medial portion of the pubic bone entering into the pubic symphysis. From it extend the superior and inferior rami.
c. os'sis sphenoida'lis [NA], body of sphenoid bone; the central portion of the sphenoid bone from which the greater and lesser wings and the pterygoid processes arise. The sphenoidal sinuses lie within it.
c. pampinifor'me, paroophoron.
c. pancre'atis [NA], body of pancreas; the part of the pancreas from the point where it crosses the portal vein to the point where it enters the lienorenal ligament.
c. papilla're, *stratum* papillare corii.
cor'pora para-aor'tica [NA], para-aortic bodies; organs of Zuckerkandl; Zuckerkandl's bodies; small masses of chromaffin tissue found near the sympathetic ganglia along the abdominal aorta; they are more prominent during fetal life.
c. paratermina'le, *gyrus* subcallosus.
c. pe'nis [NA], body of penis; scapus penis; the free pendulous portion of the penis.
c. phalan'gis [NA], body of phalanx; the shaft of each phalanx of the hand or foot.
c. pinea'le [NA], pineal body or gland; conarium; pinus; epiphysis cerebri; a small, unpaired, flattened body, shaped somewhat like a pine cone, attached at its anterior pole to the region of the posterior and habenular commissures, and lying in the depression between the two superior colliculi below the splenium of the corpus callosum; it is a glandular structure, composed of follicles containing epithelioid cells and lime concretions called brain sand; despite its attachment to the brain, it appears to receive nerve fibers exclusively from the peripheral autonomic nervous system.
c. pon'tobulba're, a collection of nerve cells in the lower part of the medulla oblongata forming a ridge which crosses the restiform body obliquely.
cor'pora quadrigem'ina, quadrigeminal bodies; the colliculus inferior and colliculus superior, together forming the lamina tecti mesencephali.
c. quadrigem'inum ante'rius, *colliculus* superior.
c. quadrigem'inum poste'rius, *colliculus* inferior.
c. ra'dii [NA], shaft of radius; the triangular body of the radius located between the expanded proximal and distal extremities of the bone.
c. restifor'me, *pedunculus* cerebellaris inferior.
c. spongio'sum pe'nis [NA], spongy body of penis; c. cavernosum urethrae; the median column of erectile tissue located between and ventral to the two corpora cavernosa penis; posteriorly it expands into the bulbus penis and anteriorly it terminates as the enlarged glans penis; it is traversed by the urethra.
c. spongio'sum ure'thrae mulie'bris, the submucous coat of the female urethra, containing a venous network that insinuates itself between the muscular layers, giving to them an erectile nature.
c. ster'ni [NA], body of sternum; mesosternum; midsternum; gladiolus; the middle and largest portion of the sternum.
c. stria'tum [NA], striate body; the caudate and lentiform (lenticular) nuclei; the striate appearance on section is caused by slender fascicles of myelinated fibers. Histologically, the c. striatum can be subdivided into the generally small-celled striatum, consisting of the nucleus caudatus and the large outer segment of the lentiform nucleus (the putamen), and a large-celled globus pallidus composed of the two inner segments.
c. ta'li [NA], body of talus; the large posterior part of the talus forming the trochlea above for articulation with the tibia and fibula and articulating below with the calcaneus.
c. tib'iae [NA], body of tibia; shaft of tibia.
c. trapezoid'eum [NA], trapezoid (4); trapezoid body; a plate of transverse fibers running over the dorsal (deep) border of the pontine nuclei; it is formed by ascending auditory fibers that cross to the opposite side of the brainstem.
c. triti'ceum, *cartilago* triticea.
c. ul'nae [NA], body of ulna; the shaft of the ulna between the proximal extremity and the head.
c. un'guis [NA], body of nail; the exposed portion of the nail distal to its root.
c. u'teri [NA], body of uterus; the part of the uterus above the isthmus, comprising about two thirds of the non-pregnant organ.
c. ventric'uli [NA], body of stomach; the part of the stomach that lies between the fundus above and the pyloric antrum below; its boundaries are poorly defined.
c. ver'tebrae [NA], body of a vertebra; the main portion of a vertebra anterior to the vertebral canal.
c. ves'icae bilia'ris [NA], c. vesicae felleae; body of gallbladder; the main part of the gallbladder terminating in the rounded fundus below and continuing into the neck of the gallbladder above.
c. ves'icae fell'eae [NA], c. vesicae biliaris.
c. ves'icae urina'riae [NA], body of urinary bladder; the portion of the bladder between the apex and fundus.
c. vit'reum [NA], vitreous (2); vitreum; vitreous or hyaloid body; a transparent jelly-like substance filling the interior of the eyeball behind the lens of the eye; it is composed of a delicate network (stroma vitreum) enclosing in its meshes a watery fluid (humor vitreus). See also subentries under vitreous.

corpuscle (kōr'pŭs-l) [L. *corpusculum,* dim. of *corpus,* body]. **1.** Corpusculum. **2.** A blood cell.
amniotic c., *corpus* amylaceum.
amylaceous c., amyloid c., *corpus* amylaceum.
articular c.'s, *corpuscula* articularia.
axis c., axile c., the central portion of a tactile c.
basal c., basal *body.*
Bizzozero's c., platelet.
blood c., blood *cell.*
bone c., osteocyte.
bridge c., desmosome.
bulboid c.'s, *corpuscula* bulboidea.

cement c., a cementocyte contained within a lacuna or crypt of the cementum of a tooth; an entrapped cementoblast.
chyle c., a cell of the same appearance as a leukocyte, present in chyle.
colloid c., *corpus* amylaceum.
colostrum c., Donné's c.; galactoblast; one of numerous bodies present in the colostrum, supposed to be modified leukocytes containing fat droplets.
concentrated human red blood c., c. prepared from one or more preparations of whole human blood which are not more than 14 days old and each of which has already been directly matched with the blood of the intended recipient.
corneal c.'s, Toynbee's or Virchow's c.'s; Virchow's cells (2); connective tissue cells found between the laminae of fibrous tissue in the cornea.
Dogiel's c., an encapsulated sensory nerve ending.
Donné's c., colostrum c.
dust c.'s, hemoconia.
Eichhorst's c.'s, the globular forms sometimes occurring in the poikilocytosis of pernicious anemia.
exudation c., inflammatory or plastic c.; exudation cell; a cell present in an exudate which assists in the organization of new tissue.
genital c.'s, *corpuscula* genitalia.
ghost c., achromocyte.
Gluge's c.'s, large pus cells containing fat droplets.
Golgi-Mazzoni c., an encapsulated sensory nerve ending similar to a pacinian c. but simpler in structure.
Grandry's c.'s, general sensory endings in the beak, mouth, and tongue of birds; similar to Merkel's c.'s.
Hassall's concentric c.'s, thymic c.'s.
Herbst's c.'s, tactile c.'s, resembling pacinian c.'s, but much smaller; found in birds.
inflammatory c., exudation c.
Key-Retzius c.'s, tactile c.'s, resembling pacinian c.'s, found in the beak of certain aquatic birds.
lamellated c.'s, *corpuscula* lamellosa.
lymph c., lymphatic c., lymphoid c., a mononuclear type of leukocyte formed in lymph nodes and other lymphoid tissue, and also in the blood.
malpighian c.'s, (1) *corpusculum* renis; **(2)** *folliculi* lymphatici lienales.
Mazzoni's c., a tactile c. apparently identical with Krause's end bulb.
Meissner's c., *corpusculum* tactus.
Merkel's c., *meniscus* tactus.
Mexican hat c., see target cell *anemia.*
milk c., one of the fat droplets in milk.
molluscum c., molluscum *body.*
Negri c.'s, Negri *bodies.*
Norris' c.'s, decolorized red blood cells that are invisible or almost invisible in the blood plasma, unless they are appropriately stained.
oval c., *corpusculum* tactus.
pacchionian c.'s, *granulationes* arachnoideales.
pacinian c.'s, *corpuscula* lamellosa.
pessary c., an elongated red blood cell with hemoglobin concentrated in the peripheral portion.
phantom c., achromocyte.
plastic c., exudation c.
Purkinje's c.'s, Purkinje's *cells.*
pus c., pus cell; pyocyte; one of the polymorphonuclear leukocytes that comprise the chief portion of the formed elements in pus.
Rainey's c.'s, rounded, ovoidal, or sickle-shaped spores or bradyzoites, 12 to 16 by 4 to 9 μm, found within the elongated cysts (Miescher's tubes) of the protozoan *Sarcocystis.*
red c., erythrocyte.
renal c., *corpusculum* renis.
reticulated c., reticulocyte.
Ruffini's c.'s, sensory end-structures in the subcutaneous connective tissues of the fingers, consisting of an ovoid capsule within which the sensory fiber ends with numerous collateral knobs.
salivary c., one of the leukocytes present in saliva.
Schwalbe's c., *caliculus* gustatorius.
shadow c., achromocyte.
splenic c.'s, *folliculi* lymphatici lienales.
tactile c., *corpusculum* tactus.
taste c., *caliculus* gustatorius.
terminal nerve c.'s, *corpuscula* nervosa terminalia.
third c., platelet.
thymic c., Hassall's concentric c.'s; Hassall's or Virchow-Hassall bodies; small spherical bodies of keratinized and usually squamous epithelial cells arranged in a concentric pattern around clusters of degenerating lymphocytes, eosinophils, and macrophages; found in the medulla of the lobules of the thymus.
touch c., *corpusculum* tactus.
Toynbee's c.'s, corneal c.'s.
Traube's c., achromocyte.
Tröltsch's c.'s, minute spaces, resembling c.'s, between the radial fibers of the drum membrane of the ear.
Valentin's c.'s, small bodies, probably amyloid, found occasionally in nerve tissue.
Vater's c.'s, *corpuscula* lamellosa.
Vater-Pacini c.'s, *corpuscula* lamellosa.
Virchow's c.'s, corneal c.'s.
white c., any type of leukocyte.
Zimmermann's c., platelet.

corpuscula (kōr-pŭs′kyū-lă). Plural of corpusculum.

corpuscular (kōr-pŭs′kyū-lăr). Relating to a corpuscle.

corpusculum, pl. **corpuscula** (kōr-pŭs′kyū-lŭm, -kyū-lă) [NA]. Corpuscle (1); a small mass or body.
corpus′cula articula′ria [NA], articular corpuscles; encapsulated nerve terminations within joint capsules.
corpus′cula bulboi′dea [NA], bulboid corpuscles; Krause's end bulbs; nerve terminals in skin, mouth, conjunctiva, and other parts, consisting of a laminated capsule of connective tissue enclosing the terminal, branched, convoluted ending of an afferent nerve fiber; generally believed to be sensitive to cold.
corpus′cula genita′lia [NA], genital corpuscles; special encapsulated nerve endings found in the skin of the genitalia and nipple.
corpus′cula lamello′sa [NA], lamellated corpuscles; pacinian, Vater's, or Vater-Pacini corpuscles; small oval bodies in the skin of the fingers, in the mesentery, tendons, and elsewhere, formed of concentric layers of connective tissue with a soft core in which the axon of a nerve fiber runs, splitting up into a number of fibrils that terminate in bulbous enlargements; they are sensitive to pressure.

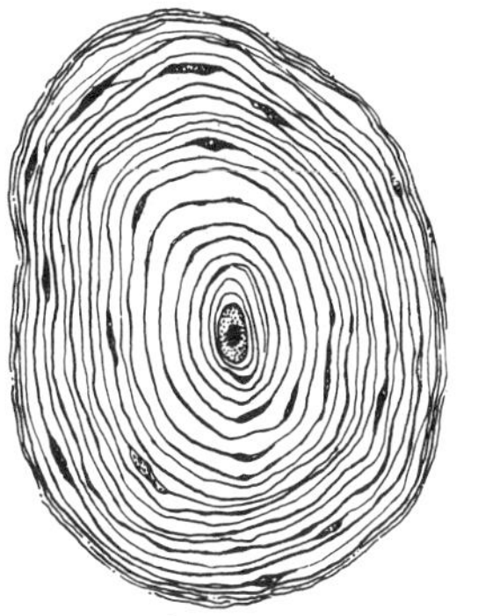

Cross Section of a Corpusculum Lamellosum (Pacinian Corpuscle)

corpus'cula nervo'sa termina'lia [NA], terminal nerve corpuscles; generic term denoting specialized encapsulated nerve endings such as the corpuscula bulboidea, lamellosa, tactus, genitalia, and articularia, and the menisci tactus.

c. re'nis, pl. **corpus'cula re'nis** [NA], renal corpuscle; malpighian corpuscles (1); the tuft of glomerular capillaries and the capsula glomeruli that encloses it.

c. tac'tus, pl. **corpus'cula tac'tus** [NA], tactile, touch, or oval corpuscle; Meissner's corpuscle; one of numerous oval bodies found in the papillae of the corium, especially those of the fingers and toes; they consist of a connective tissue capsule in which the axon fibrils terminate around and between a pile of wedge-shaped epithelioid cells.

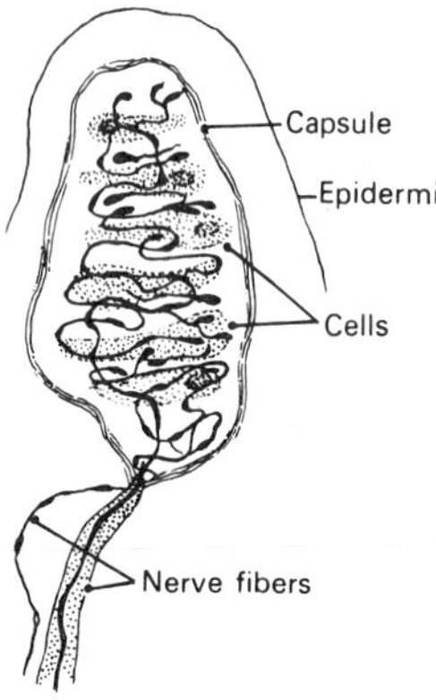

Corpusculum Tactus (Meissner's Corpuscle)

correction (kō-rek'shŭn). The act of reducing a fault; the elimination of an unfavorable quality.

occlusal c., **(1)** the c. of malocclusion, by whatever means is employed; **(2)** elimination of disharmony of occlusal contacts.

spontaneous c. of placenta previa, the upward "migration" of the placenta away from the internal os by the differential growth rates of upper and lower uterine segments.

corrective (kō-rek'tiv) [L. *cor-rigo (conr-)*, pp. *-rectus*, to set right, fr. *rego*, to keep straight]. Corrigent. **1.** Counteracting, modifying, or changing what is injurious. **2.** A drug that modifies or corrects an undesirable or injurious effect of another drug.

correlation (kōr-ĕ-lā'shŭn). **1.** The mutual or reciprocal relation of two or more items or parts. **2.** The act of bringing into such a relation.

product-moment c., a statistical procedure which yields the correlation coefficient referred to as r (-1.00 to $+1.00$) and involves the actual values, rather than the ranks (rank order) of the measurements.

rank-difference c., the relationship between paired series of measurements, each ranked according to magnitude, which yields a coefficient known as *rho;* the value of *rho* varies from zero (no relationship) to 1.00 (perfect relationship).

Correra's line. See under line.

correspondence (kōr-ĕ-spon'dens). In optics, those points on each retina that have the same visual direction.

abnormal c., anomalous c.

anomalous c., abnormal c., a condition, frequent in strabismus, in which corresponding retinal points do not have the same visual direction; the fovea of one eye corresponds to an extrafoveal area of the fellow eye.

dysharmonious c., a type of anomalous retinal c. in which the angle of the visual direction of the two retinas is different than the objective angle of the strabismus.

harmonious c., a type of anomalous retinal c. in which the angle of the visual direction of the two retinas is equal to the objective angle of strabismus.

Corrigan, Sir Dominic J., Irish pathologist and clinician, 1802–1880. See C.'s *disease, pulse.*

corrigent (kōr'i-jent). Corrective.

corrin (kōr'in) [fr. *core* (of vitamin B_{12} molecule)]. The cyclic system of four pyrrole rings forming corrinoids, which are the central structure of the vitamins B_{12} and related compounds, differing from porphin (porphyrin) in that two of the pyrrole rings are directly linked (C-19 to C-1).

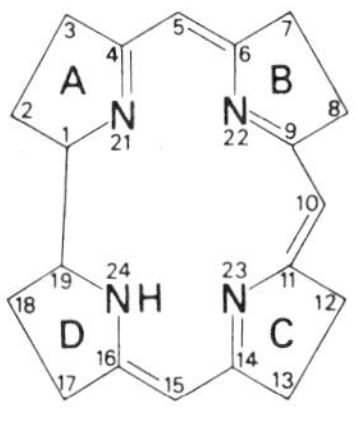

Corrin

Note that the C-20 of porphyrin is absent, hence is skipped in the numbering.

corrode (kŏ-rōd'). To cause, or to be affected by, corrosion.

corrosion (kŏ-rō'shŭn) [L. *cor-rodo (conr-)*, pp. *-rosus*, to gnaw]. **1.** Gradual deterioration or consummation of a substance by another, especially by biochemical or chemical reaction. *Cf.* erosion. **2.** The product of corroding, such as rust.

corrosive (kŏ-rō'siv). **1.** Causing corrosion. **2.** An agent that produces corrosion; *e.g.*, an acid or strong alkali.

corrugator (kōr'ŭ-gā-ter, -tōr) [L. *cor-rugo (conr-)*, pp. *-atus*, to wrinkle, fr. *ruga*, a wrinkle]. A muscle that draws together the skin, causing it to wrinkle.

CORTEX

cortex, gen. **corticis,** pl. **cortices** (kōr'teks, -ti-sis, -ti-sēz) [L. bark] [NA]. The outer portion of an organ, such as the kidney, as distinguished from the inner, or medullary, portion.

adrenal c., c. glandulae suprarenalis.

agranular c., see c. cerebri.

association c., association areas; generic term denoting the large expanses of the cerebral c. that are not sensory or motor in the customary sense, and instead are thought to be involved in advanced stages of sensory information processing, multisensory integration, or sensorimotor integration. See also c. cerebri.

auditory c., auditory area; the region of the cerebral c. that receives the auditory radiation from the medial geniculate body, a cell group of the thalamus in turn receiving the auditory pathway ascending from the cochlear nuclei in the rhombencephalon; it corresponds approximately to Brodmann's areas 41 and 42 and is tonotopically organized.

cerebellar c., c. cerebelli.

c. cerebel'li [NA], cerebellar c.; the thin gray surface layer of the cerebellum, consisting of an outer molecular layer or stratum moleculare (including a single layer of Purkinje cells, the ganglionic layer), and an inner granular layer or stratum granulosum.

cerebral c., c. cerebri.

c. cer′ebri [NA], cerebral c.; the gray cellular mantle (1 to 4 mm thick) covering the entire surface of the cerebral hemisphere of mammals; characterized by a laminar organization of cellular and fibrous components such that its nerve cells are stacked in defined layers varying in number from one, as in the archicortex of the hippocampus, to five or six in the larger neocortex, the outermost (molecular or plexiform) layer contains very few cell bodies and is composed largely of the distal ramifications of the long apical dendrites issued perpendicularly to the surface by pyramidal and fusiform cells in deeper layers. From the surface inward, the layers as classified in K. Brodmann's parcellation are: 1) molecular or plexiform layer; 2) outer granular layer; 3) pyramidal cell layer; 4) inner granular layer; 5) inner pyramidal layer (ganglionic layer); and 6) multiform cell layer, many of which are fusiform. This multilaminate organization is typical of the neocortex (homotypic c.; isocortex in O. Vogt's terminology), which in man covers the largest part by far of the cerebral hemisphere. The more primordial heterotypic c. or allocortex (Vogt) has fewer cell layers. A form of c. intermediate between isocortex and allocortex, called juxtallocortex (Vogt) covers the ventral part of the cingulate gyrus and the entorhinal area of the parahippocampal gyrus.

On the basis of local differences in the arrangement of nerve cells (cytoarchitecture), Brodmann outlined 47 areas in the cerebral c. which, in functional terms, can be classified into three categories: motor c. (areas 4 and 6), characterized by a poorly developed inner granular layer (agranular c.) and prominent pyramidal cell layers; sensory c., characterized by a prominent inner granular layer (granular c. or koniocortex) and comprising the somatic sensory c. (areas 1 to 3), the auditory c. (areas 41 and 42), and the visual c. (areas 17 to 19); and association c., the vast remaining expanses of the cerebral c.

deep c., paracortex.

dysgranular c., the region of the cerebral c. that is transitional between the agranular c. of the precentral gyrus and the granular frontal cortex (Brodmann's area 8).

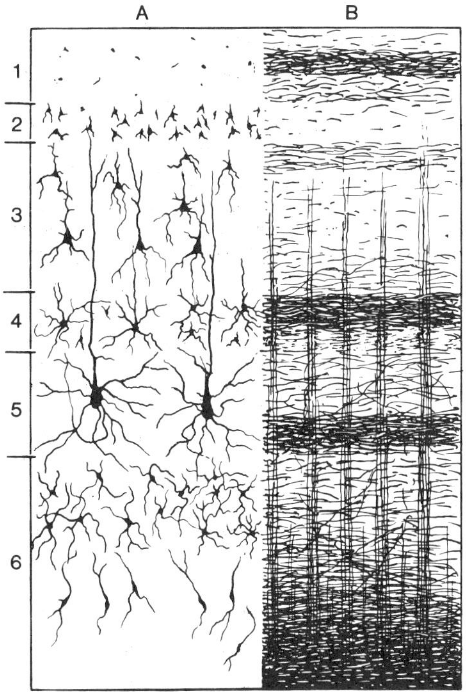

Layers of the Homotypic Cerebral Cortex

A, cells; *B*, fibers; *1* molecular layer; *2*, outer granular layer; *3*, pyramidal cell layer; *4*, inner granular layer, *5*, inner pyramidal layer, *6*, multiform cell layer. (After Brodmann.)

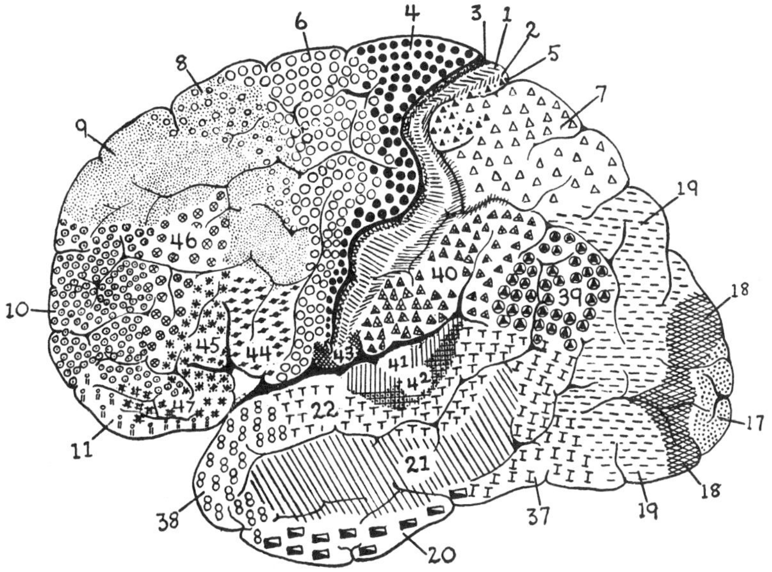

Cortex Cerebri Mapped Using Brodmann's Areas

Cytoarchitectural map of convex surface of the human cortex. The numbered patterns (47) are distinctive areas that differ from each other in total thickness, in the thickness and density of individual layers, and in the arrangement and number of cells and fibers. Investigators since Brodmann (1909) have parceled the cerebral cortex into more than 200 areas; Brodmann's map, however, is still widely used as a reference.

fetal (adrenal) c., provisional c.; fetal zone; androgenic zone (2); an extensive area of the adrenal gland present in primates during fetal life and for a short period after birth; located between the definitive cortex and the medulla, it contains large steroid-secreting cells arranged in a reticular pattern; involution of this zone in humans is largely completed by three months after birth.
frontal c., frontal area; c. of the frontal lobe of the cerebral hemisphere; **(1)** originally, the entire cortical expanse anterior to the sulcus centralis, including the agranular motor and premotor c. (Brodmann's areas 4 and 6), the dysgranular c. (area 8), and the granular frontal (prefrontal) c. anterior to the latter; **(2)** now more often refers to the granular frontal (prefrontal) c.
c. glan'dulae suprarena'lis [NA], adrenal or suprarenal c.; the outer part of the adrenal gland, consisting of three zones from without inward: zona glomerulosa, zona fasciculata, and zona reticularis; this part of the adrenal c. yields steroid hormones such as corticosterone, deoxycorticosterone, and estrone.
granular c., see c. cerebri.
c. of hair shaft, the principal structural component of the hair shaft, composed of closely packed fusiform keratinized cells and invested by the cuticula pili.
heterotypic c., allocortex.
homotypic c., isocortex.
insular c., insula (1).
laminated c., neocortex and allocortex.
c. of lens, c. lentis.
c. len'tis [NA], c. of lens; the softer, more superficial part of the lens of the eye which encloses the central part or nucleus; its refractive power is less than that of the nucleus.
c. of lymph node, c. nodi lymphatici.
motor c., motor, excitable, or Rolando's area; the region of the cerebral c. most nearly immediately influencing movements of the face, neck and trunk, and arm and leg; it corresponds approximately to Brodmann's areas 4 and 6 of the precentral gyrus; its effects upon the motor neurons innervating the skeletal musculature are mediated by the pyramidal tract and are particularly essential for man's capacity to perform finely graded movements of arm and leg.
c. no'di lymphat'ici [NA], c. of lymph node; the outer portion of the lymph node underneath its capsule, consisting of fibrous trabeculae separating densely packed masses of lymphocytes arranged in nodules and separated from the trabeculae and capsule by lymph sinuses.
olfactory c., piriform c.
orbitofrontal c., fronto-orbital area; the cerebral c. covering the basal surface of the frontal lobes.
c. ovarii [NA], c. of ovary; the layer of the ovarian stroma lying immediately beneath the tunica albuginea, composed of connective tissue cells and fibers, among which are scattered primary and secondary (antral) follicles in various stages of development; the c. varies in thickness according to the age of the individual, becoming thinner with advancing years.
c. of ovary, c. ovarii.
parastriate c., see visual c.
peristriate c., see visual c.
piriform c., piriform area; the olfactory c., corresponding to the rostral half of the uncus; receiving its major afferents from the olfactory bulb, it is classified as allocortex. See also c. cerebri.
prefrontal c., see frontal c.
premotor c., premotor area; a somewhat ill-defined term usually referring to the agranular cortex of Brodmann's area 6.
primary visual c., see visual c.
provisional c., fetal (adrenal) c.
renal c., c. renis.
c. re'nis [NA], renal c.; the part of the kidney consisting of renal lobules in the outer zone beneath the capsule and also the lobules of the renal columns which are extensions inward between the pyramids; contains the renal corpuscles and the proximal and distal convoluted tubules.
secondary sensory c., a cortical region occupying the parietal operculum (upper lip of the lateral sulcus) closely posterior to the foot of the postcentral gyrus; like the primary somatic-sensory c. of the postcentral gyrus, this region receives sensory impulses originating in face, trunk, and limbs; projections to the s.s.c. are from the ventral basal complex (ventral posteromedial and posterolateral thalamic nuclei) and from the primary somesthetic cortex.
secondary visual c., see visual c.
sensory c., formerly denoting specifically the somatic sensory c., but now used to refer collectively to the somatic sensory, auditory, visual, and olfactory regions of the cerebral c.
somatic sensory c., somatosensory c., somesthetic area; the region of the cerebral c. receiving the somatic sensory radiation from the ventrobasal nucleus of the thalamus; it represents the primary cortical processing mechanism for sensory information originating at the body surfaces (touch) and in deeper tissues such as muscle, tendons, and joint capsules (position sense); it corresponds approximately to Brodmann's areas 1 to 3 on the postcentral gyrus.
striate c., see visual c.
supplementary motor c., a region from which, by electrical stimulation, the musculature of all bodily parts can be activated, as it also can by stimulation of the motor c. of the precentral gyrus; the region corresponds approximately to the expansion of Brodmann's area 6 over the medial surface of the cerebral hemisphere; this area has largely a bilateral representation and is concerned primarily with tonic and postural motor activities.
suprarenal c., c. glandulae suprarenalis.
temporal c., *lobus* temporalis.
tertiary c., paracortex.
c. of thymus, the outer part of a lobule of the thymus; it surrounds the medulla and is composed of masses of closely packed lymphocytes.
visual c., visual area; the region of the cerebral c. occupying the entire surface of the occipital lobe, and composed of Brodmann's areas 17 to 19. Area 17 (which is also called striate c. or area because the line of Gennari is grossly visible on its surface) is the primary visual c., receiving the visual radiation from the lateral geniculate body of the thalamus. The surrounding areas 18 (parastriate c. or area) and 19 (peristriate c. or area) are probably involved in subsequent steps of visual information processing; area 18 is referred to as the secondary visual c.

Corti, Marquis Alfonso, Italian anatomist, 1822–1888. See C.'s *arch, canal, cells, ganglion, membrane, organ, pillars, rods,* auditory *teeth, tunnel;* pillar *cells* of C.

cortical (kōr'ti-kăl). Relating to a cortex.

corticalization (kōr'ti-kăl-i-zā'shŭn). Encephalization; telencephalization; in phylogenesis, the migration of function from subcortical centers to the cortex.

corticalosteotomy (kōr'ti-kăl-os-tē-ot'ō-mē). An osteotomy through the cortex at the base of the dentoalveolar segment, which serves to weaken the resistance of the bone to the application of orthodontic forces.

corticectomy (kōr-ti-sek'tō-mē). Topectomy.

cortices (kōr'ti-sēz). Plural of cortex.

corticifugal (kōr-ti-sif'yū-găl) [L. *cortex,* rind, bark, + *fugio,* to flee]. Corticoefferent; corticofugal; passing in a direction away from the outer surface; denoting especially nerve fibers conveying impulses away from the cerebral cortex.

corticipetal (kōr-ti-sip'e-tăl) [L. *cortex,* rind, bark, + *peto,* to seek]. Corticoafferent; passing in a direction toward the outer surface; denoting nerve fibers conveying impulses toward the cerebral cortex.

corticoafferent (kōr′ti-kō-af′er-ent). Corticipetal.

corticobulbar (kōr′ti-kō-bŭl′bar). Corticofugal fibers projecting to the rhombencephalon that terminate 1) directly on some motor cranial nerve nuclei, 2) in the reticular formation, and 3) on sensory relay nuclei, such as the nuclei cuneatus and gracilis and the spinal trigeminal nucleus.

corticocerebellum (kor′ti-kō-ser-ĕ-bel′ŭm). Neocerebellum.

corticoefferent (kōr′ti-kō-ef′er-ent). Corticifugal.

corticofugal (kōr′ti-kō-fyū′găl). Corticifugal.

corticoid (kōr′ti-koyd). **1.** Having an action similar to that of a hormone of the adrenal cortex. **2.** Any substance exhibiting this action.

corticoliberin (kōr′ti-kō-lib′er-in). Corticotropin-releasing factor or hormone; a peptide hormone from the hypothalamus that stimulates the anterior pituitary to release adrenocorticotropic hormone.

corticomedial (kōr′ti-kō-mē′dē-ăl). Cortical and medial; specifically used to refer to one of the two major cytological divisions of the amygdaloid complex. See corpus amygdaloideum.

corticosteroid. (kōr′ti-kō-stēr′oyd). A steroid produced by the adrenal cortex; a corticoid containing a steroid.

corticosterone (kōr-ti-kos′ter-ōn). 11β,21-Dihydroxy-4-pregnene-3,20-dione; a corticosteroid that induces some deposition of glycogen in the liver, sodium conservation, and potassium excretion.

corticothalamic (kōr′ti-kō-thal′ă-mik). Pertaining to cortex and thalamus; the term is applied to fibers projecting from the cerebral cortex to the thalamus.

corticotroph (kōr′ti-kō-trof). A cell of the adenohypophysis that produces adrenocorticotropic hormone (ACTH).

corticotropin, (kōr′ti-kō-trō′pin) [G. *tropē*, a turning]. Adrenocorticotropic *hormone.*

c.-zinc hydroxide, purified c. absorbed on zinc hydroxide; same uses as c. but with a prolonged duration of action.

β-corticotropin. Acid- or pepsin-degraded c.

Corticoviridae (kōr′ti-kō-vir′i-dē). Provisional name for a family of nonenveloped, ether-sensitive bacterial viruses of medium size, with a lipid-containing capsid and genome of cyclic, double-stranded DNA (MW 5×10^6), which accounts for about 12% of virion weight.

cortisol (kōr′ti-sol). Hydrocortisone.

c. acetate, *hydrocortisone* acetate.

cortisone (kōr′ti-sōn) [former acronym for corticosterone]. 17α, 21-Dihydroxy-4-pregnene-3,11,20-trione; 17α-hydroxy-11-dehydrocorticosterone; a glucocorticoid not normally secreted in significant quantities by the human adrenal cortex. Endogenously, it is probably a metabolite of hydrocortisone but exhibits no biological activity until converted to hydrocortisone (cortisol); it acts upon carbohydrate metabolism and influences the nutrition and growth of connective (collagenous) tissues.

α-cortol (kōr′tol). 5β-Pregnane-3α,11β,17,20α,21-pentaol; the 5β enantiomer of α-allocortol; a reduction product of cortisone, present in the urine, differing from cortisone in that the three keto groups are reduced to hydroxyls.

β-cortol. α-Cortol with a 20β–OH group; the 5β enantiomer of β-allocortol, found in urine.

α-cortolone (kōr′tō-lōn). 3α,17α,20α,21-Tetrahydroxy-5β-pregnane-11-one; the 5β enantiomer of α-allocortolone; a reduction product of cortisone, present in the urine, differing from cortisone in that two of the keto groups (at positions 3 and 20) are reduced to hydroxyls.

β-cortolone. α-Cortolone with a 20β–OH group; the 5β enantiomer of β-allocortolone, found in urine.

corundum (ko-rŭn′dŭm) [Hind. *kurand*]. Native crystalline aluminum oxide.

coruscation (kōr-ŭs-kā′shŭn) [L. *corusco*, to flash]. Psychiatric term for a subjective sensation of a flash of light before the eyes.

Corvisart des Marets, Baron Jean N., French clinician, 1755–1821. See C.'s *facies.*

corylophyline (kōr-il-ō-fī′lēn). *Glucose* oxidase.

corymbiform (kō-rim′bi-fōrm) [L. *corymbus*, cluster, garland]. Denoting the flower-like clustering configuration of skin lesions in granulomatous diseases (*e.g.*, syphilis, tuberculosis).

corynebacteria (kō-rī′nē-bak-tēr′ē-ă). Plural of corynebacterium.

corynebacteriophage (kō-rī′nē-bak-tēr′ē-ō-fāj). Any one of the bacteriophages specific for corynebacteria.

β c., β phage; a DNA-containing bacteriophage that induces toxigenicity in strains of *Corynebacterium diphtheriae* that are lysogenic for its prophage.

Corynebacterium (kō-rī′nē-bak-tēr′ē-ŭm) [G. *coryne*, a club, + *bacterium*, a small rod]. A genus of nonmotile (except for some plant pathogens), aerobic to anaerobic bacteria (family Corynebacteriaceae) containing irregularly staining, Gram-positive, straight to slightly curved, often club-shaped rods which, as a result of snapping division, show a picket fence arrangement. These organisms are widely distributed in nature. The best known species are parasites and pathogens of humans and domestic animals. The type species is *C. diphtheriae.*

C. ac′nes, *Propionibacterium acnes.*

C. bo′vis, *Bacillus pseudodiphtheria;* a nonpathogenic species of bacteria found in freshly drawn cow's milk.

C. diphthe′riae, *C. ulcerans;* Klebs-Loeffler bacillus; Loeffler's bacillus; a species which causes diphtheria and produces a powerful exotoxin causing degeneration of various tissues, notably myocardium, in man and experimental animals; virulent strains of this organism are lysogenic; it is commonly found in membranes in the pharynx, larynx, trachea, and nose in cases of diphtheria; it is also found in apparently healthy pharynx and nose in carriers, and is occasionally found in the conjunctiva and in superficial wounds; it occasionally infects the nasal passages and wounds of horses; it is the type species of the genus *C.*

C. enzy′micum, a species found in human lungs, blood, and joints; pathogenic for laboratory animals.

C. e′qui, a species found in spontaneous pneumonia of foals and in other infections of horses; also found in swine, cattle, and buffaloes.

C. hofman′nii, *C. pseudodiphtheriticum.*

C. kut′scheri, a species pathogenic to mice.

C. minutis′simum, a species that causes erythrasma in humans.

C. murisep′ticum, a species which causes septicemia in mice.

C. o′vis, *C. pseudotuberculosis.*

C. par′vum, name used for a species synonymous with *Propionibacterium acnes,* used as a reticulostimulant and immunomodulator in cancer therapy.

C. pho′cae, a species found in an erysipelas occurring in the transition between the corium and the blubber of seals.

C. pseudodiphtherit′icum, *C. hofmannii;* Hofmann's bacillus; a nonpathogenic species found in normal throats.

C. pseudotuberculo′sis, *C. ovis;* Preisz-Nocard bacillus; a species found in necrotic areas in sheep kidney, in caseous lymphadenitis in sheep, and in ulcerative lesions in horses, cattle, and other warm-blooded animals.

C. pyog′enes, a species which is probably the most frequently occurring pyogenic organism in cattle, swine, and sheep but which is not pathogenic for man; it produces a toxin and a heat-labile hemolysin and is frequently found alone, or with other bacteria, in a great variety of suppurative processes.

C. rena′le, a species of bacteria which occurs in purulent infections of the urinary tract in cattle, sheep, horses, and dogs; pathogenic to laboratory animals.

C. stria'tum, a species found in nasal mucus and in the throat; also found in udders of cows with mastitis; pathogenic to laboratory animals.

C. ul'cerans, *C. diphtheriae.*

C. xero'sis, a species found in normal and diseased conjunctiva; there is no evidence that this organism is pathogenic.

corynebacterium, pl. **corynebacteria** (kō-rī'nē-bak-tēr'ē-ŭm, -ă). A vernacular term used to refer to any member of the genus *Corynebacterium.*

coryza (kō-rī'ză) [G.]. Acute *rhinitis.*

allergic c., a rhinitis in an allergic individual due to the presence of an agent to which he is hypersensitive.

coryzavirus (kō-rī'ză-vī'rŭs). Former name for *Rhinovirus.*

cosmesis (koz-mē'sis) [G. *kosmēsis,* an adorning, fr. *kosmeō,* to order, arrange, adorn, fr. *kosmos,* order]. A concern in therapeutics, especially in surgical operations, for the appearance of the patient; *i.e.,* a resort to an operation which will improve the appearance, or avoidance of an operation which will mutilate or disfigure.

cosmetic (koz-met'ik). **1.** Relating to cosmesis. **2.** Relating to the use of cosmetics.

cosmetics (koz-met'iks). Composite term for a variety of camouflages applied to the skin, hair, and nails for purposes of beautifying in accordance with cultural dictates.

cosmid (koz'mid). A synthetic plasmid, a circular DNA containing in order: a plasmid origin of replication and a drug-resistance marker, the *cos* (cohesive end) gene from a bacteriophage λ, and a fragment of eukaryotic DNA to be cloned; c.'s are constructed to permit cloning of fragments of up to about 40,000 nucleotides long, with one or more unique restriction sites being necessary to permit cloning.

cosmopolitan (koz-mō-pol'i-tan) [G. *kosmos,* universe, + *polis,* city-state]. In the biological sciences, a term denoting worldwide distribution.

costa, gen. and pl. **costae** (kos'tă, -tē) [L.]. **1** [NA]. Rib; one of the twenty-four elongated curved bones forming the main portion of the bony wall of the chest. **2.** Basal rod; a rodlike internal supporting organelle that runs along the base of the undulating membrane of certain flagellate parasites such as *Trichomonas.*

c. cervica'lis [NA], cervical rib; a supernumerary rib articulating with a cervical vertebra, usually the seventh, but not reaching the sternum anteriorly. See also cervical rib *syndrome.*

cos'tae fluctuan'tes, costae fluitantes.

cos'tae fluitan'tes [NA], floating ribs; vertebral ribs; costae fluctuantes; the two lower ribs on either side that are not attached anteriorly.

cos'tae spu'riae [NA], false ribs; vertebrochondral ribs; five lower ribs on either side that do not articulate with the sternum directly.

cos'tae ve'rae [NA], true ribs; vertebrosternal ribs; seven upper ribs on either side whose cartilages articulate directly with the sternum.

costal (kos'tăl). Relating to a rib.

costalgia (kos-tal'jē-ă) [L. *costa,* rib, + G. *algos,* pain]. Pleurodynia.

costectomy (kos-tek'tō-mē) [L. *costa,* rib, + G. *ektomē,* excision]. Excision of a rib.

Costen, James B., U.S. otolaryngologist, 1895–1962. See C.'s *syndrome.*

costicartilage (kos-ti-kar'ti-lij). *Cartilago* costalis.

costiform (kos'ti-fōrm) [L. *costa,* rib, + *forma,* form]. Rib-shaped.

costive (kos'tiv) [contraction from L. *constipo,* to press together]. Pertaining to or causing constipation.

costiveness (kos'tiv-ness). Constipation.

costo- [L. *costa,* rib]. Combining form relating to the ribs.

costocentral (kos-tō-sen'trăl). Costovertebral.

costochondral (kos-tō-kon'drăl). Relating to the costal cartilages.

costochondritis (kos'tō-kon-drī'tis) [costo- + G. *chondros,* cartilage, + *-itis,* inflammation]. Costal chondritis; inflammation of one or more costal cartilages, characterized by local tenderness and pain of the anterior chest wall that may radiate, but without the local swelling typical of Tietze's syndrome.

costoclavicular (kos-tō-klă-vik'yū-lăr). Relating to the ribs and the clavicle.

costocoracoid (kos-tō-kōr'ă-koyd). Relating to the ribs and the coracoid process of the scapula.

costogenic (kos-tō-jen'ik). Arising from a rib.

costoinferior (kos-tō-in-fēr'ē-ōr). Relating to the lower ribs.

costoscapular (kos-tō-skap'yū-lăr). Relating to the ribs and the scapula.

costoscapularis (kos-tō-skap-yū-lā'ris). *Musculus* serratus anterior.

costosternal (kos-tō-ster'năl). Pertaining to the ribs and the sternum.

costosternoplasty (kos-tō-ster'nō-plas-tē) [costo- + G. *sternon,* chest, + *plastos,* formed]. Operation to correct a malformation of the anterior chest wall.

costosuperior (kos-tō-sū-pēr'ē-ōr). Relating to the upper ribs.

costotome (kos'tō-tōm). An instrument, knife or shears, designed for cutting through a rib.

costotomy (kos-tot'ō-mē) [costo- + G. *tomē,* a cutting]. Division of a rib.

costotransverse (kos-tō-trans-vers'). Transversocostal; relating to the ribs and the transverse processes of the vertebrae articulating with them.

costotransversectomy (kos'tō-tranz-ver-sek'tō-mē). Excision of a proximal portion of a rib and the articulating transverse process.

costovertebral (kos-tō-ver'tĕ-brăl). Costocentral; vertebrocostal (1); relating to the ribs and the bodies of the thoracic vertebrae with which they articulate.

costoxiphoid (kos-tō-zī'foyd). Relating to the ribs and the xiphoid cartilage of the sternum.

cosyntropin (kō-sin-trō'pin). Tetracosactide; tetracosactrin; α^{ACTH}; ^{24}- or β^{1-24}-corticotropin; a synthetic corticotrophic agent, comprising the first 24 amino-acid residues of human ACTH, which sequence is found in several other species and which retains the full biologic activity of the complete ACTH; the remaining 15 residues differ among species and confer specific immunologic properties.

Cotard, Jules, French neurologist, 1840–1887. See C.'s *syndrome.*

cotarnine (kō-tar'nēn). An alkaloidal principle, $C_{12}H_{15}NO_4$, derived from narcotine by oxidation; an astringent.

COTe Abbreviation of cathodal opening *tetanus.*

cothromboplastin (kō-throm'bō-plas-tin). *Factor* VII.

cotinine (kō'ti-nēn). 1-Methyl-5-(3-pyridyl)-2-pyrrolidinone; one of the major detoxication products of nicotine; eliminated rapidly and completely by the kidneys.

cotransport (kō-trans'pōrt). The transport of one substance across a membrane, coupled with the simultaneous transport of another substance across the same membrane in the same direction.

Cotte, Gaston, French surgeon, 1879–1951. See C.'s *operation.*

Cotton, Frank A., U.S. chemist, *1930. See C. *effect.*

cotton (kot'ŭn) [Ar. *qútun*]. The white, fluffy, fibrous covering of the seeds of a plant of the genus *Gossypium* (family Malvaceae); used extensively in surgical dressings.

absorbent c., c. from which all fatty matter has been extracted, so that it readily takes up fluids.

purified c., absorbent c. in which the hairs of the seed of varieties of *Gossypium* and other allied species are freed from adhering impurities, deprived of fatty matter, bleached, and sterilized; used for tampons, etc.
soluble gun c., pyroxylin.
styptic c., absorbent c. wet with a dilute solution of ferric chloride, and then dried; applied locally as a hemostatic.

cottonseed oil (kot'ŭn-sēd). The refined fixed oil obtained from the seed of cultivated plants of various varieties of *Gossypium hirsutum* or of other species of *Gossypium* (family Malvaceae); a solvent.

Cotunnius (Cotugno), Domenico, Neapolitan anatomist, 1736–1822. See C. *aqueduct, canal, disease, liquid, space; liquor* cotunnii.

cotyle (kot'i-lē) [G. *kotylē*, anything hollow, the cup or socket of a joint]. **1.** Any cup-shaped structure. **2.** Acetabulum.

cotyledon (kot-i-lē'don) [G. *kotylēdon*, any cup-shaped hollow]. **1.** Any cup-shaped hollow structure. **2.** In plants, a seed leaf, the first leaf to grow from a seed. **3.** A placental unit. See maternal c.
fetal c., a unit of the fetal placenta supplied by the vessels of a stem villus; several such c.'s may occur between two placental septa; traditionally called embryologists' c.
maternal c., a unit of the placenta made up of trophoblastic cells, fibrous tissue, and abundant blood vessels, which is visible grossly on the maternal surface as an irregularly shaped lobe circumscribed by a deep cleft and made up of a stem villus with numerous branching free villi and anchoring villi; placental vessels in the chorionic plate supply the stem villus and its branches, allowing gas and metabolite exchange across the trophoblastic layer with maternal blood in the intervillous space; traditionally called clinicians' c.

Cotylogonimus (kot-i-lō-gon'i-mŭs) [G. *kotylē*, cup, + *gonimos*, productive]. A group of heterophyid flukes, now properly included in the genus *Heterophyes*.

cotyloid (kot'i-loyd) [G. *kotylē*, a small cup, + *eidos*, appearance]. **1.** Cup-shaped; cuplike. **2.** Relating to the cotyloid cavity or acetabulum.

couching (kowch'ing) [Fr. *coucher*, to lay down, to put to bed]. An obsolete operation for cataract, consisting of displacement of the lens into the vitreous cavity out of the line of vision.

cough (kawf). **1.** A sudden explosive forcing of air through the glottis, occurring immediately on opening the previously closed glottis, and excited by mechanical or chemical irritation of the trachea or bronchi, or by pressure from adjacent structures. **2.** To force air through the glottis by a series of expiratory efforts.
brassy c., loud metallic clanging c. caused by pressure on the trachea or laryngeal nerves, as by an aneurysm of the aortic arch.
ear c., a reflex c., through the auricular branch of the vagus, excited by irritation in the external auditory canal.
hebetic c., nervous c. occurring frequently at puberty, and sometimes simulating tuberculosis.
kennel c., a highly contagious form of laryngitis, tracheitis, and bronchitis in dogs, probably caused by a virus.
privet c., an allergic c., occurring in China during May and June, supposed to be caused by inhalation of the pollen of a species of privet (*Lingustrum*); it is analogous to the laurel fever seen in New England.
reflex c., a c. excited reflexly by irritation in some distant part, as the ear or the stomach.
stomach c., a reflex c. excited at times by irritation of the gastric mucous membrane.
tooth c., c. of reflex origin, due to caries or other disease or malformation of the teeth.
trigeminal c., a reflex c. due to irritation of the terminals of the trigeminus nerve in the upper respiratory passages.
weaver's c., c., dyspnea, and sense of constriction of the chest, caused in persons working with mildewed yarns.
whooping c., pertussis.

coulomb (Q) (kū-lom') [C. A. de *Coulomb*, Fr. physicist, 1736–1806]. The amount of electricity delivered by a current of 1 ampere in 1 second; equal to 1/96,500 faraday.

coumaranone (kū-mar'ă-nōn). 3(2*H*)-Benzofuranone, the basis of many plant products; *e.g.*, aurone.

coumaric anhydride (kū-mā'rik). Coumarin.

coumarin (kū'mă-rin) [*coumarou*, native name of Tonka bean]. Cumarin; coumaric anhydride; *ortho*-oxycinnamic anhydride; 2*H*-1-benzopyran-2-one; a fragrant neutral principle obtained from the Tonka bean, *Dypterix odorata*, and made synthetically from salicylic aldehyde; it is used to disguise unpleasant odors.

coumetarol (kū-met'ă-rol). Cumetharol; cumethoxaethane; 3,3'-(2-methoxyethylidene)bis(4-hydroxycoumarin); an oral anticoagulant.

Councilman, William T., U.S. pathologist, 1854–1933. See C. (hyaline) *body*, C.'s *lesions*.

Councilmania (kown-sil-man'ē-ă) [W. *Councilman*]. Obsolete generic term for a group of amebas now recognized as *Entamoeba*.

counseling (kown'sel-ing) [L. *consilium*, deliberation]. The giving of advice, opinion, and instruction to direct the judgment or conduct of another.
genetic c., the process whereby an expert in hereditary disorders provides information to patients or relatives in families with genetic disorders as an aid to decision making concerning marriage, children, early diagnosis, and limitation of disability.
marital c., the process whereby a trained counselor assists married couples to resolve problems that arise and trouble them in their relationship; husband and wife are seen by the same counselor in separate and joint c. sessions focusing on immediate family problems.
pastoral c., the use of psychotherapeutic methods by clergymen for parishioners seeking help with personal problems.

count (kownt). **1.** A reckoning, enumeration, or accounting. **2.** To enumerate or score.
Addis c., a quantitative enumeration of the red blood c., white blood c., and casts in a 12-hr urine specimen; used to follow the progress of known renal disease.
Arneth c., the percentage distribution of polymorphonuclear neutrophils, based on the number of lobes in the nuclei (from 1 to 5). See also Arneth *index*.
blood c., see *blood count*.
epidermal ridge c., an index of the frequency of sweat pores on the fingertips by enumeration along a set of arbitrarily defined lines; a classic example of a galtonian trait determined almost exclusively by genetic factors.
filament-nonfilament c., a differential c. of the number of neutrophils showing nuclear division and those showing no such division.

counter (kown'ter). A device that counts.
automated differential leukocyte c., an instrument using digital imaging or cytochemical techniques to differentiate leukocytes.
electronic cell c., an automatic blood cell c. in which cells passing through an aperture alter resistance and are counted as voltage pulses, or in which cells passing through a flow cell deflect light; some types of c. are capable of multiple simultaneous measurements on each blood sample; *e.g.*, leukocyte count, red cell count, hemoglobin, hematocrit, and red cell indices.
Geiger-Müller c., an instrument for measuring radioactivity by counting the emission of radioactive particles; it consists of a metallic cylinder, negatively charged, in a tube containing a fine, positively charged wire at its center; radiations produce ionization of the gas molecules between the cylinder and the wire and result in an electrical discharge independent of the energy of the impinging particle or ray.

proportional c., a Geiger-Müller c. operating in the voltage range and under conditions in which pulse height is proportional to the energy of the particles being counted, thus making discrimination between particles of different energies possible.
scintillation c., scintillascope; scintillometer; spinthariscope; an instrument used for the detection of radioactivity; the radiation is absorbed by a scintillator (a crystal or a compound, such as POPOP, in solution) which results in minute flashes of light that are detected by a photomultiplier and an amplifier.
whole-body c., shielding and instrumentation, usually involving more than one detector, designed to evaluate the total-body burden of various gamma-emitting nuclides.

counter- [L. *contra,* against]. Combining form meaning opposite, opposed, against. See also contra-.

counterbalancing (kown-ter-bal'ăn-sing). A procedure in behavioral research for distributing unwanted but unavoidable influences equally among the different experimental conditions or subjects.

counterconditioning (kown'ter-kon-dish'ŭn-ing). Any of a group of specific behavior therapy techniques in which a second conditioned response is instituted for the express purpose of counteracting or nullifying a previously conditioned or learned response.

countercurrent (kown'ter-ker'ent). **1.** Flowing in an opposite direction. **2.** A current flowing in a direction opposite to another current.

countercurrent exchanger. A system in which heat or chemicals passively diffuse across a membrane separating two c. streams so that at each end the fluid leaving along one side of the membrane nearly resembles, in temperature or composition, the fluid entering the other; *e.g.,* the venae comites in the arms serve as a c. exchanger, the arterial blood serving to rewarm the cooler venous blood.

countercurrent multiplier. A system in which energy is used to transport material across a membrane separating two c. tubes connected at one end to form a hairpin shape; by this means a concentration can be achieved in the fluid in the hairpin bend, relative to the inflow and outflow fluids, that is much greater than the transport mechanism could produce between the two sides of the membrane at any point; *e.g.,* the nephronic loops in the renal medulla act as c. multipliers.

counterdepressant (kown'ter-dē-pres'ănt). **1.** A drug or agent that prevents or antagonizes the depressing action of another drug or agent. **2.** Having a counterdepressing effect.

counterdie (kown'ter-dī). The reverse image of a die, usually made of a softer and lower fusing metal than the die.

counterextension (kown'ter-eks-ten'shŭn). Countertraction.

counterimmunoelectrophoresis (kown'ter-im'yū-nō-ē-lek'trō-fō-rē'sis). A modification of immunoelectrophoresis in which antigen (*e.g.,* serum containing hepatitis B virus) is placed in wells cut in the sheet of agar gel toward the cathode, and antiserum is placed in wells toward the anode; antigen and antibody, moving in opposite directions, form precipitates in the area between the cells where they meet in concentrations of optimal proportions.

counterincision (kown'ter-in-sizh'ŭn). A second incision adjacent to a primary incision.

counterinvestment (kown'ter-in-vest'ment). Anticathexis.

counterirritant (kown-ter-ir'i-tant). **1.** An agent that causes irritation or a mild inflammation of the skin in order to relieve a deep-seated inflammatory process. **2.** Relating to or producing counter-irritation.

counterirritation (kown'ter-ir-i-tā'shŭn). Revulsion (1); irritation or mild inflammation (redness, vesication, or pustulation) of the skin excited for the purpose of relieving an inflammation of the deeper structures.

counteropening (kown'ter-ō-pen-ing). Contra-aperture; counter-puncture; a second opening made at the dependent part of an abscess or other cavity containing fluid, which is not draining satisfactorily through an opening previously made.

counterphobic (kown-ter-fō'bik). **1.** Denoting a state of actual preference, on the part of a phobic person, for the very situation of which he is afraid. **2.** Opposed to the phobic impulse, as in c. mastery of a feared action by repeated engagement in the action.

counterpulsation (kown'ter-pŭl-sā'shŭ). A means of assisting the failing heart by automatically removing arterial blood just before and during ventricular ejection and returning it to the circulation during diastole; a balloon catheter is inserted into the aorta and activated by an automatic mechanism triggered by the EKG.

counterpuncture (kown'ter-pŭnk-chūr). Counteropening.

countershock (kown'ter-shok). An electric shock applied to the heart to terminate a disturbance of its rhythm.

counterstain (kown'ter-stān). A second stain of different color, having affinity for tissues, cells, or parts of cells other than those taking the primary stain, used to render more distinct the parts taking the first stain.

countertraction (kown-ter-trak'shŭn). Counterextension; the resistance, or back-pull, made to extension on a limb; *e.g.,* in the case of extension made on the leg, c. may be effected by raising the foot of the bed so that the weight of the body pulls against the weight attached to the limb.

countertransference (kown'ter-trans-fer'ens). In psychoanalysis, the analyst's transference (often unconscious) of his emotional needs and feelings toward the patient, with personal involvement to the detriment of the desired objective analyst-patient relationship.

countertransport (kown-ter-tranz'pōrt). The transport of one substance across a membrane, coupled with the simultaneous transport of another substance across the same membrane in the opposite direction.

coup de sabre (kū-dĕ-sahb') [Fr. stroke of a sword]. Linear scleroderma usually found over the scalp or forehead.

couple (kŭ'pl). To copulate; to perform coitus; said especially of the lower animals.

coupling (kŭp'ling). **1.** Bigeminal rhythm; usually the result of the repeated pairing of a normal sinus beat with a ventricular extrasystole. **2.** See c. *phase.*
constant c., fixed c.
fixed c., constant c.; where several premature beats are seen, the interval between each of them and the preceding normal beat is constant.
variable c., where several extrasystoles are seen, the interval between each of them and the preceding sinus beat varies.

Courvoisier, Ludwig G., French surgeon, 1843–1918. See C.'s *law, sign.*

couvade (kū-vahd') [Fr. *couver,* to hatch]. A primitive custom in certain cultures in which a man develops labor pains while his wife is in labor and then submits to the same postpartum purification rites and taboos.

Couvelaire, Alexandre, French obstetrician, 1873–1948. See C. *uterus.*

couvercle (kū-ver'kl) [Fr. cover, lid]. An external coagulum, especially a blood clot formed extravascularly.

covalent (kō-vāl'ent). Denoting an interatomic bond characterized by the sharing of 2, 4, or 6 electrons.

coverslip (kŭv'er-slip). Cover *glass.*

cow (kow). A generator for short-lived isotopes based upon successively eluting or otherwise separating ("milking") a short-lived radioactive daughter from a longer-lived parent; *e.g.,* ^{99m}Tc from

^{99}Mo, ^{113m}In from ^{113}Sn.

Cowden. Surname of the family from which the condition subsequently known as Cowden's *disease* was first reported.

Cowdria ruminantium (kow'drē-ă rū-mi-nan'tē-ŭm) [E.V. *Cowdry*]. The rickettsial species causing heartwater in cattle, sheep, and goats in South Africa, transmitted by ticks of the genus *Amblyomma.*

cowdriosis (kow-drē-ō'sis). Heartwater.

Cowdry, Edmund Vincent, U.S. cytologist, 1888–1975. See C.'s type A and B inclusion *bodies.*

Cowling's rule. See under rule.

Cowper, William, British anatomist, 1666–1709. See cowperitis; C.'s *cyst, gland, ligament.*

cowperian (kow-pēr'ē-an). Relating to or described by Cowper.

cowperitis (kow-per-ī'tis). Inflammation of Cowper's gland.

cowpox (kow'poks). A disease of bovine teat skin caused by the cowpox virus, but clinically indistinguishable from bovine vaccinia mammillitis caused by the vaccinia virus.

coxa, gen. and pl. **coxae** (kok'să, -sē) [L]. **1.** *Os* coxae. **2.** *Articulatio* coxae.

c. adduc'ta, c. vara.

false c. va'ra, approximation of the head of the femur to the shaft, due not to deformity of the neck of the femur, but to curvature of the shaft.

c. flex'a, c. vara.

c. mag'na, enlargement and deformation of femoral head; usually a sequela of Legg-Calvé-Perthes disease or osteoarthritis.

c. pla'na, Legg-Calvé-Perthes *disease.*

c. val'ga, alteration of the angle made by the axis of the femoral neck to the axis of the femoral shaft, so that the angle exceeds 135°; the femoral neck is in more of a straight line relationship to the shaft of the femur.

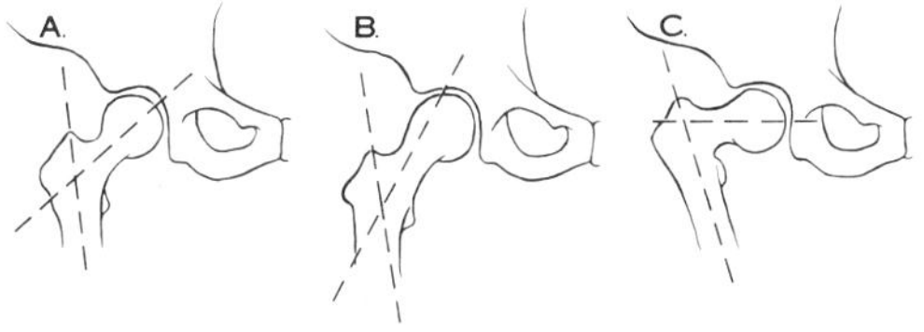

Coxa Valga and Coxa Vara
A, normal femoral neck; *B*, coxa valga; *C*, coxa vara

c. va'ra, c. adducta; c. flexa; alteration of the angle made by the axis of the femoral neck to the axis of the femoral shaft so that the angle is less than 135°; the neck becomes more horizontal.

c. va'ra lux'ans, c. vara with dislocation of the femoral head.

coxalgia (koks-al'jē-ă) [L. *coxa,* hip, + G. *algos,* pain]. Coxodynia.

c. fu'gax, transient pain in the hip.

Coxiella (kok-sē-el'ă) [H. R. *Cox,* U.S. bacteriologist, *1907]. A genus of filterable bacteria (order Rickettsiales) containing small, pleomorphic, rod-shaped or coccoid, Gram-negative cells which occur intracellularly in the cytoplasm of infected cells and possibly extracellularly in infected ticks. These organisms have not been cultivated in cell-free media; they are parasitic on man and other animals. The type species is *C. burnetii.*

C. burnet'ii, *Rickettsia burnetii;* a species which causes Q fever in man; it is the type species of the genus *C.*

coxodynia (koks-ō-din'ē-ă) [L. *coxa,* hip, + G. *odynē,* pain]. Coxalgia; pain in the hip joint.

coxofemoral (kok-sō-fem'ō-răl). Relating to the hip bone and the femur.

coxotomy (koks-ot'ō-mē) [L. *coxa,* hip, + G. *tomē,* cutting]. Obsolete term for incision into the hip joint.

coxotuberculosis (koks'ō-tū-ber-kyū-lō'sis). Tuberculous hip-joint disease.

Coxsackievirus (kok-sax'ē-vī'rŭs) [*Coxsackie,* N.Y., where first isolated]. A group of picornaviruses, included in the genus *Enterovirus,* of spherical shape and about 28 nm in diameter, causing myositis, paralysis, and death in young mice, and are responsible for a variety of diseases in man, although inapparent infections are common. They are divided antigenically into two groups, A and B, each of which includes a number of serological types, *e.g., Enterovirus* coxsackie A1 to 24 and *Enterovirus* coxsackie B1 to 6. Type A viruses cause human herpangina and hand-foot-and-mouth disease; type B viruses cause epidemic pleurodynia; both type viruses may cause aseptic meningitis, myocarditis and pericarditis, and acute onset juvenile diabetes.

cozymase (kō-zī'mās). Former name for nicotinamide adenine dinucleotide.

c.p. Abbreviation for chemically pure.

CPAP Abbreviation for continuous positive airway *pressure.*

C-peptide. C chain; the 30 amino-acid chain that connects the A and B chains of insulin in proinsulin; removed in the conversion of proinsulin to insulin.

CPK Abbreviation for *creatine* phosphokinase.

CPM Abbreviation for continuous passive *motion.*

CPPB Abbreviation for continuous positive pressure *breathing.*

CPPV Abbreviation for continuous positive pressure *ventilation.*

CPR Abbreviation for cardiopulmonary *resuscitation.*

cps Abbreviation for cycles per second.

CR Abbreviation for conditioned *reflex;* crown-rump *length.*

Cr **1.** Symbol for chromium. **2.** Abbreviation for creatinine.

crab (krab). **1.** A crustacean, many varieties of which are edible. **2.** An insect, the crab louse, *Pthirus pubis.*

Crabtree, Herbert G. See C. *effect.*

cradle (krā'dl). A frame used to keep bedclothes from coming in contact with an injured patient.

Crafoord, Clarence, Swedish surgeon, *1899. See C. *clamp.*

Craigia (krā'gē-ă) [C. *Craig*]. Obsolete generic term for a group of amebas now recognized as *Entamoeba.*

Cramer, Friedrich, German surgeon, 1847–1903. See C. wire *splint.*

cramp (kramp). **1.** A painful spasm. **2.** A professional neurosis, qualified according to the occupation of the sufferer; *e.g.,* seamstress's c., writer's c.

accessory c., torticollis.

heat c.'s, myalgia thermica; muscle spasm induced by severe exertion in intense heat, accompanied by considerable pain; sometimes related to salt deficiency, hyperventilation, or overindulgence in alcohol.

intermittent c., tetany.

miner's c.'s, stoker's c.'s; c.'s caused by excessive salt loss through perspiration.

musician's c., an occupational neurosis, affecting those who play on musical instruments, and named usually according to the instrument played upon.

pianist's c., piano-player's c., a professional neurosis affecting the muscles of the fingers and forearms in piano players.

seamstress's c., sewing spasm; an occupational neurosis occurring in the fingers of needle-women.

shaving c., keirospasm; xyrospasm; an occupational neurosis affecting barbers.

stoker's c.'s, miner's c.'s.

tailor's c., tailor's spasm; a spasmodic neurosis of the muscles of

the forearm and hand.
typist's c., an occupational neurosis affecting chiefly the long flexor muscles of the hands.
violinist's c., a professional neurosis affecting the digits of the fingering hand, or sometimes the bowing arm, in violin players.
waiter's c., an occupational neurosis characterized by spasm of the muscles of the back and dominant arm in persons who wait tables.
watchmaker's c., an occupational neurosis characterized by spasm of the orbicularis palpebrarum muscle from holding the lens to the eye and spasm of the muscles of the hand from performing the delicate movements of watch repairing.
writer's c., dysgraphia (2); mogigraphia; graphospasm; scrivener's palsy; an occupation neurosis affecting chiefly the muscles of the thumb and two adjoining fingers of the writing hand, induced by excessive use of a writing instrument; occurs in one of four main forms: spastic, paralytic, neuralgic, and tremulous.

Crampton, Charles Ward, U.S. physician, *1877. See C. *test.*

Crampton, Sir Philip, Irish surgeon, 1777–1858. See C.'s *line, muscle.*

Crandall's syndrome. See under syndrome.

crani-. See cranio-.

crania (krā'nē-ă). Plural of cranium.

craniad (krā'nē-ad). Cephalad; situated nearer the head in relation to a specific reference point; opposite of caudad. See also superior.

cranial (krā'nē-ăl). **1.** Cranialis; cephalic; relating to the cranium or head. **2.** Superior (2).

cranialis (krā-nē-ā'lis) [NA]. Cranial (1).

craniamphitomy (krā-nē-am-fit'ō-ē) [G. *kranion,* skull, + *amphi,* around, + *tomē,* cutting]. A decompression operation in which the entire circumference of the calvarium is divided.

Craniata (krā-nē-ā'tă) [Mediev. L. *cranium,* fr. G. *kranion,* skull]. Vertebrata.

craniectomy (krā'nē-ek'tō-mē) [G. *kranion,* skull, + *ektomē,* excision]. Excision of a portion of the skull, *e.g.,* subtemporal or suboccipital.
linear c., production of an artificial cranial suture.

cranio-, crani- [G. *kranion,* skull]. Combining forms denoting relation to the cranium.

cranio-aural (krā'nē-ō-aw'răl). Relating to the skull and the ear.

craniocele (krā'nē-ō-sēl) [cranio- + G. *kēlē,* hernia]. Encephalocele.

craniocerebral (krā'nē-ō-ser'ē-brăl). Relating to the skull and the brain.

cranioclasia, cranioclasis (krā-nē-ō-klā'sē-ă, krā-nē-ok'lă-sis) [cranio- + G. *klasis,* a breaking]. Formerly used operation for crushing of the fetal skull in cases of dystocia.

cranioclast (krā'nē-ō-klast) [cranio- + G. *klaō,* to break in pieces]. Instrument like a strong forceps formerly used for crushing and extracting the fetal head after perforation.

craniocleidodysostosis (krā'nē-ō-klī'dō-dis-os-tō'sis) [cranio- + G. *kleis,* clavicle, + dysostosis]. Cleidocranial *dysostosis.*

craniodidymus (krā'nē-ō-did'i-mŭs) [cranio- + G. *didymos,* twin]. Conjoined twins with fused bodies but with two heads.

craniofacial (krā'nē-ō-fā'shăl). Relating to both the face and the cranium.

craniofenestria (krā'nē-ō-fe-nes'trē-ă) [cranio- + L. *fenestra,* window]. Craniolacunia.

craniognomy (krā-nē-og'nō-mē) [cranio- + G. *gnōme,* judgment]. Phrenology.

craniograph (krā'nē-ō-graf). An instrument for making drawings to scale of the diameters and general configuration of the skull.

craniography (krā-nē-og'ră-fē) [cranio- + G. *graphō,* to write]. The art of representing, by drawings made from measurements, the configuration of the skull and the relations of its angles and craniometric points.

craniolacunia (krā'nē-ō-lă-kū'nē-ă) [cranio- + L. *lacuna,* cleft]. Craniofenestria; incomplete formation of the bones of the vault of the fetal skull so that there are nonossified areas in the calvaria.

craniology (krā-nē-ol'ō-jē) [cranio- + G. *logos,* study]. The science concerned with variations in size, shape, and proportion of the cranium, especially with the variations characterizing the different races of men.
Gall's c., phrenology.

craniomalacia (krā'nē-ō-mă-lā'shē-ă) [cranio- + G. *malakia,* softness]. Softening of the bones of the skull.
circumscribed c., craniotabes.

craniomeningocele (krā'nē-ō-mĕ-ning'gō-sēl) [cranio- + G. *mēninx,* membrane, + *kēlē,* hernia]. Protrusion of the meninges through a defect in the skull.

craniometer (krā-nē-om'ĕ-ter). An instrument for measuring the diameters of the skull.

craniometric (krā-nē-ō-met'rik). Relating to craniometry.

craniometry (krā-nē-om'ĕ-trē) [cranio- + G. *metron,* measure]. Measurement of the dry skull after removal of the soft parts, and study of its topography.

craniopagus (krā-nē-op'ă-gŭs) [cranio- + G. *pagos,* something fixed]. Conjoined twins with fused skulls. See also janiceps; syncephalus.
c. occipita'lis, iniopagus; conjoined twins united at the occipital region of the skull.
c. parasit'icus, a variety of c. in which one fetus is rudimentary in form and parasitic on the other. See also epicomus.

craniopathy (krā-nē-op'ă-thē) [cranio- + G. *pathos,* suffering]. Any pathological condition of the cranial bones.
metabolic c., Morgagni's *syndrome.*

craniopharyngeal (krā'nē-ō-fă-rin'jē-ăl). Relating to the skull and to the pharynx.

craniopharyngioma (krā'nē-ō-fă-rin-jē-ō'mă). Pituitary adamantinoma; Erdheim tumor; Rathke's pouch tumor; suprasellar cyst; a pituitary neoplasm, usually cystic, that develops from the nests of epithelium derived from Rathke's pouch; the histologic pattern, similar to that observed in adamantinomas, consists of intersecting bands of squamous epithelium bordered by radially arranged cells.
cystic papillomatous c., a form of c. characterized by large cysts within which are fungating, irregular outgrowths of stratified squamous epithelium.

craniophore (krā'nē-ō-fōr) [cranio- + G. *phoros,* bearing]. An apparatus for holding a skull while its angles and diameters are measured.

cranioplasty (krā'nē-ō-plas-tē) [cranio- + G. *plastos,* formed]. Plastic surgery of the skull.

craniopuncture (krā'nē-ō-pŭnk'chūr). Puncture of the skull.

craniorrhachidian (krā'nē-ō-ră-kid'ē-an) [cranio- + G. *rhachis,* spine]. Craniospinal.

craniorrhachischisis (krā'nē-ō-ră-kis'ki-sis) [cranio- + G. *rhachis,* spine, + *schisis,* a cleaving]. Congenitally unclosed skull and spinal column.

craniosacral (krā'nē-ō-sā'krăl). Denoting the cranial and sacral origins of the parasympathetic division of the autonomic nervous system.

cranioschisis (krā-nē-os'ki-sis) [cranio- + G. *schisis,* a cleavage]. Congenital failure of the skull to close mid-dorsally, usually accompanied by grossly defective development of the brain.

craniosclerosis (krā'nē-ō-skler-ō'sis) [cranio- + G. *sklēros,* hard,

\+ *-osis,* condition]. Thickening of the skull.

cranioscopy (krā-nē-os'kŏ-pē) [cranio- + G. *skopeō,* to view]. Examination of the skull in the living subject for craniometric or diagnostic purposes.

craniospinal (krā'nē-ō-spī'năl). Craniorrhachidian; relating to the cranium and spinal column.

craniostenosis (krā'nē-ō-sten-ō'sis) [cranio- + G. *stenōsis,* a narrowing]. Premature closure of cranial sutures resulting in malformation of the skull.

craniostosis (krā'nē-os-tō'sis) [cranio- + G. *osteon,* a bone, + -*osis,* condition]. Craniosynostosis.

craniosynostosis (krā'nē-ō-sin'os-tō'sis). Craniostosis; premature ossification of the skull and obliteration of the sutures. The particular sutures involved determine the resultant shape of the malformed head.

craniotabes (krā'nē-ō-tā'bēz) [cranio- + L. *tabes,* a wasting]. Circumscribed craniomalacia; a disease marked by the presence of areas of thinning and softening in the bones of the skull, usually of syphilitic or rachitic origin.

craniotome (krā'nē-ō-tōm). Instrument formerly used for perforation and crushing of the fetal skull.

craniotomy (krā-nē-ot'ō-mē) [cranio- + G. *tomē,* incision]. **1.** Opening into the skull, either by attached or detached c. or by trephination. **2.** Formerly used operation for perforation of the head of the fetus, removal of the contents, and compression of the empty skull, when delivery by natural means is impossible.
attached c., attached cranial section; osteoplastic c.; bone flap; c. with a segment of the calvaria and attached soft tissues turned as a flap to expose the cranial cavity.
detached c., detached cranial section; free bone flap; c. with section of cranium separated from its attachments.
osteoplastic c., attached c.

craniotonoscopy (krā'nē-ō-tō-nos'kŏ-pē) [cranio- + G. *tonos,* tone, + *skopeō,* to examine]. Auscultatory percussion of the cranium.

craniotrypesis (krā'nē-ō-tri-pē'sis) [cranio- + G. *trypēsis,* a boring]. Trephining of the skull.

craniotympanic (krā'nē-ō-tim-pan'ik). Relating to the skull and the middle ear.

cranium, pl. **crania** (krā'nē-ŭm, -ă) [Mediev. L. fr. G. *kranion*] [NA]. Skull; the bones of the head collectively. In a more limited sense, the brain pan, the bony case containing the brain, excluding the bones of the face.
c. bif'idum, bifid c., encephalocele.
c. cerebra'le, cerebral c., calvaria.
c. viscera'le, visceral c., those parts of the skull of branchial arch origin.

crapulent, crapulous (krap'yū-lent, -lŭs) [L. *crapula,* drunkenness]. Drunken; due to alcoholic intoxication.

crassamentum (kras-ă-men'tŭm) [L. thickness, fr. *crassus,* thick]. **1.** Old term for blood *clot.* **2.** Old term for coagulum.

crater (krā'ter). The most depressed, usually central portion of an ulcer.

crateriform (krā-ter'i-fōrm) [L. *crater,* bowl, + *forma,* shape]. Hollowed like a bowl or a saucer.

craterization (krā-ter-ī-zā'shŭn). Saucerization.

craw-craw (kraw'kraw). Kra-kra; a term applied in west Africa to a vesiculopustular skin eruption, attended with itching, which may lead to ulceration; some cases are caused by *Onchocerca.* The name has also been given to papular and pustular eruptions in sections of equatorial Africa.

Crawford, Brian H., British physicist, *1906. See Stiles-C. *effect.*

crazing (krā'zing). In dentistry, the appearance of minute cracks on the surface of plastic restorations such as filling materials, denture teeth, or denture bases.

CRD Abbreviation for chronic respiratory *disease.*

cream (krēm) [L. *cremor,* thick juice, broth]. **1.** The upper fatty layer which forms in milk on standing or which is separated from it by centrifugalization; it contains about the same amount of sugar and protein as milk, but from 12 to 40% more fat. **2.** Any whitish viscid fluid resembling c. **3.** A semisolid emulsion of either the oil-in-water or the water-in-oil type, ordinarily intended for topical use.
cleansing c., a form of cold c. used to remove grime and cosmetics from the skin.
cold c., a water-in-oil emulsion of various oils, waxes, and water; the standard formula, rose water ointment, contains expressed almond oil, rose water, spermaceti, white paraffin wax, and sodium borate; used as a cleansing or lubricating c.
greaseless c., vanishing c.
leukocyte c., buffy *coat.*
lubricating c., a form of cold c. used as a massage c. or night c.; it contains lanolin or its derivatives.
vanishing c., greaseless c.; an oil-in-water emulsion containing potassium, ammonium, or sodium stearate with water and holding in emulsified form more or less free stearic acid; it also contains a hygroscopic ingredient such as glycerol, and a small amount of a fatty ingredient; it leaves a protective, invisible film of stearic acid on the skin.

crease (krēs). A line or linear depression as produced by a fold. See also fold; groove; line.
flexion c., a permanent c. in the skin on the flexor aspect of a movable joint.
palmar c., any of the several flexion c.'s normally found on the palm of the hand, corresponding approximately to the metacarpophalangeal joints.
simian c., a single transverse palmar c. formed by fusion of the distal and proximal palmar c.'s, so called because of its similarity to the transverse flexion crease seen in some monkeys; a common but not pathognomonic feature of Down's syndrome.
Sydney c., Sydney line; a variation of the proximal transverse palmar flexion c. that reaches the ulnar side of the palm; associated with acute lymphocytic anemia in early childhood, rubella embryopathy, and Down's syndrome.

creatinase (krē'ă-tĭ-nās) [EC 3.5.3.3]. An enzyme catalyzing the hydrolysis of creatine to sarcosine and urea.

creatine (krē'ă-tēn, -tin). *N*-(Aminoiminomethyl)-*N*-methylglycine; $H_2N\text{-}C(NH)\text{-}N(CH_3)\text{-}CH_2\text{-}COOH$; occurs in urine, sometimes as such, but generally as creatinine, and in muscle, generally as phosphocreatine.
c. kinase (CK) [EC 2.7.3.2], an enzyme catalyzing the transfer of phosphate from phosphocreatine to ADP, forming creatine and ATP; of importance in muscle contraction.
c. phosphate, phosphocreatine.
c. phosphokinase (CPK), former name for c. kinase.

creatinemia (krē'ă-ti-nē'mē-ă) [creatine + G. *haima,* blood]. The presence of abnormal concentrations of creatine in peripheral blood.

creatininase (krē-at'i-nin-ās) [EC 3.5.2.10]. An amidohydrolase catalyzing the conversion of creatine to creatinine, with the participation of ATP.

creatinine (Cr) (krē-at'i-nēn, -nin). A component of urine and the final product of creatine catabolism; formed by the dephosphorylative cyclization of phosphocreatine by creatininase to form the internal anhydride of creatine.

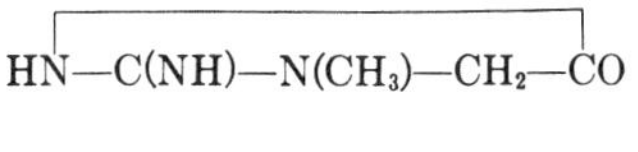

creatinuria (krē'ă-ti-nū'rē-ă) [creatine + G. *ouron*, urine]. The urinary excretion of increased amounts of creatine.

Credé, Karl S.F., German obstetrician and gynecologist, 1819–1892. See C.'s *methods.*

creep (krēp). Any time-dependent strain developing in a material or an object in response to the application of a force or stress.

cremaster (krē-mas'ter) [G. *kremastēr*, a suspender, in pl. the muscles by which the testicles are suspended, fr. *kremannymi*, to hang]. See *fascia* cremasterica; *musculus* cremaster.

cremasteric (krē-mas-ter'ik). Relating to the cremaster.

cremnocele (krem'nō-sēl) [G. *krēmnos*, overhanging cliff, labium pudendi, + *kēlē*, hernia]. A protrusion of intestine into the labium majus.

cremnophobia (krem-nō-fō'bē-ă) [G. *krēmnos*, precipice, + *phobos*, fear]. Morbid fear of precipices or steep places.

crena, pl. crenae (krē'nă, krē'nē) [L. a notch]. A V-shaped cut or the space created by such a cut; one of the notches into which the opposing projections fit in the cranial sutures.
c. a'ni [NA], anal, natal, or gluteal cleft; c. clunium; the sulcus between the nates.
c. clu'nium, c. ani.
c. cor'dis, **(1)** *sulcus* interventricularis anterior; **(2)** *sulcus* interventricularis posterior.

crenate, crenated (krē'nāt, -nā-ted) [L. *crena*, a notch]. Notched; indented; denoting the outline of a shriveled red blood cell, as observed in a hypertonic solution.

crenation (krē-nā'shŭn). The process of becoming, or state of being, crenated.

crenocyte (krē'nō-sīt) [L. *crena*, a notch, + G. *kytos*, a hollow (cell)]. A red blood cell with serrated, notched edges.

crenocytosis (krē'nō-sī-tō'sis) [crenocyte + G. *-osis*, condition]. The presence of crenocytes in the blood.

Crenosoma vulpis (krē'nō-sō-mă vŭl'pis) [G. krēnē, a (mineral) spring, + sōma, body; L. *vulpes*, fox]. A metastrongyle lungworm species of the fox, wolf, dog, raccoon, and other small carnivores in Europe, Asia, and North America; it occurs in the bronchi, causing bronchitis.

creophagy, creophagism (krē-of'ă-jē, krē-of'ă-jizm) [G. kreas, meat, + phagein, to eat]. Carnivorousness; flesh-eating. See also creophagy.

creosol (krē'ō-sol). 2-Methoxy-*p*- cresol; a slightly yellowish aromatic liquid distilled from guaiac or from beechwood tar; a constituent of creosote. *Cf.* cresol.

creosote (krē'ō-sōt) [G. *kreas*, flesh, + *sōtēr*, to preserve]. A mixture of phenols (chiefly methyl guaiacol, guaiacol, and creosol) obtained during the distillation of wood-tar, preferably that derived from beechwood; used as a disinfectant.

crepitant (krep'i-tant). **1.** Relating to or characterized by crepitation. **2.** Denoting a bubbling noise (rale) produced by air entering fluid in lung tissue; heard in pneumonia and in certain other conditions. **3.** The sensation imparted to the palpating finger by gas or air in the subcutaneous tissues.

crepitation (krep-i-tā'shŭn) [see crepitus]. Crepitus (1). **1.** Crackling; the quality of a bubbling sound (rale) which resembles noise heard on rubbing hair between the fingers. **2.** Bony crepitus; the sensation felt on placing the hand over the seat of a fracture when the broken ends of the bone are moved, or over tissue, in which gas gangrene is present. **3.** Noise or vibration produced by rubbing bone or irregular cartilage surfaces together as by movement of patella against femoral condyles in arthritis and other conditions.

crepitus (krep'i-tŭs) [L. fr. *crepo*, to rattle]. **1.** Crepitation. **2.** A noisy discharge of gas from the intestine.
articular c., the grating of a joint.
bony c., crepitation (2).

crepuscular (kre-pŭs'kyū-lăr) [L. *crepusculum*, twilight]. Pertaining to a twilight state of consciousness.

crescent (kres'ent) [L. *cresco*, pp. *cretus*, to grow]. **1.** Any figure of the shape of the moon in its first quarter. **2.** The figure made by the gray columns or cornua on cross-section of the spinal cord. **3.** Malarial c.
articular c., *meniscus* articularis.
Giannuzzi's c.'s, serous *demilunes.*
glomerular c., proliferated epithelial cells partly encircling a renal glomerulus; it occurs in glomerulonephritis.
Heidenhain's c.'s, serous *demilunes.*
malarial c., crescent (3); sickle form; the male or female gametocyte(s) of *Plasmodium falciparum,* whose presence in human red blood cells is diagnostic of falciparum malaria.
myopic c., myopic conus; a white or grayish white crescentic area in the fundus of the eye located on the temporal side of the optic disk; caused by atrophy of the choroid, permitting the sclera to become visible.
sublingual c., the crescent-shaped area on the floor of the mouth formed by the lingual wall of the mandible and the adjacent part of the floor of the mouth.

crescentic (kres-sen'tik). Shaped like a crescent.

crescograph (kres'kō-graf) [L. *cresco*, to grow, + G. *graphō*, to draw or write]. A device for recording the degree and rate of growth.

cresol (krē'sol). Tricresol; hydroxytoluene; methylphenol; HO–C_6H_4–CH_3; a mixture of the three isomeric cresols, *o*-, *m*-, and *p*-cresol, obtained from coal tar. Its properties are similar to those of phenol, but it is less poisonous; used as an antiseptic and disinfectant.

***m*-cresol.** Metacresol; a local antiseptic with a higher germicidal power than phenol and less toxicity to tissues; used in disinfectants and fumigants; its acetate derivative is used as a topical antiseptic and fungicide.

cresolase (krē'sō-lās). Monophenol monooxygenase.

cresol red. An acid-base indicator with a pK value of 8.3; yellow at pH values below 7.4, red above 9.0.

CREST Acronym for *c* alcinosis, *R* eynaud's phenomenon, *e* sophageal motility disorders, *s* clerodactyly, and *t* elangiectasia. See CREST *syndrome.*

CREST

crest (krest) [L. *crista*]. **1.** A ridge, especially a bony ridge. See also crista. **2.** The ridge of the neck of a male animal, especially of a stallion or bull. **3.** Feathers on the top of a bird's head, or finrays on the top of a fish's head.
acoustic c., *crista* ampullaris.
acousticofacial c., the part of the neural c. from which the ganglia of the seventh and eighth cranial nerves develop.
alveolar c., **(1)** the portion of the alveolar bone extending beyond the periphery of the socket, lying interproximally; **(2)** the top of the residual alveolar bone.
ampullary c., *crista* ampullaris.
anterior lacrimal c., *crista* lacrimalis anterior.
arched c., *crista* arcuata.
arcuate c., *crista* arcuata.
articular c.'s, *cristae* sacrales intermediae.

basilar c. of cochlear duct, *crista* basilaris ductus cochlearis.
buccinator c., crista buccinatoria; a ridge passing from the base of the coronoid process of the mandible to the region of the last molar tooth; it gives attachment to the buccinator muscle.
c. of cochlear opening, *crista* fenestrae cochleae.
conchal c., *crista* conchalis.
deltoid c., *tuberositas* deltoidea.
dental c., crista dentalis; a ridge on the alveolar processes of the jaw bones in the fetus.
ethmoidal c., *crista* ethmoidalis.
external occipital c., *crista* occipitalis externa.
falciform c., *crista* transversa.
frontal c., *crista* frontalis.
ganglionic c., neural c.
gingival c., gingival *margin.*
gluteal c., *tuberositas* glutea.
c. of greater tubercle, *crista* tuberculi majoris.
c. of head of rib, *crista* capitis costae.
iliac c., *crista* iliaca.
incisor c., the front part of the nasal c. of the palatine process of the maxilla.
infratemporal c., *crista* infratemporalis.
inguinal c., an elevation in the body wall of the embryo at the internal opening of the inguinal canal; part of the gubernaculum develops within it.
intermediate sacral c.'s, *cristae* sacrales intermediae.
internal occipital c., *crista* occipitalis interna.
interosseous c., *margo* interosseus.
intertrochanteric c., *crista* intertrochanterica.
lateral epicondylar c., *crista* supracondylaris lateralis.
lateral sacral c.'s, *cristae* sacrales laterales.
lateral supracondylar c., *crista* supracondylaris lateralis.
c. of lesser tubercle, *crista* tuberculi minoris.
marginal c., *crista* marginalis.
medial c., *crista* medialis.
medial epicondylar c., *crista* supracondylaris medialis.
medial supracondylar c., *crista* supracondylaris medialis.
median sacral c., *crista* sacralis mediana.
c.'s of nail bed, *cristae* matricis unguis.
nasal c., *crista* nasalis.
c. of neck of rib, *crista* colli costae.
neural c., ganglionic c.; ganglion ridge; a band of neuroectodermal cells along either side of the line of closure of the embryonic neural groove; with the closure of the neural groove to form the neural tube, these bands come to lie dorsolateral to the developing spinal cord, where they separate into clusters of cells that develop into dorsal-root ganglion cells, autonomic ganglion cells, the chromaffin cells of the adrenal medulla, Schwann cells, or integumentary pigment cells.
obturator c., *crista* obturatoria.
c. of palatine bone, palatine c., *crista* palatina.
posterior lacrimal c., *crista* lacrimalis posterior.
pubic c., *crista* pubica.
c. of ridge, the top of the alveolar ridge or residual ridge; the highest continuous surface of the ridge, but not necessarily the center of the ridge.
sacral c., *crista* sacralis.
sagittal c., a prominent ridge along the sagittal suture of the skull, present in some animals as a result of temporal muscle development.
c. of scapular spine, the posterior subcutaneous border of the spine of the scapula that expands in its medial part into a smooth triangular area.
sphenoid c., *crista* sphenoidalis.
spiral c., *crista* spiralis.
supinator c., c. of supinator muscle, *crista* musculi supinatorius.
supramastoid c., *crista* supramastoidea.
supraventricular c., *crista* supraventricularis.
terminal c., *crista* terminalis.
tibial c., *margo* anterior tibiae.
transverse c., **(1)** *crista* transversa; **(2)** *crista* transversalis.
triangular c., *crista* triangularis.
trigeminal c., that part of the cranial neural c. from which the ganglion of the fifth cranial nerve develops.
trochanteric c., *crista* intertrochanterica.
turbinated c., *crista* conchalis.
tympanic c., crista tympanica; a ridge on the tympanic ring.
urethral c., *crista* urethralis.
vestibular c., c. of vestibule, *crista* vestibuli.

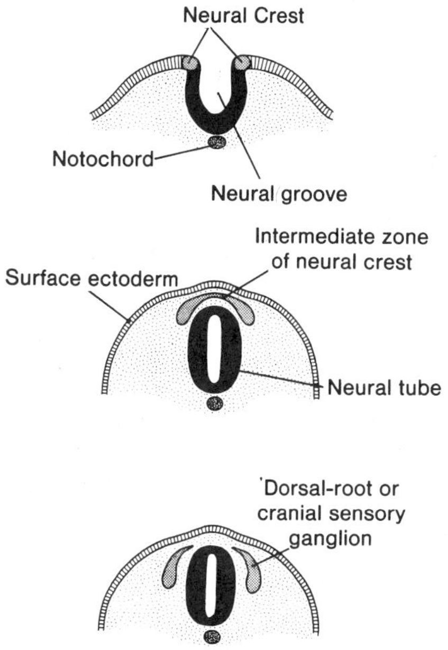

Neural Crest
Schematic representation of transverse sections of embryos showing development of neural crest into dorsal-root or cranial sensory ganglia.

cresta (kres'tă) [L. *crispus,* trembling]. A small membranous organelle characteristic of certain flagellate protozoa, located near the pelta and seen in the living organism as an independently moving structure.

cresylate (kres'i-lāt). A salt of cresylic acid, or cresol.

cresyl blue (brilliant) (kres'il) [C.I. 51010]. Aminodimethylaminoethyldiphenazonium chloride; $C_{17}H_{20}N_3OCl$; a basic oxazin dye used for staining the reticulum in young erythrocytes (reticulocytes); also used in vital staining and as a selective stain for gastric surface epithelial mucin and other acid mucopolysaccharides.

cresyl echt or **fast violet.** A metachromatic basic oxazin dye, $C_{19}H_{18}N_3O$-Cl, closely related to cresyl violet acetate and used for the same purposes.

cresyl violet acetate. A metachromatic basic oxazin dye, $C_{18}H_{15}N_3O_3$, used as a stain for nuclei and Nissl substance; related to German derived dye known as cresyl echt violet or cresyl fast violet.

creta (krē'tă) [L. orig. adj. fr. *Creta,* Crete, *i.e.* Cretan earth, chalk]. *Calcium* carbonate.

cretin (krē'tin) [Fr. *crétin*] An individual exhibiting cretinism.

cretinism (krē′tin-izm). Hypothyroid dwarfism; infantile hypothyroidism; congenital myxedema; Brissaud's, dysthyroidal, hypothyroid, or myxedematous infantilism; stunted bodily growth and mental development, appearing during the first years of life and resulting from thymic agenesis or inadequate maternal intake of iodine during gestation.

cretinistic (krē′tin-is-tik). Cretinous.

cretinoid (krē′tin-oyd). Resembling a cretin; presenting symptoms similar to those of cretinism.

cretinous (krē′tin-ŭs). Cretinistic; relating to cretinism or a cretin.

Creutzfeldt, Hans Gerhard, German neuropsychiatrist, 1885–1964. See C.-Jakob or Jakob-C. *disease;* Siemerling-C. *disease.*

crevice (krev′is) [Fr. *crevasse*] A crack or small fissure, especially in a solid substance.
gingival c., *sulcus* gingivalis.

crevicular (krē-vik′yū-lăr). **1.** Relating to any crevice. **2.** In dentistry, relating especially to the gingival crevice or sulcus.

CRF Abbreviation for corticotropin-releasing *factor.*

CRH Abbreviation for corticotropin-releasing *hormone.*

cribra (krī′bră, krib′ră). Plural of cribrum.

cribrate (krib′rāt). Cribriform.

cribration (kri-brā′shŭn). **1.** Sifting; passing through a sieve. **2.** The condition of being cribrate or numerously pitted or punctured.

cribriform (krib′ri-fōrm) [L. *cribrum,* a sieve, + *forma,* form]. Cribrate; polyporous; sievelike; containing many perforations.

cribrum, pl. **cribra** (krī′brŭm, krib′rŭm; -bră, -ra) [L. a sieve]. *Lamina* cribrosa ossis ethmoidalis.

Cricetinae (krī-sē′ti-nē). A subfamily of rodents (family Muridae) that includes the hamsters and the native American rats.

Cricetulus (kri-sē′tyū-lŭs). One of four genera of hamsters; *C. griseus,* the striped hamster native to Europe and Asia, is a reservoir for visceral leishmaniasis.

Cricetus (kri-sē′tŭs). One of four genera of hamsters; *C. cricetus* is used extensively as a research animal.

Crichton-Browne, Sir James, British physician, 1840–1938. See C.-B.'s *sign.*

Crick, Francis H.C., British biochemist and Nobel laureate, *1916. See Watson-C. *helix.*

cricoarytenoid (krī′kō-ar-i-tē′noyd). Relating to the cricoid and arytenoid cartilages.

cricoarytenoideus (krī′kō-ar-i-te-noy′dē-ŭs). See under musculus.

cricoid (krī′koyd) [L. *cricoideus,* fr. G. *krikos,* a ring, + *eidos,* form]. Ring-shaped; denoting the cricoid cartilage.

cricoidectomy (krī′koy-dek′tō-mē) [cricoid + G. excision]. Excision of the cricoid cartilage.

cricoidynia (krī′koy-din′ē-ă) [cricoid + G. *odynē,* pain]. Pain in the cricoid.

cricopharyngeal (krī′kō-fă-rin′jē-ăl). Relating to the cricoid cartilage and the pharynx; a part of the inferior constrictor muscle of the pharynx. See *musculus* constrictor pharyngis inferior.

cricothyroid (krī-kō-thī′royd). Relating to the cricoid and thyroid cartilages.

cricothyroideus (krī′kō-thī-roy′dē-ŭs). See under musculus.

cricothyroidotomy (krī′kō-thī-roy-dot′ō-mē). Cricothyrotomy.

cricothyrotomy (krī′kō-thī-rot′ō-mē) [cricoid + thyroid + G. *tomē,* incision]. Coniotomy; intercricothyrotomy; inferior laryngotomy; incision through the skin and cricothyroid membrane for relief of respiratory obstruction; used prior to tracheotomy in certain emergency respiratory obstructions.

cricotomy (krī-kot′ō-mē) [cricoid + G. *tomē,* incision]. Division of the cricoid cartilage.

Crigler, John F., U.S. physician, *1919. See C.-Najjar *disease, syndrome.*

Crile, George W., U.S. surgeon, 1864–1943. See C.'s *clamp.*

criminology (krim-i-nol′ō-jē) [L. *crimen,* crime, + G. *logos,* study]. The branch of science concerned with the physical and mental characteristics and behavior of criminals.

crinin (krin′in). Old term for a substance that will stimulate the production of secretions by specific glands.

crinis, pl. **crines** (krī′nis, -nēz) [L.]. Pilus (1).

crinogenic (krin-ō-jen′ik) [G. *krinō,* to separate, + *-gen,* to produce]. Causing secretion; stimulating a gland to increased function.

crinophagy (krin-of′ă-jē). Disposal of excess secretory granules by lysosomes.

crippled (krip′ld) [A.S. *creopan,* to creep]. Denoting a person who, owing to a physical defect or injury, is partially or completely disabled.

crisis, pl. **crises** (krī′sis, -sēz) [G. *krisis,* a separation, crisis]. **1.** A sudden change, usually for the better, in the course of an acute disease, in contrast to the gradual improvement by lysis. **2.** Tabetic c.; a paroxysmal pain in an organ or circumscribed region of the body occurring in the course of tabes dorsalis. **3.** A convulsive attack.
addisonian c., acute adrenocortical *insufficiency.*
adolescent c., the emotional turmoil often accompanying adolescence.
adrenal c., acute adrenocortical *insufficiency.*
anaphylactoid c., anaphylactoid *shock.*
blast c., a sudden alteration in the status of a patient with leukemia in which the peripheral blood cells are almost exclusively blast cells of the type causing leukemia; usually accompanied by a decrease in numbers of other formed elements of the blood, fever, and rapid clinical deterioration.
blood c., **(1)** the appearance of a large number of nucleated red blood cells in the peripheral blood, accompanied by reticulocytosis and occurring in "exhausted" bone marrow in pernicious anemia and in hemolytic icterus; **(2)** a suddenly appearing leukocytosis, indicating a change for the better in the course of a grave blood disease.
Dietl's c., incarceration symptom; paroxysmal attacks of lumbar and abdominal pain with nausea and vomiting resulting from kinking of the ureter in persons with wandering kidney.
febrile c., the stage in a febrile disease when spontaneous defervescence occurs.
gastric c., an attack, usually lasting several days, with severe pain in the abdomen or around the waist, accompanied by nausea and vomiting and occasionally diarrhea; occurs in tabes dorsalis.
glaucomatocyclitic c., a form of monocular secondary open-angle glaucoma due to recurrent mild cyclitis.
identity c., a disorientation concerning one's sense of self and role in society, often of acute onset and related to a particular and significant event in one's life.
laryngeal c., an attack of paralysis of the abductor, or spasm of the adductor, muscles of the larynx with dyspnea and noisy respiration, occurring in tabes dorsalis.
midlife c., a point in a sequence of events during the middle years of life at which certain trends of prior and subsequent events in one's life are pondered, generally involving an aggregate of personal, career, or sexual dissatisfactions.
myelocytic c., a temporary but conspicuous and sudden increase in cells of the myelocytic series in the circulating blood.
ocular c., sudden and severe pain in the eyes.
oculogyric c.'s, attacks of spasmodic eye rotation, often upward, seen in encephalitis lethargica.
sickle cell c., see sickle cell *anemia.*
tabetic c., c. (2).

therapeutic c., a turning point leading to positive or negative change in psychiatric treatment.

thyrotoxic c., thyroid c., thyroid storm; the exacerbation of symptoms that occurs in thyrotoxicosis following shock or injury or after thyroidectomy; marked by rapid pulse (140 to 170 per minute), nausea, diarrhea, fever, loss of weight, extreme nervousness, and a sudden rise in the metabolic rate; coma and death may occur; occasionally the entire clinical picture is that of profound prostration, weakness, and collapse, without the phase of muscular overactivity and tachycardia.

crispation (kris-pā'shŭn) [L. *crispo,* pp. *-atus,* to curl]. **1.** A "creepy" sensation due to slight, fibrillary muscular contractions. **2.** Retraction of a divided artery or of muscular fibers or other tissues when cut across.

CRISTA

crista, pl. **cristae** (kris'tă, -tē) [L. crest] [NA]. A ridge, crest, or elevated line projecting from a level or evenly rounded surface. See also crest.

c. ampulla'ris [NA], ampullary crest; acoustic crest; transverse septum (1); an elevation on the inner surface of the ampulla of each semicircular duct; filaments of the vestibular nerve pass through the c. to reach hair cells on its surface; the hair cells are capped by the cupula, a gelatinous protein-polysaccharide mass.

c. arcua'ta [NA], arcuate or arched crest; the ridge on the anterior surface of the arytenoid cartilage that separates the triangular from the oblong fovea.

c. basila'ris duc'tus cochlea'ris [NA], basilar crest of cochlear duct; an inward projection of the spiral ligament of the cochlea to which is attached the basilar membrane forming the floor of the cochlear duct.

c. buccinator'ia, buccinator *crest.*

c. cap'itis cos'tae [NA], crest of head of rib; the ridge that separates the superior and inferior articular surfaces of the head of a rib.

c. col'li cos'tae [NA], crest of neck of rib; the sharp upper margin of the neck of a rib.

c. concha'lis [NA], conchal crest; turbinated crest; **c. c. max'illae,** ridge of the nasal surface of the body of the maxilla that articulates with the inferior nasal concha; **c. c. os'sis palati'ni,** the ridge on the nasal surface of the perpendicular part of the palatine bone to which the inferior nasal concha attaches.

cris'tae cu'tis [NA], epidermal or skin ridges; ridges of the epidermis of the palms and soles, where the sweat pores open.

c. denta'lis, dental *crest.*

c. div'idens, the lower free edge of the septum secundum, forming the upper margin of the fetal foramen ovale.

c. ethmoida'lis [NA], ethmoidal crest; nasal concha; **c. e. max'illae,** a ridge on the upper part of the nasal surface of the frontal process of the maxilla that gives attachment to the anterior portion of the middle nasal concha; **c. e. os'sis palati'ni,** a ridge on the medial surface of the perpendicular part of the palatine bone to which the middle nasal concha attaches posteriorly.

c. fenes'trae coch'leae [NA], crest of cochlear opening; the edge of the opening of the cochlear window to which the secondary tympanic membrane is attached.

c. fronta'lis [NA], frontal crest; a ridge arising at the termination of the sagittal sulcus on the cerebral surface of the frontal bone and ending at the foramen caecum.

c. gal'li [NA], cock's comb; the triangular midline process of the ethmoid bone extending upward from the cribriform plate; it gives attachment to the falx cerebri.

c. glu'tea, *tuberositas* glutea.

c. hel'icis, *crus* helicis.

c. ilia'ca [NA], iliac crest; the long, curved upper border of the wing of the ilium.

c. infratempora'lis [NA], infratemporal crest; pterygoid ridge of sphenoid bone; a rough ridge marking the angle of union of the temporal and infratemporal surfaces of the greater wing of the sphenoid bone.

c. intertrochanter'ica [NA], intertrochanteric crest; trochanteric crest; the rounded ridge that connects the greater and lesser trochanters of the femur posteriorly and marks the junction of the neck and shaft of the bone.

c. lacrima'lis ante'rior [NA], anterior lacrimal crest; a vertical ridge on the lateral surface of the frontal process of the maxilla that forms part of the medial margin of the orbit.

c. lacrima'lis poste'rior [NA], posterior lacrimal crest; a vertical ridge on the orbital surface of the lacrimal bone which, together with the anterior lacrimal crest, bounds the fossa for the lacrimal sac.

c. margina'lis [NA], marginal crest or ridge; the rounded borders which form the mesial and distal margins of the occlusal surface of a tooth.

cris'tae ma'tricis un'guis [NA], crests of nail bed; the numerous longitudinal ridges of the nail bed distal to the lunula.

c. media'lis [NA], medial crest; a ridge of bone, on the posterior surface of the fibula, separating the attachment of the posterior tibial muscle from that of the flexor hallucis longus and soleus muscles.

cristae of mitochondria, cris'tae mitochondria'les, shelflike infoldings of the inner membrane of a mitochondrion.

c. mus'culi supinator'ius [NA], supinator crest; crest of supinator muscle; the proximal part of the interosseous border of the ulna.

c. nasa'lis [NA], nasal crest; semicrista incisiva; the midline ridge in the floor of the nasal cavity, formed by the union of the paired maxillae and palatine bones; the vomer attaches to the crest.

c. obturato'ria [NA], obturator crest; a ridge that extends from the pubic tubercle to the acetabular notch, giving attachment to the pubofemoral ligament of the hip joint.

c. occipita'lis exter'na [NA], external occipital crest; linea nuchae mediana; a ridge extending from the external occipital protuberance to the border of the foramen magnum.

c. occipita'lis inter'na [NA], internal occipital crest; a ridge running from the internal occipital protuberance to the posterior margin of the foramen magnum, giving attachment to the falx cerebelli.

c. palati'na [NA], palatine crest; crest of palatine bone; a transverse ridge near the posterior border of the bony palate, located on the inferior surface of the horizontal lamina of the palatine bone.

c. phal'lica, *crista* urethralis masculinae.

c. pu'bica [NA], pubic crest; the rough anterior border of the body of the pubis, continuous laterally with the pubic tubercle.

c. quar'ta, a ridge that projects into the posterior end of the lateral semicircular duct of the labyrinth.

c. sacra'lis [NA], sacral crest; one of five rough irregular ridges on the posterior surface of the sacrum; **c. sacra'lis median'a,** median sacral crest; an unpaired c. formed by the fused spinous processes of the upper four sacral vertebrae, **cris'tae sacra'les interme'diae,** intermediate sacral crests; articular crests; c.'s formed by the fusion of articular processes of all the sacral vertebrae; **cris'tae sacra'les latera'les,** lateral sacral crests; c.'s which are rough ridges lying lateral to the sacral foramina, represent the fused transverse processes of sacral vertebrae.

c. sphenoida'lis [NA], sphenoid crest; a vertical ridge in the midline of the anterior surface of the sphenoid bone that articulates with the perpendicular plate of the ethmoid bone.

c. spira'lis, [NA], spiral crest; ligamentum spirale; spiral ligament; the thickened periosteal lining of the bony cochlea forming the outer wall of the cochlear duct to which the basal lamina attaches.

c. supracondyla'ris latera'lis [NA], lateral supracondylar crest or ridge; lateral epicondylar crest or ridge; the distal sharp portion of the lateral margin of the humerus.
c. supracondyla'ris media'lis [NA], medial supracondylar crest or ridge; medial epicondylar crest or ridge; the distal sharp portion of the medial margin of the humerus.
c. supramastoi'dea [NA], supramastoid crest; the ridge that forms the posterior root of the zygomatic process of the temporal bone.
c. supraventricula'ris [NA], supraventricular crest; the internal muscular ridge that separates the conus arteriosus from the remaining part of the cavity of the right ventricle of the heart.
c. termina'lis [NA], terminal crest; tenia terminalis; a vertical crest on the interior wall of the right atrium that lies to the right of the sinus venarum cavarum and separates this from the remainder of the right atrium.
c. transver'sa [NA], transverse crest (1); falciform crest; a horizontal ridge that divides the fundus of the internal acoustic meatus into a superior and an inferior area. In the former are the internal opening of the facial canal and openings for the branches of the vestibular nerve to the utricle and to the ampullae of the anterior and lateral semicircular canals. In the latter are openings for the cochlear nerve, and for branches of the vestibular nerve to the saccule and to the ampulla of the posterior semicircular canal.
c. transversa'lis [NA], transverse crest (2); transverse ridge; a crest or ridge on the occlusal surface of a tooth formed by the union of two triangular crests.
c. triangula'ris [NA], triangular crest or ridge; a crest or ridge which extends from the apex of a cusp of a premolar or molar tooth toward the central part of the occlusal surface.
c. tuber'culi majo'ris [NA], crest of greater tubercle; pectoral ridge; the ridge below the greater tubercle of the humerus into which the pectoralis major muscle inserts.
c. tuber'culi mino'ris [NA], crest of lesser tubercle; the ridge below the lesser tubercle of the humerus into which the teres major muscle inserts.
c. tympan'ica, tympanic *crest.*
c. urethra'lis [NA], urethral crest; **c. u. femini'nae,** in the female, a conspicuous longitudinal fold of mucosa on the posterior wall of the urethra; **c. u. masculi'nae,** c. phallica; in the male, a longitudinal fold on the posterior wall of the urethra extending from the uvula of the bladder through the prostatic urethra; prominent in its midportion is the seminal colliculus.
c. vestib'uli [NA], crest of vestibule; vestibular crest; an oblique ridge on the inner wall of the vestibule of the labyrinth, bounding the spherical recess above and posteriorly.

---

criterion, pl. **criteria** (krī-tēr'ē-on, -ē-ă) [G. *kritērion,* a standard]. **1.** A standard or rule for judging; usually plural (criteria) denoting a set of standards or rules. **2.** In psychology, a standard against which test scores on intelligence tests or other measured behaviors are validated. **3.** A list of manifestations of a disease or disorder, a certain number of which must be present to warrant diagnosis in a given patient.
Spiegelberg's criteria (for diagnosis of ovariocyesis), 1) the oviduct on the affected side must be intact; 2) the amnionic sac must occupy the position of the ovary; 3) the amnionic sac must be connected to the uterus by the ovarian ligament; and 4) ovarian tissue must be present in the wall of the amnionic sac.

Crithidia (kri-thid'ē-ă) [Mod. L., fr. G. *krithidion,* dim. of *krithē,* barley]. A genus of asexual, monogenetic, insect-parasitizing flagellates in the family Trypanosomatidae.

crithidia (kri-thid'ē-ă) [Mod. L. fr. G. *krithidion,* dim. of *krithē,* barley]. Former term for epimastigote.

critical (krit-ĭ-kăl). **1.** Denoting or of the nature of a crisis. **2.** Denoting a morbid condition in which death is possible. **3.** In sufficient quantity as to constitute a turning point.

CRL Abbreviation for crown-rump *length.*

CRM Abbreviation for cross-reacting *material.*

C.R.N.A. Abbreviation for Certified Registered Nurse Anesthetist.

CRO Abbreviation for cathode ray *oscilloscope.*

crocidismus (krok-i-dis'mŭs) [G. *krokē,* tuft of wool]. Floccillation.

Crocq, Jean, Belgian physician, 1868–1925. See C.'s *disease.*

crocus (krō'kŭs) [L. fr. G. *krokos,* the crocus, saffron (made from its stigmas)]. Saffron; the dried stigmas of *Crocus sativus* (*C. officinalis*) (family Iridaceae), used occasionally in flatulent dyspepsia; also used as an antispasmodic in asthma and dysmenorrhea and as a coloring and flavoring agent.
autumn c., colchicum.

Crohn, Burrill, B., U.S. gastroenterologist, 1884–1983. See C.'s *disease.*

cromolyn sodium (krō'mō-lin). Sodium cromoglycate; disodium 5,5′-[(2-hydroxytrimethylene)dioxy]bis[4-oxo-4*H*-1-benzopyran-2-carboxylate]; used for the prevention of asthmatic attack.

Cronkhite, Leonard W., Jr., U.S. physician *1919. See C.-Canada *syndrome.*

Crooke, Arthur C., British pathologist, *1905. See C.'s *granules,* hyaline *change,* hyaline *degeneration.*

Crookes, Sir William, British physicist and chemist, 1832–1919. See C.'s *glass.*

Crosby, William Holmes, Jr., U.S. physician, *1914. See C. *capsule.*

cross (kros) [F. *croix,* L. *crux*]. Crux. **1.** Any figure in the shape of a c. formed by two intersecting lines. **2.** *Crux* of heart. **3.** A method of hybridization or the hybrid so produced.
back c., the mating between an animal that is homozygous at a locus of interest and an animal that is heterozygous.
double back c., a mating that is a back c. at each of two loci of interest; of special importance in linkage analysis.
hair c.'s, *cruces* pilorum.
Ranvier's c.'s, black or brown figures in the shape of a c., marking Ranvier's nodes in the longitudinal section of a nerve stained with silver nitrate.
test c., in experimental genetics, a deliberate mating designed to test claims about the pattern of inheritance of one or more traits.

crossbite (kros'bīt). An abnormal relation of one or more teeth of one arch to the opposing tooth or teeth of the other arch due to labial, buccal, or lingual deviation of tooth position, or to abnormal jaw position.

crossbreed (kros'brēd). **1.** Hybrid. **2.** To breed a hybrid.

crossbreeding (kros'brēd-ing). Hybridization.

cross-eye (kros'ī). Alternative spelling for crossed *eyes.*

crossing-over, crossover (kros-ing-ō'ver, kros'ō-ver). Reciprocal exchange of material between two paired chromosomes during meiosis, resulting in the transfer of a block of genes from each chromosome to its homologue.
somatic c., c. that occurs during the mitosis of somatic cells, in contrast to that which occurs in meiosis.
uneven c., unequal c., c. that does not occur at precisely homologous points in two chromatid strands, and hence results in localized duplication of genetic material in one chromatid and complementary deletion in the other.

cross-matching, crossmatching (kros'match-ing). **1.** A test for incompatibility between donor and recipient blood, carried out prior to transfusion to avoid potentially lethal hemolytic reactions between the donor's red blood cells and antibodies in the recipient's plasma, or the reverse; performed by mixing a sample of red blood cells of the donor with plasma of the recipient (*major crossmatch*) and the red blood cells of the recipient with the plasma of

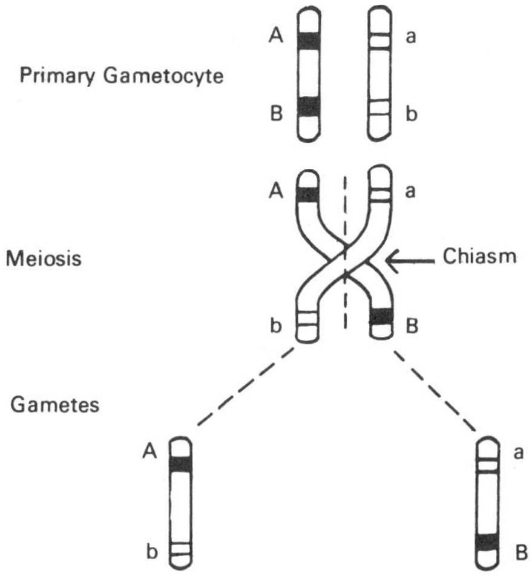

Crossing Over of Linked Genes

the donor (*minor crossmatch*). Incompatibility is indicated by clumping of red blood cells and contraindicates use of the donor's blood. **2.** In allotransplantation of solid organs (*e.g.,* kidney), a test for identification of antibody in the serum of potential allograft recipients which reacts directly with the lymphocytes or other cells of a potential allograft donor; presence of these antibodies usually, if not always, contraindicates the performance of the transplantation because virtually all such grafts will be subject to a hyperacute type of rejection.

crossway (kros'wā). The crossing of two nerve paths.

sensory c., the postlenticular portion of the posterior limb of the internal capsule of the brain.

Crosti, A., 20th century Italian dermatologist. See Gianotti-C. *syndrome.*

crotalid (krō'tă-lid). Any member of the snake family Crotalidae.

Crotalidae (krō-tal'i-dē). A family of New World vipers characterized by the presence of a heat-sensitive loreal pit between each eye and nostril, and folding, caniculated, long anterior fangs.

crotalin (krot'ă-lin) [*Crotalus,* a genus of rattlesnakes]. A protein in rattlesnake venom.

crotaline (krot'ă-lēn). Monocrotaline.

crotalism (krō'tal-izm). Crotalaria *poisoning.*

Crotalus (krot'ă-lŭs) [G. *krotalon,* a rattle, fr. *krotos,* a rattling noise]. A genus of rattlesnakes (family Crotalidae) native to North America, having large fangs that are replaced periodically throughout life and a venom that is both neurotoxic and hemolytic. The largest species are the diamondbacks of the southern states (*C. adamanteus*) and western states (*C. atrox*); the smallest are the pigmy rattlers, *Sistrurus,* of New York and several other localities.

crotamiton (krō-tam'i-ton). *N*-Ethyl-*o*-crotonotoluide; a sarcopticide for topical use in scabies.

crotaphion (krō-taf'ē-on) [G. *krotaphos,* the temple of the head]. The tip of the greater wing of the sphenoid bone; a point in craniometry.

crotonase (krō'ton-ās). Enoyl-CoA hydratase.

croton oil (krō'ton). A fixed oil expressed from the seeds of *Croton tiglium* (family Euphorbiaceae), an East Indian shrub; used as an irritant purgative, and externally as a counterirritant and vesicant.

crotonyl-ACP reductase (krō'ton-il). Enoyl-ACP reductase.

croup (krūp) [Scots, probably from A.S. *kropan,* to cry aloud]. **1.** Laryngotracheobronchitis in infants and young children caused by parainfluenza viruses 1 and 2. **2.** Any affection of the larynx in children, characterized by difficult and noisy respiration and a hoarse cough.

croupous (krū'pŭs). Relating to croup; marked by a fibrinous exudation.

croupy (krū'pē). Having the characteristics of croup, as a c. cough.

Crouzon, Octave, French physician, 1874–1938. See C.'s *disease, syndrome;* Apert-C. *syndrome.*

crowding (krowd'ing). A condition in which the teeth are crowded, assuming altered positions such as bunching, overlapping, displacement in various directions, torsiversion, etc.

Crowe, Samuel J., U.S. physician, *1883. See Davis-C. mouth *gag.*

crown (krown) [L. *corona*]. **1.** Corona. **2.** In dentistry, that part of a tooth that is covered with enamel, or an artificial substitute for that part.

anatomical c., *corona* dentis.

artificial c., a fixed restoration of the major part of the entire coronal part of a natural tooth; usually of gold, porcelain, or acrylic resin.

bell-shaped c., a c. of a tooth with an exaggerated occlusogingival contour; human deciduous molars typify the bell-shaped c.

ciliary c., *corona* ciliaris.

clinical c., *corona* clinica.

c. of head, *corona* capitis.

jacket c., a hollow c. of acrylic resin, fused porcelain or cast gold, combinations of gold and acrylic or gold and porcelain; it fits over the prepared stump of the natural c.

radiate c., *corona* radiata.

c. of tooth, *corona* dentis.

crowning (krown'ing). **1.** Preparation of the natural crown of a tooth and covering the prepared crown with a veneer of suitable dental material (gold or non-precious metal casting, porcelain, plastic, or combinations). **2.** That stage of childbirth when the fetal head has negotiated the pelvic outlet and the largest diameter of the head is encircled by the vulvar ring.

CRP Abbreviation for cAMP receptor *protein.*

CRT Abbreviation for cathode ray *tube.*

cruces (krū'sēz). Plural of crux.

cruciate (krū'shē-āt) [L. *cruciatus*]. Shaped like, or resembling, a cross.

crucible (krū'si-bl) [Mediev. L. *crucibulum,* a night lamp, later, a melting pot]. A vessel used as a container for reactions or meltings at high temperature.

crufomate (krū'fō-māt). 4-*tert*-Butyl-2-chlorophenyl methyl methylphosphoramidate; a veterinary anthelmintic.

cruor (krū'ōr) [L. blood (that flows from a wound)]. Coagulated blood.

crura (krū'ră). Plural of crus.

crural (krū'răl). Relating to the leg or thigh, or to any crus.

crureus (krū-rē'ŭs) [Mod. L.]. *Musculus* vastus intermedius.

crus, gen. cruris, pl. crura (krūs, kruris, -ră) [L.] [NA]. **1.** The leg, the segment of the inferior limb between the knee and the ankle. **2.** Any anatomical structure resembling a leg; usually (in the plural) a pair of diverging bands or elongated masses. See also limb.

c. ante'rius cap'sulae inter'nae [NA], anterior limb of the internal capsule; the portion of the internal capsule between the head of the caudate nucleus and the putamen; it lies anterior to the genu of the internal capsule.

c. ante'rius stape'dis [NA], anterior limb of stapes; the anterior of the two delicate curving limbs of the stapes that pass from the head of the bone to the base or footplate.

c. anthel'icis [NA], leg of antihelix; one of two ridges, inferior and

superior, bounding the fossa triangularis, by which the antihelix begins at the upper part of the auricle.
c. bre've incu'dis [NA], the short c. of incus; the process of the incus that fits into a depression (fossa incudis) in the epitympanic recess.
c. cer'ebri [NA], cerebral peduncle; basis or pes pedunculi; specifically, the massive bundle of corticofugal nerve fibers passing longitudinally on the ventral surface of the midbrain on each side of the midline; it consists of fibers descending from the cortex to the tegmentum of the brainstem, pontine gray matter, and spinal cord. See also *pedunculus* cerebri.
c. clitor'idis [NA], c. of clitoris; the continuation on each side of the corpus cavernosum of the clitoris which diverges from the body posteriorly and is attached to the pubic arch.
c. of clitoris, c. clitoridis.
c. cor'poris caverno'si pe'nis, c. penis.
c. dex'trum diaphrag'matis [NA], right c. of diaphragm; the muscular origin of the diaphragm from the bodies of the upper three or four lumbar vertebrae that passes upward to the right of the aorta toward the central tendon.
c. dex'trum trun'cus atrioventricula'ris [NA], the right leg or branch of the atrioventricular trunk. See also *truncus* atrioventricularis.
c. for'nicis [NA], c. of the fornix; posterior pillar of the fornix; that part of the fornix that rises in a forward curve behind the thalamus to continue forward as the corpus fornicis below the corpus callosum.
c. of fornix, c. fornicis.
c. hel'icis [NA], limb of helix; crista helicis; a transverse ridge continuing backward from the helix of the auricle, dividing the concha into an upper portion (cymba) and a lower portion (cavum conchae).
c. latera'le [NA], lateral limb; **c. l. an'uli inguina'lis superficia'lis,** the lateral limb of the superficial inguinal ring; **c. l. cartila'ginis ala'ris major'is,** the lateral limb of the greater alar cartilage of the nose.
left c. of atrioventricular trunk, c. sinistrum truncus atrioventricularis.
left c. of diaphragm, c. sinistrum diaphragmatis.
long c. of incus, c. longum incudis.
c. lon'gum incu'dis [NA], long c. of incus; the process of the incus that articulates with the stapes.
c. media'le [NA], medial limb; **c. m. ann'uli inguina'lis superficia'lis,** the medial limb of the superficial inguinal ring; **c. m. cartila'ginis ala'ris major'is,** the medial limb of the greater alar cartilage of the nose.
cru'ra membrana'cea ampulla'ria [NA], ampullary limbs of the semicircular ducts; the dilated ends of the three semicircular ducts, each of which contains a specialized thickening of the epithelium known as the crista ampullaris.
c. membrana'ceum commu'ne duc'tus semicircula'ris [NA], common limb of the membranous semicircular ducts; the united, nonampullary ends of the superior and posterior semicircular ducts.
c. membrana'ceum sim'plex duc'tus semicircula'ris [NA], simple membranous limb of the semicircular duct; the end of the lateral semicircular duct that opens into the utricle.
cru'ra os'sea cana'les semicircula'res [NA], limbs of the bony semicircular canals; the extremities of the bony semicircular canals in which the corresponding membranous limbs of the semicircular ducts are located; they are the c. osseum commune, c. osseum simplex, and crura ossea ampullaria.
c. pe'nis [NA], c. corporis cavernosi penis; the posterior portion of the corpus cavernosum penis attached to the ischiopubic ramus.
c. poste'rius cap'sulae inter'nae [NA], posterior limb of the internal capsule; that subdivision of the internal capsule caudal to the genu between the thalamus and lentiform nucleus.
c. poste'rius stape'dis [NA], posterior limb of stapes; the posterior of the two delicate limbs of the stapes that connect the head and base or footplate of the bone.
right c. of atrioventricular trunk, c. dextrum truncus atrioventricularis.
right c. of diaphragm, c. dextrum diaphragmatis.
short c. of incus, c. breve incudis.
c. sinis'trum diaphrag'matis [NA], left c. of diaphragm; the muscular origin of the diaphragm from the upper two or three lumbar vertebrae that ascends to the left of the aorta to reach the central tendon.
c. sinis'trum trun'cus atrioventricula'ris [NA], the left leg or branch of the atrioventricular trunk. See also *truncus* atrioventricularis.

crus I (krŭs). *Lobulus* semilunaris superior.

crus II (krŭs). *Lobulus* semilunaris inferior.

crush (krŭsh) [O. Fr. *cruisir*]. **1.** To squeeze injuriously between two hard bodies. **2.** A bruise or contusion from pressure between two solid bodies.

crusotomy (krūs-ot'ō-mē) [L. *crus,* leg, + G. *tomē,* incision]. (Mesencephalic) pyramidal *tractotomy.*

crust (krŭst) [L. *crusta*]. Crusta. **1.** A hard outer layer or covering. **2.** A scab.
milk c., *crusta* lactea.

crusta, pl. crustae (krŭs'tă, -tē) [L.]. Crust.
c. inflammato'ria, buffy *coat.*
c. lac'tea, milk crust, scall, or tetter; seborrhea of the scalp in an infant.
c. phlogis'tica, buffy *coat.*

Crustacea (krŭs-tā'shē-ă) [L. *crusta,* a crust]. A very large class of aquatic animals (phylum Arthropoda) with a chitinous exoskeleton and jointed appendages; *e.g.,* the crab, lobster, crayfish, shrimp, isopods, ostracods, and amphipods. Some, such as certain copepods, are parasitic; others serve as intermediate hosts for parasitic worms which cause disease in man and various vertebrates. See also Copepoda.

crutch (krŭtch) [A. S. *cryce*] A device used singly or in pairs to assist in walking when the act is impaired by a lower extremity (or trunk) disability; it transfers all or part of weight-bearing to the upper extremity.

Cruveilhier, Jean, French pathologist and anatomist, 1791–1874. See C.'s *disease, fascia, fossa, joint, ligaments, plexus;* C.-Baumgarten *disease, murmur, sign, syndrome; fossa* navicularis cruveilhier.

crux, pl. cruces (krŭks, krū'sēz) [L.]. Cross; a junction.
c. of heart, cross (2); the area of junction of the walls of the four chambers of the heart.
cru'ces pilo'rum [NA], hair crosses; crosslike figures formed by hairs growing from two directions that meet and then separate in a direction perpendicular to the original orientation.

Cruz, Oswaldo, Brazilian physician, 1872–1917. See Chagas-C. *disease,* C. *trypanosomiasis.*

cry-. See cryo-.

cryalgesia (krī-al-jē'zē-ă) [G. *kryos,* cold, + *algos,* pain]. Crymodynia; pain caused by cold.

cryanesthesia (krī'an-es-thē'zē-ă) [G. *kryos,* cold, + *an-* priv. + *aisthēsis,* sensation]. A loss of sensation or perception of cold.

cryesthesia (krī-es-thē'zē-ă) [G. *kryos,* cold, + *aisthēsis,* sensation]. **1.** A subjective sensation of cold. **2.** Sensitiveness to cold.

cry for help. Telephone calls, notes left in conspicuous places, and other behaviors which communicate extreme distress and potential suicide.

crymo- [G. *krymos,* cold]. Combining form relating to cold. See also cryo-, psychro-.

crymodynia (krī-mō-din'ē-ă) [crymo- + G. *odynē*, pain]. Cryalgesia.

crymophilic (krī-mō-fil'ik) [crymo- + G. *philos*, fond]. Cryophilic; preferring cold; denoting microorganisms which thrive best at low temperatures.

crymophylactic (krī'mō-fi-lak'tik) [crymo- + G. *phylaxis*, a guarding against]. Cryophylactic; resistant to cold, said of certain microorganisms which are not destroyed even by freezing temperatures.

crymotherapy (krī'mō-thār'ă-pē). Cryotherapy.

cryo-, cry- [G. *kryos*, cold]. Combining forms relating to cold. See also crymo-, psychro-.

cryoanesthesia (krī'ō-an-es-thē'zē-ă). Refrigeration anesthesia; localized application of cold as a means of producing regional anesthesia.

cryobiology (krī'ō-bī-ol'ō-jē). The study of the effects of low temperatures on living organisms.

cryocautery (krī'ō-kaw'ter-ē). Cold cautery; any substance, such as liquid air or carbon dioxide snow, or a low temperature instrument, the application of which causes destruction of tissue by freezing.

cryoconization (krī'ō-kon-ī-zā'shŭn). Freezing of a cone of endocervical tissue with a cryoprobe.

cryoextraction (krī'ō-ek-strak'shŭn). Removal of cataracts by the adhesion of a freezing probe to the lens.

cryoextractor (krī'ō-ek-strak'tōr, -tōr). Cryostylet; an instrument, artifically cooled, for extraction of the lens by freezing contact.

cryofibrinogen (krī'ō-fī-brin'ō-jen). An abnormal type of fibrinogen very rarely found in human plasma; it is precipitated upon cooling, but redissolves when warmed to room temperature.

cryofibrinogenemia (krī'ō-fī-brin'ō-je-nē'mē-ă). The presence in the blood of cryofibrinogens.

cryofluorane (krī-ō-flūr'ān). 1,2-Dichloro-1,1,2,2-tetrafluoroethane; used as a refrigerant and aerosol propellant; may be irritating to the respiratory tract and mildly narcotic.

cryogen (krī'ō-jen). A freezing substance used to produce very low temperatures.

cryogenic (krī-ō-jen'ik). **1.** Denoting or characteristic of a cryogen. **2.** Relating to cryogenics.

cryogenics (krī-ō-jen'iks) [cryo- + G. *-gen*, producing]. The science concerned with the production and effects of very low temperatures, particularly temperatures in the range of liquid helium (<4.2K).

cryoglobulinemia (krī'ō-glob'yū-li-nē'mē-ă). The presence of abnormal quantities of cryoglobulin in the blood plasma.
crystal c., a syndrome of repeated episodes of widespread purpura and cutaneous ulcerations in a patient whose serum contains a homogenous cryoglobulin that spontaneously forms crystals.

cryoglobulins (krī-ō-glob'yū-linz). Abnormal plasma proteins (paraproteins), now grouped with gamma globulins, characterized by precipitating, gelling, or crystallizing when serum or solutions of them are cooled; distinguished from Bence Jones proteins by their larger molecular weight (approximately 200,000 compared with 35,000 to 50,000); they may appear in patients with multiple myeloma.

cryohydrate (krī-ō-hī'drāt). A eutectic system of a salt and water.

cryohypophysectomy (krī'ō-hī-pof'i-sek'tō-mē) [cryo- + hypophysis + G. *ektomē*, excision]. Destruction of hypophysis by cold.

cryolysis (krī-ol'i-sis) [cryo- + G. *lysis*, dissolution]. Destruction by cold.

cryometer (krī-om'ĕ-ter) [cryo- + G. *metron*, measure]. A device for measuring very low temperatures.

cryopallidectomy (krī'ō-pal-i-dek'tō-mē) [cryo- + globus pallidus + G. *ektomē*, excision]. Destruction of the globus pallidus by cold.

cryopathy (krī-op'ă-thē) [cryo- + G. *pathos*, suffering]. Frigorism; a morbid condition in which exposure to cold is an important factor.

cryopexy (krī'ō-pek-sē) [cryo- + G. *pēxis*, a fixing in place]. In retinal detachment surgery, sealing the sensory retina to the pigment epithelium and choroid by a freezing probe applied to the sclera.

cryophilic (krī-ō-fil'ik) [cryo- + G. *philos*, fond]. Crymophilic.

cryophylactic (krī'ō-fī-lak'tik). Crymophylactic.

cryoprecipitate (krī'ō-prē-sip'i-tāt). Precipitate which forms when soluble material is cooled, especially with reference to the precipitate that forms in normal blood plasma which has been subjected to cold precipitation and which is rich in factor VIII.

cryoprecipitation (krī'ō-prē-sip-i-tā'shŭn). The process of forming a cryoprecipitate from solution.

cryopreservation (krī'ō-pres-er-vā'shŭn). Maintenance of the viability of excised tissues or organs at extremely low temperatures.

cryoprobe (krī'ō-prōb). An instrument used in cryosurgery.

cryoprostatectomy (krī'ō-pros-tă-tek'tō-mē) [cryo- + L. *prostata*, prostate, + G. *ektomē*, excision]. Destruction of the prostate gland by freezing, utilizing a specially designed cryoprobe.

cryoprotein (krī-ō-prō'tēn). A protein that precipitates from solution when cooled and redissolves upon warming.

cryopulvinectomy (krī'ō-pŭl-vi-nek'tō-mē) [cryo- + pulvinar + G. *ektomē*, excision]. Destruction of the pulvinar by cold.

cryoscope (krī'ō-skōp). An instrument for measuring the freezing point.

cryoscopy (krī-os'kō-pē) [cryo- + G. *skopeō*, to examine]. Algoscopy; the determination of the freezing point of a fluid, usually blood or urine, compared with that of distilled water.

cryospasm (krī'ō-spazm) [cryo- + G. *spasmos*, convulsion]. Spasm produced by cold.

cryostat (krī'ō-stat) [cryo- + G. *statos*, standing]. A freezing chamber.

cryostylet, cryostylette (krī'ō-stī'let). Cryoextractor.

cryosurgery (krī-ō-ser'jer-ē). An operation using freezing temperature (achieved by liquid nitrogen or carbon dioxide) to destroy tissue.

cryothalamectomy (krī'ō-thal-ă-mek'tō-mē) [cryo- + thalamus + G. *ektomē*, excision]. Destruction of the thalamus by cold.

cryotherapy (krī'ō-thār'ă-pē). Crymotherapy; the use of cold in the treatment of disease.

cryotolerant (krī-ō-tol'er-ant). Tolerant of very low temperatures.

cryounit (krī'ō-yū-nit). One of a variety of instruments, of various shapes and sizes, designed to grasp or destroy tissue with freezing cold.

crypt-. See crypto-.

crypt (kript). Crypta.
dental c., the space filled by the dental follicle.
enamel c., enamel niche; the narrow, mesenchymally filled space between the dental ledge and an enamel organ.
c.'s of iris, pits near the pupillary margin of the anterior surface of the iris.
Lieberkühn's c.'s, *glandulae* intestinales.
lingual c., a pit lined with epithelium in the lingual tonsil.
Morgagni's c.'s, *sinus* anales.
synovial c., a diverticulum of the synovial membrane of a joint.
tonsillar c., *crypta* tonsillaris.

crypta, pl. cryptae (krip'tă, -tē) [L. fr. G. *kryptos*, hidden] [NA]. Crypt; a pitlike depression or tubular recess.

c. tonsilla'ris, pl. **cryp'tae tonsilla'res** [NA], tonsillar crypt; one of the variable number of deep recesses that extend into the palatine and pharyngeal tonsils from the free surface where they open at the fossulae tonsillares.

cryptectomy (krip-tek'tō-mē) [crypt + G. *ektomē,* excision]. Excision of a tonsillar or other crypt.

cryptenamine acetates or **tannates** (krip-ten'ă-mēn). Acetate or tannate salts of alkaloids from a nonaqueous extract of *Veratrum viride,* containing the hypotensive alkaloids protoveratrines A and B, germitrine, neogermetrine, germerine, germidine, jervine, rubijervine, isorubijervine, and germubide; used as an antihypertensive agent. See also protoveratrines.

cryptic (krip'tik) [G. *kryptikos*] Hidden; occult; larvate.

cryptitis (krip-tī'tis). Inflammation of a follicle or glandular tubule, particularly in the rectum.

crypto-, crypt- [G. *kryptos,* hidden, concealed]. Combining forms relating to a crypt, or meaning hidden, obscure, without apparent cause.

cryptococcoma (krip'tō-kok-ō'mă). Toruloma; an infectious granuloma, typically in the brain, but also found in the lung and elsewhere, caused by *Cryptococcus neoformans.*

cryptococcosis (krip'tō-kok-ō'sis). Busse-Buschke disease; an acute, subacute, or chronic infection by *Cryptococcus neoformans,* causing a pulmonary, disseminated, or meningeal mycosis. The pulmonary form is usually transitory, mild, and unrecognized; cutaneous, skeletal, and visceral lesions may occur during dissemination; the most familiar and readily recognized form involves the central nervous system, with subacute or chronic meningitis.

Cryptococcus (krip-tō-kok'ŭs) [crypto- + G. *kokkos,* berry]. A genus of yeastlike fungi that reproduce by budding.

C. neofor'mans, a species that causes cryptococcosis in man and other mammalians and parasitizes cats in some areas, although strains vary in virulence; the cells are spherical and may bud at any point on the surface or simultaneously at several points; a prominent feature is a mucoid polysaccharide capsule which may vary in width from very thin to several times the radius of the parent cell and buds combined. Once thought to be widespread in nature, its true niche appears to be narrowing to a saprobic association with the manure and nests of pigeons; it is therefore essentially global in distribution.

cryptocrystalline (krip-tō-kris'tă-lēn). Having very minute crystals.

Cryptocystis trichodectis (krip-tō-sis'tis trī-kō-dek'tis) [crypto- + G. *kystis,* bladder; tricho- + G. *dektēs,* a beggar]. Name formerly applied to the larval form of the dog tapeworm, *Dipylidium caninum,* named for the cysticercoids found in the dog louse, *Trichodectes.*

cryptodidymus (krip'tō-did'i-mŭs) [crypto- + G. *didymos,* twin]. Conjoined twins, with the poorly developed parasitic twin concealed within the larger autosite.

Cryptogamia (krip-tō-gam'ē-ă) [crypto- + G. *gamos,* marriage]. A montaxonomic division of the plant kingdom containing all forms of plant life that do not reproduce by means of seeds; included are the algae, bacteria, fungi, lichens, mosses, liverworts, ferns, horsetails, and club mosses.

cryptogenic (krip-tō-jen'ik) [crypto- + G. *genesis,* origin]. Of obscure, indeterminate etiology or origin, in contrast to phanerogenic.

cryptolith (krip'tō-lith) [crypto- + G. *lithos,* stone]. A concretion in a gland follicle.

cryptomenorrhea (krip'tō-men-ō-rē'ă) [crypto- + G. *mēn,* month, + *rhoia,* flow]. Occurrence each month of the general symptoms of the menses without any flow of blood, as in cases of imperforate hymen.

cryptophthalmus, cryptophthalmia (krip-tof-thal'mŭs, -thal'mē-ă) [crypto- + G. *ophthalmos,* eye]. Congenital absence of eyelids with the skin passing continuously from the forehead onto the cheek over a rudimentary eye.

cryptopodia (krip-tō-pō'dē-ă) [crypto- + G. *pous,* foot]. A condition of swelling of the lower part of the leg and the foot, in such a manner that there is great distortion and the sole seems to be a flattened pad.

cryptopyrrole (krip-tō-pir'ōl). 3-Ethyl-2,4-dimethylpyrrole; one of the pyrrole derivatives obtained by the drastic reduction of heme.

cryptorchid (krip-tōr'kid) [crypto- + G. *orchis,* testis]. Relating to or characterized by cryptorchism.

cryptorchidectomy (krip'tōr-ki-dek'tō-mē) [crypto- + G. *orchis,* testis, + *ektomē,* excision]. Surgical removal of an undescended testis.

cryptorchidism (krip-tōr'ki-dizm). Cryptorchism.

cryptorchidopexy (krip-tōr'ki-dō-pek'sē) [crypto- + G. *orchis,* testis, + *pēxis,* fixation]. Orchiopexy.

cryptorchism (krip-tōr'kizm). Cryptorchidism; failure of one or both of the testis to descend.

cryptosporidiosis (krip'tō-spō-rid-ē-ō'sis). An enteric disease caused by protozoan parasites of the genus *Cryptosporidium;* characterized pathologically by villous atrophy and fusion and clinically by diarrhea in man, calves, lambs, and probably other animal species; disease in immunocompetent persons is manifest as a self-limiting diarrhea, whereas in immunocompromised persons it is manifest as a prolonged severe diarrhea which can be fatal.

Cryptosporidium (krip'tō-spō-rid'ē-ŭm). A genus of coccidian sporozoans (family Cryptosporiidae, suborder Eimeriina) that are important pathogens of calves and other domestic animals, and common opportunistic parasites of humans that flourish under conditions of compromised immune function.

Cryptostroma corticale (krip-tō-strō'mă kōr-ti-kā'lē) [crypto- + G. *stroma,* bed]. A species of fungus that is a common allergen, growing profusely under the bark of stacked maple logs; handlers who inhale the massive number of spores may develop pneumonitic as well as allergic reactions, including maple bark disease.

cryptotia (krip-tō'shē-ă) [crypto- + G. *ōtos,* ear]. A deformity, usually congenital, in which the superior portion of the auricle is hidden under the scalp.

cryptoxanthin (krip-tō-zan'thin). (3*R*)-β,β-Caroten-3-ol; β-caroten-3-ol; carotenoid yielding 1 mole of vitamin A per mole.

cryptozoite (krip'tō-zō'īt) [crypto- + G. *zōē,* life]. The exoerythrocyte stage of the malarial organism that develops directly from the sporozoite inoculated by the infected mosquito; development of the first generation of merozoites in vertebrate host tissues occurs in the liver parenchyma.

cryptozygous (krip-toz'i-gŭs, -tō-zī'gŭs) [crypto- + G. *zygon,* yoke]. Having a narrow face as compared with the width of the cranium, so that, when the skull is viewed from above, the zygomatic arches are not visible.

crystal (kris'tăl) [G. *krystallos,* clear ice, crystal]. A solid of regular shape and, for a given compound, characteristic angles, formed when an element or compound solidifies slowly enough, as a result either of freezing from the liquid form or of precipitating out of solution, to allow the individual molecules to take up regular positions with respect to one another.

asthma c.'s, Charcot-Leyden c.'s.

blood c.'s, hematoidin.

Böttcher's c.'s, small c.'s observed microscopically in prostatic fluid that is treated with a drop or two of 1% solution of ammonium phosphate.

Charcot-Leyden c.'s, asthma c.'s; Charcot-Neumann, Charcot-Robin, or Leyden's c.'s; c.'s in the shape of elongated double pyramids, formed from eosinophils, found in the sputum in bronchial asthma and in other exudates or transudates containing eosinophils.
Charcot-Neumann c.'s, Charcot-Robin c.'s, Charcot-Leyden c.'s.
chiral c., an enantiomorphic, dissymmetric, optically active c.
clathrate c., lattice-like arrangement of molecules of one substance surrounding molecules of another substance.
ear c.'s, statoconia.
Florence's c.'s, brown rhombic c.'s formed at the interface between a drop of Lugol's solution and a drop of fluid that contains semen; not a specific test for the latter.
hematoidin c.'s, hematoidin.
hydrate c., one of several possible microstructural arrangements of water molecules based on intermolecular forces; suggested as being involved in the mode of action of inhalation anesthetics.
knife-rest c., a c. of ammoniomagnesium phosphate found in alkaline urine.
Leyden's c.'s, Charcot-Leyden c.'s.
Lubarsch's c.'s, intracellular c.'s in the testis resembling sperm c.'s.
sperm c., spermin c., a c. of spermin phosphate found in the semen; possibly identical to Böttcher's c.'s.
Teichmann's c.'s, hemin.
thorn apple c.'s, ammonium urate c.'s in the shape of rounded bodies with many projecting points.
twin c., two c.'s that have grown together along a common face.
Virchow's c.'s, yellow-brown, amber, or burnt orange c.'s of hematoidin, frequently observed in extravasated blood in tissues.
whetstone c.'s, xanthine c.'s occasionally observed in urine.

crystallin (kris'tă-lin). A type of protein found in the lens of the eye; alpha (an embryonic single protein), beta, and gamma varieties are known.
gamma c., the least rapidly mobile form of c. on electrophoresis.

crystalline (kris'tă-lēn). **1.** Clear; transparent. **2.** Relating to a crystal or crystals.

crystallization (kris'tăl-i-zā'shŭn). Assumption of a crystalline form when a vapor or liquid becomes solidified, or a solute precipitates from solution.

crystallogram (kris'tă-lō-gram) [G. *crystallos,* crystal, + *gramma,* something written]. A photograph produced when x-rays are diffracted by a crystal.

crystallography (kris-tăl-log'ră-fē). The study of the shape and atomic structure of crystals.

crystalloid (kris'tăl-oyd). **1.** Resembling a crystal, or being such. **2.** A body which in solution can pass through a semipermeable membrane, as distinguished from a colloid, which cannot do so.
Charcot-Böttcher c.'s, spindle-shaped c.'s 10 to 25 μm long, found in human Sertoli cells.
Reinke c.'s, rod-shaped crystal-like structures with pointed or rounded ends present in the interstitial cells of the testis (Leydig cells) and ovary.

crystallophobia (kris'tăl-ō-fō'bē-ă) [G. *krystallon,* crystal, + *phobos,* fear]. Hyalophobia.

crystalluria (kris-tă-lū'rē-ă). The excretion of crystalline materials in the urine.

crystal violet (kris'tăl) [C.I. 42555]. Methylrosaniline chloride; hexamethylpararosanilin chloride; a compound that has been used in the external treatment of burns, wounds, and fungal infections of skin and mucous membranes, and internally for pinworm and certain fluke infections; used also as a stain for chromatin, amyloid, platelets in blood, fibrin, and neuroglia, and to differentiate among bacteria.

Cs Symbol for cesium.

C-section. See caesarian *section.*

CSF Abbreviation for cerebrospinal *fluid.*

Csillag, J. See C.'s disease.

CT Abbreviation for computed *tomography.*

Ctenocephalides (tē-nō-se-fal'i-dēz) [G. *ktenodēs,* like a cockle, + *kephalē,* head]. A genus of fleas. *C. canis* (dog flea) and *C. felis* (cat flea) are nearly universal ectoparasites of household pets; will attack man when starving owing to absence of pets.

CTP Abbreviation for cytidine 5′-triphosphate.

Cu Symbol for copper.

cubeb (kyū'beb) [Ar. and Hindu, *kababa*]. The dried unripe, nearly full-grown fruit of *Piper cubeba* (family Piperaceae), a climbing plant of the West Indies, used as stimulant, carminative, and local irritant; c. oil has been used as a mild urinary antiseptic.

cubital (kyū'bi-tăl). Relating to the elbow or to the ulna.

cubitus, gen. and pl. **cubiti** (kyū'bi-tŭs, -tī) [L. elbow] [NA]. **1.** Elbow (1). **2.** Ulna.
c. val'gus, deviation of the extended forearm to the outer (radial) side of the axis of the limb.
c. va'rus, deviation of the extended forearm to the inward (ulnar) side of the axis of the limb.

cuboid, cuboidal (kyū'boyd, kyū-boy'dăl) [G. *kybos,* cube, + *eidos,* resemblance]. **1.** Resembling a cube in shape. **2.** Relating to the os cuboideum.

cue (kyū). In conditioning and learning theory, a pattern of stimuli to which an individual has learned to respond.
response-produced c.'s, successive stimulus c.'s in a behavior chain, each response serving as a reinforcer for the previous response and as a stimulus, or c., for the next response.

cuff (kŭf). Any structure shaped like a c.
musculotendinous c., rotator c. of shoulder.
perivascular c.'s, see cuffing.
rotator c. of shoulder, musculotendinous c.; the upper half of the capsule of the shoulder joint reinforced by the tendons of insertion of the supraspinatus, infraspinatus, teres minor, and subscapularis muscles.

cuffing (kŭf'ing). A perivascular accumulation of various leukocytes seen in infectious, inflammatory, or autoimmune diseases.

cuirass (kwē-ras') [Fr. *cuirasse,* a breastplate]. The anterior surface of the thorax in relation to symptoms or disease changes.
analgesic c., tabetic c.
tabetic c., analgesic c.; Hitzig's girdle; an analgesic or hypalgesic zone in the region supplied by the third to sixth thoracic nerves; commonly found in tabes dorsalis.

cul-de-sac, pl. **culs-de-sac** (kŭl-de-sak') [Fr. bottom of a sack]. A blind pouch or tubular cavity closed at one end; *e.g.,* diverticulum; cecum.
conjunctival c., *fornix* conjunctivae.
Douglas' c., *excavatio* rectouterina.
greater c., *fundus* ventriculi.
Gruber's c., a lateral diverticulum in the suprasternal space beside the medial extremity of the clavicle behind the sternal attachment of the sternocleidomastoid muscle.
lesser c., *antrum* pyloricum.

culdocentesis (kŭl'dō-sen-tē'sis) [cul-de-sac + G. *kentesis,* puncture]. Aspiration of fluid from the cul-de-sac (rectouterine excavation) by puncture of the vaginal vault near the midline between the uterosacral ligaments. See fig. on p. 378.

culdoplasty (kŭl'dō-plas-tē) [cul-de-sac + G. *plastos,* formed]. Plastic surgery to remedy relaxation of the posterior fornix of the vagina.

culdoscope (kŭl'dō-skōp). Endoscopic instrument used in culdoscopy.

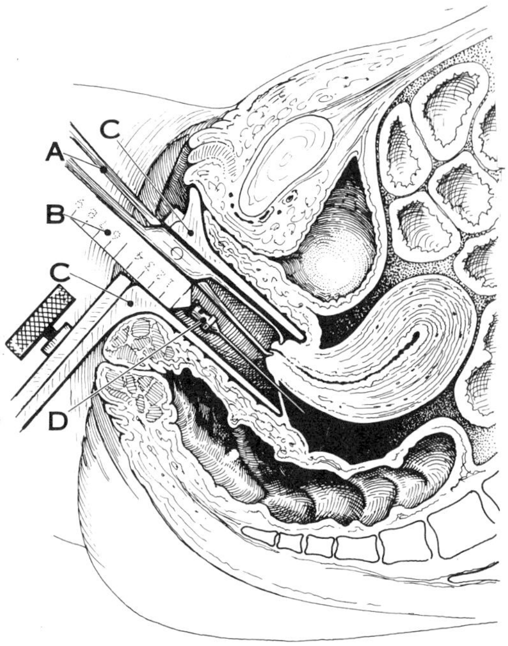

Culdocentesis
The instruments are: *A*, Allis forceps; *B*, syringe; *C*, speculum; *D*, 18-gauge spinal needle.

culdoscopy (kŭl-dos′kō-pē) [cul-de-sac + G. *skopeō*, to view]. Introduction of an endoscope through the posterior vaginal wall for viewing the rectovaginal pouch and pelvic viscera.

culdotomy (kŭl-dot′ō-mē) [cul-de-sac + G. *tomē*, incision]. Cutting into the cul-de-sac of Douglas.

Culex (kyū′leks) [L. gnat]. A genus of mosquitoes (family Culicidae) including over 2,000 species. Largely tropical but worldwide in distribution; they are vectors for a number of diseases of man and of domestic and wild animals and birds.
C. pi′piens, a subspecies complex of the abundant polytypic species, the brown house mosquito or rainbarrel mosquito of temperate climates, which breeds commonly in standing water, especially in artificial containers, and has a 5- to 6-day cycle under optimal conditions; closely related forms are found in tropical areas.
C. tarsa′lis, a species that is an important vector of St. Louis and western equine encephalomyelitis viruses and other viruses in horses, birds, and man.

Culicidae (kyū-lis′i-dē). A family of insects (order Diptera) that includes the true mosquitoes, which are all included in the subfamily Culicinae.

culicidal (kyū-li-sī′dăl) [L. *culex*, gnat, + *caedo*, to kill]. Destructive to mosquitoes.

culicide (kyū′li-sīd). An agent that destroys mosquitoes.

culicifuge (kyū-lis′i-fūj) [L. *culex*, gnat + *fugo*, to drive away]. **1.** Driving away gnats and mosquitoes. **2.** An agent that keeps mosquitoes from biting.

Culicoides (kyū-li-koy′dēz) [L. *culex*, gnat]. A genus of minute biting gnats or midges, vectors of several nonpathogenic human filariae (*Mansonella, Dipetalonema*), of *Onchocerca* in horses and cattle, and of several viral agents of domestic sheep and fowl.
C. aus′teni, species that is an intermediate host of the filarial worm, *Mansonella perstans*, chiefly in equatorial Africa.
C. fu′rens, species that is a vector of *Mansonella ozzardi*, in the West Indies.
C. milne′i, a species that is one of the vectors of *Mansonella perstans* in west Africa.
C. variipen′nis, a species that is the primary vector of bluetongue virus in the U.S.

culicosis (kyū′li-kō′sis). Dermatitis caused by *Culex* mosquitoes.

Culiseta melanura (kū-li-sē′tă mel-ă-nū′ră). A species of mosquito that is the principal endemic vector of eastern equine encephalomyelitis virus; since this species feeds primarily on birds, other mosquitoes (*Aedes* spp.) transmit the virus from birds to man and horses.

Cullen, Thomas S., U.S. gynecologist, 1868–1953. See C.'s *sign*.

culmen, pl. **cul′mina** (kul′men) [L. summit] [NA]. Lobulus culminis; the anterior prominent portion of the monticulus of the vermis of the cerebellum; vermal lobule rostral to the primary fissure.

Culp, Ormond S., U.S. urologist, 1910–1977. See C. *pyeloplasty*.

cult (kŭlt) [L. *cultus*, an honoring, adoration]. A system of beliefs and rituals based on dogma or religious teachings and characterized by devoted adherents who display a readiness to obey, an unrealistic idealization of the leader, an abandonment of personal ambition and goals, and an eschewing of traditional societal values.

cultivation (kŭl-ti-vā′shŭn) [Mediev. L. *cultivo*, pp. *-atus*, fr. L. *colo*, pp. *cultus*, to till]. Culture.

culture (kŭl′chŭr) [L. *cultura*, tillage, fr. *colo*, pp. *cultus*, to till]. Cultivation. **1.** The propagation of microorganisms on or in media of various kinds. **2.** A mass of microorganisms on or in a medium.
cell c., the maintenance or growth of dispersed cells after removal from the body, commonly on a glass surface immersed in nutrient fluid.
elective c., a method of isolating microorganisms capable of utilizing a specific substrate by incubating an inoculum in a medium containing the substrate; the medium usually contains substances or has characteristics that inhibit the growth of unwanted microorganisms.
hanging-block c., the propagation of microorganisms on a cube of solidified agar medium which is inoculated, attached to a cover glass, and inverted over a moist chamber or hollowed slide.
mixed lymphocyte c., see mixed lymphocyte culture *test*.
needle c., stab c.
neotype c., neotype *strain*.
organ c., the maintenance or growth of tissues, organ primordia, or the parts or whole of an organ *in vitro* in such a way as to allow differentiation or preservation of the architecture or function.
pure c., in the ordinary bacteriologic sense, a c. consisting of the descendants of a single cell.
roll-tube c., a c. in a tube of medium which has been melted and allowed to solidify while the tube is being spun; the inside of the tube is thereby coated with a thin layer of solidified medium.
sensitized c., a live c. of an organism to which a specific antiserum is added; after the mixture is incubated for several minutes (during which the antibody in the serum combines with the organisms), the excess serum is removed by means of centrifugation, washing in physiologic saline solution, and recentrifugation; the sensitized organisms may then be resuspended in physiologic saline solution.
shake c., a c. made by inoculating a liquefied gelatin or agar medium, distributing the inoculum thoroughly by agitation, and then allowing the medium to solidify in the tube in an upright position.
slant c., slope c.; a c. made on the slanting surface of a medium which has been solidified in a test tube inclined from the perpendicular so as to give a greater area than that of the lumen of the tube.
slope c., slant c.
smear c., a c. obtained by spreading material presumed to be infected on the surface of a solidified medium.
stab c., needle c.; a c. produced by inserting an inoculating needle

with inoculum down the center of a solid medium contained in a test tube.

stock c., a c. of a microorganism maintained solely for the purpose of keeping the microorganism in a viable condition by subculture, as necessary, into fresh medium.

streak c., a c. produced by lightly stroking an inoculating needle or loop with inoculum over the surface of a solid medium.

tissue c., the maintenance of live tissue after removal from the body, by placing in a vessel with a sterile nutritive medium.

type c., a type strain of microorganism preserved in a c. collection as the standard.

cumarin (kyū'mă-rin). Coumarin.

cumetharol (kyū-meth'ă-rol). Coumetarol.

cumethoxaethane (kyū-me-thoks'ă-eth-ān). Coumetarol.

Cummer, William E., Canadian dentist, 1879–1942. See C.'s *classification, guideline.*

cumulative (kyū'myū-lă-tiv). Tending to accumulate or pile up, as with certain drugs that may have a c. effect.

cumulus, pl. **cumuli** (kyū'myū-lŭs, -lī) [L. a heap]. A collection or heap of cells.

c. ooph'orus, discus proligerus; proligerous disk; proligerous membrane; a mass of epithelial cells surrounding the ovum in the ovarian follicle.

c. ova'ricus, rarely used term for c. oophorus.

cuneate (kyū'nē-āt) [L. *cuneus,* wedge]. Wedge-shaped.

cuneiform (kyū'nē-i-fōrm). Wedge-shaped. See entries for *os* cuneiforme.

cuneocuboid (kyū'nē-ō-kyū'boyd). Relating to the lateral cuneiform and the cuboid bones.

cuneonavicular (kyū-nē-ō-na-vik'yū-lăr). Cuneoscaphoid; relating to the cuneiform and the navicular bones.

cuneoscaphoid (kyū-nē-ō-skaf'oyd). Cuneonavicular.

cuneus, pl. **cu'nei** (kyū'nē-ŭs, kū'nē-ī) [L. wedge] [NA]. That region of the medial aspect of the occipital lobe of each cerebral hemisphere bounded by the parietooccipital fissure and the calcarine fissure.

cuniculus, pl. **cunic'uli** (kyū-nik'yū-lŭs) [L. a rabbit; an underground passage]. The burrow of the itch mite in the epidermis.

cunnilinction, cunnilinctus (kŭn-i-lingk'shŭn, -lingk'tŭs). Cunnilingus.

cunnilingus (kŭn-i-ling'gŭs) [L. *cunnus,* pudendum, + *lingo,* to lick]. Cunnilinction; cunnilinctus; oral stimulation of the vulva or clitoris; a type of oral-genital sexual activity.

Cunninghamella elegans (kŭn-ing-ha-mel'ă el'ĕ-ganz). One of several species of fungus that can cause disseminated mucormycosis in man, and possibly abortion in cattle, swine, and other animals.

cunnus (kŭn'ŭs) [L.]. Vulva.

cup (kŭp) [A.S. *cuppe*]. **1.** Poculum; an excavated or cup-shaped structure, either anatomical or pathologic. **2.** Cupping *glass.*

Diogenes c., poculum diogenis; the palm of the hand when contracted and deepened by the action of the muscles on either side.

dry c., a cupping glass formerly applied to the unbroken skin to draw blood to the area but without removing it.

eye c., a small oval receptacle used to apply a liquid to the external eye.

glaucomatous c., glaucomatous excavation; a deep depression of the optic disk combined with optic atrophy; caused by glaucoma.

ocular c., optic c.

optic c., ocular c.; caliculus ophthalmicus; the double-walled c. formed by the invagination of the embryonic optic vesicle; its inner component becomes the sensory layer of the retina, its outer layer, the pigment layer.

perilimbal suction c., a device for increasing intraocular pressure by impeding circulation and aqueous humor flow from the eye.

physiologic c., a funnel-shaped excavation of the optic disk.

suction c., one of the cupping glasses of various shapes, formerly used to produce local hyperemia according to Bier's method.

wet c., a cupping glass formerly applied to a part previously scarified or incised to draw and remove blood.

cupola (kū'pō-lă, kyū'). Cupula.

cupped (kŭpt). Hollowed; made cup-shaped.

cupping (kŭp'ing). **1.** Formation of a hollow, or cup-shaped excavation. **2.** Application of a c. glass. See also entries under cup.

cupric (kū'prik, kyū-). Pertaining to copper, particularly to copper in the form of a doubly charged positive ion.

cupric acetate (normal). Verdigris; $Cu(CH_3COOH)_2{\cdot}H_2O$; a stimulating local caustic to ulcers.

cupric arsenite. Copper arsenite; Scheele's green; $CuHAsO_3$; a poisonous green crystalline powder, obsolete as a medicinal agent; now used as an insecticide and pigment.

cupric chloride. Copper chloride; copper bichloride; copper dichloride; $CuCl_2{\cdot}2H_2O$; has been used as an antiseptic in the treatment of water supplies, ponds, and pools.

cupric citrate. Copper citrate; a salt of copper used as an astringent and antiseptic.

cupric sulfate. Copper sulfate (sulphate); $CuSo_4{\cdot}5H_2O$; it is highly poisonous to algae, is a prompt and active emetic, and is used as an irritant, astringent, and fungicide.

cupriuresis (kū'pri-yū-rē'sis, kyū'-) [L. *cuprum,* copper, + G. *ourēsis,* a urinating]. The urinary excretion of copper.

cupula, pl. **cupulae** (kū'pū-lă, kyū'pyū-lă, -lē) [L. dim. of *cupa,* a tub] [NA]. Cupola; a cup-shaped or domelike structure.

c. coch'leae [NA], the domelike apex of the cochlea.

c. cris'tae ampulla'ris [NA], cap of the ampullary crest; a gelatinous mass that overlies the hair cells of the cristae ampullares of the semicircular ducts; movement of endolymphatic fluid causes the c. to move across the hair cells of the cristae ampullaris.

c. pleu'rae [NA], cervical pleura; the dome-shaped roof of the pleural cavity extending up through the superior aperture of the thorax.

cupular (kū'pū-lăr, kyū'pyū-lăr). **1.** Relating to a cupula. **2.** Cupulate; cupuliform; dome-shaped.

cupulate (kū'pū-lāt, kyū'pyū-). Cupular (2).

cupuliform (kū'pū-lĭ-fōrm, kyū'pyū-). Cupular (2).

cupulogram (kū'pū-lō-gram). A graphic representation of vestibular function relative to normal performance.

curage (kyū'rij, kū-rahzh') [Fr. a cleansing]. Curettage by means of the finger rather than the curet.

curare (kū-rah'rē) [S. Am.]. Arrow poison; urari; an extract of various plants, especially *Strychnos toxifera, S. castelnaei, S. crevauxii,* and *Chondodendron tomentosum,* that produces nondepolarizing paralysis of skeletal muscle after intravenous injection by blocking transmission at the myoneuronal junction; used clinically (*e.g.,* as *d*-tubocurarine chloride, metocurine iodide) to provide muscle relaxation during surgical operations.

curariform (kū-rar'i-fōrm). Denoting a drug having an action like curare.

curarimimetic (kū-rar'i-mī-met'ik). Having a curare-like action.

curarine (kyū'ră-rēn). C-Curarine I; $C_{40}H_{44}N_4O^{++}$; the alkaloid principle of calabash curare.

curarization (kyū-rah-ri-zā'shŭn). Induction of muscular relaxation or paralysis by the administration of curare or of related compounds that have the ability to block nerve impulse transmission at the myoneural junction.

curative (kyūr'ă-tiv). **1.** That which heals or cures. **2.** Tending to heal or cure.

curb (kerb). Curby hock; a hard, painful, inflammatory swelling on the back part of the hock of the horse; it occurs in the plantar ligament near its insertion, is characterized by swelling and heat in the part and generally by lameness, and is believed to be caused by straining the ligament in falling, jumping, or pulling.

curd (kerd). The coagulum of milk.

cure (kyūr) [L. *curo,* to care for]. **1.** To heal; to make well. **2.** A restoration to health. **3.** A special method or course of treatment. **4.** See dental *curing.*

curet (kyū-ret′, kū-ret′). Curette.

curetment (kyū-ret′ment, kū-). Curettage.

curettage (kyū-rĕ-tahzh′, kū-). Curettement; curetment; a scraping, usually of the interior of a cavity or tract, for the removal of new growths or other abnormal tissues, or to obtain material for tissue diagnosis.
periapical c., **(1)** removal of a cyst or granuloma from its pathologic bony crypt, utilizing a curette; **(2)** the removal of tooth fragments and debris from sockets at the time of extraction or of bone sequestra subsequently.
subgingival c., apoxesis; removal of subgingival calculus, ulcerated epithelial and granulation tissues found in periodontal pockets.

curette (kyū-ret′, kū-) [Fr.]. Curet. Instrument in the form of a loop, ring, or scoop with sharpened edges attached to a rod-shaped handle, used for curettage.
Hartmann's c., a. c., cutting on the side, for the removal of adenoids.

curettement (kyū-ret′ment, kū-). Curettage.

curie (Ci) (kyū′rē) [Marie (1867–1934) and Pierre (1859–1906) *Curie,* French chemists and physicists]. A unit of measurement of radioactiviity, 3.70×10^{10} disintegrations per second (1 becquerel); 1 g of ^{226}Ra emits 1 Ci of radioactivity.

curing (kyūr′ing). **1.** The act of accomplishing a cure. **2.** A process by which something is prepared for use, as by heating, aging, etc.
dental c., the process by which plastic materials become rigid to form a denture base, filling, impression tray, or other appliance.

curium (kyū′rē-ŭm) [see curie]. An element, atomic no. 96, symbol Cm, not occurring naturally on earth, but first formed artificially in 1944 by bombarding plutonium-239 with alpha particles; the most stable of the c. isotopes is c.-247, with a half-life of approximately 16 million years.

Curling, Thomas B., British surgeon, 1811–1888. See C.'s *ulcer.*

current (ker′rĕnt) [L. *currens,* pres. p. of *curro,* to run]. A stream or flow of fluid, air, or electricity.
action c., an electrical c. induced in muscle fibers when they are effectively stimulated; normally it is followed by contraction.
after-c., see aftercurrent.
alternating c. (AC), a c. that flows first in one direction then in the other; *e.g.,* 60-cycle c.
anodal c., a c. produced in tissues under the anode when the circuit is closed.
ascending c., centripetal c.; the direction of c. flow in a nerve when the anode is placed peripheral to the cathode, in contrast to descending c.; the convention used is that c. flows from positive to negative.
axial c., the central rapidly moving portion of the bloodstream in an artery.
centrifugal c., descending c.
centripetal c., ascending c.
d'Arsonval c., high frequency c.
demarcation c., c. of injury.
descending c., centrifugal c.; the direction of c. flow in a nerve when the cathode is placed peripheral to the anode, in contrast to ascending c.
direct c. (DC), a c. that flows only in one direction; *e.g.,* that derived from a battery; sometimes referred to as galvanic c. See also galvanism.
electrotonic c., see electrotonus.
galvanic c., see direct c.; galvanism(1).
high frequency c., d'Arsonval or Tesla c.; an alternating electric c. having a frequency of 10,000 or more per second; it produces no muscular contractions and does not affect the sensory nerves.
c. of injury, demarcation c.; the c. set up when an injured part of a nerve, muscle, or other excitable tissue is connected through a conductor with the uninjured region; the injured tissue is negative to the uninjured.
labile c., an electrical c. applied to the body by means of electrodes that are constantly shifted about.
Tesla c., high frequency c.

Curschmann, Heinrich, German physician, 1846–1910. See C.'s *disease, spirals.*

curse (kers). An affliction thought to be invoked by a malevolent spirit.
Ondine's c. [*Ondine,* G. myth. char.], sleep-induced *apnea.*

Curtis, Arthur H., U.S. gynecologist, 1881–1955. See Fitz-Hugh and C. *syndrome.*

curvatura, pl. **curvatu′rae** (ker′vă-tū′ră, -tū′rē) [L.] [NA]. Curvature.
c. ventric′uli ma′jor [NA], greater curvature of stomach; the border of the stomach to which the greater omentum is attached.
c. ventric′uli mi′nor [NA], lesser curvature of stomach; the right border of the stomach to which the lesser omentum is attached.

curvature (ker′vă-chūr) [L. *curvatura,* fr. *curvo,* pp. *-atus,* to bend, curve]. Curvatura; a bending or flexure.
angular c., Pott's c.; a gibbous deformity, *i.e.,* a sharp angulation of the spine, occurring in Pott's disease.
anterior c., kyphosis.
backward c., lordosis.
gingival c., the rounding of the gum along its line of attachment to the neck of a tooth.
greater c. of stomach, *curvatura* ventriculi major.
lateral c., scoliosis.
lesser c. of stomach, *curvatura* ventriculi minor.
occlusal c., *curve* of occlusion.
Pott's c., angular c.
spinal c., see kyphosis; lordosis; scoliosis.

curve (kerv) [L. *curvo,* to bend]. **1.** A nonangular continuous bend or line. **2.** A chart or graphic representation, by means of a continuous line of shifting direction, of the course of a physiological activity, of the number of cases of a disease in a given period, or of any entity which might be otherwise presented by a table of figures.
alignment c., the line passing through the center of the teeth laterally in the direction of the c. of the dental arch.
anti-Monson c., reverse c.
Barnes' c., a c. corresponding in general with Carus' c., being the segment of a circle whose center is the promontory of the sacrum.
buccal c., the line of the dental arch from the canine, or cuspid tooth to the third molar.
Carus' c., Carus' circle; an imaginary curved line obtained from a mathematical formula, supposed to indicate the outlet of the pelvic canal.
compensating c., the anteroposterior and lateral curvature in the alignment of the occluding surfaces and incisal edges of artificial teeth; used to develop balanced occlusion.
distribution c., frequency c.; a graph of a frequency distribution.
dose-response c., a graph showing the relationship between the dose of a drug, infectious agent, etc. and the biological response.
dye-dilution c., indicator-dilution c.; graph of the serial concen-

trations (dilutions) of a dye, *e.g.*, Evans blue, following its intravascular or intracardiac injection; useful in the diagnosis of congenital cardiac shunts, measurement of cardiac output, and detection of cardiovalvular incompetence.

epidemic c., a graph in which the number of new cases of a disease is plotted against an interval of time to describe a specific epidemic or outbreak.

flow-volume c., the graph produced by plotting the instantaneous flow of respiratory gas against the simultaneous lung volume, usually during maximal forced expiration.

Frank-Starling c., Starling's c.

frequency c., distribution c.

Friedman c., a graph on which hours of labor are plotted against cervical dilation in centimeters.

gaussian c., normal *distribution.*

growth c., a graphic representation of the change in size of an individual or a population over a period of time.

indicator-dilution c., dye-dilution c.

intracardiac pressure c., c. of pressure recorded within the atrium or ventricle (intra-atrial and intraventricular pressure c.'s).

isovolume pressure-flow c., the relationship between transpulmonary pressure and respiratory air flow, expressed as a function of lung volume.

logistic c., an S-shaped c. which depicts the growth of a population in an area of fixed limits.

milled-in c.'s, milled-in *paths.*

Monson c., the c. of occlusion in which each cusp and incisal edge touches or conforms to a segment of the surface of a sphere 8 inches in diameter with its center in the region of the glabella.

muscle c., myogram.

c. of occlusion, occlusal curvature; **(1)** a curved surface which makes simultaneous contact with the major portion of the incisal and occlusal prominences of the existing teeth; **(2)** the c. of a dentition on which the occlusal surfaces lie.

Pleasure c., a c. of occlusion which when viewed in sagittal section conforms to a line that is convex upward except for the last molars.

Price-Jones c., a distribution c. of the measured diameters of red blood cells; it is to the right of the normal c. (*i.e.*, indicating larger diameters) in instances of pernicious anemia and other forms in which macrocytes are present, and to the left (*i.e.*, indicating smaller diameters) in iron deficiency and other forms of microcytic anemia.

probability c., a graph of the normal distribution representing relative probabilities.

pulse c., sphygmogram.

reverse c., anti-Monson c.; in dentistry, a c. of occlusion which is convex upward.

c. of Spee, von Spee's c.; the anatomic curvature of the mandibular occlusal plane beginning at the tip of the lower cuspid and following the buccal cusps of the posterior teeth, continuing to the terminal molar.

Starling's c., Frank-Starling c.; a graph in which cardiac output is plotted against atrial pressure; with increasing venous return and atrial pressure the output proportionately increases until further increments overload the heart and the output falls.

strength-duration c., a graph relating the intensity of an electrical stimulus to the length of time it must flow to be effective. See chronaxie and rheobase.

stress-strain c., a c. showing the ratio of deformation to load during the testing of a material in tension.

tension c., the direction of the trabeculae in cancellous bone tissue adapted to resist stress.

Traube-Hering c.'s, Traube-Hering waves; slow oscillations in blood pressure usually extending over several respiratory cycles; related to variations in vasomotor tone; rhythmical variations in blood pressure.

von Spee's c., c. of Spee.

whole-body titration c., a graphic representation of the *in vivo* changes in hydrogen ion, PA_{CO_2} and bicarbonate which occur in arterial blood in response to primary acid-base disturbances.

Curvularia (ker-vyū-lā'rē-ă). A genus of dark-colored fungi that grow rapidly on culture media. Generally regarded as contaminants, two species, *C. lunata* and *C. geniculata,* are among the true species of fungi capable of producing mycetoma in man.

Cushing, Harvey W., U.S. neurosurgeon, 1869–1939. See C.'s *basophilism, disease, syndrome;* C. *effect, phenomenon, response.*

Cushing, Hayward W., U.S. surgeon, 1854– 1934. See C.'s *suture.*

cushingoid (kush'ing-oyd). Resembling the signs and symptoms of Cushing's disease or syndrome: buffalo hump obesity, striations, adiposity, hypertension, diabetes, and osteoporosis, usually due to exogenous corticosteroids.

cushion (kush'ŭn). In anatomy, any structure resembling a pad or c.

atrioventricular canal c.'s, endocardial c.'s; a pair of mounds of embryonic connective tissue covered by endothelium, bulging into the embryonic atrioventricular canal; located one dorsally and one ventrally, they grow together and fuse, dividing the originally single canal into right and left atrioventricular orifices.

endocardial c.'s, atrioventricular canal c.'s.

c. of epiglottis, *tuberculum* epiglotticum.

eustachian c., *torus* tubarius.

levator c., *torus* levatorius.

Passavant's c., Passavant's bar, pad, or ridge; a prominence on the posterior wall of the nasal pharynx formed by contraction of the superior constrictor of the pharynx during swallowing.

pharyngoesophageal c.'s, pharyngoesophageal pads; venous plexuses on the anterior and posterior walls of the pharyngoesophageal junction.

plantar c., a dense mass of fibrofatty tissue overlying the frog in the foot of the horse; serves an important shock-absorbing function.

sucking c., *corpus* adiposum buccae.

cusp (kŭsp) [L. *cuspis,* point]. Cuspis. **1.** In dentistry, a conical elevation arising on the surface of a tooth from an independent calcification center. See also *tuberculum* dentis. **2.** A leaflet of one of the heart's valves.

anterior c., *cuspis* anterior.

c. of Carabelli, a fifth c. found on the maxillary first molars, usually located lingual to the mesiolingual c.

posterior c., *cuspis* posterior.

septal c., *cuspis* septalis.

c. of tooth, *cuspis* dentis.

cuspad (kŭs'păd) [L. *ad,* to]. In a direction toward the cusp of a tooth.

cuspal (kŭs'păl). Pertaining to a cusp.

cusparia bark (kŭs-pā'rē-ă). Angostura bark.

cuspid (kŭs'pid) [L. *cuspis,* point]. **1.** Cuspidate; having but one cusp. **2.** *Dens* caninus.

cuspidate (kŭs'pi-dāt). Cuspid (1).

cuspis, pl. **cuspides** (kŭs'pis, kŭs'pi-dēz) [L. a point] [NA]. Cusp.

c. ante'rior [NA], anterior cusp; the anterior leaflet of either the right or left atrioventricular valve.

c. coro'nae [NA], alternate term for c. dentis.

c. den'tis [NA], cusp of tooth; c. coronae; an elevation or mound on the crown of a tooth making up a part of the occlusal surface.

c. poste'rior [NA], posterior cusp; the posterior leaflet of either the right or left atrioventricular valve.

c. septa'lis [NA], septal cusp; the leaflet of the right atrioventricular valve located adjacent to the interventricular septum.

cut (kŭt). In molecular biology, a hydrolytic cleavage of two opposing phosphodiester bonds in a double-stranded nucleic acid. *Cf.* nick.

cutaneomucosal (kyū-tă'nē-ō-myū-kō'săl). Mucocutaneous.

cutaneous (kyū-tā'nē-ŭs) [L. *cutis,* skin]. Relating to the skin.

cutch (kŭtch). *Catechu* nigrum.

cutdown (kŭt'down). Venostomy; dissection of a vein for insertion of a cannula or needle for the administration of intravenous fluids or medication.

Cuterebra (kyū-te-rē'bră) [L. *cutis,* skin, + *terebro,* to bore, fr. *terebra,* an auger]. A genus of botflies with large blue or black bumblebee-like adults, whose larvae most commonly infest rodents and lagomorphs (hares and rabbits); the larvae develop into large spiny grubs, usually in the subcutaneous connective tissue of the neck. Similar grubs, probably of other species, are not uncommon in cats and are sometimes found in dogs and in man.

cuticle (kyū'ti-kl) [L. *cuticula,* dim. of *cutis,* skin]. **1.** Cuticula (1). **2.** The layer, chitinous in some invertebrates, which occurs on the surface of epithelial cells. **3.** Epidermis.
acquired c., acquired enamel c., acquired *pellicle.*
dental c., *cuticula* dentis.
enamel c., *cuticula* dentis.
c. of hair, *cuticula* pili.
Nasmyth's c., *cuticula* dentis.
posteruption c., acquired *pellicle.*
c. of root sheath, cuticula vaginae folliculi pili; a thin layer of overlapping shingle-like cells lining the hair follicle.

cuticula, pl. cuticulae (kyū-tik'yū-lă, -lē) [L. cuticle]. **1** [NA]. Cuticle (1); an outer thin layer, usually horny in nature. **2.** Epidermis.
c. den'tis [NA], dental or enamel cuticle; Nasmyth's membrane or cuticle; membrana adamantina; adamantine membrane; skin of teeth; the primary enamel cuticle, consisting of two extremely thin layers (the inner one clear and structureless, the outer one cellular), covering the entire crown of newly erupted teeth and subsequently abraded by mastication; it is evident microscopically as an amorphous material between the attachment epithelium and the tooth.
c. pi'li, cuticle of hair; a layer of overlapping shingle-like cells that invest the hair cortex and serve to lock the hair shaft in its follicle.
c. vagi'nae follic'uli pi'li, cuticle of the sheath of the follicle of the hair.

cuticularization (kyū-tik'yū-lar-ĭ-zā'shŭn). Covering an abraded area with epidermis.

cutin (kyū'tin) [L. *cutis,* skin]. A specially prepared, thin, animal membrane used as a protective covering for wounded surfaces.

cutireaction (kyū'ti-rē-ak'shŭn) [L. *cutis,* skin, + reaction]. Cutaneous reaction; the inflammatory reaction in the case of a skin test in a sensitive (allergic) subject.

cutis (kyū'tis) [L.] [NA]. Skin; the membranous protective covering of the body, consisting of the epidermis and corium (dermis).
c. anseri'na, gooseflesh; contraction of the arrectores pilorum produced by cold, fear, or other stimulus, causing the follicular orifices to become prominent.
c. hyperelas'tica, Ehlers-Danlos *syndrome.*
c. lax'a, loose skin; dermatochalasis; pachydermatocele (1); a congenital condition characterized by degeneration of elastic fibers appearing as an excessive amount of skin hanging in folds; vascular anomalies may be present; inheritance is either dominant or recessive, the latter sometimes in association with pulmonary emphysema and diverticula of the alimentary tract or bladder.
c. marmora'ta, a pink, marble-like mottling of the skin on exposure to cold, common in children and some adults; also associated with debilitating diseases.
c. rhomboida'lis nu'chae, geometric configurations of the skin of the back of the neck as a result of aging or prolonged exposure to sunlight.
c. unctuo'sa, *seborrhea* oleosa.
c. ve'ra, corium.
c. ver'ticis gyra'ta, a congenital condition in which the skin of the scalp is hypertrophied and thrown into folds forming anterior to posterior furrows.

cutisector (kyū'ti-sek'tōr) [L. *cutis,* skin, + *sector,* a cutter]. **1.** Instrument for cutting small pieces of skin for grafting. **2.** Instrument used to remove a section of skin for microscopic examination.

cutization (kyū-ti-zā'shŭn). The transition from mucous membrane to skin at the mucocutaneous margins.

cuvet, cuvette (kū-vet'). A small container or cup in which solutions are placed for photometric analysis.

Cuvier, Georges L.C.F.D. de la, French scientist, 1769–1832. See C.'s *ducts, veins.*

CV Abbreviation for *coefficient* of variation; cardiovascular; closing *volume.*

CVA Abbreviation for cerebral vascular *accident.*

CVP Abbreviation for central venous *pressure.*

cyamemazine (sī-ă-mem'ă-zēn). 10-(3-Dimethylamino-2-methylpropyl)-phenothiazine-2-carbonitrile; a sedative with antihistaminic and antispasmodic properties.

cyan- See cyano-.

cyanalcohols (sī-an-al'kō-holz). Cyanohydrins.

cyanamide (sī-an'i-mīd). An irritating and caustic water-soluble substance, H_2NCN or $NH{=}C{=}NH$; often used in referring to calcium cyanamide.

cyanate (sī'an-āt). The radical —O—C≡N or ion $(CNO)^-$.

cyanemia (sī-a-ne'mē-ă) [cyan- + G. *haima,* blood]. Obsolete term for cyanosis.

cyanide (sī'an-īd). The radical –CN or ion $(CN)^-$. The ion is extremely poisonous, forming hydrocyanic acid in water.
c. methemoglobin, cyanmethemoglobin.

cyanidenon (sī-ă-nid'ĕ-non). Luteolin.

cyanidol (sī'an-i-dol). Catechin.

cyanmethemoglobin (sī'an-met-hē'mō-glō-bin). Cyanide methemoglobin; a relatively nontoxic compound of cyanide with methemoglobin, which is formed when methylene blue is administered in cases of cyanide poisoning.

cyano-, cyan- [G. *kyanos,* a dark blue mineral] **1.** Combining forms meaning blue. **2.** Chemical prefix frequently used in naming compounds that contain the cyanide group, CN.

Cyanobacteria (sī'ă-nō-bak-tēr'ē-ă). Cyanophyceae; a division of the kingdom Procaryotae consisting of unicellular or filamentous bacteria that are either nonmotile or possess a gliding motility, reproduce by binary fission, and perform photosynthesis with the production of oxygen. These blue-green bacteria were formerly referred to as blue-green algae.

cyanochroic, cyanochrous (sī-an-ō-krō'ik, sī-an-ok'rŭs) [cyano- + G. *chroia,* color]. Cyanotic.

cyanocobalamin (sī'an-ō-kō-bal'ă-min). A complex of cyanide and cobalamin, as in vitamin B_{12}.
radioactive c., cyano[^{57}Co]cobalamin, cyano[^{58}Co]cobalamin, or cyano[^{60}Co]cobalamin produced by the growth of certain microorganisms on a medium containing cobalt-57, cobalt-58, or cobalt-60; used in the investigation of the absorption and metabolism of cyanocobalamin (vitamin B_{12}).

cyanogen (sī-an'ō-jen). Ethanedinitrile; a compound of two cyano radicals, NC-CN; its highly toxic compounds (general formula X-CN, where X is a halogen) are used in chemical syntheses and as tissue preservatives.
c. chloride, CNCl; a highly volatile liquid; a systemic poison used as a warning agent in fumigation with hydrogen cyanide.

cyanogenic (sī′an-ō-jen′ik). Capable of producing hydrocyanic acid; said of plants such as sorghum, Johnson grass, arrowgrass, and wild cherry which may cause cyanide poisoning in herbivorous animals.

cyanohydrins (sī′an-ō-hī′drinz). Cyanalcohols; R-CHOH-CN; addition compounds of HCN and aldehydes.

cyanophil, cyanophile (sī′an-ō-fil, -fīl) [cyano- + G. *philos,* fond]. A cell or element which is differentially colored blue by a staining procedure.

cyanophilous (sī-ă-nof′i-lŭs). Readily stainable with a blue dye.

Cyanophyceae (sī′ă-nō-fī′sē-ē) [cyano- + G. *phykos,* seaweed]. Cyanobacteria.

cyanopia (sī-ă-nō′pē-ă). Cyanopsia.

cyanopsia (sī-ă-nop′sē-ă) [cyano- + G. *opsis,* vision]. Cyanopia; blue vision; a condition in which all objects appear blue; may temporarily follow cataract extraction.
c. ret′inae, obsolete term for retinal venous dilation in blood hyperviscosity syndromes.

cyanose tardive (sī′ă-nōs tar′dēv). Cyanosis that is slow to appear; applied to the potentially cyanotic group of congenital heart diseases with an abnormal communication between systemic and pulmonary circulations; cyanosis is absent while the shunt is from left to right, but if the shunt reverses, as after exercise or late in the course of the disease, cyanosis appears.

cyanosed (sī′ă-nōsd). Cyanotic.

cyanosis (sī-ă-nō′sis) [G. dark blue color, fr. *kyanos,* blue substance]. A dark bluish or purplish coloration of the skin and mucous membrane due to deficient oxygenation of the blood, evident when reduced hemoglobin in the blood exceeds 5 g per 100 ml.
compression c., c. accompanied by edema and petechial hemorrhages over the head, neck, and upper part of the chest, as a venous reflex resulting from severe compression of the thorax or abdomen; the conjunctiva and retinas are similarly affected.
enterogenous c., apparent c. caused by the absorption of nitrites or other toxic materials from the intestine with the formation of methemoglobin or sulfhemoglobin; the skin color change is due to the chocolate color of methemoglobin.
false c., c. due to the presence of an abnormal pigment, such as methemoglobin, in the blood, and not resulting from a deficiency of oxygen.
hereditary methemoglobinemic c., congenital *methemoglobinemia.*
c. ret′inae, venous congestion of the retina.
tardive c., *cyanose* tardive.
toxic c., c. due to methemoglobin formation resulting from the action of certain drugs, *e.g.,* nitrites.

cyanotic (sī-ă-not′ik). Cyanochroic, cyanochrous; cyanosed; relating to or marked by cyanosis.

cyanuria (sī-ă-nū′rē-ă) [cyano- + G. *ouron,* urine]. The presence of blue urine.

cyanuric acid (sī-ă-nūr′ik). 2,4,6-Trihydroxy-1,3,5-triazine; a cyclic product formed by heating urea; used industrially and as an herbicide.

Cyathostoma (sī-ă-thos′tō-mă) [G. *kyathos,* cup, cup-shaped, + *stoma,* mouth]. A genus of gapeworms of poultry in the nematode family Syngamidae, so called because of the gaping habit of fowl infected by these worms in their upper respiratory tract.
C. bronchia′lis, a species found in wild geese and domestic ducks, geese, and swans; occurs in the larynx, trachea, and bronchi and causes distress and symptoms similar to those produced by the chicken gapeworm, *Syngamus trachea;* its life cycle is thought to be similar to that of *Syngamus trachea.*

Cyathostomum (sī-ă-thos′tō-mŭm) [see *Cyathostoma*]. A genus of strongyle nematodes (family Cyasthostomidae, formerly part of the family Strongylidae); it includes many of the small strongyles of horses formerly placed in the genus *Trichonema,* which have been variously divided into a number of genera and subgenera.

cybernetics (sī-ber-net′iks) [G. *kybernētica,* things pertaining to control or piloting]. **1.** The comparative study of electronic calculators and the human nervous system, with intent to explain the functioning of the brain. **2.** The science of control and communication in both living and nonliving systems; characteristically, control is governed by feedback, that is, by communication within the system concerning the difference between the actual and the desired result, action then being modified so as to minimize this difference. See also feedback.

cybrid (sī′brid) [cell + hybrid]. A cell with cytoplasm from two different cells as a result of cell hybridization.

cycl-. See cyclo-.

cyclamate (sī′klă-māt). A salt or ester of cyclamic acid; the calcium and sodium are noncaloric artificial sweetening agents.

cyclamic acid (sī-klam′ik). Cyclohexanesulfamic or cyclohexylsulfamic acid; a sweetening agent, usually used as sodium or calcium cyclamate.

cyclamide (sī′klă-mīd). Glycyclamide.

cyclandelate (sī-klan′de-lāt). 3,3,5-Trimethylcyclohexyl mandelate; an antispasmodic similar in action to papaverine; used for obliterative vascular diseases and vasospastic conditions.

cyclarbamate (sī-klar′bă-māt). Cyclopentaphene; 1,1-cyclopentanedimethanol dicarbanilate; a tranquilizer with antispasmodic properties.

cyclarthrodial (sī-klar-thrō′dē-ăl). Relating to a cyclarthrosis.

cyclarthrosis (sī-klar-thrō′sis) [cyclo- + G. *arthrōsis,* articulation]. A joint capable of rotation.

cyclase (sī′klās). Descriptive name applied to an enzyme that forms a cyclic compound; *e.g.,* adenylate cyclase.

cyclazocine (sī-klā′zō-sēn). A benzomorphan derivative with potent narcotic antagonist properties.

CYCLE

cycle (sī′kl) [G. *kyklos,* circle]. **1.** A recurrent series of events. **2.** A recurring period of time. **3.** One successive compression and rarefaction of a wave, as of a sound wave.
anovulatory c., a sexual c. in which no ovum is discharged.
brain wave c., the complete upward and downward excursion of a single wave, complex, or impulse as seen on an electroencephalogram.
carbon dioxide c., carbon c., the circulation of carbon as CO_2 from the expired air of animals and decaying organic matter to plant life where it is synthesized (through photosynthesis) to carbohydrate material, from which, as a result of catabolic processes in all life, it is again ultimately released to the atmosphere as CO_2. See fig. on p. 384.
cardiac c., the complete round of cardiac systole and diastole with the intervals between, or commencing with, any event in the heart's action to the moment when that same event is repeated. See fig. on p. 384.
cell c., the cyclic biochemical and structural events occurring during rapid growth of cells such as in tissue culture; the c. is divided into periods called: G_0, Gap_1 (G_1), synthesis (S_1), Gap_2 (G_2), and mitosis (M).
chewing c., a complete course of movement of the mandible during a single masticatory stroke.
citric acid c., tricarboxylic acid c.

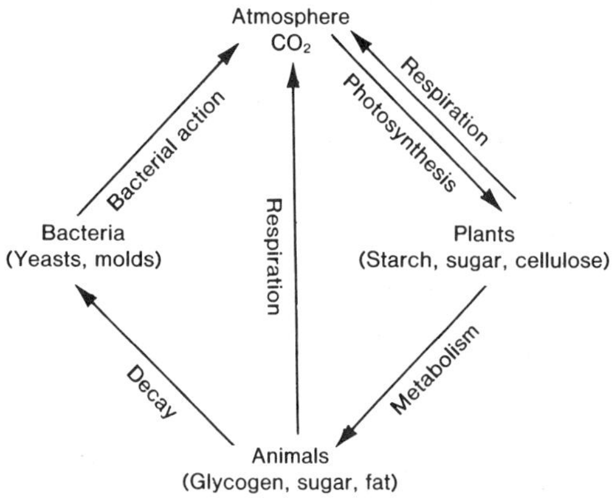

Carbon Dioxide Cycle
(After Haekle)

Estrous Cycle of Common Domesticated Animals

Species	Length		Estrus	
	Days	Average	Days	Average
Horse	19–23	21	4.5–5.5	5.3 days
Cow	18–24	21	0.5–1.0	18 hr.
Sheep	14–20	17	0.5–2.0	20 hr.
Goat	15–24	20	2–5	40 hr.
Swine	18–24	21	1–5	2 days
Dog	Usually 2 cycles per year		4–13	7–8 days
Cat	2 or 3 cycles per year		15–21	8 days

Cori c., the phases in the metabolism of carbohydrate: 1) glycogenolysis in the liver; 2) passage of glucose into the circulation; 3) deposition of glucose in the muscles as glycogen; 4) glycogenolysis during muscular activity and conversion to lactate, which is converted to glycogen in the liver.
dicarboxylic acid c., that portion of the tricarboxylic acid c. involving the dicarboxylic acids (succinic, fumaric, malic, and oxaloacetic acids).
endogenous c., the portion of a parasitic life cycle occurring within the host.
estrous c., the series of physiologic uterine, ovarian, and other changes that occur in higher animals, consisting of proestrus, estrus, postestrus, and anestrus or diestrus.
exoerythrocytic c., that nonpathogenic portion of the vertebrate phase of the life cycle of malarial organisms that takes place in liver cells, outside of the blood cells.
exogenous c., the portion of a parasitic life cycle occurring outside the host.
fatty acid oxidation c., a series of reactions involving acyl-coenzyme A compounds, whereby these undergo beta oxidation and

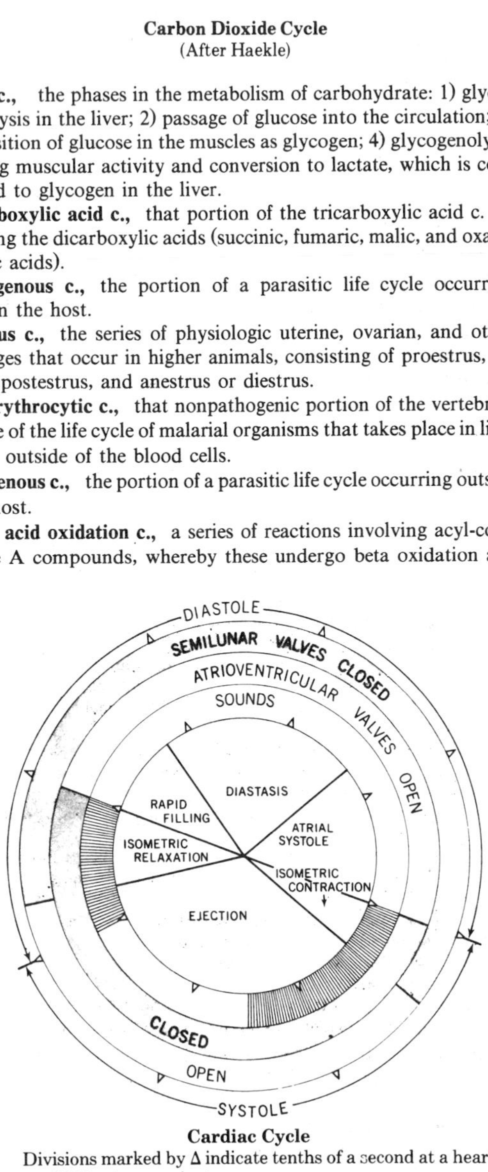

Cardiac Cycle
Divisions marked by Δ indicate tenths of a second at a heart rate of 75 beats per minute.

thioclastic cleavage, with the formation of acetylcoenzyme A; the major pathway of fatty acid catabolism in living tissue.
forced c., a cardiac c. (atrial or ventricular) that is cut short by a forced beat.
genesial c., the reproductive period of a woman's life.
glycine succinate c., a series of metabolic steps in which glycine, probably as pyruvate, is condensed with succinic acid and is then oxidized to CO_2 and H_2O with regeneration of the succinic acid.
glyoxylic acid c., a catabolic c. in plants and microorganisms like that of the tricarboxylic acid c. in animals; its key reaction is the condensation of acetate with glyoxylic acid to malic acid (analogous to the condensation of acetate and oxaloacetic acid to form citric acid in the tricarboxylic acid c.).
hair c., the cyclical phases of growth (anagen), regression (catagen), and quiescence (telogen) in the life of a hair.
Krebs c., tricarboxylic acid c.
Krebs-Henseleit c., Krebs ornithine c., Krebs urea c., urea c.
life c., the entire life history of a living organism.
masticating c.'s, the patterns of mandibular movements formed during the chewing of food.
menstrual c., the period in which an ovum matures, is ovulated, and enters the uterine lumen via the fallopian tubes; ovarian hormonal secretions effect endometrial changes such that, if fertilization occurs, nidation will be possible; in the absence of fertilization, ovarian secretions wane, the endometrium sloughs, and menstruation begins; this c. lasts an average of 28 days, with day 1 of the c. designated as that day on which menstrual flow begins.
nitrogen c., the series of events in which the nitrogen of the atmosphere is fixed, thus made available for plant and animal life, and is then returned to the atmosphere: nitrifying bacteria convert N_2 and O_2 to NO_2^- and NO_3^-, the latter being absorbed by plants and converted to protein; if plants decay, the nitrogen is in part given up to the atmosphere and the remainder is converted by microorganisms to ammonia, nitrites, and nitrates; if the plants are eaten, the animals' excreta or bacterial decay return the nitrogen to the soil and air.
ornithine c., urea c.
ovarian c., the normal sex c. which includes development of an ovarian (graafian) follicle, rupture of the follicle with discharge of the ovum, and formation and regression of a corpus luteum.
reproductive c., the c. which begins with conception and extends through gestation and parturition.
restored c., an atrial or ventricular cardiac c. that follows the returning c. and resumes the normal rhythm.
returning c., an atrial or ventricular cardiac c. that begins with an extrasystole or a forced beat.
succinic acid c., a series of oxidation reduction reactions in which succinic acid and other 4-carbon atoms acids (fumaric, malic, oxaloacetic) take part in the oxidation of pyruvic acid as part of the

tricarboxylic acid c. See also dicarboxylic acid c.

tricarboxylic acid c., citric acid or Krebs c.; the main source of energy in the mammalian body and the end toward which carbohydrate, fat, and protein metabolism are directed; a series of reactions, beginning and ending with oxaloacetic acid, during the course of which a two-carbon fragment is completely oxidized to carbon dioxide and water with the production of twelve high-energy phosphate bonds. So called because the first four substances involved (citric acid, *cis* -aconitic acid, isocitric acid, and oxalosuccinic acid) are all tricarboxylic acids; from oxalosuccinate, the others are, in order, α-ketoglutarate, succinate, fumarate, L-malate, and oxaloacetate which condenses with acetyl-CoA (from fatty acid degradation) to form citrate (citric acid) again.

urea c., Krebs ornithine or urea c.; Krebs-Henseleit c.; ornithine c.; the sequence of chemical reactions, occurring in the liver, that results in the production of urea; the key reaction is the hydrolysis of arginine by arginase to ornithine and urea; ornithine is then converted to citrulline by a carbamoylation reaction involving glutamic acid and then to arginine again by an amination reaction involving aspartic acid.

visual c., the transformation of carotenoids involved in the bleaching and regeneration of the visual pigment:

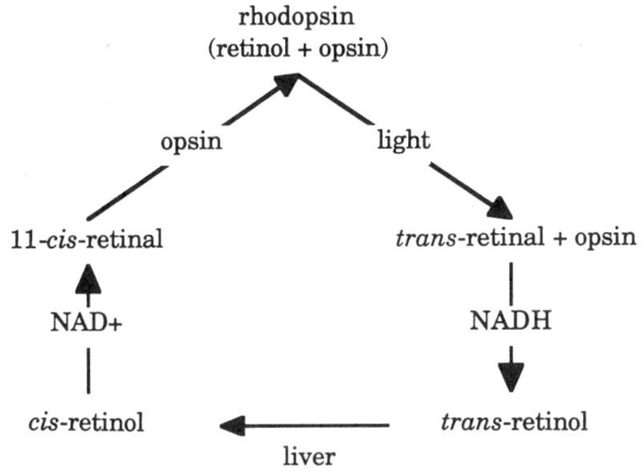

cyclectomy (sī-klek'tō-mē, sik-lek'tō-mē) [cyclo- + G. *ektomē,* excision]. Ciliectomy; excision of a portion of the ciliary body.

cyclencephaly, cyclencephalia (sī-klen-sef'ă-lē, -se-fā'lē-ă) [cyclo- + G. *enkephalos,* brain]. Cyclocephalia; cyclocephaly; condition in a malformed fetus characterized by poor development and a varying degree of fusion of the two cerebral hemispheres.

cycles per second (cps). The number of successive compressions and rarefactions per second of a sound wave. The preferred designation for this unit of frequency is hertz.

cyclic (sī'klik, sik'lik). **1.** Pertaining to, or characteristic of, a cycle; occurring periodically, denoting the course of the symptoms in certain diseases or disorders. **2.** In chemistry, continuous, without end, as in a ring; denoting a cyclic compound.

cyclic AMP (cAMP). Adenosine 3′,5′-cyclic phosphate.

3′,5′-cyclic AMP synthetase. *Adenylate* cyclase.

cyclicotomy (sī-klī-kot'ō-mē). Cyclotomy.

cyclitis (sī-klī'tis) [G. *kyklos,* circle (ciliary body), + *-itis,* inflammation]. Inflammation of the ciliary body.

heterochromic c., a chronic inflammatory c. in which the iris of the affected eye becomes atrophic.

plastic c., inflammation of the ciliary body, and usually of the entire uveal tract, with a fibrinous exudation into the anterior and vitreous chambers.

purulent c., suppurative inflammation of the ciliary body.

cyclizine hydrochloride (sī'kli-zēn). 1-Diphenylmethyl-4-methylpiperazine hydrochloride; an antihistamine agent useful in the prevention and relief of motion sickness and symptoms caused by vestibular disorders.

cyclizine lactate. An agent with the same use and action as the hydrochloride.

cyclo-, cycl- [G. *kyklos,* circle]. **1.** Combining forms relating to a circle or cycle, or denoting association with the ciliary body. **2.** In chemistry, a combining form indicating a continuous molecule, without end, or the formation of such a structure between two parts of a molecule.

cyclobarbital (sī-klō-bar'bi-tawl). 5-(1-Cyclohexen-1-yl)-5-ethylbarbituric acid; formerly used as a mild hypnotic and for pre- and postoperative sedation.

cyclobenzaprine hydrochloride (sī-klō-ben'ză-prēn). 1-Propanamine, 3-(5*H*- dibenzo[*a,d*]cyclohepten-5-ylidene)-*N,N*- diemthyl-, hydrochloride; a skeletal muscle relaxant used to relieve acute muscular spasms.

cyclocephaly, cyclocephalia (sī-klō-sef'ă-lē, -sĕ-fā'lē-ă) [cyclo- + G. *kephalē,* head]. Cyclencephaly.

cyclochoroiditis (sī'klō-kō-roy-dī'tis). Inflammation of the ciliary body and the choroid.

cyclocryotherapy (sī'klō-krī'ō-thār'ă-pē). Transscleral freezing of the ciliary body in the treatment of glaucoma.

cyclocumarol (sī-klō-kyū'mă-rol). 4-Hydroxycoumarin anticoagulant No. 63; a synthetic anticoagulant compound, related to bishydroxycoumarin.

cyclodialysis (sī'klō-dī-al'i-sis) [cyclo- + G. *dialysis,* separation]. Heine's operation; establishment of a communication between the anterior chamber and the suprachoroidal space in order to reduce intraocular pressure in glaucoma.

cyclodiathermy (sī'klō-dī-ă-ther'mē). Diathermy applied to the sclera adjacent to the ciliary body in the treatment of glaucoma.

cycloduction (sī-klō-dŭk'shŭn) [cyclo- + L. *duco,* pp. *ductus,* to draw]. Circumduction (2); rotation of the upper pole of one cornea.

cycloelectrolysis (sī'klō-ē-lek-trol'i-sis). Electrolysis applied to the ciliary body to reduce ocular pressure.

cycloguanil pamoate (sī-klō-gwahn'il). Chloroguanide triazine pamoate; 4,6-diamino-1-(*p*-chlorophenyl)-1,2-dihydro-2,2-dimethyl-*s* -triazine pamoate; a long-acting antimalarial agent that prevents the growth or survival of the pre-erythrocytic and erythrocytic parasites.

cyclohexanesulfamic acid (sī-klō-heks'an-sŭl-fam'ik). Cyclamic acid.

cyclohexatriene (sī'klō-heks-ă-trī'ēn). Benzene.

cycloheximide (sī-klō-heks'i-mīd). 3-[2-(3,5-Dimethyl-2-oxocyclohexyl)-2-hydroxyethyl]glutarimide; an antibiotic obtained from certain strains of *Streptomyces griseus;* used in biochemical research to inhibit *in vitro* protein synthesis; also a fungicide and rat repellent.

cyclohexitol (sī-klō-heks'i-tol). Inositol.

cyclohexylsulfamic acid (sī-klō-hek'sil-sŭl-fam'ik). Cyclamic acid.

cycloid (sī'kloyd) [cyclo- + G. *eidos,* resembling]. Suggesting cyclothymia; a term applied to a person who tends to have periods of marked swings of mood, but within normal limits.

cyclol (sī'klol). A cyclic dipeptide postulated as occurring in proteins; it does occur in some of the ergot alkaloids.

cyclomethycaine sulfate (sī-klō-meth'i-kān). 3-(2-Methylpiperidinyl)propyl *p*-(cyclohexyloxy)benzoate sulfate; a topical anesthetic.

cyclonamine (sī-klō-nā'mēn). Ethamsylate.

cyclopea (sī-klō'pē-ă) Cyclopia.

cyclopean (sī-klō'pē-an). Cyclopian.

cyclopentamine hydrochloride (sī-klō-pent'ă-mēn). *N*,α-dimethylcyclopentaneethylamine hydrochloride; 1-cyclopentyl-2-methylaminopropane hydrochloride; a sympathomimetic amine, similar in action to ephedrine.

cyclopentane (sī-klō-pen'tān). Pentamethylene; $(CH_2)_5$; a closed ring hydrocarbon containing 5 carbon atoms, isomeric with pentene.

cyclopenta[*a*]phenanthrene. Phenanthrene, to the *a* side of which a three-carbon fragment is fused; as the perhydro (saturated) derivative, it is the basic structure of the steroids.

cyclopentaphene (sī-klō-pen'tă-fēn). Cyclarbamate.

cyclopenthiazide (sī'klō-pen-thī'ă-zīd). $C_{13}H_{18}ClN_3O_4S_2$; a benzothiadiazide diuretic.

cyclopentolate hydrochloride (sī-klō-pen'tō-lāt). 2-(Dimethylamino) ethyl- 1-hydroxy- α-phenylcyclopentaneacetate hydrochloride; an anticholinergic, spasmolytic drug, used in refraction determinations; causes cycloplegia and mydriasis.

cyclopeptide (sī-klō-pep'tīd). A polypeptide lacking terminal —NH_2 and —COOH groups by virtue of their combination to form another peptide link, forming a ring.

cyclophenazine hydrochloride (sī-klō-fen'ă-zēn). 10-[3-(4-Cyclopropyl-1-piperazinyl)propyl]-2-(trifluoromethyl)phenothiazine dihydrochloride; a tranquilizing drug.

cyclophorases (sī-klō-fōr'ās-ez). The group of enzymes in mitochondria which catalyze the complete oxidation of pyruvic acid to carbon dioxide and water; essentially, those enzymes and coenzymes involved in the tricarboxylic acid cycle.

cyclophoria (sī-klō-fō'rē-ă) [cyclo- + G. *phora,* movement]. Abnormal tendency for the upper poles of each cornea to rotate inward or outward, the rotation being prevented by visual fusional impulses.

cyclophosphamide (sī-klō-fos'fă-mīd). *N,N*-Bis-(2-chloroethyl)-*N* '-(3-hydroxypropyl)phosphordiamidic acid cyclic ester monohydrate; an alkylating agent with antitumor activity and uses similar to those of its parent compound, nitrogen mustard (mechlorethamine hydrochloride); also a suppressor of B-cell activity and antibody formation, used to treat autoimmune diseases.

cyclophotocoagulation (sī'klō-fō'tō-kō-ag-yū-lā'shŭn) [cyclo- + photocoagulation, *q.v.*]. Photocoagulation of the ciliary processes to reduce the secretion of aqueous humor in glaucoma.

cyclophrenia (sī-klō-frē'nē-ă) [cyclo- + G. *phrēn,* the mind]. Obsolete term for manic-depressive *psychosis.*

Cyclophyllidae (sī-klō-fil'i-dē) [cyclo- + G. *phyllon,* leaf]. An order of tapeworms that includes most of the common parasites of man and domestic animals.

cyclopia (sī-klō'pē-ă) [G. *Kyklōps,* fr. *kyklos,* circle, + *ōps,* eye]. Synophthalmia; synophthalmus; a congenital defect in which the two orbits merge to form a single cavity containing one eye, its origin evidenced by fusion of the right and left optic primordia; usually combined with cyclencephaly.

cyclopian (sī-klō'pē-an). Denoting or relating to cyclopia.

cycloplegia (sī-klō-plē'jē-ă) [cyclo- + G. *plēgē,* stroke]. Paralysis of accommodation; loss of power in the ciliary muscle of the eye; may be pathologic or induced.

cycloplegic (sī-klō-plē'jik). **1.** Relating to cycloplegia. **2.** A drug that paralyzes the ciliary muscle and thus the power of accommodation.

cyclopropane (sī-klō-prō'pān). Trimethylene; $(CH_2)_3$; an explosive gas of characteristic odor, used for producing general anesthesia.

cyclops (sī'klops) [see cyclopia]. Monoculus (1); monophthalmus; monops; an individual with cyclopia.

cycloserine (sī-klō-ser'ēn). Orientomycin; D-4-amino-3-isoxazolidinone; cyclic anhydride of serine amide; an antibiotic produced by strains of *Streptomyces orchidaceus* or *S. garyphalus* with a wide spectrum of antibacterial activity.

cyclosis (sī-klō'sis) [G., fr. *kykloō,* to move around]. The movement of the protoplasm and contained plastids within the protozoan cell.

cyclosporin A (sī-klō-spōr'in). Cyclosporine.

cyclosporine (sī-klō-spōr'ēn). Cyclosporin A; $C_{62}H_{111}N_{11}O_{12}$; a cyclic oligopeptide immunosupressant produced by the fungus *Tolypocladium inflatum Gams;* used to inhibit organ transplant rejection.

cyclothiazide (sī-klō-thī'ă-zīd). 6-Chloro-3,4-dihydro-3-(2-norbornen-5-yl)-2*H*-1,2,4-benzothiadiazine-7-sulfonamide 1,1-dioxide; a diuretic and antihypertensive.

cyclothymia (sī-klō-thī'mē-ă) [cyclo- + G. *thymos,* rage]. A condition characterized by marked swings of mood, but within normal limits.

cyclothymiac, cyclothymic (sī-klō-thī'mē-ă, -thī'mik). Relating to cyclothymia.

cyclotome (sī'klō-tōm). A delicate knife for use in cyclotomy.

cyclotomy (sī-klot'ō-mē) [cyclo- + G. *tomē,* incision]. Cyclicotomy; operation of cutting the ciliary muscle.

cyclotron (sī'klō-tron). An accelerator that produces high-speed ions (*e.g.,* protons and deuterons) under the influence of an alternating magnetic field, for bombardment and disruption of atomic nuclei.

cyclotropia (sī-klō-trō'pē-ă) [cyclo- + G. *tropē,* a turn, turning]. A meridional deviation around the anterior-posterior axis of one eye with respect to the other.

cyclozoonosis (sī'klō-zō-ō-nō'sis) [cyclo- + G. *zōon,* animal, + *nosos,* disease]. A zoonosis that requires more than one vertebrate host (but no invertebrate) for completion of the life cycle; *e.g.,* various taenioid cestodes such as *Taenia saginata* and *T. solium* in which man is an obligatory host; hydatid disease, a c. in which man is not an obligatory host.

cycrimine hydrochloride (sī'kri-mēn). 1-Phenyl-1-cyclopentyl-3-piperidino-1-propanol hydrochloride; an anticholinergic drug used in the treatment of parkinsonism.

Cyd Symbol for cytidine.

cyesis (sī-ē'sis) [G. *kyēsis*] Obsolete term for pregnancy.

cyheptamide (sī-hep'tă-mīd). 10,11-Dihydro-5*H*-dibenzo-[*a,d*]cycloheptene-5-carboxamide; an anticonvulsant.

cyl. Abbreviation for cylinder, or cylindrical *lens.*

cylinder (cyl.) (sil'in-der) [G. *kylindros,* a roll]. **1.** A cylindrical *lens.* **2.** A cylindrical or rodlike renal cast. **3.** A cylindrical metal container for gases stored under high pressure.

axis c., obsolete term for axon.

Bence Jones c.'s, slightly irregular, relatively smooth, rod-shaped or cylindroid bodies of fairly tenacious, viscid proteinaceous material in the fluid of the seminal vesicles.

crossed c.'s, a lens used in refraction to determine the strength and axis of a cylindrical lens to correct astigmatism; a combination of concave and convex cylinders of like power whose axes are at right angles to each other.

Külz's c., coma *cast.*

cylindraxis (sil-in-drak'sis). Historical precursor of the term axon, based on an interpretation of the myelinated nerve fiber as a cylinder of which the axon formed the axis.

cylindrical (si-lin'dri-kăl). Shaped like a cylinder; referring to a cylinder.

cylindroadenoma (sil'in-drō-ad-ē-nō'mă). Cylindroma.

cylindroid (sil'in-droyd) [G. *kylindrōdēs,* fr. *kylindros,* roll, cylinder, + *eidos,* appearance]. False *cast.*

cylindroma (sil-in-drō'mă) [G. *kylindros,* cylinder, *-oma,* tumor]. Cylindroadenoma; a histologic type of epithelial neoplasm, frequently malignant, characterized by islands of neoplastic cells embedded in a hyalinized stroma which may represent a thickened basement membrane; may form from ducts of glands, especially in salivary glands, skin, and bronchi; in the salivary glands, also termed adenoid cystic carcinomas.

cylindrosarcoma (sil'in-drō-sar-kō'mă). Obsolete term for a sarcoma that manifests several foci of hyaline degenerative changes, such as those observed in cylindromas.

cylindruria (sil-in-drū'rē-ă). The presence of renal cylinders or casts in the urine.

cyllosoma (sil-ō-sō'mă) [G. *kyllos,* deformed, esp. clubfooted or bandylegged, + *sōma,* body]. One-sided congenital defect of the lower abdominal wall with defective development of the corresponding leg.

cymarin (sī'mă-rin). K-Strophanthin-α, a glycoside of cymarose present in the seeds of *Strophanthus kombé;* the aglycone is strophanthin; a cardiotonic.

cymba conchae (sim'bă kong'kē) [G. *kymbē,* the hollow of a vessel, a cup, bowl, a boat] [NA]. The upper, smaller part of the external ear lying above the crus helicis.

cymbocephalic, cymbocephalous (sim-bō-se-fal'ik, -sef'ă-lŭs). Relating to cymbocephaly.

cymbocephaly (sim-bō-sef'ălē) [G. *kymbē,* the hollow of a vessel, a boat-shaped structure, + *kephalē,* head]. Scaphocephaly.

cynanche (sin-ang'kē) [L. fr. G. *kynanchē,* dog quinsy, sore throat, fr. *kyōn (kym-),* dog, + *anchō,* to throttle]. Sore *throat.*

cynanthropy (sī-nan'thrō-pē) [G. *kyōn,* dog, + *anthrōpos,* man]. A delusion in which one barks and growls, imagining himself to be a dog.

cynic (sin'ik) [G. *kynikos,* doglike]. Doglike, denoting a spasm of the muscles of the face as in risus caninus.

cynocephaly (sī-nō-sef'ă-lē) [G. *kyōn,* dog, + *kephalē,* head]. Craniostenosis in which the skull slopes back from the orbits, producing a resemblance to the head of a dog.

cynodont (sī'nō-dont) [G. *kyōn,* dog, + *odous (odont-),* tooth]. **1.** A canine tooth, **2.** A tooth having one cusp or point.

cynophobia (sī-nō-fō'bē-ă) [G. *kyōn,* dog, + *phobos,* fear]. Morbid fear of dogs.

Cyon, Elie de, Russian physiologist, 1843–1912. See C.'s *nerve.*

cypridophobia (sī'pri-dō-fō'bē-ă) [G. *Kypris,* Aphrodite, + *phobos,* fear]. Morbid fear of venereal disease or of sexual intercourse.

Cyprinidae (sī-prin'i-dē) [G. *kyprinos,* a carp]. A family of bony freshwater fishes including the goldfishes, carp, chubs, and minnows.

cyproheptadine hydrochloride (sī-prō-hep'tă-dēn). 1-Methyl-4-(5-dibenzo-[a,e]-cycloheptatrienylidine)-piperidine; a potent antagonist of histamine and serotonin, with antihistaminic and antipruritic actions.

cyproterone acetate (sī-prō'ter-ōn). 6-Chloro-1β,2β-dihydro-17-hydroxy-3'*H*-cyclopropa[1,2]pregna-1,4,6-triene-3,20-dione acetate; a synthetic steroid capable of inhibiting the biological effects exerted by endogenous or exogenous androgenic hormones; an antiandrogen.

cyrtometer (ser-tom'ĕ-ter) [G. *kyrtos,* bent, + *metron,* measure]. An instrument for determining the size and shape of the chest.

Cys (Cys) Symbol for cysteine (half-cystine) or its mono- or diradical.

CYST

cyst (sist) [G. *kystis,* bladder]. Cystis. **1.** A bladder. **2.** An abnormal sac containing gas, fluid, or a semisolid material, with a membranous lining. See also pseudocyst.

adventitious c., pseudocyst (1).

allantoic c., urachal c.

alveolar hydatid c., multilocular hydatid c.; a hydatid c. of a multiloculate type, usually in the liver, caused by *Echinococcus multilocularis,* adults of which are in foxes; larvae (alveolar hydatid) are found chiefly in microtine rodents, but also among humans such as trappers and others handling pelts of infected foxes and other carnivores; growth is by exogenous budding and is not limited by an outer laminated membrane as in the hydatid c. from *E. granulosus;* necrosis, cavitation, contiguous spread, and death usually ensue.

aneurysmal bone c., benign bone aneurysm; a solitary benign osteolytic lesion expanding a long bone or within a vertebra, consisting of blood-filled spaces, and separated by fibrous tissue containing multinucleated giant cells; such c.'s cause swelling, pain, and tenderness.

apical periodontal c., periapical, radicular, or root end c.; an inflammatory odontogenic c. derived histogenetically from Malassez' epithelial rests surrounding the root apex of a nonvital tooth.

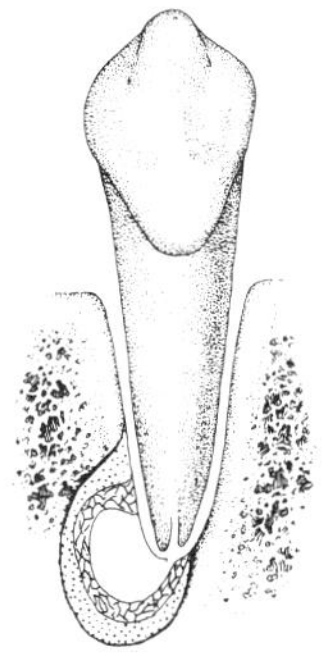

Apical Periodontal Cyst

apoplectic c., a pseudocyst formed of the effused blood in a stroke.

arachnoid c., a fluid-filled c. lined with arachnoid membrane, frequently situated near the lateral aspect of the fissure of Sylvius; usually congenital in origin.

Baker's c., a collection of synovial fluid which has escaped from the knee joint or a bursa and formed a new synovial-lined sac in the popliteal space; seen in degenerative or other joint diseases.

Bartholin's c., a c. arising from the major vestibular gland or its ducts.

bile c., *vesica* biliaris.

Blessig's c.'s, Iwanoff's c.'s; peripheral cystoid degeneration of the sensory retina found in some children and almost universal after the age of 20.

blood c., hemorrhagic c.

blue dome c., **(1)** one of a number of small dark blue nodules or c.'s in the vaginal fornix due to retained menstrual blood in endometriosis affecting this region; **(2)** a benign retention c. of the mammary gland in fibrocystic disease, containing a pale slightly yellow fluid which gives a blue color to the c. when seen through the surrounding fibrous tissue.

bone c., see solitary bone c.
Boyer's c., a subhyoid c.
branchial or **branchial cleft c.,** a cervical c. arising from persistence of ectodermal branchial cleft (groove) or endodermal pharyngeal pouches.
bronchogenic c., a c. lined by ciliated columnar epithelium believed to represent bronchial differentiation; smooth muscle and mucous glands may be present.
bursal c., a retention c. in a bursa.
calcifying and keratinizing odontogenic c., calcifying odontogenic c.
calcifying odontogenic c., calcifying and keratinizing odontogenic c.; Gorlin c.; a mixed radiolucent-radiopaque lesion of the jaws with features of both a c. and a solid neoplasm; characterized microscopically by an epithelial lining showing a palisaded layer of columnar basal cells, presence of ghost cell keratinization, dentinoid, and calcification.
cerebellar c., a c. usually occurring in the lateral cerebellar white matter; often a part of cerebellar astrocytoma.
chocolate c., c. of the ovary with intracavitary hemorrhage and formation of a hematoma containing old brown blood; often seen with endometriosis of the ovary but occasionally with other types of c.'s.
choledochal c., c. originating from common bile duct; usually becomes apparent early in life as a right upper abdominal mass in association with jaundice.
chyle c., a circumscribed dilation of a lymphatic channel of the mesentery, containing chyle.
colloid c., a c. with gelatinous contents.
compound c., multilocular c.
corpora lutea c.'s, persistent corpora lutea with c. formation.
Cowper's c., a retention c. of a bulbourethral gland.
daughter c., a secondary c., usually multiple, derived from a mother c.
dentigerous c., follicular c. (2); an odontogenic c. derived from the reduced enamel epithelium surrounding the crown of an impacted or embedded tooth.
dentinal lamina c., a small keratin-filled c., usually multiple, on the alveolar ridge of newborn infants; derived from remnants of the dental lamina.
dermoid c., sequestration c.; dermoid (2); dermoid tumor; a tumor consisting of displaced ectodermal structures along lines of embryonic fusion, the wall being formed of epithelium-lined connective tissue, including skin appendages, and containing keratin, sebum, and hair.
dermoid c. of ovary, a common benign cystic teratoma of the ovary, lined for the most part by skin, and containing hair and sebum, but also usually containing a variety of other well differentiated structures within a small inwardly projecting mass of solid tissue.
distention c., retention c.
duplication c., a congenital cystic malformation attached to or originating from any part of the alimentary canal, from the base of the tongue to the anus, which reproduces the structure of the adjacent alimentary tract.
echinococcus c., hydatid c.
endometrial c., a c. resulting from endometrial implantation outside the uterus, as in endometriosis.
endothelial c., a serous c. whose sac is lined with endothelium.
enterogenous c.'s, mediastinal cysts derived from cells sequestered from the primitive foregut; may be classified histologically as bronchogenic, esophageal, or gastric.
ependymal c., neural c.; a circumscribed distention of some portion of the central canal of the spinal cord or of the cerebral ventricles.
epidermal c., implantation c.; inclusion c. (1); implantation or sequestration dermoid; a c. formed of a mass of epidermal cells which, as a result of trauma, has been pushed beneath the epidermis; the c. is lined with stratified squamous epithelium and contains concentric layers of keratin.

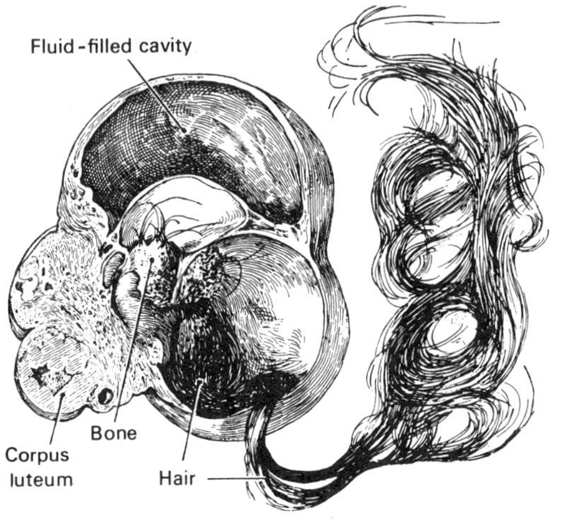

Dermoid Cyst of Ovary

epidermoid c., a spherical, firm, unilocular c. of the dermis, comprised of encysted keratin and a variable amount of sebum; the c. is lined by a keratinizing epithelium resembling the epidermis, and may be derived from the follicular infundibulum.
epithelial c., a c. lined with epithelium.
extravasation c., obsolete term for hemorrhagic c.
exudation c., a c. resulting from distention of a closed cavity, such as a bursa, by an excessive secretion of its normal fluid contents.
false c., pseudocyst (1).
fissural c., inclusion c. (2); a c. derived from epithelial remnants entrapped along the fusion line of embryonal processes.
follicular c., **(1)** a cystic graafian follicle; **(2)** dentigerous c.
Gartner's c., a c. of the chief duct in the vestigial structures of the paroophoron cervix or anterolateral vaginal wall, corresponding to the sexual portion of mesonephros.
gas c., a c. with gaseous instead of the ordinary liquid or pultaceous contents.
gingival c., a c. derived from remnants of the dental lamina situated in the attached gingiva, occasionally producing superficial erosion of the cortical plate of bone; most are located in the cuspid-premolar region.
glomerular c.'s, c.'s formed by dilatation of Bowman's capsules, found in rare cases of congenital polycystic kidneys.
Gorlin c., calcifying odontogenic c.
granddaughter c., a tertiary c. sometimes developed within a daughter c., as in the hydatid cyst of *Echinococcus.*
hemorrhagic c., sanguineous or blood c.; hematocele (1); hematocyst; a c. containing blood or resulting from the encapsulation of a hematoma.
hepatic c.'s, congenital c.'s thought to originate from an obstruction of biliary ductules; they may be solitary and range in size from small to enormous; polycystic disease may also occur.
hydatid c., echinococcus c.; hydatid (1); a c. formed in the liver, or, less frequently, elsewhere, by the larval stage of *Echinococcus,* chiefly in ruminants; two morphological forms caused by *Echinococcus granulosus* are found in man: the unilocular hydatid c. and the osseous hydatid c.; a third form in man is the alveolar hydatid c., caused by *Echinococcus multilocularis.*
implantation c., epidermal c.
inclusion c., **(1)** epidermal c.; **(2)** fissural c.

involution c., a mammary c. occurring at the menopause, due to fibrocystic disease.
iodine c.'s, obsolete term used to indicate the c.'s of *Iodamoeba butschlii,* characterized by a large iodine-positive glycogen vacuole.
Iwanoff's c.'s, Blessig's c.'s.
junctional c., a c. of the testis arising from the structures connecting the rete testis with the epididymis.
keratinous c., an epithelial c. containing keratin.
lacteal c., milk c.; a retention c. in the mammary gland resulting from closure of a lactiferous duct.
lateral periodontal c., an intraosseous c., usually encountered in the cuspid-premolar region of the mandible, derived from the remnants of the dental ledge and representing the intraosseous counterpart of the gingival c.
meibomian c., chalazion.
milk c., lacteal c.
morgagnian c., *appendix* vesiculosa.
mother c., parent c.; a hydatid c. from the inner, or germinal, layer, from which secondary c.'s containing scoleces (daughter c.'s) are developed; sometimes tertiary c.'s (granddaughter c.'s) are developed within the daughter c.'s; occurs most frequently in the liver, but may be found in other organs and tissues; symptoms are those of a tumor of the part affected.
mucous c., mucocele (1); a retention c. resulting from obstruction in the duct of a mucous gland.
multilocular c., compound c.; a c. containing several compartments formed by membranous septa.
multilocular or **multiloculate hydatid c.,** alveolar hydatid c.
myxoid c., ganglion (2).
nabothian c., nabothian follicle; a retention c. that develops when a mucous gland of the cervix uteri is obstructed, often developing in chronic inflammation of the cervix.
necrotic c., a c. due to a circumscribed encapsulated area of necrosis with subsequent liquefaction of the dead tissue.
neural c., ependymal c.
odontogenic c., a c. derived from odontogenic epithelium.
oil c., a c. resulting from loss of the epithelial lining of a sebaceous, dermoid, or lacteal c., or from the subcutaneous injection of oil or fat material.
oophoritic c., ovarian c.
osseous hydatid c., a morphological form of hydatid c. caused by *Echinococcus granulosus,* and found in the long bones or the pelvic arch of man if the embryo is filtered out in bony tissue; in this site no limiting membrane forms and the c. grows in an uncontrolled fashion, producing cancellous structures and inducing fracture, followed by spread to new sites.
ovarian c., oophoritic c.; a cystic tumor of the ovary, either non-neoplastic (follicle, lutein, germinal inclusion, or endometrial) or neoplastic; usually restricted to benign c.'s, *i.e.,* mucinous serous cystadenoma, or dermoid c.'s.
paraphysial c.'s, c.'s arising from vestigial remnants of the paraphysis; they are the possible origin of some third ventricular colloid c.'s.
parasitic c., a c. formed by the larva of a metazoan parasite, such as a hydatid or trichinal c.
parent c., mother c.
paroophoritic c., a c. arising from the paroopheron.
parvilocular c., a tumor composed of multiple small c.'s.
pearl c., a mass of epithelial cells introduced into the interior of the eye by a perforating injury.
periapical c., apical periodontal c.
phaeomycotic c., a subcutaneous cystic granuloma caused by pigmented fungi, usually solitary and located on the extremities.
pilar c., sebaceous or trichilemmal c.; steatocystoma (2); a common c. of the skin and subcutis which contains sebum and keratin, and is lined by pale-staining stratified epithelial cells derived from follicular trichilemma.
piliferous c., a dermoid c. containing hair.
pilonidal c., see pilonidal *sinus.*
pineal c., a c. of the pineal gland; rarely of clinical importance.
posttraumatic leptomeningeal c., a persistent cystic accumulation of cerebrospinal fluid with progressive loss of bone and dura, occurring at the site of a previous fracture.
primordial c., a c. which develops in place of a tooth through cystic degeneration of the enamel organ prior to formation of calcified odontogenic tissue.
proliferating tricholemmal c., pilar *tumor* of scalp.
proliferation c., proliferative c., proliferous c., a mother c. containing daughter c.'s; a c. with tumorous formation at one portion of the sac.
protozoan c., infectious form of many protozoan parasites such as *Entamoeba histolytica, Giardia lamblia, Balantidium coli,* etc., usually passed in the feces and provided with a highly condensed cytoplasm and resistant cell wall.
pseudomucinous c., a c. containing a gelatinous fluid, formerly thought to differ significantly from mucin, occurring especially in the ovary.
radicular c., apical periodontal c.
Rathke's cleft c., an intrasellar or suprasellar c. lined by cuboidal epithelium derived from remnants of Rathke's pouch.
rete c. of ovary, a c. derived from the germinal cords in the hilum of the ovary.
retention c., distention or secretory c.; a c. resulting from some obstruction to the excretory duct of a gland.
root end c., apical periodontal c.
sanguineous c., hemorrhagic c.
sebaceous c., pilar or trichilemmal c.; steatocystoma (2); wen; a common c. of the skin and subcutis containing sebum and keratin, and lined by pale-staining stratified epithelial cells derived from the pilosebaceous follicle.
secretory c., retention c.
sequestration c., dermoid c.
serous c., a c. containing clear serous fluid, such as a hygroma.
solitary bone c., unicameral bone c.; osteocystoma; a unilocular c. containing serous fluid and lined with a thin layer of connective tissue, occurring usually in the shaft of a long bone in a child.
Stafne bone c., lingual salivary gland *depression.*
static bone c., lingual salivary gland *depression.*
sterile c., a hydatid c. without brood capsules or viable scoleces.
sublingual c., ranula (2).
suprasellar c., craniopharyngioma.
synovial c., ganglion (2).
Tarlov's c., a perineural c. found in the proximal radicles of the lower spinal cord; it is usually productive of symptoms.
tarry c., a c. or collection of old blood having a tarry or black, sticky appearance; usually due to endometriosis.
tarsal c., chalazion.
teratomatous c., a c. containing structures derived from all three of the primary germ layers of the embryo.
thyroglossal duct c., thyrolingual c., a c. in the midline of the neck resulting from nonclosure of a segment of the ductus thyroglossus.
Tornwaldt's c., *bursa* pharyngea.
trichilemmal c., pilar c.
tubular c., tubulocyst.
umbilical c., vitellointestinal c.
unicameral c., unilocular c.
unicameral bone c., solitary bone c.
unilocular c., unicameral c.; a c. having a single sac.
unilocular hydatid c., the commonest form of hydatid c. in man, caused by *Echinococcus granulosus* and found in the liver, lungs, or any other site where the hexacanth embryo may settle if it passes the hepatic or pulmonary capillary filters; characterized by large

balloon-like forms lined internally with a germinative membrane, enclosed externally in a laminated membrane within a host-parasite capsule, and filled with fluid (hydatid fluid) and infectious scoleces of the young tapeworms (hydatid sand).
urachal c., allantoic c.; a c. of the urachus which may communicate with the umbilicus or bladder, or give rise to a mid-line swelling.
urinary c., a c. containing extravasated urine.
vitellointestinal c., umbilical c.; a small red sessile or pedunculated tumor at the umbilicus in an infant; it is due to the persistence of a segment of the vitellointestinal duct.
wolffian c., a c. arising from any mesonephric structure.

---

cyst-. See cysto-.

cystacanth (sis'tă-kanth) [cyst- + G. *akantha,* thorn or spine]. The fully developed larva of Acanthocephala, infective to the final host and with an inverted fully formed proboscis characteristic of the adult worm.

cystadenocarcinoma (sist-ad'en-ō-kar-si-nō'mă). A malignant neoplasm derived from glandular epithelium, in which cystic accumulations of retained secretions are formed; the neoplastic cells manifest varying degrees of anaplasia and invasiveness, and local extension and metastases occur; c.'s develop frequently in the ovaries, where pseudomucinous and serous types are recognized.

cystadenoma (sist'ad-ĕ-nō'mă). Cystoadenoma; a histologically benign neoplasm derived from glandular epithelium, in which cystic accumulations of retained secretions are formed; in some instances, considerable portions of the neoplasm, or even the entire mass, may be cystic.
papillary c. lymphomato'sum, adenolymphoma.

cystalgia (sist-al'jē-ă) [cyst- + G. *algos,* pain]. Pain in a bladder, especially the urinary bladder.

cystamine (sis'tă-mēn). Decarboxycystine; $(H_2NCH_2CH_2)_2S_2$; forms when cystine is distilled.

cystathionase (sis-tă-thī'ō-nās). Cystathionine γ-lyase.

β-cystathionase. Cystathionine β-lyase.

γ-cystathionase. Cystathionine γ-lyase.

cystathionine (sis-tă-thī'ō-nēn). $HOOC\text{-}CH(NH_2)CH_2\text{-}S\text{-}CH_2CH_2\text{-}CH(NH_2)COOH$; an intermediate in the conversion of methionine to cysteine; cleaved by cystathionases.

cystathionine β-lyase [EC 4.4.1.8]. β-Cystathionase; cystine lyase; an enzyme catalyzing cleavage of cystathionine to pyruvate, homocysteine, and NH_3. See also cystathionine γ-lyase.

cystathionine γ-lyase [EC 4.4.1.1]. γ-Cystathionase; cystathionase; cysteine desulphydrase; cystine desulphydrase; homoserine deaminase or dehydratase; a liver enzyme, requiring pyridoxal phosphate as coenzyme, that catalyzes the hydrolysis of cystathionine to cysteine and 2-ketobutyrate, releasing NH_3; also catalyzes formation of 2-ketobutyrate from homoserine, of pyruvate (and NH_3 and H_2S) from cysteine, and of thiocysteine, pyruvate, and NH_3 from cystine. See also cystathionine β-lyase.

cystathionine β-synthase [EC 4.2.1.22]. Serine sulfhydrase; cysteine synthase; methylcysteine synthase; β-thionase; an enzyme catalyzing hydrolysis of cystathionine to serine and homocysteine. See also cystathionine γ-synthase.

cystathionine γ-synthase. *O*- Succinylhomoserine (thiol)-lyase.

cystathioninuria (sis'tă-thī'ō-nin-ū'rē-ă). A disorder characterized by inability to metabolize cystathionine normally due to deficiency of cystathionase, with development of elevated concentrations of the amino acid in blood, tissue, and urine; mental retardation is an associated condition; autosomal recessive inheritance.

cystauchenitis (sis-taw-ken-ī'tis) [cyst- + G. *auchēn,* neck, + *-itis,* inflammation]. Obsolete term for *cystitis* colli.

cystauchenotomy (sis'-taw-ken-ot'ō-mē) [cyst- + G. *auchēn,* neck, + *tomē,* incision]. Cystidotrachelotomy; cystotrachelotomy; obsolete term for incision into the neck of the bladder.

cystectasia, cystectasy (sis-tek-tā'zē-ă, sis-tek'tă-sē) [cyst- + G. *ektasis,* a stretching]. Dilation of the bladder.

cystectomy (sis-tek'tō-mē) [cyst- + G. *ektomē,* excision]. **1.** Excision of the gallbladder or of the urinary bladder. **2.** Removal of a cyst.
Bartholin's c., vulvovaginal c.; removal of a cyst of a major vestibular gland.
partial c., removal of a part or segment of the bladder.
radical c., removal of the entire bladder, surrounding fatty tissues, and regional lymph nodes; in the male, including the prostate gland and seminal vesicles.
total c., removal of the entire bladder.
vulvovaginal c., Bartholin's c.

cysteic acid (sis-tē'ik). 3-Sulfoalanine; $HOOC\text{-}CH(NH_2)CH_2\text{-}SO_3H$; an oxidation product of cysteine, and a precursor of taurine and isethionic acid.

cysteine (Cys) (sis'tē-ēn). 2-Amino-3-mercaptopropionic acid; $HS\text{-}CH_2CH(NH_2)COOH$; an α-amino acid found in most proteins; especially abundant in keratin.
c. desulfhydrase, cystathionine γ-lyase.
c. synthase, cystathionine β-synthase.

cysteinesulfinic acid (sis'tē-ēn-sul-fin'ik). $HO_2S\text{-}CH_2CH(NH_2)COOH$; a natural oxidation product of cysteine; an intermediate in the formation of taurine (via cysteic acid).

cysteinyl (sis'tēn-il). Aminoacyl radical of cysteine.

cystendesis (sis-ten-de'sis) [cyst- + G. *endesis,* a binding together]. Obsolete term for suture of a wound in a bladder.

cysti-. See cysto-.

cystic (sis'tik). Cystous. **1.** Relating to the urinary bladder or gallbladder. **2.** Relating to a cyst. **3.** Containing cysts.

cysticercoid (sis-ti-ser'koyd) [cysti- + G. *kerkos,* tail, + *eidos,* resemblance]. A larval tapeworm resembling a cysticercus but having a smaller bladder, containing little or no fluid, in which scolex of the future adult tapeworm is found; the larval form is typically found in insect intermediate hosts.

cysticercosis (sis'ti-ser-kō'sis). **1.** Disease caused by encystment of cysticercus larvae (*e.g., Taenia solium* or *T. saginata*) in subcutaneous, muscle, or central nervous system tissues; c. is typically developed in swine and cattle, producing measly pork and beef. In man, it results from the hatching of the eggs of *Taenia solium* in the intestines or by accidental ingestion of eggs from human feces; encystment in the brain may cause serious nervous damage, and encystment in the eye (usually the rear chamber) may cause ophthalmic damage. **2.** Larval infections in animals with other taeniid tapeworm larvae.

Cysticercus (sis-ti-ser'kŭs) [G. *kystis,* bladder, + *kerkos,* tail]. Originally described as a genus of bladderworms, now known to be the encysted larvae of various taenioid tapeworms; the generic name is, however, retained as a convenience in referring to the larval encysted forms. See cysticercus.
C. bo'vis, the cysticercus larva of *Taenia saginata* in cattle; the cause of measly beef.
C. cellulo'sae, the cysticercus larva of *Taenia solium* in pigs; also the cause of human cysticercosis.
C. fasciola'ris, the strobilocercus larva of *Taenia taeniaeformis,* found in the liver of mice, rats, and other rodents; adult worms infect cats and canids.
C. pisifor'mis, the larva of *Taenia pisiformis;* it occurs in the liver and abdominal cavity of rabbits and hares; adult worms are found in dogs and other canids.
C. tenuicol'lis, the cystic form of *Taenia hydatigena;* it is found in

the liver and peritoneal cavity of sheep, cattle, pigs, and wild ruminants; adults are found in various predators.

cysticercus, pl. **cysticerci** (sis-ti-ser'kŭs, -ser'sē) [G. *kystis,* bladder, + *kerkos,* tail]. Bladderworm; the larval form of certain *Taenia* species, typically found in muscles of mammalian intermediate hosts that serve as a prey of various predators; it consists of a fluid-filled bladder in which the invaginated cestode scolex develops. See also *Taenia saginata; T. solium.*

cystides (sis'ti-dēz). Plural of cystis.

cystidoceliotomy (sis'ti-dō-sē-lē-ot'ō-mē) [G. *kystis,* bladder, + *koilia,* belly, + *tomē,* incision]. Obsolete term for an incision of the bladder through an incision in the abdominal wall.

cystidolaparotomy (sis'ti-dō-lap-ar-ot'ō-mē) [G. *kystis,* bladder, + *lapara,* flank, + *tomē,* incision]. Obsolete term for an incision into the bladder after a preliminary abdominal section.

cystidotrachelotomy (sis'ti-dō-trāk-ĕ-lot'ō-mē) [G. *kystis,* bladder, + *trachēlos,* neck, + *tomē,* incision]. Cystauchenotomy.

cystifelleotomy (sis'ti-fel-ē-ot'-ō-mē) [cysti- + L. *felleus,* pertaining to bile, + G. *tomē,* incision]. Cholecystotomy.

cystiform (sis'ti-fōrm). Cystoid (1).

cystigerous (sis-tij'er-ŭs). Cystopherous.

cystine (sis'tēn). Dicysteine; 3,3'-dithiobis(2-aminopropionic acid); $HOOC\text{-}CH(NH_2)\text{-}CH_2\text{-}S\text{-}S\text{-}CH_2\text{-}CH(NH_2)COOH$; an oxidation product of cysteine in which two -SH groups become one -S-S-group, which binds two peptide chains together; sometimes occurs as a deposit in the urine, or forming a vesical calculus.
c. desulfhydrase, cystathionine γ-lyase.
c. lyase, cystathionine β-lyase.

meso-**cystine.** An isomer of cystine in which the configuration about one of the α-carbons is D, about the other, L, so that the molecule as a whole possesses a plane of symmetry and is optically inactive.

cystinemia (sis-ti-nē'mē-ă) [cystine + G. *haima,* blood]. The presence of cystine in the blood.

cystinosis (sis-ti-nō'sis) [cystine + G. *-osis,* condition]. Cystine storage disease; De Toni-Fanconi or Lignac-Fanconi syndrome; the most common of a group of diseases with characteristic renal tubular dysfunction disorders, termed collectively Fanconi's *syndrome* (2). An autosomal recessive hereditary disease of early childhood characterized by widespread deposits of cystine crystals throughout the body, including bone marrow and other tissues, with slight increase in the level of plasma cystine and cystinuria; this apparent abnormality in cystine metabolism is associated with a marked generalized aminoaciduria, glycosuria, polyuria, chronic acidosis, hypophosphatemia with vitamin D-resistant rickets, and often with hypokalemia; the latter abnormalities are probably due to deficient tubular reabsorption and are accompanied by a characteristic abnormality of the proximal convoluted tubule, shown by microdissection to be narrowed at the glomerular junction (swan-neck deformity).

cystinuria (sis-ti-nū'rē-ă) [cystine + G. *ouron,* urine]. Excessive urinary excretion of cystine, along with lysine, arginine, and ornithine, arising from defective transport systems for these acids in the kidney and intestine; renal function is sometimes compromised by cystine crystalluria and nephrolithiasis; occurs in certain heritable diseases, such as Fanconi's syndrome (cystinosis) and hepatolenticular degeneration.
familial c., an inborn defect in renal tubular reabsorption of cystine, lysine, arginine, and ornithine, with recurrent cystine calculus formation; intestinal absorption of these four amino acids is also impaired.

cystinyl (sis'tin-il). Aminoacyl radical of cystine.

cystiphorous (sis-tif'er-ŭs). Cystopherous.

cystis, pl. **cystides** (sis'tis, sis'ti-dēz) [G. *kystis*] Cyst.
c. fel'lea, *vesica* biliaris.
c. urina'ria, *vesica* urinaria.

cystistaxis (sis-ti-stak'sis) [cysti- + G. *staxis,* trickling]. Cystostaxis; obsolete term for oozing of blood from the mucous membrane of the bladder.

cystitis (sis-tī'tis) [cyst- + G. *-itis,* inflammation]. Inflammation of a bladder, especially the urinary bladder.
c. col'li, inflammation of the neck of the bladder.
c. cys'tica, c. glandularis with the formation of cysts.
follicular c., chronic c. characterized by small mucosal nodules due to lymphocytic infiltration with formation of lymphoid follicles.
c. glandula'ris, chronic c. with glandlike invaginations of transitional epithelium.
interstitial c., a chronic inflammatory condition of unknown etiology involving the mucosa and muscularis of the bladder, resulting in reduced bladder capacity, pain relieved by voiding, and severe bladder irritative symptoms. See also Hunner's *ulcer.*

cysto-, cysti-, cyst- [G. *kystis,* bladder]. Combining forms relating to: **1.** The bladder. **2.** The cystic duct. **3.** A cyst.

cystoadenoma (sis'tō-ad-ĕ-nō'mă). Cystadenoma.

cystocarcinoma (sis'tō-kar-si-nō'mă) Cystoepithelioma; a carcinoma in which cystic degeneration has occurred; sometimes used incorrectly as a term for cystadenocarcinoma.

cystocele (sis'tō-sēl) [cysto- + G. *kēlē,* hernia]. Colpocystocele; vesicocele; hernia of the bladder.

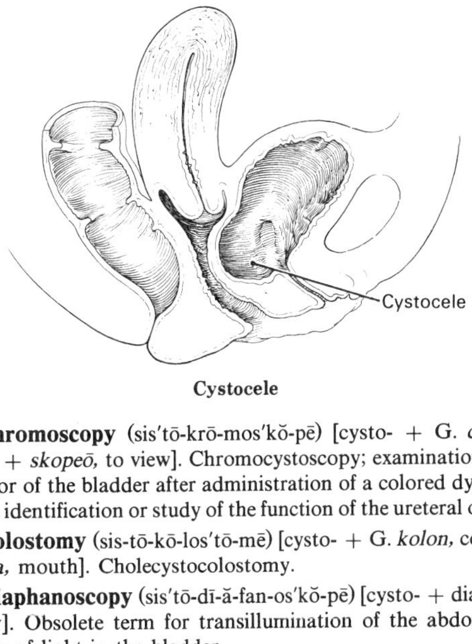

Cystocele

cystochromoscopy (sis'tō-krō-mos'kŏ-pē) [cysto- + G. *chrōma,* color + *skopeō,* to view]. Chromocystoscopy; examination of the interior of the bladder after administration of a colored dye to aid in the identification or study of the function of the ureteral orifices.

cystocolostomy (sis-tō-kō-los'tō-mē) [cysto- + G. *kolon,* colon, + *stoma,* mouth]. Cholecystocolostomy.

cystodiaphanoscopy (sis'tō-dī-ă-fan-os'kŏ-pē) [cysto- + diaphanoscopy]. Obsolete term for transillumination of the abdomen by means of light in the bladder.

cystodiverticulum (sis'tō-dī-ver-tik'yū-lŭm). Vesical *diverticulum.*

cystoduodenostomy (sis'tō-dū'ō-dē-nos'tō-mē) [cysto- + duodenum, + G. *stoma,* mouth]. Duodenocystostomy (2); drainage of a cyst into duodenum.

cystoenterocele (sis-tō-en'ter-ō-sēl) [cysto- + G. *enteron,* intestine, + *kēlē,* hernia]. Hernial protrusion of portions of the bladder and of the intestine.

cystoenterostomy (sis'tō-en-ter-os'tō-mē) [cysto- + G. *enteron,* intestine, + *stoma,* mouth]. Internal drainage of pancreatic pseudocysts into some portion of the intestinal tract.

cystoepiplocele (sis-tō-e-pip'lō-sēl) [cysto- + G. *epiploon,* omentum, + *kēle,* tumor]. Hernial protrusion of portions of the bladder and of the omentum.

cystoepithelioma (sis'tō-ep-i-thē-lē-ō'mă). Cystocarcinoma.

cystofibroma (sis'tō-fī-brō'mă). A fibroma in which cysts or cystlike foci have formed.

cystogastrostomy (sis'tō-gas-tros'tō-mē) [cysto- + G. *gastēr,* stomach, + *stoma,* mouth]. Drainage of a cyst into the stomach.

cystogram (sis'tō-gram). An x-ray demonstration of the bladder filled with contrast medium.
voiding c., cystourethrogram.

cystography (sis-tog'ră-fē) [cysto- + G. *graphō,* to write]. Roentgenography of the bladder following injection of a radiopaque substance.
antegrade c., antegrade urography in which the contrast medium is injected into the urinary bladder.

cystoid (sis'toyd) [cysto- + G. *eidos,* appearance]. **1.** Cystiform; cystomorphous; bladder-like, resembling a cyst. **2.** A tumor resembling a cyst, with fluid, granular, or pulpy contents, but without a capsule.

cystojejunostomy (sis'tō-je-jū-nos'tō-mē) [cysto- + jejunum, + G. *stoma,* mouth]. Drainage of a cyst into the jejunum.

cystolith (sis'tō-lith) [cysto- + G. *lithos,* stone]. Vesical *calculus.*

cystolithectomy (sis'tō-li-thek'tō-mē) [cysto- + G. *lithos,* stone, + *ektomē,* excision]. Cystolithotomy.

cystolithiasis (sis'tō-li-thī'ă-sis) [cysto- + G. *lithos,* stone, + *-iasis,* condition]. Vesicolithiasis; the presence of a vesical calculus.

cystolithic (sis-tō-lith'ik). Relating to a vesical calculus.

cystolithotomy (sis'tō-li-thot'ō-mē) [cysto- + G. *lithos,* stone, + *tomē,* incision]. Cystolithectomy; removal of a stone from the bladder through an incision in its wall.

cystoma (sis-tō'mă) [cyst- + G. *-oma,* tumor]. A cystic tumor; a new growth containing cysts.

cystometer (sis-tom'ĕ-ter) [cysto- + G. *metron,* measure]. A device for studying bladder function by measuring capacity, sensation, intravesical pressure, and residual urine.

cystometrogram (sis-tō-met'rō-gram) [cysto- + G. *metron,* measure, + *gramma,* a writing]. A graphic recording of urinary bladder pressure at various volumes.

cystometrography (sis'tō-mĕ-trog'ră-fē). Cystometry.

cystometry (sis-tom'ĕ-trē) [see cystometer]. Cystometrography; a method for measurement of the pressure/volume relationship of the bladder.

cystomorphous (sis-tō-mōr'fŭs) [cysto- + G. *morphē,* form]. Cystoid (1).

cystomyoma (sis'tō-mī-ō'mă). A myoma in which cysts or cystlike foci have developed.

cystomyxoadenoma (sis-tō-mik'sō-ad-ĕ-nō'mă). An adenoma in which there are cysts or cystlike foci in association with myxomatous change in the stroma.

cystomyxoma (sis'tō-mik-sō'mă). A myxoma in which cysts or cystlike foci have formed.

cystopanendoscopy (sis'tō-pan-en-dos'kō-pē) [cysto- + panendoscope]. Inspection of the interior of the bladder and urethra by means of specially designed endoscopes introduced in retrograde fashion through the urethra and into the bladder.

cystoparalysis (sis-tō-pă-ral'i-sis). Cystoplegia.

cystopexy (sis'tō-pek-sē) [cysto- + G. *pēxis,* fixation]. Ventrocystorrhaphy; vesicofixation (1); surgical attachment of the gallbladder or of the urinary bladder to the abdominal wall or to other supporting structures.

cystopherous (sis-tof'er-ŭs) [cysto- + G. *phoreō,* to carry]. Cystigerous; cystiphorous; containing cysts.

cystophotography (sis'tō-fō-tog'ră-fē). Photographing the interior of the bladder.

cystoplasty (sis'tō-plas-tē) [cysto- + G. *plastos,* formed]. Any plastic operation on the urinary bladder. *Cf.* ileocystoplasty; colocystoplasty.

cystoplegia (sis-tō-plē'jē-ă) [cysto- + G. *plēgē,* a stroke]. Cystoparalysis; paralysis of the bladder.

cystoproctostomy (sis'tō-prok-tos'tō-mē) [cysto- + G. *prōktos,* anus, + *stoma,* mouth]. Vesicorectostomy.

cystoptosis, cystoptosia (sis-tō-tō'sis, -tō'zē-ă) [cysto- + G. *ptōsis,* a falling]. Prolapse of the vesical mucous membrane into the urethra.

cystopyelitis (sis'tō-pī-el-ī'tis) [cysto- + G. *pyelos,* trough (pelvis), + *-itis,* inflammation]. Inflammation of both the bladder and the pelvis of the kidney.

cystopyelonephritis (sis-tō-pī'el-ō-nef-rī'tis) [cysto- + G. *pyelos,* trough (pelvis), + *nephros,* kidney, + *-itis,* inflammation]. Inflammation of the bladder, the pelvis of the kidney, and the kidney parenchyma.

cystoradiography (sis'tō-rā-dē-og'ră-fē). Radiography of the urinary bladder.

cystorectostomy (sis'tō-rek-tos'tō-mē) [cysto- + rectum + G. *stoma,* mouth]. Vesicorectostomy.

cystorrhagia (sis-tō-rā'jē-ă) [cysto- + G. *rhēgnymi,* to burst forth]. Hemorrhage from the bladder.

cystorrhaphy (sis-tōr'ă-fē) [cysto- + G. *raphē,* a sewing]. Suture of a wound or defect in the urinary bladder.

cystorrhea (sis'tō-rē-ă) [cysto- + G. *rhoia,* a flow]. A mucous discharge from the bladder.

cystosarcoma (sis'tō-sar-kō'mă). A sarcoma in which the formation of cysts or cystlike foci has occurred.
c. phyllo'des, phyllodes tumor; a circumscribed or infiltrating fibroadenomatous breast tumor that may be partly cystic; the stroma is cellular and resembles a fibrosarcoma, but the tumor is usually benign; the neoplasms occasionally metastasize as sarcomas.

cystoscope (sis'tō-skōp) [cysto- + G. *skopeō,* to examine]. Lithoscope; a lighted tubular endoscope for examining the interior of the bladder.

cystoscopy (sis-tos'kŏ-pē). The inspection of the interior of the bladder by means of a cystoscope.

cystospasm (sis'tō-spazm). Abnormal spasmodic contraction of the urinary bladder.

cystostaxis (sis-tō-stak'sis). Cystistaxis.

cystostomy (sis-tos'tō-mē) [cysto- + G. *stoma,* mouth]. Vesicostomy; creation of an opening into the urinary bladder.

cystotome (sis'tō-tōm). **1.** An instrument for incising the urinary bladder or gallbladder. **2.** Capsulotome; a surgical instrument used for incising the capsule of a lens.

cystotomy (sis-tot'ō-mē) [cysto- + G. *tomē,* incision]. Vesicotomy; incision into urinary bladder or gallbladder.
suprapubic c., epicystotomy; opening into the bladder through an incision above the symphysis pubis.

cystotrachelotomy (sis'tō-trā-kĕ-lot'ō-mē) [cysto- + G. *trachēlos,* neck, + *tomē,* incision]. Cystauchenotomy.

cystoureteritis (sis'tō-yū-rē-ter-ī'tis). Inflammation of the bladder and of one or both ureters.

cystoureterogram (sis'tō-yū-rē'ter-ō-gram). An x-ray demonstration of the bladder and one or both ureters.

cystoureterography (sis'tō-ū-rē'ter-og'ră-fē). Radiography of the bladder and one or both ureters.

cystourethritis (sis'tō-yū-rē-thrī'tis). Inflammation of the bladder and of the urethra.

cystourethrocele (sis'tō-yū-rē'thrō-sēl) [cysto- + urethra + G. *kēlē*, hernia]. Hernia of the urinary bladder and urethra.

cystourethrogram (sis-tō-yū-reth'rō-gram). Voiding cystogram; an x-ray picture made during voiding and with the bladder and urethra filled with contrast medium to demonstrate the urethra.

cystourethrography (sis'tō-yū'rē-throg'ră-fē). Roentgenography of the bladder and urethra after visualization by means of a radiopaque substance.

cystourethroscope (sis-tō-yū-rē'thrō-skōp). An instrument combining the uses of a cystoscope and a urethroscope, whereby both the bladder and urethra can be visually inspected.

cystous (sis'tŭs). Cystic.

Cystoviridae (sis'tō-vir'i-dē) [G. *kystis*, bladder]. Provisional name for a family of monotypic bacterial viruses, the type species of which is phage ϕ6. Virions are 73 nm in diameter, isometric, have lipid envelopes, and adsorb to the sides of pili of *Pseudomonas* species. Capsids are of cubic symmetry, and the genomes are of double-stranded RNA in three pieces (MW 13×10^6).

cystyl-aminopeptidase (sis'til-am-i-nō-pep'ti-dās) [EC 3.4.11.3]. Oxytocinase; an enzyme that degrades cystine peptides, such as oxytocin.

Cyt Symbol for cytosine.

cyt-. See cyto-.

cytapheresis (sī'tă-fē-rē'sis) [cyt- + G. *aphairesis*, a withdrawal]. A procedure in which various cells can be separated from the withdrawn blood and retained, with the plasma and other formed elements retransfused into the donor.

cytarabine (sī'tar-ă-bēn). Arabinosylcytosine.

cytase (sī'tās). Metchnikoff's term for alexin or complement, which he held to be a digestive secretion of the leukocyte.

Cytauxzoon (sī-tawk'zō-on) [cyt- + G. zōon, animal]. Theileria.

cytauxzoonosis (sī-tawks'zō-ō-nō'sis). Former name for theileriosis.

-cyte [G. *kyton*, a hollow (cell)]. Suffix meaning cell.

cytidine (C, Cyd) (sī'ti-dēn). Cytosine ribonucleoside; 1-β-D-ribofuranosylcytosine; a major component of ribonucleic acids.
c. diphosphate choline, cytidinediphosphocholine.
c. phosphate, see cytidylic acid.

cytidine 5'-diphosphate (CDP). An ester, at the 5' position, between cytidine and diphosphoric acid.

cytidinediphosphocholine (sī'ti-dēn-dī'fos-fō-kō'lēn). Cytidine disphosphate choline; an intermediate in the formation of phosphatidylcholine (lecithin); formed by the action of cytidine triphosphate on phosphocholine, linking the choline phosphate group to the α-phosphate of the cytidine triphosphate to give a pyrophosphate.

cytidine 5'-triphosphate (CTP). An ester, at the 5' position, between cytidine and triphosphoric acid.

cytidylic acid (sī-ti-dil'ik). Cytidine phosphate (five are possible, depending on the site of attachment of the phosphate to the ribosyl OH's); a constituent of ribonucleic acids.

cyto-, cyt- [G. *kytos*, a hollow (cell)]. Combining forms meaning cell.

cytoanalyzer (sī-tō-an'ă-lī-zer) [cyto- + analyzer]. An electronic optical machine that screens smears containing cells suspected of malignancy.

cytoarchitectonics (sī'tō-ar-ki-tek-ton'iks) [cyto- + G. *architektonikē*, architectural]. Cytoarchitecture.

cytoarchitectural (sī-tō-ar-ki-tek'chŭr-ăl). Pertaining to cytoarchitecture.

cytoarchitecture (sī'tō-ar'ki-tek-chŭr). Architectonics; cytoarchitectonics; the arrangement of cells in a tissue; the term commonly refers to the arrangement of nerve-cell bodies in the brain, especially the cerebral cortex.

cytobiology (sī'tō-bī-ol'ō-jē). Cytology.

cytobiotaxis (sī'tō-bī-ō-tak'sis) [cyto- + G. *bios*, life, + *taxis*, arrangement]. Cytoclesis.

cytocentrum (sī-tō-sen'trŭm) [cyto- + G. *kentron*, center]. Cell center; centrosome; central body; cinocentrum; microcentrum; kinocentrum; a zone of cytoplasm containing one or two centrioles but devoid of other organelles; usually located near the nucleus of a cell.

cytochalasins (sī-tō-kal'ă-zinz) [cyto- + G. *chalasis*, a relaxing]. A group of substances derived from molds which disaggregate the microfilaments of the cell and interfere with the division of cytoplasm, inhibit cell movement, and cause extrusion of the nucleus; used for investigations in cell biology.

cytochemistry (sī'tō-kem-is-trē). Histochemistry; the study of intracellular distribution of chemicals, reaction sites, enzymes, etc., often by means of staining reactions, radioactive isotope uptake, selective metal distribution in electron microscopy, or other methods.

cytochrome (sī'tō-krōm) [cyto- + G. *chrōma*, color]. A class of hemoprotein whose principal biological function is electron and/or hydrogen transport by virtue of a reversible valency change of the heme iron. C.'s are classified in four groups. (*a, b, c,* and *d*) according to spectrochemical characteristics; many variants exist, particularly among bacteria and in green plants and algae, one being a variant of the *c*- type cytochrome called cytochrome *f.* The mitochondrial system of c.'s provides electron transport through cytochrome *c* oxidase to molecular oxygen as the terminal electron acceptor (respiration).

cytochrome a_3. Cytochrome *c* oxidase.

cytochrome b_5 reductase [EC 1.6.2.2]. An enzyme catalyzing the reduction of ferricytochrome b_5 to ferrocytochrome b_5 at the expense of NADH.

cytochrome *cd*. Cytochrome oxidase (*Pseudomonas*).

cytochrome c_3 hydrogenase [EC 1.12.2.1]. A hydrogenase enzyme catalyzing reduction of ferricytochrome c_3 by H_2 to ferrocytochrome c_3.

cytochrome *c* oxidase [EC 1.9.3.1]. Cytochrome a_3; indophenolase; indophenol oxidase; a cytochrome of the *a* type, containing copper, that catalyzes the oxidation of ferrocytochrome *c* by molecular oxygen to ferricytochrome *c*.

cytochrome *c* reductase. NADH-dehydrogenase.

cytochrome c_2 reductase. NADPH-cytochrome c_2 reductase.

cytochrome oxidase (*Pseudomonas*) [EC 1.9.3.2]. Cytochrome *cd;* an enzyme with action identical to that of cytochrome *c* oxidase, but acting on ferrocytochrome c_2.

cytochrome P-450$_{SCC}$ [*450 nm,* the absorption maximum that the CO compound of the reduced pigment exhibits]. Cholesterol monooxygenase (side chain cleaving).

cytochrome peroxidase [EC 1.11.1.5]. A hemoprotein enzyme catalyzing the reaction between H_2O_2 and ferrocytochrome *c* to yield ferricytochrome *c*.

cytochrome reductase. NADPH-ferrihemoprotein reductase.

cytochylema (sī'tō-kī-lē'mă) [cyto- + G. *chylos*, juice]. The more fluid portion of the cytoplasm.

cytocidal (sī-tō-sī'dăl) [cyto- + L. *caedo*, to kill]. Causing the death of cells.

cytocide (sī'tō-sīd) [cyto- + L. *caedo,* to kill]. An agent that is destructive to cells.

cytocinesis (sī'tō-sin-ē'sis). Cytokinesis.

cytoclasis (sī-tok'lă-sis) [cyto- + G. *klasia,* a breaking]. Fragmentation of cells.

cytoclastic (sī-tō-klas'tik). Relating to cytoclasis.

cytoclesis (sī-tō-klē'sis) [cyto- + G. *klēsis,* a call]. Biotaxis (2); cytobiotaxis; the influence of one cell on another.

cytocuprein (sī-tō-kū'prē-in). Erythrocuprein; cerebrocuprein; hepatocuprein; hemocuprein; former terms for copper-containing proteins found in human erythrocytes and other tissues. See *superoxide* dismutase; ceruloplasmin.

cytocyst (sī'tō-sist) [cyto- + G. *kystis,* bladder]. Rarely used term for the bladder-like remains of the red blood cell or tissue cell that encloses a mature schizont.

cytodiagnosis (sī'tō-dī-ag-nō'sis). Diagnosis of the type and, when feasible, the cause of a pathologic process by means of microscopic study of cells in an exudate or other form of body fluid.

cytodieresis (sī'tō-dī-er'ē-sis). [cyto- + G. *diairesis,* division]. Cytokinesis.

cytogene (sī'tō-jēn). Plasmagene.

cytogenesis (sī-tō-jen'ĕ-sis) [cyto- + G. *genesis,* origin]. The origin and development of cells.

cytogeneticist (sī'tō-jĕ-net'i-sist). A specialist in cytogenetics.

cytogenetics (sī'tō-jĕ-net'iks). The branch of genetics concerned with the structure and function of the cell, especially the chromosomes.

cytogenic (sī-tō-jen'ik). Relating to cytogenesis.

cytogenous (sī-toj'ĕ-nŭs). Cell-forming.

cytoglucopenia (sī'tō-glū-kō-pē'nē-ă) [cyto- + glucose + G. *penia,* poverty]. An intracellular deficiency of glucose.

cytohet (sī'tō-het) [cyto- + heterozygous]. Contraction designating a cell that, in a sense, is heterozygous in having cytoplasmic genetic elements from different parental types.

cytohyaloplasm (sī-tō-hī'ă-lō-plazm). Obsolete term for hyaloplasm.

cytoid (sī'toyd) [cyto- + G. *eidos,* resemblance]. Resembling a cell.

cytokine (sī'tō-kīn) [cyto- + G. *kinēsis,* movement]. Generic term for nonantibody proteins, such as lymphokines, released by a certain cell population on contact with a specific antigen and which act as intercellular mediators, as in the generation of immune response.

cytokinesis (sī'tō-ki-nē'sis) [cyto- + G. *kinēsis,* movement]. Cytocinesis; cytodieresis; changes occurring in the protoplasm of the cell outside of the nucleus during cell division.

cytolemma (sī-tō-lem'mă) [cyto- + G. *lemma,* husk]. Cell *membrane.*

cytolipin (sī-tō-lip'in). A glycosphingolipid, specifically a ceramide oligosaccharide; **c. H,** a lactosylceramide, may display immunological properties under certain conditions; **c. K** is probably identical with globoside.

cytologic (sī-tō-loj'ik). Relating to cytology.

cytologist (sī-tol'ō-jist). One who specializes in cytology.

cytology (sī-tol'ō-jē) [cyto- + G. *logos,* study]. Cellular biology; cytobiology; the study of the anatomy, physiology, pathology, and chemistry of the cell.

exfoliative c., cytopathology (2); the examination, for diagnostic purposes, of cells denuded from a neoplasm (or other type of lesion) and recovered from the sediment of the exudate, secretions, or washings from the tissue (*e.g.,* sputum, vaginal secretion, gastric washings, urine).

cytolymph (sī'tō-limf). Obsolete term for hyaloplasm.

cytolysin (sī-tol'i-sin). An antibody that, in association with complement, effects partial or complete destruction of an animal cell.

cytolysis (sī-tol'i-sis) [cyto- + G. *lysis,* loosening]. The dissolution of a cell.

cytolysosome (sī-tō-lī'sō-sōm). Autophagic vacuole; a variety of secondary lysosome that contains mitochondria, ribosomes, or other organelles.

cytolytic (sī-tō-lit'ik). Pertaining to cytolysis; possessing a solvent or destructive action on cells.

cytoma (sī-tō'mă) [cyto- + G. *-ōma,* tumor]. An undesirable general term to indicate any neoplasm composed almost entirely of neoplastic cells, with virtually no stroma or formation of histologic structures.

cytomatrix (sī-tō-mā'triks). Cytoplasmic *matrix.*

cytomegalic (sī-tō-meg'ă-lik) [cyto- + G. *megas,* big]. Denoting or characterized by markedly enlarged cells.

cytomegalovirus (CMV) (sī-tō-meg'ă-lō-vī'rŭs) [cyto- + G. *megas,* big]. Visceral disease virus; a group of herpetoviruses infecting man and other animals, many of the viruses having special affinity for salivary glands, and causing enlargement of cells of various organs and development of characteristic inclusions in the cytoplasm or nucleus. They are all species-specific and include salivary gland virus, inclusion body rhinitis virus of pigs, and others.

cytomembrane (sī-tō-mem'brān). Cell *membrane.*

cytomere (sī'tō-mēr) [cyto- + G. *meros,* part]. The structure separating the portions of the contents of a large schizont in the course of schizogony, as in some of the sporozoans undergoing exoerythrocytic asexual division. C.'s are caused by complex invaginations of the surface of the schizont, which isolates them; ultimately, c.'s complete the budding process in the formation of large numbers of merozoites.

cytometaplasia (sī'tō-met-ă-plā'zē-ă) [cyto- + G. *metaplasis,* transformation]. Change of form or function of a cell, other than that related to neoplasia.

cytometer (sī-tom'ĕ-ter) [cyto- + G. *metron,* measure]. A standardized, usually ruled glass slide or small glass chamber of known volume, used in counting and measuring cells, especially blood cells.

cytometry (sī-tom'ĕ-trē). The counting of cells, especially blood cells, using a cytometer or hemocytometer.

cytomicrosome (sī-tō-mī'krō-sōm) [cyto- + G. *mikros,* small, + *sōma,* body]. See microsome.

cytomitome (sī-tō-mī'tōm) [cyto- + G. *mitos,* thread]. Obsolete term formerly used by cytologists to designate what appeared to be a fibrillar network in the cytoplasm of fixed cells.

cytomorphology (sī'tō-mōr-fol'ō-jē). The study of the structure of cells.

cytomorphosis (sī'tō-mōr-fō'sis) [cyto- + G. *morphōsis,* a shaping]. Changes that the cell undergoes during the various stages of its existence. See also prosoplasia.

cyton (sī'ton). Obsolete term for perikaryon.

cytopathic (sī-tō-path'ik). Pertaining to or exhibiting cytopathy.

cytopathogenic (sī'tō-path-ō-jen'ik). Pertaining to an agent or substance that causes a diseased condition in cells, in contrast to histologic changes; used especially with reference to effects observed in cells in tissue cultures.

cytopathologist (sī'tō-pa-thol'ō-jist). A physician, usually skilled in anatomical pathology, who is specially trained and experienced in cytopathology.

cytopathologic, cytopathological (sī'tō-pa-thō-loj'ik, -loj'i-kăl). **1.** Denoting cellular changes in disease. **2.** Relating to cytopathology.

cytopathology (sī'tō-pa-thol'ō-jē). **1.** The study of disease changes within individual cells or cell types. **2.** Exfoliative *cytology.*

cytopathy (sī-top'ă-thē) [cyto- + G. *pathos,* disease]. Any disorder of a cell or anomaly of any of its constituents.

cytopempsis (sī-tō-pemp'sis) [cyto- + G. *pempis,* sending through]. Transcytosis.

cytopenia (sī-tō-pē'nē-ă) [cyto- + G. *penia,* poverty]. A reduction, *i.e.,* hypocytosis, or a lack of cellular elements in the circulating blood.

cytophagous (sī-tof'ă-gŭs). Devouring, or destructive to, cells.

cytophagy (sī-tof'ă-jē) [cyto- + G. *phagein,* to devour]. Devouring of other cells by phagocytes.

cytophanere (sī'tō-fă-nēr) [cyto- + G. *phaneros,* visible, evident, open]. A radial spine seen in certain cysts of *Sarcocystis,* as in rabbit and sheep tissue cysts.

cytopharynx (sī'tō-far'inks). An organelle in certain flagellates and ciliates that serves as a gullet through which food material passes from the cytostome to the cell interior; food passed is collected in food vacuoles, into which digestive enzymes are secreted.

cytophilic (sī-tō-fil'ik) [cyto- + G. *philos,* fond]. Cytotropic.

cytophotometry (sī'tō-fō-tom'ĕ-trē) [cyto- + G. *phōs,* light + *metron,* measure]. A method of measuring the absorption of monochromatic light by stained microscopic structures (*e.g.,* chromosomes, nuclei, whole cells) with the aid of a photoelectric cell; also used to measure emitted light from such objects by fluorescence in combination with selected fluorochrome dyes.

flow c., a method of measuring fluorescence from stained cells that are in suspension and flowing through a narrow orifice, usually in combination with one or two lasers to activate the dyes; used to measure cell size, number, viability, and nucleic acid content with the aid of acridine orange, Kasten's fluorescent Feulgen stain, ethidium bromide, trypan blue, and other selected staining reagents.

cytophylactic (sī'tō-fī-lak'tik). Relating to cytophylaxis.

cytophylaxis (sī'tō-fī-lak'sis) [cyto- + G. *phylaxis,* a guarding]. Protection of cells against lytic agents.

cytophyletic (sī'tō-fī-let'ik) [cyto- + G. *phylē,* a tribe]. Relating to the genealogy of a cell.

cytopipette (sī'tō-pi-pet'). A slightly curved, blunt end pipette usually made of glass and fitted with a rubber bulb to provide gentle negative pressure for the collection of vaginal secretions for cytological examination.

cytoplasm (sī'tō-plazm) [cyto- + G. *plasma,* thing formed]. The substance of a cell, exclusive of the nucleus, which contains various organelles and inclusions within a colloidal protoplasm.

ground-glass c., uniform finely granular eosinophilic c. seen in hepatocytes in carriers of hepatitis B virus, and also in epidermal cells in keratoacanthomas.

cytoplasmic (sī-tō-plaz'mik). Relating to the cytoplasm.

cytoplast (sī'tō-plast) [cyto- + G. *plastos,* formed]. The living intact cytoplasm that remains following cell enucleation.

cytopoiesis (sī-tō-poy-ē'sis) [cyto- + G. *poiēsis,* a making]. Formation of cells.

cytopreparation (sī'tō-prep-ă-rā'shŭn). Laboratory preparation of a cellular specimen for cytologic examination.

cytopyge (sī-tō-pī'jē) [cyto- + G. *pygē,* buttocks]. The anal orifice (cell "anus") found in certain structurally complex protozoa, such as the rumen-dwelling ciliates of herbivores, through which waste matter is ejected.

cytoryctes, cytorrhyctes (sī-tō-rik'tēz) [cyto- + G. *oryktēs,* a digger]. Old term for inclusion *bodies.*

cytosides (sī'tō-sīdz). Ceramide disaccharides. See glycosphingolipid.

cytosine (Cyt) (sī'tō-sēn). 4-Amino-2(1*H*)-pyrimidinone; a pyrimidine found in nucleic acids.

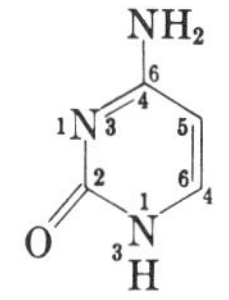

Cytosine

Inner numbering, official international (IUPAC); *outer numbering,* original Fischer (abandoned).

c. arabinoside (CA), incorrect term for arabinosylcytosine.

c. ribonucleoside, cytidine.

cytosis (sī-tō'sis) [cyto- + G. *-osis,* condition]. **1.** A condition in which there is more than the usual number of cells, as the c. of spinal fluid in acute leptomeningitis. **2.** Frequently used with a prefixed combining form as a means of describing certain features pertaining to cells; *e.g.,* isocytosis, equality in size; polycytosis, abnormal increase in number.

cytoskeleton (sī-tō-skel'ĕ-ton). The tonofilaments, keratin, desmin, neurofilaments, or other intermediate filaments serving to act as supportive cytoplasmic elements to stiffen cells or to organize intracellular organelles.

cytosmear (sī'tō-smēr). Cytologic *smear.*

cytosol (sī'tō-sol) [cyto- + "sol," abbrev. of soluble]. Cytoplasm exclusive of the mitochondria and endoplasmic reticulum components.

cytosolic (sī-tō-sol'ik). Relating to or contained in the cytosol.

cytosome (sī'tō-sōm) [cyto- + G. *sōma,* body]. **1.** The cell body exclusive of the nucleus. **2.** Multilamellar body; one of the osmiophilic bodies which are 1 μm or less in diameter, have concentric lamellae, and occur in the great alveolar cells of the lung.

cytostasis (sī-tos'tă-sis) [cyto- + G. *stasis,* standing]. The slowing of movement and accumulation of blood cells, especially polymorphonuclear leukocytes, in the capillaries, as in a region of inflammation; obstruction of a capillary as the result of accumulated leukocytes.

cytostatic (sī-tō-stat'ik). Characterized by cytostasis.

cytostome (sī'tō-stōm) [cyto- + G. *stoma,* mouth]. The cell "mouth" of certain complex protozoa, usually with a short gullet or cytopharynx leading food into the organism, where it is collected into food vacuoles, then circulated inside the body, eventually to be excreted through the cytopyge.

cytotactic (sī-tō-tak'tik). Relating to cytotaxis.

cytotaxis, cytotaxia (sī-tō-tak'sis, -tak'sē-ă) [cyto- + G. *taxis,* arrangement]. The attraction (**positive c.**) or repulsion (**negative c.**) of cells for one another.

cytothesis (sī-toth'ĕ-sis) [cyto- + G. *thesis,* a placing]. The repair of injury in a cell; the restoration of cells.

cytotoxic (sī-tō-tok'sik). Detrimental or destructive to cells; pertaining to the effect of noncytophilic antibody on specific antigen, frequently, but not always, mediating the action of complement.

cytotoxicity (sī'tō-tok-sis'i-tē). The quality or state of being cytotoxic.

lymphocyte-mediated c., the toxic or lytic activity of T-lymphocytes which is effected without mediation of antibody or of complement; there are three kinds of cytotoxic T-lymphocytes: those that are antigen-specific as a result of previous allergization (immunization), killer cells, and natural killer cells.

cytotoxin (sī'tō-tok'sin) [cyto- + G. *toxikon,* poison]. A specific substance, usually with reference to antibody, that inhibits or prevents the functions of cells, causes destruction of cells, or both.

cytotrophoblast (sī-tō-trof'ō-blast). Langhans' layer; the inner layer of the trophoblast.

cytotropic (sī-tō-trop'ik). Cytophilic; having an affinity for cells.

cytotropism (sī-tot'rō-pizm) [cyto- + G. *tropos,* a turning]. **1.** Affinity for cells. **2.** Affinity for specific cells, especially the ability of viruses to localize in and damage specific cells.

cytozoic (sī-tōzō'ik). Living in a cell; denoting certain parasitic protozoa.

cytozoon (sī-tō-zō'on) [cyto- + G. *zōon,* animal]. A protozoan cell or organism.

cytozyme (sī'tō-zīm) [cyto- + G. *zymē,* leaven]. An obsolete term for thromboplastin.

cyturia (sī-tū'rē-ă) [G. *kytos,* cell, + *ouron,* urine]. The passage of cells in unusual numbers in the urine.

Czapek, Friedrich J.F., Czechoslovakian botanist, 1868–1921. See C.'s solution *agar;* C.-Dox *medium.*

Czerny, Vincenz, German surgeon, 1842–1916. See C.'s *suture;* C.-Lembert *suture.*

D

Δ, δ **1.** Fourth letter in the Greek alphabet, delta. **2.** In chemistry, denotes a double bond, usually with a superscript to indicate position in a chain (Δ^5); application of heat in a reaction (A $\xrightarrow{\Delta}$ B); absence of heat treatment ($\not\Delta$); distance between two atoms in a molecule; or position of a substituent located on the fourth atom from the carboxyl or other primary functional group (δ).

D **1.** Symbol for the vitamin D potency of cod liver oil, multiples of which (5D, 100D, etc.) are used to designate the vitamin D potency of irradiated ergosterol (viosterol) or other substances; for deuterium; for dihydrouridine in nucleic acids; for diffusing capacity. **2.** In optics, abbreviation for diopter; for dexter (right). **3.** In electrodiagnosis, abbreviation for duration, the current flowing and the circuit being closed. **4.** In dental formulas, abbreviation for deciduous. **5.** As a subscript, refers to dead space. See physiologic dead *space.*

2,4-D Abbreviation for (2,4-dichlorophenoxy) acetic acid.

D- Prefix indicating that a chemical compound is sterically related to D-glyceraldehyde, the basis of stereochemical nomenclature. *Cf.* L.

d Symbol for deci-.

***d*-** Prefix indicating a chemical compound to be dextrorotatory. *Cf. l*-.

-*d* Suffix indicating the presence of deuterium in a compound in concentrations above normal, thus labelling the compound; subscripts (d_2, d_3, etc.) indicate the number of such atoms so fortified.

DA Abbreviation for developmental *age* (2).

dA, dAdo Abbreviation for deoxyadenosine.

da Symbol for deca-.

Daae, Anders, Norwegian physician, 1838–1910. See D.'s *disease.*

DAB Abbreviation for 3'3-diaminobenzidine HCl; in the immunoperoxidase technique, used to produce a colored complex at the site of peroxidase activity; carcinogenic.

daboia, daboya (dă-boy'ă) [Hindu fr. *dabnā,* to lurk]. Russell's *viper.*

dacarbazine (DTIC) (dă-kar'bă-zēn). 5-(3,3-Dimethyl-1-triazenyl)-1*H*- imidazole-4-carboxamide; an antineoplastic agent used in the treatment of malignant melanoma and Hodgkin's disease.

DaCosta, Jacob M., U.S. surgeon, 1833–1900. See DaC.'s *syndrome.*

dacry-. See dacryo-.

dacryadenitis (dak'rē-ad-ĕ-nī'tis). Dacryoadenitis.

dacryagogue (dak'rē-ă-gog) [dacry- + G. *agōgos,* drawing forth]. **1.** An agent that stimulates the lacrimal gland to secretion. **2.** Promoting the flow of tears. **3.** Obsolete term for *canaliculus* lacrimalis.

dacryo-, dacry- [G. *dakryon,* tear]. Combining forms relating to tears, or to the lacrimal sac or duct.

dacryoadenalgia (dak-rē-ō-ad-en-al'jē-ă) [dacryo- + G. *adēn,* gland, + *algos,* pain]. Pain in one of the lacrimal glands.

dacryoadenitis (dak-rē-ō-ad-ĕ-nī'tis) [dacryo- + G. *adēn,* gland, + *-itis,* inflammation]. Dacryadenitis; inflammation of the lacrimal gland.

dacryoblennorrhea (dak-rē-ō-blen-ō-rē'ă) [dacryo- + G. *blenna,* mucus, + *rhoia,* flow]. Dacryocystoblennorrhea; a chronic discharge of mucus from a lacrimal sac.

dacryocele (dak'rē-ō-sēl). Dacryocystocele.

dacryocyst (dak'rē-ō-sist) [dacryo- + G. *kystis,* sac]. *Saccus* lacrimalis.

dacryocystalgia (dak'rē-ō-sis-tal'jē-ă) [dacryocyst + G. *algos,* pain]. Pain in the lacrimal sac.

dacryocystectomy (dak'rē-ō-sis-tek'tō-mē) [dacryocyst + G. *ektomē,* excision]. Surgical removal of the lacrimal sac.

dacryocystitis (dak'rē-ō-sis-tī'tis) [dacryocyst + G. *-itis,* inflammation]. Inflammation of the lacrimal sac.

dacryocystoblennorrhea (dak'rē-ō-sis'tō-blen-ō-re'ă). Dacryoblennorrhea.

dacryocystocele (dak'rē-ō-sis'tō-sēl) [dacryocyst + G. *kēlē,* hernia]. Dacryocele; enlargement of the lacrimal sac with fluid.

dacryocystoethmoidostomy (dak'rē-ō-sis'tō-eth-moy-dos'tō-mē). Anastomosis of the lacrimal sac to the mucous membrane of the ethmoid sinus.

dacryocystogram (dak'rē-ō-sis'tō-gram) [dacryocyst + G. *gramma,* a writing]. A radiograph of the lacrimal apparatus obtained (after injection of radiopaque substances) for the purpose of localizing the site of obstruction; similar information is obtainable by means of a scintigraph from a gamma camera after instilling a drop of technetium-99m.

dacryocystoptosis, dacryocystoptosia (dak'rē-ō-sis'top-tō'sis, -tō'sē-ă) [dacryocyst + G. *ptōsis,* a falling]. Downward displacement of the lacrimal sac.

dacryocystorhinostenosis (dak'rē-ō-sis'tō-rī'nō-ste-nō'sis). Obstruction within the nasolacrimal duct.

dacryocystorhinostomy (dak'rē-ō-sis'tō-rī-nos'tō-mē) [dacryocyst + G. *rhis (rhin-),* nose, + *stoma,* mouth]. Dacryorhinocystotomy; an operation providing an anastomosis between the lacrimal sac and the nasal mucosa through an opening in the lacrimal bone.

dacryocystotome (dak'rē-ō-sis'tō-tōm). A small knife for incising the lacrimal sac.

dacryocystotomy (dak'rē-ō-sis-tot'ō-mē) [dacryocyst + G. *tomē,* incision]. Incision of the lacrimal sac.

dacryohemorrhea (dak'rē-ō-hem-ō-rē'ă) [dacryo- + G. *haima,* blood, + *rhoia,* flow]. The flow of bloody tears.

dacryolith (dak'rē-ō-lith) [dacryo- + G. *lithos,* stone]. Lacrimal calculus; tear stone; ophthalmolith; a concretion in the lacrimal apparatus.
Desmarres' d.'s, white pseudoconcretions, composed of masses of *Nocardia* species found in the lacrimal canaliculi.

dacryolithiasis (dak'rē-ō-li-thī'ă-sis). The formation and presence of dacryoliths.

dacryoma (dak-rē-ō'mă) [dacryo- + G. *-ōma,* tumor]. **1.** Hydrops of the lacrimal sac. **2.** A tumor of the lacrimal sac.

dacryon (dak'rē-on) [G. a tear]. The point of junction of the frontomaxillary and lacrimomaxillary sutures on the medial wall of the orbit. See fig. under craniometric *point.*

dacryops (dak'rē-ops) [dacryo- + G. *ōps,* eye]. **1.** Excess of tears in the eye. **2.** A cyst of a duct of the lacrimal gland.

dacryopyorrhea (dak'rē-ō-pī-ō-rē'ă) [dacryo- + G. *pyon,* pus, + *rhoia,* flow]. The discharge of tears containing leukocytes.

dacryopyosis (dak-rē-ō-pī-ō'sis) [dacryo- + G. *pyōsis,* suppuration]. Suppuration in the lacrimal sac or canaliculi.

dacryorhinocystotomy (dak'rē-ō-rī'nō-sis-tot'ō-mē). Dacryocystorhinostomy.

dacryorrhea (dak'rē-ō-rē'ă) [dacryo- + G. *rhoia,* flow]. An excessive secretion of tears.

dacryoscintigraphy (dak'rē-ō-sin-tig'ră-fē) [dacryo- + L. *scintilla,* spark, + G. *graphō,* to write]. A test to determine the patency of the lacrimal system by instilling a radioactive isotope, usually technetium-99, in the conjunctival sac and recording the distribution with a gamma camera.

dacryosolenitis (dak'rē-ō-sō-le-nī'tis) [dacryo- + G. *sōlēn,* a channel, + *-itis,* inflammation]. Inflammation of the lacrimal or nasal duct.

dacryostenosis (dak'rē-ō-ste-nō'sis) [dacryo- + G. *stenōsis,* narrowing]. Stricture of a lacrimal or nasal duct.

dacryosyrinx (dak'rē-ō-sir'inks) [dacryo- + G. *syrinx,* pipe]. Lacrimal *fistula.*

dactinomycin (dak'ti-nō-mī'sin). Actinomycin D; produced by several species of *Streptomyces* (*e.g., S. parvulus*); an antineoplastic antibiotic used especially for Ewing's sarcoma, rhabdomyosarcoma, and Wilms' tumor in children and for trophoblastic disease in women. See also antinomycin.

dactyl (dak'til) [G. *daktylos*] Digitus.

dactyl-. See dactylo-.

dactylagra (dak-ti-lag'ră) [dactyl- + G. *agra,* seizure]. Obsolete term meaning gout for the fingers.

dactylalgia (dak-ti-lal'jē-ă) [dactyl- + G. *algos,* pain]. Dactylodynia; pain in the fingers.

Dactylaria (dak-ti-lā'rē-ă) [G. *daktylos,* finger]. A genus of dematiaceous soil-dwelling fungi. *D. gallopava* is the causative agent of phaeohyphomycosis in chickens and turkeys.

dactyledema (dak'til-e-dē'mă) [dactyl- + G. *oidema,* swelling]. Edema of the finger.

dactylia (dak-til'ē-ă). Syndactyly.

dactylitis (dak-ti-lī'tis). Inflammation of one or more fingers.
sickle cell d., hand-and-foot *syndrome.*

dactylium (dak-til'ē-ŭm). Syndactyly.

dactylo-, dactyl- [G. *daktylos,* finger]. Combining forms relating to the fingers, and sometimes to the toes.

dactylocampsis (dak'ti-lō-kamp'sis) [dactylo- + G. *kampsis,* bending]. Permanent flexion of the fingers.

dactylocampsodynia (dak'ti-lō-kamp'sō-din'ē-ă) [dactylo- + G. *kampsis,* a bending, + *odynē,* pain]. Painful contraction of one or more fingers.

dactylodynia (dak'tĭ-lō-din'ē-ă). Dactylalgia.

dactylogryposis (dak'ti-lō-gri-pō'sis) [dactylo- + G. *grypōsis,* a crooking]. Contraction of the fingers.

dactylology (dak'ti-lol'ō-jē) [dactylo- + G. *logos,* word]. Cheirology; chirology; the use of the finger alphabet in talking.

dactylolysis spontanea (dak-ti-lol'i-sis spon-tā'nē-ă) [dactylo- + G. *lysis,* a loosening; L. *spontaneus,* willing]. Ainhum.

dactylomegaly (dak'til-ō-meg'ă-lē) [dactylo- + G. *megas,* large]. Megadactyly.

dactyloscopy (dak-ti-los'kŏ-pē) [dactylo- + G. *skopeō,* to examine]. An examination of the markings in prints made from the fingertips; employed as a method of personal identification. See Galton's system of classification of fingerprints (under fingerprint).

dactylospasm (dak'ti-lō-spazm). Spasmodic contraction of the fingers.

dactylus, pl. **dactyli** (dak'ti-lŭs, -lī) [G. *daktylos*]. Digitus.

dacuronium (dak-yū-rō'nē-ŭm). A nondepolarizing steroid neuromuscular blocking agent with more rapid onset and shorter duration of action than pancuronium.

DaFano, Corrado D., Italian-American anatomist, 1879–1927. See D.'s *stain.*

dagga (dag'ă) [aborigines' term]. Leaves of *Leonotis leonurus,* a plant found in South Africa, where it is smoked like tobacco with mild sedative effect; a term mistakenly applied to Indian hemp, *Cannabis sativa.*

Dagnini, Giuseppe, Italian physician, 1866–1928. See Aschner-D. *reflex.*

DAH Abbreviation for disordered action of heart.

dah'lin [fr. *dahlia,* after *A. Dahl,* Swedish botanist, 1751–1789]. Inulin.

dahllite (dah'līt). Podolite; $CaCO_3 \cdot 2Ca_3(PO_4)_2$; a naturally occurring calcium phosphate, similar in structure to the mineral portions of bones and teeth.

daisy (dā'zē). Colloquial term descriptive of the segmented forms (merozoites) of the mature schizont of *Plasmodium malariae.*

Dakin, Henry D., U.S. chemist, 1880–1952. See D.'s *fluid, solution;* D.-Carrel *treatment.*

Dale, Sir Henry Hallett, British pharmacologist and Nobel laureate, 1875–1968. See D. *reaction,* D.-Feldberg *law,* Schultz-D. *reaction.*

Dalen, Johan A., Swedish ophthalmologist, 1866–1940. See D.-Fuchs *nodules.*

Dalrymple, John, British oculist, 1804–1852. See D.'s *sign.*

Dalton, John, British chemist, mathematician, and natural philosopher, 1766–1844. See D.'s *law,* D.-Henry *law.*

dalton (dawl'tŏn) [J. *Dalton*]. Term unofficially used to indicate a unit of mass equal to $^1/_{12}$ the mass of a carbon-12 atom, 1.0000 in the atomic mass scale; numerically, but not dimensionally, equal to molecular or particle weight (atomic mass units).

daltonian (dawl-tō'nē-ăn). **1.** Attributed to or described by John Dalton. **2.** Pertaining to daltonism.

daltonism (dawl'tŏn-izm) [J. *Dalton*] A color vision deficiency, especially deuteranomaly or deuteranopia.

DAM Abbreviation for diacetylmonoxime.

Dam, C.P. Henrik, Danish biochemist and Nobel laureate, *1895. See D. *unit.*

dam [A.S. *fordemman,* to stop up]. **1.** Any barrier to the flow of fluid. **2.** In surgery and dentistry, a sheet of thin rubber arranged so as to shut off the part operated upon from the access of fluid.
post d., posterior palatal *seal.*
rubber d., **(1)** in surgery, thin strips of rubber used as a surgical drain. **(2)** a thin sheet of rubber with holes that is placed over teeth to isolate them from the oral cavity.

Damalinia (dam-ă-lin'ē-ă). A genus of biting lice containing a number of species found on domestic and wild animals; they are all highly host-specific, one species being confined to each species of mammal. See also *Bovicola* and *Trichodectes.*

dam'mar [Hind. *dāmar,* resin]. A resin resembling copal, obtained from various species of *Shorea* (family Dipterocarpaceae) in the East Indies; used, dissolved in chloroform, for mounting microscopic specimens.

dAMP Abbreviation for deoxyadenylic acid.

damp **1.** Humid; moist. **2.** Atmospheric moisture. **3.** Foul air in a mine; air charged with carbon oxides (black or choke d.) or with various explosive hydrocarbon vapors (firedamp).

damp'ing. Bringing a mechanism to rest with minimal oscillation; *e.g.,* in echocardiography, electrical or mechanical loading to reduce duration of echo, transmitter pulse, and transmitter complex.

Dana, Charles L., U.S. neurologist, 1852–1935. See D.'s *operation,* Putnam-D. *syndrome.*

danazol (dā'nă-zol). 17α-Pregna-2,4-dien-20-yno[2,3-*d*]isoxazol-17-ol; an anterior pituitary suppressant.

Dance, Jean B.H., French physician, 1797–1832. See D.'s *sign.*

dance (dans). Abnormal, histrionic movements related to brain damage.

hilar d., vigorous pulmonary arterial pulsations due to increased blood flow, often seen fluoroscopically in patients with congenital left-to-right shunts, especially septal defects.

Saint Anthony's d., Saint John's d., Saint Vitus d., obsolete eponyms for Sydenham's *chorea.*

dan'der. **1.** A fine scaling of the skin and scalp. See also dandruff. **2.** A normal effluvium of animal hair or coat capable of causing allergic responses in atopic persons.

dandruff (dan'drŭf). Seborrhea sicca (2); pityriasis sicca or capitis; scurf; branny tetter (1); the presence, in varying amounts, of white or gray scales in the hair of the scalp, due to the normal branny exfoliation of the epidermis. See also seborrheic *dermatitis.*

Dandy, Walter E., U.S. surgeon, 1886–1946. See D. *operation,* D.-Walker *syndrome.*

Dane, D.S., British virologist. See D. *particles.*

Dane's stain. See under stain.

Danforth, William Clark, U. S. obstetrician-gynecologist, 1878–1949. See D.'s *sign.*

Danielssen, Daniel C., Norwegian physician, 1815–1894. See D.'s *disease,* D.-Boeck *disease.*

Danlos, Henri A., French dermatologist, 1844–1912. See Ehlers-D. *syndrome.*

DANS Abbreviation for 1-dimethylaminonaphtalene-5-sulfonic acid; a green fluorescing compound used in immunohistochemistry to detect antigens.

dansyl (Dns, DNS) (dan'sil). The 5-dimethylaminonaphthalene-1-sulfonyl radical; a blocking agent for NH_2 groups, used in peptide synthesis.

dan'thron. Chrysazin; 1,8-dihydroxyanthraquinone; an anthraquinone laxative.

dantrolene sodium (dan'trō-lēn). 1-{[5-(*p*- Nitrophenyl)furfurylidene]amino}hydantoin sodium hydrate; a synthetic skeletal muscle relaxant which acts directly on muscle; also, the specific agent for prevention and treatment of malignant hyperthermia.

Danysz, Jean, Polish pathologist in France, 1860–1928. See D. *phenomenon.*

DAPI Abbreviation for 4'6-diamidino-2-phenylindole•2HCl, a fluorescent probe for DNA. See DAPI *stain.*

dapsone (dap'sōn). 4,4'Sulfonylbisbenzeneamine; 4,4'-sulfobisaniline; it is used in the treatment of leprosy and certain cutaneous diseases such as dermatitis herpetiformis, and is active against the tubercle bacillus; it is also used in the treatment of bovine coccidiosis and streptococcal mastitis.

d'Arcet, Jean, French chemist, 1725–1801. See d'A.'s *metal.*

Darier, Jean F., French dermatologist, 1856–1938. See D.'s *disease, sign.*

Darkschewitsch (Darkshevich), Liverij O., Russian neurologist, 1858–1925. See *nucleus* of D.

Darling, Samuel Taylor, U.S. physician in Panama, 1872–1925. See D.'s *disease.*

Darrow red [Mary A. *Darrow,* U.S. stain technologist, 1894–1973]. A basic oxazin dye, $C_{18}H_{14}N_3O_2Cl$, used as a substitute for cresyl violet acetate in the staining of Nissl substance.

d'Arsonval, Jacques Arsène, French biophysicist, 1851–1940. See d'A. *current, galvanometer.*

dartoic, dartoid (dar-tō'ik, dar'toyd) [G. *dartos,* flayed]. Resembling tunica dartos in its slow involuntary contractions.

dartos (dar'tōs) [G. skinned or flayed, fr. *derō,* to skin]. See *tunica* dartos.

d. mulieb'ris, a very thin layer of smooth muscle in the integument of the labia majora; less well-developed than the tunica dartos of the scrotum.

Darwin, Charles R., British biologist and evolutionist, 1809–1882. See darwinian *ear, reflex, theory, tubercle.*

darwinian (dar-win'ē-an). Relating to or ascribed to Darwin.

Dastre, Jules Albert Francois, French physician, 1844–1917. See D.-Morat *law.*

Dasyprocta (das'ē-prok'tă) [G. *dasyprōktos,* having hairy buttocks]. Agouti; a genus of rodents of the guinea pig family, a reservoir host of *Trypanosoma cruzi.*

Datura (da-tū'ră) [Hind]. A genus of solanaceous plants. Several species (*D. arborea, D. fastuosa, D. ferox,* and *D. sanguinea*) are used in Brazil, India, and Peru to produce unconsciousness. The seeds contain hyoscine (scopolamine), an alkaloid with an anticholinergic action similar to that of atropine.

D. me'tel, *D. fastuosa* L. var. *alba;* a species that contains scopolamine as its chief alkaloid and traces of hyoscyamine and atropine.

D. stramo'nium, thorn apple; jimson or stink weed; a species that is the main source of stramonium.

daturine (da-tū'rin, -rēn). Hyoscyamine.

Daubenton (D'Aubenton), Louis J.M., French physician, 1716–1799. See D.'s *angle, line, plane.*

Dauerschlaf (dow'er-shlahf) [Ger.]. Prolonged sleep induced by drugs as a treatment for certain mental disorders.

daunomycin (daw-nō-mī'sin). Daunorubicin.

daunorubicin (daw-nō-rū'bi-sin). Daunomycin; an antibiotic of the rhodomycin group, obtained from *Streptomyces peucetius;* used in the treatment of acute leukemia; also used in cytogenetics to produce Q-type chromosome bands.

Davidoff, M. von, German histologist, †1904. See D.'s *cells.*

Davidson, Edward C., U.S. surgeon, 1894–1933. See D. *syringe.*

Daviel, Jacques, French oculist, 1696–1762. See D.'s *operation, spoon.*

Davies, J.N.P., U.S. pathologist, *1915. See D.'s *disease.*

Davis, John Staige, U.S. surgeon, 1872–1946. See D. *grafts;* D.-Crowe mouth *gag.*

Davis interlocking sound. See under sound.

Dawbarn, Robert Hugh Mackay, U.S. surgeon, 1860–1915. See D.'s *sign.*

Dawson, James R., U.S. pathologist, *1908. See D.'s *encephalitis.*

Day, Richard H., U.S. physician, 1813–1892. See D.'s *test.*

Day, Richard L., U.S. pediatrician, *1905. See Riley-D. *syndrome.*

dazz'ling. The consequence of illumination too intense for adaptation by the eye; in contrast to glare, d. is alleviated by appropriate tinted glasses.

dB, db Abbreviation for decibel.

D.C. Abbreviation for Doctor of Chiropractic.

D & C Abbreviation for dilation and curettage.

dCMP Abbreviation for deoxycytidylic acid.

DDAVP Abbreviation for desmopressin acetate.

D.D.S. Abbreviation for Doctor of Dental Surgery.

DDT Abbreviation for dichlorodiphenyltrichloroethane.

de- [L. *de,* from, away] **1.** Prefix carrying often a privative or negative sense; denoting away from, cessation, without; sometimes has an intensive force. **2.** For names with this prefix not found here, see under the principal part of the name.

D & E Abbreviation for dilation and evacuation.

deacidification (dē-a-sid'i-fi-kā'shŭn). The removal or neutralization of acid.

deactivation (dē-ak-ti-vā'shŭn). The process of rendering or of becoming inactive.

deacylase (dē-as'il-ās). **1.** A member of the subclass of hydrolases (EC class 3), especially of that subclass of esterases, lipases, lactonases, and hydrolases (EC subclass 3.1). **2.** Any catalyzing the hydrolytic cleavage of an acyl group (R-CO-) in an ester linkage; also includes enzymes cleaving amide linkages (EC subclass 3.5) and similar acyl compounds.

dead (ded). **1.** Without life. See also death. **2.** Numb.

DEAE-cellulose Diethylaminoethyl *cellulose.*

deaf (def) [A.S. *deáf*]. Unable to hear; hearing indistinctly; hard of hearing.

deafferentation (dē-af'er-en-tā'shŭn) [L. *de,* from, + afferent]. A loss of the sensory nerve fibers from a portion of the body.

deaf-mute (def'myūt). An individual with deafmutism.

deafmutism (def-myū'tizm). Inability to speak, due to congenital or early acquired profound deafness.
endemic d., d. in individuals living in regions where goiter is prevalent, due to severe thyroid deficiency.

deafness (def'nes). General term for loss of the ability to hear, without designation of the degree or cause of the loss.
acoustic trauma d., boilermaker's, industrial, or occupational d.; loss of hearing due to changes in the organ of Corti secondary to overexposure to high intensity noise levels.
Alexander's d., high frequency d. due to congenital membranous cochlear dysplasia.
boilermaker's d., acoustic trauma d.
central d., d. due to disease in the auditory system of the brainstem or cerebral hemispheres.
conductive d., hearing impairment caused by interference with sound or vibratory energy in the external canal, middle ear, or ossicles.
cortical d., d. resulting from a lesion of the cerebral cortex.
functional d., psychogenic d.
high frequency d., selective loss of hearing acuity for high frequencies, usually associated with neurosensory damage, common in acoustic trauma.
hysterical d., psychogenic d.
industrial d., acoustic trauma d.
labyrinthine d., d. due to disease in the labyrinth (inner ear).
low tone d., inability to hear low notes or frequencies.
midbrain d., d. due to a lesion of the mesencephalon.
Mondini d., the hearing loss resulting from the structural aberration of Mondini dysplasia.
nerve d., neural d., former terms for sensorineural d.
occupational d., acoustic trauma d.
organic d., d. due to a pathologic process or an organic etiology, as opposed to psychogenic d.
prelingual d., hearing impairment occurring before development of speech and language skills.
postlingual d., hearing impairment occurring after speech and language skills have been developed.
perceptive d., former term for sensorineural d.
psychogenic d., functional or hysterical d.; hearing loss without evidence of organic cause or malingering; often follows severe psychic shock.
retrocochlear d., former term for nerve d.
Scheibe's d., d. (may be unilateral) due to congenital cochleosaccular dysplasia; usually autosomal recessive inheritance when associated with another syndrome.
sensorineural d., hearing impairment due to lesions or dysfunction of the cochlea or retrocochlear nerve tracts, or along the auditory pathway to the brainstem, as opposed to conductive d.
word d., auditory *aphasia.*

dealbation (dē-al-bā'shŭn) [L. *de-albo,* pp. *-atus,* to whiten]. The act of whitening, bleaching, or blanching.

dealcoholization (dē-al'kō-hol-i-zā'shŭn). The removal of alcohol from a fluid; in histologic technique, the removal of alcohol from a specimen that has been previously immersed in this fluid.

deallergize (dē-al'er-jīz). Desensitize (1).

deamidases (dē-am'i-dā-sez). Amidohydrolases.

deamidation, deamidization (dē-am-i-dā'shŭn, dē-am'i-di-zā'shŭn). The hydrolytic removal of an amide group.

deamidize (dē-am'i-dīz). Desamidize; to perform deamidation.

deaminases (dē-am'i-nā-sez) [EC group 3.5.4]. Deaminating enzymes; enzymes catalyzing simple hydrolysis of C—NH_2 bonds of purines, pyrimidines, and pterins, usually named in terms of the substrate, *e.g.,* guanine d. (EC 3.5.4.3), adenosine d. (EC 3.5.4.4), AMP d. (EC 3.5.4.6), pterin d. (EC 3.5.4.11); not generally used for deamination of noncyclic amides. D. are distinguished from ammonia-lyases (EC 4.3.1) in that the latter produce an unsaturation at the point of NH_3 removal.

deamination, deaminization (dē-am-i-nā'shŭn, dē-am'i-ni-zā'shŭn). Removal, usually by hydrolysis, of the NH_2 group from an amino compound.

deaminize (dē-am'i-nīz). To perform deamination.

Dean, Henry Trendley, U.S. dentist and epidemiologist, 1893–1962. See D.'s fluorosis *index.*

deanol acetamidobenzoate (dē'ă-nol as-ĕ-tam'i-dō-ben'zō-āt). The *p*- acetamidobenzoic acid salt of 2-dimethylaminoethanol; a central nervous system stimulant.

dearterialization (dē-ar-tēr'ē-ăl-i-zā'shŭn). Changing the character of arterial blood to that of venous blood; *i.e.,* deoxygenation of blood.

death (deth) [A.S. *dēath*]. Mors; the cessation of life. In lower multicellular organisms, d. is a gradual process at the cellular level, since tissues vary in their ability to withstand deprivation of oxygen; in higher organisms, a cessation of integrated tissue and organ functions; in man, manifested by the loss of heartbeat, by the absence of spontaneous breathing, and by cerebral d.
black d., term applied to the worldwide epidemic of the 14th century, of which some 60 million persons are said to have died; the descriptions indicate that it was pneumonic plague.
brain d., cerebral d.
cerebral d., brain d.; in the presence of cardiac activity, the permanent loss of cerebral function, manifested clinically by absence of purposive responsiveness to external stimuli, absence of cephalic reflexes, apnea, and an isoelectric electroencephalogram for at least 30 minutes in the absence of hypothermia and poisoning by central nervous system depressants.
crib d., sudden infant death *syndrome.*
fetal d., d. *in utero* of a fetus weighing 500 g or more at birth, irrespective of gestational age.
genetic d., d. of the bearer of a gene at any age before generating living offspring. See also genetic *lethal.*
infant d., d. of a liveborn infant within the first year.
local d., d. of a part of the body or of a tissue by necrosis.
maternal d., d. of a woman while pregnant or within 42 days after the termination of gestation, irrespective of the duration and site of pregnancy and the cause of d.; two periods are recognized in the 42-day interval: period 1 includes day 1 to day 7; period 2 includes day 8 to day 42. Maternal d.'s are further classified as: **direct m. d.,** d. resulting from obstetric complications of the gestation, labor, or puerperium, and from interventions, omissions, incorrect treatment, or a chain of events caused by any of the above; **indirect m. d.,** an obstetric d. resulting from previously existing disease or from disease developing during pregnancy, labor, or the puerperium; it is not directly due to obstetric causes, but to conditions aggravated by the physiological effects of pregnancy.
neonatal d., d. of a young, liveborn infant; classified as: **early n. d.,**

d. of a liveborn infant occurring less than 7 completed days (168 hours) from the time of birth; **late n. d.,** d. of a liveborn infant occurring after 7 completed days of age but before 28 completed days.

perinatal d., an inclusive term referring to both stillborn infants and neonatal d.'s.

somatic d., systemic d., d. of the entire body, as distinguished from local d.

death-rattle (deth'rat'l). A respiratory gurgling or rattling in the throat of a dying person, caused by the loss of the cough reflex and accumulation of mucus; a rare sign.

Deaver, John B., U.S. surgeon, 1855–1931. See D.'s *incision.*

debanding (dē-band'ing). The removal of fixed orthodontic appliances.

debilitant (dē-bil'i-tant). **1.** Weakening; causing debility. **2.** Obsolete term for a quieting agent or one that subdues excitement.

debilitating (dĕ-bil'i-tāt-ing). Denoting or characteristic of a morbid process that causes weakness.

debility (dĕ-bil'i-tē) [L. *debilitas,* fr. *debilis,* weak, fr. *de-* priv. + *habilis,* able]. Weakness.

debouch (dĕ-būsh') [Fr. *bouche,* mouth]. To open or empty into another part.

débouchement (dā-būsh-mon') [Fr.]. Opening or emptying into another part.

Debré, Robert, French pediatrician and bacteriologist, *1882. See D. *phenomenon.*

débridement (dā-brēd-mon') [Fr. unbridle]. Excision of devitalized tissue and foreign matter from a wound.

debrisoquine sulfate (dĕ-bris'ō-kwin). 3-4-Dihydro-2(1*H*)-isoquinolinecarboxamidine sulfate; an antihypertensive agent.

debt (det) [L. *debitum,* debt]. A deficit; a liability.

alactic oxygen d., that part of the oxygen d. that is not lactacid oxygen d.; during recovery, stores of ATP and creatine phosphate must be replenished by oxidative metabolism, and a small amount of oxygen is also needed to restore the normal oxyhemoglobin levels throughout the circulating blood.

lactacid oxygen d., that part of an oxygen d. represented by the production of lactic acid by anaerobic glycolysis during exercise and, therefore, by the need to eliminate it by oxidative metabolism during recovery.

oxygen d., the extra oxygen, taken in by the body during recovery from exercise, beyond the resting needs of the body; sometimes used as if synonymous with oxygen deficit.

deca- (da) [G. *deka,* ten] Prefix used in the SI and metric systems to signify ten. Also spelled deka-.

decagram (dek'ă-gram). Ten grams.

decalcification (dē'kal-si-fi-kā'shŭn) [L. *de-*, away, + *calx* (*calc-*), lime, + *facio,* to make]. **1.** Removal of lime salts, chiefly tricalcium phosphate, from bones and teeth, either *in vitro* or as a result of a pathologic process. **2.** Precipitation of calcium from blood as by oxalate or fluoride, or the conversion of blood calcium to an unionized form as by citrate, thus preventing or delaying coagulation.

decalcify (dē-kal'si-fī). To remove lime or calcium salts, especially from bones or teeth.

decalcifying (dē-kal'si-fī-ing). Denoting an agent, measure, or process that causes decalcification.

decaliter (dek'ă-lē-ter). Ten liters.

decalvant (dē-kal'vant) [L. *decalvare,* to make bald]. Removing the hair; making bald.

decameter (dek'ă-mē-ter). Ten meters.

decamethonium bromide (dek-ă-me-thō'nē-ŭm). Decamethylene-1,10-bis-trimethylammonium dibromide; a synthetic nondepolarizing neuromuscular blocking agent used to produce muscular relaxation during general anesthesia.

decamine (dek'ă-mēn). Dequalinium acetate.

decane (dek'ān). A paraffin hydrocarbon, $C_{10}H_{22}$.

decanoic acid (dek-ă-nō'ik). *n* -Capric acid.

decanoin (dek-ă-nō'in). Caprin.

decanormal (dek-ă-nōr'măl). Rarely used term denoting the concentration of a solution 10 times that of normal.

decant (dē-kant') [Mediev. L. *decantho,* fr. *de-* + *canthus,* the beak of a jug, fr. G. *kanthos,* corner of the eye]. To pour off gently the upper clear portion of a fluid, leaving the sediment in the vessel.

decantation (dē-kan-tā'shŭn). Pouring off the clear upper portion of a fluid.

decapacitation (dē'kă-pas-i-tā'shŭn). Prevention of capacitation by spermatozoa, and thus of their ability to fertilize ova. See also d. *factor.*

decapitate (dē-kap'i-tāt) [L. *de-,* away, + *caput,* head]. **1.** To cut off the head; specifically, to remove the head of a fetus to facilitate delivery in cases of irremediable dystocia; to cut off the head of an animal in preparation for certain physiologic experiments. **2.** Relating to an experimental animal with the head removed.

decapitation (dē-kap-i-tā'shŭn). Removal of a head. See decapitate.

decapsulation (dē-kap-sū-lā'shŭn). Incision and removal of a capsule or enveloping membrane.

d. of kidney, removing or stripping off the capsule of the kidney.

decarbonization (dē-kar'bon-i-zā'shŭn). Rarely used term denoting the process of arterialization of the blood by oxygenation and the removal of carbon dioxide in the lungs.

decarboxylase (dē-kar-boks'ē-lās). Any enzyme (EC subclass 4.1.1) that removes a molecule of carbon dioxide from a carboxylic group (*e.g.,* from an α-amino acid, converting it into an amine).

decarboxylation (dē'kar-boks-ē-lā'shŭn). A reaction involving the removal of a molecule of carbon dioxide from a carboxylic acid.

decay (dē-kā') [L. *de,* down, + *cado,* to fall]. **1.** Destruction of an organic substance by slow combustion or gradual oxidation. **2.** Putrefaction. **3.** To deteriorate; to undergo slow combustion or putrefaction. **4.** In dentistry, caries. **5.** In psychology, loss of information registered by the senses and processed into short-term memory. See also forgetting. **6.** Loss of radioactivity with time; spontaneous emission of radiation or charged particles or both from an unstable nucleus.

deceleration (dē-sel-er-ā'shŭn). **1.** The act of decelerating. **2.** The rate of decrease in velocity per unit of time. See fig. on p. 402.

early d., slowing of the fetal heart rate early in the uterine contraction phase as displayed on a graph, denoting compression of the fetal head; the fetal heart rate does not fall below 100 beats per minute.

late d., any transient fetal bradycardia exceeding 100 beats per minute, as displayed on a graph, the nadir of which occurs more than 30 seconds after the peak of the uterine contraction.

variable d., fetal bradycardia below 100 beats per minute, as displayed on a graph, denoting compression of the umbilical cord at the height of a uterine contraction.

decentration (dē-sen-trā'shŭn). Removal from the center.

decerebrate (dē-ser'ĕ-brāt). **1.** To cause decerebration. **2.** Denoting an animal so prepared, or a patient whose brain has suffered an injury which renders him in his neurologic behavior comparable to a decerebrate animal.

decerebration (dē-ser'ĕ-brā'shŭn). Removal of the brain above the lower border of the corpora quadrigemina, or a complete section of the brain at this level or somewhat below.

bloodless d., destroying the function of the cerebrum by tying the basilar artery at about the middle of the pons and the common carotid arteries in the neck.

decerebrize (dē-ser'ĕ-brīz). To remove the brain.

dechloridation (dē'klōr-i-dā'shŭn). Dechlorination; dechloruration; reduction of sodium chloride in the tissues and fluids of the body by reducing its intake or increasing its excretion.

dechlorination (dē'klōr-i-nā'shŭn). Dechloridation.

dechloruration (dē'klōr-ū-rā'shŭn). Dechloridation.

decholesterolization (dē'kō-les'ter-ol-i-zā'shŭn). Therapeutic reduction of the cholesterol concentration of the blood.

deci- (d) [L. *decimus,* tenth] Prefix used in the SI and metric systems to signify one-tenth (10^{-1}).

decibel (dB, db) (des'i-bel) [L. *decimus,* tenth, + bel]. One-tenth of a bel; unit for expressing the relative loudness of sound on a logarithmic scale.

decidua (dē-sid'yū-ă) [L. *deciduus,* falling off (qualifying *membrana,* membrane, understood)]. *Membrana* decidua.

d. basa'lis [NA], d. serotina; the area of endometrium between the implanted chorionic vesicle and the myometrium, which develops into the maternal part of the placenta.

d. capsula'ris [NA], d. reflexa; membrana adventitia (2); the layer of endometrium overlying the implanted chorionic vesicle which becomes progressively more attenuated as the chorionic vesicle enlarges; by the fourth month, it is squeezed against the d. parietalis and thereafter undergoes rapid regression.

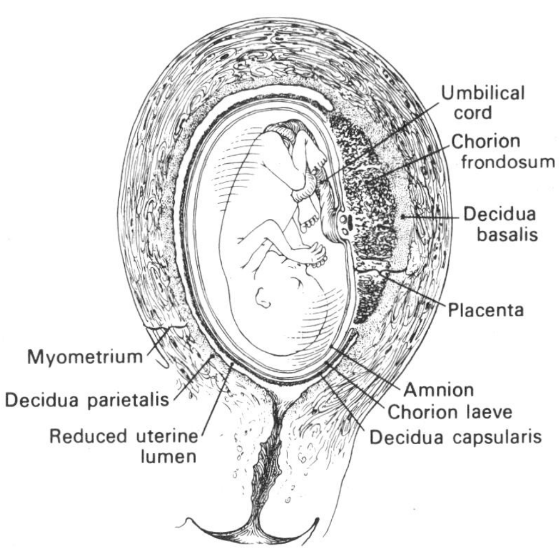

Decidua

Parts of the decidual complex as they appear early in the 5th month of pregnancy.

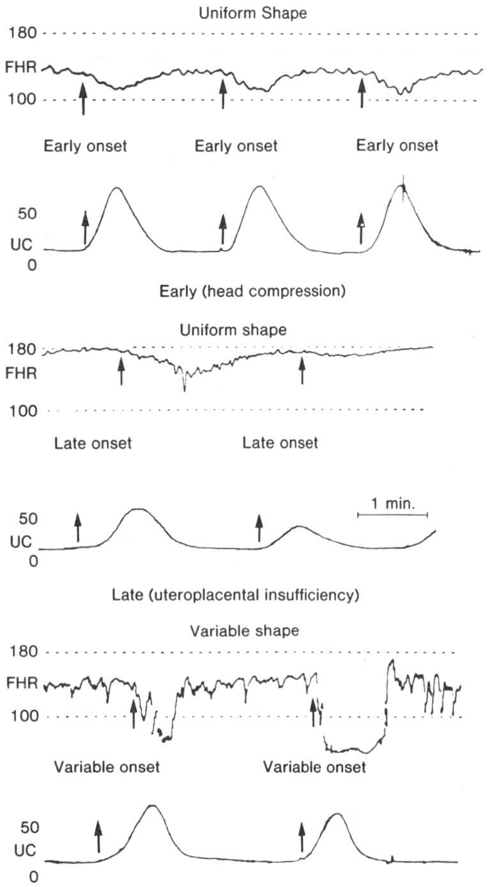

Deceleration

Fetal heart rate patterns and uterine contractions in early, late, and variable deceleration. (After E.H.G. Hon.)

ectopic d., decidual cells which may be found in the cervix, appendix, or areas other than the endometrium.

d. menstrua'lis, the succulent mucous membrane of the nonpregnant uterus at the menstrual period.

d. parieta'lis [NA], d. vera; the altered mucous membrane lining the main cavity of the pregnant uterus other than at the site of attachment of the chorionic vesicle.

d. polypo'sa, d. parietalis showing polypoid projections of the endometrial surface.

d. reflex'a, d. capsularis.

d. seroti'na, d. basalis.

d. spongio'sa, the portion of the d. basalis attached to the myometrium.

d. ve'ra, d. parietalis.

decidual (dē-sid'yū-ăl). Relating to the decidua.

deciduate (dē-sid'yū-āt) [see deciduation]. Relating to those mammals (*e.g.,* man, dog, rodent) that shed maternal uterine tissue when expelling the placenta at birth, in contrast to indeciduate mammals (horse, pig).

deciduation (dē-sid-yū-ā'shŭn) [L. *deciduus,* falling off]. Shedding of endometrial tissue during menstruation.

deciduitis (dē-sid-yū-ī'tis). Inflammation of the decidua.

deciduoma (dē-sid-yū-ō'mă). Placentoma; an intrauterine mass of decidual tissue, probably the result of hyperplasia of decidual cells retained in the uterus.

Loeb's d., mass of decidual tissue produced in the uterus, in the absence of a fertilized ovum, by means of mechanical or hormonal stimulation.

deciduous (dē-sid'yū-ŭs) [L. *deciduus,* falling off]. **1.** Not permanent; denoting that which eventually falls off. **2** (**D** in dental formulas). In dentistry, often used to designate the first or primary dentition. See *dens* deciduus.

decigram (des'i-gram). One-tenth of a gram.

deciliter (des'i-lē-ter). One-tenth of a liter.

decimeter (des'i-mē-ter). One-tenth of a meter.

decimorgan (dM) (des'i-mōr-găn). See morgan.

decinormal (des-i-nōr'măl). One-tenth of normal, denoting the concentration of a solution.

de Clerambault, G., French psychiatrist, 1872–1934. See d. C. *syndrome.*

declination (dek-li-nā'shŭn) [L. *declinatio,* a bending aside]. A bending, sloping, or other deviation from a normal vertical position.

declinator (dek'lin-ā-ter, -tōr). A retractor that holds certain structures out of the way during an operation.

declive (dē-klīv') [L. *declivis,* sloping downward, fr. *clivus,* a slope] [NA]. Declivis; lobulus clivi; the posterior sloping portion of the monticulus of the vermis of the cerebellum; vermal lobule caudal to the primary fissure.

declivis (dē-klī'vis). Declive.

decoction (dē-kok'shŭn) [L. *decoctio,* fr. *de-coquo,* pp. *-coctus,* to boil down]. **1.** The process of boiling. **2.** The pharmacopeial name for preparations made by boiling crude vegetable drugs, and then straining, in the proportion of 50 g of the drug to 1000 ml of water.

décollement (dā-kŭl-mon') [Fr. ungluing]. Surgical separation of tissues or organs which are adherent, either normally or pathologically.

decompensation (de'kom-pen-sā'shŭn). **1.** A failure of compensation in heart disease. **2.** The appearance or exacerbation of a mental disorder due to failure of defense mechanisms.

corneal d., corneal edema resulting from failure of the corneal endothelium to maintain deturgescence.

decompose (dē'kom-pōz) [L. *de,* from, down, + *com-pono,* pp. *-positus,* to put together]. **1.** To resolve a compound into its component parts; to disintegrate. **2.** To decay; to putrefy.

decomposition (dē'kom-pō-zish'ŭn). Decay; disintegration; putrefaction.

decompression (dē'kom-presh-ŭn) [L. *de-,* from, down, + *comprimo,* pp. *-pressus,* to press together]. Removal of pressure.

cardiac d., pericardial d.; incision into the pericardium to relieve pressure due to blood or other fluid in the pericardial sac.

cerebral d., removal of a piece of the cranium, usually in the subtemporal region, with incision of the dura, to relieve intracranial pressure.

explosive d., rapid d.

internal d., removal of intracranial tissue, usually tumor or brain tissue. to relieve pressure.

nerve d., release of pressure on a nerve trunk by the surgical excision of constricting bands or widening of a bony canal.

orbital d., removal of a portion of the bony orbit, usually superior (Naffziger operation), lateral (Krönlein operation), or inferior (Ogura operation).

pericardial d., cardiac d.

rapid d., explosive d.; sudden severe expansion of gases due to a reduction in ambient pressure.

spinal d., the removal of pressure upon the spinal cord as created by a tumor, cyst, hematoma, or bone; accomplished by surgical removal of the spinal laminae and spinous processes.

suboccipital d., d. of the posterior fossa by occipital craniectomy and opening of the dura.

subtemporal d., d. of the brain by temporal craniectomy and opening of the dura over the inferolateral surface of the temporal lobe.

trigeminal d., d. of the trigeminal nerve root.

decongestant (dē-kon-jes'tant). **1.** Decongestive. **2.** An agent that possesses this action.

decongestive (dē-kon-jes'tiv). Decongestant (1); having the property of reducing congestion.

decontamination (dē'kon-tam-i-nā'shŭn). Removal or neutralization of poisonous gas or other injurious agents from the environment.

decortication (dē-kōr-ti-kā'shŭn) [L. *decortico,* pp. *-atus,* to deprive of bark, fr. *de,* from, + *cortex,* rind, bark]. Decortization. **1.** Removal of the cortex, or external layer, beneath the capsule from any organ or structure. **2.** An operation for removal of the residual clot and/or newly organized scar tissue that form after a hemothorax or neglected empyema.

cerebral d., destruction of the cerebral cortex, usually due to anoxia.

reversible d., a temporary loss of function of the cerebral cortex.

decortization (dē-kōr-ti-zā'shŭn). Decortication.

decrement (dek'rē-ment) [L. *decrementum,* fr. *decresco,* to decrease]. **1.** Decrease. **2.** Decrease in conduction velocity at a particular point in a fiber; a result of altered properties at that point. See also decremental *conduction.*

decrepitation (dē-krep-i-tā'shŭn) [L. *de,* from, + *crepo,* pp. *crepitus,* to crackle]. Crackling; the snapping of certain salts when heated.

decrudescence (dē-krū-des'ens) [L. *de,* from, + *cru- desco,* to become worse, fr. *crudus,* crude]. Abatement of the symptoms of disease.

decubation (dē-kū-bā'shŭn) [L. *de,* from, + *cubo,* to lie down]. The final period of an infectious disease from the disappearance of the specific symptoms to complete restoration of health and the end of the infectious period.

decubital (dē-kyū'bi-tăl). Relating to a decubitus ulcer.

decubitus (dē-kyū'bi-tŭs) [L. *decumbo,* to lie down]. **1.** The position of the patient in bed; *e.g.,* dorsal d., lateral d. **2.** Sometimes used in referring to a decubitus ulcer.

Andral's d., position assumed by the patient who lies on the sound side in cases of beginning pleurisy.

decurrent (dē-kŭr'ent) [L. *de-curro,* pp. *-cursus,* to run down]. Extending downward.

decussate (dē'kŭ-sāt, dē-kŭs'āt) [L. *decusso,* pp. *-atus,* to make in the form of an X, fr. *decussis,* the (Roman) numeral ten (X)]. **1.** To cross. **2.** Crossed like the arms of an X.

decussatio, pl. **decussationes** (dē-kŭ-sā'shē-ō, -ō'nēz) [L. (see decussate)]. [NA]. Decussation. **1.** In general, any crossing over or intersection of parts. **2.** The intercrossing of two homonymous fiber bundles as each crosses over to the opposite side of the brain in the course of its ascent or descent through the brainstem or spinal cord.

d. bra'chii conjuncti'vi, d. pedunculorum cerebellarium superiorum.

d. fontina'lis, see *decussationes* tegmenti.

d. lemnisco'rum [NA], d. sensoria; decussation of the fillet; decussation of medial lemniscus; sensory decussation of the medulla oblongata; the intercrossing of the fibers of the left and right medial lemniscus ascending from the nuclei gracilis and cuneatus, immediately rostral to the level of the decussation of the pyramidal tracts in the medulla oblongata.

d. moto'ria [NA], official alternative for d. pyramidum.

d. nervo'rum trochlear'ium [NA], decussation of trochlear nerves; the crossing of the two trochlear nerves at their exit through the velum medullare anterius.

d. pedunculo'rum cerebella'rium superio'rum [NA], decussation of superior cerebellar peduncles; decussation of the brachia conjunctiva; Wernekinck's decussation; the decussation of the left and right superior cerebellar peduncles in the tegmentum of the mesencephalon.

d. pyram'idum [NA], d. motoria; pyramidal or motor decussation; the intercrossing of the bundles of the pyramidal tracts at the

lower border region of the medulla oblongata.
d. senso'ria [NA], official alternative for d. lemniscorum.
decussatio'nes tegmen'ti [NA], tegmental decussations; collective term denoting **(1)** the dorsal tegmental decussation (fountain or Meynert's decussation, d. fontinalis) of the left and right tectospinal and tectobulbar tracts; **(2)** the ventral tegmental decussation (rubrospinal or Forel's decussation) of the left and right rubrospinal and rubrobulbar tracts; both are located in the mesencephalon.

decussation (dē-kŭ-sā'shŭn) [L. *decussatio*]. Decussatio.
d. of brachia conjunctiva, *decussatio* pedunculorum cerebellarium superiorum.
dorsal tegmental d., see *decussationes* tegmenti (1).
d. of the fillet, *decussatio* lemniscorum.
Forel's d., see *decussationes* tegmenti (2).
fountain d., see *decussationes* tegmenti (1).
Held's d., the crossing of some of the fibers arising from the cochlear nuclei to form the lateral lemniscus.
d. of medial lemniscus, *decussatio* lemniscorum.
Meynert's d., see *decussationes* tegmenti (1).
motor d., *decussatio* pyramidum.
optic d., *chiasma* opticum.
pyramidal d., *decussatio* pyramidum.
rubrospinal d., see *decussationes* tegmenti (2).
sensory d. of medulla oblongata, *decussatio* lemniscorum.
d. of superior cerebellar peduncles, *decussatio* pedunculorum cerebellarium superiorum.
tectospinal d., dorsal tegmental d. See *decussationes* tegmenti (1).
tegmental d.'s, *decussationes* tegmenti.
d. of trochlear nerves, *decussatio* nervorum trochlearium.
ventral tegmental d., see *decussationes* tegmenti (2).
Wernekinck's d., *decussatio* pedunculorum cerebellarium superiorum.

decussationes (dē-kŭs-ā-shē-ō'nēz). Plural of decussatio.

dedentition (dē-den-tish'ŭn). Obsolete term denoting loss of teeth.

dedifferentiation (dē-dif'er-en-shē-ā'shŭn). **1.** The return of parts to a more homogeneous state. **2.** Anaplasia.

dedolation (dē-dō-lā'shŭn) [L. *de-dolo,* pp. *-atus,* to hew away]. A slicing wound made by a sharp instrument grazing the surface.

de-efferentation (dē-ef-er-en-tā'shŭn) [L. *de,* from, + efferent]. A loss of the motor nerve fibers to an area of the body.

deep (dēp). Profundus.

de-epicardialization (dē-ep-i-kar'dē-al-i-zā'shŭn). Surgical destruction of the epicardium, usually by the application of phenol, designed to promote collateral circulation to the myocardium.

Deetjen, Hermann, German physician, 1867–1915. See D.'s *bodies.*

def, DEF Abbreviation for decayed, extracted, and filled. See under index.

defatigation (dē-fat-i-gā'shŭn) [L. *de-fatigo,* pp. *-atus,* to tire out]. Weariness, exhaustion, or extreme fatigue.

defecate (def'ĕ-kāt). To perform defecation.

defecation (def-ĕ-kā'shŭn) [L. *defaeco,* pp. *-atus,* to remove the dregs, purify]. Movement (3); motion (2); the discharge of feces from the rectum.

defect (dē'fekt) [L. *deficio,* pp. *-fectus,* to fail, to lack]. An imperfection, malformation, dysfunction, or absence.
aortic or **aorticopulmonary septal d.,** a small congenital opening between the aorta and pulmonary artery about 1 cm above the semilunar valves.
atrial septal d., a congenital d. in the septum between the atria of the heart, due to failure of the foramen primum or secundum to close normally.
congenital ectodermal d., congenital ectodermal dysplasia; incomplete development of the epidermis and skin appendages; the skin is smooth and hairless, the facies abnormal, and the teeth and nails may be affected; sweating may be deficient.
coupling d., see familial *goiter.*
endocardial cushion d., persistent atrioventricular *canal.*
fibrous cortical d., nonosteogenic fibroma; a common small d. in the cortex of a bone, usually the lower femoral shaft of a child, filled with fibrous tissue.
filling d., in a region filled with contrast medium, displacement of the medium around a mass such as a colonic polyp or a gallstone in the gallbladder or intestine seen on x-ray examination as an abnormal contour of any part of the gastrointestinal tract.
iodide transport d., see familial *goiter.*
iodotyrosine deiodinase d., see familial *goiter.*
luteal phase d., luteal phase deficiency; a condition characterized by inadequate secretion of progesterone during the luteal phase of the menstrual cycle, with resultant sterility; subnormal luteal function commonly attributed to abnormal pituitary gonadotropin secretion.
metaphysial fibrous cortical d., a small (less than 2 to 3 cm in diameter) nonosteogenic fibroma of bone.
organification d., see familial *goiter.*
ventricular septal d., a congenital d. in the septum between the cardiac ventricles, usually resulting from failure of the spiral septum to close the interventricular foramen.

defective (dē-fek'tiv). Denoting or exhibiting a defect.

defemination (dē-fem-i-nā'shŭn) [L. *de-,* away, + *femina,* woman]. A weakening or loss of feminine characteristics.

defense (dē-fens') [L. *defendo,* to ward off]. The psychological mechanisms used to control anxiety, *e.g.,* rationalization, projection.
screen d., the use of falsified or incomplete memories or affects to cover repressed but associated memories and affects.
ur-d.'s, see *ur-defenses.*

deferent (def'er-ent) [L. *deferens,* pres. p. of *defero,* to carry away]. Carrying away.

deferentectomy (def'er-en-tek'tō-mē) [(ductus) deferens, + G. *ektomē,* excision]. Vasectomy.

deferential (def-er-en'shăl). Relating to the ductus deferens.

deferentitis (def'er-en-tī'tis). Vasitis; inflammation of the ductus deferens.

deferoxamine mesylate (de-fer-ok'să-mēn). Desferrioxamine mesylate; methanesulfonate of 30-amino-3,14,25-trihydroxy-3,9,14,20,25-penta-azatriacontane-2,10,13,21,24-pentaone; an iron chelate used in the treatment of iron poisoning.

defervescence (def-er-ves'ens) [L. *de-fervesco,* to cease boiling, fr. *de-* neg. + *fervesco,* to begin to boil]. Falling of an elevated temperature; abatement of fever.

defibrillation (dē-fib-ri-lā'shŭn). The arrest of fibrillation of the cardiac muscle (atrial or ventricular) with restoration of the normal rhythm.

defibrillator (dē-fib'ri-lā-ter). **1.** Any agent or measure, *e.g.,* an electric shock, that arrests fibrillation of the ventricular muscle and restores the normal beat. **2.** The machine designed to administer a defibrillating electric shock.
external d., a d. that delivers its defibrillating shock through the unopened chest wall.

defibrination (dē-fī-bri-nā'shŭn). Removal of fibrin from the blood, usually by means of constant agitation while the blood is collected in a container with glass beads or chips.

deficiency (dē-fish'en-sē) [L. *deficio,* to fail, fr. *facio,* to do]. A lack or inadequacy of something. See also deficiency *disease.* For individual d.'s or d. diseases not listed here, see the name of the disease or of the substance involved.
antitrypsin d., d. of α_1-antitrypsin, a glycoprotein of the postalbumin region of human serum, which may be moderate (40 to 60% of normal activity) or severe (less than 10% of normal) and is gene-

determined; the severe form is often associated with familial emphysema or hepatic cirrhosis; autosomal recessive inheritance.
arch length d., the difference between the available circumference of the dental arch and that required to accommodate the succedaneous teeth in proper alignment.
familial high density lipoprotein d., Tangier *disease.*
galactokinase d., an inborn error of metabolism due to congenital d. of galactokinase, resulting in increased blood galactose concentration (galactosemia), cataracts, hepatomegaly, and mental deficiency; autosomal recessive inheritance.
glucosephosphate isomerase d., phosphohexose isomerase d.; an enzyme d. characterized by chronic nonspherocytic hemolytic anemia; autosomal recessive inheritance.
immunological d., immune d., immunity d., immunodeficiency.
LCAT d., a rare condition characterized by corneal opacities, hemolytic anemia, proteinuria, renal insufficiency, and premature atherosclerosis, and very low levels of lecithin cholesterol acyltransferase (LCAT) activity; results in accumulation of unesterfied cholesterol in plasma and tissues.
luteal phase d., luteal phase *defect.*
mental d., mental *retardation.*
phosphohexose isomerase d., glucosephosphate isomerase d.
placental sulfatase d., an enzyme defect in the placenta which results in failure of conversion of 16α-hydroxydehydroepiandrosterone to estriol; primiparas with this condition fail to go into labor.
proximal femoral focal d. (PFFD), a congenital defect in which the upper end of the femur is absent.
pseudocholinesterase d., a heritable disorder manifested by exaggerated responses to drugs ordinarily hydrolyzed by serum pseudocholinesterase (*e.g.,* suxamethonium); believed to entail production of a variant enzyme that is less active than the normal enzyme in hydrolyzing appropriate substrates, but also abnormally resistant to the effects of anticholinesterases.
pyruvate kinase d., a disorder in which there is a d. of pyruvate kinase in red blood cells; characterized by hemolytic anemia varying in degree from one patient to another; autosomal recessive inheritance.
riboflavin d., see ariboflavinosis.
secondary antibody d., secondary *immunodeficiency.*
taste d., reduced or absent ability to detect a bitter taste in a group of compounds of which phenylthiourea is the prototype, due to the homozygous state of a recessive gene of high frequency. See also phenylthiourea.

deficit (def'i-sit) [L. *deficio,* to fail]. The result of temporarily using up something faster than it is being replenished.
base d., a decrease in the total concentration of blood buffer base, indicative of metabolic acidosis or compensated respiratory alkalosis.
oxygen d., the difference between oxygen uptake of the body during early stages of exercise and during a similar duration in a steady state of exercise; sometimes considered as the formation of the oxygen debt.
pulse d., **(1)** the absence of palpable pulse waves in a peripheral artery for a heart beat, as is often seen in atrial fibrillation; **(2)** the number of such missing pulse waves (usually expressed as heart rate minus pulse rate per minute).

definition (def'i-nish'ŭn) [L. *de-finio,* pp. *-finitus,* to bound, fr. *finis,* limit]. In optics, the power of a lens to give a distinct image. See also resolving *power.*

deflection (dē-flek'shŭn) [L. *de-flecto,* pp. *-flexus,* to bend aside]. **1.** A moving to one side. **2.** In the electrocardiogram, a deviation of the curve from the isoelectric base line; any wave or complex of the electrocardiogram.
intrinsic d., with the electrode in direct contact with the muscle fiber, a rapid downward d. from the peak of maximum positivity, signifying that the activation front has reached the subjacent muscle.
intrinsicoid d., the abrupt downstroke from maximum positivity when the electrode is placed not directly on the muscle but at a distance, as in the unipolar chest leads in clinical electrocardiography.

defloration (dē-flōr-ā'shŭn). [L. *defloro,* pp. *-atus,* to deflower, fr. *de-* + *flos* (*flor-*), flower]. Deflowering; depriving of virginity; the rupturing of the hymen, either in coitus or in vaginal examination.

deflores'cence (dē-flō-res'ens) [L. *de-floresco,* to fade, wither, fr. *flos* (*flor-*), flower]. Disappearance of the eruption in scarlet fever or other exanthemas.

defluoridation (dē-flūr'i-dā'shŭn). Removal of excess fluorides from a community water supply.

defluvium (dē-flū'vē-ŭm) [L., fr. *de-fluo,* pp. *-fluxus,* to flow down]. Defluxion.
d. capillo'rum, a falling (or loss) of hair.
d. ung'uium, a falling (or loss) of nails.

defluxion (dē-flŭk'shŭn) [L. *defluxio, de-fluo,* pp. *-fluxus,* to flow down]. Defluvium. **1.** A falling down or out, as of the hair. **2.** A flowing down or discharge of fluid.

deformation (dē-fōr-mā'shŭn). [L. *de-formo,* pp. *-atus,* to deform, fr. *forma,* form]. **1.** Deviation of form from the normal; specifically, an alteration in shape and/or structure of a previously normally formed part. **2.** Deformity. **3.** In rheology, the change in the physical shape of a mass by applied stress.

deforming (dē-fōrm'ing). Causing a deviation from the normal form.

deformity (dē-fōr'mi-tē). Deformation (2); a deviation from the normal shape or size, resulting in disfigurement; may be congenital or acquired.
Åkerlund d., indentation (incisura) with niche of duodenal cap as visualized radiographically.
Arnold-Chiari d., Arnold-Chiari malformation or syndrome; cerebellomedullary malformation syndrome; malformed posterior fossa structures, the result of caudad traction and displacement of the rhombencephalon due to tethering of the spinal cord with or without spina bifida and associated anomalies such as meningomyelocele.
boutonnière d., flexion of the proximal interphalangeal joint with hyperextension of the distal interphalangeal joint of the finger, caused by splitting of the extensor hood and herniation of the head of the proximal phalanx through the resulting "buttonhole."
contracture d., d. of a limb without discernable primary changes of bone.
Erlenmeyer flask d. [resemblance to an E. flask], a d. at the distal end of the femur caused by a failure of the shaft of the bone to develop to its normal tubular shape, with the result that the bone is wide for a much longer distance up the shaft than normal.
gunstock d., a form of cubitus varus resulting from condylar fracture at the elbow in which the axis of the extended forearm is not continuous with that of the arm but is displaced toward midline.
Haglund's d., Haglund's *disease.*
J-sella d., pear-shaped or J-shaped d. of sella turcica caused by increased pressure on growing sphenoid bone; noted in the mucopolysaccharide storage diseases.
keyhole d., mucosal ectropion at the posterior edge of the anus following sphincterotomy at that location.
lobster-claw d., a hand or foot suggestive of a lobster claw because of missing or fused medial digits; also called bidactyly when only the first and fifth digits are present; usually autosomal dominant inheritance.
Madelung's d., carpus curvus; an inferior radioulnar subluxation due to an anterior concave curvature of the lower extremity of the radius.
mermaid d., sirenomelia.
parachute d., parachute mitral *valve.*
pseudolobster-claw d., a condition resembling lobster-claw d. but

with less complete suppression of the medial digits.
reduction d., a congenital skeletal shortening or deficiency of one or more limbs.
seal-fin d., deflection outward of the fingers in rheumatoid arthritis.
silver-fork d., the d. resembling the curve of the back of a fork seen in Colles' fractures.
Sprengel's d., scapula elevata; congenital elevation of the scapula.
swan-neck d., narrowing of the first part of the renal proximal convoluted tubule adjoining the glomerulus, seen in cystinosis and occasionally in other renal diseases.
torsional d., in orthopedics, a d. caused by rotation of a portion of an extremity with relationship to the long axis of the entire extremity.
whistling d., d. caused by insufficient tissue in the lower border of a repaired cleft lip, giving the appearance of whistling.
Whitehead d., circumferential mucosal ectropion at the anus following Whitehead's operation.

defurfuration (dē-fer-fer-ā'shŭn) [L. *de,* away from, + *furfur,* bran]. Branny desquamation; the shedding of the epidermis in the form of fine scales.

deganglionate (dē-gang'glē-on-āt). To deprive of ganglia.

degeneracy (dē-jen'er-ă-sē) [L. *de,* from, + *genus, (gener-),* race]. A condition marked by deterioration of mental, physical, or moral processes.

degenerate 1 (dē-jen'er-āt). To pass to a lower level of mental, physical, or moral qualities; to fall below the normal or acceptable type or state. **2** (dē-jen'ĕ-răt). Below the normal or acceptable; that which has passed to a lower level. **3** (dē-jen'ĕ-răt). A person whose moral characteristics are considered to be below those of his society.

degeneratio (dē-jen-er-ā'shē-ō) [L. *degenero,* pp. *-atus,* fr. *de,* from, + *genus,* race]. Degeneration.
d. hyaloid'ea granulifor'mis, bilateral deposits of hyaline-like material in the cornea.
d. spherula'ris elaioid'es, subepithelial droplets resembling oil in the cornea near the corneoscleral limbus, occurring in the aged.

DEGENERATION

degeneration (dē-jen-er-ā'shŭn) [L. *degeneratio*]. **1.** Deterioration; passing from a higher to a lower level or type. **2.** A worsening of mental, physical, or moral qualities. **3.** A retrogressive pathologic change in cells or tissues, in consequence of which the functions may be impaired or destroyed; at some stages, the degenerative process is reversible, but usually, necrosis results.
adipose d., fatty d.
adiposogenital d., *dystrophia* adiposogenitalis.
albuminoid d., albuminous d., obsolete terms for cloudy *swelling.*
amyloid d., waxy d. (1); infiltration of amyloid between cells and fibers of tissues and organs.
angiolithic d., calcareous d. of the walls of the blood vessels.
ascending d., **(1)** retrograde d. of a severed nerve fiber; *i.e.,* toward the nerve cell of the fiber; **(2)** d. cephalad to a severed or injured spinal cord.
atheromatous d., focal accumulation of lipid material (atheroma) in the intima and subintimal portion of arteries, eventually resulting in fibrous thickening or calcification.
ballooning d., a phenomenon observed especially in cells that are infected with certain viruses, resulting in conspicuous cloudy swelling of the cell and cytoplasmic vacuolation.
basophilic d., blue staining of connective tissues when hematoxylin-eosin stain is used; found in such conditions as lupus erythematosus and solar elastosis.
calcareous d., in a precise sense, not a degenerative process *per se,* but the deposition of insoluble calcium salts in tissue that has degenerated and become necrotic, as in dystrophic calcification.
carneous d., red d.
caseous d., caseous *necrosis.*
colliquative d., obsolete term for liquefaction d.
colloid d., a d. similar to mucoid d., in which the material is inspissated.
cone d., an ocular abnormality in which color perception is severely deficient and typical changes occur in electroretinogram. See achromatopsia.
Crooke's hyaline d., Crooke's hyaline *change.*
cystoid macular d., honeycomb *macula.*
descending d., **(1)** orthograde (wallerian) d. of a severed nerve fiber; *i.e.,* distal to the section; **(2)** d. caudal to the level of section or injury of the spinal cord.
disciform d., disciform detachment of retina; foveal or parafoveal subretinal neovascularization with retinal separation and hemorrhage leading finally to a localized mass of fibrous tissue with marked loss of visual acuity.
ectatic marginal d. of cornea, marginal corneal d.
elastoid d., **(1)** elastosis (2); **(2)** hyaline d. of the elastic tissue of the arterial wall, seen during involution of the uterus.
elastotic d., elastosis (2).
familial pseudoinflammatory macular d., Sorsby's macular d.; macular d. that occurs during the fifth decade of life, with sudden development of a central scotoma in one eye followed rapidly by a similar lesion in the opposite eye; autosomal dominant inheritance.
fascicular d., neurogenic atrophy; muscular d. due to atrophy of motor neurons in the cord or brainstem.
fatty d., adipose d.; steatosis (2); abnormal formation of microscopically visible droplets of fat in the cytoplasm of cells, as a result of injury.
fibrinoid d., fibrinous d., a process resulting in poorly defined, deeply acidophilic, homogeneous refractile deposits with some staining reactions that resemble fibrin, occurring in connective tissue, blood vessel walls, and other sites.
fibrous d., not a d. *per se,* but rather a reparative process; cells and foci of tissue previously affected with degenerative processes, and necrosis, are replaced by cellular fibrous tissue.
granular d., cloudy *swelling.*
granulovacuolar d., d. of hippocampal brain cells in elderly persons, characterized by the basophilic granules surrounded by a clear zone in hippocampal neurons.
gray d., d. of the white substance of the spinal cord, the fibers of which lose their myelin sheaths and become darker in color.
hepatolenticular d., lenticular progressive d.; hepatolenticular disease; Wilson's syndrome; Wilson's disease (1); a syndrome characterized by cirrhosis, d. in the basal ganglia of the brain, and deposition of green pigment in the periphery of the cornea; the plasma levels of ceruloplasmin and copper are decreased, urinary excretion of copper is increased, and the amounts of copper in the liver, brain, kidneys, and lenticular nucleus are unusually high, while cytochrome oxidase is reduced; autosomal recessive inheritance.
heredomacular d., a group of hereditary disorders involving predominately the posterior portion of the ocular fundus, due to degeneration in the sensory layer of the retina, retinal pigment epithelium, Bruch's membrane, choroid, or a combination of these tissues.
hyaline d., a group of several degenerative processes that affect various cells and tissues, resulting in the formation of rounded masses ("droplets") or relatively broad bands of substances that are homogeneous, translucent, refractile, and moderately to deeply acidophilic; may occur in the collagen of old fibrous tissue, smooth

muscle of arterioles or the uterus, and as droplets in parenchymal cells.
hyaloideoretinal d., Wagner's disease or syndrome; progressive liquefaction and destruction of the vitreous humor with grayish-white preretinal membranes, myopia cataract, retinal detachment, and hyper- and hypopigmentation; autosomal dominant inheritance.
hydropic d., cloudy *swelling.*
infantile neuronal d., degenerative disorder of infants with widespread neuronal loss in thalamus, cerebellum, pons, and spinal cord, resembling infantile muscular atrophy.
Kuhnt-Junius d., Kuhnt-Junius disease; disciform d. of the macula retinae characterized by subretinal exudate, subretinal neovascularization, hemorrhage, and ultimately a localized mass of fibrous tissue.
lenticular progressive d., hepatolenticular d.
liquefaction d., dissolution of the basal layer by necrosis of scattered cells with edema, observed in lichen planus, lupus erythematosus, and other dermatologic conditions.
macular d., any ocular d. affecting predominately the posterior fundus.
marginal corneal d., ectatic marginal d. of cornea; Terrien's marginal d.; bilateral opacification and vascularization of the periphery of the cornea, progressing to formation of a gutter and ectasia.
Mönckeberg's d., Mönckeberg's *arteriosclerosis.*
mucinoid d., a term including both mucoid and colloid d., the essential cellular changes in both being similar, the only difference being that, in colloid d., the substance is firmer and more inspissated than in mucoid d., in which it is thin and jelly-like.
mucoid d., myxoid or myxomatous d.; myxomatosis (2); a conversion of any of the connective tissues into a gelatinous or mucoid substance.
mucoid medial d., cystic medial *necrosis.*
myelinic d., formation of myelin figures in the cytoplasm of cells, possibly by degradation or hydration of lipoprotein of self-digested organelles.
myopic d., association of crescent of the optic disk, atrophy of the choroid and macular pigment, subretinal neovascularization, hemorrhage, and pigment proliferation in pathologic myopia.
myxoid d., myxomatous d., mucoid d.
neurofibrillary d., formation of coarse, argentophilic, intracytoplasmic fibers, often in complex tangles within intracranial nerve cells that are undergoing aging. See also Alzheimer's *disease.*
Nissl d., d. of the cell body occurring after transection of the axon.
olivopontocerebellar d., olivopontocerebellar *atrophy.*
orthograde d., wallerian d.
parenchymatous d., cloudy *swelling.*
primary neuronal d., Alzheimer's *disease.*
primary pigmentary d. of retina, tapetoretinal d.
primary progressive cerebellar d., a familial ataxic condition related to cerebellar d.
pseudotubular d., a form of d. observed in adrenal glands, especially those of patients with febrile infectious disease; the shrunken, lipid-depleted cells of the zona fasciculata (and sometimes the zona glomerulosa) are arranged in a circular pattern about spaces that may be empty or partly filled with fibrin, necrotic cells, or amorphous material.
red d., carneous d.; necrosis, with staining by hemoglobin, which may occur in uterine myomas, especially during pregnancy; marked by softening and a red color resembling partly cooked meat.
reticular d., severe epidermal edema resulting in multilocular bullae.
retrograde d., retrograde cell d. with chromatolysis of Nissl bodies and peripheral displacement of the nucleus of the cell of origin of a nerve fiber injured or sectioned.
Salzmann's nodular corneal d., large and prominent nodules of a solid, opaque material that stands out from the surface of the cornea; occurs occasionally in persons previously affected by phlyctenular keratitis.
secondary d., wallerian d.
senile d., the process of involution occurring in old age.
Sorsby's macular d., familial pseudoinflammatory macular d.
spongy d., Canavan's disease or sclerosis; a rare, recessively transmitted, fatal brain disease of infancy characterized by progressive paralysis, blindness, and megalencephaly; pathologically, there is extensive spongiform demyelination of the cerebral hemispheres. See also leukodystrophy.
subacute combined d. of the spinal cord, a subacute or chronic disorder of the spinal cord, such as that occurring in certain patients with pernicious anemia, characterized by a slight to moderate degree of gliosis in association with spongiform degeneration of the posterior and lateral columns. Also called combined system disease; funicular myelitis (2); funicular myelosis; Putnam-Dana syndrome; vitamin B_{12} neuropathy.
tapetoretinal d., primary pigmentary d. of retina; a hereditary disorder of the retina mainly affecting photoreceptors and retinal pigment epithelium.
Terrien's marginal d., marginal corneal d.
transsynaptic d., transneuronal atrophy; transsynaptic chromatolysis; an atrophy of nerve cells following damage to the axons that make synaptic connection with them; noted especially in the lateral geniculate body.
Türck's d., d. of a nerve fiber and its sheath distal to the point of injury or section of the axon; usually applied to d. within the central nervous system.
vacuolar d., formation of nonlipid vacuoles in cytoplasm, most frequently due to accumulation of water by cloudy swelling.
vitelliform d., vitelliruptive d., d. in Best's disease, with the macular region of each eye occupied by a bright orange-yellow deposit followed by scarring; autosomal dominant inheritance.
wallerian d., secondary d.; orthograde d.; d. of a nerve fiber separated from its trophic center, the nerve cell characterized by proliferation of the nucleus of the interannular segment and by segmentation of the myelin, ending in atrophy and destruction of the axon; usually applied to d. of peripheral nerves.
waxy d., **(1)** amyloid d.; **(2)** Zenker's d.
xerotic d., scarring of the conjunctiva associated with keratinized epithelium.
Zenker's d., waxy d. (2); Zenker's necrosis; a form of severe hyaline d. or necrosis in skeletal muscle, occurring in severe infections.

degenerative (dē-jen′er-ă-tiv). Relating to degeneration.

degloving (dē-glov′ing). **1.** Intraoral surgical exposure of the anterior mandible used in various orthognathic surgical operations such as genioplasty or mandibular alveolar surgery. **2.** See degloving *injury.*

deglut. Abbreviation for L. *deglutiatur,* swallow.

deglutition (dē-glū-tish′ŭn) [L. *de-glutio,* to swallow]. The act of swallowing.

deglutitive (dē-glū′ti-tiv). Relating to deglutition.

Degos, R., 20th century French dermatologist. See D.'s *acanthoma, disease;* Köhlmeier-D. *disease;* D.'s *syndrome.*

degradation (deg-ră-dā′shŭn) [L. *degradatus,* degrade]. The change of a chemical compound into a less complex compound.

degranulation (dē-gran-yū-lā′shŭn). Disappearance of cytoplasmic granules (lysosomes) from a phagocytic cell when the granules fuse with, and empty their contents into, a phagosome.

degree (dĕ-grē′) [Fr. *degré;* L. *gradus,* a step]. **1.** One of the divisions on the scale of a thermometer, barometer, etc. See subentries under scale; Comparative Temperature Scales appendix. **2.** The 360th part of the circumference of a circle. **3.** A position or rank within a graded series.

d.'s of freedom, in statistics; the number of observations (*e.g.,* subjects, test items and scores, trials, conditions) minus the number of independent restrictions in the sampling undertaken.

degustation (dē-gŭs-tā'shŭn) [L. *degustatio,* fr. *de-gusto,* pp. *-atus,* to taste]. **1.** The act of tasting. **2.** The sense of taste.

dehalogenase (dē-hal'ō-jen-ās). Any enzyme (EC subclass 3.8) removing halogen atoms from organic halides.

Dehio, Karl K., Russian physician, 1851–1927. See D.'s *test.*

dehiscence (dē-his'ens) [L. *dehiscere,* to split apart or open]. A bursting open, splitting, or gaping along natural or sutured lines.

iris d., a defect of the eye characterized by multiple holes in the iris.

root d., a loss of the buccal or lingual bone overlaying the root portion of a tooth, leaving that area covered by soft tissue only.

wound d., disruption of apposed surfaces of a wound.

dehumanization (dē-hyū'măn-i-zā'shŭn) [*de-* + *humanus,* human, fr. *homo,* man]. Loss of human characteristics; brutalization by either mental or physical means; stripping one of his self-esteem.

dehydrase (dē-hī'drās). Former name for dehydratase.

dehydratase (dē-hī'drā-tās). A subclass (EC 4.2.1) of lyases (hydro-lyases) that remove H and OH as H_2O from a substrate, leaving a double bond, or add a group to a double bond by the elimination of water from two substances to form a third; synthase is sometimes used when the synthetic aspect of the reaction is emphasized. Some trivial names of enzymes in this subclass bear the generic term hydratase, emphasizing the reverse reaction.

dehydrate (dē-hī'drāt) [L. *de,* from + G. *hydōr* (*hydr-*), water]. **1.** To extract water from. **2.** To lose water.

dehydration (dē-hī-drā'shŭn). **1.** Anhydration; deprivation of water. **2.** Reduction of water content. **3.** Exsiccation (2). **4.** Desiccation.

absolute d., actual water deficit as measured by a difference from the normal or from a given water content.

relative d., water deficit relative to content of solutes contributing effective osmotic pressure; a state of increased effective osmotic pressure of body fluids.

voluntary d., that physiologic lag or deficit that results when sensations of thirst are not strong enough to bring about complete replacement of water loss, as in rapid sweating.

dehydro-. Prefix used in the names of those chemical compounds that differ from other and more familiar compounds in the absence of two hydrogen atoms; *e.g.,* dehydroascorbic acid, which resembles ascorbic acid in all structural features except for its lack of two hydrogen atoms that are present in the ascorbic acid molecule. In systematic nomenclature, didehydro- is preferred as being more exact.

dehydroacetic acid (dē-hī'drō-ă-sē'tik). 3-Acetyl-6-methyl-2*H*-pyran-2,4-(3*H*)-dione; an antimicrobial agent used as a preservative in cosmetics.

dehydroascorbic acid (dē-hī'drō-as-kōr'bik). The reversibly oxidized form of ascorbic acid; it is antiscorbutic, but is converted in the body to diketogulonic acid, which has no vitamin C activity.

dehydrobilirubin (dē-hī'drō-bil-ē-rū'bin). Biliverdine.

dehydrocholate (dē-hī-drō-kō'lāt). A salt or ester of dehydrocholic acid.

7-dehydrocholesterol (dē-hī'drō-kō-les'ter-ol). Provitamin D_3; cholest-5,7-adien-3β-ol; a sterol in skin and other animal tissues that upon activation by ultraviolet light becomes antirachitic and is then referred to as cholecalciferol (vitamin D_3).

24-dehydrocholesterol. Desmosterol.

dehydrocholic acid (dē-hī-drō-kol'ik). 3,7,12-Trioxo-5β-cholan-24-oic acid; has a stimulating effect upon the secretion of bile by the liver (choleretic), and improves the absorption of essential food materials in states associated with deficient bile formation.

11-dehydrocorticosterone (dē-hī'drō-kōr-ti-kos'ter-ōn). 21-Hydroxypregn-4-ene-3,11,20-trione; principally a metabolite of corticosterone, found in the adrenal cortex.

dehydroemetine (dē-hī-drō-em'ē-tēn). A synthetic derivative of emetine; used in the treatment of intestinal amebiasis.

d. resinate, a derivative of emetine effective orally in the treatment of leishmaniasis.

dehydro-3-epiandrosterone (dē-hī'drō-ep-i-an-dros'ter-ōn). Androstenolone; dehydroisoandrosterone; 3β-hydroxyandrost-5-ene-17-one; a weakly androgenic steroid secreted largely by the adrenal cortex, but also by the testes; one of the principal components of urinary 17-ketosteroids.

dehydrogenase (dē-hī'drō-jen-ās). Class name for those enzymes that oxidize substrates by catalyzing removal of hydrogen from metabolites (hydrogen donors) and transferring it to other substances (hydrogen acceptors), which are thus reduced; most of the oxidative enzymes (oxidoreductases, EC class 1) perform their oxidations in this manner.

aerobic d., an enzyme (usually a metalloflavoenzyme) catalyzing the transfer of hydrogen from some metabolite to oxygen, forming hydrogen peroxide in the process; usually a metalloflavoenzyme; *e.g.,* xanthine oxidase (EC 1.2.3.2) and others in sub-subclasses EC 1.1.3, 1.2.3, 1.3.3, 1.4.3, 1.5.3, 1.7.3, 1.8.3, 1.9.3, 1.10.3.

anaerobic d., an enzyme (usually a pyridinoenzyme) catalyzing the transfer of hydrogen from some metabolite to some acceptor molecule (*e.g.,* NAD, cytochrome) other than oxygen; *e.g.,* lactate d.'s (EC 1.1.1.27, 28; 1.1.2.3, 4), isocitrate d.'s (EC 1.1.1.41, 42), and others in EC class 1, excluding those listed under aerobic d.

Robison ester d., glucose 6-phosphate dehydrogenase.

dehydrogenate (dē-hī'drō-jen-āt). To subject to dehydrogenation.

dehydrogenation (dē-hī'drō-jen-ā'shŭn). Removal of a pair of hydrogen atoms from a compound by the action of enzymes (dehydrogenases) or other catalysts.

dehydroisoandrosterone (dē-hī'drō-ī-sō-an-dros'ter-ōn). Dehydro-3-epiandrosterone.

dehydropeptidase II (dē-hī-drō-pep'ti-dās). Aminoacylase.

dehydroretinaldehyde (dē-hī'drō-ret-i-nal'dē-hīd). 3-Dehydroretinaldehyde; retinene-2; vitamin A_2 aldehyde; dehydroretinol with –CHO instead of –CH_2OH at the terminal carbon of the side chain.

dehydroretinoic acid (dē-hī'drō-ret-i-nō'ik). 3-Dehydroretinoic acid; dehydroretinol with –COOH in place of –CH_2OH at the terminal carbon of the side chain.

dehydroretinol (dē-hī-drō-ret'i-nol). 3-Dehydroretinol; vitamin A_2; retinol with an additional double bond in the 3-4 position of the cyclohexane ring.

dehydrosugars (dē-hī'drō-shug-erz). Anhydrosugars.

dehydrotestosterone (dē-hī-drō-tes-tos'ter-ōn). Boldenone.

dehypnotize (dē-hip'nō-tīz). To bring out of the hypnotic state.

deiminases (dē-im'i-nās-ez). Iminohydrolases.

deinstitutionalization (dē'in-sti-tū'shŭn-ăl-i-zā-shŭn). Mainstreaming.

Deiters, Otto F.K., German anatomist, 1834–1863. See D's *cells,* terminal *frames, nucleus, process.*

déjà vu (dā-zhah-vū') [Fr. already seen]. See under phenomenon.

dejecta (dē-jek'tă). Dejection (3).

dejection (dē-jek'shŭn) [L. *dejectio,* fr. *de- jicio,* pp. *-jectus,* to cast down]. **1.** Depression (3). **2.** The discharge of excrementitious matter. **3.** Dejecta; the matter so discharged.

Dejerine, Joseph J., Paris neurologist, 1849–1917. See D.'s *disease,* hand *phenomenon,* peripheral *neurotabes, reflex, sign;* D.-Lichtheim *phenomenon;* D.-Roussy *syndrome;* D.-Sottas *disease;* Klumpke-D. *syndrome;* Landouzy-D. *dystrophy.*

deka-. See deca-.

delacrimation (dē'lak-ri-mā'shŭn) [L. *delacrimation,* fr. *lacrimo,* pp. *-atus,* to weep]. Excessive secretion of tears.

Delafield, Francis, U.S. physician and pathologist, 1841–1915. See D.'s *hematoxylin.*

delamination (dē-lam-i-nā-'shŭn) [L. *de,* from, + *lamina,* a thin plate]. Division into separate layers.

Delaney clause [James F. *Delaney,* U.S. Congressman]. A clause of the Food Additive Amendment of the U.S. Federal law specifying that no substance that has been found to induce cancer in any animal may be incorporated into food.

de Lange, Cornelia, Dutch pediatrician, 1871–1950. See de L. *syndrome.*

Delbet, Pierre, French surgeon, 1861–1925. See D.'s *sign.*

Del Castillo, E.B., 20th century Argentinian physician. See Ahumada-D. C. *syndrome,* Argonz-D. C. *syndrome,* D. C. *syndrome.*

de-lead (dē-led'). To cause the mobilization and excretion of lead deposited in the bones and other tissues, as by the administration of a chelating agent or acid salts.

DeLee, Joseph B., U.S. obstetrician and gynecologist, 1869–1942. See D.'s *maneuver.*

deleterious (del-ĕ-tēr'ē-ŭs) [G. *dēlētērios,* fr. *dēleomai,* to injure]. Injurious; noxious; harmful.

deletion (dē-lē'shŭn) [L. *deletio,* destruction]. In genetics, any spontaneous elimination of part of the normal genetic complement, whether cytogenetically visible (chromosomal d.) or inferred by phenotypic processes (point d.).

chromosomal d., a microscopically evident loss of part of a chromosome. See also monosomy.

gene d., d. of a segment of a chromosome, too small to be detected cytogenetically, inferred from the phenotype at one particular locus.

interstitial d., d. that does not involve the terminal parts of a chromosome.

nucleotide d., point d.(2); d. of a single nucleotide, which in a transcribed gene will lead to a frame-shift mutation.

point d., **(1)** d. involving a submicroscopic loss of genetic material too small to be resolved by linkage analysis; **(2)** nucleotide d.

terminal d., d. involving the terminal part of a chromosome and leading to a cohesive terminus.

delicate (del'i-kăt) [L. *delicatus,* soft, luxurious, fr. *de,* from, + *lacio,* to entice]. Of feeble resisting power.

delimitation (dē-lim-i-tā'shŭn) [L. *de-limito,* pp. *-atus,* to bound, fr. *limes,* boundary]. Putting bounds or limits; marking off; preventing the spread of a morbid process in the body or of a disease in the community.

deliquesce (del-i-kwes'). To undergo deliquescence.

deliquescence (del-i-kwes'ens) [L. *de-liquesco,* to melt or become liquid]. Becoming damp or liquid by absorption of water from the atmosphere; a property of certain salts, such as $CaCl_2$.

deliquescent (del-i-kwes'ent). Denoting a solid capable of deliquescence.

deliriant (de-lir'ē-ant). **1.** Causing delirium. **2.** A toxic agent that produces delirium.

delirious (dē-lir'ē-ŭs). In a state of delirium.

delirium (dē-lir'ē-ŭm) [L. fr. *deliro,* to be crazy, fr. *de-* + *lira,* a furrow (*i.e.,* go out of the furrow)]. A clouded state of consciousness and confusion, marked by difficulty in sustaining attention to stimuli, disordered thinking, defective perception (illusions and hallucinations), disordered sleep-wakefulness cycles, and motor disturbances.

acute d., d. of recent, rapid onset.

anxious d., d. in which the predominating symptom is an incoherent apprehension or anxiety.

collapse d., d. caused by extreme physical depression induced by a shock, profuse hemorrhage, exhausting labor, etc.

d. cor'dis, atrial *fibrillation.*

low d., d. in which there is little excitement, either mental or motor, the ideas being confused and incoherent, but following each other slowly.

d. mus'sitans, muttering d., d. common in low fevers in which the subject is unconscious, but constantly mutters incoherently.

posttraumatic d., a posttraumatic neuropsychologic disorder of the brain with disturbed consciousness, agitation, hallucinations, delusions, and/or disorientation.

senile d., d. associated with senile dementia.

toxic d., d. caused by the action of a poison.

d. tre'mens (DT) [L. pres. p. of *tremo,* to tremble], a form of acute organic brain syndrome due to alcoholic withdrawal and marked by sweating, tremor, atonic dyspepsia, restlessness, anxiety, precordial distress, mental confusion, and hallucinations.

delitescence (del-i-tes'ens) [L. *delitesco,* to lie hidden away]. **1.** Sudden subsidence of symptoms; disappearance of a tumor or a cutaneous lesion. **2.** Period of incubation of an infectious disease.

deliver (dē-liv'er) [fr. O. Fr. fr. L. *de-* + *liber,* free]. **1.** To assist a woman in childbirth. **2.** To extract from an enclosed place, as the fetus from the womb, an object or foreign body, *e.g.,* a tumor from its capsule or surroundings, or the lens of the eye in cases of cataract.

delivery (dē-liv'er-ē). Passage of the fetus and the placenta from the genital canal into the external world.

assisted cephalic d., extraction of a fetus that presents by the head.

breech d., partus agrippinus; extraction or expulsion of a fetus that presents by the buttocks or feet.

forceps d., assisted birth of the child by an instrument designed to grasp the child.

high forceps d., d. by forceps applied to the fetal head before engagement has taken place.

low forceps d., d. by forceps applied to the fetal head after it is clearly visible, the skull has reached the perineal floor, and the sagittal suture is in the anteroposterior diameter of the pelvis.

midforceps d., d. by forceps applied to the fetal head before the criteria of low forceps d. have been met, but after engagement has taken place.

postmortem d., extraction of the fetus after the death of its mother.

premature d., birth of a fetus before its proper time. See also premature *birth.*

spontaneous cephalic d., unassisted expulsion of a fetus that presents by the head.

delle (del'eh) [D. *delle,* low ground, pit]. The central lighter-colored portion of the erythrocyte, as observed in a stained film of blood.

del'len [D. pl. of *delle,* low ground, pit]. Shallow, saucer-like, clearly defined excavations at the margin of the cornea, about 1.5 by 2 mm, due to localized dehydration.

d. of Fuchs, saucer-like depressions at the corneal periphery in neuroparalytic keratitis.

delomorphous (del-ō-mōr'fŭs) [G. *dēlos,* manifest, + *morphē,* form]. Of definite form and shape; a term applied in the past to the parietal cells of the gastric glands.

delouse (dē-lows'). To remove lice from; to free from infestation with lice; used especially of prophylaxis of louse-borne diseases.

delphinine (del'fin-ēn). A toxic alkaloid, an aconine derivative, from *Delphinium staphisagria;* it resembles aconitine in its action and chemical structure.

Delphinium ajacis (del-fin'ē-ŭm ă-jā'sis) [G. *delphinion,* larkspur]. Larkspur; a species of plant (family Ranuculaceae) containing the alkaloids ajacine and ajaconine; the dried ripe seeds have been used externally as a parasiticide in pediculosis; rarely used now because of its toxicity.

delta (del'tă). **1.** Fourth letter of the Greek alphabet, Δ (capital), δ (lower case), *q.v.* **2.** In anatomy, a triangular surface.
d. for'nicis, *commissura* fornicis.
Galton's d., **(1)** a more or less well-marked triangle, in a fingerprint, on either side where the straight ridges near the joint of the distal phalanx are succeeded by arches, loops, or whorls. See also Galton's system of classification of *fingerprints;* **(2)** triradius.
d. mesoscap'ulae, the flat triangular surface at the vertebral extremity of the spine of the scapula over which glides the tendon for the lower fibers of the trapezius muscle.

deltoid (del'toyd) [G. *deltoeidēs,* shaped like the letter *delta*]. **1.** Resembling the Greek letter delta (Δ); triangular. **2.** *Musculus* deltoideus.

delusion (dē-lū'zhŭn) [L. *de-ludo,* pp. *-lusus,* to play false, deceive, fr. *ludo,* to play]. A false belief or wrong judgment held with conviction despite incontrovertible evidence to the contrary.
d. of control, d. of being controlled, d. of passivity; a d. in which one experiences his feelings, impulses, thoughts, or actions as not his own, but as being imposed on him by some external force.
expansive d., d. of grandeur.
d. of grandeur, expansive d.; a d. in which one believes himself possessed of great wealth, intellect, importance, power, etc.
d. of negation, nihilistic d.; a d. in which one imagines that the world and all that relates to it have ceased to exist.
nihilistic d., d. of negation.
d. of passivity, d. of control.
d. of persecution, persecutory d., a false notion that one is being persecuted; characteristic symptom of paranoid schizophrenia.
d. of reference, a delusional idea referring to the self.
somatic d., a d. having reference to a nonexistent lesion or alteration of some organ or part of the body; sometimes indistinguishable from hypochondriasis.
systematized d., a d. that is logically constructed from a false premise and embraces a specific sector of the patient's life.
unsystematized d., one of a group of apparently discrete, disconnected d.'s.

delusional (dē-lū'zhŭn-ăl). Relating to a delusion.

demarcation (dē-mar-kā'shŭn) [Fr. fr. L. *de,* from, + Mediev. L. *marco,* to mark]. A setting of limits; determining a boundary.

Demarquay, Jean N., French surgeon, 1811–1875. See D.'s *symptom.*

demasculinizing (dē-mas'kyū-lin-īz'ing). Depriving of male characteristics or inhibiting development of such characteristics.

Dematiaceae (dē-mat-ē-ā'sē-ē). A family of soil-inhabiting, dark-colored fungi found in decaying vegetables, rotting wood, and forest carpets, and including several of the dark-colored genera that cause chromomycosis in man, such as *Phialophora, Fonsecaea,* and *Cladosporium.*

dematiaceous (dē-mat-ē-ā'shŭs). Denoting dark conidia and/or hyphae, usually olivaceous, gray, or black; used frequently to denote dark-colored fungi.

deme (dēm) [G. demos, people]. A local, small, highly inbred group or kinship.

demecarium bromide (dem-ĕ-kar'ē-ŭm). A potent cholinesterase inhibitor used in the treatment of glaucoma and accommodative esotropia; it is stable in aqueous solution.

demeclocycline (dem'ĕ-klō-sī'klēn). Demethylchlortetracycline; 7-chloro-6-demethyltetracycline; a broad-spectrum antibiotic that is more slowly excreted and more stable in acid and alkali than are other forms of the tetracyclines; available as the hydrochloride.

demecolcine (dem-ĕ-kol'sēn). *N*-Desacetyl-*N*-methylcolchicine; an alkaloid from *Colchicum autumnale* (family Liliaceae) similar chemically to colchicine except that the acetyl group is replaced by a methyl group; used for gout and leukemia, is said to be less toxic than colchicine, and has an action upon mitosis similar to that of colchicine.

demented (dē-ment'ed). Suffering from dementia or loss of reason.

dementia (dē-men'shē-ă) [L. fr. *de-* priv. + *mens,* mind]. Amentia (2); a general mental deterioration due to organic or psychological factors; characterized by disorientation, impaired memory, judgment, and intellect, and a shallow labile affect.
Alzheimer's d., Alzheimer's *disease.*
catatonic d., d. with catatonic symptoms.
dialysis d., dialysis encephalopathy *syndrome.*
epileptic d., d. occurring in an individual afflicted with epilepsy, a result of the effects of repeated seizures over long periods.
hebephrenic d., d. with hebephrenic symptoms.
multi-infarct d., vascular d.
paralytic d., d. paralyt'ica, paresis (2).
d. paranoi'des, d. with paranoid features.
posttraumatic d., a posttraumatic neuropsychologic disorder characterized by mental impairment.
d. pre'cox [L. precocious], any one of the group of psychotic disorders known as the schizophrenias; formerly used to describe schizophrenia as a single entity.
presenile d., d. preseni'lis, **(1)** d. developing before age 65; **(2)** Alzheimer's *disease.*
primary d., d. occurring independently as a mental disorder.
primary senile d., Alzheimer's *disease.*
secondary d., chronic d. following and due to a psychosis or some other underlying disease process.
senile d., an organic brain syndrome associated with aging and marked by progressive mental deterioration, loss of recent memory, lability of affect, difficulty with novel experience, self-centeredness, and childish behavior.
toxic d., d. due to chemical poisoning, as in severe forms of drug addiction.
vascular d., multi-infarct d.; a step-like deterioration in intellectual functions with focal neurological signs, as the result of multiple infarctions of the cerebral hemispheres.

demethylase (dē-meth'i-lās). Methyltransferase.

demi- [Fr. fr. L. *dimidius,* half]. Prefix denoting half, lesser. See also hemi-, semi-.

demigauntlet (dem-ē-gawnt'let). A glovelike bandage for the fingers and hand.

demilune (dem'ē-lūn). [Fr. half-moon]. **1.** A small body with a form similar to that of a half-moon or a crescent. **2.** Term frequently used for the gametocyte of *Plasmodium falciparum.*
Giannuzzi's d.'s, serous d.'s.
Heidenhain's d.'s, serous d.'s.
serous d.'s, Gianuzzi's crescents, cells, or d.'s; Heidenhain's crescents or d.'s; the serous cells at the distal end of a mucous, tubuloalveolar secretory unit of certain salivary glands.

demineralization (dē-min'er-ăl-ī-zā'shŭn). A loss or decrease of the mineral constituents of the body or individual tissues, especially of bone.

demipenniform (dem'ē-pen'i-fōrm). Unipennate.

Demodex (dem'ō-deks) [G. *dēmos,* tallow, + *dēx,* a woodworm]. A genus of very minute (0.1 to 0.4 mm) follicular mites (family

Demodicidae) that inhabit the skin and are usually found in the sebaceous glands and hair follicles of mammals, including man. These parasites are extremely common in human populations but are rarely noted as they are seldom pathogenic.
D. bo'vis, a species that causes large swellings in the skin, filled with fluid or a cheezy material containing mites, which damages the hide of cattle.
D. ca'nis, species causing red or demodectic mange in dogs, characterized by alopecia and commonly associated with staphylococcal pyoderma.
D. ca'ti, a species causing mange in cats.
D. folliculo'rum, *Acarus folliculorum; Simonea folliculorum;* the follicular or mange mite, a very common, universally distributed, and probably nonpathogenic species that parasitizes the hair follicles and sebaceous glands of man, commonly around the nose and scalp margins but sometimes on the scalp or elsewhere on the body surface.

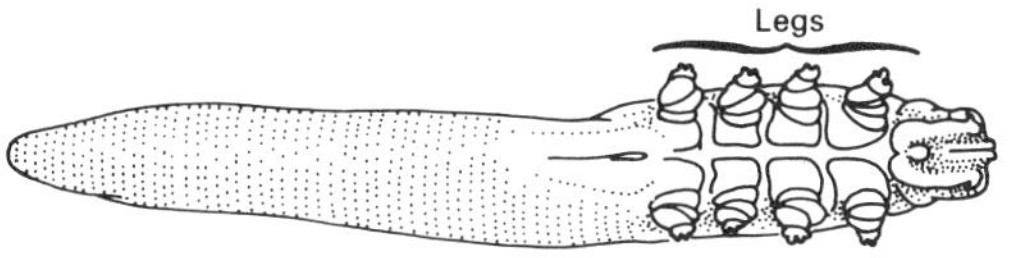

Demodex folliculorum
The follicle mite of man (×200).

demography (dĕ-mog'ră-fē) [G. *demos,* people, + *graphō,* to write]. The study of groups of people, their environment, their geographic distribution, and other characteristics.
dynamic d., a study of the functioning of a community, including statistical records.

Demoivre, Abraham, British mathematician, 1667–1754. See D.'s *formula.*

demoniac (dē-mō'nē-ak) [G. *daimōn,* a spirit]. Frenzied, fiendish, as if possessed by evil spirits.

demonstrator (dem'on-strā-ter, -tōr) [L. *de-monstro,* pp. *-atus,* to point out]. An assistant to a professor of anatomy, surgery, etc., who prepares for the lecture by dissections, collection of patients, etc., or who instructs small classes supplementary to the regular lectures; a d. corresponds in a general way to the Dozent of a German university.

De Morgan, Campbell, British physician, 1811–1876. See De M.'s *spots.*

demorphinization (dē-mōr'fin-i-zā'shŭn). **1.** Removal of morphine from an opiate. **2.** Gradual withdrawal of morphine as a method of overcoming morphine dependence.

de Morsier, G., 20th century Swiss neurologist. See de M.'s *syndrome.*

demucosation (dē-myū-kō-sā'shŭn). Excision or stripping of the mucosa of any part.

demulcent (de-mŭl'sent) [L. *de-mulceo,* pp. *-mulctus,* to stroke lightly, to soften]. **1.** Soothing; relieving irritation. **2.** An agent, such as a mucilage or oil, that soothes and relieves irritation, especially of the mucous surfaces.

demyelination, demyelinization (dē-mī'ĕ-li-nā'shŭn, dē-mī'ĕ-lin-i-za'shŭn). Destruction or loss of myelin from the medullary sheath of Schwann, as in peripheral nerve d., or of myelin associated with oligodendroglia, as in central d.

denarcotize (dē-nar'kō-tīz). To remove narcotic properties from an opiate; to deprive of narcotic properties.

denatonium benzoate (dē-nā-tō'nē-ŭm). Benzyldiethyl[(2,6-xylylcarbamoyl)methyl]ammonium benzoate; an alcohol denaturant.

denaturation (dē-na-tyū-rā'shŭn). The process of becoming denatured.

denatured (dē-nā'tyūrd). **1.** Made unnatural or changed from the normal in any of its characteristics; often applied to proteins or nucleic acids heated or otherwise treated to the point where tertiary structural characteristics are altered. **2.** Adulterated, as by addition of methyl alcohol to ethyl alcohol.

dendraxon (den-drak'son) [G. *dendron,* tree, + *axōn,* axis]. Obsolete term for telodendron.

dendriform (den'dri-fōrm) [G. *dendron,* tree, + L. *forma,* form]. Dendritic (1); dendroid; arborescent; tree-shaped, or branching.

dendrite (den'drīt) [G. *dendritēs,* relating to a tree]. **1.** Dendron; dendritic process; neurodendrite; neurodendron; one of the two types of branching protoplasmic processes of the nerve cell (the other being the axon). **2.** A crystalline treelike structure formed during the freezing of an alloy.
apical d., apical *process.*

dendritic (den-drit'ik). **1.** Dendriform. **2.** Relating to the dendrites of nerve cells.

dendrogram (den'drō-gram) [*dendron,* tree, + *gramma,* a drawing]. A treelike figure used to represent graphically a hierarchy.

dendroid (den'droyd) [G. *dendron,* tree, + *eidos,* appearance]. Dendriform.

den'dron [G. a tree]. Dendrite (1).

denervate (dē-ner'vāt). To perform denervation.

denervation (dē-ner-vā'shŭn). The act or process of cutting off a nerve supply by incision, excision, or local anesthesia.

dengue (den'gā) [Sp. corruption of "dandy" fever]. A disease of tropical and subtropical regions that occurs epidemically, is caused by dengue virus, and is transmitted by a mosquito of the genus *Aedes* (usually *A. aegypti,* but frequently *A. albopictus*). Four grades of severity are recognized: grade I, fever and constitutional symptoms; grade II, grade I plus spontaneous bleeding (of skin, gums, or gastrointestinal tract); grade III, grade II plus agitation and circulatory failure; grade IV, profound shock. Also called Aden, bouquet, breakbone, dandy, date, dengue (hemorrhagic), or polka fever; solar fever (1); scarlatina rheumatica; exanthesis arthrosia.
hemorrhagic d., a more pathogenic epidemic form of d., which has erupted in a number of epidemic outbreaks in the Pacific basin.

denial (dē-nī'ăl). Negation; an unconscious defense mechanism used to allay anxiety by denying the existence of important conflicts or troublesome impulses.

denidation (den-i-dā'shŭn) [L. *de,* from, + *nidus,* nest]. Exfoliation of the superficial portion of the mucous membrane of the uterus; stripping off of the menstrual decidua.

denitration (dē-nī-trā'shŭn). Denitrification.

denitrification (dē-nī'tri-fi-kā'shŭn). Denitration. **1.** Removal of nitrogen from any material or chemical compound; especially from the soil, as by certain (denitrifying) bacteria that render the nitrogen unavailable for plant growth. **2.** Withdrawal of nitrogen from soil by plant growth.

denitrify (dē-nī'tri-fī). To remove nitrogen from any material or chemical compound.

denitrogenation (dē-nī'trō-jĕ-nā'shŭn). Elimination of nitrogen from lungs and body tissues by breathing gases devoid of nitrogen.

Denman, Thomas, British obstetrician, 1733–1815. See D.'s spontaneous *evolution.*

Dennie's fold, Dennie's line. See under fold; line.

Denonvilliers, Charles P., Paris surgeon, 1808–1872. See D.'s *aponeurosis, ligament.*

dens, pl. **dentes** (denz, den'tēz) [L.] [NA]. **1.** Tooth, pl. teeth. **2.** Odontoid process; odontoid process of epistropheus; a strong toothlike process projecting upward from the body of the axis, or epistropheus, around which the atlas rotates. See fig. on p. 412.

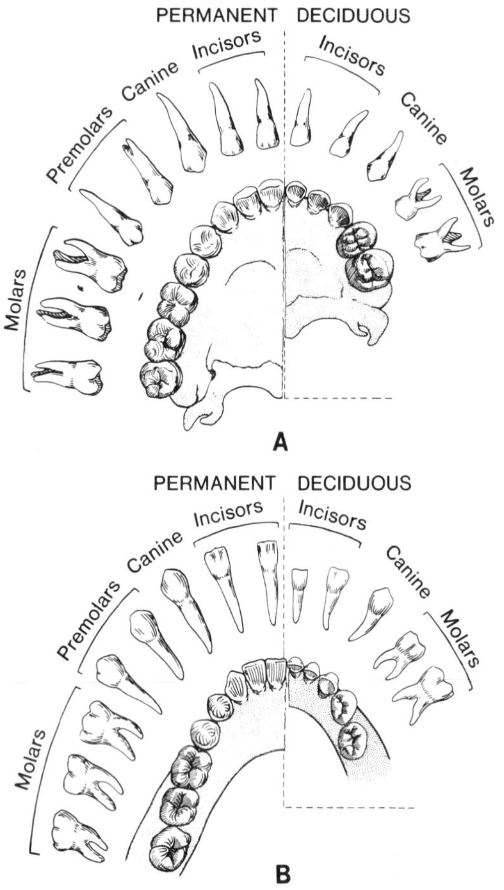

Dentes
A, Permanent and deciduous teeth, upper jaw; *B*, permanent and deciduous teeth, lower jaw.

den'tes acus'tici [NA], auditory teeth; Corti's or Huschke's auditory teeth; tooth-shaped formations or ridges occurring on the vestibular lip of the limbus lamina spiralis of the cochlear duct.
d. angula'ris, d. caninus.
d. bicus'pidus, pl. **den'tes bicus'pidi,** d. premolaris.
d. cani'nus, pl. **den'tes cani'ni** [NA], canine (3); canine tooth; cuspid, cuspidate, or eye tooth; d. angularis; d. cuspidatus; cuspid (2); a tooth having a crown of thick conical shape and a long, slightly flattened conical root; there are two canine teeth in each jaw, one on either side adjacent to the distal surface of the lateral incisors, in both the deciduous and the permanent dentition.
d. cuspida'tus, pl. **den'tes cuspida'ti,** d. caninus.
d. decid'uus, pl. **den'tes decidu'ui** [NA], baby or milk tooth; d. lacteus; primary, deciduous, or temporary tooth; first, deciduous, or primary dentition; a tooth of the first set of teeth, comprising 20 in all, that erupts between the mean ages of 6 and 28 months of life.
d. incisi'vus, pl. **den'tes incisi'vi** [NA], incisor tooth; a tooth with a chisel-shaped crown and a single conical tapering root; there are four of these teeth in the anterior part of each jaw, in both the deciduous and the permanent dentitions.
d. in den'te, a developmental disturbance in tooth formation resulting from invagination of the epithelium associated with crown development into the area destined to become pulp space; after calcification there is an invagination of enamel and dentin into the pulp space, giving the radiographic appearance of a "tooth within a tooth."
d. lac'teus, d. deciduus.
d. mola'ris, pl. **den'tes mola'res** [NA], molar tooth; molar (2); multicuspid or cheek tooth; a tooth having a somewhat quadrangular crown with four or five cusps on the grinding surface; the root is bifid in the lower jaw, but there are three conical roots in the upper jaw; there are six molars in each jaw, three on either side behind the premolars in the permanent dentition; in the deciduous dentition there are but four molars in each jaw, two on either side behind the canines. See also subentries under molar.
d. per'manens, pl. **den'tes permane'tes** [NA], second, succedaneous, or permanent tooth; d. succedaneus; secondary or succedaneous dentition; one of the 32 teeth belonging to the second or permanent dentition; eruption of the permanent teeth begins from the fifth to the seventh year, and is not completed until the seventeenth to the twenty-third year, when the last of the wisdom teeth appears.
d. premola'ris, pl. **den'tes premola'res** [NA], premolar tooth; d. bicuspidus; bicuspid tooth; a tooth usually having two tubercles or cusps on the grinding surface and a flattened root, single in the lower jaw and upper second premolar, and furrowed in the upper first premolar. There are four premolars in each jaw, two on either side between the canine and the molars; there are no premolars in the deciduous dentition.
d. sapien'tiae [L. *sapientia,* wisdom], d. serotinus.
d. seroti'nus [NA], wisdom tooth; d. sapientiae; the third molar tooth on each side in each jaw; which erupts from the seventeenth to the twenty-third year; the terminal roots are often fused, the separation being marked only by grooves.
d. succeda'neus, d. permanens.

densimeter (den-sim'ĕ-ter) [L. *densitas,* density, + G. *metron,* measure]. Densitometer (1).

densitometer (den-si-tom'ĕ-ter) [L. *densitas,* density, + G. *metron,* measure]. **1.** Densimeter; an instrument for measuring the density of a fluid. **2.** An instrument for measuring, by virtue of relative turbidity, the growth of bacteria in broth; useful in microbiologic assay of nutrients and antibiotics, phage studies, etc. **3.** An instrument for measuring the density of components (*e.g.,* protein fractions) separated by electrophoresis or chromatography, utilizing light absorption or reflection.

densitometry (den-si-tom'ĕ-trē). A procedure utilizing a densitometer.

density (den'si-tē) [L. *densitas,* fr. *densus,* thick]. **1.** The compactness of a substance; the ratio of mass to volume, usually expressed as g/ml (kg/m^3 in the SI system). **2.** The quantity of electricity on a given surface or in a given time per unit of volume. **3.** In radiology, a region of decreased transmission or reflectance of light.
count d., photon d.
flux d., flux (4).
optical d., absorbance.
photon d., count d.; the number of counted events recorded in radioisotope scanning per square centimeter or per square inch of imaged area.
vapor d., the mass per unit volume of a vapor; since the vapor d. changes with temperature and pressure, it is commonly expressed as a specific gravity, *i.e.,* the weight of the vapor divided by the weight of an equal volume of a reference gas (*e.g.,* oxygen or hydrogen) at the same temperature and pressure.

dent-, denti-, dento- [L. *dens,* tooth]. Combining forms relating to the teeth.

dental (den'tăl) [L. *dens,* tooth]. Relating to the teeth.

dental engine. The motive power of a dental handpiece that causes it to rotate.

dentalgia (den-tal'jē-ă) [L. *dens,* tooth, + G. *algos,* pain]. Toothache.

dentate (den'tāt) [L. *dentatus,* toothed]. Notched; toothed; cogged.

dentatectomy (den-tă-tek'tō-mē). [dentate (nucleus) + G. *ectomē,* excision]. Surgical destruction of the dentate nucleus of the cerebellum.

dentatum (den-tā'tŭm, den-tah'tŭm) [L. neut. of *dentatus,* toothed]. *Nucleus* dentatus cerebelli.

dentes (den'tēz) [L.]. Plural of dens.

denti-. See dent-.

denticle (den'ti-kl) [L. *denticulus,* a small tooth]. **1.** Endolith. **2.** A toothlike projection from a hard surface.

denticulate, denticulated (den-tik'yū-lāt, -lāt-ed). **1.** Finely dentated, notched, or serrated. **2.** Having small teeth.

dentiform (den'ti-fōrm) [denti- + L. *forma,* form]. Tooth-shaped; pegged. See also odontoid (1).

dentifrice (den'ti-fris) [L. *dentifricium,* fr. *dens,* tooth, + *frico,* pp. *frictus,* to rub]. Any preparation used in the cleansing of the teeth, *e.g.,* a tooth powder, toothpaste, or tooth wash.

dentigerous (den-tij'er-ŭs) [denti- + L. *gero,* to bear]. Arising from or associated with teeth, as a d. cyst.

dentilabial (den'ti-lā'bē-ăl) [denti- + L. *labium,* lip]. Relating to the teeth and lips.

dentilingual (den-ti-ling'gwăl) [denti- + L. *lingua,* tongue]. Relating to the teeth and tongue.

den'tin [L. *dens,* tooth]. Dentinum.

hereditary opalescent d., *dentinogenesis* imperfecta.

hypersensitive d., exposed d. at the cervical portion of a tooth, painful to touch, sweetness, or temperature changes.

irregular d., irritation d., tertiary d.

peritubular d., an electron-dense layer of d, observed adjacent to the odontoblastic process.

primary d., d. which forms until the root is completed.

reparative d., tertiary d.

sclerotic d., d. characterized by calcification of the dentinal tubules as a result of injury or normal aging. Also called transparent d., due to the difference in the refractive indices of the calcified dentinal tubules and the adjacent normal tubules when examined by transmitted light.

secondary d., d. formed by normal pulp function after root end formation is complete.

tertiary d., irregular, irritation, or reparative d.; morphologically irregular d. formed in response to an irritant.

transparent d., sclerotic d.

vascular d., vasodentin.

dentinal (den'ti-năl). Relating to dentin.

dentinalgia (den-ti-nal'jē-ă) [dentin + G. *algos,* pain]. Dentinal sensitivity or pain.

dentine (den'tēn). Dentinum.

dentinocemental (den'ti-nō-se-men'tăl). Cementodentinal; relating to the dentin and cementum of teeth.

dentinoenamel (den'ti-nō-ē-nam'ĕl). Amelodentinal; relating to the dentin and enamel of teeth.

dentinogenesis (den'ti-nō-jen'ĕ-sis) [dentin + G. *genesis,* production]. The process of dentin formation in the development of teeth.

d. imperfec'ta, hereditary opalescent dentin; a hereditary disorder of the teeth characterized clinically by translucent gray to yellow-brown teeth involving both primary and permanent dentition; the enamel fractures easily, leaving exposed dentin which undergoes rapid attrition; radiographically, the pulp chambers and canals appear obliterated and the roots are short and blunted; sometimes occurs in association with osteogenesis imperfecta; autosomal dominant inheritance.

dentinoid (den'ti-noyd) [dentin + G. *eidos,* resembling]. **1.** Resembling dentin. **2.** Dentinoma.

dentinoma (den'ti-nō'mă) [dentin + G. *-oma,* tumor]. Dentinoid (2); a rare benign odontogenic tumor consisting microscopically of dysplastic dentin and strands of epithelium within a fibrous stroma.

dentinum (den'ti-nŭm) [L. *dens,* tooth] [NA]. Dentin; dentine; ebur dentis; substantia eburnea; the ivory forming the mass of the tooth. About 20% is organic matrix, mostly collagen, with some elastin and a small amount of mucopolysaccharide; the inorganic fraction (70%) is mainly hydroxyapatite, with some carbonate, magnesium, and fluoride. The d. is traversed by a large number of fine tubules running from the pulp cavity outward; within the tubules are processes from the odontoblasts.

dentiparous (den-tip'ă-rŭs) [denti- + L. *pario,* to bear]. Tooth-bearing.

den'tist. A legally qualified practitioner of dentistry.

dentistry (den'tis-trē). Odontology; odontonosology; the healing science and art concerned with the embryology, anatomy, physiology, and pathology of the oral-facial complex, and with the prevention, diagnosis, and treatment of deformities, pathoses, and traumatic injuries thereof.

community d., public health d., with an academic base, emphasizing the professional obligation to foster the delivery of prevention, education, and care to populations.

forensic d., legal d.; dental jurisprudence; forensic odontology; **(1)** the relation and application of dental facts to legal problems, as in using the teeth for identifying the dead; **(2)** the law in its bearing on the practice of dentistry.

legal d., forensic d.

operative d., restorative d.; usually, the individual restoration of teeth by means of metallic or nonmetallic materials.

pediatric d., pedodontics.

preventive d., a philosophy and method of dental practice which seeks to prevent the initiation, progression, and recurrence of dental caries.

prosthetic d., prosthodontics.

public health d., that specialty of d. concerned with the prevention and control of dental diseases and promotion of oral health through organized community efforts.

restorative d., operative d.

dentition (den-tish'ŭn) [L. *dentitio,* to teethe]. The natural teeth, as considered collectively, in the dental arch; may be deciduous, permanent, or mixed.

artificial d., denture (1).

deciduous d., *dens* deciduus.

delayed d., delayed eruption of the teeth.

first d., *dens* deciduus.

mandibular d., *arcus* dentalis inferior.

maxillary d., *arcus* dentalis superior.

natural d., see d.

primary d., *dens* deciduus.

retarded d., d. in which growth phenomena such as calcification, elongation, and eruption occur later than in the average range of normal variation as a result of some systemic metabolic dysfunction (*e.g.,* hypothyroidism).

secondary d., *dens* permanens.

succedaneous d., *dens* permanens.

dento-. See dent-.

dentoalveolar (den'to-al-vē'ō-lăr). Usually, denoting that portion of the alveolar bone immediately about the teeth; used also to denote the functional unity of teeth and alveolar bone.

dentode (den'tōd). An exact reproduction of a tooth on a gnathoprаphically mounted cast.

dentoid (den'toyd) [dent- + G. *eidos,* resemblance]. Odontoid (1). See also dentiform.

dentolegal (den-tō-lē'găl). Relating to both dentistry and the law. See forensic *dentistry.*

dentoliva (den-tō-lī'vă) [L. *dens,* tooth, + *oliva,* olive]. Rarely used term for oliva.

dentulous (den'tyū-lŭs). Having natural teeth present in the mouth.

denture (den'tyūr). **1.** Artificial dentition; an artificial substitute for missing natural teeth and adjacent tissues. **2.** Sometimes used to denote the dentition of animals.
bar joint d., overlay d.
complete d., full d.; a dental prosthesis which is a substitute for the lost natural dentition and associated structures of the maxillae or mandible.
design d., a planned visualization of the form and extent of a dental prosthesis, made after a study of all factors involved.
fixed partial d., bridge (3); a restoration of one or more missing teeth which cannot be readily removed by the patient or dentist; it is permanently attached to natural teeth or roots which furnish the primary support to the appliance.
full d., complete d.
immediate d., immediate insertion d.; a complete or partial d. constructed for insertion immediately following the removal of natural teeth.
immediate insertion d., immediate d.
implant d., a d. that receives its stability and retention from a substructure which is partially or wholly implanted under the soft tissues of the d. basal seat. See also implant d. *substructure;* implant d. *superstructure;* subperiosteal *implant.*
interim d., provisional or temporary d.; a dental prosthesis to be used for a short interval of time for reasons of esthetics, mastication, occlusal support, or convenience, or to condition the patient to accept an artificial substitute for missing natural teeth until more definite prosthetic dental treatment can be provided.
overlay d., overdenture; telescopic or bar joint d.; hybrid prosthesis; a complete d. that is supported by both soft tissue and natural teeth that have been altered so as to permit the d. to fit over them. The altered teeth may have been fitted with short or long copings, locking devices, or connecting bars.
partial d., bridgework; a dental prosthesis which restores one or more, but less than all, of the natural teeth and/or associated parts and which is supported by the teeth and/or the mucosa; it may be removable or fixed.
partial d., distal extension, a removal partial d. that is retained by natural teeth at one end of the d. base segments only, and in which a portion of the functional load is carried by the residual ridge.
provisional d., interim d.
removable partial d., removable bridge; a partial d. which supplies teeth and associated structures on a partially edentulous jaw, and which can be removed from the mouth.
telescopic d., overlay d.
temporary d., interim d.
transitional d., a partial d. which is to serve as a temporary prosthesis to which teeth will be added as more teeth are lost, and which will be replaced after postextraction tissue changes have occurred; a transitional d. may become an interim d. when all of the teeth have been removed from the dental arch.
treatment d., a dental prosthesis used for the purpose of treating or conditioning the tissues which are called upon to support and retain a denture base.
trial d., wax model d.; a setup of artificial teeth so fabricated that it may be placed in the patient's mouth to verify esthetics, for the making of records, or for any other operation deemed necessary before final completion of the d.
wax model d., trial d.

denture service. Those procedures performed in the diagnosis, construction, and maintenance of artificial substitutes for missing natural teeth.

denturist (den'tyūr-ist). A person other than a dentist (usually a technician), who engages illegally in the practice of denture service.

Denucé, Jean L.P., French surgeon, 1824–1889. See D.'s *ligament.*

denucleated (dē-nū'klē-ā-ted). Deprived of a nucleus.

denudation (den-yū-dā'shŭn) [L. *de-nudo,* to lay bare, fr. *de,* from, + *nudus,* naked]. Depriving of a covering or protecting layer; the act of laying bare, as in the removal of the epithelium from an underlying surface.

denude (dē'nūd). To perform denudation.

Denys, Joseph, Belgian bacteriologist, 1857–1932. See D.-Leclef *phenomenon.*

deobstruent (dē-ob'strū-ent) [L. *de-* priv. + *obstruo,* pp. *-structus,* to build against, obstruct]. Deoppilative. **1.** Relieving or removing obstruction. **2.** An agent that removes an obstruction to flow.

deodorant (dē-ō'der-ant) [L. *de-* priv. + *odoro,* pp. *-atus,* to give an odor to, fr. *odor,* a smell]. **1.** Eliminating or masking a smell, especially an unpleasant one. **2.** Deodorizer: an agent having such an action; especially a cosmetic combined with an antiperspirant.

deodorize (dē-ō'der-īz). To use a deodorant.

deodorizer (dē-ō'der-īz-er). Deodorant (2).

deontology (dē-on-tol'ō-jē) [G. *deon* (*deont-*), that which is binding, pr. part. ntr. of *dei,* (impers.) it behooves, fr. *deō,* to bind, + *logos,* study]. A study of the field of professional etiquette and duties.

deoppilative (dē-op'pi-lā-tiv) [L. *de-* priv. + *op-pilo,* pp. *-atus,* to stop up, fr. *ob-* against, + *pilo,* to ram down]. Deobstruent.

deorsumduction (dē-ōr'sŭm-dŭk'shŭn) [L. *deorsum,* downward, + *duco,* to lead]. Infraduction; rotation of one eye downward.

deossification (dē-os'i-fi-kā'shŭn) [L. *de,* from, + *os,* bone, + *facio,* to make]. Removal of the mineral constituents of bone.

deoxidation (dē'oks-i-dā'shŭn). Depriving a chemical compound of its oxygen.

deoxidize (dē-oks'i-dīz). To remove oxygen from its chemical combination.

deoxy-. Prefix to chemical names of substances containing carbohydrate moieties to indicate replacement of an –OH by an H. The older spelling desoxy- has been retained in some instances.

deoxyadenosine (dA, dAdo) (dē-oks'ē-ă-den'ō-sēn). 2′-Deoxyribosyladenine, one of the four major nucleosides of DNA (the others being deoxycytidine, deoxyguanosine, and thymidine).

deoxyadenylic acid (dAMP) (dē-oks'ē-ad-en-il'ik). Adenine deoxyribonucleotide; deoxyadenosine phosphate, a hydrolysis product of DNA, differing from adenylic acid in containing deoxyribose in place of ribose.

deoxycholate (DOC) (dē-oks-ē-kō'lāt). A salt or ester of deoxycholic acid.

deoxycholic acid (dē-oks-ē-kō'lik). 7-Deoxycholic acid; 3α,12α-dihydroxy-5β-cholanic acid; a bile acid and choleretic; used in biochemical preparations as a detergent.

deoxycorticosterone (DOC) (dē-oks'ē-kōr-ti-kos'ter-ōn). 11-Deoxycorticosterone; deoxycortone; desoxycortone; 21-hydroxyprogesterone; 21-hydroxypregn-4-ene-3,20-dione; an adrenocortical steroid, principally a biosynthetic precursor of corticosterone and possibly aldosterone, that rarely appears in adrenocortical secretions; a potent mineralocorticoid with no appreciable glucocorticoid activity.
d. acetate, desoxycorticosterone acetate; acetate salt used for intramuscular injection for replacement therapy of the adrenocortical steroid.
d. pivalate, desoxycorticosterone pivalate; pivalate salt of the steroid.

deoxycortone (dē-oks-ē-kōr'tōn). Deoxycorticosterone.

deoxycytidine (dē-oks-ē-sī'ti-dēn). 2′-Deoxyribosylcytosine, one of the four major nucleosides of DNA (the others being deoxyadenosine, deoxyguanosine, and thymidine).

deoxycytidylic acid (dCMP) (dē-oks'ē-sī-ti-dil'ik). Deoxycytidine phosphate, a hydrolysis product of DNA.

deoxyepinephrine (dē-oks'ē-ep-i-nef'rēn). 4-[2- (Methylamino) ethyl]pyrocatechol; a sympathomimetic amine used as a vasoconstrictor.

deoxyguanosine (dē-oks-ē-gwan'ō-sēn). 2'-Deoxyribosylguanine, one of the four major nucleosides of DNA (the others being deoxyadenosine, deoxycytidine, and thymidine).

deoxyguanylic acid (dGMP) (dē-oks-ē-gwan-il'ik). Guanine deoxyribonucleotide; deoxyguanosine phosphate, a hydrolysis product of DNA.

deoxyhexose (dē-oks-ē-heks'ōs). A hexose (6-carbon sugar) in which one OH is replaced by H.

deoxypentose (dē-oks-ē-pen'tōs). A pentose (5-carbon sugar) in which one OH is replaced by H.

deoxyriboaldolase (dē-oks'ē-rī-bō-al'dō-lās). Deoxyribosephosphate aldolase.

deoxyribodipyrimidine photolyase (dē-oks'ē-rī'bō-dī-pī-rim'i-dēn) [EC 4.1.99.3]. Dipyrimidine photolyase; photoreactivating enzyme; PR enzyme (2); an enzyme in yeast which is activated by light, whereupon it can reverse a previous photochemical reaction by cleaving the cyclobutane ring of the thymine dimer.

deoxyribonuclease (DNase, DNAse, DNAase) (de-oks'ē-rī-bō-nū'klē-ās). Any enzyme (phosphodiesterase) hydrolyzing phosphodiester bonds in DNA. See also endonuclease; nuclease.

d. I, DNase I, pancreatic d.; thymonuclease; an endonuclease (EC 3.1.21.1, formerly 3.1.4.5) that cleaves DNA to a mixture of oligodeoxyribonucleotides, each ending in a 5'-phosphate; streptodornase is a similar enzyme.

d. II, DNase II, acid d.; an endonuclease (EC 3.1.22.1, formerly 3.1.4.6) that cleaves both strands of native DNA to produce a mixture of oligodeoxynucleotides, each ending in a 3'-phosphate.

acid d., d. II.

pancreatic d., d. I.

d. S_1, endonuclease S_1 (*Aspergillus*).

spleen d., former name for micrococcal *endonuclease.*

deoxyribonucleic acid (DNA) (dē-oks'ē-rī'bō-nū-klē'ik). The type of nucleic acid containing deoxyribose as the sugar component and found principally in the nuclei (chromatin, chromosomes) of animal and vegetable cells, usually loosely bound to protein (hence the term deoxyribonucleoprotein); considered to be the autoreproducing component of chromosomes and of many viruses, and the repository of hereditary characteristics.

antisense DNA, the strand of DNA complimentary to the one bearing the genetic message and from which it may be reconstructed.

competitor DNA, DNA from a test organism that is denatured and then used in *in vitro* hybridization experiments in which it competes with DNA (homologous) from a reference organism; used to determine the relationship of the test organism to the reference organism.

complementary DNA (cDNA), DNA that is complementary to messenger RNA.

DNA ligase, an enzyme that leads to the formation of a phosphodiester bond at a break of one strand in duplex DNA.

DNA nucleotidylexotransferase [EC 2.7.7.31], terminal deoxynucleotidyltransferase; terminal addition enzyme; an enzyme that can catalyze the addition of a nucleotide, presented as a nucleoside triphosphate, on a DNA or similar polydeoxynucleotide.

palindromic DNA, a segment of DNA in which the sequence is symmetrical about its midpoint and hence identical with its complimentary strand.

DNA polymerase, see nucleotidyltransferase.

recombinant DNA, see under R.

repetitive DNA, a segment of DNA that consists of a linear array of multiple copies of the same sequence of nucleotides.

satellite DNA, DNA in the satellite regions of acrocentric chromosomes.

deoxyribonucleoprotein (DNP) (dē-oks'ē-rī-bō-nū'klē-ō-prō'tēn). The complex of DNA and protein in which DNA is usually found upon cell disruption and isolation.

deoxyribonucleoside (dē-oks'ē-rī-bō-nū'klē-ō-sīd). A nucleoside component of DNA containing 2-deoxyribose; the condensation product of deoxyribose with purines or pyrimidines.

deoxyribonucleotide (dē-oks'ē-rī-bō-nū'klē-ō-tīd). A nucleotide component of DNA containing 2-deoxyribose; the phosphoric ester of deoxyribonucleoside.

deoxyribose (dē-oks-ē-rī'bōs). A deoxypentose, D-2-deoxyribose being the most common example, occurring in DNA and responsible for its name.

deoxyribosephosphate aldolase (dē-oks'ē-rī-bōs-fos'fāt) [EC 4.1.2.4]. Deoxyriboaldolase; an enzyme catalyzing cleavage of deoxyribose 5-phosphate to glyceraldehyde 3-phosphate and acetaldehyde.

deoxyriboside (dē-oks-ē-rī'bō-sīd). Deoxyribose combined via its 1-O atom with a radical derived from an alcohol, in contradistinction to deoxyribosyl, in which the entire OH on C-1 is eliminated; incorrectly used for the latter, *i.e.,* deoxyribonucleosides are deoxyribosyl compounds, not deoxyribosides.

deoxyribosyl (dē-oks-ē-rī'bō-sil). See deoxyriboside.

deoxyribotide (dē-oks-ē-rī'bō-tīd). Misnomer for deoxyribonucleotide or deoxynucleotide derived, by analogy with nucleoside-nucleotide, from incorrect usage of deoxyriboside.

deoxythymidylic acid (dTMP) (dē-oks'ē-thī-mi-dil'ik). Thymine deoxyribonucleotide; a component of DNA; originally and properly called thymidylic acid, but use of deoxy- is less ambiguous, as ribothymidylic acid is now known to exist.

deoxyvirus (dē-ok'sē-vī'rŭs). DNA *virus.*

deozonize (dē-ō'zō-nīz). To deprive of ozone.

dependence (dē-pen'dens) [L. *dependeo,* to hang from]. The quality or condition of lacking independence by relying upon, being influenced by, or being subservient to a person or object reflecting a particular need.

Dependovirus (dē-pen'dō-vī-rŭs) [L. *dependeo,* to be dependent upon, + virus]. Adeno-associated virus; adenosatellite virus; a genus of virus (family Parvoviridae) that are antigenically unrelated to adenovirus but require the presence of adenovirus in order to replicate; there are at least four serotypes, all sharing common antigens.

depersonalization (dē-per'sŏn-ăl-i-zā'shŭn). A state in which a person loses the feeling of his own identity in relation to others in his family or peer group, or loses the feeling of his own reality.

de Pezzer, O., 19th century French physician. See de P. *catheter.*

dephosphorylation (dē-fos'fōr-i-lā'shŭn). Removal of a phosphoric group, usually hydrolytically and by enzyme action, from a compound.

depigmentation (dē-pig-men-tā'shŭn). Loss of pigment which may be partial or complete.

depilate (dep'i-lāt) [L. *de-pilo,* pp. *-atus,* to deprive of hair, fr. *de-* neg. + *pilo,* to grow hair]. To remove hair by any means. *Cf.* epilate.

depilation (dep-i-lā'shŭn). Epilation.

depilatory (dē-pil'ă-tō-rē). **1.** Epilatory (1). **2.** Epilatory (2); an agent that causes the falling out of hair.

depletion (dē-plē'shŭn). **1.** The removal of accumulated fluids or solids. **2.** A reduced state of strength from too many free discharges. **3.** Excessive loss of a constituent, usually essential, of the body, *e.g.,* salt, water, etc.

chloride d., salt d.

salt d., chloride d.; excessive loss of sodium chloride from the body in urine, sweat, etc.; a cause of secondary dehydration.

water d., reduction in the total volume of body water; dehydration.

depolarization (dē-pō'lăr-i-zā'shŭn). The destruction, neutralization, or change in direction of polarity.

dendritic d., the loss of a negative charge in the dendrites of a nerve cell.

depolarize (dē-pō'lăr-īz). To deprive of polarity.

depolymerase (dē-pol'i-mer-ās). Name used originally, before hydrolytic action was understood, for an enzyme catalyzing the hydrolysis of a macromolecule to simpler components. See nuclease.

depopulation (dē-pop-yū-lā'shŭn). Humane destruction of all animals on a premises during a disease eradication program; in the U.S., used primarily in national programs established to eradicate newly introduced diseases (*e.g.,* foot-and-mouth disease) that pose serious economic threats to the livestock industries.

deposit (dē-poz'it) [L. *de-pono,* pp. *-positus,* to lay down]. A sediment or precipitate.

brickdust d., sedimentum lateritium; a sediment of urates in the urine.

depravation (dep'ră-vā'shŭn) [L. *depravatio,* fr. *depravo,* pp. *-atus,* to corrupt]. Depravity.

depraved (dē-prāvd') [L. *depravo,* to corrupt]. Deteriorated or degenerate; perverted; corrupt.

depravity (dē-prav'i-tē). Depravation; a depraved act or the condition of being depraved.

depressant (dē-pres'ănt) [L. *de-primo,* pp. *-pressus,* to press down]. **1.** Diminishing functional tone or activity. **2.** An agent that reduces nervous or functional activity, such as a sedative or anesthetic.

depressed (dē-prest'). **1.** Flattened from above downward. **2.** Below the normal level or the level of the surrounding parts. **3.** Below the normal functional level. **4.** Dejected; lowered in spirits.

depression (dē-presh'ŭn). **1.** Reduction of the level of functioning. **2.** A hollow or sunken area. **3.** Displacement of a part downward or inward. **4.** Dejection (1); a sinking of spirits so as to constitute a clinically discernible condition. See also melancholia.

agitated d., d. with excitement and restlessness.

anaclitic d., impairment of an infant's physical, social, and intellectual development following separation from its mother or from a mothering influence; characterized by listlessness, withdrawal, and anorexia. See also hospitalism.

endogenous d., endogenomorphic d., a descriptive syndrome for a cluster of symptoms and features occurring in the absence of precipitants; *e.g.,* anhedonia, psychomotor agitation or retardation, diurnal mood variation with increased severity in the morning, early morning awakening and insomnia in the middle of the night, weight loss, self-reproach or guilt, and lack of reactivity to one's environment.

lingual salivary gland d., static bone cyst; Stafne bone cyst; an indentation on the lingual surface of the mandible within which a portion of the submandibular gland lies; it appears radiographically as a sharply circumscribed ovoid radiolucency between the mandibular canal and the inferior border of the posterior mandible.

pacchionian d.'s, *foveolae* granulares.

postdrive d., slowing of the heart, often with a rate-dependent blockade of A-V and/or V-A conduction following rapid atrial stimulation.

pterygoid d., *fovea* pterygoidea.

reactive d., a psychological state occasioned directly by an intensely sad external situation (frequently loss of a loved person), relieved by the removal of the external situation (*e.g.,* reunion with a loved person).

spreading d., a decrease of activity evoked by local stimulation of the cerebral cortex and spreading slowly over the whole cortex.

depressive (dē-pres'iv). **1.** Pushing down. **2.** Pertaining to or causing depression.

depressomotor (dē-pres-ō-mō'ter). **1.** Retarding motor activity. **2.** An agent that slows or retards motion.

depressor (dē-pres'ŏr). **1.** A muscle that flattens or lowers a part. **2.** Anything that depresses or retards functional activity. **3.** An instrument or device used to push certain structures out of the way during an operation or examination. **4.** Hypotensor; an agent producing decreased blood pressure.

tongue d., an instrument with a broad flat extremity used for pressing down the tongue to facilitate examination of the fauces and pharynx.

deprivation (dep'ri-vā'shŭn). Absence, loss, or withholding of something needed.

emotional d., lack of adequate and appropriate interpersonal or environmental experiences, or both, usually in the early developmental years.

sensory d., diminution or absence of usual external stimuli or perceptual opportunities, commonly resulting in psychological distress and aberrant functioning.

depth. Distance from the surface downward.

anesthetic d., the degree of central nervous system depression produced by a general anesthetic agent; a function of potency of the anesthetic and the concentration in which it is administered.

focal d., d. of focus, penetration (3); the greatest distance through which an object point can be moved while maintaining a clear image.

deptropine citrate (dep'trō-pēn). Dibenzheptropine citrate; 3α-[(10,11-dihydro-5*H*-dibenzo[*a,d*]cyclohepten-5-yl)oxy]1αH,5αH-tropane citrate; an antihistaminic agent with anticholinergic properties.

depulization (dē-pyū'li-zā'shŭn) [L. *de,* from, + *pulex* (*pulic-*), flea]. Destruction of fleas which convey the plague bacillus from animals to man.

depurant (dep'yū-rant) [L. *de-* intens. + *puro,* pp. *-atus,* to make pure]. **1.** An agent or means used to effect purification. **2.** An agent that promotes the excretion and removal of waste material.

depuration (dep-yū-rā'shŭn). Purification; removal of waste products or foul excretions.

depurative (dep'yū-ră-tiv). Tending to depurate; depurant.

dequalinium acetate (dē-kwah-lin'ē-ŭm). Decamine; 1,1'-decamethylenebis[4-aminoquinaldinium acetate]; an antimicrobial agent.

dequalinium chloride. D. acetate, with chloride replacing acetate, used as an antimicrobial agent primarily in lozenges for the treatment of mouth and throat infections.

de Quervain, Fritz, Swiss surgeon, 1868–1940. See de Q.'s *disease, fracture, thyroiditis.*

deradelphus (dār-ă-del'fŭs) [G. *derē,* neck, + *adelphos,* brother]. Conjoined twins with a single head and neck and separate bodies below the thoracic level.

derailment (dē-rāl'ment). A symptom of a thought disorder in which one constantly gets "off the track" in his thoughts and speech; similar to loosening of association.

deranencephaly, deranencephalia (dār-an'en-sef'ă-lē, -se-fā'lē-ă) [G. *derē,* neck, + *an-,* priv., + *kephalē,* head]. Congenital malformation in which the head is absent, although there is a rudimentary neck.

derangement (dē-rānj'ment) [Fr.]. **1.** A disturbance of the regular order or arrangement. **2.** A mental disturbance or disorder.
Hey's internal d., dislocation of the semilunar cartilages of the knee joint.

Dercum, Francis X., U.S. neurologist, 1856–1931. See D.'s *disease.*

derealization (dē-rē'ă-li-zā'shŭn). An alteration in one's perception of the environment such that things that are ordinarily familiar seem strange, unreal, or two-dimensional.

dereism (dē'rē-izm) [L. *de,* away, + *res,* thing]. Mental activity in fantasy in contrast to reality.

dereistic (dē-rē-is'tik). Living in imagination or fantasy.

derencephalia (dār-en-se-fā'lē-ă). Derencephaly.

derencephalocele (dār-en-sef'ă-lō-sēl) [G. *derē,* neck, + *enkephalos,* brain, + *kēlē,* hernia]. In derencephaly, protrusion of the rudimentary brain through a defect in the upper cervical spinal canal.

derencephaly (dār-en-sef'ă-lē) [G. *derē,* neck, + *enkephalos,* brain]. Derencephalia; cervical rachischisis and anencephaly, a malformation involving an open cranial vault with a rudimentary brain usually crowded back toward bifid cervical vertebrae.

derepression (dē-rē-presh'ŭn). A homeostatic mechanism for regulating enzyme production in an inducible enzyme system: an inducer, usually a substrate of a specific enzyme pathway, combines with an active repressor (produced by a regulator gene) to deactivate the repressor; this results in activation of a previously repressed operator gene and activity of the structural genes controlled by the operator, followed by enzyme production.

deric (dār'ik) [G. *deros,* skin]. Ectodermal; to be distinguished from enteric.

derivation (dār-i-vā'shŭn) [L. *derivatio,* fr. *derivo,* pp. *-atus,* to draw off, fr. *rivus,* a stream]. **1.** Revulsion (2); the drawing of blood or the body fluids to one part to relieve congestion in another. **2.** The source or process of an evolution.

derivative (dĕ-riv'ă-tiv). **1.** Relating to or producing derivation. **2.** Something produced by modification of something preexisting. **3.** Specifically, a chemical compound that may be produced from another compound of similar structure in one or more steps, as in replacement of H by an alkyl, acyl, amino group, etc.

derm-, derma-, dermat-, dermato-, dermo- [G. *derma,* skin]. Combining forms signifying skin.

dermabrader (derm'ă-brād-er). A motor-driven device used in dermabrasion.

dermabrasion (der-mă-brā'zhŭn). Planning; operative procedure used to remove acne scars, farmer-sailor skin, and dermal nevi performed with sandpaper, wire brushes, or other abrasive materials.

Dermacentor (der-mă-sen'ter) [derm- + G. *kentōr,* a goader]. An ornate, characteristically marked genus of hard ticks (family Ixodidae) that possess eyes and 11 festoons; it consists of some 20 species whose members commonly attack dogs, man, and other mammals.
D. albopic'tus, the horse or winter tick, a species found principally on horses, elk, moose, and deer in Canada and the western United States; it is a one-host tick, but man is sometimes attacked when skinning or dressing deer.
D. anderso'ni, the Rocky Mountain spotted-fever, or wood tick; a species that is the vector of spotted fever in the Rocky Mountain regions, and also transmits tularemia and causes tick paralysis; there are characteristic black and white markings on the large scutum of the male.
D. ni'tens, the tropical horse tick, a species found primarily on horses, mules, and asses (usually on the ears), chiefly in southern

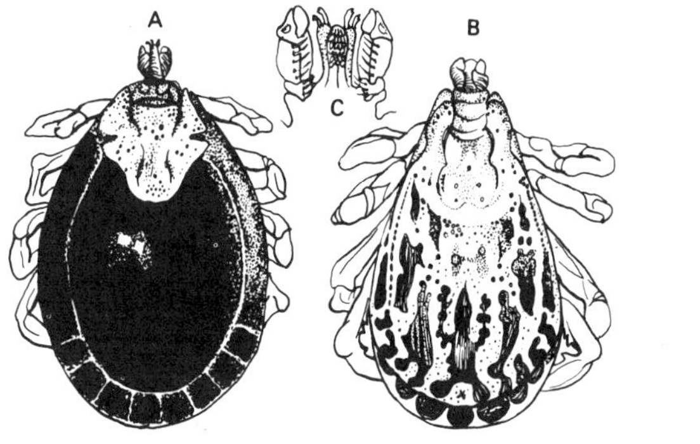

Dermacentor andersoni **(spotted fever tick)**
A, unengorged female; *B*, male; *C*, capitulum or mouthparts, showing palpi (outer pair of sensory structures), chelicerae (inner pair of cutting jaws), and hypostome (central spiny piercing and holding structure). (*A* and *B*, ×10; *C*, ×25.)

Florida, southern Texas, Mexico, Central America, and the West Indies.
D. occidenta'lis, the Pacific Cosat tick, a species found on all domestic herbivores, deer, dogs, man, and other animals in California and western Oregon; an important vector of bovine anaplasmosis.
D. reticula'tus, a common species attacking sheep, oxen, goats, and deer, and sometimes troublesome to man; it is found in Europe, Asia, and America.
D. variabi'lis, the American dog tick, a species that is a common pest of dogs (may also cause tick paralysis) along the eastern seaboard of the U.S., a vector of tularemia, and a principal vector of *Rickettsia* which causes Rocky Mountain spotted fever in the central and eastern U.S.

der'mad [derm- + L. *ad,* to]. In the direction of the outer integument.

dermagraphy (der-mag'ră-fē). Dermatographism.

dermahemia (der-mă-hē'mē-ă) [derma- + G. *haima,* blood]. Hyperemia of the skin.

dermal (der'măl). Dermatic, dermatoid (2); dermic; relating to the skin.

dermalaxia (der-mă-lak'sē-ă) [derm- + G. *malaxis,* softening]. Softening or relaxation of the skin.

dermametropathism (der'mă-me-trop' ă-thizm) [derm- + G. *metron,* measure, + *pathos,* disease]. A system that measures the intensity and nature of certain cutaneous disorders by observing the markings made by drawing a blunt instrument across the skin.

dermamyiasis (der'mă-mī-ī'ă-sis). Myiasis of the skin.

Dermanyssus gallinae (der-mă-nis'ŭs) [derm- + G. *nyssō,* to prick; L. *gallina,* hen]. *Acarus gallinae;* the red hen-mite, a parasite of chickens, pigeons, and other birds; it sometimes attacks man and causes an itching eruption, especially in sensitized individuals.

dermat- [G. *derma,* skin]. Combining form relating to the skin. See also derm-, dermato-, dermo-.

dermatalgia (der-mă-tăl'jē-ă) [dermat- + G. *algos,* pain]. Dermatodynia; localized pain, usually confined to the skin.

dermatan sulfate (der'mă-tan). Chondroitin sulfate B; a mucopolysaccharide containing alternating L-iduronic acid and *N*-acetyl-D-galactosamine 4-sulfate residues.

dermatic (der-mat'ik). Dermal.

dermatitis, pl. dermatitides (der-mă-tī'tis, -tit'i-dēz) [derm- + G. *-itis,* inflammation]. Inflammation of the skin.
actinic d., eruption of sensitivity produced by exposure to sun-

light or other light sources, usually of specific electromagnetic energy; not a burn.

d. aestiva'lis, eczema recurring during the summer.

d. ambustio'nis, d. calorica; uritis; inflammation of the skin resulting from the action of heat.

ancylostomiasis d., cutaneous *ancylostomiasis.*

d. artefac'ta, feigned eruption; d. autophytica or factitia; an eruption produced by self-inflicted trauma.

atopic d., atopic eczema; d. characterized by the distinctive phenomena of atopy, including infantile and flexural eczema.

d. atroph'icans, a diffuse idiopathic atrophy of the skin involving the appendages.

d. autophy'tica, d. artefacta.

berloque d., berlock d., a type of photosensitization resulting in deep brown pigmentation on exposure to sunlight after application of bergamot oil and other essential oils in perfume.

blastomycetic d., d. blastomycot'ica, a cutaneous form of blastomycosis.

bubble gum d., allergic contact d. developing about the lips in children who chew bubble gum; caused by plastics in the gum substance.

d. calor'ica, d. ambustionis.

caterpillar d., caterpillar rash; allergic contact d. caused by the larva of the browntail moth.

chemical d., allergic contact d. or primary irritation d. due to application of chemicals; usually characterized by erythema, edema, and vesiculation of the exposed or contacted site.

d. combustio'nis, inflammation of the skin following a burn.

d. congelatio'nis, frostbite.

contact d., a delayed type of induced sensitivity (allergy) of the skin with varying degrees of erythema, edema, and vesiculation, resulting from cutaneous contact with a specific allergen.

contact-type d., d. resembling contact d. but caused by an ingested or injected allergen, usually a drug, and with a widespread or generalized distribution.

contagious pustular d., contagious *ecthyma.*

cosmetic d., a cutaneous eruption that results from the application of a cosmetic; due to allergic sensitization or primary irritation.

dhobie mark d., dhobie or washerman's mark; an allergic contact d. due to hypersensitivity to ingredients in laundry marking ink.

diaper d., Jacquet's erythema; colloquially referred to as diaper, ammonia, or napkin rash; d. of thighs and buttocks supposedly due to ammonia produced in decomposing urine in infants' diapers.

d. exfoliati'va, exfoliative d.

d. exfoliati'va infan'tum or **neonato'rum,** impetigo neonatorum (1); a generalized pyoderma accompanied by exfoliative d., with constitutional symptoms, affecting young infants; possibly identical to toxic epidermal necrolysis caused by a toxic bacterium or a toxic drug reaction.

exfoliative d., d. exfoliativa; pityriasis rubra; Wilson's disease (2); generalized exfoliation with scaling of the skin and usually with erythema (erythroderma); may be a drug reaction or associated with various benign dermatoses or with lymphomas.

exudative discoid and lichenoid d., Sulzberger-Garbe *disease.*

d. facti'tia, d. artefacta.

d. gangreno'sa infan'tum, rupia escharotica; pemphigus gangrenosus (1); ecthyma gangrenosum; disseminated cutaneous gangrene; a bullous or pustular eruption, of uncertain origin, followed by necrotic ulcers or extensive gangrene in children under 2 years of age; if untreated, death may result from metastasis of infection, such as liver abscess.

d. herpetifor'mis, d. multiformis; Duhring's disease; herpes circinatus bullosus; hydroa herpetiforme; a chronic disease of the skin marked by a severe, extensive, itching eruption of vesicles and papules which occur in groups; relapses are common; spontaneous cure rarely occurs except in children.

d. hiema'lis, winter, frost, or lumberman's itch; pruritus hiemalis; a recurrent eczema appearing with the advent of cold weather.

infectious eczematoid d., an inflammatory reaction of skin adjacent to the site of a pyogenic infection; *e.g.,* purulent otitis, the area around a colostomy, or intranasal infection; thought to be due to a local sensitization to the resident organisms.

d. linea'ris mi'grans, **(1)** cutaneous *larva migrans;* **(2)** presence of botfly larvae in the skin.

livedoid d., a reddish blue mottled condition of the skin due to affection of the cutaneous vascular apparatus.

mango d., a perioral d. resulting from a sensitization reaction to the resinous coating on the peel of the mango fruit.

meadow d., meadow grass d., phytophlyctodermatitis; a phototoxic reaction to contact with a plant in which the bizarre configuration of the eruption is that of the streaky pattern of the plant contact; often occurs after sunbathing.

d. medicamento'sa, drug *eruption.*

d. multifor'mis, d. herpetiformis.

nickel d., allergic d. due to nickel or other metals containing nickel (*e.g.,* stainless steel) as a diluent.

d. nodo'sa, a papular eruption on legs, related to craw-craw.

d. nodula'ris necrot'ica, Werther's disease; a recurrent eruption of vesicles, papules, and papulonecrotic lesions on the buttocks and extensor surfaces of the extremities, accompanied by fever, sore throat, diarrhea, and eosinophilia; probably a variant of vasculitis, it can be of varying and increasing severity and duration, and can occasionally involve the heart, kidneys, and gastrointestinal tract.

d. papilla'ris capillit'ii, acne *keloid.*

papular d. of pregnancy, intensely pruritic papular eruption of torso and extremities occurring throughout pregnancy, with no systemic toxicity.

d. pediculoi'des ventrico'sus, straw *itch.*

plant d., see d. venenata.

primary irritant d., reaction of irritation on exposure of the skin to substances which are toxic to epidermal or connective tissue cells; lesions are usually erythematous and papular, but can be purulent or necrotic, depending on the nature of the toxic material applied.

proliferative d., a skin infection of herbivores, especially sheep, rarely of man, caused by *Dermatophilus congolensis* and characterized by extensive scabs on the legs and feet; beneath the scabs the underlying tissue is reddened and exhibits whitish points, causing the surface to resemble a strawberry.

rat mite d., an eruption of wheals, papules, or vesicles caused by the rat mite.

d. re'pens [L. creeping], *pustulosis* palmaris et plantaris.

rhus d., contact d. caused by cutaneous exposure to urushiol from species of *Toxicodendron* (*Rhus*), such as poison ivy, oak, or sumac.

sandal strap d., allergic contact on the dorsal surfaces of the feet, caused by synthetic rubber sandal straps.

Schamberg's d., progressive pigmentary *dermatosis.*

schistosome d., swimmer's itch (2); water itch (2); a sensitization response to repeated cutaneous invasion by cercariae of bird, mammal, or human schistosomes.

seborrheic d., d. seborrhe'ica, seborrheic dermatosis or eczema; seborrhea corporis; Unna's disease; dyssebacia; a scaly macular eruption that occurs primarily on the face, scalp (dandruff), interscapular area, pubic area, and about the anus; the lesions are covered with a slightly adherent oily scale.

shoe dye d., allergic contact d. of the feet, caused by sensitivity to shoe dye.

d. sim'plex, *erythema* simplex.

solar d., a d. in photosensitive persons caused by exposure to the sun's rays.

stasis d., erythema and scaling of the lower extremities due to im-

paired venous circulation.
subcorneal pustular d., subcorneal pustular *dermatosis.*
traumatic d., any d. caused by an irritant substance or by a physical agent.
trefoil d., trifoliosis.
d. veg'etans, pyoderma vegetans; a benign fungating granulomatous mass caused by chronic pyogenic infection.
d. venena'ta, a cutaneous eruption due to contact with a sensitizing agent such as urushiol in poison ivy, resins, chemicals, cosmetics, etc.; the eruption is edematous, erythematous, and vesicular.
d. verruco'sa, chromomycosis.

dermato- [G. *derma,* skin]. Combining form relating to the skin. See also derm-, dermat-, dermo-.

dermatoalloplasty (der'ma-tō-al'ō-plas-tē) [dermato- + G. *allos,* other, + *plastos,* formed]. Dermatohomoplasty; allografting of skin.

dermatoarthritis (der'mă-tō-ar-thrī'tis). Associated skin disease and arthritis.
lipoid d., a multicentric *reticulohistiocytosis.*

dermatoautoplasty (der'ma-tō-aw'tō-plas-tē) [dermato- + G. *autos,* self, + *plastos,* formed]. Autografting of skin taken from another part of the patient's own body.

Dermatobia (der-mă-tō'bē-ă) [dermato- + G. *bios,* way of living]. A genus of flies (family Oestridae) found in tropical America.
D. cyaniven'tris, *D. hominis.*
D. hom'inis, *D. cyaniventris;* human, skin, or warble botfly; a large, blue, brown-winged species whose larvae develop in boil-like cysts in the skin of man, many domestic animals, and some fowl. It is a very serious and damaging cattle parasite and frequently attacks small children. Its eggs are laid on the legs or abdomen of another insect, such as the mosquito; the eggs later hatch, when stimulated by warmth or other factors, to release the botfly larvae on the skin of the mosquito's bloodmeal host, and the larvae quickly invade the skin to initiate myiasis.

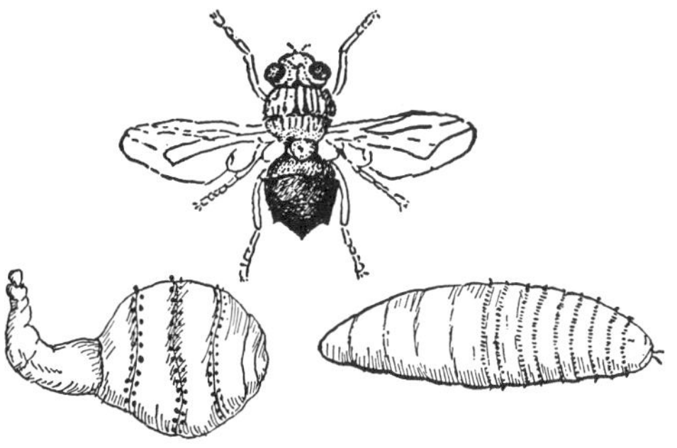

Dermatobia hominis (Dermatobia cyaniventris)
Top, adult female; *bottom,* larvae, early and late stages.

dermatobiasis (der'mă-tō-bī'ă-sis). Human botfly myiasis; infection of man and animals with larvae of the fly *Dermatobia hominis.*

dermatocele (der'mă-tō-sēl) [dermato- + G. *kēlē,* hernia]. Localized atrophy or herniation of skin that may result from a neurofibroma or a congenital defect.

dermatocellulitis (der'mă-tō-sel-yū-lī'tis). Inflammation of the skin and subcutaneous connective tissue.

dermatochalasis (der'mă-tō-kă-lā'sis) [dermato- + G. *chalaō,* to loosen]. *Cutis* laxa.

dermatoconiosis (der'mă-tō-kō-nī-o'sis) [dermato- + G. *konis,* dust, + *-osis,* condition]. An occupational dermatitis caused by local irritation from dust.

dermatocyst (der'mă-tō-sist). A cyst of the skin.

dermatodynia (der'mă-tō-din'ē-ă) [dermato- + G. *odynē,* pain]. Dermatalgia.

dermatofibroma (der'mă-tō-fī-brō'mă). A slowly growing benign skin nodule consisting of poorly demarcated cellular fibrous tissue enclosing collapsed capillaries, with scattered hemosiderin-pigmented and lipid macrophages. The following terms are considered by some to be synonymous with, and by others to be varieties of, d.: sclerosing hemangioma, histiocytoma or fibrous histiocytoma, nodular subepidermal fibrosis, fibroxanthoma, fibrous xanthoma.

dermatofibrosarcoma protuberans (der'mă-tō-fī'brō-sar-kō'mă prō-tū'ber-anz). A relatively slowly growing dermal neoplasm consisting of one or several firm nodules that are usually covered by dark red-blue skin, which tends to be fixed to the palpable masses; histologically, the neoplasm resembles a cellular dermatofibroma with a pronounced storiform pattern; metastases are unusual, but the incidence of recurrence is fairly high.
pigmented d. p., storiform neurofibroma; Bednar tumor; an uncommon variant of d. p. containing heavily pigmented dendritic melanocytes scattered between spindle cells of the tumor.

dermatofibrosis lenticularis disseminata (der'mă-tō-fī-brō'sis len-tik-yū-lā'ris di-sem-i-nā'tă). Asymmetric papules or discs of increased dermal elastic tissue appearing in early life; when osteopoikilosis is also present, the condition is called osteodermatopoikilosis; autosomal dominant inheritance.

dermatoglyphics (der'mă-tō-glif'iks) [dermato- + *glyphē,* carved work]. **1.** The configurations of the characteristic ridge patterns of the volar surfaces of the skin; in the hand of man, the distal segment of each digit has three types of configurations: whorl, loop, and arch. See also fingerprint. **2.** The science or study of these configurations or patterns.

dermatograph (der-mat'ō-graf). The linear wheal made in the skin in dermatographism.

dermatographism (der-mă-tog'ră-fizm) [dermato- + G. *graphō,* to write]. A form of urticaria in which whealing occurs in the site and in the configuration of application of stroking (pressure, friction) of the skin. Also called dermatography, dermagraphy, dermographia; dermographism; dermography; autographism; skin writing; factitious urticaria; urticaria factitia; Ebbecke's reaction.

dermatography (der-mă-tog'ră-fē). Dermatographism.

dermatoheteroplasty (der'ma-tō-het'er-ō-plas-tē) [dermato- + G. *heteros,* another, + *plastos,* formed]. Dermatoxenoplasty.

dermatohomoplasty (der'mă-tō-hō'mō-plas-tē) [dermato- + G. *homos,* same, + *plastos,* formed]. Dermatoalloplasty.

dermatoid (der'mă-toyd). **1.** Dermoid (1); resembling skin. **2.** Dermal.

dermatologist (der-mă-tol'ō-jist). A physician who specializes in the diagnosis and treatment of cutaneous lesions and the related systemic diseases.

dermatology (der-mă-tol'ō-jē) [dermato- + G. *logos,* study]. The branch of medicine concerned with the study of the skin, its chemistry, physiology, histopathology, cutaneous lesions, and the relationship of cutaneous lesions to systemic disease.

dermatolysis (der-mă-tol'i-sis) [dermato- + G. *lysis,* a loosening]. Dermolysis; loosening of the skin or atrophy of the skin by disease; erroneously used as a synonym for cutis laxa.
d. palpebra'rum, blepharochalasis.

dermatoma (der-mă-tō'mă) [dermato- + G. *-oma,* tumor]. A circumscribed thickening or hypertrophy of the skin.

dermatome (der'mă-tōm) [dermato- + G. *tomē,* a cutting]. **1.** An instrument for cutting thin slices of skin for grafting, or excising small lesions. **2.** Cutis plate; the dorsolateral part of an embryonic somite. **3.** Dermatomic area; the area of skin supplied by cutaneous

branches from a single spinal nerve; neighboring d.'s may overlap.
electric d., see electrodermatome.

dermatomegaly (der'mă-tō-meg'ă-lē) [dermato- + G. *megas,* large]. Congenital defect in which the skin hangs in folds; erroneously used as a synonym for cutis laxa.

dermatomere (der'mă-tō-mēr) [dermato- + G. *meros,* part]. A metameric area of the embryonic integument.

dermatomycosis (der'mă-tō-mī-kō'sis). Fungus infection of the skin caused by dermatophytes, yeasts, and other fungi. *Cf.* dermatophytosis.
d. ped'is, *tinea* pedis.

dermatomyoma (der'mă-tō-mī-ō'mă) [dermato- + G. *mys,* muscle, + *-oma,* tumor]. *Leiomyoma* cutis.

dermatomyositis (der'mă-tō-mī-ō-sī'tis) [dermato- + G. *mys,* muscle, + *-itis,* inflammation]. A progressive condition characterized by muscular weakness with a skin rash, typically a purplish-red heliotrope erythema on the face, and edema of the eyelids and periorbital tissue; affected muscle tissue shows degeneration of fibers with a chromic inflammatory reaction; occurs in children and adults, and in the latter may be associated with visceral cancer.

dermatoneurosis (der'mă-tō-nū-ro'sis). Dermoneurosis; any cutaneous eruption due to emotional stimuli.

dermatonosology (der'mă-tō-nō-sol'ō-jē) [dermato- + G. *nosos,* disease, + *logos,* treatise]. Dermonosology; the science of the nomenclature and classification of diseases of the skin.

dermatopathia (der'mă-tō-path'ē-ă). Dermatopathy.
d. pigmento'sa reticula'ris, *livedo* reticularis.

dermatopathology (der'mă-tō-pa-thol'ō-jē). Histopathology of skin lesions.

dermatopathy (der'mă-top'ă-thē) [dermato- + G. *pathos,* suffering]. Dermopathy; dermatopathia; any disease of the skin.

Dermatophagoides pteronyssinus (der-mă-tof-ă-goy'dēz ter-ō-ni-sī'nŭs) [dermato- + G. *phagein,* to eat; ptero- + G. *nyssō,* to prick, stab]. A common species of cosmopolitan mites found in house dust and a common contributory cause of atopic asthma.

dermatophilosis (der'mă-tō-fi-lō'sis). An infectious exudative dermatitis of cattle, sheep, goats, horses, and other animals (occasionally man) caused by *Dermatophilus congolensis;* severe (sometimes fatal) d. is seen in cattle in the Caribbean, invariable in association with *Amblyomma variegatum* infestations.

Dermatophilus congolensis (der-mă-tof'i-lŭs kon-gō-len'sis) [dermato- + G. *philos,* fond]. A species of motile, nonacid fast, aerobic to facultatively anaerobic, Gram-positive bacteria that is the etiologic agent of dermatophilosis; also causes proliferative dermatitis.

dermatophobia (der'mă-tō-fō'bē-ă) [dermatosis + G. *phobos,* fear]. Morbid fear of acquiring a skin disease.

dermatophone (der'mă-tō-fōn). An instrument used for listening to blood flow in the skin.

dermatophylaxis (der'mă-tō-fī-lak'sis) [dermato- + G. *phylaxis,* protection]. Protection of the skin against potentially harmful agents; *e.g.,* infection, excessive sunlight, noxious agents.

dermatophyte (der'mă-tō-fīt) [dermato- + G. *phyton,* plant]. A fungus that causes infections of the skin, hair, and/or nails, *i.e.,* keratinized tissues. Species of *Epidermophyton, Microsporum,* and *Trichophyton* are regarded as dermatophytes, but causative agents of tinea versicolor, tinea nigra, and cutaneous candidiasis are not so classified.

dermatophytid (der-mă-tof'i-tid). An allergic manifestation of dermatophytosis at a site distant from that of the primary fungous infection. The lesions, usually small vesicles on the hands and/or arms, are devoid of the fungus and may become extensive, covering wide areas of the body and causing extreme discomfort to the patient. See also -id (1), id *reaction.*

dermatophytosis (der'mă-tō-fī-tō'sis). An infection of the hair, skin, or nails caused by any one of the dermatophytes. The lesions may occur at any site on the body and, on the skin, are characterized by erythema, small papular vesicles, fissures, and scaling. Common sites of infection are the feet (tinea pedis), nails (onychomycosis), and scalp (tinea capitis). *Cf.* dermatomycosis.

dermatoplastic (der'ma-tō-plas'tik). Relating to dermatoplasty.

dermatoplasty (der'ma-tō-plas-tē) [dermato- + G. *plastos,* formed]. Dermoplasty; plastic surgery of the skin, as by skin grafting.

dermatopolyneuritis (der'mă-tō-pol'ē-nū-rī'tis). Acrodynia (2).

dermatorrhagia (der'mă-tō-rā'jē-ă) [dermato- + G. *rhēgnymi,* to break forth]. Hemorrhage from or into the skin.
d. parasit'ica, a disease of the horse marked by numerous localized hemorrhages into and through the skin from small nodules, due to the presence of the parasitic filarial nematode, *Parafilaria multipapillosa.*

dermatorrhea (der'mă-tō-rē'ă) [dermato- + G. *rhoia,* flow]. An excessive secretion of the sebaceous or sweat glands of the skin.

dermatorrhexis (der'mă-tō-rek'sis) [dermato- + G. *rhēxis,* rupture]. Rupture of the skin; *e.g.,* as is seen in striae cutis distensae or in Ehlers-Danlos syndrome.

dermatosclerosis (der'mă-tō-skler-ō'sis) [dermato- + G. *sclērō,* to harden]. Scleroderma.

dermatoscopy (der-mă-tos'kō-pē) [dermato- + G. *skopeō,* to view]. Inspection of the skin, usually with the aid of a lens.

dermatosis, pl. **dermatoses** (der-mă-tō'sis, -sēz) [dermato- + G. *-osis,* condition]. Nonspecific term used to denote any cutaneous lesion or group of lesions, or eruptions of any type.
acarine d., an eruption caused by one of the acarine parasites.
acute neutrophilic d., Sweet's disease; a rare d., predominant in women, of rapid onset and characterized by plaque-like lesions, usually multiple, on the face, neck, and upper extremities, accompanied by conjunctivitis, mucosal lesions, fever, malaise, and arthralgia; biopsy reveals polymorphonuclear infiltrate of the middermis; rapid remission occurs with systemic steroid therapy.
benign chronic bullous d. of childhood, linear IgA bullous disease in children; a self-limiting bullous disease, chiefly of the trunk, perioral, and pelvic areas, with onset in the first decade, successively less severe recurrences, and total remission at adolescence; linear deposit of IgA found in involved and in normal skin, but there are no identifiable circulating antibodies.
Bowen's precancerous d., Bowen's *disease.*
chick nutritional d., d. in chicks, with eruptions about the eyes, mouth, and feet; responds to pantothenic acid.
dermolytic bullous d., *epidermolysis* bullosa dystrophica.
filarial d., sorehead; a disease of sheep on high mountain ranges during the summer caused by larvae of the filarial worm, *Elaeophora schneideri,* which localize chiefly on the head, causing intense itching and loss of wool.
lichenoid d., any chronic skin eruption, characterized by induration and thickening of the skin with accentuation of skin markings.
d. medicamento'sa, drug *eruption.*
d. papulo'sa ni'gra, dark brown papular lesions, observed in blacks, on the face and upper trunk; histologically and clinically, they resemble seborrheic keratoses.
pigmented purpuric lichenoid d., Gougerot and Blum disease; an eruption comprised of lichenoid papules variously pigmented from the hemosiderin of the associated purpura; found on the legs, usually in men over 40 years of age.
progressive pigmentary d., Schamberg's disease or dermatitis; chronic purpura, especially of the legs in men, spreading to form brownish patches; associated microscopically with perivascular lymphatic infiltration, diapedesis, and hemosiderosis.
radiation d., skin changes caused by ionizing radiation, particu-

larly erythema in the acute stage and chronic changes in the epidermis and dermis resembling actinic keratosis.

seborrheic d., seborrheic *dermatitis.*

subcorneal pustular d., subcorneal pustular dermatitis; Sneddon-Wilkinson disease; a pruritic chronic annular eruption of sterile vesicles and pustules beneath the stratum corneum; bears a considerable clinical resemblance to dermatitis herpetiformis.

transient acantholytic d. (TAD), Grover's disease; a papular eruption, with histologic suprabasal acantholysis, of the chest, with scattered lesions of the back and lateral aspects of the extremities, lasting from a few weeks to several months; seen predominantly in males over 40.

ulcerative d., lip and leg ulceration; an infectious disease of sheep characterized by crusted ulcers on the skin of the face, feet, and external genitalia; thought to be caused by the orf virus.

dermatoskeleton (der'mă-tō-skel'ĕ-tŏn). Exoskeleton (1).

dermatotherapy (der'mă-tō-thār'ă-pē). Treatment of skin diseases.

dermatothlasia (der'mă-tō-thlā'zē-ă) [dermato- + G. *thlasis,* a bruising]. An uncontrollable impulse to pinch and bruise the skin.

dermatotropic (der'mă-tō-trop'ik) [dermato- + G. *trōpe,* a turning]. Dermotropic; having an affinity for the skin.

dermatoxenoplasty (der'mă-tō-zē'nō-plas-tē) [dermato- + G. *xenos,* stranger, + *plastos,* formed]. Dermatoheteroplasty; xenografting of skin.

dermatozoiasis (der'mă-tō-zō-ī'ă-sis) [dermato- + G. *zōon,* animal, + *-iasis,* condition]. Dermatozoonosis.

dermatozoon (der'mă-tō-zō'on) [dermato- + G. *zōon,* animal]. An animal parasite of the skin.

dermatozoonosis (der'mă-tō-zō-ō-nō'sis, -zō-on'ō-sis) [dermato- + G. *zōon,* animal, + nosos, disease]. Dermatozoiasis; rarely used terms for an eruption caused by an animal parasite.

dermatrophia, dermatrophy (der-mă-trō'fē-ă, der-mat'rō-fē). Atrophy or thinning of the skin.

dermenchysis (der-men'ki-sis) [derm- + G. *enchysis,* a pouring in]. Subcutaneous administration of remedies.

dermic (der'mik). Dermal.

der'mis [G. *derma,* skin] [NA]. Corium.

dermo- [G. *derma,* skin]. Combining form relating to the skin. See also derm-, dermat-, and dermato-.

dermoblast (der'mō-blast) [dermo- + G. *blastos,* germ]. One of the mesodermal cells from which the corium is developed.

dermocyma (der'mō-sī'mă) [dermo- + G. *kyma,* fetus]. Unequal conjoined twins in which the smaller parasite is buried in the integument of the autosite.

dermographia, dermographism, dermography (der-mō-graf'ē-ă, -mog'ră-fizm, -mog'ră-fē). Dermatographism.

dermoid (der'moyd) [dermo- + G. *eidos,* resemblance]. **1.** Dermatoid (1). **2.** Dermoid *cyst.*

implantation d., epidermal *cyst.*

inclusion d., a congenital cyst lined by epidermis, with skin appendages in the dermis along a line of embryonic closure.

sequestration d., epidermal *cyst.*

dermoidectomy (der-moy-dek'tō-mē) [dermoid + G. *ektomē,* excision]. Operative removal of a dermoid cyst.

dermolysis (der-mol'i-sis). Dermatolysis.

dermonecrotic (der'mō-nĕ-krot'ik). Pertaining to any application or illness which may cause necrosis of the skin.

dermoneurosis (der'mō-nū-rō'sis). Dermatoneurosis.

dermonosology (der'mō-nō-sol'ō-jē). Dermatonosology.

dermopathy (der-mop'ă-thē). Dermatopathy.

diabetic d., small macules and papules of the extensor surfaces of the extremities, most commonly the shins of diabetics, which become atrophic, hyperpigmented, and occasionally undergo ulceration with scarring.

dermophlebitis (der'mō-flĕ-bī'tis) [dermo- + G. *phleps,* vein, + *-itis,* inflammation]. Inflammation of the superficial veins and the surrounding skin.

dermoplasty (der'mō-plas-tē). Dermatoplasty.

dermoskeleton (der-mō-skel'ĕ-tŏn). Exoskeleton (1).

dermostenosis (der'mō-stĕ-nō'sis) [dermo- + G. *stenōsis,* a narrowing]. Pathologic contraction of the skin.

dermostosis (der'mos-tō'sis) [derm- + G. *osteon,* bone, + *-osis,* condition]. *Osteosis* cutis.

dermosyphilopathy (der'mō-sif-i-lop'ă-thē). Cutaneous lesions of syphilis; any syphilid.

dermotoxin (der-mō-tok'sin). A substance elaborated by a living agent, especially an exotoxin formed by bacteria, and characterized by its ability to cause pathologic changes in skin, *e.g.,* erythema, degenerative changes, necrosis.

dermotropic (der-mō-trop'ik). Dermatotropic.

dermovascular (der-mō-vas'kyū-lăr) [dermo- + L. *vasculus,* small vessel]. Pertaining to the blood vessels of the skin.

derodidymus (dār'ō-did'i-mŭs) [G. *derē,* neck, + *didymos,* twin]. *Dicephalus* diauchenos.

derotation (dē-rō-tā'shŭn) [L. *de,* away, + *rotatio,* turning]. **1.** A turning back. **2.** In orthopedics, the correction of a rotation deformity by turning or rotating the deformed structure toward a normal position.

DES Abbreviation for diethylstilbestrol.

des-. In chemistry, a prefix indicating absence of some component of the principal part of the name; largely replaced by de- (*e.g.,* deoxyribonucleic acid, dehydro-) but retained where "de" could be taken for D or *d,* as part of "desmo" (*e.g.,* desmosterol), and in such terms as desoxycortone.

desamidize (dē-sam'i-dīz). Deamidize.

De Sanctis, Carlo. See D. S.-Cacchione *syndrome.*

desaturate (dē-sat'yū-rāt). To produce desaturation.

desaturation (dē'sat-yū-rā'shŭn). The act, or the result of the act, of making something less completely saturated; more specifically, the percentage of total binding sites remaining unfilled, *e.g.,* when hemoglobin is 70% saturated with oxygen and nothing else, its d. is 30%. *Cf.* saturation (5).

Desault, Pierre J., French surgeon, 1744–1795. See D.'s *bandage, ligature.*

Descartes (Cartesius), René, French philosopher, mathematician, physiologist, 1596–1650. The founder of modern philosophy and proponent of the mechanistic or iatromathematical *school.* See D.'s *law.*

Descemet, Jean, French physician, 1732–1810. See D.'s *membrane.*

descemetitis (des'ĕ-mĕ-tī'tis). Inflammation of Descemet's membrane.

descemetocele (des-ĕ-met'ō-sēl). Hernia of Descemet's membrane through the corneal stroma.

descendens (dē-sen'denz) [L.]. Descending.

d. cervica'lis, *radix* inferior ansae cervicalis.

d. hypoglos'si, *radix* superior ansae cervicalis.

descending (dē-send'ing) [L. *de-scendo,* pp. *-scensus,* to come down, fr. *scando,* to climb]. Descendens; running downward or toward the periphery.

descensus (dē-sen'sŭs) [L.]. Descent; a falling away from a higher position. See also ptosis; procidentia.

d. ab'errans tes'tis, incomplete descent of the testis which comes to rest in the inguinal canal, femoral canal, or perineal region, or under the skin of the penis.

d. paradox'us tes'tis, the descent of the right testis to the left half of the scrotum and the left testis to the right half.

d. tes'tis [NA], descent of the testis from the abdomen into the scrotum during the seventh and eighth months of intrauterine life.

d. u'teri, *prolapse* of the uterus.

d. ventric'uli, gastroptosis.

descent (dē-sent') [L. descensus]. **1.** Descensus. **2.** In obstetrics, the passage of the presenting part of the fetus into and through the birth canal.

Deschamps, Joseph F.L., French surgeon, 1740–1824. See D.'s *needle.*

desensitization (dē-sen'si-ti-zā'shŭn). **1.** Ananaphylaxis; antianaphylaxis; the reduction or abolition of allergic sensitivity or reactions to the specific antigen (allergen). **2.** The act of removing an emotional complex.

heterologous d., stimulation by one agonist which leads to a broad pattern of unresponsiveness to further stimulation by a variety of other agonists.

homologous d., loss of sensitivity only to the class of agonist used to desensitize the tissue.

systematic d., reciprocal inhibition (2); a type of behavior therapy for eliminating phobias or anxieties: the patient and therapist construct a list of imagined scenes eliciting the phobia, ranked from least to most anxiety-producing; the patient then is trained in deep muscle relaxation, and is repeatedly asked to imagine himself in the presence of the least anxiety-producing scene on the list until he feels fully relaxed while doing so; the procedure is repeated for each scene on the list until the patient develops the capacity to feel relaxed with any of the anxiety-producing scenes; real life scenes are then substituted for the imagined scenes.

desensitize (dē-sen'si-tīz). **1.** Deallergize; to reduce or remove any form of sensitivity. **2.** To effect desensitization (1). **3.** In dentistry, to eliminate or subdue the painful response of exposed, vital dentin to irritative agents or thermal changes.

deserpidine (dē-ser'pi-dēn). 11-Desmethoxyreserpine; ester alkaloid isolated from *Rauwolfia canescens* (family Apocynaceae) with the same actions and uses as reserpine.

desferrioxamine mesylate (des'fār-ē-ok'să-mēn). Deferoxamine mesylate.

desiccant (des'i-kant) [L. *de-sicco,* pp. *-siccatus,* to dry up]. Exsiccant. **1.** Desiccative; drying; causing or promoting dryness. **2.** Desiccator (1); an agent that absorbs moisture; a drying agent.

desiccate (des'i-kāt). Exsiccate; to dry thoroughly; to render free from moisture.

desiccation (des-i-kā'shŭn). Exsiccation (1); dehydration (4); the process of being desiccated.

desiccative (des-i-kā'tiv). Desiccant (1).

desiccator (des'i-kā-ter, tōr). **1.** Desiccant (2). **2.** An apparatus, such as a glass chamber containing calcium chloride, sulfuric acid, or other drying agent, in which a material is placed for drying.

vacuum d., a d. that can be evacuated.

desipramine hydrochloride (des-ip'ră-mēn). Desmethylimipramine hydrochloride; norimipramine hydrochloride; a dibenzazepine derivative; an antidepressant similar to imipramine hydrochloride.

deslanoside (des-lan'ō-sīd). Desacetyllanatoside C; a rapidly acting steroid glycoside obtained from lanatoside C (*Digitalis lanata*) by alkaline hydrolysis; a cardiotonic.

desm-. See desmo-.

Desmarres, Louis A., French ophthalmologist, 1810–1882. See D.'s *dacryolith.*

desmectasis, desmectasia (dez-mek'tă-sis, -mek-tā'zē-ă) [desm- + G. *ektasis,* a stretching]. Ectasia of a ligament.

desmins (dez'minz). α-Amino acids, usually lysine and norleucine, condensed through their sidechains rather than through their α-amino and carboxyl groups; copolymerizes with vimentin to form constituents of connective tissue, cell walls, filaments, etc.

desmitis (dez-mī'tis) [desm- + G. *-itis,* inflammation]. Inflammation of a ligament.

desmo-, desm- [G. *desmos,* a band]. Combining forms meaning fibrous connection or ligament.

desmocranium (dez-mō-krā'nē-ŭm). The mesenchymal primordium of the cranium.

Desmodus (dez'mō-dŭs) [desmo- + G. *odous,* tooth]. A blood-feeding genus of Chiroptera, known generally as vampire bats, found in Trinidad, Mexico, and Central and South America; *D. artibaeus, D. rotundus,* and *D. rufus,* three species present in Trinidad and South America, are reservoir hosts of paralyssa.

desmodynia (dez-mō-din'ē-ă) [desmo- + G. *odynē,* pain]. Pain in a ligament.

desmogenous (dez-moj'ĕ-nŭs) [desmo- + G. *-gen,* producing]. Of connective tissue or ligamentous origin or causation; *e.g.,* denoting a deformity due to contraction of ligaments, fascia, or a scar.

desmography (dez-mog'ră-fē) [desmo- + G. *graphō,* to describe]. A description of, or treatise on, the ligaments.

desmoid (dez'moyd) [desmo- + G. *eidos,* appearance, form]. **1.** Fibrous or ligamentous. **2.** Desmoid tumor; abdominal fibromatosis; a module or relatively large mass of unusually firm scarlike connective tissue resulting from active proliferation of fibroblasts, occurring most frequently in the abdominal muscles of women who have borne children; the fibroblasts infiltrate surrounding muscle and fascia.

extra-abdominal d., a deep-seated firm tumor, most frequently occurring on the shoulders, chest, or back of young men or women, consisting of collagenous fibrous tissue that infiltrates surrounding muscle; frequently recurs but does not metastasize.

desmolases (dez'mō-lā'sez). Old and nonspecific term for enzymes catalyzing reactions other than those involving hydrolysis; *e.g.,* those involving oxidation and reduction, isomerization, the breaking of carbon-carbon bonds.

desmology (dez-mol'ō-jē) [desmo- + G. *logos,* study]. The branch of anatomy concerned with the ligaments.

desmon (dez'mon) [G. *desmos,* band, bond]. An old term for complement-fixing antibody.

desmopathy (dez-mop'ă-thē) [desmo- + G. *pathos,* suffering]. Any disease of the ligaments.

desmoplasia (dez-mō-plā'zē-ă) [desmo- + G. *plasis,* a molding]. Hyperplasia of fibroblasts and disproportionate formation of fibrous connective tissue, especially in the stroma of a carcinoma.

desmoplastic (des-mō-plas'tik). **1.** Causing or forming adhesions. **2.** Causing fibrosis in the vascular stroma of a neoplasm.

desmopressin acetate (DDAVP) (des-mō-pres'in). 1-(3-Mercaptopropionic acid)-8-D-arginine-vasopressin monoacetate trihydrate; a synthetic analog of vasopressin and an antidiuretic hormone.

desmosome (dez'mō-sōm) [desmo- + G. *sōma,* body]. Bridge corpuscle; macula adherens; a site of adhesion between two epithelial cells, consisting of a dense attachment plaque separated from a similar structure in the other cell by a thin layer of extracellular material.

desmosterol (dez-mos'ter-ol). 24-Dehydrocholesterol; postulated intermediate in cholesterol biosynthesis from lanosterol via zymosterol; accumulates after prolonged administration of substances interfering with cholesterol biosynthesis.

desomorphine (des-ō-mōr'fēn). Dihydrodeoxymorphine-D; a morphine derivative with a shorter duration of analgesic action but greater addiction liability than morphine.

desonide (des'ō-nīd). Pregna-1,4-diene-3,20-dione, 11,21-dihydroxy-16,17-[(1-methylethylidene)bis(oxy)]-, (11β,16α)-; an anti-inflammatory corticosteroid used in topical preparations.

desose (des'ōs). Obsolete term for deoxy *sugar.*

desoximetasone (des-ok-si-met'ă-sōn). Pregna-1,4-diene-3,20-dione, 9-fluoro-11,21-dihydroxy-16-methyl-, (11β,16α)-; an anti-inflammatory corticosteroid used in topical preparations.

desoxy-. See deoxy-.

desoxycortone (des-oks-ē-kōr'tōn). Deoxycorticosterone.

despeciation (dē-spē'shē-ā'shŭn). **1.** Alteration of, or loss of species characteristics. **2.** Removal of species-specific antigenic properties from a foreign protein.

D'Éspine, Jean H.A., French physician, 1846–1930. See D'É.'s *sign.*

despumation (des-pyū-mā'shŭn) [L. *de-spumo,* pp. *-atus,* to skim, fr. *spumo,* to foam, fr. *spuma,* foam]. **1.** The rising of impurities to the surface of a liquid. **2.** The skimming off of impurities on the surface of a liquid.

desquamate (des'kwă-māt) [L. *desquamo,* pp. *-atus,* to scale off, fr. *squama,* a scale]. To shred, peel, or scale off, as the casting off of the epidermis in scales or shreds, or the shedding of the outer layer of any surface.

desquamation (des-kwă-mā'shŭn). The shedding of the cuticle in scales or of the outer layer of any surface.
branny d., defurfuration.

desquamative (des-kwam'ă-tiv). Relating to or marked by desquamation.

desternalization (dē-ster'năl-i-zā'shŭn). Separation of the sternum from the costal cartilages.

desthiobiotin (des'thī-ō-bī'ō-tin). A compound derived from biotin by the removal of the sulfur atom; a precursor of biotin in bacteria and molds; it can substitute for biotin in some microorganisms, but is without effect on or is inhibitory to the growth of others.

destrudo (dē-strū'dō) [coinage on the analogy of *libido* fr. L. *destruere,* to destroy]. Energy associated with the death or destructive instinct.

desulfhydrases (dē'sulf-hī'drā-sez). Desulfurases; enzymes or groups of enzymes catalyzing the removal of a molecule of H_2S or substituted H_2S from a compound, as in the conversion of cysteine to pyruvic acid by cysteine desulfhydrase (cystathionine γ-lyase).

desulfinase (dē-sŭl'fin-ās). Term sometimes applied to the enzyme (aspartate-4-decarboxylase) removing sulfite: 1) from cysteinesulfinate, an intermediate in cysteine degradation, yielding alanine; 2) from sulfinylpyruvate, postulated to be formed by deamination of cysteinesulfinate, yielding pyruvate; degradation of sulfinylpyruvate is now considered to be spontaneous, not requiring an enzyme.

desulfurases (dē-sŭl'fyūr-ās-ez). Desulfhydrases.

desynchronous (de-sin'kron-ŭs) [de- + G. *syn,* with, + *chronos,* time]. Lack of synchrony, as in brain waves.

DET Abbreviation for diethyltryptamine.

det. Abbreviation for L. *detur,* give.

detachment (dē-tach'ment). **1.** A voluntary or involuntary feeling or sense of separation from normal associations or environment. **2.** Separation of a structure from its support.
disciform d. of retina, disciform *degeneration.*
exudative retinal d., d. of the retina without retinal breaks, arising from inflammatory disease of choroid, retinal tumors, and retinal angiomatosis.
retinal d., d. of retina, detached retina; retinal separation; loss of apposition between the sensory retina and the retinal pigment epithelium.
rhegmatogenous retinal d., retinal separation associated with a break, a hole, or a tear in the sensory retina.
vitreous d., separation of the peripheral vitreous humor from the retina.

detector (dē-tek'ter, -tōr). The component of a laboratory instrument which detects the chemical or physical signal indicating the presence of analyte.

detergent (dē-ter'jent) [L. *de-tergeo,* pp. *-tersus,* to wipe off]. Detersive. **1.** Cleansing. **2.** A cleansing or purging agent, usually salts of long-chain aliphatic bases or acids (*e.g.,* quaternary ammonium or sulfonic acid compounds) which, through a surface action that depends on their possessing both hydrophilic and hydrophobic properties, exert cleansing (oil-dissolving) and antibacterial effects; acridine derivatives (*e.g.,* acriflavine, proflavine) as well as other dyes (*e.g.,* brilliant green, crystal violet) have d. properties for the same reasons.
anionic d.'s, d.'s, such as soaps (alkali metal salts of long-chain fatty acids), that carry a negative electric charge on a lipid-like molecule and exert a limited antibacterial effect.
cationic d.'s, d.'s, such as the amine salts or quaternary ammonium or pyridinium compounds of long-chain fatty acids, that have positively charged groups attached to the larger hydrophobic portions.

deterioration (dē-tēr'i-ō-rā'shŭn) [L. *deterior,* worse]. The process or condition of becoming worse.
alcoholic d., emotional blunting, organic defects, and moral degeneration, occurring in persons chronically addicted to alcohol.
senile d., a slowly progressing decline in physical and mental health, apparently due to natural causes attendant upon the processes of aging.

determinant (dē-ter'mi-nănt) [L. *determans,* determining, limiting]. The factor that determines any given quality.
allotypic d.'s, antigenic d.'s of allotypes.
antigenic d., determinant group; the particular chemical group of a molecule that determines immunological specificity.
disease d.'s, any variables that directly or indirectly influence the frequency of occurrence and/or the distribution of any given disease; they include specific disease agents, host characteristics, and environmental factors.
genetic d., genetic marker; any antigenic d. or identifying characteristic, particularly those of allotypes.
idiotypic antigenic d., idiotype.
isoallotypic d.'s, genetic d.'s that are both isotypic and allotypic in that they appear on all members of at least one subclass of immunoglobulin but only on some members of another subclass of the same species.

determination (dē-ter-mi-nā'shŭn) [L. *de-termino,* pp. *-atus,* to limit, determine, fr. *terminus,* a boundary]. **1.** A change, for the better or for the worse, in the course of a disease. **2.** A general move toward a given point. **3.** The measurement or estimation of any quantity or quality in scientific or laboratory investigation.
sex d., d. of the sex of a fetus *in utero* by identification of sex chromatin bodies in amniotic squames obtained by amniocentesis.

determinism (dē-ter'mi-nizm). The proposition that all behavior is dependent on genetic and environmental influences, and independent of free will.
psychic d., in psychoanalysis, the concept that all psychological phenomena result from antecedent, unconsciously operating causes.

detersive (dē-ter'siv). Detergent.

De Toni, Guido. See D.T.-Fanconi *syndrome.*

detoxicate (dē-tok'si-kāt) [L. *de,* from, + *toxicum,* poison]. Detoxify; to diminish or remove the poisonous quality of any substance; to lessen the virulence of any pathogenic organism.

detoxication (dē-tok-si-kā'shŭn). Detoxification. **1.** Recovery from the toxic effects of a drug. **2.** Removal of the toxic properties from a poison. **3.** Metabolic conversion of pharmacologically active principles to pharmacologically less active principles.

detoxification (dē-tok'si-fi-kā'shŭn). Detoxication.

detoxify (dē-tok'si-fī). Detoxicate.

detrition (dē-trish'ŭn) [L. *de-tero,* pp. *-tritus,* to rub off]. A wearing away by use or friction.

detritus (dē-trī'tŭs) [L. (see detrition)]. Any broken-down material, carious or gangrenous matter, gravel, etc.

detrusor (dē-trū'ser, -sōr) [L. *detrudo,* to drive away]. A muscle that has the action of expelling a substance.
d. uri'nae, *musculus* detrusor urinae.

detumescence (dē-tū-mes'ens) [L. *de,* from, + *tumesco,* to swell up, fr. *tumeo,* to swell]. Subsidence of a swelling.

deturgescence (dē-tūr-ges'ens) [L. *de,* from, + *turgesco,* to begin to swell]. The mechanism by which the stroma of the cornea remains relatively dehydrated.

deut-. See deutero-.

deutencephalon (dū'ten-sef'ă-lon) [G. *deuteros,* second, + *enkephalos,* brain]. Rarely used term for diencephalon.

deuteranomaly (dū'ter-ă-nom'ă-lē) [G. *deuteros,* second, + *anōmalia,* anomaly]. A form of anomalous trichromatism that appears due to a deficiency of green-sensitive retinal cones.

deuteranope (dū'ter-ă-nōp). A person affected with deuteranopia.

deuteranopia (dū'ter-ă-nō'pē-ă) [G. *deuteros,* second, + anopia]. A form of dichromatism in which there are two rather than three retinal cone pigments and complete insensitivity to middle wavelengths (green).

deuteranopic (dū'ter-ă-nō'pik). Photerythrous; pertaining to or characterized by deuteranopia.

deuterio-. Prefix indicating "containing deuterium."

deuterium (D) (dū-tēr'ē-ŭm) [G. *deuteros,* second]. Hydrogen-2.
d. oxide, heavy *water.*

deutero-, deuto-, deut- [G. *deuteros,* second]. Combining forms meaning two, or second (in a series).

Deuteromycetes (dū'ter-ō-mī-sē'tēz). Fungi Imperfecti.

deuteron (dū'ter-on). Deuton; diplon; the nucleus of hydrogen-2, composed of one neutron and one proton; it thus has the one positive charge characteristic of a hydrogen nucleus.

deuteropathic (dū'ter-ō-path'ik). Relating to a deuteropathy.

deuteropathy (dū-ter-op'ă-thē) [deutero- + G. *pathos,* suffering]. A secondary disease or symptom.

deuteroplasm (dū'ter-ō-plazm) [deutero- + G. *plasma,* thing formed]. Deutoplasm.

deuteroporphyrin (dū'ter-ō-pōr'fi-rin). A porphyrin derivative resembling the protoporphyrins except that the two vinyl side chains are replaced by hydrogen.

deuterosome (dū'ter-ō-sōm). Procentriole organizer; dense spherical fibrous granules which occur in the centrosphere and act in the development of centrioles or basal bodies.

deuterotocia (dū'ter-ō-tō'sē-ă) [deutero- + G. *tokos,* childbirth]. Deuterotoky; a form of parthenogenesis in which the female has offspring of both sexes.

deuterotoky (dū-ter-ot'ō-kē). Deuterotocia.

deuto-. See deutero-.

deutogenic (dū-tō-jen'ik) [deuto- + G. *-gen,* production]. Of secondary origin following an inductive influence.

deutomerite (dū-tom'er-īt) [deuto- + L. *meros,* part]. The posterior nucleated portion of an attached cephalont in a gregarine protozoan, separated by an ectoplasmic septum from the anterior portion, or protomerite.

deuton (dū'ton). Deuteron.

deutoplasm (dū'tō-plazm) [deuto- + G. *plasma,* thing formed]. Deuteroplasm; the yolk of a meroblastic egg; the nonliving material in the cytoplasm, especially that stored in the ovum as food for the developing embryo, the commonest types being lipoid droplets and yolk granules.

deutoplasmic (dū-tō-plaz'mik). Relating to the deutoplasm.

deutoplasmigenon (dū'tō-plaz-mi-jen'on) [deutoplasm + G. *genos,* birth]. That which produces or gives rise to deutoplasm.

deutoplasmolysis (dū'tō-plaz-mol'i-sis) [deutoplasm + G. *lysis,* dissolution]. The disintegration of deutoplasm.

Deutschländer, Carl E. W., German surgeon, 1872–1942. See D.'s *disease.*

DEV Duck embryo origin *vaccine.*

devascularization (dē-vas'kyū-lăr-i-zā'shŭn) [L. *de,* away, + *vasculus,* small vessel, + G. *izo,* to cause]. Occlusion of all or most of the blood vessels to any part or organ.

development (dē-vel'ŏp-ment). The act or process of natural progression from a previous, lower, or embryonic stage to a later, more complex, or adult stage.
life-span d., development and mastery (or loss) of differing biologic, intellectual, behavioral, and social skills in different epochs of the life-span from the prenatal through the gerontological periods of growth.
psychosexual d., maturation and development of the psychic phase of sexuality from birth to adult life through the oral, anal, phallic, latency, and genital phases.

Deventer, Hendrik van, Dutch obstetrician, 1651–1724. See D.'s *pelvis.*

deviance (dē'vē-ans). Deviation (3).

deviant (dē'vē-ant). **1.** Denoting or indicative of deviation. **2.** An individual exhibiting deviation, especially sexual.

deviation (dē-vē-ā'shŭn) [L. *devio,* to turn from the straight path, fr. *de,* from, + *via,* way]. **1.** Deflection; a turning away or aside from the normal point or course. **2.** An abnormality. **3.** Deviance; in psychiatry, a departure from an accepted norm, role, or rule. **4.** A statistical measure representing the difference between an individual value in a set of values and the mean value in that set.
axis d., axis shift; deflection of the electrical axis of the heart to the right or left of the normal. See also left axis d., right axis d., and related subentries under axis.
conjugate d. of the eyes, **(1)** rotation of the eyes equally and simultaneously in the same direction, as occurs normally; **(2)** a condition in which both eyes are turned to the same side as a result of either paralysis or muscular spasm.
immune d., split tolerance; the process in which a soluble protein antigen in Freund's complete adjuvant induces a sensitivity of the cell-dependent (delayed) kind in a normal guinea pig, but induces sensitivity of the antibody-dependent (immediate) kind in a guinea pig on which sensitivity of that (immediate) kind has already been induced by a previous injection of the soluble antigen without adjuvant.
d. to the left, *shift* to the left (1).
left axis d., a mean electrical axis of the heart pointing above −30°. See hexaxial reference *system.*
primary d., the ocular deviation seen in paralysis of an ocular muscle when the nonparalyzed eye is used for fixation.
d. to the right, *shift* to the right (1).
right axis d., a mean electrical axis of the heart pointing to the right of +90°. See hexaxial reference *system.*
secondary d., ocular deviation seen in paralysis of an ocular muscle when the paralyzed eye is used for fixation.
sexual d., paraphilia; sexual perversion; a sexual practice that is

biologically or medically abnormal, morally wrong, or legally prohibited.

skew d., a hypertropia in which the eyes move in opposite directions equally.

standard d. (S.D., σ), statistical index of the degree of d. from central tendency, namely, of the variability within a distribution; the square root of the average of the squared d.'s from the mean.

Devic, Eugène, French physician, †1930. See D.'s *disease.*

device (dē-vīs'). An appliance, usually mechanical, designed to perform a specific function, such as prosthesis or orthesis.

central-bearing d., a d. which provides a central point of bearing, or support, between upper and lower record bases; it consists of a contacting point which is attached to one base and a plate attached to the other which provides the surface on which the bearing point rests or moves.

central-bearing tracing d., a central-bearing d. used for making a tracing and/or for support between upper and lower bases.

contraceptive d., a d. used to prevent pregnancy; *e.g.,* occlusive diaphragm, condom, intrauterine d.

intra-aortic balloon d., an externally and intermittently inflatable balloon placed into the descending aorta and which, on activation during diastole, augments blood pressure and organ perfusion by its pulsatile thrust; then, on deflation, decreases the cardiac work with each systole.

intrauterine d.'s (IUD), intrauterine contraceptive d.'s (IUCD), pieces of plastic or metal of various shapes (*e.g.,* coil, loop, bow) inserted into the uterus to exert a contraceptive effect.

de Vincentiis, Carlos (Charles), Italian ophthalmologist, 1849–1905. See de V. *operation.*

Devine, Sir Hugh B., Australian surgeon, 1878–1959. See D. *exclusion.*

deviometer (dē-vē-om'ĕ-ter). A form of strabismometer.

devitalization (dē-vi'tăl-i-zā'shŭn). **1.** Deprivation of vitality or of vital properties. **2.** In dentistry, the process by which tooth pulp is destroyed; *e.g.,* by chemical means, by infection, or by extirpation.

devitalize (dē-vī'tăl-īz). To deprive of vitality or of vital properties.

devitalized (dē-vī'tăl-īzd). Devoid of life; dead.

devolution (dev-ō-lū'shŭn) [L. *de-volvo,* pp. *-volutus,* to roll down]. A continuing process of degeneration or breaking down, in contrast to evolution. See also involution; catabolism.

De Vries, Hugo, botanist in Amsterdam, 1848–1935. See D. V.'s *theory.*

Dewar, Sir James, British chemist, 1842–1923. See D. *flask.*

de Wecker, Louis H., French physician, 1832–1906. See de W.'s *scissors.*

dexamethasone (dek-să-meth'ă-sōn). 9α-Fluoro-16α-methylprednisolone; a synthetic analogue of cortisol, with similar biological action; used as an anti-inflammatory agent.

dexamphetamine (deks-am-fet'ă-mēn). Dextroamphetamine sulfate.

d. sodium phosphate, the water-soluble ester of d., with the same actions and uses.

dexbrompheniramine maleate (deks'brom-fen-ir'ă-mēn). *d-* 2-[*p*-Bromo-α-(2-dimethylaminoethyl)benzyl]pyridine maleate; the dextrorotatory isomer of brompheniramine; an antihistamine.

dexchlorpheniramine maleate (deks'klōr-fen-ir'ă-mēn). *d*-2-[*p*-Chloro-α-(2-dimethylaminoethyl)benzyl]pyridine maleate; the dextrorotatory isomer of chlorpheniramine; an antihistamine.

dexiocardia (deks-ē-ō-kar'dē-ă). Dextrocardia.

dexpanthenol (deks-pan'thĕ-nol). Panthenol; pantothenyl alcohol; D-(+)-2,4-dihydroxy-*N*-(3-hydroxypropyl)-3,3-dimethylbutyramide; pantothenic acid with $-CH_2OH$ replacing the terminal $-COOH$; a cholinergic agent and a dietary source of pantothenic acid.

dexter (D) (deks'ter) [L. fr. *dextra,* neut. *dextrum*] [NA]. Located on or relating to the right side.

dextr-. See dextro-.

dextrad (deks'trad) [L. *dexter,* right, + *ad,* to]. Toward the right side.

dextral (deks'trăl). Right-handed.

dextrality (deks-tral'i-tē). Right-handedness; preference for the right hand in performing manual tasks.

dextran (deks'tran). **1.** Any of several water-soluble high molecular weight glucose polymers (average MW 75,000) produced by the action of *Leuconostoc mesenteroides* on sucrose; used in isotonic sodium chloride solution for the treatment of shock, and in distilled water for the relief of the edema of nephrosis; lower molecular weight d. (average 40,000) improves blood flow in areas of stasis by reducing cellular aggregation. **2.** Poly(α-1,6-glucose); α-1,6-glucan with branch points (1.2; 1.3; 1.4) and spacing of these characteristic of the species; used as plasma substitutes or expanders. See dextransucrase.

d. 40, d. (average MW 40,000) used as a plasma volume extender and blood flow adjuvant.

d. 70, d. (average MW 70,000) used as a plasma volume expander.

d. 75, d. (average MW 75,000) used as a plasma volume extender.

d. 110, d. (average MW 110,000) available as 5% solution in water or saline solution; used as a plasma volume expander.

animal d., glycogen.

d. sulfate, the sodium salt of sulfuric acid esters of the polysaccharide d.; it contains not less than 10 units per mg and not less than 14% of sulfate; an anticoagulant.

dextranase (deks'tran-ās) [EC 3.2.1.11]. An enzyme hydrolyzing 1,6-α-D-glucosidic linkages in dextran.

dextransucrase (deks-tran-su'krās) [EC 2.4.1.5]. A glucosyltransferase that builds poly(1,6-α-D-glucosyl), *i.e.,* polyglucoses, dextrans, or α-glucans, from sucrose, releasing D-fructose residues.

dextrase (deks'trās). Nonspecific term for the complex of enzymes that converts dextrose (glucose) into lactic acid.

dextriferron (deks-tri-fer'on). A colloidal solution of ferric hydroxide in complex with partially hydrolyzed dextrin, used in the treatment of iron-deficiency anemia; it is suitable for intravenous administration and contains 20 mg of iron per ml.

dextrin (deks'trin). British or starch gum; a mixture of oligo(α-1,4-glucose) molecules formed during the enzymic or acid hydrolysis of starch, amylopectin, or glycogen; on further hydrolysis they are converted into glucose. D.'s are of much lower molecular weight than dextrans, hence are not suitable as plasma expanders; d. (usually white d.) is used in pharmaceutical preparations.

limit d., d. limit; the polysaccharide fragments remaining at the end (limit) of exhaustive hydrolysis of amylopectin or glycogen by α-1,4-glucan maltohydrolase, which cannot hydrolyze the α-1,6 bonds at branch points.

dextrinase (deks'tri-nās). Any of the enzymes catalyzing the hydrolysis of dextrins; *e.g.,* amylo-1,6-glucosidase, dextrin dextranase.

limit d., α-dextrin endo-1,6-α-glucosidase.

dextrin dextranase [EC 2.4.1.2]. Dextrin 6-glucosyltransferase; dextrin → dextran transglucosidase; a glucosyltransferase transferring 1,4-α- D-glucosyl residues, thus catalyzing the synthesis of dextrans (with 1,6 links between monosaccharide units) from dextrins (with 1,4 links) by glucose transfer.

dextrin → dextran transglucosidase. Dextrin dextranase.

α-dextrin endo-1,6-α-glucosidase [EC 3.2.1.41]. Pullulanase; limit dextrinase; an enzyme with action similar to that of isoamylase; it cleaves 1,6-α-glucosidic linkages in pullalan, amylopectin, and glycogen, and in α- and β-amylase limit-dextrins of amylopectin and glycogen.

dextrin 6-α-D-glucosidase. Amylo-1,6-glucosidase.

dextrin 6-glucosyltransferase. Dextrin dextranase.

dextrin glycosyltransferase. 4-α-D-Glucanotransferase.

dextrin limit. Limit *dextrin.*

dextrinogenic (deks'trin-ō-jen'ik). Capable of producing dextrin.

dextrinosis (deks-trin-ō'sis). Glycogenosis.
debranching deficiency limit d., limit d., type 3 *glycogenosis.*

dextrin transglycosylase. 4-α-D-Glucanotransferase.

dextrinuria (deks-tri-nū'rē-ă). The passage of dextrin in the urine.

dextro-, dextr- [L. *dexter,* right]. **1.** Prefixes meaning right, or toward or on the right side. **2.** Chemical prefixes meaning dextrorotatory.

dextroamphetamine phosphate (deks'trō-am-fet'ă-mēn). *d*- Amphetamine phosphate; monobasic d. phosphate; monobasic *d*- α-methylphenethylamine phosphate; same actions and uses as dextroamphetamine sulfate.

dextroamphetamine sulfate. *d*- Amphetamine sulfate; dexamphetamine; (+)-α-methylphenethylamine sulfate; similar in action to racemic amphetamine sulfate, but is more stimulating to the central nervous system; sympathomimetic and appetite depressant.

dextrocardia (deks'trō-kar'dē-ă) [dextro- + G. *kardia,* heart]. Dexiocardia; displacement of the heart to the right: either as dextroposition, with simple displacement to the right, or cardiac heterotaxia, with complete transposition of the right and left chambers, presenting a mirror picture of the normal.
corrected d., false d.; type 3 d.; dextroversion of the heart; displacement and rotation of the heart into the right side of the chest but without mirror transposition of the cardiac chambers.
false d., corrected d.
isolated d., type 2 d.; d. with mirror transposition of the cardiac chambers but without displacement of the abdominal viscera.
secondary d., type 4 d.; dextroposition of the heart by some disease of the lungs, pleura, or diaphragm.
d. with si'tus inver'sus, type 1 d.; displacement of the heart to the right side of the chest with mirror transposition of the cardiac chambers together with transposition of the abdominal viscera.
type 1 d., d. with situs inversus.
type 2 d., isolated d.
type 3 d., corrected d.,
type 4 d., secondary d.

dextrocardiogram (deks'trō-kar'dē-ō-gram). That part of the electrocardiogram that is derived from the right ventricle.

dextrocerebral (deks'trō-ser'ĕ-brăl). Having a dominant right cerebral hemisphere.

dextroclination (deks'trō-kli-nā'shŭn). Dextrotorsion (2).

dextrocular (deks-trok'yū-lăr) [dextro- + L. *oculus,* eye]. Right-eyed; indicating right ocular dominance; denoting one who prefers the right eye in monocular work, such as microscopy.

dextrocycloduction (deks'trō-sī-klō-dŭk'shŭn) [dextro- + cyclo- + L. *duco,* pp. *ductus,* to lead]. Rotation of the upper pole of the cornea to the right.

dextroduction (deks-trō-dŭk'shŭn) [dextro- + L. *duco,* pp. *ductus,* to lead]. Rotation of one eye to the right.

dextrogastria (deks-trō-gas'trē-ă) [dextro- + G. *gastēr,* stomach]. Condition in which the stomach is displaced to the right; usually associated with dextrocardia.

dextroglucose (deks-trō-glū'kōs). Glucose.

dextrogram (deks'trō-gram). Electrocardiographic record in an experimental animal representing spread of impulse through the right ventricle alone.

dextrogyration (deks'trō-jī-rā'shŭn) [dextro- + L. *gyro,* pp. *-atus,* to turn in a circle, fr. *gyrus.* circle]. A twisting to the right.

dextromanual (deks-trō-man'yū-ăl) [dextro- + L. *manus,* hand]. Right-handed.

dextromethorphan hydrobromide (deks'trō-meth-ōr'fan hī-drō-brō'mīd). Hydrobromide of *d*-racemethorphan; *d*-3-methoxy-*N*-methylmorphinan hydrobromide; a synthetic morphine derivative used as an antitussive agent. It has no central depressant or analgesic action, and appears to have no addiction liability.

dextromoramide tartrate (deks-trō-mōr'ă-mīd). A narcotic analgesic related chemically and pharmacologically to methadone.

dextropedal (deks-trop'ĕ-dăl) [dextro- + L. *pes* (*ped-*), foot]. Right-footed; denoting one who uses the right leg in preference to the left.

dextroposition (deks'trō-pō-zi'shŭn). Abnormal right-sided location or origin of a normally left-sided structure, *e.g.,* origin of the aorta from the right ventricle.
d. of the heart, see dextrocardia.

dextropropoxyphene hydrochloride (deks'trō-prō-pok'sē-fēn). Propoxyphene hydrochloride.

dextropropoxyphene napsylate. Propoxyphene napsylate.

dextrorotation (deks'trō-rō-tā'shŭn). A turning or twisting to the right; especially, the clockwise twist given the plane of plane-polarized light by solutions of certain optically active substances. *Cf.* levorotation.

dextrorotatory (deks-trō-rō'tă-tōr-ē). Denoting dextrorotation, or certain crystals or solutions capable of so doing; as a chemical prefix, usually abbreviated, *d*-. *Cf.* levorotatory.

dextrose (deks'trōs). Glucose.

dextrosinistral (deks'trō-si-nis'trăl) [dextro- + L. *sinister,* left]. In a direction from right to left.

dextrosuria (deks-trō-sū'rē-ă). Obsolete term for glycosuria.

dextrothyroxine sodium (deks-trō-thī-roks'ēn). D-Thyroxine sodium salt; an antihypercholesterolemic agent.

dextrotorsion (deks-trō-tōr'shŭn) [dextro- + L. *torsio,* a twisting]. **1.** A twisting to the right. **2.** Dextroclination; in ophthalmology, rotation of the upper pole of both corneas to the right.

dextrotropic (dek-trō-trop'ik) [dextro- + G. *tropos,* a turn]. Turning to the right.

dextroversion (deks'trō-ver'zhŭn) [dextro- + L. *verto,* pp. *versus,* to turn]. **1.** Version toward the right. **2.** In ophthalmology, rotation of both eyes to the right.
d. of the heart, corrected *dextrocardia.*

df, DF Abbreviation for decayed and filled. See under index.

dGMP Abbreviation for deoxyguanylic acid.

Dharmendra antigen. See under antigen.

d'Herelle, Felix H., Canadian physician and bacteriologist, 1873–1949. See d'H. or Twort-d'H. *phenomenon.*

D. Hy. Abbreviation for Doctor of Hygiene.

di- [G. *dis,* two]. **1.** Prefix denoting two, twice. **2.** In chemistry, often used in place of bis- when not likely to be confusing; *e.g.,* dichloro-compounds. *Cf.* bi-; bis.

dia- [G. *dia,* through]. Prefix meaning through, throughout, completely.

diabetes (dī-ă-bē'tēz) [G. *diabētēs,* a compass, a siphon, diabetes]. Either d. insipidus or d. mellitus, diseases having in common the symptom polyuria; when used without qualification, refers to d. mellitus.
adult-onset d., non-insulin-dependent d. mellitus.
alimentary d., alimentary *glycosuria.*
alloxan d., experimental d. produced in animals by the adminis-

tration of alloxan, which damages the insulin-producing islet cells of the pancreas.
brittle d., d. in which there are marked fluctuations in blood glucose concentrations which are difficult to control.
bronze d., d. associated with hemochromatosis, with iron deposits in the skin, liver, pancreas, and other viscera, often with severe liver damage and glycosuria.
calcinuric d., hypercalciuria.
chemical d., latent d.
galactose d., galactosemia.
growth-onset d., insulin-dependent d. mellitus.
d. in'nocens, renal *glycosuria.*
d. insip'idus, chronic excretion of very large amounts of pale urine of low specific gravity, causing dehydration and extreme thirst; ordinarily results from inadequate output of pituitary antidiuretic hormone; may be mimicked as a result of excessive fluid intake, as in psychogenic polydipsia. See also nephrogenic d. insipidus.
insulin-dependent d. mellitus (IDDM), type I diabetes; juvenile- or growth-onset d.; severe d. mellitus, often brittle, usually of abrupt onset during the first two decades of life but can develop up to age 40; characterized by polydipsia, polyuria, increased appetite, weight loss, low plasma insulin levels, and episodic ketoacidosis; insulin therapy and dietary regulation are mandatory.
insulinopenic d., any form of d. mellitus resulting from inadequate secretion of insulin.
d. intermit'tens, d. mellitus in which there are periods of relatively normal carbohydrate metabolism followed by relapses to the previous diabetic state.
juvenile-onset d., insulin-dependent d. mellitus.
latent d., chemical d.; a mild form of d. mellitus in which the patient displays no overt symptoms, but displays certain abnormal responses to diagnostic procedures, such as an elevated fasting blood glucose concentration or reduced glucose tolerance.
lipoatrophic d., lipoatrophy.
lipogenous d., d. and obesity combined.
maturity-onset d., non-insulin-dependent d. mellitus.
d. mel'litus [L. sweetened with honey], a metabolic disease in which carbohydrate utilization is reduced and that of lipid and protein enhanced; it is caused by an absolute or relative deficiency of insulin and is characterized, in more severe cases, by chronic hyperglycemia, glycosuria, water and electrolyte loss, ketoacidosis, and coma; long-term complications include development of neuropathy, retinopathy, nephropathy, generalized degenerative changes in large and small blood vessels, and increased susceptibility to infection. See also insulin-dependent d. mellitus; non-insulin-dependent d. mellitus.
metahypophysial d., (1) d. mellitus caused by large quantities of endogenous or exogenous pituitary growth hormone; **(2)** term used to designate the irreversible phase of d. in acromegaly.
Mosler's d., inosituria with excretion of large quantities of water.
nephrogenic d. insipidus, vasopressin-resistant d.; d. insipidus due to inability of the kidney tubules to respond to antidiuretic hormone; X-linked inheritance, with full expression in males and partial defect in heterozygous females.
non-insulin-dependent d. mellitus (NIDDM), type II d.; adult- or maturity-onset d.; an often mild form of d. mellitus of gradual onset, usually in obese individuals over age 35; absolute plasma insulin levels are normal to high, but relatively low in relation to plasma glucose levels; ketoacidosis is rare, but hyperosmolar coma can occur; responds well to dietary regulation and/or oral hypoglycemic agents, but diabetic complications and degenerative changes can develop.
pancreatic d., (1) d. demonstrably dependent upon a pancreatic lesion; **(2)** d. following removal of the pancreas in an animal.
phloridzin d., marked glycosuria without hyperglycemia following the experimental administration of phloridzin, which impairs renal tubular reabsorption of glucose.
phosphate d., excessive secretion of phosphate in the urine due to a defect in tubular reabsorption; usually part of a more generalized abnormality, such as Fanconi syndrome.
piqûre d. [Fr.], puncture d.
pregnancy d., see subclinical d.
puncture d., piqûre d.; experimental d. produced in animals by puncture of the floor of the fourth ventricle of the brain.
renal d., renal *glycosuria.*
starvation d., after prolonged fasting, glycosuria following the ingestion of carbohydrate or glucose because of reduced output of insulin and/or reduced rate of glucose metabolism with a reduced ability to form glycogen.
steroid d., d. produced by pharmacological doses of steroid hormones, particularly glucocorticoids or estrogens; characterized by one or more of the typical manifestations of d. mellitus.
subclinical d., a form of d. mellitus that is clinically evident only under certain circumstances, such as pregnancy or extreme stress; persons so afflicted may, in time, manifest more severe forms of the disease.
thiazide d., impaired carbohydrate metabolism associated with the use of thiazide diuretic drugs; severe manifestations are seen in persons having d. mellitus, but impairment is mild or absent in nondiabetic individuals.
type I d., insulin-dependent d. mellitus.
type II d., non-insulin-dependent d. mellitus.
vasopressin-resistant d., nephrogenic d. insipidus.

diabetic (dī-ă-bet'ik). **1.** Relating to or suffering from diabetes. **2.** One who suffers from diabetes.

diabetogenic (dī'ă-bet-ō-jen'ik, -bē-tō-jen'ik). Causing diabetes.

diabetogenous (dī'ă-bē-toj'en-ŭs). Caused by diabetes.

diabetology (dī'ă-be-tol'ō-jē). The field of medicine concerned with diabetes.

diacele (dī'ă-sēl) [G. *dia-*, through, + *koilia*, a hollow]. *Ventriculus* tertius.

diacetate (dī-as'ē-tāt). **1.** Acetoacetate. **2.** A compound containing two acetate residues.

diacetemia (dī-as-ē-tē'mē-ă). A form of acidosis resulting from the presence of acetoacetic (diacetic) acid in the blood.

diacetic acid (dī-ă-sē'tik, -set'ik). Acetoacetic acid.

diacetonuria (dī-as'ĕ-tō-nū'rē-ă). Diaceturia.

diaceturia (dī-as-ĕ-tū'rē-ă). Diacetonuria; the urinary excretion of acetoacetic (diacetic) acid.

diacetyl (dī-as'ĕ-til). 2,3-Butanedione; a yellow liquid, $(CH_3CO)_2$, having the pungent odor of quinone and carrying the aromas of coffee, vinegar, and other foods.

diacetylcholine (dī-as'ĕ-til-kō'lēn). Succinylcholine.

diacetylmonoxime (DAM) (dī-as'ĕ-til-mon-ok'sĭm). A 2-oxo-oxime that can reactivate phosphorylated acetylcholinesterase *in vitro* and *in vivo;* it penetrates the blood-brain barrier.

diacetylmorphine (dī-as'ĕ-til-mōr'fēn). Heroin.

diacetyltannic acid (dī-as'ĕ-til-tan'ik). Acetyltannic acid.

diachronic (dī-ă-kron'ik) [dia- + G. *chronos*, time]. Systematically observed over time.

diacid (dī-as'id). Denoting a substance containing two ionizable hydrogen atoms per molecule; more generally, a base capable of combining with two hydrogen ions per molecule.

diaclasis, diaclasia (dī-ak'lă-sis, dī-ă-klā'zē-ă) [G. *diaklasis*, a breaking up, fr. *dia*, through, + *klasis*, a breaking]. Osteoclasis.

diacrinous (dī-ak'ri-nŭs) [G. *dia-krinō*, to separate one from another]. Excreting by simple passage through a gland cell.

diacrisis (dī-ak'ri-sis) [G. *dia-*, through, + *krisis*, a judgment]. Diagnosis.

diacritic, diacritical (dī-ă-krit'ik, -krit'i-kăl) [G. *diakritikos,* able to distinguish]. Distinguishing; diagnostic; allowing of distinction.

diactinic (dī'ak-tin'ik) [G. *dia,* through, + *aktis,* ray]. Having the property of transmitting light capable of bringing about chemical reactions.

diacylglycerol lipase (dī'as-il-glis'er-ol). Lipoprotein lipase.

diad (dī'ad). **1.** The transverse tubule and a cisterna in cardiac muscle fibers. **2.** Dyad (1).

diadermic (dī-ă-der'mik) [G. *dia,* through, + *derma,* skin]. Percutaneous.

diadochocinesia (dī-ad'ō-kō-si-nē'zē-ă). Diadochokinesia.

diadochokinesia, diadochokinesis (dī-ad'ō-kō-ki-nē'zē-ă, -ki-nē'sis) [G. *diadochos,* working in turn, + *kinēsis,* movement]. Diadochocinesia; the normal power of alternately bringing a limb into opposite positions, as of flexion and extention or of pronation and supination.

diadochokinetic (dī-ad'ō-kō-ki-net'ik). Relating to diadochokinesia.

diagnose (dī-ag-nōs'). To make a diagnosis.

diagnosis (dī-ag-nō'sis) [G. *diagnōsis,* a deciding]. The determination of the nature of a disease.
antenatal d., prenatal d.
clinical d., a d. made from a study of the signs and symptoms of a disease.
differential d., differentiation (2); the determination of which of two or more diseases with similar symptoms is the one from which the patient is suffering, by a systematic comparison and contrasting of the clinical findings.
d. by exclusion, a d. made by excluding those diseases to which only some of the patient's symptoms belong, leaving only one disease to which all the symptoms point.
laboratory d., a d. made by a chemical, microscopic, microbiologic, immunologic, or pathologic study of secretions, discharges, blood, or tissue.
neonatal d., systematic evaluation of the newborn for evidence of disease or malformations, and the conclusion reached.
pathologic d., a d., sometimes postmortem, made from a study of the lesions present.
physical d., a d. made by means of physical examination of the patient, or the process of a physical examination.
prenatal d., antenatal d.; d. utilizing procedures available for the recognition of diseases and malformations *in utero,* and the conclusion reached.

diagnosis-related group (DRG). A classification of patients by diagnosis or surgical procedure (sometimes including age) into major diagnostic categories (each containing specific diseases, disorders, or procedures) for the purpose of determining reimbursement of hospitalization costs, based on the premise that treatment of similar medical diagnoses would generate similar costs.

diagnostic (dī-ag-nos'tik). Relating to or aiding in diagnosis.

diagnostician (dī'ag-nos-tish'ăn). One who is skilled in making diagnoses; formerly, a name for specialists in internal medicine.

diakinesis (dī'ă-ki-nē'sis) [G. *dia,* through, + *kinēsis,* movement]. Final stage of prophase in meiosis in which the chiasmata present during the diplotene stage disappear and the chromosomes continue to shorten.

dial (dī'ăl, dīl) [L. *dies,* day]. A clock face or instrument resembling a clock face.
astigmatic d., a diagram of radiating lines, used to test for astigmatism.

Dialister (dī-ăl-is'ter). An obsolete genus of bacteria, the type species of which, *D. pneumosintes,* is now placed in the genus *Bacteroides.*

diallyl (dī-al'il). A compound containing two allyl groups.

dialysance (dī-al'i-sans) [fr. dialysis]. The number of milliliters of blood completely cleared of any substance by an artificial kidney or by peritoneal dialysis in a unit of time; conventional clearance formulas are expressed as mm/min.

dialysate (dī-al'i-sāt). Diffusate; that part of a mixture that passes through a dialyzing membrane.

dialysis (dī-al'i-sis) [G. a separation, fr. *dia- lyo,* to separate]. Diffusion (2); a form of filtration to separate crystalloid from colloid substances (or smaller molecules from larger ones) in a solution by interposing a semipermeable membrane between the solution and water; the crystalloid (smaller) substances pass through the membrane into the water on the other side, the colloids do not.
equilibrium d., in immunology, a method for determination of association constants for hapten-antibody reactions in a system in which the hapten (dialyzable) and antibody (nondialyzable) solutions are separated by semipermeable membranes. Since at equilibrium the quantity of free hapten will be the same in the two compartments, quantitative determinations can be made of hapten-bound antibody, free antibody, and free hapten.
extracorporeal d., hemodialysis performed through an apparatus outside the body.
peritoneal d., removal from the body of soluble substances and water by transfer across the peritoneum, utilizing a d. solution which is intermittently introduced into and removed from the peritoneal cavity; transfer of diffusable solutes and water between the blood and the peritoneal cavity depends on the concentration gradient between the two fluid compartments.
d. ret'inae, retinodialysis; congenital or traumatic separation of the peripheral sensory retina from the retinal pigment epithelium at the ora serrata, often causing a retinal detachment.

dialyze (dī'ă-līz). To perform dialysis; to separate a substance from a solution by means of dialysis.

dialyzer (dī'ă-lī-zer). The apparatus for performing dialysis; a membrane used in dialysis.

diamagnetic (dī'ă-mag-net'ik). Having the property of diamagnetism.

diamagnetism (dī-ă-mag'nĕ-tizm). The property of zero magnetic movement, given by molecules in which all electrons are paired; an unpaired electron yields a magnetic movement, hence the molecule containing such exhibits paramagnetism.

di-amelia (dī-ă-mē'lē-ă). Absence of two limbs.

diameter (dī-am'ĕ-ter) [G. *diametros,* fr. *dia,* through, + *metron,* measure]. **1.** A straight line connecting two opposite points on the surface of a more or less spherical or cylindrical body, or at the boundary of an opening or foramen, passing through the center of such body or opening. **2.** The distance measured along such a line.
anteroposterior d. of the pelvic inlet, conjugata.
Baudelocque's d., external *conjugate.*
biparietal d., the d. of the fetal head between the two parietal eminences.
buccolingual d., the d. of the crown of a tooth measured from the buccal to the lingual surfaces.
conjugate d. of the pelvic inlet, conjugata.
d. media'nus, conjugata.
d. obli'qua [NA], oblique d.; a measurement across the pelvic inlet from the sacroiliac joint of one side to the opposite iliopectineal eminence.
oblique d., d. obliqua.
occipitofrontal d., the d. of the fetal head from the external occipital protuberance to the most prominent point of the frontal bone in the midline.

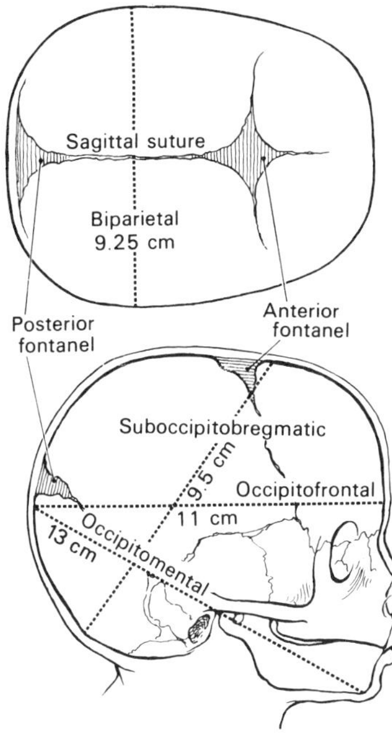

Diameters of the Fetal Skull

occipitomental d., the d. of the fetal head from the external occipital protuberance to the midpoint of the chin.
posterior sagittal d., distance from the sacrococcygeal junction to the middle of an imaginary line running between the left and right schial tuberosities.
suboccipitobregmatic d., the d. of the fetal head from the lowest posterior point of the occipital bone to the center of the anterior fontanelle.
total end-diastolic d. (TEDD), cross sectional d. of the left ventricle including the septum and posterior wall thicknesses in diastole.
total end-systolic d. (TESD), cross sectional d. of the left ventricle including the septum and posterior wall thicknesses in systole.
trachelobregmatic d., the d. of the fetal head from the middle of the anterior fontanelle to the neck.
d. transver'sa [NA], transverse d.; the transverse d. of the pelvic inlet, measured between the terminal lines.
transverse d., d. transversa.
zygomatic d., the extreme breadth of the skull at the zygomatic arches.

diamide (dī'am-id, -īd). A compound containing two amide groups.

diamidines (dī-am'i-dēnz). A group of compounds containing two amidine groups; *e.g.,* stilbamidine, propamidine.

diamine (dī'ă-mēn, -min). An organic compound containing two amine groups per molecule; *e.g.,* ethylenediamine, $NH_2CH_2CH_2NH_2$.
d. oxidase, *amine* oxidase (copper-containing) or *amine* oxidase (flavin-containing).

diamino oxyhydrase (dī-am'i-nō oks-ē-hī'drās). *Amine* oxidase (copper-containing).

diamniotic (dī-am-nē-ot'ik). Exhibiting two amniotic sacs, said of fetal membranes from multiple births.

Diamond, Louis K., U.S. physician, *1902. See D.-Blackfan *anemia, syndrome;* Gardner-D. *syndrome.*

diamthazole dihydrochloride (dī-am'thă-zōl). Dimazole dihydrochloride; 6-(2-diethylaminoethoxy)-2-dimethylaminobenzothiazole dihydrochloride; an antifungal agent for topical use.

diandry, diandria (dī'an-drē, dī-an'drē-ă) [di- + G. *andros,* male]. The phenomenon in which a single ovum is fertilized by a diploid sperm and hence produces a triploid fetus. *Cf.* digynia.

dianoetic (dī'ă-nō-et'ik) [G. *dia,* through, + *noein,* to think]. Of or pertaining to reason or other intellectual functions.

diapause (dī'ă-pawz). A period of biological quiescence or dormancy; an interval in which development is arrested or greatly slowed.
embryonic d., a d. in the course of embryogenesis; postulated to occur in instances of double parturition and possibly of delayed implantation.

diapedesis (dī'ă-pē-dē'sis) [G. *dia,* through, + *pēdēsis,* a leaping]. Migration (2); the passage of blood, or any of its formed elements, through the intact walls of blood vessels.

diaphanoscope (dī-af'ă-nō-skōp) [G. *diaphanēs,* transparent, + *skopeō,* to examine]. Polyscope; an instrument for illuminating the interior of a cavity to determine the translucency of its walls.

diaphanoscopy (dī-af-ă-nos'kō-pē). Examination of a cavity with a diaphanoscope.

diaphemetric (dī'ă-fē-met'rik) [G. *dia,* through, + *haphē,* touch, + *metron,* measure]. Relating to the determination of the degree of tactile sensibility.

diaphen hydrochloride (dī'ă-fen). 2-Diethylaminoethyl α-chlorodiphenylacetate hydrochloride; an antihistaminic agent with anticholinergic properties.

diaphorase (dī-af'ōr-ās). Originally, a series of flavoproteins with reductase activity in mitochondria; now dihydrolipoamide dehydrogenase.

diaphoresis (dī'ă-fō-rē'sis) [G. *diaphorēsis,* fr. *dia,* through, + *phoreō,* to carry]. Perspiration (1).

diaphoretic (dī-ă-fō-ret'ik). **1.** Relating to, or causing, perspiration. **2.** An agent that increases perspiration.

diaphragm (dī'ă-fram) [G. *diaphragma*]. **1.** Diaphragma (2). **2.** A thin disk pierced with an opening, used in a microscope, camera, or other optical instrument in order to shut out the marginal rays of light, thus giving a more direct illumination. **3.** A flexible metal ring covered with a dome-shaped sheet of elastic material used in the vagina to prevent pregnancy. **4.** In x-ray, grid (2).
Bucky d., in roentgenograms, a d. with moving grids that avoid grid shadows.
pelvic d., d. of pelvis, *diaphragma* pelvis.
d. of sella, *diaphragma* sellae.
urogenital d., *diaphragma* urogenitale.

diaphragma, pl. **diaphragmata** (dī-ă-frag'mă, -frag'mă-tă) [G. *diaphragma,* a partition wall, midriff] [NA]. **1.** A thin partition separating adjacent regions. **2.** Diaphragm (1); midriff; phren (1); interseptum; the musculomembranous partition between the abdominal and thoracic cavities.
d. pel'vis [NA], diaphragm of pelvis; pelvic diaphragm; the paired levator ani and coccygeus muscles together with the fascia above and below them.
d. sel'lae [NA], diaphragm of sella; tentorium of hypophysis; a fold of dura mater extending transversely across the sella turcica and roofing over the hypophyseal fossa; it is perforated in its center for the passage of the infundibulum.
d. urogenita'le [NA], urogenital diaphragm; a triangular sheet of muscle between the ischiopubic rami; composed of the sphincter urethrae, and the deep transverse perineal muscles.

diaphragmalgia (dī'ă-frag-mal'jē-ă) [diaphragm + G. *algos,* pain]. Diaphragmodynia; pain in the diaphragm.

diaphragmatic (dī'ă-frag-mat'ik). Relating to a diaphragm.

diaphragmatocele (dī'ă-frag-mat'ō-sēl) [diaphragm + G. *kēlē,* hernia]. Diaphragmatic *hernia.*

diaphragmodynia (dī'ă-frag-mō-din'ē-ă) [diaphragm + G. *odynē,* pain]. Diaphragmalgia.

diaphyseal (dī-ă-fiz'ē-ă). Diaphysial.

diaphysectomy (dī'ă-fi-sek'tō-mē) [diaphysis + G. *ektomē,* excision]. Partial or complete removal of the shaft of a long bone.

diaphysial (dī-ă-fiz'ē-ăl). Diaphyseal; relating to a diaphysis.

diaphysis, pl. **diaphyses** (dī-af'i-sis, -sēz) [G. a growing between] [NA]. The shaft of a long bone, as distinguished from the epiphyses, or extremities, and apophyses, or outgrowths.

diaphysitis (dī-af-i-sī'tis). Inflammation of the shaft of a long bone.

diapiresis (dī'ă-pī-rē'sis) [G. *diapeirō,* to drive through, fr. *peirō,* to pierce]. Passage of colloidal or other small particles of suspended matter through the unruptured walls of the blood vessels. See also diapedesis.

diaplacental (dī'ă-pla-sen'tăl). Passing through or "across" the placenta.

diaplasis (dī-ap'lă-sis) [G. a putting in shape]. Diorthosis; obsolete term for setting of a fracture or reduction of a dislocation.

diaplastic (dī-ă-plas'tik). Pertaining to diaplasis.

diaplexus (dī-ă-plek'sŭs) [G. *dia,* through, + L. *plexus,* a plaiting]. Rarely used term for *plexus* choroideus ventriculi tertii.

diapnoic, diapnotic (dī-ap-nō'ik, -not'ik). **1.** Relating to, or causing perspiration, especially insensible perspiration. **2.** A mild sudorific.

diapophysis (dī'ă-pof'i-sis) [G. *dia,* through, + *apophysis,* an offshoot]. A transverse process of a thoracic vertebra or the portion of a cervical or lumber vertebra homologous thereto. *Cf.* pleurapophysis.

Diaptomus (dī-ap'tō-mŭs). A genus of copepod crustacea, the principal intermediate host for *Diphyllobothrium latum* in North America.

diarrhea (dī-ă-rē'ă) [G. *diarrhoia,* fr. *dia,* through, + *rhoia,* a flow, a flux]. An abnormally frequent discharge of semisolid or fluid fecal matter from the bowel.

d. al'ba, pullorum *disease.*

bovine virus d., mucosal disease; a specific infectious disease of cattle, caused by a togavirus; characterized by ulceration of the mouth, pharynx, esophagus, and sometimes the stomachs and intestines; may or may not be accompanied by severe d.

choleraic d., summer d.

Cochin China d., tropical *sprue.*

colliquative d., d. associated with excessive discharge of fluid.

dysenteric d., d. in bacillary or amebic dysentery.

fatty d., pimelorrhea; d. seen in malabsorption syndromes and chronic pancreatic disease, characterized by foul smelling stools with increased fat content which usually float in water.

gastrogenous d., a d. which may occur in achylia gastrica, or which is caused by excess secretion of gastric and other intestinal juices.

lienteric d., d. in which undigested food appears in the stools.

morning d., a form in which there are several loose stools in the early morning and during the forenoon, the bowels being quiet during the remainder of the day and night.

mucous d., d. with the presence of considerable mucus in the stools.

nocturnal d., d. that occurs chiefly at night, usually in association with diabetic neuropathy; alleged to be caused by lesions of the autonomic nervous system.

pancreatogenous d., d. in which the stools are bulky, pale, foul, greasy, and oily, as a result of malabsorption of fat due to deficient secretion of pancreatic enzymes in chronic pancreatitis.

serous d., d. characterized by watery stools.

summer d., choleraic d.; d. of infants in hot weather, usually an acute gastroenteritis due to the presence of *Shigella* or *Salmonella.*

traveler's d., d. of sudden onset, often accompanied by abdominal cramps, vomiting, and fever, occurring sporadically in travelers usually during the first week of a trip; most commonly caused by enterotoxigenic *Escherichia coli.*

tropical d., tropical *sprue.*

white d., pullorum *disease.*

diarrheal, diarrheic (dī-ă-rē'ăl, -rē'ik). Relating to diarrhea.

diarthric (dī-ar'thrik) [G. *di-,* two, + *arthron,* joint]. Biarticular; diarticular; relating to two joints.

diarthrosis, pl. **diarthroses** (dī-ar-thrō'sis, -sēz) [G. articulation]. *Articulatio* synovialis.

diarticular (dī-ar-tik'yū-lăr). Diarthric.

diaschisis (dī-as'ki-sis) [G. a splitting]. A sudden inhibition of function produced by an acute focal disturbance in a portion of the brain at a distance from the original seat of injury, but anatomically connected with it through fiber tracts.

diascope (dī'ă-skōp) [G. *dia,* through, + *skopeō,* to view]. A flat glass plate through which one can examine superficial skin lesions by means of pressure.

diascopy (dī-as'kō-pē) [G. *dia,* through, + *skopeō,* to see]. Examination of superficial skin lesions with a diascope.

diastalsis (dī-ă-stal'sis) [G. an arrangement]. The type of peristalsis in which a region of inhibition precedes the wave of contraction, as seen in the intestinal tract.

diastaltic (dī-ă-stal'tik). Pertaining to diastalsis.

diastase (dī'as-tās). A mixture, obtained from malt and containing amylolytic enzymes (principally α- and β-amylases), that converts starch into dextrin and maltose; used to make soluble starches, to aid in digestion of starches in certain types of dyspepsia, and to digest glycogen in histologic sections.

diastasis (dī-as'tă-sis) [G. a separation]. **1.** Divarication; any simple separation of normally joined parts. **2.** The latter part of diastole when the blood enters the ventricle slowly and the venous pressure tends to rise.

d. rec'ti, separation of rectus abdominis muscles away from the midline, sometimes seen during or following pregnancy.

diastasuria (dī-as-tās-yū'rē-ă). Amylasuria.

diastatic (dī-ă-stat'ik). Relating to a diastasis.

diastema, pl. **diastemata** (dī'ă-stē'mă, -stē'mă-tă) [G. *diastēma,* an interval]. **1.** Fissure or abnormal opening in any part, especially if congenital. **2** [NA]. Space between two adjacent teeth in the same dental arch. **3.** Cleft or space between the maxillary lateral incisor and canine teeth, into which the lower canine is received when the jaws are closed; abnormal in man but normal in dogs and many other animals.

diastematocrania (dī-ă-stē'mă-tō-krā'nē-ă) [G. *diastēma,* an interval, + *kranion,* skull]. Congenital sagittal fissure of the skull.

diastematomyelia (dī-ă-stē'mă-tō-mī-e'lē-ă) [G. *diastēma,* interval, + *myelon,* marrow]. Complete or incomplete sagittal division of spinal cord by osseous or fibrocartilaginous septum.

diaster (dī'as-ter) [G. *di-,* two, + *astēr,* star]. Amphiaster.

diastereoisomers (dī'ă-stār-ē-ō-ī'sō-merz). Optically active isomers that are not enantiomorphs (mirror images); *e.g.,* glucose and galactose.

diastole (dī-as'tō-lē) [G. *diastolē,* dilation]. The dilation of the heart cavities, during which they fill with blood; d. of the atria precedes that of the ventricles; it alternates rhythmically with systole or contraction of the heart musculature.

cardiac d., auxocardia (2).

gastric d., a somewhat fanciful name for a phase of relaxation of stomach peristalsis seen fluoroscopically or with the gastroscope.

diastolic (dī-ă-stol'ik). Relating to diastole.

diastrophism (dī-as'trof-izm) [G. *diastrophē,* fr. *diastrephein,* distortion]. Distortion that occurs in objects as a result of bending.

diataxia (dī'ă-tak'sē-ă). Ataxia affecting both sides of the body.
cerebral d., the ataxic type of cerebral birth palsy.

diatela (dī-ă-tē'lă) [G. *dia,* through, between, + L. *tela,* web]. Rarely used term for *tela* choroidea ventriculi tertii.

diathermal (dī-ă-ther'mal) [G. *dia,* through, + *thermē,* heat]. Diathermic.

diathermancy (dī-ă-ther'man-sē). The condition of being diathermic.

diathermanous (dī-ă-ther'man-ŭs) [G. *dia-thermaino,* to heat through, fr. *thermos,* hot]. Transcalent; permeable by heat rays.

diathermic (dī-ă-ther'mik). Diathermal; relating to, characterized by, or affected by diathermy.

diathermocoagulation (dī-ă-ther'mō-kō-ag-yū-lā'shŭn). Surgical *diathermy.*

diathermy (dī'ă-ther-mē) [G. *dia,* through, + *thermē,* heat]. Transthermia; local elevation of temperature within the tissues, produced by high frequency current, ultrasonic waves, or microwave radiation.
medical d., thermopenetration; d. of mild degree causing no destruction of tissue.
short wave d., therapeutic elevation of temperature in the tissues by means of an oscillating electric current of extremely high frequency (10 to 100 million Hz) and short wavelength of 3 to 30 m.
surgical d., diathermocoagulation; electrocoagulation with a high frequency electrocautery, resulting in local tissue destruction; usually used to seal blood vessels and arrest bleeding.

diathesis (dī-ath'ĕ-sis) [G. arrangement, condition]. The constitutional or inborn state disposing to a disease, group of diseases, or metabolic or structural anomaly.
contractural d., a tendency to have contractures in hysteria.
cystic d., a condition in which multiple cysts form in the liver, kidneys, and other organs.
gouty d., inherited hyperuricemia predisposing to gout, usually appearing after puberty in males and after menopause in women.
hemorrhagic d., any tendency to spontaneous bleeding or bleeding from trivial trauma caused by a defect in clotting or a flaw in the structure of blood vessels.
spasmodic d., a constitutional tendency to convulsions, especially in childhood.
spasmophilic d., spasmophilia; a condition in which there is an abnormal mechanical or electrical excitability of the motor nerves, shown by a tendency to tetany, laryngeal spasm, or general convulsions.

diathetic (dī-ă-thet'ik). Relating to a diathesis.

diatom (dī'ă-tom) [G. *diatomos,* cut in two]. An individual of microscopic unicellular algae, the shells of which compose a sedimentary infusorial earth.

diatomaceous (dī'ă-tō-mā'shŭs). Pertaining to diatoms or their fossil remains.

diatomic (dī-ă-tom'ik). **1.** Denoting a compound with a molecule made up of two atoms. **2.** Denoting any ion or atomic grouping composed of two atoms only.

diatoric (dī'ă-tōr'ik) [G. *diatoros,* pierced]. **1.** The vertical cylindric aperture formed in the base of artificial porcelain teeth and extending into the body of the tooth, serving as a mechanical means of attaching the tooth to the denture base. **2.** Denoting teeth that contain a d.

diatrizoate sodium (dī-ă-trī-zō'āt). See under sodium.

diazepam (dī-az'ĕ-pam). 7-Chloro-1,3-dihydro-1-methyl-5-phenyl-2*H*-1,4-benzodiazepin-2-one; a skeletal muscle relaxant, sedative, and antianxiety agent; also used as an anticonvulsant, particularly in the treatment of status epilepticus.

diazines (dī'ă-zēnz). A group of synthetic tuberculostatic drugs, such as pyrazine carboxamide and pyridazine-3-carboxamide.

diazo- [G. *di-,* two, + Fr. *azote,* nitrogen]. Prefix denoting a compound containing the ⩾C–N=N–X grouping, where X is not carbon (except for CN), or the grouping N_2 attached by one atom to carbon (*e.g.,* diazomethane, CH_2N_2). *Cf.* azo-.

diazotize (dī-az'ō-tīz). To introduce the diazo group into a chemical compound, usually through the treatment of an amine with nitrous acid.

diazoxide (dī-ă-zok'sīd). 7-Chloro-3-methyl-2*H*-1,2,4-benzothiadiazine 1,1-dioxide; an antihypertensive agent.

dibasic (dī-bā'sik). Bibasic; having two replaceable hydrogen atoms, denoting an acid with two ionizable hydrogen atoms.

dibenzepin hydrochloride (dī-benz'ĕ-pin). 10-[2-(Dimethylamino)ethyl]-5,10-dihydro-5-methyl-11*H*-dibenzo[*b,e*][1,4]diazepin-11-one hydrochloride; an antidepressant.

dibenzheptropine citrate (dī-benz-hep'trō-pēn). Deptropine citrate.

dibenzopyridine (dī-ben'zō-pir'i-dēn). Acridine.

dibenzothiazine (dī-ben'zō-thī'ă-zēn). Phenothiazine.

dibenzthione (dī-benz-thī'ōn). Sulbentine; 3,5-dibenzyltetrahydro-2*H*-1,3,5-thiadiazine-2-thione; an antifungal antiseptic.

Dibothriocephalus (dī-both'rē-ō-sef'ă-lŭs) [G. *di-,* two, + *bothrion,* dim. of *bothros,* a pit, + *kephalē,* head]. Former name for *Diphyllobothrium.*
D. la'tus, *Diphyllobothrium latum.*

dibromopropamidine isethionate (dī-brō'mō-prō-pam'i-dēn). 2-Hydroxyethanesulfonic acid, a compound with 4,4'-(trimethylenedioxy)bis(3-bromobenzamidine); an antiseptic.

dibromsalan (dī-brom'să-lan). 4',5-Dibromosalicylanilide; a disinfectant.

dibucaine hydrochloride (dī-byū'kān). 2-*n*-Butoxy-*N*-[2-(diethylamino)ethyl]cinchoninamide monohydrochloride; a potent local anesthetic (surface and spinal anesthesia).

dibucaine number (DN). A test for differentiation of one of several forms of atypical pseudocholinesterases that are unable to inactivate succinylcholine at normal rates; based upon percent inhibition of the enzymes by dibucaine, normal enzyme has a DN of 75 and above, heterozygous atypical enzyme has a DN of 40-70, and homozygous atypical enzyme has a DN of less than 20. See also fluoride number.

dibutoline sulfate (dī-byū'tō-lēn). Dibutyl urethane of dimethylethyl-β-hydroxyethylammonium sulfate; an anticholinergic agent used as a mydriatic, a cycloplegic, and a gastrointestinal antispasmodic.

dibutyl phthalate (dī-byū'til thal'āt). *n*-Butyl phthalate; di-*n*-butyl ester of benzene-*o*-dicarboxylic acid; an insect repellent.

DIC Abbreviation for disseminated intravascular *coagulation.*

dicacodyl (dī-kak'ō-dil). Cacodyl.

dicelous (dī-sē'lŭs) [G. *di-,* two, + *koilos,* hollow]. Having two cavities or excavations on opposite surfaces.

dicentric (dī-sen'trik). Having two centromeres.

dicephalous (dī-sef'ă-lŭs). Having two heads.

dicephalus (dī-sef'ă-lŭs) [G. *di-,* two, + *kephalē,* head]. Bicephalus; diplocephalus; symmetrical conjoined twins with two separate heads.
d. di'auchenos, derodidymus; a d. with separate necks.
d. di'pus dibra'chius, a d. in which the merging of the bodies has obliterated the appendages on the side of the union, leaving only two arms and two legs for the double body.
d. di'pus tetrabra'chius, a d. with two legs and four separate arms.

d. di'pus tribra'chius, a d. with two legs and three arms.

d. dip'ygus, a d. with a double body below the umbilicus.

d. mon'auchenos, a d. in which fusion has involved the cervical region so that the two heads are on a single neck.

dicheilia, dichilia (dī-kī'lē-ă) [G. *di-*, two, + *cheilos*, lip]. A lip appearing to be double because of the presence of an abnormal fold.

dicheiria, dichiria (dī-kī'rē-ă) [G. *di-*, two, + *cheir*, hand]. Diplocheiria; diplochiria; complete or incomplete duplication of the digits of the hand. See also polydactyly.

dichloralphenazone (dī-klōr'al-fen-az'ōn). Dichloralantipyrine; a complex of chloral hydrate and phenazone; a sedative and hypnotic.

dichloramine-T (dī-klōr'ă-mēn). *p-* Toluenesulfonic acid dichloramide; $CH_3C_6H_4SO_2NCl_2$; used as an antiseptic in surgical dressings.

dichloride (dī-klōr'īd). Bichloride; a compound with a molecule containing two atoms of chlorine to one of another element.

dichlorisone (dī-klōr'i-sōn). 9α,11β-Dichloro-17α,21-dihydroxy-1,4-pregnadiene-3,20-dione; 9,11-dichloropredisolone; a topical antipruritic agent.

dichlorisoproterenol (dī-klōr'is-ō-prō-tār'ĕ-nol). Dichloroisoproterenol.

dichlorobenzene (dī-klōr'ō-ben'zēn). ClC_6H_4Cl; an insecticide used chiefly as a moth repellent.

dichlorodifluoromethane (dī-klōr'ō-dī-flū-rō-meth'ān). CF_2Cl_2; an easily liquefiable gas used as a refrigerant and aerosol propellant.

***p,p*'-dichlorodiphenyl methyl carbinol (DMC)** (dī-chlōr'ō-dī-fen'il). A synthetic compound found effective as a miticide.

dichlorodiphenyltrichloroethane (DDT) (dī-chlōr'ō-di-fen'il-trī-klōr-ō-eth'ān). 1,1,1-Trichloro-2,2-*bis* (*p*-chlorophenyl)ethane; dicophane; chlorophenothane; an insecticide that came into prominence during and after World War II. For a time it proved very effective, but insect populations rapidly developed tolerance for it, hence much of its original effectiveness has been lost; general usage is now widely discouraged because of the toxicity that results from the environmental persistence of this agent.

di(2-chloroethyl)sulfide. Mustard *gas.*

dichlorohydrin (dī-klōr-ō-hī'drin). Dichloroisopropyl alcohol; a colorless, odorless fluid prepared by heating anhydrous glycerin with sulfur monochloride; a solvent of resins.

2,6-**dichloroindophenol** (dī-klōr'ō-in-dō-fē'nol). A reagent for the chemical assay of ascorbic acid which depends upon the reducing properties of the latter. It is red in acid solution; in the presence of the vitamin it undergoes reduction and becomes colorless, the vitamin being oxidized to dehydroascorbic acid. Often misnamed dichlorophenol-indophenol.

dichloroisopropyl alcohol (dī-klōr'ō-is-ō-prō'pil). Dichlorohydrin.

dichloroisoproterenol (DCI) (dī-klōr'ō-is-ō-prō-tār'ĕ-nol). Dichlorisoproterenol; *dl-* 1-[3,4-dichlorophenyl]-2-isopropylaminoethanol; the congener of the adrenergic beta receptor stimulant, isoproterenol; it blocks the responses, involving beta receptors, to epinephrine and other sympathomimetic drugs.

dichlorophen (dī-klōr'ō-fen). 2,2'-Dihydroxy-5,5'methylenebix(4-chlorophenol); used topically as a fungicide and bactericide, and internally in the treatment of infections by tapeworms of man and domestic animals.

dichlorophenarsine hydrochloride (dī-klōr'ō-fen-ar'sēn). (3-Amino-4-hydroxyphenyl)dichloroarisine hydrochloride, formerly used as an arsenical antisyphilitic.

2,6-**dichlorophenol-indophenol** (dī'klōr-ō-fē'nol-in-dō-fē'nol). Misnomer for 2,6-dichloroindophenol.

(2,4-dichlorophenoxy) acetic acid (2,4-D). An herbicide, more toxic to broad-leaved dicotyledonous plants (weeds) than to monocotyledonous ones (grains and grass), used with (2,4,5-trichlorophenoxy)acetic acid as a constituent of Agent Orange.

dichlorovos (dī-klōr'ō-vos). Dichlorvos.

dichlorphenamide (dī-klōr-fen'ă-mīd). 4,5-Dichloro-*m-* benzenedisulfonamide; a carbonic anhydrase inhibitor with actions similar to those of acetazolamide.

dichlorvos (dī-klōr'vos). Dichlorovos; phosphoric acid 2,2-dichlorovinyl dimethyl phosphate; an anthelmintic in veterinary and human medicine.

dichorial, dichorionic (dī-kō'rē-ăl, dī-kō-rē-on'ik) [G. *di-*, two, + chorion]. Showing evidence of two chorions, as the placenta of diovular twins.

dichotic (dī-kot'ik). Dichotomous.

dichotomous (dī-kot'ō-mŭs). Dichotic; denoting or characterized by dichotomy.

dichotomy (dī-kot'ō-mē) [G. *dichotomia*, a cutting in two, fr. *dicha*, in two, + *tomē*, a cutting]. Division into two parts.

dichroic (dī-krō'ik). Relating to dichroism.

dichroism (dī'krō-izm) [G. *di-*, two, + *chrōa*, color]. The property of seeming to be differently colored when viewed from emitted light and from transmitted light.

circular d., the change from circular polarization to elliptical polarization of monochromatic, circularly polarized light in the immediate vicinity of the absorption band of the substance through which the light passes. See also Cotton *effect.*

dichromat (dī'krō-mat). An individual with dichromatism.

dichromate (dī-krō'māt). Bichromate; a compound containing the radical $Cr_2O_7^{=}$.

dichromatic (dī-krō-mat'ik). **1.** Having or exhibiting two colors. **2.** Relating to dichromatism (2).

dichromatism (dī-krō'mă-tizm) [G. *di-*, two, + *chrōma*, color]. **1.** The state of being dichromatic (1). **2.** Dichromatopaia; dyschromatopsia; the abnormality of color vision in which only two of the three retinal cone pigments are present, as in protanopia, deuteranopia, and tritanopia.

dichromatopsia (dī-krō-mă-top'sē-ă) [G. *di-*, two, + *chrōma*, color, + *opsis*, vision]. Dichromatism (2).

dichromic (dī-krō'mik). Having, or relating to, two colors.

dichromophil, dichromophile (dī-krō'mō-fil, dī-krō'mō-fīl) [G. *di-*, two, + *chrōma*, color, + *philos*, fond]. Taking a double stain; denoting a tissue or cell taking both acid and basic dyes in different parts.

Dick, George Frederick (1881–1967), and Gladys R.H. (1881–1963), U.S. internists. See D. *method, test,* test *toxin.*

Dickens, Frank, British biochemist, *1899. See D. *shunt;* Warburg-Lipmann-D. *shunt.*

dicloxacillin sodium (dī-klok-să-sil'in). Sodium salt of 3-(2,6-dichlorophenyl)-5-methyl-4-isoazolylpenicillin; a semisynthetic penicillin resistant to penicillinase.

dicophane (dī'kō-fān). Dichlorodiphenyltrichloroethane.

dicoria (dī-kō'rē-ă) [G. *di-*, two, + *korē*, pupil]. Diplocoria.

dicrocoeliosis (dī'krō-sē-li-ō'sis). Infection of animals and rarely man with trematodes of the genus *Dicrocoelium.*

Dicrocoelium (dīk-rō-sē'lē-ŭm) [G. *dikroos*, forked, + *koilia*, belly]. A genus of digenetic trematodes or flukes inhabiting the bile ducts and gallbladder of herbivores. The species *D. dentriticum* (lancet fluke) is rarely found in man, but is an important parasite of sheep in some localities.

dicrotic (dī-krot′ik) [G. *dikrotos,* double-beating]. Relating to dicrotism.

dicrotism (dī′krō-tizm) [G. *di-,* two, + *krotos,* a beat]. That form of the pulse in which a double beat can be felt at the wrist for each beat of the heart; due to accentuation of the dicrotic wave.

Dictyocaulus (dik′tē-ō-kaw′lŭs) [G. *diktyon,* net, + *kaulos,* stalk]. A genus of thin elongate metastrongylid nematode lungworms (subfamily Dictyocaulinae) that inhabit the air passages of herbivorous animals; the life cycle is direct, infection occurring from ingestion of infective larvae.

D. arnfiel′di, species that occurs in the bronchi of horses, mules, and donkeys; generally produces few or no symptoms, except with heavy infection.

D. fila′ria, the large or thread lungworm, a species that is the common lungworm of sheep, goats, camels, and many wild ruminants; it causes much damage, especially in younger heavily infected animals, which cough and suffer from dyspnea; emaciation and anemia often occur.

D. vivip′arus, species that is the common lungworm of cattle, deer, and other ruminants, usually found in the trachea, bronchi, and bronchioles; the chronic cough caused by this parasite is sometimes called hoose or husk, especially in Great Britain.

dictyoma (dik-tē-ō′mă) [G. *dikyton,* net (retina), + *-oma,* tumor]. Embryonal *medulloepithelioma.*

dictyotene (dik′tē-ō-tēn) [G. *diktyon,* net, + *taenia,* band]. The state of meiosis at which the oocyte is arrested during the period from late fetal life until ovulation.

dicumarol (dī-kū′mă-rol). Bishydroxycoumarin; 3,3′-methylenebis(4-hydroxycoumarin); an anticoagulant that inhibits the formation of prothrombin in the liver.

dicyclomine hydrochloride (dī-sī′klō-mēn). 2-Diethylaminoethyl bicyclohexyl-1-carboxylate hydrochloride; an anticholinergic agent.

dicysteine (dī-sis′tēn). Cystine.

didactic (dī-dak′tik) [G. *didaktikos,* fr. *didaskō,* to teach]. Instructive; denoting medical teaching by lectures or textbooks, as distinguished from clinical demonstrations with patients or laboratory exercises.

didactylism (dī-dak′ti-lizm) [G. *di-,* two, + *daktylos,* finger or toe]. Congenital condition of having two fingers on a hand or two toes on a foot.

didelphic (dī-del′fik) [G. *di-,* two, + *delphys,* womb]. Having or relating to a double uterus.

Didelphis (dī-del′fis) [G. *di-,* two, + *delphys,* womb]. A genus of marsupials, commonly called opossums, that serve as reservoir hosts of *Trypanosoma cruzi. D. marsupialis* is the common North American variety; *D. paraguayensis* is a South American form.

didym-, didymo- [G. *didymos,* twin]. Combining forms denoting relationship to the didymus, testis.

didymalgia (did-i-mal′jē-ă) [G. *didymos,* twin, pl. *didymoi,* the testes, + *algos,* pain]. Obsolete term for orchialgia.

didymitis (did-i-mī′tis) [G. *didymos,* twin, pl. *didymoi,* the testes, + *-itis,* inflammation]. Obsolete term for orchitis.

-didymus [G. *didymos,* twin]. Termination denoting a conjoined twin with the first element of the complete word designating unfused parts. See also -dymus, -pagus.

didymus (did′ē-mŭs) [G. *didymos,* a twin, pl. *didymoi,* testes]. Testis.

die (dī). In dentistry, the positive reproduction of the form of a prepared tooth in any suitable hard substance, usually in metal or specially prepared artificial stone. See also counterdie.

dieb. alt. Abbreviation for L. *diebus alternis,* every other day.

diecious (dī-ē′shŭs) [G. *di-,* two, + *oikia,* house]. Denoting animals or plants that are sexually distinct, the individuals being of one or the other sex.

Dieffenbach, Johann F., German surgeon, 1792–1847. See D.'s *method.*

Diego (Di) blood group. See Blood Groups appendix.

diel (dī′el) [irreg., fr. L. *dies,* day]. Term frequently used synonymously with diurnal (2) or circadian.

dieldrin (dī-el′drin). A chlorinated hydrocarbon used as an insecticide; may cause toxic effects in persons and animals exposed to its action through skin contact, inhalation, or food contamination.

dielectrography (dī-ē-lek-trog′ră-fē). Impedance *plethysmography.*

dielectrolysis (dī′ē-lek-trol′i-sis). Electrophoresis.

Diels, Otto, German chemist, 1876–1954. See D.'s *hydrocarbon.*

diencephalohypophysial (dī-en-sef′ă-lō-hī-pō-fiz′ē-ăl). Relating to the diencephalon and hypophysis.

diencephalon, pl. **diencephala** (dī-en-sef′ă-lon, -sef′ă-lă) [G. *dia,* through, + *enkephalos,* brain] [NA]. That part of the prosencephalon composed of the epithalamus, the dorsal thalamus, subthalamus, and hypothalamus.

diener (dē′ner) [Ger. *Diener,* servant]. A laboratory worker who assists in cleaning.

dienestrol (dī-en-es′trol). Estrodienol; 3,4-bis(*p*-hydroxyphenyl)-2,4-hexadiene; an estrogenic agent.

Dientamoeba fragilis (dī-ent-ă-mē′bă fraj′i-lis). A species of small ameba parasitic in the large intestine of man and certain monkeys; usually nonpathogenic, but believed to be capable of sometimes causing low-grade inflammation with mucous diarrhea and gastrointestinal disturbance in man.

dieresis (dī-er′ē-sis) [G. *diairesis,* a division]. *Solution* of continuity.

dieretic (dī-er-et′ik). **1.** Relating to dieresis. **2.** Dividing; ulcerating; corroding.

diesterase (dī-es′ter-ās). See phosphodiesterases.

diestrous (dī-es′trŭs). Pertaining to diestrus.

diestrus (dī-es′trŭs) [G. *dia,* between, + *oistros,* desire]. A period of sexual quiescence intervening between two periods of estrus.

diet (dī′et) [G. *diaita,* a way of life; a diet]. **1.** Food and drink in general. **2.** A prescribed course of eating and drinking in which the amount and kind of food, as well as the times at which it is to be taken, are regulated for therapeutic purposes. **3.** Reduction of caloric intake so as to lose weight. **4.** To follow any prescribed or specific d.

acid-ash d., a d. consisting largely of meat or fish, eggs, and cereals (containing a minimal quantity of milk, fruit, and vegetables) which, when catabolized, leave an acid residue to be excreted in the urine.

alkaline-ash d., basic d.; a d. consisting mainly of fruits, vegetables, and milk (with minimal amounts of meat, fish, eggs, cheese, and cereals) which, when catabolized, leave an alkaline residue to be excreted in the urine.

basal d., **(1)** a d. having a caloric value equal to the basal heat production; **(2)** in experiments in nutrition, a d. from which a given constituent (*e.g.,* a vitamin, mineral, or amino acid), the nutritional value of which is to be determined, is omitted for a period and the effects observed; the subject is observed for a second period during which the ingredient being studied is added to the d.

basic d., alkaline-ash d.

bland d., a regular d. omitting foods that mechanically or chemically irritate the gastrointestinal tract.

challenge d., a d. in which one or more specific substances are included for the purpose of determining whether an abnormal reaction occurs.

clear liquid d., a d., often used postoperatively, consisting usually of water, tea, coffee, gelatin preparations, and clear soups or broth.

diabetic d., a d. suitable for a diabetic patient; it varies very considerably in accordance with the predilection of the physician and whether or not the patient is receiving insulin.
elimination d., a d. designed to detect what ingredient of the food causes allergic manifestations in the patient; food items to which the patient may be sensitive are withdrawn separately and successively from the d. until that which causes the symptoms is discovered.
full liquid d., a d. consisting only of liquids but including cream soups, ice cream, and milk.
Giordano-Giovannetti d., a d. designed for patients with renal failure; it provides small amounts of protein, primarily as essential amino acids, along with alpha-keto derivatives of amino acids; breakdown of protein in skeletal muscle is retarded and, since transaminase reactions are reversible, a small proportion of the ammonia released by urea breakdown is utilized for synthesis of non-essential amino acids.
gout d., a d. containing a minimal quantity of purine bases (meats); liver, kidney, and sweetbread especially are excluded and replaced by dairy products, fruits, and cereals; wines and liquors are also excluded.
high calorie d., a d. containing upward of 4000 calories per day.
high fat d., a d. containing large amounts of fat.
ketogenic d., a high-fat, low-carbohydrate, and normal protein d. causing ketosis.
low calorie d., a d. of 1200 calories or less per day.
low fat d., a d. containing minimal amounts of fat.
macrobiotic d., a d. claimed to promote longevity, often by promoting an emphasis on natural foods and restrictions on non-cereal foods as well as liquids.
purine-restricted d., see gout d.
reducing d., a d. in which caloric expenditure is greater than caloric intake.
Sippy d., a d. used in the treatment of gastric ulcer; originally it consisted of hourly feedings of a mixture of milk and cream; whole or skim milk is now used because of knowledge of the effects of high fat.
smooth d., a d. containing little roughage, as used in peptic ulcer.
soft d., a normal d. limited to soft foods for those who have difficulty chewing or swallowing; there are no restrictions on seasoning or method of food preparation.

dietary (dī′ĕ-tār-ē). Relating to the diet.

Dieterle's stain. See under stain.

dietetic (dī′ĕ-tet′ik). **1.** Relating to the diet. **2.** Descriptive of food that, naturally or through processing, has a low caloric content.

dietetics (dī-ĕ-tet′iks). The practical application of diet in the prophylaxis and treatment of disease.

diethadione (dī-eth-ă-dī′ōn). 5,5-Diethyldihydro-2*H*-1,3-oxazine-2,4(3*H*)-dione; an analeptic.

diethanolamine (dī-eth-ă-nol′ă-mēn). Diethylolamine; bis(hydroxyethyl)amine; 2,2′-iminodiethanol; used as an emulsifier and as a dispersing agent in cosmetics and pharmaceuticals.
d. acetate, iodopyracet.

diethazine (dī-eth′ă-zēn). 10-(2-Diethylaminoethyl)phenothiazine; an anticholinergic agent.

diethyl (dī-eth′il). A compound containing two ethyl radicals.

5,5-diethylbarbituric acid (dī-eth′il-bar-bi-tyū′rik). Barbital.

diethylcarbamazine citrate (dī-eth′il-kar-bam′ă-zēn). *N,N*-Diethyl-4-methyl-1-piperazinecarboxamide citrate; an effective microfilaricide, although relatively ineffective against the adult filariae.

diethylenediamine (dī-eth′il-ēn-dī′ă-mēn). Piperazine.

1,4-diethylene dioxide (dī-eth′il-ēn). Dioxane.

diethylenetriamine pentaacetic acid (DTPA) (dī-eth′il-ēn-trī′ă-mēn pen-tă-a-sē′tik). Pentetic acid.

diethyl ether. Anesthetic, ethyl, or sulfuric ether; ethyl oxide; $CH_3CH_2OCH_2CH_3$; an explosive volatile liquid, the vapor of which produces inhalation anesthesia; introduced in 1846 as the first successful surgical anesthetic.

diethylmalonylurea (dī-eth′īl-mal-ō-nil-yū-rē′ă). Barbital.

diethylolamine (dī-eth-i-lol′ă-mēn). Diethanolamine.

diethylpropion hydrochloride (dī-eth-il-prō′pē-on). 1-Phenyl-2-diethylaminopropanone-1 hydrochloride; a sympathomimetic amine related chemically to amphetamine, used as an anorectic.

diethylstilbestrol (dī-eth′il-stil-bes′trol). Stilbestrol; 4,4′-dihydroxy-α, β-diethylstilbene; a synthetic crystalline compound, not a steroid, possessing estrogenic activity when given orally or by injection. Also available as the diphosphate and the dipropionate.

diethyltoluamide (dī-eth′il-tō-lū′ă-mīd). *m*-Delphene; *N,N*-diethyl-*m*-toluamide; an insect repellent.

diethyltryptamine (DET) (dī-eth-il-trip′tă-mēn). *N,N*- Diethyltryptamine; a hallucinogenic agent similar to dimethyltryptamine.

dietitian (dī-ĕ-tish′ŭn). An expert in dietetics.

Dietl, Józef, Polish physician, 1804–1878. See D.'s *crisis*.

dietogenetics (dī′ĕ-tō-jĕ-net′iks). The biologic field concerned with the interrelationship between genotype, diet, and various food requirements.

Dieulafoy, Georges, French physician, 1839–1911. See D.'s *erosion, theory*.

difarnesyl group (di-far′nĕ-sil). A 30-carbon open chain hexaisoprenoid hydrocarbon radical occurring as a side chain in vitamin K_2.

difenoxin (dī-fen-ok′sin). Difenoxylic acid; 1-(3-cyano-3,3-diphenylpropyl)-4-phenylisonipecotic acid; an antidiarrheal agent with actions similar to those of diphenoxylate.

difenoxylic acid (dī-fen-ok′si-lik). Difenoxin.

difference (dif′er-ens). The magnitude or degree by which one quality or quantity differs from another of the same kind.
alveolar-arterial oxygen d., the d. or gradient between the partial pressure of oxygen in the alveolar spaces and the arterial blood: $P_{(A-a)}O_2$. Normally in young adults this value is less than 20 mm Hg. See also alveolar gas *equation*.
arteriovenous carbon dioxide d., the d. in carbon dioxide content (in ml per 100 ml blood) between the arterial and venous bloods.
arteriovenous oxygen d., the d. in the oxygen content (in ml per 100 ml blood) between arterial and venous blood.
cation-anion d., anion *gap*.
individual d.'s, in clinical psychology, deviations of individuals from the group average or from each other.
light d., **(1)** the d. in light sensitivity of the two eyes; **(2)** brightness difference *threshold*.
standard error of d., a statistical index of the probability that a d. between two sample means is greater than zero.

differential (dif-er-en′shăl) [L. *dif-fero*, to carry apart, differ, fr. *dis*, apart]. Relating to, or characterized by, a difference; distinguishing.
threshold d., d. *threshold*.

differentiated (dif-er-en′shē-ā-ted). Having a different character or function from the surrounding structures or from the original type; said of tissues, cells, or portions of the cytoplasm.

differentiation (dif′er-en-shē-ā′shŭn). **1.** Specialization (2); the acquisition or possession of one or more characteristic or function different from that of the original type. **2.** Differential *diagnosis*. **3.** Partial removal of a stain from a histologic section to accentuate the staining differences of tissue components.
correlative d., d. due to the interaction of different parts of an organism.

echocardiographic d., the processing of a signal so that the output depends upon the rate of change of the input; *e.g.,* it will display changes in amplitude but will reduce the duration of the waveform.
invisible d., chemodifferentiation.

diffluence (dif'lū-ens) [L. *dif-fluo,* to flow in different directions, dissolve]. The process of becoming fluid.

diffraction (di-frak'shŭn) [L. *dif- fringo,* pp. *-fractus,* to break in pieces]. Deflection of the rays of light from a straight line in passing by the edge of an opaque body.

diffraction grating. A variety of filter composed of lined grooves in a thin layer of aluminum-copper alloy on a glass surface. See monochromator.

diffusate (di-fyū'zāt) [L. *dif-fundo,* pp. *-fusus,* to pour in different directions]. Dialysate.

diffuse (di-fyūs) [L. *dif-fundo,* pp. *-fusus,* to pour in different directions]. **1** (di-fyūz'). To disseminate; to spread about. **2** (di-fyūs'). Disseminated; spread about; not restricted.

diffusible (di-fyūz'i-bl). Capable of diffusing.

diffusion (di-fyū'zhŭn). **1.** The random movement of molecules or ions or small particles in solution or suspension under the influence of brownian (thermal) motion toward a uniform distribution throughout the available volume; the rate is relatively rapid among liquids and gases, but takes place very slowly among solids. **2.** Dialysis (1).
gel d., d. in a gel, as in the case of gel d. precipitin tests in which the immune reactants diffuse in agar.

diflorasone diacetate (dī-flōr'ă-sōn). Pregna-1,4-diene-3,20-dione, 17,21-bis(acetyloxy)-6,9-difluoro-11-hydroxy-16-methyl-, (6α,11β,16β)-; an anti-inflammatory corticosteroid used in topical preparations.

diflucortolone (dī-flū-kōr'ti-lōn). 6α,9-Difluoro-11β,21-dihydroxy-16α-methylpregna-1,4-diene-3,20-dione; a synthetic glucocorticoid steroid analog.

diflunisal (dī-flū'ni-saul). [1-1'-Biphenyl]-3-carboxylic acid, 2',4'-difluoro-4-hydroxy-; a salicyclic acid derivative with anti-inflammatory, analgesic, and antipyretic actions.

digametic (dī-gă-met'ik). Heterogametic.

digastric (dī-gas'trik) [G. *di-,* two, + *gastēr,* belly]. Digastricus. **1.** Biventral; having two bellies; denoting especially a muscle with two fleshy parts separated by an intervening tendinous part. See *musculus* digastricus. **2.** Relating to the d. muscle; denoting a fossa or groove with which it is in relation and a nerve supplying its posterior belly.

digastricus (dī-gas'tri-kŭs) [L.]. **1.** Digastric. **2.** Denoting the *musculus* digastricus.

Digenea (dī-jē'nē-ă) [G. *di-,* two, + *genesis,* generation]. Subclass of parasitic flatworms (class Trematoda) characterized by a complex life cycle involving developmental multiplying stages in a mollusk intermediate host, an adult stage in a vertebrate, and often involving an additional transport host or an additional intermediate host; includes all of the common flukes of man and other mammals.

digenesis (dī-jen'ĕ-sis) [G. *di-,* two, + G. *genesis,* generation]. Reproduction in distinctive patterns in alternate generations, as seen in the nonsexual (invertebrate) and the sexual (vertebrate) cycles of digenetic trematode parasites.

digenetic (dī-jĕ-net'ik). **1.** Heteroxenous; pertaining to or characterized by digenesis. **2.** Pertaining to the digenetic fluke.

DiGeorge, Angelo M., U.S. pediatrician, *1921. See D. *syndrome.*

digest [L. *digero,* pp. *-gestus,* to force apart, divide, dissolve]. **1** (di-jest', dī-). To soften by moisture and heat. **2** (di-jest', dī-). To hydrolyze or break up into simpler chemical compounds by means of hydrolyzing enzymes or chemical action, as in the action of the secretions of the alimentary tract upon food. **3** (dī'jest). The materials resulting from digestion or hydrolysis.

digestant (di-jes'tănt, dī-). **1.** Aiding digestion. **2.** Digestive (2); an agent that favors or assists the process of digestion.

digestion (di-jes'chŭn, dī-) [L. *digestio.* See digest]. **1.** The process of making a digest. **2.** The process whereby ingested food is converted into material suitable for assimilation for synthesis of tissues or liberation of energy.
gastric d., peptic d.,; that part of d., chiefly of the proteins, carried on in the stomach by the enzymes of the gastric juice.
intercellular d., d. in a cavity by means of secretions from the surrounding cells, such as occurs in the metazoa.
intestinal d., that part of d. carried on in the intestine; it affects all the foodstuffs: starches, fats, and proteins.
intracellular d., d. within the boundaries of a cell, such as occurs in the protozoa and in phagocytes.
pancreatic d., d. in the intestine by the enzymes of the pancreatic juice.
peptic d., gastric d.
primary d., d. in the alimentary tract.
salivary d., the conversion of starch into sugar by the action of salivary amylase.
secondary d., the change in the chyle effected by the action of the cells of the body, whereby the final products of d. are assimilated in the process of metabolism.

digestive (di-jes'tiv, dī-). **1.** Relating to digestion. **2.** Digestant (2).

digin (dij'in). Gitogenin.

digit (dij'it) [L. *digitus*]. Digitus.
clubbed d.'s, see clubbing.

digital (dij'i-tăl). Relating to or resembling a digit or digits or an impression made by them.

digitalgia paresthetica (dij-i-tal'jē-ă par-es-thet'i-kă). A sensory neuropathy of one or more fingers or toes, of unknown cause, that spontaneously recedes in a few months.

digitalin (dij-i-tal'in). $C_{36}H_{56}O_{14}$; a standardized mixture of digitalis glycosides used as a cardiotonic.
crystalline d., digitoxin.

Digitalis (dij-i-tal'is, -ta'lis) [L. *digitalis,* relating to the fingers; in allusion to the finger-like flowers]. Foxglove; fairy gloves; a genus of perennial flowering plants of the family Schrophulariaceae. *D. lanata,* a European species, and *D. purpurea,* purple foxglove, are the main sources of cardioactive steroid glycosides used in the treatment of certain heart diseases, especially congestive heart failure.

digitalis (dij-i-tal'is). The dried leaf of *Digitalis purpurea* dispensed as powdered d. (prepared d.) when d. is prescribed as a cardiotonic in the treatment of congestive heart failure and other cardiac disorders.

digitalism (dij'i-tal-izm). The symptoms caused by digitalis poisoning or overdosage.

digitalization (dij'i-tal-i-zā'shŭn). Administration of digitalis by any one of a number of schedules until sufficient amounts are present in the body to produce the desired therapeutic effects.

digitate (dij'i-tāt). Marked by a number of finger-like processes or impressions.

digitation (dij-i-tā'shŭn) [Mod. L. *digitatio*] A process resembling a finger.

digitationes hippocampi (dij-i-tā-shē-ō'nēz hip-ō-kam'pē) [Mod. L. pl. of *digitatio*] *Pes* hippocampi.

digiti (dij'i-tī) [L.]. Plural of digitus.

digitigrade (dij'i-ti-grād) [L. *digitus,* finger, + *gradior,* to walk]. Animals whose weight is borne on the digits only, such as the dog and cat. *Cf.* plantigrade.

digitin (dij'i-tin). Digitonin.

digitonin (dij-i-tō'nin). Digitin; a steroid glycoside obtained from *Digitalis purpurea* that has no cardiac action; used as a reagent in the determination of plasma cholesterol and steroids having a 3-hydroxyl group in beta configuration.

digitoxicity (dij'i-tok-sis'i-tē). Colloquialism for digitalis toxicity.

digitoxin (dij-i-tok'sin). Crystalline digitalin; a secondary cardioactive glycoside obtained from the leaves of *Digitalis purpurea;* it is more completely absorbed from the gastrointestinal tract than is digitalis.

digitus, pl. **digiti** (dij'i-tŭs, -tī) [L.] [NA]. Digit; dactyl; dactylus; a finger or toe.
d. annula'ris [NA], d. quartus; ring or fourth finger.
d. auricula'ris, d. minimus.
dig'iti hippocrat'ici, clubbed digits or fingers. See clubbing.
dig'iti ma'nus [NA], fingers.
d. me'dius [NA], d. tertius; middle or third finger.
d. min'imus [NA], d. quintus; d. auricularis; the little or fifth finger.
dig'iti ped'is [NA], toes.
d. pri'mus [NA], pollex.
d. quin'tus [NA], d. minimus.
d. secun'dus [NA], index (1).
d. ter'tius [NA], d. medius.
d. val'gus, permanent deviation of one or more fingers to the radial side.
d. va'rus, permanent deviation of one or more fingers to the ulnar side.

diglossia (dī-glos'ē-ă) [G. *di-,* two, + *glōssa,* tongue]. A developmental condition that results in a longitudinal split in the tongue. See bifid *tongue.*

diglyceride lipase (dī-glis'er-īd). Lipoprotein lipase.

diglycocoll hydroiodide-iodine (dī-glī'kō-kol hī-drō-ī'ō-dīd-ī'ō-dīn). Two moles of diglycocoll hydroiodide combined with two atomic weights of iodine; an antibacterial agent used in tablet form to disinfect drinking water.

dignathus (dī-nath'ŭs) [G. *di-,* two, + *gnathos,* jaw]. Augnathus; a malformed fetus with a double mandible.

digoxin (di-jok'sin). A cardioactive steroid glycoside obtained from *Digitalis lanata.*

Di Guglielmo, Giovanni, Italian physician, 1886–1961. See D.'s *disease, syndrome.*

digyny, digynia (dī'ji-nē, dī-jin'ē-ă) [di- + G. *gyne,* woman]. Fertilization of a diploid ovum by a sperm, which results in a triploid zygote. *Cf.* diandry.

diheterozygote (dī-het'er-ō-zī'gōt). An individual heterozygous for two different gene pairs at two different loci.

dihybrid (dī-hī'brid) [G. *di-,* two, + L. *hybrida,* offspring of a tame sow and a wild boar]. The offspring of parents differing in two characters.

dihydralazine (dī-hī-drăl'ă-zēn). 1,4-Dihydrazinophthalazine; an antihypertensive agent.

dihydrate (dī-hī'drāt). A compound with two molecules of water of crystallization.

dihydrazone (dī-hī'dră-zōn). Osazone.

dihydro-. Prefix indicating the addition of two hydrogen atoms.

dihydroascorbic acid (di-hī'drō-as-kōr'bik). L-Gulonolactone.

dihydrocholesterol (dī-hī'drō-kō-les'ter-ol). Cholesterol.

dihydrocodeine tartrate (dī-hī-drō-kō'dēn). 6-Hydroxy-3-methoxy-*N*- methyl-4,5-epoxymorphinan bitartrate; an analgesic derivative of codeine, about one-sixth as potent as morphine; a narcotic antitussive.

dihydrocodeinone (dī-hī-drō-kō'dēn-ōn). Hydrocodone.

4,5α-dihydrocortisol (dī-hī-drō-kōr'ti-sol). Hydrallostane.

dihydrocortisone (dī-hī-drō-kōr'ti-sōn). 17α,21-Dihydroxy-5β-pregnane-3,11,20-trione; a metabolite of cortisone, reduced at the 4,5 double bond.

dihydroergocornine (dī-hī'drō-er-gō-kōr'nīn). An ergot alkaloid derivative prepared by the hydrogenation of ergocornine and less toxic than the latter. See dihydroergotoxine mesylate.

dihydroergocristine (dī-hī'drō-er-gō-kris'tēn). An ergot alkaloid derivative prepared by the hydrogenation of ergocristine and less toxic than the latter. See dihydroergotoxine mesylate.

dihydroergocryptine (dī-hī'drō-er-gō-krip'tēn). An ergot alkaloid derivative prepared by the hydrogenation of ergocryptine and less toxic than the latter. See dihydroergotoxine mesylate.

dihydroergotamine (dī-hī'drō-er-got'ă-mēn). An ergot alkaloid derivative prepared by the hydrogenation of ergotamine; used in the treatment of migraine; less toxic and less oxytocic than ergotamine.

dihydroergotoxine mesylate (dī-hī'drō-er-gō-tok'sēn). A mixture of dihydroergocornine methanesulfate, dihydroergocristine methanesulfate, and dihydroergocryptine methane sulfate; used as an α-adrenergic blocking agent for relief of cardiovascular insufficiency.

dihydrofolate reductase (dī-hī-drō-fō'lāt) [EC 1.5.1.3]. An enzyme oxidizing tetrahydrofolate to dihydrofolate with $NADP^+$.

7,8-dihydrofolic acid (dī-hī-drō-fō'lik). Intermediate between folic acid and 5,6,7,8-tetrahydrofolic acid, oxidation of the latter requiring $NADP^+$ and dehydrofolate reductase.

dihydrolipoamide acetyltransferase (dī-hī'drō-lip-ō-am'id) [EC 2.3.1.12]. Lipoate acetyltransferase; thioltransacetylase A; an enzyme transferring acetyl from S^6-acetyldihydrolipoamide to coenzyme A.

dihydrolipoamide dehydrogenase [EC 1.8.1.4]. Coenzyme factor; diaphorase; lipoamide dehydrogenase; lipoamide reductase (NADH); lipoyl dehydrogenase; an enzyme oxidizing dihydrolipoamide at the expense of NAD^+; completes the oxidative decarboxylation of pyruvate.

dihydrolipoic acid (dī-hī'drō-lip-ō'ik). Reduced lipoic acid, formed by cleavage of the —S—S— bond as a result of the acceptance of two hydrogens.

dihydromorphinone hydrochloride (dī-hī-drō-mōr'fi-nōn). Hydromorphone hydrochloride.

dihydro-orotase (dī-hi'drō-ōr-ō'tās) [EC 3.5.2.3]. Carbamoylaspartate dehydrase; an enzyme catalyzing ring closure of *N*- carbamoyl-L-aspartate to form L-5,6-dihydroorotate.

dihydro-orotate (dī-hī'drō-ōr-ō'tāt). An intermediate in the biosynthesis of pyrimidines.

dihydropteroic acid (dī-hī'drō-te-rō'ik). An intermediate in the formation of folic acid; a compound of 6-hydroxymethylpterin and *p*-aminobenzoic acid, the combining of which is inhibited by sulfonamides.

dihydrostreptomycin (dī-hī'drō-strep-tō-mī'sin). An antiobiotic similar in action to streptomycin but with a higher risk of ototoxicity.

dihydrotachysterol (dī-hī'drō-tă-kis'ter-ōl). See tachysterol.

dihydrotestosterone (dī-hī'drō-tes-tos'ter-ōn). Stanolone.

dihydrouracil (dī-hī-drō-yūr'ă-sil). 5,6-Dihydrouracil; a reduction product of uracil and one of the intermediates of uracil catabolism.

dihydrouridine (D) (dī-hī-drō-yūr'i-dēn). Uridine in which the 5,6-double bond has been saturated by addition of two hydrogen atoms; a rare constituent of transfer ribonucleic acids.

dihydroxy-. Prefix denoting addition of two hydroxyl groups; as a suffix, becomes -diol.

dihydroxyacetone (dī'hī-drok-sē-as'e-tōn). Glyceroketone; glycerone; glycerulose; 1,3-dihydroxy-2-propanone; $HOCH_2$–CO–CH_2OH; the simplest ketose; as d. phosphate, one of the intermediates in the glycolytic pathway of glucose catabolism and fat synthesis.

dihydroxyaluminum aminoacetate (dī-hī-drok'sē-ă-lū'mi-nŭm am'i-nō-as'ĕ-tāt). Dihydroxy(glycinato)aluminum; (glycinato-*N,O*) dihydroxyaluminum; basic aluminum glycinate, a basic aluminum salt of aminoacetic acid containing small amounts of aluminum hydroxide and aminoacetic acid; used as an antacid in hyperchlorhydria and peptic ulcer.

dihydroxyaluminum sodium carbonate. Aluminum sodium carbonate hydroxide; a gastric antacid.

3,4-dihydroxyphenylalanine (dī-hī-droks'e-fen-il-al'ă-nēn). Dopa.

diiodide (dī-ī'ō-dīd). A compound containing two atoms of iodine per molecule.

diiodo-. Prefix indicating two atoms of iodine.

diiodohydroxyquin (dī-ī-ō'dō-hī-drok'si-kwin). Diodoquin; 5,7-diiodo-8-quinolinol; diiodohydroxyquinoline; $C_9H_5I_2NO$; an antiprotozoal agent, used in the treatment of intestinal amebiasis.

diiodopyramine (dī-ī-ō-dō-pir'ă-mēn). A radiopaque compound used in salpingography.

diisopromine (dī-ī-sō-prō'mēn). Disopromine; *N,N*-diisopropyl-3,3-diphenylpropylamine; a cholagogue.

diisopropyl fluorophosphate (dī-ī-sō-prō'pil flūr-ō-fos'fāt). Isoflurophate.

diketohydrindylidene-diketohydrindamine (dī-kē'tō-hī-drin-dil'i-dēn dī-kē'tō-hī-drind'ă-mēn). The colored product formed in the reaction of an α-amino acid and ninhydrin (triketohydrindene hydrate); a reaction used in the quantitative assay of α-amino acids.

diketone (dī-kē'tōn). A molecule containing two carbonyl groups; *e.g.*, acetylacetone ($CH_3COCH_2COCH_3$).

diketopiperazines (dī-kē'tō-pī-per'ă-zēnz). A class of organic compounds with a closed ring structure formed from two α-amino acids by the joining of the α-amino group of each to the carboxyl group of the other, with the loss of two molecules of water.

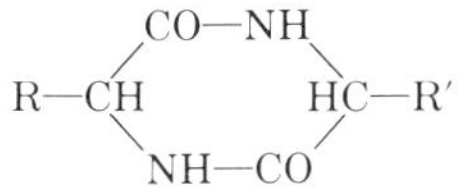

Diketopiperazine

dil. Abbreviation for L. *dilue,* dilute, or L. *dilutus,* diluted.

dilaceration (dī-las-er-ā'shŭn) [L. *di-lacero,* pp. *laceratus,* to tear in pieces, fr. *lacer,* mangled]. **1.** Discission of a cataractous lens. **2.** Displacement of some portion of a developing tooth which is then further developed in its new relation, resulting in a tooth with sharply angulated root(s).

dilatancy (dī-lā'tan-sē) [L. *dilato,* to dilate]. An increasing viscosity with increasing rate of shear accompanied by volumetric expansion.

dilatation (dil-ă-tā'shŭn). Dilation.

dilatator (dil'ă-tā-tĕr, -tōr). Dilator.

dilate (dī'lāt). To perform or undergo dilation.

dilation (dī-lā'shŭn) [L. *dilato,* pp. *dilatatus,* to spread out, dilate]. Dilatation. **1.** Physiologic or artificial enlargement of a hollow structure or opening. **2.** The act of stretching or enlarging an opening or the lumen of a hollow structure.

urethral d., increasing the caliber of the urethra by passage of a dilator.

dilation and curettage (D & C). Dilation of the cervix and curettement of the endometrium.

dilation and evacuation (D & E). Dilation of the cervix and removal of the early products of conception.

dilator (dī'lā-tĕr). Dilatator. **1.** An instrument designed for enlarging a hollow structure or opening. **2.** A muscle that pulls open an orifice. **3.** A substance that causes dilation or enlargement of an opening or the lumen of a hollow structure.

Goodell's d., a uterine d. used for dilating the cervix.

Hanks d.'s, uterine d.'s of solid metal construction.

Hegar's d.'s, a series of cylindrical bougies of graduated sizes used to dilate the cervical canal.

hydrostatic d., an instrument for dilating esophageal strictures; fluid pressure is delivered into a flexible area of the instrument placed in the stricture to establish a uniform dilating pressure.

d. ir'idis, *musculus* dilator pupillae.

Kollmann's d., a metallic expandable instrument used to dilate urethral strictures.

Plummer's d., Plummer's bag; an instrument for dilating the lower end of the esophagus in cardiospasm; it consists of a rubber tube with a perforated metal tip, and a dilatable elongated balloon near its lower end; in difficult cases the tube is threaded along a guiding thread swallowed by the patient.

d. of pupil, *musculus* dilator pupillae.

d. tu'bae, *musculus* tensor veli palatini.

Tubbs' d., a surgical instrument used to dilate the stenotic mitral valve.

Walther's d., a gently curved instrument that tapers to an increased diameter, used to dilate the female urethra.

dildo, dildoe (dil'dō). An artificial penis; an object having the approximate shape and size of an erect penis, and commonly made of wood, plastic, or rubber; utilized for sexual pleasure by vaginal insertion.

dill oil. A volatile oil distilled from the fruit of *Anethum graveolens* (family Umbelliferae); a carminative.

diloxanide furoate (dī-lok'să-nīd fyū'rō-āt). 2,2-Dichloro-4′-hydroxy-*N*-methylacetanilide furoate; an amebicide used in the treatment of dysentery.

diltiazem hydrochloride (dil-tī'ă-zem). 1,5-Benzothiazepin-4(5*H*)one, 3-(acetyloxy)-5-[2-(dimethylamino)ethyl]-2,3-dihydro-2-(4-methoxyphenyl)-monohydrochloride, (+)-*cis-;* a calcium channel blocking agent used as a coronary vasodilator.

diluent (dil'ū-ent). **1.** Diluting; denoting that which dilutes. **2.** An agent that dilutes a solution or mixture.

dilute (dī-lūt') [L. *di-luo,* to wash away, dilute]. **1.** To reduce a solution or mixture in concentration, strength, quality, or purity. **2.** Diluted; denoting a solution or mixture so effected.

dilution (dī-lū'shŭn). **1.** The act of being diluted. **2.** A diluted solution or mixture. **3.** In microbiologic techniques, a method for counting the number of viable cells in a suspension; a sample is diluted to the point where an aliquot, when plated, yields a countable number of separate colonies.

dim. Abbreviation for L. *dimidus,* one-half.

dimazole dihydrochloride (dī'mă-zōl). Diamthazole dihydrochloride.

dimazon (dī-mā'zon). 4-*o*-Tolylazo-*o*-diacetotoluide; an azo compound occurring in red crystals; used with petrolatum as an ointment to stimulate epithelial cell proliferation and thus promote the healing of superficial wounds.

dimelia (dī-mē'lē-ă) [G. *di-,* two, + *melos,* limb]. Congenital duplication of the whole or a part of a limb.

dimenhydrinate (dī-men-hī'dri-nāt). An amine salt of a theophyllinic acid; an antihistaminic, antinauseant, and antiemetic; used for motion sickness.

dimension (di-men'shŭn). Scope, size, magnitude; denoting, in the plural, linear measurements of length, width, and height.
buccolingual d., the diameter or d. of a bicuspid or molar tooth from buccal to lingual surface.
occlusal vertical d., the vertical d. of the face when the teeth or occlusion rims are in contact in centric occlusion; *decrease* in occlusal vertical d. may result from modification of tooth form by attrition or grinding, drifting of teeth, or, in edentulous patients, by resorption of residual ridges; *increase* may result from modifications of tooth form, tooth position, height of occlusion rims, rebasing or relining, or occlusal splints.
rest vertical d., the vertical d. of the face with the jaws in rest relation; *decrease* in rest vertical d. may or may not accompany a decrease in occlusal vertical d.; it may occur without a decrease in occlusal vertical d. in patients with a preponderant activity of the jaw-closing musculature, as in patients with muscular hypertenseness or in chronic gum chewers; *increase* in rest vertical d. may or may not accompany an increase in occlusal vertical d.; it sometimes occurs after the removal of remaining occlusal contacts, perhaps as a result of the removal of noxious reflex stimuli.
vertical d., vertical opening; a vertical measurement of the face between any two arbitrarily selected points which are conveniently located, one above and one below the mouth, usually in the midline.

dimer (dī'mer) [G. *di-*, two, + -mer]. A compound or unit produced by the combination of two like molecules; in the strictest sense, without loss of atoms (thus nitrogen tetroxide, N_2O_4, is the d. of nitrogen dioxide, NO_2), but usually by elimination of H_2O or a similar small molecule between the two (*e.g.*, a disaccharide), or by simple noncovalent association (as of two identical protein molecules; higher orders of complexity are called trimers, tetramers, oligomers, and polymers.
thymine d., a product of ultraviolet irradiation of thymine (free in ice or bound in nucleic acids) in which two thymine residues become linked by formation of a cyclobutane ring involving both C-5's and both C-6's at the expense of the two double bonds; several stereoisomeric forms are possible.

dimercaprol (dī-mer-kap'rol). Antilewisite; British anti-Lewisite; BAL; 2,3-dimercaptopropanol; $HSCH_2CH(SH)CH_2OH$; a chelating agent, developed as an antidote for lewisite and other arsenical poisons. It acts by competing for the metal with the essential —SH groups in the pyruvate oxidase system of the cells and forms, with arsenic, a stable, relatively nontoxic cyclic compound, the metal having a greater affinity for it than for the —SH groups of the cell proteins; also used as an antidote for antimony, bismuth, chromium, mercury, gold, and nickel.

dimercurion (dī-mer'kyūr-ī'on). The mercuric ion, Hg^{2+}.

dimeric (dī'mer-ik). Having the characteristics of a dimer.

dimerous (dim'er-ŭs) [G. *di-*, two, + *meros*, part]. Consisting of two parts.

dimetacrine tartrate (dī-met'ă-krēn). 10-[3-(Dimethylamino)propyl]-9,9-dimethylacridan tartrate; an antidepressant.

dimethicone (dī-meth'i-kōn). A silicone oil consisting of dimethylsiloxane polymers, usually incorporated into a petrolatum base or a nongreasy preparation and used for the protection of normal skin against various, chiefly industrial, skin irritants; may also be used to prevent diaper dermatitis.

dimethindene maleate (dī-meth'in-dēn). 2-[1-[2-(2-Dimethylaminoethyl)inden-3-yl]ethyl]pyridine maleate; an antihistamine also used as an antipruritic.

dimethisoquin hydrochloride (dī-me-thī'sō-kwin). 3-Butyl-1-(2-dimethylaminoethoxy)isoquinoline; an active surface anesthetic used to relieve itching and pain.

dimethisterone (dī-me-this'ter-ōn). 6α-Methyl-17-(1-propynyl)testosterone; 6α,21-dimethylethisterone; a modified testosterone or ethisterone; an orally effective synthetic progestin used alone or in combination with ethynyl estradiol as a contraceptive agent.

dimethothiazine mesylate (dī-meth-ō-thī'ă-zēn). Fonazine mesylate.

dimethoxanate hydrochloride (dī'me-thok'să-nāt). 2-Dimethylaminoethoxyethyl phenothiazine-10-carboxylate hydrochloride; a non-narcotic antitussive agent, less effective than codeine.

2,5-dimethoxy-4-methylamphetamine (DOM). An hallucinogenic agent chemically related to amphetamine and mescaline, a drug of abuse.

dimethylaminoazobenzene (dī-meth'il-ă-mē-nō-az-ō-ben'zēn) [C.I. 11160]. *Butter* yellow.

dimethylarsinic acid (dī-meth'il-ar-sin'ik). Cacodylic acid.

dimethylbenzene (dī-meth-il-ben'zēn). Xylol.

dimethylcarbinol (dī-meth-il-kar'bi-nol). Isopropyl alchohol.

dimethyl-1-carbomethoxy-1-propen-2-yl phosphate. An organic phosphorus compound used as a systemic poison for the extermination of such pests as mites, aphids, and houseflies.

β, *β*-**dimethylcysteine** (dī-meth-il-sis'tē-ēn). Penicillamine.

dimethylethylcarbinol (dī-meth'ĭl-eth-ĭl-kar'bi-nol). *Amylene* hydrate.

dimethylethylcarbinolchloral (dī-meth'ĭl-eth-ĭl-kar'bi-nō-klōr'ăl). *Amylene* chloral.

dimethyl ketone (dī-meth'il kē'tōn). Acetone.

dimethylphenol (dī-meth-il-fē'nol). Xylenol.

dimethylphenylpiperazinium (DMPP) (dī-meth'il-fen'il-pi-păr-ă-zin'ē-ŭm). A highly selective stimulant of autonomic ganglionic cells; used experimentally.

dimethyl phthalate (dī-meth'il thal'āt). Dimethyl ester of phthalic acid; an insect repellent.

dimethylpiperazine tartrate (dī-meth'il-pi-păr'ă-zēn). A diuretic, also used as a uric acid solvent.

dimethyl sulfoxide (DMSO) (dī-meth'il). Methyl sulfoxide; Me_2SO; a penetrating solvent, enhancing absorption of therapeutic agents from the skin; an industrial solvent that has been proposed as an effective analgesic and anti-inflammatory agent in arthritis and bursitis.

N,N-**dimethyltryptamine (DMT)** (dī-meth'il-trip'tă-mēn). A psychotomimetic agent present in several South American snuffs (*e.g.*, cohoba snuff) and in the leaves of *Prestonia amazonica* (family Apocynaceae). Effects are similar to those of LSD, but with more rapid onset, greater likelihood of a panic reaction, and a shorter duration (1 to 2 hours, "businessman's trip"); it produces pronounced autonomic effects, including a marked increase in blood pressure.

dimethyl *d*-tubocurarine. Metocurine iodide.

dimethyl tubocurarine chloride. Dimethyl ether of *d*-tubocurarine chloride; a skeletal muscle relaxant. See tubocurarine chloride.

dimethyl tubocurarine iodide. Metocurine iodide.

dimetria (dī-mē'trē-ă) [G. *di-*, two, + *mētra*, womb]. Obsolete term for *uterus* didelphys.

dimidiate (dī-mid'ē-āt) [L. *dimidiatus*, divided into halves]. To divide or be divided into halves.

Dimmer, Friedrich, Austrian ophthalmologist, 1855–1926. See D.'s *keratitis*.

dimorphic (dī-mōr'fik). **1.** Dimorphous (2); in fungi, a term referring to growth and reproduction in either the mold or yeast form. **2.** Dimorphous (1).

dimorphism (dī-mōr′fizm) [G. *di-*, two, + *morphē*, shape]. Existence in two shapes or forms; denoting a difference of crystal form exhibited by the same substance, or a difference in form or outward appearance between individuals of the same species.

sexual d., the somatic differences between male and female individuals that arise as a consequence of sexual maturation; inclusive of, but not restricted to, the secondary sexual characters.

dimorpholamine (dī-mōr-fol′ă-mēn). *N,N*′-1,2-Ethanediylbis [*N*-butyl-4-morpholinecarboxamide]; an analeptic.

dimorphous (dī-mōr′fŭs). **1.** Dimorphic (2); having the property of dimorphism. **2.** Dimorphic (1).

dimple (dim′pl). **1.** An indentation, usually circular and of small area, in the chin, cheek, or sacral region; probably due to some developmental fault in the subcutaneous connective tissue or in underlying bone. **2.** A depression of similar appearance to a d., resulting from trauma or the contraction of scar tissue. **3.** To cause d.'s.

coccygeal d., *foveola* coccygea.

dimp′ling. 1. Causing dimples. **2.** A condition marked by the formation of dimples, natural or artificial.

dineric (dī-ner′ik) [di- + G. *nerōn*, water]. Denoting the interface between two mutually immiscible liquids (*e.g.*, oil and water) in the same container.

dinitrocellulose (dī-nī-trō-sel′yū-lōs). Pyroxylin.

4,6-dinitro-*o*-cresol. 2-Methyl-4,6-dinitrophenol; an insecticide used against mites in the form of a spray or dust; also used as a weed killer.

dinitrogen monoxide (dī-nī′trō-jen). Nitrous oxide.

2,4-dinitrophenol (DNP, Dnp) (dī-nī-trō-fē′nol). N_2pH-OH; a toxic dye, chemically related to trinitrophenol (picric acid), used in biochemical studies of oxidative processes; it is also a metabolic stimulant.

dinoflagellate (dī′nō-flaj′ĕ-lāt) [G. *dinos*, whirling, + L. *flagellum*, a whip]. A plantlike flagellate of the subclass Phytomastigophorea, some species of which (*e.g., Gonyaulax cantanella*) produce a potent neurotoxin that may cause severe food intoxication following ingestion of parasitized shellfish.

dinoprost (dī′nō-prost). Prostaglandin $F_{2\alpha}$; 7-[3α,5α-dihydroxy-2β-[(3*S*)-hydroxy-*trans*- 1-octenyl]cyclopentyl]-*cis*- 5-heptenoic acid; an oxytocic agent.

d. tromethamine, prostaglandin $F_{2\alpha}$ tromethamine; an oxytocic agent.

dinoprostone (dī-nō-pros′tōn). Prostaglandin E_2; Prosta-5,13-dien-1-oic acid, 11,15-dihydroxy-9-oxo, (5*Z*,11α,13*E*,15*S*)-; an oxytocic agent used as an abortifacient.

dinormocytosis (dī-nōr′mō-sī-tō′sis). Obsolete term for isonormocytosis.

Dioctophyma (dī-ok-tō-fī′mă) [L. fr. G. *dionkoun*, to distend, + *phyma*, growth]. A genus of very large nematode worms infecting the kidney.

D. rena′le, a large blood red nematode found in the pelvis of the kidney and the peritoneal cavity of the dog; fairly common in wild carnivores like the mink, but rarely found in man; the life cycle is via leeches ectoparasitic on crayfish, which are then eaten by various fishes and finally by man or any of a number of other mammalian fish-eating hosts.

dioctophymiasis (dī-ok′tō-fi-mī′ă-sis). Infection of animals and rarely man with the giant kidney worm, *Dioctophyma renale*.

dioctyl calcium sulfosuccinate (dī-ok′til kal′sē-ŭm sŭl-fō-sŭk′si-nāt). Docusate calcium.

dioctyl sodium sulfosuccinate. Docusate sodium.

Diodon (dī′ō-don) [G. *di-*, two, + *odous* (*odont-*), tooth]. A genus of porcupine fishes related to balloon fish, globefish, and puffers. Although the common puffer is widely eaten as "sea squab" in the United States, many puffers, especially in the Pacific, are poisonous because of the presence of a neurotoxin, tetrodotoxin, in the liver and ovary.

diodone (dī′ō-dōn). Iodopyracet.

diodoquin (dī-ō′dō-kwin). Diiodohydroxyquin.

Diogenes, Greek philosopher, 412–323 B.C. See D. *cup; poculum* diogenis.

-diol. Suffix form of the prefix dihydroxy-.

diolamine (dī-ōl′ă-mēn). USAN-approved contraction for diethanolamine.

diopter (D) (dī-op′ter) [G. *dioptra*, a leveling instrument]. The unit of refracting power of lenses, denoting the reciprocal of the focal length expressed in meters.

prism d. (p.d.), the unit of measurement of the deviation of light in passing through a prism, being a deflection of 1 cm at a distance of 1 m.

dioptric (dī-op′trik). Obsolete term: **(1)** relating to dioptrics; **(2)** for refractive; **(3)** for diopter.

dioptrics (dī-op′triks). The branch of optics concerned with the refraction of light.

diorthosis (dī′ōr-thō′sis) [G. a making straight, fr. *di-orthoō*, to make straight, fr. *orthos*, straight]. Diaplasis.

diose (dī′ōs). Glycolaldehyde.

diosgenin (dī′-os-jen′in). (25*R*)-Spirost-5-en-3β-ol; a sapogenin derived from the saponins dioscin and trillin found in the roots of plants such as the yam; its steroid portion serves as a source from which pregnenolone and progesterone can be prepared.

diovular (dī′ov-yū-lar) [di- + Mod. L. *ovulum*, dim. of L. *ovum*, egg]. Relating to two ova.

diovulatory (dī-ō′vyū-lă-tō′rē). Releasing two ova in one ovarian cycle.

dioxane (dī-oks′ān). 1,4-Dioxane; 1,4-diethylene dioxide; a colorless liquid used as a solvent for cellulose esters and in histology as a drying agent.

dioxide (dī-oks′īd). A molecule containing two atoms of oxygen; *e.g.*, carbon dioxide, CO_2.

dioxin (dī-oks′in). **1.** A ring consisting of two oxygen atoms, four CH groups, and two double bonds; the positions of the oxygen atoms are specified by prefixes, as in 1,4-dioxin. **2.** Abbreviation for dibenzo[*b,e*][1,4]dioxin which may be visualized as an anhydride of two molecules of 1,2 benzenediol (pyrocatechol), thus forming two oxygen bridges between two benzene moieties, or as a 1,4-dioxin with a benzene ring fused to catch each of the two CH= CH groups. **3.** 2,3,7,8-Tetrachlorodibenzo[*b,e*][1,4]dioxin; a contaminant in the herbicide, 2,4,5-T; it is potentially toxic, teratogenic, and carcinogenic.

dioxybenzone (dī-ok-sē-ben′zōn). 2,2′-Dihydroxy-4-methoxybenzophenone; an ultraviolet screen for topical application to the skin.

dioxygenase (dī-oks′ĕ-jen-ās). An oxidoreductase that incorporates two atoms of oxygen (from one molecule of O_2) into the (reduced) substrate.

D.I.P. Abbreviation for desquamative interstitial *pneumonia*.

dip [M.E. *dippen*]. **1.** A downward inclination or slope. **2.** A preparation for coating a surface by submersion, as for the destruction of skin parasites.

Couranand's d., in constrictive pericarditis, rapid protodiastolic fall and reascent of the ventricular pressure curve with an elevated plateau.

type I d., early deceleration of the fetal heart rate at the height of uterine contraction, as displayed on a fetal monitor graph.

type II d., late deceleration of the fetal heart rate, 30 seconds or more after the height of uterine contraction, as displayed on a fetal monitor graph.

dipeptidase (dī-pep′ti-dās) [EC 3.4.13.11.]. A hydrolase catalyzing the hydrolysis of a dipeptide to its constituent amino acids.
methionyl d. [EC 3.4.13.13], a hydrolase catalyzing the hydrolysis of a methionyl-aminoacid.

dipeptide (dī-pep′tīd). A combination of two amino acids by means of a peptide (–CO–NH–) link.

dipeptidyl carboxypeptidase (dī-pep′ti-dil). Peptidyl dipeptidase A.

dipeptidyl peptidase. A hydrolase occurring in two forms: **I** (EC 3,4,14,1), dipeptidyl transferase, cleaving dipeptides from polypeptides; **II** (EC 3.4.14.2), with properties similar to those of I.

dipeptidyl transferase. Dipeptidyl peptidase-I.

diperodon hydrochloride (dī-per′ō-don). 3-Piperidino-1,2-propanediol dicarbanilate hydrochloride; a local anesthetic used topically on various mucous membranes and for ocular operations.

Dipetalonema (dī-pet′ă-lō-nē′mă) [G. *di-*, two, + *petalon,* leaf, + *nema,* thread]. A genus of nematode filariae with species in man and many other mammals; as with other filarial worms, it produces microfilariae in blood or tissue fluids, with adults found in deep connective tissue, membranes, or visceral surfaces.
D. recondi′tum, a filarial species found in dogs, transmitted by fleas and lice, in contrast to the canine heartworm, *Dirofilaria immitis,* which is transmitted by mosquitoes.
D. streptocer′ca, former name for *Mansonella streptocerca.*

diphallus (dī-fal′ŭs) [G. *di-*, two, + *phallos,* penis]. Double or bifid penis; a rare congenital anomaly in which the penises may be symmetrical, or placed one above the other; often with associated urogenital or other anomalies.

diphasic (dī-fā′zik). Occurring in or characterized by two phases or stages.

diphemanil methylsulfate (dī-fē′mă-nil). 4-Diphenylmethylene-1,1-dimethyl piperidinium methyl sulfate; an anticholinergic agent.

diphemethoxidine (dī-fem-ĕ-thok′si-dēn). 2-(Diphenylmethyl)-1-piperidineethanol; an anorexigenic drug.

diphenadione (dī-fen-ă-dī′ōn). 2-Diphenylacetyl-1,3-indandione; an orally effective anticoagulant with actions and uses similar to those of bishydroxycoumarin.

diphenan (dī′fen-ăn, dī-fen′an). *p*-Benzylphenylcarbamate; used as a vermicide in oxyuriasis.

diphenhydramine hydrochloride (dī-fen-hī′dră-mēn). 2-(Diphenylmethoxy)-*N,N-* dimethylethylamine hydrochloride; an antihistaminic.

diphenidol (dī-fen′i-dol). α,α-Diphenyl-1-piperidinebutanol; an antiemetic.

o-**diphenolase** (dī-fen′ō-lās). *Catechol* oxidase.

diphenol oxidase (dī-fen′ol). *Catechol* oxidase.

diphenoxylate hydrochloride (dī-fen-ok′si-lāt). 1-(3-Cyano-3,3-diphenylpropyl)-4-phenylpiperidine-4-carboxylic acid ethyl ester hydrochloride; an antidiarrheal agent, chemically related to meperidine, that inhibits rhythmic contraction of smooth muscle; it has some addiction liability.

diphenyl-. Prefix indicating two independent phenyl groups attached to a third atom or radical, as in diphenylamine.

diphenylchlorarsine (dī-fen′il-klōr-ar′sēn). A sternutator, inhalation of which causes violent sneezing, cough, salivation, headache, and retrosternal pain.

diphenylenimine (dī′fen-il-ēn′i-mēn). Carbazole.

5,5-**diphenylhydantoin** (dī-fen′il-hī-dan′tō-in). Phenytoin.

2,5-**diphenyloxazole (PPO)** (dī′fen-il-oks′ă-zōl). A scintillator used in radioactivity measurements by scintillation counting.

diphenylpyraline hydrochloride (dī-fen-il-pir′ă-lēn). 4-Diphenylmethoxy-1-methylpiperidine hydrochloride; an antihistaminic similar in action and use to diphenhydramine.

diphosgene (dī-fos′jēn). Trichloromethyl chloroformate; $ClCOOCCl_3$; a poison gas used in World War I.

1,3-**diphosphoglycerate (1,3-P$_2$Gri)** (dī-fos′fō-glis′er-āt). An intermediate in glycolysis which reacts with ADP to generate ATP and 3-phosphoglycerate.

2,3-**diphosphoglycerate (2,3-P$_2$Gri).** An intermediate in the Rapoport-Luebering shunt, formed between 1,3-P_2Gri and 3-phosphoglycerate; an important regulator of the affinity of hemoglobin for oxygen.

diphosphopyridine nucleotide (DPN) (dī′fos-fō-pir′i-dēn). Former name for nicotinamide adenine dinucleotide.

diphosphothiamin (dī′fos-fō-thī′ă-min). *Thiamin* pyrophosphate.

diphtheria (dif-thēr′ē-ă) [G. *diphthera,* leather]. Diphtheritis; a specific infectious disease due to *Corynebacterium diphtheriae* and its highly potent toxin; marked by severe inflammation of the pharynx, with formation of a fibrinous exudate, and of the mucous membrane of the throat, the nose, and sometimes the tracheobronchial tree; the toxin produces degeneration in peripheral nerves, heart muscle, and other tissues.
avian (fowl) d., an infection by the fowlpox virus in which tracheal involvement is especially severe. See also fowlpox.
calf d., a necrotic oropharyngolaryngitis of calves associated with *Fusobacterium necrophorum* infection that may spread to the lungs.
cutaneous d., d. resulting from infection of the skin by *Corynebacterium diphtheriae.*
false d., diphtheroid (1).

diphtherial, diphtheritic (dif-thēr′ē-ăl, dif-thĕ-rit′ik). Relating to diphtheria, or the membranous exudate characteristic of this disease.

diphtheritis (dif-thĕ-rī′tis). Diphtheria.

diphtheroid (dif′thĕ-royd) [diphtheria + G. *eidos,* resemblance]. **1.** Pseudodiphtheria; false diphtheria; Epstein's disease; one of a group of local infections suggesting diphtheria, but caused by microorganisms other than *Corynebacterium diphtheriae.* **2.** Any microorganism resembling *Corynebacterium diphtheriae.*

diphtherotoxin (dif′thēr-ō-tok′sin). The toxin of diphtheria.

diphyllobothriasis (dī-fil′ō-both-rī′ă-sis). Bothriocephaliasis; infection with the cestode *Diphyllobothrium lkatum;* human infection is caused by ingestion of raw or inadequately cooked fish infected with the plerocercoid larva. Leukocytosis and eosinophilia may occur; if the worm is high enough in the alimentary canal, it may preempt the supply of vitamin B_{12} or alter its absorption, leading to hyperchromic macrocytic anemia resembling pernicious anemia, although the condition is rare, even in hyperendemic areas.

Diphyllobothrium (dī-fil-lō-both′rē-ŭm) [G. *di-*, two, + *phyllon,* leaf, + *bothrion,* little ditch]. A large genus of tapeworms (order Pseudophyllidea) characterized by a spatulate scolex with dorsal and ventral sucking grooves or bothria. Several species are found in man, although only one, *D. latum,* is of widespread importance.
D. corda′tum, a species found in dogs, sea mammals, and occasionally man, in Greenland.
D. la′tum, *Dibothriocephalus latus;* the broad or broad fish tapeworm, a species that causes diphyllobothriasis, found in man and fish-eating mammals in many parts of northern Europe, Japan and elsewhere in Asia, and in Scandinavian populations of the American north central states; it often has 3 or 4 thousand segments, broader than long; the head has typical bothria characteristic of the genus.
D. linguloi′des, *Spirometra mansoni.*
D. man′soni, *Spirometra mansoni.*

D. mansonoi'des, *Spirometra mansonoides.*

diphyodont (dif'ē-ō-dont) [G. *di-,* two, + *phyō,* to produce, + *odous (odont-),* tooth]. Possessing two sets of teeth, as occurs in man and most mammals.

dipipanone (dī-pip'ă-nōn). Phenylpiperone; *dl-* 4,4-diphenyl-6-piperidinoheptan-3-one; a narcotic congener of methadone, less potent than methadone.

dipiproverine (dī-pī-prō'ver-ēn). α-Phenyl-1-piperidineacetic acid 2-piperidinoethyl ester; an intestinal antispasmodic.

dipivefrin hydrochloride (dī-piv'ĕ-frin). Propanoic acid, 2,2-dimethyl-, 4-[1-hydroxy-2-methylamino)ethyl]-1,2-phenylene ester, hydrochloride, (±)-; an adrenergic epinephrine prodrug used in drop form in initial therapy for control of intraocular pressure in chronic open-angle glaucoma.

diplacusis (dip-lă-kū'sis) [G. *diplous,* double, + *akousis,* a hearing]. A difference of perception of sound by the two ears, either in time or in pitch, so that one sound is heard as two.
d. binaura'lis, a condition in which the same sound is heard differently by the two ears.
d. dysharmon'ica, a condition in which the same sound is heard with a different pitch in each ear.
d. echo'ica, a condition in which sound heard in the affected ear is repeated.
d. monaura'lis, a condition in which one sound is perceived as two in the same ear.

diplegia (dī-plē'jē-ă) [G. *di-,* two, + *plēgē,* a stroke]. Double hemiplegia; paralysis of corresponding parts on both sides of the body.
congenital facial d., Möius' *syndrome.*
facial d., paralysis of both sides of the face.
infantile d., birth *palsy.*
masticatory d., paralysis of all the muscles of mastication.
spastic d., hypertonic double hemiplegia, usually congenital. Also called Erb-Charcot disease; Little's disease; spastic spinal paralysis; tabes spasmodica.

diplo- [G. *diploos,* double]. Combining form meaning double or twofold.

diploalbuminuria (dip'lō-al-byū-mi-nū'rē-ă). The coexistence of nephritic, or pathologic, and nonnephritic, or physiologic, albuminuria.

diplobacillus (dip'lō-bă-sil'ŭs). Two rod-shaped bacterial cells linked end to end.
Morax-Axenfeld d., *Moraxella lacunata.*

diplobacteria (dip'lō-bak-tēr'ē-ă). Bacterial cells linked together in pairs.

diploblastic (dip-lō-blas'tik) [diplo- + G. *blastos,* germ]. Formed of two germ layers.

diplocardia (dip-lō-kar'dē-ă) [diplo- + G. *kardia,* heart]. A condition in which the two lateral halves of the heart are separated to varying degrees by a central fissure.

diplocephalus (dip-lō-sef'ă-lŭs). Dicephalus.

diplocheiria, diplochiria (dip'lō-kī'rē-ă) [diplo- + G. *cheir,* hand]. Dicheiria.

diplococcemia (dip-lō-kok-sē'mē-ă). The presence of diplococci in the blood; used especially in referring to *Neisseria meningitidis* (meningococci) in circulating blood.

diplococci (dip'lō-kok'sī). Plural of diplococcus.

diplococcin (dip-lō-kok'sin). An antibiotic crystalline substance isolated from cultures of lactic acid-producing cocci present in milk active against lactobacilli and certain Gram-positive cocci, but inactive against Gram-negative bacteria.

diplococcoid (dip'lō-kok'oyd). Resembling a diplococcus.

Diplococcus (dip'lō-kok'ŭs) [diplo- + G. *kokkos,* berry]. *Streptococcus. D. pneumoniae,* the type species of *D.,* is a member of the genus *Streptococcus.*

diplococcus, pl. **diplococci** (dip'lō-kok'ŭs, -kok'sī) [diplo- + G. *kokkos,* berry]. **1.** Spherical or ovoid bacterial cells joined together in pairs. **2.** Common name of any organism belonging to the bacterial genus *Diplococcus.*

diplocoria (dip-lō-kō'rē-ă) [diplo- + G. *korē,* pupil]. Dicoria; discoria; the occurrence of two pupils in the eye.

diploë (dip'lō-ē) [G. *diploē,* fem. of *diplous,* double] [NA]. The central layer of spongy bone between the two layers of compact bone, outer and inner plates, or tables, of the flat cranial bones.

diplogenesis (dip-lō-jen'ĕ-sis) [diplo- + G. *genesis,* production]. Production of a double fetus or of one with some parts doubled.

Diplogonoporus (dip'lō-gō-nop'ō-rŭs) [diplo- + G. *gonos,* seed, + *poros,* pore]. A genus of tapeworms found in Japan (*D. grandis*) and probably also in Rumania (*D. brauni*).

diploic (dip-lō'ik). Relating to the diploë.

diploid (dip'loyd) [diplo- + G. *eidos* resemblance]. Denoting the state of a cell containing twice the normal gametic number of chromosomes, one member of each chromosome pair derived from the father and one from the mother; the normal chromosome complement of somatic cells (in man, 46 chromosomes).

diplokaryon (dip'lō-kar'ē-on) [diplo- + G. *karyon,* nut (nucleus)]. A cell nucleus containing twice the normal diploid number of chromosomes; *i.e.,* a tetraploid nucleus. See also polyploidy.

diplomelituria (dip'lō-mel-i-tū'rē-ă) [diplo- + G. *meli,* honey, + *ouron,* urine]. The occurrence of diabetic and nondiabetic glycosuria in the same individual.

diplomyelia (dip-lō-mī-ē'lē-ă) [diplo- + G. *myelon,* marrow]. Complete or incomplete doubling of the spinal cord that may be accompanied by a bony septum of the vertebral canal.

diplon (dip'lon). Deuteron.

diplonema (dip-lō-nē'mă) [diplo- + G. *nema,* thread]. The doubled form of the chromosome strand visible at the diplotene stage of meiosis.

diploneural (dip-lō-nū'răl) [diplo- + G. *neuron,* nerve]. Supplied by two nerves from different sources, said of certain muscles.

diplopagus (dip-lop'ă-gŭs) [diplo- + G. *pagos,* something fixed]. General term for conjoined twins, each with fairly complete bodies, although one or more internal organs may be in common.

diplopia (di-plō'pē-ă) [diplo- + G. *ōps,* eye]. Double vision; the condition in which a single object is perceived as two objects.
crossed d., heteronymous d.
direct d., homonymous d.
heteronymous d., crossed d.; d. in which the false image is on the same side as the sound eye; due to divergent squint or paralysis of the medial rectus muscle.
homonymous d., simple d.; direct d.; d. in which the false image is on the same side as the affected eye; due to convergent squint or paralysis of the external or lateral rectus muscle.
monocular d., monodiplopia; a form of d. in which two objects are seen with the same eye, due to an opacity in the visual axis.
simple d., homonymous d.

diplopodia (dip-lō-pō'dē-ă) [diplo- + G. *pous,* foot]. Duplication of digits of the foot.

diplosome (dip'lō-sōm) [diplo- + G. *sōma,* body]. Paired allosome; the pair of centrioles of mammalian cells.

diplosomia (dip-lō-sō'mē-ă) [diplo- + G. *somā,* body]. Condition in which twins, seemingly functionally independent, are joined at one or more points.

diplotene (dip'lō-tēn) [diplo- + G. *tainia,* band]. The late stage of prophase in meiosis in which the paired homologous chromosomes begin to repel each other and move apart, but are usually held together by regions of crossing or intertwining called chiasmata. The chiasmata are associated with breakage of two chromatids at corresponding points followed by refusion of the broken ends with exchange of segments between the chromatids; this is considered to be the cytologic basis for the crossing-over of genes.

diploteratology (dip'lō-tār-ă-tol'ō-jē). The division of teratology concerned with conjoined twins.

dipodia (dī-pō'dē-ă) [G. *di-*, two, + *pous (pod-)*, foot]. **1.** A developmental anomaly involving complete or incomplete duplication of a foot. **2.** In conjoined twins and sirenomyelia, a degree of fusion leaving two feet evident.

dipole (dī'pōl). Doublet (2); a pair of separated electrical charges, one positive and one negative.

dipotassium phosphate (dī-pō-tas'ē-ŭm). *Potassium* phosphate.

dipropyltryptamine (DPT) (dī-prō-pil-trip'tă-mēn). *N,N-* Dipropyltryptamine; a hallucinogenic agent similar to dimethyltryptamine.

diprosopus (dī-pros'ō-pŭs, dī-prō-sō'pus) [G. *di-*, two + *prosōpon*, face]. Conjoined twins with almost complete fusion of the bodies but duplication of the face or a part of it.

dipsesis (dip-sē'sis) [G. *dipsein*, to thirst]. Dipsosis; morbid thirst; an abnormal or excessive thirst, or a craving for unusual forms of drink.

dipsogen (dip'sō-jen) [G. *dipsa*, thirst, + *-gen*, producing]. A thirst-provoking agent.

dipsomania (dip-sō-mā'nē-ă) [G. *dipsa*, thirst, + *mania*, madness]. A recurring compulsion to drink alcoholic beverages to excess.

dipsosis (dip-sō'sis) [G. *dipsa*, thirst, + *-osis*, condition]. Dipsesis.

dipsotherapy (dip'sō-thār'ă-pē). Treatment of certain diseases by abstention, as far as possible, from liquids.

Diptera (dip'ter-ă) [G. *di-*, two, + *pteron*, wing]. An important order of insects (the two-wing flies and gnats), including many important disease vectors such as the mosquito, tsetse fly, sandfly, and biting midge.

dipteran (dip'ter-an). Denoting insects of the order Diptera.

dipterous (dip'ter-ŭs). Relating to or characteristic of the order Diptera.

Dipus sagitta (dī'pŭs saj'i-tă) [G. *dipous*, jerboa, two-footed; L. *sagitta*, arrow]. A small rodent of southern Russia that serves as a vector, through fleas, of *Yersinia pestis* (plague bacillus).

dipygus (dī-pī'gŭs, dip'ē-gŭs) [G. *di-*, two, + *pyge*, buttocks]. Conjoined twins with the head and thorax completely merged, and the pelvis and lower extremities duplicated; when the duplications of the lower parts are symmetrical, usually called duplicitas posterior.

dipylidiasis (dip'i-li-dī'ă-sis). Infection of carnivores and man with the cestode *Dipylidium caninum*.

Dipylidium caninum (dī-pī-lid'ē-ŭm kā-nī'nŭm) [G. *dipylos*, with two entrances; L. ntr. of *caninus*, pertaining to *canis*, dog]. The commonest species of dog tapeworm, the double-pored tapeworm, the larvae of which are harbored by dog fleas or lice; the worm occasionally infects man, especially children licked by dogs that have recently nipped infected fleas.

dipyridamole (dī-pī-rid'ă-mōl). 2,2′,2″,2‴-[4,8- Dipiperidino-pyrimidino [5,4-d] pyrimidine- 2,6-diyldinitrilo] tetraethanol; a coronary vasodilator that also reduces platelet aggregation.

dipyrimidine photolyase (dī-pi-rim'i-dēn). Deoxyribodipyrimidine photolyase.

dipyrine (dī-pī'rēn). Aminopyrine.

dipyrone (dī-pī'rōn). Methampyrone; $C_{13}H_{16}N_3NaO_4S{\cdot}H_2O$; an analgesic, anti-inflammatory, and antipyretic agent rarely used because of a high incidence of agranulocytosis.

director (di-rek'ter, -tōr; dī-) [L. *dirigo*, pp. *-rectus*, to arrange, set in order]. **1.** Staff (2); a smoothly grooved instrument used with a knife to limit the incision of tissues. **2.** The head of a service or specialty division.

dirigation (dir'i-gā'shŭn) [L. *dis-*, apart, + *rigare*, to draw off, sleuce off]. Development of voluntary control over functions that are ordinarily involuntary.

dirigomotor (dir'i-gō-mō'ter). Directing muscular movement.

Dirofilaria (dī-rō-fi-lā'rē-ă) [L. *dirus*, dread, + *filum*, thread]. A genus of filaria (family Onchocercidae, superfamily Filarioidea); *D.* species are usually found in mammals other than man, but rare examples of human infection are known, as by *D. immitis*.
D. conjuncti'vae, name assigned to filarial worms removed from tumors and abscesses in various sites in human cases, especially palpebral conjunctivae and other eye tissues, but also subcutaneous tissues from other sites; probably caused by a number of species of animal origin.
D im'mitis, heartworm; a species of filarial worms of dogs and other canids in tropical and subtropical areas, found chiefly in the right ventricle and pulmonary arteries of dogs; sometimes a serious pathogen of racing and show dogs, especially in the southern U.S. where mosquito vectors are common; *D. immitis* and its canine host have been used to test chemotherapeutic agents, and an extract of *D. immitis* may be used as a nonspecific intradermal antigen in the diagnosis of human filariasis and in complement-fixation tests. See also *Dipetalonema reconditum*.

dirofilariasis (dir'ō-fil-ă-rī'ă-sis). Infection of animals and rarely man with nematodes of the genus *Dirofilaria*.

dir. prop. Abbreviation for L. *directione propria*, with proper direction.

dirt-eating. Geophagia.

dis- [L. an inseparable particle denoting separation, taking apart, sundering in two]. Prefix having the same force as the original Latin preposition. *Cf.* dys-.

disability (dis-ă-bil'i-tē). **1.** An impairment or defect of one or more organs or members. **2.** Impairment or loss of function(s) severe enough to be a handicap.
developmental d., a category of cognitive, emotional, or physically handicapping conditions that appear in infancy or childhood and are related directly to abnormal sensory or motor development, maturation, or function; the resultant impairment involves a failure or delay in progressing through the normal developmental milestones of childhood.
learning d., a disorder in one or more of the basic cognitive and psychological processes involved in understanding or using written or spoken language; may be manifested in age-related impairment in the ability to read, write, spell, speak, or perform mathematical calculations.

disaccharide (dī-sak'ă-rīd). Bioside; a condensation product of two monosaccharides by elimination of water (usually between an alcoholic OH and a hemiacetal OH); *e.g.*, sucrose, lactose, maltose.

disaggregation (dis'ag-grē-gā'shŭn) [L. *dis-*, separating, + *aggrego (adg-)*, pp. *-gregatus*, to add to something]. **1.** A breaking up into component parts. **2.** An inability to coordinate various sensations and failure to comprehend their mutual relations.

disarticulation (dis-ar-tik-yū-lā'shŭn) [L. *dis-*, apart, + *articulus*, joint]. Exarticulation; amputation of a limb through a joint, without cutting of bone.

disassimilation (dis'ă-sim-i-lā'shŭn). Dissimilation; destructive or retrograde metabolism.

disassociation (dis'ă-sō-sē-ā'shŭn). Dissociation.

disc (disk). See disk; discus.

disc-. See disco-.

discectomy (dis-ek'tō-mē) [disco- + G. *ektomē*, excision]. Discotomy; excision, in part or whole, of an intervertebral disk.

discharge (dis'charj). **1.** That which is emitted or evacuated, as an excretion or a secretion. **2.** The activation or firing of a neuron.
after-d., see afterdischarge.

Dische, Zacharias, 20th century U.S. biochemist. See D. *reaction.*

dischronation (dis-krō-nā'shŭn) [L. *dis-*, apart, + G. *chronos,* time]. A disturbance in the consciousness of time.

disci (dis'kī). Plural of discus.

disciform (dis'i-fōrm). Disk-shaped.

discission (di-sish'ŭn) [L. *di- scindo,* pp. *-scissus,* to tear asunder]. **1.** Incision or cutting through a part. **2.** In ophthalmology, opening of the capsule and breaking up of the cortex of the lens with a needle knife or laser.

discitis (dis-kī'tis). Diskitis; nonbacterial inflammation of an intervertebral disk or disk space.

disclination (dis-klin-ā'shŭn). Obsolete term for extorsion (2).

disco-, disc- [G. *diskos,* disk]. Combining forms indicating relation to, or similarity to, a disk.

discoblastic (dis-kō-blas'tik). Denoting a discoblastula.

discoblastula (dis'kō-blas'tyū-lă). A blastula of the type produced by the meroblastic discoidal cleavage of a large-yolked ovum.

discogastrula (dis'kō-gas'trū-lă). A gastrula of the type formed after the discoidal cleavage of a large-yolked ovum.

discogenic (dis'kō-gen'ik) [disco- + G. *genesis,* origin]. Denoting a disorder originating in or from an intervertebral disk.

discogram (dis'kō-gram). The graphic record, usually roentgenographic, of discography.

discography (dis-kog'ră-fē) [disco- + G. *graphō,* to write]. Radiographic visualization of intervertebral disk space by injection of contrast media.

discoid (dis'koyd) [disco- + G. *eidos,* appearance]. **1.** Resembling a disk. **2.** In dentistry, an excavating or carving instrument having a circular blade with a cutting edge around the periphery.

discopathy (dis-kop'ă-thē) [disco- + G. *pathos,* disease]. Disease of a disk, particularly of an invertebral disk.
traumatic cervical d., an injury characterized by fissuration, laceration and/or fragmentation of a cervical disk or surrounding ligaments, with or without displacement of fragments against spinal cord, nerve roots, or ligaments.

discoplacenta (dis-kō-pla-sen'tă). A placenta of discoid shape.

discordance (dis-kōr'dans). Dissociation of two characteristics in the members of a sample from a population; used as a measure of dependence. *Cf.* concordance.

discoria (dis-kōr'ē-ă) [G. *dis,* double, + *korē,* pupil]. Diplocoria.

discotomy (dis-kot'ō-mē) [disco- + G. *tomē,* incision]. Discectomy.

discrete (dis-krēt') [L. *dis- cerno,* pp. *-cretus,* to separate]. Separate; distinct; not joined to or incorporated with another; denoting especially certain lesions of the skin.

discrimination (dis'krim-i-nā'shŭn) [L. *discrimino,* pp. *-atus,* to separate]. In conditioning, responding differentially, as when an organism makes one response to a reinforced stimulus and a different response to an unreinforced stimulus.

discus, pl. **disci** (dis'kŭs, -kī) [L. fr. G. *diskos,* a quoit, disk] [NA]. Disk (1); any approximately flat circular surface.
d. articula'ris [NA], articular disk; intra-articular cartilage; interarticular fibrocartilage; fibrocartilago interarticularis; fibroplate; a plate or ring of fibrocartilage attached to the joint capsule and separating the articular surfaces of the bones for a varying distance, sometimes completely; it serves to adapt two articular surfaces that are not entirely congruent.
d. articula'ris acromioclavicula'ris [NA], acromioclavicular disk; Weitbrecht's cartilage; the articular disk of fibrocartilage usually found between the acromial end of the clavicle and the medial border of the acromion.
d. articula'ris radioulna'ris [NA], radioulnar articular disk; triquetrous cartilage (1); triangular disk of wrist; triangular cartilage; radioulnar disk; the disk that holds together the distal ends of the radius and ulna; it is attached by its apex to a depression between the styloid process and distal surface of the head of the ulna, and by its base to the ridge separating the ulnar notch from the carpal surface of the radius.
d. articula'ris sternoclavicula'ris [NA], sternoclavicular articular disk; sternoclavicular disk; the fibrocartilaginous disk that subdivides the sternoclavicular joint into two cavities.
d. articula'ris temporomandibula'ris [NA], temporomandibular articular disk; mandibular disk; the fibrocartilaginous plate that separates the joint into upper and lower cavities.

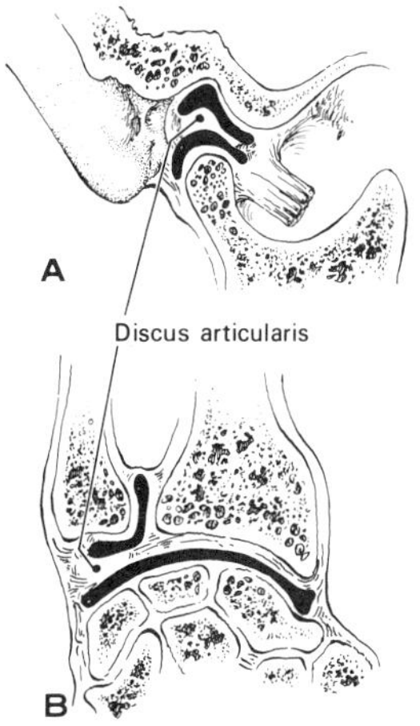

Discus Articularis
Articular disk of: *A*, temporomandibular joint; *B*, distal radioulnar joint.

d. interpu'bicus [NA], interpubic disk; lamina fibrocartilaginea interpubica; the disk of fibrocartilage that unites the pubic bones at the pubic symphysis.
d. intervertebra'lis [NA], intervertebral disk or cartilage; fibrocartilago intervertebralis; a disk interposed between the bodies of adjacent vertebrae. It is composed of an outer fibrous part (annulus fibrosus) that surrounds a central gelatinous mass (nucleus pulposus).
d. lentifor'mis, rarely used term for *nucleus* subthalamicus.
d. ner'vi op'tici [NA], an oval area of the ocular fundus devoid of light receptors, where retinal ganglion cell axons converge to form the optic nerve. Also called blind spot (3); Mariotte's blind spot; papilla nervi optici; optic disk or papilla; porus opticus.
d. prolig'erus, *cumulus* oophorus.

discussive (di-skŭ'siv). Discutient.

discutient (di-skyū'shē-ent) [L. *dis-cutio,* pp. *-cussus,* to strike asunder, shatter]. Discussive. **1.** Scattering or dispersing a pathologic accumulation. **2.** An agent that causes the dispersal of a tumor or pathologic collection of any sort.

disdiaclast (dis-dī'ă-klast) [G. *dis,* twice, + *dia,* through, + *klastos,* broken]. A doubly refractive element in striated muscular tissue.

DISEASE

disease (di-zēz′) [Eng. *dis*- priv. + ease]. **1.** Morbus; illness; sickness; an interruption, cessation, or disorder of body functions, systems, or organs. **2.** A morbid entity characterized usually by at least two of these criteria: recognized etiologic agent(s), identifiable group of signs and symptoms, or consistent anatomical alterations. See also syndrome.

aaa d., endemic anemia of ancient Egypt, ascribed in the Papyrus Ebers to intestinal infestation with ancylostoma; now called ancylostomiasis.

ABO hemolytic d. of the newborn, erythroblastosis fetalis due to maternal-fetal incompatibility with respect to an antigen of the ABO blood group; the fetus possesses A or B antigen which is lacking in the mother, and the mother produces immune type antibody which causes hemolysis of fetal erythrocytes.

Acosta's d., altitude *sickness* (1).

Adams-Stokes d., Adams-Stokes *syndrome.*

adaptation d.'s, d.'s falling theoretically into Selye's concept of the general-adaptation syndrome.

Addison's d., chronic adrenocortical *insufficiency.*

Addison-Biermer d., pernicious *anemia.*

adenoid d., **(1)** adenoids; **(2)** obsolete term for Hodgkin's d.

akamushi d. (ak-kă-mū′shē), tsutsugamushi d.

Akureyri d., epidemic *neuromyasthenia.*

Albers-Schönberg d., osteopetrosis.

Albert's d., Swediauer's d.; achillobursitis involving inflammation of the bursa between the Achilles tendon and the os calcis.

Albright's d., McCune-Albright *syndrome.*

Aleutian d. of mink, anorexia, diarrhea, weight loss, and death caused by an unclassified virus resistant to formalin (0.3%); it occurs chiefly in mink homozygous for the recessive Aleutian gene.

Alexander's d., a d. of the brain, probably due to defective astrocytic metabolism, developing rapidly in young children and characterized by mental deterioration, stooped posture, seizures, and paralysis, terminating fatally before the age of five; megaloencephaly is associated with widespread leukodystrophic change and eosinophilic deposits at cerebral interfaces.

alkali d., a term applied to various animal poisonings of plant and mineral origin in arid regions under the belief that they were caused by the ingestion of alkaline waters; *e.g.,* botulism of wild ducks, caused by feeding on decayed vegetation in nearly dried-up lakes.

Almeida's d., paracoccidioidomycosis.

Alpers d., *poliodystrophia* cerebri progressiva infantalis.

Alzheimer's d., Alzheimer's dementia; presenile dementia (2); primary senile dementia; dementia presenilis (2); primary neuronal degeneration; progressive mental deterioration manifested by memory loss, confusion, and disorientation beginning in late middle life and resulting in death in 5-10 years. Pathologically, the brain is atrophic, especially in the frontal occipital and temporal regions; histologically, it is characterized by thickening, conglutination, and distortion of the intracellular neurofibrils (neurofibrillary tangles) and by senile plaques composed of granular or filamentous argentophilic masses with an amyloid core, found predominately in the cerebral cortex, amygdala, and hippocampus; the cerebral cortex has few and shrunken neurons which may contain cytoplasmic vacuoles and argentophilic granules displacing the nucleus to the periphery; granulovacuolar degeneration of this kind seen mainly in the anterior hippocampus.

anarthritic rheumatoid d., rheumatoid d. without arthritis.

Anders' d., *adiposis* dolorosa.

Andersen's d., type 4 *glycogenosis.*

antibody deficiency d., antibody deficiency *syndrome.*

aortoiliac occlusive d., Leriche's syndrome; obstruction of the abdominal aorta and its main branches by atherosclerosis.

Aran-Duchenne d., progressive muscular *atrophy.*

Aujeszky's d., pseudorabies.

Australian X d., Murray Valley *encephalitis.*

autoimmune d., any disorder in which destruction of normal tissue arises from humoral or cellular immune responses of the individual to his own tissue constituents; may be systemic, as systemic lupus erythematosus, or organ specific, as thyroiditis.

aviator's d., term sometimes applied to a disorder in pilots flying at high altitudes, analogous to decompression *sickness.*

Ayerza's d., Ayerza's *syndrome.*

Azorean d., Machado-Joseph d.

Baelz' d., *cheilitis* glandularis.

Ballet's d., *ophthalmoplegia* externa.

Baló's d., *encephalitis* periaxialis concentrica.

Bamberger's d., **(1)** saltatory *spasm;* **(2)** polyserositis.

Bamberger-Marie d., hypertrophic pulmonary *osteoarthropathy.*

Bang's d., bovine *brucellosis.*

Bannister's d., angioneurotic *edema.*

Banti's d., Banti's *syndrome.*

Barclay-Baron d., vallecular *dysphagia.*

Barlow's d., infantile *scurvy.*

Barraquer's d., progressive *lipodystrophy.*

Basedow's d., Graves' d.

Batten-Mayou d., cerebral *sphingolipidosis,* late juvenile type.

Bayle's d., paresis (2).

Bazin's d., *erythema* induratum.

Bechterew's d., *spondylitis* deformans.

Becker's d., an obscure South African cardiomyopathy leading to rapidly fatal congestive heart failure and idiopathic mural endomyocardial d.

Begbie's d., localized chorea.

Béguez César d., Chédiak-Steinbrink-Higashi *syndrome.*

Behçet's d., Behçet's *syndrome.*

Behr's d., Behr's *syndrome.*

Benson's d., asteroid *hyalosis.*

Bernhardt's d., *meralgia* paraesthetica.

Besnier-Boeck-Schaumann d., sarcoidosis.

Best's d., autosomal dominant retinal degeneration beginning during the first years of life. See also vitelliruptive *degeneration.*

Bielschowsky's d., cerebral *sphingolipidosis,* early juvenile type.

Biermer's d., pernicious *anemia.*

big liver d., see avian *lymphomatosis* (2).

Binswanger's d., Binswanger's encephalopathy; encephalitis subcorticalis chronica; subcortical arteriosclerotic encephalopathy; an organically caused dementia, found in chronic hypertensives; characterized by recurrent edema of cerebral white matter, with secondary demyelination.

bird-breeder's d., bird-breeder's *lung.*

black d., infectious necrotic *hepatitis* of sheep.

black-tongue d., a d. of dogs similar to human pellagra and due to niacin deficiency.

blinding d., onchocerciasis.

Bloch-Sulzberger d., *incontinentia* pigmenti.

Blocq's d., astasia-abasia.

Blount's d., Blount-Barber d.; nonrachitic bowlegs in children.

Blount-Barber d., Blount's d.

blue d., Rocky Mountain spotted *fever.*

bluecomb d. of chickens, avian monocytosis; an acute or subacute d. of young laying chickens characterized by lowered egg production, diarrhea, frequently cyanosis of the head, and pathologic changes involving chiefly the liver and kidney; etiology is not definitely established.

bluecomb d. of turkeys, transmissible enteritis; mud fever (2); an

acute or chronic d. of young turkeys caused by bluecomb virus, with diarrhea, loss of weight, and often cyanosis of the head.
Boeck's d., sarcoidosis.
Borna d. [*Borna,* Saxony where a severe epidemic occurred], enzootic encephalomyelitis; an infectious encephalomyelitis of horses, cattle, and sheep caused by Borna disease virus and occurring in Germany and several other European countries; affected animals show depression, then excitement and spasms, and finally paralysis.
Bornholm d. [*Bornholm,* Danish island in the Baltic where the d. was first described], epidemic *pleurodynia.*
Bouchard's d., myopathic dilation of the stomach.
Bouillaud's d., obsolete eponym for acute rheumatic fever with carditis.
Bourneville's d., tuberous *sclerosis.*
Bourneville-Pringle d., tuberous sclerosis with adenoma sebaceum.
Bowen's d., Bowen's precancerous dermatosis; a form of intraepidermal carcinoma characterized by the development of pinkish or brownish papules covered with a thickened horny layer; microscopically, there is dyskeratosis with large round epidermal cells with large nuclei and pale-staining cytoplasm which are scattered through all levels of the epidermis.
Brailsford-Morquio d., Morquio's *syndrome.*
Breda's d., espundia.
Bright's d., **(1)** nonsuppurative nephritis with albuminuria and edema, associated in fatal cases with large white kidneys; or with hematuria and red kidneys; or with contracted granular kidneys, corresponding to the stages of glomerulonephritis now termed subacute or membranous, acute, and chronic, respectively; **(2)** an eponym sometimes used in general reference to kidney d. without specifying the kind.
Brill's d., Brill-Zinsser d.
Brill-Symmers d., nodular *lymphoma.*
Brill-Zinsser d., Brill's d.; recrudescent typhus fever; recrudescent typhus; an endogenous infection associated with the "carrier state" in persons who previously had epidemic typhus fever; it is a rather mild d. and may be mistaken for endemic (murine) typhus; first described by Brill in New York City but not recognized as a recrudescent form of epidemic typhus until after the work of Zinsser.
brisket d., a d. of cattle, characterized by edematous swelling of the brisket and the tissues of the neck; the body cavities also contain large quantities of clear straw-colored transudate; this d. results from right heart failure as a consequence of increased pulmonary resistance, which is in some way associated with movement of animals to high altitudes.
Brissaud's d., tic.
Brocq's d., a variety of parapsoriasis.
Brodie's d., **(1)** Brodie's *knee;* **(2)** hysterical arthralgia; **(3)** hysterical spinal neuralgia, simulating Pott's disease, following a trauma.
bronzed d., see chronic adrenocortical *insufficiency;* hemochromatosis; bronze *diabetes.*
Brooke's d., **(1)** the multiple form of trichoepithelioma; **(2)** *keratosis* follicularis contagiosa.
Bruck's d., a d. marked by osteogenesis imperfecta, ankylosis of the joints, and muscular atrophy.
Brushfield-Wyatt d., nevoid amentia; mental retardation probably associated with Sturge-Weber syndrome.
Bruton's d., X-linked *hypogammaglobulinemia.*
Buerger's d., *thromboangiitis* obliterans.
bulging eye d., gedoelstiosis.
Bury's d., *erythema* elevatum diutinum.
Buschke's d., **(1)** *scleredema* adultorum; **(2)** obsolete eponym for cryptococcosis.
Busquet's d., an osteoperiostitis of the metatarsal bones, leading to exostoses on the dorsum of the foot.
Buss d., bovine sporadic *encephalomyelitis.*
Busse-Buschke d., cryptococcosis.
Byler d. [*Byler,* an Amish kindred], familial intrahepatic cholestasis, with early onset of loose, foul-smelling stools, jaundice, hepatosplenomegaly, and dwarfism, due to an error in conjugated bile salt metabolism; autosomal recessive inheritance.
Caffey's d., infantile cortical *hyperostosis.*
caisson d. (kā'son) [Fr. *caisson* (fr. *caisse,* a chest), a water-tight box or cylinder containing air under high pressure, used in sinking structural pilings underwater], decompression *sickness.*
Calvé-Perthes d., Legg-Calvé-Perthes d.
Canavan's d., spongy *degeneration.*
canine parvovirus d., an acute d. of dogs with a variable mortality rate caused by the canine parvovirus; seen in three distinct clinical forms; a generalized neonatal d., a severe nonsuppurative myocarditis, and a frequently fatal enteritis.
Caroli's d., congenital cystic dilation of the intrahepatic bile ducts, sometimes associated with intrahepatic stones and biliary obstruction.
Carrión's d., Oroya *fever.*
Castleman's d., benign mediastinal lymph node *hyperplasia.*
cat-bite d., cat-bite fever; rat-bite fever, presumably spread from rats to cats and thus to man.
cat-scratch d., cat-scratch fever; regional granulomatous lymphadenitis; benign inoculation lymphoreticulosis or reticulosis; an ulceroglandular d. of man that frequently follows the scratch or bite of a cat, although some cases have occurred when there has been no contact with a cat; a seemingly specific infection, producing regional lymphadenitis, indolent reaction, and benign low grade infection; diagnosis is based on the Foshay test.
celiac d., gluten enteropathy; a disease occurring in children and adults characterized by sensitivity to gluten, with chronic inflammation and atrophy of the mucosa of the upper small intestine; manifestations include diarrhea, malabsorption, steatorrhea, and nutritional and vitamin deficiencies.
central core d., a congenital myopathy characterized by hypotonia, delay of motor development in infancy, and nonprogressive or slowly progressive muscle weakness; on biopsy the central core of muscle fibers stains abnormally, myofibrils are abnormally compact, and there is virtual absence of mitochondria and sarcoplasmic reticulum; histochemically, the cores are devoid of oxidative enzyme, phosphorylase, and ATPase activity; autosomal dominant inheritance with reduced penetrance.
cerebrovascular d., a brain dysfunction due to an abnormality of the blood supply.
Chagas' d., Chagas-Cruz d., South American *trypanosomiasis.*
Charcot's d., amyotrophic lateral *sclerosis.*
Charcot-Marie-Tooth d., peroneal muscular *atrophy.*
Charlouis' d., yaws.
Cheadle's d., infantile *scurvy.*
Chédiak-Higashi d., Chédiak-Steinbrinck-Higashi *syndrome.*
Chiari's d., Chiari's *syndrome.*
cholesterol ester storage d., a lipidosis due to deficiency of lysosomal acid lipase activity, resulting in accumulation of cholesterol esters in liver and adrenal glands with variable accumulation of triglycerides; autosomal recessive inheritance.
Christensen-Krabbe d., *poliodystrophia* cerebri progressiva infantalis.
Christian's d., **(1)** Hand-Schüller-Christian d.; **(2)** nodular nonsuppurative *panniculitis.*
Christmas d., *hemophilia* B.
chronic active liver d., chronic *hepatitis.*
chronic granulomatous d., granulomatous d.; congenital dysphagocytosis; a congenital defect in the killing of phagocytosed bacteria by polymorphonuclear leukocytes, resulting in increased susceptibility to severe infection; inheritance is usually by X-linked

transmission.
chronic hypertensive d., the chronic accumulative effects of long-standing high blood pressure on such vital organs as the heart, kidney, and brain.
chronic obstructive pulmonary d. (COPD), general term used for those diseases in which forced expiratory flow is slowed, especially when no etiologic or other more specific term can be applied.
chronic respiratory d. (CRD), a common and serious d. of the respiratory tract of chickens caused by *Mycoplasma gallinarum;* secondary infection with *Escherichia coli* is common.
circling d., listeriosis in sheep.
Civatte's d., *poikiloderma* of Civatte.
clover d., trifoliosis.
Coats' d., exudative *retinitis.*
Cockayne's d., Cockayne's *syndrome.*
cold hemagglutinin d., a condition associated with the presence of cold hemagglutinating autoantibody active *in vivo;* when the concentration of IgM antibody is high there may be increased serum viscosity, but clinical manifestations (due to hemagglutination) usually appear following exposure to cold; hemolysis usually is mild but may be severe, resulting in autoimmune hemolytic anemia, cold antibody type.
collagen d.'s, collagen-vascular d.'s, a group of generalized d.'s affecting connective tissue and frequently characterized by fibrinoid necrosis or vasculitis; in some collagen d.'s, auto-immunization, particularly antinuclear antibodies, has been shown and circulating immune complexes are found. The term is not entirely acceptable because there is no evidence that collagen is primarily involved; "collagen" was once synonymous with "connective tissue" rather than describing a specific fibrinous protein in that tissue. See also connective-tissue d.'s.
combined system d., subacute combined *degeneration* of the spinal cord.
communicable d., any d. that is transmissible by infection or contagion directly or through the agency of a vector.
Concato's d., polyserositis.
connective-tissue d.'s, a group of generalized d.'s affecting connective tissue, especially those not inherited as mendelian characteristics; rheumatic fever and rheumatoid arthritis were first proposed as such d.'s, and other so-called collagen d.'s have been added.
Conradi's d., chondrodystrophia congenita punctata; congenital shortening of the humerus and femur, with stippled epiphyses, high arched palate, cataracts, erythroderma in the newborn, and scaling followed by follicular atrophoderma; autosomal recessive inheritance, but may occur in either dominant or recessive forms.
constitutional d., obsolete term for a d. related to diathesis, disposition, or constitution, often inherited as an inborn error of structure or metabolism.
contagious d., an infectious d. transmissible by direct or indirect contact; now used synonymously with communicable d.
Cori's d., type 3 *glycogenosis.*
corn-meal d., see *Besnoitia tarandi.*
corridor d., a highly pathogenic disease of cape buffaloes (*Syncerus caffer*) and cattle in eastern and southern Africa caused by *Theileria parva lawrencei* and transmitted primarily by the tick *Rhipicephalus appendiculatus;* lesions and symptoms are similar to those of East Coast fever.
Corrigan's d., aortic *regurgitation.*
Cotunnius d., sciatica.
Cowden's d., multiple hamartoma syndrome; hypertrichosis and gingival fibromatosis from infancy, accompanied by postpubertal fibroadenomatous breast enlargement; papules of the face are characteristic of multiple trichilemmomas.
crazy chick d., nutritional *encephalomalacia* of chicks.
Creutzfeldt-Jakob d., Jakob-Creutzfeldt d.; a form of subacute spongiform encephalopathy caused by a slow virus, characterized by dementia, myoclonus, ataxia, and other neurologic disturbances, and which progresses rapidly to coma and death.
Crigler-Najjar d., Crigler-Najjar *syndrome.*
Crocq's d., acrocyanosis.
Crohn's d., regional *enteritis.*
Crouzon's d., craniofacial *dysostosis.*
Cruveilhier's d., progressive muscular *atrophy.*
Cruveilhier-Baumgarten d., Cruveilhier-Baumgarten *syndrome.*
Csillag's d., chronic atrophic and lichenoid dermatitis.
Curschmann's d., frosted *liver.*
Cushing's d., Cushing's syndrome associated with an ACTH-producing adenoma.
cystic d. of the breast, fibrocystic d. of the breasts.
cystic d. of renal medulla, microcystic d. of renal medulla; presence of small cysts in the renal medulla associated with anemia, sodium depletion, and chronic renal failure. It is of two types: 1) autosomal recessive or juvenile type (also called familial juvenile nephrophthisis), beginning at about age 10 with an average duration of 6 to 8 years; 2) autosomal dominant or adult type, beginning at about age 30 but with a more fulminant course.
cystine storage d., cystinosis.
cytomegalic inclusion d., inclusion body d.; cytomegalovirus disease; the presence of inclusion bodies within the cytoplasm and nuclei of enlarged cells of various organs of newborn infants dying with jaundice, hepatomegaly, splenomegaly, purpura, thrombocytopenia, and fever; the condition also occurs, at all ages, as a complication of other d.'s in which immune mechanisms are severely depressed, and has been found incidentally in salivary gland epithelium, apparently as a localized or mild infection (salivary gland virus d.).
cytomegalovirus d., cytomegalic inclusion d.
Daae's d., epidemic *pleurodynia.*
dancing d., procursive *chorea.*
Danielssen's d., Danielssen-Boeck d., anesthetic *leprosy.*
Darier's d., *keratosis* follicularis.
Darling's d., histoplasmosis.
Davies' d., endomyocardial *fibrosis.*
decompression d., decompression *sickness.*
deer-fly d., tularemia.
deficiency d., any d. resulting from undernutrition or an inadequacy of calories, proteins, essential amino acids, fatty acids, vitamins, or trace minerals.
degenerative joint d., osteoarthritis.
Degos' d., malignant atrophic *papulosis.*
Dejerine's d., Déjérine-Sottas d., hereditary hypertrophic *neuropathy.*
demyelinating d., one of a group of d.'s of unknown cause in which there is extensive loss of the myelin sheaths of nerve fibers, as in multiple sclerosis and Schilder's disease.
dense-deposit d., membranoproliferative *glomerulonephritis,* type 2.
de Quervain's d., radial styloid tendovaginitis; fibrosis of the sheath of a tendon of the thumb.
Dercum's d., *adiposis* dolorosa.
Deutschländer's d., (1) tumor of one of the metatarsal bones; (2) march *fracture.*
Devic's d., *neuromyelitis* optica.
diamond skin d., a form of swine erysipelas, caused by *Erysipelothrix rhusiopathiae,* in which rhomboidal erythematous areas appear on the skin.
Di Guglielmo's d., the acute form of erythremic myelosis.
disappearing bone d., Gorham's d.; extensive decalcification of a single bone; of unknown cause, sometimes associated with angioma.
dog d., phlebotomus *fever.*
dominantly inherited Lévi's d., snub-nose *dwarfism.*
Donohue's d., leprechaunism.

drug-induced d., a morbid condition resulting from the administration of a drug.
Dubini's d., electric *chorea* (1).
Dubois' d., Dubois' *abscesses.*
Duchenne's d., **(1)** pseudohypertrophic muscular *dystrophy;* **(2)** progressive bulbar *paralysis.*
Duchenne-Aran d., progressive muscular *atrophy.*
Duhring's d., *dermatitis* herpetiformis.
Dukes' d., fourth d.
Duncan's d., an X-linked recessive immunodeficiency and lymphoproliferative disease occurring in boys.
Duplay's d., subacromial *bursitis.*
Dupuytren's d. of the foot, plantar *fibromatosis.*
Duroziez' d., congenital stenosis of the mitral valve.
Dutton's d., Dutton's relapsing fever; African tick-borne relapsing fever caused by *Borrelia duttonii* and spread by the soft tick, *Ornithodoros moubata.*
dynamic d., functional *disorder.*
Eales' d., peripheral retinal periphlebitis causing recurrent retinal or intravitreous hemorrhages in young adults.
Ebstein's d., Ebstein's *anomaly.*
Eisenmenger's d., Eisenmenger's *complex.*
emotional d., see mental *illness.*
Engelmann's d., diaphysial *dysplasia.*
English d., obsolete term for rickets.
Epstein's d., diphtheroid (1).
Erb's d., progressive bulbar *paralysis.*
Erb-Charcot d., spastic *diplegia.*
Erdheim d., cystic medial *necrosis.*
Eulenburg's d., congenital *paramyotonia.*
exanthematous d., see exanthema.
extramammary Paget d., Paget's d. (3); an intraepidermal form of mucinous adenocarcinoma which may be secondary to an internal malignancy or occur as a carcinoma in situ, most commonly in the anogenital region.
extrapyramidal d., degenerative d. affecting the corpus striatum or other part of the extrapyramidal system, *e.g.,* parkinsonism, paralysis agitans, chorea, hepatolenticular degeneration.
Fabry's d., angiokeratoma corporis diffusum; glycolipid lipidosis; an X-linked recessive disorder due to deficiency of α-galactosidase and characterized by abnormal accumulations of neutral glycolipids in histiocytes in blood vessel walls, with angioperatomas on the thighs, buttocks, and genitalia, hypohidrosis, paresthesia in extremities, cornea verticillata, and spokelike posterior subcapsular cataracts; death results from renal, cardiac, or cerebrovascular complications.
Fahr's d., progressive calcific deposition in the walls of cerebral blood vessels, occasionally associated with mental retardation and extrapyramidal symptoms.
Farber's d., disseminated *lipogranulomatosis.*
Feer's d., Selter's d.; an affection marked by recurrent sweating, cyanosis of the extremities, motor weakness, tremor, rapid pulse, and insomnia.
femoropopliteal occlusive d., obstruction of the femoral and popliteal arteries by atherosclerosis.
Fenwick's d., idiopathic gastric atrophy. See atrophic *gastritis.*
fibrocystic d. of the breast, cystic hyperplasia of the breast; chronic cystic mastitis; mammary dysplasia; cystic d. of the breast; a benign d. common in women of the third, fourth, and fifth decades characterized by formation, in one or both breasts, of small cysts containing fluid which may appear as blue dome cysts; associated with stromal fibrosis and with variable degrees of intraductal epithelial hyperplasia and sclerosing adenosis.
fibrocystic d. of the pancreas, cystic *fibrosis.*
fifth d. [after scarlatina, morbilli, rubella, and fourth d.], *erythema* infectiosum.
Filatov's d., fourth d.
Flatau-Schilder d., adrenoleukodystrophy.
Flegel's d., *hyperkeratosis* lenticularis perstans.
flint d., chalicosis.
Folling's d., phenylketonuria.
foot-and-mouth d. (FMD), contagious aphthae; aphthous fever; aftosa; a highly infectious disease of wide distribution and great economic importance, occurring in cattle, swine, and sheep, caused by a picornavirus (genus *Rhinovirus*) and characterized by vesicular eruptions in the mouth, tongue, hoofs, and udder; man is rarely affected.
Forbes' d., type 3 *glycogenosis.*
Fordyce's d., Fordyce's *spots.*
Forrestier's d., diffuse idiopathic skeletal *hyperostosis.*
Fothergill's d., **(1)** trigeminal *neuralgia;* **(2)** anginose *scarlatina.*
Fournier's d., Fournier's gangrene; syphiloma of Fournier; infective gangrene involving the scrotum.
fourth d., Dukes' or Filatov's d.; scarlatinoid (2); scarlatinella; an exanthematous affection of childhood bearing a resemblance to scarlatina analogous to that of German measles to measles; it runs a mild course and the etilogy is unknown. Filatov subscribed to the existence of three primary specific fevers, scarlatina, morbilli, and rubella, and believed that there also was a scarlatiniform type of rubella which constituted a distinct febrile illness (fourth d.).
Fox-Fordyce d., apocrine miliaria; a rare chronic eruption of dry papules and distended ruptured apocrine glands, with follicular hyperkeratosis of the nipples, axillae, and pubic and sternal regions, and with intense pruritus.
Franklin's d., γ-heavy chain d.
Freiberg's d., epiphysial ischemic (aseptic) necrosis of second metatarsal head.
Friedmann's d., narcolepsy.
Friedreich's d., *myoclonus* multiplex.
Friend d., mouse leukemia caused by the Friend strain of virus.
Fuerstner's d., pseudospastic paralysis with tremor.
functional d., functional disorder.
fusospirochetal d., infection of the mouth and/or pharynx occurring in debilitated persons and associated with fusiform bacilli and spirochetes, commonly part of the normal flora of the mouth. See also necrotizing ulcerative *gingivitis.*
Gairdner's d., angor pectoris (1); angina pectoris sine dolore; attacks of cardiac distress accompanied by apprehension.
Gamna's d., a form of chronic splenomegaly characterized by conspicuous thickening of the capsule and the presence of multiple, small, rustlike, brown foci (Gamna-Gandy bodies), which contain iron; this condition may be observed in fibrocongestive splenomegaly, sickle cell d., and some examples of hemochromatosis.
Gandy-Nanta d., siderotic splenomegaly, probably the same as Gamna's d.
garapata d., tick fever occurring in Spain.
Garré's d., sclerosing *osteitis.*
gasping d., infectious avian *bronchitis.*
Gaucher's d., familial splenic anemia; cerebrosidosis; cerebroside lipidosis; a storage d. resulting from glycocerebroside accumulation in macrophages due to a genetic deficiency of glucocerebrosidase; may occur in adults but occurs most severely in infants, in whom cerebroside also accumulates in neurons; marked by hepatosplenomegaly, lymphadenopathy, and bone destruction by characteristic cells containing cytoplasmic tubules; autosomal recessive inheritance.
Gerhardt's d., erythromelalgia.
Gerlier's d., epidemic *vertigo.*
Gierke's d., type 1 *glycogenosis.*
Gilbert's d., familial nonhemolytic *jaundice.*
Gilchrist's d., blastomycosis.
Gilles de la Tourette's d., Gilles de la Tourette's *syndrome.*
Glanzmann's d., Glanzmann's *thrombasthenia.*
glycogen-storage d., glycogenosis.

Goldflam d., *myasthenia* gravis.
Gorham's d., disappearing bone d.
Gougerot and Blum d., pigmented purpuric lichenoid *dermatosis.*
Gougerot-Ruiter d., cutaneous *vasculitis.*
Gougerot-Sjögren d., Sjögren's *syndrome.*
Gowers d., **(1)** saltatory *spasm;* **(2)** a distal type of progressive muscular dystrophy.
Graefe's d., *ophthalmoplegia* progressiva.
graft versus host d., graft versus host reaction; GVH d.; a kind of incompatibility reaction (which may be fatal) in a subject (host) of low immunological competence (deficient lymphoid tissue) who has been the recipient of immunologically competent lymphoid tissue from a donor who lacks at least one antigen possessed by the recipient host; the reaction, or disease, is the result of action of the transplanted cells against those host tissues that possess the antigen not possessed by the donor.
granulomatous d., chronic granulomatous d.
Graves' d., Basedow's or Parry's d.; toxic goiter characterized by diffuse hyperplasia of the thyroid gland, a form of hyperthyroidism; exophthalmos is a common, but not invariable, concomitant.
greasy pig d., a generalized exudative epidermitis of young pigs, characterized by high mortality and thought to be caused by *Staphylococcus hyicus.*
Greenfield's d., former eponym for the late infantile form of metachromatic leukodystrophy.
Greenhow's d., parasitic *melanoderma.*
Griesinger's d., bilious typhoid of Griesinger, a severe form of louse-borne relapsing fever caused by *Borrelia recurrentis* and causing high fever, epistaxis, dyspnea, intense jaundice, purpura, and splenomegaly.
Grover's d., transient acantholytic *dermatosis.*
Guinon's d., Gilles de la Tourette's *syndrome.*
Gumboro d., infectious bursal d.
Günther's d., obsolete eponym for congenital erythropoietic *porphyria.*
GVH d., graft versus host d.
H d., Hartnup d.
Haff d. [*Haff,* an arm of the Baltic Sea in East Prussia], hemoglobinuria, muscular weakness, and pains in the limbs, occurring in persons living in the vicinity of the inlet, caused by arsenic poisoning from waste in a celluloid factory.
Haglund's d., Haglund's deformity; an abnormal prominence of the posterior superior lateral aspect of the os calcis, caused by a gait disorder.
Hailey and Hailey d., familial benign chronic *pemphigus.*
Hallervorden-Spatz d., see Hallervorden-Spatz, Hallervorden *syndrome.*
Hallopeau's d., **(1)** *pustulosis* palmaris et plantaris; **(2)** *pemphigus* vegetans (2).
Hamman's d., Hamman's *syndrome.*
Hammond's d., athetosis.
hand-foot-and-mouth d., an exanthematous eruption of small, pearl-gray vesicles of the fingers, toes, palms, and soles, accompanied by often painful vesicles and ulceration of the buccal mucous membrane and the tongue and by slight fever; the d. lasts 4 to 7 days, and is usually caused by *Enterovirus* coksackie type A-16, but others, including A-5, have been identified with this d.
Hand-Schüller-Christian d., Schüller's d. or syndrome; Christian's syndrome; Christian's disease (1); generalized histiocytosis of bones, especially the skull, with bone destruction by accumulation of Langerhans' cells and eosinophil leukocytes; may cause loosening and exfoliation of the teeth.
Hansen's d., leprosy (2).
Harada's d., Harada's *syndrome.*
hard pad d., a form of canine distemper characterized by hyperkeratosis of the foot pads and nose.
Hartnup d., H d.; Hartnup syndrome; a congenital metabolic disorder consisting of aminoaciduria due to a defect in renal tubular absorption of neutral α-amino acids and urinary excretion of tryptophan derivatives because defective intestinal absorption leads to bacterial degradation of unabsorbed tryptophan in the gut; characterized by a pellagra-like, light-sensitive skin rash with temporary cerebellar ataxia; autosomal recessive inheritance.
Hashimoto's d., Hashimoto's *thyroiditis.*
heavy chain d., a term used for a group of d.'s, the paraproteinemias, characterized by production of homogenous immunoglobulins or fragments, and associated with malignant disorders of the plasmacytic and lymphoid cell series. Three types have been recognized: γ-heavy-chain d., α-heavy-chain d., and μ-heavy-chain d.; each is diagnosed by the finding of the appropriate heavy-chain fragment in the serum, urine, or both.
α-heavy-chain d., the most common form of heavy-chain d., characterized by a finding in the serum of a protein reactive with antisera to α-chains by not light chains; clinical features include diarrhea, steatorrhea, and severe malabsorption.
γ-heavy-chain d., Franklin's d.; heavy-chain d. characterized by a finding in the serum and urine of a broad protein peak that is reactive with antisera to γ-chains and unreactive with antisera to light chains; common features include anemia, lymphocytosis, eosinophilia, thrombocytopenia, hyperuricemia, lymphadenopathy, and hepatosplenomegaly.
μ-heavy-chain d., the rarest form of heavy-chain d., primarily seen in patients with long-standing chronic lymphatic leukemia; diagnosis is made on immunoelectrophoresis by finding a component reactive with antisera to μ-chains but not to light chains.
Hebra's d., **(1)** *erythema* multiforme; **(2)** familial nonhemolytic *jaundice.*
Heck's d., focal epithelial *hyperplasia.*
Heerfordt's d., uveoparotid *fever.*
hemoglobin C d., the homozygous state of hemoglobin C.
hemoglobin H d., see *hemoglobin* H.
hemolytic d. of newborn, *erythroblastosis* fetalis.
hemorrhagic d. of deer, deer hemorrhagic *fever.*
hemorrhagic d. of the newborn, a syndrome characterized by spontaneous internal or external bleeding accompanied by hypoprothrombinemia, slightly decreased platelets, and markedly elevated bleeding and clotting times, usually occurring between the third and sixth days of life and effectively treated with vitamin K.
hepatolenticular d., hepatolenticular *degeneration.*
herring-worm d., anisakiasis.
Hers' d., type 6 *glycogenosis.*
hidebound d., scleroderma (usually applied to extensive involvement).
Hippel's d., Hippel-Lindau d., Lindau's d.
Hirschsprung's d., congenital *megacolon.*
Hjärre's d., coli granuloma; a granulomatous d. of the intestines and liver of chickens, due to coliform organisms.
Hodgkin's d., a d. marked by chronic enlargement of the lymph nodes, often local at the onset and later generalized, together with enlargement of the spleen and often of the liver, no pronounced leukocytosis, and commonly anemia and continuous or remittent (Pel-Ebstein) fever; considered to be a malignant neoplasm of lymphoid cells of uncertain origin (Reed-Sternberg cells), associated with inflammatory infiltration of lymphocytes and eosinophilic leukocytes and fibrosis; can be classified into lymphocytic predominant and nodular sclerosing types (with a better prognosis), mixed cellularity type, and lymphocytic depletion type (with the worst prognosis); a similar disease occurs in domestic cats.
Hodgson's d., dilation of the arch of the aorta associated with insufficiency of the aortic valve.
hoof-and-mouth d., an incorrect but often used term for foot-and-mouth d.
hookworm d., see ancylostomiasis; necatoriasis.
Hoppe-Goldflam d., *myasthenia* gravis.

Huntington's d., hereditary *chorea.*
Hurler's d., Hurler's *syndrome.*
Hutchinson-Gilford d., progeria.
hyaline membrane d. of the newborn, respiratory distress syndrome of the newborn; a d. seen especially in premature neonates with respiratory distress; characterized postmortem by atelectasis and alveolar ducts lined by an eosinophilic membrane; also associated with reduced amounts of lung surfactant.
hydatid d., infection of man, sheep, and most other herbivorous and omnivorous mammals with larvae of *Echinococcus.*
Hyde's d., *prurigo* nodularis.
Iceland d., epidemic *neuromyasthenia.*
I-cell d., *mucolipidosis* II.
idiopathic Bamberger-Marie d., acropachyderma.
immune complex d., immune complex disorder; an immunologic category of d.'s evoked by the deposition of antigen-antibody or antigen-antibody-complement complexes on cell surfaces, with subsequent involvement of breakdown products of complement, platelets, and polymorphonuclear leukocytes, and development of vasculitis; nephritis is common. Arthus phenomenon and serum sickness are classic examples, but many other disorders, including most of the connective tissue d.'s, may belong in this immunologic category; immune complex d.'s can also occur during a variety of d.'s of known etiology, such as subacute bacterial endocarditis.
immunoproliferative small intestinal d., Mediterranean lymphoma; diffuse lymphoplasmacytic infiltration of the proximal small bowel mucosa and mesenteric lymph nodes resulting in diarrhea, weight loss, abdominal pain, and clubbing of fingers and toes; seen in poor people in developing countries.
inclusion body d., cytomegalic inclusion d.
inclusion cell d., *mucolipidosis* II.
industrial d., a morbid condition resulting from exposure to an agent discharged by a commercial enterprise into the environment. *Cf.* occupational d.
infectious d., infective d., a d. resulting from the presence and activity of a microbial agent.
infectious bursal d., Gumboro d.; a highly contagious acute d. of chickens caused by an unclassified virus and characterized by whitish diarrhea, dehydration, prostration, and destruction of the bursa of Fabricius, compromising the bird's immune system.
interstitial d., a d. occurring chiefly in the connective-tissue framework of an organ, the parenchyma suffering secondarily.
iron-storage d., the storage of excess iron in the parenchyma of many organs, as in idiopathic hemochromatosis or transfusion hemosiderosis.
island d., tsutsugamushi d.
Itai-Itai d., a form of cadmium poisoning described in Japanese people, characterized by renal tubular dysfunction, osteomalacia, pseudofractures, and anemia, caused by ingestion of contaminated shellfish or other sources containing cadmium.
Jaffe-Lichtenstein d., fibrous *dysplasia* of bone.
Jakob-Creutzfeldt d., Creutzfeldt-Jakob d.
Jansky-Bielschowsky d., cerebral *sphingolipidosis,* early juvenile type.
Jembrana d. [*Jembrana,* county in Bali, Indonesia, where disease first recognized], a febrile d. of cattle thought to be caused by a rickettsia of the genus *Ehrlichia.*
Jensen's d., *retinochoroiditis* juxtapapillaris.
Johne's d., chronic dysentery of cattle; a d. occurring in cattle and sheep, usually manifested by thickening of the wall of the intestine, particularly of the ileum; caused by infection with *Mycobacterium paratuberculosis.*
jumper d., jumper d. of Maine, a nervous affliction found in isolated parts of the world characterized by sudden muscular contractions (producing jumps if the muscles of the legs are the ones affected). See also Gilles de la Tourette's *syndrome;* latah; miryachit; palmus (2).
Jüngling's d., *osteitis* tuberculosa multiplex cystica.
Kashin-Bek d., a form of generalized osteoarthrosis limited to areas of Asia, including the Urov river; believed to result from ingestion of wheat infected with the fungus *Fusarium sporotrichiella.*
Katayama d. [town in Japan where the d. is common], *schistosomiasis* japonica.
Kawasaki d., mucocutaneous lymph node *syndrome.*
Kienböck's d., lunatomalacia; osteolysis of the lunate bone following trauma to the wrist.
Kimmelstiel-Wilson d., Kimmelstiel-Wilson *syndrome.*
Kimura's d., angiolymphoid *hyperplasia* with eosinophilia.
kinky-hair d., Menkes syndrome; congenital metabolic defect manifested in short, sparse, poorly pigmented kinky hair; associated with failure to thrive, physical and mental retardation, and progressive severe deterioration of the brain; X-linked recessive inheritance.
Klippel's d., arthritic general *pseudoparalysis.*
Köhler's d., epiphysial aseptic necrosis of the tarsal navicular bone or of the patella.
Köhlmeier-Degos d., malignant atrophic *papulosis.*
Krabbe's d., former eponym for globoid cell *leukodystrophy.*
Kufs d., cerebral *sphingolipidosis,* adult type.
Kugelberg-Welander d., juvenile muscular *atrophy.*
Kuhnt-Junius d., Kuhnt-Junius *degeneration.*
Kussmaul's d., *polyarteritis* nodosa.
Kyasanur Forest d., a d. occurring among forest workers in the Kyasanur Forest and in Mysore, India, caused by a group B arbovirus (*Flavivirus*) transmitted chiefly by *Haemaphysalis spinigera,* although other ticks have been implicated as well; symptoms include fever, headache, back and limb pains, diarrhea, and intestinal bleeding; central nervous system symptoms do not occur.
Kyrle's d., *hyperkeratosis* follicularis et parafollicularis.
Lafora body d., Lafora's d., myoclonus epilepsy beginning at 11 to 18 years of age with progressive mental impairment; characterized by EEG focal posterior discharges and periodic acid-Schiff-positive inclusions in various tissues including brain and skin in which the inclusion bodies are found; death occurs within 10 years of onset.
Lane's d., *erythema* palmare hereditarium.
Larrey-Weil d., Weil's disease.
Lasègue's d., obsolete eponym for delusions of persecution.
laughing d., **(1)** a disabling state of hypnosis or narcosis induced by witch doctors and characterized by involuntary laughing; **(2)** the compulsive mirthless laughter of schizophrenics.
L-chain d., Bence Jones *myeloma.*
Legg-Calvé-Perthes, Legg-Perthes, or **Legg's d.,** epiphysial aseptic necrosis of the upper end of the femur. Also called pseudocoxalgia; coxa plana; osteochondritis deformans juvenilis; Perthes or Calvé-Perthes d.; quiet hip d.
Legionnaires' d. [American *Legion* convention, 1976, at which many delegates were so affected], legionellosis; an acute infectious d., caused by *Legionella pneumophila,* with prodromal influenza-like symptoms and a rapidly rising high fever, followed by severe pneumonia and production of usually nonpurulent sputum, mental confusion, hepatic fatty changes, and renal tubular degeneration.
Leigh's d., necrotizing *encephalomyelopathy.*
Leiner's d., *erythroderma* desquamativum.
Lenègre's d., Lenègre's *syndrome.*
Leri-Weill d., dyschondrosteosis.
Letterer-Siwe d., nonlipid *histiocytosis.*
Lev's d., Lev's *syndrome.*
Lewandowski-Lutz d., *epdermodysplasia* verruciformis.
Lhermitte-Duclos d., dysplastic hypertrophy of the cerebellum characterized clinically by signs and symptoms of increased intracranial pressure; usually seen in adults.
Lindau's d., (von) Hippel-Lindau or Hippel's d.; von Hippel-Lindau syndrome; retinocerebral angiomatosis; a type of phacomato-

sis, consisting of hemangiomas of the retina, which may be multiple and bilateral, associated with hemangiomas or hemangioblastomas primarily of the cerebellum and walls of the fourth ventricle, occasionally involving the spinal cord; sometimes associated with cysts or hamartomas of kidney, adrenal, or other organs; autosomal dominant inheritance.
linear IgA bullous d. in children, benign chronic bullous *dermatosis* of childhood.
Little's d., spastic *diplegia.*
Lobo's d., lobomycosis.
locoweed d., loco.
Löffler's d., Löffler's *endocarditis.*
Lorain's d., idiopathic *infantilism.*
Luft's d., a metabolic d. due to relative uncoupling of phosphorylation in skeletal muscle with myopathic syndromes and general hypermetabolism.
lumpy skin d., an infectious d. of cattle in Africa, manifested by an acute febrile illness followed by the appearance of lumps and plaques under the skin and on some of the mucous membranes; caused by a poxvirus related to the African sheep pox virus.
Lutz-Splendore-Almeida d., paracoccidioidomycosis.
Lyell's d., staphylococcal scalded skin *syndrome.*
Lyme d. [Lyme, CT, where first reported], an inflammatory disorder typically occurring during the summer months and caused by *Borrelia burgdorferi,* a non-pyogenic, penicillin-sensitive spirochete transmitted by *Ixodes dammini* in the eastern U.S. and *I. pacificus* in the western U.S.; the characteristic lesion, erythema chronicum migrans, usually is preceded or accompanied by fever, malaise, fatigue, headache, and stiff neck; neurologic or cardiac manifestations, or arthritis (Lyme arthritis) may occur weeks to months later.
lysosomal d., a d. due to inadequate functioning of a lysosomal enzyme; most such d.'s are associated with a storage d.
Machado-Joseph d., Azorean or Portuguese d.; a condition characterized by signs of spinocerebellar and extrapyramical disease associated with progressive external ophthalmoplegia, dystonia, and, often, peripheral amyotrophy; found predominately in people of Azorean ancestry; autosomal dominant inheritance.
Madelung's d., multiple symmetric *lipomatosis.*
Majocchi's d., *purpura* annularis telangiectodes.
Malherbe's d., pilomatrixoma.
Manson's d., *schistosomiasis* mansoni.
maple bark d., hypersensitivity pneumonitis caused by spores of *Cryptostroma corticale* growing under the bark of stacked maple logs.
maple syrup urine d., branched chain ketoaciduria or ketonuria; a disorder caused by deficient oxidative decarboxylation of α-keto acid metabolites of leucine, isoleucine, and valine which are present in blood and urine in elevated concentrations, the urine having an odor similar to that of maple syrup; neonatal death is common; survivors usually exhibit gross brain damage; autosomal recessive inheritance.
marble bone d., osteopetrosis.
Marburg virus d., human infection by Marburg virus, causing fever, diarrhea, a maculopapular rash, and disseminated intravascular coagulation with high mortality.
Marchiafava-Bignami d., a degenerative process involving the corpus callosum that occurs predominately in chronic alcoholics, particularly in wine drinkers.
Marek's d., avian *lymphomatosis* (2).
Marfan's d., Marfan's *syndrome.*
margarine d., a toxic multiform erythema caused by a substance used in the manufacture of margarine.
Marie-Strümpell d., ankylosing *spondylitis.*
Marion's d., a congenital obstruction of the posterior urethra.
Martin's d., a periosteoarthritis of the foot from excessive walking.
McArdle's d., McArdle-Schmid-Pearson d., type 5 *glycogenosis.*
Mediterranean-hemoglobin E d., thalassemia with hemoglobin E in the blood.
Meige's d., the congenital type of hereditary lymphedema with onset at about the age of puberty.
Ménétrièr's d., Ménétrièr's syndrome; hypertrophic gastritis; giant hypertrophy of the gastric mucosa; gastric mucosal hyperplasia, either mucoid or glandular; the latter type may be associated with the Zollinger-Ellison syndrome.
Ménière's d., Ménière's syndrome; endolymphatic hydrops; auditory or labyrinthine vertigo; an affection characterized clinically by vertigo, nausea, vomiting, tinnitus, and progressive deafness.
mental d., see mental *illness.*
Merzbacher-Pelizaeus d., Pelizaeus-Merzbacher d.
Meyenburg's d., relapsing *polychondritis.*
Meyer's d., adenoids.
mianeh d., Persian relapsing *fever.*
Mibelli's d., porokeratosis.
microcystic d. of renal medulla, cystic d. of renal medulla.
micrometastatic d., the condition of a patient who has had all clinically evident cancer removed, but who may be expected to have a recurrence from metastases that are too small to be apparent.
Mikulicz' d., benign swelling of the lacrimal, and usually also of the salivary glands in consequence of an infiltration of and replacement of the normal gland structure by lymphoid tissue. See also Mikulicz' *syndrome;* Sjögren's *syndrome.*
Milian's d., ninth-day *erythema.*
Milroy's d., Nonne-Milroy d.; the congenital type of hereditary lymphedema.
Milton's d., angioneurotic *edema.*
Minamata d., a toxic d., first described in the inhabitants of Minamata Bay, Japan, as the result of eating fish contaminated with mercury; characterized by peripheral paresthesis, dysarthria, ataxia, and the loss of peripheral vision, all of which may be severe and permanent, even resulting in death.
miner's d., **(1)** ancylostomiasis; **(2)** miner's *nystagmus.*
minimal-change d., lipoid *nephrosis.*
Mitchell's d., erythromelalgia.
mixed connective-tissue d., d. with overlapping features of various systemic connective-tissue d.'s and with serum antibodies to nuclear ribonucleoprotein.
Möbius d., ophthalmoplegic migraine or periodic oculomotor paralysis.
molecular d., a d. in which the manifestations are due to alterations in molecular structure and function.
Mondor's d., thrombophlebitis of the thoracoepigastric vein of the breast and chest wall.
Monge's d., chronic mountain *sickness.*
Morgagni's d., Adams-Stokes *syndrome.*
Morquio's d., Morquio-Ullrich d., Morquio's *syndrome.*
Morvan's d., syringomyelia.
Moschcowitz' d., thrombotic thrombocytopenic *purpura.*
motor neuron d., a general term including progressive muscular atrophy (infantile, juvenile, and adult), amyotrophic lateral sclerosis, progressive bulbar paralysis, and primary lateral sclerosis; frequently a familial d.
moyamoya d. [Jap. hazy], a cerebrovascular disorder occurring predominantly in Japanese, in which the vessels of the base of the brain become occluded and revascularized with a fine network of vessels; it occurs commonly in young children and is manifested by convulsions, hemiplegia, mental retardation, and subarachnoid hemorrhage; the diagnosis is made by the angiographic picture.
Mucha-Habermann d., *pityriasis* lichenoides et varioliformis acuta.
mucosal d., bovine virus *diarrhea.*
multicore d., nonprogressive congenital myopathy characterized

clinically by weakness of proximal muscles with multifocal degeneration of the muscle fibers, and pathologically by eccentric areas of decreased or absent oxidative enzyme activity.

Nairobi sheep d., a d. of sheep in east Africa caused by Nairobi sheep d. virus, transmitted by *Rhipicephalus appendiculatus,* and characterized by hemorrhagic gastroenteritis with high fever.

navicular d., navicularthritis; a common cause of lameness in horses, especially light racing animals; it is essentially a chronic osteitis of the navicular bone associated with bursitis and inflammation of the plantar aponeurosis; occurs most frequently in the forefeet and is believed to be due to damage from frequent and severe strain.

Neftel's d., paresthesia of the head and trunk, and extreme discomfort in any but the recumbent position.

Neumann's d., *pemphigus* vegetans (1).

neutral lipid storage d., Dorfman-Chanarin *syndrome.*

Newcastle d. [*Newcastle* upon Tyne, England, where first reported], Ranikhet d.; an acute febrile, and contagious d. of fowls resembling fowl plague, caused by a *Paramyxovirus* (Newcastle d. virus) and characterized by high infectivity and respiratory and nervous symptoms; it is readily transmissible to man, in whom it causes a severe but transient conjunctivitis.

Nicolas-Favre d., venereal *lymphogranuloma.*

Niemann-Pick d., sphingomyelin lipidosis; lipid histiocytosis with accumulation of phospholipid (sphingomyelin) in histiocytes in the liver, spleen, lymph nodes and bone marrow; cerebral involvement may occur at a late stage, with red macular spots less common than in Tay-Sachs d.; occurs most commonly in Jewish infants and leads to early death; a more benign form may occur rarely in adults; autosomal recessive inheritance.

nil d., lipoid *nephrosis.*

nodular d., oesophagostomiasis in herbivores and primates, characterized by nodules in the wall of the large intestine, cecum, and occasionally, the ileum; the nodules are filled with caseous material and result from host response to encystment of the larvae of *Oesophagostomum* species.

Nonne-Milroy d., Milroy's d.

Norrie's d., atrophia bulborum hereditaria; congenital bilateral masses of tissue arising from the retina or vitreous and resembling glioma (pseudoglioma), usually with atrophy of iris and development of cataract; X-linked recessive inheritance.

notifiable d., reportable d; a d. that, by statutory requirements, must be reported to the public health or veterinary authorities when the diagnosis is made because of its importance to human or animal health.

oasthouse urine d. [*oast,* kiln for drying hops, malt, or tobacco], an inherited metabolic defect in the absorption of methionine in which unabsorbed methionine is converted by intestinal bacteria to α-hydroxybutyric acid; characterized by diarrhea, tachypnea, and marked urinary excretion of α-hydroxybutyric acid (causing an odor like that of an oasthouse).

occupational d., a morbid condition resulting from exposure to an agent during the usual performance of one's occupation. *Cf.* industrial d.

Oguchi's d., congenital nonprogressive night blindness with yellow or gray coloration of fundus; after 2 or 3 hours in total darkness, normal color of fundus returns; autosomal recessive inheritance.

Ollier's d., enchondromatosis.

Oppenheim's d., *amyotonia* congenita.

organic d., a d. in which there are anatomical or pathophysiological changes in some bodily tissue or organ, in contrast to a functional disorder.

Ormond's d., idiopathic retroperitoneal *fibrosis.*

Osgood-Schlatter d., Schlatter's or Schlatter-Osgood d.; apophysitis tibialis adolescentium; epiphysial aseptic necrosis of the tibial tubercle.

Osler's d., **(1)** erythremia; **(2)** hereditary hemorrhagic *telangiectasia.*

Osler-Vaquez d., erythremia.

Otto's d., Otto pelvis; arthrokatadysis; protrusio acetabuli; a d. characterized by an inward bulging of the acetabulum into the pelvic cavity, accompanied by arthritis of the hip joints, usually due to rheumatoid arthritis.

Owren's d., parahemophilia; a congenital deficiency of factor V, resulting in prolongation of prothrombin time and coagulation time.

Paas' d., a familial, and perhaps hereditary, skeletal deformation marked by coxa valga, double patella, shortening of the middle and terminal phalanges of fingers and toes, deformities of the elbows, scoliosis, and spondylitis deformans of the lumbar vertebrae; all of these manifestations may be unilateral or bilateral.

Paget's d., **(1)** osteitis deformans; a generalized skeletal disease, frequently familial, of older persons in which bone resorption and formation are both increased, leading to thickening and softening of bones (*e.g.,* the skull), and bending of weight-bearing bones; **(2)** a d. of elderly women, characterized by an infiltrated, somewhat eczematous lesion surrounding and involving the nipple and areola, and associated with subjacent intraductal cancer of the breast and infiltration of the lower epidermis by malignant cells; **(3)** extramammary Paget d.

Panner's d., epiphysial aseptic necrosis of the capitellum of the humerus.

paper mill worker's d., extrinsic allergic alveolitis caused by moldy wood pulp containing spores of Alternaria fungi.

parasitic d., a d. due to the presence and vital activity of a parasite, or as a reaction to a parasite.

Parkinson's d., parkinsonism (1).

parrot d., psittacosis.

Parrot's d., **(1)** pseudoparalysis in infants, due to syphilitic osteochondritis; **(2)** achondroplasia; **(3)** marasmus.

Parry's d., Graves' d.

Pauzat's d., osteoplastic periostitis or fatigue fractures of the metatarsal bones, caused by excessive marching.

Pavy's d., cyclic or recurrent physiologic albuminuria.

Paxton's d., *trichomycosis* axillaris.

pearl-worker's d., inflammatory hypertrophy of the bones affecting grinders of mother-of-pearl.

Pel-Ebstein d., Pel-Ebstein *fever.*

Pelizaeus-Merzbacher d., Merzbacher-Pelizaeus d.; former eponym for an early infantile form of progressive familial leukodystrophy.

Pellegrini's d., Pellegrini-Stieda d., a calcific density in the medial collateral ligament and/or bony growth at the internal condyle of the femur.

pelvic inflammatory d. (PID), acute or chronic inflammation in the pelvic cavity, particularly, suppurative lesions of the female genital tract; *e.g.,* salpingitis and its complications.

periodic d., any condition or d. in which episodes tend to recur at regular intervals; many such cases are manifestations of familial Mediterranean fever; the cause of the periodicity is usually unknown.

perna d. [*per* chlor*na* phthalin], halogen or chloric acne occurring in workers in perchlornaphthalin.

Perthes d., Legg-Calvé-Perthes d.

Pette-Döring d., nodular *panencephalitis.*

Peyronie's d., van Buren's d.; penile fibromatosis; a d. of unknown cause in which there are plaques or strands of dense fibrous tissue surrounding the corpus cavernosum of the penis, causing deformity and painful erection; sometimes associated with Dupuytren's contracture.

Pick's d., **(1)** [F. Pick] Pick's syndrome; a form of multiple serositis (or polyserositis) characterized by chronic congestive hepatomegaly, persistent or recurrent ascites, sometimes recurrent pleural

effusion, peritonitis, and pleuritis, occurring in a patient with previous (or concurrent) hyalinizing pericarditis; **(2)** [A. Pick] Pick's *atrophy.*
pink d., acrodynia (2).
plaster of Paris d., atrophy of bone in a limb which has been encased for some time in a plaster of Paris splint.
Plummer's d., eponym sometimes applied to hyperthyroidism resulting from a nodular toxic goiter, usually not accompanied by exophthalmos.
polycystic d. of kidneys, polycystic *kidney.*
polycystic liver d., polycystic *liver.*
Pompe's d., type 2 *glycogenosis.*
Portuguese-Azorean d., Machado-Joseph d.
Posadas d., coccidioidomycosis.
Pott's d., tuberculous *spondylitis.*
Potter's d., Potter's *facies.*
poultry handler's d., extrinsic allergic alveolitis similar to bird-breeder's lung, caused by inhalation of particulate emanations from domesticated fowl such as chickens and turkeys.
pregnancy d. of sheep, lambing paralysis; lambing sickness; a highly fatal metabolic d. of well-nourished ewes in the late stages of pregnancy, especially in ewes carrying twin lambs; it is caused by carbohydrate depletion of the blood and tissues, and is characterized by hypoglycemia, ketonuria, fatty infiltration of the liver, rapid emaciation, coma, and a high death rate.
primary d., a d. that arises spontaneously and is not associated with or caused by a previous disease, injury, or event, but which may lead to a secondary d.
Pringle's d., *adenoma* sebaceum.
Profichet's d., obsolete eponym for *calcinosis* circumscripta.
pullorum d., diarrhea alba; white diarrhea; an infectious d. of chicks and other young birds caused by salmonellae which are carried in the ovaries of adult hens and appears in the eggs; in incubator-hatched birds, the d. usually involves the lungs and air sacs, but often spreads in flocks of young birds as an alimentary tract infection manifested by severe diarrhea followed by septicemia and death.
pulpy kidney d., enterotoxemia.
pulseless d., Takayasu's syndrome or disease; a progressive obliterative arteritis of the vessels arising from the arch of the aorta. See also aortic arch *syndrome.*
Purtscher's d., transient traumatic retinal angiopathy after compression injuries to body or cranial trauma; ocular fundi show large white patches associated with the retinal veins about the disk or macula, hemorrhages, and retinal edema.
quiet hip d., Legg-Calvé-Perthes d.
Quincke's d., angioneurotic *edema.*
Quinquaud's d., *folliculitis* decalvans.
rag-sorter's d., pulmonary *anthrax.*
Ranikhet d. [Ranikhet, town in northern India], Newcastle d.
Rayer's d., biliary *xanthomatosis.*
Raynaud's d., Raynaud's *syndrome.*
Recklinghausen's d., neurofibromatosis (1).
Recklinghausen's d. of bone, *osteitis* fibrosa cystica.
Refsum's d., Refsum's syndrome; heredopathia atactica polyneuritiformis; a rare degenerative disorder transmitted as an autosomal recessive trait and caused by an absence of phytanic acid α-hydroxylase; clinically characterized by retinitis pigmentosa, polyneuritis, deafness, nystagmus, and cerebellar signs.
Reiter's d., Reiter's *syndrome.*
Rendu-Osler-Weber d., hereditary hemorrhagic *telangiectasia.*
reportable d., notifiable d.
rhesus d., sensitization of the mother during pregnancy to Rh factor in fetal blood, leading to erythroblastosis fetalis.
rheumatic d., see rheumatism.
rheumatic heart d., d. of the heart resulting from rheumatic fever, chiefly manifested by abnormalities of the valves.
rheumatoid d., rheumatoid *arthritis,* referring particularly to nonarticular lesions such as subcutaneous nodules.
Riedel's d., Riedel's *thyroiditis.*
Riga-Fede d., ulceration of the lingual frenum in teething infants, related to abrasion of the tissue against the new central incisors.
Ritter's d., **(1)** staphylococcal scalded skin *syndrome;* **(2)** *icterus* neonatorum.
Robinson's d., hidrocystoma(s) occurring in the skin of the face, especially in the region of the eyes.
Robles' d., ocular *onchocerciasis.*
Roger's d., maladie de Roger; a congenital cardiac anomaly consisting of a small isolated defect of the interventricular septum.
Rokitansky's d., **(1)** acute yellow *atrophy* of the liver; **(2)** Chiari's *syndrome.*
Romberg's d., facial *hemiatrophy.*
Rosenbach's d., **(1)** Heberden's *nodes;* **(2)** erysipeloid.
Roth's d., *meralgia* paresthetica.
Roth-Bernhardt d., *meralgia* paresthetica.
Rougnon-Heberden d., *angina* pectoris.
Roussy-Lévy d., Roussy-Lévy syndrome; a type of cerebellar ataxia regularly associated with wasting of the calves and intrinsic muscles of the hands and with absent tendon reflexes; pes cavus and claw toes develop; autosomal dominant inheritance.
Rubarth's d., infectious canine *hepatitis.*
runt d., wasting d.; a graft versus host reaction in mice first observed following intravenous injection of allogeneic spleen cells into newly born animals.
Rust's d., spondylarthrocace (2); malum vertebrale suboccipitale; tuberculosis of the two upper cervical vertebrae and their articulations.
salivary gland virus d., see cytomegalic inclusion d.
salmon d., salmon *poisoning.*
Sandhoff's d., an infantile form of G_{M2} gangliosidosis characterized by a defect in the production of hexosaminidases A and B; it resembles Tay-Sachs disease, but occurs predominantly (if not entirely) in non-Jewish children.
sandworm d., an inflammatory eruption on the inner side of the sole, observed in certain parts of Australia, marked by a patch of erythema spreading in spirals, and disappearing spontaneously; probably a form of creeping eruption similar to larva migrans.
Schamberg's d., progressive pigmentary *dermatosis.*
Schaumberg's d., adrenoleukodystrophy.
Schenck's d., sporotrichosis.
Scheuermann's d., adolescent round back; juvenile kyphosis; osteochondritis deformans juvenilis dorsi; epiphysial aseptic necrosis of vertebral bodies.
Schilder's d., adrenoleukodystrophy.
Schlatter's d., Schlatter-Osgood d., Osgood-Schlatter d.
Scholz' d., former eponym for the juvenile form of metachromatic leukodystrophy.
Schönlein's d., Henoch-Schönlein *purpura.*
Schottmüller's d., paratyphoid *fever.*
Schüller's d., Hand-Schüller-Christian d.
sclerocystic d. of the ovary, polycystic ovary *syndrome.*
sea-blue histiocyte d., splenomegaly and mild thrombocytopenia, with histiocytes in the bone marrow which contain cytoplasmic granules that stain bright blue; sometimes familial.
secondary d., **(1)** a d. that follows and results from an earlier disease, injury, or event; **(2)** a wasting disorder that follows successful transplantation of bone marrow into a lethally irradiated host; frequently severe and usually associated with fever, anorexia, diarrhea, dermatitis, and desquamation. See also graft versus host d.
Seitelberger's d., infantile neuroaxonal *dystrophy.*
Selter's d., Feer's d.
Senear-Usher d., *pemphigus* erythematosus.
senile hip d., *malum* coxae senile.
serum d., serum *sickness.*

sexually transmitted d. (STD), see venereal d.
Shaver's d., bauxite *pneumoconiosis.*
shimamushi d. (shē-mă-mū'shē), tsutsugamushi d.
sickle cell d., sickle cell *anemia.*
sickle cell C d., a d. resulting from abnormal sickle-shaped erythrocytes (containing hemoglobin C and S) in response to a lowering of the partial pressure of oxygen; characterized by anemia, crises due to hemolysis or vascular occlusion, chronic leg ulcers and bone deformities, and infarcts of bone or of the spleen.
sickle cell-thalassemia d., microdrepanocytic *anemia.*
Siemerling-Creutzfeldt d., adrenoleukodystrophy.
silo-filler's d., a pulmonary lesion produced by oxides of nitrogen produced by fresh silage; in its acute form it may lead to death from pulmonary edema or may go on to a subacute or chronic proliferative pulmonary disease sometimes leading to chronic pulmonary invalidism.
Simmonds' d., hypophysial or pituitary cachexia; anterior pituitary insufficiency due to trauma, vascular lesions, or tumors; usually developing postpartum as a result of pituitary necrosis caused by ischemia during a hypotensive episode during delivery; characterized clinically by asthenia, loss of weight and body hair, arterial hypotension, and manifestations of thyroid, adrenal, and gonadal hypofunction.
Simons' d., progressive *lipodystrophy.*
sixth d., *exanthema* subitum.
sixth venereal d., venereal *lymphogranuloma.*
Sjögren's d., Sjögren's *syndrome.*
skinbound d., scleroderma (usually applied to extensive involvement).
slipped tendon d., a manganese-deficiency perosis in the young chick, which allows the tendons on the caudal aspect of the tarsus to displace medially and laterally, so that the chick squats and walks on the plantar surface of the limbs.
slow virus d., a d. that follows a slow, progressive course, such as visna and maedi of sheep, caused by viruses of the subfamily Lentivirinae (family Retroviridae), and subacute sclerosing panencephalitis, seemingly caused by the measles virus; spongiform encephalopathy and kuru of man, scrapie of sheep, and transmissible encephalopathy of mink may also belong in this group, but the respective etiologic agents have escaped definitive characterization.
Sneddon-Wilkinson d., subcorneal pustular *dermatosis.*
social d.'s, obsolete term used to designate venereal d.'s, especially gonorrhea and syphilis.
specific d., a d. produced by the action of a special pathogenic microorganism.
Spielmeyer-Sjögren d., cerebral *sphingolipidosis,* late juvenile type.
Spielmeyer-Stock d., retinal atrophy in amaurotic familial idiocy.
Spielmeyer-Vogt d., Vogt-Spielmeyer d.; cerebral *sphingolipidosis,* late juvenile type.
Stargardt's d., fundus flavimaculitus initiated with atrophic macular lesions.
Steele-Richardson-Olszewski d., Steele-Richardson-Olszewski *syndrome.*
Steinert's d., myotonic *dystrophy.*
Sticker's d., *erythema* infectiosum.
stiff lamb d., a muscular dystrophy occurring in young lambs fed on ewe's milk or on feed that is deficient in vitamin E or selenium, or both; see also white muscle d. of calves.
Still's d., a form of juvenile arthritis characterized by high fever and signs of systemic illness which can exist for months before the onset of arthritis.
Stokes-Adams d., Adams-Stokes *syndrome.*
stone-masons' d., silicosis.
storage d., accumulation of a specific substance within tissues, generally because of congenital deficiency of an enzyme necessary for further metabolism of the substance; *e.g.,* glycogen-storage d.'s.
Strümpell's d., **(1)** *spondylitis* deformans; **(2)** acute epidemic *leukoencephalitis.*
Strümpell-Marie d., ankylosing *spondylitis.*
Strümpell-Westphal d., pseudosclerosis (2).
Sturge's d., Sturge-Weber d., Sturge-Weber *syndrome.*
Stuttgart d., the uremic form of canine leptospirosis, usually caused by a leptospire.
Sulzberger-Garbe d., Sulzberger-Garbe syndrome; exudative discoid and lichenoid dermatitis; a type of disseminated lichenified eczema, associated with a variety of other cutaneous and systemic manifestations.
Sutton's d., **(1)** [R.L. Sutton], halo *nevus;* **(2)** [R.L. Sutton, Jr.], *aphthae* major.
Swediauer's d., Albert's d.
sweet clover d., a hemorrhagic d., due to dicumarol which causes marked reduction in prothrombin, occurring in cattle fed on sweet clover fodder, spoiled during curing.
Sweet's d., acute neutrophilic *dermatosis.*
Swift's d., acrodynia (2).
swine edema d., a clinical entity of unknown etiology but thought to be due to *Escherichia coli* toxins; it is characterized by edema of various parts of the body but particularly of the walls of the stomach and intestines.
swineherd's d., a leptospirosis caused by a leptospire occurring in those who attend swine or who are occupied in the slaughtering or processing of pork, and characterized by aches and pains throughout the body, fever, headache, dizziness, and nausea.
swine vesicular d., a contagious disease of swine caused by a porcine enterovirus of the family Picornaviridae, closely related to the human enterovirus Coxsackie B-5, and characterized by vesicular lesions and erosions of the epithelium of the mouth, nares, snout, and feet; human infections have been reported in laboratory workers.
Sydenham's d., Sydenham's *chorea.*
Sylvest's d., epidemic *pleurodynia.*
systemic autoimmune d.'s, a group of connective tissue (collagen) d.'s characterized by the presence of autoantibodies responsible for immunopathologically mediated tissue lesions; systemic lupus erythematosus in the prototype.
systemic febrile d.'s, undifferentiated type *fevers.*
Takahara's d., acatalasemia.
Takayasu's d., pulseless d.
Talma's d., *myotonia* acquisita.
Tangier d. [an island in the Chesapeake Bay, home of the family of first cases described], analphalipoproteinemia; familial high density lipoprotein deficiency; a heritable disorder of lipid metabolism characterized by almost complete absence from plasma of high density lipoproteins, and by storage of cholesterol esters in foam cells, tonsillar enlargement, an orange or yellow-gray color of the pharyngeal and rectal mucosa, hepatosplenomegaly, lymph node enlargement, corneal opacity, and peripheral neuropathy; autosomal recessive inheritance.
Taussig-Bing d., Taussig-Bing *syndrome.*
Tay's d., drusen.
Taylor's d., diffuse idiopathic cutaneous atrophy.
Tay-Sachs d., cerebral *sphingolipidosis,* infantile type.
Teschen d. [*Teschen,* Silisia], infectious porcine encephalomyelitis; an epizootic picornavirus (Teschen d. virus) infection of hogs resembling human poliomyelitis; it is characterized by stiffness, convulsions, paralysis, and prostration, and is widespread in Europe, with most serious losses occurring in Poland and Czechoslovakia.
Theiler's d., **(1)** mouse *encephalomyelitis;* **(2)** equine serum *hepatitis.*
third d., rubella.
Thomsen's d., *myotonia* congenita.
Thornwaldt's d., see Tornwaldt's d.

Thygeson's d., superficial punctate *keratitis.*
thyrocardiac d., heart d. resulting from hyperthyroidism.
Tommaselli's d., hemoglobinuria and pyrexia due to quinine intoxication.
Tornwaldt's d., Thornwaldt's d.; inflammation or obstruction of the pharyngeal bursa or an adenoid cleft with the formation of a cyst containing pus.
Tourette's d., Gilles de la Tourette's *syndrome.*
tsutsugamushi d. (sū'sū-gă-mū'shē) an acute infectious disease, caused by *Rickettsia tsutsugamushi* and transmitted by *Trombicula akamushi* and *T. deliensis,* that occurs in harvesters of hemp in some parts of Japan; characterized by fever, painful swelling of the lymphatic glands, a small blackish scab on the genitals, neck, or axilla, and an eruption of large dark red papules. Also called shimamushi, akamushi, or island d.; scrub, mite, or tropical typhus; tsutsugamushi, flood, Japanese river, kedani, inundation, or island fever.
tunnel d., ancylostomiasis.
Underwood's d., *sclerema* neonatorum.
Unna's d., seborrheic *dermatitis.*
Unverricht's d., myotonic and tonic-clonic seizures with progressive neurological and intellectual decline with age of onset between 8 and 13 years of age; autosomal recessive inheritance.
Urbach-Wiethe d., lipid *proteinosis.*
vagabond's d., parasitic *melanoderma.*
vagrant's d., parasitic *melanoderma.*
van Bogaert's d., former eponym for metachromatic *leukodystrophy.*
van Buren's d., Peyronie's d.
Vaquez' d., erythremia.
venereal d., any contagious d. acquired during sexual contact; *e.g.,* syphilis, gonorrhea, chancroid.
veno-occlusive d. of the liver, obliterating endophlebitis of small hepatic vein radicles, described in Jamaican children, associated with ingestion of toxic plant substances in bush tea; causes ascites which may progress to cirrhosis.
Vidal's d., *lichen* simplex.
Vincent's d., necrotizing ulcerative *gingivitis.*
Virchow's d., **(1)** acute congenital encephalitis; **(2)** *leontiasis* ossea.
virus X d., a term applied to a number of virus d.'s of obscure etiology, *e.g.,* Australian X d. (Murray Valley encephalitis).
Vogt-Spielmeyer d., Spielmeyer-Vogt d.
Voltolini's d., d. of the labyrinth, leading to deafmutism, in young children.
von Economo's d., encephalitis lethargica; epidemic encephalitis; polioencephalitis infectiva; the basis for postencephalic parkinsonism, suspected to be of viral origin.
von Gierke's d., type 1 *glycogenosis.*
von Hippel-Lindau d., Lindau's d.
von Meyenburg's d., relapsing *polychondritis.*
von Recklinghausen's d., neurofibromatosis.
von Willebrand's d., von Willebrand's syndrome; angiohemophilia; hereditary pseudohemophilia; constitutional thrombopathy (1); vascular hemophilia; a hemorrhagic diathesis characterized by tendency to bleed primarily from mucous membranes, prolonged bleeding time, normal platelet count, normal clot retraction, partial and variable deficiency of factor VIII, and possibly a morphologic defect of platelets; autosomal dominant inheritance with reduced penetrance and variable expressivity.
Voorhoeve's d., *osteopathia* striata.
Wagner's d., hyaloideoretinal *degeneration.*
Wardrop's d., *onychia* maligna.
wasting d., runt d.
Weber-Christian d., nodular nonsuppurative *panniculitis.*
Wegner's d., syphilitic *osteochondritis.*
Weil's d., Larrey-Weil d.; infectious icterus; infectious jaundice (1); leptospirosis caused by a leptospire and believed to be acquired by contact with the urine of infected rats; characterized clinically by fever, jaundice, muscular pains, conjunctival congestion, and albuminuria; agglutinins regularly appear in the serum.
Werdnig-Hoffmann d., infantile muscular *atrophy.*
Werlhof's d., idiopathic thrombocytopenic *purpura.*
Wernicke's d., Wernicke's *syndrome.*
Werther's d., *dermatitis* nodularis necrotica.
Wesselsbron d., Wesselsbron *fever.*
Westphal's d., pseudosclerosis (2).
Whipple's d., intestinal lipodystrophy; lipodystrophia intestinalis; lipophagia granulomatosis; a rare d. characterized by steatorrhea, frequently generalized lymphadenopathy, arthritis, fever, and cough; many "foamy" macrophages are found in the jejunal lamina propria; lymph nodes contain periodic acid-Schiff positive particles that appear bacilliform by electron microscopy.
white muscle d., a nutritional myopathy of young animals, manifested by stiffness and soreness; cardiac muscle damage is frequent, and affected muscles exhibit whitish, chalklike streaks, which are degenerated fibers; it is due to a deficiency of vitamin E or selenium, or both, and is seen most frequently in calves and lambs but has also been reported in other species.
white spot d., *morphea* guttata.
Wilkie's d., superior mesenteric artery *syndrome.*
Wilson's d., **(1)** [S.A.K. Wilson] hepatolenticular *degeneration;* **(2)** [Sir W.J.E. Wilson] exfoliative *dermatitis.*
Winiwarter-Buerger d., *thromboangiitis* obliterans.
Winkelman's d., progressive pallidal degeneration.
Winkler's d., *chondrodermatitis* nodularis chronica helicis.
Wohlfart-Kugelberg-Welander d., juvenile muscular *atrophy.*
Wolman's d., a lipidosis caused by deficiency of lysosomal acid lipase activity resulting in widespread accumulation of cholesterol esters and triglycerides in viscera with xanthomatosis, adrenal calcification, hepatosplenomegaly, foam cells in bone marrow and other tissues, and vacuolated lymphocytes in peripheral blood; autosomal recessive inheritance.
wool-sorters' d., pulmonary *anthrax.*
Woringer-Kolopp d., pagetoid reticulosis; a benign localized form of lymphoma with solitary or closely grouped cutaneous tumors consisting of epidermal infiltrations of mononuclear cells resembling those found in mycosis fungoides.
X d. of cattle, bovine *hyperkeratosis.*
yellow d., xanthochromia.
Ziehen-Oppenheim d., *dystonia* musculorum deformans.

disengagement (dis-en-gāj'ment) [Fr.]. **1.** The act of setting free or extricating; in childbirth, the emergence of the head from the vulva. **2.** Ascent of the presenting part from the pelvis after the inlet has been negotiated.

disequilibrium (dis-ē'kwi-lib'rē-ŭm). A disturbance or absence of equilibrium.
genetic d., a state in the genetic composition of a population which may be expected under selection to change toward an equilibrium or absorbing state.
linkage d., a state involving two loci in which the probability of a joint gamete is not equal to the product of the probabilities of the constituent genes.

disgerminoma (dis-jer-mi-nō'mă). Dysgerminoma.

dish. A shallow container, usually concave.
Petri d., a small, shallow, circular d. made of thin glass or clear plastic with a loosely fitting, overlapping cover used especially in microbiology for the cultivation of microorganisms on solid media; it is frequently referred to as a plate.
Stender d., a flat shallow vessel used in staining sections.

disharmony (dis-har'mō-nē). The state of being deranged or lacking

in orderliness.
occlusal d., **(1)** contacts of opposing occlusal surfaces of teeth which are not in harmony with other tooth contacts and with the anatomic and physiologic control of the mandible; **(2)** occlusions which do not coincide with their respective jaw relations. See also deflective occlusal *contact.*

disimpaction (dis′im-pak′shŭn). Separation of impaction in a fractured bone.

disinfect (dis-in-fekt′). To destroy pathogenic microorganisms in or on any substance or to inhibit their growth and vital activity.

disinfectant (dis-in-fek′tănt). **1.** Capable of destroying pathogenic microorganisms or inhibiting their growth activity. **2.** An agent that possesses this property.
complete d., a d. that kills both vegetative forms and spores.
incomplete d., a d. that kills only the vegetative forms, leaving the spores uninjured.

disinfection (dis-in-fek′shŭn). Destruction of pathogenic microorganisms or their toxins or vectors.

disinhibition (dis′in-hi-bish′ŭn). Inhibition of an inhibition; removal of an inhibitory effect by a stimulus, as when a conditioned reflex has undergone extinction; may be restored by some extraneous stimulus.

disinsection, disinsectization (dis-in-sek′shŭn, dis′in-sek-ti-zā′shŭn) [L. *dis-*, apart, + insect]. Freeing an area from insects.

disintegration (dis-in-tĕ-grā′shŭn). **1.** Loss or separation of the component parts of a substance, as in catabolism or decay. **2.** Disorganization of psychic processes.

disinvagination (dis′in-vaj-i-nā′shŭn). Relieving an invagination.

disjugate (dis′jū-gāt) [L. *dis-*, apart, + *jugatus,* yoked]. Not paired in action or joined together; the opposite of conjugate. See disjugate *movement.*

disjunction (dis-jŭnk′shŭn) [L. *dis-*, apart, + *junctura,* juncture]. Separation of pairs of chromosomes at the anaphase stage of cell division.

disk [L. *discus;* G. *diskos,* a quoit, disk]. **1.** Discus. **2.** In dentistry, a circular piece of thin paper or other material, coated with an abrasive substance, used for cutting and polishing teeth and fillings. **3.** Lamella (2).
A d.'s, A *bands.*
acromioclavicular d., *discus* articularis acromioclavicularis.
anisotropic d.'s, A *bands.*
articular d., *discus* articularis.
blastodermic d., the aggregation of blastomeres of a telolecithal ovum after cleavage has occurred.
blood d., platelet.
Bowman's d.'s, d.'s resulting from transverse segmentation of striated muscular fiber treated with weak acids, certain alkaline solutions, or freezing.
Burlew d., Burlew wheel; an abrasive-impregnated rubber wheel used in dentistry for polishing.
choked d., papilledema.
ciliary d., *orbiculus* ciliaris.
cone d.'s, membranous d.'s of flattened sacs about 140 Å thick that occur in the outer segment of cones of the retina.
cuttlefish d., a circle of paper or thin plastic coated with ground cuttlefish bone; used, when attached to a mandrel and rotated by a dental handpiece, for fine smoothing and finishing of dental materials and tooth.
diamond d., a steel d. with the cutting surface(s) covered with fine diamond chips, for use in a dental handpiece.
embryonic d., germinal d.
emery d.'s, d.'s of paper or other materials coated with emery powder used in surfacing teeth or fillings.
germinal d., germ d., embryonic d.; the point in a telolecithal ovum where the embryo begins to be formed.
H d., H *band.*
hair d., a richly innervated area of skin around a hair follicle, consisting of a thickened layer of epithelial cells in which ramify unmyelinated terminals of a single axon.
Hensen's d., H *band.*
herniated d., protruded or ruptured d.; protrusion of a degenerated or fragmented intervertebral d. into the intervertebral foramen compressing the nerve root or into the spinal canal compressing the cauda equina in the lumbar region and the spinal cord at higher levels.

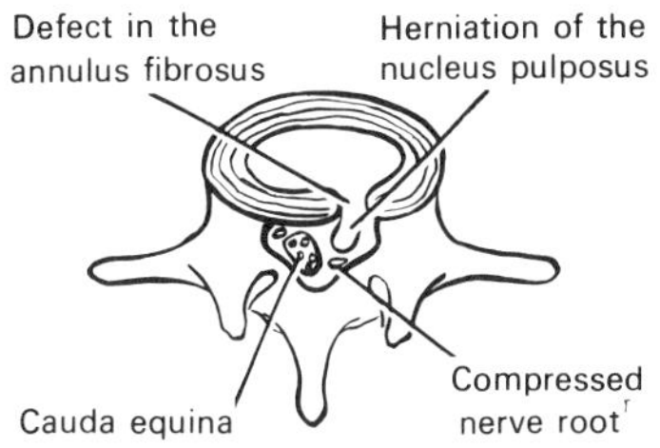

Herniated Disk
Horizontal section of posterolateral herniation of the intervertebral disk.

I d., I *band.*
intercalated d., a specialized intercellular attachment of cardiac muscle comprising gap junctions, fascia adherens, and occasionally desmosomes.
intermediate d., Z *line.*
interpubic d., *discus* interpubicus.
intervertebral d., *discus* intervertebralis.
isotropic d., I *band.*
mandibular d., *discus* articularis temporomandibularis.
Merkel's tactile d., *meniscus* tactus.
Newton's d., a d. on which are seven colored sectors, each occupying proportionally the same space as the corresponding primary color in the spectrum; when the disk is rapidly rotated it appears white.
optic d., *discus* nervi optici.
Placido's d., keratoscope.
proligerous d., *cumulus* oophorus.
protruded d., herniated d.
Q d.'s, A *bands.*
radioulnar d., radioulnar articular d., *discus* articularis radioulnaris.
Ranvier's d.'s, tactile nerve endings, of cupped disklike form, in the skin.
rod d.'s, membranous d.'s of flattened sacs about 140 Å thick that occur in the outer segment of rods of the retina.
ruptured d., herniated d.
sacrococcygeal d., a thin plate of fibrocartilage interposed between the sacrum and coccyx.
sandpaper d.'s, d.'s of paper coated with various grits of silica; used for surfacing teeth or dental materials.
stenopeic d., stenopaic d., a metallic or other opaque d. with a narrow slit through which one looks; used as a test for astigmatism.
sternoclavicular d., sternoclavicular articular d., *discus* articularis sternoclavicularis.
stroboscopic d., a revolving d. that gives successive views of a moving object.
tactile d., *meniscus* tactus.
temporomandibular articular d., *discus* articularis temporomandibularis.

transverse d., one of the dark transverse bands seen on examining a striated muscular fiber under the microscope.
triangular d. of wrist, *discus* articularis radioulnaris.
Z d., Z *line.*

diskitis (dis-kī'tis). Discitis.

disko-. See disco-.

dislocate (dis'lō-kāt). To luxate; to put out of joint.

dislocatio (dis-lō-kā'shē-ō) [L.]. Dislocation.
d. erec'ta, a subglenoid dislocation of the shoulder in which the arm is held vertically with the hand on top of the head; the head of the humerus is inferiorly placed.

dislocation (dis-lō-kā'shŭn) [L. *dislocatio,* fr. *dis-,* apart, + *locatio,* a placing]. Luxation; displacement of an organ or any part; specifically a disturbance or disarrangement of the normal relation of the bones entering into the formation of a joint.

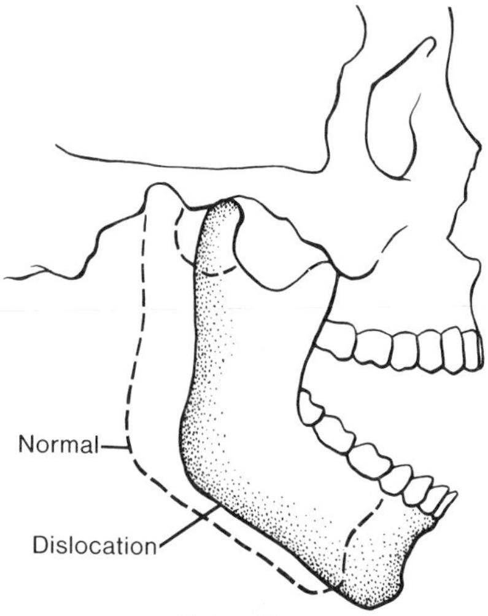

Dislocation

d. of articular processes, locked facets; complete d. of one or both articular processes, usually with overriding of the inferior articular process of the vertebra above into a position anterior to the superior articular process of the vertebra below.
closed d., simple d.; a d. not complicated by an external wound.
compound d., open d.
fracture d., dislocation associated with or accompanied by a fracture.
Kienböck's d., d. of semilunar bone.
Nélaton's d., wedging of the astragalus between the widely separated tibia and fibula, usually complicated with fracture.
open d., compound d.; a d. complicated by a wound opening from the surface down to the affected joint.
simple d., closed d.

dismember (dis-mem'ber). To amputate an arm or leg.

dismutase (dis'myū-tās). Generic name for enzymes catalyzing the reaction of two identical molecules to produce two molecules in differing states of oxidation (*e.g.,* superoxide dismutase) or of phosphorylation (*e.g.,* glucose 1-phosphate phosphodismutase).

dismutation (dis'myū-tā'shŭn). A reaction involving a single substance but producing two products; *e.g.,* two molecules of acetaldehyde may react, producing an oxidation product (acetic acid) and a reduction product (ethyl alcohol).

disomic (dī-sō'mik). Relating to disomy.

disomy (dī'sō-mē) [G. *dis,* two, + *sōma,* body]. The state of an individual or cell having two members of a pair of homologous chromosomes; the normal state in man, in contrast to monosomy and trisomy; can also apply to an abnormal chromosome represented twice in a single cell.

disopromine (di-sō-prō'mēn). Diisopromine.

disopyramide (dī-sō-pir'ă-mīd). α-[2-(Diisopropylamino)ethyl]-α-phenyl-2-pyridineacetamide; an antiarrhythmic drug.

disorder (dis-ōr'der). A disturbance of function, structure, or both, resulting from a genetic or embryologic failure in development or from exogenous factors such as poison, trauma or disease.
adjustment d.'s, a class of mental d.'s in which the development of symptoms is related to the presence of some environmental stressor.
affective d.'s, a class of mental d.'s characterized by a disturbance in mood.
antisocial personality d., a personality d. characterized by a history of continuous and chronic antisocial behavior with disregard for and violation of the rights of others, beginning before the age of 15; early childhood signs include chronic lying, stealing, fighting, and truancy; in adolescence there may be unusually early or aggressive sexual behavior, excessive drinking, and use of illicit drugs, such behavior continuing in adulthood.
attention deficit d., minimal brain dysfunction; a mental d., with onset in childhood, characterized by developmentally inappropriate inattention, impulsiveness, and varying hyperactivity.
autonomic d., disorganization of autonomic processes.
behavior d., general term used to denote mental illness or psychological dysfunction, specifically those mental, emotional, or behavioral subclasses for which organic correlates do not exist.
bipolar d., manic-depressive psychosis; an affective d. characterized by the occurrence of alternating periods of euphoria (mania) and depression.
borderline personality d., a mental d. in which the symptoms are not continually psychotic yet are not strictly neurotic: may include impulsivity and unpredictability, unstable interpersonal relationships, inappropriate or uncontrolled anger, identity disturbances, rapid shifts of mood, self-damaging behavior, chronic feelings of emptiness or boredom, and intolerance of being alone.
character d., a term referring to a group of behavioral d.'s, now replaced by a more general term, personality d., of which character d.'s are now a subclass.
conduct d., a mental d. of childhood or adolescence characterized by a pattern of conduct in which either the basic rights of others or the major age-appropriate societal norms or rules are violated.
conversion d., a mental d. in which an unconscious emotional conflict is expressed as an alteration or loss of physical functioning, usually controlled by the voluntary nervous system.
cyclothymic d., an affective d. characterized by mood swings including periods of hypomania and depression.
dysthymic d., a chronic disturbance of mood characterized by mild depression or loss of interest in usual activities.
emotional d., see mental *illness.*
functional d., functional disease or illness; dynamic disease; a physical d. with no known or detectable organic basis to explain the symptoms.
generalized anxiety d., anxiety neurosis or state; chronic, repeated episodes of anxiety reactions.
identity d., a mental d. of childhood or adolescence in which one suffers severe distress regarding one's ability to reconcile aspects of the self into a coherent acceptable sense of self.
immune complex d., immune complex *disease.*
immunoproliferative d.'s, d.'s in which there is a continuing proliferation of cells of the immunocyte complex associated with autoallergic disturbances and γ-globulin abnormalities such as in chronic lymphocytic leukemia, "macroglobulinemias," and multiple myeloma, with the implication that the etiologic factor concerned might be immunologic (allergic).

impulse control d., a class of mental d.'s characterized by an individual's failure to resist an impulse to perform some act harmful to himself or to others; includes pathological gambling, kleptomania, pyromania, intermittent and isolated explosive d.'s.
intermittent explosive d., a d. of impulse control characterized by several discrete episodes of loss of control of aggressive impulses which result in serious assault or destruction of property.
isolated explosive d., a d. of impulse control characterized by a single episode of failure to resist a violent, externally directed act which had serious impact on others.
mental d., a psychological syndrome or behavioral pattern that is associated with either subjective distress or objective impairment. See also mental *illness.*
neuropsychologic d., a disturbance of mental function due to trauma, associated with one of more of the following: psychotic, neurotic, behavioral, or psychophysiologic manifestations, or mental impairment. See also mental *illness.*
oppositional d., a mental d. of childhood or adolescence marked by a pattern of disobedient, negativistic, and provocative opposition to authority figures.
organic mental d., a psychological or behavioral abnormality associated with transient or permanent dysfunction of the brain, usually characterized by the presence of an organic mental *syndrome* (*q.v.*).
overanxious d., a mental d. of childhood or adolescence marked by excessive worrying and fearful behavior not related specifically to separation or due to recent stress.
panic d., recurrent panic attacks that occur unpredictably.
personality d., general term for a group of behavioral d.'s characterized by usually lifelong, ingrained, maladaptive patterns of deviant behavior, life style, and social adjustment that are different in quality from psychotic and neurotic symptoms; former designations for individuals with these personality d.'s were psychopath and sociopath. See also subentries under personality.
pervasive developmental d., a class of mental disorders of infancy, childhood, or adolescence characterized by distortions in the development of the multiple basic psychological functions involved in the development of social skills and language.
plasma iodoprotein d., see familial *goiter.*
posttraumatic stress d., development of characteristic symptoms following a psychologically traumatic event that is generally outside the range of usual human experience; symptoms include numbed responsiveness to environmental stimuli, a variety of autonomic and cognitive dysfunctions, and dysphoria.
psychogenic pain d., a d. in which the principal complaint is pain that is out of proportion to objective findings and that is related to psychological factors.
psychosomatic d., psychophysiologic d., a d. characterized by physical symptoms of psychic origin, usually involving a single organ system innervated by the autonomic nervous system; physiological and organic changes stem from a sustained disturbance.
schizophreniform d., a mental d. resembling schizophrenia, but having a duration of less than six months.
somatization d., a mental d. characterized by presentation of a complicated medical history and of physical symptoms referring to a variety of organ systems, but without a detectable or known organic basis.
somatoform d.'s, a group of mental d.'s characterized by presentation of physical symptoms which represent emotional conflicts or mental disorders; includes somatization d., conversion d., psychogenic pain d., and hypochondriasis.
substance abuse d.'s, a class of mental disorders in which behavioral and biological changes are associated with regular use of substances that affect the central nervous system.
thought process d., an intellectual function symptom of schizophrenia, manifested by irrelevance and incoherence of verbal productions ranging from simple blocking and mild circumstantiality to total loosening of associations.
visceral d., nomenclature used in reference to psychosomatic d.

disorganization (dis-ōr'gan-i-zā'shŭn). Destruction of an organ or tissue with consequent loss of function.

disorientation (dis'ōr-ē-en-tā'shŭn). Loss of the sense of familiarity with one's surroundings; loss of one's bearings.

disparate (dis'pa-răt) [L. *dis-paro,* pp. *-atus,* to separate, fr. *paro,* to prepare]. Unequal; not alike.

disparity (dis-par'i-tē) [L. *disparis,* dissimilar]. The condition of being disparate.
conjugate d., difference in the sizes of the retinal images in each eye, caused by asymmetrical convergence.
fixation d., the amount of heterophoria possible with fusion present.
retinal d., the slight difference in retinal images that arises because of the lateral separation of the two eyes that stimulates stereoscopic vision.

dispensary (dis-pen'ser-ē) [L. *dis-penso,* pp. *-atus,* to distribute by weight, fr. *penso,* to weigh]. **1.** A physician's office, especially the office of one who dispenses his own medicines. **2.** The office of a hospital pharmacist, where medicines are given out on the physicians' orders. **3.** An outpatient department of a hospital.

dispensatory (dis-pen'să-tō-rē) [L. *dispensator,* a manager, steward; see dispensary]. A work originally intended as a commentary on the Pharmacopeia, but now more of a supplement to that work which contains an account of the sources, mode of preparation, physiologic action, and therapeutic uses of most of the agents, official and nonofficial; used in the treatment of disease.

dispense (dis-pens'). To give out medicine and other necessities to the sick; to fill a medical prescription.

dispermy, dispermia (dī'sper-mē, dī-sperm'ē-ă). Entrance of two sperms into one ovum.

dispersal (dis-per'săl). Dispersion (1).
flash d., the property of rapid disintegration of a tablet when placed on the tongue.

disperse (dis-pers'). To dissipate, to cause disappearance of, to scatter, to dilute.

dispersion (dis-per'zhŭn) [L. *dispersio*]. **1.** Dispersal; the act of dispersing or of being dispersed. **2.** Incorporation of the particles of one substance into the mass of another, including solutions, suspensions, and colloidal dispersions (solutions). **3.** Specifically, what is usually called a colloidal *solution.*
coarse d., suspension (4).
colloidal d., colloidal *solution.*
molecular d., d. in which the dispersed phase consists of individual molecules; if the molecules are of less than colloidal size, the result is a true solution.
optical rotatory d. (ORD), the change in optical rotation with the wavelength of the incident monochromatic polarized light; the displacement of the former from zero within the absorption band is known as the Cotton *effect.*
temporal d., asynchronous repolarization of myocardial fibers that predisposes to abnormal current flow and ectopy (especially with bradyarrhythmias)

dispersity (dis-per'si-tē). The extent to which the dimensions of particles have been reduced in colloid formation.

dispersoid (dis-per'soyd). Dispersion colloid; molecular dispersed solution; a colloidal solution in which the dispersed phase can be concentrated by centrifugation.

dispireme (dī-spī'rēm) [G. *di-,* twice, + *speirēma,* coil, convolution]. The double chromatin skein in the telophase of mitosis.

displaceability (dis-plās-ă-bil'i-tē). The capability of, or susceptibility to, displacement.

tissue d., compression of tissue; the property of tissue that permits it to be moved from an initial or relaxed position or form.

displacement (dis-plās'ment). **1.** Removal from the normal location or position. **2.** The adding to a fluid (particularly a gas) in an open vessel one of greater density whereby the first is expelled. **3.** In chemistry, a change in which one element, radical, or molecule is replaced by another, or in which one element exchanges electric charges with another by reduction or oxidation. **4.** In psychiatry, the transfer of impulses from one expression to another, as from fighting to talking.
affect d., a shift of feeling from the object originally arousing it to some associated object.
mesial d., mesioplacement.
tissue d., the change in the form or position of tissues as a result of pressure.

Disse, Josef, German anatomist, 1852–1912. See D.'s *spaces.*

dissect (di-sekt', dī-) [L. *dis-seco,* pp. *-sectus,* to cut asunder]. **1.** To cut apart or separate the tissues of the body for study. **2.** In an operation, to separate the different structures along natural lines by dividing the connective tissue framework.

dissection (di-sek'shŭn, dī-). Anatomy (3); necrotomy (1); the act of dissecting.

disseminated (di-sem'i-nā-ted) [L. *dis-semino,* pp. *-atus,* to scatter seed, fr. *semen (-min-),* seed]. Widely scattered throughout an organ, tissue, or the body.

dissepiment (di-sep'i-ment) [L. *dis- sepio,* pp. *-septus,* to divide by a fence]. A separating tissue, partition, or septum.

dissimilation (di-sim-i-lā'shŭn). Disassimilation.

dissimulation (di-sim-yū-lā'shŭn). Concealment of the truth about a situation, especially about a state of health, as by a malingerer.

dissociation (di-sō-sē-ā'shŭn, -shē-ā'shŭn) [L. *dis-socio,* pp. *-atus,* to disjoin, separate, fr. *socius,* partner, ally]. **1.** Disassociation; separation, or a dissolution of relations. **2.** The change of a complex chemical compound into a simpler one by any lytic reaction or by ionization. **3.** An unconscious process by which a group of mental processes is separated from the rest of the thinking processes, resulting in an independent functioning of these processes and a loss of the usual relationships.
albuminocytologic d., increased protein in the cerebrospinal fluid without increase in cell count, characteristic of the Guillain-Barré syndrome; it is also associated with spinal block and with intracranial neoplasia, and is seen in the last phases of poliomyelitis.
atrial d., mutually independent beating of the two atria or of parts of the atria.
atrioventricular (A-V) d., **(1)** any situation in which atria and ventricles are activated and contract independently, as in complete A-V block; **(2)** interference d.; more specifically, the d. between atria and ventricles that results from slowing of the atrial pacemaker or acceleration of the ventricular pacemaker.
complete atrioventricular (A-V) d., **(1)** A-V d. not interrupted by ventricular captures; **(2)** complete A-V *block.*
electromechanical d., persistence of electrical activity in the heart without associated mechanical contraction; often a sign of cardiac rupture.
incomplete atrioventricular (A-V) d., A-V d. interrupted by ventricular captures.
interference d., d. with interference; A-V d. interrupted from time to time by ventricular captures.
isorhythmic d., A-V d. characterized by equal or closely similar atrial and ventricular rates.
longitudinal d., d. between parallel chambers of the heart, as between one atrium and the other or between one ventricle and the other, in contrast to d. between atria and ventricles.
sleep d., sleep *paralysis.*
syringomyelic d., loss of pain and temperature sensation with relative retention of tactile sensation, related to a cavity in the central portion of the cord interrupting the decussation of nerve fibers.
tabetic d., loss of sensation of proprioceptive type due to involvement of the posterior columns of the spinal cord.

dissolve (di-zolv) [L. *dis-solvo,* pp. *-solutus,* to loose asunder, to dissolve]. To change or cause to change from a solid to a dispersed form by immersion in a fluid of suitable properties.

dissonance (di'sō-nans) [L. *dissonus,* discordant, confused]. In social psychology and attitude theory, an aversive state which arises when an individual is aware of inconsistency or conflict within himself.

dissymmetry (di-sim'ĕ-trē) [dis- + symmetry]. Absence of symmetry.

distad (dis'tad). Toward the periphery; in a distal direction.

distal (dis'tăl) [L. *distalis*]. Distalis. **1.** Situated away from the center of the body, or from the point of origin; specifically applied to the extremity or distant part of a limb or organ. **2.** In dentistry, away from the median sagittal plane of the face, following the curvature of the dental arch.

distalis (dis-tā'lis) [NA]. Distal (1, 2).

distance (dis'tans) [L. *distantia,* fr. *di-sto,* to stand apart, be distant]. The measure of space between two objects.
focal d., the d. from the center of a lens to its focus.
infinite d., infinity; the limit of distant vision, the rays entering the eyes from an object at that point being practically parallel.
interarch d., interridge d.; interalveolar space; **(1)** the vertical d. between the maxillary and mandibular arches under conditions of vertical dimensions which must be specified; **(2)** the vertical d. between maxillary and mandibular ridges.
interocclusal d., interocclusal rest space; **(1)** the vertical d. between the opposing occlusal surfaces, assuming rest relation unless otherwise designated; **(2)** freeway *space.*
interridge d., interarch d.
large interarch d., open bite; a large d. between the maxillary and mandibular arches; may also imply an excessive vertical dimension.
pupillary d., the d. between the center of each pupil; the major reference points in measuring for fitting of spectacle frames and lenses.
reduced interarch d., closed bite; an occluding vertical dimension which results in an excessive interocclusal d. when the mandible is in rest position, and in a reduced interridge d. when the teeth are in contact.
small interarch d., close bite; a small d. between the maxillary and mandibular arches.
sociometric d., some measurable degree of mutual or social perception; hypothetically, greater sociometric d. is associated with more inaccuracy in evaluating a relationship.

distemper (dis-tem'per) [L. *dis-* priv. + *tempero,* to qualify, temper, fr. *tempus,* time]. **1. Canine d.,** a specific disease of young dogs that is highly contagious and highly fatal, caused by canine d. virus. **2. Feline d.,** panleukopenia.

distensibility (dis-ten-si-bil'i-tē) [L. *dis- tendo,* to stretch apart]. The capability of being distended or stretched.

distention, distension (dis-ten'shŭn) [L. *dis-tendere,* to stretch apart]. The act or state of being distended or stretched. See also dilation.

distichia, distichiasis (dis-tik'ē-ă; dis-ti-kī'ă-sis) [G. *di-,* double, + *stichos,* row]. A congenital, abnormal, accessory row of eyelashes.
acquired d., aberrant eyelashes arising from metaplasia of tarsal glands.

distill (dis-til'). To extract a substance by distillation.

distillate (dis'ti-lāt). The product of distillation.

distillation (dis-ti-lā'shŭn) [L. *de- (di-)stillo,* pp. *-atus,* to drop down]. Volatilization of a liquid by heat and subsequent condensation of the vapor; a means of separating the volatile from the nonvolatile, or the more volatile from the less volatile, part of a liquid mixture.

destructive d., dry d.

dry d., destructive d.; submission of an organic substance to heat in a closed vessel so that oxygen is absent and combustion prevented, with the objective of effecting its decomposition with release of volatile constituents and the formation of new substances.

fractional d., d. of a compound liquid at varying degrees of heat whereby the components of different boiling points are collected separately.

molecular d., d. in high vacuum, intended to make possible use of low temperatures to minimize damage to thermally labile molecules that would be decomposed by boiling at higher temperatures.

distobuccal (dis-tō-bŭk'kăl). Relating to the distal and buccal surfaces of a tooth; denoting the angle formed by their junction.

distobucco-occlusal (dis'tō-bŭk'ō-ō-klū'săl). Relating to the distal, buccal, and occlusal surfaces of a bicuspid or molar tooth; denoting especially the angle formed by the junction of these surfaces.

distobuccopulpal (dis'tō-bŭk'ō-pŭl'păl). Relating to the point (trihedral) angle formed by the junction of a distal, buccal, and pulpal wall of a cavity.

distocervical (dis-tō-ser'vi-kăl). Relating to the line angle formed by the junction of the distal and cervical (gingival) walls of a class V cavity.

distoclusal (dis-tō-klū'săl). Disto-occlusal. **1.** Relating to or characterized by distoclusion. **2.** Denoting a compound cavity or restoration involving the distal and occlusal surfaces of a tooth. **3.** Denoting the line angle formed by the distal and occlusal walls of a class V cavity.

distoclusion (dis-tō-klū'zhŭn). Distal occlusion (2); a malocclusion in which the mandibular arch articulates with the maxillary arch in a position distal to normal; in Angle's classification, a Class II malocclusion.

distogingival (dis-tō-jin'ji-văl). Relating to the junction of the distal surface with the gingival line of a tooth.

distoincisal (dis'tō-in-sī'zăl). Relating to the line (dihedral) angle formed by the junction of the distal and incisal walls of a class V cavity in an anterior tooth.

distolabial (dis-tō-lā'bē-ăl). Relating to the distal and labial surfaces of a tooth; denoting the angle formed by their junction.

distolabiopulpal (dis'tō-lā'bē-ō-pŭl'păl). Relating to the point (trihedral) angle formed by the junction of distal, labial and pulpal walls of the incisal part of a class IV (mesioincisal) cavity.

distolingual (dis-tō-ling'gwăl). Relating to the distal and lingual surfaces of a tooth; denoting the angle formed by their junction.

distolinguo-occlusal (dis'tō-ling'gwō-ō-klū'zăl). Relating to the distal, lingual, and occlusal surfaces of a bicuspid or molar tooth; denoting especially the angle formed by the junction of these surfaces.

Distoma (dis'tō-mă) [G. *di-*, two, + *stoma,* mouth]. Distomum; obsolete term for various digenetic flukes, now referred to other genera; *e.g., Fasciola, Fasciolopsis, Paragonimus, Opisthorchis, Clonorchis, Dicrocoelium, Heterophyes,* and *Schistosoma.*

distomiasis, distomatosis (dis'tō-mī'ă-sis, -mă-tō'sis). Presence in any of the organs or tissues of digenetic flukes formerly classified as Distoma or Distomum; in general, infection by any parasitic trematode or fluke.

hemic d., schistosomiasis.

pulmonary d., paragonimiasis.

distomolar (dis-tō-mō'lăr). A supernumerary tooth located in the region posterior to the third molar tooth.

Distomum (dis'tō-mŭm). Distoma.

disto-occlusal (dis'tō-ō-klū'săl). Distoclusal.

disto-occlusion (dis'tō-ō-klū'zhŭn). Distal *occlusion* (1).

distoplacement (dis'tō-plās-ment). Distoversion.

distopulpal (dis-tō-pŭl'păl). Relating to the line (dihedral) angle formed by the junction of the distal and pulpal walls of a cavity.

distortion (dis-tōr'shŭn). **1.** In psychiatry, a defense mechanism that helps to repress or disguise unacceptable thoughts. **2.** In dental impressions, the permanent deformation of the impression material after the registration of an imprint. **3.** A twisting out of normal shape or form.

parataxic d., an attitude toward another person based on a distorted evaluation of him, usually because of too close an identification of that person with emotionally significant figures in the patient's past life.

distoversion (dis'tō-ver-zhŭn). Distoplacement; malposition of a tooth distal to normal, in a posterior direction following the curvature of the dental arch.

distractibility (dis-trak-tĭ-bil'i-tē). A disorder of attention in which the mind is easily diverted by inconsequential occurrences; seen in mania.

distraction (dis-trak'shŭn) [L. *dis-traho,* pp. *-tractus,* to pull in different directions]. **1.** Difficulty or impossibility of concentration or fixation of the mind. **2.** Extension of a limb to separate bony fragments or joint surfaces.

distress (dis-tres') [L. *distringo,* to draw asunder]. Mental or physical suffering or anguish.

fetal d., any threatening or adverse condition of the fetus, caused by stress; some of the criteria for recognition of fetal d. are cardiac arrhythmia, bradycardia, tachycardia, passage of meconium.

distribution (dis-tri-byū'shŭn) [L. *dis-tribuo,* pp. *-tributus,* to distribute, fr. *tribus,* a tribe]. **1.** The passage of the branches of arteries or nerves to the tissues and organs. **2.** The area in which the branches of an artery or a nerve terminate, or the area supplied by such an artery or nerve. **3.** The relative numbers of individuals in various categories or populations.

binomial d., a d. obtained by expansion of the binomial $(q + p)^n$, where p is the probability of an event occurring in one of two possible ways, q is the alternative probability, and n is the number of occurrences.

countercurrent d., a method of separation of two or more substances by repeated distribution between two immiscible liquid phases that move past each other in opposite directions; a form of liquid-liquid chromatography.

epidemiological d., see histogram.

exponential d., the time until failure of a process at constant hazard.

frequency d., a statistical description of raw data in terms of the number or frequency of items characterized by each of a series or range of values of a continuous variable.

gaussian d., normal d.

normal d., gaussian d. or curve; a specific bell-shaped frequency d. commonly assumed by statisticians to represent the infinite population of measurements from which a sample has been drawn; characterized by two parameters, the mean (x) and the standard deviation (σ), in the equation:

$$y = \frac{1}{\sigma\sqrt{2\pi}}\, e^{-\frac{(x-\bar{x})^2}{2\sigma^2}}$$

Poisson d., a discontinuous d. important in statistical work and defined by the equation $p(x) = e^{-\mu}\mu^x/x!$, where e is the base of natural logarithms, x is the sequence of integers, μ is the mean, and *x*! represents the factorial of *x*.

districhiasis (dis-tri-kī'ă-sis) [G. *dis*, double, + *thrix* (*trich-*), hair]. Growth of two hairs in a single follicle.

distrix (dis'triks) [G. *dis*, twice, + *thrix*, hair]. Splitting of the hairs at their ends.

disturbance (dis-ter'bans). Deviation from, interruption of, or interference with a normal state.
emotional d., mental d., see mental *illness*.
psychographic d.'s, obsolete term for the use of a bombastic and inflated style as a symptom of a psychiatric disorder.

disulfamide (dī-sul'fă-mīd). 5-Chlorotoluene-2,4-disulfonamide; a diuretic.

disulfate (dī-sŭl'fāt). A molecule containing two sulfates.

disulfide (dī-sŭl'fīd). **1.** A molecule containing two atoms of sulfur to one of the reference element, *e.g.*, CS_2, carbon disulfide. **2.** A compound containing the –S–S–group, *e.g.*, cystine.

disulfiram (dī-sŭl'fi-ram). Tetraethylthiuram disulfide; bis(diethylthiocarbamyl)disulfide; an antioxidant that interferes with the normal metabolic degradation of alcohol in the body, resulting in increased acetaldehyde concentrations in blood and tissues. Used in the treatment of chronic alcoholism; when a small quantity of alcohol is consumed an unpleasant reaction results. Also used as a chelator in copper and nickel poisoning.

diterpenes (dī-ter'pēnz). Hydrocarbons or their derivatives containing 4 isoprene units, hence containing 20 carbon atoms and 4 branched methyl groups; *e.g.*, vitamin A, retinene.

dithiazanine iodide (dī-thī-az'ă-nēn). 3-Ethyl-2-[5-(3-ethyl-2(3*H*)-benzothiazolylidene)-1,3-pentadienyl]benzothiazolium iodide; a broad spectrum anthelmintic, effective against *Strongyloides*.

dithranol (dith'ră-nol). Anthralin.

Dittrich, Franz, German pathologist, 1815–1859. See D.'s *plugs*, *stenosis*.

diuresis (dī-yū-rē'sis) [G. *dia*, throughout, completely, + *ourēsis*, urination]. Excretion of urine; commonly denotes production of unusually large volumes of urine.
alcohol d., d. following the ingestion of alcoholic beverages; due, in part, to inhibition of the output of antidiuretic hormone by the neurohypophysis.
osmotic d., d. due to a high concentration of osmotically active substances in the renal tubules (*e.g.*, urea, sodium sulfate), which limit the reabsorption of water.
water d., d. following the drinking of water; due to reduced secretion of the antidiuretic hormone of the neurohypophysis in response to the lowered osmotic pressure of the blood.

diuretic (dī-yū-ret'ik). **1.** Promoting the excretion of urine. **2.** An agent that increases the amount of urine excreted.
cardiac d., a d. which acts by increasing function of the heart, and thereby improves renal perfusion.
direct d., a d. whose primary effect is on renal tubular function.
indirect d., a d. that acts by increasing cardiac function or by increasing the state of hydration.
loop d., a class of d. agents that act by inhibiting reabsorption of sodium and chloride, not only in the proximal and distal tubules but also in Henle's loop.

diurnal (dī-er'năl) [L. *diurnus*, of the day]. **1.** Pertaining to the daylight hours; opposite of nocturnal. **2.** Repeating once each 24 hours, *e.g.*, a d. variation or a d. rhythm. *Cf.* circadian.

diurnule (dī-er'nūl) [L. *diurnus*, daily, fr. *dies*, day]. A pill, tablet, or capsule containing the maximum daily dose of a drug.

divagation (dī-vă-gā'shŭn) [L. *divagare*, to wander about]. Rarely used term for rambling speech or thought.

divalence, divalency (dī-vā'lens, dī-vā'len-sē). Bivalence.

divalent (dī-vā'lent, div'ă-). Bivalent (1).

divalproex sodium (dī-val'prō-eks). Pentanoic acid, 2-propyl-, sodium salt (2:1); an anticonvulsant used in petit mal and related seizure disorders.

divarication (dī'var-i-kā'shŭn) [L. *divaricare*, to spread asunder]. Diastasis (1).

divergence (dī-ver'jens) [L. *di-*, apart, + *vergo*, to incline]. **1.** A moving or spreading apart or in different directions. **2.** The spreading of branches of the neuron to form synapses with several other neurons.

divergent (dī-ver'jent). Moving in different directions; radiating.

diverticula (dī-ver-tik'yū-lă). Plural of diverticulum.

diverticular (dī-ver-tik'yū-lăr). Relating to a diverticulum.

diverticulectomy (dī'ver-tik-yū-lek'tō-mē). Excision of a diverticulum.

diverticulitis (dī'ver-tik-yū-lī'tis). Inflammation of a diverticulum, especially of the small pockets in the wall of the colon which fill with stagnant fecal material and become inflamed; rarely, they may cause obstruction, perforation, or bleeding.

diverticuloma (dī'ver-tik-yū-lō'mă) [diverticulum + G. *-oma*, tumor]. Development of a granulomatous mass in the wall of the colon.

diverticulopexy (dī-ver-tik'yū-lō-pek-sē) [diverticulum + G. *pēxis*, fixation]. A plastic operation to obliterate a diverticulum.

diverticulosis (dī'ver-tik-yū-lō'sis). Presence of a number of diverticula of the intestine, common in middle age; the lesions are acquired pulsion diverticula.

diverticulum, pl. **diverticula** (dī-ver-tik'yū-lŭm, yū-lă) [L. *deverticulum* (or *di-*), a by-road, fr. *de-verto*, to turn aside] [NA]. A pouch or sac opening from a tubular or saccular organ, such as the gut or bladder.
allantoenteric d., allantoic d.
allantoic d., allantoenteric d.; an endodermally lined outpouching of the hindgut (in humans, the yolk sac of a very young embryo); in most amniotes, the primordium of the allantois later grows into the extraembryonic celom; in humans, the distal part of the allantoic lumen is rudimentary, not extending beyond the body stalk.
diverticula ampul'lae duc'tus deferen'tis [NA], diverticula of the ampulla of the ductus deferens; the irregular sacculations of the ampullary part of the ductus deferens near its termination in the ejaculatory duct.
cervical d., a d. in the neck derived from retention of part of one of the pharyngeal pouches (endodermal) or branchial grooves (ectodermal) of the embryo.
duodenal d., a d. of the duodenum, often of large size, that is occasionally found projecting from the duodenum near the duodenal papilla.
epiphrenic d., a d. which originates just above the cardioesophageal junction and usually protrudes to the right side of the lower meadiastinum.
false d., a d. of the intestine that passes through a defect in the muscular wall of the gut and thus does not include a layer of muscle in its wall.
Heister's d., see *bulbus* venae jugularis superior.
hypopharyngeal d., pharyngoesophageal d.
Meckel's d., the remains of the yolk stalk of the embryo, which, when persisting abnormally as a blind sac or pouch in the adult, is located on the ileum a short distance above the cecum; it may be attached to the umbilicus and, if the lining includes gastric mucosa, peptic ulceration and bleeding may result.
metanephric d., an outgrowth from the caudal portion of the mesonephric duct on either side, which grows cephalodorsally to make contact with the masses of metanephrogenous tissue giving rise to the tubules of the permanent kidney; it gives rise to the epi-

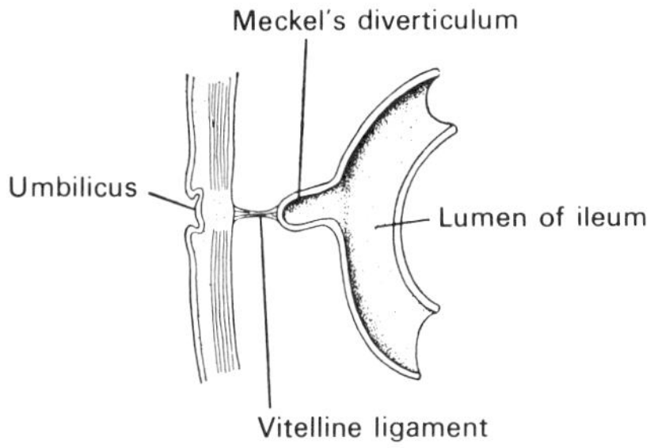

Meckel's Diverticulum
Combined with fibrous cord (vitelline ligament).

thelial lining of the ureter, the pelvis, and the collecting tubules of the kidney.
Nuck's d., *processus* vaginalis peritonei.
pancreatic diverticula, the ventral and dorsal endodermal buds from the embryonic foregut which constitute the primordia of the parenchyma of the pancreas.
Pertik's d., an abnormally deep recessus pharyngeus.
pharyngoesophageal d., hypopharyngeal d.; Zenker's d.; most common d. of the esophagus, arises between the inferior pharyngeal constrictor and the crico-pharyngeus muscles.
pituitary d., Rathke's d., pocket, or pouch; craniopharyngeal canal; hypophyseal pouch; a tubular outgrowth of ectoderm from the stomodeum of the embryo; it grows dorsad toward the infundibular process of the diencephalon, around which it forms a cup-like mass, giving rise to the pars distalis and pars juxtaneuralis of the hypophysis.
pulsion d., a d. formed by pressure from within, frequently causing herniation of mucosa through the muscularis.
Rathke's d., pituitary d.
thyroid d., thyroglossal d., the endodermal bud from the floor of the embryonic pharynx; the primordium of the parenchyma of the thyroid gland.
traction d., a d. formed by the pulling force of contracting bands of adhesion, occurring mainly in the esophagus, from tuberculous hilar or mediastinal lymphadenitis.
true d., a term denoting a d. that includes all the layers of the wall from which it protrudes.
urethral d., a sac-like outpouching of the urethral wall, either from a congenital defect or, more commonly, as a result of chronic penetrating inflammation.
ventricular d., a congenital outpouching of the right or left ventricle.
vesical d., cystodiverticulum; a d. of the bladder wall; may be either true or false type.
Zenker's d., pharyngoesophageal d.

divicine (dī-vis-ēn). A base with alkaloidal properties present in *Lathyrus sativus* which is responsible, in part at least, for the latter's poisonous action. See lathyrism.

div. in p. aeq. Abbreviation for L. *divide in partes aequales,* divide into equal parts.

divinyl ether (dī-vī'nil). Vinyl ether; $O(CH{=}CH_2)_2$; a volatile liquid, the vapor of which produces rapid induction of general anesthesia; prolonged administration is associated with adverse side effects on the liver and central nervous system.

division (di-vizh'ŭn). A separating into two or more parts.
anterior primary d., *ramus* ventralis nervi spinalis.
cleavage d., the rapid mitotic d. of the zygote with decrease in size of individual cells or blastomeres and the formation of a morula. See also cleavage (1).
conjugate d., simultaneous d. of haploid nuclei, as in Basidiomycetes.
direct nuclear d., amitosis.
equation d., nuclear d. in which each chromosome divides equally.
indirect nuclear d., mitosis.
meiotic d., meiosis.
mitotic d., mitosis.
multiplicative d., reproduction by simultaneous d. of a mother cell into a number of daughter cells. If the process occurs without fertilization of the mother cell, or encystment, the daughter cells are called merozoites; if they develop within a cyst, and usually after fertilization, they are called sporozoites.
posterior primary d., *ramus* dorsalis nervi spinalis.
reduction d., see *reduction* of chromosomes.
Remak's nuclear d., amitosis.

divulse (di-vŭls') [L. *di-vello,* pp. *-vulvus,* to pull apart]. To tear away or apart.

divulsion (di-vŭl'shŭn). **1.** Removal of a part by tearing. **2.** Forcible dilation of the walls of a cavity or canal.

divulsor (di-vŭl'sĕr, -sōr). An instrument for forcible dilation of the urethra or other canal or cavity.

dixyrazine (dī-zir'ă-zēn). 2-{2-[4-(2-Methyl-3(10*H*- Phenothiazin-10-yl)propyl)-1-piperazinyl]ethoxy}ethanol; a phenothiazine compound used as an antipsychotic.

dizygotic, dizygous (dī'zī-got'ik, dī-zī'gŭs) [G. *di-*, two, + *zygotos,* yoked together]. Relating to twins derived from two separate zygotes.

dizziness (diz'i-nes) [A. S. *dyzig,* foolish]. Imprecise term commonly used by patients in an attempt to describe various peculiar subjective symptoms such as faintness, giddiness, light-headedness, or unsteadiness. See also vertigo.

djenkolic acid (jeng-kol'ik) [*djenkol,* bean in which first isolated]. *S,S'*-Methylenebiscysteine; $CH_2[S{-}CH_2CH(NH_2)COOH]_2$; a sulfur-containing amino acid, resembling cystine but with a methylene bridge between the two sulfur atoms.

DL-. Prefix (in small capital letters) denoting a substance consisting of equal quantities of the two enantiomorphs, D and L; replaces the older *dl-* (in lower case italics) as a more exact definition of structure.

dM Symbol for decimorgan.

DMC Abbreviation for *p,p'*-dichlorodiphenyl methyl carbinol.

D.M.D. Abbreviation for Doctor of Dental Medicine.

dmf, DMF Abbreviation for decayed, missing, and filled. See under index.

dmfs, DMFS Abbreviation for decayed, missing, and filled surfaces. See under index.

DMPP Abbreviation for dimethylphenylpiperazinium.

DMSO Abbreviation for dimethyl sulfoxide.

DMT Abbreviation for dimethyltryptamine.

DN Abbreviation for dibucaine number.

DNA Abbreviation for deoxyribonucleic acid. For terms bearing this abbreviation, see subentries under deoxyribonucleic acid.

DNAse, DNAase, DNase Abbreviations for deoxyribonuclease.

DNP **1.** Dnp; abbreviation for 2,4-dinitrophenol. **2.** Abbreviation for deoxyribonucleoprotein.

Dnp DNP (1).

DNR Abbreviation for "do not resuscitate."

Dns, DNS Abbreviations for dansyl.

D.O. Abbreviation for Doctor of Osteopathy.

DOA Abbreviation for dead on admission (arrival).

dobutamine (dō-byū'tă-mēn). (±)-4-[2-[[(3-(*p*- Hydroxyphenyl)-1-methylpropyl]amino]ethyl]pyrocatechol hydrochloride; a synthetic derivative of dopamine characterized by prominent inotropic but weak chronotropic and arrhythmogenic properties; a cardiotonic agent.

DOC Abbreviation for deoxycorticosterone; deoxycholate.

d'Ocagne, Philbert M., French mathematician, 1862–1938. See d'O. *nomogram.*

dock (dok). **1.** The amputation of a part of the tail of horses, sheep, or dogs. **2.** The base of the tail left after docking.

docosanoic acid (dō'kō-san-ō'ik). Behenic acid.

doctor (dok'ter) [L. a teacher, fr. *doceo,* pp. *doctus,* to teach]. **1.** A title conferred by a university on one who has followed a prescribed course of study, or given as a title of distinction; as d. of medicine, laws, philosophy, etc. **2.** A physician, especially one upon whom has been conferred the degree of M.D. by a university or medical school.

doctrine (dok'trin) [L. *doceo,* to teach]. A particular system of principles taught or advocated.

Arrhenius d., Arrhenius law; the theory of electrolytic dissociation (1887) that became the basis of our modern understanding of electrolytes: in an electrically conductive solution (*e.g.,* acid, base, or salt), free ions are present before electrolysis, and the proportion of molecules dissociated into ions can be calculated from measurements of electrical conductivity as well as of osmotic pressure.

humoral d., fluidism; humoralism; humorism; the ancient Greek theory of the four body humors (blood, yellow and black bile, and phlegm) that determined health and disease. The humors were associated with the four elements (air, fire, earth, and water), which in turn corresponded each to a pair of the qualities (hot, cold, dry, and moist). A proper and evenly balanced mixture of the humors was characteristic of health of body and mind; an imperfect balance resulted in disease. Temperament of body or mind also was supposed to be determined, *e.g.,* sanguine blood), choleric (yellow bile), melancholic (black bile), or phlegmatic (phlegm).

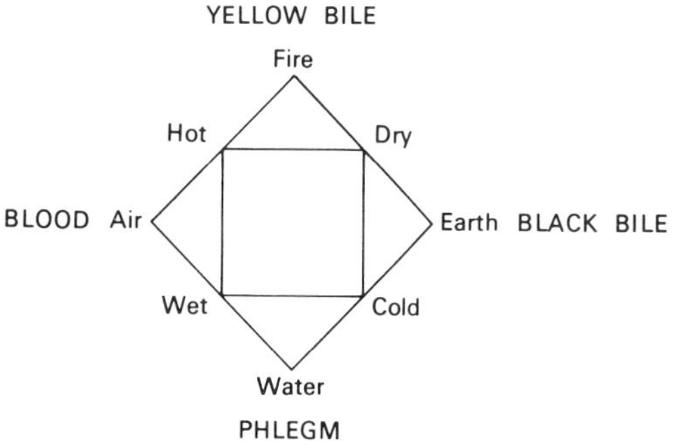

Diagram Illustrating Ancient Humoral Doctrine

Monro's d., Monro-Kellie d., a d. that states that the cranial cavity is a closed rigid box and that therefore a change in the quantity of intracranial blood can occur only through the displacement of or replacement by cerebrospinal fluid.

docusate calcium (dok'yū-sāt). Dioctyl calcium sulfosuccinate; calcium salt of bis(2-ethylhexyl)sulfosuccinate; a surface-active agent used in the treatment of constipation as a nonlaxative fecal softener.

docusate sodium. Dioctyl sodium sulfosuccinate (2); bis-2-ethylhexyl sodium sulfosuccinate; a surface-active agent used as a dispersing agent in topically applied preparations. After oral administration it lowers the surface tension of the gastrointestinal tract and is used in the treatment of constipation.

dodecane (dō'dĕ-kān). $n\text{-}C_{12}H_{26}$; a straight, unbranched, saturated hydrocarbon containing 12 carbon atoms; the 12th member of the alkane series that begins with methane.

dodecanoic acid (dō-dek'ă-nō-ik). Lauric acid.

dodecarbonium chloride (dō-dē-kar-bō'nē-ŭm). Benzyl(dodecycarbamoylmethyl)dimethyl ammonium chloride; an antiseptic.

dodecyl (dō'dĕ-sil). The radical of dodecane.

d. gallate, dodecyl 3,4,5-trihydroxybenzoate; an antioxidant.

d. sulfate, see *sodium* dodecyl sulfate.

Döderlein, Albert, S.G., German obstetrician, 1860–1941. See D.'s *bacillus.*

Doerfler, Leo. See D.-Stewart *test.*

Dogiel, Alexander S., Russian histologist, 1852–1922. See D.'s *corpuscle.*

Dogiel, Jan von, Russian anatomist and physiologist, 1830–1905. See D.'s *cells.*

dogmatic (dog-mat'ik) [G. *dogmatikos,* concerning opinions; *d. iatroi,* physicians who go by general principles; fr. *dogma,* an opinion]. See dogmatic *school.*

dogmatist (dog'mă-tist). A follower of the dogmatic *school.*

Döhle, Karl G.P., German histologist and pathologist, 1855–1928. See D. *bodies, inclusions.*

Doisy, Edward A., U.S. biochemist and Nobel laureate, *1893. See Allen-D. *test, unit.*

dol (dōl) [L. *dolor,* pain]. A unit measure of pain.

dolicho- [G. *dolichos,* long]. Combining form meaning long.

dolichocephalic, dolichocephalous (dol-i-kō-sĕ-fal'ik, -sef'ă-lŭs) [dolicho- + G. *kephalē,* head]. Dolichocranial; having a disproportionately long head; denoting a skull with a cephalic index below 75.

dolichocephaly, dolichocephalism (dol-i-kō-sef'ă-lē, sef'ă-lizm). The condition of being dolichocephalic.

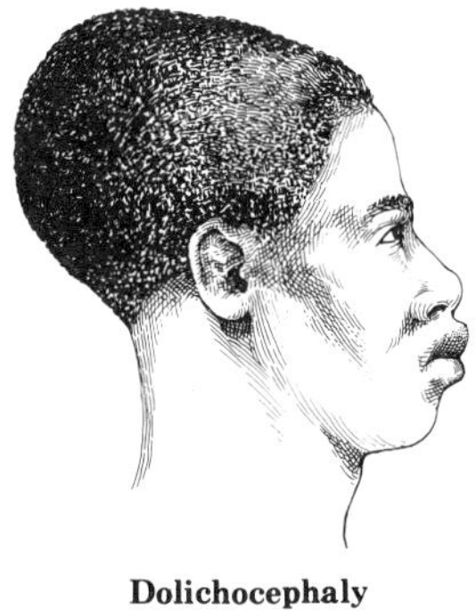

Dolichocephaly

dolichocolon (dol-i-kō-kō'lōn) [dolicho- + G. *kolon,* colon]. A colon of abnormal length.

dolichocranial (dol-i-kō-krā'nē-ăl). Dolichocephalic.

dolichofacial (dol-i-kō-fā'shăl). Dolichoprosopic.

dolichol (dol'i-kol). Polyisoprenes in which the terminal member is saturated and oxidized to an alcohol, usually phosphorylated and often glycosylated; found in nuclear membranes, but not in mitochondrial or plasma membranes; urinary levels are elevated in disorders exhibiting abnormal skin, rectal, or brain profiles in electron microscopy of biopsies.

dolichopellic, dolichopelvic (dol-i-kō-pel'ik, -pel'vik) [dolicho- + G. *pellis,* bowl (pelvis)]. Having a disproportionately long pelvis.

dolichoprosopic, dolichoprosopous (dol-i-kō-pros-ō'pik, -kō-pros'ō-pŭs) [dolicho- + G. *prosōpikos,* facial]. Dolichofacial; having a disproportionately long face.

dolichostenomelia (dol′i-kō-sten′ō-mē′lē-ă) [dolicho- + G. *stenos,* narrow, + *melos,* limb]. Arachnodactyly.

dolichouranic, dolichuranic (dol′i-kō-yū-ran′ik, dol-ik-yū-) [dolicho- + G. *ouranos,* vault of the palate]. Having a long palate, with a palatal index below 110.

dolor (dō′lōr) [L.]. Pain, as one of the four signs of inflammation (d., calor, rubor, tumor) enunciated by Celsus.

d. cap′itis, headache, especially due to changes in the scalp or bones rather than in the intracranial structures.

dolorific (dō-lōr-if′ik). Pain-producing.

dolorimetry (dō-lō-rim′ĕ-trē) [L. *dolor,* pain, + G. *metron,* measure]. The measurement of pain.

dolorology (dō-lōr-ol′ō-jē) [L. *dolor,* pain, + G. *logos,* study]. The study and treatment of pain.

DOM Abbreviation for 2,5-dimethoxy-4-methylamphetamine.

domains (dō-mānz′). Homologous units of approximately 110 to 120 amino acids each which comprise the light and heavy chains of the immunoglobulin molecule and which serve specific functions. The light chain has two d.'s, one in the variable region and one in the constant region of the chain; the heavy chain has four to five d.'s, depending upon the class of immunoglobulin, one in the variable region and the remaining ones in the constant region.

Dombrock blood group. See Blood Groups appendix.

domiciliated (dō-mi-sil′ē-āt-ed) [L. *domicilium,* a dwelling]. A state of close association of an organism within human abodes or activities, such that partial domestication results, leading to the organism's dependence on continued association with the human environment; this frequently results in the d. organism becoming a noxious pest, a vector, or an intermediate host of human disease.

dominance (dom′i-nans). The state of being dominant.

false d., quasidominance.

d. of genes, an expression of the apparent physiologic relationship existing between two or more genes that may occupy the same chromosome locus (alleles). At a specific paired locus there are three possible combinations of two allelic genes, *A* and *a:* the pair may consist of both genes of one type (*AA*), both of contrasting type (*aa*), or one of each (*Aa*). If both are alike (*AA* or *aa*), the individual or cell is homozygous with respect to the gene concerned; if they are different (*Aa*), the individual or cell is heterozygous. If a heterozygous individual presents only the hereditary characteristic determined by gene *A,* while the effect of gene *a* is not apparent, gene *A* is said to be dominant and gene *a* is said to be recessive; in this case, the dominant homozygote, *AA,* and the heterozygote, *Aa,* should be indistinguishable. If both genes produce a recognizable or intermediate effect in the heterozygote, the three classes *AA, Aa,* and *aa* are distinguishable each from the others, and there is intermediate d. or no d. between the alleles.

genetic d., denoting a pattern of inheritance of an autosomal mendelian trait due to a gene that always manifests itself phenotypically; generally, the phenotype in the homozygote is more severe than in the heterozygote, but details depend on what criterion of phenotyping is used.

dominant (dom′i-nant) [L. pres. p. of *dominor,* pp. *-atus,* to rule, fr. *dominus,* a master]. **1.** Ruling or controlling. **2.** In genetics, denoting an allele possessed by one of the parents of a hybrid which is expressed in the latter to the exclusion of a contrasting allele (the recessive) from the other parent.

Dominici, Henri, French physician, 1867–1919. See D. *tube.*

domiphen bromide (dō′mi-fen). Dodecyldimethyl(2-phenoxyethyl)ammonium bromide; an antiseptic.

Donath, Julius, German physician, 1870–1950. See D.-Landsteiner *phenomenon,* D.-Landsteiner cold *autoantibody,* Landsteiner-D. *test.*

Donders, Franz C., Dutch ophthalmologist, 1818–1889. See D.'s *glaucoma, law, pressure, rings; space* of D.

Don Juan (wahn) [legendary Spanish nobleman]. In psychiatry, a term used to denote males with compulsive sexual overactivity, usually with a succession of female partners.

Donnan, Frederick G., British physical chemist, 1870–1956. See D. or Gibbs-D. *equilibrium.*

Donné, Alfred, French physician, 1801–1878. See D.'s *corpuscle.*

Donohue, William L., Canadian pathologist, *1906. See D.'s *disease.*

donor (dō′ner) [L. *dono,* pp. *donatus,* to donate, to give]. **1.** An individual from whom blood, tissue, or an organ is taken for transplantation. **2.** A compound that will transfer an atom or a radical to an acceptor; *e.g.,* methionine is a methyl d. **3.** An atom that readily yields electrons to an acceptor; *e.g.,* nitrogen, which will donate both electrons to a shared pool in forming a coordinate bond.

hydrogen d., a metabolite from which hydrogen is removed (by a dehydrogenase system) and transferred by a hydrogen carrier to another metabolite, which is thus reduced.

universal d., in blood grouping, a person belonging to group O; *i.e.,* one whose erythrocytes do not contain either agglutinogen A or B and are, therefore, not agglutinated by plasma containing either of the ordinary isoagglutinins, alpha or beta.

Donovan, Charles, Irish surgeon, 1863–1951. See D. *body;* Leishman-D. *body.*

donovanosis (don′ō-vă-nō′sis). Granuloma inguinale, caused by *Calymmatobacterium granulomatis,* which is observed intracellularly (in macrophages in the lesion) as Donovan bodies.

Doose, H., 20th century German pediatrician and epileptologist. See D. *syndrome.*

dopa, Dopa, DOPA (dō′pă). 3,4-Dihydroxyphenylalanine; an intermediate in the catabolism of phenylalanine and tyrosine, and in the biosynthesis of norepinephrine, epinephrine, and melanin; the L form, levodopa, is biologically active.

d. decarboxylase, aromatic L-amino-acid decarboxylase.

decarboxylated d., dopamine.

d. oxidase, provisional name given the enzyme(s) catalyzing the formation of melanins from d.; it now appears that the copper-containing monophenol monooxygenases and/or catechol oxidases are responsible for the oxidation of tyrosine to d. and d. quinone.

d. quinone, an oxidation product of d. and an intermediate in the formation of melanin from tyrosine.

L-dopa. Levodopa.

dopamine (dō′pă-mēn). 3-Hydroxytyramine; decarboxylated dopa; an intermediate in tyrosine metabolism and precursor of norepinephrine and epinephrine; its presence in the central nervous system and localization in the basal ganglia (caudate and lentiform nuclei) suggest that d. may have other functions.

d. hydrochloride, a biogenic amine and neural transmitter substance, used as a vasopressor agent for treatment of shock.

dopamine β-hydroxylase. Dopamine β-monooxygenase.

dopamine β-mono-oxygenase [EC 1.14.17.1]. Dopamine β-hydroxylase; an enzyme catalyzing oxidation of ascorbate and dihydroxyphenylethylamine simultaneously by O_2 to yield norepinephrine and dehydroascorbate.

dopaminergic (dō′pă-min-er′jik) [dopamine + G. *ergon,* work]. Relating to nerve cells or fibers that employ dopamine as their neurotransmitter.

dope (dōp) [Dutch, *doop,* sauce]. **1.** Any drug, either stimulating or depressing, administered for its temporary effect, or taken habitually or addictively. **2.** To administer or take such a drug.

Doppler, Christian J., Austrian mathematician and physicist in U.

S., 1803–1853. See D. *echocardiography, effect, phenomenon, shift, ultrasonography.*

doraphobia (dō-rā-fō'bē-ă) [G. *dora,* hide, skin, + *phobos,* fear]. Morbid fear of touching the skin or fur of animals.

Dorello, P., Italian anatomist, *1872. See D's *canal.*

Dorendorf, H., German physician, *1866. See D.'s *sign.*

Dorfman, Maurice L., 20th century dermatologist. See D.-Chanarin *syndrome.*

Döring, G., German neurologist. See Pette-D. *disease.*

dornase (dōr'nās). Obsolete contraction of deoxyribonuclease. See also streptodornase.

pancreatic d., a stabilized deoxyribonuclease preparation from beef pancreas; used by inhalation in the form of aerosols to reduce thick mucopurulent secretions in certain bronchopulmonary infections.

Dorno, Carl, Swiss climatologist, 1865–1942. See D. *rays.*

doromania (dō-rō-mā'nē-ă) [G. *doron,* gift, + *mania,* insanity]. An abnormal desire to give presents.

dorsa (dōr'să). Plural of dorsum.

dorsabdominal (dōr-sab-dom'i-nal). Relating to the back and the abdomen.

dorsad (dor'sad) [L. *dorsum,* back, + *ad,* to]. Toward or in the direction of the back.

dorsal (dōr'săl) [Mediev. L. *dorsalis,* fr. *dorsum,* back]. **1.** Tergal; pertaining to the back or any dorsum. **2.** In human anatomy, posterior (2). **3.** In veterinary anatomy, pertaining to the back or upper surface of an animal. Often used to indicate the position of one structure relative to another; *i.e.,* nearer the back surface of the body. **4.** Old term meaning thoracic, in a limited sense; *e.g.,* d. vertebrae.

dorsalgia (dōr-sal'jē-ă) [L. *dorsum,* back, + G. *algos,* pain]. Dorsodynia; pain in the upper back.

dorsalis (dōr-sā'lis) [L.] [NA]. Posterior (2).

Dorset, Marion, U.S. bacteriologist, *1872. See D.'s egg culture *medium.*

dorsiduct (dōr'si-dŭkt) [L. *dorsum,* back, + *duco,* pp. *ductus,* to draw]. To draw backward or toward the back.

dorsiflexion (dōr-si-flek'shŭn). Turning upward of the foot or toes or of the hand or fingers.

dorsiscapular (dōr'si-skap'yū-lăr). Relating to the dorsal surface of the scapula.

dorsispinal (dōr'si-spī'năl). Relating to the vertebral column, especially to its dorsal aspect.

dorsocephalad (dōr'sō-sef'ă-lad) [L. *dorsum,* back, + G. *kephalē,* head, + L. *ad,* to]. Toward the occiput, or back of the head.

dorsodynia (dōr-sō-din'ē-ă) [L. *dorsum,* back, + G. *odynē,* pain]. Dorsalgia.

dorsolateral (dōr-sō-lat'er-ăl). Relating to the back and the side.

dorsolumbar (dōr-sō-lŭm'bar). Referring to the back in the region of the lower thoracic and upper lumbar vertebrae.

dorsoventrad (dōr-sō-ven'trad). In a direction from the dorsal to the ventral aspect.

dorsum, gen. **dorsi,** pl. **dorsa** (dōr'sŭm, -sī, -să) [L. back] [NA]. Tergum. **1.** The back of the body. **2** The upper or posterior surface, or the back, of any part.

d. ephip'ii, d. sellae.

d. lin'guae [NA], the back of the tongue; the upper surface of the tongue divided by the sulcus terminalis into an anterior two-thirds, the pars presulcalis, and a posterior one-third, the pars postsulcalis.

d. ma'nus [NA], the back of the hand.

d. na'si [NA], the external ridge of the nose, looking forward and upward.

d. pe'dis [NA], the back, or upper surface, of the foot.

d. pe'nis [NA], the aspect of the penis opposite to that of the urethra.

d. scap'ulae, the posterior surface of the scapula.

d. sel'lae [NA], d. ephipii; a square portion of bone on the body of the sphenoid posterior to the sella turcica or hypophysial fossa.

dosage (dō'sij). **1.** The giving of medicine or other therapeutic agent in prescribed amounts. **2.** The determination of the proper dose of a remedy. *Cf.* dose.

dose (dōs) [G. *dosis;* see dosis]. The quantity of a drug or other remedy to be taken or applied all at one time or in fractional amounts within a given period. *Cf.* dosage (2).

absorbed d., the amount of energy absorbed per unit mass of irradiated material at the target site; in radiation therapy, the unit for absorbed d. is the rad.

air d., the radiation d., expressed in roentgens, delivered at a point in free air.

booster d., a d. given at some time after an initial d. to enhance the effect, said usually of antigens for the production of antibodies.

cumulative d., the total d. resulting from repeated exposures to radiation of the same part of the body or of the whole body.

curative d., the quantity of any substance required to effect the cure of a disease or that will correct the manifestations of a deficiency of a particular factor in the diet.

daily d., the total amount of a remedy that is to be taken within 24 hours.

depth d., the amount of radiation received beneath the surface in proportion to the amount recorded at the surface.

divided d., fractional d.; a definite fraction of a full d.; given repeatedly at short intervals so that the full d. is taken within a specified period, usually one day.

effective d. (ED), the d. which produces the desired effect; when followed by a subscript (generally "ED_{50}"), it denotes the d. having such an effect on a certain percentage (*e.g.,* 50%) of the test animals.

epilation d., the minimum amount of radiation sufficient to produce hair loss, usually in 10 to 14 days.

equianalgesic d., the qualitative ratio between actual milligram potency of comparable analgesics required to achieve the equivalent therapeutic effect.

erythema d., the minimum amount of x-rays or other form of radiation sufficient to produce erythema after the application; this d. is indicated by the Sabouraud meter as the B tint, the Holzkhecht as 5(5H), the Hampson as 4, and the Kienbock as 10.

exit d., the amount of radiation leaving a body opposite the area of entry.

fractional d., divided d.

initial d., loading d.; a comparatively large d. given at the beginning of treatment to get the patient under the influence of the drug.

L d.'s ["L" for *limes*], a group of terms that indicate the relative activity or potency of diphtheria toxin; the L d.'s are distinctly different from the minimal lethal d. and minimal reacting d., inasmuch as the latter two represent the direct effects of toxin, whereas the L d.'s pertain to the combining power of toxin with specific antitoxin.

L^+ d., L_+ d., alternate for L† the limes tod d. of diphtheria toxin, *i.e.,* the smallest amount of toxin that, when mixed with one unit of antitoxin and injected subcutaneously into a 250-g guinea pig, results in death of the animal within 96 hours (based on the average in a series); on theoretical grounds, one might expect that the difference between the L_+ and L_0 d.'s would be identical to 1 MLD, but this is not so in actual practice; with various toxic filtrates, the difference may range from several to more than 100 MLD's, indicating that the toxin-antitoxin combination is *not* a firm chemical

union that occurs in constant proportions.
lethal d. (LD), the d. of a chemical or biologic preparation (*e.g.*, a bacterial exotoxin or a suspension of bacteria) that is likely to cause death; it varies in relation to the type of animal and the route of administration; when followed by a subscript (generally "LD_{50}" or median lethal d.), it denotes the d. likely to cause death in a certain percentage (*e.g.*, 50%) of the test animals.
Lf, L_f d., the limes flocculation d. of diphtheria toxin, *i.e.*, the smallest amount of toxin that, when mixed with one unit of antitoxin, yields the most rapid flocculation in the Ramon test (*in vitro*); in general, the L_f d. is slightly less than the L_r d.
Lo, L_0 d., the limes nul d. of diphtheria toxin, *i.e.*, the largest amount of toxin that, when mixed with one unit of antitoxin and injected subcutaneously into a 250-g guinea pig, yields no recognizable reaction in the average of a series; actually, the L_0 d. is usually recorded as the one that causes a barely perceptible local edema at the site of inoculation.
loading d., initial d.
Lr, L_r d., the limes reacting d. of diphtheria toxin, *i.e.*, the smallest amount of toxin that, when mixed with one unit of antitoxin and injected intracutaneously in the shaved skin of a susceptible guinea pig, yields a minimal, positive reaction and inflammation localized to the region of the injection; the L_r d. closely approximates the L_0 d., as would be expected, inasmuch as a slight excess of unneutralized toxin results in a reaction.
maintenance d., see maintenance drug *therapy*.
maximal d., the largest amount of a drug that an adult can take with safety.
maximal permissible d. (MPD), the greatest d. of radiation to which members of a population may be exposed without harmful effects; further defined in terms of acute or chronic exposure of the whole body or of organs, systems, or regions of the body.
minimal d., the smallest amount of a drug that will produce a physiologic effect in an adult.
minimal infecting d. (M.I.D.), the smallest quantity of infectious material regularly producing infection; usually expressed as $I.D._{50}$, the quantity causing infection in 50% of a suitable series of animals or cells (cell cultures).
minimal lethal d. (MLD, mld), the minimal d. of a toxic substance or infectious agent that is lethal, as assayed in various experimental animals (*e.g.*, the least amount diphtheria toxin that, on an average, kills a 250-g guinea pig within 96 hours after subcutaneous inoculation); when followed by a subscript (generally "MLD_{50}"), denotes the minimal dose that is lethal to a certain percentage (*e.g.*, 50%) of animals so assayed.
minimal reacting d. (MRD, mrd), the minimal d. of a toxic substance causing a reaction, as manifested in the skin of a series of susceptible test animals; the assay is based on the development of a characteristic, minimal but definite, "standard," focal inflammation (congestion and edema, induration, degenerative changes, and desquamation of epidermal cells), becoming apparent in 18 to 24 hours after intracutaneous injection of the toxin, and attaining a peak in approximately 96 hours.
optimum d., the d. of a drug or radiation that will produce the desired effect with minimum likelihood of undesirable symptoms.
preventive d., the smallest amount of any substance that will prevent occurrence of symptoms of a disease or the consequences of a lack of a particular factor in the diet.
sensitizing d., in experimental anaphylaxis, the antigenic inoculum that renders an animal susceptible (sensitive) to anaphylactic shock following a subsequent inoculum (shocking d.) of the same antigen (anaphylactogen).
shocking d., in experimental anaphylaxis, the inoculum of antigen that causes anaphylactic shock in an animal sensitized by a previous inoculum (sensitizing d.) of the same antigen.
skin d., the quantity of radiation delivered to the skin surface.
tissue culture infectious d. ($TCID_{50}$, TCD_{50}), the quantity of a cytopathogenic agent, such as a virus, that will produce a cytopathic effect in 50% of the cultures inoculated.
tolerance d., the largest d. of a remedy that can be accepted without the production of injurious symptoms.

dosimetry (dō-sim'ĕ-trē) [G. *dosis*, dose, + *metron*, measure]. The accurate determination of dosage.
thermoluminescence d., the calculation of a radiation dose by measuring the light output after heating a special absorbent material (*e.g.*, lithium fluoride) placed in the radiation beam; the light output is proportional to the amount of radiation exposure.
x-ray d., roentgenometry.

dot. A small spot.
Gunn's d.'s, minute, highly glistening, white or yellowish specks usually seen in the posterior part of the fundus; nonpathologic.
Horner-Trantas d.'s, evanescent white cellular infiltrates occurring in the bulbar form of vernal keratoconjunctivitis.
Maurer's d.'s, Maurer's clefts; finely granular precipitates or irregular cytoplasmic particles that usually occur diffusely in red blood cells infected with the trophozoites of *Plasmodium falciparum*, occasionally those of *P. malariae;* rarely observed in *P. falciparum* blood smears because its trophozoites seldom are seen in peripheral blood.
Schüffner's d.'s, Schüffner's granules; fine, round, uniform red or red-yellow d.'s (as colored with Romanovsky stains) characteristically observed in erythrocytes infected with *Plasmodium vivax* and *P. ovale*, but not ordinarily found in *P. malariae* and *P. falciparum* infections.
Trantas' d.'s, pale, grayish red, uneven nodules of gelatinous aspect at the limbal conjunctiva in vernal conjunctivitis.
Ziemann's d.'s, Ziemann's stippling; fine d.'s seen in erythrocytes in malariae malaria.

dotage (dō'tij). Anility; dotardness; the deterioration of previously intact mental powers, common in old age.

dotardness (dō'tard-nes). Dotage.

doublet (dŭb'let). **1.** A combination of two lenses designed to correct the chromatic and spherical aberration. **2.** Dipole.
Wollaston's d., a combination of two planoconvex lenses in the eyepiece of a microscope designed to correct the chromatic aberration.

douche (dūsh) [Fr. fr. *doucher*, to pour]. **1.** A current of water, gas, or vapor directed against a surface or projected into a cavity. **2.** An instrument for giving a d. **3.** To apply a d.

Douglas, Beverly, U.S. surgeon, *1891. See D. *graft*.

Douglas, Claude G., British physiologist, 1882–1963. See D. *bag*.

Douglas, James, Scottish anatomist in London, 1675–1742. See D.'s *abscess, cul-de-sac, fold, line, pouch, cavum* douglasi.

Douglas, John C., Irish obstetrician, 1777–1850. See D.'s spontaneous *evolution, mechanism*.

dourine (dū'rēn) [Fr.]. Equine syphilis; a venereally transmitted trypanosomiasis of horses caused by *Trypanosoma equiperdum* and characterized by inflammation of the genitals, glandular swelling, and paralysis of the hind quarters.

dovetail (dŭv'tāl). A widened portion of a cavity preparation usually established to increase the retention and resistance form.

dowel (dow'l). **1.** A cast gold or preformed metal pin placed into a root canal for the purpose of providing retention for a crown. **2.** A preformed metal pin placed in a copper-plated die to provide a die stem.

Down, John Langdon H., British physician, 1828–1896. See D.'s *syndrome*.

down. Fine, soft hair.
malignant d., *hypertrichosis* lanuginosa acquisita.

Downey, H., U.S. hematologist, 1877–1959. See D. *cell*.

down-regulation. Rapid development of a refractory or tolerant state consequent upon repeated administration of a pharmacologically or physiologically active substance; often accompanied by an initial decrease in affinity of receptors for the agent and a subsequent diminution in the number of receptors.

Downs, William B., U.S. orthodontist, 1899–1966. See D.'s *analysis.*

Dox, Arthur W., U.S. chemist, *1882. See Czapek-D. *medium.*

doxapram hydrochloride (doks'ă-pram). 1-Ethyl-4-(2-morpholinoethyl)-3,3-diphenyl-2-pyrrolidone monohydrochloride (or hydrochloride hydrate); a central nervous system stimulant, advocated but infrequently used as a respiratory stimulant in anesthesia.

doxepin hydrochloride (dok'sĕ-pin). *N,N*- Dimethyldibenz[*b,e*]oxepin-$\Delta^{11(6H),\gamma}$-propylamine hydrochloride; an antidepressant and antianxiety agent.

doxorubicin (dok'sō-rū'bi-sin). Adriamycin; an antineoplastic antibiotic isolated from *Streptomyces peucetius;* also used in cytogenetics to produce Q-type chromosome bands.

doxycycline (dok-sē-sī'klēn). α-6-Deoxy-5-hydroxytetracycline; an antibiotic.

doxylamine succinate (dok-sil'ă-mēn). Mereprine; 2-[α-(2-dimethylaminoethoxy)-α-methylbenzyl]pyridine succinate; an antihistaminic.

Doyère, Louis, French physiologist, 1811–1863. See D.'s *eminence.*

Doyle, J.B., U.S. gynecologist, *1907. See D.'s *operation.*

Doyne, Robert Walter, British ophthalmologist, 1857–1916. See D.'s honeycomb *choroidopathy,* guttate *iritis.*

D.P. Abbreviation for Doctor of Podiatry.

D.P.H. Abbreviation for Department of Public Health; Doctor of Public Health.

D.P.M. Abbreviation for Doctor of Podiatric Medicine.

DPN Abbreviation for diphosphopyridine nucleotide.

DPN$^+$ Abbreviation for oxidized diphosphopyridine nucleotide.

DPNase NAD$^+$ nucleosidase.

DPNH Abbreviation for reduced diphosphopyridine nucleotide.

DPNH → aldehyde transhydrogenase. Alcohol dehydrogenase.

DPT Abbreviation for dipropyltryptamine.

DR Abbreviation for *reaction* of degeneration.

dr Abbreviation for dram.

drachm (dram) [G. *drachmē,* an ancient Greek weight, equivalent to about 60 gr]. Dram.

dracontiasis (drak-on-tī'ă-sis) [G. *drakōn* (*drakont-*), dragon]. Dracunculiasis; dracunculosis; infection with *Dracunculus medinensis.*

dracunculiasis, dracunculosis (dra-kŭng-kyū-lī'ă-sis, -kyū-lō'sis). Dracontiasis.

Dracunculus (dra-kŭng'kyū-lŭs) [L. dim. of *draco,* serpent]. A genus of nematodes (superfamily Dracunculoidea) that have some resemblances to true filarial worms; however, adults are larger (females being as long as 1 m), and the intermediate host is a freshwater crustacean rather than an insect.
D. loa, old incorrect term for *Loa loa.*
D. medinen'sis [L. of Medina], a species of skin-infecting, yard-long nematodes, formerly incorrectly classed as *Filaria;* adult worms live anywhere in the body of man and various semi-aquatic mammals; the females migrate along fascial planes to subcutaneous tissues, where troublesome chronic ulcers are formed in the skin; when the host enters water, larvae are discharged from the ulcers, from which the head of the female worm protrudes; these larvae, if ingested by *Cyclops* species, develop in the intermediate host to the infective stage; man and various animals contract the infection from accidental ingestion of infected *Cyclops* in drinking water. Popularly known as guinea, Medina, serpent, or dragon worm, and frequently thought to be the "fiery serpent" that plagued the Israelites.
D. oc'uli, old incorrect term for *Loa loa.*
D. persa'rum [L. of the Persians], old term for *D. medinensis.*

draft. Draught. **1.** A current of air in a confined space. **2.** A quantity of liquid medicine ordered as a single dose.

drag. 1. The lower or cast side of a denture flask. **2.** Any tendency for one moving thing to pull something else along with it.
solvent d., the influence exerted by a flow of solvent through a membrane on the simultaneous movement of a solute through the membrane.

dragée (dra-zhā') [Fr.]. A sugar-coated pill or capsule.

Dragendorff, Georg J.N., German physician and pharmaceutical chemist, 1836–1898. See D.'s *test.*

Drager, Glenn A., U.S. neurologist, *1917. See Shy-D. *syndrome.*

Dräger, Heinrich, German manufacturer of industrial and diving respiratory apparatus, *1898. See D. *respirometer.*

drain (drān) [A. S. *drehnian,* to draw off]. **1.** To draw off fluid from a cavity as it forms. **2.** A device, usually in the shape of a tube or wick, for removing fluid as it collects in a cavity, especially a wound cavity.
cigarette d., a wick of gauze wrapped in rubber tissue, providing capillary drainage.
Mikulicz' d., a d. made of several strings of gauze held together by a single layer of gauze.
Penrose d., a cigarette d. of soft rubber tubing.
stab d., a d. passed into a cavity through a puncture made at a dependent part away from the wound of operation, designed to prevent infection of the wound.
sump d., a d. consisting of an outer tube with a smaller tube within it which is attached to a suction pump; the outer tube has multiple perforations that allow fluid to pass into its interior and be carried away through the suction tube.

drainage (drān'ij). Continuous withdrawal of fluids from a wound or other cavity.
capillary d., d. by means of a wick of gauze or other material.
closed d., d. of a body cavity via a water- or air-tight system.
dependent d., downward d.; d. from the lowest part and into a receptacle at a level lower than the structure being drained.
downward d., dependent d.
infusion-aspiration d., drip-suck irrigation; a type of d. in which antibiotics are continuously infused into a cavity at the same time fluid is being drained (aspirated) from the cavity.
open d., d. allowing air to enter.
postural d., d. used in bronchiectasis and lung abscess in which the patient's head is lowered backwards with the trachea inclined downward and below the affected chest area.
suction d., closed drainage of a cavity, with a suction apparatus attached to the drainage tube.
through d., d. obtained by the passage of a perforated tube, open at both extremities, through a cavity; in addition, the cavity can be washed out by a solution passed through the tube.
tidal d., d. of the urinary bladder by means of an intermittent filling and emptying apparatus.
Wangensteen d., continuous d. by suction through an indwelling gastric or duodenal tube.

dram (dr) [see drachm]. Drachm; a unit of weight: $^1/_8$ oz.; 60 gr, apothecaries' weight; $^1/_{16}$ oz., avoirdupois weight.

drape (drāp). **1.** To cover parts of the body other than those to be examined or operated upon. **2.** The cloth or materials used for such cover.

Draper, John W., British chemist, 1811–1882. See D.'s *law.*

drapetomania (drap'ĕ-tō-mā'nē-ă) [G. *drapetēs,* runaway, + *mania,* insanity]. An uncontrollable desire to run away from home.

draught (draft). Draft.

draw-sheet (draw'shēt). A narrow sheet placed crosswise on the bed under the patient, with a rubber sheet of the same width beneath it; used to assist in moving the patient or in changing soiled bed coverings.

dream (drēm). Ideas or images formed in the mind during sleep.
anxiety d., a d. (or nightmare) of which anxiety forms an important part.
wet d., a true physiologic orgasm during sleep including, in males, a nocturnal seminal emission (oneirogmus), usually accompanying a d. with sexual content.

dream-work. In psychoanalysis, the process by which the change from latent to manifest content of a dream is effected.

Drechslera (dresh'ler-ă). A saprobic genus of fungi, frequently recovered in the clinical laboratory, characterized by conidia attached to a zigzagged conidiophore. *D. spicifera* causes phaeohyphomycosis in man, cats, and horses.

drench. 1. The pouring of a liquid medicinal agent from a bottle into the mouth of an animal while holding its head high, thus forcing it to swallow. **2.** The liquid medicinal agent intended for giving to an animal by drenching.

drepanidium (drep-ă-nid'ē-ŭm) [G. *drepanē,* a sickle]. A young sickle-shaped or crescentic form of a gregarine.

drepanocyte (drep'ă-nō-sīt) [G. *drepanē,* sickle, + *kytos,* a hollow (cell)]. Sickle *cell.*

drepanocythemia (drep'ă-nō-sī-thē'mē-ă) [drepanocyte + G. *haima,* blood]. Obsolete term for sickle cell *anemia.*

drepanocytic (drep'ă-nō-sit'ik). Relating to or resembling a sickle cell.

drepanocytosis (drep'ă-nō-sī-tō'sis) [drepanocyte + G. *-osis,* condition]. Obsolete term for sickle cell *anemia.*

dresser (dres'ĕr). In Great Britain, a surgical assistant whose primary duty is bandaging and dressing wounds.

dressing (dres'ing). The material applied, or the application itself of material, to wound for protection, absorbance, drainage, etc.
adhesive absorbent d., a sterile individual d. consisting of a plain absorbent compress affixed to a film of fabric coated with a pressure-sensitive adhesive.
antiseptic d., a sterile d. of gauze impregnated with an antiseptic.
bolus d., tie-over d.
dry d., dry gauze or other material applied to a wound.
fixed d., a d. stiffened with a substance that produces immobilization when it dries.
Lister's d., the first type of antiseptic d., one of gauze impregnated with carbolic acid.
occlusive d., a d. that hermetically seals a wound.
pressure d., a d. by which pressure is exerted on the area covered to prevent the collection of fluids in the underlying tissues; most commonly used after skin grafting and in the treatment of burns.
tie-over d., bolus d.; a d. placed over a skin graft or other sutured wound and tied on by the sutures which have been left of sufficient length for that purpose.
water d., an application of gauze or other material that is kept wet with sterilized water or saline solution.

Dressler, William, U.S. physician, †1969. See D. *beat;* D.'s *syndrome.*

Drew-Smythe, Henry James, British obstetrician and gynecologist, *1891. See D.-S. *catheter.*

Dreyer, Georges, Oxford pathologist, 1873–1934. See D.'s *formula.*

DRG Abbreviation for diagnosis related group.

dribble (dri'bl). **1.** To drool, slaver, drivel. **2.** To fall in drops, as the urine from a distended bladder.

drift. A gradual movement, as from an original position.
antigenic d., a continuous change with time of the antigenic structure of a virus, as in the recurrence of epidemics of influenza A at two or three year intervals. *Cf.* antigenic *shift.*
genetic d., a change in the frequencies of genetic traits over generations.

drift'ing. Random movement of a tooth to a position of greater stability.

drifts. Drift movements; slow ocular movements of greater amplitude than flicks, occurring during ocular fixation.

Drigalski, Wilhelm von, German bacteriologist, 1871–1950. See D.-Conradi or Conradi-D. *agar.*

drill. 1. To make a hole in bone or other hard substance. **2.** An instrument for making or enlarging a hole in bone or in a tooth.
bur d., see bur.
dental d., a rotary power-driven instrument into which cutting points may be inserted. See also handpiece.

Drinker, Philip, U.S. industrial hygienist, 1894–1972. See D. *respirator.*

drip. 1. To flow a drop at a time. **2.** A flowing in drops.
alkaline milk d., a variable mixture of sodium bicarbonate in whole milk dripped into the stomach through a small oral or nasal tube to produce constant achlorhydria; used in the treatment of certain ulcers.
intravenous d., the slow but continuous introduction of solutions intravenously, a drop at a time.
Murphy d., proctoclysis.
postnasal d., term sometimes used to describe sensation of excessive mucoid or mucopurulent discharge from the posterior nares.

drive. 1. A basic compelling urge. **2.** In psychology, classified as either innate (*e.g.,* hunger) or learned (*e.g.,* hoarding) and appetitive (*e.g.,* hunger, thirst, sex) or aversive (*e.g.,* fear, pain, grief). See also motive; motivation.
acquired d.'s, secondary d.'s.
exploratory d., the d. to investigate the unfamiliar or unknown.
kinetic d., excessive excitation of the kinetic system.
learned d., motive (1).
meiotic d., a form of genetic load due to a selective force operating on the gametes produced by one of the sexes.
physiological d.'s, primary d.'s; those d.'s which stem from the biological needs of an organism.
primary d.'s, physiological d.'s.
secondary d.'s, acquired d.'s; those d.'s not directly related to biological needs; a secondary d. can be learned as an offshoot of a primary d., in which case it is often referred to as a motive.

driving (drīv'ing). The induction of a frequency in the electroencephalogram by sensory stimulation at this frequency.
photic d., a change in the alpha frequency corresponding to a flicker.

dromic (drō'mik) [G. *dromos,* a running, race-course]. Orthodromic.

dromograph (drom'ō-graf) [G. *dromos,* a running, + *graphō,* to record]. An instrument for recording the rapidity of the blood circulation.

dromomania (drom-ō-mā'nē-ă) [G. *dromos,* a running, + *mania,* insanity]. An uncontrollable impulse to wander or travel.

dromostanolone propionate (drō-mos'tan-ō-lōn, drō-mō-stan'ō-lōn). 17β-Hydroxy-2α-methyl-5α-androstan-3-one propionate; an antineoplastic agent.

dromotropic (drō-mō-trop'ik) [G. *dromos,* a running, + *tropē,* a turn]. Influencing the velocity of conduction of excitation, as in nerve or cardiac muscle fibers.
negatively d., acting to diminish conduction velocity.

positively d., acting to increase conduction velocity.

dronabinol (drō-nab'i-nol). 6*H*- Dibenzo[*b,d*]pyran-l-ol, 6a,7,8,10a-tetrahydro-6,6,9-trimethyl-3-pentyl-, (6a*R*-*trans*)-; the principal psychoactive substance present in *Cannabis sativa,* used therapeutically as an antinauseant to control the nausea and vomiting associated with cancer chemotherapy.

drop [A.S. *droppan*]. **1.** To fall, or to be dispensed or poured in globules. **2.** A liquid globule. **3.** A volume of liquid regarded as a unit of dosage, equivalent in the case of water to about 1 minim. See also drops. **4.** A solid confection in globular form, usually directed to be allowed to dissolve in the mouth.
hanging d., a d. of liquid on the undersurface of the object glass for examination under the microscope.

dropacism (drop'ă-sizm) [G. *dropakizein,* to apply a depilatory]. Epilation of hair by use of wax or plaster.

droperidol (drō-per'i-dol). A butyrophenone drug used in neuroleptanalgesia and preanesthetic medication.

drop'per. Instillator.

drops. A popular term for a medicine taken in doses measured by d.'s, usually a tincture, or applied by dropping, as an eyewash.
eye d., see eyewash; ophthalmic *solution.*
knock-out d., a popular name for chloral alcoholate given with criminal intent to produce unconsciousness rapidly; it is formed by adding chloral hydrate to beer or some stronger alcoholic liquor.
stomach d., a stomachic tonic, usually tincture of gentian, alone or with other stomachics.

dropsical (drop'si-kăl). Hydropic.

dropsy (drop'sē) [G. *hydrōps*]. Old term for edema.
abdominal d., ascites.
epidemic d., a disease causing occasional epidemics in India and Mauritius; marked by edema, anemia, eruptive angiomatosis, and mild fever; may be associated with nutritional deficiency.

drowsiness (drow'zē-nes). Hypnesthesia; a state of impaired awareness associated with a desire or inclination to sleep.

Dr.P.H. Abbreviation of Doctor of Public Health.

drug (drŭg). **1.** Therapeutic agent; any substance, other than food, used in the prevention, diagnosis, alleviation, treatment, or cure of disease. For types or classifications of d.'s, see the specific name. See also subentries under agent. **2.** To administer or take a d., usually implying an overly large quantity or a narcotic. **3.** General term for any substance, stimulating or depressing, that can be habituating or addictive, especially a narcotic.
crude d., an unrefined preparation, usually of plant origin, that occurs either in the entire, nearly entire, broken, cut, or powdered state.
orphan d.'s, see orphan *products.*
recreational d., any d. used non-medically for personal enjoyment.
scheduled d., a d. assigned to any of the five schedules in the Controlled Substances Act (1970). See also controlled *substance.*

drug-fast. Pertaining to microorganisms that resist or become tolerant to an antibacterial agent.

druggist (drŭg'ist). Old common term for pharmacist.

drug interactions. The pharmacological result, either desirable or undesirable, of drugs interacting with themselves or other drugs, with endogenous physiologic chemical agents (*e.g.,* MAOI with epinephrine), with components of the diet, and with chemicals used in diagnostic tests or the results of such tests.

drum, drumhead (drŭm, drŭm'hed). *Membrana* tympani.

Drummond, Sir David, British physician, 1852–1932. See D.'s *sign.*

drunkenness (drŭnk'en-nes). Intoxication, usually alcoholic. See also acute *alcoholism.*
sleep d., somnolentia (2); a half-waking condition in which the faculty of orientation is in abeyance, and under the influence of nightmare-like ideas the person may become actively excited and violent.

drusen (drū'sen) [Ger. pl. of *druse,* stony nodule, geode]. Guttate, senile guttate, or Doyne's honeycomb choroidopathy; Tay's disease; hyaline or colloid bodies that contain sialomucin and cerebroside and are located in degenerated retinal pigment cells.
giant d., optic nerve glial hamartomas composed of astrocytes.
d. of optic disk, laminated, concentric, noncellular, calcium-containing masses within the optic nerve that may simulate papilledema and/or cause visual field defects.
optic nerve d., basophilic, calcareous, laminated acellular bodies within the optic nerve anterior to the scleral lamina cribrosa.

dry ice (drī īs). *Carbon* dioxide snow.

DT Abbreviation for *delirium* tremens; duration *tetany.*

dT Abbreviation for thymidine.

DT-diaphorase. NAD(P)H dehydrogenase (quinone).

dTDP Abbreviation for thymidine 5′-diphosphate.

dThd Abbreviation for thymidine.

DTIC Abbreviation for dacarbazine.

dTMP Abbreviation for deoxythymidylic acid.

DTP Abbreviation for distal tingling on percussion (see Tinel's *sign*); diphtheria, tetanus toxoids, and pertussis *vaccine.*

DTPA Abbreviation for diethylenetriamine pentaacetic acid.

dTTP Abbreviation for thymidine 5′-triphosphate.

dualism (dū'ăl-izm) [L. *dualis,* relating to two, fr. *duo,* two]. **1.** In chemistry, a theory advanced by Berzelius that every compound, no matter how many elements enter into it, is composed of two parts, one electrically negative, the other positive; still applicable, with modification, to polar compounds, but inapplicable to nonpolar compounds. **2.** In hematology, the concept that blood cells have two origins, *i.e.,* lymphogenous or myelogenous. **3.** The theory that the mind and body are two distinct systems, independent and different in nature.

Duane, Alexander, U.S. ophthalmologist, 1858–1926. See D.'s *syndrome.*

Dubin, I.N., U.S. pathologist, *1913. See D.-Johnson *syndrome.*

Dubini, Angelo, Milan physician, 1813–1902. See D.'s *disease.*

DuBois. See Meeh-DuBois *formula.*

DuBois, Eugene F., U.S. physiologist, 1882–1959. See D.'s *formula;* Aub-D. *table.*

Dubois, Paul, French obstetrician, 1795–1871. See D.'s *abscesses, disease.*

duboisine (dū-boy'sēn). An alkaloid obtained from the leaves of *Duboisia myoporoides* (family Solanaceae). See hyoscyamine.

Du Bois-Reymond, Emil H., German physiologist, 1818–1896. See D.B.-R.'s *law.*

Duboscq, Jules, Paris optician, 1817–1886. See D.'s *colorimeter.*

Dubowitz, Victor, 20th century English pediatrician. See D. *score.*

Dubreuil-Chambardel, Louis, French dentist, 1879–1927. See D.-C. *syndrome.*

Dubreuilh, M.W., French dermatologist. See precancerous *melanosis* of D.

Duchenne, Guillaume B.A., French neurologist, 1806–1875. See D.'s *disease, dystrophy, paralysis, sign, syndrome;* D.-Aran or Aran-D. *disease;* D.-Erb *paralysis.*

Duckworth, Sir Dyce, British physician, 1840–1928. See D.'s *phenomenon.*

Duclos, D., French neurologist. See Lhermitte-D. *disease.*

Ducrey, Augusto, Italian dermatologist, 1860–1940. See D.'s *bacillus,* D. *test.*

DUCT

duct (dŭkt) [L. *duco,* pp. *ductus,* to lead]. Ductus; a tubular structure giving exit to the secretion of a gland, or conducting any fluid. See also canal.

aberrant d., *ductulus* aberrans.

aberrant bile d.'s, small d.'s occasionally present in the ligaments of the liver or originating from the surface of the liver.

accessory pancreatic d., *ductus* pancreaticus accessorius.

alveolar d., **(1)** *ductulus* alveolaris; **(2)** the smallest of the intralobular d.'s in the mammary gland, into which the secretory alveoli open.

amniotic d., the transitory opening between the seroamniotic folds in birds just before they fuse to form the seroamniotic raphe.

anal d.'s, short d.'s lined with simple columnar to stratified columnar epithelium which extend from the valvulae anales to the sinus anales.

arterial d., *ductus* arteriosus.

Bartholin's d., *ductus* sublingualis major.

Bellini's d.'s, papillary d.'s.

Bernard's d., *ductus* pancreaticus accessorius.

bile d., biliary or gall d.; any of the d.'s conveying bile between the liver and the intestine, including hepatic, cystic, and common bile d.

biliary d., bile d.

Blasius' d., *ductus* parotideus.

Botallo's d., *ductus* arteriosus.

branchial d., the lumen of one of the pharyngeal pouches of the young embryo, elongated and narrowed by later differential growth.

bucconeural d., craniopharyngeal d.

d. of bulbourethral gland, *ductus* glandulae bulbourethralis.

canalicular d.'s, **(1)** *ductus* lactiferi; **(2)** *ductuli* biliferi.

carotid d., *ductus* caroticus.

cervical d., see branchial d. and cervical *diverticulum.*

choledoch d., *ductus* choledochus.

cochlear d., *ductus* cochlearis.

common bile, gall d., *ductus* choledochus.

common hepatic d., *ductus* hepaticus communis.

craniopharyngeal d., bucconeural or hypophysial d.; the slender tubular part of the hypophysial diverticulum; the stalk of Rathke's pocket.

Cuvier's d.'s, obsolete term for the common cardinal veins.

cystic d., cystic gall d., *ductus* cysticus.

deferent d., *ductus* deferens.

efferent d., *ductulus* efferens testis.

ejaculatory d., *ductus* ejaculatorius.

endolymphatic d., *ductus* endolymphaticus.

d. of epididymis, *ductus* epididymidis.

excretory d., ductus excretorius; a d. carrying the secretion from a gland or a fluid from any reservoir.

excretory d. of seminal vesicle, *ductus* excretorius vesiculae seminalis.

frontonasal d., the passage that leads downward from the frontal sinus to open into the ethmoidal infundibulum.

galactophorous d.'s, *ductus* lactiferi.

gall d., bile d.

Gartner's d., *ductus* epoophori longitudinalis.

genital d., genital *tract.*

guttural d., *tuba* auditiva.

hemithoracic d., ductus hemithoracicus; an accessory thoracic duct, usually emptying into the thoracic duct but sometimes discharging independently into the right subclavian vein.

Hensen's d., *ductus* reuniens.

hepatic d., see *ductus* hepaticus communis, dexter and sinister.

hepatocystic d., *ductus* hepaticus communis.

Hoffmann's d., *ductus* pancreaticus.

hypophysial d., craniopharyngeal d.

incisive d., *ductus* incisivus.

intercalated d.'s, the minute d.'s of glands, such as the salivary and the pancreas, that lead from the acini; they are lined by low cuboidal cells.

interlobar d., a d. draining the secretion of the lobe of a gland and formed by the junction of a number of interlobular d.'s.

interlobular d., any d. leading from a lobule of a gland and formed by the junction of the fine d.'s draining the acini.

intralobular d., a d. that lies within a lobule of a gland.

jugular d., *truncus* jugularis.

lacrimal d., *canaliculus* lacrimalis.

lactiferous d.'s, *ductus* lactiferi.

left d. of caudate lobe, *ductus* lobi caudati sinister.

left hepatic d., *ductus* hepaticus sinister.

longitudinal d. of epoophoron, *ductus* epoophori longitudinalis.

Luschka's d.'s, glandlike tubular structures in the wall of the gallbladder, especially in the part covered with peritoneum.

lymphatic d., one of the two large lymph channels, *ductus* lymphaticus dexter, or *ductus* thoracicus.

major sublingual d., *ductus* sublingualis major.

mamillary d.'s, *ductus* lactiferi.

mammary d.'s, *ductus* lactiferi.

mesonephric d., *ductus* mesonephricus.

metanephric d., the slender tubular portion of the metanephric diverticulum; the primordium of the epithelial lining of the ureter.

milk d.'s, *ductus* lactiferi.

minor sublingual d.'s, *ductus* sublinguales minores.

Müller's d., müllerian d., *ductus* paramesonephricus.

nasal d., *ductus* nasolacrimalis.

nasolacrimal d., *ductus* nasolacrimalis.

nephric d., pronephric d.

omphalomesenteric d., obsolete term for yolk *stalk.*

pancreatic d., *ductus* pancreaticus.

papillary d.'s, Bellini's d.'s; the principal straight excretory d.'s in the kidney medulla and papillae whose openings form the area cribrosa.

paramesonephric d., *ductus* paramesonephricus.

paraurethral d.'s, *ductus* paraurethrales.

parotid d., *ductus* parotideus.

Pecquet's d., *ductus* thoracicus.

perilymphatic d., *ductus* perilymphaticus.

pharyngobranchial d.'s, see *ductus* pharyngobranchialis III and IV.

pronephric d., nephric d.; the d. of the pronephros.

prostatic d.'s, *ductuli* prostatici.

right d. of caudate lobe, *ductus* lobi caudati dexter.

right hepatic d., *ductus* hepaticus dexter.

right lymphatic d., *ductus* lymphaticus dexter.

Rivinus' d.'s, *ductus* sublinguales minores.

salivary d., striated d.

Santorini's d., *ductus* pancreaticus accessorius.

Schüller's d.'s, *ductus* paraurethrales.

secretory d., striated d.

semicircular d.'s, *ductus* semicirculares.

seminal d., gonaduct (1); any one of the d.'s conveying semen from the epididymis to the urethra, ductus deferens, or ejaculatory d.

d.'s of Skene's glands, *ductus* paraurethrales.

spermatic d., *ductus* deferens.

Stensen's d., Steno's d., *ductus* parotideus.

striated d., salivary or secretory d.; a type of intralobular d. found in some salivary glands and which modifies the secretory product.
subclavian d., *truncus* subclavius.
submandibular d., *ductus* submandibularis.
submaxillary d., *ductus* submandibularis.
sudoriferous d., *ductus* sudoriferus.
sweat d., *ductus* sudoriferus.
testicular d., *ductus* deferens.
thoracic d., *ductus* thoracicus.
thyroglossal d., *ductus* thyroglossus.
thyrolingual d., *ductus* thyroglossus.
uniting d., *ductus* reuniens.
utriculosaccular d., *ductus* utriculosaccularis.
vitelline d., vitellointestinal d., archaic terms for yolk stalk.
Walther's d.'s, *ductus* sublinguales minores.
Wharton's d., *ductus* submandibularis.
Wirsung's d., *ductus* pancreaticus.
wolffian d., *ductus* mesonephricus.

ductal (dŭk'tăl). Relating to a duct.

ductile (dŭk'tĭl) [L. *ductilis,* capable of being led or drawn]. Denoting the property of a material that allows it to be bent, drawn out (as a wire), or otherwise deformed without breaking.

duction (dŭk'shŭn) [L. *duco,* to lead]. **1.** The act of leading, bringing, conducting. **2.** In ophthalmology, ocular rotations with reference to one eye; usually additionally designating direction of movement of the eye; *e.g.,* rotation toward the nose, adduction; toward the temple, abduction; upward, supra- or sursumduction; downward, deorsumduction; of the upper pole of one cornea, cycloduction; of the upper pole of one cornea outward, excycloduction; of the upper pole of one cornea inward, incycloduction.
F d., sexduction; transfer of chromosomal fragments from one bacterium to another by means of F′ carriers.
forced d., passive d.
passive d., forced d.; a maneuver to determine whether a mechanical obstruction is present in the eye; with forceps grasping an eye muscle, an attempt is made to passively move the eyeball in the direction of restricted rotation.

ductless (dŭkt'les). Having no duct; denoting certain glands having only an internal secretion.

ductular (dŭk'tū-lăr). Relating to a ductule.

ductule (dŭk'tūl). Ductulus.
aberrant d., *ductulus* aberrans.
biliary d.'s, *ductuli* biliferi.
excretory d.'s of lacrimal gland, *ductuli* excretorii glandulae lacrimalis.
interlobular d.'s, *ductuli* interlobulares.
prostatic d.'s, *ductuli* prostatici.
transverse d.'s of epoophoron, *ductuli* transversi epoophori.

ductulus, pl. **ductuli** (dŭk'tū-lŭs, -tū-lī) [Mod. L. dim. of L. *ductus,* duct] [NA]. Ductule; a minute duct.
d. aber'rans, pl. **duc'tuli aberran'tes** [NA], aberrant ductule or duct; ductus aberrans; vas aberrans; one of the diverticula of the epididymis: **d. a. supe'rius,** a diverticulum from the head of the epididymis; **d. a. infe'rius,** Haller's vas aberrans, which extends from the tail of the epididymis.
d. alveola'ris, pl. **duc'tuli alveola'res** [NA], alveolar duct (1); the part of the respiratory passages beyond a respiratory bronchiole; from it arise alveolar sacs and alveoli.
duc'tuli bilif'eri [NA], biliary ductules; ductus biliferi; canalicular ducts (2); tubuli biliferi; the excretory ducts of the liver that connect the interlobular ductules to the right (or left) hepatic duct.
d. ef'ferens tes'tis, pl. **duc'tuli efferen'tes tes'tis** [NA], efferent duct; one of 12 to 14 of small seminal ducts leading from the testis to the head of the epididymis.
duc'tuli excreto'rii glan'dulae lacrima'lis [NA], excretory ductules of lacrimal gland; the multiple (6 to 10) excretory ducts of the lacrimal gland that open into the superior fornix of the conjunctival sac.
duc'tuli interlobula'res [NA], interlobular ductules; bile ductules occupying portal canals between hepatic lobules which open into the ductuli biliferi.
duc'tuli parooph'ori, tubuli paroophori; tubular remnants of the embryonic mesonephros forming the paroophoron.
duc'tuli prostat'ici [NA], prostatic ductules or ducts; ductus prostatici; about 20 minute canals which receive the prostatic secretion from the glandular tubules and discharge it through openings on either side of the urethral crest in the posterior wall of the urethra.
duc'tuli transver'si epooph'ori [NA], transverse ductules of the epoophoron; tubuli epoophori; a series of 10 to 15 short tubules opening into the longitudinal duct of the epoophoron. See also epoophoron.

DUCTUS

ductus, gen. and pl. **ductus** (dŭk'tŭs) [L. a leading, fr. *duco,* pp. *ductus,* to lead] [NA]. Duct (3).
d. aber'rans, *ductulus* aberrans.
d. arterio'sus [NA], Botallo's duct; arterial canal or duct; a fetal vessel connecting the left pulmonary artery with the descending aorta; in the first two months after birth, it normally changes into a fibrous cord, the ligamentum arteriosum; occasional postnatal failure to close causes a surgically correctable cardiovascular handicap.
d. bilif'eri, *ductuli* biliferi.
d. carot'icus, carotid duct; a portion of the embryonic dorsal aorta between points of juncture with the third and fourth arch arteries; it disappears early in development.
d. choled'ochus [NA], common bile or gall duct; choledoch duct; choledoch; choledochus; a duct formed by the union of the hepatic and cystic ducts; it discharges at the duodenal papilla.
d. cochlea'ris [NA], cochlear duct; Löwenberg's scala or canal; membranous cochlea; scala media; a spirally arranged membranous tube suspended within the cochlea, occupying the lower portion of the vestibular scala; it begins by a blind extremity, the cecum vestibulare, in the cochlear recess of the vestibule, terminating in another blind extremity, the cecum cupulare or lagena, at the cupola of the cochlea; it contains endolymph and communicates with the sacculus by the ductus reuniens; the spiral organ (of Corti), the neuroepithelial receptor organ for hearing, occupies the floor of the duct.
d. cys'ticus [NA], cystic duct; cystic gall duct; the d. leading from the gallbladder; it joins the hepatic duct to form the common bile duct.
d. def'erens [NA], deferent duct or canal; spermatic or testicular duct; vas deferens; spermiduct (1); the secretory duct of the testicle, running from the epididymis, of which it is the continuation, to the prostatic urethra where it terminates as the ejaculatory duct.
d. def'erens vestigia'lis [NA], d. epoophori longitudinalis.
d. dorsopancreat'icus, d. pancreaticus accessorius.
d. ejaculato'rius [NA], ejaculatory duct; spermiduct (2); the duct formed by the union of the deferent duct and the excretory duct of the seminal vesicle, which opens into the prostatic urethra.
d. endolymphat'icus [NA], endolymphatic duct; aqueductus vestibuli (2); a small membranous canal, connecting with both saccule and utricle of the membranous labyrinth, passing through the aqueductus vestibuli, and terminating in a dilated blind extremity, the saccus endolymphaticus, on the posterior surface of the petrous

portion of the temporal bone beneath the dura mater.
d. epididym'idis [NA], duct of epididymis; a convoluted tube into which the efferent ductules open and which itself terminates in the deferent duct.
d. epooph'ori longitudina'lis [NA], longitudinal duct of epoophoron; d. deferens vestigialis; Gartner's duct or canal; a rudimentary vestige of the mesonephric duct in the female into which the tubules of the epoophoron open; it is located in the broad ligament of the uterus, parallel with the lateral part of the uterine tube, and in the lateral walls of the cervix and vagina. See also epoophoron.
d. excreto'rius, excretory *duct.*
d. excreto'rius vesic'ulae semina'lis [NA], excretory duct of seminal vesicle; duct of seminal vesicle; the passage leading from a seminal vesicle to the ejaculatory duct.
d. glan'dulae bulbourethra'lis [NA], duct of bulbourethral gland; the long slender duct on each side passing down through the inferior fascia of the urogenital diaphragm to enter the bulb of the penis and course forward 2 or 3 cm before terminating in the urethra.
d. hemithorac'icus, hemithoracic *duct.*
d. hepat'icus commu'nis [NA], common hepatic duct; hepatocystic duct; the part of the biliary duct system that is formed by the confluence of right and left hepatic ducts. At the porta hepatis it is joined by the cystic duct to become the common bile duct.
d. hepat'icus dex'ter [NA], right hepatic duct; the duct that transmits bile to the common hepatic duct from the right half of the liver and the right part of the caudate lobe.
d. hepat'icus sinis'ter [NA], left hepatic duct; the duct that drains bile from the left half of the liver, including the quadrate lobe and the left part of the caudate lobe.
d. incisi'vus [NA], incisive duct; a rudimentary duct, or protrusion of the mucous membrane into the incisive canal, on either side of the anterior extremity of the nasal crest.
d. lactif'eri [NA], lactiferous ducts; milk ducts; galactophorous canals or ducts; canalicular ducts (1); mamillary or mammary ducts; galactophores; tubuli galactophori; tubuli lactiferi; the ducts, numbering 15 or 20, which drain the lobes of the mammary gland; they open at the nipple.
d. lingua'lis, a pit on the upper surface of the tongue at the apex of the sulcus terminalis; it marks the point of origin of the d. thyroglossus of the embryo; known more commonly as the foramen cecum.
d. lo'bi cauda'ti dex'ter [NA], right duct of caudate lobe; the bile duct from the right half of the caudate lobe, a tributary to the right hepatic duct.
d. lo'bi cauda'ti sinis'ter [NA], left duct of caudate lobe; a tributary to the left hepatic duct draining bile from the left half of the caudate lobe.
d. lymphat'icus dex'ter [NA], right lymphatic duct; d. thoracicus dexter; one of the two terminal lymph vessels, a short trunk, about 2 cm in length, formed by the union of the right jugular lymphatic vessel and vessels from the lymph nodes of the right superior limb, thoracic wall, and both lungs; it lies on the right side of the root of the neck and empties into the right brachiocephalic vein.
d. mesoneph'ricus [NA], mesonephric or wolffian duct; a duct in the embryo draining the mesonephric tubules; in the male it becomes the ductus deferens; in the female it becomes vestigial. See also *ductus* epoophori longitudinalis.
d. nasolacrima'lis [NA], nasolacrimal duct; nasal duct; the passage leading downward from the lacrimal sac on each side to the anterior portion of the inferior meatus of the nose, through which tears are conducted into the nasal cavity.
d. om'phalomesenter'icus, obsolete term for yolk *stalk.*
d. pancreat'icus [NA], pancreatic duct; Wirsung's canal or duct; Hoffmann's duct; the excretory duct of the pancreas which extends through the gland from tail to head where it empties into the duodenum at the greater duodenal papilla.
d. pancreat'icus accesso'rius [NA], accessory pancreatic duct; d. dorsopancreaticus; Bernard's or Santorini's canal or duct; the excretory duct of the head of the pancreas, one branch of which joins the pancreatic duct, the other opening independently into the duodenum at the lesser duodenal papilla.
d. paramesoneph'ricus [NA], paramesonephric duct; Müller's or müllerian duct; either of the two paired embryonic tubes extending along the mesonephros roughly parallel to the mesonephric duct and emptying into the cloaca; in the female, the upper parts of the ducts form the uterine tubes, while the lower fuse to form the uterus and part of the vagina; in the male, vestigial as the vagina masculina and the appendix testis.
d. paraurethra'les [NA], paraurethral ducts; Schüller's ducts; ducts of Skene's glands; inconstant ducts along the side of the female urethra that convey the mucoid secretion of Skene's glands to the vestibule.
d. parotid'eus [NA], parotid duct; Steno's or Stensen's duct; Blasius' duct; the duct of the parotid gland opening from the cheek into the vestibule of the mouth opposite the neck of the superior second molar tooth.
patent d. arterio'sus, see d. arteriosus.
d. perilymphat'icus [NA], perilymphatic duct; cochlear aqueduct; aqueductus cochleae; a fine canal connecting the perilymphatic space of the cochlea with the subarachnoid space.
d. pharyngobranchia'lis III, a narrow communication between the third branchial pouch and the pharynx in the embryo.
d. pharyngobranchia'lis IV, a narrow communication between the fourth branchial pouch and the pharynx in the embryo.
d. prostat'ici, *ductuli* prostatici.
d. reun'iens [NA], uniting canal or duct; Hensen's canal or duct; canaliculus or canalis reuniens; a short membranous tube passing from the lower end of the saccule to the cochlear duct of the membranous labyrinth.
d. semicircula'res [NA], semicircular ducts; three small membranous tubes in the bony semicircular canals that lie within the bony labyrinth and form loops of about two-thirds of a circle. The three (**d. semicircula'ris ante'rior, d. semicircula'ris latera'lis,** and **d. semicircula'ris poste'rior**) lie in planes at right angles to each other and open into the vestibule by five openings of which one is common to the anterior and lateral ducts. Each duct has an ampulla at one end within which filaments of the vestibular nerve terminate.
d. sublingua'les mino'res [NA], minor sublingual ducts; Walther's canals or ducts; Rivinus' ducts; from 8 to 20 small ducts of the sublingual salivary gland which open into the mouth on the surface of the sublingual fold; a few join the submandibular ducts.
d. sublingua'lis ma'jor [NA], major sublingual duct; Bartholin's duct; the duct that drains the anterior portion of the sublingual gland; it opens at the sublingual papilla.
d. submandibula'ris [NA], submandibular duct; d. submaxillaris; submaxillary duct; Wharton's duct; the duct of the submandibular salivary gland; it opens at the sublingual papilla near the frenulum of the tongue.
d. submaxilla'ris, d. submandibularis.
d. sudorif'erus, sudoriferous duct; sweat duct; the superficial portion of the sweat gland which passes through the corium and epidermis, opening on the surface by the porus sudoriferus or sweat pore.
d. thorac'icus [NA], thoracic duct; van Horne's canal; Pecquet's duct; the largest lymph vessel in the body, beginning at the cisterna chyli at about the level of the second lumbar vertebra; the pars abdominalis extends superiorly to pass through the aortic opening of the diaphragm, where it becomes the pars thoracica and crosses the posterior mediastinum to form the arcus ductus thoracici and discharge into the left brachiocephalic vein at its origin.
d. thorac'icus dex'ter [NA], *ductus* lymphaticus dexter.
d. thyroglos'sus, thyroglossal or thyrolingual duct; a transitory endodermal tube in the embryo, carrying thyroid-forming tissue at its caudal end; normally, the duct disappears after the thyroid has

moved to its definitive location in the neck; its point of origin is regularly marked on the root of the adult tongue by the foramen cecum; occasionally, its incomplete regression results in the formation of cysts along its embryonic course. See also *lobus* pyramidalis glandulae thyroidae.

d. utric'ulosaccula'ris [NA], utriculosaccular duct; Böttcher's canal; a duct that connects the inner aspect of the utricle with the endolymphatic duct a short distance from its origin from the saccule.

d. veno'sus [NA], in the fetus, continuation of the umbilical vein through the liver to the vena cava inferior; after birth, its lumen becomes obliterated, forming the ligamentum venosum.

d. veno'sus aran'tii, rarely used term for d. venosus.

Duddell, Benedict, 18th century British oculist. See D.'s *membrane.*

Duffy blood group. See Blood Groups appendix.

Dugas, Louis A., U.S. physician, 1806–1884. See D.'s *test.*

Duhring, Louis A., U.S. dermatologist, 1845–1913. See D.'s *disease.*

Dührssen, Alfred, German obstetrician-gynecologist, 1862–1933. See D.'s *incisions.*

Dukes, Clement, British physician, 1845–1925. See D.'s *disease.*

Dukes, Cuthbert E., British pathologist, 1890–1977. See D. *classification.*

dulcin (dŭl'sin). *p*-Phenetol carbamide; 4-ethoxyphenylurea; has been used as a substitute for sugar, being 200 times as sweet as cane sugar. Because of hydrolysis to aminophenol, it may produce an injurious effect when used over long periods of time.

dulcite, dulcitol, dulcose (dŭl'sīt, -si'tol, -kōs). Galactitol.

dull (dŭl). Not sharp or acute, in any sense; qualifying a surgical instrument, the action of the mind, pain, a sound (especially the percussion note), etc.

dullness, dulness (dŭl'nes). The character of the sound obtained by percussing over a solid part which is incapable of resonating; usually applied to an area containing less air than those which can resonate.

shifting d., a sign of free peritoneal fluid wherein the d. of percussion shifts, generally from one to the other, as the patient is turned from side to side.

Dulong, Pierre L., French chemist, 1785–1838. See D.-Petit *law.*

dumas (dū'mas). Foot *yaws.*

dummy (dŭm'ē). Pontic.

Dumontpallier, Alphonse, French physician, 1827–1899. See D.'s *pessary.*

dumping (dŭmp'ing). See dumping *syndrome.*

Duncan. Surname of boys afflicted with what is now known as Duncan's *disease.*

Duncan, James M., Scottish gynecologist, 1826–1890. See D.'s *folds, mechanism, ventricle.*

Dunn, R.L. See Lison-D. *stain.*

duocrinin (dū-ō-krin'in). A postulated gastrointestinal hormone that is liberated by the contact of gastric contents with the intestine and that stimulates the secretory activity of the duodenal glands (Brunner's glands).

duodenal (dū'ō-dē'năl, dū-od'ĕ-năl). Relating to the duodenum.

duodenectomy (dū-ō-dĕ-nek'tō-mē) [duodenum + G. *ektomē,* excision]. Excision of the duodenum.

duodenitis (dū-od-ĕ-nī'tis). Inflammation of the duodenum.

duodeno- [L. *duodenum, q.v.*]. Combining form relating to the duodenum.

duodenocholangitis (dū-ō-dē'nō-kō-lan-jī'tis) [duodeno- + G. *cholē,* bile, + *angeion,* vessel, + *-itis,* inflammation]. Inflammation of the duodenum and common bile duct.

duodenocholecystostomy (dū-ō-dē'nō-kō-lē-sis-tos'tō-mē) [duodeno- + G. *cholē,* bile, + *kystis,* bladder, + *stoma,* mouth]. Cholecystoduodenostomy.

duodenocholedochotomy (dū-ō-dē'nō-kō-led-ō-kot'ō-mē) [duodeno- + G. *cholēdochus,* bile duct, + *tomē,* incision]. Incision into the common bile duct and the adjacent portion of the duodenum.

duodenocystostomy (dū-ō-dē'nō-sis-tos'tō-mē). **1.** Cholecystoduodenostomy. **2.** Cystoduodenostomy.

duodenoenterostomy (dū-ō-dē'nō-en-ter-os'tō-mē) [duodeno- + G. *enteron,* intestine, + *stoma,* mouth]. Establishment of communication between the duodenum and another part of the intestinal tract.

duodenojejunostomy (dū-ō-dē'nō-jĕ-jū-nos'tō-mē) [duodeno- + jejunum, + G. *stoma,* mouth]. Operative formation of an artificial communication between the duodenum and the jejunum.

duodenolysis (dū-ō-dĕ-nol'i-sis) [duodeno- + G. *lysis,* a freeing]. Incision of adhesions to the duodenum.

duodenorrhaphy (dū-ō-dĕ-nōr'ă-fē) [duodeno- + G. *rhaphē,* a seam]. Suture of a tear or incision in the duodenum.

duodenoscopy (dū-ō-dĕ-nos'kō-pē) [duodeno- + G. *skopeō,* to examine]. Inspection of the interior of the duodenum through an endoscope.

duodenostomy (dū-ō-dĕ-nos'tō-mē) [duodeno- + G. *stoma,* mouth]. Establishment of a fistula into the duodenum.

duodenotomy (dū-ō-dĕ-not'ō-mē) [duodeno- + G. *tomē,* incision]. Incision of the duodenum.

duodenum, gen. **duodeni,** pl. **duodena** (dū-ō-dē'nŭm, dū-od'ĕ-nŭm; -dē'nă, -od'ĕ-nă) [Mediev. L. fr. L. *duodeni,* twelve] [NA]. The first division of the small intestine, about 25 cm or 12 fingerbreadths (hence the name) in length, extending from the pylorus to the junction with the jejunum at the level of the first or second lumbar vertebra on the left side. It is divided into the pars superior, the first part of which is the duodenal cap, the pars descendens, into which the bile and pancreatic ducts open, the pars horizontalis (inferior) and the pars ascendens, terminating at the duodenojejunal junction.

duovirus (dū'ō-vī'rŭs). Rotavirus.

Duplay, Emanuel Simon, French surgeon, 1836–1924. See D.'s *disease.*

duplication (dū-pli-kā'shŭn). **1.** A doubling. See also reduplication. **2.** The inclusion of two copies of the same genetic material in a genome; an important step in diversification of genomes, as in the evolution of the (non-allelic) hemoglobin chains from a common ancestor.

d. of chromosomes, a chromosome aberration resulting from unequal crossing over or exchange of segments between two homologous chromosomes; one chromosome of the pair loses a small segment, while the other gains this segment; the chromosome gaining the segment has undergone d. while its homologue has undergone deletion.

duplicitas (dū-plis'i-tahs) [L. a doubling, fr. *duplex* (*duplic-*), twofold]. Doubling of a part.

d. ante'rior, anadidymus; conjoined twins in which fusion has united the pelvis and lower extremities, leaving the thoraces and head separate. See also cephalodidymus.

d. poste'rior, catadidymus; ileadelphus; iliadelphus; conjoined twins in which the heads and upper parts of the bodies have become fused, leaving the buttocks and legs separate. See also dipygus.

Dupré, 17th century Paris surgeon and anatomist. See D.'s *muscle.*

Dupuy-Dutemps, Louis, French ophthalmologist, 1871–1946. See D.-D. *operation.*

Dupuytren, Baron Guillaume, French surgeon and surgical pathologist, 1777–1835. See D.'s *amputation, canal, contracture, disease* (of the foot), *fascia, fracture, hydrocele, sign, suture, tourniquet.*

dura (dū'ră) [L. fem. of *durus,* hard]. Dura mater.

dural (dū'răl). Duramatral; relating to the dura mater.

duralumin (dūr-al'ū-min). An alloy of aluminum slightly heavier than this metal but nearly as strong as steel and noncorrodible; used in the manufacture of surgical and orthopedic appliances, *e.g.,* splints; not for internal use in the body as screws, plates.

dura mater (dū'ră mā'ter) [L. hard mother]. Dura; pachymeninx (as distinguished from leptomeninx, the combined pia mater and arachnoidea); a tough, fibrous membrane forming the outer envelope of the brain (the d.m. encephali) and the spinal cord (the d.m. spinalis).

d. m. of the brain, d. m. encephali.

d. m. enceph'ali [NA], d. m. of the brain, the intracranial dura, consisting of two layers, the outer one of which adheres to the periosteum of the cranial bones; the inner layer is fused with the outer except that locally the two layers separate to enclose large venous ducts, the sinus durae matris.

d. m. of the spinal cord, d. m. spinalis.

d. m. spina'lis [NA], d. m. of the spinal cord; endorrhachis; does not (in contrast to the d. m. encephali) adhere to the enveloping bony structures (vertebrae), and is separated from the latter by a considerable space, the epidural space, containing the plexus venosi vertebrales interni and variable amounts of fatty tissue.

duramatral (dū-ră-mā'trăl). Dural.

Duran-Reynals, Francisco, U.S. bacteriologist, 1899–1958. See D.-R. permeability *factor.*

duraplasty (dū'ră-plas-tē) [dura (mater) + G. *plastos,* formed]. A plastic or reconstructive operation on the dura mater.

duration (dū-rā'shŭn). A continuous period of time.

half amplitude pulse d., the time, in milliseconds, required for a wave form to reach half of its full magnitude.

pulse d., the interval between the leading and trailing edges of an output pulse.

Dürck, Hermann, Munich pathologist, 1869–1941. See D.'s *nodes.*

dur. dolor. Abbreviation for L. *duarte dolare,* while pain lasts.

Duret, Henri, French neurosurgeon, 1849–1921. See D.'s *lesion.*

Durham, Arthur E., British surgeon, 1834–1895. See D.'s *tube.*

Duroziez, Paul L., Paris physician, 1826–1897. See D.'s *disease, murmur, symptom.*

Dutton, Joseph Everett, British physician, 1877–1905. See D.'s *disease,* relapsing *fever.*

Duverney, Joseph G., French anatomist, 1648–1730. See D.'s *fissure, foramen, gland, muscle.*

D.V.M. Abbreviation for Doctor of Veterinary Medicine. This degree is now standard in the United States. The University of Pennsylvania uses the abbreviation V.M.D.

dwarf (dwōrf) [A.S. *dweorh*] Nanus; an abnormally undersized person. See subentries under dwarfism.

dwarfishness (dwōrf'ish-nes). Dwarfism.

dwarfism (dwōrf'izm). Dwarfishness; nanism; the condition of being abnormally undersized.

achondroplastic d., see achondroplasia.

acromelic d., acromelia.

aortic d., underdevelopment of physical stature associated with severe aortic stenosis.

asexual d., d. in which adult sexual development is deficient.

ateliotic d., idiopathic d.; d. of unknown cause characterized by normal proportions and, by currently available criteria, functional normality but with abnormally short stature.

camptomelic d., d. with shortening of the lower limbs, due to anterior bending of the femur and tibia.

chondrodystrophic d., see chondrodystrophy.

diastrophic d., an autosomal recessive form of d. characterized in its complete form by scoliosis, hitchhiker thumb, absent interphalangeal joints, cleft palate, chondritis followed by calcification of the ears, shortening of the Achilles tendon, clubbed foot, and characteristic radiologic findings; a milder variant may be allelic.

Fröhlich's d., d. with Fröhlich's syndrome.

hypothyroid d., cretinism.

idiopathic d., ateliotic d.

infantile d., infantilism (1).

Laron type d., d. associated with an absence of somatomedin and with high plasma levels of somatotropin.

lethal d., d. leading to intrauterine or neonatal death.

Lorain-Lévi d., pituitary d.

mesomelic d., d. with shortness of the forearms and lower legs.

metatropic d., congenital skeletal dysplasia characterized by a changing pattern of d. in which there is lengthening of the trunk (relative to the limbs) at birth but with subsequent shortening.

micromelic d., d. with abnormally short or small limbs.

phocomelic d., d. in which the diaphyses of the long bones are abnormally short or the intermediate parts of the limbs are absent.

physiologic d., primordial or true d.; d. characterized by normal development that is at a lesser rate than that for members of the same family, race, or other races.

pituitary d., Lorain-Lévi d., infantilism, or syndrome; pituitary infantilism; a rare form of d. caused by the absence of a functional anterior pituitary gland; may be present at birth or develop during early childhood.

polydystrophic d., Maroteaux-Lamy *syndrome.*

primordial d., physiologic d.

Seckel d., Seckel *syndrome.*

senile d., d. characterized by craniofacial anomalies with progeroid appearance.

sexual d., d. with normal sexual development.

Silver-Russell d., Silver-Russell *syndrome.*

snub-nose d., dominantly inherited Lévi's disease; d. characterized by low birth weight, snub nose, and stocky build; autosomal dominant inheritance.

thanatophoric d., a lethal d. characterized by micromelia, bowed long bones, enlarged head, flattened vertebral bodies, and muscular hypotonia; lack of pulmonary ventilation causes respiratory difficulties with cyanosis leading to death within days after birth.

true d., physiologic d.

Dy Symbol for dysprosium.

dyad (dī'ad) [G. *dyas,* the number two, duality]. **1.** Diad (2); a pair. **2.** In chemistry, a bivalent element. **3.** A pair of peronsin an interactional situation, *e.g.,* patient and therapist, husband and wife. **4.** The double chromosome resulting from the splitting of a tetrad during meiosis.

dyclonine hydrochloride (dī'klō-nēn). 4'-Butoxy-3-piperidinopropiophenone hydrochloride; a topical local anesthetic.

dydrogesterone (dī-drō-jes'ter-ōn). 9β,10α-pregna-4,6-diene-3,20-dione; a synthetic steroid, derived from retroprogesterone, with progestational effects.

dye (dī) [A.S. *deah, deag*]. A stain or coloring matter; a compound consisting of chromophore and auxochrome groups attached to one or more benzene rings, its color being due to the chromophore and its dyeing affinities to the auxochrome. D.'s are used for intravital coloration of living cells, staining tissues and microorganisms, as antiseptics and germicides, and some as stimulants of epithelial growth. For individual d.'s, see the specific names.

acidic d.'s, d.'s which ionize in solution to produce negatively charged ions or anions; they consist of sodium salts of phenols and carboxylic acid dyes; their solutions tend to be neutral or slightly alkaline; examples are eosin and aniline blue.

acridine d.'s, derivatives of the compound acridine which is closely related to xanthene; important as fluorochromes in histology, cytochemistry, and chemotherapy; examples include acriflavine, acridine orange, and quinacrine mustard.
azin d.'s, d. derivatives of phenazine, $C_6H_4{\cdot}N_2{\cdot}C_6H_4$ that include important histologic stains, such as neutral red, azocarmine G., and safranin O.
azo d.'s, d.'s in which the azo group is the chromophore and joins benzene or naphthalene rings; they include a large number of biologic stains, such as Congo red and oil red O; also used clinically to promote epithelial growth in the treatment of ulcers, burns, and other wounds; many have anticoagulant action.
azocarmine d.'s, d.'s giving a dark purplish red color as histologic stains.
basic d.'s, d.'s which ionize in solution to give positively charged ions or cations; the auxochrome group is an amine which can form a salt with an acid like HCl; solutions are usually slightly acidic; examples include basic fuchsin and toluidine blue O.
diphenylmethane d.'s, d.'s in which the central carbon connecting two phenyl groups lacks an amino or imino group; the chromophore is the quinoid ring; an alternative formulation is as a ketonimide; the most common example is auramine O.
ketonimine d.'s, d.'s in which the chromophore is $\geq C{=}NH$ connected to two benzene rings; alkylamino groups are added para to the methane carbon on both rings. The most important member for biological purposes is auramine O; an alternative formulation is as a diphenylmethane dye.
natural d.'s, d.'s obtained from animals or plants; examples include carmine, obtained from cochineal in the dried female insect *Dactylopius cacti* of Central America, and hematoxylin, extracted from the bark of the logwood tree *Haematoxylon campechianum* in the Caribbean area.
nitro d.'s, d.'s in which the chromophore is $-NO_2$, which is so acidic that all dyes in this group are of the acid type; important examples in cytoplasmic staining are picric acid and naphthol yellow S.
oxazin d.'s, similar to azin d.'s except that one of the connecting N atoms is replaced by O; most important representatives are brilliant cresyl blue, orcein, litmus, and cresyl violet.
rosanilin d.'s, several triaminotriphenylmethane d.'s or mixtures of them often sold under the name of basic fuchsin; rosanilin d.'s differ from other triphenylmethane d.'s in that the amino groups are unsubstituted, and they may have methyl groups introduced directly onto the benzene rings; the four possible such dyes are pararosanilin, rosanilin, new fuchsin, and magenta II.
salt d., neutral *stain.*
synthetic d.'s, organic d. compounds originally derived from coal-tar derivatives; presently produced by synthesis from benzene and its derivatives; examples include eosin, methylene blue, and fluorescein.
thiazin d.'s, similar to azin d.'s except that one of the connecting N atoms is replaced by S; includes many important biological stains, especially in hematology, *e.g.,* azure A, azure B, and methylene blue.
triphenylmethane d.'s, a group of d.'s that includes pararosanilin, as well as many others used in histology and cytology; employed as nuclear, cytoplasmic, and connective tissue stains; important in histochemistry as in the preparation of Schiff's reagent.
xanthene d.'s, derivatives of the compound xanthene; include the pyronins, rhodamines, and fluoresceins.

Dyggve. See D.-Melchior-Clausen *syndrome.*

-dymus [G. *-dymos,* fold]. **1.** Suffix to be combined with number roots; *e.g.,* didymus, tridymus, tetradymus. **2.** Occasionally used shortened form for -didymus.

dynamics (dī-nam′iks) [G. *dynamis,* force]. **1.** The science of motion in response to forces. **2.** In psychiatry, the determination of how behavior patterns and emotional reactions develop. **3.** In the behavioral sciences, any of the numerous intrapersonal and interpersonal influences or phenomena associated with personality development and interpersonal processes.
group d., a term used to represent the study of underlying features of group behavior, *e.g.,* motives, attitudes; it is concerned with group change rather than with static characteristics.

dynamo- [G. *dynamis,* force]. Combining form relating to force or energy.

dynamogenesis (dī′nă-mō-jen′ĕ-sis) [dynamo- + G. *genesis,* production]. Dynamogeny; the production of force, especially of muscular or nervous energy.

dynamogenic (dī′nă-mō-jen′ik). Producing power or force, especially nervous or muscular power or activity.

dynamogeny (dī-nă-moj′ĕ-nē). Dynamogenesis.

dynamograph (dī-nam′ō-graf) [dynamo- + G. *graphō,* to write]. An instrument for recording the degree of muscular power.

dynamometer (dī-nă-mom′ĕ-ter) [dynamo- + G. *metron,* measure]. Ergometer; an instrument for measuring the degree of muscular power.

dynamoscope (dī-nam′ō-skōp) [dynamo- + G. *skopeō,* to examine]. A modified stethoscope for auscultation of the muscles.

dynamoscopy (dī-nă-mos′kō-pē). Auscultation of a contracting muscle.

dynatherm (dī′nă-therm) [G. *dynamis,* force, + *thermē,* heat]. An apparatus for inducing diathermy.

dyne (dīn) [G. *dynamis,* force]. The unit of force in the CGS system, replaced in the SI system by the newton (1 newton = 10^5 dynes), that gives a body of 1 g mass an acceleration of 1 cm/sec^2; expressed as F (dynes) = m (grams) × a (cm/sec^2).

dynein (dīn′ēn) [dyne + protein]. A protein associated with motile structures, exhibiting adenosine triphosphatase activity; it forms "arms" on the outer tubules of cilia and flagella. See also tubulin; dynein *arm.*

dyphylline (dī-fil′in). 7-(2,3-Dihydroxypropyl)theophylline; exhibits characteristic peripheral vasodilator and bronchodilator actions of other theophylline compounds.

dys- [G.]. Prefix meaning bad or difficult. *Cf.* dis-.

dysacousia, dysacusia (dis-ă-kū′sē-ă). Dysacusis.

dysacusis (dis-ă-kū′sis) [dys- + G. *akousis,* hearing]. Dysacousia; dysacusia. **1.** Any impairment of hearing that is not primarily a lessening of the ability to perceive sound; involves difficulty in processing details of sound as opposed to any loss of sensitivity to sound. **2.** Pain or discomfort in the ear from exposure to sound.

dysadaptation (dis′ad-ap-tā′shŭn). Dysaptation.

dysantigraphia (dis′an-tē-graf′ē-ă) [dys- + G. *antigraphō,* to write back]. A form of agraphia in which the subject is unable to copy written or printed matter.

dysaphia (dis-ā′fē-ă, dis-af′ē-ă) [dys- + G. *haphē,* touch]. Impairment of the sense of touch.

dysaphic (dis-ā′fik). Relating to impaired tactile sensibility.

dysaptation (dis′ap-tā′shŭn). Dysadaptation; inability of the retina and iris to accommodate well to varying intensities of light.

dysarteriotony (dis-ar-tēr-ē-ot′ō-nē) [dys- + G. *artēria,* artery, + *tonos,* tension]. Abnormal blood pressure, either too high or too low.

dysarthria (dis-ar′thrē-ă) [dys- + G. *arthroō,* to articulate]. Dysarthrosis (1); a disturbance of articulation due to emotional stress, to brain injury, or to paralysis, incoordination, or spasticity of the muscles used for speaking.
d. litera′lis, seldom used term for stammering.
d. syllaba′ris spasmod′ica, seldom used term for stuttering.

dysarthric (dis-ar'thrik). Relating to dysarthria.

dysarthrosis (dis-ar-thrō'sis) [dys- + G. *arthrōsis,* joint]. **1.** Dysarthria. **2.** Malformation of a joint. **3.** A false joint.

dysautonomia (dis'aw-tō-nō'mē-ă) [dys- + G. *autonomia,* self-government]. Abnormal functioning of the autonomic nervous system.
familial d., Riley-Day syndrome; a congenital syndrome with specific disturbances of the nervous system and aberrations in autonomic nervous system function such as indifference to pain, diminished lacrimation, poor vasomotor control, motor incoordination, labile cardiovascular reactions, hyporeflexia, frequent attacks of bronchial pneumonia, hypersalivation with aspiration and difficulty in swallowing, hyperemesis, emotional instability, and an intolerance for anesthetics; autosomal recessive inheritance.

dysbarism (dis'bar-izm) [dys- + G. *baros,* weight]. General term for the symptom complex resulting from exposure to decreased or changing barometric pressure, including all physiologic effects resulting from such changes with the exception of hypoxia, and including the effects of rapid decompression.

dysbasia (dis-bā'zē-ă) [dys- + G. *basis,* a step]. **1.** Difficulty in walking. **2.** The difficult or distorted walking that occurs in persons with certain mental disorders.
d. angiosclerot'ica, d. angiospas'tica, obsolete terms meaning intermittent difficulty in walking due to peripheral vascular causes.
d. lordot'ica progressi'va, torsion neurosis; an affection characterized by lordoscoliosis of the lower portion of the vertebral column, occurring when the patient stands or walks and usually disappearing when he lies down.

dysbolism (dis'bō-lizm) [dys- + G. *bolē* (*metabolē*), + *-ismos,* metabolism]. Abnormal, but not necessarily morbid, metabolism, as in alkaptonuria.

dysbulia (dis-bū'lē-ă) [dys- + G. *boulē,* will]. Weakness and uncertainty of volition.

dysbulic (dis-bū'lik). Relating to, or characterized by, dysbulia.

dyscalculia (dis-kal-kyū'lē-ă). Difficulty in performing simple mathematical problems; commonly seen in parietal lobe lesions.

dyscephalia (dis-sĕ-fā'lē-ă) [dys- + G. *kephalē,* head]. Dyscephaly; malformation of the head and face.
d. mandib'ulo-oculofacia'lis, a syndrome of bony anomalies of the calvaria, face, and jaw, with brachygnathia, narrow curved nose, and multiple ocular defects including microphthalmia, microcornea, and cataract, often with alopecia overlying skull sutures, or alopecia areata and hypoplasia, or absence of eyebrows. Also called congenital sutural alopecia; progeria with cataract or with microphthalmia; mandibulo-oculofacial dysmorphia or syndrome; oculomandibulodyscephaly; Hallermann-Streiff syndrome.

dyscephaly (dis-sef'ă-lē). Dyscephalia.

dyscheiral, dyschiral (dis-kī'răl). Relating to dyscheiria.

dyscheiria, dyschiria (dis-kī'rē-ă) [dys- + G. *cheir,* hand]. A disorder of sensibility in which, although there is no apparent loss of sensation, the patient is unable to tell which side of the body has been touched (acheiria), or refers it to the wrong side (allocheiria), or to both sides (syncheiria).

dyschezia (dis-kē'zē-ă) [dys- + G. *chezō,* to defecate]. Difficulty in defecation.

dyschiria (dis-kī'rē-ă). Dyscheiria.

dyschondrogenesis (dis-kon-drō-jen'ĕ-sis) [dys- + G. *chondros,* cartilage, + *genesis,* production]. Abnormal development of cartilage.

dyschondroplasia (dis-kon-drō-pla'zē-ă) [dys- + G. *chondros,* cartilage, + *plasis,* a forming]. Enchondromatosis.
d. with hemangiomas, Maffuci's *syndrome.*

dyschondrosteosis (dis'kon-dros-tē-ō'sis) [dys- + G. *chondros,* cartilage, + *osteon,* bone, + *-osis,* condition]. Leri-Weill disease or syndrome; Leri's pleonosteosis; a bone dysplasia characterized by bowing of the radius, dorsal dislocation of the distal ulna and proximal carpal bones, and mesomelic dwarfism; autosomal dominant inheritance.

dyschroia, dyschroa (dis-kroy'ă, -krō'ă) [dys- + G. *chroia, chroa,* color]. A bad complexion; discoloration of the skin.

dyschromatopsia (dis'krō-mă-top'sē-ă) [dys- + G. *chrōma,* color, + *opsis,* vision]. Dichromatism (2).

dyschromatosis (dis-krō-mă-tō'sis) [dys- + G. *chrōma,* color, + *-osis,* condition]. An asymptomatic anomaly of pigmentation occurring among the Japanese; may be localized or diffuse.

dyschromia (dis-krō'mē-ă) Any abnormality in the color of the skin.

dyscinesia (dis'si-nē'zē-ă). Dyskinesia.

dyscoimesis (dis-koy-mē'sis) [dys- + G. *koimēsis,* a sleeping, fr. *koimaō,* to put to sleep]. A form of insomnia marked by difficulty or delay in falling asleep.

dyscontrol (dis-kon-trōl'). Episodes of violence, without adequate cause but assumed to be related to an epileptic discharge in the amygdala.

dyscoria (dis-kō'rē-ă) [dys- + G. *korē,* pupil of eye]. Abnormality in the shape of the pupil.

dyscrasia (dis-krā'zē-ă) [G. bad temperament, fr. dys- + *krasis,* a mixing]. **1.** A morbid general state resulting from the presence of abnormal material in the blood, usually applied to diseases affecting blood cells or platelets. **2.** Old term indicating disease.
blood d., a diseased state of the blood; usually refers to abnormal cellular elements of a permanent character.

dyscrasic, dyscratic (dis-krā'sik, krat'ik). Pertaining to or affected with dyscrasia.

dysdiadochokinesia, dysdiadochocinesia (dis-dī-ad'ō-kō-ki-nē'zē-ă) [dys- + G. *diadochos,* working in turn, + *kinēsis,* movement]. Impairment of the ability to perform rapidly alternating movements.

dysembryoma (dis-em-brē-ō'mă). A teratoid tumor with its tissues showing more irregular arrangement than the typical embryomas.

dysembryoplasia (dis-em'brē-ō-plā'zē-ă) [dys- + G. *embryon,* fetus, + *plasis,* a molding]. Prenatal malformation.

dysemia (dis-ē'mē-ă) [dys- + G. *haima,* blood]. Any abnormal condition or disease of the blood.

dysencephalia splanchnocystica (dis'en-se-fā'lē-ă splangk-nō-sis'ti-kă). Gruber's or Meckel syndrome; a malformation syndrome, lethal in the perinatal period, and characterized by intrauterine growth retardation, sloping forehead, occipital exencephalocele, ocular anomalies, cleft palate, polydactyly, polycystic kidney, and other malformations; autosomal recessive inheritance.

dyseneia (dis'ĕ-nē'ă) [dys- + G. *ania,* bridle; *dysēnios,* refractory]. Defective articulation secondary to deafness.

dysenteric (dis-en-tăr'ik). Relating to or suffering from dysentery.

dysentery (dis-en-tăr-ē) [G. *dysenteria,* fr. *dys-,* bad, + *entera,* bowels]. A disease marked by frequent watery stools, often with blood and mucus, and characterized clinically by pain, tenesmus, fever, and dehydration.
amebic d., diarrhea resulting from ulcerative inflammation of the colon, caused chiefly by infection with *Entamoeba histolytica;* may be mild or severe and may also be associated with amebic infection of other organs.
bacillary d., Japanese d.; infection with *Shigella dysenteriae, S. flexneri,* or other organisms.
balantidial d., a type of colitis resembling in many respects amebic d.; caused by the parasitic ciliate, *Balantidium coli.*
bilharzial d., d. due to infection with *Schistosoma mansoni, S. haematobium,* or *S. japonicum.*
chronic d. of cattle, Johne's *disease.*

fulminating d., malignant d.
helminthic d., d. caused by infection with parasitic worms.
Japanese d., bacillary d.
lamb d., enterotoxemia of lambs caused by type B toxins of *Clostridium perfringens.*
malignant d., fulminating d.; d. in which the symptoms are intensely acute, leading to prostration, collapse, and often death.
Sonne d., d. due to infection by *Shigella sonnei;* sometimes milder than other types of bacterial d. caused by *Shigella.*
spirillar d., a form of d. or diarrhea, described as occurring in the south of France, believed to be caused by a spirillum present in great numbers in the intestinal epithelia.
swine d., an acute hemorrhagic colitis of swine, often accompanied by gastritis; the small intestines usually are not involved; its primary cause is *Treponema hyodysenteriae,* and it has a high mortality rate, especially among feeder pigs.
viral d., profuse watery diarrhea due to, or thought to be due to, infection by a virus.
winter d. of cattle, a specific, highly contagious and severe disease of unknown origin; the disease is seen in the cold months of the year, outbreaks generally abate after a few days; the death rate is low, but the loss in flesh and milk is often high.

dyserethism (dis-er′ĕ-thizm) [dys- + G. *erethismos,* irritation]. A condition of slow response to stimuli.

dysergia (dis-er′jē-ă) [dys- + G. *ergon,* work]. Lack of harmonious action between the muscles concerned in executing any definite voluntary movement.

dysesthesia (dis-es-thē′zē-ă) [G. *dysaisthesia,* fr. *dys-,* hard, difficult, + *aisthēsis,* sensation]. **1.** Impairment of sensation short of anesthesia. **2.** A condition in which a disagreeable sensation is produced by ordinary stimuli.

dysfibrinogenemia (dis′fī-brin′ō-jĕ-nē′mē-ă). A familial disorder of qualitatively abnormal fibrinogens, with various types classified as follows: 1) Amsterdam, Bethesda II, Cleveland, Los Angeles, Saint Louis, Zurich I and II: major defect, aggregation of fibrin monomers; thrombin time prolonged; inhibitory effect on normal clotting; asymptomatic; 2) Bethesda I and Detroit: major defect, fibrinopeptide release; thrombin time prolonged; inhibitory effect on normal clotting; abnormal bleeding; 3) Baltimore: major defect, fibrinopeptide release; thrombin time prolonged; no inhibitory effect on normal clotting; bleeding and thrombosis; 4) Leuven: major defect, questionable aggregation of fibrin monomers; thrombin time prolonged; slight inhibitory effect on normal clotting; abnormal bleeding; 5) Metz: major defect unreported; thrombin time infinite; effect on normal clotting unreported; abnormal bleeding; 6) Nancy: major defect, aggregation of fibrin monomers; thrombin time prolonged; slight inhibitory effect on normal clotting; asymptomatic; 7) Oklahoma: major defect unreported; thrombin time normal; no effect on normal clotting; abnormal bleeding; 8) Oslo: major defect unreported; thrombin time shortened; effect on normal clotting unreported; abnormal thrombosis; 9) Parma: major defect unreported; thrombin time infinite; no inhibitory effect on normal clotting; abnormal bleeding; 10) Paris I: major defect unreported; thrombin time infinite; inhibitory effect on normal clotting; asymptomatic; 11) Paris II: major defect unreported; thrombin time prolonged; inhibitory effect on normal clotting; asymptomatic; 12) Troyes: major defect unreported; thrombin time prolonged; effect on normal clotting unreported; asymptomatic; 13) Vancouver: major defect unreported; thrombin time prolonged; no effect on normal clotting; abnormal bleeding; 14) Wiesbaden: major defect, aggregation of fibrin monomers; thrombin time prolonged; inhibitory effect on normal clotting; bleeding and thrombosis.

dysfunction (dis-fŭnk′shŭn). Difficult or abnormal function.
constitutional hepatic d., familial nonhemolytic *jaundice.*
dental d., abnormal functioning of dental structures.
minimal brain d., attention deficit *disorder.*
papillary muscle d., papillary muscle syndrome; impaired function of a papillary muscle, usually due to ischemia or infarction, with resulting incompetence of the mitral valve.
psychosexual d., sexual d., a disturbance of sexual functioning, *e.g.,* impotence, premature ejaculation, anorgasmia, presumed to be of predominantly psychological rather than physical etiology.
temporomandibular joint d. (TMJ), chronic or impaired function of the temporomandibular articulation. See temporomandibular *arthrosis;* myofacial pain-dysfunction *syndrome.*

dysgammaglobulinemia (dis-gam′ă-glob′yū-li-nē′mē-ă). An immunoglobulin abnormality, especially a disturbance of the percentage distribution of γ-globulins.

dysgenesis (dis-jen′ĕ-sis) [dys- + G. *genesis,* generation]. Defective embryonic development.
gonadal d., defective gonadal development, varying types and degrees of which have been identified, including gonadal aplasia or agenesis, rudimentary gonads, congenitally defective gonads, and true hermaphroditism; the character of the external genitalia, genital ducts, and secondary sexual development are only sometimes uniquely related to a given type of gonadal d. **XO g.d.** is the formation of monosomy X with a gonadal streak rather than a true ovary, notably in Turner's syndrome; **XX g.d.** is an autosomal recessive disorder with a female karyotype, streaked gonads, and primary amenorrhea, but with no body features of Turner's syndrome; **XY g.d.** is an X-linked disorder associated with a male karyotype and a female habitus, streaked gonads, and absence of secondary sexual characteristics.
iridocorneal mesodermal d., Rieger's anomaly; mesodermal d. of cornea and iris, producing pupillary anomalies, posterior embryotoxon, and secondary glaucoma.
seminiferous tubule d., germinal aplasia; a disorder in which the seminiferous tubules exhibit an abnormal cytoarchitecture and extensive hyalinization; the testes are small, and few spermatozoa are formed; the body habitus may be eunuchoid, and gynecomastia may be present; urinary gonadotropin output is usually elevated, and the incidence of mental deficiency and illness is above normal; sex chromatin may be male or female, and androgen secretion ranges from subnormal to normal. It is a constant feature of (and is often used synonymously with) Klinefelter's *syndrome.*
testicular d., a congenital derangement of seminiferous tubular structure and function, resulting in male infertility; the defect in spermatogenesis may be incomplete, as in maturational arrest or premature sloughing, or spermatogenesis may be completely absent, as in the Sertoli-cell-only syndrome.

dysgenic (dis-jen′ik). Applying to factors that have a detrimental effect upon hereditary qualities, physical or mental.

dysgerminoma (dis-jer-mi-nō′mă) [dys- + L. *germen,* a bud or sprout, + G. *-ōma,* tumor]. Disgerminoma; a rare malignant neoplasm of the ovary (counterpart of seminoma of the testis), composed of undifferentiated gonadal germinal cells and occurring more frequently in patients less than 20 years of age. The neoplasms are gray-yellow and firm, contain foci of necrosis and hemorrhage, and tend to be encapsulated; characteristically, they spread by way of lymphatic vessels, but widespread metastases also occur.

dysgeusia (dis-gū′sē-ă) [dys- + G. *geusis,* taste]. Impairment or perversion of the gustatory sense.

dysgnathia (dis-nath′ē-ă) [dys- + G. *gnathos,* jaw]. Any abnormality that extends beyond the teeth and includes the maxilla or mandible, or both.

dysgnathic (dis-nath′ik). Pertaining to or characterized by abnormality of the maxilla and mandible.

dysgnosia (dis-nō′sē-ă) [G. *dysgnōsia,* difficulty of knowing]. Any cognitive disorder, *i.e.,* any mental illness.

dysgonic (dis-gon'ik) [dys- + G. *gonikos,* relating to the seed or offspring]. A term used to indicate that the growth of a bacterial culture is slow and relatively poor; used especially in reference to the growth of cultures of the bovine tubercle bacillus (*Mycobacterium bovis*). See also eugonic.

dysgraphia (dis-graf'ē-ă) [dys- + G. *graphē,* writing]. **1.** Difficulty in writing. **2.** Writer's *cramp.*

dyshematopoiesis (dis-hē'mă-tō-poy-ē'sis) [dys- + G. *haima (haimat-),* blood, + *poiēsis,* making]. Dyshemopoiesis; defective formation of the blood.

dyshematopoietic (dis-hē'mă-tō-poy-et'ik). Dyshemopoietic; pertaining to or characterized by dyshematopoiesis.

dyshemopoiesis (dis-hē'mō-poy-ē'sis). Dyshematopoiesis.

dyshemopoietic (dis-hē'mō-poy-et'ik). Dyshematopoietic.

dyshidria (dis-hid'rē-ă) Dyshidrosis.

dyshidrosis (dis-i-drō'sis) [dys- + G. *hidrōs,* sweat]. Pompholyx; cheiropompholyx; chiropompholyx; dyshidria; dysidria; dysidrosis; a vesicular or vesicopustular eruption that occurs primarily on the hands and feet; the lesions spread peripherally but have a tendency to central clearing.

dysidria (dis-id'rē-ă). Dyshidrosis.

dysidrosis (dis-i-drō'sis). Dyshidrosis.

dyskaryosis (dis-kar-ē-ō'sis) [dys- + G. *karyon,* nucleus, + *-ōsis,* condition]. Abnormal maturation seen in exfoliated cells which have normal cytoplasm but hyperchromatic nuclei, or irregular chromatin distribution; may be followed by the development of a malignant neoplasm.

dyskaryotic (dis-kar-ē-ot'ik). Pertaining to or characterized by dyskaryosis.

dyskeratoma (dis-ker-ă-tō'mă) [dys- + G. *keras,* horn, + *-oma,* tumor]. A skin tumor exhibiting dyskeratosis.
warty d., isolated dyskeratosis follicularis; a benign solitary tumor of the skin, usually of the scalp, face, or neck, with a central keratotic plug; it appears to arise from a hair follicle, and microscopically resembles a lesion of keratosis follicularis but is larger, with more extensive epithelial downgrowth.

dyskeratosis (dis'ker-ă-tō'sis) [dys- + G. *keras,* horn, + *-osis,* condition]. **1.** Premature keratinization of epithelial cells that have not reached the keratinizing surface layer; dyskeratotic cells are generally rounded and separated from adjacent cells by apoptosis. **2.** Epidermalization of the conjunctival and corneal epithelium. **3.** A disorder of keratinization.
benign d., d. that may occur in congenital and bullous diseases of the skin.
d. congen'ita, nail dystrophy, oral leukokeratosis, and reticular pigmentation of the skin, with anemia progressing to pancytopenia; X-linked recessive inheritance.
intraepithelial d., d. of oral, conjunctival, and corneal epithelium; autosomal dominant inheritance.
isolated d. follicula'ris, warty *dyskeratoma.*
malignant d., d. that may occur in precancerous or malignant lesions.

dyskeratotic (dis'ker-a-tot'ik). Relating to or characterized by dyskeratosis.

dyskinesia (dis-ki-nē'zē-ă) [dys- + G. *kinēsis,* movement]. Dyscinesia; difficulty in performing voluntary movements.
d. al'gera, a hysterical condition in which active movement causes pain.
biliary d., abnormal mobility (spasm) of the gallbladder or its ducts impairing filling or emptying due to intrinsic (inflammatory) or extrinsic (calculi) disease.
extrapyramidal d.'s, abnormal involuntary movements attributed to pathological states of one or more parts of the corpus striatum (see extrapyramidal motor system) and characterized by insuppressible, stereotyped, automatic movements that cease only during sleep; *e.g.,* Parkinson's disease; chorea; athetosis; hemiballism.
d. intermit'tens, intermittent disability of the limbs due to impairment of circulation.
tardive oral d., abnormal grimacing about the mouth occurring some weeks after taking certain psychotropic drugs.
tracheobronchial d., degeneration of elastic and connective tissue of bronchi and trachea.

dyskinetic (dis-ki-net'ik). Denoting or characteristic of dyskinesia.

dyslalia (dis-lā'lē-ă, -lal'ē-ă) [dys- + G. *lalia,* talking]. Disorder of articulation due to structural abnormalities of the articulatory organs or impaired hearing.

dyslexia (dis-lek'sē-ă) [dys- + G. *lexis,* word, phrase]. Incomplete alexia; a level of reading ability markedly below that expected on the basis of the individual's level of over-all intelligence or ability in skills.

dyslexic (dis-lek'sik). Relating to, or characterized by, dyslexia.

dyslipidosis (dis'lip-i-dō'sis). Rarely used term for an inborn disorder of lipid metabolism.

dyslogia (dis-lō'jē-ă) [dys- + G. *logos,* speaking, reason]. **1.** Impairment of speech as the result of a brain lesion. **2.** Impairment of the reasoning faculty.

dysmasesis (dis-mă-sē'sis) [dys- + G. *masēsis,* chewing]. Difficulty in mastication.

dysmature (dis'mă-tyūr). **1.** Denoting faulty development or ripening; often connoting structural and/or functional abnormalities. **2.** In obstetrics, denoting an infant whose birth weight is inappropriately low for its gestational age.

dysmaturity (dis'mă-chūr-i-tē). Syndrome of an infant born with relative absence of subcutaneous fat, wrinkling of the skin, prominent finger and toe nails, and meconium staining of the infant's skin and of the placental membranes; often associated with postmaturity or placental insufficiency.

dysmegalopsia (dis-meg-ă-lop'sē-ă) [dys- + G. *magas,* great, + *opsis,* vision]. Difficulty in perception of the size of objects; an abnormality in which objects appear larger than they are.

dysmelia (dis-mē'lē-ă) [dys- + G. *melos,* limb]. Congenital abnormality characterized by missing or foreshortened extremities, sometimes with associated spine abnormalities; caused by metabolic disturbance at the time of primordial limb development.

dysmenorrhea (dis-men-ōr-ē'ă) [dys- + G. *mēn,* month, + *rhoia,* a flow]. Menorrhalgia; difficult and painful menstruation.
essential d., primary d.
functional d., primary d.
intrinsic d., primary d.
mechanical d., obstructive d.; d. due to obstruction of discharge of menstrual blood, as in cervical stenosis.
membranous d., d. accompanied by an exfoliation of the menstrual decidua.
obstructive d., mechanical d.
ovarian d., a form of secondary d. due to disease of an ovary.
primary d., essential, functional, or intrinsic d.; d. due to a functional disturbance and to inflammation, new growths, or anatomic factors.
secondary d., d. due to inflammation, infection, tumor, or anatomical or orthopedic factors.
spasmodic d., d. accompanied by painful contractions of the uterus.
tubal d., a form of secondary d. due to stenosis or other abnormal condition of the fallopian tubes.
ureteric d., a form of secondary d. characterized by pain due to spasm of the ureter occurring at the time of the menses.
uterine d., a form of secondary d. resulting from disease of the

uterus.

vaginal d., a form of secondary d. due to obstruction or other abnormal condition in the vagina.

dysmetria (dis-mē'trē-ă, -met'rē-ă) [dys- + G. *metron,* measure]. A form of dysergia in which the subject is unable to arrest a muscular movement at the desired point. See also hypermetria; hypometria.

ocular d., abnormality of ocular movements in which the eyes overshoot on attempting to fixate an object.

dysmimia (dis-mim'ē-ă) [dys- + G. *mimeomai,* to mimic]. Obsolete term for an impairment of expression by gestures or of imitation.

dysmnesia (dis-nē'zē-ă) [dys- + G. *mnēmē, mnēsi-,* memory]. Obsolete term for a naturally poor or an impaired memory.

dysmorphia (dis-mōr'fē-ă). Dysmorphism.

mandibulo-oculofacial d., *dyscephalia* mandibulo-oculofacialis.

dysmorphism (dis-mōr'fizm) [G. *dysmorphia,* badness of form]. Abnormality of shape.

dysmorphogenesis (dis'mōr-fō-jen'ĕ-sis) [dys- + G. *morphē,* form, + *genesis,* production]. The process of abnormal tissue formation.

dysmorphology (dis-mōr-fol'ō-jē) [dys- + G. *morphē,* form, + *logos,* study]. General term for the study of, or the subject of, abnormal development of tissue form.

dysmorphophobia (dis'mōr-fō-fō'bē-ă) [dys- + G. *morphē,* form, + *phobos,* fear]. Preoccupation with some imagined defect in physical appearance which is out of proportion to any actual deformity that may exist.

dysmyelination (dis-mī-ĕ-li-nā'shŭn). Improper laying down or breakdown of a myelin sheath of a nerve fiber, caused by abnormal myelin metabolism.

dysmyotonia (dis-mī-ō-tō'nē-ă) [dys- + G. *mys,* muscle, + *tonos,* tension, tone]. Abnormal muscular tonicity (either hyper- or hypo). See dystonia.

dysnystaxis (dis-nis-tak'sis) [dys- + G. *nystaxis,* drowsiness]. Light sleep; a condition of half sleep.

dysodontiasis (dis'ō-don-tī'ă-sis) [dys- + G. *odous,* tooth, + *-iasis,* condition]. Difficulty or irregularity in the eruption of the teeth.

dysontogenesis (dis'on-tō-jen'ĕ-sis) [dys- + G. *ōn,* being, + *genesis,* origin]. Defective development of the individual.

dysontogenetic (dis'on-tō-jĕ-net'ik). Characterized by dysontogenesis.

dysorexia (dis-ō-rek'sē-ă) [dys- + G. *orexis,* appetite]. Diminished or perverted appetite.

dysosmia (dis-oz'mē-ă) [dys- + G. *osmē,* smell]. Impaired sense of smell.

dysosteogenesis (dis'os-tē-ō-jen'ĕ-sis) [dys- + G. *osteon,* bone, + *genesis,* production]. Dysostosis; defective bone formation.

dysostosis (dis-os-tō'sis) [dys- + G. *osteon,* bone, + *-osis,* condition]. Dysosteogenesis.

acrofacial d., acrofacial syndrome; mandibulofacial d. associated with malformations of the extremities such as defective radius and thumbs, and radioulnar synostosis.

cleidocranial d., clidocranial d., craniocleidodysostosis; cleidocranial dysplasia; a development defect characterized by absence or rudimentary development of the clavicles, abnormal shape of the skull with depression of the sagittal suture, frontal bosses, many wormian bones, and aplasia or hypoplasia of teeth; autosomal dominant inheritance.

craniofacial d., Crouzon's disease or syndrome; craniostosis with widening of the skull and high forehead, ocular hypertelorism, exophthalmos, beaked nose, and hypoplasia of the maxilla; usually autosomal dominant inheritance.

mandibuloacral d., an autosomal recessive disorder characterized by dental crowding, acro-osteolysis, stiff joints, and atrophy of the skin of the hands and feet; clavicals are hypoplastic, cranial suture are wide, and multiple wormian bones are present.

mandibulofacial d., mandibulofacial dysplasia; mandibulofacial dysostosis syndrome; a variable syndrome of malformations primarily of derivatives of the first branchial arch; characterized by palpebral fissures sloping outward and downward with notches or coloboma in the outer third of the lower lids, bony defects or hypoplasia of malar bones and zygoma, hypoplasia of the mandible, macrostomia with high or cleft palate and malposition and malocclusion of teeth, low-set malformed external ears, atypical hair growth, and occasional pits or clefts between mouth and ear. Also called Franceschetti's syndrome (if complete or nearly complete), or Treacher Collins syndrome (if limited to orbit and malar region).

metaphysial d., a rare developmental abnormality of the skeleton in which metaphyses of tubular bones are expanded by deposits of cartilage.

d. mul'tiplex, Hurler's *syndrome.*

orodigitofacial d., an inherited syndrome, lethal in males, with varying combinations of defects of the oral cavity, face, and hands, including lobulated or bifid tongue, cleft or pseudocleft palate, tongue tumors, missing or malpositioned teeth, pug-nose, depressed nasal bridge, brachydactyly, clinodactyly, incomplete syndactyly, and, frequently, mental retardation; X-linked dominant inheritance. Also called, OFD, orofaciodigital, or Papillon-Léage and Psaume syndrome.

otomandibular d., otomandibular syndrome; hypoplasia of the mandible, often with malformation of the temporomandibular joint, associated with malformations of the ear but not of the eye or with malar defects.

peripheral d., d. of the metacarpals and metatarsals, accompanied by variable facial features; possibly autosomal dominant inheritance.

dyspallia (dis-pal'ē-ă) [dys- + L. *pallium,* cloak]. Developmental distortion of the brain mantle.

dyspareunia (dis-pa-rū'nē-ă) [dys- + G. *pareunos,* lying beside, fr. *para,* beside, + *eunē,* a bed]. Occurrence of pain during sexual intercourse.

dyspepsia (dis-pep'sē-ă) [dys- + G. *pepsis,* digestion]. Gastric indigestion; impaired gastric function or "upset stomach" due to some disorder of the stomach; characterized by epigastric pain, sometimes burning, nausea, and gaseous eructation.

acid d., d. associated with excess gastric acidity.

adhesion d., pain, d., and other symptoms alleged to result from perigastric adhesions.

atonic d., functional d. (1); d. with impaired tone in the muscular walls of the stomach.

fermentative d., d. accompanied by fermentation of the contents of the stomach, usually occurring in gastric dilation.

flatulent d., d. with frequent eructations of swallowed air, sometimes without underlying organic disease.

functional d., (1) atonic d.; **(2)** nervous d.

nervous d., functional d. (2); d. associated with nervousness, tension, or anxiety.

reflex d., functional d. excited by reflex irritation from disease elsewhere than in the stomach or intestines.

dyspeptic (dis-pep'tik). Relating to or suffering from dyspepsia.

dysphagia, dysphagy (dis-fā'jē-ă, dis'fă-jē) [dys- + G. *phagein,* to eat]. Aglutition; aphagia; difficulty in swallowing.

d. luso'ria [coinage from L. *lusus naturae,* a sport of nature], d. said to be due to compression by the right subclavian artery arising abnormally from the thoracic aorta and passing behind the esophagus.

d. nervo'sa, nervous d., esophagism.

sideropenic d., Plummer-Vinson *syndrome.*

vallecular d., Barclay-Baron disease; d. caused by food becoming lodged above the epiglottis.

dysphagocytosis (dis-fag'ō-sī-tō'sis). Disordered phagocytosis, especially failure of cells to ingest and digest bacteria.
congenital d., chronic granulomatous *disease.*

dysphasia (dis-fā'zē-ă) [dys- + G. *phasis,* speaking]. Dysphrasia; lack of coordination in speech, and failure to arrange words in an understandable way.

dysphemia (dis-fē'mē-ă) [dys- + G. *phēmē,* speech]. Disordered phonation, articulation, or hearing due to emotional or mental deficits.

dysphonia (dis-fō'nē-ă) [dys- + G. *phōnē,* voice]. Difficulty or pain in speaking.
d. pli'cae ventricula'ris, phonation with the ventricular bands rather than with the vocal cords, one of the causes of hoarseness.
d. pu'berum, the breaking of the voice in boys at puberty.
d. spas'tica, phonic spasm; a spasmodic contraction of the adductor muscles of the larynx excited by attempted phonation, occurring chiefly in public speakers and seemingly analogous to writer's cramp.

dysphoria (dis-fōr'ē-ă) [dys- + G. *phora,* a bearing]. A feeling of unpleasantness or discomfort.

dysphrasia (dis-frā'zē-ă) [dys- + G. *phrasis,* speaking]. Dysphasia.

dysphylaxia (dis-fī-lak'sē-ă) [dys- + G. *phylaxis,* watching]. A form of insomnia marked by awakening too early.

dyspigmentation (dis'pig-men-tā'shŭn). Any abnormality in the formation or distribution of pigment, especially in the skin; usually applied to an abnormal reduction in pigmentation (depigmentation).

dyspinealism (dis-pin'ē-ăl-izm). Obsolete term for the syndrome supposed to result from the deficiency of pineal gland secretion.

dyspituitarism (dis-pi-tū'i-ter-izm). The complex of phenomena due to excessive or deficient secretion by the pituitary gland

dysplasia (dis-plā'zē-ă) [dys- + G. *plasis,* a molding]. Abnormal tissue development. See also heteroplasia.
anhidrotic ectodermal d., hypohidrotic ectodermal d.; Christ-Siemens syndrome; congenital defective or absent sweat glands, smooth finely wrinkled skin, sunken nose, malformed and missing teeth, sparse fragile hair, and sometimes with deformed nails, absent breast tissue, mental retardation, or syndactyly; X-linked recessive inheritance.
anterofacial, anteroposterior, or **anteroposterior facial d.,** abnormal growth of the face or cranium in an anteroposterior direction as seen and measured with a cephalogram.
asphyxiating thoracic d., hereditary hypoplasia of the thorax, associated with pelvic skeletal abnormality. Also called Jeune's syndrome; thoracic-pelvic-phalangeal dystrophy; asphyxiating thoracic chondrodystrophy.
atriodigital d., Holt-Oram *syndrome.*
bronchopulmonary d., chronic pulmonary insufficiency arising from long-term artificial pulmonary ventilation; seen more frequently in premature infants than in mature infants.
cerebral d., abnormal development of the telencephalon.
cervical d., d. of the uterine cervix, epithelial atypia involving part of the thickness of cervical squamous epithelium, occurring most often in young women; appears to regress frequently, but may progress over a long period to carcinoma; marked d. may be microscopically difficult to distinguish from carcinoma in situ.
chondroectodermal d., Ellis-van Crevald syndrome; triad of chondrodysplasia, ectodermal d., and polydactyly, with congenital heart defects in over half of patients; autosomal recessive inheritance.
cleidocranial d., clidocranial d., cleidocranial *dysostosis.*
congenital ectodermal d., congenital ecotodermal *defect.*
craniodiaphysial d., small stature and thickening of the cranial bones with sclerosis and diaphysial widening of tubular bones; autosomal recessive inheritance.
craniocarpotarsal d., craniocarpotarsal *dystrophy.*
craniometaphysial d., syndrome of metaphysial d. associated with severe sclerosis and overgrowth of bones of the skull (leontiasis ossea).
dentin d., a hereditary disorder of the teeth, involving both primary and permanent dentition, in which the clinical morphology and color of the teeth are normal, but the teeth radiographically exhibit short roots, obliteration of the pulp chambers and canals, and mobility and premature exfoliation; autosomal dominant inheritance.
diaphysial d., Engelmann's disease; progressive, symmetrical fusiform enlargement of the shafts of long bones characterized by the formation of excessive new periosteal and endosteal bone and irregular conversion of this cortical bone into cancellous bone; anemia does not occur as a rule, as in osteopetrosis.
ectodermal d., a congenital defect of the ectodermal tissues, including the skin and its appendages. See anhidrotic ectodermal d. and hidrotic ectodermal d.
enamel d., *amelogenesis* imperfecta.
encephalo-ophthalmic d., Krause's syndrome; retinopathy of prematurity combined with cerebral dysplasia.
d. epiphysia'lis hemime'lia, tarsomegaly.
d. epiphysia'lis mul'tiplex, multiple epiphysial d.; a dominantly inherited abnormality of epiphyses characterized by difficulty in walking, pain and stiffness of joints, stubby fingers, and often dwarfism of short-limb type; on x-ray examination, the epiphyses are mottled and irregular; ossification centers are late in appearance and may be multiple, but the vertebrae are normal.
d. epiphysia'lis puncta'ta, chondrodystrophia calcificans congenita; chondrodysplasia punctata; stippled epiphysis; a developmental error of the epiphyses characterized by severe deformities, epiphyses ossified from several discrete centers and with a stippled appearance, and thickened shafts of the long bones; congenital cataract and mental retardation are often present.
epithelial d., nonmalignant disorders of differentiation of epithelial cells.
faciodigitogenital d., Aarskog-Scott syndrome; a syndrome of ocular hypertelorism, anteverted nostrils, broad upper lip, saddle-bag scrotum, and laxity of ligaments resulting in genu recurvatum, flat feet, and hyperextensible fingers; X-linked recessive inheritance.
familial fibrous d. of jaws, cherubism.
familial white folded d., white sponge *nevus.*
fibromuscular d., idiopathic nonatherosclerotic disease leading to stenosis of arteries, usually the renal arteries, and hypertension; two varieties are fibromuscular hyperplasia and perimuscular fibrosis.
fibrous d. of bone, Jaffe-Lichtenstein disease; a disturbance of medullary bone maintenance in which bone undergoing physiologic lysis is replaced by abnormal proliferation of fibrous tissue, resulting in asymmetric distortion and expansion of bone; may be confined to a single bone (monostotic fibrous d.) or involve multiple bones (polyostotic fibrous d.).
florid osseous or **cemental d.,** sclerotic cemental *mass.*
hereditary renal-retinal d., a disorder characterized by tapetoretinal degeneration, nephrogenic diabetes insipidus, and progressive azotemia; probable autosomal recessive inheritance.
hidrotic ectodermal d., congenital dystrophy of the nails and hair with thickened nails and sparse or absent scalp hair; often associated with keratoderma of the palms and soles; teeth and sweat gland function are normal; autosomal dominant inheritance.
hypohidrotic ectodermal d., anhidrotic ectodermal d.
lymphopenic thymic d., thymic *alymphoplasia.*
mammary d., fibrocystic *disease* of the breast.
mandibulofacial d., mandibulofacial *dysostosis.*
metaphysial d., a failure of remodeling to normal tubular structure of new bone at the metaphyses of long bones; the ends of long

bones appear to be expanded and porotic, with thin cortex; there may be an associated overgrowth of cranial bones (craniometaphysial d.).

Mondini d., congenital anomaly of osseus and membranous labyrinth characterized by aplastic cochlea, and deformity of the vestibule and semicircular canals with partial or complete loss of auditory and vestibular function; may be associated with spontaneous cerebrospinal fluid otorrhoea resulting in meningitis. See also Mondini *deafness.*

monostotic fibrous d., fibrous d. of a single bone.

mucoepithelial d., an epithelial cell dyshesive disease characterized by red, periorificial mucosal lesions of oral, nasal, vaginal, urethral, anal, bladder, and conjunctival mucosa, with cataracts, follicular keratosis, non-scarring alopecia, frequent pulmonary infections, pneumothorax, and sometimes cor pulmonale; autosomal dominant inheritance.

multiple epiphysial d., d. epiphysialis multiplex.

oculoauriculovertebral (OAV) d., OAV or Goldenhar's syndrome; a syndrome characterized by epibulbar dermoids, preauricular appendages, micrognathia, and vertebral and other anomalies.

oculodentodigital (ODD) d., ODD, oculodentodigital, or Meyer-Schwickerath and Weyers syndrome; microphthalmia, coloboma, or anomalies of the iris associated with malformed and malpositioned teeth, and anomalies of the fingers including syndactyly, camptodactyly, or absent phalanges.

oculovertebral d., oculovertebral or Weyers-Thier syndrome; microphthalmia, colobomas or anophthalmia with small orbit, twisted face due to unilateral d. of maxilla, macrostomia with malformed teeth and malocclusion, vertebral malformations, and branched and hypoplastic ribs.

odontogenic d., odontodysplasia.

ophthalmomandibulomelic (OMM) d., OMM syndrome; an autosomal dominant disorder with corneal clouding and multiple abnormalities of the mandible and limbs.

periapical cemental or **fibrous d.,** cementoma; periapical osteofibrosis; a benign, painless, non-neoplastic condition of the jaws which occurs almost exclusively in middle-aged black females; lesions are usually multiple, most frequently involve vital mandibular anterior teeth, surround the root apices, and are initially radiolucent (becoming more opaque as they mature).

polyostotic fibrous d., multifocal osteitis fibrosa; osteitis fibrosa disseminata; the occurrence of lesions of fibrous d. in multiple bones, commonly on one side of the body; may occur with areas of pigmentation and endocrine dysfunction (McCune-Albright syndrome).

pseudoachondroplastic spondyloepiphysial d., severe dwarfism with onset at 2 to 4 years of age characterized by short limbs, a relatively long trunk, and normal skull and facies.

retinal d., an overgrowth of glial tissue compensating for aplasia of sensory elements.

septo-optic d., de Morsier's syndrome; congenital optic nerve hypoplasia as the result of aplasis of the retinal ganglia cells and their axons.

spondyloepiphysial d., a group of conditions characterized by growth insufficiency of the vertebral column, with flattening of vertebrae, and often involving the epiphyses at the hip and shoulder; results in dwarfism of the short trunk type, often also with short extremities, sometimes with other malformations; types with dominant, recessive, and X-linked recessive inheritance have been described in different families.

ventriculoradial d., a congenital syndrome consisting of a ventricular septal defect with associated absence of thumb or radius.

dysplastic (dis-plas'tik). Pertaining to or marked by dysplasia.

dyspnea (disp-nē'ă) [G. *dyspnoia,* fr. *dys-,* bad, + *pnoē,* breathing]. Shortness of breath, a subjective difficulty or distress in breathing, usually associated with disease of the heart or lungs; occurs normally during intense physical exertion or at high altitude.

paroxysmal nocturnal d., acute d. appearing suddenly at night, usually waking the patient after an hour or two of sleep; caused by pulmonary congestion and edema which result from left-sided heart failure.

Traube's d., obsolete eponym for inspiratory d. with maximal expansion of the chest and a slow respiratory rhythm.

dyspneic (disp-nē'ik). "out of breath;" relating to or suffering from dyspnea.

dyspraxia (dis-prak'sē-ă) [dys- + G. *praxis,* a doing]. Impaired or painful functioning in any organ.

dysprosium (dis-prō'sē-ŭm). A metallic element of the lanthanide (rare earth) series, symbol Dy, atomic No. 66, atomic weight 162.50.

dysproteinemia (dis-prō'tēn-ē'mē-ă, -prō'tē-in-). An abnormality in plasma proteins, usually in immunoglobulins.

dysproteinemic (dis-prō-tēn-ē'mik). Relating to dysproteinemia.

dysraphism, dysraphia (dis'ră-fizm, dis-raf'ē-ă) [dys- + G. *raphē,* suture]. Defective fusion, especially of the neural folds, resulting in status dysraphicus.

dysrhythmia (dis-rith'mē-ă) [dys- + G. *rhythmos,* rhythm]. Defective rhythm. *Cf.* arrhythmia. See also entries under rhythm.

cardiac d., any abnormality in the rate, regularity, or sequence of cardiac activation.

electroencephalographic d., a diffusely irregular brain wave tracing.

paroxysmal cerebral d., a diffusely abnormal electroencephalogram considered by some to indicate epilepsy.

dyssebacia (dis-sĕ-bā'shē-ă) [dys- + L. *sebum,* grease]. Seborrheic *dermatitis.*

dyssomnia (dis-som'nē-ă). Disturbance of normal sleep or rhythm pattern.

dysspondylism (dis-spon'di-lizm) [dys- + G. *spondylos,* vertebra]. An abnormality of development of the spine or vertebral column.

dysstasia (dis-stā'sē-ă) [dys- + G. *stasis,* standing]. Difficulty in standing.

dysstatic (dis-tat'ik). Marked by difficulty in standing.

dyssyllabia (dis-il-lā'bē-ă) [dys- + G. *syllabē,* syllable]. Syllable-stumbling.

dyssynergia (dis-in-er'jē-ă) [dys- + G. *syn,* with, + *ergon,* work]. Ataxia.

d. cerebella'ris myoclon'ica, a disorder with symptoms similar to those of Hunt's syndrome (1), as well as those of myoclonus and epilepsy.

d. cerebellar'is progressi'va, Hunt's *syndrome* (1).

detrusor sphincter d., a disturbance of the normal relationship between bladder (detrusor) contraction and sphincter relaxation during voluntary or involuntary voiding efforts.

dystaxia (dis-tak'sē-ă) [dys- + G. *taxis,* order]. A mild degree of ataxia.

dystelephalangy (dis-tel'ē-fă-lan'jē) [dys- + G. *telos,* end, + phalanx]. Bowing of the distal phalanx of the little finger.

dysthymia (dis-thī'mē-ă) [dys- + G. *thymos,* mind, emotion]. Any disorder of mood.

dysthymic (dis-thī'mik). Relating to dysthymia.

dystocia (dis-tō'sē-ă) [G. *dystokia,* fr. *dys-,* difficult, + *tokos,* childbirth]. Difficult childbirth.

fetal d., d. due to an abnormality of the fetus.

maternal d., d. caused by an abnormality or physical problem in the mother.

placental d., retention or difficult delivery of the placenta.

dystonia (dis-tō'nē-ă) [dys- + G. *tonos,* tension]. A state of abnormal (either hypo- or hyper-) tonicity in any of the tissues.
d. lenticula'ris, d. resulting from a lesion of the lenticulate nucleus.
d. musculo'rum defor'mans, torsion d.; Ziehen-Oppenheim disease; progressive torsion spasm; a genetic, environmental, or idiopathic disorder, usually beginning in childhood or adolescence, children, marked by muscular contractions producing abnormal distortions of the spine and hips; the musculature is hypertonic when in action, hypotonic when at rest. Hereditary forms usually begin with involuntary posturing of the foot or hand (autosomal recessive form) or of the neck or trunk (autosomal dominant form); both forms may progress to produce contortions of the entire body.
torsion d., d. musculorum deformans.

dystonic (dis-ton'ik). Pertaining to dystonia.

dystopia (dis-tō'pē-ă) [dys- + G. *topos,* place]. Allotopia; malposition; faulty or abnormal position of a part or organ.
d. cantho'rum, Waardenburg *syndrome.*
d. transver'sa exter'na tes'tis, crossing over of the testis under the skin of the dorsum of the penis to the contralateral half of the scrotum. See also *descensus* paradoxus testis.
d. transver'sa inter'na tes'tis, passage of each testis into a contralateral inguinal canal within the pelvis, each coming to lie in the corresponding half of the scrotum. See also *descensus* paradoxus testis.

dystopic (dis-top'ik). Pertaining to, or characterized by, dystopia. See also ectopic.

dystrophia (dis-trō'fē-ă) [L. fr. G. *dys-,* bad, + *trophē,* nourishment]. Dystrophy.
d. adipo'sogenita'lis, adiposogenital degeneration, dystrophy, or syndrome; hypophysial s.; adiposis orchica; a disorder characterized primarily by obesity and hypogonadotrophic hypogonadism in adolescent boys; dwarfism is rare, and when present is thought to reflect hypothyroidism. Fröhlich's syndrome is often used synonymously for this disorder, although the original case involved a pituitary tumor; most cases are thought to result from hypothalamic dysfunction in areas regulating appetite and gonadal development.
d. brevicol'lis, a condition marked by symptoms of d. adiposogenitalis together with a deforming shortness of the neck, but without synostosis of the cervical vertebrae seen in Klippel-Feil syndrome.
d. myoton'ica, myotonic *dystrophy.*
d. un'guium, dystrophy of the nails.

dystrophic (dis-trof'ik). Relating to dystrophy.

dystrophoneurosis (dis-trof'ō-nū-rō'sis) [dys- + G. *trophē,* nourishment, + *neuron,* nerve, + *-osis,* condition]. Any nervous disease associated with faulty nutrition.

dystrophy (dis'trō-fē) [dys- + G. *trophē,* nourishment]. Dystrophia; progressive changes that may result from defective nutrition of a tissue or organ.
adiposogenital d., *dystrophia* adiposogenitalis.
adult pseudohypertrophic muscular d., Becker type tardive muscular d.; muscular d. of late onset, often in the second or third decade, with relatively mild course; X-linked recessive inheritance.
Barnes' d., a rare type of muscular d., in which muscles are often hypertrophic and stronger than normal, but later become weak and atrophic.
Becker type tardive muscular d., adult pseudohypertrophic muscular d.
childhood muscular d., pseudohypertrophic muscular d.
corneal d., central corneal opacification, usually bilateral, symmetrical, and often hereditary, involving predominantly epithelial, stromal, or endothelial layers, often in a typical pattern.
craniocarpotarsal d., craniocarpotarsal dysplasia; Freeman-Sheldon or whistling face syndrome; congenital association of skeletal defects (ulnar deviation of hands with camptodactyly, talipes equinovarus, and frontal bone defects) and characteristic facies (protrusion of lips as in whistling, sunken eyes with hypertelorism, and small nose); autosomal dominant inheritance.
Duchenne's d., pseudohypertrophic muscular d.
endothelial d. of cornea, spontaneous loss of corneal endothelium leading to edema of the corneal stroma and epithelium.
epithelial d., corneal d. affecting primarily the epithelium and its basement membrane. See also juvenile epithelial d.
facioscapulohumeral muscular d., facioscapulohumeral atrophy; Landouzy-Dejerine d.; a relatively benign type of d. commencing in childhood and characterized by wasting and weakness, mainly of the muscles of the face, shoulder girdle, and arms; autosomal dominant inheritance.
Favre's d., vitreo-tapetoretinal d.
fingerprint d., a condition wherein fine parallel lines in a fingerprint configuration area are seen in the basal epithelial layer and basement membrane of the corneal epithelium. See also map-dot-fingerprint d.
fleck d. of cornea, a bilateral occurrence of subtle spots in the corneal stroma; the spots vary in size and shape, and have sharp margins and clear centers; photophobia may occur; autosomal dominant inheritance.
Fuchs' epithelial dystrophy, epithelial edema secondary to endothelial d. of the cornea.
Groenouw's corneal d., (1) a granular type of corneal d., with autosomal dominant inheritance; **(2)** a macular type of corneal d., with autosomal recessive inheritance.
gutter d. of cornea, keratoleptynsis (1); a marginal furrow usually inferiorly about 1 mm from the limbus; and sometimes bilateral.
infantile neuroaxonal d., Seitelberger's disease; slowly progressive mental and neurological deterioration, with upper and lower motor neuron dysfunction, in an infant or young child; characterized pathologically by spheroids in severely dystrophic axons in central and peripheral nervous tissue.
juvenile epithelial d., Meesman d.; epithelial d. characterized by progressive cysts and opacities of the corneal epithelium, with onset in infancy; autosomal dominant inheritance with incomplete penetrance.
Landouzy-Dejerine d., facioscapulohumeral muscular d.
lattice corneal d., a reticular type of d. manifest at puberty and progressing slowly until eventually useful vision is lost; autosomal dominant inheritance.
Leyden-Möbius muscular d., limb-girdle muscular d.
limb-girdle muscular d., Leyden-Möbius muscular or pelvofemoral muscular d.; a progressive disorder that usually begins in the preadolescent period; manifestations include those of childhood and facioscapulohumeral muscular d.; commonly, the pelvic girdle is most severely involved; autosomal recessive inheritance.
map-dot-fingerprint d., fingerprint d. accompanied by map-like patterns and microcystic epithelial inclusions.
Meesman d., juvenile epithelial d.
microcystic epithelial d., bilateral, symmetrical intraepithelial cysts in the central area of the cornea of healthy women, without hereditary predisposition.
muscular d., myodystrophia; myodystrophy; inborn abnormality of muscle associated with dysfunction and ultimately with deterioration.
myotonic d., dystrophia myotonica; myotonia atrophica or dystrophica; Steinert's disease; a chronic, slowly progressing disease, with onset usually in the third decade, marked by atrophy of the muscles, failing vision, lenticular opacities, ptosis, slurred speech, and general muscular weakness; there may be atelectasis of the lungs and cyanosis due to involvement of the diaphragm; autosomal dominant inheritance.

pelvofemoral muscular d., limb-girdle muscular d.
progressive muscular d., Erb's or idiopathic muscular atrophy; a form of progressive muscular atrophy in which the disease begins in the muscle and not in the spinal centers.
progressive tapetochoroidal d., choroideremia (2).
pseudohypertrophic muscular d., a type of muscular d. occurring in males with onset between the ages of 2 and 6 years; muscular weakness first appears in the pelvic girdle and spreads with relative rapidity to the musculature of the pectoral girdle, trunk, and extremities; muscular pseudohypertrophy (enlarged, weakened, inelastic masses) is a common finding, as are contractures of muscle and tendon; X-linked recessive inheritance. Also called childhood muscular d.; pseudohypertrophic muscular atrophy or paralysis; Duchenne's d., disease (1), or paralysis; pseudomuscular hypertrophy.
reticular d. of cornea, bilateral, progressive, superficial degeneration of the corneal epithelium and adjacent Bowman's membrane.
ring-like corneal d., thread-like opacities of the anterior corneal stroma, with acute, painful onset followed by decreased vision; autosomal dominant inheritance.
sympathetic reflex d., diffuse superficial and deep burning pain in an extremity associated with vasomotor disturbances, trophic changes, and limitation or immobility of joints as the result of some local injury. See also causalgia.
thoracic-pelvic-phalangeal d., asphyxiating thoracic *dysplasia.*
twenty-nail d., sudden onset of linear ridging of all of the nails, with occasional thinning and splitting; seen in generalized lichen planus.
vitreo-tapetoretinal d., Favre's d.; autosomal recessive bilateral peripheral and central retinoschisis with pigmentary degeneration of the retina, chorioretinal atrophy, vitreous degeneration, and night blindness.

dystropy (dis'trō-pē) [dys- + G. *tropos,* a turning]. Abnormal or eccentric behavior.

dysuria (dis-yū'rē-ă) [dys- + G. *ouron,* urine]. Dysury; difficulty or pain in urination.

dysuric (dis-yū'rik). Relating to or suffering from dysuria.

dysury (dis'yū-rē). Dysuria.

dysversion (dis-ver'zhŭn) [dys- + L. *verto,* to turn]. A turning in any direction, less than inversion; particularly d. of the optic nerve head (situs inversus of the optic disk).

E

ϵ **1.** Fifth letter of the Greek alphabet, episilon. **2.** Symbol for molar absorption *coefficient.* For terms beginning with this prefix, see the specific term.

E **1.** Symbol for exa-; extraction *ratio.* **2.** As a subscript, refers to expired *gas.*

E_0+, E^0, E_h Symbols for oxidation-reduction *potential.*

EAE Abbreviation for experimental allergic *encephalitis.*

Eagle, Harry, U.S. physician and cell biologist, *1905. See E.'s basal *medium.*

Eagle, W., 20th century U.S. otolaryngologist. See E. *syndrome.*

Eales, Henry, British ophthalmologist, 1852–1913. See E.'s *disease.*

ear (ēr) [A.S. *eáre*]. Auris; the organ of hearing: composed of the **external e.,** which includes the auricle and the external acoustic, or auditory, meatus; the **middle e.,** or the tympanic cavity with its ossicles; and the **internal** or **inner e.,** or labyrinth, which includes the semicircular canals, vestibule, and cochlea. See also auricula.
aviator's e., *aerotitis* media.
Aztec e., an auricle with the lobule absent.
Blainville e.'s, asymmetry in size or shape of the auricles.
boxer's e., cauliflower e.
Cagot e., (kă-gō′) [a people in the Pyrenees among whom physical stigmata are common], an auricle having no lobulus.
cauliflower e., boxer's e.; thickening and induration of the e. with distortion of contours following extravasation of blood within its tissues.
darwinian e., an auricle in which the upper border is not rolled over to form the helix, but projects upward as a flat, sharp edge.
lop e., see lop-ear.
Morel's e., a large, misshapen, outstanding auricle, with obliterated grooves and thinned edges.
Mozart e. [Wolfgang Amadeus Mozart, composer, said to have had this deformity], a deformity of the pinna where the two crura of the antihelix and the crus of the helix are fixed, giving a bulging appearance of the superior part of the pinna.
scroll e., a deformity of the external e. in which the pinna is rolled forward.
Stahl's e., a deformed external e., in which the fossa ovalis and upper portion of the scaphoid fossa are covered by the helix; regarded as a stigma of degenerate constitution.
Wildermuth's e., an e. in which the helix is turned backward and the anthelix is prominent.

earache (ēr′āk). Otalgia; otodynia; pain in the ear.

eardrum (ēr′drŭm). *Membrana* tympani.

Earle, Wilton R., U.S. pathologist, 1902–1962. See Earle L *fibrosarcoma.*

Earle's solution. See under solution.

earth (erth) [A.S. *eorthe*]. **1.** Soil; dirt; the soft material of the land, as opposed to rock and sand. **2.** An easily pulverized mineral. **3.** An insoluble oxide of aluminum or of certain other elements characterized by a high melting point.
alkaline e.'s, see alkaline earth *elements.*

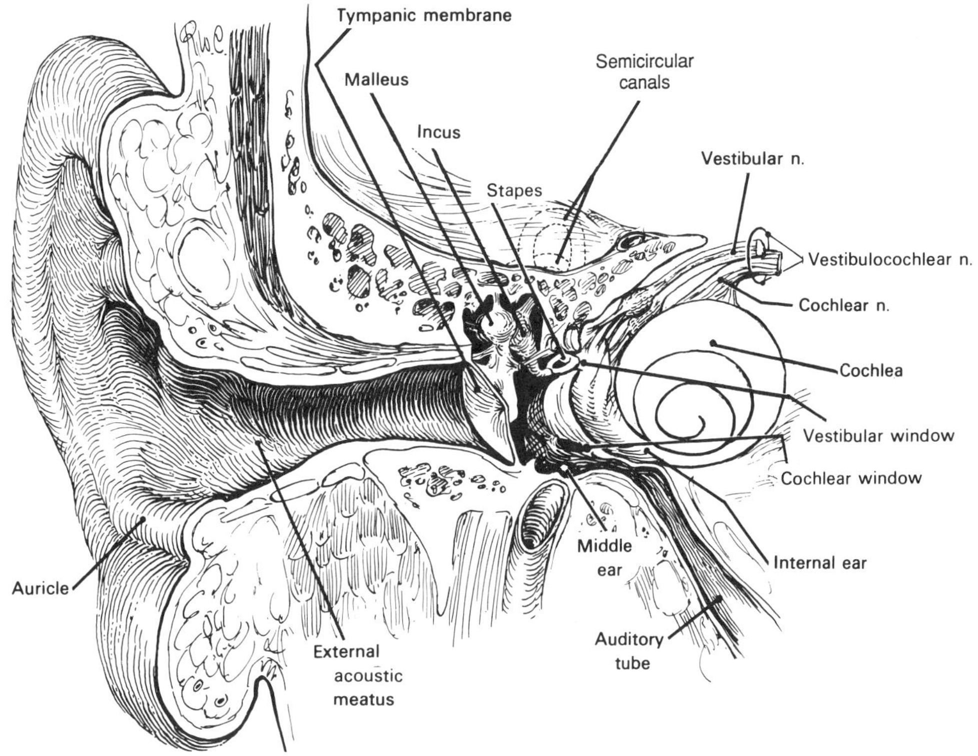

Ear
Section through the petrous part of the temporal bone to show the outer, middle, and inner ear.

diatomaceous e., a powder made of desiccated diatom material; used as a filtering agent, adsorbent, and abrasive in many chemical operations.
fuller's e. [fr. *fulling,* an old process of cleaning wool, with earth or clay], a refined clay sometimes used as a dusting powder or applied moistened with water as a form of poultice.
rare e.'s, see lanthamides.

earth-eating. Geophagia.

earwax (ēr'waks). Cerumen.

eat (ēt) [A.S. *etan*] **1.** To take solid food. **2.** To chew and swallow any substance as one would food. **3.** To corrode.

Eaton, Lee M., U.S. neurologist, 1905–1958. See E.-Lambert, Lambert-E. *syndrome.*

Eaton, Monroe D., U.S. microbiologist, *1904. See E. *agent,* E. agent *pneumonia.*

E.B., EB Abbreviation for elementary *body* (1).

Ebbecke's reaction. See under reaction.

Ebbinghaus, Hermann, German, 1850–1909. See E. *test.*

Eberth, Karl J., German physician, 1835–1926. See E.'s *bacillus, lines, perithelium.*

Eberthella (ā-ber-tel'lă) [K. J. *Eberth*]. An obsolete name of a genus of bacteria. The type species, *E. typhi,* is a member of the genus *Salmonella* (*S. typhi*).

Ebner, Victor von. See von Ebner, Victor.

ebonation (ē-bō-nā'shŭn). Removal of loose fragments of bone from a wound.

ébranlement (ā-brahn-la-mon') [Fr.]. Twisting a polyp on its stalk to cause atrophy.

Ebstein, Wilhelm, German physician, 1836–1912. See E.'s *anomaly, disease, sign;* Armanni-E. *kidney;* Pel-E. *disease, fever.*

ebullism (eb'yū-lizm) [L. *ebullire,* to boil out]. Formation of water vapor bubbles in the tissues brought on by an extreme reduction in barometric pressure; occurs if the body is exposed to pressures which are found above an altitude of 63,000 feet.

ebur (ē'bŭr) [L. ivory]. A tissue resembling ivory in outward appearance or structure.
e. den'tis, dentinum.

eburnation (ē-bŭr-nā'shŭn) [L. *eburneus,* of ivory]. Bone sclerosis; a change in exposed subchondral bone in degenerative joint disease in which it is converted into a dense substance with a smooth surface like ivory.
e. of dentin, a condition observed in arrested dental caries wherein decalcified dentin is burnished and takes on a polished, often brown-stained appearance.

eburneous (ē-bŭr'nē-ŭs). Resembling ivory, especially in color.

eburnitis (ē-bŭr-nī'tis) [L. *eburneus,* of ivory, + G. -itis, inflammation]. Increased density and hardness of dentin, which may occur after the dentin is exposed.

EBV Abbreviation for Epstein-Barr *virus.*

EC Abbreviation for Enzyme Commission of the International Union of Biochemistry, used in conjunction with a unique number to define a specific enzyme in the Enzyme Commission's list [*Enzyme Nomenclature Recommendations, (1978)*]; *e.g.,* EC 1.1.1.1 defines an alcohol dehydrogenase; EC 2.6.1.1. defines aspartate aminotransferase, popularly known as glutamic-oxalacetic transaminase (GOT).

ec-. Prefix fr. G. preposition meaning out of, away from.

écarteur (ā-kar-ter') [Fr. *écarter,* to separate]. A type of retractor.

ecaudate (ē-kaw'dāt) [L. *e-* priv. + *cauda,* tail]. Tailless.

ecboline (ek'bō-lēn). Ergotoxine.

eccentric (ek-sen'trik) [G. *ek,* out, + *kentron,* center]. **1.** Erratic (1); abnormal or peculiar in ideas or behavior. **2.** Proceeding from a center. *Cf.* centrifugal (2). **3.** Peripheral.

eccentrochondroplasia (ek-sen'trō-kon-drō-plā'zē-ă) [G. *ek,* out + *kentron,* center, + *chondros,* cartilage, + *plasis,* a molding]. Abnormal epiphysial development from eccentric centers of ossification.

eccentropiesis (ek-sen'trō-pī-ē'sis) [G. *ek,* out, + *kentron,* center, + *piesis,* pressure]. Pressure exerted from within outward.

ecchondroma (ek-kon-drō'mă) [G. *ek,* from, + *chondros,* cartilage, + *-oma,* tumor]. Ecchondrosis. **1.** A cartilaginous neoplasm arising as an overgrowth from normally situated cartilage, as a mass protruding from the articular surface of a bone, in contrast to enchondroma. **2.** An enchondroma which has burst through the shaft of a bone and become pedunculated.

ecchondrosis (ek-kon-drō'sis). Ecchondroma.
e. physalifor'mis, e. physaliph'ora, a notochordal rest of the cranial clivus which may form a small tumor.

ecchondrotome (ek-kon'drō-tōm) [G. *ek,* out, + *chondros,* cartilage, + *tomē,* incision]. Chondrotome.

ecchymoma (ek-i-mō'mă) [G. *ek,* out, + *chymos,* juice, + *-oma,* tumor]. A slight hematoma following a bruise.

ecchymosed (ek'i-mōsd). Characterized by or affected with ecchymosis.

ecchymosis, pl. **ecchymoses** (ek-i-mō'sis, -sēz) [G. *ekchymōsis,* ecchymosis, fr. *ek,* out, + *chymos,* juice]. A purplish patch caused by extravasation of blood into the skin, differing from petechiae only in size.
Tardieu's ecchymoses, Tardieu's petechiae or spots; subpleural and subpericardial petechiae or ecchymoses (or both), as observed in the tissues of persons who have been strangled, or otherwise asphyxiated.

ecchymotic (ek-i-mot'ik). Relating to an ecchymosis.

Eccleston. See Paget-E. *stain.*

eccrine (ek'rin) [G. *ek-krino,* to secrete]. **1.** Exocrin (1). **2.** Denoting the flow of sweat.

eccrinology (ek-ri-nol'ō-jē) [G. *ek-drino,* to secrete, + *logos,* study]. The branch of physiology and of anatomy concerned with the secretions and the secreting (exocrine) glands.

eccrisis (ek'ri-sis) [G. separation]. **1.** The removal of waste products. **2.** Any waste product; excrement.

eccritic (e-krit'ik). **1.** Promoting the expulsion of waste matters. **2.** An agent that promotes excretion.

eccyesis (ek-sī-ē'sis) [G. *ek,* out, + *kyēsis,* pregnancy]. Ectopic *pregnancy.*

ecdemic (ek-dem'ik) [G. *ekdēmos,* foreign, from home, fr. *dēmos,* people]. Denoting a disease brought into a region from without.

ecdysiasm (ek-diz'ē-azm) [fr. G. *ekdysiazesthai,* to remove one's clothes]. A morbid tendency to undress to produce sexual desire in others.

ecdysis (ek'di-sis) [G. *ekdysis,* shedding]. Desquamation, sloughing, or molting as a necessary phenomenon to permit growth in arthropods and skin renewal in amphibians and reptiles.

ECF Abbreviation for extracellular *fluid.*

ECF-A Abbreviation for eosinophil chemotactic *factor* of anaphylaxis.

ECG Abbreviation for electrocardiogram.

ecgonine (ek'gō-nēn, -nin). 3β-Hydroxy-1αH,5αH-tropane-2β-carboxylic acid; the important part of the cocaine molecule.

echeosis (ek-ē-ō'sis) [G. *ēchein,* to suffer from noises in ears]. Rarely used term for a mental disturbance caused by continuous disturbing noises.

Echidnophaga gallinacea (ek-id-nof'ă-gă gal-i-nā'sē-ă). The stick-tight flea, a serious pest of poultry in subtropical America; also frequently attacks domestic mammals and man.

echin-. See echino-.

echinate (ek'i-nāt). Echinulate.

echino-, echin- [G. *echinos,* hedgehog, sea urchin]. Combining forms meaning prickly or spiny.

Echinochasmus (ĕ-kī-nō-kaz'mŭs) [echino- + G. *chasma,* open mouth]. A genus of digenetic flukes (family Echinostomatidae), particularly common in wading and fish-eating birds; the species *E. perfoliatus* var. *japonicus* is reported as a rare intestinal parasite of man in Japan.

echinococcosis (ĕ-kī'nō-kok-kō'sis). Infection with *Echinococcus;* larval infection is called hydatid *disease.*

Echinococcus (ĕ-kī'nō-kok'ŭs) [echino- + G. *kokkos,* a berry]. A genus of very small taeniid tapeworms, two to five segments in adult worms; adults are found in various carnivores but not in man; larvae, in the form of hydatid cysts, are found in the liver and other organs of ruminants, pigs, horses, rodents, and, under certain epidemiological circumstances, man (*e.g.,* sheep herders living closely with their infected dogs).

E. granulo'sus, hydatid tapeworm; a species in which adults infect canids and the larval form (osseous and unilocular hydatid cysts) infects sheep and other ruminants, pigs, and horses; may also occur in man, giving rise to a large cyst in the liver or other organs and tissues.

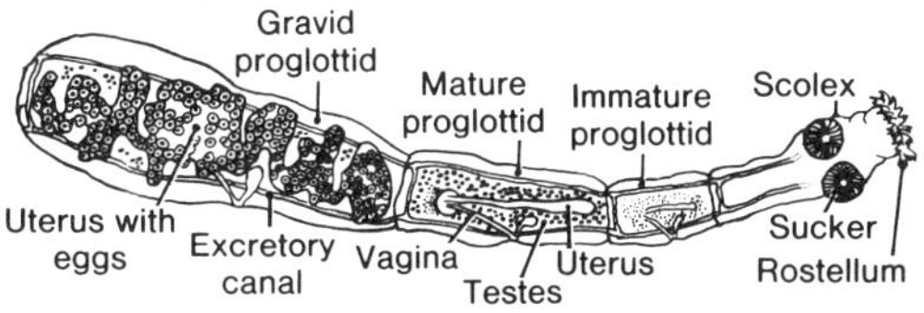

Echinococcus granulosus
(Magnification, ×12)

E. multilocula'ris, a species that occurs, in the adult form, in the north temperate and arctic regions in foxes; the larva (alveolar hydatid cyst) is found in the liver of microtine rodents and in man; it produces a proliferative, often slow-growing cyst in the liver that, in man, is usually fatal.

echinocyte (ek'i-nō-sīt) [echino- + G. *kytos,* cell]. A crenated red blood cell.

echinoderm (e-kī'nō-derm). A member of the phylum Echinodermata.

Echinodermata (e-kī-nō-der'mă-tă) [echino- + G. *derma,* skin]. A phylum of Metazoa which includes starfish, sea urchins, sea lilies, and other classes. All but the sea cucumbers (Holothuroidea) are basically radially symmetrical and most possess a calcareous endoskeleton with external spines. They inhabit the sea bottom, some near shore, others in deep water.

Echinorhynchus (e-kī-nō-ring'kŭs) [echino- + G. *rhynchos,* snout]. A genus of acanthocephalid (thorny-headed) worms which originally included species now contained in *Macracanthorhynchus, Gigantorhynchus,* and other genera.

echinosis (ek-i-nō'sis) [echino- + G. *-osis,* condition]. A condition in which the red blood cells have lost their smooth outlines, resembling an echinus or sea urchin.

Echinostoma (ĕ-kī-nō-stō'mă, ek-i-nos'tō-mă) [echino- + G. *stoma,* mouth]. A genus of digenetic flukes (family Echinostomatidae) with characteristic oral spines; widely distributed and parasitic in a broad range of bird and mammal hosts; several species have been reported from man from Southeast Asia.

E. iloca'num, a species reported from man in the Philippines.

E. malay'anum, a species typically found in the pig, but reported occasionally from man in Malaysia; infection results from ingestion of snails with infective cysts (metacercariae).

echinostomiasis (ĕ-kī'nō-stō-mī'ă-sis). Infection of birds and mammals, including man, with trematodes of the genus *Echinostoma.*

echinulate (e-kin'yū-lāt) [Mod. L. *echinulus,* dim. of L. *echinus,* hedgehog]. Echinate; prickly or spinous.

Echis (ek'is, ē'kis) [G. *echis,* a viper]. The saw-scaled or carpet viper, a genus of small (under 1 m), irritable, and alert snakes with a highly toxic venom; they are responsible for numerous snakebite cases with many fatalities.

echo (ek'ō) [G.]. A reverberating sound sometimes heard in auscultation of the chest.

atrial e., electrical reactivation of the atrium by a retrograde impulse returning from the A-V node while the antegrade impulse continues to the ventricle; characterized electrocardiographically, by a pair of P waves enclosing a QRS complex, the second P wave being inverted, indicating that it is the reverse (the retrograde pathway) of the pathway of the first P wave (the antegrade pathway).

nodus sinuatrialis (NS) e., a postectopic sinus beat occurring earlier than would be expected from the preceding sinus node discharge interval; *i.e.,* the interval following a premature beat of superventricular origin is less than the ordinary cycle length between sinus beats, whereas ordinarily the interval would be expected to exceed cycle length.

echoacousia (ek'ō-ă-kū'zē-ă) [echo + G. *akouō,* to hear]. A subjective disturbance of hearing in which a sound appears to be repeated.

echoaortography (ek'ō-ā-ōr-tog'ră-fē) [echo + aortography]. Application of ultrasound techniques to the diagnosis and study of the aorta, particularly the abdominal aorta.

echocardiogram (ek-ō-kar'dē-ō-gram). The ultrasonic record obtained by echocardiography. See ultrasonography.

echocardiography (ek'ō-kar-dē-og'ră-fē) [echo + cardiography]. Ultrasound cardiography; the use of ultrasound in the investigation of the heart and great vessels and diagnosis of cardiovascular lesions, especially mitral disease, pericardial effusion, and abdominal aortic aneurysm.

cross-sectional e., two-dimensional e.

Doppler e., use of Doppler ultrasonography techniques to augment two-dimensional e. by allowing velocities to be registered within the echocardiographic image.

two-dimensional e., cross-sectional e.; e. in which visualization is produced by reconstructed multiple B-mode echoes of ultrasonic beams that create a spacially oriented two-dimensional image.

echoencephalography (ek'ō-en-sef-ă-log'ră-fē) [echo + encephalography]. The use of reflected ultrasound in the diagnosis of intracranial processes.

echo-free (ek'ō-frē). Sonolucent.

echogenic (ek-ō-jen'ik). Containing internal interfaces which reflect high frequency sound waves.

echogram (ek'ō-gram) [echo + G. *gramma,* a diagram]. Ultrasonic display of reflection techniques appropriate for any field of application, but applied especially to the heart; *e.g.,* echocardiogram. See also ultrasonogram.

echograph (ek'ō-graf) [echo + G. *graphō,* to write]. Ultrasonograph.

echographer (e-kog'ră-fer). Ultrasonographer.

echographia (ek-ō-graf'ē-ă) [echo + G. *graphō,* to write]. A form of agraphia in which one cannot write spontaneously, but can write from dictation or copy.

echography (e-kog'ră-fē) [echo + G. *graphō,* to write]. Ultrasonography.

echokinesis, echokinesia (ek'ō-ki-nē'sis, -nē'zē-ă) [echo + G. *kinēsis,* movement]. Echopraxia.

echolalia (ek-ō-lā'lē-ă) [echo + G. *lalia,* a form of speech]. Echophrasia; echo reaction or speech; involuntary repetition of a word or sentence just spoken by another person.

echolocation (ek'ō-lō-kā'shŭn). Term applied to the method by which bats direct their flight and avoid solid objects. The creatures emit high-pitched cries which, though inaudible to human ears, are heard by the bats themselves as reflected sounds (echoes) from objects in their path.

echomatism (e-kō'mă-tizm) [echo + G. *matizō,* to strive to do]. Echopraxia.

echomimia (ek-ō-mim'ē-ă) [echo + G. *mimēsis,* imitation]. Echopathy.

echomotism (ek'ō-mō'tizm) [echo + L. *motio,* motion]. Echopraxia.

echopathy (ĕ-kop'ă-thē) [echo + G. *pathos,* suffering]. Echomimia; a form of psychopathology, usually associated with schizophrenia, in which the words (echolalia) or actions (echopraxia) of another are imitated and repeated.

echophony, echophonia (ĕ-kof'ō-nē, ek-ō-fō'nē-ă) [echo + G. *phōnē,* voice]. A duplication of the voice sound occasionally heard in auscultation of the chest.

echophotony (ek-ō-fot'ō-nē) [echo + G. *phōs* (*phōt-*), light, + *tonos,* tone]. The mental association of sound tones with particular colors.

echophrasia (ek-ō-frā'zē-ă) [echo + *phrasis,* speech]. Echolalia.

echopraxia (ek'ō-prak'sē-ă) [echo + G. *praxis,* action]. Echokinesia; echokinesis; echomatism; echomotism; involuntary imitation of movements made by another.

echoscope (ek'ō-skōp) [echo + G. *skopeō,* to view]. Instrument for displaying echoes by means of ultrasonic pulses on an oscilloscope to demonstrate structures lying at depths within the body.

echothiophate iodide (ek-ō-thī'ō-fāt). Diethoxyphosphorylthiocholine iodide; a potent organophosphorus compound and cholinesterase inhibitor, used in the treatment of glaucoma.

echovirus (ek'ō-vī-rŭs). ECHO *virus.*

Eck, Nikolai V., Russian physiologist, 1849–1917. See E. *fistula;* reverse E. *fistula.*

Ecker, Alexander, German anatomist, 1816–1887. See E.'s *fissure.*

Ecker, Enrique E., U.S. bacteriologist, 1887–1966. See Rees-E. *fluid.*

eclabium (ek-lā'bē-ŭm) [G. *ek,* out, + L. *labium,* lip]. Eversion of a lip.

eclampsia (ek-lamp'sē-ă) [G. *eklampsis,* a shining forth]. Occurrence of one or more convulsions, not attributable to other cerebral conditions such as epilepsy or cerebral hemorrhage, in a patient with preeclampsia.

puerperal e., puerperal convulsions; convulsions and coma associated with hypertension, edema, or proteinuria occurring in a woman following delivery.

superimposed e., superimposed *preeclampsia.*

eclamptic (ek-lamp'tik). Relating to eclampsia.

eclamptogenic, eclamptogenous (ek-lamp-tō-jen'ik, -tog'ĕ-nŭs). Causing eclampsia.

eclectic (ek-lek'tik) [G. *eklektikos,* selecting, fr. *ek,* out, + *lego,* to select]. Picking out from different sources what appears to be the best.

eclecticism (ek-lek'ti-sizm). **1.** A now defunct system of medicine that advocated use of indigenous plants to effect specific cures of certain signs and symptoms. **2.** A system of medicine practiced by ancient Greek and Roman physicians who were not affiliated with a medical sect but who adopted the practice and teachings which they considered best from other systems.

ecmnesia (ek-nē'zē-ă) [G. *ek,* out, + *mnēsios,* relating to memory]. Obsolete term for a loss of memory for recent events.

eco- [G. *oikos,* house, household, habitation]. Combining form denoting relationship to environment.

ecoid (e'koyd) [eco- + G. *eidos,* resemblance]. The framework of a red blood cell.

ecology (ē-kol'ō-jē) [eco- + G. *logos,* study]. Bioecology; bionomics (2); the branch of biology concerned with the total complex of interrelationships among living organisms, encompassing the relations of organisms to each other, to the environment, and to the entire energy balance within a given ecosystem.

human e., the relations of persons to their total (biologic and social) environment.

ecomania (ē-kō-mā'nē-ă) [eco- + G. *mania,* frenzy]. Obsolete term for a syndrome of domineering behavior at home and humility toward persons in authority.

econazole (e-kōn'ă-zōl). 1-2-[(4-chlorophenyl)methoxy]-2-(2,4-dichlorophenyl)ethyl]-1*H*- imidazole; a broad spectrum antifungal agent used in the treatment of tinea pedis and related fungal infections.

Economo. See von Economo.

economy (ē-kon'ō-mē) [G. *oikonomia,* management of the house, fr. *oikos,* house, + *nomos,* usage, law]. The system; the body regarded as an aggregate of functioning organs.

ecophobia (ē-kō-fō'bē-ă) [eco- + G. *phobos,* fear]. Obsolete term for a morbid fear of one's home surroundings. See also nostrophobia.

ecospecies (ē-kō-spē'shēz). Two or more populations of a species isolated by ecological barriers, theoretically able to exchange genes and interbreed, but partially separated from one another by differences in habitat or behavior.

ecosystem (ē'kō-sis-tem). Ecological system; a biocenosis (biotic community) and its biotope.

parasite-host e., parasitocenose.

ecotaxis (ē-kō-tak'sis). Migration of lymphocytes from the thymus and bone marrow into tissues possessing an appropriate microenvironment.

écouteur (ā-kū-ter') [Fr. a listener-in]. One who obtains erotic gratification through listening to sexual accounts.

écouvillon (ā-kū-vē-yō-hn') [Fr., cleaning brush]. A brush with firm bristles for freshening sores or abrading the interior of a cavity.

ecphoria (ek-fōr'ē-ă) [G. *ek,* out, + *phora,* a carrying]. The recall of memory.

ecphorize (ek'fōr-īz) [see ecphoria]. To revive a memory.

ecphyma (ek-fī'mă) [G. a pimply eruption]. A warty growth or protuberance.

écraseur (ā-krah-zer') [Fr. *écraser,* to crush]. Obsolete term for a snare, especially one of enough strength to cut through the base or pedicle of a tumor.

ECS Abbreviation for electrocerebral silence.

ecstasy (ek'stă-sē) [G. *ekstasis*]. Status raptus; mental exaltation, with some degree of sensory anesthesia and a rapturous expression.

ecstatic (ek-stat'ik). Relating to or marked by ecstasy.

ecstrophe (ek'strō-fē). Exstrophy.

ECT Abbreviation for electroconvulsive (electroshock) *therapy.*

ect-. See ecto-.

ectacolia (ek-tă-kō'lē-ă) [G. *ektasis,* a stretching, + *kolon,* colon]. Colectasia.

ectad (ek'tad) [G. *ektos,* outside, + L. *ad,* to]. Outward.

ectal (ek'tăl) [G. *ektos,* outside]. Outer; external.

-ectasia, -ectasis [G. *ektasis,* a stretching]. Combining forms in suffix position used to denote dilation or expansion.

ectasia, ectasis (ek-tā'zē-ă, ek'tă-sis) [G. *ektasis,* a stretching]. Dilation of a tubular structure.
e. cor'dis, dilation of the heart.
corneal e., anterior herniation of the cornea.
diffuse arterial e., spontaneous enlargement with dilation of the vessels in a circumscribed area.
hypostatic e., dilation of a blood vessel, usually a vein, in a dependent portion of the body, as in varicose veins of the leg.
mammary duct e., dilation of mammary ducts by lipid and cellular debris in older women; rupture of ducts may result in granulomatous inflammation and infiltration by plasma cells. See also plasma cell *mastitis.*
papillary e., senile *hemangioma.*
scleral e., sclerectasia.
senile e., senile *hemangioma.*
e. ventric'uli paradox'a, hourglass *stomach.*

ectatic (ek-tat'ik). Relating to, or marked by, ectasis.

ectental (ek-ten'tăl) [G. *ektos,* outside, + *entos,* within]. Ectoental; relating to both ectoderm and endoderm; denoting the line where these two layers join.

ECTEOLA-cellulose. Cellulose treated with epichlorhydrin and triethanolamine to add tertiary amine groups to the cellulose and convert it to an anion-exchange material.

ectethmoid (ekt-eth'moyd) [G. *ektos,* outside, + ethmoid]. *Labyrinthus* ethmoidalis.

ecthyma (ek-thī'mă) [G. a pustule]. A pyogenic infection of the skin due to staphylococci or streptococci and characterized by adherent crusts beneath which ulceration occurs; the ulcers may be single or multiple, and heal with scar formation.
contagious e., orf; soremouth; contagious pustular dermatitis; a specific disease of sheep and goats, caused by a poxvirus (*Parapoxvirus*), that is transmissible to man and characterized by vesiculation and ulceration of the infected site.
e. gangreno'sum, *dermatitis* gangrenosa infantum.

ecthymatiform, ecthymiform (ek-thī-mat'i-fōrm, ek-thī'mi-fōrm). Resembling ecthyma.

ectiris (ek-tī'ris) [G. *ektos,* outside, + iris]. The outer layer of the iris.

ecto-, ect- [G. *ektos,* outside]. Combining forms denoting outer, on the outside. See also exo-.

ectoantigen (ek-tō-an'ti-jen). Exoantigen; any toxin or other excitor of antibody formation, separate or separable from its source.

ectoblast (ek'tō-blast) [ecto- + G. *blastos,* germ]. **1.** Ectoderm. **2.** As used by some experimental embryologists, the original outer cell layer from which the primary germ layers are formed; in this sense, synonymous with protoderm.

ectocardia (ek-tō-kar'dē-ă) [ecto- + G. *kardia,* heart]. Exocardia; congenital displacement of the heart.

ectocardiac, ectocardial (ek-tō-kar'dē-ak, -dē-ăl). Relating to ectocardia.

ectocervical (ek'tō-ser'vi-kăl). Pertaining to the pars vaginalis of the cervix uteri lined with stratified squamous epithelium.

ectochoroidea (ek'tō-kō-roy'dē-ă). *Lamina* suprachoroidea.

ectocornea (ek-tō-kōr'nē-ă). The outer layer of the cornea.

ectocrine (ek'tō-krin) [ecto- + G. *krinō,* to separate]. **1.** Relating to substances, either synthesized or arising by decomposition of organisms, that affect plant life. **2.** A compound with ectocrine properties. **3.** An ectohormone. *Cf.* endocrine; exocrine.
ecological e., a chemical substance that undergoes biosynthesis in one species and that exerts an effect on the function of another species through mechanisms of the external environment; *e.g.,* the biosynthesis of vitamins by ruminants and their subsequent ingestion by other animals. See also ectohormone.

ectocyst (ek'tō-sist) [ecto- + G. *kystis,* bladder]. The outer layer of a hydatid cyst.

ectoderm (ek'tō-derm) [ecto- + G. *derma,* skin]. Ectoblast (1); the outer layer of cells in the embryo, after establishment of the three primary germ layers (ectoderm, mesoderm, endoderm).
epithelial e., superficial e.; that part of the e. separating from the neuroectoderm at about the fourth week of embryonic life; the epidermis and its specialized derivatives develop from it.
superficial e., epithelial e.

ectodermal (ek-tō-der'măl). Ectodermic; deric; relating to the ectoderm.

ectodermatosis (ek'tō-der-mă-tō'sis). Ectodermosis.

ectodermic (ek-tō-der'mik). Ectodermal.

ectodermosis (ek'tō-der-mō'sis). Ectodermatosis; a disorder of any organ or tissue developed from the ectoderm.
e. ero'siva plu'riorificia'lis, Stevens-Johnson *syndrome.*

ectoentad (ek-tō-en'tad). From without inward.

ectoental (ek-tō-en'tăl). Ectental.

ectoenzyme (ek-tō-en'zīm). An enzyme that is excreted externally and that acts outside the organism.

ectoethmoid (ek-tō-eth'moyd). *Labyrinthus* ethmoidalis.

ectogenous (ek-toj'e-nŭs) [ecto- + G. *-gen,* producing]. Exogenous.

ectoglobular (ek-tō-glob'yū-lăr). Not within a globular body; specifically not within a red blood cell.

ectohormone (ek'tō-hōr-mōn). A parahormonal chemical mediator of ecological significance which is secreted, largely by an organism (usually an invertebrate) into its immediate environment (air or water); it can alter the behavior or functional activity of a second organism, often of the same species as that secreting the e. See also ecological *ectocrine.*

ectomeninx (ek-tō-mē'ningks, -men'ingks) [ecto- + G. *mēninx,* membrane]. A primitive condensation of mesenchyme surrounding the embryonic brain.

ectomere (ek'tō-mēr) [ecto- + G. *meros,* part]. One of the blastomeres involved in formation of ectoderm.

ectomerogony (ek'tō-mĕ-rog'-ō-nē) [ecto- + G. *meros,* part, + *gonē,* generation]. The production of merozoites in the asexual reproduction of sporozoan parasites at the surface of schizonts and of blastophores, or by infolding into the schizont, as contrasted with endomerogony; e. has been observed in various species of *Eimeria.*

ectomesenchyme (ek-tō-mes'en-kīm) [ecto- + G. *mesos,* middle, + *enkyma,* infusion]. Mesectoderm (2).

ectomorph (ek'tō-mōrf) [ecto- + G. *morphē,* form]. Longitype; a constitutional body type or build (biotype or somatotype) in which tissues originating from the ectoderm predominate; from a morphological standpoint, the limbs predominate over the trunk.

ectomorphic (ek-tō-mōrf'ik). Relating to ectomorph.

-ectomy [G. *ektomē,* excision]. Combining form used as a suffix to denote removal of any anatomical structure. See also -tomy.

ectopagus (ek-top'ă-gŭs) [ecto- + G. *pagos,* something fixed]. Conjoined twins in which the bodies are joined laterally.

ectoparasite (ek-tō-par'ă-sīt). A parasite that lives on the surface of the host body.

ectoparasiticide (ek'tō-par-ă-sit'i-sīd). An agent that is applied directly to the host to kill ectoparasites.

ectoparasitism (ek'tō-par'ă-sī-tizm). Infestation.

ectoperitonitis (ek'tō-pār-i-tō-nī'tis). Inflammation beginning in the deeper layer of the peritoneum which is next to the viscera or the abdominal wall.

ectophyte (ek'tō-fīt) [ecto- + G. *phyton,* plant]. A plant parasite of the skin.

ectopia (ek-tō'pē-ă) [G. *ektopos,* out of place, fr. *ektos,* outside, + *topos,* place]. Ectopy; heterotopia (1); congenital displacement of any organ or part of the body.
e. cloa'cae, *exstrophy* of the cloaca.
e. cor'dis, congenital condition in which the heart is exposed on the chest wall because of maldevelopment of the sternum and pericardium.
e. len'tis, displacement of the lens of the eye.
e. mac'ulae, heterotropia maculae; a condition in which the fovea centralis is displaced to an optically wrong position.
e. pupil'lae congen'ita, displacement of the pupil present at birth.
e. re'nis, displacement of the kidney.
e. tes'tis, aberratio testis; ectopic testis; parorchidium; cryptorchidism with the testis positioned other than along the normal path of descent.
e. ves'icae, *exstrophy* of the bladder.

ectopic (ek-top'ik) [see ectopia]. **1.** Aberrant (3); heterotopic (1); out of place; said of an organ not in its proper position, or of a pregnancy occurring elsewhere than in the cavity of the uterus. **2.** In cardiography, denoting a heart beat that has its origin in some abnormal focus; developing from a focus other than the sinoatrial node.

ectoplacental (ek'tō-pla-sen'tăl). **1.** Outside, beyond, or surrounding the placenta; in primates, referring especially to the parts of the trophoblast not directly involved in the formation of the placenta. **2.** In rodents, referring to the actively growing part of the trophoblast involved in the formation of the placenta.

ectoplasm (ek'tō-plazm) [ecto- + G. *plasma,* something formed]. Exoplasm; the peripheral, more viscous cytoplasm of a cell; it contains microfilaments but is lacking in other organelles.

ectoplasmatic, ektoplasmic, ektoplastic (ek-tō-plas-mat'ik, -plas'mik, -plas'tik). Relating to the ectoplasm.

ectopy (ek'tō-pē). Ectopia.

ectoretina (ek'tō-ret'i-nă). *Stratum* pigmenti retinae.

ectosarc (ek'tō-sark) [ecto- + G. *sarx,* flesh]. The outer membrane, or ectoplasm, of a protozoon.

ectoscopy (ek-tos'kŏ-pē) [ecto- + G. *skopeō,* to examine]. An obsolete method of diagnosis of disease of any of the internal organs by a study of movements of the abdominal wall or thorax caused by phonation.

ectosteal (ek-tos'tē-ăl) [ecto- + G. *osteon* bone]. Relating to the external surface of a bone.

ectostosis (ek-tos-tō'sis) [ecto- + G. *osteon,* bone, + *-osis,* condition]. Ossification in cartilage beneath the perichondrium, or formation of bone beneath the periosteum.

ectothrix (ek'tō-thriks) [ecto- + G. *thrix,* hair]. A sheath of macroconidia on the outside of a hair as well as mycelium within the hair shaft; a characteristic of some of the dermatophytes.

ectotoxin (ek-tō-tok'sin). Extracellular *toxin.*

ectozoon (ek-tō-zō'on) [ecto- + G. *zōon,* animal]. An animal parasite living on the surface of the body.

ectro- [G. *ektrōsis,* miscarriage]. Combining form denoting congenital absence of a part.

ectrocheiry, ectrochiry (ek-trō-kī'rē) [ectro- + G. *cheir,* hand]. Total or partial absence of a hand.

ectrodactyly, ectrodactylia, ectrodactylism (ek-trō-dak'ti-lē, -dak-til'i-ă, -dak'ti-lizm) [ectro- + G. *daktylos,* finger]. Congenital absence of one or more fingers or toes.

ectrogenic (ek-trō-jen'ik). Relating to ectrogeny.

ectrogeny (ek-troj'ĕ-nē) [ectro- + G. *-gen,* producing]. Congenital absence of any part.

ectromelia (ek-trō-mē'lē-ă) [ectro- + G. *melos,* limb]. **1.** Congenital absence of one or more limbs. **2.** Mousepox; infectious e.; a disease of mice caused by a species of (*Orthopoxvirus*); characterized by gangrenous loss of feet and necrotic areas in the internal organs; in laboratory mouse colonies, it usually results in high mortality rates.

ectromelic (ek-trō-mel'ik). Pertaining to, or characterized by, ectromelia.

ectropion, ectropium (ek-trō'pē-on, -pē-ŭm) [G. *ek,* out, + *tropē,* a turning]. A rolling outward of the margin of a part, *e.g.,* of an eyelid.
atonic e., flaccid or paralytic e.; e. of the lower eyelid following paralysis of the orbicularis oculi muscle.
cicatricial e., e. of the eyelids after burns, lacerations, or skin infection.
flaccid e., atonic e.
paralytic e., atonic e.
spastic e., e. of the lower eyelid as a result of ocular irritation.
e. u'veae, iridectropium; eversion of the anterior edge of the secondary optic vesicle at the pupillary margin.

ectropody (ek-trop'ō-dē) [ectro- + G. *pous,* foot]. Total or partial absence of a foot.

ectrosyndactyly (ek'trō-sin-dak'ti-lē) [ectro- + G. *syn,* together, + *daktylos,* finger]. Congenital deformity marked by the absence of one or more digits and the fusion of others.

ectrotic (ek-trot'ik) [G. *ektrōtikos,* relating to abortion, fr. *ektrōsis,* miscarriage]. Obsolete term for abortive (1).

ectylurea (ek'til-yū-rē'ă). 2-Ethyl-*cis*-crotonylurea; a mild sedative used in the treatment of nervous tension and anxiety.

ectype (ek'tīp) [G. *ek,* out, + *typos,* stamp, model]. Extreme somatotype, such as ectomorph (longitype) or endomorph (brachytype).

ecuresis (ek-yū-rē'sis) [G. *ek,* out, + *ourēsis,* urination]. A condition in which urinary excretion and intake of water act to produce an absolute dehydration of the body. See also emuresis.

eczema (ek'zĕ-mă, eg'zĕ-mă, eg-zē'mă) [G. fr. *ekzeō,* to boil over]. Generic term for acute or chronic inflammatory conditions of the skin, typically erythematous, edematous, papular, vesicular, and crusting; followed often by lichenification and scaling and occasionally by duskiness of the erythema and, infrequently, hyperpigmentation; often accompanied by sensations of itching and burning; the vesicles form by intraepidermal spongiosis. Sometimes referred to colloquially as tetter, dry tetter, scaly tetter.
allergic e., macular, papular, or vesicular eruption due to an allergic reaction.
atopic e., atopic *dermatitis.*
baker's e., allergic e. due to contact with flour, yeast, or other ingredients handled by bakers.
chronic e., lichenoid e.
e. craquelé, winter e.
e. diabetico'rum, e. occurring in diabetes.
e. ep'ilans, e. with hair loss.
e. erythemato'sum, a dry form of e. marked by extensive areas of redness with scaly desquamation.
facial e., a photosensitivity disease of sheep in New Zealand associated with ingestion of plants during periods when autumn rains produce lush growth following seasons of dryness and close grazing; the predisposing cause is hepatic disease, which results from toxins of the fungus *Pithomyces chartarum,* which grows on the plants.

flexural e., e. of skin at the flexures of elbow, knees, wrists, etc.
hand e., e. that predominantly and persistently affects the hands; of multiple causation, including allergic, industrial, dyshidrotic, bacterial, and atopic mechanisms.
e. herpet'icum, Kaposi's varicelliform eruption; pustulosis vacciniformis acuta; a febrile condition caused by herpesvirus type 1, occurring most commonly in children, consisting of a widespread eruption of vesicles rapidly becoming umbilicated pustules; clinically, it is indistinguishable from a generalized vaccinia, but the two may be distinguished by electron microscopy or demonstration of inclusion bodies in smears, which are intranuclear in e. herpeticum and intracytoplasmic in e. vaccinatum.
e. hypertroph'icum, e. marked by papillary hypertrophy of the skin.
infantile e., e. in infants; the clinical appearance varies according to the dominant causative mechanism, *e.g.,* contact-type hypersensitivity, candidiasis, atopy, seborrhea, or a combination including skin maceration in folds of skin and in the diaper area.
e. intertri'go, see intertrigo.
lichenoid e., chronic e.; thickening of skin in e.
e. mad'idans, weeping e.; humid, moist, or wet tetter; a moist eczematous eruption.
e. margina'tum, *tinea* cruris.
e. nummula're, discrete, coin-shaped patches of e.
e. papulo'sum, a dermatitis marked by an eruption of discrete or aggregated reddish excoriated papules.
e. parasit'icum, eczematous eruption precipitated by parasite infestation.
e. pustulo'sum, impetigo eczematodes; a later stage of vesicular e., in which the vesicles have become secondarily infected; the lesions become covered with purulent crusts.
e. ru'brum, a stage of vesicular e., presenting red, excoriated, weeping areas.
seborrheic e., seborrheic *dermatitis.*
e. squamo'sum, a form of dry, scaly e.
stasis e., eczematous eruption on legs due to or aggravated by vascular stasis.
tropical e., e. occurring in plaques on extensors of the extremities; of common occurrence and unknown etiology.
e. tylot'icum, eczematous eruption of palms and soles with marked hyperkeratosis, thickening, and cracking of the skin.
e. vaccina'tum, a form of generalized vaccinia supervening upon an existing atopic e., characterized by crops of vesicles and vesicopustules appearing on the face, neck, extremities, and trunk, with even minimal atopic involvement; accompanied by a high fever, malaise, and enlargement of the lymph nodes.
varicose e., e. occurring over areas in which the skin has been compromised by varicosities.
e. verruco'sum, e. with hyperkeratosis; chronic lichenified e.
e. vesiculo'sum, dermatitis marked by an eruption of vesicles upon erythematous patches that rupture and exude serum.
weeping e., e. madidans.
winter e., e. craquelé; e. resulting from accelerated evaporation of moisture (including insensitive sweat) from the cutaneous surface; occurs as dry crackled plaques, usually on the extremities, but not infrequently also on the trunk in any season under circumstances (occupational, environmental) of excessively rapid drying out of the skin.

eczematization (ek-zem'ă-ti-zā'shŭn). **1.** Formation of an eruption resembling eczema. **2.** Occurrence of eczema secondary to a preexisting dermatosis.

eczematoid (ek-zem'ă-toyd). Resembling eczema in appearance.

eczematous (ek-zem'ă-tŭs). Marked by or resembling eczema.

ED Abbreviation for effective *dose.*

edathamil (ĕ-dath'ă-mil). Ethylenediaminetetraacetic acid.

EDB Abbreviation for *ethylene* dibromide.

EDC Abbreviation for estimated date of confinement. See Nägele's *rule.*

edea (e-dē'ă) [G. *aidoia,* genitals]. The external genitals.

Edebohls, George M., U.S. surgeon, 1853–1908. See E.'s *position.*

edema (e-dē'mă) [G. *oidēma,* a swelling]. An accumulation of an excessive amount of watery fluid in cells, tissues, or serous cavities.
angioneurotic e., periodically recurring episodes of noninflammatory swelling of skin, mucous membranes, viscera, and brain, of sudden onset and lasting hours to days, occasionally with arthralgia, purpura, or fever; cerebral or glottal e. may cause death; seems to be associated with food allergies, urticaria, and possibly with stress and emotional factors. Also called angioedema; atrophedema; Bannister's, Milton's, or Quincke's disease; circumscribed, periodic, or Quincke's e.; giant urticaria or hives; urticaria gigans, gigantea, or tuberosa.
Berlin's e., retinal e. after anterior ocular concussion.
blue e., the swelling and cyanosis of an extremity in hysterical paralysis.
brain e., cerebral e.
brown e., e. of the lungs associated with chronic passive congestion.
bullous e., a reddened, swollen appearance of the ureteral orifice in the bladder wall, frequently observed in tuberculosis of the ureter.
bullous e. ves'icae, a prominent area of focal e. involving the bladder mucosa, consisting of elevated masses of edematous tissue or clusters of clear fluid-filled vesicles; often associated with chronic inflammation or irritation secondary to tubes, foreign bodies, or perivesical inflammation.
cachectic e., marantic e.; e. occurring in diseases characterized by wasting and hypoproteinemia; due to low plasma oncotic pressure.
cardiac e., e. resulting from congestive heart failure.
cerebral e., brain e.; brain swelling due to increased volume of the extravascular compartment from the uptake of water in the neuropile and white matter. See also brain *swelling.*
circumscribed e., angioneurotic e.
cystoid macular e., e. of the posterior pole of the eye secondary to abnormal permeability of capillaries of the central sensory retina.
dependent e., a clinically detectable increase in extracellular fluid volume localized in a dependent area, as of a limb, characterized by swelling or pitting.
gestational e., occurrence of a generalized and excessive accumulation of fluid in the tissues of greater than 1+ pitting after 12 hours' bed rest, or of a weight gain of 5 pounds or more in 1 week due to the influence of pregnancy.
e. glot'tidis, e. of the larynx.
heat e., e. caused by excessively high external temperature.
hereditary angioneurotic e. (HANE), a relatively rare hereditary form of angioneurotic e. associated with either a deficiency of C1 esterase inhibitor or a functionally inactive form of the inhibitor, either of which permits uncontrolled activation of early complement components and production of a kinin-like factor which induces the angioedema; autosomal dominant inheritance.
hydremic e., obsolete term for e. occurring in states marked by pronounced hydremia.
inflammatory e., a swelling due to effusion of fluid in the soft parts surrounding a focus of inflammation.
lymphatic e., leukophlegmasia; e. due to stasis in the lymph channels.
malignant e., a form of anthrax in which the eyelids, lips, and other parts of the face, the neck, and the upper extremities are the seats of marked e., with an eruption of vesicles and bullae, which is prone to become gangrenous; the constitutional symptoms are those characteristic of extreme sepsis.
marantic e., cachectic e.

menstrual e., retention of water and increase in weight, which occurs during or preceding menstruation.
e. neonato'rum, a diffuse, firm, and commonly fatal e. occurring in the newborn, usually beginning in the legs and spreading upward.
noninflammatory e., e. due to mechanical or other causes, not marked by inflammation or congestion.
nutritional e., a form of swelling caused by insufficient protein intake together with resulting hypoproteinemia.
e. of the optic disk, papilledema.
periodic e., angioneurotic e.
pitting e., e. that retains for a time the indentation produced by pressure.
premenstrual e., see menstrual e.
pulmonary e., e. of lungs usually resulting from mitral stenosis or left ventricular failure.
Quincke's e., angioneurotic e.
salt e., e. from excessive intake or retention of sodium chloride.
solid e., infiltration of the subcutaneous tissues by mucoid material, as in myxedema.
Yangtze e., gnathostomiasis.

edematization (e-dem'ă-ti-zā'shŭn). Making edematous.

edematous (e-dem'ă-tŭs). Marked by edema.

edentate (ē-den'tāt) [L. *edentatus*]. Edentulous.

edentulous (ē-den'tyū-lŭs) [L. *edentulus,* toothless]. Edentate; toothless, having lost the natural teeth.

edestin (ĕ-des'tin). A globulin derived from the castor oil bean, hemp seed, and other seeds.

edetate (ed'ĕ-tāt). USAN-approved contraction for ethylenediaminetetraacetate, the anion of ethylenediaminetetraacetic acid; various e.'s are used as chelating agents to carry cations in (*e.g.,* ferric sodium e. as an iron carrier) or out (*e.g.,* sodium e. for calcium or heavy metal removal).

edetic acid (ĕ-det'ik). Ethylenediaminetetraacetic acid.

edge (ej). A line at which a surface terminates. See also border, margin, margo.
cutting e., **(1)** the beveled, knifelike, sharpened working angle of a dental hand instrument; **(2)** *margo* incisalis.
denture e., denture *border.*
incisal e., *margo* incisalis.
leading e., the initial part of a wave form at maximum slope.
shearing e., *margo* incisalis.

Edinger, Ludwig, German anatomist, 1855–1918. See E.-Westphal *nucleus.*

edisylate (e-dis'i-lāt). USAN-approved contraction for 1,2-ethanedisulfonate, $^{-}O_3S(CH_2)_2SO_3{}^{-}$.

Edlefsen, Gustav J.F., German physician, 1842–1910. See E.'s *reagent.*

Edman, P., contemporary Australian scientist. See E.'s *reagent.*

Edridge-Green, Frederick W., British ophthalmologist, 1863–1953. See E.-G. *lamp.*

edrophonium chloride (ed-rō-fō'nē-ŭm). Dimethylethyl (3-hydroxyphenyl)ammonium chloride; a competitive antagonist of skeletal muscle relaxants (curare derivatives and gallamine triethiodide), used as an antidote for curariform drugs, as a diagnostic agent in myasthenia gravis, and in myasthenic crisis.

EDTA Abbreviation for ethylenediaminetetraacetic acid.

educt (ē'dŭkt). An extract.

edulcorant (e-dŭl'kō-rant). Sweetening.

edulcorate (e-dŭl'kō-rāt) [L. *e-* intensive, + *dulcoro,* to sweeten, fr. *dulcor,* sweetness, fr. *dulcis,* sweet]. To sweeten or render less acrid.

Edwards, J.H., 20th century British physician. See E.'s *syndrome.*

Edwardsiella (ed'ward-sē-el'lă). A genus of Gram-negative, facultatively anaerobic bacteria (family Enterobacteriaceae) containing motile, peritrichous, nonencapsulated rods. The type species is *E. tarda,* which is occasionally isolated from the stools of healthy humans and those with diarrhea, from the blood of humans and other animals, and from human urine.

EEE Abbreviation for eastern equine *encephalomyelitis.*

EEG Abbreviation for electroencephalogram.

EENT Abbreviation for eye, ear, nose, and throat. See also ENT.

effect (e-fekt') [L. *ef-ficio,* pp. *effectus,* to accomplish, fr. *facio,* to do]. The result or consequence of an action.
abscopal e., a reaction produced following irradiation but occurring outside the zone of actual radiation absorption.
additive e., an e. wherein two or more substances or actions used in combination produce a total e. the same as the arithmetic sum of the individual e.'s.
after-e., see aftereffect.
Arias-Stella e., Arias-Stella *phenomenon.*
autokinetic e., in psychology, the apparent drifting about of a small, fixed, spot of light which is being observed in a dark room.
Bernoulli e., the decrease in fluid pressure that occurs in converting potential to kinetic energy when motion of the fluid is accelerated, in accordance with Bernoulli's law; applied in water aspirators, atomizers, and humidifiers in which a gas is accelerated across the end of a narrow, fluid-filled orifice.
Bohr e., the influence exerted by carbon dioxide on the oxygen dissociation curve of blood, *i.e.,* the curve is shifted to the right, which means a reduction in the affinity of hemoglobin for oxygen.
clasp-knife e., clasp-knife *spasticity.*
Compton e., in electromagnetic radiations of medium energy, a change in wavelength of the bombarding photon with the dislodgement of an orbital electron, usually from an outer shell.
Cotton e., the positive and negative displacement from zero of the rotation of plane polarized monochromatic light and the change of monochromatic circularly polarized light into elliptically polarized light in the immediate vicinity of the absorption band of the substance through which the light passes. See also optical rotatory *dispersion.*
Crabtree e., inhibition of cellular respiration of isolated systems by high concentrations of glucose; a "reciprocal" of Pasteur's e.
cumulative e., cumulative action; the condition in which repeated administration of a drug may produce e.'s that are more pronounced than those produced by the first dose.
Cushing e., Cushing *phenomenon.*
cytopathic e. degenerative changes in cells (especially in tissue culture) associated with the multiplication of certain viruses; when, in tissue culture, spread of virus is restricted by an overlay of agar (or other suitable substance) the cytopathic e. may lead to formation of plaque.
Doppler e., Doppler phenomenon; a change in frequency is observed when the sound and observer are in relative motion away from or toward each other. See also Doppler *shift.*
electrophonic e., the sensation of hearing produced when an alternating current of suitable frequency and magnitude is passed from an external source through a person.
experimenter e.'s, the influence of the experimenter's behavior, personality traits, or expectancies on the results of his own research.
Fahraeus-Lindqvist e., sigma e.; the decrease in apparent viscosity that occurs when a suspension, such as blood, is made to flow through a tube of smaller diameter; observed in tubes less than about 0.3 mm in diameter.
Fenn e., the increased liberation of heat in a stimulated muscle when it is allowed to do mechanical work; the amount of heat liberated is increased in proportion to the distance the muscle is allowed to shorten and in proportion to the tension it must develop (*e.g.,*

the weight it lifts) during shortening; thus increased chemical energy is consumed both to liberate increased heat and to do increased mechanical work.

founder e., an unusually high frequency of a gene in a population derived from a small set of ancestors, perpetuating the result of the high variance due to the small size of the sample they comprise.

gene dosage e., in perfectly codominant alleles, the linear relationship between the phenotypic value and the number of genes of one type substituted by another type.

Haldane e., the promotion of carbon dioxide dissociation by oxygenation of hemoglobin.

Orbeli e., the fatigue of a muscle stimulated by its nerve (*i.e.,* indirectly) is reduced by concurrent stimulation of sympathetic fibers to the muscle; thought to be caused by norepinephrine diffusing from adrenergic fibers which innervate blood vessels in the muscle.

oxygen e., enhancement of radiosensitivity of cells in a high concentration of oxygen.

Pasteur's e., the inhibition of fermentation by oxygen, first observed by Pasteur.

photechic e., Russell e.; the ability of an agent, other than light, to make a developable latent image in a photographic film emulsion.

photoelectric e., the loss of electrons from the surface of a metal upon exposure to light.

position e., a change in the phenotypic expression of one or more genes due to a change in position with respect to other genes; may result from change in chromosome structure or from crossing-over.

Raman e., a change in frequency undergone by monochromatic light scattered in passage through a transparent substance whose characteristics determine the amount of change, yielding a spectrum in which the incident wavelength band is flanked by small satellite bands of greater and lesser wavelengths.

Rivero-Carvallo e., inspiratory increase in the systolic murmur of tricuspid insufficiency; the characteristic distinguishing tricuspid insufficiency from mitral insufficiency.

Russell e., photechic e.

second gas e., when a constant concentration of an anesthetic like halothane is inspired, the rise in alveolar concentration is accelerated by concomitant administration of nitrous oxide, because alveolar uptake of the latter creates a potential subatmospheric intrapulmonary pressure that leads to increased tracheal inflow.

sigma e., Fahraeus-Lindquist e.

Somogyi e., in diabetes, a rebound phenomenon of reactive hyperglycemia in response to a preceding period of relative hypoglycemia that has increased secretion of hyperglycemic agents (epinephrine, norepinephrine, glucagon, cortisol, and growth hormone; described in diabetic patients given too much insulin who developed unrecognized nocturnal hypoglycemia that made them hyperglycemic (suggesting insufficient insulin) when tested the next morning.

Staub-Traugott e., in normal persons, a drop in blood glucose which follows a second oral dose of glucose given 30 minutes or so after the first.

Stiles-Crawford e., light that enters through the center of the pupil produces a greater visual effect than light that enters obliquely.

Venturi e., term applied to the operation of a Venturi tube and similar systems.

Vulpian's e., after section and degeneration of the hypoglossal nerve, stimulation of the chorda tympani going to the tongue causes a slow and prolonged contraction of the lingual muscles and vasodilation.

Wedensky e., a relatively long enhancing e. following application of a maximal shock or stimulus to a neuromuscular preparation during which a subthreshold stimulation, otherwise too small to evoke a response, will produce a response; a relatively prolonged lowered threshold of excitability following a maximal shock.

Wolff-Chaikoff e., Wolff-Chaikoff *block.*

Zeeman e., the splitting of spectral lines into three or more symmetrically placed lines when the light source is subjected to a magnetic field.

effector (ē-fek'tŏr, -tōr) [L. producer]. **1.** C. Sherrington's term for a peripheral tissue that receives nerve impulses and reacts by contraction (muscle), secretion (gland), or a discharge of electricity (electric organ of certain bony fishes). **2.** A small metabolic molecule that by combining with a repressor gene depresses the activity of an operon.

effemination (e-fem-i-nā'shŭn) [L. *ef-femino,* pp. *-atus,* to make feminine, fr. *ex,* out, + *femina,* woman]. Acquisition of feminine characteristics, either physiologically as part of female maturation, or pathologically by individuals of either sex.

efferent (ef'er-ent) [L. *efferens,* fr. *effero,* to bring out]. Conducting (fluid or a nerve impulse) outward from a given organ or part thereof; *e.g.,* the efferent connections of a group of nerve cells, efferent blood vessels, or the excretory duct of an organ.

gamma e., the thin axon of a gamma motor neuron innervating the intrafusal muscle fibers of a muscle spindle.

effervesce (ef-er-ves') [L. *ef-fervesco,* to boil up, from *ferveo,* to boil]. To boil up or form bubbles rising to the surface of a fluid in large numbers, as in the evolution of CO_2 from aqueous solution when the pressure is reduced.

effervescent (ef-er-ves'ent). **1.** Boiling; bubbling; effervescing. **2.** Causing to effervesce, as an e. powder. **3.** Tending to effervesce when freed from pressure, as an e. solution.

efficiency (ĕ-fish'en-sē). **1.** The production of the desired effects or results with minimum waste of time, effort, or skill. **2.** A measure of effectiveness; specifically, the useful work output divided by the energy input.

visual e., a rating used in computing compensation for industrial ocular injuries, incorporating measurements of central acuity, visual field, and ocular motility.

effleurage (e-fler-ahz') [Fr. *effleurer,* to touch lightly]. A stroking movement in massage.

effloresce (e-flō-es') [L. *ef-floresco* (*exf-*), to blossom, fr. *flos* (*flor-*), flower]. To become powdery by losing the water of crystallization on exposure to a dry atmosphere.

efflorescent (e-flō-es'ent). Denoting a crystalline body that gradually changes to a powder by losing its water of crystallization on exposure to a dry atmosphere.

effluvium, pl. effluvia (e-flū'vē-ŭm, -ē-ă) [L. a flowing out, fr. *ef-fluo,* to flow out]. **1.** A shedding, especially of hair. **2.** Obsolete term for an exhalation, especially one of bad odor or injurious influence.

telogen e., shedding of normal club hairs by premature development of telogen in anagen follicles, resulting from various kinds of stress, *e.g.,* difficult childbirth, shock, drug intake, fever.

effort (ef'ert). Deliberate exertion of physical or mental power.

distributed e., in psychology, learning that involves small units of work and interpolated rest periods, as contrasted with massed learning, in which the individual works continually until the skill is mastered.

effuse (e-fūs') [L. *ef-fundo,* pp. *-fusus;* to pour out]. Thin and widely spread; denoting the surface character of a bacterial culture.

effusion (e-fū'zhŭn) [L. *effusio,* a pouring out]. **1.** The escape of fluid from the blood vessels or lymphatics into the tissues or a cavity. **2.** The fluid effused.

eflornithine hydrochloride (ē-flōr'ni-thēn). 2-(Difluoromethyl)-DL-ornithine monohydrochloride, monohydrate; an antineoplastic and antiprotozoal orphan drug used in the treatment of *Pneumocystis carinii* pneumonia in AIDS and of *Trypanosoma brucei gambiense* sleeping sickness.

egersis (ē-ger′sis) [G. a waking]. Extremely alert wakefulness.

egesta (ē-jes′tă) [L. *e-gero,* pp. *-gestus,* to carry out, discharge]. Unabsorbed food residues that are discharged from the digestive tract.

egg (eg) [A.S. *aeg*]. The female sexual cell or gamete; after fertilization and fusion of the pronuclei it is a zygote and no longer an egg, although some authors refer to a 2-celled or 4-celled "egg." In the reptile and bird the egg is provided with a protective shell, membranes, albumin, and yolk for the nourishment of the embryo. See also oocyte, ovum.
centrolecithal e., an e. in which the yolk is concentrated near the center of the e. cell, as is the case in many of the insects.
homolecithal e., isolecithal e.; an e. in which the total amount of yolk is small and fairly uniformly distributed throughout the cytoplasm.
isolecithal e., homolecithal e.
microlecithal e., an e. containing a small amount of deutoplasm.
telolecithal e., an e. containing a relatively large quantity of deutoplasm concentrated at the abapical pole; *e.g.,* e.'s of reptiles and birds.

egg cluster. One of the clumps of cells resulting from the breaking up of the gonadal cords in the ovarian cortex; these clumps later develop into primary ovarian follicles.

Egger, Fritz, Swiss internist, 1863–1938. See E.'s *line.*

Eggleston, Cary, U.S. physician, 1884–1966. See E. *method.*

egg′shell. Testa (1); the calcareous envelope of a bird's egg.

egilops (ē′ji-lops) [G. *aigilōps,* a lacrimal fistula, fr. *aix* (*aig-*), goat, + *ops,* eye]. Obsolete term for a swelling, abscess, or fistula at the inner canthus of the eye.

eglandulous (ē-glan′dū-lŭs) [L. *e,* without, + gland or glandula]. Without glands.

Eglis glands. See under gland.

ego (ē′gō) [L. I]. In psychoanalysis, one of the three components of the psychic apparatus in the freudian structural framework, the other two being the id and superego. Although the e. has some conscious components, many of its functions are learned and automatic. It occupies a position between the primal instincts (pleasure principle) and the demands of the outer world (reality principle), and therefore mediates between the person and external reality by performing the important functions of perceiving the needs of the self, both physical and psychological, and the qualities and attitudes of the environment. It evaluates, coordinates, and integrates these perceptions so that internal demands can be adjusted to external requirements, and is also responsible for certain defensive functions to protect the person against the demands of the id and superego.

ego-alien (ē′gō-ā′lē-en). Egodystonic.

egobronchophony (ē′gō-brong-kof′ō-nē) [G. *aix* (*aig-*), goat, + *bronchos,* bronchus, + *phōnē,* voice]. Egophony with bronchophony.

egocentric (ē-gō-sen′trik) [ego + G. *kentron,* center]. Egotropic; marked by extreme concentration of attention upon oneself, *i.e.,* self-centered. *Cf.* allocentric.

egocentricity (ē′gō-sen-tris′i-tē). The condition of being egocentric.

ego-dystonic (ē′gō-dis-ton′ik) [ego + G. *dys,* bad, + *tonos,* tension]. Ego-alien; repugnant to or at variance with the aims of the ego.

egomania (ē-gō-mā′nē-ă) [ego + G. *mania,* frenzy]. Extreme self-appreciation or self-content.

egophonic (ē-gō-fon′ik). Relating to egophony.

egophony (ē-gof′ō-nē) [G. *aix* (*aig-*), goat, + *phōnē,* voice]. Tragophony; capriloquism; a peculiar broken quality of the voice sounds, like the bleating of a goat, heard about the upper level of the fluid in cases of pleurisy with effusion.

ego-syntonic (ē′gō-sin-ton′ik) [ego + G. *syn,* together, + *tonos,* tension]. Acceptable to the aims of the ego.

egotropic (ē-gō-trop′ik) [ego + G. *tropē,* a turning]. Egocentric.

Ehlers, Edward L., Danish dermatologist, 1863–1937. See E.-Danlos *syndrome.*

Ehrenritter, Johann, Austrian anatomist, †1790. See E.'s *ganglion.*

Ehret, Heinrich, German physician, *1870. See E.'s *phenomenon.*

Ehrlich, Paul, German bacteriologist, immunologist, and Nobel laureate, 1854–1915. See *Ehrlichia;* E.'s *anemia,* inner *body, phenomenon, postulate, reactions,* diazo *reagent, stains,* (side-chain) *theory;* E.-Türk *linc.*

Ehrlichia (er-lik′ē-ă) [P. *Ehrlich*]. A genus of small, often pleomorphic, coccoid to ellipsoidal, nonmotile, Gram-negative bacteria (order Rickettsiales) that occur either singly or in compact inclusions in circulating mammalian leukocytes; species are the etiologic agents of ehrlichiosis and are transmitted by ticks. The type species is *E. canis.*
E. ca′nis, the species causing canine ehrlichiosis in dogs; it is the type species of the genus *E.*
E. ristic′ii, the species causing equine monocytic ehrlichiosis.
E. sennet′su, the species causing Sennetsu fever in man.

ehrlichiosis (er-lik-ē-ō′sis). Infection with parasitic leukocytic rickettsiae of the genus *Ehrlichia;* in man, especially by *E. sennetsu* which produces manifestations similar to those of Rocky Mountain spotted fever.
canine e., tropical canine pancytopenia; a fatal disease of dogs in Asia, Africa, and the U.S. caused by *Ehrlichia canis,* transmitted by the tick *Rhipicephalus sanguineus,* and characterized by hemorrhage, pancytopenia, and emaciation.
equine monocytic e., Potomac horse fever; a febrile disease of horses in the U.S. caused by *Ehrlichia risticii* and characterized by anorexia, leukopenia, and occasional diarrhea.

Eichhorst, Hermann L., Swiss physician, 1849–1921. See E.'s *corpuscles, neuritis.*

Eicken, Karl von, German laryngologist, 1873–1960. See E.'s *method.*

***n*-eicosanoic acid** (ī′kō-să-nō′ik). Arachidic acid.

9-eicosenoic acid. Gadoleic acid.

eicosanoids (ī′kō-să-noydz) [G. *eicosa-,* twenty, + *eidos,* form]. The physiologically active substances derived from arachidonic acid, *i.e.,* the prostaglandins, leukotrienes, and thromboxanes. Also known as the arachidonic acid cascade.

eidetic (ī-det′ik) [G. *eidon,* saw (aorist of verb)]. **1.** Relating to the power of visualization of objects previously seen or imagined. **2.** A person possessing this power to a high degree.

eidoptometry (ī-dop-tom′ĕ-trē) [G. *eidos,* form, + *optikos,* referring to vision, + *metron,* measure]. Obsolete term for measurement of the acuteness of form vision.

Eikenella corrodens (ī-kĕ-nel′ă kōr-rō′denz) [M. *Eiken,* 1958]. A species of nonmotile, rod-shaped, Gram-negative, facultatively anaerobic bacteria that is part of the normal flora of the adult human oral cavity but may be an opportunistic pathogen, especially in immuno-compromised hosts.

eikonometer, eiconometer (ī-kō-nom′ĕ-ter) [G. *eikon,* image, + *metron,* measure]. **1.** An instrument for determining the magnifying power of a microscope, or the size of a microscopic object. **2.** An instrument for determining the degree of aniseikonia.

eiloid (ī′loyd) [G. *eilō,* to roll up, + *eidos,* appearance]. Resembling a coil or roll.

Eimer, Gustav Heinrich Theodor, German zoologist, 1843–1898. See Eimeria.

Eimeria (ī-mē′rē-ă) [G.H.T. *Eimer*]. The largest, most economically important, and most widespread genus of the coccidial protozoa (family Eimeriidae, class Sporozoea). The mature oocyst contains four sporocysts, each of which contains two sporozoites. *E.* may be highly pathogenic, especially in young hosts. Many species are known that infect wild vertebrates; domesticated mammals and birds commonly are infected with one or more species. Domestic animals and fowl suffer from *E.* infections (coccidiosis) most acutely under conditions of overcrowding with fecal contamination.

E. or **coccidia of cattle,** *E. zuernii,* the species most often associated with clinical cases of coccidiosis in calves and young adults; found in the cecum and lower bowel, and sometimes in the small intestine. *E. bovis,* a species that occurs principally in the small intestine and causes clinically recognizable disease; many less common species have been described.

E. or **coccidia of chickens,** *E. tenella,* a species producing cecal coccidiosis of young chicks; *E. necatrix,* producing severe disease in the small intestine and ceca; *E. acervulina, E. hagani,* and *E. praecox,* which localize in the duodenum; *E. mitis* localizes in the small intestine, *E. brunetti* in the lower small intestine and rectum, and *E. maxima* in the lower small intestine.

E. or **coccidia of geese,** *E. truncata,* a species occurring in the kidney tubules where it causes much damage and considerable mortality in young birds; *E. anseris, E. nocens,* and *E. parvula,* occurring in the small intestine where *E. anseris* can produce hemorrhagic enteritis.

E. or **coccidia of pheasants,** *E. phasiani* and *E. dispersa,* species which infect the small intestine; coccidiosis of pheasants in captivity under overcrowded conditions may be very destructive.

E. or **coccidia of rabbits,** *E. stiedae,* the most common species in rabbits, affecting the bile ducts; *E. perforans,* affecting the small intestine and cecum; *E. media, magna,* and *E. irresidua* which infect the small intestine.

E. or **coccidia of sheep and goats,** *E. ovina (arloingi),* the most common and destructive species in sheep, principal losses being in young lambs; *E. minakolyakimovae,* a highly pathogenic parasite of sheep; *E. parva* and *E. pallida* are frequently found but believed to be of low virulence; *E. faurei, E. intricata, E. granulosa, E. ahsata, E. hawkins, E. gilruthi, E. gonzalezi, E. christenseni, E. punctata, E. crandallis,* and *E. honessi,* are found in sheep or goats, and are probably of low pathogenicity. All of these species invade the epithelium of the small intestine.

E. or **coccidia of swine,** *E. debliecki,* the most common and most pathogenic species, involving the small intestine, cecum, and colon; *E. scabra,* involving the small intestine; *E. perminuta, E. spinosa, E. scrofae, E. suis, E. cerdonis, E. porci,* and *E. neodebliecki* believed to have little pathogenicity. See *Isospora* for other species in swine.

E. or **coccidia of turkeys,** *E. meleagridis,* a species which localizes in the cecum, *E. dispersa* and *E. innocua* in the small intestine, *E. adenoeides* in the lower ileum, cecum, and rectum, and *E. gallopavonis* in the ileum and rectum.

E. sardi'nae, species that occurs in sardines and herring, and has been found in the feces of men who have eaten these fish; it was once erroneously believed to be a coccidium of man.

Eimeriidae (ī-mĕr-ī'i-dē) [see *Eimeria*]. A family of sporozoan coccidia; important genera are *Eimeria* and *Isospora,* infections by *Eimeria* being by far the most common and most serious in domesticated animals.

Einarson's gallo cyanin-chrome alum stain. See under *stain.*

einstein (īn'stīn) [A. *Einstein,* German-born theoretical physicist in U.S., 1879–1955]. A unit of energy equal to 1 mol quantum, hence to 6.02×10^{23} quanta.

einsteinium (īn-stīn'ē-ŭm) [A. *Einstein,* German-born theoretical physicist in U.S., 1879–1955]. An artificially prepared transuranium element, atomic no. 99, atomic symbol Es (formerly E); it has many isotopes, all of which are radioactive.

Einthoven, Willem, Dutch physiologist, 1860-1927. See E.'s *equation, galvanometer, law, triangle.*

Eisenlohr, Carl, German physician, 1847–1896. See E.'s *syndrome.*

Eisenmenger, Victor, German physician, 1864–1932. See E.'s *complex, disease, tetralogy;* E. *syndrome.*

eisodic (ī-sod'ik) [G. *eis,* into, + *hodos,* a way]. Rarely used term for afferent.

ejaculate (ē-jak'yū-lāt) [see ejaculation]. **1.** To expel suddenly, as of semen. **2.** Semen expelled in ejaculation.

ejaculatio (ē-jak-yū-lā'shē-ō). Ejaculation.

e. defic'iens, absence of ejaculation.

e. pre'cox, premature *ejaculation.*

e. retarda'ta, unusually delayed ejaculation.

ejaculation (ē-jak-yū-lā'shŭn) [L. *e-iaculo,* pp. *-atus,* to shoot out]. Ejaculatio; emission of seminal fluid.

premature e., ejaculatio precox; prospermia; during sexual intercourse, too rapid achievement of climax and e. in the male relative to his own or his partner's wishes.

ejaculatory (ē-jak'yū-lă-tōr-ē). Relating to an ejaculation.

ejecta (ē-jek'tă) [L. ntr. pl. of *ejectus,* pp. of *ejicio,* to throw out]. Ejection (2).

ejection (ē-jek'shŭn) [L. *ejectio,* from *ejicio,* to cast out]. **1.** The act of driving or throwing out by physical force from within. **2.** Ejecta; that which is ejected.

ejector (ē-jek'tŏr, -tōr). A device used for forcibly expelling (ejecting) a substance.

saliva e., dental or saliva pump; a hollow, perforated suction tube used in the evacuation of saliva or liquid debris from the oral cavity.

Ejrup, Erick E., 20th century Swedish internist. See E. *maneuver.*

eka- [Sanskrit *eka,* one]. Prefix used to denote an undiscovered or just discovered element in the periodic system before a proper and official name is assigned by authorities; *e.g.,* eka-osmium, now plutonium.

Ekbom, K. A., Swedish neurologist, *1907. See E. *syndrome.*

EKG Abbreviation for electrocardiogram.

ekiri (ē-kī'rī) [Jap.]. An acute, toxic form of dysentery of infants seen in Japan and due to *Shigella sonnei.*

EKY Abbreviation for electrokymogram.

elaboration (ē-lab'ōr-ā'shŭn) [L. *e-laborō,* pp. *-atus,* to labor, endeavor, fr. *labor,* toil, to work out]. The process of working out in detail by labor and study.

secondary e., the mental process occurring partly during dreaming and partly during the recalling or telling of a dream by means of which the latent (relatively organized) content of the dream is brought into increasingly more coherent and logical order, resulting in the manifest content of the dream; an aspect of dream work.

Elaeophora schneideri (ē-lē-of'ō-ră schnī'der-ī) [Mod. L. *elaea,* fr. G. *elaia,* olive, + *agnos,* sheep, + *phoros,* to bear]. The bloodworm of sheep; a species of nematodes causing filarial dermatosis.

elaidic acid (el-ā-id'ik). *Trans-* 9-octadecenoic acid; $CH_3(CH_2)_7CH{=}CH(CH_2)_7COOH$; an unsaturated monobasic *trans-* isomer of oleic acid.

elaiopathia (el'ā-ō-path'ē-ă) [G. *elaion,* oil, + *pathos,* suffering]. Eleopathy.

elapid (el'ă-pid). Any member of the snake family Elapidae.

Elapidae (ē-lap'i-dē) [G. *elops,* a serpent]. A family of highly venomous snakes characterized by a pair of comparatively short, permanently erect deeply grooved fangs at the front of the mouth. There are over 150 species, including the cobra, krait, mamba, and coral snakes.

elasmobranch (ē-las'mō-brank) [G. *elasmos,* a metal plate, + *bran-*

chia, gills]. Cartilaginous fish of the class Chondrichthyes that have platelike gills, with each gill slit opening independently on the body surface.

elastance (ē-las'tans). A measure of the tendency of a structure to return to its original form after removal of a deforming force. In medicine and physiology, usually a measure of the tendency of a hollow viscus (*e.g.* lung, urinary bladder, gall bladder) to recoil toward its original dimensions upon removal of a distending or compressing force, the recoil pressure resulting from a unit distention or compression of the viscus; the reciprocal of compliance. The relationship between elasticity and e. is of the same nature as that between the specific inductive capacity of an insulator material and the capacitance of a particular condenser made from that material.

elastase (ĕ-las'tās). Former name for a serine proteinase (EC 3.4.21.11, formerly 3.4.4.7) hydrolyzing elastin; now divided into pancreatic e. (pancreatopeptidase E) (EC 3.4.21.36) and leukocyte e. (lysosomal or neutrophil e.) (EC 3.4.21.37).

elastic (ĕ-las'tik) [G. *elastreō,* epic form of *elaunō,* drive, push]. **1.** Having the property of returning to the original shape after being compressed, bent, or otherwise distorted. **2.** A rubber or plastic band used in orthodontics as either a primary or adjunctive source of force to move teeth. The term is generally modified by an adjective to describe the direction of the force or the location of the terminal connecting points.
intermaxillary e., material used to provide e. traction between the upper and lower teeth.
vertical e., e. material used in a direction perpendicular to the occlusal plane, connecting one arch wire to the other, and usually used to improve intercuspation.

elastica (ĕ-las'ti-kă). **1.** The elastic layer in the wall of an artery. **2.** Elastic *tissue.*

elasticin (ĕ-las'ti-sin). Elastin.

elasticity (ĕ-las-tis'i-tē). The quality or condition of being elastic.
physical e. of muscle, the quality of muscle that enables it to yield to passive physical stretch.
physiologic e. of muscle, the biologic quality, unique for muscle, of being able to change and resume size under neuromuscular control.
total e. of muscle, the combined effect of physical and physiologic e. of muscle.

elastin (ĕ-las'tin). Elasticin; a yellow elastic fibrous mucoprotein that is the major connective tissue protein of elastic structures (*e.g.,* large blood vessels).

elastofibroma (ĕ-las'tō-fī-brō'mă). A nonencapsulated slow-growing mass of poorly cellular, collagenous, fibrous tissue and elastic tissue; occurs usually in subscapular adipose tissue of old persons.

elastoidin (ĕ-las'toy-din). A complex collagen.

elastoma (ĕ-las-tō'mă). Pseudoxanthoma elasticum.
juvenile e., a connective tissue nevus characterized by an increase in the number and size of the elastic fibers, and often by increased vascularity.
Miescher's e., circinate groups of hyperkeratotic papules that become dislodged, leaving a small bloody depression; associated with pseudoxanthoma elasticum.

elastometer (ĕ-las-tom'ĕ-ter). A device for measuring the elasticity of any body or of the animal tissues.

elastomucin (ĕ-las-tō-myū'kin). The mucoprotein of connective tissue; *e.g.,* elastin.

elastorrhexis (ĕ-las-tō-rek'sis) [G. *rhēxis,* rupture]. Fragmentation of elastic tissue in which the normal wavy strands appear shredded and clumped, and take a basophilic stain.

elastosis (ĕ-las-tō'sis). **1.** Degenerative change in elastic tissue. **2.** Elastoid degeneration (1); elastotic degeneration; degeneration of collagen fibers, with altered staining properties resembling elastic tissue.
e. colloida'lis conglomera'ta, colloid milium or acne; colloid degeneration of the elastic tissue of the dermis in persons who are repeatedly or constantly exposed to sunlight over a period of many years.
e. dystroph'ica, angioid streaks of the retina due to rupture of Bruch's membrane.
e. per'forans serpigino'sa, circinate groups of asymptomatic keratotic papules; the epidermis is thickened around a central plug of dermal elastic tissue which is extruded through the epidermis.
solar e., e. seen histologically in the sun-exposed skin of the elderly or in those who have chronic actinic damage.

elation (ē-lā'shŭn) [L. *elatio,* fr. *ef-fero,* pp. *e-latus,* to lift up]. The feeling or expression of excitement or gaiety; if prolonged and inappropriate, a characteristic of mania.

Elaut, Leon J.S., 20th century Belgian pathologist. See E.'s *triangle.*

elbow (el'bō) [A.S. *elnboga*]. **1.** Ancon; cubitus (1); the joint between the arm and the forearm. **2.** An angular body resembling a flexed e.
capped e., shoe *boil.*
Little Leaguer's e., an epicondylitis of the medial epicondyle at the origin of the flexor muscles of the forearm; related to throwing and usually seen in children or adolescents.
miner's e., inflammation with fluid distention of the olecranon bursa.
nursemaid's e., Malgaigne's luxation; longitudinal subluxation of the radial bone into the articular ligament.
tennis e., epicondylalgia externa; lateral humeral epicondylitis; chronic inflammation at the origin of the extensor muscles of the forearm from the lateral epicondyle of the humerus, as a result of unusual strain (not necessarily from playing tennis).

elbowed (el'bōd). Angular; kneed.

el'der, el'der flowers. Sambucus.

electro- [G. *ēlektron,* amber (on which static electricity can be generated by friction)]. Prefix denoting electric or electricity.

electroanalgesia (ē-lek'trō-an-ăl-jē'zē-ă). Analgesia induced by the passage of an electric current.

electroanalysis (ē-lek'trō-ă-nal'i-sis). Quantitative analysis of metals by electrolysis.

electroanesthesia (ē-lek'trō-an-es-thē'zē-ă). Anesthesia produced by an electric current.

electroaxonography (ē-lek'trō-ak-son-og'ră-fē). Axonography.

electrobasograph (ē-lek-trō-bā'sō-graf) [electro- + G. *basis,* walking, + *graphō,* to write]. An apparatus for recording gait.

electrobasography (ē-lek-trō-bā-sog'ră-fē). The graphic process by which an electrobasograph is made; used for gait analysis.

electrobioscopy (ē-lek'trō-bī-os'kō-pē) [electro- + G. *bios,* life, + *skopeō,* to examine]. Use of electricity as a means of determining whether life is present or not.

electrocardiogram (ECG, EKG) (ē-lek-trō-kar'dē-ō-gram) [electro- + G. *kardia,* heart, + *gramma,* a drawing]. Graphic record of the heart's action currents obtained with the electrocardiograph.

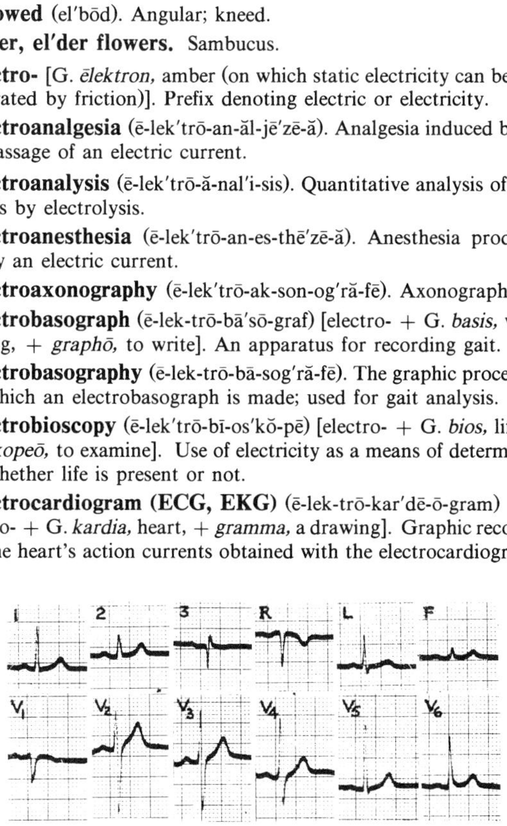

Normal 12-Lead Electrocardiogram

unipolar e., an e. taken with the exploring electrode placed on the chest overlying the heart or upon a single limb, the indifferent electrode being the central terminal.

electrocardiograph (ē-lek-trō-kar'dē-ō-graf). An instrument for recording the potential of the electrical currents that traverse the heart and initiate its contraction.

electrocardiography (ē-lek'trō-kar-dē-og'ră-fē). **1.** A method of recording electrical currents traversing the heart muscle just prior to each heart beat. **2.** The study and interpretation of electrocardiograms.

fetal e., recording the electrocardiogram of the fetus *in utero.*

electrocardiophonogram (ē-lek'trō-kar-dē-ō-fōn'ō-gram). The record obtained by electrocardiophonography.

electrocardiophonography (ē-lek'trō-kar-dē-ō-fō-nog'ră-fē) [electro- + G. *kardia,* heart, + *phōnē,* sound, + *graphō,* to write]. Method of electrically recording the heart sounds.

electrocauterization (ē-lek'trō-caw'ter-i-zā'shŭn). Cauterization by passage of high frequency current through tissue or by metal that has been electrically heated.

electrocautery (ē-lek'trō-caw'ter-ē). Electric cautery. **1.** An instrument for directing a high frequency current through a local area of tissue. **2.** A metal cauterizing instrument heated by an electric current.

electrocerebral silence (ECS) (ē-lek'trō-ser-ē'brăl sī'lens). Flat or isoelectric encephalogram; an electroencephalogram with absence of potentials of cerebral origin over 2 μv from symmetrically placed electrode pairs 10 or more centimeters apart, and with interelectrode resistance between 100 and 10,000 ohms; if such a record is present for 30 minutes in a comatose, apneic adult and if drug intoxication, hypothermia, and hypotension have been ruled out, cerebral death is indicated.

electrochemical (ē-lek'trō-kem'i-kăl). Denoting chemical reactions involving electricity, and the mechanisms involved.

electrocholecystectomy (ē-lek'trō-kō-lē-sis-tek'tō-mē). Removal of gallbladder by electrosurgery.

electrocholecystocausis (ē-lek'trō-kō-lē-sis'tō-kaw-sis). Cauterization of gallbladder mucosa by electrosurgery.

electrocoagulation (ē-lek'trō-kō-ag-yū-lā'shŭn). Coagulation produced by an electrocautery.

electrocochleogram (ē-lek'trō-kok'lē-ō-gram). The record obtained by electrocochleography.

electrocochleography (ē-lek'trō-kok-lē-og'ră-fē) [electro- + L. *cochlea,* snail shell, + G. *graphō,* to write]. A measurement of the electrical potentials generated in the inner ear as a result of sound stimulation.

electrocontractility (ē-lek'trō-kon-trak-til'i-tē). The power of contraction of muscular tissue in response to an electrical stimulus.

electroconvulsive (ē-lek'trō-kon-vŭl'siv). Denoting a convulsive response to an electrical stimulus. See electroshock *therapy.*

electrocorticogram (ē-lek-trō-kōr'ti-kō-gram). A record of electrical activity derived from the cerebral cortex.

electrocorticography (ē-lek'trō-kōr-ti-kog'ră-fē). The technique of surveying the electrical activity of the cerebral cortex.

electrocute (ē-lek'trō-kyūt) [electro- + execute]. To cause death by the passage of an electric current through the body.

electrocution (ē-lek-trō-kyū'shŭn). Electrothanasia; death caused by electricity. See electrocute.

electrocystography (ē-lek'trō-sis-tog'ră-fē). Recording of electric currents or changes in electric potential from the urinary bladder.

electrode (ē-lek'trōd). [electro- + G. *hodos,* way]. **1.** One of the two extremities of an electric circuit; one of the two poles of an electric battery or of the end of the conductors connected thereto. **2.** An electrical terminal specialized for a particular electrochemical reaction.

active e., exciting, localizing, or therapeutic e.; a small e. whose exciting effect is used to stimulate or record potentials from a localized area.

calomel e., an e. in which the wire is connected through a pool of mercury to a paste of mercurous chloride (Hg_2Cl_2, calomel) in a potassium chloride solution covered by more potassium chloride solution; commonly used as a reference e.

carbon dioxide e., Severinghaus e.; a glass e. in a film of bicarbonate solution covered by a thin plastic membrane permeable to carbon dioxide but impermeable to water and electrolytes; the carbon dioxide pressure of a gas or liquid sample quickly equilibrates through the membrane and is measured in terms of the resulting pH of the bicarbonate solution, as sensed by the glass e.; commonly used to analyze arterial blood samples.

central terminal e., in electrocardiography, an e. in which connections from the three limbs (right arm, left arm, and left leg) are joined and led to the electrocardiograph to form the indifferent e.

Clark e., an oxygen e. consisting of the tip of a platinum wire exposed to a thin film of electrolyte covered by a plastic membrane permeable to oxygen but not to water or the electrolyte. When a certain voltage is applied, oxygen is destroyed at the platinum surface; the flow of current is then proportional to the rate at which oxygen can diffuse to the platinum surface from the gas or liquid sample outside the membrane, and is thus a measure of the oxygen pressure in the sample; commonly used to measure oxygen pressure in arterial blood samples.

dispersing e., indifferent e.

exciting e., active e.

exploring e., an e. placed on or near an excitable tissue; in unipolar elecrocardiography, the e. is placed on the chest in the region of the heart and paired with an indifferent electrode.

glass e., a thin-walled glass bulb containing a standard buffer solution, a little quinhydrone, and a platinum wire; when immersed in an unknown solution, a potential difference develops that varies with the pH of the unknown solution; this difference can be made to give the pH; used in pH meters.

hydrogen e., the ultimate standard of reference in all pH determinations, limited and technically difficult to use, consisting of a piece of spongy platinum black partly immersed in a solution in a small glass tube; the tube above the solution is filled with hydrogen gas that is bubbled through the solution and absorbed by the platinum; the electrode thus measures the potential between H_2 and H^+, the "standard" potential of which (1 atmosphere, 1 molar) is taken as zero; hence, the hydrogen e. potential measures $[H^+]$ or pH.

indifferent e., dispersing or silent e.; in unipolar electrocardiography, a remote e. placed either upon a single limb or connected with the central terminal and paired with an exploring e.; the indifferent e. is supposed to contribute little or nothing to the resulting record.

ion-selective e.'s, glass, liquid ion-exchange, or solid state e.'s used to measure electrolyte and calcium ion activity in biological fluids.

localizing e., active e.

negative e., cathode.

oxidation-reduction e., redox e.; an e. capable of measuring oxidation-reduction potential. See quinhydrone e.

oxygen e., an e., usually consisting of a platinum wire or dropping mercury, used to measure the oxygen concentration in a solution by polarography.

positive e., anode.

quinhydrone e., one of several oxidation-reduction e.'s in which the ratio of the two forms (quinone-quinhydrone), determined by the hydrogen ion concentration, sets up a potential that can be measured and converted to a pH value (fails above pH 8).

redox e., oxidation-reduction e.

reference e., an e. expected to have a constant potential, such as a calomel e., and used with another e. to complete an electrical circuit through a solution; *e.g.,* when a reference e. is used with a glass e. for pH measurement, changes in voltage between the two e.'s can be attributed to the effects of pH on the glass e. alone.
Severinghaus e., carbon dioxide e.
silent e., indifferent e.
therapeutic e., active e.

electrodermal (ē-lek'trō-der'măl) [electro- + G. *derma,* skin]. Pertaining to electric properties of the skin, usually referring to altered resistance.

electrodermatome (ē-lek'trō-der'mă-tōm). Any dermatome powered by electricity.

electrodesiccation (ē-lek'trō-des-i-kā'shŭn) [electro- + L. *desicco,* to dry up]. Destruction of lesions or sealing off of blood vessels (usually of the skin, but also of available surfaces of mucous membrane) by monopolar high frequency electric current.

electrodiagnosis (ē-lek'trō-dī-ag-nō'sis). Determination of the nature of a disease through observation of changes in electrical activity.

electrodialysis (ē-lek'trō-dī-al'i-sis). In an electric field, the removal of ions from larger molecules and particles. *Cf.* electro-osmosis.

electroencephalogram (EEG) (ē-lek'trō-en-sef'ă-lō-gram). The record obtained by means of the electroencephalograph.

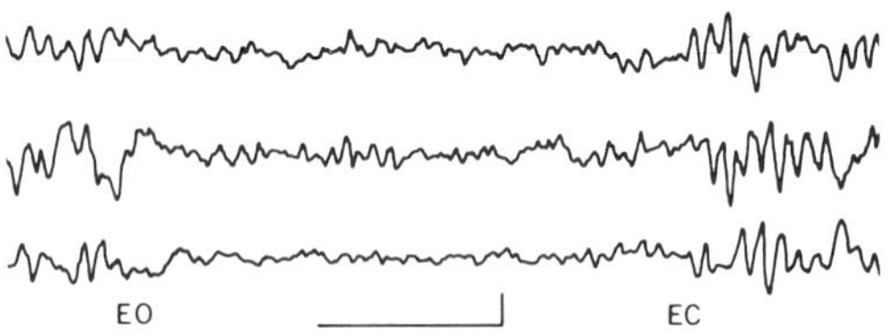

Electroencephalogram
EEG from left occipital, midline occipital, and right occipital leads to show the effect of opening (*EO*) and closing (*EC*) the eyes on the alpha rhythm; the horizontal line at the base indicates a time interval of 1 second and the vertical arm a calibration of 50 microvolts.

flat e., isoelectric e., electrocerebral silence.

electroencephalograph (ē-lek'trō-en-sef'ă-lō-graf) [electro- + G. *encephalon,* brain, + *graphō,* to write]. An apparatus consisting of amplifiers and a system for recording the electric potentials of the brain derived from electrodes attached to the scalp.

electroencephalography (ēlek'trō-en-sef'ă-log'ră-fē). Registration of the electrical potentials recorded by an electroencephalograph.

electroendosmosis (ē-lek'trō-en-dos-mō'sis). Endosmosis produced by means of an electric field.

electrogastrogram (ē-lek'trō-gas'trō-gram). The record obtained with the electrogastrograph.

electrogastrograph (ē-lek'trō-gas'trō-graf). An instrument used in electrogastrography.

electrogastrography (ē-lek'trō-gas-trog'ră-fē). The recording of the electrical phenomena associated with gastric secretion and motility.

electrogram (ē-lek'trō-gram). **1.** Any record on paper or film made by an electrical event. **2.** In electrophysiology, a recording taken directly from the surface by unipolar or bipolar leads.
His bundle e., an e. recorded from the His bundle, either in the experimental animal or in man during cardiac catheterization.

electrohemostasis (ē-lek'trō-hē-mos'tă-sis, -hē-mō-stā'sis) [electro- + G. *haima,* blood, + *stasis,* halt]. Arrest of hemorrhage by means of an electrocautery.

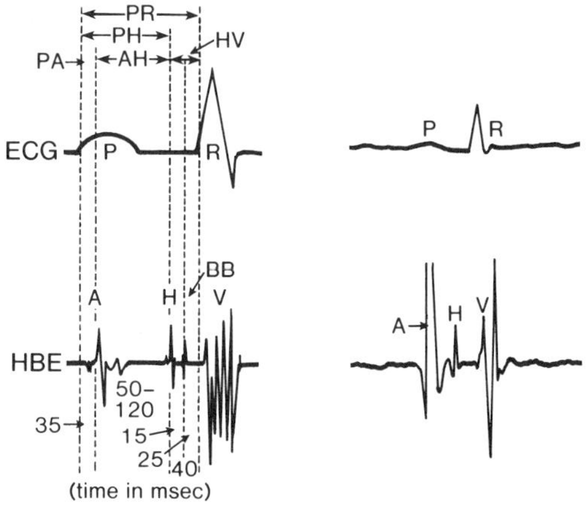

Electrogram
His bundle electrogram demonstrating mean values for conduction intervals in normal hearts.

electrohysterograph (ē-lek'trō-his'ter-ō-graf) [electro- + G. *hystera,* womb, + *graphō,* to write]. Instrument that records uterine electrical activity.

electroimmunodiffusion (ē-lek'trō-im'yū-nō-di-fyū'zhŭn). An immunochemical method that combines electrophoretic separation with immunodiffusion by incorporating antibody into the support medium.

electrokymogram (EKY) (ē-lek-trō-kī'mō-gram). Graphic record of the heart's movements produced by the electrokymograph.

electrokymograph (ē-lek-trō-kī'mō-graf). An apparatus for recording, from changes in the x-ray silhouette, the movements of the heart and great vessels; consists of a fluoroscope, x-ray tube, and a photomultiplier tube together with an electrocardiograph.

electrokymography (ē-lek-trō-kī-mog'ră-fē) [electro- + G. *kyma,* wave, + *graphō,* to write]. **1.** Registration of the movements of the heart and great vessels by means of the electrokymograph. **2.** The science and technique of interpreting electrokymograms.

electrolysis (ē-lek-trol'i-sis) [electro- + G. *lysis,* dissolution]. **1.** Decomposition of a salt or other chemical compound by means of an electric current. **2.** Destruction of certain of the body tissues (*e.g.,* hair) by means of galvanic electricity.

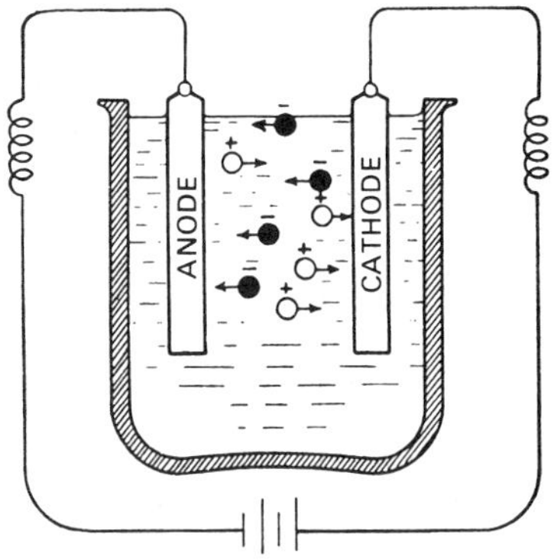

Chemical Electrolysis
The liquid contains a crystalloid such as sodium chloride. The circles represent anions (*black*) and cations (*clear*).

electrolyte (ē-lek′trō-līt) [electro- + G. *lytos,* soluble]. Any compound that, in solution, conducts electricity and is decomposed (electrolyzed) by it; an ionizable substance in solution.
amphoteric e., ampholyte; an e. that can either give up or take on a hydrogen ion and can thus behave as either an acid or a base.

electrolytic (ē-lek-trō-lit′ik). Referring to or caused by electrolysis.

electrolyze (ē-lek′trō-līz). To decompose chemically by means of an electric current.

electrolyzer (ē-lek′trō-līz-er). An obsolete apparatus for the treatment of strictures, fibromas, etc., by electrolysis.

electromagnet (ē-lek-trō-mag′net). A bar of soft iron rendered magnetic by an electric current encircling it.

electromassage (ē-lek′trō-mas-sazh′). Massage combined with the application of electricity.

electromicturation (ē-lek′trō-mik-tū-rā′shŭn) [electro- + L. *micturio,* to desire to make water]. Electrical stimulation of the conus medullaris to empty the urinary bladder of paraplegics.

electromorph (ē-lek′trō-mōrf) [electro- + G. *morphē,* form, shape]. A mutant form of a protein, phenotypically distinguished by its electrophoretic mobility.

electromyogram (EMG) (ē-lek-trō-mī′ō-gram). A graphic representation of the electric currents associated with muscular action.

electromyograph (ē-lek-trō-mī′ō-graf). An instrument for recording electrical currents generated in an active muscle.

electromyography (ē-lek′trō-mī-og′ră-fē) [electro- + G. *mys,* muscle, + *graphō,* to write]. A method of recording the electrical currents generated in an active muscle.

electron (ē-lek′tron). One of the negatively charged subatomic particles that are distributed about the positive nucleus and with it constitute the atom; in mass they are estimated to be $^{1}/_{1838}$ of the hydrogen atom; when emitted from inside the nucleus of a radioactive substance, e.'s are called beta particles.
Auger e., an e. released following displacement of an orbital e. by energy absorbed from impinging x- or γ-rays; the kinetic energy of the e. is equal to the net energy change of the transition; the release of an Auger e. competes with emission of characteristic x-rays for energy release in orbital electron transitions.
conversion e., an internal conversion e.
emission e., a beta particle or similar e. resulting from radioactive decay.
internal conversion e., conversion e.; an e., similar to an Auger e., released from one of the e. orbits of the atom upon activation by a γ-ray from that atom's nucleus; the e. has kinetic energy equal to the net energy transition of the disintegration.
positive e., positron.
valence e., one of the e.'s that take part in chemical reactions of an atom.

electronarcosis (ē-lek′trō-nar-kō-sis). Production of insensibility to pain by the use of electrical current.

electronegative (ē-lek-trō-neg′ă-tiv). Relating to or charged with negative electricity; referring to an element whose uncharged atoms have a tendency to ionize by adding electrons, thus becoming anions (*e.g.,* oxygen, fluorine, chlorine).

electroneurography (ē-lek′trō-nū-rog′ră-fē). A method of recording the electrical changes and nerve conduction velocities associated with the passing of impulses along peripheral nerves.

electroneurolysis (ē-lek′trō-nū-rol′i-sis). Destruction of nerve tissue by electricity.

electroneuromyography (ē-lek′trō-nūr′ō-mī-og′ră-fē). A method of measuring changes in a peripheral nerve by combining electromyography of a muscle with electrical stimulation of the nerve trunk carrying fibers to and from the muscle.

electronic (ē-lek-tron′ik). **1.** Pertaining to electrons. **2.** Denoting devices or systems utilizing the flow of electrons in a vacuum, gas, or semiconductor.

electron-volt (eV, ev). The energy imparted to an electron by a potential of 1 volt; equal to 1.6×10^{-12} erg in the CGS system, or 1.6×10^{-19} joule in the SI system.

electronystagmography (ENG) (ē-lek′trō-nis′tag-mog′ră-fē) [electro- + nystagmus + G. *graphō,* to write]. A method of nystagmography based on electro-oculography; skin electrodes are placed at outer canthi to register horizontal nystagmus or above and below each eye for vertical nystagmus.

electro-oculogram (ē-lek′trō-ok′yū-lō-gram). A record on paper or film of electric currents in electro-oculography.

electro-oculography (EOG) (ē-lek′trō-ok′yū-log′ră-fē). Oculography in which electrodes placed on the skin adjacent to the eyes measure changes in standing potential between the front and back of the eyeball as the eyes move; a sensitive electrical test for detection of retinal pigment epithelium dysfunction.

electro-olfactogram (EOG) (ē-lek′trō-ol-fak′tō-gram). Ottoson potential; osmogram; an electronegative wave of potential occurring on the surface of the olfactory epithelium in response to stimulation by an odor.

electro-osmosis (ē-lek′trō-os-mō′sis). The diffusion of a substance through a membrane in an electric field. *Cf.* Electrodialysis.

electropathology (ē-lek-trō-pa-thol′ō-jē). The study of pathologic conditions in their relation to electrical reactions.

electropherogram (ē-lek-trō-fer′ō-gram). Electrophoretogram; ionogram; ionopherogram; the densitometric or colorimetric pattern obtained from filter paper or similar porous strips on which substances have been separated by electrophoresis; may also refer to the strips themselves.

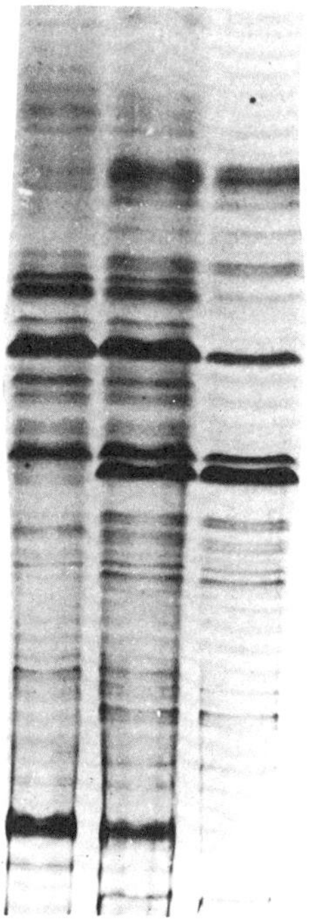

Electropherogram
Electrophoretic separation of cytoskeletal proteins of certain hamster cells on a polyacrylate gel in the presence of sodium dodecyl sulfate and stained with a blue dye. Migration is from top to bottom and is related to particle mass.

electrophil, electrophile (ē-lek'trō-fil, -fīl) [electro- + G. *philos,* fond]. **1.** The electron-attracting atom or agent in an organic reaction. *Cf.* nucleophil. **2.** Electrophilic; relating to an electrophil.

electrophilic (ē-lek-trō-fil'ik). Electrophil (2).

electrophobia (ē-lek-trō-fō'bē-ă) [electro- + G. *phobos,* fear]. Morbid fear of electricity.

electrophoresis (ē-lek-trō-fōr'ē-sis) [electro- + G. *phorēsis,* a carrying]. Dielectrolysis; ionophoresis; phoresis (1); the movement of particles in an electric field toward one or other electric pole, anode, or cathode.

disc e., a modification of gel e. in which a discontinuity (pH, gel pore size) is introduced near the origin to produce a lamina (disc) of the materials being separated; the separating bands retain their disc-like shape as they move through the gel.

gel e., e. through a gel, usually contained in a cylindrical tube.

isoenzyme e., electrophoretic separation of serum enzymes; separation of lactate dehydrogenase and creatine phosphokinase is commonly used for diagnosis of acute myocardial infarction.

lipoprotein e., electrophoretic separation of plasma lipoproteins.

thin-layer e. (TLE), electrophoretic migrations (separations) through a thin layer of inert material, such as cellulose, supported on a glass or plastic plate.

electrophoretic (ē-lek'trō-phōr-et'ik). Ionophoretic; relating to electrophoresis, as an e. separation.

electrophoretogram (ē-lek'trō-fōr-et'ō-gram). Electropherogram.

electrophototherapy (ē-lek'trō-fō'tō-ther'ă-pē). Phototherapy in which the source of the rays is the electric light.

electrophrenic (ē-lek'trō-fren'ik). Denoting electrical stimulation of the phrenic nerve usually at its motor point in the neck. See also e. *respiration.*

electrophysiology (ē-lek'trō-fiz-ē-ol'ō-jē). The branch of science concerned with electrical phenomena that are associated with physiologic processes. Electrical phenomena are prominent in neurons and effectors.

electropneumograph (ē-lek-trō-nū'mō-graf). An electric apparatus used for recording breathing. See pneumograph.

electropositive (ē-lek-trō-pos'i-tiv). Relating to or charged with positive electricity; referring to an element whose atoms tend to lose electrons; *e.g.,* sodium, potassium, calcium.

electropuncture (ē-lek-trō-pŭnk'chūr). Passage of an electrical current through needle electrodes piercing the tissues.

electroradiology (ē-lek'trō-rā-dē-ol'ō-jē). The use of electricity and x-ray in treatment.

electroradiometer (ē-lek'trō-rā-dē-om'ĕ-ter) [electro- + L. *radius,* ray, + G. *metron,* measure]. A modified electroscope designed for the differentiation of radiant energy.

electroretinogram (ERG) (ē-lek'trō-ret'i-nō-gram) [electro- + retina + G. *gramma,* something written]. A record of the retinal action currents produced in the retina by an adequate light stimulus.

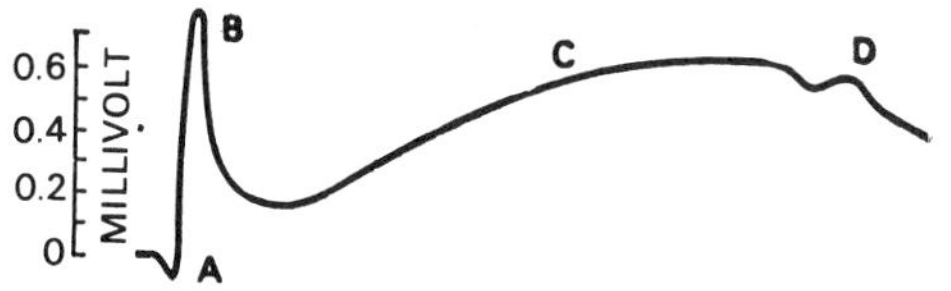

Electroretinogram
The A wave reflects photoreceptor activity; the B wave originates from nerve cells of the inner nuclear layer; the C wave is initiated by light absorption by photoreceptors but is generated by the retinal pigment epithelium; the D wave occurs when the light stimulus is removed.

electroretinography (ē-lek'trō-ret'i-nog'rā-fē). The recording and study of the retinal action currents.

electroscission (ē-lek'trō-si-shŭn) [electro- + L. *scissio,* to cleave]. Division of tissues by means of an electrocautery knife.

electroscope (ē-lek'trō-skōp) [electro- + G. *skopeō,* to examine]. An instrument for the detection of electrical charges or gaseous ions (*e.g.,* from *β* or x-rays); consists of two strips of gold leaf suspended from an insulated conductor and enclosed in an airtight container viewed with a low-power microscope.

electroshock (ē-lek'trō-shok). See electroshock *therapy.*

electrosol (ē-lek'trō-sol). Colloidal *metal.*

electrospectrography (ē-lek'trō-spek-trog'ră-fē). The recording, study, and interpretation of electroencephalographic wave patterns.

electrospinogram (ē-lek-trō-spī'nō-gram). The record obtained by electrospinography.

electrospinography (ē-lek'trō-spī-nog'ră-fē). The recording of spontaneous electrical activity of the spinal cord.

electrostenolysis (ē-lek'trō-stĕ-nol'i-sis). The precipitation of metals in membrane pores in the course of electrolysis.

electrostethograph (ē-lek'trō-steth'ō-graf) [electro- + G. *stēthos,* chest, + *graphō,* to record]. Electrical instrument that amplifies or records the respiratory and cardiac sounds of the chest.

electrostriction (ē-lek-trō-strik'shŭn). The contraction in volume in a protein solution during proteolysis due to the formation of new charged groups.

electrosurgery (ē-lek-trō-ser'jer-ē). Electrotomy; division of tissues by high frequency current applied locally with a metal instrument or needle.

electrotaxis (ē-lek-trō-tak'sis) [electro- + G. *taxis,* orderly arrangement]. Electrotropism; galvanotaxis; galvanotropism; reaction of plant or animal protoplasm to either an anode or a cathode. See also tropism.

negative e., e. by which an organism is attracted toward an anode or repelled from a cathode.

positive e., e. by which an organism is attracted toward a cathode or repelled from an anode.

electrothanasia (ē-lek'trō-thă-nā'zē-ă) [electro- + G. *thanatos,* death]. Electrocution.

electrotherapeutics, electrotherapy (ē-lek'trō-thār-ă-pyū'tiks, -thār'ă-pē). Use of electricity in the treatment of disease.

electrotherm (ē-lek'trō-therm) [electro- + G. *thermē,* heat]. A flexible sheet of resistance coils used for applying heat to the surface of the body.

electrotome (ē-lek'trō-tōm). An electric scalpel.

electrotomy (ē-lek-trot'ō-mē) [electro- + G. *tomē,* incision]. Electrosurgery.

electrotonic (ē-lek-trō-ton'ik). Relating to electrotonus.

electrotonus (ē-lek-trot'ō-nŭs) [electro- + G. *tonos,* tension]. Galvanotonus (1); changes in excitability and conductivity in a nerve or muscle cell caused by the passage of a constant electric current. See also catelectrotonus; anelectrotonus.

electrotropism (ē-lek-trot'rō-pizm, ē-lek-trō-trō'pizm) [electro- + G. *tropē,* a turning]. Electrotaxis.

electuary (ē-lek'chū-ā-rē) [G. *eleikton,* a medicine that melts in the mouth, fr. *ekleichō,* to lick up]. Confection.

eledoisin (el-ē-doy'sin). An undecapeptide toxin that is formed in the venom gland of cephalopods of the genus *Eledone* and causes vasodilation and contraction of extravascular smooth muscle.

eleidin (ē-lē'ī-din). A refractile and weakly staining keratin present in the cells of the stratum lucidum of the palmar and plantar epidermis.

element (el′ĕ-ment) [L. *elementum,* a rudiment, beginning]. **1.** A substance composed of atoms of only one kind, *i.e.,* of identical atomic (proton) number, that therefore cannot be decomposed into two or more elements, and that can lose its chemical properties only by union with some other e. or by a nuclear reaction changing the proton number. **2.** An indivisible structure or entity. **3.** A functional entity, frequently exogenous, within a bacterium, such as an extrachromosomal e.
actinide e.'s, actinides.
alkaline earth e.'s, those e.'s in the family Be, Mg, Ca, Sr, Ba, and Ra, the hydroxides of which are highly ionized and hence alkaline in water solution.
amphoteric e., an e. one or more of whose oxides unite with water to form hydroxides that may act as acids or as bases (*e.g.,* aluminum).
anatomical e., morphologic e.; any anatomical unit, such as a cell.
electronegative e., an e. whose atoms have a tendency to accept electrons and form negative ions (*e.g.,* oxygen).
electropositive e., an e. whose atoms have a tendency to lose electrons and form positive ions (*e.g.,* sodium).
extrachromosomal e., extrachromosomal genetic e., plasmid.
labile e.'s, tissue cells, as of epithelium, connective tissue, etc., that continue to multiply by mitosis during the life of the individual.
morphologic e., anatomical e.
neutral e., an e. of the zero group of the periodic system comprising the rare gases, He, Ne, Kr, etc.
noble e., noble *metal.*
picture e., see pixel.
rare earth e.'s, lanthanides.
trace e.'s., e.'s present in minute amounts in the body, many of which are essential in metabolism or for the manufacture of essential compounds.
transposable e., a transposon.
volume e., see voxel.

eleo- [G. *elaion,* oil]. Combining form relating to oil. See also oleo-.

eleoma (el-ē-ō′mă) [G. *elaion,* oil, + *-oma,* tumor]. Lipogranuloma.

eleometer (el-ē-om′ĕ-ter) [G. *elaion,* oil, + *metron,* measure]. Oleometer.

eleopathy (el-ē-op′ă-thē). Elaiopathia; a rare condition in which there is boggy swelling of the joints, said to be due to a fatty deposit following contusion; or possibly a condition resulting from the injection of paraffin oil as a form of malingering.

eleostearic acid (el-ē-ō-stē′ă-rik, -stēr′ik). An 18-carbon fatty acid with three double bonds (at carbons 9, 11, and 13); isomeric with linolenic acid; found in plant fats.

eleotherapy (el-ē-ō-ther′ă-pē) [G. *elaion,* oil]. Oleotherapy.

eleothorax (el-ē-ō-thōr′aks) [G. *elaion,* oil]. Oleothorax.

elephantiac, elephantiasic (el-ĕ-fan′tē-ak, fan-tē-as′ik). Relating to elephantiasis.

elephantiasis (el-ĕ-fan-tī′ă-sis) [G. fr. *elephas,* elephant]. Barbados or elephant leg; Malabar leprosy; mal de Cayenne or de San Lazaro; pes febricitans; phlegmasia malabarica; hypertrophy and fibrosis of the skin and subcutaneous tissue, especially of the lower extremities and genitalia, due to long-standing obstructed lymphatic vessels, caused chiefly by the presence of the filarial worms *Wuchereria bancrofti* or *Brugia malayi.*
e. congen′ita angiomato′sa, Klippel-Trenaunay-Weber *syndrome.*
congenital e., congenital enlargement of one or more of the limbs or other parts, due to dilation of the lymphatics.
gingival e., a fibrous hyperplasia of the gingiva.
e. neuromato′sa, enlargement of a limb due to diffuse neurofibromatosis of the skin and subcutaneous tissue.
nevoid e., thickening of skin, usually unilateral, involving a small area or the entire extremity, due to congenital enlargement of lymph vessels and lymph vessel obstruction.
e. nos′tras, a solid persisting edema of the eyelids and face that follows recurrent erysipelas or that may result from injury.
e. scro′ti, parasitic chylocele; chyloderma; lymph scrotum; brawny swelling of the scrotum as a result of chronic lymphatic obstruction.
e. telangiecto′des, hypertrophy of the skin and subcutaneous tissues accompanied by and dependent upon dilation of the blood vessels.
e. vul′vae, chronic hypertrophic *vulvitis.*

eleutheromania (ē-lū′ther-ō-mā′nē-ă) [G. *eleutheros,* free, + *mania,* madness]. Rarely used term for an excessive passion for freedom.

elevation (el-ĕ-vā′shŭn). A raised place. See also eminence; eminentia.
frontonasal e., frontonasal process; forebrain eminence or prominence; the unpaired embryonic prominence between the medial nasal elevations, which eventually merges with them to contribute to the bridge of the nose and the underlying nasal septum.
lateral nasal e., lateral nasal fold or process; an ectodermally covered mesenchymal swelling separating the embryonic olfactory pit from the developing eye.
medial nasal e., medial nasal fold or process; an ectodermally covered mesenchymal swelling lying medial to the olfactory placode or pit in the embryo.
tactile e.'s, *toruli* tactiles.

elevator (el′ĕ-vā-tĕr) [L. fr. *e-levo,* pp. *-atus,* to lift up]. **1.** An instrument for prying up a sunken part, as the depressed fragment of bone in fracture of the skull, or for elevating tissues. **2.** Dental lever; a surgical instrument used to luxate and remove teeth and roots that cannot be engaged by the beaks of a forceps, or to loosen teeth and roots prior to forceps application.
periosteal e., an instrument used for separating the periosteum from the bone.
screw e., a dental instrument with a threaded extremity used for extracting the root of a broken tooth.

elfwort (elf′wōrt). Elecampane.

eliminant (ē-lim′i-nant). **1.** An evacuant that promotes excretion or the removal of waste. **2.** An agent that increases excretion.

elimination (ē-lim-i-nā′shŭn) [L. *elimino,* pp. *-atus,* to turn out of doors, fr. *limen,* threshold]. Expulsion; removal of waste material from the body; the getting rid of anything.
carbon dioxide e., ($\dot{V}CO_2$), the rate at which carbon dioxide enters the alveolar gas from the blood, equal in the steady state to the metabolic production of carbon dioxide by tissue metabolism throughout the body; units: ml/min STPD or mmol/min.

elinguation (ē-ling-gwā′shŭn) [L. *e,* out, + *lingua,* tongue]. Glossectomy.

elinin (el′i-nin). A lipoprotein fraction of red blood cells that contains the Rh and A and B factors.

ELISA Abbreviation for enzyme-linked immunosorbent *assay.*

elixir (ē-lik′ser) [Mediev. L., fr. Ar. *al- iksir,* the philosopher's stone]. A clear, sweetened, hydroalcoholic liquid intended for oral use; e.'s contain flavoring substances and are used either as vehicles or for the therapeutic effect of the active medicinal agents.

Ellik, Milo, U.S. urologist, *1905. See E. *evacuator.*

Elliot, John W., U.S. surgeon, 1852–1925. See E.'s *position.*

Elliot, Robert H., British ophthalmologist, 1864–1936. See E.'s *operation.*

Elliott, Thomas R., British physician, 1877–1961. See E.'s *law.*

ellipsis (ē-lip′sis) [G. *ek-,* out, + *leipsis,* leaving]. Omission of words or ideas, leaving the whole to be completed by the reader or listener.

ellipsoid (ē-lip′soyd) [G. *ellips,* oval, + *eidos,* form]. **1.** Sheath of Schweigger-Seidel; a spherical or spindle-shaped condensation of phagocytic macrophages in a reticular stroma investing the wall of the splenic arterial capillaries shortly before they release their blood in the cords of red pulp. **2.** The outer end of the inner segment of the retinal rods and cones. **3.** Having the shape of an ellipse or oval.

elliptocyte (ē-lip′tō-sīt) [G. *elleipsis,* a leaving out, an ellipse, + *kytos,* cell]. Cameloid cell; ovalocyte; an elliptical red blood corpuscle found normally in the lower vertebrates with the exception of Cyclostomata; in mammals it occurs normally only among the camels (family Camelidae), hence cameloid cell.

elliptocytosis (ē-lip′tō-sī-tō′sis). Ovalocytosis; a relatively rare hereditary abnormality of hemopoiesis in which 50 to 90% of the red blood cells consist of rod forms and elliptocytes, frequently with an associated hemolytic anemia. See also elliptocytic *anemia.*

Ellis, Richard W.B., 20th century British physician. See E.-van Creveld *syndrome.*

Ellis types 1 and 2 nephritis or **glomerulonephritis.** See under nephritis, glomerulonephritis.

Ellison, Edwin H., U.S. physician, *1918. See Zollinger-E. *syndrome, tumor.*

Ellsworth, Read McLane, U.S. physician, *1899. See E.-Howard *test.*

Eloesser, Leo, U.S. thoracic surgeon, 1881–1976. See E. *procedure.*

elongation (ē-lon-gā′shŭn). The increase in the gauge length measured after fracture in tension within the gauge length, expressed in percentage of original gauge length.

Elschnig, Anton, German ophthalmologist, 1863–1939. See E.'s *pearls, spots.*

eluant (el′yū-ant). Eluent.

eluate (el′yū-āt) [see elution]. The material washed out of paper or out of a column of adsorbent in chromatography.

eluent (el′yū-ent) [see elution]. Eluant; the liquid used in the process of elution.

elute (ē-lūt′). Elutriate; to perform or accomplish an elution.

elution (ē-lū′shŭn) [L. *e-luo,* pp. *lutus,* to wash out]. Elutriation. **1.** The separation, by washing, of one solid from another. **2.** The removal, by means of a suitable solvent, of one material from another that is insoluble in that solvent, as in column chromatography.

elutriate (ē-lū′trē-āt). Elute.

elutriation (ē-lū-trē-ā′shŭn) [L. *elutrio,* pp. *-atus,* to wash out, decant, fr. *e-luo,* to wash out]. Elution.

elytro- [G. *elytron,* sheath (vagina)]. Obsolete combining form denoting the vagina. See also colpo-, vagino-.

em-. See en-.

emaciation (ē-mā-sē-ā′shŭn) [L. *e-macio,* pp. *-atus,* to make thin]. Wasting (1); becoming abnormally thin from extreme loss of flesh.

emaculation (ē-mak-yū-lā′shŭn) [L. *emaculo,* pp. *-atus,* to clear from spots, fr. *e-,* out, + *macula,* spot]. Removal of spots or other blemishes from the skin.

emanation (em-ă-nā′shŭn) [L. *e- mano,* pp. *-atus,* to flow out]. **1.** Any substance that flows out or is emitted from a source or origin. **2.** The radiation from a radioactive element.
- **actinium e.,** radon-219. See emanon.
- **radium e.,** radon-222. See emanon.
- **thorium e.,** radon-220. See emanon.

emanatorium (em′ă-nă-tōr′ē-ŭm). An institution where, formerly, radiation treatment now considered dangerous (using radioactive waters and the inhalation of radium emanations) was administered.

emancipation (ē-man-si-pā′shŭn). In embryology, delimitation of a specific area in an organ-forming field, giving definite shape and limits to the organ primordium.

emanon (em′ă-non). Radon; archaic term once used to denote all radon isotopes collectively, when the term radon was restricted to the isotope radon-222, the naturally occurring intermediate of the uranium-238 radioactive series; so called because original names for radon-219, radon-220, and radon-222 were, respectively, "actinium emanation," "thorium emanation," and "radium emanation."

emanotherapy (em′ă-nō-thār′ă-pē). Treatment of various diseases by means of radium emanation (radon), or other emanation.

emarginate (ē-mar′ji-nāt) [L. *emargino,* to deprive of its edge, fr. *e-* priv. + *margo* (*margin-*), edge]. Notched; nicked; with broken margin.

emargination (ē-mar′ji-nā′shŭn). Incisura (2).

emasculation (ē-mas-kyū-lā′shŭn) [L. *emasculo,* pp. *-atus,* to castrate, fr. *e-* priv. + *masculus,* masculine]. Eviration (1); castration of the male by removal of the testis and/or penis.

Embadomonas (em-bă-dom′ō-nas, em′bă-dō-mō′nas) [G. *embadon,* surface, + *monas,* unit, monad]. Old name for *Retortamonas.*

embalm (em-bahlm′) [L. *in,* in, + *balsamum,* balsam]. To treat a dead body with balsams or other chemicals to preserve it from decay.

Embden, Gustav G., German biochemist, 1874–1933. See E. *ester,* Robison-E. *ester,* E.-Meyerhof *pathway,* E.-Meyerhof-Parnas *pathway.*

embed (em-bed′). Imbed; to surround a pathological or histological specimen with a firm and sometimes hard medium such as paraffin, wax, celloidin, or a resin, in order to make possible the cutting of thin sections for microscopic examination.

embelin (em′bĕ-lin). 2,5-Dihydroxy-3-undecyl-*p*- benzoquinone; the active principle from the dried fruit of *Embelia ribes* and *E. robusta* (family Myrsinaceae); has been used as a teniacide.

emboitement (awm-bwaht-mawn′) [Fr., encasement]. Preformation *theory.*

embolalia (em-bō-lā′lē-ă). Embololalia.

embole (em′bō-lē) [G. *embolē,* insertion]. Embolia; emboly; formation of the gastrula by invagination.

embolectomy (em-bō-lek′tō-mē) [G. *embolos,* a plug (embolus), + *ektomē,* excision]. Removal of an embolus.

embolemia (em-bō-lē′mē-ă) [G. *embolos,* a plug (embolus), + *haima,* blood]. The presence of septic emboli in the circulating blood, leading to the formation of abscesses and pyemia.

emboli (em′bō-lī). Plural of embolus.

embolia (em-bō′lē-ă). Embole.

embolic (em-bol′ik). Relating to an embolus or to embolism.

emboliform (em-bol′i-fōrm) [G. *embolos,* plug (embolus), + L. *forma,* form]. Shaped like an embolus.

embolism (em′bō-lizm) [G. *embolisma,* a piece or patch; lit. something thrust in]. Obstruction or occlusion of a vessel by an embolus.
- **air e.,** aeremia; gas e.; the presence of bubbles of a gas in the vascular system; occurrence is related to the entry of air into the venous circulation following trauma or surgery.
- **amniotic fluid e.,** obstruction of small blood vessels by epithelial squames in amniotic fluid entering the maternal circulation, causing obstetric shock. See also amniotic fluid *syndrome.*
- **atheroma e.,** cholesterol e.
- **bland e.,** e. by simple nonseptic material.
- **cellular e.,** e. due to a mass of cells transported from disintegrating tissue.

cholesterol e., atheroembolism; atheroma e.; e. of lipid debris from an ulcerated atheromatous deposit, generally from a large artery to small arterial branches; it is usually small and rarely causes infarction.
cotton-fiber e., e. by cotton fibers from sterile gauze used in intravenous medication or transfusion; may form as foreign body granulomas in small pulmonary arteries.
crossed e., paradoxical e.; **(1)** obstruction of a systemic artery by an embolus originating in the venous system which passes through a septal defect or patent foramen ovale to the arterial system; **(2)** obstruction by a minute embolism that passes through the pulmonary capillaries from the venous to the arterial system.
direct e., e. occurring in the direction of the blood current.
fat e., oil e.; the occurrence of fat globules in the circulation following fractures of a long bone, in burns, in parturition, and in association with fatty degeneration of the liver; the emboli most commonly block pulmonary or cerebral vessels when symptoms referable to either or both of these regions appear.
gas e., air e.
hematogenous e., e. occurring in a blood vessel.
infective e., pyemic e.
lymph e., lymphogenous e., e. occurring in a lymphatic vessel.
miliary e., multiple e. (1); e. occurring simultaneously in a number of capillaries.
multiple e., **(1)** miliary e.; **(2)** e. caused by the arrest of a number of small emboli.
obturating e., complete closing of the lumen of a vessel by an embolism.
oil e., fat e.
pantaloon e., saddle e.
paradoxical e., crossed e.
pulmonary e., e. of pulmonary arteries, most frequently by detached fragments of thrombus from a leg or pelvic vein, especially when thrombosis has followed an operation or confinement to bed.
pyemic e., infective e.; plugging of an artery by an embolus detached from a suppurating thrombus.
retinal e., e. of an artery of the retina.
retrograde e., venous e.; e. of a vein by an embolus carried in a direction opposite to that of the normal blood current, after being diverted into a smaller vein.
riding e., straddling e.
saddle e., pantaloon e.; a straddling e. at the bifurcation of the aorta which occludes both common iliac arteries.
straddling e., riding e.; e. occurring at the bifurcation of an artery and blocking more or less completely both branches.
tumor e., e. by neoplastic tissue transported from a tumor site and which may grow as a metastasis.
venous e., retrograde e.

embolization (em'bol-i-zā'shŭn). Therapeutic introduction of various substances into the circulation to occlude vessels, either to arrest or prevent hemorrhaging or to devitalize a structure or organ by occluding its blood supply.

embololalia (em'bō-lō-lā'lē-ă) [G. *embolos,* something thrown in, fr. *emballo,* to throw in, + *lalia,* speaking]. Embolalia; embolophasia; embolophrasia; interjection of meaningless words into a sentence when speaking.

embolomycotic (em'bō-lō-mī-kot'ik) [G. *embolos,* a plug (embolus), + *mykēs,* fungus]. Relating to or caused by an infective embolus.

embolophasia (em'bō-lō-fā'zē-ă) [G. *embolos,* something thrown in, + *phasis,* a saying]. Embololalia.

embolophrasia (em'bō-lō-frā'zē-ă) [G. *embolos,* something thrown in, + *phrasis,* phrase]. Embololalia.

embolus, pl. emboli (em'bō-lŭs, -lī) [G. *embolos,* a plug, wedge or stopper]. **1.** A plug, composed of a detached thrombus or vegetation, mass of bacteria, or other foreign body, occluding a vessel. **2.** *Nucleus* emboliformis.
catheter e., coiled worm-shaped platelet and fibrin aggregates produced during vascular catheterization, originating on the catheter or its guide wire.

emboly (em'bō-lē). Embole.

embouchement (ahm-būsh-mon') [Fr.]. The opening of one blood vessel into another.

embrasure (em-brā'shūr) [Fr. an opening in a wall for cannon]. In dentistry, an opening that widens outwardly or inwardly; specifically, that space adjacent to the interproximal contact area that spreads toward the facial, gingival, lingual, occlusal, or incisal aspect.
buccal e., a space existing on the facial aspect of the interproximal contact area between adjacent posterior teeth.
gingival e., a space existing cervical to the interproximal contact area between adjacent teeth.
incisal e., a space existing on the incisal aspect of the interproximal contact area between adjacent anterior teeth.
labial e., a space existing on the facial aspect of the interproximal contact area between adjacent anterior teeth.
lingual e., a space existing on the lingual aspect of the interproximal contact area between adjacent teeth.
occlusal e., a space existing on the occlusal aspect of the interproximal contact areas between adjacent posterior teeth.

embrocation (em-brō-kā'shŭn) [G. *embrochē,* a fomentation]. Rarely used term for liniment or for the application of a liniment.

embry-. See embryo-.

embryatrics (em-brē-at'riks) [embryo- + G. *iatros,* physician]. Rarely used term for fetology.

embryo-, embry- [G. *embryon,* embryo]. Combining forms relating to the embryo.

embryo (em'brē-ō) [G. *embryon,* fr. *en,* in, + *bryō,* to be full, swell]. **1.** An organism in the early stages of development. **2.** In man, the developing organism from conception until approximately the end of the second month; developmental stages from this time to birth are commonly designated as fetal. **3.** A primordial plant within a seed. See fig. on p. 502.
heterogametic e., a male e. with XY sex chromosomes.
hexacanth e., oncosphere e.; the e. of tapeworms of the subclass Cestoda, such as *Taenia saginata,* characterized by three pairs of hooks used for penetration through the gut of an intermediate host.
homogametic e., a female e. with XX sex chromosomes.
oncosphere e., hexacanth e.
presomite e., an e. prior to the appearance of the first pair of somites, about 20 to 21 days after fertilization in humans.
previllous e., the e. of a placental mammal prior to the formation of chorionic villi.

embryoblast (em'brē-ō-blast) [embryo- + G. *blastos,* germ]. Inner cell *mass;* the cells at the embryonic pole of the blastocyst concerned with formation of the body of the embryo *per se.*

embryocardia (em'brē-ō-kar'dē-ă) [embryo- + G. *kardia,* heart]. Tic-tac rhythm or sounds; pendulum rhythm; a condition in which the cadence of the heart sounds resembles that of the fetus, the first and second sounds becoming alike and evenly spaced; a sign of serious myocardial disease.
jugular e., atrial *flutter.*

embryogenesis (em'brē-ō-jen'ĕ-sis) [embryo- + G. *genesis,* origin]. That phase of prenatal development involved in establishment of the characteristic configuration of the embryonic body; in humans, e. is usually regarded as extending from the end of the second week, when the embryonic disk is formed, to the end of the eighth week, after which the conceptus is usually spoken of as a fetus.

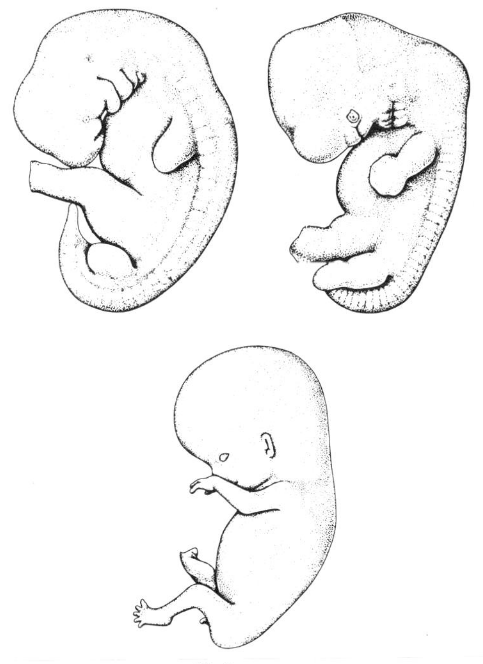

Embryo
Schematic drawing of human embryos at 5, 6, and 8 weeks.

embryogenic, embryogenetic (em-brē-ō-jen'ik, -jĕ-net'ik). Producing an embryo; relating to the formation of an embryo.

embryogeny (em-brē-oj'ĕ-nē). The origin and growth of the embryo.

embryoid (em'brē-oyd). Embryonoid.

embryologist (em-brē-ol'ō-jist). One who specializes in embryology.

embryology (em-brē-ol'ōjē) [embryo- + G. *logos,* study]. Science of the origin and development of the organism from fertilization of the ovum to extrauterine or extraovular life.

embryoma (em-brē-ō'mă). Embryonal *tumor.*
e. of the kidney, Wilms' *tumor.*

embryomorphous (em'brē-ō-mōr'fŭs) [embryo- + G. *morphē,* shape]. **1.** Relating to the formation and structure of the embryo. **2.** Applied to structures or tissues in the body similar to those in the embryo, or embryonal rests.

embryonal (em'brē-ō-năl). Embryonate (1); relating to an embryo.

embryonate (em'brē-ō-nāt). **1.** Embryonal. **2.** Containing an embryo.

embryonic (em-brē-on'ik). Of, pertaining to, or in the condition of an embryo.

embryoniform (em-brē-on'i-fōrm). Embryonoid.

embryonization (em'brē-on-i-zā'shŭn). Reversion of a cell or tissue to an embryonic form.

embryonoid (em'brē-ō-noyd) [embryo- + G. *eidos,* appearance]. Embryoid; embryoniform; resembling an embryo or a fetus.

embryony (em'brē-ō-nē). The condition of being an embryo.

embryopathy (em-brē-op'ă-thē) [embryo- + G. *pathos,* disease]. Fetopathy (1); a morbid condition in the embryo or fetus.

embryophore (em'brē-ō-fōr) [embryo- + G. *phoros,* bearing]. A membrane or wall around the hexacanth embryo of tapeworms, forming the inner portion of the eggshell. In the genus *Taenia,* the e. is exceptionally thick, with radial striations that form a highly protective structure; in the genus *Diphyllobothrium,* the e. is ciliated and enhances the aquatic life cycle of this and other pseudophyllid cestodes. See also coracidium.

embryoplastic (em-brē-ō-plas'tik) [embryo- + G. *plassō,* to form]. **1.** Producing an embryo. **2.** Relating to the formation of an embryo.

embryoscope (em'brē-ō-skōp) [embryo- + G. *skopeō,* to examine]. An instrument for examining the embryos in hens' eggs at different stages of development.

embryotomy (em-brē-ot'ō-mē) [embryo- + G. *tomē,* cutting]. Any mutilating operation on the fetus to make possible its removal when delivery is impossible by natural means.

embryotoxicity (em'brē-ō-tok-sis'i-tē). Injury to the embryo, which may result in death or abnormal development of a part, due to substances that enter the maternal and placental circulation.

embryotoxon (em'brē-ō-tok'son) [embryo- + G. *toxon,* bow]. Congenital opacity of the periphery of the cornea.
anterior e., *arcus* cornealis.
posterior e., a developmental abnormality marked by a prominent white ring of Schwalbe and iris strands that partially obscure the chamber angle.

embryotroph (em'brē-ō-trōf) [embryo- + G. *trophē,* nourishment]. **1.** Histotroph; nutritive material supplied to the embryo during development. **2.** In the implantation stages of deciduate placental mammals, fluid adjacent to the blastodermic vesicle; a mixture of the secretion of the uterine glands, cellular debris resulting from the trophoblastic invasion of the endometrium, and exudated plasma.

embryotrophic (em'brē-ō-trof'ik). Relating to any process or agency involved in the nourishment of the embryo.

embryotrophy (em'brē-ot'rō-fē) [embryo- + G. *trophē,* nourishment]. The nutrition of the embryo.

emedullate (ē-med'yū-lāt) [L. *e-,* from, + *medulla,* marrow]. To extract any marrow or pith.

emeiocytosis (ē'mē-ō-sī-tō'sis) [L. *emitto,* to send forth, + G. *kytos,* cell, + *-osis,* condition]. Exocytosis (2).

emergence (ē-mer'jens). Recovery of normal function following a period of unconsciousness, especially that associated with a general anesthetic.

emergency (ē-mer'jen-sē) [L. *e-mergo,* pp. *-mersus,* to rise up, emerge, fr. *mergo,* to plunge into, dip]. An unexpeced development or happening; a sudden need for action.

emergent (ē-mer'jent). **1.** Arising suddenly and unexpectedly, calling for quick judgment and prompt action. **2.** Coming out; leaving a cavity or other part.

Emerson method. See under method.

emery (em'er-ē). An abrasive containing aluminum oxide and iron.

emesis (em'ĕ-sis) [G. fr. *emeō,* to vomit]. Vomiting. Also used as a combining form in a suffix position.

emetic (ĕ-met'ik) [G. *emetikos,* producing vomiting, fr. *emeō,* to vomit]. Vomitive. **1.** Relating to or causing vomiting. **2.** Vomitory; an agent that causes vomiting.

emetine (em'ĕ-tēn). Cephaeline methyl ether; $C_{29}H_{40}N_2O_4$; the principal alkaloid of ipecac, used as an emetic; its salts are used in amebiasis; available as the hydrochloride.

emetocathartic (em'ĕ-tō-kă-thar'tik). **1.** Both emetic and cathartic. **2.** An agent that causes vomiting and purging of the lower intestines.

EMF Abbreviation for electromotive *force.*

EMG Abbreviation for electromyogram.

-emia [G. *haima,* blood]. Suffix meaning blood.

emiction (ē-mik'shŭn). Rarely used term for urination.

emigration (em-i-grā'shŭn). [L. *e-migro,* pp. *-atus,* to emigrate]. The passage of white blood cells through the endothelium and wall of small blood vessels.

eminence (em'i-nens) [L. *eminentia*]. Eminentia.
arcuate e., *eminentia* arcuata.
articular e., *tuberculum* articulare.
canine e., canine prominence; an elevation on the maxilla corresponding to the socket of the canine tooth.
collateral e., *eminentia* collateralis.
e. of concha, *eminentia* conchae.
cruciate or cruciform e., *eminentia* cruciformis.
deltoid e., *tuberositas* deltoidea.
Doyère's e., the slightly elevated area of the striated muscle fiber's surface that corresponds to the site of the motor *endplate.*
facial e., *colliculus* facialis.
forebrain e., frontonasal *elevation.*
frontal e., *tuber* frontale.
genital e., in very young embryos, the vaguely outlined median elevation immediately cephalic to the proctodeum; its central part develops into the genital tubercle.
hypobranchial e., copula linguae; His' copula; a median elevation in the floor of the embryonic pharynx caudal to the tuberculum impar; it merges laterally with the ventral part of the second and third branchial arches, and in later development is incorporated in the root of the tongue.
hypoglossal e., *trigonum* nervi hypoglossi.
hypothenar e., hypothenar (1).
ileocecal e., *valva* ileocecalis.
iliopectineal e., *eminentia* iliopubica.
iliopubic e., *eminentia* iliopubica.
intercondylar or **intercondyloid e.,** *eminentia* intercondylaris.
maxillary e., *tuber* maxillae.
medial e., *eminentia* medialis.
median e., eminentia mediana; the slightly prominent lower segment of the infundibulum of the hypothalamus, immediately proximal to the hypophysial stalk; the region is characterized by the capillary tufts of the infundibular arteries, from which the hypothalamohypophysial portal system of veins arises.
olivary e., oliva.
orbital e., orbital *tubercle.*
parietal e., *tuber* parietale.
pyramidal e., *eminentia* pyramidalis.
radial e. of wrist, eminentia carpi radialis; a rather large flat e. on the radial side of the palmar aspect of the wrist, due to the tuberosity of scaphoid and the ridge on the trapezium.
restiform e., *eminentia* restiformis.
round e., *eminentia* medialis.
e. of scapha, *eminentia* scaphae.
thenar e., thenar (1).
thyroid e., *prominentia* laryngea.
e. of triangular fossa, *eminentia* fossae triangularis.
ulnar e. of wrist, eminentia carpi ulnaris; an e. smaller than the radial, on the ulnar side of the palmar aspect of the wrist, due to presence of the pisiform bone.

EMINENTIA

eminentia, pl. **eminentiae** (em-i-nen'shē-ă, -shē-ē) [L. prominence, fr. *e-mineo,* to stand out, project] [NA]. Eminence; a circumscribed area raised above the general level of the surrounding surface, particularly on a bone surface.
e. abducen'tis, *colliculus* facialis.
e. arcua'ta [NA], arcuate eminence; a prominence on the anterior surface of the petrous portion of the temporal bone indicating the position of the superior semicircular canal.
e. articula'ris, *tuberculum* articulare.
e. car'pi radia'lis, radial *eminence* of the wrist.
e. car'pi ulna'ris, ulnar *eminence* of the wrist.
e. collatera'lis [NA], collateral eminence; a longitudinal elevation of the floor of the collateral trigone of the lateral ventricle of the brain, between the hippocampus and the calcar avis, caused by the proximity of the floor of the collateral fissure.
e. con'chae [NA], eminence of the concha; apophysis conchae; the prominence on the cranial surface of the auricle corresponding to the concha.
e. crucifor'mis [NA], cruciate or cruciform eminence; a figure on the internal surface of the occipital bone formed by ridges running forward and backward from the protuberance and by the margins of the groove for the transverse sinus on either side; it divides the surface of the bone into four fossae, a cerebral and a cerebellar on each side.
e. facia'lis, *colliculus* facialis.
e. fos'sae triangula'ris [NA], eminence of triangular fossa; e. triangularis; agger perpendicularis; the prominence on the cranial surface of the auricle corresponding to the triangular fossa.
e. fronta'lis [NA], official alternate term for *tuber* frontale.
e. hypoglos'si, *trigonum* nervi hypoglossi.
e. iliopu'bica [NA], iliopubic or iliopectineal eminence; a rounded elevation on the superior surface of the hip bone at the junction of the ilium and the superior ramus of the pubis.
e. intercondyla'ris [NA], e. intercondyloidea; intercondylar or intercondyloid eminence; spinous process of tibia; an elevation on the proximal extremity of the tibia between the two articular surfaces.
e. intercondyloid'ea, e. intercondylaris.
e. maxil'lae [NA], official alternate term for *tuber* maxillae.
e. media'lis [NA], medial or round eminence; e. or funiculus teres; longitudinal elevation of the fossa rhomboidea, extending along either side of the midline throughout the length of the rhombencephalon.
e. media'na, median *eminence.*
e. orbita'lis, orbital *tubercle.*
e. parieta'lis, *tuber* parietale.
e. pyramida'lis [NA], pyramidal eminence; pyramid of tympanum; pyramis tympani; a conical projection posterior to the vestibular window in the middle ear; it is hollow and contains the stapedius muscle.
e. restifor'mis, restiform eminence; a prominence of the dorsolateral surface of the medulla oblongata corresponding to the inferior cerebellar peduncle.
e. sca'phae [NA], eminence of scapha; the prominence on the cranial surface of the auricle corresponding to the scapha.
e. sym'physis, *tuberculum* mentale.
e. te'res, e. medialis.
e. triangula'ris, e. fossae triangularis.

emiocytosis (ē'mē-ō-sī-tō'sis) [L. *emitto,* to send forth, + G. *kytos,* cell, + *-osis,* condition]. Exocytosis (2).

emissarium (em-i-sā'rē-ŭm) [L. an outlet, fr. *e-mitto,* pp. *-missus,* to send out]. *Vena* emissaria.
e. condyloid'eum, *vena* emissaria condylaris.
e. mastoid'eum, *vena* emissaria mastoidea.
e. occipita'le, *vena* emissaria occipitalis.
e. parieta'le, *vena* emissaria parietalis.

emissary (em'i-sār-ē) [see emissarium]. **1.** Relating to, or providing, an outlet or drain. **2.** *Vena* emissaria.

emission (ē-mish'ŭn) [L. *emissio,* fr. *e- mitto,* to send out]. A discharge; referring usually to a seminal discharge occurring during sleep (**nocturnal e.**).

emissivity (ē-mi-siv′i-tē). The giving off of heat rays; a perfect "black body" has an e. of 1, a highly polished metallic surface may have an e. as low as 0.02.

EMIT Abbreviation for enzyme-multiplied *immunoassay.*

emmenagogic (ĕ-men′ă-goj′ik). Relating to or acting as an emmenagogue.

emmenagogue (ĕ-men′ă-gog) [G. *emmēnos,* monthly, fr. *en,* in, + *mēn,* month, + *agōgos,* leading]. Hemagogue (2); an agent that induces or increases menstrual flow.

emmenia (ĕ-men′ē-ă, ĕ-mē′nē-ă) [G. *emmēnos,* monthly]. Menses.

emmenic (ĕ-men′ik). Menstrual.

emmeniopathy (ĕ-men′ē-op′ă-thē) [G. *emmēnos,* monthly, + *pathos,* suffering]. Any disorder of menstruation.

emmenology (em-ĕ-nol′ō-jē) [G. *emmēnos,* monthly, + *logos,* study]. Branch of medicine concerned with the physiology and pathology of menstruation.

Emmens S/L test. See under test.

Emmet, Thomas A., U.S. gynecologist, 1828–1919. See E.'s *needle, operation.*

emmetropia (em-ĕ-trō′pē-ă). [G. *emmetros,* according to measure, + *ōps,* eye]. The state of refraction of the eye in which parallel rays, when the eye is at rest, are focused exactly on the retina.

emmetropic (em-ĕ-trop′ik). Pertaining to or characterized by emmetropia.

emmetropization (em′ĕ-trōp-i-zā′shŭn). The process by which the refraction of the anterior ocular segment and the axial length of the eye tend to balance each other to produce emmetropia.

Emmonsiella capsulata (e-mon-sī-el′ă kap-sū-lā′tă). *Ajellomyces capsulatum.*

emodin (em′ō-din). Archin; frangulic acid; 1,3,8-trihydroxy-6-methylanthraquinone; a crystalline substance (cathartic) found in rhubarb, senna, cascara sagrada, and other purgative drugs.

emollient (ē-mol′ē-ent) [L. *emolliens,* pres. p. of *e- mollio, emollire,* to soften]. Malactic. **1.** Soothing to the skin or mucous membrane. **2.** An agent that softens the skin or soothes irritation in the skin or mucous membrane.

emotion (ē-mō′shŭn) [L. *e-moveo,* pp. *-motus,* to move out, agitate]. A strong feeling, aroused mental state, or intense state of drive or unrest directed toward a definite object and evidenced in both behavior and in psychologic changes, with accompanying autonomic nervous system manifestations.

emotional (ē-mō′shŭn-ăl). Relating to or marked by an emotion.

emotiovascular (ē-mō′shē-ō-vas′kyū-ler). Relating to the vascular changes, such as pallor and blushing, caused by emotions of various kinds.

e.m.p. Abbreviation for L. *ex modo praescripto,* in the manner prescribed.

empasm, empasma (em′pazm, em-paz′mă) [G. *empasma,* fr. *empasso,* to sprinkle on]. A dusting powder.

empathic (em-path′ik). Relating to or marked by empathy.

empathize (em′pă-thīz). To feel empathy in relation to another person; to put oneself in another's place.

empathy (em′pă-thē) [G. *en (em),* in, + *pathos,* feeling]. **1.** The intellectual and occasionally emotional sensing and identification with another person's mental and emotional states. *Cf.* sympathy (3). **2.** The anthropomorphization or humanizing of objects and the feeling of oneself as being in and part of them.

generative e., the inner experience of sharing in and comprehending the momentary psychologic state of another person.

emperipolesis (em-pār′i-pō-lē′sis) [G. *en (em),* inside, + *peri,* around, + *poleomai,* to wander about]. Active penetration of one cell by another, which remains intact; observed in tissue cultures in which polymorphonuclear leukocytes have entered macrophages and subsequently left.

emphlysis (em′fli-sis) [G. *en,* in, + *phlysis,* an eruption, fr. *phlyō,* to boil over]. A vesicular eruption, such as pemphigus.

emphractic (em-frak′tik). Relating to emphraxis.

emphraxis (em-frak′sis) [G. a stoppage]. **1.** A clogging or obstruction of the mouth of the sweat gland. **2.** An impaction.

emphysema (em-fi-sē′mă) [G. inflation of stomach, etc. fr. *en,* in, + *physēma,* a blowing, fr. *physa,* bellows]. **1.** Presence of air in the interstices of the connective tissue of a part. **2.** Pulmonary e.; a condition of the lung characterized by increase beyond the normal in the size of air spaces distal to the terminal bronchiole (those parts containing alveoli), with destructive changes in their walls and reduction in their number. Clinical manifestation is undue breathlessness on exertion, due to the combined effect (in varying degrees) of reduction of alveolar surface for gas exchange, ventilation-perfusion imbalance, and collapse of smaller airways with trapping of alveolar gas occurring predominantly in expiration; this causes the chest to be held in the position of inspiration ("barrel chest"), with prolonged expiration and increased residual volume; symptoms of chronic bronchitis often, but not necessarily, coexist. Two structural varieties are described: panlobular e. and centrilobular e.

centri-acinar e., centrilobular e.

centrilobular e., centri-acinar e.; e. affecting the lobules around their central bronchioles, causally related to bronchiolitis, and seen in coal-miner's pneumoconiosis.

compensating e., compensatory e., increase in the air capacity of a portion of the lung when another portion is consolidated, shrunken, or unable to perform its respiratory function; the alveoli are distended, but there is no destruction of alveolar walls, and hence, no true e., as this term is now defined.

cutaneous e., subcutaneous e.

diffuse e., panlobular e.

familial e., e. inherited in association with severe antitrypsin deficiency.

gangrenous e., gas *gangrene.*

generalized e., panlobular e.

interlobular e., interstitial e. in the connective tissue septa between the pulmonary lobules.

interstitial e., **(1)** presence of air in the pulmonary tissues consequent upon rupture of the air cells; **(2)** presence of air or gas in the connective tissue.

intestinal e., *pneumatosis* cystoides intestinalis.

mediastinal e., deflection of air, usually from a ruptured emphysematous bleb in the lung, into the mediastinal tissue.

panacinar e., panlobular e.

panlobular e., diffuse, generalized, or panacinar e.; e affecting all parts of the lobules, in part, or usually the whole, of the lungs.

paraseptal e., e. involving the periphery of the pulmonary lobules.

pulmonary e., emphysema (2).

senile e., e. consequent upon the physiologic atrophy of old age.

subcutaneous e., aerodermectasia; cutaneous e.; pneumoderma; pneumohypoderma; the presence of air or gas in the subcutaneous tissues.

subgaleal e., extracranial *pneumatocele.*

surgical e., subcutaneous e. from air trapped in the tissues by an operation or injury.

emphysematous (em-fi-sem′ă-tŭs). Relating to or affected with emphysema.

empiric (em-pir′ik) [see empirical]. **1.** Empirical. **2.** A member of a school of Graeco-Roman physicians, late B.C. to early A.D., who placed their confidence in and their practice purely on experience, avoiding all speculation, theory, or abstract reasoning; they were little concerned with causes or with correlating symptoms in order to gain a true understanding of a disease, even holding basic knowledge, physiology, pathology, and anatomy in low esteem and of no value in practice.

empirical (em-pir'i-kăl) [G. *empeirikos;* fr. *empeiria,* experience, fr. *en,* in, + *peira,* a trial]. **1.** Empiric (1); founded on practical experience but not proved scientifically, in contrast to rational (1). **2.** Relating to an empiric (2).

empiricism (em-pir'i-sizm). A looking to experience as a guide to practice or to the therapeutic use of any remedy.

emprosthotonos (em'pros-thot'ō-nŭs) [G. *emprosthen,* forward, + *tonos,* tension]. Tetanus anticus; a tetanic contraction of the flexor muscles, curving the back with concavity forward.

empyema (em-pī-ē'mă, -pi-ē'mă) [G. *empyēma,* suppuration, fr. *en,* in, + *pyon,* pus]. Pus in a body cavity; when used without qualification, refers specifically to pyothorax.

e. artic'uli, obsolete term for suppurative *arthritis.*

e. benig'num, latent e.

latent e., e. benignum; the presence of pus in a cavity, especially one of the accessory sinuses, unattended by subjective symptoms.

loculated e., pyothorax in which pleural adhesions form one or more pockets containing pus.

mastoid e., mastoiditis.

e. necessita'tis, a form of pyothorax in which the pus burrows to the outside, producing a subcutaneous abscess which finally ruptures; it may result in spontaneous recovery without requiring an operation.

e. of the pericardium, pyopericardium.

pulsating e., a large, tense collection of pus in the pleural cavity through which the cardiac pulsations are transmitted to the chest wall.

empyemic (em-pī-ē'mik). Relating to empyema.

empyesis (em-pī-ē'sis) [G. suppuration]. A pustular eruption.

empyocele (em'pī-ō-sēl) [G. *en,* in, + *pyon,* pus, + *kēlē,* tumor]. A suppurating hydrocele; a collection of pus in the scrotum.

empyreuma (em-pī-rū'mă) [G. a banked fire]. Characteristic odor given off by organic substances when charred or subjected to destructive distillation in closed vessels.

emu Abbreviation for electromagnetic *unit.*

emulgent (ē-mŭl'jent) [L. *e- mulgeo,* pp. *-mulsus,* to milk out, drain out]. Denoting a straining, extracting, or purifying process.

emulsifier (ē-mŭl'si-fī-er). An agent, such as gum arabic or the yolk of an egg, used to make an emulsion of a fixed oil.

emulsify (ē-mŭl'si-fī). To make in the form of an emulsion.

emulsin (ē-mŭl'sin). **1.** A preparation, derived from almonds, that contains β-glucosidase. **2.** Sometimes used as a synonym for β-glucosidase; "emulsin" was one of the earliest enzymes to be studied (*ca.* 1830).

emulsion (ē-mŭl'shŭn) [Mod. L. fr. *e-mulgeo,* pp. *-mulsus,* to milk or drain out]. A system containing two immiscible liquids in which one is dispersed, in the form of very small globules (internal phase), throughout the other (external phase).

emulsive (ē-mŭl'siv). **1.** Denoting a substance that can be made into an emulsion. **2.** Denoting a substance, such as a mucilage, by which a fat or resin can be emulsified. **3.** Making soft or pliant. **4.** Yielding a fixed oil on pressure.

emulsoid (ē-mŭl'soyd). Emulsion, hydrophil, hydrophilic, or lyophilic colloid; a colloidal dispersion in which the dispersed particles are more or less liquid and exert a certain attraction on and absorb a certain quantity of the fluid in which they are suspended.

emuresis (em-yū-rē'sis) [G. *en (em),* in, + *ourēsis,* urination]. A condition in which urinary excretion and intake of water act to produce an absolute hydration of the body. See also ecuresis.

emylcamate (ē-mil'kă-māt, em-il-kam'āt). 1-Ethyl-1-methylpropyl carbamate; a mild sedative, used to control tension and anxiety and to relieve pain and muscular spasm.

en-. Prefix fr. G. preposition meaning in; appears as em- before b, p, or m.

enalapril maleate (e-nal'ă-pril). L-Proline, 1-[*N*- [1-(ethoxycarbonyl)-3-phenylpropyl]-L-alanyl]-, (*S*)-, (*Z*)-2-butenedioate (1:1); an angiotensin converting enzyme inhibitor used as an anti-hypertensive agent.

enamel (ē-nam'ĕl). Enamelum.

dwarfed e., nanoid e.

mottled e., alterations in e. structure due to excessive fluoride ingestion during tooth formation; varies in appearance from small white opacities to yellow and black spotting.

nanoid e., dwarfed e.; a condition of abnormal thinness of the e.

whorled e., e. in which the rods assume a spiral or twisting course.

enamelogenesis (ē-nam'ĕl-ō-jen'ĕ-sis). Amelogenesis.

e. imperfec'ta, *amelogenesis* imperfecta.

enameloma (ē-nam-ĕl-ō'mă). Enamel pearl; a developmental anomaly in which there is a small nodule of enamel below the cemento-enamel junction, usually at the bifurcation of molar teeth.

enamelum (ē-nam'ĕ-lŭm) [NA]. Enamel; substantia adamantina or vitrea; the hard glistening substance covering the exposed portion of the tooth. In its mature form, it is composed of an inorganic portion made up of hydroxyapatite with small amounts of carbonate, magnesium, fluoride, and an organic matrix of protein and glycoprotein; structurally, it is made up of oriented rods each of which consists of a stack of rodlets encased in an organic prism sheath.

enanthal (ē-nan'thăl). Heptanal.

enanthate (e-nan'thāt). USAN-approved contraction for heptanoate, $CH_3(CH_2)_5COO^-$.

enanthem, enanthema (en-an'them, en-an-thē'mă) [G. *en,* in, + *anthēma,* bloom, eruption, fr. *antheō,* to bloom]. A mucous membrane eruption, especially one occurring in connection with one of the exanthemas.

enanthematous (en-an-them'ă-tŭs). Relating to an enanthem.

enanthesis (en-an-thē'sis) [G. *en,* in, + *anthēsis,* full bloom]. The skin eruption of a general disease, such as scarlatina or typhoid fever.

enantio- [G. *enantios,* opposite] Combining form meaning opposite, opposed, or opposing.

enantiomer (ē-nan'tē-ō-mer) [enantio- + G. *meros,* part]. Antimer; optical antipode; one of a pair of molecules that are mirror images of each other.

enantiomeric (ē-nan'tē-ō-mer'ik). Pertaining to enantiomerism.

enantiomerism (ē-nan-tē-om'er-izm). In chemistry, isomerism in which the molecules in their configuration are related to one another like an object and its mirror image (enantiomers), and consequently are not superimposable; e. entails optical activity, both enantiomers rotating the plane of plane polarized light equally, but in opposite directions.

enantiomorph (ē-nan'tē-ō-mōrf). An enantiomer in crystal form.

enantiomorphic (ē-nan'tē-ō-mōr'fik) [enantio- + G. *morphē,* form]. Enantiomorphous. **1.** Relating to two objects, each of which is the mirror image of the other. **2.** In chemistry, relating to isomers, the optical activities of which are equal in magnitude but opposite in sign.

enantiomorphism (ē-nan'tē-ō-mōr'fizm) [enantio- + G. *morphē,* form]. The relation of two objects similar in form but not superposable, as the two hands or an object and its mirror image.

enantiomorphous (ē-nan'tē-ō-mōr'fŭs). Enantiomorphic.

enarthrodial (en-ar-thrō'dē-al). Relating to an enarthrosis.

enarthrosis (en-ar-thrō'sis) [G. *en-arthrōsis,* a jointing where the ball is deep set in the socket]. *Articulatio* spheroidea.

encainide hydrochloride (en-kā'nīd). Benzamide, 4-methoxy-*N*-[2-[2-(1-methyl-2-piperidinyl)ethyl]phenyl]-, monohydrochloride, (±)-; an anti-arrhythmic.

encanthis (en-kan'this) [G. *en,* in, + *kanthos,* canthus]. Obsolete term for a minute tumor or excrescence at the inner angle of the eye.

encapsulated (en-kap'sū-lā-ted). Encapsulated; enclosed in a capsule or sheath.

encapsulation (en-kap-sū-lā'shŭn) [L. *in* + capsula, dim. of *capsa,* box]. Enclosure in a capsule or sheath.

encapsuled (en-kap'sūld). Encapsulated.

encarditis (en-kar-dī'tis). Endocarditis.

encatarrhaphy (en-kă-tar'ră-fē) [G. *enkatarrhaptō,* to sew in]. Rarely used term for the artificial implantation of an organ or tissue in a part where it does not naturally occur.

encelitis, enceliitis (en-sē-lī'tis, -lē-ī'tis) [G. *en,* in, + *koilia,* belly, + *-itis,* inflammation]. Inflammation of any of the abdominal viscera.

encephal-. See encephalo-.

encephalalgia (en-sef-ă-lal'jē-ă) [encephalo- + G. *algos,* pain]. Headache.

encephalatrophic (en-sef-ă-lă-trof'ik). Relating to encephalatrophy.

encephalatrophy (en-sef-ă-lat'rō-fē) [encephalo- + G. *a-* priv. + *trophē,* nourishment]. Atrophy of the brain.

encephalauxe (en-sef-ă-lawk'sē) [encephalo- + G. *auxē,* increase]. Hypertrophy of the brain.

encéphale isolé (ahn-sef-al' ē-sō-lā') [Fr. isolated brain]. An animal with its caudal medulla transected and its respiration maintained artificially; it remains alert, has sleep-wake cycles, normal pupillary reactions, and a normal electroencephalogram. *Cf.* cerveau isolé.

encephalemia (en-sef-ă-lē'mē-ă) [encephalo- + G. *haima,* blood]. Brain *congestion.*

encephalic (en'se-fal'ik). Relating to the brain, or to the structures within the cranium.

encephalitic (en-sef-ă-lit'ik). Relating to encephalitis.

encephalitides (en-sef-ă-lit'ĭ-dēz). Plural of encephalitis.

encephalitis, pl. **encephalitides** (en-sef-ă-lī'tis, en-sef-ă-lit'i-dēz) [G. *enkephalos,* brain,+ *-itis,* inflammation]. Cephalitis; inflammation of the brain.

acute hemorrhagic e., e. hemorrhagica.

acute necrotizing e., an acute form of e., usually caused by herpes simplex virus and affecting largely the temporal lobes and limbic system.

Australian X e., Murray Valley e.

bunyavirus e., California e.; e. of abrupt onset, with severe frontal headache and low-grade to moderate fever, caused by members of the genus *Bunyavirus* (Bunyamwera supergroup); infections also occur in rodents, lagomorphs, and domestic animals.

California e., bunyavirus e.

Coxsackie e., an inflammation of the brain, seen mainly in infants and involving principally the gray matter of the medulla and cord, caused by *Enterovirus* Coxsackie B.

Dawson's e., inclusion body e.

epidemic e., von Economo's *disease.*

equine e., equine *encephalomyelitis.*

experimental allergic e. (EAE), experimental allergic *encephalomyelitis.*

Far East Russian e., tick-borne e. (Eastern subtype).

fox e., e. in foxes, caused by the infectious canine hepatitis virus and characterized by paralysis and death.

e. hemorrhag'ica, acute hemorrhagic e.; e. of apoplectoid character due to blood extravasation.

herpes e., e. caused by the herpes simplex virus.

hyperergic e., e. as a result of an immunologic allergic reaction of the nervous system to antigenic stimuli.

Ilhéus e., an e. caused by the Ilhéus virus (genus *Flavivirus*) and endemic to eastern Brazil and other parts of South and Central America.

inclusion body e., Dawson's or subacute inclusion body e.; subacute sclerosing leukoencephalitis or panencephalitis; a usually fatal disease that seems to result from persistent measles virus infection and causes varying types of inflammatory reaction in both the white and gray matter; it is characterized by the presence of Cowdry type A nuclear inclusion bodies; the clinical course progresses from personality change to mental deterioration and progressive paralysis.

Japanese B e., e. japonica; Russian autumn e.; an epidemic e. or encephalomyelitis of Japan, Siberian Russia, and other parts of Asia; due to the Japanese B e. virus (genus *Flavivirus).*

e. japon'ica, Japanese B e.

lead e., lead *encephalopathy.*

e. lethar'gica, von Economo's *disease.*

Mengo e., an e. occurring in Africa, due to the Mengo strain of encephalomyocarditis virus (an enterovirus).

Murray Valley e., Australian X disease or e.; a severe e. with a high mortality rate occurring in the Murray Valley of Australia; the disease is most severe in children and is characterized by headache, fever, malaise, drowsiness or convulsions, and rigidity of the neck; extensive brain damage may result; it is caused by the Murray Valley encephalitis virus (genus *Flavivirus).*

necrotizing e., an e. with extensive necrosis in the cerebral cortex, and with lesser damage in the basal ganglia and brainstem.

e. neonato'rum, e. of the newborn, described by R. Virchow as marked by the presence of fat-laden cells in the brain.

opossum e., e. of opossum caused by *Chlamydia psittaci.*

e. periaxia'lis concen'trica, Baló's disease; e. that is clinically similar to adrenoleukodystrophy (e. periaxialis diffusa), but pathologically characterized by concentric globes or circles of demyelination of cerebral white matter separated by normal tissue.

e. periaxia'lis diffu'sa, adrenoleukodystrophy.

postvaccinal e., demyelinating e. following vaccination.

Powassan e., an acute disease of children varying clinically from undifferentiated febrile illness to e.; caused by the Powassan virus and transmitted by ixodid ticks.

purulent e., e. pyogenica.

e. pyogen'ica, suppurative or purulent e.; a form marked by the occurrence of numerous miliary abscesses (disseminated cerebral microabscesses) and minute blood extravasations in the brain substance.

Russian autumn e., Japanese B e.

Russian spring-summer e. (Eastern subtype), tick-borne e. (Eastern subtype).

Russian spring-summer e. (Western subtype), tick-borne e. (Central European subtype).

Russian tick-borne e., tick-borne e. (Eastern subtype).

secondary e., e., usually demyelinating, following vaccination for smallpox or during convalescence from measles, mumps, varicella, and certain other infectious diseases.

subacute inclusion body e., inclusion body e.

e. subcortical'is chron'ica, Binswanger's *disease.*

suppurative e., e. pyogenica.

tick-borne e. (Central European subtype), biundulant meningoencephalitis; Central European tick-borne fever; diphasic milk fever; Russian spring-summer e. (Western subtype); tick-borne meningoencephalitis caused by a flavivirus closely related to the virus causing the Far Eastern type; it is transmitted by *Ixodes ricinus,* also by infected raw milk, especially that of goats.

tick-borne e. (Eastern subtype), a severe form of e. caused by a flavivirus and transmitted by ticks (*Ixodes pertulcatus* and *I. ricinus*). Also called Far East Russian e.; Russian spring-summer e. (Eastern subtype); Russian tick-borne e.; vernal e.; woodcutter's e.

varicella e., e. occurring as a complication of chickenpox.

vernal e., tick-borne e. (Eastern subtype).

woodcutter's e., tick-borne e. (Eastern subtype).

encephalitogen (en-sef'ă-lĭ'tō-jen) [encephalitis + G. *-gen,* producing]. An agent which evokes encephalitis, particularly with reference to the antigen which produces experimental allergic encephalomyelitis.

encephalitogenic (en-sef'ă-li-tō-jen'ik). Producing encephalitis; typically by hypersensitivity mechanisms. See encephalitogen.

Encephalitozoon (en-sef'ă-li-tō-zō'on) [encephalitis + G. *zōon,* animal]. A genus of protozoan parasites, formerly considered part of the family Toxoplasmatidae, class Sporozoea, but now recognized as a member of the protozoan phylum Microspora, family Nosematidae. *E. cuniculi* is considered the primary microsporan parasite of mammals, commonly found in the brain and kidney tubules of rodents and carnivores.

encephalization (en-sef'ă-li-zā'shŭn). Corticalization.

encephalo-, encephal- [G. *enkephalos,* brain]. Combining forms indicating the brain or some relationship thereto.

encephalocele (en-sef'ă-lō-sēl) [encephalo- + G. *kēlē,* hernia]. Cephalocele; craniocele; cranium bifidum; bifid cranium; a congenital gap in the skull with herniation of brain substance.

encephalodynia (en-sef'ă-lō-din'ē-ă) [encephalo- + G. *odynē,* pain]. Headache.

encephalodysplasia (en-sef'ă-lō-dis-plā'zē-ă) [encephalo- + G. *dys,* bad, + *plastos,* formed]. Any congenital abnormality of the brain.

encephalogram (en-sef'ă-lō-gram) [encephalo- + G. *gramma,* a drawing]. The record obtained by encephalography.

encephalography (en-sef-ă-log'ră-fē) [encephalo- + G. *graphō,* to write]. Graphic representation of the brain, usually by roentgenograms.

gamma e., visualization of the encephalon by the administration of small amounts of gamma-emitting radionuclides; commonly called a brain scan.

encephaloid (en-sef'ă-loyd) [encephalo- + G. *eidos,* resemblance]. Resembling brain substance; denoting a carcinoma of soft, brain-like consistency, with reference to gross features.

encephalolith (en-sef'ă-lō-lith) [encephalo- + G. *lithos,* stone]. Cerebral calculus; a concretion in the brain or one of its ventricles.

encephalology (en-sef-ă-lol'ō-jē) [encephalo- + G. *logos,* study]. The branch of medicine dealing with the brain in all its relations.

encephaloma (en-sef-ă-lō'mă). Cerebroma; herniation of brain substance.

encephalomalacia (en-sef'ă-lō-mă-lā'shē-ă) [encephalo- + G. *malakia,* softness]. Cerebromalacia; infarction of brain tissue, usually caused by vascular insufficiency.

nutritional e. of chicks, crazy chick disease; a d. of young chicks caused by vitamin E deficiency.

encephalomeningitis (en-sef'ă-lō-men-in-jī'tis) [encephalo- + G. *mēninx,* membrane, + *-itis,* inflammation]. Meningoencephalitis.

encephalomeningocele (en-sef'ă-lō-me-nin'gō-sēl) [encephalo- + G. *mēninx,* membrane, + *kēlē,* hernia]. Meningoencephalocele.

encephalomeningopathy (en-sef'ă-lō-men-in-gop'ă-thē). Meningoencephalopathy.

encephalomere (en-sef'ă-lō-mēr) [encephalo- + G. *meros,* a part]. A neuromere.

encephalometer (en-sef-ă-lom'ĕ-ter) [encephalo- + G. *metron,* measure]. An apparatus for indicating on the skull the location of the cortical centers.

encephalomyelitis (en-sef-ă-lō-mī'ĕ-lī'tis) [encephalo- + G. *myelon,* marrow, + *-itis,* inflammation]. Acute inflammation of the brain and spinal cord.

acute disseminated e., a diffuse inflammation of the brain and spinal cord usually caused by a perivascular hypersensitivity response.

avian infectious e., epidemic tremor; a disease of very young chicks caused by a picornavirus and characterized by tremor, ataxia, somnolence, and finally death.

benign myalgic e., epidemic *neuromyasthenia.*

bovine sporadic e., Buss disease; an acute, septic e., pleuritis, and peritonitis of cattle caused by *Chlamydia psittaci;* it occurs in the north central United States.

eastern equine e. (EEE), a form of equine e. seen in the eastern U.S. and caused by the eastern equine e. virus, a species of *Alphavirus;* initial fever and viremia are followed by signs of central nervous system involvement (excitement, then somnolence, paralysis, and death); the incidence of clinical infection in man is low but case fatality may be high.

enzootic e., Borna *disease.*

epidemic myalgic e., epidemic *neuromyasthenia.*

equine e., equine encephalitis; an acute, often fatal, virus disease of horses and mules characterized by central nervous system disturbances; in the U.S., this disease in typically caused by one of two arthropod-borne viruses, and their resulting diseases are designated western equine or eastern equine e.; these viruses also may cause neurologic disease in man.

experimental allergic e., experimental allergic encephalitis; a demyelinating allergic e. produced by the injection of brain tissue, usually with an adjuvant.

granulomatous e., a disease causing necrosis and granulomas in the substance of the brain.

infectious porcine e., Teschen *disease.*

mouse e., Theiler's disease (1); mouse poliomyelitis; e. due to the mouse encephalomyelitis virus (a species of *Enterovirus*) which is not pathogenic in monkeys or in man, but attacks mouse colonies and causes a flaccid paralysis, usually of the hind limbs.

Venezuelan equine e. (VEE), a form of equine e. found in parts of South America, Panama, and Trinidad, caused by the Venezuelan equine e. virus (a species of *Alphavirus*), and characterized by less central nervous system involvement than occurs in either eastern or western equine e.; fever, diarrhea, and depression are common; in man, there is fever and severe headache after an incubation period of 2 to 5 days, and in a few cases there has been central nervous system involvement.

virus e., an acute e. due to a neurotropic virus.

western equine e. (WEE), an equine e. found in the western U.S. and parts of South America, caused by the western equine e. virus (a species of *Alphavirus*); the infection is similar to but milder than eastern equine e. in man is, as a rule, inapparent, but some cases with central nervous system involvement have been fatal.

zoster e., inflammation of the brain and spinal cord caused by varicella-zoster virus.

encephalomyelocele (en-sef'ă-lō-mī'ĕ-lō-sēl) [G. *enkephalos,* brain, + *myelon,* marrow, + *kēlē,* hernia]. Congenital defect in the occipital region with herniation of the meninges, medulla, and spinal cord.

encephalomyeloneuropathy (en-sef'ă-lō-mī'ĕ-lō-nū-rop'ă-thē). A disease involving the brain, spinal cord, and peripheral nerves.

nonspecific e., a syndrome of abdominal complaints followed by the subacute onset of neurological manifestations due to the ingestion of clioquinol.

encephalomyelopathy (en-sef′ă-lō-mī-ĕ-lop′ă-thē) [G. *enkephalos*, brain, + *myelon*, marrow, + *pathos*, suffering]. Any disease of both brain and spinal cord.

carcinomatous e., paracarcinomatous e.; degeneration of spinal cord tracts, brainstem, and cerebellar parenchyma associated with a carcinoma.

epidemic myalgic e., a disease superficially resembling poliomyelitis, characterized by diffuse involvement of the nervous system associated with myalgia.

necrotizing e., Leigh's disease; subacute e. affecting infants, causing dementia, spasticity, and optic atrophy; autosomal recessive inheritance.

paracarcinomatous e., carcinomatous e.

encephalomyeloradiculitis (en-sef′ă-lō-mī′ĕ-lō-ră-dik′yū-lī-tis). Inflammation involving the brain, spinal cord, and peripheral nerves. See also Guillain-Barré *syndrome*.

encephalomyeloradiculopathy (en-sef′ă-lō-mī′ĕ-lō-ră-dik′yū-lop-ă-thē). A disease process involving the brain, spinal cord, and spinal roots.

encephalomyocarditis (en-sef′ă-lō-mī′ō-kar-dī′tis). Associated encephalitis and myocarditis.

encephalon, pl. encephala (en-sef′ă-lon, lă) [G. *enkephalos*, brain, fr. *en*, in, + *kephalē*, head] [NA]. Brain; that portion of the cerebrospinal axis contained within the cranium, comprised of the prosencephalon, mesencephalon, and rhombencephalon.

encephalonarcosis (en-sef′ă-lō-nar-kō′sis) [encephalo- + G. *narkē*, stupor]. Stupor or coma from brain disease.

encephalopathia (en-sef′ă-lō-path′ē-ă). Encephalopathy.

e. addiso′nia, apathy, somnolence, or rarely psychic irritative symptoms, occurring in the course of Addison's disease, probably related to electrolyte imbalance.

encephalopathy (en-sef′ă-lop′ă-thē) [encephalo- + G. *pathos*, suffering]. Cephalopathy; cerebropathia; cerebropathy; encephalopathia; any disease of the brain.

bilirubin e., e. due to the toxic effects of bilirubin. See also *icterus* neonatorum; kernicterus.

Binswanger's e., Binswanger's *disease*.

demyelinating e., progressive subcortical e.; extensive idiopathic loss of myelin sheaths in the brain, as occurs in encephalitis periaxialis concentrica, adrenoleukodystrophy, and types of leukodystrophy.

familial e., a progressive form of e. occurring in young members of the same family; characterized by headache, vertigo, ataxia, drowsiness and stupor, and sometimes convulsions.

hepatic e., portal-systemic e.

hypernatremic e., subarachnoid and subdural effusions in infants with hypernatremic dehydration.

hypertensive e., cerebral symptoms such as headache, somnolence, convulsions, and vomiting, occurring in advanced stages of arterial hypertension.

lead e., lead encephalitis; saturnine e.; a rapidly developing e., caused by the ingestion of lead compounds and seen particularly in early childhood; it is characterized pathologically by extensive cerebral edema, status spongiosus, neurocytolysis, and some reactive inflammation; clinical manifestations are convulsions, delirium, hallucinations, and other cerebral symptoms due to chronic lead poisoning. See also lead *poisoning*.

metabolic e., e. characterized by memory loss, vertigo, and generalized weakness, resulting from a jejunal bypass for obesity.

palindromic e., recurrent e.; a relatively mild form which tends to recur.

pancreatic e., an e. associated with extensive pancreatic necrosis; the cerebral lesions consist of capillary necrosis, perivascular bleeding, and focal gliosis.

portal-systemic e., hepatic e.; an e. associated with cirrhosis of the liver, attributed to the passage of toxic nitrogenous substances from the portal to the systemic circulation; cerebral manifestations may include coma.

progressive subcortical e., demyelinating e.

recurrent e., palindromic e.

saturnine e., lead e.

spongiform e., e. characterized by progressive diffuse vacuolation.

subacute spongiform e., transmissible e.; a form of spongiform e. that is associated with a slow virus, is transmissible, and has a rapidly progressive, fatal course; *e.g*, Creutzfeldt-Jakob disease, kuru, Gerstmann-Sträussler syndrome, scrapie.

subcortical arteriosclerotic e., Binswanger's *disease*.

thyrotoxic e., a rare condition arising in severe cases of thyrotoxicosis, marked by bulbar symptoms (disturbances in deglutition, mastication, and speech) and loss of consciousness merging into deep coma.

transmissible e. of mink, a slow virus disease of mink very similar to scrapie of sheep.

traumatic e., disturbance of structure of cerebral nerve cells, glia, or intracranial vessels resulting from injury.

traumatic progressive e., chronic brain damage resulting from multiple brain injuries.

Wernicke's e., Wernicke's *syndrome*.

Wernicke-Korsakoff e., see Wernicke's *syndrome;* Korsakoff's *syndrome*.

encephalopsy (en-sef′ă-lop-sē) [encephalo- + G. *opsis*, sight]. The association of special colors with words or other sensory data.

encephalopyosis (en-sef′ă-lō-pī-ō′sis) [encephalo- + G. *pyōsis*, suppuration]. Purulent inflammation of the brain.

encephalorrhachidian (en-sef′ă-lō-ră-kid′ē-an) [encephalo- + G. *rhachis*, spine]. Cerebrospinal.

encephalorrhagia (en-sef′ă-lō-rā′jē-ă) [encephalo- + G. *rhēgnymi*, to burst forth]. Cerebral *hemorrhage*.

encephaloschisis (en-sef-ă-los′ki-sis) [encephalo- + G. *schisis*, fissure]. Developmental failure of closure of the rostral part of the neural tube.

encephalosclerosis (en-sef′ă-lō-sklĕr-o′sis) [encephalo- + G. *sklērōsis*, hardening]. A sclerosis, or hardening, of the brain. See also cerebrosclerosis.

encephaloscope (en-sef′ă-lō-skōp) [encephalo- + G. *skopeō*, to view]. Any instrument used to view the interior of a brain abscess or other cerebral cavity through an opening in the skull.

encephaloscopy (en-sef-ă-los′kō-pē). Cerebroscopy; examination of the brain or the cavity of a cerebral abscess by direct inspection.

encephalosis (en-sef-ă-lō′sis). Cerebrosis; any organic disease of the brain.

encephalospinal (en-sef′ă-lō-spī′năl). Cerebrospinal.

encephalothlipsis (en-sef′ă-lō-thlip′sis) [encephalo- + G. *thlipsis*, pressure]. Compression of the brain.

encephalotome (en-sef′ă-lō-tōm). An instrument for use in performing encephalotomy.

encephalotomy (en-sef-ă-lot′ō-mē) [encephalo- + G. *tomē*, incision]. Dissection or incision of the brain.

enchondral (en-kon′drăl). Intracartilaginous.

enchondroma (en-kon-drō′mă) [Mod. L. fr. G. *en*, in, + *chondros*, cartilage, + *-oma*, tumor]. A benign cartilaginous growth starting within the medullary cavity of a bone originally formed from cartilage; e.'s may distend the cortex, especially of small bones, and may be solitary or multiple (endochondromatosis).

enchondromatosis (en-kon′drō-ma-tō′sis). Asymmetrical chondrodystrophy; dyschondroplasia; Ollier's disease; a rarely familial, and probably nonmendelian hamartomatous proliferation of cartilage in the metaphyses of several bones, most commonly of the hands and feet, causing distorted growth in length or pathological fractures; chondrosarcoma frequently develops.

enchondromatous (en-kon-drō'mă-tŭs). Relating to or having the elements of enchondroma.

enchondrosarcoma (en-kon'drō-sar-kō'mă). A malignant neoplasm of cartilage cells derived from an enchondroma, as may occur in enchondromatosis.

enclave (en-klāv, ahn-klahv') [Fr. fr. L. *clavis,* key]. An enclosure; a detached mass of tissue enclosed in tissue of another kind; seen especially in the case of isolated masses of gland tissue detached from the main gland.

encoding (en-kōd'ing). The first stage in the memory process, followed by storage and retrieval, involving processes associated with receiving or briefly registering stimuli through one or more of the senses and modifying that information; a decay process or loss of this information (a type of forgetting) occurs rapidly unless the next two stages, storage and retrieval, are activated.

encopresis (en-kō-prē'sis) [G. *enkopros,* full of manure]. Involuntary passage of feces.

encranial (en-krā'nē-ăl). Endocranial.

encranius (en-krā'nē-ŭs) [G. *en,* in, + *kranion,* skull]. In conjoined twins, a form of fetal inclusion in which the smaller parasite lies partly or wholly within the cranial cavity of the larger autosite.

encu Acronym for *e*quivalent *n*ormal *c*hild *u*nit, that amount of information that will have the conditional probability that a consultand is a carrier for an autosomal dominant trait; *e.,g.,* each normal child contributes one encu.

encysted (en-sis'ted) [G. *kystis,* bladder]. Encapsulated by a membranous bag.

encystment (en-sist'ment). The condition of being or becoming encysted.

end. An extremity, or the most remote point of an extremity.
distal e., heel (2); the posterior extremity of a dental appliance.

end-. See endo-.

Endamoeba (end'ă-mē'bă) [endo- + G. *amoibē,* change]. A genus of amebae parasitic in invertebrates; originally described from cockroaches.

endangiitis, endangeitis (end-an-jē-ī'tis) [endo- + G. *angeion,* vessel, + *-itis,* inflammation]. Endoangiitis; endovasculitis; inflammation of the intima of a blood vessel.
e. oblit'erans, inflammation of the intima of a vessel with resulting occlusion of its lumen.

endaortitis (end'ā-ōr-tī'tis). Endo-aortitis; inflammation of the intima of the aorta.

endarterectomy (end-ar-ter-ek'tō-mē) [endo- + artery + G. *ektomē,* excision]. Excision of diseased endothelial lining of an artery and also of occluding atheromatous deposits, so as to leave a smooth lining.
carotid e., excision of occluding material, including intima, from the carotid a.
coronary e., excision of occluding material, including intima, from the coronary artery.

endarteritis (end'ar-ter-ī'tis). Endoarteritis; inflammation of the intima of an artery.
bacterial e., implantation and growth of bacteria with formation of vegetations on the arterial wall, such as may occur in a patent ductus arteriosus or arteriovenous fistula.
e. defor'mans, e. with atheromatous patches and calcareous deposits.
e. oblit'erans, obliterating e., arteritis obliterans; obliterating arteritis; an extreme degree of e. proliferans closing the lumen of the artery.
e. prolif'erans, proliferating e., chronic e. accompanied by a marked increase of fibrous tissue in the intima.

endaural (end-aw'răl) [endo- + L. *auris,* ear]. Within the ear.

end'brain. Telencephalon.

end-brush (end'brŭsh). Telodendron.

end-bulb. See under bulb.

end-diastolic (end'dī-ă-stol'ik). **1.** Occurring at the end of diastole, immediately before the next systole, as in end-diastolic pressure. **2.** Interrupting the final moments of diastole, barely premature, as in end-diastolic extrasystole.

endemia (en-dē'mē-ă). Rarely used term for an endemic disease.

endemic (en-dem'ik) [G. *endēmos,* native, fr. *en,* in, + *dēmos,* the people]. **1.** Present in a community or among a group of people; said of a disease prevailing continually in a region. *Cf.* epidemic **2.** Enzootic.

endemoepidemic (en-dem'ō-ep-i-dem'ik). Denoting a temporary large increase in the number of cases of an endemic disease.

endergonic (en-der-gon'ik) [endo- + G. *ergon,* work]. Referring to a chemical reaction that takes place with absorption of energy from its surroundings. *Cf.* exergonic.

endermic, endermatic (en-der'mik, en-der-mat'ik) [G. *en,* in, + *derma (dermat-),* skin]. In or through the skin; denoting a method of treatment, as by inunction; the remedy produces its constitutional effect when absorbed through the skin surface to which it is applied.

endermism (en-der'mizm). Treatment with endermic medication.

endermosis (en-der-mō'sis). Any eruptive disease of the mucous membrane.

end-feet. Axon *terminals.*

end'gut. Hindgut.

end'ing. 1. A termination or conclusion. **2.** A nerve e.
annulospiral e., annulospiral organ; one of two types of sensory nerve e. associated with a neuromuscular spindle (the other being the flower-spray e.); after entering the muscle spindle, the fiber divides into two flat ribbon-like branches that wind themselves in rings or spirals about the intrafusal muscle fibers.
calyciform e., caliciform e., a synaptic e. in relation to certain neuroepithelial hair cells of the inner ear.
epilemmal e., a nerve e. in close relation to the outer surface of the sarcolemma.
flower-spray e., flower-spray organ of Ruffini; one of the two types of sensory nerve e. associated with the neuromuscular spindle (the other being the annulospiral e.); in this type, the fiber branches spread out upon the surface of the intrafusal fibers like a spray of flowers.
free nerve e.'s, *terminationes* nervorum liberae.
grape e.'s, an autodescriptive term applied to synaptic terminals at the ends of short, stalklike axon branches.
hederiform e., a type of free sensory ending in the skin.
nerve e., any one of the specialized terminations of peripheral sensory or motor nerve fibers. See motor *endplate,* and various listings under corpuscle and bulb.
sole-plate e., motor *endplate.*
synaptic e.'s, axon *terminals.*

Endo, Shigeru, Japanese bacteriologist, 1869–1937. See E.'s *agar, medium.*

endo-, end- [G. *endon,* within]. Prefixes indicating within, inner, absorbing, containing. See also ento-.

endoabdominal (en'dō-ab-dom'i-năl). Within the abdomen.

endoaneurysmoplasty (en'dō-an-yū-riz'mō-plas-tē). Aneurysmoplasty.

endoaneurysmorrhaphy (en'dō-an-yū-riz-mōr'ă-fē) [endo- + G. *aneurysma,* aneurysm, + *raphe,* suture]. Aneurysmoplasty.

endoangiitis (en'dō-an-jē-ī'tis). Endangiitis.

endo-aortitis (en'dō-ā-ōr-tī'tis). Endaortitis.

endoappendicitis (en'dō-ă-pen-di-sī'tis). Simple catarrhal inflammation, limited more or less strictly to the mucosal surface of the vermiform appendix.

endoarteritis (en'dō-ar-ter-ī'tis). Endarteritis.

endoauscultation (en'dō-aws-kŭl-tā'shŭn). Auscultation of the thoracic organs, especially the heart, by means of a stethoscopic tube passed into the esophagus or into the heart.

endobasion (en'dō-bā'sē-on). A cephalometric and craniometric point located in the midline at the most posterior point of the anterior border of the foramen magnum on the contour of the foramen; it is slightly posterior and internal to basion.

endobiotic (en-dō-bī-ot'ik). Living as a parasite within the host.

endoblast (en'dō-blast) [endo- + G. *blastos,* germ]. Entoblast; a potential endoderm.

endobronchial (en-dō-brong'kē-ăl). Intrabronchial.

endocardiac, endocardial (en-dō-kar'dē-ak, -dē-ăl). **1.** Intracardiac. **2.** Relating to the endocardium.

endocardiography (en'dō-kar-dē-og'ră-fē). Electrocardiography with the exploring electrode within the chambers of the heart. See also intracardiac *catheter.*

endocarditic (en'dō-kar-dit'ik). Relating to endocarditis.

endocarditis (en'dō-kar-dī'tis). Encarditis; inflammation of the endocardium.

abacterial thrombotic e., nonbacterial thrombotic e.

acute bacterial e., see bacterial e.

atypical verrucous e., Libman-Sacks e.

bacteria-free stage of bacterial e., e. described prior to the antibiotic era and presumably due to spontaneous healing of the bacterial vegetations.

bacterial e., e. caused by the direct invasion of bacteria and leading to deformity of the valve leaflets; **acute b. e.** is caused by pyogenic organisms such as hemolytic streptococci or staphylococci; **subacute b. e.** is usually due to *Streptococcus viridans* or *S. fecalis.*

cachectic e., nonbacterial thrombotic e.

e. chorda'lis, e. affecting particularly the chordae tendineae.

constrictive e., endomyocardial fibroelastosis producing a clinical picture identical with constrictive pericarditis.

infectious e., infective e., e. due to infection by microorganisms.

isolated parietal e., fibrous thickening of the endocardium of the left ventricle without valvular involvement.

Libman-Sacks e., atypical verrucous or nonbacterial verrucous e.; Libman-Sacks syndrome; verrucous e. sometimes associated with disseminated lupus erythematosus.

Löffler's e.; Löffler's fibroplastic e., Löffler's syndrome (2) or disease; fibroplastic parietal e. with eosinophilia, an e. of obscure cause characterized by progressive congestive heart failure, multiple systemic emboli, and eosinophilia.

malignant e., septic e.; acute bacterial e., usually secondary to suppuration elsewhere and running a fulminating course.

marantic e., nonbacterial thrombotic e. associated with cancer and other debilitating diseases.

mural e., inflammation of the endocardium involving the walls of the chambers of the heart.

nonbacterial thrombotic e., abacterial thrombotic e.; cachectic or terminal e.; thromboendocarditis; verrucous endocardial lesions occurring in the terminal stages of many chronic infectious and wasting diseases.

nonbacterial verrucous e., Libman-Sacks e.

polypous e., bacterial e. with the formation of pedunculated masses of fibrin, or thrombi, attached to the ulcerated valves.

rheumatic e., endocardial involvment as part of rheumatic heart disease, recognized clinically by valvular involvement; in the acute stage, there may be tiny fibrin vegetations along the lines of closure of the valve leaflets, with subsequent fibrous thickening and shortening of the leaflets.

septic e., malignant e.

subacute bacterial e. (SBE), see bacterial e.

terminal e., nonbacterial thrombotic e.

valvular e., inflammation confined to the endocardium of the valves.

vegetative e., verrucous e., e. associated with the presence of fibrinous clots (vegetations) forming on the ulcerated surfaces of the valves.

endocardium, pl. **endocardia** (en-dō-kar'dē-ŭm, -ē-ă) [endo- + G. *kardia,* heart]. [NA]. The innermost tunic of the heart, which includes endothelium and subendothelial connective tissue; in the atrial wall, smooth muscle and numerous elastic fibers also occur.

endoceliac (en-dō-sē'lē-ak) [endo- + G. *koilia,* cavity, ventricle]. Intracelial; within one of the body cavities.

endocervical (en'dō-ser'vi-kăl). **1.** Intracervical; within any cervix, specifically within the cervix uteri. **2.** Relating to the endocervix.

endocervicitis (en'dō-ser-vi-sī'tis). Endotrachelitis; inflammation of the mucous membrane of the cervix uteri.

endocervix (en-dō-ser'viks). The mucous membrane of the cervical canal.

endochondral (en-dō-kon'drăl) [endo- + G. *chondros,* cartilage]. Intracartilaginous.

endocolitis (en'dō-kō-lī'tis). Simple catarrhal inflammation of the colon.

endocolpitis (en'dō-kol-pī'tis) [endo- + G. *colpos,* vagina, + *-itis,* inflammation]. Inflammation of the vaginal mucous membrane.

endocranial (en-dō-krā'nē-ăl). Encranial; entocranial. **1.** Within the cranium. **2.** Relating to the endocranium.

endocranium (en'dō-krā'nē-ŭm). Entocranium; the lining membrane of the cranium, or dura mater of the brain.

endocrine (en'dō-krin) [endo- + G. *krinō,* to separate]. **1.** Secreting internally, most commonly into the systemic circulation; of or pertaining to such secretion. **2.** The internal or hormonal secretion of a ductless gland. **3.** Denoting a gland that furnishes an internal secretion.

endocrinolgist (en'dō-kri-nol'ō-jist). One who specializes in endocrinology.

endocrinology (en'dō-kri-nol'ō-jē) [endocrine + G. *logos,* study]. The science and medical specialty concerned with the internal or hormonal secretions and their physiologic and pathologic relations.

endocrinoma (en'dō-kri-nō'mă). A tumor with endocrine tissue that retains the function of the parent organ, usually to an excessive degree.

multiple e., familial endocrine *adenomatosis,* type 1.

endocrinopathic (en'dō-kri-nō-path'ik). Relating to or suffering from an endocrinopathy.

endocrinopathy (en'dō-kri-nop'ă-thē). A disorder in the function of an endocrine gland and the consequences thereof.

multiple e., familial endocrine *adenomatosis,* type 1.

endocrinotherapy (en'dō-kri-nō-ther'ă-pē). Treatment of disease by the administration of extracts of endocrine glands.

endocyclic (en-dō-sī'klik, -sik'lik). Within a cycle or ring; *e.g.,* the 6 C atoms of the benzene ring in toluene. *Cf.* exocyclic.

endocyma (en-dō-sī'mă) [endo- + G. *kyma,* fetus]. A teratoma (sometimes identifiable as an included parasitic twin) which develops in a visceral location.

endocyst (en'dō-sist). The inner layer of a hydatid cyst.

endocystitis (en'dō-sis-tī'tis) [endo- + G. *kystis,* bladder, + *-itis,* inflammation]. Inflammation of the mucous membrane of the bladder.

endocytosis (en'dō-sī-tō'sis) [endo- + G. *kytos,* cell, + *-osis,* condition]. The process, including pinocytosis and phagocytosis, whereby materials are taken into a cell by the invagination of the plasma membrane, which it breaks off as a boundary membrane of the part engulfed. *Cf.* exocytosis (2).

endoderm (en'dō-derm) [endo- + G. *derma,* skin]. Entoderm; hypoblast; the innermost of the three primary germ layers of the embryo (ectoderm, mesoderm, endoderm) from which are derived the epithelial lining of the primitive gut tract, its glands, and the epithelial component of structures developing as outgrowths from the gut.

Endodermophyton (en'dō-der-mof'i-ton) [endo- + G. *derma,* skin, + *phyton,* plant]. Former name for *Trichophyton,* especially for the species causing tinea imbricata, *T. concentricum.*

endodiascope (en'dō-dī'ă-skōp). An x-ray tube that may be placed within a cavity of the body.

endodiascopy (en'dō-dī-as'kō-pē) [endo- + G. *dia,* through, + *skopeō,* to view]. X-ray visualization by means of an endodiascope.

endodontia (en-dō-don'shē-ă). Endodontics.

endodontics (en-dō-don'tiks) [endo- + G. *odous,* tooth]. Endodontia; endodontology; a field of dentistry concerned with the biology and pathology of the dental pulp and periapical tissues, and with the prevention, diagnosis, and treatment of pathoses and traumatic injuries in these tissues.

endodontist (en-dō-don'tist). Endodontologist; one who specializes in the practice of endodontics.

endodontologist (en'dō-don-tol'ō-jist). Endodontist.

endodontology (en'do-don-tol'ō-jē). Endodontics.

endodyocyte (en'dō-dī'ō-sīt) [endo- + G. *dys,* two, + *kytos,* cell]. **1.** A trophozoite formed by endodyogeny. **2.** Merozoite.

endodyogeny (en'dō-dī-oj'ĕ-nē) [endo- + G. *dys,* two, + *genesis,* creation]. A process of asexual development seen among certain coccidia, such as *Toxoplasma* and *Frenkelia,* in which no separate nuclear division occurs, as in schizogony; the two daughters develop internally within the parent, without nuclear conjugation.

endoenteritis (en'dō-en-ter-ī'tis) [endo- + G. *enteron,* intestine, *-itis,* inflammation]. Inflammation of the intestinal mucous membrane.

endoenzyme (en-dō-en'zīm). Intracellular *enzyme.*

endoesophagitis (en'dō-ē-sof-ă-jī'tis). Inflammation of the internal lining of the esophagus.

endofaradism (en-dō-far'ă-dizm). Application of an alternating electric current to the interior of any cavity of the body. See fulguration.

endogalvanism (en-dō-gal'van-izm). Application of a direct electric current to the interior of any cavity of the body. See fulguration.

endogamy (en-dog'ă-mē) [endo- + G. *gamos,* marriage]. Reproduction by conjugation between sister cells, the descendants of one original cell.

endogastric (en-dō-gas'trik). Within the stomach.

endogastritis (en'dō-gas-trī'tis) [endo- + G. *gastēr,* stomach, + *-itis,* inflammation]. Inflammation of the mucous membrane of the stomach.

endogenic (en-dō-jen'ik). Endogenous.

endogenote (en-dō-jē'nōt). In microbial genetics, the original genome of a merozygote.

endogenous (en-doj'ĕ-nŭs) [endo- + G. *-gen,* production]. Endogenic; originating or produced within the organism or one of its parts.

endoglobular, endoglobar (en-dō-glob'yū-lăr, -glō'bar). Within a globular body; specifically, within a red blood cell.

endognathion (en-dog-nath'ē-on, en-dō-nā'thē-on) [endo- + G. *gnathos,* jaw]. The medial of the two segments constituting the incisive bone. See mesognathion.

endoherniotomy (en'dō-her-nē-ot'ō-mē). An obsolete procedure for closure, by sutures, of the interior lining of a hernial sac.

endointoxication (en'dō-in-tok-si-kā'shŭn). Poisoning by an endogenous toxin.

endolaryngeal (en'dō-lă-rin'jē-ăl). Within the larynx.

Endolimax (en-dō-lī'maks) [endo- + G. *leimax,* a meadow or garden]. A genus of small nonpathogenic amebae parasitic in the large intestine of man and other animals.

endolith (en'dō-lith) [endo- + G. *lithos,* stone]. Denticle (1); pulp calcification, calculus, or stone; a calcified body found in the pulp chamber of a tooth; may be composed of irregular dentin (true denticle) or due to ectopic calcification of pulp tissue (false denticle).

endolymph (en'dō-limf). Endolympha.

endolympha (en'dō-lim'fă) [endo- + L. *lympha,* a clear fluid] [NA]. Endolymph; Scarpa's liquor; the fluid contained within the membranous labyrinth of the inner ear.

endolymphic (en-dō-lim'fik). Relating to the endolymph.

endomeninx (en'dō-mē'ningks, -men'ingks) [endo- + G. *meninx,* membrane]. Inner membrane surrounding the embryonic neural tube; involved in the formation of the leptomeninges.

endomerogony (en'dō-me-rog'ō-nē) [endo- + G. *meros,* part, + *gonē,* generation]. Production of merozoites in the asexual reproduction of sporozoan protozoa by a process originating in the interior of the schizont (as contrasted with ectomerogony); observed in species of *Eimeria.*

endometria (en-dō-mē'trē-ă). Plural of endometrium.

endometrial (en-dō-mē'trē-ăl). Relating to or composed of endometrium.

endometrioid (en-dō-mē'trē-oyd). Microscopically resembling endometrial tissue.

endometrioma (en'dō-mē-trē-ō'mă). Circumscribed mass of ectopic endometrial tissue in endometriosis.

endometriosis (en'dō-mē-trē-ō'sis). Ectopic occurrence of endometrial tissue, frequently forming cysts containing altered blood.

endometritis (en'dō-mē-trī'tis). Inflammation of the endometrium.
decidual e., inflammation of the decidual mucous membrane of the gravid uterus.
e. dis'secans, e. with ulceration and exfoliation of the mucous membrane.

endometrium, pl. **endometria** (en'dō-mē'trē-ŭm, -trē-ă) [endo- + G. + *mētra,* uterus] [NA]. Tunica mucosa uteri; the mucous membrane comprising the inner layer of the uterine wall; it consists of a simple columnar epithelium and a lamina propria that contains simple tubular uterine glands.
Swiss cheese e., glandular hyperplasia of the e. with cyst formation, so-called because of the appearance of the cysts in histologic sections.

endometropic (en'dō-mē-trop'ik) [endo- + G. *metra,* uterus, + *tropē,* a turning]. Denoting an external stimulus capable of producing a response of the uterus, specifically the endometrium.

endomitosis (en'dō-mī-tō'sis). Endopolyploidy.

endomorph (en'dō-mōrf) [endo- + G. *morphē,* form]. Brachytype; a constitutional body type or build (biotype or somatotype) in which tissues that originated in the endoderm prevail; from a morphological standpoint, the trunk predominates over the limbs.

endomorphic (en'dō-mōr'fik). Relating to, or having the characteristics of, an endomorph.

endomotorsonde (en'dō-mō'tŏr-sond') [endo- + L. *motor,* mover, + Fr. *sonde,* sounding line]. Radiotelemetering capsule for studying the interior of the gastrointestinal tract.

Endomyces geotrichum (en-dō-mī'sez jē-ot'ri-kŭm). A species of yeastlike fungus that is the perfect state of *Geotrichum candidum* and the cause of geotrichosis.

Endomycetales (en'dō-mī-sē-tā'lēz). Saccharomycetales; an order of Ascomycetes that includes the yeasts.

endomyocardial (en'dō-mī-ō-kar'dē-ăl). Relating to the endocardium and the myocardium.

endomyocarditis (en-dō-mī'ō-kar-dī'tis). Inflammation of both endocardium and myocardium.

endomyometritis (en'dō-mī-ō-mē-trī-tis) [endo- + G. *mys,* muscle, + *mētra,* uterus, + *-itis,* inflammation]. Postcesarean section sepsis involving the tissues of the uterus.

endomysium (en'dō-miz'ē-ŭm, -mis'ē-ŭm) [endo- + G. *mys,* muscle]. The fine connective tissue sheath surrounding a muscle fiber.

endoneuritis (en'dō-nū-rī'tis). Inflammation of the endoneurium.

endoneurium (en-dō-nū'rē-ŭm) [endo- + G. *neuron,* nerve]. Henle's sheath; sheath of Key and Retzius; the delicate connective tissue enveloping individual nerve fibers within a peripheral nerve.

endonuclease (en-dō-nū'klē-ās). A nuclease (phosphodiesterase) that cleaves polynucleotides (nucleic acids) at interior bonds, thus producing poly- or oligonucleotide fragments of varying size. *Cf.* exonuclease.

micrococcal e. [EC 3.1.31.1], micrococcal nuclease; spleen e., deoxyribonuclease, or phosphodiesterase; an enzyme that cleaves nucleic acids to oligonucleotides terminating in 3'-phosphates.

nucleate e., endonuclease (*Serratia marcescens*).

restriction e., restriction enzyme; one of many e.'s isolated from bacteria that hydrolyze (cut) double-stranded DNA chains at specific (usually hexanucleotide) sequences, thus inactivating a foreign (viral or other) DNA and restricting its activity; these e.'s have become standard laboratory tools for making specific cuts in DNA as a first step in deducing sequences and are sometimes referred to as a "chemical knife;" usually named by a three- or four-letter abbreviation of the name of the organism from which isolated (*e.g.,* EcoB from *Escherichia coli,* strain B).

single-stranded nucleate e., endonuclease S_1 (*Aspergillus*).

spleen e., micrococcal e.

endonuclease (Serratia marcescens) [EC 3.1.30.2]. *Azotobacter* nuclease; nucleate e.; a nuclease (a nucleate oligonucleotidohydrolse) that forms oligonucleotides ending in 5'-phosphates from RNA and DNA.

endonulcease S_1 (Aspergillus) [EC 3.1.30.1]. Single-stranded nucleate endonuclease; deoxyribo-nuclease S_1; mung bean nuclease; an enzyme cleaving RNA or DNA to 5'-ended mono- or oligonucleotides.

endonucleolus (en'dō-nū-klē'ō-lŭs). A minute unstainable spot near the center of a nucleolus.

endoparasite (en-dō-par'ă-sīt). A parasite living within the body of its host.

endoparasitism (en-dō-par'ă-sī-tizm). Infection.

endopeptidase (en-dō-pep'ti-dās). An enzyme catalyzing the hydrolysis of a peptide chain at points well within the chain, not near termini; *e.g.,* pepsin, trypsin. *Cf.* exopeptidase.

endoperiarteritis (en'dō-păr'i-ar-ter-ī'tis) [endo- + G. *peri,* around, + arteritis]. Panarteritis.

endopericardiac (en'dō-păr-ē-kar'dē-ak). Intrapericardiac.

endopericarditis (en'dō-păr'i-kar-dī'tis) [endo- + G. *peri,* around, + *kardia,* heart, + *-itis,* inflammation]. Simultaneous inflammation of the endocardium and pericardium.

endoperimyocarditis (en'dōpăr'i-mī'ō-kar-dī'tis) [endo- + G. *peri,* around, + *mys,* muscle, + *kardia,* heart, + *-itis,* inflammation]. Perimyoendocarditis; simultaneous inflammation of the heart muscle and of the endocardium and pericardium.

endoperineuritis (en'dō-păr'i-nū-rī'tis). Inflammation of both endoneurium and perineurium.

endoperitonitis (en'dō-păr'i-tō-nī'tis). Superficial inflammation of the peritoneum.

endoperoxide (en'dō-per-ok'sīd). A peroxide (–O–O–) group that bridges two atoms that are both parts of a larger molecule.

endophlebitis (en'dō-fle-bī'tis) [endo- + G. *phleps (phleb-),* vein, + *-itis,* inflammation]. Inflammation of the intima of a vein.

endophthalmitis (en-dof-thal-mī'tis) [endo- + G. *ophthalmos,* eye, + *-itis,* inflammation]. Inflammation of the tissues of the eyeball.

granulomatous e., a diffuse, chronic inflammation of intraocular tissues.

e. ophthal'mia nodo'sa, e. due to intraocular caterpillar hairs.

e. phacoanaphylac'tica, iridocyclitis anaphylactica; inflammation of the uveal tract as a result of sensitization by the lens cortex; simulates sympathetic ophthalmia.

endophyte (en'dō-fīt) [endo- + G. *phyton,* plant]. A plant parasite living within another organism.

endophytic (en-dō-fit'ik). **1.** Pertaining to an endophyte. **2.** Referring to an infiltrative, invasive tumor.

endoplasm (en'dō-plazm). Entoplasm; the inner or medullary part of the cytoplasm, as opposed to the ectoplasm, containing the cell organelles.

endoplast (en'dō-plast) [endo- + G. *plastos,* formed]. Former name for endosome.

endoplastic (en-dō-plas'tik). Relating to the endoplasm.

endopolygeny (en'dō-pō-lij'ĕ-nē) [endo- + G. *polys,* many, + *genesis,* creation]. Asexual reproduction in which more than two offspring are formed within the parent organism and in which two or possibly more nuclear divisions occur before merozoite formation begins; a form of internal budding observed in *Toxoplasma gondii. Cf.* endodyogeny.

endopolyploid (en-dō-pol'ē-ployd). Relating to endopolyploidy.

endopolyploidy (en-dō-pol'ē-ploy-dē). Endomitosis; the process or state of duplication of the chromosomes without accompanying spindle formation or cytokinesis, resulting in a polyploid nucleus.

endoradiography (en'dō-rā-dē-og'ră-fē). Study of organs or cavities by use of x-ray and a radiopaque substance.

endoreduplication (en'dō-rē-dū'pli-kā'shŭn). A form of polyploidy or polysomy characterized by a redoubling of chromosomes, giving rise to four-stranded chromosomes at prophase and metaphase.

end organ. See under organ.

endorphinergic (en'dōr-fin-er'jik) [endorphin + G. *ergon,* work]. Relating to nerve cells or fibers that employ an endorphin as their neurotransmitter.

endorphins (en'dōr-finz) [fr. *endogenous morphine*]. Opioid peptides originally isolated from the brain but now found in many parts of the body; in the brain, e.'s bind to the same receptors that bind exogenous opiates. A variety of e.'s (*e.g.,* alpha and beta) that vary not only in their physical and chemical properties but also in physiologic action have been isolated. See also enkephalins.

endorrhachis (en-dō-rā'kis) [endo- + G. *rhachis,* the spine]. *Dura mater* spinalis.

endosalpingiosis (en'dō-sal-pin-jē-ō'sis). Aberrant mucous membrane in the ovary or elsewhere consisting of ciliated tubal mucosa without stroma of endometrial type.

endosalpingitis (en'dō-sal-pin-jī'tis) [endo- + G. *salpinx (salping-),* tube, + *-itis,* inflammation]. Inflammation of the lining membrane of the eustachian or the fallopian tube.

endosarc (en'dō-sark) [endo- + G. *sarx (sark-),* flesh]. Entosarc; the endoplasm of a protozoan.

endoscope (en'dō-skōp) [endo- + G. *skopeō,* to examine]. An instrument for the examination of the interior of a canal or hollow viscus.

endoscopist (en-dos'kŏ-pist). A specialist trained in the use of an endoscope.

endoscopy (en-dos'kŏ-pē) [see endoscope]. Examination of the interior of a canal or hollow viscus by means of a special instrument, such as an endoscope.

endoskeleton (en-dō-skel'ĕ-tŏn). The internal bony framework of the body; the skeleton in its usual context as distinguished from exoskeleton.

endosmosis (en-dos-mō'sis). Obsolete term for osmosis in a direction toward the interior of a cell or a cavity; the inward direction is not self-evident in all systems.

endosome (en'dō-sōm) [endo- + G. *soma,* body]. A more or less central body in the vesicular nucleus of certain Feulgen-negative (DNA−) protozoa (*e.g.,* trypanosomes, parasitic amebae, and phytoflagellates), with the chromatin (DNA+) lying between the nuclear membrane and the e. *Cf.* nucleolus.

endosonoscopy (en-dō-son'ŏ-skŏ-pē). A sonographic study carried out by transducers inserted into the body as miniature probes in the urethra, bladder, or rectum.

endospore (en'dō-spōr) [endo- + G. *sporos,* seed]. **1.** A resistant body formed within the vegetative cells of some bacteria, particularly those belonging to the genera *Bacillus* and *Clostridium.* **2.** A fungus spore borne within a cell or within the tubular end of a sporophore.

endosteal (en-dos'tē-ăl). Relating to the endosteum.

endosteitis, endostitis (en'dos-tē-ī'tis, en'dos-tī'tis). Perimyelitis; central osteitis (2); inflammation of the endosteum or of the medullary cavity of a bone.

endosteoma (en-dos'tē-ō'mă) [endo- + G. *osteon,* bone, + *-ōma,* tumor]. Endostoma; a benign neoplasm of bone tissue in the medullary cavity of a bone.

endostethoscope (en-dō-steth'ō-skōp) [endo- + G. *stēthos,* chest, + *skopeō,* to examine]. A stethoscopic tube used in endoauscultation.

endosteum (en-dos'tē-ŭm) [endo- + G. *osteon,* bone] [NA]. Medullary membrane; perimyelis; a layer of cells lining the inner surface of bone in the central medullary cavity.

endostoma (en-dō-stō'mă). Endosteoma.

endotendineum (en'dō-ten-din'ē-ŭm) [endo- + L. *tendon,* tendon, + *-eus,* adj.; the whole, in its neuter form, used substantively]. The fine connective tissue surrounding secondary fascicles of a tendon.

endothelia (en-dō-thē'lē-ă). Plural of endothelium.

endothelial (en-dō-thē'lē-ăl). Relating to the endothelium.

endotheliocyte (en-dō-thē'lē-ō-sīt). Endothelial *leukocyte.*

endothelioid (en-dō-thē'lē-oyd). Resembling endothelium.

endothelioma (en'dō-thē-lē-ō'mă). Generic term for a group of neoplasms, particularly benign tumors, derived from the endothelial tissue of blood vessels or lymphatic channels; e.'s may be benign or malignant.

endotheliosis (en'dō-thē-lē-ō'sis). Proliferation of endothelium.

endothelium, pl. **endothelia** (en-dō-thē'lē-ŭm, -lē-ă) [endo- + G. *thēlē,* nipple]. A layer of flat cells lining especially blood and lymphatic vessels and the heart.
e. of anterior chamber, e. camerae anterioris.
e. cam'erae anterio'ris [NA], endothelium of the anterior chamber; a single layer of large, squamous cells that covers the posterior surface of the cornea.

endothermic (en-dō-ther'mik) [endo- + G. *thermē,* heat]. Denoting a chemical reaction during which heat is absorbed. *Cf.* exothermic (1).

endothrix (en'dō-thriks) [endo- + G. *thrix,* hair]. A trichophyton (notably *Trichophyton violaceum* and *T. tonsurans*) whose arthroconidia and, occasionally, mycelia characteristically invade the interior of the hair shaft; there is no conspicuous external sheath of spores, as there is with ectothrix.

endotoxemia (en'dō-tok-sē'mē-ă). Presence in the blood of endotoxins, which, if derived from Gram-negative rod-shaped bacteria, may cause a generalized Shwartzman phenomenon with shock.

endotoxic (en-dō-tok'sik). Denoting an endotoxin.

endotoxicosis (en'dō-tok-si-kō'sis). Poisoning by an endotoxin.

endotoxin (en-dō-tok'sin). Intracellular toxin. **1.** A bacterial toxin not freely liberated into the surrounding medium, in contrast to exotoxin. **2.** The complex phospholipid-polysaccharide macromolecules which form an integral part of the cell wall of a variety of relatively avirulent as well as virulent strains of Gram-negative bacteria. The toxins are relatively heat-stable, are less potent than most exotoxins, are less specific, and do not form toxoids; on injection, they may cause a state of shock accompanied by severe diarrhea, and, in smaller doses, fever and leukopenia followed by leukocytosis; they have the capacity of eliciting the Shwartzman and the Sanarelli-Shwartzman phenomena.

endotracheal (en'dō-trā'kē-ăl). Within the trachea.

endotrachelitis (en'dō-trak-el-ī'tis). Endocervicitis.

endovaccination (en'dō-vak-si-nā'shŭn). Oral administration of vaccines.

endovasculitis (en'dō-vas'kyū-lī'tis). Endangiitis.
hemorrhagic e., endothelial and medial hyperplasia of placental blood vessels with thrombosis, fragmentation, and diapedesis of red blood cells resulting in stillbirth or fetal developmental disorders.

endovenous (en-dō-vē'nŭs). Intravenous.

end-piece. The terminal part of the tail of a spermatozoon consisting of the axoneme and the flagellar membrane.

endplate, end-plate (end'plāt). The ending of a motor nerve fiber in relation to a skeletal muscle fiber.
motor e., sole-plate ending; the large and complex end-formation by which the axon of a motor neuron establishes synaptic contact with a striated muscle fiber (cell); several terminal branches of a motor axon end in irregular, club-shaped synaptic end-formations which are bedded in a single trough-like depression of the muscle fiber's surface; the postsynaptic membrane, the sarcolemma that forms the bottom of the trough, is greatly increased in surface area by deep infoldings protruding into the underlying cytoplasm of the muscle fiber; the subsynaptic interval between the plasma membrane of the axon terminals and the sarcolemma is filled with an amorphous substance; the trough is closed off toward the surface by the Schwann sheath, which peels away from the axons as the latter enter the trough and thus forms a lid over the trough; the slight bulge of this closure plate corresponds to Doyère's eminence.

end-tidal (end-tī'dăl). At the end of a normal expiration.

endyma (en'di-mă) [G. a garment]. Ependyma.

E.N.E. Abbreviation for ethylnorepinephrine.

-ene. Suffix applied to a chemical name indicating the presence of a carbon-carbon double bond; *e.g.,* propene (unsaturated propane, $CH_3—CH=CH_2$).

enediol (ēn-dī'ōl). The atomic arrangement –C(OH=C(OH–) produced by proton migration from the CH of a —CHOH group that is attached to a –CO– group to the oxygen of the –CO– group (usually induced by alkali), giving rise to doubly bonded carbon atoms (the -ene group), each bearing a –CHOH group (a diol); a special case of enolization.

enema (en'ĕ-mă) [G.]. A rectal injection for clearing out the bowel, or administering drugs or food.

analeptic e., an e. of a pint of lukewarm water with one-half teaspoonful of table salt.

barium e., a type of contrast e.; administration of barium, a radiopaque medium, for radiographic study of the lower intestinal tract.

blind e., the introduction into the rectum of a rubber tube to facilitate the expulsion of flatus.

contrast e., e. using barium or another contrast medium.

double contrast e., after evacuation of a barium e. and injection of air into the rectum, radiographic study will show finer details of mucosa of the rectum and colon.

flatus e., an e. of magnesium sulfate in glycerin and warm water.

high e., enteroclysis; an e. instilled high up into the colon.

nutrient e., a rectal injection of predigested food.

oil retention e., a rectal injection of mineral oil, introduced at low pressure and retained for several hours before expelling, to soften feces.

soapsuds e., an e. of shredded or powdered soap in warm water.

turpentine e., an e. of turpentine and olive oil in soapsuds.

enemator (en-ĕ-mā'ter, -tōr). An appliance used to give an enema.

enemiasis (en-ĕ-mī'ă-sis). The use of enemas.

energetics (en-er-jet'iks). The study of the energy changes involved in physical and chemical changes.

energometer (en-er-gom'ĕ-ter) [G. *energeia,* energy, + *metron,* measure]. An apparatus for measuring blood pressure.

energy (en'er-jē) [G. *energeia,* fr. *en,* in, + *ergon,* work]. Dynamic force; the exertion of power; the capacity to do work, taking the forms of kinetic e., potential e., chemical e., electrical e., etc.

e. of activation, e. that must be added to that already possessed by a molecule or molecules in order to initiate a reaction; usually expressed in the Arrhenius equation relating a velocity constant to absolute temperature.

binding e., fusion e.; e. that would be released if a particular atomic nucleus were formed through the combination of individual protons and neutrons.

chemical e., e. liberated by a chemical reaction, *e.g.,* oxidation of carbon, or absorbed in the formation of a chemical compound.

free e., a thermodynamic function symbolized as *F,* or *G* (Gibbs free e.), $= H - TS$, where *H* is the enthalpy of a system, *T* the absolute temperature, and *S* the entropy; chemical reactions proceed spontaneously in the direction that involves a net decrease in the free e. of the system.

fusion e., binding e.

Gibbs free e. (*G*), see free e.

kinetic e., the e. of motion.

latent e., potential e.

nuclear e., e. given off in the course of nuclear reaction or stored in the formation of an atomic nucleus.

nutritional e., trophodynamics.

e. of position, potential e.

potential e., latent e.; e. of position; the e., existing in a body by virtue of its position or state of existence, which is not being exerted at the time.

psychic e., psychic force; in psychoanalysis, a hypothetical mental force, analogous to the physical concept of e., which enables and vitalizes an individual's psychological activity. See also libido.

radiant e., e. contained in light rays or any other form of radiation.

solar e., e. derived from sunlight.

total e., the sum of kinetic and potential e.'s.

enervation (en-er-vā'shŭn) [L. *enervo,* pp. *-atus,* to enervate, fr. *e-* priv. + *nervus,* nerve]. Failure of nerve force; weakening.

enflurane (en-flūr'ān). 2-Chloro-1,1,2-trifluoroethyl difluoromethyl ether; a potent volatile inhalation anesthetic that is nonflammable and nonexplosive.

ENG Abbreviation for electronystagmography.

engagement (en-gāj'ment). In obstetrics, the mechanism by which the biparietal diameter of the fetal head enters the plane of the inlet.

engastrius (en-gas'trē-ŭs) [G. *en,* in, + *gastēr,* belly]. Unequal conjoined twins in which the smaller parasite is wholly or partly within the abdomen of the larger autosite.

Engelmann, Guido, German surgeon, *1876. See E.'s *disease.*

Engelmann, Theodor W., German physiologist, 1843–1909. See E.'s basal *knobs.*

engineering (en-jin-ēr'ing). The practical application of physical, mechanical, and mathematical principles.

biomedical e., application of e. principles to obtain solutions to biomedical problems.

dental e., application of e. principles to dentistry.

genetic e., manipulation of basic genetic material of an organism to modify biologic heredity or to produce peptides of high purity, such as hormones or antigens.

Englisch, Josef, Austrian physician, 1835–1915. See E.'s *sinus.*

englobe (en-glōb'). To take in by a spheroidal body; said of the ingestion of bacteria and other foreign bodies by the phagocytes.

englobement (en-glōb'ment). The process of inclusion by a spheroidal body, such as by a phagocyte.

engorged (en-gōrjd') [O. Fr. fr. Mediev. L. *gorgia,* throat, narrow passage, fr. L. *gurges,* a whirlpool]. Absolutely filled; distended with fluid. See also congested; hyperemic.

engorgement (en-gōrj'ment). Distention with fluid or other material. See also congestion; hyperemia.

engram (en'gram) [G. *en,* in, + *gramma,* mark]. In the mnemic hypothesis, a physical habit or memory trace made on the protoplasm of an organism by the repetition of stimuli.

engraphia (en-graf'ē-ă). The formation of engrams.

en grappe (ahn-grap') [Fr. *en,* in, + *grappe,* bunch of grapes]. Denoting the grapelike cluster arrangement of microconidia of certain dermatophytes.

enhancement (en-hans'ment). **1.** The act of augmenting. **2.** In immunology, the prolongation of a process or event by suppressing an opposing process.

contrast e., the intravenous administration of water-soluble iodinated contrast material, which increases the CT number of the vascular pool, as well as some lesions (particularly in the brain), due to abnormal leakage into the interstitium.

immunological e., immunoenhancement.

enhematospore, enhemospore (en-hem'ă-tō-spōr, en-hem'ō-spōr) [G. *en,* in, + *haima,* blood, + *sporos,* seed]. Obsolete terms for merozoite.

enkephalinergic (en-kef'ă-lin-er'jik) [enkephalin + G. *ergon,* work]. Relating to nerve cells or fibers that employ an enkephalin as their neurotransmitter.

enkephalins (en-kef'ă-linz). Pentapeptide endorphins, found in many parts of the brain, that bind to specific receptor sites, some of which may be pain-related opiate receptors; hypothesized as endogenous neurotransmitters and nonaddicting analgesics. Metenkephalin is Tyr-Gly-Gly-Phe-Met; leuenkephalin has Leu in place of Met; proenkephalin has Pro in place of Met.

enlargement (en-larj'ment). **1.** An increase in size. **2.** An intumescence or swelling.

cervical e. of spinal cord, *intumescentia* cervicalis.

gingival e., an overgrowth (localized or diffuse) of gingival tissue, nonspecific in nature. See also gingival *hyperplasia,* gingival *hypertrophy.*

lumbar e. of spinal cord, *intumescentia* lumbalis.

-enoic [-ene + -ic]. Suffix indicating an unsaturated acid.

enol (ē'nol) [-ene + -ol]. A compound possessing a hydroxyl group (alcohol) attached to a doubly bonded (ethylenic) carbon atom (–CH=CH(OH)–); properly italicized when attached as a prefix or infix to an otherwise complete name; *e.g., enol* pyruvate; phospho*enol* pyruvate.

enolase (ē'nol-ās) (EC 4.2.1.11). Phosphopyruvate hydratase; an enzyme catalyzing the dehydration of 2-phospho-D-glycerate to phospho*enol* pyruvate.

enolization (ē'nol-i-zā'shŭn). Conversion of a keto to an enol form; *e.g.,* CH_3-CO-COOH → CH_2=C(OH)COOH.

***enol* pyruvate** (ē-nol-pī'rūvāt). CH_2=C(OH)–COO^-, the form of pyruvate encountered in the biologically important phospho*enol* -pyruvate (*enol* pyruvate phosphate), not in the free form.

enophthalmia (en-of-thal'mē-ă). Enophthalmos.

enophthalmos (en'of-thal'mos) [G. *en,* in, + *ophthalmos,* eye]. Enophthalmia; recession of the eyeball within the orbit.

enorganic (en-ōr-gan'ik). Rarely used term denoting that which occurs as an innate characteristic of an organism.

enosimania (en'ō-si-mā'nē-ă) [G. *enosis,* a quaking, + *mania,* insanity]. Rarely used term for the obsessive belief of having committed an unpardonable offense.

enostosis (en-os-tō'sis) [G. *en,* in, + *osteon,* bone, + *-osis,* condition]. A mass of proliferating bone tissue within a bone.

enoyl (ēn'ō-il) [-ene + -oyl]. The acyl radical of an unsaturated aliphatic acid.

enoyl-ACP reductase [EC 1.3.1.9]. Crotonyl-ACP reductase; an enzyme catalyzing hydrogenation of acyl-ACP complexes to 2,3-dehydroacyl-ACP's, with NAD^+ as hydrogen acceptor; important in fatty acid metabolism.

enoyl-ACP reductase (NADPH) [EC 1.3.1.10]. Acyl-ACP dehydrogenase or red uctase; an enzyme carrying out the same reaction as enoyl-ACP reductase, but with $NADP^+$ as hydrogen acceptor.

enoyl-CoA hydratase [EC 4.2.1.17]. Enoyl hydrase; crotonase; an enzyme catalyzing a reversible reaction between an L-3-hydroxyacyl-CoA and a 2,3- (or 3,4) *trans-* enoyl-CoA.

2-enoyl-CoA reductase. Acyl-CoA dehydrogenase ($NADP^+$).

enoyl hydrase. Enoyl-CoA hydratase.

Enroth, Emil E., Finnish ophthalmologist, 1879–1953. See E.'s *sign.*

E.N.S. Abbreviation for ethylnorepinephrine.

ensiform (en'si-fōrm) [L. *ensis,* sword, + *forma,* appearance]. Xiphoid.

ensisternum (en'sis-ter'nŭm) [L. *ensis,* sword, + sternum]. *Processus* xiphoideus.

enstrophe (en'strō-fē) [G. *en,* in, + *strophē,* a turning]. Entropion (2).

ensu Acronym for *e*quivalent *n*ormal *s*on *u*nit, that amount of information which will half the conditional probability that a female consultand is a carrier for an X-linked trait; each normal son contributes one ensu.

ENT Abbreviation for ears, nose, and throat. See otorhinolaryngology.

ent-. See ento-.

en'tad [G. *entos,* within, + L. *ad,* to]. Toward the interior.

ental (en'tăl) [G. *entos,* within]. Relating to the interior; inside.

entamebiasis (ent-ă-mē-bi'ă-sis). Infection with *Entamoeba histolytica.* See amebiasis; amebic *dysentery.*

Entamoeba (ent-ă-mē'bă) [G. *entos,* within + *amoibē,* change]. *Paramoeba;* a genus of ameba parasitic in the cecum and large bowel of man and other primates and in many domestic and wild mammals and birds; with the exception of *E. histolytica,* members of the genus appear to be relatively harmless inhabitants of the host.

E. bucca'lis, *E. gingivalis.*

E. co'li, *Amoeba coli;* nonpathogenic species that occurs in the large intestine of man, other primates, dogs, and possibly pigs; often confused with *E. histolytica,* but distinguished by nuclear details and by the number of nuclei and the form of chromatoidals in the cyst.

E. gingiva'lis, *E. buccalis; Amoeba buccalis; A. dentalis;* a species found in the oral cavity of man, other primates, dogs, and cats; in man, it is frequently associated with poor oral hygiene and its resultant diseases.

E. hartman'ni, species found in the large intestine of man, other primates, and dogs; now considered to be a distinct strain or species that is nonpathogenic and smaller than *E. histolytica* but otherwise indistinguishable from it; formerly called the "small race" of *E. histolytica.*

E. histoly'tica, *Amoeba dysenteriae; A. histolytica;* a species that is the only distinct pathogen of the genus, the so-called "large race" of *E. histolytica,* causing tropical or amebic dysentery in man and also in dogs (man is the reservoir for canine infections). In man, the organism, though usually nonpathogenic, may penetrate the epithelial tissues of the colon, causing ulceration (amebic dysentery); in a small proportion of these cases, the organism may reach the liver by the portal bloodstream and produce abscesses (hepatic amebiasis); in a fraction of these cases it may then spread to other organs, such as the lungs, brain, kidney, or skin and frequently be fatal.

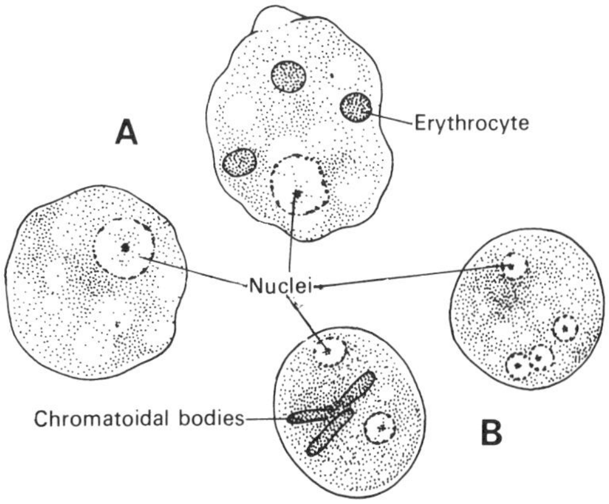

Entamoeba histolytica

A, trophozoites, one ameba having ingested erythrocytes (×1000); *B,* cysts, one of which has chromatoidal bodies (×1500).

E. moshkov'skii, a species of ameba very similar to *E. histolytica,* probably not infective to man, but a cause of diagnostic difficulties since it has been recovered from human sewage and may be responsible for false-positive results in tests of sewage plant effluents.

entasia, entasis (en-tā'zē-ă, en'tă-sis) [G. distention]. Tonic *spasm.*

entatic (en-tat'ik) [G. *enteinein,* to stretch; metaphorically, to intensify]. **1.** Pertaining to entasia. **2.** Rarely used synonym of aphrodisiac.

enter-. See entero-.

enteral (en'ter-ăl) [G. *enteron,* intestine]. Within, or by way of, the intestine or gastrointestinal tract, especially as distinguished from parenteral.

enteralgia (en-ter-al'jē-ă) [entero- + G. *algos,* pain]. Enterdynia; severe abdominal pain accompanying spasm of the bowel.

enteramine (en-ter-am'ēn). Serotonin.

enterectasis (en-ter-ek'tă-sis) [entero- + G. *ektasis,* a stretching]. Dilation of the bowel.

enterectomy (en-ter-ek'tō-mē) [entero- + G. *ektomē,* excision]. Resection of a segment of the intestine.

enterelcosis (en-ter-el-kō'sis) [entero- + G. *helkos,* ulcer]. Ulceration of the bowel.

enteric (en-ter'ik) [G. *enterikos,* from *entera,* bowels]. Relating to the intestine.

enteritis (en-ter-ī'tis) [entero- + G. *-itis,* inflammation]. Inflammation of the intestine, especially of the small intestine.
e. anaphylac'tica, chronic anaphylaxis; a hemorrhagic and necrotizing inflammation developing in the ileum (and also the colon) of sensitized dogs when they are fed a second dose of the sensitizing material.
chronic cicatrizing e., regional e.
diphtheritic e., e. with the formation of a membrane or a false membrane. See also pseudomembranous *enterocolitis.*
feline infectious e., panleukopenia.
granulomatous e., regional e.
e. of mink, a highly contagious enteric disease of mink similar to panleukopenia and caused by mink enteritis virus.
mucomembranous e., mucoenteritis (2); an affection of the intestinal mucous membrane characterized by constipation or diarrhea, sometimes alternating, colic, and the passage of pseudomembranous shreds or incomplete casts of the intestine.
e. necrot'icans, e. with necrosis of the bowel wall caused by *Clostridium welchii.*
phlegmonous e., severe acute inflammation of the intestine, with edematous bowel walls that are infiltrated with pus.
e. polypo'sa, e. associated with polyp formation.
pseudomembranous e., pseudomembranous *enterocolitis.*
regional e., Crohn's disease; distal, regional or terminal ileitis; granulomatous or chronic cicatrizing e.; a subacute chronic e., of unknown cause, involving the terminal ileum and less frequently other parts of the gastrointestinal tract; characterized by patchy deep ulcers that may cause fistulas, and narrowing and thickening of the bowel by fibrosis and lymphocytic infiltration, with noncaseating tuberculoid granulomas which may also be found in regional lymph nodes; symptoms include fever, diarrhea, cramping abdominal pain, and weight loss.
transmissible e., bluecomb *disease* of turkeys.
tuberculous e., enteric tuberculosis occurring in the absence of obvious pulmonary t.; may be caused by bovine tuberculosis contracted through drinking of unpasteurized milk.

entero-, enter- [G. *enteron,* intestine]. Combining forms relating to the intestines.

enteroanastomosis (en'ter-ō-an-as-tō-mō'sis). Enteroenterostomy.

enteroanthelone (en-ter-ō-an'thĕ-lōn). Enterogastrone.

enteroapocleisis (en'ter-ō-ap'ō-klī'sis) [entero- + G. *apokleisis,* exclusion, fr. *apo,* from, + *kleiō,* to close]. Exclusion of a segment of the intestine by forming an anastomosis between the parts above and below.

Enterobacter (en'ter-ō-bak'ter). A genus of aerobic, facultatively anaerobic, nonsporeforming, motile bacteria (family Enterobacteriaceae) containing Gram-negative rods. The cells are peritrichous, and some strains have encapsulated cells. Glucose is fermented with the production of acid and gas. The Voges-Proskauer test is usually positive. Gelatin is slowly liquefied by the most commonly occurring forms (*E. cloacae*). These organisms occur in the feces of man and other animals and in sewage, soil, water, and dairy products; occasionally they are found in urine and pus and in other pathologic materials from animals. The type species is *E. cloacae.*
E. aerog'enes, a species found in water, soil, sewage, dairy products, and the feces of man and other animals. Organisms previously identified as motile strains of *Aerobacter aerogenes* are now placed in this species.
E. clo'acae, a species found in the feces of man and other animals and in sewage, soil, and water; it is occasionally found in urine and pus and in other pathologic materials from animals; it is the type species of the genus *E.*

enterobacteria (en'ter-ō-bak-tēr'ē-ă). Plural of enterobacterium.

Enterobacteriaceae (en'ter-ō-bak-tēr-ē-ā'sē-ē). A family of aerobic, facultatively anaerobic, nonsporeforming bacteria (order Eubacteriales) containing Gram-negative rods. Some species are nonmotile, and nonmotile variants of motile species occur; the motile cells are peritrichous. These organisms grow well on artificial media. They reduce nitrates to nitrites and utilize glucose fermentatively with the production of acid or acid and gas. Indophenol oxidase is not produced by these organisms. They do not liquefy alginate, and pectate is liquefied only by members of one genus, *Pectobacterium.* This family includes many animal parasites and some plant parasites causing blights, galls, and soft rots. Some of these organisms occur as saprophytes which decompose carbohydrate-containing plant materials. The type genus is *Escherichia.*

enterobacterium, pl. **enterobacteria** (en'ter-ō-bak-tēr'ē-ŭm, -ă). A member of the family Enterobacteriaceae.

enterobiasis (en'ter-ō-bī'ă-sis). Infection with *Enterobius vermicularis,* the human pinworm.

Enterobius (en-ter-ō'bī-ŭs) [entero- + G. *bios,* life]. A genus of nematode worms, formerly included with the genus *Oxyuris,* which includes the pinworms (*E. vermicularis*) of man and primates.

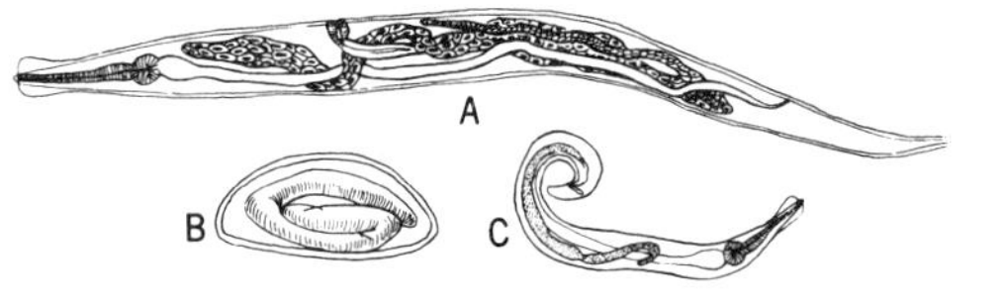

Enterobius vermicularis

A, gravid female; *B,* egg; *C,* male (original magnification, *A* and *C,* ×15; *B,* ×500).

enterobrosis, enterobrosia (en'ter-ō-brō'sis, -brō'zhē-ă) [entero- + G. *brōsis,* corrosion]. Perforation of the intestine.

enterocele (en'ter-o-sēl) **1** [entero- + G. *kēlē,* hernia]. A hernial protrusion through a defect in the rectovaginal or vesicovaginal pouch. **2** [entero- +G. *koilia,* a hollow]. *Cavitas* abdominalis. **3** [see 1]. An intestinal hernia.
partial e., parietal *hernia.*

enterocentesis (en'ter-ō-sen-tē'sis) [entero- + G. *kentēsis,* puncture]. Puncture of the intestine with a hollow needle (trocar and cannula) to withdraw substances.

enterocholecystostomy (en'ter-ō-kō-lē-sis-tos'tō-mē) [entero- + G. *cholē,* bile, + *kystis,* bladder, + *stoma,* mouth]. Cholecystenterostomy.

enterocholecystotomy (en'ter-ō-kō-lē-sis-tot'ō-mē) [entero- + G. *cholē,* bile, + *kystis,* bladder, + *tomē,* a cutting]. Cholecystenterotomy.

enterocleisis (en-ter-ō-klī'sis) [entero- + G. *kleisis,* a closing]. Occlusion of the lumen of the alimentary canal.
omental e., use of omentum to aid closure of an opening in intestine.

enteroclysis (en-ter-ok'li-sis) [entero- + G. *klysis,* a washing out]. High *enema.*

enterococcus, pl. **enterococci** (en'ter-ō-kok'ŭs, -kok'sī) [entero- + G. *kokkos,* a berry]. A streptococcus which inhabits the intestinal tract.

enterocolitis (en'ter-ō-kō-lī'tis) [entero- + G. *kolon,* colon, + *-itis,* inflammation]. Coloenteritis; inflammation of the mucous membrane of a greater or lesser extent of both small and large intestines.
antibiotic e., e. caused by oral administration of broad spectrum antibiotics, resulting from overgrowth of antibiotic-resistant staphylococci or yeasts and fungi, when the normal fecal Gram-negative organisms are suppressed.
necrotizing e., extensive ulceration and necrosis of the ileum and colon in premature infants in the neonatal period; possibly due to perinatal intestinal ischemia and bacterial invasion.
pseudomembranous e., pseudomembranous colitis or enteritis; e. with the formation and passage of pseudomembranous material in the stools; occurs most commonly as a sequel to antibiotic therapy.
regional e., the changes of regional enteritis involving both the colon and the small intestine.

enterocolostomy (en'ter-ō-kō-los'tō-mē) [entero- + G. *kōlon,* colon, + *stoma,* mouth]. Establishment of an artificial opening between the small intestine and the colon.

enterocyst (en'ter-ō-sist) [entero- + G. *kystis,* bladder]. Enterocystoma; a cyst of the wall of the intestine.

enterocystocele (en'ter-ō-sis'tō-sēl) [entero- + G. *kystis,* bladder, + *kēlē,* hernia]. A hernia of both intestine and bladder wall.

enterocystoma (en'ter-ō-sis-tō'mă). Enterocyst.

enterodynia (en'ter-ō-din'ē-ă) [entero- + G. *odynē,* pain]. Enteralgia.

enteroenterostomy (en'ter-ō-en-ter-os'tō-mē). Enteroanastomosis; intestinal anastomosis; establishment of a new communication between two segments of intestine.

enterogastritis (en'ter-ō-gas-trī'tis) [entero- + G. *gastēr,* belly, + *-itis,* inflammation]. Gastroenteritis.

enterogastrone (en'ter-ō-gas'trōn). Anthelone E; enteroanthelone; a hormone, obtained from intestinal mucosa, that inhibits gastric secretion and motility; secretion of e. is stimulated by exposure of duodenal mucosa to dietary lipids.

enterogenous (en-ter-oj'ĕ-nŭs) [entero- + G. *-gen,* producing]. Of intestinal origin.

enterograph (en'ter-ō-graf). An instrument designed for use in enterography.

enterography (en-ter-og'ră-fē) [entero- + G. *graphō,* to write]. The making of a graphic record delineating the intestinal muscular activity.

enterohepatitis (en'ter-ō-hep-ă-tī'tis) [entero- + G. *hēpar* (*hēpat-*), liver, + *-itis,* inflammation]. Inflammation of both the intestine and the liver.
infectious e., histomoniasis.

enterohepatocele (en'ter-ō-hep'ă-tō-sēl) [entero- + G. *hēpar* (*hēpat-*), liver, + *kēlē,* hernia]. Congenital umbilical hernia containing intestine and liver.

enteroidea (en-ter-oy'dē-ă) [entero- + G. *eidos,* resemblance]. Fevers due to infection caused by any of the intestinal bacteria, including the enteric fevers (typhoid and paratyphoid A and B) and the parenteric fevers.

enterokinase (en'tĕr-ō-kī'nās). Enteropeptidase.

enterokinesis (en'ter-ō-ki-nē'sis) [entero- + G. *kinēsis,* movement]. Muscular contraction of the alimentary canal. See also peristalsis.

enterokinetic (en'ter-ō-ki-net'ik). Relating to, or producing, enterokinesis.

enterolith (en'ter-ō-lith) [entero- + G. *lithos,* stone]. An intestinal calculus formed of layers of soaps and earthy phosphates surrounding a nucleus of some hard body such as a swallowed fruit stone or other indigestible substance.

enterolithiasis (en'ter-ō-li-thī'ă-sis). Presence of calculi in the intestine.

enterology (en-ter-ol'ō-jē) [entero- + G. *logos,* study]. The branch of medical science concerned especially with the intestinal tract.

enterolysis (en-ter-ol'i-sis) [entero- + G. *lysis,* dissolution]. Division of intestinal adhesions.

enteromegaly, enteromegalia (en-ter-ō-meg'ă-lē, -ō-me-gā'lē-ă) [entero- + G. *megas,* great]. Megaloenteron.

enteromenia (en-ter-ō-mē'nē-ă) [entero- + G. *emmēnos,* monthly]. Vicarious menstruation in the intestine.

enteromerocele (en'ter-ō-mēr'ō-sēl) [entero- + G. *mēros,* thigh, + *kēlē,* hernia]. Femoral *hernia.*

enterometer (en-ter-om'ĕ-ter) [entero- + G. *metron,* measure]. An instrument used in measuring the diameter of the intestine.

Enteromonas (en'ter-ō-mō'nas, en-ter-om'ō-nas) [entero- + G. *monas,* monad]. A genus of flagellate protozoa, one species of which, *E. hominis,* is found as a rare nonpathogenic resident in the human large intestine.

enteromycosis (en'ter-ō-mī-kō'sis) [entero- + G. *mykēs,* fungus, + *-osis,* condition]. An intestinal disease of fungal origin.

enteronitis (en'ter-ō-nī'tis) [entero- + G. *-itis,* inflammation]. Obsolete term for enteritis.

enteroparesis (en'ter-ō-pă-rē'sis, -par'i-sis) [entero- + G. *paresis,* slackening, relaxation]. A state of diminished or absent peristalsis with flaccidity of the muscles of the intestinal walls.

enteropathogen (en'ter-ō-path'ō-jen). An organism capable of producing disease in the intestinal tract.

enteropathogenic (en'ter-ō-path-ō-jen'ik). Capable of producing disease in the intestinal tract.

enteropathy (en-ter-op'ă-thē) [entero- + G. *pathos,* suffering]. An intestinal disease.
gluten e., celiac *disease.*
protein-losing e., increased fecal loss of serum protein, especially albumin, causing hypoproteinemia.

enteropeptidase (en'ter-ō-pep'ti-dās) [EC 3.4.21.9]. Enterokinase; an intestinal proteolytic enzyme from the duodenal mucosa that converts trypsinogen into trypsin.

enteropexy (en'ter-ō-pek-sē). [entero- + G. *pēxis,* fixation]. Fixation of a segment of the intestine to the abdominal wall.

enteroplasty (en'ter-ō-plas-tē) [entero- + G. *plastos,* formed]. Plastic surgery of the intestine.

enteroplegia (en'ter-ō-plē'jē-ă) [entero- + G. *plēgē,* stroke]. Rarely used term for adynamic *ileus.*

enteroplex (en-ter-ō-pleks). An instrument for use in effecting union of the divided ends of the intestine.

enteroplexy (en'ter-ō-plek-sē) [entero- + G. *plexis,* weaving]. Joining the divided ends of the intestine.

enteroproctia (en'ter-ō-prok'shē-ă) [entero- + G. *prōktos,* anus]. The presence of an artifical anus, as by a colostomy.

enteroptosis, enteroptosia (en'ter-ō-tō'sis, -tō'sē-ă) [entero- + G. *ptōsis,* a falling]. Abnormal descent of the intestines in the abdominal cavity, usually associated with falling of the other viscera.

enteroptotic (en'ter-ō-tot'ik). Relating to or suffering from enteroptosis.

enterorenal (en'ter-ō-rē'năl). Relating to both the intestines and the kidneys.

enterorrhagia (en-ter-ō-rā'jē-ă) [entero- + G. *rhēgnymi,* to burst forth]. Intestinal hemorrhage; bleeding within the intestinal tract.

enterorrhaphy (en-ter-ōr'ă-fē) [entero- + G. *rhaphē,* suture]. Suture of the intestine.

enterorrhexis (en'ter-ō-rek'sis) [entero- + G. *rhēxis,* rupture]. Rupture of the gut or bowel.

enteroscope (en'ter-ō-skōp) [entero- + G. *skopeō,* to view]. A speculum for inspecting the inside of the intestine in operative cases.

enterosepsis (en'ter-ō-sep'sis) [entero- + G. *sēpsis,* putrefaction]. Sepsis occurring in or derived from the alimentary canal.

enterospasm (en'ter-ō-spazm) [entero- + G. *spasmos,* spasm]. Increased, irregular, and painful peristalsis.

enterostasis (en-ter-os'tă-sis) [entero- + G. *stasis,* a standing]. Intestinal stasis; a retardation or arrest of the passage of the intestinal contents.

enterostaxis (en'ter-ō-stak'sis) [entero- + G. *staxis,* a dripping]. Oozing of blood from the mucous membrane of the intestine.

enterostenosis (en'ter-ō-sten-ō'sis) [entero- + G. *stenōsis,* narrowing]. Narrowing of the lumen of the intestine.

enterostomy (en-ter-os'tō-mē) [entero- + G. *stoma,* mouth]. An artificial anus or fistula into the intestine through the abdominal wall.
double e., e. in which both proximal and distal openings of divided intestine are sutured to the abdomen wall.

enterotome (en'ter-ō-tōm) [entero- + G. *tomē,* a cutting]. An instrument for incising the intestine, especially in the creation of an artificial anus.

enterotomy (en-ter-ot'ō-mē). Incision into the intestine.

enterotoxemia (en'ter-ō-tok-sē'mē-ă) [entero- + toxemia]. Pulpy kidney disease; milk colic; acute, highly fatal diseases, chiefly of cattle and sheep, caused by toxins produced in the intestine by various types of *Clostridium perfringens.*

enterotoxication (en'ter-ō-tok-si-kā'shŭn). Autointoxication.

enterotoxigenic (en'ter-ō-tok-si-jen'ik). Denoting an organism containing or producing a toxin specific for cells of the intestinal mucosa.

enterotoxin (en'ter-ō-tok'sin). Intestinotoxin; a cytotoxin specific for the cells of the intestinal mucosa.
cytotonic e., an e. which morphologically changes, but does not kill, the target cell.
Escherichia coli e., e. produced by certain strains (serotypes) of *Escherichia coli,* seemingly associated with a transferable plasmid.
staphylococcal e., a soluble exotoxin produced by some strains of *Staphylococcus aureus,* and a cause of food poisoning.

enterotoxism (en'ter-ō-tok'sizm). Autointoxication.

enterotropic (en'ter-ō-trop'ik) [entero- + G. *tropikos,* turning]. Attracted by or affecting the intestine.

Enterovirus (en'ter-ō-vī'rŭs). A genus of viruses (family Picornaviridae) that includes poliovirus types 1 to 3, Coxsackievirus A and B, echoviruses, and the enteroviruses identified since 1969 and assigned type numbers. They are transient inhabitants of the alimentary canal and are stable at pH 3.0 to 5.0 for 1 to 3 hours.

enterozoic (en'ter-ō-zō'ik). Relating to an enterozoon.

enterozoon (en'ter-ō-zō'on) [entero- + G. *zōon,* animal]. An animal parasite in the intestine.

enthalpy (en'thal-pē) [G. *enthalpein,* to warm in]. Heat content, symbolized as H; a thermodynamic function, defined as $E + PV$, where E is the internal energy of a system, P the pressure, and V the volume.

enthesis (en'thĕ-sis) [G. an insertion, fr. *en,* in, + *thesis,* a placing]. Rarely used term for the insertion of synthetic or other inorganic material to replace lost tissue.

enthesitis (en-thĕ-sī'tis) [G. *enthetos,* implanted, + *-itis,* inflammation]. Traumatic disease occurring at the insertion of muscles where recurring concentration of muscle stress provokes inflammation with a strong tendency toward fibrosis and calcification.

enthesopathic (en-thē-sō-path'ik). Denoting or characteristic of enthesopathy.

enthesopathy (en-thē-sop'ă-thē) [G. *en,* in, + *thesis,* a placing, + *pathos,* suffering]. A disease process occurring at the site of insertion of muscle tendons and ligaments into bones or joint capsules.

enthetic (en-thet'ik). **1.** Rarely used term denoting enthesis. **2.** Exogenous.

enthlasis (en'thlă-sis) [G. a dent, fr. *en,* in, + *thlaō,* to crush]. Depressed fracture of the skull.

en thyrse (ahn tirs') [Fr., fr. G. *en-,* in, + *thyrsos,* a stalk, wand]. Microconidia of certain dermatophytes arranged singly along both sides of a hypha.

entire (en-tīr'). Having a smoothly continuous edge or border without indentations or projections; denoting a margin, as of a bacterial colony.

entity (en'ti-tē) [L. *ens (ent-),* being, pres. p. of *esse,* to be]. An independent thing; that which contains in itself all the conditions essential to individuality; that which forms of itself a complete whole; denoting a separate and distinct disease or condition.

ento-, ent- [G. *entos,* within]. Prefixes meaning inner, or within. See also endo-.

entoblast (en'tō-blast) [ento- + G. *blastos,* germ]. Endoblast.

entocele (en'tō-sēl) [ento- + G. *kēlē,* hernia]. An internal hernia.

entochoroidea (en'tō-kō-roy'dē-ă) [ento- + G. *chorioeidēs,* choroid]. *Lamina* choroidocapillaris.

entocone (en-tō-kōn) [ento- + G. *kōnos,* cone]. The mesiolingual cusp of a maxillary molar tooth.

entoconid (en-tō-kō'nid) [ento- + G. *kōnos,* cone]. The inner posterior cusp of a mandibular molar tooth.

entocornea (en-tō-kōr'nē-ă). *Lamina* limitans posterior corneae.

entocranial (en'tō-krā'nē-ăl). Endocranial.

entocranium (en'tō-krā'nē-ŭm). Endocranium.

entoderm (en'tō-derm) [ento- + G. *derma,* skin]. Endoderm.

entoectad (en-tō-ek'tad) [G. *entos,* within, + *ektos,* without, + L. *ad,* to]. From within outward.

Entoloma sinuatum (en-tō-lō'mă sī-nyū-ā'tum). A species of mushroom capable of producing mycetismus gastrointestinalis.

entomion (en-tō'mē-on) [G. *entomē,* notch]. The tip of the mastoid angle of the parietal bone.

entomology (en-tō-mol'ō-jē) [G. *entomon,* insect, + *logos,* study]. The science concerned with the study of insects.

entomophobia (en'tō-mō-fō'bē-ă) [G. *entomon,* insect, + *phobos,* fear]. Morbid fear of insects.

Entomophthora (en-tō-mof'thō-ră) [G. *entomē,* insect, + *phthora,* destruction]. A genus of fungi (family Entomophthorales) that are parasitic on insects. Several species are currently used in the control of pests on fruits and vegetable crops in place of, or in conjunction with, chemical pesticides. One species, *E. coronata,* can also cause nasal polyps in horses and entomophthoramycosis conidiobolae in humans.

entomophthoramycosis (en-tō-mof'thō-ră-mī-kō'sis). Rhinomucormycosis; rhinophycomycosis; a disease caused by fungi of the genus *Entomopthora;* tissues are invaded by broad nonseptate hyphae which become surrounded by eosinophilic material.
e. basidiobo'lae, a subcutaneous zygomycosis due to the fungus *Basidiobolus haptosporus,* characterized by the development of flat, firm subcutaneous granulomas which do not ulcerate; occa-

sionally, lesions may extend to muscles and lymph nodes and other deep tissues; the disease is found in Indonesia and in Uganda and other tropical African countries, but has not been seen in tropical America.

e. conidiobo'lae, a zygomycosis caused by *Conidiobolus coronatus* which is seen in horses but may be transmitted to man, or by *Entomophthora coronata* in humans, characterized by large nasal polyps and granulomas of the nasal cavity; it has been reported from Texas, the West Indies, the Congo, Nigeria, and other African states, Colombia, and Brazil.

Entomopoxvirus (en'tō-mō-poks-vī'rŭs) [G. *entomon,* insect]. The genus of viruses (family Poxviridae) that comprises the poxviruses of insects; they seem not to multiply in vertebrates.

entopic (en-top'ik) [G. *en,* within, + *topos,* place]. Placed within; occurring or situated in the normal place; opposed to ectopic.

entoplasm (en'tō-plasm). Endoplasm.

entoptic (en-top'tik) [ento- + G. *optikos,* relating to vision]. Within the eyeball.

entoretina (en-tō-ret'i-nă). Henle's nervous layer; the layers of the retina from the outer plexiform to the nerve fiber layer inclusive.

entosarc (en'tō-sark). Endosarc.

Entozoa (en-tō-zō'ă) [ento- + G. *zōon,* animal]. A nontaxonomic name for the branch of the kingdom Animalia, whose members possess a digestive cavity or tract; includes all vertebrates and higher invertebrate forms.

entozoal (en-tō-zō'ăl). Relating to entozoa.

entozoon, pl. **entozoa** (en-tō-zō'on, -ă) [ento- + G. *zōon,* animal]. An animal parasite whose habitat is any of the internal organs or tissues.

entrails (en'trālz). The viscera of an animal.

entropion, entropium (en-trō'pē-on, -pē-ŭm) [G. *en,* in, + *tropē,* a turning]. **1.** Inversion or turning inward of a part. **2.** Enstrophe; the infolding of the margin of an eyelid.

atonic e., e. that follows loss of tone of the orbicularis oculi muscle or elasticity of the skin.

cicatricial e., e. that follows scarring of the palpebral conjunctiva.

spastic e., e. that arises from excessive contracture of the orbicularis oculi muscle.

entropionize (en-trō'pē-on-īz). To invert a part.

entropy (en'trō-pē) [G. *entropia,* a turning towards]. That fraction of heat (energy) content not available for the performance of work, usually because (in a chemical reaction) it has been used to increase the random motion of the atoms or molecules in the system; thus, e. is a measure of randomness or disorder. E. occurs in the free energy (F) equation: $F = H - TS$ (H, enthalpy or heat content; T, absolute temperature; S, entropy) which, applied to the free energy available in a reaction at a given temperature (ΔF), becomes $\Delta F = \Delta H - T\Delta S$; at equilibrium, $\Delta H = T\Delta S$. See also second *law* of thermodynamics.

entypy (en'ti-pē) [G. *entypē,* pattern]. The condition in an early mammalian embryo in which the endoderm covers the embryonic and amniotic ectoderm; part of the preplacental trophoblast may also be covered.

enucleate (ē-nū'klē-āt). To remove entirely; to shell like a nut, as in the removal of an eye from its capsule or a tumor from its enveloping capsule.

enucleation (ē-nū-klē-ā'shŭn) [L. *enucleo,* to remove the kernel, fr. *e,* out, + *nucleus,* nut, kernel]. **1.** Removal of an entire structure (such as an eyeball or tumor), without rupture, as one shells the kernel of a nut. **2.** Removal or destruction of the nucleus of a cell.

enuresis (en-yū-rē'sis) [G. *en-oureō,* to urinate in]. Involuntary loss of urine.

nocturnal e., bed-wetting; incontinence during sleep.

envelope (en'vĕ-lōp). In anatomy, a structure that encloses or covers.

corneocyte e., subplasmalemmal dense zone; an electron-dense, 10-15 nm thick layer of highly cross-linked protein on the cytoplasmic surface of the cell membrane of epidermal corneocytes; it is highly resistant to proteolytic agents.

nuclear e., nuclear membrane; karyotheca; caryotheca; the double membrane at the boundary of the nucleoplasm; it has regularly spaced pores covered by a disklike nuclear pore complex and a space or cisterna about 150 Å wide between the two layers; the outer membrane is continuous at intervals with the endoplasmic reticulum.

viral e., the outer structure that encloses the nucleocapsids of some viruses.

envenomation (en-ven-ō-mā'shŭn). The act of injecting a poisonous material (venom) by sting, spine, bite, or other venom apparatus.

environment (en-vī'ron-ment) [Fr. *environ,* around]. The milieu; the aggregate of all of the external conditions and influences affecting the life and development of an organism.

envy (en'vē). One's feeling of discontent or jealousy resulting from comparison with another person.

penis e., the psychoanalytic concept in which a female envies male characteristics or capabilities, especially the possession of a penis.

enzootic (en-zō-ot'ik) [G. *en,* in, + *zōon,* animal]. Endemic (2); denoting a disease of animals which is indigenous to a certain locality; more precisely, the temporal pattern of occurrence of a disease in a population of animals which has a predictable regularity with only minor changes in its incidence with time. *Cf.* epizootic, sporadic.

enzygotic (en-zī-got'ik) [G. *eis* (*en*), one, + zygote]. Derived from a single fertilized ovum; denoting twins so derived.

enzymatic (en-zī-mat'ik). Enzymic; relating to an enzyme.

enzyme (en'zīm) [G. en, in, + *zymē,* leaven]. Organic catalyst; a protein, secreted by cells, that acts as a catalyst to induce chemical changes in other substances, itself remaining apparently unchanged by the process. E.'s, with the exception of those discovered long ago (*e.g.,* pepsin, emulsin), are generally named by adding -ase to the name of the substrate on which the e. acts (*e.g.,* glucosidase), the substance activated (*e.g.,* hydrogenase), and/or the type of reaction (*e.g.,* oxidoreductase, transferase, hydrolase, lyase, isomerase, ligase or synthetase—these being the six main groups in the Enzyme Nomenclature Recommendations of the International Union of Biochemistry). For individual enzymes not listed below, see the specific name.

acetyl-activating e., acetate-CoA ligase.

acyl-activating e., **(1)** long-chain fatty acid–CoA ligase; **(2)** butyrate-CoA ligase.

adaptive e., induced e.

angiotensin-converting e., peptidyl dipeptidase A.

autolytic e., an e. capable of causing lysis of the cell forming it.

branching e., 1,4-α- glucan branching enzyme.

β-carotene cleavage e., β-carotene 15,15′-dioxygenase.

condensing e., *citrate* synthase.

D e., 4-α-D-glucanotransferase.

deamidizing e.'s, amidohydrolases.

deaminating e.'s, deaminases.

debranching e.'s, debranching factors; e.'s that bring about destruction of branches in glycogen; formerly considered to be one enzyme, now known to be a mixture of transferases (4-α-D-glucanotransferase) and hydrolases (amylo-1,6-glucosidase).

disproportionating e., 4-α-D-glucanotransferase.

extracellular e., exoenzyme; lyoenzyme; an e. performing its functions outside a cell; *e.g.,* the various digestive e.'s.

hydrolyzing e.'s, hydrolases.

induced e., inducible e., adaptive e.; an e. that can be detected in a growing culture of a microorganism, after the addition of a particular substance (inducer) to the culture medium, but was not detectable prior to the addition and can act on the inducer. A prototype is the β-galactosidase of *Escherichia coli,* synthesized upon the addition of various galactosides, whether or not these are good substrates.

intracellular e., endoenzyme; an e. that performs its functions within the cell that produces it; most e.'s are intracellular e.'s.

malate-condensing e., malate synthase.

malic e., malate dehydrogenase.

methionine-activating e., *methionine* adenosyltransferase.

new yellow e. [EC 1.4.3.3], D-amino-acid oxidase, a flavoenzyme found in yeast, which contains FAD as coenzyme instead of FMN as does NADPH dehydrogenase; so-called to distinguish it from Warburg's old yellow e.

old yellow e., NADPH dehydrogenase.

P e., phosphorylase.

pantoate-activating e., *pantothenate* synthetase.

phosphorylase-rupturing e., *phosphorylase* phosphate.

photoreactivating e., deoxyribodipyrimidine photolyase.

PR e., **(1)** phosphorylase-rupturing e. (see phosphorylase phosphatase); **(2)** photoreactivating e. (see deoxyribodipyrimidine photolyase).

Q e., 1,4-α-glucan branching e. in plants.

R e., α-dextrin endo-1,6-α-glucosidase.

reducing e., reductase.

repressible e., an e. that is produced continuously unless production is repressed by excess of a product (corepressor). See also inactive *repressor.*

respiratory e., one of those e.'s in tissues that is a part of an oxidation-reduction system accomplishing the conversion of substrates to CO_2 and H_2O and the transfer of the electrons removed to O_2.

restriction e., restriction *endonuclease.*

Schardinger e., *xanthine* oxidase.

splitting e.'s, e.'s that, like aldolases, catalyze the conversion of a molecule into two smaller molecules without the addition or subtraction of any atoms.

T e., 1,4-α-D-glucan 6-α-D-glucosyltransferase.

terminal addition e., DNA nucleotidylexotransferase.

transferring e.'s, transferases.

Warburg's old yellow e., NADPH dehydrogenase.

Warburg's respiratory e., Atmungsferment.

Enzyme Commission. See EC.

enzymic (en-zī'mik). Enzymatic.

enzymologist (en-zī-mol'ō-jist). Zymologist; a specialist in enzymology.

enzymology (en-zī-mol'ō-jē) [enzyme + G. *logos,* study]. Zymology; the branch of chemistry concerned with the properties and actions of enzymes.

enzymolysis (en-zī-mol'i-sis) [enzyme + G. *lysis,* dissolution]. **1.** The splitting or cleavage of a substance into smaller parts by means of enzymatic action. **2.** Lysis by the action of an enzyme.

enzymopathy (en-zī-mop'ă-thē) [enzyme + G. *pathos,* disease]. Any disturbance of enzyme function, including genetic deficiency of specific enzymes.

enzymosis (en-zī-mō'sis) [enzyme + G. *-osis,* condition]. Obsolete term for fermentation (enzymic digestion).

EOG Abbreviation for electro-oculography; electro-olfactogram.

eosin (ē'ō-sin) [G. *ēōs,* dawn]. A derivative of fluorescein used as a fluorescent acid dye for cytoplasmic stains and counterstains in histology and in Romanovsky-type blood stains.

alcohol-soluble e., *ethyl* eosin.

e. B [C.I. 45400], e. I bluish; acid red 91; the disodium salt of 4',5'-dibromo-2',7'-dinitrofluorescein.

ethyl e., see under ethyl.

e. I bluish, e. B.

e. y, e. Ys [C.I. 45380], e. yellowish; acid red 87; the disodium salt of 2',4',5',7'-tetrabromofluorescein.

e. yellowish, e. Y.

eosinocyte (ē-ō-sin'ō-sīt). Eosinophilic *leukocyte.*

eosinopenia (ē'ō-sin-ō-pē'nē-ă) [eosino(phil) + G. *penia,* poverty]. Hypoeosinophilia; the presence of eosinophils in an abnormally small number in the peripheral bloodstream.

eosinophil, eosinophile (ē-ō-sin'ō-fil, -fīl) [eosin + G. *philos,* fond]. Eosinophilic *leukocyte.*

eosinophilia (ē'ō-sin-ō-fil'ē-ă). Eosinophilic *leukocytosis.*

simple pulmonary e., Löffler's syndrome (1); pulmonary infiltrates seen as transient migratory shadows on the chest x-ray, accompanied by blood e.; often symptomless, but there may be cough, fever, and breathlessness; most cases are due to worm infestation, especially by *Ascaris lumbricoides;* a few cases follow administration of drugs.

tropical e., e. associated with cough and asthma, caused by occult filarial infection without evidence of microfilaremia, occurring most frequently in India and Southeast Asia.

eosinophilic (ē-ō-sin-ō-fil'ik). Staining readily with eosin dyes; denoting such cell or tissue elements.

eosinophiluria (ē-ō-sin'ō-fil-yū'rē-ă). Presence of eosinophils in the urine.

eosinotactic (ē'ō-sin-ō-tak'tik) [eosino(phile) + G. *taktikos,* in orderly arrangement]. Exerting a force of attraction or repulsion on eosinophile cells.

eosinotaxis (ē'ō-sin-ō-tak'sis). Movement of eosinophils with reference to a stimulus which attracts or repels them.

eosophobia (ē-ō-sō-fō'bē-ă) [G. *ēōs,* dawn, + *phobos,* fear]. Morbid dread of the dawn.

epactal (ē-pak'tăl) [G. *epaktos,* imported, fr. *epagō,* to bring on or in]. Supernumerary.

epamniotic (ep'am-nē-ot'ik) [G. *epi,* upon, + amnion]. Upon or above the amnion.

eparsalgia (ep-ar-sal'jē-ă) [G. *epairo,* to lift up, + *algos,* pain]. Epersalgia; pain and soreness from overuse or unaccustomed use of a part, as a joint or muscle.

eparterial (ep'ar-tēr-ē-ăl) [G. *epi,* upon, + *artēia,* artery]. Upon or over an artery.

epaxial (ep-ak'sē-ăl) [G. *epi,* upon, + L. *axis,* axis]. Above or behind any axis, such as the spinal axis or the axis of a limb.

ependyma (ep-en'di-mă) [G. *ependyma,* an upper garment] [NA]. Endyma; the cellular membrane lining the central canal of the spinal cord and the brain ventricles.

ependymal (ep-en'di-măl). Relating to the ependyma.

ependymitis (ep-en-di-mī'tis). Inflammation of the ependyma.

ependymoblast (ep-en'di-mō-blast) [ependyma + G. *blastos,* germ]. An embryonic ependymal cell.

ependymoblastoma (ep-en'di-mō-blas-tō'mă) [ependymoblast + G. *-ōma,* tumor]. A glial neoplasm of the central nervous system, occurring typically in childhood; the prototype tumor cells resemble ependymoblasts.

ependymocyte (ep-en'di-mō-sīt) [ependyma + G. *kytos,* cell]. An ependymal cell.

ependymoma (ep-en-di-mō'mă). A glioma derived from relatively undifferentiated ependymal cells, comprising approximately 1 to 3% of all intracranial neoplasms; e.'s occur in all age groups and may originate from the lining of any of the ventricles or, more commonly, from the central canal of the spinal cord; histologically, the neoplastic cells tend to be arranged radially about blood vessels, to

which they are attached by means of fibrillary processes.
myxopapillary e., a slow-growing e. of the filum terminale, occurring most often in young adults, consisting of cuboidal cells in papillary arrangement around a mucinous vascular core.

epersalgia (ep-er-sal'jē-ă). Eparsalgia.

Eperythrozoon (ep'ĕ-rith'rō-zō'on) [G. *epi,* upon + *erythros,* red, + *zōon,* animal]. A genus of minute, rickettsia-like bacterial parasites (family Bartonellaceae, order Rickettsiales) of animals occurring upon the surface of erythrocytes and in the plasma; they appear as rings, coccoids, and short rods when clustered on the surface of the red cells in stained films. Some species cause anemia and icterus.
E. coccoi'des, a species present in mice, but usually requiring splenectomy to reveal infections; rats and hamsters may be artificially infected; bloodsucking arthropods, especially lice, have been implicated as biological vectors, and mechanical transmission by bloodsucking flies has been demonstrated; the pathogenic effect is slight except when combined with other disease-producing agents.
E. o'vis, a species rarely causing disease in sheep.
E. su'is, a species that produces icterus and anemia in young pigs and icteroanemia of swine.
E. wenyo'ni, a species rarely causing disease in cattle.

eperythrozoonosis (ep'ĕ-rith'rō-zō-ō-nō'sis). Infection with any species of *Eperythrozoon.*

ephapse (ef'aps) [G. *ephapsis,* contact]. A place where two or more nerve cell processes (axons, dendrites) touch without forming a typical synaptic contact; the possibility of some form of neural transmission at such nonsynaptic contact sites has often been suggested.

ephaptic (e-fap'tik). Relating to an ephapse.

ephebiatrics (ĕ-fē'bē-at'riks) [G. *ephebos,* Athenian youth of military age]. Adolescent *medicine.*

ephebic (ĕ-fē'bik) [G. *ephēbikos,* relating to youth, fr. *hēbē,* youth]. Rarely used term relating to the period of puberty or to a youth.

ephebology (ef-ĕ-bol'ō-jē) [G. *ephēbos,* puberty, + *logos,* study]. Rarely used term for the study of the morphologic and other changes incidental to puberty.

ephedrine (ĕ-fed'rin, ef'ĕ-drin). 2-Methylamino-1-phenyl-1-propanol; an alkaloid from the leaves of *Ephedra equisetina, E. sinica,* and other species (family Gnetaceae), or produced synthetically; an adrenergic (sympathomimetic) agent with actions similar to those of epinephrine; used as a bronchodilator, mydriatic, pressor agent, and topical vasoconstrictor. Generally used salts are e. hydrochloride and e. sulfate.

ephelis, pl. **ephelides** (ef-ē'lis, ef-ē'li-dēz) [G.]. Freckle.

epi-. G. preposition, used as a prefix, meaning upon, following, or subsequent to.

epiandrosterone (ep'i-an-dros'ter-ōn). Isoandrosterone; 3β-hydroxy-5α-androstan-17-one; inactive isomer (3β instead of 3α) of androsterone; found in urine and in testicular and ovarian tissue.

epiblast (ep'i-blast) [epi- + G. *blastos,* germ]. A potential ectoderm.

epiblastic (ep-i-blas'tik). Relating to epiblast.

epiblepharon (ep'i-blef'ă-ron) [epi- + G. *blepharon,* eyelid]. A congenital horizontal skin fold near the margin of the eyelid, due to abnormal insertion of muscle fibers. In the upper lid, it simulates blepharochalasis; in the lower lid, it causes a turning inward of the lashes.

epiboly, epibole (ē-pib'ō-lē) [G. *epibolē,* a throwing or laying on]. **1.** A process involved in gastrulation of telolecithal eggs in which, as a result of differential growth, some of the cells of the protoderm move over the surface toward the lips of the blastopore. **2.** Growth of epithelium in an organ culture to surround the underlying mesenchymal tissue.

epibulbar (ep-i-bŭl'bar). Upon a bulb of any kind; specifically, upon the eyeball.

epicanthus (ep-i-kan'thŭs) [epi- + G. *kanthos,* canthus]. *Plica* palpebronasalis.
e. inver'sus, a crescentic upward fold of skin from the lower eyelid at the inner canthus; frequent in congenital blepharoptosis.
e. palpebra'lis, e. arising from the upper lid above the tarsal portion and extending to the lower portion of the orbit.
e. supracilia'ris, e. arising from the region of the eyebrows and extending toward the tear sac.
e. tarsa'lis, e. arising from the tarsal fold and disappearing in the skin close to the inner canthus.

epicardia (ep-i-kar'dē-ă) [epi- + G. *kardia,* heart]. The portion of the esophagus from where it passes through the diaphragm to the stomach.

epicardial (ep-i-kar'dē-ăl). **1.** Relating to the epicardia. **2.** Relating to the epicardium.

epicardium (ep-i-kar'dē-ŭm) [epi- + G. *kardia,* heart]. [NA]. *Lamina* visceralis (1).

epichordal (ep-i-kōr'dăl) [epi- + G. *chordē,* a chord]. On the dorsal side of the notochord; applicable particularly to that part of the brain developing dorsal to the cephalic part of the notochord.

epicomus (ep-i-kō'mŭs, ē-pik'ō-mŭs) [epi- + G. *komē,* hair of the head]. Unequal conjoined twins in which the smaller parasite is joined to the larger autosite at the occiput.

epicondylalgia (ep'i-kon-di-lal'jē-ă) [epicondyle + G. *algos,* pain]. Pain in an epicondyle of the humerus or in the tendons or muscles originating therefrom.
e. exter'na, tennis *elbow.*

epicondyle (ep-i-kon'dīl) [epi- + G. *kondylos,* a knuckle]. Epicondylus.
lateral e., *epicondylus* lateralis.
lateral e. of femur, *epicondylus* lateralis ossis femoris.
lateral e. of humerus, *epicondylus* lateralis humeri.
medial e., *epicondylus* medialis.
medial e. of femur, *epicondylus* medialis ossis femoris.
medial e. of humerus, *epicondylus* medialis humeri.

epicondyli (ep-i-kon'di-lī). Plural of epicondylus.

epicondylian (ep-i-kon-dil'ē-an). Epicondylic.

epicondylic (ep-i-kon-dil'ik). Epicondylian; relating to an epicondyle or to the part above a condyle.

epicondylitis (ep'i-kon-di-lī'tis). Infection or inflammation of an epicondyle.
lateral humeral e., tennis *elbow.*

epicondylus, pl. **epicondyli** (ep-i-kon'di-lŭs, -lī) [L.] [NA]. Epicondyle; a projection from a long bone near the articular extremity above or upon the condyle.
e. latera'lis [NA], lateral epicondyle; **e. l. hu'meri,** lateral epicondyle of humerus; the e. situated at the lateral side of the distal end of the bone; **e. l. os'sis fem'oris,** lateral epicondyle of femur; lateral femoral tuberosity; the e. located proximal to the lateral condyle.
e. media'lis [NA], medial epicondyle; **e. m. hu'meri,** medial epicondyle of humerus; epitrochlea; the e. situated proximal and medial to the condyle; **e. m. os'sis fem'oris,** medial epicondyle of femur; medial femoral tuberosity; the e. located proximal to the medial condyle.

epicoracoid (ep-i-kōr'ă-koyd). Upon or above the coracoid process.

epicorneascleritis (ep-i-kōr'nē-ă-skle-rī'tis). A superficial transient inflammatory infection of the cornea and sclera.

epicranium (ep-i-krā'nē-ŭm) [epi- + G. *kranion,* skull]. The muscle, aponeurosis, and skin covering the cranium.

epicrisis (ep-i-krī'sis). A secondary crisis; a crisis terminating a recrudescence of morbid symptoms following a primary crisis.

epicritic (ep-i-krit'ik) [G. *epikritikos,* adjudicatory, fr. *epi,* on, + *krinō,* to separate, judge]. That aspect of somatic sensation which permits the discrimination and the topographical localization of the finer degrees of touch and temperature stimuli. *Cf.* protopathic.

epicystitis (ep'i-sis-tī'tis) [epi- + G. *kystis,* bladder, + *-itis,* inflammation]. Inflammation of the cellular tissue around the bladder.

epicystotomy (ep'i-sis-tot'ō-mē) [epi- + G. *kystis,* bladder, + *tomē,* incision]. Suprapubic *cystotomy.*

epicyte (ep'i-sīt) [epi- + G. *kytos,* cell]. A cell membrane, especially of protozoa; the external layer of cytoplasm in gregarines.

epidemic (ep-i-dem'ik) [epi- + G. *dēmos,* the people]. **1.** A disease whose frequency of occurrence is in excess of the expected frequency in a population during a given time interval; distinguished from endemic, since the disease is not continuously present but has been introduced from outside. **2.** A temporary increase in number of cases of an endemic disease.

point e., an e. where a pronounced clustering of cases of disease occurs within a very short period of time (within a few days or even hours) due to exposure of persons or animals to a common source of infection such as food or water.

epidemicity (ep'i-dem-is'i-tē). The state of prevailing disease in epidemic form.

epidemiography (ep'i-dem-ē-og'ră-fē) [G. *epidēmios,* epidemic, + *graphē,* a writing]. A descriptive treatise of epidemic diseases or of any particular epidemic.

epidemiologist (ep'i-dē-mē-ol'ō-jist). One who specializes in epidemiology.

epidemiology (ep-i-dē-mē-ol'ō-jē) [G. *epidēmios,* epidemic, + *logos,* study]. The study of the relationships between the various factors that determine the frequency and distribution of diseases in human and other animal populations.

epiderm, epiderma (ep'i-derm, ep-i-der'mă). Epidermis.

epidermal, epidermatic (ep-i-der'măl, -der-mat'ik). Epidermic; relating to the epidermis.

epidermalization (ep-i-der'mal-i-zā'shŭn). Squamous *metaplasia.*

epidermatoplasty (ep-i-der'ma-tō-plas-tē) [epidermis + G. *plastos,* formed]. Rarely used term for skin grafting by means of strips or small patches of epidermis with the underlying outer layer of the corium.

epidermic (ep-i-der'mik). Epidermal.

epidermidosis (ep'i-der-mi-dō'sis). Epidermosis.

epidermis, pl. **epidermides** (ep-i-derm'is, -derm'i-dēz) [G. *epidermis,* the outer skin, fr. *epi,* on, + *derma,* skin] [NA]. Cuticle (3); cuticula (2); epiderm; epiderma; the outer epithelial portion of the skin (cutis). The e. of the palms and soles has the following strata: stratum corneum (horny layer), stratum lucidum (clear layer), stratum granulosum (granular layer), stratum spinosum (prickle cell layer), and stratum basale (basal cell layer); in other parts of the body, the stratum lucidum may be absent.

epidermitis (ep-i-der-mī'tis). Inflammation of the epidermis or superficial layers of the skin.

epidermization (ep'i-der-mi-zā'shŭn). **1.** Skin grafting. **2.** The covering of an area with epidermis.

epidermodysplasia (ep-i-der'mō-dis-plā'zē-ă) [epidermis + G. *dys-,* bad, + *plasis,* a molding]. Faulty growth or development of the epidermis.

e. verrucifor'mis, Lewandowski-Lutz disease; numerous flat warts on the hands and feet, sometimes familial, in which intranuclear viral particles with the appearance of infectious wart virus have been demonstrated; skin carcinoma sometimes develops.

epidermoid (ep-i-der'moyd) [epidermis + G. *eidos,* appearance]. **1.** Resembling epidermis. **2.** A cholesteatoma or other cystic tumor arising from aberrant epidermic cells.

epidermolysis (ep'i-der-mol'i-sis) [epidermis + G. *lysis,* loosening]. A condition in which the epidermis is loosely attached to the corium, readily exfoliating or forming blisters.

e. bullo'sa, a group of inherited chronic noninflammatory skin diseases in which large bullae and erosions result from slight mechanical trauma; a dominant form localized on the hands and feet is also called Weber-Cockayne syndrome.

e. bullo'sa dystroph'ica, dermolytic bullous dermatosis; a form of e. bullosa in which scarring develops after separation of the entire epidermis with blistering; it is inherited as a dominant (appearing in infancy or childhood) or recessive (present at birth or appearing in early infancy) trait, the latter including lethal and nonlethal types.

e. bullo'sa letha'lis, Herlitz syndrome; e. bullosa in which the bullae are persistent, nonhealing, and often present in the oral mucosa and trachea, but not on the palms and soles, leading to death in the absence of adequate treatment.

e. bullo'sa sim'plex, e. bullosa in which lesions heal rapidly without scarring and there is separation through the cytoplasm of basal epidermal cells; occurs most frequently on the feet in adults after unaccustomed trauma such as long marches; autosomal dominant inheritance.

Epidermophyton (ep'i-der-mof'i-ton, -der'mō-fī'ton) [epidermis + G. *phyton,* plant]. A genus of fungi, separated by Sabouraud from *Trichophyton* on the basis that it never invades the hair follicles, whose macroconidia are clavate and smooth-walled. The only species, *E. floccosum,* is an anthropophilic species that is a common cause of tinea pedis.

epidermosis (ep-i-der-mō'sis). Epidermidosis; a skin disease affecting only the epidermis.

epidermotropism (ep-i-der-mot'rō-pizm) [epidermis + G. *tropē,* a turning]. Movement towards the epidermis, as in the migration of T-lymphocytes into the epidermis in mycosis fungoides.

epidialysis (ep'i-dī-al'i-sis) [epi- + G. *dialysis,* a separation]. Dehiscence of the pigmentary layer of the iris.

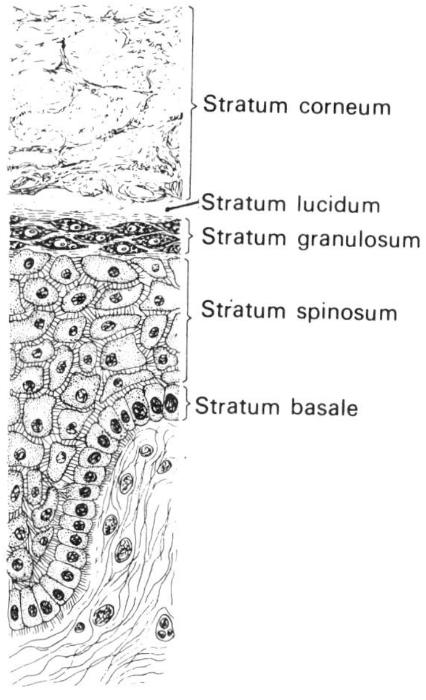

Epidermis

Microscopic section of epidermis of thick skin and a small part of the corium.

epidiascope (ep-i-dī'ă-skō-p) [epi- + G. *dia,* through, + *skopeō,* to view]. A projector by which images are reflected by a mirror through a lens, or lenses, onto a screen, using reflected light for opaque objects and transmitted light for translucent or transparent ones.

epididymal (ep-i-did'i-măl). Relating to the epididymis.

epididymectomy (ep'i-did-i-mek'tō-mē) [epididymis + G. *ektomē,* excision]. Epididymidectomy; operative removal of the epididymis.

epididymidectomy (ep'i-did-i-mid-ek'tō-mē). Epididymectomy.

epididymis, gen. **epididymidis,** pl. **epididymides** (ep-i-did'i-mis, -di-dim'i-dis, -di-dim'i-dēz) [Mod. L. fr. G. *epididymis,* fr. *epi,* on, + *didymos,* twin, in pl. testes] [NA]. Parorchis; an elongated structure connected to the posterior surface of the testis, consisting of the caput epididymidis (globus major), corpus epididymidis, and cauda epididymidis (globus minor) which turns sharply upon itself to become the ductus deferens; the main component is the very convoluted duct (ductus epididymidis) which in the tail and the beginning of the ductus deferens is a reservoir for spermatozoa.

epididymisoplasty (ep-i-did'i-mis-ō-plas-tē). Epididymoplasty.

epididymitis (ep-i-did-i-mī'tis). Inflammation of the epididymis.

epididymo-orchitis (ep-i-did'i-mō-ōr-kī'tis) [epididymis + G. *orchis,* testis]. Simultaneous inflammation of both epididymis and testis.

epididymoplasty (ep-i-did'i-mō-plas-tē) [epididymis + G. *plastos,* formed]. Epididymisoplasty; surgical repair of the epididymis.

epididymotomy (ep'i-did-i-mot'ō-mē) [epididymis + G. *tomē,* a cutting]. Incision into the epididymis, as in preparation for epididymovasostomy or for drainage of purulent material.

epididymovasectomy (ep-i-did'i-mō-va-sek'tō-mē) [epididymis + vasectomy]. Surgical removal of the epididymis and vas deferens, usually proximal to its entry into the inguinal canal.

epididymovasostomy (ep-i-did'i-mō-va-sos'tō-mē) [epididymis + vasostomy]. Surgical anastomosis of the vas deferens to the epididymis.

epidural (ep-i-dū'răl). Peridural; upon (or outside) the dura mater.

epidurography (ep-i-dū-rog'ră-fē). Radiographic visualization of the epidural space following the regional instillation of a radiopaque contrast medium.

epiestriol (ep-i-es'trē-ol). See estriol.

epifascial (ep-i-fash'ē-ăl). Upon the surface of a fascia, denoting a method of injecting drugs in which the solution is put on the fascia lata instead of injected into the substance of the muscle.

epigastralgia (ep'i-gas-tral'jē-ă) [epigastrium + G. *algos,* pain]. Pain in the epigastric region.

epigastric (ep-i-gas'trik). Relating to the epigastrium.

epigastrium (ep-i-gas'trē-ŭm) [G. *epigastrion*] [NA]. *Regio* epigastrica.

epigastrius (ep-i-gas'trē-ŭs). Unequal conjoined twins in which the smaller parasite is attached to the larger autosite in the epigastric region.

epigastrocele (ep-i-gas'trō-sēl) [epigastrium + G. *kēlē,* hernia]. A hernia in the epigastric region.

epigenesis (ep-i-jen'ĕ-sis) [epi- + G. *genesis,* creation]. **1.** Development of offspring as a result of the union of the ovum and sperm. *Cf.* preformation *theory.* **2.** Regulation of the expression of gene activity without alteration of genetic structure.

epigenetic (ep'i-jĕ-net'ik). Relating to epigenesis.

epiglottic, epiglottidean (ep-i-glot'ik, ep-i-glo-tid'ē-an). Relating to the epiglottis.

epiglottidectomy (ep'i-glot-i-dek'tō-mē) [epiglottis + G. *ektomē,* excision]. Excision of the epiglottis.

epiglottiditis (ep'i-glot-i-dī'tis). Epiglottitis.

epiglottis (ep-i-glot'is) [G. *epiglōttis,* fr. *epi,* on, + *glōttis,* the mouth of the windpipe] [NA]. A leaf-shaped plate of elastic cartilage, covered with mucous membrane, at the root of the tongue, which serves as a diverter valve over the superior aperture of the larynx during the act of swallowing; it stands erect when liquids are being swallowed, but is passively bent over the aperture by solid foods being swallowed.

epiglottitis (ep-i-glot-ī'tis). Epiglottiditis; inflammation of the epiglottis, which may cause respiratory obstruction, especially in children; frequently due to infection by *Haemophilus influenzae* type b.

epignathus (e-pig'nă-thŭs) [epi- + G. *gnathos,* jaw]. Unequal conjoined twins in which the smaller, incomplete parasite is attached to the larger autosite at the lower jaw.

epihyal (ep-i-hī'ăl). Above the hyoid arch.

epihyoid (ep-i-hī'oyd). Upon the hyoid bone; denoting certain accessory thyroid glands lying above the geniohyoid muscle.

epikeratophakia (ep'i-ker'ă-tō-phak'ē-ă) [epi- + G. *keras,* horn, + *phakos,* lens]. Epikeratophakic keratoplasty; modification of refractive error by application of a donor cornea to the anterior surface of the patient's cornea from which epithelium has been removed.

epikeratoprosthesis (ep'i-ker'ă-tō-pros'thē-sis) [epi- + G. *keras,* horn, + *prosthesis,* an addition]. A contact lens attached to the corneal stroma to replace the epithelium.

epilamellar (ep'i-lă-mel'ăr) [epi- + L. *lamella,* dim. of *lamina,* a thin metal plate]. Upon or above a basement membrane.

epilate (ep'i-lāt) [L. *e,* out, + *pilus,* a hair]. To extract a hair; to remove the hair from a part by forcible extraction, electrolysis, or loosening at the root by chemical means. *Cf.* depilate.

epilation (ep-i-lā'shŭn). Depilation; the act or result of removing hair.

epilatory (e-pil'ă-tō-rē). **1.** Depilatory (1); psilotic (2); having the property of removing hair; relating to epilation. See also decalvant. **2.** Depilatory (2).

epilemma (ep-i-lem'ă) [epi- *lemma,* husk]. The connective tissue sheath of nerve fibers near their termination.

epilepidoma (ep'i-lep-i-dō'mă) [epi- + G. *lepis,* rind, + *-ōma,* tumor]. A tumor resulting from hyperplasia of tissue derived from the true epiblast.

epilepsia (ep-i-lep'sē-ă) [G.]. Epilepsy.

e. nu'tans, head nodding attacks in children, usually part of another type of seizure; *e.g.,* atonic epilepsy.

e. partia'lis contin'ua, Kojewnikoff's epilepsy; a form of epilepsy marked by repetitive clonic muscular contractions with or without major convulsions.

epilepsy (ep'i-lep'sē) [G. *epilēpsia,* seizure]. Epilepsia; falling sickness; convulsive state; status convulsius; seizure; fit; a chronic disorder characterized by paroxysmal brain dysfunction due to excessive neuronal discharge, and usually associated with some alteration of consciousness. The clinical manifestations of the attack may vary from complex abnormalities of behavior including generalized or focal convulsions to momentary spells of impaired consciousness. These clinical states have been subjected to a variety of classifications, none universally accepted to date and, accordingly, the terminologies used to describe the different types of attacks remain purely descriptive and nonstandardized; they are variously based on 1) the clinical manifestations of the seizure (motor, sensory, reflex, psychic or vegetative), 2) the pathological substrate (hereditary, inflammatory, degenerative, neoplastic, traumatic, or cryptogenic), 3) the location of the epileptogenic lesion (rolandic, temporal, diencephalic regions), and 4) the time of

life at which the attacks occur (nocturnal, diurnal, menstrual, etc.).
activated e., iatrogenically induced seizures, particularly to determine their clinical pattern and EEG characteristics; commonly used methods are hyperventilation, intermittent photic stimulation, and sleep and convulsant drugs.
akinetic e., epileptic manifestations without movement, usually with loss of consciousness.
anosognosic e., e. characterized by attacks of which the person is unaware.
atonic e., e. characterized by loss of muscular tone.
audiogenic e., a form of reflex e. precipitated by sounds.
automatic e., psychomotor e.
autonomic e., diencephalic, vasomotor, or vasovagal e.; episodes of autonomic dysfunction presumably due to diencephalic irritation.
centrencephalic e., an imprecise term for e. characterized electroencephalographically by bilateral synchronous discharges, and clinically by absence or generalized tonic-clonic e.
complex precipitated e., a form of reflex e. initiated by specialized sensory stimuli, *e.g.,* certain visual patterns.
cortical e., focal e.
diencephalic e., autonomic e.
early posttraumatic e., convulsions beginning a few minutes to one month after head injury; recurrent attacks are unlikely.
eating e., seizures provoked by complete acts of eating a meal; a form of complex precipitated e.
focal e., cortical, local, or partial e.; partial seizure; an epileptic attack beginning with an isolated disturbance of cerebral function such as a twitching of a limb, a somatosensory or special sense phenomenon, or a disturbance of higher mental function.
generalized tonic-clonic e., generalized, major, or grand mal e.; idiopathic e. (2); grand mal; a seizure characterized by loss of consciousness and tonic muscular spasm, followed by clonic convulsive movements of all limbs; frequently preceded by an aura or warning.
grand mal e., generalized tonic-clonic e.
idiopathic e., **(1)** an e. without evident cause; **(2)** generalized tonic-clonic e.
jacksonian e., a convulsive attack beginning with twitching of the peripheral part of a limb extending to involve the proximal muscles; may spread to entire side and become generalized.
juvenile myoclonic e., myoclonic jerks of the shoulder muscles and clonic-tonic-clonic seizures of teenagers on awakening.
Kojewnikoff's e., *epilepsia* partialis continua.
laryngeal e., a form of reflex e. precipitated by coughing.
late e., tardy e.; e. beginning in middle age.
local e., focal e.
major e., generalized tonic-clonic e.
masked e., a form of e. characterized by a paroxysmal disturbance, such as headache or vomiting, associated with an epileptic electroencephalographic pattern.
matutinal e., a form of e. which occurs on awakening.
myoclonic astatic e., a petit mal variant characterized by atonic (drop attacks) and tonic or tonic-clonic attacks in neurologically disabled (hemiplegic, ataxic, etc.) children with mental retardation; characterized in EEG by 2/sec spike and wave discharges; usually progresses in spite of medication.
myoclonus e., Unverricht's or Lafora's disease; a seizure characterized by sporadic or continuous clonus of muscle groups; it is of familial origin and is associated with progressive mental deterioration.
nocturnal e., a form of e. in which the attacks occur at night.
partial e., focal e.
pattern sensitive e., a form of reflex e. precipitated by seeing certain patterns.
petit mal e., absence.
photogenic e., a form of reflex e. precipitated by light.
posttraumatic e., a convulsive state following and causally related to head injury; with brain damage either manifested clinically or ascertained by special examinations such as computed tomography. To assume causal relationship, the individual must have had no previous epilepsy, no cerebral disease, and no other brain trauma. The attacks should have started, depending on the severity of the wounding, within 3 months to 2 years of the alleged trauma and be of a type compatible with the site of injury and the EEG abnormalities.
primary generalized e., generalized tonic-clonic e.
procursive e., a psychomotor attack initiated by whirling or running.
psychomotor e., automatic e.; temporal lobe e.; complex partial seizure; attacks with elaborate and multiple sensory, motor, and/or psychic components, the common feature being a clouding or loss of consciousness and amnesia for the event; clinical manifestations may take the form of automatisms; emotional outbursts of temper, anger or show of fear; motor or psychic disturbances; or may be related to any sphere of human activity. Electroencephalographically, the attack is characterized by spike discharges in the temporal spiking, especially in sleep. See also terms used to designate aspects of this seizure type: procursive, visceral, uncinate e.
reflex e., sensory precipitated e.; seizures which are induced by peripheral stimulation; may be triggered by audiogenic, laryngeal, photogenic, or other stimulation.
rolandic e. [Luigi *Rolando],* a benign, autosomal, dominant form of e. occurring in children characterized clinically by arrest of speech, by muscular contractions of the side of the face and arm and electroencephalographically by high voltage spikes followed by slow waves in the rolandic area leads.
secondary generalized e., e. with focal manifestations progressing to a generalized convulsion; partial seizures that become generalized.
sensory e., focal e. initiated by a somatosensory phenomenon.
sensory precipitated e., reflex e.
sleep e., incorrect term for narcolepsy.
somnambulic e., postictal automatism in which the patient walks or runs about exhibiting natural behavior of which he or she has no subsequent remembrance.
startle e., a form of reflex e. precipitated by sudden noises.
symptomatic e., an acquired form of e., usually focal in nature, due to brain disease.
tardy e., late e.
temporal lobe e., psychomotor e.
tonic e., an attack in which the body is rigid.
tornado e., a type of focal e. or partial seizure with an aura of severe vertigo and a feeling of being drawn up into space.
uncinate e., uncinate attack; uncinate fit; a form of psychomotor e. or complex partial seizure initiated by a dreamy state and hallucinations of smell and taste, usually the result of a medial temporal lesion.
vasomotor e., autonomic e.
vasovagal e., autonomic e.
visceral e., e., usually psychomotor, in which the attacks are initiated by visceral symptoms or sensations; most cases have their focus in the temporal lobe.

epileptic (ep-i-lep'tik). Relating to, characterized by, or suffering from epilepsy.

epileptiform (ep-i-lep'ti-fōrm). Epileptoid.

epileptogenic, epileptogenous (ep-i-lep-tō-jen'ik, ep-i-lep-toj'ĕ-nŭs). Causing epilepsy.

epileptoid (ep-i-lep'toyd) [G. *epilēpsia,* seizure, epilepsy, + *eidos,* resemblance]. Epileptiform; resembling epilepsy; denoting certain convulsions, especially of functional nature.

epiloia (ep-i-loy'ă) [contrived term coined by Sherloc (1911)]. Tuberous *sclerosis.*

epimandibular (ep-i-man-dib'yū-lăr) [epi- + L. *mandibulum,* mandible]. Upon the lower jaw.

epimastical (ep-i-mast'i-kăl) [G. *epakmastikos,* coming to a height]. Increasing steadily until an acme is reached, then declining; said of a fever.

epimastigote (ep-i-mas'ti-gōt) [epi- + G. *mastix,* whip]. Term replacing "crithidial stage," to avoid confusion with the insect-parasitizing flagellates of the genus *Crithidia.* In the e. stage the flagellum arises from the kinetoplast alongside the nucleus and emerges from the anterior end of the organism; an undulating membrane is present.

epimenorrhagia (ep-i-men-ō-rā'jē-ă). Too prolonged and too profuse menstruation occurring at any time, but most frequently at the beginning and end of menstrual life.

epimenorrhea (ep-i-men-ō-rē'ă). Too frequent menstruation, occurring at any time, but particularly at the beginning and end of menstrual life.

epimer (ep'i-mer) [epi- + G. *meros,* part]. One of two molecules differing only in the spatial arrangement about a single carbon atom; *e.g.,* glucose and galactose (with respect to carbon-4). *Cf.* anomer. See also sugars.

epimerase (ep'i-mer-ās) [EC 5.1]. A class of enzymes catalyzing epimeric changes.

epimere (ep'i-mēr) [epi- + G. *meros,* part]. The dorsal part of the myotome. See myotome (3).

epimerite (ep-i-mēr'īt) [epi- + G. *meros,* part]. The hooklike anchoring structure at the anterior end of a cephaline gregarine sporozoan; it is left embedded in tissues when the rest of the cephalont is freed in the lumen of the intestine of the invertebrate host.

epimicroscope (ep-i-mī'krō-skōp). Opaque microscope; a microscope with a condenser built around the objective; used for the investigation of opaque, or only slightly translucent, minute specimens.

epimorphosis (ep'i-mōr-fō'sis) [epi- + G. *morphē,* shape]. Regeneration of a part of an organism by growth at the cut surface.

epimysiotomy (ep'i-mis-ē-ot'ō-mē) [epimysium + G. *tomē,* a cutting]. Incision of the sheath of a muscle.

epimysium (ep-i-mis'ē-ŭm) [epi- + G. *mys,* muscle]. Perimysium externum; the fibrous envelope surrounding a skeletal muscle.

epinephrine (ep'i-nef'rin). Adrenaline; 3,4-dihydroxy-α[methylaminomethyl]benzyl alcohol; a catecholamine that is the chief neurohormone of the adrenal medulla of most species. It is the most potent stimulant (sympathomimetic) of adrenergic α- and β-receptors, resulting in increased heart rate and force of contraction, vasoconstriction or vasodilation, relaxation of bronchiolar and intestinal smooth muscle, glycogenolysis, lipolysis, and other metabolic effects; used in the treatment of bronchial asthma, acute allergic disorders, open-angle glaucoma, and heart block, and as a topical and local vasoconstrictor. Generally used salts are e. hydrochloride and e. bitartrate, the latter most frequently used in topical preparations.

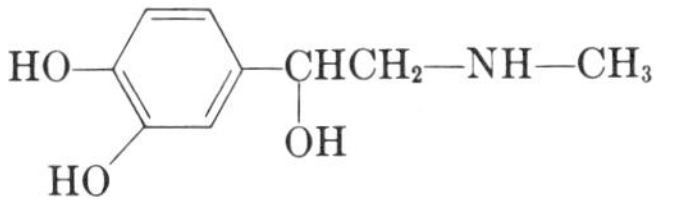

Epinephrine

epinephros (ep-i-nef'ros) [epi- + G. *nephros,* kidney]. *Glandula* suprarenalis.

epineural (ep-i-nū'răl). On a neural arch of a vertebrae.

epineurial (ep-i-nū'rē-ăl). Relating to the epineurium.

epineurium (ep-i-nū'rē-ŭm) [epi- + G. *neuron,* nerve]. The connective tissue encapsulating a nerve trunk and binding together the fascicles; it contains the blood vessels and lymphatics supplying the nerves.

epinosic (ep-i-nō'sik). Relating to epinosis.

epinosis (ep-i-nō'sis) [epi- + G. *nosos,* disease]. An imaginary feeling of illness following a real illness.

epionychium (ep-i-ō-nik'ē-ŭm). Eponychium.

epiotic (ep'i-ot'ik, -ō'tik) [epi- + G. *ous,* ear]. One of the components of the otic capsule of some vertebrates; in the mammal the petrosal or petrous temporal bone incorporates the various otic elements seen in lower vertebrates.

epipastic (ep-i-pas'tik) [G. *epi-passō,* to sprinkle over]. **1.** Usable as a dusting powder. **2.** A dusting powder.

epipericardial (ep'i-per-i-kar'dē-ăl). Upon or about the pericardium.

epipharynx (ep'i-far'ingks) [G. *epi,* on, over, + pharynx]. *Pars* nasalis pharyngis.

epiphenomenon (ep'i-fē-nom'ĕ-non). A symptom appearing during the course of a disease, not of usual occurrence, and not necessarily associated with the disease.

epiphora (ē-pif'ō-ră) [G. a sudden flow, fr. *epi,* on, + *pherō,* to bear]. Watery eye (1); tearing; an overflow of tears upon the cheek, due to imperfect drainage by the tear-conducting passages.

atonic e., e. arising from weakness of the orbicularis oculi muscle.

epiphrenic, epiphrenal (ep'i-fren'ik, -frē'năl) [epi- + G. *phrēn,* diaphragm]. Upon or above the diaphragm.

epiphysial, epiphyseal (ep-i-fiz'ē-ăl). Relating to an epiphysis.

epiphysiodesis (ep'i-fiz-ē-od'ĕ-sis) [epiphysis + G. *desis,* bind]. **1.** Premature union of the epiphysis with the diaphysis, resulting in cessation of growth. **2.** An operative procedure which partially or totally destroys an epiphysis and may incorporate a bone graft to produce fusion of the epiphysis or premature cessation of its growth; generally undertaken to equalize leg length.

epiphysiolysis (ep-i-fiz-ē-ol'i-sis) [epiphysis + G. *lysis,* loosening]. Loosening or separation, either partial or complete, of an epiphysis from the shaft of a bone.

epiphysiopathy (ep-i-fiz-ē-op'ă-thē) [epiphysis + G. *pathos,* suffering]. Any disorder of an epiphysis of the long bones.

epiphysis, pl. epiphyses (e-pif'i-sis, -sēz) [G. an excrescence, fr. *epi,* upon, + *physis,* growth] [NA]. A part of a long bone developed from a center of ossification distinct from that of the shaft and separated at first from the latter by a layer of cartilage. See fig. on p. 526.

atavistic e., a bone that is independent phylogenetically but is now fused with another bone, *e.g.,* coracoid process of the scapula.

e. cer'ebri, *corpus* pineale.

pressure e., a secondary center of ossification in the articular end of a long bone.

stippled e., *dysplasia* epiphysialis punctata.

traction e., a secondary center of ossification at the site of attachment of a tendon.

epiphysitis (e-pif-i-sī'tis). Inflammation of an epiphysis.

epipial (ep'i-pī'ăl). On the pia mater.

epiplo- [G. *epiploon,* omentum]. Combining form relating to the omentum. See also omento-.

epiplocele (e-pip'lō-sēl) [epiplo- + G. *kēlē,* hernia]. Rarely used term for hernia of the omentum.

epiploic (ep'i-plō'ik). Omental.

epiploon (e-pip'lō-on) [G.]. *Omentum* majus.

epiplopexy (e-pip'lō-pek-sē) [epiplo- + G. *pēxis,* fixation]. Obsolete synonym of omentopexy.

epipteric (ep'i-ter'ik). In the neighborhood of the pterion.

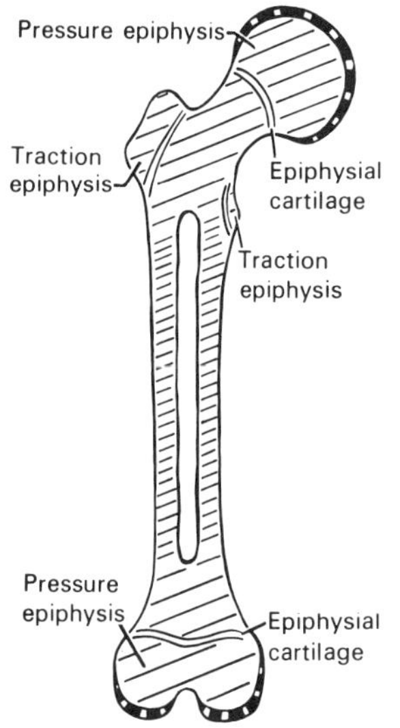

Epiphyses of the Femur

epipygus (ep-i-pī'gŭs) [epi- + G. *pygē,* buttocks]. Unequal conjoined twins in which the smaller, incomplete parasite is attached to the buttock of the larger autosite.

D-epirhamnose (ep-i-ram'nōz). Quinovose; 6-deoxy-D-glucose; occurs in plants and bacteria in combination with diacylglycerol and is sulfated (at C-6) as a glycolipid.

episclera (ep'i-sklĕr'ă) [epi- + sclera]. The connective tissue between the sclera and the conjunctiva.

episcleral (ep-i-sklĕr'ăl). **1.** Upon the sclera. **2.** Relating to the episclera.

episcleritis (ep-i-skle-rī'tis). Inflammation of the episcleral connective tissue. See also scleritis.

e. multinodula'ris, e. with numerous nodules near the corneoscleral limbus.

nodular e., e. with localized inflammation foci in episcleral tissues.

e. periodi'ca fu'gax, subconjunctivitis; hot eye; diffuse transient e., with a tendency to recur at regular intervals.

episio- [G. *episeion,* pudenda]. Combining form relating to the vulva. See also vulvo-.

episioperineorrhaphy (e-piz'ē-ō-per'i-nē-ōr'ă-fē, e-pis') [episio- + G. *perinaion,* perineum, + *rhaphē,* a stitching]. Repair of a ruptured perineum and lacerated vulva or repair of a surgical incision of the vulva and perineum; made for obstetrical purposes.

episioplasty (e-piz'ē-ō-plas-tē, e-pis') [episio- + G. *plastos,* formed]. Plastic surgery of the vulva.

episiorrhaphy (e-piz-i-ōr'ră-fē, e-pis-) [episio- + G. *rhaphē,* a stitching]. Repair of a lacerated vulva or an episiotomy.

episiostenosis (e-piz'i-ō-stĕ-nō'sis, e-pis') [episio- + G. *stenōsis,* narrowing]. Narrowing of the vulvar orifice.

episiotomy (e-piz-ē-ot'ō-mē, e-pis-) [episio- + G. *tomē,* incision]. Surgical incision of the vulva to prevent laceration at the time of delivery or to facilitate vaginal surgery.

episome (ep'i-sōm) [epi- + G. *sōma,* body (chromosome)]. An extrachromosomal element (plasmid) that may either integrate into the bacterial chromosome of the host or replicate and function stably when physically separated from the chromosome.

resistance-transferring e.'s, resistance *plasmids.*

epispadia (ep-i-spā'dē-ă). Epispadias.

epispadial (ep-i-spā'dē-ăl). Relating to an epispadias.

epispadias (ep-i-spā'dē-ăs) [epi- + G. *spadōn* a rent]. Epispadia; a malformation in which the urethra opens on the dorsum of the penis; frequently associated with extrophy of the bladder.

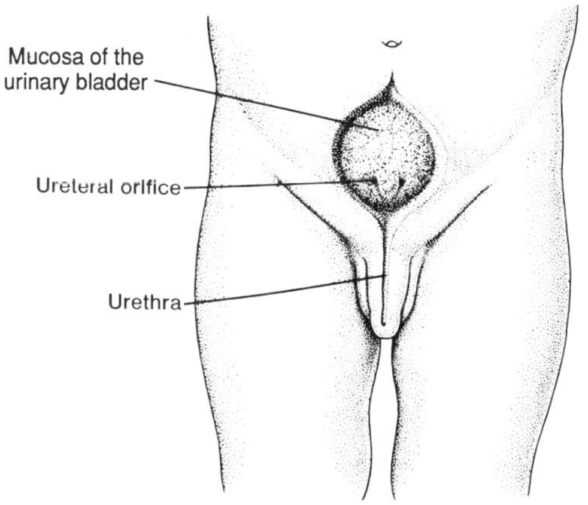

Epispadias and Ectopia of the Bladder

epispastic (ep-i-spas'tik). Vesicant.

epispinal (ep-i-spī'năl). Upon the vertebral column or spinal cord, or upon any structure resembling a spine.

episplenitis (ep-i-splē-nī'tis). Inflammation of the capsule of the spleen.

epistasis (e-pis'tă-sis) [G. scum; epi- + G. *stasis,* a standing]. Epistasy. **1.** The formation of a pellicle or scum on the surface of a liquid, especially as on standing urine. **2.** A form of gene interaction whereby one gene masks or interferes with the phenotypic expression of one or more genes at other loci; the gene whose phenotype is expressed is said to be "epistatic," while the gene or genes whose phenotype is altered or suppressed is said to be "hypostatic."

epistasy (e-pis'tă-sē). Epistasis.

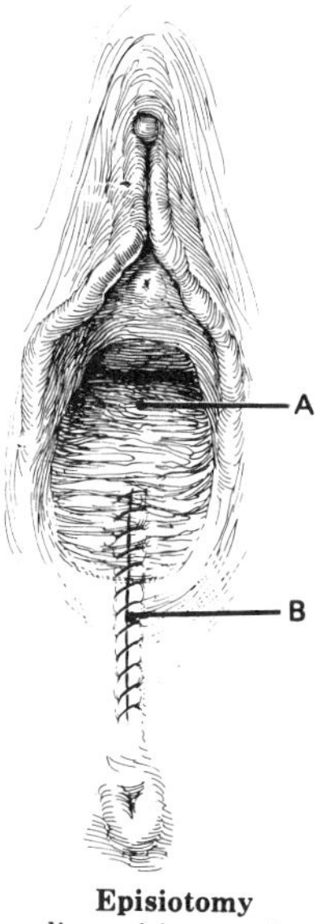

Episiotomy

A, vagina; *B,* median episiotomy closed by continuous suture.

epistatic (ep-is-tat'ik). Relating to epistasis.

epistaxis (ep'i-stak'sis) [G. fr. *epistazō,* to bleed at the nose, fr. *epi,* on, + *stazō,* to fall in drops]. Nosebleed; nasal hemorrhage; profuse bleeding from the nose.
renal e., hematuria occurring without a detectable lesion.

epistemophilia (ĕ-pis'tē-mō-fil'ē-ă) [G. *epistēmē,* knowledge, + *philos,* fond]. Love, especially excessive, of knowledge.

episternal (ep-i-ster'năl). **1.** Over or on the sternum. **2.** Relating to the episternum.

episternum (ep-i-ster'nŭm) [epi- + L. *sternum,* chest]. *Manubrium* sterni.

epistropheus (ep-i-strō'fē-ŭs) [G. the pivot]. Axis (5).

epitarsus (ep-i-tar'sŭs) [epi- + G. *tarsos,* flat mat, edge of eyelid]. A fold of conjunctiva arising on the tarsal surface of the lid and losing itself in the skin close to the medial angle of the eye.

epitaxy (ep-i-tak'sē) [epi- + G. *taxis,* arrangement]. The growth of one crystal in one or more specific orientations on the substrate of another kind of crystal, with a close geometric fit between the networks in contact; seen in the alternating layers of different composition in stones from the kidney and gallbladder, indicating an abrupt change of composition during formation.

epitendineum (ep'i-ten-din'ē-ŭm) [L.]. Epitenon; the white fibrous sheath surrounding a tendon.

epitenon (ĕ-pit'ĕ-non, ep-i-ten'on). Epitendineum.

17-epitestosterone (ep'i-tes-tos'ter-ōn). 17α-Hydroxyandrost-4-en-3-one; 17α epimer of testosterone; a biologically inactive steroid found in testes and ovaries; may be a metabolite of 4-androstene-3,17-dione and a precursor of 17α-estradiol.

epithalamus (ep'i-thal'ă-mŭs) [epi- + thalamus] [NA]. A small dorsomedial area of the thalamus corresponding to the habenula and its associated structures, the stria medullaris and the pineal body.

epithalaxia (ep'i-thă-lak'sē-ă) [epithelium + G. *allaxis,* exchange]. Shedding of any surface epithelium, but especially of that lining the intestine.

epithelia (ep-i-thē'lē-ă). Plural of epithelium.

epithelial (ep-i-thē'lē-ăl). Relating to or consisting of epithelium.

epithelialization (ep-i-thē'lē-ăl-i-zā'shŭn). Epithelization; formation of epithelium over a denuded surface.

epitheliocyte (ep-i-thē'lē-ō-sīt) [epithelium + G. *kytos,* cell]. An *in vitro* tissue culture epithelial cell.

epitheliofibril (ep-i-thē'lē-ō-fī'bril). Tonofibril.

epithelioglandular (ep-i-thē'lē-ō-glan'dyū-lăr). Relating to glandular epithelium.

epithelioid (ep-i-thē'lē-oyd) [epithelium + G. *eidos,* resemblance]. Resembling or having some of the characteristics of epithelium.

epitheliolytic (ep-i-thē'lē-ō-lit'ik). Destructive to epithelium.

epithelioma (ep'i-thē-lē-ō'mă) [epithelium + G. *-ōma,* tumor]. **1.** An epithelial neoplasm or hamartoma of the skin, especially of skin appendage origin. **2.** A carcinoma of the skin derived from squamous, basal, or adnexal cells.
e. adenoi'des cys'ticum, trichoepithelioma.
basal cell e., basal cell *carcinoma.*
Borst-Jadassohn type intraepidermal e., precancerous lesions clinically suggestive of actinic or seborrheic keratosis, with nests of immature or abnormal keratinocytes within the epidermis.
chorionic e., choriocarcinoma.
e. contagio'sum, fowlpox.
e. cunicula'tum, verrucous carcinoma occurring uncommonly on the sole of the foot, forming a slowly growing warty mass that may invade deeply but which rarely metastasizes.
Malherbe's calcifying e., pilomatrixoma.
malignant ciliary e., adult medulloepithelioma; malignant hyperplasia of ciliary epithelium with frequent involvement of the pigmented layer.
multiple self-healing squamous e., multiple skin tumors, most frequently on the head, each resembling a well-differentiated squamous carcinoma or keratoacanthoma; individual tumors resolve spontaneously after several months, leaving deep-pitted scars with irregular crenellated borders, and are usually replaced by additional new tumors; autosomal dominant inheritance.
sebaceous e., a benign tumor of the sebaceous gland epithelium in which small basaloid or germinative cells predominate.

epitheliomatous (ep-i-thē-lē-ō'mă-tŭs). Pertaining to epithelioma.

epitheliopathy (ep'i-thē-lē-op'ă-thē) [epithelium + G. *pathos,* suffering]. Disease involving epithelium.
pigment e., an acute disease manifested by rapid loss of vision, and multifocal, cream-colored placoid lesions of the retinal pigment epithelium; resolves with restoration of vision.

epitheliosis (ep-i-thē-lē-ō'sis). Proliferation of epithelial cells, as seen in ducts of the breast in fibrocystic disease.

epithelite (ep-i-thē'līt). A skin lesion resulting from excessive irradiation.

epithelium, pl. **epithelia** (ep-i-thē'lē-ŭm, -ă) [G. *epi,* upon, + *thēlē,* nipple, a term applied originally to the thin skin covering the nipples and the papillary layer of the border of the lips] [NA]. The purely cellular avascular layer covering all the free surfaces, cutaneous, mucous, and serous, including the glands and other structures derived therefrom.

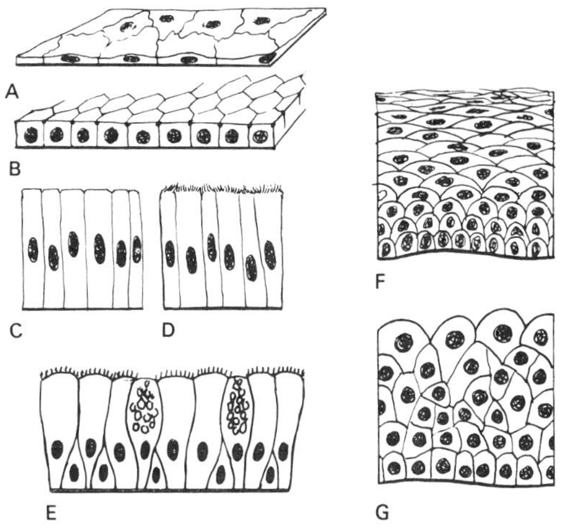

Types of Epithelium
A, simple squamous; *B,* simple cuboidal; *C,* simple columnar; *D,* ciliated columnar; *E,* pseudostratified ciliated columnar with goblet cells; *F,* stratified squamous; *G,* transitional.

anterior e. of cornea, e. anterius corneae.
e. ante'rius cor'neae [NA], anterior e. of the cornea; the stratified squamous e. covering the outer surface of the cornea; it is smooth, consists usually of five layers of cells, and contains numerous free nerve endings.
Barrett's e., columnar esophageal e. seen in Barrett syndrome.
ciliated e., any e. having motile cilia on the free surface.
columnar e., cylindrical e.; e. formed of a single layer of prismatic cells taller than they are wide.
crevicular e., sulcular e.; the stratified squamous e. lining the inner aspect of the soft tissue wall of the gingival sulcus.
cuboidal e., simple e. with cells appearing as cubes in a vertical section but as polyhedra in surface view.

cylindrical e., columnar e.
e. duc'tus semicircula'ris [NA], the simple squamous e. of the semicircular ducts.
enamel e., reduced enamel e.; the several layers of the enamel organ remaining on the enamel surface after formation of enamel is completed.
external dental or **enamel e.,** the cuboidal cells of the outer layer of the odontogenic organ of a developing tooth.
germinal e., a cuboidal layer of peritoneal e. covering the gonads, once thought to be the source of germ cells.
gingival e., a stratified squamous e. that undergoes some degree of keratinization and covers the free and attached gingiva.
glandular e., e. composed of secretory cells.
inner dental or **enamel e.,** the columnar epithelial layer of enamel matrix, secreting ameloblasts, of the odontogenic organ of a developing tooth.
junctional e., epithelial attachment; a collar of epthelial cells attached to the tooth surface and subepithelial connective tissue found at the base of the gingival crevice.
laminated e., stratified e.
e. of lens, e. lentis.
e. lentis [NA], e. of the lens; the layer of cuboidal cells lying on the anterior surface of the crystalline lens inside the lens capsule. At the equator the cells elongate and give rise to the lens fibers.
mesenchymal e., the flat e. derived from mesenchymal cells found lining certain connective tissue spaces such as the anterior chamber of eye, perilymph spaces in the ear, and subdural and subarachnoid spaces.
muscle e., myoepithelium.
olfactory e., an e. of the pseudostratified type which contains olfactory, receptor, nerve cells whose axons extend to the olfactory bulb of the brain.
pavement e., simple squamous e.
pigment e., e. composed of cells containing granules of pigment or melanin, as in the retinal or iris pigment layer.
pseudostratified e., an e. which gives a superficial appearance of being stratified because the cell nuclei are at different levels, but in which all cells reach the basement membrane, hence it is classed as a simple e.
reduced enamel e., enamel e.
respiratory e., the pseudostratified ciliated e. that lines the conducting portion of the airway, including part of the nasal cavity and larynx, the trachea, and bronchi.
seminiferous e., the e. lining the convoluted tubules of the testis where spermatogenesis and spermiogenesis occur.
simple e., an e. having one layer of cells.
simple squamous e., pavement e.; e. composed of a single layer of flattened scalelike cells, such as mesothelium, endothelium, and that in the pulmonary alveoli.
stratified e., laminated e.; a type of e. composed of a series of layers, the cells of each varying in size and shape. It is named more specifically according to the type of cells at the surface, *e.g.,* stratified squamous e., stratified columnar e., stratified ciliated columnar e.
stratified ciliated columnar e., an e. consisting of several layers of cells with the deeper cells being polyhedral in form and the surface ones columnar with motile cilia, such as lines the fetal esophagus.
stratified squamous e., an e. consisting of several layers in which the surface cells are flattened and scalelike and the deeper cells are polyhedral in form; the surface may be cornified and dry, or noncornified and moist.
sulcular e., crevicular e.
surface e., **(1)** a layer of celomic epithelial cells covering the gonadal ridges as they are formed on the medial border of the mesonephroi near the root of the mesentery; **(2)** the mesothelial covering of the definitive ovary.
transitional e., a highly distensible stratified e. with large polyploid superficial cells which are cuboidal in the relaxed state but broad and squamous in the distended state; occurs in the kidney, ureter, and bladder.

epithelization (ep-i-thē-li-zā'shŭn). Epithelialization.

epithem (ep'i-them) [G. *epithēma,* a cover]. An external application, such as a poultice, but not a plaster or ointment.

epithesis (ĕ-pith'ĕ-sis) [epi- + G. *tithenai,* to place]. **1.** Orthopedic correction of a deformed extremity. **2.** A splint or other apparatus applied to an extremity.

epithet (ep'i-thet) [G. *epithetos,* added, fr. epi- + *tithenai,* to place]. Characterizing term or name.
specific e., in bacteriology, the second part of the name of a species; it is not, by itself, a name; the name of a bacterial species consists of two parts, the generic name and the specific e.

epithiazide (ep-i-thī'ă-zīd). 6-Chloro-3,4-dihydro-3-{[(2,2,2-trifluoroethyl)-thio] methyl}-2*H*- 1,2,4-benzothiadiazine-7-sulfonamide 1,1-dioxide; a diuretic.

epitope (ep'i-tōp). An antigenic determinant, in simplest form, of a complex antigenic molecule.

epitoxoid (ep-i-tok'soyd). A toxoid that has less affinity for specific antitoxin than that manifested by the toxin.

epitrichial (ep-i-trik'ē-ăl). Relating to the epitrichium.

epitrichium (ep-i-trik'ē-ŭm) [epi- + G. *trichion,* dim. of *thrix,* (*trich-*), hair]. Periderm.

epitrochlea (ep-i-trok'lē-ă) [epi- + L. *trochlea,* a pulley, block, contr. fr. G. *trochilia*]. *Epicondylus* medialis humeri.

epitrochlear (ep-i-trok'lē-ăr). Relating to the epitrochlea.

epituberculosis (ep'i-tū-ber-kyū-lō'sis). The occurrence of glandular swelling or pulmonary infiltration in the area of a focus of pulmonary tuberculosis or of enlarged bronchial glands.

epitympanic (ep-i-tim-pan'ik). Above, or in the upper part of, the tympanic cavity or membrane.

epitympanum (ep'i-tim'pă-nŭm). *Recessus* epitympanicus.

epizoic (ep-i-zō'ik). Living as a parasite on the skin surface.

epizoology (ep'i-zō-ol'ō-jē) [epi- + G. *zōon,* animal, + *logos,* study]. Epizootiology.

epizoon, pl. **epizoa** (ep-i-zō'on, -zō'ă) [epi- + G. *zōon,* animal]. An animal parasite living on the body surface.

epizootic (ep'i-zō-ot'ik) [epi- + G. *zōon,* animal]. **1.** Denoting a disease of animals which is attacking a large number of animals simultaneously. **2.** The temporal pattern of occurrence of a disease in a population of animals where the disease frequency is clearly in excess of the expected frequency during a given time interval. *Cf.* enzootic, sporadic.

epizootiology (ep'i-zō-ot'ē-ol'ō-jē) [epi- + G. *zōon,* animal, + *logos,* study]. Epizoology; epidemiology of disease in animal populations.

épluchage (ā-plū-shazh') [F. picking, cleaning]. The removal of all contaminated tissue in infected wounds.

eponychia (ep-ō-nik'ē-ă). Infection involving the proximal nail fold.

eponychium (ep-ō-nik'ē-ŭm) [G. *epi,* upon, + *onyx* (*onych-*), nail]. Epionychium. **1.** The condensed eleidin-rich areas of the epidermis preceding the formation of the nail in the embryo. **2** [NA]. Perionychium; nail skin; the epidermis forming the ungual wall behind and at the sides of the nail. **3.** The thin skin adherent to the nail at its proximal portion.

eponym (ep'ō-nim) [G. *epōnymos,* named after]. The name of a disease, structure, operation, or procedure, usually derived from the name of the person who discovered or described it first.

eponymic (ep-ō-nim'ik). **1.** Relating to an eponym. **2.** An eponym.

epoophorectomy (ep-ō-of'ō-rek'tō-mē) [G. *epi,* upon, + *ōophoros,* bearing eggs, + *ektomē,* excision]. Removal of the epoophoron.

epoöphoron (ep′ō-of′ŏ-ron) [epi- + G. *ōophoros,* egg-bearing] [NA]. Organ of Rosenmüller; pampiniform body; a collection of rudimentary tubules in the mesosalpinx between the ovary and the uterine tube; composed of two portions, the ductus epoophori longitudinalis and the ductuli transversi epoophori, they are vestiges of tubules of the middle portion of the mesonephros and the homologue of the ductuli aberrantes and proximal ductus epididymidis in the male.

epoprostenol, epoprostenol sodium (e-pō-prost′en-ol). Prostacyclin.

epoxy (ē-pok′sē). Chemical term describing an oxygen atom bound to two linked carbon atoms (—CH—CH—, with O bridging the two carbons); produced from peracids acting on alkenes. E.'s are important chemical intermediates, and the basis of e. resins (polymers) formed from e. monomers.

EPS Abbreviation for exophthalmos-producing *substance.*

epsilon (ep′si-lon). Fifth letter of the Greek alphabet, ϵ (*q.v.*).

Epsom salt [*Epsom,* England]. *Magnesium* sulfate.

EPSP Abbreviation for excitatory postsynaptic *potential.*

Epstein, Alois, German pediatrician, 1849–1918. See E.'s *disease, pearls, symptom.*

Epstein, M. Anthony, 20th century British virologist. See E.-Barr *virus.*

epulis (ep-yū′lis) [G. *epoulis,* a gumboil]. A nonspecific exophytic gingival mass.

congenital e. of newborn, a congenital benign nodular tumor of the alveolar ridge, of unknown histogenesis; histologically, it is composed of large cells with a granular cytoplasm similar to that of a granular cell tumor (myoblastoma).

e. fissura′tum, inflammatory fibrous *hyperplasia.*

giant cell e., giant cell *granuloma.*

e. gravida′rum, a gingival pyogenic granuloma that develops during pregnancy.

pigmented e., melanotic neuroectodermal *tumor.*

epuloid (ep′yū-loyd). A gingival mass that resembles an epulis.

equation (ē-kwā′zhŭn) [L. *aequare,* to make equal]. A statement expressing the equality of two things, usually with the use of mathematical or chemical symbols.

alveolar gas e., the e. defining the steady state relation of the alveolar oxygen pressure to the barometric pressure, inspired gas composition, alveolar carbon dioxide pressure, and respiratory exchange ratio; the e. is used in various forms depending upon which simplifying assumptions are acceptable for different applications.

Arrhenius e., an e. relating chemical reaction rate (k) to the absolute temperature (T) by the e.: $(d \ln k/dT) = (\Delta E/RT^2)$.

Bohr's e., an e. to calculate the respiratory dead space from the fact that gas expired from the lungs is a mixture of gas from the dead space and gas from the alveoli, *i.e.,* the dead space volume divided by the tidal volume equals the difference between alveolar and mixed expired gas composition, divided by the difference between alveolar and inspired gas composition; gas composition can be expressed in any consistent units of concentration or partial pressure of oxygen or carbon dioxide.

chemical e., an e. on one side of which are the reactants and on the other side the products of a chemical reaction; the two halves may be separated by an equal sign or by arrows.

constant field e., Goldman e.

Einthoven's e., Einthoven's *law.*

Gibbs-Helmholtz e., an e. expressing the relationship in a galvanic cell between the chemical energy transformed and the maximal electromotive force obtainable.

Goldman e., constant field e.; Goldman-Hodgkin-Katz (GHK) e.; an e. derived to predict membrane potentials in terms of the membrane's permeability to ions and their concentrations on either side.

Goldman-Hodgkin-Katz (GHK) e., Goldman e.

Hasselbalch's e., Henderson-Hasselbalch e.

Henderson-Hasselbalch e., Hasselbalch's e.; a formula relating the pH of a solution to the ratio of bicarbonate ion concentration to free carbon dioxide in solution: pH = pK′ + log $([HCO_3^-]/[CO_2])$. The value of pK′ for blood plasma is 6.10 and includes the first dissociation constant of H_2CO_3, the relation between $[H_2CO_3]$ and $[CO_2]$, and other corrections. The partial pressure of CO_2 multiplied by its solubility in plasma at 38°C (0.0301 mM/mm Hg) is commonly substituted for $[CO_2]$; *e.g.,* when the plasma bicarbonate concentration is 24 mEq/liter and the P_{CO_2} is 40 mm Hg, the pH = 6.10 + log (24/0.0301 × 40) = 7.40.

Hill's e., the e.: $y/100 = Kx^n/(1 + Kx^n)$, where y is the percent saturation of blood, x the oxygen pressure, and K and n are constants; represents the shape of the oxygen dissociation curve of hemoglobin, which would be hyperbolic if n equaled 1, but which becomes increasingly sigmoid with higher values of n (for human blood, n equals 2.5).

Hufner's e., an e. expressing the relationship between myoglobin dissociation and oxygen partial pressure: $([MBO_2]/[Mb]) = (K \times pO_2)$.

Lineweaver-Burk e., a rearrangement of the Michaelis-Menten constant, $K_m = [S](V_{max} - V)/V$, to $[S]/V = [S]/V_{max} + K_m/V_{max}$, in which form a plot of $[S]/V$ versus $[S]$ gives a straight line of slope $1/V_{max}$ and intercept K_m.

Michaelis-Menten e., see Michaelis-Menten *constant.*

Nernst's e., the e. relating the equilibrium potential of electrodes to ion concentrations; the e. relating the electrical potential and concentration gradient of an ion across a permeable membrane at equilibrium: $E = [RT/nF] [\ln (C_1/C_2)]$, where E = potential, R = absolute gas constant, T = absolute temperature, n = valence, F = the Faraday, ln = the natural logarithm, and C_1 and C_2 are the ion concentrations on the two sides; in nonideal solutions, concentration should be replaced by activity. See also Nernst's theory; activity (2).

personal e., a slight error in judgment, perceptual response, or action peculiar to the individual and so constant that it is usually possible to allow for it in accepting the person's statements or conclusions, thus arriving at approximate exactness; observed in persons whose work involves readings of events in time, such as navigators and air traffic controllers.

Rayleigh e., Rayleigh test; a ratio of red to green required by each observer to match spectral yellow.

equator (ē-kwā′ter) [Mediev. L. *aequator,* fr. L. *aequo,* to make equal] [NA]. A line encircling a globular body, equidistant at all points from the two poles; the periphery of a plane cutting a sphere at the midpoint of, and at right angles to, its axis.

e. bul′bi oc′uli [NA], e. of eyeball; an imaginary line encircling the globe of the eye equidistant from the anterior and posterior poles.

e. of eyeball, e. bulbi oculi.

e. of lens, e. lentis.

e. len′tis [NA], e. of the lens; the periphery of the lens lying between the two layers of the zonula ciliaris.

equatorial (ē-kwă-tō′rē-ăl). Situated, like the earth's equator, equidistant from each end.

equiaxial (ē′kwi-ak′sē-ăl). Having axes of equal length.

equicaloric (ē′kwi-kă-lōr′ik). [L. *aequus,* equal, + *calor,* heat]. Equal in heat value. See also isodynamic.

equilenin (ek-wi-len′in). 3-Hydroxyestra-1,3,5(10),6,8-pentaen-17-one; an estrogenic steroid isolated from pregnant mare's urine.

equilibration (ē′kwi-li-brā′shŭn, e-kwil-ĭ-). **1.** The act of maintaining an equilibrium or balance. **2.** The act of exposing a liquid, *e.g.,* blood or plasma, to a gas at a certain partial pressure until the partial pressures of the gas within and without the liquid are equal. **3.** In dentistry, modification of occlusal forms of the teeth by grinding, with the intent of equalizing occlusal stress, producing simultaneous occlusal contacts, or harmonizing cuspal relations.

equilibrium (ē-kwi-lib′rē-ŭm) [L. *aequilibrium,* a horizontal position, fr. *aequus,* equal, + *libra,* a balance]. **1.** The condition of being evenly balanced; a state of repose between two or more antagonistic forces that exactly counteract each other. **2.** Dynamic e.; in chemistry, a state of apparent repose created by two reactions proceeding in opposite directions at equal speed; in chemical equations, sometimes indicated by two opposing arrows ($\rightleftarrows$) instead of the equal sign. See also equilibrium *constant.*

acid-base e., acid-base *balance.*

Donnan e., Gibbs-Donnan e.; when a semipermeable membrane or its equivalent (*e.g.,* a solid ion-exchanger) separates a nondiffusible substance, such as protein, from diffusible substances, the diffusible anions and cations are distributed on the two sides of the membrane so that 1) the products of their concentrations are equal, and 2) the sum of the diffusible and nondiffusible anions on either side of the membrane is equal to the sum of the concentrations of diffusible and nondiffusible cations; the unequal distribution of diffusible ions thus produced creates a potential difference across the membrane (membrane potential).

dynamic e., equilibrium (2).

genetic e., the condition of a dynamic genetic system in which the several rates of change between all possible pairs of parts are such that the composition is invariant.

Gibbs-Donnan e., Donnan e.

Hardy-Weinberg e., random mating e.; that state in which the genetic structure of the population conforms to the prediction of the Hardy-Weinberg law; it is not a stable e., although for a large mating population it may be approximated.

homeostatic e., see homeostasis.

nitrogenous e., a condition in which the amount of nitrogen excreted from the body equals that taken in with the food; nutritive e. so far as protein is concerned.

nutritive e., physiologic e.; condition in which there is a perfect balance between intake and excretion of nutritive material, so that there is no increase or loss in weight.

physiologic e., nutritive e.

radioactive e., a situation (not a true e.) in which a particular atom is being produced by the radioactive breakdown of a precursor while it is itself breaking down, the two breakdowns matching so that the amount of the atom in question remains temporarily constant.

random mating e., Hardy-Weinberg e.

stable e., e. in which, after a small perturbation, the original state will tend to be restored.

unstable e., e. in which the response to a small perturbation will tend to make the perturbation greater.

equilin (ek′wi-lin). 3-Hydroxyestra-1,3,5(10),7-tetraen-17-one; an estrogenic steroid occurring in the urine of pregnant mares.

equimolar (ē-kwi-mō′ler). Containing an equal number of moles or having the same molarity, as in two or more substances.

equimolecular (ē′kwi-mō-lek′yū-ler). Containing an equal number of molecules, as in two or more solutions.

equine (ē′kwīn) [L. *equinus,* fr. *equus,* horse]. Relating to, derived from, or resembling the horse, mule, ass, or other members of the genus *Equus.*

equinovalgus (ē-kwī-nō-val′gŭs, ek′wi-nō-). *Talipes* equinovalgus.

equinovarus (ē-kwī-nō-vā′rŭs, ek′wi-nō-). *Talipes* equinovarus.

equisetosis (ē′kwi-se-tō′sis). A toxicosis in horses caused by eating horsetail (*Equisetum arvense,* a weed).

equitoxic (ē-kwi-tok′sik). Of equivalent toxicity.

equivalence, equivalency (ē-kwiv′ă-lens, -len-sē) [L. *aequus,* equal, + *valentia,* strength (valence)]. The property of an element or radical of combining with or displacing, in definite and fixed proportion, another element or radical in a compound.

equivalent (ē-kwiv′ă-lent) [see equivalence]. **1.** Equal in any respect. **2.** That which is equal in size, weight, force, or any other quality to something else.

combustion e., the heat value of a gram of carbohydrate or fat oxidized outside the body.

gold e., gold number; a unit of power of the protective colloids; the number of milligrams of protective colloid just sufficient to prevent the precipitation of 10 ml of a 0.0053 to 0.0058% gold solution by the action of 1 ml of a 10% sodium chloride solution.

gram e., combining or equivalent weight; **(1)** the weight in grams of an element that combines with or replaces 1 gram of hydrogen; **(2)** the atomic or molecular weight in grams of an atom or group of atoms involved in a chemical reaction divided by the number of electrons donated, taken up, or shared by the atom or group of atoms in the course of that reaction; **(3)** the weight of a substance contained in 1 liter of 1 normal solution, a variant of (1).

Joule's e. (J), the dynamic e. of heat; the amount of work converted to heat that will raise the temperature of 1 pound of water 1°F is 778 foot-pounds; in metric units, 1 calorie, which raises 1 gram of water 1°C, equals 4.187×10^7 dyne-centimeters, which equals 4.187 joules (J).

lethal e., a combination of selective effects that on average have the same impact on the composition of the gene pool as one death; *e.g.,* two carriers at 50% risk of dying would be the lethal e. of one carrier at 100% risk.

metabolic e. (MET), the oxygen cost of energy expenditure measured at supine rest (1 MET = 3 to 4 ml O per kg of body weight per minute); multiples of MET are used to estimate the oxygen cost of activity, *e.g.,* 3 to 5 METs for light work; more than 9 METs for heavy work.

nitrogen e., the nitrogen content of protein; used in calculating the protein breakdown in the body from the nitrogen excreted in the urine, 1 g of nitrogen considered as having originated in 6.25 g of protein catabolized.

starch e., the amount of oxygen consumed in the combustion of a given weight of fat as compared with that consumed in the combustion of an equal weight of starch; the figure is about 2.38, that for starch being taken as 1.

toxic e., the amount of toxin or other poison per kilogram of body weight necessary to kill an animal.

ER Abbreviation for endoplasmic *reticulum.*

Er Symbol for erbium.

ERA Abbreviation for evoked response *audiometry.*

Eranko, Eino, Finnish anatomist, *1924. See E.'s fluorescence *stain.*

erasion (ē-rā′zhŭn) [L. *eradere,* to erase]. Obsolete term for the scraping away of tissue, especially of bone.

Erb, Wilhelm H., German neurologist, 1840–1921. See E.'s *atrophy, disease, palsy, paralysis,* spinal *paralysis, sign;* E.-Charcot *disease;* Duchenne-E. *paralysis;* E.-Westphal *sign;* Westphal-E. *sign.*

ERBF Abbreviation for effective renal blood *flow.*

erbium (er′bē-ŭm). A rare earth (lanthanide) element, symbol Er, atomic no. 68, atomic weight 167.26.

ercalcidiol (er-kal-sid′ē-ol). 25-Hydroxyergocalciferol.

ercalciol (er-kal′sē-ol). Ergocalciferol.

ercalcitriol (er-kal-sit′rē-ol). 1,25-Dihydroxyergocalciferol.

ERCP Abbreviation for endoscopic retrograde *cholangiopancreatography.*

Erdheim, Jakob, Austrian physician, 1874–1937. See E. *disease, tumor.*

Erdmann, Hugo, German chemist, 1862–1910. See E.'s *reagent.*

erectile (ē-rek'tīl). Capable of erection.

erection (ē-rek'shŭn) [L. *erectio,* fr. *erigo,* pp. *erectus,* to set up]. The condition of erectile tissue when filled with blood, which then becomes hard and unyielding; denoting especially this state of the penis.

erector (ērek'tŏr, -tōr) [Mod. L.]. Arrector. **1.** One who or that which raises or makes erect. **2.** Denoting specifically certain muscles having such action.

eremophilia (er'ē-mō-fil'ē-ă) [G. *erēmia,* solitude, + *philos,* fond]. Morbid desire to be alone.

eremophobia (er'ē-mō-fō'bē-ă) [G. *erēmia,* solitude, + *phobos,* fear]. Morbid fear of deserted places or of solitude.

erethism (er'ĕ-thizm) [G. *erethismos,* irritation]. An abnormal state of excitement or irritation, either general or local.

erethismic, erethistic, erethitic (er-ĕ-thiz'mik, -this'tik, -thit'ik). Marked by or causing erethism; excited; irritable.

ereuthophobia (er'ū-thō-fō'bē-ă) [G. *ereuthos,* blushing, + *phobos,* fear]. Morbid fear of blushing.

ERG Abbreviation for electroretinogram.

erg [G. *ergon,* work]. The unit of work in the CGS system; the amount of work done by 1 dyne acting through 1 centimeter, 1 g cm^2 s^{-2}; In the SI system, 1 erg equals 10^{-7} joule.

ergasia (er-gā'zē-ă) [G. work]. **1.** Any form of activity, especially mental. **2.** The total of functions and reactions of an individual.

ergasiomania (er-gas'ē-ō-mā'nē-ă) [G. *ergasia,* work, + *mania,* insanity]. Morbid or obsessive need to work.

ergasiophobia (er-gas'ē-ō-fō'bē-ă) [G. *ergasia,* work, + *phobos,* fear]. Aversion to work of any kind.

ergasthenia (er-gas-thē'nē-ă) [G. *ergasia,* work, + *astheneia,* weakness, disease]. Rarely used term for debility or any morbid symptoms due to overexertion.

ergastoplasm (er-gas'tō-plazm) [G. *ergastēr,* a workman, + *plasma,* something formed]. Granular endoplasmic *reticulum.*

ergin (er'jin). A hypothetical substance in the blood or tissue fluids presumed to lead to the allergic phenomenon, as a result of the union of the e. with allergen. See also reagin.

ergine (erg'ēn). Lysergic acid amide.

ergo- [G. *ergon,* work]. Combining form relating to work.

ergobasine (er-gō-bā'sēn). Ergonovine.

ergocalciferol (er'gō-kal-sif'er-ol). Vitamin D_2; calciferol; ercalciol; viosterol; (5*Z,* 7*E,* 22*E*)-(3*S*)-9,10-secoergosta-5,7,10(19),22-tetraen-3-ol; activated ergosterol, the vitamin D of plant origin; it arises from ultraviolet irradiation of ergosterol, which is cleaved at the 9,10 bond and develops a double bond between C-10 and C-19; used in prophylaxis and treatment of vitamin D deficiency.

ergocornine (er-gō-kōr'nēn). $C_{31}H_{39}N_5O_5$; an alkaloid isolated from ergot.

ergocristine (er'gō-kris'tēn). $C_{35}H_{39}N_5O_5$; an alkaloid isolated from ergot.

ergocryptine (er-gō-krip'tēn). $C_{32}H_{41}N_5O_5$; an alkaloid isolated from ergot.

ergodynamograph (er'gō-dī-nam'ō-graf) [ergo- + G. *dynamis,* force, + *graphō,* to write]. An instrument for recording both the degree of muscular force and the amount of the work accomplished by muscular contraction.

ergoesthesiograph (er'gō-es-thē'zē-ō-graf) [ergo- + G. *aisthēsis,* sensation, + *graphō,* to record]. An apparatus for recording graphically muscular aptness as shown in the ability to counterbalance variable resistances.

ergogenic (er-gō-jen'ik). Tending to increase work.

ergograph (er'gō-graf) [ergo- + G. *graphō,* to write]. An instrument for recording the amount of work done by muscular contractions, or the amplitude of contraction.

Mosso's e., an instrument consisting of pulleys, weights, and a recording lever, which is used to obtain a graphic record of flexion of a finger, hand, or arm.

ergographic (er-gō-graf'ik). Relating to the ergograph and the record made by it.

ergometer (er-gom'ĕ-ter) [ergo- + G. *metron,* measure]. Dynamometer.

ergometrine (er-gō-met'rēn). Ergonovine.

e. maleate, *ergonovine* maleate.

ergonomics (er-gō-nom'iks) [ergo- + G. *nomos,* law]. A branch of ecology concerned with human factors in the design and operations of machines and the physical environment.

ergonovine (er-gō-nō'vēn, -vin). Ergometrine, ergobasine, ergostetrine; an alkaloid from ergot; on hydrolysis it yields D-lysergic acid and L-2-aminopropanol.

e. maleate, ergometrine maleate; a powerful oxytocic agent; this action is more prominent, and other actions of ergot (vasoconstriction, central nervous system stimulation, adrenergic blockade, etc.) are less prominent than for other ergot alkaloids; effective orally and parenterally.

ergosine (er'gō-sēn, -sin). An alkaloid from ergot with actions similar to those of ergotamine.

ergostat (er'gō-stat) [ergo- + G. *statos,* standing, placed]. A form of machine for exercising the muscles.

ergosterin (er-gos'ter-in). Ergosterol.

ergosterol (er-gos'ter-ol). Ergosterin; 7,22-didehydrocholesterol; ergosta-5,7,22-trien-3β-ol; the most important of the provitamins D_2; ultraviolet irradiation converts e. to lumisterol, tachysterol, and ergocalciferol.

ergostetrine (er-gō-stet'rēn, -rin). Ergonovine.

er'got. Rye smut; the resistant, overwintering stage of the parasitic ascomycetous fungus *Claviceps purpurea,* a pathogen of rye grass that transforms the seed of rye into a compact spurlike mass of fungal pseudotissue (the sclerotium) containing five or more optically isomeric pairs of alkaloids. The levorotary isomers induce uterine contractions, control bleeding, and alleviate certain localized vascular disorders (migraine headaches). E. exemplifies fungal products with profound toxic effects at appropriate levels.

corn e., *Ustilago* maydis.

ergotamine (er-got'ă-mēn). $C_{33}H_{35}N_5O_5$; an alkaloid from ergot, used for the relief of migraine; it is a potent stimulant of smooth muscle, particularly of the blood vessels and the uterus, and produces adrenergic blockade (chiefly of the alpha receptors); hydrogenated e., dihydroergotamine, is less toxic and has fewer side effects. Also available as e. tartrate.

ergotaminine (er-got-am'i-nēn). An isomer of ergotamine but practically inert.

ergotherapy (er-gō-thār'ă-pē) [G. *ergon,* work, + *therapeia,* therapy]. Treatment of disease by muscular exercise.

ergothioneine (er'gō-thī-ō-nē'in). Thioneine; thiohistidylbetaine; 2'-thiolhistidine betaine; the betaine of a sulfur-containing derivative of histidine, present in blood and other mammalian tissue and in ergot.

ergotism (er'got-izm). Poisoning by a toxic substance contained in the sclerotia of the fungus, *Claviceps purpura,* growing on rye grass; characterized by necrosis of the extremities due to contraction of the peripheral vascular bed.

ergotoxine (er'gō-tok'sēn, -sin). Ecboline; a mixture of alkaloids obtained from ergot, consisting of 1:1:1 ergocristine, ergocornine and ergocryptine, more toxic than other natural and semisynthetic ergot alkaloids; a potent stimulant of smooth muscle, particularly of the blood vessels and uterus, and produces adrenergic blockade (chiefly of the alpha receptors).

ergotropic (er'gō-trop'ik) [ergo- + G. *tropos*, a turning]. The term introduced by W.R. Hess to denote those mechanisms and the functional status of the nervous system that favor the organism's capacity to expend energy, as distinguished from the trophotropic mechanisms promoting rest and reconstitution of energy stores. In general, the balance between ergotropic and trophotropic nervous mechanisms corresponds in large part to that between the sympathetic and parasympathetic subdivisions of the autonomic nervous system.

Erichsen, Sir John E., British surgeon, 1818–1896. See E.'s *sign*.

eriodictyon (ār'ē-ō-dik'tē-on). Mountain balm; yerba santa; the dried leaves of *Eriodictyon californicum* (family Hydrophyllaceae); the fluidextract and the syrup have been used as an expectorant and to mask the taste of bitter substances.

erisophake (e-ris'ō-fāk) [G. *erysis*, a drawing, + *phakos*, lentil]. A surgical instrument designed to hold the lens by suction in cataract extraction.

Erlenmeyer, Emil, German chemist, 1825–1909. See E. *flask*, flask *deformity*.

Ernst, Paul, German pathologist, 1859–1937. See Babès-E. *bodies*.

erode (ē-rōd') [L. *erodere*, to gnaw away]. **1.** To cause, or to be affected by, erosion. **2.** To remove by ulceration.

erogenous (ĕ-roj'ĕ-nŭs) [G. *eros*, love, + *genos*, birth]. Capable of producing sexual excitement when stimulated.

eros (ē'ros, ār'os) [G. love]. In psychoanalysis, the life principle representing all instinctual tendencies toward procreation and life. *Cf.* thanatos. See also subentries under instinct.

erose (ē-rōs') [L. *erodo*, pp. *erosus*, to gnaw away]. Denoting an edge or margin which is irregularly notched or indented, as if gnawed away; used especially in reference to bacterial colonies.

erosion (ē-rō'zhŭn) [L. *erosio*, fr. *erodere*, to gnaw away]. **1.** A wearing away or a state of being worn away, as by friction or pressure. *Cf.* corrosion. **2.** A shallow ulcer; in the stomach and intestine, an ulcer limited to the mucosa, with no penetration of the muscularis mucosa. **3.** Odontolysis; the wearing away of a tooth by chemical or abrasive action; when the cause is unknown, it is referred to as idiopathic e.

Dieulafoy's e., acute ulcerative gastroenteritis complicating pneumonia, possibly caused by overproduction of adrenal steroid hormones.

recurrent corneal e., repeated vesiculation followed by exfoliation of the corneal epithelium.

erosive (ē-rō'siv). **1.** Having the property of eroding or wearing away. **2.** An eroding agent.

erotic (ĕ-rot'ik) [G. *erōtikos*, relating to love, fr. *erōs*, love]. Relating to sexual passion; lustful; having the quality to produce sexual arousal.

erotism, eroticism (er'ō-tizm, ĕ-rot'i-sizm). A condition of sexual excitement.

anal e., pleasurable experience centered around the anal zone, especially during the anal phase in children.

erotization (er'ō-ti-zā'shŭn). Libidinization; the act of sexual arousal or the state of being sexually excited.

erotogenesis (er'ō-tō-jen'ĕ-sis) [G. *erōs*, love, + *genesis*, origin]. The origin or genesis of sexual impulses.

erotogenic (er'ō-tō-jen'ik) [G. *erōs*, love, + *-gen*, production]. Causing sexual excitement.

erotomania (er'ō-tō-mā'nē-ă) [G. *erōs*, love, + *mania*, frenzy]. Excessive or morbid inclination to erotic thoughts and behavior.

erotopathic (er'ō-tō-path'ik). Relating to erotopathy.

erotopathy (er-ō-top'ă-thē) [G. *erōs*, love, + *pathos*, suffering]. Any abnormality of the sexual impulse.

erotophobia (er'ō-tō-fō'bē-ă) [G. *erōs*, love, + *phobos*, fear]. Morbid aversion to the thought of sexual love and to its physical expression.

ERP Abbreviation for early receptor *potential*.

ERPF Abbreviation for effective renal plasma *flow*.

erratic (ĕ-rat'ik) [L. *erro*, pp. *erratus*, to wander]. **1.** Eccentric. **2.** Denoting symptoms that vary in intensity, frequency, or location.

error (er'ōr). **1.** A defect in structure or function. **2.** In biostatistics: 1) a mistaken decision, as in hypothesis testing or classification by a discriminant function; 2) the difference between the true value and the observed value of a variate, ascribed to randomness or observer misreading.

inborn e.'s of metabolism, a group of disorders each of which involves a disorder of a single unique enzyme, genetic in origin, and operating from birth; effects are ascribable to accumulation of the substrate on which the enzyme normally acts (*e.g.*, phenylketonuria), to deficiency of the product of the enzyme (*e.g.*, albinism), or to forcing metabolism through an auxilliary pathway (*e.g.*, oxaluria).

ertacalciol (er-tă-kal'sē-ol). See tachysterol.

erubescence (er-ū-bes'ens) [L. *erubescere*, to redden]. A reddening of the skin.

erubescent (er-ū-bes'ent). Denoting reddening of the skin.

erucic acid (ĕ-rū'sik). 13-Docosenoic acid; a 22-carbon unsaturated fatty acid present in the seeds of nasturtium (Indian cress) and of several *Cruciferae* species (rape, mustard, and wallflower); thought to be toxic to cardiac muscle.

eructation (ē-rŭk-tā'shŭn) [L. *eructo*, pp. *-atus*, to belch]. Belching; ructus; the voiding of gas or of a small quantity of acid fluid from the stomach through the mouth.

eruption (ē-rŭp'shŭn) [L. *e-rumpo*, pp. *-ruptus*, to break out]. **1.** A breaking out, especially the appearance of lesions on the skin. **2.** A rapidly developing dermatosis of the skin or mucous membranes, especially when appearing as a local manifestation of a general disease, such as typhoid fever or one of the exanthemata; an e. is characterized, according to the nature of the lesion, as macular, papular, vesicular, pustular, bullous, nodular, erythematous, etc. **3.** The passage of a tooth through the alveolar process and perforation of the gums.

accelerated e., a dental e. pattern which is chronologically advanced in comparison with the average pattern of dental e.; e. of the first tooth occurs at an earlier age than the average, and the intervals of time between subsequent dental e.'s are shorter than the average.

butterfly e., butterfly (2).

clinical e., development of the crown of a tooth that can be observed clinically.

continuous e., the e. of a tooth into the mouth and its continuous movement in a vertical direction.

creeping e., cutaneous *larva migrans*.

delayed e., a dental e. pattern which is chronologically late in comparison with the average pattern of dental e.; e. of the first tooth occurs at a later age than the average, and the intervals of time between subsequent dental e.'s are longer than the average.

drug e., dermatitis or dermatosis medicamentosa; drug rash; medicinal eruption; any e. caused by the ingestion, injection, inhalation, or insertion of a drug, most often the result of allergic sensitization; reactions to drugs applied to the cutaneous surface are not generally designated as drug e., but as contact-type dermatitis.

feigned e., *dermatitis* artefacta.

fixed drug e., a type of drug e. that recurs at a fixed site (or sites) following the administration of a particular drug; the lesions usually consist of intensely erythematous and purplish, sharply demarcated macules, and occasionally of herpetic vesicles; the affected areas undergo gradual involution, but flare and enlarge on readministration of the offending drug.

iodine e., an acneform or follicular e. or granulomatous lesion caused by a reaction to systemic iodine or iodide administration.

Kaposi's varicelliform e., *eczema* herpeticum.

medicinal e., drug *eruption.*

passive e., the apparent continued e. of the teeth, actually the result of apical migration of the gingivae and crestal bone.

polymorphic light e., a papular, sometimes eczematous, e. appearing in a few hours and lasting up to several days on skin exposed to shortwave ultraviolet light; subepidermal edema and deep perivascular lymphocytic infiltration is seen microscopically.

serum e., urticaria seen in serum sickness.

surgical e., the uncovering of an unerupted tooth to permit its further e. into the oral cavity by surgically removing overlying soft tissue, bone, and sometimes teeth.

eruptive (ē-rŭp'tiv). Characterized by eruption.

ERV Abbreviation for expiratory reserve *volume.*

erysipelas (er-i-sip'ĕ-las) [G., fr. *erythros,* red + *pella,* skin]. Rose (1); fire (1); a specific, acute, cutaneous inflammatory disease caused by a hemolytic streptococcus and characterized by hot, red, edematous, brawny, and sharply defined eruptions; usually accompanied by severe constitutional symptoms.

ambulant e., e. migrans.

coastal e., onchocerciasis.

e. inter'num, an erysipelatous eruption in the vagina, uterus, and peritoneum, occurring in the puerperium.

e. mi'grans, ambulant or wandering e.; a widely spreading form involving the entire face, or even the surface of the body.

e. per'stans fa'ciei, chronic, dusky red eruption of erysipelas on the face.

phlegmonous e., a form marked by invasion of the subcutaneous tissues, with the formation of deep-seated abscesses.

e. pustulo'sum, development of pustules over the area of e.

surgical e., e. caused by infection of the wound following a surgical procedure.

swine e., a destructive disease of swine, occurring in both acute and chronic forms, caused by *Erysipelothrix rhusiopathiae.*

e. verruco'sum, development of verrucous or warty lesions on the area of e.

wandering e., e. migrans.

erysipelatous (er'i-si-pel'ă-tŭs). Relating to erysipelas.

erysipeloid (er-i-sip'ĕ-loyd) [G. *erysipelas* + *eidos,* resemblance]. Rosenbach's disease (2); crab hand; pseudoerysipelas; a specific, usually self-limiting, cellulitis of the hand caused by *Erysipelothrix rhusiopathiae;* appears as a dusky erythema with diamondlike configuration of the skin at the site of a wound sustained in handling fish or meat and may become generalized, with plaques of erythema and bullae, and severe toxemia; occasionally may become a protracted illness with acute exacerbations.

Erysipelothrix (ăr-i-sip'ĕ-lō-thriks, -si-pel'ō-thriks) [erysipelas + G. *thrix,* hair]. A genus of bacteria (family Corynebacteriaceae) containing nonmotile, Gram-positive, rod-shaped organisms which have a tendency to form long filaments; older cells tend to become Gram-negative. They produce acid but no gas from glucose. They are facultatively anaerobic and catalase-negative. Members of this genus are parasitic on mammals, birds, and fish. The type species is *E. rhusiopathiae.*

E. insidio'sa, *E. rhusiopathiae.*

E. rhusiopath'iae, *E. insidiosa;* a species which causes swine erysipelas, human erysipeloid, and septicemia in mice, and commonly infects fish handlers; it is the type species of the genus *E.*

erysipelotoxin (ăr-i-sip'ĕ-lō-tok'sin). A toxin produced by types of *Streptococcus pyogenes* (group A hemolytic streptococci), the bacterial cause of erysipelas.

erythema (er-i-thē'mă) [G. *erythēma,* flush]. Inflammatory redness of the skin.

e. ab ig'ne, e. caloricum.

acrodynic e., acrodynia (2).

e. annula're, rounded or ringed lesions.

e. annula're centrif'ugum, e. figuratum perstans; a chronic recurring erythematous eruption consisting of small and large annular lesions, both discrete and confluent; there is usually a scant marginal scale.

e. annula're rheumat'icum, a variant of e. multiforme associated with rheumatic fever.

e. arthrit'icum epidem'icum, Haverhill *fever.*

e. bullo'sum, e. multiforme with formation of large vesicles or bullae.

e. calor'icum, e. ab igne; toasted shins; a reticulated, pigmented, macular eruption that occurs, mostly on the shins, of bakers, stokers, and others exposed to radiant heat.

e. chron'icum mi'grans, a raised erythematous ring with advancing indurated borders and central clearing, radiating from the site of a tick bite such as that by *Ixodes dammini;* the characteristic skin lesion of Lyme disease.

e. circina'tum, e. multiforme in which the lesions are grouped in more or less circular fashion.

e. dyschro'micum per'stans, variously sized gray or red, slightly elevated macular lesions that tend to coalesce on the trunk, extremities, and face, clinically resembling pinta but with no demonstrable treponeme and with negative serology.

e. eleva'tum diu'tinum, Bury's disease; a chronic symmetrical eruption of flattened nodules, of a pinkish or purplish color, occurring in plaques on the buttocks and extensors of wrists, elbows, and knees, becoming fibrotic and finally scarring; early lesions show leukocytic angiitis with fibrinoid or lipid deposits in vessel walls.

e. exfoliati'va, *keratolysis* exfoliativa.

e. figura'tum per'stans, e. annulare centrifugum.

e. fu'gax, a diffuse and fleeting e. occurring most commonly in erethistic persons from a variety of, and often minimal, emotional stimuli.

e. gyra'tum, e. circinatum in which the various ringed lesions overlap each other.

hemorrhagic exudative e., Henoch-Schönlein *purpura.*

e. indura'tum, Bazin's disease; nodular tuberculid; recurrent hard subcutaneous nodules that frequently break down and form necrotic ulcers, usually on the calves and less frequently on the thighs or arms of middle-aged women; they are associated with erythrocyanotic changes in cold weather; although microscopically granulomatous and necrotizing, the disease is not tuberculous.

e. infectio'sum, fifth or Sticker's disease; a mild infectious disease characterized by an erythematous maculopapular eruption, accompanied by little or no fever; caused by parvovirus B-19.

e. intertri'go, see intertrigo.

e. i'ris, herpes iris (1); concentric rings of e. varying in intensity, characteristic of e. multiforme.

Jacquet's e., diaper *dermatitis.*

e. kerato'des, keratodermia with an erythematous border.

macular e., roseola.

e. margina'tum, a variant of e. multiforme seen in rheumatic fever; occasionally has a configuration to suggest the designation e. migrans (geographic tongue).

e. mi'grans, e. mi'grans ling'uae, geographic *tongue.*

Milian's e., ninth-day e.

e. multifor'me, Hebra's disease (1); herpes iris (2); e. polymorphe; an acute eruption of macules, papules, or subdermal vesicles presenting a multiform appearance, the characteristic lesion being the

target or iris lesion over the dorsal aspect of the hands and forearms; its origin may be allergic, seasonal, or from drug sensitivity, and the eruption may be recurrent or may run a severe course with fatal termination (Stevens-Johnson syndrome).
e. multifor'me bullo'sum or **exudati'vum,** Stevens-Johnson *syndrome.*
necrolytic migratory e., an erythematous, scaling, and sometimes bullous and erosive dermatitis occurring irregularly in plaques chiefly on the lower trunk, buttocks, perineum, and thighs; associated with weight loss, anemia, stomatitis, and elevation of plasma glucagon in glucagonoma of the pancreas.
e. neonato'rum, e. toxicum neonatorum.
ninth-day e., Milian's e. or disease; a nontoxic eruption which simulates measles or a toxic erythema, occurring usually on the ninth day of a course of medication; first described as a reaction to arsenical treatment of syphilis.
e. nodo'sum, nodal fever; a dermatosis marked by the sudden formation of painful nodes on the extensor surfaces of the lower extremities, with lesions that are self-limiting but tend to recur; associated with arthralgia and fever, or may be the result of drug sensitivity or associated with sarcoidosis and various infections.
e. nodo'sum lepro'sum, an acute type of lepromatous reaction with generalized systemic involvement and tender deep nodules of the face, thighs, and arms; usually seen in undiagnosed, untreated, or neglected cases of leprosy.
e. nodo'sum mi'grans, subacute migratory *panniculitis.*
e. palma're heredita'rium, Lane's disease; a condition characterized by asymptomatic symmetrical palmar e.; autosomal dominant inheritance.
e. papula'tum, the papular form of e. multiforme.
e. paratrim'ma, e. due to stasis over pressure points.
e. per'nio, chilblain.
e. per'stans, probably a chronic form of e. multiforme in which the relapses recur so persistently that the eruption is almost permanent.
e. polymorphe, e. multiforme.
scarlatiniform e., e. scarlatinoi'des, an erythematous macular eruption accompanied by slight constitutional symptoms and followed by desquamation.
e. sim'plex, dermatitis simplex; blushing or redness of the skin caused by a toxic reaction or a neurovascular phenomenon.
e. sola're, sunburn.
symptomatic e., a general term applied to various e.'s associated with systemic disease, fevers, allergic states, etc.
e. tox'icum, flushing of the skin due to allergic reaction to some toxic substance.
e. tox'icum neonato'rum, e. neonatorum; a common transient eruption of erythema, small papules, and occasionally pustules filled with eosinophilic leukocytes overlying hair follicles of the newborn.
e. tubercula'tum, e. multiforme in which the papules are of large size.

erythematous (er-i-them'ă-tŭs, -thē'mă-tŭs). Relating to or marked by erythema.

erythematovesicular (er-i-thē'mă-tō-ve-sik'yū-lăr). Denoting a condition characterized by edema, erythema, and vesiculation, as in allergic contact dermatitis.

erythermalgia (er'i-ther-mal'jē-ă). Erythromelalgia.

erythr-. See erythro-.

erythralgia (ăr-i-thral'jē-ă) [erythro- + G. *algos,* pain]. Painful redness of the skin. See also erythromelalgia.

erythrasma (er-i-thraz'mă) [G. *erythrainō,* to redden]. An eruption of reddish brown patches, in the axillae and groins especially, due to the presence of *Corynebacterium minutissimum.*

erythredema (ĕ-rith-rē-dē'mă) [erythro- + G. *oidēma,* swelling]. Acrodynia (2).

erythremia (er-i-thrē'mē-ă) [erythro- + G. *haima,* blood]. A chronic form of polycythemia of unknown cause; characterized by bone marrow hyperplasia, an increase in blood volume as well as in the number of red cells, redness or cyanosis of the skin, and splenomegaly. Also called Osler's disease (1); Vaquez' or Osler-Vaquez disease; polycythemia rubra, vera, or rubra vera.
altitude e., chronic mountain *sickness.*

erythrism (er'i-thrizm, ĕ-rith'rizm) [G. *erythros,* red]. Redness of the hair with a ruddy, freckled complexion.

erythristic (er-i-thris'tik). Rufous; relating to or marked by erythrism; having a ruddy complexion and reddish hair.

erythrite (ĕ-rith'rīt). Erythritol.

erythritol (ĕ-rith'ri-tol). Erythrite; erythrol; tetrahydroxybutane (1,2,3,4-butanetetrol); the 4-carbon sugar alcohol obtained by the reduction of erythrose, notable for its sweetness (twice that of sucrose); found in lichens, algae, and fungi; a coronary vasodilator.

erythrityl tetranitrate (ĕ-rith'ri-til tet-ră-nī'trāt). Erythrol tetranitrate; tetranitrol; a vasodilator used in angina pectoris and hypertension.

erythro-, erythr- [G. *erythros,* red]. **1.** Combining forms meaning red or denoting relationship to redness. **2.** Prefixes indicating the structure of erythrose in a larger sugar; used as such, it is italicized (*e.g.,* 2-deoxy-D-*erythro*-pentose).

erythroblast (ĕ-rith'rō-blast) [erythro- + G. *blastos,* germ]. Erythrocytoblast; originally, a term denoting all forms of human red blood cells containing a nucleus, both pathologic (*i.e.,* megaloblastic) and normal (*i.e.,* normoblastic). The pathologic or megaloblastic series is observed in pernicious anemia in relapse. The term megaloblast is also used to indicate the first generation of cells in the red blood cell series which can be distinguished from precursor endothelial cells; hence with this usage, megaloblast denotes both a normal and an abnormal cell. In the *normoblastic series* of maturation four stages of development can be recognized: 1) pronormoblast, 2) basophilic normoblast, 3) polychromatic normoblast, and 4) orthochromatic normoblast. In the *megaloblastic series* of maturation, stages similar to those found in the normoblastic series are seen: 1) promegaloblast, 2) basophilic megaloblast, 3) polychromatic megaloblast, and 4) orthochromatic megaloblast. In the *normal series* of maturation, after loss of the nucleus, young erythrocytes are called *reticulocytes;* these cells may be recognized with supravital stains such as brilliant cresyl blue; ultimately the reticulocytes become erythrocytes, or mature red blood cells.

erythroblastemia (ĕ-rith'rō-blas-tē'mē-ă) [erythroblast + G. *haima,* blood]. The presence of nucleated red cells in the peripheral blood.

erythroblastopenia (ĕ-rith'rō-blas-tō-pē'nē-ă) [erythroblast + G. *penia,* poverty]. A primary deficiency of erythroblasts in bone marrow, seen in aplastic anemia.

erythroblastosis (ĕ-rith'rō-blas-tō'sis) [erythroblast + *-osis,* condition]. The presence of erythroblasts in considerable number in the blood.
avian e., fowl e.; an expression of disease of the avian leukosis-sarcoma complex; characterized by severe anemia and large numbers of erythroblasts in the blood; chickens are most susceptible but fatal natural infections have been reported in guinea fowl.
e. feta'lis, fetal e., hemolytic anemia of newborn (1); hemolytic disease of newborn; congenital or neonatal anemia; anemia neonatorum; a grave hemolytic anemia that, in most instances, results from development in the mother of anti-Rh antibody in response to the Rh factor in the (Rh-positive) fetal blood; it is characterized by many erythroblasts in the circulation, and often generalized edema (hydrops fetalis) and enlargement of the liver and spleen; the disease is sometimes caused by antibodies for blood factors other than

Rh and, in rare examples, the cause is not conclusively known. See also hemolytic *anemia* of newborn (2).

fowl e., avian e.

erythroblastotic (ĕ-rith'rō-blas-tot'ik). Pertaining to erythroblastosis, especially erythroblastosis fetalis.

erythrocatalysis (ĕ-rith'rō-kă-tal'i-sis) [erythro- + G. *katalysis,* dissolution]. Phagocytosis of the red blood cells.

erythrochromia (ĕ-rith'rō-krō'mē-ă) [erythro- + G. *chrōma,* color]. A red coloration or staining.

erythroclasis (er-i-throk'lă-sis) [erythro- + G. *klasis,* a breaking]. Fragmentation of the red blood cells.

erythroclastic (ĕ-rith'rō-klas'tik). Pertaining to erythroclasis; destructive to red blood cells.

erythrocuprein (ĕ-rith'rō-kū'prē-in). Cytocuprein.

erythrocyanosis (ĕ-rith'rō-sī-ă-nō'sis) [erythro- + G. *kyanos,* blue, + *-osis,* condition]. A condition seen in children, girls, and women particularly, in which exposure of the limbs to cold causes them to become swollen and dusky red; it results from direct exposure to cold, but not freezing, temperatures.

erythrocyte (ĕ-rith'rō-sīt) [erythro- + G. *kytos,* cell]. Red blood cell or corpuscle; a mature red blood cell.

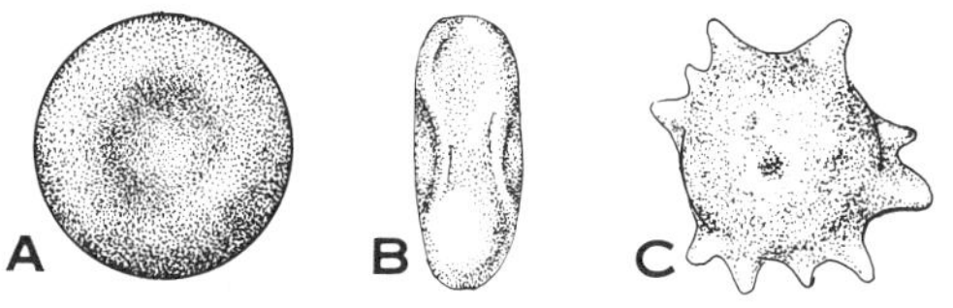

Erythrocyte
Erythrocytes in 0.9 per cent sodium chloride solution. *A*, viewed from broad surface; *B*, profile; *C*, crenated. (After Broderson.)

erythrocythemia (ĕ-rith'rō-sī-thē'mē-ă) [erythro- + G. *kytos,* cell, + *haima,* blood]. Polycythemia.

erythrocytic (ĕ-rith-rō-sit'ik). Pertaining to an erythrocyte.

erythrocytoblast (ĕ-rith-rō-sī'tō-blast) [erythro- + G. *kytos,* cell, + *blastos,* germ]. Erythroblast.

erythrocytolysin (ĕ-rith'rō-sī-tol'i-sin). Hemolysin (1).

erythrocytolysis (ĕ-rith'rō-sī-tol'i-sis) [erythrocyte + G. *lysis,* loosening]. Hemolysis.

erythrocytometer (ĕ-rith'rō-sī-tom'ĕ-ter) [erythrocyte + G. *metron,* measure]. An instrument for counting the red blood cells; Hayden used this term to denote an instrument to measure the diameter of red blood cells.

erythrocytopenia (ĕ-rith'rō-sī-tō-pē'nē-ă). Erythropenia.

erythrocytopoiesis (ĕ-rith'rō-sī'tō-poy-ē'sis). Erythropoiesis.

erythrocytorrhexis (ĕ-rith'rō-sī-tō-rek'sis) [erythrocyte + G. *rhēxis,* rupture]. Erythrorrhexis; a partial erythrocytolysis in which particles of protoplasm escape from the red blood cells, which then become crenated and deformed.

erythrocytoschisis (ĕ-rith'rō-sī-tos'ki-sis) [erythrocyte + G. *schisis,* a splitting]. A breaking up of the red blood cells into small particles that morphologically resemble platelets.

erythrocytosis (ĕ-rith'rō-sī-tō'sis). Polycythemia, especially that which occurs in response to some known stimulus.

erythrocyturia (ĕ-rith'rō-sī-tū'rē-ă). Red blood cells in urine.

erythrodegenerative (ĕ-rith'rō-de-jen'er-ă-tiv). Pertaining to or characterized by degeneration of the red blood cells.

erythroderma (ĕ-rith-rō-der'mă) [erythro- + G. *derma,* skin]. Erythrodermatitis; a nonspecific designation for intense and usually widespread reddening of the skin, often preceding, or associated with exfoliation.

congenital ichthyosiform e., ichthyosiform e.; keratoma malignum; a genodermatosis characterized by diffuse chronic erythema and scale formation with hyperkeratosis of palms and soles, and associated in varying degrees with other defects, including ocular and neural changes.

e. desquamati'vum, Leiner's disease; severe, extensive seborrheic dermatitis in the newborn; frequently occurs in undernourished, cachectic children.

e. exfoliati'va, *keratolysis* exfoliativa.

ichthyosiform e., congenital ichthyosiform e.

maculopapular e., pityriasis lichenoides; lichen variegatus; an eruption of macules and papules of reddish color.

e. psoriat'icum, extensive exfoliative dermatitis simulating psoriasis.

Sézary e., Sézary *syndrome.*

erythrodermatitis (ĕ-rith'rō-der-mă-tī'tis). Erythroderma.

erythrodontia (ĕ-rith-rō-don'shē-ă) [erythro- + G. *odous,* tooth]. Reddish discoloration of the teeth, as may occur in porphyria.

erythrogenesis imperfecta (ĕ-rith-rō-jen'ĕ-sis im-per-fek'tă). Congenital hypoplastic *anemia.*

erythrogenic (ĕ-rith-rō-jen'ik) [erythro- + *-gen,* producing]. **1.** Producing red, as causing an eruption or a red color sensation. **2.** Pertaining to the formation of red blood cells.

erythrogonium, pl. **erythrogonia** (ĕ-rith-rō-gō'nē-ŭm, -nē-ă) [erythro- + G. *gonē,* generation]. The precursor of an erythrocyte; occasionally refers to the erythropoietic tissue as a whole.

erythroid (er'i-throyd, ĕ-rith'royd). Reddish in color.

erythrokeratoderma (ĕ-rith'rō-kār-ă-tō-der'mă). The association of erythoderma and hyperkeratosis, which may be symptomatic at sites of chronic injury or inherited; symmetrical progressive e. is inherited as an autosomal dominant gene and does not involve the palms and soles.

e. variabi'lis, keratosis rubra figurata; a dermatosis characterized by hyperkeratotic plaques of bizarre, geographic configuration, associated with erythrodermic areas that may vary remarkably in size, shape, and position from day to day; onset is usually in the first year of life; autosomal dominant inheritance.

erythrokinetics (ĕ-rith'rō-ki-net'iks) [erythro- + G. *kinēsis,* movement]. A consideration of the kinetics of erythrocytes from their generation to destruction; erythrokinetic studies are sometimes made in cases of anemia to evaluate the balance between erythrocyte production and destruction.

erythrol (er'i-throl). Erythritol.

e. tetranitrate, erythrityl tetranitrate.

erythroleukemia (ĕ-rith'rō-lū-kē'mē-ă). Simultaneous neoplastic proliferation of erythroblastic and leukoblastic tissues.

erythroleukosis (ĕ-rith'rō-lū-kō'sis). A condition resembling leukemia in which the erythropoietic tissue is affected in addition to the leukopoietic tissue.

erythrolysin (er-i-throl'i-sin). Hemolysin (1).

erythrolysis (er-i-throl'i-sis). Hemolysis.

erythromelalgia (ĕ-rith'rō-mel-al'jē-ă) [erythro- + G. *melos,* limb, + *algos,* pain]. Erythermalgia; Gerhardt's or Mitchell's disease; red neuralgia; rodonalgia; paroxysmal throbbing and burning pain in the skin, affecting one or both legs and feet, sometimes one or both hands, accompanied by a dusky mottled redness of the parts; associated with polycythemia vera, thrombocythemia, gout, neurological disease, or heavy-metal poisoning.

erythromelia (ĕ-rith-rō-mē'lē-ă) [erythro- + G. *melos,* limb]. Diffuse idiopathic erythema and atrophy of the skin of the lower limbs.

erythromycin (ĕ-rith-rō-mī'sin). An antibiotic agent obtained from cultures of a strain of *Streptomyces erythraeus* found in soil; it is active against *Corynebacterium diphtheriae* and several other species of *Corynebacterium*, Group A hemolytic streptococci, *Streptococcus pneumoniae*, and *Bordetella pertussis*. Gram-positive bacteria are in general more susceptible to its action than are Gram-negative bacteria, although *neisseriae* and *brucellae* are susceptible to its action. Available as the estolate, ethylcarbonate, ethylsuccinate, gluceptate, lactobionate, stearate, and salts.

erythron (er'i-thron). The total mass of circulating red blood cells, and that part of the hematopoietic tissue from which they are derived.

erythroneocytosis (ĕ-rith'rō-nē-ō-sī-tō'sis) [erythrocyte + G. *neos*, new, + *kytos*, cell, + *-osis*, condition]. The presence in the peripheral circulation of regenerative forms of red blood cells.

erythropenia (ĕ-rith-rō-pē'nē-ă) [erythrocyte + G. *penia*, poverty]. Erythrocytopenia; deficiency in the number of red blood cells.

erythrophagia (ĕ-rith-rō-fā'jē-ă). Phagocytic destruction of red blood cells.

erythrophagocytosis (ĕ-rith'rō-fag'ō-sī-tō'sis). Phagocytosis of erythrocytes.

erythrophil (ĕ-rith'rō-fil) [erythro- + G. *philos*, fond]. **1.** Erythrophilic; staining readily with red dyes. **2.** A cell or tissue element that stains red.

erythrophilic (ĕ-rith-rō-fil'ik). Erythrophil (1).

erythrophore (ĕ-rith'rō-fōr) [erythro- + G. *phoros*, bearing]. Allophore; a chromatophore containing granules of a red or brown pigment.

erythroplakia (ĕ-rith-rō-plā'kē-ă) [erythro- + G. *plax*, plate]. A red velvety plaque-like lesion of mucous membrane which often represents malignant change.

erythroplasia (ĕ-rith-rō-plā'zē-ă) [erythro- + G. *plassō*, to form]. Erythema and dysplasia of the epithelium.
e. of Queyrat, carcinoma *in situ* of the glans penis.
Zoon's e., *balanitis* of Zoon.

erythropoiesis (ĕ-rith'rō-poy-ē'sis) [erythrocyte + G. *poiēsis*, a making]. Erythrocytopoiesis; the formation of red blood cells.

erythropoietic (ĕ-rith'rō-poy-et'ik). Pertaining to or characterized by erythropoiesis.

erythropoietin (ĕ-rith-rō-poy'ĕ-tin). Erythropoietic hormone (2); hematopoietin; hemopoietin; a sialic acid-containing protein that enhances erythropoiesis by stimulating formation of proerythroblasts and release of reticulocytes from bone marrow; it is secreted by the kidney, and possibly by other tissues, and can be detected in human plasma and urine.

erythroprosopalgia (ĕ-rith'rō-pros-ō-pal'jē-ă) [erythro- + G. *prosōpon*, face, + *algos*, pain]. A disorder similar to erythromelalgia, but with the pain and redness occurring in the face.

erythropsia (ĕ-rith-rop'sē-ă) [erythro- + G. *ōps*, eye]. Red vision; an abnormality of vision in which all objects appear to be tinged with red.

erythropyknosis (ĕ-rith'rō-pik-nō'sis) [erythro- + G. *pyknos*, dense]. Alteration of red blood cells to develop the so-called "brassy bodies," under the influence of the malarial parasite.

erythrorrhexis (er'i-thrō-rek'sis, ĕ-rith-rō-rek'sis) [erythrocyte + G. *rhēxis*, rupture]. Erythrocytorrhexis.

erythrose (ĕ-rith'rōs). A tetrose isomeric with threose.

erythrosin B (ĕ-rith'rō-sin) [C.I. 45430]. Tetraiodofluorescein, a fluorescent red acid dye, used as a counterstain in histology and as a fluorescent indicator.

erythroxyline (er-i-throk'si-lēn). Name given to cocaine by its discoverer, Gaedeke, in 1855.

erythrulose (ĕ-rith'rū-lōs). The 2-keto analog of erythrose.

erythruria (er-i-thrū'rē-ă) [erythro- + G. *ouron*, urine]. The passage of red urine.

Es Symbol for einsteinium.

Esbach, Georges H., French physician, 1843–1890. See E.'s *reagent*.

escape (es-kāp'). Term used to describe the situation when a higher pacemaker defaults or A-V conduction fails and a lower pacemaker assumes the function of pacemaking for one or more beats.
nodal e., e. with the A-V node as pacemaker.
ventricular e., e. with an ectopic ventricular focus as pacemaker.

eschar (es'kar) [G. *eschara*, a fireplace, a scab caused by burning]. A thick, coagulated crust or slough which develops following a thermal burn or chemical or physical cauterization of the skin.

escharotic (es-kă-rot'ik) [G. escharōtikos]. Caustic or corrosive.

escharotomy (es-kă-rot'ō-mē) [eschar + G. *tomē*, incision]. Surgical incision in an eschar to lessen constriction, as might be done following a burn.

Escherich, Theodor, German physician, 1857–1911. See *Escherichia coli;* E.'s *sign*.

Escherichia (esh-er-ik'ē-ă) [T. *Escherich*]. A genus of aerobic, facultatively anaerobic bacteria containing short, motile or nonmotile, Gram-negative rods. Motile cells are peritrichous. Glucose and lactose are fermented with the production of acid and gas. These organisms are found in feces; occasionally they are pathogenic to man, causing enteritis, peritonitis, cystitis, etc. It is the type genus of the family Enterobacteriaceae. The type species is *E. coli*.
E. au'rescens, a species commonly found in fecal matter; also found in an infected eye and in contaminated water supplies.
E. co'li, a species that occurs normally in the intestines of man and other vertebrates, is widely distributed in nature, and is a frequent cause of infections of the urogenital tract and of diarrhea in infants; enteropathogenic strains (serovars) of *E. coli* cause diarrhea due to enterotoxin, the production of which seems to be associated with a transferable episome; the type species of the genus.
E. freun'dii, *Citrobacter freundii*.

escorcin, escorcinol (es-kōr'sin, -sin-ol). A brown powder derived from esculetin; used for the detection of defects in the cornea and conjunctiva, which it marks by a red coloration.

esculapian (es-kyū-lā'pē-ăn). Aesculapian.

esculent (es'kyū-lent) [L. *esculentus*, edible]. Edible; fit for eating.

esculin (es'kyū-lin) [L. *aesculus*, the Italian oak]. Aesculin; bicolorin; enallachrome; esculoside; polychrome; 6,7-dihydroxycoumarin 6-glucoside; a glucoside from horse-chestnut bark; used as a sunburn protective.

escutcheon (es-kŭch'ŭn) [through Old Fr., fr. L. *scutum*, shield]. The region of the skin in quadrupeds (usually cattle) between the hind legs above the udder and below the anus; the hair in this region generally grows upward.

ESEP Abbreviation for extreme somatosensory evoked *potential*.

eseridine (es-er'i-dēn). Eserine aminoxide; eserine oxide; an alkaloid from the seed of *Physostigma;* a parasympathomimetic agent.

eserine (es'er-ēn). Physostigmine.
e. aminoxide, eseridine.
e. oxide, eseridine.
e. salicylate, *physostigmine* salicylate.

-esis [G. *-esis*, condition or process]. Suffix meaning condition, action, or process.

Esmarch, Johann F.A. von, German surgeon, 1823–1908. See E.'s *tourniquet*.

esmolol hydrochloride (es'mō-lol). Benzene propanoic acid, 4-[2-hydroxy-3-[(1-methylethyl)amino]propoxy]-, methyl ester, hydrochloride; a β-adrenergic blocking agent used to treat supraventricular tachycardia and noncompensatory tachycardia.

esodeviation (es'ō-dē-vē-ā'shŭn). **1.** Esophoria. **2.** Esotropia.

esodic (e-sod'ik) [G. *esō,* inward, + *hodos,* way]. Afferent.

esoethmoiditis (es'ō-eth-moy-dī'tis) [G. *esō,* within, + ethmoid, + *-itis,* inflammation]. Obsolete term for inflammation of the lining membrane of the ethmoid cells.

esogastritis (es'ō-gas-trī'tis) [G. *esō,* within, + *gastēr,* stomach, + *-itis,* inflammation]. Obsolete term for catarrhal inflammation of the mucous membrane of the stomach.

esophagalgia (ē-sof-ă-gal'jē-ă) [esophagus + G. *algos,* pain]. Esophagodynia; pain in the esophagus.

esophageal (ē-sof'ă-jē'ăl, ē'-sŏ-faj'ē-ăl). Relating to the esophagus.

esophagectasis, esophagectasia (ē-sof-ă-jek'tă-sis, -jek-tā'zē-ă) [esophagus + G. *ektasis,* a stretching]. Dilation of the esophagus.

esophagectomy (ē-sof-ă-jek'tō-mē) [esophagus + G. *ektomē,* excision]. Excision of any part of the esophagus.

transhiatal e., resection of the esophagus by blunt dissection from a cervical incision from above and transhiatal approach through an abdominal incision.

transthoracic e., resection of the esophagus through a thoracotomy incision.

esophagi (ē-sof'ă-jī, -gī). Plural of esophagus.

esophagism (ē-sof'ă-jizm). Dysphagia nervosa; nervous dysphagia; esophageal spasm causing dysphagia.

esophagitis (ē-sof-ă-jī'tis). Inflammation of the esophagus.

reflux e., peptic e., inflammation of the lower esophagus from regurgitation of acid gastric contents, usually due to malfunction of the lower esophageal sphincter; symptoms include substernal pain, heartburn, and regurgitation of acid juice.

esophagocardioplasty (ē-sof'ă-gō-kar'dē-ō-plas-tē). Plastic surgery of the esophagus and cardiac end of the stomach.

esophagocele (ē-sof'ă-gō-sēl) [esophagus + G. *kēlē,* hernia]. Protrusion of the mucous membrane of the esophagus through a tear in the muscular coat.

esophagodynia (ē-sof'ă-gō-din'ē-ă) [esophagus + G. *odynē,* pain]. Esophagalgia.

esophagoenterostomy (ē-sof'ă-gō-en-ter-os'tō-mē) [esophagus + G. *enteron,* intestine, + *stoma,* mouth]. Surgical formation of a direct communication between the esophagus and intestine.

esophagofiberscope (ē-sof'ă-gō-fī'ber-skōp). A flexible instrument for examination of the esophagus.

esophagogastrectomy (ē-sof'ă-gō-gas-trek'tō-mē). Removal of a portion of the lower esophagus and proximal stomach for treatment of neoplasms or strictures of those organs, especially those lesions located at or near the cardioesophageal junction.

esophagogastroanastomosis (ē-sof'ă-gō-gas'trō-ă-nas-tō-mō'sis). Esophagogastrostomy.

esophagogastromyotomy (ē-sof'ă-gō-gas'trō-mī-ot'ō-mē). Esophagomyotomy.

esophagogastroplasty (ē-sof'ă-gō-gas'trō-plas-tē). Cardioplasty.

esophagogastrostomy (ē-sof'ă-gō-gas-tros'tō-mē) [esophagus + G. *gastēr,* stomach, + *stoma,* mouth]. Esophagogastroanastomosis; gastroesophagostomy; anastomosis of esophagus to stomach, usually following esophagogastrectomy.

esophagogram (e-sof'ă-gō-gram). A roentgenogram of the esophagus.

esophagography (ē-sof-ă-gog'ră-fē) [esophagus + G. *graphō,* to write]. Roentgenography of the esophagus using swallowed radiopaque contrast media; the technique of obtaining an esophagogram.

esophagomalacia (ē-sof'ă-gō-mă-lā'shē-ă) [esophagus + G. *malakia,* softness]. Softening of the walls of the esophagus.

esophagomycosis (ē-sof'ă-gō-mī-kō'sis) [esophagus + G. *mykēs,* fungus, + *-osis,* condition]. A fungous infection of the esophagus.

esophagomyotomy (ē-sof'ă-gō-mī-ot'ō-mē) [esophagus + G. *mys,* muscle, + *tomē,* incision]. Cardiomyotomy; esophagogastromyotomy; treatment of esophageal achalasia by longitudinal division of the lowest part of the esophageal muscle down to the submucosal layer; some muscle fibers of the cardia may also be divided.

esophagoplasty (ē-sof'ă-gō-plas-tē) [esophagus + G. *plastos,* formed]. Plastic surgery of the wall of the esophagus.

esophagoplication (ē-sof'ă-gō-pli-kā'shŭn) [esophagus + L. *plico,* to fold]. Reduction in size of a dilated esophagus or of a pouch in it by making longitudinal folds or tucks in its wall.

esophagoptosis, esophagoptosia (ē-sof'ă-gō-tō'sis, -tō'sē-ă) [esophagus + G. *ptōsis,* a falling]. Relaxation and downward displacement of the walls of the esophagus.

esophagoscope (ē-sof'ă-gō-skōp) [esophagus + G. *skopeō,* to examine]. An endoscope for inspecting the interior of the esophagus.

esophagoscopy (ē-sof-ă-gos'kŏ-pē) [esophagus + G. *skopeō,* to examine]. Inspection of the interior of the esophagus by means of an endoscope.

esophagospasm (ē-sof'ă-gō-spazm). Spasm of the walls of the esophagus.

esophagostenosis (ē-sof'ă-gō-stĕ-nō'sis) [esophagus + G. *stenōsis,* a narrowing]. Stricture or a general narrowing of the esophagus.

esophagostomiasis (ē-sof'ă-gō-stō-mī'ă-sis) [esophagus + G. *stoma,* mouth, + *-iasis,* condition]. Oesophagostomiasis.

esophagostomy (ē-sof-ă-gos'tō-mē) [esophagus + G. *stoma,* mouth]. Surgical formation of an opening directly into the esophagus from without.

esophagotomy (ē-sof-ă-got'ō-mē) [esophagus + G. *tomē,* an incision]. An incision through the wall of the esophagus.

esophagus, pl. **esophagi** (ē-sof'ă-gŭs, -jī, -gī) [G. *oisophagos,* gullet] [NA]. The portion of the digestive canal between the pharynx and stomach. It is about 25 cm long and consists of three parts: pars cervicalis, from the cricoid cartilage to the thoracic inlet; pars thoracica, from thoracic inlet to the diaphragm; and pars abdominalis, below the diaphragm to the cardiac opening of the stomach.

Barrett e., Barrett *syndrome.*

esophoria (es-ō-fō'rē-ă) [G. *esō,* inward, + *phora,* a carrying]. Esodeviation (1); a tendency for the eyes to turn inward, prevented by binocular vision.

esophoric (es-ō-fōr'ik). Relating to or marked by esophoria.

esophylaxis (es'ō-fī-lak'sis) [G. *eso,* within, + *phylaxis,* a guarding]. Old term denoting protection against disease by the biologic action of the cells and fluids of the body.

esosphenoiditis (es'ō-sfē'noyd-ī'tis) [G. *esō,* within, + sphenoid, + *-itis,* inflammation]. Obsolete term for osteomyelitis of the sphenoid bone.

esotropia (es-ō-trō'pē-ă) [G. *esō,* inward, + *tropē,* turn]. Esodeviation (2); internal or convergent squint; convergent or internal strabismus; the form of strabismus in which the visual axes converge; may be paralytic or concomitant, monocular or alternating, accommodative or nonaccommodative.

A-e., convergent strabismus greater in upward than in downward gaze.

basic e., nonaccommodative e.

consecutive e., e. that follows surgical correction of exotropia.

cyclic e., alternate day strabismus; periodic convergent strabismus often occurring every 48 hours.

mixed e., that type of e. in which both accommodative and nonaccommodative factors are present.

nonaccommodative e., basic e.; that type of e. not influenced by correction of refractive error.

nonrefractive accommodative e., that type of e. in which an abnormality of the accommodative-convergence mechanism is not eliminated by correction of refractive error.
refractive accommodative e., that type of e. eliminated by correction of hypermetropic refractive error.
V-e., convergent strabismus greater in downward than in upward gaze.
X-e., increasing convergence from the primary position in both upward and downward gaze.

esotropic (es-ō-trop'ik). Relating to or marked by esotropia.

ESP Abbreviation for extrasensory *perception.*

espundia (es-pūn'dē-ă) [Sp., fr. L. *spongia,* sponge]. Bubas braziliana; Breda's disease; a type of American leishmaniasis caused by *Leishmania braziliensis* that affects the mucous membranes, particularly in the nasal and oral region, resulting in grossly destructive changes; particularly common in Brazil where a significant proportion of persons infected with *L. braziliensis* develop this condition; may develop metastatically from sores originally found elsewhere on the body.

esquinancea (es-kwi-nan'sē-ă) [Fr. *esquinancie,* quinsy]. Sense of suffocation caused by an inflammatory swelling in the throat, as in suppurative tonsillitis or pharyngitis.

ESR Abbreviation for erythrocyte sedimentation *rate;* electron spin *resonance.*

essence (es'ens) [L. *essentia,* fr. *esse,* to be]. **1.** The true characteristic or substance of a body. **2.** An element. **3.** A fluidextract. **4.** An alcoholic solution, or spirit, of the volatile oil of a plant. **5.** Any volatile substance responsible for odor or taste of the organism (usually a plant) producing it; by extension, synthetic perfumes or flavors.

essential (ē-sen'shăl). **1.** Necessary, indispensable (*e.g.,* e. amino acids). **2.** Characteristic of. **3.** Determining. **4.** Idiopathic; of unknown etiology. **5.** Relating to an essence (*e.g.,* e. oil). **6.** Inherent; intrinsic.

Esser, Johannes F.S., Dutch surgeon, 1877–1946. See E. *graft, operation.*

Essick, C., 20th century U.S. anatomist. See E.'s cell *bands.*

Essig splint. See under splint.

ester (es'ter). An organic compound containing the grouping, $-X(0)-O-R$ (X = carbon, sulfur, phosphorus, etc.; R = radical of an alcohol), formed by the elimination of H_2O between the –OH of an acid group and the –OH of an alcohol group; usually written as in ethyl acetate (from acetic acid and ethyl alcohol), $CH_3CO—OC_2H_5$ or $CH_3COOC_2H_5$.
Cori e., glucose 1-phosphate; important intermediate in sugar metabolism.
Embden e., hexose phosphate; an equilibrium mixture of glucose 6-phosphate and fructose 6-phosphate; significant in the understanding of sugar metabolism.
Harden-Young e., fructose 1,6-bisphosphate; important intermediate in sugar metabolism.
Robison e., Robison-Emden e., D-glucose 6-phosphate; important intermediate in sugar metabolism.

esterase (es'ter-ās). A generic term for enzymes (EC class 3.1, hydrolases) that catalyze the hydrolysis of esters.
C1 e., the activated first component of complement (C1).

esterification (es'ter'i-fi-kā'shŭn). The process of forming an ester, as in the reaction of ethanol and acetic acid to form ethyl acetate.

Estes, William L., Jr., U.S. surgeon, 1885–1940. See E. *operation.*

esthematology (es-thē-mă-tol'ō-jē) [G. *aisthēma,* perception, + *logos,* study]. The science concerned with the senses and sense organs.

esthesia (es-thē'zē-ă) [G. *aisthesis,* sensation]. **1.** Perception. **2.** Sensitivity (2).

esthesic (es-thē'sik) [G. *aisthēsis,* sensation]. Relating to the mental perception of the existence of any part of the body.

esthesio- [G. *aesthēsis,* sensation]. Combining form relating to sensation or perception.

esthesiodic (es-thē-zē-od'ik) [esthesio- + G. *hodos,* way]. Esthesodic; conveying sensory impressions.

esthesiogenesis (es-thē'zē-ō-jen'ĕ-sis) [esthesio- + G. *genesis,* origin]. The production of sensation, especially of nervous erethism.

esthesiogenic (es-thē-zē-ō-jen'ik). Producing a sensation.

esthesiography (es-thē-zē-og'ră-fē) [esthesio- + G. *graphē,* a writing]. **1.** A description of the organs of sense and of the mechanism of sensation. **2.** Mapping out on the skin the areas of tactile and other forms of sensibility.

esthesiology (es-thē-zē-ol'ō-jē) [esthesio- + G. *logos,* study]. The science concerned with sensory phenomena.

esthesiometer (es-thē-zē-om'ĕ-ter) [esthesio- + G. *metron,* measure]. Tactometer; an instrument for determining the state of tactile and other forms of sensibility.

esthesiometry (es-thē-zē-om'ĕ-trē). Measurement of the degree of tactile or other sensibility.

esthesioneuroblastoma (es-thē'zē-ō-nūr'ō-blas-tō'mă). A neoplasm of immature, poorly differentiated neuronal cells believed to arise from spinal or cranial ganglia.
olfactory n., olfactory *neuroblastoma.*

esthesioneurocytoma (es-thē'zē-ō-nur'ō-sī-tō'mă). A neoplasm composed of nearly mature neuron-like cells believed to arise from a spinal or cranial ganglia.

esthesioneurosis (es-thē'zē-ō-nū-rō'sis). Esthesionosus; any sensory neurosis; *e.g.,* anesthesia, hyperesthesia, paresthesia.

esthesionosus (es-thē'zē-on'ō-sŭs) [esthesio- + G. *nosos,* disease]. Esthesioneurosis.

esthesiophysiology (es-thē'zē-ō-fiz-ē-ol'ō-jē). The physiology of sensation and the sense organs.

esthesioscopy (es-thē-zē-os'kŏ-pē) [esthesio- + G. *skopeō,* to view]. Examination into the degree and extent of tactile and other forms of sensibility.

esthesodic (es'thē-zod'ik). Esthesiodic.

esthetic (es-thet'ik) [G. *aisthēsis,* sensation]. **1.** Pertaining to the sensations. **2.** Pertaining to esthetics (*i.e.,* beauty).

esthetics (es-thet'iks). The branch of philosophy concerned with beauty, especially with the components thereof.
denture e., **(1)** the cosmetic effect produced by a dental prosthesis; **(2)** the qualities involved in the appearance of a given restoration.

esthiomene (es-thē-om'ĕ-nē) [G. *esthiomenos,* eaten, eroded]. Obsolete term for an ulcerative lesion of the vulva surrounded by fibrous induration and edema, associated with lymphogranuloma inguinale.

esthiomenous (es-thē-om'ĕ-nŭs) [see esthiomene]. Obsolete term for corroding, ulcerating, or phagedenic.

estival (es'ti-văl) [L. *aestivus,* summer (adj.)]. Aestival; relating to or occurring in the summer.

estivation (es-ti-vā'shŭn). Living through the summer in a quiescent, torpid state. *Cf.* hibernation.

estivoautumnal (es'ti-vō-aw-tŭm'năl) [L. *aestivus,* summer (adj.), + *autumnalis,* autumnal]. Relating to or occurring in summer and autumn.

Estlander, Jakob A., Finnish surgeon, 1831–1881. See E. *flap, operation.*

estradiol (es-tră-dī'ol). Estrogenic hormone; β-estradiol; 17β-estradiol; 1,3,5(10)-estratriene-3,17β-diol; the most potent naturally occurring estrogen in mammals, formed by the ovary, placenta, testis, and possibly the adrenal cortex; therapeutic indications for e. are those typical of an estrogen. α-Estradiol, 17α-estradiol, exhibits considerably less biologic activity.

e. benzoate, fatty acid esters of 17β-estradiol usually dissolved in oil for injection purposes; such esters exhibit a longer duration of action than does the unesterified steroid.

e. cypionate, has the same actions and uses as e. but a prolonged duration of action; administered in oil by intramuscular injection.

e. dipropionate, an esterified natural estrogen for parenteral use.

ethinyl e., ethynyl e.

ethynyl e., ethinyl e.; 17α-ethynyl-1,3,5-estratriene-3,17-diol; a semisynthetic derivative of 17β-estradiol; active by mouth, it is among the most potent of known estrogenic compounds.

e. undecylate, an esterified natural estrogen for parenteral use.

e. valerate, estradiol 17-valerate; estra-1,3,5(10)-triene-3,17β-diol 17-valerate; same actions and uses as e., but with a prolonged duration of action; administered in sesame oil by intramuscular injection.

estragon oil (es'tră-gon). Tarragon oil.

estramustine phosphate sodium (es-tră-mŭs'tēn). Estra-1,3,5(10)-triene-3,17-diol(17β)-, 3-[bis(2-chloroethyl)carbamate] 17-(dihydrogen phosphate), disodium salt; an antineoplastic agent that combines the actions of estrogen and nitrogen mustard in the treatment of carcinoma of the prostate.

estrane (es'trān). Hypothetical parent hydrocarbon of the (steroid) estrogenic compounds whose names begin with "estr-" (estradiol, estrone, estriol); conceived to establish a systematic nomenclature.

estratriene (es-tră-trī'ēn). 1,3,5(10)-Estratriene; the hypothetical triply-unsaturated estrane that is the nucleus of most naturally occurring estrogenic steroids in animals.

estrin (es'trin). Estrogen.

estriol (es'trē-ol). Folliculin hydrate; trihydroxyestrin; estra-1,3,5(10)-triene-3,16α,17β-triol; an estrogenic metabolite of estradiol, usually the predominant estrogenic metabolite found in urine; epimers at C-16, C-17, or both are known as 16-epiestriol, etc.

estrodienol (es-trō-dē'nol). Dienestrol.

estrogen (es'trō-jen) [ability to induce estrus]. Estrin; generic term for any substance, natural or synthetic, that exerts biological effects characteristic of estrogenic hormones such as estradiol. E.'s are formed by the ovary, placenta, testes, and possibly the adrenal cortex, as well as by certain plants; stimulate secondary sexual characteristics, and exert systemic effects, such as growth and maturation of long bones; and are used therapeutically in any disorder attributable to e. deficiency or amenable to e. therapy.

conjugated e., an amorphous preparation of naturally occurring, water-soluble, conjugated forms of mixed e.'s obtained from the urine of pregnant mares; the principal e. present is sodium estrone sulfate; suitable for parenteral, oral, and topical administration, and used in conditions responsive to e. therapy.

esterified e.'s, a mixture of the sodium salts of sulfate esters of estrogenic substances; used for oral e. therapy.

estrogenic (es-trō-jen'ik). **1.** Causing estrus in animals. **2.** Having an action similar to that of an estrogen.

estrone (es'trōn). Folliculin; follicular hormone; ketohydroxyestrin; 3-hydroxyestra-1,3,5(10)-trien-17-one; a metabolite of 17β-estradiol, commonly found in urine, with considerably less biological activity than the parent hormone.

estrous (es'trŭs). Estrual; pertaining to estrus.

estrual (es'trū-ăl). Estrous.

estrus (es'trŭs) [G. *oistros,* mad desire]. Heat (2); that portion or phase of the sexual cycle of female animals characterized by willingness to permit coitus; readily detectable behavioral and other signs are exhibited by animals during this period.

postpartum e., e. with ovulation and corpus luteum production which occurs in some animals (*e.g.,* the fur seal) immediately following the birth of the young.

esu Abbreviation for electrostatic *unit.*

esylate (es'ī-lāt). USAN-approved contraction for ethanesulfonate, $CH_3CH_2SO_3^-$.

etafedrine hydrochloride (et-ă-fed'rēn). *l-N*-Ethylephedrine hydrochloride; a sympathomimetic drug for treatment of bronchial asthma.

etafenone (e-taf'ĕ-nōn). 2'-[2-(Diethylamino)ethoxy]-3-phenylpropiophenone hydrochloride; a coronary vasodilator.

etamsylate (e-tam'si-lāt). Ethamsylate.

état (ā-tah') [Fr. state]. A condition or state.

e. criblé (ā-tah'kri-blā) [Fr. sieve], in neuropathology, a term describing perivascular atrophy of cerebral tissue, producing lacunae.

e. mamelonné [Fr. knobby, tubercular], the condition of the gastric mucous membrane in chronic inflammation, when it presents numerous nodular projections.

ethacridine lactate (eth-ak'ri-dēn). Acrinol; 6,9-diamino-2-ethoxyacridine lactate; an antiseptic for treatment of wounds.

ethacrynate sodium (eth-ă-krī'nāt). Sodium salt of ethacrynic acid for parenteral use.

ethacrynic acid (eth-ă-krin'ik). [2,3-Dichloro-4-(2-methylenebutyryl)phenoxy]acetic acid; an unsaturated ketone derivative of aryloxyacetic acid; a potent diuretic and a weak antihypertensive; used in the treatment of severe edema in heart failure or cirrhosis.

ethadione (eth-ă-dī'ōn). 3-Ethyl-5,5-dimethyl-2,4-oxazolidinedione; an anticonvulsant.

ethaldehyde (eth-al'dĕ-hīd). Acetaldehyde.

ethambutol hydrochloride (eth-am'bū-tol). (+)-2,2'-(Ethylenedimino)-di(1-butanol) dihydrochloride; a tuberculostatic, effective against organisms resistant to other tuberculostatic drugs; a serious reaction is visual impairment which, however, appears to be reversible.

ethamivan (eth-am'i-van). *N,N*-Diethylvanillamide; 3-methoxyl-4-hydroxybenzoic acid diethylamide; a central nervous system stimulant and analeptic, used as an adjunctive agent in the treatment of severe respiratory depression due to barbiturates and carbon dioxide retention.

ethamoxytriphetol (eth-ă-moks'ē-trī-fē'tol). 1-[*p*-(2-Diethylaminoethoxy)phenyl]-2-(*p*-methoxyphenyl)-1-phenylethanol; the prototype antiestrogen that inhibits the effects of estrogen to its specific cellular receptors; the two most widely structurally related antiestrogens are clomiphene citrate and tamoxifen.

ethamsylate (e-tham'si-lāt). Cyclonamine; etamsylate; 2,5-dihydroxybenzenesulfonic acid compound with diethylamine; a hemostatic agent.

ethanal (eth'ă-nal). Acetaldehyde.

ethane (eth'ān). CH_3CH_3; a constituent of natural and "bottled" gases.

ethanedial (eth-ān-dī'al). Glyoxal.

ethanediamine (eth-ān-dī'ă-mēn). Ethylenediamine.

ethanedinitrile (eth'ān-dī-nī'tril). Cyanogen.

ethanoic acid (eth-ă-nō'ik). Acetic acid.

ethanol (eth'an-ol). Alcohol (2).

ethanolamine (eth-an-ol'ă-mēn). β-Hydroxyethylamine; colamine; 2-aminoethanol; $HO(CH_2)_2NH_2$; used to prepare e. oleate, a sclerosing agent used for treatment of varicose veins.

ethanolaminephosphotransferase (eth-ă-nol'ă-mēn-fos-fō-trans'-

fer-ās) [EC 2.7.8.1]. Phosphorylethanolamine glyceride-transferase; a transferase that catalyzes the reaction of CDP-ethanolamine with a 1,2-diacylglycerol to yield CMP and a phosphatidylethanolamine.

ethaverine hydrochloride (eth-av'ĕ-rēn, eth-ă-ver'ēn). Ethylpapaverine hydrochloride; 6,7-diethoxy-1-(3,4-diethoxybenzyl)-isoquinoline hydrochloride; a smooth muscle relaxant.

ethchlorvynol (eth-klōr'vī-nol). Ethyl β-chlorovinyl ethynyl carbinol; a hypnotic and anticonvulsant; used for the induction of sleep in simple insomnia and as a daytime sedative.

ethene (eth'ēn). Ethylene.

ethenyl (eth'en-il). Vinyl.

ethenylbenzene (eth-en-il-ben'zēn). Styrene.

ethenylene (eth-en'il-ēn). Vinylene.

ether (ē'ther) [G. *aithēr,* the pure upper air]. **1.** Any organic compound in which two carbon atoms are independently linked to a common oxygen atom, thus containing the group –C–O–C–. **2.** Loosely used to refer to diethyl e. or an anesthetic e., although a large number of e.'s have anesthetic properties. For individual e.'s, see the specific name.
anesthetic e., diethyl e.; also increasingly regarded as a general designation for many e.'s.
solvent e., a fairly pure form of e. ($C_4H_{10}O$) but not sufficiently pure for anesthesia; used as a solvent.
xylostyptic e., styptic *collodion.*

ethereal (ē-thēr'ē-ăl) [G. *aitherios,* etherial, fr. *aithēr,* the upper air]. Relating to or containing ether.

etherification (ē-ther'i-fi-kā'shŭn). Conversion of an alcohol into an ether.

etherization (ē'ther-i-zā'shŭn). Administration of diethyl ether to produce anesthesia.

ethiazide (e-thī'ă-zīd). Aethiazidum; 6-chloro-3-ethyl-3,4-dihydro-2*H*-1,2,4-benzothiadiazine-7-sulfonamide 1,1-dioxide; a diuretic.

ethical (eth'i-kăl). Relating to ethics; in conformity with the rules governing personal and professional conduct.

ethics (eth'iks) [G. *ethikos,* arising from custom, fr. *ethos,* custom]. The discipline concerned with morality and moral obligations.
medical e., the principles of proper professional conduct concerning the rights and duties of the physician himself, his patients, and his fellow practitioners, as well as his actions in the care of patients and in relations with their families.

ethidene (eth'i-dēn). Ethylidene.

Ethidium (eth-id'ē-ŭm). Homidium bromide.

ethidium bromide (ĕ-thid'ē-ŭm). A sensitive fluorochrome that binds to DNA; used in cytochemistry and electrophoresis.

ethinamate (e-thin'ă-māt). 1-Ethynylcyclohexyl carbamate; a mild central nervous system depressant used for induction of sleep in simple insomnia and as a daytime sedative.

ethindrone (e-thin'drōn). Ethisterone.

ethinyl (e-thī'nil). Ethynyl.
e. trichloride, trichloroethylene.

ethinylestrenol (eth'i-nil-es'tre-nol). Lynestrenol.

ethiodized oil (eth-ī'ō-dīzd). An iodine addition product of the ethyl ester of the fatty acid of poppyseed oil; a radiopaque medium that can be sterilized.

ethionamide (ĕ-thī'on-ă-mīd). 2-Ethylisothionicotinamide; a drug used in the treatment of pulmonary tuberculosis; given only with other antituberculous agents because bacterial resistance develops when it is administered alone.

ethionine (e-thī'ō-nēn). *S*-Ethyl-L-homocysteine; a methionine analogue and antagonist, differing in the presence of an S- ethyl group in place of the S- methyl group.

ethisterone (e-this'ter-ōn). Ethindrone; pregneninolone; 17α-ethynyltestosterone; an orally effective semisynthetic steroid that has biological effects similar to those of progesterone.

ethmo- [G. *ēthmos,* sieve]. Combining form denoting: **1.** Ethmoid. **2.** The ethmoid bone.

ethmocranial (eth-mō-krā'nē-ăl). Relating to the ethmoid bone and the cranium as a whole.

ethmofrontal (eth-mō-fron'tăl). Relating to the ethmoid and the frontal bones.

ethmoid (eth'moyd) [G. *ēthmos,* sieve, + *eidos,* resemblance]. Ethmoidal. **1.** Resembling a sieve. **2.** Relating to the e. bone, *os* ethmoidale.

ethmoidal (eth-moy'dăl). Ethmoid.

ethmoidale (eth-moy-da'lē). A cephalometric point in the anterior cranial fossa located at the lowest sagittal point of the cribriform plate of the ethmoid bone.

ethmoidectomy (eth-moy-dek'tō-mē) [ethmo- + G. *ektomē,* excision]. Removal of all or part of the mucosal lining and bony partitions between the ethmoid sinuses.

ethmoiditis (eth-moy-dī'tis). Inflammation of the ethmoid sinuses.

ethmolacrimal (eth-mō-lak'ri-măl). Relating to the ethmoid and the lacrimal bones.

ethmomaxillary (eth-mō-mak'si-lā-rē). Relating to the ethmoid and the maxillary bones.

ethmonasal (eth-mō-nā'săl). Relating to the ethmoid and the nasal bones.

ethmopalatal (eth-mō-pal'ă-tăl). Relating to the ethmoid and the palate bones.

ethmosphenoid (eth-mō-sfē'noyd). Relating to the ethmoid and sphenoid bones.

ethmoturbinals (eth-mō-ter'bi-nalz). The conchae of the ethmoid bone; the superior and middle conchae; occasionally a third, the supreme concha, exists.

ethmovomerine (eth'mō-vō'mer-in). Relating to the ethmoid bone and the vomer.

ethnocentrism (eth-nō-sen'trizm) [G. *ethnos,* race, tribe, + *kentron,* center of a circle]. The tendency to evaluate other groups according to the values and standards of one's own ethnic group, especially with the conviction that one's own ethnic group is superior to the other groups.

ethoheptazine citrate (eth-ō-hep'tă-zēn). Ethyl hexahydro-1-methyl-4-phenylazepinecarboxylate citrate; an analgesic.

ethohexadiol (eth'ō-hek-să-dī'ol, -hek-să'dī-ol). 2-Ethyl-1,3-hexanediol; octylene glycol; used as an insect repellant, in compound dimethyl phthalate solution.

ethologist (ē-thol'ō-jist). A specialist in ethology.

ethology (ē-thol'ō-jē) [G. *ethos,* character, habit, + *logos,* study]. The study of animal behavior.

ethomoxane (eth-ō-mok'sān). Ethoxybutamoxane; 2-(butylaminomethyl)-8-ethoxy-1,4-benzodioxan; an antianxiety agent.

ethopharmacology (eth'ō-far-mă-kol'ō-jē) [G. *ethos,* character, habit, + pharmacology]. The study of drug effects on behavior, relying on observation and description of species-specific elements (acts and postures during social encounters).

ethopropazine hydrochloride (eth-ō-prō'pă-zēn). Profenamine hydrochloride; 10-(2-diethylaminopropyl)-phenothiazine hydrochloride; an anticholinergic agent with some antihistaminic and ganglionic blocking activity; used in the symptomatic treatment of Parkinson's disease.

ethosuximide (eth-ō-sŭk'si-mīd). 2-Ethyl-2-methylsuccinimide;

α,α-ethylmethylsuccinimide; an anticonvulsant used in the control of petit mal epilepsy; bone marrow damage and aplastic anemia may occasionally occur.

ethotoin (eth-ō-tō'in). 3-Ethyl-5-phenylhydantoin; an anticonvulsant used in the treatment of grand mal epilepsy.

ethotrimeprazine (eth'ō-trī-mep'ră-zēn). Etymemazine.

ethoxazene hydrochloride (e-thok'să-zēn). 4-[(*p*-Ethoxyphenyl)azo]-*m*-phenylenediamine monohydrochloride; an azo compound used as a urinary antiseptic and as an acid-base indicator that changes the color of the urine to orange or red.

ethoxy (e-thok'sē). The monovalent radical, CH_3CH_2O–.

ethoxybutamoxane (eth-ok'si-byū-tă-mok'sān). Ethomoxane.

ethoxyzolamide (eth-ok-sē-zol'ă-mīd). 6-Ethoxy-2-benzothiazolesulfonamide; a diuretic related chemically and pharmacologically to acetazolamide; also used as an adjunct in the treatment of glaucoma and epilepsy.

ethyl (eth'il). The hydrocarbon radical, CH_3CH_2–.
e. alcohol, alcohol (2).
e. aminobenzoate, benzocaine.
e. biscoumacetate, ethyl 4,4′-dihydroxydicoumarin-3,3′-ylacetate; an anticoagulant chemically related to bishydroxycoumarin.
e. butyrate, $CH_3CH_2CH_2COOCH_2CH_3$; used in perfumery.
e. carbamate, urethan.
e. chloride, chloroethane; chlorethyl; a very volatile explosive liquid (under increased pressure); produces local anesthesia by superficial freezing, but also is a potent inhalation anesthetic.
e. eosin, alcohol-soluble eosin; the e. ester of tetrabromofluorescein, a fluorescent red acid dye used as a counterstain in histology.
e. formate, a volatile, flammable liquid used as a fumigant, agricultural larvicide, and fungicide; also used as a flavor.
e. oleate, an alternative vehicle in BP injections of deoxycorticosterone acetate, menaphthone, etc.
e. oxide, diethyl ether.
e. salicylate, the salicylic acid ester of e. alcohol, with the same action as methyl salicylate.

ethylate (eth'i-lāt). A compound in which the hydrogen of the hydroxyl group of ethanol is replaced by a metallic atom, usually sodium or potassium; *e.g.*, C_2H_5ONa, sodium ethylate.

ethylbenztropine (eth'il-benz-trō'pēn). 3-Diphenylmethoxy-8-ethyl-1α*H*,5α*H*-nortropane; an anticholinergic agent.

ethylcellulose (eth-il-sel'yū-lōs). An ethyl ether of cellulose, used as a tablet binder.

ethylene (eth'i-lēn). Ethene; olefiant gas; CH_2CH_2; an explosive constituent of ordinary illuminating gas; an inhalation anesthetic, now infrequently used, which is slightly more potent than nitrous oxide.
e. dibromide (EDB), a pesticide and gasoline additive shown to be carcinogenic in rats and mice.
e. oxide, a fumigant, used for sterilizing surgical instruments.
e. tetrachloride, tetrachlorethylene.

ethylenediamine (eth'i-lēn-dī'ă-mēn). Ethanediamine; $H_2N(CH_2)_2NH_2$; a volatile colorless liquid of ammoniacal odor and caustic taste; the dihydrochloride is used as a urinary acidifier.

ethylenediaminetetraacetic acid (EDTA) (eth'il-ēn-dī'ă-mēn-tet-ră-ă-sē'tik). Edetic acid; edathamil; $(HOOC–CH_2)_2N(CH_2)_2N(CH_2–COOH)_2$; a chelating agent used to remove multivalent cations from solution as chelates, and used in biochemical research to remove Mg^{2+}, Fe^{2+}, etc., from reactions affected by such ions. As the sodium salt, used as a water softener, to stabilize drugs rapidly decomposed in the presence of traces of metal ions, and as an anticoagulant; as the sodium calcium salt, used to remove radium, lead, strontium, plutonium, and cadmium from the skeleton, forming stable un-ionized soluble compounds that are excreted by the kidneys.

ethylene glycol. See glycol(2).

ethylestrenol (eth-il-es'tre-nol). 17α-Ethyl-4-estren-17β-ol; a semisynthetic orally effective anabolic steroid used to accelerate anabolism or to retard excessive catabolism; it also can exert typically androgenic effects.

ethyl ether. Diethyl ether.

ethyl green. Brilliant green.

ethylidene (eth-il'i-dēn). Ethidene; the radical $CH_3CH=$.

ethylidyne (eth-il'i-dīn). The radical $CH_3C\equiv$.

ethylisobutrazine (eth'il-ī-sō-byū'tră-zēn). Etymemazine.

ethylmorphine hydrochloride (eth-il-mōr'fēn). The ethyl ether of morphine; an antispasmodic, antitussive, and analgesic, used locally as an irritant lymphagogue in chronic catarrhal middle ear disease, atrophic rhinitis, and painful ocular diseases (iritis, corneal ulcer, etc.).

ethylnorepinephrine (E.N.E., E.N.S.) (eth'il-nōr-ep-i-nef'rin). α-(1-Aminopropyl)-3,4-dihydroxybenzyl alcohol; a sympathomimetic, used in asthma; it does not raise the blood pressure.

ethylpapaverine hydrochloride (eth'il-pa-pav'er-ēn). Ethaverine hydrochloride.

ethylparaben (eth-il-par'ă-ben). Ethyl *p*- hydroxybenzoate; an antifungal preservative.

ethylphenacemide (eth-il-fen-as'-ĕ-mīd). (2-Phenylbutyryl)urea; an anticonvulsant.

ethylphenylephrine hydrochloride (eth'il-fen-il-ef'rēn). Etilefrine hydrochloride.

ethylstibamine (eth-il-stib'ă-mēn). Fourneau 693; a synthetic organic compound of antimony; used in the treatment of several protozoal diseases, and for the relief of pain in multiple myeloma.

ethylvinyl ether (eth'il-vī'nil). Vinylethyl ether; $CH_3CH_2OCHCH_2$; a rarely used flammable inhalation anesthetic of moderate potency.

ethynodiol (ĕ-thī-nō-dī'ōl). 17α-Ethynyl-4-estrene-3β, 17β-diol; a semisynthetic orally effective steroid with biological effects that largely resemble those of progesterone; in addition, it is weakly estrogenic and androgenic; administered in combination with an estrogen as an oral contraceptive.
e. diacetate, 3,17-diacetate of ethynodiol; an antifertility agent, usually used in combination with mestranol.

ethynyl (e-thī'nil). Ethinyl; acetenyl; the monovalent radical $HC\equiv C$–.
e. estradiol, see under estradiol.

etiane (ē'ti-ān). Etiocholane; testane; the 5β isomer of androstane.

etianic acids (ē'ti-an-ik). Androstane-17-carboxylic acids. See etio-(1).

etidocaine (e-tī'dō-kān). (±)-2-(Ethylpropylamino)-2′,6′-butyroxylidide; a local anesthetic.

etidronate disodium (e-ti-drō'nāt). Phosphoric acid, (1-hydroxyethylidene)-bis-, disodium salt; a drug that affects bone resorption, used in the treatment of Paget's disease, heterotopic ossification, and hypercalcemia of malignancy.

etidronic acid (e-ti-dron'ik). (1-Hydroxyethylidene)bis(phosphonic acid); used as a calcium regulator, usually as the salt etidronate disodium.

etilefrine hydrochloride (et-il-ef'rin). Ethylphenylephrine hydrochloride; a sympathomimetic amine vasopressor agent.

etio-. 1. Prefix used with (for example) cholane to indicate replacement of the C-17 side chain by H; thus, etiocholane is the 5β isomer of androstane. **2** [G. *aitia,* cause]. Combining form meaning cause.

etioallocholane (ē'tē-ō-al-ō-kō'lān). The 5α isomer of androstane.

etiocholane (ē'tē-ō-kō'lān). The 5β isomer of androstane.

etiocholanolone (ē'tē-ō-kō-lan'ō-lōn). 3α-Hydroxy-5β-androstan-17-one; a metabolite of adrenocortical and testicular hormones, and an important urinary 17-ketosteroid; produces fever when given to human beings.

etiogenic (ē'tē-ō-jen'ik) [G. *aitia,* cause, + *genesis,* production]. Of a causal nature.

etiolated (ē'tē-ō-lāt-ed). Subjected to, or characterized by, etiolation.

etiolation (ē-tē-ō-lā'shŭn) [Fr. *étioler,* to blanch]. **1.** Paleness or pallor resulting from absence of light, as in persons confined because of illness or imprisonment, or in plants bleached by being deprived of light. **2.** The process of blanching, bleaching, or making pale by withholding light.

etiologic (ē'tē-ō-loj'ik). Relating to etiology.

etiology (ē-tē-ol'ō-jē) [G. *aitia,* cause, + *logos,* treatise, discourse]. The science and study of the causes of disease and their mode of operation. *Cf.* pathogenesis.

etiopathic (ē'tē-ō-path'ik) [G. *aitia,* cause, + *pathos,* disease]. Relating to specific lesions concerned with the cause of a disease.

etioporphyrin (ē'tē-ō-pōr'fi-rin). A porphyrin derivative characterized by the presence on each of the four pyrrole rings of one methyl group and one ethyl group; four isomeric forms are thus possible.

etiotropic (ē'tē-ō-trop'ik) [G. *aitia,* cause, + *tropē,* a turning]. Directed against the cause; denoting a remedy that attenuates or destroys the causal factor of a disease.

etomidate (ē-tom'i-dāt). R-(+)-1-(α-Methylbenzyl)imidazole-5-carboxylate; a potent intravenous depressant used for induction of general anesthesia.

etoposide (e-tō-pō'sīd). 4'-Demethylpipodohyllotoxin 9-[4,6-*O*-(*R*)-ethylidene-β-D-glucopyranoside; a semisynthetic derivative of podophyllotoxin; a mitotic inhibitor used in the treatment of refractory testicular tumors and small cell lung cancer.

etorphine (et-ōr'fēn). Tetrahydro-7α-(1-hydroxy-1-methylbutyl)-6,14-*endo*-ethenooripavine; a narcotic analgesic.

etozolin (et-ō-zō'lin). 3-Methyl-4-oxo-5-piperidino-$\Delta^{2,\alpha}$-thiazolidineacetic acid ethyl ester; a diuretic.

etretinate (e-tret'i-nāt). 2,4,6,8-Nonatetraenoic acid; a retinoid used in the treatment of severe recalcitrant psoriasis.

etymemazine (et-i-mem'ă-zēn). Ethotrimeprazine; ethylisobutrazine; 10-(3-dimethylamino-2-methylpropyl)-2-ethylphenothiazine; an antihistaminic.

Eu Symbol for europium.

eu-. G. particle, used as a prefix, meaning good, well, often in the sense of normal.

eualleles (yū'ă-lēlz). Genes that have undergone different nucleotide substitutions at the same position. *Cf.* heteroalleles.

Eubacteriales (yū'bak-tē-rē-ā'lēz). An obsolete order of bacteria which contained simple, undifferentiated, rigid cells which were either spheres or straight rods. It contained motile (peritrichous) and nonmotile, Gram-negative and Gram-positive, and sporeforming and nonsporeforming species. The order contained 13 families: Achromobacteraceae, Azotobacteraceae, Bacillaceae, Bacteroidaceae, Brevibacteriaceae, Brucellaceae, Corynebacteriaceae, Enterobacteriaceae, Lactobacillaceae, Micrococcaceae, Neisseriaceae, Propionibacteriaceae, and Rhizobacteriaceae.

Eubacterium (yū'bak-tēr'ē-ŭm). A genus of anaerobic, nonsporeforming, nonmotile bacteria containing straight or curved Gram-positive rods which usually occur singly, in pairs, or in short chains. Usually these organisms attack carbohydrates. They may be pathogenic. The type species is *E. foedans.*

E. aerofa'ciens, a species infrequently found in human intestines; pathogenic for mice.

E. bifor'me, a species that occurs infrequently in human intestines; pathogenic for rabbits but not for mice.

E. combe'si, a species from forest soil found in an area then called French West Africa; it is not pathogenic for guinea pigs or mice. Formerly called *Cillobacterium combesi.*

E. contor'tum, *Catenabacterium contortum;* a species found in cases of putrid, gangrenous appendicitis and in the intestines.

E. crispa'tum, a species found in pus from a dental abscess.

E. discifor'mans, a species found in cases of fetid suppurations in empyema, pulmonary gangrene, liver abscess, and dermatosis; occurs commonly in the respiratory system, the liver, and the skin; pathogenic for man, rabbits, guinea pigs, and mice.

E. ethyl'icum, a species found in a case of gastritis; occurs infrequently in the human stomach.

E. filamento'sum, *Catenabacterium filamentosum;* a species found in the intestines of rats; it is also found in cases of acute appendicitis, lung abscess, putrid pleurisy, and uterine suppuration.

E. foe'dans, a species found in spoiled, salted ham; it is the type species of the genus.

E. len'tum, a species occurring commonly in the feces of normal persons.

E. limo'sum, a species that occurs in human feces and presumably in the feces of other warm-blooded animals.

E. minu'tum, a species that occurs infrequently in the intestines of breast-fed infants; it was originally found in a case of infant diarrhea; it is pathogenic for mice.

E. monilifor'me, a species found rarely in the human respiratory system; it is pathogenic for guinea pigs, causing death in eight days. Formerly called *Cillobacterium moniliforme.*

E. multifor'me, a species isolated from the feces of a dog and from soil from equatorial Africa; it is not pathogenic for guinea pigs. Formerly called *Cillobacterium multiforme.*

E. nio'sii, a species that occurs in the respiratory tract; pathogenic for rabbits and guinea pigs.

E. par'vum, a species found in the large intestine of a horse and in a case of acute appendicitis; it occurs infrequently in the intestines of foals and of humans, and is not pathogenic for laboratory animals.

E. poeciloi'des, a species infrequently found in human intestines; originally found in a case of intestinal occlusion; it is pathogenic for guinea pigs and rabbits.

E. pseudotortuo'sum, a species found in a case of purulent, acute appendicitis; occurs uncommonly in the intestines.

E. quar'tum, a species found in cases of infantile diarrhea; occurs in the intestines of children, but is rather uncommon.

E. quin'tum, a species found in cases of infantile diarrhea; pathogenic for guinea pigs.

E. recta'le, a species found in association with a rectal ulcer; occurs in the rectum.

E. ten'ue, a species isolated from dog feces; its pathogenicity is unknown; formerly called *Cillobacterium tenue.*

E. tortuo'sum, a species found infrequently in the intestines of humans.

eubiotics (yū-bī-ot'iks) [eu- + G. *biotikos,* relating to life]. The science of hygienic living.

eubolism (yū'bō-lizm). Obsolete word for normal body metabolism.

eucaine (yū'kān). β-Eucaine; 2,2,6-trimethyl-4-piperidinol benzoate; a local anesthetic for topical anesthesia.

eucalyptol (yū-kă-lip'tol). Cineole.

eucalyptus (yū-kă-lip'tŭs). The dried leaves of *Eucalyptus globulus* (family Myrtaceae), the blue gum or Australian fever tree; it has been used in the treatment of malaria, bronchitis, asthma, and chronic gonorrhea.

e. oil, the volatile oil distilled with steam from the fresh leaf of *Eucalyptus globulus* or some other species of *Eucalyptus;* contains not less than 70% of eucalyptol; used as an antiseptic, stimulant, and expectorant.

eucapnia (yū-kap'nē-ă) [eu- + G. *kapnos,* vapor]. A state in which the arterial carbon dioxide pressure is optimal. See also normocapnia.

eucaryote (yū-kar'ē-ōt) [eu- + G. *karyon,* kernel, nut]. Eukaryote.

eucaryotic (yū-kar-ē-ot'ik). Eukaryotic.

eucasin (yū-kā'sin). Ammonium caseinate prepared by passing ammonia gas over finely powdered dry casein; added as a concentrated food to bouillon, chocolate, etc.

eucatropine hydrochloride (yū-kat'rō-pēn). 1,2,2,6-Tetramethyl-4-piperidinol mandelate hydrochloride; a mydriatic; it produces no anesthesia, pain, or increased intraocular pressure.

Eucestoda (yū-ses-tō'dă). Cestoda.

euchlorhydria (yū-klōr-hi'drē-ă). A condition in which free hydrochloric acid exists in normal amount in the gastric juice.

eucholia (yū-kō'lē-ă) [eu- + G. *cholē,* bile]. A normal state of the bile as regards quantity and quality.

euchromatic (yū-krō-mat'ik). **1.** Orthochromatic. **2.** Characteristic of euchromatin.

euchromatin (yū-krō'mă-tin). The parts of chromosomes which, during interphase, are uncoiled dispersed threads and not stained by ordinary dyes; metabolically active, in contrast to the inert heterochromatin.

euchromosome (yū-krō'mō-sōm). Autosome.

eucorticalism (yū-kōr'ti-kăl-izm). Normal functioning of the adrenal cortex.

eucrasia (yū-krā'zhē-ă) [G. *eukrasia,* good temperament, fr. *eu,* well, + *krasis,* a mixing]. **1.** Obsolete term for homeostasis. **2.** A condition of reduced susceptibility to the adverse effects of certain drugs, articles of diet, etc.

eucupine (yū'kū-pēn). Euprocin hydrochloride.

eudemonia (yū-dē-mō'nē-ă) [eu- + G. *daimon,* destiny]. A feeling of well-being or happiness.

eudiaphoresis (yū-dī'ă-fō-rē'sis) [eu- + G. *diaphorēsis,* perspiration]. Normal free sweating.

eudipsia (yū-dip'sē-ă) [eu- + G. *dipsa,* thirst]. Ordinary mild thirst.

Euflagellata (yū-flaj'ĕ-lā'tă). Former term for the protozoan flagellates now included in the subphylum Mastigophora.

eugenic (yū-jen'ik). Relating to eugenics.

eugenic acid. Eugenol.

eugenics (yū-jen'iks) [G. *eugeneia,* nobility of birth, fr. *eu,* well, + *genesis,* production]. Aristogenics; a term coined by Galton to denote practices and policies, as of mate selection or of sterilization, that tend to better the innate qualities of man and to develop them to the highest degree.

eugenism (yū'jen-izm). "The aggregate of the most favorable conditions for healthy and happy existence" (Galton).

eugenol (yū'je-nol). Eugenic acid; 4-allyl-2-methoxyphenol; obtained from oil of cloves; used in dentistry with zinc oxide as an analgesic and as a base for impression materials; also used in perfumery as a substitute for oil of cloves.

Euglena (yū-glē'nă) [eu- + G. *glēnē,* eyeball]. A widespread genus of photosynthesizing free-living fresh water flagellates (family Euglinidae).

E. grac'ilis, an abundant species sometimes used in assaying vitamin B_{12} concentrations of serum and urine in various types of anemia.

E. vir'idis, a species that inhabits stagnant pools, often in great numbers.

Euglenidae (yū-glē'ni-dē). A family of green (phytomonad) flagellates (subphylum Mastigophora, class Phytomastigophorea).

euglobulin (yū-glob'yū-lin). That fraction of the serum globulin less soluble in $(NH_4)_2SO_4$ solution than the pseudoglobulin fraction.

euglycemia (yū-glī-sē'mē-ă) [eu- + G. *glykys,* sweet, + *haima,* blood]. Normoglycemia; a normal blood glucose concentration.

euglycemic (yū-glī-sē'mik). Normoglycemic; denoting, characteristic of, or promoting euglycemia.

eugnathia (yū-nā'thē-ă, -nath'ē-ă) [eu- + G. *gnathos,* jaw]. Eugnathic anomaly; an abnormality that is limited to the teeth and their immediate alveolar supports.

eugnosia (yū-nō'sē-ă) [eu- + G. *gnōsis,* perception]. Normal ability to synthesize sensory stimuli.

eugonic (yū-gon'ik) [G. *eugonos,* productive, fr. *eu,* well, + *gonos,* seed, offspring]. A term used to indicate that the growth of a bacterial culture is rapid and relatively luxuriant; used especially in reference to the growth of cultures of the human tubercle bacillus (*Mycobacterium tuberculosis*). See also dysgonic.

Eugregarinida (yū'greg-ă-rin'i-dă) [eu- + L. *gregarius,* gregarious]. An order of gregarines (subclass Gregarinia), reproducing only by sporogony, in which schizogony is absent; they are parasites of annelids and arthropods.

euhydration (yū-hī-drā'shŭn). Normal state of body water content; absence of absolute or relative hydration or dehydration.

Eukaryotae (yū-kar-ē-ō'tē). Eucaryotae; a superkingdom of organisms characterized by eukaryotic cells; acellular members (kingdom Protoctista) are characterized by a single eukaryotic unit; more complex (multicellular) members have been assigned to the kingdoms Fungi, Plantae, and Animalia.

eukaryote (yū-kar'ē-ōt) [eu- + G. *karyon,* kernel, nut]. Eucaryote. **1.** A cell containing a membrane-bound nucleus with chromosomes of DNA, RNA, and proteins, mostly large (10-100μm), with cell division involving a form of mitosis in which mitotic spindles (or some microtubule arrangement) are involved; mitochondria are present, and, in photosynthetic species, plastids are found; undulipodia (cilia or flagella) are of the complex 9+2 organization of tubulin and various proteins. Possession of a e. type of cell characterizes the four kingdoms above the Monera or prokaryote level of complexity: Protoctista, Fungi, Plantae, and Animalia, combined into the superkingdom Eukaryotae. **2.** Common name for members of the Eukaryotae.

eukaryotic (yū'kar-ē-ot'ik). Eucaryotic; pertaining to or characteristic of a eukaryote.

eukeratin (yū-kār'ă-tin). Hard keratin present in hair, wool, horn, nails, etc.

eukinesia (yū-ki-nē'zē-ă) [eu- + G. *kinēsis,* movement]. Normal movement.

Eulenburg, Albert, German neurologist, 1840–1917. See E.'s *disease.*

eumelanin (yū-mel'ă-nin) [eu- + G. *melos* (*melan-*), black]. The most abundant type of human melanin, found in brown and black hair.

eumelanosome (yū-mel'ă-nō-sōm). Melanosome.

eumetria (yū-mē'trē-ă) [G. moderation, goodness of meter]. Graduation of the strength of nerve impulses to match the need.

eumorphism (yū-mōr'fizm) [eu- + G. *morphē,* shape]. Preservation of the natural form of a cell.

eumycetes (yū-mī-sē'tēz) [eu- + G. *mykēs,* fungus]. The true fungi.

Eumycetozoea (yū'mī-sē-tō-zō'ē-ă) [eu- + G. *mykēs* (*mykēt-*), fungus, + *zōon,* animal]. Microscopic animal forms, frequently known as slime animals, that consist of an irregular semifluid mass of multinucleated ameboid protoplasm; although grouped as a class of the superclass Rhizopoda (subphylum Sarcodina), some of the mycetozoan forms closely resemble certain species of pseudomycetes and are sometimes classified as members of the Myxomycetes, the slime molds. See also Proteomyxidia.

eunoia (yū-noy'ă) [G. goodwill, fr. *eu,* well, + *nous,* mind]. Rarely used term denoting a normal mental state.

eunuch (yū'nŭk) [G. *eunouchos,* chamberlain, fr. *eunē,* bed, + *echein,* to have]. An individual whose testes have been removed or have never developed.

eunuchism (yū'nŭk-izm). **1.** The state of being a eunuch; absence of the testes with consequent lack of reproductive and sexual function and of development of secondary sex characteristics. **2.** Eunuchoidism.

eunuchoid (yū'nŭ-koyd) [G. *eunouchos,* eunuch, + *eidos,* resembling]. Resembling, or having the general characteristics of, a eunuch; usually indicating the physical habitus of a male in whom hypogonadism occurred before puberty.

eunuchoidism (yū'nŭ-koyd-izm). Eunuchism (2); male hypogonadism; a state in which testes are present but fail to function normally; may be of gonadal or pituitary origin.

hypergonadotropic e., e. of gonadal origin, commonly accompanied by enhanced levels of pituitary gonadotropins in the blood and urine, as in Klinefelter's syndrome.

hypogonadotropic e., hypogonadotropic *hypogonadism.*

euosmia (yū-oz'mē-ă) [eu- + G. *osmē,* smell]. **1.** A pleasant odor. **2.** Normal olfaction.

eupancreatism (yū-pan'krē-ă-tizm). The state of normal pancreatic digestive function.

euparal (yū'pa-răl). A medium for mounting histologic specimens, composed of sandarac, eucalyptol, paraldehyde, camphor, and phenyl salicylate.

Euparyphium (yū-pa-rif'ē-ŭm) [eu- + G. *paryphē,* a border]. A genus of nonpathogenic flukes (family Echinostomatidae), several species of which have been reported from the intestines of man.

eupaverin (yū-pav'ĕ-rin). 1-Benzyl-3-ethyl-6,7-dimethoxyisoquinoline; a smooth muscle relaxant.

eupepsia (yū-pep'sē-ă) [G., fr. *eu,* well, + *pepsis,* digestion]. Good digestion.

eupeptic (yū-pep'tik). Digesting well; having a good digestion.

euphenics (yū-fē'niks) [eu- + G. *phainō,* to show forth]. Modification of the internal or external environment of an individual so as to prevent or modify the phenotypic expression of a genetic defect, without modifying the genotype.

Euphorbia pilulifera (yū-fōr'bē-ă pil-ŭ-lif'ĕ-ră). Asthma-weed (2); a species of plant (family Euphorbiaceae); the dried herb is used in asthma, coryza and other respiratory affections, in angina pectoris, and as an antispasmodic.

euphoretic (yū-fō-ret'ik). Euphoriant.

euphoria (yū-fōr'ē-ă) [eu- + G. *pherō,* to bear]. A feeling of well-being, commonly exaggerated and not necessarily well founded.

euphoriant (yū-fōr'ē-ant). Euphoretic. **1.** Having the capability to produce a sense of well-being. **2.** An agent with such a capability.

euplasia (yū-plā'zē-ă) [eu- + G. *plassō,* form]. The state of cells or tissue which is normal or typical for that particular type.

euplastic (yū-plas'tik) [G. *euplastos,* easily molded; *eu,* well, + *plastos,* formed]. **1.** Relating to euplasia. **2.** Healing readily and well.

euploid (yū'ployd). Relating to euploidy.

euploidy (yū'ploy-dē) [eu- + G. *-ploos,* -fold]. The state of a cell whose number of chromosomes is an exact multiple of the haploid number normal for the species.

eupnea (yūp-nē'ă) [G. *eupnoia,* fr. *eu,* well, + *pnoia,* breath]. Easy, free respiration; the type observed in a normal individual under resting conditions.

eupraxia (yū-prak'sē-ă) [eu- + G. *praxis,* a doing]. Normal ability to perform coordinated movements.

euprocin hydrochloride (yū'prō-sin). Eucupine; isopentylhydrocupreine; hydrocupreine isopentyl ether; a derivative of quinine used as an antiseptic and local anesthetic.

Euproctis (yū-prok'tis) [eu- + G. *prōktos,* rump]. A genus of moths. The hairs of the cocoon and caterpillar of the species *E. chrysorrhoea,* the brown-tail moth, cause caterpillar dermatitis.

eurhythmia (yū-rith'mē-ă) [eu- + G. *rhythmos,* rhythm]. Harmonious body relationships of the separate organs.

europium (yū-rō'pē-ŭm) [L. *Europa,* Europe]. An element of the rare earth (lanthanide) group, symbol Eu, atomic no. 63, atomic weight 151.96.

eury- [G. *eurys,* wide]. Combining form meaning wide or broad.

eurycephalic, eurycephalous (yū'rē-se-fal'ik, -sef'ă-lŭs) [eury- + G. *kephalēs,* head]. Having an abnormally broad head; sometimes used in reference to a brachycephalic head.

eurygnathic (yū-rig-nath'ik). Eurygnathous; having a wide jaw.

eurygnathism (yū-rig'nă-thizm) [eury- + G. *gnathos,* jaw]. The condition of having a wide jaw.

eurygnathous (yū-rig'nă-thŭs). Eurygnathic.

euryon (yū'rē-on) [G. *eurys,* broad]. The extremity, on either side, of the greatest transverse diameter of the head; a point used in craniometry.

euryopia (yū-rē-ō'pē-ă) [eury- + G. *ops,* eye]. A wide intraocular distance.

eurysomatic (yū'rē-sō-mat'ik) [eury- + G. *soma,* body]. Having a thick-set body.

euscope (yū'skōp) [eu- + G. *skopeō,* to view]. An instrument for showing on a screen an enlarged image from a microscope.

Eusimulium (yū-si-myū'lē-ŭm) [eu- + L. *simulo,* to simulate]. *Simulium.*

eustachian (yū-stā'shŭn, yū-stā'kē-ăn). Described by or attributed to Eustachio.

Eustachio, Bartolommeo E., Italian anatomist, 1520–1574. See eustachian *catheter, cushion, tonsil, tube, tuber, valve.*

eustachitis (yū-stā-kī'tis). Inflammation of the mucous membrane of the eustachian tube.

eusthenia (yū-sthē'nē-ă) [eu- + G. *sthenos,* strength]. Normal strength.

Eustrongylus (yū-stron'ji-lŭs) [eu- + G. *strongylos,* rounded]. Former name for *Dioctophyma.*

eusystole (yū-sis'tō-lē) [eu- + systole]. A condition in which the cardiac systole is normal in force and time.

eusystolic (yū-sis-tol'ik). Relating to eusystole.

eutectic (yū-tek'tik) [eu- + G. *tēxis,* a melting away]. **1.** Easily melted; denoting specifically mixtures of certain chemical compounds that have a lower melting point than any of their ingredients; *e.g.,* a solid, such as menthol, that when triturated with another solid of the same class, such as camphor, unites with it to form a liquid, the mixture having a lower melting point than either of its components. **2.** The alloy that freezes at a constant temperature; the lowest of the series.

eutelegenesis (yū'tel-ĕ-jen'ĕ-sis) [eu- + G. *tēle,* end, + *genesis,* production]. Artificial insemination by semen from a donor selected because of certain desirable characteristics for the development of superior offspring.

euthanasia (yū-thă-nā'zē-ă) [eu- + G. *thanatos,* death]. **1.** A quiet, painless death. **2.** The intentional putting to death of a person with an incurable or painful disease.

euthenics (yū-then'iks) [G. *euthenein,* to thrive]. The science concerned with establishing optimum living conditions for plants, animals, or humans, especially through proper provisioning and environment.

eutherapeutic (yū'thăr-ă-pyū'tik). Having excellent curative properties.

Eutheria (yū-thē'rē-ă) [eu- + G. *thērion,* animal]. A subclass of mammals, excluding monotremes and marsupials, having a placenta through which the young are nourished.

euthermic (yū-ther'mik) [eu- + G. *thermos,* warm]. At an optimal temperature.

euthymia (yū-thī'mē-ă) [eu- + G. *thymos,* mind]. Joyfulness; mental peace and tranquility.

euthymic (yū-thī'mik). Relating to, or characterized by, euthymia.

euthyroidism (yū-thī'roy-dizm). A condition in which the thyroid gland is functioning normally, its secretion being of proper amount and constitution.

euthyscope (yū'thi-skōp) [G. *euthys,* straight, + *skopeō,* to view]. A modified ophthalmoscope with which the site of excentric fixation may be dazzled by a bright light while the true fovea is simultaneously shielded by an opaque disk; used in pleoptics.

euthyscopy (yū-this'kŏ-pē). Examination with the euthyscope.

eutonic (yū-ton'ik) [eu- + G. *tonus,* tone]. Normotonic (1).

eutrichosis (yū-tri-kō'sis) [eu- + G. *thrix,* hair]. A normal growth of healthy hair.

eutrophia (yū-trō'fē-ă) [G. fr. *eu,* well, + *trophē,* nourishment]. Eutrophy; a state of normal nourishment and growth.

eutrophic (yū-trof'ik). Relating to, characterized by, or promoting eutrophia.

eutrophy (yū'trō-fē). Eutrophia.

euvolia (yū-vō'lē-ă). Normal water content or volume of a given compartment; *e.g.,* extracellular e.

eV, ev Abbreviation for electron-volt.

evacuant (ē-vak'yū-ant). **1.** Promoting an excretion, especially of the bowels. **2.** An agent that increases excretion, especially a cathartic.

evacuate (ē-vak'yū-āt) [L. *e-vacuo,* pp. *-vacuatus,* to empty out]. To accomplish evacuation.

evacuation (ē-vak-yū-ā'shŭn). **1.** Removal of waste material, especially from the bowels by defecation. **2.** Stool (2). **3.** Removal of air from a closed vessel; production of a vacuum.

evacuator (ē-vak'yū-ā-tŏr). A mechanical evacuant; an instrument for the removal of fluid or small particles from a body cavity, or of impacted feces from the rectum.
Ellik e., a special instrument with glass receptacle, latex or plastic bulb, and flexible tubing, used to evacuate tissue fragments, blood clots, or calculi from the urinary bladder.

evagination (ē-vaj-i-nā'shŭn) [L. *e,* out, + *vagina,* sheath]. Protrusion of some part or organ from its normal position.

evanescent (ev-ă-nes'ent) [L. *e,* out, + *vanescere,* to vanish]. Of short duration.

Evans, Robert S., U.S. physician, *1912. See E.'s *syndrome.*

Evans blue [H.M. *Evans,* U.S. anatomist, 1882–1971] [C.I. 23860]. Azovan blue; tetrasodium salt of 4,4'-bis[7-(1-amino-8-hydroxy-2,4-disulfo)naphthylazo]-3,3'-bitolyl; $C_{34}H_{24}N_6Na_4O_{14}S_4$; a diazo dye used for the determination of the blood volume on the basis of the dilution of a standard solution of the dye in the plasma after its intravenous injection; it binds to proteins and is also used as a vital stain for following diffusion through blood vessel walls.

Evans forceps. See under forceps.

evaporate (ē-vap'ōr-āt). Volatilize; to cause or undergo evaporation.

evaporation (ē-vap-ŏ-ra'shŭn) [L. *e,* out, + *vaporare,* to emit vapor]. Volatilization. **1.** A change from liquid to vapor form. **2.** Loss of volume of a liquid by conversion into vapor.

evasion (ē-vā'zhŭn). The act of escaping or avoiding.
macular e., *horror* fusionis.

eventration (ē'ven-trā'shŭn) [L. *e,* out, + *venter,* belly]. **1.** Evisceration (3); protrusion of omentum and/or intestine through an opening in the abdominal wall. **2.** Removal of the contents of the abdominal cavity.
e. of the diaphragm, extreme elevation of a half or part of the diaphragm, which is usually atrophic and abnormally thin.

eversion (ē-ver'zhŭn) [L. *e-everto,* pp. *-versus,* to overturn]. A turning outward, as of the eyelid or foot.

evert (ē-vert') [L. *e-verto,* to overturn]. To turn outward.

evidement (e-vēd-mon') [Fr. *évider,* to scoop out]. Obsolete term for the scraping out of morbid tissue from a natural or pathologic cavity.

evil (ē'vil). Disease, especially of animals.
joint e., joint *ill.*
king's e., historic term for cervical tuberculous lymphadenitis (scrofula) which was formerly thought to be curable by the touch of a king.
poll e., suppurative inflammation of the cranial nuchal (atlantal) bursa that lies between the atlas and the cranial end of the ligamentum nuchae in the horse.
quarter e., blackleg.

eviration (ev-i-rā'shŭn, ē-vī-rā'shŭn) [L. *e,* out, + *vir,* man]. **1.** Emasculation. **2.** Loss or absence of the masculine, with acquirement of feminine characteristics; a type of effemination. **3.** Delusional belief of a man that he has become a woman.

evisceration (ē-vis-er-ā'shŭn) [L. *eviscero,* to disembowel]. **1.** Exenteration. **2.** Removal of the contents of the eyeball, leaving the sclera and sometimes the cornea. **3.** Eventration (1).

evisceroneurotomy (ē-vis'er-ō-nū-rot'ō-mē) [L. *eviscero,* to disembowel, + G. *neuron,* nerve, + *tomē,* a cutting]. Evisceration of the eye with division of the optic nerve.

evocation (ev-ō-kā'shŭn, ē-vō-kā'shŭn) [L. *evoco,* pp. *evocatus,* to call forth, evoke]. Induction of a particular tissue produced by the action of an evocator during embryogenesis.

evocator (ev'ō-kā-ter, -tōr). The substance discharged from an orga-

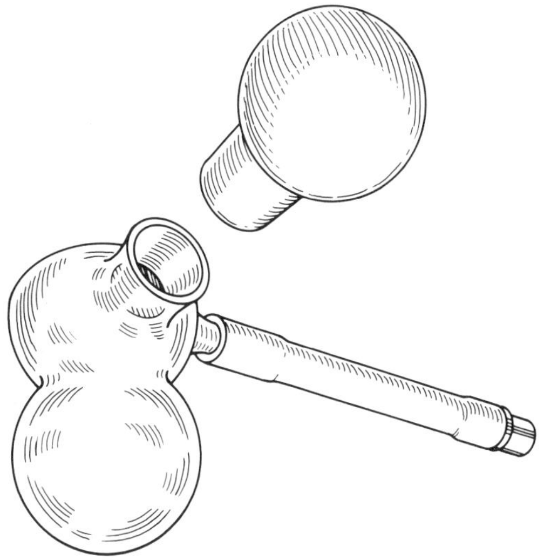

Ellik Evacuator

nizer; a factor in the control of morphogenesis in the early embryo.

evolution (ev-ō-lū'shŭn) [L. *e-volvo*, pp. *-volutus*, to roll out]. A continuing process of change from one state, condition or form to another.
bathmic e., orthogenic e.; a change of type due to something inherent in the constitution, independent of the environment.
biologic e., organic e.; the doctrine that all forms of animal or plant life have been derived by gradual changes from simpler forms or from a single cell.
convergent e., the evolutionary development of similar structures in two or more species, often widely separated phylogenetically, in response to similarities of environment.
Denman's spontaneous e., a mechanism of spontaneous molding of the fetus and impaction of the shoulder with prolapse of the arm noted in some cases of transverse lie; vaginal delivery is achieved with the breech appearing at the vulva immediately after the prolapsed shoulder.
Douglas' spontaneous e., a mechanism whereby molding of the fetus and impaction of the shoulder and prolapsed arm occurs in transverse lie, allowing vaginal delivery with the lateral aspect of the thorax following the prolapsed shoulder.
emergent e., a character appearing suddenly due to a mutation.
organic e., biologic e.
orthogenic e., bathmic e.
saltatory e., the theory that e. of a new species from an older one may occur as a large "jump," such as a major repatterning of chromosomes, rather than by gradual accumulation of small "steps" or mutations.
spontaneous e., the unaided delivery of the fetus from a transverse lie.

evulsion (ē-vŭl'shŭn) [L. *evulsio*, fr. *e-vello*, pp. *-vulsus*, to pluck out]. A forcible pulling out or extraction. *Cf.* avulsion.

Ewart, William, British physician, 1848–1929. See E.'s *procedure, sign.*

ewe (yew). A female sheep of breeding age.

Ewing, James, U.S. pathologist, 1866–1943. See E.'s *sarcoma, tumor.*

Ewing, James H., 1798–1827. See E.'s *sign.*

ex- [L. and G. out of]. Prefix denoting out of, from, away from.

exa- (E) Prefix used in the SI and metric systems to signify one quintillion (10^{18}).

exacerbation (eg-zas-er-bā'shŭn, -ek-sas-) [L. *ex- acerbo*, pp. *-auts*, to exasperate, increase, fr. *acerbus*, sour]. An increase in the severity of a disease or any of its signs or symptoms.

examination (eg-zam-i-nā'shŭn). Any investigation or inspection made for the purpose of diagnosis; usually qualified by the method used.
cytologic e., microscopic examination of cells, especially for diagnosis of disease.
Papanicolaou e., see Pap *test.*
physical e., e. by means such as visual inspection, palpation, percussion, and auscultation to collect information for diagnosis.
postmortem e., autopsy.

examiner (eg-zam'in-er) [L. *examino*, to weigh, examine]. One who performs an examination.
medical e., **(1)** a physician who examines a person and reports upon his physical condition to the company or individual at whose request the examination was made; **(2)** in states or municipalities where the office of coroner has been abolished, a physician appointed to investigate all cases of sudden or violent death.

exanthem (eg-zan'them). Exanthema.

exanthema (eg-zan-thē'mă) [G. efflorescence, an eruption, fr. *anthos*, flower]. Exanthem; a skin eruption occurring as a symptom of an acute viral or coccal disease, as in scarlet fever or measles.
Boston e. [after the city in which an epidemic occurred], a viral disease resembling e. subitum, with the e. appearing after the fever has subsided; it is caused by strain 16 of ECHO virus.
epidemic e., epidemic *polyarthritis.*
keratoid e., a symptom occurring in the secondary stage of yaws: patches of fine, light colored, furfuraceous desquamation, scattered irregularly over limbs and trunk.
e. subi'tum, pseudorubella; roseola infantilis or infantum; sixth disease; a viral disease of infants and young children, marked by sudden onset with fever lasting several days (sometimes with convulsions) and followed by a fine macular (sometimes maculopapular) rash that appears within a few hours to a day after the fever has subsided.
vesicular e., a disease of swine and probably of certain marine mammals, caused by vesicular e. virus of swine; it closely resembles foot-and-mouth disease and, in swine, is characterized by fever, loss of weight, and vesicles on the snout, tongue, and feet.

exanthematous (eg-zan-them'ă-tŭs). Relating to an exanthema.

exanthesis (eg-zan-thē'sis) [G.]. **1.** A rash or exanthem. **2.** The coming out of a rash or eruption.
e. arthro'sia, dengue.

exanthrope (ek'zan-thrōp) [G. *ex*, out of, + *anthrōpos*, man]. An external cause of disease, one not originating in the body.

exanthropic (ek-zan-throp'ik). Originating outside of the human body.

exarteritis (eks-ar-ter-ī'tis). Periarteritis.

exarticulation (eks-ar-tik-yū-lā'shŭn) [L. *ex*, out, + *articulus*, joint]. Disarticulation.

excalation (eks-kă-lā'shŭn) [G. *ex*, from, + *chalān*, to abate, release]. Absence, suppression, or failure of development of one of a series of things, as of a digit.

excavatio (eks-kă-vā'shē-ō) [L. fr. *ex-cavo*, pp. *-cavatus*, to hollow out, fr. *ex*, out, + *cavus*, hollow] [NA]. Excavation (1).
e. dis'ci [NA], excavation of optic disk; e. papillae; physiologic excavation; the normally occurring depression or pit in the center of the optic disk.
e. papil'lae, e. disci.
e. rectouteri'na [NA], rectouterine pouch; rectovaginouterine pouch; cavum douglasi; Douglas' cul-de-sac; Douglas' pouch; a pocket formed by the deflection of the peritoneum from the rectum to the uterus.
e. rectovesica'lis [NA], rectovesical pouch; Proust's space; a pocket formed by the deflection of the peritoneum from the rectum to the bladder in the male.
e. vesicouteri'na [NA], uterovesical or vesicouterine pouch; cavum vesicouterinum; a pocket formed by the deflection of the peritoneum from the bladder to the uterus in the female.

excavation (eks-kă-vā'shŭn). **1.** Excavatio; a natural cavity, pouch, or recess. **2.** A cavity formed artificially or as the result of a pathologic process.
atrophic e., an exaggeration of the normal or physiologic cupping of the optic disk (excavatio disci) caused by atrophy of the optic nerve.
glaucomatous e., glaucomatous *cup.*
e. of optic disk, *excavatio* disci.
physiologic e., *excavatio* disci.

excavator (eks'că-vā-tŏr, -tōr). **1.** An instrument like a large sharp spoon or scoop, used in scraping out pathologic tissue. **2.** In dentistry, an instrument, generally a small spoon or curette, for cleaning out and shaping a carious cavity preparatory to filling.
hatchet e., see hatchet.
hoe e., a single-beveled dental e., with the blade at an angle to the axis of the handle and the cutting edge perpendicular to the plane of the angle.

excementosis (ek'sē-men-tō'sis). A nodular outgrowth of cementum on the root surface of a tooth.

excentric (ek-sen'trik). Alternative spelling for eccentric (2, 3).

excess (ek'ses). That which is more than the usual or specified amount.

antibody e., in a precipitation test, the presence of antibody in an amount greater than that required to combine with all of the antigen present.

antigen e., (1) in a precipitation test, the presence of uncombined antigen above that required to combine with all of the antibody; precipitation may be inhibited because the presence of excess antigen gives rise to soluble antigen-antibody complexes; **(2)** *in vivo,* the resultant antigen-antibody interaction in such an antigen e. may give rise to immune complexes, which have a potential to induce cellular damage; such injury underlies the pathologic changes seen in certain immune complex diseases.

base e., a measure of metabolic alkalosis, usually predicted from the Siggaard-Andersen nomogram; the amount of strong acid that would have to be added per unit volume of whole blood to titrate it to pH 7.4 while at 37°C and at a carbon dioxide pressure of 40 mm Hg.

convergence e., that condition in which an esophoria or esotropia is greater for near vision than for far vision.

negative base e., a measure of metabolic acidosis, usually predicted from the Siggaard-Andersen nomogram; the amount of strong alkalai that would have to be added per unit volume of whole blood to titrate it to pH 7.4 while at 37°C and at a carbon dioxide pressure of 40 mm Hg.

exchange (eks-chānj'). To substitute one thing for another, or the act of such substitution.

sister chromatid e., the e. during mitosis of homologous genetic material between sister chromatids; increased as a result of inordinate chromosomal fragility due to genetic or environmental factors.

excipient (ek-sip'ē-ent) [L. *excipiens;* pres. p. of *ex- cipio,* to take out]. A more or less inert substance added in a prescription as a diluent or vehicle or to give form or consistency when the remedy is given in pill form; *e.g.,* simple syrup, aromatic powder, honey, and various elixirs.

excise (ek-sīz'). Exsect; to cut out. See also resect.

excision (ek-sizh'ŭn) [L. *excidere,* to cut out]. **1.** Exsection; exeresis; the act of cutting out; the surgical removal of part or all of a structure or organ. See also resection. **2.** In molecular biology, a recombination event in which a genetic element is removed.

excitability (ek-sī'tă-bil'i-tē). Having the capability of being excitable.

supranormal e., at the end of phase three of the cardiac action potential, the successful stimulation threshold falls below the level necessary to produce excitation during the rest of the phase of diastole, so that an ordinary subthreshold stimulus becomes effective. *Cf.* supranormal *conduction.*

excitable (ek-sī'tă-bl). **1.** Capable of quick response to a stimulus; having potentiality for emotional arousal. *Cf.* irritable. **2.** In neurophysiology, referring to a tissue, cell, or membrane capable of undergoing excitation in response to an adequate stimulus.

excitant (ek-sī'tănt) [L. *excito,* pp. *-atus,* pres. p. *-ans,* to arouse]. Stimulant.

excitation (ek-sī-tā'shŭn). **1.** The act of increasing the rapidity or intensity of the physical or mental processes. **2.** In neurophysiology, the complete all-or-none response of a nerve or muscle to an adequate stimulus, ordinarily including propagation of e. along the membranes of the cell or cells involved. See also stimulation.

excitatory (ek-sī'tă-tō-rē). Tending to produce excitation.

excitement (ek-sīt'ment). An emotional state characterized by its potential for impulsive or poorly controlled activity.

catatonic e., an excited catatonic state. See catatonia.

manic e., an excited mental state characterized by hyperactivity, talkativeness, flight of ideas, pressured speech, grandiosity, and, occasionally, grandiose delusions.

excitoglandular (ek-sī'tō-glan'dyū-lăr). Increasing the secretory activity of a gland.

excitometabolic (ek-sī'tō-met-ă-bol'ik). Increasing the activity of the metabolic processes.

excitomotor (ek-sī'tō-mō'ter). Centrokinetic (2); causing or increasing the rapidity of motion.

excitomuscular (ek-sī'tō-mŭs'kyū-lăr). Causing muscular activity.

excitor (ek-sī'ter, -tōr). Stimulant (2).

excitosecretory (ek-sī'tō-sē-krē'tō-rē). Stimulating to secretion.

excitovascular (ek-sī'tō-vas'kyū-lăr). Increasing the activity of the circulation.

exclave (eks-klāv') [L. *ex,* out, + *-clave* (in enclave, *q.v.*)]. An outlying, detached portion of a gland or other part, such as the thyroid or pancreas; an accessory gland.

exclusion (eks-klū'zhŭn) [L. *ex- cludo,* pp. *-clusus,* to shut out]. A shutting out; disconnection from the main portion.

allelic e., in each cell of an individual heterozygous at an autosomal locus, the non-preferential supression of the phenotypic manifestation of one or other of the alleles; the phenotype of the body is thus mosaic.

Devine e., e. of the lower part of the stomach, followed by gastrojejunostomy, for treatment of duodenal ulcer.

e. of pupil, seclusion of pupil; the condition resulting from posterior annular synechia, in which the iris is bound down throughout the entire pupillary margin, but the pupil is not occluded.

exconjugant (eks-kon'jū-gant) [ex- + L. *conjugo,* to join]. A member of a conjugating pair of protozoan ciliates after separation and prior to the subsequent mitotic division of each of the e.'s. See also conjugant; conjugation (3).

excoriate (eks-kō'rē-āt). To scratch or otherwise denude the skin by physical means.

excoriation (eks-kō'rē-ā'shŭn) [L. *excorio,* to skin, strip, fr. *corium,* skin, hide]. A scratch mark; a linear break in the skin surface, usually covered with blood or serous crusts.

neurotic e., repeated self-induced e., with or without underlying skin lesions, associated with compulsive or neurotic behavioral problems.

excrement (eks'krē-ment) [L. *ex- cerno,* pp. *-cretus,* to separate]. Waste matter or any excretion cast out of the body; *e.g.,* feces.

excrementitious (eks'krē-men-tish'ŭs). Relating to any excrement.

excrescence (eks-kres'ens) [L. *ex- cresco,* pp. *-çretus,* to grow forth]. Any outgrowth from a surface.

excreta (eks-krē'tă) [L. neut. pl. of *excretus,* pp. of *ex-cerno,* to separate]. Excretion (2).

excrete (eks-krēt'). To separate from the blood and cast out; to perform excretion.

excretion (eks-krē'shŭn) [see excrement]. **1.** The process whereby the undigested residue of food and the waste products of metabolism are eliminated, material is removed to regulate the composition of body fluids and tissues, or substances are expelled to perform functions on an exterior surface. **2.** Excreta; the product of a tissue or organ that is material to be passed out of the body. *Cf.* secretion.

excretory (eks-krē'tō-rē). Relating to excretion.

excursion (eks-ker'zhŭn). Any movement from one point to another, usually with the implied idea of returning again to the original position.

lateral e., movement of the mandible to the right or left side.
protrusive e., movement of the mandible to a position forward of the centric position.

excycloduction (ek-sī-klō-dŭk'shŭn). Rotation of the upper pole of one cornea outward.

excyclophoria (ek-sī-klō-fō'rē-ă). The tendency toward outward rotation of the upper pole of the cornea, prevented by visual fusional impulses.

excyclovergence (ek-sī-klō-ver'jens). Rotation of the upper pole of each cornea outwards.

excystation (ek-sis-tā'shŭn). Removal from a cyst; denoting the action of certain encysted organisms in escaping from their envelope.

exemia (ek-sē'mē-ă) [G. *ex*, out of, + *haima*, blood]. A condition, as in shock, in which a considerable portion of the blood is removed from the main circulation but remains within blood vessels in certain areas where it is stagnant.

exencephalia (eks'en-se-fā'lē-ă). Exencephaly.

exencephalic (eks'en-se-fal'ik). Exencephalous; relating to exencephaly.

exencephalocele (eks'en-sef'ă-lō-sēl) [*ex*, out, + G. *enkephalos*, brain, + *kēlē*, tumor]. Herniation of the brain.

exencephalous (eks-en-sef'ă-lŭs). Exencephalic.

exencephaly (eks-en-sef'ă-lē) [G. *ex*, out, + *enkephalos*, brain]. Exencephalia; condition in which the skull is defective with the brain exposed or extruding.

exenteration (eks-en-ter-ā'shŭn) [G. *ex*, out, + *enteron*, bowel]. Evisceration (1); removal of internal organs and tissues, usually radical removal of the contents of a body cavity.
anterior pelvic e., removal of the urinary bladder, lower parts of the ureters, vagina, uterus, adnexa, and adjacent lymph nodes; a urinary diversion is necessary.
orbital e., removal of the entire contents of the orbit.
pelvic e., removal of all of the organs and adjacent structures of the pelvis; usually performed to surgically ablate cancer involving urinary bladder, uterine cervix, or rectum.
posterior pelvic e., removal of the vagina, uterus, adnexa, rectum, anus, and adjacent lymph nodes; a colostomy is necessary.
total pelvic e., Brunschwig's operation; removal of the urinary bladder, lower parts of the ureters, vagina, uterus, adnexa, rectum, anus, and adjacent lymph nodes; a colostomy and urinary diversion are necessary.

exenteri'tis (eks-en-ter-ī'tis) [G. *exō*, on the outside, + enteritis]. Inflammation of the peritoneal covering of the intestine.

exercise (ek'ser-sīz). **1.** *Active:* bodily exertion for the sake of restoring the organs and functions to a healthy state or keeping them healthy. **2.** *Passive:* motion of limbs without effort by the patient.
isometric e., e. consisting of muscular contractions without movement of the involved parts of the body.
Kegel's e.'s, alternate contraction and relaxation of perineal muscles for treatment of urinary stress incontinence.

exeresis (ek-ser'ĕ-sis) [G. *exairesis*, a taking out, fr. *haireō*, to take, grasp]. Excision.

exergonic (ek-ser-gon'ik) [exo- + G. *ergon*, work]. Referring to a chemical reaction that takes place with release of energy to its surroundings. *Cf.* endergonic.

exflagellation (eks-flaj-ĕ-lā'shŭn). Polymitus; the extrusion of rapidly waving flagellum-like microgametes from microgametocytes; in the case of human malaria parasites, this occurs in the blood meal taken by the proper anopheline vector within a few minutes after ingestion of the infected blood by the mosquito.

exfoliation (eks-fō-lē-ā'shŭn) [Mod. L. fr. L. *ex*, out, + *folium*, leaf]. **1.** Detachment and shedding of superficial cells of an epithelium or from any tissue surface. **2.** Scaling or desquamation of the horny layer of epidermis, which varies in amount from minute quantities to shedding the entire integument. **3.** Loss of deciduous teeth following physiological loss of root structure. **4.** Extrusion of permanent teeth as a result of disease or loss of their antagonists.
e. of lens, sheetlike separation of the capsule of the lens; it may occur if the eyes are exposed to intense heat.

exfoliative (eks-fō'lē-ā-tiv) [Mod. L. *exfoliativus*]. Marked by exfoliation, desquamation, or profuse scaling.

exhalation (eks-hă-lā'shŭn) [L. *ex-halo*, pp. *-halatus*, to breathe out]. **1.** Expiration; breathing out. **2.** The giving forth of gas or vapor. **3.** Any exhaled or emitted gas or vapor.

exhale (eks'hāl). **1.** Expire (1); to breathe out. **2.** To emit a gas or vapor or odor.

exhaustion (ek-zos'chŭn) [L. *ex-haurio*, pp. *-haustus*, to draw out, empty]. **1.** Extreme fatigue; inability to respond to stimuli. **2.** Removal of contents; using up of a supply of anything. **3.** Extraction of the active constituents of a drug by treating with water, alcohol, or other solvent.
heat e., a form of reaction to heat, marked by prostration, weakness, and collapse, resulting from severe dehydration.

exhibitionism (ek-si-bish'ŭn-izm). A morbid compulsion to expose a part of the body, especially the genitals, to a person of the opposite sex with the intent of provoking sexual interest in the viewer.

exhibitionist (ek-si-bish'ŭn-ist). One who engages in exhibitionism.

exhilarant (eg-zil'ar-ant) [L. *ex-hilero*, pp. *-atus*, pres. p. *-ans*, to gladden]. Mentally stimulating.

existential (eg-zi-sten'shăl). Pertaining to a branch of philosophy, existentialism, concerned with the search for the meaning of one's one existence, that has been extended into e. *psychotherapy*.

exitus (eks'i-tŭs) [L. fr. *ex-eo*, pp. *-itus*, to go out]. An exit or outlet.

Exner, Siegmund, Austrian physiologist, 1846–1926. See Call-E. *bodies*, E.'s *plexus*.

exo- [G. *exō*, outside]. Prefix meaning exterior, external, or outward. See also ecto-.

exoantigen (ek-sō-an'ti-jen). Ectoantigen.

exocardia (ek-sō-kar'dē-ă). Ectocardia.

exocrine (ek'sō-krin) [exo- + G. *krinō*, to separate]. **1.** Eccrine (1); denoting glandular secretion delivered to an apical or lumenal surface. **2.** Denoting a gland that secretes outwardly through excretory ducts.

exocyclic (ek-sō-sī'klik, -sik'lik). Relating to atoms or groups attached to a cyclic structure but not themselves cyclic; *e.g.*, the $—CH_3$ group of toluene. *Cf.* endocyclic.

exocytosis (ek'sō-sī-to'sis) [exo- + G. *kytos*, cell, + *-osis*, condition]. **1.** The appearance of migrating inflammatory cells in the epidermis. **2.** Emiocytosis; emeiocytosis; the process whereby secretory granules or droplets are released from a cell; the membrane around the granule fuses with the cell membrane, which ruptures, and the secretion is discharged. *Cf.* endocytosis.

exodeviation (ek'sō-dē-vē-ā'shŭn). **1.** Exophoria. **2.** Exotropia.

exodontia (ek-sō-don'shē-ă) [exo- + G. *odous*, tooth]. The branch of dental practice concerned with the extraction of teeth.

exodontist (ek-sō-don'tist). One who specializes in the extraction of teeth.

exoenzyme (ek-sō-en'zīm). Extracellular *enzyme*.

exogamy (ek-sog'ă-mē) [exo- + G. *gamos*, marriage]. Sexual reproduction by means of conjugation of two gametes of different ancestry, as in certain protozoan species.

exogastrula (eks-ō-gas'trū-lă). An abnormal embryo in which the primitive gut has been everted.

exogenetic (ek'sō-je-net'ik). Exogenous.

exogenote (ek-sō-jē'nōt). In microbial genetics, the fragment of genetic material that has been transferred from a donor to the recipient and is homologous for a region of the recipient's original genome (endogenote), producing in the homologous region a condition analogous to diploidy.

exogenous (eks-oj'ĕ-nŭs) [exo- + G. *-gen,* production]. Exogenetic; ectogenous; enthetic (2); originating or produced outside of the organism.

exo-1,4-α-D-glucoidase [EC 3.2.1.3]. Glucoamylase; amyloglucosidase; γ-amylase; acid maltase; a hydrolase removing terminal 1,4-linked glucose residues from nonreducing ends of chains, with release of *β*-glucose.

exolever (ek'sō-lē'ver) [exo- + L. *levare,* to raise]. A modified elevator for the extraction of tooth roots.

exometer (eks-om'ĕ-ter) [exo- + G. *metron,* measure]. A device for recording the fluorescence of x-ray as compared to candle power.

exomphalos (eks-om'fă-lŭs) [G. *ex,* out, + *omphalos,* umbilicus]. Exumbilication. **1.** Protrusion of the umbilicus. **2.** Umbilical *hernia.* **3.** Omphalocele.

exon (ek'son). A portion of a DNA that codes for a section of the mature messenger RNA from that DNA, and is therefore expressed ("translated" into protein) at the ribosome.

exon shuffle. The variation in the patterns by which RNA may produce diverse sets of exons from a single gene.

exonuclease (ek-sō-nū'klē-ās). A nuclease that releases one nucleotide at a time, serially, beginning at one end of a polynucleotide (nucleic acid); several have been prepared from *Escherichia coli,* designated e. I, e. II, etc. *Cf.* endonuclease.

exopeptidase (ek-sō-pep'ti-dās). An enzyme that catalyzes the hydrolysis of the terminal amino acid of a peptide chain; *e.g.,* carboxypeptidase. *Cf.* endopeptidase.

Exophiala (ek-sō-fī'ă-lă) [*exo* + G. *phiale,* a broad flat vessel]. A genus of pathogenic fungi having dematiaceous conidiophores with one- or two-celled annelloconidia. They cause mycetoma or phaeohyphomycosis; in cases of mycetoma, black granules develop in subcutaneous abscesses; in cases of phaeohyphomycosis, sclerotic bodies are found in tissues.

E. jeansel'mei, a species found in cases of mycetoma or phaeohyphomycosis.

E. wernec'kii, Cladosporidium werneckii; a species that causes tinea nigra.

exophoria (ek'so-fō'rē-ă) [exo- + G. *phora,* a carrying]. Exodeviation (1); tendency of the eyes to deviate outward when fusion is suspended.

exophoric (ek-sō-fōr'ik). Relating to exophoria.

exophthalmic (ek-sof-thal'mik). Relating to exophthalmos; marked by prominence of the eyeball.

exophthalmometer (ek-sof-thal-mom'ĕ-ter) [exophthalmos + G. *metron,* measure]. Proptometer; statometer; an instrument to measure the distance between the anterior pole of the eye and a fixed reference point, often the zygomatic bone.

exophthalmos, exophthalmus (ek-sof-thal'mos) [G. *ex,* out, + *ophthalmos,* eye]. Protrusion of one or both eyeballs; can be congenital and familial, or due to pathology, such as a retro-orbital tumor (usually unilateral) or thyroid disease (usually bilateral).

endocrine e., e. associated with thyroid gland disorders.

malignant e., relentless, progressive protrusion of the eyeballs.

exophyte (ek'sō-fīt) [exo- + G. *phyton,* plant]. An exterior or external plant parasite.

exophytic (ek-sō-fit'ik). **1.** Pertaining to an exophyte. **2.** Denoting a neoplasm or lesion that grows outward from an epithelial surface.

exoplasm (ek'sō-plazm). Ectoplasm.

exoserosis (ek'sō-se-rō'sis). Serous exudation from the skin surface, as in eczema or abrasions.

exoskeleton (ek-sō-skel'ĕ-tŏn). **1.** Dermoskeleton; dermatoskeleton; all hard parts, such as hair, teeth, nails, feathers, dermal plates, scales, etc., developed from the ectoderm or mesoderm in vertebrates. **2.** Outer chitinous envelope of an insect, or the chitinous or calcareous covering of certain Crustacea and other invertebrates.

exosmosis (ek-sos-mō'sis). Obsolete term for osmosis from within outward, as from the interior of a blood vessel; the outward direction is not self-evident in all systems.

exospore (ek'sō-spōr) [exo- + G. *sporos,* seed]. An exogenous spore, not encased in a sporangium.

exosporium (ek-sō-spō'rē-um). The outer envelope of a spore.

exostectomy (ek-sos-tek'tō-mē) [exostosis + G. *ektomē,* excision]. Exostosectomy; removal of an exostosis.

exostosectomy (ek-sos-tō-sek'tō-mē). Exostectomy.

exostosis, pl. exostoses (eks-os-tō'sis, -sēz) [exo- + G. *osteon,* bone, + *-osis,* condition]. Hyperostosis; poroma (2); a cartilage-capped bony projection arising from any bone that develops from cartilage. See also osteochondroma.

e. bursa'ta, an e. arising from the joint surface of a bone and covered with cartilage and a synovial sac.

e. cartilagin'ea, an ossified chondroma arising from the epiphysis or joint surface of a bone.

diaphysial juxtaepiphysial e., hereditary multiple exostoses.

hereditary multiple exostoses, diaphysial aclasis; hereditary deforming chondrodystrophy; diaphysial juxtaepiphysial e.; osteochondromatosis; a disturbance of enchondral bone growth in which multiple osteochondromas of long bones appear during childhood, with shortening of the radius and fibula; autosomal dominant inheritance.

ivory e., a small, rounded, eburnated tumor arising from a bone, usually one of the cranial bones.

multiple e., hereditary multiple exostoses.

solitary osteocartilaginous e., osteochondroma.

exoteric (ek-sō-tār'ik) [G. *exōterikos,* outer]. Of external origin; arising outside the organism.

exothermic (ek-sō-ther'mik) [exo- + G. *thermē,* heat]. **1.** Denoting a chemical reaction during which heat is emitted. *Cf.* endothermic. **2.** Relating to the external warmth of the body.

exotoxic (ek-sō-tok'sik). **1.** Relating to an exotoxin. **2.** Relating to the introduction of an exogenous poison or toxin.

exotoxin (ek-sō-tok'sin). Extracellular toxin; ectotoxin; a specific, soluble, antigenic, usually heat labile, injurious substance elaborated by certain Gram-positive bacteria (rarely by Gram-negative species); it is formed within the cell, but is released into the environment where it is rapidly active in extremely small amounts; most e.'s are protein in nature (MW 70,000 to 900,000) and can have the toxic portion of the molecule destroyed by heat, prolonged storage, or chemicals; the nontoxic but antigenic form is a toxoid.

exotropia (ek-sō-trō'pē-ă) [exo- + G. *tropē,* turn]. Exodeviation; divergent or external strabismus; external squint; wall-eye (1); that type of strabismus in which the visual axes diverge; may be paralytic or concomitant, monocular or alternating, constant or intermittent.

A-e., divergent strabismus greater in downward than in upward gaze.

basic e., e. in which the strabismus is the same for near and far vision.

divergence excess e., e. in which the strabismus is notably greater for far vision than for near vision.

divergence insufficiency e., e. in which the strabismus is notably greater for near vision than for far vision.

V-e., divergent strabismus greater in upward than in downward gaze.

X-e., increasing divergence from primary position in both upward and downward gaze.

expansion (eks-pan'shŭn) [L. *ex-pando,* pp. *-pansus,* to spread out]. **1.** An increase in size as of chest or lungs. **2.** The spreading out of any structure, as a tendon. **3.** An expanse; a wide area.

hygroscopic e., **(1)** e. due to the absorption of moisture; **(2)** in dental casting, the addition of water to the surface of the casting investment during setting to increase the size of the mold.

perceptual e., development of an ability to recognize and interpret sensory stimuli through associations with past similar stimuli; perceptual e. by relaxation of defenses is a goal of psychotherapy.

setting e., the dimensional increase that occurs concurrently with the hardening of various materials, such as plaster of Paris.

wax e., in dentistry, a method of expanding wax patterns to compensate for the shrinkage of gold during the casting process.

expansiveness (ek-span'siv-nes). A state of optimism, loquacity, and reactivity.

expectorant (ek-spek'tō-rănt) [L. *ex,* out, + *pectus,* chest]. **1.** Promoting secretion from the mucous membrane of the air passages or facilitating its expulsion. **2.** An agent that increases bronchial secretion and facilitates its expulsion.

expectorate (ek-spek'tō-rāt). To spit; to eject saliva, mucus, or other fluid from the mouth.

expectoration (ek-spek-tō-rā'shŭn). **1.** Mucus and other fluids formed in the air passages and upper food passages (the mouth), and expelled by coughing. See also sputum (1). **2.** The act of spitting; the expelling from the mouth of saliva, mucus, and other material from the air or upper food passages.

prune-juice e., prune-juice *sputum.*

experience (ek-spēr'ē-ens). The feeling of emotions and sensations, as opposed to thinking; involvement in what is happening rather than abstract reflection on an event or interpersonal encounter.

corrective emotional e., reexposure under favorable circumstances to an emotional situation with which one could not cope in the past.

experiment (eks-per'i-ment). A test or trial.

control e., an e. used to check another, to verify the result, or to demonstrate what would have occurred had the factor under study been omitted. See also control; control *animal.*

delayed reaction e., a method of measuring memory: a stimulus is presented and removed before the organism is permitted to respond to it; the interval during which the stimulus is absent, providing the organism responds correctly, is an indication of the length of memory.

double blind e., an e. conducted with neither experimenter nor subjects knowing which e. is the control; prevents bias in recording results. See also double-masked e.

double-masked e., a double-blind study conducted so neither the subject nor the observer know the identity of the control or variable.

factorial e.'s, an experimental design in which two or more series of treatments are tried in all combinations.

hertzian e.'s, e.'s demonstrating that electromagnetic induction is propagated in waves, analogous to waves of light but not affecting the retina.

Mariotte's e., an e. in which one looks fixedly with one eye (the other being closed), at a black dot on a card, on which is also marked a black cross; as the card is moved to or from the eye, at a certain distance the cross becomes invisible but appears again as the card is moved further; this proves the absence of photoreceptors where the optic nerve enters the eye.

Nussbaum's e., exclusion of the glomeruli of the kidney from the circulation by ligation of the renal artery in animals, such as the frog, that have a renal portal system to maintain circulation to the tubules.

Scheiner's e., a demonstration of accommodation; through two minute holes in a card, separated from each other by less than the diameter of the pupil, one looks at a pin; at a short distance from the eye the pin appears double; as it is moved from the eye a point is found where it appears single, and beyond which it remains single for the eye, but for the myopic eye it soon again becomes double.

Stensen's e., compression of the abdominal aorta of an animal promptly causes paralysis of the posterior portions of the body since the blood supply to the lumbar cord is almost entirely shut off.

Toynbee's e., swallowing when the mouth and nose are closed causes rarefaction of air in the tympanum.

Weber's e., if the peripheral end of the divided vagus nerve is stimulated the heart is arrested in diastole.

expiration (eks-pi-rā'shŭn) [L. *expiro* or *ex-spiro,* pp. *-atus,* to breathe out]. Exhalation (1).

expiratory (ek-spī'ră-tō-rē). Relating to expiration.

expire (ek-spīr'). **1.** Exhale (1). **2.** To die.

explant (eks'plant). Living tissue transferred from an organism to an artificial medium for culture.

explantation (eks-plan-tā'shŭn). The act of transferring an explant.

exploration (eks-plōr-ā'shŭn) [L. *ex-ploro,* pp. *-ploratus,* to explore]. An active examination, usually involving endoscopy or a surgical procedure, to ascertain conditions present as an aid in diagnosis.

exploratory (eks-plōr'ă-tōr-ē). Relating to, or with a view to, exploration.

explorer (ek'splōr'er). A sharp pointed probe used to investigate natural or restored teeth surfaces in order to detect caries or other defects.

explosion (eks-plō'zhŭn) [L. *explosio,* fr. *explodo,* to drive away by clapping]. A sudden and violent increase in volume accompanied by noise and release of energy, as from a chemical change, nuclear reaction, or escape of gases or vapors under pressure.

expose (eks-pōz'). To perform or undergo exposure.

exposure (eks-pō'zhūr). **1.** A displaying, revealing, exhibiting, or making accessible. **2.** In dentistry, loss of hard tooth structure covering the dental pulp due to caries, dental instrumentation, or trauma.

express (eks-pres') [L. *ex-premo,* pp. *-pressus,* to press out]. To press or squeeze out.

expression (eks-presh'ŭn). **1.** Squeezing out; expelling by pressure. **2.** Facies (3); mobility of the features giving a particular emotional significance to the face. **3.** Any act determined by the nature of an individual.

expressivity (eks-pres-siv'i-tē). In clinical genetics, the form in which a penetrant gene is manifested.

expulsive (eks-pŭl'siv) [L. *ex-pello,* pp. *-pulsus,* to drive out]. Tending to expel.

exquisite (eks-kwiz'it) [L. *exqueiro,* pp. *exquisitus,* to search out]. Extremely intense, keen, sharp; said of pain or tenderness in a part.

exsanguinate (ek-sang'gwi-nāt) [L. *ex,* out, + *sanguis (-guin),* blood]. **1.** To remove or withdraw the circulating blood; to make bloodless. **2.** Exsanguine.

exsanguination (ek-sang'gwi-nā'shŭn). Removal of blood; making exsanguine.

exsanguine (ek-sang'gwin). Exsanguinate (2); deprived of blood.

exsect (ek-sekt') [L. *ex- seco,* pp. *-sectus,* to cut out]. Excise.

exsection (ek-sek'shŭn). Excision.

exsiccant (ek-sik'ant). Desiccant.

exsiccate (ek'si-kāt). Desiccate.

exsiccation (ek-si-kā'shŭn) [L. *ex sicco,* pp. *siccatus,* to dry up]. **1.** Desiccation. **2.** Dehydration (3); the removal of water of crystallization.

exsomatize (ek-sō'mă-tīz) [G. *ex,* out of, + *sōma,* body]. To remove from the body.

exsorption (ek-sōrp'shŭn) [G. *ex,* out, + *sorbēre,* to suck]. Movement of substances from the blood into the lumen of the gut.

exstrophy (ek'strō-fē) [G. *ex,* out, + *strophē,* a turning]. Ecstrophe; congenital eversion of a hollow organ.
e. of the bladder, ectopia vesicae; a congenital gap in the anterior wall of the bladder and the abdominal wall in front of it, the posterior wall of the bladder being exposed.
e. of the cloaca, ectopia cloacae; a developmental anomaly in which an area of intestinal mucosa is interposed between two separate areas of the urinary bladder.

extend (eks-tend') [L. *ex- tendo,* pp. *-tensus,* to stretch out]. To straighten a limb, to diminish or extinguish the angle formed by flexion; to place the distal segment of a limb in such a position that its axis is continuous with that of the proximal segment.

extension (eks-ten'shŭn) [L. *extensio,* to stretch out]. **1.** The act of bringing the distal portion of a joint in continuity (though only parallel) with the long axis of the proximal portion. **2.** A pulling or dragging force exerted on a limb in a distal direction. **3.** Obsolete term for traction.
Buck's e., Buck's traction; apparatus for applying longitudinal skin traction on the leg through contact between the skin and adhesive tape; friction between the tape and skin permits application of force, which is applied through a cord over a pulley, suspending a weight; elevation of the foot of the bed allows the body to act as a counterweight.
nail e., an obsolete method of e., by a weight on a nail or pin (Steinmann pin) in the distal fragment of a fracture.
ridge e., an intraoral surgical operation for deepening the labial, buccal, and/or lingual sulci; it is performed to increase the intraoral height of the alveolar ridge in order to assist denture retention.
skeletal e., skeletal *traction.*

extensor (eks-ten'ser, -sōr) [L. one who stretches, fr. *ex-tendo,* to stretch out] [NA]. A muscle the contraction of which tends to straighten a limb; the antagonist of a flexor. See under musculus.

exterior (eks-tē'rē-ōr) [L.]. Outside; external.

exteriorize (eks-tēr'ē-ōr-īz). **1.** To direct a patient's interests, thoughts, or feelings into a channel leading outside himself, to some definite aim or object. **2.** To expose an organ temporarily for observation, or permanently for purposes of physiologic experiment, *e.g.,* fixation of a segment of bowel with blood supply intact to the outer aspect of the abdominal wall.

extern (eks'tern) [F. *externe,* outside, a day scholar]. An advanced student or recent graduate who assists in the medical or surgical care of hospital patients; formerly, one who lived outside of the institution.

external (eks-ter'năl) [L. *externus*]. Externus; exterior; on the outside or farther from the center; often incorrectly used to mean lateral.

externus (eks-ter'nŭs). External.

exteroceptive (eks'ter-ō-sep'tiv) [L. *exterus,* outside, + *capere,* to take]. Relating to the exteroceptors; denoting the surface of the body containing the end organs adapted to receive impressions or stimuli from without.

exteroceptor (eks'ter-ō-sep'ter, -tōr) [L. *exterus,* external, + *receptor,* receiver]. One of the peripheral end organs of the afferent nerves in the skin or mucous membrane, which respond to stimulation by external agents.

exterofective (eks'ter-ō-fek'tiv) [L. *extero,* from outside, + *affectus,* affected]. Pertaining to the response of the nervous system to external stimuli.

extima (eks'ti-mă) [L. fem. of *extimus,* outermost]. Rarely used term for the adventitia of a blood vessel.

extinction (eks-tingk'shŭn) [L. *extinguo,* to quench]. **1.** In behavior modification or operant conditioning, a progressive decrease in the frequency of a response that is not positively reinforced; the withdrawal of reinforcers known to maintain an undesirable behavior. **2.** Absorbance.
specific e., specific absorption *coefficient.*
visual e., pseudo- *hemianopsia.*

extinguish (eks-ting'gwish) [L. *extinguo,* to quench]. **1.** To quench, as a flame; to abolish; to cause loss of identity; to destroy. **2.** In psychology, to progressively abolish a previously conditioned response.

extirpation (eks-tir-pā'shŭn) [L. *extirpo,* to root out, fr. *stirps,* a stalk, root]. Partial or complete removal of an organ or diseased tissue.

Exton, William G., U.S. physician, 1876–1943. See E. *reagent.*

extorsion (eks-tōr'shŭn) [L. *extorsio,* fr. *ex- torqueo,* to twist out]. **1.** Outward rotation of a limb or of an organ. **2.** Conjugate rotation of the upper poles of each cornea outward.

extortor (eks-tōr'ter, -tōr). An outward rotator.

extra-. L. preposition, used as a prefix, meaning without, outside of.

extra-articular (eks-tră-ar-tik'yū-lăr). Outside of a joint.

extrabuccal (eks-tră-bŭk'ăl). Outside or not part of the cheek.

extrabulbar (eks-tra-bul'bar). Outside of or unrelated to any bulb, such as the bulb of the urethra, or the medulla oblongata.

extracaliceal (eks'tră-kă-lis'ē-ăl). Outside of a calix.

extracapsular (eks'tră-kap'sū-lăr). Outside of the capsule of a joint.

extracarpal (eks-tră-kar'păl). **1.** Outside of, having no relation to, the carpus. **2.** On the outer side of the carpus.

extracellular (eks-tră-sel'yū-lăr). Outside of the cells.

extrachromosomal (eks'tră-krō-mō-sōm'ăl). Outside of, or separated from, a chromosome (usually bacterial).

extracorporeal (eks'tră-kōr-pō'rē-ăl). Outside of, or unrelated to, the body or any anatomical "corpus."

extracorpuscular (eks'tră-kōr-pŭs'kyū-lăr). Outside of the corpuscles, especially the blood corpuscles.

extracranial (eks-tră-krā'nē-ăl). Outside of the cranial cavity.

extract (eks'trakt). **1** (ek'strakt). A concentrated preparation of a drug obtained by removing the active constituents of the drug with suitable solvents, evaporating all or nearly all of the solvent, and adjusting the residual mass or powder to the prescribed standard. **2** (ek-strakt'). To remove part of a mixture with a solvent. **3.** To perform extraction.
alcoholic e., a solid e. obtained by extracting the alcohol-soluble principles of a drug, followed by the evaporation of the alcohol.
allergenic e., allergic e., e. (usually containing protein) from various sources, *e.g.,* food, bacteria, pollen, and the like, suspected of specific action in stimulating manifestations of allergy.
Buchner e., a cell-free e. of yeast, such as was prepared by Eduard and Hans Buchner and observed to catalyze alcoholic fermentation; this observation essentially eliminated "vitalism" as being responsible for biological chemical reactions and initiated the beginnings of modern biochemistry (enzymology).
equivalent e., valoid; a fluidextract of the same strength, weight for weight, as the original drug.
fluid e., see fluidextract.
hydroalcoholic e., a solid e. obtained by extracting the soluble principles of the drug with alcohol and water, followed by evaporation of the solution.

liquid e., fluidextract.
pollen e., liquid obtained by extracting the protein from the pollen of plants.

extractant (ek-strak'tant). An agent used to isolate or extract a substance from a mixture or combination of substances, from the tissues, or from a crude drug.

extraction (ek-strak'shŭn) [L. *ex-traho,* pp. *-tractus,* to draw out]. **1.** Luxation and removal of a tooth from its alveolus. **2.** Partitioning of material (solute) into a solvent. **3.** The active portion of a drug; the making of an extract. **4.** Surgical removal by pulling out. **5.** Removal of the fetus from the uterus or vagina at or near the end of pregnancy, either manually or with instruments. **6.** Removal by suction of the product of conception before a menstrual period has been missed.
Baker's pyridine e., hot pyridine treatment of tissues fixed in dilute Bouin's solution, used to extract phospholipids from tissues as a control in the histochemical staining of this material.
breech e., obstetrical e. of the baby by the buttocks.

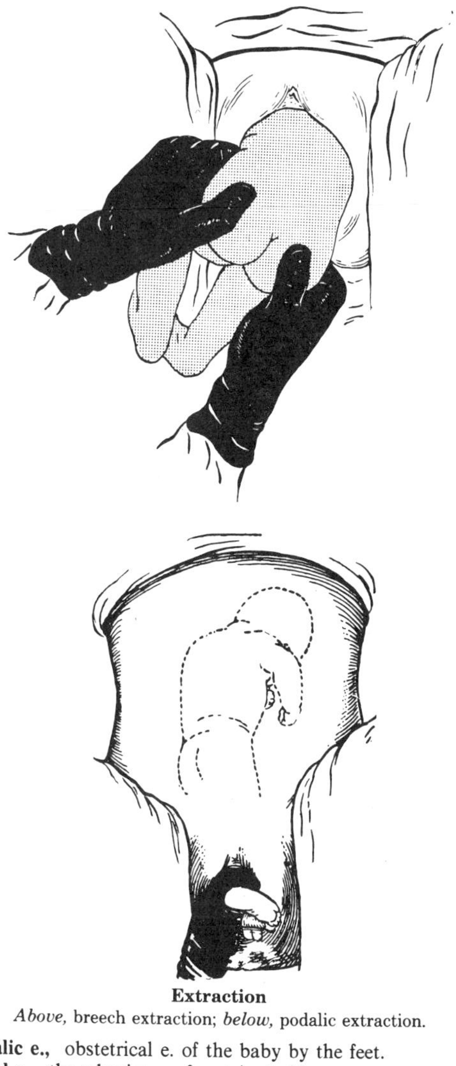

Extraction
Above, breech extraction; *below,* podalic extraction.

podalic e., obstetrical e. of the baby by the feet.
serial e., the selective e. of certain deciduous or permanent teeth, or both, during the early years of dental development, usually with the eventual e. of the first, or occasionally the second, premolars, to encourage autonomous adjustment of moderate to severe crowding of anterior teeth; it may or may not require subsequent orthodontic treatment.

extractives (ek-strak'tivs). Substances present in vegetable or animal tissue that can be separated by successive treatment with solvents and recovered by evaporation of the solution.

extractor (ek-strak'ter, tōr). Instrument for use in drawing or pulling out any natural part, as a tooth, or a foreign body.
vacuum e., device for producing traction upon the head of a fetus by means of a soft cup held by a vacuum.

extracystic (eks-tră-sis'tik). Outside of, or unrelated to, the gallbladder or urinary bladder or any cystic tumor.

extradural (eks-tră-dū'răl). **1.** On the outer side of the dura mater. **2.** Unconnected with the dura mater.

extraembryonic (eks'tră-em-brē-on'ik). Outside the embryonic body; *e.g.,* those membranes involved with the embryo's protection and nutrition which are discarded at birth without being incorporated in its body.

extraepiphysial (eks'tră-ep-i-fiz'ē-ăl). Not relating to, or connected with, an epiphysis.

extragenital (eks'tră-jen'i-tăl). Outside of, away from, or unrelated to, the genital organs.

extrahepatic (eks-tră-he-pat'ik). Outside of, or unrelated to, the liver.

extrajection (eks-tră-jek'shŭn) [L. *ex,* out of, + *jacio,* to cast]. Attributing or projecting one's own psychic process to another person.

extraligamentous (eks-tră-lig-ă-men'tŭs). Outside of, or unconnected with, a ligament.

extramalleolus (eks-tră-mal-ē'ō-lŭs). *Malleolus* lateralis.

extramedullary (eks-tră-med'yū-lăr-ē). Outside of, or unrelated to, any medulla, especially the medulla oblongata.

extramural (eks-tră-myū'răl) [extra- + L. *murus,* wall]. Outside, not in the substance, of the wall of a part.

extraneous (eks-tră'nē-ŭs) [L. *extraneus*]. Outside of the organism and not belonging to it.

extranuclear (eks-tră-nū'klē-er). Located outside of, or not involving, a cell nucleus.

extraocular (eks-tră-ok'yū-lăr). Adjacent to but outside the eyeball.

extraoral (eks-tră-ō'răl). Outside of the oral cavity; external to the oral cavity. In its usual use it includes anything external to the lips and cheeks also.

extraovular (eks'tră-ov'yū-lăr, -ōv'yū-lăr). Outside the egg; existence after hatching from the egg, as in reptiles and birds.

extrapapillary (eks-tră-pap'i-lā-rē). Unconnected with any papillary structure.

extraparenchymal (eks'tră-pă-reng'kī-măl). Unrelated to the parenchyma of an organ.

extraperineal (eks-tră-per-i-ne'al). Not connected with the perineum.

extraperiosteal (eks-tră-per-ē-os'tē-ăl). Not connected with, or unrelated to, the periosteum.

extraperitoneal (eks-tră-per-i-tō-nē'ăl). Outside of the peritoneal cavity.

extraphysiologic (eks'tră-fiz-ē-ō-loj'ik). Outside of the domain of physiology; more than physiologic, therefore pathologic.

extraplacental (eks-tră-pla-sen'tăl). Unrelated to the placenta.

extraprostatic (eks-tră-pros-tat'ik). Outside of, or independent of, the prostate.

extraprostatitis (eks-tră-pros-tă-tī'tis). Obsolete term for paraprostatitis.

extrapulmonary (eks-tră-pŭl′mō-năr-ē). Outside of, or having no relation to, the lungs.

extrapyramidal (eks-tră-pi-ram′i-dăl). Other than the pyramidal tract. See extrapyramidal motor *system*.

extrasensory (eks-tră-sen′sōr-ē). Outside or beyond the ordinary senses, not limited to the senses, as in e. *perception*.

extraserous (eks-tră-sē′rŭs). Outside of a serous cavity.

extrasomatic (eks-tră-sō-mat′ik). Outside of, or unrelated to, the body.

extrasystole (eks′tră-sis′tō-lē). Premature beat; premature systole; an ectopic, usually premature, contraction of the heart; such beats arise from the atrium, the A-V node, or the ventricle and interrupt the dominant, usually sinus, rhythm.

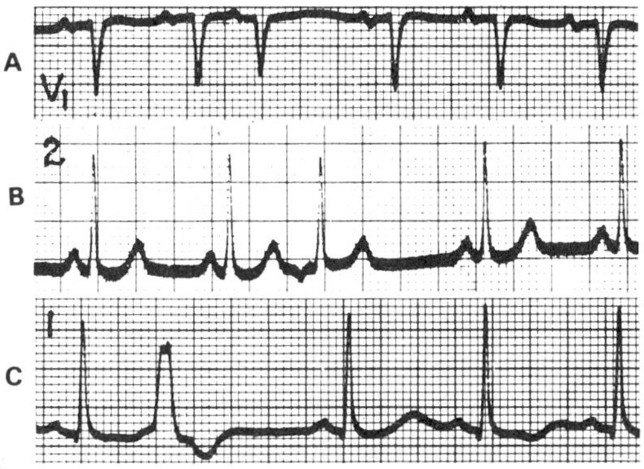

Extrasystoles
A, atrial; *B*, A-V nodal; *C*, ventricular

atrial e., auricular e.; a premature contraction of the heart arising from an ectopic atrial focus.
atrioventricular (A-V) e., junctional e.; an e. arising from the "junctional" tissues, either the A-V node or A-V bundle.
atrioventricular (A-V) nodal e., nodal e.; a premature beat arising from the A-V node and leading to a simultaneous or almost simultaneous contraction of atria and ventricles.
auricular e., atrial e.
infranodal e., ventricular e.
interpolated e., a ventricular e. which, instead of being followed by a compensatory pause, is sandwiched between two consecutive sinus cycles.
junctional e., atrioventricular e.
lower nodal e., a nodal e. supposed to arise from the lower part of the A-V node, recognized in the electrocardiogram by the retrograde P wave that follows the QRS complex.
midnodal e., a nodal e. supposed to arise from the midportion of the A-V node and recognized in the electrocardiogram by absence of the P wave that is lost within the normal QRS complex.
nodal e., atrioventricular nodal e.
return e., a form of reciprocal rhythm in which the impulse having arisen in the ventricle ascends toward the atria, but before reaching the atria is reflected back to the ventricles to produce a second ventricular contraction.

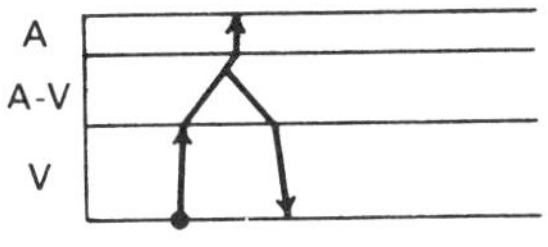

Return Extrasystole

supraventricular e., an e. arising from a center above the ventricle, *i.e.*, arising from the atrium or A-V node.
upper nodal e., a nodal e. supposed to arise from the upper part of the A-V node; recognized in the electrocardiogram by a retrograde P wave preceding the QRS complex by an abnormally short P-R interval.
ventricular e., infranodal e.; a premature contraction of the ventricle.

extratarsal (eks-tră-tar′săl). **1.** Outside of, having no relation to, the tarsus. **2.** On the outer side of the tarsus.

extratracheal (eks-tră-tră′kē-ăl). Outside of the trachea.

extratubal (eks-tră-tū′băl). Outside of any tube; specifically, not in the auditory (eustachian) or uterine (fallopian) tubes.

extrauterine (eks-tră-yū′ter-in). Outside of the uterus.

extravaginal (eks-tră-vaj′i-năl). Outside of the vagina.

extravasate (eks-trav′ă-sāt) [L. *extra*, out of, + *vas*, vessel]. **1.** To exude from or pass out of a vessel into the tissues, said of blood, lymph, or urine. **2.** Extravasation (2); suffusion (4); the substance thus exuded.

extravasation (eks-trav′ă-sā′shŭn). **1.** The act of extravasating. **2.** Extravasate (2).

extravascular (eks-tră-vas′kyū-lăr). Outside of the blood vessels or lymphatics or of any special blood vessel.

extraventricular (eks-tră-ven-trik′yū-lăr). Outside of any ventricle, especially of one of the ventricles of the heart.

extraversion (eks-tră-ver′zhŭn, -shŭn). Extroversion.

extravisual (ek-stră-vizh′ū-ăl). Outside the field of vision, or beyond the visible spectrum.

extremital (eks-trem′i-tăl). Relating to an extremity. See also distal.

extremitas (eks-trem′i-tas) [L. fr. *extremus*, last, outermost] [NA]. Extremity; one of the ends of an elongated or pointed structure. Incorrectly used to mean limb. See membrum.
e. acromia′lis clavic′ulae [NA], acromial extremity of clavicle; the flattened lateral extremity of the clavicle that articulates with the acromion and is anchored to the coracoid process by the conoid and trapezoid ligaments.
e. ante′rior [NA], anterior extremity; specifically, the anterior end of the spleen.
e. infe′rior [NA], inferior extremity; inferior pole; **e. i. ren′is,** the inferior end of the kidney; **e. i. tes′tis,** the inferior end of the testis.
e. poste′rior [NA], posterior extremity; specifically, the posterior end of the spleen.
e. sterna′lis clavic′ulae [NA], sternal extremity of clavicle; the enlarged medial end of the clavicle that articulates with the manubrium sterni.
e. supe′rior [NA], superior extremity; superior pole; **e. s. ran′is,** the superior end of the kidney; **e. s. tes′tis,** the superior end of the testis.
e. tuba′ria [NA], tubal extremity; lateral pole; the rounded lateral end of the ovary.
e. uteri′na [NA], uterine extremity; medial pole; the rounded medial end of the ovary.

extremity (eks-trem′i-tē). Extremitas.
acromial e. of clavicle, *extremitas* acromialis claviculae.
anterior e., *extremitas* anterior.
anterior e. of caudate nucleus, *caput* nuclei caudati.
inferior e., *extremitas* inferior.
lower e., *membrum* inferius.
posterior e., *extremitas* posterior.
sternal e. of clavicle, *extremitas* sternalis claviculae.
superior e., *extremitas* superior.
tubal e., *extremitas* tubaria.
upper e., *membrum* superius.
upper e. of fibula, *caput* fibulae.
uterine e., *extremitas* uterina.

extrinsic (eks-trin'sik) [L. *extrinsecus,* from without]. Originating outside of the part where found or upon which it acts; denoting especially a muscle.

extrogastrulation (eks'trō-gas-trū-lā'shŭn). Evagination during gastrulation, of the primitive gut material instead of the normal invagination, as the result of some environmental or experimental manipulation of the developing embryo or its environment.

extrospection (eks-trō-spek'shŭn) [ex- + L. *spectō,* pp. *-atus,* to look at, inspect]. Constant examination of the skin because of fear of parasites or dirt.

extroversion (eks'trō-ver'zhŭn, -shŭn) [incorrectly formed fr. L. *extra,* outside, + *verto,* pp. *versus,* to turn]. Extraversion. **1.** A turning outward. **2.** A trait involving social intercourse, as practiced by an extrovert. *Cf.* introversion.

extrovert (eks'trō-vert). A gregarious person whose chief interests lie outside himself, and who is socially self-confident and involved in the affairs of others. *Cf.* introvert.

extrude (eks-trūd'). To thrust, force, or press out.

extrusion (eks-trū'zhŭn). **1.** A thrusting or forcing out of a normal position. **2.** The overeruption or migration of a tooth beyond its normal occlusal position.

e. of a tooth, elongation of a tooth; movement of a tooth in an occlusal or incisal direction.

extubate (eks'tū-bāt). To accomplish extubation.

extubation (eks'tū-bā'shŭn) [L. *ex,* out, + *tuba,* tube]. Removal of a tube from an organ, structure, or orifice; specifically, removal of the tube after intubation.

exuberant (ek-zū'ber-ănt) [L. *exubero,* to abound, be abundant]. Denoting excessive proliferation or growth, as of a tissue or granulation.

exudate (eks'ū-dāt) [L. *ex,* out, + *sudare,* to sweat]. Exudation (2); any fluid that has exuded out of a tissue or its capillaries, more specifically because of injury or inflammation (*e.g.,* peritoneal pus in peritonitis, or the e. that forms a scab over a skin abrasion) in which case it is characteristically high in protein and white blood cells. *Cf.* transudate.

exudation (eks-ū-dā'shŭn). **1.** The act or process of exuding. **2.** Exudate.

exudative (eks-ū'dă-tiv). Relating to the process of exudation or to an exudate.

exude (ek-zūd') [L. *ex,* out, + *sudo,* to sweat]. In general, to ooze or pass gradually out of a body structure or tissue; more specifically, restricted to a fluid or semisolid that so passes and may become encrusted or infected, because of injury or inflammation.

exulcerans (eks-ŭl'ser-anz). Ulcerating.

exumbilication (eks'ŭm-bil-i-kā'shŭn) [L. *ex,* out, + *umbilicus,* navel]. Exomphalos.

exuviae (ex-ū'vē-ē) [L. clothing, etc., stripped from the body, fr. *exuo,* pp. *exutus,* to strip off]. Obsolete term for any cast off parts, as desquamated epidermis.

eye (ī) [A.S. *eāge*]. Oculus; the organ of vision. See also oculus.

amaurotic cat's e., a yellow reflex from the pupil in cases of retinoblastoma or pseudoglioma.

aphakic e., the e. from which the lens is absent.

artificial e., a curved disk of opaque glass or plastic, containing an imitation iris and pupil in the center, inserted beneath the eyelids and supported by the stump left after evisceration or enucleation; it may be ready-made (stock) or custom-made.

black e., ecchymosis of the lids and their surroundings.

blear e., lippitude; blepharitis accompanied by a viscid discharge that tends to cause the lid edges to cling together.

bovine cancer e., a malignant squamous cell carcinoma of cattle, especially the Hereford breed, that originates in the conjunctival

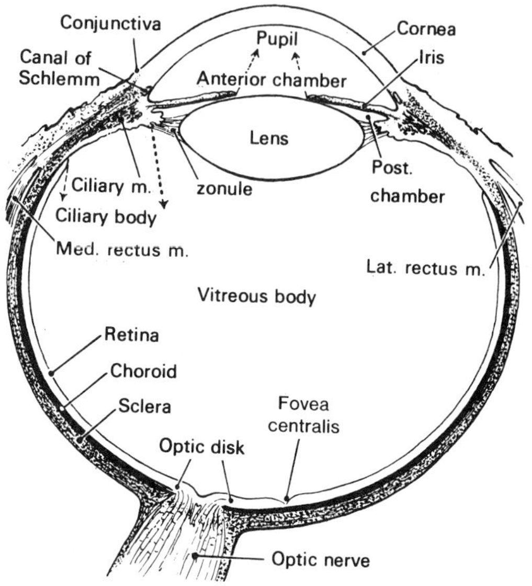

Human Eye (Right)

mucous membranes or the surrounding skin; it occurs principally in range cattle having unpigmented skin around the eye and living in regions of intense sunlight.

compound e., the eye of arthropods, most highly developed in insects and crustaceans; the e. consists of a group of functionally related visual elements (ommatidia) whose corneal surfaces collectively form a segment of a sphere.

crossed e.'s, strabismus.

cyclopian e., cyclopean e., see cyclopia.

dark-adapted e., scotopic e.; an e. that has been in darkness or semidarkness and has undergone regeneration of rhodopsin (visual purple), which renders it more sensitive to reduced illumination.

dominant e., master or master-dominant e.; the e. that is customarily used for monocular tasks.

epiphysial e., pineal e.

exciting e., the injured e. in sympathetic ophthalmia.

fixing e., the e., in cases of strabismus, that is directed toward the object looked at.

hare's e., lagophthalmos.

heavy e., in severe uniocular myopia, the affected e., which is lower.

hot e., *episcleritis* periodica fugax.

light-adapted e., photopic e.; an e. that has been exposed to light, with bleaching of rhodopsin (visual purple) and insensitivity to low illumination.

Listing's reduced e., a representation that simplifies calculations of retinal imagery: radius of anterior refracting surface, 5.1 mm; total length, 20 mm; distance of nodal point to retina, 15 mm.

master e., master-dominant e., dominant e.

parietal e., pineal e.

phakic e., an e. containing the natural lens.

photopic e., light-adapted e.

pineal e., epiphysial or parietal e.; an e. in or near the median line in certain crustacea and lower vertebrates; homologue of pineal gland in higher forms.

pink e., see pinkeye.

raccoon e.'s, descriptive term for the appearance produced by subconjunctival hemorrhages.

reduced e., a simplified design of the ocular optical system, represented as having a single refracting surface and a uniform index of

refraction; a model based on this concept is used in retinoscopy and ophthalmoscopy.
schematic e., the representation of the optical system of an ideal normal eye in which are listed the curvatures and indices of refraction of the refracting elements and their intervening distances.
scotopic e., dark-adapted e.
spectacle e.'s, a condition in rats caused by pantothenic acid deficiency, and possibly lack of inositol as well, in which a hairless ring of inflamed skin surrounds the e.'s.
squinting e., the e., in cases of strabismus, that is not directed toward the object looked at.
sympathizing e., the uninjured e. in sympathetic ophthalmia that is later implicated in the disease process.
watery e., **(1)** epiphora; **(2)** excessive lacrimation.
web e., pterygium (1).

eyeball (ī'bawl). *Bulbus* oculi.

eye bank. A place where corneas of eyes removed after death are preserved for subsequent keratoplasty.

eye'brow. Supercilium (1).

eye'glasses. Spectacles.

eyegrounds (ī'growndz). The fundus of the eye as seen with the ophthalmoscope.

eye'lash. Cilium (1).
ectopic e., the condition in which the e.'s grow from the eyelid at a site other than the lid margin.
piebald e., canities circumscripta; an isolated bundle of white e.'s among normally pigmented e.'s.

eye'lid. Palpebra.
lower e., *palpebra* inferior.
third e., *plica* semilunaris conjunctivae (2).
upper e., *palpebra* superior.

eyepiece (ī'pēs). The compound lens at the end of the microscope tube nearest the eye; it magnifies the image made by the objective.

eye'spot. **1.** A colored spot or plastid (chromatophore) in a unicellular organism. **2.** Ocellus (1).

eye'stone. A small smooth shell or other object that is inserted beneath the eyelid for the purpose of removing a foreign body.

eye'strain. Asthenopia.

eye'wash. A soothing solution used for bathing the eye.

F

F **1.** Symbol for fractional *concentration,* followed by subscripts indicating location and chemical species; free *energy;* Fahrenheit; faraday; visual *field;* fluorine; force; filial *generation,* followed by subscript numerals indicating first, second, third, etc. **2.** Abbreviation for focus (1).

f Symbol for femto-; respiratory *frequency.*

F.A.A.N. Abbreviation for Fellow of the American Academy of Nursing.

Fab See Fab *fragment.*

fabella (fa-bel'lă) [Mod. L. dim of *faba,* bean]. A sesamoid bone in the tendon of the lateral head of the gastrocnemius muscle.

Faber, Knud H., Danish physician, 1862–1956. See F.'s *anemia, syndrome.*

fabism (fā'bizm) [L. *faba,* bean]. Favism.

fabrication (fab-ri-kā'shŭn). Fabulation; telling false tales as true; *e.g.,* the malingering of symptoms or illness.

Fabricius (Fabrizzi), Giralamo (Hieronymus ab Aquapendente), Italian anatomist and embryologist, 1533–1619. See *bursa* fabricii, F.'s *ship.*

Fabry, Johannes, German dermatologist, 1860–1930. See F.'s *disease.*

fabulation (fab-yū-lā'shŭn) [L. *fabulatio,* fr. *fabulo,* pp. *-atus,* to speak]. Fabrication.

F.A.C.C.P. Abbreviation for Fellow of the American College of Chest Physicians.

F.A.C.D. Abbreviation for Fellow of the American College of Dentists.

face (fās). Facies (1); the front portion of the head; the visage including eyes, nose, mouth, forehead, cheeks, and chin; excludes ears.
bird f., brachygnathia.
cow f., *facies* bovina.
dish f., *facies* scaphoidea.
frog f., the appearance caused by broadening of the nose which occurs in certain cases of nasal polyps.
hippocratic f., hippocratic *facies.*
masklike f., Parkinson's *facies.*
moon f., the round, usually red face, with large jowls, seen in Cushing's disease or in hyperadrenocorticalism.

face-bow. Hinge-bow; a caliper-like device used to record the relationship of the jaws to the temporomandibular joints; the record may then be used to orient the maxillary cast to the opening and closing axis of the articulator.
adjustable axis f.-b., kinematic f.-b.; a f.-b. whose caliper ends can be adjusted to permit location of the axis of rotation of the mandible.
kinematic f.-b., adjustable axis f.-b.

face-lift. See rhytidectomy.

facet, facette (fas'et, fă-set') [Fr. *facette*]. **1.** A small smooth area on a bone or other firm structure. **2.** A worn spot on a tooth, produced by chewing or grinding.
clavicular f., *incisura* clavicularis.
corneal f., a corneal depression following loss of stroma.
Lenoir's f., the medial articular surface of the patella.
locked f.'s, *dislocation* of articular processes.

facetectomy (fas-ĕ-tek'tō-mē) [facet + G. *ektomē,* excision]. Excision of a facet.

facial (fā'shăl). Facialis; relating to the face.

facialis (fā-shē-ā'lis) [L.] [NA]. Facial.

-facient [L. *facio,* to make]. Suffix meaning one who or that which brings about.

FACIES

facies, pl. **facies** (fā'shē-ēz, fash'ē-ēz) [L.]. **1** [NA]. Face. **2** [NA]. Surface. **3.** Expression (2).
acromial articular f. of clavicle, *facies* articularis acromialis claviculae.
adenoid f., the open-mouthed and often stupid appearance in children with adenoid hypertrophy, associated with a pinched nose and narrow nares.
f. antebrachia'lis ante'rior [NA], alternate term for *regio* antebrachialis anterior.
f. antebrachia'lis poste'rior [NA], alternate term for *regio* antebrachialis posterior.
f. ante'rior [NA], anterior surface; the surface of a structure or part of the body that faces forward. The NA recognizes an anterior surface without qualification on the following structures: pancreas; patella; prostate; radius; suprarenal gland; ulna.
f. ante'rior antebra'chii [NA], the anterior surface of the forearm.
f. ante'rior bra'chii [NA], the anterior surface of the arm.
f. ante'rior cor'neae [NA], the anterior surface of the cornea.
f. ante'rior cor'poris maxil'lae [NA], anterior surface of the maxilla; the surface of the maxilla below the orbit and lateral to the nasal aperture.
f. ante'rior cru'ris [NA], anterior surface of the leg; the anterior surface of the inferior limb between the knee and the ankle.
f. ante'rior glan'dulae suprarena'lis [NA], the anterior surface of the suprarenal gland.
f. ante'rior ir'idis [NA], the anterior surface of the iris of the eye.
f. ante'rior latera'lis hu'meri [NA], anterolateral surface of humerus; the surface of the humerus lateral to the intertubercular groove.
f. ante'rior len'tis [NA], the anterior surface of the lens of the eye.
f. ante'rior media'lis hu'meri [NA], anteromedial surface of humerus; the surface of the humerus between the anterior and medial margins of the bone.
f. ante'rior mem'bri inferio'ris [NA], the anterior surface of the inferior limb.
f. ante'rior palpebra'rum [NA], anterior surface of eyelids.
f. ante'rior pancrea'tis [NA], the anterior surface of the pancreas.
f. ante'rior par'tis petro'sae [NA], anterior surface of petrous part; the surface of the petrous part of the temporal bone contrib-

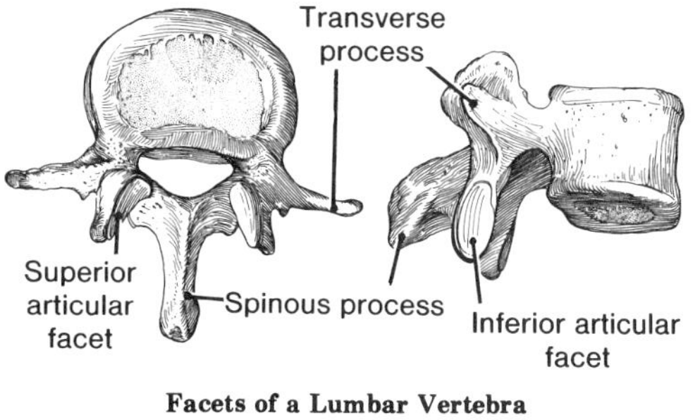

Facets of a Lumbar Vertebra

uting to the floor of the middle cranial fossa.
f. ante'rior patel'lae [NA], the anterior surface of the patella.
f. ante'rior pros'tatae [NA], the anterior surface of the prostate.
f. ante'rior ra'dii [NA], the anterior surface of the radius.
f. ante'rior re'nis [NA], the anterior surface of the kidney.
f. ante'rior ul'nae [NA], the anterior surface of the ulna.
f. antoni'na, a facial expression due to alteration in the eyelids and anterior segment of the eye; found in leprosy.
aortic f., the pale sallow complexion of one suffering from incompetence of the aortic valve.
f. articular'is [NA], articular surface; any articular surface. The NA recognizes without qualification an articular surface on the following bones or cartilages: the inferior surface of the arytenoid cartilage; the posterior surface of the patella; and in the mandibular surface of the temporal bone.
f. articula'ris acromia'lis clavic'ulae [NA], acromial articular surface of clavicle; a small oval facet on the lateral end of the clavicle for articulation with the acromion.
f. articula'ris acro'mii [NA], articular surface of acromion; a small oval facet on the medial border of the acromion for articulation with the lateral end of the clavicle.
f. articula'ris ante'rior den'tis [NA], anterior articular surface of dens; the curved articular facet on the anterior aspect of the dens of the axis that articulates with the anterior arch of the atlas.
f. articula'ris arytenoi'dea cricoi'deae [NA], arytenoidal articular surface of cricoid; one of two oval facets on the superior margin of the cricoid lamina for articulation with the arytenoid cartilages.
f. articula'ris calca'nea ta'li [NA], calcaneal articular surface of talus; one of three articular surfaces on the talus for union with the calcaneus; **f. a. c. poste'rior,** posterior calcaneal articular surface; an oval facet on the underside of the talus which participates in the subtalar joint; **f. a. c. me'dia,** middle calcaneal articular surface and **f. a. c. ante'rior,** anterior calcaneal articular surface, both of which underlie the head of the talus and contribute to the talocalcaneonavicular joint.
f. articula'ris cap'itis cos'tae [NA], articular surface of head of rib; an articular surface on the head of a rib that articulates with the body of a vertebra.
f. articula'ris cap'itis fib'ulae [NA], articular surface of head of fibula; the flat circular surface on the head of the fibula for articulation with the corresponding facet on the lateral condyle of the tibia.
f. articula'ris car'pi ra'dii [NA], carpal articular surface of radius; the biconcave distal surface of the radius for articulation with the scaphoid bone laterally and the lunate medially.
f. articula'ris cartila'ginis arytenoi'deae [NA], articular surface of arytenoid cartilage; the oval surface on the undersurface of the muscular process of the arytenoid for articulation with the cricoid cartilage.
f. articula'ris cuboi'dea calca'nei [NA], cuboidal articular surface of calcaneus; the saddle-shaped surface on the anterior end of the calcaneus for articulation with the cuboid bone.
f. articula'ris fibula'ris tib'iae [NA], fibular articular surface of tibia; the flat circular articular facet on the inferior and lateral aspect of the lateral condyle of the tibia for articulation with the head of the fibula.
f. articula'ris infe'rior atlan'tis [NA], fovea articularis inferior atlantis; inferior articular pit of atlas; one of two concave surfaces on the lateral masses of the atlas that articulate with corresponding surfaces on the axis.
f. articula'ris infe'rior tib'iae [NA], inferior articular surface of tibia; the quadrilateral surface on the distal end of the tibia for articulation with the talus; it is concave anteroposteriorly and broader anteriorly.
f. articula'ris malle'oli fib'ulae [NA], malleolar articular surface of fibula; the surface on the medial aspect of the lateral malleolus that articulates with the talus.
f. articula'ris malle'oli tib'iae [NA], malleolar articular surface of tibia; the articular facet on the lateral surface of the medial malleolus for articulation with the side of the talus; it is continuous with the inferior articular surface of the tibia.
f. articula'ris navicula'ris ta'li [NA], navicular articular surface of talus; the large convex surface on the head of the talus for articulation with the navicular bone.
f. articula'ris os'sis tempora'lis [NA], articular surface of temporal bone; the smooth portion of the mandibular fossa of the temporal bone that articulates with the disk of the temporomandibular joint.
f. articula'ris patel'lae [NA], articular surface of patella; the posterior surface of the patella, covered with hyaline cartilage and subdivided by a vertical ridge into a larger lateral and a smaller medial surface for articulation with the corresponding condyles of the femur.
f. articula'ris poste'rior den'tis [NA], posterior articular surface of dens; the facet on the posterior surface of the dens of the axis that articulates with the transverse ligament of the atlas.
f. articula'ris sterna'lis clavic'ulae [NA], sternal articular surface of clavicle; the oval surface on the sternal end of the clavicle that articulates with the fibrocartilaginous disk of the sternoclavicular joint.
f. articula'ris sup'erior atlan'tis [NA], fovea articularis superior atlantis; superior articular pit of atlas; one of two concave articular surfaces on the superior aspect of the lateral masses of the atlas that articulate with the occipital condyles.
f. articula'ris supe'rior tib'iae [NA], superior articular surface of the tibia; the articular surface on the proximal end of the tibia that is divided into medial and lateral portions for articulation with the condyles of the femur.
f. articula'ris tala'ris calca'nei [NA], talar articular surface of calcaneus; one of three facets of the calcaneus that articulate with the overlying talus; the **f. a. t. ante'rior** and **f. a. t. me'dia** contribute to the talocalcaneonavicular joint and are separated by the tarsal sinus from the **f. a. t. poste'rior** which enters into the subtalar joint.
f. articula'ris thyroi'dea cricoi'deae [NA], thyroidal articular surface of cricoid; one of two small circular facets on the cricoid cartilage near the inferior margin of the junction of the arch and lamina for articulation with the inferior horns of the thyroid cartilage.
f. articula'ris tuber'culi cos'tae [NA], articular surface of tubercle of rib; an oval facet on the inferomedial part of the tubercle of a rib for articulation with a pit on the transverse process of a vertebra.
f. auricula'ris os'sis il'ii [NA], auricular surface of ilium; the irregular, L-shaped articular surface on the medial aspect of the ilium that articulates with the sacrum.
f. auricula'ris os'sis sac'ri [NA], auricular surface of sacrum; the rough articular surface on the lateral aspect of the sacrum that articulates with the ilium on each side.
f. bovi'na, cow face; the cowlike face of ocular hypertelorism.
f. brachia'lis ante'rior [NA], alternate term for *regio* brachialis anterior.
f. brachia'lis poste'rior [NA], alternate term for *regio* brachialis posterior.
f. bucca'lis, f. vestibularis dentis.
f. cerebra'lis, cerebral surface; the internal surface of certain cranial bones; they are the greater wing of the sphenoid and the squamous part of the temporal bone.
cherubic f., the characteristic child-like f. seen in cherubism; also seen in glycogenosis, particularly type 2.
f. co'lica sple'nis [NA], colic surface of the spleen; the surface of the spleen in contact with the colon.
f. contac'tus den'tis [NA], contact surface of tooth; the surface of a tooth that faces the adjacent tooth in the dental arch; opposite to the f. distalis dentis and f. mesialis dentis.
Corvisart's f., the characteristic f. seen in cardiac insufficiency or aortic regurgitation; a swollen, purplish, cyanotic face with shiny eyes and puffy eyelids.

f. costa'lis [NA], costal surface; the surface of certain structures that face the ribs; they are the lungs and the scapula.
f. costa'lis pulmo'nis [NA], costal surface of lung; the surface of each lung that lies in contact with the costal pleura.
f. costa'lis scap'ulae [NA], costal surface of scapula; the concave aspect of the body of the scapula that faces the thorax and that principally lodges the subscapularis muscle.
f. crura'lis ante'rior [NA], alternate term for *regio* cruralis anterior.
f. crura'lis poste'rior [NA], alternate term for *regio* cruralis posterior.
f. cubita'lis ante'rior [NA], alternate term for *regio* cubitalis anterior.
f. cubita'lis poste'rior [NA], alternate term for *regio* cubitalis posterior.
f. diaphragmat'ica [NA], diaphragmatic surface; the surface of an organ in contact with the diaphragm, as of the heart, liver, lungs, and spleen.
f. digita'lis dorsa'lis [NA], dorsal surface of digit; the dorsal surface of a finger or toe.
f. digita'lis ventra'lis [NA], ventral surface of digit; the palmar surface of the hand.
f. dista'lis den'tis [NA], distal surface of tooth; the contact surface of a tooth that is directed away from the median plane of the dental arch; opposite to the f. mesialis dentis.
f. doloro'sa, facial expression of a sick or unhappy person.
f. dorsa'lis [NA], dorsal surface; the dorsal surface of a structure such as the sacrum and the scapula.
f. dorsa'lis os'sis sac'ri [NA], dorsal surface of sacrum; the posterosuperior aspect of the sacrum marked by a median and two lateral sacral crests between which four dorsal sacral foramina are located on each side.
f. dorsa'lis scap'ulae [NA], dorsal surface of scapula; the outer aspect of the body of the scapula, subdivided by the prominent spine of the scapula into a smaller supraspinous fossa and a larger infraspinous fossa.
elfin f., f. characterized by a short, upturned nose, wide mouth, widely spaced eyes, and full cheeks; it may be associated with hypercalcemia, supravalvar aortic stenosis, and mental retardation.
f. exter'na [NA], external surface; the outer convex surface of either the frontal or the parietal bone.
f. exter'na os'sis fronta'lis [NA], external surface of frontal bone; the convex outer surface of the frontal bone.
f. exter'na os'sis parieta'lis [NA], external surface of parietal bone; the convex outer surface of the parietal bone.
f. facia'lis den'tis [NA], f. vestibularis dentis.
f. femora'lis ante'rior [NA], alternate term for *regio* femoralis anterior.
f. femora'lis poste'rior [NA], alternate term for *regio* femoralis posterior.
f. gas'trica sple'nis [NA], gastric surface of the spleen; the surface of the spleen in contact with the stomach.
f. glu'tea os'sis il'ii [NA], gluteal surface of ilium; the external surface of the ala of the ilium marked by the anterior, posterior and inferior gluteal lines that separate the origins of the gluteal muscles.
hippocratic f., f. hippocra'tica, hippocratic face; a pinched expression of the face, with sunken eyes, hollow cheeks and temples, relaxed lips, and leaden complexion; observed in one dying after severe and prolonged illness.
hound-dog f., the facial appearance in cutis laxa, with loose facial skin hanging in folds.
hurloid f., the coarse gargoyle-like facial appearance characteristically seen in the mucopolysaccharidoses and mucolipidoses.
Hutchinson's f., the peculiar facial expression produced by the drooping eyelids and motionless eyes in ophthalmoplegia.
f. infe'rior cer'ebri [NA], basis cerebri; base of brain; the inferior surface of the brain visible when seen from below.
f. infe'rior hemisphe'rii cerebel'li [NA], inferior surface of the cerebellar hemisphere; it rests in the posterior cranial fossa and overlies the medulla; it includes the semilunaris inferior, lobulus biventer, tonsilla cerebelli, and flocculus.
f. infe'rior lin'guae [NA], inferior surface of tongue; the surface of the tongue that faces the floor of the oral cavity, its mucosa being thin, smooth and devoid of papillae.
f. infe'rior pancrea'tis [NA], inferior surface of pancreas; the surface of the body of the pancreas that faces downward.
f. infe'rior par'tis petro'sae [NA], inferior surface of petrous part of the temporal bone; the portion of the petrous part of the temporal bone that contributes to the external base of the skull.
f. inferolatera'lis pros'tatae [NA], inferolateral surface of prostate; the surface of the prostate facing the body of the pubis and the pelvic diaphragm.
f. infratempora'lis maxil'lae [NA], infratemporal surface of maxilla; the posterolateral surface of the body of the maxilla that faces the infratemporal fossa.
f. interloba'res pulmo'nis [NA], interlobar surfaces of lung; the pulmonary surfaces in the interlobar fissures of the lung.
f. inter'na [NA], internal surface; the internal concave surface of either the frontal or the parietal bone.
f. inter'na os'sis fronta'lis [NA], internal surface of frontal bone; the surface of the frontal bone that contributes to the boundary of the cranial cavity.
f. inter'na os'sis parieta'lis [NA], internal surface of parietal bone; the concave surface of the parietal bone forming part of the wall of the cranial cavity.
f. intestina'lis u'teri [NA], intestinal surface of uterus; the posterosuperior surface of the uterus with which loops of intestine come in contact.
f. labia'lis, f. vestibularis dentis.
f. latera'lis [NA], lateral surface; the surface of a part of the body that faces away from the midline. The NA recognizes a lateral surface on the following structures: fibula; ovary; radius; testis; tibia; zygomatic bone.
f. latera'lis bra'chii [NA], the lateral surface of the arm.
f. latera'lis cru'ris [NA], lateral surface of leg; f. fibularis cruris; the lateral surface of the part of the inferior limb between the knee and the ankle.
f. latera'lis dig'iti ma'nus [NA], the lateral surface of a finger.
f. latera'lis dig'iti pe'dis [NA], the lateral surface of a toe.
f. latera'lis fib'ulae [NA], the lateral surface of the fibula.
f. latera'lis mem'bri inferior'is [NA], the lateral surface of the inferior limb.
f. latera'lis os'sis zygomat'ici [NA], the lateral surface of the zygomatic bone.
f. latera'lis ova'rii [NA], lateral surface of ovary; the surface of the ovary facing the pelvic wall.
f. latera'lis tes'tis [NA], the lateral surface of the testis.
f. latera'lis tib'iae [NA], the lateral surface of the tibia.
leonine f., leontiasis.
f. lingua'lis den'tis [NA], lingual surface of tooth, the surface of a tooth that faces the tongue; opposite to the f. vestibulum dentis.
f. luna'ta acetab'uli [NA], lunate surface of acetabulum; the curved articular surface that surrounds the acetabular fossa and articulates with the head of the femur.
f. malleola'ris latera'lis ta'li [NA], lateral malleolar surface of talus; that surface of the trochlea of the talus that articulates with the lateral malleolus of the fibula.
f. malleola'ris media'lis ta'li [NA], medial malleolar surface of talus; the surface of the trochlea of the talus that articulates with the medial malleolus of the tibia.
f. masticato'ria, f. occlusalis dentis.
f. maxilla'ris os'sis palati'ni [NA], **(1)** maxillary surface of the palatine bone; the lateral surface of the perpendicular plate of the

palatine bone; **(2)** the part of the anterior surface of the greater wing of the sphenoid bone that is perforated by the foramen rotundum and forms the posterior boundary of the pterygopalatine fossa.

f. media'lis [NA], medial surface; the surface of a part of the body that faces toward the midline. The NA recognizes a medial surface on the following structures: arytenoid cartilage; fibula; lung; ovary; testis; tibia; ulna.

f. media'lis cartilag'inis arytenoi'deae [NA], medial surface of arytenoid cartilage.

f. media'lis cer'ebri [NA], medial surface of the cerebral hemisphere; it faces, above as well as anterior and posterior to the corpus callosum, the falx cerebri; below it are the mesencephalon and the dura-covered medial wall of the middle cranial fossa.

f. media'lis dig'iti pe'dis [NA], the medial surface of a toe.

f. media'lis fib'ulae [NA], medial surface of fibula.

f. media'lis ova'rii [NA], medial surface of ovary, the surface of the ovary that faces the pelvic cavity.

f. media'lis pulmo'nis [NA], medial surface of lung; it consists of a vertebral part and a mediastinal part.

f. media'lis tes'tis [NA], medial surface of testis.

f. media'lis tib'iae [NA], medial surface of tibia.

f. media'lis ul'nae [NA], medial surface of ulna.

f. mesia'lis den'tis [NA], mesial surface of tooth; the contact surface of a tooth that is directed toward the median plane of the dental arch; opposite to the f. distalis dentis.

mitral f., the pink, slightly cyanosed cheeks of patients with mitral valve disease.

myasthenic f., the facial expression in myasthenia gravis, caused by drooping of the eyelids and corners of the mouth, and weakness of the muscles of the face.

myopathic f., a peculiar facial appearance characterized by protrusion of the lips, drooping of the lids, and general relaxation of the muscles of the face; caused by muscular weakness.

f. nasa'lis maxil'lae [NA], nasal surface of maxilla; the surface of the maxilla that forms part of the lateral nasal wall with a large defect (hiatus maxillaris) posteriorly and the lacrimal sulcus in its midportion.

f. nasa'lis os'sis palanti'ni [NA], nasal surface of palatine bone; **(1)** the nasal surface of the perpendicular lamina of the palatine bone that forms part of the lateral wall of the nasal cavity; **(2)** the nasal surface of the horizontal lamina of the palatine bone that forms part of the floor of the nasal cavity.

f. occlusa'lis den'tis [NA], occlusal surface (1); f. masticatoria; masticating, masticatory, or grinding surface; the surface of a tooth that occludes with or contacts an opposing surface of a tooth in the opposing jaw.

f. orbita'lis [NA], orbital surface; the surface of a bone which contributes to the walls of the orbit. The NA recognizes an orbital surface on the following bones: greater wing of the sphenoid bone; the maxilla; the frontal bone; the zygomatic bone.

f. palati'na [NA], palatine surface; the inferior surface of the horizontal plate of the palatine bone.

Parkinson's f., masklike face; the expressionless or masklike f. characteristic of parkinsonism (1).

f. patella'ris fem'oris [NA], patellar surface of femur; trochlea femoris; the depression between the femoral condyles anteriorly that accommodates the patella.

f. pelvi'na os'sis sa'cri [NA], pelvic surface of sacrum; the surface of the sacrum that faces downward and forward forming part of the posterior wall of the pelvic cavity.

f. poplit'ea fem'oris [NA], popliteal plane or surface of the femur; planum popliteum; the posterior surface of the lower end of the femur between the diverging lips of the linea aspera.

f. poste'rior [NA], posterior surface; the surface of a part of the body that faces toward the posterior part of the body. The NA recognizes a posterior surface without qualification on the following structures: arytenoid cartilage; cornea; fibula; humerus; iris; kidney; pancreas; prostate; radius; suprarenal gland; ulna.

f. poste'rior cartilag'inis arytenoi'deae [NA], the posterior surface of the arytenoid cartilage.

f. poste'rior cor'neae [NA], the posterior surface of the cornea.

f. poste'rior cru'ris [NA], the posterior surface of the leg.

f. poste'rior fib'ulae [NA], the posterior surface of the fibula.

f. poste'rior glan'dulae suprarena'lis [NA], the posterior surface of the suprarenal gland.

f. poste'rior hu'meri [NA], the posterior surface of the humerus.

f. poste'rior ir'idis [NA], the posterior surface of the iris.

f. poste'rior len'tis [NA], the posterior surface of the lens of the eye.

f. poste'rior mem'bri inferio'ris [NA], the posterior surface of the inferior limb.

f. poste'rior palpebra'rum [NA], posterior surface of eyelids; the internal surface of the eyelids, covered with conjunctiva.

f. poste'rior pancrea'tis [NA], the posterior surface of the pancreas.

f. poste'rior par'tis petro'sae [NA], posterior surface of petrous part; the surface of the petrous part of the temporal bone that contributes to the posterior cranial fossa.

f. poste'rior pros'tatae [NA], the posterior surface of the prostate.

f. poste'rior ra'dii [NA], the posterior surface of the radius.

f. poste'rior re'nis [NA], the posterior surface of the kidney.

f. poste'rior tib'iae [NA], the posterior surface of the tibia.

f. poste'rior ul'nae [NA], the posterior surface of the ulna.

Potter's f., Potter's disease; characteristic f. seen in bilateral renal agenesis and other severe renal malformations, exhibiting ocular hypertelorism, low-set ears, receding chin, and flattening of the nose. See also Potter's *syndrome.*

f. pulmona'lis cor'dis [NA], pulmonary surface of heart; the lateral surface of the heart, directed toward the lungs; on the left it is principally the left ventricle; on the right it is the right atrium and the upper part of the right ventricle.

f. rena'lis [NA], renal surface; **f. r. glan'dulae suprarena'lis** [NA], the surface of the suprarenal gland in contact with the kidney; **f. r. sple'nis** [NA], the surface of the spleen in contact with the left kidney.

f. sacropelvi'na os'sis il'ii [NA], sacropelvic surface of ilium; the medial surface of the ilium behind and below the iliac fossa; it includes the iliac tuberosity, the auricular surface and the smooth pelvic surface below and in front of the auricular surface.

f. scaphoi'dea, dish face; a facial malformation characterized by protuberant forehead, depressed nose and maxilla, and prominence of the chin.

f. sternocosta'lis cor'dis [NA], sternocostal surface of heart; the anterior aspect of the heart, formed mostly by the right ventricle and to a lesser extent the left ventricle.

f. supe'rior hemisphe'rii cerebel'li [NA], superior (upper) surface of the cerebellar hemisphere; it lies against the under surface of the tentorium and includes the ala lobuli centralis, lobulus quadrangularis, lobulus simplex, and lobulus semilunaris superior.

f. supe'rior ta'li [NA], superior surface of talus; the surface of the trochlea of the talus in contact with the inferior articular surface of the tibia.

f. superolatera'lis cer'ebri [NA], superolateral surface of the cerebrum; cortical convexity; the aspect of the cerebral hemisphere that lies in contact with the flat bones of the skull; it includes parts of the frontal, parietal, temporal, and occipital lobes.

f. symphy'sialis [NA], symphysial surface of pubis.

f. tempora'lis [NA], temporal surface; the surface of a bone which contributes to the temporal fossa, namely, the greater wing of the sphenoid, the squamous part of the temporal, frontal and zygomatic bones.

f. urethra'lis pe'nis [NA], urethral surface of penis; the surface of the penis opposite to the dorsum penis.

f. vesica'lis u'teri [NA], vesical surface of uterus; the surface of the uterus facing the bladder and separated from it by the uterovesical pouch of peritoneum.

f. vestibula'ris den'tis [NA], vestibular surface of tooth; facial surface of tooth; f. facialis dentis; buccal or labial surface (1); f. buccalis or labialis; the surface of a tooth that faces the buccal or labial mucosa of vestibule of the mouth; opposite to the f. lingualis dentis.

f. viscera'lis hep'atis [NA], visceral surface of liver; the posteroinferior surface of the liver that faces adjacent abdominal organs; the porta hepatis and gallbladder are located on this surface.

f. viscera'lis lie'nis [NA], visceral surface of spleen; the surface of the spleen in contact with adjacent viscera. See also f. colica lienis, f. gastrica lienis, and f. renalis lienis.

---

facilitation (fă-sil'i-tā'shŭn) [L. *facilitas,* fr. *facilis,* easy]. Enhancement or reinforcement of a reflex or other nervous activity by the arrival at the reflex center of other excitatory impulses.

Wedensky f., the arrival of an impulse at a blocked zone, enhancing the excitability of the nerve beyond the block and indicating that the neuromuscular preparation distal to the block has been changed even though the enhancing stimulus is not conducted through the blocked zone.

facing (fās'ing). A tooth-colored material (usually plastic or porcelain) used to hide the buccal or labial surface of a gold crown to give the outward appearance of a natural tooth.

facio- [L. *facies,* face]. Combining form relating to the face. See also prosopo-.

faciocephalalgia (fā'shē-ō-sef'ă-lal'jē-ă). Neuralgic pain in the face.

faciolingual (fā'shē-ō-ling'gwăl). Relating to the face and the tongue, often denoting a paralysis affecting these parts.

facioplasty (fā'shē-ō-plas-tē) [facio- + G. *plastos,* formed]. Plastic surgery involving the face.

facioplegia (fā'shē-ō-plē'jē-ă) [facio- + G. *plēgē,* a stroke]. Facial *palsy.*

F.A.C.O.G. Abbreviation for Fellow of the American College of Obstetricians and Gynecologists.

F.A.C.P. Abbreviation for Fellow of the American College of Physicians, or of Prosthodontists.

F.A.C.R. Abbreviation for Fellow of the American College of Radiologists.

F.A.C.S. Abbreviation for Fellow of the American College of Surgeons.

F.A.C.S.M. Abbreviation for Fellow of the American College of Sports Medicine.

F-actin. See under actin.

factitious (fak-tish'ŭs) [L. *factitius,* made by art, fr. *facio,* to make]. Artificial; self-induced; not natural.

FACTOR

---

factor (fak'ter) [L. maker, causer, fr. *facio,* to make]. **1.** One of the contributing causes in any action. **2.** One of the components that by multiplication makes up a number or expression. **3.** Gene. **4.** A vitamin or other essential element.

f. I, in the clotting of blood, fibrinogen.

f. II, **(1)** in the clotting of blood, prothrombin; **(2)** lipoic acid.

f. III, in the clotting of blood, tissue thromboplastin. See thromboplastin.

f. IV, in the clotting of blood, calcium ions.

f. V, in the clotting of blood, also known as: proaccelerin (Owren), labile or plasma labile f. (Quick), plasma accelerator globulin (Ware and Seegars), thrombogene (Nolf), prothrombokinase (Milstone), plasmin prothrombins conversion f. (Stefanini), component A of prothrombin (Quick), prothrombin accelerator (Fantl and Nance), cofactor of thromboplastin (Honorato), and accelerator f. Deficiency of this f. leads to a rare hemorrhagic tendency known as parahemophilia or hypoproaccelerinemia, with autosomal recessive inheritance; heterozygous individuals are recognized by reduced levels of f. V but have no bleeding tendency.

f. V_{1a}, cobyric acid.

f. VII, in the clotting of blood, also known as: proconvertin (Owren), convertin, serum prothrombin conversion accelerator (de Vries, Alexander), stable f. (Stefanini), cofactor V (Owren), prothrombinogen (Quick), cothromboplastin (Mann and Hurn), serum accelerator (Jacox). F. VII is known to be involved in: 1) the congenital deficiency of f. VII, with purpura and bleeding from mucous membranes, autosomal recessive inheritance; 2) the acquired deficiency of f. VII in association with a deficiency of vitamin K, the neonatal period, and the administration of prothrombinopenic drugs; 3) the acquired excess of f. VII in some patients with thromboembolism. It accelerates the conversion of prothrombin to thrombin, in the presence of tissue thromboplastin, calcium, and f. V.

f. VIII, in the clotting of blood, also known as: antihemophilic f. A (Brinkhous), antihemophilic globulin (1) (Patek and Taylor), antihemophilic globulin A (Cramer), plasma thromboplastin f. (Ratnoff), plasma thromboplastin f. A (Aggeler), thromboplastic plasma component (Shinowara), thromboplastinogen (Quick), prothrombokinase (Feissly), platelet cofactor (Johnson), plasmokinin (Laki), thrombokatilysin (Leggenhager), and proserum prothrombin conversion accelerator. F. VIII is converted to its active form, f. VIII', by f. IXa, f. Xa, and thrombin; deficiency of f. VIII is associated with classic hemophilia A. **F. VIII:C** is the coagulant component of f. VIII which, in normal persons, circulates in the plasma complexed with **f. VIIIR** (von Willebrand f.), the plasma f. VIII related protein, a large glycoprotein component that is synthesized by endothelial cells and megakaryocytes, and circulates in the plasma where it binds to arteries that have lost their endothelial cell linings, creating a surface to which platelets adhere.

f. IX, in the clotting of blood, also known as: Christmas f. (Biggs and Macfarlane), plasma thromboplastin component (Aggeler), antihemophilic globulin B (Cramer), plasma thromboplastin f. B (Aggeler), plasma f. X (Shulman), antihemophilic f. B, and platelet cofactor II. F. IX is required for the formation of intrinsic blood thromboplastin and affects the amount formed (rather than the rate). Its active form, f. IXa (EC 3.4.21.22), is a serine proteinase converting f. X to f. Xa by cleaving an arginine-isoleucine bond. Deficiency of f. X causes hemophilia B.

f. X, in the clotting of blood, also known as: Stuart f., Stuart-Prower f., prothrombase, and prothrombinase. Its active form, f. Xa (EC 3.4.21.6), is formed from f. X by limited proteolysis and assists in the conversion of prothrombin to thrombin.

f. X for Haemophilus, hemin.

f. XI, in the clotting of blood, also known as plasma thromboplastin antecedent, a component of the contact system which is absorbed from plasma and serum by glass and similar surfaces. Its active form, f. XIa (EC 3.4.21.27) is a serine proteinase converting f. IX to f. IXa. Deficiency of f. XI results in a hemorrhagic tendency and is caused by an autosomal recessive gene.

f. XII, in the clotting of blood, also known as glass f. and Hageman f. When activated by glass or otherwise to its active form, f. XIIa (EC 3.4.21.38), a serine proteinase, it activates f.'s VII and XI and converts f. XI to its active form, f. XIa. Deficiency of f. XII results in great prolongation of the clotting time of venous blood,

but only rarely in a hemorrhagic tendency; deficiency is caused by an autosomal recessive gene.
f. XIII, in the clotting of blood, also known as: fibrin-stabilizing f., Laki-Lorand f., and L-L f. It is catalyzed by thrombin into its active form, f. XIIIa, which cross-links subunits of the fibrin clot to form insoluble fibrin.
f. 3, (1) operational name given to an incompletely characterized selenium-containing natural product which, in minute amounts, prevents liver damage in rats due to deficiency of vitamin E; **(2)** f. I (capital I); f. III in the vitamin B_{12} series, 5-hydroxybenzimidazole, analogue of the usual B_{12} nucleotide components.
f. A, see properdin f. A.
ABO f.'s, see Blood Groups appendix.
accelerator f., f. V.
acetate replacement f., lipoic acid.
adrenal weight f., a postulated substance of adenohypophysial origin responsible for maintenance of the weight of the adrenal cortex.
angiogenesis f., a substance of 2000 to 20,000 MW which is secreted by macrophages and stimulates neovascularization in healing wounds or in the stroma of tumors.
animal protein f. (APF), vitamin B_{12}.
antialopecia f., inositol.
antiberiberi f., thiamin.
anti-black-tongue f., nicotinic acid.
anticomplementary f., zymosan.
antihemophilic f. A (AHF), f. VIII.
antihemophilic f. B, f. IX.
antihemorrhagic f., vitamin K.
antineuritic f., thiamin.
antinuclear f. (ANF), a f. present in serum with strong affinity for nuclei and detected by fluorescent antibody technique; present in lupus erythematosus, rheumatic arthritis, and certain other conditions.
antipellagra f., nicotinic acid.
antipernicious anemia f. (APA), vitamin B_{12}.
antisterility f., vitamin E (2).
atrial natriuretic f., atriopeptin; a peptide hormone released from cardiac atrial tissue in response to stretching, which causes increased elimination of sodium by the kidney; increased in heart failure and other states of volume overload.
f. B, see properdin f. B.
B_T f., carnitine.
bacteriocin f.'s, bacteriocinogenic *plasmids.*
bifidus f., an unidentified substance associated with *Lactobacillus bifidus* subsp. *pennsylvanicus,* present in mammalian milk.
biotic f.'s, environmental f.'s or influences resulting from the activities of living organisms, as contrasted to those resulting from climatic, geological, or other f.'s.
Bittner's milk f., mammary tumor *virus* of mice.
blood f., the outmoded concept that blood group antigens (agglutinogens) are subdivided into blood f.'s, each with a specificity for an antibody; a single antigen, produced by a single gene, was thought to consist of a set of blood f.'s and to react with a corresponding set of antisera. See also Blood Groups appendix.
branching f., 1,4-α-glucan-branching enzyme.
C f.'s, coupling f.'s.
CAMP f., see CAMP *test.*
capillary permeability f., *vitamin* P.
Castle's intrinsic f., intrinsic f.
Christmas f., f. IX.
citrovorum f. (CF), folinic acid.
clearing f.'s, lipoprotein lipases that appear in plasma during lipemia and catalyze hydrolysis of triglycerides only when the latter are bound to protein and when an acceptor (*e.g.,* serum albumin) is present, thus "clearing" the plasma.
clotting f., coagulation f.; any of the various plasma components involved in the clotting process.
coagulation f., clotting f.
cobra venom f., a component of cobra venom that renders C3 proactivator (properdin factor B) susceptible to factor D of the properdin system, leading to activation of C3 and other components of complement and lysis of unsensitized erythrocytes. See also *component* of complement.
coenzyme f., dihydrolipoamide dehydrogenase.
complement chemotactic f., the activated complex of the fifth, sixth, and seventh components of complement (C567) which induces chemotaxis in the case of polymorphonuclear leukocytes.
corticotropin-releasing f. (CRF), corticoliberin.
coupling f.'s (CF), C f.'s; proteins that restore phosphorylating ability to mitochondria that have lost it, *i.e.,* have become "uncoupled" so that oxidation no longer produces ATP. Usually termed coupling factor F_1, F_2, etc.
f. D, see properdin f. D.
debranching f.'s, debranching *enzymes.*
decapacitation f., a f., postulated to be present in epididymal fluid and seminal plasma, that prevents the capacitation of spermatozoa.
diabetogenic f., rarely used term for a f. in crude extracts of the anterior lobe of the hypophysis that produces degenerative changes in the islet cells of the pancreas and causes permanent diabetes.
diffusing f., hyaluronidase (1).
direct lytic f. of cobra venom, cobrotoxin.
Duran-Reynals permeability f., Duran-Reynals spreading f., hyaluronidase (1).
f. E, see properdin f. E.
eosinophil chemotactic f. of anaphylaxis, (ECF-A), a peptide (MW 500 to 600) that is chemotactic for eosinophilic leukocytes and is released from disrupted mast cells.
epidermal growth f., a heat-stable antigenic protein isolated from the submaxillary glands of male mice; when injected into newborn animals it accelerates eyelid opening and tooth eruption, stimulates epidermal growth and keratinization, and, in larger doses, inhibits body growth and hair development and produces fatty livers.
erythrocyte maturation f., vitamin B_{12}.
essential food f.'s, those substances required in the diet: certain amino acids and unsaturated fatty acids, vitamins, essential minerals, etc.
extrinsic f., dietary vitamin B_{12}.
F f., F *plasmid.*
F′ f., F′ *plasmid.*
fermentation Lactobacillus casei f., pteropterin.
fertility f., F *plasmid.*
fibrin-stabilizing f., f. XIII.
filtrate f., former term for pantothenic acid.
follicle-stimulating hormone-releasing f. (FRF, FSH-RF), folliberin.
G f., the single common variance or f. that is common to (*i.e.,* empirically intercorrelates) different intelligence tests (general).
galactagogue f., a f. in extracts of the posterior lobe of the hypophysis which, by stimulating the smooth muscle of the lobuloalveolar system of the mammary gland, causes a flow of milk from the nipple.
galactopoietic f., prolactin.
glass f., f. XII.
glycotropic f., insulin-antagonizing f.; a principle in extracts of the anterior lobe of the hypophysis which raises the blood sugar and antagonizes the action of insulin; purified pituitary growth hormone produces an identical effect.
f. Gm, a f. that determines certain of the allotypes of human immunoglobulins; found only on the γ chains of IgG (γ-globulin).
gonadotropin-releasing f., gonadoliberin (1).
growth hormone-releasing f. (GHRF, GH-RF), somatoliberin.
f. H, (1) former designation for biotin; **(2)** vitamin B_{12} analogue or

precursor.
Hageman f., f. XII.
HG f., glucagon.
human antihemophilic f., human antihemophilic fraction; antihemophilic globulin (2); a lyophilized concentrate of f. VIII, obtained from fresh normal human plasma; used as a hemostatic agent in hemophilia.
hyperglycemic-glycogenolytic f. (HGF), glucagon.
f. I, f. 3 (2).
inhibition f., migration-inhibitory f.
initiation f. (IF), one of several soluble proteins involved in the initiation of protein synthesis, then released from the ribosome as it progresses into chain elongation.
insulin-antagonizing f., glycotropic f.
insulin-like growth f. (IGF), somatomedin.
intrinsic f. (IF), Castle's intrinsic f.; a relatively small mucoprotein (MW about 50,000) secreted by the neck cell of the gastric glands and required for adequate absorption of vitamin B_{12}; deficiency results in pernicious anemia.
f. Inv, a f. that determines certain of the allotypes of human immunoglobulins; found on the κ chains of IgG, IgA, IgM, and Bence Jones protein.
labile f., f. V.
Lactobacillus bulgaricus f. (LBF), pantetheine.
Lactobacillus casei f., folic acid (2).
lactogenic f., prolactin.
Laki-Lorand f., f. XIII.
LE f.'s, antinuclear immunoglobulins in plasma of persons with disseminated lupus erythematosus, associated with positive LE tests.
lethal f., a gene mutation or chromosomal structural change which, when expressed, causes death prior to sexual maturity or totally precludes reproduction.
leukocytosis-promoting f., a substance obtained by Menkin from inflammatory exudates; it stimulates leukocytosis.
leukopenic f., a principle obtained by Menkin from inflammatory exudates; it causes leukopenia when injected into normal animals.
lipotropic f., choline.
liver filtrate f., former term for pantothenic acid.
liver Lactobacillus casei f., folic acid (2).
L-L f., f. XIII.
luteinizing hormone/follicle-stimulating hormone-releasing f. (LH/FSH-RF), gonadoliberin (2).
luteinizing hormone-releasing f. (LRF, LH-RF), former name for luteinizing hormone-releasing *hormone*.
lymph node permeability f. (LNPF), a substance, released by lymphocytes when stimulated or damaged, that increases capillary permeability and the accumulation of mononuclear cells.
mammotropic f., prolactin.
maturation f., vitamin B_{12}.
migration-inhibitory f., inhibition f.; a soluble, nondialyzable substance that is produced by sensitized lymphocytes (*i.e.,* lymphocytes from a sensitized animal) when exposed to the specific antigen, and that causes adherence and inhibition of migration of macrophages.
milk f., mammary tumor *virus* of mice.
mouse antialopecia f., inositol.
müllerian regression f., müllerian duct inhibitory f., a nonsteroidal substance of fetal testicular origin which acts unilaterally to inhibit development of the müllerian ducts and acts with testosterone to promote development of the vas deferens and related structures.
myocardial depressant f. (MDF), a toxic f. in shock which impairs cardiac contractility; probably a peptide released with underperfusion of the splanchnic area at the release of proteolytic enzymes from the pancreas.
nephritic f., a serum protein (possibly an IgG autoantibody), found in some patients with membranoproliferative glomerulonephritis and hypocomplementemia, which, together with the cofactors of the alternate pathway of complement activation, cleaves the third component of complement (C3).
nerve growth f. (NGF), a protein (MW about 26,000) that controls the development of sympathetic postganglionic neurons and possibly also sensory (dorsal root) ganglion cells in mammals; similar, but not identical, factors have been isolated from the venoms of several species of snakes; it has been isolated from the submaxillary glands of male mice, and when injected into newborn animals, sympathetic ganglia become hyperplastic and hypertrophic.
osteoclast activating f., a lymphokine that stimulates bone resorption and inhibits bone-collagen synthesis.
f. P, a chemical (postulated by T. Lewis), formed in ischemic skeletal or cardiac muscle, held to be responsible for the pain of intermittent claudication and angina pectoris.
P f., see P blood group, Blood Groups appendix.
pellagra-preventing (P-P) f., nicotinic acid.
plasma f. X, f. IX.
plasma labile f., f. V.
plasma thromoplastin f. (PTF), f. VIII.
plasma thromboplastin f. B, f. IX.
plasmin prothrombins conversion f. (PPCF), f. V.
platelet f. 3, a blood coagulation factor derived from platelets; chemically, a phospholipid lipoprotein that acts with certain plasma thromboplastin f.'s to convert prothrombin to thrombin.
platelet-aggregating f., platelet-activating f. (PAF), a substance released from rabbit basophilic leukocytes that causes aggregation of platelets and also is involved in the deposition of immune complexes.
platelet-derived growth f., a f. in platelets that is mitogenic for cells at the site of a wound, *e.g.,* causing endothelial proliferation.
platelet tissue f., thromboplastin.
prolactin inhibiting f. (PIF), prolactostatin.
prolactin releasing f. (PRF), prolactoliberin.
properdin f. A, a component of the properdin system; a hydrazine-sensitive β_1-globulin (mw about 180,000), now known to be C3 (third component of complement).
properdin f. B, C3 proactivator; cobra venom cofactor; glycine-rich β-glycoprotein; β_2-glycoprotein II; a normal serum protein (mw 95,000) and a component of the properdin system.
properdin f. D, C3 proactivator convertase; glycine-rich β-glycoproteinase; a normal serum α-globulin (mw about 25,000) required in the properdin system.
properdin f. E, a serum protein (mw 160,000) required for activation of C3 (third component of complement) by cobra venom factor. See also properdin *system*.
protein f., the f. (6.25) by which the nitrogen content of a protein is multiplied to give the amount of protein.
pyruvate oxidation f., lipoic acid.
R f.'s, resistance *plasmids*.
recognition f.'s, f.'s which effect "recognition" of target antigens by polymorphonuclear neutrophil leukocytes; apparently the Fc portion of antibody molecules and the activated third component of complement (C3), for both of which phagocytes have receptor sites.
relaxation f., substance presumably involved in the return of muscle fibrils to the resting state after nervous stimulation ceases, postulated to act by withdrawing Ca^{2+} from myosin-ATPase sites.
releasing f. (RF), releasing hormone; a substance of hypothalamic origin capable of accelerating the rate of secretion of a given hormone by the anterior pituitary gland.
resistance f.'s, resistance *plasmids*.
resistance-inducing f., an agent from normal chick embryos that interferes with multiplication of the avian leukosis-sarcoma virus, and is seemingly an avirulent leukosis virus antigenically related to the avian leukosis-sarcoma virus.

resistance-transfer f., the transfer gene of the resistance plasmid.
rheumatoid f.'s (RF), globulins in the serum of individuals with rheumatoid arthritis that enhance agglutination of suspended particles coated with pooled human γ-globulin.
risk f., a single characteristic statistically associated with, although not necessarily causally related to, an increased risk of morbidity or mortality.
S f., the individual variables, or empirically most minute subclusters of intercorrelations or common variance, found in different intelligence tests (specific).
secretor f., an inherited capacity to secrete antigens of the ABO blood group in saliva and other body fluids, controlled by a pair of allelic genes designated *Se* and *se* (or *S* and *s*), with *Se* dominant to *se;* the saliva of secretors (genotype *SeSe* or *Sese*) contains the blood group substances A, B, or H found in their erythrocytes; the saliva of nonsecretors (genotype *sese*) contains no blood group substance; tests for ABH secretion are useful in genetic linkage and population studies; the secretor phenomenon is also closely associated with the Lewis blood group.
sex f., F *plasmid.*
slow-reacting f. of anaphylaxis (SRF-A), slow-reacting *substance* (of anaphylaxis).
SLR (Streptococcus lactis R) f., rhizopterin.
somatotropin release-inhibiting f. (SRIF), somatostatin.
somatotropin-releasing f. (SRF), somatoliberin.
spreading f., hyaluronidases (1).
stable f., f. VII.
Stuart f., Stuart-Prower f., f. X.
sulfation f., somatomedin.
sun protection f. (SPF), the ratio of the minimal ultraviolet dose required to produce erythema with and without a sunscreen; the most effective sunscreens have an SPF of 15.
thymic lymphopoietic f., thymin; thymopoietin; thymosin; a glycoprotein (MW about 12,000) that has been extracted from thymus; there is ground for the belief that this thymus-produced humoral factor(s) or hormone(s) confers immunological competence on thymus-dependent cells and induces lymphopoiesis.
thyroid-stimulating hormone-releasing f. (TSH-RF), thyroliberin.
thyrotoxic complement-fixation f., a form of thyrotoxin; an antigen found most readily in thyroid tissue from thyrotoxic individuals; known to be chemically and immunologically distinct from thyroglobulin, and fixes complement when combined with antibody related to the γ-globulin fraction of serum. With the exception of extremely small concentrations, the antigen is rarely found in normal glands or in diseased glands that are not associated with thyrotoxicosis; it is probably an intracellular substance (possibly a constituent of the "microsomal fraction"), and does not contain iodine in significant quantity. Not related to the complement-fixation reaction occurring with serum in Hashimoto's disease, in which the antigen is thyroglobulin.
thyrotropin-releasing f. (TRF), former name for thyrotropin-releasing *hormone.*
transfer f., **(1)** the transfer gene of a conjugative plasmid, especially of the resistance plasmid; **(2)** a substance, free of nucleic acid and antibody, that is obtained from the leukocytes of a person with a delayed-type sensitivity and that will, following injection into the skin of a nonsensitive person, transfer the specific sensitivity to the recipient.
transforming f., the DNA responsible for bacterial transformation.
transmethylation f., choline.
tumor angiogenic f. (TAF), a substance released by solid tumors which induces formation of new blood vessels to supply the tumor.
tumor necrosis f., cachectin.
uncoupling f.'s, uncouplers.
von Willebrand f., f. VIIIR.
W f., biotin.
Y f., yeast eluate f., obsolete terms for pyridoxine.

---

factorial (fak-tōr'ē-ăl). **1.** Pertaining to a statistical factor or factors. **2.** Of an integer, that integer multiplied by each smaller integer in succession down to one; *e.g.,* 5! equals 5 × 4 × 3 × 2.

facultative (fak-ŭl-tā'tiv). Able to live under more than one specific set of environmental conditions; possessing an alternative pathway.

faculty (fak'ŭl-tē). A natural or specialized power of a living organism.

FAD Abbreviation for *flavin* adenine dinucleotide.

Faget, Jean C., French physician, 1818–1884. See F.'s *sign.*

fagopyrism (fag-ō-pī'rizm, fă-gop'i-rizm). Photosensitization, mainly in cattle and sheep, caused by ingestion of buckwheat (*Fagopyrum esculentum*) and characterized by irritation of the skin, edema, and a serous exudate.

Fahr, Theodore, German physician, 1877–1945. See F.'s *disease.*

Fahraeus, Robert (Robin) Sanno, Swedish pathologist, 1888–1968. See F.-Lindqvist *effect.*

Fahrenheit, Gabriel D., German physicist, 1686–1736. See F. *scale.*

failure (fāl'yūr). The state of insufficiency or nonperformance.
backward heart f., a theory that maintains that the phenomena of congestive heart f. result from passive engorgement of the veins caused by a "backward" rise in pressure proximal to the failing cardiac chambers.
cardiac f., heart f. (1).
congestive heart f., heart f. (1).
coronary f., acute coronary insufficiency.
electrical f., f. in which the cardiac inadequacy is secondary to disturbance of the electrical impulse. *Cf.* pump f.
forward heart f., a theory that maintains that the phenomena of congestive heart f. result from the inadequate cardiac output, and especially from the consequent inadequacy of renal blood flow with resulting retention of sodium and water.
heart f., **(1)** congestive heart f.; cardiac f. or insufficiency; myocardial insufficiency; mechanical inadequacy of the heart so that as a pump it fails to maintain the circulation of blood, with the result that congestion and edema develop in the tissues. See also forward f., backward f., right and left ventricular f.; **(2)** the resulting clinical syndrome consisting of shortness of breath, pitting edema, enlarged tender liver, engorged neck veins, and pulmonary rales.
high output f., heart f. in which, despite relative myocardial insufficiency and consequent congestive heart f., the cardiac output is maintained at normal or supernormal levels, as is sometimes seen in emphysema, thyrotoxicosis, etc.
left ventricular f., congestive heart f. manifested by signs of pulmonary congestion and edema, *i.e.,* dyspnea, basal rales, pulmonary edema, etc.
low output f., heart f. in which the cardiac output is subnormal, as is usually seen in f. due to coronary, hypertensive, or rheumatic heart disease.
pacemaker f., f. of an artificial pacemaker to generate or deliver effective stimuli to the myocardium.
power f., pump f.
pump f., power f.; a term used to emphasize default of the heart as a mechanical pump; in acute myocardial infarction, pump f. signifies congestive heart failure, pulmonary edema, or cardiogenic shock. *Cf.* electrical f.
right ventricular f., congestive heart f. manifested by distention of the neck veins, enlargement of the liver, and dependent edema.
secondary f., **(1)** f. of the function of an organ as a result of antecedent pathology elsewhere; **(2)** decreasing responsiveness to a drug after an initial satisfactory response, usually occurring several

months after initiation of treatment.

faint (fānt). **1.** Extremely weak; threatened with syncope. **2.** An attack of syncope.

falcate (fal'kāt). Falciform.

falces (fal'sēz). Plural of falx.

falcial (fal'shăl). Falcine; relating to the falx cerebelli or falx cerebri.

falciform (fal'si-fōrm) [L. *falx,* sickle, + *forma,* form]. Falcate; having a crescentic or sickle shape.

falcine (fal'sēn). Falcial.

falcula (fal'kyū-lă) [L. dim. of *falx*]. *Falx* cerebelli.

falcular (fal'kyū-lăr). **1.** Resembling a sickle or falx. **2.** Relating to the falx cerebelli or cerebri.

fallopian (fa-lō'pē-an). Described by or attributed to Fallopius.

Fallopius (Fallopio), Gabriele, Italian anatomist, 1523–1562. See fallopian *aqueduct, arch, canal, hiatus, ligament, neuritis, pregnancy, tube.*

Fallot, Étienne-Louis A., French physician, 1850–1911. See F.'s *tetrad, tetralogy, triad; pentalogy* of F.

false negative (fawls neg'ă-tiv). **1.** A test result which erroneously excludes an individual from a specific diagnostic or reference group, due particularly to insufficiently exact methods of testing. **2.** An individual whose test results exclude him from a particular diagnostic group though he may truly belong to such a group. **3.** Term used to denote a false-negative *result.*

false positive (fawls pos'i-tiv). **1.** A test result which erroneously assigns an individual to a specific diagnostic or reference group, due particularly to insufficiently exact methods of testing. **2.** An individual whose test results include him in a particular diagnostic group though he may not truly belong to such a group. **3.** Term used to denote a false-positive *result.*

falsification (fawl'si-fi-kā'shŭn). The deliberate act of misrepresentation so as to deceive.

retrospective f., unconscious distortion of past experience to conform to present psychological needs.

falx, pl. **falces** (falks, fal'sēz) [L. sickle] [NA]. A sickle-shaped structure.

f. aponeurot'ica, f. inguinalis.

f. cerebel'li [NA], falcula; a short process of dura mater projecting forward from the internal occipital crest below the tentorium; it occupies the posterior cerebellar notch and the vallecula, and bifurcates below into two diverging limbs passing to either side of the foramen magnum.

f. cer'ebri [NA], the scythe-shaped fold of dura mater in the longitudinal fissure between the two cerebral hemispheres; it is attached anteriorly to the crista galli of the ethmoid bone and caudally to the upper surface of the tentorium.

f. inguina'lis [NA], tendo conjunctivus; inguinal aponeurotic fold; conjoined or conjoint tendon; f. aponeurotica; common tendon of insertion of the transversus and obliquus internus muscles into the crest and spine of the pubis and iliopectineal line; it is frequently muscular rather than aponeurotic and may be poorly developed.

f. sep'ti [NA], official alternative term for *valvula* foraminis ovalis.

familial (fa-mil'ē-ăl) [L. *familia,* family]. Affecting several members of the same family, usually within a single sibship; commonly but incorrectly used to mean genetic.

family (fam'ĭ-lē). [L. *familia*]. **1.** A group of blood relatives, or, more strictly, the parents and their children. **2.** In biologic classification, a division between the order and the tribe or genus.

cancer f., a group of blood relatives in which cancer has been reported; the mode of aggregation may be genetic, as in familial polyposis of the colon, or due to common exposure to a carcinogenic or oncogenic agent, such as a virus.

nuclear f., in genetics, two parents and their progeny in common.

famotidine (fă-mō'ti-dēn). Propanimidamide, *N*'-(aminosulfonyl)-3-[[[2-[(diaminomethylene)amino]-4-thiazdyl]methyl]thio]-; a histamine H_2 antagonist used in the treatment of duodenal ulcers.

famotine hydrochloride (fam'ō-tēn). 1-[(*p*-Chlorophenoxy)methyl]-3,4-dihydroisoquinoline hydrochloride; an antiviral agent.

Fañanás, J., Spanish physician. See F. *cell.*

Fanconi, Guido, Swiss pediatrician, *1892. See F.'s *anemia, pancytopenia, syndrome;* De Toni-F. *syndrome;* Lignac-F. *syndrome.*

fang [A.S. *fōhan,* to seize]. **1.** A long tooth or tusk, usually a canine. **2.** The hollow tooth of a snake through which the venom is ejected.

fango (fang'gō) [It. mud]. Mud from the Battaglio thermal springs in Italy, applied externally in the treatment of rheumatism and other diseases of the joints and muscles.

Fannia (fan'ē-ă). A genus of flies of the family Muscidae. Species include *F. canicularis* (the lesser housefly), commonly observed in kitchens or near food, which resembles *Musca domestica* (the common housefly) but is somewhat smaller and has three brown stripes on the thorax, and *F. scalaris* (the latrine fly) which commonly lays eggs in liquid feces of humans and animals and is distinguished from *F. canicularis* by two brown stripes on its thorax.

fantasy (fan'tă-sē) [G. *phantasia,* idea, image]. Phantasia; imagery that is more or less coherent, as in dreams and daydreams, yet unrestricted by reality.

Farabeuf, Louis H., Paris surgeon, 1841–1910. See F.'s *amputation, triangle.*

farad (fa'rad) [M. *Faraday*]. A practical unit of electrical capacity; the capacity of a condenser having a charge of 1 coulomb under an electromotive force of 1 volt.

faradaic (fa-ră-dā'ik). Faradic.

Faraday, Michael, British physicist and chemist, 1791–1867. See farad, faraday; F.'s *constant, laws;* F. *space.*

faraday (F) (fa'ră-dā) [M. *Faraday*]. 96,500 coulombs, the amount of electricity required to reduce one equivalent of (*e.g.*) silver ion.

faradic (fa-rad'ik). Faradaic; relating to induced electricity.

faradism (fa'ră-dizm). Faradic (induction) electricity.

surging f., a current of gradually increasing and decreasing amplitude obtained by interposing a rhythmic resistance to the alternating current produced by the induction coil.

faradization (fa'rad-i-zā'shŭn). Therapeutic application of the faradic (induced) electrical current.

faradocontractility (fa'ră-dō-kon'trak-til'i-tē). Contractility of muscles under the stimulus of a faradic (induced) electric current.

faradomuscular (fa'ră-dō-mŭs'kyū-lăr). Denoting the effect of applying a faradic (induced) electric current directly to a muscle.

faradopalpation (fa'ră-dō-pal-pā'shŭn). Esthesiometry by means of a sharp-pointed electrode through which a feeble alternating current passes to an indifferent electrode.

faradotherapy (fa'ră-dō-thār'ă-pē). Treatment of disease or paralysis by means of faradic (induced) electric current.

Farber, Sidney, U.S. pediatric pathologist, 1903–1973. See F.'s *disease, syndrome.*

farcy (far'sē) [L. *farcio,* to stuff]. **1.** A lymphatic disease of cattle caused by *Nocardia farcinica.* **2.** The skin form of glanders.

fardel (far-del'). The total measurable penalty that is incurred as a result of the occurrence of a genetic disease in an individual; one of two major quantitative considerations in the prognostic aspects of genetic counseling, the other being risk of occurrence. The f. roughly measures the duration and the severity of the penalty, *i.e.,* the total integral of the time-intensity function; *e.g.,* color blindness has a low intensity of penalty throughout life, anencephaly causes intense distress for a brief time, Alzheimer's disease is intermediate in both respects but the f. is greater.

farfara (far'far-ă) [L. *farfarus,* coltsfoot]. Coltsfoot or tussilago leaves; the dried leaves of *Tussilago farfara* (family Compositae); used as a demulcent to relieve irritable coughing.

farina (fă-rē'nă) [L.]. Flour or meal, as prepared from cereal grains such as *Avena sativa* or *Triticum sativum;* used as a starchy food.

farinaceous (far-i-nā'shŭs). **1.** Relating to farina or flour. **2.** Starchy.

α-farnesene (far'nĕ-sēn). 3,7,11-Trimethyl-1,3,6,10-dodecatetraene; a straight open-chain hydrocarbon built up of three isoprene units; one of the four isomeric forms occurs in the natural coating of apples.

β-farnesene. 7,11-Dimethyl-3-methylene-1,6,10-dodecatriene; one of the two isomers (*trans*) that occurs in the alarm pheramone of some aphids and also in various essential oils.

farnesene alcohol. Farnesol.

farnesol (far'nĕ-sol). Farnesene alcohol; a difarnesyl group that occurs in the side chain of vitamin K_2 and constitutes squalene; found in oil of citronella.

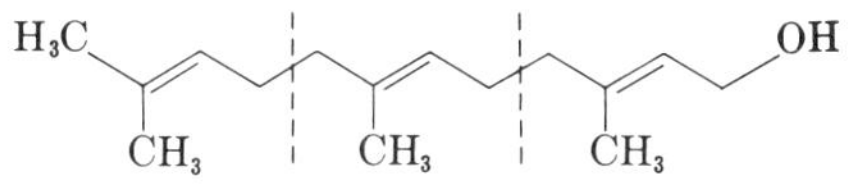

Farnesol
(Dotted lines indicate formal division into isoprenyl groups)

Farnsworth, Dean, U.S. naval officer, 1902–1959. See F.-Munsell color *test.*

Farr, William, British medical statistician, 1807–1883. See F.'s *law.*

Farrant's mounting fluid. See under fluid.

Farre, Arthur, British obstetrician and gynecologist, 1811–1887. See F.'s *line.*

farsightedness (far'sīt'ed-nes). Hyperopia.

FASCIA

fascia, pl. **fasciae** (fash'ē-ă, -ē-ē) [L. a band or fillet] [NA]. A sheet of fibrous tissue that envelops the body beneath the skin; it also encloses muscles and groups of muscles, and separates their several layers or groups.

Abernethy's f., a layer of subperitoneal areolar tissue in front of the external iliac artery.

f. adhe'rens, a broad intercellular junction in the interculated disk of cardiac muscle which anchors actin filaments.

anal f., f. diaphragmatis pelvis inferior.

antebrachial f., f. antebrachii.

f. antebra'chii [NA], antebrachial f.; deep f. of forearm; it is continuous with the brachial f.; in the region of the wrist it forms two thickened bands, the extensor and flexor retinacula.

f. axilla'ris [NA], axillary f.; the f. that forms the floor of the axilla. It is continuous with the pectoral and clavipectoral f. anteriorly, with the brachial f. laterally, and with the f. of the latissimus dorsi and serratus anterior muscles posteriorly and medially.

axillary f., f. axillaris.

bicipital f., *aponeurosis* musculi bicipitis brachii.

brachial f., f. brachii.

f. bra'chii [NA], brachial f.; the deep f. of the arm; it is continuous proximally with the pectoral f. and the f. covering the deltoid; distally it is continuous with the antebrachial f.

broad f., f. lata.

f. buc'copharyn'gea [NA], buccopharyngeal f.; the f. that covers the muscular layer of the pharynx and is continued forward onto the buccinator muscle.

buccopharyngeal f., f. buccopharyngea.

Buck's f., f. penis profunda.

f. bul'bi, *vagina* bulbi.

Camper's f., superficial layer of the tela subcutanea of the abdomen.

cervical f., f. cervicalis.

f. cervica'lis [NA], cervical f.; f. of neck; it is divided into an external or investing layer (lamina superficialis) that surrounds the neck and encloses the trapezius and sternocleidomastoid muscles, a pretracheal or middle layer (lamina pretrachealis) in relation to the infrahyoid muscles, and a prevertebral layer (lamina prevertebralis) applied to the vertebrae and axial muscles.

f. cine'rea, *gyrus* fasciolaris.

clavipectoral f., f. clavipectoralis.

f. clavipectora'lis [NA], clavipectoral f.; a f. that extends between the coracoid process, the clavicle, and the thoracic wall. It envelops the subclavius and pectoralis minor muscles and forms a strong membrane in the interval between them.

f. clitor'idis [NA], f. of clitoris; fibrous tissue comparable to the f. of the penis.

f. of clitoris, f. clitoridis.

Colles' f., f. perinei superficialis.

Cooper's f., f. cremasterica.

cremasteric f., f. cremasterica.

f. cremaster'ica [NA], cremasteric f.; Cooper's f.; Scarpa's sheath; one of the coverings of the spermatic cord, formed of delicate connective tissue and of muscular fibers derived from the internal oblique muscle.

cribriform f., f. cribosa.

f. cribro'sa [NA], cribriform f.; Hesselbach's f.; the part of the superficial f. of the thigh that covers the saphenous opening.

f. cru'ris [NA], f. of leg; deep f. of leg; it is continuous with the f. lata and is attached proximally to the patella, ligamentum patellae, the tubercle and condyles of the tibia, and the head of the fibula; distally it is thickened to form the flexor and extensor retinacula.

Cruveilhier's f., f. perinei superficialis.

deep f., a thin fibrous membrane, devoid of fat, that invests the muscles, separating the several groups and the individual muscles, forms sheaths for the nerves and vessels, becomes specialized around the joints to form or strengthen ligaments, envelops various organs and glands, and binds all the structures together into a firm compact mass.

deep f. of arm, f. brachii.

deep f. of forearm, f. antebrachii.

deep f. of leg, f. cruris.

f. denta'ta hippocam'pi, *gyrus* dentatus.

dentate f., *gyrus* dentatus.

f. diaphragma'tis pel'vis infe'rior [NA], inferior f. of pelvic diaphragm; anal f.; the f. that covers the inferior aspect of the levator ani and coccygeus muscles.

f. diaphragma'tis pel'vis supe'rior [NA], superior f. of pelvic diaphragm; the f. on the superior aspect of the levator ani and coccygeus muscles.

f. diaphragma'tis urogenita'lis infe'rior [NA], alternate term for *membrana* perinei.

f. diaphragma'tis urogenita'lis supe'rior, superior f. of urogenital diaphragm.

dorsal f. of foot, f. dorsalis pedis.

dorsal f. of hand, f. dorsalis manus.

f. dorsa'lis ma'nus [NA], dorsal f. of hand; the deep f. of the back of the hand continuous proximally with the extensor retinaculum.

f. dorsa'lis pe'dis [NA], dorsal f. of foot; the f. that encloses the

extensor tendons of the toes and blends with the inferior extensor retinaculum.
Dupuytren's f., *aponeurosis* palmaris.
endopelvic f., f. pelvis visceralis.
endothoracic f., f. endothoracica.
f. endothora'cica [NA], endothoracic f.; the extrapleural f. that lines the wall of the thorax; it extends over the cupula of the pleura as the suprapleural membrane and also forms a thin layer between the diaphragm and pleura (f. phrenicopleuralis).
external spermatic f., f. spermatica externa.
f. of extraocular muscles, f. muscularis musculorum bulbi.
extraperitoneal f., f. subperitonealis.
f. of forearm, f. antebrachii.
Gerota's f., f. renalis.
Godman's f., an extension of the pretracheal f. into the thorax and on to the pericardium.
Hesselbach's f., f. cribrosa.
iliac f., f. iliaca.
f. ili'aca [NA], iliac f.; the f. covering the iliacus and psoas muscles.
iliopectineal f., a f. formed by the union of the fasciae covering the iliacus and pectinus muscles which cover the floor of the iliopectineal fossa.
inferior f. of pelvic diaphragm, f. diaphragmatis pelvis inferior.
inferior f. of urogenital diaphragm, *membrana* perinei.
infraspinatus f., f. in'fraspina'ta, the f. attached to the borders of the infraspinous fossa and covering the infraspinatus muscle; it is continuous with the f. covering the deltoid.
infundibuliform f., f. spermatica interna.
intercolumnar fasciae, *fibrae* intercrurales.
internal spermatic f., f. spermatica interna.
interosseous f., the f. covering the interosseous muscles of the hand or foot; it consists of a dorsal layer and a palmar or plantar layer.
lacrimal f., that part of the periorbita that bridges across the fossa for lacrimal sac.
f. la'ta [NA], broad f.; the strong f. enveloping the muscles of the thigh.
f. of leg, f. cruris.
lumbodorsal f., f. thoracolumbalis.
masseteric f., f. masseterica.
f. massete'rica [NA], masseteric f.; the f. that covers the lateral surface of the masseter muscle.
middle cervical f., *lamina* pretrachealis.
muscular f. of extraocular muscle, f. muscularis musculorum bulbi.
f. muscula'ris musculo'rum bul'bi [NA], muscular f.; f. of extraocular muscles; the part of the orbital f. that encloses the extraocular muscles; it is thin posteriorly but becomes thicker where it is continuous with the bulbar sheath.
f. of neck, f. cervicalis.
f. nu'chae [NA], nuchal f.; the f. that encloses the posterior muscles of the neck.
nuchal f., f. nuchae.
obturator f., f. obturatoria.
f. obturato'ria [NA], obturator f.; the portion of the pelvic f. that covers the obturator internus muscle.
orbital fasciae, fasciae orbitales.
fas'ciae orbita'les [NA], orbital fasciae; the fascial layers in the orbit consisting of periorbita, septum orbitale, f. muscularis musculorum bulbi, and vagina bulbi.
palmar f., *aponeurosis* palmaris.
parotid f., f. parotidea.
f. parotid'ea [NA], parotid f.; the part of the cervical f. that ensheaths the parotid gland and is fixed above to the zygomatic arch.
f. parotid'eomasseter'ica, a dense membrane covering both the lateral and medial surfaces of the parotid gland, continuous anteriorly with the f. covering the masseter muscle. See f. parotidea and f. masseterica.
pectoral f., f. pectoralis.
f. pectora'lis [NA], pectoral f.; the f. that covers the pectoralis major muscle; it is attached to the sternum and to the clavicle; laterally and below it is continuous with the f. of the shoulder, axilla, and thorax.
f. pel'vis [NA], f. of the pelvis; it includes parietal and visceral components: **f. p. parieta'lis,** including the f. obturatoria, covers the muscles that pass from the interior of the pelvis to the thigh; **f. p. viscera'lis,** endopelvic f.; covers the pelvic organs and surrounds vessels and nerves in the subperitoneal space.
f. pe'nis [NA], f. of the penis; it is divided into two layers: **f. p. superficia'lis,** a superficial layer continuous with f. perinei superficialis; **f. p. profun'da,** Buck's f.; a deep layer which surrounds the three erectile bodies of the penis.
f. perine'i superficia'lis [NA], superficial f. of perineum; Colles' or Cruveilhier's f.; the membranous layer of the subcutaneous tissue in the urogenital region attaching posteriorly to the border of the urogenital diaphragm, at the sides to the ischiopubic rami, and continuing anteriorly onto the abdominal wall.
perirenal f., f. renalis.
pharyngobasilar f., f. pharyngobasilaris.
f. pharyngobasila'ris [NA], pharyngobasilar f.; tela submucosa pharyngis; aponeurosis pharyngea; the fibrous coat of the pharyngeal wall situated between the mucous and muscular coats; it is attached above to the basilar part of the occipital bone, and the petrous part of the temporal bone.
phrenicopleural f., f. phrenicopleuralis.
f. phrenicopleura'lis [NA], phrenicopleural f.; the thin layer of endothoracic f. intervening between the diaphragmatic pleura and the diaphragm.
plantar f., *aponeurosis* plantaris.
popliteal f., the f. that covers the popliteal fossa.
Porter's f., *lamina* pretrachealis.
pretracheal f., *lamina* pretrachealis.
prevertebral f., *lamina* prevertebralis.
f. pros'tatae [NA], f. of prostate; the condensation of pelvic visceral f. that encloses the prostate gland.
f. of prostate, f. prostatae.
rectovesical f., *septum* rectovesicale.
renal f., f. renalis.
f. rena'lis [NA], renal f.; perirenal f.; Gerota's f. or capsule; the condensation of the fibroareolar tissue and fat surrounding the kidney to form a sheath for the organ.
Scarpa's f., the deeper, membranous or lamellar part of the subcutaneous tissue of the lower abdominal wall; it is continuous with the superficial perineal (Colles') f.
semilunar f., *aponeurosis* musculi bicipitis brachii.
Sibson's f., *membrana* suprapleuralis.
f. spermat'ica exter'na [NA], external spermatic f.; the outer fascial covering of the spermatic cord; it is continuous at the superficial inguinal ring with the f. covering the external oblique muscle.
f. spermat'ica inter'na [NA], internal spermatic f.; infundibuliform f.; tunica vaginalis communis; the inner covering of the spermatic cord, continuous above the deep inguinal ring with f. transversalis.
subperitoneal f., f. subperitonealis.
f. subperitonea'lis [NA], subperitoneal f.; extraperitoneal f.; the thin layer of f. and adipose tissue between the peritoneum and f. transversalis.
superficial f., *tela* subcutanea.
superficial f. of perineum, f. perinei superficialis.
superior f. of pelvic diaphragm, f. diaphragmatis pelvis superior.
superior f. of urogenital diaphragm, f. diaphragmatis urogenitalis superior; a layer of f. that has been described on the superior surface of the sphincter urethrae and the deep transverse perineal mus-

cles. Its presence is doubted by some anatomists.
temporal f., f. temporalis.
f. tempora'lis [NA], temporal f.; temporal aponeurosis; the f. covering the temporal muscle; it is composed of two layers, lamina superficialis and lamina profunda; both attach above to the superior temporal line but diverge inferiorly to attach to the lateral and medial surfaces of the zygomatic arch.
f. thoracolumba'lis [NA], thoracolumbar f.; thoracolumbar aponeurosis; lumbodorsal f.; the f. which covers the deep muscles of the back; it is attached to the angles of the ribs and to the spines of the thoracic, lumbar, and sacral vertebrae, to the transverse processes of the lumbar vertebrae, to the lower border of the twelfth rib and to the iliac crest, as well as to the lumbocostal, iliolumbar, intertransverse, and supraspinous ligaments.
Toldt's f., continuation of Treitz's f. behind the body of the pancreas.
f. transversa'lis [NA], transversalis f.; the lining f. of the abdominal cavity, between the inner surface of the abdominal musculature and the peritoneum.
Treitz's f., f. behind the head of the pancreas.
triangular f., *ligamentum* reflexum.
f. triangula'ris abdom'inis, *ligamentum* reflexum.
Tyrrell's f., *septum* rectovesicale.
umbilical prevesical f., the thin fascial layer interposed between the transversalis f. and the umbilicovesical f. It extends between the medial umbilical ligaments from the umbilicus downward in front of the bladder, forming the posterior boundary of the retropubic space.
umbilicovesical f., a thin fascial layer that extends between the medial umbilical ligaments and is continuous with f. enclosing the bladder.
Zuckerkandl's f., the posterior layer of the renal f.

fascial (fash'ē-ăl). Relating to any fascia.

fascicle (fas'i-kl). Fasciculus.
muscle f., a bundle of muscle fibers surrounded by perimysium.
nerve f., a bundle of nerve fibers surrounded by perineurium.

fascicular (fa-sik'yū-lăr). Fasciculate; fasciculated; relating to a fasciculus; arranged in the form of a bundle or collection of rods.

fasciculate, fasciculated (fa-sik'yū-lāt, -lā-ted). Fascicular.

fasciculation (fa-sik-yū-lā'shŭn). **1.** An arrangement in the form of fasciculi. **2.** Involuntary contractions, or twitchings, of groups (fasciculi) of muscle fibers, a coarser form of muscular contraction than fibrillation.

fasciculi (fa-sik'yū-lī). Plural of fasciculus.

FASCICULUS

fasciculus, gen. and pl. **fasciculi** (fă-sik'yū-lŭs, fă-sik'yū-lī) [L. dim. of *fascis,* bundle] [NA]. Fascicle; a band or bundle of fibers, usually of muscle or nerve fibers; a nerve fiber tract.
f. ante'rior pro'prius, anterior ground bundle; the ground bundle of the anterior column of the spinal cord. See fasciculi proprii.
arcuate f., **(1)** f. longitudinalis superior; **(2)** f. uncinatus.
f. at'rioventricula'ris, *truncus* atrioventricularis.
Burdach's f., f. cuneatus.
calcarine f., a group of short association fibers beneath the calcarine fissure of the occipital lobe of the cerebrum.
central tegmental f., *tractus* tegmentalis centralis.
f. cir'cumoliva'ris pyram'idis, an anomalous bundle of nerve fibers on the anterior surface of the medulla oblongata that emerges from the pyramid and curves forward and dorsally over the lower pole of the olive; it is variously interpreted as an aberrant bundle of pontocerebellar fibers or corticopontine fibers.
f. corticospina'lis ante'rior, *tractus* pyramidalis anterior.
f. corticospina'lis latera'lis, *tractus* pyramidalis lateralis.
cuneate f., f. cuneatus.
f. cunea'tus [NA], cuneate or wedge-shaped f.; Burdach's f., column, or tract; cuneate funiculus; the larger lateral subdivision of the funiculus posterior.
dorsal longitudinal f., f. longitudinalis dorsalis.
dorsolateral f., f. dorsolateralis.
f. dorsolatera'lis [NA], tractus dorsolateralis; dorsolateral f. or tract; f. marginalis; Lissauer's f., bundle, tract, or marginal zone; Spitzka's marginal tract or zone; Waldeyer's tract or zonal layer; a longitudinal bundle of thin, unmyelinated and poorly myelinated fibers capping the apex of the posterior horn of the spinal gray matter, composed of posterior root fibers and short association fibers that interconnect neighboring segments of the posterior horn.
Flechsig's fasciculi, f. anterior proprius and f. lateralis proprius. See fasciculi proprii.
Foville's f., *stria* terminalis.
fronto-occipital f., f. occipitofrontalis.
f. grac'ilis [NA], slender f.; column or tract of Goll; funiculus gracilis; the smaller medial subdivision of the funiculus posterior.
hooked f., f. uncinatus.
inferior longitudinal f., f. longitudinalis inferior.
interfascicular f., f. semilunaris.
f. interfascicula'ris [NA], official alternative term for f. semilunaris.
intersegmental fasciculi, fasciculi proprii.
f. latera'lis plex'us brachia'lis [NA], lateral cord of the brachial plexus; in the brachial plexus, the bundle of nerve fibers formed by the anterior divisions of the superior and middle trunks, this cord gives off the lateral pectoral nerve and terminates by dividing into the musculocutaneous nerve and the lateral root of the median nerve.
f. latera'lis pro'prius, lateral ground bundle. See fasciculi proprii.
f. lenticula'ris, see *ansa* lenticularis.
Lissauer's f., f. dorsolateralis.
f. longitudina'lis dorsa'lis [NA], dorsal longitudinal f.; Schütz' bundle; tract of Schütz; a bundle of thin, poorly myelinated nerve fibers reciprocally connecting the periventricular zone of the hypothalamus with ventral parts of the central gray substance of the midbrain.
f. longitudina'lis infe'rior [NA], inferior longitudinal f.; a well marked bundle of long association fibers running the whole length of the occipital and temporal lobes of the cerebrum, in part parallel with the inferior horn of the lateral ventricle.
f. longitudina'lis media'lis [NA], medial longitudinal f.; posterior longitudinal bundle; Collier's tract; a longitudinal bundle of fibers extending from the upper border of the mesencephalon into the cervical segments of the spinal cord, located close to the midline and ventral to the central gray matter; it is composed largely of fibers from the vestibular nuclei ascending to the motor neurons innervating the external eye muscles (abducens, trochlear, and oculomotor nuclei), and descending to spinal cord segments innervating the musculature of the neck.
fascic'uli longitudina'les pon'tis, longitudinal pontine bundles; the massive bundles of corticofugal fibers passing longitudinally through the pars ventralis pontis; they are composed of corticopontine, corticobulbar, and corticospinal fibers.
f. longitudina'lis supe'rior [NA], superior longitudinal f.; arcuate f. (1); long association fiber bundle lateral to the centrum ovale of the cerebral hemisphere, connecting the frontal, occipital, and temporal lobes; the fibers pass from the frontal lobe through the operculum to the posterior end of the lateral sulcus where many fibers radiate into the occipital lobe and others turn downward and for-

ward around the putamen and pass to anterior portions of the temporal lobe.
f. macula'ris, the collection of fibers in the optic nerve directly connected with the macula lutea.
mamillotegmental f., f. mamillotegmentalis.
f. mamillotegmenta'lis [NA], mamillotegmental f.; a small bundle of fibers that passes dorsalward from the mamillary body for a short distance with the mamillothalamic tract, then turns down the brainstem to reach the dorsal and ventral tegmental nuclei of the mesencephalon.
mamillothalamic f., f. mamillothalamicus.
f. mamillothalam'icus [NA], mamillothalamic tract or f.; f. thalamomamillaris; bundle of Vicq d'Azyr; a compact, thick bundle of nerve fibers that passes dorsalward from the mamillary body on either side to terminate in the anterior nucleus of the thalamus.
f. margina'lis, *fasciculus* dorsolateralis.
f. media'lis plex'us brachia'lis [NA], medial cord of the brachial plexus; in the brachial plexus, the bundle of nerve fibers formed by the anterior division of the inferior trunk, it gives off the medial pectoral nerve, the medial brachial cutaneous, medial antebrachial cutaneous, ulnar, and the medial root of the median nerves.
medial longitudinal f., f. longitudinalis medialis.
Meynert's f., f. retroflexus.
f. obli'quus pon'tis, oblique bundle of the pons; a bundle of fibers in the ventral surface of the pons running from the anterior mesial portion outward and backward.
occipitofrontal f., f. occipitofrontalis.
f. occip'itofronta'lis, occipitofrontal f.; fronto-occipital f.; a bundle of association fibers extending from the frontal to the occipital lobes of the cerebrum.
oval f., see f. semilunaris.
f. pedun'culomamilla'ris, *pedunculus* corporis mamillaris.
perpendicular f., a bundle of association fibers running vertically and interconnecting regions of the temporal, occipital, and parietal lobes.
f. poste'rior plex'us brachia'lis [NA], posterior cord of the brachial plexus; in the brachial plexus, the bundle of nerve fibers formed by the posterior divisions of the upper, middle and lower trunks, it gives rise to the subscapular, thoracodorsal, axillary, and radial nerves.
proper fasciculi, fasciculi proprii.
fascic'uli pro'prii [NA], proper fasciculi; ground bundles; Flechsig's fasciculi or ground bundles (f. anterior proprius and f. lateralis proprius); intersegmental fasciculi; ascending and descending association fiber systems of the spinal cord which lie deep in the anterior, lateral, and posterior funiculi adjacent to the gray matter.
f. pyramida'lis ante'rior, *tractus* pyramidalis anterior.
f. pyramida'lis latera'lis, *tractus* pyramidalis lateralis.
retroflex f., f. retroflexus.
f. retroflex'us [NA], retroflex f.; Meynert's f. or retroflex bundle; habenulointerpeduncular tract; tractus habenulopeduncularis; a compact bundle of fibers arising in the habenula and passing ventralward to the interpeduncular nucleus at the base of the midbrain; part of its fibers bypass this nucleus and terminate in the raphe nuclei of the caudal mesencephalic tegmentum.
f. rotun'dus, *tractus* solitarius.
fasciculi rubroreticula'res [NA], bundles of fibers that connect the red nucleus to the pontine and midbrain reticular nuclei.
semilunar f., f. semilunaris.
f. semiluna'ris [NA], f. interfascicularis; semilunar or interfascicular f.; comma bundle or comma tract of Schultze; a compact bundle composed of descending branches of posterior root fibers located near the border between the fasciculi gracilis and cuneatus of the cervical and thoracic spinal cord; it corresponds to the septomarginal f., Hoche's tract, or oval area of Flechsig in the lumbar, and to the triangle of Philippe-Gombault in the sacral spinal segments; like these, it can be demonstrated only in cases of demyelination resulting from dorsal root lesions.
septomarginal f., f. septomarginalis. See f. semilunaris.
f. septomargina'lis [NA], septomarginal f. or tract. See f. semilunaris.
slender f., f. gracilis.
f. solita'rius, *tractus* solitarius.
subcallosal f., f. subcallosus.
f. subcallo'sus [NA], subcallosal f.; a bundle of thin nerve fibers running longitudinally beneath the corpus callosum in the angle between the latter and the caudate nucleus; it forms an anterior continuation of the tapetum of the temporal lobe and appears to consist largely of fibers projecting from the cerebral cortex to the caudate nucleus.
superior longitudinal f., f. longitudinalis superior.
f. thalam'icus, see *fields* of Forel.
f. thal'amomamilla'ris, f. mamillothalamicus.
transverse fasciculi, fasciculi transversi.
fascic'uli transver'si [NA], transverse fasciculi; the transversely directed fibers in the distal portions of the palmar and plantar aponeuroses.
unciform f., uncinate f., f. uncinatus.
uncinate f. of Russell, uncinate *bundle* of Russell.
f. uncina'tus [NA], uncinate, unciform, or hooked f.; arcuate f. (2); frontotemporal or temporofrontal tract; a band of long association fibers reciprocally connecting the frontal and temporal lobes of the cerebrum, running caudally through the white matter of the frontal lobe, sharply curving ventrally under the stem of the sylvian fissure, and then fanning out to the cortex of the anterior half of the superior and middle temporal gyri.
wedge-shaped f., f. cuneatus.

fasciectomy (fash-ē-ek'tō-mē) [fascia + G. *ektomē,* excision]. Excision of strips of fascia.

fasciitis (fas-ē-ī'tis, fash-). Fascitis. **1.** Inflammation in fascia. **2.** Reactive proliferation of fibroblasts in fascia.
eosinophilic f., Shulman's syndrome; induration and edema of the connective tissues of the extremities, usually appearing following exertion; associated with elevated sedimentation rate, elevated IgG, and eosinophilia.
necrotizing f., a rare soft-tissue infection primarily involving the superficial fascia and resulting in extensive undermining of surrounding tissues; progress is often fulminant and may involve all soft-tissue components, including the skin; usually occurs postoperatively, after minor trauma, or after inadequate care of abscesses or cutaneous ulcers.
nodular f., pseudosarcomatous f.; a rapidly-growing tumor-like proliferation of fibroblasts, not thought to be neoplastic, with mild inflammatory exudation occurring in fascia; the fibrosis may infiltrate surrounding tissue but does not progress indefinitely or metastasize.
parosteal f., a rare form of nodular f. arising from the periosteum, and which may be associated with reactive cortical bone formation.
proliferative f., a benign rapidly-growing subcutaneous nodule characterized by proliferation of fibroblasts and basophilic giant cells slightly resembling ganglion cells.
pseudosarcomatous f., nodular f.

fascio- [L. *fascia,* a band or fillet]. Combining form denoting a fascia.

fasciodesis (fas-ē-od'ĕ-sis, fas-) [fascio- + G. *desis,* a binding together]. Surgical attachment of a fascia to another fascia or a tendon.

Fasciola (fa-sē'ō-lă, fa-sī'ō-lă) [L. dim. of *fascia,* a band]. A genus of large, leaf-shaped, digenetic liver flukes (family Fasciolidae, class Trematoda) of mammals.
F. gigan'tica, a species, resembling *F. hepatica* but of larger size,

found in herbivores, especially in Africa.

F. hepat'ica, the liver or sheep liver fluke, the common liver fluke inhabiting the bile ducts of sheep and cattle; the intermediate hosts are aquatic snails, *Lymnaea* or related genera; after the cercariae escape, they become encysted on watercress, lettuce, and other water plants by which they gain access to the intestinal canal; rarely, this fluke is reported from humans, in whom it may cause considerable biliary damage.

fasciola, pl. fasciolae (fa-sē'ō-lă, fa-sī'ō-lă; -ō-lē) [L. dim. of *fascia,* band, fillet]. A small band or group of fibers.

f. cine'rea, *gyrus* fasciolaris.

fasciolar (fa-sē'ō-lăr, fa-sī'). Relating to the gyrus fasciolaris.

fascioliasis (fas'ē-ō-lī'ă-sis, fa-sī'ō-lī'ă-sis). Infection with a species of *Fasciola.*

fasciolid (fa-sē'ō-lid, fa-sī'). A member of the family Fasiolidae.

Fascioloides magna (fas'ē-ō-loy'dēz mag'nă, fa-sī'o-). A species of fasciolid flukes found in the lungs and liver of deer and sometimes cattle in North America; it is not known to infect man.

fasciolopsiasis (fas'ē-ō-lop-sī'ă-sis, fa-sī'o-). Parasitization by any of the flukes of the genus *Fasciolopsis.*

Fasciolopsis (fas'ē-ō-lop'sis, fa-sī'ō-) [*Fasciola* + G. *opsis,* form, appearance]. A genus of very large intestinal fasciolid flukes.

F. bus'ki, the large intestinal fluke, a species found in the intestine of humans in eastern and southern Asia; transmitted via ingestion of water chestnuts or other vegetation contaminated with infective metacercariae.

F. rathoui'si, a species reported from China in a few cases in the intestine or liver; possibly the same as *F. buski.*

fascioplasty (fash'ē-ō-plas-tē). Plastic surgery of a fascia.

fasciorrhaphy (fash-ē-ōr'ă-fē) [fascio- + G. *raphē,* suture]. Aponeurorrhaphy; suture of a fascia or aponeurosis.

fasciotomy (fash-ē-ot'ō-mē) [fascio- + G. *tomē,* incision]. Incision through a fascia; used in the treatment of certain vascular disorders and injuries when marked swelling is anticipated which could compromise blood flow; f. is often combined with embolectomy in the treatment of acute arterial embolism.

fascitis (fa-sī'tis). Fasciitis.

fast [A.S. *foest,* firm, fixed]. Durable; resistant to change; applied to stained microorganisms which cannot be decolorized. See also acid-fast.

fast green FCF [C.I. 42053]. An acid arylmethane dye widely used in histology and cytology and less subject to fading than light green FCF which it has replaced in many procedures; used as a quantitative cytochemical stain for histones at alkaline pH after acid extraction of DNA, and also in electrophoresis as a protein stain.

fastidious (fas-tid'ē-ŭs). In bacteriology, having complex nutritional requirements.

fastidium cibi (fas-tid'ē-ŭm kib'ī) [L.]. Rarely used term for fickle or finicky appetite, caused by distaste for food.

fastigatum (fas-ti-gā'tŭm) [L. *fastigatus,* pointed]. *Nucleus* fastigii.

fastigium (fas-tij'ē-ŭm) [L. top, as of a gable; a pointed extremity]. **1.** Apex of the roof of the fourth ventricle of the brain, an angle formed by the anterior and posterior medullary vela extending into the substance of the vermis. **2.** The acme or period of full development of a disease.

fastness (fast'nes). The state of tolerance exhibited by bacteria to a drug or other agent. See fast.

fat [A.S. *faet*]. **1.** Adipose *tissue.* **2.** Obese; corpulent. **3.** A greasy, soft-solid material, found in animal tissues and many plants, composed of a mixture of glycerol esters; together with oils they comprise the homolipids.

brown f., hibernating or interscapular gland; interscapular hibernoma; multilocular f. or adipose tissue; thermogenic tissue that is composed of cells containing numerous small fat droplets; lobular masses are found in the interscapular and mediastinal regions and other locations; although found most frequently in certain hibernating animals, it is also found in pigs, rodents, and the newborn of man.

caul f., the f. contained in the caul.

multilocular f., brown f.

neutral f., a triester of fatty acids and glycerol.

saturated f., see saturated *fatty acid.*

split f., free fatty acids, as reduced by the action of lipases, neutral fats, or phospholipids.

unilocular f., white fat (2); adipose tissue in which the fat is present in a single droplet within the fat cells.

unsaturated f., see unsaturated *fatty acid.*

white f., **(1)** adipose *tissue;* **(2)** unilocular f.

fatal (fā'tăl) [L. *fatalis,* of or belonging to fate]. Pertaining to or causing death; denoting especially inevitability or inescapability of death.

fatality (fā-tal'i-tē). **1.** A condition, disease, or disaster ending in death. **2.** An individual instance of death.

fatigability (fat'i-gă-bil'i-tē). A condition in which fatigue is easily induced.

fatigable (fat'i-gă-bl) [L. *fatigabilis,* easily tired, fr. *fatigo,* to tire]. Tiring on very slight exertion.

fatigue (fă-tēg') [Fr., fr. L. *fatigo,* to tire]. **1.** That state, following a period of mental or bodily activity, characterized by a lessened capacity for work and reduced efficiency of accomplishment, usually accompanied by a feeling of weariness, sleepiness, or irritability; may also supervene when, from any cause, energy expenditure outstrips restorative processes and may be confined to a single organ. **2.** Sensation of boredom and lassitude due to absence of stimulation, monotony, or lack of interest in one's surroundings.

auditory f., temporary shift of threshold sensitivity following exposure to sound.

battle f., shell shock; a term used to denote psychiatric illness consequent to the stresses of battle. See also war *neurosis.*

functional vocal f., phonasthenia.

fat-pad. An accumulation of somewhat encapsulated adipose tissue.

Bichat's f.-p., *corpus* adiposum buccae.

Imlach's f.-p., fat surrounding the round ligament of the uterus in the inguinal canal.

fatty (fat'ē). Oily or greasy; relating in any sense to fat.

fatty acid. Any acid derived from fats by hydrolysis (*e.g.,* oleic, palmitic, or stearic acids); any long-chain monobasic organic acid.

diethenoid f. a., a f. a. containing two double bonds, *e.g.,* linoleic acid.

saturated f. a., a f. a., the carbon chain of which contains no ethylenic or other unsaturated linkages between carbon atoms (*e.g.,* stearic acid and palmitic acid); called saturated because it is incapable of absorbing any more hydrogen.

f. a. thiokinase, **(1)** long chain: long-chain fatty acid–CoA ligase; **(2)** medium chain: butyrate-CoA ligase.

unsaturated f. a., a f. a., the carbon chain of which possesses one or more double or triple bonds (*e.g.,* oleic acid, with one double bond in the molecule, and linoleic acid, with two); called unsaturated because it is capable of absorbing additional hydrogen.

fauces, gen. faucium (faw'sēz, faw'sē-ŭm) [L. the throat] [NA]. The space between the cavity of the mouth and the pharynx.

faucial (faw'shăl). Relating to the fauces.

faucitis (faw-sī'tis). Inflammation of the fauces.

fauna (faw'nă) [Mod. L. application of *Fauna,* sister of *Faunus,* a rural deity]. The animal forms of a continent, district, locality, or habitat.

faveolate (fā-vē′ō-lāt). Pitted.

faveolus, pl. **faveoli** (fā-vē′ō-lŭs, -ō-lī) [Mod. L. dim. of *favus,* honeycomb]. A small pit or depression.

favic chandeliers (fā′vik shan-dĕ-lērz′). Specialized fungal hyphae that are curved, branched, and antler-like in appearance, formed by the pathogens *Trichophyton schoenleinii* and *T. concentricum.*

favid (fā′vid). An allergic reaction in the skin observed in patients who have favus.

favism (fā′vizm) [Ital. *favismo,* from *fava,* bean]. Fabism; an acute condition seen chiefly in Italy, following the ingestion of certain species of beans, *e.g., Vicia faba,* or inhalation of the pollen of its flower; characterized by fever, headache, abdominal pain, severe anemia, prostration, and coma; it occurs in certain individuals with genetic erythrocytic deficiency of glucose 6-phosphate dehydrogenase.

Favre, Maurice, French physician, 1876–1954. See Gamna-F. *bodies;* Nicolas-F. *disease.*

Favre's dystrophy. See under dystrophy.

favus (fā′vŭs, fah′vŭs) [L. honeycomb]. Tinea favosa; porrigo scutulata, favosa, or lupinosa; crusted or honeycomb ringworm; honeycomb tetter; a severe type of chronic ringworm of the scalp and nails caused by three dissimilar dermatophytes, *Trichophyton schoenleinii, T. violaceum,* and *Microsporum gypseum;* it occurs more frequently in the Mediterranean countries, southeastern Europe, southern Asia, northern Africa, and the Orient. Differences in severity are related to hygiene.

Fc See Fc *fragment.*

F.C.A.P. Abbreviation for Fellow of the College of American Pathologists.

FDA Abbreviation for Food and Drug Administration of the United States Department of Health and Human Services.

FDNB Abbreviation for fluoro-2,4-dinitrobenzene.

FDP Abbreviation for fibrin/fibrinogen degradation *products.*

Fe [L. *ferrum,* iron] Symbol for iron.

fear (fēr) [A.S. *faer*]. Apprehension; dread; alarm; by having an identifiable stimulus, f. is differentiated from anxiety which has no easily identifiable stimulus.

features (fē′chūrz) [through Old Fr., fr. L. *factura,* a making, fr. *facio,* to do]. The various parts of the face, forehead, eyes, nose, mouth, chin, cheeks, and ears, that give to it its individuality and character.

febricant (feb′ri-kant). Febrifacient.

febricula (fē-brik′yū-lă) [L. dim. of *febris,* fever]. A simple continued fever; a mild fever of short duration, of indefinite origin, and without any distinctive pathology.

febrifacient (feb-ri-fā′shĕnt) [L. *febris,* fever, + *facio,* to make]. Febricant. **1.** Febrific; febriferous; causing or favoring the development of fever. **2.** Anything that produces fever. See also pyrogenic.

febriferous (fē-brif′er-ŭs) [L. *febris,* fever, + *fero,* to bear, + *-ous*]. Febrifacient (1).

febrific (fē-brif′ik). Febrifacient (1).

febrifugal (fē-brif′yū-găl). Antipyretic (1).

febrifuge (feb′ri-fyūj) [L. *febris,* fever, + *fugo,* to put to flight]. Antipyretic (2).

febrile (feb′ril, fē′bril). Feverish (1); pyretic; pyrectic; denoting or relating to fever.

febris (fē′bris) [L.]. Fever.

fecal (fē′kăl). Relating to feces.

fecalith (fē′kă-lith) [L. *faeces,* feces, + G. *lithos,* stone]. Coprolith.

fecaloid (fē′kă-loyd) [L. *faeces,* feces, + G. *eidos,* resemblance]. Resembling feces.

fecaloma (fē′kă-lō-mă). Coproma.

fecaluria (fē-kă-lū′rē-ă) [L. *faeces,* feces, + G. *ouron,* urine]. The commingling of feces with urine passed from the urethra in persons with a fistula connecting the intestinal tract and bladder, often noticed most dramatically by the passage of flatus through the urethra.

feces (fē′sēz) [L., pl. of *faex (faec-),* dregs]. Stercus; the matter discharged from the bowel during defecation, consisting of the undigested residue of the food, epithelium, the intestinal mucus, bacteria, and waste material from the food.

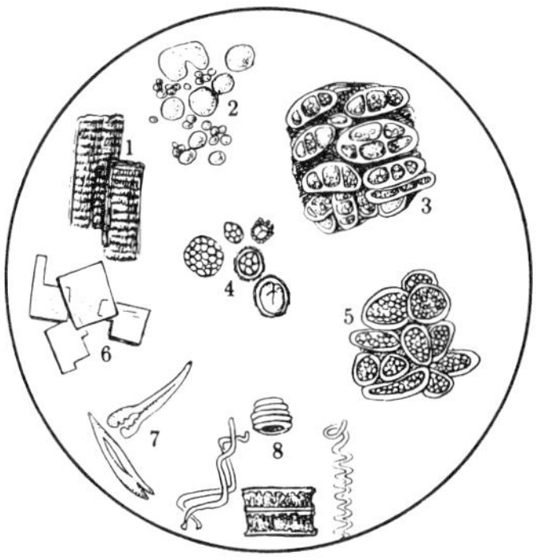

Feces

Microscopic appearance of common objects in the feces; original magnification ×800. *1,* Muscle fibers (meat); *2,* casein and fat droplets; *3,* portions of cereal husks; *4,* spores of fung; *5,* endosperm of rice; *6,* cholesterol crystals; *7,* hairs of wheat grain; *8,* vegetable spirals.

Fechner, Gustav T., German physicist, 1801–1887. See Weber-F. *law;* F.-Weber *law.*

feculent (fek′yū-lent). Excrementitious; fecal; foul.

fecund (fē′kŭnd, fek′ŭnd) [L. *fecundus,* fruitful]. Fertile (1).

fecundate (fē′kŭn-dāt) [L. *fecundo,* pp. *-atus,* to make fruitful, fertilize]. To impregnate; to make fertile.

fecundation (fē-kŭn-dā′shŭn). The act of rendering fertile. See also fertilization, impregnation.

fecundity (fē-kŭn′di-tē). Pronounced fertility; capability of repeated fertilization.

Fede, Francesco, Italian physician, 1832–1913. See Riga-F. *disease.*

feedback (fēd′bak). **1.** In a given system, the return, as input, of some of the output, as a regulatory mechanism; *e.g.,* regulation of a furnace by a thermostat. **2.** An explanation for the learning of motor skills: sensory stimuli set up by muscle contractions modulate the activity of the motor system. **3.** The feeling evoked by another person's reaction to oneself.

negative f., that which occurs if the sign or sense of the returned signal results in reduced amplification.

positive f., that which occurs when the sign or sense of the returned signal results in increased amplification or leads to instability.

feeding (fēd′ing). Giving food or nourishment.

fictitious f., sham f.

forced f., forcible f., forced alimentation; **(1)** giving liquid food through a nasal tube passed into the stomach; **(2)** forcing a person to eat more food than he desires.

gastric f., giving of nutriment directly into the stomach by means of a tube which may be inserted via the nasopharynx and esophagus or directly through the abdominal wall.

nasal f., the giving of nourishment through a flexible rubber tube passed through the nasal passages into the stomach.

sham f., fictitious f.; a procedure used in the study of the psychic phase of gastric secretion: in experiments on dogs, the food, after being eaten, does not enter the stomach but issues from an esophageal fistula made in the neck; the chewing and swallowing of food causes an abundant secretion of gastric juice.

feeling (fēl'ing). **1.** Any kind of conscious experience of sensation. **2.** The mental perception of a sensory stimulus. **3.** A quality of any mental state, whereby it is recognized as pleasurable or the reverse.

Feer, Emil, Swiss pediatrician, 1864–1955. See F.'s *disease.*

FEF Abbreviation for forced expiratory *flow.*

Fehling, Hermann von, German chemist, 1812–1885. See F.'s *reagent, solution.*

Feil, André, French physician, *1884. See Klippel-F. *syndrome.*

Feiss, Henry O., 20th century American orthopedic surgeon. See F. *line.*

Feldberg, Wilhelm, British physiologist, *1900. See Dale-F. *law.*

Feldman, Harry Alfred, U.S. epidemiologist, *1914. See Sabin-F. dye *test.*

Felidae (fē'li-dē) [L. *felis,* cat]. A family of carnivora embracing the cats, tigers, lions, etc.

feline (fē'līn) [L. *felis,* cat]. Pertaining or relating to cats.

Felix, Arthur, Polish bacteriologist, 1887–1956. See Weil-F. *reaction, test.*

fellatio (fĕ-lā'shē-ō) [L.]. Fellation; fellatorism; irrumation; oral stimulation of the penis; a type of oral-genital sexual activity.

fellation (fĕ-lā'shŭn). Fellatio.

fellatorism (fel'ă-tōr-izm). Fellatio.

fellatrix (fel-ă-triks'). A female who takes the oral part in fellatio.

felon (fel'ŏn) [M.E. *feloun,* malignant]. Whitlow; a purulent infection or abscess involving the bulbous distal end of a finger.

felt'work. 1. A fibrous network. **2.** A close plexus of nerve fibrils. See neuropile.

Felty, Augustus R., U.S. physician, *1895. See F.'s *syndrome.*

FeLV Abbreviation for feline leukemia *virus.*

felypressin (fel-i-pres'in). Octapressin; [Phe^2,Lys^8]vasopressin; lysine vasopressin with phenylalanine at position 2.

female (fē'māl). In zoology, denoting the sex that bears the young or the sexual cell which develops into a new organism.

genetic f., **(1)** an individual with a normal female karyotype, including two X chromosomes; **(2)** an individual whose cell nuclei contain Barr sex chromatin bodies, which are normally present in f.'s and absent in males; patients with ambiguous sexual development or Turner's syndrome are classed as genetic males or genetic f.'s by absence or presence of Barr bodies even though their sex chromosome complement may be abnormal.

XO f., the genetic f. in Turner's syndrome.

XXX f., see triple X *syndrome.*

feminization (fem'i-ni-zā'shŭn). Development of female characteristics by a male.

testicular f., see testicular feminization *syndrome.*

femoral (fem'ŏ-răl). Relating to the femur or thigh.

femorocele (fem'ŏ-rō-sēl) [L. *femur,* thigh, + G. *kēlē,* hernia]. Femoral *hernia.*

femorotibial (fem'ŏ-rō-tib'ē-ăl). Relating to the femur and the tibia.

femto- (f) [Danish *femten,* fifteen]. Prefix used in the SI and metric systems to signify one-quadrillionth (10^{-15}).

femur, gen. **femoris,** pl. **femora** (fē'mŭr, fem'ŏ-ris, -ă) [L. thigh] [NA]. **1.** The thigh. **2.** *Os femoris.*

fencamine (fen'kă-mēn). 8-({2-[Methyl(α-methylphenethyl) amino]ethyl}amino)caffeine; a central nervous system stimulant.

fenclonine (fen'klō-nēn). DL-3-(*p*-Chlorophenyl)alanine; a serotonin inhibitor.

Fendt, H., 19th century Austrian dermatologist. See Spiegler-F. *pseudolymphoma, sarcoid.*

fenestra, pl. **fenestrae** (fe-nes'tră, -trē) [L. window]. **1** [NA]. An anatomical aperture, often closed by a membrane. **2.** An opening left in a plaster of Paris or other form of fixed dressing in order to permit access to a wound or inspection of the part. **3.** The opening in one of the blades of an obstetrical forceps. **4.** A lateral opening in the sheath of an endoscopic instrument that allows lateral viewing or operative maneuvering through the sheath. **5.** Openings in the wall of a tube, catheter, or trocar designed to promote better flow of air or fluids.

f. of the cochlea, f. cochleae.

f. coch'leae [NA], f. of the cochlea; f. rotunda; cochlear or round window; an opening on the medial wall of the middle ear leading into the cochlea, closed in life by the secondary tympanic membrane.

f. nov-ova'lis, artificial opening through the otic capsule of the lateral semicircular canal, connecting the membranous labyrinth with the mastoid cavity produced during fenestration surgery.

f. ova'lis, f. vestibuli.

f. rotun'da, f. cochleae.

f. of the vestibule, f. vestibuli.

f. vestib'uli [NA], f. of the vestibule; f. ovalis; oval or vestibular window; an oval opening on the medial wall of the tympanic cavity leading into the vestibule, closed in life by the foot of the stapes.

fenestrated (fen'es-trā'ted). Having fenestrae or window-like openings.

fenestration (fen-es-trā'shŭn). **1.** The presence of openings or fenestrae in a part. **2.** Making openings in a dressing to allow inspection of the parts. **3.** In dentistry, a surgical perforation of the mucoperiosteum and alveolar process to expose the root tip of a tooth to permit drainage of tissue exudate.

tracheal f., a surgical procedure to create an epithelialized mucocutaneous opening from the neck into the trachea.

fenethylline hydrochloride (fen-eth'ĭ-lēn). 7-{2-[(α-Methylphenethyl)amino]ethyl}theophylline hydrochloride; an analeptic.

fenfluramine hydrochloride (fen-flū'ră-mēn). *N*-Ethyl-α-methyl-*m*-(trifluoromethyl)phenethylamine hydrochloride; an anorexigenic agent.

Fenn, Wallace Osgood, U.S. physiologist, 1893–1971. See F. *effect.*

fennel (fen'l) [through Old Fr., fr. L. *faeniculum,* fennel, dim. of *faenum,* hay]. Fennel seed, the dried ripe fruit of cultivated varieties of *Foeniculum vulgare* (family Umbelliferae), an herb native to southern Europe and Asia, used as a diaphoretic and carminative; a volatile oil distilled from the fruit is used as a flavoring.

fenoprofen calcium (fen-ō-prō'fen). Calcium (±)-*m*-phenoxyhydratropate dihydrate; an anti-inflammatory analgesic used in the treatment of rheumatoid arthritis.

fenpipramide (fen-pip'ră-mīd). α,α-Diphenyl-1-piperidinebutyramide; an antispasmodic.

fentanyl citrate (fen'tă-nil). *N*-(1-Phenethyl-4-piperidyl)propionanilide citrate; a narcotic analgesic used as a supplementary analgesic in general anesthesia.

fenticlor (fen'ti-klōr). 2,2'-Thiobis[4-chlorophenol]; a topical anti-infective agent.

fenugreek (fen'yū-grēk) [L. *faenum graecum,* fenugreek, fr. *faenum,* hay, + *Graecus,* Greek]. *Trigonella faenumgraecum* (family Leguminosae); an annual plant indigenous to western Asia and cultivated in Africa and parts of Europe; the mucilaginous seeds are used as food and in the preparation of culinary spices (curry).

Fenwick, Edwin Hurry, British urologist, 1856–1944. See F.-Hunner *ulcer.*

Fenwick, Samuel, British physician, 1821–1902. See F.'s *disease.*

Féréol, Louis H.F., Paris physician, 1825–1891. See F.-Graux *palsy.*

Fergusson, Sir William, British surgeon, 1808–1877. See F.'s *incision.*

ferment (fer-ment'). To cause or to undergo fermentation.

ferment (fer'ment) [L. *fermentum,* leaven]. Obsolete term for enzyme.

fermentable (fer-ment'ă-bl). Capable of undergoing fermentation.

fermentation (fer-men-tā'shŭn) [L. *fermento,* pp. *-atus,* to ferment]. **1.** A chemical change induced in a complex organic compound by the action of an enzyme, whereby the substance is split into simpler compounds. **2.** In bacteriology, the anaerobic dissimilation of substrates with the production of energy and reduced compounds; the mechanism of f. does not involve a respiratory chain or cytochrome, hence oxygen is not the final electron acceptor as it is in oxidation.

acetic f., acetous f., f., as of wine or beer, whereby the alcohol is oxidized to acetic acid (vinegar).

amylic f., f. of potato or corn mash, or other starchy material, by which fusel oil is produced.

lactic acid f., the production of lactic acid in milk, or other carbohydrate-containing media, caused by the presence of any one of a number of lactic acid bacteria.

fermentative (fer-ment'ă-tiv). Causing or having the ability to cause fermentation.

fermium (fer'mē-ŭm) [E. *Fermi,* It. physicist in U.S., 1901–1954]. Radioactive element, artificially prepared in 1955, atomic symbol Fm, atomic no. 100.

Fernandez reaction. See under reaction.

Fernbach, Auguste, French microbiologist, 1860–1939. See F. *flask.*

fern'ing. A term used to describe the pattern of arborization produced by cervical mucus, secreted at midcycle, upon crystallization, which resembles somewhat a fern or a palm leaf.

ferratin (fer'ă-tin). Sodium iron albuminate; a hematinic.

ferredoxins (fer-ĕ-dok'sinz). Proteins containing iron and (labile) sulfur in equal amounts, displaying electron-carrier activity but no classical enzyme function; differentiated from rubredoxins but, generally, not from high potential iron-sulfur proteins. F.'s are found in green plants, algae, and anaerobic bacteria, and are involved in several oxidation-reduction reactions in living organisms (*e.g.,* nitrogen fixation).

Ferrein, Antoine, French anatomist, 1693–1769. See F.'s *canal, cords, foramen, ligament, pyramid, tube, vasa* aberrantia hepatis; *processus* ferreini.

ferri- [L. *ferrum,* iron]. Prefix designating the presence of a ferric ion in a compound.

ferric (fer'ik). Relating to iron, especially denoting a salt containing iron in its higher (triad) valence, Fe^{3+}.

ferric ammonium citrate. Soluble ferric citrate; brown ferric ammonium citrate; a compound used in hypochromic anemia; it is relatively free of astringent and irritant action.

ferric ammonium citrate, green. A compound used in hypochromic anemia.

ferric ammonium sulfate. Iron alum; ferric alum; ammonium ferric sulfate; an astringent and styptic.

ferric chloride. Iron trichloride or perchloride; an astringent and styptic.

ferric citrate. A compound used in anemia.

ferric fructose. A potassium-iron-fructose used as a hematinic drug.

ferric glycerophosphate. A tonic and a source of iron.

ferric hydroxide. Hydrated iron oxide; a compound used, freshly prepared, as an antidote to arsenic poisoning.

ferric oxide. A compound used as a coloring material; red f. o. (together with yellow f. o.) is so used in preparations designed for application to the skin.

ferric phosphate. A compound used as a feed and as a food supplement.

soluble f. p., f. phosphate with sodium citrate; used for iron deficiency anemia.

ferric sodium edetate. See under edetate.

ferric sulfate. Iron persulfate, tersulfate, or sesquisulfate; an astringent and styptic.

ferricyanide (fe-rī-sī'ă-nīd, fer-ē-). The anion $Fe(CN)_6{}^{3-}$.

ferricytochrome (fe-rī-sī'tō-krōm, fer-ē-). A cytochrome containing oxidized (ferric) iron.

ferriheme (fe'rī-hēm, fer'ē-). Hematin.

f. chloride, hemin.

ferrihemoglobin (fer'ī-hē-mō-glō'bin, fer'ē-). Methemoglobin.

ferriporphyrin (fe-rī-pōr'fi-rin, fer-ē-). The compound formed between a ferric ion and a porphyrin; *e.g.,* ferriprotoporphyrin (hemin).

f. chloride, hemin.

ferriprotoporphyrin (fer'i-prō-tō-pōr'fi-rin, fer'ē-). Hemin.

ferritin (fer'ī-tin, fer'ē-). An iron protein complex, containing up to 23% iron, formed by the union of ferric iron with apoferritin; it is found in the intestinal mucosa, spleen, and liver, and regulates iron transport from the intestinal lumen to plasma.

ferro- [L. *ferrum,* iron]. Prefix designating the presence of metallic iron or of the divalent ion Fe^{2+}.

ferrochelatase (fār-ō-kē'lă-tās) [EC 4.9.9.1.1]. A lyase that catalyzes the acid hydrolysis of heme, forming protoporphyrin and free ferrous iron.

ferrocholinate (fār'ō-kō'li-nāt). Iron choline citrate chelate, used for oral administration in the treatment and prevention of iron deficiency anemias.

ferrocyanide (fār-ō-sī'ă-nīd). Ferrocyanogen; a compound containing the anion $Fe(CN)_6{}^{4-}$.

ferrocyanogen (fār'ō-sī-an'ō-jen). Ferrocyanide.

ferrocytochrome (fār-ō-sī'tō-krōm). A cytochrome containing reduced (ferrous) iron.

ferroheme (fār'ō-hēm). Heme.

ferrokinetics (fār-ō-ki-net'iks) [L. *ferrum,* iron, + G. *kinēsis,* movement]. The study of iron metabolism using radioactive iron.

ferroporphyrin (fār-ō-pōr'fi-rin). The compound formed between a ferrous ion and a porphyrin; *e.g.,* ferroprotoporphyrin (heme).

ferroproteins (fār-ō-prō'tēnz). Proteins containing iron in a prosthetic group; *e.g.,* heme, cytochrome.

ferroprotoporphyrin (fār'ō-prō-tō-pōr'fi-rin). Heme.

ferrosoferric (fār-ō'sō-fār'ik). Denoting a combination of a ferrous compound with a ferric compound, as in Fe_3O_4.

ferrotherapy (fār'ō-thār'ă-pē) [L. *ferrum,* iron]. Therapeutic use of iron.

ferrous (fār'ŭs) [L. *ferreus,* made of iron]. Relating to iron, especially denoting a salt containing iron in its lowest valence state, Fe^{2+}.

ferrous bromide. Iron bromide; a compound that has been used in the treatment of chorea.

ferrous citrate. A compound that occurs in several forms, two of which are monoferrous acid citrate monohydrate and triferrous dicitrate decahydrate; used in iron deficiency anemia. The radiopharmaceutical ferrous citrate, containing ^{59}Fe, is also used.

ferrous fumarate. Iron fumarate; a hematinic.

ferrous gluconate. A compound used in the treatment of anemia.

ferrous lactate. A relatively nonastringent chalybeate.

ferrous succinate. A compound used in the prevention and treatment of iron deficiency anemia.

ferrous sulfate. Iron sulfate; iron vitriol; a compound used in anemia; the commercial impure variety (copperas) is used as a deodorant and disinfectant.
dried f. s., exsiccated iron sulfate; a hematinic.

ferrugination (fe-rū'ji-nā'shŭn) [L. *ferrugo,* iron-rust]. Deposition of ferric salts in the walls of small blood vessels, typically within the basal ganglia and cerebellum.

ferruginous (fe-rū'ji-nŭs) [L. *ferrugineus,* iron rust, rust-colored]. **1.** Iron-bearing; associated with or containing iron. **2.** Of the color of iron rust.

ferrule (fer'ūl) [corrupted through O. Fr. and Medieval L., fr. L. *viriola,* a small bracelet]. A metal band or ring used around the crown or root of a tooth.

Ferry, Erwin S., U.S. physicist, 1868–1956. See F.-Porter *law.*

fertile (fer'til) [L. *fertilis,* fr. *fero,* to bear]. **1.** Fecund; fruitful; capable of conceiving and bearing young. **2.** Impregnated; fertilized.

fertility (fer-til'i-tē). The state of being fertile; specifically, the ability to produce young.

fertilization (fer'til-i-zā'shŭn). The process beginning with penetration of the secondary oocyte by the spermatozoon and completed by fusion of the male and female pronuclei.
in vitro f., a process whereby (usually multiple) ova, obtained by laparotomy, are placed in a medium to which sperm are added for fertilization, the zygote thus produced then being introduced into the uterus and allowed to develop to term; used both in laboratories and in human reproduction clinics.
in vivo f., f. of a ripe egg within the uterus of a fertile donor female (rather than in an artificial medium), for subsequent nonsurgical transfer to an infertile recipient.

fertilizin (fer-til'i-zin). An acid polysaccharide-amino acid complex associated with the female gamete membrane of several organisms; provides receptor groups that agglutinate sperm and bind them to ova.

Ferula (făr'ū-lă) [L. giant plant]. A genus of plants of the family Umbelliferae. *F. assa-foetida, F. rubricaulis* and *F. foetida* furnish asafetida; *F. galbaniflua* and *F. rubricaulis,* galbanium; and *F. sumbul,* sumbul.

fervescence (fer-ves'ens) [L. *fervesco,* to begin to boil, fr. *ferveo,* to boil]. An increase of fever.

fes'ter [L. *fistula*]. **1.** To ulcerate. **2.** An ulcer. **3.** To form pus or putrefy.

festinant (fes'ti-nant) [L. *festino,* to hasten]. Rapid; quick; hastening; accelerating.

festination (fes-ti-nā'shŭn) [L. *festino,* to hasten]. The peculiar acceleration of a shuffling gait noted in parkinsonism (1) and some other nervous affections.

festoon (fes-tūn') [thr. Fr. fr. L. *festum,* festival, hence festive decorations]. **1.** A carving in the base material of a denture that simulates the contours of the natural tissue that is being replaced by the denture. **2.** A distinguishing characteristic of certain hard tick species, consisting of small rectangular areas separated by grooves along the posterior margin of the dorsum of both males and females.
gingival f., an arcuate enlargement of the marginal gingiva.

festooning (fes-tūn'ing). Undulating, like the pattern of dermal papillae beneath a subepidermal blister.

FET Abbreviation for forced expiratory *time.*

fetal (fē'tăl). Relating to a fetus.

fetalism (fē'tăl-izm). Presence of certain fetal structures or characteristics in the body after birth.

fetal reticularis (fē'tăl re-tik-yū-lā'ris). Term sometimes used as a synonym for: **1.** Fetal (adrenal) *cortex.* **2.** Androgenic *zone* (2). **3.** X *zone* (2).

fetation (fē-tā'shŭn). Pregnancy.

feticide (fē'ti-sīd) [L. *fetus* + *caedo,* to kill]. Destruction of the embryo or fetus in the uterus.

fetid (fet'id, fē'tid) [L. *foetidus*]. Foul-smelling.

fetish (fet'ish, fē'tish) [Fr. *fétiche,* fr. L. *factitius,* made by art, artificial]. An inanimate object or nonsexual body part that is regarded as endowed with magic or erotic qualities.

fetishism (fet'ish-izm, fē'tish-). The act of worshipping or using for sexual arousal and gratification that which is regarded as a fetish.

fetlock (fet'lok). The metacarpophalangeal and metatarsophalangeal joints of ungulates; also the cushion-like caudal projection above the hoof of the horse and similar animals, and the tuft of hair in this region.

fetoglobulins (fē-tō-glob'yū-linz). Plasma globulins of unknown function. α-F. occurs in small amounts in normal adults and in larger amounts in the fetus, especially in the second trimester; elevated levels have been detected in adult patients with liver disease and neoplasms and in pregnant women.

fetography (fē-tog'ră-fē) [L. *fetus* + G. *graphō,* to write]. Radiography of the fetus *in utero,* using an oil-soluble medium. *Cf.* amniography.

fetology (fē-tol'ō-jē) [L. *fetus* + G. *logos,* study]. Fetal *medicine.*

fetometry (fē-tom'ĕ-trē) [L. *fetus* + G. *metron,* measure]. Estimation of the size of the fetus, especially of its head, prior to delivery.

fetopathy (fē-top'ă-thē) [L. *fetus* + G. *pathos,* suffering, disease]. Embryopathy.
diabetic f., f. resulting from maternal diabetes, which may cause macrosomia and fetal death.

fetoplacental (fē'tō-pla-sen'tăl). Relating to the fetus and its placenta.

fetoproteins (fē-tō-prō'tēnz). Fetal proteins found in small amounts in adults in the following forms: α**-f.** (AFP) increases in maternal blood during pregnancy and, when detected by amniocentesis, is an important indicator of open neural tube defects; β**-f.,** although a fetal liver protein, has been detected in adult patients with liver disease; γ**-f.** occurs in various neoplasms. See also fetoglobulins.

fetor (fē'tōr) [L. an offensive smell, fr. *feteo,* to stink]. A very offensive odor.
f. hepat'icus, a peculiar odor to the breath in persons with severe liver disease; caused by volatile aromatic substances that accumulate in the blood and urine due to defective hepatic metabolism.
f. o'ris, halitosis.

fetoscope (fē'tō-skōp). A fiberoptic endoscope used in fetology.

fetoscopy (fē-tos'kŏ-pē). Use of a fiberoptic endoscope to view the fetus and the fetal surface of the placenta transabdominally, and also for collection of fetal blood from the umbilical vein for antenatal diagnosis of fetal disorders.

fetotoxicity (fē'tō-tok-sis'i-tē). Injury to the fetus, that may result in death or retardation of growth or development, due to a substance that enters the maternal and placental circulation.

fetus, pl. **fetuses** (fē'tŭs, fē'tŭs-ez) [L. offspring]. **1.** The unborn young of a viviparous animal after it has taken form in the uterus. **2** [NA]. In man, the product of conception from the end of the eighth week to the moment of birth.
harlequin f., ichthyosis fetalis (1); a severe form of collodian baby in a newborn, usually premature, infant; *i.e.,* a form of ichthyosi-

form erythroderma characterized by encasement of the body in grayish brown, often fissured plaques resembling plates of armor, and by grotesque deformity of the face, hands, and feet; usually fatal within a few days.

impacted f., a f. which, because of its large size or narrowing of the pelvic canal, has become wedged and incapable of spontaneous advance or recession.

f. in fe'tu, condition in which a small imperfectly formed fetus is contained within a fetus.

f. papyra'ceus, one of twin f.'s that has died and been pressed flat against the uterine wall by the growth of the living f.

Feulgen, Robert, German nucleic acid biochemist and cytochemist, 1884–1955. First to detect DNA in cells by a specific cytochemical test.

FEV Abbreviation for forced expiratory *volume.*

FEVER

fever (fē'ver) [A.S. *fefer*]. Pyrexia; febris. **1.** A bodily temperature above the normal of 98.6°F (37°C). **2.** A disease in which there is an elevation of the body temperature above the normal.

absorption f., an elevation of temperature often occurring, without other untoward symptoms, shortly after childbirth, assumed to be due to absorption of uterine discharges through abrasions of the vaginal wall.

acclimating f., elevated temperature with malaise that occurs upon working in a very hot environment.

Aden f., dengue.

aestivoautumnal f., falciparum *malaria.*

African hemorrhagic f., hemorrhagic f. associated with the morphologically similar but antigenically distinct Marburg and Ebola viruses. See also viral hemorrhagic f.

African swine f. (ASF), a highly fatal disease of swine caused by African swine f. virus having its reservoir in wild wart hogs and bush pigs; it is characterized by high f., cough, diarrhea, and high mortality; clinically, it closely resembles hog cholera (swine f.), but the viruses of these diseases do not cross-immunize.

algid pernicious f., a pernicious malarial attack in which the patient presents symptoms of collapse and shock.

aphthous f., foot and mouth *disease.*

ardent f., heat apoplexy (2); a term sometimes applied to hyperpyrexia occurring in intermittent malarial f.

Argentinian hemorrhagic f., a form of hemorrhagic f. observed in South America, seemingly transmitted by contact from rodents to man and caused by the Junin virus.

aseptic f., f. accompanied by malaise due to absorption of dead but not infected tissue following an injury.

Assam f., visceral *leishmaniasis.*

autumn f., seven-day f.; **(1)** a f. resembling dengue occurring at the end of the summer in India; **(2)** hasamiyami.

biliary f. of dogs, a form of babesiosis (piroplasmosis) of the dog characterized by fever and icterus and caused by *Babesia canis.*

biliary f. of horses, equine *babesiosis.*

bilious remittent f., **(1)** old term for relapsing f.; **(2)** malarial "bilious" vomiting associated with marked increase of serum bilirubin in severe subtertian f.

black f., Rocky Mountain spotted f.

blackwater f., hemoglobinuria resulting from severe hemolysis occurring in falciparum malaria.

blue f., Rocky Mountain spotted f.

Bolivian hemorrhagic f., a disease similar to Argentinian hemorrhagic f. but caused by the Machupo virus.

bouquet f., dengue.

boutonneuse f., tick typhus in tropical and South Africa, and Asia, caused by *Rickettsia conori.*

bovine ephemeral f., ephemeral f. of cattle.

breakbone f., dengue.

bullous f., *pemphigus* acutus.

Bunyamwera f., a febrile illness of humans in Africa caused by the Bunyamwera virus and transmitted by culicine mosquitoes.

Burdwan f., visceral *leishmaniasis.*

Bwamba f., a febrile illness of humans in Africa caused by virus of the Bwamba serologic group and transmitted by mosquitoes.

cachectic f., visceral *leishmaniasis.*

camp f., typhus.

canefield f., field f.

canicola f., a disease of man caused by the *canicola* serovar of *Leptospira interrogans* and transmitted by infective urine, usually from dogs but rarely from cattle and swine.

Carter's f., an Asiatic relapsing f. caused by *Borrelia carteri.*

catarrhal f., old term for the group of diseases including the common cold, influenza, and lobular and lobar pneumonia.

cat-bite f., cat-bite *disease.*

catheter f., urinary f.

cat-scratch f., cat-scratch *disease.*

Central European tick-borne f., tick-borne *encephalitis* (Central European subtype).

cerebrospinal f., meningococcal *meningitis.*

Charcot's intermittent f., f., chills, right upper quadrant pain, and jaundice associated with intermittently obstructing common duct stones.

childbed f., puerperal f.

Colorado tick f., tick f. (5); an infection caused by Colorado tick f. virus and transmitted to humans by *Dermacentor andersoni;* the symptoms are mild, there is no rash, the temperature is not excessive, and the disease is rarely, if ever, fatal.

Congolian red f., murine *typhus.*

continued f., a f. of some duration in which there are no intermissions or marked remissions in the temperature.

cotton-mill f., byssinosis.

Crimean-Congo hemorrhagic f., a form of hemorrhagic f. distinct from Omsk hemorrhagic f., occurring in central Russia, transmitted by species of the tick *Hyalomma,* and caused by Crimean-Congo hemorrhagic fever virus; horses are the chief reservoir of human infection.

dandy f., dengue.

date f., dengue.

deer-fly f., tularemia.

deer hemorrhagic f., hemorrhagic disease of deer; a hemorrhagic disease of certain deer of the central and eastern United States, caused by an orbivirus and characterized by multiple hemorrhages, shock, and trauma; infection is thought to be arthropod-borne.

dehydration f., thirst f.

dengue f., dengue hemorrhagic f., dengue.

desert f., primary *coccidioidomycosis.*

digestive f., a slight rise of body temperature occurring during the period of digestion.

diphasic milk f., tick-borne *encephalitis* (Central European subtype).

double quotidian f., malaria in which two paroxysms of f. occur daily.

Dumdum f., visceral *leishmaniasis.*

Dutton's relapsing f., Dutton's *disease.*

East Coast f., a serious disease of cattle, chiefly in eastern Africa, caused by *Theileria parva parva* and characterized by high fever, swelling of the lymph nodes, and high case fatality; transmitted by *Rhipicephalus appendiculatus* and other ticks of the genus *Rhipicephalus.*

Ebola hemorrhagic f., viral hemorrhagic f.

elephantoid f., lymphangitis and an elevation of temperature marking the beginning of endemic elephantiasis (filariasis).
enteric f., **(1)** typhoid f.; **(2)** the group of typhoid and paratyphoid f.'s.
entericoid f., a f., neither paratyphoid nor typhoid, resembling the latter.
ephemeral f., a febrile episode lasting no more than a day or two.
ephemeral f. of cattle, bovine ephemeral f.; an acute febrile disease of cattle in many African and Asian countries and Australia, caused by a rhabdovirus and characterized by stiffness and lameness.
epidemic hemorrhagic f., hemorrhagic f. with renal syndrome; a condition characterized by acute onset of headache, chills and high f., sweating, thirst, photophobia, coryza, cough, myalgia, arthralgia, and abdominal pain with nausea and vomiting; this phase lasts from three to six days and is followed by capillary and renal interstitial hemorrhages, edema, oliguria, azotemia, and shock; most varieties are caused by arboviruses (togaviruses, arenaviruses, and possibly bunyaviruses), and are being rodent-borne.
epimastical f., a f. increasing steadily until its acme is reached, then declining by crisis or lysis.
equine biliary f., equine *babesiosis.*
eruptive f., tick *typhus.*
essential f., f. without known infectious disease.
exanthematous f., fever associated with an exanthem.
exsiccation f., thirst f.
falciparum f., falciparum *malaria.*
familial Mediterranean f., familial paroxysmal *polyserositis.*
famine f., relapsing f.
fatigue f., an elevation of the body temperature, lasting sometimes several days, following excessive and long continued muscular exertion.
field f., canefield f.; a leptospirosis caused by *leptospire.*
five-day f., trench f.
flood f., tsutsugamushi *disease.*
food f., a disorder seen primarily in childhood, consisting of a sudden rise of temperature accompanied by marked digestive disturbances, which lasts from a few days to several weeks; believed to be a form of food poisoning.
Fort Bragg f., pretibial f.
Gambian f., an irregular relapsing f., lasting one to four days with intermissions of two to five days, marked by enlargement of the spleen, frequent pulse, and rapid breathing; due to the presence in the blood of *Trypanosoma gambiense,* the pathogenic microorganism of Gambian or West African sleeping sickness.
glandular f., infectious *mononucleosis.*
Haverhill f. [*Haverhill,* MA, where an epidemic occurred in 1926], erythema arthriticum epidemicum; an infection by *Streptobacillus moniliformis* marked by initial chills and high f. (gradually subsiding), by arthritis usually in the larger joints and spine, and by a rash occurring chiefly over the joints and on the extensor surfaces of the extremities; "Haverhill f." is used to indicate *Streptobacillus moniliformis* infections not associated with rat bite, in contradistinction to rat-bite f.
hay f., autumnal catarrh; rhinitis nervosa; a form of atopy characterized by an acute irritative inflammation of the mucous membranes of the eyes and upper respiratory passages accompanied by itching and profuse watery secretion, followed occasionally by bronchitis and asthma; the episode recurs annually at the same or nearly the same time of the year, in spring, summer, or late summer and autumn, caused by an allergic reaction to the pollen of trees, grasses, weeds, flowers, etc.
hematuric bilious f., hematuria due to renal lesions caused by the malarial hematozoon, *Plasmodium falciparum.*
hemoglobinuric f., malarial *hemoglobinuria.*
hemorrhagic f., a syndrome that occurs in perhaps 20 to 40% of infections by arboviruses of the hemorrhagic f. group: alphaviruses, flaviviruses, bunyaviruses, and arenaviruses; some types of hemorrhagic f. are tick-borne, others mosquito-borne, and some seem to be zoonoses; clinical manifestations are high f., scattered petechiae, gastrointestinal tract and other organ bleeding, hypotension, and shock; kidney damage may be severe, especially in Korean hemorrhagic f., and neurologic signs may appear, especially in the Argentinian-Bolivian types. See also epidemic hemorrhagic f.
hemorrhagic f. with renal syndrome, epidemic hemorrhagic f.
hepatic intermittent f., ague-like paroxysms of f. occurring in cases of one or more stones in the common bile duct.
herpetic f., a disease of short duration, apparently infectious, marked by chills, nausea, elevation of temperature, sore throat, and a herpetic eruption on the face and other areas.
hospital f., classical epidemic typhus.
Ilhéus f., a febrile illness caused by the Ilhéus virus, an arborvirus (genus *Flavivirus*), and transmitted by a mosquito. See also Ilhéus *encephalitis.*
inanition f., thirst f.
intermittent malarial f., see intermittent *malaria.*
inundation f., tsutsugamushi *disease.*
island f., tsutsugamushi *disease.*
jail f., typhus.
Japanese river f., tsutsugamushi *disease.*
jungle f., malaria.
jungle yellow f., a form occurring in South America, transmitted by *Aedes leucocelaenus* and various treetop mosquitoes of the *Haemagogus* complex; transmitted normally to primates, occasionally by chance to man to set off a human outbreak of classical yellow fever transmitted by *Aedes aegypti.*
kedani f., tsutsugamushi *disease.*
Kew Gardens f. [*Kew Gardens,* area in Queens, NYC, where first reported], rickettsialpox.
Kinkiang f., *schistosomiasis* japonica.
Korean hemorrhagic f., Manchurian hemorrhagic f.; a form of epidemic hemorrhagic f. caused by the Hantaan virus.
Lassa (hemorrhagic) f., a severe form of epidemic hemorrhagic f. first recognized in Lassa, Nigeria, caused by Lassa virus, and characterized by high f., sore throat, severe muscle aches, skin rash with hemorrhages, headache, abdominal pain, vomiting, and diarrhea; the multimammate rat *Mastomys natalensis* serves as reservoir, but person-to-person transmission also is common.
laurel f., an affection of the same nature as hay f., occurring at the time of flowering of laurel.
low f., f. associated with psychological depression and dulling of mental processes.
malarial f., see malaria and subentries.
malignant catarrhal f., malignant catarrh of cattle; a highly fatal, sporadic disease of cattle caused by malignant catarrhal f. virus and characterized by inflammation, ulceration, and exudation of the oral and upper respiratory mucous membranes, and sometimes eye lesions and nervous system disturbances.
malignant tertian f., falciparum *malaria.*
Malta f., brucellosis.
Manchurian f., a f. closely resembling typhus that prevails from September to December in South Manchuria; the probable pathogen is *Rickettsia manchuriae.*
Manchurian hemorrhagic f., Korean hemorrhagic f.
Marseilles f., tick *typhus.*
marsh f., malaria.
Mediterranean f., **(1)** brucellosis; **(2)** familial paroxysmal *polyserositis.*
Mediterranean exanthematous f., an affection occurring sporadically in the Mediterranean littoral marked by a severe chill with abrupt rise of temperature, pains in the joints, tonsillitis, diarrhea, vomiting, and, on the third to fifth day, a rash of elevated nonconfluent macules beginning on the thighs and spreading to the entire

body; lasts from ten days to two weeks and then disappears by rapid lysis without desquamation.
meningotyphoid f., typhoid f. marked by symptoms of irritation or inflammation of the cerebral or spinal meninges.
metal fume f., an occupational disease, characterized by malaria-like symptoms, due to inhalation of particles and fumes of metallic oxides.
Mexican spotted f., Rocky Mountain spotted f.
mianeh f., Persian relapsing f.
miliary f., **(1)** an infectious disease characterized by profuse sweating and the production of sudamina, occurring formerly in severe epidemics; **(2)** miliaria.
milk f., **(1)** a slight elevation of temperature following childbirth, said to be due to the establishment of the secretion of milk, but probably the same as absorption f.; **(2)** parturient paresis or paralysis; an afebrile metabolic disease, occurring shortly after parturition in dairy cattle, characterized by hypocalcemia and manifested by loss of consciousness and general paralysis.
mill f., byssinosis.
miniature scarlet f. [L. *minio,* pp. *atus,* to color with *minium,* red-lead], a reaction consisting of f., nausea, vomiting, and a transient scarlatiniform rash which appears in a susceptible person when injected with the toxin of *Streptococcus pyogenes.*
monoleptic f., a continued f. having but one paroxysm. *Cf.* polyleptic f.
Mossman f., a f., noted especially among sugar cane cutters in the Mossman District of North Queensland, caused by a leptospira.
mud f., **(1)** a leptospirosis caused by the *grippotyphosa* serovar of *Leptospira interrogans;* **(2)** bluecomb *disease* of turkeys.
mumu f., Samoan term for elephantoid f.
nanukayami f., nanukayami; a form of leptospirosis known in Japan and caused by a leptospire normally found in the field mouse or vole.
nodal f., *erythema* nodosum.
North Queensland tick f., a mild form of tick typhus with eschar, adenopathy, rash, and fever, caused by *Rickettsia australis* and thought to be transmitted by the tick, *Ixodes holocyclus.*
Omsk hemorrhagic f., a form of epidemic hemorrhagic fever found in central Russia, caused by the Omsk hemorrhagic f. virus and transmitted by Dermacentor ticks; associated with gastrointestinal symptoms and hemorrhages but little or no central nervous system involvement.
O'nyong-nyong f., a dengue-like disease caused by the O'nyong-nyong virus and transmitted by a mosquito, characterized by joint pains and notable lymphadenopathy followed by a maculopapular eruption of the face which extends to the trunk and extremities but fades in several days without desquamation.
Oroya f., Carrion's disease; a generalized, acute, febrile, endemic, and systemic form of bartonellosis; marked by high fever, rheumatic pains, progressive, severe anemia, and albuminuria.
Pahvant Valley f., tularemia.
paludal f., malaria.
pappataci f., phlebotomus f.
papular f., an affection characterized by mild f., rheumatoid pains, and a maculopapular eruption.
paratyphoid f., paratyphoid; Schottmüller's disease; an acute infectious disease with symptoms and lesions resembling those of typhoid f., though milder in character; associated with the presence of the paratyphoid organism of which at least three varieties (types A, B, and C) have been described. See *Salmonella paratyphi, S. schotmülleri,* and *S. hirschfeldii.*
parenteric f., one of a group of f.'s clinically resembling typhoid and paratyphoid A and B, but caused by bacteria differing specifically from those of either of these diseases.
parrot f., psittacosis.
Pel-Ebstein f., Pel-Ebstein disease; the remittent fever common in Hodgkin's disease.
Persian relapsing f., mianeh f. or disease; a tick-borne relapsing f., occurring in the Middle East, caused by *Borrelia persica* and transmitted by *Ornithodoros tholozani* and possibly by *Ornithodoros lahorensis.*
petechial f., *purpura* hemorrhagica (2).
pharyngoconjunctival f., a disease characterized by pharyngitis and conjunctivitis, and due to an adenovirus, often type 3 but occasionally other types.
phlebotomus f., pappataci, sandfly, three-day, or Pym's f.; dog disease; an infectious but not contagious disease occurring in the Balkan Peninsula and other parts of southern Europe, caused by an arbovirus (family Bunyaviridae) apparently introduced by the bite of the sandfly, *Phlebotomus papatasii;* symptoms resemble those of dengue but are less severe and of shorter duration.
polka f., dengue.
polyleptic f., a f. occurring in two or more paroxysms; *e.g.,* smallpox, relapsing f., intermittent f. *Cf.* monoleptic f.
polymer fume f., an occupational disease marked by f., pain in the chest, and cough caused by the inhalation of fumes given off by a plastic, polytetrafluorethylene, when heated.
Potomac horse f., equine monocytic *ehrlichiosis.*
pretibial f., Fort Bragg f.; a mild disease first observed among military personnel at Fort Bragg, NC, characterized by f., moderate prostration, splenomegaly, and a rash on the anterior aspects of the legs; due to the *autumnalis* serovar of *Leptospira interrogans.*
protein f., f. produced by the injection of foreign protein, such as milk.
puerperal f., childbed f.; puerperal sepsis; postpartum sepsis with a rise in f. after the first 24 hours following delivery, but before the eleventh postpartum day.
Pym's f., phlebotomus f.
pyogenic f., pyemia.
Q f. [*Q,* for "query," so named because etiologic agent was unknown], a disease caused by *Coxiella burnetii,* which is propagated in sheep and cattle, where it produces no symptoms; human infections occur as a result of contact not only with such animals but also with humans, air and dust, wild reservoir hosts, and other sources.
quartan f., malariae *malaria.*
quintan f., trench f.
quotidian f., quotidian *malaria.*
rabbit f., tularemia.
rat-bite f., sodoku, sokosho; a single designation for two bacterial diseases associated with rat bites; one caused by *Streptobacillus moniliformis,* the other by *Spirillum minus;* both diseases are characterized by relapsing f., chills, headache, arthralgia, lymphadenopathy, and a maculopapular rash on the extremities.
recrudescent typhus f., Brill-Zinsser *disease.*
recurrent f., relapsing f.
red f., red f. of the Congo, murine *typhus.*
redwater f., **(1)** bovine *babesiosis;* **(2)** a highly fatal disease of cattle and occasionally of sheep caused by infection with *Clostridium haemolyticum.*
relapsing f., famine, spirillum, or recurrent f.; bilious typhoid of Griesinger; typhinia; an acute infectious disease caused by any one of a number of strains of *Borrelia,* marked by a number of febrile attacks lasting about six days and separated from each other by apyretic intervals of about the same length; the microorganism is found in the blood during the febrile periods but not during the intervals, the disappearance being associated with specific antibodies and previously evoked antibodies. There are two epidemiologic varieties: 1) the louse-borne variety, occurring chiefly in Europe, northern Africa, and India, and caused by strains of *B. recurrentis;* 2) the tick-borne variety, occurring in Africa, Asia, and North and South America, caused by various species of *Borrelia,* each of which is transmitted by a different species of the soft tick, *Ornithodoros.*

remittent malarial f., see remittent *malaria.*
rheumatic f., f. following infection of the throat with group A streptococci, occurring primarily in children and young adults, and variably associated with acute migratory polyarthritis, Sydenham's chorea, subcutaneous nodules over bony prominences, myocarditis with formation of Aschoff bodies (which may cause acute cardiac failure), and endocarditis (frequently followed by scarring of valves, causing stenosis or incompetence); relapses are common if repeated streptococcal infections occur.
ricefield f., a disease occurring in Indonesia, caused by a leptospire.
Rift Valley f. [*Rift Valley* in Kenya], a fatal endemic disease of sheep, caused by Rift Valley f. virus, which is also pathogenic for man and cattle, producing in man f. of an undifferentiated type.
Rocky Mountain spotted f., an acute infectious disease of high mortality, characterized by frontal and occipital headache, intense lumbar pain, malaise, a moderately high continuous f., and a rash on wrists and ankles from the second to the fifth day, later spreading to all parts of the body; it occurs in the spring of the year primarily in the southeast U.S. and the Rocky Mountain region, although it is also endemic elsewhere in the U.S., in parts of Canada, in Mexico, and in South America; the pathogenic organism is *Rickettsia rickettsii,* transmitted by two or more tick species of the genus *Dermacentor;* in the U.S. it is spread by *D. andersoni* in the western states and *D. variabilis* (a dog tick) in the eastern states. Also called black, blue, Mexican spotted, São Paulo, or Tobia f.; tick f. (4); blue disease; black measles (2).
Roman f., malignant tertian, falciparum, or aestivoautumnal f., formerly prevalent in the Roman Campagna and in the city of Rome; caused by *Plasmodium falciparum.*
Ross River f., epidemic *polyarthritis.*
sakushu f., hasamiyami.
salt f., elevated temperature in an infant, following a rectal injection of a salt solution. See also thirst f.
sandfly f., phlebotomus f.
San Joaquin f., primary *coccidioidomycosis.*
São Paulo f., Rocky Mountain spotted f.
scarlet f., scarlatina.
Sennetsu f., a disease of man in western Japan caused by the rickettsia *Ehrlichia sennetsu* and characterized by fever, malaise, anorexia, backache, and lymphadenopathy.
septic f., septicemia.
seven-day f., autumn f.
ship f., typhus.
shipping f., **(1)** in horses, synonymous with pinkeye or influenza; **(2)** in cattle, a common syndrome seen especially during or after shipping in cold weather or other stressful circumstances, manifested by acute inflammation of the upper respiratory tract usually terminating in pneumonia; caused by parainfluenza virus type 3, although some of the infections are associated with *Pasteurella.*
Sindbis f., a febrile illness of humans in Africa, Australia, and other countries, characterized by arthralgia, rash, and malaise; caused by the Sindbis virus and transmitted by culicine mosquitoes.
slow f., a continued f. of long duration.
snail f., schistosomiasis.
solar f., **(1)** dengue; **(2)** sunstroke.
South African tick-bite f., a typhus-like f. of South Africa caused by *Rickettsia rickettsii,* and usually characterized by primary eschar and regional adenitis, rigors, and maculopapular rash on the fifth day, often with severe central nervous system symptoms.
spirillum f., relapsing f.
spotted f., tick typhus caused by *Rickettsia rickettsii* in North and South America and Siberia.
steroid f., f. presumably caused by elevated plasma concentrations of certain pyrogenic steroids; can be produced by administration of etiocholanolone.
swamp f., **(1)** equine infectious *anemia;* **(2)** malaria.
swine f., hog *cholera.*
symptomatic f., traumatic f.
syphilitic f., the elevation of temperature often present in the early roseolous stage of secondary syphilis.
tertian f., vivax *malaria.*
Texas f., bovine *babesiosis.*
therapeutic f., see pyretotherapy (1).
thermic f., heatstroke.
thirst f., dehydration, exsiccation, or inanition f.; an elevation of temperature in infants after reduction of fluid intake, diarrhea, or vomiting; probably caused by reduced available body water, with reduced heat loss by evaporation; an analogous condition in adults is seen when exertion is continued in the face of dehydration.
three-day f., phlebotomus f.
tick f., **(1)** any infectious disease of man or the lower animals caused by a protozoan blood parasite transmitted through the agency of a tick; **(2)** the tick-borne variety of relapsing f.; **(3)** bovine *babesiosis;* **(4)** Rocky Mountain spotted f.; **(5)** Colorado tick f.
Tobia f., Rocky Mountain spotted f.
traumatic f., symptomatic or wound f.; elevation of temperature following an injury.
trench f., five-day or quintan f.; an uncommon rickettsial d. caused by *Rochalimaea quintans* and transmitted by the louse *Pediculus humanus,* first appearing as an epidemic during the trench warfare of World War I; characterized by the sudden onset of chills and fever, myalgia (especially of the back and legs), headache, and general malaise which typically last five days but may also recur.
trypanosome f., the febrile stage of sleeping sickness.
tsutsugamushi f., tsutsugamushi *disease.*
typhoid f., enteric f. (1); typhia; typhoid (2); abdominal typhoid; an acute infectious disease caused by *Salmonella typhi* and characterized by a continued f., rising in a steplike curve the first week, severe physical and mental depression, an eruption of rose-colored spots on the chest and abdomen, tympanites, often diarrhea, and sometimes intestinal hemorrhage or perforation of the bowel; average duration is four weeks, although aborted forms and relapses are not uncommon; the lesions are located chiefly in the lymph follicles of the intestines, the mesenteric glands, and the spleen; antibody titer of the Widal test rises during the infection, and early positive blood and urine cultures become negative.
undifferentiated type f.'s, systemic febrile diseases; a term applied to illnesses resulting from infection by any one of the arboviruses pathogenic for man, in which the only constant manifestation is f.; rash, lymphadenopathy, or arthralgia (alone, or in combination) may occur in some individuals but not in others; some arboviruses may induce infections in which undifferentiated type f. is the only manifestation, whereas other arboviruses may induce in some persons only undifferentiated f. and in other persons similar f. followed by secondary manifestations, *e.g.* a hemorrhagic f. or encephalitis.
undulant f. [referring to the wavy appearance of the long temperature curve], brucellosis.
urethral f., urinary f.
urinary f., catheter or urethral f.; an elevation of temperature, usually slight and transitory, following catheterization of the urethra, or the passage of blood clots, gravel, or a calculus.
urticarial f., *schistosomiasis* japonica.
uveoparotid f., Heerfordt's disease; chronic enlargement of the parotid glands and inflammation of the uveal tract accompanied by a long-continued f. of low degree; now recognized as a form of sarcoidosis.
Uzbekistan hemorrhagic f., a viral f. in central Asia probably transmitted by *Hyalomma anatolicum.*
valley f., primary *coccidioidomycosis.*
viral hemorrhagic f., Ebola hemorraghic f.; an epidemic disease, not highly transmissible, observed in southern Sudan and Zaire,

notably along the Ebola river; it is caused by Ebola virus and is associated with fever, malaise, muscular pain, respiratory tract symptoms, vomiting, and diarrhea; epistaxis, hemoptysis, hematemesis, and subconjunctival hemorrhages occur in severe cases, and body rash and tremors occur in some instances.
vivax f., vivax *malaria.*
Wesselsbron f. [*Wesselsbron,* town in South Africa where causative agent first isolated], Wesselsbron disease; a mosquito-borne disease of sheep and man caused by the Wesselsbron virus and characterized by abortion and lamb mortality in sheep and by fever, headache, muscular pains, and mild rash in man.
West African f., malarial *hemoglobinuria.*
West Nile f., a febrile illness caused by West Nile virus and characterized by headache, fever, maculopapular rash, myalgia, lymphadenopathy, and leukopenia; spread by *Culex* mosquitoes from a reservoir in birds.
wound f., traumatic f.
Yangtze Valley f., *schistosomiasis* japonica.
yellow f., a tropical mosquito-borne viral hepatitis, due to yellow f. virus, with an urban form transmitted by *Aedes aegypti,* and a rural, jungle, or sylvatic form from tree-dwelling mammals by various mosquitoes of the *Haemagogus* species complex; characterized clinically by fever, slow pulse, albuminuria, jaundice, congestion of the face, and hemorrhages, especially hematemesis (hence the synonym, "black vomit"); immunity to reinfection accompanies recovery.
Zika f., an acute degenerative disease, clinically resembling dengue, of the central nervous system, especially involving the hippocampus; caused by Zika virus.

feverish (fē'ver-ish). **1.** Febrile. **2.** Having a fever.

Fevold, Harry Leonard, U.S. biochemist, *1902. See under *test.*

Fevold test. See under test.

FF Abbreviation for filtration *fraction.*

FIBER

fiber (fī'ber) [L. *fibra*]. Fibra; fibre; a slender thread or filament. **1.** Extracellular filamentous structures such as collagenic or elastic connective tissue f.'s. **2.** The nerve cell axon with its glial envelope. **3.** Elongated, hence threadlike cells such as muscle cells and the epithelial cells composing the major part of the eye lens.
A f.'s, myelinated nerve f.'s in somatic nerves, measuring 1 to 22 μm in diameter, conducting nerve impulses at a rate of 6 to 120 m/sec.
accelerator f.'s, augmentor f.'s; postganglionic sympathetic nerve f.'s originating in the superior, middle, and inferior cervical ganglia of the sympathetic trunk, conveying nervous impulses to the heart that increase the rapidity and force of the cardiac pulsations.
adrenergic f.'s, nerve f.'s that transmit nervous impulses to other nerve cells (or smooth muscle or gland cells) by the medium of the adrenaline-like transmitter substance norepinephrine (noradrenaline).
afferent f.'s, those that convey impulses to a ganglion or to a nerve center in the brain or spinal cord.
alpha f.'s, large somatic motor or proprioceptive nerve f.'s conducting impulses at rates near 100 m/sec.
anastomosing f.'s, anastomotic f.'s, individual f.'s passing from one nerve trunk or muscle bundle to another.
arcuate f.'s, nervous or tendinous f.'s passing in the form of an arch from one part to another. See *fibrae* arcuatae subentries.
argyrophilic f.'s, reticular connective tissue f.'s that react with silver salts and appear black microscopically.
association f.'s, intrinsic or endogenous f.'s; nerve f.'s interconnecting subdivisions of the cerebral cortex of the same hemisphere or different segments of the spinal cord on the same side.

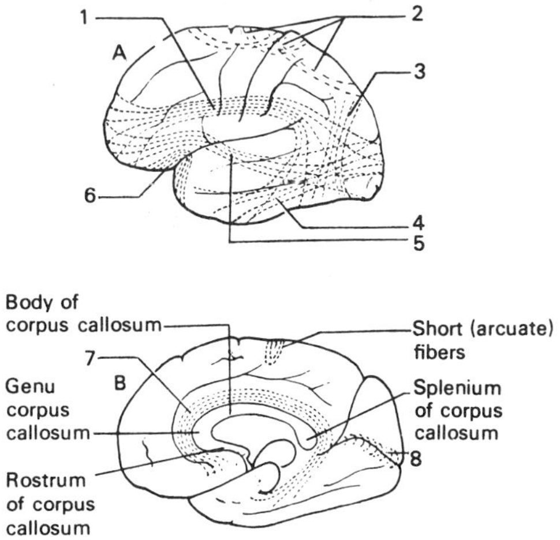

Association Fibers of the Cerebrum
A, projected onto the lateral surface of the hemisphere; *B,* onto the medial surface; *1,* superior longitudinal fasciculus; *2,* short association bundles; *3,* vertical occipital fasciculus; *4,* inferior longitudinal fasciculus; *5,* occipitofrontal fasciculus; *6,* uncinate fasciculus; *7,* cingulum; *8,* calcarine fasciculus. (After Dr. Murray Barr, modified.)

astral f.'s, f.'s (fibrils) radiating from the centrosphere as seen with a light microscope; revealed as microtubules under the electron microscope.
augmentor f.'s, accelerator f.'s.
B f.'s, myelinated f.'s autonomic nerves, with a diameter of 2 μm or less, conducting at a rate of 3 to 15 m/sec.
Bergmann's f.'s, filamentous glia f.'s traversing the cerebellar cortex perpendicular to the surface.
beta f.'s, nerve f.'s having conduction velocities of about 40 m/sec.
C f.'s, unmyelinated f.'s, 0.4 to 1.2 μm in diameter, conducting nerve impulses at a velocity of 0.7 to 2.3 m/sec.
cholinergic f.'s, nerve f.'s that transmit impulses to other nerve cells, muscle fibers, or gland cells by the medium of the transmitter substance acetylcholine.
chromatic f., chromonema.
circular f.'s, *fibrae* circulares.
climbing f.'s, nerve f.'s in the cerebellar cortex that synapse upon smooth branchlets of Purkinje cell dendrites.
collagen f., collagenous f., white f. (2); an individual f. that varies in diameter from less than 1 μm to about 12 μm and is composed of fibrils; the f.'s, which are usually arranged in bundles, undergo some branching and are of indefinite length; chemically the f. is a glycoprotein, collagen, which yields gelatin upon boiling; they make up the principal element of irregular connective tissue, tendons, aponeuroses, and most ligaments, and occur in the matrix of cartilage and osseous tissue.
commissural f.'s, nerve f.'s crossing the midline and connecting two corresponding parts or regions of the nervous system.
cone f., a part of the cone cell of the retina; the **inner c. f.** is a slender axon-like part of the cone extending from the cell body to the pedicle located in the outer plexiform layer of the retina; in the outer fovea, where the cones are much elongated, they narrow to an **outer c. f.,** located between the inner segment and the cell body.
corticobulbar f.'s, nerve f.'s projecting from the motor and soma-

tic sensory cortex to the rhombencephalon; included in this corticofugal f. system are corticoreticular f.'s terminating in the reticular formation of the rhombencephalon, and corticonuclear f.'s to the motor nuclei innervating the musculature of the face, tongue, and jaws, and to some f.'s of the rhombencephalic sensory relay nuclei. See also *tractus* corticobulbaris.
corticonuclear f.'s, *fibrae* corticonucleares.
corticopontine f.'s, *fibrae* corticopontinae.
corticoreticular f.'s, *fibrae* corticoreticulares.
corticospinal f.'s, *fibrae* corticospinales.
dentinal f.'s, dental f.'s, **(1)** Tomes's f.'s; the processes of the pulpal cells, the odontoblasts, which extend in radial fashion through the dentin to the dentoenamel junction and are contained within the dentinal tubules; **(2)** the intertubular fine collagenous f.'s which with the dentinal ground substance infiltrated with calcium salts constitutes the dentinal matrix.
depressor f.'s, sensory nerve f.'s having pressure-sensitive nerve endings in the wall of certain arteries capable of activating blood pressure-lowering brainstem mechanisms when stimulated by an increase in intra-arterial pressure.
dietary f., the plant polysaccharides and lignin that are resistant to hydrolysis by the digestive enzymes in humans.
elastic f.'s, yellow f.'s; f.'s that are 0.2 to 2 μm in diameter but may be larger in some ligaments; they branch and anastomose to form networks and fuse to form fenestrated membranes; the f.'s and membranes consist of microfibrils about 110 Å wide and an amorphous substance containing elastin.
enamel f.'s, *prismata* adamantina.
endogenous f.'s, association f.'s.
exogenous f.'s, nerve f.'s by which a given region of the central nervous system is connected with other regions; the term applies to both afferent and efferent fiber connections.
external arcuate f.'s, *fibrae* arcuatae externae.
gamma f.'s, nerve f.'s that have a conduction rate of about 20 m/sec. See also gamma *efferent.*
Gerdy's f.'s, *ligamentum* metacarpale transversum superficiale.
Gratiolet's f.'s, *radiatio* optica.
gray f.'s, unmyelinated f.'s.
inhibitory f.'s, nerve f.'s that inhibit the activity of the nerve cells with which they have synaptic connections, or of the effector tissue (smooth muscle, heart muscle, glands) in which they terminate.
intercolumnar f.'s, *fibrae* intercrurales.
intercrural f.'s, *fibrae* intercrurales.
internal arcuate f.'s, *fibrae* arcuatae internae.
intrafusal f.'s, muscle f.'s present within a neuromuscular spindle.
intrinsic f.'s, association f.'s.
James f.'s, atrio-His bundle connections thought to be the basis for the short P-R interval syndrome; these f.'s should be distinguished from the internodal tracts of the atrium, sometimes referred to as "James tracts."
Korff's f.'s, argyrophilic f.'s that pass between odontoblasts at the periphery of the dental pulp and fan out into the dentin.
Kühne's f., artificial muscle f. made by filling the intestine of an insect with a growth of myxomycetes; used to demonstrate the contractility of protoplasm.
f.'s of lens, *fibrae* lentis.
Mahaim f.'s, paraspecific f.'s originating from the A-V node, the His bundle, or the bundle branches and inserting into the ventricular myocardium; they are potential pathways for reentrant dysrhythmias.
medullated nerve f., myelinated nerve f.
meridional f.'s, *fibrae* meridionales.
mossy f.'s, highly branched nerve f.'s in the cerebellar cortex that terminate in rosette formations and synapse upon granule cell dendrites.
motor f.'s, nerve f.'s that transmit impulses that activate effector cells, *e.g.,* in muscle or gland tissue.
Müller's f.'s, **(1)** *fibrae* circulares; **(2)** Müller's radial cells; sustentacular f.'s of retina; sustentacular neuroglial cells of the retina, running through the thickness of the retina from the internal limiting membrane to the bases of the rods and cones where they form a row of junctional complexes.
myelinated nerve f., medullated nerve f.; an axon enveloped by a myelin sheath formed by oligodendroglia cells (in brain and spinal cord) or Schwann cells (in peripheral nerves).
Nélaton's f.'s, Nélaton's *sphincter.*
nerve f., the axon of a nerve cell, ensheathed by oligodendroglia cells in brain and spinal cord, and by Schwann cells in peripheral nerves.
nonmedullated f.'s, unmyelinated f.'s.
nuclear bag f., the largest type of intrafusal muscle f.'s in a neuromuscular spindle, containing a central aggregation of nuclei (nuclear bag).
nuclear chain f., the shortest and most numerous type of intrafusal muscle f.'s in a neuromuscular spindle, containing a single row of centrally positioned nuclei.
oblique f.'s of stomach, *fibrae* obliquae ventriculi.
osteocollagenous f.'s, fine collagenous f.'s in the matrix of osseous tissue.
osteogenetic f.'s, the f.'s in the osteogenetic layer of the periosteum.
pectinate f.'s, *musculi* pectinati.
perforating f.'s, Sharpey's f.'s; bundles of collagenous f.'s that pass into the outer circumferential lamellae of bone or the cementum of teeth.
periodontal ligament f.'s, the collagen f.'s, running from the cementum to the alveolar bone, that suspend a tooth in its socket; they include apical, oblique, horizontal, and alveolar crest f.'s, indicating that the orientation of the f.'s varies at different levels.
periventricular f.'s, *fibrae* periventriculares.
pilomotor f.'s, nerve f.'s that innervate the arrectores pilorum muscles of hair follicles responsible for piloerection.
precollagenous f.'s, immature, argyrophilic f.'s.
pressor f.'s, sensory nerve f.'s whose stimulation causes vasoconstriction and rise of blood pressure.
projection f.'s, nerve f.'s connecting the cerebral cortex with other centers in the brain or spinal cord; fibers arising from cells in the central nervous system that pass to distant loci.
Prussak's f.'s, elastic and connective tissue f.'s bounding the pars flaccida membranae tympani.
Purkinje's f.'s, interlacing f.'s formed of modified cardiac muscle cells with central granulated protoplasm containing one or two nuclei and a transversely striated peripheral portion; they are found beneath the endocardium of the ventricles. See also conducting *system* of the heart.
pyramidal f.'s, *fibrae* pyramidales.
red f.'s, red mammalian muscle f.'s that have numerous large mitochondria and that are smaller in diameter and contract more slowly than white f.'s.
Reissner's f., a rodlike, highly refractive f. running caudally from the subcommissural organ throughout the length of the central canal of the brainstem and spinal cord.
Remak's f.'s, unmyelinated f.'s.
reticular f.'s, the collagen (type III) f.'s forming the distinctive loose connective tissue stroma of embryonic tissues, mesenchyme, red pulp of the spleen, cortex and medulla of lymph nodes, and the hematopoietic compartments of bone marrow and comprising a substantial portion of the collagen f.'s of the skin, blood vessels, synovial membrane, uterine tissue, and granulation tissue; characterized by its organization as a reticular meshwork of fine filaments and an affinity for silver and for periodic acid-Schiff stains.
Retzius' f.'s, stiff f.'s in Deiters' cells.
rod f., a part of the rod cell of the retina which extends to either side of the cell body; the inner rod f. terminates in the spherule, a

synaptic ending located in the outer plexiform layer.
Rosenthal f., an oval or elongated eosinophilic mass believed to represent a modified process of an astrocyte; seen in large numbers in certain slowly growing astrocytomas and areas of chronic reactive gliosis.
Sappey's f.'s, nonstriated muscular f.'s in the check ligaments of the eyeball.
Sharpey's f.'s, perforating f.'s.
skeletal muscle f.'s, multinucleated contractile cells varying from less than 10 to 100 μm in diameter and from less than 1 mm to several centimeters in length; the f. consists of sarcoplasm and cross-striated myofibrils which in turn consist of myofilaments; human skeletal muscles are a mixture of red, white, and intermediate type f.'s; the red f.'s are smaller, have more mitochondria and myoglobin, and contract more slowly.
spindle f., see mitotic *spindle.*
sudomotor f.'s, postganglionic and cholinergic sympathetic nerve f.'s that innervate the sweat glands.
sustentacular f.'s of retina, Müller's f.'s (2).
tautomeric f.'s, nerve f.'s of the spinal cord that do not extend beyond the limits of the spinal cord segment in which they originate.
Tomes' f.'s, dentinal f.'s (1).
transseptal f.'s, nonelastic f.'s running from tooth to tooth over the crest of the alveolus.
transverse f.'s of pons, *fibrae* pontis transversae.
unmyelinated f.'s, Remak's f.'s; gray or nonmedullated f.'s; nerve f.'s (axons) lacking a myelin sheath but, in common with others, enveloped by a sheath of Schwann cells.
Weitbrecht's f.'s, *retinaculum* capsulae articularis coxae.
white f., **(1)** white mammalian muscle f.'s that are larger in diameter, have fewer mitochondria, and contract more quickly than red f.'s; **(2)** collagen f.'s.
yellow f.'s, elastic f.'s.
zonular f.'s, *fibrae* zonulares.

---

fiberoptic (fī-ber-op'tik). Pertaining to fiberoptics.

fiberoptics (fī-ber-op'tiks). An optical system whereby the image is conveyed by a compact bundle of small diameter, flexible, glass or plastic fibers.

fiberscope (fī'ber-skōp). An optical instrument that transmits images through a flexible bundle of glass or plastic fibers. See also fiberoptics.

fibr-. See fibro-.

fibra, pl. **fibrae** (fī'bră, fī'brē) [L.] [NA]. Fiber.
fi'brae arcua'tae cer'ebri [NA], arcuate fibers of the cerebrum; short association fibers that connect adjacent gyri in the cerebral cortex.
fi'brae arcua'tae exter'nae [NA], external arcuate fibers; they include: 1) dorsal external arcuate fibers that arise from cells in the accessory or lateral cuneate nucleus and pass to the cerebellum as components of the inferior cerebellar peduncle; 2) ventral external arcuate fibers that arise from the arcuate nuclei at the base of the medulla oblongata and pass around the lateral surface of the medulla to enter the inferior cerebellar peduncle.
fi'brae arcua'tae inter'nae [NA], internal arcuate fibers; fibers that arise in the nucleus gracilis and cuneatus, pass in a curving course across the midline of the medulla oblongata, and form the contralateral medial lemniscus; also designates other fibers such as those of the olivocerebellar tract that arch through the substance of the medulla.
fi'brae circula'res [NA], circular fibers; Müller's fibers (1); Rouget's muscle; Müller's muscle (2); the circular fibers of the ciliary muscle.
fi'brae corticonuclea'res [NA], corticonuclear fibers; the fibers that compose the tractus corticobulbaris.
fi'brae corticopon'tinae, corticopontine fibers; the fibers that compose the *tractus* corticopontini.
fi'brae corticoreticula'res [NA], corticoreticular fibers; corticofugal fibers distributed to the reticular formation of the mesencephalon and rhombencephalon. See also corticobulbar *fibers.*
fi'brae corticospina'les [NA], fibrae pyramidalis.
fi'brae intercrura'les [NA], intercrural fibers; intercolumnar fibers or fasciae; horizontal arched fibers that pass from the inguinal ligament across the medial and lateral crura of the superficial inguinal ring.
fi'brae len'tis [NA], fibers of the lens; the elongated cells of ectodermal origin forming the substance of the crystalline lens of the eye.
fi'brae meridiona'les [NA], meridional fibers; the longitudinal fibers of the ciliary muscle.
fi'brae obli'quae ventric'uli [NA], oblique fibers of the stomach; the smooth muscle fibers of the innermost layer of the tunica muscularis of the stomach; the fibers occur chiefly at the cardiac end of the stomach and spread over the anterior and posterior surfaces.
fi'brae periventricula'res [NA], periventricular fibers; a heterogeneous system of thin nerve fibers in the periventricular gray matter of the hypothalamus; the dorsal longitudinal fasciculus is a caudal continuation of the system.
fi'brae pon'tis transver'sae [NA], transverse fibers of the pons; fibers arising from the nuclei pontis, decussate and pass into the cerebellum as the middle cerebellar peduncles.
fi'brae pyramida'les, fibrae corticospinalis; pyramidal or corticospinal fibers; the fibers that compose the tractus pyramidalis (corticospinalis).
fi'brae zonula'res [NA], zonular fibers; delicate fibers that pass from the equator of the lens to the ciliary body, collectively known as the zonula ciliaris.

fibre (fī'ber). Fiber.

fibremia (fī-brē'mē-ă) [fibrin + G. *haima,* blood]. Inosemia (2); presence of formed fibrin in the blood, causing thrombosis or embolism.

fibril (fī'bril) [Mod. L. *fibrilla*]. A minute fiber or component of a fiber.
collagen f.'s, unit f.'s.
muscular f., myofibril.
subpellicular f., subpellicular *microtubule.*
unit f.'s, collagen f.'s; the f.'s which comprise a collagen fiber, ranging from 20 to 200 nm and averaging about 100 nm in diameter (substantially larger in tendons), with cross-striations averaging 640 Å.

fibrilla, pl. **fibrillae** (fī-bril'ă, -ē) [Mod. L. dim. of L. *fibra,* a fiber]. Fibril.

fibrillar, fibrillary (fī'bri-lăr, -lar-ē). **1.** Filar (1); relating to a fibril. **2.** Denoting the fine rapid contractions or twitchings of fibers or of small groups of fibers in skeletal or cardiac muscle.

fibrillate (fī'bri-lāt). **1.** To make or to become fibrillar. **2.** Fibrillated. **3.** To be in a state of fibrillation (3).

fibrillated (fī'bri-lā-ted). Fibrillate (2); composed of fibrils.

fibrillation (fī-bri-lā'shŭn, fib-rĭ-). **1.** The condition of being fibrillated. **2.** The formation of fibrils. **3.** Exceedingly rapid contractions or twitching of muscular fibrils, but not of the muscle as a whole. **4.** Vermicular twitching, usually slow, of individual muscular fibers; commonly occurs in atria or ventricles of the heart as well as in recently denervated skeletal muscle fibers.
atrial f., auricular f., ataxia cordis; delirium cordis; f. in which the normal rhythmical contractions of the cardiac atria are replaced by rapid irregular twitchings of the muscular wall; the ventricles respond irregularly to the dysrhythmic bombardment from the atria.

ventricular f., fine, rapid, fibrillary movements of the ventricular muscle that replace the normal contraction.

fibrillogenesis (fī'bril-ō-jen'ĕ-sis). The development of fine fibrils (as seen with the electron microscope) normally present in collagenous fibers of connective tissue.

fibrin (fī'brin) [L. *fibra,* fiber]. An elastic filamentous protein derived from fibrinogen by the action of thrombin, which releases fibrinopeptides A and B from fibrinogen in coagulation of the blood; a component of thrombi, vegetations, and acute inflammatory exudates such as in diphtheria and lobar pneumonia.

fibrinase (fī'brin-ās). **1.** Former term for *factor* XIII. **2.** Plasmin.

fibrino- [L. *fibra,* fiber]. Combining form relating to fibrin.

fibrinocellular (fī'bri-nō-sel'yū-lăr). Composed of fibrin and cells, as in certain types of exudates resulting from acute inflammation.

fibrinogen (fī-brin'ō-jen). Factor I (blood clotting); a globulin of the blood plasma that is converted into fibrin by the action of thrombin in the presence of ionized calcium to produce coagulation of the blood.

human f., f. prepared from normal human plasma; a coagulant (clotting factor), used as an adjunct in the management of acute, congenital, or acquired chronic hypofibrinogenemia.

fibrinogenase (fī-brin'ō-je-nās). Thrombin.

fibrinogenemia (fī-brin'ō-jĕ-nē'mē-ă). Hyperfibrinogenemia.

fibrinogenesis (fī'bri-nō-jen'ĕ-sis). Formation or production of fibrin.

fibrinogenic, fibrinogenous (fī'brin-ō-jen'ik, fī'bri-noj'ĕ-nŭs). **1.** Pertaining to fibrinogen. **2.** Producing fibrin.

fibrinogenolysis (fī-brin'ō-jen-ol'i-sis) [fibrinogen + G. *lysis,* dissolution]. The inactivation or dissolution of fibrinogen in the blood.

fibrinogenopenia (fī-brin'ō-jen-ō-pē'nē-ă) [fibrinogen + G. *penia,* poverty]. A concentration of fibrinogen in the blood that is less than the normal.

fibrinoid (fī'bri-noyd) [fibrin + G. *eidos,* resemblance]. **1.** Resembling fibrin. **2.** A deeply or brilliantly acidophilic, homogeneous, refractile, proteinaceous material that: 1) is frequently formed in the walls of blood vessels and in connective tissue of patients with such diseases as disseminated lupus erythematosus, polyarteritis nodosa, scleroderma, dermatomyositis, and rheumatic fever; 2) is sometimes observed in healing wounds, chronic peptic ulcers, the placenta, necrotic arterioles of malignant hypertension, and other unrelated conditions.

fibrinokinase (fī'brin-ō-kī'nās). Fibrinolysokinase; name proposed for the enzyme that converts plasminogen to plasmin; subsequently called urokinase, but now called plasminogen *activator.*

fibrinolysin (fī-brin-ō-lī'sin). Plasmin.

streptococcal f., streptokinase.

fibrinolysis (fī-bri-nol'i-sis) [fibrino- + G. *lysis,* dissolution]. Hydrolysis of fibrin.

fibrinolysokinase (fī'brin-ō-lī-sō-kī'nās). Fibrinokinase.

fibrinolytic (fī-brin-ō-lit'ik). Denoting, characterized by, or causing fibrinolysis.

fibrinopeptide (fī'brin-ō-pep'tīd). One of two peptides (A and B) released from fibrinogen by the action of thrombin to form fibrin.

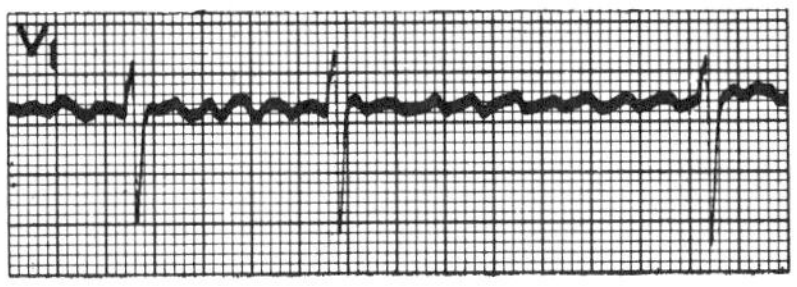

Atrial Fibrillation

fibrinopurulent (fī'bri-nō-pyū'rū-lent). Pertaining to pus or suppurative exudate that contains a relatively large amount of fibrin.

fibrinoscopy (fī-bri-nos'k-ō-pē) [fibrino- + G. *skopeō,* to view]. The chemical and physical examination of the fibrin of exudates, blood clots, etc.

fibrinous (fī'brin-ŭs). Pertaining to or composed of fibrin.

fibrinuria (fī-bri-nū'rē-ă) [fibrin + G. *ouron,* urine]. The passage of urine that contains fibrin.

fibro-, fibr- [L. *fibra,* fiber]. Combining forms denoting fiber.

fibroadenoma (fī'brō-ad-ĕ-nō'mă). Adenoma fibrosum; fibroid adenoma; a benign neoplasm derived from glandular epithelium, in which there is a conspicuous stroma of proliferating fibroblasts and connective tissue elements; commonly occurs in breast tissue.

giant f., a massive benign f. seen mostly in adolescent girls.

intracanalicular f., a f. of the breast consisting of nodules of fibrous tissue which invaginate and compress the ducts.

pericanalicular f., a f. of the breast consisting of an increased number of small ducts surrounded by concentric bands of fibrous tissue.

fibroadipose (fī-brō-ad'i-pōz). Fibrofatty; relating to or containing both fibrous and fatty structures.

fibroareolar (fī'brō-ă-rē'ō-lăr). Denoting connective tissue that is both fibrous and areolar in character.

fibroblast (fī'brō-blast). A stellate or spindle-shaped cell with cytoplasmic processes present in connective tissue, capable of forming collagen fibers; an inactive f. is sometimes called a fibrocyte.

fibroblastic (fī-brō-blas'tik). Relating to fibroblasts.

fibrocarcinoma (fī'brō-kar-si-nō'mă). Scirrhous *carcinoma.*

fibrocartilage (fī-brō-kar'ti-lij). Fibrocartilago; a variety of cartilage that contains visible collagen fibers; appears as a transition between tendons or ligaments or bones.

circumferential f., a ring of f. around the articular end of a bone, serving to deepen the joint cavity. See also *labrum* acetabulare and *labrum* glenoidale.

external semilunar f., *meniscus* lateralis.

interarticular f., *discus* articularis.

internal semilunar f. of knee joint, *meniscus* medialis.

semilunar f., see *meniscus* lateralis; *meniscus* medialis.

stratiform f., a layer of f. in the bottom of a groove in a bone through which a tendon runs.

fibrocartilaginous (fī'brō-kar-ti-laj'i-nŭs). Relating to or composed of fibrocartilage.

fibrocartilago (fī'brō-kar-ti-lā'gō). Fibrocartilage.

f. basa'lis, basilar *cartilage.*

f. interarticula'ris, *discus* articularis.

f. intervertebra'lis, *discus* intervertebralis.

fibrocellular (fī-brō-sel'yū-lăr). Both fibrous and cellular.

fibrochondritis (fī'brō-kon-drī'tis). Inflammation of a fibrocartilage.

fibrochondroma (fī'brō-kon-drō'mă). A benign neoplasm of cartilaginous tissue, in which there is a relatively unusual amount of fibrous stroma.

fibrocongestive (fī'brō-kon-jes'tiv). Term sometimes used to indicate the general condition of an organ or tissue in which acute or chronic, persistent congestion has resulted in degeneration and necrosis of cells and replacement with connective tissue elements, as in chronic congestive splenomegaly.

fibrocyst (fī'brō-sist). Any cystic lesion circumscribed by or situated within a conspicuous amount of fibrous connective tissue.

fibrocystic (fī-brō-sis'tik). Pertaining to or characterized by the presence of fibrocysts.

fibrocystoma (fī'brō-sis-tō'mă). A benign neoplasm, usually derived from glandular epithelium, characterized by cysts within a conspicuous fibrous stroma.

fibrocyte (fī'brō-sīt) [fibro- + G. *kytos*, cell]. Designation sometimes applied to an inactive fibroblast.

fibrodysplasia (fī'brō-dis-plā'zē-ă). Abnormal development of fibrous connective tissue.

f. ossif'icans progres'siva, a generalized disorder of connective tissue in which bone replaces tendons, fasciae, and ligaments; genetic lethal and presumed to be autosomal dominant inheritance. See also fibrous *dysplasia* of bone.

fibroelastic (fī'brō-ē-las'tik). Composed of collagen and elastic fibers.

fibroelastosis (fī'brō-ē-las-tō'sis). Excessive proliferation of collagenous and elastic fibrous tissue.

endocardial f., endomyocardial f., **(1)** endocardial sclerosis; a congenital condition characterized by thickening of the left ventricular mural endocardium (chiefly due to fibrous and elastic tissue), thickening and malformation of the cardiac valves, subendocardial changes in the myocardium, and hypertrophy of the heart; chief symptoms are cyanosis, dyspnea, anorexia, and irritability; **(2)** endomyocardial *fibrosis*.

fibroenchondroma (fī'brō-en-kon-drō'mă). An enchondroma in which the neoplastic cartilage cells are situated within an abundant fibrous stroma.

fibroepithelioma (fī'brō-ep-i-thē-lē-ō'mă). A skin tumor composed of fibrous tissue intersected by thin anastomosing bands of basal cells of the epidermis; may give rise to basal cell carcinoma of the nodular type.

fibrofatty (fī-brō-fat'ē). Fibroadipose.

fibrofolliculoma (fī'brō-fō-lik-yū-lō'mă). Neoplastic proliferation of the fibrous sheath of the hair follicle, with solid extensions of the epithelium of the follicular infundibulum; multiple f.'s may be familial.

fibrogenesis (fī-brō-jen'ĕ-sis). The production or development of fibers.

fibrogliosis (fī'brō-glī-ō'sis) [fibro- + G. *glia*, glue, + *-osis*, condition]. A cellular reaction within the brain, usually in response to a penetrating injury, in which both astrocytes and fibroblasts participate and which culminates in a fibrous and glial scar.

fibroid (fī'broyd) [fibro- + G. *eidos*, resemblance]. **1.** Resembling or composed of fibers or fibrous tissue. **2.** Old term for certain types of leiomyoma, especially those occurring in the uterus. **3.** Fibroleiomyoma.

fibroidectomy (fī-broy-dek'tō-mē) [fibroid + G. *ektomē*, excision]. Fibromectomy; removal of a fibroid tumor.

fibroin (fī'brō-in). A white insoluble protein forming the primary constituent (70%) of cobweb and silk.

fibrokeratoma (fī'brō-ker-ă-tō'mă). A keratotic cutaneous polyp containing abundant connective tissue.

fibroleiomyoma (fī'brō-lī'ō-mī-ō'mă). Leiomyofibroma; fibroid (3); a leiomyoma containing non-neoplastic collagenous fibrous tissue, which may make the tumor hard; f.'s usually arise in the myometrium, and the proportion of fibrous tissue increases with age.

fibrolipoma (fī'brō-li-pō'mă). Lipoma fibrosum; a lipoma with an abundant stroma of fibrous tissue.

fibroma (fī-brō'mă) [fibro- + G. *-oma*, tumor]. A benign neoplasm derived from fibrous connective tissue.

ameloblastic f., a benign mixed odontogenic tumor characterized by neoplastic proliferation of both epithelial and mesenchymal components of the tooth bud without the production of dental hard tissue; presents clinically as a slow-growing painless radiolucency occurring most commonly in the mandible of children and adolescents.

aponeurotic f., a calcifying recurrent non-metastasizing fibromatosis seen most frequently on the palms of young people as small nodules not attached to the overlying skin.

central cementifying f., a microscopic variant of a central ossifying f.

central ossifying f., a painless, slow-growing, expansile, sharply circumscribed benign fibro-osseus tumor of the jaws that is derived from cells of the periodontal ligament; presents initially as a radiolucency that becomes progressively more opaque as it matures. See also central cementifying f.

chondromyxoid f., chondrofibroma; chondromyxoma; an uncommon benign bone tumor, occurring most frequently in the tibia of adolescents and young adults, composed of lobulated myxoid tissue with scanty chondroid foci.

concentric f., a benign neoplasm, actually a leiomyoma, that occupies the entire circumference of the wall of the uterus.

desmoplastic f., a benign fibrous tumor of bone affecting children and young adults; cortical destruction may result.

giant cell f., a variant of irritation f., occurring most frequently on the gingiva of young adults, composed of fibroblasts with large stellate or multiple nuclei.

irritation f., slow-growing nodules on the oral mucosa, composed of fibrous tissue covered by epithelium, resulting from mechanical irritation by dentures, fillings, cheek biting, etc.

f. mol'le, skin *tag*.

f. mol'le gravida'rum, molluscum fibrosum gravidarum; skin tags or polyps that develop on women during pregnancy and often disappear at term.

f. myxomato'des, myxofibroma.

nonossifying f., a loculated osteolytic focus of cellular fibrous tissue, slightly expanding a bone, usually near the end of a long bone in older children; similar to fibrous cortical defect, although larger.

nonosteogenic f., fibrous cortical *defect*.

peripheral ossifying f., odontogenic f., cementifying f., a reactive focal gingival overgrowth derived histogenetically from cells of the periodontal ligament and usually developing in response to local irritants (plaque and calculus) on associated teeth; consists microscopically of a hyperplastic cellular fibrous stroma supporting deposits of bone, cementum, or dystrophic calcification.

periungual f., Koenen's tumor; multiple smooth firm nodules formed at the nail folds, often over 10 mm in length, which appear at or after puberty in tuberous sclerosis.

rabbit f., Shope f.

recurring digital f.'s of childhood, infantile digital fibromatosis; multiple fibrous flesh-colored nodules on the extensor aspect of the terminal phalanges of adjacent digits of infants and young children which often recur after attempted excision, do not metastasize, and may spontaneously regress in two to three years; composed of spindle cells containing cytoplasmic inclusions believed to be derived from myofibrils.

senile f., skin *tag*.

Shope f., rabbit f.; a connective tissue tumor of cottontail rabbits caused by a poxvirus of the genus *Leporipoxvirus* and found by Shope to be transmissible with cellular suspensions or Berkefeld filtrates; it is related to myxomatosis and is used in Europe as a vaccine to protect against the myxoma virus.

telangiectatic f., angiofibroma; a benign neoplasm of fibrous tissue in which there are numerous, small and large, frequently dilated, vascular channels.

fibromatoid (fī-brō'mă-toyd). A focus, nodule, or mass (of proliferating fibroblasts) that resembles a fibroma but is not regarded as neoplastic.

fibromatosis (fī'brō-mă-tō'sis). **1.** A condition characterized by the occurrence of multiple fibromas, with a relatively large distribution. **2.** Abnormal hyperplasia of fibrous tissue.

abdominal f., desmoid (2).

aggressive infantile f., a childhood counterpart of abdominal or extra-abdominal desmoid tumors, characterized by firm subcutaneous nodules that grow rapidly in any part of the body but do not metastasize.
f. col'li, congenital *torticollis.*
congenital generalized f., multiple subcutaneous and visceral fibrous tumors present at birth; a rare disorder often fatal in the first week of life, although sometimes undergoing spontaneous remission.
infantile digital f., recurring digital *fibromas* of childhood.
juvenile hyalin f., systemic hyalinosis; a rare recessively inherited disorder of generalized cutaneous nodules or tumors in children with normal mentality; the lesions consist of fibroblasts separated by an eosinophilic hyalin stroma composed mostly of glycosaminoglycans.
juvenile palmo-plantar f., f. that occurs in children from birth to adolescence as a single poorly demarcated nodule of the thenar or hypothenar eminence or overlying the calcaneus of the mid-sole.
palmar f., nodular fibroplastic proliferation in the palmar fascia of one or both hands, preceding or associated with Dupuytren's contracture.
penile f., Peyronie's *disease.*
plantar f., Dupuytren's disease of the foot; nodular fibroblastic proliferation in plantar fascia of one or both feet; rarely associated with contracture.

fibromatous (fī-brō'mă-tŭs). Pertaining to, or of the nature of, a fibroma.

fibromectomy (fī-brō-mek'tō-mē). Fibroidectomy.

fibromuscular (fī'brō-mŭs'kyū-lăr). Both fibrous and muscular; relating to both fibrous and muscular tissues.

fibromyectomy (fī'brō-mī-ek'tō-mē). Excision of a fibromyoma.

fibromyoma (fī'brō-mī-ō'mă). A leiomyoma that contains a relatively abundant amount of fibrous tissue.

fibromyositis (fī'brō-mī-ō-sī'tis) [fibro- + G. *mys,* muscle, + *-itis,* inflammation]. Chronic inflammation of a muscle with an overgrowth, or hyperplasia, of the connective tissue.

fibromyxoma (fī'brō-mik-sō'mă) [fibro- + G. *myxa,* mucus, + *-ōma,* tumor]. A myxoma that contains a relatively abundant amount of mature fibroblasts and connective tissue.

fibronectin (fī-brō-nek'tin) [L. *fibra,* fiber, + *nexus,* interconnection]. A fibrous linking glycoprotein widely distributed in connective tissue and basement membranes, and present on cell surfaces; acts as an adhesive and as a reticuloendothelial mediated host defense mechanism which is impaired by surgery and other trauma, burns, infection, neoplasia, and disorders of the immune system.
plasma f., a circulating α_2-glycoprotein that functions as an opsonin, mediating reticuloendothelial and macrophage clearance of fibrin microaggregates, collagen debris, and bacterial particulates, protecting microvascular perfusion and lymphatic drainage.

fibroneuroma (fī'brō-nū-rō'mă). Neurofibroma.

fibro-osteoma (fī'brō-os-tē-ō'mă). An osteoma in which the neoplastic bone-forming cells are situated within a relatively abundant stroma of fibrous tissue.

fibropapilloma (fī'brō-pap-i-lō'mă). A papilloma characterized by a conspicuous amount of fibrous connective tissue at the base and forming the cores upon which the neoplastic epithelial cells are massed.

fibroplasia (fī-brō-plā'zē-ă) [fibro- + G. *plasis,* a molding]. Production of fibrous tissue, usually implying an abnormal increase of non-neoplastic fibrous tissue.
retrolental f., *retinopathy* of prematurity.

fibroplastic (fī-brō-plas'tik) [fibro- + G. *plastos,* formed]. Producing fibrous tissue.

fibroplate (fī'brō-plāt). *Discus* articularis.

fibropolypus (fī-brō-pol'i-pŭs). A polypus composed chiefly of fibrous tissue.

fibropsammoma (fī'brō-sam-mō'mă). A psammoma that has an unusually abundant, dense stroma of fibrous tissue; a form of meningioma.

fibroreticulate (fī'brō-re-tik'yū-lāt). Relating to or consisting of a network of fibrous tissue.

fibrosarcoma (fī'brō-sar-kō'mă). A malignant neoplasm derived from deep fibrous tissue, characterized by bundles of immature proliferating fibroblasts with variable collagen formation, which tends to invade locally and metastasize by the bloodstream.
ameloblastic f., ameloblastic sarcoma; a rapidly growing, painful, destructive, radiolucent odontogenic tumor that usually arises through malignant change in the mesenchymal component of a pre-existing ameloblastic fibroma.
Earle L f., a transplantable f. derived from subcutaneous tissue of a mouse of C3H strain, grown in tissue culture to which 20-methylcholanthrene had been added.
infantile f., a rapidly growing but infrequently metastasizing f. which usually appears on the extremities in the first year of life.

fibrose (fī-brōs'). To form fibrous tissue.

fibroserous (fī-brō-sē'rŭs). Composed of fibrous tissue with a serous surface; denoting any serous membrane.

fibrosis (fī-brō'sis). Formation of fibrous tissue as a reparative or reactive process, as opposed to formation of fibrous tissue as a normal constituent of an organ or tissue.
cystic f. (of the pancreas), fibrocystic disease of the pancreas; mucoviscidosis; Clarke-Hadfield syndrome; viscidosis; a congenital metabolic disorder, inherited as a recessive trait, in which secretions of exocrine glands are abnormal; excessively viscid mucus causes obstruction of passageways (including pancreatic and bile ducts, intestines, and bronchi) and the sodium and chloride content of sweat are increased throughout the patient's life; symptoms usually appear in childhood and include meconium ileus, poor growth despite good appetite, malabsorption and foul bulky stools, chronic bronchitis with cough, recurrent pneumonia, bronchiectasis, emphysema, clubbing of the fingers, and salt depletion in hot weather; the underlying metabolic defect is unknown and survival is shortened.
endomyocardial f., endocardial fibroelastosis (2); Davids' disease; thickening of the ventricular endocardium by f., involving the subendocardial myocardium, and sometimes the atrioventricular valves, with mural thrombosis, leading to progressive right and left ventricular failure with mitral and tricuspid insufficiency; occurs in adults and is endemic in parts of Africa.
idiopathic retroperitoneal f., retroperitoneal f.; Ormond's disease; idiopathic fibrous retroperitonitis; periureteritis plastica; f. of retroperitoneal structures commonly involving and often obstructing the ureters; the cause is usually unknown, although some cases have followed methysergide treatment.
leptomeningeal f., a fibrous reaction within the subarachnoid space; sometimes a sequel to infectious or chemical meningitis. See also adhesive *arachnoiditis.*
mediastinal f., idiopathic fibrous mediastinitis; idiopathic f. obstructing the superior vena cava or other superior mediastinal structures.
nodular subepidermal f., see dermatofibroma.
pericentral f., f. occurring around the central veins in the hepatic lobules.
perimuscular f., subadventitial f.; f. in the outer media of arteries, usually the renal arteries of young women, where it causes segmental stenosis and hypertension; a variety of fibromuscular dysplasia.
pipestem f., Symmers' clay pipestem f.; Symmers' f.; a characteristic pipe-shaped f. formed around hepatic portal veins in some cases

of long-continued heavy infection with *Schistosoma mansoni;* thought to be induced by the presence of large numbers of schistosome eggs in the hepatic tissues.
replacement f., the formation of fibrous tissue that occupies sites where various other cells and tissues have become atrophied, or degenerated and necrotic.
retroperitoneal f., idiopathic retroperitoneal f.
subadventitial f., perimuscular f.
Symmers' clay pipestem f., Symmers' f., pipestem f.

fibrositis (fī-brō-sī'tis) [fibro- + G. *-itis,* inflammation]. **1.** Inflammation of fibrous tissue. **2.** Muscular rheumatism; term used to denote aching, soreness, or stiffness, with multiple tender foci (trigger points); thought to be due to a sleep disturbance preventing normal muscle relaxation.
cervical f., posttraumatic neck *syndrome.*

fibrothorax (fī-brō-thō'raks). Fibrosis of the pleural space.

fibrotic (fī-brot'ik). Pertaining to or characterized by fibrosis.

fibrous (fī'brŭs). Composed of or containing fibroblasts, and also the fibrils and fibers of connective tissue formed by such cells.

fibroxanthoma (fī'brō-zan-thō'mă). See dermatofibroma.
atypical f., a solitary, often ulcerated, small cutaneous benign tumor composed of foamy histiocytes, spindle cells, and bizarre giant cells; usually found on the exposed skin of older people; microscopically, atypical f. closely resembles malignant fibrous histiocytoma.

fibula (fib'yū-lă) [L. *fibula* (contr. fr. *figibula*), that which fastens, a clasp, buckle, fr. *figo,* to fix, fasten] [NA]. Calf bone; peroneal bone; splint bone (2); perone; the lateral and smaller of the two bones of the leg; it articulates with the tibia above and the tibia and talus below.

fibular (fib'yū-lăr) [L. *fibularis*]. Relating to the fibula.

fibularis (fib-yū-lā'ris) [Mod. L.] [NA]. Fibular.

fibulocalcaneal (fib'yū-lō-kal-kā'nē-ăl). Relating to the fibula and the calcaneus.

ficin (fī'sin) [EC 3.4.22.3]. A proteolytic enzyme isolated from figs (*Ficus carica, globata,* and *doliaria*); used as an anthelmintic and in industry as a protein digestant.

Fick, Adolf, German physician, 1829–1901. See F. *principle.*

ficosis (fī-kō'sis) [L. *ficus,* fig]. Sycosis.

Fiedler, Carl L.A., German physician, 1835–1921. See F.'s *myocarditis.*

field (fēld) [A.S. *feld*]. A definite area of plane surface, considered in relation to some specific object.
auditory f., the space included within the limits of hearing of a definite sound, as of a tuning fork.
Broca's f., Broca's *center.*
Cohnheim's f., Cohnheim's *area.*
f. of consciousness, see under consciousness.
f. of fixation, in ophthalmology, the angular distance around which the line of fixation can be turned.
f.'s of Forel, tegmental f.'s of Forel; campi foreli; three circumscript, myelin-rich regions of the subthalamus known as H fields (from Haubenfelder); 1) field H_1, corresponding to the fasciculus thalamicus, a horizontal fiber stratum at the junction of the subthalamus and the overlying thalamus, is composed of pallidothalamic and cerebellothalamic fibers (brachium conjunctivum) and is separated by the zona incerta from the more ventrally placed field H_2; 2) field H_2, formed by the fasciculus lenticularis and arching over the dorsal border of the subthalamic nucleus, is composed largely of pallidothalamic fibers; 3) field H or prerubral field, is a large field of intermingling gray and white matter immediately rostral to the red nucleus, uniting fields H_1 and H_2 around the medial margin of the zona incerta; its gray matter forms the prerubral nucleus. See also *ansa* lenticularis.
free f., a f. (three-dimensional space) in a homogeneous, isotropic medium free from boundaries; in practice, a f. in which boundary effects are negligible.
H f.'s, see f.'s of Forel.
individuation f., the f. within which an organizer can bring about the rearrangement of primordial tissues in such a manner that a complete embryo is formed.
magnetic f., the sphere of influence of a magnet.
microscopic f., the area within which objects are visible with microscope oculars and objectives of various magnifying powers.
nerve f., the regional distribution of nerve terminals.
prerubral f., see f.'s of Forel.
tegmental f.'s of Forel, f.'s of Forel.
visual f. (F), the area simultaneously visible to one eye without movement; often measured by means of an arc (perimeter) located 330 mm from the eye.
Wernicke's f., Wernicke's *center.*

Field's rapid stain. See under stain.

Fielding, George H., British anatomist, 1801–1871. See F.'s *membrane.*

field-vole. A species of field mouse (*Microtus montebelloi*), normal host of *Leptospira hebdomadis,* the cause of autumn fever or nanukayami fever.

Fiessinger, Noël Armand, French physician, 1881–1946. See F.-Leroy-Reiter *syndrome.*

fig [L. *ficus;* A.S. *fic*]. Ficus, the partially dried fruit of *Ficus carica* (family Moraceae); used as a nutrient, mild laxative, and demulcent.

FIGLU Abbreviation for formiminoglutamic acid.

Figueira, Fernandes, Brazilian pediatrician, †1928. See F.'s *syndrome.*

figuratus (fig-yū-rā'tŭs) [L. *figuro,* pp. *-atus,* to form, fashion]. Figured; a term descriptive of certain skin lesions.

figure (fig'yūr). **1.** A form or shape. **2.** A person representing the essential aspects of a particular role.
authority f., a real or projected person in a position of power; during the transference phase of psychoanalysis, the psychoanalyst becomes an authority f.
flame f., a small area of dermal necrosis with intense eosinophil staining of collagen bundles; seen in the lesions of Well's syndrome.
fortification f.'s, fortification *spectrum.*
mitotic f., the microscopic appearance of a cell undergoing mitosis; a cell whose chromosomes are visible with the light microscope.
myelin f., myelin body; a rolled-up or scroll-like arrangement of a lipid bilayer within a cell, superficially resembling the myelin sheath of nerves; observed with the electron microscope in the cytoplasm or as inclusion in mitochondria and antiphagic vacuoles where they may represent artifacts of lipid fixation.
Purkinje's f.'s, shadows of the retinal vessels, seen as dark lines on a reddish field when a light enters the eye through the sclera and not the pupil.

figure and ground. That aspect of perception wherein the perceived is separated into at least two parts, each with different attributes but influencing one another. Figure is the most distinct; ground the least formed; *e.g.,* a bird (figure) seen against the sky (ground).

fila (fī'lă) [L.]. Plural of filum.

filaceous (fī-lā'shŭs) [L. *filum,* a thread]. Filamentous.

filaggrin (fil-ag'grin) [filament aggregating]. A major protein of the keratohyalin granule, composed of histadine, lysine, and arginine (stratum corneum basic proteins).

filamen (fil'ă-men). A high-molecular-weight, actin-binding protein that is part of the intracellular filamentous structure of fibroblastic cells; its distribution in cells is derived from its interaction with polymerized actin.

filament (fil'ă-ment) [L. *filamentum,* fr. *filum,* a thread]. **1.** Filamentum. **2.** In bacteriology, a fine threadlike form, unsegmented or segmented without constrictions.

actin f., one of the contractile elements in muscular fibers and other cells; in skeletal muscle, the actin f.'s are about 50 Å wide and 100 μm long, and attach to the transverse Z f.'s.

axial f., axoneme (2); the central f. of a flagellum or cilium; with the electron microscope it is seen as a complex of nine peripheral diplomicrotubules and a central pair of microtubules.

cytokeratin f.'s, keratin f.'s.

keratin f.'s, cytokeratin f.'s; a class of intermediate f.'s that form a network within epithelial cells and anchor to desmosomes, thus imparting tensile strength to the tissue.

intermediate f.'s, a class of tough protein f.'s (including keratin f.'s, neurofilaments, desmin, and vimentin) which measure 8-10 nm in thickness and comprise part of the cytoskeleton of the cytoplasm of most eukaryotic cells; so named because they are intermediate in thickness between actin f.'s and microtubules.

myosin f., one of the contractile elements in skeletal, cardiac, and smooth muscle fibers; in skeletal muscle, the f. is about 100 Å thick and 1.5 μm long.

parabasal f., term formerly used for rhizoplast.

root f.'s, *fila* radicularia.

spermatic f., a spermatozoon, especially the tail of a spermatozoon.

Z f., the thin zig-zag structure at the Z line of striated muscle fibers to which the actin f.'s attach.

filamentous (fil-ă-men'tŭs). Filaceous; filar (2). **1.** Filiform (1); threadlike in structure. **2.** Composed of filaments or threadlike structures.

filamentum, pl. **filamenta** (fil-ă-men'tŭm, -tă) [L.]. Filament (1); a fibril, fine fiber, or threadlike structure.

filar (fī'lăr) [L. *filum,* a thread]. **1.** Fibrillar. **2.** Filamentous.

Filaria (fī-lar'ē-ă). Former genus of nematodes now classified in several genera and species of the family Onchocercidae; *e.g., Wuchereria bancrofti* (*F. bancrofti, F. diurna,* or *F. nocturna*), *Brugia malayi* (*F. malaya*), *Onchocerca volvulus* (*F. volvulus*), *Mansonella perstans* (*F. perstans* or *F. sanguinis hominis*), *M. streptocerca, M. ozzardi* (*F. demarquayi* or *F. ozzardi*), *Loa loa* (*F. extraocularis, F. lentis, F. loa,* or *F. oculi humani*), and *Dracunculus medinensis* (*F. medinensis*). See also filaria.

filaria, pl. **filariae** (fi-lar'ē-ă, -ē-ē) [L. *filum,* a thread]. Common name for nematodes of the family Onchocercidae, which live as adults in the blood, tissue fluids, tissues, or body cavities of many vertebrates. The females lay partially embryonated eggs, the embryos uncoil and circulate in blood or tissue fluids as microfilariae; if ingested by an appropriate bloodsucking arthropod, larval stages develop; later, infective larvae may be deposited on another vertebrate host's skin when the arthropod seeks another blood meal.

filarial (fi-lā'rē-ăl). Pertaining to a filaria (or filariae), including the microfilaria stage.

filariasis (fil-ă-rī'ă-sis). Presence of filariae in the tissues of the body, or in blood (microfilaremia) or tissue fluids (microfilariasis), occurring in tropical amd subtropical regions; living worms cause minimal tissue reaction, which may be asymptomatic, but death of the adult worms leads to granulomatous inflammation and permanent fibrosis causing obstruction of the lymphatic channels from dense hyalinized scars in the subcutaneous tissues; the most serious consequence is elephantiasis or pachyderma.

bancroftian f., f. caused by *Wuchereria bancrofti.*

periodic f., a form of f. in which microfilariae appear in the peripheral blood at regular 24-hr intervals; usually refers to the nocturnal periodicity of bancroftian filariasis.

filaricidal (fi-lar-i-sī'dăl). Fatal to filariae.

filaricide (fi-lar'i-sīd) [filaria + L. *caedo,* to kill]. An agent that kills filariae.

filariform (fi-lar'i-fōrm). **1.** Resembling filariae or other types of small nematode worms. **2.** Thin or hairlike.

Filariicae (fi-lar'ē-i-sē). Filarioidea.

Filarioidea (fi-lar'ē-oy'dē-ă). Filariicae; a superfamily of filarial nematodes parasitic in many animal species, including man; includes the families Filariidae, Diplotraenidae, Onchocercidae, and Stephanofilariidae. See *Filaria,* also *Dipetalonema, Dirofilaria, Loa loa, Mansonella, Onchocerca, Wuchereria,* and *Brugia.*

Filaroides (fil'ă-roy'dēz). A genus of nematode parasites occurring in the lungs, bronchi, and trachea of dogs. *F. osleri* is a small, widely distributed species that causes a chronic disease of dogs, manifested by small (usually less than 1 cm in diameter), gray-white or pink nodules; the most marked symptom is a harsh cough.

Filatov, Nil F., Russian pediatrician, 1847–1902. See F.'s *disease, spots.*

Filatov, Vladimir P., Russian ophthalmologist, 1875–1956. See F. *flap;* F. 's *operation;* F.-Gillies *flap,* tubed *pedicle.*

file (fīl). A tool for smoothing, grinding, or cutting.

Hedström f., a coarse root canal f. similar to a rasp.

periodontal f., an instrument with a series of ridges or points arranged in rows on its surface, used for scaling or removing dental calculus from the teeth.

root canal f., a pointed, flexible, steel intracanal instrument used in rasping canal walls.

filial (fil'ē-ăl) [L. *filialis,* fr. *filius,* son, *filia,* daughter]. Denoting the relationship of offspring to parents. See filial *generation.*

filiform (fil'i-fōrm) [L. *filum,* thread]. **1.** Filamentous (1). **2.** In bacteriology, denoting an even growth along the line of inoculation, either stroke or stab.

filioparental (fil'ē-ō-pă-ren'tăl). Pertaining to a child-parent relationship.

filipuncture (fil'i-pŭnk-chūr) [L. *filum,* thread]. Treatment of an aneurysm by the insertion of a coil of slender wire to induce coagulation.

fillet (fil'et) [Fr. *filet,* a band]. **1.** Lemniscus. **2.** A skein, loop of cord, or tape used for making traction on a part of the fetus.

lateral f., *lemniscus* lateralis.

medial f., *lemniscus* medialis.

filling (fil'ing). Lay term for a dental restoration.

film. 1. A light-sensitive or x-ray-sensitive substance used in taking photographs or radiographs. **2.** A thin layer or coating.

absorbable gelatin f., a sterile, nonantigenic, absorbable, water-insoluble, thin sheet of gelatin prepared by drying a gelatin-formaldehyde solution on plates; used in the closure and repair of defects in membranes such as the dura mater or the pleura; it undergoes absorption over a period of 1 to 6 months.

bitewing f., a special packaging of roentgenographic f. that allows an appendage of one f. package to be held between the occlusal surfaces of the teeth.

panoramic x-ray f., in dentistry, a radiograph taken to give a panoramic view of the entire upper and lower dental arch as well as the temporomandibular joint.

plain f., X-ray taken without use of a contrast medium. See flat *plate.*

precorneal f., a protective f., 7 to 9 nm thick, consisting of external oily, intermediate watery, and deep mucoprotein layers.

tear f., the layer of mucin, fluid, and lipid that forms the anterior surface of the cornea and conjunctiva.

filopodia (fil-ō-pō'dē-ă). Plural of filopodium.

filopodium, pl. **filopodia** (fī-lō-pō'dē-ŭm, -ă) [L. *filum,* thread, +

G. *pous,* foot]. A slender filamentous pseudopodium of certain free-living amebae.

filopressure (fī-lō-presh'ŭr) [L. *filum,* thread]. Temporary pressure on a blood vessel by a ligature, which is removed when the flow of blood has ceased.

filovaricosis (fī'lō-var-ē-kō'sis) [L. *filum,* thread, + *varix,* dilation of vein]. A series of swellings along the course of the axon of a nerve fiber.

filter (fil'ter) [Mediev. L. *filtro,* pp. *-atus,* to strain through felt, fr. *filtrum,* felt]. **1.** Filtrum; a porous substance through which a liquid or gas is passed in order to separate it from contained particulate matter or impurities. **2.** To use or to subject to the action of a f. **3.** A radiolucent screen, used in both diagnostic and therapeutic radiology, that permits the passage of certain rays and inhibits the passage of others which have a lower and less desirable energy. **4.** A device used in spectrophotometric analysis to isolate a segment of the spectrum.

filtrable, filterable (fil'tră-bl, fil'ter-ă-bl). Capable of passing a filter; frequently applied to smaller viruses and some bacteria.

filtrate (fil'trāt). That which has passed through a filter.

filtration (fil-trā'shŭn). **1.** Percolation (1); the process of passing a liquid or gas through a filter. **2.** In radiology, the process of attenuating a radioactive or electromagnetic beam by interposing some absorber, frequently metal, between the source and the target, thus permitting passage of only certain particles or wavelengths. F. that results from interposing necessary parts of the equipment, such as the glass envelope of an emitter, is called inherent f.

gel f., separation of molecular sizes by passage of a mixture through columns of beads of cross-linked dextrans or similar relatively inert material of a well defined pore size range; the larger the molecule, the less time it spends in the interior of the beads, thus emerging earlier from the column than smaller molecules.

filtrum (fil'trŭm) [Mediev. L.]. Filter (1).

Merkel's f. ventric'uli, f. ventriculi.

f. ventric'uli, Merkel's f. ventriculi; a groove between the two prominences, in each lateral wall of the vestibule of the larynx, formed by the cuneiform and the arytenoid cartilages.

filum, pl. **fila** (fī'lŭm, -lă) [L. thread] [NA]. A structure of filamentous or threadlike appearance.

f. du'rae ma'tris spina'lis [NA], the termination of the spinal dura mater, surrounding the f. terminale of the cord, and attached to the deep dorsal sacrococcygeal ligament.

fi'la olfacto'ria, *nervi* olfactorii.

fi'la radicula'ria [NA], root filaments; nerve rootlets; the small, individual fiber fascicles into which the roots of all of the spinal nerves and several cranial nerves (hypoglossus, vagus, oculomotorius) divide in fanlike fashion before entering or leaving the spinal cord or brainstem; the spinal dorsal root may divide into 8 to 12 such rootlets.

terminal f., f. terminale.

f. termina'le [NA], terminal f.; terminal thread; nervus impar; a long, slender connective tissue strand extending from the extremity of the conus medullaris to the coccygeal ligament.

fimbria, pl. **fimbriae** (fim'brē-ă, -brē-ē) [L. fringe]. **1** [NA]. Fringe; any fringelike structure. **2.** Pilus (2).

f. hippocam'pi [NA], corpus fimbriatum (1); tenia hippocampi; a narrow sharp-edged crest of white fiber matter, continuous with the alveus hippocampi, attached to the medial border of the hippocampus; composed of efferent fibers of the hippocampus that form the fornix, fibers of the hippocampal commissure, and septohippocampal fibers.

ovarian f., f. ovarica.

f. ova'rica [NA], ovarian f.; infundibulo-ovarian ligament; the longest of the fimbriae of the uterine tube; it extends from the infundibulum to the ovary.

fim'briae tu'bae uteri'nae [NA], fimbriae of uterine tube; Richard's fringes; laciniae tubae; the irregularly branched or fringed processes surrounding the ampulla at the abdominal opening of the uterine tube; most of the epithelial cells have cilia which beat toward the uterus.

fimbriae of uterine tube, fimbriae tubae uterinae.

fimbriate, fimbriated (fim'brē-āt, -ā-ted). Having fimbriae.

fimbriectomy (fim'brē-ek'tō-mē) [L. *fimbria,* fringe, + G. *ektomē,* excision]. Excision of fimbriae.

fimbriocele (fim'brē-ō-sēl) [L. *fimbria,* fringe, + G. *kēlē,* hernia]. Hernia of the corpus fimbriatum of the oviduct.

fimbrioplasty (fim'brē-ō-plas-tē) [L. *fimbria,* fringe, + G. *plastos,* formed]. Corrective operation upon the tubal fimbriae.

Finckh, Johann, German psychiatrist, *1873. See F. *test.*

fineness (fīn'nes). A designator used to indicate gold content of an alloy, 1000 fine being 24-carat or pure gold.

finger (fing'ger) [A.S.]. *Digitus* manus; one of the digits of the hand.

baseball f., drop, hammer, or mallet f.; an avulsion, partial or complete, of the long finger extensor from the base of the distal phalanx.

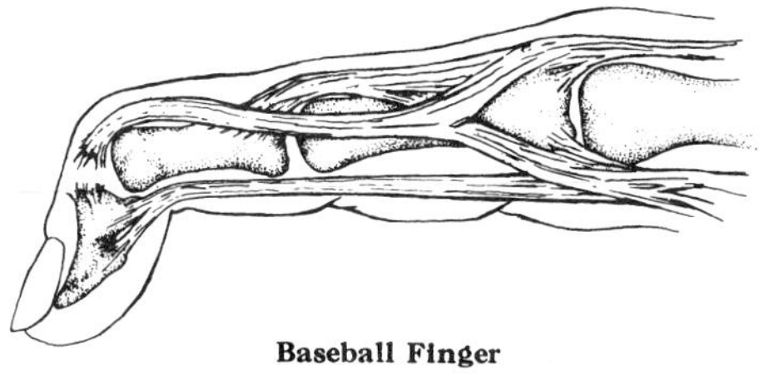

Baseball Finger

bolster f., monilial infection of the nail fold.

clubbed f.'s, see clubbing.

dead f.'s, acroasphyxia.

drop f., baseball f.

drumstick f.'s, see clubbing.

fifth f., *digitus* minimus.

first f., pollex.

fourth f., *digitus* annularis.

hammer f., baseball f.

hippocratic f.'s, see clubbing.

index f., index (1).

jerk f., trigger f.

little f., *digitus* minimus.

lock f., trigger f.

mallet f., baseball f.

middle f., *digitus* medius.

ring f., *digitus* annularis.

sausage f.'s, the thick, short f.'s of acromegaly.

second f., index (1).

snap f., trigger f.

spade f.'s, the course, thick f.'s of acromegaly or myxedema.

spider f., arachnodactyly.

spring f., trigger f.

stuck f., trigger f.

third f., *digitus* medius.

trigger f., jerk, lock, snap, spring, or stuck f.; an affection in which the movement of the f. is arrested for a moment in flexion or extension and then continues with a jerk.

waxy f.'s, acroasphyxia.

webbed f.'s, two or more f.'s united and enclosed in a common sheath of skin.

white f.'s, an occupational disease occurring in operators of pneumatic hammers who are exposed to cold, affecting usually the f.'s of the left hand.

fingernail (fing'ger-nāl). See unguis.

fingerprint (fing'ger-print'). **1.** An impression of the inked bulb of the distal phalanx of a finger, showing the configuration of the ridges, used as a means of identification. See also dermatoglyphics; Galton's system of classification of f.'s. **2.** Term, sometimes used informally, referring to any analytical method capable of making fine distinctions between similar compounds; *e.g.*, the pattern of an infrared absorption curve or of a two-dimensional paper chromatograph.

Galton's system of classification of f.'s, a system of classification based on the variations in the patterns of the ridges, which are grouped into arches, loops, and whorls (A.L.W. or arch-loop-whorl system). "Arches are formed when the ridges run from one side to the other of the bulb of the digit, without making any backward turn, but no twist; whorls, when there is a turn through at least one complete circle; they are also considered to include all duplex spirals." The abbreviations used in making a record of f.'s are: *a,* arch; *l,* loop; *w,* whorl; *i,* loop with an inner (thumb side) slope; *o,* loop with an outer (little-finger side) slope. The ten digits are registered in four groups as follows, distinguished by capital letters: *A,* the fore, middle, and ring fingers of the right hand; *B,* the fore, middle, and ring fingers of the left hand; *C,* the thumb and little finger of the right hand; *D,* the thumb and little finger of the left hand.

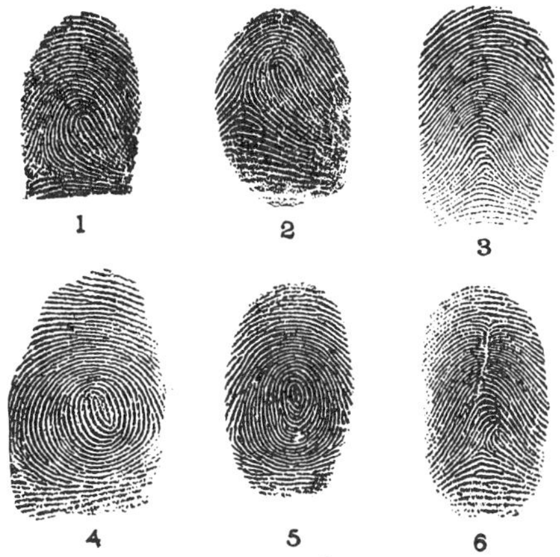

Fingerprints
1 and *2*, loops showing Galton's delta; *3*, arches; *4*, whorls; *5*, circles; *6*, showing the mark of a scar.

Fink, R.P., 20th century U.S. anatomist. See F.-Heimer *stain.*

Finkeldey, Wilhelm, 20th century German pathologist. See Warthin-F. *cells.*

Finney, John M.T., U.S. surgeon, 1863–1942. See F.'s *operation;* F. *pyloroplasty.*

Finsen, Niels R., Danish physician and Nobel laureate, 1860–1904. See F. *light.*

fire (fīr). **1.** In dermatology, erysipelas. **2.** In dentistry, the fusing of water and a powder containing kaolin, feldspar, and other substances to produce porcelain used in restorations and artificial teeth.

firedamp (fīr'damp). Methane or other light hydrocarbons forming an explosive mixture when mixed with 7 or 8 volumes of air.

first aid. Immediate assistance administered in the case of injury or sudden illnes by a bystander or other lay person, before the arrival of trained medical personnel.

Fischer, Emil, German chemist, 1852–1919. See F. projection formulas of sugars (under *sugars*).

Fischer, Louis, U.S. pediatrician, 1864–1944. See F.'s *sign, symptom.*

Fishberg, Arthur M., U.S. physician, *1898. See F.'s concentration *test.*

Fisher, Miller, U.S. neurologist, *1910. See F.'s *syndrome.*

Fishman-Lerner unit. See under unit.

fission (fish'ŭn) [L. *fissio,* a cleaving, fr. *findo,* pp. *fissus,* to cleave]. **1.** The act of splitting, *e.g.*, amitotic division of a cell or its nucleus. **2.** Splitting of the nucleus of an atom.

binary f., simple f. in which the two new cells are approximately equal in size.

bud f., gemmation.

multiple f., sporulation; division of the nucleus, simultaneously or successively, into a number of daughter nuclei, followed by division of the cell body into an equal number of parts, each containing a nucleus.

simple f., division of the nucleus and then the cell body into two parts. See also binary f.

fissiparity (fis-i-par'i-tē) [L. *findo,* pp. *fissus,* split, + *pario,* pp. *paritus,* to bring forth]. Schizogenesis.

fissiparous (fi-sip'ă-rŭs) [L. *findo,* pp. *fissus,* split, + *pario,* to produce]. Reproducing or propagating by fission.

Fissipedia (fis-i-pē'dē-ă) [L. *fissus,* cloven, + *pes* (*ped-*), foot]. A suborder of the carnivora with separated toes, *e.g.*, dogs, cats, bears.

FISSURA

fissura, pl. **fissurae** (fi-sū'ră, -sū'rē) [L. fr. *findo,* to cleave]. [NA]. **1.** A deep fissure, cleft, or slit. **2.** In neuroanatomy, a particularly deep sulcus of the surface of the brain or spinal cord.

f. antitragohelici'na [NA], antitragohelicine fissure; a fissure in the auricular cartilage between the cauda helicis and the antitragus.

f. calcari'na, *sulcus* calcarinus.

fissu'rae cerebel'li [NA], cerebellar fissures; the deep furrows which divide the lobules of the cerebellum. See also postcentral *fissure;* f. prima cerebelli; f. secunda cerebelli.

f. cer'ebri latera'lis, *sulcus* lateralis cerebri.

f. choroi'dea, **(1)** [NA], choroid fissure (1); the narrow cleft along the medial wall of the lateral ventricle along the margins of which the choroid plexus is attached; it lies between the upper surface of the thalamus and lateral edge of the fornix in the central part of the ventricle and between the stria terminalis and fimbria hippocampi in the inferior horn; **(2)** optic *fissure.*

f. collatera'lis, *sulcus* collateralis.

f. denta'ta, *sulcus* hippocampi.

f. hippocam'pi, *sulcus* hippocampi.

f. horizonta'lis cerebel'li [NA], horizontal fissure of the cerebellum; great horizontal fissure; horizontal fissure that divides the ansiform lobule into its major parts, crus I (superior semilunar lobule) and crus II (inferior semilunar lobule).

f. horizonta'lis pulmo'nis dex'tri [NA], horizontal fissure of right lung; transverse fissure of the lung; the deep fissure that separates the upper and middle lobes of the right lung.

f. ligamen'ti tere'tis [NA], fissure of the round ligament; fissure for ligamentum teres; umbilical fissure; umbilical fossa; fossa venae umbilicalis; a cleft on the inferior surface of the liver, running from the inferior border to the left extremity of the porta hepatis; it lodges the ligamentum teres hepatis.

f. ligamen'ti veno'si [NA], fissure of the venous ligament; a deep cleft extending from the porta hepatis and the inferior vena cava between the left lobe and the caudate lobe; it lodges the ligamentum venosum.

f. longitudina'lis cer'ebri [NA], longitudinal fissure of the cerebrum; great longitudinal fissure; the deep cleft separating the two hemispheres of the cerebrum.

f. media'na ante'rior medul'lae oblonga'tae [NA], anterior median fissure or anteromedian groove of the medulla oblongata; the longitudinal groove in the midline of the anterior aspect of the medulla oblongata; it is the medullary equivalent of the f. mediana anterior of the spinal cord and ends at the foramen cecum posterius; its caudal part is obliterated by the decussation of the pyramids.

f. media'na ante'rior medul'lae spina'lis [NA], anterior median fissure or anteromedian groove of the spinal cord; sulcus ventralis; a deep median fissure on the anterior surface of the spinal cord.

f. obli'qua [NA], oblique fissure; the deep fissure in each lung that runs obliquely downward and forward. It divides the upper and lower lobes of the left lung and separates the upper and middle lobes from the lower lobe of the right lung.

f. orbita'lis infe'rior [NA], inferior orbital fissure; sphenomaxillary fissure; a cleft between the greater wing of the sphenoid and the orbital plate of the maxilla, through which pass the maxillary division and the orbital branch of the trigeminal nerve, fibers from the pterygopalatine (Meckel's) ganglion, and the infraorbital vessels.

f. orbita'lis supe'rior [NA], superior orbital fissure; sphenoidal fissure; foramen lacerum anterius; a cleft between the greater and the lesser wings of the sphenoid establishing a channel of communication between the middle cranial fossa and the orbit, through which pass the oculomotor and trochlear nerves, the ophthalmic division of the trigeminal nerve, the abducens nerve, and the ophthalmic veins.

f. parietooccipita'lis, *sulcus* parietooccipitalis.

f. petro-occipita'lis [NA], petro-occipital fissure; Ecker's fissure; a fissure between the petrous part of the temporal bone and the basilar part of the occipital bone that extends anteromedially from the jugular foramen.

f. petrosquamo'sa [NA], petrosquamous fissure; a shallow fissure indicating externally the line of fusion of the petrous and squamous portions of the temporal bone.

f. petrotympan'ica [NA], petrotympanic fissure; glaserian fissure; a fissure between the tympanic and petrous portions of the temporal bone; it transmits the chorda tympani nerve.

f. posterolatera'lis [NA], posterolateral fissure; prenodular f.; the earliest fissure to appear in the development of the cerebellum; it separates the flocculus and nodulus from the uvula and tonsil.

f. pri'ma cerebel'li [NA], primary fissure of the cerebellum; the deepest fissure of the cerebellum; demarcates the division of anterior and posterior lobes of the cerebellum.

f. pterygoid'ea, *incisura* pterygoidea.

f. pterygomaxilla'ris [NA], pterygomaxillary fissure; f. pterygopalatina; the narrow gap between the lateral pterygoid plate and the maxilla through which the infratemporal fossa communicates with the pterygopalatine fossa.

f. pterygopalati'na, f. pterygomaxillaris.

f. puden'di, *rima* pudendi.

f. secun'da cerebel'li [NA], secondary fissure of the cerebellum; a fissure that separates the uvula of the inferior vermis of the cerebellum from the pyramid.

f. sphenopetro'sa [NA], sphenopetrosal fissure; a narrow fissure between the undersurface of the greater wing of the sphenoid and the petrous portion of the temporal bone.

f. transver'sa cerebel'li, transverse fissure of the cerebellum; the cleft caused by the protrusion of the anterior lobe of the cerebellum over the superior and middle cerebellar peduncles.

f. transver'sa cer'ebri [NA], transverse fissure of the cerebrum; the triangular space between the corpus callosum and fornix above and the dorsal surface of the thalamus below, which is bounded laterally by the choroid fissure of the lateral ventricle, lined by pia mater, and opens caudally into the cisterna ambiens of the subarachnoid space.

f. tympanomastoid'ea [NA], tympanomastoid fissure or suture; auricular fissure; a fissure separating the tympanic portion from the mastoid portion of the temporal bone; it transmits the auricular branch of the vagus nerve.

f. tympanosquamo'sa [NA], tympanosquamous fissure; squamotympanic fissure; the fissure separating the tympanic part of the temporal bone from the squamous part; it is continuous medially with the petrotympanic fissure and the petrosquamous fissure.

fissural (fish'ŭ-răl). Relating to a fissure.

fissuration (fish'ŭ-rā'shŭn). State of being fissured.

FISSURE

fissure (fish'ŭr) [L. *fissura*]. **1.** A deep furrow, cleft, or slit. For the normal anatomical f.'s, see under fissura; for most of the brain f.'s, see under sulcus. **2.** In dentistry, a developmental break or fault in the tooth enamel.

abdominal f., congenital failure of the ventral body wall to close. See also celosomia.

Ammon's f., a pearl-shaped opening in the sclera during early embryogenesis.

anal f., a crack or slit in the mucous membrane of the anus, very painful and difficult to heal.

anterior median f. of medulla oblongata, *fissura* mediana anterior medullae oblongatae.

anterior median f. of spinal cord, *fissura* mediana anterior medullae spinalis.

antitragohelicine f., *fissura* antitragohelicina.

ape f., *sulcus* lunatus cerebri.

auricular f., *fissura* tympanomastoidea.

Bichat's f., the nearly circular f. corresponding to the medial margin of the cerebral (pallial) mantle, marking the hilus of the cerebral hemisphere, consisting of the fissura (sulcus) callosomarginalis and fissura choroidea along the hippocampus, both of which are continuous with the stem of the f. of Sylvius at the anterior extremity of the temporal lobe.

branchial f., a persistent branchial cleft.

Broca's f., the f. surrounding Broca's convolution.

calcarine f., *sulcus* calcarinus.

callosomarginal f., *sulcus* cinguli.

caudal transverse f., *porta* hepatis.

cerebellar f.'s, *fissurae* cerebelli.

cerebral f.'s, see separately named f.'s. See also sulci.

choroid f., **(1)** *fissura* choroidea (1); **(2)** optic f.

Clevenger's f., *sulcus* temporalis inferior.

collateral f., *sulcus* collateralis.

decidual f., a cleft in the decidua basalis or placenta.

dentate f., *sulcus* hippocampi.

Duverney's f.'s, *incisurae* cartilaginis meatus acustici externi.

Ecker's f., *fissura* petrooccipitalis.

enamel f., a deep cleft between adjoining cusps affording retention to caries-producing agents.

glaserian f., *fissura* petrotympanica.

great horizontal f., *fissura* horizontalis cerebelli.

great longitudinal f., *fissura* longitudinalis cerebri.

Henle's f.'s, minute spaces filled with connective tissue between the muscular fasciculi of the heart.

hippocampal f., *sulcus* hippocampi.
horizontal f. of cerebellum, *fissura* horizontalis cerebelli.
horizontal f. of right lung, *fissura* horizontalis pulmonis dextri.
inferior orbital f., *fissura* orbitalis inferior.
lateral cerebral f., *sulcus* lateralis cerebri.
left sagittal f., a sagittal groove on the undersurface of the liver formed by the fissura ligamenti teretis anteriorly and the fissura ligamenti venosi posteriorly.
f. for ligamentum teres, *fissura* ligamenti teretis.
linguogingival f., a f. sometimes occurring on the lingual surface of one of the upper incisors and extending into the cementum.
f.'s of liver, see left sagittal f., right sagittal f., *porta* hepatis.
longitudinal f. of cerebrum, *fissura* longitudinalis cerebri.
lunate f., *sulcus* lunatus cerebri.
f.'s of lung, see *fissura* horizontalis and *fissura* obliqua.
oblique f., *fissura* obliqua.
optic f., choroid f. (2); fissura choroidea (2); in the embryo, the temporary gap in the ventral margin of the developing optic cup.
oral f., *rima* oris.
palpebral f., *rima* palpebrarum.
Pansch's f., a cerebral f. running from the lower extremity of the central f. nearly to the end of the occipital lobe.
paracentral f., a curved f. on the medial surface of the cerebral hemisphere, bounding the paracentral gyrus and separating it from the precuneus and the gyrus cinguli.
parieto-occipital f., *sulcus* parieto-occipitalis.
petro-occipital f., *fissura* petro-occipitalis.
petrosquamous f., *fissura* petrosquamosa.
petrotympanic f., *fissura* petrotympanica.
portal f., *porta* hepatis.
postcentral f., a f. on the superior surface of the cerebellum separating the culmen from the central lobule.
posterior median f. of the medulla oblongata, *sulcus* medianus posterior medullae oblongatae.
posterior median f. of spinal cord, *sulcus* medianus posterior medullae spinalis.
posterolateral f., *fissura* posterolateralis.
posthippocampal f., *sulcus* calcarinus.
postlingual f., a transverse f. on the superior vermis of the cerebellum separating the lingula from the central lobule.
postlunate f., a transverse f. on the superior vermis of the cerebellum separating the posterior lunate lobule in front from the ansiform lobule behind.
postpyramidal f., a f. that separates the pyramid of the cerebellum from the tuber.
postrhinal f., a f. separating the hippocampal from the collateral gyrus.
prenodular f., *fissura* posterolateralis.
primary f. of the cerebellum, *fissura* prima cerebelli.
pterygoid f., *incisura* pterygoidea.
pterygomaxillary f., *fissura* pterygomaxillaris.
rhinal f., *sulcus* rhinalis.
right sagittal f., a sagittal groove on the undersurface of the liver formed by the fossa vesicae felleae anteriorly and the sulcus venae cavae posteriorly.
f. of Rolando, *sulcus* centralis.
f. of round ligament, *fissura* ligamenti teretis.
Santorini's f.'s, *incisurae* cartilaginis meatus acustici externi.
secondary f. of the cerebellum, *fissura* secunda cerebelli.
simian f., *sulcus* lunatus cerebri.
sphenoidal f., *fissura* orbitalis superior.
sphenomaxillary f., *fissura* orbitalis inferior.
sphenopetrosal f., *fissura* sphenopetrosa.
squamotympanic f., *fissura* tympanosquamosa.
superior orbital f., *fissura* orbitalis superior.
superior temporal f., *sulcus* temporalis superior.
sylvian f., f. of Sylvius, *sulcus* lateralis cerebri.
transverse f. of cerebellum, *fissura* transversa cerebelli.
transverse f. of cerebrum, *fissura* transversa cerebri.
transverse f. of the lung, *fissura* horizontalis pulmonis dextri.
tympanomastoid f., *fissura* tympanomastoidea.
tympanosquamous f., *fissura* tympanosquamosa.
umbilical f., *fissura* ligamenti teretis.
f. of venous ligament, *fissura* ligamenti venosi.
vestibular f. of cochlea, a fine f. in the lower part of the first turn of the cochlea, formed by a spiral lamina which projects from the outer wall of the cochlea but does not quite reach the osseous spiral lamina, thus leaving a narrow gap.
zygal f., a figure formed by two nearly parallel cerebral f.'s connected by a short f. at right angles, forming an H.

FISTULA

fistula, pl. **fistulae** or **fistulas** (fis'tyū-lă, -tyū-lē, -tyū-lăs) [L. a pipe, a tube]. An abnormal passage from a hollow organ to the surface, or from one organ to another.

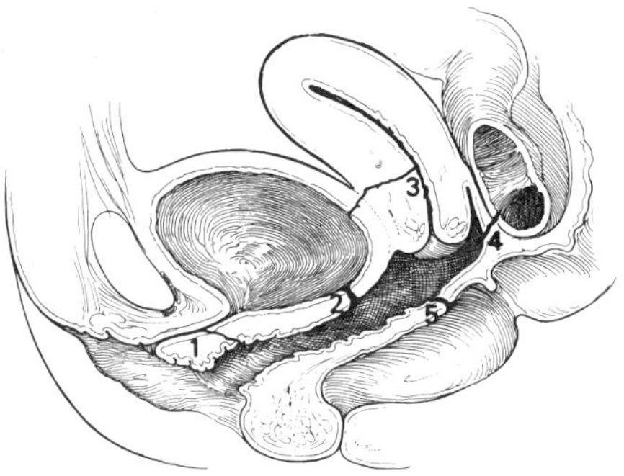

Fistulas
1, Urethrovaginal; *2*, vesicovaginal; *3*, vesicouterine; *4*, enterovaginal; *5*, rectovaginal.

abdominal f., a tract leading from one of the abdominal viscera to the external surface.
amphibolic f., amphibolous f., a complete anal f. opening both externally and internally.
anal f., a f. opening at or near the anus; usually, but not always, opening into the rectum above the internal sphincter.
arteriovenous f., an abnormal communication between an artery and a vein, usually resulting in the formation of an arteriovenous aneurysm.
f. au'ris congen'ita, a congenital f. resulting from a defect in the formation of the auricle of the ear.
biliary f., a f. leading to some portion of the biliary tract.
f. bimuco'sa, a complete f., both ends of which open on the mucous surface.
blind f., incomplete f.; a f. that ends in a cul-de-sac, being open at one extremity only.
branchial f., a congenital f. in the neck resulting from incomplete closure of a branchial cleft.
Brescia-Cimino f., a direct, surgically created, arteriovenous f.; used to facilitate chronic hemodialysis.
bronchoesophageal f., communication between a bronchus and the esophagus; may occur in association with either infection or tumors involving a bronchus or the esophagus.
bronchopleural f., communication between a bronchus and the pleural cavity.

carotid-cavernous f., arteriovenous communication resulting from rupture of the intracavernous portion of the carotid artery.
cervical f., a f. that opens into the external neck, as from thyroglossal cysts, abscesses, bronchial fistulas, etc.; may occur midline, from thyroglossal cysts, or elsewhere.
cholecystoduodenal f., communication between gallbladder and duodenum secondary to severe cholecystitis with perforation and abscess formation; stones erode through adjacent duodenal wall, and large stones may cause gallstone ileus.
coccygeal f., a fistulous opening of a dermoid cyst in the coccygeal region.
f. col'li congen'ita, a congenital f. of the neck leading to the pharynx, larynx, or trachea.
colocutaneous f., a f. between the colon and the skin.
coloileal f., a f. between the colon and the ileum.
colonic f., **(1)** internal, a f. between the colon and a hollow viscus; **(2)** external, a f. between the colon and the skin.
colovaginal f., a f. between colon and vagina.
colovesical f., vesicocolic f.; a f. between colon and urinary bladder.
complete f., a f. that is open at both ends.
craniosinus f., a f. between the intracranial space and a nasal sinus.
dental f., gingival f.
duodenal f., an opening through the duodenal wall and into the peritoneal cavity, into another organ, or through the abdominal wall.
Eck f., transposition of the portal circulation to the systemic by making an anastomosis between the vena cava and portal vein and then ligating the latter close to the liver.
enterocutaneous f., a f. between intestine and skin of abdomen.
enterovaginal f., a fistulous passage connecting the intestine and the vagina.
enterovesical f., a f. connecting the intestine and the bladder.
ethmoidal-lacrimal f., internal lacrimal f.; a fistulous communication between the lacrimal sac and the ethmoidal sinus.
external f., a f. between a hollow viscus and the skin.
fecal f., intestinal f.
gastric f., a fistulous tract from the stomach to the abdominal wall.
gastrocolic f., a fistulous communication between the stomach and the colon.
gastrocutaneous f., a f. between the stomach and the skin.
gastroduodenal f., an abnormal opening between the stomach and the duodenum.
gastrointestinal f., a fistulous tract connecting the stomach with the intestine.
genitourinary f., urogenital f.; a fistulous opening into the urogenital tract.
gingival f., dental f.; a sinus tract originating in a peripheral abscess and opening into the oral cavity on the gingiva.
hepatic f., a f. leading to the liver.
hepatopleural f., a f. between the liver and the pleural space.
horseshoe f., an anal f. partially encircling the anus and opening at both extremities on the cutaneous surface.
incomplete f., blind f.
internal f., a f. between hollow viscera.
internal lacrimal f., ethmoidal-lacrimal f.
intestinal f., fecal or stercoral f.; a tract leading from the lumen of the bowel to the exterior.
lacrimal f., **f. lacrima'lis**, dacryosyrinx; an abnormal opening into a tear duct or the lacrimal sac.
lacteal f., mammary f.; a fistulous opening into one of the lactiferous ducts.
lymphatic f., a congenital f. in the neck connecting with a lymphatic vessel and giving exit to lymph.
mammary f., lacteal f.
Mann-Bollman f., a f. used in experimental investigations; a loop of ileum is isolated, the distal (aboral) end is anastomosed laterally to the duodenum or the small intestine, and the open proximal (oral) end is sutured to the abdominal wall; peristaltic waves travel from oral to aboral end, with leakage to the exterior thus reduced to a minimum.
metroperitoneal f., uteroperitoneal f.
oroantral f., a pathologic communication between the maxillary antrum and the oral cavity, most commonly a complication of maxillary or molar tooth extraction.
orofacial f., a pathologic communication between the cutaneous surface of the face and the oral cavity.
oronasal f., a pathologic communication between the nasal cavity and the oral cavity.
parietal f., thoracic f.; a f., either blind or complete, opening on the wall of the thorax or abdomen.
perineovaginal f., a f. through the perineum, opening into the vagina.
pharyngeal f., a form of f. colli congenita.
pilonidal f., pilonidal *sinus*.
pulmonary f., a parietal f. communicating with the lung.
rectolabial f., rectovulvar f.; a f. opening into the rectum and on the surface of a labium majus.
rectourethral f., a f. connecting the rectum and the urethra.
rectovaginal f., a fistulous opening between the rectum and the vagina.
rectovesical f., a fistulous communication between the rectum and the bladder.
rectovestibular f., a f. between rectum and vestibule of the vagina.
rectovulvar f., rectolabial f.
reverse Eck f., side-to-side anastomosis of the portal vein with the inferior vena cava and ligation of the latter above the anastomosis but below the hepatic veins; the blood from the lower part of the body is thus directed through the hepatic circulation.
salivary f., a pathologic communication between a salivary duct or gland and the cutaneous surface or the oral mucus.
sigmoidovesical f., a f. between sigmoid colon and urinary bladder.
spermatic f., a f. communicating with the testis or any of the seminal passages.
stercoral f., intestinal f.
Thiry's f., an artificial f. for collecting the intestinal secretions of a dog or other animal for experimental purposes; a loop of intestine is isolated, its vascular and nervous connections are preserved, and the continuity of the intestinal tract is restored by anastomosis; one end of the isolated segment is closed, the other attached to the skin of the abdomen.
Thiry-Vella f., Vella's f.; experimental isolation of a segment of intestine in a dog or other animal; the mesenteric attachment is preserved, the divided intestine at each end of the segment is joined by anastomosis, and the ends of the segment are stitched to openings in the abdominal wall.
thoracic f., parietal f.
tracheal f., a form of f. colli congenita.
tracheobiliary f., a rare congenital anastomosis between an accessory bronchus and aberrant biliary duct system.
tracheoesophageal f., congenital abnormality involving a communication between the trachea and esophagus; often associated with esophageal atresia, but may also be acquired; in the adult, etiology is similar to that of bronchoesophageal f.
umbilical f., a f. of intestine or urachus at the umbilicus.
urachal f., a f. connecting the urachus with a hollow organ.
ureterocutaneous f., a f. between the ureter and the skin.
ureterovaginal f., a f. between the lower ureter and vagina.
urethrovaginal f., a f. between the urethra and the vagina.
urinary f., a f. resulting in abnormal drainage of urine to the skin or into another organ.

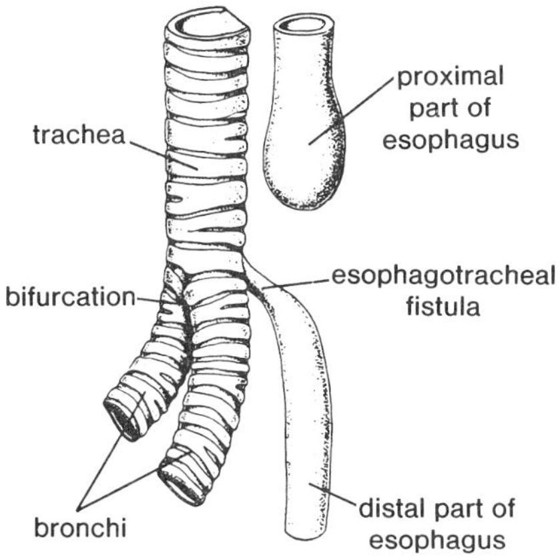

Tracheoesophageal Fistula

urogenital f., genitourinary f.
uteroperitoneal f., metroperitoneal f.; a fistulous tract through the uterine wall opening into the peritoneal cavity.
Vella's f., Thiry-Vella f.
vesical f., a f. from the urinary bladder.
vesicocolic f., colovesical f.
vesicocutaneous f., a f. between the bladder and the skin.
vesicointestinal f., a f. between urinary bladder and small intestine.
vesicouterine f., a f. between the bladder and the uterus.
vesicovaginal f., f. between the bladder and the vagina.
vesicovaginorectal f., an abnormal opening between the vagina and the bladder and rectum.
vitelline f., a f. between the umbilicus and the terminal ileum along the course of a persistent vitelline cord. See Meckel's *diverticulum.*

---

fistulation, fistulization (fis-tyū-lā'shŭn, -tyū-li-zā'shŭn). Formation of a fistula in a part; becoming fistulous.

fistulatome (fis'tyū-lă-tōm) [fistula + G. *tomē,* a cutting]. Syringotome; fistula knife; a long, thin-bladed, probe-pointed knife for slitting open a fistula.

fistulectomy (fis-tyū-lek'tō-mē) [fistula + G. *ektomē,* excision]. Syringectomy; excision of a fistula.

fistuloenterostomy (fis'tyū-lō-en-ter-os'tō-mē) [fistula + G. *enteron,* intestine, + *stoma,* mouth]. An operation connecting a fistula with the intestine.

fistulotomy (fis-tyū-lot'ō-mē) [fistula + G. *tomē,* incision]. Syringotomy; incision or surgical enlargement of a fistula.

fistulous (fis'tyū-lŭs). Relating to or containing a fistula.

fit [A.S. *fitt*]. **1.** An attack of an acute disease, or the sudden appearance of some symptom, such as coughing. **2.** A convulsion. **3.** Epilepsy. **4.** In dentistry, the adaptation of any dental restoration, *e.g.,* of an inlay to the cavity preparation in a tooth, or of a denture to its basal seat.
uncinate f., uncinate *epilepsy.*

fitness (fit'nes). **1.** Well-being. **2.** Suitability.
clinical f., absence of frank disease or of subclinical precursors.
evolutionary f., the probability that the line of descent from an individual with a specific trait will not die out.
genetic f., in a phenotype, the mean mumber of surviving offspring that it generates in its lifetime, usually expressed as a fraction or percentage of the average genetic f. of the population.
physical f., a state of well-being in which performance is optimal.

Fitz-Hugh, T., Jr., U.S. physician, 1894–1963. See F.-H. and Curtis *syndrome.*

fixation (fik-sā'shŭn) [L. *figo,* pp. *fixus,* to fix, fasten]. **1.** The condition of being firmly attached or set. **2.** Fixing; in histology, the rapid killing of tissue elements and their preservation and hardening to retain as nearly as possible the same relations they had in the living body. **3.** In chemistry, the conversion of a gas into solid or liquid form by chemical reactions, with or without the help of living tissue. **4.** In psychoanalysis, the quality of being firmly attached to a particular person or object. **5.** In physiological optics, the coordinated positioning and accommodation of both eyes that results in bringing or maintaining a sharp image of a stationary or moving object on the fovea of each eye.
bifoveal f., binocular f.
binocular f., bifoveal f.; a condition in which both eyes are simultaneously directed to the same target.
circumalveolar f., stabilization of a fracture segment or surgical splint by wire passed through and around the dental alveolar process.
circummandibular f., stabilization of a fracture segment or surgical splint by wire passed around the mandible.
circumzygomatic f., stabilization of a fracture segment or surgical splint by wire passed around the zygomatic arch.
complement f., f. of complement in a serum by an antigen-antibody combination whereby it is rendered unavailable to complete a reaction in a second antigen-antibody combination for which complement is necessary; the second system usually serves as an indicator (red blood cells plus specific hemolysin); if complement is fixed with the first antigen-antibody union, hemolysis does not occur, but, if complement is not so removed, it causes hemolysis in the second system. See also Bordet-Gengou *phenomenon;* Wassermann *test.*
craniofacial f., stabilization of facial fractures to the cranial base by direct wiring or by external skeletal pin fixation.
crossed f., in convergent strabismus, the use of the right inturned eye for the left visual field, and the left inturned eye for the right visual field to avoid ocular rotation.
eccentric f., a monocular condition in which the line of sight connects the object and an extrafoveal retinal area.
elastic band f., the stabilization of fractured segments of the jaws by means of intermaxillary elastics applied to splints or appliances.
external f., f. of fractured bones by splints, plastic dressings, or transfixion pins.
external pin f., in oral surgery, stabilization of fractures of the mandible, maxilla, or zygoma by pins or screws drilled into the bony part through the overlying skin and connected by a metal bar.
external pin f., biphase, pin f. by replacing the rigid metal bar connector with an acrylic bar adapted at the time of reduction of the fracture.
freudian f., see fixation (5).
genetic f., the increase of the frequency of a gene by genetic drift such that no other allele is preserved in a specific finite population.
intermaxillary f., mandibulomaxillary or maxillomandibular f.; f. of fractures of the mandible or maxilla by applying elastic bands or stainless steel wire between the maxillary and mandibular arch bars or other types of splint.
internal f., intraosseous f.; stabilization of fractured bony parts by direct f. to one another with surgical wires, screws, pins, plates, or methylmethacrylate.
intraosseous f., internal f.
mandibulomaxillary f., intermaxillary f.
maxillomandibular f., intermaxillary f.
nasomandibular f., mandibular immobilization, especially for edentulous jaws, with maxillomandibular splints, attached by connecting a circum-mandibular wire with an intraoral interosseous wire passed through a hole drilled into the anterior nasal spine of the maxillae.

fixative (fik'să-tiv). **1.** Serving to fix, bind, or make firm or stable. **2.** A substance used for the preservation of gross and histologic specimens of tissue, or individual cells, usually by denaturing and precipitating or cross-linking the protein constituents. See also fluid; solution.

acetone f., acetone used at low temperatures to fix enzymes, particularly phosphatases; it removes fat and glucogen.

Altmann's f., a bichromate-osmic acid f.

Bouin's f., a solution of glacial acetic acid, formalin, and picric acid, useful for soft and delicate tissues (as those of embryos) and small pieces of tissues; it preserves glycogen and nuclei and permits brilliant staining, but penetrates slowly, distorts kidney tissue and mitochondria, and does not permit Feulgen stain for DNA.

Carnoy's f., ethanol, chloroform, and acetic acid (6:3:1) or ethanol and acetic acid (3:1), an extremely rapid f. used for glucogen preservation and as a nuclear f.

Champy's f., a mixture of potassium bichromate, chromic acid, and osmic acid, considered an excellent cytologic f. with advantages and disadvantages similar to those of Flemming's f.; it differs from Flemming's f. in substituting bichromate for acetic acid.

Flemming's f., a mixture of chromic acid, osmic acid, and acetic acid that makes an excellent cytoplasmic and chromosomal f., especially when acetic acid is omitted; disadvantages are that it penetrates poorly, requires lengthy washing, and deterioriates rapidly.

formaldehyde f., a widely used fixing agent for pathologic histology; the commercial solution is 37-40% formaldehyde and is known as 100% formalin or formol; a common impurity is formic acid, which must be neutralized or the f. made in buffer solution; tissues fixed may have a pigment artifact precipitated.

formol-calcium f., a f. for preservation of lipids.

formol-Müller f., Müller's f. containing 2% commercial formalin.

formol-saline f., a general f. for histologic and histochemical preparations.

formol-Zenker f., Zenker's f. in which glacial acetic acid has been replaced by formalin.

glutaraldehyde f., a f. used in phosphate or cacodylate buffer for electron microscopy, and as a chromatin and enzyme f.; may be used preceding osmic acid as a second f. to add membrane preservation for electron microscopy.

Golgi's osmiobichromate f., an osmic-bichromate mixture used to demonstrate nerve cells and their processes.

Helly's f., a combination of potassium dichromate, mercuric chloride, formaldehyde, and distilled water, used as a microanatomic f. for cytoplasmic granules and nuclear staining; has the same disadvantages as Zenker's f.

Hermann's f., a hardening f. of glacial acetic acid, osmic acid, and platinum chloride.

Kaiserling's f., a method of preserving histologic and pathologic specimens without altering the color, by immersing them in an aqueous solution of potassium nitrate, potassium acetate, and formalin.

Luft's potassium permanganate f., a f. useful in electron microscopy for cytologic preservation of lipoprotein complexes in membranes and myelin, because of its oxidative properties.

Marchi's f., a mixture of Müller's f. with osmium tetroxide, with potassium chlorate substituted for the potassium dichromate of Müller's f. for better results; used to demonstrate degenerating myelin. See also Marchi's *stain.*

methanol f., a f. used with dry blood films, and often incorporated into the stain used.

Müller's f., a hardening f. composed of potassium dichromate, sodium sulfate, and distilled water, similar to Regaud's f.

neutral buffered formalin f., a general histologic f. less likely to leave formalin deposits in tissue than formol-saline f.

Newcomer's f., a f. containing isopropanol, propionic acid, and dioxane, recommended as a substitute for Carnoy's f. in preservation of chromatin; also useful for fixing polysaccharides; small pieces of tissue must be used, although excessive shrinkage may still occur.

Orth's f., formalin added to Müller's f., used for bringing out chromaffin, studying early degenerative processes and necrosis, and for demonstrating rickettsiae and bacteria.

osmic acid f., a f. used alone in buffer or as a postfixative after a glutaraldehyde f. in electron microscopy; an excellent membrane f. but a poor preservative of chromatin.

Park-Williams f., a f. for spirochetes, comprised of a 2% solution of osmic acid to the fumes of which the bacteria are exposed for a few seconds.

picroformol f., a f. containing formalin and picric acid.

Regaud's f., a f. containing formaldehyde and sodium dichromate, used to preserve mitochondria but not fat; requires afterchroming and extensive washing.

Schaudinn's f., a solution of mercuric chloride, sodium chloride, alcohol, and glacial acetic acid, used on wet smears for cytologic fixation.

Thoma's f., nitric acid in 95% alcohol, used for decalcifying bone in the preparation of histologic specimens.

Zenker's f., a rapid f. consisting of mercuric chloride, potassium dichromate, sodium sulfate, glacial acetic acid, and water, useful for trichrome stains; must be washed to remove potassium dichromate and treated with iodine solution to remove mercuric chloride; tissues tend to become brittle if left in the f. for more than 24 hours.

fixator (fik-sā'ter). A device providing rigid immobilization through external skeletal fixation by means of rods (f.'s) attached to pins which are placed in or through the bone.

fixing (fik'sing). Fixation (2).

flaccid (flak'sid, flas'id) [L. *flaccidus*]. Relaxed, flabby, or without tone.

flaccidity (flă-sid'i-tē). The condition or state of being flaccid.

Flack, Martin, British physiologist, 1882–1931. See F.'s *node;* Keith and F. *node.*

flagella (flă-jel'ă). Plural of flagellum.

flagellar (fla-jel'ăr). Relating to a flagellum or to the extremity of a protozoan.

Flagellata (flaj'ĕ-lā'tă). Former name for Mastigophora.

flagellate (flaj'ĕ-lāt). **1.** Possessing one or more flagella. **2.** Common name for a member of the class Mastigophora.

collared f., choanomastigote.

flagellated (flaj'ĕ-lā-ted). Possessing one or more flagella.

flagellation (flaj'ĕ-lā'shŭn) [L. *flagellatus,* fr. *flagellāre,* to whip or scourge]. Whipping either one's self or another as a means of arousing or heightening sexual feeling.

flagellin (flaj'ĕ-lin). A protein (MW about 20,000) containing the amino acid, ϵ-*N*-methyllysine; found in the flagella of bacteria.

flagellosis (flaj'ĕ-lō'sis). Infection with flagellated protozoa in the intestinal or genital tract, *e.g.,* trichomoniasis.

flagellum, pl. **flagella** (flă-jel'ŭm, -ă) [L. dim. of *flagrum,* a whip]. A whiplike locomotory organelle of constant structural arrangment consisting of nine double peripheral microtubules and two single central microtubules; it arises from a deeply staining basal granule, often connected to the nucleus by a fiber, the rhizoplast. Though characteristic of the protozoan class Mastigophora, comparable structures are commonly found in many other groups, *e.g.,* in spermatozoa.

flammable (flam'ă-bl) [L. *flamma,* flame]. Inflammable; the property of burning readily and quickly.

flange (flanj). That part of the denture base which extends from the cervical ends of the teeth to the border of the denture.

buccal f., the portion of the f. of a denture that occupies the buccal vestibule of the mouth.

denture f., **(1)** the essentially vertical extension from the body of the denture into one of the vestibules of the oral cavity; also, on the lower denture, the essentially vertical extension along the lingual side of the alveololingual sulcus; **(2)** the buccal and labial vertical extension of the upper or lower denture base, and the lingual vertical extension of the lower one; the buccal and labial denture f.'s have two surfaces: the buccal or labial surface and the basal seat surface; the lower lingual f. also has two surfaces: the basal seat surface and the lingual surface.

labial f., the portion of the f. of a denture which occupies the labial vestibule of the mouth.

lingual f., the portion of the f. of a mandibular denture that occupies the space adjacent to the tongue.

flank. Latus.

flap. **1.** Mass or tongue of tissue for transplantation, vascularized by a pedicle or stem; specifically, a pedicle f. **2.** An uncontrolled movement, as of the hands. See asterixis.

Abbe f., a full-thickness f. of the middle portion of the lower lip that is transferred into the upper lip, or vice versa.

advancement f., sliding f.

arterial f., axial pattern f.

axial pattern f., arterial f.; a f. that includes a direct specific artery within its longitudinal axis.

bilobed f., a f. consisting of two lobes at approximately right angles, based on a common pedicle.

bipedicle f., double pedicle f.; a f. with two pedicles, one at each end.

bone f., attached *craniotomy.*

buried f., a f. denuded of both surface epithelium and superficial dermis and transferred into the subcutaneous tissues.

caterpillar f., waltzed f.; a tubed f. transferred end-over-end (in stages) from the donor area to a distant recipient area.

cellulocutaneous f., a f. of skin and subcutaneous tissue.

composite f., compound f., a skin f. incorporating underlying muscle, bone, or cartilage.

cross f., a skin f. transferred from one part of the body to a corresponding part, as from one arm to the other.

delayed f., a f. raised in its donor area in two or more stages to increase its chances of survival after transfer.

deltopectoral f., an arterial skin f. of the deltoid and pectoral regions, based on the internal mammary vessels.

direct f., immediate f.; a f. raised completely and transferred at the same stage.

distant f., a f. in which the donor site is distant from the recipient area.

double pedicle f., bipedicle f.

envelope f., a mucoperiosteal f. retracted from a horizontal incision along the free gingival margin.

Estlander f., a full-thickness f. of the lip, transferred from the side of one lip to the same side of the other lip.

Filatov f., Filatov-Gillies f., tubed f.

flag f., a flag-shaped f. on a proximal pedicle, transferred from one surface to another of the same finger or from one finger to an adjacent finger.

flat f., open f.; a f. in which during transfer the pedicle is left flat or open, *i.e.,* untubed.

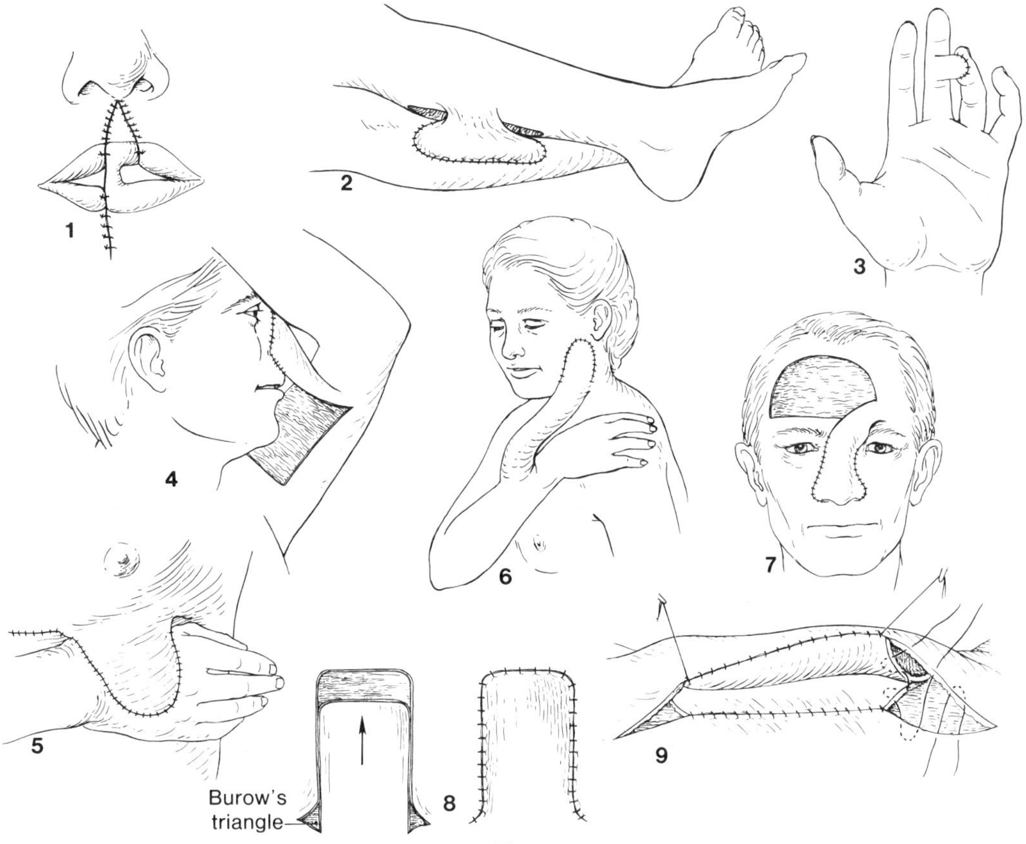

Flaps

1, Abbe; *2*, cross-leg; *3*, flag; *4*, distant; *5*, direct flat; *6*, jump; *7*, rotation; *8*, sliding; *9*, tubed.

free f., island f. in which the donor vessels are severed proximally, the f. is transported as a free object to the recipient area, and the f. is revascularized by anastomosing its supplying vessels to vessels there.
free bone f., detached *craniotomy.*
French f., sliding f.
full-thickness f., a f. of the full thickness of mucosa and submucosa or of skin and subcutaneous tissues.
gingival f., a portion of the gingiva whose coronal margin is surgically detached from the tooth and the alveolar process.
hinged f., a turnover f. transferred by lifting it over on its pedicle as though the pedicle was a hinge.
immediate f., direct f.
island f., a f. in which the pedicle consists solely of the supplying artery and vein(s), sometimes including a nerve.
jump f., a distant f. transferred in stages via an intermediate carrier; *e.g.,* an abdominal f. is attached to the wrist, then at a later stage the wrist is brought to the face.
lined f., a f. covered with epithelium on both sides; *e.g.,* a folded skin f.
lingual f., tongue f.
liver f., see asterixis.
local f., a f. transferred to an adjacent area.
mucoperichondrial f., a f. composed of mucosa and perichondrium, as from the nasal septum.
mucoperiosteal f., a f. composed of mucosa and periosteum, as from the hard palate or gingiva.
musculocutaneous f., myocutaneous f.
myocutaneous f., musculocutaneous or myodermal f.; a pedicle skin f., often an island f., with an attached subjacent muscle and its investments and blood supply.
myodermal f., myocutaneous f.
neurovascular f., a f. containing a sensory nerve, one purpose of which is to restore sensation to the recipient area.
open f., flat f.
parabiotic f., a skin f. bridging from one animal to another.
partial-thickness f., split-thickness f.
pedicle f., **(1)** a skin f. sustained by a blood-carrying stem from the donor site during transfer; **(2)** in periodontal surgery, a f. used to increase the width of attached gingiva, or to cover a root surface, by moving the attached gingiva, which remains joined at one side, to an adjacent position and suturing the free end.
pericoronal f., a f. of gingiva covering an unerupted tooth, especially the lower third molar.
permanent pedicle f., a pedicle f. in which the pedicle is not severed at the time of transfer, so that it continues to supply blood from the donor site to the recipient area.
pharyngeal f., a f. from the posterior wall of the pharynx to the soft palate, as a speech aid in cleft palate.
random pattern f., a f. in which the pedicle blood supply is derived randomly from the network of vessels in the area, rather than from a single longitudinal artery as in an axial pattern f.
rope f., tubed f.
rotation f., a pedicle f. that is rotated from the donor site to an adjacent recipient area, usually as a direct f.
sickle f., a sickle-shaped f. from the anterior scalp and one side of the forehead, based on the opposite temporal artery.
skin f., a f. comprised of skin and its subjacent subcutaneous tissue.
sliding f., advancement or French f.; a rectangular f. raised in an elastic area, with its free end adjacent to a defect; the defect is covered by stretching the f. longitudinally until the end comes over it.
split-thickness f., partial-thickness f.; a f. of a portion of the skin, *i.e.,* the epidermis and part of the dermis, or of part of the mucosa and submucosa, but not including the periosteum.
subcutaneous f., a pedicle f. in which the pedicle is denuded of epithelium and buried in the subcutaneous tissue of the recipient area.
tongue f., lingual f.; a f. derived from the tongue; used to close a defect in an adjacent part, such as the lip or palate.
tubed f., Filatov, Filatov-Gillies, or rope f.; Filatov-Gillies tubed pedicle f.; tubed pedicle f.; a f. in which the sides of the pedicle are sutured together to create a tube, with the entire surface covered by skin.
tubed pedicle f., tubed f.
turnover f., a hinged f. that is turned over 180°, usually to receive a second (covering) f.
waltzed f., caterpillar f.

flare (flār). **1.** A gradual tapering or spreading outward. **2.** A diffuse redness of the skin extending beyond the local reaction to the application of an irritant; it is due to dilation of the arterioles and capillaries; depends upon an axon reflex set up by the liberation of a histamine-like substance in skin when injured. See also triple *response.*
aqueous f., Tyndall phenomenon observed in the fluid of the anterior chamber of the eye.

flarimeter (flă-rim'ĕ-ter) [L. *flare,* to blow, + G. *metron,* measure]. Obsolete device for use in evaluating cardiopulmonary fitness; pulse rate and blood pressure were measured during attempts to expire the vital capacity through calibrated orifices while maintaining a mouth pressure of 20 mm Hg.

flash. 1. A sudden and brief burst of light or heat. **2.** Excess material extruded between the sections of a flask in the process of molding denture bases or other dental restorations.
hot f., colloquialism for one of the vasomotor symptoms of the climacteric that may involve the whole body as a f. of heat, but occurs less frequently than hot flushes; also used interchangeably with hot *flush.*

flashback. An involuntary recurrence of some aspect of a hallucinatory experience or perceptual distortion occurring some time after taking the hallucinogen that produced the original effect and without subsequent ingestion of the substance.

flask. A small receptacle, usually of glass, used for holding liquids, powder, or gases.
casting f., refractory f.
crown f., denture f.
denture f., crown f.; a sectional metal boxlike case in which a sectional mold is made of plaster of Paris or artificial stone for the purpose of compressing and curing dentures or other resinous restorations.
Dewar f., vacuum f.; a glass vessel, often silvered, with two walls, the space between which is evacuated; used for maintaining materials at constant temperature or, more usually, at low temperature.
Erlenmeyer f., a f. with a broad base, conical body, and narrow neck; so shaped that its liquid content can be shaken laterally without spilling.
Fernbach f., a f. used in microbial fermentations where a large surface area of the liquid substrate is required.
Florence f., a globular long-necked bottle of thin glass used for holding water or other liquid in laboratory work.
injection f., a denture f. designed so as to permit the forced flow of denture base material from a reservoir into the mold after the flask is closed and during curing.
refractory f., casting f. or ring; a metal tube in which a refractory mold is made for casting metal dental restorations or appliances.
vacuum f., Dewar f.
volumetric f., a f. calibrated to contain or to deliver a definite amount of liquid.

flask'ing. The process of investing the cast and a wax denture in a flask preparatory to molding the denture-base material into the form of the denture.

Flatau, Edward, Polish neurologist, 1869–1932. See F.-Schilder *disease,* F.'s *law.*

flatfoot (flat'fut). *Talipes* planus.

flatulence (flat'yū-lens) [Mod. L. *flatulentus,* fr. L. *flatus,* a blowing, fr. *flo,* pp. *flatus,* to blow]. Presence of an excessive amount of gas in the stomach and intestines.

flatulent (flat'yū-lent). Relating to or suffering from flatulence.

flatus (flā'tŭs) [L. a blowing]. Gas or air in the gastrointestinal tract which may be expelled through the anus.

f. vagina'lis, expulsion of gas from the vagina.

flatworm (flat'werm). A member of the phylum Platyhelminthes, including the parasitic tapeworms and flukes.

flavedo (fla-vē'dō) [L. *flavus,* yellow]. Yellowness or sallowness of the skin.

flavianic acid (flā-vē-an'ik) [C.I. 10316]. A naphthol derivative dye, 8-hydroxy-5,7-dinitro-2-naphthalenesulfonic acid, useful in the precipitation (and subsequent determination) of arginine and other basic substances.

flavin(e) (flā'vin, -vēn, flav'in, -ēn) [L. *flavus,* yellow]. **1.** Riboflavin. **2.** A yellow acridine dye, preparations of which are used as antiseptics.

f. adenine dinucleotide (FAD), a condensation product of riboflavin and adenosine diphosphate; the coenzyme of various aerobic dehydrogenases, *e.g.,* D-amino-acid oxidase (EC 1.4.3.3.) and L-amino-acid oxidase (EC 1.4.3.2).

f. mononucleotide (FMN), riboflavin 5'-phosphate; half of f. adenine dinucleotide.

Flavivirus (flā'vi-vī-rŭs) [L. *flavus,* yellow, + virus]. A genus of viruses (family Togaviridae) formerly classified as group B arboviruses; the type species is the yellow fever virus.

Flavobacterium (flā-vō-bak-tēr'ē-ŭm) [L. *flavus,* yellow]. A genus of aerobic to facultatively anaerobic, nonsporeforming, motile and nonmotile bacteria (family Achromobacteraceae) containing Gram-negative rods; motile cells are peritrichous. These organisms characteristically produce yellow, orange, red, or yellow-brown pigments. They are found in soil and fresh and salt water. Some species are pathogenic. The type species is *F. aquatile.*

F. aquati'le, a species found in water containing a high percentage of calcium carbonate; it is the type species of *F.*

F. bre've, a species found in sewage; pathogenic for laboratory animals.

F. piscici'da, a species pathogenic for fish.

flavoenzyme (flā-vō-en'zīm). Any enzyme that possesses a flavin nucleotide as coenzyme; *e.g.,* xanthine oxidase (EC 1.2.3.2), succinate dehydrogenase (EC 1.3.99.1).

flavokinase (flā-vō-kī'nās). *Riboflavin* kinase.

flavone (flā'vōn). 2-Phenyl-4*H*-1-benzopyran-4-one or 2-phenylchromone; a plant pigment that is the basis of the flavonoids.

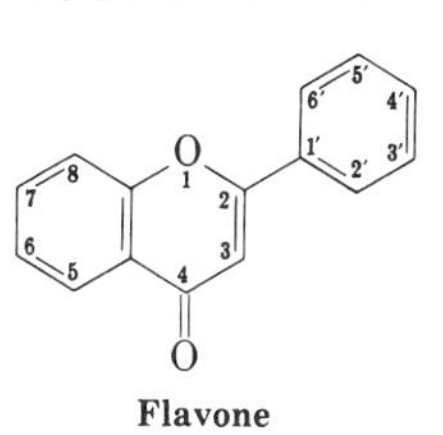

Flavone

flavonoids (flā'vō-noydz). Substances of plant origin containing flavone in various combinations (anthoxanthins, apigenins, flavones, quercitins, etc.) and with varying biological activities.

flavonol (flā'vō-nol). Reduced flavone.

flavoprotein (flā'vō-prō'tēn). A compound protein (enzyme) possessing a flavin as prosthetic group.

flavor (flā'ver). **1.** The quality affecting the taste or odor of any substance. **2.** A therapeutically inert substance added to a prescription to give an agreeable taste to the mixture.

flavoxate hydrochloride (flā-vok'sāt). 2-Piperidinoethyl 3-methyl-4-oxo-2-phenyl-4*H*-1-benzopyran-8-carboxylate hydrochloride; a smooth muscle relaxant for the urinary tract.

flavus (flā'vŭs) [L.]. Yellow.

flaxseed (flaks'sēd). Linseed.

f. oil, linseed oil.

flea (flē). An insect of the order Siphonaptera, marked by lateral compression, sucking mouthparts, extraordinary jumping powers, and ectoparasitic adult life in the hair and feathers of warm-blooded animals. Important f.'s include *Ctenocephalides felis* (cat f.), or *C. canis* (dog f.), *Pulex irritans* (human f.), *Tunga penetrans* (chigger, chigoe, or sand f.), *Echidnophaga gallinacea* (sticktight f.), *Xenopsylla* (rat f.), and *Ceratophyllus.* See also Copepoda (the so-called water f.'s).

flecainide acetate (flē-kā'nīd). *N*-(2-Piperidylmethyl)-2,5-bis(2,2,2-trifluoroethoxy)benzamide monoacetate; a member of the membrane-stabilizing group of antiarrhythmics, with local anesthetic activity, used in the treatment of ventricular arrhythmias.

Flechsig, Paul E., German neurologist, 1847– 1929. See F.'s *areas,* ground *bundles, fasciculi, tract;* oval *area* of F.; semilunar *nucleus* of F.

flection (flek'shŭn). Flexion.

Flegel, H., 20th century German dermatologist. See Flegel's *disease.*

Fleisch, Alfred, Swiss physician and physiologist, *1892. See F. *pneumotachograph.*

Fleischer, Bruno, German ophthalmologist, 1874–1965. See F.'s *ring,* Kayser-F. *ring.*

Fleischmann, Friedrich Ludwig, 19th century German anatomist. See F.'s *bursa.*

Fleischner, Felix, Austrian-American radiologist, 1893–1969. See F. *lines.*

Fleitmann, Theodore, 19th century German chemist. See F.'s *test.*

Flemming, Walther, German anatomist, 1843–1905. See intermediate *body* of F.; germinal *center* of F.; F.'s *fixative,* triple *stain.*

Flesch, Rudolf, Austrian educator, *1911. See F. *formula.*

flesh [A.S. *flaesc*]. **1.** The meat of animals used for food. **2.** Muscular *tissue.*

proud f., exuberant granulations in the granulation tissue on the surface of a wound.

fleshflies (flesh'flīz). Members of the order Diptera, whose larvae (maggots) develop in putrefying or living tissues. Maggots of the latter group produce myiasis; these include screw-worms (both primary and secondary invaders); wool maggots of sheep; botflies or skin maggots of man and domestic animals (including warble or heel flies); head or nasal botflies of sheep and goats, horses, camels, and deer; and horse botflies (or gadflies) whose larvae develop in the stomach, duodenum, or rectum of horses.

flex (fleks) [L. *flecto,* pp. *flexus,* to bend]. To bend; to move a joint in such a direction as to approximate the two parts which it connects.

flexibilitas cerea (flek-si-bil'i-tas sē'rē-ă) [L. waxy flexibility]. The rigidity of catalepsy which may be overcome by slight external force, but which returns at once, holding the limb firmly in the new position.

fleximeter (flek-sim'ĕ-ter). Goniometer (3).

flexion (flek'shŭn) [L. *flecto,* pp. *flectus,* to bend]. Flection. **1.** The act of flexing or bending, *e.g.,* bending of a joint so as to approximate the parts it connects; bending of the spine so that the concavity of the curve looks forward. **2.** The condition of being flexed or bent.

palmar f., turning the hand or fingers toward the palmar surface.
plantar f., turning the foot or toes toward the plantar surface.

Flexner, Simon, U.S. pathologist, 1863–1946. See F.'s *bacillus.*

flexor (flek'ser, -sōr). A muscle the action of which is to flex a joint.

flexura, pl. **flexu'rae** (flek-shyūr'ă, -shyūr'ē) [L. a bending] [NA]. Flexure; a bend, as in an organ or structure.

f. co'li dex'tra [NA], right colic flexure; hepatic flexure; the bend of the colon at the juncture of its ascending and transverse portions.
f. co'li sinis'tra [NA], left colic flexure; splenic flexure; the bend at the junction of the transverse and descending colon.
f. duode'ni infe'rior [NA], inferior flexure of the duodenum; the bend at the junction of the descending and horizontal parts of the duodenum. Occasionally a bend, the left inferior duodenal flexure, occurs at the junction of the horizontal and ascending parts.
f. duode'ni supe'rior [NA], superior flexure of the duodenum; the flexure at the junction of the superior and descending parts of the duodenum.
f. duode'nojejuna'lis [NA], duodenojejunal flexure or angle; an abrupt bend in the small intestine at the junction of the duodenum and jejunum.
f. perinea'lis rec'ti [NA], perineal flexure of the rectum; the anteroposterior curve with convexity anteriorward of the last portion of the rectum.
f. sacra'lis rec'ti [NA], sacral flexure of the rectum; the anteroposterior curve with concavity anteriorward of the first portion of the rectum.
f. sigmoid'ea, *colon* sigmoideum.

flexural (flek'sher-ăl). Relating to a flexure.

flexure (flek'sher) [L. *flexura*]. Flexura.

basicranial f., pontine f.
caudal f., sacral f.; the bend in the lumbosacral region of the embryo.
cephalic f., cranial, cerebral, or mesencephalic f.; the sharp, ventrally concave bend in the developing midbrain of the embryo.
cerebral f., cephalic f.
cervical f., the ventrally concave bend at the juncture of the brainstem and spinal cord in the embryo.
cranial f., cephalic f.
dorsal f., a f. in the mid-dorsal region in the embryo.
duodenojejunal f., *flexura* duodenojejunalis.
hepatic f., *flexura* coli dextra.
inferior f. of duodenum, *flexura* duodeni inferior.
left colic f., *flexura* coli sinistra.
lumbar f., the normal ventral curve of the vertebral column in the lumbar region.
mesencephalic f., cephalic f.
perineal f. of rectum, *flexura* perinealis recti.
pontine f., basicranial f.; transverse rhombencephalic f.; the dorsally concave curvature of the rhombencephalon in the embryo.
right colic f., *flexura* coli dextra.
sacral f., caudal f.
sacral f. of rectum, *flexura* sacralis recti.
sigmoid f., *colon* sigmoideum.
splenic f., *flexura* coli sinistra.
superior f. of duodenum, *flexura* duodeni superior.
telencephalic f., a f. appearing in the embryonic forebrain region.
transverse rhombencephalic f., pontine f.

flick'er. The visual sensation caused by stimulation of the retina by a series of intermittent light flashes occurring at a certain rate. See also flicker *fusion;* critical flicker-fusion *frequency.*

flicks. Flick movements; rapid, involuntary fixation movements of the eye of 5 to 10 minutes of arc.

Flieringa, Henri J., Dutch ophthalmologist, *1891. See F.'s *ring.*

flight into disease. Gain through falling ill or assuming the sick role. See primary *gain,* secondary *gain.*

flight into health. In psychoanalysis, the early but often only temporary disappearance of the symptoms that ostensibly brought the patient into therapy; a defense against the anxiety engendered by the prospect of further psychoanalytic exploration of the patient's conflicts.

Flint, Austin, U.S. physician, 1812–1886. See F.'s *murmur.*

Flint, Austin, Jr., U.S. physiologist, 1836–1915. See F.'s *arcade.*

flip. A burn occurring on one side only of the entrance site in a pistol wound of the soft parts.

floater (flōt'er). An object in the field of vision that originates in the vitreous body. See also muscae volitantes.

floating (flōt'ing). **1.** Free or unattached. **2.** Out of the normal position; unduly movable; wandering; denoting an occasional abnormal condition of certain organs, such as the kidneys, liver, spleen, etc.

floc (flok). A colloquial term for the product of a flocculation, *i.e.,* the separation of the disperse phase of a colloidal suspension into discrete, usually visible particles, as in certain serologic precipitin tests.

floccillation (flok-si-lā'shŭn) [Mod. L. *flocculus*]. Carphologia; carphology; crocidismus; an aimless plucking at the bedclothes, as if one were picking off threads or tufts of cotton.

floccose (flok'ōs) [L. *floccus,* a flock of wool]. In bacteriology, applied to a growth of short, curving filaments or chains closely but irregularly disposed.

flocculable (flok'yū-lă-bl). Capable of undergoing flocculation.

floccular (flok'yū-lăr). Relating to a flocculus of any sort; specifically to the flocculus of the cerebellum.

flocculate (flok'yū-lāt). To become flocculent.

flocculation (flok-yū-lā'shŭn). Flocculence; precipitation from solution in the form of fleecy masses; the process of becoming flocculent.

floccule (flok'yūl). Flocculus.

flocculence (flok'yū-lens). Flocculation.

flocculent (flok'yū-lent). **1.** Resembling tufts of cotton or wool; denoting a fluid, such as the urine, containing numerous shreds or fluffy particles of gray-white or white mucus or other material. **2.** In bacteriology, denoting a fluid culture in which there are numerous colonies either floating in the fluid medium or loosely deposited at the bottom.

flocculonodular (flok'yū-lō-nod'yū-lăr). See flocculonodular *lobe.*

flocculus, pl. **flocculi** (flok'yū-lŭs, -lī) [Mod. L. dim. of L. *floccus,* a tuft of wool]. Floccule. **1.** A tuft or shred of cotton or wool or anything resembling it. **2** [NA]. A small lobe of the cerebellum at the posterior border of the brachium pontis anterior to the lobulus biventer; it is associated with the nodulus of the vermis; together, these two structures compose the vestibular part of the cerebellum.

accessory f., an occasional small lobule of the cerebellum in the immediate neighborhood of the flocculus.

Flocks, Milton, U.S. ophthalmologist, *1914. See Harrington-F. *test.*

Flood, Valentine, Irish anatomist and surgeon, 1800–1847. See F.'s *ligament.*

flood (flŭd) [A.S. *flōd*] **1.** To bleed profusely from the uterus, as after childbirth or in cases of menorrhagia. **2.** Colloquialism for a profuse menstrual discharge.

flooding (flŭd'ing). **1.** Bleeding profusely from the uterus, especially after childbirth or in severe cases of menorrhagia. **2.** Profuse uterine hemorrhage. **3.** A type of behavior therapy; a therapeutic strategy at the beginning of therapy, in which the patients imagine the most anxiety-producing scene and fully immerse (flood) themselves in it. *Cf.* systematic *desensitization.*

floor (flōr). The lower inner surface of an open space or hollow organ.

flora (flō'ră) [L. *Flora,* goddess of flowers, fr. *flos (flor-),* a flower]. **1.** Plant life, usually of a certain locality or district. **2.** Microbial associates; the population of microorganisms inhabiting the internal and external surfaces of healthy conventional animals.

florantyrone (flor-an'ti-rōn). γ-Oxy-γ-(8-fluoranthene)butyric acid; used in chronic cholecystitis and cholangitis; it increases the volume of bile without increasing the quantity of bile solids or stimulating evacuation of the gallbladder.

Florence, Albert, French physician, 1851–1927. See F.'s *crystals.*

Florence flask. See under flask.

Florey, Sir Howard W., British pathologist and Nobel laureate, 1898–1968. See F. *unit.*

florid (flōr'id) [L. *floridus,* flowery]. Of a bright red color; denoting certain cutaneous lesions.

Florschütz, Georg, German physician, *1859. See F.'s *formula.*

floss. 1. Dental f. **2.** To use dental f. in oral hygiene.
dental f., floss silk; an untwisted thread made from fine, short, silk fibers, frequently waxed; used for cleansing interproximal spaces and between contact areas of the teeth.

flotation (flō-tā'shŭn). A process for separating solids by their tendency to float upon or sink into a liquid.

Flourens, Marie J.P., French physiologist, 1794–1867. See F.'s *theory.*

flow (flō) [A.S. *flōwan*]. **1.** To bleed from the uterus less profusely than in flooding. **2.** The menstrual discharge. **3.** Movement of a fluid or gas; specifically, the volume of fluid or gas passing a given point per unit of time. In respiratory physiology, the symbol for gas flow is $\dot{V}$ and for blood flow is $\dot{Q}$, followed by subscripts denoting location and chemical species. **4.** In rheology, a permanent deformation of a body which proceeds with time.
Bingham f., the f. characteristics exhibited by a Bingham plastic.
effective renal blood f. (ERBF), the amount of blood flowing to the parts of the kidney that are involved with production of constituents of urine.
effective renal plasma f. (ERPF), the amount of plasma flowing to the parts of the kidney that have a function in the production of constituents of urine; the clearance of substances such as iodopyracet and *p*-aminohippuric acid, assuming that the extraction ratio in the peritubular capillaries is 100%.
forced expiratory f. (FEF), expiratory f. during measurement of forced vital capacity; subscripts specify the exact parameter measured, *e.g.,* peak instantaneous f., the instantaneous f. at some specified point on the curve of volume expired versus time, or on the flow-volume curve, the mean f. between two expired volumes.
gene f., changes over time in the genetic composition of a population as a result of migration rather than of mutation and selection.
laminar f., the relative motion of elements of a fluid along smooth parallel paths.
newtonian f., the type of f. characteristic of a newtonian fluid.
peak expiratory f., the maximum f. at the outset of forced expiration, which is reduced in proportion to the severity of airway obstruction, as in asthma.
shear f., a f. of a material in which parallel planes in the material are displaced in a direction parallel to each other.

Flower, Sir William H., British surgeon and anatomist, 1831–1899. See F.'s *bone,* dental *index.*

flower basket of Bochdalek. Part of the plexus choroideus of the fourth ventricle protruding through Luschka's foramen and resting on the dorsal surface of the glossopharyngeal nerve.

flower of paradise. *Catha edulis.*

flowers (flow'erz). A mineral substance in a powdery state after sublimation.
f. of antimony, *antimony* trioxide.
f. of benzoin, benzoic acid.
f. of sulfur, sublimed *sulfur.*
f. of zinc, *zinc* oxide.

flowmeter (flō'mē-ter). A device for measuring velocity or volume of flow of liquids or gases.
electromagnetic f., a f. in which a magnetic field is applied to a blood vessel to measure flow in terms of the voltage developed by the blood as a conductor moving through the magnetic field.

floxuridine (flok-sū'ri-dēn). 5-Fluoro-2'-deoxyuridine (5-FUDR); the deoxynucleoside of fluorouracil; an antineoplastic agent. Fluorouracil is metabolized to f. and this, in turn, to 5-fluoro-2'-deoxyuridine 5'-monophosphate. The latter agent inhibits thymidylic synthetase; uridine phosphatase is also inhibited.

flu (flū). Influenza.

fluanisone (flū-an'i-sōn). Haloanisone; 4'-fluoro-4-[4-(*o*-methoxyphenyl)-1-piperazinyl]butyrophenone; an antianxiety agent.

flucrylate (flū'kri-lāt). 2,2,2-Trifluoro-1-methylethyl-2-cyanoacrylate; a tissue adhesive used in surgery.

fluctuate (flŭk'tyū-āt) [L. *fluctuo,* pp. *-atus,* to flow in waves]. **1.** To move in waves. **2.** To vary, to change from time to time, as in referring to any quantity or quality, *e.g.,* height of blood pressure, concentration of substance in urine or blood, secretory activity, etc.

fluctuation (flŭk-tyū-ā'shŭn). **1.** The act of fluctuating. **2.** A wave-like motion felt on palpating a cavity with nonrigid walls, especially one containing fluid.

flucytosine (flū-sī'tō-sēn). 5-Fluorocytosine; an antifungal drug for the treatment of cryptococcosis.

fludrocortisone acetate (flū-drō-kōr'ti-sōn). 9α-Fluorohydrocortisone acetate; 9α-fluorocortisol; 9α-fluoro-17-hydroxycorticosterone; 9α-fluoro-11β,17α,21-trihydroxypregn-4-ene-3,20-dione 21-acetate; a mineralocorticoid too potent for systemic use except in cases of adrenocortical insufficiency; otherwise used only topically.

flufenamic acid (flū-fen-am'ik). *N*-(α,α,α-Trifluoro-*m*-tolyl)anthranilic acid; an anti-inflammatory agent for the treatment of arthritis.

fluid (flū'id) [L. *fluidus,* fr. *fluo,* to flow]. **1.** Flowing; liquid; gaseous. **2.** A nonsolid substance, either liquid or gas.
allantoic f., the f. within the allantoic cavity.
amniotic f., liquor amnii; a liquid within the amnion that surrounds the fetus and protects it from mechanical injury.
Brodie f., an aqueous salt solution used in manometers designed for testing gas evolution or uptake, as in cell respiration.
Callison's f., a diluting f. for counting red blood cells, consisting of 1 ml of Loeffler's alkaline methylene blue, 1 ml of formalin, 10 ml of glycerol, 1 g of neutral ammonium oxalate, and 2.5 g of sodium chloride added to 90 ml of distilled water, mixed well, and permitted to stand until the solids are dissolved and the reagent is clear; the preparation is filtered prior to use.
cerebrospinal f. (CSF), *liquor* cerebrospinalis.
crevicular f., gingival f.
Dakin's f., Dakin's *solution.*
dentinal f., dental lymph; the lymph or f. of dentin which appears on the surface of freshly cut dentin, especially in young teeth; it is a transudate of extracellular f., mainly cytoplasm of odontoblastic processes, from the dental pulp via the dentinal tubules.
extracellular f. (ECF), (1) the interstitial f. and the plasma, constituting about 20% of the weight of the body; **(2)** sometimes used to mean all f. outside of cells, usually excluding transcellular f.

extravascular f., all f. outside the blood vessels, *i.e.,* intracellular, interstitial, and transcellular f.'s; it constitutes about 48 to 58% of the body weight.
Farrant's mounting f., an aqueous solution containing gum arabic, arsenic trioxide, glycerol, and water, used in mounting histologic sections directly from water; some modifications involve addition of potassium acetate to bring the pH up to neutrality and substitution of other preservatives like cresol or thymol for arsenic trioxide.
gingival f., crevicular or sulcular f.; f. containing plasma proteins, which is present in increasing amounts in association with gingival inflammation.
infranatant f., clear f. which, after the settling out of an insoluble liquid or solid by the action of normal gravity or of centrifugal force, takes up the lower portion of the contents of a vessel.
interstitial f., tissue f.; the f. in spaces between the tissue cells, constituting about 16% of the weight of the body; closely similar in composition to lymph.
intracellular f. (ICF), the f. within the tissue cells, constituting about 30 to 40% of the body weight.
intraocular f., *humor* aquosus.
newtonian f., a f. in which flow and rate of shear are always proportional to the applied stress; such f. precisely obeys Poiseuille's law. *Cf.* non-newtonian f.
non-newtonian f., a f. in which flow and rate of shear are not always proportional to the applied stress and which does not obey Poiseuille's law. For examples, see also anomalous *viscosity;* Fahraeus-Lindqvist *effect;* Bingham *plastic. Cf.* newtonian f.
pleural f., the thin film of f. between the visceral and parietal pleurae.
prostatic f., succus prostaticus; a whitish secretion that is one of the constituents of the semen.
pseudoplastic f., a f. which exhibits shear thinning.
Rees-Ecker f., an aqueous solution of sodium citrate, sucrose, and brilliant cresyl blue used in platelet counts.
Scarpa's f., endolympha.
seminal f., semen (1).
sulcular f., gingival f.
supernatant f., clear f. which, after the settling out of an insoluble liquid or solid by the action of normal gravity or of centrifugal force, takes up the upper portion of the contents of a vessel.
synovial f., synovia.
thixotropic f., a liquid which tends to turn into a gel when left standing, but which turns back into a liquid if agitated, as by vibrations or subjection to adequate shear.
tissue f., interstitial f.
transcellular f.'s, the f.'s that are not inside cells, but are separated from plasma and interstitial f. by cellular barriers; *e.g.,* cerebrospinal f., synovial f., pleural f.
ventricular f., the portion of the cerebrospinal f. that is contained in the ventricles of the brain.

fluidextract (flū-id-eks'trakt). Liquid extract; pharmacopeial liquid preparation of vegetable drugs, made by percolation, containing alcohol as a solvent or as a preservative, or both, and so made that each milliliter contains the therapeutic constituents of 1 g of the standard drug that it represents.

fluidglycerates (flū-id-glis'er-āts). Pharmaceutical preparations, formerly official in the NF, containing approximately 50% by volume of glycerin but no alcohol, and of the same drug strength as fluidextracts.

fluidism (flū'i-dizm). Humoral *doctrine.*

fluidity (flū-id'i-tē). The reciprocal of viscosity; unit: rhe = poise^{-1}.

fluidounce (flū'id-owns'). A measure of capacity: 8 fluidrams. The imperial f. is a measure containing 1 avoirdupois ounce, 437.5 grains, of distilled water at 15.6°C, and equals 28.4 ml; the U.S. f. is $^{1}/_{128}$ gallon, contains 454.6 grains of distilled water at 25°C, and equals 29.57 ml.

fluidrachm, fluidram (flū'i-dram'). A measure of capacity: $^{1}/_{8}$ of a fluidounce; a teaspoonful. The imperial f. contains 54.8 grains of distilled water, and equals 3.55 ml; the U.S. f. contains 57.1 grains of distilled water and equals 3.70 ml.

fluke (flūk) [A.S. *flōc,* flatfish]. Common name for members of the class Trematoda (phylum Platyhelminthes). All f.'s of mammals (subclass Digenea) are internal parasites in the adult stage and are characterized by complex digenetic life cycles involving a snail initial host, in which larval multiplication occurs, and the release of swimming larvae (cercariae) which directly penetrate the skin of the final host (as in schistosomes), encyst on vegetation (as in *Fasciola*), or encyst in or on another intermediate host (as in *Clonorchis* and other fish-borne f.'s). F.'s of lower vertebrates (order Monogenea), especially fish, are frequently monogenetic ectoparasites or gill parasites. Blood f.'s live in the mesenteric-portal bloodstream and associated vesical and pelvic venous plexuses; they include *Schistosoma haematobium* (the vesical blood f.), *S. mansoni* (Manson's intestinal blood f.), and *S. japonicum* (the Oriental blood f.). Other important f.'s are *Paragonimus westermani* (bronchial or lung f.), *Opisthorchis felineus* (cat liver f.), *Clonorchis sinensis* (Chinese liver or Oriental f.), *Heterophyes heterophyes* (Egyptian or small intestinal f.), *Fasciolopsis buski* (large intestinal f.), *Dicrocoelium dendriticum* (lancet f.), *Fasciola hepatica* (liver or sheep liver f.), and *Paramphistomum* (rumen f.).

flumen, pl. **flumina** (flū'men, flū'min-ă) [L.]. A flowing, or stream.
flumina pilo'rum [NA], hair streams; the curved lines along which the hairs are arranged on the head and various parts of the body, especially noticeable in the fetus.

flumethasone (flū-meth'ă-sōn). 6α,9α-Difluoro-11β,17α,21-trihydroxy-16α-methylpregna-1,4-diene-3,20-dione; a synthetic corticosteroid; the 21-pivalate salt and acetate are also available.

flumethiazide (flū'me-thī'ă-zīd). 6-Trifluoromethyl-7-sulfamoyl-4*H*-1,2,4-benzothiadiazine 1,1-dioxide; an orally effective diuretic agent, related chemically to chlorothiazide and with similar pharmacologic actions and uses; it inhibits carbonic anhydrase.

flumina (flū'mi-nă). Plural of flumen.

flunisolide (flū-nis'ō-lid). Pregna-1,4-diene-3,20-dione, 6-fluoro-11,21-dihydroxy-16,17[(1-methylethylidene)bis(oxy)]-, hemihydrate, (6α,11β,16α)-; an anti-inflammatory corticosteroid used intranasally or by inhalation in the treatment of allergies and asthma.

fluo- [L. *fluo,* pp. *fluxus,* to flow]. **1.** Combining form denoting flow. **2.** Prefix often used to denote fluorine in the generic names of drugs. See also fluor-; fluoro-.

fluocinolone acetonide (flū-ō-sin'ō-lōn as'ĕ-tō-nīd). 6α,9α-Difluoro-11β,16α,17α,21-tetrahydroxy-1,4-pregnadiene-3,20-dione cyclic 16,17-acetal with acetone; 6α,9α-difluoro-16α-hydroxyprednisolone 16,17-acetonide; a fluorinated corticosteroid for topical use in the treatment of selected dermatoses.

fluocinonide (flū-ō-sin'ō-nīd). Pregna-1,4-diene-3,20-dione, 21-(acetyloxy)-6,9-difluoro-11-hydroxy-16,17-[(methylethylidene)-bis(oxy)]-, (6α,11β,16β)-; an anti-inflammatory corticosteroid used in topical preparations.

fluocortolone (flū-ō-kōr'tō-lōn). 6α-Fluoro-11β,21-dihydroxy-16α-methylpregna-1,4-diene-3,20-dione; a glucocorticoid used as an anti-inflammatory agent.
f. caproate, f. hexanoate; ester of f. used topically in the treatment of skin diseases.
f. hexanoate, f. caproate.
f. pivalate, ester of f. used topically.

fluor-, fluoro-. Prefixes denoting fluorine.

fluorapatite (flūr-ap'ă-tīt). $3Ca_3(PO_4)_2 \cdot CaF_2$; a naturally occurring fluorophosphate of calcium.

9*H*-**fluorene** (flūr'ēn). Diphenylenemethane; parent compound of 2-acetylaminofluorene; occurs in coal tar.

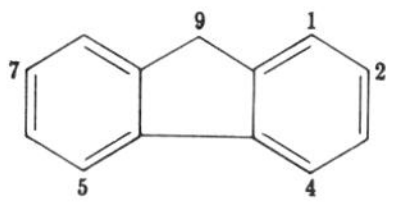

9*H*-**Fluorene**

fluorescein (flūr-es'ē-in) [C.I. 45350]. Resorcinolphthalein; resorcinol phthalic anhydride; 9-(*o*-carboxyphenyl)-6-hydroxy-3*H*-xanthen-3-one; an orange-red crystalline powder that yields a bright green fluorescence in solution, and is reduced to fluorescin; a nontoxic, water-soluble indicator used diagnostically to trace water flow.

f. isothiocyanate, a derivative of f., used as a fluorescent label for specific proteins to permit histologic observation of their distribution.

f. sodium, resorcinolphthalein sodium; uranin; a dye used for diagnosis of certain ocular diseases, differentiation or delineation of organ parts in surgery, and determination of circulation time.

fluorescence (flūr-es'ens). Emission of a longer wavelength radiation by a substance as a consequence of absorption of energy from a shorter wavelength radiation, continuing only as long as the stimulus is present; distinguished from phosphorescence in that, in the latter, emission persists for a perceptible period of time after the stimulus has been removed.

fluorescent (flūr-es'ent). Possessing the quality of fluorescence.

fluorescin (flūr'-es-in). Reduced fluorescein, with similar uses as fluorescein.

fluoridation (flūr'i-dā'shŭn). Addition of fluorides to a community water supply, usually 1 ppm, to reduce incidence of dental decay.

fluoride (flūr'īd). A compound of fluorine with a metal, a nonmetal, or an organic radical; the anion of fluorine.

fluoride number. The percent inhibition of pseudocholinesterase produced by fluorides; used to differentiate normal from atypical pseudocholinesterases. See also dibucaine number.

fluoridization (flūr'i-di-zā'shŭn). Therapeutic use of fluorides to reduce the incidence of dental decay; sometimes used to refer to the topical application of fluoride agents to the teeth.

fluorine (flūr'ēn). A gaseous chemical element, symbol F, atomic no. 9, atomic weight 19.00.

fluoro-. See fluor-.

fluorochrome (flūr'ō-krōm). Any fluorescent dye used to stain tissues and cells for examination by fluorescence microscopy.

fluorochroming (flūr'ō-krōm-ing). **1.** Tagging or "labeling" of antibody with a fluorescent dye so that it may be observed with a microscope (using ultraviolet light), as a means of studying the origin, distribution, and sites of reaction (with antigen) in tissues. **2.** Microscopic detection of cellular and tissue chemical components (DNA, RNA, proteins, polysaccharides) with the aid of fluorochromes bound to these components.

9α-**fluorocortisol** (flūr-ō-kōr'ti-sol). Fludrocortisone acetate.

fluorocyte (flūr'ō-sīt). Term used occasionally for a reticulocyte that exhibits fluorescence.

fluoro-2,4-dinitrobenzene (FDNB) (flūr'ō-dī-nī-trō-ben'zēn). Sanger's reagent; used to combine with the free NH_2 group of the NH_2-terminal amino acid residue in a peptide, thus marking this residue; the combined forms are known as DNP-proteins, Dnp-aminoacyl, etc., the fluorine having been replaced to leave a dinitrophenyl residue (DNP, Dnp, or N_2ph-) attached to the NH_2 group.

fluorography (flūr-og'ră-fē). Photofluorography.

9α-**fluorohydrocortisone acetate** (flūr'ō-hī-drō-kōr'ti-sōn). Fludrocortisone acetate.

fluorometer (flūr-om'ĕ-ter). A device employing an ultraviolet source, monochromators for selection of wavelength, and a detector of visible light; used in fluorometry.

fluorometholone (flūr-ō-meth'ō-lōn). 9α-Fluoro-11β,17α-dihydroxy-6α-methyl-1,4-pregnadiene-3,20-dione; a glucocorticoid for topical use.

fluorometry (flūr-om'ĕ-trē) [fluoro- + G. *metron,* measure]. An analytic method for determining fluorescent compounds, using a beam of ultraviolet light which excites the compounds and causes them to emit visible light.

fluorophotometry (flūr'ō-fō-tom'ĕ-trē). Photomultiplier tube measurement of fluorescence emitted from the interior of the eye after intravenous administration of fluorescein; used to measure the rate of formation of aqueous humor or integrity of the retinal vasculature.

fluororoentgenography (flūr'ō-rent-gen-og'ră-fē). Photofluorography.

fluoroscope (flūr'ō-skōp) [fluorescence + G. *skopeō,* to examine]. Roentgenoscope; an apparatus for rendering visible the shadows of the x-rays which, after passing through the body under examination, are projected on a surface containing a fluorescent material such as calcium tungstate.

fluoroscopic (flūr-ō-skop'ik). Relating to or effected by means of fluoroscopy.

fluoroscopy (flūr-os'kŏ-pē). Roentgenoscopy; examination of the tissues and deep structures of the body by x-ray, using the fluoroscope.

fluorosis (flūr-ō'sis). **1.** A condition caused by an excessive intake of fluorides (2 or more p.p.m. in drinking water), characterized mainly by mottling, staining, or hypoplasia of the enamel of the teeth, although the skeletal bones are also affected. **2.** Chronic poisoning of livestock with fluorides which blacken and soften developing teeth and reduce bones to a chalky brittleness; most often caused by ingestion of forage contaminants near large aluminum plants.

chronic endemic f., f. caused by excessive fluorine in the natural water supply, as seen in parts of India; osteosclerosis with ankylosis of the spine may develop.

fluorouracil (flūr-ō-yū'ră-sil). 5-Fluorouracil; a pyrimidine analogue; an antineoplastic effective in the treatment of some carcinomas; the cells of certain neoplasms incorporate uracil into ribonucleic acid more readily than do normal tissue cells. See also floxuridine.

fluoxetine hydrochloride (flū-oks'ĕ-tēn). Benzenepropanamine, *N*-methyl-γ-[4-(trifluoromethyl)-phenoxy]-; an oral antidepressant chemically unrelated to other antidepressants.

fluoxymesterone (flū-ok-sē-mes'ter-ōn). 9α-Fluoro-11β,17β-dihydroxy-17α-methyl-4-androstene-3-one; an orally effective synthetic halogenated steroid, related in chemical structure and pharmacologic action to methyltestosterone, but more potent.

flupentixol (flū-pen-tik'sol). 4-{3-[2-(Trifluoromethyl)thioxanthen-9-ylidene]propyl}-1-piperazineethanol; a neuroleptic.

fluperolone acetate (flū-per'ō-lōn). 9α-Fluoro-11β,17α,21-trihydroxy-21-methylpregna-1,4-diene-3,20-dione 21-acetate; a synthetic corticosteroid used as an anti-inflammatory agent.

fluphenazine (flū-fen'ă-zēn). 4-[3-[2-(Trifluoromethyl)-phenothiazin-10-yl]propyl]-1-piperazine ethanol; a phenothiazine-piperazine compound; a tranquilizer.

f. enanthate, a long-acting antipsychotic, used parenterally.

f. hydrochloride, an antipsychotic, used in the management of acute and chronic schizophrenia, involutional, senile, and toxic psychoses, and the manic phase of manic-depressive psychosis.

fluprednisolone (flū-pred-nis'ō-lōn). 6α-Fluoro-$11\beta,17\alpha$,21-trihydroxy-1,4-pregnadiene-3,20-dione; a glucocorticoid with anti-inflammatory activity and toxicity similar to those of cortisol.

flurandrenolide (flūr-an-dren'ō-līd). Pregn-4-ene-3,20-dione, 6-fluoro-11,21-dihydroxy-16,17-[(1-methylethylidene)bis(oxy)]-, ($6\alpha,11\beta,16\alpha$)-; an anti-inflammatory glucocorticoid used in topical preparations.

flurazepam hydrochloride (flūr-az'ĕ-pam). 7-Chloro-1-[2-(diethylamino)ethyl]-5-(*o*- fluorophenyl)-1,3-dihydro-2*H*-1,4-benzodiazepin-2-one dihydrochloride; an oral hypnotic and sedative.

flurbiprofen (flūr-bi'prō-fen). [1,1'-Biphenyl]-4-acetic acid, 2-fluoro-α-methyl-, (±)-; a nonsteroidal anti-inflammatory agent with analgesic, anti-inflammatory, and antipyretic actions.

flurogestone acetate (flūr-ō-jes'tōn). 9-Fluoro-11β,17-dihydroxypregn-4-ene-3,20-dione 17-acetate; a progestational agent.

flurothyl (flūr'ō-thil). Bis(2,2,2-trifluoroethyl) ether; a convulsant, administered by inhalation for the same indications as electroconvulsive therapy; produces grand mal convulsions.

fluroxene (flūr-ok'sēn). 2,2,2-Trifluoroethyl vinyl ether; a volatile, halogenated inhalation anesthetic.

flush (flŭsh). **1.** To wash out with a full stream of fluid. **2.** A transient erythema due to heat, exertion, stress, or disease. **3.** Flat, or even with another surface, as a f. stoma.

hectic f., redness of the face associated with a rise of temperature in various fevers.

hot f., colloquialism for a vasomotor symptom of the climacteric characterized by sudden vasodilation with a sensation of heat, usually involving the face and neck, and upper part of the chest; sweats, often profuse, frequently follow the f. *Cf.* hot *flash.*

malar f., localized hectic f. and warmth of the malar eminences, often occurring in tuberculosis and sometimes seen in rheumatic fever.

flutter (flŭt'er) [A.S. *floterian,* to float about]. Agitation; tremulousness.

atrial f., auricular f., jugular embryocardia; rapid regular atrial contractions occurring usually at rates between 250 and 400 per minute and often producing "saw-tooth" waves in the electrocardiogram.

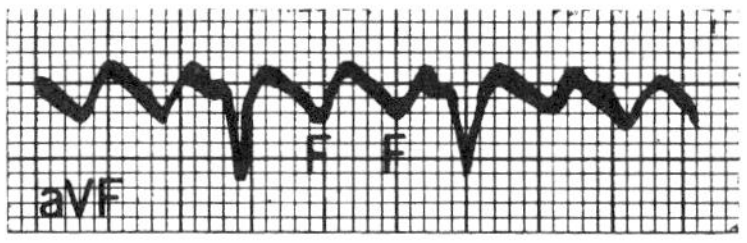

Atrial Flutter

diaphragmatic f., rapid rhythmical contractions (average, 150 per minute) of the diaphragm, simulating atrial f. clinically and sometimes electrocardiographically.

impure f., mixture of atrial flutter (FF) waves and fibrillation (ff) waves in the electrocardiogram.

ocular f., a spontaneous, brief, intermittent, horizontal oscillation of the eyes occurring during fixation; it often coexists with ocular dysmetria in cerebellar syndromes.

ventricular f., a form of rapid ventricular tachycardia in which the electrocardiographic complexes assume a regular undulating pattern with an absence of distinct QRS and T waves.

flutter-fibrillation. An electrocardiographic pattern of atrial activity with features of both fibrillation and flutter.

flux (flŭks) [L. *fluxus,* a flow]. **1.** The discharge of a fluid material in large amount from a cavity or surface of the body. See also diarrhea. **2.** Material discharged from the bowels. **3.** A material used to remove oxides from the surface of molten metal and to protect it when casting; serves a similar purpose in soldering operations. Also, an ingredient in dental porcelain which by its lower melting temperature helps to bond the silica particles. **4.** (*J*). Flux density; the moles of a substance crossing through a unit area of a boundary layer or membrane per unit of time.

luminous f., the quantity of light emitted from a point source in a given time; its unit is the lumen.

net f., the difference between the two unidirectional f.'s.

unidirectional f., the f. of a substance from one surface of a boundary layer or membrane to the other, disregarding any counterbalancing f. in the other direction, as measured by tracer technique.

fly (flī) [A.S. *fleóge*]. A two-winged insect in the order Diptera. Typical flies of the housefly type and similar forms are in the family Muscidae. Important f.'s include *Simulium* (black f.), *Calliphora* (bluebottle f.), *Piophila casei* (cheese f.), *Chrysops* (deer f.), *Siphona irritans* (horn f.), *Fannia scolaris* (latrine f.), *Oestrus ovis* and *Gasterophilus hemorrhoidalis* (nose f.), *Cochliomyia hominivorax* (primary screw-worm f.) and *C. macellaria* (secondary screw-worm f.), *Stomoxys calcitrans* (stable f.), *Glossina* (tsetse f.), and members of the insect order Trichoptera. For some types of flies not listed as subentries here (usually written as one word), see the full name (*e.g.,* blowfly, botfly, gadfly, horsefly, housefly).

heel f., see botfly.

louse f.'s, pupiparous, dorsoventrally flattened dipterous ectoparasites of the family Hippoboscidae. See also *Hippobosca* and *Melophagus.*

mangrove f., species of *Chrysops* in Africa, vectors of *Loa loa; e.g., Chrysops silacea.*

Russian f., Spanish f., cantharis.

warble f., see botfly.

Flynn, P. See F.-Aird *syndrome.*

Fm Symbol for fermium.

FMD Abbreviation for foot-and-mouth *disease.*

FMN Abbreviation for *flavin* mononucleotide.

foam (fōm). **1.** Masses of small bubbles on the surface of a liquid. **2.** To produce such bubbles. **3.** Masses of air cells in a solid or semisolid, as in f. rubber.

human fibrin f., a dry artificial sponge of human fibrin prepared by clotting with thrombin a f. of a solution of human fibrinogen; the clotted f. is dried from the frozen state and heated; used as a topical anticoagulant.

focal (fō'kăl). **1.** Denoting a focus. **2.** Relating to a localized area.

foci (fō'sī). Plural of focus.

focimeter (fō-sim'ĕ-ter). Lensometer.

focus, pl. **foci** (fō'kŭs, fō'sī) [L. a hearth]. **1** (**F**). The point at which the light rays meet after passing through a convex lens. **2.** The center, or the starting point, of a disease process.

conjugate foci, two points so related to a lens or concave mirror that an image at one point is focused at the other, and vice versa.

Ghon's f., Ghon's *tubercle.*

natural f. of infection, an ecosystem in which an infectious agent normally persists in nature; *e.g.,* yellow fever virus in a jungle-monkey-*Haemagogus* mosquito ecosystem.

principal f., the real or virtual meeting point of rays passing into a lens parallel to its axis.

real f., the point of meeting of convergent rays.

virtual f., the point from which divergent rays seem to proceed, or that at which they would meet if prolonged backward.

Fogarty, Thomas J., U.S. thoracic surgeon, *1934. See F. *catheter, clamp.*

fogging (fog'ing). A method of refraction in which accommodation is relaxed by overcorrection with a convex spherical lens.

fogo selvagem (fō'gō sel'vă-jem) [Pg. wild fire]. Brazilian pemphigus; wildfire; a form of pemphigus foliaceus, occurring in southern Brazil, in which the lesions are bullous, appear localized to the face and upper trunk, become widespread, variegated, erythrodermic, and exfoliative, and are immunologically indistinguishable from pemphigus foliaceus or vulgaris.

foil (foyl). An extremely thin pliable sheet of metal.

Foix, Charles, French neurologist, 1882–1927. See F.'s *syndrome;* F.-Alajouanine *myelitis.*

folacin (fō'lă-sin). Folic acid or any derivative thereof that has the biological (vitamin) activity of folic acid.

folate (fō'lāt). A salt or ester of folic acid.

FOLD

fold (fōld). **1.** A ridge or margin apparently formed by the doubling back of a lamina. See also plica. **2.** In the embryo, a transient elevation or reduplication of tissue in the form of a lamina.

adipose f.'s of the pleura, *plicae* adiposae.
alar f.'s, *plicae* alares.
amniotic f., Schultze's f.; a f. of amniotic membrane enclosing the yolk stalk and extending from the point of insertion of the umbilical cord to the yolk sac; in reptiles and birds it is the reflected edge of the amnion where it folds over to cover the embryo during early development.
aryepiglottic f., arytenoepiglottidean f., *plica* aryepiglottica.
axillary f., *plica* axillaris; one of the folds of skin and muscular tissue bounding the axilla anteriorly and posteriorly.
caval f., a f. near the base on the right side of the dorsal mesentery, in which a primordial segment of the inferior vena cava develops between the right subcardinal vein and vessels within the liver.
cecal f.'s, *plicae* cecales.
f. of chorda tympani, *plica* chordae tympani.
ciliary f.'s, *plicae* ciliares.
circular f.'s, *plicae* circulares.
Dennie's infraorbital f., Dennie's *line.*
Douglas' f., *plica* rectouterina.
Duncan's f.'s, the f.'s on the peritoneal surface of the uterus immediately after delivery.
duodenojejunal f., *plica* duodenalis superior.
duodenomesocolic f., *plica* duodenalis inferior.
epigastric f., *plica* umbilicalis lateralis.
falciform retinal f., a congenital f. from the disk to the ciliary region in the inferior temporal quadrant of the retina.
fimbriated f., *plica* fimbriata.
gastric f.'s, *plicae* gastricae.
gastropancreatic f.'s, *plicae* gastropancreaticae.
genital f., urogenital *ridge.*
giant gastric f.'s, enlarged gastric submucosal ridges covered by hyperplastic mucosa, as seen in Zollinger-Ellison syndrome, Ménétrièr's disease, and hypertrophic hypersecretory gastropathy.
glossopalatine f., *arcus* palatoglossus.
gluteal f., a prominent f. that marks the upper limit of the thigh from the lower limit of the buttock; it coincides with the lower border of the gluteus maximus muscle.
Guérin's f., *valvula* fossae navicularis.
Hasner's f., *plica* lacrimalis.
head f., a ventral folding of the cephalic extremity in the embryonic disk, so that the brain lies rostrad to the mouth and pericardium.
Houston's f.'s, *plicae* transversales recti.
ileocecal f., *plica* ileocecalis.
incudal f., *plica* incudis.
inferior duodenal f., *plica* duodenalis inferior.
infrapatellar synovial f., *plica* synovialis infrapatellaris.
inguinal f., *plica* inguinalis.
inguinal aponeurotic f., *falx* inguinalis.
interureteric f., *plica* interureterica.
f.'s of iris, *plicae* iridis.
Kerckring's f.'s, *plicae* circulares.
labioscrotal f.'s, lateral f.'s at either side of the embryonic cloacal membrane that develop into either the scrotum or the labia majora.
lacrimal f., *plica* lacrimalis.
f. of laryngeal nerve, *plica* nervi laryngei.
lateral f.'s, ventral foldings of the lateral margins of the embryonic disk, thus establishing the definitive embryonic body form.
lateral glossoepiglottic f., *plica* glossoepiglottica lateralis.
lateral nasal f., lateral nasal *elevation.*
lateral umbilical f., *plica* umbilicalis lateralis.
f. of left vena cava, *plica* venae cavae sinistrae.
longitudinal f. of duodenum, *plica* longitudinalis duodeni.
malar f., an ill-defined groove in the skin that extends downward and medially from the lateral canthus.
mallear f., *plica* mallearis.
mammary f., mammary *ridge.*
Marshall's vestigial f., *plica* venae cavae sinistrae.
medial nasal f., medial nasal *elevation.*
medial umbilical f., *plica* umbilicalis medialis.
mesonephric f., urogenital *ridge.*
middle glossoepiglottic f., *plica* glossoepiglottica mediana.
middle umbilical f., *plica* umbilicalis mediana.
mongolian f., *plica* palpebronasalis.
Morgan's f., a single wrinkle or f. beneath the margin of the lower lid of both eyes, present from birth (or shortly thereafter) in patients with atopic dermatitis.
mucobuccal f., the line of flexure of the mucous membrane as it passes from the mandible or maxillae to the cheek.
mucosal f.'s of gallbladder, *plicae* tunicae mucosae vesicae felleae.
nail f., *vallum* unguis.
nasojugal f., a shallow groove in the skin that extends downward and laterally from the medial canthus.
neural f.'s, the elevated margins of the neural groove.
opercular f., tissue forming a bridge or an adhesion between the tonsil and the anterior pillar of the fauces.
palmate f.'s, *plicae* palmatae.
palpebronasal f., *plica* palpebronasalis.
paraduodenal f., *plica* paraduodenalis.
pericardiopleural f., a f. formed in the embryonic pericardiopleural opening; it eventually closes off the pleural from the pericardial cavity.
pharyngoepiglottic f., *plica* glossoepiglottica lateralis.
pleuroperitoneal f., pleuroperitoneal *membrane.*
presplenic f., a fan-shaped f. of peritoneum that passes from the gastrosplenic ligament near the lower end of the spleen to the phrenicocolic ligament with which it blends. It contains branches of the splenic or the left gastroepiploic artery.
rectal f.'s, *plicae* transversales recti.
rectouterine f., *plica* rectouterina.
rectovaginal f., *plica* rectovaginalis.
rectovesical f., the f. of peritoneum in the male that bounds the rectovesical pouch laterally.
retinal f., a congenital or secondary f., secondary to membrane contraction, producing star-shaped, meridional, or circular f.'s on the retina.
retrotarsal f., *fornix* conjunctivae.
Rindfleisch's f.'s, semilunar f.'s of the serous surface of the pericardium, embracing the beginning of the aorta.
sacrogenital f.'s, peritoneal f.'s that extend backward from the sides of the bladder, on either side of the rectum, to the sacrum; they form the lateral boundaries of the rectovesical pouch.

salpingopalatine f., *plica* salpingopalatina.
salpingopharyngeal f., *plica* salpingopharyngea.
Schultze's f., amniotic f.
semilunar f., *plica* semilunaris.
semilunar f. of colon, *plica* semilunaris coli.
semilunar conjunctival f., *plica* semilunaris conjunctivae.
spiral f. of cystic duct, *plica* spiralis ductus cystici.
stapedial f., *plica* stapedis.
sublingual f., *plica* sublingualis.
superior duodenal f., *plica* duodenalis superior.
synovial f., *plica* synovialis.
tail f., the ventral folding of the caudal extremity of the embryonic disk.
tarsal f., the f. marking the attachment of the levator palpebrae superioris muscle into the skin of the upper eyelid.
transverse f.'s of rectum, *plicae* transversales recti.
transverse vesical f., *plica* vesicalis transversa.
Treves' f., *plica* ileocecalis.
triangular f., *plica* triangularis.
Tröltsch's f., *plica* mallearis.
urachal f., *plica* umbilicalis mediana.
ureteric f., *plica* interureterica.
urorectal f., urorectal *septum.*
uterovesical f., vesicouterine *ligament.*
vascular f. of the cecum, *plica* cecalis vascularis.
Vater's f., a f. of mucous membrane in the duodenum just above the greater duodenal papilla.
ventricular f., *plica* vestibularis.
vestibular f., *plica* vestibularis.
vestigial f., *plica* venae cavae sinistrae.
vocal f., *plica* vocalis.

Foley, Frederic E.B., U.S. urologist, 1891–1966. See F. *catheter, operation,* Y-plasty *pyeloplasty.*

folia (fō'lē-ă). Plural of folium.

foliaceous (fō-lē-ā'shŭs). Foliate.

foliar (fō'lē-ăr). Foliate.

foliate (fō'lē-āt). Foliaceous; foliar; foliose; pertaining to or resembling a leaf or leaflet.

folic acid (fō'lik). **1.** Collective term for pteroylglutamic acids and their oligoglutamic acid conjugates. **2.** Specifically, pteroylmonoglutamic acid; Lactobacillus casei or liver Lactobacillus casei factor; *N*-[*p*-[[(2-amino-4-hydroxypteridin-6-yl)methyl]amino]benzoyl]-L(+)-glutamic acid; the growth factor for *Lactobacillus casei,* and a member of the vitamin B complex necessary for the normal production of red blood cells. It is a hemopoietic vitamin present, with or without L(+)-glutamic acid moieties, in peptide linkages in liver, green vegetables, and yeast; used to treat folate deficiency and megaloblastic anemia.

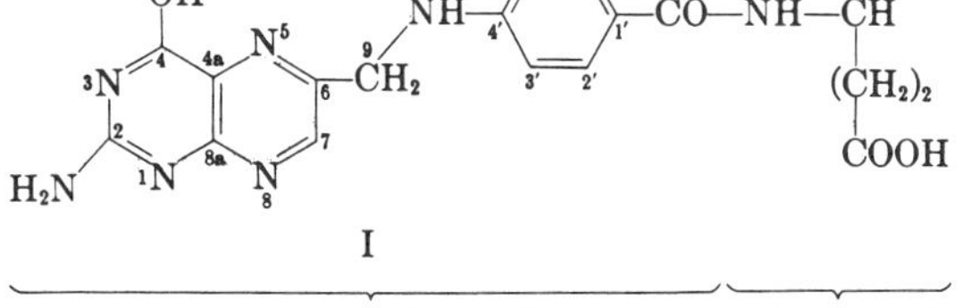

Folic acid

folie (fō-lē') [Fr. folly]. Old term for madness or insanity.
f. à deux (ā-du) [Fr. two], identical or similar mental disorders, such as a paranoid fixation, usually affecting two members of the same family living together.
f. du doute (du-dūt) [F. from doubt], an excessive doubting about all the affairs of life and a morbid scrupulousness concerning minutiae.
f. gémellaire (zha-mel-ār') [Fr. relating to twins], a psychosis appearing simultaneously, or nearly so, in twins, who are not necessarily living together or intimately associated at the time.
f. de pourquoi (pūr-kwah') [Fr. why], a psychopathologic tendency to ask questions.

Folin, Otto K.O., U.S. biochemist, 1867–1934. See F.'s *reaction, test;* F.-Looney *test.*

folinate (fō'li-nāt). A salt or ester of folinic acid.

folinic acid (fō-lin'ik). Citrovorum factor; leucovorin; 5-formyl-5,6,7,8-tetrahydrofolic acid; the active form of folic acid which acts as formyl group carrier in transformylation reactions; the calcium salt, leucovorin calcium, has therapeutic use.

foliose (fō'lē-ōs). Foliate.

folium, pl. folia (fō'lē-ŭm, -lē-ă) [L. a leaf] [NA]. A broad, thin, leaflike structure.
fo'lia cerebel'li [NA], folia of the cerebellum; the narrow, leaf-like gyri of the cerebellar cortex. See also f. vermis, superior to the horizontal fissure.
fo'lia lin'guae, *papillae* foliatae.
f. ver'mis [NA], a small posterior subdivision of the superior vermis of the cerebellum.

Folli (Folius), Cecilio (Caesilius), Venice anatomist, 1615–1660. See F.'s or follian *process.*

folliberin (fol-lib'er-in). Follicle-stimulating hormone-releasing factor or hormone; a decapeptide of hypothalamic origin which is capable of accelerating pituitary secretion of follitropin.

follicle (fol'i-kl) [L. *folliculus,* a small sac, dim. of *follis,* a pair of bellows]. Folliculus.
aggregated lymphatic f.'s, *folliculi* lymphatici aggregati.
anovular ovarian f., a f. that does not contain an ovum.
atretic ovarian f., corpus atreticum; a f. that degenerates before coming to maturity; great numbers of such atretic f.'s occur in the ovary before puberty; in the sexually mature woman, several are formed each month.
dental f., the dental sac with its enclosed odontogenic organ and developing tooth.
gastric f.'s, *glandulae* gastricae.
gastric lymphatic f., *folliculus* lymphaticus gastricus.
graafian f., vesicular ovarian f.
growing ovarian f., a f. having several layers of proliferating follicular cells surrounding the ovum, but separated from it by an extracellular glycoprotein layer (zona pellucida).
hair f., *folliculus* pili.
intestinal f.'s, *glandulae* intestinales.
Lieberkühn's f.'s, *glandulae* intestinales.
lingual f.'s, *folliculi* linguales.
lymph f., lymphatic f., *folliculus* lymphaticus.
lymphatic f.'s of larynx, *folliculi* lymphatici laryngei.
lymphatic f.'s of rectum, *folliculi* lymphatici recti.
mature ovarian f., a f. ready for ovulation; in the human ovary its antrum attains a diameter of 6 to 8 mm and presents a surface bulge; a first maturation division of the ovum usually occurs just prior to the rupture of the f.
Montgomery's f.'s, *glandulae* areolares.
nabothian f., nabothian *cyst.*
ovarian f., one of the spheroidal cell aggregations in the ovary containing an ovum.
polyovular ovarian f., a f. containing more than one ovum.
primary ovarian f., folliculus ovaricus primarius; an ovarian f. before the appearance of an antrum; marked by developmental changes in the oocyte and follicular cells so that the latter form one

or more layers of cuboidal or columnar cells; the f. becomes surrounded by a sheath of stroma, the theca.
primordial ovarian f., a f. in which the primordial oocyte is surrounded by a single layer of flattened follicular cells.
sebaceous f.'s, *glandulae* sebaceae.
secondary f., vesicular ovarian f.
solitary f.'s, *folliculi* lymphatici solitarii.
splenic lymph f.'s, *folliculi* lymphatici lienales.
f.'s of thyroid gland, *folliculi* glandulae thyroideae.
vesicular ovarian f., folliculus ovaricus vesiculosa; graafian or secondary f.; a f. in which the oocyte attains its full size and is surrounded by an extracellular glycoprotein layer (zona pellucida) which separates it from a peripheral layer of follicular cells permeated by one or more fluid filled antra; the theca of the f. develops into internal and external layers.

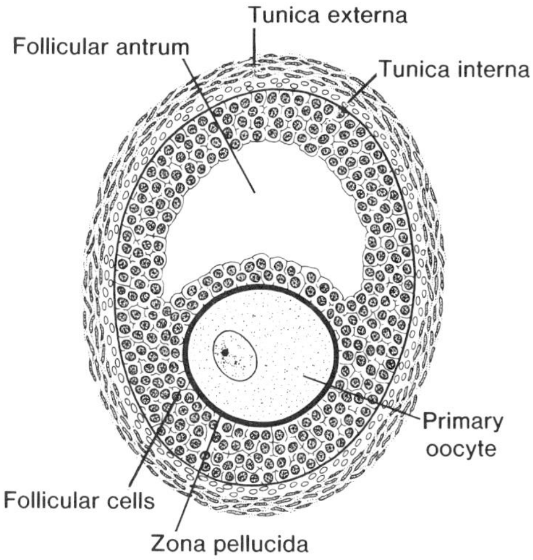

Schematic Representation of Maturing Follicle
The oocyte surrounded by the zona pellucida is eccentrically located and the follicular antrum has developed by coalescence of intercellular spaces.

folliclis (fol-i-klē') [Fr.]. Obsolete term for *lupus* miliaris disseminatus faciei.

follicular (fŏ-lik'yū-lăr). Relating to a follicle or follicles.

folliculi (fŏ-lik'yū-lī). Plural of folliculus.

folliculin (fŏ-lik'yū-lin). Estrone.
f. hydrate, estriol.

folliculitis (fŏ-lik-yū-lī'tis). An inflammatory reaction in hair follicles; the lesions may be papules or pustules.
f. absce'dens et suffo'diens, a chronic progressive follicular-pustular eruption in the scalp.
f. bar'bae, *tinea* barbae.
f. decal'vans, alopecia follicularis; Quinquaud's disease; acne decalvans; a papular or pustular inflammation of the hair follicles of the scalp, resulting in scarring and loss of hair in the affected area.
eosinophilic pustular f., a dermatosis characterized by sterile pruritic papules and pustules that coalesce to form plaques with papulovesicular borders; spontaneous exacerbations and remissions may be accompanied by peripheral leukocytosis, eosinophilia, or both, and may result in eventual destruction of hair follicles and formation of eosinophilic abscesses.
f. exter'na, *blepharitis* follicularis.
f. inter'na, *blepharitis* follicularis.
f. keloida'lis, acne *keloid.*
f. na'res per'forans, inflammation of a hair follicle in the nose; the infection extends to, and perforates, the cutaneous surface.
perforating f., erythematous papules with a central keratin plug which are scattered on the arms, thighs, and buttocks; the follicular epithelium is ruptured by follicular extrusion of dermal fibers.
f. ulerythemato'sa reticula'ta, atrophoderma vermiculatum; erythematous "ice-pick" or pitted scars on the cheeks; a scarring type of folliculitis.

folliculoma (fŏ-lik-yū-lō'-mă). **1.** Granulosa cell *tumor.* **2.** Cystic enlargement of a graafian follicle.

folliculosis (fŏ-lik-yū-lō'sis). Presence of lymph follicles in abnormally great numbers.

folliculus, pl. folliculi (fŏ-lik'yū-lŭs, -yū-lī) [L. a small sac, dim. of *follis,* bellows]. [NA]. Follicle. **1.** A more or less spherical mass of cells usually containing a cavity. **2.** A crypt or minute cul-de-sac or lacuna, such as the depression in the skin, from which the hair emerges.
follic'uli glan'dulae thyroi'deae, follicles of the thyroid gland; the small spherical vesicular components of the thyroid gland lined with epithelium and containing colloid in varying amounts; the colloid serves for storage of the thyroid hormone precursor, thyroglobulin.
follic'uli lingua'les, lingual follicles; lenticular papillae; collections of lymphoid tissue in the mucosa of the pharyngeal part of the tongue posterior to the terminal sulcus collectively forming the lingual tonsil.
follic'uli lymphat'ici aggrega'ti [NA], aggregated lymphatic follicles or nodules; aggregate, agminate, or agminated glands; Peyer's patches or glands; agmen peyerianum; collections of many lymphoid follicles closely packed together, forming oblong elevations on the mucous membrane of the small intestine.
follic'uli lymphat'ici aggrega'ti appen'dicis vermifor'mis [NA], masses of lymphoid tissue in the submucous coat of the vermiform appendix.
follic'uli lymphat'ici laryn'gei, lymphatic follicles of the larynx; laryngeal tonsils; small follicles located on the posterior aspect of the epiglottis and in the ventricle of the larynx.
follic'uli lymphat'ici liena'les [NA], splenic lymph follicles or nodules; splenic corpuscles; malpighian corpuscles (2); malpighian bodies, glands, or nodules; small nodular masses of lymphoid tissue attached to the sides of the smaller arterial branches.
follic'uli lymphat'ici rec'ti, lymphatic follicles of the rectum; scattered collections of lymphoid tissue in the wall of the rectum.
follic'uli lymphat'ici solita'rii [NA], solitary follicles; solitary glands; solitary nodules of the intestine; minute collections of lymphoid tissue in the mucosa of the small and large intestines, being especially numerous in the cecum and appendix.
f. lymphat'icus, lymph or lymphatic follicle; nodulus lymphaticus; lymph nodule; one of the spherical masses of lymphoid cells frequently having a more lightly staining center.
f. lymphat'icus gas'tricus, gastric lymphatic follicle; one of the numerous small masses of lymphoid tissue in the gastric mucosa.
f. ovar'icus prima'rius [NA], primary ovarian *follicle.*
f. ovar'icus vesiculo'sus [NA], vesicular ovarian *follicle.*
f. pi'li [NA], hair follicle; a tube-like invagination of the epidermis from which the hair shaft develops and into which the sebaceous glands open; the follicle is lined by a cellular inner and outer root sheath of epidermal origin and is invested with a fibrous sheath derived from the dermis.

Folling, Ivar A., Norwegian physician, 1888–1973. See F.'s *disease.*

follitropin (fol-i-trō'pin). Follicle-stimulating hormone or principle; gametokinetic hormone; a glycoprotein hormone of the anterior pituitary that stimulates the graafian follicles of the ovary and assists subsequently in follicular maturation and the secretion of estradiol; in the male, it stimulates the epithelium of the seminiferous tubules and is partially responsible for inducing spermatogenesis.

Foltz, Jean C.E., French anatomist and ophthalmologist, 1822–1876. See F. *valvule.*

fomentation (fō-men-tā'shŭn) [L. *fomento,* pp. *-atus,* to foment, fr. *fomentum,* a poultice, fr. *foveo,* to keep warm]. **1.** A warm application. See also poultice; stupe. **2.** Application of warmth and moisture in the treatment of disease.

fomes, pl. **fomites** (fō'mēz, fō'mi-tēz) [L. tinder, fr. *foveo,* to keep warm]. Fomite; a substance, such as clothing, capable of absorbing and transmitting the agent of disease; usually used in the plural.

fomite (fō'mīt). Fomes.

fomites (fō'mi-tēz). Plural of fomes.

fonazine mesylate (fō'nă-zēn). Dimethothiazine mesylate; 10-[2-(dimethylamino)propyl]-*N,N*-dimethylphenothiazine-2-sulfonamide monomethanesulfonate; a serotonin inhibitor.

Fonio, Anton, Swiss physician, *1889. See F.'s *solution.*

Fonsecaea (fon-sē-sē'ă). A genus of fungi of which at least two species, *F. pedrosoi* and *F. compacta,* cause chromoblastomycosis.

Fontan, Francois, French thoracic surgeon, *1929. See F. *procedure, operation.*

Fontana, Arturo, Italian dermatologist, 1873–1950. See F.'s *stain;* Fontana-M. silver *stain;* Masson-F. ammoniacal silver *stain.*

Fontana, Felice, Italian physiologist, 1730–1805. See F.'s *canal, spaces.*

fontanel, fontanelle (fon'tă-nel') [Fr. dim. of *fontaine,* fountain, spring]. Fonticulus.

anterior f., *fonticulus* anterior.
anterolateral f., *fonticulus* sphenoidalis.
bregmatic f., *fonticulus* anterior.
Casser's f., *fonticulus* mastoideus.
cranial f.'s, *fonticuli* cranii.
frontal f., *fonticulus* anterior.
Gerdy's f., sagittal f.
mastoid f., *fonticulus* mastoideus.
occipital f., *fonticulus* posterior.
posterior f., *fonticulus* posterior.
posterolateral f., *fonticulus* mastoideus.
sagittal f., Gerdy's f.; an occasional f.-like defect in the sagittal suture in the newborn.
sphenoidal f., *fonticulus* sphenoidalis.

fonticulus, pl. **fonticuli** (fon-tik'yū-lŭs, -lī) [L. dim. of *fons (font-),* fountain, spring] [NA]. Fontanel; one of several membranous intervals at the angles of the cranial bones in the infant. See f. cranii.

f. ante'rior [NA], anterior fontanel; frontal or bregmatic fontanel; a diamond-shaped membranous interval at the junction of the coronal, sagittal, and metopic sutures where the frontal angles of the parietal bones meet the two ununited halves of the frontal bone.

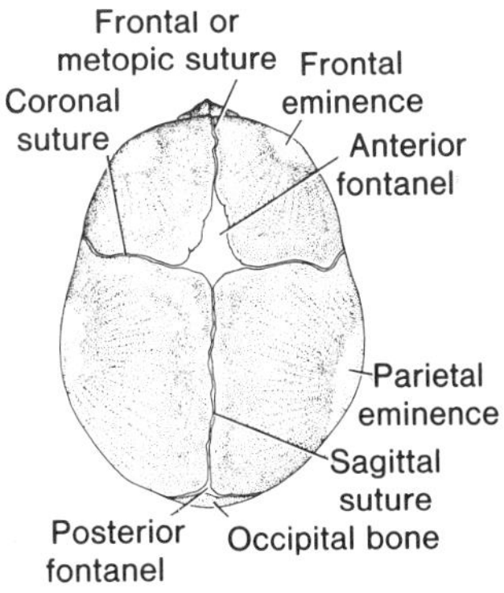

Fonticuli (Fontanels) in Skull of Newborn

f. anterolatera'lis [NA], official alternate term for f. sphenoidalis.

fontic'uli cra'nii [NA], cranial fontanels; the membranous intervals between the angles of the cranial bones in the infant; they include the midline f. anterior and f. posterior, and the paired f. sphenoidalis and f. mastoideus.

f. mastoi'deus [NA], f. posterolateralis; mastoid fontanel; Casser's or posterolateral fontanel; the membranous interval on either side between the mastoid angle of the parietal bone, the petrous portion of the temporal bone, and the occipital bone.

f. poste'rior [NA], posterior fontanel; occipital fontanel; a triangular interval at the union of the lambdoid and sagittal sutures where the occipital angles of the parietal bones meet the occipital.

f. posterolatera'lis [NA], official alternate term for f. mastoideus.

f. sphenoida'lis [NA], f. anterolateralis; sphenoidal fontanel; anterolateral fontanel; an irregularly shaped interval on either side where the frontal, sphenoidal angle of the parietal, squamous portion of the temporal and greater wing of the sphenoid meet.

food (fūd) [A.S. *fōda*]. That which is eaten to supply necessary nutritive elements.

Foot, N.C., 20th century U.S. pathologist. See F.'s reticulin impregnation *stain.*

foot (fut) [A.S. *fōt*]. **1.** Pes (1); the lower, pedal, podalic, extremity of the leg. **2 (ft.).** A unit of length, containing 12 inches, equal to 30.48 cm.

athlete's f., *tinea* pedis.
buttress f., a condition of the horse's f. in which there is exostosis of the extensor process of the third phalanx, with swelling and chronic inflammation at the coronary band on the anterior surface of the f.
claw f., see clawfoot.
club f., see *talipes* equinovarus.
contracted f., **(1)** *talipes* cavus; **(2)** contracted heel; a condition of the horse in which a part of the foot, often a heel, is contracted and shrunken as a result of loss of moisture in the hoof.
drop f., see foot-drop.
fescue f., fescue poisoning; poisoning by a toxic principle in tall fescue grass; mainly a disease of cattle, but sheep are sometimes affected; lameness in the hind feet is first noticed, followed by necrosis of the extremities.
flat f., *talipes* planus.
fungous f., mycetoma (1).
f. of hippocampus, *pes* hippocampi.
Hong Kong f., *tinea* pedis.
immersion f., trench f.; a condition resulting from prolonged exposure to damp and cold; the extremity is initially cold and anesthetic, but on rewarming becomes hyperemic, paresthetic, and hyperhidrotic; recovery is often slow.
Madura f., mycetoma (1).
Morand's f., a f. having eight toes.
mossy f., lymphedematous keratoderma; lymphostatic verrucosis; a profuse velvety papillomatous growth that develops large warty projections; caused by chronic lymphedema and stasis with maceration and associated infection.
pumiced f., a condition of the horse's hoof, frequently associated with chronic laminitis, in which the sole is level with or extends beyond the bearing surface of the hoof wall, causing lameness, particularly when the animal moves on hard surfaces; the sole becomes thick and flaky.
reel f., *talipes* equinovarus.
sandal f., a wide space between the first and second toes seen in Down's syndrome.
spastic flat f., eversion of the f. with spasm of the muscles (peroneal) on the outer side; often associated with abnormal bars of bone between the calcaneum and the navicular (scaphoid) or between the navicular and the talus.
trench f., immersion f.

footcandle (fut'kan-dl). Illumination or brightness equivalent to 1 lumen per square foot; replaced in the SI system by the candela.

foot-drop (fut'drop). Paralysis or weakness of the dorsiflexor muscles of the foot and ankle, as a consequence of which the foot falls, the toes dragging on the ground in walking, usually due to injury of the peroneal nerve.

footplate, foot-plate (fut'plāt). **1.** *Basis* stapedis. **2.** Pedicel.

foot-pound (fut'pownd). Energy expended, or work done, in raising a mass of 1 pound a height of 1 foot vertically against gravitational force.

foot-poundal (fut'pownd-ăl). Energy exerted, or work done, when a force of 1 poundal displaces a body 1 foot in the direction of the force.

forage (fōr-ahzh') [Fr. boring]. The operation of cutting a channel by surgical diathermy through an enlarged prostate.

FORAMEN

foramen, pl. **foramina** (fō-rā'men, fō-ram'i-nă) [L. an aperture, fr. *foro,* to pierce] [NA]. Trema (1); an aperture or perforation through a bone or a membranous structure.

alveolar foramina, foramina alveolaria.

foram'ina alveola'ria [NA], alveolar foramina; openings of the posterior dental canals on the infratemporal surface of the maxilla.

anterior condyloid f., *canalis* hypoglossalis.

anterior palatine foramina, foramina palatina minora.

aortic f., *hiatus* aorticus.

apical dental f., f. apicis dentis.

f. ap'icis den'tis [NA], apical dental f.; root f.; the opening at the apex of the root of a tooth that gives passage to the nerve and blood vessels.

arachnoid f., *apertura* mediana ventriculi quarti.

f. of Arnold, f. petrosum.

Bichat's f., *cisterna* venae magnae cerebri.

blind f. of frontal bone, f. cecum ossis frontalis.

blind f. of the tongue, f. cecum linguae.

Bochdalek's f., pleuroperitoneal *hiatus.*

Botallo's f., the orifice of communication between the two atria of the fetal heart. See also f. ovale.

f. bur'sae omenta'lis major'is, a f. produced by two folds of peritoneum that encroach upon and constrict the lesser sac of peritoneum; it forms a communication between the superior recess of the lesser sac which lies above it and the inferior recess below.

carotid f., the opening at each extremity of the carotid canal in the petrous portion of the temporal bone; the external carotid f. is on the inferior surface of the pyramid; the internal is at the apex.

cecal f. of frontal bone, f. cecum ossis frontalis.

cecal f. of the tongue, f. cecum linguae.

f. ce'cum lin'guae [NA], blind or cecal f. of the tongue; Morgagni's f. (1); a median pit on the dorsum of the posterior part of the tongue, from which the limbs of a V-shaped furrow run forward and outward; it is the site of origin of the thyroid gland in the embryo.

f. ce'cum medul'lae oblonga'tae, f. cecum posterius; Vicq d'Azyr's f.; small triangular depression at the lower boundary of the pons that marks the upper limit of the median fissure of the medulla oblongata.

f. ce'cum os'sis fronta'lis [NA], blind or cecal f. of the frontal bone; the f. formed by a notch at the lower end of the frontal crest and its articulation with the ethmoid bone.

f. ce'cum poste'rius, f. cecum medullae oblongatae.

conjugate f., a f. formed by the notches of two bones in apposition.

f. costotransversa'rium [NA], costotransverse f.; an opening between the neck of a rib and the transverse process of a vertebra, occupied by the costotransverse ligament.

costotransverse f., f. costotransversarium.

f. diaphrag'matis sel'lae, a hole in the center of the diaphragm of the sella giving passage to the infundibulum of the hypothalamus.

Duverney's f., f. epiploicum.

emissary sphenoidal f., f. venosum.

epiploic f., f. epiploicum.

f. epiplo'icum [NA], epiploic f.; Duverney's or Winslow's f.; aditus ad saccum peritonaei minorum; the passage, below and behind the portal fissure of the liver, connecting the two sacs of the peritoneum.

ethmoidal f., f. ethmoidale.

f. ethmoida'le [NA], ethmoidal f.; either of two foramina formed by grooves on either edge of the ethmoidal notch of the frontal bone, and completed by similar grooves on the ethmoid bone: **f. e. ante'rius,** located in an anterior position; **f. e. poste'rius,** located in a posterior position.

external acoustic f., *porus* acusticus externus.

external auditory f., *porus* acusticus externus.

Ferrein's f., *hiatus* canalis nervi petrosi majoris.

frontal f., f. frontale.

f. fronta'le [NA], frontal f.; an occasional small opening in the supraorbital margin of the frontal bone medial to the supraorbital foramen. See also *incisura* frontalis.

great f., f. magnum.

greater palatine f., f. palatinum majus.

Huschke's f., an opening in the floor of the bony meatus acusticus, usually closed in the adult.

Hyrtl's f., *porus* crotaphytico-buccinatorius.

incisive f., f. incisivum.

f. incisi'vum [NA], incisive f.; incisor f.; Stensen's f.; one of several (usually four) openings of the incisive canals into the incisive fossa.

incisor f., f. incisivum.

inferior dental f., f. mandibulae.

infraorbital f., f. infraorbitale.

f. infraorbita'le [NA], infraorbital f.; the external opening of the infraorbital canal, on the anterior surface of the body of the maxilla.

interatrial f. pri'mum, primary interatrial f.; ostium primum; f. subseptale; **(1)** in the embryonic heart, the temporary opening between right and left atria situated between the lower margin of the septum primum and the atrioventricular canal cushions; **(2)** in an adult heart, the abnormal persistence of the so-named communication which is normal in young embryos.

interatrial f. secun'dum, secondary interatrial f.; ostium secundum; a secondary opening appearing in the upper part of the septum primum in the sixth week of embryonic life, just prior to the closure of the interatrial f. primum.

internal acoustic f., *porus* acusticus internus.

internal auditory f., *porus* acusticus internus.

interventricular f., f. interventriculare.

f. interventricula're [NA], interventricular f.; Monro's f.; porta (2); the short, often slitlike passage that, on both the left and right side, connects the third brain ventricle (in the diencephalon) with the lateral ventricles (in the cerebral hemispheres); the passage is bounded anteriorly by the columna fornicis and posteriorly by the anterior pole of the thalamus.

intervertebral f., f. intervertebrale.

f. intervertebra'le [NA], intervertebral f.; one of a number of openings into the vertebral canal bounded by the pedicles of adjacent vertebrae above and below, the vertebral bodies anteriorly, and the articular processes posteriorly.

f. ischiad'icum [NA], sciatic f.; either of two foramina formed by the sacrospinous and sacrotuberous ligaments crossing the sciatic

notches of the hip bone: **f.i. ma'jus,** the greater f.i. and **f.i. mi'nus,** the lesser f.i.
jugular f., f. jugulare.
f. jugula're [NA], jugular f.; f. lacerum posterius; a passage between the petrous portion of the temporal bone and the jugular process of the occipital, sometimes divided into two by the intrajugular processes; it contains the internal jugular vein, inferior petrosal sinus, the glossopharyngeal, vagus, and accessory nerves, and meningeal branches of the ascending pharyngeal and occipital arteries.
f. of Key-Retzius, *apertura* lateralis ventriculi quarti.
lacerated f., f. lacerum.
f. lac'erum [NA], lacerated f.; f. lacerum medium; sphenotic f.; an irregular aperture, filled with cartilage in the living, located between the apex of the petrous part of the temporal bone, the body of the sphenoid, and the basilar part of the occipital bones. Several structures pass along the margins of the f. but no structures pass through.
f. lac'erum ante'rius, *fissura* orbitalis superior.
f. lac'erum me'dium, f. lacerum.
f. lac'erum poste'rius, f. jugulare.
Lannelongue's foramina, foramina venarum minimarum.
f. latera'lis ventric'uli quar'ti, *apertura* lateralis ventriculi quarti.
lesser palatine foramina, foramina palatina minora.
f. of Luschka, *apertura* lateralis ventriculi quarti.
Magendie's f., *apertura* mediana ventriculi quarti.
f. mag'num [NA], great f.; the large opening in the basal part of the occipital bone through which the spinal cord becomes continuous with the medulla oblongata.
malar f., f. zygomaticofaciale.
f. mandib'ulae [NA], mandibular f.; inferior dental f.; the opening into the mandibular canal on the medial surface of the ramus of the mandible.
mandibular f., f. mandibulae.
mastoid f., f. mastoideum.
f. mastoi'deum [NA], mastoid f.; an opening at the posterior portion of the mastoid process, transmitting the mastoid branch of the occipital artery to the dura and an emissary vein to the sigmoid sinus.
mental f., f. mentale.
f. menta'le [NA], mental f.; mental canal; the anterior opening of the mandibular canal on the body of the mandible lateral to and above the mental tubercle.
Monro's f., f. interventriculare.
Morgagni's f., **(1)** f. cecum linguae; **(2)** congenital defect in the fusion of sternal and costal elements of the diaphragmatic anlage that is the site of a parasternal hernia.
nasal f., vascular f. opening on the outer surface of each nasal bone.
foram'ina nervo'sa [NA], habenulae perforata; zona perforata; the perforations along the tympanic lip of the spiral lamina giving passage to the cochlear nerves.
f. nutric'ium [NA], nutrient f.; the external opening of the canalis nutricius in a bone.
nutrient f., f. nutricium.
obturator f., f. obturatum.
f. obtura'tum [NA], obturator f.; a large, oval or irregularly triangular aperture in the hip bone, the margins of which are formed by the pubis and the ischium; it is closed in the natural state by the obturator membrane, except for a small opening for the passage of the obturator vessels and nerve.
olfactory f., one of the openings in the cribriform plate of the ethmoid bone, transmitting the olfactory nerves.
optic f., *canalis* opticus.
f. op'ticum, *canalis* opticus.
f. ova'le, oval f., **(1)** [NA] in the fetal heart, the oval opening in septum secundum; the persistent part of septum primum acts as a valve for this interatrial communication during fetal life and postnatally becomes fused to septum secundum to close it; **(2)** [NA] a large oval opening in the greater wing of the sphenoid bone, transmitting the mandibular nerve and a small meningeal artery; **(3)** valvular incompetence of the f. ovale of the heart; a condition contrasting with probe patency of the f. ovale in that the valvula foraminis ovalis has abnormal perforations in it, or is of insufficient size to afford adequate valvular action at the f. ovale prenatally, or effect a complete closure postnatally.
foram'ina palati'na mino'ra [NA], lesser palatine foramina; anterior palatine foramina; openings on the hard palate of palatine canals passing vertically through the tuberosity of the palatine bone and transmitting the smaller palatine nerves and vessels.
f. palati'num ma'jus [NA], greater or posterior palatine f.; an opening in the posterolateral corner of the hard palate opposite the last molar tooth, marking the lower end of the pterygopalatine canal.
foram'ina papilla'ria re'nis [NA], papillary foramina of the kidney; numerous minute openings, the apertures of the collecting tubules, in the summit of each renal papilla.
papillary foramina of kidney, foramina papillaria renis.
parietal f., f. parietale.
f. parieta'le [NA], parietal f.; a f. in the parietal bone near the sagittal margin posteriorly; it transmits an emissary vein to the superior sagittal sinus.
petrosal f., f. petrosum.
f. petro'sum [NA], petrosal f.; canaliculus innominatus; f. of Arnold; an occasional opening in the greater wing of the sphenoid bone, between the f. spinosum and f. ovale, which transmits the lesser petrosal nerve.
posterior condyloid f., *canalis* condylaris.
posterior palatine f., f. palatinum majus.
postglenoid f., a small f. that is sometimes present in the temporal bone immediately in front of the external acoustic meatus.
primary interatrial f., interatrial f. primum.
f. proces'sus transver'si [NA], f. of transverse process; f. vertebroarterialis; transverse of vertebroarterial f.; f. transversarium; the f. in the transverse process of a cervical vertebra for the passage of the vertebral artery and vein and the sympathetic nerve plexus.
f. quadra'tum, f. venae cavae.
Retzius' f., *apertura* lateralis ventriculi quarti.
root f., f. apicis dentis.
f. rotun'dum [NA], round f.; an opening in the greater wing of the sphenoid bone, transmitting the maxillary nerve.
round f., f. rotundum.
sacral f., f. sacrale.
f. sacra'le [NA], sacral f.; one of the openings between the fused sacral vertebrae transmitting the sacral nerves. The anterior foramina, **foram'ina sacra'lia pelvi'na,** transmit ventral branches of the sacral nerves. The posterior foramina, **foram'ina sacra'lia dorsa'lia,** give passage to dorsal branches of the sacral nerves.
Scarpa's foramina, two openings in the line of the intermaxillary suture; the anterior f. transmits the left nasopalatine nerve, the posterior the right.
sciatic f., f. ischiadicum.
secondary interatrial f., interatrial f. secundum.
f. singula're [NA], solitary f.; a f. in the internal acoustic meatus, posterior to the area cochlearis, that transmits the nerves to the ampulla of the posterior semicircular duct.
foramina of the smallest veins, foramina venarum minimarum.
solitary f., f. singulare.
sphenopalatine f., f. sphenopalatinum.
f. sphenopalati'num [NA], sphenopalatine f.; the f. formed from the sphenopalatine notch of the palatine bone in articulation with the sphenoid bone; it transmits the sphenopalatine artery and accompanying nerves.
sphenotic f., f. lacerum.

f. spino'sum [NA], an opening in the great wing of the sphenoid bone, anterior to the spine, transmitting the middle meningeal artery.
Stensen's f., f. incisivum.
stylomastoid f., f. stylomastoideum.
f. stylomastoid'eum [NA], stylomastoid f.; an opening on the inferior surface of the petrous portion of the temporal bone, between the styloid and mastoid processes; it transmits the facial nerve and stylomastoid artery.
f. subsepta'le, interatrial f. primum.
supraorbital f., f. supraorbitale.
f. supraorbita'le [NA], supraorbital f.; a f. in the supraorbital margin of the frontal bone at the junction of the medial and intermediate thirds. See also *incisura* supraorbitalis.
thebesian foramina, foramina venarum minimarum.
thyroid f., (1) f. thyroideum; **(2)** an obsolete term for f. obturatum.
f. thyroid'eum [NA], thyroid f. (1); an opening occasionally existing in one or both of the plates of the thyroid cartilage.
f. transversa'rium, f. processus transversus.
transverse f., f. processus transversus.
f. of transverse process, f. processus transversus.
f. of vena cava, f. venae cavae.
f. ve'nae ca'vae [NA], f. of the vena cava; f. quadratum; an opening in the right lobe of the central tendon of the diaphragm which transmits the inferior vena cava and branches of the right phrenic nerve.
foram'ina vena'rum minima'rum [NA], foramina of the smallest veins; Lannelongue's, Vieussens', or thebesian foramina; a number of fossae in the wall of the right atrium, containing the openings of minute intramural veins.
f. veno'sum [NA], venous f.; Vesalius' f.; emissary sphenoidal f.; a minute inconstant f. in the greater wing of the sphenoid bone, anterior and medial to the f. ovale, transmitting a small emissary vein from the cavernous sinus.
vertebral f., f. vertebrale.
f. vertebra'le [NA], vertebral f.; the f. formed by the union of the vertebral arch with the body.
f. vertebroarteria'lis [NA], official alternate term for f. processus transversi.
vertebroarterial f., f. processus transversi.
Vesalius' f., f. venosum.
Vicq d'Azyr's f., f. cecum medullae oblongatae.
Vieussens' foramina, foramina venarum minimarum.
Weitbrecht's f., an opening in the articular capsule of the shoulder joint, communicating with the subtendinous bursa of the subscapularis muscle.
Winslow's f., f. epiploicum.
zygomaticofacial f., f. zygomaticofaciale.
f. zygomaticofacia'le [NA], zygomaticofacial f.; malar f.; the opening on the lateral surface of the zygomatic bone below the orbital margin that transmits the zygomaticofacial nerve.
zygomatico-orbital f., f. zygomatico-orbitale.
f. zygomat'ico-orbita'le [NA], zygomatico-orbital f.; the common opening on the orbital surface of the zygomatic bone of the canals transmitting the zygomaticofacial and zygomaticotemporal nerves; sometimes each of these canals has a separate opening on the orbital surface.
zygomaticotemporal f., f. zygomaticotemporale.
f. zygomat'icotempora'le [NA], zygomaticotemporal f.; the opening, on the temporal surface of the zygomatic bone, of the canal that gives passage to the zygomaticotemporal nerve.

foramina (fō-ram'i-nă). Plural of foramen.

Foraminifera (fō-ram-i-nif'er-ă, for'ă-mi-nif'er-ă) [L. *foramen,* aperture, + *fero,* to carry]. A subclass of Rhizopoda possessing anastomosing pseudopodia; these form a network around the cell which usually develops into a complex calcareous shell; an important component of the ocean bottom and of rockbeds overlying oil deposits.

foraminiferous (fō-ram-i-nif'er-ŭs, fōr'ă-mi-nif'er-ŭs). **1.** Possessing openings or foramina. **2.** Relating to the Foraminifera.

foraminotomy (fōr'am-i-not'ō-mē) [L. *foramen,* aperture, + G. *tomē,* a cutting]. An operation upon an aperture, usually to open it, *e.g.,* surgical enlargement of the intervertebral foramen.

foraminulum, pl. **foraminula** (fōr'ă-min'yū-lŭm, yū-lă) [Mod. L. dim. of *foramen*]. A very minute foramen.

Forbes, A.P. See F.-Albright *syndrome.*

Forbes, Gilbert B., U.S. pediatrician, *1915. See F. *disease.*

Forbes, Thomas R. See Hooker-F. *test.*

force (F) (fōrs) [L. *fortis,* strong]. Power; strength; that which tends to produce motion in a body.
animal f., muscular power.
chewing f., the degree of f. applied by the muscles of mastication during the mastication of food. See also masticatory f.
dynamic f., energy.
electromotive f. (EMF), the f. (measured in volts) that causes the flow of electricity from one point to another.
G f., inertial f. produced by accelerations or gravity, expressed in gravitational units; one G is equal to the pull of gravity at the earth's surface at sea level and 45° latitude (32.2 ft./sec^2; 980.6 cm/sec^2). See also *g.*
London f.'s, interactions between atoms caused by dipoles created by electron distribution; the same as Van der Waals' f.'s.
f. of mastication, masticatory f.; biting strength; the motive f. created by the dynamic action of the muscles during the physiologic act of mastication.
masticatory f., f. of mastication.
nerve f., nervous f., obsolete terms denoting the property of nerve tissue to conduct stimuli.
occlusal f., the result of muscular f. applied on opposing teeth.
psychic f., psychic *energy.*
reciprocal f.'s, in dentistry, f.'s whereby the resistance of one or more teeth is utilized to move one or more opposing teeth.
reserve f., the energy residing in the organism or any of its parts above that required for its normal functioning.
van der Waals' f.'s, first postulated by van der Waals in 1873 to explain deviations from ideal gas behavior seen in real gases; the attractive f.'s between atoms or molecules other than electrostatic (ionic), covalent (sharing of electrons), or hydrogen bonding (sharing a proton); generally ascribed to dipolar and dispersion effects, π-electrons, etc.; these relatively nondescript f.'s contribute to the mutual attraction of organic molecules.
vital f., see vitalism.

forceps (fōr'seps) [L. a pair of tongs]. **1.** An instrument for seizing a structure, and making compression or traction. *Cf.* clamp. **2** [NA]. Bands of white fibers in the brain, f. major and f. minor.
Adson f., a small thumb f. with two teeth on one tip and one tooth on the other.
alligator f., a long f. with a small hinged jaw on the end.
Allis f., a straight grasping f. with serrated jaws, used to forcibly grasp or retract tissues or structures.
f. anterior, f. minor.
Arruga's f., f. for the intracapsular extraction of a cataract.
arterial f., a locking f. with sloping blades for grasping the end of a blood vessel until a ligature is applied.
axis-traction f., obstetrical f. provided with a second handle so attached that traction can be made in the line in which the head must move in the axis of the pelvis.
Barton's f., an obstetrical f. with one fixed curved blade and a hinged anterior blade for application to a high transverse head.
bone f., a strong f. used for seizing or removing fragments of bone.

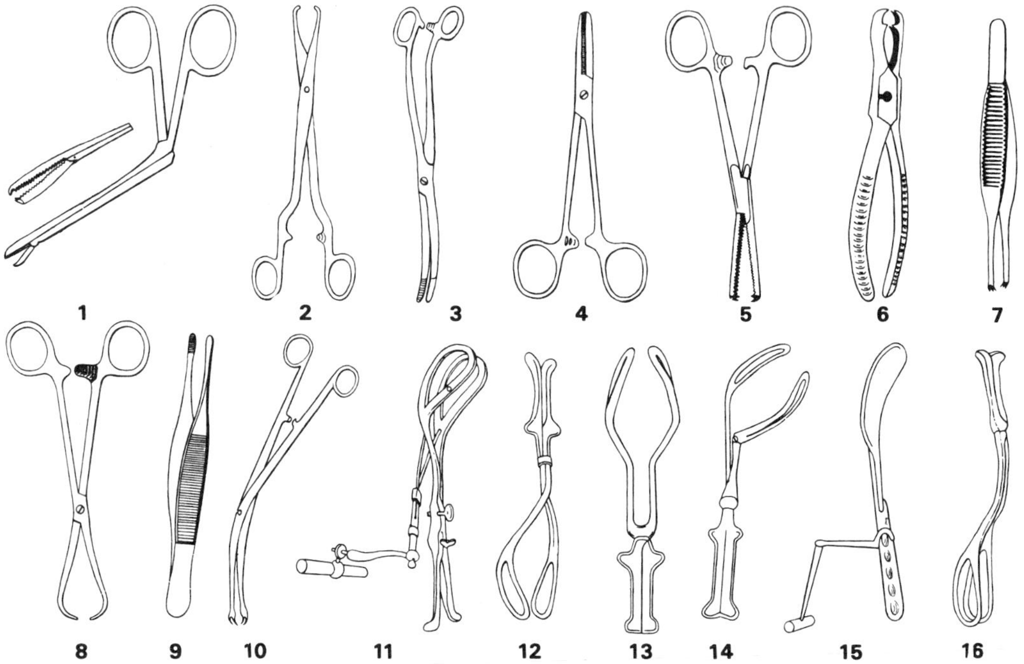

Forceps
Some types of forceps: *1,* alligator; *2,* bullet; *3,* dressing; *4,* hemostatic; *5,* Kocher's; *6,* lion-jaw bone-holding; *7,* mouse-tooth; *8,* tenaculum; *9,* thumb; *10,* vulsella; *11,* Tarnier's axis-traction; *12,* Kjelland's; *13,* Simpson's; *14,* Barton's; *15,* Tucker-McLean axis-traction; *16,* Piper's.

Brown-Adson f., an Adson f. with about 16 delicate teeth on each tip.
bulldog f., a f. for occluding a blood vessel.
bullet f., a f. with thin curved blades with serrated grasping surfaces, for extracting a bullet from tissues.
capsule f., f. used for removing the capsule of the lens in extracapsular extraction of cataract.
Chamberlen f., the original obstetrical f., without a curvature.
clamp f., rubber dam clamp f.; a f. with pronged jaws designed to engage the jaws of a rubber dam clamp so that they may be separated to pass over the widest buccolingual contour of a tooth.
clip f., a small f. with spring catch to hold a bleeding vessel.
cup biopsy f., a slender flexible f. with movable cup-shaped jaws, used to obtain biopsy specimens by introduction through a specially designed endoscope.
cutting f., labitome.
dental f., extracting f.; f. used to luxate teeth and remove them from the alveolus.
dressing f., a f. for general use in dressing wounds, removing fragments of necrosed tissue, small foreign bodies, etc.
Evans f., a thumb f. with points designed to resemble a needle holder, used to grasp curved needles during various suture procedures.
extracting f., dental f.
Graefe f., a small thumb f. with one horizontal row of six or eight delicate teeth across each tip.
hemostatic f., a f. with a catch for locking the blades, used for seizing the end of a blood vessel to control hemorrhage.
jeweller's f., a small thumb f. with very fine pointed blades, used to grasp tissues in microsurgical procedures.
Kjelland's f., an obstetrical f. having a sliding lock, and little pelvic curve.
Lahey f., thyroid f. used to deliver the uterus in vaginohysterectomy.
Laplace's f., a f. for approximating intestine during surgical anastomosis.
Levret's f., a modification of the Chamberlen f., curved to correspond to the curve of the parturient passage.
lion-jaw bone-holding f., a sturdy f. with strong sharp teeth in the jaws, used for holding bone fragments.
Löwenberg's f., f. with short curved blades ending in rounded grasping extremities devised for the removal of adenoid growths in the nasopharynx.
f. ma'jor [NA], f. posterior; pars occipitalis corporis callosi; occipital radiation of the corpus callosum; that part of the fiber radiation of the corpus callosum which bends sharply backward into the occipital lobe of the cerebrum.
f. mi'nor [NA], f. anterior; pars frontalis corporis callosi; frontal radiation of the corpus callosum; that part of the fiber radiation of the corpus callosum which bends forward toward the frontal pole of the cerebrum.
mosquito f., mosquito *clamp.*
mouse-tooth f., a f. with one or two fine points at the tip of each blade, fitting into hollows between the points on the opposite blade.
needle f., needle-holder.
nonfenestrated f., obstetrical f. without openings in the blades, thus facilitating rotation of the head.
obstetrical f., f. used for grasping and applying traction to or for rotation of the fetal head; the blades are introduced separately into the genital canal, permitting the fetal head to be grasped firmly but with minimal compression, and then are articulated after being placed in correct position.
O'Hara f., two slender clamp f.'s held together by a serrefine, used in intestinal anastomosis.
Piper's f., obstetrical f. used to facilitate delivery of the head in breech presentation.

f. poste'rior, f. major.
Randall stone f., a f. with variably curved slender blades and serrated jaws, used to extract calculi from the renal pelvis or calices.
rubber dam clamp f., clamp f.
Simpson's f., an obstetrical f.
speculum f., a tubular f. for use through a speculum.
Tarnier's f., a type of axis-traction f.
tenaculum f., a f. with jaws armed each with a sharp, straight hook like a tenaculum.
thumb f., a spring f. used by compression with thumb and forefinger.
tubular f., a long slender f. intended for use through a cannula or other tubular instrument.
Tucker-McLean f., a type of axis-traction f.
vulsella f., vulsellum f., volsella; vulsella; vulsellum; a f. with hooks at the tip of each blade.
Willett's f., Willett's clamp; a traction f. used to treat placenta previa by pulling the fetal head down against the placenta.

Forchheimer, Frederick, U.S. physician, 1853–1913. See F.'s *sign.*

forcipate (fōr'si-pāt). Shaped like a forceps.

forcipressure (fōr'si-presh-ŭr). A method of arresting hemorrhage by compressing a blood vessel with forceps.

Fordyce, John A., U.S. dermatologist, 1858–1925. See F.'s *angiokeratoma, disease, granules, spots;* Fox-F. *disease.*

forearm (fōr'arm). Antebrachium; the segment of the superior limb between the elbow and the wrist.

forebrain (fōr'brān). Prosencephalon.

foreconscious (fōr'kon-shŭs). Denoting memories, not at present in the consciousness, which can be evoked from time to time, or an unconscious mental process which becomes conscious only on the fulfillment of certain conditions. *Cf.* preconscious.

forefinger (fōr'fing'ger). Index (1).

forefoot (fōr'fut). A front foot of a quadruped.

foregut (fōr'gŭt). Headgut; the cephalic portion of the primitive digestive tube in the embryo. From its endoderm arises the epithelial lining (of the pharynx, trachea, lungs, esophagus, and stomach), the first part and cranial half of the second part of the duodenum, and the parenchyma of the liver and pancreas.

forehead (fōr'ed, fōr'hed). Frons.
olympian f., the abnormally prominent, high, and broad f. in hereditary syphilis.

forekidney (fōr'kid-nē). Pronephros.

Forel, Auguste H., Swiss neurologist, 1848–1931. See F.'s *decussation, field;* tegmental *fields* of F.

foremilk (fōr'milk). Colostrum.

forensic (fō-ren'sik) [L. *forensis,* of a forum]. Pertaining or applicable to legal proceedings.

foreplay (fōr'plā). Stimulative sexual activity preceding sexual intercourse.

forepleasure (fōr'plezh'er, plā'zher). Sexual pleasure resulting from the foreplay that precedes the genital-orgastic pleasure in sexual intercourse.

foreskin (fōr'skin). Preputium.

forestomach (fōr'stŭm'ŭk). *Antrum* cardiacum.

forewaters (fōr'wah-terz). Colloquialism for the bulging fluid-filled amniotic membrane presenting in front of the fetal head.

forget'ting. Being unable to retrieve or recall information that was once registered, learned, and stored in short- or long-term memory.

fork (fōrk). **1.** A pronged instrument used for holding or lifting. **2.** An instrument resembling a f. in that it has tines or prongs.
bite f., face-bow f.
face-bow f., bite f.; that part of the face-bow assemblage used to attach the maxillary trial base to the face-bow proper.
tuning f., a steel or magnesium instrument roughly resembling a two-pronged f., the vibrations of the prongs of which, when struck, give a musical note; used to test the hearing, especially bone conduction.

form (fōrm) [L. *forma*]. Shape; structure; mold.
accolé f.'s (ak-ōlā'), appliqué f.'s.
appliqué f.'s (ap-li-kā'), accolé f.'s; a term applied to the manner in which the ring stage of *Plasmodium falciparum* parasitizes the marginal portion of erythrocytes.
arch f., the shape and contour of the dental arch, or of an orthodontic wire formed to the shape of that arch.
boat f., the less stable of two conformations assumed by 6-membered cyclic sugars (pyranoses), as opposed to chair f. See also Haworth conformational formulas of cyclic *sugars.*
cavity preparation f., the configuration or shape of a cavity preparation.
chair f., the more stable of two conformations assumed by 6-membered cyclic sugars (*e.g.,* the pyranoses), as opposed to boat f. See also Haworth conformational formulas of cylic *sugars.*
convenience f., the changes needed outside the basic outline f. to enable proper instrumentation for the cavity preparation and insertion of a dental restoration.
extension f., the extension of the cavity preparation outline f. to include areas of incipient carious lesions; this extension provides a dental restoration with margins that are self-cleansing or easily cleaned.
face f., **(1)** the outline f. of the face; **(2)** the outline f. of the face from an anterior view.
half-chair f., see Haworth conformational formulas of cyclic *sugars.*
involution f., an irregular or atypical bacterial cell produced as a result of exposure to unfavorable conditions.
L f., see L-phase *variants.*
occlusal f., occlusal pattern; the f. of the occlusal surface of a tooth or a row of teeth.
outline f., the shape of the area of the tooth surface included within the cavosurface margins of the cavity preparation of a dental restoration.
posterior tooth f., the distinguishing contours of the occlusal surface of the various posterior teeth.
replicative f. (RF), the altered, double-stranded f. to which single-stranded coliphage DNA is converted after infection of a susceptible bacterium, formation of the complementary ("minus") strand being mediated by enzymes that were present in the bacterium before entrance of the viral ("plus") strand.
resistance f., the shape given to a cavity preparation that enables the dental restoration to withstand masticatory forces.
retention f., the shape of a cavity preparation that prevents displacement of the dental restoration by lateral or tipping forces as well as masticatory forces.
sickle f., malarial *crescent.*
skew f., see Haworth conformational formulas of cyclic *sugars.*
tooth f., the characteristics of the curves, lines, angles, and contours of various teeth which permit their identification and differentiation.
twist f., see Haworth conformational formulas of cyclic *sugars.*
wave f., waveshape; the f. of a pulse; *e.g.,* of the pacemaker pulse as demonstrated on the oscilloscope under a specified load.
wax f., wax *pattern.*

-form [L. *-formis*]. Suffix denoting in the form or shape of; equivalent to -oid.

Formad, Henry F., U.S. physician, 1847–1892. See F.'s *kidney.*

formaldehyde (fōr-mal'dĕ-hīd) [form(ic) + aldehyde]. Formic aldehyde; methyl aldehyde; a pungent gas, H-CHO; used as an antiseptic, disinfectant, and histologic fixative.

Formalin (fŏr'mă-lin). Formol; a 37% aqueous solution of formaldehyde.

formalinize (fŏr-mă-li-nīz). To add formalin solution to inactivate vaccines without destroying their immunizing power.

formamidase (fŏr-mam'i-dās) [EC 3.5.1.9]. Formylase; kynurenine formamidase; an enzyme catalyzing the hydrolysis of formylkynurenine to kynurenine and formate, a reaction of significance in tryptophan catabolism.

formate (fōr'māt). A salt or ester of formic acid; *i.e.*, the monovalent radical H-COO–or the anion $HCOO^-$.

formatio, pl. formationes (fōr-mā'shē-ō, -ō'nēz) [L. fr. *formo*, pp. *-atus*, to form] [NA]. A formation; a structure of definite shape or cellular arrangement.

f. hippocampa'lis, hippocampal formation. See hippocampus.

f. reticula'ris [NA], reticular formation; reticular substance (2); substantia reticularis (2); a massive but vaguely delimited neural apparatus composed of closely intermingled gray and white matter and extending throughout the central core of the brainstem into the diencephalon; the term refers to the large neuronal population of the brainstem that do not compose motoneuronal cell groups or cell groups forming part of specific sensory conduction systems; its neurons generally have long dendrites and heterogeneous afferent connections, the reason why the formation is often called "nonspecific;" the f. reticularis has complex, largely polysynaptic ascending and descending connections that play a role in the central control of autonomic (respiration, blood pressure, thermoregulation, etc.) and endocrine functions, as well as in bodily posture, skeletomuscular reflex activity, and general behavioral states such as alertness and sleep. See also reticular activating *system.*

formation (fōr-mā'shŭn). **1.** Formatio. **2.** That which is formed. **3.** The act of giving form and shape.

concept f., in psychology, the learning to conceive and respond in terms of abstract ideas based upon an action or object.

personality f., the life history associated with the development of individual patterns and of one's individuality.

reaction f., in psychoanalysis, a postulated defense mechanism in which attitudes and behaviors that are adopted are the opposites of that which the individual would ordinarily be expected to express.

reticular f., *formatio* reticularis.

rouleaux f. [Fr. pl. of *rouleau,* a roll], pseudoagglutination (2); the arrangement of red blood cells in fluid blood (or in diluted suspensions) with their biconcave surfaces in apposition, thereby forming groups that resemble stacks of coins.

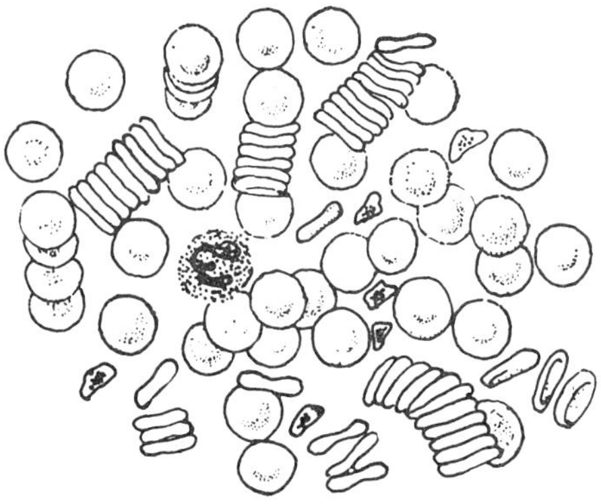

Red Blood Cells in Rouleaux Formation

symptom f., symptom *substitution.*

formationes (fōr-mā'shē-ō'nēz). Plural of formatio.

formazan (fōr'mă-zan). A water-insoluble colored compound of the general structure, RNH—N=CR'—N=NR", formed by reduction of a tetrazolium salt in the histochemical demonstration of oxidative enzymes; the R's are usually phenyl groups; examples include neotetrazolium, blue tetrazolium, and nitro blue tetrazolium.

formboard (fōrm'bōrd). A board containing cut-outs in various shapes, into which blocks of corresponding shape are to be fitted; an intelligence test.

forme fruste, pl. **formes frustes** (fōrm' frūst') [Fr. from L. *forma,* form; *frustra,* without effect]. A partial or arrested form of disease.

formic (fōr'mik) [L. *formica,* ant]. **1.** Pertaining to f. acid. **2.** Relating to ants.

formic acid. H-COOH; the smallest carboxylic acid; a strong caustic, used as an astringent and counterirritant.

formic aldehyde. Formaldehyde.

formication (fōr-mi-kā'shŭn) [L. *formica,* ant]. A form of paresthesia or tactile hallucination in which one feels a sensation as of small insects creeping under the skin; usually seen in substance-induced organic mental syndromes.

formiminoglutamic acid (FIGLU) (fōr-mim'i-nō-glū-tam'ik). $HN{=}CH\text{-}NH\text{-}CH(COOH)CH_2CH_2COOH$; an intermediate metabolite in histidine catabolism in the conversion of histidine to glutamic acid, with the formimino group being transferred to tetrahydrofolic acid, it may appear in the urine of patients with folic acid or vitamin B_{12} deficiency, or liver disease.

formocresol (fōr-mō-krē'sol). An aqueous solution containing cresol, formaldehyde, and glycerine, used in vital primary teeth needing coronal pulpotomy.

formol (fōr'mol). Formalin.

formosulfathiazole (fōr'mō-sŭl-fă-thī'ă-zol). N^1-(2-Thiazolyl)sulfanilamide condensation product with formaldehyde; an antimicrobial agent for treatment of intestinal infections.

FORMULA

formula, pl. **formulas, formulae** (fōr'myū-lă, -lăz, -lē) [L. dim. of *forma,* form]. **1.** A recipe or prescription containing directions for the compounding of a medicinal preparation. **2.** In chemistry, a symbol or collection of symbols expressing the number of atoms of the element or elements forming one molecule of a substance, together with, on occasion, information concerning the arrangement of the atoms within the molecule, their electronic structure, their charge, the nature of the bonds within the molecule, etc. **3.** An expression by symbols and numbers of the normal order or arrangement of parts or structures.

Arneth f., the normal, approximate ratio of polymorphonuclear neutrophils, based on the number of lobes in the nuclei, as follows: 1 lobe, 5%; 2 lobes, 35%; 3 lobes, 41%; 4 lobes, 17%; 5 lobes, 2%.

Bazett's f., a f. for correcting the observed Q-T interval in the electrocardiogram for cardiac rate: corrected Q-T = Q-T sec/ $\sqrt{\text{R-R sec.}}$

Bernhardt's f., a f. used to calculate the ideal weight, in kilograms, for an adult; it is the height in centimeters times the chest circumference in centimeters divided by 240.

Black's f., a translation of Pignet's f. into British measurements: $F = (W + C) - H$; F is the empirical factor, W is the weight in pounds, C the chest girth in inches at full inspiration, and H the height in inches; a man is classed as very strong when F is over 120, strong between 110 and 120, good 100 to 110, fair 90 to 100, weak 80 to 90, very weak under 80.

Broca's f., a fully developed man (30 years old) should weigh as many kilograms as he is centimeters in height over and above 1 meter.
chemical f., a statement of the structure of a molecule expressed in chemical symbols.
Christison's f., Häser's f.
constitutional f., structural f.
Demoivre's f., an obsolete f. for calculating life expectancy.
dental f., a statement in tabular form of the number of each kind of teeth in the jaw; the dental f. for man is, for the deciduous teeth:

$$\text{i.}\ \frac{2\text{–}2}{2\text{–}2},\ \text{c.}\ \frac{1\text{–}1}{1\text{–}1},\ \text{m.}\ \frac{2\text{–}2}{2\text{–}2} = 20$$

for the permanent teeth:

$$\text{i.}\ \frac{2\text{–}2}{2\text{–}2},\ \text{c.}\ \frac{1\text{–}1}{1\text{–}1},\ \text{bic.}\ \frac{2\text{–}2}{2\text{–}2},\ \text{m.}\ \frac{3\text{–}3}{3\text{–}3} = 32.$$

Dreyer's f., an obsolete f. indicating relationship between vital capacity and body surface area.
DuBois' f., a f. for predicting a man's surface area from weight and height: $A = 71.84W^{0.425}H^{0.725}$, where A = surface area in cm^2, W = weight in kg, and H = height in cm.
electrical f., a graphic representation by means of symbols of the reaction of a muscle to an electrical stimulus.
empirical f., molecular f.; in chemistry, a f. indicating the kind and number of atoms in the molecules of a substance, or its composition, but not the relation of the atoms to each other or the intimate structure of the molecule.
Fischer's projection f.'s, see under sugars.
Flesch f., a method of determining the difficulty of a written passage by a formulation that provides an estimate of how many people in the U.S. would be able to read and understand the passage; used in determining patient comprehension of hospital consent forms.
Florschütz' f., the correct relation of height to the abdominal circumference: L: $(2B - L)$, L representing the individual's height, and B the circumference of the abdomen; the normal value so determined would be 5, and any below that would indicate obesity.
Gorlin f., a f. for calculating the area of the orifice of a cardiac valve, based on flow across the valve and the mean pressures in the chambers on either side of the valve.
graphic f., structural f.
Häser's f., Christison's f.; Trapp's f.; Trapp-Häser f.; a f. to determine the number of grams of urinary solids per liter, obtained by multiplying 2.33 by the last two figures of the specific gravity of the urine.
Haworth perspective and conformational f.'s, see under sugars.
Long's f., Long's coefficient; a f. for estimating from the specific gravity of a specimen of urine the approximate amount of solids in grams per liter; the last two figures of the value for specific gravity are multiplied by 2.6.
Mall's f., the age (in days) of an embryo calculated by the square root of its length (measured from vertex to breech) in millimeters multiplied by 100.
Meeh f., Meeh-DuBois f.
Meeh-Dubois f., Meeh f.; a f. for predicting surface area, assuming that it is proportional to the $^2/_3$ power of the body weight.
molecular f., empirical f.
official f., a f. contained in the Pharmacopeia or the National Formulary.
Pignet's f., see Black's f.
Poisson-Pearson f., a f. to determine the statistical error in calculating the endemic index of malaria: let N = total number of children under 15 years in a locality; n = total number examined for the spleen-rate; x = number found with enlarged spleen; $(x/n)\,100$ = spleen-rate; $e\%$ = percentage of error; then the percentage error will be, by this f.:

$$e\% = \frac{200}{n}\sqrt{\frac{2x(n-x)}{n}}\ \sqrt{1 - \frac{n-1}{N-1}}.$$

Ranke's f., A = grams of albumin per liter of a serous fluid: then, A = (sp. gr. − 1000) × 0.52 − 5.406.
rational f., in chemistry, a f. that indicates the constitution as well as the composition of a substance.
Reuss' f., a means of estimating the approximate amount of albumin in a transudate or exudate; $^3/_8$ (sp. gr. − 1.000) − 2.8 results in a value that is a practicable indication of the percentage of albumin in the fluid.
Runeberg's f., a f. for estimating the percentage of albumin in a serous fluid, similar to Reuss' f. except that, instead of 2.8, 2.73 is subtracted in the instance of a transudate, and 2.88 in that of an inflammatory exudate.
spatial f., stereochemical f.
stereochemical f., spatial f.; a chemical f. in which the arrangement of the atoms or atomic groupings in space are indicated.
structural f., constitutional or graphic f.; a f. in which the connections of the atoms and groups of atoms, as well as their kind and number, are indicated.
Trapp's f., Trapp-Häser f., Häser's f.
Van Slyke's f., standard urea *clearance.*
vertebral f., a f. indicating the number of vertebrae in each segment of the spinal column; for man it is C. 7, T. 12, L. 5, S. 5, Co. 4 = 33, the letters standing for cervical, thoracic, lumbar, sacral, and coccygeal.

formulary (fōr′myū-lā-rē). A collection of formulas for the compounding of medicinal preparations. See *National Formulary; Pharmacopeia.*
hospital f., a continually revised compilation of pharmaceuticals, plus important ancillary information, that reflects the current clinical judgment of the institution's medical staff.

formyl (fōr′mil). The radical, H-CO–.
active f., the f. group taking part in transformylation reactions with a folic acid derivative in the role of carrier.

formylase (fōr′mi-lās). Formamidase.

formylkynurenine (fōr′mil-ki-nūr′ĕ-nēn). The product of the oxidative cleavage of the indole ring in tryptophan; the intermediate first formed in tryptophan catabolism.

formylmethionine (fōr′mil-me-thī′ō-nēn). Methionine acylated on the NH_2 group by a formyl (–CHO) group. See also initiating *codon.*

Forney, William R., U.S. pediatrician, *1931. See F.'s *syndrome.*

fornicate (fōr′ni-kāt). **1** [L. *fornicatus,* arched, fr. *fornix,* vault, arch]. Vaulted or arched; resembling a fornix. **2** [see fornication]. To commit fornication.

fornication (fōr-ni-kā′shŭn) [L. *fornicatio,* an arched or vaulted basement (brothel)]. Sexual intercourse, especially between unmarried partners.

fornices (fōr′ni-sēz). Plural of fornix.

fornix, gen. **fornicis,** pl. **fornices** (fōr′niks, -ni-sis, -ni-sēz) [L. arch, vault]. **1** [NA]. In general, an arch-shaped structure; often the arch-shaped roof (or roof portion) of an anatomical space. **2** [NA]. Trigonum cerebrale; the compact, white fiber bundle by which the hippocampus of each cerebral hemisphere projects to the contralateral hippocampus and to the septum, anterior nucleus of the thalamus, and mamillary body. Arising from pyramidal cells of Ammon's horn, the fibers of the f. form the alveus hippocampi and the fimbria hippocampi, and in their further course compose, sequentially, the crus fornicis, corpus fornicis, commissura fornicis, and columna fornicis; the f. fibers to the septum issue from the upper part of the columna fornicis, passing in part anterior to the commissura anterior as the precommissural f., while all others follow the compact postcommissural f. bundle to the anterior thalamic nucleus and corpus mamillare.

f. conjuncti'vae [NA], conjunctival cul-de-sac; retrotarsal fold; the space formed by the junction of the bulbar and palpebral portions of the conjunctiva, that of the upper lid being the **f. c. supe'rior** and that of the lower lid the **f. c. infe'rior.**

f. pharyn'gis [NA], vault of the pharynx; the upper end of the nasopharynx where the pharyngeal mucosa is firmly applied to the body of the sphenoid bone.

f. sac'ci lacrima'lis [NA], fornix of the lacrimal sac; the upper, blind end of the lacrimal sac that extends above the openings of the lacrimal canaliculi.

transverse f., *commissura* fornicis.

f. u'teri, f. vaginae.

f. vagi'nae [NA], f. uteri; the recess at the vault of the vagina; it is divided into a pars anterior, pars posterior, and pars lateralis with respect to its relation to the cervix of the uterus.

Forrestier, J., 20th century rheumatologist. See F.'s *disease.*

Forssman, Hans, Swedish physician, *1912. See Börjeson-F.-Lehmann *syndrome.*

Forssman, John, Swedish bacteriologist and pathologist, 1868–1947. See F. *antibody, antigen, reaction,* antigen-antibody *reaction.*

Förster, Richard, German ophthalmologist, 1825–1902. See F.'s *uveitis.*

foscarnet (fos-kar'net). Trisodium phosphonoformate; a pyrophosphate analogue used to treat herpes simplex infections.

Fosdick, Leonard S., U.S. chemist, *1903. See F.-Hansen-Epple *test.*

Foshay, Lee, U.S. bacteriologist, 1896–1961. See F. *test.*

FOSSA

fossa, gen. and pl. **fossae** (fos'ă, fos'ē) [L. a trench or ditch] [NA]. A depression usually more or less longitudinal in shape below the level of the surface of a part.

acetabular f., f. acetabuli.

f. acetab'uli [NA], acetabular f.; a depressed area in the floor of the acetabulum above the acetabular notch.

adipose fossae, subcutaneous spaces containing accumulations of fat in the mamma.

amygdaloid f., f. tonsillaris.

anconal f., f. olecrani.

anterior cranial f., f. cranii anterior.

f. anthel'icis [NA], f. of the anthelix; periconchal sulcus; the depression on the medial surface of the auricle that corresponds to the anthelix.

f. of anthelix, f. anthelicis.

articular f. of temporal bone, f. mandibularis.

f. axilla'ris [NA], axillary f. or space; axilla; axil; ala (2); axillary cavity; armpit; the space below the shoulder joint, bounded by the pectoralis major anteriorly, the latissimus dorsi posteriorly, the serratus anterior medially, and the humerus laterally; it has a superior opening between the clavicle, scapula, and first rib, and an inferior opening covered by the axillary fascia; it contains the axillary artery and vein, the infraclavicular part of the brachial plexus, lymph nodes and vessels, and areolar tissue.

axillary f., f. axillaris.

Bichat's f., f. pterygopalatina.

Biesiadecki's f., iliacosubfascial f.

Broesike's f., parajejunal f.

f. cani'na [NA], canine f.; a depression on the anterior surface of the maxilla below the infraorbital foramen and on the lateral side of the canine eminence.

canine f., f. canina.

f. carot'ica, *trigonum* caroticum.

Claudius' f., f. ovarica.

condylar f., f. condylaris.

f. condyla'ris [NA], condylar f.; a depression behind the condyle of the occipital bone in which the posterior margin of the superior facet of the atlas lies in extension.

coronoid f., f. coronoidea.

f. coronoi'dea [NA], coronoid f.; a hollow on the anterior surface of the distal end of the humerus, just above the trochlea, in which the coronoid process of the ulna rests when the elbow is flexed.

f. cra'nii ante'rior [NA], anterior cranial f.; anterior cranial base; the portion of the internal base of the skull, anterior to the lesser wings of the sphenoid bone, in which the frontal lobes of the brain rest.

f. cra'nii me'dia [NA], middle cranial f.; the internal base of the skull between the lesser wings of the sphenoid bone and the ridge of the petrous part of the temporal bones, where the temporal lobes of the brain and the hypophysis rest.

f. cra'nii poste'rior [NA], posterior cranial f.; the internal base of the skull between the ridge of the petrous part of the temporal bones and the grooves for the transverse sinuses, where the cerebellum, pons, and medulla oblongata rest.

crural f., *fovea* femoralis.

Cruveilhier's f., f. scaphoidea.

cubital f., f. cubitalis.

f. cubita'lis [NA], cubital f.; chelidon; antecubital space; the f. in front of the elbow.

digastric f., f. digastrica.

f. digas'trica [NA], digastric f.; a hollow on the posterior surface of the base of the mandible, on either side of the median plane, giving attachment to the anterior belly of the digastric muscle.

digital f., **(1)** f. trochanteria; **(2)** f. malleoli lateralis.

f. duc'tus veno'si, a wide groove located posteriorly on the undersurface of the fetal liver between the caudate and the left lobes; it lodges the ductus venosus.

duodenal fossae, see *recessus* duodenalis inferior and *recessus* duodenalis superior.

duodenojejunal f., *recessus* duodenalis superior.

epigastric f., f. epigastrica; scrobiculus cordis; pit of the stomach; the slight depression in the midline just inferior to the xiphoid process of the sternum.

f. epigas'trica, epigastric f.

femoral f., *fovea* femoralis.

floccular f., f. subarcuata.

gallbladder f., f. vesicae felleae.

Gerdy's hyoid f., *trigonum* caroticum.

f. glan'dulae lacrima'lis [NA], f. of the lacrimal gland; lacrimal f.; a hollow in the orbital plate of the frontal bone, formed by the overhanging margin and zygomatic process, lodging the lacrimal gland.

glenoid f., **(1)** *cavitas* glenoidalis; **(2)** f. mandibularis.

greater supraclavicular f., *trigonum* omoclaviculare.

Gruber-Landzert f., *recessus* duodenalis inferior.

f. of helix, scapha (2).

hyaloid f., f. hyaloidea.

f. hyaloi'dea [NA], hyaloid f.; lenticular f.; patellar f. of vitreous; a depression on the anterior surface of the vitreous body in which lies the lens.

hypophysial f., f. hypophysialis.

f. hypophysia'lis [NA], hypophysial f.; pituitary f.; f. of the sphenoid bone housing the pituitary gland.
iliac f., f. iliaca.
f. ilia'ca [NA], iliac f.; the smooth inner surface of the ilium above the arcuate line, giving attachment to the iliacus muscle.
iliacosubfascial f., f. iliacosubfascialis; Biesiadecki's f.; a peritoneal recess between the psoas muscle and the crest of the ilium.
f. iliacosubfascia'lis, iliacosubfascial f.
iliopectineal f., a hollow between the iliopsoas and pectineus muscles in the center of the femoral (Scarpa's) triangle, lodging the femoral vessels and nerve.
f. incisi'va [NA], incisive fossa; the depression in the midline of the bony palate behind the central incisors into which the incisive canals open.
incisive f., f. incisiva.
incudal f., f. incudis.
f. in'cudis [NA], incudal f.; f. for the incus; a small depression in the lower and posterior part of the epitympanic recess that lodges the short limb of the incus.
f. for incus, f. incudis.
inferior duodenal f., *recessus* duodenalis inferior.
infraclavicular f., f. infraclavicularis.
f. infraclavicula'ris [NA], infraclavicular f. or triangle; Mohrenheim's f. or space; regio infraclavicularis; deltoideopectoral triangle or trigone; trigonum deltoideopectorale; a triangular depression bounded by the clavicle and the adjacent borders of the deltoid and pectoralis major muscles.
infraduodenal f., *recessus* retroduodenalis.
f. infraspina'ta [NA], infraspinous f.; the hollow on the dorsal aspect of the scapula inferior to the spine, giving attachment chiefly to the infraspinatus muscle.
infraspinous f., f. infraspinata.
infratemporal f., f. infratemporalis.
f. infratempora'lis [NA], infratemporal f.; zygomatic f.; the cavity on the side of the skull bounded laterally by the zygomatic arch and ramus of the mandible, medially by the lateral pterygoid plate, anteriorly by the zygomatic process of the maxilla, posteriorly by the articular eminence of the temporal bone and the posterior border of the lateral pterygoid plate, and above by the squama of the temporal bone and the infratemporal crest on the greater wing of the sphenoid bone.
inguinal f., see f. inguinalis lateralis and f. inguinalis medialis.
f. inguina'lis latera'lis [NA], lateral inguinal f.; a depression on the peritoneal surface of the anterior abdominal wall lateral to the ridge formed by the inferior epigastric artery; it corresponds to the position of the deep inguinal ring.
f. inguina'lis media'lis [NA], medial inguinal f.; fovea inguinalis interna; a depression on the peritoneal surface of the anterior abdominal wall between the ridges formed by the inferior epigastric artery and the medial umbilical ligament; it corresponds to the position of the superficial inguinal ring.
f. innomina'ta, innominate f.
innominate f., f. innominata; a shallow depression between the false vocal cord and the aryepiglottic fold on either side.
intercondylar f., f. intercondylaris.
f. intercondyla'ris [NA], intercondylar f.; intercondyloid or intercondylic f. (2); intercondyloid or popliteal notch; the deep f. between the femoral condyles in which the cruciate ligaments are attached.
intercondyloid f., intercondylic f., (1) see *area* intercondylaris anterior and *area* intercondylaris posterior; **(2)** f. intercondylaris.
f. intermesocol'ica transver'sa, a f. occupying the position of the superior duodenal recess but extending transversely from right to left for about the length of a finger.
interpeduncular f., f. interpeduncularis.
f. interpeduncula'ris [NA], interpeduncular f.; deep depression on the inferior surface of the mesencephalon, between the crura cerebri, the floor of which is formed by the posterior perforated substance.
intrabulbar f., the dilated commencement of the spongy part of the male urethra lying within the bulb of the penis.
ischiorectal f., f. ischiorectalis.
f. ischiorecta'lis [NA], ischiorectal f.; Velpeau's f.; a wedge-shaped space with its base toward the perineum between the tuberosity of the ischium and the obturator internus muscle laterally and the external anal sphincter and the levator ani muscle medially.
Jobert de Lamballe's f., the hollow just above the knee formed by the adductor magnus and the sartorius and gracilis.
Jonnesco's f., *recessus* duodenalis superior.
jugular f., f. jugularis.
f. jugula'ris, jugular f.; **(1)** [NA]; an oval depression near the posterior border of the petrous portion of the temporal bone, medial to the styloid process, in which lies the beginning of the internal jugular vein; **(2)** the depression in the anterior part of the neck just superior to the jugular notch of the manubrium sterni.
lacrimal f., f. glandulae lacrimalis.
f. of lacrimal gland, f. glandulae lacrimalis.
f. of lacrimal sac, f. sacci lacrimalis.
Landzert's f., a f. formed by two peritoneal folds, enclosing the left colic artery and the inferior mesenteric vein, respectively, at the side of the duodenum; it is smaller than the paraduodenal recess which is sometimes found in the same region.
lateral f. of brain, f. lateralis cerebri.
lateral cerebral f., f. lateralis cerebri.
lateral inguinal f., f. inguinalis lateralis.
f. of lateral malleolus, f. malleoli lateralis.
f. latera'lis cer'ebri [NA], lateral cerebral f.; lateral f. of the brain; f. of Sylvius; vallecula sylvii; the deep depression of the basal surface of the forebrain that corresponds in position to the anterior perforated substance. Bounded medially by the optic tract and rostrally by the orbital surface of the frontal lobe, it extends laterally around the overhanging pole of the temporal lobe into the Sylvian fissure (sulcus lateralis).
lenticular f., f. hyaloidea.
lesser supraclavicular f., f. supraclavicularis minor.
little f. of the cochlear window, *fossula* fenestrae cochleae.
little f. of the vestibular (round) window, *fossula* fenestrae vestibuli.
Malgaigne's f., *trigonum* caroticum.
f. malle'oli fib'ulae, f. malleoli lateralis.
f. malle'oli latera'lis [NA], f. of the lateral malleolus; digital f. (2); f. malleoli fibulae; a large rough depression on the medial aspect of the lower end of the fibula just behind the articular facet for the talus giving attachment to the posterior talofibular and the transverse tibiofibular ligaments.
mandibular f., f. mandibularis.
f. mandibula'ris [NA], mandibular f.; glenoid f. (2); articular f. of temporal bone; a deep hollow in the squamous portion of the temporal bone at the root of the zygoma, in which rests the condyle of the mandible.
mastoid f., f. mastoi'dea, *foveola* suprameatica.
medial inguinal f., f. inguinalis medialis.
Merkel's f., a groove in the posterolateral wall of the vestibule of the larynx between the corniculate and cuneiform cartilages.
mesentericoparietal f., parajejunal f.
middle cranial f., f. cranii media.
Mohrenheim's f., f. infraclavicularis.
Morgagni's f., f. navicularis urethrae.
mylohyoid f., *sulcus* mylohyoideus.
navicular f. of urethra, f. navicularis urethrae.
f. navicula'ris auric'ulae, f. triangularis.
f. navicula'ris au'ris, scapha (2).
f. navicula'ris cruveil'hier, f. scaphoidea.
f. navicula'ris ure'thrae [NA], navicular f. of the urethra; Mor-

gagni's f. or fovea; f. terminalis urethrae; the terminal dilated portion of the urethra in the glans penis.
f. navicula'ris vestib'ulae vagi'nae, f. vestibuli vaginae.
f. olecra'ni [NA], olecranon f.; anconal f.; a hollow on the dorsum of the distal end of the humerus, just above the trochlea, in which the olecranon process of the ulna rests when the elbow is extended.
olecranon f., f. olecrani.
oval f., f. ovalis.
f. ova'lis, oval f.; **(1)** [NA], an oval depression on the lower part of the septum of the right atrium; its floor corresponds to the septum primum of the fetal heart; **(2)** *hiatus* saphenus.
ovarian f., f. ovarica.
f. ova'rica [NA], ovarian f.; Claudius' f.; a depression in the parietal peritoneum of the pelvis; it is bounded in front by the obliterated umbilical artery, and behind by the ureter and the uterine vessels; it lodges the ovary.
paraduodenal f., *recessus* paraduodenalis.
parajejunal f., f. parajejunalis; mesentericoparietal f. or recess; Broesike's f.; a peritoneal f. that has been seen in a few cases in which the jejunum has no mesentery but is attached to the posterior parietal peritoneum; the f. begins at the point where the mesentery ends, and is seen on raising up the knuckle of free intestine.
f. parajejuna'lis, parajejunal f.
pararectal f., a depression on either side of the rectum formed by the reflection of the peritoneum to the posterior pelvic wall.
paravesical f., f. paravesicalis.
f. paravesica'lis [NA], paravesical f.; a depression formed by the peritoneum on each side of the urinary bladder.
patellar f. of vitreous, f. hyaloidea.
peritoneal f.'s, depressions or pouches formed between various peritoneal folds; they may be the sites of internal hernias.
petrosal f., *fossula* petrosa.
piriform f., *recessus* piriformis.
pituitary f., f. hypophysialis.
f. poplit'ea [NA], popliteal f. or space; the lozenge-shaped space posterior to the knee joint bounded superiorly by the biceps femoris and the semimembranosus muscle and inferiorly by the two heads of the gastrocnemius muscle.
popliteal f., f. poplitea.
posterior cranial f., f. cranii posterior.
f. provesica'lis, Hartmann's *pouch.*
pterygoid f., f. pterygoidea.
f. pterygoi'dea [NA], pterygoid f.; the f. formed by the divergence posteriorly of the plates of the pterygoid process of the sphenoid bone; it lodges the medial pterygoid and the tensor palati muscles.
pterygomaxillary f., f. pterygopalatina.
f. pterygopalati'na [NA], pterygopalatine f.; pterygomaxillary f.; Bichat's f.; sphenomaxillary f., a small pyramidal space, housing the pterygopalatine ganglion, between the pterygoid process, the maxilla, and the palatine bone.
pterygopalatine f., f. pterygopalatina.
radial f., f. radialis.
f. radia'lis [NA], radial f.; a shallow depression above the capitulum of the humerus in front, in which the margin of the head of the radius rests when the elbow is in extreme flexion.
retroduodenal f., *recessus* retroduodenalis.
retromandibular f., f. retromandibularis; the depression beneath the auricle behind the angle of the jaw.
f. retromandibula'ris, retromandibular f.
retromolar f., a triangular depression in the mandible posterior to the third molar tooth.
rhomboid f., f. rhomboidea.
f. rhomboi'dea [NA], rhomboid f.; the floor of the fourth ventricle of the brain, formed by the ventricular surface of the rhombencephalon.
Rosenmüller's f., *recessus* pharyngeus.
f. sac'ci lacrima'lis [NA], f. of the lacrimal sac; a f. formed by the lacrimal bone and the frontal process of the maxilla, lodging the lacrimal sac.
scaphoid f., **(1)** f. scaphoidea; **(2)** scapha (2).
f. scaphoid'ea [NA], scaphoid f. (1); Cruveilhier's f.; f. navicularis cruveilhier; a hollow on the posterior surface of the medial lamina of the pterygoid process; it gives origin to the tensor muscle of the soft palate.
f. scar'pae ma'jor, *trigonum* femorale.
sigmoid f., *sulcus* sinus sigmoidei.
sphenomaxillary f., f. pterygopalatina.
f. subarcua'ta [NA], subarcuate f.; floccular f.; hiatus subarcuatus; an irregular depression on the posterior surface of the petrous portion of the temporal bone, above and a little lateral to the internal acoustic meatus. In the fetus, the flocculus of the cerebellum rests here; in the adult, a small vein enters the bone here.
subarcuate f., f. subarcuata.
subcecal f., Treitz's f.; an inconstant depression in the peritoneum extending posterior to the cecum.
subinguinal f., the depression on the anterior surface of the thigh beneath the groin.
sublingual f., *fovea* sublingualis.
submandibular f., *fovea* submandibularis.
f. submandibula'ris, *fovea* submandibularis.
submaxillary f., *fovea* submandibularis.
subscapular f., f. subscapularis.
f. subscapula'ris [NA], subscapular f.; the concave ventral aspect of the body of the scapula giving attachment to the subscapularis muscle.
superior duodenal f., *recessus* duodenalis superior.
f. supraclavicula'ris ma'jor [NA], *trigonum* omoclaviculare.
f. supraclavicula'ris mi'nor [NA], lesser supraclavicular f.; a triangular space between the two heads of origin of the sternocleidomastoid muscle.
supramastoid f., *foveola* suprameatica.
f. supraspina'ta [NA], supraspinous f.; the hollow on the dorsal aspect of the scapula above the spine, lodging the supraspinatus muscle.
supraspinous f., f. supraspinata.
supratonsillar f., f. supratonsillaris.
f. supratonsilla'ris [NA], supratonsillar f. or recess; Tourtual's sinus; the interval between the palatoglossal and palatopharyngeal arches above the tonsil.
supravesical f., f. supravesicalis.
f. supravesica'lis [NA], supravesical f.; fovea supravesicalis; the depression on the peritoneal surface of the anterior abdominal wall between the median and medial umbilical folds.
f. of Sylvius, f. lateralis cerebri.
temporal f., f. temporalis.
f. tempora'lis [NA], temporal f.; the space on the side of the cranium bounded by the temporal lines and terminating below at the level of the zygomatic arch.
f. termina'lis ure'thrae, f. navicularis urethrae.
tonsillar f., f. tonsillaris.
f. tonsilla'ris [NA], tonsillar f.; amygdaloid f.; sinus tonsillaris; the depression between the palatoglossal and palatopharyngeal arches occupied by the palatine tonsil.
Treitz's f., subcecal f.
triangular f., f. triangularis.
f. triangula'ris [NA], triangular f.; f. navicularis auriculae; the depression at the upper part of the auricle between the two crura of the anthelix.
trochanteric f., f. trochanterica.
f. trochanter'ica [NA], trochanteric f.; digital f. (1); a depression at the root of the neck of the femur beneath the curved tip of the great trochanter; it gives attachment to the tendon of the obturator externus.
trochlear f., *fovea* trochlearis.

f. trochlea'ris, *fovea* trochlearis.
umbilical f., *fissura* ligamenti teretis.
Velpeau's f., f. ischiorectalis.
f. ve'nae ca'vae, *sulcus* venae cavae.
f. ve'nae umbilica'lis, *fissura* ligamenti teretis.
f. veno'sa, *recessus* paraduodenalis.
vermian f., a small depression near the lower part of the internal occipital crest which lodges part of the inferior vermis of the cerebellum.
f. vesi'cae fel'leae [NA], gallbladder f.; a depression on the visceral surface of the liver anteriorly, between the quadrate and the right lobes, lodging the gallbladder.
vestibular f., f. vestibuli vaginae.
f. of vestibule of vagina, f. vestibuli vaginae.
f. vestib'uli vagi'nae [NA], f. of the vestibule of the vagina; vestibular f.; f. navicularis vestibulae vaginae; the portion of the vestibule of the vagina between the frenulum of the pudendal lips and the posterior commissure of the vulva.
Waldeyer's fossae, see *recessus* duodenalis inferior and *recessus* duodenalis superior.
zygomatic f., f. infratemporalis.

---

fossette (fo-set') [Fr. dim. of *fosse,* a ditch]. **1.** Fossula. **2.** A deep corneal ulcer of small diameter.

fossula, pl. **fossulae** (fos'yū-lă, -lē) [L. dim. of *fossa,* ditch]. **1.** [NA]. Fossette (1); a small fossa. **2.** A minor fissure or slight depression on the surface of the cerebrum.
f. fenes'trae coch'leae [NA], little fossa of the cochlear window; f. rotunda; a depression on the medial wall of the middle ear at the bottom of which is the cochlear (round) window.
f. fenes'trae vestib'uli [NA], little fossa of the vestibular window; Huguier's sinus; a depression on the medial wall of the middle ear at the bottom of which is the vestibular (oval) window.
f. petro'sa [NA], petrosal fossa; receptaculum ganglii petrosi; a small and often only faintly marked depression on the inferior surface of the petrous portion of the temporal bone, between the jugular fossa and the opening of the carotid canal; here opens the canaliculus tympanicus transmitting the tympanic nerve.
f. rotun'da, f. fenestrae cochleae.
tonsillar fossulae, fossulae tonsillares.
fos'sulae tonsilla'res [NA], tonsillar fossulae; the small pits at the openings of the tonsillar crypts onto the medial surface of the tonsil.

fossulate (fos'yū-lāt). Containing a fossula or small fossa; grooved; hollowed out.

Foster frame. See under frame.

Foster Kennedy. See Kennedy, Robert Foster.

Fothergill, John, British physician, 1712–1780. See F.'s *disease, neuralgia, sign.*

Fothergill, William E., British gynecologist, 1865–1926. See F.'s *operation.*

Fouchet, A., French physician, *1894. See F.'s *reagent, stain.*

foudroyant (fū-droy'ant) [Fr. *foudroyer,* to strike by lightning]. Fulminant.

foulage (fū-lahzh') [Fr. impression]. Kneading and pressure of the muscles, constituting a form of massage.

foundation (fown-dā'shŭn). A base; a supporting structure.
denture f., denture-supporting or tissue-bearing area; supporting area (2); stress-bearing area (1); basal seat; that portion of the oral structures which is available to support a denture. See also denture f. *area;* denture f. *surface;* mean f. *plane.*

founder (fown'der). **1.** A person who contributes to the initial genetic structure of a population. **2.** Laminitis (2).

fourchette (fūr-shet') [Fr. dim. of *fourché,* fr. L. *furca,* fork]. *Frenulum* labiorum pudendi.

Fourneau 693 [after Ernest F.A. *Fourneau,* French chemist, 1872–1949]. Ethylstibamine.

Fourneau 710 [E.F.A. *Fourneau*]. A synthetic quinoline; an antimalarial agent.

Fourneau 933 [E.F.A. *Fourneau*]. Piperoxan hydrochloride.

Fournier, Jean A., French syphilographer, 1832–1914. See F.'s *disease, gangrene; syphiloma* of F.

fovea, pl. **foveae** (fō'vē-ă, fō'vē-ē) [L. a pit] [NA]. A cup-shaped depression or pit.
f. ante'rior, f. superior.
f. articula'ris cap'itis ra'dii [NA], articular pit of head of the radius; the depression in the center of the head of the radius for articulation with the capitulum of the humerus.
f. articula'ris infe'rior atlan'tis, *facies* articularis inferior atlantis.
f. articula'ris supe'rior atlan'tis, *facies* articularis superior atlantis.
f. cap'itis os'sis fem'oris [NA], pit of the head of the femur; a depression on the extremity of the head of the femur giving attachment to the ligamentum teres.
f. cardi'aca, anterior intestinal portal; the opening of the foregut into the midgut.
f. centra'lis ret'inae [NA], central pit; a depression in the center of the macula retinae containing only cones and lacking blood vessels.
f. coc'cygis, postnatal pit of the newborn; it marks the site where the embryonic spinal cord attaches to the skin.
f. costa'lis infe'rior [NA], inferior costal pit; demifacet on the lower edge of the body of a vertebra articulating with the head of a rib.
f. costa'lis proces'sus transver'sus [NA], costal pit of the transverse process; a facet on the transverse process of a vertebra for articulation with the tubercle of a rib.
f. costa'lis supe'rior [NA], superior costal pit; a demifacet on the upper edge of the body of a vertebra articulating with the head of a rib; a single rib articulates with the f. costalis inferior and f. costalis superior of the adjacent vertebrae.
f. den'tis atlan'tis [NA], pit for dens; a circular facet on the posterior (inner) surface of the anterior arch of the atlas which articulates with the dens of the axis.
f. ellip'tica, *recessus* ellipticus.
f. ethmoida'lis, the portion of the frontal bone comprising the roof of the anterior superior ethmoid cells.
f. femora'lis, femoral or crural fossa; a depression on the peritoneal surface of the abdominal wall, inferior to the inguinal ligament, corresponding to the situation of the femoral ring.
f. hemiellip'tica, *recessus* ellipticus.
f. hemisphe'rica, *recessus* sphericus.
f. infe'rior [NA], a triangular area of the rhomboidal fossa below the striae medullares of either side.
f. inguina'lis inter'na, *fossa* inguinalis medialis.
Morgagni's f., *fossa* navicularis urethrae.
f. oblon'ga cartilag'inis arytenoid'eae [NA], oblong pit of the arytenoid cartilage; a broad shallow depression on the anterolateral surface of the arytenoid cartilage, for attachment of the thyroarytenoid muscle.
f. pterygoid'ea [NA], pterygoid pit or depression; a depression on the medial side of the neck of the condylar process of the mandible, giving attachment to the lateral pterygoid muscle.
f. sphe'rica, *recessus* sphericus.
f. sublingua'lis [NA], sublingual pit or fossa; a shallow depression on either side of the mental spine, on the inner surface of the body of the mandible, superior to the mylohyoid line, lodging the sublingual gland.
f. submandibula'ris [NA], submandibular fossa; submaxillary fossa; fossa submandibularis; f. submaxillaris; the depression on

the medial surface of the body of the mandible inferior to the mylohyoid line in which the submandibular gland is lodged.

f. submaxilla'ris, f. submandibularis.

f. supe'rior [NA], f. anterior; a slight depression on either side of the rhomboidal fossa, above the striae medullares.

f. supravesica'lis, *fossa* supravesicalis.

f. triangula'ris cartilag'inis arytenoid'eae [NA], triangular pit of arytenoid cartilage; a deep depression in the upper portion of the anterolateral surface of the arytenoid cartilage, lodging glands.

f. trochlea'ris [NA], trochlear pit or fossa; fossa trochlearis; a shallow depression in the roof of the orbit close to the medial margin to which is attached the pulley for the superior oblique tendon.

foveate, foveated (fō'-vē-āt, -ā-ted). Pitted; having foveas or depressions on the surface.

foveation (fō-vē-ā'shŭn) [L. *fovea,* a pit]. Pitted scar formation, as in smallpox, chickenpox, or vaccinia.

foveola, pl. **foveolae** (fō-vē'ō-lă, -lē) [Mod. L. dim. of L. *fovea,* pit] [NA]. A minute fovea or pit.

f. coccyge'a [NA], coccygeal f.; coccygeal dimple; a depression in the skin over the coccyx caused by the caudal retinaculum.

coccygeal f., f. coccygea.

f. gas'trica [NA], gastric pit; one of the numerous small pits in the mucous membrane of the stomach which are the mouths of the gastric glands.

foveolae granula'res [NA], granular pits; pacchionian depressions; pits on the inner surface of the skull, along the course of the superior sagittal sinus, in which are lodged the arachnoidal granulations.

f. ocula'ris, the central portion of the fovea centralis that contains cones only.

f. papilla'ris, the minute depression sometimes seen at the apex of a papilla of the kidney where a collecting duct opens into a calix.

f. suprameа'tica [NA], suprameatal pit; mastoid or supramastoid fossa; fossa mastoidea; a small depression on the mastoid part of the temporal bone, posterior to the suprameatal spine.

foveolar (fō-vē'ō-lăr). Pertaining to a foveola.

foveolate (fō'vē-ō-lāt, fō-vē'ō-lāt). Having minute pits (foveolae) or small depressions on the surface.

Foville, Achille L., French neurologist, 1799–1878. See F.'s *fasciculus, syndrome.*

Fowler, George R., U.S. surgeon, 1848–1906. See F.'s *position.*

fowlpox (fowl'poks). Epithelioma contagiosum; a disease of fowl, worldwide in distribution, caused by fowlpox virus and characterized by proliferative nodular dermal lesions followed by scabbing, chiefly on the head but sometimes involving the feet and vent; there may also be eye lesions or involvement of the trachea (so-called fowl diphtheria); transmission is by contact, or mechanically by mosquitoes.

Fox, George H., U.S. dermatologist, 1846–1937. See F.-Fordyce *disease.*

Fox, Lewis, U.S. periodontist, *1903. See Goldman-F. *knives.*

foxglove (foks'glŭv). *Digitalis.*

FPS, fps Abbreviation for foot-pound-second. See under system; unit.

Fr 1. Symbol for francium. **2.** Abbreviation for French *scale.*

Fraccaro, M. See Schmid-F. *syndrome.*

fraction (frak'shŭn). **1.** The quotient of two quantities. **2.** An aliquot portion or any portion.

amorphous f. of adrenal cortex, noncrystalline residue of an acetone extract of the adrenal cortex after crystalline steroids, *e.g.,* corticosterone, deoxycorticosterone, etc., have been isolated.

blood plasma f.'s, portions of the blood plasma as separated by electrophoresis or other technique.

dried human plasma protein f., freeze-dried human plasma protein f.

ejection f. (systolic), the f. of the blood contained in the ventricle at the end of diastole that is expelled during its contraction, *i.e.,* the stroke volume divided by end-diastolic volume, normally 0.67 or greater; with the onset of congestive heart failure, the ejection f. decreases, sometimes to as little as 0.10 in severe cases.

filtration f. (FF), the f. of the plasma entering the kidney that filters into the lumen of the renal tubules, determined by dividing the glomerular filtration rate by the renal plasma flow; normally, it is around 0.17.

human antihemophilic f., human antihemophilic *factor.*

human plasma protein f., a sterile solution of selected proteins derived from the blood plasma of adult human donors, containing 4.5 to 5.5 g of protein per 100 ml, of which 83 to 90% is albumin and the remainder is α- and β-globulins; used as a blood volume supporter.

mole f., the ratio of the moles of one component of a system to the total moles of all the components present.

recombination f., the proportion of progeny of a mating pair of specific genotype and coupling phase that are recombinant; there must be no differential selection among the possible types of progeny, and the recombination f. should be the same regardless of the alleles involved.

regurgitant f., the amount of blood regurgitated into the heart or between its chambers as divided by the stroke output; normally, no blood regurgitates, but in patients with severe valvular lesions such as mitral insufficiency, regurgitation can approach 80%; this f. affords a quantitative measure of the severity of the valvular lesion.

fractionation (frak-shŭn-ā'shŭn). **1.** To separate components of a mixture. **2.** The protraction of a total therapeutic radiation dose over a period of time, ordinarily days or weeks, in order to minimize untoward radiation effects on normal contiguous tissue.

FRACTURE

fracture (frak'chŭr) [L. *fractura,* a break]. **1.** To break. **2.** A break, especially the breaking of a bone or cartilage.

apophysial f., separation of apophysis from bone.

articular f., a f. involving the joint surface of a bone.

avulsion f., a f. that occurs when a joint capsule, ligament, or muscle insertion of origin is pulled from the bone as a result of a sprain dislocation or strong contracture of the muscle against resistance; as the soft tissue is pulled away from the bone, a fragment or fragments of the bone may come away with it.

Barton's f., f. dislocation of the radiocarpal joint.

basal skull f., a f. involving the base of the cranium.

bending f., an injury in which a long bone or bones, usually the radius and ulnar, are bent due to multiple microfractures, none of which can be seen by x-ray imaging.

Bennett's f., f. dislocation of the first metacarpal bone at the carpal-metacarpal joint.

birth f., f. occurring during the trauma of delivery or, occasionally, before delivery in infants with osteogenesis imperfecta.

blow-out f., a f. of the floor of the orbit, without a fracture of the rim, produced by a blow on the globe with the force being transmitted via the globe to the orbital floor.

boxer's f., f. of first metacarpal bone.

capillary f., hairline f.

Chance f., a transverse f., usually in the lumbar spine, through the body of the vertebra extending posteriorly through the pedicles and the spinous process.

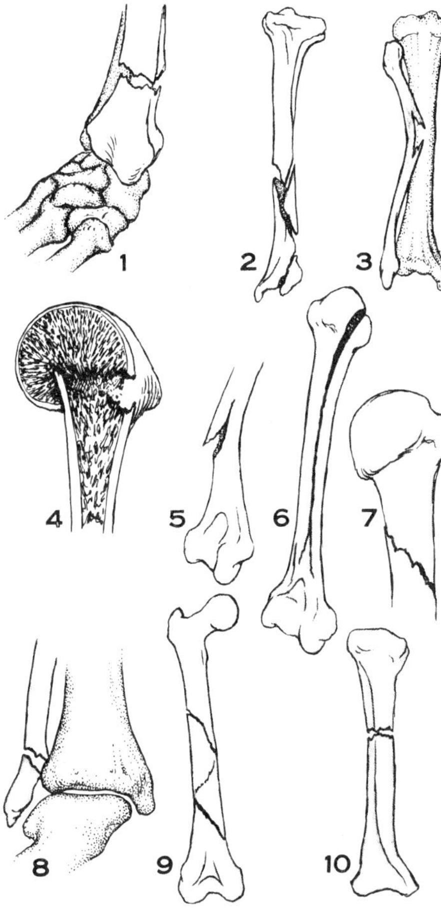

Types of Fractures
1, Colles'; *2*, comminuted; *3*, greenstick; *4*, impacted; *5*, incomplete; *6*, linear; *7*, oblique; *8*, Pott's; *9*, spiral; *10*, transverse.

closed f., simple f.; a f. in which skin is intact at site of f.
closed skull f., simple skull f.; f. with intact overlying scalp and/or mucous membranes.
Colles' f., a f. of the lower end of the radius with displacement of the distal fragment dorsally; sometimes called a reversed Colles' f., or Smith's f. when volar displacement of the distal fragment occurs in the same location.
comminuted f., a f. in which the bone is broken into pieces.
comminuted skull f., a f. of the skull with fragmentation of bone.
complicated f., a f. with significant soft tissue injury (in neurovascular injury).
compound f., open f.
compound skull f., open skull f.
f. by contrecoup, contrafissura.
cough f., a f. of a rib, usually the fifth or seventh, from vigorous coughing.
craniofacial dysjunction f., Le Fort III f.; transverse facial f.; a complex f. in which the facial bones are separated from the cranial bones.
dentate f., a f. in which the opposing surfaces are rough, with toothed or serrate projections fitting into corresponding indentations.
depressed f., depressed skull f.
depressed skull f., depressed f.; a f. with inward displacement of a part of the calvarium; the so-called dishpan, derby hat, and ping-pong f.'s consist of regular cranial concavity in infants, and may or may not be associated with f.
de Quervain's f., f. of navicular bone with dislocation of lunar bone.
derby hat f., see depressed skull f.
diastatic skull f., **(1)** separation of cranial bones at a suture; **(2)** f. with marked separation of bone fragments.
direct f., a f., especially of the skull, occurring at the point of injury.
dishpan f., see depressed skull f.
dislocation f., a f. of a bone near an articulation with its concomitant dislocation from that joint.
double f., segmental f.; a f. in two parts of the same bone.
Dupuytren's f., f. of lower part of fibula, with dislocation of ankle.
dyscrasic f., obsolete term for a f. occurring in general malnutrition.
epiphysial f., separation of the epiphysis of a long bone, caused by trauma.
expressed skull f., a f. with outward displacement of a part of the cranium.
extracapsular f., a f. at the articular extremity of a bone, but outside of the line of attachment of the capsular ligament of the joint.
fatigue f., f. that occurs in bone subject to repeated or unusual subliminal, endogenous stress, most often transverse in configuration.
fetal f., intrauterine f.
fissured f., linear f.
folding f., torus f.
Galeazzi's f., f. of the shaft of the radius with dislocation of the distal radioulnar joint.
Gosselin's f., v-shaped f. of distal end of tibia.
greenstick f., the bending of a bone with incomplete f. involving the convex side of the curve only.
growing f., linear skull f. in a young child which increases in size, usually as the result of an associated dural tear and arachnoid cyst formation.
Guérin's f., Le Fort I f.; horizontal f.; a f. of the facial bones in which there is a horizontal f. at the base of the maxillae above the apices of the teeth.
gutter f., a long, narrow, depressed f. of the skull.
hairline f., capillary f.; a f. without separation of the fragments, the line of break being hairlike, as seen sometimes in the skull.
hangman's f., a f. or f. dislocation of the cervical spine at the level of C-2 and C-3 and through the pedicles of C-2.
horizontal f., Guérin's f.
impacted f., a f. in which one of the fragments is driven into the cancellous tissue of the other fragment.
incomplete f., a f. in which the line of f. does not include the entire bone.
indirect f., a f., especially of the skull, that occurs at a point not at the site of impact.
intra-articular f., f. occurring within a joint capsule.
intracapsular f., a f. at the articular extremity of a bone within the line of insertion of the capsular ligament of the joint.
intraperiosteal f., a f. in which the periosteum is not ruptured.
intrauterine f., fetal f.; a f. of one or more bones of a fetus occurring before birth.
Le Fort I f. Guérin's f.
Le Fort II f., pyramidal f.
Le Fort III f., craniofacial dysjunction f.
linear f., -fissured f.; a f. running parallel with the long axis of the bone.
linear skull f., a skull f. resembling a line.
longitudinal f., a f. involving the bone in the line of its axis.
march f., Deutschländer's disease (2); a fatigue f. of one of the

metatarsals.
Monteggia's f., f. of the ulna with dislocation of the head of the radius.
multiple f., **(1)** f. at two or more places in a bone; **(2)** f. of several bones occurring simultaneously.
neurogenic f., a f. in bone weakened by disease of the nerve supply.
oblique f., a f. the line of which runs obliquely to the axis of the bone.
occult f., a condition in which there are clinical signs of f. but no x-ray evidence; after 3 or 4 weeks x-ray imaging shows new bone formation.
open f., compound f.; f. in which the skin is perforated and there is an open wound down to the f.
open skull f., compound skull f.; a f. with laceration of overlying scalp and/or mucous membrane.
parry f., rarely used synonym for Monteggia's f.
pathologic f., a f. occurring at a site weakened by preexisting disease, especially neoplasm or necrosis, of the bone.
pertrochanteric f., a f. through the great trochanter of the femur; a form of extracapsular hip f.
pilon f., a f. of the distal metaphysis of the tibia extending into the ankle joint.
ping-pong f., see depressed skull f.
pond f., a circular depressed skull f.
Pott's f., f. of the lower part of the fibula and of the malleolus of the tibia, with outward displacement of the foot.
pyramidal f., Le Fort II f.; a f. of the midfacial skeleton with the principal f. lines meeting at an apex at or near the superior aspect of the nasal bones.
segmental f., double f.
sentinel spinous process f., f. of the spinous process with undetected deeper f.'s of the vertebral arch.
Shepherd's f., a f. of the external tubercle (posterior process) of the talus, sometimes mistaken for a displacement of the os trigonum.
silver-fork f., a Colles' f. of the wrist in which the deformity has the appearance of a fork in profile.
simple f., closed f.
simple skull f., closed skull f.
Skillern's f., f. of distal radius with greenstick f. of neighboring portion of ulna.
skull f., a break of the cranium resulting from trauma.
Smith's f., reversed Colles' f.; f. of the radius near its lower articular surface with displacement of the fragment toward the palmar (volar) aspect.
spiral f., a f. the line of which is helical in the bone.
splintered f., a comminuted f. in which the fragments are long and sharp-pointed.
spontaneous f., a f. occurring without any external injury.
sprain f., an avulsion f. in which a small portion of adjacent bone has been pulled or pushed off.
stable f., a f. that does not tend to displace once it has been reduced and immobilized.
stellate f., a f. in which the lines of break radiate from a central point.
stellate skull f., a multiple radiating linear f.
strain f., the tearing off, by a sudden force, of a piece of bone attached to a tendon, ligament, or capsule; the force may be exogenous or endogenous.
stress f., a fatigue f. occurring usually from sudden, strong, violent, endogenous force (*e.g.,* a simple f. of fibula in a runner); distinguished from strain f. in that stress f. is not at the point of connective tissue attachment, but usually at the point of muscular attachment.
subcapital f., an intracapsular f. of the neck of the femur, at the point where the neck of the femur joins the head.
subperiosteal f., a f. occurring beneath the periosteum, and without displacement.
supracondylar f., a f. of the distal end of the humerus.
torsion f., a f. resulting from twisting of the limb.
torus f., folding f.; a deformity in children consisting of a local bulging caused by the longitudinal compression of the soft bone; it occurs in the radius or ulna or both.
transcervical f., a f. through the neck of the femur.
transcondylar f., a f. through condyles of the humerus or femur.
transverse f., a f. the line of which forms a right angle with the axis of the bone.
transverse facial f., craniofacial dysjunction f.
trimalleolar f., a f. through both malleoli and the posterior process of the tibia.
unstable f., a f. with an intrinsic tendency to slip out of place after reduction.
ununited f., a f. in which union fails to occur, the ends of the bone becoming rounded and eburnated, and a false joint occurs.
Wagstaffe's f., f., with displacement, of the inner malleolus.

Fraenkel, Albert, German physician, 1848–1916. See F.'s *pneumococcus,* F.-Weichselbaum *pneumococcus.*

fragilitas (fră-jil'i-tas) [L.]. Fragility.
f. crin'ium, brittleness of the hair; a condition in which the hair of the head or face tends to split or break off.
f. os'sium, obsolete term for *osteogenesis* imperfecta.
f. san'guinis, *fragility* of the blood.

fragility (fră-jil'i-tē) [L. *fragilitas*]. Brittleness; liability to break, burst, or disintegrate.
f. of the blood, fragilitas sanguinis; increased susceptibility of the red blood cells to break down when the proportion of the saline content of the fluid is altered.

fragilocyte (fra-jil'ō-sīt) [L. *fragilis,* brittle, + G. *kytos,* hollow (cell)]. A red blood cell that is unusually fragile when subjected to a hypotonic salt solution.

fragilocytosis (fra-jil'ō-sī-tō'sis) A condition of the blood in which the red blood cells are abnormally fragile.

fragment (frag'ment). A small part broken from a larger entity.
butterfly f., a broad triangular f. that is commonly present in comminuted fractures of the diaphysis.
Fab f., Fab portion or piece; the antigen-binding f. of an immunoglobulin molecule.
Fc f., Fc portion or piece; the crystallizable f. of an immunoglobulin molecule.
one-carbon f., The formyl group or the methyl group that takes part in transformylation or transmethylation reactions; by means of these reactions, a group containing a single carbon atom is added to a compound being biosynthesized, adding a methyl group (as in thymidine formation), adding a hydroxymethyl group (as in serine biosynthesis), or closing a ring (as in purine formation).
two-carbon f., the acetyl group (CH_3CO–) that takes part in transacetylation reactions with coenzyme A as carrier; commonly referred to as acetate or acetic acid, from which it is derived.

fragmentation (frag-men-tā'shŭn). The breaking of an entity into smaller parts.
f. of the myocardium, a transverse rupture of the muscular fibers of the heart, especially those of the papillary muscles.

fraise (frāz) [Fr. strawberry]. A burr in the shape of a hemispherical button with cutting edges, used to enlarge a trephine opening in the skull or to cut osteoplastic flaps; the smooth convexity of the button prevents injury to the dura.

Fraley, Elwin E., U.S. urologist, *1934. See F. *syndrome.*

frambesia (fram-be'zē-ă) [Fr. *framboise,* raspberry]. Yaws.

frambesiform (fram-bē'zi-fōrm). Resembling the lesion of frambesia.

frambesioma (fram-bē-zē-ō'mă) [frambesia + *-oma,* tumor]. Mother *yaw.*

frame (frām). A structure made of parts fitted together.
Balkan f., Balkan beam or splints, an overhead f., supported on uprights attached to the bedposts or to a separate stand, from which a splinted limb is slung in the treatment of fracture or joint disease.
Bradford f., an oblong rectangular f. made of pipe, over which are stretched transversely two strips of canvas; permits trunk and lower extremities to move as a unit.
Deiters' terminal f.'s, platelike structures in the organ of Corti uniting the outer phalangeal cells with Hensen's cells.
Foster f., a reversible bed similar to a Stryker f.
occluding f., articulator.
reading f., the grouping of nucleotides by threes into codons.
Stryker f., a f. that holds the patient and permits turning in various planes without individual motion of parts.
trial f., a type of spectacle f. with variable adjustments, for holding trial lenses during refraction.
Whitman's f., a f. similar to the Bradford f., but with curved sides.

framework (frām'wŏrk). **1.** See stroma. **2.** In dentistry, the skeletal prosthesis (usually metal) around which and to which are attached the remaining portions of the prosthesis to produce the finished appliance (partial denture).

Franceschetti, Adolphe, Swiss ophthalmologist, *1896. See F.'s *syndrome.*

Francisella (fran'si-sel'lă). A genus of nonmotile, nonsporeforming, aerobic bacteria that contain small, Gram-negative cocci and rods. Capsules are rarely produced and the cells may show bipolar staining. These organisms are highly pleomorphic; they do not grow on plain agar or in liquid media without special enrichment; they are pathogenic and cause tularemia in man. The type species is *F. tularensis.*
F. novici'da, a species pathogenic for some species of animals but not known to infect man.
F. tularen'sis, *Pasteurella tularensis;* a species that causes tularemia in man, transmitted to man from wild animals by bloodsucking insects, by contact with infected animals, or by drinking water; it can penetrate unbroken skin to cause infection; it is the type species of the genus *F.*

francium (fran'sē-ŭm) [*France,* native country of Mlle. M. Perey, the discoverer]. Radioactive element of the alkali metal series; symbol Fr; atomic no. 87; half-life of most stable known isotope, ^{223}Fr, is 21 minutes.

Francke, Karl E., German physician, 1859– 1920. See F.'s *needle.*

frangula (frang'gū-lă). The bark of *Rhamnus frangula* (family Rhamnaceae); a laxative or cathartic.

frangulic acid (frang'yū-lik) [see frangula]. Emodin.

frangulin (frang'yū-lin). Rhamnoxanthin; emodine-*l*-rhamnoside; $C_{21}H_{20}O_9$; a glycoside from frangula; has been used as a purgative.

Frank, Otto, German physiologist, 1865–1944. See F.-Starling *curve.*

frank. Unmistakable; manifest; clinically evident.

Frankenhäuser, Ferdinand, German gynecologist, 1832–1894. See F.'s *ganglion.*

Frankfort [*Frankfurt*-am-Main, Germany]. See F. horizontal *plane,* F.-mandibular incisor *angle.*

frankincense (frangk'in-sens) [Mediev. L. *francum incensum,* pure incense]. Olibanum.

Franklin, Benjamin, U.S. physicist and statesman, 1706–1790. See franklinic; F. *spectacles.*

Franklin, Edward C., U.S. physician, *1928. See F.'s *disease.*

franklinic (frank'lin-ik) [B. *Franklin*]. Denoting static or frictional electricity.

Fräntzel's murmur. See under murmur.

Fraser, Alexander, Canadian pathologist, 1869–1939. See F.-Lendrum *stain* for fibrin.

Fraser, G. R., 20th century British geneticist. See F.'s *syndrome.*

Fraumeni, Joseph F., Jr., 20th century epidemiologist. See Li-F. cancer *syndrome.*

Fraunhofer, Joseph von, German optician, 1787–1826. See F.'s *lines.*

Frazier, Charles H., U.S. surgeon, 1870–1936. See F.'s *needle,* F.-Spiller *operation.*

FRC Abbreviation for functional residual *capacity.*

F.R.C.P. Abbreviation for Fellow of the Royal College of Physicians (of England).

F.R.C.P.(C) Abbreviation for Fellow of the Royal College of Physicians (Canada).

F.R.C.P.(E) or **(Edin)** Abbreviation for Fellow of the Royal College of Physicians (Edinburgh).

F.R.C.P.(I) Abbreviation for Fellow of the Royal College of Physicians (Ireland).

F.R.C.S. Abbreviation for Fellow of the Royal College of Surgeons (of England).

F.R.C.S.(C) Abbreviation for Fellow of the Royal College of Surgeons (Canada).

F.R.C.S.(E) or **(Edin)** Abbreviation for Fellow of the Royal College of Surgeons (Edinburgh).

F.R.C.S.(I) Abbreviation for Fellow of the Royal College of Surgeons (Ireland).

freckle (frek'l) [O. E. *freken*]. Ephelis; yellowish or brownish macules developing on the exposed parts of the skin, especially in persons of light complexion; the lesions increase in number on exposure to the sun; the epidermis is microscopically normal except for increased melanin. See also lentigo.
Hutchinson's f., malignant *lentigo.*
iris f.'s, small, pigmented clusters of uveal melanocytes on the surface of the iris.
melanotic f., malignant *lentigo.*

Fredet, Pierre, French surgeon, 1870–1946. See F.-Ramstedt *operation.*

Freeman, E.A. See F.-Sheldon *syndrome.*

freemartin (frē'mar-tin) [(?) Sc. *fear* or *fearr,* sterile and dry cow, + *martin,* fr. Martinmas when cattle, especially if sterile and unproductive of milk, were slaughtered]. A masculinized, sterile female twin calf, developing from twin fetuses of opposite sexes in which the chorionic blood vessels become fused at an early stage of embryonic development, with the result that the hormones of the male twin are conveyed in the circulation to the female twin and influence its sexual development. F.'s are a type of hermaphrodite with underdeveloped uterus, enlarged penis-like clitoris, and, sometimes, structures resembling the ductus deferens and seminal vesicles.

freeze-drying (frēz'drī-ing). Lyophilization.

freezing (frē'zing). Congelation (1); congealing, stiffening, or hardening by exposure to cold.
gastric f., treatment for peptic ulcer designed to reduce or eliminate the production of acid gastric juice by freezing the secretory cells with a supercooled fluid introduced into a balloon positioned in the stomach.

Frei, Wilhelm S., German dermatologist, 1885–1943. See F. *test;* F.-Hoffman *reaction.*

Freiberg, Albert Henry, U.S. surgeon, 1869–1940. See F.'s *disease.*

Frejka, B., 20th century Czech orthopedist. See F. pillow *splint.*

fremitus (frem'i-tŭs) [L. a dull roaring sound, fr. *fremo,* pp. *-itus,* to roar, resound]. A vibration imparted to the hand resting on the chest or other part of the body. See also thrill.

bronchial f., adventitious pulmonary sounds or voice sounds perceptible to the hand resting on the chest, as well as by the ear.

hydatid f., hydatid *thrill.*

pericardial f., vibration in the chest wall produced by the friction of opposing roughened surfaces of the pericardium.

pleural f., vibration in the chest wall produced by a friction rub resulting from the rubbing together of the roughened inflamed opposing surfaces of the pleura.

rhonchal f., f. produced by vibrations from the passage of air in the bronchial tubes partially obstructed by mucous secretion.

subjective f., vibration felt within the chest by the patient himself, when humming with the mouth closed; or f. felt when there is a rough, pericardial or pleural friction rub, particularly when pain is minimal.

tactile f., vibration felt with the hand on the chest during vocal f.

tussive f., a form of f. similar to the vocal, produced by a cough.

vocal f., the vibration in the chest wall, felt on palpation, produced by the spoken voice.

frena (frē'nă). Plural of frenum.

frenal (frē'năl). Relating to any frenum.

frenectomy (frē-nek'tō-mē) [frenum + G. *ektomē,* excision]. Removal of any frenum.

Frenkel, Heinrich S., Swiss neurologist, 1860–1931. See F.'s *symptom.*

Frenkel, Henri, French ophthalmologist, 1864–1934. See F.'s anterior ocular traumatic *syndrome.*

frenoplasty (frē'nō-plas-tē) [frenum + G. *plastos,* formed]. Correction of an abnormally attached frenum by surgically repositioning it.

frenotomy (frē-not'ō-mē) [frenum + G. *tomē,* a cutting]. Division of any frenum or frenulum, especially that of the tongue.

frenulum, pl. **frenula** (fren'yū-lŭm, -lă) [Mod. L. dim. of L. *frenum,* bridle] [NA]. A small frenum or bridle.

f. cerebell'i, f. veli medullaris superius.

f. clitor'idis [NA], f. or bridle of the clitoris; f. preputii clitoridis; the line of union of the inner portions of the labia minora on the undersurface of the glans clitoridis.

f. of clitoris, f. clitoridis.

f. epiglot'tidis, *plica* glossoepiglottica mediana.

f. of Giacomini, uncus *band* of Giacomini.

f. of ileocecal valve, f. valvae ileocecalis.

f. la'bii inferio'ris, f. la'bii superio'ris [NA], f. of the lower lip, f. of the upper lip; the folds of mucous membrane extending from the gum to the middle line of the lower and upper lips, respectively.

f. labio'rum mino'rum, f. labiorum pudendi.

f. labio'rum puden'di [NA], f. of the pudendal lips; f. labiorum minorum; f. pudendi; fourchette; the fold connecting the two labia minora posteriorly.

f. lin'guae [NA], f. of the tongue; vinculum linguae; a fold of mucous membrane extending from the floor of the mouth to the midline of the undersurface of the tongue.

frenulum of lower lip, frenulum of upper lip, f. labii inferioris and superioris.

f. of M'Dowel, tendinous fasciculi passing from the tendon of the pectoralis major muscle across the bicipital groove.

f. of Morgagni, f. valvae ileocecalis.

f. of prepuce, f. preputii.

f. prepu'tii [NA], f. of the prepuce; vinculum preputii; a fold of mucous membrane passing from the undersurface of the glans penis to the deep surface of the prepuce.

f. prepu'tii clitor'idis, f. clitoridis.

f. of pudendal lips, f. labiorum pudendi.

f. puden'di, f. labiorum pudendi.

f. of superior medullary velum, f. veli medullaris superius.

synovial frenula, *vincula* tendinum.

f. of tongue, f. linguae.

f. val'vae ileoceca'lis [NA], f. of the ileocecal valve; Morgagni's frenum or retinaculum; f. of Morgagni; a fold, more evident in cadavers, running from the junction of the two commissures of the ileocecal valve on either side along the inner wall of the cecocolic junction.

f. ve'li medulla'ris supe'rius [NA], f. of the superior medullary velum; f. cerebelli; a band passing from the longitudinal groove between the corpora quadrigemina on to the superior medullary velum.

frenum, pl. **frena, frenums** (frē'nŭm, -nă, -nŭmz) [L. a bridle, curb]. Bridle (1). **1.** A narrow reflection or fold of mucous membrane passing from a more fixed to a movable part, serving to check undue movement of the part. **2.** An anatomical structure resembling such a fold.

Morgagni's f., *frenulum* valvae ileocecalis.

synovial frena, *vincula* tendinum.

frenzy (fren'zē) [thr. Old Fr. and L. fr. G. *phrenēsis,* inflammation of the brain, fr. *phrēn,* mind]. Extreme mental or emotional excitement.

frequency (frē'kwen-sē) [L. *frequens,* repeated, often, constant]. The number of regular recurrences in a given time, *e.g.,* heartbeats, sound vibrations.

critical flicker fusion f., the minimal number of flashes of light per second at which an intermittent light stimulus no longer stimulates a continuous visual sensation.

dominant f., the f. occurring most often in an electroencephalogram.

fundamental f., **(1)** the principal component of a sound wave, which has the greatest wavelength; **(2)** tone produced by the vibration of the vocal folds before the air reaches any cavities.

gene f., **(1)** the probability that a gene picked at random from a defined population is of a particular type; **(2)** epidemiologically, the proportion of genes in a population that are of the particular type; **(3)** statistically, the estimate of either of the above two quantities.

f. of micturition, micturition at short intervals; it may result from increased urine formation or decreased bladder capacity.

respiratory f. (f), the number of breaths per minute.

Frerichs, Friedrich T. von, German pathologist and clinician, 1819–1885. See F.'s *theory.*

freshening (fresh'ĕn-ing). Preparation of an open, partially healed wound for secondary closure by removal of fibrin, granulations, and early scar tissue.

Fresnel, Augustin Jean, French physicist, 1788–1827. See F. *lens, prism.*

fressreflex (fres'rē-fleks) [Ger fr. *fressen,* to feed, said of animals]. Sucking and chewing movements elicited by stimulation of the face and lips.

fretting (fret'ing). Abrasive polishing and wear of two metallic surfaces at their interface due to repetitive motion.

fretum, pl. **freta** (frē'tŭm, -tă) [L.]. A strait; a constriction.

Freud, Sigmund, Austrian neurologist and psychiatrist, 1856–1939, founder of psychoanalysis.

freudian (froy'dē-ăn). Relating to or described by Freud.

freudian slip. A mistake which presumably suggests some underlying motive, often sexual or aggressive in nature.

Freund, Jules, U.S. bacteriologist, 1891–1960. See F.'s complete *adjuvant,* incomplete *adjuvant.*

Freund, Wilhelm A., German gynecologist, 1833–1918. See F.'s *anomaly, operation.*

Frey, Lucie, Polish physician, 1852–1932. See F.'s *syndrome.*

Frey, Max von, German physician, 1852–1932. See F.'s irritation *hairs.*

FRF Abbreviation for follicle-stimulating hormone-releasing *factor.*

friable (frī'ă-bl) [L. *friabilis,* fr. *frio,* to crumble]. **1.** Easily reduced to powder. **2.** In bacteriology, denoting a dry and brittle culture falling into powder when touched or shaken.

fricative (frik'ă-tiv). Speech sound made by forcing the air stream through a narrow orifice.

friction (frik'shŭn). **1.** The act of rubbing the surface of an object against that of another; especially rubbing the limbs of the body to aid the circulation. **2.** The force required for relative motion of two bodies that are in contact.

dynamic f., the force that must be overcome to maintain steady motion of one body relative to another because they remain in contact. *Cf.* starting f.

starting f., static f.; the force that must be overcome to initiate the motion of one body relative to another because they have been resting in contact. *Cf.* dynamic f.

static f., starting f.

Fridenberg, Percy H., U.S. ophthalmologist, 1868–1960. See F.'s stigmometric card *test.*

Friderichsen, Carl, Danish physician, *1886. See Waterhouse-F. *syndrome,* F.-Waterhouse *syndrome.*

Friedländer, Carl, German pathologist, 1847–1887. See F.'s *bacillus, pneumonia, stain* (for capsules).

Friedman, Emanuel A., U.S. obstetrician, *1926. See F. *curve.*

Friedmann, Max, German neurologist, 1858–1925. See F.'s *disease.*

Friedreich, Nikolaus, German neurologist, 1825–1882. See F.'s *ataxia, disease, phenomenon, sign.*

Friend, Charlotte, U.S. microbiologist, *1921. See F. *disease, virus,* leukemia *virus.*

frigid (frij'id) [L. *frigidus,* cold]. **1.** Cold. **2.** Temperamentally, especially sexually, cold or irresponsive.

frigidity (fri-jid'i-tē). **1.** Impotence in the female. **2.** The state of being frigid (2); female sexual inadequacy ranging from the freudian concept of inability to achieve orgasm to any degree of sexual response considered unsatisfactory by either the female or her partner.

frigorific (frig-ō-rif'ik) [L. *frigus,* cold, + *facio,* to make]. Producing cold.

frigorism (frig'ō-rizm) [L. *frigus,* cold]. Cryopathy.

fringe (frinj). Fimbria (1).

cervical f., hairlike wisps or linear strands of blood vessels seen on the neck.

costal f., zona corona; an irregularly disposed collection of visible veins seen in the skin of people usually of or past middle age; it has no specific connection with any deep structure, such as the diaphragm, and no necessary connection with underlying pulmonary or cardiac disease.

Richard's f.'s, *fimbriae* tubae.

synovial f., *villi* synoviales.

frit [Fr. *frit,* fried]. **1.** The material from which the glaze for artificial teeth is made. **2.** A powdered pigment material used in coloring the porcelain of artificial teeth.

Fritsch, Heinrich, German gynecologist, 1844–1915. See Bozeman-F. *catheter.*

Froehde, A., 19th century German chemist. See F.'s *reagent.*

frog [A.S. *frogge*]. **1.** An amphibian in the order Anura, which includes the toads; the commonest frog genera are *Rana* (grass frogs) and *Hyla* (tree frogs). **2.** A specialized portion of the hoof of the horse; a wedge-shaped, horny mass lying between the bars and the sole on the ground surface of the foot.

Fröhlich, Alfred, Austrian neurologist and pharmacologist, 1871–1953. See F.'s *dwarfism, syndrome.*

Frohn, Damianus, German physician, *1843. See F.'s *reagent.*

Froin, Georges, French physician, *1874. See F.'s *syndrome.*

frôlement (frol-mon') [Fr.]. **1.** Light friction or massage with the palm of the hand. **2.** A rustling sound heard in auscultation.

Froment, Jules, Lyon physician, *1878. See F.'s *sign.*

Frommel, Richard, German gynecologist, 1854–1912. See Chiari-F. *syndrome.*

frons, gen. **frontis** (fronz, fron'tis) [L.] [NA]. Forehead; brow (2); the part of the face between the eyebrows and the hairy scalp.

frontad (frŭn'tad). Toward the front.

frontal (frŭn'tăl). **1.** In front; relating to the anterior part of a body. **2.** Frontalis.

frontalis (frŭn-tā'lis) [L.] [NA]. Frontal (2); referring to the frontal (coronal) plane or to the frontal bone or forehead.

frontomalar (frŭn'tō-mā'lăr). Frontozygomatic.

frontomaxillary (frŭn'tō-mak'si-lā-rē). Relating to the frontal and the maxillary bones.

frontonasal (frŭn'tō-nā'săl). Relating to the frontal and the nasal bones.

fronto-occipital (frŭn'tō-ok-sip'i-tăl). Relating to the frontal and the occipital bones, or to the forehead and the occiput.

frontoparietal (frŭn'tō-pa-rī'ĕ-tăl). Relating to the frontal and the parietal bones.

frontotemporal (frŭn-tō-tem'pō-răl). Relating to the frontal and the temporal bones.

frontotemporale (frŭn'tō-tem-pō-rā'lē). A craniometric point located at the most anterior point of the temporal line on the frontal bone.

frontozygomatic (frŭn'tō-zī'gō-mat'ik). Frontomalar; relating to the frontal and zygomatic bones.

Froriep, August von, German anatomist, 1849–1917. See F.'s *ganglion, induration.*

Frost, Albert D., U.S. ophthalmologist, 1889–1945. See F. *suture.*

Frost, William A., British ophthalmologist, 1853–1935. See F.-Lang *operation.*

frost. A deposit resembling that of frozen vapor or dew.

urea f., uremic f., uridrosis crystallina; powdery deposits on the skin, especially the face, of urea and uric acid salts due to excretion of nitrogenous compounds in the sweat; seen in severe uremia.

frostbite (frost'bīt). Congelation (2); dermatitis congelationis; local tissue destruction resulting from exposure to extreme cold or contact with extremely cold objects; in mild cases, it results in erythema and slight pain; in severe cases, it can be painless or paresthetic and result in blistering, deep-seated destruction, and gangrene.

frottage (frō-tahzh') [F. a rubbing]. **1.** The rubbing movement in massage. **2.** Production of sexual excitement by rubbing against someone.

frotteur (frō-tuhr'). One who gets sexual excitement through frottage.

FRS Abbreviation for first rank *symptoms.*

F.R.S. Abbreviation for Fellow of the Royal Society.

F.R.S.C. Abbreviation for Fellow of the Royal Society (Canada).

Fru Symbol for fructose.

fructo- [L. *fructus,* fruit]. Prefix indicating the fructose configuration.

fructofuranose (frŭk-tō-fūr'ă-nōs, fruk-) D-Fructose in furanose form.

β-fructofuranosidase (frŭk'tō-fūr-ă-nō-sīd'ās, fruk-) [EC 3.2.1.26]. Invertase; invertin; saccharase; β-*h*-fructosidase; an enzyme hydrolyzing β-D-fructofuranosides and releasing free fructose; if the substrate is sucrose, the product is glucose plus fructose (invert sugar).

fructokinase (frŭk-tō-kī'nās, fruk-) [EC 2.7.1.4]. A liver enzyme that catalyzes the reaction of ATP and D-fructose to form fructose 6-phosphate.

fructosan (frŭk'tō-san, fruk-). A polysaccharide of fructose (*e.g.*, inulin) containing small amounts of other sugars; present in certain tubers. Also called levan; levulin; levulan; levulosan; polyfructose.

fructose (Fru) (frŭk'tōs, fruk-). Fruit sugar; levulose; levoglucose; D-*arabino*-2-hexulose; a 2-ketohexose that in D form is physiologically the most important of the ketohexoses and one of the two products of sucrose hydrolysis, and is metabolized or converted to glycogen in the absence of insulin; used intravenously when either oral carbohydrate or fluid intake requires replacement or supplement.

fructose-bisphosphatase [EC 3.1.3.11]. Hexosebisphosphatase; hexosediphosphatase; a hydrolase that catalyses conversion of fructose 1,6-bisphosphate to fructose 6-phosphate in gluconeogenesis; AMP is an allosteric inhibitor.

fructose-bisphosphate aldolase [EC 4.1.2.13]. Fructose-diphosphate aldolase; 1-phosphofructaldolase; ketose-1-phosphate aldolase; zymohexase; fructose-1,6-bisphosphate triophosphate-lyase; an enzyme cleaving fructose 1,6-bisphosphate to dihydroxyacetone (glyceroketone) phosphate and glyceraldehyde 3-phosphate; also acts on certain ketose 1-phosphates.

fructose-diphosphate aldolase. Fructose-bisphosphate aldolase.

fructosemia (frŭk-tō-sē'mē-ă, fruk-). Levulosemia; presence of fructose in the circulating blood. See also hereditary fructose *intolerance.*

fructoside (frŭk'tō-sīd, fruk'). Fructose in -C-O- linkage where the -C-O- group is the original 2 group of the fructose.

fructosuria (frŭk-tō-sū'rē-ă, fruk-) [fructose + G. *ouron,* urine]. Levulosuria; excretion of fructose in the urine.
essential f., a benign, asymptomatic metabolic abnormality due to deficiency of fructokinase, the first enzyme in the specific fructose pathway; fructose appears in the blood and urine, but is simply excreted unchanged; autosomal recessive inheritance. See also hereditary fructose *intolerance.*

fructosyl-. Prefix indicating fructose in -C-R- (not -C-O-R-) linkage through its carbon-2 (R usually C).

frusemide (frū'sĕ-mīd). Furosemide.

frustration (frŭs'trā'shŭn) [L. *frustro,* pp. *-atus,* to deceive, disappoint, fr. *frustra* (adv.), in vain]. A psychologic or psychiatric term indicating the thwarting of or inability to gratify a desire or to satisfy an urge or need.

FSH Abbreviation for follicle-stimulating *hormone.*

FSH-RF Abbreviation for follicle-stimulating hormone-releasing *factor.*

FSH-RH Abbreviation for follicle-stimulating hormone-releasing *hormone.*

ft. Abbreviation for L. *fiat,* let it be done (made).

FTI Abbreviation for free thyroxine *index.*

Fuchs, Ernst, Austrian ophthalmologist, 1851–1930. See F.'s *adenoma, coloboma,* epithelial *dystrophy, uveitis,* black *spot, spur, stomas, syndrome;* Dalen-F. *nodules; angle* of F., *dellen* of F.

fuchsin (fuk'sin) [Leonhard *Fuchs,* German botantist, 1501–1506]. A nonspecific term referring to any of several red rosanilin dyes used as stains in histology and bacteriology.
acid f. [C.I. 42685], rubin s; a mixture of the sodium salts bi- and trisulfonic acids of rosanilin and pararosanilin; used as an indicator dye and for staining of cytoplasm and collagen.
aldehyde f., a stain developed by Gomori, utilizing basic f. paraldehyde and hydrochloric acid; it produces violet staining of elastic fibers, mast cell granules, gastric chief cells, beta cells of the pancreatic islets, and certain hypophyseal beta granules; other pituitary granules and cells stain in other colors. See also Gomori's aldehyde fuchsin *stain.*
aniline f., a mixture of aniline and basic f. in 30% ethanol with a trace of phenol, as in Goodpasture's stain.
basic f. [C.I. 42500], diamond f.; a triphenylmethane dye whose dominant component is pararosanilin; an important stain in histology, histochemistry, and bacteriology.
carbol f., (1) see carbol-fuchsin *paint;* **(2)** see Ziehl's *stain.*
diamond f., basic f.

fuchsinophil (fuk'si-nō-fil) [fuchsin + G. *philos,* fond]. **1.** Fuchsinophilic; staining readily with fuchsin dyes. **2.** A cell or histologic element that stains readily with fuchsin.

fuchsinophilia (fuk'si-nō-fil'ē-ă). The property of staining readily with fuchsin.

fuchsinophilic (fuk'si-nō-fil'ik). Fuchsinophil (1).

fucose (fyū'kōs). Rhodeose; 6-deoxygalactose; a methylpentose, the L-configuration of which occurs in the mucopolysaccharides of the blood group substances, in human milk (as a polysaccharide), and elsewhere in nature.

fucosidosis (fyū'kō-sī-dō'sis). A metabolic storage disease characterized by accumulation of fucose-containing glycolipids and deficiency of the enzyme α-fucosidase; progressive neurologic deterioration begins after the first year of life, accompanied by spasticity, tremor, and mild skeletal changes; autosomal recessive inheritance.

FUDR Abbreviation for fluorodeoxyuridine. See floxuridine.

Fuerstner, Carl German psychiatrist, 1848–1906. See F.'s *disease.*

fugacity (fū-gas'i-tē) [L. *fuga,* flight]. The tendency of the molecules in a fluid, as a result of all forces acting on them, to leave a given site in the body; the escaping tendency of a fluid, as in diffusion, evaporation, etc.

-fugal [L. *fugio,* to flee]. Suffix denoting movement away from the part indicated by the main portion of the word.

-fuge [L. *fuga,* flight]. Suffix meaning flight, denoting the place from which flight takes place or that which is put to flight.

fugitive (fyū'ji-tiv) [L. *fugitivus,* fleeing, fr. *fugio,* pp. *fugitus,* to flee]. **1.** Temporary; transient. **2.** Wandering; fleeting; denoting certain inconstant symptoms.

fugue (fūg) [Fr. fr. L. *fuga,* flight]. A condition in which an individual suddenly abandons a present activity or lifestyle and starts a new and different one for a period of time; afterward, the individual alleges amnesia for events occurring during the f. period, although earlier events are remembered and habits and skills are usually unaffected.

fugutoxin (fū'gū-tok-sin). The potent poison derived from the ovaries and skin of the Pacific pufferfish.

fulcrum, pl. **fulcra, fulcrums** (ful'krŭm, -kră, -krŭmz) [L. a bedpost, fr. *fulcio,* to prop up]. A support or the point thereon on which a lever turns.

fulgurant (ful'gŭ-rănt) [L. *fulgur,* flashing lightning]. Fulgurating (1); sharp and piercing. *Cf.* fulminant.

fulgurating (ful'gŭ-rā-ting). **1.** Fulgurant. **2.** Relating to fulguration.

fulguration (ful-gŭ-rā'shŭn) [L. *fulgur,* lightning stroke]. Destruction of tissue by means of a high-frequency electric current: **direct f.** utilizes an insulated electrode with a metal point, which is connected to the uniterminal of the high-frequency apparatus, from which a spark of electricity is allowed to impinge on the area to be treated; **indirect f.** involves directly connecting the patient by a metal handle to the uniterminal and utilizing an active electrode to complete an arc from the patient.

fulminant (ful'mi-nănt) [L. *fulmino*, pp. *-atus*, to hurl lightning, fr. *fulmen*, lightning]. Occurring suddenly, with lightning-like rapidity, and with great intensity or severity; applied to certain pains, *e.g.*, those of tabes dorsalis. *Cf.* fulgurant.

fulminating (ful'mi-nā'ting). Running a speedy course, with rapid worsening.

fumarase (fyū'mă-rās). Fumarate hydratase.

fumarate hydratase (fyū'mă-rāt) [EC 4.2.1.2]. Fumarase; an enzyme catalyzing the interconversion of fumaric acid and malic acid, a reaction of importance in the tricarboxylic acid cycle.

fumarate reductase. *Succinate* dehydrogenase.

fumarate reductase (NADH) [EC 1.3.1.6]. An oxidoreductase catalyzing the reduction of fumarate to succinate.

fumaric acid (fyū-mar'ik). Allomaleic or boletic acid; *trans*-butanedioic acid; an unsaturated dicarboxylic acid occurring as an intermediate in the tricarboxylic acid cycle.

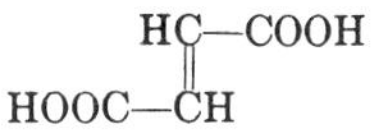

Fumaric acid

fumaric aminase. *Aspartate* ammonia-lyase.

fumaric hydrogenase. *Succinate* dehydrogenase.

fumigant (fyū'mi-gănt) [see fumigate]. Any vaporous substance used as a disinfectant or pesticide.

fumigate (fyū'mi-gāt) [L. *fumigo* pp. *-atus*, to fumigate, fr. *fumus*, smoke, + *ago*, to drive]. To expose to the action of smoke or of fumes of any kind as a means of disinfection or eradication.

fumigation (fyū-mi-gā'shŭn). The act of fumigating; the use of a fumigant.

fuming (fyūm'ing) [L. *fumus*, smoke]. Giving forth a visible vapor, a property of concentrated nitric, sulfuric, and hydrochloric acids, and certain other substances.

functio laesa (fŭngk'shē-ō lē'să) [L.]. Loss of function; a fifth sign of inflammation added by Galen to those enunciated by Celsus (rubor, tumor, calor, and dolor).

function (fŭngk'shŭn) [L. *functio*, fr. *fungor*, pp. *functus*, to perform]. **1.** The special action or physiologic property of an organ or other part of the body. **2.** To perform its special work or office, said of an organ or other part of the body. **3.** The general properties of any substance, depending on its chemical character and relation to other substances, according to which it may be grouped among acids, bases, alcohols, esters, etc. **4.** A particular reactive grouping in a molecule; *e.g.*, a functional group, such as the –OH group of an alcohol.

allomeric f., the combined f. of the several segments of the spinal cord and medulla, communicating with each other by means of the white matter.

arousal f., the ability of a sensory event to arouse the cortex to vigilance or readiness.

atrial transport f., the role of the atria in filling and stretching the ventricles by their presystolic contraction, without which the force of ventricular contraction and the cardiac output may significantly decrease.

discriminant f., a particular combination of continous variable test results designed to achieve separation of groups; *e.g.*, a single number representing a combination of weighted laboratory test results designed to discriminate between clinical classes.

isomeric f., the individual f. of an isolated segment of the spinal cord.

modulation transfer f. (MTF), in depicting radionuclide distribution or radiographic systems, the efficiency, at a given spatial frequency, of transferring the modulation of the object to that of the image; it is a more complete expression of spatial resolution and is used to evaluate imaging systems and their components.

functional (fŭnk'shŭn-ăl). **1.** Relating to a function. **2.** Not organic in origin; denoting a disorder with no known or detectable organic basis to explain the symptoms.

functionalism (fŭnk'shŭn-ăl-ism). A branch of psychology concerned with the function of mental processes in man and animals, especially the role of the mind, intellect, emotions, and behavior in an individual's adaptation to his environment. *Cf.* structuralism.

function corrector. A removable orthodontic appliance utilizing oral and facial muscle forces to move teeth and possibly change the relationship of the dental arches.

fundament (fŭn'dă-ment) [L. *fundamentum*, foundation, fr. *fundus*, bottom]. **1.** A foundation. **2.** The anus.

fundectomy (fŭn-dek'tō-mē) [fundus + G. *ektomē*, excision]. Fundusectomy.

fundic (fŭn'dik). Relating to a fundus.

fundiform (fŭn'di-fōrm) [L. *funda*, a sling, + *forma*, shape]. Looped; sling-shaped.

fundoplication (fŭn'dō-pli-kā'shŭn) [fundus + L. *plico*, to fold]. Nissen's operation; suture of the fundus of the stomach around the esophagus to prevent reflux in repair of hiatal hernia.

Fundulus (fŭn'dŭ-lŭs) [Mod. L. fr. L. *fundus*, bottom]. A genus of marine and freshwater fish, of many species, native to the U.S.; commonly called killifish, mumichog, or mudfish. They are widely used as bait fish, experimental fish, or in mosquito-control programs.

fundus, pl. fundi (fŭn'dŭs, dī) [L. bottom] [NA]. Bas-fond; the bottom or lowest part of a sac or hollow organ; that part farthest removed from the opening or exit; occasionally a broad cul-de-sac.

f. albipuncta'tus, a nonprogressive disorder of the retinal pigment epithelium characterized by numerous discrete, white dots.

f. diabet'icus, the retinal involvement of capillary microaneurysms, hemorrhages, deposits, and neovascularization, occurring in diabetes mellitus.

f. flavimacula'tus, a genetic disorder of the pigment epithelium of the retina manifested by yellowish white flecks.

f. of gallbladder, f. vesicae felleae.

f. of internal acoustic (auditory) meatus, f. meatus acustici interni.

leopard f., tessellated f.

f. mea'tus acus'tici inter'ni [NA], f. of the internal acoustic (auditory) meatus; the thin cribriform plate of bone separating the cochlea and vestibule from the internal acoustic meatus; a transverse crest divides it into two regions; in the superior region are located the area nervi facialis and the area vestibularis superior; in the inferior region are located the area cochleae, area vestibularis inferior, and foramen singulare.

f. oc'uli, the portion of the interior of the eyeball around the posterior pole, visible through the ophthalmoscope. See eyegrounds.

pepper and salt f., ophthalmoscopic appearance of the f. caused by choriocapillaris atrophy and pigment proliferation.

f. polycythe'micus, the engorged, dilated veins, with cyanotic retina, occurring in erythremia.

f. of stomach, f. ventriculi.

tessellated f., f. tigré, leopard or tigroid f. or retina; a normal f. to which a deeply pigmented choroid gives the appearance of dark polygonal areas between the choroidal vessels, especially in the periphery.

f. tigré, tessellated f.

tigroid f., tessellated f.

f. tym'pani, *paries* jugularis cavi tympani.
f. of urinary bladder, f. vesicae urinariae.
f. u'teri [NA], f. of the uterus; the upper rounded extremity of the uterus above the openings of the uterine (fallopian) tubes.
f. of uterus, f. uteri.
f. ventric'uli [NA], f. of the stomach; greater cul-de-sac; the portion of the stomach that lies above the cardiac notch.
f. vesi'cae fel'leae [NA], f. of the gallbladder; the wide closed end of the gallbladder situated at the inferior border of the liver.
f. vesi'cae urina'riae [NA], f. of the urinary bladder; base of bladder; the f. is formed by the posterior wall which is somewhat convex.

funduscope (fŭn'dŭs-skōp) [L. *fundus,* bottom, + G. *skopeō,* to view]. Ophthalmoscope.

funduscopy (fŭn-dŭs'kŏ-pē). Ophthalmoscopy.

fundusectomy (fŭn-dŭ-sek'tō-mē) [L. *fundus,* cardia, + G. *ektomē,* excision]. Fundectomy; excision of the fundus of an organ.

fungal (fŭng'găl). Fungous.

fungate (fŭng'gāt). To grow exuberantly like a fungus or spongy growth.

fungemia (fŭn-jē'mē-ă). Fungal infection disseminated by way of the bloodstream.

fungi (fŭn'jī). Plural of fungus.

Fungi (fŭn'jī) [L. *fungus,* a mushroom]. A division of eukaryotic organisms that grow in irregular masses, without roots, stems, or leaves, and are devoid of chlorophyll or other pigments capable of photosynthesis. Each organism (thallus) is unicellular to filamentous, and possesses branched somatic structures (hyphae) surrounded by cell walls containing cellulose or chitin or both, and containing true nuclei. They reproduce sexually or asexually (spore formation), and may obtain nutrition from other living organisms as parasites or from dead organic matter as saprobes (saprophytes).

fungicidal (fŭn-ji-sī'dăl) [fungus + L. *caedo,* to kill]. Having a killing action on fungi.

fungicide (fŭn'ji-sīd). Mycocide; any substance that has a destructive killing action upon fungi.

fungicidin (fŭn-ji-sī'din). Nystatin.

fungiform (fŭn'ji-fōrm). Fungilliform; shaped like a fungus or mushroom; applied to any structure with a broad, often branched, free portion and a narrower base.

Fungi Imperfecti (fŭn'jī im-per-fek'tī). Deuteromycetes; a class of fungi in which sexual reproduction is not known or in which one of the mating types has not yet been discovered. Formerly, most fungi causing disease in man were considered asexual and were placed in this class, but studies have revealed that they are not imperfect and that in their sexual forms they can be classified as ascomycetes or basidiomycetes.

fungilliform (fŭn-jil'i-fōrm) [Mod L. *fungillus,* dim. of L. *fungus*]. Fungiform.

fungistatic (fŭn-ji-stat'ik) [fungus + G. *statos,* standing]. Mycostatic; having an inhibiting action upon the growth of fungi.

fungitoxic (fŭn-ji-tok'sik). Poisonous or in any way deleterious to the growth of fungi.

fungitoxicity (fŭn'ji-tok-sis'i-tē). The property of being fungitoxic.

fungoid (fŭng'goyd). Resembling a fungus; denoting an exuberant morbid growth on the surface of the body.

fungosity (fŭng-gos'i-tē). A fungoid growth.

fungous (fŭng'gŭs). Fungal; relating to a fungus.

fungus, pl. fungi (fŭng'gŭs, fŭn'jī) [L. *fungus,* a mushroom]. A general term used to encompass the diverse morphological forms of yeasts and molds. Originally classified as primitive plants without chlorophyll, the fungi are being placed increasingly in the kingdom protista, along with the algae (all but the blue-green algae), the protozoa, and the slime molds. Fungi share with bacteria the important ability to break down complex organic substances of almost every type (cellulose) and are essential to the recycling of carbon and other elements in the cycle of life. Fungi are important as foods and to the fermentation process in the development of substances of industrial and medical importance, including alcohol, the antibiotics, other drugs, and antitoxins. Relatively few fungi are pathogenic for man, whereas most plant diseases are caused by fungi.
f. cer'ebri, an ulcerated cerebral hernia with granulation tissue protruding from scalp wound.
fission fungi, Schizomycetes.
imperfect f., a f. in which the means of sexual reproduction is not yet recognized; these fungi generally reproduce by means of conidia.
mosaic f., rarely used term for intercellular deposits of cholesterol in scrapings from skin lesions thought to resemble the branching of fungi.
perfect f., a f. possessing both sexual and asexual means of reproduction, and in which both mating forms are recognized.
ray f., a bacterium which is a member of the order Actinomycetales.
slime f., see mycetozoa.
thrush f., *Candida albicans.*
umbilical f., a mass of granulation tissue on the stump of the umbilical cord in the newborn.
yeast f., obsolete term for *Saccharomyces.*

funic (few'nik). Funicular; relating to the funis, or umbilical cord.

funicle (fyū'ni-kl). Funiculus.

funicular (fyū-nik'yū-lăr). **1.** Relating to a funiculus. **2.** Funic.

funiculitis (fyū-nik'yū-lī'tis) [funiculus + G. *-itis,* inflammation]. **1.** Inflammation of a funiculus, especially of the spermatic cord. **2.** Inflammation of that portion of a spinal nerve that lies within the intervertebral canal.
endemic f., filarial f.
filarial f., endemic f.; cellulitis of the spermatic cord due to filariasis; occurs endemically in Sri Lanka and Egypt, and probably elsewhere in the East.

funiculopexy (fyū-nik'yū-lō-pek-sē) [funiculus + G. *pēxis,* a fixing]. Suturing of the spermatic cord to the surrounding tissue in the correction of an undescended testicle.

funiculus, pl. funiculi (fyū-nik'yū-lŭs, -lī) [L. dim. of *funis,* cord] [NA]. Funicle; a small, cordlike structure composed of several to many longitudinally oriented fibers, vessels, ducts, or combinations thereof.
f. am'nii, amniotic cord found in several domestic animals.
anterior f., f. anterior.
f. ante'rior [NA], anterior f.; anterior white column of spinal cord; a column or bundle of white matter on either side of the anterior median fissure, between that and the anterolateral sulcus.
cuneate f., *fasciculus* cuneatus.
dorsal f., f. posterior.
f. dorsa'lis, f. posterior.
f. gra'cilis, *fasciculus* gracilis.
lateral f. of spinal cord, f. lateralis.
f. latera'lis [NA], lateral f. of spinal cord; anterolateral column of spinal cord; the lateral white column of the spinal cord between the lines of exit and entrance of the anterior and posterior nerve roots.
funic'uli medu'lae spina'lis [NA], any of the columns of the spinal cord.
posterior f., f. posterior.
f. poste'rior [NA], dorsal or posterior f.; f. dorsalis; posterior white column of the spinal cord, the large wedge-shaped fiber bun-

dle lying between the posterior gray column and the posterior median septum, and composed largely of dorsal root fibers.

f. sep'arans, an oblique ridge in the floor of the fourth ventricle of the brain, separating the area postrema from the ala cinerea, or trigonum vagi.

f. solita'rius, *tractus* solitarius.

f. spermat'icus [NA], spermatic cord; chorda spermatica; testicular cord; the cord formed by the ductus deferens and its associated structures extending from the deep inguinal ring through the inguinal canal into the scrotum.

f. te'res, *eminentia* medialis.

f. umbilica'lis [NA], umbilical cord; chorda umbilicalis; funis (1); the definitive connecting stalk between the embryo or fetus and the placenta; at birth it consists of Wharton's jelly in which the umbilical vessels are embedded.

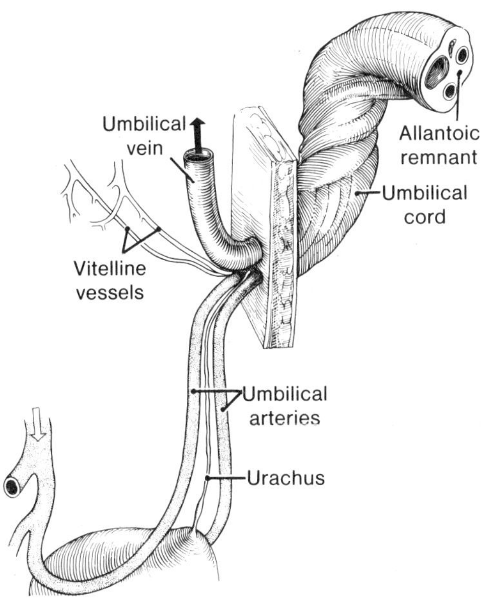

Funiculus Umbilicalis (Umbilical Cord)

funiform (fyū'ni-fōrm) [L. *funis,* cord, + *forma,* shape]. Ropelike.

funis (fyū'nis) [L. a rope, cord]. **1.** *Funiculus* umbilicalis. **2.** A cordlike structure.

funnel (fŭn'ĕl). **1.** A hollow conical vessel with a tube of variable length proceeding from its apex, used in pouring fluids from one container to another, in filtering, etc. **2.** In anatomy, an infundibulum.

Buchner f., a porcelain f. that contains a perforated porcelain plate upon which filter paper can be laid.

Martegiani's f., Martegiani's area; the funnel-shaped dilation of the posterior extremity of the hyaloid canal.

pial f., the pia-lined channel in which each blood vessel entering the brain lies suspended; essentially, the pial f.'s are perivascular extensions of the subarachnoid space.

FUO Abbreviation for fever of unknown origin.

fur (fer). **1.** The coat of soft, fine hair of some mammals. **2.** A layer of epithelium, mucus, and debris on the dorsum of the tongue. Its relation to underlying disease or disturbance of the alimentary canal is not proved.

furaltadone (fyū-ral'tă-dōn). Furmethonol; nitrofurmethone; a complex morpholino-furfuryl-oxazolidone; an antibacterial agent.

furan (fyūr'an). A cyclic compound found, usually in saturated form, in those sugars with an oxygen bridge between carbon atoms 1 and 4, or 2 and 5, or 3 and 7, for which reason they are known as furanoses.

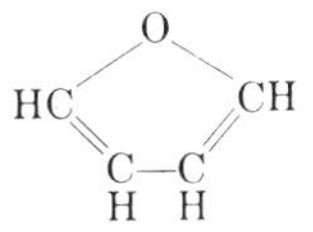

Furan

furanose (fyūr'ă-nōs) [furan + -ose(1)]. A saccharide unit or molecule containing the furan grouping; specific examples are preceded by prefixes indicating the configuration, *e.g.,* fructofuranose, ribofuranose.

furazolidone (fyū-ră-zol'i-dōn). 3-(5-Nitro-2-furfurylideneamino)-2-oxazolidione; has antibacterial and antiprotozoal activity against enteric organisms; used in the treatment of bacterial enteritis and diarrhea, and topically in vaginal trichomonal infections.

furcal (fer'kăl). Forked.

furcation (fŭr-kā'shŭn) [L. *furca,* fork]. **1.** A forking, or a forklike part or branch. **2.** In dental histology, the region of a multirooted tooth at which the roots divide.

furcula (fer'kyū-lă) [L. a forked prop, dim. of *furca,* a fork]. **1.** The fused clavicles which form V-shaped bone (wishbone) of the bird's skeleton. **2.** In the embryo, an inverted U-shaped elevation that appears on the ventral wall of the pharynx, being formed by the two linear ridges and the caudal part of the hypobranchial eminence; the depression enclosed by the U is the laryngotracheal groove.

furfur, pl. **furfures** (fer'fer, fer'fyū-rēz) [L. bran]. An epidermal scale; *e.g.,* dandruff.

furfuraceous (fer-fyū-rā'shŭs) [L. *furfuraceus,* fr. *furfur,* bran]. Pityroid; branny, or composed of small scales; denoting a form of desquamation.

furfural (fer'fyūr-ăl). C_4H_3O-CHO; C_4H_3O-CHO; a colorless, aromatic, irritating fluid obtained in the distillation of bran with dilute sulfuric acid; used in the manufacture of medicinal agents.

furfurol (fer'fyūr-ol). Misnomer for furfural and furfuryl alcohol.

furfuryl (fer'fyū-ril). The monovalent radical derived from f. alcohol by loss of the OH group.

f. alcohol, 2-furanmethanol; 2-hydroxymethylfuran; a solvent and wetting agent.

furnace (fŭr'năs). A stovelike apparatus containing a chamber for heating, melting, or fusing.

dental f., **(1)** a f. used to eliminate the wax pattern from the investment mold prior to casting in gold or semiprecious metal; **(2)** a f. used to fuse and glaze dental porcelains.

muffle f., **(1)** an electric f. heated by direct transfer of heat from a resistant muffle; **(2)** a dental f. heated by a muffle.

furor epilepticus (fyū'rōr ep-i-lep'ti-kŭs). Attacks of anger to which epileptic individuals are occasionally subject, occurring without apparent provocation and without disturbance of consciousness.

furosemide (fyū-rō'sĕ-mid, -mīd). Frusemide; 4-chloro-*N*-furfuryl-5-sulfamoylanthranilic acid; a diuretic.

furrow (fer'rō) [A.S. *furh*] A groove or sulcus.

digital f., one of the grooves on the palmar surface of a finger, at the level of an interphalangeal joint.

genital f., a groove on the genital tubercle in the embryo, appearing toward the end of the second month.

gluteal f., *sulcus* gluteus.

mentolabial f., *sulcus* mentolabialis.

primitive f., the groove in the primitive streak.

Fürth, Otto von, German physician, *1867. See F.'s *myosin.*

furuncle (fyū'rŭng-kl) [L. *furunculus,* a petty thief]. Furunculus;

boil; a localized pyogenic infection originating in a hair follicle.

furuncular (fyū-rŭng'kyū-lăr). Furunculous; relating to a furuncle.

furunculoid (fyū-rŭng'kyū-loyd) [furunculus + G. *eidos,* resemblance]. Resembling a furuncle.

furunculosis (fyū-rŭng-kyū-lō'sis). A condition marked by the presence of furuncles.

f. orienta'lis, the lesion occurring in cutaneous leishmaniasis.

furunculous (fyū-rŭng'kyū-lŭs). Furuncular.

furunculus, pl. furunculi (fyū-rŭng'kyū-lŭs, -lī) [L. a petty thief, a boil, dim. of *fur,* a thief]. Furuncle.

Fusarium (fyū-zā'rē-ŭm) [L. *fusus,* spindle]. A genus of rapidly growing fungi producing characteristic sickle-shaped, multiseptate macroconidia which can be mistaken for those produced by some dermatophytes. Usually saprobic, a few species such as *F. oxysporum* and *F. solani* can produce corneal ulcers; some species are common colonizers of burned skin.

fusel oil (fyū'zel). A mixture, in varying proportions, of amyl, butyl, hexyl, and propyl alcohols; present in newly distilled spirits.

fusidate sodium (fyū'si-dāt). Sodium fusidate; the sodium salt of fusidic acid; has antibacterial properties.

fusidic acid (fyū-sid'ik). Ramycin; 3α,11α,16β-trihydroxy-4α,8,14-trimethyl-18-nor-5α,8α,9β,13α,14β-cholesta-17(20),24-dien-21-oic 16-acetate; a fermentation product of *Fusidium coccineum,* a parasitic fungus on the plant *Veronica.* See fusidate sodium.

fusiform (fyū'zi-fōrm, fyū'si-) [L. *fusus,* a spindle, + *forma,* form]. Spindle-shaped; tapering at both ends.

Fusiformis (fyū-si-fōr'mis) [see fusiform]. An obsolete generic name sometimes used for the anaerobic fusiform bacteria found in the human mouth; these organisms are closely related to the anaerobic organisms found in the human intestine and have been placed in the genus *Fusobacterium.*

fusimotor (fyū'zē-mō'ter) [L. *fusus,* spindle, + *movere,* to move]. Pertaining to the efferent innervation of intrafusal muscle fibers by gamma motor neurons. See also neuromuscular *spindle.*

fusion (fyū'zhŭn) [L. *fusio,* a pouring, fr. *fundo,* pp. *fusus,* to pour]. **1.** Liquefaction, as by melting by heat. **2.** Union, as by joining together. **3.** The blending of slightly different images from each eye into a single perception. **4.** The joining of two or more adjacent teeth during their development by a dentinal union. See also concresence.

cell f., the merging of the contents of two cells by artificial means without the destruction of either, resulting in a heterokaryon that, for at least a few generations, will reproduce its kind; an important method in assignment of loci to chromosomes.

centric f., robertsonian *translocation.*

flicker f., see critical flicker-fusion *frequency.*

nuclear f., the formation of more complex atomic nuclei from less complex nuclei with release of energy, as in the formation of helium nuclei from hydrogen nuclei (hydrogen f.).

spinal f., spine f., vertebral f.; spondylosyndesis; an operative procedure to accomplish bone ankylosis between two or more vertebrae.

vertebral f., spinal f.

Fusobacterium (fyū'zō-bak-tēr'ē-ŭm) [L. *fusus,* a spindle, + bacterium]. A genus of bacteria (family Bacteroidaceae) containing Gram-negative, nonsporeforming, obligately anaerobic rods which produce butyric acid as a major metabolic product. Nonmotile and motile organisms occur; motile cells are peritrichous. These organisms are found in cavities of man and other animals; some species are pathogenic. The type species is *F. nucleatum.*

F. fusifor'me, F. nucleatum.

F. mortif'erum, *Sphaerophorus mortiferus;* a species found in various infections in man.

F. necropho'rum, *Sphaerophorus necrophorus;* necrosis bacillus; Schmorl's bacillus; a species causing or associated with several necrotic conditions in animals, such as calf diphtheria, labial necrosis of rabbits, necrotic rhinitis of pigs, foot rot of cattle, sheep, and goats, and occasionally necrotic lesions in man; it is the type species of *F.*

F. nuclea'tum, *F. fusiforme;* a species (probably Plaut's or Vincent's bacillus) found in the mouth and in infections of the upper respiratory tract, pleural cavity, and occasionally the lower intestinal tract; it is the type species of the genus *F.*

F. plau'ti, a species found in the buccal cavity; also found in cultures of *Entamoeba histolytica.*

fusocellular (fyū'zō-sel'yū-lăr). Spindle-celled.

fusospirochetal (fyū-zō-spī-rō-kē'tăl). Referring to the associated fusiform and spirochetal organisms such as those found in the lesions of Vincent's angina.

fustic (fŭs'tik). A complex of natural dyes derived from certain West Indian, Central, and South American trees, *Rhus cotinus* and *Chlorophora tinctoria;* used as mordant dyes for textiles. An important dye in the complex is morin, which is associated with the dye maclurin.

fustigation (fŭs'ti-gā'shŭn) [L. *fustigo,* pp. *-atus,* to beat with a cudgel]. A form of massage consisting in beating the surface with light rods.

Futcher's line. See under line.

FVC Abbreviation for forced vital *capacity.*

Fy blood group. See Duffy blood group, Blood Groups appendix.

G

γ **1.** Third letter in the Greek alphabet, gamma. **2.** In chemistry, denotes the third in a series, the fourth carbon in an aliphatic acid, or position 2 removed from the α position in the benzene ring. **3.** Symbol for 10^{-4} gauss. For terms having this prefix, see the specific term.

γ-Abu Abbreviation for γ-aminobutyric acid.

G Abbreviation or symbol for newtonian *constant* of gravitation or gravitational *unit;* gap (3) gauss; giga-; glucose, as in UDPG; guanosine, as in GDP.

G Symbol for Gibbs free *energy.*

g Abbreviation for gram.

g Unit of acceleration based on the acceleration produced by the earth's gravitational attraction, where $1\,g = 980.6$ cm/sec^2 (about 32 ft./sec^2) at sea level and 45° latitude.

Ga Symbol for gallium.

GABA Abbreviation for γ-aminobutyric acid.

G acid. 2-Naphthol-6,8-disulfonic acid.

G-actin. See under actin.

Gaddum, John H., British biochemist, *1900. See G.-Schild *test.*

gadfly (gad'flī). See *Tabanus.*

gadoleic acid (gad-ō-lē'ik). 9-Eicosenoic acid; an unsaturated fatty acid from cod liver oil and other sources.

gadolinium (gad-ō-lin'ē-ŭm) [Johan *Gadolin,* Finnish chemist, 1760–1852]. An element of the lanthanide group, symbol Gd, atomic no. 64, atomic weight 157.25.

Gaenslen, Frederick J., U.S. surgeon, 1877–1937. See G.'s *sign.*

Gaffky, Georg T.A., German hygienist, 1850–1918. See G. *scale, table.*

gag. **1.** To retch; to cause to retch or heave. **2.** To prevent from talking. **3.** An instrument adjusted between the teeth to keep the mouth from closing during operations in the mouth or throat.
Davis-Crowe mouth g., instrument used for opening the mouth, depressing the tongue, maintaining the airway, and transmitting volatile anesthetics during tonsillectomy or oropharyngeal surgery.

gage (gāj). Gauge.

gain (gān). Increase; profit; advantage.
primary g., alleviation of anxiety derived from the conversion of emotional concerns into demonstrably organic illnesses (*e.g.,* hysterical blindness or paralysis). *Cf.* secondary g.
secondary g., interpersonal or social advantages (*e.g.,* assistance, attention, sympathy) gained indirectly from organic illness. *Cf.* primary g.
time compensation g. (TCG), time-varied gain *control.*
time-varied g. (TVG), time-varied gain *control.*

Gairdner, Sir William T., Scottish physician, 1824–1907. See G.'s *disease.*

Gaisböck, Felix, German physician, 1868–1955. See G.'s *syndrome.*

gait (gāt). Manner of walking.
antalgic g., a characteristic g. resulting from pain on weightbearing in which the stance phase of g. is shortened on the affected side.
ataxic g., an unsteady, staggering, or irregular g.
calcaneal g., a g. disturbance due to paralysis of the calf muscles, seen following poliomyelitis and in some other neurologic diseases.
cerebellar g., a staggering g., often with a tendency to fall to one or other side, forward or backward.
Charcot's g., the g. of hereditary ataxia.
equine g., high steppage g.
festinating g., see festination.
gluteus maximus g., compensatory backward propulsion of trunk to maintain center of gravity over support.
gluteus medius g., compensatory list of body (or throw of trunk) to weak gluteal side, to put center of gravity over the femur.
helicopod g., helicopodia; a g., seen in some conversion reactions or hysterical disorders, in which the feet describe half circles.
hemiplegic g., the walk of hemiplegics characterized by swinging the affected leg in a half circle.
high steppage g., equine g.; a g. in which the foot is raised high to avoid catching a drooping foot and brought down suddenly in a flapping manner; often seen in peroneal nerve palsy and tabes.
scissor g., one leg swings across the other instead of straight forward, producing a criss-cross motion of the legs in walking, with the foot imprints reversed.
spastic g., a g. characterized by stiffness of legs, feet, and toes.
steppage g., see high steppage g.

Gal Symbol for galactose.

galact-. See galacto-.

galactacrasia (gă-lak'tă-krā'zē-ă) [galact- + G. *akrasia,* bad mixture, fr. *a-* priv. + *krasis,* a mixing]. Abnormal composition of mother's milk.

galactagogue (gă-lak'tă-gog) [galact- + G. *agōgos,* leading]. An agent that promotes the secretion and flow of milk.

galactans (gă-lak'tanz). Galactosans; polymers of galactose occurring naturally, along with galacturonans and arabans, in pectins.

galactic (gă-lak'tik). Pertaining to milk; promoting the flow of milk.

galactidrosis (gă-lak-ti-drō'sis) [galact- + G. *hidrōs,* sweat, + *-osis,* condition]. Sweating of a milky fluid.

galacto- galact- [G. *gala,* milk]. Combining forms indicating milk.

galactoblast (gă-lak'tō-blast) [galacto- + *blastos,* germ]. Colostrum *corpuscle.*

galactobolic (gă-lak-tō-bol'ik) [galacto- + G. *bole,* throwing]. Causing the release or ejection of milk from the breast.

galactocele (gă-lak'tō-sēl) [galacto- + G. *kēlē,* tumor]. Lactocele; retention cyst caused by occlusion of a lactiferous duct.

galactogen (gă-lak'tō-jen) [galacto- + G. *-gen,* producing]. A polysaccharide containing galactose in various forms.

galactokinase (gă-lak-tō-kī'nās) [EC 2.7.1.6]. An enzyme (phosphotransferase) that, in the presence of ATP, catalyzes the phosphorylation of galactose to galactose 1-phosphate, the first step in the metabolism of galactose.

galactolipid, galactolipin (gă-lak-tō-lip'id, -lip'in). Cerebroside.

galactometer (gal'ak-tom'ĕ-ter) [galacto- + G. *metron,* measure]. Lactometer; a form of hydrometer for determining the specific gravity of milk as an indication of its fat content.

galactophagous (gal'ak-tof'ă-gŭs) [galacto- + G. *phagein,* to eat]. Subsisting on milk.

galactophore (gă-lak'tō-fōr) [galacto- + G. *phoros,* bearing]. *Ductus* lactiferi.

galactophoritis (gă-lak'tō-fō-rī'tis) Inflammation of the milk ducts.

galactophorous (gal-ak-tof'ŏ-rŭs). Conveying milk.

galactopoiesis (gă-lak'tō-poy-ē'sis) [galacto- + G. *poiesis,* forming]. Milk production.

galactopoietic (gă-lak'tō-poy-et'ik). Pertaining to galactopoiesis.

galactopyranose (gă-lak-tō-pir'ă-nōs). D-Galactose in pyranose form.

galactorrhea (gă-lak-tō-rē′ă) [galacto- + G. *rhoia,* a flow]. Lactorrhea; incontinence of milk. **1.** Any white discharge from the nipple that is persistent and looks like milk. **2.** Continued discharge of milk from the breasts between intervals of nursing or after the child has been weaned.

galactosamine (gă-lak-tō-sam′ēn). Chondrosamine; the 2-amino-2-deoxy derivative of galactose, NH_2 replacing the 2-OH group; occurs in various mucopolysaccharides, notably of chondroitin sulfuric acid and of B blood group substance.

galactosaminoglycan (gă-lak′tōs-am-i-nō-glī′kan). See mucopolysaccharide.

galactosans (gă-lak′tō-sanz). Galactans.

galactoscope (gă-lak′tō-skōp) [galacto- + G. *skopeō,* to examine]. Lactoscope; an instrument for judging of the richness and purity of milk by the translucency of a thin layer.

galactose (Gal) (gă-lak′tōs). Cerebrogalactose; cerebrose; brain sugar; a hexose found (in D form) as a constituent of lactose, cerebrosides, mucoproteins, etc., in galactoside or galactosyl combination

galactosemia (gă-lak-tō-sē′mē-ă) [galactose + G. *haima,* blood]. Galactose diabetes; an inborn error of galactose metabolism due to congenital deficiency of the enzyme galactosyl-1-phosphate uridyltransferase, resulting in tissue accumulation of galactose 1-phosphate; manifested by nutritional failure, hepatosplenomegaly with cirrhosis, cataracts, mental retardation, galactosuria, aminoaciduria, and albuminuria which regress or disappear if galactose is removed from the diet; autosomal recessive inheritance.

galactose-1-phosphate uridylyltransferase [EC 2.7.7.10]. An enzyme catalyzing the reaction of UTP and α-D-galactose 1-phosphate to form UDPgalactose, the second and most important step in the metabolism of galactose.

α-D-galactosidase (gă-lak-tō-sīd′ās) [EC 3.2.1.22]. Melibiase; an enzyme catalyzing the hydrolysis of α-D-galactosides to D-galactose.

β-D-galactosidase [EC 3.2.1.23]. Lactase; a sugar-splitting enzyme that catalyzes the hydrolysis of lactose into glucose and galactose, and that of other β-D-galactosides; it also catalyzes galactotransferase reactions.

galactoside (gă-lak′tō-sīd). A compound in which the H of the OH group on carbon-1 of galactose is replaced by an organic radical.

galactosis (gal-ak-tō′sis) [galacto- + G. *-osis,* condition]. Formation of milk by the lacteal glands.

galactosuria (gă-lak-tō-sū′rē-ă) [galactose + G. *ouron,* urine]. The excretion of galactose in the urine.

galactosyl (gă-lak′tō-sil). A compound in which the -OH attached to carbon-1 of galactose is replaced by an organic radical.

galactotherapy (gă-lak′tō-thār′ă-pē). Lactotherapy; treatment of disease by means of an exclusive or nearly exclusive milk diet.

galactowaldenase (gă-lak-tō-wal′dĕ-nās). UDPglucose 4-epimerase.

galactozymase (gă-lak-tō-zī′mās). Obsolete term for an amylase in milk.

galacturonan (gă-lak′tūr-ō-nan). A polysaccharide that yields galacturonic acid on hydrolysis; a constituent of some pectins.

galacturonic acid (gă-lak-tūr-on′ik). Galacturonose; pectic acid; an oxidation product of galactose, in which the 6-CH_2OH group has become a –COOH group; occurs in many natural products (*e.g.,* pectins).

galacturonose (gă-lak′tūr-ō-nōs). Galacturonic acid.

galangal, galanga (ga-lan′găl, -gă) [Mediev. L. *galanga,* mild ginger, fr. Chinese]. Galingal; Chinese ginger; the rhizome of *Alpinia offcinarum* (family Zingiberaceae); an aromatic stimulant and carminative.

Galant, Nikolay Fedorovich, Russian hygienist, *1893. See G.'s *reflex.*

Galassi's pupillary phenomenon. See under phenomenon.

galea (gā′lē-ă) [L. a helmet]. **1** [NA]. A structure shaped like a helmet. **2.** G. aponeurotica. **3.** A form of bandage covering the head. **4.** Caul (1).

g. aponeurot′ica [NA], epicranial aponeurosis; aponeurosis epicranialis; galea (2); the aponeurosis connecting the frontalis and occipitalis muscles to form the epicranius.

Galeati, Domenico, Italian physician, 1686–1775. See G.'s *glands.*

galeatomy (gā-lē-at′ō-mē) [galea + G. *tomē,* incision]. Incision of the galea aponeurotica.

Galeazzi, Riccardo, Italian surgeon, 1886–1952. See G.'s *fracture.*

Galen (Galenius, Galenos), Claudius (Clarissmus), Greek physician and medical scientist in Rome, *c.* 130–201 A.D. See G.'s *anastomosis, nerve, vein;* great *vein* of G.

galena (gă-lē′nă). *Lead* sulfide.

galenic (gā-len′ik). Relating to Galen or to his theories.

galenicals (gā-len′i-kălz) [Claudius *Galen*]. **1.** Herbs and other vegetable drugs, as distinguished from the mineral or chemical remedies. **2.** Crude drugs and the tinctures, decoctions, and other preparations made from them, as distinguished from the alkaloids and other active principles. **3.** Remedies prepared according to an official formula.

Gall, Franz J., Austrian anatomist, 1758–1828. See G.'s *craniology.*

gall (gawl) [A.S. *gealla*]. **1.** Bile. **2.** An excoriation or erosion. **3.** Nutgall.

galla (gal′ă) [L.]. Nutgall.

gallamine triethiodide (gal′ă-mēn trī-eth-ī′ō-dīd). [ν-Phenenyltris(oxyethylene)]tris[triethylammonium iodide]; a triple quaternary ammonium compound with action comparable to that of tubocurarine to produce relaxation during surgical operations.

Gallavardin, Louis, French physician, *1875. See G.'s *phenomenon.*

gallbladder (gawl′blad-er). *Vesica* bilaris.

sandpaper g., a roughened condition of the mucous membrane of the g., associated usually with the presence of gallstones.

strawberry g., a g. of which the mucosa is dotted with yellowish cholesterol deposits contrasting with the red hyperemic background.

Gallego's differentiating solution. See under solution.

gallein (gal′ē-in). Pyrogallolphthalein; 3′,4′,5′,6′-tetrahydroxyfluoran; structurally related to fluorescein and used as an indicator, turning rose-red above pH 6.6, yellowish brown below pH 4.

gallic acid (gal′ik). 3,4,5-Trihydroxybenzoic acid; usually made from tannic acid or nutgalls; used locally as an astringent, for the same purpose as tannic acid.

Gallie, William E., Canadian surgeon, 1882–1959. See G.'s *transplant.*

Galliformes (gal-i-fōr′mēz) [L. *gallus,* a cock, + *forma,* form]. An order of birds embracing the pheasant, turkey, and chicken.

gallinaceous (gal-i-nā′shŭs) [L. *gallinaceus,* fr. *gallina,* a hen]. Pertaining to the order Galliformes.

gallium (gal′ē-ŭm) [L. *Gallia,* France]. A rare metal, symbol Ga, atomic no. 31, atomic weight 69.7.

gallium-67 (^{67}Ga). A cyclotron-produced radionuclide with a physical half-life of 78 hours and major gamma ray emissions of 93, 184, and 296 kiloelectron volts; used in the citrate form as a tumor- and inflammation-localizing radiotracer.

gallium-68 (^{68}Ga). A positron emitter with a radioactive half-life of 68 minutes.

gallocyanin, gallocy'anine (gal-ō-sī'ă-nin, ă-nēn) [C.I. 51030]. A blue phenoxazin dye, $C_{15}H_{13}N_2O_5Cl$, used as a stain for nucleic acids after boiling with chrome alum, and is applicable for quantitative cytophotometric determination of these moieties.

gallon (gal'ŭn). A measure of liquid capacity containing 4 quarts, 231 cubic inches, or 8.3389 pounds of distilled water; it is the equivalent of 3.7853 liters. The British imperial g. contains 277.274 cubic inches.

gal'lop. Cantering rhythm; g. rhythm; bruit de galop; Traube's bruit; a triple cadence to the heart sounds at rates of 100 beats per minute or more; due to an abnormal third or fourth heart sound being heard in addition to the first and second sounds, and usually indicative of serious disease.
atrial g., presystolic g.
presystolic g., atrial g.; g. rhythm in which the g. sound occurs in late diastole and is an audible fourth heart sound.
protodiastolic g., g. rhythm in which the g. sound occurs in early diastole and is an abnormal third heart sound.
summation g., g. rhythm in which the g. sound is due to superimposition of third and fourth heart sounds; sometimes heard in normal subjects with tachycardia, but usually indicative of myocardial disease.
systolic g., a triple cadence to the heart sounds in which the extra sound occurs during systole, usually in the form of a systolic "click."

gallstone (gal'stōn). Cholelith; chololith; biliary calculus; a concretion in the gallbladder or a bile duct, composed chiefly of a mixture of cholesterol, calcium bilirubinate, and calcium carbonate, occasionally as a pure stone composed of just one of these substances.
opacifying g.'s, g.'s becoming roentgenographically opaque after prolonged exposure to cholecystographic contrast mediums.
silent g.'s, g.'s that cause no symptoms and are discovered by x-ray examination, at the time of operation, or autopsy.

Gallus (gal'ŭs) [L. *gallus,* a cock]. A genus of gallinaceous birds including *G. domestica,* the domestic chicken.

Galton, Sir Francis, British scientist, 1822–1911. See G.'s *delta,* system of classification of *fingerprints, law, whistle.*

galtonian (gahl-tō'nē-ăn). Attributed to or described by Sir Francis Galton.

galvanic (gal-van'ik). Pertaining to galvanism.

galvanism (gal'vă-nizm) [Luigi *Galvani,* It. physician and anatomist, 1737–1798]. Voltaism. **1.** Direct current electricity produced by chemical action, as by a battery. **2.** Oral manifestations of direct current electricity occurring when dental restorations with dissimilar electric potentials (such as silver and gold) are placed in the mouth; characterized by pain or development of small areas of leukoplakia.

galvanization (gal'va-ni-zā'shŭn). Application of direct current (galvanic) electricity, as in galvanizing (electroplating).

galvano- [see galvanism]. Prefix meaning electrical, denoting primarily direct current.

galvanocautery (gal'vă-nō-kaw'ter-ē). A form of electrocautery using a wire heated by a galvanic current.

galvanocontractility (gal'vă-nō-kon-trak-til'i-tē). The capability of a muscle of contracting under the stimulus of a galvanic (direct) current.

galvanofaradization (gal'vă-nō-far'ă-di-zā'shŭn). Simultaneous application of a galvanic and a faradic current.

galvanometer (gal'vă-nom'ĕ-ter). An instrument for measuring the strength of an electric current.
d'Arsonval g., a sensitive g. consisting of a moving coil suspended in a permanent magnetic field between delicate metallic wires or ribbons that serve as both torsion springs and conductors; a mirror on the coil deflects a beam of light along the scale.

galvanomuscular (gal'vă-nō-mŭs'kyū-lăr). Denoting the effect of the application of a galvanic (direct) current to a muscle.

galvanopalpation (gal'vă-nō-pal-pā'shŭn). Esthesiometry by means of a sharp-pointed electrode through which a feeble direct current passes to the cathode applied to an indifferent part.

galvanoscope (gal'vă-nō-skōp) [galvano- + G. *skopeō,* to view]. An instrument for detecting the presence of a galvanic current.

galvanosurgery (gal'vă-nō-ser'jer-ē). An operation in which direct electric current is utilized.

galvanotaxis (gal'vă-nō-tak'sis). Electrotaxis.

galvanotherapy (gal'van-ō-thār'ă-pē). Treatment of disease by application of direct (galvanic) current.

galvanotonus (gal-vă-not'ō-nŭs) [galvano- + G. *tonos,* tension]. **1.** Electrotonus. **2.** Tonic muscular contraction in response to a galvanic stimulus.

galvanotropism (gal-vă-not'rō-pizm) [galvano- + G. *tropē,* a turning]. Electrotaxis.

gamabufagin (gam-ă-bū'fă-jin). Gamabufotalin.

gamabufogenin (gam-ă-bū'fō-jen-in). Gamabufotalin.

gamabufotalin (gam-ă-bū'fō-tal-in). Gamabufagin; gamabufogenin; a trihydroxybufadienolide, present in the venoms of toads (family Bufonidae), which chemically and pharmacologically resembles digitalis.

gambir (gam'bēr). Catechu; an extract from the leaves of *Uncaria (Ourouparia)* gambier (family Rubiaceae); used as an astringent. Commercial g. is known as terra japonica.

game (gām). A contest, physical or mental, conducted according to set rules, played for amusement or for a stake.
language g., in philosophy, all the operations and behaviors contained in and expressed by symbols, language rules, and the social customs concerning language use.
model g., the use of g.'s, especially of g.'s of strategy, for the explanation of human behavior (both normal and abnormal).

gametangium (gam-ĕ-tan'jē-ŭm). A structure in which gametes are produced.

gamete (gam'ēt) [G. *gametēs,* husband; *gametē,* wife]. **1.** One of two cells undergoing karyogamy. **2.** Any germ cell, whether ovum, spermatozoon, or pollen cell.
joint g., the set of (nonallelic) genes inherited in a single germinal cell.

gameto- [see gamete]. Combining form relating to a gamete.

gametocide (gă-mē'tō-sīd) [gameto- + L. *caedo,* to kill]. An agent destructive of gametes, specifically the malarial gametocytes.

gametocyst (ga-mē'tō-sist) [gameto- + G. *kystis,* bladder]. A cyst formed around a pair of united gregarine gamonts in which gametes are produced.

gametocyte (gă-mē'tō-sīt) [gameto- + G. *kytos,* cell]. Gamont; a cell capable of dividing to produce gametes, *e.g.,* a spermatocyte or oocyte.

gametogenesis (gam'ĕ-tō-jen'ĕ-sis) [gameto- + G. *genesis,* production]. The process of formation and development of gametes.

gametogonia (gam'ĕ-tō-gō'nē-ă). Gametogony.

gametogony (gam-ĕ-tog'ō-nē) [gameto- + G. *gonus,* a begetting]. Gametogonia; gamogony; a stage in the sexual cycle of sporozoans in which gametes are formed, often by schizogony.

gametoid (gam'ĕ-toyd). Pertaining to certain biologic features that resemble those characteristic of gametes or reproductive cells.

gametokinetic (gam'ĕ-tō-ki-net'ik) [gameto- + G. *kinēsis,* movement]. Moving toward, or causing, karyogamy or true conjugation.

gametophagia (gam′ĕ-tō-fā′jē-ă) [gameto- + G. *phagein*, to eat]. Gamophagia; the disappearance of the male or female element in zygosis.

Gamgee, Joseph Sampson, British surgeon, 1828–1886. See G. *tissue.*

gamic (gam′ik) [G. *gamikos*, pert. to marriage]. Relating to or derived from sexual union; usually used as a suffix.

gamma (gam′ă) [G.]. Third letter of the Greek alphabet, γ(*q.v.*).

gamma-benzene hexachloride. Lindane.

gammacism (gam′ă-sizm) [G. *gamma*, equivalent of the letter g]. Mispronunciation of, or trouble articulating, the "g" sound.

gammagram (gam′ă-gram). Scintiscan.

gammopathy (gă-mop′ă-thē). A primary disturbance in immunoglobulin (γ-globulin) synthesis.
biclonal g., a g. in which the serum contains two distinct monoclonal immunoglobulins.
monoclonal g., any one of a group of disorders due to proliferation of a single clone of lymphoid or plasma cells (visible on electrophoresis as a single peak) and characterized by the presence of monoclonal immunoglobulin in serum or urine.

Gamna, Carlos, Italian physician, *1896. See G.'s *disease;* G.-Favre *bodies;* Gandy-G. *bodies;* G.-Gandy *bodies, nodules.*

gamogenesis (gam-ō-jen′ĕ-sis) [G. *gamos*, marriage, + *genesis*, production]. Sexual reproduction.

gamogony (gam-og′ō-nē). Gametogony.

gam′ont [G. *gamos*, marriage, + *ōn* (*ont-*), being]. Gametocyte.

gamophagia (gam-ō-fā′jē-ă). Gametophagia.

gamophobia (gam-ō-fō′bē-ă) [G. *gamos*, marriage, + *phobos*, fear]. Morbid fear of marriage.

ganciclovir (gan-sī′klō-vir). 9-[[Hydroxy-1-(hydroxymethyl)ethoxy]methyl]guanine; an antiviral agent used in the treatment of opportunistic cytomegalovirus infections.

Gandy, Charles, French physician, *1872. See Gamna-G. *bodies, nodules;* G.-Gamna *bodies;* G.-Nanta *disease.*

ganga (gang′gă). An extract of the flowers of *Cannabis sativa* (Indian hemp or hashish) which grows in India, Persia, and Arabia. See also cannabis.

ganglia (gang′glē-ă). Plural of ganglion.

ganglial (gang′glē-ăl). Ganglionic.

gangliate, gangliated (gang′glē-āt, gang′glē-ā-ted). Ganglionated; having ganglia.

gangliectomy (gang-glē-ek-tō-mē). Ganglionectomy.

gangliform (gang′glē-fōrm). Ganglioform; having the form or appearance of a ganglion.

gangliitis (gang-glē-ī′tis). Ganglionitis.

ganglioblast (gang′glē-ō-blast) [ganglion + G. *blastos*, germ]. An embryonic cell from which develop ganglion cells.

gangliocyte (gang′glē-ō-sīt). Ganglion *cell.*

gangliocytoma (gang′glē-ō-sī-tō′mă). Ganglioneuroma.

ganglioform (gang′glē-ō-fōrm). Gangliform.

ganglioglioma (gang′glē-ō-glē-ō′mă). Central *ganglioneuroma.*

gangliolysis (gang-glē-ol′i-sis). The dissolution or breaking up of a ganglion.
percutaneous radiofrequency g., g. produced by radiofrequency currents applied to a ganglion by a needle passed through the skin.

ganglioma (gang-glē-ō′mă). Ganglioneuroma.

GANGLION

ganglion, pl. **ganglia, ganglions** (gang′glē-on, -glē-ă, -glē-onz) [G. a swelling or knot]. **1** [NA]. Neural or nerve g.; neuroganglion; originally, any group of nerve cell bodies in the central or peripheral nervous system; currently, an aggregation of nerve cell bodies located in the peripheral nervous system. **2.** Myxoid or synovial cyst; a cyst containing mucopolysaccharide-rich fluid within fibrous tissue or, occasionally, muscle or a semilunar cartilage; usually attached to a tendon sheath in the hand, wrist, or foot, or connected with the underlying joint.
aberrant g., a collection of nerve cells sometimes found on a posterior spinal nerve root between the spinal g. and the spinal cord.
acousticofacial g., a primordial ganglionic cell mass in young embryos which later separates into the acoustic or spiral g. of the vestibulocochlear (eighth cranial) nerve and the geniculate g. of the facial (seventh cranial) nerve.
Acrel's g., (1) pseudoganglion on the posterior interosseous nerve on the dorsal aspect of the wrist joint; **(2)** a cyst on a tendon of an extensor muscle at the level of the wrist.
Andersch's g., g. inferius nervi glossopharyngei.
aorticorenal ganglia, ganglia aorticorenalia.
gang′lia aorticorena′lia [NA], aorticorenal ganglia; a semidetached portion of the celiac ganglia, at the origin of each renal artery; contains the sympathetic neurons innervating the vasculature of the kidney.
Arnold's g., g. oticum.
auditory g., g. spirale cochleae.
Auerbach's ganglia, collections of parasympathetic nerve cells in the myenteric plexus. See *plexus* myentericus.
auricular g., g. oticum.
autonomic ganglia, visceral ganglia. See *systema* nervosum autonomicum.
ganglia of autonomic plexuses, ganglia plexuum autonomicorum.
basal ganglia, originally, all of the large masses of gray matter at the base of the cerebral hemisphere; currently, the corpus striatum (caudate and lentiform nuclei) and cell groups associated with the corpus striatum, such as the subthalamic nucleus and substantia nigra.
Bezold's g., an aggregation of nerve cells in the interatrial septum.
Bochdalek's g., a g. of the plexus of the dental nerve lying in the maxilla just above the root of the canine tooth.
Bock's g., carotid g.
Böttcher's g., g. on the cochlear nerve in the internal acoustic meatus.
cardiac ganglia, ganglia cardiaca.
gang′lia cardi′aca [NA], cardiac ganglia; Wrisberg's ganglia; parasympathetic ganglia of the cardiac plexus lying between the arch of the aorta and the bifurcation of the pulmonary artery.
carotid g., Bock's or Laumonier's g.; a small ganglionic swelling on filaments from the internal carotid plexus, lying on the undersurface of the carotid artery in the cavernous sinus.
celiac ganglia, ganglia celiaca.
gang′lia celia′ca [NA], celiac ganglia; solar ganglia; semilunar g. (2); Willis' centrum nervosum; the largest and highest group of sympathetic prevertebral ganglia, located on the superior part of the abdominal aorta, on either side of the celiac artery; contains sympathetic neurons whose unmyelinated postganglionic axons innervate the stomach, liver, gallbladder, spleen, kidney, small intestine, and ascending and transverse colon.
g. cervica′le infe′rius, g. cervicothoracicum.
g. cervica′le me′dium [NA], middle cervical g.; a sympathetic g.,

of small size and sometimes absent; located at the level of the cricoid cartilage.
g. cervica'le supe'rius [NA], superior cervical g.; the uppermost and largest of the ganglia of the sympathetic trunk, lying near the base of the skull between the internal carotid artery and the internal jugular vein.
cervicothoracic g., g. cervicothoracicum.
g. cer'vicothora'cicum [NA], cervicothoracic g.; g. stellatum; g. cervicale inferius; stellate or inferior cervical g.; a sympathetic trunk g. lying behind the subclavian artery near the origin of the vertebral artery, at the level of the seventh cervical vertebra, close to the first thoracic g. with which it is usually fused.
g. cilia're [NA], ciliary, lenticular, or Schacher's g.; a small parasympathetic g. lying in the orbit between the optic nerve and the lateral rectus muscle; it receives preganglionic innervation from the Edinger-Westphal nucleus by way of the oculomotor nerve, and in turn gives rise to postganglionic fibers that innervate the ciliary muscle and the sphincter of the iris.
ciliary g., g. ciliare.
coccygeal g., g. impar.
Corti's g., g. spirale cochleae.
diffuse g., a cystic swelling due to inflammatory effusion into one or several adjacent tendon sheaths.
dorsal root g., g. spinale.
Ehrenritter's g., g. superius nervi glossopharyngei.
g. extracrania'le, g. inferius nervi glossopharyngei.
g. of facial nerve, g. geniculi.
Frankenhäuser's g., *plexus* uterovaginalis.
Froriep's g., a temporary collection of nerve cells on the dorsal aspect of the hypoglossal nerve in the embryo; it represents a rudimentary sensory g.
gasserian g., g. trigeminale.
geniculate g., g. geniculi.
g. genic'uli [NA], geniculate g.; intumescentia ganglioformis; g. of facial or intermediate nerve; a g. of the intermediate nerve, located within the facial canal and containing the sensory neurons innervating the taste buds on the anterior two-thirds of the tongue.
Gudden's g., *nucleus* interpeduncularis.
g. haben'ulae, *nucleus* habenulae.
hypogastric ganglia, ganglia pelvina.
g. im'par [NA], coccygeal g.; Walther's g.; the most inferior, unpaired g. of the sympathetic trunk.
inferior cervical g., g. cervicothoracicum.
inferior g. of glossopharyngeal nerve, g. inferius nervi glossopharyngei.
inferior mesenteric g., g. mesentericum inferius.
inferior g. of vagus, g. inferius nervi vagi.
g. infe'rius ner'vi glossopharyn'gei [NA], inferior g. of glossopharyngeal nerve; petrosal or petrous g.; g. extracraniale; Andersch's g.; the lower of two sensory g.'s on the glossopharyngeal nerve as it traverses the jugular foramen.
g. infe'rius ner'vi va'gi [NA], inferior g. of vagus; nodose g.; g. of trunk of vagus; a large sensory g. of the vagus, anterior to the internal jugular vein.
intercrural g., *nucleus* interpeduncularis.
gang'lia interme'dia [NA], intermediate ganglia; small sympathetic ganglia most commonly found on the rami communicantes in the cervical and lumbar region.
intermediate ganglia, ganglia intermedia.
g. of intermediate nerve, g. geniculi.
interpeduncular g., *nucleus* interpeduncularis.
intervertebral g., g. spinale.
intracranial g., g. superius nervi glossopharyngei.
g. isth'mi, *nucleus* interpeduncularis.
jugular g., **(1)** g. superius nervi glossopharyngei; **(2)** g. superius nervi vagi.
Laumonier's g., carotid g.
Lee's g., *plexus* uterovaginalis.
lenticular g., g. ciliare.
Lobstein's g., g. splanchnicum.
Ludwig's g., a small collection of parasympathetic nerve cells in the interatrial septum.
gang'lia lumba'lia [NA], lumbar ganglia; four or more ganglia on the medial border of the psoas major muscle on either side; they form, with the sacral and coccygeal ganglia and their connecting cords, the abdominopelvic sympathetic trunk.
lumbar ganglia, ganglia lumbalia.
Meckel's g., g. pterygopalatinum.
g. mesenter'icum infe'rius [NA], inferior mesenteric g.; the lowest of the sympathetic prevertebral ganglia, located at the origin of the inferior mesenteric artery from the aorta and containing the sympathetic neurons innervating the descending and sigmoid colon.
g. mesenter'icum supe'rius [NA], superior mesenteric g.; a paired sympathetic g. located at the origin of the superior mesenteric artery from the aorta.
middle cervical g., g. cervicale medium.
nasal g., g. pterygopalatinum.
nerve g., neural g., ganglion (1).
nodose g., g. inferius nervi vagi.
otic g., g. oticum.
g. o'ticum [NA], otic g.; auricular g.; Arnold's g.; otoganglion; an autonomic g. situated below the foramen ovale medial to the mandibular nerve; its postganglionic, parasympathetic fibers are distributed to the parotid gland.
parasympathetic ganglia, those ganglia of the autonomic nervous system composed of cholinergic neurons receiving afferent fibers from preganglionic visceral motor neurons in either the brainstem or the middle sacral spinal segments (S2 to S4); on the basis of their location with respect to the organs they innervate, parasympathetic ganglia can be categorized as juxtamural or intramural ganglia. See also *systema* nervosum autonomicum.
paravertebral ganglia, ganglia trunci sympathetici.
pelvic ganglia, ganglia pelvina.
gang'lia pelvi'na [NA], pelvic ganglia; hypogastric ganglia; the parasympathetic ganglia scattered through the pelvic plexus on either side.
periosteal g., a flattened subperiosteal cavity containing clear, yellow, viscid synovia-like fluid.
petrosal g., petrous g., g. inferius nervi glossopharyngei.
phrenic ganglia, ganglia phrenica.
gang'lia phren'ica [NA], phrenic ganglia; several small autonomic ganglia contained in the plexuses accompanying the inferior phrenic arteries.
gang'lia plex'uum autonomico'rum [NA], ganglia of autonomic plexuses; autonomic ganglia lying in plexuses of autonomic fibers, *e.g.,* the celiac and inferior mesenteric ganglia of the sympathetic, and the small parasympathetic ganglia of the myenteric plexus.
prevertebral ganglia, the sympathetic ganglia (celiac, aorticorenal, superior and inferior mesenteric) lying in front of the vertebral column, as distinguished from the ganglia of the sympathetic trunk (paravertebral ganglia).
pterygopalatine g., g. pterygopalatinum.
g. pterygopalati'num [NA], pterygopalatine g.; sphenopalatine or nasal g.; Meckel's g.; a small parasympathetic g. in the upper part of the pterygopalatine fossa whose postsynaptic fibers supply the lacrimal and nasal glands.
Remak's ganglia, **(1)** groups of nerve cells in the wall of the venous sinus where it joins the right atrium of the heart; **(2)** autonomic ganglia in nerves of the stomach.
renal ganglia, ganglia renalia.
gang'lia rena'lia [NA], renal ganglia; small scattered sympathetic ganglia along the renal plexus.
Ribes' g., a small sympathetic g. situated on the anterior communicating artery of the brain.

sacral ganglia, ganglia sacralia.
gang'lia sacra'lia [NA], sacral ganglia; three or four ganglia on either side constituting, with the g. impar and the connecting cords, the pelvic portion of the sympathetic trunk.
Scarpa's g., g. vestibulare.
Schacher's g., g. ciliare.
semilunar g., **(1)** g. trigeminale; **(2)** ganglia celiaca.
sensory g., a cluster of primary sensory neurons forming a usually visible swelling in the course of a peripheral nerve or its dorsal root; such nerve cells establish the sole afferent neural connection between the sensory periphery (skin, mucous membranes of the oral and nasal cavities, muscle tissue, tendons, joint capsules, special sense organs, blood vessel walls, tissues of the internal organs) and the central nervous system; they are the cells of origin of all sensory fibers of the peripheral nervous system.
Soemmering's g., *substantia* nigra.
solar ganglia, ganglia celiaca.
sphenopalatine g., g. pterygopalatinum.
spinal g., g. spinale.
g. spina'le [NA], spinal g.; dorsal root g.; intervertebral g.; the g. of the posterior root of each spinal segmental nerve; contains the cell bodies of the pseudounipolar primary sensory neurons whose peripheral axonal branches become part of the mixed segmental nerve, while the central axonal branches enter the spinal cord as a component of the sensory posterior root.
spiral g. of cochlea, g. spirale cochleae.
g. spira'le coch'leae [NA], spiral g. of cochlea; Corti's g.; auditory g.; an elongated g. of bipolar sensory nerve cell bodies on the cochlear part of the vestibulocochlear nerve in the spiral canal of the modiolus; each g. cell gives rise to a peripheral process that passes between the layers of the lamina spiralis ossea to the organ of Corti, and a central axon that enters the hindbrain as a component of the inferior (cochlear) root of the eighth nerve.
splanchnic g., g. splanchnicum.
g. splanch'nicum [NA], splanchnic g.; Lobstein's g. a small sympathetic g. often present in the course of the greater splanchnic nerve.
stellate g., g. cervicothoracicum.
g. stella'tum [NA], an official alternate term for g. cervicothoracicum.
sublingual g., g. sublinguale; a tiny g. occasionally found anterior to the g. submandibulare, of which it is a displaced portion; innervates the sublingual gland.
g. sublingua'le, sublingual g.
submandibular g., g. submandibulare.
g. submandibula're [NA], submandibular g.; submaxillary g.; a small parasympathetic g. suspended from the lingual nerve; its postganglionic branches go to the submandibular and sublingual glands; its preganglionic fibers come from the nucleus salivatorius by way of the chorda tympani.
submaxillary g., g. submandibulare.
superior cervical g., g. cervicale superius.
superior g. of glossopharyngeal nerve, g. superius nervi glossopharyngei.
superior mesenteric g., g. mesentericum superius.
superior g. of the vagus nerve, g. superius nervi vagi.
g. supe'rius ner'vi glossopharyn'gei [NA], superior g. of glossopharyngeal nerve; Ehrenritter's g.; intracranial g.; jugular g. (1); the upper and smaller of two ganglia on the glossopharyngeal nerve as it traverses the jugular foramen.
g. supe'rius ner'vi va'gi [NA], superior g. of the vagus nerve; jugular g. (2); a small sensory g. on the vagus as it traverses the jugular foramen.
sympathetic ganglia, those ganglia of the autonomic nervous system that receive afferent fibers originating from preganglionic visceral motor neurons in the intermediolateral cell column of thoracic and upper lumbar spinal segments (Th 1–L 2). On the basis of their location, the sympathetic ganglia can be classified as paravertebral ganglia (ganglia trunci sympathici) and prevertebral ganglia (ganglia celiaca). See also *systema* nervosum autonomicum.
ganglia of sympathetic trunk, ganglia trunci sympathici.
terminal g., g. terminale.
g. termina'le, terminal g.; **(1)** [NA] one of the cells located along the nervi terminales; **(2)** one of the scattered postganglionic autonomic neurons located in or close to the wall of the organ innervated; they are usually parasympathetic.
thoracic ganglia, ganglia thoracica.
gang'lia thorac'ica [NA], thoracic ganglia; ganglia, 11 or 12 on either side, at the level of the head of each rib, constituting with the connecting nerve cords the thoracic portion of the sympathetic trunk.
trigeminal g., g. trigeminale.
g. trigemina'le [NA], trigeminal g.; semilunar g. (1); gasserian g.; the large flattened sensory g. of the trigeminal nerve lying close to the cavernous sinus along the medial part of the middle cranial fossa in laminae of the dura mater (*i.e.,* cavity of Meckel).
Troisier's g., Troisier's node; historic term for a lymph node immediately above the clavicle, especially on the left side, that is palpably enlarged as the result of a metastasis from a malignant neoplasm; the presence of such a node indicates that the probable site of primary involvement is in an abdominal organ. See also signal *node.*
gang'lia trun'ci sympath'ici [NA], ganglia of sympathetic trunk; paravertebral ganglia; the clusters of postganglionic neurons located at intervals along the sympathetic trunks, including the superior cervical, middle cervical, and cervicothoracic (stellate) g., the thoracic, lumbar, and sacral ganglia, and the g. impar.
g. of trunk of vagus, g. inferius nervi vagi.
tympanic g., g. tympanicum.
g. tympan'icum [NA], tympanic g.; a small g. on the tympanic nerve during its passage through the petrous portion of the temporal bone.
Valentin's g., a g. on the superior alveolar nerve.
vertebral g., g. vertebrale.
g. vertebra'le [NA], vertebral g.; a small g. located along the sympathetic trunk or one of the nerve cords connecting the middle cervical g. and the cervicothoracic g.; it usually lies near the vertebral artery.
vestibular g., g. vestibulare.
g. vestibula're [NA], vestibular g., Scarpa's g.; a collection of bipolar nerve cell bodies forming a swelling on the vestibular part of the eighth nerve in the internal acoustic meatus; consists of a pars superior and a pars inferior connected by a narrow isthmus.
Vieussens' g., *plexus* celiacus.
Walther's g., g. impar.
Wrisberg's ganglia, ganglia cardiaca.

---

ganglionated (gang'glē-ō-nā'ted). Gangliate.

ganglionectomy (gang'glē-ō-nek'tō-mē) [ganglion + G. *ektomē,* excision]. Gangliectomy; excision of a ganglion.

ganglioneuroma (gang'glē-ō-nū-rō'mă). Gangliocytoma; ganglioma; neurocytoma; a benign neoplasm composed of mature ganglionic neurons, in varying numbers, scattered singly or in clumps within a relatively abundant and dense stroma of neurofibrils and collagenous fibers; usually found in the posterior mediastinum and retroperitoneum, sometimes in relation to the adrenal glands.
central g., ganglioglioma; a rare form of glioma composed of nearly mature, slowly growing neuron-like cells; found in the optic chasm or cerebral white matter.
dumbbell g., a g. in which the gross configuration resembles a dumbbell, *e.g.,* two spheroidal masses connected by a narrow portion, usually the result of the neoplasm being somewhat molded by a resistant structure such as two ribs.

ganglioneuromatosis (gang'glē-ō-nūr'ō-mă-tō'sis). The condition of having many widespread ganglioneuromas.

ganglionic (gang-glē-on'ik). Ganglial; relating to a ganglion.

ganglionitis (gang'glē-ō-nī'tis). Gangliitis. **1.** Inflammation of a lymphatic ganglion. **2.** Inflammation of a nerve ganglion.

ganglionostomy (gang'glē-ō-nos'tō-mē) [ganglion + G. *stoma*, mouth]. Making an opening into a ganglion (2).

ganglioplegic (gang'glē-ō-plē'jik) [ganglion + G. *plēgē*, stroke, shock]. A pharmacologic compound that paralyzes an autonomic ganglion, usually for a relatively short period of time.

ganglioside (gang'glē-ō-sīd). A glycosphingolipid chemically similar to cerebrosides but containing one or more sialic (*N*-acetylneuraminic or *N*-glycolylneuraminic) acid residues; found principally in nerve tissue and the spleen.

gangliosidosis (gang'glē-ō-si-dō'sis). Ganglioside lipidosis; any disease characterized, in part, by the abnormal accumulation within the nervous system of specific gangliosides; such gangliosides are normally present only in trace quantities.

G_{M1} g., generalized g.; g. characterized by accumulation of a specific monosialoganglioside, G_{M1}; resembles Tay-Sachs disease, except that visceral mucopolysaccharidosis is also present.

G_{M2} g., cerebral *sphingolipidosis*, infantile type.

generalized g., G_{M1} g.

gangosa (gang-gō'să) [Sp. *gangoso*, snuffling; fem. to agree with *enfermedad*, disease]. Rhinopharyngitis mutilans; a destructive ulceration beginning on the soft palate and extending thence to the hard palate, nasopharynx, and nose, resulting in mutilating cicatrices. The disease, so far as is known, occurs only in certain portions of the tropics, especially the islands of the Pacific, and is generally regarded as a sequel to yaws.

gangrene (gang'grēn) [G. *gangraina*, an eating sore, fr. *graō*, to gnaw]. Mortification; necrosis due to obstruction, loss, or diminution of blood supply; it may be localized to a small area or involve an entire extremity or organ (such as the bowel), and may be wet or dry.

arteriosclerotic g., dry g. resulting from sclerotic changes in the arteries, with subsequent occlusion, as in the aged, due to arteriosclerosis.

cold g., dry g.

cutaneous g., g. of the skin characterized by sloughing; may occur in shingles or in any acute infection that interferes with superficial circulation.

decubital g., decubitus *ulcer*.

diabetic g., g. resulting from arteriosclerosis associated with diabetes.

disseminated cutaneous g., *dermatitis* gangrenosa infantum.

dry g., cold g.; mummification (1); mummification necrosis; a form of g. in which the involved part is dry and shriveled.

embolic g., g. resulting from obstruction of an artery by an embolus.

emphysematous g., gas g.

Fournier's g., Fournier's *disease*.

gas g., emphysematous g.; emphysematous or gas phlegmon; gangrenous emphysema; progressive emphysematous necrosis; clostridial myonecrosis; g. occurring in a wound infected with various anaerobic sporeforming bacteria, especially *Clostridium perfringens* and *C. novyi*, which cause crepitation of the surrounding tissues, due to gas liberated by bacterial fermentation, and constitutional septic symptoms.

hemorrhagic g., **(1)** hemorrhagic *infarct;* **(2)** g. occurring rarely in meningococcal septicemia.

hospital g., decubitus *ulcer*.

hot g., g. following inflammation of the part.

Meleney's g., Meleney's ulcer; g. of the skin and subcutaneous tissues, usually following an operation, caused by a synergistic interaction between microaerophilic nonhemolytic streptococci and aerobic hemolytic staphylococci which produces extensive tissue necrosis with undermining ulcers.

moist g., a form of g. in which the necrosed part is moist and soft.

nosocomial g., decubitus *ulcer*.

Pott's g., senile g.

presenile spontaneous g., g. occurring in middle life as a result of thromboangiitis obliterans.

pressure g., decubitus *ulcer*.

progressive bacterial synergistic g., superficial death of tissue due to bacterial infection.

senile g., Pott's g.; dry g. occurring in the aged in consequence of occlusion of an artery, particularly affecting the extremities.

spontaneous g. of newborn, g. due to vascular occlusion of unknown cause, usually in marasmic or dehydrated infants.

static g., venous g.; moist g. due to obstruction in the return circulation.

symmetrical g., g. affecting the extremities of both sides of the body; it is seen particularly in severe arteriosclerosis, myocardial infarction, and ball-valve thrombus.

thrombotic g., g. due to occlusion of an artery by a thrombus.

trophic g., g. due to disorder of the trophic nerves of the part.

venous g., static g.

wet g., ischemic necrosis of an extremity with bacterial infection, producing cellulitis adjacent to the necrotic areas.

white g., leukonecrosis; death of a part accompanied by the formation of grayish white sloughs.

gangrenous (gang'grĕ-nŭs). Mortified; relating to or affected with gangrene.

Ganong, William F., U.S. physiologist, *1924. See Lown-G.-Levine *syndrome*.

Ganser, Siegbert J.M., German psychiatrist, 1853–1931. See G.'s *commissures, syndrome; nucleus* basalis of G.

Gant, Samuel G., U.S. surgeon, 1870–1944. See G.'s *clamp*.

gantry (gan'trē). A movable frame housing the x-ray tube, collimators, and detectors in a CT machine.

Gantzer, Carol F.L., 17th century German anatomist. See G.'s accessory *bundle, muscle*.

Ganz, William, U.S. cardiologist, *1919. See Swan-G. *catheter*.

gap. 1. A hiatus or opening in a structure. **2.** An interval or discontinuity in any series or sequence. **3 (G).** A period in the cell cycle.

g. 1 (G 1), in the somatic cell cycle, the g. that follows mitosis and is followed by synthesis for the next cycle.

g. 2 (G 2), in the somatic cell cycle, a pause between completion of synthesis and the onset of cell division.

air-bone g., the difference between the threshold for hearing acuity by bone conduction and by air conduction.

anion g., cation-anion difference; the difference between the sum of the measured cations and anions in the plasma or serum calculated as follows: $(Na + K) - (Cl + HCO_3) = < 20$ MMOL/l. Elevated values may occur in diabetic or lactic acidosis; normal or low values occur in bicarbonate-losing metabolic acidoses.

auscultatory g., silent g.; the period during which Korotkoff sounds indicating true systolic pressure fade away and reappear at a lower pressure point; responsible for errors made in recording falsely low systolic blood pressure, especially in hypertensive patients, of up to 25 mm Hg, and avoided by pumping the cuff 30 mm Hg beyond palpable systolic pressure.

Bochdalek's g., vertebrocostal *trigone*.

chromosomal g., a localized area of thinning in a chromatid which may simulate a complete break.

DNA g., a localized loss of one of the two strands in the double helix of DNA.

interocclusal g., freeway *space*.

silent g., auscultatory g.

gapes (gāps). A disease of young chickens, turkeys, and other birds caused by the gapeworm, *Syngamus trachea,* which localizes in the trachea and causes gasping and choking; infection is either direct, by ingestion of infective eggs, or indirect, by ingestion of transport hosts such as land snails, slugs, or earthworms.

gapeworm (gāp'wŏrm). See *Syngamus.*

Garbe, William, Canadian dermatologist, *1908. See Sulzberger-G. *disease, syndrome.*

Gardner, Eldon J., U.S. geneticist, *1909. See G. 's *syndrome.*

Gardner, F.H. See G.-Diamond *syndrome.*

gargle (gar'gl) [thru Old Fr. fr. L. *gurgulio,* gullet, windpipe]. **1.** To rinse the fauces with fluid in the mouth through which expired breath is forced to produce a bubbling effect while the head is held far back. **2.** A medicated fluid used for gargling; a throat wash.

gargoylism (gar'goyl-izm) [gargoyle, fr. L. *gurgulio,* gullet]. Old term denoting the gargoyle-like facies and related characteristics of Hurler's syndrome and Hunter's syndrome.

Gariel, Maurice, French physician, 1812–1878. See G.'s *pessary.*

Garland, G.M., U.S. physician, 1848–1926. See G.'s *triangle.*

Garland, Hugh, British neurologist. See Marinesco-G. *syndrome.*

garlic (gar'lik). Allium.

g. oil, a volatile oil from the bulb or entire plant of *Allium sativum* (family Liliaceae); contains diallyl disulfide and allyl propyl disulfide; has been used as an anthelmintic and rubefacient.

Garré, Carl, Swiss surgeon, 1857–1928. See G.'s *disease.*

Gärtner, August, German physician, 1848–1934. See G.'s *bacillus, method,* vein *phenomenon, tonometer.*

Gartner, Herman T., Danish anatomist and surgeon, 1785–1827. See G.'s *canal, cyst, duct.*

gas [coined by Van Helmont, 17th century Belgian chemist]. **1.** A thin fluid, like air, capable of indefinite expansion but convertible by compression and cold into a liquid and, eventually, a solid. **2.** In clinical practice, a liquid entirely in its vapor phase at one atmosphere of pressure because ambient temperature is above its boiling point.

alveolar g. (symbol subscript A), alveolar air; the g. in the pulmonary alveoli, where O_2-CO_2 exchange with pulmonary capillary blood occurs.

anesthetic g., see inhalation *anesthetic.*

blood g.'s, a clinical expression for the determination of the partial pressures of oxygen and carbon dioxide in blood.

carbonic acid g., *carbon* dioxide.

expired g., (1) any g. that has been expired from the lungs; **(2)** often used synonymously with mixed expired g.

hemolytic g., a poisonous g., such as arsine, inhalation of which causes hemolysis with hemoglobinuria, jaundice, gastroenteritis, and nephritis.

ideal alveolar g., the uniform composition of g. that would exist in all alveoli for a given total respiratory exchange if all alveoli had identical ventilation-perfusion ratios and achieved perfect equilibrium with the blood leaving the pulmonary capillaries.

inert g.'s, noble g.'s.

inspired g. (symbol subscript I), **(1)** any g. that is being inhaled; **(2)** specifically, that g. after it has been humidified at body temperature.

laughing g. [so called because its inhalation sometimes excites a hilarious delirium preceding insensibility], nitrous oxide.

marsh g., methane.

mixed expired g., one or more complete breaths of expired g. coming thoroughly mixed from the dead space and the alveoli.

mustard g., sulfur mustard; bis- or di(2-chloroethyl)sulfide; $S(CH_2CH_2Cl)_2$; a poisonous vesicating gas introduced in World War I; it is the progenitor of the so-called nitrogen mustards.

noble g.'s, inert g.'s; elements in the zero group in the periodic series: helium, neon, argon, krypton, xenon, and radon.

olefiant g. [see olefin], ethylene.

sewer g., g., probably mostly methane, resulting from decomposition of organic matter in sewers; potentially explosive and toxic.

sneezing g., sternutator.

suffocating g., a g., such as chlorine or phosgene, that causes intense irritation of the bronchial tubes and lungs, resulting in pulmonary edema.

tear g., a g., such as acetone, benzene bromide, and xylol, that causes irritation of the conjunctiva and profuse lacrimation. See also lacrimator.

vesicating g., a g., such as mustard g., which upon contact with the skin causes vesication and sloughing; inhalation may result in bronchopneumonia.

vomiting g., a g., such as chloropicrin, that can cause vomiting and gastrointestinal disorders such as colic and diarrhea.

water g., an illuminating and fuel g. produced by passing steam over red-hot coal; consists chiefly of hydrogen, hydrocarbons, and carbon monoxide.

gaseous (gas'ē-ŭs). Of the nature of gas.

Gaskell, Walter H., British physiologist, 1847–1914. See G.'s *bridge, clamp, nerves.*

gasometer (gas-om'ĕ-ter). A calibrated instrument or vessel for measuring the volumes of gases. See also spirometer.

gasometric (gas-ō-met'rik). Relating to gasometry.

gasometry (gas-om'ĕ-trē). Measurement of gases; determination of the relative proportion of gases in a mixture.

Gass, J. Donald M., U.S. ophthalmologist, *1928. See Irvine-G. *syndrome.*

Gasser (Gasserio), Johann L., Vienna anatomist 1723–1765. See gasserian *ganglion.*

gasserian (ga-ser'ē-an). Relating to or described by Johann L. Gasser.

gassing (gas'ing). Poisoning by irrespirable or otherwise noxious gases.

Gastaut, H. See Lennox-G. *syndrome.*

gas'ter [G. *gastēr,* belly]. [NA]. Stomach.

Gasterophilidae (gas'ter-ō-fil'i-dē) [G. *gastēr,* belly, stomach, + *philos,* fond]. Gastrophilidae; a family of botflies (or warble flies) that produce enteric myiasis in members of the horse family (genus *Gasterophilus*), in rhinoceroses (genus *Gyrostigma*), and in elephants (genera *Cobboldia, Platycobboldia,* and *Rodhainomyia*).

Gasterophilus (gas-ter-of'i-lŭs) [G. *gastēr,* belly, stomach, + *philos,* fond]. *Gastrophilus;* a genus of botflies (horse botflies or warble flies) that cause enteric myiasis in domestic and wild horses and other equids. The bee-like adult attaches eggs to the hairs of the legs or body of the horse; infective eggs hatch when contacted by the lips of the horse, and the larvae attach to, penetrate, and are swallowed or burrow through the tissues to the stomach, where they adhere. After some months, the larvae pass out with the feces, pupate, and emerge as adults. Moderate infection produces little or no symptomatology; heavy infection can cause severe digestive disorders. Important species include *G. hemorrhoidalis* (the red-tailed botflies, a nose fly); *G. intestinalis* (the common horse botfly or nit fly), whose larvae are found in the esophageal portion of the stomach; *G. nasalis* or *G. veterinus* (chin fly or throat botfly), found in the throat or under the jaws of the horse, the larvae migrating to the pyloric portion of the stomach or the anterior duodenum; and *G. pecuorum* (the dark-winged horsefly), the most common and pathogenic species in Europe (absent in the U.S.).

gastr-. See gastro-.

gastradenitis (gas'trad-ĕ-nī'tis) [gastr- + G. *adēn,* gland, + *-itis,* inflammation]. Gastroadenitis; inflammation of the glands of the stomach.

gastralgia (gas-tral'jē-ă) [gastr- + G. *algos,* pain]. Stomach *ache.*

gastrectasis, gastrectasia (gas-trek'tă-sis, gas-trek-tā'zē-ă) [gastr- + G. *ektasis,* extension]. Dilation of the stomach.

gastrectomy (gas-trek'tō-mē) [gastr- + G. *ektomē,* excision]. Excision of a part or all of the stomach.
Pólya g., Pólya's *operation.*

gastric (gas'trik). Relating to the stomach.

gastric cardia (gas'trik kar'dē-ă). *Pars* cardiaca ventriculi.

gastricsin (gas-trik'sin) Former term for a human peptidase (EC 3.4.4.22) now termed pepsin C (EC 3.4.23.3).

gastricus (gas'tri-kŭs) [L.] [NA]. Gastric.

gastrinoma (gas-tri-nō'mă). A gastrin-secreting tumor associated with the Zollinger-Ellison syndrome.

gastrins (gas'trinz). Hormones secreted in the pyloric-antral mucosa of the mammalian stomach that stimulate secretion of HCl by the parietal cells of the gastric glands; there are two types (one sulfated, the other not), both heptadecapeptides, the terminal tetrapeptide (Trp-Met-Asp-Phe-NH_2) being as active as the whole molecule.

gastritis (gas-trī'tis) [gastr- + G. *-itis,* inflammation]. Inflammation, especially mucosal, of the stomach.
atrophic g., chronic g. with atrophy of the mucous membrane and destruction of the peptic glands, sometimes associated with pernicious anemia or gastric carcinoma; also applied to gastric atrophy without inflammatory changes.
catarrhal g., g. with excessive secretion of mucus.
g. cys'tica polypo'sa, large sessile mucosal polyps arising in the stomach proximal to an old gastroenterostomy.
exfoliative g., g. with excessive shedding of nucosal epithelial cells.
g. fibroplas'tica, g. with fibrosis and sclerosis.
hypertrophic g., Ménétrièr's *disease.*
interstitial g., inflammation of the stomach involving the submucosa and muscle coats.
phlegmonous g., severe inflammation, chiefly of the submucous coat, with purulent infiltration of the wall of the stomach.
polypous g., a form of chronic g., in which there is irregular atrophy of the mucous membrane with cystic glands giving rise to a knobby or polypous appearance of the surface.
pseudomembranous g., g. characterized by the formation of a false membrane.
sclerotic g., a fibrous thickening of the walls of the stomach with diminution in the capacity of the organ.
traumatic g., "hardware disease"; a condition of cattle, caused by the penetration of the stomach wall, usually the reticulum, by any kind of sharp object (usually metallic) which has been swallowed.

gastro-, gastr- [G. *gastēr,* stomach]. Combining forms denoting the stomach.

gastroacephalus (gas'trō-ă-sef'ă-lŭs) [gastro- + G. *a-* priv. + *kephalē,* head]. Unequal conjoined twins in which an acephalous parasite is attached to the abdomen of the autosite.

gastroadenitis (gas'trō-ad-ĕ-nī'tis). Gastradenitis.

gastroalbumorrhea (gas'trō-al-byū-mō-rē'ă) [gastro- + albumin, + G. *rhoia,* flow]. Loss of albumin into the stomach.

gastroamorphus (gas'trō-ă-mōr'fŭs) [gastro- + G. *amorphos,* unshapely]. An included amorphous parasitic twin within the abdomen of the autosite.

gastroanastomosis (gas'trō-an-as-tō-mō'sis). Gastrogastrostomy; anastomosis of the cardiac and antral segments of the stomach, for relief from marked hour-glass contraction of the stomach.

gastroatonia (gas'trō-ă-tō'nē-ă) [gastro- + G. *atonia,* languor]. Obsolete term for loss of tone in the stomach musculature.

gastroblennorrhea (gas'trō-blen-ō-rē'ă) [gastro- + blennorrhea]. Excessive proliferation of mucus by the stomach.

gastrocardiac (gas'trō-kar'dē-ak). Relating to both the stomach and the heart.

gastrocele (gas'trō-sēl) [gastro- + G. *kēlē,* hernia]. **1.** Archenteron; celenteron; subgerminal cavity; the primitive cavity formed by the invagination of the blastula. **2.** Hernia of a portion of the stomach.

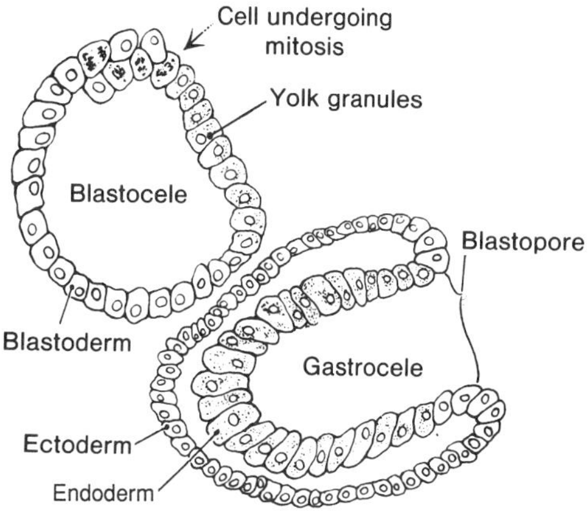

Formation of the Gastrocele

gastrochronorrhea (gas'trō-kron-ō-rē'ă) [gastro- + G. *chronos,* time (chronic), + *rhoia,* a flow]. Excessive continuous gastric secretion.

gastrocnemius (gas-trok-nē'mē-ŭs) [G. *gastroknēmia,* calf of the leg, fr. *gaster (gastr-),* belly, + *knēmē,* leg]. *Musculus* gastrocnemius.

gastrocolic (gas'trō-kol'ik). Relating to the stomach and the colon.

gastrocolitis (gas'trō-kō-lī'tis). Inflammation of both stomach and colon.

gastrocoloptosis (gas'trō-kō-lō-tō'sis) [gastro- + G. *kōlon,* colon, + *ptōsis,* a falling]. Displacement downward of stomach and colon.

gastrocolostomy (gas'trō-kō-los'tō-mē) [gastro- + G. *kōlon,* colon, + *stoma,* mouth]. Establishment of a communication between stomach and colon.

gastrodialysis (gas'trō-dī-al'i-sis). Dialysis across the mucous membrane of the stomach.

Gastrodiscoides hominis (gas'trō-dis-koy'dēz hom'i-nis) [gastro- + G. *diskos,* disk; L. *homo,* gen. *hominis,* man]. *Gastrodiscus hominis;* a species of trematode sometimes found in the intestinal canal of man in India, Southeast Asia, and China; its normal host is the pig.

Gastrodiscus hominis (gas-trō-dis'kŭs). *Gastrodiscoides hominis.*

gastroduodenal (gas'trō-dū'ō-dē'năl, -du-od'ĕ-nal). Relating to the stomach and duodenum.

gastroduodenitis (gas'trō-dū-ō-dē-nī'tis). Inflammation of both stomach and duodenum.

gastroduodenoscopy (gas'trō-dū-ō-dĕ-nos'kō-pē) [gastro- + duodenum, + G. *skopeō,* to view]. Visualization of the interior of the stomach and duodenum by a gastroscope.

gastroduodenostomy (gas'trō-dū-ō-dĕ-nos'tō-mē) [gastro- + duodenum + G. *stoma,* mouth]. Establishment of a communication between the stomach and the duodenum.

gastrodynia (gas-trō-din'ē-ă) [gastro- + G. *odynē,* pain]. Stomach *ache.*

gastroenteric (gas'trō-en-ter'ik). Gastrointestinal.

gastroenteritis (gas'trō-en-ter-ī'tis) [gastro- + G. *enteron,* intestine, + *-itis,* inflammation]. Enterogastritis; inflammation of the

mucous membrane of both stomach and intestine.
acute infectious nonbacterial g., epidemic nonbacterial g.
endemic nonbacterial infantile g., infantile g.; an endemic viral g. of young children (6 months to 12 years) that is especially widespread during winter, caused by strains of rotavirus; the incubation period is 2 to 4 days, with symptoms lasting 3 to 5 days, including abdominal pain, diarrhea, fever, and vomiting.
epidemic nonbacterial g., acute infectious nonbacterial g.; an epidemic, highly communicable but rather mild disease of sudden onset, caused by the epidemic gastroenteritis virus (especially Norwalk agent), with an incubation period of 16 to 48 hours and a duration of 1 to 2 days, which affects all age groups; infection is associated with some fever, abdominal cramps, nausea, vomiting, diarrhea, and headache, one or another of which may be predominant.
infantile g., endemic nonbacterial infantile g.
porcine transmissible g., transmissible g. of swine.
transmissible g. of swine (TGE), porcine transmissible g.; a rapidly spreading disease of swine, caused by a coronavirus and characterized by severe diarrhea and vomiting; case fatality rate in pigs younger than 10 days is high; in older pigs it is low.
viral g., see endemic nonbacterial infantile g.; epidemic nonbacterial g.

gastroenteroanastomosis (gas'trō-en-ter-ō-an-as-tō-mō'sis). Gastroenterostomy.

gastroenterocolitis (gas'trō-en'ter-ō-kō-lī'tis) [gastro- + G. *enteron,* intestine, + *kolon,* colon, + *-itis,* inflammation]. Inflammatory disease involving the stomach and intestines.

gastroenterocolostomy (gas'trō-en-ter-ō-kō-los'tō-mē) [gastro- + G. *enteron,* intestine, + *kolon,* colon + *stoma,* mouth]. Formation of direct communication between the stomach and the large and small intestines.

gastroenterologist (gas'trō-en-ter-ol'ō-jist). A specialist in gastroenterology.

gastroenterology (gas'trō-en-ter-ol'ō-jē) [gastro- + G. *enteron,* intestine, + *logos,* study]. The medical specialty concerned with the function and disorders of the stomach and intestines.

gastroenteropathy (gas'trō-en-ter-op'ă-thē) [gastro- + G. *enteron,* intestine, + *pathos,* suffering]. Any disorder of the alimentary canal.

gastroenteroplasty (gas'trō-en-ter-ō-plas'tē) [gastro- + G. *enteron,* intestine, + *plassō,* to form]. Operative repair of defects in the stomach and intestine.

gastroenteroptosis (gas'trō-en-ter-ō-tō'sis) [gastro- + G. *enteron,* intestine, + *ptōsis,* a falling]. Downward displacement of the stomach and a portion of the intestine.

gastroenterostomy (gas'trō-en-ter-os'tō-mē) [gastro- + G. *enteron,* intestine, + *stoma,* mouth]. Establishment of a new opening between the stomach and the intestine, either anterior or posterior to the mesocolon.

gastroenterotomy (gas'trō-en-ter-ot'ō-mē) [gastro- + G. *enteron,* intestine, + *tomē,* incision]. Section into both stomach and intestine.

gastroepiploic (gas'trō-ep'i-plō'ik). Relating to the stomach and the greater omentum (epiploon).

gastroesophageal (gas'trō-ē-sof'ă-jē'ăl) [gastro- + G. *oisophagos,* gullet (esophagus)]. Relating to both stomach and esophagus.

gastroesophagitis (gas'trō-ē-sof-ă-jī'tis). Inflammation of the stomach and esophagus.

gastroesophagostomy (gas'trō-ē-sof-ă-gos'tō-mē) [gastro- + G. *oisophagos,* gullet (esophagus), + *stoma,* mouth]. Esophagogastrostomy.

gastrogastrostomy (gas'trō-gas-tros'tō-mē). Gastroanastomosis.

gastrogavage (gas-trō-gă-vahzh'). Gavage (1).

gastrogenic (gas-trō-jen'ik). Deriving from or caused by the stomach.

gastrograph (gas'trō-graf) [gastro- + G. *graphē,* a writing]. Gastrokinesograph; an instrument for recording graphically the movements of the stomach.

gastrohepatic (gas'trō-he-pat'ik) [gastro- + G. *hēpar* (*hēpat-*), liver]. Relating to the stomach and the liver.

gastrohydrorrhea (gas'trō-hī-drō-rē'ă) [gastro- + G. *hydōr,* water, + *rhoia,* a flow]. Excretion into the stomach of a large amount of watery fluid containing neither hydrochloric acid, chymosin nor pepsin ferments.

gastroileitis (gas'trō-il-ē-ī'tis). Inflammation of the alimentary canal in which the stomach and ileum are primarily involved.

gastroileostomy (gas'trō-il-ē-os'tō-mē). A surgical joining of stomach to ileum; a technical error in which the ileum instead of jejunum is selected for the site of a gastrojejunostomy.

gastrointestinal (GI) (gas'trō-in-tes'tin-ăl). Gastroenteric; relating to the stomach and intestines.

gastrojejunocolic (gas'trō-jē-jū'nō-kol'ik). Referring to the stomach, jejunum, and colon.

gastrojejunostomy (gas'trō-jē-jū-nos'tō-mē) [gastro- + jejunum G. *stoma,* mouth]. Gastronesteostomy; establishment of a direct communication between the stomach and the jejunum.

gastrokinesograph (gas'trō-ki-nē'sō-graf) [gastro- + G. *kinēsis,* motion, + *graphē,* a writing]. Gastrograph.

gastrolavage (gas-trō-lă-vahzh'). Lavage of the stomach.

gastrolienal (gas-trō-lī'ē-năl) [gastro- + L. *lien,* spleen]. Gastrosplenic.

gastrolith (gas'trō-lith) [gastro- + G. *lithos,* stone]. Gastric calculus; a concretion in the stomach.

gastrolithiasis (gas'trō-li-thī'ă-sis). Presence of one or more calculi in the stomach.

gastrologist (gas-trol'ō-jist). A specialist in gastrology.

gastrology (gas-trol'ō-jē) [gastro- + G. *logos,* study]. The branch of medicine concerned with the stomach and its diseases.

gastrolysis (gas-trol'i-sis) [gastro- + G. *lysis,* loosening]. Division of perigastric adhesions.

gastromalacia (gas'trō-mă-lā'shē-ă) [gastro- + G. *malakia,* softness]. Softening of the walls of the stomach.

gastromegaly (gas'trō-meg'ă-lē) [gastro- + G. *megas* (*megal-*), large]. **1.** Enlargement of the abdomen. **2.** Enlargement of the stomach.

gastromelus (gas-trom'ĕ-lē) [gastro- + G. *melos,* a limb]. A condition in which an individual has a supernumerary limb attached to the abdomen.

gastromyxorrhea (gas'trō-mik-sō-rē'ă) [gastro- + G. *myxa,* mucus, + *rhoia,* a flow]. Myxorrhea gastrica; excessive secretion of mucus in the stomach.

gastronesteostomy (gas'trō-nes-tē-os'tō-mē) [gastro- + G. *nēstis,* jejunum, + *stoma,* mouth]. Gastrojejunostomy.

gastropagus (gas-trop'ă-gŭs) [gastro- + -pagus]. Conjoined twins united at the abdomen.

gastroparalysis (gas'trō-pă-ral'i-sis). Paralysis of the muscular coat of the stomach.

gastroparasitus (gas'trō-par-ă-sī'tŭs). Unequal conjoined twins in which the incomplete parasite is attached to, or within, the abdomen of the autosite.

gastroparesis (gas-trō-pă-rē'sis, -par'ĕ-sis) [gastro- + G. *paresis,* a letting go, paralysis]. A slight degree of gastroparalysis.
g. diabetico'rum, dilation of the stomach with gastric retention in

diabetics, commonly seen in association with severe acidosis or coma.

gastropathic (gas-trō-path'ik). Denoting gastropathy.

gastropathy (gas-trop'ă-thē) [gastro- + G. *pathos,* disease]. Any disease of the stomach.
hypertrophic hypersecretory g., nodular thickenings of gastric mucosa with acid hypersecretion and frequently peptic ulceration, not associated with a gastrin-secreting tumor.

gastropexy (gas'trō-pek-sē) [gastro- + G. *pēxis,* fixation]. Attachment of the stomach to the abdominal wall or diaphragm.

Gastrophilidae (gas-trō-fil'i-dē). Gasterophilidae.

Gastrophilus (gas-trof'i-lŭs). *Gasterophilus.*

gastrophrenic (gas'trō-fren'ik) [gastro- + G. *phrēn,* diaphragm]. Relating to the stomach and the diaphragm.

gastroplasty (gas'trō-plas-tē) [gastro- + G. *plastos,* formed]. Operative treatment of a defect in the stomach or lower esophagus which utilizes the stomach wall for the reconstruction.
Collis g., a technique for lengthening a "short" esophagus; a full-thickness incision of the gastric cardia is made parallel to the lesser curvature, to allow transverse closure and so lengthen the esophagus by making tubular the upper part of the stomach.
vertical banded g., a g. for treatment of morbid obesity in which an upper gastric pouch is formed by a vertical staple line, with a cloth band applied to prevent dilation at the outlet into the main pouch.

gastroplication (gas'trō-pli-kā'shŭn) [gastro- + L. *plico,* to fold]. Gastroptyxis; gastrorrhaphy (2); stomach reefing; an operation for reducing the size of the stomach by suturing a longitudinal fold with the peritoneal surfaces in apposition.

gastropneumonic (gas'trō-nū-mon'ik) [gastro- + G. *pneumōn,* lung]. Pneumogastric.

gastropod (gas'trō-pod). Common name for members of the class Gastropoda.

Gastropoda (gas-trop'ŏ-dă) [gastro- + G. *pous (pod-),* foot]. A class of the phylum Mollusca that includes the snails, whelks, slugs, and limpets.

gastroptosis, gastroptosia (gas-trō-tō'sis, -tō'sē-ă) [gastro- + G. *ptosis,* a falling]. Bathygastry; descensus ventriculi; ventroptosis; downward displacement of the stomach.

gastroptyxis (gas-trō-tik'sis) [gastro- + G. *ptyxis,* a fold]. Gastroplication.

gastropulmonary (gas-trō-pŭl'mo-nar-ē). Pneumogastric.

gastropylorectomy (gas'trō-pī-lōr-ek'tō-mē). Pylorectomy.

gastropyloric (gas'trō-pī-lōr'ik). Relating to the stomach as a whole and to the pylorus.

gastrorrhagia (gas-trō-rā'jē-ă) [gastro- + G. *rhēgnymi,* to burst forth]. Gastric hemorrhage; hemorrhage from the stomach.

gastrorrhaphy (gas-trōr'ă-fē) [gastro- + G. *rhaphē,* a stitching]. **1.** Suture of a perforation of the stomach. **2.** Gastroplication.

gastrorrhea (gas-trō-rē'ă) [gastro- + G. *rhoia,* a flow]. Excessive secretion of gastric juice or of mucus (gastromyxorrhea) by the stomach.

gastrorrhexis (gas'trō-rek'sis) [gastro- + G. *rhēxis,* a bursting]. A tear or bursting of the stomach.

gastroschisis (gas-tros'ki-sis) [gastro- + G. *schisis,* a fissure]. A defect in the abdominal wall resulting from rupture of the amniotic membrane during physiological gut-loop herniation or later due to delayed umbilical ring closure; usually accompanied by protrusion of viscera.

gastroscope (gas'trō-skōp) [gastro- + G. *skopeō,* to examine]. An endoscope for inspecting the inner surface of the stomach.

gastroscopic (gas-trō-skop'ik). Relating to gastroscopy.

gastroscopy (gas-tros'kŏ-pē). Inspection of the inner surface of the stomach through an endoscope.

gastrospasm (gas'trō-spazm). Spasmodic contraction of the walls of the stomach.

gastrosplenic (gas-trō-splen'ik). Gastrolienal; relating to the stomach and the spleen.

gastrostaxis (gas'trō-stak'sis) [gastro- + G. *staxis,* trickling]. Oozing of blood from the mucous membrane of the stomach.

gastrostenosis (gas-trō-ste-nō'sis) [gastro- + G. *stenosis,* narrowing]. Diminution in size of the cavity of the stomach.

gastrostogavage (gas-tros'tō-gă-vahzh'). Gavage (1).

gastrostolavage (gas-tros'tō-lă-vahzh'). Lavage of the stomach through a gastric fistula.

gastrostomy (gas-tros'tō-mē) [gastro- + G. *stoma,* mouth]. Establishment of a new opening into the stomach.

gastrothoracopagus (gas'trō-thōr-ă-kop'ă-gŭs) [gastro- + G. *thōrax,* chest, + *pagos,* something fixed]. Conjoined twins united at thorax and abdomen.

gastrotome (gas'trō-tōm). A knife for incising the stomach.

gastrotomy (gas-trot'ō-mē) [gastro- + G. *tomē,* incision]. Incision into the stomach.

gastrotonometer (gas'trō-tō-nom'ĕ-ter). An apparatus used in gastrotonometry.

gastrotonometry (gas'trō-tō-nom'ĕ-trē) [gastro- + G. *tonos,* tension, + *metron,* measure]. The measurement of intragastric pressure.

gastrotoxic (gas-trō-tok'sik). Poisonous to the stomach.

gastroxin (gas-trō-tok'sin). A cytotoxin specific for the cells of the mucous membrane of the stomach.

gastrotropic (gas-trō-trop'ik) [gastro- + G. *tropikos,* turning]. Affecting the stomach.

gastroxia (gas-trok'sē-ă) [gastro- + G. *oxys,* keen, acid]. Gastroxynsis.

gastroxynsis (gas-trok-sin'sis) [gastro- + G. *oxynō,* to make sharp, acid]. Gastroxia; intermittent excessive secretion of the gastric juice.

gastrula (gas'trū-lă) [Mod. L. dim. of G. *gastēr,* belly]. Invaginate planula; the embryo in the stage of development following the blastula; in lower forms with minimal yolk, it is a simple double-layered structure consisting of ectoderm and endoderm enclosing the archenteron which opens to the outside by way of the blastopore; in forms with considerable yolk, the configuration of the g. is greatly modified due to the persistence of the yolk throughout the gastrulation process; in the human embryo, the absence of yolk allows for a more rapid direct "putting in place" of the germ layers which are derived from the pluripotential embryonic disc.

gastrulation (gas-trū-lā'shŭn). Transformation of the blastula into the gastrula; the development and invagination of the embryonic germ layers.

Gatch, Willis D., U.S. surgeon, 1878–1961. See G. *bed.*

gate (gāt). **1.** To close an ion channel by electrical (*e.g.,* membrane potential) or chemical (*e.g.,* neurotransmitter) action. **2.** Action of a special nerve fiber to block the transmission of impulses through a synapse, *e.g.,* gating of pain impulses at synapses in the dorsal horns.

Gaucher, Philippe C.E., French physician, 1854–1918. See G. *cells,* G.'s *disease;* pseudo-G. *cell.*

Gauer, Otto Hans, German physiologist, 1909–1979. See Henry-G. *response.*

gauge (gāj). Gage; a measuring device.
bite g., gnathodynamometer.

Boley g., a caliper-type g. graduated in millimeters used to measure the thickness of various dental materials.

catheter g., a metal plate with holes of graduated diameter used to determine the size of a catheter.

strain g., a device, employing the Wheatstone bridge principle, used for accurate measurement of forces such as strain, stress, or pressure.

undercut g., a device, used with a surveyor, to precisely locate areas for the placement of the retentive components of clasps when designing removable partial dentures.

Gaule, J., German physician, 1849–1939. See G.'s *spots.*

gaultheria oil (gawl-thēr'ē-ă). Checkerberry or wintergreen oil; a volatile oil distilled from the leaves of *Gaultheria procumbens* (family Ericaceae). See also *methyl* salicylate.

gaultherin (gawl'thĕ-rin). A glycoside from the bark of several species of *Betula* (birch); it yields methyl salicylate, D-glucose, and D-xylose on hydrolysis.

gauntlet (gawnt'let). A glove. See under bandage.

gauss (G) (gows) [J. K. F. *Gauss*]. A unit of magnetic field intensity, equal to $^{-4}$T.

Gauss, Johann K.F., German physicist, 1777–1855. See gauss; gaussian *curve, distribution.*

Gauss, Karl J., German gynecologist, 1875–1957. See G.'s *sign.*

Gaussel, A., French physician, 1871–1937. See Grasset-G. *phenomenon.*

gaussian (gows'ē-ăn). Relating to or described by Johann K.F. Gauss.

gauze (gawz). A bleached cotton cloth of plain weave, used for dressings, bandages, and absorbent sponges; petrolatum g. is saturated with petrolatum.

gavage (gă-vahzh') [Fr. *gaver,* to gorge fowls]. **1.** Gastrogavage; gastrostogavage; forced feeding by stomach tube. **2.** Therapeutic use of a high-potency diet.

Gavard, Hyacinthe, French anatomist, 1753–1802. See G.'s *muscle.*

Gay, Alexander H., Russian anatomist, 1842–1907. See G.'s *glands.*

gay (gā). **1.** A homosexual, especially male. **2.** Denoting a homosexual or the lifestyle thereof.

Gay-Lussac, Joseph L., French naturalist, 1778–1850. See G.-L.'s *law.*

gaze (gāz). The act of looking steadily at an object.

conjugate g., movement of both eyes with the visual axes parallel.

dysconjugate g., failure of the eyes to rotate simultaneously in the same direction.

ping-pong g., spontaneous, alternating conjugate deviation to the right and left caused by disorders of the brainstem and cerebellum.

G-banding. See G-banding *stain.*

Gd Symbol for gadolinium.

GDP Abbreviation for guanosine 5'-diphosphate.

GDPmannose phosphorylase. Mannose-1-phosphate guanylyltransferase(GDP).

Ge Symbol for germanium.

Gedoelstia (ge-del'stē-ă). A genus of nasal botflies (family Oestridae) that includes the species *G. cristata* and *G. haessleri* which parasitize wildebeest, hartebeeste, and other African antelopes, and may also cause an ophthalmomyiasis in sheep and humans.

gedoelstiosis (ge-del-sti-ō'sis). Bulging eye disease; infection of herbivores and rarely man with larvae of flies of the genus *Gedoelstia,* causing ophthalmomyiasis in man.

Geigel, Richard, German physician, 1859–1930. See G.'s *reflex.*

Geiger, Hans, German physicist, 1882–1945. See G.-Müller *counter tube.*

gel (jel) [Mod. L. *gelatum*]. **1.** Gelatum; a jelly, or the solid or semisolid phase of a colloidal solution. **2.** To form a g. or jelly; to convert a sol into a g.

colloidal g., a colloid that has developed resistance to flow because of chemical or thermal change.

pharmacopeial g., a suspension, in a water medium, of an insoluble drug in hydrated form wherein the particle size approaches or attains colloidal dimensions.

gelasmus (jĕ-laz'mŭs) [Gr. *gelasma,* a laugh, fr. *gelaō,* to laugh]. Spasmodic, hysterical laughter.

gelate (jel'āt). Gelatinize.

gelatin (jel'ă-tin) [L. *gelo,* pp. *gelatus,* to freeze, congeal]. A derived protein formed from the collagen of tissues by boiling in water; it swells up when put in cold water, but dissolves only in hot water; used as a hemostat, plasma substitute, and protein food adjunct in malnutrition.

glycerinated g., glycerogelatin; glycogelatin; glycerin jelly; a preparation made of equal parts of g. and glycerin; a firm mass liquefying at gentle heat; it is used as a vehicle for suppositories and urethral bougies.

Irish moss g., g. extracted from Irish moss; used to make the mucilage of Irish moss that is used as a substitute for gum arabic in making emulsions.

vegetable g., a substance similar to g., obtained from gluten.

zinc g., see under zinc.

gelatiniferous (jel'ă-ti-nif'er-ŭs) [gelatin + L. *fero,* to bear]. Producing or containing gelatin.

gelatinization (jĕ-lat'i-ni-zā'shŭn). Conversion into gelatin or a substance resembling it.

gelatinize (jĕ-lat'i-nīz). Gelate. **1.** To convert into gelatin. **2.** To become gelatinous.

gelatinoid (jĕ-lat'i-noyd). Gelatinous (2).

gelatinous (jĕ-lat'i-nŭs). **1.** Pertaining to or characteristic of gelatin. **2.** Gelatinoid; jelly-like or resembling gelatin.

gelation (jĕ-lā'shŭn). In colloidal chemistry, the transformation of a sol into a gel.

gelatum (jĕ-lā'tŭm) [Mod. L.]. Gel (1).

Gélineau, Jean Baptiste Edouard, French physician, 1859–1906. See G.'s *syndrome.*

Gell, P.G., British immunologist. See G. and Coombs *reactions.*

Gellé, Marie-Ernst, French otologist, 1834–1923. See G. *test.*

Gellerstedt, Niles, *1896. See Ceelen-G. *syndrome.*

gelosis (jĕ-lō'sis) [L. *gelo,* to freeze, congeal, + G. *-osis,* condition]. An extremely firm mass in tissue (especially in a muscle), with a consistency resembling that of frozen tissue.

gelotripsy (jel'ō-trip-sē) [gelosis + G. *tripsis,* a rubbing, fr. *tribō,* to rub]. Nerve-point massage; rubbing away an indurated swelling or tender point in neuralgia and myalgia.

gelsemine (jel'sĕ-mēn) [Mod. L. *gelsemium,* fr. Pers. *yāsmin,* jasmine]. A crystallizable alkaloid derived from gelsemium; a mydriatic and central nervous system stimulant.

Gély, Jules A., French surgeon, 1806–1861. See G.'s *suture.*

gem- [shortened form of L. *geminus,* twin]. Prefix denoting twin substitutions on a single atom; *e.g.,* the *gem*-dimethyl substitution on carbon-4 of lanosterol.

Gemella (jĕ-mel'ă) [L. dim. of *geminus,* twin]. A genus of motile, aerobic, facultatively anaerobic, coccoid bacteria (family Streptococcaceae) which occur singly or in pairs, with flattened adjacent sides. They are Gram-indeterminate but have a cell wall like that of Gram-positive bacteria, and are parasitic on mammals. The type species is *G. haemolysans,* which is found in bronchial secretions and in mucus from the respiratory tract.

gemellipara (jem-ĕ-lip'ără) [L. *gemellus,* twin, + *pario, to bear*]. A woman who has given birth to twins.

gemellology (jem-el-ol'ō-jē) [L. *gemellus,* twin-born, + G. *logos,* study]. The study of twins and the phenomenology of twinning.

gemellus (jĕ-mel'ŭs) [L. dim. of *geminus,* twin]. *Musculus* gemellus.

gemfibrozil (jem-fī'brō-zil). Pentanoic acid, 5-(2,5-dimethylphenoxy)-2,2-dimethyl-; an antihyperlipidemic agent used in the treatment of hypertriglyceridemia.

geminate (jem'i-nāt) [L. *gemino,* pp. *-atus,* to double, fr. *geminus,* twin]. Occurring in pairs.

gemination (jem-i-nā'shŭn) [L. *geminatio,* a doubling]. Embryologic partial division of a primordium, as of a single tooth germ, resulting in two partially or completely separated crowns.

geminous (jem'i-nŭs). Relating to gemination.

gemistocyte (jĕ-mis'tō-sīt). Protoplasmic *astrocyte* (1).

gemistocytoma (jĕ-mis'tō-sī-tō'mă). Protoplasmic *astrocytoma.*

gemma (jem'ă) [L. bud]. Any budlike or bulblike body, especially a taste bud or end bulb.

gemmation (jem-ā'shŭn) [L. *gemma,* a bud]. Budding; bud fission; a form of fission in which the parent cell does not divide, but puts out a small budlike process (daughter cell) with its proportionate amount of chromatin; the daughter cell then separates to begin independent existence.

gemmule (jem'yūl) [L. *gemmula,* dim. of *gemma,* bud]. **1.** A small bud that projects from the parent cell, and finally becomes detached, forming a cell of a new generation. **2.** Dendritic *spine.* **3.** Hypothetical particles which, according to Darwin's theory of inheritance, were transferred from the body cells to germ cells of the parent organism; thus characteristics were transmitted to the offspring.
Hoboken's g.'s, Hoboken's *nodules.*

gen-, -gen [G. *genos,* birth]. **1.** Combining form, used as a prefix or suffix, meaning "producing" or "coming to be." **2.** In chemistry, used as a suffix to indicate "precursor of." See also pro- (2).

gena (jē'nă) [L.]. Cheek.

genal (jē'năl). Relating to the gena, or cheek.

gender (jen'der). The sex of assignment by oneself or those who raise the individual. *Cf.* sex; gender *role.*

gene (jēn) [G. *genos,* birth]. Factor (3); a functional unit of heredity which occupies a specific place or locus on a chromosome, is capable of reproducing itself exactly at each cell division, and is capable of directing the formation of an enzyme or other protein. The g. as a functional unit probably consists of a discrete segment of a giant DNA molecule containing the proper number of purine (adenine and guanine) and pyrimidine (cytosine and thymine) bases in the correct sequence to code the sequence of amino acids needed to form a specific peptide. Protein synthesis is mediated by molecules of messenger-RNA formed on the chromosome with the g. unit of DNA acting as a template, which then pass into the cytoplasm and become oriented on the ribosomes where they in turn act as templates to organize a chain of amino acids to form a peptide. G.'s normally occur in pairs in all cells except gametes as a consequence of the fact that all chromosomes are paired except the sex chromosomes (X and Y) of the male.
allelic g., see allele; *dominance* of g.'s.
autosomal g., a g. located on any chromosome other than a sex chromosome (X or Y).
condominant g., a set of two or more alleles such that each is expressed despite the presence of one of the others.
control g., see operator g., regulator g.
dominant g., see *dominance* of genes.
H g., histocompatibility g.
histocompatibility g., H g.; in laboratory animals, a g. whose product can elicit an immune response and thereby cause rejection of a homograft when tissue is transplanted from one individual to another; in man, H g.'s control HLA antigens.
holandric g., Y-linked g.
immune response g.'s, Ir g.'s; g.'s in the HLA-D region of the histocompatibility complex of human chromosome 6 which seem to control the immune response to specific antigens.
Ir g.'s, immune response g.'s.
jumping g., a g. associated with transposable elements.
lethal g., a g. that produces a genotype that leads to death of the organism before reproduction is possible or that precludes reproduction; for a recessive lethal g., homozygosity is necessary to express it.
mimic g.'s, nonallelic (independent) g.'s with closely similar effects.
mitochondrial g., a functioning g. located not in the nucleus of a cell but in the mitochondria.
modifier g., a nonallelic g. that controls or changes the manifestation of a g. by interfering with its transcription.
mutant g., a g. that has been changed from an ancestral type, not necessarily in the current generation. See also subentries at mutant and mutation.
operator g., a g. with the function of activating the production of messenger-RNA by one or more adjacent structural g.'s; part of the feedback system for determining the rate of production of an enzyme.
penetrant g., a g. that in the appropriate genotypes is phenotypically manifest; strictly, it is the trait that is penetrant, not the g.
pleiotropic g., polyphenic g.; a g. that has multiple, apparently unrelated, phenotypic manifestations.
polyphenic g., pleiotropic g.
recessive g., see *dominance* of g.'s.
regulator g., a g. with the function of producing a repressor substance capable of combining with an operator g. and inhibiting the ability of the operator g. to activate one or more structural g.'s, thus preventing the production of a specific enzyme; when the enzyme is again demanded, a specific regulatory metabolite combines with the repressor substance and removes its inhibiting effect on the operator g., and thus starts production of the enzyme.
repressor g., a g. that prevents a nonallele from being transcribed.
sex-linked g., a g. located on a sex chromosome, in usual usage, the X chromosome.
split g., a g. that is assembled from discontinuous parts.
structural g., a g. with the function of determining the structure (amino acid sequence) of a specific protein or peptide.
suppressor g., a g. that can reverse the effect of a specific type of mutation in other g.'s.
transfer g.'s, g.'s carried by a conjugative plasmid, essential for fertility and establishment of the bacterial donor state.
transforming g., oncogene.
X-linked g., a g. located on an X chromosome.
Y-linked g., holandric g.; a g. located on a Y chromosome.

genealogy (jē-nē-awl'ō-jē) [G. *genea,* descent, + *logos,* study]. The history of the descent of a person or family.

gene library. A random assembly of cloned DNA fragments inside of a vector which may or may not contain all the genetic information of a species.

gene mapping. See genetic map.

genera (jen'er-ă). Plural of genus.

generalist (jen'er-ăl-ist) A general physician or family physician; a physician trained to take care of the majority of nonsurgical diseases, sometimes including obstetrics.

generalization (jen'er-ăl-i-zā'shŭn). **1.** The rendering or becoming general, diffuse, or widespread, as when a primarily local disease becomes systemic. **2.** The reasoning by which a basic conclusion is reached which applies to different items, each having some common factor.

stimulus g., in conditioning, the eliciting of a conditioned response by stimuli never before experienced but which are similar to a particular conditioned stimulus.

generalized (jen'er-ă-līzd). Involving the whole of an organ, as when an epileptic seizure involves all parts of the brain.

generate (jen'er-āt) [L. *genero,* pp. *-atus,* to beget]. **1.** To produce. **2.** To procreate.

generation (jen-er-ā'shŭn) [L. *generatio,* fr. *genero,* pp. *-atus,* to beget]. **1.** Reproduction (2). **2.** A stage in succession of descent; *e.g.,* father, son, and grandson are three g.'s.

asexual g., nonsexual g.; reproduction by fission, gemmation, or in any other way without union of the male and female cell, or conjugation. See also parthenogenesis.

filial g., the offspring resulting from a genetically specified mating: first filial g. (symbol F_1), the offspring resulting from mating of parents of contrasting genotypes; second filial g. (F_2), the offspring resulting from the mating of two F_1 individuals; third filial g. (F_3), fourth filial g. (F_4), etc., the offspring in succeeding g.'s of continued inbreeding of F_1 descendents.

nonsexual g., asexual g.

parental g. (P_1), the parents of a mating, usually experimental, involving contrasting genotypes; the original mating of a genetic experiment; parents of the F_1 g.

sexual g., reproduction by conjugation, or the union of male and female cells.

skipped g., a phenomenon of pedigrees in which a gene is transmitted from one affected person to another through a phenotypically unaffected person, as by recessivity (especially for X-linked traits), epistasis, variable expressivity, or absence of an environmental challenge such as a toxin.

spontaneous g., heterogenesis; the supposed origin of living matter *de novo,* or from the vitalization of nonliving matter. See also biogenesis.

virgin g., parthenogenesis.

generative (jen'er-ă-tiv). Relating to generation.

generator (jen'er-ā-ter) [*generator,* a begetter, producer]. An apparatus for conversion of chemical, mechanical, atomic, or other forms of energy into electricity.

aerosol g., a device for producing airborne suspensions of small particles for inhalation therapy or experimental work; *e.g.,* a La Mer g., spinning disk, or vibrating reed, each of which produces a monodisperse aerosol.

asynchronous pulse g., fixed rate pulse g.; a g. in which the rate of discharge is independent of the natural activity of the heart.

atrial synchronous pulse g., atrial triggered pulse g.; a ventricular stimulating pulse whose rate of discharge is directly determined by the atrial rate.

atrial triggered pulse g., atrial synchronous pulse g.

demand pulse g., ventricular inhibited pulse g.

fixed rate pulse g., asynchronous pulse g.

pulse g., a device that produces an electrical discharge with a regular or rhythmical wave form in which the electromotive force varies in a specific pattern in relation to time; *e.g.,* in an electronic pacemaker, it produces an electrical discharge at regular intervals, and these intervals may be modified by a sensory circuit which can reset the time-base for subsequent discharge on the basis of other electrical activity, such as that produced by spontaneous cardiac beating.

radionuclide g., a column containing a large amount of a particular radionuclide that decays down to a second radionuclide of shorter physical half-life; the daughter radionuclide is separated from the parent by the process of elution and affords a continuing supply of relatively short-lived radionuclides for laboratory use; the elution is loosely termed "milking" with the generator referred to as a "radioactive cow."

standby pulse g., ventricular inhibited pulse g.

ventricular inhibited pulse g., demand pulse g.; standby pulse g.; a g. which suppresses its output in response to natural ventricular activity but which, in the absence of such activity, functions as an asynchronous pulse.

ventricular synchronous pulse g., ventricular triggered pulse g.; a pulse which delivers its output synchronously with naturally occurring ventricular activity but which, in the absence of such activity, functions as an asynchronous pulse.

ventricular triggered pulse g., ventricular synchronous pulse g.

generic (jĕ-năr'ik) [L. *genus* (*gener-*), birth]. **1.** Relating to or denoting a genus. **2.** General. **3.** Characteristic or distinctive.

generic name. 1. In chemistry, a noun that indicates the class or type of a single compound; *e.g.,* salt, saccharide (sugar), hexose, alcohol, aldehyde, lactone, acid, amine, alkane, steroid, vitamin. "Class" is more appropriate and more often used than is "generic." **2.** In the pharmaceutical and commercial fields, a misnomer for nonproprietary name. **3.** In the biologic sciences, the first part of the scientific name (Latin binary combination or binomial) of an organism; written with an initial capital letter and in italics. In bacteriology, the species name consists of two parts (comprising one name): the g. n. and the specific epithet; in other biologic disciplines, the species name is regarded as being composed of two names: the g. n. and the specific name.

genesial (je-nē'sē-ăl). Relating to generation.

genesiology (je-nē-sē-ol'ō-jē) [G. *genesis,* generation, + *logos,* study]. The branch of science concerned with generation or reproduction.

genesis (jen'ĕ-sis) [G.]. An origin or beginning process; also used as combining form in suffix position.

gene splicing. Splicing (1).

genetic (jĕ-net'ik). Relating to 1) genetics; 2) ontogeny.

genetic burden. A measurement of the cost (mainly in genetic deaths) incurred in the discharge of genetic load; burden and load are broadly related, but while the load is enduring, it may otherwise be discharged (*e.g.,* by genetic drift) or the burden may be postponed indefinitely.

geneticist (jĕ-net'i-sist). A specialist in genetics.

genetic map. An abstract representation of the array of genetic loci such that the scale of distance is proportional to the expected number of crossings over between them; *e.g.,* on a g. m. the combined distance between locus A and locus C is the algebraic sum of the two distances between loci A and B, and B and C.

genetics (jĕ-net'iks) [G. *genesis,* origin or production]. The branch of science concerned with heredity.

behavior g., the study of heritable factors in behavioral patterns, as by pedigree analysis, biochemical abnormality, or karyotypic analysis.

biochemical g., the study of g. in terms of the chemical (biochemical) events involved, as in the elucidation of the manner in which DNA molecules replicate and control the synthesis of specific enzymes by way of the genetic code.

clinical g., g. applied to the diagnosis, prognosis, management, and prevention of genetic diseases.

galtonian g., the g. of quantitative traits by analysis of the first two moments of unresolved data; the preferred method for analysis of multivariate gaussian distribution.

human g., the study of the genetic aspects of man as a species.

mathematical g., the study of genetic traits by formal analysis, *e.g.,* quantitative g., population dynamics, genetic epidemiology.

medical g., the study of the etiology, pathogenesis, and natural history of human diseases which are at least partially genetic in origin.

mendelian g., the study of the pattern of segregation of phenotypes under the control of a single genetic locus.
microbial g., the study of hereditary mechanisms of microbes.
molecular g., molecular biology applied to g.
population g., the study of genetic influences on the somatic characteristics of populations.
quantitative g., the formal study of measurable genetic traits.
somatic cell g., the study of the structure, organization, and function of a genome by the techniques of cell hybridization.
statistical g., the study of the applications of principles of statistics to problems in genetics.
transplantation g., g. as applied to the transplanting of tissues from one animal to another.

genetotrophic (jĕ-net-ō-trof′ik) [G. *genesis,* origin, + *trophē,* nourishment]. Relating to inherited individual distinctions in nutritional requirements.

Geneva Convention. An international agreement formed at meetings in Geneva, Switzerland, in 1864 and 1906, relating (among medical subjects) to the safeguarding of the wounded in battle, of those having the care of them, and of the buildings in which they are being treated. The direct outcome of the first of these meetings was the establishment of the Red Cross Society.

Geneva lens measure [*Geneva,* Switzerland]. A device for measuring the radii of the curvature of a spectacle lens.

Gengou, Octave, French bacteriologist 1875–1957. See G. *phenomenon;* Bordet-G. potato blood *agar, bacillus, phenomenon.*

genial, genian (jĕ-nī′ăl, -nī′an) [G. *geneion,* chin]. Mental (2).

-genic. Suffix denoting producing or forming, produced or formed by.

genicula (je-nik′yū-lă). Plural of geniculum.

genicular (je-nik′yū-lăr). Commonly used to mean genual, *q.v.*

geniculate (je-nik′yū-lāt) [L. *geniculo,* pp. *-atus,* to bend the knee, fr. *genu,* knee]. **1.** Geniculated; bent like a knee. **2.** Referring to the geniculum of the facial nerve, denoting the ganglion there present. **3.** Denoting the corpus geniculatum laterale or mediale.

geniculated (je-nik′yū-lā-ted). Geniculate (1).

geniculum, pl. genicula (je-nik′yū-lŭm, -lă) [L. dim. of *genu,* knee]. **1** [NA]. A small genu or angular kneelike structure. **2.** A knotlike structure.
g. cana′lis facia′lis [NA], g. of facial canal; the bend in the facial canal corresponding to the g. nervi facialis.
g. of facial canal, g. canalis facialis.
g. of facial nerve, g. nervi facialis.
g. ner′vi facia′lis [NA], g. of facial nerve; **(1)** a rectangular bend of the facial nerve in the facial canal where it turns posterior in the medial wall of the middle ear. **(2)** complex loop of facial nerve fibers around abducens nucleus.

-genin. Suffix used to denote the basic steroid unit of the toxic substance, usually a steroid glycoside.

genioglossus (jĕ′nī-ō-glos′ŭs) [G. *geneion,* chin, + *glōssa,* tongue]. *Musculus* genioglossus.

geniohyoid (jĕ-nī′ō-hī′oyd). *Musculus* geniohyoideus.

geniohyoideus (jĕ-nī′ō-hī-oyd′ē-ŭs) [G. *geneion,* chin, + *hyoeidēs,* y-shaped, hyoid]. *Musculus* geniohyoideus.

genion (jĕ-nī′on) [G. *geneion,* chin]. The tip of the mental spine, a point in craniometry.

genioplasty (jĕ′nī-ō-plas-tē) [G. *geneion,* chin, cheek, + *plastos,* formed]. Mentoplasty.

genital (jen′i-tăl). **1.** Relating to reproduction or generation. **2.** Relating to the genitals. **3.** Relating to or characterized by genitality.

genitalia (jen′i-tā′lē-ă) [L. neut. pl. of *genitalis,* genital]. *Organa* genitalia.
ambiguous external g., external g. not clearly of either sex; most commonly designates external g. that are incompletely masculinized.
external g., the vulva in the female, and the penis and scrotum in the male.

genitality (jen-i-tal′i-tē). In psychoanalysis, a term referring to the genital components of sexuality (*i.e.,* the penis and vagina), as opposed, for example, to orality and anality.

genitals (jen′i-tălz) [see genitalia]. *Organa* genitalia.

genitocrural (jen′i-tō-krū′răl). Genitofemoral.

genitofemoral (jen′i-tō-fem′ō-răl). Genitocrural; relating to the genitalia and the thigh; denoting the g. nerve.

genitourinary (GU) (jen′i-tō-yū′ri-nar-ē). Urogenital; urinogenital; urinosexual; relating to the organs of reproduction and urination.

genius (jēn′yŭs, jēn′ē-ŭs). [L.]. **1.** Markedly superior intellectual or artistic abilities or exceptional creative power. **2.** A person so endowed.

genius epidemicus (ep-i-dem′i-kŭs) [Mod. L.]. The influence, atmospheric, telluric, or cosmic, or the combination of any two or three, anciently regarded as the cause of epidemic and endemic diseases.

Gennari, Francesco, Italian anatomist, 1750–1795. See G.'s *band, stria; line* of G., *stripe* of G.

genocopy (jen′ō-kop-e). A genotype at one locus that produces a phenotype which simulates that produced by another genotype; *e.g.,* two types of elliptocytosis that are g.'s of each other, but are distinguished by the fact that one is linked to the Rh blood group locus and the other is not.

genodermatology (jen′ō-der-mă-tol′ō-jē) [G. *genos,* birth, descent, + *derma,* skin, + *logos,* theory]. Study of the hereditary aspects of cutaneous disorders.

genodermatosis (jen′ō-der-mă-tō′sis). A skin condition of genetic origin.

genome (je′nōm, -nom) [gene + chromosome]. **1.** A complete set of chromosomes derived from one parent, the haploid number of a gamete. **2.** The total gene complement of a set of chromosomes found in higher life forms, or the functionally similar but simpler linear arrangements found in bacteria and viruses.

genomic (jĕ-nom′ik). Relating to a genome.

genospecies (jĕ′nō-spē-sēz, jen′). A group of organisms in which interbreeding is possible, as evidenced by genetic transfer and recombination.

genote (jē′nōt). In microbial genetics, an element of recombination when one of the pair is not a complete chromosome; commonly used as a suffix (*e.g.,* endogenote, exogenote, F genote).
F g., F-genote, F′ *plasmid.*

genotoxic (jē-nō-toks′ik). Denoting a substance that is damaging to DNA and thereby may cause mutation or cancer.

genotype (jen′ō-tīp) [G. *genos,* birth, descent, + *typos,* type]. The genetic constitution of an individual, used with respect to gene combination at one specified locus or with respect to any specified combination of loci. For specific blood group genotypes, see Blood Groups appendix.

genotypical (jen-ō-tip′i-kăl). Relating to the genotype.

gentamicin, gentamycin (jen-tă-mī′sin). A broad spectrum antibiotic complex, obtained from *Micromonospora purpurea* and *M. echinospora,* that inhibits the growth of both Gram-positive and Gram-negative bacteria; the sulfate salt is used medicinally.

gentian (jen′shŭn). Gentian root; the dried rhizome and roots of *Gentiana lutea* (family Gentianaceae), an herb of southern and central Europe; a simple bitter.

gentianophil, gentianophile (jen′shŭn-o-fil, -fīl) [gentian + G. *philos,* fond]. Gentianophilous; staining readily with gentian violet.

gentianophilous (jen-shŭn-of′i-lŭs). Gentianophil.

gentianophobic (jen′shŭn-ō-fō′bik) [gentian + G. *phobos,* fear]. Not taking a gentian violet stain, or taking it poorly.

gentian violet. An unstandardized dye mixture of violet rosanilins, now superceded by crystal violet or methyl violet 2B.

gentiobiase (jen′shi-ō-bī′ās). β-D-Glucosidase.

genu, gen. **ge′nus,** pl. **genua** (jē′nū, jē′nŭs, jen′ū-ă) [L.] [NA]. **1.** Knee. **2.** Any structure of angular shape resembling a flexed knee.

g. cap′sulae inter′nae [NA], g., or knee, of the internal capsule; the obtuse angle, opening laterally in the horizontal plane, formed by the union of the two limbs (crus anterius and crus posterius) of the internal capsule.

g. cor′poris callo′si [NA], g. or knee of the corpus callosum; the anterior extremity of the corpus callosum that folds downward and backward on itself, terminating in the rostrum.

g. of corpus callosum, g. corporis callosi.

g. of facial nerve, g. nervi facialis.

g. of internal capsule, g. capsulae internae.

g. ner′vi facial′lis [NA], g. of facial nerve; the curve which the fibers of the root of the facial nerve describe around the abducens nucleus in the pontine tegmentum; the internal g. of the facial nerve.

g. recurva′tum, back-knee; hyperextension of the knee, the lower extremity having a forward curvature.

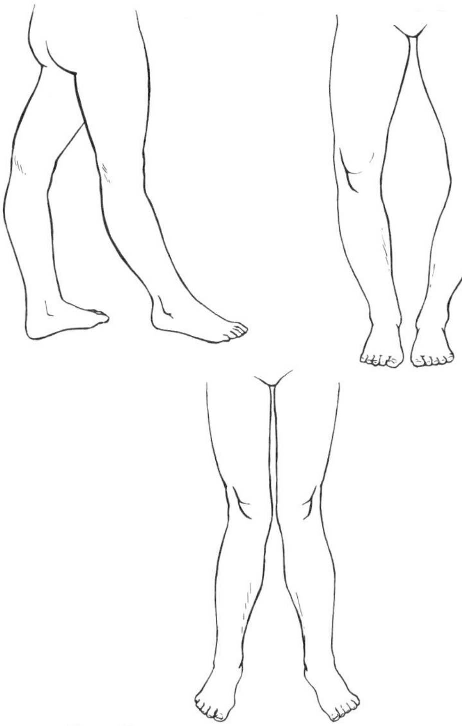

Genu Recurvatum, Valgum, and Varum

g. val′gum, knock-knee; tibia valga; a deformity marked by abduction of the leg in relation to the thigh.

g. va′rum, bowleg; bandy-leg; tibia vara; an outward bowing of the legs.

genual (jen′yū-ăl) [L. *genu,* knee]. Genicular; relating to the knee.

genus, pl. **genera** (jē′nŭs, jen′er-ă) [L. birth, descent]. In natural history classification, the division between the family, or tribe, and the species; a group of species alike in the broad features of their organization but different in detail.

genyantrum (jen-ē-an′trŭm) [G. *genys,* cheek, + *antron,* cave]. *Sinus* maxillaris.

geo- [G. *gē,* earth]. Combining form relating to the earth, or to soil.

geode (jē′ōd). A cystlike space (or spaces) with or without an epithelial lining, observed radiologically in subarticular bone, usually in arthritic disorders.

geomedicine (jē-ō-med′i-sin). Nosochthonography; nosogeography; the science concerned with the influence of climatic and environmental conditions on health and disease.

geopathology (jē′ō-pă-thol′ō-jē). The study of disease in relation to regions, climates, and other environmental influences.

geophagia, geophagism, geophagy (jē-ō-fā′jē-ă, jē-of′ă-jizm, -of′ă-jē) [geo- + G. *phagein,* to eat]. The practice of eating dirt or clay. Also known as earth-eating; dirt-eating.

geophilic (jē-ō-fil′ik) [geo- + G. *phileō,* to love]. Soil seeking or soil preferring; designates preference of a parasite for soil rather than a human or animal host.

Geophilus (jē-of′i-lŭs). A genus of centipedes, characterized by very large numbers of legs (47 to 67 pairs); includes *G. californius, G. rubens,* and *G. umbraticus,* in the U.S.

Georgi, Walter, German bacteriologist, 1889–1920. See Sachs-G. *test.*

geotaxis (jē-ō-tak′sis) [geo- + G. *taxis,* orderly arrangement]. Geotropism; a form of positive barotaxis in which there is a tendency to growth or movement toward or into the earth.

geotrichosis (jē′ō-tri-kō′sis) [geo- + G. *thrix,* hair, + *-osis,* condition]. A systemic mycosis allegedly caused by *Geotrichum candidum;* ascribed symptoms are diverse and suggestive of secondary or mixed infections.

Geotrichum (jē-ot′ri-kŭm). A genus of yeastlike fungi which produce arthroconidia but rarely blastoconidia. One species, *G. candidum* (perfect state *Endomyces geotrichum*), is said by some to cause lesions in the pulmonary and alimentary tracts of man; others consider these lesions to be secondary to an underlying condition. See also geotrichosis.

geotropism (jē-ot′rō-pizm) [geo- + G. *tropē,* a turning]. Geotaxis.

gephyrophobia (jĕ-fī-rō-fō′bē-ă) [G. *gephyra,* bridge, + *phobos,* fear]. Fear of crossing a bridge.

Geraghty, John T., U.S. physician, 1876–1924. See G.'s *test,* Rowntree and G.'s *test.*

geratology (jār-ă-tol′ō-jē). Gerontology.

gerbil (jer′bil) [Mod. L. *gerbillus,* fr. Arab.]. A name applied to any of 13 genera of small rodents (subfamily Gerbillinae) from Africa and Asia; they resemble jerboas or kangaroo rats and can survive without drinking water.

Gerdy, Pierre N., French surgeon, 1797–1856. See G.'s *fibers, fontanel,* hyaloid *fossa, ligament,* interatrial *loop, tubercle.*

Gerhardt, Carl J., German physician, 1833–1902. See G.'s *disease, reaction, sign, test* for acetoacetic acid; G.-Semon *law.*

Gerhardt, Charles F., French chemist, 1816–1856. See G.'s *test* for urobilin in the urine.

geriatric (jār-ē-at′rik). Relating to old age or to geriatrics.

geriatrics (jār-ē-at′riks) [G. *gēras,* old age, + *iatrikos,* healing]. The branch of medicine concerned with the medical problems and care of old people.

dental g., gerodontics; gerodontology; treatment of dental problems peculiar to advanced age.

Gerlach, Joseph, German anatomist, 1820–1896. See G.'s annular *tendon, tonsil, valve, valvula.*

Gerlier, Felix, Swiss physician, 1840–1914. See G.'s *disease.*

germ (jerm) [L. *germen,* sprout, bud, germ]. **1.** A microbe; a microorganism. **2.** A primordium; the earliest trace of a structure within an embryo.

dental g., tooth g.

enamel g., the enamel organ of a developing tooth; one of a series of knoblike projections from the dental lamina, later becoming bell-shaped and receiving in its hollow the dental papilla.

reserve tooth g., enamel organ and papilla of a permanent tooth.

tooth g., dental g.; the enamel organ and dentin papilla, constituting the developing tooth.

germanium (jer-măn'ē-ŭm) [L. *Germania,* Germany]. A metallic element, symbol Ge, atomic no. 32, atomic weight 72.59.

germicidal (jer-mi-sī'dăl). Germicide (1).

germicide (jer'mi-sīd) [germ + L. *caedo,* to kill]. **1.** Germicidal; destructive to germs or microbes. **2.** An agent with this action.

germinal (jer'mi-năl). Relating to a germ or, in botany, to germination.

germinoma (jer-mi-nō'mă). A neoplasm of the germinal tissue of gonads, mediastinum, or pineal region; the degree of differentiation to form adult cell types (*e.g.,* sperm, ova, teratoma) varies.

gero-, geront-, geronto- [G. *gerōn,* old man]. Combining forms denoting old age. See also presby-.

geroderma (jăr-ō-der'mă) [gero- + G. *derma,* skin]. **1.** The atrophic skin of the aged. **2.** Any condition in which the skin is thinned and wrinkled, resembling the integument of old age.

gerodontics, gerodontology (jăr-ō-don'tiks, -don-tol'ō-jē) [gero- + G. *odous,* tooth]. Dental *geriatrics.*

geromarasmus (jăr'ō-mă-raz'mŭs) [gero- + G. *marasmos,* a wasting]. Senile *atrophy.*

geromorphism (jăr-ō-mōr'fizm) [gero- + G. *morphē,* form]. Obsolete term for a condition of premature senility.

gerontal (jăr-on'tăl). Relating to old age.

gerontine (jăr'on-tēn). Spermine.

geronto-, geront-. See gero-.

gerontologist (jăr-on-tol'ō-jist). One who specializes in gerontology.

gerontology (jăr-on-tol'ō-jē) [geronto- + G. *logos,* study]. Geratology; the scientific study of the process and problems of aging.

gerontophilia (jăr'on-tō-fil'ē-ă) [geronto- + G. *philos,* fond]. Morbid love for old persons.

gerontophobia (jăr'on-tō-fō'bē-ă) [geronto- + G. *phobos,* fear]. Morbid fear of old persons.

gerontotherapeutics (jăr-on'tō-thăr-ă-pyū'tiks). The science concerned with treatment of the aged.

gerontotherapy (jăr-on'tō-thăr-ă-pē). Geriatric therapy: treatment of disease in the aged.

gerontoxon (jăr'on-tok'son) [geronto- + G. *toxon,* bow]. *Arcus* cornealis.

Gerota, Dimitru, Roumanian anatomist and surgeon, 1867–1939. See G.'s *capsule, fascia, method.*

Gersh, Isidore, U.S. histologist, *1907. See Altmann-G. *method.*

Gerstmann, Josef, Austrian neurologist, *1887. See G. *syndrome; G. -Straüssler syndrome.*

gestagen (jes'tă-jen). Inclusive term used to denote any one of several gestagenic substances, which are usually steroid hormones.

gestagenic (jes-tă-jen'ik). Inducing progestational effects in the uterus.

gestalt (ge-stahlt) [Ger. shape]. A system of phenomena so integrated as to constitute a functional unit with properties not derivable from its parts.

gestaltism (ge-stahlt'izm) [see gestalt]. The theory in psychology that the objects of mind come as complete forms or configurations which cannot be split into parts; *e.g.,* a square is perceived as such rather than as four discrete lines.

gestation (jes-tā'shŭn) [L. *gestatio,* from *gesto,* pp. *gestatus,* to bear]. Pregnancy. Considerable breed variation exists within the species, in addition to individual variation, in the length of the g. period.

Gestation periods of common domesticated animals (in days)

Species	Range	Average
Ass	365–375	370
Horse	329–346	340
Cow	273–291	282
Sheep	143–152	148
Goat	148–156	148
Swine	111–116	114
Dog	58–63	60
Cat	56–65	63
Rabbit	30–32	32
Guinea pig	67–68	68
Rat	21–22	22
Mouse	18–20	

gestosis, pl. **gestoses** (jes-tō'sis, -sēz) [L. *gesto,* to carry, to bear, + G. *-osis,* condition]. Any disorder of pregnancy.

gesture (jes'chŭr) [L. *gestus,* movement, gesture]. Any movement expressive of an idea, opinion, or emotion.

suicide g., an apparent attempt at suicide by someone wishing to attract attention, gain sympathy, or achieve some goal other than self-destruction.

Gey's solution. See under solution.

GFR Abbreviation for glomerular filtration *rate.*

GH Abbreviation for growth *hormone.*

ghee (gē) [Eng. spelling of Hind. *ghi*]. A clarified butter in India made from cow or buffalo milk that has been coagulated before churning; used as an emollient, a dressing for wounds, and a food.

Gheel colony. See under colony.

Ghon, Anton, Prague pathologist, 1866–1936. See G.'s *focus,* primary *lesion, tubercle;* G.-Sachs *bacillus.*

GHRF, GH-RF Abbreviation for growth hormone-releasing *factor.*

GHRH, GH-RH Abbreviation for growth hormone-releasing *hormone.*

GI Abbreviation for gastrointestinal; Gingival Index.

Giacomini, Carlo, Italian anatomist, 1841–1898. See *band* of G., *frenulum* of G., uncus *band* of G.

Giannuzzi, Italian anatomist, 1839–1876. See G.'s *cells, crescents, demilunes.*

Gianotti, F., 20th century Italian dermatologist. See G.-Crosti *syndrome.*

giantism (jī'an-tizm). Gigantism.

Giardia (jē-ar'dē-ă) [Alfred *Giard,* Fr. biologist, 1846–1908]. A genus of parasitic flagellates that parasitize the small intestine of many mammals, including most domestic animals and man; *e.g., G. bovis* in cattle, *G. canis* in dogs, and *G. cati* in cats. Many species have been described, but recent workers have suggested that these should be reduced to only two or three.

G. lam'blia, a flattened, heart-shaped organism (10 to 20 μm in length) with 8 flagella; it attaches itself to the intestinal mucosa by means of a pair of sucking organs; it is usually asymptomatic except in heavy infections, when it may interfere with absorption of fats and produce flatulence, steatorrhea, and acute discomfort; it is the common species of *G.* in man, but is also found in pigs.

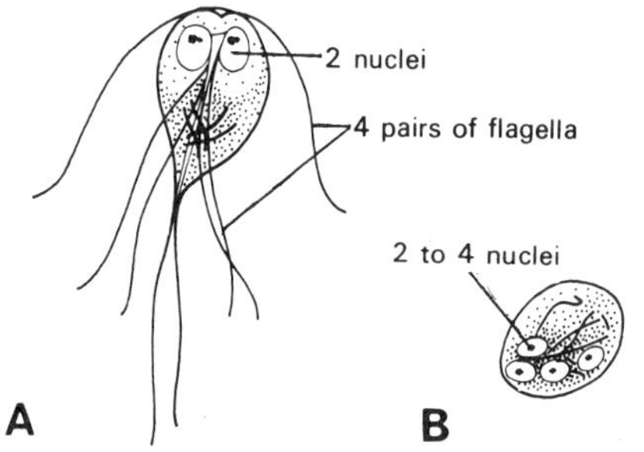

Giardia lamblia
A, trophozoite; *B*, cyst.

giardiasis (jē-ar-dī'ă-sis). Lambliasis; infection with *Giardia; G.* lamblia may cause diarrhea, dyspepsia, and occasionally malabsorption in man.
chinchilla g., an intestinal infection of chinchilla characterized by diarrhea, anorexia, lassitude, and frequently death, believed to be caused by the presence of large numbers of *Giardia.*

gibbon (gib'on) [Fr.]. A genus of anthropoid apes, *Hylobates,* of the superfamily Hominoidea.

gibbous (gib'ŭs) [L. *gibbosus*] Humped; humpbacked; denoting a sharp angle in the flexion of the spine.

Gibbs, J. Willard, U.S. mathematician and physicist, 1839–1903. See G.-Donnan *equilibrium,* G.-Helmholtz *equation,* Helmholtz-G. *theory;* G.'s *theorem,* free *energy.*

gibbus (gib'ŭs) [L. a hump]. Extreme kyphosis, hump, or hunch; a deformity of spine in which there is a sharply angulated segment, the apex of the angle being posterior.

Gibney, Virgil P., U.S. orthopedist, 1847–1927. See G.'s fixation *bandage.*

Gibson, George A., Scottish physician, 1854–1913. See G. *murmur.*

Gibson, Kasson C., U.S. dentist, 1849–1925. See G.'s *bandage.*

gid. Staggers (2).

Giemsa, Gustav, German bacteriologist, 1867–1948. See G. *stain,* G. chromosome banding *stain.*

Gierke, Edgar von, German pathologist, 1877–1945. See G.'s *disease,* von G's *disease.*

Gierke, Hans P.B., German anatomist, 1847–1886. See G.'s respiratory *bundle.*

Gifford, Harold, U.S. ophthalmologist, 1858–1929. See G.'s *operation, reflex, sign.*

giga- (G) [G. *gigas,* giant]. Prefix used in the SI and metric systems to signify one billion (10^9).

gigantism (jī'gan-tizm) [G. *gigas,* giant]. Giantism; gigantosoma; hypersomia; somatomegaly; a condition of abnormal size or overgrowth of the entire body or of any of its parts.
acromegalic g., a form of pituitary g. in which the signs of acromegaly accompany abnormal height.
cerebral g., a syndrome characterized by increased birth weight and length (above 90th percentile), accelerated growth rate for the first 4 or 5 years without elevation of serum growth hormone levels, and then reversion to normal growth rate; characteristic facies include prognathism, hypertelorism, antimongoloid slant, and dolichocephalic skull; moderate mental retardation and impaired coordination are also associated.
eunuchoid g., g. with deficient development of sexual organs; may be of pituitary or gonadal origin.
pituitary g., a form of g. caused by hypersecretion of pituitary growth hormone; a rare disorder commonly the result of a pituitary adenoma.
primordial g., unusually large size from birth due to familial or genetic factors and not to hyperpituitarism.

giganto- [G. *gigas,* giant]. Combining form meaning huge, or gigantic.

gigantomastia (jī-gan'tō-mas'tē-ă) [giganto- + G. *mastos,* breast]. Massive hypertrophy of the breast.

Gigantorhynchus (ji-gan'to-ring'kŭs) [giganto- + G. *rhynchos,* snout]. A genus of very large acanthocephalan worms. See also *Macracanthorynchus* and *Moniliformis.*

gigantosoma (jī-gan-tō-sō'mă) [giganto- + G. *sōma,* body]. Gigantism.

Gigli, Leonardo, Italian gynecologist, 1863–1908. See G.'s *operation, saw.*

Gila monster (hē'lă) [*Gila,* a river in Arizona]. A large poisonous lizard, *Heloderma suspectum* and *H. horridum,* of New Mexico, Arizona, and northern Mexico.

Gilbert, Nicholas A., French physician, 1858–1927. See G.'s *disease, syndrome.*

gilbert [W. *Gilbert,* English physicist, 1544–1603]. The unit of magnetomotive force or magnetic potential.

Gilchrist, Thomas C., U.S. physician, 1862–1927. See G.'s *disease, mycosis.*

Gilford, Hastings, British physician, 1861–1941. See Hutchinson-G. *disease, syndrome.*

Gilles de la Tourette, Georges, French physician, 1857–1904. See G. de la T.'s *disease, syndrome.*

Gillette, Eugène P., French surgeon, 1836–1886. See G.'s suspensory *ligament.*

Gilliam, David Tod, U.S. gynecologist, 1844–1923. See G.'s *operation.*

Gillies, Sir Harold D., British plastic surgeon, 1882–1960. See G.'s *operation;* Filatov-G. *flap,* tubed *pedicle.*

Gillmore needle. See under needle.

Gilmer, Thomas L., U.S. oral surgeon, 1849–1931. See G. *wire.*

Gil-Vernet, Jose Maria G.-V. Vila, Spanish urologist, *1922. See G.-V. *operation.*

Gimbernat, Don Manuel L.A. de, Spanish anatomist and surgeon, 1734–1816. See G.'s *ligament.*

ginger (jin'jer). Zingiber; the dried rhizome of *Zingiber officinale* (family Zingiberaceae), known in commerce as Jamaica g., African g., and Cochin g. The outer cortical layers are often either partially or completely removed; used as a carminative and flavoring agent.
Chinese g., galangal.
Indian g., *Asarum canadense.*
g. oleoresin, a carminative, stimulant, and flavoring agent.
wild g., *Asarum canadense.*

gingili oil (jin'ji-lē). Sesame oil.

gingiva, gen. and pl. **gingivae** (jin'ji-vă, -vē) [L.] [NA]. Gum (2); the dense fibrous tissue, covered by mucous membrane, that envelops the alveolar processes of the upper and lower jaws and surrounds the necks of the teeth.
alveolar g., gingival tissue applied to the alveolar bone.
attached g., that part of the oral mucosa which is firmly bound to the tooth and alveolar process.
buccal g., that portion of the g. that covers the buccal surfaces of the teeth and alveolar process.
free g., that portion of the g. that surrounds the tooth and is not

directly attached to the tooth surface; the outer wall of the gingival sulcus.
labial g., that portion of the g. that covers the labial surfaces of the teeth and the alveolar process.
lingual g., that portion of the g. that covers the lingual surfaces of the teeth and the alveolar process.
septal g., that portion of the g. that covers the septum.

gingival (jin'ji-văl). Relating to the gums.

Gingival Index (GI). An index of periodontal disease based upon the severity and location of the lesion.

Gingival-Periodontal Index (GPI). An index of gingivitis, gingival irritation, and advanced periodontal disease.

gingivectomy (jin-ji-vek'tō-mē) [gingiva + G. *ektomē,* excision]. Gum resection; surgical resection of unsupported gingival tissue.

gingivitis (jin-ji-vī'tis) [gingiva + G. *-itis,* inflammation]. Inflammation of the gingiva as an inflammatory response to bacterial plaque on adjacent teeth; characterized by erythema, edema, and fibrous enlargement of the gingiva without resorption of the underlying alveolar bone.
acute necrotizing g. (ANUG), see necrotizing ulcerative g.
chronic desquamative g., gingivosis; a gingival condition of unknown etiology, usually encountered in middle-aged and older women, characterized by localized patches or generalized erythema, mucosal atrophy, and desquamation, and usually accompanied by a burning sensation and pain; desquamation occurs at the level of the epithelial basement membrane, with chronic inflammation of the adjacent connective tissue.
diabetic g., g. in which the host response to bacterial plaque is presumably modified by the metabolic alterations encountered in the uncontrolled diabetic patient.
diphenylhydantoin g., g. exacerbated by long-term therapy with diphenylhydantoin; the host response to bacterial plaque is characterized by marked hyperplasia of the fibrous connective tissue and, to a lesser degree, of the surface epithelium, resulting in gross enlargement of interdental papillae which may coalesce and obscure the clinical crowns of the teeth.
fusospirochetal g., necrotizing ulcerative g.
hormonal g., g. in which the host response to bacterial plaque is presumably exacerbated by hormonal alterations occurring during puberty, pregnancy, oral contraceptive use, or menopause.
hyperplastic g., proliferative g.; g. of long-standing duration in which the gingiva becomes enlarged and firm due to proliferation of fibrous connective tissue.
leukemic hyperplastic g., enlarged gingiva due to infiltration of leukemic cells.
marginal g., g. in which the clinical alterations are confined to the marginal gingiva and do not involve the attached gingiva.
necrotizing ulcerative g. (NUG), Vincent's disease or infection; fusospirochetal or ulceromembranous g.; trench mouth; an acute or recurrent g. of young and middle-aged adults characterized clinically by gingival erythema and pain, fetid odor, and necrosis and sloughing of interdental papillae and marginal gingiva which gives rise to a gray pseudomembrane; fever, regional lymphadenopathy, and other systemic manifestations also may be present. A fusiform bacillus and *Treponema vincentii* can be isolated from the gingival tissues in large numbers and are felt to play a significant but poorly defined role in the pathogenesis.
proliferative g., inflammatory changes in the gingiva characterized by proliferation of the gingival components.
suppurative g., g. in which a purulent exudate can be expressed from the gingival surface.
ulceromembranous g., necrotizing ulcerative g.

gingivo- [L. *gingiva*]. Combining form relating to the gingivae.

gingivoaxial (jin'ji-vō-ak'sē-ăl). Pertaining to the line angle formed by the gingival and axial walls of a cavity.

gingivoglossitis (jin'ji-vō-glos-sī'tis). Inflammation of both the tongue and gingival tissues. See also stomatitis.

gingivolabial (jin'ji-vō-lā'bē-ăl). Referring to the line angle formed by the junction of the gingival and labial walls of a (class III or IV) cavity.

gingivolinguoaxial (jin'ji-vō-ling'gwō-ak'sē-ăl). Referring to the point angle formed by the gingival, lingual, and axial walls of a cavity.

gingivo-osseous (jin'ji-vō-os'ē-ŭs). Referring to the gingiva and its underlying bone.

gingivoplasty (jin'ji-vō-plas-tē). A surgical procedure that reshapes and recontours the gingival tissue in order to attain esthetic, physiologic, and functional form.

gingivosis (jin-ji-vō'sis). Chronic desquamative *gingivitis.*

gingivostomatitis (jin'ji-vō-stō'mă-tī'tis) [gingivo- + G. *stoma,* mouth, + *-itis,* inflammation]. Inflammation of the gingiva and other oral mucous membranes.

ginglyform (jing'gli-fōrm, ging-) [G. *ginglymos,* a hinge joint, + L. *forma,* form]. Ginglymoid.

ginglymoarthrodial (jing'gli-mō-ar-thrō'dē-ăl, ging-). Denoting a joint having the form of both ginglymus and arthrodia, or hinge joint and sliding joint.

ginglymoid (jing'gli-moyd, ging-) [G. *ginglymos,* a hinge joint, + *eidos,* resembling]. Ginglyform; relating to or resembling a hinge joint.

ginglymus (jing'gli-mŭs, ging-) [G. *ginglymos*] [NA]. Hinge or ginglymoid joint; a uniaxial joint in which a broad, transversely cylindrical convexity on one bone fits into a corresponding concavity on the other, allowing of motion in one plane only, as in the elbow.
helicoid g., *articulatio* trochoidea.
lateral g., *articulatio* trochoidea.

ginseng (jin'seng) [Ch.]. The roots of several species of *Panax* (family Araliaceae), esteemed as of great medicinal virtue by the Chinese, but not often used in western medicine.

Giordano-Giovannetti diet. See under diet.

GIP Abbreviation for gastric inhibitory *polypeptide.*

Girard, A. See G.'s *reagent.*

girdle (ger'dl) [A.S. *gyrdel*] A belt; a zone. See also cingulum (1).
Hitzig's g., tabetic *cuirass.*
Neptune's g., a wet pack applied around the abdomen.
pelvic g., *cingulum* membri inferioris.
shoulder g., *cingulum* membri superioris.
thoracic g., *cingulum* membri superioris.

Girdlestone, Gathorne Robert, British orthopedist, *1881. See G. *procedure.*

gitalin (jit'ă-lin). An extract of *Digitalis purpurea* containing a mixture of glycosides and aglycons, with action and uses similar to those of digitalis.

githagism (gith'ă-jism) [L. *gith,* a plant, Roman coriander, + *ago,* to drive]. A disease similar to lathyrism, believed to be due to poisoning by seeds of the corn cockle, *Lychnis githago.*

gitogenin (jit'ō-jen-in). Digin; (25*R*)-5α-spirostan-2α,3β-diol; the genin of gitonin; a cardiotonic agent.

gitonin (jit'ō-nin). A gitogenin tetraglycoside composed of two galactoses, one glucose, and one xylose; F-gitogenin has one galactose, two glucoses, and 1 xylose. Both are cardiotonic agents.

gitoxin (ji-tok'sin). Anhydrogitalin; bigitalin; pseudodigitoxin; $C_{41}H_{64}O_{14}$; a secondary cardiac glycoside from *Digitalis purpurea* and *D. lanata.*

gitterzelle (git'er-zel-e) [Ger. fr. *Gitter,* lattice, + *Zelle,* cell]. Compound granule *cell.*

Giuffrida-Ruggieri, Vincenzo, Italian anthropologist, 1872–1922. See G.-R. *stigma.*

glabella (glă-bel'ă) [L. *glabellus,* hairless, smooth, dim. of *glaber*]. Intercilium. **1** [NA]. A smooth prominence, most marked in the male, on the frontal bone above the root of the nose. **2.** Mesophryon; the most forward projecting point of the forehead in the midline at the level of the supraorbital ridges.

glabellad (glă-bel'ad). Toward the glabella.

glabrous, glabrate (glā'brŭs, glā'brāt) [L. *glaber,* smooth]. Smooth or hairless; denoting areas of the body where hair does not normally grow, *i.e.,* palms or soles.

gladiate (glad'ē-āt) [L. *gladius,* a sword]. Xiphoid.

gladiolus (glă-dī'ō-lŭs, glad'ē-ō'lŭs) [L. dim. of *gladius,* a sword]. *Corpus* sterni.

GLAND

gland [L. *glans,* acorn]. An organized aggregation of cells functioning as a secretory or excretory organ.

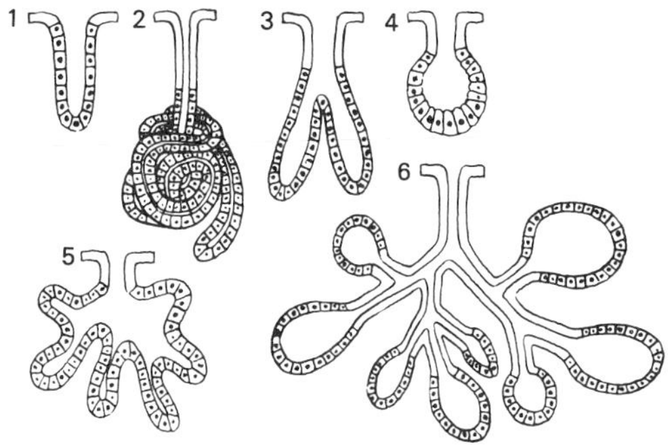

Types of Glands
1, Simple tubular; *2,* simple coiled tubular; *3,* branched tubular; *4,* simple alveolar; *5.* branched alveolar; *6,* compound alveolar.

accessory g., a small mass of glandular structure, detached from but lying near another and larger g., to which it is similar in structure and probably in function.
accessory lacrimal g.'s, *glandulae* lacrimales accessoriae.
accessory parotid g., *glandula* parotidea accessoria.
accessory suprarenal g.'s, *glandulae* suprarenales accessoriae.
accessory thyroid g., *glandula* thyroidea accessoria.
acid g., oxyntic g.; one of the gastric g.'s secreting the hydrochloric acid of the gastric juice.
acinotubular g., tubuloacinar g.
acinous g., a g. in which the secretory unit(s) has a grapelike shape and a very small lumen; *e.g.,* the exocrine part of the pancreas.
admaxillary g., *glandula* parotidea accessoria.
adrenal g., *glandula* suprarenalis.
aggregate g.'s, *folliculi* lymphatici aggregati.
agminate g.'s, agminated g.'s, *folliculi* lymphatici aggregati.
Albarran's g.'s, Albarran y Dominguez' tubules; minute submucosal glands or branching tubules in the subcervical region of the prostate g., emptying for the most part into the posterior portion of the urethra.
albuminous g., a g. that secretes a watery fluid.
alveolar g., a g. in which the secretory unit(s) has a saclike form and an obvious lumen; *e.g.,* the active mammary gland.
anal g., **(1)** one of a number of large sudoriferous g.'s in the mucous membrane of the anus; **(2)** an incorrect synonym for anal *sac.*
anterior lingual g., *glandula* lingualis anterior.
apical g., *glandula* lingualis anterior.
apocrine g., **(1)** a g. whose secretion contains the apical portion of the secretory cell; **(2)** a sweat g. whose duct opens into the hair follicle above the sebaceous duct; such g.'s are usually confined to skin of the perianal and genital area, axillae, and areolae of the breasts.
areolar g.'s, *glandulae* areolares.
arteriococcygeal g., *corpus* coccygeum.
arytenoid g.'s, *glandulae* laryngeae.
Aselli's g., Aselli's pancreas; a single large lymph node ventral to the abdominal aorta that receives all the lymph from the intestines in many smaller mammals.
g.'s of auditory tube, *glandulae* tubariae.
axillary g.'s, *lymphonodi* axillares.
axillary sweat g.'s, sudoriferous g.'s of the axilla which develop in association with hair follicles and differ from eccrine g.'s in undergoing enlargement and secretory development at puberty; formerly thought to be apocrine.
Bartholin's g., *glandula* vestibularis major.
Bauhin's g., *glandula* lingualis anterior.
Baumgarten's g.'s, Henle's g.'s.
g.'s of biliary mucosa, *glandulae* mucosae biliosae.
Blandin's g., *glandula* lingualis anterior.
Boerhaave's g.'s, *glandulae* sudoriferae.
Bowman's g., see *glandulae* olfactoriae.
brachial g., one of the lymph nodes of the arm.
bronchial g.'s, **(1)** *lymphonodi* bronchopulmonales; **(2)** *glandulae* bronchiales.
Bruch's g.'s, trachoma g.'s; lymph nodes in the palpebral conjunctiva.
Brunner's g.'s, *glandulae* duodenales.
buccal g.'s, *glandulae* buccales.
bulbourethral g., *glandula* bulbourethralis.
cardiac g., a coiled tubular g. located in the cardiac region of the stomach; secretes primarily mucus.
cardiac g.'s of esophagus, g.'s located in the lamina propria of the uppermost and lowermost levels of the esophagus; they resemble cardiac g.'s of the stomach in that they are branched tubules of mucous cells.
celiac g.'s, *lymphonodi* coeliaci.
ceruminous g.'s, *glandulae* ceruminosae.
cervical g.'s, **(1)** see *lymphonodi* cervicales anteriores and laterales **(2)** *glandulae* cervicales uteri.
cervical g.'s of uterus, *glandulae* cervicales uteri.
Ciaccio's g.'s, see *glandulae* lacrimales accessoriae.
ciliary g.'s, *glandulae* ciliares.
circumanal g.'s, *glandulae* circumanales.
coccygeal g., *corpus* coccygeum.
coil g., convoluted g.; a g. whose secretory part is convoluted.
compound g., a g. whose larger excretory ducts branch repeatedly into smaller ducts which ultimately drain secretory units.
conjunctival g.'s, *glandulae* conjunctivales.
convoluted g., coil g.
Cowper's g., *glandula* bulbourethralis.
crop g., cells in the crop of male and female pigeons and doves that secrete a caseous or milklike material with which the bird feeds its young; it is stimulated to secrete by prolactin, the lactogenic hormone of the anterior hypophysis, and is used as a test object for assaying the activity of this hormone.
ductless g.'s, *glandulae* endocrinae.
duodenal g.'s, *glandulae* duodenales.
Duverney's g., *glandula* vestibularis major.
Ebner's g.'s, serous g.'s of the tongue opening in the bottom of the trough surrounding the circumvallate papillae.
eccrine g., a coiled tubular sweat g. (other than apocrine g.'s) that occurs in the skin on almost all parts of the body.

ecdysial g.'s, prothoracic, thoracic, peritracheal, or ventral g.'s; insect structures that originate from the ectoderm of the ventrocaudal part of the head and serve as a source of ecdysone.
Eglis' g.'s, small, inconstant mucous g.'s of the ureter and renal pelvis.
endocrine g.'s, *glandulae* endocrinae.

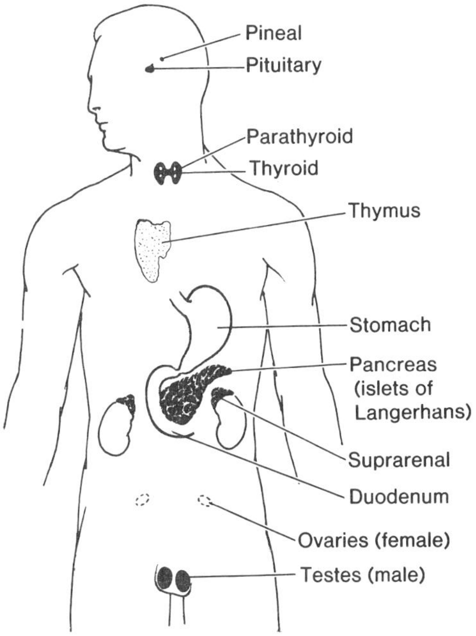

Positions of the Endocrine Glands

esophageal g.'s, *glandulae* esophageae.
g.'s of eustachian tube, *glandulae* tubariae.
excretory g., a g. separating excrementitious or waste material from the blood.
exocrine g., a g. from which secretions reach a free surface of the body by ducts.
external salivary g., *glandula* parotidea.
follicular g., a g. consisting of follicles.
fundus g.'s, *glandulae* gastricae.
Galeati's g.'s, *glandulae* intestinales.
gastric g.'s, *glandulae* gastricae.
Gay's g.'s, *glandulae* circumanales.
genal g.'s, *glandulae* buccales.
genital g., **(1)** testis; **(2)** ovarium.
Gley's g.'s, see *glandula* parathyroidea.
greater vestibular g., *glandula* vestibularis major.
Guérin's g.'s, *glandulae* urethrales femininae.
Harder's g., harderian g., **(1)** the deep g. of the semilunar conjunctival fold or "third eyelid" found in animals such as pig and deer; **(2)** misnomer for the superficial g. of the semilunar conjunctival fold in the dog; not present in man.
Havers' g.'s, synovial g.'s; collections of adipose tissue in the hip, knee, and other joints, covered by synovial membrane, thought by Havers to be g.'s secreting the synovia.
hemal g., hemal *node.*
hematopoietic g., a blood-forming organ, such as the spleen.
hemolymph g., hemal *node.*
Henle's g.'s, Baumgarten's g.'s; accessory lacrimal g.'s located near the fornices in the medial part of the palpebral conjunctiva; they open on the conjunctiva surface.
hibernating g., brown *fat.*
holocrine g., a g. whose secretion consists of disintegrated cells of the g. itself, *e.g.,* a sebaceous g., in contrast to a merocrine g.
inguinal g.'s, see *lymphonodi* inguinales profundi and superficiales.
internal salivary g., the sublingual and submandibular g.'s regarded as one.
g.'s of internal secretion, *glandulae* endocrinae.
interrenal g.'s, interrenal *bodies.*
interscapular g., brown *fat.*
interstitial g., see interstitial *cells.*
intestinal g.'s, *glandulae* intestinales.
intraepithelial g.'s, accumulations of glandular cells that lie within an epithelium, as those of the urethra.
jugular g., signal *node.*
Knoll's g.'s, g.'s in the ventricular folds of the larynx (false vocal cords).
Krause's g.'s, **(1)** see *glandulae* lacrimales accessoriae; **(2)** g.'s in the mucous membrane of the tympanic cavity.
labial g.'s, *glandulae* labiales.
lacrimal g., *glandula* lacrimalis.
lactiferous g., *glandula* mammaria.
laryngeal g.'s, *glandulae* laryngeae.
lesser vestibular g.'s, *glandulae* vestibulares minores.
Lieberkühn's g.'s, *glandulae* intestinales.
Littre's g.'s, *glandulae* urethrales masculinae.
Luschka's g., **(1)** *tonsilla* pharyngea; **(2)** former name for *corpus* coccygeum.
Luschka's cystic g.'s, *glandulae* mucosae biliosae.
lymph g., lymphonodus.
major salivary g.'s, a category of salivary g.'s that includes the three largest g.'s of the oral cavity which also secrete most of the saliva: the parotid, submandibular, and sublingual g.'s.
malpighian g.'s, *folliculi* lymphatici lienales.
mammary g., *glandula* mammaria.
marrow-lymph g., a type of hemal node, resembling the bone marrow in structure and probable function.
master g., hypophysis.
maxillary g., *glandula* submandibularis.
meibomian g.'s, *glandulae* tarsales.
merocrine g., a g. that releases only an acellular secretory product, in contrast to a holocrine g.
Méry's g., *glandula* bulbourethralis.
mesenteric g.'s, see *lymphonodi* mesenterici.
metrial g., collections of granular epithelial cells in the uterine muscle beneath the placenta that develop during pregnancy in certain animals (*e.g.,* mouse, rat). The cells are thought to disintegrate and pass (as a holocrine secretion) into the afferent placental vessels to furnish nutriment for the embryo.
milk g., *glandula* mammaria.
minor salivary g.'s, the smaller, largely mucous-secreting, exocrine g.'s of the oral cavity, consisting of the labial, buccal, molar, lingual, and palatine g.'s.
mixed g., **(1)** a g. that contains both serous and mucous secretory units; **(2)** a g. that is both exocrine and endocrine, *e.g.,* the pancreas.
molar g.'s, *glandulae* molares.
Moll's g.'s, *glandulae* ciliares.
Montgomery's g.'s, *glandulae* areolares.
g.'s of mouth, *glandulae* oris.
mucilaginous g., one of the synovial villi, supposed by Havers to secrete the synovia.
muciparous g., *glandula* mucosa.
mucous g., *glandula* mucosa.
mucous g.'s of auditory tube, *glandulae* tubariae.
nasal g.'s, *glandulae* nasales.
Nuhn's g., *glandula* lingualis anterior.
odoriferous g., **(1)** a g., such as Tyson's g., the secretion of which

has a strong odor; (2) see scent g.'s.
oil g.'s, (1) *glandulae* sebaceae; (2) uropygial g.
olfactory g.'s, *glandulae* olfactoriae.
oxyntic g., acid g.
pacchionian g.'s, *granulationes* arachnoideales.
palatine g.'s, *glandulae* palatinae.
palpebral g.'s, *glandulae* tarsales.
parathyroid g., *glandula* parathyroidea.
paraurethral g.'s, *glandulae* urethrales femininae.
parotid g., *glandula* parotidea.
pectoral g.'s, see *lymphonodi* axillares.
peptic g., a pepsin-secreting g. See *glandulae* gastricae.
perianal odoriferous g.'s, see scent g.'s.
peritracheal g.'s, ecdysial g.'s.
perspiratory g.'s, *glandulae* sudoriferae.
Peyer's g.'s, *folliculi* lymphatici aggregati.
pharyngeal g.'s, *glandulae* pharyngeae.
Philip's g.'s, enlarged deep g.'s just above the clavicle, found in children with pulmonary tuberculosis and occasionally in others.
pileous g., a sebaceous g. emptying into the hair follicle.
pineal g., *corpus* pineale.
pituitary g., hypophysis.
Poirier's g., a lymph node on the uterine artery where it crosses the ureter.
preen g., uropygial g.
prehyoid g., *glandula* thyroidea accessoria.
preputial g.'s, *glandulae* preputiales.
prostate g., prostata.
prothoracic g.'s, ecdysial g.'s.
pyloric g.'s, *glandulae* pyloricae.
racemose g., a g. that has the appearance of a bunch of grapes if viewed as a three-dimensional reconstruction; *e.g.,* a compound acinous or alveolar g.
Rivinus' g., *glandula* sublingualis.
Rosenmüller's g., *node* of Cloquet.
saccular g., a single alveolar g.
salivary g., *glandula* salivaria.
salivary g. of abdomen, pancreas.
scent g.'s, cutaneous g.'s producing odoriferous secretions (pheromones or recognition odors); they may be located on different parts of the body, *e.g.,* under the chin (rabbit); between the digits (goat); on the medial surface of the metatarsus (deer), in the preorbital fold (antelope); in the occipital region (camel); on the flank (hamster); in the perianal region and on the dorsum of the tail base (carnivores).
sebaceous g.'s, *glandulae* sebaceae.
seminal g., *vesicula* seminalis.
sentinel g., a single enlarged lymph node in the omentum that may be an indication of an ulcer opposite to it in the greater or lesser curvature of the stomach.
seromucous g., *glandula* seromucosa.
serous g., *glandula* serosa.
Serres' g.'s, epithelial cell rests found in the subepithelial connective tissue in the palate of the newborn, similar to those found in the gingivae.
sexual g., See gonad.
Skene's g.'s, *glandulae* urethrales femininae.
solitary g.'s, *folliculi* lymphatici solitarii.
sublingual g., *glandula* sublingualis.
submandibular g., *glandula* submandibularis.
submaxillary g., *glandula* submandibularis.
sudoriferous g.'s, *glandulae* sudoriferae.
suprahyoid g., *glandula* thyroidea accessoria.
suprarenal g., *glandula* suprarenalis.
Suzanne's g., a small mucous g. in the floor of the mouth.
sweat g.'s, *glandulae* sudoriferae.
synovial g.'s, Havers' g.'s.
target g., the effector that functions when stimulated by the internal secretion of another gland or by some other stimulus.
tarsal g.'s, *glandulae* tarsales.
Terson's g.'s, *glandulae* conjunctivales.
Theile's g.'s, *glandulae* mucosae biliosae.
thoracic g.'s, ecdysial g.'s.
thymus g., thymus.
thyroid g., *glandula* thyroidea.
Tiedemann's g., *glandula* vestibularis major.
tracheal g.'s, *glandulae* tracheales.
trachoma g.'s, Bruch's g.'s.
tubular g., a g. composed of one or more tubules ending in a blind extremity.
tubuloacinar g., acinotubular g.; a g. whose secretory elements are elongated acini.
tubuloalveolar g., a g. that has secretory units of short tubules.
tympanic g., tympanic body; one of the mucous g.'s in the mucosa of the tympanic cavity.
Tyson's g.'s, *glandulae* preputiales.
unicellular g., a single secretory cell such as a mucous goblet cell.
urethral g.'s, see *glandulae* urethrales.
uropygial g., glandula uropygius; oil g. (2); preen g.; a compound alveolar g. of birds located on the dorsum of the tail or pygostyle; the secretion of this g. (fatty acids and wax) exits from a papilla on the dorsal surface at the base of the tail feathers; the bird applies the substance to its feathers by means of the bill when preening. The uropygial g. is lacking in some species but its waterproofing ability is essential to water birds.
uterine g.'s, *glandulae* uterinae.
vaginal g., one of the mucous g.'s in the mucous membrane of the vagina.
vascular g., hemal *node.*
ventral g.'s, ecdysial g.'s.
vesical g., one of a number of mucous follicles, not true g.'s, in the mucous membrane near the neck of the bladder.
vestibular g.'s, see *glandula* vestibularis major and *glandulae* vestibulares minores.
vulvovaginal g., *glandula* vestibularis major.
Waldeyer's g.'s, coil g.'s near the margins of the eyelids.
Wasmann's g.'s, *glandulae* gastricae.
Weber's g.'s, muciparous g.'s at the border of the tongue on either side posteriorly.
Wepfer's g.'s, *glandulae* duodenales.
Wölfler's g., *glandula* thyroidea accessoria.
Wolfring's g.'s, see *glandulae* lacrimales accessoriae.
Zeis' g.'s, sebaceous g.'s opening into the follicles of the eyelashes.

---

glanders (glan′derz) [O. Fr. *glandres,* glands]. A chronic debilitating disease of horses and other equids, as well as some members of the cat family, caused by *Pseudomonas mallei* and transmissible to man. It attacks the mucous membranes of the nostrils of the horse, attended with an increased and vitiated secretion and discharge of mucus, and enlargement and induration of the glands of the lower jaw.

glandes (glan′dēz). Plural of glans.

glandilemma (glan-di-lem′ă) [L. *glandula,* gland, + G. *lemma,* sheath]. The capsule of a gland.

GLANDULA

---

glandula, pl. **glandulae** (glan′dū-lă, -lē) [L. gland, dim. of *glans,*

acorn] [NA]. A glandule or small gland.
glan'dulae areola'res [NA], areolar glands; Montgomery's follicles or glands; a number of mammary glands forming small rounded projections from the surface of the areola of the breast.
g. atrabilia'ris, g. suprarenalis.
g. basila'ris, hypophysis.
glan'dulae bronchia'les [NA], bronchial glands (2); mucous and seromucous glands whose secretory units lie outside of the muscle of the bronchi.
glan'dulae bucca'les [NA], buccal glands; genal glands; numerous racemose, mucous, or serous glands in the submucous tissue of the cheeks.
g. bulbourethra'lis [NA], bulbourethral gland; antiparastata; anteprostate; antiprostate; Cowper's or Méry's gland; one of two small compound racemose glands, which produce a mucoid secretion, lying side by side along the membranous urethra just above the bulb of the corpus spongiosum; they discharge through a small duct into the spongy portion of the urethra.
glan'dulae cerumino'sae [NA], ceruminous glands; apocrine sudoriferous glands in the external acoustic meatus.
glan'dulae cervica'les uteri [NA], cervical glands of the uterus; cervical glands (2); branched mucus-secreting glands in the mucosa of the cervix.
glan'dulae cilia'res [NA], ciliary glands; Moll's glands; a number of modified apocrine sudoriferous glands in the eyelids, with ducts that usually open into the follicles of the eyelashes.
glan'dulae circumana'les [NA], circumanal glands; Gay's glands; large apocrine sweat glands surrounding the anus.
glan'dulae conjunctiva'les [NA], conjunctival glands; Terson's glands; clusters of mucous cells in the conjunctival epithelium, most numerous on the bulbar conjunctiva.
glan'dulae cu'tis [NA], any of the glands of the skin.
glan'dulae duodena'les [NA], duodenal glands; Brunner's or Wepfer's glands; small, branched, coiled tubular glands which occur mostly in the submucosa of the first part of the duodenum; they secrete a mucoid substance.
glan'dulae endocri'nae [NA], endocrine glands; ductless glands; glands of internal secretion; glandulae sine ductibus; glands that have no ducts, their secretions being absorbed directly into the blood.
glan'dulae esopha'geae [NA], esophageal glands; a variable number of small compound mucous glands in the submucosa of the esophagus.
glan'dulae gas'tricae [NA], gastric glands; glandulae propriae; gastric follicles; fundus glands; Wasmann's glands; branched tubular glands lying in the mucosa of the fundus and body of the stomach; such glands contain parietal cells which secrete hydrochloric acid, zymogen cells which produce pepsin, and mucous cells.
glan'dulae glomifor'mes [NA], **(1)** glomus (2); **(2)** tubular glands of the skin, the blind extremity of which is coiled in the form of a ball or glomerulus.
glan'dulae intestina'les [NA], intestinal glands or follicles; Lieberkühn's crypts, follicles, or glands; Galeati's glands; the tubular glands in the mucous membrane of the small and large intestines.
glan'dulae labia'les [NA], labial glands; mucous glands in the submucous tissue of the lips.
glan'dulae lacrima'les accesso'riae [NA], accessory lacrimal glands; small compound, branched, tubular glands located near the upper end of the tarsus mainly in the medial half of the lid (Wolfring's and Ciaccio's glands) and near the fornix (Krause's glands (1)).
g. lacrima'lis [NA], lacrimal gland; the gland that secretes tears; it consists of 6 to 12 separate compound tubuloalveolar serous glands, located in the upper lateral part of the orbit, and is partially divided into a smaller pars palpebralis and a larger pars orbitalis by the aponeurosis of the levator palpebrae muscle.
glan'dulae laryn'geae [NA], laryngeal or arytenoid glands; a large number of mixed glands in the mucous membrane of the larynx; they are called, according to their situation, anterior, middle, and posterior.
g. lingua'lis ante'rior [NA], anterior lingual gland; apical gland; Bauhin's, Blandin's, or Nuhn's gland; one of the small mixed glands deeply placed near the apex of the tongue on each side of the frenulum.
g. mamma'ria [NA], mammary gland; lactiferous gland; milk gland; the compound alveolar apocrine secretory gland that forms the breast. It consists of 15 to 24 lobes, each consisting of many lobules, separated by adipose tissue and fibrous septa; The parenchyma of the resting gland consists of ducts; the alveoli develop only during pregnancy. See also mamma.
glan'dulae mola'res [NA], molar glands; four or five large buccal glands in the neighborhood of the last molar tooth.
g. muco'sa [NA], mucous gland; muciparous gland; a gland that secretes mucus.
glan'dulae muco'sae bilio'sae [NA], glands of the biliary mucosa; Luschka's cystic glands; Theile's glands; small, mucous, tubuloalveolar glands in the mucosa of the larger bile ducts and especially in the neck of the gallbladder.
glan'dulae nasa'les [NA], nasal glands; seromucous glands in the respiratory region of the nasal mucous membrane.
glan'dulae olfacto'riae [NA], olfactory glands; branched tubuloalveolar serous secreting glands (of Bowman) in the mucous membrane of the olfactory region of the nasal cavity.
glan'dulae o'ris [NA], glands of mouth; glands that empty into the oral cavity.
glan'dulae palati'nae [NA], palatine glands; a number of racemose mucous glands in the posterior half of the submucous tissue covering the hard palate.
g. parathyroi'dea [NA], parathyroid gland; epithelial body; parathyroid; one of Gley's glands or Sandström's bodies; one of two small paired endocrine glands, superior and inferior, usually found embedded in the connective tissue capsule on the posterior surface of the thyroid gland; they are concerned with the metabolism of calcium and phosphorus. The parenchyma is composed of chief and oxyphilic cells arranged in anastomosing cords.
g. parotid'ea [NA], parotid gland; g. parotis; external salivary gland; the largest of the salivary glands, one of two compound acinous glands situated below and in front of the ear, on either side, extending from the angle of the jaw to the zygomatic arch and backward to the sternocleidomastoid muscle; it is subdivided into a pars superficialis and a pars profunda by emerging branches of the facial nerve, and discharges through the parotid duct.
g. parotid'ea accesso'ria [NA], g. parotis accessoria; accessory parotid gland; admaxillary gland; socia parotidis; an occasional islet of parotid tissue separate from the mass of the gland, lying anteriorly just above the commencement of the parotid duct.
g. paro'tis, g. parotidea.
g. paro'tis accesso'ria, g. parotidea accessoria.
glan'dulae pharyn'geae [NA], pharyngeal glands; racemose mucous glands beneath the mucous membrane of the pharynx.
g. pituita'ria [NA], hypophysis.
glan'dulae preputia'les [NA], preputial glands; Tyson's glands; sebaceous glands of the corona glandis and inner surface of the prepuce.
glan'dulae pro'priae [NA], alternate term for glandulae gastricae.
g. prosta'tica, prostata.
glan'dulae pylor'icae [NA], pyloric glands; the coiled, tubular glands of the pylorus whose cells secrete mucus.
g. saliva'ria [NA], salivary gland; any of the saliva-secreting exocrine glands of the oral cavity. See major salivary *glands;* minor salivary *glands.*
glan'dulae seba'ceae [NA], sebaceous glands, crypts, or follicles; oil glands (1); numerous holocrine glands in the dermis that usually open into the hair follicles and secrete an oily semifluid sebum.

g. semina'lis [NA], *vesicula* seminalis.
g. seromuco'sa [NA], seromucous gland; **(1)** a gland in which some of the secretory cells are serous and some mucous; **(2)** a gland whose cells secrete a fluid intermediate between a watery and a viscous mucoid substance.
g. sero'sa [NA], serous gland; a gland that secretes a watery substance that may or may not contain an enzyme.
glan'dulae sine duc'tibus [NA], an alternative term for glandulae endocrinae.
g. sublingua'lis [NA], sublingual gland; Rivinus' gland; one of two salivary glands in the floor of the mouth beneath the tongue, discharging through the sublingual ducts; most of the secretory units in the human gland are mucus-secreting with serous demilunes.
g. submandibula'ris [NA], submandibular gland; submaxillary or maxillary gland; one of two salivary glands in the neck, located in the space bounded by the two bellies of the digastric muscle and the angle of the mandible; it discharges through the submandibular duct; the secretory units are predominantly serous although a few mucous alveoli, some with serous demilunes, occur.
glan'dulae sudorif'erae [NA], sudoriferous glands; sweat or perspiratory glands; Boerhaave's glands; the coil glands of the skin that secrete the sweat.
glan'dulae suprarena'les acceso'riae [NA], accessory suprarenal glands; isolated, often minute, masses of suprarenal tissue sometimes found near the main glands or in the broad ligament or the epididymis.
g. suprarena'lis [NA], suprarenal gland, body, or capsule; adrenal gland, body, or capsule; g. atrabiliaris; atrabiliary capsule; epinephros; paranephros; butterfly adrenal; a flattened, roughly triangular body resting upon the upper end of each kidney; it is one of the ductless glands furnishing internal secretions (epinephrine and norepinephrine from the medulla and steroid hormones from the cortex).

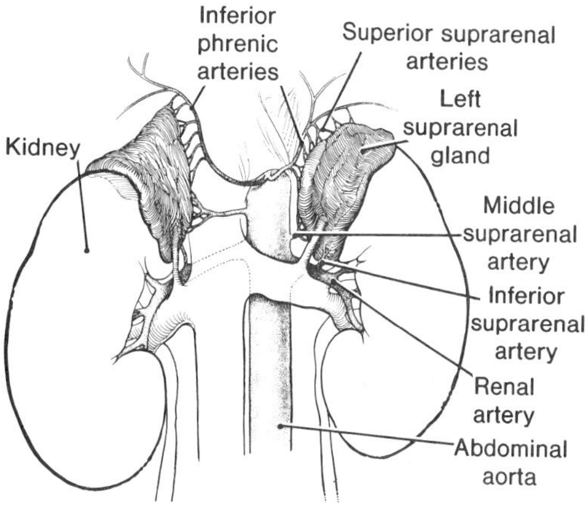

Glandula Suprarenalis

glan'dulae tarsa'les [NA], tarsal or palpebral glands; meibomian glands; sebaceous glands embedded in the tarsal plate of each eyelid, discharging at the edge of the lid near the posterior border.
g. thyroi'dea [NA], thyroid gland or body; a ductless gland, consisting of irregularly spheroidal follicles, lying in front and to the sides of the upper part of the trachea, and of horseshoe shape, with two lateral lobes connected by a narrow central portion, the isthmus; occasionally an elongated offshoot, the pyramidal lobe, passes upward from the isthmus in front of the trachea. It is supplied by branches from the external carotid and subclavian arteries, and its nerves are derived from the middle cervical and cervicothoracic ganglia of the sympathetic system. It secretes thyroid hormone and calcitonin.
g. thyroi'dea accesso'ria, pl. **glan'dulae thyroi'deae accesso'riae** [NA], accessory thyroid gland; prehyoid or suprahyoid gland; Wölfler's gland; accessory thyroid; thyroidea accessoria; thyroidea ima; an isolated mass, or one of several such masses, of thyroid tissue, sometimes present in the side of the neck, or just above the hyoid bone (suprahyoid accessory thyroid gland), or even as low as the arch of the aorta.
glan'dulae trachea'les [NA], tracheal glands; numerous tubuloalveolar mixed glands located principally in the submucosa of the trachea; they open into the tracheal lumen through short ducts.
glan'dulae tuba'riae [NA], glands of the eustachian tube; glands of auditory tube; mucous glands of the auditory tube; glands located principally near the pharyngeal end of the auditory tube.
glan'dulae urethra'les [NA], urethral glands; **g. u. fem'inae** [NA], paraurethral glands; Skene's or Guérin's glands; numerous mucous glands in the wall of the female urethra; **g. u. masculi'nae** [NA], Littre's glands; numerous mucous glands in the wall of the penile urethra.
g. uropy'gius, uropygial *gland.*
glan'dulae uteri'nae [NA], uterine glands; numerous simple tubular glands in the uterine mucosa which secrete a glycogen-rich mucous fluid during the luted phase of the menstrual cycle.
g. vestibula'ris ma'jor [NA], greater vestibular gland; Bartholin's, Tiedemann's, or Duverney's gland; vulvovaginal gland; one of two mucoid-secreting tubuloalveolar glands on either side of the lower part of the vagina, the equivalent of the bulbourethral glands in the male.
glan'dulae vestibula'res mino'res [NA], lesser vestibular glands; a number of minute mucous glands opening on the surface of the vestibule between the orifices of the vagina and urethra.

glandular (glan'dū-lăr). Glandulous; relating to a gland.
glandule (glan'dūl) [L. *glandula*]. A small gland.
glandulous (glan'dū-lŭs). Glandular.
glans, pl. **glandes** (glanz, glan'dēz) [L. acorn] [NA]. A conical acorn-shaped structure.
g. clito'ridis [NA], a small mass of erectile tissue capping the body of the clitoris.
g. pe'nis [NA], balanus; the conical expansion of the corpus spongiosum which forms the head of the penis.
Glanzmann, Eduard, Swiss clinician, 1887–1959. See G.'s *disease, thrombasthenia;* G.-Riniker *syndrome.*
glaphenine (gla-fen'ēn). *N*-(7-Chloro-4-quinolyl)anthranilic acid 2,3-dihydroxypropyl ester; an anti-inflammatory agent with analgesic properties.
glare (glār). A sensation caused by brightness within the visual field that is sufficiently greater than the luminance to which the eyes are adapted; results in annoyance, discomfort, and decreased visual performance.
blinding g., veiling g.; g. resulting from excessive illumination.
dazzling g., g. produced by excessive illumination in the peripheral field.
peripheral g., g. occurring when the surrounding brightness is greater than the brightness of the object of attention.
specular g., g. arising from specularly reflected light.
veiling g., blinding g.
glarometer (glā-rom'ĕ-ter). An instrument that measures sensitivity to central glare from the headlights of an approaching vehicle.
Glaser (Glaserius), Johann H., Swiss anatomist, 1629–1675. See glaserian *artery, fissure.*
glaserian (gla-ser'ē-an). Relating to or described by Johann H. Glaser.

Glasgow, William C., U.S. physician, 1845–1907. See G.'s *sign.*

Glasgow coma scale. See coma *scale.*

glass [A.S. *glaes*]. A transparent substance composed of silica and oxides of various bases.

cover g., coverslip; a thin g. disk or plate covering an object examined under the microscope.

Crookes' g., a spectacle lens combined with metallic oxides to absorb ultraviolet or infrared rays.

crown g., a compound of lime, potash, alumina, and silica; commonly used in lenses; has a low dispersion (52.2) relative to index of refraction (1.523).

cupping g., cup (2); a g. vessel, from which the air has been exhausted by heat or a special suction apparatus, formerly applied to the skin in order to draw blood to the surface. See also cupping, and entries under cup.

flint g., g. that contains lead oxide instead of lime to increase index of refraction; used in reading segments of fused bifocal lenses.

object g., objective (1).

quartz g., a transparent, colorless crystal, made by fusing pure quartz sand, which transmits ultraviolet light.

soluble g., water g.; a silicate of potassium or sodium, soluble in hot water but solid at ordinary temperatures; used for fixed dressings.

vita g., a specially prepared g. that is transparent to ultraviolet rays of the spectrum.

water g., soluble g.

Wood's g., a g. containing nickel oxide, used in Wood's lamp.

glasses (glas'ez). **1.** Spectacles. **2.** Lenses for correcting refractive errors in the eyes.

Glauber, Johann R., German chemist, 1604–1668. See G.'s *salt.*

glaucoma (glaw-kō'mă) [G. *glaukōma,* opacity of the crystalline lens, fr. *glaukos,* bluish green]. A disease of the eye characterized by increased intraocular pressure, excavation, and atrophy of the optic nerve; produces defects in the field of vision.

absolute g., the final stage of blindness in g.

acute g., angle-closure g.

angle-closure g., narrow-angle, closed-angle, or acute g.; primary g. in which contact of the iris with the peripheral cornea excludes acqueous humor from the trabecular drainage meshwork.

aphakic g., g. following cataract removal.

capsular g., g. occurring in association with widespread deposition of cellular organelles on the lens capsule, ocular blood vessels, iris, and ciliary body. See also *pseudoexfoliation* of lens capsule.

chronic g., open-angle g.

α-chymotrypsin-induced g., transient secondary g. following the use of α-chymotrypsin in cataract extraction.

closed-angle g., angle-closure g.

combined g., g. with angle-closure and open-angle mechanisms in the same eye.

compensated g., open-angle g.

congenital g., buphthalmos.

corticosteroid-induced g., g. caused by a hereditary predisposition in which local instillation of eyedrops containing corticosteroid causes increased intraocular pressure.

Donders' g., obsolete eponym for open-angle g.

g. ful'minans, acute angle-closure g. rapidly followed by blindness.

ghost cell g., g. occurring after vitrectomy, arising from erythrocyte membranes blocking outflow channels of aqueous humor.

hemorrhagic g., secondary g. after formation of new blood vessels in the iris.

hypersecretion g., g. caused by excessive formation of the aqueous humor.

low tension g., optic nerve atrophy and excavation with typical field defects of g. but without abnormal increase in intraocular pressure.

malignant g., secondary g. caused by forward displacement of the iris and lens, obliterating the anterior chamber; usually follows a filtering operation for primary glaucoma.

narrow-angle g., angle-closure g.

neovascular g., g. occurring in rubeosis iridis.

open-angle g., chronic, compensated, or simple g.; g. simplex; primary g. in which the aqueous humor has free access to the trabecular meshwork.

phacogenic g., phacomorphic g.

phacolytic g., g. secondary to hypermature cataract and occlusion of the trabecular drainage meshwork by lens material.

phacomorphic g., phacogenic g.; secondary g. caused by either excessive size or spherical shape of the lens.

pigmentary g., g. associated with accumulation of pigment particles in the trabecular meshwork.

pseudoexfoliative capsular g., secondary g. incident to a degenerative cyclitis producing deposits on anterior lens capsule.

pupillary block g., g. secondary to failure of the aqueous humor to pass through the pupil to the anterior chamber.

secondary g., g. occurring as a sequel of preexisting ocular disease or injury.

simple g., g. sim'plex, open-angle g.

glaucomatocyclitic (glaw-kō'mă-tō-si-klit'ik). Denoting increased intraocular pressure associated with evidences of cyclitis. See also glaucomatocyclitic *crisis.*

glaucomatous (glaw-kō'mă-tŭs). Relating to glaucoma.

glaucosuria (glaw'kō-sū'rē-ă) [G. *glaukos,* bluish green, + *ouron,* urine]. Obsolete term for indicanuria.

GLC Abbreviation for gas-liquid *chromatography.*

Glc, GlcA, GlcN, GlcNAc, GlcUA Symbols for the radicals of glucose, gluconic acid, glucosamine, *N*-acetylglucosamine, and glucuronic acid.

Gleason, Donald F., U.S. pathologist, *1920. See G.'s tumor *grade, score.*

gleet (glēt). Medorrhea; a slight chronic discharge of thin mucus from the urethra, following gonorrhea.

gleety (glē'tē). Relating to gleet.

Glenner, George B., U.S. pathologist and histologist, *1927. See G.-Lillie *stain* for pituitary.

glenohumeral (glē'nō-hyū'mer-ăl). Relating to the glenoid cavity and the humerus.

glenoid (glē'noyd, glen'oyd) [G. *glēnoeidēs,* fr. *glēnē,* pupil of eye, socket of joint, honeycomb, + *eidos,* appearance]. Resembling a socket; denoting the articular depression of the scapula entering into the formation of the shoulder joint.

Gley, Marcel E. E., French physiologist, 1857–1930. See G.'s *glands.*

glia (glī'ă) [G. glue]. Neuroglia.

gliacyte (glī'ă-sīt) [G. *glia,* glue, + *kytos,* cell]. A neuroglia cell. See neuroglia.

gliadin (glī'ă-din). A class of protein, separable from wheat and rye glutens, that contains up to 40% glutamine; a member of the prolamins, which are insoluble in water, absolute alcohol, and neutral solvents, but soluble in 70 to 80% alcohol.

glial (glī'ăl). Pertaining to glia or neuroglia.

glide (glīd). A smooth, or effortless, continuous movement.

mandibular g., the side-to-side, protrusive, and intermediate movement of the mandible occurring when the teeth or other occluding surfaces are in contact.

glio- [G. *glia,* glue]. Combining form meaning glue or gluelike, relating specifically to the neuroglia.

glioblast (glī'ō-blast) [glio- + G. *blastos,* germ]. An early neural cell developing, like the neuroblast, from the early ependymal cell of the neural tube.

glioblastoma (glī'ō-blas-tō'mă) [G. *glia,* glue, + *blastos,* germ, + *-oma,* tumor]. Grade IV astrocytoma; a glioma consisting chiefly of undifferentiated anaplastic cells that are precursors of astrocytes and that vary greatly in size, shape, and staining reactions; frequently, they are arranged radially about an irregular focus of necrosis, and pseudorosettes are sometimes formed; these neoplasms grow rapidly and invade extensively, occurring most frequently in the cerebrum of adults.

glioblastosis cerebri (glī'ō-blas-tō'sis ser'ĕ-brī). Astrocytosis cerebri; a diffuse intracranial neoplasm of astrocytic origin.

glioma (glī-ō'mă) [G. *glia,* glue, + *-oma,* tumor]. Any neoplasm derived from one of the various types of cells that form the interstitial tissue of the brain, spinal cord, pineal gland, posterior pituitary gland, and retina.
gigantocellular g., a histologic form of glioblastoma with large, often multinucleated, bizarre, tumor cells.
mixed g., astroependymoma.
nasal g., term for a lesion that is probably not a true neoplasm, but an unusual anomaly consisting of glial tissue with bizarre astrocytes, ganglionic neurons, and ependymal cells in small nodules at the base of the nose.
g. of optic chiasm, a slow-growing tumor, usually an astrocytoma, of the optic chiasm in children.
g. of the spinal cord, a glial tumor of the spinal cord, commonly an ependymoma; neoplasms of the spinal cord are relatively rare, but g.'s constitute approximately one-fourth of the total.
telangiectatic g., g. telangiecto'des, a g. in which the stroma has numerous, conspicuous, frequently dilated small blood vessels and capillaries, as well as large, endothelium-rimmed lakes of blood.

gliomatosis (glī-ō-mă-tō'sis). Neurogliomatosis; neoplastic growth of neuroglial cells in the brain or spinal cord; the term is used especially with reference to a relatively large neoplasm or to multiple foci.

gliomatous (glī-ō'mă-tŭs). Pertaining to or characterized by a glioma.

gliomyxoma (glī'ō-mik-sō'mă). A myxoma that contains a considerable amount of proliferating glial cells and fibers.

glioneuroma (glī'ō-nū-rō'mă). A ganglioneuroma derived from neurons, with numerous glial cells and fibers in the matrix.

gliosarcoma (glī'ō-sar-kō'mă). A glioma consisting of immature, undifferentiated, pleomorphic, spindle-shaped cells with relatively large, hyperchromatic, frequently bizarre nuclei and poorly formed fibrillary processes. Sometimes used as a term for a malignant neoplasm derived from connective tissue (*e.g.,* that associated with blood vessels in the brain) in which there are proliferating glial cells. See also spongioblastoma.

gliosis (glī-ō'sis). Overgrowth of the neuroglia.
isomorphous g., a scar in which the previous arrangement of neuroglial fibers is preserved. See also brain *cicatrix.*
piloid g., an area of chronic, reactive astrocytosis composed of thin, hairlike cells in vaguely parallel array.
g. u'teri, fetal neural tissue persisting or recurring locally as a benign condition in the endometrium or cervix; possibly derived from a homograft of fetal glial stroma.

glipizide (glip'i-zīd). 1-Cyclohexyl-3-[[*p*- [21(5-methylpyrazinecarboxyamido)ethyl]-phenyl]-sulfonyl]-urea; an oral sulfonylurea.

Glisson, Francis, British physician, anatomist, physiologist and pathologist, 1597–1677. See G.'s *capsule, cirrhosis, disease, sphincter.*

glissonitis (glis-ō-nī'tis). Inflammation of Glisson's capsule, or the connective tissue surrounding the portal vein and the hepatic artery and bile ducts.

Gln Symbol for glutamine or its acyl radical, glutaminyl.

global (glō'băl). The complete, generalized, overall, or total aspect.

globe (glōb). Globus.
g. of eye, *bulbus* oculi.
pale g., *globus* pallidus.

globi (glō'bī). **1.** Plural of globus. **2.** Brown bodies sometimes found in the granulomatous lesions of leprosy, in addition to the macrophages that contain the acid-fast bacilli; thought to be degenerate forms of such cells, in which the organisms are no longer viable and have become granular or amorphous.

globin (glō'bin). Hematohiston; the protein of hemoglobin.

Globocephalus (glō-bō-sef'ă-lŭs). A genus of hookworm (subfamily Uncinariinae, family Ancylostomatidae) consisting of about five species, found chiefly in the small intestine of pigs. The species *G. urosubalatus,* of worldwide distribution, is a common hookworm of wild and domestic pigs.

globoside (glō'bō-sīd). A glycosphingolipid; specifically, a ceramide tetrasaccharide (tetraglycosylceramide), isolated from kidney and erythrocytes, of the structure: *N*-acetylgalactosaminyl ($\beta 1 \rightarrow {}^1 3$)galactosyl($\alpha 1 \rightarrow 4$)galactosyl($\beta 1 \rightarrow 4$)glucosylceramide.

globule (glob'yūl) [L. *globulus,* dim. of *globus,* a ball]. Globulus. **1.** A small spherical body of any kind. **2.** A fat droplet in milk.
dentin g., calcospherites formed by calcification or mineralization of the dentin occurring in globular areas.
Morgagni's g.'s, Morgagni's spheres; vesicles beneath the capsule and between lens fibers in early cataract.
polar g., polar *body.*

globuliferous (glob-yū-lif'er-ŭs) [L. *globulus,* globule, + *fero,* to bear]. Containing globules or corpuscles, especially red blood cells.

globulin (glob'yū-lin) [L. *globulus,* globule]. Name for a family of proteins precipitated from plasma (or serum) by half-saturation with ammonium sulfate (*i.e.,* addition of an equal volume of saturated ammonium sulfate). G.'s may be further fractionated by solubility, electrophoresis, ultracentrifugation, and other separation methods into many subgroups, the main groups being α-, β-, and γ-g.; these differ with respect to associated lipids or carbohydrates and in their content of many physiologically important factors. Among the latter are immunoglobulins (antibodies) in the β and γ fractions, lipoproteins in the α and β fractions, gluco- or mucoproteins (orosomucoid, haptoglobin), and metal-binding and metal-transporting proteins (transferrin, siderophilin, ceruloplasmin). Other substances found in g. fractions are: macroglobulin, plasminogen, prothrombin, euglobulin, antihemophilic g., fibrinogen, cryoglobulin.
β_{1C} g., the third component (C3) of complement. See *component* of complement.
β_{1E} g., the fourth component (C4) of complement. See *component* of complement.
β_{1F} g., the fifth component (C5) of complement. See *component* of complement.
accelerator g. (AcG, ac-g), accelerin; a g. in serum that hastens the conversion of prothrombin to thrombin in the presence of thromboplastin and ionized calcium. See *factor* V (plasma accelerator g.); serum accelerator g.
antihemophilic g. (AHG), **(1)** *factor* VIII; **(2)** human antihemophilic *factor.*
antihemophilic g. A, *factor* VIII.
antihemophilic g. B, *factor* IX
antihuman g., Coombs' serum; serum from a rabbit or other animal previously immunized with purified human g. to prepare antibodies directed against IgG and complement; used in the direct and indirect Coombs' tests.
chickenpox immune g. (human), chickenpox immunoglobulin; g. fraction of serum from persons recently recovered from herpes zoster infection; used to prevent infection of high-risk children.
corticosteroid-binding g. (CBG), transcortin.

human gamma g., human normal immunoglobulin; a preparation of the proteins of liquid human plasma, containing the antibodies of normal adults; it is obtained from pooled liquid human plasma from a number of donors and may be prepared by precipitation with organic solvents under controlled conditions of pH, ionic strength, and temperature.

immune serum g. (human), a sterile solution of g.'s that contains many antibodies normally present in adult human blood; a passive immunizing agent.

measles immune g. (human), measles immunoglobulin; a sterile solution of g.'s derived from the blood plasma of normal adult human donors; it is prepared from immune serum g. that complies, after dilution if necessary, with the measles antibody reference standard; a passive immunizing agent.

pertussis immune g., pertussis immunoglobulin; a sterile solution of g.'s derived from the plasma of adult human donors who have been immunized with pertussis vaccine; used both prophylactically and therapeutically.

plasma accelerator g., *factor* V.

poliomyelitis immune g. (human), poliomyelitis immunoglobulin; a sterile solution of g.'s that contains those antibodies normally present in adult human blood; it is a passive immunologic agent that attenuates or prevents poliomyelitis, measles, and infectious hepatitis, and confers temporary but significant protection against paralytic polio.

rabies immune g. (human), rabies immunoglobulin; g. fraction of pooled plasma of high anti-rabies virus titer from immunized persons.

RH_0 (D) immune g., anti-D or Rh_0 (D) immunoglobulin; a g. fraction of antibody specific for the most common antigen, Rh_0 (D), of the Rh group; used to prevent Rh-sensitization of an Rh-negative woman after delivery of an Rh-positive fetus.

serum accelerator g., a substance in serum that accelerates the conversion of prothrombin to thrombin in the presence of thromboplastin and calcium; produced by the action of traces of thrombin upon plasma accelerator g.

specific immune g. (human), g. fraction of pooled serums (or plasma) selected for high titer of antibodies specific for a particular antigen, or from persons specifically immunized.

tetanus immune g., tetanus immunoglobulin; a sterile solution of g.'s derived from the blood plasma of adult human donors who have been immunized with tetanus toxoid; a passive immunizing agent.

thyroxine-binding g. (TBG), thyroxine-binding protein(1); an α-globulin of blood with a strong binding affinity for thyroxine; triiodothyronine is bound to it much less firmly.

zoster immune g., a g. fraction of pooled plasma from individuals who have recovered from herpes zoster; used prophylactically and therapeutically for varicella.

globulinuria (glob'yū-li-nū'rē-ă). The excretion of globulin in the urine, usually, if not always, in association with serum albumin.

globulus (glob'yū-lŭs) [L.]. Globule.

globus, pl. **globi** (glō'bŭs, -bī) [L.]. Globe. **1** [NA]. A round body; sphere; ball. **2.** See globi.

g. hyster'icus, spheresthesia; a sensation as of a ball in the throat or as if the throat were compressed; a symptom of hysteria.

g. ma'jor, *caput* epididymidis.

g. mi'nor, *cauda* epididymidis.

g. pal'lidus [NA], pale globe; pallidum; the inner and lighter gray portion of the lentiform nucleus. See also paleostriatum.

glomal (glō'măl). Relating to or involving a glomus.

glomangioma (glō-man-jē-ō'mă). Glomus *tumor.*

glomangiosis (glō-man-jē-ō'sis). The occurrence of multiple complexes of small vascular channels, each resembling a glomus.

pulmonary g., g. occurring within small pulmonary arteries in severe pulmonary hypertension and congenital heart disease.

glome (glōm). Glomus.

glomectomy (glō-mek'tō-mē) [L. *glomus* + G. *ektomē,* cutting out]. Excision of a glomus tumor.

glomera (glom'er-ă). Plural of glomus.

glomerular (glō-mār'yū-lăr). Glomerulose; relating to or affecting a glomerulus or the glomeruli.

glomerule (glom'er-yūl). Glomerulus.

glomerulitis (glō-mār'yū-lī'tis). Inflammation of a glomerulus, specifically of the renal glomeruli, as in glomerulonephritis.

glomerulonephritis (glō-mār'yū-lō-nef-rī'tis) [glomerulus + G. *nephros,* kidney, + *-itis,* inflammation]. Glomerular nephritis; renal disease characterized by bilateral inflammatory changes in glomeruli which are not the result of infection of the kidneys.

acute g., acute hemorrhagic or post-streptoccal g.; acute nephritis; g. that frequently occurs as a late complication of pharyngitis, especially due to type 12 β-hemolytic streptococci, characterized by abrupt onset of hematuria, edema of the face, oliguria, and variable azotemia and hypertension; the renal glomeruli usually show cellular proliferation or infiltration by polymorphonuclear leukocytes.

acute crescentic g., rapidly progressive g.

acute hemorrhagic g., acute g.

acute post-streptococcal g., acute g.

anti-basement membrane g., g. resulting from anti-basement membrane antibodies, characterized by smooth linear deposits of IgG and C3 along glomerular capillary walls; includes rapidly progressive g. and g. in Goodpasture's syndrome.

Berger's focal g., focal g.

chronic g., chronic nephritis; g. that presents with persisting proteinuria, chronic renal failure, and hypertension, of insidious onset or as a late sequel of acute g.; the kidneys are symmetrically contracted and granular, with scarring and loss of glomeruli and the presence of tubular atrophy and interstitial fibrosis.

diffuse g., g. affecting most of the renal glomeruli; it may lead to azotemia.

Ellis type 1 g., Ellis type 1 nephritis; obsolete designation for g. presenting as acute g., followed by complete recovery in most cases, or the development of rapidly progressive g., or incomplete remission with persistent proteinuria and subsequent development of chronic g.

Ellis type 2 g., Ellis type 2 nephritis; obsolete designation for g. which is usually not related to preceding bacterial infection; characterized by an insidious onset of the nephrotic syndrome, failure of complete remission, and eventual development of chronic renal failure. The kidneys usually show membranous g.

exudative g., g. with infiltration of glomeruli by polymorphonuclear leukocytes, occurring in acute g.

focal g., Berger's focal g.; focal nephritis; IgA nephropathy; g. affecting a small proportion of renal glomeruli which commonly presents with hematuria and may be associated with acute upper respiratory infection in young males, not usually due to streptococci; associated with IgA deposits in the glomerular mesangium and may also be associated with systemic disease, as in Henoch-Schönlein purpura.

focal embolic g., g. associated with subacute bacterial endocarditis, frequently producing microscopic hematuria without azotemia.

hypocomplementemic g., membranoproliferative g.

lobular g., membranoproliferative g.

local g., segmental g.

membranoproliferative g., hypocomplementemic, lobular, or mesangiocapillary g.; chronic g. characterized by mesangial cell proliferation, increased lobular separation of glomeruli, thickening of glomerular capillary walls and increased mesangial matrix, and low serum levels of ccmplement; occurs mainly in older children,

with a variably slow progressive course, episodes of hematuria or edema, and hypertension. It is classified into three types: type 1, the commonest, in which there are subendothelial electron-dense deposits; type 2, dense-deposit disease, in which the lamina densa is greatly thickened by extremely electron-dense material; type 3, in which there are both subendothelial and subepithelial deposits.
membranous g., g. characterized by diffuse thickening of glomerular capillary basement membranes, due in part to subepithelial deposits of immunoglobulins separated by spikes of basement membrane material, and clinically by an insidious onset of the nephrotic syndrome and failure of disappearance of proteinuria; the disease is most commonly idiopathic but may be secondary to malignant tumors, drugs, infections, or systemic lupus erythematosus.
mesangial proliferative g., diffuse mesangial proliferation; IgM nephropathy; g. characterized clinically by the nephrotic syndrome and histologically by diffuse glomerular increases in endocapillary and mesangial cells and in mesangial matrix; in some cases, there are mesangial deposits of IgM and complement.
mesangiocapillary g., membranoproliferative g.
proliferative g., g. with hypercellularity of glomeruli due to proliferation of endothelial or mesangial cells, occurring in acute g. and membranoproliferative g.
rapidly progressive g., acute crescentic g.; g. usually presenting insidiously, without preceding streptococcal infection, with increasing renal failure leading to death within a few months; at autopsy the kidneys are normal in size, numerous glomerular capsular epithelial crescents are present, and antiglomerular basement membrane antibodies are frequently found.
segmental g., local g.; g. affecting only part of a glomerulus or glomeruli.
subacute g., subacute nephritis; undesirable term for g. with proteinuria, hematuria and azotemia persisting for many weeks; renal changes are variable, including those of rapidly progressive and membranoproliferative g.

glomerulopathy (glō-mār-yū-lop'ă-thē) [glomerulus + G. *pathos,* suffering]. Glomerular disease of any type.
focal sclerosing g., focal, segmental glomerulosclerosis reported in adults and children with normal serum complement, progressing to chronic glomerulonephritis.

glomerulosclerosis (glo-mār'yū-lō-sklĕ-rō'sis) [glomerulus + G. *sklērōsis,* hardness]. Glomerular sclerosis; hyaline deposits or scarring within the renal glomeruli, a degenerative process occurring in association with renal arteriosclerosis or diabetes.
diabetic g., intercapillary g.; rounded hyaline or laminated nodules in the periphery of the glomeruli with capillary basement membrane thickening and increased mesangial matrix.
focal segmental g., segmental collapse of glomerular capillaries with thickened basement membranes and increased mesangial matrix; seen in some glomeruli of patients with nephrotic syndrome or mesangial proliferative glomerulonephritis.
intercapillary g., diabetic g.

glomerulose (glō-mār'yū-lōs). Glomerular.

glomerulus, pl. **glomeruli** (glō-mār'yū-lŭs, -yū-lī) [Mod. L. dim. of L. *glomus,* a ball of yarn] [NA]. Glomerule. **1.** A plexus of capillaries. **2.** Malpighian g. or tuft; a tuft formed of capillary loops at the beginning of each uriniferous tubule in the kidney; this tuft with its capsule (Bowman's capsule) constitutes the corpusculum renis (malpighian body). **3.** The twisted secretory portion of a sweat gland. **4.** A cluster of dendritic ramifications and axon terminals forming a complex synaptic relationship and surrounded by a glial sheath.
malpighian g., g. (2).
g. of mesonephros, one of the tufts of capillary vessels within the mesonephros derived from a lateral branch of the primary aorta; each g. is connected to a tubule.
olfactory g., one of the small spherical territories in the olfactory bulb in which dendrites of mitral and tufted cells synapse with axons of olfactory receptor cells.
g. of pronephros, one of the tufts of capillary vessels in the pronephros derived from a lateral branch of the aorta.

glomus, pl. **glomera** (glō'mŭs, glom'er-ă) [L. *glomus,* a ball]. Glome. **1** [NA]. A small globular body. **2.** Glomus body; glandulae glomiformes (1); a highly organized arteriolovenular anastomosis forming a tiny nodular focus in the nailbed, pads of the fingers and toes, ears, hands, and feet and many other organs of the body. The afferent arteriole enters the connective tissue capsule of the g., becomes devoid of an internal elastic membrane, and develops a relatively thick epithelioid muscular wall and small lumen; the anastomosis may be branched and convoluted, richly innervated with sympathetic and myelinated nerves, and connected with a short, thin-walled vein that drains into a periglomic vein and then into one of the veins of the skin. The g. functions as a shunt or bypass regulating mechanism in the flow of blood, temperature, and conservation of heat in the part as well as in the indirect control of the blood pressure and other functions of the circulatory system.
g. aor'ticum, aortic body; corpus aorticum; one of the small bilateral structures, similar to the g. caroticum, attached to a small branch of the aorta near its arch; they contain chemoreceptors that respond primarily to decreases in blood oxygen tension; less sensitive to decreases in blood pH or increases in carbon dioxide tension.
g. carot'icum [NA], carotid body; intercarotid body; nodulus caroticus; a small epithelioid structure located just above the bifurcation of the common carotid artery on each side. It consists of granular principal cells and nongranular supporting cells, a sinusoidal vascular bed and a rich network of sensory fibers of the glossopharyngeal nerve. It serves as a chemoreceptor organ responsive to oxygen lack, carbon dioxide excess, and increased hydrogen ion concentration.

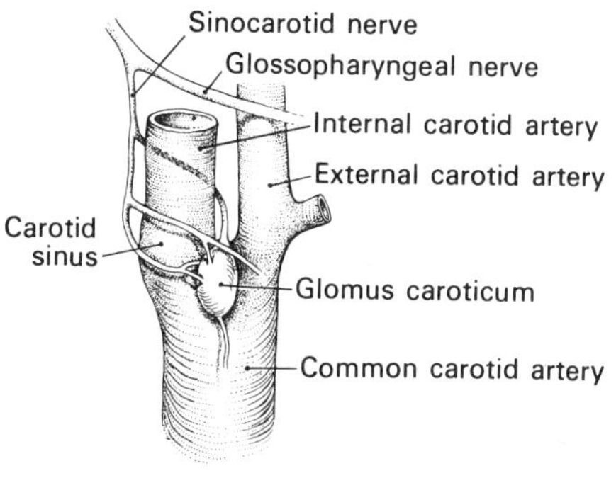

Glomus Caroticum

choroid g., g. choroideum.
g. choroide'um [NA], choroid g.; choroid skein; a marked enlargement of the choroid plexus of the lateral ventricle at the junction of the central part with the inferior horn.
g. coccyge'um, *corpus* coccygeum.
g. intravaga'le, a minute collection of chemoreceptor cells on the auricular branch of the vagus nerve. A tumor of this g. may cause deafness and tinnitus.
g. jugula're, a microscopic collection of chemoreceptor tissue in the adventitia of the jugular bulb; a tumor of this g. may cause paralysis of the vocal cords, attacks of dizziness, blackouts, and nystagmus.
g. pulmona'le, a structure similar to the g. caroticum, found in relation to the pulmonary artery.

glonoin (glō'nō-in). Nitroglycerin.

gloss-. See glosso-.

glossa (glos'ă) [G.]. Lingua (1).

glossagra (glos-ag'ră) [gloss- + G. *agra,* a seizure]. Glossalgia of gouty origin.

glossal (glos'ăl). Lingual (1).

glossalgia (glos-al'jē-ă) [gloss- + G. *algos,* pain]. Glossodynia.

glossectomy (glo-sek'tō-mē) [gloss- + G. *ektomē,* excision]. Elinguation; glossosteresis; lingulectomy (1); excision or amputation of the tongue.

Glossina (glo-sī'nă) [G. *glōssa,* tongue]. A genus of bloodsucking Diptera (tsetse flies) confined to Africa; they serve as vectors of the pathogenic trypanosomes that cause various forms of African sleeping sickness in humans and in domestic and wild animals.

G. mor'sitans, a species originally thought to be the sole transmitter of *Trypanosoma brucei,* the cause of nagana in central Africa; this species transmits this disease in some regions, but it is not the sole or even always the principal transmitting agent; it is the vector of *T. rhodesiense,* one of the pathogenic agents of East African, Rhodesian, or acute sleeping sickness.

G. pallid'ipes, a species that is the principal transmitter of nagana; it also transmits *Trypanosoma rhodesiense.*

G. palpa'lis, a species of *G.* that transmits *Trypanosoma gambiense,* one of the pathogenic parasites of West African, Gambian, or chronic sleeping sickness.

glossitis (glo-sī'tis) [gloss- + G. *-itis,* inflammation]. Inflammation of the tongue.

g. area'ta exfoliati'va, geographic *tongue.*

atrophic g., bald tongue; an erythematous, edematous, and painful tongue which appears smooth due to loss of the filiform and sometimes the fungiform papillae secondary to certain nutritional deficiencies, or disorders such as pernicious anemia (Hunter's or Moeller's g.) and chronic recurrent pellagra.

benign migratory g., geographic *tongue.*

g. desic'cans, a painful affection of the tongue, of unknown origin, in which the surface becomes raw and fissured.

Hunter's g., see atrophic g.

median rhomboid g., an asymptomatic, ovoid or rhomboid, macular or mamellated, erythematous lesion with papillary atrophy on the dorsum of the tongue just anterior to the circumvalate papillae; due to infection with *Candida albicans.*

Moeller's g., see atrophic g.

glosso-, gloss- [G. *glōssa,* tongue]. Combining forms relating to the tongue.

glossocele (glos'ō-sēl) [glosso- + G. *kēlē,* tumor, hernia]. Protrusion of the tongue from the mouth, owing to its excessive size. See also macroglossia.

glossocinesthetic (glos'ō-sin-es-thet'ik). Glossokinesthetic.

glossodontotropism (glos-ō-don'tō-trō-pizm) [glosso- + G. *odous (odont-),* tooth, + *tropē,* a turning]. A manifestation of tension or anxiety in which the tongue is attracted to the teeth or to dental faults.

glossodynamometer (glos'ō-dī-nă-mom'ĕ-ter) [glosso- + G. *dynamis,* power, + *metron,* measure]. An apparatus for estimating the contractile force of the tongue muscles.

glossodynia (glos'ō-din'ē-ă) [glosso- + G. *odynē,* pain]. Glossalgia; glossopyrosis; a condition characterized by burning or painful tongue.

glossodyniotropism (glos-ō-din'ē-ō-trō-pizm) [glosso- + G. *odynē,* pain, + *tropē,* a turning]. Apparent satisfaction from subjecting the tongue to a pain-inducing dental fault; considered by some to be a masochistic behavior or manifestation.

glossoepiglottic, glossoepiglottidean (glos'ō-ep-i-glot'ik, glos'ō-ep-i-glo-tid'ē-an). Relating to the tongue and the epiglottis.

glossograph (glos'ō-graf) [glosso- + G. *graphō,* to write]. An instrument for recording the movements of the tongue in speaking.

glossohyal (glos-ō-hī'ăl). Hyoglossal.

glossokinesthetic (glos'ō-kin-es-thet'ik) [glosso- + G. *kinēsis,* movement, + *aisthētikos,* perceptive]. Glossocinesthetic; denoting the subjective sensation of the movements of the tongue.

glossolalia (glos-ō-lā'lē-ă) [glosso- + G. *lalia,* talk, chat]. Unintelligible jargon or babbling.

glossology (glos-ol'ō-jē) [glosso- + G. *logos,* study]. Glottology; the branch of medical science concerned with the tongue and its diseases.

glossolysis (glos-ol'i-sis) [glosso- + G. *lysis,* a loosening]. Glossoplegia; paralysis of the tongue.

glossoncus (glos-ong'kŭs) [glosso- + G. *onkos,* mass, tumor]. Any swelling involving the tongue, including neoplasms.

glossopalatinus (glos'ō-pal-ă-tī'nŭs) [glosso- + Mod. L. *palatinus,* fr. L. *palatum,* palate]. *Musculus* palatoglossus.

glossopathy (glos-op'ă-thē) [glosso- + G. *pathos,* suffering]. A disease of the tongue.

glossopharyngeal (glos'ō-fă-rin'jē-ăl). Relating to the tongue and the pharynx.

glossopharyngeus (glos'ō-fă-rin'jē-ŭs). *Musculus* glossopharyngeus.

glossoplasty (glos'ō-plas-tē) [glosso- + G. *plastos,* formed]. Plastic surgery of the tongue.

glossoplegia (glos-ō-plē'jē-ă) [glosso- + G. *plēgē,* stroke]. Glossolysis.

glossoptosis, glossoptosia (glos-op-tō'sis, -op-tō'sē-ă) [glosso- + G. *ptōsis,* a falling]. Downward displacement of the tongue.

glossopyrosis (glos-ō-pī-rō'sis) [glosso- + G. *pyrosis,* a burning]. Glossodynia.

glossorrhaphy (glo-sōr'ă-fē) [glosso- + G. *rhaphē,* suture]. Suture of a wound of the tongue.

glossoscopy (glos-os'kŏ-pē) [glosso- + G. *skopeō,* to view]. Examination of the tongue.

glossospasm (glos'ō-spazm). Spasmodic contraction of the tongue.

glossosteresis (glos'ō-ste-rē'sis). Glossectomy.

glossotomy (glo-sot'ō-mē) [glosso- + G. *tomē,* incision]. Any cutting operation on the tongue.

glossotrichia (glos-ō-trik'ē-ă) [glosso- + G. *thrix,* hair]. Hairy *tongue.*

glottal (glot'ăl). Relating to the glottis.

glottic (glot'ik). Relating to (1) the tongue or (2) the glottis.

glottidospasm (glot'i-dō-spazm). Laryngospasm.

glottis, pl. glottides (glot'is, glot'i-dēz) [G. *glōttis,* aperture of the larynx] [NA]. The vocal apparatus of the larynx, consisting of the vocal folds of mucous membrane investing the vocal ligament and vocal muscle on each side, the free edges of which are the vocal cords, and of a median fissure, the rima glottidis.

false g., *rima* vestibuli.

g. respirato'ria, *pars* intercartilaginea rimae glottidis.

g. spu'ria, *rima* vestibuli.

true g., *rima* glottidis.

g. ve'ra, *rima* glottidis.

g. voca'lis, *pars* intermembranacea rimae glottidis.

glottitis (glo-tī'tis). Inflammation of the glottic portion of the larynx.

glottology (glo-tol'ō-jē) [G. *glōssa, glōtta,* tongue, + *logos,* study]. Glossology.

Glu Symbol for glutamic acid or its acyl radical, glutamyl.

glucagon (glū'kă-gon). Hyperglycemic-glycogenolytic factor; HG factor; pancreatic hyperglycemic hormone; a hormone consisting of a straight-chain polypeptide of 29 residues (bovine g.), extracted from pancreatic alpha cells. Parenteral administration of 0.5 to 1 mg results in prompt mobilization of hepatic glycogen, thus elevating blood glucose concentration. It activates hepatic phosphorylase, thereby increasing glycogenolysis, decreases gastric motility and gastric and pancreatic secretions, and increases urinary excretion of nitrogen and potassium; it has no effect on muscle phosphorylase. As the hydrochloride, it is used in the treatment of glycogen storage disease (von Gierke's) and hypoglycemia, particularly hypoglycemic coma due to exogenously administered insulin.

gut g., a substance of intestinal origin that is secreted into the blood following ingestion of glucose and is a potent stimulus to the secretion of insulin; its chemical structure and the biologic effects that it produces are different from those of g., and it cross-reacts with antibodies to g.

glucagonoma (glu'kă-gon-ō'mă). a glucagon-secreting tumor, usually derived from pancreatic islet cells.

glucal (glū'kăl). Glycal.

glucan (glū'kan). A polyglucose; *e.g.*, callose, cellulose, starch amylose, glycogen amylose.

1,4-α-glucan branching enzyme [EC 2.4.1.18]. α-Glucan branching glycosyltransferase; branching enzyme or factor; amylo-(1,4→1,6)-transglucosylase or transglucosidase; an enzyme in muscle and in plants (Q enzyme) that cleaves α-1,4 linkages in glycogen or starch, transferring the fragments into α-1,6 linkages, creating branches in the polysaccharide molecules; in plants, it converts amylose to amylopectin.

α-glucan branching glycosyltransferase. 1,4-α-Glucan branching enzyme.

1,4-α-D-glucan 6-α-D-glucosyltransferase [EC 2.4.1.24]. Oligoglucan-branching glycosyltransferase; T enzyme; a glucosyltransferase that transfers an α-glucosyl residue in a 1,4-α-glucan to the primary hydroxyl group of glucose in a 1,4-α-glucan. See also 1,4-α-glucan branching enzyme.

4-α-D-glucanotransferase [EC 2.4.1.25]. Dextrin transglycosylase or glycosyltransferase; D enzyme; disproportionating enzyme; amylomaltase; a 4-glycosyltransferase converting maltodextrins into amylose and glucose by transferring parts of 1,4-glucan chains to new 4-positions on glucose or other 1,4-glucans.

α-glucan phosphorylase. Phosphorylase.

glucases (glū'cās-ez). Obsolete term for enzymes cleaving starch to glucose.

glucemia (glū-sē'mē-ă). Obsolete term for glycemia.

gluceptate (glū-sep'tat). USAN-approved contraction for glucoheptonate.

glucide (glū'sīd). Obsolete term at one time suggested to embrace the carbohydrates and the glucosides; modern equivalent is saccharide.

glucinium (glū-sin'ē-ŭm). Former name for beryllium.

gluciphore (glū'si-fōr) [G. *glykys*, sweet, + *phoros*, bearing]. Term coined for chemical groups believed to be responsible for sweet taste.

gluco-. Combining form denoting relationship to glucose. See also glyco-.

glucoamylase (glū-kō-am'i-lās). Exo-1,4-α-D-glucosidase.

glucoascorbic acid (glū'kō-as-kōr'bik). 3-Keto-D-glucoheptonofuranolactone; a compound resembling ascorbic acid but with an additional –CHOH– between C-5 and C-6 of ascorbic acid; shows toxic effects on addition to diet which apparently are not caused by ascorbic acid antagonism.

glucocerebroside (glū-kō-ser'ĕ-brō-sīd). Glucosylceramide.

glucocoid (glū'kō-koyd). Obsolete term for glucocorticoid.

glucocorticoid (glū-kō-kōr'ti-koyd). Glycocorticoid. **1.** Any steroid-like compound capable of significantly influencing intermediary metabolism such as promotion of hepatic glycogen deposition, and of exerting a clinically useful anti-inflammatory effect. Cortisol is the most potent of the naturally occurring g.'s; most semisynthetic g.'s are cortisol derivatives. **2.** Denoting this type of biological activity.

glucocorticotrophic (glū'kō-kōr'ti-kō-trōf'ik). Denoting a principle of the anterior hypophysis that stimulates the production of glucocorticoid hormones of the adrenal cortex; no hormone exerting only this effect has been identified.

glucocyamine (glū-kō-sī'ă-mēn). Glycocyamine.

glucofuranose (glū-kō-fūr'ă-nōs). D-Glucose in furanose form.

glucogenesis (glū-kō-jen'ĕ-sis) [gluco- + G. *genesis*, production]. Formation of glucose.

glucogenic (glū-kō-jen'ik). Giving rise to or producing glucose.

glucohemia (glū-kō-hē'mē-ă). Obsolete term for glycemia.

glucoinvertase (glū-kō-in'ver-tās). α-D-Glucosidase.

glucokinase (glū-kō-kī'nās) [EC 2.7.1.2]. A hexokinase or phosphotransferase that catalyzes the conversion of glucose to glucose 6-phosphate by ATP.

glucokinetic (glū'kō-ki-net'ik). Tending to mobilize glucose; usually evidenced by a reduction of the glycogen stores in the tissues to produce an increase in the concentration of glucose circulating in the blood.

glucolipids (glū-kō-lip'idz). Glycosphingolipids that contain glucose.

glucolysis (glū-kol'i-sis). Glycolysis.

gluconeogenesis (glū'kō-nē-ō-jen'ĕ-sis). Glyconeogenesis.

gluconic acid (glū-kon'ik). The hexonic (aldonic) acid derived from glucose by oxidation of the –CHO group to –COOH.

gluconolactonase (glū'kon-o-lak'tō-nās) [EC 3.1.1.17]. Lactonase; an enzyme catalyzing the hydrolysis of gluconolactone to gluconic acid.

glucopenia (glū-kō-pē'nē-ă) [gluco- + G. *penia*, poverty]. Hypoglycemia.

glucoprotein (glū-kō-prō'tēn). A glycoprotein in which the sugar is glucose.

glucopyranose (glū-kō-pir'ă-nōs). D-Glucose in its pyranose form.

glucosamine (glū'kō-să-mēn). Chitosamine; 2-amino-2-deoxyglucose; an amino sugar found in chitin, cell membranes, and mucopolysaccharides generally; used as a pharmaceutic aid.

glucosans (glū'kō-sanz). Polysaccharides yielding glucose upon hydrolysis; *e.g.*, cellulose, glycogen, starch, dextrins.

glucose (glū'kōs). D-Glucose; cellohexose; dextrose; dextroglucose; blood, corn, grape, or starch sugar; a dextrorotatory monosaccharide (hexose) found in the free state in fruits and other parts of plants, and combined in glucosides, disaccharides (often with fructose in sugars), oligosaccharides, and polysaccharides; it is the product of complete hydrolysis of cellulose, starch, and glycogen. Free g. also occurs in the blood (normal human concentration, 80 to 120 mg per 100 ml); in diabetes mellitus, it appears in the urine.

g. dehydrogenase [EC 1.1.1.47], converts β-D-glucose to D-glucono-1,5-lactone, transferring hydrogen to NAD or NADP. *Cf.* g. oxidase.

liquid g., a pharmaceutic aid consisting of dextrose, dextrins, maltose, and water, obtained by the incomplete hydrolysis of starch.

g. oxidase [EC 1.1.3.4], corylophyline; g. oxyhydrase; microcide; notatin; an antibacterial flavoprotein enzyme, obtained from *Penicillum notatum* and other fungi, which is antibacterial only in the presence of glucose and oxygen, its effect being due to the oxidation of glucose to glucono-δ-lactone, with conversion of

O_2 to H_2O_2.

g. oxyhydrase, g. oxidase.

g. phosphomutase, phosphoglucomutase.

glucose 6-phosphatase [EC 3.1.3.9]. A liver enzyme catalyzing the hydrolysis of glucose 6-phosphate to glucose and inorganic phosphate.

glucose 6-phosphate dehydrogenase [EC 1.1.1.49]. Zwischenferment; Robison ester dehydrogenase; an NADP enzyme catalyzing the dehydrogenation (oxidation) of glucose 6-phosphate to 6-phosphogluconolactone, this reaction initiating the Dickens shunt.

glucosephosphate isomerase (glū'kōs-fos'fāt) [EC 5.3.1.9]. Phosphohexose isomerase; phosphohexomutase; hexosephosphate isomerase; an enzyme that catalyzes the interconversion of fructose 6-phosphate and glucose 6-phosphate.

glucose 1-phosphate kinase. Phosphoglucokinase.

glucose 1-phosphate phosphodismutase [EC 2.7.1.41]. A phosphotransferase catalyzing the transfer of a phosphate residue from one glucose-1-phosphate to another, yielding glucose 1,6-bisphosphate.

α-D-glucosidase (glū'kō-si-dās) [EC 3.2.1.20]. Maltase; glucoinvertase; a glucohydrolase removing terminal nonreducing 1,4-linked α-glucose residues by hydrolysis, yielding α-glucose.

β-glucosidase [EC 3.2.1.21]. Gentiobiase; cellobiase; amygdalase; a glucohydrolase similar to α-glucosidase, but attacking β-glucosides and releasing β-glucose.

glucosidases (glū'kō-sid-ās-ez). Enzymes that hydrolyze glucosides.

glucoside (glū'kō-sīd). A compound of glucose with an alcohol or other R–OH compound involving loss of the H atom of the 1-OH (hemiacetal) group of the glucose, yielding a –C–O–R link from the C-1 of the glucose; a glycoside of glucose.

glucosone (glū'kō-sōn) [glucose + -one]. A 2-dehydrogenation (2-keto) product of glucose; a possible intermediate in the formation of glucosamine from glucose.

glucosulfone sodium (glū-kō-sŭl'fōn). *p,p'*-Sulfonyldianiline *N,N'*-diglucoside disodium; a chemotherapeutic agent used in the treatment of leprosy; parenteral administration is better tolerated than oral administration.

glucosuria (glū-kō-sū'rē-ă) [glucose + G. *ouron*, urine]. Glycosuria (1); the urinary excretion of glucose, usually in enhanced quantities.

glucosyl (glū'kō-sil). The radical of glucose that has lost its hemiacetal (C-1) OH.

glucosylceramide (glū'kō-sil-ser'ă-mīd). Glucocerebroside; a neutral glycolipid containing equimolar amounts of fatty acid, glucose, and sphingosine (or a derivative thereof).

glucosyltransferase (glū'kō-sil-trans'fer-ās). Transglucosylase; any enzyme transferring glucosyl groups from one compound to another; g.'s are in EC subclass 2.4 (glycosyltransferases).

glucuronate (glū-kūr'ō-nāt). A salt or ester of glucuronic acid.

glucurone (glū'kū-rōn). D-Glucuronolactone.

glucuronic acid (glū-kū-ron'ik). Glucuronose; the uronic acid of glucose in which C-6 is oxidized to a carboxyl group; it detoxicates or inactivates various substances (*e.g.*, benzoic acid, phenol, camphor, and the female sex hormones) undergoing conjugation with such substances in the liver, the glucuronides so formed being excreted in the urine.

β-D-glucuronidase (glū-kū-ron'i-dās) [EC 3.2.1.31]. Glusulase; glycuronidase; an enzyme catalyzing the hydrolysis of various β-D-glucuronides, liberating free glucuronic acid.

glucuronide (glū-kū'ron-īd). A glycoside of glucuronic acid; many foreign chemicals, as well as catabolic products of normal body constituents (*e.g.*, steroid hormones), are commonly excreted in the urine as g.'s, the conjugation taking place in the liver.

D-glucuronolactone (glū'kū-rō'nō-lak'tōn). Glucurone; lactone of D-glucofuranuronic acid; used as a means of orally administering glucuronic acid in the management of collagen and joint diseases.

glucuronose (glū-kū'ron-ōs) Glucuronic acid.

glucuronosyltransferase (glū-kū-ron'ō-sil-trans'fer-ās). Any of a family of enzymes that transfer glucuronate to the acceptor named, forming glucuronosides; *e.g.*, UDPglucuronate—bilirubin glucuronosyltransferase.

glue-sniffing (glū'snif-ing). Inhalation of fumes from plastic cements; the solvents, which include toluene, xylene, and benzene, induce central nervous system stimulation followed by depression. See also solvent *inhalation*.

Gluge, Gottlieb, German histologist, 1812–1898. See G.'s *corpuscles*.

glusulase (glū'sŭl-ās). β-Glucuronidase.

glutamate (glū'tă-māt). A salt or ester of glutamic acid.

g. acetyltransferase [EC 2.3.1.35], ornithine acetyltransferase; an enzyme catalyzing transfer of acetyl from α-N-acetylornithine to g.

g. decarboxylase [EC 4.1.1.15], aspartate 1-decarboxylase; a carboxy-lyase converting L-glutamate to 4-aminobutyrate and L-aspartate to 3-aminopropanoate.

g. dehydrogenases [EC 1.4.1.2, 3, and 4], glutamic acid dehydrogenases; pyridine-containing catalyzing the deamination of glutamic acid to α-ketoglutaric acid (2-oxoglutarate) with reduction of NAD^+ or $NADP^+$.

γ-glutamate (glutamate γ-) carboxypeptidase. γ-Glutamyl hydrolase.

glutamic acid (Glu) (glū-tam'ik). An amino acid, $HOOC\text{-}CH_2\text{-}CH_2\text{-}CH(NH_2)\text{-}COOH$, occurring in proteins; the sodium salt is monosodium glutamate.

g. a. dehydrogenases, *glutamate* dehydrogenases.

g. a. hydrochloride, a gastric acidifier alleged to aid in digestion; also used for gastric HCl replacement therapy.

glutamic-aspartic transaminase. *Aspartate* aminotransferase.

glutamic-oxaloacetic transaminase (GOT). *Aspartate* aminotransferase.

glutamic-pyruvic transaminase (GPT). Alanine aminotransferase.

glutaminase (glū-tam'in-ās) [EC 3.5.1.2]. An enzyme in kidney and other tissues that catalyzes the breakdown of glutamine to ammonia and glutamic acid.

glutamine (Gln) (glū'tă-mēn, -tă-min, glū-tam'in). Glutaminic acid; 2-aminoglutaramic acid; the δ-amide of glutamic acid, derived by oxidation from proline in the liver or by the combination of glutamic acid with ammonia; it is present in proteins and in blood and other tissues, and is an important source of urinary ammonia, being broken down in the kidney by the action of the enzyme glutaminase.

g. synthetase [EC 6.3.1.2], an enzyme that catalyzes the amination of glutamic acid to g. with the concomitant hydrolysis of ATP to ADP and P_i.

glutaminic acid (glū-tă-min'ik). Glutamine.

glutaminyl (Gln) (glū-tam'i-nil). The acyl radical of glutamine.

glutamoyl (glū-tam'ō-il). The radical of glutamic acid from which both α- and δ-hydroxyl groups have been removed.

glutamyl (Glu) (glū-tam'il, glū'tă-mil). The radical of glutamic acid from which either the α- or the δ-hydroxyl group has been removed.

g. transpeptidase, γ-glutamyltransferase.

γ-glutamyl hydrolase [EC 3.4.22.12]. Carboxypeptidase G; conjugase; γ-glutamate (glutamate γ-) carboxypeptidase; *N*-pteroyl-L-glutamate hydrolase; an enzyme cleaving glutamate residues from pteridine oligoglutamates.

γ-glutamyltransferase (glū-tam'il-trans'fer-ās) [EC 2.3.2.2]. Glutamyl transpeptidase; an enzyme that catalyzes the transfer of a γ-glutamyl group from a γ-glutamyl peptide to another peptide or amino acid.

glutaral (glū'tă-ral). Glutaraldehyde.

glutaraldehyde (glū-tă-ral'dĕ-hīd). Glutaral; pentanedial; $C_5H_8O_2$; a dialdehyde used as a fixative for electron microscopy, especially for nuclear morphology and for localization of enzyme activity; also used as a germicidal agent for disinfection and sterilization of instruments or equipment that cannot be heat sterilized.

glutaric acid (glū-tar'ik). Pentanedioic acid; $HOOC(CH_2)_3COOH$; an intermediate in tryptophan catabolism.

glutaryl-CoA synthetase (glū'tă-ril) [EC 6.2.1.6]. An enzyme similar to acyl-CoA synthetase, but which splits ATP, GTP, or ITP to the diphosphate in acting on glutarate.

glutathione (glū-tă-thī'ōn). γ-L-Glutamyl-L-cysteinylglycine; a tripeptide of glycine, cystine, and glutamic acid, the glutamic acid being attached through its γ-carboxyl group, a mode of attachment differing from its usual α-carboxyl (peptide) link in proteins.
Oxidized g. (GSSG) acts in cells as a hydrogen acceptor and **reduced g. (GSH)** acts as a hydrogen donor; oxidized g. is reduced by **g. reductase** (EC 1.6.4.2) which appears to be a ubiquitous reducing agent involved in many redox reactions.

gluteal (glū'tē-ăl) [G. *gloutos,* buttock]. Relating to the buttocks.

glutelins (glū'tĕ-linz). A class of simple proteins occurring in the seeds of grain; soluble in dilute acids and alkalies, but not in neutral solutions (*e.g.,* glutenin from wheat).

gluten (glū'tĕn) [L. *gluten,* glue]. Wheat gum; the insoluble protein constituent of wheat and other grains; a mixture of gliadin, glutenin, and other proteins.
g. casein, a protein resembling casein, present in g.

glutenin (glū'tĕ-nin). A glutelin in wheat.

gluteofemoral (glū'tē-ō-fem'ō-răl). Relating to the buttock and the thigh.

gluteoinguinal (glū'tē-ō-ing'gwi-năl). Relating to the buttock and the groin.

glutethimide (glū-teth'i-mīd). 2-Ethyl-2-phenylglutarimide; a central nervous system depressant used as a hypnotic in simple insomnia and formerly as a daytime sedative.

gluteus (glū-tē'ŭs). *Musculus* gluteus.

glutinoid (glū'ti-noyd). Albuminoid (3).

glutinous (glū'tin-ŭs). Adhesive; sticky.

glutitis (glū-tī'tis) [G. *gloutos,* buttock, + *-itis,* inflammation]. Inflammation of the muscles of the buttock.

Glx Symbol for glutamyl (Glu) and/or glutaminyl (Gln) to denote uncertainty between them.

Gly Symbol for glycine or its acyl radical, glycyl.

glyburide (glī'byū-rīd). Glybenzycydamide; 1-[[*p*-[2-(5-chloro-*o*-anisamido)ethyl]phenyl]sulfonyl]-3-cyclohexylurea; an oral hypoglycemic drug.

glycal (glī'kăl). Glucal; an unsaturated sugar derivative in which the adjacent hydroxyl groups are removed, one of which is that upon the carbon-1 of the aldose (or carbon-2 of the ketose), yielding a CH=CH between these two positions.

glycan (glī'kan). Polysaccharide.

glycanohydrolases (glī'kan-ō-hī'drō-lā-sez) [EC group 3.2.1]. Hydrolases acting on glycans; *e.g.,* chitinase, hyaluronoglucosidase.

glycate (glī'kāt). The product of the nonenzymic reaction between a sugar and the free amino group(s) of proteins in which it is not known if the sugar is attached by a glycosyl or a glycoside linkage, or has formed a Schiff base.

glycation (glī-kā'shŭn). The nonenzymic reaction that forms a glycate.

glycemia (glī-sē'mē-ă) [G. *glykys,* sweet, + *haima,* blood]. The presence of glucose in the blood.

glyceraldehyde (glis-er-al'dĕ-hīd). Glyceric aldehyde; glycerose; $HOCH_2$-CHOH-CHO; a triose and the simplest optically active monosaccharide; the dextrorotatory isomer is taken as the structural reference point for all D compounds, the levorotatory isomer for all L compounds.

glyceraldehyde 3-phosphate. HCO-CHOH-CH_2-OPO_3H_2; an intermediate in the glycolytic breakdown of glucose; one of the products of the splitting of fructose 1,6-bisphosphate under the catalytic influence of fructose-bisphosphate aldolase.

glyceric acid (gli-ser'ik, glis'er-ik). $HOCH_2$-CHOH-COOH; the fatty acid analogue of glycerol; occurs particularly in the form of phosphorylated derivatives, as an intermediate in glycolysis.

L-glyceric aciduria. Excretion of L-glyceric acid in the urine; a primary metabolic error due to deficiency of D-glyceric dehydrogenase resulting in excretion of L-glyceric and oxalic acids, leading to the clinical syndrome of oxalosis with frequent formation of oxalate renal calculi.

glyceric aldehyde. Glyceraldehyde.

glyceridases (glis'er-ĭ-dās-ez). General term for enzymes catalyzing the hydrolysis of glycerol esters (glycerides); *e.g.,* triacylglycerol lipase.

glyceride (glis'er-id, -īd). An ester of glycerol. The term is usually used in combination with phospho- (phosphoglyceride). The use of mono-, di-, and triglyceride is being replaced by the more precise terms mono-, di-, and triacylglycerol, respectively.
mixed g.'s, g.'s which, on hydrolysis, yield more than one variety of fatty acid.

glycerin (glis'er-in). Glycerol.
g. jelly, glycerinated *gelatin.*

glycerite (glis'er-īt). **1.** Glycerol. **2.** A pharmaceutical preparation made by triturating the active medicinal substance with glycerol.
starch g., a preparation containing 100 g of starch, 2 g of benzoic acid, 200 ml of purified water, and 700 g of glycerin in each 1000 g; a topical emollient.
tannic acid g., g. of tannin, containing tannic acid, sodium citrate, exsiccated sodium sulfite, and glycerin; an astringent.

glycerogelatin (glis'er-ō-jel'ă-tin). Glycerinated *gelatin.*

glyceroketone (glis'er-ō-kē'tōn). Dihydroxyacetone.

glycerokinase (glis'er-ō-kī'nās). *Glycerol* kinase.

glycerol (glis'er-ol). Glycerin; glycerite (1); glyceryl alcohol; 1,2,3-propanetriol; a sweet oily fluid obtained by the saponification of fats and fixed oils; used as a solvent, as a skin emollient; by injection or in the form of suppository for constipation, orally to reduce ocular tension, and as a vehicle and sweetening agent.
iodinated g., isopropylidene g.; an isomeric mixture of 2-(1-iodoethyl)-1,3-dioxolane-4-methanol and 2-(2-iodoethyl)-1,3-dioxolane-4-methanol; a mucolytic agent.
g. kinase [EC 2.7.1.30], glycerokinase; an enzyme that catalyzes a reaction between ATP and glycerol to yield glycerol phosphate and ADP.
g. phosphate, glycerophosphate; the anion of a phosphoric ester of g.; the central component of phosphatidates.

glycerol-3-phosphate dehydrogenase (NAD^+) [EC 1.1.1.8]. α-Glycerol phosphate dehydrogenase; 3-phosphoglycerol dehydrogenase; an oxidoreductase that catalyzes the interconversion of dihydroxyacetone phosphate and glycerol 3-phosphate, with the participation of NAD; its action provides the glycerol moiety from carbohydrate during lipogenesis.

glycerone (Grn) (glis′er-ōn) [contraction of glyceroketone]. Dihydroxyacetone.

glycerophosphate (glis′er-ō-fos′fāt). *Glycerol* phosphate.

glycerophosphocholine (glis′er-ō-fos-fō-kō′lēn). Glycerophosphorylcholine; $HOCH_2$-CHOH-CH_2-OP(O_2H)-OCH_2CH_2-$[N(CH_3)_3]^+$; a component of phosphatidylcholines (lecithins), in which the two OH's of g. are esterified with fatty acids.

glycerophosphoric acid (glis′er-ō-fos-fōr′ik). A phosphoric ester of glycerol. See also *glycerol* phosphate.

glycerophosphorylcholine (glis′er-ō-fos′fōr-il-kō′lēn). Glycerophosphocholine.

glycerose (glis′er-ōs). Glyceraldehyde.

glycerulose (glis′er-yū-lōs). Dihydroxyacetone.

glyceryl (glis′er-il). The trivalent radical, $C_3H_5\equiv$, of glycerol; often used in error for glycero- or glycerol.
g. alcohol, glycerol.
g. borate, boroglycerin.
g. ether, *glycerol* ether.
g. guaiacolate, guaifenesin.
g. monostearate, the ester of glycerol and one molecule of stearic acid; used in the manufacture of cosmetic creams and dermatologic preparations.
g. triacetate, triacetin.
g. tributyrate, Tributyrin.
g. tricaprate, caprin.
g. trinitrate, nitroglycerin.

glycinate (glī′sin-āt). A salt of glycine.

glycine (Gly) (glī′sēn). Glycocin; glycocoll; gelatin sugar; aminoacetic acid; $NH_2.CH_2.COOH$; the simplest amino acid in proteins; a major component of gelatin and silk fibroin; used as a nutrient and dietary supplement, and in solution for irrigation.
g. amidinotransferase [EC 2.1.4.1], g. transamidinase; an enzyme catalyzing the transfer of an amidine group from arginine to glycine, forming guanidinoacetate and ornithine; an important reaction in creatine synthesis.
g. betaine, betaine.
g. dehydrogenases, enzymes (EC 1.4.1.10 and 1.4.2.1) that catalyze the conversion of glycine to glyoxylate and ammonia.
g. transamidinase, g. amidinotransferase.

glycineamide ribonucleotide (glī′sin-ă-mīd). An intermediate in purine biosynthesis, in which the amide N of glycineamide is linked to the C-1 of a ribosyl moiety.

glycinemia (glī-si-nē′mē-ă). *Hyperglycinuria* with hyperglycinemia.

glycine-rich β-glycoprotein. Properdin *factor* B.

glycinuria (glī-si-nū′rē-ă) [glycine + G. *ouron,* urine]. The excretion of glycine in the urine.
familial g., a metabolic disorder believed to be due to defective renal glycine reabsorption; it may or may not be accompanied by oxalate urolithiasis; autosomal dominant inheritance.

glyco- [G. *glykys,* sweet]. Combining form denoting relationship to sugars (*e.g.,* glycogen) or to glycine (*e.g.,* glyocholate). See also gluco-.

glycobiarsol (glī-kō-bī′ar-sol). Oxo(hydrogen *N*- glycoloylarsanilato)bismuth; a pentavalent arsenical containing bismuth; used in the treatment of milder forms of intestinal amebiasis or as subsequent therapy.

glycocalyx (glī-kō-kā′liks) [glyco- + G. *kalyx,* husk, shell]. A PAS-positive filamentous coating on the apical surface of certain epithelial cells, composed of carbohydrate moieties of proteins that protrude from the free surface of the plasma membrane.

glycocholate (glī-kō-kō′lāt). A salt or ester of glycocholic acid.
g. sodium, a normal constituent of bile of man and herbivores; g. sodium from herbivores is purified and used as a choleretic and cholagogue.

glycocholic acid (glī-kō-kō′lik). *N*-cholylglycine; one of the major bile acid conjugates, formed by condensation of the —COOH group of cholic acid and the NH_2 group of glycine; water-soluble and a powerful detergent.

glycocin (glī′kō-sin). Glycine.

glycocoll (glī′kō-kol). Glycine.

glycocorticoid (glī′kō-kōr′ti-koyd). Glucocorticoid.

glycocyamine (glī-kō-sī′ă-mēn). Glucocyamine; 2-guanidinoacetic acid; $HN=C(NH_2)NH-CH_2COOH$; formed by the transfer of the amidine group from arginine to glycine.

glycogelatin (glī-kō-jel′ă-tin). Glycerinated *gelatin.*

glycogen (glī′kō-jen). Animal dextran; animal or liver starch; hepatin; zoamylin; a glucosan of high molecular weight, resembling amylopectin in structure but even more highly branched, found in most of the tissues of the body, especially those of the liver and muscle; as the principal carbohydrate reserve, it is readily converted into glucose.
g. posphorylase, phosphorylase.
g. (starch) synthase [EC 2.4.1.11], a glucosyltransferase catalyzing the incorporation of glucose from UDPglucose into 1,4-α-D-glucosyl chains.

glycogenase (gli′kō-jĕ-nās). α- and β-Amylase.

glycogenesis (glī-kō-jen′ĕ-sis) [glyco- + G. *genesis,* production]. Formation of glycogen from glucose by means of glycogen synthase and dextrin dextranase; the first enzyme catalyzes formation of a polyglucose with α-1,4 links from UDPglucose, the second cleaves fragments from one chain and transfers them to an α-1,6 linkage in another.

glycogenetic (glī′kō-jĕ-net′ik). Glycogenous; glycogenic (2); relating to glycogenesis.

glycogenolysis (glī′kō-jĕ-nol′i-sis). The hydrolysis of glycogen to glucose.

glycogenosis (glī′kō-jĕ-nō′sis). Glycogen storage disease; dextrinosis; any of the glycogen deposition diseases characterized by accumulation of glycogen of normal or abnormal chemical structure in tissue; also may be enlargement of the liver, heart, or striated muscle, including the tongue, with progressive muscular weakness. Six types (Cori classification) are recognized, depending on the enzyme deficiency involved, all of autosomal recessive inheritance, but with a different gene for each enzyme deficiency.
generalized g., type 2 g.
glucose 6-phosphatase hepatorenal g., type 1 g.
hepatophosphorylase deficiency g., type 6 g.
myophosphorylase deficiency g., type 5 g.
type 1 g., Gierke's or von Gierke's disease; glucose 6-phosphatase hepatorenal g.; g. due to glucose 6-phosphatase deficiency resulting in accumulation of excessive amounts of glycogen of normal chemical structure, particularly in liver and kidney.
type 2 g., generalized g.; Pompe's disease; g. due to lysosomal α-1,4-glucosidase deficiency resulting in accumulation of excessive amounts of glycogen of normal chemical structure in heart, muscle, liver and nervous system.
type 3 g., Cori's disease; Forbes' disease; limit dextrinosis; debranching deficiency limit dextrinosis; g. due to amylo-1,6-glucosidase deficiency resulting in accumulation of abnormal glycogen with short outer chains in liver and muscle.
type 4 g., Andersen's disease; branching deficiency amylopectinosis; familial cirrhosis of the liver with storage of abnormal glycogen; g. due to deficiency of 1,4-α-glucan branching enzyme resulting in accumulation of abnormal glycogen with long inner and outer chains in liver, kidney, muscle, and other tissues.
type 5 g., McArdle's disease; McArdle-Schmid-Pearson disease; myophosphorylase deficiency g.; g. due to muscle glycogen phos-

phorylase deficiency resulting in accumulation of glycogen of normal chemical structure in muscle.
type 6 g., hepatophosphorylase deficiency g.; Hers' disease; g. due to hepatic glycogen phosphorylase deficiency resulting in accumulation of glycogen of normal chemical structure in liver and leukocytes.

glycogenous (glī-koj'ĕ-nŭs). Glycogenetic.

glycogeusia (glī-kō-gū'sē-ă) [glyco- + G. *geusis,* taste]. A subjective sweet taste.

glycoglycinuria (glī'kō-glī-si-nū'rē-ă). A metabolic disorder characterized by glucosuria and hyperglycinuria; autosomal dominant inheritance.

glycol (glī'kol). **1.** A compound containing adjacent alcohol groups. **2.** Ethylene g., $CH_2OH–CH_2OH$, the simplest g.

glycolaldehyde (glī-kol-al'dĕ-hīd). Biose; diose; $CH_2OH–CHO$; the simplest (2-carbon) sugar; the aerobic deamination product of ethanolamine.

glycolaldehydetransferase (glī-kol-al'dĕ-hīd-trans'fer-ās). Transketolase.

glycoleucine (glī'kō-lū-sin). Norleucine.

glycolic acid (glī-kol'ik). $CH_2OH–COOH$; an intermediate in the interconversion of glycine and ethanolamine.

glycolic aciduria. Excessive excretion of glycolic acid in the urine; a primary metabolic defect due to deficiency of 2-hydroxy-3-oxoadipate carboxylase, resulting in excretion of glycolic and oxalic acids, leading to the clinical syndrome of oxalosis.

glycolipid (glī-kō-lip'id). Glycosphingolipid.

glycolyl (glī'kō-lil). $CH_2OH–CO–$; the acyl radical of glycolic acid, replacing acetyl in some sialic acids; the products are called *N*-glycolylneuraminic acids.

glycolylurea (glī'kō-lil-yū-rē'ă). Hydantoin.

glycolysis (glī-kol'i-sis) [glyco- + G. *lysis,* a loosening]. Glucolysis; the energy-yielding conversion of glucose to lactic acid (instead of pyruvate oxidation products) in various tissues, notably muscle, when sufficient oxygen is not available (as in an emergency situation); since molecular oxygen is not consumed in the process, this is frequently referred to as "anaerobic g."

glycolytic (glī-kō-lit'ik). Relating to glycolysis.

glyconeogenesis (glī'kō-nē-ō-jen'ĕ-sis) [glyco- + G. *neos,* new, + *genesis,* production]. Gluconeogenesis; the formation of glycogen from noncarbohydrates, such as protein or fat, by conversion of the latter to glucose. See also glycogenesis.

glyconic acids (glī-kon'ik). Aldonic acids.

glycopenia (glī-kō-pē'nē-ă) [glyco- + G. *penia,* poverty]. A deficiency of any or all sugars in an organ or tissue.

glycopeptide (glī-kō-pep'tīd). A compound containing sugar(s) linked to amino acids (or peptides), with the latter preponderant, as in bacterial cell walls. *Cf.* peptidoglycan.

Glycophagus (glī-kof'ă-gŭs) [glyco- + G. *phagein,* to eat]. A common genus of grain mites, frequently implicated in dermatitis among food handlers. See also *Tyrophagus putrescentiae.*

glycophilia (glī-kō-fil'ē-ă) [glyko- + G. *phileō,* to love]. A condition in which there is a distinct tendency to develop hyperglycemia, even after the ingestion of a relatively small quantity of glucose.

glycoprotein (glī-kō-prō'tēn). **1.** One of a group of protein-carbohydrate compounds (conjugated proteins), among which the most important are the mucins, mucoid, and amyloid. **2.** Sometimes restricted to proteins containing small amounts of carbohydrate, in contrast to mucoids or mucoproteins, usually measured as hexosamine; such conjugated proteins are found in many places, notably γ-globulins, α_1-globulins, α_2-globulins, transferrin, etc., and are contained in mucus and mucins. See also mucoprotein.
α_1-acid g., orosomucoid.

β_2-glycoprotein II. Properdin *factor* B.

glycoptyalism (glī-kō-tī'ă-lizm) [glyco- + G. *ptyalon,* saliva]. Glycosialia.

glycopyrrolate (glī-kō-pī'rō-lāt). 3-Hydroxy-1,1-dimethylpyrrolidinium bromide; a parasympatholytic compound used as premedication prior to general anesthesia, as an antagonist to the bradycardic effects of neostigmine during curare reversal, and as an adjunct in the treatment of peptic ulcer.

glycorrhachia (glī-kō-rā'kē-ă, -rak-ē-ă) [glyco- + G. *rhachis,* spine]. Presence of sugar in the cerebrospinal fluid.

glycorrhea (glī-kō-rē'ă) [glyco- + G. *rhoia,* a flow]. A discharge of sugar from the body, as in glucosuria, especially in unusually large quantities.

glycosaminoglycan (glī'kōs-am-i-nō-glī'kan). See mucopolysaccharide.

glycosecretory (glī'kō-sē-krē'tō-rē). Causing or involved in the secretion of glycogen.

glycosialia (glī'kō-sī-al'ē-ă, -ā'lē-ă) [glyco- + G. *sialon,* saliva]. Glycoptyalism; the presence of sugar in the saliva.

glycosialorrhea (glī'kō-sī'ă-lō-rē'ă) [glyco- + G. *sialon,* saliva, + *rhoia,* a flow]. An excessive secretion of saliva that contains sugar.

glycoside (glī'kō-sīd). Condensation product of a sugar with any other radical involving the loss of the H of the hemiacetal OH of the sugar, leaving the O of this OH as the link; thus, the condensation through the O-1 with an alcohol, which loses its OH, yields an alcohol-glycoside (or a glycosido-alcohol); links involving loss of the entire sugar 1-OH, as in condensation with a purine or pyrimidine –NH– group, yield glycosyl compounds.

***N*-glycoside.** Misnomer for glycosyl.

glycosphingolipid (glī'kō-sfing-gō-lip'id). Ceramide saccharide; glycolipid; a ceramide linked to one or more sugars via the terminal OH group; included as g.'s are cerebrosides, gangliosides, and ceramide oligosaccharides (oligoglycosylceramides). The prefix glyc- may be replaced by gluc-, galact-, lact-, etc.

glycostatic (glī-kō-stat'ik). Indicating the property of certain extracts of the anterior hypophysis that permits the body to maintain its glycogen stores in muscle, liver, and other tissues.

glycosuria (glī-kō-sū'rē-ă) [glyco- + G. *ouron,* urine]. Glycuresis. **1.** Glucosuria. **2.** Urinary excretion of carbohydrates.
alimentary g., alimentary diabetes; digestive g.; g. developing after the ingestion of a moderate amount of sugar or starch, which normally is disposed of without appearing in the urine, because renal absorption exceeds capacity of the liver and the other tissues to remove the glucose, thus allowing blood glucose levels to become high enough for renal excretion to occur.
benign g., g. not associated with diabetes mellitus but resulting from a low renal threshold for sugar.
digestive g., alimentary g.
normoglycemic g., renal g.
pathologic g., chronic excretion of relatively large amounts of sugar in the urine.
phloridzin g., phlorizin g., the presence of sugar in the urine after the experimental administration of phloridzin, which results in a lower renal threshold for reabsorption of glucose.
renal g., diabetes innocens; renal diabetes; normoglycemic g.; the recurring or persistent excretion of glucose in the urine, in association with blood glucose levels that are in the normal range; results from the failure of renal tubules to reabsorb glucose at a normal rate from the glomerular filtrate (low renal threshold).

glycosyl (glī'kō-sil). The radical resulting from detachment of the OH of the hemiacetal of a saccharide. *Cf.* glycoside.

glycosylation (glī'kō-si-lā'shŭn). Formation of linkages with glycosyl groups, as between glucose and the hemoglobin chain to form the fraction hemoglobin A_{Ic}, whose level rises in association with the raised blood glucose concentration in poorly controlled or uncontrolled diabetes mellitus. See also glycosylated *hemoglobin.*

glycosyltransferase (glī'kō-sil-trans'fer-ās). Transglycosylase; any enzyme (EC subclass 2.4) transferring glycosyl groups from one compound to another.

glycotropic, glycotrophic (glī-kō-trop'ik, -trof'ik) [glyco- + G. *trophē,* nourishment; *tropē,* a turning]. Pertaining to a principle in extracts of the anterior lobe of the pituitary that antagonizes the action of insulin and causes hyperglycemia. See glycotropic *factor.*

glycuresis (glī-kū-rē'sis) [glyco- + G. *ourēsis,* urination]. Glycosuria.

glycuronate (glī-kūr'on-āt). A salt or ester of a glyuronic acid.

glycuronic acid (glī-kūr-on'ik). Glycuronose; the uronic acid of a sugar in which the terminal carbon is oxidized to a carboxyl group.

glycuronidase (glī-kūr-on'i-dās). β-D-glucuronidase.

glycuronide (glī-kūr'on-īd). A glycoside of a uronic acid; *e.g.,* glucuronide.

glycuronose (glī-kūr'on-ōs). Glycuronic acid.

glycuronuria (glī-kū-rō-nū'rē-ă). The presence of glucuronic acid in the urine.

glycyclamide (glī-sī'klă-mīd). Cyclamide; tolcyclamide; tolhexamide; 1-cyclohexyl-3-*p*- tolylsulfonylurea; an oral hypoglycemic agent.

glycyl (Gly) (glī'sil). The acyl radical of glycine.

g. betaine, betaine.

glycyrrhiza (glis-ĭ-rī'ză) [G. fr. *glykys,* sweet, + *rhiza,* root]. Liquorice; licorice; the dried rhizome and root of *Glycyrrhiza glabra* (family Leguminoseae) and allied species; a demulcent, mild laxative, and expectorant; also used to disguise the taste of other remedies; its action appears to depend upon glycyrrhizic acid, a salt-retaining glycoside that mimics the action of aldosterone.

glyoxal (glī-oks'ăl). Ethanedial; oxalaldehyde; CHO–CHO; the simplest dialdehyde.

glyoxalase (glī-oks'ă-lās). Enzymes, lactoylglutathione lyase (g. I) or hydroxyacylglutathione hydrolase (g. II), in red cells and other tissues that convert glyoxal and substituted glyoxals bound to glutathione into the corresponding free hydroxy acids (g. II) or glyoxals (g. I).

glyoxaline (glī-oks'ă-lin). Imidazole.

glyoxylate transacetylase (glī-oks'i-lāt). *Malate* synthase.

glyoxyldiureide (glī-oks-il-dī'yū-rīd). Allantoin.

glyoxylic acid (glī-oks-il'ik). CHO–COOH; produced by the action of glycine dehydrogenases upon glycine or sarcosine, or from allantoic acid by allantoicase.

glysobuzole (glī-sō-byū'zōl). Isobuzole.

gm Former abbreviation for gram.

Gmelin, Leopold, German physiologist and chemist, 1788–1853. See G.'s *test,* Rosenbach-G. *test.*

GMP Abbreviation for guanylic acid.

GMS Abbreviation for Gomori's methenamine-silver (stain).

gnashing (nash'ing). The grinding together of the teeth as a nonmasticatory function; usually associated with emotional tension. See also bruxism.

gnat (nat) [A.S. *gnaet*]. A midge; general term applied to several species of minute insects, including species of *Simulium* (buffalo g.) and *Hippelates* (eye g.). British authors sometimes include mosquitoes in this group, but this is not done in the U.S.

gnath-. See gnatho-.

gnathic (nath'ik) [G. *gnathos,* jaw]. Relating to the jaw or alveolar process.

gnathion (nath'ē-on) [G. *gnathos,* jaw] [NA]. The most inferior point of the mandible in the midline. In cephalometrics, it is the midpoint between the most anterior and inferior point on the bony chin, measured at the intersection of the mandibular baseline and the nasion-pogonion line.

gnatho-, gnath- [G. *gnathos,* jaw]. Combining forms relating to the jaw.

gnathocephalus (nath-ō-sef'ă-lŭs) [*gnatho-* + G. *kephalē,* head]. A fetal malformation with little of the head formed except the jaws.

gnathodynamics (nath'ō-dī-nam'iks) [gnatho- + G. *dynamis,* power]. The study of the relationship of the magnitude and direction of the forces developed by and upon the components of the masticatory system during function.

gnathodynamometer (nath'ō-dī-nă-mom'ĕ-ter) [gnatho- + dynamometer]. Bite gauge; occlusometer; a device for measuring biting pressure.

gnathography (nă-thog'ră-fē). The recording of the action of the masticatory apparatus in function.

gnathological (nath-ō-loj'i-kăl). Pertaining to gnathodynamics.

gnathology (nă-thol'ō-jē). The science of the masticatory system, including physiology, functional disturbances, and treatment.

gnathopalatoschisis (nath'ō-pal-ă-tos'ki-sis). Clefts of prepalate and palate.

gnathoplasty (nath'ō-plas-tē) [gnatho- + G. *plastos,* formed]. Plastic surgery of the jaw.

gnathoschisis (nă-thos'ki-sis) [gnatho- + G. *schisis,* a cleaving]. Alveoloschisis.

gnathostatics (nath-ō-stat'iks) [gnatho- + G. *statikos,* causing to stand]. In orthodontic diagnosis, a technical procedure for orienting the dentition to certain cranial landmarks.

Gnathostoma (nă-thos'tō-mă) [gnatho- + G. *stoma,* mouth]. A genus of spiruroid nematode worms (family Gnathostomatidae) characterized by several rows of cuticular spines about the head and by multiple-host aquatic life cycles; it includes pathogenic parasites of cats, cattle, and swine.

G. siamen'se, invalid name for *G. spinigerum.*

G. spinig'erum, a parasite of cats, dogs, and wild carnivores, but it has occasionally been found in man in the Far East; it is transmitted via copepods and fish; human infection is usually confined to the skin, but several cases have been reported of eye or brain infection with wandering larvae of this species.

gnathostomiasis (nath-ō-stō-mī'ă-sis). Yangtze edema; a migrating edema, or creeping eruption, caused by cutaneous infection by larvae of *Gnathostoma spinigerum.*

gnoscopine (nos'kō-pēn). α-Gnoscopine; *dl*-narcotine; an opium alkaloid, $C_{22}H_{23}NO_7$, obtained by racemization of noscapine; an antitussive.

gnosia (nō'sē-ă) [G. *gnōsis,* knowledge]. The perceptive faculty enabling one to recognize the form and the nature of persons and things.

gnotobiology (nō'tō-bī-ol'ō-jē) [G. *gnotos,* known, + *bios,* life, + *logos,* study]. The study of animals in the absence of contaminating microorganisms; *i.e.,* of "germ-free" animals.

gnotobiota (nō'tō-bī-ō'tă) [G. *gnotos,* known, + Mod. L. *biota,* fr. G. *bios,* life]. Living colonies or species, assembled from pure isolates.

gnotobiote (nō-tō-bī'ōt). An individual organism from a group assembled from pure isolates (gnotobiota).

gnotobiotic (nō'tō-bī-ot'ik) [see gnotobiota]. Denoting germ-free or formerly germ-free organisms in which the composition of any associated microbial flora, if present, is fully defined.

GnRH Abbreviation for gonadotropin-releasing *hormone*.

goal (gōl). In psychology, any object or objective that an organism seeks to attain or achieve.

goatpox (gōt'poks). Variola caprina; an acute infectious disease of goats caused by a strain of *Capripoxvirus* and characterized by generalized vesicular eruptions on the skin and frequently the respiratory mucous membranes; it occurs chiefly in southern and eastern Europe and North Africa.

Godélier, Charles P., French physician, 1813–1877. See G.'s *law*.

Godman, John D., U.S. anatomist, 1794–1830. See G.'s *fascia*.

Godwin, John T., U.S. pathologist, *1917. See G. *tumor*.

Goeckerman, William H., U.S. dermatologist, 1884–1954. See G. *treatment*.

Goethe, Johann W. von, German poet, philosopher, and scientist, 1749–1832. See G.'s *bone*.

Gofman, Moses, German physician, *1887. See G. *test*.

Goggia, Carlo P., 20th century Italian physician. See G.'s *sign*.

goggle (gog'gl). **1.** A screen cover for the eye. **2.** A type of spectacle with auxiliary shields for protecting the eyes.
plethysmographic g., a specially designed g. to serve as an ophthalmodynamometer while permitting subjective visual and objective ocular changes during transient increased intraocular pressure.

goiter (goy'ter) [Fr. from L. *guttur*, throat]. Struma (1); a chronic enlargement of the thyroid gland, not due to a neoplasm, occurring endemically in certain localities, especially mountainous regions, and sporadically elsewhere.
aberrant g., struma aberrata; enlargement of a supernumerary thyroid gland.
acute g., a g. that develops very rapidly.
adenomatous g., an enlargement of the thyroid gland due to the growth of one or more encapsulated adenomas or multiple nonencapsulated colloid nodules within its substance.
cabbage g., g. due to ingestion of cabbage or other goitrogenic foodstuff.
colloid g., a form of g. in which the contents of the follicles increase greatly, causing pressure atrophy of the epithelium so that the gelatinous matter predominates in the tumor.
cystic g., an enlargement in the thyroid region due to the presence of one or more cysts within the gland.
diffuse g., g. in which the morbid process involves the whole gland, as opposed to nodular g. or thyroid adenoma.
diving g., wandering g.; a freely movable g. that is sometimes above and sometimes below the sternal notch.
endemic g., g., usually of simple type, prevalent in certain regions where dietary intake of iodine is suboptimal.
exophthalmic g., any of the various forms of hyperthyroidism in which the thyroid gland is enlarged and exophthalmos is present.
familial g., a group of heritable thyroid disorders in which g. is commonly apparent first during childhood; often associated with skeletal and/or mental retardation, and with other signs of hypothyroidism which may develop with age. Various types of familial g. have been identified: 1) iodide transport defect, in which the gland is unable to concentrate iodide; 2) organification defect, in which the iodination of tyrosine is defective; 3) Pendred's *syndrome;* 4) coupling defect, in which cretinism results from defective coupling of iodotyrosines to form iodothyronines; 5) iodotyrosine deiodinase defect, in which deiodination of iodotyrosine is defective and there is considerable glandular loss of these hormonal precursors and cretinism may be present; 6) plasma iodoprotein disorder, in which an abnormal iodinated serum protein is present that is insoluble in acidic butanol.
fibrous g., a firm hyperplasia of the thyroid and its capsule.
follicular g., parenchymatous g.
lingual g., a tumor of thyroid tissue involving the embryonic rudiment at the base of the tongue.
lymphadenoid g., Hashimoto's *thyroiditis*.
microfollicular g., g. in which the glandular tissue consists of unusually small colloid filled follicles and areas of undifferentiated tissue with indistinct follicle formation.
multinodular g., adenomatous g. with several colloid nodules.
nontoxic g., g. not accompanied by hyperthyroidism.
parenchymatous g., follicular g.; a form of g. in which there is a great increase in the follicles with proliferation of the epithelium.
simple g., thyroid enlargement unaccompanied by constitutional effects, *e.g.,* hypo- or hyperthyroidism, commonly caused by inadequate dietary intake of iodine.
substernal g., enlargement of the thyroid gland, chiefly of the lower part of the isthmus, palpable with difficulty or not at all.
suffocative g., a g. that by pressure causes extreme dyspnea.
thoracic g., enlargement of accessory thyroid tissue in the thorax with or without hyperthyroidism.
toxic g., a g. that forms an excessive secretion, causing signs and symptoms of hyperthyroidism.
wandering g., diving g.

goitrogen (goy'trō-jen). Any substance that induces goiter, *e.g.,* cabbage, rapeseed, etc.

goitrogenic (goy-trō-jen'ik). Causing goiter.

goitrous (goy'trŭs). Denoting or characteristic of a goiter.

gold. Aurum; a yellow metallic element, symbol Au, atomic no. 79, atomic weight 196.97.
cohesive g., nearly pure g. so treated as to be free of adsorbed surface gases and impurities so that it will weld under pressure at room temperature; in dentistry, used as a restorative material placed directly into a prepared cavity and welded by pressure.
colloidal radioactive g., radiogold colloid.
mat g., powdered g. formed by electrolytic precipitation, compressed into strips, and sintered.
noncohesive g., g. that will not weld because gases adsorb to the surface; some forms may be made cohesive by heat treatment; in dentistry, used as a direct filling material.
powdered g., g. formed by atomizing or by chemical precipitation, lightly precondensed, and wrapped with g. foil so as to form pellets.
g. sodium thiomalate, sodium aurothiomalate; used in the treatment of rheumatoid arthritis.
g. sodium thiosulfate, sodium aurothiosulfate; used in the treatment of lupus erythematosus and some cases of rheumatoid arthritis.
g. thioglucose, aurothioglucose.

Goldberg, Minnie B., U.S. internist, *1900. See G.-Maxwell *syndrome*.

Goldblatt, Harry, U.S. pathologist, 1891–1977. See G.'s *clamp, hypertension, kidney, phenomenon*.

Goldenhar, M., French physician. See G.'s *syndrome*.

golden seal (gold'n sēl). Hydrastis.

Goldflam, Samuel V., Polish neurologist, 1852–1932. See G. *disease*, Hoppe-G. *disease*.

gold foil. Pure gold rolled into extremely thin sheets; used in the restoration of carious or fractured teeth. See also cohesive *gold*, noncohesive *gold*.

Goldman, David E., U.S. physiologist, *1911. See G. *equation;* G.-Hodgkin-Katz *equation*.

Goldman, Henry M., U.S. periodontist, *1911. See G.-Fox *knives*.

Goldmann, Hans, Swiss ophthalmologist, *1899. See G. *perimeter*, G.'s applanation *tonometer*.

Goldscheider, J.K.A.E. Alfred, German neurologist, 1858–1935. See G.'s *test*.

Goldstein, Hyman I., U.S. physician, 1887–1954. See G.'s toe *sign.*

Goldthwait, Joel E., U.S. surgeon, 1866–1961. See G.'s *sign.*

Golgi, Camillo, Italian histologist and Nobel laureate, 1843–1926. See G. *apparatus, complex,* tendon *organ,* internal *reticulum, zone;* G.'s *cells,* osmiobichromate *fixative, stain;* G.-Mazzoni *corpuscle;* Holmgren-G. *canals.*

golgiokinesis (gol'jē-ō-ki-nē'sis). In mitosis, the process of division of the Golgi apparatus and its distribution to the two daughter cells.

Goll, Friedrich, Swiss anatomist, 1829–1903. See G.'s *column; nucleus* of G. *tract* of G.

Goltz, Robert W., U.S. dermatologist, *1923. See G. *syndrome.*

Gombault, François A.A., French neurologist and pathologist, 1844–1904. See G.'s *triangle.*

gomenol (gō'mĕ-nol) [*Gomen,* a locality in New Caledonia, + L. *oleum,* oil]. Oleogomenol; an ethereal oil obtained from a plant, *Melaleuca viridiflora;* the chief constituent is cineole. It has germicidal action, is free from irritating properties, and has been used in chronic inflammations of the pulmonary mucous membrane and as a vermifuge.

gomitoli (gom-i'tō-lē) [It. *gomitolo,* coil]. Intricately coiled and looped capillary vessels present largely in the upper infundibular stem of the stalk of the pituitary gland; they comprise a portion of the pituitary portal circulation.

Gomori, George, Hungarian histochemist in the U.S., 1904–1957. See G.'s *stains;* G.-Jones periodic acid-methenamine-silver *stain;* Grocott-G. methenamine-silver *stain.*

Gompertz, Benjamin, British actuary, 1779–1865. See G.'s *hypothesis.*

gomphosis (gom-fō'sis) [G. *gomphos,* bolt, nail, + *-osis,* condition] [NA]. Peg-and-socket articulation or joint; articulatio dentoalveolaris; dentoalveolar or gompholic joint; a form of fibrous joint in which a peglike process fits into a hole, as the root of a tooth into the socket in the alveolus.

gonad-. See gonado-.

gonad (gō'nad) [Mod. L. fr. G. *gonē,* seed]. An organ that produces sex cells; a testis or an ovary.
female g., ovary.
indifferent g., the primordial organ in an embryo before its differentiation into testis or ovary.
male g., testis.
streaked g., gonadal *streak.*

gonadal (gō-nad'ăl). Relating to a gonad.

gonadectomy (gō-nad-ek'tō-mē) [gonado- + G. *ektomē,* excision]. Excision of ovary or testis.

gonado-, gonad- [G. *gonē,* seed]. Combining forms relating to the gonads.

gonadocrins (gō-nad'ō-krinz). Peptides which stimulate release of both follicle-stimulating hormone and luteinizing hormone from the pituitary; found in ovarian follicular fluid in rats.

gonadoliberin (gō'nad-ō-lib'er-in). **1.** Gonadotropin-releasing factor or hormone; a hypothalamic substance causing the release of gonadotropin. **2.** Luteinizing hormone/follicle-stimulating hormone-releasing factor; a decapeptide from pig hypothalami which induces release of both lutropin and follitropin in constant proportions and thus acts as both luliberin and folliberin.

gonadopathy (gon-ă-dop'ă-thē) [gonado- + G. *pathos,* suffering]. Disease affecting the gonads.

gonadorelin hydrochloride (gō-nad-ō-rel'in). $C_{55}H_{75}N_{17}O_{13} \cdot x$ HCl; a gonadotropin releasing hormone obtained from sheep, pigs, or other animals and used to evaluate the functional capacity of the gonadotrophs of the anterior pituitary.

gonadotroph (gō-nad'ō-trōf, -gon'ă-dō-). A cell of the adenohypophysis that affects certain cells of the ovary or testis.

gonadotrophic (gō'nad-o-trōf'ik, gon'ă-dō-) [gonado- + G. *trophē,* nourishment]. Gonadotropic.

gonadotrophin (gō'nad-ō-trō'fin, gon'ă-dō-). Gonadotropin.

gonadotropic (gō'nad-ō-trōp'ik, gon'ă-dō-) [gonado- + G. *tropē,* a turning]. Gonadotrophic. **1.** Descriptive of or relating to the actions of a gonadotropin. **2.** Promoting the growth and/or function of the gonads.

gonadotropin (gō'nad-ō-trō'pin, gon'ă-dō-). Gonadotrophin; gonadototropic hormone; a hormone capable of promoting gonadal growth and function; such effects, as exerted by a single hormone, are usually limited to discrete functions or histological components of a gonad, such as stimulation of follicular growth or of androgen formation; most g.'s exert their effects in both sexes, although the effect of a given g. will be very different usually in males and in females.
anterior pituitary g., pituitary gonadotropic hormone; any g. of hypophysial origin; formerly used to designate a single hormone, because it was thought that the anterior hypophysis secreted only one g.
chorionic g. (CG), anterior pituitary-like hormone; chorionic gonadotropic hormone; choriogonadotropin; a glycoprotein with a carbohydrate fraction composed of galactose and hexosamine, extracted from the urine of pregnant women and produced by the placental trophoblastic cells; its most important role appears to be stimulation, during the first trimester, of ovarian secretion of the estrogen and progesterone required for the integrity of conceptus; it appears to play no significant role in the last two trimesters of pregnancy, as the estrogen and progesterone are then formed by the placenta.
equine g., pregnant mare's serum g.; formed by the equine placenta. Its activity in animals is similar to that of the follicle-stimulating hormone; relatively ineffective in human beings.
human chorionic g. (HCG), see chorionic g.
human menopausal g. (HMG), a pituitary hormone obtained from the urine of menopausal women (urogonadotropin); biological activity is similar to that of follicle-stimulating hormone, but also weakly mimics the effects of luteinizing hormone; used in conjunction with human chorionic g. to induce ovulation. See also menotropins.
pregnant mare's serum g. (PMSG), equine g.

gonaduct (gon'ă-dŭkt) [gonado- + duct]. **1.** Seminal *duct.* **2.** *Tuba* uterina.

gonalgia (gō-nal'jē-ă) [G. *gony,* knee, + *algos,* pain]. Pain in the knee.

gonane (gon'ān). The hypothetical parent hydrocarbon molecule of gonadal steroid hormones, such as estrane or androstane, which was conceived to achieve forms of systematic nomenclature.

gonangiectomy (gon-an-jē-ek'tō-mē) [G. *gonē,* seed, + *angeion,* vessel, + *ektomē,* excision]. Obsolete term for vasectomy.

gonarthritis (gon-ar-thrī'tis) [G. *gony,* knee, + *arthron,* joint, + *-itis,* inflammation]. Inflammation of the knee joint.

gonarthrotomy (gon-ar-throt'ō-mē) [G. *gony,* knee, + *arthron,* joint, + *tomē,* incision]. Incision into the knee joint.

gonatagra (gon-ă-tag'ră) [G. *gony,* knee, + *agra,* seizure]. Obsolete term for gout in the knee.

gonatocele (gō-nat'ō-sēl) [G. *gony,* knee, + *kēlē,* tumor]. Obsolete term for tumor of the knee.

gonecyst, gonecystis (gon'ĕ-sist, gon-ĕ-sis'tis) [G. *gonē,* seed, + *kystis,* bladder]. *Vesicula* seminalis.

gonecystolith (gon-ĕ-sis'tō-lith) [gonecyst + G. *kystis,* bladder, + *lithos,* stone]. Obsolete term for a concretion or calculus in a seminal vesicle.

Gongylonema (gon'ji-lō-nē'mă) [Gr. *gongylos,* round, + *nēma,* thread]. An important genus of spiruroid nematodes that parasitize the alimentary canal of birds and mammals; transmitted via various insects, especially beetles, carrying the encysted infective larvae. Several species are of veterinary importance, and one is also known to parasitize man.

G. ingluvic'ola, species parasitic in the mucosa of the crop, esophagus, and proventriculus of chickens, turkeys, and quail; transmitted by beetles, it tunnels into the crop wall but is relatively nonpathogenic.

G. neoplas'ticum, species parasitic in the stomach or esophagus epithelium of various rodents, rabbits, and sheep and transmitted by coprophagous beetles; it is often associated with benign proliferations, once thought to be neoplastic, in the stomach and esophagus of infected, malnourished rats.

G. pul'chrum, the gullet worm of cattle; a species that penetrates the submucosa of the esophagus or rumen of many domestic and wild ruminants, pigs, bears, and man (human cases are chiefly caused by immature worms); it is transmitted by coprophagous beetles and is of worldwide distribution.

gongylonemiasis (gon'ji-lō-nē-mī'ă-sis). Infection of animals and rarely man with nematodes of the genus *Gongylonema.*

gonia (gō'nē-ă). Plural of gonion.

gonio- [G. *gōnia,* angle]. Combining form meaning angle.

goniocraniometry (gō'nē-ō-krā-nē-om'ĕ-trē) [G. *gōnia,* angle, + *kranion,* skull, + *metron,* measure]. Measurement of the angles of the cranium.

goniodysgenesis (gō'nē-ō-dis-jen'ĕ-sis) [G. *gōnia,* angle, + dysgenesis]. Developmental aberration of the anterior ocular segment.

gonioma (gon-ē-ō'mă) [G. *gonē,* seed, + *-oma,* tumor]. Former term for a malignant neoplasm of the testis thought to be derived from the first stages of spermatogenetic cells; probably the same as embryonal carcinoma of the testis.

goniometer (gō-nē-om'ĕ-ter) [G. *gōnia,* angle, + *metron,* measure]. **1.** An instrument for measuring angles, as of crystals. **2.** An appliance for the static test of labyrinthine disease, which consists of a plank, one end of which may be raised to any desired height; as one end of the plank is gradually raised, the point at which a patient loses balance is noted. **3.** Arthometer; fleximeter; pronometer; a calibrated device designed to measure the arc or range of motion of a joint.

gonion, pl. gonia (gō'nē-on, gō'nē-ă) [G. *gōnia,* an angle] [NA]. The lowest posterior and most outward point of the angle of the mandible. In cephalometrics, it is measured by bisecting the angle formed by the tangents to the lower and the posterior borders of the mandible; when the angles of both sides of the mandible appear on the profile roentgenogram, the point midway between the right and left side is used.

goniopuncture (gō'nē-ō-pŭnk-chūr). An operation for congenital glaucoma in which a puncture is made in the filtration angle of the anterior chamber.

gonioscope (gō'nē-ō-skōp) [G. *gōnia,* angle, + *skopeō,* to examine]. A lens designed to study the angle of the anterior chamber of the eye.

gonioscopy (gō-nē-os'kŏ-pē). Examination of the angle of the anterior chamber of the eye with a gonioscope or with a contact prism lens.

goniospasis (gō-nē-os'pă-sis) [gonio- + G. *spasis,* a drawing in]. A procedure to relieve glaucoma in which traction is exerted on the angle of the anterior chamber of the eye by means of a wire passed through the iris.

goniosynechia (gō'nē-ō-si-nek'ē-ă) [G. *gōnia,* angle, + *synechis,* holding together]. Peripheral anterior synechia; adhesion of the iris to the posterior surface of the cornea in the angle of the anterior chamber; associated with angle-closure glaucoma.

goniotomy (gō-nē-ot'ō-mē) [G. *gōnia,* angle, + *tomē,* incision]. Surgical opening of the trabecular meshwork in congenital glaucoma.

gonitis (gō-nī'tis) [G. *gony,* knee, + *-itis,* inflammation]. Obsolete term for inflammation of the knee.

gonoblennorrhea (gon'ō-blen-ō-rē'ă) [G. *gonē,* seed, + *blennos,* mucus, + *rhoia,* a flow]. Obsolete term for gonorrhea.

gonocele (gon'ō-sēl) [G. *gonē,* seed, + *kēlē,* tumor]. A cystic lesion of the epididymis or rete testis, resulting from obstruction and containing secretions from the testis.

gonochorism, gonochorismus (gon-ok'ō-rizm, -ō-riz'mŭs) [G. *gonē,* seed, sex, + *chōrizō,* to separate]. Normal gonadal differentiation appropriate to the sex.

gonocide (gon'ō-sīd). Gonococcicide. **1.** Destructive to the gonococcus. **2.** An agent that kills gonococci.

gonococcal (gon'ō-kok'ăl). Gonococcic; relating to the gonococcus.

gonococcemia (gon'ō-kok-sē'mē-ă) [gonococcus + G. *haima,* blood]. Gonohemia; the presence of gonococci in the circulating blood.

gonococci (gon-ō-kok'sī). Plural of gonococcus.

gonococcic (gon'ō-kok'sik). Gonococcal.

gonococcicide (gon-ō-kok'si-sīd) [gonococcus + L. *caedo,* to kill]. Gonocide.

gonococcus, pl. gonococci (gon-ō-kok'ŭs, -sī) [G. *gonē,* seed, + *kokkos,* berry]. *Neisseria gonorrhoeae.*

gonocyte (gon'ō-sīt) [G. *gonē,* seed, + *kytos,* hollow (cell)]. Primordial germ *cell.*

gonohemia (gon-ō-hē'mē-ă). Gonococcemia.

gonomery (gon-om'er-ē) [G. *gonē,* seed, + *meros,* part]. A condition in which paternal and maternal chromosomes remain in two distinct groups in the zygote.

gono-opsonin (gon-ō-op'sō-nin). A specific gonococcal opsonin.

gonophage (gon'ō-fāj). A gonocidal bacteriophage.

gonophore, gonophorus (gon'ō-fōr, gō-nof'ō-rŭs) [G. *gonē,* seed, + *phoros,* bearing]. Any structure serving to store up or conduct the sexual cells; oviduct, spermatic duct, uterus, or seminal vesicle; an accessory generative organ.

gonorrhea (gon-ō-rē'ă) [G. *gonorrhoia,* fr. *gonē,* seed, + *rhoia,* a flow]. Specific urethritis; urethritis venera; a contagious catarrhal inflammation of the genital mucous membrane, transmitted chiefly by coitus and due to *Neisseria gonorrhoeae;* may involve the lower or upper genital tract, especially the uterine tubes, or spread to the

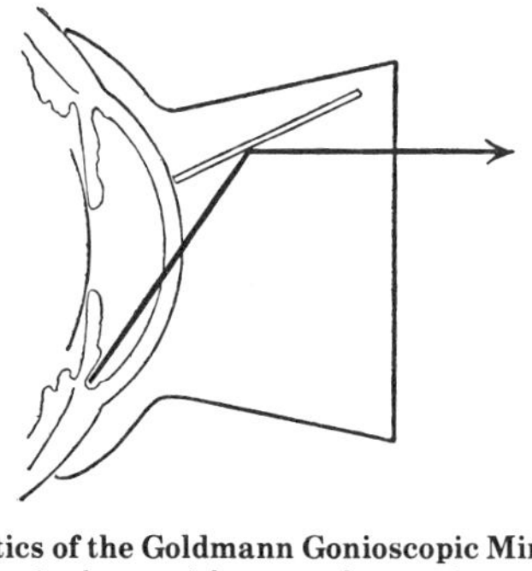

Optics of the Goldmann Gonioscopic Mirror

The mirror in the special contact lens makes an angle of 64 degrees with the front surface of the contact lens. The rays of light which emanate from the angle of the anterior chamber are reflected by the mirror into the observer's eye. The lower chamber angle is seen when the mirror is placed above, and *vice versa.*

peritoneum and rarely to the heart, joints, or other structures by way of the bloodstream.

gonorrheal (gon-ō-rē'ăl). Relating to gonorrhea.

gonosome (gon'ō-sōm) [G. gonē, seed + *sōma,* body]. Sex *chromosome.*

gonotoxemia (gon'ō-tok-sē'mē-ă). Toxic condition resulting from the hematogenous dissemination of gonococci and the effects of the absorbed endotoxin.

gonotoxin (gon-ō-tok'sin). The endotoxin elaborated by the gonococcus, *Neisseria gonorrhoeae.*

gonotyl (gon'ō-til) [G. *gonos,* offspring, + *tylē,* knob]. A sucker-like structure enclosing the genital pore of flukes of the family Heterophyidae.

Gonyaulax catanella (gon-ē-aw'laks kat-ă-nel'ă) [G. *gony,* knee, + *aulakos,* a furrow]. A marine dinoflagellate protozoan that produces a powerful toxin that accumulates in the tissues of mussels and other filter-feeding shellfish and may cause fatal mussel poisoning in man.

gonycampsis (gon-ē-kamp'sis) [G. *gony,* knee, + *kampsis,* a bending or curving]. Ankylosis or any abnormal curvature of the knee.

Goodell, William, U.S. gynecologist, 1829–1894. See G.'s *dilator, sign.*

Goodpasture, Ernest W., U.S. pathologist, 1886–1960. See G.'s *stain, syndrome.*

Goormaghtigh, Norbert, Belgian physician, 1890–1960. See G.'s *cells.*

gooseflesh (gūs'flesh). *Cutis* anserina.

Gopalan, C., 20th century Indian biochemist. See G.'s *syndrome.*

Goppert's sign. See under sign.

Gordius (gōr'dē-ŭs) [L., fr. G. *Gordios,* king of Gordium in Phrygia; an allusion to the knotlike twistings of these worms]. An old name for the nematode genus *Dracunculus,* properly applied to members of the phylum Nematomorpha, commonly called the gordian or horsehair worms, hair worms, or hair snakes.

Gordon, Alfred, U.S. neurologist, 1874–1953. See G.'s *reflex, sign, symptom.*

Gordon and Sweet stain. See under *stain.*

gorget (gōr'jet). A director or guide with wide groove for use in lithotomy.
probe g., a g. with a probe-pointed tip.

Gorham, Lemuel W., U.S. physician, 1885–1968. See G.'s *disease.*

Goriaew's rule. See under rule.

Gorlin, Richard, U.S. physiologist and cardiologist, *1926. See Gorlin *formula.*

Gorlin, Robert J., U.S. oral pathologist, *1923. See G.'s *sign, syndrome;* G.-Chaudhry-Moss *syndrome.*

Gorman's syndrome. See under syndrome.

gorondou (gō-ron'dū). Goundou.

Gosselin, Léon Athanese, French surgeon, 1815–1887. See G.'s *fracture.*

gossypine (gos'i-pēn). Obsolete name for choline.

gossypol (gos'i-pol). $C_{30}H_{30}O_8$; a toxic principle isolated from the seed of the cotton plant *(Gossypium)* which reduces sperm count; used in China as an oral male contraceptive.

gossypose (gos'i-pōs). Raffinose.

GOT Abbreviation for glutamic-oxaloacetic transaminase.

Göthlin, Gustaf F., Swedish physiologist, 1874–1949. See G.'s *test.*

Gottron, H.A., German physician. See Arndt-G. *syndrome.*

gouge (gowj). A strong curved chisel used in operation on bone.

Gougerot, Henri, French physician, 1881–1955. See G.-Sjögren's *disease;* G. and Blum *disease;* G.-Carteaud *syndrome.*

Gould, Sir Alfred P., British surgeon, 1852–1922. See G.'s *suture.*

Gouley, John W.S., U.S. urologist, 1832–1920. See G.'s *catheter.*

goundou (gūn'dū) [native name]. Henpuye; gorondou; dog nose; anákhré; a disease, endemic in West Africa, characterized by exostoses from the nasal processes of the maxillary bones, producing a symmetrical swelling on each side of the nose; believed to be an osteitis connected with yaws.

gout (gowt) [L. *gutta,* drop]. Arthritis nodosa (2) or uratica; an inherited disorder of purine metabolism, occurring especially in men, characterized by a raised but variable blood uric acid level and severe recurrent acute arthritis of sudden onset resulting from deposition of crystals of sodium urate in connective tissues and articular cartilage.
abarticular g., g. involving structures other than the joints.
articular g., the usual form of g. attacking one or more of the joints.
calcium g., pseudogout.
interval g., an asymptomatic phase between acute attacks of g.
latent g., masked g.; hyperuricemia without symptoms of gout. Often used synonymously with interval g.
lead g., saturnine g.
masked g., latent g.
retrocedent g., obsolete term for the occurrence of severe gastric, cardiac, or cerebral symptoms during an attack of g., especially when the joint symptoms at the same time suddenly subside.
saturnine g., lead g.; g. occurring in a person with lead poisoning.
secondary g., g. resulting from increased serum uric acid levels as a result of antecedent diseases such as those of the blood and bone marrow, lead poisoning, and chronic renal failure on dialysis.
tophaceous g., g. in which deposits of uric acid and urates occur as gouty tophi.

gouty (gow'tē). Relating to or characteristic of gout.

Gowers, Sir William R., British neurologist, 1845–1915. See G. *column, contraction, disease, syndrome, tract.*

GPI Abbreviation for Gingival-Periodontal Index.

GPT Abbreviation for glutamic-pyruvic transaminase.

gr Abbreviation for grain (3).

Graaf, Reijnier de, Dutch physiologist and histologist, 1641–1673. See graafian *follicle.*

graafian, Relating to or described by R. de Graaf.

gracilis (gras'i-lis) [L.]. Slender; denoting a thin or slender structure.

grad. Abbreviation for L. *gradatim,* by degrees, gradually.

grade (grād) [L. *gradus,* step]. **1.** A rank, division, or level on the scale of a value system. **2.** In cancer pathology, a classification of the degree of malignancy or differentation of tumor tissue; *e.g.,* well, moderately well, or poorly differentiated, and undifferentiated or anaplastic. **3.** In exercise testing, the measurement of a vertical rise or fall as a percent of the horizontal distance travelled.
Gleason's tumor g., a classification of adenocarcinoma of the prostate by evaluation of the pattern of glandular differentiation; the tumor g., know as Gleason's score, is the sum of the dominant and secondary patterns, each numbered on a scale of 1 to 5.

Gradenigo, Giuseppe, Italian physician, 1859–1926. See G.'s *syndrome.*

gradient (grā'dē-ent). Rate of change of temperature, pressure, or other variable as a function of distance, time, etc.
atrioventricular g., the diastolic pressure difference between the atrium and ventricle.
concentration g., density g.
density g., concentration g.; a solution in which the concentration (density) of a solute increases in a continuous fashion from top to

bottom, or end to end, of a container (*e.g.,* the centrifuge tube in density-gradient centrifugation).

electrochemical g., a measure of the tendency of an ion to move passively from one point to another, taking into consideration the differences in its concentration and in the electrical potentials between the two points; commonly expressed as the additional voltage needed to achieve equilibrium.

mitral g., the diastolic pressure difference between the left atrium and left ventricle.

systolic g., the difference in pressure during systole between two communicating cardiovascular chambers, *e.g.,* between the left ventricle and aorta in aortic stenosis.

ventricular g., the algebraic sum of (*i.e.,* the net electrical difference between) the area enclosed within the QRS complex and that within the T wave in the electrocardiogram.

graduate (grad'yū-āt) [Mediev. L. *graduatus,* fr. L. *gradus,* step]. A vessel, usually of glass and suitably marked, used for measuring the volume of liquids.

graduated (grad'yū-āt'ed). **1.** Marked by lines or in other ways to denote capacity, degrees, percentages, etc. **2.** Divided or arranged in levels, grades, or successive steps.

Graefe, Albrecht von, German ophthalmologist, 1828–1870. See G. *forceps;* G.'s *disease, knife, operation, sign, spots;* pseudo-G's *phenomenon, sign;* von G.'s *sign.*

Graefenberg, Ernst, German gynecologist in America, 1881–1957. See G. *ring.*

Graffi, Arnold, German pathologist, *1910. See G.'s *virus.*

graft [A.S. *graef*]. **1.** Any free (unattached) tissue or organ for transplantation. **2.** To transplant such structures. See also flap; implant; transplant.

accordion g., mesh g.; a skin g. in which multiple slits have been made, so it can be stretched to cover a large area.

adipodermal g., dermal-fat g.

allogeneic g., allograft.

anastomosed g., a g. in which circulation is established by surgical anastomoses of blood vessels.

animal g., zoograft.

augmentation g., a g. of material used to increase the size, shape, or volume of a structure.

autodermic g., a skin autograft.

autogeneic, autologous, or **autoplastic g.,** autograft.

Blair-Brown g., a split-thickness g. of intermediate thickness.

bone g., bone transplanted from a donor site to a recipient site. See also osteoplasty.

brephoplastic g., a g. from an embryo or newborn to an adult.

cable g., a multiple strand nerve g. arranged as a pathway for regeneration of axons.

chessboard g.'s, obsolete synonym for postage stamp g.'s.

chip g., a g. utilizing small pieces of cartilage or bone which is packed into a bone defect.

chorioallantoic g., transplanting of living material to the chorioallantoic membrane of the embryonic chick.

composite g., a g. composed of several structures, such as skin and cartilage or a full-thickness segment of the ear.

corneal g., keratoplasty.

cutis g., a g. of corium, from which epidermis and subcutaneous tissue have been separated.

Davis g.'s, small pieces (2 to 3 mm) of full-thickness skin.

delayed g., application of a skin g. after waiting several days for healthy granulations to form.

dermal g., a g. of dermis, made from skin by cutting away a thin split-thickness g.

dermal-fat g., adipodermal g.; a dermal g. with attached subcutaneous fat.

Douglas g., obsolete eponym for sieve g.

epidermic g., a g. supposed to contain only epidermis.

Esser g., inlay g.

fascia g., a g. of fibrous tissue, usually the fascia lata.

fascicular g., a nerve g. in which each bundle of fibers is approximated and sutured separately.

fat g., a free g. of fat.

filler g., a g. used for the filling of defects, *e.g.,* filling a cyst with bone chips.

free g., a g. transplanted without its normal attachments, or a pedicle, from one site to another.

full-thickness g., a g. of the full thickness of mucosa and submucosa or of skin and subcutaneous tissue.

funicular g., a nerve g. in which each funiculus (composed of two or more fasciculi) is approximated and sutured separately.

H g., H *shunt.*

heterologous g., heteroplastic g., heterospecific g., xenograft.

heterotopic g., transplantation of a tissue or organ into a position it normally does not occupy.

homologous g., homoplastic g., allograft.

hyperplastic g., a g. in active proliferation.

implantation g., placing of Davis g.'s deep into the interstices of granulation tissue.

infusion g., transplantation by injection of a suspension of cells.

inlay g., epithelial inlay; Esser g.; a skin g. wrapped (raw side out) around a bolus of dental compound and inserted into a prepared surgical pocket.

interspecific g., xenograft.

isogeneic g., isologous g., isoplastic g., syngraft.

Krause g., a full-thickness skin g.

mesh g., accordion g.

mucosal g., a g. of mucous membrane, usually the full-thickness of the lining of the cheek or lower lip.

nerve g., a nerve, or part of a nerve, used as a g.

Ollier g., Ollier-Thiersch g., Thiersch g.; a thin split-thickness g., usually in small pieces.

omental g., a segment of omentum, with its supplying blood vessels, transplanted as a free flap to a distant area and revascularized by arterial and venous anastomoses.

onlay g., a bone g. applied on the outside of the recipient bone(s).

orthotopic g., transplantation of a tissue or organ into its normal anatomical position.

osteoperiosteal g., a g. of bone with its attached periosteum.

partial-thickness g., split-thickness g.

pedicle g., see pedicle *flap.*

periosteal g., a g. of periosteum, usually placed on bare bone.

Phemister g., an autogenous onlay bone graft used in treating delayed union of fractures.

pinch g., Reverdin g.; small bits of skin, of partial or full thickness, removed from a healthy area and seeded in a site to be covered.

porcine g., a split-thickness g. from a pig, applied to a raw area on a human as a temporary dressing.

postage stamp g.'s, small pieces cut from a sheet of split-thickness g.

primary skin g., a skin g. transferred immediately after the creation of a raw area.

punch g.'s, small full-thickness g.'s of the scalp, removed with a circular punch and transplanted to a bald area to grow hair.

Reverdin g., pinch g.

sieve g., a full-thickness skin g. taken after cutting multiple holes in it with a circular punch, thus leaving islands of skin in the donor area to heal it.

skin g., a piece of skin transplanted from one part of the body to another to cover a denuded area.

sleeve g., a g. for repairing a severed nerve by connecting central and peripheral ends with a sleevelike structure, commonly, a segment of vein.

split-skin g., split-thickness g.
split-thickness g., partial-thickness g.; split-skin g.; a g. of portions of the skin, *i.e.,* the epidermis and part of the dermis, or of part of the mucosa and submucosa, but not including the periostium.
Stent g., an inlay skin g., or a skin g. held in place by a tie-over dressing.
syngeneic g., syngraft.
tendon g., a g. of tendon, as in tendon transplantation.
Thiersch g., Ollier g.
vascularized g., the state of a g. after the recipient vasculature has been connected with the vessels in the g.
white g., rejection of a skin allograft so acute that vascularization never occurs.
Wolfe g., Wolfe-Krause g., a full-thickness skin g. without any subcutaneous fat.
xenogeneic g., xenograft.
zooplastic g., zoograft.

graft'ing. Transplanting a graft.

Graham, Thomas, British chemist, 1805–1869. See G.'s *law.*

Grahamella (grā-am-el'ă) [G. S. *Graham-Smith*]. A genus of aerobic, nonmotile microorganisms (order Rickettsiales) containing long or short, rod-shaped, Gram-negative cells which resemble those of *Bartonella* but which are less pleomorphic. These organisms occur within the erythrocytes of lower mammals, but they appear to be nonpathogenic and do not affect the health of the host.

Graham Little, Sir Ernest Gordon, British physician, 1867–1950. See G.L. *syndrome.*

Graham Steell, British physician, 1851–1942. See G. S.'s *murmur.*

grain (grān) [L. *granum*]. **1.** Cereal plants, such as corn, wheat, rye, or a seed of one of them. **2.** A minute, hard particle of any substance, as of sand. **3 (gr).** A unit of weight, $^1/_{60}$ dram, $^1/_{437.5}$ avoirdupois ounce, $^1/_{480}$ Troy ounce, $^1/_{5760}$ Troy pound, $^1/_{7000}$ avoirdupois pound; the equivalent of 0.0648 g.

grains (grānz). Hyaline bodies within the horny layer of the epidermis, found in keratosis follicularis.

Gram, Hans C.J., Danish bacteriologist, 1853–1938. See G.'s *iodine, stain;* Weigert-G. *stain* for bacteria in tissues.

-gram [G. *gramma,* character, mark]. Suffix denoting a recording, usually by an instrument. *Cf.* -graph.

gram (g). A unit of weight in the metric or centesimal system, the equivalent of 15.432 grains.

gram-centimeter. The energy exerted, or work done, when a mass of 1 g is raised a height of 1 cm; equal to 9.807×10^{-5} joules or newton-meters.

gramicidin (gram-i-sī'din). One of a group of polypeptides produced by *Bacillus brevis* that are primarily bacteriostatic in action against gram-positive cocci and bacilli. Commercial preparations contain several g.'s known as g. A, B, C, and D; g. S (for Soviet) is cyclic, the others are linear.

gram-ion. The weight in grams of an ion that is equal to the sum of the atomic weights of the atoms making up the ion.

gram-meter. A unit of energy equal to 100 gram-centimeters.

gram-molecule. The amount of a substance with a mass in grams equal to its molecular weight; *e.g.,* a g.-m. of hydrogen weighs 2 g, that of water 18 g.

Gram-negative. See Gram's *stain.*

Gram-positive. See Gram's *stain.*

grana (grā'nă) [pl. of L. *granum,* grain]. Bodies within the chloroplasts of plant cells that contain layers composed of chlorophyll and phospholipids.

granatum (gra-nā'tum) [L. *granatus,* having many seeds]. Pomegranate.

grandiose (gran'dē-ōs). Pertaining to feelings of great importance, expansiveness, or delusions of grandeur.

grand mal (grawn mahl). Tonic-clonic generalized *epilepsy.*

Grandry, M., 19th century French anatomist. See G.'s *corpuscles.*

Granger, Amedee, U.S. radiologist, 1879–1939. See G.'s *line.*

Granit, Ragnar A., Finnish-Swedish neurophysiologist and Nobel laureate, *1900. See G.'s *loop.*

granular (gran'yū-lăr). **1.** Composed of or resembling granules or granulations. **2.** particles with strong affinity for nuclear stains, seen in many bacterial species.

granulatio, pl. **granulationes** (gran-yū-lā'shē-ō, -shē-o'nēz) [L.]. Granulation.
granulatio'nes arachnoidea'les [NA], arachnoidal granulations; pacchionian bodies, granulations; tufted prolongations of pia-arachnoid, composed of numerous arachnoid villi that penetrate dural venous sinuses and effect transfer of cerebrospinal fluid to the venous system. At advanced age these are more numerous and tend to calcify. See also arachnoid *villi.*

granulation (gran'yū-lā'shŭn) [L. *granulatio*]. **1.** Formation into grains or granules; the state of being granular. **2.** A granular mass in or on the surface of any organ or membrane; or one of the individual granules forming the mass. **3.** The formation of minute, rounded, fleshy connective tissue projections on the surface of a wound, ulcer, or inflamed tissue surface in the process of healing; one of the fleshy granules composing this surface. See also granulation *tissue.* **4.** In pharmacy, the formation of crystals by constant agitation of a supersaturated solution of a salt.
arachnoidal g.'s, *granulationes* arachnoideales.
pacchionian g.'s, *granulationes* arachnoideales.

granulationes (gran-yū-lā-shē-ō'nēz) Plural of granulatio.

granule (gran'yūl) [L. *granulum,* dim. of *granum,* grain]. **1.** A grain-like particle; a granulation; a minute discrete mass. **2.** A very small pill, usually gelatin coated or sugar coated, containing a drug to be given in small dose. **3.** A colony of the bacterium or fungus causing a disease or simply colonizing the tissues of the patient. In compromised patients the differentiation is difficult.
acidophil g., oxyphil g.; a g. staining with an acid dye such as eosin.
acrosomal g., the single g. within an acrosomal vesicle which results from the coalescence of proacrosomal g.'s.
alpha g., a g. of an alpha cell which was named as the first of several kinds or because it was acidophilic.
Altmann's g., **(1)** fuchsinophil g.; **(2)** mitochondrion.
amphophil g., a g. that stains with both acid and basic dyes.
argentaffin g.'s, g.'s that reduce silver ions from an ammoniacal silver nitrate staining solution.
azurophil g., kappa g.; a g. that stains a reddish purple color with an azure dye; such g.'s are seen in dry smears of certain mature and developing blood cells, and are membrane-bound primary lysosomes containing enzymes.
basal g., basal *body.*
basophil g., a g. that stains readily with a basic dye.
Bensley's specific g.'s, g.'s in the cells of the islands of Langerhans in the pancreas.
beta g., a g. of a beta cell.
Birbeck's g., Langerhans' g.
Bollinger g.'s, **(1)** relatively small, but frequently microscopically visible, pale yellow or yellow-white g.'s observed in the granulomatous lesion, or the exudate, in botryomycosis; the g.'s consist of irregular aggregates or colonizations of Gram-positive cocci, usually staphylococci; **(2)** term sometimes incorrectly used synonymously with Bollinger bodies.
chromatic g., chromophil g. (2).
chromophil g., **(1)** any readily stainable g.; **(2)** chromatic g.; a g. of

chromophil (Nissl) substance.
chromophobe g.'s, g.'s that do not stain or stain poorly with the ordinary dyes; such g.'s are present in some cells in the anterior lobe of the pituitary.
cone g., nucleus of a retinal cell connecting with one of the cones.
Crooke's g.'s, lumpy masses of basophilic material in the basophil cells of the anterior lobe of the pituitary, associated with Cushing's disease, or following the administration of ACTH.
delta g., a g. of a delta cell.
elementary g., a particle of blood dust, or hemoconia.
eosinophil g., a g. that stains with eosin.
Fordyce's g.'s, Fordyce's *spots.*
fuchsinophil g., Altmann's g (1); a g. that has an affinity for fuchsin.
glycogen g., glycogen occurring in cells as beta g.'s which average about 300 Å in diameter, or as alpha g.'s which are aggregates measuring 900 Å of smaller particles.
iodophil g., a g. that stains brown with iodine; found in many of the polymorphonuclear leukocytes in pneumonia, erysipelas, scarlet fever, and various other acute diseases.
juxtaglomerular g.'s, stainable osmophilic secretory g.'s present in the juxtaglomerular cells, closely resembling zymogen g.'s.
kappa g., azurophil g.
keratohyalin g.'s, irregularly shaped basophilic g.'s in the cells of the stratum granulosum of the epidermis.
lamellar g., keratinosome.
Langerhans' g., Birbeck's g.; a small membrane-bound g. with characteristic plate-like interval ultrastructure; first reported in Langerhans' cells of the epidermis.
Langley's g.'s, g.'s in serous secreting cells.
membrane-coating g., keratinosome.
metachromatic g.'s, **(1)** g.'s that stain a color different from that of the dye used. See also metachromasia; **(2)** term sometimes used as a synonym for volutin.
mucinogen g.'s, g.'s that produce mucin, as in cells of the salivary glands and in the gastric and intestinal mucosae.
Neusser's g.'s, tiny basophilic g.'s sometimes observed in an indistinct zone about the nucleus of a leukocyte.
neutrophil g., a g. stainable with the neutral component of stains, *e.g.,* the Romanovsky-type blood stains.
Nissl g.'s, Nissl *substance.*
oxyphil g., acidophil g.
Palade g., ribosome.
proacrosomal g.'s, small carbohydrate-rich g.'s appearing in vesicles of the Golgi apparatus of spermatids; they coalesce into a single acrosomal g. contained within an acrosomal vesicle.
prosecretion g.'s, g.'s in the cytoplasm of a cell indicative of a preliminary step in the formation of a secretory product.
rod g., the nucleus of a retinal cell connecting with one of the rods.
Schüffner's g.'s, Schüffner's *dots.*
secretory g., a membrane-bound particle, usually protein, formed in the granular endoplasmic reticulum and the Golgi complex.
seminal g., one of the minute granular bodies present in the semen.
volutin g.'s, volutin.
Zimmermann's g., platelet.

granulo- [L. *granulum,* granule]. Combining form meaning granular, or denoting relationship to granules.

granuloblast (gran'yū-lō-blast) [granulo- + G. *blastos,* germ]. Rarely used term for an immature hematopoietic cell capable of giving rise to granulocytes.

granuloblastosis (gran'yū-lō-blas-tō'sis). A leukemic form of leukosis in the chicken characterized by an increase of immature, granular blood cells in the circulating blood and frequently infiltration of the parenchymatous organs.

granulocyte (gran'yū-lō-sīt) [granulo- + G. *kytos,* cell]. A mature granular leukocyte, including neutrophilic, acidophilic, and basophilic types of polymorphonuclear leukocytes, *i.e.,* respectively, neutrophils, eosinophils, and basophils.
immature g., an immature neutrophil, except that it may be neutrophilic, acidophilic, or basophilic in character.

granulocytopenia (gran'yū-lō-sī-tō-pē'nē-ă) [granulocyte + G. *penia,* poverty]. Granulopenia; hypogranulocytosis; less than the normal number of granular leukocytes in the blood.

granulocytopoiesis (gran'yū-lō-sī'tō-poy-ē'sis). Granulopoiesis.

granulocytopoietic (gran'yū-lō-sī'tō-poy-et'ik) [granulocyte + G. *poieō,* to make]. Granulopoietic.

granulocytosis (gran'yū-lō-sī-tō'sis). A condition characterized by more than the normal number of granulocytes in the circulating blood or in the tissues.

granuloma (gran-yū-lō'mă) [granulo- + G. *-oma,* tumor]. Indefinite term applied to nodular inflammatory lesions, usually small or granular, firm, persistent, and containing compactly grouped mononuclear phagocytes. See also granulomatosis.
actinic g., an annular eruption on sun-exposed skin which microscopically shows phagocytosis of dermal elastic fibers by giant cells and histiocytes.
amebic g., ameboma.
g. annula're, lichen annularis; a chronic or recurrent papular eruption that tends to develop on the distal portions of the extremities and over prominences, although the condition may be generalized; waxy papules tend to form annular lesions characterized microscopically by foci of dermal necrosis with mucin deposits, bordered by fibrous histiocytes.
apical g., periapical g.
beryllium g., a sarcoid-like granulomatous reaction to exposure to beryllium.
bilharzial g., schistosome g.
canine venereal g., transmissible venereal tumor; a rapidly growing, soft, easily bleeding, infectious, connective tissue tumor occurring in the vagina of the female dog and on the penis and sheath of the male; ordinarily transmitted by coitus.
coccidioidal g., secondary *coccidioidomycosis.*
coli g., Hjärre's *disease.*
dental g., periapical g.
g. endem'icum, the lesion occurring in cutaneous leishmaniasis.
eosinophilic g., a lesion observed more frequently in children and adolescents, occasionally in young adults, which occurs chiefly as a solitary focus in one bone, although multiple involvement is sometimes observed and similar foci may develop in the lung; characterized by numerous Langerhans cells and eosinophils, and occasional foci of necrosis; may be related to Hand-Schüller-Christian disease, possibly representing a benign clinical form.
g. facia'le, persistent well demarcated nodules that usually appear on the face and consist of a dense dermal infiltrate of eosinophils and neutrophils, with fibrinoid vasculitis and later mononuclear infiltration and fibrosis.
foreign body g., a g. caused by the presence of foreign particulate material in tissue, characterized by a histiocytic reaction with foreign body giant cells.
g. gangrenes'cens, lethal midline g.
giant cell g., giant cell epulis; a non-neoplastic lesion characterized by a proliferation of granulation tissue containing numerous multinucleated giant cells; it occurs on the gingiva and alveolar mucosa (occasionally on other soft tissues) where it presents as a soft red-blue hemorrhagic nodular swelling; it also occurs within the mandible or maxilla as a unilocular or multilocular radiolucency; microscopically similiar lesions occur in the tubular bones of the hands and feet, are considered neoplastic, and may have a malignant course. See also giant cell *tumor* of bone.
g. gravida'rum, pregnancy tumor; a pyogenic g. developing on the gingiva during pregnancy; thought to be related to hormonically

altered response of the oral mucous membranes to local irritants such as bacterial plaque on adjacent teeth.
infectious g., any granulomatous lesion known to be caused by a living agent; *e.g.,* bacteria, fungi, helminths.
g. inguina'le, g. pudendi or venereum; ulcerating g. of pudenda; pudendal ulcer; a specific g., classified as a venereal disease and caused by *Calymmatobacterium granulomatis;* the ulcerating granulomatous lesions occur in the inguinal regions and the genitalia; peripheral extension of the lesions produces extensive destruction.
g. inguina'le trop'icum, groin ulcer; an elongated ulcer, with elevated papillary edges, sometimes occurring in the groin in persons in the tropics.
laryngeal g., a polypoid granulomatous projection of granulomatous tissue into the lumen of the larynx, commonly following a traumatic tracheal intubation.
lethal midline g., g. gangrenescens; malignant g.; destructive granulomatous lesion usually arising in the nose or paranasal sinuses and ending fatally; may be distinguished from Wegener's granulomatosis by the absence of angiitis and of involvement of other organs.
lipoid g., g. characterized by aggregates or accumulations of fairly large mononuclear phagocytes that contain lipid.
lipophagic g., a lesion formed as a result of the inflammatory reaction provoked by foci of necrosis in subcutaneous fat, as in certain types of traumatic injury; the central focus of necrotic material is surrounded by an irregular zone of numerous macrophages, many of which become laden with tiny globules of lipid.
Majocchi g.'s, papules due to a deep follicular fungal infection with rupture of the hair follicles; most frequently seen on shaved legs of women.
malignant g., lethal midline g.
g. multifor'me, a chronic granulomatous annular eruption of the skin on the upper body in older adults in central Africa; of unknown cause.
oily g., reaction to inclusion of a bulky, insoluble liquid (often an oily substance) which occurs several months, but sometimes years, after injection of the material.
paracoccidioidal g., paracoccidioidomycosis.
parasitic g., cutaneous leishmaniasis manifested as warty papules affecting primarily the lower limbs.
periapical g., apical, dental, or root end g.; a proliferation of granulation tissue surrounding the apex of a nonvital tooth and arising in response to pulpal necrosis.
g. puden'di, g. inguinale.
pyogenic g., g. pyogen'icum, g. telangiectaticum; a small rounded mass of highly vascular granulation tissue, frequently with an ulcerated surface, projecting from the skin; histologically, the mass resembles a capillary hemangioma; occurs also in the gingiva, usually on the labial or lingual surface.
reparative giant cell g., see giant cell g.
reticulohistiocytic g., reticulohistiocytoma.
root end g., periapical g.
sarcoidal g., a non-necrotizing epithelioid cell g. similar to those seen in sarcoidosis.
schistosome g., bilharzial g.; a granulomatous lesion formed around schistosome eggs embedded in tissues in cases of schistosomiasis (bilharziasis); typically these granulomata are found in intestinal tissues (*Schistosoma japonicum* or *S. mansoni* infection), bladder tissue (*S. haematobium*), and hepatic tissue (all three human schistosomes).
sea urchin g., granulomatous nodules, either foreign-body type or composed of epitheliod cells, from the retention of the spine of the sea urchin, occurring several months after the wounding of the skin.
silicon g., eruption of granulomatous lesions due to traumatic inoculation of the skin with sand, or materials that contain silicon; this condition may follow dermabrasion using sandpaper technique.
swimming pool g., a chronic, low grade, infectious, verrucous lesion most commonly seen on the knees; although due to an acid-fast mycobacterium, it is not tuberculous.
g. telangiecta'ticum, pyogenic g.
g. trop'icum, yaws.
ulcerating g. of pudenda, g. inguinale.
g. vene'reum, g. inguinale.
zirconium g., g. from zirconium salts, usually occurring in the axillae, from antiperspirants containing this material; may also be caused by intradermal injection of antigens containing the lactate salt.

granulomatosis (gran'yū-lō-mă-tō'sis). Any condition characterized by multiple granulomas.
allergic g., Churg-Strauss *syndrome.*
bronchocentric g., a severe form of allergic bronchopulmonary aspergillosis.
g. discifor'mis chron'ica et progress'iva, Miescher's g.
lipid g., lipoid g., xanthomatosis.
lipophagic intestinal g., obsolete term for Whipple's *disease.*
lymphomatoid g., polymorphic reticulosis; a disease related to Wegener's g., but more widespread and diffuse, most frequently affecting male adults; characterized initially by nodular lower lung lesions which are granulomatous proliferations of atypical lymphocytes, plasma cells, and histiocytes, notably perivascular with destruction of small arteries; eventually the skin, kidneys, and nervous system are often involved; pulmonary lymphomatoid g. may be followed by the development of malignant lymphoma.
Miescher's g., g. disciformis chronica et progressiva; a variant of necrobiosis lipoidica.
g. siderot'ica, a form in which firm, brown foci that contain iron pigment (Gamna bodies) are present in an enlarged spleen.
Wegener's g., a disease, occurring mainly in the fourth and fifth decades, characterized by necrotizing granulomas and ulceration of the upper respiratory tract, with purulent rhinorrhea, nasal obstruction, and sometimes with otorrhea, hemoptysis, pulmonary infiltration and cavitation, and fever; exophthalmos, involvement of the larynx and pharynx, and glomerulonephritis may occur; the underlying condition is a vasculitis affecting small vessels, and is possibly due to an immune disorder. See also lymphomatoid g.

granulomatous (gran-yū-lom'ă-tŭs). Having the characteristics of a granuloma.

granulomere (gran'yū-lō-mēr) [granulo- + G. *meros,* a part]. Chromomere (2); the central part of a blood platelet.

granulopenia (gran'yū-lō-pē'nē-ă). Granulocytopenia.

granuloplasm (gran'yū-lō-plazm). The inner substance of an ameba, or other unicellular organism, within the ectoplasm and surrounding the nucleus.

granuloplastic (gran'yū-lō-plas'tik). Forming granules.

granulopoiesis (gran'yū-lō-poy-ē'sis) [granulo(cyte) + G. *poiēsis,* a making]. Granulocytopoiesis; production of granulocytes. In adults, granulocytes are produced chiefly in the red bone marrow of flat bones.

granulopoietic (gran'yū-lō-poy-et'ik). Granulocytopoietic; pertaining to granulopoiesis.

granulosa (gran-yū-lō'să). *Stratum* granulosum folliculi ovarici vesiculosi.

granulosis (gran-yū-lō'sis). Granulosity; a mass of minute granules of any character.
g. ru'bra na'si, erythema, papules, and occasional vesicles of the tip of the nose and extending upward and laterally to the cheeks, resulting from occlusion and chronic inflammation of sweat ducts.

granulosity (gran-yū-los'i-tē). Granulosis.

granum (grā′nŭm). Singular of grana.

-graph [G. *graphō,* to write]. Suffix denoting: **1.** Something written, as in monograph, radiograph. **2.** The instrument for making a recording, as in kymograph. *Cf.* -gram.

graph (graf) [G. *graphō,* to write]. A line or tracing denoting varying values of commodities, temperatures, urinary output, etc.; more generally, any geometric or pictorial representation of measurements that might otherwise be expressed in tabular form.

graphanesthesia (graf′an-es-thē′zē-ă) [G. *graphē,* writing + *anaisthēsia,* fr. *an-* priv. + *aisthēsis,* perception]. Tactual inability to recognize figures or letters written on the skin; may be due to spinal cord or brain disease.

graphesthesia (graf-es-thē′zē-ă) [G. *graphē,* writing, + *aisthēsis,* perception]. Ability to recognize writing on the skin.

graphite (graf′īt). Plumbago; black lead; a crystallizable soft black form of carbon.

grapho-. [G. *graphō,* to write]. Combining form denoting a writing or description.

graphology (gră-fol′ō-jē) [grapho- + G. *logos,* study]. The study of handwriting as an indication of temperament or character.

graphomania (graf-ō-mā′ne-ă) [grapho- + G. *mania,* insanity]. Morbid and excessive impulse to write.

graphomotor (graf-ō-mō′ter) [grapho- + L. *motus,* fr. *movere,* to move]. Relating to the movements used in writing.

graphopathology (graf′ō-path-ol′ō-jē) [grapho- + pathology]. Interpretation of personality disorders from a study of handwriting.

graphophobia (graf-ō-fō′bē-ă) [grapho- + G. *phobos,* fear]. Morbid fear of writing.

graphorrhea (graf-ō-rē′ă) [grapho- + G. *rhoia,* flow]. The writing of long lists of meaningless words.

graphospasm (graf′ō-spazm). Writer's *cramp.*

-graphy [G. *graphō,* to write]. Suffix denoting a writing or description.

grasp. Grip (2).
palm g., holding an object by wrapping the palm and the fingers around it.
pen g., a method, similar to that of holding a pen in writing, of grasping an instrument.

Grasset, Joseph, French physician, 1849–1918. See G.'s *law, phenomenon, sign;* G.-Gaussel *phenomenon;* Landouzy-G. *law.*

Gratiolet, Louis P., French anatomist, physiologist, and physician, 1815–1865. See G.'s *fibers, radiation.*

grattage (gră-tazh′) [Fr. scraping]. Scraping or brushing an ulcer or surface with sluggish granulations to stimulate the healing process.

Gräupner, Sigurd C., German physician, 1861–1916. See G.'s *method.*

grave (grāv) [L. *gravis,* heavy, grave]. Denoting symptoms of a serious or dangerous character.

gravel (grav′l). Uropsammus (1); small concretions, usually of uric acid, calcium oxalate, or phosphates, formed in the kidney and passed through the ureter, bladder, and urethra.

Graves, Robert J., Irish physician, 1796–1853. See G. *disease.*

grav′id. Pregnant.

gravida (grav′i-dă) [L. *gravidus* (adj.), fem. *gravida,* fr. *gravis,* heavy]. A pregnant woman. Gravida followed by a roman numeral or preceded by a Latin prefix (primi-, secundi-, *etc.*) designates the pregnant woman by number of pregnancies; *e.g.,* **gravida I,** primigravida; a woman in her first pregnancy; **gravida II,** secundigravida; a woman in her second pregnancy. *Cf.* para.

gravidic (grav-id′ik). Relating to pregnancy or a pregnant woman.

gravidism (grav′id-izm). Pregnancy.

graviditas (grav-vid′i-tas) [L.]. Pregnancy.
g. examnia′lis, extraamniotic *pregnancy.*
g. exochoria′lis, extrachorial *pregnancy.*

gravidity (gra-vid′i-tē) [L. *graviditas,* pregnancy]. Number of pregnancies.

gravimeter (gră-vim′ĕ-ter) [L. *gravis,* heavy, + G. *metron,* measure]. Hydrometer.

gravimetric (grav-i-met′rik). Relating to or determined by weight.

gravireceptors (grav′i-rē-sep′terz). Highly specialized receptor organs and nerve endings in the inner ear, joints, tendons, and muscles that give the brain information about body position, equilibrium, direction of gravitational forces, and the sensation of "down" or "up."

gravitation (grav-i-tā′shŭn) [L. *gravitas,* weight]. The force of attraction between any two bodies in the universe, varying directly as the product of their masses and inversely as the square of the distance between their centers; expressed as $F = G \cdot m_1 m_2 \cdot l^2$, where G (gravitational constant) $= 6.672 \times 10^{-11}\ m^3 \cdot kg^{-1} \cdot s^{-2}$.

gravity (grav′i-tē) [L. *gravitas*]. The attraction toward the earth that makes any mass exert downward force or have weight. Strictly speaking, g. is the algebraic sum of the gravitational attraction of the earth and the opposing centrifugal effect of the mass's rotation around the earth; thus, g. equals gravitational attraction at the north and south poles but becomes progressively less as one approaches the equator. A satellite in a stable orbit has zero g. because the centrifugal effect of orbital motion exactly balances the gravitational attraction of the earth.
specific g. (sp. gr.), the weight of any body compared with that of another body of equal volume regarded as the unit; usually the weight of a liquid compared with that of distilled water.
zero-g., see zerogravity.

Grawitz, Paul, German pathologist, 1850–1932. See G.'s *basophilia, tumor.*

gray (Gy) (grā) [Louis H. *Gray,* British radiologist, 1905–1965]. The SI unit of absorbed dose of ionizing radiation, equivalent to one joule per kilogram of tissue; 1 Gy = 100 rad.

Greeff, C. Richard, German ophthalmologist, 1862–1938. See Prowazek-G. *bodies.*

green (grēn). A color between blue and yellow in the spectrum. For individual green dyes, see specific names.
Scheele's g., cupric arsenite.

Greenfield, J. Godwin, British neuropathologist, 1884–1958. See G.'s *disease.*

Greenhow, Edward H., British physician, 1814–1888. See G.'s *disease.*

Greenough microscope. See under microscope.

greffotome (gref′ō-tōm) [Fr. *greff,* graft, + G. *tōme,* incision]. An instrument for slicing off bits of epidermis to use in grafting.

gregaloid (greg′ă-loyd) [L. *grex* (*greg-*), a flock]. Denoting a loose colony of protozoa formed by the chance union of independent cells, especially among sarcodines with pseudopodial adherence.

Gregarina (greg-ă-rī′nă) [L. *gregarius,* gregarious, fr. *grex* (*greg-*), a flock]. A genus of sporozoan protozoa (phylum Apicomplexa, subclass Gregarinia), parasitic in annelids and arthropods, and lacking schizogony and endodyogeny in the life cycle.

gregarine (greg′ă-rēn). A member of the subclass Gregarinia.

Gregarinia (greg′ă-rin′i-ă). A sporozoan subclass consisting of a number of parasites of the body cavity and intestinal tract of invertebrates, especially annelids and arthropods; typical genera include *Gregarina* in insects and *Monocystis* in earthworms.

gregarinosis (greg′ă-ri-nō′sis). A disease due to the presence of gregarines.

Greig, David M., Scottish physician, 1864–1936. See G.'s *syndrome.*

gression (gres'shŭn) [L. *grador,* pp. *gressus,* to walk, fr. *gradus,* a step]. Displacement of a tooth backward.

Greville bath. See under bath.

Grey Turner, See Turner, George Grey.

grid. **1.** A chart with horizontal and perpendicular lines for plotting curves. **2.** Diaphragm (2); in x-ray imaging, a device formed of lead strips for preventing scattered radiation from reaching the x-ray film.

Wetzel g., chart of growth, plotting height, weight, physical fitness and related aspects of young and adolescent children during growth.

Gridley, Mary F., U.S. medical technologist, 1908–1954. See G.'s *stain;* G.'s *stain* for fungi.

grief (grēf). A normal emotional response to an external loss; distinguished from depression since it usually subsides after a reasonable time.

Griesinger, Wilhelm, German neurologist, 1817–1868. See G.'s *disease, symptom;* bilious *typhoid* of G.

Griffith's sign. See under sign.

grindelia (grin-dē'lē-ă) [David H. *Grindel,* German botanist, 1776–1836]. The dried leaves and flowering tops of *Grindelia camporum, G. humilius,* and *G. squarrosa* (family Compositae); used as an expectorant; a fluidextract has been used externally in the treatment of rhus poisoning.

grinding (grīnd'ing). Abrasion (3).

selective g., the modification of the occlusal forms of teeth by g. according to a plan or by g. at selected places marked by articulating ribbon or paper.

grinding-in. A term used to denote the act of correcting occlusal disharmonies by grinding the natural or artificial teeth.

grip. **1.** Influenza. **2.** Grasp.

devil's g., epidemic *pleurodynia.*

grippe (grip) [Fr. *gripper,* to seize]. Influenza.

griseofulvin (gris'ē-ō-fŭl'vin). A fungistatic antibiotic produced by *Penicillium griseofulvin* and *P. patulum;* used in the systemic treatment of superficial fungal infections caused by the dermatophytes *Microsporum, Trichophyton,* and *Epidermophyton.*

griseus (gris'ē-ŭs) [L.]. Gray.

Grisolle, Augustin, French physician, 1811–1869. See G.'s *sign.*

Grisonella ratellina (gri-sŏ-nel'ă ra-te-lī'nă). A South American weasel, a reservoir host of *Trypanosoma cruzi.*

gristle (gris'l) [A.S.]. Cartilage.

Gritti, Rocco, Italian surgeon, 1828–1920. See G.'s *operation;* G.-Stokes *amputation.*

Grn Abbreviation for glycerone.

Grocco, Pietro, Italian physician, 1857–1916. See G.'s *sign, triangle;* Orsi-G. *method.*

Grocott-Gomori methenamine-silver stain. See under stain.

Groenouw, Arthur, German ophthalmologist, 1862–1945. See G.'s corneal *dystrophy.*

groin (groyn). *Regio* inguinalis. Sometimes used to indicate just the crease in the junction of the thigh with the trunk.

Grönblad, Ester E., Swedish ophthalmologist, *1898. See G.-Strandberg *syndrome.*

GROOVE

groove (grūv). A narrow elongated depression or furrow on any surface. See also sulcus.

alveolobuccal g., alveolobuccal sulcus; gingivobuccal g. or sulcus; the upper and lower half of the buccal vestibule on each side.

alveololabial g., alveololabial sulcus; gingivolabial g. or sulcus; **(1)** the upper and lower half of the labial vestibule; **(2)** in the embryo, the g. formed by the deepening of the labial sulcus; its inner wall becomes incorporated with the alveolar process of the mandible or the maxilla, and its outer wall with the lips and cheeks.

alveololingual g., alveololingual sulcus; gingivolingual g. or sulcus; **(1)** that part of the oral cavity proper, on each side of the frenulum linguae, between the tongue and the mandibular alveolar process or ridge; **(2)** in the embryo, the g. on each side between the lingual primordium and the alveolar elevations of the mandible.

anterior auricular g., *incisura* anterior auris.

anterior intermediate g., *sulcus* intermedius anterior.

anterior interventricular g., *sulcus* interventricularis anterior.

anterolateral g. *sulcus* lateralis anterior.

anteromedian g., **(1)** *fissura* mediana anterior medullae oblongatae; **(2)** *fissura* mediana anterior medullae spinalis.

arterial g.'s, *sulci* arteriosi.

atrioventricular g., *sulcus* coronarius.

g. for auditory tube, *sulcus* tubae auditivae.

auriculoventricular g., *sulcus* coronarius.

bicipital g., *sulcus* intertubercularis.

branchial g., an external embryonic g. between contiguous branchial arches. See also branchial *clefts.*

carotid g., *sulcus* caroticus.

carpal g., *sulcus* carpi.

cavernous g., *sulcus* caroticus.

costal g., *sulcus* costae.

g. of crus of the helix, *sulcus* cruris helicis.

dental g., a transitory depression in the gingival surface of the embryonic jaw along the line of ingrowth of the dental lamina.

developmental g.'s, developmental lines; fine lines found in the enamel of a tooth that mark the junction of the lobes of the crown in its development.

digastric g., *incisura* mastoidea.

ethmoidal g., *sulcus* ethmoidalis.

frontal g.'s, see entries under *sulcus* frontalis.

gingivobuccal g., alveolobuccal g.

gingivolabial g., alveololabial g.

gingivolingual g., alveololingual g.

greater palatine g., *sulcus* palatinus major.

g. of greater petrosal nerve, *sulcus* nervi petrosi majoris.

Harrison's g., a deformity of the ribs which results from the pull of the diaphragm on ribs weakened by rickets or other softening of the bone.

inferior petrosal g., *sulcus* sinus petrosi inferioris.

infraorbital g., *sulcus* infraorbitalis.

interosseous g., **(1)** *sulcus* calcanei; **(2)** *sulcus* tali.

intertubercular g., *sulcus* intertubercularis.

interventricular g.'s, see *sulcus* interventricularis anterior and *sulcus* interventricularis posterior.

lacrimal g., *sulcus* lacrimalis.

laryngotracheal g., the depression in the floor of the posterior part of the pharynx, continued downward on the ventral wall of the foregut; from it are developed the lower part of the larynx and the trachea, bronchi, and lungs.

lateral bicipital g., *sulcus* bicipitalis lateralis.

g. of lesser petrosal nerve, *sulcus* nervi petrosi minoris.
linguogingival g., a g. separating the embryonic mandibular portion of the tongue from the remainder of the mandibular process.
Lucas' g., *stria* spinosa.
mastoid g., *incisura* mastoidea.
medial bicipital g., *sulcus* bicipitalis medialis.
median g. of tongue, *sulcus* medianus linguae.
medullary g., neural g.
musculospiral g., *sulcus* nervi radialis.
mylohyoid g., *sulcus* mylohyoideus.
g. of nail matrix, *sulcus* matricis unguis.
nasolabial g., *sulcus* nasolabialis.
nasopalatine g., a g. on the vomer lodging the nasopalatine nerve.
nasopharyngeal g., an indistinct line marking the boundary between the nasal cavities and the nasal part of the pharynx.
neural g., medullary g.; the gutter-like g. formed in the midline of the embryo's dorsal surface by the progressive elevation of the lateral margins of the neural plate; the ultimate dorsal fusion of the margins results in the formation of the neural tube.
obturator g., *sulcus* obturatorius.
occipital g., *sulcus* arteriae occipitalis.
olfactory g., *sulcus* olfactorius.
optic g., *sulcus* prechiasmatis.
palatine g., *sulcus* palatinus.
palatovaginal g., *sulcus* palatovaginalis.
paraglenoid g., preauricular g.
pharyngeal g.'s, embryonic endodermal or ectodermal g.'s between successive pharyngeal arches.
pharyngotympanic g., *sulcus* tubae auditivae.
pontomedullary g., the transverse g. on the ventral aspect of the brainstem that demarcates the pons from the medulla oblongata; from its bottom the sixth, seventh, and eighth cranial nerves emerge.
popliteal g., sulcus popliteus; a g. on the lateral condyle of the femur between the epicondyle and the articular margin. Its anterior end gives origin to the popliteus muscle; its posterior end lodges the tendon of the muscle when the knee is fully flexed.
posterior auricular g., *sulcus* auriculae posterior.
posterior intermediate g., *sulcus* intermedius posterior.
posterior interventricular g., *sulcus* interventricularis posterior.
posterolateral g., *sulcus* lateralis posterior.
preauricular g., preauricular sulcus; paraglenoid g. or sulcus; sulcus paraglenoidalis; a g. on the pelvic surface of the ilium just lateral to the auricular surface; it is more pronounced in the female.
primary labial g., labial *sulcus.*
primitive g., the median depression in the primitive streak flanked by the primitive ridges.
pterygopalatine g., *sulcus* palatinus major.
g. for radial nerve, *sulcus* nervi radialis.
retention g., one of the g.'s forming opposing vertical constrictions in a tooth to aid in retention of a dental restoration.
rhombic g.'s, seven pairs of transverse furrows in the floor of the embryonic hindbrain.
sagittal g., *sulcus* sinus sagittalis superioris.
Sibson's g., a g. occasionally seen on the outer side of the thorax formed by the prominent lower border of the pectoralis major muscle.
sigmoid g., *sulcus* sinus sigmoidei.
skin g.'s, *sulci* cutis.
g. for spinal nerve, *sulcus* nervi spinalis.
spiral g., *sulcus* nervi radialis.
subclavian g., *sulcus* musculi subclavii.
g. for subclavian artery, *sulcus* arteriae subclaviae.
g. for subclavian vein, *sulcus* venae subclaviae.
subcostal g., *sulcus* costae.
g. for superior sagittal sinus, *sulcus* sinus sagittalis superioris.
supplemental g., a curvilinear depression normally found on each side of a triangular ridge (crista triangularis).
supra-acetabular g., *sulcus* supra-acetabularis.
g. for tendon of flexor hallucis longus, *sulcus* tendinis musculi flexoris hallucis longi.
g. for tendon of long peroneal muscle, *sulcus* tendinis musculi peronei longi.
tracheobronchial g., a median ventral diverticulum of the embryonic foregut that gives rise to the epithelial component of the respiratory system.
transverse nasal g., *stria* nasi transversa.
tympanic g., *sulcus* tympanicus.
g. for ulnar nerve, *sulcus* nervi ulnaris.
urethral g., the g. on the undersurface of the embryonic penis which ultimately is closed to form the penile portion of the urethra.
venous g.'s, *sulci* venosi.
vertebral g., the depression bounded by the spinous processes and laminae of the vertebrae, in which lie the deep muscles of the back.
vomeral g., *sulcus* vomeris.
vomerovaginal g., *sulcus* vomerovaginalis.

Gross, Ludwik, 20th century U.S. oncologist. See G.'s *virus,* leukemia *virus.*

group (grūp). **1.** A number of similar or related objects. **2.** In chemistry, a radical. For individual chemical groups, see the specific name.
blood g., see *blood group.*
characterizing g., a g. of atoms in a molecule that distinguishes the class of substances in which it occurs from all other classes; thus carbonyl (CO) is the characterizing g. of ketones; COOH, of organic acids, etc.
connective tissue g., a collective name for mucous tissue, dentin, bone, cartilage, and ordinary connective tissue, all derived from the mesenchyme.
control g., a g. of subjects participating in the same experiment as another g. of subjects, but which is not exposed to the variable under investigation.
cytophil g., the atom g. in the antibody (amboceptor) that binds it to the cell.
determinant g., antigenic *determinant.*
encounter g., a form of psychological sensitivity training that emphasizes the experiencing of individual relationships within the g. and minimizes intellectual and didactic imput; the g. focuses on the present rather than concerning itself with the past or outside problems of its members. See also sensitivity training g.
experimental g., task-oriented g.; a g. of subjects exposed to the variable of an experiment, as opposed to the control g.
functional g., see function (4).
linkage g., a set of two or more loci, not yet assigned to specific chromosomes, that have been shown by linkage analysis to be physically close in the genome.
matched g.'s, a method of experimental control in which subjects in one g. are matched on a one-to-one basis with subjects in other g.'s concerning all organism variables (*e.g.,* age, sex, height, weight) which the experimenter deems important.
partial g.'s, an old, infrequently used term for the sum of the different antibodies (in an immune serum) that correspond to various antigenic fractions of the microorganism.
prosthetic g., a non-amino acid compound attached to a protein, usually in a reversible fashion, that confers new properties upon the conjugated protein thus produced. See also coenzyme.
sensitivity training g., a g. in which members seek to develop self-awareness and an understanding of g. processes rather than to obtain therapy for an emotional disturbance. See also encounter g.; personal growth *laboratory.*
symptom g., **(1)** see syndrome; **(2)** see complex (1).
T g., abbreviation for training g.

task-oriented g., experimental g.
therapeutic g., any g. of patients meeting together for mutual psychotherapeutic goals.
training (T) g., any g. emphasizing training in self-awareness and group dynamics.

Grover, Ralph W., U.S. dermatologist, *1920, See G.'s *disease.*

growth (grōth). The increase in size of a living being or any of its parts occurring in the process of development.
accretionary g., g. by an increase of intercellular material.
appositional g., g. accomplished by the addition of new layers on those previously formed; *e.g.,* the addition of lamellae in the formation of bone; it is the characteristic method of g. when rigid materials are involved.
auxetic g., intussusceptive g.; g. by increase in the size of component cells.
differential g., different rates of g. in associated tissues or structures; used especially in embryology when the differences in g. rates result in changing the original proportions or relations.
interstitial g., g. from a number of different centers within an area; in contrast with appositional g., it can occur only when the materials involved are nonrigid.
intussusceptive g., auxetic g.
multiplicative g., g. by an increase in the number of cells.
new g., neoplasm.

grub (grŭb). Wormlike larva or maggot of certain insects, particularly in the orders Coleoptera, Diptera, and Hymenoptera, and the genus *Hypoderma.*

Gruber, George B., 20th century German physician. See G.'s *syndrome;* Meckel-G. *syndrome.*

Gruber, Josef, Austrian otologist, 1827–1900. See G.'s *method.*

Gruber, Max von, German hygienist, 1853–1927. See G.'s *reaction,* G.-Widal *reaction.*

Gruber, Wenzel (Wenaslaus) L., Russian anatomist, 1814–1890. See G.'s *cul-de-sac,* G.-Landzert *fossa.*

gruel (grū'ĕl) [thru O. Fr., fr. Mediev. L. *grutum,* meal]. A semiliquid food of oatmeal or other cereal boiled in water; thin porridge.

grumous (grū'mŭs) [L. *grumus,* a little heap]. Thick and lumpy, as clotting blood.

Grunert's spur. See under spur.

Grunstein-Hogness assay. See under assay.

Grünwald. See May-G. *stain.*

Grütz, O. See Bürger-G. *syndrome.*

Grynfeltt, Joseph C., French surgeon, 1840–1913. See G.'s *triangle.*

gryochrome (grī'ō-krōm) [G. *gry,* something insignificant, + *chrōma,* color]. A term applied by Nissl to nerve cells in which the stainable portion is present in the form of minute granules without definite arrangement.

gryposis (gri-pō'sis) [G. *grypos,* hooked, + *-osis,* condition]. An abnormal curvature.
g. un'guium, onychogryposis.

GSH Abbreviation for reduced *glutathione.*

GSR Abbreviation for galvanic skin *response.*

GSSG Abbreviation for oxidized *glutathione.*

gt. Abbreviation for gutta.

g-tolerance, The tolerance of a person or a piece of equipment to forces that develop as a result of acceleration or deceleration.

GTP Abbreviation for guanosine 5′-triphosphate.

gtt. Abbreviation for guttae.

GU Abbreviation for genitourinary.

guaiac (gwī'ak) [Sp. *guayaco,* imitating the native Carib name]. Guaiac gum; the resin of *Guiacum officinale* or *G. sanctum* (family Zygophyllaceae); a nauseant, diaphoretic, stimulant, and reagent in testing for occult blood.

guaiacin (gwī'ă-sin). Guaiac saponin, a constituent of guiac used as a reagent for oxidases, with which it gives a blue color.

guaiacol (gwī'ă-kol). *o*-Methoxyphenol; methylcatechol; catecholmonomethyl ether; $C_6H_4(OH)(OCH_3)$; has been used as an expectorant and intestinal disinfectant; also available as g. carbonate.
g. glyceryl ether, guaifenesin.
g. phosphate, phosphoric guaiacyl ether, a white crystalline powder, insoluble in water; used as an intestinal antiseptic and in fever.

guaifenesin (gwī-fen'ĕ-sin). Glyceryl guaiacolate; guaiacol glyceryl ether; 3-(*o* -methoxyphenoxy)-1,2-propanediol; an expectorant that reduces the viscosity of sputum.

guanabenz acetate (gwahn-ă-benz). [(2,6-Dichlorobenzylidene)amino]guaridine monoacetate; a centrally acting antiadrenergic antihypertensive.

guanacline sulfate (gwahn'ă-klēn). Cyclazenin sulfate; [2-(3,6-Dihydro-4-methyl-1(2*H*)-pyridinyl)ethyl]guanidine sulfate dihydrate; an antihypertensive.

guanadrel sulfate (gwahn'ă-drel). (1,4-Dioxaspiro[4,5]dec-2-ylmethyl)guanidine sulfate; an antihypertensive drug.

guanase (gwahn'ās). *Guanine* deaminase.

guanazolo (gwahn-ă-zōl'ō). 8-Azaguanine.

guanethidine sulfate (gwahn-eth'i-dēn). [2-(Octahydro-1-azocinyl)-ethyl]-guanidine sulfate; a potent antihypertensive agent. It appears to interfere with the release of the chemical mediator (norepinephrine) at the sympathetic neuroeffector junction; it does not produce ganglionic or parasympathetic blockade with recommended doses. In ophthalmology, it is used topically for the treatment of glaucoma and to counteract eyelid retraction in Graves' disease.

guanidine (gwahn'i-dēn, -din). NH_2-C(NH)-NH_2; a strongly basic compound, usually found (in some plants and lower animals) as the hydrochloride; a constituent of creatine; administered as a cholinergic striated muscle stimulant.

guanidinoacetate methyltransferase (gwahn'i-din-ō-as'e-tāt) [EC 2.1.1.2]. The enzyme catalyzing the transfer of a methyl group from *S*-adenosylmethionine ("active methionine") to guanidinoacetate (glycocyamine), forming creatine.

guanine (gwahn'ēn, -in). 2-Amino-6-oxypurine; one of the two major purines (the other being adenine) occurring in all nucleic acids.

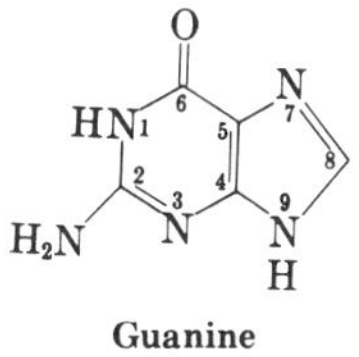

Guanine

g. aminase, g. deaminase.
g. deaminase [EC 3.5.4.3], guanase; guanine aminase; a deaminase of the liver that catalyzes the conversion of guanine into xanthine.
g. deoxyribonucleotide, deoxyguanylic acid.
g. ribonucleotide, guanylic acid.

guanochlor sulfate (gwahn'ō-klōr). {[2-(2,6-Dichlorophenoxy) ethyl]amino}guanidine sulfate; used as an α-adrenergic blocking agent for the treatment of essential hypertension.

guanophores (gwahn-ō-fōrz) [guanine + G. *phoros,* bearing]. Cells in the skin of some cold-blooded vertebrates (particularly fishes) which contain granules composed of guanine and give the creatures a metallic (gold or silver) luster.

guanosine (Guo) (gwahn'ō-sēn, -sin). 9-β-D-Ribofuranosylguanine; 9-β-D-ribosylguanine (guanine combined through its N-9 with the C-1 of β-D-ribose); a major constituent of RNA and of guanine nucleotides.

guanosine 5'-diphosphate (GDP). Guanosine esterfied at its 5' position with diphosphoric acid.

guanosine 5'-phosphate. Guanylic acid.

guanosine 5'-triphosphate (GTP). An immediate precursor of guanine nucleotides in RNA; similar to ATP.

guanoxan sulfate (gwahn-ok'san). (1,4-Benzodioxan-2-ylmethyl)-guanidine sulfate; an antihypertensive agent.

guanyl (gwahn'il). The radical of guanine.
g. cyclase, guanylate cyclase.

guanylate cyclase (gwahn'i-lāt) [EC 4.6.1.2]. Guanylyl cyclase; guanyl cyclase; analogous to adenylate (adenylyl) cyclase, but cyclizing guanosine triphosphate to guanosine 3':5'-cyclic phosphate.

guanylic acid (GMP) (gwă-nil'ik). Guanine ribonucleotide; guanosine 5'-phosphate; a major component of ribonucleic acids.

guanyloribonuclease (gwahn'i-lō-rī-bō-nū'klē-ās). *Ribonuclease* T_1.

guanylyl (gwahn'i-lil). The radical of guanylic acid.
g. cyclase, Guanylate cyclase.

guarana (gwah-rah-nah') [Native Brazilian word]. A dried paste of the crushed seeds of *Paullinia cupana* (family Sapindaceae), a vine extensively cultivated in Brazil. It contains guaranine (caffeine), saponin, a volatile oil, and paullinitannic acid. Has been used for the relief of headache.

guaranine (gwahr'ă-nēn). Caffeine.

guarding (gard'ing). A spasm of muscles to minimize motion or agitation of sites affected by injury or disease.
abdominal g., a spasm of abdominal wall muscles, detected on palpation, to protect inflamed abdominal viscera from pressure; usually a result of inflammation of the peritoneal surface as in appendicitis, diverticulitis, or generalized peritonitis.

Guarnieri, Giuseppi, Italian physician, 1856–1918. See G.'s gelatin *agar, bodies.*

gubernaculum (gū'ber-nak'yū-lŭm) [L. a helm]. A fibrous cord connnecting two structures.
g. den'tis, a connective tissue band uniting the tooth sac with the gum.
Hunter's g., obsolete term for g. testis.
g. tes'tis [NA], a mesenchymal column of tissue that connects the fetal testis to the developing scrotum; it appears to play a significant role in testicular descent.

Gubler, Adolphe, French physician, 1821–1879. See G.'s *hemiplegia, line, paralysis, syndrome, tumor;* Millard-G. *syndrome.*

Gudden, Bernhard A. von, German neurologist 1824–1886. See G.'s *commissures, ganglion,* tegmental *nuclei.*

Guéneau de Mussy, Noël F.O., French physician, 1813–1885. See G. de M.'s *point.*

Guérin, Alphonase F.M., French surgeon, 1816–1895. See G's *fold, fracture, glands, sinus, valve.*

Guérin, Camille, French bacteriologist, 1872–1961. See Bacille bilié de Calmette-G.; Calmette-G. *vaccine.*

guidance (gī'dăns). **1.** The act of guiding. **2.** A guide.
condylar g., condylar guide; the mechanical device on an articulator which is intended to produce g. in articulator movement, similar to those produced by the paths of the condyles in the temporomandibular joints. See also condylar guidance *inclination.*
incisal g., incisal path; the influence on mandibular movements caused by the contacting surfaces of the mandibular and maxillary anterior teeth during eccentric excursions.

guide (gīd). **1.** To lead in a set course. **2.** Any device or instrument by which another is led into its proper course, *e.g.,* a grooved director, a catheter g.
anterior g., incisal g.
catheter g., a flexible metallic wire or thin sound over which a catheter is passed to advance it into its proper position, as in a blood vessel or the urethra. See also stylet.
condylar g., condylar *guidance.*
incisal g., anterior g.; in dentistry, that part of an articulator on which the anterior g. pin rests to maintain the vertical dimension of occlusion and the incisal g. angle as established by the incisal guidance; may be adjustable, with a superior surface that may be changed to provide variations in the incisal g. angle, or customized, being individually formed in plastic to allow other than straight line incisal guidance in eccentric movements.
mold g., a g. used to specify the shape of artificial teeth, or of an artificial tooth.

guideline (gīd'līn). A marking in the form of a line that serves as a guide or reference.
clasp g., survey *line.*
Cummer's g., survey *line.*

Guillain, Georges, French neurologist, 1876–1961. See G.-Barré *reflex, syndrome;* Landry-Guillain-Barré *syndrome.*

guillotine (gil'ō-tēn, gē'ō-tēn) [Fr. an instrument for execution by decapitation]. An instrument in the shape of a metal ring through which runs a sliding knifeblade, used in cutting off an enlarged tonsil.

guinea green B (gin'ē) [C.I. 42085]. An acid diaminotriphenylmethane dye, used as an indicator for H-ion determinations (changing at pH 6.0 from magenta to green) and as a fiber cytoplasmic stain in certain Masson trichrome staining procedures.

guinea pig (gin'ē). *Cavia porcellus.*

Guinon, Georges, French physician, 1859–1929. See G.'s *disease.*

Guldberg, C., Norwegian chemist, 1862–1902. See G.-Waage *law.*

gullet (gŭl'et) [L. *gula,* throat]. Throat (1).

L-gulonic acid (gū-lon'ik). Oxidation product (–CHO → -COOH) of L-gulose; reduction product of glucuronic acid (–CHO → CH_2OH); a precursor (except in primates and guinea pigs) of ascorbic acid via L-gulonolactone.

L-gulonolactone (gū-lon'ō-lak-tōn). Dihydroascorbic acid; the immediate precursor of ascorbic acid in those animals capable of ascorbic acid biosynthesis.

gulose (gū'lōs). One of the eight pairs (D and L) of aldoses.

gum (gŭm). **1** [L. *gummi*]. The dried exuded sap from a number of trees and shrubs, forming an amorphous brittle mass; it usually forms a mucilaginous solution in water. **2** [A.S. *goma,* jaw]. Gingiva.
g. arabic, acacia. See also arabin.
Bassora g., a g. from Iran and Turkey, resembling tragacanth, acacia, and the gummy exudate of cherry and plum trees; used in making storax.
g. benjamin, g. benzoin, benzoin.
British g., dextrin.
eucalyptus g., red g.; a dried gummy exudation from *Eucalyptus rostrata* and other species of *Eucalyptus* (family Myrtaceae); used as an astringent (in gargles and troches) and as an antidiarrheal agent.
ghatti g., Indian g.
guaiac g., guaiac.
guar g., the ground endosperms of *Cyamopsis tetragonolobus;* used in pharmaceutical jelly formulations.
Indian g., ghatti g.; an exudation from *Anogeisus latifolia* (family Combrettaceae); the mucilage is used as a substitute for acacia mucilage.

karaya g., sterculia g.
locust g., algaroba.
g. opium, opium.
red g., eucalyptus g.
senegal g., the g. of *Acacia senegal.* See acacia.
starch g., dextrin.
sterculia g., karaya g.; the dried gummy exudation from *Sterculia urens, S. villosa, S. tragacantha,* or other species of *Sterculia,* or from *Cochlospermum gossypium* or other species of *Cochlospermum* (family Bixaceae); used as a hydrophilic laxative and in the manufacture of lotions and pastes.
wheat g., gluten.

gumboil (gŭm'boyl). Gingival *abscess.*

gumma, pl. **gummata** or **gummas** (gŭm'ă, ăz, -ă-tă) [L. *gummi,* gum, fr. G. *kommi*] Gummatous or nodular syphilid; syphiloma; an infectious granuloma that is characteristic of tertiary syphilis, but does not always develop, and that may be solitary (as large as 8 to 10 cm in diameter) or multiple and diffusely scattered (1 mm or less in diameter). G.'s are characterized by an irregular central portion that is firm, sometimes partially hyalinized, and consisting of coagulative necrosis in which "ghosts" of structures may be recognized; a poorly defined middle zone of epithelioid cells, with occasional multinucleated giant cells; and a peripheral zone of fibroblasts and numerous capillaries, with infiltrated lymphocytes and plasma cells. As g.'s become older, an irregular scar or rounded fibrous nodule persists.

gummatous (gŭm'ă-tŭs). Syphilomatous; pertaining to or characterized by the features of a gumma.

gummy (gŭm'ē). **1.** Resembling or of the consistency of gum. **2.** Pertaining to the gross consistency of or resembling a gumma.

Gumprecht, Ferdinand, German physician, *1864. See Klein-G. shadow *nuclei,* G.'s *shadows.*

Gunn, Robert Marcus, British ophthalmologist, 1850–1909. See G. *phenomenon;* G.'s or Marcus G.'s *dots, sign, syndrome;* Marcus G. *pupil.*

Günning, Jan W., Dutch chemist, 1827–1901. See G.'s *reaction.*

Gunning, Thomas B., U.S. dentist, 1813–1889. See G. *splint.*

Günther, Hans, German physician, 1884–1956. See G.'s *disease.*

Günz, Justus G., German anatomist, 1714–1751. See G.'s *ligament.*

Günzberg, Alfred, German physician, *1861. See G.'s *reagent, test.*

Guo Symbol for guanosine.

gurney (gŭr'nē) [Scottish *gurn,* to grimace in pain; Sir Goldsworthy *Gurney,* British physician and inventor, 1793–1875]. A stretcher or cot with wheels used to transport hospital patients.

Gussenbauer, Carl, German surgeon, 1842–1903. See G.'s *suture.*

gustation (gŭs-tā'shŭn) [L. *gustatio,* fr. *gusto,* pp. *-atus,* to taste]. **1.** The act of tasting. **2.** The sense of taste.

gustatory (gŭs'tă-tōr-ē). Relating to gustation, or taste.

gut (gŭt) [A.S.]. **1.** Intestinum. **2.** Embryonic digestive tube. **3.** Abbreviated term for catgut. See also suture.
blind g., cecum.
postanal g., postcloacal g.; tailgut; an extension of the hindgut caudal to the point at which the anal opening is formed.
postcloacal g., postanal g.
preoral g., Seessel's *pocket.*

Guthrie, George J., British ophthalmologist, 1785–1856. See G.'s *muscle.*

Guthrie, R., U.S. pediatrician, *1916. See G. *test.*

Gutmann, Carl, German physician, *1872. See Michaelis-G. *body.*

gutta (gt.), pl. **guttae (gtt.)** (gŭt'ă, -ē) [L.]. A drop.
g. sere'na, amaurosis.

gutta-percha (gut'ă-per'chă) [Malay *gatah,* gum, + *percha,* the name of a tree]. The coagulated, purified, dried, milky juice of trees of the genera *Palaguium* and *Payena* (family Sapotaceae); used as a temporary filling material in dentistry, and in the manufacture of splints and electrical insulators; a solution is used as a substitute for collodion, as a protective, and to seal incised wounds.

guttat. Abbreviation for L. *guttatim,* drop by drop.

guttate (gŭt'tāt). Of the shape of, or resembling, a drop, characterizing certain cutaneous lesions.

guttural (gŭt'er-ăl). Relating to the throat.

gutturotetany (gŭt'er-ō-tet'ă-nē) [L. *guttur,* throat, + G. *tetanos,* convulsive tension]. Laryngeal spasm causing a temporary stutter.

Gutzeit, Max A.G., German chemist, 1847–1915. See G.'s *test.*

Guyon, Felix J.C., French surgeon, 1831–1920. See G.'s *amputation, isthmus, sign.*

Gy Abbreviation for gray.

Gymnamoebida (jim-nă-mē'bi-dă) [G. *gymnos,* naked, + *amoibē,* change (ameba)]. An order of naked amebae lacking a shell (testa), although there may be an enveloping layer of condensed ectoplasm; includes the genus *Amoeba.*

gymnastics (jim-nas'tiks) [G. *gymnos,* naked]. Muscular exercise, performed indoors, as distinguished from athletics, and usually by means of special apparatus.
Swedish g., Swedish *movements.*

Gymnoascaceae (jim'nō-as-kā'sē-ē). A family of fungi which includes the ascomycetous state of many of the dermatophytes and several of the systemic pathogens for man (*Histoplasma capsulatum, Blastomyces dermatitidis,* etc.). Until the sexual forms were recognized, these pathogens were classified with Fungi Imperfecti.

gymnocyte (jim'nō-sīt) [G. *gymnos,* naked, + *kytos,* hollow (cell)]. Obsolete term referring to a cell without a limiting membrane.

gymnophobia (jim-nō-fō'bē-ă) [G. *gymnos,* naked, + *phobos,* fear]. Morbid dread of the sight of a naked person or of an uncovered part of the body.

GYN Abbreviation for gynecology.

gyn-, gyne-, gyneco-, gyno- [G. *gynē,* woman]. Combining forms denoting relationship to a woman.

gynandrism (ji-nan'drizm, gī'nan-drizm) [gyn- + G. *anēr* (*andr-*), man]. A developmental abnormality characterized by hypertrophy of the clitoris and union of the labia majora, simulating in appearance the penis and scrotum.

gynandroblastoma (ji-nan'drō-blas-tō'mă, gī-). **1.** Arrhenoblastoma. **2.** A rare variety of arrhenoblastoma of the ovary, containing granulosa or theca cell elements and producing simultaneous androgenic and estrogenic effects.

gynandroid (gī-nan'droyd, jī-) [gyn- + G. *anēr* (*andr-*), man, + *eidos,* resemblance]. An individual exhibiting gynandrism.

gynandromorphism (gī-nan-drō-mōr'fizm, jī-) [gyn- + G. *anēr* (*andr-*), man, + *morphē,* form]. An abnormal combination of male and female characteristics.

gynandromorphous (gī-nan-drō-mōr'fŭs, jī-). Having both male and female characteristics.

gynatresia (gī-nă-trē'zē-ă, jī-). [gyn- + G. *a-* priv. + *trēsis,* a hole]. Occlusion of some part of the female genital tract, especially occlusion of the vagina by a thick membrane.

gyne-, gyneco-. See gyn-.

gynecic (gī-nē'sik, jī-). Pertaining to or associated with women.

gynecogenic (gī'nĕ-kō-jen'ik, jin'ĕ-). **1.** Giving birth predominantly to females. **2.** Obsolete term meaning productive of female characteristics.

gynecography (gī-nĕ-kog'ră-fē, jin'ĕ-) [gyne- + G. *graphō,* to write]. Hysterosalpingography.

gynecoid (gī'nĕ-koyd, jin'ĕ-) [gyneco- + G. *eidos,* resemblance]. Resembling a woman in form and structure.

gynecologic, gynecological (gī'nĕ-kō-loj'ik, -loj'i-kăl, jin'ĕ-). Relating to gynecology.

gynecologist (gī-nĕ-kol'ō-jist, jī-nĕ-). A physician specializing in gynecology.

gynecology (GYN) (gī-nĕ-kol'ō-jē, jin-ĕ-) [gyneco- + G. *logos,* study]. The medical specialty concerned with diseases of the female genital tract, as well as endocrinology and reproductive physiology of the female.

gynecomania (gī'nĕ-kō-mā'nē-ă, jin'ĕ-) [gyneco- + G. *mania,* frenzy]. Morbid or excessive desire for women.

gynecomastia, gynecomasty (gī'nĕ-kō-mas'tē-ă, -mas'tē; jin'ĕ-) [gyneco- + G. *mastos,* breast]. Excessive development of the male mammary glands, due mainly to ductal proliferation with periductal edema; frequently secondary to increased estrogen levels, but mild g. may occur in normal adolescence.

gynephobia (gī-nĕ-fō'bē-ă, jin-ĕ-) [gyne- + G. *phobos,* fear]. Morbid fear of women or of the female sex.

gyniatrics (gī-nē-at'riks, jin-ē-) [gyn- + G. *iatrikos,* of medicine or surgery]. Gyniatry; treatment of the diseases of women.

gyniatry (gī-nē-at'rē,jin-ē). Gyniatrics.

gyno-. See gyn-.

gynocardia oil (gī-nō-kar'dē-ă). Chaulmoogra oil.

gynogenesis (gī-nō-jen'ĕ-sis, jin-ō-) [gyno- + G. *genesis,* production]. Egg development activated by a spermatozoon, but to which the male gamete contributes no genetic material.

gynopathy (gī-nop'ă-thē, jī-) [gyno- + G. *pathos,* suffering]. Any disease peculiar to women.

gynoplasty, gynoplastics (gī'nō-plas-tē, jin'ō-; gī'nō-plas-tiks, jīn'ō-) [gyno- + G. *plassō,* to form]. Reparative or plastic surgery of the female genital organs.

gypsum (jip'sŭm) [L. fr. G. *gypsos*] $CaSO_4 \cdot 2H_2O$; the natural hydrated form of calcium sulfate; a component of the stones, plasters, and investments used in dentistry.

gyrate (jī'rāt) [L. *gyro,* pp. *gyratus,* to turn round in a circle, *gyrus*] **1.** Of a convoluted or ring shape. **2.** To revolve.

gyration (jī-rā'shŭn). **1.** A circular motion or revolution. **2.** Arrangement of convolutions or gyri in the cerebral cortex.

gyrectomy (jī-rek'tō-mē) [G. *gyros,* ring, + *ektomē,* excision]. Excision of a cerebral gyrus.
frontal g., topectomy.

gyrencephalic (jī'ren-sĕ-fal'ik) [G. *gyros,* ring (gyrus), + *enkaphalē,* brain]. Denoting brains, such as that of man, in which the cerebral cortex has convolutions, in contrast to the lissencephalic (smooth) brains of small mammals such as the rodents.

gyri (jī'rī) [L.]. Plural of gyrus.

gyrochrome (jī'rō-krōm) [G. *gyros,* a ring, circle, + *chrōma,* a color]. Denoting a nerve cell in which the chromophil substance is arranged roughly in rings.

Gyromitra esculenta (gī-rō-mē'tră es-kyū-len'tă). *Helvella esculenta;* a species of mushroom that may produce a monomethylhydrazine toxin which causes nausea, diarrhea, and other symptoms; in severe cases death may occur.

gyrosa (jī-rō'să) [L.]. Sham-movement *vertigo.*

gyrose (jī'rōs) [G. *gyros,* circle]. Marked by irregular curved lines like the surface of a cerebral hemisphere.

gyrospasm (jī'rō-spazm) [G. *gyros,* circle, + *spasmos,* spasm]. Spasmodic rotary movements of the head.

GYRUS

gyrus, gen. and pl. **gy'ri** (jī'rŭs, -rī) [L. fr. G. *gyros,* circle] [NA]. Convolution (2); one of the prominent rounded elevations that form the cerebral hemispheres, each consisting of an exposed superficial portion and a portion hidden from view in the wall and floor of the sulcus.
angular g., g. angularis.
g. angula'ris [NA], angular g. or convolution; a folded convolution in the inferior parietal lobule formed by the union of the posterior ends of the superior and middle temporal gyri.
annectent g., transitional g.
anterior central g., g. precentralis.
anterior piriform g., prepiriform g.
ascending frontal g., g. precentralis.
ascending parietal g., g. postcentralis.
gy'ri bre'ves in'sulae [NA], short gyri of insula; several short, radiating gyri converging toward the base of the insula, composing the anterior two-thirds of the insular cortex.
callosal g., g. cinguli.
central gyri, the gyri precentralis and postcentralis.
gy'ri cer'ebri [NA], **gyri of cerebrum,** the gyri or convolutions of the cerebral cortex.
cingulate g., g. cinguli.
g. cin'guli [NA], cingulate g. or convolution; callosal g. or convolution; falciform lobe; lobus falciformis; a long, curved convolution of the medial surface of the cortical hemisphere, arched over the corpus callosum from which it is separated by the deep sulcus corporis callosi; together with the g. parahippocampalis, with which it is continuous behind the corpus callosum, it forms the g. fornicatus.
deep transitional g., the transverse g. of the embryo which in development becomes buried in the depth of the central sulcus of the cerebral hemisphere.
dentate g., g. dentatus.
g. denta'tus [NA], dentate g. or fascia; fascia dentata hippocampi; one of the two interlocking gyri composing the hippocampus, the other one being the cornu ammonis.
fasciolar g., g. fasciolaris.
g. fasciola'ris [NA], fasciolar g.; fascia cinerea; fasciola cinerea; a small paired band that passes around the splenium of the corpus callosum from the lateral longitudinal stria to the g. dentatus.
g. fornica'tus, (1) the horseshoe-shaped cortical convolution bordering the hilus of the cerebral hemisphere; its upper limb is formed by the g. cinguli, its lower by the g. parahippocampalis; **(2)** used previously to refer to the entire limbic system.
g. fronta'lis infe'rior [NA], inferior frontal g. or convolution; a broad convolution on the convexity of the frontal lobe of the cerebrum between the inferior frontal sulcus and the sylvian fissure; divided by branches of the sylvian fissure into three parts: pars basilaris (opercularis), pars triangularis, and pars orbitalis; the first two constitute a portion of the frontal operculum.
g. fronta'lis me'dius [NA], middle frontal g. or convolution; a convolution on the convexity of each frontal lobe of the cerebrum running in an anteroposterior direction between the superior and inferior frontal sulci.
g. fronta'lis supe'rior [NA], superior frontal g. or convolution; marginal g.; a broad convolution running in an anteroposterior direction on the medial edge of the convex surface and of each frontal lobe.
fusiform g., g. fusiformis.
g. fusifor'mis, g. occipitotemporalis lateralis; fusiform g.; lateral

occipitotemporal g.; lobulus fusiformis; an extremely long convolution extending lengthwise over the inferior aspect of the temporal and occipital lobes, demarcated medially by the sulcus collateralis from the lingual g. and the anterior part of the parahippocampal g., laterally by the sulcus temporalis inferior from the inferior temporal g.
Heschl's gyri, gyri temporales transversi.
hippocampal g., g. parahippocampalis.
inferior frontal g., g. frontalis inferior.
inferior occipital g., a g. situated below the lateral occipital sulcus on the lower part of the lateral surface of the occipital lobe.
inferior parietal g., *lobulus* parietalis inferior.
inferior temporal g., g. temporalis inferior.
gy'ri in'sulae [NA], the gyri breves insulae and g. longus insulae.
interlocking gyri, several small gyri in the walls of the central sulcus of the hemisphere; the opposed gyri interlock with one another.
lateral occipitotemporal g., g. fusiformis.
lingual g., g. lingualis.
g. lingua'lis [NA], g. occipitotemporalis medialis; lingual g.; medial occipitotemporal g.; a relatively short horizontal convolution on the inferomedial aspect of the occipital and temporal lobes, demarcated from the lateral occipitotemporal or fusiform g. by the deep sulcus collateralis, from the cuneus by the calcarine sulcus; its anterior extreme abuts the isthmus of the parahippocampal g.; the medial or upper strip of the g. forming the lower bank of the calcarine sulcus corresponds to the inferior half of the area striata or primary visual cortex and represents the contralateral upper quadrant of the binocular field of vision.
long g. of insula, g. longus insulae.
g. lon'gus in'sulae [NA], long g. of the insula; the most posterior and longest of the slender straight gyri that compose the insula.
marginal g., g. frontalis superior.
medial occipitotemporal g., g. lingualis.
middle frontal g., g. frontalis medius.
middle temporal g., g. temporalis medius.
occipital gyri, see inferior occipital g. and superior occipital g.
g. occip'itotempora'lis latera'lis [NA], g. fusiformis.
g. occip'itotempora'lis media'lis [NA], g. lingualis.
orbital gyri, gyri orbitales.
gy'ri orbita'les [NA], orbital gyri; a number of small, irregular convolutions occupying the concave inferior surface of each frontal lobe of the cerebrum.
parahippocampal g., g. parahippocampalis.
g. par'ahippocampa'lis [NA], parahippocampal g.; hippocampal g. or convolution; a long convolution on the medial surface of the temporal lobe, forming the lower part of the g. fornicatus, extending from behind the splenium corporis callosi forward along the g. dentatus of the hippocampus from which it is demarcated by the hippocampal fissure. The anterior extreme of the g. curves back upon itself, forming the uncus, the major location of the olfactory cortex. See also entorhinal *area.*
paraterminal g., g. paraterminalis.
g. paratermina'lis [NA], paraterminal g. See g. subcallosus.
postcentral g., g. postcentralis.
g. postcentra'lis [NA], postcentral g.; posterior central g. or convolution; ascending parietal g. or convolution; the anterior convolution of the parietal lobe, bounded in front by the central sulcus (fissure of Rolando) and posteriorly by the interparietal sulcus.
posterior central g., g. postcentralis.
precentral g., g. precentralis.
g. precentra'lis [NA], anterior central g. or convolution; ascending frontal g. or convolution; the posterior convolution of the frontal lobe bounded posteriorly by the central sulcus and anteriorly by the precentral sulcus.
prepiriform g., anterior piriform g.; a g. covering deeply placed amygdaloid nucleus; concerned with olfactory function.
g. rec'tus [NA], straight g.; a g. running along the medial part of the orbital surface of the frontal lobe of the cerebral hemisphere. It is bounded laterally by the olfactory sulcus.
Retzius' g., the intralimbic g. in the cortical portion of the rhinencephalon.
short gyri of the insula, gyri breves insulae.
splenial g., the band of cortex on the medial surface of the cerebral hemisphere which passes around the splenium of the corpus callosum, narrowing anteriorly and finally blending with the indusium griseum.
straight g., g. rectus.
subcallosal g., g. subcallosus.
g. subcallo'sus [NA], g. paraterminalis; pedunculus corporis callosi; area subcallosa; subcallosal g. or area; peduncle of the corpus callosum; paraterminal g. or body; corpus paraterminale; Zuckerkandl's convolution; a slender vertical whitish band immediately anterior to the lamina terminalis and anterior commissure; contrary to its name, it is not a cortical convolution but is the ventral continuation of the septum pellucidum.
superior frontal g., g. frontalis superior.
superior occipital g., a g. lying above the lateral occipital sulcus on the lateral surface of the occipital lobe.
superior parietal g., *lobulus* parietalis superior.
superior temporal g., g. temporalis superior.
supracallosal g., *indusium* griseum.
supramarginal g., g. supramarginalis.
g. supramargina'lis [NA], supramarginal g. or convolution; a folded convolution capping the posterior extremity of the lateral (sylvian) sulcus; together with the g. angularis, it forms the inferior half of the parietal lobe.
g. tempora'lis infe'rior [NA], inferior temporal g. or convolution; third temporal convolution; a sagittal convolution on the inferolateral border of the temporal lobe of the cerebrum, separated from the middle temporal g. by the inferior temporal sulcus. On the inferior surface of the temporal lobe it is separated from the medial occipitotemporal g. by the occipitotemporal sulcus. It includes the lateral occipitotemporal g.
g. tempora'lis me'dius [NA], middle temporal g. or convolution; second temporal convolution; a longitudinal g. on the lateral surface of the temporal lobe, between the superior and inferior temporal sulci.
g. tempora'lis supe'rior [NA], superior temporal g. or convolution; first temporal convolution; a longitudinal g. on the lateral surface of the temporal lobe between the lateral (sylvian) fissure and the superior temporal sulcus.
gy'ri tempora'les transver'si [NA], transverse temporal gyri or convolutions; Heschl's gyri; two or three convolutions running transversely on the upper surface of the temporal lobe bordering on the lateral (sylvian) fissure, separated from each other by the transverse temporal sulci.
transitional g., annectent g.; transitional convolution; a small convolution connecting two lobes or two main gyri in the depth of a sulcus.
transverse temporal gyri, gyri temporales transversi.
uncinate g., uncus (2).

H

H Abbreviation or symbol for hyperopia or hyperopic; horizontal; Hauch; Holzknecht *unit;* henry; hydrogen; the Fraunhofer line at λ 3968 due to calcium.

H Symbol for enthalpy, heat content, in the equation for free energy.

H^+ Symbol for hydrogen ion, the proton.

^1H, ^2H, ^3H Symbol for hydrogen-1, hydrogen-2, and hydrogen-3 respectively.

h Symbol for hecto-.

h Symbol for Planck's *constant.*

Ha Symbol proposed for hahnium.

HAA Abbreviation for hepatitis-associated *antigen.*

Haab, Otto, Swiss ophthalmologist, 1850–1931. See H.'s *magnet, reflex.*

Haase's rule. See under rule.

Habel, Karl, U.S. physician and virologist, *1908. See H. *test.*

habena, pl. **habenae** (hă-bē'nă, -bē'nē) [L. strap]. **1.** A frenum or restricting fibrous band. **2.** A restraining bandage. **3.** Habenula (2).

habenal, habenar (hab'ĕ-năl, hă-bē'năr). Relating to a habena.

habenula, pl. **habenulae** (ha-ben'yū-lă, -lē) [L.]. **1.** Frenulum. **2** [NA]. Habena (3); in neuroanatomy, the term originally denoted the stalk of the pineal gland (pineal habenula; pedunculus of pineal body), but gradually came to refer to a neighboring group of nerve cells with which the pineal gland was believed to be associated, the nucleus habenulae. Currently, the NA term refers exclusively to this circumscript cell mass in the dorsomedial thalamus, embedded in the posterior end of the stria medullaris from which it receives most of its afferent fibers. By way of the fasciculus retroflexus (habenulointerpeduncular tract) it projects to the interpeduncular nucleus and other paramedian cell groups of the midbrain tegmentum. Despite its proximity to the pineal stalk, no habenulopineal fiber connection is known to exist. It is a part of the epithalamus.
h. of cecum, extension of the mesocolic tenia, dorsal or ventral to the terminal ileum.
Haller's h., Scarpa's h.; rarely used term for the cordlike remains of the vaginal process of the peritoneum.
haben'ulae perfora'ta, *foramina* nervosa.
pineal h., the peduncle or stalk of the pineal gland. See habenula (2).
Scarpa's h., Haller's h.
h. urethra'lis, one of two fine, whitish lines running from the meatus urethrae to the clitoris in girls and young women; the vestiges of the anterior part of the corpus spongiosum.

habenular (hă-ben'yū-lăr). Relating to a habenula, especially the stalk of the pineal body.

Haber, Henry, 20th century British dermatologist. See H.'s *syndrome.*

Habermann, R., German dermatologist, *1884. See Mucha-H. *disease, syndrome.*

hab'it [L. *habec,* pp. *habitus,* to have]. **1.** An act, behavioral response, practice, or custom established in one's reportoire by frequent repetition of the same act. See also addiction. **2.** A basic variable in the study of conditioning and learning used to designate a new response learned either by association or by being followed by a reward or reinforced event.

habituation (ha-bit-chū-ā'shŭn). **1.** The process of forming a habit, referring generally to psychological dependence on the continued use of a drug to maintain a sense of well-being, which can result in drug addiction. **2.** The method by which the nervous system reduces or inhibits responsiveness during repeated stimulation.

habitus (hab'i-tŭs) [L. habit]. The physical characteristics of a person.
fetal h., fetal attitude; relationship of one fetal part to another.
gracile h., a frail, underweight appearance, characteristic of the child with an atrial septal defect.

habromania (hab-rō-mā'nē-ă) [G. *habros,* graceful, + *mania,* insanity]. Morbid impulse toward gaiety.

Habronema (ha-brō-nē'mă) [G. *habros,* graceful, delicate, + *nēma,* a thread]. A genus of spiruroid nematodes inhabiting the stomach of horses. The larvae develop in housefly and stable fly maggots living in manure, become infective when the fly larvae pupate, and are carried by adult flies to open wounds on horses, where they are left and cause cutaneous habronemiasis; reinfection of the horse's stomach by *H.* occurs by accidental ingestion of infected flies or from licking wounds in which infective larvae are found.
H. ma'jus, one of two species (the other being *H. microstoma*) similar in appearance, hosts, distribution, and life cycle to *H. muscae;* the intermediate host is the stable fly, *Stomoxys calcitrans.*
H. megas'toma, a species that causes tumors in gastric mucosa containing large numbers of the small nematodes; the larvae cause cutaneous habronemiasis; the intermediate host is the common housefly, *Musca domestica.*
H. micros'toma, see *H. majus.*
H. mus'cae, a species that occurs in the stomach of the horse, mule, ass, or zebra; the intermediate host is the common housefly, *Musca domestica,* or related flies.

habronemiasis (hab'rō-nē-mī'ă-sis). Infection of horses with any species of *Habronema;* commonly denotes wound infections that contain the larvae of this worm.
cutaneous h., summer sores; chronic granulomatous sores on the skin of horses caused by fly-borne larvae of *Draschia megastoma* (primarily), *Habronema muscae,* and *H. majus* which are deposited in skin wounds; the lesions are characterized by being pulpy and persistent but usually regress spontaneously in winter.

hacking (hak'ing). A chopping stroke made with the edge of the hand in massage.

Hadfield, Geoffrey, British physician, *1889. See Clarke-H. *syndrome.*

Hadrurus (hă-drū'rŭs) [G. *hadros,* thick, stout, + *ouro,* tail]. A genus of scorpions found in the southwestern U.S., characterized by numerous setae on the stinger; the commonest species is *H. arizonensis,* the olive hairy scorpion. See also Scorpionida.

Haeckel, Ernst H., German naturalist, 1834–1919. See H.'s gastrea *theory, law.*

haem-. For words so beginning, and not found here, see under hem-.

Haemadipsa ceylonica (hē-mă-dip'să sā-lon'i-kă) [G. *haima,* blood, + *dipsa,* thirst]. A species of land leech found in Sri Lanka; it attaches itself to the skin of animals or man. Its bite is painful, and numerous bites may cause anemia.

Haemamoeba (hē-mă-mē'bă) [G. *haima,* blood, + *amoibē,* change]. Old term for ameboid protozoa now classified in the suborder Haemosporina, blood parasites that include the genus *Plasmodium.*

Haemaphysalis (hē-mă-fī'să-lis) [G. *haima,* blood, + *physaleos,* full of wind]. A genus of small, eyeless, inornate ticks that have festoons and a characteristic basis capituli. As larvae and nymphs, they are found chiefly on small mammals and birds; as adults, they are found on larger mammals and some birds. They are important as vectors of protozoa and viruses, (e.g., Kyasanur Forest disease virus), and may be carried long distances on migrating birds.

H. chordei'lis, the bird tick, a common tick of turkeys and upland game birds in North America.

H. cinnabar'ina [G. *kinnabarinos,* like cinnabar, vermilion]. a tick that occurs chiefly in the dry district of British Columbia; this species can cause ascending paraplegia or tick paralysis in both man and animals.

H. cinnabar'ina puncta'ta, a race of *H.* in Europe, North Africa, and Japan; larvae and nymphs feed on terrestrial reptiles, and adults on various domestic herbivores, rabbits, and hedgehogs; it transmits bovine babesiosis and anaplasmosis.

H. concin'na, common rodent tick species of the U.S.S.R. that is a vector and reservoir of tick typhus.

H. leach'i, a species of Africa, Asia, and Australia that occurs on domestic and wild carnivores, on small rodents, and occasionally on cattle; it transmits canine babesiosis and boutonneuse fever.

H. leporis-palus'tris [L. fem. of *paluster,* marshy], the rabbit tick, a tick species that occurs in all species of rabbits and on many wild birds in all parts of North America from Alaska to Mexico, and is important in the spread of Rocky Mountain spotted fever and tularemia among rabbits; it does not attack man or most domestic animals and does not spread these diseases to them, but serves to maintain the infection in reservoir hosts.

H. spiniger'a, a tropical forest species in India that is a vector of Kyasanur Forest disease; various rodents and insectivores serve as hosts of immature ticks of this species, which carry an arbovirus of the Russian spring-summer B group complex; monkeys act as reservoirs of human infection.

Haematopinus (hē'mă-tō-pī'nŭs) [G. *haima,* blood, + L. *pinus,* pine tree]. An important genus of sucking lice (family Haematopinidae) affecting swine and other domestic and wild animals; it is normally nonpathogenic. *H. asini* affects horses, mules, and asses; *H. eurysternus* and *H. quadripertusus,* cattle; and *H. suis,* swine.

Haemobartonella (hē'mō-bar-tō-nel'ă) [G. *haima,* blood, + dim. of A.S. *beretūn,* courtyard, grange, fr. *bere,* barley, + *tūn,* enclosure]. A genus of parasitic bacteria (order Rickettsiales) found in and on the surface of erythrocytes, but which rarely produce disease in animals without splenectomy. They are identical to *Eperythrozoon* species, except that *H.* species are not found free in the plasma nor are ring forms seen on the surface of infected erythrocytes. Species are found in laboratory rats and in dogs, cats, and other domestic animals. The type species is *H. muris.*

H. mu'ris, a species found in rats, mice, and hamsters; ectoparasites such as the rat louse, the flea, and possibly the bedbug are vectors; it is the type species of *H.*

Haemococcidium (hē'mō-kok-sid'ē-ŭm) [G. *haima,* blood, + *kokkos,* berry]. Old name for *Plasmodium* species.

Haemodipsus ventricosus (hē-mō-dip'sŭs ven-tri-kō'sŭs) [G. *haima,* blood, + *dipsos,* thirst; L. *venter* (*ventr-*), belly]. The rabbit louse, a transmitter of *Pasteurella tularensis.*

Haemogregarina (hē'mō-greg-ă-rī'nă) [G. *haima,* blood, + L. *grex,* a flock]. A sporozoan coccidian genus (order Eucoccidiida, family Haemogregarinidae) that parasitizes the blood cells of cold-blooded animals and the digestive system of invertebrate primary hosts in an obligatory two-host cycle.

Haemonchus (hē-mong'kŭs) [G. *haima,* blood, + *onchos,* spear]. An economically important genus of nematode parasites (family Trichostrongylidae) occurring in the abomasum of ruminant animals and causing severe anemia, especially in younger or previously unexposed animals. Some significant species are *H. placei* (in cattle, sheep, and goats), *H. similis* (in cattle and sheep), and *H. contortus,* the stomach, barberpole, or twisted wire worm of cattle, sheep, goats, and other ruminants, of which a few cases have been reported from man.

Haemophilus (hē-mof'i-lŭs) [G. *haima,* blood, + *philos,* fond]. *Hemophilus;* a genus of aerobic to facultatively anaerobic, nonmotile bacteria (family Brucellaceae) containing minute, Gram-negative, rod-shaped cells which sometimes form threads and are pleomorphic. These organisms are strictly parasitic, growing best, or only, on media containing blood. They may or may not be pathogenic. They occur in various lesions and secretions, as well as in normal respiratory tracts, of vertebrates. The type species is *H. influenzae.*

H. aegyp'ticus, a species that causes acute or subacute infectious conjunctivitis in warm climates.

H. aphroph'ilus, a species found in the blood and, rarely, on the heart valve as a cause of endocarditis.

H. ducrey'i, Ducrey's bacillus; a species which causes soft chancre (chancroid).

H. gallina'rum, a species that causes fowl coryza.

H. haemoglobinoph'ilus, a species which occurs in large numbers in preputial secretions of dogs.

H. haemolyt'icus, a species which is usually nonpathogenic but which, on rare occasions, causes subacute endocarditis.

H. influen'zae, influenza bacillus; Pfeiffer's or Weeks' bacillus; Koch-Weeks bacillus; a species found in the respiratory tract that causes acute respiratory infections, acute conjunctivitis, and purulent meningitis in children, rarely in adults; originally considered to be the cause of influenza, it is the type species of the genus *H.*

H. influen'zae-mur'ium, a species that causes conjunctivitis and respiratory infections in mice.

H. o'vis, a species that causes bronchial pneumonia and generalized hemorrhagic involvement in sheep.

H. parahaemoly'ticus, a species found in the upper respiratory tract and associated frequently with pharyngitis; occasionally causes subacute endocarditis.

H. parainfluen'zae, a species which is usually nonpathogenic but which occasionally causes subacute endocarditis.

H. pertus'sis, *Bordetella pertussis.*

H. su'is, a species, related to *H. influenzae,* found in swine and associated with influenza virus in the pnemonia of swine influenza.

Haemoproteus (hē'mō-prō'tē-ŭs) [G. *haima,* blood, + *Proteus,* a sea god who had the power of assuming different shapes]. A genus of sporozoa (suborder Haemosporina) parasitic in birds and reptiles, combined with *Leucocytozoon, Hepatocystis,* and other genera in the family Haemoproteidae. Schizogony occurs in endothelial cells of blood vessels, especially in the lungs of the host, while halter-shaped gametocytes are found in the red blood cells. Infection is transmitted by pupiparous Diptera, such as louse flies (Hippoboscidae) and by bloodsucking midges (*Culicoides*).

Haemosporina (hē'mō-spō-rī'nă) [G. *haima,* blood, + *sporos,* seed]. A suborder of coccidia (class Sporozoea) that lack syzygy, with separate development of macrogamete and microgamont, the latter producing eight flagellated microgametes; heteroxenous with merogany in vertebrates and sporogony in bloodsucking insects; includes the genera *Haemoproteus, Leucocytozoon,* and *Plasmodium.*

Haemostrongylus vaso'rum (hē'mō-stron'ji-lŭs) [G. *haima,* blood, + *strongylos,* round]. *Angiostrongylus vasorum.*

Haenel, Hans G., German neurologist, 1874–1942. See H.'s *symptom.*

Haffkine, Waldemar M.W., Russian physician, 1860–1930. See H.'s *vaccine.*

hafnium (haf'nē-ŭm) [L. *Hafniae,* Copenhagen]. A rare chemical element, symbol Hf, atomic no. 72, atomic weight 178.50.

Hagedorn, Werner, German surgeon, 1831–1894. See H. *needle.*

Hageman. Surname of person in whom deficiency of Hageman *factor* (*q.v.*) first observed.

hagiotherapy (hag'ē-ō-thăr'ă-pē) [G. *hagios,* sacred]. Treatment of the sick by contact with relics of the saints, visits to shrines, and other religious observances.

Haglund, S.E. Patrick, Swedish orthopedist, 1870–1937. See H.'s *deformity, disease.*

Hahn's oxine reagent. See under reagent.

hahnemannian (hah-nĕ-mahn'ē-an) [C.F.S. Hahnemann, Ger. physician and founder of homeopathy, 1755–1843]. Relating to homeopathy as taught by Hahnemann.

hahnium (Ha) (hahn'ē-ŭm) [Otto *Hahn,* Ger. physical chemist, 1879–1968]. Name proposed for the artificially made element 105.

Haidinger, Wilhelm von, Austrian mineralogist, 1795–1871. See H.'s *brushes.*

Hailey, Hugh E., U.S. dermatologist, *1909. See Hailey and H. *disease.*

Hailey, W. Howard, U.S. dermatologist, *1898. See H. and Hailey *disease.*

hair (hār) [A.S. *haer*]. **1.** Pilus (1). **2.** One of the fine hairlike processes of the auditory cells of the labyrinth, and of other sensory cells, called auditory h.'s, sensory h.'s, etc.

auditory h.'s, cilia on the free surface of the auditory cells.

bamboo h., trichorrhexis invaginata; h. with nodules along the shaft caused by intermittent fracturing and telescoping of the h., with intervening lengths of normal h., giving the appearance of bamboo; seen in Netherton's syndrome.

bayonet h., a spindle-shaped developmental defect occurring at the tapered end of the h.

beaded h., monilethrix.

burrowing h.'s, ingrown h.'s.

club h., a h. in resting state, prior to shedding, in which the bulb has become a club-shaped mass.

exclamation point h., the type of h. found at margins of patches of alopecia areata; the bulb is absent.

Frey's irritation h.'s, short h.'s of varying degrees of stiffness, set at right angles into the end of a light wooden handle; used for determining the presence and degree of irritability of pressure points in the skin.

ingrown h.'s, burrowing h.'s; pili cuniculati or incarnati; h.'s that grow at more acute angles than is normal, and in all directions; they incompletely clear the follicle, turn back in, and cause formation of pustules and papules; most commonly found on the bearded portion of the face and neck.

kinky h., tightly curled or bent h.

lanugo h., lanugo.

moniliform h., monilethrix.

nettling h.'s, sharp-pointed barbed h.'s of certain caterpillars which cause a dermatitis when brought in contact with the skin.

ringed h., thrix annulata; pili annulati; leukotrichia annularis; trichonosus versicolor; a condition in which the h. shows alternate pigmented and white segments.

Schridde's cancer h.'s, thick lusterless h.'s scattered in the beard and the temporal region, said to occur in cancerous patients but found also in persons with other cachectic conditions.

stellate h., h. split in several strands at the free end.

tactile h., the vibrissae or whiskers of animals such as rats and cats which have especially well developed touch endings in the follicular wall.

taste h.'s, hairlike projections of gustatory cells of taste buds; electron micrographs show them to be clusters of microvilli.

terminal h., a mature h.

twisted h.'s, *pili* torti.

vellus h., soft, downy h.

woolly h., tightly coiled h. with the texture of wool.

hair cast. A small, nodular accretion of epithelial cells and keratinous debris resulting from failure of the internal root sheath to disintegrate; it appears for 3 to 7 mm along the hair shaft.

hairworm (hār'werm). See *Trichostrongylus; Gordius.*

hairy (hār'ē). Pilar; pilary; pileous; pilose. **1.** Of or resembling hair. **2.** Covered with hair. See also hirsutism.

halation (hă-lā'shŭn). Blurring of the visual image by glare.

halazepam (hal-az'e-pam). 7-Chloro-1,3-dihydro-5-phenyl-1-(2,2,2-trifluoroethyl)-2*H*- 1,4-benzodiazepin-2-one; a benzodiazepine used in the management of anxiety disorders and for short-term relief of symptoms of anxiety.

halazone (hal'ă-zōn). *N,N-* (*N,N*-Dichlorosulfamyl)benzoic acid; a chloramine used for the sterilization of drinking water.

Halbeisen, William A. See Stryker-H. *syndrome.*

Halberstaedter, Ludwig, German physician, 1876–1949. See H.-Prowazek *bodies.*

halcinonide (hal-sin'ō-nīd). Pregn-4-ene-3,20-dione, 21-chloro-9-fluoro- 11-hydroxy- 16,17- [(1-methylethylidene)bis(oxy)]-, (11β, 16α)-; an anti-inflammatory corticosteroid used in topical preparations.

Haldane, John S., Scottish physiologist at Oxford, 1860–1936. See H. *chamber, effect, transformation, tube;* H.'s *apparatus,* H.-Priestley *sample.*

Hale's colloidal iron stain. See under stain.

Hales, Stephen, British physiologist, 1677–1761. See H.'s *piesimeter.*

halethazole (hă-leth'ă-zōl). 5-Chloro-2-[*p*-(diethylamino-ethoxy)phenyl]benzothiazole; an antiseptic with antifungal properties.

half-life (haf'līf). The period during which the radioactivity of a radioactive substance decreases to half of its original value; similarly applied to the decrease in activity of any unstable active substance with time. *Cf.* half-time.

biological h.-l., the time required for one-half of an administered radioactive substance to be lost through biological processes.

effective h.-l., the time required for one-half of an administered dose of radioactivity to be dissipated through a combination of physical decay and biological turnover.

physical h.-l., the time required for half of a given number of atoms, of a specific radionuclide, to undergo disintegration.

half-moon (haf'mūn). Lunula (1).

red h.-m., irregular red discoloration of the usually pale demilune at the base of the fingernail; may be seen in congestive failure, malignant disease, or liver disease, but not specific for any of these.

half-time (haf'tīm). The time, in a first-order chemical (or enzymic) reaction, for half of the substance (substrate) to be converted or to disappear. *Cf.* half-life.

halfway house (haf'wā hows). A facility for individuals who no longer require the complete facilities of a hospital or institution but are not yet prepared to return to their communities.

halibut liver oil (hal'i-bŭt). The fixed oil obtained from the fresh or suitably preserved livers of halibut species of the genus *Hippoglossus* (family Pleuronectidae); a supplementary source of vitamins A and D.

halide (hal'īd). A salt of a halogen.

haliphagia (hal-i-fā'jē-ă) [G. *hals,* salt, + *phagein,* to eat]. Ingestion of an excessive quantity of a salt or salts, especially of sodium chloride, calcium, magnesium, or potassium salts, or of sodium bicarbonate.

halisteresis (hă-lis-ter-ē'sis) [G. *hals,* salt, + *sterēsis,* privation, fr. *stereō,* to deprive]. Halosteresis; a deficiency of lime salts in the bones.

halisteretic (hă-lis-ter-et'ik). Relating to or marked by halisteresis.

halitosis (hal-i-tō'sis) [L. *halitus,* breath, + G. *-osis,* condition]. Fetor oris; ozostomia; stomatodysodia; a foul odor from the mouth.

halitus (hal'i-tŭs) [L., fr. *halo,* to breathe]. Any exhalation, as of a breath or vapor.

hallachrome (hal'ă-krōm). A quinone intermediate, derived from dopa, in the formation of melanin from tyrosine.

Hallé, Adrien J.M.N., French physician, 1859–1947. See H.'s *point.*

Haller, Albrecht v., Swiss physiologist, 1708–1777. See H.'s *ansa, annulus, arches, circle, cones, habenula, insula, line, plexus, rete,* vascular *tissue, tripod, tunica* vasculosa, *unguis, vas* aberrans.

Hallermann, Wilhelm, German ophthalmologist. See H.-Streiff *syndrome.*

Hallervorden, Julius, German neurologist, 1882–1965. See H. *syndrome;* H.-Spatz *disease.*

hallex, pl. **hallices** (hal'eks, hal'i-sēz) [L.]. Hallux.

Hallgren, Bertil. See H.'s *syndrome.*

Hallion, L., French physiologist, 1862–1940. See H.'s *test.*

Hallopeau, François H., French dermatologist, 1842–1919. See H.'s *acrodermatitis* continua, *disease.*

hallucal (hal'ū-kăl). Relating to the hallux.

hallucination (ha-lū'si-nā'shŭn) [L. *alucinari,* to wander in mind]. The apparent, often strong subjective perception of an object or event when no such situation is present.

formed visual h., h. composed of scenes, often landscapes.

hypnagogic h., h. occurring in the period between wakefulness and sleep.

lilliputian h., h. of reduced size of objects or persons.

stump h., phantom *limb.*

unformed visual h., h. composed of sparks, lights, or bursting spheres of light.

hallucinogen (ha-lū'si-nō-jen) [L. *alucinari,* to wander in mind, + G. *-gen,* producing]. A mind-altering chemical, drug, or agent, specifically a chemical whose most prominent pharmacologic action is on the central nervous system (*e.g.,* mescaline); in normal subjects, it elicits optical or auditory hallucinations, depersonalization, perceptual disturbances, and disturbances of thought processes.

hallucinogenic (ha-lū'si-nō-jen'ik). Relating to a hallucinogen.

hallucinosis (ha-lū-si-nō'sis). A syndrome, usually of organic origin, characterized by more or less persistent hallucinations.

hallus (hal'ŭs). Hallux.

hallux, pl. **halluces** (hal'ŭks, hal'yū-sēz) [a Mod. L. form for L. *hallex* (*hallic-*), great toe] [NA]. Hallex; hallus; pollex pedis; the great toe; the first digit of the foot.

h. doloro'sus, painful toe; a condition, usually associated with flatfoot, in which walking causes severe pain in the metatarsophalangeal joint of the great toe.

h. exten'sus, a deformity in which the great toe is held rigidly in the extended position.

h. flex'us, hammer toe involving the first toe.

h. mal'leus, hammer toe involving the first toe.

h. rig'idus, stiff toe; a condition in which there is stiffness in the first metatarsophalangeal joint; the joint may be the site of a hypertrophic arthritis.

h. val'gus, a deviation of the tip of the first toe, or main axis of the toe, toward the outer or lateral side of the foot.

h. va'rus, deviation of the main axis of the great toe to the inner side of the foot away from its neighbor.

halo (hā'lō) [G. *halōs,* threshing floor on which oxen trod a circle; the halo round the sun or moon]. **1.** A reddish yellow ring surrounding the optic disk, due to a widening of the scleral ring making the deeper structures visible. **2.** An annular flare of light surrounding a luminous body. **3.** Areola (4). **4.** A circular metal band used in a h. cast, attached to the skull with pins.

anemic h., pale, relatively avascular areas in the skin seen around vascular spiders, cherry angiomas, and sometimes in acute macular eruptions.

glaucomatous h., **(1)** glaucomatous ring; a yellowish white ring surrounding the optic disk, indicating atrophy of the choroid in glaucoma; **(2)** rainbow symptom; a h. surrounding lights, caused by corneal edema in glaucoma.

senile h., circumpapillary h. seen in choroidal atrophy of the aged.

haloanisone (hal-ō-an'i-sōn). Fluanisone.

halodermia (hal-ō-der'mē-ă) [halogen + G. *derma,* skin]. Dermatosis caused by ingestion or injection of halogens, most notably bromides and iodides.

halogen (hal'ō-jen) [G. *hals,* salt, + *-gen,* producing]. One of the chlorine group (fluorine, chlorine, bromine, iodine, astatine) of elements; h.'s form monobasic acids with hydrogen, and their hydroxides (fluorine forms none) are also monobasic acids.

halogenation (hal'ō-jĕ-nā'shŭn). Incorporation of one or more halogen atoms into a molecule.

Halogeton (hal-ō-jē'ton). A genus of plants (family Chenopodiaceae) on range lands in the western U.S. and other arid regions of the world; it causes poisoning in cattle and sheep because of the presence of soluble oxalates.

halometer (hal-om'ĕ-ter). An instrument used to measure the diffraction halo of a red blood cell; based on the premise that the halo of the large erythrocyte of pernicious anemia is smaller than that of the normal cell; the hazy colorless halo of normal size is characteristic of secondary anemia.

haloperidol (hal-ō-per'i-dol). A butyrophenone used as an antipsychotic; also used in Huntington's chorea and Gilles de la Tourette's disease.

halophil, halophile (hal'ō-fil, -fīl) [G. *hals,* salt, + *philos,* fond]. A microorganism whose growth is enhanced by or dependent on a high salt concentration.

halophilic (hal-ō-fil'ik). Requiring a high concentration of salt for growth.

haloprogin (hal-ō-prō'jin). 3-Iodo-2-propynyl 2,4,5-trichlorophenyl ether; an antifungal agent.

halosteresis (hă-los-tē-rē'sis). Halisteresis.

halothane (hal'ō-thān). 2-Bromo-2-chloro-1,1,1-trifluoroethane; a widely used potent nonflammable and nonexplosive inhalation anesthetic, with rapid onset and reversal; side effects include respiratory and cardiovascular depression, and sensitization to epinephrine-induced arrhythmias.

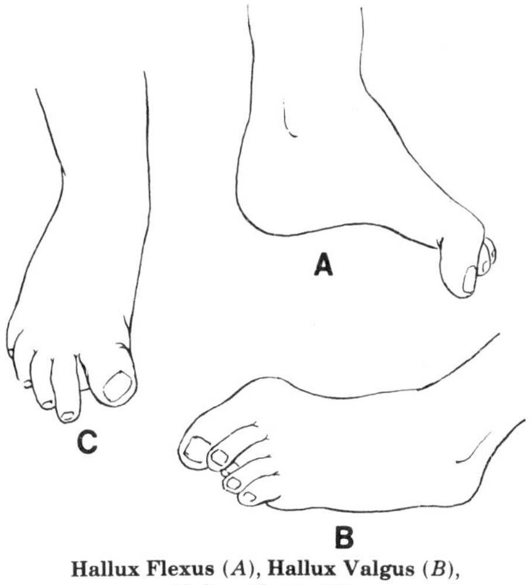

Hallux Flexus (*A*), **Hallux Valgus** (*B*), **Hallux Varus** (*C*)

Halstead, Ward C., U.S. psychologist, 1908–1968. See H.-Reitan *battery.*

Halsted, William Stewart, U.S. surgeon, 1852–1922. See H.'s *law, operation, suture.*

Halteridium (hawl-tĕ-rid'ē-ŭm) [G. *haltēres,* weights held in the hand in leaping]. Former name for *Haemoproteus.*

halzoun (hal'zūn) [Ar., snail]. Local name of a buccopharyngeal infection occurring in Lebanon, probably caused by pentastomid larvae of the dog tongue worm, *Linguatula serrata,* which wander into the throat of the human host after ingestion of infected raw sheep, or goat liver or lymph nodes.

Ham, Thomas Hale, U.S. physician, *1905. See H.'s *test.*

ham [A.S.]. **1.** Poples. **2.** The buttock and back part of the thigh.

hamamelis (ham'ă-mē'lis) [Mod. L., fr. G. *hama- mēlis,* fr. *hama,* together with, + *mēlon,* apple]. Witch hazel; a shrub or small tree, *Hamamelis virginiana* (family Harmarmelidaceae), whose bark and dried leaves have been used externally as an application to contusions and other injuries, in headache, and for the cure of noninflammatory hemorrhoids; the water, popularly known as "extract of witch hazel," is made from the bark.

hamartia (ham-ar'shē-ă) [G. *hamartion,* a bodily defect]. A localized developmental disturbance characterized by abnormal arrangement and/or combinations of the tissues normally present in the area.

hamartoblastoma (hă-mar'tō-blas-tō'mă) [hamartoma + blastoma]. A malignant neoplasm of undifferentiated anaplastic cells thought to be derived from a hamartoma.

hamartochondromatosis (ham-ar'tō-kon'drō-mă-tō'sis) [G. *hamartion,* bodily defect, + *chondros,* cartilage, + *-osis,* condition]. Neoplasm-like foci of cartilaginous tissue in sites where cartilage is a normal constituent, but in which the growth of cartilage cells is out of proportion to the other elements of the organ.

hamartoma (ham-ar-tō'mă) [G. *hamartion,* a bodily defect, + *-oma,* tumor]. A focal malformation that resembles a neoplasm, grossly and even microscopically, but results from faulty development in an organ; composed of an abnormal mixture of tissue elements, or an abnormal proportion of a single element, normally present in that site which develop and grow at virtually the same rate as normal components, and are not likely to result in compression of adjacent tissue (in contrast to a neoplasm).

fibrous h. of infancy, a tumor appearing usually in the upper arm or shoulder in the first two years of life and consisting of cellular fibrous tissue infiltrating the subcutis.

pulmonary h., adenochondroma; h. of the lung, producing a coin lesion composed primarily of cartilage and bronchial epithelium.

hamartomatous (ham-ar-tō'mă-tŭs). Relating to hamartoma.

hamartophobia (ham'ar-tō-fō'bē-ă) [G. *hamartia,* fault, + *phobos,* fear]. Morbid fear of error or sin.

hamatum (ha-mā'tŭm) [L. neut. of *hamatus,* hooked, fr. *hamus,* a hook]. *Os* hamatum.

hamaxophobia (hă-maks'ō-fō'bē-ă). Amaxophobia.

Hamburger, Hartog J., Dutch physiologist, 1859–1924. See H.'s *law, phenomenon.*

Hamilton, Frank Hastings, U.S. surgeon, 1813–1886. See H.'s *pseudophlegmon.*

Hamman, Louis, U.S. physician, 1877–1946. See H.'s *disease, sign, syndrome;* H.-Rich *syndrome.*

Hammarsten, Olof, Swedish physiological chemist, 1841–1932. See H.'s *reagent.*

hammer (ham'er). Malleus.

Hammerschlag, Albert, Austrian physician, 1863–1935. See H.'s *method.*

Hammond, William A., U.S. neurologist, 1828–1900. See H.'s *disease.*

Hampson unit. See under unit.

Hampton, Aubrey Otis, U.S. radiologist, 1900–1955. See H. *hump, line, maneuver, technique.*

ham'ster. Any of four genera (subfamily Cricetinae, family Muridae) of small rodents widely used in research and as pets: *Cricetus, Cricetulus, Mesocricetus, and Phodopus.* All hamsters are seed and plant feeders, store food, hibernate in winter, and breed throughout the year under laboratory conditions.

ham'string. 1. One of the tendons bounding the popliteal space on either side; the **medial h.** comprises the tendons of the semimembranosus, semitendinosus, gracilis, and sartorius muscles; the **lateral h.** is the tendon of the biceps femoris muscle. **2.** In domestic animals, the combined tendons of the superficial digital flexor, triceps surae, biceps femoris, and semitendinosus muscles which are referred to as the common calcanean tendon (tendo calcaneus communis); it is attached to the tuber calcis of the hock.

hamular (ham'yū-lăr) [L. *hamulus, q.v.*]. Hook-shaped; unciform.

hamulus, gen. and pl. **hamuli** (ham'yū-lŭs, -lī) [L. dim. of *hamus,* hook] [NA]. Any hooklike structure.

h. coch'leae, h. laminae spiralis.

lacrimal h., h. lacrimalis.

h. lacrima'lis [NA], lacrimal h.; hamular process of lacrimal bone; the hooklike lower end of the lacrimal crest, curving between the frontal process and orbital surface of the maxilla to form the upper aperture of the bony portion of the nasolacrimal canal.

h. lam'inae spira'lis [NA], hook of spiral lamina; h. cochleae; the upper hooklike termination of the bony spiral lamina at the apex of the cochlea.

h. os'sis hama'ti [NA], hook of hamate bone; a hooklike process on the distal and medial part of the palmar surface of the hamate bone.

pterygoid h., h. pterygoideus.

h. pterygoid'eus [NA], pterygoid h.; hamular process of sphenoid bone; the inferior, hook-shaped extremity of the medial plate of the pterygoid process.

Hancock, Henry, British surgeon, 1809–1880. See H.'s *amputation.*

Hand, Alfred, U.S. pediatrician, 1868–1949. See H.-Schüller-Christian *disease.*

hand [A.S.]. Manus.

accoucheur's h., obstetrical h.; main d'accoucheur; position of the h. in tetany or in muscular dystrophy; the fingers are flexed at the metacarpophalangeal joints and extended at the phalangeal joints, with the thumb flexed and adducted into the palm; in resemblance to the position of the physician's hand in making a vaginal examination.

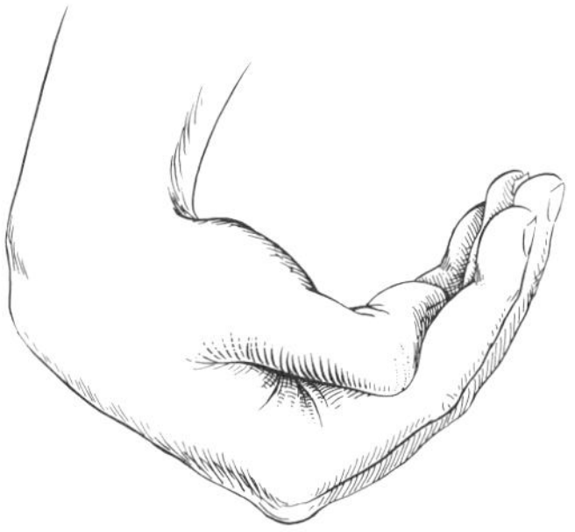

Accoucheur's Hand

ape h., a deformity marked by extension of the thumb at nearly a right angle with the axis of the h.

claw h., see clawhand.
cleft h., split h.; main fourché; a congenital deformity in which the division between the fingers, especially between the third and fourth, extends into the metacarpal region. See also lobster-claw *deformity.*
club h., see talipomanus.
crab h., erysipeloid.
drop h., wrist-drop.
flat h., *manus* plana.
ghoul h., a condition seen in African blacks, probably a manifestation of tertiary yaws, marked by depigmentation of the palms and contraction of the skin which give a clawlike and corpselike appearance to the h.'s.
Marinesco's succulent h., edema of the h. with coldness and lividity of the skin, observed in syringomyelia.
obstetrical h., accoucheur's h.
opera-glass h., main en lorgnette; a deformity of the h. seen in chronic absorptive arthritis, the fingers and wrists being shortened and the covering skin wrinkled into transverse folds; the phalanges appear to be retracted into one another like an opera glass or miniature telescope.
skeleton h., extension of fingers with atrophy of tissues; occurs in progressive muscular atrophy.
spade h., the coarse, thick, square h. of acromegaly or myxedema.
split h., cleft h.
trench h., frostbite of the h.
trident h., a h. in which the fingers are of nearly equal length and deflected at the first interphalangeal joint, so as to give a forklike shape; seen in achondroplasia.
writing h., a contraction of the h. muscles in parkinsonism, bringing the fingers somewhat in the position of holding a pen.

handedness (hand'ed-nes). Preference for the use of one hand, most commonly the right, associated with dominance of the opposite cerebral hemisphere; may also be the result of training or habit.

handicap (hand'i-kap). A physical, mental, or emotional condition that interferes with an individual's normal functioning. See also disability.

handpiece (hand'pēs). A powered dental instrument held in the hand, used to hold rotary cutting, grinding, or polishing implements while they are being revolved.

HANE Acronym for hereditary angioneurotic *edema.*

hangnail (hang'nāl). Agnail; a loose tag of epidermis attached at the proximal portion in the medial or lateral nail fold.

Hanhart, Ernst. See H.'s *syndrome.*

Hanks, Horace Tracy, U.S. surgeon, 1837–1900. See H. *dilators.*

Hanks' solution. See under solution.

Hanlon, C. Rollins, U.S. cardiovascular and thoracic surgeon, *1915. See Blalock-H. *operation.*

Hannover, Adolph, Danish anatomist, 1814–1894. See H.'s *canal.*

Hanot, Victor C., French physician, 1844–1896. See H.'s *cirrhosis.*

Hansemann macrophage. See under macrophage.

Hansen, Gerhard A., Norwegian physician, 1841–1912. See H.'s *bacillus, disease.*

hapalonychia (hap'ă-lō-nik'ē-ă) [hapalo- + G. *onyx* (*onych-*), nail]. Eggshell nails; thinning of nails resulting in bending and breaking of the free edge, with longitudinal fissures.

haphalgesia (haf-al-jē'zē-ă) [G. *haphē,* touch, + *algēsis,* sense of pain]. Pitres sign (1); pain or an extremely disagreeable sensation caused by the merest touch.

haphephobia (haf-ē-fō'bē-ă) [G. *haphē,* touch, + *phobos,* fear]. Aphephobia; a morbid dislike or fear of being touched.

haplo- [G. *haplous,* simple, single]. Combining form meaning simple or single.

haplodont (hap'lō-dont) [haplo- + G. *odous,* tooth]. Having molar teeth with simple crowns, *i.e.,* simple conical teeth without ridges or tubercles.

haploid (hap'loyd) [haplo- + G. *ploides,* in form]. Monoploid; denoting the number of chromosomes in sperm or ova, which is half the number in somatic (diploid) cells; the h. number in man is 23.

haplology (hap-lol'ō-jē) [haplo- + G. *logos,* study]. The omission of syllables because of excessive speed of utterance.

haploprotein (hap-lō-prō'tēn). The functional complex between an apoprotein and the prosthetic group that together are responsible for biological activity.

haploscope (hap'lō-skōp) [haplo- + G. *skopeō,* to view]. An instrument for presenting separate views to each eye so that they may be seen as one.
mirror h., a h. using mirrors to displace the field of view of the two eyes, as in Worth's amblyoscope and the synoptophore.

haploscopic (hap-lō-skop'ik). Relating to a haploscope.

Haplosporidia (hap'lō-spō-rid'ē-ă) [haplo- + G. *sporos,* seed]. An order of sporozoans, now placed in the protozoan phylum Ascetospora, class Stellatosporea, that reproduce asexually by schizogony and produce spores but no flagella, though pseudopodia may be present.

haplotype (hap'lō-tīp) [haplo- + G. *typos,* impression, model]. **1.** The genetic constitution of an individual with respect to one member of a pair of allelic genes; individuals are of the same h. (but of different genotypes) if alike with respect to one allele of a pair but different with respect to the other allele of a pair. **2.** In immunogenetics, that portion of the phenotype determined by closely linked genes inherited as a unit from one parent (*i.e.,* genes located on one of the pair of chromosomes). The human major histocompatability complex comprises 4 recognized gene loci (A, B, C, and D) for which there are more than 50 alleles that control the corresponding antigens, 4 of which (one from each of the 4 loci) compose each HLA h. Similarly, the allotypic markers (antigens) of the immunoglobulin subclasses IgG1, IgG2, IgG3, and IgA2 occur in combinations and are inherited as units; the alleles that control these various h.'s are not linked to those controlling the antigens of the κ type L chains.

hap'ten [G. *haptō,* to fasten, bind]. Incomplete or partial antigen; an antigen that is incapable, alone, of causing the production of antibodies but is capable of combining with specific antibodies. See also hapten *inhibition* of precipitation.
conjugated h., conjugated antigen; a h. that may cause the production of antibodies when it has been covalently linked to protein.

haptics (hap'tiks) [G. *haptō,* to grasp, touch]. The science concerned with the tactile sense.

haptodysphoria (hap'tō-dis-fō'rē-ă) [G. *haptō,* to touch, + dysphoria]. An unpleasant sensation derived from touching certain objects.

haptoglobin (hap-tō-glō'bin). A group of α_2-globulins in human serum, so called because of their ability to combine with hemoglobin; variant types form a polymorphic system, with α- and β-polypeptide chains controlled by separate genetic loci.

haptometer (hap-tom'ĕ-ter) [G. *haptō,* to touch, + *metron,* measure]. Instrument for measuring sensitivity to touch.

Harada, Einosuke, Japanese surgeon, 1892–1947. See H.'s *disease, syndrome.*

Harden, Sir Arthur, British biochemist, 1865–1940. See H.-Young *ester.*

Harder, Johann J., Swiss anatomist, 1656–1711. See H.'s *gland.*

Harding, Harold E., 20th century British pathologist. See H.-Passey *melanoma.*

hardness (hard'nes). The degree of firmness of a solid, as determined

by its resistance to deformation, scratching, or abrasion. See also hardness *scale;* relevant subentries under *number.*
indentation h., a number related to the size of the impression made by an indenter (or tool) of specific size and shape under a known load.

Hardy, G.H., 20th century British mathematician. See H.-Weinberg *equilibrium, law.*

Hardy, LeGrand H., U.S. ophthalmologist, 1895–1954. See H.-Rand-Ritter *test.*

harelip (hār'lip). Cleft *lip.*

harmaline (har'mă-lēn). Harmidine; 4,9-dihydro-7-methoxy-1-methyl-3*H*-pyrido[3,4-*b*]indole; 3,4-dihydroharmine; an amine oxidase inhibitor and a central nervous system stimulant; obtained from the seeds of *Peganum harmala* (family Zygophyllaceae) and from *Banisteria caapi* (family Malpighiaceae); has been used in parkinsonism.

harmidine (har'mi-dēn). Harmaline.

harmine (har'mēn). Banisterine; telepathine; leucoharmine; 7-methoxy-1-methyl-9*H*- pyrido[3,4-*b*]indole; obtained from *Peganum harmala* (family Zygophyllaceae) and *Banisteria caapi* (family Malpighaceae); a central nervous system stimulant and potent monoamine oxidase inhibitor; psychic effects resemble those of LSD, but sedative and depressive qualities may predominate over hallucinatory manifestations.

harmonia (har-mō'nē-ă) [L. and G. a joining]. *Sutura* plana.

harmonic (har-mon'ik). A component of complex sound whose frequency is a multiple of the fundamental frequency of the sound. This fundamental frequency is called the first harmonic; the second harmonic has twice the frequency of the fundamental, and so forth.

harmony (har'mō-nē). Agreement; accord; in dentistry, denotes occlusal h.
functional occlusal h., such occlusal relationship of opposing teeth in all functional ranges and movements as will provide the greatest masticatory efficiency without causing undue strain or trauma upon the supporting tissues, teeth, and muscles.
occlusal h., occlusion without deflective or interceptive occlusal contacts in centric jaw relation as well as eccentric movements.

harpaxophobia (har'paks-ō-fō'bē-ă) [G. *harpax,* robber, + *phobos,* fear]. Morbid fear of robbers.

harpoon (har-pūn'). A small, sharp-pointed instrument with a barbed head used for extracting bits of tissue for microscopic examination.

Harrington, David O., U.S. ophthalmologist, *1904. See H.-Flocks *test.*

Harris, Henry A., British anatomist, 1886–1968. See H.'s *lines.*

Harris, Henry F., U.S. physician, 1867–1926. See H.'s *hematoxylin.*

Harris, R.I., 20th century Canadian orthopedist. See Salter-H. *classification* of epiphysial fractures.

Harris, Wilfred, British physician, 1869–1960. See H.'s *migraine.*

Harris and Ray test. See under test.

Harrison, Edward, British physician, 1766–1838. See H.'s *groove.*

Hartel, Fritz, 20th century German surgeon. See H.'s *technique.*

Hartman, Alexis F., U.S. pediatrician, 1898–1964. See Shaffer-H. *method.*

Hartman, LeRoy L., U.S. dentist, 1893–1951. See H.'s *solution.*

Hartmann, Alexis F., U.S. pediatrician, 1898–1964. See H.'s *solution.*

Hartmann, Arthur, German laryngologist, 1849–1931. See H.'s *curette.*

Hartmann, Henri A.C.A., French surgeon, 1860–1952. See H.'s *operation, pouch.*

Hartmannella (hart-mă-nel'ă). A common free-living ameba found in soil, sewage, and water, known to invade invertebrates (snails, grasshoppers, oysters); suspected but not established as an agent of human primary amebic meningoencephalitis.

Hartnup. Surname of British family in which the disease was first described. See H. *disease, syndrome.*

hartshorn (harts'hōrn). Crude ammonium carbonate; a mixture of ammonium bicarbonate and ammonium carbamate obtained from ammonium sulfate and calcium carbonate by sublimation; used as an expectorant and in smelling salts; so called because originally obtained from deer antlers.

harvest bug. The larva of *Trombicula* species.

hasamiyami (has'ă-mē-yah'mē). Autumn fever (2); akiyami; sakushu fever; a fever occurring in Japan in the autumn; resembles Weil's disease, but is milder and is caused by the *autumnalis* serovar of *Leptospira interrogans.*

Häser, Heinrich, German physician, 1811–1884. See H.'s *formula,* Trapp-H. *formula.*

Hashimoto, H., Japanese surgeon, 1881–1934. See H.'s *disease, struma, thyroiditis.*

hashish (hash'ish) [Ar. hay]. Hasheesh; a form of cannabis that consists largely of resin from the flowering tops and sprouts of cultivated female plants; contains the highest concentration of cannabinols among the preparations derived from cannabis.

Hasner, Joseph Ritter von, Prague ophthalmologist, 1819–1892. See H.'s *fold, valve.*

Hassall, Arthur H., British physician, 1817–1894. See H.'s *bodies,* concentric *corpuscles;* H.-Henle *bodies;* Virchow-H. *bodies.*

Hasselbalch, Karl, Danish biochemist and physician, 1874–1962. See H.'s *equation;* Henderson-H. *equation.*

hatch'et. A dental instrument with an end cutting blade set at an angle to the axis of the handle and having one or two bevels; in the former case, made as right and left pairs called enamel h.'s; used for removing enamel and dentin on posterior teeth where access with a chisel is difficult.

Haubenfelder (how'ben-fel'der) [Ger.]. See *fields* of Forel.

Hauch (H) (howkh) [Ger. breath]. A term used to designate the flagellar antigen of bacteria. See also H *antigen.*

Haudek, Martin, Austrian roentgenologist, 1880–1931. See H.'s *niche.*

Hauser, G.A., 20th century German gynecologist. See Mayer-Rokitansky-Küster-H. syndrome; Rokitansky-Küster-H. syndrome.

haustorium, pl. **haustoria** (haw-stō'rē-ŭm, -stō'rē-ă) [Mod. L. fr. L. *haustus,* a drinking]. An organ for the absorption of nutriment.

haustra (haw'stră) [L.]. Plural of haustrum.

haustral (haw'străl). Relating to a haustrum.

haustration (haw-strā'shŭn). **1.** The process of formation of a haustrum. **2.** An increase in prominence of the haustra.

haustrum, pl. **haustra** (haw'strŭm, haw'stră) [L. a machine for drawing water, fr. *haurio,* pp. *haustus,* to draw up, drink up]. One of a series of saccules or pouches, so-called because of a fancied resemblance to the buckets on a water wheel.
haus'tra co'li [NA], cellulae coli; the sacculations of the colon, caused by the teniae, or longitudinal bands, which are slightly shorter than the gut so that the latter is thrown into tucks or pouches.

haustus (haws'tŭs) [L. a drink, draft]. A potion or medicinal draft.

HAV Abbreviation for hepatitis A *virus.*

Haverhillia multiformis (ha-ver-hil'ē-ă mŭl-ti-fōr'mis). An organism, which may be identical with *Streptobacillus moniliformis,* originally identified as the cause of Haverhill fever.

Havers, Clopton, British anatomist, 1650–1702. See H.'s (haversian) *canals, glands, lamellae, spaces, system.*

haversian (ha-ver'shan). Relating to Clopton Havers and the various osseous structures described by him.

hawkinsin (hawk'in-sin) [*Hawkins,* surname of family from which first reported]. 2-*L*- Cystein-*S*- yl-1,4-dihydroxycyclohex-5-en-1-yl acetic acid; a sulfur-containing amino acid present in the urine in patients with hawkinsinuria.

hawkinsinuria (hawk'in-si-nū'rē-ă) [see hawkinsin]. A rare metabolic disease manifested in infancy by a failure to thrive, acidosis, and presence of hawkinsin in the urine; autosomal dominant inheritance.

Hawley, C.A., U.S. orthodontist. See H. *appliance, retainer.*

Haworth, Walter Norman, British chemist, 1883–1950. See H. conformational formulas of and perspective formulas of cyclic *sugars.*

Hayem, Georges, French physician, 1841–1933. See H's *hematoblast, solution;* H.-Widal *anemia, syndrome.*

Hayflick, Leonard, U.S. microbiologist, *1928. See H.'s *limit.*

Haygarth, John, British physician, 1740–1827. See H.'s *nodes, nodosities.*

hazelwort (hā'zel-wōrt). *Asarum europaeum.*

Hb Abbreviation for hemoglobin.

HB_cAb Abbreviation for antibody to the hepatitis B core antigen.

HB_eAb Abbreviation for antibody to the hepatitis B e antigen.

HB_sAb Abbreviation for antibody to the hepatitis B surface antigen.

HB_cAg Abbreviation for hepatitis B core *antigen.*

HB_sAg Abbreviation for hepatitis B surface *antigen.*

Hb AS Abbreviation indicating heterozygosity for hemoglobin A and hemoglobin S, the sickle cell trait.

HBe, HB_eAg Abbreviation for hepatitis B e *antigen.*

HbCO Abbreviation for carboxyhemoglobin.

HbO_2 Abbreviation for oxyhemoglobin.

Hb S Abbreviation for sickle cell *hemoglobin.*

HBV Abbreviation for hepatitis B *virus.*

HCG Abbreviation for human chorionic *gonadotropin.*

HCS Abbreviation for human chorionic somatomammotropic *hormone;* human chorionic *somatomammotropin.*

Hct Abbreviation for hematocrit (2).

h.d. Abbreviation for L. *hora decubitus,* at bedtime.

HDL Abbreviation for high density lipoprotein. See lipoprotein.

HDRV Abbreviation for human diploid cell rabies *vaccine.*

HDV Abbreviation for human delta *virus.*

He Symbol for helium.

^3He, ^4He Symbols for helium-3 and helium-4 respectively.

Head, Sir Henry, British neurologist, 1861–1940. See H.'s *areas, lines, zones.*

head (hed) [A.S. *heāfod*]. Caput.
- **bulldog h.,** the broad h. with high vault occurring in achondroplasia.
- **deep h.,** *caput* profundum.
- **h. of epididymis,** *caput* epididymidis.
- **h. of femur,** *caput* ossis femoris.
- **h. of fibula,** *caput* fibulae.
- **hourglass h.,** in congenital syphilis, a skull with depressed coronal suture.
- **humeral h.,** *caput* humerale.
- **humeroulnar h.,** *caput* humeroulnare.
- **h. of humerus,** *caput* humeri.
- **lateral h.,** *caput* laterale.
- **little h. of humerus,** *capitulum* humeri.
- **long h.,** *caput* longum.
- **h. of malleus,** *caput* mallei.
- **h. of mandible,** *caput* mandibulae.
- **Medusa h.,** *caput* medusae.
- **h. of metacarpal bone,** *caput* ossis metacarpalis.
- **h. of metatarsal bone,** *caput* ossis metatarsalis.
- **oblique h.,** *caput* obliquum.
- **h. of pancreas,** *caput* pancreatis.
- **h. of phalanx,** *caput* phalangis.
- **radial h.,** *caput* radiale.
- **h. of radius,** *caput* radii.
- **h. of rib,** *caput* costae.
- **saddle h.,** clinocephaly.
- **short h.,** *caput* breve.
- **h. of stapes,** *caput* stapedis.
- **superficial h.,** *caput* superficiale.
- **swelled h.,** Paget's disease of the skull.
- **h. of talus,** *caput* tali.
- **h. of thigh bone,** *caput* ossis femoris.
- **transverse h.,** *caput* transversum.
- **h. of ulna,** *caput* ulnae.
- **ulnar h.,** *caput* ulnare.

headache (hed'āk). Cephalalgia; cephalea; cerebralgia; encephalalgia; encephalodynia; diffuse pain in various parts of the head, not confined to the area of distribution of any nerve. See also cephalodynia.
- **bilious h.,** migraine.
- **blind h.,** migraine.
- **cluster h.,** probably a migraine variant, may be precipitated by the injection of histamine; characterized by recurrent, severe, unilateral orbitotemporal h.'s associated with conjunctival injection. Also called histaminic or Horton's h,; histaminic or Horton's cephalalgia.
- **fibrositic h.,** h. centered in the occipital region due to fibrositis of the occipital muscles; tender areas are present and, commonly, tender nodules are found in the scalp in the lower occipital region.
- **histaminic h.,** cluster h.
- **Horton's h.,** cluster h.
- **migraine h.,** see migraine.
- **nodular h.,** radiating pain in the head accompanied by nodular swellings in the splenius, frontalis, trapezius, and other muscles.
- **organic h.,** h. due to disease of the brain or its coverings.
- **reflex h.,** symptomatic h.
- **sick h.,** migraine.
- **spinal h.,** h., usually frontal or occipital, following dural puncture; precipitated by sitting up, relieved by lying down; postulated to be due to leakage of cerebrospinal fluid from subarachnoid space through the site of the puncture.
- **symptomatic h.,** reflex h.; a h. secondary to another organic condition.
- **tension h.,** h. associated with nervous tension, anxiety, etc., often related to chronic contraction of the scalp muscles. See also post-traumatic neck *syndrome.*
- **vacuum h.,** h. due to closure of the frontal sinus.
- **vascular h.,** migraine.

headgear (hed'gēr). A removable extraoral appliance used as a source of traction to apply force to the teeth and jaws.

headgut (hed'gŭt). Foregut.

head-nodding (hed'nod-ing). Head tremors; head movements associated with congenital nystagmus, spasmus nutans, and miner's nystagmus.

head-tilt (hed'tilt). An abnormal position of the head adopted to prevent double vision resulting from underaction of the vertical ocular muscles.

heal (hēl) [A.S. *healan*]. **1.** To restore to health, especially to cause an ulcer or wound to cicatrize or unite. **2.** To become well, to be cured; to cicatrize or close, said of an ulcer or wound.

healer (hē'ler). **1.** A physician; one who heals or cures. **2.** One who claims to cure by prayer, mysticism, new thought, or other form of suggestion.

healing (hēl'ing). **1.** Curing; restoring to health; promoting the closure of wounds and ulcers. **2.** The process of a return to health. **3.** Closing of a wound. See also union.

faith h., a psychotherapeutic treatment based upon prayer and a profound belief in divine intervention in human affairs.

h. by first intention, primary adhesion or union; h. by fibrous adhesion, without suppuration or granulation tissue formation.

h. by second intention, secondary adhesion or union; delayed closure of two granulating surfaces.

h. by third intention, the slow filling of a wound cavity or ulcer by granulations, with subsequent cicatrization.

health (helth) [A.S. *haelth*]. The state of the organism when it functions optimally without evidence of disease or abnormality.

mental h., emotional, behavioral, and social maturity or normality; the absence of a mental or behavioral disorder; a state of psychological well-being in which the individual has achieved a satisfactory integration of his instinctual drives acceptable to both himself and his social milieu.

public h., the art and science of community health, concerned with statistics, epidemiology, hygiene, and the prevention and eradication of epidemic diseases.

Health Maintenance Organization (HMO). A comprehensive prepaid system of health care with emphasis on the prevention and early detection of disease, and continuity of care.

healthy (helth'ē). Well; in a state of normal functioning; free from disease.

Heaney, Noble Sproat, U.S. gynecological surgeon and obstetrician, 1880–1955. See H.'s *operation.*

hear (hēr) [A.S. *hēran*]. To perceive sounds; denoting the function of the ear.

hearing (hēr'ing). The ability to perceive sound; the sensation of sound as opposed to vibration.

color h., pseudochromesthesia (2); chromatic audition; a subjective perception of color produced by certain sounds.

normal h., acusis.

hearing aid (hēr'ing ād). An electronic amplifying device designed to bring sound more effectively into the ear; it consists of a microphone, amplifier, and receiver.

hearing impairment, hearing loss. A reduction in the ability to perceive sound; may range from slight to complete deafness. See also deafness; threshold *shift.*

heart (hart) [A.S. *heorte*]. Cor; a hollow muscular organ which receives the blood from the veins and propels it into the arteries. It is divided by a musculomembranous septum into two halves—right or venous and left or arterial—each of which consists of a receiving chamber (atrium) and an ejecting chamber (ventricle).

armored h., Panzerherz; calcareous deposits in the pericardium occurring in subacute or chronic inflammation.

artificial h., a mechanical pump used to replace the function of a damaged heart, either temporarily or as a permanent internal prosthesis.

athletic h., hypertrophy of the h. supposedly due to overindulgence in athletics.

beer h., beer-drinker's *cardiomyopathy.*

bony h., the presence of extensive calcareous patches in the pericardium and walls of the h.

drop h., cardioptosia.

fatty h., **(1)** fatty degeneration of the myocardium; **(2)** adiposis cardiaca; cor adiposum; accumulation of adipose tissue on the external surface of the h. with occasional infiltration of fat between the muscle bundles of the h. wall; associated with obesity.

frosted h., icing h.; hyaloserositis involving the pericardium.

hairy h., fibrinous *pericarditis.*

hanging h., suspended h.

horizontal h., description of the h.'s electrical axis when this is directed at approximately −30°; recognized in the electrocardiogram when the QRS in lead aVL is positive while that in aVF is negative.

hypoplastic h., a small h., as seen in Addison's disease.

icing h., frosted h.

intermediate h., description of the h.'s electrical axis when this is directed at approximately +30°; recognized in the electrocardiogram when the QRS complexes in both lead aVL and aVF are mainly positive.

irritable h., neurocirculatory *asthenia.*

left h., hemicardia sinistra; the left atrium and left ventricle.

luxus h., a German term for combined dilation and hypertrophy of the h., especially of the left ventricle.

movable h., *cor* mobile.

myxedema h., the enlarged h. associated with severe hypothyroidism.

parchment h., right ventricular hypoplasia; a congenital or acquired condition in which there is thinning of the right ventricular myocardium.

pendulous h., *cor* pendulum.

pulmonary h., the right atrium and ventricle, receiving the venous blood and propelling it to the lungs. See also *cor* pulmonale.

right h., hemicardia dextra; the right atrium and right ventricle.

sabot h., *coeur* en sabot.

semihorizontal h., description of the h.'s electrical axis when this is directed at approximately 0°; recognized in the electrocardiogram when the QRS complex in lead aVL is positive while that in aVF is isodiphasic.

semivertical h., description of the h.'s electrical axis when this is directed at approximately +60°; recognized in the electrocardiogram when the QRS complex in lead aVF is positive while that in aVL is isodiphasic.

skin h., the peripheral blood vessels.

soldier's h., neurocirculatory *asthenia.*

stone h., ischemic *contracture* of the left ventricle.

suspended h., hanging h.; a h. which gives the appearance on x-ray visualization of being suspended from the great vessels, its lower surface not resting upon the diaphragm.

systemic h., the left atrium and ventricle, receiving the aerated

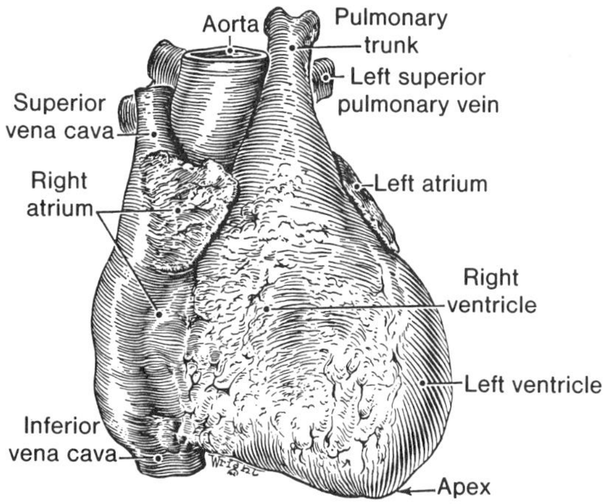

Anterior View of Normal Heart

blood from the lungs and propelling it throughout the body.

teardrop h., h. presenting a symmetrical vertically elongated appearance on x-ray.

tiger h., a fatty degenerated h. in which the fat is disposed in the form of broken stripes in the subendocardial myocardium.

tobacco h., cardiac irritability marked by irregular action, palpitation, and sometimes pain, occurring as a result of the excessive use of tobacco.

venous h., the right side, including both the atrium and ventricle, of the h.

vertical h., description of the h.'s electrical axis when this is directed at approximately +90°; recognized in the electrocardiogram when the QRS complex in lead aVL is negative while that in aVF is positive.

wooden-shoe h., *coeur* en sabot.

heartbeat (hart'bēt). A single complete cycle of contraction and dilation of heart muscle.

heartburn (hart'bern). Pyrosis.

heartwater (hart'wah-ter). Cowdriosis; an acute febrile disease of cattle, sheep, and goats in sub-Saharan Africa and certain Caribbean islands (Guadeloupe and Antigua), caused by the rickettsial organism *Cowdria ruminantium* which is transmitted by ticks of the genus *Amblyomma;* some species of African antelope and European and American deer also are susceptible.

heartworm. *Dirofilaria immitis.*

heat (hēt) [A.S. *haete*]. **1.** A high temperature; the sensation produced by proximity to fire or an incandescent object, as opposed to cold. The basis of h. is the kinetic energy of atoms and molecules, which becomes zero at absolute zero. **2.** Estrus.

atomic h., the amount of h. required to raise an atom from 0° to 1°C; approximately the same for all elements (about 6 Cal per gram-atom).

h. of combustion, the quantity of h. liberated per gram-molecule when a substance undergoes complete oxidation.

h. of compression, h. produced when a gas is compressed.

conductive h., h. transmitted by direct contact, as by an electric pad or hot water bottle.

convective h., h. conveyed by a warm medium, such as air or water, in motion from its source.

conversive h., h. produced in a body by the absorption of waves which are not in themselves hot, such as the sun's rays or infrared radiation.

h. of crystallization, the quantity of h. liberated or absorbed per mol when a substance passes into the crystalline state.

h. of dissociation, the h. (expressed in calories) expended in the dissociation of 1 mole of a substance into specified products.

h. of evaporation, h. of vaporization; the h. absorbed in the evaporation of water, sweat or other liquid; for water it amounts to 540 cal per g at 100°C.

h. of formation, the h. (expressed in calories) absorbed or liberated during the (hypothetical) reaction in which a mole of a compound is formed from the necessary elements, in elemental form.

initial h., the first burst of h. produced after the beginning of a muscle twitch, described by A. V. Hill.

innate h., in ancient Greek medicine, the h. of the heart sustained by the pneuma and distributed by the arteries throughout the body.

latent h., the amount of h. that a substance may absorb without an increase in temperature, as in conversion from solid to liquid state (ice to water at 0°C), or from liquid to gaseous state (water to steam at 100°C). *Cf.* sensible h.

molecular h., the product of the specific h. of a body multiplied by its molecular weight.

prickly h., *miliaria* rubra.

radiant h., h. given off from any body in the form of waves, similar to light waves but of greater wavelength.

sensible h., the amount of h. that, when absorbed by a substance, causes a rise in temperature. *Cf.* latent h.

h. of solution, the quantity of h. absorbed or evolved when a solid is dissolved in a liquid.

specific h., the amount of h. required to raise any substance through 1° of temperature, compared with that raising the same volume of water 1°.

h. of vaporization, h. of evaporation.

heat-labile (hēt'lā'bl). Destroyed or altered by heat.

heatstroke (hēt'strōk). Heat apoplexy (1); heat or malignant hyperpyrexia; thermic fever; a severe and often fatal illness produced by exposure to excessively high temperatures, especially when accompanied by marked exertion; characterized by headache, vertigo, confusion, hot dry skin, and a slight rise in body temperature; in severe cases collapse and coma, very high fever, and tachycardia develop.

heaves (hēvz). A chronic pulmonary emphysema of horses; symptoms include a wheezy cough and dyspnea, especially when exercised.

Hebeloma (heb-ĕ-lō'mă). A genus of mushrooms that is a source of gastrointestinal toxins.

hebephrenia (hē-bĕ-frē'nē-ă, heb'ĕ-) [G. *hēbē,* puberty, + *phrēn,* the mind]. A syndrome characterized by shallow and inappropriate affect, giggling, and silly, regressive behavior and mannerisms.

hebephrenic (hē-bĕ-frĕn'ik, heb-ē-). Relating to or characterized by hebephrenia.

Heberden, William, British physician, 1710–1801. See H.'s *angina, nodes, nodosities;* Rougnon-H. *disease.*

hebetic (hē-bet'ik) [G. *hēbētikos,* youthful, fr. *hēbē,* youth]. Pertaining to youth.

hebetude (heb'ĕ-tūd) [L. *hebetudo,* fr. *hebeo,* to be dull]. Moria (1).

hebiatrics (hē-bē-at'riks) [G. *hēbē,* youth, + *iatrio,* to heal]. Adolescent *medicine.*

Hebra, Ferdinand von, Austrian dermatologist, 1816–1880. See H.'s *disease, prurigo.*

hecateromeric (hek'ă-ter-ō-mer'ik) [G. *hekateros,* each of two, + *meros,* part]. Hecatomeric; hecatomeral; denoting a spinal neuron whose axon divides and gives off processes to both sides of the cord; usually the same as a heteromeric neuron.

hecatomeral, hecatomeric (hek'ă-tom'er-ăl, hek'ă-tō-mer'ik). Hecateromeric.

Hecht, Victor, early 20th century Austrian pathologist. See H.'s *pneumonia.*

Heck, John W., U.S. dentist, *1923. See H.'s *disease.*

hectic (hek'tik) [G. *hektikos,* habitual, hectic, consumptive, fr. *hexis,* habit]. Denoting a daily afternoon rise of temperature, accompanied by a flush on the cheeks, occurring in active tuberculosis and other infections; use of the term is based on the appearance of the temperature chart.

hecto- (h) [G. *hekaton,* one hundred]. Prefix used in the SI and metric systems to signfy one hundred (10^2).

hectogram (hek'tō-gram). One hundred grams, the equivalent of 1543.7 grains.

hectoliter (hek'tō-lē-ter). One hundred liters, the equivalent of 105.7 quarts or 26.4 American (22 imperial) gallons.

hedeoma (he-dē-ō'mă). See pennyroyal.

hederiform (hed'er-i-fōrm) [L. *hedera,* ivy, + *forma,* shape]. Ivy-shaped; a term used for certain sensory endings in the skin.

hedonophobia (hē'dō-nō-fō'bē-ă) [G. *hēdonē,* delight, + *phobos,* fear]. Morbid fear of pleasure.

hedrocele (hed'rō-sēl) [G. *hedra,* a seat, the fundament, + *kēlē,* hernia]. Prolapse of the intestine through the anus.

Hedström file. See under file.

heel (hēl) [A.S. *hēla*]. **1.** Calx (2). **2.** Distal *end.*

contracted h., contracted *foot* (2).

cracked h., *keratoderma* plantare sulcatum.

grease h., **(1)** initially, lesions of horsepox occurring in the skin of the flexor surface of the fetlock of the horse; **(2)** scratches; now frequently applied to any weeping, eczematous condition of that area.

painful h., calcodynia; calcaneodynia; a condition in which bearing the weight on the h. causes pain of varying severity.

prominent h., a condition marked by a tender swelling on the os calcis due to a thickening of the periosteum or fibrous tissue covering the back of the os calcis.

Heerfordt, Christian Frederick, Danish ophthalmologist, *1871. See H.'s *disease.*

Hegar, Alfred, German gynecologist, 1830–1914. See H.'s *dilators, sign.*

Hegglin, Robert M.P., Swiss physician, 20th century. See H.'s *anomaly, syndrome;* May-H. *anomaly.*

Hehner, Otto, British chemist, 1853–1924. See H. *number.*

Heidenhain, Rudolph P., German histologist and physiologist, 1834–1897. See H.'s *crescents, demilunes, law,* azan *stain,* iron hematoxylin *stain;* H. *pouch;* Biondi-H. *stain.*

height (hīt). Vertical measurement.

anterior facial h. (AFH), in cephalometrics, the linear measurement from the nasion to the menton.

h. of contour, the line encircling a tooth or other structure at its greatest bulge or diameter with respect to a selected path of insertion.

cusp h., **(1)** the shortest distance between the tip of a cusp and its base plane; **(2)** the shortest distance between the deepest part of the central fossa of a posterior tooth and a line connecting the points of the cusps of the tooth.

facial h., the linear dimension in the midline from the hairline to the menton.

nasal h., the distance between the nasion and the lower border of the nasal aperture.

orbital h., the distance between the midpoints of the upper and lower margins of the orbit.

Heilbronner, Karl, Dutch physician, 1869–1914. See H.'s *thigh.*

Heim, Ernst L., German physician, 1747–1834. See H.-Kreysig *sign.*

Heim, Friedrich L.K., German physician, 1770–1839. See H.-Kreysig *sign.*

Heimlich, Harry J., U.S. thoracic surgeon, *1920. See H. *maneuver.*

Heine, Leopold, German ophthalmologist, 1870–1940. See H.'s *operation.*

Heineke, Walter H., German surgeon, 1834–1901. See H.-Mikulicz *pyloroplasty.*

Heinz, Robert, German pathologist, 1865–1924. See H. *bodies,* H. body *test;* H.-Ehrlich *bodies.*

Heister, Lorenz, German anatomist, 1683–1758. See H.'s *diverticulum, valve.*

Helbings' sign. See under sign.

helcomenia (hel-kō-mē'nē-ă) [G. *helkos,* ulcer, + *emmēnos,* monthly]. Occurrence of ulcers at the time of a menstruation.

helcoplasty (hel'kō-plas-tē) [G. *helkos,* ulcer, + *plastos,* formed]. Obsolete term for plastic surgery of ulcers.

Held, Hans, German anatomist, 1866–1942. See H.'s *bundle, decussation.*

helianthine (hē-li-an'thin). Methyl orange.

helical (hel'i-kăl) [G. *helix,* a coil]. **1.** Helicine (2); relating to a helix. **2.** Helicoid.

helices (hel'i-sēz). Plural of helix.

helicine (hel'i-sēn) [G. *helix,* a coil]. **1.** Coiled. **2.** Helical (1).

helicoid (hel'i-koyd) [G. *helix,* a coil, + *eidos,* resemblance]. Helical (2); resembling a helix.

helicopodia (hel'i-kō-pō'dē-ă) [G. *helix,* a coil, + *pous,* foot]. Helicopod *gait.*

helicotrema (hel'i-kō-trē'mă) [G. *helix,* a spiral, + *trēma,* a hole] [NA]. Breschet's or Scarpa's hiatus; a semilunar opening at the apex of the cochlea through which the scala vestibuli and the scala tympani of the cochlea communicate with one another.

Helie, Louis T., French gynecologist, 1804–1867. See H.'s *bundle.*

heliencephalitis (hē-lē-en-sef-ă-lī'tis) [G. *helios,* sun, + *enkephalos,* brain, + *-itis,* inflammation]. Inflammation of the brain following sunstroke.

helio- [G. *hēlios,* sun]. Combining form relating to the sun.

helioaerotherapy (hē'lē-ō-ār-ō-thār'ă-pē). Treatment of disease by exposure to sunshine and fresh air.

heliopathy (hē-lē-op'ă-thē) [helio- + G. *pathos,* suffering]. Injury from exposure to sunlight.

heliophobia (hē'lē-ō-fō'bē-ă) [helio- + G. *phobos,* fear]. Morbid fear of exposure to the sun's rays.

heliosis (hē-lē-ō'sis) [helio- + G. *-osis,* condition]. Sunstroke.

heliotaxis (hē-lē-ō-tak'sis) [helio- + G. *taxis,* orderly arrangement]. Heliotropism; a form of phototaxis, and perhaps of thermotaxis, in which there is a tendency to growth or movement toward (positive h.) or away from (negative h.) the sun or the sunlight.

heliotropism (hē-lē-ot'rō-pizm) [helio- + G. *tropē,* a turning]. Heliotaxis.

Heliozoea (hē'lē-ō-zō'ē-ă) [helio- + G. *zōon,* animal]. A class of protozoans (subphylum Sarcodina) distinguished by stiff radiating axopodia on all sides, usually naked, though some have a skeleton of siliceous scales and spines, but without a central capsule. They are mostly fresh water dwellers, and colonial forms are common.

helium (hē'lē-ŭm) [G. *hēlios,* the sun]. A gaseous element present in minute amounts in the atmosphere; symbol He, atomic no. 2, atomic weight 4.0026; used as a diluent of medicinal gases.

helium-3 (^{3}He). The rare stable isotope of h. (1 part in a million of ordinary h.); produced by the beta-decay of tritium.

helium-4 (^{4}He). The common h. isotope, making up 99.999% of natural h.; it is emitted in the form of alpha rays (which are h. nuclei), from a variety of radioactive nuclides.

helix, pl. helices (hē'liks, hel'i-sēz) [L. fr. G. *helix,* a coil]. **1** [NA]. The margin of the auricle; a folded rim of cartilage forming the upper part of the anterior, the superior, and the greater part of the posterior edges of the auricle. **2.** A line in the shape of a coil (or a spring, or the threads on a bolt), each point being equidistant from a straight line that is the axis of the cylinder in which each point of the h. lies; often, mistakenly, applied to a spiral (the threads on a screw).

α h., Pauling-Corey h.; the right-handed helical form assumed by many proteins, deduced by Pauling and Corey from x-ray diffraction studies of collagen; the h. is stabilized by hydrogen bonds between, *e.g.,* $>C=O$ and $HN<$ groups (symbolized by the center dot in $>CO{\cdot}HN<$).

DNA h., Watson-Crick h.

double h., Watson-Crick h.

Pauling-Corey h., α h.

twin h., Watson-Crick h.

Watson-Crick h., DNA, double, or twin h.; the helical structure assumed by two strands of deoxyribonucleic acid, held together throughout their length by hydrogen bonds between bases on opposite strands.

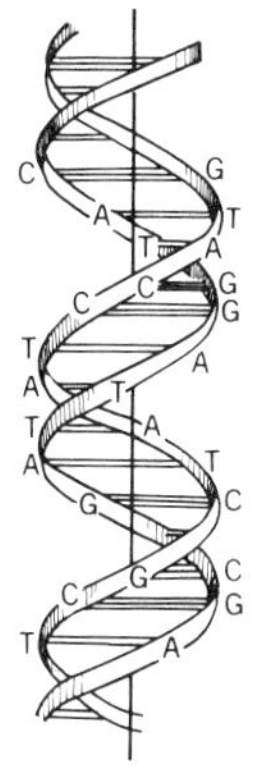

Watson-Crick Helix
Schematic drawing of the double helix of DNA. The two vertical ribbons represent the deoxyribose-phosphate chains; the horizontal bands represent the hydrogen-bonded base pairs that bridge the gap between the chains; the vertical line indicates the fiber axis.

hellebore (hel'ĕ-bōr) [G. *helleboros*]. A plant of the genus *Helleborus,* especially *H. niger* (black h.). See also *Veratrum album* (European or white h.) and *V. viride* (American or green h.).

helleborin (hĕ-leb'o-rin, hel-ĕ-bō'rin). A toxic glycoside from *Veratrum viride* (green hellebore); a narcotic.

helleborism (hel'ĕ-bōr-izm). A condition resulting from poisoning by *Veratrum Helleborus.*

helleborus (he-leb'ō-rŭs) [G. *helleboros*]. Black hellebore, the dried rhizome and roots of *Helleborus niger* (family Ranunculaceae); used as a cardiac and arterial tonic, diuretic, and cathartic.

Heller, Arnold L.G., German pathologist, 1840–1913. See H.'s *plexus.*

Heller, Ernst, German surgeon, 1877–1964. See H. *operation.*

Hellin, Dyonizy, Polish pathologist, 1867–1935. See H.'s *law.*

Helly, Konrad, Swiss pathologist, *1875. See H.'s *fixative.*

Helmholtz, Hermann L.F. von, German physician, physicist, and physiologist, 1821–1894. See H.'s axis *ligament, theory of accommodation, color vision, hearing;* H.-Gibbs *theory;* Gibbs-H. *equation;* Young-H. *theory* of color vision.

hel'minth [G. *helmins,* worm]. An intestinal vermiform parasite, primarily nematodes, cestodes, trematodes, and acanthocephalans.

helminthagogue (hel-minth'ă-gog) [G. *helmins,* worm, + *agōgos,* leading]. Anthelmintic (1).

helminthemesis (hel-min-them'ĕ-sis) [G. *helmins,* a worm, + *emesis,* vomiting]. The vomiting or expulsion through the mouth of intestinal worms.

helminthiasis (hel-min-thī'ă-sis). Helminthism; invermination; the condition of having intestinal vermiform parasites.

helminthic (hel-min'thik). Anthelmintic (1).

helminthism (hel'min-thizm). Helminthiasis.

helminthoid (hel-min'thoyd) [G. *helminthōdēs,* wormlike, fr. *helmins,* worm, + *eidos,* resemblance]. Wormlike.

helminthology (hel-min-thol'ō-jē) [G. *helmins,* worm, + *logos,* study]. Scolecology; the branch of science concerned with worms; especially the branch of zoology and of medicine concerned with intestinal vermiform parasites.

helminthoma (hel-min-thō'mă) [G. *helmins,* worm, + *-oma,* tumor]. A discrete nodule of granulomatous inflammation (including the healed stage) caused by a helminth or its products, so termed on the basis of certain gross resemblances to a neoplasm.

helminthophobia (hel'min-thō-fō'bē-ă) [G. *helmins,* worm, + *phobos,* fear]. Morbid fear of worms.

Helminthosporium (hel-min-thō-spōr'ē-ŭm). A saprobic fungus, commonly misapplied to isolates of *Drechslera,* which is usually isolated in clinical laboratories; it has determinant parallel-walled conidiophores.

helmintic (hel-min'tik). Anthelmintic (1).

Heloderma (hē-lō-der'mă) [G. *hēlos,* nail, + *derma,* skin]. The only genus of poisonous lizards, such as the Gila monster, so named because of the tubercular scales which cover their bodies. They are native to Mexico and the southwestern U.S.

heloma (hē-lō'mă) [G. *hēlos,* nail, + *-oma,* tumor]. Clavus (1).
h. dur'um, hard *corn.*
h. mol'le, soft *corn.*

helosis (hē-lō'sis) [G. *hēlousthai,* to become callous]. Rarely used term denoting the condition of having corns.

helotomy (hē-lot'ō-mē) [heloma + G. *tomē,* cutting]. Surgical treatment of corns.

Helvella esculenta (hel-vel'ă es-kyū-len'tă). *Gyromitra esculenta.*

Helweg, Hans K.S., Danish physician, 1847–1901. See H.'s *bundle.*

Helweg-Larssen, H.F., 20th century Danish dermatologist. See H.-L. *syndrome.*

hem-, hema- [G. *haima,* blood]. Combining forms meaning blood. See also hemat-, hemato-, hemo-.

hemachromatosis (hē'mă-krō-mă-tō'sis, hem'ă-). Hemochromatosis.

hemachrome (hē'mă-krōm, hem'ă-) [hema- + G. *chrōma,* color]. The coloring matter of the blood, hemoglobin or hematin.

hemachrosis (hē-mă-krō'sis, hem-ă) [hema- + G. *chrōsis,* coloration]. An intensified redness of the blood.

hemacytometer (hē'mă-sī-tom'ĕ-ter, hem'ă-). Hemocytometer.

hemacytozoon (hē'mă-sī-tō-zō'on, hem'ă). Hemocytozoon.

hemadostenosis (hē'mă-dō-ste-nō'sis, hem'ad-ō) [G. *haimas (haimad-),* a stream of blood, + *stenōsis,* a narrowing]. Contraction of the arteries.

hemadrometer (hē-mă-drom'ĕ-ter, hem-ă). Hemodromometer.

hemadromograph (hē-mă-drō'mō-graf, hem-ă-) [hema- + G. *dromos,* a course + *graphō,* to record]. Hemodromograph.

hemadromometer (hē'mă-drō-mom'ĕ-ter, hem-ă-). Hemodromometer.

hemadsorption (hē'mad-sōrp-shŭn, hem'ad-). A phenomenon manifested by an agent or substance adhering to or being adsorbed on the surface of a red blood cell, as tuberculin (for example) can be adsorbed on red blood cells under certain conditions.

hemadynamometer (hē'mă-dī-nă-mom'ĕ-ter, hem'ă-). Hemodynamometer.

hemafacient (hē-mă-fā'shē-ent, hem-ă-). Hemopoietic.

hemagglutination (hē-mă-glū'ti-nā'shŭn, hem-). Hemoagglutination; the agglutination of red blood cells; may be immune as a result of specific antibody either for red blood cell antigens per se or other antigens which coat the red blood cells, or may be nonimmune as in h. caused by viruses or other microbes.
passive h., indirect h. test; a kind of passive agglutination in which erythrocytes, usually modified by mild treatment with tannic acid or other chemicals, are used to adsorb soluble antigen onto their surface, and which then agglutinate in the presence of antiserum specific for the adsorbed antigen.
reverse passive h., a diagnostic technique for virus infection using agglutination by viruses of red blood cells that previously have been coated with antibody specific to the virus.
viral h., the nonimmune agglutination of suspended red blood cells by certain of a wide range of otherwise unrelated viruses, usually by the virion itself but in some instances by products of viral

growth, the species of erythrocyte agglutinated differing with the different viruses. See also hemagglutination *inhibition.*

hemagglutinin (hē'mă-glū'ti-nin, hem-). Hemoagglutinin; a substance, antibody or other, that causes hemagglutination.

hemagogic (hē-mă-goj'ik, hem-ă-). Promoting a flow of blood.

hemagogue (hē'mă-gog, hem'ă-) [hem- + G. *agogos,* leading]. **1.** An agent that promotes a flow of blood. **2.** Emmenagogue.

hemal (hē'măl) [G. *haima,* blood]. **1.** Relating to the blood or blood vessels. **2.** Referring to the ventral side of the vertebral bodies or their precursors, where the heart and great vessels are located, as opposed to neural (2).

hemalum (hē-mal'ŭm, hem-). A solution of hematoxylin and alum used as a nuclear stain in histology, especially with eosin as a counterstain.

hemamebiasis (hē'mă-mē-bī'ă-sis, hem'ă-). Any infection with ameboid forms of parasites in red blood cells, as in malaria.

hemanalysis (hē-mă-nal'ĭ-sis, hem-) [G. *haima,* blood, + analysis]. Analysis of the blood; an examination of blood, especially with reference to chemical methods.

hemangiectasis, hemangiectasia (hē-man-jē-ek'tăsis, -ek-tā'zē-ă, hem-an-) [G. *haima,* blood, + *angeion,* vessel, + *ektasis,* a stretching]. Dilation of blood vessels.

hemangio- [G. *haima,* blood, + *angeion,* vessel]. Combining form relating to the blood vessels.

hemangioblast (he-man'jē-ō-blast) [hemangio- + G. *blastos,* germ]. A primitive embryonic cell of mesodermal origin producing cells from which are derived vascular endothelium, reticuloendothelial elements, and blood-forming cells of all types.

hemangioblastoma (he-man'jē-ō-blas-tō'mă). Angioblastoma; Lindau's tumor; a benign cerebellar neoplasm composed of capillary vessel-forming endothelial cells; a slowly growing tumor that affects, primarily, middle-aged individuals.

hemangioendothelioblastoma (he-man'jē-ō-en-dō-thē'-lē-ō-blas-tō'mă) [hemangio- + endothelium + G. *blastos,* germ, + *-oma,* tumor]. Hemangioendothelioma in which the endothelial cells seem to be especially immature forms.

hemangioendothelioma (he-man'jē-ō-en-dō-thē-lē-ō'mă) [hemangio- + endothelium + G. *-oma,* tumor]. Hemendothelioma; a neoplasm derived from blood vessels, characterized by numerous prominent endothelial cells that occur singly, in aggregates, and as the lining of congeries of vascular tubes or channels; in the elderly, may be malignant (angiosarcoma or hemangiosarcoma), but in children are benign and probably represent a growing stage of capillary hemangioma.

h. tubero'sum mul'tiplex, an eruption of pinkish papules, caused by hyperplasia of the endothelium of the superficial blood vessels.

hemangiofibroma (he-man'jē-ō-fī-brō'mă). A hemangioma with an abundant fibrous tissue framework.

juvenile h., juvenile *angiofibroma.*

hemangioma (he-man'jē-ō'mă) [hemangio- + G. *-oma,* tumor]. A congenital anomaly, in which a proliferation of vascular endothelium leads to a mass that resembles neoplastic tissue; it can occur anywhere in the body but is most frequently noticed in the skin and subcutaneous tissues.

arterial h., capillary h.

capillary h., arterial h.; h. congenitale or simplex; a congenital malformation consisting of numerous, variably sized but predominantly small, closely packed capillaries. See also *nevus* vascularis.

cavernous h., cavernous angioma; nevus cavernosus; a vascular malformation containing large blood-filled spaces, due apparently to dilation and thickening of the walls of the capillary loops; in the skin, extends more deeply than a capillary h. and is less likely to regress spontaneously.

h. congenital'le, capillary h.

h. pla'num exten'sum, a benign, flat, cutaneous hemangioma of considerable size.

racemose h., cirsoid *aneurysm.*

sclerosing h., see dermatofibroma.

senile h., a red papule due to weakening of the capillary wall, seen in most persons over 30 years of age. Also called cherry angioma; papillary or senile ectasia; De Morgan's or ruby spots.

h. sim'plex, capillary h.

verrucous h., a variant of the angiomatous nevus, appearing at birth or in early childhood, situated on the lower extremities with bluish-red nodules and warty surface; they enlarge and sometimes have satellite lesions.

hemangiomatosis (he-man'jē-ō-mă-tō'sis). A condition in which there are numerous hemangiomas.

hemangiopericytoma (he-man'jē-ō-per'i-sī-tō'mă) [hemangio- + pericyte + G. *-oma,* tumor]. Perithelioma; an uncommon vascular, usually benign, neoplasm composed of round and spindle cells that are derived from the pericytes and surround endothelium-lined vessels; malignant h.'s are difficult to distinguish microscopically from the benign.

hemangiosarcoma (he-man'jē-ō-sar-kō'mă). A rare malignant neoplasm characterized by rapidly proliferating, extensively infiltrating, anaplastic cells derived from blood vessels and lining irregular blood-filled or lumpy spaces.

hemapheic (hē-mă-fē'ik, hem-ă-). Pertaining to or containing hemaphein.

hemaphein (hē-mă-fē'in, hem-ă-) [G. *haima,* blood, + *phaios,* dusky]. A brown pathologic pigment derived from hemoglobin; said to be a combination of indican and urobilin.

hemapheism (hē-mă-fē'izm, hem-ă-). The presence of hemaphein in the blood plasma and urine.

hemarthron, hemarthros (he-mar'thron, he-mar'thrōs). Hemarthrosis.

hemarthrosis (hē'mar-thrō'sis, hem'ar-) [G. *haima,* blood, + *arthron,* joint]. Hemarthron; hemarthros; blood in a joint.

hemastrontium (hē-mă-stron'shē-ŭm, hem-ă-). A stain made by adding strontium chloride to a solution of hematein and aluminum chloride in citric acid and alcohol; used in histology.

hemat- [G. *haima* (*haimat-*), blood]. Combining form meaning blood. See also hem-, hemato-, hemo-.

hematachometer (hē'mă-tă-kom'ĕ-ter, hem'ă-). Hemotachometer.

hematapostema (hē'mat-ă-pos-tē'mă, hem'at-) [hemat- + G. *apostēma,* abscess]. An abscess into which blood has effused.

hematein (hē-mă-tē'in, hem-ă). An oxidation product of hematoxylin.

Baker's acid h., an acidic solution of oxidized hematoxylin used on frozen sections for staining phospholipids.

hematemesis (hē-mă-tem'ĕ-sis, hem-ă-) [hemat- + G. *emesis,* vomiting]. Vomitus cruentes; vomiting of blood.

hematencephalon (hē'mat-en-sef'ă-lon, hem'at-) [hemat- + G. *enkephalos,* brain]. Cerebral *hemorrhage.*

hematherapy (hē'mă-thār'ă-pē, hem'ă-). Hemotherapy.

hematherm (hē'mă-therm, hem'ă-) [G. *haima,* blood, + *thermos,* warm]. Homeotherm.

hemathermal (hē-mă-ther'măl, hem-ă-) [G. *haima,* blood, + *thermos,* warm]. Homeothermic.

hemathermous (hē-mă-ther'mŭs, hem-ă-). Homeothermic.

hemathidrosis (hē'mat-hī-drō'sis, hem'at-). Hematidrosis.

hemathorax (hē-mă-thōr'aks, hem-ă-). Hemothorax.

hematic (hē-mat'ik). **1.** Hemic; relating to blood. **2.** Hematinic (2).

hematid (hē'mă-tid, hem'a-) [hemat- + *-id*]. **1.** A red blood cell.

2. Infrequently used as a term for a cutaneous eruption presumed to be caused by a substance in the circulating blood.

hematidrosis (hē'mat-i-drō'sis, hem'at-) [hemat- + G. *hidrōs*, sweat]. Hemathidrosis; hemidrosis (1); sudor sanguineus; excretion of blood or blood pigment in the sweat; an extremely rare disorder.

hematimeter (hē-mă-tim'ĕ-ter, hem-ă-). Hemocytometer.

hematin (hē'mă-tin, hem'ă-). Ferriheme; hematosin; hydroxyhemin; oxyheme; oxyhemochromogen; phenodin; heme in which the iron is Fe(III) (Fe^{3+}); the prosthetic group of methemoglobin.

h. chloride, hemin.

reduced h., heme.

hematinemia (hē'mă-ti-nē'mē-ă, hem'ă-) [hematin + G. *haima*, blood]. The presence of heme in the circulating blood.

hematinic (hē-mă-tin'ik, hem-a-). Hematonic. **1.** Improving the condition of the blood. **2.** Hematic (2); an agent that improves the quality of blood by increasing the number of erythrocytes and/or the hemoglobin concentration.

hemato- [G. *haima* (*haimat-*), blood]. Combining form meaning blood. See also hem-, hemat-, hemo-.

hematobilia (hē'mă-tō-bil'ē-ă, hem'ă-). Hemobilia.

hematobium (hē-mă-tō'bē-ŭm, hem-ă-) [hemato- + G. *bios*, life]. Any microorganism that is parasitic in the blood, especially an animal form or hemozoon.

hematoblast (hē'mă-tō-blast, hem'ă-) [hemato- + G. *blastos*, germ]. A primitive, undifferentiated form of blood cell from which erythroblasts, lymphoblasts, myeloblasts, and other immature blood cells are derived; probably identical or closely similar to hemocytoblast and hemohistioblast; in normal bone marrow, present only in small numbers and difficult to identify in smears, inasmuch as h.'s are fragile and easily disintegrated; when marrow is hyperplastic, they may be observed in small groups.

Hayem's h., platelet.

hematocele (hē'mă-tō-sēl, hem'ă-) [hemato- + G. *kēlē*, tumor]. **1.** Hemorrhagic *cyst*. **2.** Effusion of blood into a canal or a cavity of the body. **3.** Swelling due to effusion of blood into the tunica vaginalis testis.

pelvic h., intraperitoneal effusion of blood into the pelvis.

pudendal h., effusion of blood into the labium majus.

hematocelia (hē'mă-tō-sē'lē-ă, hem'a-). Obsolete term for hematocele (2).

hematocephaly (hē'mă-tō-sef'ă-lē, hem'ă-) [hemato- + G. *kephalē*, head]. Intracranial effusion of blood, commonly in a fetus.

hematochezia (hē'mă-tō-kē'zē-ă, hem'ă-) [hemato- + G. *chezō*, to go to stool]. Passage of bloody stools, in contradistinction to melena, or tarry stools.

hematochlorin (hē'mă-tō-klō'rin, hem'ă). A green coloring matter derived from hemoglobin obtained from the placenta.

hematochyluria (hē'mă-tō-kī-lū'rē-ă, hem'a-) [hemato- + G. *chylos*, juice, + *ouron*, urine]. Presence of blood as well as chyle in the urine.

hematocolpometra (hē'mă-tō-kol'pō-mē'tră, hem'ă-) [hemato- + G. *kolpos*, vagina, + *mētra*, womb]. Accumulation of blood in the uterus and vagina resulting from an imperforate hymen or other lower vaginal obstruction.

hematocolpos (hē'mă-tō-kol'pos, hem'ă-) [hemato- + G. *kolpos*, vagina]. Retained menstruation; an accumulation of menstrual blood in the vagina in consequence of imperforate hymen or other obstruction.

hematocrit (hē'mă-tō-krit, hem'ă-) [hemato- + G. *krinō*, to separate]. **1.** A centrifuge or device for separating the cells and other particulate elements of the blood from the plasma. **2 (Hct).** Percentage of the volume of a blood sample occupied by cells, as determined by a h. *Cf.* plasmacrit.

hematocryal (hē-mă-tok'rē-ăl, hem-ă-) [hemato- + G. *kryos*, cold]. Poikilothermal.

hematocyst (hē'mă-tō-sist, hem'ă-). Hemorrhagic *cyst*.

hematocystis (hē'mă-tō-sis'tis, hem'ă-) [hemato- + G. *kystis*, bladder]. An effusion of blood into the bladder.

hematocyte (hē'mă-tō-sīt, hem'ă-). Hemocyte.

hematocytoblast (hē'mă-tō-sī'tō-blast, hem'ă-). Hemocytoblast.

hematocytolysis (hē'mă-tō-sī-tol'ĕ-sis, hem'ă-). Hemocytolysis.

hematocytometer (hē'mă-tō-sī-tom'ĕ-ter, hem'ă-). Hemocytometer.

hematocytozoon (hē'mă-tō-sī'tō-zō'on, hem'ă-). Hemocytozoon.

hematocyturia (hē'mă-tō-sī-tū'rē-ă, hem'ă-) [hemato- + G. *kytos*, cell, + *ouron*, urine]. Presence of red blood cells in the urine; true hematuria as distinguished from hemoglobinuria.

hematodyscrasia (hē'mă-tō-dis-krā'zē-ă, hem'ă-). Hemodyscrasia.

hematodystrophy (hē'mă-tō-dis'trō-fē, hem'ă-). Hemodystrophy.

hematogenesis (hē'mă-tō-jen'ĕ-sis, hem'ă-) [hemato- + G. *genesis*, production]. Hemopoiesis.

hematogenic, hematogenous (hē'mă-tō-jen'ik, hem-ă-toj'en-ŭs, hem'ă-). **1.** Hemopoietic. **2.** Pertaining to anything produced from, derived from, or transported by the blood.

hematohistioblast (hē'mă-tō-his'tē-ō-blast, hem'ă-). Hemohistioblast.

hematohiston (hē'mă-tō-his'tōn, hem'ă-). Globin.

hematoid (hē'mă-toyd, hem'ă-) [hemato- + G. *eidos*, resemblance]. Resembling blood.

hematoidin (hē-mă-toy'din). Blood or h. crystals; a pigment derived from hemoglobin which contains no iron but is closely related to or similar to bilirubin. H. is formed intracellularly, presumably within reticuloendothelial cells, but is often found extracellularly after 5 to 7 days in foci of previous hemorrhage. It occurs as refractile, yellow-brown and orange-red granules, but more characteristically as rhomboid plates arranged in a radial pattern, so-called h. burrs.

hematologist (hē-mă-tol'ō-jist, hem-ă-). A physician trained and experienced in hematology, *i.e.*, skilled in performing diagnostic examinations of blood and bone marrow, or in treatment of such diseases, or both.

hematology (hē-mă-tol'ō-jē, hem-ă-) [hemato- + G. *logos*, study]. Hemology; the medical specialty that pertains to the anatomy, physiology, pathology, symptomatology, and therapeutics related to the blood and blood-forming tissues.

hematolymphangioma (hē'mă-tō-limf'an-jē-ō'-mă, hem'ă-). A congenital anomaly consisting of numerous, closely packed, variably sized lymphatic vessels and larger channels, in association with a moderate number of blood vessels of a similar type.

hematolysis (hē-mă-tol'ĭ-sis, hem-ă-). Hemolysis.

hematolytic (hē'ma-tō-lit'ik, hem'ă). Hemolytic.

hematoma (hē-mă-tō'mă, hem-ă-) [hemato- + G. *-oma*, tumor]. A localized mass of extravasated blood that is relatively or completely confined within an organ or tissue, a space, or a potential space; the blood is usually clotted (or partly clotted), and, depending on how long it has been there, may manifest various degrees of organization and decolorization.

h. au'ris, othematoma.

corpus luteum h., *corpus* hemorrhagicum.

epidural h., extradural *hemorrhage*.

intracranial h., see intracranial *hemorrhage*, and related entries under hemorrhage.

intramural h., a h. in the wall of a structure, such as the bowel or bladder, usually resulting from trauma.

subdural h., subdural *hemorrhage*.

hematomanometer (hē′mă-tō-mă-nom′ĕ-ter, hem′ă-). Hemomanometer.

hematometra (hē′mă-tō-mē′tră, hem′ă-) [hemato- + G. *mētra,* uterus]. Hemometra; a collection or retention of blood in the uterine cavity.

hematometry (hē-mă-tom′ĕ-trē, hem-ă) [hemato- + G. *metron,* measure]. Hemometry; examination of the blood in order to determine any or all of the following: 1) the total number, types, and relative proportions of various blood cells; 2) the number or proportion of other formed elements; 3) the percentage of hemoglobin. In some instances, h. is used to include a determination of blood pressure.

hematomphalocele (hē′mat-om-fal′ō-sēl, hem′at-) [hemato- + G. *omphalos,* umbilicus, + *kēlē,* hernia]. Umbilical hernia into which an effusion of blood has taken place.

hematomyelia (hē′mă-tō-mī-ē′lē-ă, hem′ă-) [hemato- + G. *myelos,* marrow]. Hematorrhachis interna; myelapoplexy; myelorrhagia; hemorrhage into the substance of the spinal cord; it is usually a posttraumatic lesion but may also be encountered in instances of spinal cord capillary telangiectases.

hematomyelopore (hē′mă-tō-mī′ĕ-lō-pōr, hem′ă-) [hemato- + G. *myelos,* marrow, + *poros,* a pore]. Formation of porosities in the spinal cord as a result of hemorrhages.

hematonic (hē-mă-ton′ik, hem-ă-). Hematinic.

hematopathology (hē′mă-tō-path-ol′ō-jē, hem′ă-) [hemato- + G. *pathos,* suffering, + *logos,* study]. Hemopathology; the division of pathology concerned with diseases of the blood and of hemopoietic and lymphoid tissues.

hematopathy (hē-mă-top′ă-thē, hem-ă-). Hemopathy.

hematopenia (hē′mă-tō-pē′nē-ă, hem′ă-) [hemato- + G. *penia,* poverty]. Deficiency of blood, including hypocytosis or cytopenia.

hematophagia (hē′mă-tō-fā′jē-ă, hem′ă-) [hemato- + G. *phagein,* to eat]. Hemophagia; living on the blood of another animal, as does the vampire bat or a leech.

hematophagous (hē′mă-tof′ă-gŭs, hem′ă-) [hemato- + G. *phagein,* to eat]. Subsisting on blood.

hematophagus (hē′mă-tof′ă-gŭs, hem′ă-) [hemato- + G. *phagein,* to eat]. A blood eater, especially bloodsucking insects.

hematophilia (hē′mă-tō-phil′ē-ă, hem′ă-). Obsolete term for hemophilia.

hematoplastic (hē′mă-tō-plas′tik, hem′ă) [hemato- + G. *plassō,* to form]. Hemopoietic.

hematopoiesis (hē′mă-tō-poy-ē′sis, hem′ă-). Hemopoiesis.

hematopoietic (hē′mă-tō-poy-et′ik). Hemopoietic.

hematopoietin (hē′mă-tō-poy′ĕ-tin, hem′ă-). Erythropoietin.

hematoporphyria (hē′mă-tō-pōr-fir′ē-ă, hem′ă-) [hemato- + G. *porphyra,* purple]. Obsolete term for any disorder of porphyrin metabolism, regardless of the cause.

hematoporphyrin (hē′mă-tō-pōr′fi-rin, hem′ă-). Hemoporphyrin; 3,8-bis(α-hydroxyethyl)-2,7,12,18-tetramethylporphyrin-13,17-bis-propionic acid; a dark red, almost purple, porphyrin resulting from the decomposition of hemoglobin; chemical composition is that of heme with the iron removed and the two vinyl ($-CH{=}CH_2$) groups hydrated to hydroxyethyl ($-CHOH-CH_3$).

hematoporphyrinemia (hē′mă-tō-pōr′fi-ri-nē′mē-ă, hem′ă-). Older term used to designate the occurrence of hematoporphyrin in the circulating blood.

hematoporphyrinuria (hē′mă-tō-pōr′fi-ri-nū′rē-ă, hem′ă-). Older term used to designate enhanced urinary excretion of porphyrins.

hematopsia (hē-mă-top′sē-ă, hem-ă-) [hemato- + G. *opsis,* vision]. Hemorrhage into the eye.

hematorrhachis (hē-mă-tōr′ă-kis, hem-ă-) [hemato- + G. *rhachis,* spine]. Hemorrhachis; spinal apoplexy; a spinal hemorrhage.
h. exter′na, extradural or subdural h.; hemorrhage into the spinal canal external to the cord, either within or outside the dura.
extradural h., h. externa.
h. inter′na, hematomyelia.
subdural h., h. externa.

hematosalpinx (hē′mă-tō-sal′pinks, hem′ă-) [hemato- + G. *salpinx,* a trumpet]. Hemosalpinx; collection of blood in a tube, often associated with a tubal pregnancy.

hematosepsis (hē′mă-tō-sep′sis, hem′ă). Septicemia.

hematosin (hē-mă-tō′sin, hem-ă-). Hematin.

hematosis (hē-mă-tō′sis, hem-ă-). **1.** Hemopoiesis. **2.** Oxygenation of the venous blood in the lungs.

hematospectroscope (hē′mă-tō-spek′trō-skōp, hem′ă-). A spectroscope especially adapted to examination of the blood.

hematospectroscopy (hē′mă-tō-spek-tros′kō-pē, hem′ă-). Examination of the blood by means of a spectroscope.

hematospermatocele (hē′mă-tō-sper′mă-tō-sēl, hem′ă-). A spermatocele that contains blood.

hematospermia (hē′mă-tō-sper′mē-ă, hem′ă-). Hemospermia.

hematostatic (hē′mă-tō-stat′ik, hem′ă-). **1.** Hemostatic. **2.** Due to stagnation or arrest of blood in the vessels of the part.

hematostaxis (hē′mă-tō-stak′sis, hem′ă-) [hemato- + G. *staxis,* a dripping]. Spontaneous bleeding due to a disease of the blood.

hematosteon (hē-mă-tos′tē-on, hem-ă) [hemato- + G. *osteon,* bone]. Bleeding in the medullary cavity of a bone.

hematothermal (hē′mă-tō-ther′măl, hem′ă-). Homeothermic.

hematotoxic (hē′mă-tō-toks′ik, hem′ă-). Hemotoxic.

hematotoxin (hē′mă-tō-toks′in, hem′ă-). Hemotoxin.

hematotrachelos (hē′mă-tō-tră-kē′lŭs, hem′ă-) [hemato- + G. *trachēlos,* neck]. Distention of the cervix uteri with accumulated blood.

hematotropic (hē′mă-tō-trop′ik, hem′ă-). Hemotropic.

hematotympanum (hē′mă-tō-tim′pan-ŭm, hem′ă-). Hemotympanum.

hematoxic (hē-mă-toks′ik, hem-ă-). Hemotoxic.

hematoxin (hē-mă-toks′in, hem-ă). Hemotoxin.

hematoxylin (hē-mă-toks′i-lin, hem-ă-) [C.I. 75290]. A dark yellow or orange crystalline compound, $C_{16}H_{14}O_6 \cdot 3H_2O$, containing the coloring matter of *Haematoxylon campechianum* (logwood), from which it is obtained by extraction with ether. It is used as a dye in histology, especially for cell nuclei and chromosomes, muscle cross-striations, and enterochromaffin cells; its staining properties depend upon its oxidation to hematein and mordanting with chrome and iron alums. It is also used as an indicator (red to yellow at pH 0.0 to 1.0, yellow to violet at pH 5.0 to 6.0).
Boehmer's h., an alum type of h. in which natural ripening occurs in about 8 to 10 days, and the solution is good for many months.
Delafield's h., an alum type of h. used in histology; natural ripening takes about 2 months and the solution is good for years.
Harris' h., an alum type of h. similar to Delafield's h., but which uses chemical ripening to produce oxidation of h. for immediate use.
iron h., unique ferric lakes of hematein that produce deep blue-black stains; useful for studies of cytologic detail, such as chromosomes, spindle fibers, Golgi apparatus, myofibrils, and mitochrondria; also useful to demonstrate *Entamoeba histolytica.* See also Heidenhain's iron h. *stain;* Weigert's iron h. *stain.*
phosphotungstic acid h. (PTAH), Mallory's phosphotungstic acid h. stain; a s. with broad application in cytology and histology; nuclei, mitochrondria, fibrin, neuroglial fibrils, and cross-striations of skeletal and cardiac muscle stain blue; cartilage ground substance,

bone reticulum, and elastin appear in shades of yellow-orange and brownish red; also useful for demonstrating abnormal or diseased astrocytes, often in combination with periodic acid-Schiff stain and Luxol fast blue.

hematozoic (hē'ma-tō-zō'ik, hem'ă). Hemozoic.

hematozoon (hē'ma-tō-zō'on, hem'ă-). Hemozoon.

hematuresis (hē'mă-tū-rē'sis, hem'ă-). Hematuria, especially with reference to unusually large amounts of blood in urine.

hematuria (hē-mă-tū'-rē-ă, hem-ă-) [hemato- + G. *ouron,* urine]. Any condition in which the urine contains blood or red blood cells.
angioneurotic h., obsolete term for renal *epistaxis.*
Egyptian h., *schistosomiasis* haematobium.
endemic h., *schistosomiasis* haematobium.
essential h., a h. in which the cause and source are not recognized.
false h., pseudohematuria.
gross h., the presence of blood in the urine in sufficient quantity to be visible to the naked eye.
initial h., the presence of blood only in the first fraction of voided urine, usually indicating a urethral or prostatic source of bleeding.
microscopic h., presence of blood cells in uncatheterized urine, visible only under the microscope.
painful h., h. associated with dysuria, usually indicating the coexistence of infection, trauma, calculi, or foreign bodies within the lower urinary tract.
painless h., h. not associated with dysuria, often connoting a vascular or neoplastic etiology.
renal h., h. resulting from extravasation of blood into the glomerular spaces, or tubules, or pelves of the kidneys.
terminal h., the presence of blood only in the last fraction of voided urine, usually indicating a prostatic source of bleeding.
total h., uniform mixing of blood in the entire voided urine, commonly indicating an upper or mid-urinary tract source of bleeding.
urethral h., h. in which the site of bleeding is in the urethra.
vesical h., h. in which the site of bleeding is in the urinary bladder.

heme (hēm). Ferroheme; reduced hematin; ferroprotoporphyrin; protoheme; the tetrapyrrole chelate of iron in which the iron is Fe(II) (Fe^{2+}); the oxygen-carrying, color-furnishing, prosthetic group of hemoglobin.

hemelytrometra (hē-mel'i-trō-mē'tră, hem-el') [G. *haima,* blood, *elytron,* sheath (vagina), + *mētra,* uterus]. Obsolete term for hematocolpometra.

hemendothelioma (hē-men'dō-thē-lē-ō'mă, hem'en-dō-). Hemangioendothelioma.

hemeralopia (hem'er-al-ō'pē-ă) [G. *hēmera,* day, + *alaos,* obscure, + *ōps,* eye]. Day blindness; hemeranopia; night sight; inability to see as distinctly in a bright light as in reduced illumination.

hemeranopia (hem'er-ă-nō'pē-ă) [G. *hemera,* day, + *an-,* priv., + *ōps,* eye]. Hemeralopia.

hemerythrins (hē-mē-rith'rinz, hem-ē-). Iron-containing, oxygen-binding proteins in some worms, with molecular weights approximately that of hemoglobin but differing from hemoglobin in that the molecules do not contain porphyrin groups.

hemi- [G.]. Prefix signifying one-half; corresponds to Latin *semi-.*

hemiacardius (hem'ē-ă-kar'dē-ŭs) [hemi- + G. *a-* priv. + *kardia,* heart]. One of twin fetuses, in which only a part of the circulation is effected by its own heart, the rest by the heart of the other twin.

hemiacetal (hem'ē-as'e-tăl). A hydrated aldehyde, $RCH(OH)_2$, in which one of the hydroxyl groups is esterified with an alcohol, yielding RCH(OH)OR′ (in an acetal, both hydroxyl groups are so esterified). In the aldose sugars, the esterification is internal (R is R′) and labile, brought about by the migration of the H of the 4-OH or 5-OH to the carbonyl O, yielding the furanose or pyranose structures; the h. forms of the sugars are involved in all polysaccharides, as glycosyls or glycosides. See also hemiketal.

hemiacrosomia (hem'ē-ak-rō-sō'mē-ă) [hemi- + G. *akron,* extremity, + *sōma,* body]. A congenital form of hemihypertrophy of an extremity.

hemiageusia (hem'ē-ă-gū'sē-ă) [hemi- + G. *a-* priv. + *geusis,* taste]. Hemiageustia; hemigeusia; loss of taste from one side of the tongue.

hemiageustia (hem'ē-ă-gūs'tē-ă). Hemiageusia.

hemialgia (hem-ē-al'jē-ă) [hemi- + G. *algos,* pain]. Pain affecting one entire half of the body.

hemiamyosthenia (hem'ē-ă-mī'os-thē'nē-ă) [hemi- + G. *a-* priv. + *mys* (*myo-*), muscle, + *stheneia,* strength]. Hemiparesis.

hemianalgesia (hem'ē-an'al-jē'zē-ă). Analgesia affecting one side of the body.

hemianencephaly (hem'ē-an-en-sef'ă-lē). Anencephaly on one side only, or involving one side much more extensively than the other.

hemianesthesia (hem'ē-an-es-thē'-zē-ă). Unilateral anesthesia; anesthesia on one side of the body.
alternate h., crossed h.; h. affecting the head on one side and the body and extremities on the other side.
crossed h., alternate h.

hemianopia (hem'ē-ă-nō'pē-ă). Hemianopsia.

hemianopsia (hem'ē-an-op'sē-ă) [hemi- + G. *an-* priv. + *opsis,* vision]. Hemianopia; loss of vision for one half of the visual field of one or both eyes.
absolute h., h. in which the affected field is totally insensitive to all visual stimuli.
altitudinal h., a defect in the visual field in which the upper or lower half is lost; may be unilateral or bilateral.
bilateral h., binocular h.; h. affecting both eyes.
binasal h., blindness in the nasal field of vision of both eyes.
binocular h., bilateral h.
bitemporal h., blindness in the temporal field of vision of both eyes.
complete h., h. involving one-half of the visual field.
congruous h., h. in which the visual field defects in both eyes are completely symmetrical in extent and intensity.
crossed h., heteronymous h.; altitudinal h. involving the upper field of one eye and the lower field of the other.
heteronymous h., crossed h.
homonymous h., blindness in the corresponding (right or left) field of vision of each eye.
incomplete h., h. involving less than half the visual field of each eye.
incongruous h., an incomplete or asymmetric homonymous h.
pseudo-h., visual extinction; a condition in which individual stimuli are seen correctly, but when the nasal visual field of one eye and the temporal visual field of the fellow eye are stimulated simultaneously, one field is blind.
quadrantic h., quadrantanopsia; loss of vision in a quarter section of the visual field of one or both eyes; if bilateral, it may be homonymous or heteronymous, binasal or bitemporal, or crossed, *i.e.,* involving the upper quadrant in one eye and the lower quadrant in the other.
relative h., h. in which color sense, form sense, or both are retained.
unilateral h., uniocular h., loss of sight in one-half of the visual field of one eye only.

hemianoptic (hem'ē-an-op'tik). Pertaining to hemianopsia.

hemianosmia (hem'ē-an-oz'mē-ă) [hemi- + G. *an-* priv. + *osmē,* smell]. Loss of the sense of smell on one side.

hemiaplasia (hem'ē-ă-plā'zē-ă) [hemi- + aplasia]. Absence of one lobe of a bilobed organ; used especially with reference to the thyroid gland.

hemiapraxia (hem'ē-ă-prak'sē-ă). Apraxia affecting one side of the body.

hemi-arthroplasty (hem-ē-ar'thrō-plas-tē). Arthroplasty in which one joint surface is replaced with artificial material, usually metal.

hemiasynergia (hem'ē-ă-sin-er'jē-ă). Asynergia affecting one side of the body.

hemiataxia (hem'ē-ă-tak'sē-ă). Ataxia affecting one side of the body.

hemiathetosis (hem'ē-ath'ē-tō'sis). Athetosis affecting one hand, or one hand and foot, only.

hemiatrophy (hem-ē-at'rō-fē). Atrophy of one lateral half of a part or of an organ, as the face or tongue.
facial h., Romberg's disease, trophoneurosis, or syndrome; facial trophoneurosis; atrophy, usually progressive, affecting the tissues of one side of the face; saber-cut depression on forehead, heterochromia iridis, or bullous keratopathy may be present.
progressive lingual h., lingual trophoneurosis; atrophy of one lateral half of the tongue.

hemiballism (hem-ē-bal'izm) [hemi- + G. *ballismos,* jumping about]. Hemiballismus.

hemiballismus (hem-ē-bal-iz'mŭs) [hemi- + G. *ballismos,* jumping about]. Hemiballism; violent writhing and choreic movements involving one side of the body, usually related to damage to the subthalamic nucleus of the opposite side of the brain.

hemiblock (hem'ē-blok). Arrest of the impulse in one of the two main divisions of the left branch of the bundle of His; *i.e.,* in either the anterior (superior) division or the posterior (inferior) division.

hemic (hē'mik). Hematic (1).

hemicardia (hem-ē-kar'dē-ă) [hemi- + G. *kardia,* heart]. **1.** Either lateral half, including atrium and ventricle, of the heart. **2.** A congenital malformation of the heart in which only two of the usual four chambers are formed.
h. dex'tra, right *heart.*
h. sinis'tra, left *heart.*

hemicellulose (hem-ē-sel'yū-lōs). Cellulosan; plant cell-wall polysaccharides closely associated with cellulose, such as xylans, mannans, and galactans.

hemicentrum (hem'ē-sen'trŭm) [hemi- + G. *kentron,* center]. One of the two lateral halves of the body of the vertebra.

hemicephalalgia (hem'ē-sef'ă-lal'jē-ă) [hemi- + G. *kephalē,* head, + *algos,* pain]. Hemicrania (2); the unilateral headache characteristic of typical migraine.

hemicephalia (hem-ē-se-fā'lē-ă) [hemi- + G. *kephalē,* head]. Partial anencephaly; congenital failure of the cerebrum to develop normally; usually the cerebellum and basal ganglia are represented at least in rudimentary form.

hemicerebrum (hem'ē-ser'ē-brŭm). A cerebral hemisphere.

Hemichorda (hem-ē-kōr'dă). Hemichordata.

Hemichordata (hem'ē-kōr-dā'tă) [hemi- + Mod. L. *chordata,* having a notochord, fr. G. chordē, string]. Hemichorda; a phylum comprised of soft-bodied, bilaterally symmetrical wormlike marine animals with gill-slits to the pharynx and a conical proboscis; a ciliated larval stage resembles that of echinoderms.

hemichorea (hem'ē-kōr-ē'ă). Chorea dimidiata; hemilateral chorea; chorea involving the muscles on one side only.

hemichromosome (hem'i-krō'mō-sōm). A lateral half of a chromosome.

hemicolectomy (hem'ē-kō-lek'tō-mē) [hemi- + G. *kolon,* colon, + *ektomē,* excision]. Removal of the right or left side of the colon.

hemicorporectomy (hem'ē-kōr-pō-rek'tō-mē) [hemi- + L. *corpus,* body, + G. *ektomē,* excision]. Surgical removal of the lower half of the body, including the lower extremities, bony pelvis, genitalia, and various of the pelvic contents including the lower part of the rectum to the anus.

hemicrania (hem-ē-krā'nē-ă) [hemi- + G. *kranion,* skull]. **1.** Migraine. **2.** Hemicephalalgia.

hemicraniectomy (hem'ē-krā-nē-ek'tōmē) [hemi- + G. *kranion,* skull, + *ektomē,* excision]. Hemicraniotomy.

hemicraniosis (hem'ē-krā-nē-ō'sis). Enlargement of one side of the cranium.

hemicraniotomy (hem'ē-krā-nē-ot'ō-mē) [hemi- + G. *kranion,* skull, + *tomē,* cut]. Hemicraniectomy; separation and reflection of the greater part or all of one half of the cranium, as a preliminary to an operation upon the brain.

hemidesmosomes (hem-ē-des'mō-sōmz). Half desmosomes that occur on the basal surface of the stratum basalis of stratified squamous epithelium.

hemidiaphoresis (hem'ē-dī-ă-fō-rē'sis). Hemihidrosis; hemidrosis (2); diaphoresis, or sweating, on one side of the body.

hemidrosis (hem-ē-drō'sis). **1.** Hematidrosis. **2.** Hemidiaphoresis.

hemidysesthesia (hem'ē-dis-es-thē'-zē-ă). Dysesthesia affecting one side of the body.

hemidystrophy (hem-ē-dis'trō-fē) [hemi- + G. *dys-,* ill, + *trophē,* nourishment, growth]. Underdevelopment of one lateral half of the body.

hemiectromelia (hem'ē-ek-trō-mē'lē-ă) [hemi- + ectromelia]. Defective development of the limbs on one side of the body.

hemiepilepsy (hem-ē-ep'i-lep-sē). Unilateral convulsive movements.

hemifacial (hem-ē-fā'shăl). Pertaining to one side of the face.

hemigastrectomy (hem'ē-gas-trek-tō-mē). Excision of the distal one-half of the stomach.

hemigeusia (hem'ē-gū'sē-ă). Hemiageusia.

hemiglobin (hem'ē-glō-bin). Obsolete term for methemoglobin.

hemiglossal (hem'ē-glos'ăl) [hemi- + G. *glōssa,* tongue]. Hemilingual.

hemiglossectomy (hem'ē-glos-ek'tō-mē) [hemi- + G. *glōssa,* tongue, + *ektomē,* excision]. Surgical removal of one-half of the tongue.

hemiglossitis (hem'ē-glos-ī'tis) [hemi- + G. *glōssa,* tongue, + *-itis,* inflammation]. A vesicular eruption on one side of the tongue and the corresponding inner surface of the cheek, probably herpetic.

hemignathia (hem-ē-nath'ē-ă) [hemi- + G. *gnathos,* jaw]. Defective development of one side of the mandible.

hemihepatectomy (hem'ē-hep-ă-tek'tō-mē). Surgical removal of one-half or a lobe of the liver.

hemihidrosis (hem'ē-hī-drō'sis). Hemidiaphoresis.

hemihydranencephaly (hem-ē-hī'dran-en-sef'ă-lē). A unilateral form of hydranencephaly.

hemihypalgesia (hem'ē-hī-pal-je'zē-ă). Hypalgesia affecting one side of the body.

hemihyperesthesia (hem'ē-hī'per-es-thē'zē-ă). Hyperesthesia, or increased tactile and painful sensibility, affecting one side of the body.

hemihyperhidrosis (hem'ē-hī-per-hī-drō'sis) [hemi- + G. *hyper,* over, + *hidrōsis,* sweating]. Hemihyperidrosis; excessive sweating confined to one side of the body.

hemihyperidrosis (hem'ē-hī-per-i-drō'sis). Hemihyperhydrosis.

hemihypertonia (hem'ē-hī-per-tō'nē-ă) [hemi- + G. *hyper,* over, + *tonos,* tone]. Hemitonia; exaggerated muscular tonicity on one side of the body.

hemihypertrophy (hem'ē-hī-per'trō-fē). Muscular or osseous hypertrophy of one side of the face or body.

hemihypesthesia (hem'ē-hī-pes-thē'zē-ă) [hemi- + G. *hypo,* under, + *aesthēses,* sensation]. Hemihypoesthesia; diminished sensibility in one side of the body.

hemihypoesthesia (hem'ē-hī-pō-es-thē'zē-ă) [hemi- + G. *hypo,* under, + *aisthēses,* sensation]. Hemihypesthesia.

hemihypotonia (hem'ē-hī-pō-tō'nē-ă) [hemi- + G. *hypo,* under, + *tonos,* tone]. Partial loss of muscular tonicity on one side of the body.

hemikaryon (hem-i-kar'i-on) [hemi- + G. *karyon,* nut (nucleus)]. A cell nucleus containing the haploid number of chromosomes.

hemiketal (hem'ē-kē-tăl). A hydrated ketone, $R_2C(OH)OR'$, in which one of the hydroxyl groups is esterified with an alcohol (in a ketal, both hydroxyl groups are so esterified). In the ketose sugars, migration of an alcoholic H from the δ or ϵ OH to the keto O leads to intramolecular cyclization (furanose or pyranose), R and R′ thus being the same carbon chain; the h. forms of the sugars are involved in polysaccharide formation, as glycosyls or glycosides. See also hemiacetal.

hemilaminectomy (hem'ē-lam-i-nek'tō-mē) [hemi- + L. *lamina,* layer, + G. *ektomē,* excision]. Removal of a portion of a vertebral lamina, usually performed for exploration of, access to, or decompression of the intraspinal contents; often used to denote unilateral laminectomy.

hemilaryngectomy (hem'ē-lar-in-jek'tō-mē) [hemi- + G. *larnyx* (*laryng-*), larynx, + *ektomē,* excision]. Excision of one lateral half of the larynx.

hemilateral (hem-ē-lat'er-ăl). Relating to one lateral half.

hemilesion (hem-ē-lē'zhŭn). A unilateral lesion.

hemilingual (hem-ē-ling'gwăl) [hemi- + L. *lingua,* tongue]. Hemiglossal; relating to one lateral half of the tongue.

hemimacroglossia (hem'ē-mak'rō-glos'ē-ă) [hemi- + G. *makros,* large, + *glōssa,* tongue]. Enlargement of half the tongue.

hemimandibulectomy (hem'ē-man-dib'yū-lek'tō-mē). Resection of one-half of the mandible.

hemimetabolous (hem'ē-me-tab'ō-lŭs) [hemi- + G. *metabolē,* change]. Pertaining to a member of the series of insect orders, the Hemimetabola, in which simple or incomplete metamorphosis is found.

hemin (hēm'in). The chloride of heme in which Fe^{2+}has become Fe^{3+}. Also called hematin chloride; chlorohemin; ferriheme chloride, ferriprotoporphyrin; ferriporphyrin chloride; Teichmann's crystals; factor X for *Haemophilus.*

hemiopalgia (hem'ē-ō-pal'jē-ă) [hemi- + G. *ōps,* eye, + *algos,* pain]. Pain in one eye, usually accompanied by hemicrania.

hemipagus (hem-ip'ă-gŭs) [hemi- + G. *pagos,* something fixed]. Conjoined twins united laterally at the thorax, or at the thorax and neck, and sometimes also at the jaws.

hemiparanesthesia (hem'ē-par-an-es-thē'zē-ă). Anesthesia of one lower extremity, or of the lower part of one side of the body.

hemiparaplegia (hem'ē-par-ă-plē'jē-ă). Paralysis of one leg.

hemiparesis (hem-ē-pa-rē'sis, -par'ē-sis). Hemiamyosthenia; slight paralysis affecting one side of the body.

hemipelvectomy (hem'ē-pel-vek'tō-mē) [hemi- + L. *pelvis,* basin (pelvis), + G. *ektomē,* excision]. Hindquarter, interilioabdominal, interpelviabdominal, or Jaboulay's amputation; amputation of an entire leg together with the os coxae.

hemiplegia (hem-ē-plē'jē-ă) [hemi- + G. *plēgē,* a stroke]. Paralysis of one side of the body.

alternating h., crossed h. or paralysis; stauroplegia; h., as the result of a brainstem lesion, occurring on the contralateral side (with reference to the lesion) with paralysis of a motor cranial nerve on the ipsilateral side.

contralateral h., paralysis occurring on the side opposite to the causal central lesion.

crossed h., alternating h.

double h., diplegia.

facial h., paralysis of one side of the face, the muscles of the extremities being unaffected.

Gubler's h., Gubler's *syndrome.*

infantile h., birth *palsy.*

spastic h., a h. with increased tone in the antigravity muscles of the affected side.

hemiplegic (hem-ē-plē'jik). Relating to hemiplegia.

Hemiptera (hem-ip'ter-ă) [hemi- + G. *pteron,* wing]. An arthropod order of the class Insecta that includes many plant lice and other true bugs; those of the subfamily Triatominae are bloodsuckers and of medical importance. The best known species is *Cimex lectularius,* the common bedbug.

hemipyonephrosis (hem'ē-pī-ō-ne-frō'sis). Obsolete term for unilateral pyonephrosis, or pyonephrosis of half a kidney.

hemisection (hem-ē-sek'shŭn). Surgical removal of a root of a multirooted tooth and its related coronal portion.

hemisensory (hem'ē-sen'sōr-ē). Loss of sensation on one side of the body. *Cf.* hemianesthesia.

hemiseptum (hem-ē-sep'tŭm). A lateral half of any septum.

hemispasm (hem'ē-spazm). A spasm affecting one or more muscles of one side of the face or body.

hemisphere (hem'i-sfēr) [hemi- + G. *sphaira,* ball, globe]. Hemispherium; half of a spherical structure.

cerebellar h., **(1)** hemispherium (2); **(2)** *hemispherium* cerebelli.

cerebral h., **(1)** hemispherium (1); **(2)** *hemispherium* cerebri.

dominant h., that cerebral hemisphere containing the representation of speech and controlling the arm and leg used preferentially in skilled movements.

hemispherectomy (hem'ē-sfēr-ek'tō-mē). Excision of one cerebral hemisphere; undertaken for malignant tumors, intractable epilepsy usually associated with infantile hemiplegia due to birth injury, and other cerebral conditions.

hemispherium (hem'i-sfēr'ē-ŭm) [G. *hemisphairion*] [NA]. Hemisphere. **1.** H. cerebri. **2.** H. cerebelli.

h. bul'bi ure'thrae, one of the lateral halves of the bulb of the urethra that are separated by a median groove on the posterior part of the undersurface.

h. cerebel'li [NA], cerebellar hemisphere; hemispherium (2); the large part of the cerebellum lateral to the vermis cerebelli.

h. cer'ebri [NA], cerebral hemisphere; hemispherium (1); the large mass of the telencephalon, on either side of the midline, consisting of the cerebral cortex and its associated fiber systems, together with the deeper-lying subcortical telencephalic nuclei (*i.e.,* basal ganglia). See fig. on p. 696.

Hemispora (hem'ē-spō'ră) [hemi- + G. *sporos,* seed]. Generic name for certain species of *Fungi Imperfecti* in which chains of conidia develop from tubular structures that form as the result of a constriction at the end of each of a series of short hyphal branches; close septations divide the contents of the tube into relatively square, thick-walled, deeply staining segments that eventually separate and become rounded, thick-walled spores with rough surfaces. *H.* organisms occur fairly frequently as contaminants in cultures for other fungi; they are usually regarded as nonpathogenic forms, but there are a few reported instances in which they were apparently the causal agents of disease.

hemistrumectomy (hem'ē-strū-mek'tō-mē) [hemi- + L. *struma,* + G. *ektomē,* excision]. Excision of approximately one-half of a goiter.

hemisyndrome (hem'ē-sin-drōm). A condition in which one-half of the body is atrophied or hypertrophied.

hemisystole (hem-ē-sis'tō-lē). Systole alternans; contraction of the left ventricle following every second atrial contraction only, so that there is but one pulse beat to every two heart beats.

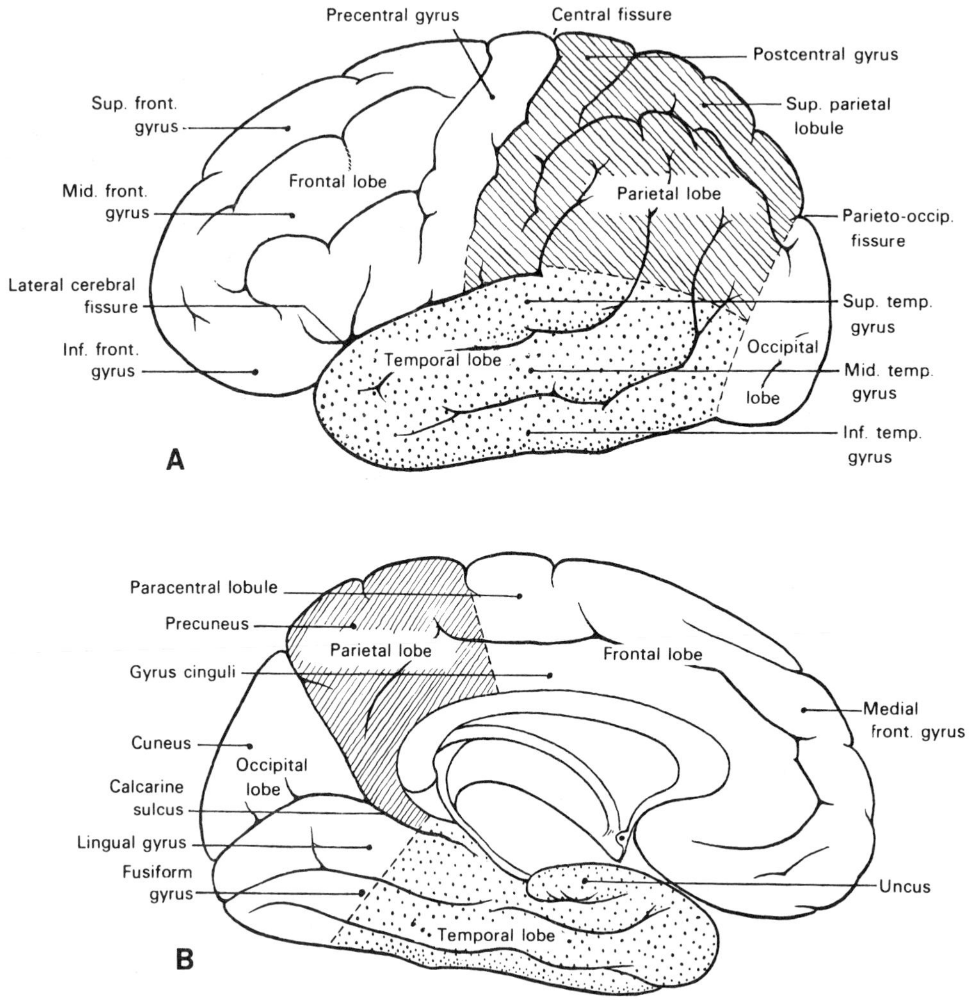

Hemispherium Cerebri (Cerebral Hemisphere)
The lateral (*A*) and medial (*B*) aspects of the cerebral hemisphere with principal gyri.

hemiterpene (hem-ē-ter′pēn). Isoprene.

hemithermoanesthesia (hem′ē-ther′mō-an-es-thē′zē-ă). Loss of sensibility to heat and cold affecting one side of the body.

hemithorax (hem-ē-thō′raks). One side of the thorax.

hemitonia (hem-ē-tō′nē-ă). Hemihypertonia.

hemitremor (hem′ē-trem′er, -trē′mer). Tremor affecting the muscles of one side of the body.

hemivertebra (hem-ē-ver′tē-bră). A congenital defect of the spine in which one side of a vertebra fails to develop completely.

hemizygosity (hem′i-zī-gos′i-tē). The state of being hemizygous.

hemizygote (hem-i-zī′gōt) [hemi- + G. *zygōtos,* yoked]. An individual hemizygous with respect to one or more specified genes; *e.g.,* a hemophilic male is a h. with respect to the gene for hemophilia.

hemizygotic (hem′i-zī-got′ik). Hemizygous.

hemizygous (hem-i-zī′gŭs). Hemizygotic; having unpaired genes in an otherwise diploid cell; males are normally h. for genes on the X chromosome.

hemlock (hem′lok). Conium.

hemo- [G. *haima,* blood]. Combining form signifying blood. See also hem-, hemat-, hemato-.

hemoagglutination (hē′mō-ă-glū′ti-nā′shŭn). Hemagglutination.

hemoagglutinin (hē′mō-ă-glū′ti-nin). Hemagglutinin.

hemoantitoxin (hē′mō-an-ti-tok′sin). An antibody that neutralizes the effects of a hemotoxin, such as the hemolytic material in cobra venom.

Hemobartonella (hē′mō-bar-tō-nel′ă). See *Haemobartonella.*

hemobilia (hē-mō-bil′ē-ă). Hematobilia; bleeding into the biliary passages, usually as a result of hepatic trauma or a neoplasm in the liver or biliary tract.

hemoblast (hēm′ō-blast). Hemocytoblast.
lymphoid h. of Pappenheim, pronormoblast. See also discussion under erythroblast.

hemoblastosis (hē′mō-blas-tō′sis). A proliferative condition of the hematopoietic tissues in general.

hemocatharsis (hē′mō-kă-thar′sis) [hemo- + G. *katharsis,* a cleansing]. Cleansing the blood.

hemocatheresis (hē′mō-kath-e-rē′sis) [hemo- + G. *kathairesis*, destruction]. Destruction of the blood cells, especially of erythrocytes (hemocytocatheresis).

hemocatheretic (hē′mō-kath-ĕ-ret′ik). Pertaining to or characterized by hemocatheresis.

hemocele (hē′mō-sēl) [hemo- + G. *koilōma*, cavity]. The system of blood-containing spaces pervading the body in arthropods.

hemocholecyst (hē′mō-kō′lē-sist, -kol′ē-sist) [hemo- + G. *cholē*, bile, + *kystis*, bladder]. **1.** A cyst containing blood and bile. **2.** Nontraumatic hemorrhage or old blood accumulated in the gallbladder.

hemocholecystitis (hē′mō-kō′lē-sis-tī′tis). Hemorrhagic cholecystitis.

hemochromatosis (hē′mō-krō-mă-tō′sis) [hemo- + G. *chrōma*, color, + *-osis*, condition]. Hemachromatosis; a disorder of iron metabolism characterized by excessive absorption of ingested iron, saturation of iron-binding protein, and deposition of hemosiderin in tissue, particularly in the liver, pancreas, and skin; cirrhosis of the liver, diabetes (bronze diabetes), bronze pigmentation of the skin, and eventual heart failure may occur; can also result from administration of large amounts of iron orally, by injection, or in forms of blood transfusion therapy.
exogenous h., hemosiderosis due to repeated blood transfusions; it can progress to pigmentary cirrhosis.
hereditary h., idiopathic h., primary h.
primary h., hereditary or idiopathic h.; a specific inherited metabolic defect with increased absorption and accumulation of iron on a normal diet; autosomal dominant inheritance with reduced penetrance in females; juvenile h. may represent a homozygous state of the same gene.
secondary h., increased intake and accumulation of iron secondary to known cause, such as oral iron therapy or multiple transfusions.

hemochrome (hē′mō-krōm). Hemochromogen.

hemochromogen (hē-mō-krō′mō-jen) [hemo- + G. *chrōma*, color, + *-gen*, producing]. Hemochrome; term originally used for combinations of ferro- or ferriporphyrins with 2 moles of a nitrogenous base, *e.g.*, pyridine ferroporphyrin.

hemoclasis, hemoclasia (hē-mok′lă-sis, hē′mō-klā′zē-ă) [hemo- + G. *klasis*, a breaking]. Rupture, dissolution (hemolysis), or other type of destruction of red blood cells.

hemoclastic (hē′mō-klas′tik). Pertaining to hemoclasis.

hemoconcentration (hē′mō-kon-sen-trā′shŭn). Decrease in the volume of plasma in relation to the number of red blood cells; increase in the concentration of red blood cells in the circulating blood.

hemoconia (hē-mō-kō′nē-ă) [hemo- + G. *konis*, dust]. Blood dust or motes; dust corpuscles; small refractive particles in the circulating blood, probably lipid material associated with fragmented stroma from red blood cells.

hemoconiosis (hē′mō-kō-nē-ō′sis). A condition in which there is an abnormal amount of hemoconia in the blood.

hemocryoscopy (hē′mō-krī-os′kŏ-pē) [hemo- + G. *kryos*, cold, + *skopeō*, to examine]. Determination of the freezing point of blood.

hemocuprein (hē-mō-kū′prē-in). Cytocuprein.

hemocyanin (hē-mō-sī′ă-nin). An oxygen-carrying pigment (molecular weights between 0.5 and 10 $\times$ 10^6) of lower sea animals; copper is an essential component, but it contains no heme; used as an experimental antigen.

hemocyte (hē′mō-sīt) [hemo- + G. *kytos*, a hollow (cell)]. Hematocyte; any cell or formed element of the blood.

hemocytoblast (hē′mō-sī′tō-blast) [hemo- + G. *kytos*, cell, + *blastos*, germ]. Hematocytoblast; hemoblast; a blood cell derived from embryonic mesenchyme, characterized by basophilic cytoplasm and a relatively large nucleus with a spongy, loose network of chromatin and several nucleoli; mitochondria are extremely fine and delicate. H.'s represent the primitive stem cells of the monophyletic theory of the origin of blood and have the potentiality of developing into erythroblasts, young forms of the granulocytic series, megakaryocytes, etc.

hemocytocatheresis (hē′mō-sī′tō-kă-ther′ē-sis) [hemo- + G. *kytos*, a hollow (cell), + *kathairesis*, destruction]. Hemolysis, or other type of destruction of red blood cells.

hemocytolysis (hē′mō-sī-tol′i-sis) [hemo- + G. *kytos*, cell, + *lysis*, dissolution]. Hematocytolysis; the dissolution of blood cells, including hemolysis.

hemocytometer (hē′mō-sī-tom′ĕ-ter) [hemo- + G. *kytos*, cell, + *metron*, measure]. Hemacytometer; hematimeter; hematocytometer; an apparatus for estimating the number of blood cells in a quantitatively measured volume of blood; it consists of a glass pipette with an ampulla for collecting and diluting the blood, and a counting chamber marked in squares.

hemocytometry (hē′mō-sī-tom′ĕ-trē). The counting of red blood cells.

hemocytotripsis (hē′mō-sī-tō-trip′sis) [hemo- + G. *kytos*, + *tripsis*, a grinding]. Fragmentation or disintegration of blood cells by means of mechanical trauma, *e.g.*, compression between hard surfaces.

hemocytozoon (hē′mō-sī-tō-zō′on) [hemo- + G. *kytos*, cell, + *zōon*, animal]. Hemacytozoon; hematocytozoon; a protozoon parasite of the blood cells.

hemodiagnosis (hē′mō-dī-ag-nō′sis). Diagnosis by means of examination of the blood.

hemodialysis (hē′mō-dī-al′i-sis). Dialysis of soluble substances and water from the blood by diffusion through a semipermeable membrane; separation of cellular elements and colloids from soluble substances is achieved by pore size in the membrane and rates of diffusion.

hemodialyzer (hē-mō-dī′ă-lī-zer). Artificial kidney; a machine for hemodialysis in acute or chronic renal failure; toxic substances in the blood are removed by exposure to dialyzing fluid across a semipermeable membrane.
ultrafiltration h., a h. that uses fluid pressure differentials to bring about loss (usually) of protein-free fluid from the blood to the bath, as in certain edematous conditions.

hemodiastase (hē-mō-dī′as-tās). Blood amylase.

hemodilution (hē′mō-di-lū′shŭn). Increase in the volume of plasma in relation to red blood cells; reduced concentration of red blood cells in the circulation.

hemodromograph (hē-mō-drō′mō-graf) [hemo- + G. *dromos*, course, + *graphō*, to record]. Hemadromograph; rarely used term(s) for an instrument for recording the rapidity of the blood circulation.

hemodromometer (hē′mō-drō-mom′ĕ-ter) [hemo- + G. *dromos*, course, + *metron*, measure]. Hemadrometer; hemadromometer; rarely used term(s) for an instrument for measuring the rapidity of the blood circulation.

hemodynamic (hē′mō-dī-nam′ik). Relating to the physical aspects of the blood circulation.

hemodynamics (hē′mō-dī-nam′iks) [hemo- + G. *dynamis*, power]. The study of the dynamics of the blood circulation.

hemodynamometer (hē′mō-dī-nă-mom′ĕ-ter) [hemo- + G. *dynamis*, force, + *metron*, measure]. Hemadynamometer; an instrument for determining the blood pressure.

hemodyscrasia (hē′mō-dis-krā′zē-ă) [hemo- + G. *dyscrasia*, bad temperament]. Hematodyscrasia; any abnormal condition or disorder of the blood and hemopoietic tissue, used especially with reference to those resulting in changes in the formed elements.

hemodystrophy (hē-mō-dis'trō-fē). Hematodystrophy; any disease or abnormal condition of the blood and hemopoietic tissues, exclusive of simple transitory changes.

hemofiltration (hē'mō-fil-trā'shŭn). A process, similar to hemodialysis, by which blood is dialyzed using ultrafiltration and simultaneous reinfusion of physiologic saline solution.

hemoflagellates (hē-mō-flaj'ĕ-lāts) [hemo- + L. *flagellum,* dim. of *flagrum,* a whip]. Protozoan flagellates in the family Trypanosomatidae that are parasitic in the blood of many species of domestic and wild animals and birds, and of man; they include the genera *Leishmania* and *Trypanosoma,* several species of which are important pathogens.

hemofuscin (hē-mō-fŭs'in). A brown pigment derived from hemoglobin which occurs in urine occasionally along with hemosiderin, usually indicative of increased red blood cell destruction; occurs also in the liver with hemosiderin in cases of hemochromatosis.

hemogenesis (hē-mō-jen'ĕ-sis). Hemopoiesis.

hemogenic (hē-mō-jen'ik). Hemopoietic.

HEMOGLOBIN

hemoglobin (Hb) (hē-mō-glō'bin). The red respiratory protein of erythrocytes, consisting of approximately 6% heme and 94% globin, with a molecular weight of 68,000, which as oxyhemoglobin (HbO_2) transports oxygen from the lungs to the tissues where the oxygen is readily released and HbO_2 becomes Hb. When Hb is exposed to certain chemicals, its normal respiratory function is blocked; *e.g.,* the oxygen in HbO_2 is easily displaced by carbon monoxide, thereby resulting in the formation of fairly stable carboxyhemoglobin (HbCO), as in asphyxiation resulting from inhalation of exhaust fumes from gasoline engines. When the iron in Hb is oxidized from the ferrous to ferric state, as in poisoning with nitrates and certain other chemicals, a nonrespiratory compound, methemoglobin (MetHb), is formed.

In man there are four kinds of normal Hb: embryonic (Hb Gower-2), fetal (Hb F), and two adult types (Hb A, Hb A_2), each consisting of two α globin chains containing 141 amino acid residues, and two of another kind (β, γ, δ, or ϵ), each containing 146 amino acid residues. The production of each kind of globin chain is controlled by a structural gene of similar Greek letter designation; normal individuals are homozygous for the normal gene at each of five loci. Mutations, resulting in the substitution of one amino acid for another in the polypeptide chain, can occur at any codon in any of the five loci and have resulted in production of more than 550 types of abnormal Hb, most of no known clinical significance. In addition, deletions of one or more amino acid residues are known, and gene rearrangements due to unequal crossing over between homologous chromosomes.

The listing of Hb types below includes only the abnormal types known to be of clinical significance. Newly discovered abnormal Hb types are first assigned a name, usually the location where discovered, and a molecular formula is added when determined. The formula consists of Greek letters to designate the basic chains, with subscript 2 if there are two identical chains; a superscript letter (^{A} if normal for adult Hb, etc.) is added, or the superscript may designate the site of amino acid substitution (numbering amino acid residues from the N terminus of the polypeptide) and specifying the change, using standard abbreviations for the amino acids.

h. A, normal adult Hb (Hb A) with molecular formula $\alpha_2{}^A\beta_2{}^A$.
h. A$_{Ic}$, the major fraction of glycosylated h.
h. A$_2$, the normal Hb (Hb A_2) of the molecular formula $\alpha_2{}^A\ \delta_2$, which makes up approximately 1.5 to 3% of the total h. concentration.
aberrant h., a mutant Hb that functions abnormally. *Cf.* variant h.
h. Bart's, a Hb homotetramer (all four polypeptides identical) of molecular formula γ_4, found in the early embryo and in α-thalassemia; not effective in oxygen transport.
bile pigment h., choleglobin.
h. C, an abnormal Hb with substitution of lysine for glutamic acid at the 6th position of the β chain, of molecular formula $\alpha_2{}^A\beta_2{}^{6\ \mathrm{Glu \rightarrow Lys}}$; this type reduces the normal plasticity of erythrocytes. Heterozygotes: Hb C trait, about 28 to 44% of total Hb is Hb C, no anemia. Homozygotes: nearly all Hb is Hb C, moderate normocytic hemolytic anemia. Individuals heterozygous for both Hb C and Hb S (Hb SC disease) and for Hb C and thalassemia are known, and have atypical hemolytic anemias.
h. C$_{Georgetown}$, h. C$_{Harlem}$, two abnormal Hb's, both with the substitution of valine for glutamic acid at the 6th position of the β chain as in Hb S, and in addition each has a second substitution; Hb C_{Harlem} has substitution of asparagine for aspartic acid at position 73 of the β chain; Hb $C_{Georgetown}$ has a second substitution in one of the core residues (positions 83 through 120); both types cause sickling of erythrocytes similar to Hb S.
carbon monoxide h., carboxyhemoglobin.
h. Chesapeake, an abnormal Hb with a single α chain substitution, molecular formula $\alpha_2{}^{92\ \mathrm{Arg \rightarrow Leu}}\beta_2{}^A$; heterozygotes have polycythemia, apparently to compensate for the increased oxygen affinity of this Hb, resulting in decreased liberation of oxygen in the tissues.
h. D$_{Punjab}$, an abnormal Hb with a single β chain substitution, molecular formula $\alpha_2{}^A\beta_2{}^{121\ \mathrm{Glu \rightarrow Gln}}$; heterozygotes are asymptomatic, homozygotes have mild hemolytic anemia.
h. E, an abnormal Hb with a single β chain substitution, molecular formula $\alpha_2{}^A\beta_2{}^{26\ \mathrm{Glu \rightarrow Lys}}$, common in Southeast Asia, especially Thailand; heterozygotes are asymptomatic with 35 to 45% Hb E; homozygotes have mild to moderate hemolytic anemia with 90 to 100% Hb E and the remainder Hb F.
h. F, fetal h.; normal fetal Hb (Hb F) of molecular formula $\alpha_2{}^A\gamma_2{}^F$, which is the major Hb component during intrauterine life, decreasing rapidly during infancy to reach a concentration of less than 0.5% in normal children and adults; the concentration of Hb

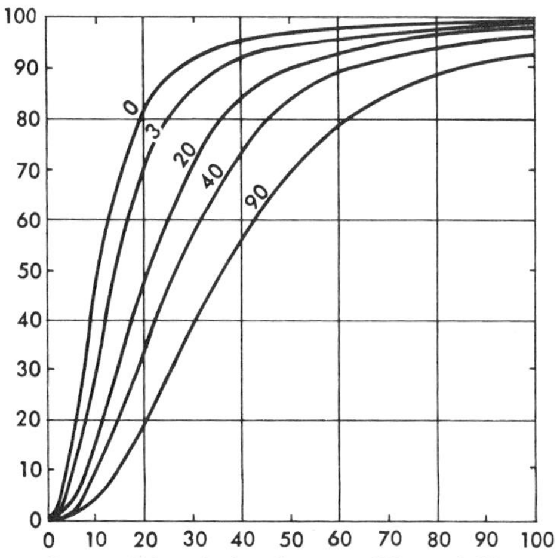

Oxygen Dissociation Curves of Hemoglobin
Hemoglobin exposed to 0, 3, 20, 40, and 90 mm CO_2 pressures. *Ordinates,* per cent saturation with oxygen; *abscissae,* oxygen pressures. (After Barcroft.)

F is increased in some hemoglobinopathies and in some cases of hypoplastic anemia, pernicious anemia, and leukemia.

h. F (hereditary persistence of), a condition due to a gene that depresses synthesis of β and δ chains (as in thalassemia), but this is fully compensated by increased γ chain synthesis and there is no anemia; there are 3 types: 1) African type, no β or δ chain synthesis by the chromosome with the abnormal gene, heterozygotes have 20 to 30% Hb F and Hb A_2 slightly decreased, homozygotes form no Hb A or Hb A_2; 2) Greek type, reduced β and δ chain synthesis, heterozygotes have 10 to 20% Hb F and normal Hb A_2; 3) Swiss type, heterozygotes have only 1 to 3% Hb F and normal Hb A_2.

fetal h., h. F.

glycosylated h., any one of four h. A fractions (A_{Ia1}, A_{Ia2}, A_{Ib}, or A_{Ic}) to which glucose and related monosaccharides bind; concentrations are increased in the erythrocytes of patients with diabetes mellitus, and can be used as a retrospective index of glucose control over time in such patients.

h. Gower-1, a Hb of molecular formula $\delta_2\epsilon_2$, found as a minor Hb in the early embryo.

h. Gower-2, a normal Hb of molecular formula $\alpha_2{}^A\epsilon_2$, which is a major Hb component of the early embryo; production of ϵ chains normally ceases at about the third month of fetal development.

green h., choleglobin.

h. H, a homotetramer of Hb (all four polypeptides identical) of molecular formula β_4, found only when α chain synthesis is depressed and not effective in oxygen transport. Hb H disease is a thalassemia-like syndrome in individuals heterozygous for both severe and mild genes for α-thalassemia; moderate anemia and red cell abnormalities with 25 to 35% Hb Bart's at birth, but with Hb Bart's later replaced by Hb H and with Hb A_2 decreased.

h. I, an abnormal Hb with a single α chain substitution, molecular formula $\alpha_2{}^{16\ \mathrm{Lys}\rightarrow\mathrm{Glu}}\beta_2{}^A$; a thalassemia-like syndrome has been found in individuals heterozygous for both Hb I and α-thalassemia genes, with formation of about 70% Hb I.

h. J$_{\text{Capetown}}$, an abnormal Hb with a single α chain substitution, molecular formula $\alpha_2{}^{92\ \mathrm{Arg}\rightarrow\mathrm{Gln}}\beta_2{}^A$; heterozygotes have polycythemia because of increased oxygen affinity of this Hb.

h. Kansas, an abnormal Hb of molecular formula $\alpha_2{}^A\beta_2{}^{102\ \mathrm{Asn}\rightarrow\mathrm{Thr}}$; found in association with familial cyanosis due to decreased oxygen affinity of this Hb.

h. Lepore, a group of abnormal Hb's with normal α chains but the non-α chains consist of the N-terminal portion of the δ chain joined to the C-terminal portion of the β chain, apparently as the result of nonhomologous pairing and crossing over between the genes for β and δ chains. The major types are Hb Lepore$_{\text{Boston}}$, Hb Lepore$_{\text{Hollandia}}$, and Hb Lepore$_{\text{Baltimore}}$, which differ in the region of crossing over. Heterozygotes form about 10% Hb Lepore, normal amounts of Hb A_2; and moderately increased amounts of Hb F, and usually have mild anemia, microcytosis, and hypochromia; homozygotes form only Hb Lepore and Hb F and have severe anemia.

h. M, a group of abnormal Hb's in which a single amino acid substitution favors the formation of methemoglobin in spite of normal quantities of methemoglobin reductase. Heterozygotes have congenital methemoglobinemia; the homozygous state of these genes is unknown and is presumably lethal. Specific types include: Hb M_{Iwate}, $\alpha^{87\ \mathrm{His}\rightarrow\mathrm{Tyr}}$ (α chain, position 87, histidine replaced by tyrosine); Hb $M_{\text{Hyde Park}}$, $\beta^{92\ \mathrm{His}\rightarrow\mathrm{Tyr}}$; Hb M_{Boston}, $\alpha^{58\ \mathrm{His}\rightarrow\mathrm{Tyr}}$; Hb $M_{\text{Saskatoon}}$, $\beta^{63\ \mathrm{His}\rightarrow\mathrm{Tyr}}$; Hb $M_{\text{Milwaukee-1}}$, $\beta^{67\ \mathrm{Val}\rightarrow\mathrm{Glu}}$.

mean cell h. (MCH), the h. content of the average red cell, calculated from the h. therein and the red cell count, in erythrocyte indices.

muscle h., myoglobin.

oxygenated h., oxyhemoglobin.

h. Rainier, an abnormal Hb of the molecular formula $\alpha_2{}^A\beta_2{}^{145\ \mathrm{Tyr}\rightarrow\mathrm{His}}$; heterozygotes have polycythemia because of increased oxygen affinity of this Hb.

reduced h., the form of Hb in red blood cells after the oxygen of oxyhemoglobin is released in the tissues.

h. S, sickle cell h.; an abnormal Hb with substitution of valine for glutamic acid at the 6th position of the β chain; molecular formula $\alpha_2{}^A\beta_2{}^S$, or more specifically $\alpha_2{}^A\beta_2{}^{6\ \mathrm{Glu}\rightarrow\mathrm{Val}}$. Heterozygous state: sickle cell trait, no anemia, Hb S 20 to 45% of total, the rest Hb A. Homozygous state: sickle cell anemia, Hb S 75 to 100% of total, the rest Hb F or Hb A_2.

sickle cell h. (Hb S), h. S.

unstable h.'s, a group of rare Hb's with amino acid substitutions (or amino acid deletions in three types) that alter the three-dimensional shape of the globin in a manner that renders the molecule unstable; they have an increased but variable tendency to autooxidation and Heinz body formation and are associated with congenital nonspherocytic hemolytic anemia. The unstable β chain abnormalities include Hb's Freiburg, Genova, Gun Hill, Hammersmith, Köln, Philly, Sabine, Santa Ana, Sydney, Wien, and Zürich; unstable α chain abnormalities include Hb's Bibba, Sinai, and Torino.

variant h., a harmless mutant form of Hb.

h. Yakima, an abnormal Hb of the molecular formula $\alpha_2{}^A\beta_2{}^{99\ \mathrm{Asp}\rightarrow\mathrm{His}}$; heterozygotes have polycythemia because of increased oxygen affinity of this Hb.

---

hemoglobinemia (hē'mō-glo-bi-nē'mē-ă). The presence of free hemoglobin in the blood plasma, as when intravascular hemolysis occurs.

h. paralyt'ica, *azoturia* of horses.

puerperal h., postparturient *hemoglobinuria.*

hemoglobinocholia (hē'mō-glō'bi-nō-kō'lē-ă) [hemoglobin + G. *cholē,* bile]. The presence of hemoglobin in the bile.

hemoglobinolysis (hē'mō-glō-bi-nol'i-sis) [hemoglobin + G. *lysis,* dissolution]. Hemoglobinopepsia; destruction or chemical splitting of hemoglobin.

hemoglobinopathy (hē'mō-glō-bi-nop'ă-thē) [hemoglobin + G. *pathos,* disease]. A disorder or disease caused by or associated with the presence of hemoglobins in the blood, *e.g.,* sickle cell disease, thalassemia, hemoglobin C, D, E, H, or I disorders. Occasionally, combinations of abnormal hemoglobins are seen in hemoglobinopathies.

hemoglobinopepsia (hē-mō-glō'bi-nō-pep'sē-ă) [hemoglobin + G. *pepsis,* digestion]. Hemoglobinolysis.

hemoglobinophilic (hē'mō-glō'bi-nō-fil'ik) [hemoglobin + G. *phileō,* to love]. Denoting certain microorganisms that cannot be cultured except in the presence of hemoglobin.

hemoglobinuria (hē'mō-glō-bi-nū'rē-ă) [hemoglobin + G. *ouron,* urine]. The presence of hemoglobin in the urine, including certain closely related pigments that are formed from slight alteration of the hemoglobin molecule; when present in sufficient quantities, they result in the urine being colored varying shades from light red-yellow to fairly dark red; due to the Donath-Lansteiner cold autoantibody.

bovine h., bovine *babesiosis.*

epidemic h., the presence of hemoglobin, or of pigments derived from it, in the urine of young infants, attended with cyanosis, jaundice, and other conditions; may be due to secondary methemoglobinemia.

malarial h., West African or hemoglobinuric fever; a condition, now uncommon, resulting from *Plasmodium falciparum* infection (malignant tertian malaria); frequently seen in Caucasians after interrupted treatment with quinine.

march h., a form occurring after marathon races, protracted marching, or heavy physical exercise.

paroxysmal nocturnal h., Marchiafava-Micheli syndrome or anemia; an infrequent disorder with insidious onset (usually in the third or fourth decade) and chronic course, characterized by episodes of hemolytic anemia, hemoglobinuria (chiefly at night), pallor, icterus or bronzing of the skin, a moderate degree of splenomegaly, and sometimes hepatomegaly; red blood cells are usually macrocytic and vary considerably in size, but there is no evidence of spherocytosis, erythrophagocytosis, or abnormal leukocytes.

postparturient h., puerperal h. or hemoglobinemia; a sudden, severe hemolytic disease that appears sporadically in well nourished dairy cows 2 to 4 weeks after calving, and usually occurs in stabled animals in the winter and early spring; the cause is not known, although the disease is often associated with hypophosphatemia.

puerperal h., postparturient h.

toxic h., h. occurring after the ingestion of various poisons, in certain blood diseases, and in certain infections.

hemoglobinuric (hē'mō-glō-bi-nū'rik). Relating to or marked by hemoglobinuria.

hemogram (hē'mō-gram) [hemo- + G. *gramma,* a drawing]. A complete detailed record of the findings in a thorough examination of the blood, especially with reference to the numbers, proportions, and morphologic features of the formed elements.

hemohistioblast (hē'mō-his'tē-ō-blast) [hemo- + G. *histion,* web, + *blastos,* germ]. Hematohistioblast; a primitive mesenchymal cell believed to be capable of developing into all types of blood cells, including monocytes, and into histiocytes.

hemolamella (hē'mō-lă-mel'ă). Platelet.

hemoleukocyte (hē-mō-lū'kō-sīt). Obsolete term for leukocyte.

hemolipase (hē-mō-lip'ās). Blood lipase.

hemolith (hē'mō-lith) [hemo- + G. *lithos,* stone]. A concretion in the wall of a blood vessel.

hemology (hē-mol'ō-jē). Hematology.

hemolymph (hē'mō-limf) [hemo- + L. *lympha,* clear water]. **1.** The blood and lymph, in the sense of a "circulating tissue." **2.** The nutrient fluid of certain invertebrates.

hemolysate (hē-mol'i-sāt). Preparation resulting from the lysis of erythrocytes.

hemolysin (hē-mol'i-sin). **1.** Erythrocytolysin; erythrolysin; any substance elaborated by a living agent and capable of causing lysis of red blood cells and liberation of their hemoglobin. **2.** A sensitizing (complement-fixing) antibody that combines with red blood cells of the antigenic type that stimulated formation of the h., affecting the cells in such a manner that complement fixes with the antibody-cell union and causes dissolution of the cells, with liberation of their hemoglobin.

α h., see α *hemolysis.*

α' h., see α' *hemolysis.*

β h., see β *hemolysis.*

bacterial h., any hemolytic agent elaborated by various species of bacteria, or by certain strains within a species.

cold h., Donath-Landsteiner cold *autoantibody.*

heterophil h., a sensitizing antibody that can combine with red blood cells of various species (in addition to those used as the antigen in stimulating the formation of the h.), resulting in hemolysis when the proper amount of complement is present.

immune h., a sensitizing, complement-fixing, hemolytic antibody formed in an animal as the result of parenteral administration of red blood cells or whole blood from another species; immune h. may also be formed in human beings who are transfused with human blood that is antigenic in the recipient, *e.g.,* the formation of anti-Rh antibody in an Rh-negative person who is treated with Rh-positive red blood cells.

natural h., h. occurring in the plasma of an animal of one species, *e.g.,* a dog, which fixes complement with the red blood cells of some other species, *e.g.,* a rabbit, thereby causing hemolysis of the cells of the rabbit, although the dog was not previously exposed to antigenic stimulation with such cells.

specific h., a sensitizing, complement-fixing, hemolytic antibody that reacts totally or completely with red blood cells of the antigenic type used to stimulate the formation of the h.

warm-cold h., h. which combines with red blood cells at temperatures below 20°C and are eluted at warmer temperatures, *e.g.,* 30 to 37°C. See Donath-Landsteiner cold *autoantibody,* hemagglutinating cold *autoantibody.*

hemolysinogen (hē'mō-lī-sin'ō-jen). The antigenic material in red blood cells that stimulates the formation of hemolysin.

hemolysis (hē-mol'i-sis) [hemo- + G. *lysis,* destruction]. Erythrolysis; erythrocytolysis; hematolysis; alteration, dissolution, or destruction of red blood cells in such a manner that hemoglobin is liberated into the medium in which the cells are suspended, *e.g.,* by specific complement-fixing antibodies, toxins, various chemical agents, tonicity, alteration of temperature.

α h., an incomplete type of h. observed in blood agar, with many erythrocytes being destroyed (*i.e.,* no longer recognizable) in an irregular, indistinctly outlined, comparatively narrow zone (*e.g.,* 1 or 2 mm) immediately surrounding a bacterial colony, whereas moderate numbers of erythrocytes remain apparently intact; the agar and recognizable erythrocytes are usually discolored, green to relatively dark green-brown; around the discolored zone, there is a second, irregular, vaguely delimited, narrow, peripheral zone of fairly clear agar in which there are only a few intact erythrocytes, the others having been lysed; when the typical discoloration occurs, α h. is termed viridans h., but it may occur without the greening change.

α' h., h. observed infrequently in blood agar cultures of occasional strains of streptococci; the zone of h. about the colony is not as clear, or wide, or distinctly outlined as it is in β h.; there are a few apparently intact erythrocytes throughout the zone, but they are more numerous in the immediate vicinity of the colony, and there is no discoloration as there is in α h.; the unique feature is that the zone becomes wider, *i.e.,* the process is stimulated, when the culture is incubated at refrigerator temperatures (not true for β h.); some strains of streptococci that are α'-hemolytic on horse blood agar cause typical α h. on rabbit blood agar.

β h., complete or "true" h. observed in blood agar cultures of various bacteria, especially hemolytic streptococci and staphylococci; virtually all of the erythrocytes are destroyed in a relatively wide, regularly circumscribed, circular zone about the colony, thereby resulting in a clear "halo" of transparent agar; the zone of h. is frequently much wider than the diameter of the colony; the degree of change varies with species of erythrocytes, *e.g.,* those of sheep and rabbits are usually more easily hemolyzed than those of man, and so on; the hemolysin acts extracellularly (in the absence of the bacterial cells) and may be quantitatively estimated by means of tube-dilution tests of a bacteria-free filtrate (containing the hemolytic substance) with a suspension of erythrocytes.

γ h., a term sometimes used to indicate that there is no h. in relation to bacterial colonies in or on blood agar; thus, nonhemolytic organisms may be referred to as producing γ h.

biologic h., h. caused by agents elaborated by various animal and plant forms.

conditioned h., immune h.

immune h., conditioned h.; h. caused by complement when erythrocytes have been sensitized by specific complement-fixing antibody.

venom h., that caused by hemolytic material in the venom of various species of snakes or other venomous animals.

viridans h., see α h.

hemolytic (hē-mō-lit'ik). Hematolytic; hemotoxic (2); destructive to blood cells, resulting in liberation of hemoglobin.

hemolyzation (hē'mol-i-zā'shŭn). The production or occurrence of hemolysis.

hemolyze (hē'mō-līz). To produce hemolysis or liberation of the hemoglobin from red blood cells.

hemomanometer (hē'mō-mă-nom'ĕ-ter). Hematomanometer; a manometer constructed and calibrated in such a manner that it is suitable for determining blood pressure.

hemomediastinum (hē'mō-mē-dē-ă-stī'nŭm). Blood in the mediastinum.

hemometra (hē-mō-mē'tră). Hematometra.

hemometry (hē-mom'ĕ-trē). Hematometry.

hemonchosis (hē-mong-kō'sis). Infection of sheep or other ruminants with *Haemonchus contortus.*

hemonephrosis (hē'mō-ne-frō'sis) [hemo- + G. *nephros,* kidney]. Obsolete term for blood in the pelvis of the kidney.

hemopathology (hē'mō-pa-thol'ō-jē). Hematopathology.

hemopathy (hē-mop'ă-thē) [hemo- + G. *pathos,* suffering]. Hematopathy; any abnormal condition or disease of the blood or hemopoietic tissues.

hemoperfusion (hē'mō-per-fyū'zhŭn) [hemo- + L. *perfusio,* to pass through]. Passage of blood through columns of adsorptive material, such as activated charcoal, to remove toxic substances from the blood.

hemopericardium (hē'mō-păr'-i-kar'dē-ŭm). Blood in the pericardial sac.

hemoperitoneum (hē'mō-păr-i-tō-nē'ŭm). Blood in the peritoneal cavity.

hemopexin (hēm-ō-peks'in). A serum protein related to β-globulins, with molecular weight around 57,000, containing 22% carbohydrate; important in binding heme and porphyrins, preventing excretion, and perhaps regulating heme in drug metabolism.

hemophagia (hē-mō-fā'jē-ă) [hemo- + G. *phagein,* to eat]. Hematophagia.

hemophagocytosis (hē'mō-fag'ō-sī-tō'sis). The process of engulfment (and usually destruction) of blood cells by the various types of phagocytic cells; used especially with reference to the engulfment of erythrocytes and others of the erythroid series.

hemophil, hemophile (hē'mō-fil, -fīl) [hemo- + G. *philos,* fond]. A microorganism growing preferably in media containing blood.

hemophilia (hē-mō-fil'ē-ă) [hemo- + G. *philos,* fond]. An inherited disorder of blood coagulation characterized by a permanent tendency to hemorrhages, spontaneous or traumatic, due to a defect in the blood coagulating mechanism.

h. A., h. due to deficiency of factor VIII; an X-linked recessive condition, occurring almost exclusively in human males and also affecting several breeds of dogs, characterized by prolonged clotting time, decreased formation of thromboplastin, and diminished conversion of prothrombin.

h. B., Christmas disease; a clotting disorder resembling h. A, caused by hereditary deficiency of factor IX; also seen as an X-linked recessive condition in cairn terrier breed of dogs.

renal h., obsolete term for renal *epistaxis.*

vascular h., von Willebrand's *disease.*

hemophiliac (hē-mō-fil'ē-ak). A person suffering from hemophilia.

hemophilic (hē-mō-fil'ik). Relating to hemophilia.

Hemophilus (hē-mof'i-lŭs). *Haemophilus.*

hemophobia (hē-mō-fō'bē-ă) [hemo- + G. *phobos,* fear]. Morbid fear of blood or of bleeding.

hemophoresis (hē'mō-fō-rē'sis) [hemo- + G. *phoreō,* to bear]. Blood convection or irrigation of tissues.

hemophthalmia, hemophthalmus (hē-mof-thal'mē-ah, -mof-thal'mŭs) [hemo- + G. *ophthalmos,* eye]. A blood-filled eye.

hemophthisis (hē-mof'thi-sis, hē-mof-thī'sis) [hemo- + G. *phthisis,* a wasting away]. Anemia resulting from abnormal degeneration or destruction, or a deficiency in the formation of red blood cells.

hemoplastic (hē-mō-plas'tik). Hemopoietic.

hemoplasty (hē'mō-plas-tē) [hemo- + G. *plassō,* to form]. Formation or elaboration of blood by the hemopoietic tissues.

hemopneumopericardium (hē'mō-nū'mō-păr-i-kar'dē-ŭm). Pneumohemopericardium; the occurrence of blood and air in the pericardium.

hemopneumothorax (hē'mō-nū-mō-thō'raks) [hemo- + G. *pneuma,* air, + thorax]. Pneumohemothorax; accumulation of air and blood in the pleural cavity.

hemopoiesis (hē'mō-poy-ē'sis) [hemo- + G. *poiēsis,* a making]. Hematogenesis; hematopoiesis; hematosis (1); hemogenesis; sanguification; the process of formation and development of the various types of blood cells and other formed elements.

hemopoietic (hē'mō-poy-et'ik). Hemafacient; hematogenic (1); hematogenous (1); hematopoietic; hematoplastic; hemogenic; hemoplastic; sanguifacient; pertaining to or related to the formation of blood cells.

hemopoietin (hē-mō-poy'ĕ-tin). Erythropoietin.

hemoporphyrin (hē-mō-pōr'fi-rin). Hematoporphyrin.

hemoprecipitin (hē'mō-prē-sip'i-tin). An antibody that combines with and precipitates soluble antigenic material from erythrocytes.

hemoprotein (hē-mō-prō'tēn). Protein linked to a metal-porphyrin compound.

hemoptysis (hē-mop'ti-sis) [hemo- + G. *ptysis,* a spitting]. The spitting of blood derived from the lungs or bronchial tubes as a result of pulmonary or bronchial hemorrhage.

cardiac h., h. secondary to heart disease or tachycardia.

endemic h., parasitic h.

parasitic h., endemic h.; the clinical expression of paragonimiasis, marked by a cough and spitting of blood from the lungs.

hemopyelectasis, hemopyelectasia (hē'mō-pī'ĕ-lek'tă-sis, -lek-tā'zē-ă) [hemo- + pyelectasia]. Dilation of the pelvis of the kidney with blood and urine.

hemorepellant (hē'mō-rē-pel'ant). **1.** A substance or surface that discourages the adherence of blood. **2.** Having such an action.

hemorheology (he'mō-rē-ol'ō-jē) [hemo- + G. *rheos,* stream, flow, + *logos,* study]. The science of the flow of blood in relation to the pressures, flow, volumes, and resistances in blood vessels, especially in terms of blood viscosity and red cell deformation in the microcirculation.

hemorrhachis (hē-mōr'ă-kis). Hematorrhachis.

hemorrhage (hem'ŏ-rij) [G. *haimorrhagia,* fr. *haima,* blood, + *rhēgnymi,* to burst forth]. **1.** Hemorrhea; bleeding; an escape of blood through ruptured or unruptured vessel walls. **2.** To bleed.

brainstem h., h. into the pons or mesencephalon, often secondary to brainstem distortion by transtentorial herniations due to rapidly expanding intracranial lesions.

cerebral h., encephalorrhagia (1); hematencephalon; intracerebral h.; h. into the substance of the cerebrum, usually in the region of the internal capsule by the rupture of the lenticulostriate artery.

concealed h., internal h.

extradural h., epidural hematoma; an accumulation of blood between the skull and the dura mater.

gastric h., gastrorrhagia.

intermediate h., h. that is recurrent.

internal h., concealed h.; bleeding into organs or cavities of the body.

intestinal h., enterorrhagia.

intracerebral h., cerebral h.

intracranial h., escape of blood within the cranium due to loss of

integrity of vascular channels, frequently forming hematoma.
intrapartum h., h. occurring in the course of normal labor and delivery.
intraventricular h., extravasation of blood into the ventricular system of the brain.
nasal h., epistaxis.
parenchymatous h., bleeding into the substance of an organ.
h. per rhex'is, h. due to the rupture of a blood vessel.
petechial h., punctate h.; capillary h. into the skin that forms petechiae.
pontine h., h. occurring in the substance of the pons, typically in hypertensive patients.
postpartum h., h. from the birth canal in excess of 500 ml during the first 24 hours after birth.
primary h., h. immediately after an injury or operation, as distinguished from intermediate or secondary h.
punctate h., petechial h.
renal h., gross hematuria, the source of which is in the kidney.
secondary h., h. at an interval after an injury or an operation.
serous h., obsolete term for a profuse transudation of plasma through the walls of the capillaries.
splinter h., linear subungual h. typically seen in but not diagnostic of bacterial endocarditis.
subarachnoid h., extravasation of blood into the subarachnoid space, usually due to aneurysm and usually spreading throughout the cerebrospinal fluid pathways.
subdural h., subdural hematoma; hemorrhagic pachymeningitis; extravasation of blood between the dural and arachnoidal membranes; chronic hematomas may become encapsulated by neomembranes.
subgaleal h., collection of blood beneath the galea aponeurotica.
syringomyelic h., h. into a syringomyelic cavity.
unavoidable h., h. occurring during labor in cases of placenta previa, as distinguished from accidental h.

hemorrhagenic (hem-ŏ-ră-jen'ik) [hemorrhage + G. *genesis,* origin]. Hemorrhagiparous; causing hemorrhage.

hemorrhagic (hem-ŏ-raj'ik). Relating to or marked by hemorrhage.

hemorrhagins (hem-ŏ-raj'inz, -rā'jins). A group of toxins found in certain venoms and poisonous material from some plants, *e.g.,* rattlesnake venom and ricin; h. cause degeneration and lysis of endothelial cells in capillaries and small vessels, thereby resulting in numerous small hemorrhages in the tissues.

hemorrhagiparous (hem'ŏ-ră-jip'ă-rŭs) [hemorrhage + L. *pario,* to produce]. Hemorrhagenic.

hemorrhea (hem-ō-rē'ă) [G. *haimorrhoia,* fr. *haima,* blood, + *rhoia,* a flow]. Hemorrhage.

hemorrhoid (hem'ŏ-royd). Denoting one of the tumors or varices constituting hemorrhoids.

hemorrhoidal (hem-ŏ-roy'dăl). **1.** Relating to hemorrhoids. **2.** Applied to certain arteries and veins supplying the region of the rectum and anus. See entries for *arteria* rectalis; *vena* rectales.

hemorrhoidectomy (hem'ŏ-roy-dek'tō-mē) [hemorrhoids + G. *ektomē,* excision]. Surgical removal of hemorrhoids; accomplished by excision of hemorrhoidal tissues by sharp dissection, or by application of elastic ligature at the base of the hemorrhoidal bundles to produce ischemic necrosis and ultimate ablation of the h.

hemorrhoids (hem'ŏ-roydz) [G. *haimorrhois,* pl. *haimorrhoides,* veins likely to bleed, fr. *haima,* blood, + *rhoia,* a flow]. Piles; a varicose condition of the external hemorrhoidal veins causing painful swellings at the anus.
cutaneous h., hyperplasia of the connective tissue in one or more of the normal radiating folds of the skin immediately surrounding the anus.
external h., dilated veins forming tumors at the outer side of the external sphincter.
internal h., dilated veins beneath the mucous membrane within the sphincter.

hemosalpinx (hē'mō-sal'pinks). Hematosalpinx.

hemosialemesis (hē'mō-sī-ăl-em'ĕ-sis) [hemo- + G. *sialon,* saliva, + *emesis,* vomiting]. Vomiting of blood and saliva.

hemosiderin (hē-mō-sid'er-in). A golden yellow or yellow-brown insoluble protein produced by phagocytic digestion of hematin; found in most tissues, especially in the liver, in the form of granules much larger than ferritin molecules (of which they are believed to be aggregates), but with a higher content, as much as 37%, of iron; stains blue with Perl's Prussian blue stain.

hemosiderosis (hē'mō-sid-er-ō'sis). Accumulation of hemosiderin in tissue. See hemochromatosis.
idiopathic pulmonary h., Ceelen-Gellerstadt syndrome; repeated sudden attacks of dyspnea and hemoptysis leading to diffuse pulmonary h., seen most commonly in children; of unknown cause, but some cases may be associated with Goodpasture's syndrome.
nutritional h., a disease seen in black South Africans which results from ingestion of iron in foodstuffs prepared in iron vessels; excessive absorption of iron chiefly affects the liver.
pulmonary h., h. usually associated with mitral stenosis and marked by an accumulation of macrophages loaded with hemosiderin within the alveoli.

hemospermia (hē'mō-sper'mē-ă) [hemo- + G. *sperma,* seed]. Hematospermia; the presence of blood in the seminal fluid.
h. spu'ria, h. occurring in the prostatic urethra.
h. ve'ra, h. in which the bleeding is from the seminal vesicles.

hemosporidium (hē'mō-spō-rid'ē-ŭm) [hemo- + Mod. L. dim. of G. *sporos,* seed]. A blood parasite of the order Haemosporidia.

hemosporines (hē'mō-spō-rēnz). Common term for members of the order Haemosporidia.

hemostasia (hē-mō-stā'zē-ă). Hemostasis.

hemostasis (hē'mō-stā-sis, hē-mos'tă-sis) [hemo- + G. *stasis,* a standing]. Hemostasia. **1.** The arrest of bleeding. **2.** The arrest of circulation in a part. **3.** Stagnation of blood.

hemostat (hē'mō-stat). **1.** Any agent that arrests, chemically or mechanically, the flow of blood from an open vessel. **2.** An instrument for arresting hemorrhage by compression of the bleeding vessel.

hemostatic (hē-mō-stat'ik). Hematostatic (1). **1.** Arresting the flow of blood within the vessels. **2.** Antihemorrhagic.

hemostyptic (hē-mo-stip'tik) [hemo- + G. *styptikos,* astringent]. Styptic (2).

hemotachometer (hē'mō-tă-kom'ĕ-ter) [hemo- + G. *tachos,* swiftness, + *metron,* measure]. Hematachometer; an instrument for measuring the rapidity of the flow of blood in the arteries.

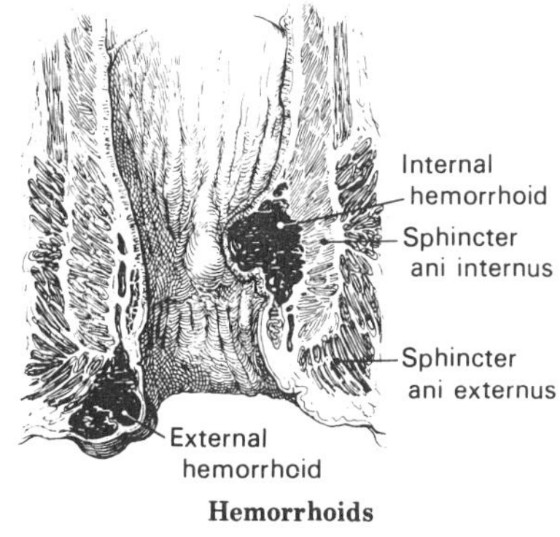

Hemorrhoids

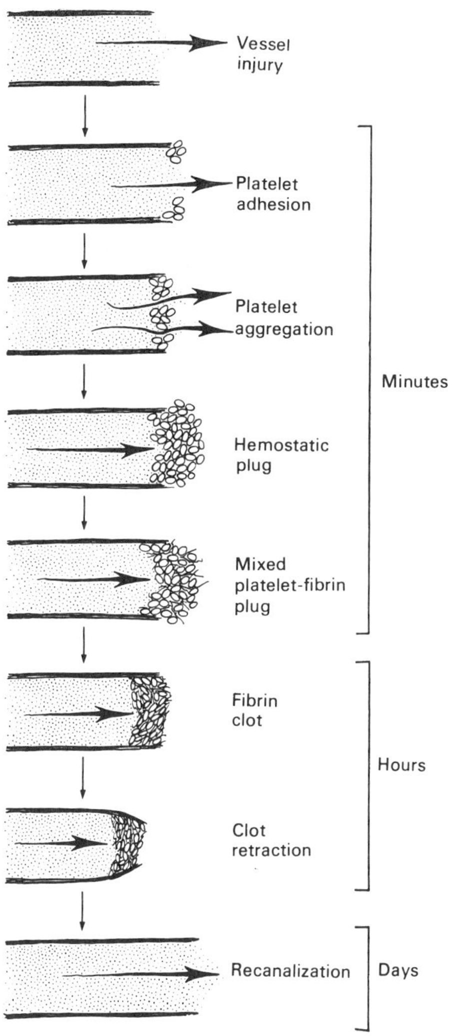

Hemostasis
Morphological events of hemostasis.

hemotherapy, hemotherapeutics (hē'mō-thār'ă-pē, thār-ă-pyū'-tiks). Hematherapy; treatment of disease by the use of blood or blood derivatives, as in transfusion.

hemothorax (hē-mō-thōr'aks). Hemathorax; blood in the pleural cavity.

hemothymia (hē-mō-thī'mē-ă) [hemo- + G. *thymos,* desire, anger]. A passion for blood; a morbid impulse to commit murder.

hemotoxic (hē-mō-tok'sik). Hematotoxic; hematoxic. **1.** Causing blood poisoning. **2.** Hemolytic.

hemotoxin (hē-mō-tok'sin). Hematotoxin; hematoxin; any substance that causes destruction of red blood cells, including various hemolysins; usually used with reference to substances of biologic origin, in contrast to chemicals.

cobra h., the constituent in cobra venom that hemolyzes the red blood cells of various species.

hemotroph, hemotrophe (hēm'ō-trof) [hemo- + G. *trophē,* food]. The materials supplied to the embryos of placental mammals through the maternal bloodstream.

hemotropic (hē-mō-trop'ik) [hemo- + G. *tropos,* a turning]. Hematotropic; pertaining to the mechanism by which a substance in or on blood cells, especially the erythrocytes, attracts phagocytic cells; the latter change direction and migrate toward the h. cells.

hemotympanum (hē'mō-tim'pă-nŭm). Hematotympanum; the presence of blood in the middle ear.

hemozoic (hē-mō-zō'ik). Hematozoic; parasitic in the blood of vertebrates; denoting certain protozoa.

hemozoon (hē-mō-zō'on) [hemo- + G. *zōon,* animal]. Hematozoon; a blood-dwelling parasitic animal such as the trypanosomes or microfilariae of *Wuchereria* or *Brugia.*

HEMPAS Abbreviation for *h*ereditary *e*rythroblastic *m*ultinuclearity associated with *p*ositive *a*cidified *s*erum. See HEMPAS *cells.*

hemuresis (hem-yū-rē'sis). Obsolete term for hematuria.

henbane (hen'bān). Hyoscyamus.

Henderson, Lawrence J., U.S. biochemist, 1879–1942. See H.-Hasselbalch *equation.*

Hendersonula toruloidea (hen-der-sō-nyū'lă tōr-yū-loy'dē-ă). A species of black yeast capable of producing infections of the nails as well as of the skin of the feet.

Henke, Wilhelm, German anatomist, 1834–1896. See H.'s *space.*

Henle, Friedrich G.J., German anatomist, pathologist, and histologist, 1809–1885. See H.'s *ampulla, ansa, fissures,* fiber *layer,* nervous *layer, loop, membrane,* fenestrated elastic *membrane, reaction, sheath, spine, tubules, warts;* Hassall-H. *bodies.*

henna (hen'ă) [Ar. *hennā*]. The leaves of Egyptian privet, *Lawsonia inermis;* used as a cosmetic and hair dye.

Henoch, Eduard H., German pediatrician, 1820–1910. See H.'s *chorea;* H.-Schönlein *purpura.*

henpuye (hen-pū'yē) [native term on the Gold Coast (Ghana) meaning "dog-nose"]. Goundou.

Henry, James Paget, German-American physiologist, *1914. See H.-Gauer *response.*

Henry, Joseph, U.S. physicist, 1797–1878. See henry; Dalton-H. *law.*

Henry, William, British chemist, 1775–1837. See H.'s *law.*

henry (H) (hen'rē) [J. *Henry*]. The unit of electrical inductance, when 1 volt is induced by a change in current of 1 ampere/sec.

Henseleit, K., German internist, *1907. See Krebs-H. *cycle.*

Hensen, Victor, German anatomist and physiologist, 1835–1924. See H.'s *band, canal, cell, disk, duct, knot, line, node, stripe.*

Hensing, Friedrich W., German anatomist, 1719–1745. See H.'s *ligament.*

hepar, gen. hepatis (hē'par, hē'pah-tis) [L. borrowed fr. G. *hēpar,* gen. *hēpatos,* the liver] [NA]. Liver.

h. loba'tum, a fissured liver, from the scars of healed syphilitic gummas.

heparan sulfate (hep'ă-ran). Heparitin sulfate.

heparin (hep'ă-rin). Heparinic acid; an anticoagulant principle that is a component of various tissues (especially liver and lung) and mast cells in man and several mammalian species; its principle and active constituent is a mucopolysaccharide comprised of D-glucuronic acid and D-glucosamine, both sulfated, in 1,4-α linkage, of molecular weight 6,000 to 20,000. In conjunction with a serum protein cofactor (the so-called heparin cofactor), h. acts as an antithrombin and an antiprothrombin by preventing platelet agglutination and consequent thrombus formation; it also enhances activity of "clearing factors" (lipoprotein lipases).

h. eliminase, h. lyase.

h. lyase [EC 4.2.2.7], h. eliminase; heparinase; an enzyme eliminating Δ-4,5-D-glucuronate residues from heparin and similar 1,4-linked polyglucuronates.

h. sodium, a mixture of active principles (usually obtained from various tissues of domestic animals) having the properties of prolonging the clotting time of human blood; used in the treatment of angina pectoris, intermittent claudication, coronary thrombosis, and similar conditions.

heparinase (hep'ă-rin-ās). *Heparin* lyase.

heparinemia (hep'ă-ri-nē'mē-ă). The presence of demonstrable levels of heparin in the circulating blood.

heparinic acid (hep-ă-rin'ik). Heparin.

heparinize (hep'ă-rin-īz). To perform therapeutic administration of heparin.

heparitin sulfate (hep'ă-rit-in). Heparan sulfate; a heteropolysaccharide that has the same repeating disaccharide as heparin but with fewer sulfates and more acetyl groups.

hepat-, hepatico-, hepato- [G. *hēpar* (*hēpat-*), liver]. Combining forms denoting the liver.

hepatalgia (hep-ă-tal'jē-ă) [hepat- + G. *algos,* pain]. Hepatodynia; pain in the liver.

hepatatrophia, hepatatrophy (hep'ă-tă-trō'fē-ă, hep-ă-tat'rō-fē). Atrophy of the liver.

hepatectomy (hep-ă-tek'tō-mē) [hepat- + G. *ektomē,* excision]. Removal of the liver, whole or in part.

hepatic (he-pat'ik) [G. *hēpatikos*]. Relating to the liver.

hepatico-. See hepat-.

hepaticodochotomy (he-pat'i-kō-dō-kot'ō-mē). Combined hepaticotomy and choledochotomy.

hepaticoduodenostomy (he-pat'i-kō-dū'ō-de-nos'tō-mē) [hepatico- + duodenostomy]. Hepatoduodenostomy; establishment of a communication between the hepatic ducts and the duodenum.

hepaticoenterostomy (he-pat'i-kō-en-ter-os'tō-mē) [hepatico- + enterostomy]. Hepatocholangioenterostomy; establishment of a communication between the hepatic ducts and the intestine.

hepaticogastrostomy (he-pat'i-kō-gas-tros'tō-mē) [hepatico- + gastrostomy]. Establishment of a communication between the hepatic duct and the stomach.

hepaticolithotomy (he-pat'i-kō-li-thot'ō-mē) [hepatico- + G. *lithos,* stone, + *tomē,* a cutting]. Removal of a stone from a hepatic duct.

hepaticolithotripsy (he-pat'i-kō-lith'ō-trip-sē) [hepatico- + G. *lithos,* stone, + *tripsis,* a rubbing]. The crushing of a biliary calculus in the hepatic duct.

hepaticopulmonary (he-pat'i-kō-pul'mŏ-nār-ē). Hepatopneumonic.

hepaticostomy (he-pat-i-kos'tō-mē) [hepatico- + G. *stoma,* mouth]. Establishment of an opening into the hepatic duct.

hepaticotomy (he-pat-i-kot'ō-mē) [hepatico- + G. *tomē,* incision]. Incision into the hepatic duct.

hepatin (hep'ă-tin). Glycogen.

hepatitic (hep-ă-tit'ik). Relating to hepatitis.

hepatitis (hep-ă-tī'tis) [hepat- + G. *-itis,* inflammation]. Inflammation of the liver; usually from a viral infection, but sometimes from toxic agents.

h. A, viral h. type A.

active chronic h., subacute h.; juvenile or posthepatitic cirrhosis; h. with chronic portal inflammation that extends into the parenchyma, with piecemeal necrosis and fibrosis which usually progresses to a coarsely nodular postnecrotic cirrhosis.

acute parenchymatous h., acute yellow *atrophy* of the liver.

anicteric virus h., a relatively mild h., without jaundice, due to a virus; the principal physical signs and symptoms are enlargement of the liver, lymph nodes, and often the spleen, together with headache, continuous fatigue, nausea, anorexia, sudden distaste for smoking, abdominal pains, and sometimes mild fever.

h. B, viral h. type B.

cholangiolitic h., h. with inflammatory changes around small bile ducts, producing mainly obstructive jaundice; may be due to viral infection.

cholestatic h., jaundice with bile stasis in inflamed intrahepatic bile ducts; usually due to toxic effects of a drug.

chronic h., subacute h.; chronic active liver disease; any of several types of h. persisting for more than six months, often progressing to cirrhosis.

chronic interstitial h., obsolete term for cirrhosis of the liver.

h. contagio'sa ca'nis, infectious canine h.

delta h., viral h. type D.

drug-induced h., hepatocellular damage produced by a drug.

epidemic h., viral h. type A.

equine serum h., Theiler's disease (2); an acute hepatic disease of the horse, often associated with prior administration of biological products; neurologic signs and jaundice are usually prominent signs; etiology is unknown.

h. exter'na, perihepatitis.

giant cell h., neonatal h.

halothane h., hepatocellular damage said to result from the administration of halothane anesthesia.

infectious h. (IH), viral h. type A.

infectious canine h., h. contagiosa canis; Rubarth's disease; a disease of dogs, caused by the infectious canine h. virus and characterized by fever, leukopenia, abdominal pain, diarrhea, vomiting, edema, and transient corneal opacities.

infectious necrotic h. of sheep, black disease (so named because of the extensive hemorrhages seen on the inner surface of the pelt when it is removed); German braxy; a disease of sheep caused by *Clostridium novyi,* which invades livers damaged by *Fasciola hepatica* and causes severe necrosis and death; this disease occurs in nearly all parts of the world, including the United States.

long incubation h., viral h. type B.

lupoid h., plasma cell h.; jaundice with evidence of liver cell damage and positive L.E. cell tests, but without evidence of systemic lupus erythematosus; liver biopsies usually show active chronic h. with infiltration by plasma cells, or postnecrotic cirrhosis; serum is negative for h. B antigen.

mouse h., murine h., a form of h. in mice due to synergism between the mouse h. virus and *Eperythrozoon coccoides.*

NANB h., non-A, non-B h.

neonatal h., giant cell h.; h. of unknown cause, characterized by onset of obstructive jaundice in the neonatal period, hepatocellular degeneration, and appearance of multinucleated giant cells; may be difficult to distinguish from biliary atresia, but is more likely to end with recovery, although cirrhosis may develop.

non-A, non-B h., NANB h.; h. caused by two or more infectious agents not detectable by methods which reveal the presence of h. viruses A and B; may be sporadic or epidemic, and may follow blood transfusion; in the acute stage, generally milder than h. B, but a greater proportion of such infections become chronic and progress to cirrhosis.

peliosis h., a rare condition in which the liver contains very numerous small blood-filled spaces, sometimes lined with endothelium; it may be found incidentally or rupture may cause intraperitoneal hemorrhage.

persistent chronic h., a benign chronic h. which may follow acute viral h. A or B, or complicate bowel diseases; after six months, liver biopsy changes are mild, unlike active chronic h.; rarely, if ever, progresses to cirrhosis, portal hypertension, or liver failure.

plasma cell h., lupoid h.

serum h. (SH), viral h. type B.

short incubation h., viral h. type A.

subacute h., active chronic h.

suppurative h., h. with abscess formation; often amebic in origin.

transfusion h., viral h. type B.
viral h., virus h.; **(1)** h. caused by any one of three immunologically unrelated viruses: h. A virus, h. B virus, and non-A, non-B virus; **(2)** h. caused by a viral infection, including that by Epstein-Barr virus and cytomegalovirus.
viral h. type A, epidemic or infectious h.; virus A h.; h. A; short incubation h.; a virus disease with a short incubation period (usually 15 to 50 days), caused by h. A virus often transmitted by fecal-oral route; may be inapparent, mild, severe, or occasionally fatal and occurs sporadically or in epidemics, commonly in school-age children and young adults; necrosis of periportal liver cells with lymphocytic and plasma cell infiltration is characteristic and jaundice is a common symptom.
viral h. type B, serum or transfusion h.; virus B h.; h. B; long incubation h.; a virus disease with a long incubation period (usually 50 to 160 days), caused by hepatitis B virus usually transmitted by injection of infected blood or blood derivatives or by use of contaminated needles, lancets, or other instruments; clinically and pathologically similar to viral h. type A, but there is no cross-protective immunity; HB_sAg is found in the serum and the hepatitis delta virus occurs in some patients.
viral h. type D, delta h.; acute or chronic h. caused by the human delta virus. The acute type occurs in two forms: 1) coinfection, the simultaneous occurrance of h. B virus and h. delta virus infections, which usually is self-limiting; 2) superinfection, the appearance of h. delta virus infection in a h. B virus carrier, which often leads to chronic h. The chronic type appears to be more severe than other types of viral h.
virus h., viral h.
virus A h., viral h. type A.
virus B h., viral h. type B.
virus h. of ducks, a disease of very young ducklings, caused by the duck h. virus (*Enterovirus*) and manifested by an acute illness of several days followed by death; the principal lesions are an enlarged necrotic liver filled with ecchymotic hemorrhages.

hepatization (hep'ă-ti-ză'shŭn). Conversion of a loose tissue into a firm mass like the substance of the liver macroscopically, denoting especially such a change in the lungs in the consolidation of pneumonia.
gray h., the second stage of h. in pneumonia, when the exudate is beginning to degenerate prior to breaking down; the color is a yellowish gray or mottled.
red h., the first stage of h. in which the exudate is blood-stained.
yellow h., the final stage of h. in which the exudate is becoming purulent.

hepato-. See hepat-.

hepatoblastoma (hep'ă-tō-blas-tō'mă). A malignant neoplasm occurring in young children, primarily in the liver, composed of tissue resembling embryonal or fetal hepatic epithelium, or mixed epithelial and mesenchymal tissues.

hepatocarcinoma (hep'ă-tō-kar-si-nō'mă). Malignant *hepatoma.*

hepatocele (hep'ă-tō-sēl, he-pat'ō-sēl) [hepato- + G. *kēlē,* hernia]. Hernia of the liver; protrusion of part of the liver through the abdominal wall or the diaphragm.

hepatocholangioenterostomy (hep'ă-tō-kō-lan'jē-ō-en-ter-os'tō-mē) [hepato- + G. *cholē,* bile, + *angeion,* vessel, + *enteron,* intestine, + *stoma,* mouth]. Hepaticoenterostomy.

hepatocholangiojejunostomy (hep'ă-tō-kō-lan'jē-ō-jē-jū-nos'tō-mē) [hepato- + G. *cholē,* bile, + *angeion,* vessel, + jejunostomy]. Union of the hepatic duct to the jejunum.

hepatocholangiostomy (hep'ă-tō-kō-lan-jē-os'tō-mē). Creation of an opening into the common bile duct to establish drainage.

hepatocholangitis (hep'ă-tō-kō-lan-jī'tis). Inflammation of the liver and biliary tree.

hepatocuprein (hep'ă-tō-kū'prē-in). Cytocuprein.

hepatocystic (hep'ă-tō-sis'tik) [hepato- + G. *kystis,* bladder]. Relating to the gallbladder, or to both liver and gallbladder.

Hepatocystis (hep'ă-tō-sis'tis) [hepato- + G. *kystis,* bladder]. A genus of blood-parasitizing hemosporines (family Plasmodiidae) with gametocytes in red cells and cystlike exoerythrocytic schizonts in the liver parenchyma; parasitic in Old World primates, bats, and squirrels, but not in domestic animals or in the western hemisphere. The species *H. kochi,* a common parasite of African baboons and other monkeys, is transmitted by the biting midge, *Culicoides.*

hepatocyte (hep'ă-tō-sīt). A parenchymal liver cell.

hepatoduodenostomy (hep'ă-tō-dū-ō-de-nos'tō-mē). Hepaticoduodenostomy.

hepatodynia (hep'ă-tō-din'ē-ă) [hepato- + G. *odynē,* pain]. Hepatalgia.

hepatodysentery (hep'ă-tō-dis'en-ter-ē). Dysentery associated with liver disease.

hepatoenteric (hep'ă-tō-en-tĕr'ik) [hepato- + G. *enteron,* intestine]. Relating to the liver and the intestine.

hepatofugal (hep'ă-tō-fyū'găl). Away from the liver, usually referring to portal blood flow.

hepatogastric (hep'ă-tō-gas'trik). Relating to the liver and the stomach.

hepatogenic, hepatogenous (hep-ă-tō-jen'ik, -toj'en-ŭs). Of hepatic origin; formed in the liver.

hepatography (hep-ă-tog'ră-fē) [hepato- + G. *graphē,* a writing]. Roentgenography of the liver.

hepatohemia (hep'ă-tō-hē'mē-ă) [hepato- + G. *haima,* blood]. Rarely used term for congestion of the liver.

hepatoid (hep'ă-toyd) [hepato- + G. *eidos,* resemblance]. Resembling or like the liver.

hepatojugularometer (hep'ă-tō-jŭg'yū-lă-rom'ĕ-ter) [hepato- + L. *jugulum,* throat, + G. *metron,* measure]. An apparatus for the quantitative control and measurement of the pressure and force applied over the liver to test the hepatojugular reflux.

hepatolienography (hep'ă-tō-lī-en-og'ră-fē) [hepato- + L. *lien,* spleen, + G. *graphē,* a writing]. Hepatosplenography.

hepatolienomegaly (hep'ă-tō-lī'ē-nō-meg'ă-lē). Hepatosplenomegaly.

hepatolith (hep'ă-tō-lith) [hepato- + G. *lithos,* stone]. A concretion in the liver.

hepatolithectomy (hep'ă-tō-li-thek'tō-mē) [hepato- + G. *lithos,* stone, + *ektomē,* excision]. Removal of a calculus from the liver.

hepatolithiasis (hep'ă-tō-li-thī'ă-sis) [hepato- + G. *lithiasis,* presence of a calculus]. Presence of calculi in the liver.

hepatologist (hep-ă-tol'ō-jist). A specialist in hepatology.

hepatology (hep-ă-tol'ō-jē) [hepato- + G. *logos,* study]. The branch of medicine concerned with diseases of the liver.

hepatolysin (hep-ă-tol'i-sin). A cytolysin that destroys parenchymal cells of the liver.

hepatoma (hep-ă-tō'mă) [hepato- + G. *-oma,* tumor]. See malignant h.
malignant h., hepatocellular or liver cell carcinoma; hepatocarcinoma; a carcinoma derived from parenchymal cells of the liver.

hepatomalacia (hep'ă-tō-mă-lā'shē-ă) [hepato- + G. *malakia,* softening]. Softening of the liver.

hepatomegaly, hepatomegalia (hep'ă-tō-meg'ă-lē, -mĕ-gā'lē-ă) [hepato- + G. *megas,* large]. Megalohepatia; enlargement of the liver.

hepatomelanosis (hep'ă-tō-mel'ă-nō'sis) [hepato- + G. *melas,* black, + *-osis,* condition]. Deep pigmentation of the liver.

hepatomphalocele (hep'ă-tom-fal'ō-sēl, hep-ă-tom'fă-lō-sēl) [hepato- + omphalocele]. Hepatomphalos; umbilical hernia with involvement of the liver.

hepatomphalos (hep-ă-tom'fă-lōs). Hepatomphalocele.

hepatonecrosis (hep'ă-tō-ne-krō'sis). Death of liver cells.

hepatonephric (hep'ă-tō-nef'rik). Hepatorenal.

hepatonephromegaly (hep'ă-tō-nef'rō-meg'ă-lē) [hepato- + G. *nephros,* kidney, + *megas,* great]. Enlargement of both liver and kidney or kidneys.

hepatopathic (hep'ă-tō-path'ik). Damaging the liver.

hepatopathy (hep-ă-top'ă-thē) [hepato- + G. *pathos,* suffering]. Disease of the liver.

hepatoperitonitis (hep'ă-tō-păr'i-tō-nī'tis). Perihepatitis.

hepatopetal (hep'ă-tō-pet'al). Toward the liver, usually referring to the normal direction of portal blood flow.

hepatopexy (hep'ă-tō-pek-sē) [hepato- + G. *pēxis,* fixation]. Anchoring of the liver to the abdominal wall.

hepatophyma (hep'ă-tō-fī'mă) [hepato- + G. *phyma,* tumor]. Rounded or nodular tumor of the liver.

hepatopneumonic (hep'ă-tō-nū-mon'ik) [hepato- + G. *pneumonikos,* pulmonary]. Hepaticopulmonary; hepatopulmonary; relating to the liver and the lungs.

hepatoportal (hep'ă-tō-pōr'tăl). Relating to the portal system of the liver.

hepatoptosis (hep'ă-top-tō'sis, tō-tō'sis) [hepato- + G. *ptōsis,* a failing]. Wandering liver; a downward displacement of the liver.

hepatopulmonary (hep'ă-tō-pŭl'mō-năr'ē). Hepatopneumonic.

hepatorenal (hep-ă-tō-rē'năl) [hepato- + L. *renalis,* renal, fr. *renes,* kidneys]. Hepatonephric; relating to the liver and the kidney.

hepatorrhagia (hep'ă-tō-ră'jē-ă) [hepato- + G. *rhēgnymi,* to burst forth]. Hemorrhage into or from the liver.

hepatorrhaphy (hep-ă-tōr'ă-fē) [hepato- + G. *rhaphē,* a suture]. Suture of a wound of the liver.

hepatorrhea (hep'ă-tō-rē'ă) [hepato- + G. *rhoia,* a flow]. Obsolete term for cholorrhea.

hepatorrhexis (hep'ă-tō-rek'sis) [hepato- + G. *rhēxis,* rupture]. Rupture of the liver.

hepatoscopy (hep-ă-tos'kō-pē) [hepato- + G. *skopeō,* to examine]. Examination of the liver.

hepatosplenitis (hep'ă-tō-splē-nī'tis). Inflammation of the liver and spleen.

hepatosplenography (hep'ă-tō-splē-nog'ră-fē). Hepatolienography; the use of a contrast medium to outline or depict the liver and spleen roentgenographically.

hepatosplenomegaly (hep'ă-tō-splē-nō-meg'ă-lē) [hepato- + G. *splēn,* spleen, + *megas,* large]. Hepatolienomegaly; enlargement of the liver and spleen.

hepatosplenopathy (hep'ă-tō-splē-nop'ă-thē). Disease of the liver and spleen.

hepatostomy (hep-ă-tos'tō-mē) [hepato- + G. *stoma,* mouth]. Establishment of a fissure into the liver.

hepatotherapy (hep'ă-tō-thăr'ă-pē). **1.** Treatment of disease of the liver. **2.** Therapeutic use of liver extract or of the raw substance of the liver.

hepatotomy (hep-ă-tot'ō-mē) [hepato- + G. *tomē,* incision]. Incision into the liver.

hepatotoxemia (hep'ă-tō-tok-sē'mē-ă) [hepato- + G. *toxikon,* poison, + *haima,* blood]. Autointoxication assumed to be due to improper functioning of the liver.

hepatotoxic (hep'ă-tō-tok'sik). Relating to an agent that damages the liver, or pertaining to any such action.

hepatotoxin (hep'ă-tō-tok'sin). A toxin that is destructive to parenchymal cells of the liver.

Hepatozoon (hep'ă-tō-zō'on) [hepato- + G. *zōon,* animal]. A genus of coccidian parasites (family Haemogregarinidae), in which schizogony occurs in the visceral organs, gametogony in the leukocytes or erythrocytes of vertebrate animals, and sporogony in certain ticks and other blood-sucking invertebrates. *H. canis* occurs in dogs, cats, jackals, and hyenas, but is most pathogenic in dogs, in which it may cause serious disease and death; other species have been described from rats, mice, rabbits, and squirrels.

hepta- [G. *hepta,* seven]. Prefix denoting seven.

heptabarbital (hep-tă-bar'bi-tawl). 5-(1-Cyclohepten-1-yl)-5-ethylbarbituric acid; a short-acting barbiturate that produces sedation, hypnosis, or anesthesia, depending upon the dose administered.

heptad (hep'tad). A septivalent chemical element or radical.

heptaminol (hep-tam'i-nol). 6-Amino-2-methyl-2-heptanol; a sympathomimetic, vasoconstrictor, and cardiotonic.

heptanal (hep'tă-năl). Enanthal; heptaldehyde; $CH_3(CH_2)_5CHO$; obtained from the ricinoleic acid of castor oil by chemical means; used in the manufacture of ethyl oenanthate, a constituent of many artificial essences (flavors).

heptazone hydrochloride (hep'tă-zōn). Phenadoxone hydrochloride.

heptose (hep'tōs). A sugar with 7 carbon atoms in its molecule; *e.g.,* sedoheptulose.

heptulose (hep'tū-lōs). Ketoheptose.

D-*altro*-2-heptulose. Sedoheptulose.

D-*manno*-heptulose. A ketoheptose of the mannose configuration, occurring in the urine of individuals who have eaten a large quantity of avocados.

Herbert, Herbert, British ophthalmic surgeon, 1865–1942. See H.'s *operation.*

herbivorous (her-biv'ō-rŭs) [L. *herba,* herb, + *voro,* to devour]. Feeding on plants.

Herbst, Ernst F.G., German anatomist, 1803–1893. See H.'s *corpuscles.*

herd. **1.** A group of people or animals in a given area. **2.** An immunologic concept of an ecologic composite that includes susceptible animal species (including man), vectors, and environmental factors.

hereditary (hĕ-red'i-ter-ē) [L. *hereditarius;* fr. *heres* (*hered-*), an heir]. Transmitted from parent to offspring; derived from ancestry; obtained by inheritance.

heredity (hĕ-red'i-tē) [L. *hereditas,* inheritance, fr. *heres* (*hered-*), heir]. The transmission of characters from parent to offspring.

heredo- [L. *heres,* an heir]. Prefix denoting heredity.

heredoataxia (her'ĕ-dō-ă-tak'sē-ă). Hereditary spinal *ataxia.*

heredofamilial (her'ĕ-dō-fă-mil'ē-ăl). Obsolete term denoting an inherited condition present in more than one member of a family.

heredopathia atactica polyneuritiformis (her'ĕ-dō-path'ē-ă ă-tak'ti-kă pol'ē-nū-rī-ti-fōr'mis). Refsum's *disease.*

Herelle, Felix H. See d'Herelle, Felix H.

Herellea (hĕ-rel'ē-ă). A bacterial generic name which has been officially rejected because its type species, *H. vaginicola,* is a member of the genus *Acinetobacter.*

Hering, Heinrich Ewald, German physiologist, 1866–1948. See sinus *nerve* of H; H.-Breuer *reflex;* Traube-H. *curve.*

Hering, Karl E.K., German physiologist, 1834–1918. See H.'s *test, theory; canal* of H.; Traube-H. *curves, waves;* Semon-H. *theory.*

heritability (her'i-tă-bil'i-tē) [see heredity]. **1.** In intelligence or personality testing, a statistical term used to denote the extent of variance of an individual's total score or response which is attributable to a presumed genetic component, in contrast to an acquired component. **2.** In genetics, a statistical term used to denote the proportion of phenotypic variance due to variance in genotypes.

heritage (her'i-tij) [O. Fr]. The total of all the inherited characters.

Herlitz, Carl G., Swedish pediatrician, *1902. See H. *syndrome.*

Herman. See Padykula-H. *stain* for myosin ATPase.

Hermann, Friedrich, German anatomist, 1859–1920. See H.'s *fixative.*

hermaphrodism (her-maf'rō-dizm). Hermaphroditism.

hermaphrodite (her-maf'rō-dīt) [G. *Hermaphroditus,* the son of *Hermēs,* Mercury, + *Aphroditē,* Venus]. An individual with hermaphroditism.

hermaphroditism (her-maf'rō-dīt-izm). Hermaphrodism; the presence in one individual of both ovarian and testicular tissue; *i.e.,* true h.

adrenal h., altered appearance of the genitalia due to disorders of adrenocortical function, most often female virilization; not an example of true h.

bilateral h., true h. with ovotestis on both sides.

dimidiate h., lateral h.

false h., pseudohermaphroditism.

female h., more correctly designated as female pseudohermaphroditism, as the term is commonly used; however, it can designate an instance of true h., in which bodily characteristics are predominantly female.

lateral h., dimidiate h.; a form in which a testis is present on one side and an ovary on the other.

male h., more correctly designated as male pseudohermaphroditism, as the term is commonly used; however, it can designate an instance of true h. in which bodily characteristics are predominantly male.

transverse h., pseudohermaphroditism in which the external genitalia are characteristic of one sex and the gonads are characteristic of the other sex.

true h., h. in which both ovarian and testicular tissue are present.

unilateral h., h. in which the doubling of sex characteristics occurs only on one side: ovotestis on one side and either ovary or testis on the other.

hermetic (her-met'ik). Airtight; denoting a vessel closed or sealed in such a way that air can neither enter it nor issue from it.

HERNIA

hernia (her'nē-ă) [L. rupture]. Rupture (1); protrusion of a part or structure through the tissues normally containing it.

abdominal h., laparocele; a h. protruding through or into any part of the abdominal wall.

antevesical h., an interstitial h. projecting medially from the internal inguinal ring.

Barth's h., a loop of intestine between a persistent vitelline duct and the abdominal wall.

Béclard's h., a h. through the opening for the saphenous vein.

bilocular femoral h., Cooper's h.

h. en bissac, properitoneal inguinal h.

Bochdalek's h., congenital diaphragmatic h.

h. of the broad ligament of the uterus, a coil of intestine contained in a pouch projecting into the substance of the broad ligament.

cecal h., a h. containing cecum.

cerebral h., protrusion of brain substance through a defect in the skull.

Cloquet's h., a femoral h. perforating the aponeurosis of the pectineus and insinuating itself between this aponeurosis and the muscle, lying therefore behind the femoral vessels.

complete h., an indirect inguinal h. in which the contents extend into the tunica vaginalis.

concealed h., a h. not found on inspection or palpation.

congenital diaphragmatic h., Bochdalek's h.; absence of the pleuroperitoneal membrane (usually on the left) or an enlarged foramen of Morgagni which allows protrusion of abdominal viscera into the chest.

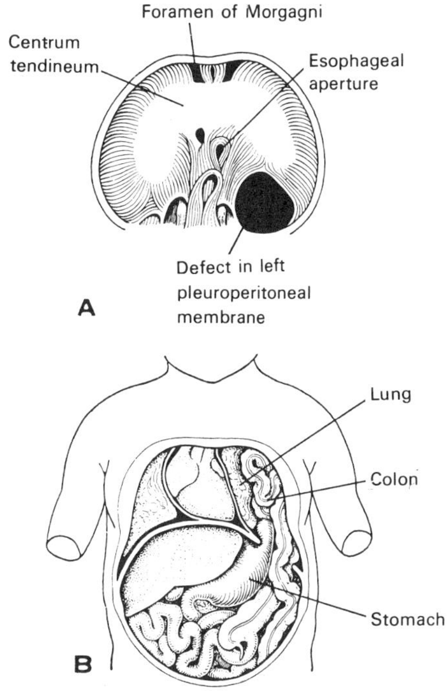

Congenital Diaphragmatic Hernia

A, Caudal surface of the diaphragm, showing a large defect of the pleuroperitoneal membrane on the left side. *B,* hernia of the intestinal loops and part of the stomach into the left pleural cavity; the heart and mediastinum are frequently pushed to the right, while the left lung is compressed.

Cooper's h., Hey's h.; bilocular femoral h.; a femoral h. with two sacs, the first being in the femoral canal, and the second passing through a defect in the superficial fascia and appearing immediately beneath the skin.

crural h., femoral h.

diaphragmatic h., diaphragmatocele; protrusion of abdominal contents into the chest through a weakness in the respiratory diaphragm; a common type is the hiatal h.

direct inguinal h., see inguinal h.

double loop h., "w" h.

dry h., a h. with adherent sac and contents.

duodenojejunal h., Treitz' h.; retroperitoneal h.; a h. in the subperitoneal tissues.

epigastric h., h. through the linea alba above the navel.

extrasaccular h., sliding h.

fascial h., a bulging of muscle through a defect in its fascia.

fatty h., pannicular h.

femoral h., enteromerocele; femorocele; merocele; crural h.; h. through the femoral ring.

gastroesophageal h., a hiatal h. into the thorax.

gluteal h., sciatic h.
Hesselbach's h., h. with diverticula through the cribriform fascia, presenting a lobular outline.
Hey's h., Cooper's h.
hiatal h., hiatus h., h. of a part of the stomach through the esophageal hiatus of the diaphragm.
Holthouse's h., inguinal h. with extension of the loop of intestine along Poupart's ligament.
iliacosubfascial h., a h. the sac of which passes through the iliac fascia and lies in the iliac fossa in contact with the iliacus muscle.
incarcerated h., irreducible h.
incisional h., h. occurring through a surgical incision or scar.
indirect inguinal h., see inguinal h.
infantile h., a h. in which an intestinal loop descends behind the tunica vaginalis, having, therefore, three peritoneal layers in front of it.
inguinal h., a h. at the inguinal region: **direct i. h.** involves the abdominal wall between the deep epigastric artery and the edge of the rectus muscle; **indirect i. h.** involves the internal inguinal ring and passes into the inguinal canal.

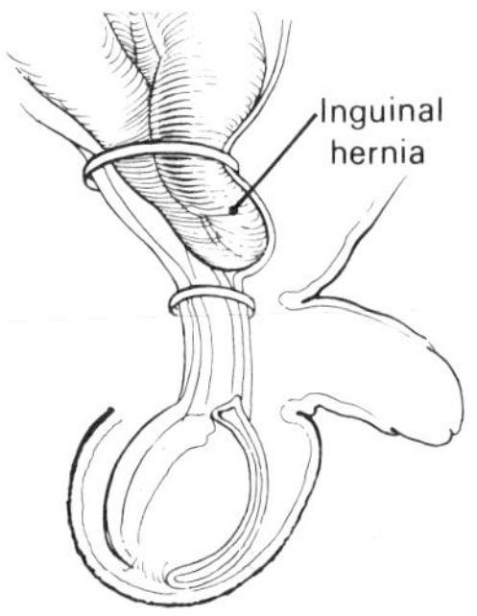

Inguinal Hernia

inguinocrural h., inguinofemoral h., a bilocular or double h., both inguinal and femoral.
inguinolabial h., an inguinal h. descending into the labium.
inguinoscrotal h., an inguinal h. descending into the scrotum.
inguinosuperficial h., an inguinal h. that has turned cephalad away from the scrotum and lies subcutaneously on the abdominal wall.
intersigmoid h., a h. into the intersigmoid fossa on the under surface of the root of the mesosigmoid near the inner border of the psoas magnus muscle.
interstitial h., a h. in which the protrusion is between any two of the layers of the abdominal wall.
intraepiploic h., a coil of intestine incarcerated in an omental sac.
intrailiac h., an interstitial h. projecting from the internal inguinal ring.
intrapelvic h., an interstitial h. projecting into the pelvis from the internal inguinal ring.
irreducible h., incarcerated h.; a h. that cannot be reduced without operation.
ischiatic h., a h. through the sacrosciatic foramen.
Krönlein's h., properitoneal inguinal h.
labial h., h. through the canal of Nuck.
lateral ventral h., spigelian h.
Laugier's h., a h. passing through an opening in the lacunar ligament.
levator h., pudendal h.
Littre's h., **(1)** parietal h.; **(2)** h. of Meckel's diverticulum.
lumbar h., a protrusion between the last rib and the iliac crest where the aponeurosis of the transversus muscle is covered only by the latissimus dorsi.
Malgaigne's h., infantile inguinal h. prior to the descent of the testis.
meningeal h., herniation of meninges through a spina bifida.
mesenteric h., h. through a hole in the mesentery.
obturator h., h. through the obturator foramen.
orbital h., displacement of orbital fat through a defect in the orbital septum or Tenon's capsule into the subcutaneous tissues of the eyelid or subconjunctivally.
pannicular h., fatty h.; the escape of subcutaneous fat through a gap in a fascia or an aponeurosis.
paraesophageal h., h. through the esophageal hiatus of the diaphragm.
paraperitoneal h., a vesical h. in which only a part of the protruded organ is covered by the peritoneum of the sac.
parasaccular h., sliding h.
parasternal h., Morgagni's *foramen (2).*
parietal h., Richter's h.; Littre's h. (1); partial enterocele; a h. in which only a portion of the wall of the intestine is engaged.
perineal h., perineocele; levator or pudendal h.; a h. protruding through the pelvic diaphragm.
Petit's h., lumbar h., occurring in Petit's triangle.
posterior vaginal h., downward displacement of Douglas' pouch.
properitoneal inguinal h., h. en bissac; Krönlein's h.; a complicated h. having a double sac, one part in the inguinal canal, the other projecting from the internal inguinal ring in the subperitoneal tissues.
pudendal h., perineal h.
reducible h., a h. in which the contents of the sac can be returned to their normal location.
retrograde h., a double loop h. the central loop of which lies in the abdominal cavity.
retroperitoneal h., duodenojejunal h.
retropubic h., a h. projecting downward, in the subperitoneal tissues, from the internal inguinal ring.
retrosternal h., a diaphragmatic h. protruding through Morgagni's foramen.
Richter's h., parietal h.
Rokitansky's h., a separation of the muscular fibers of the bowel allowing protrusion of a sac of the mucous membrane.
sciatic h., gluteal h.; ischiocele; protrusion of intestine through the great sacrosciatic foramen.
scrotal h., oscheocele (1); scrotocele; complete inguinal h., located in the scrotum.
sliding h., extrasaccular, parasaccular, or slipped h.; a h. in which an abdominal viscus forms part of the sac.
sliding esophageal hiatal h., displacement of the cardioesophageal junction and the stomach through the esophageal hiatus.
sliding hiatal h., a h. of the esophagus through the diaphragm into the posterior mediastinum, with partial peritoneal sac anteriorly.
slipped h., sliding h.
spigelian h., lateral ventral h.; abdominal h. through the semilunar line.
strangulated h., an irreducible h. in which the circulation is arrested; gangrene occurs unless relief is prompt.
synovial h., protrusion of a fold of the stratum synoviale through a rent in the stratum fibrosum of a joint capsule.
Treitz' h., duodenojejunal h.
umbilical h., exomphalos (2); a h. in which bowel or omentum protrudes through the abdominal wall under the skin at the umbilicus.
Velpeau's h., femoral h. in which the intestine is in front of the blood vessels.
ventral h., an abdominal incisional h.
vesicle h., protrusion of a segment of the bladder through the abdominal wall or into the inguinal canal and into the scrotum.
vitreous h., prolapse of the vitreous humor into the anterior chamber; may follow removal or displacement of the lens from the

lenticular space.
"w" h., double loop h.; the presence of two loops of intestine in a hernial sac.

hernial (her'nē-ăl). Relating to hernia.

herniated (her'nē-ā-ted). Denoting any structure protruded through a hernial opening.

herniation (her-nē-ā'shŭn). Formation of a protrusion.
caudal transtentorial h., uncal h.; displacement of medial temporal structures into incisura, with or without rostrocaudal brainstem shift.
cingulate h., displacement of the cingulate gyrus beneath the falx.
foraminal h., tonsillar h.; displacement of cerebellar tonsils through the foramen magnum.
rostral transtentorial h., displacement of anterior cerebellar structures into incisura, with or without caudorostral brainstem shift.
sphenoidal h., displacement of ventral frontal lobar tissue over the sphenoid ridge.
subfalcial h., h. beneath the falx cerebri.
tonsillar h., foraminal h.
transtentorial h., h. into the incisura, either from above (rostral h.) or below (caudal h.).
uncal h., caudal transtentorial h.

hernio- [L. *hernia,* rupture]. Combining form relating to hernia.

hernioenterotomy (her'nē-ō-en-ter-ot'ō-mē). Incision of the intestine following the reduction of a hernia.

herniography (her-nē-og'ră-fē). Radiographic examination of a hernia following injection of a contrast medium into the hernial sac.

hernioid (her'nē-oyd) [hernio- + G. *eidos,* resemblance]. Resembling hernia.

herniolaparotomy (her'nē-ō-lap-ă-rot'ō-mē). Laparotomy for correction of hernia.

hernioplasty (her'nē-ō-plas-tē) [hernio- + G. *plastos,* formed]. Herniorrhaphy.

herniopuncture (her'nē-ō-pŭnk'chūr). Insertion of a hollow needle into a hernia in order to reduce the size of the tumor by withdrawing gas or liquid.

herniorrhaphy (her'nē-ōr'ă-fē) [hernio- + G. *rhaphē,* a seam]. Hernioplasty; surgical repair of a hernia.

herniotome (her'nē-ō-tōm). Hernia *knife.*
Cooper's h., a slender bistoury with short cutting edge for dividing the constricting tissues at the neck of a hernial sac.

herniotomy (her-nē-ot'ō-mē) [hernio- + G. *tomē,* a cutting]. Celotomy; surgical division of the constriction or strangulation of a hernia, often followed by herniorrhaphy.
Petit's h., h. without incision into the sac.

heroic (hē-rō'ik) [G. *hērōikos,* pertaining to a hero]. Denoting an aggressive, daring procedure which in itself may endanger the patient but which also has a possibility of being successful, whereas lesser action would result in failure.

heroin (her'ō-in). Diacetylmorphine; an alkaloid, $C_{17}H_{17}(OC_2H_3O)_2ON$, prepared from morphine by acetylation; formerly used for the relief of cough. Except for research, its use in the United States is prohibited by Federal law because of its potential for abuse.

Herophilus. Greek physician and anatomist of the Alexandrian school, circa 300 B.C. See torcular herophili.

herpangina (her-pan'ji-nă, herp-an-jī'nă). A disease caused by types of coxsackievirus and marked by vesiculopapular lesions about 1 to 2 mm in diameter which are present around the fauces and soon break down to form grayish yellow ulcers; accompanied by sudden onset of fever, loss of appetite, dysphagia, pharyngitis, and sometimes abdominal pain, nausea, and vomiting.

herpes (her'pēz) [G. *herpēs,* a spreading skin eruption, shingles, fr. *herpō,* to creep]. Serpigo (2); an eruption of groups of deep-seated vesicles on erythematous bases.
h. catarrha'lis, h. simplex.
h. circina'tus bullo'sus, *dermatitis* herpetiformis.
h. cor'neae, herpetic *keratitis.*
h. desqua'mans, *tinea* imbricata.
h. digita'lis, h. simplex.
h. facia'lis, h. simplex.
h. febri'lis, h. simplex.
h. generalisa'tus, generalized h. simplex virus infection.
h. genita'lis, genital h., h. simplex.
h. gestatio'nis, hydroa gestationis; a polymorphous, bullous eruption, more common on the extremities than on the trunk, with the appearance of pemphigoid or dermatitis herpetiformis; recurrent during each subsequent pregnancy after onset.
h. i'ris, **(1)** *erythema* iris; **(2)** *erythema* multiforme.
h. labia'lis, h. simplex.
neonatal h., herpesvirus type 2 infection transmitted to the newborn infant during passage through an infected birth canal; severity varies from mild to fatal generalized infection, and premature infants are more susceptible than others.
h. sim'plex, a variety of infections caused by herpesvirus types 1 and 2; type 1 infections are marked by the eruption of one or more groups of vesicles on the vermilion border of the lips or at the external nares, type 2 by such lesions on the genitalia; both types commonly are recrudescent and reappear during other febrile illnesses or even physiologic states such as menstruation. Also called h. catarrhalis; h. digitalis; h. facialis; h. febrilis; h. genitalis; h. labialis; hydroa febrile.
traumatic h., h. simplex infection at the site of trauma or of a burn, sometimes accompanied by temperature elevation and malaise.
h. zos'ter, zona (2); zona ignea; zona serpiginosa; zoster; shingles; an infection caused by a herpetovirus (varicella-zoster virus), characterized by an eruption of groups of vesicles on one side of the body following the course of a nerve due to inflammation of ganglia and dorsal nerve roots resulting from activation of the virus which in many instances has remained latent for years; the condition is self-limited but may be accompanied by or followed by severe postherpetic pain.
h. zo'ster ophthal'micus, a herpetic involvement of the ophthalmic branch of the trigeminal nerve.
h. zo'ster varicello'sus, h. zoster associated with disseminated varicelliform lesions.

Herpesvirus (her'pēz-vī'rŭs). A genus of the family Herpetoviridae including herpes simplex and closely related viruses. The former system of classification included in this genus all of the viruses now included in the family Herpetoviridae.
H. su'is, the causative agent of pseudorabies.
H. varicel'lae, varicella-zoster *virus.*

herpesvirus (her'pēz-vī'rŭs). **1.** Herpes simplex virus; a virus of the genus *Herpesvirus* (family Herpetoviridae), divided into two types: **h. type 1,** the pathogen of herpes simplex in humans, causing acute stomatitis, especially in children, fever blisters, usually on the lips and external nares, and also eczema herpeticum and herpetic gingivostomatitis, keratoconjunctivitis, and meningoencephalitis; **h. type 2,** the cause of genital herpes and neonatal herpes. **2.** Formerly, any virus of the genus *Herpesvirus,* which then included those viruses now grouped in the family Herpetoviridae; herpetovirus is now used in this general sense.

herpetic (her-pet'ik). **1.** Relating to or characterized by herpes. **2.** Relating to or caused by a herpetovirus or herpesvirus.

herpetiform (her-pet'i-fōrm). Resembling herpes.

Herpetomonas (her-pĕ-tom′ō-nas) [G. *herpeton*, a reptile (fr. *herpō*, to creep), + *monas*, unit (one of the *Monadidae*)]. A genus of asexual monogenetic flagellates (family Trypanosomatidae) that are strictly insect parasites, with a variety of body forms including promastigote (leptomad), epimastigote (crithidial), amastigote (leishmanial), and trypomastigote (trypanosome-like); infective forms are passed in the host feces. *H. muscae domesticae*, the type species, is found in the common housefly.

Herpetoviridae (her′pĕ-tō-vir′i-dē). A heterogeneous family of morphologically similar viruses, all of which contain double-stranded DNA and which infect man and a wide variety of other vertebrates. Infections produce type A inclusion bodies; in many instances, infection may remain latent for many years, even in the presence of specific circulating antibodies. Virions are enveloped, ether-sensitive, and vary up to 200 nm in diameter; the nucleocapsids are 100 nm in diameter and of icosahedral symmetry, with 162 capsomeres. Only one genus, *Herpesvirus*, has been established, but the family includes herpes simplex virus, varicella-zoster virus, cytomegalovirus, and EB virus (all of which infect man), pseudorabies virus of swine, equine rhinopneumonitis virus, infectious bovine rhinotracheitis virus, canine herpesvirus, B virus of Old World monkeys, several viruses of New World monkeys, virus III of rabbits, infectious laryngotracheitis virus of fowl, Marek's disease virus of chickens, Lucké tumor virus of frogs, and many others.

herpetovirus (her′pĕ-tō-vī′rŭs). Any virus belonging to the family Herpetoviridae. See also herpesvirus (2).

canine h., a h. causing an upper respiratory tract infection which becomes generalized in puppies under 1 week of age, terminating invariably in death; infection is milder in older puppies and asymptomatic in adult dogs; the latter may become convalescent viral shedders.

caprine h., a h. that causes a severe generalized and fatal infection of newborn kids, characterized by fever, depression, inappetence, and mild to severe enteritis; the infection in adult goats is clinically mild, with abortion a frequent sequela.

Herring, Percy T., British physiologist, 1872–1967. See H. *bodies*.

Herrmann, C., Jr., 20th century. See H.'s *syndrome*.

Hers, H.G. See H.'s *disease*.

hersage (ār-sahzh′) [Fr. (from L. *hirpex*, a large rake), a harrowing]. Separating the individual fibers of a nerve trunk.

Hertwig, Richard, German zoologist, 1850–1937. See Magendie-H. *sign, syndrome*.

Hertwig, Wilhelm A.O., German embryologist, 1849–1922. See H.'s *sheath*.

Hertz, Heinrich R., German physicist, 1857–1894. See hertz; hertzian *experiments, rays*.

hertz (Hz) (herts′) [H.R. *Hertz*]. A unit of frequency equivalent to 1 cycle per second.

hertzian (hert′zē-an). Attributed to or described by Heinrich R. Hertz.

Herxheimer, Karl, German dermatologist, 1861–1944. See H.'s *reaction*; Jarisch-H. *reaction*.

herzstoss (hārz′stos) [Ger. heart thrust]. Cardiac systole characterized by a massive diffuse precordial heave without any definite point of maximal impulse.

Heschl, Richard L., Austrian pathologist, 1824–1881. See H.'s *gyri*.

hesitancy (hez′i-tăn-sē). An involuntary delay or inability in starting the urinary stream.

hesperetin (hes-per′ĕ-tin). 3′,5,7-Trihydroxy-4′-methoxyflavanone; a flavone aglycon of hesperidin.

hesperidin (hes-per′i-din). Cirantin; hesperetin 7-rutinoside; hesperetin 7-rhamnoglucoside; a flavone diglycoside obtained from unripe citrus fruit which reputedly possesses vitamin P activity.

Hess, Alfred F., U.S. physician, 1875–1933. See H.'s *test*.

Hess, Carl von, German ophthalmologist, 1863–1923. See H. *screen*.

Hess, Walter R., Swiss physiologist and Nobel laureate, *1881. See trophotropic *zone* of H.

Hesselbach, Franz K., German anatomist and surgeon, 1759–1816. See H.'s *fascia, hernia, ligament, triangle*.

hetacillin (het-ă-sil′in). Phenazacillin; 6-(2,2-dimethyl-5-oxo-4-phenyl-1-imidazolidinyl)penicillanic acid; a semisynthetic penicillin compound with antimicrobial properties.

heter-. See hetero-.

heteradelphus (het-er-ă-del′fŭs) [heter- + G. *adelphos*, brother]. Unequal conjoined twins in which the smaller incomplete parasite is attached to the larger, more nearly normal autosite.

heterakid (het′er-ā′kid). Common name for members of the family Heterakidae.

Heterakis (het-er-ā′kis). A genus of important nematode parasites (family Heterakidae, order Ascaridida) *H. gallinarum* is the cecal worm of chickens, turkeys, and many gallinaceous birds, and is the vector of *Histomonas meleagridis*, a protozoan that causes histomoniasis. Other species are *H. brevispiculum, H. dispar, H. isolonche*, and *H. spumosa*, the latter an abundant cecal parasite of rats and other rodents.

heteralius (het-er-ā′lē-ŭs) [heter- + G. *halios*, useless]. Unequal conjoined twins in which the parasite appears as little more than an excrescence on the autosite.

heteraxial (het-er-ak′sē-ăl). Having mutually perpendicular axes of unequal length.

heterecious (het-er-ē′shŭs) [heter- + G. *oikion*, home]. Metoxenous; having more than one host; said of a parasite passing different stages of its life cycle in different animals.

heterecism (het′er-ē-sizm) [heter- + G. *oikion*, home]. Metoxeny (1); the occurrence, in a parasite, of two cycles of development passed in two different hosts.

heteresthesia (het-er-es-thē′zē-ă) [heter- + G. *aisthēsis*, sensation]. A change occurring in the degree (either plus or minus) of the sensory response to a cutaneous stimulus as the latter crosses a certain line on the surface.

hetero-, heter- [G. *heteros*, other]. Combining forms meaning other, or different.

heteroagglutinin (het′er-ō-ă-glū′ti-nin). A form of hemagglutinin, one that agglutinates the red blood cells of species other than that in which the h. occurs. See also hemagglutinin.

heteroalleles (het′er-ō-ă-lēlz′). Genes that have undergone mutation at different nucleotide positions. *Cf.* eualleles.

heteroantibody (het′er-ō-an′ti-bod-ē). Antibody that is heterologous with respect to antigen, in contradistinction to isoantibody.

heteroantiserum (het′er-ō-an′ti-sē-rŭm). Antiserum developed in one animal species against antigens or cells of another species.

heteroatom (het′er-ō-at′ŏm). An atom, other than carbon, located in the ring structure of an organic compound, as the N in pyridines or pyrimidines (heterocyclic compounds).

heteroblastic (het-er-ō-blas′tik) [hetero- + G. *blastos*, germ]. Developing from more than a single type of tissue.

heterocellular (het′er-ō-sel′yū-lăr). Formed of cells of different kinds.

heterocentric (het′er-ō-sen′trik) [hetero- + G. *kentron*, center]. **1.** Having different centers; said of rays that do not meet at a common focus. *Cf.* homocentric. **2.** Allocentric.

heterocephalus (het-er-ō-sef′ă-lŭs) [hetero- + G. *kephalē*, head]. Conjoined twins with heads of unequal size.

heterocheiral, heterochiral (het-er-ō-kī'răl) [hetero- + G. *cheir,* hand]. Relating to or referred to the other hand.

heterochromatic (het'er-ō-krō-mat'ik). Characteristic of heterochromatin.

heterochromatin (het'er-ō-krō'mă-tin). Heteropyknotic chromatin; the part of the chromonema that remains tightly coiled and condensed during interphase and thus stains readily.
constitutive h., repetitive h. that lies in secondary constrictions in the nucleolar organizers.
facultative h., non-repetitive h. that comprises translatable sequences of DNA.
satellite-rich h., h. that codes for 18S and 28S components of ribosomal RNA and is located close to the centromeres of certain chromosomes.

heterochromia (het'er-ō-krō'mē-ă) [hetero- + G. *chrōma,* color]. A difference in coloration in two structures or two parts of the same structure which are normally alike in color.
atrophic h., h. iridis after trauma or inflammation, or in old age.
binocular h., a congenital defect of pigmentation, with or without extraocular pigmentary defects.
h. i'ridis, h. of iris, a difference in coloration of the irides, or different parts of the same iris. See binocular h.; monocular h.
monocular h., nevi of the iris; a variegated iris.
simple h., h. iridis appearing as a developmental defect.
sympathetic h., h. iridis occurring after lesions of the cervical sympathetic nerves.

heterochromosome (het'er-ō-krō'mō-sōm). Allosome.

heterochromous (het'er-ō-krō'mŭs). Having an abnormal difference in coloration.

heterochron (het'er-ō-kron) [hetero- + G. *chronos,* time]. Having varying chronaxies.

heterochronia (het-er-ō-krō'nē-ă) [hetero- + G. *chronos,* time]. Origin or development of tissues or organs at an unusual time or out of the regular sequence. *Cf.* synchronia.

heterochronic (het-er-ō-kron'ik). Heterochronous.

heterochronous (het-er-ok'rō-nŭs). Heterochronic; relating to heterochronia.

heterocladic (het'er-ō-klad'ik) [hetero- + G. *klados,* a twig]. Denoting an anastomosis between branches of different arterial trunks, as distinguished from homocladic.

heterocrine (het'er-ō-krin) [hetero- + G. *krinō,* to separate]. Denoting the secretion of two or more kinds of material.

heterocrisis (het'er-ō-krī'sis). Rarely used term for an irregular crisis, one occurring at an abnormal time or with unusual symptoms.

heterocytotropic (het'er-ō-sī'tō-trop'ik) [hetero- + G. *kytos,* cell, + *tropē,* a turning toward]. Having an affinity for cells of a different species.

heterodermic (het'er-ō-der'mik) [hetero- + G. *derma,* skin]. Denoting skin grafting in which the grafts are taken from the skin of an animal of another species (dermatoheteroplasty).

heterodisperse (het'er-ō-dis-pers'). Of varying size; describing aerosols whose particles are not uniform in size.

heterodont (het'er-ō-dont) [hetero- + G. *odous,* tooth]. Having teeth of varying shapes, such as those of humans and the majority of mammals, in contrast to homodont.

Heterodoxus spiniger (het-er-ō-dok'sŭs spī'ni-ger). A biting louse of the dog, sometimes called the kangaroo louse.

heterodromous (het-er-ŏd'rō-mŭs) [hetero- + G. *dromos,* running]. Moving in the opposite direction.

heteroduplex (het'er-ō-dū'pleks) [hetero- + L. *duplex,* two-fold]. A DNA molecule, the two constitutive strands of which are derived from distinct sources and hence are likely to be somewhat mismatched.

heterodymus (het-er-od'i-mŭs) [hetero- + G. *didymos,* twin]. Unequal conjoined twins in which the incomplete parasite, consisting of head and neck and, to some extent, thorax, is attached to the anterior surface of the autosite.

heteroerotic (het'er-ō-ĕ-rot'ik). Alloerotic.

heteroerotism (het'er-ō-ār'ō-tizm). Alloerotism.

heterogametic (het'er-ō-gă-met'ik) [hetero- + G. *gametikos,* connubial]. Digametic; relating to production of gametes of contrasting types with respect to sex chromosomes; human males are h.

heterogamous (het-er-og'ă-mŭs). Relating to heterogamy.

heterogamy (het-er-og'ă-mē) [hetero- + G. *gamos,* marriage]. **1.** Conjugation of unlike gametes. **2.** Bearing different types of flowers. **3.** Reproduction by indirect methods of pollination.

heterogenic, heterogeneic (het'er-ō-jen'ik, -jĕ-nē'ik). Pertaining to different gene constitutions, especially with respect to different species.

heterogeneity (het'er-ō-jĕ-nē'i-tē). Heterogeneous state or quality.
genetic h., h. characterized by a phenotype that may be produced by diverse mechanisms which can be distinguished by special methods such as linkage analysis.

heterogeneous (het'er-ō-jē'nē-ŭs). Composed of parts having various and dissimilar characteristics or properties.

heterogenesis (het'er-ō-jen'ĕ-sis) [hetero- + G. *genesis,* production]. Spontaneous *generation.*

heterogenetic (het'er-ō-jĕ-net'ik). Relating to heterogenesis.

heterogenote (het'er-ō-jē'nōt). In microbial genetics, an organism that contains an exogenous piece of genetic material that differs somewhat from the corresponding region of its own original genome, but in a very limited way resembles a heterozygote.

heterogenous (het-er-oj'ĕ-nŭs). Having a different or dissimilar origin.

heterograft (het'er-ō-graft). Xenograft.

heterohypnosis (het'er-ō-hip-nō'sis). Hypnosis induced by or in another, as opposed to autohypnosis.

heterokaryon (het'er-ō-kar'ē-on) [hetero- + G. *karyon,* kernel, nut]. Genetically different nuclei in a common cytoplasm, usually resulting from the artificial fusion of two cells from different species.

heterokaryotic (het'er-ō-kar-ē-ot'ik). Exhibiting the properties of a heterokaryon.

heterokeratoplasty (het'er-ō-ker'ă-tō-plas-tē). Keratoplasty in which the cornea from one species of animal is grafted to the eye of another species.

heterokinesia (het'er-ō-ki-nē'zē-ă) [hetero- + G. *kinēsis,* movement]. Heterokinesis (2); executing movements the reverse of those one is told to make.

heterokinesis (het'er-ō-ki-nē'sis). **1.** Differential distribution of X and Y chromosomes during meiotic cell division. **2.** Heterokinesia.

heterolalia (het'er-ō-lā'lē-ă) [hetero- + G. *lalia,* speech]. Heterophasia; heterophemia; heterophemy; the habitual substitution of meaningless or inappropriate words for those intended; a form of aphasia.

heterolateral (het'er-ō-lat'er-ăl) [hetero- + L. *latus,* side]. Contralateral.

heterolipids (het'er-ō-lip'idz). Compound lipids; lipids containing N and P atoms in addition to the usual C, H, and O. *Cf.* homolipids.

heteroliteral (het'er-ō-lit'er-ăl) [hetero- + L. *litera,* letter]. Relating to stammering or the substitution of one letter for another in the pronunciation of certain words.

heterologous (het-er-ol'ō-gŭs) [hetero- + G. *logos,* ratio, relation].

1. Pertaining to cytologic or histologic elements occurring where they are not normally found. 2. Derived from an animal of a different species, as the serum of a horse is h. for a rabbit.

heterology (het-er-ol'ō-jē). A departure from the normal in structure, arrangement, or mode or time of development.

heterolysin (het-er-ol'i-sin). A lysin that is formed in one species of animal and manifests lytic activity on the cells of a different species.

heterolysis (het-er-ol'i-sis) [hetero- + G. *lysis*, a loosening]. Dissolution or digestion of cells or protein components from one species by a lytic agent from a different species.

heterolytic (het'er-ō-lit'ik). Pertaining to heterolysis or to the effect of a heterolysin.

heteromastigote (het-er-ō-mas'ti-gōt) [hetero- + G. *mastix*, a whip]. A flagellate having two flagella, one anterior and one posterior.

heteromeral (het'er-om'er-ăl). Heteromeric (2).

heteromeric (het'er-ō-mār'ik) [hetero- + G. *meros*, part]. **1.** Having a different chemical composition. **2.** Heteromeral; heteromerous; denoting spinal neurons that have processes passing over to the opposite side of the cord.

heteromerous (het'er-om'er-ŭs). Heteromeric (2).

heterometabolous (het'er-ō-me-tab'ō-lŭs) [hetero- + G. *metabolē*, change]. Pertaining to a member of the Heterometabola, a superorder sometimes used for a series of insect orders in which incomplete metamorphosis is found.

heterometaplasia (het'er-ō-met-ă-plā'zē-ă). Tissue transformation resulting in production of a tissue foreign to the part where produced.

heterometric (het'er-ō-met'rik) [hetero- + G. *metron*, measure]. Involving or depending upon a change in size.

heterometropia (het'er-ō-me-trō'pē-ă) [hetero- + G. *metron*, measure, + *ōps*, eye]. A condition in which the refraction is different in the two eyes.

heteromorphism (het'er-ō-mōrf'izm) [hetero- + G. *morphē*, shape]. In cytogenetics, a difference in shape or size between the two members of a pair of metaphase chromosomes (*i.e.*, between homologous chromosomes).

heteromorphosis (het'er-ō-mōr-fō'sis) [hetero- + G. *morphōsis*, a molding]. **1.** Development of one tissue from a tissue of another kind or type. **2.** Embryonic development of tissue or an organ inappropriate to its site.

heteromorphous (het'er-ō-mōr'fŭs). Differing from the normal type.

heteronomous (het-er-on'ō-mŭs) [hetero- + G. *nomos*, law]. **1.** Different from the type; abnormal. **2.** Subject to the direction or control of another; not self-governing. *Cf.* autonomous.

heteronomy (het-er-on'ō-mē) [hetero- + G. *nomos*, law]. The condition or state of being heteronomous.

heteronuclear (het'er-ō-nū'klē-er). Denoting a heterokaryon that has lost some of the nuclear material from which the cell line was originally constituted.

heteronymous (het-er-on'i-mŭs) [G. *heterōnymos*, having a different name, fr. *onyma*, or *onoma*, name]. Having different names or expressed in different terms.

hetero-osteoplasty (het'er-ō-os'tē-ō-plas-tē). Bone transplantation from one species to another; formerly used to denote transplants from one person to another.

heteropagus (het-er-op'ă-gŭs) [hetero- + G. *pagos*, fixed]. Unequal conjoined twins in which the imperfectly developed parasite is attached to the ventral portion of the autosite. See also epigastrius.

heteropathy (het'er-op'ă-thē) [hetero- + G. *pathos*, suffering]. **1.** Abnormal sensitivity to stimuli. **2.** Allopathy.

heterophagy (het-er-of'ă-jē) [hetero- + G. *phagein*, to eat]. Digestion within a cell of an exogenous substance phagocytosed from the cell's environment.

heterophasia (het'er-ō-fā'zē-ă) [hetero- + G. *phasis*, speech]. Heterolalia.

heterophemia, heterophemy (het'er-ō-fē'mē-ă, het-er-of'ĕ-mē) [hetero- + G. *phēmē*, a speech]. Heterolalia.

heterophil, heterophile (het'er-ō-fil, -fīl) [hetero- + G. *philos*, fond]. **1.** The neutrophilic leukocyte in man; in some animals the granules vary in size and staining reaction. **2.** Pertaining to heterogenetic antigens and related antibody.

heterophonia (het'er-ō-fō'nē-ă) [hetero- + G. *phōnē*, voice]. Heterophthongia. **1.** The change of voice at puberty. **2.** Any abnormality in the voice sounds.

heterophoria (het'er-ō-fō'rē-ă) [hetero- + G. *phora*, movement]. A tendency for deviation of the eyes from parallelism, prevented by binocular vision.

heterophthalmus (het'er-of-thal'mŭs) [hetero- + G. *ophthalmos*, eye]. Allophthalmia; a difference in the appearance of the two eyes, usually due to heterochromia iridis.

heterophthongia (het-er-of-thon'jē-ă) [G. *heterophthongos*, fr. *heteros*, different, + *phthongos*, sound, voice]. Heterophonia.

Heterophyes (het-er-of'i-ēz) [hetero- + G. *phyē*, stature, form]. A genus of digenetic flukes (family Heterophyidae) parasitic in fish-eating birds and mammals, including man; cercariae from infected snails penetrate and encyst in fish, which are eaten by the final hosts.

H. brevicae'ca, a species reported from man in the Philippines and implicated in heart lesions caused by the eggs of this minute fluke, carried from the intestinal mucosa to obstruct coronary capillaries.

H. heteroph'yes, the Egyptian intestinal or small intestinal fluke, a species infecting the small intestine and cecum in man and other fish-eating mammals in Egypt and the Far East.

H. katsura'dai, a species, somewhat smaller than *H. heterophyes*, found in Japan.

heterophyiasis (het'er-ō-fī-ī'ă-sis). Heterophyidiasis; infection with a heterophyid trematode, particularly *Heterophyes heterophyes*.

heterophyid (het'er-o-fī'id). Common name for a member of the family Heterophyidae.

Heterophyidae (het'er-ō-fī'i-dē). A family of tiny fish-borne trematodes, including the genus *Heterophyes* and its common human parasite, *H. heterophyes*.

heterophyidiasis (het'er-ō-fī-id-ī'ă-sis). Heterophyiasis.

heteroplasia (het'er-ō-plā'zē-ă) [hetero- + G. *plasis*, a forming]. Alloplasia. **1.** Development of cytologic and histologic elements that are not normal for the organ or part in question, as the growth of bone in a site where there is normally fibrous connective tissue. **2.** Malposition of tissue or a part that is otherwise normal, as a ureter that develops at the lower pole of a kidney.

heteroplastic (het'er-ō-plas'tik). **1.** Pertaining to or manifesting heteroplasia. **2.** Relating to heteroplasty.

heteroplastid (het'er-ō-plas'tid). The graft in heteroplasty.

heteroplasty (het'er-ō-plas-tē) [hetero- + G. *plastos*, formed]. **1.** Heterotransplantation. **2.** Formerly, transplantation of any graft other than an autograft.

heteroploid (het'er-ō-ployd). Relating to heteroploidy.

heteroploidy (het'er-ō-ploy'dē) [hetero- + G. *ploides*, in form]. The state of a cell possessing some number of haploid sets other than the normal diploid number (in man, 46).

heteropolysaccharide (het'er-ō-pol-ē-sak'ă-rīd). A polysaccharide composed of two or more different types of monosaccharides.

heteroproteose (het'er-ō-prō'tē-ōs). See primary *proteose.*

heteropsychologic (het'er-ō-sī-kō-loj'ik). Relating to ideas developed from without or derived from another's consciousness.

heteropyknosis (het'er-ō-pik-nō'sis) [hetero- + G. *pyknos,* dense]. Any state of variable density or condensation, usually referring to differences in degree of density between different chromosomes or between different regions of the same chromosome; may be attentuated (**negative p.**) or accentuated (**positive p.**).

heteropyknotic (het'er-ō-pik-not'ik). Relating to or characterized by heteropyknosis.

heterosaccharide (het'er-ō-sak'ă-rīd). A glycoside in which a sugar group is attached to a nonsugar group; *e.g.,* amygdalin.

heterosexual (het'er-ō-sek'shū-ăl). **1.** Relating to or characteristic of heterosexuality. **2.** One whose interests and behavior are characteristic of heterosexuality.

heterosexuality (het'er-ō-sek-shū-al'i-tē). Erotic attraction, predisposition, or activity, including sexual congress between persons of the opposite sex.

heterosis (het-er-ō'sis). The beneficial effect of crossing (hybridization) upon growth, vigor, and physical or mental qualities in a strain of plants or in animal stock, as measured by the mid-parent mean and F_1.

heterosome (het'er-ō-sōm) [hetero- + G. *sōma,* body]. In genetics, the chromosome pair that is different in the two sexes. See sex *chromosome.*

heterospecific (het'er-ō-spe-sif'ik). Heterologous, as pertains to grafts.

heterosuggestion (het'er-ō-sŭg-jes'chŭn). Suggestion received from another person; opposed to autosuggestion.

heterotaxia (het'er-ō-taks'ē-ă) [hetero- + G. *taxis,* arrangement]. Heterotaxis; heterotaxy; abnormal arrangement of organs or parts of the body in relation to each other.
cardiac h., see dextrocardia.

heterotaxic (het-er-ō-taks'ik). Abnormally placed or arranged.

heterotaxis, heterotaxy (het-er-ō-taks'is, het'er-ō-taks-ē). Heterotaxia.

heterothallic (het'er-ō-thal'ik) [hetero- + G. *thallos,* a young shoot]. In fungi, denoting a kind of sexual reproduction in which a sexual spore is produced only by fusion with a nucleus of another mating type. *Cf.* homothallic.

heterotherm (het'er-ō-therm). A heterothermic animal.

heterothermic (het'er-ō-ther'mik). Having partial regulation of body temperature; between poikilothermic and homeothermic.

heterotic (het-er-ot'ik). Relating to heterosis.

heterotonia (het'er-ō-tō'nē-ă) [hetero- + G. *tonos,* tension]. Abnormality or variation in tension or tonus.

heterotopia (het-er-ō-tō'pē-ă) [hetero- + G. *topos,* place]. **1.** Ectopia. **2.** In neuropathology, displacement of gray matter, typically into the deep cerebral white matter.

heterotopic (het-er-ō-top'ik). **1.** Ectopic (1). **2.** Relating to heterotopia (2).

heterotopous (het-er-ot'ō-pŭs). Heterotopic, especially in reference to teratomas composed of tissues that are out of place in the region where found.

heterotransplantation (het'er-ō-tranz-plan-tā'shŭn). Heteroplasty (1); transfer of a heterograft (xenograft).

heterotrichosis (het'er-ō-tri-kō'sis) [hetero- + G. *trichōsis,* growth of hair]. A condition characterized by hair growth of variegated color.

heterotroph (het'er-ō-trof, -trōf) [hetero- + G. *trophē,* nourishment]. A microorganism that obtains its carbon, as well as its energy, from organic compounds. See also autotroph.

heterotrophic (het'er-ō-trof'ik). Relating to a heterotroph.

heterotropia, heterotropy (het'er-ō-trō'pē-ă, het-er-ot'rō-pē) [hetero- + G. *tropē,* a turning]. Strabismus.
h. mac'ulae, *ectopia* maculae.

heterotypic (het'er-ō-tip'ik). Of a different or unusual type or form.

heteroxanthine (het'er-ō-zan'thin). 7-Methylxanthine; one of the alloxuric bases in urine, representing end products of purine metabolism.

heteroxenous (het-er-oks'ĕ-nŭs) [hetero- + G. *xenos,* stranger]. Digenetic (1).

heterozoic (het-er-ō-zō'ik) [hetero- + G. *zōikos,* relating to an animal]. Relating to another animal or another species of animal.

heterozygosity, heterozygosis (het'er-ō-zī-gos'i-tē, -zī-gō'sis) [hetero- + G. *zygon,* a yoke]. The state of being heterozygous.

heterozygote (het'er-ō-zī'gōt) [hetero- + G. *zygotos,* yoked]. A heterozygous individual.
compound h., genetic compound; in medical genetics, the presence of two different, harmful, mutant alleles at the same loci.
manifesting h., manifesting carrier; an organism heterozygous for what is ordinarily a recessive condition which, as a result of special mechanisms (such as lyonization), has phenotypic manifestations.

heterozygous (het'er-ō-zī'gŭs). Having different allelic genes at one or more paired loci in homologous chromosomes.
doubly h., in the analysis of linkage between two loci, denoting that genotype in which a parent is h. at both loci, the state that on average contains the maximum information about the linkage.

Heubner, Johann O.L., German pediatrician, 1843–1926. See H.'s *disease; artery* of H.

Heurenius, Johannes. See van Horne, Jan.

Heuser, Chester, U.S. embryologist, 1885–1965. See H.'s *membrane.*

hexa-, hex- [G. *hex,* six]. Prefixes meaning six.

hexabione (hek-să-bī'ōn). Obsolete term for pyridoxine.

hexacanth (hek'să-kanth) [hexa- + G. *akantha,* hook or thorn]. Oncosphere; the motile six-hooked first-stage larva of cyclophyllidean cestodes; it emerges from the egg and actively claws its way through the intermediate host's intestine prior to development into the next larval stage; *e.g.,* the h. of *Taenia saginata,* which penetrates the intestine of a cow that ingested the egg, then forms a cysticercus in the muscles of the intermediate host.

hexacarbacholine bromide (hek'să-kar-bă-kō'lēn). Hexamethylene-1,6-bis(carbamoylcholine bromide); a neuromuscular blocking agent with depolarizing and nondepolarizing actions.

hexachlorocyclohexane (hek-să-klō'rō-sī-klō-hek'sān). Lindane.

hexachlorophane (hek-să-klō'rō-fān). Hexachlorophene.

hexachlorophene (hek-să-klo'rō-fēn). Hexachlorophane; 2,2′-methylenebis(3,4,6-trichlorophenol); an antibacterial; used in soaps and detergents to inhibit bacterial growth; excessive use causes neurological lesions.

hexacosanol (heks-ă-kō'să-nol). See ceryl.

hexacosyl (heks-ă-kō'sil). Ceryl.

hexad (heks'ad). A sexivalent element or radical.

hexadactyly, hexadactylism (hek'să-dak'ti-lē, -lizm) [hexa- + G. *daktylos,* finger]. The presence of six fingers or six toes on one or both hands or feet.

hexadecanoic acid (hek'să-dek-ă-nō'ik). Palmitic acid.

1-hexadecanol (hek-să-dek'ă-nol). *Cetyl* alcohol.

hexadiphane (hek-să-dī'fān). Prozapine.

hexafluorenium bromide (hek'să-flū-rēn'ē-ŭm). Hexamethylenebis[fluoren-9-yldimethylammonium bromide]; a potentiator for succinylcholine in anesthesiology by producing a mild nondepolarizing neuromuscular blockade; also inhibits plasma cholinesterase.

hexamer (hek'să-mer) [hexa- + G. *meros,* part]. See virion.

hexamethone bromide (hek-să-meth'ōn). Hexamethonium chloride.

hexamethonium chloride (hek'să-me-thō'nē-ŭm). Hexamethone bromide; hexamethylenebis(trimethylammonium chloride); a ganglionic blocking agent used in the treatment of hypertension, usually in combination with other hypotensive drugs; also used as the bromide and the tartrate.

hexamidine isethionate (hek-sam'i-dēn). *p,p*'- (Hexamethylenedioxy)dibenzamidine bis(β-hydroxyethanesulfonate); a topical antiseptic.

hexamine (hek'să-mēn). Methenamine.

Hexamita (hek-sam'i-tă) [hexa- + G. *mitos,* thread]. A genus of protozoan flagellates (order Diplomonadida, class Zoomastigophorea), related to *Giardia,* which have a symmetrical body, two anterior nuclei, six anterior and two posterior flagella, and two separate axostyles; they are parasitic in the small intestine of many gallinaceous birds and of certain mammals. *H. meleagridis* is a species that occurs in the turkey, peafowl, pheasant, quail, and Chukkar partridge; it is most pathogenic in turkeys, causing outbreaks of hexamitiasis.

hexamitiasis (hek-sam-i-tī'ă-sis). An infectious catarrhal enteritis of turkeys, quail, Chukkar partridges, and other gallinaceous birds caused by *Hexamita meleagridis* and manifested by diarrhea. Adult birds are symptomless carriers, but poults under 10 weeks often are severely affected.

hexane (hek'sān). A saturated hydrocarbon, C_6H_{14}, of the paraffin series.

hexanoate (hek'să-nō-āt). Caproylate.

hexanoic acid (hek-să-nō'ik). *n*-Caproic acid.

hexanoyl (hek'să-nō-il). Caproyl.

hexaploidy (heks'ă-ploy-dē). See polyploidy.

Hexapoda (hek-sap'ō-dă) [hexa- + G. *pous,* foot]. Insecta.

hexestrol (hek-ses'trol). *p,p*'-(1,2-Diethylethylene)diphenol; dihydrodiethylstilbestrol; a synthetic compound with estrogenic activity.

hexetidine (hek-set'i-dēn). 5-Amino-1,3-bis-(2-ethylhexyl)-hexahydro-5-methylpyrimidine; a local anti-infective agent used in the treatment of vaginitis and cervicitis due to fungal and protozoan organisms.

hexitol (heks'i-tol). The polyol (sugar alcohol) obtained on the reduction of a hexose.

hexobarbital sodium (hek-sō-bar'bi-tal). Sodium 5-(1-cyclohexen-1-yl)-1,5-dimethylbarbiturate; a barbiturate sedative and hypnotic of short duration.

hexobendine (hek-sō-ben'dēn). 3,4,5-Trimethoxybenzoic acid ester with 3,3'-[ethylenebis(methylamino)]-di-1-propanol; a coronary and cerebral vasodilator.

hexocyclium methylsulfate (hek-sō-sik'lē-ŭm meth'il-sŭl-fāt). N^4-(β-Cyclohexyl-β-hydroxy-β-phenylethyl)-N^1-methylpiperazine dimethylsulfate; an anticholinergic agent.

hexokinase (heks-ō-kī'nās) [EC 2.7.1.1]. A phosphotransferase present in yeast, muscle, and other tissues which catalyzes the phosphorylation of glucose and other hexoses to form hexose 6-phosphate (phosphate is transferred from ATP, which is converted to ADP).

hexon (heks'on). A hexagonal capsomere (hexamer unit) of adenovirus capsids. Antigenically, h.'s as a group differ from the penton base and also from its protruding fiber.

hexonic acid (heks-on'ik). The aldonic acid obtained on the oxidation of the aldehyde group of an aldohexose to a carboxylic acid (*e.g.,* gluconic acid from glucose).

hexosamine (hek'sō-sam'ēn). The amine derivative (NH_2 replacing OH) of a hexose; *e.g.,* glucosamine.

hexosaminidase (hek'sō-sa-min'i-dās). General term for enzymes cleaving *N*-acetylhexose (glucose or galactose) residues from ganglioside-like oligosaccharides. At least four specific enzymes carrying out this type of reaction are known: α-N-acetylgalactosaminidase (EC 3.2.1.49), α-N-acetylglucosaminidase (EC 3.2.1.50), β-N-acetylhexosaminidase (EC 3.2.1.52), and β-N-acetylgalactosaminidase (EC 3.2.1.53), each being specific for the configuration and type of sugar included in the name.

hexosans (hek'sō-sanz). Polyhexoses; polysaccharides with the general formula $(C_6H_{10}O_5)_x$ which, on hydrolysis, yield hexoses; included are glucosans, mannans, galactans, and fructosans.

hexose (hek'sōs). A monosaccharide containing six carbon atoms in the molecule ($C_6H_{12}O_6$); glucose is the principal h. in nature.

hexosebisphosphatase, hexosediphosphatase (hek'sōs-bis-fos'fă-tās, -dī-). Fructose-bisphosphatase.

hexose phosphatase. An enzyme catalyzing the hydrolysis of a hexose phosphate to a hexose (*e.g.,* glucose 6-phosphatase).

hexosephosphate isomerase (hek-sōs-fos'fāt). Glucosephosphate isomerase.

hexose-1-phosphate uridylyltransferase. UDPglucose—hexose-1-phosphate uridylyltransferase.

hexulose (hek'syū-lōs). Ketohexose.

hexuronic acid (hek-syūr-on'ik). The uronic acid of a hexose.

hexyl (hek'sil). The radical of hexane, $CH_3(CH_2)_4CH_2$–.

hexylcaine hydrochloride (hek'sil-kān). Cyclohexylamino-2-propylbenzoate hydrochloride; a local anesthetic agent suitable for surface application, infiltration, or nerve block.

hexylresorcinol (hek'sil-re-sōr'si- nol). 4-Hexyl-1,3-dihydroxybenzene; a broad spectrum anthelmintic.

Hey, William, British surgeon, 1736–1819. See H.'s *amputation,* internal *derangement, hernia, ligament.*

Heyer, W.T., U.S. scientist, *1902. See H.-Pudenz *valve.*

Heyns, O.S., 20th century South African obstetrician. See H.'s abdominal decompression *apparatus.*

Hf Symbol for hafnium.

Hg Symbol for mercury (hydrargyrum).

HGF Abbreviation for hyperglycemic-glycogenolytic *factor.*

HGH Abbreviation for human growth hormone. See somatotropin.

hiatal (hī-ā'tăl). Relating to a hiatus.

hiatus, pl. hiatus (hī-ā'tŭs) [L. an aperture, fr. *hio,* pp. *hiatus,* to yawn] [NA]. An aperture, opening, or foramen.

h. adducto'rius [NA], an alternate term for h. tendineus.

h. aor'ticus [NA], aortic opening or foramen; the opening in the diaphragm bounded by the two crura, the vertebral column, and the median arcuate ligament, through which pass the aorta and thoracic duct.

Breschet's h., helicotrema.

h. of canal for greater petrosal nerve, h. canalis nervi petrosi majoris.

h. cana'lis facia'lis, h. canalis nervi petrosi majoris.

h. of canal of lesser petrosal nerve, h. canalis nervi petrosi minoris.

h. cana'lis ner'vi petro'si majo'ris [NA], h. of canal for greater petrosal nerve; h. of the facial canal; h. canalis facialis; fallopian h.; Ferrein's foramen; the opening on the anterior aspect of the petrous part of the temporal bone which leads to the facial canal and gives passage to the greater petrosal nerve.

h. cana'lis ner'vi petro'si mino'ris [NA], h. of canal of lesser petrosal nerve; canalis nervi petrosi superficialis minoris; Arnold's canal; the small opening in the petrous bone lateral to the h. for the greater petrosal nerve that gives passage to the lesser petrosal nerve.

h. esophage'us [NA], esophageal opening; the opening in the diaphragm, between the central tendon and the h. aorticus, through which pass the esophagus and the two vagus nerves.

h. ethmoida'lis, h. semilunaris.

fallopian h., h. canalis nervi petrosi majoris.

h. maxilla'ris [NA], maxillary h.; the large opening into the maxillary sinus on the nasal surface of the maxilla.

maxillary h., h. maxillaris.

pleuropericardial h., an opening connecting the pleural and pericardial cavities; usually the result of incomplete development of the pleuropericardial fold of the embryo.

pleuroperitoneal h., Bochdalek's foramen; an opening through the diaphragm, connecting pleural and peritoneal cavities, usually the result of defective development of the pleuroperitoneal membrane in the embryo; if the defect is extensive there may be herniation of digestive organs into the pleural cavity. See also diaphragmatic *hernia.*

sacral h., h. sacralis.

h. sacra'lis [NA], sacral h.; a gap at the lower end of the sacrum, exposing the vertebral canal, due to failure of the laminae of the last sacral segment to coalesce.

h. saphe'nus [NA], saphenous opening; fossa ovalis (2); the opening in the fascia lata inferior to the medial part of the inguinal ligament through which the saphenous vein passes to enter the femoral vein.

Scarpa's h., helicotrema.

semilunar h., h. semilunaris.

h. semiluna'ris [NA], semilunar h.; h. ethmoidalis; a deep, narrow groove in the lateral wall of the middle meatus of the nasal cavity, into which the maxillary sinus, the frontonasal duct, and the middle ethmoid cells open.

h. subarcua'tus, *fossa* subarcuata.

h. tendin'eus [NA], tendinous opening; h. adductorius; femoral opening; the aperture in the tendon of insertion of the adductor magnus that transmits the femoral artery and vein from the adductor canal to the popliteal space.

h. tota'lis sacra'lis, incomplete development of sacral vertebrae.

hibernation (hī-ber-nā'shŭn) [L. *hibernus,* relating to winter]. Winter sleep; a torpid condition in which certain animals pass the cold months. True hibernators, such as woodchucks, ground squirrels, dormice, and some others, have body temperatures reduced to near the freezing point, with a very slow heartbeat, low metabolism, and infrequent respirations. Partial hibernators, such as bears, skunks, and raccoons, have reduced physiologic activity during the cold months, but they are not comatose. *Cf.* estivation.

artificial h., the use of a mixture of drugs, including antihistamines, narcotics, hypnotics, and adrenolytic compounds, to induce sleep or a dormant state analogous to that observed in hibernating animals; once used as an adjuvant to anesthesia.

hibernoma (hī'ber-nō'mă) [L. *hibernus,* pertaining to winter, + G. *-ōma,* tumor]. A rare type of benign neoplasm in human beings, consisting of brown fat that resembles the fat in certain hibernating animals; individual tumor cells contain multiple lipid droplets. See also brown *fat.*

interscapular h., brown *fat.*

hiccup, hiccough (hik'ŭp). A diaphragmatic spasm causing a sudden inhalation which is interrupted by a spasmodic closure of the glottis, producing a noise.

epidemic h., a persistent h. occurring as a complication of influenza.

Hicks, John Braxton, British gynecologist, 1823–1897. See B. H. *contractions, sign, version.*

hidr-, See hidro-.

hidradenitis (hī-drad'ĕ-nī'tis) [G. *hidrōs,* sweat, + *adēn,* gland, + *-itis,* inflammation]. Hidrosadenitis; hydradenitis; inflammation of the sweat glands; more specifically, of the apocrine glands.

h. axilla'ris of Verneuil, an axillary abscess.

h. suppurati'va, spiradenitis; inflammation of the apocrine sweat glands secondary to folliculitis of the perianal, axillary, and genital areas or under the breasts, producing chronic abscesses or sinuses.

hidradenoma (hī-drad-ĕ-nō'mă) [G. *hidrōs,* sweat, + *adēn,* gland, + *-oma,* tumor]. Hydradenoma; a benign neoplasm derived from epithelial cells of sweat glands.

clear cell h., eccrine *acrospiroma.*

nodular h., eccrine *acrospiroma.*

papillary h., apocrine adenoma; a solitary tumor occurring usually in the labia majora, cystic and papillary, and composed of epithelium resembling that of apocrine glands.

hidro-, hidr- [G. *hidrōs,* sweat]. Combining forms relating to sweat or sweat glands.

hidroa (hī-drō'ă). Hydroa.

hidrocystoma (hī'drō-sis-tō'mă) [hidro- + G. *kystis,* bladder, + *-ōma,* tumor]. Hydrocystoma (2); syringocystoma; a cystic form of hidradenoma, usually apocrine.

hidromeiosis (hī'drō-mī-ō'sis) [hidro- + G. *meiōsis,* a lessening]. A decline in the rate of sweating during exposure to heat, especially that from warm baths.

hidropoiesis (hī'drō-poy-ē'sis, hid'rō-) [hidro- + G. *poiēsis,* formation]. The formation of sweat.

hidropoietic (hī'drō-poy-et'ik, hid'rō-). Relating to hidropoiesis.

hidrosadenitis (hī'drō-sad-ĕ-nī'tis, hid'rō-). Hidradenitis.

hidroschesis (hī-dros'kĕ-sis, hid-ros') [hidro- + G. *schesis,* a checking]. Suppression of sweating.

hidrosis (hi-drō'sis, hī-) [G. *hidrōs,* sweat, + *-osis,* condition]. Idrosis; the production and excretion of sweat.

hidrotic (hi-drot'ik, hī-). Relating to or causing hidrosis.

hierarchy (hī'er-ar-kē, hī-rar'kē) [G. *hierarchia,* rule or power of the high priest]. **1.** Any system of persons or things ranked one above the other. **2.** In psychology and psychiatry, an organization of habits or concepts in which simpler components are combined to form increasingly complex integrations.

dominance h., a social situation in which one organism dominates all below it, the next all below it, and so on down to the organism dominated by all; *e.g.,* the pecking order in barnyard hens.

Maslow's h., a ranking of needs which man presumably fills successively in the order of lowest to highest: physiological needs, love and belonging, self-esteem, and self-actualization.

response h., alternative reactions or modes of adjustment to a given situation arranged in the probable order of prior effectiveness; *e.g.,* a mother attempting to discipline an unruly child may first cajole, then plead, scold, and finally punish; her behaviors can be ordered along a response h. for further monitoring of effectiveness.

hieromania (hī'er-ō-mā'nē-ă) [G. *hieros,* holy, + *mania,* insanity]. Obsolete term for pathologic religious fervor characterized by delusions with a religious content.

hierophobia (hī'er-ō-fō'bē-ă) [G. *hieros,* holy, + *phobos,* fear]. Morbid fear of religious or sacred objects.

hierotherapy (hī'er-ō-thār'ă-pē) [G. hieros, holy, + *therapeia,* therapy]. Faith healing; treatment of disease by prayer and religious practices.

Higashi, Ototaka. See Chédiak-H. *disease,* Chédiak-Steinbrinck-H. *anomaly, syndrome.*

Highmore, Nathaniel, British anatomist, 1613–1685. See H.'s *body; antrum* of H.

Higoumenakia sign. See under sign.

hila (hī'lă). Plural of hilum.

hilar (hī'lăr). Pertaining to a hilum.

hilitis (hī-lī'tis). Inflammation of the lining membrane of any hilus.

Hill, Archibald V., British biophysicist and Nobel laureate, 1886–1977. See H.'s *equation.*

Hill, Harold A., 20th century U.S. radiologist. See H.-Sachs *lesion.*

Hill, Sir Leonard Erskine, British physiologist, 1866-1952. See H.'s *sign, phenomenon.*

Hill, Lucius, U.S. thoracic surgeon, *1921. See H. *operation.*

Hill, Robert Hill, British plant physiologist, *1899. See H. *reaction.*

Hillis, David S., U.S. obstetrician-gynecologist, 1873–1942. See H.-Müller *maneuver.*

hillock (hil'lok). In anatomy, any small elevation or prominence.

axon h., implantation cone; the conical area of origin of the axon from the nerve cell body; it contains parallel arrays of microtubules and is devoid of Nissl substance.

facial h., *colliculus* facialis.

seminal h., *colliculus* seminalis.

Hilton, John, British surgeon, 1804–1878. See H.'s *law,* white *line, method, sac.*

hilum, pl. **hila** (hī'lŭm, hī'lă) [L. a small bit or trifle] [NA]. **1.** Porta (1); the part of an organ where the nerves and vessels enter and leave. **2.** A depression or slit resembling the h. in the olivary nucleus of the brain.

h. of dentate nucleus, h. nuclei dentati.

h. of kidney, h. renalis.

h. li'enis [NA], h. splenicum.

h. of lung, h. pulmonis.

h. of lymph node, h. lymphonodi; the depressed area of the surface of a lymph node through which the efferent lymphatics emerge from the medulla and through which blood vessels enter and leave the node.

h. lymphono'di, h. of lymph node.

h. nu'clei denta'ti [NA], h. of dentate nucleus; the mouth of the flasklike dentate nucleus of the cerebellum, directed inward, and giving exit to many of the fibers which compose the pedunculus cerebellaris superior or brachium conjunctivum.

h. nu'clei oliva'ris [NA], h. of the olivary nucleus; the medially oriented opening in the folded cell layer composing the inferior olivary nucleus through which the efferent fibers of the nucleus make their exit.

h. of olivary nucleus, h. nuclei olivaris.

h. ova'rii [NA], h. of ovary; the depression along the mesovarian margin, at the insertion of the mesovarium, where vessels and nerves enter or leave the ovary.

h. of ovary, h. ovarii.

h. pulmo'nis [NA], h. of lung; porta pulmonis; a wedge-shaped depression on the mediastinal surface of each lung, where the bronchus, blood vessels, nerves, and lymphatics enter or leave the viscus.

h. rena'lis [NA], h. of kidney; porta renis; the depression on the medial border of the kidney through which pass the vessels and nerves and which contains the apex of the renal pelvis.

h. of spleen, h. splenicum.

h. sple'nicum [NA], h. of spleen; h. lienis; porta lienis; a fissure on the gastric surface of the spleen, giving passage to the splenic vessels and nerves.

hilus (hī'lŭs) [an Eng. variant of L. *hilum*]. Former incorrect NA designation for hilum.

himantosis (hī-man-tō'sis) [G. *himas,* strap, + *-osis,* condition]. An unusually long uvula.

hindbrain (hīnd'brān). Rhombencephalon.

hindgut (hīnd'gŭt). Endgut. **1.** The large intestine, rectum, and anal canal. **2.** The caudal or terminal part of the embryonic gut.

hindwater (hīnd'wah-ter). Colloquialism for amniotic fluid *in utero* behind the presenting part of the fetus.

Hines, Marion, U.S. neurologist, *1889. See strip *area* of H.

hinge-bow (hinj'bō). Face-bow.

Hinman, Frank, Jr., U.S. urologist, *1915. See H. *syndrome.*

Hinton, William A., U.S. physician, 1883–1959. See H. *test.*

hip [A.S. *hype*]. Coxa (2); the lateral prominence of the pelvis from the waist to the thigh; more strictly the h. joint.

snapping h., a condition in which a tendon under tension, moving over the greater trochanter of the proximal end of the femur, causes a click.

Hippel, Eugen von. See von Hippel, Eugen.

Hippelates (hip-ĕ-lā'tēz) [G. *hippelatēs,* driver of horses]. The eye gnats, a genus of flies in the family Chloropidae (fruit flies) that are attracted to the body secretions and fluids of animals and man, particularly those in the eyes. *H.* is suspected of transmitting certain types of conjunctivitis (such as pinkeye), bovine mastitis, and yaws (frambesia tropica).

Hippobosca (hip-ō-bos'kă) [G. *hippos,* horse, + *boskein,* to feed]. A genus of pupiparous louse flies (family Hippoboscidae) related to the tsetse flies; they are ectoparasites on birds and mammals. See also *Melophagus.*

Hippoboscidae (hip-ō-bos'ki-dē, -bos'i-dē). A family of winged and wingless flies (order Diptera) that are parasitic on birds and mammals; it includes the genera *Hippobosca* and *Melophagus.*

hippocampal (hip-ō-kam'păl). Relating to the hippocampus.

hippocampus (hip-ō-kam'pŭs) [G. *hippocampos,* seahorse] [NA] . Hippocampus major; the complex, internally convoluted structure that forms the medial margin ("hem") of the cortical mantle of the cerebral hemisphere, bordering the choroid fissure of the lateral ventricle, and composed of two gyri (Ammon's horn and the dentate gyrus), together with their white matter, the alveus and fimbria hippocampi. In monkeys, apes, and man the h. is confined to the temporal lobe by the massive development of the corpus callosum. Cytoarchitecturally a unique form of allocortex (archicortex), the h. forms part of the limbic system (formerly rhinencephalon). Its major afferent connections are with the entorhinal area of the parahippocampal gyrus, and septum pellucidum; by way of the fornix it projects to the septum, anterior nucleus of the thalamus, and mamillary body.

h. ma'jor, hippocampus.

h. mi'nor, *calcar* avis.

Hippocrates of Cos. Greek physician, called the "Father of Medicine," circa 460–377 B.C. See hippocratic *facies, fingers, nails, school, succussion.*

hippocratic (hip-ŏ-krat'ik). Relating to, described by, or attributed to Hippocrates.

Hippocratic Oath. An oath demanded of the physician about to enter upon the practice of his profession, the composition of which, though usually attributed to Hippocrates of Cos, is probably an ancient oath of the Aesclepiads. It appears in a book of the hippocratic collection as follows:

"I swear by Apollo the physician, by Aesculapius, Hygeia, and Panacea, and I take to witness all the gods, all the goddesses, to keep according to my ability and my judgment the following Oath:

"To consider dear to me as my parents him who taught me this art; to live in common with him and if necessary to share my goods with him; to look upon his children as my own brothers, to teach them this art if they so desire without fee or written promise; to impart to my sons and the sons of the master who taught me and the disciples who have enrolled themselves and have agreed to the rules of the profession, but to these alone, the precepts and the instruction. I will prescribe regimen for the good of my patients according to my ability and my judgment and never do harm to anyone. To please no one will I prescribe a deadly drug, nor give advice which may cause his death. Nor will I give a woman a pessary to procure abortion. But I will preserve the purity of my life and my art. I will not cut for stone, even for patients in whom the disease is manifest; I will leave this operation to be performed by practitioners (specialists in this art). In every house where I come I will enter only for the good of my patients, keeping myself far from all intentional ill-doing and all seduction, and especially from the pleasures of love with women or with men, be they free or slaves. All that may come to my knowledge in the exercise of my profession or outside of my profession or in daily commerce with men, which ought not to be spread abroad, I will keep secret and will never reveal. If I keep this oath faithfully, may I enjoy my life and practice my art, respected by all men and in all times; but if I swerve from it or violate it, may the reverse be my lot."

hippocratism (hi-pok'ră-tizm). A system of medicine, attributed to Hippocrates and his disciples, based on the imitation of nature's processes in the therapeutic management of disease.

hippurate (hip'yū-rāt). A salt or ester of hippuric acid.

hippuria (hi-pyū'rē-ă). The excretion of an abnormally large amount of hippuric acid in the urine.

hippuric acid (hi-pyūr'ik). *N*-Benzoylglycine; a detoxification and excretory product of benzoic acid found in the urine of man and many herbivorous animals; used therapeutically in the form of its salts (hippurates of calcium and ammonium).

hippuricase (hi-pyūr'i-cās). Aminoacylase.

hippus (hip'ŭs) [G. *hippos,* horse, from a fancied suggestion of galloping movements]. Spasmodic, rhythmical pupillary dilation and constriction, independent of illumination, convergence, or psychic stimuli.

respiratory h., dilation of the pupils occurring during inspiration, and contraction during expiration.

hirci (her'sī). Plural of hircus.

hircismus (her-siz'mŭs) [L. *hircus,* goat]. Offensive odor of the axillae.

hircus, gen. and pl. **hirci** (her'kŭs, her'sī) [L. he-goat]. **1.** The odor of the axillae. **2** [NA]. One of the hairs growing in the axillae. **3.** Tragus (1).

Hirschberg, Julius, German ophthalmologist, 1843–1925. See H.'s *method.*

Hirschfeld, Isador, U.S. dentist, 1881–1965. See H.'s *canals.*

Hirschowitz syndrome. See under syndrome.

Hirsch-Peiffer stain. See under *stain.*

Hirschsprung, Harald, Danish physician, 1830–1916. See H.'s *disease.*

hirsute (her-sūt') [L. *hirsutus,* shaggy]. Relating to or characterized by hirsutism.

hirsuties (her-su'tē-ēz) [Mod. L. fr. L. *hirsutus,* shaggy]. Hirsutism.

hirsutism (her'sū-tizm) [L. *hirsutus,* shaggy]. Hirsuties; pilosis; presence of excessive bodily and facial hair, in a male pattern, especially in women; may be present in normal adults as an expression of an ethnic characteristic or may develop in children or adults as the result of a metabolic disorder, usually endocrine in nature.

Apert's h., h. caused by a virilizing disorder of adrenocortical origin.

constitutional h., mild to moderate degree of h. present in an individual exhibiting otherwise normal endocrine and reproductive function; it appears to be a heritable form of h. and commonly is an expression of an ethnic characteristic.

idiopathic h., h. of uncertain origin in women, who may additionally exhibit menstrual abnormalities and sterility; may reflect hypersecretion of adrenocortical androgens.

hirtellous (hĭr'tĕ-lŭs) [L. *hirtus,* hairy, shaggy]. Having or resembling fine hairs; term describing the filamentous protein polysaccharide coating of microvilli. See glycocalyx.

hirudicide (hi-rū'di-sīd) [L. *hirudo,* leech, + *caedo,* to kill]. An agent that kills leeches.

hirudin (hir'yū-din) [L. *hirudo,* leech]. An antithrombin substance extracted from the salivary glands of the leech that has the property of preventing coagulation of the blood.

Hirudinea (hir'ū-din'ē-ă) [L. *hirudo,* leech]. The leeches, a class of worms (phylum Annelida) with flat, segmented bodies, a sucker at the posterior end, and often a smaller sucker at the anterior end; they are predatory on invertebrate tissues, or feed on blood and tissue exudates of vertebrates.

hirudiniasis (hi-rū-di-nī'ă-sis) [L. *hirudo,* leech, + G. *-iasis,* condition]. A condition resulting from leeches attaching themselves to the skin or being taken into the mouth or nose while drinking.

Hirudo (hi-rū'dō) [L. leech]. A genus of leeches (class Hirudinea, family Gnathobdellidae). Species previously used in medicine are: *H. australis,* Australian leech; *H. decora,* American leech; *H. interrupta* or *H. troctina,* a leech of northern Africa; *H. medicinalis,* speckled, Swedish, or German leech, the species previously in most general use; *H. m. officinalis,* a variety of the preceding; *H. provincialis,* the green or Hungarian leech; *H. quinquestriata,* five-striped leech.

His, His-, -His Symbols for histidine, histidyl, and histidino respectively.

His, Wilhelm, Sr., Swiss anatomist and embryologist in Germany, 1831–1904. See H.'s *copula, line, rule;* H.'s perivascular *space; isthmus* of His.

His, Wilhelm, Jr., German physician, 1863–1934. See H.'s *band, bundle, spindle;* Kent-H. *bundle;* H.-Tawara *system.*

Hiss, Philip H., U.S. bacteriologist, 1868–1913. See H.'s *stain.*

histaminase (his-tam'i-nās). *Amine* oxidase (copper-containing).

histamine (his'tă-mēn). 2-(4-Imidazolyl)ethylamine; a depressor amine derived from histidine by histidine decarboxylase and present in ergot and in animal tissues. It is a powerful stimulant of gastric secretion, a constrictor of bronchial smooth muscle and a vasodilator (capillaries and arterioles) that causes a fall in blood pressure. H., or a substance indistinguishable in action from it, is liberated in the skin as a result of injury. When pricked into the skin in high dilution, it causes the triple response.

h. phosphate, used in the treatment of certain allergies, cephalalgia, and acute multiple sclerosis with varying results; also used to test gastric secretory function, in the diagnosis of pheochromocytoma and in the treatment of Ménière's disease; also available as h. acid phosphate.

histamine-fast. Indicating the absence of the normal response to histamine, especially in speaking of true gastric anacidity.

histaminemia (his'tă-mi-nē'mē-ă) [histamine + G. *haima,* blood]. The presence of histamine in the circulating blood.

histaminuria (his'tă-mi-nū'rē-ă) [histidine + G. *ouron,* urine]. The excretion of histamine in the urine.

histangic (his-tan'jik). Histoangic.

histidase (his'ti-dās). *Histidine* ammonia-lyase.

histidinal (his'ti-din-ăl). The aldehyde analogue of histidine (–CHO replacing –COOH).

histidinase (his'ti-di-nās). *Histidine* ammonia-lyase.

histidine (His) (his'ti-dēn). α-Amino-β-(4-imidazolyl)propionic acid; a basic amino acid in proteins.

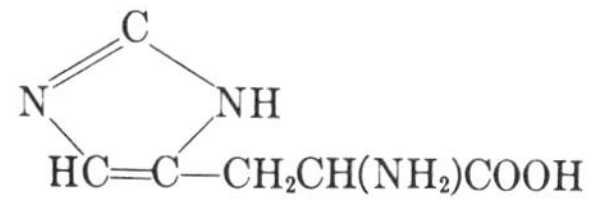

Histidine

h. ammonia-lyase [EC 4.3.1.3], histidase; histidinase; h. deaminase; an enzyme catalyzing deamination of histidine to urocanate.
h. deaminase, h. ammonia-lyase.
h. decarboxylase [EC 4.1.1.22], an enzyme catalyzing the decarboxylation of histidine to histamine.

histidinemia (his'ti-di-nē'mē-ă). Elevation of blood histidine level and excretion of histidine and related imidazole metabolites in urine due to deficiency of histidine transport protein; speech defects and mild mental retardation are associated conditions in about half of the patients, growth retardation occurs in some; autosomal recessive inheritance.

histidino (-His) (his'ti-din-ō). The radical of histidine produced by removal of a hydrogen from a nitrogen atom; prefixed by N^{α}, N^{τ}, or N^{π}.

histidinol (his'ti-di-nol). The alcohol analogue of histidine (–COOH becomes $-CH_2OH$).

histidinuria (his'ti-di-nū'rē-ă). Excretion of considerable amounts of histidine in the urine; frequently observed in later months of pregnancy, and in histidinemia.

histidyl (His-) (his'ti-dil). The acyl radical of histidine.

histio- [G. *histion,* web (tissue)]. Combining form relating to tissue.

histioblast (his'tē-ō-blast) [histio- + G. *blastos,* germ]. Histoblast; a tissue-forming cell.

histiocyte (his'tē-ō-sīt) [histio- + G. *kytos,* cell]. Histocyte; a macrophage present in connective tissue.
cardiac h., caterpillar cell; Anitschkow cell or myocyte; a large mononuclear cell found in connective tissue of the heart wall in inflammatory conditions, especially in the Aschoff body. The ovoid nucleus contains a central chromatin mass appearing as a wavy bar in longitudinal section.
sea-blue h., a h. containing cytoplasmic granules that stain bright blue with hematologic stains such as Wright-Giemsa; found in bone marrow and in the spleen, associated with hepatosplenomegaly and thrombocytopenic purpura and in other blood diseases.

histiocytoma (his'tē-ō-sī-tō'mă) [histio- + G. *kytos,* cell, + *-ōma,* tumor]. A tumor composed of histiocytes. See also dermatofibroma.
fibrous h., see dermatofibroma.
generalized eruptive h., nodular non-X histiocytosis; a rare recurring generalized eruption in adults of flesh colored or erythematous papules remaining localized to the skin and consisting of dermal nodules of mononuclear histiocytes that do not stain for lipid.
malignant fibrous h., a deeply situated tumor, especially on the extremities of adults, frequently recurring after surgery and metastasizing to the lungs; shows partial fibroblastic and histiocytic differentiation with a variable storiform pattern, myxoid areas, and giant cells.

histiocytosis (his'tē-ō-sī-tō'sis). Histocytosis; a generalized multiplication of histiocytes.
kerasin h., obsolete term for Gaucher's *disease.*
lipid h., h. with cytoplasmic accumulation of lipid, either phospholipid (Niemann-Pick disease) or glucocerebroside (Gaucher's disease).
malignant h., histiocytic medullary reticulosis; a rapidly fatal form of lymphoma, characterized by fever, jaundice, pancytopenia, and enlargement of the liver, spleen, and lymph nodes; the affected organs show focal necrosis and hemorrhage, with proliferation of histiocytes and phagocytosis of red blood cells.
nodular non-X h., generalized eruptive *histiocytoma.*
nonlipid h., Letterer-Siwe disease; an acute progressive generalized disease in young children, characterized by a purpuric rash, enlargement of lymph glands and spleen, and invasion of the spleen, liver, and bone marrow by Langerhans' cells.
regressing atypical h., a rare disease characterized clinically by multiple ulcerating cutaneous papules and nodules which show spontaneous regression; the skin is infiltrated by malignant-appearing histiocytes.
sinus h. with massive lymphadenopathy, a chronic disease occurring in children and characterized by massive painless cervical lymphadenopathy due to distension of the lymphatic sinuses by macrophages containing ingested lymphocytes, and by capsular and pericapsular fibrosis.
h. X, proliferation of Langerhans' cells of undetermined clinical type, possibly Hand-Schüller-Christian d., Letterer-Siwe disease, and eosinophilic granuloma.
h. Y, verrucous *xanthoma.*

histiogenic (his'tē-ō-jen'ik). Histogenous.

histioid (his'tē-oyd). Histoid.

histioma (his-tē-ō'mă). Histoma.

histionic (his-tē-on'ik). Relating to any tissue.

histo- [G. *histos,* web (tissue)]. Combining form denoting relationship to tissue.

histoangic (his-tō-an'jik) [histo- + G. *angeion,* vessel]. Histangic; relating to the structure of blood vessels, especially in terms of their function.

histoblast (his'tō-blast). Histioblast.

histochemistry (his'tō-kem'is-trē). Cytochemistry.

histocompatibility (his'tō-kom-pat-i-bil'i-tē). A state of immunologic similarity or identity of tissues sufficient to permit successful homograft transplantation; implies identity of histocompatibility genes in donor and recipient with respect to the particular tissue.

histocompatibility testing. A testing system for HLA antigens, of major importance in transplantation.

histocyte (his'tō-sīt). Histiocyte.

histocytosis (his'tō-sī-tō'sis). Histiocytosis.

histodifferentiation (his'tō-dif-er-en-shē-ā'shŭn). The morphologic appearance of tissue characteristics during development.

histofluorescence (his-tō-flūr-es'ens). Fluorescence of the tissues under exposure to ultraviolet rays following the injection of a fluorescent substance or as a result of a natural fluorescing substance.

histogenesis (his-tō-jen'ĕ-sis) [histo- + G. *genesis,* origin]. Histogeny; the origin of a tissue; the formation and development of the tissues of the body.

histogenetic (his-tō-jĕ-net'ik). Relating to histogenesis.

histogenous (his-toj'ĕ-nŭs) [histo- + G. *-gen,* producing]. Histiogenic; formed by the tissues; *e.g.,* the h. cells in an exudate arising from proliferation of the fixed tissue cells.

histogeny (his-toj'ĕ-nē). Histogenesis.

histogram (his'tō-gram) [histo- + G. *gramma,* a writing]. A graphic columnar or bar representation to compare the magnitudes of frequencies or numbers of items.

histoid (his'toyd) [histo- + G. *eidos,* resemblance]. Histioid. **1.** Resembling in structure one of the tissues of the body. **2.** Sometimes used with reference to the histologic structure of a neoplasm derived from and consisting of a single, relatively simple type of neoplastic tissue that closely resembles the normal, as in certain fibromas and leiomyomas.

histoincompatibility (his'tō-in'kom-pat-i-bil'i-tē). A state of immunologic dissimilarity of tissues sufficient to cause rejection of a homograft when tissue is transplanted from one individual to another; implies a difference in histocompatibility genes in donor and recipient.

histologic, histological (his-to-loj'ik, i-kăl). Pertaining to histology.

histologist (his-tol'ō-jist). Microanatomist; one who specializes in the science of histology.

histology (his-tol'ō-jē) [histo- + G. *logos,* study]. Microanatomy; the science concerned with the minute structure of cells, tissues, and organs in relation to their function. See microscopic *anatomy.*
pathologic h., histopathology.

histolysis (his-tol'i-sis) [histo- + G. *lysis,* dissolution]. Disintegration of tissue.

histoma (his-tō'mă) [histo- + G. *-oma,* tumor]. Histioma; a benign neoplasm in which the cytologic and histologic elements are closely similar to those of normal tissue from which the neoplastic cells are derived.

histometaplastic (his'tō-met-ă-plas'tik). Exciting tissue metaplasia.

Histomonas meleagridis (hi-stom'ō-nas me-lē-ag'ri-dis). *Amoeba meleagridis;* a protozoan flagellate (order Trichomonadida) parasitizing the intestine and liver of turkeys, chickens, and many other domestic and wild gallinaceous birds; it is nearly ubiquitous but rarely pathogenic in chickens; in the turkey, it causes histomoniasis. It is now considered to be in a family (Monocercomonadidae) that includes *Dientamoeba.*

histomoniasis (hi-stom'ō-nī'ă-sis). Blackhead (2); infectious enterohepatitis; a disease chiefly affecting turkeys, caused by *Histomonas meleagridis* and characterized by ulcerative and necrotic lesions of the liver and cecum, acute onset, and a high mortality rate. It is transmitted inside the eggs of the nematode *Heterakis gallinae,* which is primarily responsible for maintaining and spreading the infection.

histomorphometry (his'tō-mōr-fom'ĕ-trē) [histo- + G. *morphē,* shape, + *metron,* measure]. The quantitative measurement and characterization of microscopical images using a computer; manual or automated digital image analysis typically involves measurements and comparisons of selected geometric areas, perimeters, length angle of orientation, form factors, center of gravity coordinates, as well as image enhancement.

histone (his'tōn). One of a number of simple proteins that contains a high proportion of basic amino acids, are soluble in water, dilute acids, and alkalies, and are not coagulable by heat; *e.g.,* the proteins associated with nucleic acids in the nuclei of plant and animal tissues.

histonectomy (his-tō-nek'tō-mē) [histo- + G. *ektomē,* excision]. Periarterial *sympathectomy.*

histoneurology (his-tō-nū-rol'ō-jē). Neurohistology.

histonomy (his-ton'ō-mē) [histo- + G. *nomos,* law]. A law of the development and structure of the tissues of the body.

histonuria (his-tō-nū'rē-ă) [histone + G. *ouron,* urine]. The excretion of histone in the urine, as observed in certain instances of leukemia, febrile illnesses, and wasting diseases.

histopathogenesis (his'tō-path-ō-jen'ĕ-sis) [histogenesis + pathogenesis]. Abnormal embryonic development or growth of tissue.

histopathology (his'tō-pa-thol'ō-jē). Pathologic histology; the science or study dealing with the cytologic and histologic structure of abnormal or diseased tissue.

histophysiology (his'tō-fiz-ē-ol'ō-jē). The microscopic study of tissues in relation to their functions.

Histoplasma capsulatum (his-tō-plaz'mă kap-sū-lā'tŭm) [histo- + G. *plasma,* something formed]. A dimorphic fungus species of worldwide distribution that causes histoplasmosis in man and other mammals; its ascomycetous state is *Ajellomyces capsulatum.* The organism's natural habitat is soil fertilized with bird and bat droppings, where it grows as a mold, fragments of which, following inhalation, produce the primary pulmonary infection; within the mammalian host tissues, inhaled mycelial fragments grow as uninuclear yeasts that reproduce by budding. This parasitic form may also be induced in the laboratory by culturing the mycelial phase at 37°C on a blood-enriched medium; growth reverts to the mycelial form when the temperature is below 37°C. *H.c.* var. *duboisii* causes a clinically distinct disease, African histoplasmosis, in which large yeast cells with thicker walls are found in tissues, in contrast to the small yeast cells of *H.c.* var. *farciminosum,* which causes epizootic lymphangitis.

histoplasmin (his'tō-plas'min). An antigenic extract of *Histoplasma capsulatum,* used in immunological tests for the diagnosis of histoplasmosis; also used in skin test surveys of populations to determine the geographic distribution of the fungus and to predict those that are endemic for histoplasmosis.

histoplasmoma (his'tō-plaz-mō'mă). An infectious granuloma caused by *Histoplasma capsulatum.*

histoplasmosis (his'tō-plaz-mō'sis). Darling's disease; a widely distributed infectious disease caused by *Histoplasma capsulatum* and occurring frequently in epidemics; normally acquired and manifested by a inhalation of spores of the fungus in soil dust and manifested by a primary benign pneumonitis similar in clinical features to primary tuberculosis; occasionally, the primary disease progresses to produce localized lesions in lung, such as pulmonary cavitation, or the typical disseminated disease of the reticuloendothelial system which is manifested by fever, emaciation, splenomegaly, and leukopenia.
African h., a form of h. caused by *Histoplasma capsulatum* var. *duboisii,* observed only in tropical Africa; the organism grows chiefly in giant cells, causing lesions localized to skin, bone, or lacrimal glands, or is disseminated with multiple foci of osteomyelitis and visceral disorders; generalized forms produce lesions in lymph nodes, spleen, liver, bone, and lungs, although lung involvement is uncommon.
presumed ocular h., subretinal neovascularization in the macular region associated with chorioretinal atrophy and pigment proliferation adjacent to the optic disk, and peripheral chorioretinal atrophy ("histo-spots").

historadiography (his'tō-rā-dē-og'ră-fē). Roentgenography of tissue; refers specifically to microscopic sections of tissue.

historrhexis (his-tō-rek'sis) [histo- + G. *rhēxis,* rupture]. Breakdown of tissue by some agency other than infection.

histotome (his'tō-tōm) [histo- + G. *tomē,* cut]. Microtome.

histotomy (his-tot'ō-mē). Microtomy.

histotoxic (his-tō-tok'sik). Relating to poisoning of the respiratory enzyme system of the tissues.

histotroph (his'tō-trof). Embryotroph (1).

histotrophic (his-tō-trof'ik) [histo- + G. *trophē,* nourishment]. Providing nourishment for or favoring the formation of tissue.

histotropic (his-tō-trop'ik) [histo- + G. *tropikos,* turning]. Attracted toward the tissues; denoting certain parasites, stains, and chemical compounds.

histozoic (his-tō-zō'ik) [histo- + G. *zōikos,* relating to an animal]. Living in the tissues outside of a cell body; denoting certain parasitic protozoa.

histozyme (his'tō-zīm). Aminoacylase.

hitchhiker (hitch'hīk-er). A gene that has no selective advantage, or may even be harmful, but that nevertheless temporarily becomes widespread because it is closely linked and coupled with a highly advantageous gene that is strongly selected.

Hitzig. Eduard, German psychiatrist, 1838–1907. See H.'s *girdle.*

HIV Abbreviation for human immunodeficiency *virus.*

hives (hīvz). Urticaria.
giant h., angioneurotic *edema.*

Hjärre, A., German pathologist, 1897–1958. See H.'s *disease.*

Hl Abbreviation for latent *hyperopia.*

HLA Abbreviation for human lymphocyte *antigens.*

Hm Abbreviation for manifest *hyperopia.*

HMG Abbreviation for human menopausal *gonadotropin.*

HMO Abbreviation for hypothetical mean *organism;* Health Maintenance Organization.

HMS Abbreviation for hypothetical mean *strain.*

HN2 Symbol for nitrogen mustard.

Ho Symbol for holmium.

hoarse (hōrs) [A.S. *hās*]. Having a rough, harsh voice.

hoarseness (hōrs'nes). An unnaturally deep and harsh quality of the voice.

Hoboken, Nicholas van, Dutch anatomist and physician, 1632–1678. See H.'s *gemmules, nodules, valves.*

Hoche, Alfred E., German psychiatrist, 1865–1943. See H.'s *bundle, tract.*

hock (hok). The tarsus in the horse and other quadrupeds; the joint of the hind limb between the stifle and the fetlock; corresponds to the ankle in man.
capped h., calcaneal *bursitis.*
curby h., curb.

Hodge, Hugh L., U.S. gynecologist, 1796–1873. See H.'s *forceps, pessary.*

Hodgen, John T., U.S. surgeon, 1826–1882. See H. *splint.*

Hodgkin, Alan L., British physiologist and Nobel laureate, *1914. See Goldman-H.-Katz *equation.*

Hodgkin, Thomas, British physician, 1798–1866. See H.'s *disease.*

Hodgkin-Key murmur. See under murmur.

Hodgson, Joseph, British physician, 1788–1869. See H.'s *disease.*

hodoneuromere (hō-dō-nū'rō-mēr) [G. *hodos,* path, + *neuron,* nerve, + *meros,* part]. In embryology, obsolete term for a metameric segment of the neural tube with its pair of nerves and their branches.

hodophobia (hō-dō-fō'bē-ă) [G. *hodos,* path, + *phobos,* fear]. Morbid fear of traveling.

HOECHST 33258. A bisbenzimidazole dye employed in cytochemistry and fluorescence microscopy as a sensitive indicator of DNA in chromosomes, specifically constitutive heterochromatin.

Hoeppli, Reinhard J.C., German parantologist, *1893. See Splendore-H. *phenomenon.*

hof (hōf) [Ger. court]. The hollow in the cytoplasm of a cell that lodges the nucleus.

Hofbauer, J. Isfred I., U.S. gynecologist, 1878–1961. See H. *cell.*

Hoffa, Albert, German surgeon, 1859–1908. See H.'s *operation.*

Hoffman. See Frei-H. *reaction.*

Hoffmann, Johann, German neurologist, 1857–1919. See H.'s muscular *atrophy, phenomenon, reflex, sign;* Werdnig-H. *disease.*

Hoffmann, Moritz, German anatomist, 1622–1698. See H.'s *duct.*

Hofmann (Hofmann-Wellenhof), Georg von, Austrian bacteriologist, 1843–1890. See H.'s *bacillus.*

Hofmeister, Franz, German biochemist, 1850–1922. See H. *series.*

Hofmeister, Franz von, German surgeon, 1867–1926. See H.'s *operation;* H.-Pólya *anastomosis.*

Hoglund's sign. See under sign.

Hogness, D.S., U.S. molecular biologist, *1925. See H. *assay, box.*

holandric (hol-an'drik) [G. *holos,* entire, + *aner,* man]. Related to genes located on the Y chromosome.

holarthritic (hol-ar-thrit'ik). Relating to holarthritis.

holarthritis (hol-ar-thrī'tis) [G. *holos,* entire, + *arthron,* joint, + *-itis,* inflammation]. Inflammation of all or a great number of the joints.

Holden, Luther, British anatomist, 1815–1905. See H.'s *line.*

Holder. See Virchow-H. *angle.*

hole of retina. A break in the continuity of the sensory retina, permitting separation between the stratum pigmenti retinae and the stratum cerebrale retinae.

holism (hō'lizm) [G. *holos,* entire]. The approach to the study of a psychological phenomenon through the analysis of a phenomenon as a complete entity in itself. *Cf.* atomism.

holistic (hō-lis'tik). Pertaining to the characteristics of holism or h. psychologies.

Holl, Mortiz, Austrian surgeon, 1852–1920. See H.'s *ligament.*

Hollander, Franklin, U.S. physiologist, *1899. See H.'s *test.*

Hollenhorst, Robert W., U.S. ophthalmologist, *1913. See H. *plaques.*

hollow (hol'ō). A concavity or depression.
Sebileau's h., depression between the inferior aspect of the tongue and the sublingual glands.

Holmes, Sir Gordon M., British neurologist, 1876–1965. See H.-Adie *pupil, syndrome;* Stewart-H. *sign.*

Holmes, Thomas H., U.S. psychiatrist, *1918. See H.-Rahe *questionnaire.*

Holmes, W. See H.'s *stain.*

Holmgren, Alarik F., Swedish physiologist, 1831–1897. See H. *method;* H.'s *test.*

Holmgren, Emil A., Swedish histologist, 1866–1922. See H.-Golgi *canals.*

holmium (hol'mē-ŭm) [G.E.A. *Holm,* Swedish geologist, 1891–1927]. An element of the lanthanide group, symbol Ho, atomic no. 67, atomic weight 164.94.

holo- [G. *holos,* whole, entire, complete]. Combining form denoting entirety or relationship to a whole.

holoacardius (hol'ō-ă-kar'dē-ŭs) [holo- + G. *a-* priv. + *kardia,* heart]. A separate, grossly defective twin lacking a heart of its own, its blood supply being dependent on a shunt from the placental circulation of a more nearly normal twin; a placental parasitic twin or omphalosite. *Cf.* acardius.
h. aceph'alus, a h. also lacking a head.
h. amor'phus, a h. in which the body of the parasite is represented by only a shapeless mass.

holo-ACP synthase [EC 2.7.8.7]. An enzyme catalyzing transfer of 4'-phosphopantetheinyl residue from CoA to a serine of apo-ACP to form holo-ACP, releasing adenosine 3',5'-bisphosphate.

holoacrania (hol'ō-ă-krā'nē-ă) [holo- + G. *a-* priv. + *kranion,* skull]. A congenital skull defect in which bones of the vault are absent.

holoanencephaly (hol'ō-an-en-sef'ă-lē) [holo- + G. *an-* priv. + *enkephalos,* brain]. Complete absence of cranium and brain.

holoblastic (hol-ō-blas'tik) [holo- + G. *blastos,* germ]. Denoting the involvement of the entire (isolecithal or moderately telolecithal) ovum in cleavage.

holocephalic (hol'ō-sĕ-fal'ik) [holo- + G. *kephalē,* head]. Denoting a fetus with a complete head but having deficiencies in other body parts.

holocord (hol'ō-kōrd). Relating to the entire spinal cord, extending from the cervico-medullary junction to the conus medullaris.

holocrine (hol'ō-krin) [holo- + G. *krinō,* to separate]. See holocrine *gland.*

holodiastolic (hol'ō-dī-ă-stol'ik). Relating to or occupying the entire diastole.

holoendemic (hol'ō-en-dem'ik). Endemic in the entire population, as trachoma in the villages of Saudi Arabia.

holoenzyme (hol-ō-en'zīm). A complete enzyme, *i.e.,* apoenzyme plus coenzyme.

hologastroschisis (hol'ō-gas-tros'ki-sis) [holo- + G. *gastēr,* belly, + *schisis,* cleaving]. A congenital malformation in which a cleft extends the entire length of the abdomen.

hologram (hol'ō-gram) [holo- + G. *gramma,* something written]. A three-dimensional image.

hologynic (hol-ō-jin'ik) [holo- + G. *gynē,* woman]. Related to sex-limited characters manifest only in females.

holomastigote (hol-ō-mas'ti-gōt) [holo- + G. *mastix,* whip]. Possessing flagella over the entire surface.

holometabolous (hol'ō-me-tab'ō-lŭs) [holo- + G. *metabolē,* change]. Pertaining to a member of the Holometabola, a series of insect orders in which complex or complete metamorphosis is found.

holomorphosis (hol'ō-mōr-fō'sis) [holo- + G. *morphosis,* shaping]. Attainment or reestablishment of physical wholeness.

holophytic (hol-ō-fit'ik) [holo- + G. *phyton,* plant]. Having a plant-like mode of obtaining nourishment; denoting certain photosynthesizing protozoans, *e.g., Euglena.*

holoprosencephaly (hol'ō-pros-en-sef'ă-lē) [holo- + G. *prosō,* forward, + *enkephalos,* brain]. Failure of the forebrain to divide into hemispheres or lobes.

holorachischisis (hol'ō-rā-kis'ki-sis) [holo- + G. *rhachis,* spine, + *schisis,* fissure]. Araphia; rachischisis totalis; spina bifida of the entire spinal column.

holosystolic (hol'ō-sis-tol'ik). Pansystolic.

holotelencephaly (hol'ō-tel-en-sef'ă-lē) [holo- + telencephalon]. Congenital absence of one cerebral ventricle with no separation of the cerebral hemispheres; associated with arrhinencephaly.

holotrichous (ho-lot'ri-kŭs) [holo- + G. *thrix,* hair]. Possessing cilia over the entire surface.

holozoic (hol-ō-zō'ik) [holo- + G. *zōon,* animal]. Animal-like in mode of obtaining nourishment, lacking photosynthetic capacity; denoting certain protozoans, in distinction to others that are holophytic.

Holt, M. See H.-Oram *syndrome.*

Holter, Norman, U.S. biophysicist, 1914–1983. See H. *monitor.*

Holter monitor. See under monitor.

Holth, Sören, Norwegian ophthalmologist, 1863–1937. See H.'s *operation.*

Holthouse, Carsten, British surgeon, 1810–1901. See H.'s *hernia.*

Holzknecht, Guido, Austrian radiologist, 1872–1931. See H. *unit.*

homalocephalous (hom'ă-lō-sef'ă-lŭs) [G. *homalos,* level, + *kephalē,* head]. Having a flattened head.

Homalomyia (hom'ă-lō-mī'yă) [G. *homalos,* even, + *myia,* a fly]. A genus of flies the larvae of which sometimes infect human or animal intestines.

homaluria (hom-ă-lū'rē-ă) [G. *homalos,* level, + *ouron,* urine]. Rarely used term for normal urine flow.

Homans, John, U.S. surgeon, 1877–1954. See H.'s *sign.*

homatropine (hō-mat'rō-pēn). Tropine mandelate; mandelytropine; an anticholinergic, mydriatic, and cycloplegic agent; available as the hydrobromide and the methylbromide.

homaxial (hō-mak'sē-ăl) [G. *homos,* the same, + axis]. Having all the axes alike, as a sphere.

Home, Sir Everard, British surgeon, 1756–1832. See H.'s *lobe.*

homeo- [G. *homoios,* like]. Combining form meaning the same, or alike. See also homo-(1).

homeocyte (hō'mē-ō-sīt) [homeo- + G. *kytes,* cell]. Obsolete term for a lymphocyte.

homeometric (hō'mē-ō-met'rik) [homeo- + G. *metron,* measure]. Without change in size.

homeomorphous (hō'mē-ō-mōr'fŭs) [homeo- + G. *morphē,* shape]. Of similar shape, but not necessarily of the same composition.

homeopath (hō'mē-ō-path). Homeopathist.

homeopathic (hō'mē-ō-path'ik). **1.** Homeotherapeutic (1); relating to homeopathy. **2.** Denoting an extremely small dose of a pharmacological agent, such as might be used in homeopathy; more generally, a dose believed to be too small to produce the effect usually expected from that agent. *Cf.* pharmacologic (2), physiologic (4), supraphysiologic.

homeopathist (hō-mē-op'ă-thist). Homeopath; a medical practitioner of homeopathy.

homeopathy (hō-mē-op'ă-thē) [homeo- + G. *pathos,* suffering]. A system of therapy developed by Samuel Hahnemann based on the "law of similia," from the aphorism, *similia similibus curantur* (likes are cured by likes), which holds that a medicinal substance that can evoke certain symptoms in healthy individuals may be effective in the treatment of illnesses having symptoms closely resembling those produced by the substance.

homeoplasia (hō'mē-ō-plā'zē-ă) [homeo- + G. *plasis,* a molding]. Homoioplasia; the formation of new tissue of the same character as that already existing in the part.

homeoplastic (hō'mē-ō-plas'tik). Relating to or characterized by homeoplasia.

homeorrhesis (hō'mē-ō-rē'sis) [homeo- + G. *rheos,* stream, current]. Ontogenic or waddington homeostasis; the set of processes by which imbalances and other defects in ontogeny are corrected before development is completed.

homeosis (hō-mē-ō'sis) [homeo- + G. *-osis,* condition]. Formation of a body part having characteristics normally found in a related or homologous part at another location in the body.

homeostasis (hō'mē-ō-stā'sis, -os'tă-sis) [homeo- + G. *stasis,* a standing]. **1.** The state of equilibrium (balance between opposing pressures) in the body with respect to various functions and to the chemical compositions of the fluids and tissues. **2.** The processes through which such bodily equilibrium is maintained.

Bernard-Cannon h., physiological h.; the set of mechanisms responsible for the cybernetic adjustment of physiological and biochemical states in postnatal life.

genetic h., Lerner h.

Lerner h., genetic h.; the restorative mechanisms that tend to correct perturbations in the genetic composition of a population.

ontogenic h., homeorrhesis.

physiological h., Bernard-Cannon h.

waddingtonian h. [C.H. *Waddington,* British embryologist and geneticist, 1905–1975], homeorrhesis.

homeostatic (hō'mē-ō-stat'ik). Relating to homeostasis.

homeotherapeutic (hō'mē-ō-thār-ă-pyū'tik). **1.** Homeopathic (1). **2.** Relating to homeotherapy.

homeotherapy, homeotherapeutics (hō'mē-ō-thār'ă-pē, -thār-ă-pyū'tiks). Treatment or prevention of a disease utilizing the principles of homeopathy.

homeotherm (hō'mē-ō-therm) [homeo- + G. *thermos,* warm]. Warm-blooded animal; hematherm; any of the animals, including mammals and birds, that tend to maintain a constant body temperature.

homeothermal (hō′mē-ō-ther′măl). Homeothermic.

homeothermic (hō′mē-ō-ther′mik). Hemathermal; hemathermous; hematothermal; homeothermal; homoiothermal; homothermal; warm-blooded; pertaining to, or having the essential characteristic of, homeotherms. *Cf.* poikilothermic, heterothermic.

homeotic (hō-mē-ot′ik). Pertaining to or characterized by homeosis.

homeotypical (hō′mē-ō-tip′i-kăl). Of or resembling the usual type.

homergy (hom′er-jē) [G. *homos,* same, + *ergon,* work]. Obsolete term for normal metabolism and its results.

homicidal (hom-i-sī′dăl). Having a tendency toward homicide.

homicide (hom′i-sīd) [L. *homo,* man, + *caedo,* to kill]. The killing of one human being by another.

homidium bromide (hō-mid′ē-ŭm). Ethidium; a trypanocide used in veterinary medicine.

Hominidae (hō-min′i-dē). The Primate family which includes modern man (*Homo sapiens*) and several groups of fossil men.

Hominoidea (hom-i-noy′dē-ă) [L. *homo* (*homin-*), man, + G. *eidos,* form]. A superfamily of the Primates including the anthropoid apes and man. Divided into the families Pongidae (anthropoid apes) and Hominidae (man).

Homo (hō′mō) [L. man]. The genus of Primates that includes man. **H. sa′piens** [L. wise man], modern man.

homo- [G. *homos,* the same]. **1.** Combining form meaning the same or alike. See also homeo-. **2.** In chemistry, prefix used to indicate insertion of one more carbon atom in a chain.

homobiotin (hō-mō-bī′ō-tin). A compound resembling biotin except for the substitution of an oxygen atom for the sulfur and the presence of an additional CH_2 group in the side chain; an active biotin antagonist.

homoblastic (hō-mō-blas′tik) [homo- + G. *blastos,* germ]. Developing from a single type of tissue.

homocarnosine (hō-mō-kar′nō-sēn). *N*[2]-(4-Aminobutyryl)histidine; a constituent of the brain formed from histidine and γ-aminobutyric acid.

homocentric (hō′mō-sen′trik). Having the same center; denoting rays that meet at a common focus. *Cf.* heterocentric (1).

homochlorcyclizine (hō′mō-klōr-sī′kli-zēn). 1-[(4-Chlorophenyl)-phenylmethyl]hexahydro-4-methyl-1*H*-1,4-diazepine; an antihistaminic with antiserotonin properties.

homochronous (hō-mŏk′rō-nŭs) [homo- + G. *chronos,* time]. **1.** Synchronous. **2.** Occurring at the same age in each generation.

homocladic (hō-mō-klad′ik) [homo- + G. *klados,* a branch]. Denoting an anastomosis between branches of the same arterial trunk, as distinguished from heterocladic.

homocysteine (hō-mō-sis′tē-ēn). $HSCH_2CH_2CHNH_2COOH$; a homologue of cysteine, produced by the demethylation of methionine, and an intermediate in the biosynthesis of cysteine from methionine via cystathionine.

homocystine (hō-mō-sis′tēn). The disulfide resulting from the mild oxidation of homocysteine; an analogue of cystine.

homocystinemia (hō′mō-sis-ti-nē′mē-ă). Presence of an excess of homocystine in the plasma, as in homocystinuria.

homocystinuria (hō′mō-sis-ti-nū′rē-ă). A disorder characterized by excretion of homocystine in urine, mental retardation, ectopia lentis, sparse blond hair, genu valgum, convulsive tendency, failure to thrive, thromboembolic episodes, and fatty changes of liver; associated with defective formation of cystathionine synthetase; autosomal recessive inheritance.

homocytotropic (hō′mō-sī′tō-trop′ik) [homo- + G. *kytos,* cell, + *tropē,* a turning toward]. Having an affinity for cells of the same or a closely related species.

homodont (hō′mō-dont) [homo- + G. *odous,* tooth]. Having teeth all alike in form, as those of the lower vertebrates, in contrast to heterodont.

homodromous (hō-mod′rō-mŭs) [homo- + G. *dromos,* running]. Moving in the same direction.

homoeo-. See homeo-.

homoerotism, homoeroticism (hō-mō-er′ō-tizm, -ĕ-rot′i-sizm) [homo- + G. *erōs,* love]. Homosexuality.

homogametic (hō′mō-gă-met′ik) [homo- + G. *gametikos,* connubial]. Monogametic; producing only one type of gamete with respect to sex chromosomes; in man and most animals, the female is h.

homogamy (hō-mog′ă-mē) [homo- + G. *gamos,* marriage]. Similarity of husband and wife in a specific trait.

homogenate (hŏ-moj′ĕ-nāt). Tissue ground into a creamy consistency in which the cell structure is disintegrated (so-called "cell-free"). *Cf.* brei.

homogeneous (hō-mō-jē′nē-ŭs) [homo- + G. *genos,* race]. Of uniform structure or composition throughout.

homogenesis (hō-mō-jen′ĕ-sis) [homo- + G. *genesis,* production]. Homogeny; production of offspring similar to the parents, in contrast to heterogenesis.

homogenization (hŏ-moj′ĕ-ni-zā′shŭn). The process by which a material is made homogeneous.

homogenize (hŏ-moj′ĕ-nīz). To make homogeneous.

homogenous (hŏ-moj′ĕ-nŭs) [homo- + G. *genos,* family, kind]. Having a structural similarity because of descent from a common ancestor.

homogentisate 1,2-dioxygenase (hō-mō-jen′tis-āt) [EC 1.13.11.5]. Homogentisicase; homogentisic acid oxidase; an iron-containing enzyme that catalyzes the oxidative cleavage of the benzene ring by O_2 in homogentisic acid, forming 4-maleylacetoacetic acid.

homogentisic acid (hō′mō-jen-tis′ik). Alcapton; alkapton; glycosuric acid; (2,5-dihydroxyphenyl)acetic acid; an intermediate in phenylalanine and tyrosine catabolism; if made alkaline, it oxidizes rapidly in air to a quinone that polymerizes to a melanin-like material.
h. a. oxidase, homogentisate 1,2-dioxygenase.

homogentisicase (hō′mō-jen-tis′i-kās). Homogentisate 1,2-dioxygenase.

homogentisuria (hō′mō-jen-ti-sū′rē-ă). Alkaptonuria.

homogeny (hō-moj′ĕ-ne). Homogenesis.

homograft (hō′mō-graft). Allograft.

homoioplasia (hō′moy-ō-plā′zē-ă). Homeoplasia.

homoiothermal (hō-moy-ō-ther′măl). Homeothermic.

homokaryon (hō-mō-kar′ē-on) [homo- + G. *karyon,* kernel, nut]. Genetically identical nuclei in a common cytoplasm, usually resulting from fusion of two cells from the same species.

homokaryotic (hō′mō-kar-ē-ot′ik). Exhibiting the properties of a homokaryon.

homokeratoplasty (hō′mō-ker′ă-tō-plas-tē). Corneal transplant between members of the same species.

homolateral (hō-mō-lat′er-ăl) [homo- + L. *latus,* side]. Ipsilateral.

homolipids (hō-mō-lip′idz). Simple lipids; lipids containing only C, H, and O. *Cf.* heterolipids.

homologous (hŏ-mol′ō-gŭs) [see homologue]. Corresponding or alike in certain critical attributes. **1.** In biology or zoology, denoting organs or parts corresponding in evolutionary origin and similar to some extent in structure, but not necessarily similar in function. **2.** In chemistry, denoting a single chemical series, differing by fixed increments. **3.** In genetics, denoting chromosomes or chromosome parts identical with respect to their genetic loci. **4.** In immunology, denoting serum or tissue derived from members of a single species, or an antibody with respect to the antigen that produced it.

homologue (hom'ō-log) [homo- + G. *logos,* word, ratio, relation]. A member of a homologous pair or series.

homology (hŏ-mol'ō-jē). The state of being homologous.
h. of chains, h. of strands; the degree of similarity between the base sequences of strands of two DNAs.
DNA h., the degree (or percentage) of hybridization capable between the DNA of different microorganisms.
h. of strands, h. of chains.

homolysin (hō-mol'i-sin). A sensitizing hemolytic antibody (hemolysin) formed as the result of stimulation by an antigen derived from an animal of the same species.

homolysis (hō-mol'i-sis). Lysis of red blood cells by a homolysin and complement.

homomorphic (hō-mō-mōr'fik) [homo- + G. *morphē,* shape, appearance]. Denoting two or more structures of similar size and shape.

homonomous (hō-mon'ō-mŭs) [G. *homonemos,* under the same laws, fr. *homos,* same, + *nomos,* law]. Denoting parts, having similar form and structure, arranged in a series, as the fingers or toes.

homonomy (hō-mon'ō-mē). The condition of being homonomous.

homonuclear (hō-mō-nū'klē-er). Denoting a cell line that still has the original chromosome complement.

homonymous (hō-mon'i-mŭs) [G. *homōnymous,* of the same name, fr. *onyma,* name]. Having the same name or expressed in the same terms, *e.g.,* the corresponding halves (right or left, superior or inferior) of the retinas.

homophenes (hō'mō-fēnz). Words in which the visible organs of speech behave the same, *e.g.,* tug, tongue, tuck.

homophil (hō'mō-fil) [homo- + G. *philos,* fond]. Denoting an antibody that reacts only with the specific antigen which induced its formation.

homoplastic (hō-mō-plas'tik) [homo- + G. *plastos,* formed]. Similar in form and structure, but not in origin.

homoplasty (hō'mō-plas'-tē). Repair of a defect by a homograft.

homopolymer (hō-mō-pol'i-mer). A polymer composed of a series of identical radicals; *e.g.,* polylysine, poly(adenylic acid), polyglucose.

homoproline (hō-mō-prō'lēn). Pipecolic acid.

homoprotocatechuic acid (hō'mō-prō'tō-kat-ĕ-chū'ik). (3,4-Dihydroxyphenyl)acetic acid; an isomer of homogentisic acid found in urine; a degradation product of tyrosine, dopa, and hydroxytyramine.

homorganic (hom-ōr-gan'ik). Produced by the same organs, or by homologous organs.

homosalate (hō-mō-sal'āt). 3,3,5-Trimethylcyclohexyl salicylate; an ultraviolet screening agent for topical application to the skin.

homoserine (hō-mō-ser'ēn). 2-Amino-4-hydroxybutyric acid; $HOCH_2CH_2CH(NH_2)COOH$; a hydroxyamino acid differing from serine in the possession of an additional CH_2 group; formed in the conversion of methionine to cysteine.
h. deaminase, cystathionine γ-lyase.
h. dehydratase, cystathionine γ-lyase.

homosexual (hō-mō-sek'shū-ăl). **1.** Relating to or characteristic of homosexuality. **2.** One whose interests and behavior are characteristic of homosexuality.

homosexuality (hō'mō-sek-shū-al'i-tē). Homoeroticism; homoerotism; erotic attraction, predisposition, or activity, including sexual congress, between individuals of the same sex, especially past puberty.
ego-dystonic h., a psychological or psychiatric disorder in which an individual experiences persistent distress associated with same-sex preference and a strong need to change the behavior or, at least, to alleviate the distress associated with the h.
latent h., unconscious h.; an erotic inclination toward members of the same sex not consciously experienced or expressed in overt action, as opposed to overt h. Use of this term is disappearing because of both its potentially iatrogenic effect and the inability to validate the phenomenon by techniques outside of psychoanalytic theory.
overt h., homosexual inclinations consciously experienced and expressed in actual homosexual behavior.
unconscious h., latent h.

D-homosteroid (hō-mō-stēr'oyd). A steroid in which the D ring is made up of six carbon atoms instead of the usual five.

4-homosulfanilamide hydrochloride (hō'mō-sŭl-fă-nil'ă-mīd). Mafenide.

homothallic (hō-mō-thal'ik) [homo- + G. *thallos,* a young shoot]. In fungi, denoting a kind of sexual reproduction in which a nucleus of a thallus is capable of fusing with another nucleus from the same thallus or mating type. *Cf.* heterothallic.

homothermal (hō-mō-ther'măl) [homo- + G. *thermē,* heat]. Homeothermic.

homotonic (hō-mō-ton'ik). Of uniform tension or tonus.

homotopic (hō-mō-top'ik) [homo- + G. *topos,* place]. Pertaining to or occurring at the same place or part of the body.

homotransplantation (hō'mō-tranz-plan-tā'shŭn). Allotransplantation.

homotype (hō'mō-tīp) [homo- + G. *typos,* type]. Any part or organ of the same structure or function as another, especially as one on the opposite side of the body.

homotypic, homotypical (hō-mō-tip'ik, i-kăl). Of the same type or form; corresponding to the other one of two paired organs or parts.

homovanillic acid (hō'mō-vă-nil'ik). A phenol found in human urine; produced through the methylation of homoprotocatechuic acid on the meta-OH group.

homozoic (hō-mō-zō'ik) [homo- + G. *zōikos,* relating to an animal]. Relating to the same animal or the same species of animal.

homozygosity, homozygosis (hō'mō-zī-gos'i-tē, -zī-gō'sis) [homo- + G. *zygon,* yoke]. The state of being homozygous.

homozygote (hō-mō-zī'gōt) [homo- + G. *zygōtos,* yoke]. A homozygous individual.

homozygous (hō-mō-zī'gŭs). Having identical genes at one or more paired loci in homologous chromosomes.

homozygous by descent. Possessing two genes at a given locus which are descended from a single source, as may occur in consanguineous mating.

homunculus (hō-mŭngk'yū-lŭs) [L. dim. of *homo,* man]. **1.** An exceedingly minute body which, according to the views of development held by medical scientists of the 16th and 17th centuries, was contained in a sex cell. From this preformed but infinitely small structure the human body was supposed to be developed. See also preformation *theory.* **2.** The figure of a human sometimes superimposed on pictures of the surface of the brain to represent the motor or sensory regions of the body represented there.

Honduras bark (hon-dū'răs). Cascara amara.

honey (hŏn'ē) [A.S. *hunig*]. Mel (1); clarified h., a saccharine substance deposited in the honeycomb by the honeybee, *Apis mellifera;* used as an excipient, as a flavor in gargles and cough remedies, and as a food.

honk (hawnk). **1.** In medical terms, a sound that can be likened to the call of a goose. **2.** Sometimes specifically used to denote a sound of laryngeal origin which is often due to redundant vocal cords vibrating in a forced expiration.
systolic h., systolic whoop; a somewhat musical systolic murmur likened to the honking of a goose; sometimes of innocent but unexplained origin, at other times a sign of mitral insufficiency.

hood (hud) [O.E. *hōd,* hat]. The anterior part of the integument of soft ticks (family Argasidae) that extends over the capitulum and forms the roof of the camerostome.

hoof (huf) [A.S. *hōf*]. The horny covering of the ends of the digits or feet in many animals; it consists, like nails and horns, of thickened and modified epidermis or cuticle.

hook (huk) [A.S. *hōk*]. **1.** An instrument curved or bent near its tip, used for fixation of a part or traction. **2.** A hooklike structure.
calvarial h., an instrument used in prying off the top of the skull after it has been sawed around, at autopsies and dissections.
h. of hamate bone, *hamulus* ossis hamati.
palate h., an instrument for pulling forward the soft palate in order to facilitate posterior rhinoscopy.
sliding h., a movable attachment used on an orthodontic wire for the application of elastic traction or headgear force.
h. of spiral lamina, *hamulus* laminae spiralis.
squint h., a surgical instrument used in operations on muscles of the eye.
tracheotomy h., right-angled h. used in holding the trachea steady during tracheotomy.

Hooke, Robert, British experimental physicist, 1635–1703. See hookean *behavior;* H.'s *law.*

Hooker, Charles W. See H.-Forbes *test.*

hooklets (huk'letz). **1.** Clawlike, retractile chitinous hooks that encircle or line the rostellum of the scolex of certain taenioid tapeworms for attachment to the intestinal mucosa, with the additional aid of suckers; the h.'s can be withdrawn and the rostellum inverted when the tapeworm moves. Various arrangements and forms of the h.'s characterize the families of taenioid cestodes. **2.** H.'s of degenerated scoleces of *Echinococcus* species in the fluids of the hydatid cyst. **3.** The h.'s of the oncosphere, by which it claws out of its membrane sheath after hatching and penetrates the host gut wall; these h.'s can later be found in the cercomer of the procercoid or cysticercoid.

hookworm (huk'werm). Common name for bloodsucking nematodes of the family Ancyclostomatidae, chiefly members of the genera *Ancylostoma* (the Old World hookworm), *Necator,* and *Uncinaria,* and including the species *A. caninum* (dog h.) and *N. americanus* (New World h.).

hoose (hūs). Verminous *bronchitis.*

Hoover, Charles F., U.S. physician, 1865–1927. See H.'s *signs.*

Hopkins, Sir Frederick G., British biochemist and Nobel laureate, 1861–1947. See Benedict-H.-Cole *reagent.*

Hoplopsyllus anomalus (hop-lō-sil'ŭs ă-nom'ă-lŭs) [G. *hoplo,* tool, weapon, + *psyll,* flea]. A species of flea parasitic on ground squirrels of the western U.S., and a vector of plague.

Hopmann, Carl M., German rhinologist, 1849–1925. See H.'s *papilloma, polyp.*

Hoppe, Hermann H., U.S. physician, 1867–1929. See H.-Goldflam *disease.*

hops. Humulus.

hor. decub. Abbreviation for L. *hora decubitus,* at bedtime.

hordeolum (hōr-dē'ō-lŭm) [Mod. L., *hordeolus,* a sty in the eye, dim. of *hordeum,* barley]. A suppurative inflammation of a gland of the eyelid.
h. exter'num, sty; inflammation of the sebaceous gland of an eyelash.
h. inter'num, acute chalazion; h. meibomianum; meibomian sty; an acute purulent infection of a meibomian (tarsal) gland.
h. meibomia'num, h. internum.

horizontalis (hōr-i-zon-tā'lis) [L.] [NA]. Horizontal, referring to the plane of the body, perpendicular to the vertical plane, at right angles both to the median and coronal planes, that separates the body into upper and lower parts.

hormion (hōr'mē-on) [G. *hormos,* cord, chain, necklace]. A craniometric point at the junction of the posterior border of the vomer with the sphenoid bone.

Hormodendrum (hōr-mō-den'drŭm) [G. *hormos,* chain, + *dendron,* tree]. One of several generic names once used for the causative agents of chromomycosis; however, most species of this genus are rapidly growing fungus contaminants on laboratory media, whereas the organisms causing chromomycosis grow very slowly on laboratory media. See *Fonsecaea; Phialophora; Cladosporium.*

hormonal (hōr-mōn'ăl). Pertaining to hormones.

HORMONE

hormone (hōr'mōn) [G. *hormōn,* pres. part. of *hormaō,* to rouse or set in motion]. A chemical substance, formed in one organ or part of the body and carried in the blood to another organ or part; depending on the specificity of their effects, h.'s can alter the functional activity, and sometimes the structure, of just one organ or of various numbers of them. A number of h.'s are formed by ductless glands, but secretin and pancreozymin, formed in the gastrointestinal tract, by definition are also h.'s. For h.'s not listed below, see specific names.
adipokinetic h., adipokinin.
adrenocortical h.'s, h.'s secreted by the human adrenal cortex; *e.g.,* cortisol, aldosterone, corticosterone.
adrenocorticotropic h. (ACTH), corticotropin; adrenocorticotropin; adrenotropin; corticotropic or adrenotropic h.; the h. of the anterior lobe of the hypophysis which governs the nutrition and growth of the adrenal cortex, stimulates it to functional activity, and also possesses extraadrenal adipokinetic activity; it is a polypeptide containing 39 amino acids, but exact structure varies from one species to another; sometimes prefixed by α to distinguish it from β-corticotropin.
adrenotropic h., adrenocorticotropic h.
androgenic h., any h. that produces a masculinizing effect; of the naturally occurring androgenic h.'s, testosterone is the most potent.
anterior pituitary-like h., chorionic *gonadotropin.*
antidiuretic h. (ADH), vasopressin.
cardiac h., herz h.
chorionic gonadotropic (-trophic) h., chorionic *gonadotropin.*
chorionic "growth h.-prolactin," human placental *lactogen.*
chromatophorotropic h., see melanotropin.
corpus luteum h., progesterone.
cortical h.'s, steroid h.'s produced by the adrenal cortex.
corticotropic h., adrenocorticotropic h.
corticotropin-releasing h. (CRH), corticoliberin.
ectopic h., inappropriate h.; a h. formed by tissue outside the normal endocrine site of production; *e.g.,* adrenocorticotropic h. produced by a bronchogenic carcinoma.
erythropoietic h., **(1)** generally, any h. that promotes the formation of red blood cells, *e.g.,* testosterone; **(2)** erythropoietin.
estrogenic h., estradiol.
follicle-stimulating h. (FSH), follitropin.

follicle-stimulating h.-releasing h. (FSH-RH), folliberin.
follicular h., estrone.
galactopoietic h., prolactin.
gametokinetic h., follitropin.
gastrointestinal h., any secretion of the gastrointestinal mucosa affecting the timing and quantity of various digestive secretions (*e.g.,* secretin) or causing enhanced motility of the target organ (*e.g.,* cholecystokinin).
gonadotropic h., gonadotropin.
gonadotropin-releasing h. (GnRH), gonadoliberin (1).
growth h. (GH), somatotropin.
growth h.-releasing h. (GH-RH), somatoliberin.
heart h., herz h.
herz h., cardiac or heart h.; a substance present in extracts of cardiac tissue that augments cardiac contraction; possibly adenosine, a catecholamine, or some nonspecific stimulant present generally in tissues.
human chorionic somatomammotropic h. (HCS), human placental *lactogen.*
hypophysiotropic h., a h. that stimulates the rate of secretion of hypophysial h.'s; *e.g.,* a releasing factor.
inappropriate h., ectopic h.
interstitial cell-stimulating h. (ICSH), lutropin.
lactogenic h., prolactin.
lipid-mobilizing h., lipotropin.
lipotropic h., lipotropic pituitary h. (LPH), lipotropin.
luteinizing h. (LH), lutropin.
luteinizing h.-releasing h. (LH-RH, LRH), luliberin.
luteotropic h. (LTH), luteotropin.
mammotropic h., prolactin.
melanocyte-stimulating h. (MSH), melanotropin.
pancreatic hyperglycemic h., glucagon.
parathyroid h. (PTH), parathormone; parathyrin; a peptide h. formed by the parathyroid glands; it raises the serum calcium when administered parenterally by causing bone resorption.
pituitary gonadotropic h., anterior pituitary *gonadotropin.*
pituitary growth h., somatotropin.
placental growth h., human placental *lactogen.*
progestational h., progesterone.
prolactin inhibiting h., prolactostatin.
prolactin releasing h., prolactoliberin.
releasing h. (RH), releasing *factor.*
salivary gland h., parotin.
sex h.'s, a general term covering those steroid h.'s that are formed by testicular, ovarian, and adrenocortical tissues, and that are androgens or estrogens.
somatotropic h. (STH), somatotropin.
steroid h.'s, those h.'s possessing the steroid ring system; *e.g.,* androgens, estrogens, adrenocortical h.'s.
sympathetic h., sympathin.
thyroid-stimulating h. (TSH), thyrotropin.
thyrotropic h., thyrotropin.
thyrotropin-releasing h. (TRH), thyroliberin.
tropic (trophic) h.'s, those h.'s of the anterior lobe of the pituitary that affect the growth, nutrition, or function of other endocrine glands.

hormonogenesis (hōr'mō-nō-jen'ĕ-sis). Hormonopoiesis; the formation of hormones.

hormonogenic (hōr'mō-nō-jen'ik). Hormonopoietic; pertaining to the formation of a hormone.

hormonopoiesis (hōr'mō-nō-poy-ē'sis) [hormone + G. *poiēsis,* production]. Hormonogenesis.

hormonopoietic (hōr'mō-nō-poy-et'ik). Hormonogenic.

hormonoprivia (hōr'mō-nō-priv'ē-ă) [hormone + G. *privus,* deprived of]. Obsolete term meaning partial or total deprivation of hormones.

hormonotherapy (hōr'mō-nō-thăr'ă-pē). Treatment with hormones.

horn (hōrn) [A.S.]. Cornu.
Ammon's h. [G. *Ammōn,* the Egyptian deity *Amūn],* cornu ammonis; one of the two interlocking gyri composing the hippocampus, the other being the gyrus dentatus.
anterior h., *cornu* anterius.
cicatricial h., a keratinous h. projecting outward from a scar.
coccygeal h., *cornu* coccygeum.
cutaneous h., cornu cutaneum; warty h.; a protruding keratotic growth of the skin; the base may show changes of actinic keratosis or carcinoma.
dorsal h., *cornu* posterius.
frontal h., *cornu* inferius ventriculi lateralis. See under *cornu* inferius.
greater h., *cornu* majus.
horns of hyoid bone, see *cornu* majus; *cornu* minus.
iliac h., bony spur of posterior part of ilium, often found in nail-patella syndrome.
inferior h., *cornu* inferius.
inferior h. of lateral ventricle, cornu inferius ventriculi lateralis. See under *cornu* inferius (3).
inferior h. of saphenous opening, *cornu* inferius hiatus saphenus.
inferior h. of thyroid cartilage, *cornu* inferius cartilaginis thyroideae.
lateral h., *cornu* laterale.
lesser h., *cornu* minus.
nail h., overgrown nail.
occipital h., cornu posterius ventriculi lateralis. See under *cornu* posterius (1).
posterior h., *cornu* posterius.
pulp h., a prolongation of the pulp extending toward the cusp of a tooth.
sacral h., *cornu* sacrale.
sebaceous h., a solid outgrowth from a sebaceous cyst.
superior h., *cornu* superius.
superior h. of saphenous opening, *cornu* superius (2).
superior h. of thyroid cartilage, *cornu* superius (1).
temporal h., cornu inferius ventriculi lateralis. See under *cornu* inferius (3).
uterine h., h. of uterus, *cornu* uteri.
ventral h., *cornu* anterius.
warty h., cutaneous h.

Horner, Johann F., Swiss ophthalmologist, 1831–1886. See H.'s *syndrome, pupil;* Bernard-H. *syndrome;* H.- Trantas *dots.*

Horner, William E., U.S. anatomist, 1793–1853. See H.'s *muscle, teeth.*

hornification (hōr'ni-fi-kā'shŭn). Keratinization.

horny (hōrn'ē). Corneous; keratic; keratinous (2); keratoid (1); keroid; of the nature or structure of horn.

horopter (hō-rop'ter) [G. *horos,* limit, + *optēr,* one who sees, fr. *ops,* eye]. The sum of the points in space, the images of which for a given fixation point fall on corresponding retinal points. If the fixation point is 2 meters, the horopter is a straight line; if less, a curve concave to the face; if more, a convex curve.

horripilation (ho-rip-i-lā'shŭn) [L. *horreo,* to bristle, + *pilus,* hair]. Erection of the fine hairs on contraction of the arrectores pilorum.

horror (hor'er) [L.]. Dread; fear.
h. autotox'icus [L., dread of self-poisoning], a term introduced by Ehrlich, meaning that immunity is directed against foreign materials but not against the constituents of one's own body; exceptions to this concept are the autoallergic reactions and diseases.
h. fusio'nis, [L., dread of intermingling], macular evasion; simulta-

neous projection into consciousness of retinal images so different that fusion is impossible.

horsefly (hōrs'flī). See *Tabanus; Anthomyia canicularis.*

horsepower (hōrs'pow-er). A unit of power, 550 foot-pounds per second, or 746 watts.

horsepox (hōrs'poks). A disease, now rare, that usually appears as typical eruptions, first papular, then vesicular, in the mouth or on the lips and buccal mucosa, sometimes on the skin of the fetlocks; caused by the horsepox virus.

Horsfall, Frank L., Jr., U.S. physician, 1906–1971. See Tamm-H. *mucoprotein, protein.*

Horsley, Sir Victor A.H., British surgeon, 1857–1916. See H.'s bone *wax.*

hor. som. Abbreviation for L. *hora somni,* before sleep, at bedtime.

Hortega, Pio del Rio, Spanish neurohistologist in South America, 1882–1945. See H. *cell; H.'s* neuroglia *stain.*

Horton, Bayard T., U.S. physician, *1895. See H.'s *arteritis, cephalalgia, headache.*

hospice (hos'pis) [L. *hospes,* a host, a guest]. An institution that provides a centralized program of palliative and supportive services to dying persons and their families, in the form of physical, psychological, social, and spiritual care; such services are provided by an interdisciplinary team of professionals and volunteers who are available at home and in inpatient settings.

hospital (hos'pi-tăl) [L. *hospitalis,* for a guest, fr. *hospes* (*hospit-*), a host, a guest]. An institution for the treatment, care, and cure of the sick and wounded, for the study of disease, and for the training of physicians, nurses, and allied health personnel.
closed h., a h. that restricts membership on its attending or consulting staff, and thereby limits who may admit and treat patients.
day h., a special facility, or an arrangement within a h. setting, that enables the patient to come to the h. for treatment during the day and return home or to another facility at night. *Cf.* night h.
general h., any large civilian h. that is equipped to care for medical, surgical, maternity, and psychiatric cases, and usually has a resident medical staff.
government h., public h.; a h. administered by officials of the city, county, state, or nation.
group h., a private h. organized and controlled by a group of physicians and restricted to the reception and care of their own patients.
maternity h., a special h. for the care of women in childbirth.
mental h., a medical institution for the care and treatment of persons with psychiatric disorders.
municipal h., a government h. administered by city officials.
night h., a special facility, or an arrangement within a h. setting, providing treatment and lodging at night for patients able to work in the community during the day. *Cf.* day h.
open h., a h. where all physicians, not members of the regular staff, are permitted to send their patients and control their treatment.
philanthropic h., voluntary h.
private h., proprietary h.; **(1)** a h. similar to a group h. except that it is controlled by a single practitioner or by him and the associates in his office; **(2)** a h. operated for profit.
proprietary h., private h.
public h., government h.
special h., a h. for the medical and surgical care of patients with specific types of diseases, as of the ear, nose, and throat, eyes, mental.
state h., a h. supported by taxpayers and administered by state government officials.
teaching h., a h. that also functions as a formal center of learning for the training of physicians, nurses, and allied health personnel.
Veterans Administration h., a h. operated at federal government expense and administered by the Veterans Administration for care of veterans of U.S. wars and retired military personnel.
voluntary h., philanthropic h.; a h. supported in part by voluntary contributions and under the control of a local, usually self-appointed, board of managers; a non-profit h.
weekend h., a special facility, or an arrangement within a h. setting, which enables a patient to work in the community during the work week and receive treatment in the hospital during the weekend.

hospitalism (hos'pi-tăl-ism). The second stage of a depression observed in the first year of human life, following anaclitic depression, characterized by stupor and a wasting away; usually caused by prolonged hospitalization in which an infant is separated from its mother or a mothering influence.

hospitalization (hos'pi-tăl-i-zā'shŭn). Confinement in a hospital as a patient for diagnostic study and treatment.

host [L. *hospes,* a host]. The organism in or on which a parasite lives, deriving its body substance or energy from the h.
amplifier h., a h. in which infectious agents multiply rapidly to high levels, providing an important source of infection for vectors in vector-borne diseases.
dead-end h., a h. from which infectious agents are not transmitted to other susceptible h.'s.
definitive h., final h.; one in which a parasite reaches the adult or sexually mature stage.
final h., definitive h.
intermediate h., intermediary h., secondary h.; one in which larval or developmental stages occur.
paratenic h., transport h.; an intermediate h. in which no development of the parasite occurs, although its presence may be required as an essential link in the completion of the parasite's life cycle; *e.g.,* the successive fish h.'s that carry the plerocercoid of *Diphyllobothrium latum,* the broad fish tapeworm, to larger food fish eventually eaten by man or other final h.'s.
reservoir h., the h. of an infection in which the infectious agent multiplies and/or develops, and upon which the agent is dependent for survival in nature; the h. essential for the maintenance of the infection during times when active transmission is not occurring.
secondary h., intermediate h.
transport h., paratenic h.

hotfoot. Ignipedites.

Hottentot apron (hot'en-tot ā'prŭn) [fr. Hottentot, because of frequency of the condition in this group of people]. *Velamen* vulvae.

hottentotism (hot'en-tot'izm) [D. fr. Hottentot, (D. *hateren* to stammer, *tateren* to stutter), a people in South Africa named by the Dutch for the sounds of their speech]. A form of stammering.

Hotz, Ferdinand Carl, U.S. ophthalmologist, 1843–1908. See H.-Anagnostakis *operation.*

Hounsfield, Godfrey N., 20th century British electronics engineer. See H. *unit.*

housefly (hows'flī). See *Musca domestica* (common housefly), and *Fannia canicularis* (lesser housefly).

house officer. An intern or resident employed by a hospital to provide service to patients while receiving training in a medical specialty.

Houssay, Bernardo A., Argentine physiologist and Nobel laureate, 1887–1971. See H. *animal, phenomenon, syndrome.*

Houston, John, Dublin physician, 1802–1845. See H.'s *folds, muscle, valves.*

Hovius, Jacob, Dutch ophthalmologist, *1675. See *canal* of H.

Howard, John Eager, U.S. internist and endocrinologist, *1902. See H. *test;* Ellsworth-H. *test.*

Howell, William H., U.S. physiologist, 1860–1945. See H. *unit,* H.-

Jolly *bodies.*

Howship, John, British surgeon, 1781–1841. See H.'s *lacunae;* Romberg-H. *symptom.*

Hoyer, Heinrich F., Polish anatomist and histologist, 1834–1907. See H.'s *anastomosis, canals;* Sucquet-H. *canals.*

HPL Abbreviation for human placental *lactogen.*

HPV Abbreviation for human papilloma *virus.*

H_2Q Symbol for ubiquinol.

h.s. Abbreviation for L. *hora somni,* before sleep, at bedtime.

HSV Abbreviation for herpes simplex *virus.*

Ht Abbreviation for total *hyperopia.*

5-HT Abbreviation for 5-hydroxytryptamine.

H-tetanase (tet'ă-nās). Behring's term for the hemolytic constituent of tetanus toxin.

HTLV-III Abbreviation for human T-cell lymphotropic *virus* type III.

Hubrecht, Ambrosius A.W., Dutch zoologist and comparative anatomist, 1853–1915. See H.'s protocordal *knot.*

Hucker-Conn stain. See under stain.

Hudson, Arthur Cyril, British ophthalmologist, 1875–1962. See H.'s *line;* H.-Stähli *line.*

hue (hū). One of the three qualities of color; that property by which colors of the spectrum are distinguished from each other and from grays or similar brightness; determined by the wavelength or a combination of wavelengths of light.

Hueck, Alexander F., German anatomist, 1802–1842. See H.'s *ligament.*

Huët, G.J., Dutch physician, *1879. See Pelger-H. nuclear *anomaly.*

Hueter, Karl, German surgeon, 1838–1882. See H.'s *maneuver, sign.*

Hüfner, Carl Gustav von, German physician, 1840–1908. See H.'s *equation.*

Huggins, Charles B., U.S. surgeon and Nobel laureate, *1901. See H.'s *operation.*

Huguier, Pierre C., French surgeon, 1804–1873. See H.'s *canal, circle, sinus.*

Huhner, Max, U.S. urologist, 1873–1947. See H. *test.*

Hull's triad. See under triad.

hum (hŭm). A low continuous murmur.

venous h., bruit de diable; nun's murmur; brief noise originating from the neck veins that may be confused with cardiac murmurs, particularly with the continuous murmur of patent ductus arteriosus.

humectant (hyū-mek'tănt). **1.** Moistening. **2.** A substance used to obtain a moistening effect.

humectation (hyū-mek-tā'shŭn) [L. *humecto,* pp. *-mectus,* to moisten, fr. *humeo,* to be damp]. **1.** Therapeutic application of moisture. **2.** Serous infiltration of the tissues. **3.** Soaking of a crude drug in water preparatory to the making of an extract.

humeral (hyū'mer-ăl). Relating to the humerus.

humeroradial (hyū'mer-ō-rā'dē-ăl). Relating to both humerus and radius; denoting especially the ratio of length of one to the other.

humeroscapular (hyū'mer-ō-skap'yū-lăr). Relating to both humerus and scapula.

humeroulnar (hyū'mer-ō-ŭl'năr). Relating to both humerus and ulna; denoting especially the ratio of length of one to the other.

humerus, gen. and pl. **humeri** (hyū'mer-ŭs, -ī) [L. shoulder] [NA]. The bone of the arm, articulating with the scapula above and the radius and ulna below.

humidity (hyū-mid'i-tē) [L. *humiditas,* dampness]. Moisture or dampness, as of the air.

absolute h., the weight of water vapor actually present per unit volume of gas or air.

relative h., the actual amount of water vapor present in the air or in a gas, divided by the amount necessary for saturation at the same temperature and pressure; expressed as a percentage.

humin (hyū'min). An insoluble brownish residue obtained upon acid hydrolysis of protein.

Hummelsheim, Eduard K.M.J., German ophthalmologist, 1868–1952. See H.'s *operation.*

humor, gen. **humoris** (hyū'mer, hyū-mōr'is) [L. correctly, *umor,* liquid]. **1** [NA]. Any clear fluid or semifluid hyaline anatomical substance. **2.** One of the elemental body fluids that were the basis of the physiologic and pathologic teachings of the hippocratic school: blood, yellow bile, black bile, and phlegm. See also humoral *doctrine.*

aqueous h., h. aquosus.

h. aquo'sus [NA], aqueous h.; intraocular fluid; the watery fluid that fills the anterior and posterior chambers of the eye. It is secreted by the ciliary processes, and passes through the posterior chamber and the pupil into the anterior chamber where it passes through the trabecular meshwork and is reabsorbed into the venous system at the iridocorneal angle by way of the sinus venosus of the sclera.

Morgagni's h., Morgagni's *liquor.*

ocular h., one of the two h.'s of the eye: aqueous and vitreous.

peccant h.'s, based on the historic humoral theory of disease, such h.'s or deranged fluids in the body were regarded as the direct causes of various illnesses.

thunder h., an obstinate skin eruption.

vitreous h., h. vitreus.

h. vit'reus [NA], vitreous h.; the fluid component of the corpus vitreum.

humoral (hyū'mōr-ăl). Relating to a humor in any sense.

humoralism, humorism (hyū'mōr-ăl-izm, -mōr-izm) [L. *umor, humor,* moisture]. Humoral *doctrine.*

hump (hŭmp). A rounded protuberance or bulge.

Hampton h., a pleura-based density usually at a costophrenic angle and convex toward the pulmonary hilum; seen in pulmonary infarct.

humpback (hŭmp'bak). Nonmedical term for kyphosis or gibbus.

Humphry, Sir George M., British surgeon, 1820–1896. See H.'s *ligament.*

humulin (hyū'mū-lin). Lupulin.

humulus (hyū'mū-lŭs) [Mediev. L.]. Hops; the dried fruits (strobiles) of *Humulus lupulus* (family Moraceae), a climbing herb of central and northern Asia, Europe, and North America; an aromatic bitter, mildly sedative, and a diuretic; primarily used in the brewing industry for giving aroma and flavor to beer.

hunchback (hŭnch'bak). Nonmedical term for kyphosis or gibbus.

Hung's method. See under method.

hunger (hŭn'ger) [A.S.]. **1.** A desire or need for food. **2.** Any appetite, strong desire, or craving.

affect h., emotional h. for maternal love and feelings of protection and care implied in the mother-child relationship.

narcotic h., the physiological craving for narcotics.

Hunner, Guy L., U. S. surgeon, 1868–1957. See H.'s *stricture, ulcer;* Fenwick-H. *ulcer.*

Hunt, James Ramsay, U.S. neurologist, 1872–1937. See H.'s *atrophy, neuralgia,* paradoxical *phenomenon, syndrome;* Ramsay H.'s *syndrome.*

Hunt, W.E., U.S. neurosurgeon, *1921. See Tolosa-H. *syndrome.*

Hunter, Charles. See H.'s *syndrome.*

Hunter, John, Scottish surgeon, anatomist, physiologist and pathologist, 1728–1793. See H.'s *canal, gubernaculum, operation;* H.-Schreger *bands, lines.*

Hunter, William, Scottish anatomist and obstetrician, 1718–1783. See H.'s *ligament, line, membrane.*

Hunter, William, British pathologist, 1861–1937. See H.'s *glossitis.*

hunting (hŭnt'ing). The oscillation of a controlled variable, such as the temperature of a thermostat, around its set point. See hunting *reaction.*

Huntington, George, U.S. physician, 1850–1916. See H.'s *chorea, disease.*

Hurler, Gertrud, 20th century Austrian pediatrician. See H.'s *disease, syndrome;* hurloid *facies;* Pfaundler-H. *syndrome.*

Hurst bougies. See under bougie.

Hürthle, Karl W., German histologist, 1860–1945. See H.'s *cell;* H. cell *adenoma, carcinoma,* cell *tumor.*

Huschke, Emil, German anatomist, 1797–1858. See H.'s *cartilages, foramen,* auditory *teeth* (under tooth), *valve.*

Hutchinson, Sir Jonathan, British surgeon, 1828–1913. See H.'s *facies, freckle, mask,* crescentic *notch, patch, pupil, teeth,* (see under tooth), *triad;* H.-Gilford *disease, syndrome.*

Hutchison, Sir Robert, British pediatrician, 1871–1960. See H.'s *syndrome.*

Huxley, Thomas H., British biologist, physiologist, and comparative anatomist, 1825–1895. See H.'s *layer, membrane, sheath.*

Huygens, Christian, Dutch physicist, 1629–1695. See H.'s *ocular.*

HVL Abbreviation for half-value *layer.*

hyal-. See hyalo-.

hyalin (hī'ă-lin) [G. *hyalos,* glass]. A clear, eosinophilic, homogeneous substance occurring in degeneration; *e.g.,* in arteriolar walls in arteriolar sclerosis and in glomerular tufts in diabetic glomerulosclerosis.

alcoholic h., Mallory *bodies.*

hyaline (hī'ă-lin, -lēn) [G. *hyalos,* glass]. Hyaloid; of a glassy, homogeneous, translucent appearance, a characteristic gross and microscopic appearance.

hyalinization (hī'ă-lin-i-zā'shŭn). The formation of hyalin.

hyalinosis (hī'ă-li-nō'sis). Hyaline *degeneration,* especially that of relatively extensive degree.

systemic h., juvenile hyalin *fibromatosis.*

hyalinuria (hī-ă-li-nū'rē-ă) [hyalin + G. *ouron,* urine]. The excretion of hyalin or casts of hyaline material in the urine.

hyalitis (hī-ă-lī'tis). Vitreitis.

suppurative h., purulent vitreous humor due to exudation from adjacent structures, as in panophthalmitis.

hyalo-, hyal- [G. *hyalos,* glass]. Combining forms meaning glassy, or relating to hyalin.

hyalobiuronic acid (hī'ă-lō-bī-yūr-on'ik). A disaccharide made up of *N*-acetylglucosamine and glucuronic acid in a 1,3-linkage; occurs in hyaluronic acid as the repeating unit.

hyalocyte (hī'ă-lō-sīt) [hyalo- + G. *kytos,* cell]. Vitreous *cell.*

hyalogens (hī-al'ō-jenz). Substances similar to mucoids that are found in many animal structures (*e.g.,* cartilage, vitreous humor, hydatid cysts) and yield sugars on hydrolysis.

hyalohyphomycosis (hī'ă-lō-hī'fō-mī-kō'sis) [hyalo- + G. *hyphe,* web, + *mykēs,* fungus, + *-osis,* condition]. An infection caused by a fungus with hyaline (colorless) mycelium, *e.g.,* species of *Fusarium, Penicillium,* and *Scopulariopsis;* circumstances for infections usually involve a decrease in body resistance due to surgery, indwelling catheters, steroid therapy, or immunosuppressive drugs or cytotoxins.

hyaloid (hī'ă-loyd) [hyalo- + G. *eidos,* resemblance]. Hyaline.

hyalomere (hī'ă-lō-mēr) [hyalo- + G. *meros,* part]. The clear periphery of a blood platelet.

Hyalomma (hī-ă-lom'ă) [hyalo- + G. *omma,* eye]. An Old World genus (about 21 species) of large ixodid ticks with submarginal eyes, coalesced festoons, an ornate scutum, and a long rostrum. Adults parasitize all domestic animals and a wide variety of wild animals; larvae or nymphs may parasitize small mammals, birds, and reptiles. Species harbor a great variety of pathogens of humans and animals, and also cause considerable mechanical injury.

H. anato'licum, a species of tick of cattle, horses, and other ruminants; it is a major vector of tropical theileriosis of cattle, a probable vector of Uzbekistan hemorrhagic fever, and possibly a vector of a Near Eastern variety of equine encephalomyelitis from horses, donkeys, and sheep in Egypt and Syria.

H. margina'tum, a particularly common species of tick carried by birds migrating between Europe and Asia and Africa, and the probable vector of the virus of Crimean hemorrhagic fever.

H. variega'tum, species that is the vector of the viral agent of lymphocytic choriomeningitis in Ethiopia.

hyalophagia, hyalophagy (hī'ă-lō-fā'jē-ă, hī-ă-lof'ă-jē) [hyalo- + G. *phagein,* to eat]. The eating or chewing of glass.

hyalophobia (hī'ă-lō-fō'bē-ă) [hyalo- + G. *phobos,* fear]. Crystallophobia; morbid fear of glass objects.

hyaloplasm, hyaloplasma (hī'ă-lō-plazm, -plaz'mă) [hyalo- + G. *plasma,* thing formed]. The protoplasmic fluid substance of a cell.

nuclear h., karyolymph.

hyaloserositis (hī'ă-lō-ser-ō-sī'tis) [hyalo- + Mod. L. *serosa,* serous membrane, + *-itis,* inflammation]. Inflammation of a serous membrane with a fibrinous exudate that eventually becomes hyalinized, resulting in a relatively thick, dense, opaque, glistening, white or gray-white coating; when the process involves the visceral serous membranes of various organs, the grossly apparent condition is sometimes colloquially termed icing liver, sugar-coated spleen, frosted heart, and so on, depending on the site.

hyalosis (hī-ă-lō'sis) [hyalo- + G. *-osis,* condition]. Degenerative changes in the corpus vitreum.

asteroid h., Benson's disease; numerous small spherical bodies ("snowball" opacities) in the corpus vitreum, visible ophthalmoscopically; an age change, usually unilateral, and not affecting vision.

punctate h., a condition marked by minute opacities in the vitreous.

hyalosome (hī-al'ō-sōm) [hyalo- + G. *sōma,* body]. An oval or round structure within a cell nucleus that stains faintly but otherwise resembles a nucleolus.

hyalurate (hī-ă-lū'rāt). Hyaluronate.

hyaluronate (hī-ă-lū'ron-āt). Hyalurate; a salt or ester of hyaluronic acid.

h. lyase [EC 4.2.2.1], hyaluronic lyase; a lyase cleaving hyaluronic acids. See also hyaluronidase (1).

hyaluronic acid (HA) (hī'ă-lū-ron'ik). A mucopolysaccharide made up of alternating 1,4-linked residues of hyalobiuronic acid, forming a gelatinous material in the tissue spaces and acting as an intercellular cement substance generally throughout the body; it is hydrolyzed to disaccharide or tetrasaccharide units by hyaluronidase.

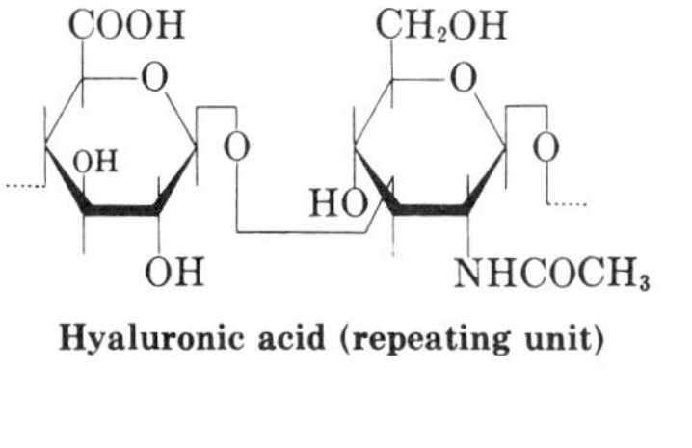

Hyaluronic acid (repeating unit)

hyaluronic lyase. *Hyaluronate* lyase.

hyaluronidase (hī'ă-lū-ron'i-dās). **1.** Term used loosely for hyaluronate lyase, hyaluronoglucosaminidase, and hyaluronoglucuronidase, one or more of which are present in testis, sperm, bee and snake venoms, type II pneumonococci, certain hemolytic streptococci, etc. Also called diffusing or spreading factor; Duran-Reynals spreading or permeability factor; invasin. **2.** A soluble enzyme product prepared from mammalian testes; it is used to increase the effect of local anesthetics and to permit wider infiltration of subcutaneously administered fluids, is suggested in the treatment of certain forms of arthritis to promote resolution of redundant tissue, is used to speed the resorption of traumatic or postoperative edema and hematoma, is used in combination with collagenase to dissociate organs such as liver and heart into viable cell suspensions, and in histochemistry is used on tissue secretions to verify the presence of hyaluronic acid or chondroitin sulfates.

hyaluronoglucosaminidase (hī-ă-lū'ron-ō-glū'kō-să-min'i-dās) [EC 3.2.1.35]. An enzyme hydrolyzing 1,4 linkages in hyaluronates. See also hyaluronidase (1).

hyaluronoglucuronidase (hī-ă-lū'ron-ō-glū-kur-on'i-dās) [EC 3.2.1.36]. An enzyme hydrolyzing 1,3 linkages in hyaluronates. See also hyaluronidase (1).

hybaroxia (hī-bă-rok'sē-ă) [G. *hyper,* above, + *baros,* pressure, + *oxys,* acute]. Oxygen therapy with pressures greater than 1 atmosphere or ambient oxygen pressure applied to the entire body in a chamber or room.

hybenzate (hī-ben'zāt). USAN-approved contraction for *o*-(4-hydroxybenzoyl)benzoate.

hybrid (hī'brid) [L. *hybrida,* offspring of a tame sow and a wild boar, fr. G. *hybris,* violation, wantonness]. **1.** Crossbreed (1); an individual (plant or animal) whose parents are different varieties of the same species or belong to different but closely allied species. **2.** Fused tissue culture cells, as in a hybridoma.
SV40-adenovirus h., a virion consisting of SV40 genetic material encased in an adenovirus capsid.

hybridism (hī'brid-izm). The state of being hybrid.

hybridization (hī'brid-i-zā'shŭn). Crossbreeding; the process of breeding a hybrid.
cell h., fusion of two or more dissimilar cells, leading to formation of a synkaryon.
cross h., annealing of a DNA probe to an imperfectly matching DNA molecule.
DNA h., a technique used to determine the relatedness of microorganisms by the speed and efficiency of the reassociation of single-stranded DNA to form double-stranded DNA when one of the strands originates from one organism and the other strand from another organism; occurs when the base sequences are complementary or nearly so.
somatic cell h., production of a heterokaryon.

hybridoma (hī-brid-ō'mă) [G. *hybris,* violation, wantonness, + *-ōma,* tumor]. A tumor of hybrid cells used in the *in vitro* production of specific monoclonal antibodies; produced by fusion of an established tissue culture line of lymphocyte tumor cells (*e.g.,* mouse plasmacytoma cells) and specific antibody-producing cells (*e.g.,* splenocytes from specifically immunized mice); fusions are accomplished by use of polyethylene glycol.

hycanthone (hī-kan'thōn). 1-[[2-(Diethyl]amino)ethyl]amino]-4-(hydroxymethyl)thioxanthen-9-one; an antischistosomal drug.

hyclate (hī'klāt). USAN-approved contraction for monohydrochloride hemiethanolate hemihydrate, $HCl\cdot{}^1/_2\ C_2H_5OH\cdot{}^1/_2\ H_2O$.

hydantoin (hī-dan'tō-in). Glycolylurea; 2,4-imidazolidinedione; derived from urea or from allantoin; the $NH–CH_2–CO$ group is prototypical of *α*-amino acids:

$$\overline{NH—CH_2—CO—NH—CO}$$

hydantoinate (hī-dan-tō'in-āt). A salt of hydantoin.

hydatid (hī'da-tid). [G. *hydatis,* a drop of water, a hyatid]. **1.** Hydatid *cyst.* **2.** A vesicular structure resembling an *Echinococcus* cyst.
Morgagni's h., *appendix* vesiculosa.
nonpedunculated h., *appendix* testis.
pedunculated h., *appendix* epididymidis.
sessile h., *appendix* testis.
stalked h., *appendix* vesiculosa.

hydatidiform (hī-da-tid'i-form). Having the form or appearance of a hydatid.

hydatidocele (hī-da-tid'ō-sēl) [hydatid + G. *kēlē,* tumor]. A cystic mass composed of one or more hydatids formed in the scrotum.

hydatidoma (hī'da-ti-dō'mă) [hydatid + G. *-oma,* tumor]. A benign neoplasm in which there is prominent formation of hydatids.

hydatidosis (hī'da-ti-dō'sis). The morbid state caused by the presence of hydatid cysts.

hydatidostomy (hī'da-ti-dos'tō-mē) [hydatid + G. *stoma,* mouth]. Surgical evacuation of a hydatid cyst.

Hydatigera taeniaeformis (hī-da-tij'er-ă tē-ni-ē-fōr'mis). *Taenia taeniaeformis.*

hydatoid (hī'da-toyd) [G. *hydōr* (*hydat-*), water, + *eidos,* resemblance]. **1.** The aqueous humor. **2.** The hyaloid membrane. **3.** Relating to the aqueous humor. **4.** Watery or resembling water.

Hyde, James N., U.S. dermatologist, 1840–1910. See H.'s *disease.*

hydnocarpus oil (hid-nō-kar'pŭs). Chaulmoogra oil.

hydr-. See hydro-.

hydracetin (hī-dras'ĕ-tin). Pure form of acetylphenylhydrazine.

hydradenitis (hī'drad-ĕ-nī'tis). Hidradenitis.

hydradenoma (hī'drad-ĕ-nō'mă). Hidradenoma.

hydragogue (hī'dră-gog) [hydr- + G. *agōgos,* drawing forth]. Producing a discharge of watery fluid; denoting a class of cathartics that retain fluids in the intestine and aid in the removal of edematous fluids, *e.g.,* saline cathartics.

hydralazine hydrochloride (hī-dral'ă-zēn). 1-Hydrazinophthalazine hydrochloride; a vasodilating antihypertensive agent.

hydrallostane (hī-dral'ō-stān). 4,5*α*-Dihydrocortisol; 11*β*,17*α*,21-trihydroxy-5*β*-pregnane-3,20-dione; a metabolite of cortisole, reduced at the 4,5 double bond.

hydramine (hī'dră-mēn). Rarely used contraction of hydroxylamine.

hydramitrazine tartrate (hī-dră-mī'tră-zēn). 2,4-Bis(diethylamino)-6-hydrazino-*s*-triazine tartrate; an intestinal antispasmodic.

hydramnion, hydramnios (hī-dram'nē-on, -nē-os) [G. *hydōr,* water, + amnion]. Presence of an excessive amount of amniotic fluid.

hydranencephaly (hī'dran-en-sef'ă-lē) [hydr- + G. *an-* priv. + *enkephalos,* brain]. Congenital absence of cerebral hemispheres; a fluid-filled cavity; the basal ganglia and remnants of mesencephalon are covered by leptomeninges, dura, skull bones, and skin, in contrast to anencephaly.

hydrargyria, hydrargyrism (hī-drar-jir'ē-ă, hī-drar'jir-izm) [L. *hydrargyrum,* mercury]. Mercury *poisoning.*

hydrargyrum (hī-drar'ji-rŭm) [G. *hydrargyros,* quicksilver, fr. *hydōr,* water, + *argyros,* silver]. Mercury.

hydrarthrodial (hī-drar-thrō'dē-ăl). Relating to hydrarthrosis.

hydrarthron (hī-drar'thron). Hydrarthrosis.

hydrarthrosis (hī-drar-thrō'sis) [hydr- + G. *arthron,* joint]. Hydrarthron; hydrarthrus; hydrops articuli; effusion of a serous fluid into a joint cavity.
intermittent h., a disorder characterized by a periodically recurring serous effusion into the cavity of a joint; the articulation may be the seat of a chronic arthritis or may apparently be normal in the intervals of the attacks.

hydrarthrus (hī-drar'thrŭs). Hydrarthrosis.

hydrase (hī'drās). Former name for hydratase.

hydrastine (hī-dras'tēn). An alkaloid of hydrastis; an isoquinoline chemically related to narcotine. As the hydrochloride, used locally in the treatment of catarrhal inflammation of the mucous membranes, and internally in the treatment of gastric inflammation, as a uterine stimulant, and to check uterine hemmorrhage.

hydrastinine (hī-dras'ti-nēn). A semisynthetic alkaloid prepared from hydrastine; the hydrochloride has been used in uterine hemorrhage and as an oxytocic; in large doses, it is a powerful depressant of the entire motor tract (motor cortex, nerve, and muscle).

hydrastis (hī-dras'tis) [Mod. L. fr. G. *hydōr* (*hydro-*), water, + *draō,* to accomplish]. Golden seal; jaundice or yellow root; Indian turmeric; the dried rhizome of *Hydrastis canadensis* (family Ranunculaceae), a native of the eastern U.S.; used in the treatment of chronic catarrhal states of the mucous membranes and in metrorrhagia.

hydratase (hī'dră-tās). Trivial name applied, together with dehydratase, to certain hydro-lyases (EC class 4.2.1) catalyzing hydration-dehydration; *e.g.,* fumarate-malate interconversion by fumarate hydratase.

hydrate (hī'drāt). An aqueous solvate (in older terminology, a hydroxide); a compound crystallizing with one or more molecules of water; *e.g.,* $CuSO_4.5H_2O$.

hydrated (hī'drāt-ed). Hydrous; combined with water, forming a hydrate.

hydration (hī-drā'shŭn). **1.** Chemically, the addition of water; differentiated from hydrolysis, where the union with water is accompanied by a splitting of the original molecule and the water molecule. See also solvation. **2.** Clinically, the taking in of water; used commonly in the sense of reduced h. or dehydration.
absolute h., actual water excess as measured by a difference from the normal or from a given water content.

hydrazide (hī'dră-zīd). An organic compound of the general formula $RCO–NHNH_2$; an acyl derivative of hydrazine.

hydrazine (hī'dră-zēn). $H_2N–NH_2$, from which phenylhydrazine and similar products are derived.

hydrazine yellow. Tartrazine.

hydrazinolysis (hī'dră-zi-nol'i-sis). Cleavage of chemical bonds by hydrazine ($NH_2\_NH_2$); applied in protein and nucleic acid degradations.

hydrazone (hī'dră-zōn). A substance derived from aldehydes and ketones by reaction with hydrazine or a hydrazine derivative to give the grouping $\geq C=N–NH_2$.

hydremia (hī-drē'mē-ă) [hydr- + G. *haima,* blood]. Dilution anemia; polyplasmia; a condition in which the blood volume is increased as a result of an increase in the water content of plasma, with or without a reduction in the concentration of protein; there is an excess of plasma in proportion to the formed elements and a corresponding decrease in hematocrit.

hydrencephalocele (hī-dren-sef'ă-lō-sēl) [hydr- + G. *enkephalos,* brain, + *kēlē,* tumor]. Hydrocephalocele; hydroencephalocele; protrusion, through a cleft in the skull, of brain substance expanded into a sac containing fluid.

hydrencephalomeningocele (hī'dren-sef'ă-lō-me-ning'gō-sēl). Protrusion, through a defect in the skull, of a sac containing meninges, brain substance, and cerebrospinal fluid.

hydrencephalus (hī-dren-sef'ă-lŭs) [hydr- + G. *enkephalos,* brain]. Rarely used term for internal *hydrocephalus.*

hydriatric, hydriatic (hī-drē-at'rik, -at'ik) [hydr- + G. *iatrikos,* relating to medicine]. Relating to the obsolete use of water to treat or cure disease.

hydric (hī'drik). Relating to hydrogen in chemical combination.

hydride (hī'drīd). A compound of hydrogen in which it assumes a formal negative charge, *e.g.,* sodium borohydride, $NaBH_4$.

hydrindantin (hī-drin-dan'tin). The reduced form of ninhydrin.

hydro-, hydr- [G. *hydōr,* water]. Combining forms denoting: **(1)** water or association with water; **(2)** hydrogen.

hydroa (hī-drō'ă) [hydro + G. *ōon,* egg]. Hidroa; any bullous eruption.
h. aestiva'le, h. vacciniforme.
h. fe'brile, *herpes* simplex.
h. gestatio'nis, *herpes* gestationis.
h. herpetifor'me, *dermatitis* herpetiformis.
h. puero'rum, h. vacciniforme.
h. vaccinifor'me, h. aestivale; h. puerorum; a hereditary recurrent eruption of umbilicated bullae, occurring on exposure to the sun and affecting chiefly male children or young men.
h. vesiculo'sum, obsolete term for erythema multiforme with iris or vesicular lesions.

hydroadipsia (hī'drō-ă-dip'sē-ă) [hydro- + G. *a-* priv. + *dipsa,* thirst]. Absence of thirst for water.

hydroappendix (hī'drō-ă-pen'diks). Distention of the vermiform appendix with a serous fluid.

hydrobilirubin (hī'drō-bil-i-rū'bin). A dark brown-red pigment that may be formed when bilirubin is reduced.

hydroblepharon (hī-drō-blef'ă-ron) [hydro- + G. *blepharon,* eyelid]. Edematous swelling of the eyelid.

hydrobromate (hī-drō-brō'māt). A salt of hydrobromic acid.

hydrobromic acid (hī-drō-brō'mik). An aqueous solution of hydrogen bromide; its salts are bromides.

hydrocalycosis (hī'drō-kal-i-kō'sis) [hydro- + G. *kalyx,* cup of a flower]. A rare, usually symptomless, anomaly of the renal calix which is dilated from obstruction of the infundibulum; usually discovered incidentally at pyelography or autopsy; may become infected.

hydrocarbon (hī-drō-kar'bŏn). A compound containing only hydrogen and carbon.
Diels h., a phenanthrene derivative obtained by the dehydrogenation of various steroids.
saturated h., a h. that contains the greatest possible number of hydrogen atoms, so that the molecule contains neither rings nor multiple bonds.

hydrocele (hī'drō-sēl) [hydro- + G. kēlē, hernia]. A collection of serous fluid in a sacculated cavity; specifically, such a collection in the tunica vaginalis testis, or in a separate pocket along the spermatic cord.
cervical h., h. colli; a cyst formed by secretion into a persistent duct or fissure of the neck; when it involves lymph channels, it is usually a lymphangioma.
h. col'li, cervical h.
congenital h., a collection of fluid in the unobliterated canal leading from the abdominal cavity to the investing sac of the testis.
Dupuytren's h., bilocular h. in which the sac fills the scrotum and also extends into the abdominal cavity beneath the peritoneum.
h. fem'inae, h. muliebris; Nuck's h.; accumulation of serous fluid in the labium majus or in Nuck's canal.
filarial h., h. due to microfilaria (chiefly of *Wuchereria bancrofti*) in the tunica vaginalis.

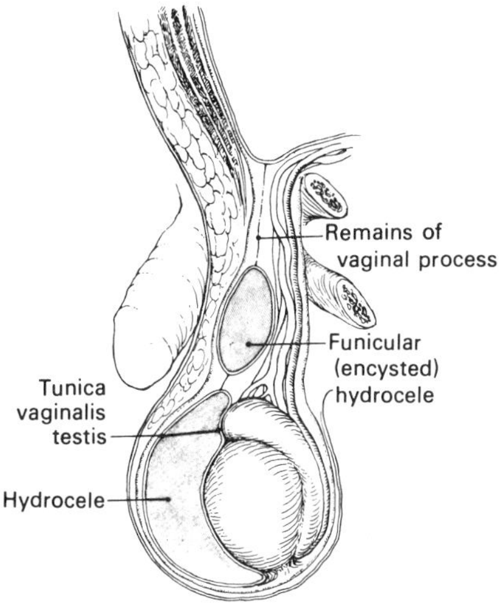

Hydrocele

funicular h., fluid in a portion of the tunica vaginalis shut off from both testis and abdominal cavity.
h. mulie'bris, h. feminae.
Nuck's h., h. feminae.
h. spina'lis, *spina* bifida.

hydrocelectomy (hī'drō-sē-lek'tō-mē) [hydrocele + G. *ektomē,* excision]. Excision of a hydrocele.

hydrocephalic (hī'drō-se-fal'ik). Relating to or suffering from hydrocephalus.

hydrocephalocele (hī-drō-sef'ă-lō-sēl). Hydrencephalocele.

hydrocephaloid (hī-drō-sef'ă-loyd). **1.** Resembling hydrocephalus. **2.** A condition in infants suffering from diarrhea or other debilitating disease, in which there are general symptoms resembling those of hydrocephalus without, however, any abnormal accumulation of cerebrospinal fluid.

hydrocephalus (hī-drō-sef'ă-lŭs) [hydro- + G. *kephalē,* head]. Hydrocephaly. **1.** A condition marked by an excessive accumulation of fluid dilating the cerebral ventricles, thinning brain tissues, and causing separation of cranial bones; termed obstructive h. when caused by obstruction of the third or fourth ventricle or communicating h. when caused by blockage of absorption by pacchionian granulations. **2.** In infants, an accumulation of fluid in the subarachnoid or subdural space.
communicating h., h. in which there is a patent connection between the ventricles of the brain and the subarachnoid space.
congenital h., primary h.; h. due to developmental defect of the brain.
double compartment h., independent supra- and infra-tentorial h. usually due to a veil occlusion of the aqueduct of Sylvius.
external h., **(1)** accumulation of fluid in the subarachnoid spaces of the brain; **(2)** accumulation of fluid in the subdural space due to a persistent communication between the subarachnoid and subdural spaces.
h. ex vac'uo, h. due to loss or atrophy of brain tissue.
internal h., Whytt's disease; h. in which the accumulation of fluid is confined to the ventricles; also occurs as autosomal recessive condition in Hereford and Holstein breeds of cattle.
noncommunicating h., obstructive h.
normal pressure h., occult h.; a type of h. developing usually in older people, due to failure of cerebrospinal fluid to be absorbed by the pacchionian granulations, and characterized clinically by progressive dementia, unsteady gait, and usually a normal spinal fluid pressure.
obstructive h., noncommunicating h.; h. with ventricular block.
occult h., normal pressure h.
otitic h., a form of thrombotic h. associated with otitis media and thrombosis of one or both transverse sinuses of the dura.
postmeningitic h., ventricular dilation following meningitis and secondary to obstruction of cerebrospinal fluid pathways.
posttraumatic h., ventricular dilation following injury, due either to impaired circulation and/or absorption of cerebrospinal fluid or due to loss of brain substance (h. ex vacuo).
primary h., congenital h.
secondary h., an accumulation of fluid in the cranial cavity, due to meningitis or obstruction to the venous flow.
thrombotic h., increase in cerebrospinal fluid and of intracranial pressure following thrombosis of the cerebral veins or sinuses; caused by septic infection, dehydration, tuberculosis, typhoid, leukemia, and other conditions.
toxic h., thrombotic h. associated with some general infection or toxic state.

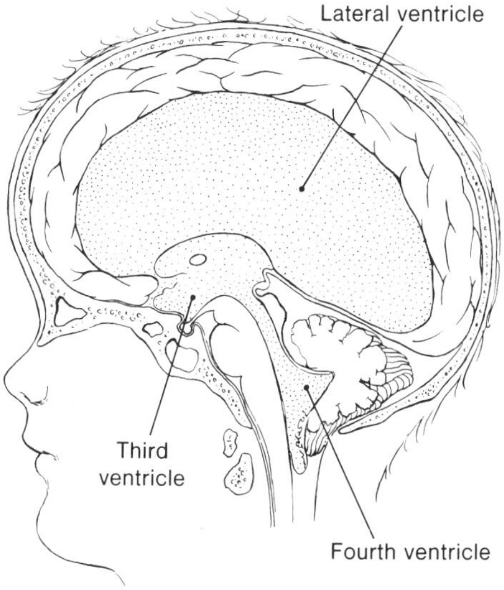

Hydrocephalus

hydrocephaly (hī-drō-sef'ă-lē). Hydrocephalus.

hydrochloric acid (hī-drō-klōr'ik). Muriatic acid; HCl; the acid of gastric juice. The commercial product is used as an escharotic; the gas and the concentrated solution are strong irritants.
diluted h. a., a preparation that contains, in each 100 ml, 10 g of HCl; used internally for achlorhydria.

hydrochloride (hī-drō-klōr'īd). A compound formed by the addition of a hydrochloric acid molecule to an amine or related substance; *e.g.,* guanine hydrochloride.

hydrochlorothiazide (hī'drō-klōr-ō-thī'ă-zīd). 6-Chloro-3,4-dihydro-2*H*-1,2,4-benzothiadiazine-7-sulfonamide 1,1-dioxide; a potent orally effective diuretic and antihypertensive agent related to chlorothiazide.

hydrocholecystis (hī'drō-kō-lē-sis'tis) [hydro- + G. *cholē,* bile, + *kystis,* bladder]. An effusion of serous fluid into the gallbladder.

hydrocholeresis (hī'drō-kō-ler-ē'sis, -kol-er-) [hydro- + G. *cholē,* bile, + *hairesis,* a taking]. Increased output of a watery bile of low specific gravity, viscosity, and solid content.

hydrocholeretic (hī'drō-kō-ler-et'ik). Pertaining to hydrocholeresis.

hydrocirsocele (hī-drō-sir'sō-sēl) [hydro- + G. *kirsos,* varix, + *kēlē,* tumor]. Obsolete term for hydrocele complicated with varicocele.

hydrocodone (hī-drō-kō'dōn). Dihydrocodeinone; a weak analgesic derivative of codeine used principally as an antitussive.

hydrocolloid (hī-drō-kol'oyd). A gelatinous colloid in unstable equilibrium with its contained water, useful in dentistry for impressions because of its dimensional stability under controlled conditions.
irreversible h., a h. whose physical state is changed by an irreversible chemical reaction when water is added to a powder and an insoluble substance is formed.
reversible h., a h. composed of a base substance whose physical state may be changed to that of a liquid by the application of heat and then changed to that of an elastic gel by cooling.

hydrocolpocele, hydrocolpos (hī-drō-kol'pō-sēl, -kol'pos) [hydro- + G. *kolpos,* bosom (vagina)]. Accumulation of mucus or other nonsanguineous fluid in the vagina.

hydrocortamate hydrochloride (hī-drō-kōr'tă-māt). 17-Hydroxycorticosterone-21-diethylaminoacetate hydrochloride; cortisol 21-(*N,N*-diethyl)glycinate hydrochloride; an ester-salt of hydrocortisone, used topically in the treatment of acute and chronic dermatoses.

hydrocortisone (hī-drō-kōr'ti-sōn). Cortisol; 17α-hydroxycorticosterone; 11β,17,21-trihydroxy-4-pregnene-3,20-dione; a reduction product (at C-11) of cortisone; a steroid hormone secreted by the adrenal cortex (the active hormone secreted in the greatest quantity by the adrenals) and the most potent of the naturally occurring glucocorticoids.
h. acetate, cortisol acetate; hydrocortisone 21-acetate; similar actions and uses as h.
h. cyclopentylpropionate, an ester of h.
h. cypionate, the cyclopentanepropionic ester of cortisone, for oral administration.
h. hydrogen succinate, a form of h. administered intravenously.
h. sodium phosphate, hydrocortisone 21-(disodium phosphate); an anti-inflammatory agent for intravenous or intramuscular administration.
h. sodium succinate, a very soluble ester salt of h. (cortisol), used parenterally in the management of emergencies resulting from acute adrenal insufficiency.

hydrocotarnine (hī'drō-kō-tar'nēn). 5,6,7,8-Tetrahydro-4-methoxy-6-methyl-1,3-dioxolo[4,5-*g*]isoquinoline; an alkaloidal principle derived from cotarnine; it is the basic hydrolytic product of narcotine; also obtained from the mother liquors of thebaine.

hydrocupreine (hī-drō-kū'prē-ēn). 10,11-Dihydro-6'-hydroxycinchonan-9-ol; its 6' ethers are used as antiseptics, *e.g.,* euprocin hydrochloride.

hydrocyanic acid (hī'drō-sī-an'ik). Prussic acid; hydrogen cyanide; HCN; a colorless, very toxic liquid, with the odor of bitter almonds, present in bitter almonds (amygdalin), the stones of peaches, plums and other fruits, and laurel leaves; inhalation of 300 p.p.m. causes death.

hydrocyanism (hī-drō-sī'an-izm). Poisoning with hydrocyanic acid.

hydrocyst (hī'drō-sist) [hydro- + G. *kystis,* bladder]. A cyst with clear, watery contents.

hydrocystoma (hī'drō-sis-tō'mă) [hydro- + G. *kystis,* bladder, + -*ōma,* tumor]. **1.** An eruption of deeply seated vesicles, due to retention of fluid in the sweat follicles. **2.** Hidrocystoma.

hydrodipsia (hī-drō-dip'sē-ă) [hydro- + G. *dipsa,* thirst]. Water thirst, a characteristic of animals that ordinarily drink water.

hydrodipsomania (hī'drō-dip'sō-mā'nē-ă) [hydro- + G. *dipsa,* thirst, + *mania,* frenzy]. Periodic episodes of uncontrollable thirst, occasionally found in epileptic patients.

hydrodiuresis (hī'drō-dī-yū-rē'sis). Diuresis effected by water.

hydrodynamics (hī'drō-dī-nam'iks) [hydro- + G. *dynamis,* force]. The branch of physics concerned with the flow of liquids.

hydroencephalocele (hī'drō-en-sef'ă-lō-sēl). Hydrencephalocele.

hydroflumethiazide (hī'drō-flū-mĕ-thī'ă-zīd). 3,4-Dihydro-6-(trifluoromethyl)-2*H*-1,2,4-benzothiadiazine-7-sulfonamide 1,1-dioxide; a diuretic and antihypertensive agent.

hydrofluoric acid (hī-drō-flūr'ik). A solution of hydrogen fluoride gas in water; a poisonous, caustic, foaming liquid that is used to clean metals; extremely irritating to skin and lungs.

hydrogel (hī'drō-jel). A colloid in which the particles are in the external or dispersion phase and water in the internal or dispersed phase. *Cf.* hydrosol.

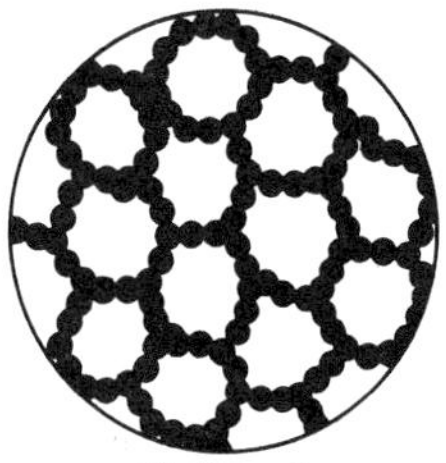

Hydrogel

hydrogen (hī'drō-jen) [hydro- + G. *-gen,* producing]. A gaseous element, symbol H, atomic no. 1, atomic weight 1.0079.
activated h., h. removed by a dehydrogenase, *e.g.,* a flavoprotein, from a metabolite for transference to another substance with which it combines.
arseniureted h., arsine.
h. bromide, HBr; a colorless gas that has a very irritating odor and fumes in moist air; in aqueous solution, it is hydrobromic acid.
h. chloride, HCl; a very soluble gas which, in solution, forms hydrochloric acid.
h. cyanide, hydrocyanic acid.
h. dehydrogenase [EC 1.12.1.2], a hydrogenase enzyme catalyzing the conversion of NAD^+ to NADH by molecular hydrogen (H_2).
h. dioxide, h. peroxide.
heavy h., hydrogen-2.
h. peroxide, h. dioxide; hydroperoxide; H_2O_2; an unstable compound readily broken down to water and oxygen, a reaction catalyzed by various powdered metals and by the enzyme, catalase; a 3% solution is used as a mild antiseptic for skin and mucous membranes.
h. phosphide, phosphine.
phosphureted h., phosphine.
h. sulfide, sulfureted h.; H_2S; a colorless, flammable, toxic gas with a familiar "rotten egg" odor, formed in the decomposition of organic matter containing sulfur; used as a reagent, and in the manufacture of chemicals.
sulfureted h., h. sulfide.

hydrogen-1 (^1H). Protium; the common h. isotope, making up 99.985% of the h. atoms occurring in nature.

hydrogen-2 (^2H). Heavy hydrogen; deuterium; the isotope of h. of atomic weight 2; the less common stable isotope of h. making up 0.015% of the h. atoms occurring in nature.

hydrogen-3 (^3H). Tritium; a hydrogen isotope of mass number 3; weakly radioactive, emitting beta particles to become the stable helium-3; half-life, 12.5 years.

hydrogenase (hī'drō-je-nās, hī-droj'ĕ-nās). Hydrogenlyase; any enzyme that removes molecular hydrogen (H_2) from NADH or adds it to ferricytochrome or to ferredoxin.

hydrogenation (hī'drō-jĕ-nā'shŭn, hī-droj'ĕ-nā-shŭn). Addition of hydrogen to a compound, especially to an unsaturated fat or fatty acid; thus, soft fats or oils are solidified or "hardened."

hydrogen exponent. The logarithm of the hydrogen ion concentration in blood or other fluid; its negative is the pH of that fluid.

hydrogenlyase (hī'drō-gen-lī'ās). Hydrogenase.

hydrokinetic (hī'drō-ki-net'ik). Pertaining to the motion of fluids and the forces giving rise to such motion.

hydrokinetics (hī'drō-ki-net'iks). That branch of kinetics concerned with fluids in motion.

hydrolabile (hī-drō-lā'bil). Unstable in the presence of water.

hydrolability (hī'drō-lă-bil'i-tē). A state in which the fluid in the tissues readily changes in amount.

hydrolabyrinth (hī'drō-lab'i-rinth). Hydrops labyrinthi; excess of endolymph in the inner ear.

hydrolases (hī'drō-lās-ez). Hydrolyzing enzymes (EC class 3); enzymes cleaving substrates with addition of H_2O at the point of cleavage; *e.g.*, esterases, phosphatases, nucleases, peptidases.

hydro-lyases (hī-drō-lī'ās-ēz). A class of lyases (EC 4.2.1) comprising enzymes removing H and OH as water, leading to formation of new double bonds within the affected molecule; the trivial names usually contain dehydratase or hydratase.

hydrolymph (hī'drō-limf). The circulating fluid in many of the invertebrates.

hydrolysate (hī-drol'i-sāt). A solution containing the products of hydrolysis.

hydrolysis (hī-drol'i-sis) [hydro- + G. *lysis*, dissolution]. Hydrolytic cleavage; a chemical process whereby a compound is cleaved into two or more simpler compounds with the uptake of the H and OH parts of a water molecule on either side of the chemical bond cleaved; h. is effected by the action of acids, alkalies, or enzymes. *Cf.* hydration.

hydrolytic (hī-drō-lit'ik). Referring to or causing hydrolysis.

hydrolyze (hī'drō-līz). To subject to hydrolysis.

hydroma (hī-drō'mă). Hygroma.

hydromassage (hī'drō-mă-sahzh). Massage produced by streams of water.

hydromeningocele (hī'drō-men-ing'gō-sēl) [hydro- + G. *mēninx*, membrane, + *kēlē*, hernia]. Protrusion of the meninges of brain or spinal cord through a defect in the bony wall, the sac so formed containing fluid.

hydrometer (hī-drom'ĕ-ter) [hydro- + G. *mĕron*, measure]. Areometer; gravimeter; an instrument for determining the specific gravity of a liquid.

hydrometra (hī-drō-mē'tră) [hydro- + G. *mētra*, uterus]. Accumulation of thin mucus or other watery fluid in the cavity of the uterus.

hydrometric (hī-drō-met'rik). Relating to hydrometry or the hydrometer.

hydrometrocolpos (hī'drō-mē-trō-kol'pos) [hydro- + G. *mētra*, uterus, + *kolpos*, bosom (vagina)]. Distention of uterus and vagina by fluid other than blood or pus.

hydrometry (hī-drom'ĕ-trē). Determination of the specific gravity of a fluid by means of a hydrometer.

hydromicrocephaly (hī'drō-mī-krō-sef'ă-lē). Microcephaly associated with an increased amount of cerebrospinal fluid.

hydromorphone hydrochloride (hī-drō-mōr'fōn). Dihydromorphinone hydrochloride; a synthetic derivative of morphine, with analgesic potency about 10 times that of morphine.

hydromphalus (hī-drom'fă-lŭs) [hydro- + G. *omphalos*, umbilicus]. A cystic tumor at the umbilicus, most commonly a vitello-intestinal cyst.

hydromyelia (hī-drō-mī-ē'lē-ă) [hydro- + G. *myelos*, marrow]. An increase of fluid in the dilated central canal of the spinal cord, or in congenital cavities elsewhere in the cord substance.

hydromyelocele (hī-drō-mī'ĕ-lō-sēl) [hydro- + G. *myelos*, marrow, + *kēlē*, tumor, hernia]. Protrusion of a portion of cord, thinned out into a sac distended with cerebrospinal fluid, through a spina bifida.

hydromyoma (hī'drō-mī-ō'mă). A leiomyoma that contains cystlike foci of proteinaceous fluid; h.'s occur more frequently in leiomyomas of the uterus, as a result of degenerative changes.

hydronephrosis (hī'drō-ne-frō'sis) [hydro- + G. *nephros*, kidney, + *-osis*, condition]. Nephrohydrosis; uronephrosis; dilation of the pelvis and calices of one or both kidneys resulting from obstruction to the flow of urine.

hydronephrotic (hī'drō-ne-frot'ik). Relating to hydronephrosis.

hydroparasalpinx (hī'drō-par-ă-sal'pinks) [hydro- + G. *para*, beside, + *salpinx*, trumpet]. Accumulation of serous fluid in the accessory tubes of the oviduct.

hydropathic (hī-drō-path'ik). Relating to hydropathy.

hydropathy (hī-drop'ă-thē). The obsolete use of water to treat and cure disease.

hydropenia (hī-drō-pē'nē-ă) [hydro- + G. *penia*, poverty]. Reduction or deprivation of water.

hydropenic (hī-drō-pē'nik). Pertaining to or characterized by hydropenia.

hydropericarditis (hī'drō-pār-i-kar-dī'tis). Pericarditis with a large serous effusion.

hydropericardium (hī'drō-pār-i-kar'dē-ŭm). Cardiac dropsy; a noninflammatory accumulation of fluid in the pericardial sac.

hydroperitoneum, hydroperitonia (hī'drō-pār-i-tō-nē'ŭm, -tō'nē-ă) [hydro- + peritoneum]. Ascites.

hydroperoxidases (hī'drō-per-oks'i-dā-sez). Those oxidoreductases that require H_2O_2 as hydrogen acceptors; *e.g.*, peroxidases, catalase.

hydroperoxide (hī'drō-per-ok'sīd). *Hydrogen* peroxide.

hydrophil, hydrophile (hī'drō-fil, -fīl). Hydrophilic.

hydrophilia (hī-drō-fil'ē-ă) [hydro- + G. *philos*, fond]. A tendency of the blood and tissues to absorb fluid.

hydrophilic (hī-drō-fil'ik). Hydrophil; hydrophile; hydrophilous; denoting the property of attracting or associating with water molecules, possessed by polar radicals or ions, as opposed to hydrophobic (2).

hydrophilous (hī-drof'i-lŭs). Hydrophilic.

hydrophobia (hī-drō-fō'bē-ă) [hydro- + G. *phobos*, fear]. Rabies in humans; a coinage based on exaggerated folklore depictions.

hydrophobic (hī-drō-fōb'ik). **1.** Relating to or suffering from hydrophobia. **2.** Lacking an affinity for water molecules, as opposed to hydrophilic.

hydrophorograph (hī'drō-fōr'ō-graf) [G. *hydrophoros*, carrying water, + *graphō*, to record]. An instrument for recording the flow or pressure of a fluid; *e.g.*, the flow of urine or the pressure of spinal fluid.

hydrophthalmia, hydrophthalmos, hydrophthalmus (hī'drof-thal'mē-ă, -thal'mos) [hydro- + G. *ophthalmos*, eye]. Bupthalmia.

Hydrophyidae (hī-drō-fī'i-de). A family of snakes, the true sea snakes, characterized hydrophobia. a vertically compressed tail, giving it a paddle- or oarlike appearance; their fangs, like those of cobras, are small, grooved, and permanently erect. They are common in shallow waters along coastal margins in many regions of the Pacific basin and are important medically in western Malaysia and coastal Vietnam. There are 52 known species, all venomous, but few bite humans.

hydropic (hī-drop′ik). Dropsical; containing an excess of water or of watery fluid.

hydropneumatosis (hī-drō-nū-mă-tō′sis) [hydro- + G. *pneuma,* breath, spirit]. Combined emphysema and edema; the presence of liquid and gas in tissues.

hydropneumogony (hī′drō-nū-mō′gō-nē) [hydro- + G. *pneuma,* air, + *gony,* knee]. Injection of air into a joint to determine the amount of effusion.

hydropneumopericardium (hī-drō-nū′mō-per-i-kar′dē-ŭm) [hydro- + G. *pneuma,* air, + pericardium]. Pneumohydropericardium; the presence of a serous effusion and of gas in the pericardial sac.

hydropneumoperitoneum (hī-drō-nū′mō-păr-i-tō-nē′ŭm) [hydro- + G. *pneuma,* air, + peritoneum]. Pneumohydroperitoneum; the presence of gas and serous fluid in the peritoneal cavity.

hydropneumothorax (hī′drō-nū-mō-thōr′aks) [hydro- + G. *pneuma,* air, + thorax]. Pneumohydrothorax; pneumoserothorax; the presence of both gas and fluids in the pleural cavity.

hydroposia (hī-drō-pō′zē-ă) [hydro- + G. *posis,* drinking]. Water-drinking, a characteristic of animals that ordinarily drink water.

hydrops (hī′drops) [G. *hydrōps*]. An excessive accumulation of clear, watery fluid in any of the tissues or cavities of the body; synonymous, according to its character and location, with ascites, anasarca, edema, etc.
h. artic′uli, hydrarthrosis.
endolymphatic h., Ménière's *disease.*
fetal h., h. fetal′is, abnormal accumulation of serous fluid in the fetal tissues, as in erythroblastosis fetalis.
h. follic′uli, accumulation of fluid in a graafian follicle.
immune fetal h., fetal edema and ascites secondary to maternal/-fetal blood group incompatibility.
h. labyrin′thi, hydrolabyrinth.
nonimmune fetal h., fetal edema and ascites unrelated to maternal/fetal blood group incompatibilities.
h. ova′rii, hydrovarium.
h. tu′bae, hydrosalpinx.
h. tu′bae pro′fluens, intermittent hydrosalpinx.

hydropyonephrosis (hī′drō-pī′ō-ne-frō′sis) [hydro- + G. *pyon,* pus, + nephrosis]. Presence of purulent urine in the pelvis and calices of the kidney following obstruction of the ureter.

hydroquinol (hī-drō-kwin′ol). Hydroquinone.

hydroquinone (hī-drō-kwin′ōn). Hydroquinol; quinol; 1,4-benzenediol; *p*-dihydroxybenzene; an antioxidant used in ointment.

hydrorchis (hī-drōr′kis) [hydro- + G. *orchis,* testicle]. A collection of water (hydrocele) in the testis, as in the tunica vaginalis or along the spermatic cord.

hydrorheostat (hī-drō-rē′ō-stat). A rheostat in which resistance to the flow of electric current is provided by water.

hydrorrhea (hī-drō-rē′ă) [hydro- + G. *rhoia,* flow]. A profuse discharge of watery fluid from any part.
h. grav′idae, h. gravida′rum, discharge of a watery fluid from the vagina during pregnancy.
nasal h., seldom used term for rhinorrhea.

hydrosalpinx (hī-drō-sal′pinks) [hydro- + G. *salpinx,* trumpet]. Hydrops tubae; accumulation of serous fluid in the fallopian tube, often an end result of pyosalpinx.
intermittent h., hydrops tubae profluens; intermittent discharge of watery fluid from the oviduct.

hydrosarca (hī-drō-sar′kă) [hydro- + G. *sarx,* flesh]. Anasarca.

hydrosarcocele (hī-drō-sar′kō-sēl) [hydro- + G. *sarx,* flesh, + *kēlē,* tumor]. A chronic swelling of the testis complicated with hydrocele.

hydrosol (hī′dro-sol). A colloid in aqueous solution, the particles being in the dispersed or internal phase and the water in the external or dispersion phase. *Cf.* hydrogel.

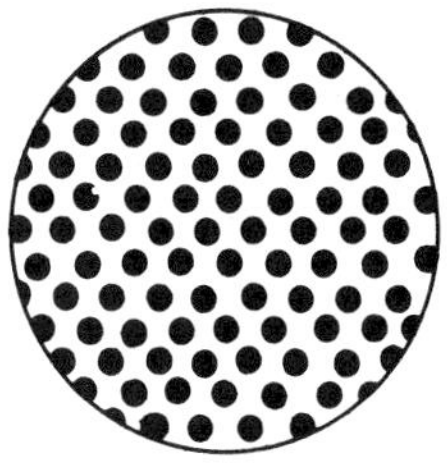

Hydrosol

hydrosphygmograph (hī-drō-sfig′mō-graf). A sphygmograph in which the pulse beat is transmitted to the recorder through a column of water.

hydrostat (hī′drō-stat) [hydro- + G. *statikos,* causing to stand]. A device for regulating water level.

hydrostatic (hī-drō-stat′ik). Relating to the pressure of fluids or to their properties when in equilibrium.

hydrosudopathy (hī′drō-sū-dop′ă-thē) [hydro- + L. *sudor,* sweat, + G. *pathos,* suffering]. Hydrosudotherapy.

hydrosudotherapy (hī′drō-sū′dō-thār′ă-pē). Hydrosudopathy; hydrotherapy combined with induced sweating, as in the Turkish bath.

hydrosyringomyelia (hī′drō-sĭ-rin′gō-mī-ē′lē-ă) [hydro- + G. *hydōr,* water, + *syrinx,* a tube, + *myelos,* marrow]. Syringomyelia.

hydrotaxis (hī-drō-tak′sis) [hydro- + G. *taxis,* arrangement]. The movement of cells or organisms in relation to water.

hydrotherapeutic (hī′drō-thār′ă-pyū′tik). Hydriatric.

hydrotherapeutics (hī′drō-thār′ă-pyū′tiks). Hydrotherapy.

hydrotherapy (hī-drō-thār′ă-pē) [hydro- + G. *therapeia,* therapy]. Hydrotherapeutics; therapeutic use of water by external application, either for its pressure effect or as a means of applying physical energy to the tissues.

hydrothermal (hī-drō-ther′măl) [hydro- + G. *thermē,* heat]. Relating to hot water.

hydrothionemia (hī′drō-thī-ō-nē′mē-ă) [hydro- + G. *theion,* sulfur, + *haima,* blood]. The presence of hydrogen sulfide in the circulating blood.

hydrothionuria (hī′drō-thī-ō-nū′rē-ă) [hydro- + G. *theion,* sulfur, + *ouron,* urine]. The excretion of hydrogen sulfide in the urine.

hydrothorax (hī-drō-thōr′aks). Pleurorrhea; serothorax; presence of serous fluid in one or both pleural cavities, usually resulting from cardiac failure and passive congestion of the lungs; h. is not considered to include conditions in which the effusion is associated with inflammatory reactions.
chylous h., chylothorax.

hydrotomy (hī-drot′ō-mē) [hydro- + G. *tomē,* a cutting]. In histology, tearing apart the tissue elements by injection of water.

hydrotropism (hī-drot′rō-pizm, hī-drō-trō′pizm) [hydro- + G. *tropos,* a turning]. The property in growing organisms of turning toward a moist surface (**positive h.**) or away from a moist surface (**negative h.**).

hydrotubation (hī′drō-tū-bā′shŭn). Injection of a liquid medication or saline solution through the cervix into the uterine cavity and fallopian tubes for dilation and medication of the tubes.

hydroureter (hī′drō-yū-rē′ter, -yūr′ē-ter). Uroureter; distention of the ureter with urine, due to blockage from any cause.

hydrous (hī′drŭs). Hydrated.

hydrovarium (hī-drō-vā'rē-ŭm). Hydrops ovarii; a collection of fluid in the ovary.

hydroxamic acids (hī-drok-sam'ik). R-CO-NH-OH; hydroxylamine derivatives of carboxylic acids, including amino acids, formed by the action of hydroxylamine.

hydroxide (hī-drok'sīd). A compound containing a potentially ionizable hydroxyl group; particularly a compound that liberates OH^- upon dissolving in water.

hydroxocobalamin (hī-drok'sō-kō-bal'ă-min). Hydroxocobemine; vitamin B_{12b}, differing from cyanocobalamin (vitamin B_{12}) in the presence of a hydroxyl ion in place of the cyanide ion. See also *vitamin* B_{12}.

hydroxocobemine (hī-drok'sō-kō-bē-mēn). Hydroxocobalamin.

hydroxy-. Prefix indicating addition or substitution of the –OH group to or in the compound whose name follows. See also oxa-, oxo-, oxy- (6).

hydroxy acid (hī-drok'sē). An organic acid containing both OH and COOH groups; *e.g.,* lactic acid.

3-**hydroxyacyl-CoA dehydrogenase** (hī-drok'sē-as'il) [EC 1.1.1.35]. β-Ketoreductase; β-ketohydrogenase; β-hydroxyacyl dehydrogenase; enzyme catalyzing the oxidation of a 3-hydroxyacyl-CoA to a 3-ketoacyl-CoA with reduction of NAD; one of the enzymes of the fatty acid oxidation cycle.

hydroxyacylglutathione hydrolase (hī-drok'sē-as'il-glū-tă-thī'ōn) [EC 3.1.2.6]. Glyoxalase II; an enzyme with catalytic activity similar to that of lactoylglutathione lyase, but more general.

hydroxyamphetamine hydrobromide (hī-drok'sē-am-fet'ă-mēn hī-drō-brō'mīd). α-Methyltyramine hydrobromide; *p*-(2-aminopropyl)phenol hydrobromide; a sympathomimetic, decongestant, and mydriatic.

hydroxyapatite (hī-drok'sē-ap-ă-tīt). Hydroxylapatite; $3Ca_3(PO_4)_2 \cdot Ca(OH)_2$; a natural mineral structure that the crystal lattice of bones and teeth closely resembles; used in chromatography of nucleic acids.

γ-**hydroxybutyric acid** (hī-drok'sē-byū-tir'ik). 4-Hydroxybutyric acid; $HOCH_2(CH_2)_2COOH$; a sedative and hypnotic formerly used as an intravenous anesthetic, especially in Europe.

hydroxycarbamide (hī-drok'sē-kar'bă-mīd). Hydroxyurea.

hydroxychloroquine sulfate (hī-drok'sē-klōr'ō-kwīn). A quinoline derivative; an antimalarial agent whose actions and uses resemble those of chloroquine phosphate; also used in the treatment of lupus erythematosus and rheumatoid arthritis.

25-**hydroxycholecalciferol** (hī-drok'sē-kō'lē-kal-sif'er-ol). Calcidiol.

hydroxychroman (hī-drok-sē-krō'man). Chromanol.

hydroxychromene (hī-drok-sē-krō'mēn). Chromenol.

hydroxyephedrine (hī-drok'sē-fed'rēn). *p*-Hydroxy-α[1-(methylamino)ethyl]benzyl alcohol; a sympathomimetic agent for the treatment of shock.

hydroxyhemin (hī-drok-sē-hē'min). Hematin.

hydroxykynureninuria (hī-drok'sē-kī-nū'rē-ni-nū'rē-ă). An abnormality in tryptophan metabolism, probably due to a defect in kynureninase, characterized by mild mental retardation, migrane-like headaches, and urinary excretion of large amounts of kynurenine, kynurenine-3-monooxygenase, and xanthurenic acid; autosomal recessive inheritance.

hydroxyl (hī-drok'sil). The radical, –OH.

hydroxylamine (hī-drok'sil-ă'mēn). Oxammonium; NH_2OH; a partially oxidized derivative of ammonia; reacts with carbonyl groups to produce oximes; forms acid salts, *e.g.,* h. hydrochloride ($HONH_2.HCl$ or $HONH_3Cl$).

h. reductase [EC 1.7.99.1], an enzyme catalyzing reduction of h. to ammonia with a variety of donors (*e.g.,* methylene blue, flavin). See also NADH-hydroxylamine reductase.

hydroxylamino (hī-drok'sil-am-i-nō). The monovalent group, –NH-OH.

hydroxylapatite (hī-drok'sil-ap-ă-tīt). Hydroxyapatite.

hydroxylases (hī-drok'si-lā-sez). Enzymes catalyzing formation of hydroxyl groups by addition of an oxygen atom, hence oxidizing the substrate; most are found in EC subclass 1.14.

hydroxylation (hī-drok-si-lā'shŭn). Placing of a hydroxyl group on a compound in a position where one did not exist before.

p-**hydroxymercuribenzoate** (hī-drok'sē-mer'kyū-rē-ben'zō-āt). An organic mercurial, $HOHgC_6H_4COO^-$, formed spontaneously by hydrolysis of the *p*-chloro compound. See also *p*-mercuribenzoate.

hydroxynervone (hī-drok-sē-ner'vōn). Oxynervone; a cerebroside containing α-hydroxynervonic acid.

hydroxyphenamate (hī-drok'sē-fen'ă-māt). 2-Hydroxy-2-phenylbutyl carbamate; a tranquilizer.

hydroxyphenyluria (hī-drok'sē-fen-il-ū'rē-ă). Urinary excretion of tyrosine and phenylalanine, as a result of ascorbic acid deficiency; occurs notably in those premature infants who lack this vitamin.

17α-**hydroxyprogesterone** (hī-drok'sē-prō-jes'ter-ōn). 17α-Hydroxy-4-pregnen-3,20-dione; medical use is similar to that of progesterone. The acetate is an orally effective derivative, useful in conditions in which parenterally administered progesterone or the caproate is indicated; it possesses some androgenic potency and may cause virilizing changes in a female fetus. The caproate or hexanoate has essentially the same actions and uses as progesterone, but is more potent and has a longer duration of action.

21-**hydroxyprogesterone.** Deoxycorticosterone.

hydroxyprogesterone hexanoate. 17α-Hydroxyprogesterone caproate.

hydroxyproline (hī-drok-sē-prō'lēn). 4-Hydroxy-2-pyrrolidinecarboxylic acid; an imino acid found among the hydrolysis products of collagen; not found in proteins other than those of connective tissue.

hydroxyprolinemia (hī-drok'sē-prō-li-nē'mē-ă). A metabolic disorder characterized by enhanced plasma concentrations and urinary excretion of free hydroxyproline, and associated with severe mental retardation; autosomal recessive inheritance.

15-**hydroxyprostaglandin dehydrogenase** (hī-drok'sē-pros-tă-glan'din) [EC 1.1.1.141]. An enzyme that catalyzes the oxidation of prostaglandins, rendering them inactive, by converting the 15-hydroxyl group to a keto group.

8-**hydroxyquinoline sulfate** (hī-drok'sē-kwin'ō-lēn). An antiseptic, antiperspirant, and deodorant.

hydroxystilbamidine isethionate (hī-drok'sē-stil-bam'i-dēn). 2-Hydroxy-4,4'-stilbenedicarboxamidine di-β-hydroxyethanesulfonate; an antifungal and antiprotozoan agent used in the treatment of the nonprogressive cutaneous form of blastomycosis.

hydroxytoluic acid (hī-drok'sē-tō-lū'ik). Mandelic acid.

5-**hydroxytryptamine (5HT)** (hī-drok-sē-trip'tă-mēn). Serotonin.

hydroxytryptophan decarboxylase (hī-drok-sē-trip'tō-fan). Aromatic L-amino-acid decarboxylase.

3-**hydroxytyramine** (hī-drok-sē-tī'ră-mēn). Dopamine.

hydroxyurea (hī-drok'sē-yū-rē'ă). Hydroxycarbamide; H_2NO-CONHOH; an antineoplastic agent.

hydroxyzine (hī-drok'si-zēn). $C_{21}H_{27}ClN_2O_2$; a mild sedative and minor tranquilizer used in neuroses; available as the hydrochloride and pamoate.

Hydrozoa (hī-drō-zō'ă) [hydro- + G. *zōon,* animal]. A class of coelenterates or jellyfishes, including *Hydra,* a freshwater polyp, *Phy-*

salia, the "Portuguese man-of-war," *Millepora,* a stinging coral, and the sea wasps, *Chironex Heckeri* and *Chiropsalmus quadrigatus,* whose stings can cause severe wheals, pain, and skin necrosis, and occasionally rapid death from respiratory and cardiac depression.

hydruria (hī-drū'rē-ă) [hydro- + G. *ouron,* urine]. Polyuria.

hydruric (hī-drū'rik). Relating to polyuria.

hygieiolatry (hī-jē-yol'ă-trē) [G. *hygieia,* health, + *latreia,* worship]. Rarely used term for an extreme observance of the principles of hygiene.

hygieiology (hī-jē-yol'ō-jē) [G. *hygieia,* health, + *-logia*]. The science of hygiene and sanitation, and the practice thereof.

hygieist (hī'jē-ist) [G. *hygieia,* health]. Hygienist.

hygiene (hi'jēn) [G. *hygieinos,* healthful, fr. *hygiēs,* healthy]. **1.** The science of health and its maintenance. **2.** Cleanliness that promotes health and well being, especially of a personal nature.
criminal h., the branch of mental h. or penology devoted to the study of the causes and prevention of criminality and the treatment of criminals.
mental h., the science and practice of maintaining and restoring mental health; a branch of psychiatry that has become an interdisciplinary field including subspecialties in psychology, nursing, social work, law, and other professions.
oral h., the cleaning of the mouth by means of brushing, flossing, irrigating, massaging, or the use of other devices. See also oral *physiotherapy.*

hygienic (hī-jen'ik, hī-jē-en'ik). Healthful; relating to hygiene; tending to maintain health.

hygienist (hī-jē'nist, hī'jē-en-ist). Hygiest; one who is skilled in the science of health.
dental h., a licensed, professional auxiliary in dentistry who is both an oral health educator and clinician, and who uses preventive, therapeutic, and educational methods for the control of oral diseases.

hygr-. See hygro-.

hygric (hī'grik) [G. *hygros,* moist]. Relating to moisture.

hygric acid. *N*-methylproline, the methylbetaine of which is stachydrine.

hygro-, hygr- [G. *hygros,* moist]. Combining forms meaning moist, relating to moisture or humidity.

hygroma (hī-grō'mă) [hygro- + G. *-oma,* tumor]. Hydroma; a cystic swelling containing a serous fluid, such as cystic lymphangioma, housemaid's knee, etc.
h. axilla're, h. of the axillary region.
cervical h., h. colli cysticum.
h. col'li cys'ticum, cervical h.; a benign cystic overgrowth of lymphatics of the neck, present at birth, which may form a large tumor-like mass.
subdural h., accumulation in the subdural space of proteinaceous fluid, usually derived from serum, or of cerebrospinal fluid due to a tear in the arachnoid membrane.

hygrometer (hī-grom'ĕ-ter) [hygro- + G. *metron,* measure]. Any device for measuring the water vapor in the atmosphere, usually indicating relative humidity directly.

hygrometry (hī-grom'ĕ-trē). Psychrometry.

hygrophobia (hī-grō-fō'bē-ă) [hygro- + G. *phobos,* fear]. Morbid fear of dampness or moisture.

hygroscopic (hī-grō-skop'ik). Denoting a substance capable of readily absorbing and retaining moisture; *e.g.,* NaOH, $CaCl_2$.

hygrostomia (hī'grō-stō'mē-ă) [hygro- + G. *stoma,* mouth]. Sialism.

Hyl Symbol for hydroxylysine or hydroxylysyl.

hyla (hī'lă). A lateral extension of the cerebral (or sylvian) aqueduct.

hylephobia (hī-lē-fō'bē-ă) [G. *hylē,* forest, + *phobos,* fear]. Morbid fear of forests.

hylic (hī'lik) [G. *hylikos* fr. *hylē,* matter]. Of or pertaining to essential matter; obsolete term denoting the pulp tissue of the embryo.

hyloma (hī-lō'mă) [G. *hylē,* stuff, crude matter, + *-oma,* tumor]. Hylic tumor; a neoplasm of pulp tissue, resulting from proliferation of elements derived from the embryonic pulp of epiblastic origin.
mesenchymal h., a neoplasm of tissue derived from the mesoblastic pulp or mesenchyme.
mesothelial h., a neoplasm derived from tissue of mesothelial origin.

hymen (hī'men) [G. *hymēn,* membrane] [NA]. Virginal membrane; a thin crescentic or annular membranous fold partly occluding the vaginal external orifice in the virgin.

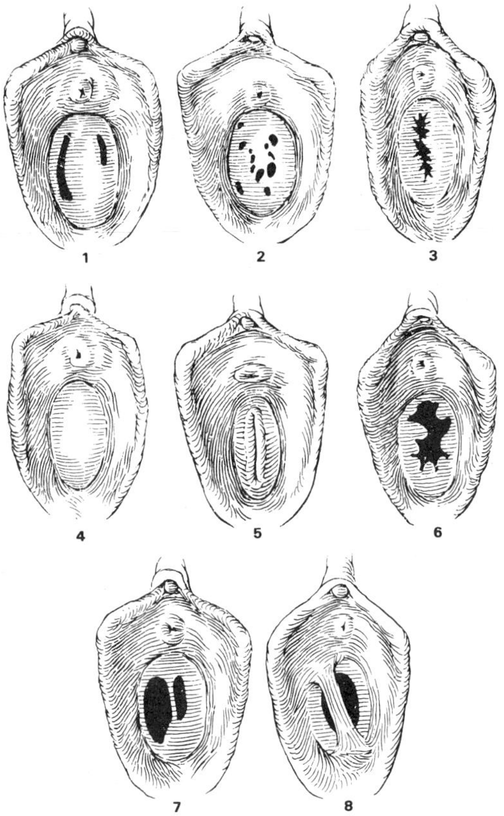

Various Forms of the Hymen
1, Bifenestratus; *2,* cribriform; *3,* denticulate; *4,* imperforate; *5,* infundibuliform; *6,* sculptatus; *7,* septate; *8,* subseptus.

h. bifenestra'tus, h. bifo'ris, a h. in which there are two openings separated by a wide septum. *Cf.* h. septus.
cribriform h., a h. with a number of small perforations.
denticulate h., a h. with markedly serrated edges.
imperforate h., a h. in which there is no opening, the membrane completely occluding the vagina.
infundibuliform h., a projecting, funnel-shaped h. with a central opening with sloping edges.
h. sculpta'tus, a h. with markedly uneven and ragged edges.
septate h., a h. in which there are two openings separated by a narrow band of tissue. *Cf.* h. bifenestratus.

h. subsep'tus, a h. in which the opening is partly closed by a septum.

vertical h., a h. in which the opening is perpendicular.

hymenal (hī'men-ăl). Relating to the hymen.

hymenectomy (hī-me-nek'tō-mē) [G. *hymēn,* membrane, + *ektomē,* excision]. Excision of the hymen.

hymenitis (hī-me-nī'tis). Inflammation of the hymen.

hymenoid (hī'men-oyd). **1.** Membranous. **2.** Resembling the hymen.

hymenolepiasis (hī'me-nō-lĕ-pī'ă-sis). Illness produced by infection with *Hymenolepis.*

hymenolepidid (hī'men-ō-lep'i-did). Common name for tapeworms of the family Hymenolepididae.

Hymenolepididae (hī'men-ō-lep'i-did-ē) [G. *hymēn,* membrane, + *lepis,* rind]. A family of tapeworms (order Cyclophyllidea) that includes the medically important genus *Hymenolepis.*

Hymenolepis (hī-me-nol'ĕ-pis) [G. *hymēn,* membrane, + *lepis,* rind]. The largest genus (family Hymenolepididae) of tapeworms in the order Cyclophyllidea; especially common parasites of rodents, shrews, and aquatic birds.

H. diminu'ta, a tapeworm species of rats and mice, rarely found in man; its cysticercoid larvae are harbored by beetles, fleas, caterpillars, and other insects.

H. lanceola'ta, a tapeworm of aquatic birds, rarely found in man.

H. na'na, the dwarf or dwarf mouse tapeworm; a small tapeworm of man, sometimes found in great numbers in the intestine; the cysticercoid can develop by two pathways: in the final host, with the egg from one human directly infective to another human host, in which both larval and adult stages occur, or through two hosts, an insect (or crustacean) intermediate and a vertebrate final host, the obligate two-host cycle of most cyclophylidean cestodes; in addition, *H. nana,* can internally reinfect the same human or rodent host, producing a massive reinfection.

H. na'na, var. **frater'na,** a race, strain, or subspecies of *H. nana* adapted to mice, although infectivity to humans may remain; the human form, *H. nana,* presumably is derived from the rodent strain.

hymenology (hī-mĕ-nol'ō-jē) [G. *hymēn,* membrane, + *logos,* study]. The branch of anatomy and physiology concerned with the membranes of the body.

Hymenoptera (hī-me-nop'ter-ă) [G. *hymēn,* membrane, + *pteron,* wing]. An order of insects, including bees, wasps, and ants, characterized by locked pairs of membranous wings and high development of social or colonial behavior.

hymenorrhaphy (hī-me-nōr'ă-fē) [G. *hymēn,* membrane, + *raphē,* a suture]. Suture of the hymen in order to close the vagina.

hymenotomy (hī-me-not'ō-mē) [G. *hymēn,* membrane, + *tomē,* incision]. Surgical division of a hymen.

Hynes, Wilfred, British plastic surgeon, *1903. See Anderson-H. *pyeloplasty.*

hyo- [G. *hyoeides,* shaped like the letter upsilon, υ]. Combining form meaning U-shaped, or hyoid.

hyoepiglottic (hī'ō-ep-i-glot'ik). Hyoepiglottidean; relating to the hyoid bone and the epiglottis; denoting the elastic h. ligament connecting the two structures.

hyoepiglottidean (hī'ō-ep-i-glo-tid'ē-an). Hyoepiglottic.

hyoglossal (hī'ō-glos'ăl). Glossohyal; relating to the hyoid bone and the tongue.

hyoglossus (hī'ō-glos'ŭs). *Musculus* hyoglossus.

hyoid (hī'oyd) [G. *hyoeidēs,* shaped like the letter upsilon, υ]. U-shaped or V-shaped; denoting the *os* hyoideum and the *apparatus* hyoideus.

hyopharyngeus (hī'ō-far'in-jē'ŭs). See *musculus* constrictor pharyngis medius.

hyoscine (hī'ō-sēn). Scopolamine.

h. hydrobromide, *scopolamine* hydrobromide.

hyoscyamine (hī-ō-sī'ă-mēn). Daturine; *l*- tropine tropate; an alkaloid found in hyoscyamus, belladonna, duboisine, and stramonium; the levorotatory component of the racemic mixture, atropine; used as an antispasmodic, analgesic, and sedative; h. hydrobromide is used for the same purposes.

h. sulfate, an antispasmodic, hypnotic, and sedative, also used in parkinsonism to relieve tremor, rigidity, and excessive salivation.

***dl*-hyoscyamine.** Atropine.

hyoscyamus (hī-ō-sī'ă-mŭs) [G. *hyoskyamos,* henbane or hog's bean, fr. *hys,* gen. *hyos,* a hog, + *kyamos,* a bean]. Henbane; the leaves and flowering tops of *Hyoscyamus niger* (family Solanaceae); it contains hyoscyamine and hyoscine (scopolamine); an anticholinergic and antispasmodic.

Hyostrongylus rubidus (hī-ō-stron'ji-lŭs rū'bi-dŭs) [G. *hys,* gen. *hyos,* a hog, + *strongylos,* round]. The red stomach worm of swine; a small reddish trichostrongyle nematode that burrows into the mucosa of the fundus of the pig stomach and sucks blood; moderate numbers appear to cause little damage unless the animal's resistance is lowered by other factors.

hyothyroid (hī'ō-thī'royd). See *membrana* thyrohyoidea.

hyp-. Variation of the prefix hypo-, often used before a vowel.

hypacusia (hī'pă-kū'zē-ă, hip'ă-). Hypacusis.

hypacusis (hī'pă-kū'sis, hip'ă-) [hypo- + G. *akousis,* hearing]. Hypacusia; hypoacusis; hearing impairment of a conductive or neurosensory nature.

hypalbuminemia (hī'pal-byū-mi-nē'mē-ă, hip'al-) [G. *hypo,* under, + albuminemia]. Hypoalbuminemia.

hypalgesia (hī'pal-jē'zē-ă, hīp'al-) [G. *hypo,* under, + *algēsis,* sense of pain]. Hypalgia; hypoalgesia; decreased sensibility to pain.

hypalgesic, hypalgetic (hī'pal-jē'sik, -jet'ik, hip'al-). Relating to hypalgesia; having diminished sensitiveness to pain.

hypalgia (hī-pal'jē-ă, hip-al') [G. *hypo,* under, + *algos,* pain]. Hypalgesia.

hypamnion, hypamnios (hī-pam'nē-on, -nē-os) [G. *hypo,* under, + amnion]. Presence of an abnormally small amount of amniotic fluid.

hypanakinesia, hypanakinesis (hī-pan'ă-ki-nē'sē-ă, -kin-ē'sis) [G. *hypo,* under, + *anakinēsis,* a to- and fro- movement]. Diminution in the normal gastric or intestinal movements.

hyparterial (hī'par-tēr'ē-ăl, hip'-ar-) [G. *hypo,* beneath, + *artēria,* artery]. Below or beneath an artery.

hypaxial (hī-pak'sē-ăl, hip-ak') [G. *hypo,* beneath, + axis]. Below any axis, such as the spinal axis or the axis of a limb.

hypazoturia (hī'paz-ō-tū'rē-ă). Hypoazoturia.

hypencephalon (hī'pen-sef'ă-lon) [G. *hypo,* under, + *enkephalos,* brain]. The midbrain, pons, and medulla.

hypengyophobia (hī-pen'gī-ō-fō'bē-ă) [G. *hypengyos,* responsible, + *phobos,* fear]. Morbid fear of responsibility.

hyper- [G. *hyper,* above, over]. Prefix denoting excessive or above the normal; corresponds to L. *super-.*

hyperacanthosis (hī'per-ă-kan-thō'sis). Acanthosis.

hyperacid (hī-per-as'id). Superacid; having an excessive concentration of acid.

hyperacidity (hī'per-a-sid'i-tē). An abnormally high degree of acidity, as of the gastric juice.

hyperactivity (hī'per-ak-tiv'i-tē). **1.** Superactivity. **2.** General restlessness or excessive movement such as that characterizing children with attention deficit disorder or hyperkinesis.

hyperacusis, hyperacusia (hī'per-ă-kū'sis, -kū'sē-ă) [hyper- + G. *akousis*, a hearing]. Auditory hyperesthesia; abnormal acuteness of hearing due to increased irritability of the sensory neural mechanism.

hyperadenosis (hī'per-ad-ĕ-nō'sis) [hyper- + G. *adēn*, gland, + *-ōsis*, condition]. Glandular enlargement, especially of the lymphatic glands.

hyperadiposis, hyperadiposity (hī'per-ad-i-pō'sis, -pos'i-tē). An extreme degree of adiposis or fatness.

hyperadrenalcorticalism (hī'per-ă-drē'năl-kōr'ti-kăl-izm). Hypercorticoidism.

hyperadrenocorticalism (hī'per-ă-drē'nō-kōr'ti-kăl-izm). Hypercorticoidism.

hyperaldosteronism (hī'per-al-dos'ter-on-izm). Aldosteronism.

hyperalgesia (hī-per-al-jē'zē-ă) [hyper- + G. *algos*, pain]. Hyperalgia; extreme sensitiveness to painful stimuli.
auditory h., painful reaction to noises not ordinarily unpleasant.

hyperalgesic, hyperalgetic (hī'per-al-jē'sik, -jet'ik). Relating to hyperalgesia.

hyperalgia (hī'per-al'jē-ă). Hyperalgesia.

hyperalimentation (hī'per-al'i-men-tā'shŭn). Superalimentation; suralimentation; administration or consumption of nutrients beyond minimum normal requirements, in an attempt to replace nutritional deficiencies.
parenteral h., h. by intravenous administration of nutrients in greater than normal concentrations.

hyperallantoinuria (hī'per-ă-lan'tō-i-nū'rē-ă). Increased excretion of allantoin in the urine.

hyperaminoaciduria (hī'per-am'i-nō-as-i-dū'rē-ă). Aminoaciduria.

hyperammonemia (hī'per-am-ō-nē'mē-ă). See ammoniemia.
cerebroatrophic h., Rett's *syndrome*.

hyperamylasemia (hī'per-am'i-lā-sē'mē-ă) [hyper- + amylase, + G. *haima*, blood]. Elevated serum amylase, usually seen as one of the manifestations of acute pancreatitis.

hyperanacinesia, hyperanacinesis (hī'per-an-ă-si-nē'zē-ă, -nē'sis). Hyperanakinesia.

hyperanakinesia, hyperanakinesis (hī'per-an-ă-ki-nē'zē-ă, -ki-nē'sis) [hyper- + G. *anakinēsis*, to-and-fro movement]. Hyperanacinesia; hyperanacinesis; excessive to-and-fro movement, *e.g.*, of the stomach or intestine.

hyperaphia (hī'per-ă'fē-ă) [hyper- + G. *haphē*, touch]. Tactile hyperesthesia; oxyaphia; extreme sensitiveness to touch.

hyperaphic (hī-per-af'ik). Marked by hyperaphia.

hyperbaric (hī-per-bar'ik) [hyper- + G. *baros*, weight]. **1.** Pertaining to pressure of ambient gases greater than 1 atmosphere. **2.** Concerning solutions, more dense than the diluent or medium; *e.g.*, in spinal anesthesia, a h. solution has a specific gravity greater than that of spinal fluid.

hyperbarism (hī-per-bar'izm) [hyper- + G. *baros*, weight]. Disturbances in the body resulting from the pressure of ambient gases at greater than 1 atmosphere; *e.g.*, nitrogen narcosis, oxygen toxicity.

hyperbetalipoproteinemia (hī'per-bet-ă-lip'ō-prō-tē-nē'mē-ă). Enhanced concentration of β-lipoproteins in the blood.
familial h., type II familial *hyperlipoproteinemia*.
familial h. and hyperprebetalipoproteinemia, type III familial *hyperlipoproteinemia*.

hyperbilirubinemia (hī'per-bil'i-rū-bi-nē'mē-ă). An abnormally large amount of bilirubin in the circulating blood, resulting in clinically apparent icterus or jaundice when the concentration is sufficient.

hyperbrachycephaly (hī'per-brak-ē-sef'ă-lē) [hyper- + G. *brachys*, short, + *kephalē*, head]. An extreme degree of brachycephaly, with a cephalic index of over 85.

hypercalcemia (hī'per-kal-sē'mē-ă). An abnormally high concentration of calcium compounds in the circulating blood; commonly used to indicate an elevated concentration of calcium ions in the blood.
idiopathic h. of infants, persistent h. of unknown cause in very young children, associated with osteosclerosis, renal insufficiency, and sometimes hypertension; may also be associated with supravalvular aortic stenosis, elfin facies, and mental retardation.

hypercalcinuria (hī'per-kal-si-nū'rē-ă). Hypercalciuria.

hypercalciuria (hī'per-kal-sē-yu'rē-ă). Hypercalcinuria; hypercalcuria; calcinuric diabetes; excretion of abnormally large amounts of calcium in the urine, as in hyperparathyroidism.

hypercalcuria (hī'per-kal-kyū'rē-ă). Hypercalciuria.

hypercapnia (hī-per-kap'nē-ă) [hyper- + G. *kapnos*, smoke, vapor]. Hypercarbia; abnormally increased arterial carbon dioxide tension.

hypercarbia (hī-per-kar'bē-ă). Hypercapnia.

hypercardia (hī-per-kar'dē-ă) [hyper- + G. *kardia*, heart]. Hypertrophy of the heart.

hypercatharsis (hī'per-kă-thar'sis) [hyper- + G. *katharsis*, a cleansing]. Excessive and frequent defecation.

hypercathartic (hī'per-kă-thar'tik). **1.** Causing excessive purgation. **2.** An agent having an excessive purgative action.

hypercathexis (hī'per-kă-thek'sis) [hyper- + G. *kathexis*, a holding in, retention]. In psychoanalysis, excessive investment of an object with libido or interest.

hypercementosis (hī'per-sē-men-tō'sis) [hyper- + L. *caementum*, a rough quarry stone, + *-osis*, condition]. Cementum hyperplasia; excessive deposition of secondary cementum on the root of a tooth which may be caused by localized trauma or inflammation, excessive tooth eruption, or osteitis deformans, or occur idiopathically.

hyperchloremia (hī'per-klō-rē'mē-ă). An abnormally large amount of chloride ions in the circulating blood.

hyperchlorhydria (hī'per-klōr-hī'drē-ă) [hyper- + chlorhydric (acid)]. Chlorhydria; hyperhydrochloria; presence of an excessive amount of hydrochloric acid in the stomach.

hyperchloride (hī-per-klōr'īd). Perchloride.

hyperchloruria (hī'per-klōr-yū'rē-ă). Increased excretion of chloride ions in the urine.

hypercholesteremia (hī'per-kō-les'ter-ē'mē-ă). Hypercholesterolemia.

hypercholesterinemia (hī'per-kō-les'ter-i-nē'mē-ă). Hypercholesterolemia.

hypercholesterolemia (hī'per-kō-les'ter-ol-ē'mē-ă). Hypercholesteremia; hypercholesterinemia; the presence of an abnormally large amount of cholesterol in the cells and plasma of the circulating blood.
familial h., type II familial *hyperlipoproteinemia*.
familial h. with hyperlipemia, type III familial *hyperlipoproteinemia*.

hypercholesterolia (hī'per-kō-les'ter-ō'lē-ă). The presence of an abnormally large quantity of cholesterol in the bile.

hypercholia (hī-per-kō'lē-ă) [hyper- + G. *cholē*, bile]. A condition in which an abnormally large amount of bile is formed in the liver.

hyperchromasia (hī'per-krō-mā'zē-ă). Hyperchromatism.

hyperchromatic (hī'per-krō-mat'ik) [hyper- + G. *chrōma*, color]. **1.** Hyperchromic (1); abnormally highly colored, excessively stained, or overpigmented. **2.** Showing increased chromatin.

hyperchromatism (hī'per-krō'mă-tizm) [hyper- + G. *chrōma*, color]. Hyperchromasia; hyperchromia. **1.** Excessive pigmentation. **2.** Increased staining capacity, especially of cell nuclei for hematoxylin. **3.** An increase in chromatin in cell nuclei.

hyperchromia (hī-per-krō'mē-ă). Hyperchromatism.

macrocytic h., so-called hyperchromatic macrocythemia; inasmuch as the red blood cells are larger than normal, the total amount of hemoglobin per cell is increased, but the percentage of hemoglobin per cell is usually in the normochromic range.

hyperchromic (hī-per-krōm'ik). **1.** Hyperchromatic (1). **2.** Denoting increased light absorption.

hyperchylia (hī-per-kī'lē-ă) [hyper- + G. *chylos,* juice]. Excessive secretion of gastric juice.

hyperchylomicronemia (hī'per-kī'lō-mī-krō-nē'mē-ă). Increased plasma concentrations of chylomicrons.

familial h., type I familial *hyperlipoproteinemia.*

familial h. with hyperprebetalipoproteinemia, type V familial *hyperlipoproteinemia.*

hypercinesis, hypercinesia (hī'per-si-nē'sis, -si-nē'zē-ă). Hyperkinesis.

hypercorticoidism (hī'per-kōr'ti-koyd-izm). Hyperadrenalcorticalism; hyperadrenocorticalism; hypercorticalism; excessive secretion of one or more steroid hormones of the adrenal cortex; sometimes used also to designate the state produced by therapeutic administration of large quantities of steroids having glucocorticoid activity, *e.g.,* hydrocortisone. See also Cushing's *syndrome.*

hypercortisolism (hī'per-kōr'ti-sol-izm). See hyperadrenocorticalism.

hypercryalgesia (hī'per-krī-al-jē'zē-ă) [hyper- + G. *kryos,* cold, + *algēsis,* the sense of pain]. Hypercryesthesia.

hypercryesthesia (hī'per-krī-es-thē'zē-ă) [hyper- + G. *kryos,* cold, + *aisthēsis,* sensation]. Hypercryalgesia; extreme sensibility to cold.

hypercupremia (hī'per-kū-prē'mē-ă) [hyper- + L. *cuprum,* copper, + G. *haima,* blood]. An abnormally high level of plasma copper.

hypercyanotic (hī'per-sī-ă-not'ik). Marked by extreme cyanosis.

hypercyesis, hypercyesia (hī'per-sī-ē'sis, -ē'zē-ă) [hyper- + G. *kyēsis,* pregnancy]. Superfetation.

hypercythemia (hī'per-sī-thē'mē-ă) [hyper- + G. *kytos,* cell, + *haima,* blood]. Hypererythrocythemia; the presence of an abnormally high number of red blood cells in the circulating blood.

hypercytochromia (hī'per-sī-tō-krō'mē-ă) [hyper- + G. *kytos,* cell, + *chrōma,* color]. Increased intensity of staining of a cell, especially blood cells.

hypercytosis (hī'per-sī-tō'sis). Old term for any condition in which there is an abnormal increase in the number of cells in the circulating blood or the tissues; frequently used synonymously with leukocytosis.

hyperdactyly, hyperdactylia, hyperdactylism (hī-per-dak'ti-lē, -dak-til'ē-ă, -dak'ti-lizm) [hyper- + G. *daktylos,* finger or toe]. Polydactyly.

hyperdiastole (hī'per-dī-as'tō-lē). Extreme cardiac diastole.

hyperdicrotic (hī'per-dī-krot'ik). Superdicrotic; pronouncedly dicrotic.

hyperdicrotism (hī-per-dik'rō-tizm, -dī'krō-tizm). Extreme dicrotism.

hyperdipsia (hī-per-dip'sē-ă) [hyper- + G. *dipsa,* thirst]. Intense thirst that is relatively temporary.

hyperdistention (hī'per-dis-ten'shŭn). Superdistention; extreme distention.

hyperdynamia (hī'per-dī-nā'mē-ă, -nam'ē-ă) [hyper- + G. *dynamis,* force]. Extreme violence or muscular restlessness.

h. u'teri, excessive uterine contractions in childbirth.

hyperdynamic (hī-per-dī-nam'ik). Marked by hyperdynamia.

hyperechema (hī'per-ē-kē'mă) [hyper- + G. *ēchēma,* sound]. Auditory magnification or exaggeration.

hyperemesis (hī-per-em'ĕ-sis) [hyper- + G. *emesis,* vomiting]. Excessive vomiting.

h. gravida'rum, pernicious vomiting in pregnancy.

h. lacten'tium, vomiting by nursing infants with pyloric stenosis.

hyperemetic (hī'per-ĕ-met'ik). Marked by excessive vomiting.

hyperemia (hī-per-ē'mē-ă) [hyper- + G. *haima,* blood]. The presence of an increased amount of blood in a part or organ. See also congestion.

active h., arterial or fluxionary h.; h. due to an increased afflux of arterial blood into dilated capillaries.

arterial h., active h.

Bier's h., obsolete term for h. produced by Bier's *method* (2).

collateral h., the increased blood flow through collateral channels when the circulation through the main artery to a part is arrested, as when the blood supply to one lung or to a portion of it is occluded the blood flow to the other lung or portion of a lung is increased.

constriction h., obsolete term for h. produced by Bier's *method* (2).

fluxionary h., active h.

passive h., venous h.; h. due to an obstruction in the flow of blood from the affected part, the venous radicles becoming distended.

peristatic h., peristasis.

reactive h., h. following the arrest and subsequent restoration of the blood supply to a part.

venous h., passive h.

hyperemic (hī-per-ē'mik). Denoting hyperemia.

hyperencephaly (hī'per-en-sef'ă-lē) [hyper- + G. *enkephalos,* brain]. A fetal developmental deficiency of the vault of the cranium, exposing the poorly formed brain.

hypereosinophilia (hī'per-ē-ō-sin-ō-fil'ē-ă). A greater degree of abnormal increase in the number of eosinophilic granulocytes in the circulating blood or the tissues; *e.g.,* in diseases where the degree of eosinophilia usually ranges from 10 to 30%, an increase to 50 or 60% (or more) might be regarded as h.

hyperephidrosis (hī'per-ef-i-drō'sis) [hyper- + G. *ephidrōsis,* perspiration]. Hyperhidrosis.

hyperepithymia (hī'per-ep'i-thī'mē-ă) [hyper- + G. *epithymia,* yearning]. Inordinate desire.

hyperergasia (hī-per-er-gā'zē-ă) [hyper- + G. *ergasia,* work]. Increased or excessive functional activity.

hyperergia (hī'per-er'jē-ă). Hypergia; an allergic hypersensitivity.

hyperergic (hī-per-er'jik). Hypergic; relating to hyperergia.

hypererythrocythemia (hī'per-ē-rith'rō-sī-thē'mē-ă). Hypercythemia.

hyperesophoria (hī'per-es-ō-fō'rē-ă) [hyper- + G. *esō,* inward, + *phora,* movement]. A tendency of one eye to deviate upward and inward, prevented by binocular vision.

hyperesthesia (hī'per-es-thē'zē-ă) [hyper- + G. *aisthēsis,* sensation]. Oxyesthesia; abnormal acuteness of sensitivity to touch, pain, or other sensory stimuli.

auditory h., hyperacusis.

cerebral h., h. due to some central lesion in the brain.

cervical h., the hypersensitivity of teeth in the cervical area due to exposure of the dentin.

gustatory h., hypergeusia.

muscular h., hypermyesthesia; sensitiveness of the muscles to pressure.

olfactory h., h. olfacto'ria, hyperosmia.

h. op'tica, extreme sensitiveness of the eyes to light. See photophobia (1).

tactile h., hyperaphia.

hyperesthetic (hī'per-es-thet'ik). Marked by hyperesthesia.

hypereuryprosopic (hī'per-yū'ri-prō-sop'ik) [hyper- + G. *eurys*, wide, + *prosōpon*, face]. Pertaining to or characterized by a very low and wide face.

hyperexophoria (hī'per-ek-sō-fō'rē-ă) [hyper- + G. *exō*, outward, + *phora*, movement]. A tendency of one eye to deviate upward and outward, prevented by binocular vision.

hyperextension (hī'per-eks-ten'shŭn). Overextension; superextension; extension of a limb or part beyond the normal limit.

hyperferremia (hī'per-fer-ē'mē-ă). High serum iron level; found in hemochromatosis.

hyperfibrinogenemia (hī'per-fī-brin'ō-jĕ-nē'mē-ă). Fibrinogenemia; an increased level of fibrinogen in the blood.

hyperfibrinolysis (hī'per-fī-brin-ol'i-sis). Markedly increased fibrinolysis, as in subdural hematomas.

hyperflexion (hī-per-flek'shŭn). Superflexion; flexion of a limb or part beyond the normal limit.

hyperfolliculoidism (hī-per-fō-lik'yū-loyd-izm). Excessive production of estradiol, as seen in new growths derived from the graafian follicles; a cause of abnormal uterine bleeding, *e.g.*, metropathia hemorrhagica.

hypergalactosis (hī'per-ga-lak-tō'sis) [hyper- + G. *gala*, milk, + -*ōsis*, condition]. Excessive secretion of milk.

hypergammaglobulinemia (hī'per-gam-ă-glob'yū-li-nē'mē-ă). An increased amount of the γ-globulins in the plasma, such as that frequently observed in chronic infectious diseases.

hypergasia (hī'per-gā'zē-ă) [G. *hypo* (*hyp-*), under, + *ergasia*, work]. Diminished functional activity.

hypergenesis (hī-per-jen'ĕ-sis) [hyper- + G. *genesis*, production]. Excessive development or redundant production of parts or organs of the body.

hypergenetic (hī-per-jĕ-net'ik). Relating to hypergenesis.

hypergenitalism (hī-per-jen'i-tăl-izm). Abnormally overdeveloped genitalia in adults or for the individual's age.

hypergeusia (hī-per-gū'sē-ă, -jū'sē-ă) [hyper- + G. *geusis*, taste]. Gustatory hyperesthesia; oxygeusia; abnormal acuteness of the sense of taste.

hypergia (hī-per'jē-ă). Hyperergia.

hypergic (hī-per'jik). Hyperergic.

hyperglandular (hī-per-glan'dyū-lăr). Characterized by overactivity or increased size of a gland.

hyperglobulia, hyperglobulism (hī'per-glob-yū'lē-ă, -glob'yū-lizm) [hyper- + L. *globulus*, globule]. Old term for polycthemia.

hyperglobulinemia (hī'per-glob'yū-lin-ē'mē-ă). An abnormally large amount of globulins in the circulating blood plasma.

hyperglycemia (hī'per-glī-sē'mē-ă) [hyper- + G. *glykys*, sweet, + *haima*, blood]. Hyperglycosemia; an abnormally high concentration of glucose in the circulating blood, especially with reference to a fasting level.

nonketotic h., a rare inborn error of glycine metabolism characterized by severe h., plasma hyperosmolality, dehydration, and, in some cases, focal motor seizures and severe mental retardation; no ketoacidosis is present; autosomal recessive inheritance.

posthypoglycemic h., Somogyi *phenomenon*.

hyperglyceridemia (hī'per-glis'er-i-dē'mē-ă). Elevated plasma concentration of glycerides, which usually are present within chylomicrons; normal if transiently present after absorption of a meal containing lipids, abnormal if a persistent state.

endogenous h., type IV familial hyperlipoproteinemia or, more commonly, a nonfamilial sporadic variety.

exogenous h., persistent h. due to retarded rate of removal from plasma of chylomicrons of dietary origin; occurs in alcoholism, hypothyroidism, insulinopenic diabetes mellitus, types I and V hyperlipoproteinemia, and during acute pancreatitis.

hyperglycinemia (hī'per-glī-si-nē'mē-ă). Elevated plasma glycine concentration. See also *hyperglycinuria* with hyperglycinemia.

hyperglycinuria (hī'per-glī-si-nū'rē-ă). Enhanced urinary excretion of glycine.

h. with hyperglycinemia, glycinemia; a metabolic disorder of unknown nature generally appearing in the neonatal period and commonly fatal; characterized by vomiting, metabolic acidosis, ketonuria, osteoporosis, periodic thrombocytopenia, neutropenia, mental retardation, and neuropsychiatric dysfunction; autosomal recessive inheritance.

hyperglycogenolysis (hī'per-glī'kō-jĕ-nol'i-sis). Excessive glycogenolysis.

hyperglycorrhachia (hī'per-glī-kō-rak'ē-ă) [hyper- + G. *glykys*, sweet, + *rhachis*, spine]. Excessive sugar in the cerebrospinal fluid.

hyperglycosemia (hī'per-glī-kō-sē'mē-ă). Hyperglycemia.

hyperglycosuria (hī'per-glī-kō-sū'rē-ă). Persistent excretion of unusually large amounts of glucose in the urine; *i.e.*, an extreme degree of glucosuria.

hyperglyoxylemia (hī'per-glī-ok'si-lē'mē-ă). Enhanced plasma (and possibly tissue) concentrations of glyoxylate; may develop during thiamine deficiency.

hypergnosis (hī-per-nō'sis) [hyper- + G. *gnosis*, knowledge]. **1.** Projection of inner conflicts into the environment. **2.** Exaggerated perception, such as the expansion of an isolated thought.

hypergonadism (hī-per-gō'nad-izm). A clinical state resulting from enhanced secretion of gonadal hormones.

hypergonadotropic (hī'per-gō'nă-dō-trop'ik). Indicating an increased production or excretion of gonadotropic hormones.

hypergranulosis (hī'per-gran-yū-lō'sis). Increased thickness of the granular layer of the epidermis, associated with hyperkeratosis.

hyperguanidinemia (hī'per-gwan'i-di-nē'mē-ă). A condition in which there is an abnormally large amount of guanidine in the circulating blood.

hypergynecosmia (hī'per-gī-nĕ-koz'mē-ă) [hyper- + G. *gyne*, woman, + *kosmeō*, to decorate]. Overdevelopment of secondary sex characteristics of the mature female or their precocious development in the young girl.

hyperhedonia, hyperhedonism (hī'per-hē-dō'nē-ă, -hē'don-izm) [hyper- + G. *hēdonē*, pleasure]. **1.** The feeling of an abnormally great pleasure in any act or from any happening. **2.** Sexual erethism.

hyperhemoglobinemia (hī'per-hē'mō-glō-bi-nē'mē-ă). An unusually large amount of hemoglobin in the circulating blood plasma; *i.e.*, much more than that ordinarily observed in most examples of hemoglobinemia.

hyperheparinemia (hī'per-hep'ar-in-ē'mē-ă). Elevated plasma concentrations of heparin; believed to be the cause of a heritable bleeding tendency.

hyperhidrosis (hī'per-hī-drō'sis) [hyper- + hidrosis]. Hyperidrosis; hyperephidrosis; polyhidrosis; polyidrosis; sudorrhea; excessive or profuse sweating.

gustatory h., excessive sweating of the lips, nose, and forehead after eating certain foods; it is physiologic in many persons, but sometimes occurs after parotid surgery or as a result of damage to the parasympathetic or sympathetic nerves of the head and neck.

h. oleo'sa, *seborrhea* oleosa.

hyperhydration (hī'per-hī-drā'shŭn). Overhydration; excess water content of the body; may result from the intravenous administration of unduly large amounts of glucose solution.

hyperhydrochloria (hī'per-hī-drō-klōr'ē-ă). Hyperchlorhydria.

hyperhydropexy, hyperhydropexis (hī-per-hī'drō-pek-sē, hī'per-hī-drō-pek'sis) [hyper- + G. *hydōr,* water, + *pēgnynai,* to fasten]. Increased fixation of water in tissues.

hypericin (hī-per'i-sin). A photosensitizing substance present in *Hypericum perforatum,* St. John's wart, which can cause a photosensitivity similar to fagopyrism in grazing animals.

hyperidrosis (hī'per-i-drō'sis). Hyperhidrosis.

hyperindicanemia (hī'per-in'di-kan-ē'mē-ă). An unusually large amount of indican in the circulating blood; *i.e.,* greater than that observed in most instances of indicanemia.

hyperinfection (hī'per-in-fek'shŭn). Infection by very large numbers of organisms as a result of immunologic deficiency.

hyperinosemia (hī'per-i'nō-sē'mē-ă, hī'per-in'ō-) [hyper- + G. *is (in-),* fiber, + *haima,* blood]. A greatly increased quantity of fibrinogen in the circulating blood; under certain conditions, unusually large amounts of fibrin may be formed, thereby resulting in a greater degree of coagulability of the blood.

hyperinosis (hī-per-i-nō'sis). Hyperinosemia.

hyperinsulinemia (hī'per-in'sū-lin-ē'mē-ă). Hyperinsulinism.

hyperinsulinism (hī'per-in'sū-lin-izm). Hyperinsulinemia; increased levels of insulin in the plasma due to increased secretion of insulin by the beta cells of the pancreatic islets; decreased hepatic removal of insulin is a cause in some patients, although h. usually is associated with insulin resistance and is commonly found in obesity in association with varying degrees of hyperglycemia.

alimentary h., elevated levels of insulin in the plasma following ingestion of meals by individuals with abnormally rapid gastric emptying (*e.g.,* following gastroenterostomy or vagotomy); rapid glucose absorption leads to excessive insulin release which in turn can lead to a marked fall in blood glucose to hypoglycemic levels.

hyperinvolution (hī'per-in'vō-lū'shŭn). Superinvolution.

hyperisotonic (hī'per-ī-sō-ton'ik). Hypertonic.

hyperkalemia (hī'per-kă-lē'mē-ă) [hyper- + Mod. L. *kalium,* potash, + G. *haima,* blood]. Hyperkaliemia; hyperpotassemia; a greater than normal concentration of potassium ions in the circulating blood.

hyperkaliemia (hī'per-kal-i-ē'mē-ă). Hyperkalemia.

hyperkaluresis (hī'per-kal-yū-rē'sis) [hyper- + Mod. L. *kalium,* potassium, + G. *oureō,* to urinate]. Excessive urinary excretion of potassium.

hyperkeratinization (hī'per-ker'at-i-ni-zā'shŭn). Hyperkeratosis.

hyperkeratomycosis (hī'per-ker'ă-tō-mī-kō'sis). Thickening of the horny layer of the skin due to mycotic infection.

hyperkeratosis (hī'per-ker-ă-tō'sis). Hyperkeratinization; hypertrophy of the horny layer of the epidermis or mucous membrane. See also keratoderma; keratosis.

bovine h., X disease of cattle; a specific disease characterized by thickening and hardening of the skin and proliferation of the epithelium of some of the mucous membranes; caused by poisoning (*e.g.,* from processed feed grains contaminated with certain highly chlorinated naphthalenes used as wood preservatives and constituents of lubricating greases).

h. congen'ita, *ichthyosis* vulgaris.

h. eccen'trica, porokeratosis.

epidermolytic h., ichthyosis hystrix or spinosa; porcupine skin; a bullous form of congenital ichthyosiform erythroderma inherited as an autosomal dominant trait and present at birth; characterized by coarse, verruciform scaling most prominent in the flexural areas, and associated with blister formation; histologically, there is hyperkeratosis, granular reticular spaces in the upper epidermis, acanthosis, and rapid epidermal cell turnover.

h. figura'ta centrif'uga atroph'ica, porokeratosis.

h. follicula'ris et parafollicula'ris, Kyrle's disease; h. penetrans; discrete and confluent horny follicular plugs on crateriform base, usually occurring on the arms and legs.

h. lenticula'ris per'stans, Flegel's disease; small keratotic papules of the dorsa of the feet, on the legs, and occasionally elsewhere, with pinpoint keratotic papules of the palms and soles; onset in the fourth and fifth decades; possibly an autosomal dominant trait.

h. pen'etrans, h. follicularis et parafollicularis.

h. subungua'lis, h. affecting the nailbeds of the fingers or toes.

hyperketonemia (hī'per-kē'tō-nē'mē-ă). Elevated concentrations of ketone bodies in the blood.

hyperketonuria (hī'per-kē'tō-nū'rē-ă). Increased urinary excretion of ketonic compounds.

hyperkinemia (hī'per-ki-nē'mē-ă) [hyper- + G. *kineō,* to move, + *haima,* blood]. Increased volume flow through the circulation; increased circulation rate; supernormal cardiac output.

hyperkinesis, hyperkinesia (hī'per-ki-nē'sis, -nē'zē-ă) [hyper- + G. *kinēsis,* motion]. Hypercinesis; hypercinesia. **1.** Supermotility; excessive motility. **2.** Excessive muscular activity.

hyperkinetic (hī'per-ki-net'ik). Pertaining to or characterized by hyperkinesia.

hyperlactation (hī'per-lak-tā'shŭn). Superlactation.

hyperleukocytosis (hī'per-lū'kō-sī-tō'sis). An unusually great increase in the number and proportion of leukocytes in the circulating blood or the tissues; *i.e.,* much more than that ordinarily observed in most instances of leukocytosis.

hyperlexia (hī-per-lek'sē-ă) [hyper- + G. *lexis,* word, phrase]. In retarded children, the presence of advanced reading ability.

hyperlipemia (hī'per-li-pē'mē-ă) [hyper- + G. *lipos,* fat, + *haima,* blood]. Lipemia.

carbohydrate-induced h., type III and type IV familial *hyperlipoproteinemia.*

combined fat- and carbohydrate-induced h., type V familial *hyperlipoproteinemia.*

familial fat-induced h., type I familial *hyperlipoproteinemia.*

idiopathic h., type I familial *hyperlipoproteinemia.*

mixed h., type V familial *hyperlipoproteinemia.*

hyperlipidemia (hī'per-lip-i-dē'mē-ă). Lipemia.

hyperlipoidemia (hī'per-lip-oy-dē'mē-ă). Lipemia.

hyperlipoproteinemia (hī'per-lip'ō-prō'tē-in-ē'mē-ă, -prō'tēn-). An increase in the lipoprotein concentration of the blood.

acquired h., nonfamilial h. that develops as a consequence of some primary disease, such as thyroid deficiency.

familial h., a group of diseases characterized by changes in concentration of β-lipoproteins and pre-β-lipoproteins and the lipids associated with them. See types I through V familial h.

type I familial h., Bürger-Grütz syndrome; familial fat-induced hyperlipemia; familial hyperchylomicronemia; familial hypertriglyceridemia (1); idiopathic hyperlipemia; h. characterized by the presence of large amounts of chylomicrons and triglycerides in the plasma on a normal diet, and disappearance on a fat-free diet; low α- and β-lipoproteins on a normal diet, with increase on fat-free diet; decreased plasma postheparin lipolytic activity; and low tissue lipoprotein lipase activity. It is accompanied by bouts of abdominal pain, hepatosplenomegaly, pancreatitis, and eruptive xanthomas; autosomal recessive inheritance.

type II familial h., familial hyperbetalipoproteinemia or hypercholesterolemia; familial hypercholesteremic xanthomatosis; h. characterized by increased plasma levels of β-lipoproteins, cholesterol, and phospholipids, but normal triglycerides; heterozygotes have mild lipid changes and are susceptible to atherosclerosis in middle age, but homozygotes have severe changes often with generalized xanthomatosis and xanthelasma, and atherosclerosis as young adults. The primary defect is a deficiency of apoprotein of

VLDL and the disorder is divided into two classes: 1) type IIA, which has elevated LDL; type IIB which has elevated LDL and VLDL; both autosomal inheritance.

type III familial h., familial hyperbetalipoproteinemia and hyperprebetalipoproteinemia; familial hypercholesterolemia with hyperlipemia; carbohydrate-induced hyperlipemia; h. characterized by increased plasma levels of LDL, β-lipoproteins, pre-β-lipoproteins, cholesterol, phospholipids, and triglycerides; hypertriglyceridemia is endogenous, induced by high carbohydrate diet, and glucose tolerance is abnormal; frequently accompanied by eruptive xanthomas and atheromatosis, particularly coronary artery disease; biochemical defect is a deficiency of LDL receptor; autosomal recessive inheritance.

type IV familial h., familial hyperprebetalipoproteinemia; familial hypertriglyceridemia (2); carbohydrate-induced hyperlipemia; plasma levels of VLDL, pre-β-lipoproteins and triglycerides are increased on a normal diet, but β-lipoproteins, cholesterol, and phospholipids are normal; hypertriglyceridemia is endogenous, induced by high carbohydrate diet; may be accompanied by abnormal glucose tolerance and susceptibility to ischemic heart disease; probably autosomal recessive inheritance.

type V familial h., familial hyperchylomicronemia with hyperprebetalipoproteinemia; mixed hyperlipemia; combined fat- and carbohydrate-induced hyperlipemia; h. characterized by increased plasma levels of chylomicrons, VLDL, pre-β-lipoproteins, and triglycerides, and slight elevation of cholesterol on a normal diet, with β-lipoproteins normal; may be accompanied by bouts of abdominal pain, hepatosplenomegaly, susceptibility to atherosclerosis, and abnormal glucose tolerance; probably autosomal recessive inheritance.

hyperliposis (hī'per-li-pō'sis) [hyper- + G. *lipos,* fat]. **1.** Excessive adiposity. **2.** An extreme degree of fatty degeneration.

hyperlithuria (hī'per-li-thu'rē-ă). An excessive excretion of uric (lithic) acid in the urine.

hyperlogia (hī-per-lō'jē-ă) [hyper- + G. *logios,* eloquent]. Morbid verbosity or loquacity.

hyperlordosis (hī'per-lōr-dō'sis). Extreme lordosis.

hyperlysinemia (hī'per-lī-si-nē'mē-ă). Abnormal increase of the amino acid lysine in the circulating blood; associated with mental retardation, convulsions, anemia, and asthenia; autosomal recessive inheritance.

hyperlysinuria (hī'per-lī-si-nū'rē-ă). The presence of abnormally high concentrations of lysine in the urine; a form of aminoaciduria that occurs in cystinuria, hepatolenticular degeneration, and the Fanconi syndrome.

hypermagnesemia (hī'per-mag-nē-sē'mē-ă). An abnormally large concentration of magnesium in the blood serum.

hypermastia (hī-per-mas'tē-ă) [hyper- + G. *mastos,* breast]. **1.** Polymastia. **2.** Excessively large mammary glands.

hypermenorrhea (hī'per-men-ō-rē'ă) [hyper- + G. *mēn,* month, + *rhoia,* flow]. Menorrhagia; menostaxis; excessively prolonged or profuse menses.

hypermetabolism (hī'per-me-tab'ō-lizm). Heat production by the body above normal, as in thyrotoxicosis.

hypermetamorphosis (hī'per-met-ă-mōr'fō-sis) [hyper- + G. *metamorphōsis,* transformation]. Excessive and rapid change of ideas occurring in a mental disorder.

hypermetria (hī-per-mē'trē-ă) [hyper- + G. *metron,* measure]. Ataxia characterized by overreaching a desired object or goal. *Cf.* hypometria.

hypermetrope (hī-per-met'rōp). Hyperope.

hypermetropia (hī'per-me-trō'pē-ă) [hyper- + G. *metron,* measure, + *ōps,* eye]. Hyperopia.

index h., h. arising from decreased refractivity of the lens.

hypermimia (hī-per-mim'ē-ă) [hyper- + G. *mimeia,* farce]. Excessive mimetic movements.

hypermnesia (hī-per-nē'zē-ă) [hyper- + G. *mnēmē,* memory]. **1.** Extreme power of memory. **2.** A capacity under hypnosis for immediate registration and precise recall of many more individual items than is thought possible under ordinary circumstances.

hypermobility (hī'per-mō-bil'i-tē). Increased range of movement of joints, joint laxity, occurring normally in young children or as a result of disease, *e.g.,* Marfan's or Ehlers-Danlos syndrome; h. may result in degenerative joint disease.

hypermorph (hī'per-mōrf) [hyper- + G. *morphē,* form]. Person whose sitting height is low in proportion to the standing height, owing to excessive length of limb. *Cf.* hypomorph; ectomorph.

hypermyesthesia (hī'per-mī'es-thē'zē-ă) [hyper- + G. *mys,* muscle, + *aisthēsis,* feeling]. Muscular *hyperesthesia.*

hypermyotonia (hī'per-mī-ō-tō'nē-ă) [hyper- + G. *mys,* muscle, + *tonos,* tension]. Extreme muscular tonus.

hypermyotrophy (hī'per-mī-ot'rō-fē) [hyper- + G. *mys,* muscle, + *trophē,* nourishment]. Muscular hypertrophy.

hypernatremia (hī'per-nă-trē'mē-ă) [hyper- + natrium, + G. *haima,* blood]. An abnormally high plasma concentration of sodium ions.

hyperneocytosis (hī'per-nē'ō-sī-tō'sis) [hyper- + G. *neos,* new, + *kytos,* cell, + *-osis,* condition]. Hyperskeocytosis; hyperleukocytosis in which there are considerable numbers of immature and young cells (especially in the granulocytic series); *i.e.,* a "shift to the left" in the hemogram.

hypernephroid (hī-per-nef'royd) [hyper- + G. *nephros,* kidney, + *eidos,* appearance]. Resembling or of the type of the adrenal gland.

hypernephroma (hī'per-ne-frō'mă) [hyper- + G. *nephros,* kidney, + *-oma,* tumor]. Renal *adenocarcinoma.*

hypernoia (hī-per-noy'ă) [hyper- + G. *noeō,* to think]. **1.** Great rapidity of thought. **2.** Excessive mental activity or imagination.

hypernomic (hī-per-nom'ik) [hyper- + G. *nomos,* law]. Uncontrolled to excess.

hypernutrition (hī'per-nū-trish'ŭn). Supernutrition.

hyperoncotic (hī'per-on-kot'ik). Indicating an oncotic pressure higher than normal, *e.g.,* of blood plasma.

hyperonychia (hī'per-ō-nik'ē-ă) [hyper- + G. *onyx,* (*onych-*), nail]. Hypertrophy of the nails.

hyperope (hī'per-ōp). Hypermetrope; one suffering from hyperopia.

hyperopia (H) (hī-per-ō'pē-ă) [hyper- + G. *ōps,* eye]. Hypermetropia; farsightedness; longsightedness; long or far sight; that optical condition in which only convergent rays can be brought to focus on the retina.

absolute h., manifest h. that cannot be overcome by an effort of accommodation.

axial h., h. due to shortening of the anteroposterior diameter of the globe of the eye.

curvature h., h. due to decreased refraction of the anterior ocular segment.

facultative h., manifest h.

latent h. (Hl), the difference between total and manifest h.

manifest h. (Hm), faculative h.; h. that can be compensated by accommodation.

total h. (Ht), that which can be determined after complete paralysis of accommodation by means of a cycloplegic.

hyperopic (H) (hī-per-ō'pik). Pertaining to hyperopia.

hyperorality (hī'per-ō-ral'i-tē) [hyper- + L. *os* (*or-*), mouth]. A condition in which unlikely objects are placed in the mouth.

hyperorchidism (hī-per-ōr'ki-dizm) [hyper- + G. *orchis,* testis]. Obsolete term for increased size or functioning of the testes.

hyperorexia (hī'per-ō-rek'sē-ă) [hyper- + G. *orexis,* appetite]. *Bulimia* nervosa.

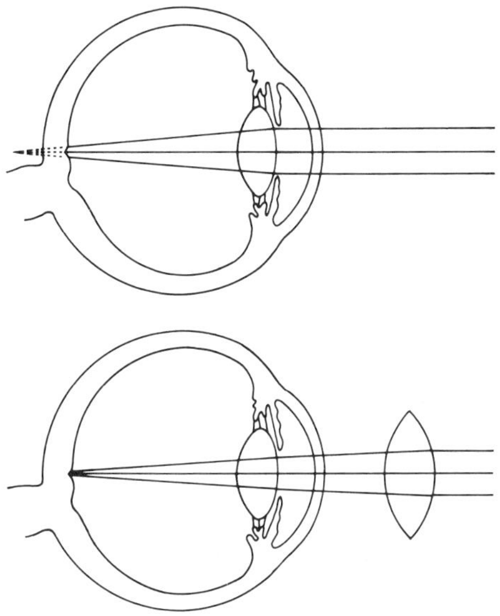

Hyperopia
Top, light rays in the hyperopic eye; *bottom*, after correction by means of a convex lens.

hyperorthocytosis (hī'per-ōr'thō-sī-tō'sis) [hyper- + G. *orthos*, correct, + *kytos*, cell, + *-osis*, condition]. Hyperleukocytosis in which the relative percentages of the various types of white blood cells are within the normal range and immature forms are not observed.

hyperosmia (hī-per-oz'mē-ă) [hyper- + G. *osmē*, sense of smell]. Olfactory hyperesthesia; hyperesthesia olfactoria; hyperosphresia; hyperosphresis; oxyosmia; oxyosphresia; an exaggerated or abnormally acute sense of smell.

hyperosmolality (hī'per-oz-mō-lal'i-tē). Increased concentration of a solution expressed as osmoles of solute per kilogram of serum water.

hyperosmolarity (hī'per-oz-mō-lar'i-tē). An increase in the osmotic concentration of a solution expressed as osmols of solute per liter of solution.

hyperosmotic (hī'per-oz-mot'ik). **1.** Having an osmolality greater than another fluid, ordinarily assumed to be plasma or extracellular fluid. **2.** Relating to increased osmosis.

hyperosphresia, hyperosphresis (hī'per-os-frē'sē-ă, hī'per-os-frē'sis) [hyper- + G. *osphrēsis*, smell]. Hyperosmia.

hyperosteoidosis (hī'per-os-tē-oy-dō'sis). Excessive formation of osteoid, as seen in rickets and osteomalacia.

hyperostosis (hī'per-os-tō'sis) [hyper- + G. *osteon*, bone, + *-ōsis*,]. **1.** Hypertrophy of bone. **2.** Exostosis.

ankylosing h., diffuse idiopathic skeletal h.

h. cortica'lis defor'mans, marked irregular thickening of the skull and bone cortex, with thickening and widening of the shafts of long bones and elevated serum alkaline phosphatase; autosomal recessive inheritance.

diffuse idiopathic skeletal h., ankylosing h.; hyperostotic spondylosis; Forrestier's disease; a generalized spinal and extraspinal articular disorder characterized by calcification and ossification of ligaments, particularly of the anterior longitudinal ligament; distinct from ankylosing spondylitis or degenerative joint disease.

flowing h., rheostosis.

h. frontal'is inter'na, abnormal deposition of bone on the inner aspect of the os frontale, visible by x-ray; may be a part of Morgagni's syndrome.

generalized cortical h., Van Buchem's *syndrome*.

infantile cortical h., Caffey's disease or syndrome; Caffey-Silverman syndrome; familial subperiosteal bone formation over many bones, especially the mandible and clavicles and the shafts of long bones; it follows fever, usually appearing before 6 months of age and disappearing during childhood.

streak h., rheostosis.

hyperovarianism (hī'per-ō-vā'rē-an-izm). Sexual precocity in young girls due to premature development of ovaries accompanied by the secretion of ovarian hormones.

hyperoxaluria (hī'per-ok-să-lū'rē-ă). Oxaluria; presence of an unusually large amount of oxalic acid or oxalates in the urine.

primary h. and oxalosis, a metabolic disorder characterized by calcium oxalate nephrocalcinosis and nephrolithiasis, extrarenal oxalosis, and increased urinary output of oxalic and glycolic acids; usually evident clinically in the first decade of life, with progressive renal failure and uremia; autosomal recessive inheritance.

hyperoxia (hī-per-ok'sē-ă). **1.** An increased amount of oxygen in tissues and organs. **2.** A greater oxygen tension than normal, such as that produced by breathing air or oxygen at pressures greater than 1 atmosphere.

hyperoxidation (hī'per-oks-i-dā'shŭn). Excessive oxidation.

hyperoxide (hī-per-oks'īd). Superoxide.

hyperpancreatism (hī'per-pan'krē-ă-tizm). A condition of increased activity of the pancreas, trypsin being in excess among the enzymes.

hyperparasite (hī-per-par'ă-sīt). A secondary parasite capable of development within a previously existing parasite.

hyperparasitism (hī-per-par'ă-sīt-izm). Biparasitism; a condition in which a secondary parasite develops within a previously existing parasite.

hyperparathyroidism (hī'per-par-ă-thī'royd-izm). A condition due to an increase in the secretion of the parathyroids, causing generalized osteitis fibrosa cystica, elevated serum calcium, decreased serum phosphorus, and increased excretion of both calcium and phosphorus.

primary h., h. due to neoplasms or idiopathic hyperplasia of the parathyroid glands.

secondary h., h. that arises as a result of disordered metabolism producing hypocalcemia, as in chronic uremia due to renal disease, malabsorption, rickets, or osteomalacia; associated with hyperplasia of the parathyroid glands.

hyperparotidism (hī'per-pa-rot'i-dizm). Increased activity of the parotid glands.

hyperpathia (hī-per-path'ē-ă) [hyper- + G. *pathos*, suffering]. Exaggerated subjective response to painful stimuli, with a continuing sensation of pain after the stimulation has ceased.

hyperpepsia (hī-per-pep'sē-ă) [hyper- + G. *pepsis*, digestion]. **1.** Abnormally rapid digestion. **2.** Impaired digestion with hyperchlorhydria.

hyperpepsinia (hī'per-pep-sin'ē-ă). An excess of pepsin in the gastric juice.

hyperperistalsis (hī'per-per-i-stal'sis). Excessive rapidity of the passage of food through the stomach and intestine.

hyperphagia (hī-per-fā'jē-ă) [hyper- + G. *phagein*, to eat]. Gluttony; overeating.

hyperphalangism (hī'per-fă-lan'jizm). Polyphalangism; presence of a supernumerary phalanx in a finger or toe.

hyperphenylalaninemia (hī'per-fen'il-al-ă-ni-nē'mē-ă). The presence of abnormally high blood levels of phenylalanine, which may or may not be associated with elevated tyrosine levels, in newborn infants (premature and full-term), associated with the heterozygous state of phenylketonuria, maternal phenylketonuria, or transient deficiency of phenylalanine hydroxylase or *p*-hydroxyphenylpyruvic acid oxidase.

hyperphonesis (hī'per-fō-nē'sis) [hyper- + G. *phōnēsis,* a sounding]. An increase in the percussion sound, or of the voice sound in auscultation

hyperphonia (hī'per-fō'nē-ă) [hyper- + G. *phōnē,* sound, voice]. Overuse of the voice, as by excessive loudness or tension of the vocal muscles.

hyperphoria (hī-per-fō'rē-ă) [hyper- + G. *phora,* motion]. A tendency of the visual axis of one eye to deviate upward, prevented by binocular vision.

hyperphosphatasemia (hī'per-fos'fă-tă-sē'mē-ă). Abnormally high content of alkaline phosphatase in the circulating blood. See also hyperphosphatasia.

hyperphosphatasia (hī'per-fos-fă-tā'zē-ă). Elevated alkaline phosphatase, with dwarfism, macrocranium, blue sclerae, and expansion of the diaphyses of tubular bones with multiple fractures; autosomal recessive inheritance.

hyperphosphatemia (hī'per-fos-fă-tē'mē-ă). Abnormally high concentration of phosphates in the circulating blood.

hyperphosphaturia (hī'per-fos-fă-tū'rē-ă). An increased excretion of phosphates in the urine.

hyperphrenia (hī-per-frē'nē-ă) [hyper- + G. *phrēn,* mind]. An excessive degree of intellectual activity; a form of mania.

hyperpiesis, hyperpiesia (hī'per-pī-ē'sis, -pī-ē'zē-ă) [hyper- + G. *piesis,* pressure]. Essential *hypertension.*

hyperpietic (hī-per-pī-et'ik). Relating to or marked by high blood pressure.

hyperpigmentation (hī'per-pig-men-tā'shŭn). Superpigmentation; an excess of pigment in a tissue or part.

hyperpipecolatemia (hī-per-pip'ĕ-kō-lă-tē'mē-ă). A metabolic disorder in which serum concentrations of pipecolic acid are greatly increased; characterized by hepatomegaly and progressive, generalized demyelination of the nervous system.

hyperpituitarism (hī'per-pi-tū'i-tă-rizm). Excessive production of anterior pituitary hormones, especially growth hormone; may result in gigantism or acromegaly.

hyperplasia (hī-per-plā'zē-ă) [hyper- + G. *plasis,* a molding]. Numerical or quantitative hypertrophy; an increase in number of cells in a tissue or organ, excluding tumor formation, whereby the bulk of the part or organ may be increased. See also hypertrophy.

angiofollicular mediastinal lymph node h., benign mediastinal lymph node h.

angiolymphoid h. with eosinophilia, Kimura's disease; solitary or multiple small benign cutaneous erythematous nodules, occurring mainly on the head and neck, characterized by immature and mature vascular structures with vacuolated endothelial cells and with a varied infiltrate of eosinophiles, lymphocytes which may form follicles, and histiocytes.

atypical melanocytic h., proliferation of melanocytes showing nuclear atypicality, especially as scattered single cells high in the epidermis; interpreted by some pathologists as malignant melanoma in situ.

basal cell h., increase in the number of cells in an epithelium resembling the basal cells; a variety of epithelial dysplasia.

benign mediastinal lymph node h., angiofollicular mediastinal lymph node h.; Castleman's disease; solitary masses of lymphoid tissue containing concentric perivascular aggregates of lymphocytes, occurring usually in the mediastinum or hilar region of young adults; similar changes have been reported outside the mediastinum and, if associated with interfollicular sheets of plasma cells, may progress to lymphoma or plasmacytoma.

cementum h., hypercementosis.

congenital adrenal h., a group of diseases arising from specific enzymatic defects in corticosteroid biosynthesis; adrenal h. with excessive secretion of adrenal androgens develops as a result of these defects. There are four major types, with clinical similarities but distinct genetic and biochemical differences: 1) simple virilizing form; 2) sodium-losing form; 3) hypertensive form; 4) 3β-hydroxysteroid dehydrogenase defect; autosomal recessive inheritance.

congenital sebaceous h., misnomer for *nevus* sebaceus.

cystic h., formation of multiple retention cysts from obstruction of ducts or glands by h. of the lining epithelium, as in fibrocystic disease of the breast and metropathia hemorrhagica.

cystic h. of the breast, fibrocystic *disease* of the breast.

denture h., inflammatory fibrous h.

ductal h., h. characterized by intraductal proliferation of epithelial cells, *e.g.,* in the breast.

fibromuscular h., thickening of arterial media by fibrosis and muscular h., usually involving the renal arteries and causing multifocal stenosis and hypertension; a variety of fibromuscular dysplasia.

focal epithelial h., Heck's disease; multiple soft nodular lesions of the lips, buccal mucosa, tongue, and other oral sites in children and adolescents; lesions spontaneously regress after a period of several months, and have been attributed etiologically to papovaviruses.

gingival h., gingival enlargement due to proliferation of fibrous connective tissue.

inflammatory fibrous h., denture h.; epulis fissuratum; overgrowth of tissue in the mucobuccal or labial fold, induced by chronic trauma from ill-fitting dentures.

inflammatory papillary h., palatal papillomatosis; closely arranged papules of the palatal mucosa underlying an ill-fitting denture.

intravascular papillary endothelial h., Masson's *pseudoandiosarcoma.*

nodular h. of prostate, benign prostatic hypertrophy; glandular and stromal h. occurring very commonly in the middle and lateral lobes of older men, forming nodules that may increasingly obstruct the urethra.

nodular regenerative h., nodular *transformation* of the liver.

pseudoepitheliomatous h., pseudocarcinomatous h., a benign increase in epidermal cells, observed in chronic inflammatory dermatoses; microscopically, it resembles squamous cell carcinoma.

senile sebaceous h., h. of mature sebaceous glands, forming a nodule on the skin of the face or forehead in elderly persons.

verrucous h., a non-invasive precursor of verrucous or squamous carcinoma of the oral mucosa, occurring in the elderly, characterized by sharp or blunt upward papillary projections of squamous epithelium.

hyperplastic (hī-per-plas'tik). Relating to hyperplasia.

hyperploid (hī'per-ployd). Relating to hyperploidy.

hyperploidy (hī'per-ploy-dē) [hyper- + G. *ploides,* in form]. The state of a cell or individual possessing one or more chromosomes in addition to the normal number.

hyperpnea (hī-per-nē'ă, hī-perp'nē-ă) [hyper- + G. *pnoē,* breathing]. Breathing that is deeper and more rapid than is normal at rest.

hyperpolarization (hī'per-pō'lăr-i-zā'shŭn). An increase in polarization of membranes or nerves or muscle cells; the reverse change from that associated with excitatory action.

hyperponesis (hī'per-pō-nē'sis) [hyper- + G. *ponos,* toil]. Exaggerated activity within the motor portion of the nervous system.

hyperpotassemia (hī'per-pō-tas-ē'mē-ă). Hyperkalemia.

hyperpragia (hī-per-prā'jē-ă) [hyper- + G. *prassō,* to do]. Excessive mental activity, as in the manic phase of bipolar disorder.

hyperpraxia (hī-per-prak'sē-ă) [hyper- + G. *praxis*, action]. Excessive activity.

hyperprebetalipoproteinemia (hī'per-prē-ba'tă-lip-ō-prō'tē-in-ē'mē-ă, -prō'tēn-). Increased concentrations of pre-β-lipoproteins in the blood.

familial h., type IV *hyperlipoproteinemia*.

hyperprochoresis (hī'per-prō-kōr-ē'sis) [hyper- + G. *pro-chōreō*, to go forward]. Rarely used term for hyperperistalsis.

hyperproinsulinemia (hī'per-prō-in'sŭl-i-nē'mē-ă). Elevated plasma levels of proinsulin or proinsulin-like material.

hyperprolactinemia (hī'per-prō-lak-ti-nē'mē-ă). Elevated levels of prolactin in the blood, which is a normal physiological reaction during lactation, but pathological otherwise; prolactin may also be elevated in cases of certain pituitary tumors, and amenorrhea is often present.

hyperprolinemia (hī'per-prō-li-nē'mē-ă). A metabolic disorder characterized by enhanced plasma proline concentrations and urinary excretion of proline, hydroxyproline, and glycine; associated with mental retardation, renal anomalies, and renal disease; autosomal recessive inheritance.

hyperprosexia (hī'per-prō-sek'sē-ă) [hyper- + G. *prosexis*, attention]. Fixation of the mind on one idea.

hyperproteinemia (hī'per-prō'tē-in-ē'mē-ă, -prō'tēn-). An abnormally large concentration of protein in plasma.

hyperproteosis (hī'per-prō-tē-ō'sis). The condition due to an excessive amount of protein in the diet.

hyperpyretic (hī'per-pī-ret'ik). Hyperpyrexial; relating to hyperpyrexia.

hyperpyrexia (hī'per-pī-rek'sē-ă) [hyper- + G. *pyrexis*, feverishness]. Extremely high fever.

fulminant h., malignant *hyperthermia*.

heat h., heatstroke.

malignant h., heatstroke.

hyperpyrexial (hī'per-pī-rek'sē-ăl). Hyperpyretic.

hyperreflexia (hī'per-rē-flek'sē-ă). A condition in which the reflexes are exaggerated.

hyperresonance (hī-per-rez'ō-nans). **1.** An extreme degree of resonance. **2.** Resonance increased above the normal, and often of lower pitch, on percussion of an area of the body; occurs in the chest due to overinflation of the lung as in emphysema or pneumothorax and in the abdomen over a distended bowel.

hypersalemia (hī'per-sal-ē'mē-ă). An increase in the salt content of the circulating blood.

hypersaline (hī-per-sā'lēn, -sā'līn). Marked by increased salt in a saline solution.

hypersalivation (hī'per-sal-i-vā'shŭn). Increased salivation.

hypersarcosinemia (hī'per-sar-kō-si-nē'mē-ă). Sarcosinemia.

hypersensitiveness (hī-per-sen'si-tiv-nes). A term introduced into immunologic terminology because of the original misconception that repeated inoculations of toxin-containing preparations produced an increase in the already existing sensitivity to the toxin per se; usage continued in some areas even though it was soon learned that the reactions were allergic (immunologic) in nature, *i.e.*, the result of newly induced sensitivity to previously innocuous substances. See hypersensitivity.

hypersensitivity (hī'per-sen-si-tiv'i-tē). Abnormal sensitivity, a condition in which there is an exaggerated response by the body to the stimulus of a foreign agent. See allergy.

delayed h., cellular *immunity*.

hypersensitization (hī'per-sen'si-ti-zā'shŭn). The immunological process by which hypersensitivity is induced.

hyperserotonemia (hī'per-sēr'ō-tō-nē'mē-ă). Unusually large amounts of serotonin in the circulating blood, probably a causal factor in the carcinoid syndrome.

hyperskeocytosis (hī'per-skē'ō-sī-tō'sis) [G. *skaios*, left, + *kytos*, cell, + *-osis*, condition]. Hyperneocytosis.

hypersomatotropism (hī'per-sō'mă-tō-trō'pizm). A state characterized by abnormally enhanced secretion of pituitary growth hormone (somatotropin).

hypersomia (hī-per-sō'mē-ă) [hyper- + G. *sōma*, body]. Gigantism.

hypersomnia (hī-per-som'nē-ă) [hyper- + L. *somnus*, sleep]. A condition in which sleep periods are excessively long, but the person responds normally in the intervals; distinguished from somnolence.

hypersonic (hī-per-son'ik) [hyper- + L. *sonus*, sound]. Pertaining to or characterized by supersonic speeds of Mach 5 or greater. While any speed above the speed of sound may be referred to as supersonic, speeds of Mach 5 or greater are specifically referred to as h.

hypersphyxia (hī-per-sfik'sē-ă) [hyper- + G. *sphyxis*, pulse]. A condition of high blood pressure and increased circulatory activity.

hypersplenism (hī-per-splēn'izm). A condition, or group of conditions, in which the hemolytic action of the spleen is greatly increased.

hypersteatosis (hī'per-stē-ă-tō'sis). Excessive sebaceous secretion.

hyperstereoroentgenography (hī'per-ster-ē-ō-rent-gen-og'ră-fē). Roentgenography with the two positions from which the x-rays are projected rather widely separated.

hypersthenia (hī-per-sthē'nē-ă) [hyper- + G. *sthenos*, strength]. Excessive tension or strength.

hypersthenic (hī-per-sthen'ik). Pertaining to or marked by hypersthenia.

hypersthenuria (hī'per-sthen-yū'rē-ă) [hyper- + G. *sthenos*, strength, + *ouron*, urine]. Excretion of urine of unusually high specific gravity and concentration of solutes, resulting usually from loss or deprivation of water.

hypersusceptibility (hī'per-sŭ-sep-ti-bil'i-tē). Inordinate response to an infective, chemical, or other agent.

hypersystole (hī-per-sis'tō-lē). Abnormal force or duration of the cardiac systole.

hypersystolic (hī'per-sis-tol'ik). Relating to or marked by hypersystole.

hypertarachia (hī'per-tă-rak'ē-ă) [hyper- + G. *tarachē*, disorder, confusion]. Exaggerated irritability of the nervous system.

hypertelorism (hī-per-tel'ōr-izm) [hyper- + G. *tele*, far off, + *horizō*, to separate, fr. *horos*, a boundary]. Abnormal distance between two paired organs.

canthal h., telecanthus.

ocular h., Greig's syndrome; extreme width between the eyes due to an enlarged sphenoid bone; other congenital deformities and mental retardation may be associated.

hypertensin (hī-per-ten'sin). Former name for angiotensin.

hypertensinase (hī-per-ten'si-nās). Former name for angiotensinase.

hypertensinogen (hī'per-ten-sin'ō-jen). Former name for angiotensinogen.

hypertension (hī'per-ten'shŭn) [hyper- + L. *tensio*, tension]. High blood pressure.

adrenal h., h. due to a pheochromocytoma.

benign h., essential h. that runs a relatively long and symptomless course.

essential h., hyperpiesis; primary h.; idiopathic h.; h. without preexisting renal disease or known cause.

Goldblatt's h., Goldblatt *phenomenon.*
idiopathic h., essential h.
malignant h., severe h. that runs a rapid course, causing necrosis of arteriolar walls in kidney, retina, etc.; hemorrhages occur, and death most frequently is caused by uremia or rupture of a cerebral vessel.
pale h., h. with pallor of the skin, a severe form with pronounced constriction of peripheral vessels.
portal h., h. in the portal system as seen in cirrhosis of the liver and other conditions causing obstruction to the portal vein.
postpartum h., increased blood pressure during the six weeks immediately following the completion of labor.
primary h., essential h.
pulmonary h., h. in the pulmonary circuit; may be primary, or secondary to pulmonary or cardiac disease, *e.g.,* fibrosis of the lung or mitral stenosis.
renal h., h. secondary to renal disease.
renovascular h., h. produced by renal arterial obstruction.

hypertensive (hī-per-ten'siv). **1.** Marked by an increased blood pressure. **2.** Denoting a person suffering from high blood pressure.

hypertensor (hī-per-ten'ser, -sōr). Pressor.

hypertestoidism (hī-per-tes'toyd-izm). Hypergonadism in the male, characterized by proliferation of Leydig cells with excessive production of testosterone.

hyperthecosis (hī'per-thē-kō'sis). Diffuse hyperplasia of the theca cells of the graafian follicles.
stromal h., condition in which luteinized cells are present in ovarian stroma at a distance from follicular structures.
testoid h., hyperplasia of Leydig cells of the testis.

hyperthelia (hī-per-thē'lē-ă) [hyper- + G. *thēlē,* nipple]. Polythelia.

hyperthermalgesia (hī'per-ther-măl-jē'zē-ă) [hyper- + G. *thermē,* heat, + *algēsis,* pain]. Extreme sensitiveness to heat.

hyperthermia (hī-per-ther'mē-ă) [hyper- + G. *thermē,* heat]. Therapeutically induced hyperpyrexia.
malignant h., fulminant hyperpyrexia; rapid onset of extremely high fever with muscle rigidity, precipitated in genetically susceptible persons, especially by halothane or succinylcholine.

hyperthermoesthesia (hī-per-ther'mō-es-thē'zē-ă) [hyper- + G. *thermē,* heat, + *aisthēsis,* feeling]. Extreme sensitiveness to heat.

hyperthrombinemia (hī'per-throm-bi-nē'mē-ă). An abnormal increase of thrombin in the blood, frequently resulting in a tendency to intravascular coagulation.

hyperthymia (hī-per-thī'mē-ă) [hyper- + G. *thymos,* soul, thought]. Excessive emotivity.

hyperthymic (hī-per-thī'mik). **1.** Pertaining to hyperthymia. **2.** Pertaining to hyperthymism.

hyperthymism (hī-per-thī'mizm). Hyperthymization; excessive activity of the thymus gland; formerly postulated to be a causal factor in certain instances of unexpected and sudden death, such as status thymicolymphaticus.

hyperthymization (hī'per-thī-mi-zā'shŭn). Hyperthymism.

hyperthyroidism (hī-per-thī'royd-izm). An abnormality of the thyroid gland in which secretion of thyroid hormone is usually increased and is no longer under regulatory control of hypothalamic-pituitary centers; characterized by a hypermetabolic state, usually with weight loss, tremulousness, elevated plasma levels of thyroxin and/or triiodothyronine, and sometimes exophthalmos; may progress to severe weakness, wasting, hyperpyrexia, and other manifestations of thyroid storm.
iodine-induced h., Jod-Basedow *phenomenon.*
ophthalmic h., hyperthyroidism with exophthalmos.
primary h., h. due to a disorder originating within the thyroid gland, in contrast to one of pituitary origin; may be due to generalized overactivity of the gland or to a localized hyperactive nodule.
secondary h., h. due to stimulation of the thyroid gland by an excess of thyrotrophin secreted by the pituitary gland.

hyperthyroxinemia (hī'per-thī-rok-si-nē'mē-ă). An elevated thyroxine concentration in the blood.

hypertonia (hī-per-tō'nē-ă) [hyper- + G. *tonos,* tension]. Hypertonicity (1); extreme tension of the muscles or arteries.
h. polycythe'mica, a form of polycythemia without a prominent degree of splenomegaly, but with increased blood pressure.
sympathetic h., overfunction of the sympathetic nervous system, often manifested as anxiety.

hypertonic (hī-per-ton'ik). Hyperisotonic. **1.** Spastic (1); having a greater degree of tension. **2.** Having a greater osmotic pressure than a reference solution, which is ordinarily assumed to be blood plasma or interstitial fluid; more specifically, refers to a fluid in which cells shrink.

hypertonicity (hī'per-tō-nis'i-tē). **1.** Hypertonia. **2.** An increased effective osmotic pressure of body fluids.

hypertrichiasis (hī'per-tri-kī'ă-sis). Hypertrichosis.

hypertrichophrydia (hī'per-trik-ō-fri'dē-ă) [hyper- + G. *thrix,* hair, + *ophrys,* eyebrow]. Excessively thick eyebrows.

hypertrichosis (hī'per-tri-kō'sis) [hyper- + G. *trichōsis,* a being hairy]. Hypertrichiasis; growth of hair in excess of the normal.
h. lanugino'sa, a rare congenital condition in which there is excessive growth of fine hair over the entire body.
h. lanugino'sa acquis'ita, malignant down; the sudden growth of silky lanugo-like hairs, especially on the face in adults; usually associated with visceral carcinoma.
nevoid h., congenital growth of hair abnormal for its site, texture, color, or length; often associated with other nevoid abnormalities.
h. partia'lis, abnormally excessive hair growth in patches in unusual areas.
h. universa'lis, generalized excessive hair growth.

hypertriglyceridemia (hī'per-trī-glis'er-i-dē'mē-ă). Elevated triglyceride concentration in the blood.
familial h., **(1)** type I familial *hyperlipoproteinemia;* **(2)** type IV familial *hyperlipoproteinemia.*

hypertroph (hī'per-trof). A microorganism that requires living cells to supply the enzyme systems necessary for growth and reproduction.

hypertrophia (hī-per-trō'fē-ă). Hypertrophy.

hypertrophic (hī-per-trof'ik). Relating to or characterized by hypertrophy.

hypertrophy (hī-per'trō-fē) [hyper- + G. *trophē,* nourishment]. Hypertrophia; general increase in bulk of a part or organ, not due to tumor formation. Use of the term may be restricted to denote greater bulk through increase in size, but not in number, of the individual tissue elements. See also hyperplasia.
adaptive h., thickening of the walls of a hollow organ, like the urinary bladder, when there is obstruction to outflow.
benign prostatic h., nodular *hyperplasia* of prostate.
compensatory h., increase in size of an organ or part of an organ or tissue, when called upon to do additional work or perform the work of destroyed tissue or of a paired organ.
compensatory h. of the heart, thickening of the walls of the heart in response to vascular, valvular, or other heart disease.
complementary h., increase in size or expansion of part of an organ or tissue to fill the space left by the destruction of another portion of the same organ or tissue.
concentric h., thickening of the walls of the heart or any cavity with apparent diminution of the capacity of the cavity.
eccentric h., thickening of the wall of the heart or other cavity, with dilation.
endemic h., enlargement of the calcaneus preceded by fever and pain in the heel, reported from the Gold Coast (now Ghana) and in

Taiwan among the native population.
false h., pseudohypertrophy.
functional h., physiologic h.
giant h. of gastric mucosa, Ménétrièr's *disease.*
hemangiectatic h., Klippel-Trenaunay-Weber *syndrome.*
lipomatous h., lipomatous *infiltration.*
numerical h., hyperplasia.
physiologic h., functional h.; temporary increase in size of an organ or part to provide for a natural increase of function, such as the kind that occurs in the walls of the uterus and in the mammae during pregnancy.
pseudomuscular h., pseudohypertrophic muscular *dystrophy.*
quantitative h., hyperplasia.
simple h., increase in size of cells.
simulated h., increased size of a part due to continued growth unrestrained by attritions, as is seen in the case of the teeth of certain animals when the opposing teeth have been destroyed.
true h., an increase in size involving all the different tissues composing the part.
vicarious h., h. of an organ following failure of another organ because of a functional relationship between them; *e.g.,* enlargement of the pituitary gland, after destruction of the thyroid.

hypertropia (hī'per-trō'pē-ă) [hyper- + G. *tropē,* a turn]. *Strabismus* sursum vergens.

hypertyrosinemia (hī'per-tī'rō-si-nē'mē-ă). Tyrosinemia.

hyperuresis (hī'per-yū-rē'sis) [hyper- + G. *oureō,* to urinate]. Obsolete term for polyuria.

hyperuricemia (hī'per-yū-rē-sē'mē-ă). Enhanced blood concentrations of uric acid.

hyperuricemic (hī'per-yū-ri-sē'mik). Relating to or characterized by hyperuricemia.

hyperuricuria (hī'per-yū-ri-kyū'rē-ă). Increased urinary excretion of uric acid.

hypervaccination (hī'per-vak-si-nā'shŭn). Repeated inoculation of an individual already immunized; used as a means of preparing a highly potent antiserum.

hypervalinemia (hī'per-val-i-nē'mē-ă). Abnormally high plasma concentrations of valine, a common finding in maple syrup urine disease.

hypervascular (hī'per-vas'kyū-ler) [hyper- + L. *vas,* a vessel]. Abnormally vascular; containing an excessive number of blood vessels.

hyperventilation (hī'per-ven-ti-lā'shŭn). Overventilation; increased alveolar ventilation relative to metabolic carbon dioxide production, so that alveolar carbon dioxide pressure decreases to below normal.

hypervitaminosis (hī'per-vī'tă-mi-nō'sis). A condition resulting from the ingestion of an excessive amount of a vitamin preparation, symptoms varying according to the particular vitamin implicated; serious effects may be caused by overdosage with fat-soluble vitamins, especially A or D, and rarely with water-soluble vitamins.

hypervolemia (hī'per-vō-lē'mē-ă) [hyper- + L. *volumen,* volume, + G. *haima,* blood]. Plethora (1); abnormally increased volume of blood.

hypervolemic (hī'per-vō-lē'mik). Pertaining to or characterized by hypervolemia.

hypervolia (hī-per-vō'lē-ă). Augmented water content or volume of a given compartment; *e.g.,* cellular h.

hypesthesia (hī-pes-thē'zē-ă) [G. *hypo,* under, + *aisthēsis,* feeling]. Hypoesthesia; diminished sensitivity to stimulation.
olfactory h., hyposmia.

hypha, pl. **hyphae** (hī'fă, hī'fē) [G. *hyphē,* a web]. A branching tubular cell characteristic of the growth of filamentous fungi (molds). In most species the hyphae are divided by cross-walls (septa) into multicellular hyphae; intercommunicating hyphae constitute a mycelium, the visible colony on natural substrates or artificial laboratory media. The terms hypha and mycelium often are used interchangeably.
racquet h., a vegetative h. with distal ends of successive cells inflated, resembling a string of elongated snowshoes or tennis racquets; seen in some mycelial strains of *Coccidioides immitis* in addition to arthroconidia.
spiral hyphae, hyphae that end in a flat or helical coil, as in laboratory colonies of *Trichophyton mentagrophytes.*

hyphedonia (hīp-hē-dō'nē-ă) [G. *hypo,* under, + *hēdonē,* pleasure]. A habitually lessened or attenuated degree of pleasure from that which should normally give great pleasure.

hyphema (hī-fē'mă) [G. *hyphaimos,* suffused with blood]. Blood in the anterior chamber of the eye.

hyphemia (hī-fē'mē-ă) [hypo- + G. *haima,* blood]. Hypovolemia.
intertropical h., tropical h., ancylostomiasis.

hyphidrosis (hip-hī-drō'sis). Hypohidrosis.

Hyphomyces destruens (hī-fō-mī'sēs des'trū-enz). *Pythium insidiosum.*

Hyphomycetes (hī'fō-mī-sē'tēs) [G. *hyphe,* web, + *mykēs,* fungus]. A class of fungi that includes all of the filamentous members of the Fungi Imperfecti which form neither acervuli nor pycnidia. No sexual reproduction occurs; most members of this group produce asexual spores.

hyphomycosis (hī'fō-mī-kō'sis). Pythiosis; swamp cancer; a disease of horses and mules (rarely of man) caused by *Pythium insidiosum* (*Hyphomyces destruens*), characterized by granulomatous and necrotic lesions that appear on the head and lower legs, ulcerate, and enlarge by subcutaneous extension.

hypn-. See hypno-.

hypnagogic (hip-nă-goj'ik) [hypno- + G. *agōgos,* leading]. Denoting a transitional state, related to the hypnoidal, preceding the oncome of sleep; applied also to various hallucinations that may manifest themselves at that time.

hypnagogue (hip'nă-gog) [hypno- + G. *agōgos,* leading]. An agent that induces sleep.

hypnalgia (hip-nal'jē-ă) [hypno- + G. *algos,* pain]. Dream pain; pain occurring during sleep.

hypnapagogic (hip-nap-ă-goj'ik) [hypno- + G. *apo,* from, + *agōgos,* leading]. Denoting a state similar to the hypnagogic, through which the mind passes in coming out of sleep; denoting also hallucinations experienced at such time.

hypnesthesia (hip-nes-thē'zē-ă) [hypno- + G. *aisthēsis,* sensation]. Drowsiness.

hypnic (hip'nik) [G. *hypnikos,* relating to sleep]. Relating to or causing sleep.

hypno-, hypn- [G. *hypnos,* sleep]. Combining forms relating to sleep or hypnosis.

hypnoanalysis (hip'nō-ă-nal'i-sis). Psychoanalysis or other psychotherapy which employs hypnosis as an adjunctive technique.

hypnoanalytic (hip'nō-an-ă-lit'ik). Pertaining to hypnoanalysis.

hypnocatharsis (hip'nō-kă-thar'sis) [hypno- + G. *katharsis,* purification]. Ventilation of emotional tension and anxiety under hypnosis.

hypnocinematograph (hip'nō-sin-ĕ-mat'ō-graf) [hypno- + G. *kinēma,* movement, + *graphē,* a record]. Somnocinematograph.

hypnocyst (hip'nō-sist) [hypno- + G. *kystis,* bladder (cyst)]. A quiescent or "sleeping" cyst; an encysted protozoon, the reproductive activity of which is in abeyance.

hypnodontics (hip-nō-don'tiks) [hypno- + G. *odous,* tooth]. Hypnosis as applied to the practice of dentistry.

hypnogenesis (hip-nō-jen'ĕ-sis) [hypno- + G. *genesis*, production]. The induction of sleep or of the hypnotic state.

hypnogenic, hypnogenous (hip-nō-jen'ik, -noj'ĕ-nŭs). Relating to hypnogenesis.

hypnoidal (hip-noy'dăl) [hypno- + G. *eidos*, resemblance]. Resembling hypnosis; denoting the subwaking state, a mental condition intermediate between sleeping and waking.

hypnolepsy (hip'nō-lep-sē) [hypno- + G. *lēpsis*, a seizing]. Narcolepsy.

hypnologist (hip-nol'ō-jist). **1.** A student of hypnology. **2.** Hypnotist.

hypnology (hip-nol'ō-jē) [hypno- + G. *logos*, study]. The branch of scientific inquiry regarding sleep or hypnosis and its phenomena.

hypnophobia (hip-nō-fō'bē-ă) [hypno- + G. *phobos*, fear]. Morbid fear of falling asleep.

hypnopompic (hip-nō-pom'pik) [hypno- + G. *pompē*, procession]. Denoting the occurrence of visions or dreams during the drowsy state following sleep.

hypnosis (hip-nō'sis) [G. *hypnos*, sleep, + *-osis*, condition]. Hypnotic state or sleep; status hypnoticus; an artificially induced trancelike state, resembling sonambulism, in which the subject is highly susceptible to suggestion, oblivious to all else, and responds readily to the commands of the hypnotist.

lethargic h., trance coma; the deep sleep following major h.

major h., a state of extreme suggestibility in h. in which the subject is insensible to all outside impressions except the commands of the hypnotist.

minor h., an induced state resembling normal sleep in which the subject is susceptible to suggestion, though not to the extent of catalepsy or somnambulism.

hypnotherapy (hip-nō-thăr'ă-pē). **1.** Treatment of disease by inducing prolonged sleep. **2.** Psychotherapeutic treatment by means of hypnotism.

hypnotic (hip-not'ik) [G. *hypnōtikos*, causing one to sleep]. **1.** Causing sleep. **2.** An agent that promotes sleep. **3.** Relating to hypnotism.

hypnotism (hip'nō-tizm) [G. *hypnos*, sleep]. **1.** Somnipathy; somnolism; the process or act of inducing hypnosis. **2.** The practice or study of hypnosis.

hypnotist (hip'nō-tist). Hypnologist (2); one who practices hypnotism.

hypnotize (hip'nō-tīz). To induct one into hypnosis.

hypnotoid (hip'nō-toyd). Resembling hypnosis.

hypnozoite (hip-nō-zō'īt). Exoerythrocytic schizozoite of *Plasmodium vivax* or *P. ovale* in the human liver, characterized by delayed primary development; thought to be responsible for malarial relapse.

hypo- [G. *hypo*, under]. **1.** Prefix denoting deficient or below the normal; corresponds to the Latin *sub-*. See also hyp-. **2.** In chemistry, denoting the lowest, or least rich in oxygen, of a series of chemical compounds.

hypoacidity (hī'pō-a-sid'i-tē). A lower than normal degree of acidity, as of the gastric juice.

hypoacusis (hī'pō-ă-kū'sis). Hypacusis.

hypoadenia (hī-pō-ă-dē'nē-ă) [hypo- + G. *adēn*, gland]. Any deficiency in the function of a glandular organ or tissue.

hypoadrenalism (hī'pō-ă-drē'năl-izm). Reduced adrenocortical function.

hypoalbuminemia (hī'pō-al-bū-mi-nē'mē-ă). Hypalbuminemia; an abnormally low concentration of albumin in the blood.

hypoaldosteronism (hī'pō-al-dos'ter-on-izm). A condition due to deficient secretion of aldosteron; can occur in two forms: 1) as part of generalized adrenocortical insufficiency; 2) as a selective deficiency caused by a primary defect of the adrenal gland or a defect in control of aldosterone secretion.

hyporeninemic h., selective aldosterone deficiency resulting from renin deficiency.

selective h., isolated h., aldosterone deficiency without a concomitant deficiency of glucocorticoid hormones.

hypoaldosteronuria (hī'pō-al-dos'ter-on-ū'rē-ă). Abnormally low levels of aldosterone in the urine.

hypoalgesia (hī-pō-al-jē'zē-ă) [hypo- + G. *algēsis*, a sense of pain]. Hypalgesia.

hypoalimentation (hī'pō-al-i-men-tā'shŭn). Subalimentation.

hypoazoturia (hī'pō-az-ō-tū'rē-ă) [hypo- + Fr. *azote*, nitrogen, + G. *ouron*, urine]. Hypazoturia; excretion of abnormally small quantities of nonprotein nitrogenous material (especially urea) in the urine.

hypobaria (hī-pō-bar'ē-ă). Hypobarism.

hypobaric (hī-pō-bar'ik) [hypo- + G. *baros*, weight]. **1.** Pertaining to pressure of ambient gases below 1 atmosphere. **2.** With respect to solutions, less dense than the diluent or medium; *e.g.*, in spinal anesthesia, a h. solution has a specific gravity lower than that of spinal fluid.

hypobarism (hī-pō-bar'izm). Hypobaria; dysbarism resulting from decreasing barometric pressure on the body without hypoxia; gas in body cavities tends to expand, and gases dissolved in body fluids tend to come out of solution as bubbles. *Cf.* decompression *sickness*.

hypobaropathy (hī'pō-ba-rop'ă-thē) [hypo- + G. *baros*, weight, + *pathos*, suffering]. Sickness produced by reduced barometric pressure; not always distinguished from hypobarism and altitude sickness.

hypobetalipoproteinemia (hī'pō-bā'tă-lip'ō-prō'tēn-ē'mē-ă). Abnormally low levels of β-lipoproteins in the plasma. See also abetalipoproteinemia.

hypoblast (hī'pō-blast) [hypo- + G. *blastos*, germ]. Endoderm.

hypoblastic (hī-pō-blas'tik). Relating to or derived from the hypoblast.

hypobranchial (hī-pō-brang'kē-ăl). Located beneath the branchial apparatus.

hypobromite (hī-pō-brō'mīt). A salt of hypobromous acid.

hypobromous acid (hī-pō-brō'mŭs). An acid, HOBr, the aqueous solution of which possesses oxidizing and bleaching properties.

hypocalcemia (hī'pō-kal-sē'mē-ă). Abnormally low levels of calcium in the circulating blood; commonly denotes subnormal concentrations of calcium ions.

hypocalcification (hī'pō-kal-si-fi-kā'shŭn). Deficient calcification of bone or teeth.

enamel h., a defect of enamel maturation, caused by local, systemic, or hereditary factors, and characterized by low mineral content. See also amelogenesis imperfecta.

hypocapnia (hī-pō-kap'nē-ă) [hypo- + G. *kapnos*, smoke, vapor]. Hypocarbia; abnormally decreased arterial carbon dioxide tension.

hypocarbia (hī-pō-kar'bē-ă). Hypocapnia.

hypocelom (hī-pō-sē'lom) [hypo- + G. *koilos*, hollow]. Rarely used term for the ventral portion of the celom, or body cavity, of the embryo.

hypochloremia (hī'pō-klō-rē'mē-ă). An abnormally low level of chloride ions in the circulating blood.

hypochloremic (hī'pō-klō-rē'mik). Pertaining to or characterized by hypochloremia.

hypochlorhydria (hī'pō-klōr-hī'drē-ă, -hid'rī-ah). Hypohydrochloria; presence of an abnormally small amount of hydrochloric acid in the stomach.

hypochlorite (hī-pō-klōr'īt). A salt of hypochlorous acid.

hypochlorous acid (hī-pō-klōr'ŭs). An acid, HOCl, having oxidizing and bleaching properties.

hypochloruria (hī'pō-klōr-yū'rē-ă). Excretion of abnormally small quantities of chloride ions in the urine.

hypocholesteremia (hī'pō-kō-les-tĕ-rē'mē-ă). Hypocholesterolemia.

hypocholesterinemia (hī'pō-kō-les'tĕ-ri-nē'mē-ă). Hypocholesterolemia.

hypocholesterolemia (hī'pō-kō-les'ter-ol-ē'mē-ă). Hypocholesteremia; hypocholesterinemia; the presence of abnormally small amounts of cholesterol in the circulating blood.

hypocholia (hī-pō-kō'lē-ă). Oligocholia.

hypochondria (hī-pō-kon'drē-ă). Hypochondriasis.

hypochondriac (hī-pō-kon'drē-ak). **1.** Hypochondriacal. **2.** A person manifesting hypochondriasis. **3.** Beneath the ribs; relating to the hypochondrium.

hypochondriacal (hī'pō-kon-drī'ă-kăl). Hypochondriac (1); relating to or suffering from hypochondriasis.

hypochondriasis (hī'pō-kon-drī'ă-sis) [fr. hypochondrium, regarded as the site of hypochondria, + G. *-iasis,* condition]. Hypochondria; a morbid concern about one's own health and exaggerated attention to any unusual bodily or mental sensations; a delusion that one is suffering from some disease.

hypochondrium, pl. **hypochondria** (hī-pō-kon'drē-ŭm, -ă) [L. fr. G. *hypochondrion,* abdomen, belly, from *hypo,* under, + *chondros,* cartilage (of ribs)]. *Regio* hypochondriaca.

hypochondroplasia (hī'pō-kon-drō-plā'zē-ă) [hypo- + G. *chondros,* cartilage, + *plasis,* a molding]. Dwarfism similar to but milder than achondroplasia and neither seen with achondroplasia in the same families nor evident until mid-childhood; the skull and facies are normal; autosomal dominant inheritance.

hypochordal (hī-pō-kōr'dăl) [hypo- + G. *chordē,* cord]. On the ventral side of the spinal cord.

hypochromasia (hī'pō-krō-mā'zē-ă). Hypochromia.

hypochromatic (hī'-pō-krō-mat'ik) [hypo- + G. *chrōma,* color]. Hypochromic (1); containing a small amount of pigment, or less than the normal amount for the individual tissue.

hypochromatism (hī-pō-krō'mă-tizm). **1.** The condition of being hypochromatic. **2.** Hypochromia.

hypochromia (hī-pō-krō'mē-ă) [hypo- + G. *chrōma,* color]. Hypochromasia; hypochromatism (2); hypochrosis; an anemic condition in which the percentage of hemoglobin in the red blood cells is less than the normal range.

hypochromic (hī-pō-krō'mik). **1.** Hypochromatic. **2.** Denoting decrease in light absorption.

hypochrosis (hī-pō-krō'sis) [hypo- + G. *chrōsis,* a tinting]. Hypochromia.

hypochylia (hī-pō-kī'lē-ă) [hypo- + G. *chylos,* juice]. Oligochylia.

hypocinesis, hypocinesia (hī'pō-si-nē'sis, -nē'zē-ă). Hypokinesis.

hypocitraturia (hī'pō-si-trā-tūr'ē-ă). Abnormally low concentration of citrate in the urine.

hypocomplementemia (hī'pō-kom'plĕ-men-tē'mē-ă). A hereditary or acquired condition of the blood in which one or another component of complement is lacking or reduced in amount; associated with immune complex diseases and cases of membranoproliferative glomerulonephritis in which nephritic factor is present.

hypocone (hī'pō-kōn) [hypo- + G. *kōnos,* pine cone]. The distolingual cusp of an upper molar tooth.

hypoconid (hī-pō-kon'id). The distobuccal cusp of a lower molar tooth.

hypoconule (hī-pō-kon'yūl) [hypo- + Mod. L. dim. of L. *conus,* cone]. The distal, or fifth, cusp of an upper molar tooth.

hypoconulid (hī-pō-kon'yū-lid) [hypo- + Mod. L. dim. of *conus,* cone]. The distal, fifth, cusp of a lower molar tooth.

hypocorticoidism (hī-pō-kōr'ti-koyd-izm). Adrenocortical *insufficiency.*

hypocupremia (hī'pō-kū-prē'mē-ă) [hypo- + L. *cuprum,* copper, + G. *haima,* blood]. Reduced copper content of the blood; found in Wilson's disease because ceruloplasmin is depressed, even though serum albumin-attached copper is increased.

hypocystotomy (hī'pō-sis-tot'ō-mē). Perineal cystotomy.

hypocythemia (hī'pō-sī-thē'mē-ă) [hypo- + G. *kytos,* cell, + *haima,* blood]. Hypocytosis of the circulating blood, such as that observed in aplastic anemia.

progressive h., refractory anemia.

hypocytosis (hī'pō-sī-tō'sis) [hypo- + G. *kytos,* cell, + *-osis,* condition]. Varying degrees of abnormally low numbers of red and white cells and other formed elements of the blood; in some instances, the term is also used to indicate a paucity of component cells of any tissue. See also cytopenia; pancytopenia.

hypodactyly, hypodactylia, hypodactylism (hī'pō-dak'ti-lē, -dak-til'ē-ă, -dak'til-izm) [hypo- + G. *daktylos,* finger]. Less than the full normal complement of digits.

hypoderm (hī'pō-derm) [hypo- + G. *derma,* skin]. *Tela* subcutanea.

Hypoderma (hī-pō-der'mă) [hypo- + G. *derma,* skin]. A genus of botflies whose larvae are the cause of a tropical form of myiasis linearis (cutaneous larva migrans) of man; occasionally they invade the interior of the eye. Two species, *H. bovis* and *H. lineatum,* are botflies of cattle. The ova of *H. bovis* are deposited on hairs of the legs, and the larvae penetrate the skin and migrate through the tissues to the skin of the back, where they appear during late winter as the common warbles; these ulcerate to the surface and mature larvae escape in early summer, fall to the ground, pupate, and give rise to a new generation of flies.

hypodermatic (hī'pō-der-mat'ik). Subcutaneous.

hypodermatoclysis (hī'pō-der-mă-tok'li-sis). Rarely used spelling of hypodermoclysis.

hypodermatomy (hī'pō-der-mat'ō-mē) [hypo- + G. *derma,* skin, + *tomē,* incision]. Subcutaneous division of a structure.

hypodermatosis (hī'pō-der-mă-tō'sis). Infection of herbivores and man with larvae of flies of the genus *Hypoderma.*

hypodermic (hī'pō-der'mik). **1.** Subcutaneous. **2.** Hypodermic *injection.* **3.** Hypodermic *syringe.*

hypodermis (hī-pō-der'mis). *Tela* subcutanea.

hypodermoclysis (hī'pō-der-mok'li-sis) [hypo- + G. *derma,* skin, + *klysis,* a washing out]. Subcutaneous injection of a saline or other solution.

hypodermolithiasis (hī'pō-der'mō-li-thī'ă-sis) [hypo- + G. *derma,* skin, + lithiasis]. Subcutaneous deposits of calcium. See also *calcinosis* cutis.

hypodipsia (hī-pō-dip'sē-ă) [hypo- + G. *dipsa,* thirst]. Insensible or subliminal thirst; a physiologic condition, perhaps caused by hypertonicity of body fluids, insufficient to initiate drinking but at times sufficient to sustain drinking when started; loosely, oligodipsia.

hypodontia (hī-pō-don'shē-ă) [hypo- + G. *odous,* tooth]. Partial anodontia; oligodontia; a condition of having fewer than the normal compliment of teeth, either congenital or acquired.

hypodynamia (hī'pō-dī-nā'mē-ă, -dī-nam'ē-ă) [hypo- + G. *dynamis,* force]. Diminished power.

h. cor'dis, diminished force of cardiac contraction.

hypodynamic (hī'pō-dī-nam'ik). Possessing or exhibiting subnormal power or force.

hypoeccrisis (hī'pō-ek'ri-sis) [hypo- + G. *eccrisis,* separation]. Reduced excretion of waste matter.

hypoeccritic (hī'pō-ĕ-krit'ik). Characterized by hypoeccrisis.

hypoeosinophilia (hī'pō-ē'ō-sin-ō-fil'ē-ă). Eosinopenia.

hypoergia, hypoergy (hī'pō-er'jē-ă, hī-pō-er'jē) [hypo- + G. *(en)ergeia,* from *ergon,* work]. Hyposensitiveness.

hypoesophoria (hī'pō-es-ō-fō'rē-ă) [hypo- + G. *esō,* within, + *phoros,* bearing]. A tendency of the visual axis of one eye to deviate downward and inward, prevented by binocular vision.

hypoesthesia (hī'pō-es-thē'zē-ă). Hypesthesia.

hypoexophoria (hī'pō-ek-sō-fō'rē-ă) [hypo- + G. *exō,* without, + *phoros,* bearing]. A tendency of the visual axis of one eye to deviate downward and outward, prevented by binocular vision.

hypoferremia (hī'pō-fer-ē'mē-ă). A deficiency of iron in the circulating blood.

hypofibrinogenemia (hī'pō-fī-brin'ō-jĕ-nē'mē-ă). Abnormally low concentration of fibrinogen in the circulating blood plasma.

hypofunction (hī'pō-fŭnk-shŭn). Reduced, low, or inadequate function.

hypogalactia (hī'pō-ga-lak'shē-ă) [hypo- + G. *gala,* milk]. Less than normal milk secretion.

hypogalactous (hī'pō-ga-lak'tŭs). Producing or secreting a less than normal amount of milk.

hypogammaglobinemia (hī'pō-gam'ă-glō'bi-nē'mē-ă). Hypogammaglobulinemia.

hypogammaglobulinemia (hī'pō-gam'ă-glob'yū-li-nē'mē-ă). Hypogammaglobinemia; decreased quantity of the gamma fraction of serum globulin; sometimes used loosely to denote decreased quantity of immunoglobulins in general; associated with increased susceptibility to pyogenic infections.

acquired h., common variable *immunodeficiency.*

primary h., h. due to a primary immunodeficiency of immunoglobulin-forming cells (B-lymphocytes).

secondary h., secondary *immunodeficiency.*

transient h. of infancy, transient agammaglobulinemia; a type of primary immunodeficiency that occurs in infants of both sexes, usually before the sixth month of life, probably resulting from immaturity of lymphoid tissue.

X-linked h., X-linked infantile h., Glanzmann-Riniker syndrome; Bruton type, congenital, or X-linked agammaglobulinemia; Bruton's disease; a congenital, X-linked recessive, primary immunodeficiency characterized by decreased numbers (or absence) of circulating B-lymphocytes with corresponding decrease in immunoglobulins of the five classes; associated with marked susceptibility to infection by pyogenic bacteria (notably, pneumococci and *Haemophilus influenzae*) beginning after loss of maternal antibodies.

hypoganglionosis (hī'pō-gang-lē-on-ō'sis). A reduction in the number of ganglionic nerve cells.

hypogastric (hī-pō-gas'trik). Relating to the hypogastrium.

hypogastrium (hī'pō-gas'trē-ŭm) [G. *hypogastrion,* lower belly, fr. *hypo,* under, + *gastēr,* belly] [NA]. *Regio* pubica.

hypogastrocele (hī'pō-gas'trō-sēl) [hypogastrium + G. *kēlē,* hernia]. Hernia of the lower part of the abdomen.

hypogastropagus (hī'pō-gas-trop'ă-gŭs) [hypogastrium + G. *pagos,* fr. *pēgnynai,* to fasten]. Twins joined at the hypogastrium.

hypogastroschisis (hī'pō-gas-tros'ki-sis) [hypogastrium + G. *schisis,* cleaving]. Congenital fissure in the hypogastric region.

hypogenesis (hī'pō-jen'ĕ-sis) [hypo- + G. *genesis,* origin]. General underdevelopment of parts or organs of the body.

polar h., less than normal degree of development at the cephalic or caudal extremity of the embryo.

hypogenetic (hī'pō-jĕ-net'ik). Relating to hypogenesis.

hypogenitalism (hī-pō-jen'i-tăl-izm). Partial or complete failure of maturation of the genitalia; commonly, a consequence of hypogonadism.

hypogeusia (hī-pō-gū'sē-ă) [hypo- + G. *geusis,* taste]. Blunting of the sense of taste.

hypoglobulia (hī'pō-glo-byū'lē-ă) [hypo- + G. *globulus,* globule]. Old term for abnormally low numbers of red blood cells in the circulating blood; also used infrequently with reference to abnormally decreased proportions of erythroid elements in the bone marrow.

hypoglossal (hī-pō-glos'ăl) [L. *hypoglossus* fr. hypo- + *glossus,* tongue]. Subglossal. **1.** Below the tongue. **2.** Relating to the twelfth cranial nerve, nervus hypoglossus.

hypoglossis (hī-pō-glos'is). Hypoglottis.

hypoglossus (hī'pō-glos'ŭs) [L.] [NA]. Hypoglossal.

hypoglottis (hī'pō-glot'is) [G. *hypoglōssis,* or *-glōttis,* undersurface of tongue, fr. *hypo,* under, + *glōssa,* tongue]. Hypoglossis; ranula (1); the undersurface of the tongue.

hypoglycemia (hī'pō-glī-sē'mē-ă). Glucopenia; an abnormally small concentration of glucose in the circulating blood, *i.e.,* less than the minimum of the normal range.

leucine h., reduction in blood glucose concentration produced by administration of leucine; believed to reflect the ability of this amino acid to stimulate insulin secretion.

neonatal h., familial onset of symptomatic h. during infancy, with persistently low blood glucose, leucine-induced hyperinsulinism, and variable mental retardation.

hypoglycemic (hī'pō-glī-sē'mik). Pertaining to or characterized by hypoglycemia.

hypoglycogenolysis (hī'pō-glī'kō-jĕ-nol'i-sis). Deficient glycogenolysis.

hypoglycorrhachia (hī'pō-glī-kō-rak'ē-ă) [hypo- + G. *glykys,* sweet, + *rhachis,* spine]. Depressed concentration of glucose in the cerebrospinal fluid; a characteristic of bacterial, fungal, and tuberculous meningitis.

hypognathous (hī'pō-nath'ŭs, hī-pog'na-thŭs) [hypo- + G. *gnathos,* jaw]. Having a congenitally defectively developed lower jaw.

hypognathus (hī'pō-nath'ŭs, hī-pog'na-thŭs) [hypo- + G. *gnathos,* jaw]. Unequal conjoined twins in which the rudimentary parasite is attached to the mandible of the autosite.

hypogonadism (hī'pō-gō'nad-izm). Inadequate gonadal function, as manifested by deficiencies in gametogenesis and/or the secretion of gonadal hormones; results in atrophy or deficient development of secondary sexual characteristics and, when occurring in prepubertal males, in altered body habitus characterized by a short trunk and long limbs.

h. with anosmia, Kallmann's syndrome; failure of sexual development secondary to inadequate secretion of pituitary gonadotropins, associated with anosmia due to agenesis of the olfactory lobes of the brain; probably X-linked inheritance.

familial hypogonadotropic h., a disorder characterized by failure of sexual development, owing to inadequate secretion of pituitary gonadotropins; probably autosomal recessive inheritance.

hypogonadotropic h., hypogonadotropic eunuchoidism; secondary h.; defective gonadal development or function, or both, resulting from inadequate secretion of pituitary gonadotropins.

male h., eunuchoidism.

primary h., defective gonadal development or function, or both, due to abnormality or loss of the gonad itself.

secondary h., hypogonadotropic h.

hypogonadotropic (hī'pō-gon'ă-dō-trop'ik). Indicating inadequate secretion of gonadotrophins and the consequences thereof.

hypogranulocytosis (hī'pō-gran'yū-lō-sī-tō'sis). Granulocytopenia.

hypohepatia (hī'pō-hĕ-pat'ē-ă) [hypo- + G. *hēpar,* liver]. Rarely used term for underfunctioning of the liver.

hypohidrosis (hī'pō-hī-drō'sis). Hypoidrosis; hyphidrosis; diminished perspiration.

hypohidrotic (hī'pō-hi-drot'ik). Characterized by diminished sweating.

hypohydremia (hī'pō-hī-drē'mē-ă) [hypo- + G. *hydōr,* water, + *haima,* blood]. Any deficiency in the amount of fluid in the blood.

hypohydrochloria (hī'pō-hī-drō-klōr'ē-ă). Hypochlorhydria.

hypohyloma (hī'pō-hī-lō'mă) [hypo- + G. *hylē,* substance, + *-oma,* tumor]. A neoplasm resulting from abnormal proliferation of tissue derived from the embryonic pulp of hypoblastic origin.

hypohypnotic (hī'pō-hip-not'ik) [hypo- + G. *hypnos,* sleep]. Denoting incomplete or light slumber.

hypoidrosis (hī'pō-id-rō'sis). Hypohidrosis.

hypoisotonic (hī'pō-ī-sō-ton'ik). Hypotonic.

hypokalemia (hī'pō-ka-lē'mē-ă) [hypo- + Mod. L. *kalium,* potassium, + G. *haima,* blood]. Hypopotassemia; the presence of an abnormally small concentration of potassium ions in the circulating blood; occurs in familial periodic paralysis and in potassium depletion due to excessive loss from the gastrointestinal tract or kidneys. The changes of h. may include vacuolation of renal tubular epithelial cytoplasm with impairment of urinary concentrating power and acidification, flattening of the T wave of the electrocardiogram, and muscle weakness.

hypokinemia (hī'pō-ki-nē'mē-ă) [hypo- + G. *kineo,* to move, + *haima,* blood]. Reduced volume flow through the circulation; reduced circulation rate; subnormal cardiac output.

hypokinesis, hypokinesia (hī'pō-ki-nē'sis, -nē'zē-ă) [hypo- + G. *kinēsis,* movement]. Hypocinesis; hypocinesia; hypomotility; diminished or slow movement.

hypokinetic (hī'pō-ki-net'ik). Relating to or characterized by hypokinesis.

hypolepidoma (hī'pō-lep-i-dō'mă) [hypo- + G. *lepis,* rind, + *-oma,* tumor]. A neoplasm resulting from abnormal proliferation of one of the tissues derived from the hypoblast.

hypoleukemia (hī'pō-lū-kē'mē-ă). Subleukemic *leukemia.*

hypoleydigism (hī-pō-lī'dig-ism). Subnormal secretion of androgens by the interstitial (Leydig's) cells of the testes.

hypoliposis (hī'pō-li-pō'sis). Presence of an abnormally small amount of fat in the tissues.

hypologia (hī'pō-lō'jē-ă) [hypo- + G. *logos,* word]. Lack of ability for speech.

hypolymphemia (hī'pō-lim-fē'mē-ă). Abnormally small numbers of lymphocytes in the circulating blood.

hypomagnesemia (hī'pō-mag-nē-sē'mē-ă). Subnormal blood serum concentration of magnesium; may cause convulsions and concurrent hypocalcemia.

hypomania (hī'pō-mā'nē-ă). A mild degree of mania.

hypomastia (hī'pō-mas'tē-ă) [hypo- + G. *mastos,* breast]. Hypomazia; atrophy or congenital smallness of the breasts.

hypomazia (hī-pō-mā'zē-ă). Hypomastia.

hypomelancholia (hī'pō-mel-an-kō'lē-ă). A mild degree of mental depression.

hypomelanosis (hī'pō-mel-ă-nō'sis). Leukoderma.
h. of Ito, *incontinentia* pigmenti achromiens.

hypomelia (hī-pō-mē'lē-ă) [hypo- + G. *melos,* limb]. General term for hypoplasia of some or all parts of one or more limbs.

hypomenorrhea (hī'pō-men-ō-rē'ă) [hypo- + G. *mēn,* month, + *rhoia,* flow]. Diminution of the flow or a shortening of the duration of menstruation.

hypomere (hī'pō-mēr) [hypo- + G. *meros,* part]. **1.** The portion of the myotome that extends ventrolaterally to form body-wall muscle, innervated by the primary ventral ramus of a spinal nerve. **2.** Less commonly, the somatic and splanchnic layers of the lateral mesoderm which give rise to the lining of the celom.

hypometabolism (hī'pō-me-tab'ō-lizm). Reduced metabolism. See also hypometabolic *state.*
euthyroid h., an unusual condition resembling myxedema but with an apparently normal thyroid gland.

hypometria (hī-pō-mē'trē-ă) [hypo- + G. *metron,* measure]. Ataxia characterized by underreaching an object or goal. *Cf.* hypermetria.

hypomnesia (hī-pō-nē'zē-ă) [hypo- + G. *mnēmē,* memory]. Impaired memory.

hypomorph (hī'pō-mōrf) [hypo- + G. *morphē,* form]. A person whose standing height is short in proportion to the sitting height, owing to shortness of the limbs. *Cf.* hypermorph; endomorph.

hypomotility (hī'pō-mō-til'i-tē). Hypokinesis.

hypomyelination, hypomyelinogenesis (hī'pō-mī'ē-lin-ā-shun, -ō-jen'ē-sis). Defective formation of myelin in the spinal cord and brain; the basis for a number of demyelinating diseases.

hypomyotonia (hī'pō-mī-ō-tō'nē-ă) [hypo- + G. *mys* (*myo-*) muscle, + *tonos,* tension]. A condition of diminished muscular tonus.

hypomyxia (hī'pō-mik'sē-ă) [hypo- + G. *myxa,* mucus]. A condition in which the secretion of mucus is diminished.

hyponatremia (hī'pō-nă-trē'mē-ă) [hypo- + natrium, + G. *haima,* blood]. Abnormally low concentrations of sodium ions in the circulating blood.

hyponeocytosis (hī'pō-nē'ō-sī-tō'sis) [hypo- + G. *neos,* new, + *kytos,* cell, + *-osis,* condition]. Hyposkeocytosis; leukopenia associated with the presence of immature and young leukocytes (especially in the granulocytic series), *i.e.,* a "shift to the left" in the hemogram.

hyponoia (hī'pō-noy'-ă) [hypo- + G. *noeō,* to think]. Deficient or sluggish mental activity or imagination.

hyponychial (hī'pō-nik'ē-ăl). **1.** Subungual. **2.** Relating to the hyponychium.

hyponychium (hī'pō-nik'ē-ŭm) [hypo- + G. *onyx,* nail] [NA]. The epithelium of the nail bed, particularly its posterior part in the region of the lunula.

hyponychon (hī-pon'i-kon) [hypo- + G. *onyx,* nail]. An ecchymosis beneath a fingernail or toenail.

hypooncotic (hī'pō-on-kot'ik). Indicating an oncotic pressure less than normal, *e.g.,* of blood plasma.

hypoorthocytosis (hī'pō-ōr'thō-sī-tō'sis) [hypo- + G. *orthos,* correct, + *kytos,* cell, + *-osis,* condition]. Leukopenia in which the relative numbers of the various types of white blood cells are within the normal range, and no immature cells are found in the circulating blood.

hypoovarianism (hī'pō-ō-vā'rē-an-izm). Hypovarianism; inadequate ovarian function, commonly referring to reduced secretion of ovarian hormones.

hypopancreatism (hī'pō-pan'krē-ă-tizm). A condition of diminished activity of digestive enzyme secretion by the pancreas.

hypopancreorrhea (hī'pō-pan'krē-ō-rē'ă) [hypo- + pancreas + G. *rhoia,* flow]. Reduced delivery of pancreatic digestive enzyme secretions.

hypoparathyroidism (hī'pō-par-ă-thī'royd-izm). Parathyroid insufficiency; a condition due to diminution or absence of the secretion of the parathyroid hormones. See also pseudohypoparathyroidism;

pseudo-pseudohypoparathyroidism.

familial h., idiopathic h. in members of the same family, with low serum calcium and tetany, and sometimes with increased bone density.

hypopepsia (hī-pō-pep'sē-ă) [hypo- + G. *pepsis,* digestion]. Oligopepsia; impaired digestion, especially that due to a deficiency of pepsin.

hypoperistalsis (hī'pō-per-i-stal'sis). Reduced or inadequate peristalsis.

hypophalangism (hī'pō-fă-lan'jizm). Congenital absence of one or more of the phalanges of a finger or toe.

α-hypophamine (hī-pof'ă-mēn). Oxytocin.

β-hypophamine. Vasopressin.

hypopharyngoscope (hī'pō-fa-ring'ō-skōp). Instrument used for examination of the hypopharynx.

hypopharynx (hī'pō-far'inks). *Pars* laryngea pharyngis.

hypophonesis (hī'pō-fō-nē'sis) [hypo- + G. *phōnēsis,* a sounding]. In percussion or auscultation, a sound that is diminished or fainter than usual.

hypophonia (hī'pō-fō'nē-ă) [hypo- + G. *phōnē,* voice]. Leptophonia; microphonia; microphony; an abnormally weak voice due to incoordination of the muscles concerned in vocalization.

hypophoria (hī'pō-fō'rē-ă) [hypo- + G. *phora,* motion]. A tendency of the visual axis of one eye to deviate downward, prevented by binocular vision.

hypophosphatasemia (hī'pō-fos'fă-tă-sē'mē-ă). Hypophosphatasia.

hypophosphatasia (hī'pō-fos'fă-tā'zē-ă). Hypophosphatasemia; an abnormally low content of alkaline phosphatase in the circulating blood.

congenital h., a rare disorder associated with a low level of serum alkaline phosphatase, hyperphosphaturia, hypercalcemia, skeletal abnormalities, pathologic fractures, craniostenosis, and often early death; eyes may show blue sclerae, lid retraction, band-shaped keratopathy, cataracts, papilledema, and optic atrophy.

hypophosphatemia (hī'pō-fos-fă-tē'mē-ă). Abnormally low concentrations of phosphates in the circulating blood.

hypophosphaturia (hī'pō-fos'fă-tū'rē-ă). Reduced urinary excretion of phosphates.

hypophosphorous acid (hī-pō-fos'fō-rŭs). An aqueous solution containing 31% HPH_2O_2; used as a stabilizing reducing agent in pharmaceutical preparations.

hypophrasia (hī'pō-frā'zē-ă) [hypo- + G. *phrasis,* speaking]. Slowness or lack of speech associated with a psychosis.

hypophyseal (hī'pō-fiz'ē-ăl). Hypophysial.

hypophysectomize (hī'pof-i-sek'tō-mīz). To remove the hypophysis cerebri.

hypophysectomy (hī'pof-i-sek'tō-mē). Excision or destruction of the pituitary gland by means of craniotomy or stereotaxy.

hypophyseoprivic (hī'pō-fiz'ē-ō-priv'ik). Hypophysioprivic.

hypophyseotropic (hī'pō-fiz'ē-ō-trop'ik). Hypophysiotropic.

hypophysial (hī'pō-fiz'ē-ăl). Hypophyseal; relating to a hypophysis.

hypophysin (hī-pof'i-sin). An aqueous extract of the posterior lobe of the fresh hypophysis of cattle; contains oxytocin and vasopressin.

hypophysioprivic (hī'pō-fiz'ē-ō-priv'ik) [hypophysis + L. *privus,* deprived of]. Hypophyseoprivic; denoting the condition in which the pituitary gland may be functionally inactive or may be absent, as after hypophysectomy.

hypophysiotropic (hī'pō-fiz'ē-ō-trop'ik). Hypophyseotropic; denoting a hormone that acts on the pituitary gland (hypophysis).

hypophysis (hī-pof'i-sis) [G. an undergrowth] [NA]. Glandula pituitaria or basilaris; pituitary or master gland; h. cerebri; an unpaired compound gland suspended from the base of the hypothalamus by a short extension of the infundibulum, the infundibular or pituitary stalk. The h. consists of two major subdivisions: 1) the neurohypophysis, comprising the infundibulum and its bulbous termination, the pars nervosa or infundibular process (posterior lobe), which is composed of neuroglia-like pituicytes, blood vessels, and unmyelinated nerve fibers of the hypothalamohypophyseal tract whose cell bodies reside in the supraoptic and paraventricular nuclei of the hypothalamus, and convey to the lobe for storage and release the neurosecretory hormones oxytocin and antidiuretic hormone; 2) the adenohypophysis, comprising the larger pars distalis, a sleeve-like extension of this lobe (pars tuberalis) which invests the infundibular stalk, and a thin pars intermedia (poorly developed in man) between the anterior and posterior lobes; the anterior lobe consists of cords of cells of several different types interspersed with capillaries of the hypothalamohypophysial portal system; secretion of somatotropins, prolactin, thyroid-stimulating hormone, gonadotropins, adrenal corticotropin, and other related peptides in the adenohypophysis is regulated by releasing and inhibiting factors elaborated by neurons in the hypothalamus which are taken up by a primary plexus of capillaries in the median eminence and transported via portal vessels in the pars infundibularis and infundibular stem to a secondary plexus of capillaries in the pars distalis. See also hypothalamus.

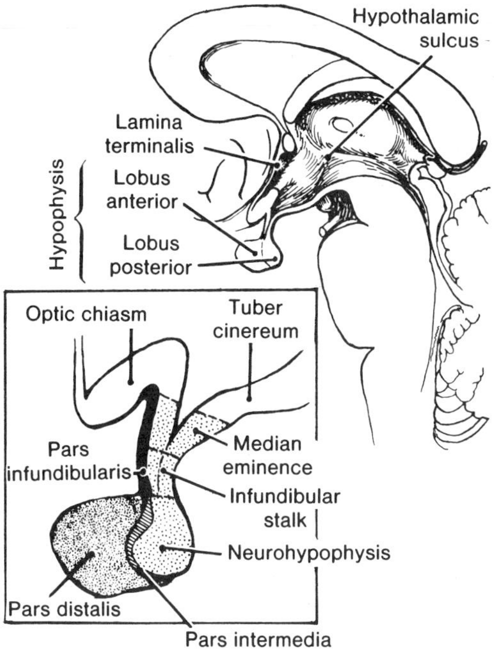

Hypophysis and Hypothalamus

h. cere'bri, hypophysis.

pharyngeal h., *pars* pharyngea hypophyseos; residual tissue derived from the hypophysial diverticulum which lies in the lamina propria of the nasopharynx; its cells and their arrangement are identical with those of the pars distalis.

h. sic'ca, posterior *pituitary.*

hypophysitis (hī-pof-i-sī'tis). Inflammation of the hypophysis.

lymphoid h., an acute anterior pituitary lymphocytic reaction characterized clinically by signs and symptoms of anterior pituitary insufficiency; probably an autoimmune disorder because antipituitary antibodies are present in the serum.

hypopiesis (hī'pō-pī-ē'sis) [hypo- + G. *piesis,* pressure]. Hypotension (1).
orthostatic h., orthostatic *hypotension.*

hypopituitarism (hī'pō-pi-tū'i-tă-rizm). A condition due to diminished activity of the anterior lobe of the hypophysis, with inadequate secretion, to varying degrees, of one or more anterior pituitary hormones.

hypoplasia (hī'pō-plā'zē-ă) [hypo- + G. *plasis,* a molding]. **1.** Underdevelopment of tissue or an organ, usually due to a decrease in the number of cells. **2.** Atrophy due to destruction of some of the elements and not merely to their general reduction in size.
cartilage-hair h., an inherited form of dwarfism characterized by shortness of the extremities without skull defects, and with sparse, brittle hair of light color.
enamel h., a developmental disturbance of teeth characterized by deficient or defective enamel matrix formation; may be hereditary, as in amelogenesis imperfecta, or acquired, as encountered in dental fluorosis, local infection, childhood fevers, and congenital syphilis.
focal dermal h., Goltz syndrome; a rare congenital condition characterized by irregular linear streaks of skin atrophy with skeletal malformations, and papillomas of the lips.
optic nerve h., congenitally small optic disk due to failure of development of retinal ganglion cells, with a reduced number of axons; visual impairment may be marked.
renal h., an abnormally small kidney that is morphologically normal but has either a reduced number of nephrons or smaller nephrons.
right ventricular h., parchment *heart.*
thymic h., *immunodeficiency* with hypoparathyroidism.

hypoplastic (hī'pō-plas'tik). Pertaining to or characterized by hypoplasia.

hypopnea (hī-pop'nē-ă) [hypo- + G. *pnoē,* breathing]. Oligopnea; breathing that is shallower, slower, or both, than normal.

hypoposia (hī'pō-pō'sē-ă) [hypo- + G. *posis,* drinking]. Hypodipsia, with emphasis on tendency to drink rather than on the reduced sensation of thirst.

hypopotassemia (hī'pō-pō-ta-sē'mē-ă). Hypokalemia.

hypopraxia (hī-pō-prak'sē-ă) [hypo- + G. *praxis,* action, + *-ia,* condition]. Deficient activity.

hypoproaccelerinemia (hī'pō-prō-ak-sel'er-i-nē'mē-ă). Abnormally low concentration of blood-clotting factor V, *i.e.,* proaccelerin, in the circulating blood.

hypoproconvertinemia (hī'pō-prō-kon-ver'ti-nē'mē-ă). Abnormally low concentration of blood-clotting factor VII, *i.e.,* proconvertin, in the circulating blood; a deficiency causes a quantitative prolongation of the prothrombin time.

hypoproteinemia (hī'pō-prō'tē-in-ē'mē-ă, -prō-tēn-). Abnormally small amounts of total protein in the circulating blood plasma.

hypoproteinosis (hī'pō-prō'tē-in-o'sis, -prō'tēn-). A condition, especially in children, due to a dietary deficiency of protein; characterized by anorexia, vomiting, retardation of growth, anemia, and increased susceptibility to infections.

hypoprothrombinemia (hī'pō-prō-throm'bin-ē'mē-ă). Prothrombinopenia; abnormally small amounts of prothrombin in the circulating blood.

hypoptyalism (hī'pō-tī'ă-lizm) [hypo- + G. *ptyalon,* saliva]. Hyposalivation.

hypopyon (hī-pō'pi-on) [hypo- + G. *pyon,* pus]. The presence of leukocytes in the anterior chamber of the eye.
recurrent h., Behçet's *syndrome.*

hyporeflexia (hī'pō-rē-flek'sē-ă). A condition in which the reflexes are weakened.

hyporeninemia (hī'pō-ren-i-nē'mē-ă). Low levels of renin in the circulating blood.

hyporeninemic (hī'pō-ren-i-nē'mik). Denoting or characterized by hyporeninemia.

hyporiboflavinosis (hī'pō-rī'bō-flā-vi-nō'sis). A more correct term than the more commonly used ariboflavinosis (*q.v.*).

hyposalemia (hī-pō-să-lē'mē-ă) [hypo- + L. *sal,* salt, + G. *haima,* blood]. Obsolete term meaning abnormally small amounts of various salts in the circulating blood; sometimes was used as a synonym for hypochloremia.

hyposalivation (hī'pō-sal'i-vā'shŭn). Hypoptyalism; reduced salivation.

hyposarca (hī'pō-sar'kă) [hypo- + G. *sarx* (*sark-*), flesh]. Extreme anasarca of the subcutaneous connective tissue.

hyposcheotomy (hī-pos-kē-ot'ō-mē) [hypo- + G. *oscheon,* scrotum, + *tomē,* incision]. Incision or puncture into a hydrocele at its most dependent point.

hyposcleral (hī-pō-sklēr'ăl). Beneath the sclerotic coat of the eyeball.

hyposensitivity (hī'pō-sen-si-tiv'i-tē). Hypoergia; hypoergy; a condition of subnormal sensitivity, in which the response to a stimulus is unusually delayed or lessened in degree.

hyposialadenitis (hī'pō-sī'al-ad-ĕ-nī'tis) [hypo- + G. *sialon,* saliva, + *adēn,* gland, + *-itis,* inflammation]. Inflammation of a salivary gland or glands.

hyposkeocytosis (hī'pō-skē'ō-sī-tō'sis) [hypo- + *skaios,* left, + *kytos,* cell, + *-osis,* condition]. Hyponeocytosis.

hyposmia (hī-poz'mē-ă) [hypo- + G. *osmē,* smell]. Hyposphresia; olfactory hypesthesia; diminished sense of smell.

hyposmosis (hī-pos-mō'sis). A reduction in the rapidity of osmosis.

hyposmotic (hī-pos-mot'ik). Having an osmolality less than another fluid, ordinarily assumed to be plasma or extracellular fluid.

hyposomatotropism (hī'pō-sō'mă-tō-trō'pizm). A state characterized by deficient secretion of pituitary growth hormone (somatotropin).

hyposomia (hī'pō-sō'mē-ă) [hypo- + G. *sōma,* body]. Inadequate development of the body.

hyposomniac (hī'pō-som'nē-ak) [hypo- + L. *somnus,* sleep]. Pertaining to reduction in time of sleeping.

hypospadiac (hī'pō-spā'dē-ak). Relating to hypospadias.

hypospadias (hī'pō-spā'dē-ăs) [G. one having the orifice of the penis too low, fr. *hypospaō,* to draw away from under]. A developmental anomaly characterized by a defect on the ventrum of the penis so that the urethral canal is open for a variable distance on the undersurface of the penis and may be associated with chordee; also a similar defect in the female in which the urethra opens into the vagina. See fig. on p. 754.
balanic h., male h. involving the glans penis.
penoscrotal h., h. with the opening at the junction of the penis and scrotum.
perineal h., h. in which the urethral defect continues along the perineum to near the anus; the scrotum is usually cleft, the testes undescended, and the penis rudimentary.

hyposphresia (hī'pos-frē'zē-ă) [hypo- + G. *osphrēsis,* smell]. Hyposmia.

hyposphyxia (hī'pō-sfik'sē-ă) [hypo- + G. *sphyxis,* pulse]. Abnormally low blood pressure with sluggishness of the circulation.

hypostasis (hi-pos'tă-sis) [G. *hypo-stasis,* a standing under, sediment]. **1.** Formation of a sediment at the bottom of a liquid. **2.** Hypostatic *congestion.* **3.** The phenomenon whereby the pheno-

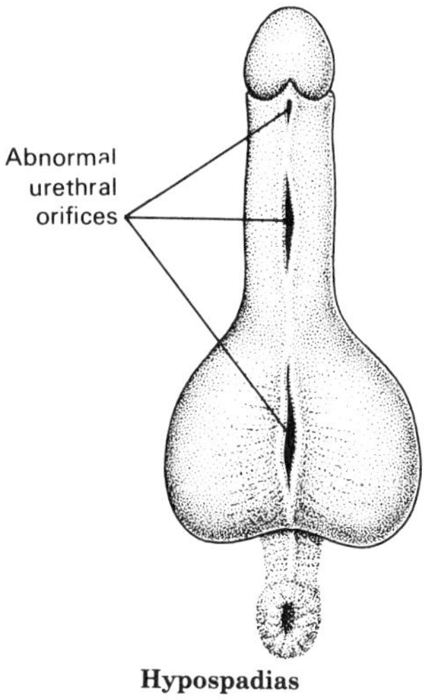

Hypospadias

type that would ordinarily be manifested at one locus is obscured by the genotype at another locus (epistasis); *e.g.*, in man, observed in the Bombay blood group phenomenon.

postmortem h., postmortem *livedo.*

pulmonary h., hydrostatic congestion of the lung.

hypostatic (hī-pō-stat'ik). **1.** Sedimentary; resulting from a dependent position. **2.** Relating to hypostasis.

hyposthenia (hī'pos-thē'nē-ă) [hypo- + G. *sthenos,* strength]. Weakness. See asthenia.

hypostheniant (hī'pos-thē'nē-ant). **1.** Weakening. **2.** An agent that reduces strength.

hyposthenic (hī-pos-then'ik). Weak.

hyposthenuria (hī'pos-thĕ-nū'rē-ă) [hypo- + G. *sthenos,* strength, + *ouron,* urine]. Secretion of urine of low specific gravity, due to inability of the tubules of the kidneys to produce a concentrated urine or occurs following excessive water ingestion in diabetes insipidus.

hypostome (hī'pō-stōm) [hypo- + G. *stoma,* mouth]. The central unpaired holdfast organ of the tick capitulum; the h. is covered with recurved spines that enable it to serve as an anchoring device while the tick feeds.

hypostomia (hī'pō-stō'mē-ă) [hypo- + G. *stoma,* mouth]. A form of microstomia in which the oral opening is a small vertical slit.

hypostosis (hīp-os-tō'sis) [hypo- + G. *osteon,* bone, + *-osis,* condition]. Deficient development of bone.

hypostypsis (hī'pō-stip'sis) [hypo- + G. *stypsis,* astringence]. A state of mild astringence.

hypostyptic (hī'pō-stip'tik). Mildly styptic or astringent.

hyposystole (hī'pō-sis'tō-lē). A weak or incomplete cardiac systole.

hypotaxia (hī'pō-tak'sē-ă) [hypo- + G. *taxis,* order]. A condition of weak or imperfect coordination.

hypotelorism (hī-pō-tel'ōr-izm) [hypo- + G. *tēle,* far off, + *horizō,* to separate, fr. *horos,* boundary]. Abnormal closeness of eyes.

hypotension (hī'pō-ten'shŭn) [hypo- + L. *tensio,* a stretching]. **1.** Hypopiesis; subnormal arterial blood pressure. **2.** Reduced pressure or tension of any kind.

arterial h., see hypotension (1).

induced h., controlled h., deliberate acute reduction of arterial blood pressure to reduce operative blood loss by pharmacologic means during anesthesia and surgery.

intracranial h., subnormal pressure of cerebrospinal fluid; most commonly following lumbar puncture and associated with headache, nausea, vomiting, stiffness of the neck, and sometimes fever; intracranial h. may also result from dehydration, and may occur in diabetic coma, during hyperpnea, or after the injection of a hypertonic solution.

orthostatic h., orthostatic hypopiesis; postural h.; a form of low blood pressure that occurs in a standing posture.

postural h., orthostatic h.

hypotensive (hī'pō-ten'siv). Characterized by low blood pressure or causing reduction in blood pressure.

hypotensor (hī-pō-ten'ser, -sōr). Depressor (4).

hypothalamohypophysial (hī'pō-thal'ă-mō-hī'pō-fiz'ē-ăl). Relating to both the hypothalamus and the hypophysis.

hypothalamus (hī'pō-thal'ă-mŭs) [hypo- + thalamus] [NA]. The ventral and medial region of the diencephalon forming the walls of the ventral half of the third ventricle; it is delineated from the thalamus by the hypothalamic sulcus, lying medial to the internal capsule and subthalamus, continuous with the precommissural septum anteriorly and with the mesencephalic tegmentum and central gray substance posteriorly. Its ventral surface is marked by, from before backward, the optic chiasma, the unpaired infundibulum which extends by way of the infundibular stalk into the posterior lobe of the hypophysis, and the paired mamillary bodies. The nerve cells of the h. are grouped into the supraoptic paraventricular, lateral preoptic, lateral hypothalamic, tuberal, anterior hypothalamic, ventromedial, dorsomedial, arcuate, posterior hypothalamic, and premamillary nuclei and the mamillary body. It has afferent fiber connections with the mesencephalon and limbic system and efferent fiber connections with the same structures and with the posterior lobe of the hypophysis; its functional connection with the anterior lobe of the hypophysis is established by the hypothalamohypophysial portal system. The h. is prominently involved in the functions of the autonomic nervous system and, through its vascular link with the anterior lobe of the hypophysis, in endocrine mechanisms; it also appears to play a role in neural mechanisms underlying moods and motivational states. See also hypophysis.

hypothenar (hī'pō-thē'nar, hī-poth'ĕ-nar) [hypo- + G. *thenar,* the palm]. **1** [NA]. Antithenar; hypothenar eminence or prominence; the fleshy mass at the medial side of the palm. **2.** Denoting any structure in relation with this part.

hypothermal (hī-pō-ther'măl). Denoting hypothermia.

hypothermia (hī'pō-ther'mē-ă) [hypo- + G. *thermē,* heat]. A body temperature significantly below 98.6°F (37°C).

accidental h., unintentional decrease in body temperature, especially in the newborn, infants, and elderly, particularly during operations.

moderate h., a body temperature of 23–32° C. induced by surface cooling.

profound h., a body temperature of 12–20° C.

regional h., reduction of the temperature of an extremity or organ by external cold or perfusion with cold blood or solutions.

total body h., the deliberate reduction of total body temperature, in order to reduce tissue metabolism.

hypothesis (hī-poth'ĕ-sis) [L. fr. G. *hypotithenai,* to propose or suppose]. A supposition or assumption advanced as a basis for reasoning or argument, or as a guide to experimental investigation; a tentative theory unsupported by the essential facts that would prove its truth. See also postulate; theory.

autocrine h., that tumor cells containing viral oncogenes may have encoded a growth factor, normally produced by other cell types, and thereby produce the factor autonomously, leading to uncontrolled proliferation.

Avogadro's h., Avogadro's *law.*

frustration-aggression h., the theory that frustration may lead to aggression, but that aggression is always the result of some form of frustration.

gate-control h., gate-control *theory.*

Gompertz' h., a theory that the force of mortality increases in geometrical progression, being based on the assumption that the average exhaustion of a person's power to avoid death is such that at the end of equal infinitely small intervals of time he loses equal proportions of the power to oppose destruction which he had at the commencement of each of these intervals.

insular h., obsolete theory of the origin of diabetes mellitus from destruction or loss of function of the islets of Langerhans in the pancreas.

Lyon h., the concept that one X-chromosome is inactive during interphase in normal females, and is represented in interphase cell nuclei as the sex chromatin body; as either X-chromosome may be inactivated, females heterozygous for an X-linked mutant gene may show patches of tissue expressing the phenotype of the mutant gene while the majority of tissue remains normal. See also sex *chromatin; lyonization.*

Makeham's h., a development of Gompertz' h. as to the force of mortality following some mathematical law. Makeham assumed that death was the consequence of two generally coexisting causes: 1) chance; 2) a deterioration or increased inability to withstand destruction. The first of these is constant, the second is an increasing geometrical progression.

Michaelis-Menten h., that a complex is formed between an enzyme and its substrate, which complex then decomposes to yield free enzyme and the reaction products, the latter rate determining the overall rate of substrate-product conversion. See also Michaelis-Menten *constant.*

mnemic h., mnemism; mnemic or Semon-Hering theory; the theory that stimuli or irritants leave definite traces (engrams) on the protoplasm of the animal or plant, and when these stimuli are regularly repeated they induce a habit which persists after the stimuli cease; assuming that the germ cells share with the nerve cells in the possession of engrams, acquired habits may thus be transmitted to the descendants.

null h., that the results observed in a study, experiment, or test are not different from those that might have occurred by chance alone.

sequence h., that the amino acid sequence of a protein is determined by a particular sequence of nucleotides (the cistron) in the DNA of the organism producing the protein.

sliding filament h., the theory that the contracting muscle shortens because two sets of filaments slide past each other.

Starling's h., the principle that net filtration through capillary membranes is proportional to the transmembrane hydrostatic pressure difference minus the transmembrane oncotic pressure difference; although well established, it is called Starling's h. to distinguish it from Starling's law of the heart.

zwitter h., that an amphoteric molecule (*e.g.*, an amino acid) has, at its isoelectric point, equal numbers of positive and negative charges, thus becoming a zwitterion.

hypothrombinemia (hī'pō-throm-bin-ē'mē-ă). Abnormally small amounts of thrombin in the circulating blood, thereby resulting in bleeding tendency.

hypothromboplastinemia (hī'pō-throm'bō-plas-ti-nē'mē-ă). Abnormally small amounts of blood-clotting factor III, *i.e.*, thromboplastin, in the blood, as a result of deficient quantities being released from the tissues.

hypothymia (hī'pō-thī'me-ă) [hypo- + G. *thymos,* mind, soul]. Depression of spirits; the "blues."

hypothymic (hī'pō-thī'mik). **1.** Denoting or characteristic of hypothymia. **2.** Pertaining to hypothymism.

hypothymism (hī'pō-thī'mizm). Inadequate function of the thymus.

hypothyroid (hī'pō-thī'royd). Marked by reduced thyroid function.

hypothyroidism (hī'pō-thī'royd-izm) [hypo- + G. *thyreoeidēs,* thyroid]. Diminished production of thyroid hormone, leading to clinical manifestations of thyroid insufficiency, including low metabolic rate, tendency to weight gain, somnolence and sometimes myxedema.

infantile h., cretinism.

secondary h., h. that arises as a consequence of inadequate thyrotropin secretion by the anterior pituitary gland.

hypothyroxinemia (hī'pō-thī-rok-sin-ē'mē-ă). A subnormal thyroxine concentration in the blood.

hypotonia (hī'pō-tō'nē-ă) [hypo- + G. *tonos,* tone]. Hypotonicity (1); hypotonus; hypotony. **1.** Reduced tension in any part, as in the eyeball. **2.** Relaxation of the arteries. **3.** A condition in which there is a diminution or loss of muscular tonicity, in consequence of which the muscles may be stretched beyond their normal limits.

hypotonic (hī-pō-ton'ik). Hypoisotonic. **1.** Having a lesser degree of tension. **2.** Having a lesser osmotic pressure than a reference solution, which is ordinarily assumed to be blood plasma or interstitial fluid; more specifically, refers to a fluid in which cells would swell.

hypotonicity (hī'pō-tō-nis'i-tē). **1.** Hypotonia. **2.** A decreased effective osmotic pressure.

hypotonus, hypotony (hī'pō-tō'nŭs, hī-pot'ō-nē). Hypotonia.

hypotoxicity (hī'pō-toks-is'i-tē). Reduced toxicity; the quality of being only slightly poisonous.

hypotrichiasis (hī'pō-tri-kī'ă-sis). **1.** Hypotrichosis. **2.** *Alopecia* congenitalis.

hypotrichosis (hī'pō-tri-kō'sis) [hypo- + G. *trichōsis,* hairiness]. Oligotrichosis; oligotrichia; hypotrichiasis (1); a less than normal amount of hair on the head and/or body.

h. congen'ita, autosomal recessive condition seen in Guernsey and Holstein cattle.

hypotropia (hī-pō-trō'pē-ă) [hypo- + G. *tropē,* turn]. *Strabismus* deorsum vergens.

hypotympanotomy (hī'pō-tim-pă-not'ō-mē) [hypo- + G. *tympanon,* tympanum, + *tomē,* incision]. Operative procedure for the complete surgical extirpation, without sacrifice of hearing, of small tumors confined to the lower tympanic cavity.

hypotympanum (hī'pō-tim'pă-nŭm). The lower part of the tympanic cavity. It is separated by a bony wall from the jugular bulb.

hypouresis (hī'pō-yū-rē'sis). Reduced flow of urine.

hypouricemia (hī'pō-yū-ri-sē'mē-ă). Reduced blood concentration of uric acid.

hypouricuria (hī'pō-yū'ri-kyū'rē-ă). Reduced excretion of uric acid in the urine.

hypovarianism (hī'pō-vā'rē-an-izm). Hypoovarianism.

hypoventilation (hī'pō-ven-ti-lā'shŭn). Underventilation; reduced alveolar ventilation relative to metabolic carbon dioxide production, so that alveolar carbon dioxide pressure increases above normal.

hypovitaminosis (hī'pō-vī'tă-min-ō'sis). A nutritional deficiency state characterized by insufficiency of one or more vitamins in the diet; manifested first by depletion of tissue levels, then by functional changes, and finally by appearance of morphologic lesions.

hypovolemia (hī'pō-vō-lē'mē-ă) [hypo- + L. *volumen,* volume, + G. *haima,* blood]. Hyphemia; a decreased amount of blood in the body.

hypovolemic (hī'pō-vō-lē'mik). Pertaining to or characterized by hypervolemia.

hypovolia (hī-pō-vō'lē-ă) [hypo- + L. *volumen,* volume]. Diminished water content or volume of a given compartment; *e.g.*, extracellular h.

hypoxanthine (hī-pō-zan'thin). Sarcine (1); 6-oxypurine; purine-6(1*H*)-one; a purine present in the muscles and other tissues, formed during purine catabolism by deamination of adenine.

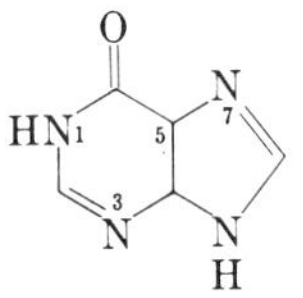

Hypoxanthine

h. guanine phosphoribosyltransferase, h. phosphoribosyltransferase.

h. oxidase, *xanthine* oxidase.

h. phosphoribosyltransferase [EC 2.4.2.8], h. guanine phosphoribosyltransferase; an enzyme present in human tissue that converts h. and guanine to their respective 5′ nucleotides, with 5-phosphoribose 1-diphosphate as the ribose-phosphate donor.

hypoxemia (hī-pok-sē′mē-ă) [hypo- + oxygen, + G. *haima,* blood]. Subnormal oxygenation of arterial blood, short of anoxia.

hypoxia (hī-pok′sē-ă) [hypo- + oxygen]. Decrease below normal levels of oxygen in inspired gases, arterial blood, or tissue, short of anoxia.

anemic h., h. resulting from a decreased concentration of functional hemoglobin or a reduced number of erythrocytes; it is caused by hemorrhage or anemia of various types, or by poisoning with CO, nitrites, or chlorates.

diffusion h., abrupt transient decrease in alveolar oxygen tension when room air is inhaled at the conclusion of a nitrous oxide anesthesia, because nitrous oxide diffusing out of the blood dilutes the alveolar oxygen.

hypoxic h., h. resulting from a defective mechanism of oxygenation in the lungs; may be caused by a low tension of oxygen, abnormal pulmonary function or respiratory obstruction, or a right-to-left shunt in the heart.

ischemic h., tissue h. characterized by tissue oligemia and caused by arterial or arteriolar obstruction or vasoconstriction.

oxygen affinity h., h. due to reduced ability of hemoglobin to release oxygen.

stagnant h., tissue h. characterized not by tissue oligemia (tissue blood volume being normal or even increased), but by intravascular stasis due to impairment of venous outflow or (in some instances) to decreased arterial inflow.

hypoxic (hī-pok′sik). Denoting or characterized by hypoxia.

hypsarhythmia, hypsarrhythmia (hip′să-rith′mē-ă) [G. *hypsi,* high, + *a-* priv. + *rhythmos,* rhythm]. The abnormal and characteristically chaotic electroencephalogram commonly found in patients with infantile spasms.

hypsi-, hypso- [G. *hýpsos,* height]. Combining forms meaning high or denoting relationship to height.

hypsibrachycephalic (hip-sē-brak′ē-sĕ-fal′ik) [hypsi- + G. *brachys,* broad, + *kephalē,* head]. Having a high broad head.

hypsicephalic (hip-si-sĕ-fal′ik). Oxycephalic.

hypsicephaly (hip-si-sef′ă-lē) [hypsi- + G. *kephalē,* head]. Oxycephaly.

hypsiconchous (hip-si-kon′kŭs) [hypsi- + G. *konchos,* a shell, the upper part of the skull]. Having a high orbit, with an orbital index above 85.

hypsiloid (hip′si-loyd) [G. *upsilon (ypsilon)*]. Upsiloid; ypsiliform; Y-shaped; U-shaped.

hypsistaphylia (hip′si-stă-fil′ē-ă) [hypsi- + G. *staphylē,* uvula]. A condition in which the palate is high and narrow.

hypsistenocephalic (hip-si-sten′ō-sĕ-fal′ik) [hypsi- + G. *stenos,* narrow, + *kephalē,* head]. Having a high, narrow head.

hypso-. See hypsi-.

hypsocephaly (hip-sō-sef′ă-lē) [hypso- + G. *kephalē,* head]. Oxycephaly.

hypsochromic (hip-sō-krōm′ik) [hypso- + G. *chroma,* color]. Denoting the shift of an absorption spectrum maximum to a shorter wavelength (greater energy).

hypsodont (hip′sō-dont) [hypso- + G. *odous,* tooth]. Having long teeth.

hypurgia (hī-per′jē-ă) [G. *hypourgia,* help, service, fr. *hypo,* + *ergon,* work]. Any minor factor(s) modifying the course of a disease for good or for ill, especially the former.

Hyrtl, Joseph, Austrian anatomist, 1810–1894. See H.'s *anastomosis, foramen, loop,* epitympanic *recess, sphincter.*

hyster-. See hystero-.

hysteralgia (his′ter-al′jē-ă) [hystero- + G. *algos,* pain]. Pain in the uterus. Also called hysterodynia; metrodynia.

hysteratresia (his′ter-ă-trē′zē-ă). Atresia of the uterine cavity, usually resulting from inflammatory endocervical adhesions.

hysterectomy (his-ter-ek′tō-mē) [hystero- + G. *ektomē,* excision]. Uterectomy; removal of the uterus; unless otherwise specified, usually denotes complete removal of the uterus (corpus and cervix).

abdominal h., celiohysterectomy; abdominohysterectomy; laparohysterectomy; removal of the uterus through an incision in the abdominal wall.

abdominovaginal h., a combined vaginal and abdominal surgical approach that allows partial or complete removal of vagina, vulva, rectum, and perineum (abdominoperineal approach), as well as pelvic organs; usually done in cases of advanced pelvic cancer.

cesarean h., Porro h. or operation; cesarean section followed by h.

modified radical h., TeLinde operation; an extended h. in which a portion of the upper vagina is removed; the ureters are exposed and pulled back laterally without dissection from the ureteral bed.

paravaginal h., removal of the uterus through a perineal incision involving only the lower two-thirds of the vaginal wall.

Porro h., cesarean h.

radical h., complete removal of the uterus, upper vagina, and parametrium.

subtotal h., supracervical h.

supracervical h., subtotal h.; removal of the fundus of the uterus, leaving the cervix *in situ.*

vaginal h., vaginohysterectomy; colpohysterectomy; removal of the uterus through the vagina without incising the wall of the abdomen.

hysteresis (his-ter-ē′sis) [G. *hysterēsis,* a coming later]. **1.** Failure of either one of two related phenomena to keep pace with the other; or any situation in which the value of one depends upon whether the other has been increasing or decreasing. **2.** Magnetic inertia; the lag of a magnetic effect behind its cause. **3.** The temperature differential that exists when a substance, such as reversible hydrocolloid, melts at one temperature and solidifies at another.

static h., the difference in the value reached by a dependent variable at a particular constant value of the independent variable, depending on whether the latter value had been approached from above or below; *e.g.,* in measuring the pressure volume relations of the lungs, if one completely expires and then inspires to a particular volume and holds it constant, the transpulmonary pressure required to maintain that lung volume is greater than if one had completely inspired and then expired to the same volume and held it constant.

hystereurysis (his-ter-yū′rē-sis) [hystero- + G. *eurynein,* to dilate, fr. *eurys,* wide]. Dilation of the lower segment and cervical canal of the uterus.

hysteria (his-ter′ē-ă, his-tēr′) [G. *hystera,* womb, from the original notion of womb-related disturbances in women]. A diagnostic term, referable to a wide variety of psychogenic symptoms involving disorder of function, which may be mental, sensory, motor, or visceral.

anxiety h., h. characterized by manifest anxiety.

canine h., syndrome in dogs caused in ingestion of nitrogen trichloride, formerly in common use as a bleaching agent for flour.

conversion h., conversion h. neurosis; conversion reaction; h. characterized by the substitution, through psychic transformation, of physical signs or symptoms for anxiety; generally restricted to such major symptoms as blindness, deafness, and paralysis, or lesser ones such as blurred vision and numbness.

epidemic h., mass h.

major h., a syndrome, now rarely seen, described by Charcot and characterized by a first stage of aura, a second stage of epileptoid convulsions, a third stage of tonic and clonic spasms, a fourth stage of dramatic behavior, and a fifth stage of delirium; the entire attack may last from a few minutes to half an hour. Sometimes used as a synonym for hysteroepilepsy.

mass h., epidemic h.; **(1)** spontaneous, en masse development of identical physical and/or emotional symptoms among a group of individuals, as seen in a classroom of schoolchildren; **(2)** a socially contagious frenzy of irrational behavior in a group of people as a reaction to an event.

minor h., a mild form of h. characterized chiefly by subjective pains, nervousness, undue sensitiveness, and sometimes episodes of emotional excitement, but without paralysis or other such symptoms.

hysterical, hysteric (his-ter'ē-kăl, -ter'ik). Relating to or characterized by hysteria.

hystericoneuralgic (his-ter'i-kō-nū-ral'jik). Relating to neuralgic pains of hysterical origin.

hysterics (his-ter'iks). An expression of emotion accompanied often by crying, laughing, and screaming.

hystero-, hyster-. 1 [G. *hystera,* womb (uterus)]. Combining forms denoting: 1) the uterus (See also metra-, metro-, utero-.); 2) hysteria. **2** [G. *hysteros,* later]. Combining forms meaning late or following.

hysterocatalepsy (his'ter-ō-kat'ă-lep-sē). Hysteria with cataleptic manifestations.

hysterocele (his'ter-ō-sēl) [hystero- + G. *kēlē,* hernia]. **1.** An abdominal or perineal hernia containing part or all of the uterus. **2.** Protrusion of uterine contents into a weakened, bulging area of uterine wall.

hysterocleisis (his'ter-ō-klī'sis) [hystero- + G. *kleisis,* closure]. Operative occlusion of the uterus.

hysterocolposcope (his'ter-ō-kol'pō-skōp) [hystero- + G. *kolpos,* vagina, + *skopeō,* to view]. Instrument for inspection of the uterine cavity and vagina.

hysterocystopexy (his'ter-ō-sis'tō-pek-sē) [hystero- + G. *kystis,* bladder, + *pēxis,* fixation]. Attachment of both uterus and bladder to the abdominal wall to correct prolapse.

hysterodynia (his'ter-ō-din'ē-ă) [hystero- + G. *odynē,* pain]. Hysteralgia.

hysteroepilepsy (his'ter-ō-ep'i-lep-sē). Hysterical convulsions. See major *hysteria.*

hysterogenic, hysterogenous (his-ter-ō-jen'ik, his-ter-oj'ĕ-nŭs). Causing hysterical symptoms or reactions.

hysterogram (his'ter-ō-gram). **1.** X-ray examination of the uterus, usually using a contrast medium. **2.** A recording of the strength of uterine contractions.

hysterograph (his'ter-ō-graf). Apparatus for recording the strength of uterine contractions.

hysterography (his'ter-og'ră-fē) [hystero- + G. *graphō,* to write]. Metrography. **1.** X-ray examination of the uterine cavity filled with a contrast medium. **2.** Graphic procedure used to record uterine contractions.

hysteroid (his'ter-oyd) [hystero- + G. *eidos,* resemblance]. Resembling or simulating hysteria.

hysterolith (his'ter-ō-lith) [hystero- + G. *lithos,* stone]. Uterine *calculus.*

hysterolysis (his-ter-ol'i-sis) [hystero- + G. *lysis,* dissolution]. Breaking up of adhesions between the uterus and neighboring parts.

hysterometer (his-ter-om'ĕ-ter) [hystero- + G. *metron,* measure]. Uterometer; a graduated sound for measuring the depth of the uterine cavity.

hysteromyoma (his'ter-ō-mī-ō'mă) [hystero- + G. *mys,* muscle, + *-oma,* tumor]. A myoma of the uterus.

hysteromyomectomy (his'ter-ō-mī-ō-mek'tō-mē) [hysteromyoma + G. *ektomē,* excision]. Operative removal of a uterine myoma.

hysteromyotomy (his'ter-ō-mī-ot'ō-mē) [hystero- + G. *mys,* muscle, + *tomē,* incision]. Incision into the muscles of the uterus.

hysteronarcolepsy (his'ter-ō-nar'kō-lep-sē). Narcolepsy of emotional origin.

hystero-oophorectomy (his'ter-ō-ō'of-ō-rek'tō-mē) [hystero- + G. *ōon,* egg, + *phoros,* bearing, + *ektomē,* excision]. Surgical removal of the uterus and ovaries.

hysteropathy (his-ter-op'ă-thē) [hystero- + G. *pathos,* suffering]. Any disease of the uterus.

hysteropexy (his'ter-ō-pek-sē) [hystero- + G. *pēxis,* fixation]. Uteropexy; uterofixation; fixation of a misplaced or abnormally movable uterus.

abdominal h., laparohysteropexy; attachment of the uterus to the anterior abdominal wall.

hysterophore (his'ter-ō-fōr) [hystero- + G. *phoros,* bearing]. A pessary or other support for a prolapsed or displaced uterus.

hysteropia (his-ter-ō'pē-ă) [hystero- + G. *ōps* (*ōp-*), eye]. A visual defect of hysterical origin.

hysteroplasty (his'ter-ō-plas-tē). Uteroplasty.

hysterorrhaphy (his-ter-ōr'ă-fē) [hystero- + G. *raphē,* suture]. Sutural repair of a lacerated uterus.

hysterorrhexis (his'ter-ō-rek'sis) [hystero- + G. *rhēxis,* rupture]. Metrorrhexis; rupture of the uterus.

hysterosalpingectomy (his'ter-ō-sal-pin-jek'tō-mē) [hystero- + G. *salpinx,* a trumpet, + *ektomē,* excision]. Operation for the removal of the uterus and one or both uterine tubes.

hysterosalpingography (his'ter-ō-sal-ping-gog'ră-fē) [hystero- + G. *salpinx,* a trumpet, + *graphō,* to write]. Gynecography; hysterotubography; uterosalpingography; uterotubography; roentgenography of the uterus and oviducts after the injection of radiopaque material.

hysterosalpingo-oophorectomy (his'ter-ō-sal-ping'gō-ō-of-ō-rek'-tō-mē) [hystero- + G. *salpinx,* trumpet, + *ōon,* egg, + *phoros,* bearing, + *ektomē,* excision]. Excision of the uterus, oviducts, and ovaries.

hysterosalpingostomy (his'ter-ō-sal-ping-gos'tō-mē) [hystero- + G. *salpinx,* trumpet, + *stoma,* mouth]. Metrosalpingography; operation to restore patency of a uterine tube.

hysteroscope (his'ter-ō-skōp) [hystero- + G. *skopeō,* to view]. Uteroscope; metroscope; an endoscope used in direct visual examination of the uterine cavity.

hysteroscopy (his-ter-os'kŏ-pē). Uteroscopy; visual instrumental inspection of the uterine cavity.

hysterospasm (his'ter-ō-spazm). Spasm of the uterus.

hysterosystole (his-ter-ō-sis'tō-lē) [G. *hysteros,* following, after, +

systolē, a contracting]. A delayed contraction of the heart; opposed to premature contraction or extrasystole.

hysterothermometry (his'ter-ō-ther-mom'ĕ-trē). Measurement of uterine temperature.

hysterotomy (his-ter-ot'ō-mē) [hystero- + G. *tomē,* incision]. Uterotomy; metrotomy; incision of the uterus.

abdominal h., transabdominal incision into the uterus. Also variously called abdominohysterotomy; celiohysterotomy; laparohysterotomy; laparouterotomy.

vaginal h., colpohysterotomy; incision into the uterus via the vagina.

hysterotonin (his'ter-ō-tō'nin) [hystero- + G. *tonos,* tension]. Pressor substance found in decidua and amniotic fluid of patients with toxemia of pregnancy.

hysterotrachelectomy (his'ter-ō-trak-el-ek'tō-mē) [hystero- + G. *trachēlos,* neck, + *ektomē,* excision]. Removal of the cervix uteri.

hysterotracheloplasty (his'ter-ō-trak'ĕ-lō-plas-tē) [hystero- + G. *trachēlos,* neck, + *plastos,* formed, shaped]. Plastic surgery of the cervix uteri.

hysterotrachelorrhaphy (his'ter-ō-trak-ĕ-lōr'ă-fē) [hystero- + G. *trachēlos,* neck, + *rhaphē,* a seam]. Sutural repair of a lacerated cervix uteri.

hysterotrachelotomy (his'ter-ō-trak-ĕ-lot'ō-mē) [hystero- + G. *trachēlos,* neck, + *tomē,* incision]. Incision of the cervix uteri.

hysterotrismus (his'ter-ō-tris'mŭs). Symptoms of lockjaw with a functional basis.

hysterotubography (his'ter-ō-tū-bog'ră-fē). Hysterosalpingography.

Hz Abbreviation for hertz.

I

I **1.** Symbol for iodine; luminous *intensity.* **2.** Abbreviation for intensity of electrical current, expressed in amperes. **3.** As a subscript, symbol for inspired *gas.* **4.** Designation for I blood group (see Blood Groups appendix).

-ia [G. *-ia,* a primitive substantive-forming suffix, denoting action or an abstract]. Suffix denoting condition, used in formation of names of many diseases. *Cf.* -ism.

IANC Abbreviation for International Anatomical Nomenclature Committee. See *Nomina Anatomica.*

IAP Abbreviation for intermittent acute *porphyria.*

-iasis [G. verb-nominalizing suffix]. Suffix denoting a condition or state, particularly morbid; in medical neologisms it has the same value as, and is sometimes interchangeable with, G. *-osis.*

iatraliptic (ī'ă-tră-lip'tik) [G. *iatros,* physician, + *aleiptēs,* an anointer]. Denoting treatment by inunction.

iatraliptics (ī'ă-tră-lip'tiks). Method of treatment by inunction.

iatric (ī-at'rik) [G. *iatros,* physician]. Pertaining to medicine or to a physician.

iatro- [G. *iatros,* physician]. Combining form denoting relation to physicians, medicine, treatment.

iatrochemical (ī-at-rō-kem'i-kăl). Denoting a school of medicine practicing iatrochemistry.

iatrochemist (ī-at-rō-kem'ist). A member of the iatrochemical school.

iatrochemistry (ī-at-rō-kem'is-trē). Chemiatry; the study of chemistry in relation to physiologic and pathologic processes, and the treatment of disease by chemical substance as practiced by a school of medical thought in the 17th century.

iatrogenic (ī-at-rō-jen'ik) [iatro- + G. *-gen,* producing]. Denoting an unfavorable response to medical or surgical treatment, induced by the treatment itself.

iatrology (ī-a-trol'ō-jē) [iatro- + G. *logos,* study]. Rarely used term for medical science.

iatromathematical (ī-at'rō-math-ĕ-mat'i-kăl). Iatrophysical.

iatromechanical (ī-at'rō-mĕ-kan'i-kăl). Iatrophysical.

iatrophysical (ī-at'rō-fiz'i-kăl). Iatromathematical; iatromechanical; denoting a school of medical thought in the 17th century which explained all physiologic and pathologic phenomena by the laws of physics.

iatrophysicist (ī-at'rō-fiz'-i-sist). A member of the iatrophysical school.

iatrophysics (ī-at'rō-fiz'iks). Physics as applied to medicine.

iatrotechnique (ī-at'rō-tek-nēk') [iatro- + G. *technē,* art]. The art of medicine and surgery; the technique or mode of application of medical science.

IBC Abbreviation for iron-binding *capacity.*

IBR Abbreviation for infectious bovine *rhinotracheitis.*

ibufenac (ī-byū'fe-nak). (*p*-Isobutylphenyl)acetic acid; an analgesic with anti-inflammatory properties.

ibuprofen (ī-bū'prō-fen). *dl-p*-Isobutylhydratropic acid; an anti-inflammatory agent.

IBV Abbreviation for infectious bronchitis *virus.*

-ic [L. *-icus,* fr. G. *-ikos*]. **1.** Suffix denoting of or pertaining to. **2.** Chemical suffix denoting that the element to the name of which it is attached is in combination in one of its higher valencies. *Cf.* -ous (1). **3.** Suffix indicating an acid.

ICD Abbreviation for *International Classification of Diseases of the World Health Organization.*

ICDA Abbreviation for *International Classification of Diseases, Adapted for Use in the United States;* includes a classification of surgical operations and other therapeutic and diagnostic procedures.

ICF Abbreviation for intracellular *fluid.*

ichnogram (ik'nō-gram) [G. *ichnos,* footstep, + *gramma,* a drawing, fr. *graphō,* to write]. Imprint of the soles of the feet, taken standing.

ichor (ī'kōr) [G. *ichōr,* serum]. A thin watery discharge from an ulcer or unhealthy wound.

ichoremia (ī-kō-rē'mē-ă). Ichorrhemia.

ichoroid (ī'kō-royd) [G. *ichōr,* serum, + *eidos,* resemblance]. Denoting a thin purulent discharge.

ichorous (ī'kōr-ŭs). Relating to or resembling ichor.

ichorrhea (ī'kō-rē'ă) [G. *ichōr,* serum, + *rhoia,* a flow]. A profuse ichorous discharge.

ichorrhemia (ī-kō-rē'mē-ă) [G. *ichōr,* serum, + *rhoia,* a flow, + *haima,* blood]. Ichoremia; blood poisoning from the absorption of an ichorous discharge.

ichthammol (ik'tham-mol). Ammonium ichthosulfonate; sulfonated bitumen; ammonium sulfoichthyolate; a viscous fluid, reddish brown to brownish black in color, with a strong, characteristic, empyreumatic odor, soluble in water and in glycerin; obtained by the destructive distillation of certain bituminous schists, sulfonating the distillate and neutralizing the product with ammonia. It is used in skin disorders; its beneficial effect is due to its mild irritant, stimulant, antiseptic, and analgesic action.

ichthyism (ik'thi-izm). [G. *ichthys,* fish]. Ichthyismus; poisoning by eating stale or otherwise unfit fish.

ichthyismus (ik-thi-iz'mŭs) [G. *ichthys,* fish]. Ichthyism.

i. exanthemat'icus, toxic erythematous eruption due to ingestion of spoiled fish.

ichthyo- [G. *ichthys,* fish]. Combining form relating to fish.

ichthyoacanthotoxism (ik'thi-ō-ă-kan'thō-tok'sizm) [ichthyo- + G. *akantha,* thorn, + *toxikon,* poison]. Poisoning from the stings or spines of venomous fishes.

ichthyocolla (ik-thē-ō-kol'ă) [ichthyo- + G. *kolla,* glue]. Isinglass; fish gelatin obtained from sounds or swim bladders of fish such as the hake, cod, and sturgeon; used as a glue, a food substitute, and a clarifying agent.

ichthyohemotoxin (ik'thē-ō-hē'mō-tok'sin) [ichthyo- + G. *haima,* blood, + *toxikon,* poison]. The toxic substance in the blood of certain fishes.

ichthyohemotoxism (ik'thē-ō-hē'mō-tok'sizm). Poisoning resulting from the ingestion of fish containing the toxic substance, ichthyohemotoxin.

ichthyoid (ik'thē-oyd) [ichthyo- + G. *eidos,* resemblance]. Fish-shaped.

ichthyootoxin (ik'thē-ō-ō-tok'sin) [ichthyo- + G. *ōon,* egg, + *toxikon,* poison]. Toxic substance restricted to the roe of fishes.

ichthyophagous (ik-thē-of'ă-gŭs) [ichthyo- + G. *phagein,* to eat]. Fish-eating; subsisting on fish.

ichthyophobia (ik'thē-ō-fō'bē-ă) [ichthyo- + G. *phobos,* fear]. Morbid fear of fish.

ichthyosarcotoxin (ik'thē-ō-sar'kō-tok'sin) [ichthyo- + G. *sarx,* flesh, + *toxikon,* poison]. Toxic substance found in the flesh or organs of fishes.

ichthyosarcotoxism (ik'thē-ō-sar'kō-tok'sizm) [ichthyo- + G. *sarx,* flesh, + *toxikon,* poison]. Poisoning caused by the toxic substance (ichthyosarcotoxin) in the flesh or organs of fish.

ichthyosis (ik-thē-ō'sis) [ichthyo- + G. *-osis,* condition]. Congenital disorder of keratinization characterized by dryness and fish-skin-like scaling of the skin, often associated with other defects; distinguishable genetically, clinically, microscopically, and by epidermal cell kinetics. Also called alligator or fish skin; i. sauroderma; sauriasis; sauriderma; sauriosis; sauroderma.
acquired i., a thickening and scaling of the skin associated with some malignant diseases (*e.g.,* Hodgkin's disease, lymphosarcoma), leprosy, and severe nutritional deficiencies.
i. congen'ita neonato'rum, generalized i. with parchment-like skin seen in premature babies.
i. cor'nea, an ocular complication of a congenital abnormality of the skin with corneal keratinization, dryness, and scaling.
i. feta'lis, **(1)** harlequin *fetus;* **(2)** recessive condition in Holstein and Norwegian red poll cattle resembling harlequin fetus in man.
i. follicula'ris, a form of autosomal dominant type of i., with horny follicular plugging of the extensor surfaces of the extremities; onset in early childhood.
i. hys'trix [G. *hystrix,* hedgehog], epidermolytic *hyperkeratosis.*
i. intrauteri'na, i. vulgaris.
lamellar i., a dry form of congenital ichthyosiform erythroderma inherited as an autosomal recessive trait and present at birth; characterized by large, coarse scales over most of the body and thickened palms and soles, and associated with ectropion; histologically, there is hyperkeratosis, a prominent granular layer in the epidermis, slight acanthosis, many mitotic figures, and rapid epidermal cell turnover. See also collodion baby; harlequin fetus.
i. linea'ris circumscrip'ta, congenital or infantile migratory erythema and scaling that shows a peripheral double margin; persists throughout life and may be associated with trichorrhexis invaginata in Netherton's syndrome; autosomal recessive inheritance.
nacreous i., a variant of i. characterized by dry pearly scales.
i. palma'ris et planta'ris, palmoplantar *keratoderma.*
i. sauroder'ma, ichthyosis.
i. scutula'ta, i. marked by diamond-shaped or shield-shaped lesions.
i. seba'cea, the presence of an unusual amount of vernix caseosa.
i. seba'cea cor'nea, a type of i. with vernix caseosa as seen in the newborn.
i. sim'plex, i. vulgaris.
i. spino'sa, epidermolytic *hyperkeratosis.*
i. u'teri, transformation of the columnar epithelium of the endometrium into stratified squamous epithelium.
i. vulga'ris, hyperkeratosis congenita; i. intrauterina or simplex; keratosis diffusa fetalis; a form of i. inherited as an autosomal dominant trait, with onset in childhood of fine scales on the trunk and extremities but not on the flexural areas, and associated with atopy and prominent palmar and plantar markings; histologically, there is hyperkeratosis, absence of a granular layer in the epidermis, and normal epidermal cell turnover.
X-linked i., a form of i., due to steroid sulphatase deficiency, that appears at birth or in early infancy and affects only males; characterized by scaling predominantly on the neck and trunk but not on the palms and soles, and associated with small cataracts; histologically, there is hyperkeratosis, a granular layer in the epidermis, and normal epidermal cell turnover.

ichthyotic (ik-thē-ot'ik). Relating to ichthyosis.

ichthyotoxicology (ik'thē-ō-tok-si-kol'ō-jē) [ichthyo- + G. *toxikon,* poison, + *logos,* study]. The study of the poisons produced by fishes, and their recognition, effects, and antidotes.

ichthyotoxicon (ik-thē-ō-tok'si-kon) [ichthyo- + G. *toxikon,* poison]. Fish poison (1); a toxic principle in certain fishes.

ichthyotoxin (ik'thē-ō-tok'sin) [ichthyo- + G. *toxicon,* poison]. The hemolytic active principle of eel serum.

ichthyotoxism (ik'thē-ō-tok'sizm) [ichthyo- + G. *toxikon,* poison]. Poisoning by fish.

iconomania (ī'kon-ō-mā'nē-ă) [G. *eikōn,* image, + *mania,* insanity]. Morbid impulse to worship images.

icosahedral (ī'kō-să-hē'drăl) [G. *eikosi,* twenty, + *-edros,* having sides or bases]. Having 20 equal triangular surfaces, as do most viruses with cubic symmetry.

***n*-icosanoic acid** (ī'kō-să-nō'ik). Arachidic acid.

ICP Abbreviation for intracranial *pressure.*

-ics [-ic + -s]. Suffix denoting organized knowledge, practice, or treatment.

ICSH Abbreviation of interstitial cell-stimulating *hormone.*

ictal (ik'tăl) [L. *ictus,* a stroke]. Relating to or caused by a stroke or seizure.

icteric (ik-ter'ik) [G. *ikterikos,* jaundiced]. Relating to or marked by jaundice.

ictero- [G. *ikteros,* icterus, jaundice]. Combining form relating to icterus.

icteroanemia (ik'ter-ō-ă-nē'mē-ă). Hayem-Widal *syndrome.*
swine i., an infectious disease of swine manifested by icterus, anemia, and emaciation; caused by *Eperythrozoon suis.*

icterogenic (ik'ter-ō-jen'ik) [ictero- + G. *-gen,* producing]. Causing jaundice.

icterohematuric (ik'ter-ō-hē'mă-tū'rik) [ictero- + G. *haima,* blood, + *ouron,* urine]. Denoting jaundice with the passage of blood in the urine.

icterohemoglobinuria (ik'ter-ō-hē'mō-glō-bi-nū'rē-ă). Jaundice with hemoglobin in the urine.

icterohepatitis (ik'ter-ō-hep-ă-tī'tis) [ictero- + G. *hēpar,* liver, + *-itis,* inflammation]. Inflammation of the liver with jaundice as a prominent symptom.

icteroid (ik'ter-oyd) [ictero- + G. *eidos,* resemblance]. Yellow-hued, or seemingly jaundiced.

icterus (ik'ter-ŭs) [G. *ikteros*] Jaundice.
acquired hemolytic i., Hayem-Widal *syndrome.*
benign familial i., familial nonhemolytic *jaundice.*
chronic familial i., hereditary *spherocytosis.*
congenital hemolytic i., hereditary *spherocytosis.*
cythemolytic i., i. caused by absorption of bile produced in excess through stimulation by free hemoglobin caused by the destruction of red blood corpuscles.
i. gra'vis, malignant jaundice; jaundice associated with high fever and delirium; seen in severe hepatitis with acute yellow atrophy and other extensive diseases of the liver.
infectious i., Weil's *disease.*
i. mel'as, a form in which the skin assumes a dirty dark brown color.
i. neonato'rum, Ritter's disease (2); jaundice of the newborn; pedicterus; **(1)** a temporary physiologic jaundice or excessive hemolysis, such as occurs in sepsis, neonatal hepatitis, or erythroblastosis fetalis; **(2)** a severe and often fatal form due to congenital atresia of the biliary system.
physiologic i., physiologic jaundice; mild jaundice of the newborn due mainly to functional immaturity of the liver.
i. pre'cox, a relatively innocent but rapidly developing type of jaundice with mild anemia in the newborn, most frequently caused by ABO incompatibility between mother and fetus.

ictometer (ik-tom'ĕ-ter) [L. *ictus,* stroke, + G. *metron,* measure]. An apparatus for determining the force of the apex beat of the heart.

ictus (ik'tŭs) [L.]. **1.** A stroke or attack. **2.** A beat.

i. cor'dis, heart *beat.*
i. epilep'ticus, an epileptic convulsion.
i. paralyt'icus, a paralytic stroke.
i. so'lis, sunstroke.

ICU Abbreviation for intensive care *unit.*

I.D. Abbreviation for infecting dose. See minimal infecting *dose.*

-id. 1 [G. *-eidēs,* resembling, through Fr. *-id*]. Suffix indicating a state of sensitivity of the skin in which a part remote from the primary lesion reacts ("-id reaction") to substances of the pathogen, giving rise to a secondary inflammatory lesion; the lesion manifesting the reaction is designated by the use of -id as a suffix. 2 [G. *-idion,* a diminutive ending]. Suffix indicating a small or young specimen.

id [L. *id,* that]. **1.** In psychoanalysis, one of three components of the psychic apparatus in the freudian structural framework, the other two being the ego and superego. It is completely in the unconscious realm, is unorganized, is the reservoir of psychic energy or libido, and is under the influence of the primary processes. **2.** The total of all psychic energy available from the innate drives and impulses in a newborn infant; through socialization this diffuse undirected energy becomes channeled in less egocentric and more socially responsive directions (development of the ego from the id).

IDDM Abbreviation for insulin-dependent *diabetes* mellitus.

-ide. **1.** Suffix denoting the more electronegative element in a binary chemical compound; formerly denoted by the qualification, -ureted; *e.g.,* hydrogen sulfide was sulfureted hydrogen. **2.** Suffix to a sugar name indicating substitution for the H of the hemiacetal OH; *e.g.,* glycoside.

idea (ī-dē'ă) [G. semblance]. Any mental image or concept.
autochthonous i.'s, thoughts that suddenly burst into awareness as if they are vitally important, often as if they have come from an outside source.
compulsive i., a fixed and inappropriate i.
dominant i., an i. that governs all one's actions and thoughts.
fixed i., **(1)** permanent dominant i.; idée fixe; an exaggerated notion, belief, or delusion that persists, despite evidence to the contrary, and controls the mind; **(2)** the obstinate conviction of a psychotic person regarding the correctness of his delusion.
hyperquantivalent i., an i. that dominates all thought and cannot easily be changed.
permanent dominant i., fixed i.
i. of reference, the misinterpretation that other people's statements or acts pertain to one's self when, in fact, they do not.

ideal (ī-dēl'). A standard of perfection.
ego i., the part of the personality that comprises the goals and aims of the self, usually referring to the emulation of significant persons with whom one has identified.

ideation (ī-dē-ā'shŭn). The formation of ideas or thoughts.

ideational (ī-dē-ā'shŭn-ăl). Relating to ideation.

idée fixe (ē-dā'fēks') [Fr. obsession]. Fixed *idea.*

identification (ī-den'ti-fi-kā'shŭn) [Mediev. L. *identicus,* fr. L. *idem,* the same, + *facio,* to make]. Incorporation; a sense of oneness, or psychic continuity with another person or group.

identity (ī-den'ti-tē). The social role of the person and his perception of it.
ego i., the ego's sense of its own identity.
gender i., the anatomical and biological sexual i. of the person. *Cf.* gender *role.*
sense of i., one's sense of his own identity or selfhood.

ideo- [G. *idea,* form, notion]. Combining form pertaining to ideas or ideation. *Cf.* idio-.

ideokinetic (ī'dē-ō-ki-net'ik). Ideomotor.

ideology (ī-dē-ol'ō-jē, id-ē-) [ideo- + G. *logos,* study]. The composite system of ideas, beliefs, and attitudes that constitutes an individual's or group's organized view of others.

ideomotion (ī-dē-ō-mō'shŭn). Muscular movement executed under the influence of a dominant idea, being practically automatic and not volitional.

ideomotor (ī'dē-ō-mō'ter). Ideokinetic; relating to ideomotion.

ideophobia (ī'dē-ō-fō'bē-ă). Morbid fear of new or different ideas.

ideoplastia (ī'dē-ō-plas'tē-ă) [ideo- + G. *plassō,* to form]. The receptive condition in a hypnotized person in which he is thought to be completely open to suggestion.

idio- [G. *idios,* one's own]. Combining form meaning private, distinctive, peculiar to. *Cf.* ideo-.

idioagglutinin (id'ē-ō-ă-glū'tin-in). An agglutinin that occurs naturally in the blood of a person or an animal, without the injection of a stimulating antigen or the passive transfer of antibody.

idiochromosome (id'ē-ō-krō'mō-sōm). Sex *chromosome.*

idiocy (id'ē-ō-sē) [G. *idiōteria,* awkwardness, uncouthness]. Obsolete term for a subclass of mental *retardation.*
amaurotic familial i., obsolete term for cerebral *sphingolipidosis.*

idiodynamic (id'ē-ō-dī-nam'ik). Independently active.

idiogamist (id'ē-og'ă-mist) [idio- + G. *gamos,* marriage]. Rarely used term for one who is capable of sexual union with only one or a few individuals of the opposite sex, being impotent in the presence of any others.

idiogenesis (id'ē-ō-jen'ĕ-sis) [idio- + G. *genesis,* production]. Origin without evident cause; denoting especially that of an idiopathic disease.

idioglossia (id'ē-ō-glos'ē-ă) [idio- + G. *glōssa,* tongue, speech]. An extreme form of lalling or vowel or consonant substitution, by which the speech of a child may be made unintelligible and appear to be another language to one who has not the key to the literal changes.

idioglottic (id'ē-ō-glot'ik). Relating to idioglossia.

idiogram (id'ē-ō-gram) [idio- + G. *gramma,* something written]. **1.** Karyotype. **2.** Diagrammatic representation of chromosome morphology characteristic of a species or population.

idiographic (id'ē-ō-graf'ik) [idio- + G. *graphō,* to write]. Pertaining to the behavior of a particular individual as an individual, as opposed to nomothetic.

idioheteroagglutinin (id'ē-ō-het'er-ō-ă-glū'tin-in) [idio- + G. *heteros,* another, + agglutinin]. An idioagglutinin occurring in the blood of one animal, but capable of combining with the antigenic material from another species.

idioheterolysin (id'ē-ō-het-er-ol'i-sin). An idiolysin occurring in the blood of an animal of one species, but capable of combining with the red blood cells of another species, thereby causing hemolysis when complement is present.

idiohypnotism (id'ē-ō-hip'nō-tizm). Autohypnosis.

idioisoagglutinin (id'ē-ō-ī'sō-ă-glū'tin-in) [idio- + G. *isos,* equal, + agglutinin]. An idioagglutinin occurring in the blood of an animal of a certain species, capable of agglutinating the cells from animals of the same species.

idioisolysin (id'ē-ō-ī-sol'i-sin). An idiolysin occurring in the blood of an animal of a certain species, capable of combining with the red blood cells from animals of the same species, thereby causing hemolysis when complement is present.

idiolalia (id'ē-ō-lā'lē-ă) [idio- + G. *lalia,* talk]. Use of a language invented by the person himself.

idiolysin (id-ē-ol'i-sin). A lysin that occurs naturally in the blood of a person or an animal, without the injection of a stimulating antigen or the passive transfer of antibody.

idiomuscular (id'ē-ō-mŭs'kyū-lăr). Relating to the muscles alone, independent of the nervous control.

idionodal (id′ē-ō-nō′dăl). Arising from the A-V node itself; applied to the ventricular rhythm in complete S-A or A-V block, or in other forms of A-V dissociation, when the A-V node rather than an ectopic ventricular focus controls the ventricles. See also idioventricular.

idiopathetic (id′ē-ō-pă-thet′ik). Idiopathic.

idiopathic (id′ē-ō-path′ik) [idio- + G. *pathos,* suffering]. Idiopathetic. **1.** Agnogenic; denoting a disease of unknown cause. **2.** Denoting a primary disease.

idiopathy (id-ē-op′ă-thē) [idio- + G. *pathos,* suffering]. An idiopathic disease.

idiophrenic (id′ē-ō-fren′ik) [idio- + G. *phrēn,* mind]. Relating to, or originating in, the mind or brain alone, not reflex or secondary.

idiopsychologic (id′ē-ō-sī-kō-loj′ik). Relating to ideas developed within one's own mind, independent of suggestion from without.

idioreflex (id-ē-ō-rē′fleks). A reflex due to a stimulus or irritation originating in the organ or part in which the reflex occurs.

idiosome (id′ē-ō-sōm) [idio- + G. *sōma,* body]. **1.** The attraction sphere of a spermatid or of an oocyte. **2.** The indivisible element of living matter.

idiospasm (id′ē-ō-spazm). A localized spasm.

idiosyncrasy (id′ē-ō-sin′kră-sē) [G. *idiosynkrasia,* fr. *idios,* one's own, + *synkrasis,* a mixing together]. An individual mental, behavioral, or physical characteristic or peculiarity.

idiosyncratic (id′ē-ō-sin-krat′ik). Relating to or marked by an idiosyncrasy.

idiot (id′ē-ōt) [G. *idiōtēs,* an ignorant, uncouth person]. Obsolete term for a subclass of mental retardation or an individual classified therein.

idiot-prodigy (id′ē-ōt prod′i-jē). Idiot-savant.

idiotrophic (id′ē-ō-trof′ik) [idio- + G. *trophē,* food]. Capable of choosing its own food.

idiotropic (id′ē-ō-trop′ik) [idio- + G. *tropē,* a turning]. Turning inward upon one's self.

idiot-savant (ē-dē-ō′ sah-vahn′) [Fr.] Idiot-prodigy; a person of low general intelligence who possesses an unusual faculty in performing certain mental tasks of which most normal persons are incapable.

idiotype (id′ē-ō-tīp). Idiotypic antigenic determinant; a determinant that confers on an immunoglobulin molecule an antigenic "individuality" analogous to the "individuality" of the molecule's antibody activity and that seems to reflect the antigenic properties of the receptor (combining site) confering specificity of antibody activity.

idiovariation (id′ē-ō-va-rē-ā′shŭn). The process of constant change in the hereditary qualities of a strain of organism; mutation.

idioventricular (id-ē-ō-ven-trik′yū-lăr). Pertaining to or associated with the cardiac ventricles alone, when dissociated from the atria.

iditol (ī′di-tol). Reduction product of the hexose idose.

idose (ī′dōs). One of the aldohexoses, isomeric with glucose and galactose. See formulas under sugar.

idoxuridine (IDU) (ī-doks-yū′ri-dēn). 2′-Deoxy-5-iodouridine; 5-iododeoxyuridine; a pyrimidine analogue that produces both antiviral and anticancer effects by interference with DNA synthesis; used locally in the eye for the treatment of keratitis from herpes simplex or vaccinia.

IDP Abbreviation for inosine 5′-diphosphate.

idrosis (ī-drō′sis) [G. *hidrōs,* sweat]. Hidrosis.

IDU Abbreviation for idoxuridine.

iduronic acid (ī-dūr-on′ik). The uronic acid of idose; a constituent of dermatan sulfate.

IF Abbreviation for initiation *factor;* intrinsic *factor.*

IFN Abbreviation for interferon.

Ig Abbreviation for immunoglobulin.

IGF Abbreviation for insulin-like growth *factor.*

ignatia (ig-nā′shē-ă) [*St. Ignatius*]. Ignatia amara; St. Ignatius' bean; the dried ripe seed of *Strychnos ignatii* (family Loganiaceae). It is similar in its properties to nux vomica and is a source of strychnine.

ignipedites (ig′ni-pe-dī′tēz) [L. *ignis,* fire, + *pes (ped-),* foot, + G. *itēs*]. Hotfoot; burning pain in the soles of the feet, in multiple neuritis.

ignipuncture (ig′ni-pŭngk-chūr) [L. *ignis,* fire, + puncture]. The original procedure of closing a retinal break in retinal separation by transfixation of the break with cautery.

ignotine (ig′nō-tēn). Carnosine.

IH Abbreviation for infectious *hepatitis.*

ikota (ī-kō′tă). A neurosis, similar to latah, affecting married women among the Samoyeds of Siberia.

IL Abbreviation for interleukin.

ILA Abbreviation for insulin-like *activity.*

Ile Symbol for isoleucine or its acyl radical, isoleucyl.

ileac (il′ē-ak). **1.** Relating to the ileus. **2.** Relating to the ileum.

ileadelphus (il′ē-ă-del′fŭs). *Duplicitas* posterior.

ileal (il′ē-ăl). Of or pertaining to the ileum.

ileectomy (il-ē-ek′tō-mē) [ileum + G. *ektomē,* excision]. Removal of the ileum.

ileitis (il-ē-ī′tis). Inflammation of the ileum.

backwash i., involvement of the terminal ileum by the inflammatory and ulcerative changes seen in chronic ulcerative colitis; distinguished from involvement of ileum and proximal colon by regional (granulomatous) enteritis (*i.e.,* Crohn's disease of terminal ileum and proximal colon).

distal i., regional i., terminal i., regional *enteritis.*

ileo- [ileum]. Combining form denoting relationship to the ileum.

ileocecal (il′ē-ō-sē′kăl). Relating to both ileum and cecum.

ileocecostomy (il′ē-ō-sē-kos′tō′mē). Cecoileostomy; anastomosis of the ileum to the cecum.

ileocecum (il-ē-ō-sē′kŭm). The combined ileum and cecum.

ileocolic (il′ē-ō-kol′ik). Ileocolonic; relating to the ileum and the colon.

ileocolitis (il′ē-ō-kō-lī′tis). Inflammation to a varying extent of the mucous membrane of both ileum and colon.

ileocolonic (il′ē-ō-kō-lon′ik). Ileocolic.

ileocolostomy (il′ē-ō-kō-los′tō-mē) [ileo- + colostomy]. Establishment of a new communication between the ileum and the colon.

ileocystoplasty (il′ē-ō-sis′tō-plas-tē) [ileo- + G. *kystis,* bladder, + *plastos,* formed]. Surgical reconstruction of the bladder involving the use of an isolated intestinal segment to augment bladder capacity.

ileoentectropy (il′ē-ō-en-tek′trō-pē) [ileo- + G. *entos,* within, + *ek,* out, + *tropē,* a turning]. Eversion of a segment of the ileum.

ileoileostomy (il′ē-ō-il-ē-os′tō-mē) [ileum + ileum + G. *stoma,* mouth]. **1.** Establishment of a communication between two segments of the ileum. **2.** The opening so established.

ileojejunitis (il′ē-ō-je-jū-nī′tis). A chronic inflammatory condition involving the jejunum and parts or most of the ileum; occurs in different forms: a granulomatous state resembling regional ileitis, pseudodiverticula, or cicatricial stenosis of the bowel.

ileopexy (il′ē-ō-pek′sē) [ileo- + G. *pēxis,* fixation]. Surgical fixation of ileum.

ileoproctostomy (il'ē-ō-prok-tos'tō-mē) [ileo- + G. *prōktos,* anus (rectum), + *stoma,* mouth]. Ileorectostomy; establishment of a communication between the ileum and the rectum.

ileorectostomy (il'ē-ō-rek-tos'tō-mē) [ileum + rectum + G. *stoma,* mouth]. Ileoproctostomy.

ileorrhaphy (il'ē-ōr'ă-fē) [ileo- + G. *raphe,* suture]. Suturing the ileum.

ileosigmoidostomy (il'ē-ō-sig'moyd-os'tō-mē) [ileo- + sigmoid, + G. *stoma,* mouth]. Establishment of a communication between the ileum and the sigmoid colon.

ileostomy (il'ē-os'tō-mē) [ileo- + G. *stoma,* mouth]. Establishment of a fistula through which the ileum discharges directly to the outside of the body.
Brooke i., i. in which the divided proximal ileum, brought through the abdominal wall, is evaginated and its edge is sutured to the dermis; a 2 cm protrusion is maintained by additional suturing.
Kock i., Kock *pouch.*

ileotomy (il'ē-ot'ō-mē) [ileo- + G. *tomē,* incision]. Incision into the ileum.

ileotransversostomy (il'ē-ō-tranz-vers-os'tō-me) [ileum + transverse colon, + G. *stoma,* mouth]. Anastomosis of the ileum to the transverse colon.

ileum (il'ē-ŭm) [L. fr. G. *eileō,* to roll up, twist] [NA]. The third portion of the small intestine, about 12 feet in length, extending from the junction with the jejunum to the ileocecal opening.
i. du'plex, tubular or cystic segmental duplications of alimentary tract.

ileus (il'ē-ŭs) [G. *eileos,* intestinal colic, from *eilō,* to roll up tight]. Mechanical, dynamic, or adynamic obstruction of the bowel; may be accompanied by severe colicky pain, abdominal distention, vomiting, absence of passage of stool, and often fever and dehydration.
adynamic i., paralytic i.; obstruction of the bowel due to paralysis of the bowel wall, usually as a result of localized or generalized peritonitis or shock.
dynamic i., spastic i.; intestinal obstruction due to spastic contraction of a segment of the bowel.
gallstone i., obstruction of the small intestine produced by passage of a gallstone from the biliary tract (usually the gallbladder as a result of cholecystitis) into the intestinal tract (usually by means of a fistulous connection between the gallbladder and the duodenum); occurrence and site of obstruction depend upon size of the stone, but the usual location is at or near the ileocecal junction.
mechanical i., obstruction of the bowel due to some mechanical cause, *e.g.,* volvulus, gallstone, adhesions.
meconium i., intestinal obstruction in the newborn following inspissation of meconium due to lack of trypsin; associated with cystic fibrosis of pancreas.
occlusive i., complete mechanical blocking of the intestinal lumen.
paralytic i., adynamic i.
spastic i., dynamic i.
i. subpar'ta, obstruction of the large bowel by pressure of the pregnant uterus.
terminal i., obstruction of the lower part of the small bowel.
verminous i., obstruction due to masses of intestinal parasites.

iliac (il'ē-ak). Relating to the ilium.

iliacus (il-ī'ă-kŭs). See *musculus* iliacus.

iliadelphus (il'ē-ă-del'fŭs) [L. *ilium* + G. *adelphos,* brother]. *Duplicitas* posterior.

ilio- [L. *ilium*]. Combining form denoting relationship to the ilium.

iliococcygeal (il'ē-ō-kok-sij'ē-ăl). Relating to the ilium and the coccyx.

iliocolotomy (il'ē-ō-kō-lot'ō-mē) [ilio- + G. *kolon,* colon, + *tomē,* incision]. The operation of opening into the colon in the inguinal (iliac) region.

iliocostal (il'ē-ō-kos'tăl). Relating to the ilium and the ribs; denoting muscles passing between the two parts.

iliocostalis (il'ē-ō-kos-tā'lis). See *musculus* iliocostalis.

iliofemoral (il'ē-ō-fem'ō-răl). Relating to the ilium and the femur.

iliofemoroplasty (il-ē-o-fem'ōr-ō-plas-tē). An obsolete method of securing a hip fusion by an extra-articular technique (a joint bypass procedure) in which a turned down bone flap from the ilium is placed into a split in the greater trochanter.

iliohypogastric (il'ē-ō-hī-pō-gas'trik). Relating to the iliac and the hypogastric regions.

ilioinguinal (il'ē-ō-ing'gwi-năl). Relating to the iliac region and the groin.

iliolumbar (il-ē-ō-lŭm'băr). Relating to the iliac and the lumbar regions.

iliometer (il-ē-om'ĕ-ter) [ilio- + G. *metron,* measure]. An instrument for measuring exact position of iliac spines and lower vertebrae.

iliopagus (il-ē-op'ă-gŭs) [ilio- + G. *pagos,* something fixed]. Conjoined twins in which the fusion is restricted to the iliac region.

iliopectineal (il'ē-ō-pek-tin'ē-ăl). Relating to the ilium and the pubis.

iliopelvic (il'ē-ō-pel'vik). Relating to the iliac region and the cavity of the pelvis.

iliosacral (il'ē-ō-sā'krăl). Relating to the ilium and the sacrum.

iliosciatic (il'ē-ō-sī-at'ik). Relating to the ilium and the ischium.

iliospinal (il'ē-ō-spī'năl). Relating to the ilium and the spinal column.

iliothoracopagus (il'ē-ō-thōr-ă-kop'ă-gŭs) [ilio- + G. *thorax,* chest, + *pagos,* fixed]. Ischiothoracopagus; conjoined twins in which union occurs through the ilia and extends to involve the thoraces.

iliotibial (il'ē-ō-tib'ē-ăl). Relating to the ilium and the tibia.

iliotrochanteric (il'ē-ō-trō-kan-ter'ik). Relating to the ilium and the great trochanter of the femur.

ilioxiphopagus (il'ē-ō-zī-fop'ă-gŭs) [ilio- + xiphoid, + G. *pagos,* fixed]. Conjoined twins in which the fusion extends from the xiphoid to the iliac region.

ilium, pl. ilia (il'ē-ŭm, il'ē-ă) [L. groin, flank]. *Os* ilium.

ill. In veterinary medicine, a term used in the common names of several diseases.
joint i., joint evil; a chronic suppurative inflammation of the joints of foals and other newly born animals, due to umbilical infection with pyogenic bacteria, one of the commonest being *Actinobacillus equuli.*
louping i., a highly virulent viral encephalomyelitis of sheep in Great Britain characterized by cerebellar ataxia; caused by a flavivirus (louping-ill virus) and transmitted by the hard tick, *Ixodes ricinus.*
navel i., a term applied to any kind of acute generalized infections of young mammals having their origin in a wound infection occurring in the stump of the umbilical cord; these infections generally are pyemic, and liver and lung abscesses and multiple acute arthritis are characteristic.

illicium (il-lis'ē-ŭm) [L. an allurement, fr. *il-licio,* to allure]. Chinese or star anise; the dried fruit of *Ilicium verum* (family Magnoliaceae), an evergreen shrub or small tree of southern China; used as a stimulating carminative.

illinition (il-in-ish'ŭn) [L. *il-lino,* pp. *-litus,* to smear on (*in* + *lino*)]. The friction of a surface to facilitate absorption of an ointment.

illness (il'nes). Disease (1).
functional i., functional *disorder.*
mental i., **(1)** a broadly inclusive term, generally denoting one or all of the following: 1) a disease of the brain, with predominant behavioral symptoms, as in paresis or acute alcoholism; 2) a disease of the "mind" or personality, evidenced by abnormal behavior, as in hysteria or schizophrenia; also called mental or emotional disease, disturbance, or disorder, or behavior disorder; **(2)** any psychiatric illness listed in *Current Medical Information and Terminology* of the American Medical Association or in the *Diagnostic and Statistical Manual for Mental Disorders* of the American Psychiatric Association. See also behavior *disorder.*

illumination (i-lū'mi-nā'shŭn) [L. *il-lumino,* pp. -atus, to light up]. **1.** Throwing light on the body or a part or into a cavity for diagnostic purposes. **2.** Lighting an object under a microscope.
axial i., central i.; the transmission or reflection of light in the direction of the axis of an optical system.
central i., axial i.
contact i., i. of the eye by means of an instrument in contact with the cornea or bulbar conjunctiva.
critical i., the precise focusing of the light source directly upon the object being examined.
dark-field i., dark-ground i.; a procedure in which a black circular shield is used to block the majority of the vertically directed rays of light (*i.e.,* the field is dark), and a circumferential, suitably angled, mirrored surface is used to direct the peripheral rays horizontally against the object, thereby reflecting the light vertically through the objective lens and along the optical axis; thus, the object is well illuminated in a contrasting dark background.
dark-ground i., dark-field i.
direct i., erect or vertical i.; an i. in which the rays of light are directed downward, almost perpendicularly onto the upper surface of the object, which reflects the rays upward into the optical system.
erect i., direct i.
focal i., lateral or oblique i.; i. in which a beam of light is directed diagonally to an object so that it is brilliantly illuminated while the surrounding area is in shadow.
Köhler i., i. of microscopic objects in which the light source is focused on the substage condenser diaphragm and the diaphragm of the light source is in focus with the object to be observed; minimizes both the brightness and uniformity of the illuminated field.
lateral i., focal i.
oblique i., focal i.
vertical i., direct i.

illuminism (i-lū'mi-nizm). A psychotic state of exaltation in which one has delusions and hallucinations of communion with supernatural or exalted beings.

illusion (i-lū'zhŭn) [L. *illusio,* fr. *il- ludo,* pp. *-lusus,* to play at, mock]. A false perception; the mistaking of something for what it is not.
i. of doubles, Capgras' *syndrome.*
i. of movement, successive stimulation of neighboring retinal points which causes the sensation of movement.
oculogravic i., apparent movement of the visual field when the body is subjected to acceleration; due to gravity.
oculogyral i., an i. occurring in angular acceleration in which the position of fixed light appears to drift.
optical i., a false interpretation of the color, form, size, or movement of a visual sensation.

illusional (i-lū'zhŭn-ăl). Relating to or of the nature of an illusion.

Ilosvay, Lajos de, Hungarian chemist, *1851. See I. *reagent.*

IM Abbreviation for internal medicine.

I.M., i.m. Abbreviation for intramuscular, or intramuscularly.

ima (ī'mă) [L.]. Lowest. See also imus.

image (im'ij) [L. *imago,* likeness]. **1.** Representation of an object made by the rays of light emanating or reflected from it. **2.** Representation produced by x-rays, ultrasound, tomography, thermography, radioisotpes, etc.; as a verb, to produce such representations.
accidental i., afterimage.
body i., body schema; **(1)** the cerebral representation of all body sensation organized in the parietal cortex; **(2)** personal conception of one's own body as distinct from the actual, anatomic body or the conception of other persons of one's own body.
catatropic i., Purkinje-Sanson i.
direct i., virtual i.
eidetic i., vivid mental i. in the form of a dream, fantasy, or an unusual power of memory and visualization of objects previously seen or imagined.
false i., the i. in the deviating eye in strabismus.
heteronymous i., a double i. in physiological diplopia, when fixation is directed beyond an object; the right i. arises from the left eye, while the left i. arises from the right eye.
homonymous i.'s, double i.'s produced by stimuli arising from points proximal to the horopter.
hypnagogic i., imagery occurring between wakefulness and sleep.
hypnopompic i., imagery occurring after the sleeping state and before complete wakefulness; similar to hypnagogic imagery except for the time of occurrence.
incidental i., afterimage.
inverted i., real i.
mental i., a picture of an object not present, produced in the mind by memory or imagination.
mirror i., a representation of an object or part thereof as its reflected i. in a glass mirror.
motor i., the i. of body movements.
optical i., an i. formed by the refraction or reflection of light.
Purkinje i.'s, Purkinje-Sanson i.'s.
Purkinje-Sanson i.'s, catatropic, Purkinje, or Sanson's i.'s; the two images formed by the anterior and posterior surfaces of the cornea and the two images formed by the anterior and posterior surfaces of the lens.
real i., inverted i.; an i. formed by the convergence of the actual rays of light from an object.
retinal i., a real i. formed on the retina.
Sanson's i.'s, Purkinje-Sanson i.'s.
sensory i., an i. based on one or more types of sensation.
specular i., the i. of a source of light made visible by the reflection from a mirror.
tactile i., an i. of an object as perceived by the sense of touch.
unequal retinal i., aniseikonia.
virtual i., direct i.; an erect i. formed by projection of divergent rays from an optical system.
visual i., a collection of foci corresponding to all the luminous points of an object.

imagery (im'ij-rē). A technique in behavior therapy in which the client or patient is conditioned to use pleasant fantasies to counter the unpleasant feelings associated with anxiety.

imaginal (ĭ-maj'i-năl). Relating to an image or to the process of imagining.

imaging (im'ă-jing) [see image]. Production of an image by x-rays, ultrasound, tomography, thermography, radioisotopes, etc.
magnetic resonance i. (MRI), nuclear magnetic resonance (NMR) i.; a diagnostic i. modality, using nuclear magnetic resonance technology, in which the patient's body is placed in a magnetic field and its nuclei (hydrogen) are excited by radiofrequency pulses at angles to the field's axis; resulting signals from the hydrogen ions, varying in strength where hydrogen is in greater or lesser concentrations in the body, are processed through a computer to produce an image; by varying the radiofrequency pulse sequences,

the apparent contrast of adjacent tissues and of black and white values can be altered.

nuclear magnetic resonance (NMR) i., magnetic resonance i.

imago, pl. imagines (i-mā'gō, i-maj'i-nēz) [L. image]. **1.** The last stage of an insect after it has completed all its metamorphoses through the egg, larva, and pupa; the adult insect form. **2.** Archetype (2).

imbalance (im-bal'ans) [L. *in-* neg. + *bi-lanx* (*-lanc-*), having two scales, fr. *bis,* twice, + *lanx,* dish, scale of a balance]. **1.** Lack of equality between opposing forces. **2.** Lack of equality in some aspect of binocular vision, such as muscle balance, image size, and/or image shape.

autonomic i., vasomotor i.; a lack of balance between sympathetic and parasympathetic nervous systems, especially in relation to the vasomotor disturbances.

occlusal i., an inharmonious relationship between the teeth of the maxilla and mandible during closing or functional movements of the jaw.

sex chromosome i., any abnormal pattern of sex chromosomes; *e.g.,* XXY in men with seminiferous tubule dysgenesis, XO in women with Turner's syndrome; rarer patterns of i. are XXX, XXXY, and XYY.

sympathetic i., vagotonia.

vasomotor i., autonomic i.

imbecile (im'bē-sil) [L. *imbecillus,* weak, silly]. An obsolete term for a subclass of mental *retardation* or the individual classified therein.

imbed'. Embed.

imbibition (im-bi-bish'ŭn) [L. *im-bibo,* to drink in (*in* + *bibo*)]. **1.** Absorption of fluid by a solid body without resultant chemical change in either. **2.** Taking up of water by a gel, thereby increasing its size.

imbricate, imbricated (im'bri-kāt, im'bri-kā-ted) [L. *imbricatus,* covered with tiles]. Overlapping like shingles.

imbrication (im'bri-kā'shŭn) [see imbricate]. The operative overlapping of layers of tissue in the closure of wounds or the repair of defects.

imidazole (im-id-az'ōl). Glyoxaline; iminazole; 1,3-diazole; 1,3-diaza-2,4-cyclopentadiene; a five-membered heterocyclic compound occurring in histidine and other biologically important compounds.

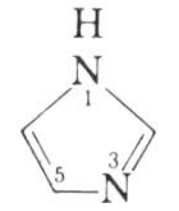

Imidazole

imidazolyl (im-id-az'ō-lil). Iminazolyl; the radical of imidazole.

imide (im'īd). The radical or group, =NH, attached to two –CO– groups.

imido-. Prefix denoting the radical of an imide, formed by the loss of the H of the =NH group.

imidodipeptidase (im'i-dō-dī-pep'ti-dās). *Proline* dipeptidase.

imidole (im'i-dōl). Pyrrole.

iminazole (im-in-az'ōl). Imidazole.

iminazolyl (im-in-az'ō-lil). Imidazolyl.

-imine. Suffix denoting the group, =NH.

imino-. Prefix denoting the group, =NH.

imino acids (im'i-nō, i-mē'nō). Compounds with molecules containing both an acid group (usually the carboxyl, –COOH) and an imino group (=NH); *e.g.,* proline, hydroxyproline.

iminocarbonyl (im'i-nō-kar'bon-il). See carboxamide.

iminodipeptidase (im'i-nō-dī-pep'ti-dās). *Prolyl* dipeptidase.

iminoglycinuria (im'i-nō-glī-si-nū'rē-ă). A benign inborn error of amino acid transport; glycine, proline, and hydroxyproline are excreted in the urine.

iminohydrolases (im'i-nō-hī'drō-lās-ez) [EC 3.5.3]. Deiminases; enzymes hydrolyzing imino groups; *e.g.,* arginine deiminase.

imipenem (im-i-pen'em). $C_{12}H_{17}N_3O_4S \cdot H_2O$; a thienamycin antibiotic with broad spectrum activity used, in combination with cilastin, to treat a variety of infections.

imipramine hydrochloride (im-ip'ră-mēn). 5-(3-Dimethylaminopropyl)-10,11-dihydro-5*H*- dibenz (*b,f*)azepine hydrochloride; an antidepressant.

Imlach, Francis, Scottish anatomist and surgeon, 1819–1891. See I.'s *fat-pad, ring.*

immedicable (im-med'i-kă-bl) [L. *in-* neg. + *medicabilis,* curable]. Obsolete term meaning not curable by medicinal remedies.

immersion (i-mer'zhŭn) [L. *im-mergo,* pp. *-mersus,* to dip in (*in* + *mergo*)]. **1.** The placing of a body under water or other liquid. **2.** In microscopy, filling the space between the objective lens and the top of the cover glass with a fluid, such as water or oil, in order to reduce spherical aberration and increase effective numerical aperture by elimination of refractive effects which result from an air-glass interface; the best resolution is achieved when the space between the condenser lens and the specimen slide is also filled with the fluid.

homogeneous i., in i. microscopy, use of a fluid, such as oil, that has a refractive index virtually identical to that of glass, providing the highest possible numerical aperture.

oil i., water i., see immersion (2).

immiscible (i-mis'i-bl) [L. *im-misceo,* to mix in (*in* + *misceo*)]. Incapable of mutual solution; *e.g.,* oil and water.

immittance (i-mit'ans) [L. *immitto,* to send in]. In audiology, a general term describing measurements made of tympanic membrane impedance, compliance, or admittance.

immobilization (i-mo'bi-li-zā'shŭn) [see immobilize]. The act of making immovable.

immobilize (i-mō'bi-līz) [L. *in-* neg. + *mobilis,* movable]. To render fixed or incapable of moving.

immortalization (i-mōr'tăl-i-zā'shŭn). Conferring on normal cells cultured *in vitro* the property of an infinite lifespan, as from spontaneous mutation, by exposure to chemical carcinogens, or by viral infection. I. of primary cells in culture is the first of several steps in the expression of transforming genes of DNA tumor viruses, of retrovirus oncogenes, and cellular oncogenes derived from human cancer cells.

immune (i-myūn') [L. *immunis,* free from service, fr. *in,* neg., + *munus* (*muner-*), service]. **1.** Free from the possibility of acquiring a given infectious disease; resistant to an infectious disease. **2.** Pertaining to the mechanism of sensitization in which the reactivity is so altered by previous contact with an antigen that the responsive tissues respond quickly upon subsequent contact, or to *in vitro* reactions with antibody-containing serum from such sensitized individuals.

immunifacient (im'yū-ni-fā'shent) [L. *immunis,* exempt, + *faciens,* making, pr. part. of *facio*]. Making immune; said of a semelincident disease or of a prophylactic serum or vaccine.

immunity (i-myū'ni-tē) [L. *immunitas* (see immune)]. Insusceptibility; the status or quality of being immune (1).

acquired i., resistance resulting from previous exposure of the individual in question to an infectious agent or antigen; it may be *active* and *specific,* as a result of naturally acquired (apparent or inapparent) infection or intentional vaccination (artificial active i.); or it may be *passive,* being acquired from transfer of antibodies from another person or from an animal, either naturally, as from mother to fetus, or by intentional inoculation (artificial passive i.), and, with respect to the particular antibodies transferred, it is *specific.* Passive, cell-mediated i. produced by the transfer of living lymphoid cells from an immune (allergic or sensitive) animal to a normal one is sometimes referred to as adoptive i.

active i., see acquired i.

adoptive i., see acquired i.

antiviral i., i. resulting from virus infection, either naturally acquired or produced by intentional vaccination; compared to some bacterial i.'s, it is of relatively long duration, but this may be the result of infection-immunity rather than being peculiar to virus infection per se, since it occurs also in bacterial i. after infections such as typhoid fever.

artificial active i., see acquired i.

artificial passive i., see acquired i.

bacteriophage i., the state induced in a bacterium by lysogenization, the lysogenic bacterium being insusceptible to further lysogenization or to a lytic cycle by a superinfecting bacteriophage, in contradistinction to bacteriophage resistance.

cell-mediated i. (CMI), cellular i., delayed hypersensitivity; i. associated with cellular elements (including T-lymphocytes), in contradistinction to humoral i.

concomitant i., infection i.

general i., i. associated with widely diffused mechanisms that tend to protect the body as a whole, as compared with local i.

genetic i., innate i.

group i., herd i.

herd i., group i.; **(1)** a concept that there is resistance or relative resistance to the spread of infectious disease in a herd or group, irrespective of the presence or absence of a significant degree of i. in the individual members; *e.g.,* the ecologic composite (animal species including man, vector, and environmental factors) is not such to allow spread of an infectious agent along natural routes even though individuals of the population might be fully susceptible if in another herd structure; **(2)** the immunologic status of a population as a whole, determined by the ratio of resistant to susceptible members and their distribution.

humoral i., i. associated with circulating antibodies, in contradistinction to cellular i.

infection i., concomitant i.; premunition; the paradoxical immune status in which resistance to reinfection coincides with the persistence of the original infection.

inherent i., innate i.

innate i., genetic, inherent, natural, or nonspecific i.; resistance manifested by a species (or by races, families, and individuals in a species) that has not been immunized (sensitized, allergized) by previous infection or vaccination; it results from body mechanisms that are poorly understood, but are different from those responsible for the altered reactivity (see immune (2)) associated with the specific nature of acquired i.; in general, innate i. is nonspecific and is not stimulated by specific antigens.

local i., a natural or acquired i. to certain infectious agents, as manifested by an organ or a tissue, as a whole or in part.

natural i., nonspecific i., innate i.

passive i., see acquired i.

relative i., a modified, not completely effective resistance that results when there is a sort of "fluctuating equilibrium" between the defense mechanisms of the host and the infective agent.

specific i., the immune status (see immune (2)) in which there is an altered reactivity directed solely against the antigenic determinants (infectious agent or other) that stimulated it. See acquired i.

specific active i., see acquired i.

specific passive i., see acquired i.

stress i., insusceptibility or resistance to the effects of emotional strain.

immunization (im'yū-ni-zā'shŭn). The process or procedure by which an individual is rendered immune. See also vaccination, allergization.

active i., the production of active immunity.

passive i., the production of passive immunity.

immunize (im'yū-nīz). To render immune.

immuno- [L. *immunis,* immune]. Combining form meaning immune, or relating to immunity.

immunoadjuvant (im'yū-nō-ad'jū-vant). See adjuvant (2).

immunoagglutination (im'yū-nō-ă-glū-ti-nā'shŭn). Specific agglutination effected by antibody.

immunoassay (im'yū-nō-as'ā). Immunochemical assay; detection and assay of hormones, or other substances, by serological (immunological) methods; in most applications the hormone (or other substance) in question serves as antigen, both in antibody production and in measurement of antibody by the test substance. See also radioimmunoassay; radioimmunoelectrophoresis; immunologic pregnancy *test.*

double antibody i., double antibody *precipitation.*

enzyme-multiplied i. (EMIT), a type of i. in which the ligand is labeled with an enzyme, and the enzyme-ligand-antibody complex is enzymatically inactive, allowing quantitation of unlabeled ligand. See also competitive binding *assay;* enzyme-linked immunosorbent *assay;* radioimmune *assay.*

solid phase i., i. in which the antigen or serum is bound to a solid surface, such as a microplate wall or the sides of a tube, the other reactants being free in solution.

thin-layer i., a method for detection of antigen-antibody reactions, applicable to detection of either antigen or antibody, based on the fact that either reactant, when added to a polystyrene surface (such as a well in a polystyrene plate) is adsorbed as a thin layer and acts as an immunosorbent capable of binding with the second reactant.

immunoblast (im'yū-nō-blast) [immuno- + G. *blastos,* germ]. An antigenically stimulated lymphocyte; a large cell with well-defined basophilic cytoplasm, a large nucleus with prominent nuclear membrane, distinct nucleoli, and clumped chromatin. See also lymphocyte *transformation.*

immunochemistry (im'yū-nō-kem'is-trē). Chemoimmunology; the field of chemistry concerned with chemical aspects of immunologic phenomena, *e.g.,* chemical reactions related to antigen stimulation of tissues, chemical studies of antigens and antibody.

immunocompetence (im'yū-nō-kom'pĕ-tens). Immunological competence; the ability to produce a normal immune response.

immunocompetent (im'yū-nō-kom'pĕ-tent). Possessing the ability to mount a normal immune response.

immunocompromised (im'yū-nō-kom'pro-mīzd). Denoting an individual whose immunologic mechanism is deficient either because of an immunodeficiency disorder or because it has been rendered so by immunosuppressive agents.

immunoconglutinin (im'yū-nō-kon-glū'ti-nin). An autoantibody-like immunoglobulin (IgM) formed in animals (or man) against their own complement following injection of complement-containing complexes or sensitized bacteria.

immunocyte (im'yū-nō-sīt) [immuno- + G. *kytos,* cell]. A leukocyte capable, actively or potentially, of producing antibodies.

immunocytochemistry (im'yū-nō-sī-tō-kem'is-trē). The study of cell constituents by immunologic methods, such as the use of fluorescent antibodies.

immunodeficiency (im'yū-nō-dē-fish'en-sē). Immunological, immunity, or immune deficiency; a condition resulting from a defective immunological mechanism; may be *primary* (due to a defect in the immune mechanism itself) or *secondary* (dependent upon another disease process), *specific* (due to defect in either the B-lymphocyte or the T-lymphocyte system, or both) or *nonspecific* (due to defect in one or another component of the nonspecific immune mechanism: the complement, properdin, or phagocytic system).

cellular i. with abnormal immunoglobulin synthesis, Nezelof type of thymic alymphoplasia; Nezelof syndrome; an ill-defined group of sporadic disorders of unknown cause, occurring in both males and females and associated with recurrent bacterial, fungal, protozoal, and viral infections; there is thymic hypoplasia with depressed cellular (T-lymphocyte) immunity combined with defective humoral (B-lymphocyte) immunity, although immunoglobulin levels may be normal.

combined i., i. of both the B-lymphocytes and T-lymphocytes.

common variable i., acquired hypogammaglobulinemia; i. of unknown cause, and usually unclassifiable, which may occur at any age (usually after age 15 years) in either sex; the total quantity of immunoglobulin is commonly less than 300 mg/dl, with the number of B-lymphocytes frequently within normal limits but with a lack of plasma cells in lymphoid tissue; cellular (T-lymphocyte) immunity may also be abnormal but usually is intact; associated with increased susceptibility to pyogenic infection and, not infrequently, with autoimmune disease.

i. with hypoparathyroidism, congenital aplasia of the thymus; thymic hypoplasia; pharyngeal pouch syndrome; a condition arising from developmental failure of the third and fourth pharyngeal pouches, resulting in absence or underdevelopment of the thymus and parathyroid gland, among other structures; associated with facial deformity, hypoparathyroidism, and deficiency in cellular (T-lymphocyte) immunity, but humoral (B-lymphocyte) immunity is normal; ordinarily, if the tetany is survived, death ensues from overwhelming infection. See also DiGeorge *syndrome*.

secondary i., secondary agammaglobulinemia or hypogammaglobulinemia; secondary antibody deficiency; i. in which there is no evident defect in the lymphoid tissues, but rather hypercatabolism or loss of immunoglobulins such as occurs in familial idiopathic hypercatabolic hypoproteinemia or in defects associated with the nephrotic syndrome.

severe combined i., absence of both humoral (antibody) and cellular immunity with alymphoplasia or marked lymphopenia (both B-type and T-type lymphocytes), associated with marked susceptibility to infection by bacteria, fungi, protozoa, and viruses, and to progressive disease from live vaccines; death occurs usually before the end of the first year of life, although bone marrow transplants have been effective; may be X-linked recessive or autosomal recessive (Swiss type agammaglobulinemia).

immunodeficient (im'yū-nō-dē-fish'ent). Lacking in some essential function of the immune system.

immunodepressant (im'yū-nō-dē-pres'ănt). Immunosuppressant.

immunodepressor (im'yū-nō-dē-pres'ŏr, -ōr). Immunosuppressant.

immunodiagnosis (im'yū-nō-dī-ag-nō'sis). The process of determining specified immunologic characteristics of individuals or of cells, serum, or other biologic specimens.

immunodiffusion (im'yū-nō-di-fyū'zhŭn, i-myū'nō-). A technique of study of antigen-antibody reactions by observing precipitates formed by combination of specific antigen and antibodies which have diffused in a gel in which they have been separately placed.

double i., see gel diffusion precipitin *tests* in two dimensions.

radial i. (RID), see gel diffusion precipitin *tests* in two dimensions.

single i., see gel diffusion precipitin *tests* in one dimension, and in two dimensions.

immunoelectrophoresis (im'yū-nō-ē-lek'trō-fō-rē'sis, i-myū'nō-). A kind of precipitin test in which the components of one group of immunological reactants (usually a mixture of antigens) are first separated on the basis of electrophoretic mobility in agar or other medium, the separated components then being identified, by means of the technique of double diffusion, on the basis of precipitates formed by reaction with components of the other group of reactants (antibodies).

crossed i., two-dimensional i.

rocket i., a quantitative method for serum proteins which involves electrophoresis of antigen into a gel containing antibody; the technique is restricted to detection of antigens that move to the positive pole on electrophoresis. See electroimmunodiffusion.

two-dimensional i., crossed i.; a combination of conventional electrophoretic separation and electroimmunodiffusion; electrophoresis is first carried out, then the electrophoretic strip is placed on a second slide and an antibody-containing agarose solution is allowed to solidify adjacent to it; electrophoresis is then performed at right angles to the original separation.

immunoenhancement (im'yū-nō-en-hans'ment). Immunological enhancement; in immunology, the potentiating effect of specific antibody in establishing and in delaying rejection of a tumor allograft; aside from antibody, nonspecific substances may also act to enhance immune response.

immunoenhancer (im'yū-nō-en-hans'er). Any specific or nonspecific substance that increases the degree of the immune response.

immunoferritin (im'yū-nō-fer'i-tin). Antibody-ferritin conjugate used to identify specific antigen by electron microscopy.

immunofluorescence (im'yū-nō-flūr-es'ens, i-myū'nō-). Labeling of antibodies by fluorescein, or rhodamine, isothiocyanates to identify bacterial, viral, or other antigenic material specific for the labeled antibody; the specific binding of antibody can be determined microscopically through the production of a characteristic visible light by the application of ultraviolet rays to the preparation. See also fluorescent antibody *technique*.

immunogen (i-myū'nō-jen). Antigen.

behavioral i., the personal habits and lifestyle of an individual which are associated with a decreased risk of physical illness and dysfunction, and with greater longevity.

immunogenetics (im'yū-nō-jĕ-net'iks). The branch of genetics concerned with inheritance of differences in antigens or antigenic responses.

immunogenic (im'yū-nō-jen'ik). Antigenic.

immunogenicity (im'yū-nō-jĕ-nis'i-tē). Antigenicity.

immunoglobulin (Ig) (im'yū-nō-glob'yū-lin). One of a class of structurally related proteins consisting of two pairs of polypeptide chains, one pair of light (L) [low molecular weight] chains (κ or λ), and one pair of heavy (H) chains (γ, α, or μ, and more recently, δ and ϵ), all four linked together by disulfide bonds. On the basis of the structural and antigenic properties of the H chains, Ig's are classified (in order of relative amounts present in normal human serum) as IgG (7S in size, 80%), IgA (10 to 15%), IgM (19 S, a pentameter of the basic unit, 5 to 10%), IgD (less than 0.1%), and IgE (less than 0.01%). All of these classes are homogeneous and susceptible to amino acid sequence analysis. Each class of H chain can associate with either κ or λ L chains. Subclasses of Ig's, based on differences in the H chains, are referred to as IgG1, etc.

When split by papain, IgG yields three pieces: the Fc piece, consisting of the C-terminal portion of the H chains, with no antibody activity but capable of fixing complement, and crystallizable; and two identical Fab pieces, carrying the antigen-binding sites and each consisting of an L chain bound to the remainder of an H chain.

Antibodies are Ig's, and all Ig's probably function as antibodies. However, Ig refers not only to the usual antibodies, but also to a great number of pathological proteins classified as myeloma proteins, which appear in multiple myeloma along with Bence Jones proteins, myeloma globulins, and Ig fragments.

From the amino-acid sequences of Bence Jones proteins, it is known that all L chains are divided into a region of variable sequence (V_L) and one of constant sequence (C_L), each comprising about half the length of the L chain. The constant regions of all human L chains of the same type (κ or λ) are identical except for a single amino acid substitution, under genetic controls. H chains are similarly divided, although the V_H region, while similar in length to the V_L region, is only one-third or one-fourth the length of the C_H region. Binding sites are a combination of V_L and V_H protein regions. The large number of possible combinations of L and H chains make up the "libraries" of antibodies of each individual.

Light chain (κ or λ) ≡ Bence Jones protein

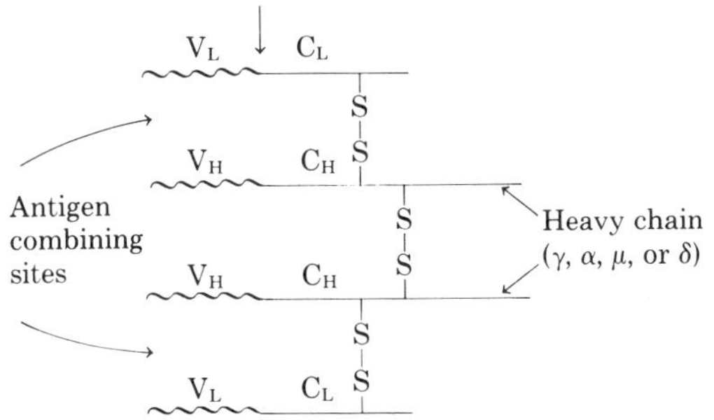

anti-D i., Rh_0 (D) immune *globulin.*
chickenpox i., chickenpox immune *globulin* (human).
human normal i., human gamma *globulin.*
measles i., measles immune *globulin* (human).
monoclonal i., monoclonal protein; M protein (2); paraprotein (2); a homogenous i. resulting from the proliferation of a single clone of plasma cells and which during electrophoresis of serum appears as a narrow band or "spike;" it is characterized by heavy chains of a single class and subclass, and light chains of a single type.
pertussis i., pertussis immune *globulin.*
poliomyelitis i., poliomyelitis immune *globulin* (human).
rabies i., rabies immune *globulin* (human).
Rh_0(D) i., Rh_0(D) immune *globulin.*
tetanus i., tetanus immune *globulin.*

immunohematology (im'yū-nō-hē-mă-tol'ō-jē, i-myū'nō-). That division of hematology concerned with immune, or antigen-antibody, reactions, and with related changes in the blood.

immunohistochemistry (im'yū-nō-his'tō-kem'is-trē). Demonstration of specific antigens in tissues by the use of markers that are either fluorescent dyes or enzymes, especially horseradish peroxidase.

immunologist (im-yū-nol'ō-jist). A specialist in the science of immunology.

immunology (im'yū-nol'ō-jē) [immuno- + G. *logos,* study]. The science concerned with the various phenomena of immunity, induced sensitivity, and allergy.

immunopathology (im'yū-nō-pă-thol'ō-jē, i-myū'nō-). The study of diseases or conditions resulting from reactions of immunity.

immunopotentiation (im'yū-nō-pō-ten-shē-ā'shŭn). Enhancement of the immune response by increasing the rate at, or degree to, which it develops and by prolongation of its duration.

immunopotentiator (im'yū-nō-pō-ten'shē-ā-tōr). Any of a wide variety of specific or nonspecific substances which on innoculation elicit a generalized immune response.

immunoprecipitation (im'yū-nō-prē-sip-i-tā'shŭn). Immune precipitation; the phenomenon of aggregation of sensitized antigen upon addition of specific antibody (precipitin) to antigen in solution.

immunoreaction (im'yū-nō-rē-ak'shŭn). An immunologic reaction, especially *in vitro* between antigen and antibody.

immunoreactive (im'yū-nō-rē-ak'tiv). Denoting or exhibiting immunoreaction.

immunoselection (im'yū-nō-se-lek'shŭn). Selective death or survival of fetuses of different genotypes depending on immunologic incompatibility with the mother.

immunosorbent (im'yū-nō-sōr'bent). An antibody (or antigen) used to remove specific antigen (or antibody) from solution or suspension; commonly used with reference to antibody bound to a particulate substance such as a dextran polymer used to remove soluble antigen (*e.g.,* insulin) from solution.

immunosuppressant (im'yū-nō-sŭ-pres'ant). Immunosuppressive (2); immunodepressant; immunodepressor; an agent that induces immunosuppression.

immunosuppression (im'yū-nō-sŭ-presh'ŭn). Prevention or interference with the development of immunologic response; may reflect natural immunologic unresponsiveness (tolerance), may be artificially induced by chemical, biological, or physical agents, or may be caused by disease.

immunosuppressive (im'yū-nō-sŭ-pres'iv). **1.** Denoting or inducing immunosuppression. **2.** Immunosuppressant.

immunosympathectomy (im'yū-nō-sim'pă-thek'tō-mē). Inhibition of development of sympathetic ganglia induced in newborn animals by injection of antiserum specific for the protein which selectively enhances growth of sympathetic neurons.

immunotherapy (im'yū-nō-ther'ă-pē). Originally, therapeutic administration of serum or gamma globulin containing preformed antibodies produced by another individual; currently, i. includes nonspecific systemic stimulation, adjuvants, active specific i., and adoptive i.
adoptive i., passive transfer of immunity from an immune donor through inoculation of sensitized lymphocytes, transfer factor, immune RNA, or antibodies in serum or gamma globulin.

immunotolerance (im'yū-nō-tol'er-ăns). Immunological *tolerance.*

immunotransfusion (im'yū-nō-trans-fyū'zhŭn, i-myū'nō-). An indirect transfusion in which the donor is first immunized by means of injections of an antigen prepared from microorganisms isolated from the recipient; later, the donor's blood is collected, defibrinated, and then administered to the patient; the latter is then presumably passively immunized by means of antibody formed in the donor, *i.e.,* antibody that reacts with the microorganisms in the patient.

imolamine (i-mol'ă-mēn). 4-[2-(Diethylamino)ethyl]-5-imino-3-phenyl-Δ^2-1,2,4-oxadiazoline; used for relief of angina pectoris.

IMP Abbreviation for inosine monophosphate.

impact (im'pakt) [L. *impingo,* pp. *-pactus,* to strike at (*in* + *pango*), fasten, drive in]. The forcible striking of one body against another.

impact (im-pakt'). **1.** To forcibly strike against another body. **2.** To press closely together so as to render immovable.

impacted (im-pak'ted). Wedged or pressed closely together so as to be immovable.

impaction (im-pak'shŭn). The process or condition of being impacted.
dental i., confinement of a tooth in the alveolus and prevention of its eruption into normal position. See also impacted *tooth.*
fecal i., coprostasis; an immovable collection of compressed or hardened feces in the colon or rectum.
food i., the forcible wedging of food between adjacent teeth during mastication, producing gingival recession and pocket formation.
mucus i., filling of the proximal bronchi, and also the bronchioles, with mucus.

impairment (im-pār'ment). Weakening, damage, or deterioration; *e.g.,* as a result of injury or disease.

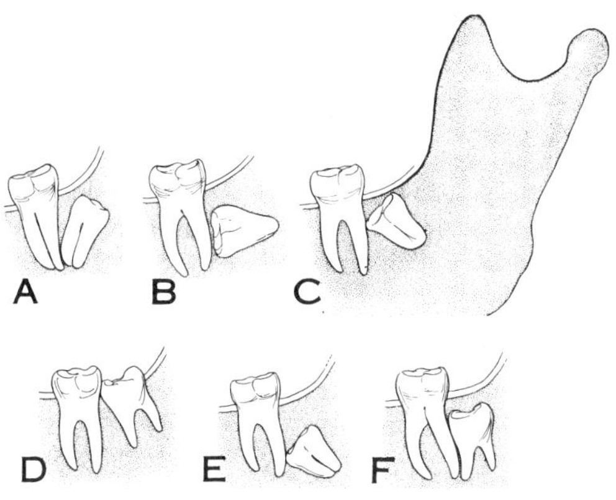

Impacted Mandibular Third Molar
A, distoangular; *B*, horizontal; *C*, mesioangular; *D*, high level; *E*, low level; *F*, vertical.

functional aerobic i., the degree of observed duration of the test and duration expected for a healthy person of the same age, sex, and habitual activity status, expressed as a percent of the normal.
mental i., a disorder characterized by the display of an intellectual defect, as shown or determined by diminished cognitive, interpersonal, social, and vocational effectiveness and by psychological examination and assessment.

imparidigitate (im-par-i-dij'i-tāt) [L. *impar,* unequal, + *digitus,* digit]. Perissodactyl; perissodactylous (1).

IMP-aspartate ligase. Adenylosuccinate synthase.

impatent (im-pat'ent, im-pā'tent). Not patent; closed.

impedance (im-pē'dăns). **1.** Total opposition to flow. When flow is steady, i. is simply the resistance, *i.e.,* the driving pressure per unit flow; when flow is changing, i. also includes the factors that oppose changes in flow. Thus, deviations of i., from simple ohmic resistance because of the effects of capacitance and inductance, become more important in alternating current as the frequency of oscillations increases. In fluid analogies (*e.g.,* pulsatile flow of blood, to-and-fro flow of respiratory gas), i. depends not only on viscous resistance but also upon compressibility, compliance, inertance, and the frequency of imposed oscillations. **2.** Resistance of an acoustic system to being set in motion.

imperception (im-per-sep'shŭn) [L. *in-,* not, + *per- cipio,* pp. *-ceptus,* to perceive]. Inability to form a mental image of an object by combining the sensory data obtained therefrom.

imperforate (im-per'fōr-āt). Atretic.

imperforation (im-per-fōr-ā'shŭn) [L. *im-* neg. + *per-foro,* pp. *-atus,* to bore through]. Condition of being atretic, occluded, or closed; indicated in compound words by the prefix *atreto-* or the suffix *-atresia.*

impermeable (im-per'mē-ă-bl) [L. *im- permeabilis,* not to be passed through]. Impervious, not permeable; not permitting passage of substances (*e.g.,* liquids, gases, heat) through a membrane or other structure.

impermeant (im-per'mē-ant) [L. *im-,* neg., + *permano,* to penetrate]. Unable to pass through a particular semipermeable membrane.

impersistence (im-per-sis'tens) [L. *im-,* neg. + *persisto,* to persist]. A transitory existence or occurrence, lasting only a short time.
motor i., inability to sustain a movement.

impervious (im-per'vē-ŭs). Impermeable.

impetiginization (im'pe-tij'i-ni-zā'shŭn). The occurrence of impetigo in an area of preexisting dermatosis.

impetiginous (im-pe-tij'i-nŭs). Relating to impetigo.

impetigo (im-pe-tī'gō) [L. a scabby eruption, fr. *im-peto* (*inp-*), to rush upon, attack]. I. contagiosa; i. vulgaris; crusted tetter; a contagious superficial pyoderma, caused by staphylococci and streptococci, that begins with a superficial flaccid vesicle which ruptures and forms a thick yellowish crust, most commonly occurring on the face.
Bockhart's i., follicular i.
i. bullo'sa, i. with lesions of large size, forming bullae.
bullous i. of newborn, i. neonatorum (2); pemphigus gangrenosus (2); usually, widely disseminated bullous lesions appearing soon after birth, caused by infection with staphylococci, occasionally mixed with streptococci.
i. circina'ta, a ringlike configuration of bullous lesions of i. formed by confluence of several bullae or by the rupture of a single lesion with crusting of the periphery.
i. contagio'sa, impetigo.
i. eczemato'des, *eczema* pustulosum.
follicular i., Bockhart's i.; superficial pustular perifolliculitis; a follicular pustular eruption involving the scalp or other hairy area.
i. herpetifor'mis, a rare pyoderma, occurring most commonly in pregnant women, as an eruption of small closely aggregated pustules developing upon an inflammatory base and accompanied by severe constitutional symptoms.
i. neonato'rum, **(1)** *dermatitis* exfoliativa infantum; **(2)** bullous i. of newborn.
i. vulga'ris, impetigo.

impetus (im'pe-tŭs) [L. an onset, fr. *im-peto,* to attack]. In psychoanalysis, the motor element of an instinct; the amount of force of the individual's energy which the instinctive impulse demands.

implant [L. *im-,* in, + *planto,* pp. *-atus,* to plant, fr. *planta,* a sprout, shoot]. **1** (im-plant'). To graft or insert. **2** (im'plant). Material inserted or grafted into tissues. See also graft, transplant. **3.** In dentistry, a graft or insert set firmly or deeply, or onto the alveolar recess prepared for its insertion. See also i. *denture.* **4.** In orthopedics, a metallic or plastic device employed in joint reconstruction.
bag-gel i., an i. composed of a silicone rubber bag containing a silicone gel; used in augmentation mammaplasty.
carcinomatous i.'s, transference of carcinoma cells from a primary tumor to adjacent tissues where growth continues.
cochlear i., cochlear prothesis; an electronic device implanted under the skin with electrodes in the middle ear on the promontory or cochlear window or in the inner ear in the cochlea to create sound sensation in total sensory deafness.
endometrial i.'s, fragments of endometrial mucosa implanted on pelvic structure following retrograde transference through the oviducts.
endo-osseous i., an i. into alveolar bone inserted through the prepared root canal of a tooth in order to increase effective root length.
endosteal i., an i. that is inserted into the alveolar and/or basal bone and protrudes through the mucoperiosteum.
inflatable i., an i. consisting of an empty silicone rubber bag with an inlet tube and a valve; after insertion into or behind the breast, the bag is inflated with a liquid to the desired size; used in augmentation mammaplasty.
intraocular i., a plastic lens placed in the anterior or posterior chamber of the eye to substitute for the lens removed in cataract extraction.
magnetic i., a tissue-tolerated, magnetized metal placed within the bone to aid in denture retention; a similar magnet is placed in the overlying denture to complete the field.
orbital i., the glass, plastic, or metal device placed in the muscle cone after enucleation of an eye.
penile i., a rigid, flexible, or inflatable device surgically placed in

the corpora cavernosa to produce an erection.

pin i., a type of i. usually rod-shaped, used in the area of the maxillary sinuses.

post i., that portion of an i. substructure that protrudes through the mucosa to connect with the restoration.

submucosal i., an i. resting beneath the mucosa. See also i. *denture.*

subperiosteal i., an artificial metal appliance made to conform to the shape of a bone and placed on its surface beneath the periosteum. See i. denture *substructure.*

supraperiosteal i., an alloplastic graft inserted superficial to the periosteum to change the contour of an area.

triplant i., a combination of three pin i.'s to form a single abutment to support or retain a dental prosthesis.

implantation (im-plan-tā'shŭn). **1.** Attachment of the fertilized ovum (blastocyst) to the endometrium, and its subsequent embedding in the compact layer, occurring 6 or 7 days after fertilization of the ovum. **2.** Insertion of a natural tooth into an artificially constructed alveolus. **3.** Tissue grafting. See also transplantation.

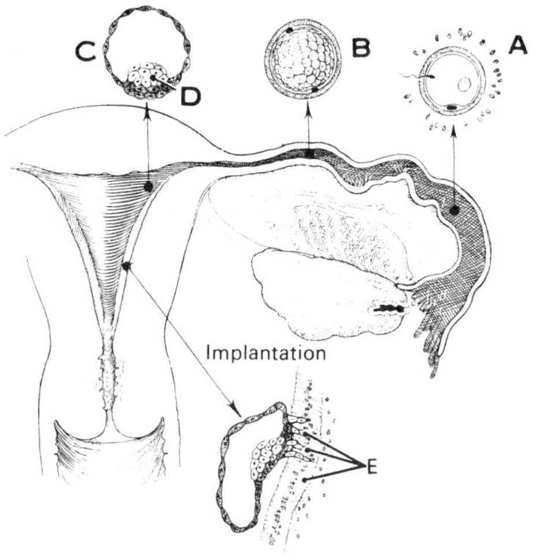

Implantation

A, sperm entering ovum; B, morula; C, blastocyst (enters uterus at about 5th day); D, inner cell mass of blastocyst; E, implantation, with trophoblastic cells penetrating between cells of uterine epithelium.

central i., circumferential or superficial i.; i. in which the blastocyst remains in the uterine cavity, as in carnivores, rhesus monkeys, and rabbits.

circumferential i., central i.

cortical i., i. of blastocyst in the ovarian cortex, causing an ovarian pregnancy.

delayed i., a phenomenon characterized by an interval ranging from a few weeks to approximately 6 months between the time an ovum is fertilized and subsequent i. of the zygote, as in the marten and the armadillo.

eccentric i., i. in which the blastocyst lies in a uterine crypt, as in the mouse, rat, and hamster.

interstitial i., i. in which the blastocyst lies within the substance of the endometrium, as in humans and guinea pigs.

nerve i., planting one nerve into the sheath of another nerve.

pellet i., intramuscular or subcutaneous insertion of an active therapeutic agent in pellet form to provide protracted absorption at a rate slower than subcutaneous or intramuscular injection and as a means of providing a sustained therapeutic effect with agents not active when ingested.

periosteal i., insertion of a normal tendon into a periosteum as part of a tendon transplantation operation.

subcutaneous i., insertion of material under the skin.

superficial i., central i.

impletion (im-plē'shŭn) [L. *implere,* to fill up]. Obsolete term denoting the normal lack of awareness of the blind spot in the temporal field of each eye, even with one eye closed, due to cortical mediation.

implosion (im-plō'shŭn). **1.** A sudden collapse, as of an evacuated vessel, in which there is a bursting inward rather than outward as in explosion. **2.** A type of behavior therapy, similar to flooding, during which the patient is given massive exposure to extreme anxiety-arousing stimuli by being asked to describe, and thus relive in his imagination, those life events or situations typically producing these overwhelming emotional reactions. As the patient does so, the therapist attempts to extinguish the future influence of such unconscious material over the patient's behavior and feelings, and previous avoidance responses to the stimuli are replaced by more appropriate responses.

impotence, impotency (im'pō-tens, -ten-sē) [L. *impotentia,* inability, fr. *in-* neg. + *potentia,* power]. **1.** Weakness; lack of power. **2.** Specifically, inability of the male to achieve and/or maintain penile erection and thus engage in copulation; a manifestation, usually, of a neurological or psychomotor dysfunction.

atonic i., i. caused by paralysis of the motor nerves.

paretic i., i. caused by a lesion of the nervous system.

psychic i., that caused by psychologic factors.

symptomatic i., i. caused by disturbance of the sensory perineal reflexes.

impregnate (im-preg'nāt) [L. *im-,* in, + *praegnans,* with child]. **1.** To fecundate; to cause to conceive. **2.** To diffuse or permeate with another substance. See also saturate.

impregnation (im-preg-nā'shŭn). **1.** The act of making pregnant. **2.** The process of diffusing or permeating with another substance, as in metallic i. of tissue components with silver nitrate or ammoniacal silver. See also saturation.

impressio, pl. **impressiones** (im-pres'ē-ō, im-pres-ē-ō'nēz) [L.] [NA]. Impression (1); a mark seemingly made by pressure of one structure or organ on another.

i. cardi'aca hep'atis [NA], cardiac impression of liver; a depression on the superior area of the diaphragmatic surface of the liver corresponding to the position of the heart.

i. cardi'aca pulmo'nis [NA], cardiac impression of the lung; the depression on the medial surface of each lung produced by the presence of the heart. It is more pronounced on the left lung.

i. col'ica [NA], colic impression; a hollow on the visceral surface of the right lobe of the liver anteriorly, corresponding to the situation of the right flexure and beginning of the transverse colon.

impressio'nes digita'tae [NA], digitate impressions; the depressions on the inner surface of the skull which correspond to the convolutions of the brain.

i. duodena'lis [NA], duodenal impression; a hollow on the visceral surface of the right lobe of the liver alongside the gallbladder, marking the situation of the duodenum.

i. esophage'a [NA], esophageal impression; the marking of the esophagus on the back of the left lobe of the liver.

i. gas'trica [NA], gastric impression; a hollow on the visceral surface of the left lobe of the liver corresponding to the location of the stomach.

i. ligamen'ti costoclavicula'ris [NA], impression for the costoclavicular ligament; rhomboid impression; tuberositas costalis; costal tuberosity; an irregular pitted area on the inferior surface of the clavicle at its sternal end, giving attachment to the costoclavicular ligament.

i. petro'sa pal'lii, petrosal impression of the pallium; a shallow impression on the inferior surface of the cerebral hemisphere made

by the superior margin of the petrous part of the temporal bone.
i. rena'lis [NA], renal impression; a hollow on the visceral surface of the right lobe of the liver, in which lies the right kidney.
i. suprarena'lis [NA], suprarenal impression; a hollow on the visceral surface of the right lobe of the liver, adjoining the sulcus venae cavae, in which lies the right suprarenal gland.
i. trigem'inales [NA], trigeminal impression; a depression on the anterior surface of the petrous portion of the temporal bone, near the apex, lodging the trigeminal ganglion.

impression (im-presh'ŭn) [L. *impressio,* fr. *im- primo,* pp. *-pressus,* to press upon]. **1.** Impressio. **2.** Mental i.; an effect produced upon the mind by some external object acting through the organs of sense. **3.** An imprint or negative likeness; especially, the negative form of the teeth and/or other tissues of the oral cavity, made in a plastic material which becomes relatively hard or set while in contact with these tissues, made in order to reproduce a positive form or cast of the recorded tissues; classified, according to the materials of which they are made, as reversible and irreversible hydrocolloid i., modeling plastic i., plaster i., and wax i.
basilar i., an invagination of the base of the skull into the posterior fossa with compression of the brainstem and cerebellar structures into the foramen magnum. *Cf.* platybasia.
cardiac i. of liver, *impressio* cardiaca hepatis.
cardiac i. of lung, *impressio* cardiaca pulmonis.
colic i., *impressio* colica.
complete denture i., **(1)** an i. of an edentulous arch made for the purpose of constructing a complete denture; **(2)** a negative registration of the entire denture-bearing, stabilizing area of either the maxillae or mandible; **(3)** a negative registration of the entire denture foundation and border seal areas present in the edentulous mouth.
i. for costoclavicular ligament, *impressio* ligamenti costoclavicularis.
deltoid i., *tuberositas* deltoidea.
digitate i.'s, *impressiones* digitatae.
direct bone i., an i. of denuded bone, used in the construction of subperiosteal denture implants.
duodenal i., *impressio* duodenalis.
esophageal i., *impressio* esophagea.
final i., in dentistry, the i. that is used to make the master cast.
gastric i., *impressio* gastrica.
mental i., i. (2).
partial denture i., an i. or negative copy of all or a part of the partially edentulous dental arch or area, made for the purpose of designing or constructing a partial denture.
petrosal i. of the pallium, *impressio* petrosa pallii.
preliminary i., primary i., in dentistry, one made for the purpose of diagnosis or the construction of a tray.
renal i., *impressio* renalis.
rhomboid i., *impressio* ligamenti costoclavicularis.
sectional i., an i. that is made in sections.
suprarenal i., *impressio* suprarenalis.
trigeminal i., *impressio* trigeminalis.

im'print. In congenital cataract, a superficial opacity separated from a deep opacity by a clear interval.

imprint'ing. A particular kind of learning characterized by its occurrence in the first few hours of life, and which determines species-recognition behavior.

impulse (im'pŭls) [L. *im-pello,* pp. *-pulsus,* to push against, impel (*inp-*)]. **1.** A sudden pushing or driving force. **2.** A sudden, often unreasoning, determination to perform some act. **3.** The action potential of a nerve fiber.
cardiac i., movement of the chest wall produced by cardiac contraction.
ectopic i., an electrical i. from an area of the heart other than the sinus node.
escape i., one or two i.'s (atrial, junctional, or ventricular) arising as a result of delay in the formation or arrival of the prevailing pacemaker.
irresistible i., a compulsion to act such that one feels or claims it cannot be resisted.
morbid i., an i that drives one to commit some act, usually of a deviant or forbidden nature, notwithstanding efforts to restrain oneself.

impulsion (im-pŭl'shŭn). An abnormal urge to perform a certain activity.

impulsive (im-pŭl'siv). Relating to or actuated by an impulse, rather than controlled by reason or careful deliberation.

imus (ī'mŭs) [L.]. Lowest; the most inferior or caudal of several similar structures.

IMV Abbreviation for intermittent mandatory *ventilation.*

IMViC Acronym for *i* ndole production, *m* ethyl red, *V* oges-Proskauer reaction, and ability to use *c* itrate as a sole source of carbon (*i* inserted for euphony); used primarily to differentiate *Escherichia coli* from *Enterobacter aerogenes* and related organisms.

In Symbol for indium.

in- [L.]. **1.** Prefix conveying a sense of negation, akin to G. *a-, an-* or Eng. *un-*. **2.** Prefix denoting in, within, inside. **3.** Prefix denoting an intensive action; appears as im- before b, p, or m.

inaction (in-ak'shŭn). Inactivity, rest, or lack of response to a stimulus.

inactivate (in-ak'ti-vāt). To destroy the activity or the effects of an agent or substance, as the activity of complement is destroyed when serum is heated.

inactivation (in-ak-ti-vā'shŭn). The process of destroying or removing the activity or the effects of an agent or substance; *e.g.,* the complementary effect of a serum may be destroyed by means of i. at 56°C for 30 min.

inanimate (in-an'i-māt) [L. *in-* neg. + *anima,* breath, soul]. Not alive.

inanition (in'ă-nish'ŭn) [L. *inanis,* empty]. Severe weakness and wasting as occurs from lack of food, defect in assimilation, or neoplastic disease.

inapparent (in'ă-pār'ent). Not apparent; latent; beneath the threshold of clinical recognition, as an inapparent infection.

inappetence (in-ap'ĕ-tens) [L. *in-* neg. + *ap-peto,* pp. *-petitus,* to strive after, long for (*adp-*)]. Lack of desire or of craving.

inarticulate (in-ar-tik'yū-lit). **1.** Not articulate in the form of intelligible speech. **2.** Unable to satisfactorily express oneself in words.

inassimilable (in-ă-sim'il-ă-bl). Not assimilable; not capable of undergoing assimilation.

inattention (in-ă-ten'shŭn). Lack of attention; negligence.
selective i., an aspect of attentiveness in which a person attempts to ignore or avoid that which generates anxiety.
sensory i., the inability to feel a tactile stimulus when a similar stimulus, presented simultaneously in a homologous area of the body, is perceived.
visual i., the inability to perceive a photic stimulus in a visual field when a similar but perceived stimulus is presented simultaneously in the homologous field.

inborn (in'bōrn). Innate; inherited; implanted during development *in utero.*

in'bred. Denoting populations (groups, genetic lines, etc.) derived from small sets of ancestors.

inbreeding (in'brēd-ing). **1.** Mating between organisms that are genetically more closely related than organisms selected at random from the population. **2.** A practice of mating animals that are closely related.

incarcerated (in-kar'ser-ā-ted) [L. *in,* in, + *carcero,* pp. *-atus,* to imprison, fr. *carcer,* prison]. Confined; imprisoned; trapped.

incarnant (in-kar'nant) [L. *incarno,* fr. *in* + *caro* (*carn-*), flesh]. Promoting or accelerating the granulation of a wound.

incarnative (in-kar'nă-tiv). Incarnant.

incendiarism (in-sen'di-ă-rizm) [L. *incendiarius,* causing a conflagration]. Pyromania.

incentive (in-sen'tiv) [LL. *incentivus,* provocative]. In experimental psychology, an object or goal of motivated behavior.

incertae sedis (in-ser'tē sē'dis) [L.]. Of uncertain or doubtful affiliation or doubtful position, said of organisms in taxonomic classifications.

incest (in'sest) [L. *incestus,* unchaste, fr. *in-,* not, + *castus,* chaste]. **1.** Sexual relations between persons closely related by blood, especially between parents and children, brother and sister. **2.** The crime of sexual relations between persons related by blood, where such cohabitation is prohibited by law.

incestuous (in-ses'chū-ŭs). **1.** Pertaining to incest. **2.** Guilty of incest.

incidence (in'si-dens) [L. *incido,* to fall into or upon, to happen]. **1.** The number of new cases of a disease in a defined population over a specific period of time. **2.** In optics, intersection of a ray of light with a surface.

incident (in'si-dent) [L. *incido,* pp. *-casus,* to fall into, to meet with]. Going toward; impinging upon, as incident rays.

incisal (in-sī'zăl) [L. *incido,* pp. *-cisus,* to cut into]. Cutting; relating to the cutting edges of the incisor and cuspid teeth.

incise (in-sīz'). To cut with a knife.

incision (in-sizh'ŭn) [L. *incisio*]. A cut; a surgical wound; a division of the soft parts made with a knife.

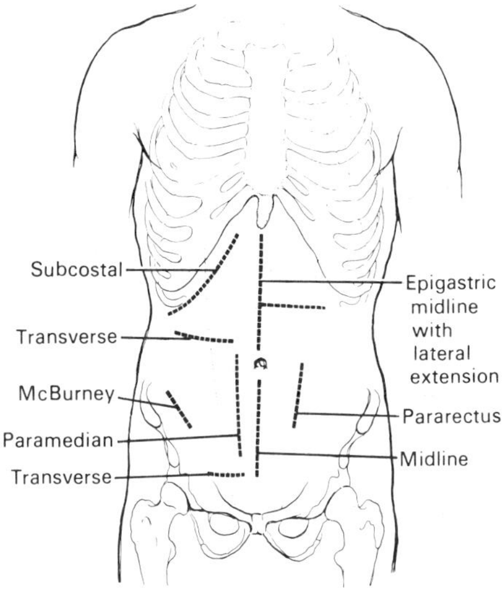

Abdominal Incisions

Agnew-Verhoeff i., obsolete procedure for release of pus in the lacrimal sac in acute phlegmonous dacryocystitis.
bucket-handle i., a bilateral subcostal abdominal i.
celiotomy i., an i. through the abdominal wall.
chevron i., a bilateral subcostal i. in the abdomen, in the shape of an inverted "V"; used in upper gastrointestinal, renal, or adrenal surgery.
Deaver's i., an i. in right lower abdominal quadrant, with medial displacement of the rectus muscle.
Dührssen's i.'s, three surgical i.'s of an incompletely dilated cervix, corresponding roughly to 2, 6, and 10 o'clock, used as a means of effecting immediate delivery of the fetus.
endaural i., i. through the external auditory canal to permit mastoid surgery.
Fergusson's i., an i. used in maxillectomy, along the junction of cheek and nose, to bisect the upper lip.
flank i., an i. usually made near and parallel to the twelfth rib between the iliac crest on the lower side and the ribs on the upper.
Kocher's i., an i. parallel with right costal margin.
McBurney's i., an i. parallel with the course of the external oblique muscle, one or two inches cephaled to the anterior superior spine of the ilium.
paramedian i., an i. lateral to the midline.
Pfannenstiel's i., an i. made transversely, and through the external sheath of the recti muscles, about an inch above the pubes, the muscles being split or separated in the direction of their fibers.

incisive (in-sī'siv). **1.** Cutting; having the power to cut. **2.** Relating to the incisor teeth.

incisor (in-sī'zŏr) [L. *incido,* to cut into]. One of the cutting teeth, i. teeth, four in number in each jaw at the apex of the dental arch.
central i., the first tooth in the maxilla and mandible on either side of the midsagittal plane of the head.
lateral i., second i.
scalpriform i.'s, the cutting or gnawing i.'s of a rodent.
second i., lateral i.; second maxillary or mandibular permanent or deciduous tooth on either side of the midsagittal plane of the head.

INCISURA

incisura, pl. **incisurae** (in'sī-sū'ră, in'si-sū'rē) [L. a cutting into] [NA]. Incisure; notch; emargination; an indentation at the edge of any structure.
i. acetab'uli [NA], acetabular notch; cotyloid notch; a gap in the lower part of the margin of the acetabulum.
i. angula'ris [NA], angular notch; sulcus angularis; a sharp angular depression in the lesser curvature of the stomach at the junction of the body with the pyloric canal.
i. ante'rior au'ris [NA], anterior notch of the ear; auricular notch (1); anterior auricular groove; sulcus auriculae anterior; a notch between the tuberculum supratragicum and the crus helicis.
i. ap'icis cor'dis [NA], notch of the apex of the heart; a slight notch near the apex of the heart where the anterior interventricular sulcus reaches the diaphragmatic surface of the heart.
i. cardi'aca [NA], cardiac notch; a deep notch between the esophagus and fundus of the stomach.
i. cardi'aca pulmo'nis sinis'tri [NA], cardiac notch of the left lung; the notch in the anterior border of the superior lobe of the left lung which accommodates the pericardium.
incisurae cartilag'inis mea'tus acus'tici exter'ni [NA], notches in cartilage of external acoustic meatus; incisurae santorini; Santorini's incisures or fissures; Duverney's fissures; (usually) two vertical fissures in the anterior portion of the cartilage of the external auditory meatus, filled by fibrous tissue.
i. cerebel'li ante'rior, anterior notch of the cerebellum; semilunar notch (1); a wide, shallow notch on the anterior surface of the cerebellum occupied laterally by the superior cerebellar peduncles and the inferior quadrigeminal medially bodies.
i. cerebel'li poste'rior, posterior notch of the cerebellum; marsupial notch; a narrow notch between the cerebellar hemispheres posteriorly, occupied by the falx cerebelli.
i. clavicula'ris [NA], the clavicular notch or facet; a hollow on

either side of the upper surface of the manubrium sterni which articulates with the clavicle.
i. costa'lis [NA], costal notch; one of the notches or facets on the lateral edge of the sternum for articulation with a costal cartilage.
i. ethmoida'lis [NA], ethmoidal notch; an oblong gap between the orbital parts of the frontal bone in which the ethmoid bone is lodged.
i. fibula'ris [NA], fibular notch; a hollow on the lateral surface of the lower end of the tibia in which the fibula is lodged.
i. fronta'lis [NA], frontal notch; a small notch, sometimes a foramen, on the orbital margin of the frontal bone medial to the supraorbital notch.
i. interarytenoi'dea [NA], interarytenoid notch; the posterior portion of the aditus laryngis between the two arytenoid cartilages.
i. intertrag'ica [NA], intertragic notch; i. tragica; the deep notch in the lower part of the auricle between the tragus and antitragus.
i. ischiad'ica ma'jor [NA], greater sciatic notch; iliosciatic or sacrosciatic notch; the deep indentation in the posterior border of the hip bone at the point of union of the ilium and ischium.
i. ischiad'ica mi'nor [NA], lesser sciatic notch; the notch in the posterior border of the ischium below the ischial spine.
i. jugula'ris [NA], jugular notch; **i. j. os'sis occipita'lis** [NA], the notch in the occipital bone which forms one boundary of the jugular foramen; **i. j. os'sis tempora'lis** [NA], the notch in the temporal bone which forms one boundary of the jugular foramen; **i. j. sterna'lis** [NA], sternal notch; suprasternal, presternal, or interclavicular notch; the large notch in the superior margin of the sternum.
i. lacrima'lis [NA], lacrimal notch; the notch on the frontal process of the maxilla into which the lacrimal bone fits.
i. ligamen'ti tere'tis hep'atis [NA], notch for the round ligament of the liver; umbilical notch; i. umbilicalis; the notch in the inferior border of the liver that accommodates the round ligament.
i. mandib'ulae [NA], mandibular notch; sigmoid notch; the deep notch between the condylar and coronoid processes of the mandible.
i. mastoi'dea [NA], mastoid or digastric notch or groove; the groove medial to the mastoid process of the temporal bone from which the digastric muscle originates.
i. nasa'lis [NA], nasal notch; the notch in the medial border of the maxilla anteriorly which, with its fellow, forms most of the piriform opening of the nasal cavity.
i. pancre'atis [NA], pancreatic notch; a notch separating the uncinate process of the head of the pancreas from the neck.
i. parieta'lis [NA], parietal notch; the angle posteriorly between the squamous and petrous parts of the temporal bone.
i. preoccipita'lis [NA], preoccipital notch; an indentation in the ventrolateral border of the temporal lobe of the cerebral hemisphere.
i. pterygoi'dea [NA], pterygoid notch; pterygoid fissure; fissura pterygoidea; the cleft between the medial and lateral laminae of the pterygoid process of the sphenoid bone into which the pyramidal process of the palatine bone is fitted.
i. radia'lis [NA], radial notch; the concavity on the lateral aspect of the coronoid process of the ulna which articulates with the head of the radius.
i. rivi'ni, i. tympanica.
incisurae santori'ni, incisurae cartilaginis meatus acustici externi.
i. scap'ulae [NA], scapular or suprascapular notch; a notch on the superior border of the scapula through which the suprascapular nerve passes.
i. semiluna'ris ul'nae, i. trochlearis.
i. sphenopalati'na [NA], sphenopalatine notch; the deep notch between the orbital and sphenoidal processes of the palatine bone which is converted into the foramen of the same name by the undersurface of the sphenoid bone.
i. supraorbita'lis [NA], supraorbital notch; a groove in the orbital margin of the frontal bone, about the junction of the medial and intermediate thirds, through which pass the supraorbital nerve and artery. See also *foramen* supraorbitale.
i. tento'rii [NA], notch of the tentorium; the triangular opening in the tentorium cerebelli through which the brainstem extends from the posterior into the middle cranial fossa.
i. termina'lis au'ris [NA], terminal notch of the auricle; auricular notch (2); a deep notch separating the lamina tragi and cartilage of the external auditory meatus from the main auricular cartilage, the two being connected below by the isthmus.
i. thyroi'dea infe'rior [NA], inferior thyroid notch; a shallow notch in the middle of the lower border of the thyroid cartilage.
i. thyroi'dea supe'rior [NA], superior thyroid notch; a deep notch in the middle of the upper border of the thyroid cartilage.
i. trag'ica, i. intertragica.
i. trochlea'ris [NA], trochlear notch; i. semilunaris ulnae; semilunar notch (2); the large semicircular notch at the proximal extremity of the ulna between the olecranon and coronoid processes that articulates with the trochlea of the humerus.
i. tympan'ica [NA], tympanic incisure or notch; Rivinus' incisure or notch; i. rivini; the notch in the superior part of the tympanic ring bridged by the flaccid part of the tympanic membrane.
i. ulna'ris [NA], ulnar notch; the concave surface on the medial side of the distal end of the radius which articulates with the head of the ulna.
i. umbilica'lis, i. ligamenti teretis hepatis.
i. vertebra'lis [NA], vertebral notch; intervertebral notch; one of the two concavities above (superior) and below (inferior) the pedicle of a vertebra; the notches of two adjacent vertebrae form an intervertebral foramen.

---

incisure (in-sī'zhūr) [L. *incisura*]. Incisura (2).
Lanterman's i.'s, Schmidt-Lanterman i.'s.
Rivinus' i., *incisura* tympanica.
Santorini's incisures, *incisurae* cartilaginis meatus acustici externi.
Schmidt-Lanterman i.'s, Schmidt-Lanterman clefts; Lanterman's i.'s; funnel-shaped interruptions in the regular structure of the myelin sheath of nerve fibers, formerly interpreted as actual breaks in the sheath but shown by electron microscopy to correspond each to a strand of cytoplasm locally separating the two otherwise fused oligodendroglial (or, in peripheral nerves, Schwann cell) membranes composing the myelin sheath.
tympanic i., *incisura* tympanica.

inclinatio, pl. **inclinationes** (in'kli-nā'shē-ō, -nā-shē-ō'nēz) [L.]. Inclination.
i. pel'vis [NA], inclination of the pelvis; the angle which the plane of the pelvic inlet makes with the horizontal plane.

inclination (in-kli-nā'shŭn) [L. *inclinatio,* a leaning]. **1.** A leaning or sloping. **2.** In dentistry, deviation of the long axis of a tooth from the perpendicular.
condylar guidance i., the angle of i. of the condylar guidance to an accepted horizontal plane.
enamel rod i., the direction of the enamel rods with reference to the outer surface of the enamel of a tooth.
lateral condylar i., the direction of the lateral condyle path.
i. of pelvis, *inclinatio* pelvis.

inclinometer (in'kli-nom'ĕ-ter) [L. *in- clino,* to incline, + G. *metron,* measure]. Obsolete instrument for determining the direction of the ocular axes in astigmatism.

inclusion (in-klū'zhŭn) [L. *inclusio,* a shutting in, fr. *in- cludo,* pp. *-clusis,* to close in]. **1.** Any foreign or heterogenous substance contained in a cell or in any tissue or organ, not introduced as a result of trauma. **2.** The process by which a foreign or heterogenous structure is misplaced in another tissue.
cell i.'s, **(1)** metaplasm; the residual elements of the cytoplasm

which are metabolic products of the cell, *e.g.*, pigment granules or crystals; **(2)** storage materials such as glycogen or fat; **(3)** engulfed material such as carbon or other foreign substances. See also inclusion *body*.

Döhle i.'s, Döhle *bodies*.

fetal i., unequal conjoined twins in which the incompletely developed parasite is wholly inclosed within the autosite.

leukocyte i.'s, Döhle *bodies*.

incoercible (in-kō-er'si-bl) [L. *in-* neg. + *coerceo,* pp. *-ercitus,* to hold together, restrain, fr. *arceo,* to shut up]. Impossible to control, to restrain, or to stop.

incoherent (in-kō-hēr'ent) [L. *in-* neg. + *co-haereo,* pp. *-haesus,* to cling together, fr. *haereo,* to stick]. Not coherent; disjointed; confused; denoting a lack of connectedness or organization of parts during verbal expression.

incompatibility (in'kom-pat-i-bil'i-tē). The quality of being incompatible.

physiologic i., therapeutic i.; a form of i. in which the substances in a mixture exert opposing physiologic actions.

therapeutic i., physiologic i.

incompatible (in-kom-pat'i-bl) [L. *in-* neg., + *con-,* with, + *patior,* pp. *passus,* to suffer]. **1.** Not of suitable composition to be combined or mixed with another agent or substance, without resulting in an undesirable reaction (including chemical alteration or destruction). **2.** Denoting persons who are unable to freely associate with one another without resulting anxiety and conflict.

incompetence, incompetency (in-kom'pe-tens, in-kom'pĕ-ten-sē) [L. *in-,* neg. + *com-peto,* strive after together]. **1.** Insufficiency (2); the quality of being incompetent or incapable of performing the allotted function, especially failure of cardiac or venous valves to close completely. **2.** In psychiatry, the inability to distinguish right from wrong or to manage one's affairs.

aortic i., defective closure of the aortic valve permitting regurgitation into the left ventricle during diastole.

cardiac i., inability of the ventricles to pump out the blood returning to the atria fast enough to prevent an abnormal rise in atrial pressure.

mitral i., defective closure of the mitral valve permitting regurgitation into the left atrium during systole.

muscular i., imperfect closure of an anatomically normal cardiac valve, in consequence of defective action of the papillary muscles.

pulmonary i., pulmonic i., defective closure of the pulmonic valve permitting regurgitation into the right ventricle during diastole.

pyloric i., a patulous state or want of tone of the pylorus that allows the passage of food into the intestine before gastric digestion is completed.

relative i., imperfect closure of a cardiac valve, in consequence of excessive dilation of the corresponding cavity of the heart.

tricuspid i., defective closure of the tricuspid valve permitting regurgitation into the right atrium during systole.

valvular i., a leaky state of one or more of the cardiac valves, the valve not closing tightly and blood therefore regurgitating through it.

inconstant (in-kon'stant). **1.** Variable; irregular. **2.** In anatomy, denoting a structure, such as an artery, nerve, etc., that may or may not be present.

incontinence (in-kon'ti-nens) [L. *in-continentia,* fr. *in-* neg. + *contineo,* to hold together, fr. *teneo,* to hold]. Incontinentia. **1.** Inability to prevent the discharge of any of the excretions, especially of urine or feces. **2.** Lack of restraint of the appetites, especially sexual. *Cf.* intemperance.

i. of milk, galactorrhea.

overflow i., paradoxical i.; involuntary loss of urine associated with overdistention of the bladder, with or without a detrusor contraction.

paradoxical i., overflow i.

passive i., dribbling of urine by reason of inability of the bladder to empty itself and of consequent overdistention. See also overflow i.

i. of pigment, loss of melanin from the epidermis, and accumulation in melanophores in the upper dermis; seen in several inflammatory diseases of the skin and in incontinentia pigmenti.

reflex i., in neurogenic disorders, loss of urine due to detrusor hyperreflexia and/or involuntary urethral relaxation in the absence of the desire to void.

urge i., urgency i., leakage of urine during a strong desire to void.

urinary exertional i., urinary stress i.

urinary stress i., urinary exertional i.; leakage of urine as a result of coughing, straining, or some sudden voluntary movement, due to weakness of the muscles around the neck of the bladder and surrounding the vagina, resulting in an incompetent internal vesical sphincter.

incontinentia (in-kon'ti-nen'shē-ă) [L.]. Incontinence.

i. pigmen'ti, Bloch-Sulzberger disease or syndrome; an inherited developmental defect of the skin which may also involve other structures; characterized by pigmented lesions in linear, zebra-stripe, and other bizarre configurations, sometimes preceded by vesicles and bullae, and often followed by verrucous lesions; occasionally accompanied by other developmental abnormalities.

i. pigmen'ti achro'miens, hypomelanosis of Ito; inherited hypopigmented macules in a "marble-cake" pattern, variably associated with epidermal nevi, alopecia, and ocular, skeletal, and neural abnormalities.

incontinent (in-kon'ti-nent). Denoting incontinence.

incoordination (in-kō-ōr-di-nā'shŭn) [L. *in-* neg. + coordination]. Ataxia.

incorporation (in-kōr-pō-rā'shŭn) [L. *in-,* in, + *corporare,* pp. *corporatus,* to make into a body]. Identification.

increase (in'krēs). Any growth in quantity.

absolute cell i., an actual i. in one of the types of leukocytes, the absolute number of leukocytes in 1 cu mm of blood being obtained by multiplying the total leukocyte count by the percentage of the cell types in question.

increment (in'kre-ment) [L. *incrementum,* increase]. A change in the value of a variable; usually an increase, with "decrement" applied to a decrease, though "increment" can also correctly be applied to both.

incretion (in-krē'shŭn) [L. *in,* within, + *secernere,* to separate]. **1.** The functional activity of an endocrine gland. **2.** Rarely used term for the product of the activity of an endocrine gland.

incrustation (in'krŭs-tā'shŭn) [L. *in- crusto,* pp. *-atus,* to incrust, fr. *crusta,* crust]. **1.** Formation of a crust or a scab. **2.** A coating of some adventitious material or an exudate; a scab.

incubation (in'kyū-bā'shŭn) [L. *incubo,* to lie on]. **1.** Act of maintaining controlled environmental conditions for the purpose of favoring growth or development of microbial or tissue cultures. **2.** Maintenance of an artificial environment for an infant, usually a premature or hypoxic one, by providing proper temperature, humidity, and, usually, oxygen. **3.** The development, without sign or symptom, of an infection from the time the infectious agent gains entry until the appearance of the first signs or symptoms.

incubator (in'kyū-bā'tōr). **1.** A container in which controlled environmental conditions may be maintained; *e.g.,* for culturing microorganisms. **2.** An apparatus for maintaining an infant (usually premature) in an environment of proper oxygenation, humidity, and temperature.

incubus (in'kū-bŭs) [L. fr. *incubo,* to lie on]. **1.** Originally, an evil spirit which lay upon and oppressed sleeping persons; especially, a male spirit which copulated with sleeping women. *Cf.* succubus.

2. Nightmare.

incudal (in'kū-dăl). Relating to the incus.

incudectomy (in-kū-dek'tō-mē) [incus + G. *ektomē,* excision]. Removal of the incus of the tympanum.

incudes (in-kū'dēz) [L.]. Plural of incus.

incudiform (in-kū'di-fōrm) [L. *incus* (*incud-*), anvil]. Shaped like an anvil.

incudomalleal (in-kū'dō-mal'lē-ăl). Relating to the incus and the malleus; denoting the articulation between the incus and the malleus in the middle ear.

incudostapedial (in-kū'dō-stā-pē'dē-ăl). Relating to the incus and the stapes; denoting the articulation between the incus and the stapes in the middle ear.

incurable (in-kyūr'ă-bl). Denoting a disease or morbid process that is unresponsive to medical or surgical treatment.

incurvation (in'ker-vā'shŭn). An inward curvature; a bending inward.

incus, gen. **incudis,** pl. **incudes** (ing'kŭs, in-kū'dis, in-kū'dēz) [L. anvil] [NA]. Anvil; ambos; the middle of the three ossicles in the middle ear; it has a body (corpus incudis) and two limbs or processes (crus longum incudis and crus breve incudis); at the tip of the long limb is a small knob, processus lenticularis, which articulates with the head of the stapes.

incycloduction (in-sī-klō-dŭk'shŭn). Rotation of the upper pole of one cornea inward.

incyclophoria (in-sī'klō-fō'rē-ă) [L. *in,* + *cyclo-* + G. *phora,* movement]. The tendency toward inward rotation of the upper pole of the cornea, prevented by fusion.

in d. Abbreviation for L. *in dies,* daily.

indanediones (in-dān'ĕ-dī-ōnez). A class of orally effective indirect-acting anticoagulants of which phenindione is representative.

indapamide (in-dap'ă-mīd). 4-Chloro-*N*- (2-methyl-1-indolinyl)-3-sulfamoylbenzamide; a loop diuretic used to treat edema associated with congestive heart failure, hepatic cirrhosis, and renal disease.

indeciduate (in-dē-sid'yū-āt). Relating to the mammals (Indecidua) that do not shed any maternal uterine tissue when expelling the placenta at birth (horse, pig) in contrast to deciduate mammals (man, dog, rodent).

indenization (in-den-i-zā'shŭn) [*in-* + denizen]. Innidiation.

indentation (in-den-tā'shun) [Mediev. L. *in-dento,* pp. *-atus,* to make notches like teeth, fr. L. *dens* (*dent-*), tooth]. **1.** The act of notching or pitting. **2.** A notch. **3.** A state of being notched.

INDEX

index, gen. **indicis,** pl. **indices** or **indexes** (in'deks, -di-sis, -di-sēz, -dek-sĕz) [L. one that points out, an informer, the forefinger, an index, fr. *in-dico,* pp. *-atus,* to declare]. **1** [NA]. Forefinger; index finger; digitus secundus; second finger (the thumb being counted as the first). **2.** A guide, standard, indicator, symbol, or number denoting the relation in respect to size, capacity, or function, of one part or thing to another. See also quotient; ratio. **3.** A core or mold used to record or maintain the relative position of a tooth or teeth to one another and/or to a cast. **4.** A guide, usually made of plaster, used to reposition teeth, casts, or parts.

absorbancy i., specific absorption *coefficient.*

alveolar i., **(1)** gnathic i.; **(2)** basilar i.

anesthetic i., ratio of the number of units of anesthetic required for anesthesia to the number of units of anesthetic required to produce respiratory or cardiovascular failure.

antitryptic i., an obsolete term for the relative retardation in loss of viscosity of a solution of casein incubated with trypsin, to which a drop of abnormal blood serum (as from a cancerous patient) has been added, compared with that in a similar solution to which normal serum has been added; if the former drips through the tube of the viscosimeter in 100 seconds, and the latter in 104 seconds, the antitryptic i. is 4.

Arneth i., an expression based on adding the percentages of polymorphonuclear neutrophils with 1 or 2 lobes in their nuclei, plus one-half the percentage with 3 lobes; the normal value is 60%. See also Arneth *formula;* Arneth *count.*

auricular i., relation of the width to the height of the auricle or pinna: (width of pinna × 100)/length of pinna.

Ayala's i., Ayala's quotient; spinal quotient; the cerebrospinal i. when 10 ml cerebrospinal fluid have been removed.

basilar i., alveolar i. (2); ratio between the basialveolar line and the maximum length of the cranium, according to the formula: (basialveolar line × 100)/length of cranium.

Bödecker i., a modification of the DMF caries i.

body mass i., weight in kilograms divided by height in meters squared; a method of determining obesity.

buffer i., buffer *value.*

cardiac i., the amount of blood ejected by the heart in a unit of time divided by the body surface area; usually expressed in liters per minute per square meter.

cardiothoracic i., cardiothoracic *ratio.*

centromeric i., the ratio of the length of the short arm of the chromosome to that of the total chromosome; ordinarily expressed as a percentage.

cephalic i., length-breadth i.; the ratio of the maximal breadth to the maximal length of the head, obtained by the formula: (breadth × 100)/length.

cephalo-orbital i., the ratio of the cubic content of the two orbits to that of the cranial cavity multiplied by 100.

cephalorrhachidian i., cerebrospinal i.

cerebral i., the ratio of the transverse to the anteroposterior diameter of the cranial cavity multiplied by 100.

cerebrospinal i., cephalorrhachidian i.; the figure obtained by multiplying the pressure of the cerebrospinal fluid, after fluid has been withdrawn by spinal puncture, by the quantity of fluid withdrawn and then dividing by the original pressure.

chemotherapeutic i., the ratio of the minimal effective dose of a chemotherapeutic agent to the maximal tolerated dose. Originally used by Ehrlich to express the relative toxicity of a chemotherapeutic agent to a parasite and to its host.

chest i., thoracic i.

color i. (C.I.), blood quotient; globular value; the ratio between the amount of hemoglobin and the number of red blood cells, obtained by dividing the concentration of hemoglobin (expressed as per cent of normal) by the relative number of red blood cells (expressed as per cent, on the basis of 5,000,000 per cu mm as normal); the average color i. is approximately 0.85.

cranial i., the ratio of the maximal breadth to the maximal length of the skull, obtained by the formula: (breadth × 100)/length.

Dean's fluorosis i., an i. that measures the degree of mottled enamel (fluorosis) in teeth; used most often in epidemiological field studies.

def or **DEF caries i.,** an i. of past caries experience based upon the number of decayed, extracted, and filled deciduous (indicated by lower case letters) or permanent (indicated by capital letters) teeth.

degenerative i., the percentage of granulocytes that contain toxic granules in the cytoplasm, as compared with the total percentage of granulocytes.

dental i., Flower's dental i.; relation of the dental length (distance from the anterior surface of the first premolar to the posterior sur-

face of the third molar) to the basinasal (basion to nasion) length: (dental length $\times 100$)/basinasal length.
df or **DF caries i.,** an i. of past caries experience based upon the number of decayed and filled deciduous (indicated by lower case letters) or permanent (indicated by capital letters) teeth.
dmf or **DMF caries i.,** an i. of past caries experience based upon the number of decayed, missing, and filled deciduous (indicated by lower case letters) or permanent (indicated by capital letters) teeth.
dmfs or **DMFS caries i.,** an i. of past caries experience based upon the number of decayed, missing, and filled surfaces of deciduous (indicated by lower case letters) or permanent (indicated by capital letters) teeth.
effective temperature i., a composite i. of environmental comfort which is compared after exposure to different combinations of air temperature, humidity, and movement.
empathic i., the degree of empathy experienced by one person concerning another person, more particularly of a sufferer from some emotional or somatic condition.
endemic i., the percentage of children infected with malaria or other endemic disease, in any given locality.
erythrocyte indices, calculations for determining the average size, hemoglobin content, and concentration of red blood cells, including mean cell volume, mean cell hemoglobin, and mean cell hemoglobin concentrate.
facial i., relation of the length of the face to its maximal width between the zygomatic prominences; to get **superior facial i.,** length of the face is measured from the nasion to the alveolar point: (nasialveolar length $\times$ 100)/bizygomatic width; **total facial i.,** length is measured from the nasion to the mental tubercle: (nasimental length $\times$ 100)/bizygomatic width.
Flower's dental i., dental i.
free thyroxine i. (FTI), an arbitrary value obtained by multiplying the triiodothyronine uptake by the serum thyroxine concentration; it largely corrects for variations in thyroid-bound globulin concentration by providing a clinically valid estimate of the physiologically active free thyroxine; direct assay or laboratory measurement of free serum thyroxine yields a more accurate value.
gnathic i., alveolar i. (1); relation between the basialveolar (basion to alveolar point) and basinasal (basion to nasion) lengths: (basialveolar length $\times$ 100)/basinasal length; the result indicates the degree of projection of the maxilla or upper jaw.
height-length i., vertical i.
icteric i., see icterus i.
icterus i., the value that indicates the relative level of bilirubin in serum or plasma; calculated by comparing (in a colorimeter) the intensity of the color of the specimen with that of a standard solution (potassium dichromate, 0.05 g, in 500 ml of water, plus 0.2 ml of sulfuric acid); the normal range is 3 to 5, and values greater than 15 are usually associated with clinically apparent jaundice; an i. less than 3 is observed in various examples of secondary anemia, aplastic anemia, and chlorosis. Sometimes erroneously called icteric i.: it is an i. of jaundice, not a jaundiced i.
iron i., an obsolete i. of iron obtained by dividing the figure for the average content of iron in normal blood (42.74 mg) by the red cell count in millions; it normally varies between 8 and 9; in pernicious anemia, the i. is usually greater than 10, but it tends to be normal in chronic secondary anemia.
karyopyknotic i., an i. used to monitor the hormonal status of the patient as reflected by exfoliated vaginal cells and their morphology; an expression of the percentage of intermediate and superficial cells from squamous cells of vaginal epithelium which have pyknotic nuclei.
length-breadth i., cephalic i.
length-height i., vertical i.
leukopenic i., a significant decrease in the white blood count after ingestion of food to which a patient is hypersensitive, a count made during the normal fasting state being used as the basis for evaluation of the postprandial count.
maturation i., an i. indicating the degree of maturation attained by the vaginal epithelium as adjudged by the cell types being exfoliated therefrom; serves as an objective means of evaluating hormonal secretion or response; represents the percentage of parabasal cells/intermediate cells/superficials, in that order; "shift to the left" is used to indicate more immature cells on the surface (atrophy), while "shift to the right" indicates more mature epithelium.
metacarpal i., the average ratio of length to breadth of metacarpals II to V; this ratio is increased in the Marfan syndrome.
mitotic i., the proportions of cells in a tissue that are undergoing mitosis, often expressed as the number of cells in each square nm of tissue section or a percentage of the total cell sample.
molar absorbancy i., molar absorption *coefficient.*
nasal i., relation of the greatest width of the nasal aperture to the length of a line from the nasion to the lower border of the nasal aperture: (nasal width $\times$ 100)/nasal height.
nucleoplasmic i., the quotient of the nuclear volume divided by the cytoplasmic volume.
obesity i., body weight divided by body volume.
opsonic i., a value that indicates the relative content of opsonin in the blood of a person with an infectious disease, as evaluated *in vitro* in comparison with presumably normal blood; the opsonic i. is calculated from the following equation: phagocytic i. of normal serum $\div$ phagocytic i. of test serum $= 1 \div x$, where x represents the opsonic i.
orbital i., relation of the height of the orbit to its width: (orbital height $\times$ 100)/orbital width.
orbitonasal i., the ratio of the width between the lateral angles of the eyes, measured with a tape measure passing over the root of the nose times 100, to the width between the lateral angles of the eyes measured with a caliper.
palatal i., palatine i., palatomaxillary i.
palatomaxillary i., palatal or palatine i.; relation of the palatomaxillary width, measured between the outer borders of the alveolar arch just above the middle of the second molar tooth, and the palatomaxillary length, measured from the alveolar point to the middle of a transverse line touching the posterior borders of the two maxillae = (palatomaxillary width $\times$ 100)/palatomaxillary length; it notes the varying forms of the dental arcade and palate.
pelvic i., the ratio of the conjugate to the transverse diameters of the pelvis: (conjugate diameter $\times$ 100)/transverse diameter.
phagocytic i., the average number of bacteria observed in the cytoplasm of polymorphonuclear leukocytes after mixing and incubating, at 37°C, 1) a suspension of washed, presumably normal leukocytes, 2) the serum to be tested for opsonin, and 3) a young culture of microorganisms that are causing disease in the patient.
PMA i., an i. which measures the presence or absence of gingival inflammation as occurring on the papillae or the marginal or attached gingivae.
ponderal i., cube root of body weight times 100 divided by stature.
pressure-volume i., method of evaluating the cerebrospinal fluid hydrodynamics.
refractive i. (n), the relative velocity of light in another medium compared to the velocity in air; *e.g.,* in the case of air to crown glass, $n = 1.52$; in the case of air to water, $n = 1.33$. See also *law* of refraction.
Robinson i., an i. used to calculate heart work load. See double *product.*
Röhrer's i., body weight in grams times 100 divided by the cube of height in centimeters.
root caries i., the ratio of the number of teeth with carious lesions of the root, and/or restorations of the root, to the number of teeth with exposed root surfaces.
sacral i., a ratio obtained by multiplying the greatest breadth of

the sacrum by 100 and dividing by the length.
saturation i., an indication of the relative concentration of hemoglobin in the red blood cells, calculated as: g of hemoglobin per 100 ml (expressed as percent of normal) ÷ hematocrit value (expressed as percent of normal) = saturation i. The normal i. for adults and infants is 0.97 to 1.02; in primary and secondary anemia, the i. is usually considerably less than 0.97.
Schilling's i., Schilling's *blood count.*
shock i., the quotient of the cardiac rate divided by the systolic blood pressure; normally approximately 0.5, but in shock (*i.e.,* rising pulse rate with falling blood pressure), the i. may reach 1.0.
small increment sensitivity i., see SISI *test.*
spiro-i., see *spiro-index.*
splenic i., a rough indication of the salubrity, or the reverse, in regard to malaria of a particular district, judged by the relative absence or prevalence of enlarged spleens among the population.
staphylo-opsonic i., the opsonic i. calculated in relation to a staphylococcal infection, with a young culture of *Staphylococcus aureus* or the strain of staphylococcus from the patient being used in the test.
stroke work i., a measure of the work done by the heart with each contraction, adjusted for body surface area; equal to the stroke volume of the heart multiplied by the arterial pressure and divided by body surface area; the normal stroke work i. does not exceed 40 gram-meters per square meter.
therapeutic i., the ratio of LD_{50} to ED_{50}, used in quantitative comparison of drugs.
thoracic i., chest i.; anteroposterior diameter of the thorax times 100 divided by the transverse diameter of the thorax.
tibiofemoral i., the ratio obtained by multiplying the length of the tibia by 100 and dividing by the length of the femur.
transversovertical i., vertical i.
tuberculo-opsonic i., the opsonic i. calculated in relation to tuberculous infection, with an actively growing culture of *Mycobacterium tuberculosis* or the strain of tubercle bacillus from the patient being used in the test.
uricolytic i., the percentage of uric acid oxidized to allantoin before being secreted.
vertical i., height-length or length-height i.; transversovertical i.; the relation of the height to the length of the skull: (height × 100)/length.
vital i., the ratio of births to deaths within a population during a given time.
volume i., an indication of the relative size (*i.e.,* volume) of erythrocytes, calculated as follows: hematocrit value, expressed as per cent of normal ÷ red blood cell count, expressed as per cent of normal = volume i.
zygomaticoauricular i., the ratio between the zygomatic and the auricular diameters of the skull or head.

indican (in'di-kan). **1.** Plant i.; indoxyl *β*- D-glucoside from *Indigofera* species; a source of indigo. **2.** Metabolic i.; uroxanthin; 3-indoxylsulfuric acid, a substance found (as its salts) in sweat and in variable amounts in urine; indicative, when in quantity, of protein putrefaction in the intestine (indicanuria).
metabolic i., indican (2).
plant i., indican (1).

indicanidrosis (in'di-kan-i-drō'sis) [indican + G. *hidrōs,* sweat]. Excretion of indican in the sweat.

indicant (in'di-kant) [L. *in-dico,* pres. p. *-ans* (*-ant*), to point out]. **1.** Pointing out; indicating. **2.** An indication; especially a symptom indicating the proper line of treatment.

indicanuria (in'di-kan-yū'rē-ă). An increased urinary excretion of indican, a derivative of indol formed chiefly in the intestine when protein is putrefied; indol is also formed during the putrefaction of protein in other sites.

indication (in-di-kā'shŭn) [L. fr. *in- dico,* pp. *-atus,* to point out, fr. *dico,* to proclaim]. The basis for initiation of a treatment for a disease or of a diagnostic test; may be furnished by a knowledge of the cause (**causal i.**), by the symptoms present (**symptomatic i.**), or by the nature of the disease (**specific i.**).

indicator (in'di-kā-ter, -tōr) [L. one that points out]. In chemical analysis, a substance that changes color within a certain definite range of pH or oxidation potential, or in any way renders visible the completion of a chemical reaction; *e.g.,* litmus, phenolsulfonphthalein.
alizarin i., a solution consisting of 1 g sodium alizarin sulfonate dissolved in 100 cc distilled water; used as an i. for free acidity in gastric contents.
oxidation-reduction i., redox i.; a substance that undergoes a definite color change at a specific oxidation potential.
redox i., oxidation-reduction i.

indices (in'di-sēz). Alternative plural of index.

Indiella (in-dē-el'ă). Old name for *Madurella.*

indigenous (in-dij'ĕ-nŭs) [L. *indigenus,* born in fr. *indu,* within (old form of *in*), + G. *-gen,* producing]. Native; natural to the country where found.

indigestion (in-di-jes'chŭn). Nonspecific term for a variety of symptoms resulting from a failure of proper digestion and absorption of food in the alimentary tract.
acid i., i. resulting from hyperchlorhydria; often used by the laity as a synonym for pyrosis.
fat i., steatorrhea (1).
gastric i., dyspepsia.
nervous i., i. caused by emotional upsets or stress.

indigo (in'dĭ-gō) [L. *indicum,* fr. G. *indikon,* indigo, ntr. of *Indikos,* Indian] [C.I. 73000]. Indigo blue; indigotin; ($\Delta^{2,2'}$-biindoline)-3,3'-dione; $C_{16}H_{10}N_2O_2$; a blue dyestuff obtained from *Indigofera tinctoria,* and other species of *Indigofera* (family Leguminosae); also made synthetically.

indigo blue. Indigo.

indigo carmine [C.I. 73015]. Sodium indigotindisulfonate; sodium indigotin 5,5'-disulfonate; $C_{16}H_8N_2O_8S_2Na$; a blue dye used for measurement of kidney function and as a special stain for Negri bodies.

indigotin (in-dig'ō-tin, in-di-gō'-tin). Indigo.

indigouria, indiguria (in'dĭ-gō-yū'rē-ă, in-di-gū'rē-ă). The excretion of indigo in the urine.

indisposition (in-dis-pō-zish'ŭn) [L. *in* neg. + *dispositio,* an arrangement, fr. *dis-pono,* pp. *-positus,* to place apart]. A slight illness; malaise.

indium (in'dē-ŭm) [*indigo,* because it gives a blue line in the spectrum]. A metallic element, symbol In, atomic no. 49, atomic weight 114.82.

indium-111 (^{111}**In**). A cyclotron-produced radionuclide with a physical half-life of 2.8 days and with gamma ray emissions of 173 and 247 kiloelectron volts. In a chloride form, it is used as a bone marrow and tumor-localizing tracer; in a chelate form, as a cerebrospinal fluid tracer.
i. chloride, i. trichloride, Cl_3In; used in electron microscopy to stain nucleic acids in thin tissue sections.

individuation (in'di-vid-yū-ā'shŭn). **1.** Development of the individual from the specific. **2.** In jungian psychology, the process by which one's personality is differentiated, developed, and expressed.

indocyanine green (in-dō-sī'ă-nēn). A tricarbocyanine dye that binds to serum albumin and is used in blood volume determinations and in liver function tests.

indocybin (in-dō-sī'bin). Psilocybin.

indolaceturia (in'dōl-as-ĕ-tū'rē-ă). Excretion of an appreciable amount of indoleacetic acid in the urine; a manifestation of Hartnup disease.

indolamine (in-dol'ă-mēn). General term for an indole or indole derivative containing a primary, secondary, or tertiary amine group (*e.g.*, serotonin).

indole (in'dōl). Ketole; 2,3-benzopyrrole; basis of many biologically active substances (*e.g.*, serotonin, tryptophan).

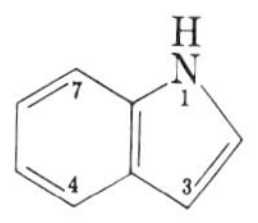

Indole

indolent (in'dō-lent) [L. *in-* neg. + *doleo,* pr. p. *dolens* (*-ent-*), to feel pain]. Inactive; sluggish; painless or nearly so, said of a morbid process.

indolic acids (in-dōl'ik). Metabolites of tryptophan formed within the body or by intestinal microorganisms; the principal i. a. encountered in urine are indoleacetic acid, indoleacetylglutamine, 5-hydroxyindoleacetic acid, and indolelactic acid.

indologenous (in'dō-loj'ĕ-nŭs). Producing or causing the production of indole.

indoluria (in-dō-lū'rē-ă). Excretion of indole in the urine; actual reference commonly is to indolic acids and indoxyl, as indole itself rarely appears in the urine.

indolyl (in'dō-lil). The radical of indole.

indomethacin (in-dō-meth'ă-sin). 1-(*p*-Chlorobenzoyl)-5-methoxy-2-methylindole-3-acetic acid; an analgesic, antipyretic, and anti-inflammatory nonsteroidal agent used in the management of rheumatoid arthritis and in the treatment of osteoarthritis, ankylosing spondylitis, and gout.

indophenolase (in-dō-fē'nol-ās). Cytochrome *c* oxidase.

indophenol oxidase (in-dō-fē'nol). Cytochrome *c* oxidase.

indoprofen (in-do-prō'fen). *p*-(1-Oxo-2-isoindolinyl)hydratropic acid; a nonsteroidal anti-inflammatory agent with analgesic and antipyretic properties.

indoxyl (in-dok'sil). The radical of 3-hydroxyindole; a product of intestinal bacterial degradation of indoleacetic acid, excreted in the urine as indoleaceturic acid (conjugated with glycine), as a sulfate (urinary indican), or as a glucuronide (glucosiduronate); increased amounts are excreted in phenylketonuria.

indoxyluria (in-dok-sil-yū'rē-ă). The excretion of indoxyl, especially indoxyl sulfate, in the urine; i. may be associated with indicanuria, inasmuch as hydrolysis of indican results in formation of indoxyl.

induce (in-dūs'). To cause or bring about. See induction.

inducer (in-dūs'er). A molecule, usually a substrate of a specific enzyme pathway, that combines with active repressor (produced by a regulator gene) to deactivate the repressor; this results in activation of a previously repressed operator gene and initiates activity of the structural genes controlled by the operator, which in turn results in enzyme production; a homeostatic mechanism for regulating enzyme production in an inducible enzyme system.

inductance (in-dŭk'tans) [see induction]. The coefficient of electromagnetic induction; the unit of inductance is the henry.

induction (in-dŭk'shŭn) [L. *inductio,* a leading in]. **1.** Production or causation. **2.** Production of an electric current or magnet in a body by electricity or magnetism in another body in close proximity to the first body. **3.** The period from the start of anesthesia to the establishment of a depth of anesthesia adequate for a surgical procedure. **4.** In embryology, the influence exerted by an organizer or evocator on the differentiation of adjacent cells or on the development of an embryonic structure. **5.** A modification imposed upon the offspring by the action of environment on the germ cells of one or both parents. **6.** In microbiology, the change from probacteriophage to vegetative phage that may occur spontaneously or after stimulation by certain physical and chemical agents. **7.** In enzymology, the process of increasing the amount or the activity of an enzyme. See also inducer. **8.** A stage in the process of hypnosis.

electromagnetic i., electromagnetic waves propagated by i. in an electromagnetic field.

lysogenic i., i. that occurs when prophage is transferred to a nonlysogenic bacterium by conjugation or by transduction.

spinal i., the manner in which one sensory stimulus lowers the threshold for another.

inductor (in-dŭk'ter, -tōr). **1.** That which brings about induction. **2.** In embryology, an evocator or an organizer.

inductorium (in-dŭk-tō'rē-ŭm). An instrument formerly used in physiologic experiments to generate pulses of induced electricity for stimulating nerve or muscle.

inductotherm (in-dŭk'tō-therm). The apparatus used in inductothermy.

inductothermy (in-dŭk'tō-ther-mē) [induction + G. *thermē,* heat]. Artificial fever production by means of electromagnetic induction.

indulin (in'dū-lin) [C.I. 50400-50415]. A blue quinone-imine dye related to nigrosin; occasionally used as a stain in histology and bacteriology.

indulinophil, indulinophile (in-dū-lin'ō-fil, -fīl) [indulin + G. *philos,* fond]. Taking an indulin stain readily.

indurated (in'dū-rāt-ed) [L. *in-duro,* pp. *-duratus,* to harden, fr. *durus,* hard]. Hardened, usually used with reference to soft tissues becoming extremely firm but not as hard as bone.

induration (in-dū-rā'shŭn) [L. *induratio* (see indurated)]. **1.** The process of becoming extremely firm or hard, or having such physical features. **2.** Scelrosis (1); a focus or region of indurated tissue.

brown i. of the lung, pigment i. of the lung; a condition characterized by firmness of the lungs, and a brown color associated with hemosiderin-pigmented macrophages in alveoli, consequent upon long-continued congestion due to heart disease.

cyanotic i., i. related to persistent, chronic venous congestion in an organ or tissue, frequently resulting in fibrous thickening of the walls of the veins and eventual fibrosis of adjacent tissue; the affected tissue becomes firmer than normal, and tends to have an unusual, red-blue color.

Froriep's i., *myositis* fibrosa.

gray i., a condition occurring in lungs during and after pneumonic processes in which there is failure of resolution; there is a conspicuous increase in fibrous connective tissue in the walls of the alveoli, and also within the alveoli (*i.e.*, fibrous organization of exudate); in contrast to brown i., there is usually not a prominent degree of pigmentation, unless chronic passive congestion is also present.

pigment i. of the lung, brown i. of the lung.

plastic i., sclerosis of corpus cavernosum of penis.

red i., a condition observed in lungs in which there is an advanced degree of acute passive congestion, or acute pneumonitis (sometimes termed interstitial pneumonia), or a similar pathologic process.

indurative (in'dū-rā-tiv). Pertaining to, causing, or characterized by induration.

indusium, pl. **indusia** (in-dū'zē-ŭm, -zē-ă) [L. a woman's undergarment, fr. *induo,* to put on]. **1.** A membranous layer or covering. **2.** The amnion.

i. gris'eum [NA], supracallosal gyrus; a thin layer of gray matter on the dorsal surface of the corpus callosum in which the striae longitudinalis medialis and lateralis (striae lancisi) lie embedded. The i. griseum is a rudimentary component of the hippocampus, continuous caudally around the splenium of the corpus callosum with the gyrus fasciolaris or fasciola cinerea, a slender convolution in turn continuous with the dentate gyrus or fascia dentata of the hippocampus; rostrally the i. griseum curves around the genu and rostrum corporis callosi, and extends ventralward to the olfactory trigone as the tenia tecta or rudimentum hippocampi, hidden in the depth of the sulcus parolfactorius posterior that marks the anterior border of the gyrus subcallosus or precommissural septum.

inebriant (in-ē'brē-ant) [see inebriety]. **1.** Making drunk; intoxicating. **2.** An intoxicant, such as alcohol.

inebriation (in-ē-brē-ā'shŭn) [see inebriety]. Intoxication, especially as by alcohol.

inebriety (in-ē-brī'ĕ-tē) [L. *in-* intensive + *ebrietas,* drunkenness]. Habitual indulgence in alcoholic beverages in excessive amounts.

inert (in-ert') [L. *iners,* unskillful, sluggish, fr. *in,* neg. + *ars,* art]. **1.** Slow in action; sluggish; inactive. **2.** Devoid of active chemical properties, as the inert gases. **3.** Denoting a drug or agent having no pharmacologic or therapeutic action.

inertia (in-er'shē-ă, in-er'shăh) [L. want of skill, laziness]. **1.** The tendency of a physical body to oppose any force tending to move it from a position of rest or to change its uniform motion. **2.** Denoting inactivity or lack of force, lack of mental or physical vigor, or sluggishness of thought or action.

magnetic i., hysteresis (2).

psychic i., a psychiatric term denoting resistance to any change in ideas or to progress; fixation of an idea.

uterine i., absence of effective uterine contractions during labor; **primary u. i., true u. i.,** u. i. that occurs when the uterus fails to contract with sufficient force to effect continuous dilation or effacement of the cervix or descent or rotation of the fetal head, and when the uterus is easily indentable at the acme of contraction; **secondary u. i.,** u. i. that occurs when the uterine contractions are vigorous but, as a result of the exhaustion or dehydration of the patient, decrease in vigor, and the progress of labor ceases.

in extremis (in eks-trē'mis) [L. *extremus,* last]. At the point of death.

infancy (in'fan-sē). Babyhood, the earliest period of extrauterine life; roughly, the first year of life.

in'fant [L. *infans,* not speaking]. A child under the age of 1 year; more specifically, a newborn baby.

i. Hercules, term applied to young children with precocious sexual and muscular development due to a virilizing adrenocortical disorder.

liveborn i., the product of a livebirth; an i. who shows evidence of life after birth; life is considered to be present after birth if any one of the following is observed: 1) if the infant breathes; 2) if the infant shows beating of the heart; 3) if pulsation of the umbilical cord occurs; or 4) if there is definite movement of voluntary muscles.

post-term i., an i. with a gestational age of 42 completed weeks or more (294 days or more).

preterm i., an i. with gestational age of less than 37 completed weeks (259 completed days).

stillborn i., an i. who shows no evidence of life after birth. *Cf.* liveborn i.

term i., an i. with gestational age of 37 completed weeks (259 completed days) to less than 42 completed weeks (less than 294 completed days).

infanticide (in-fan'ti-sīd) [infant + L. *caedo,* to kill]. **1.** The killing of an infant. **2.** One who murders an infant.

infantile (in'făn-tīl). **1.** Relating to, or characteristic of, infants or infancy. **2.** Denoting childish behavior.

infantilism (in-fan'ti-lizm). **1.** Infantile dwarfism; a state marked by extremely slow development of mind and body. **2.** Childishness, as in a temper tantrum by an adolescent or adult.

Brissaud's i., cretinism.

dysthyroidal i., cretinism.

hepatic i., delayed development as a result of liver disease.

hypothyroid i., cretinism.

idiopathic i., Lorain's disease; proportionate or universal i.; dwarfism generally associated with hypogonadism; may be caused by deficient secretion of anterior pituitary hormones.

Lorain-Lévi i., pituitary *dwarfism.*

myxedematous i., cretinism.

pancreatic i., i. associated with deficiency or absence of pancreatic secretion.

pituitary i., pituitary *dwarfism.*

proportionate i., idiopathic i.

renal i., renal *rickets.*

sexual i., failure to develop secondary sexual characteristics after the normal time of puberty.

static i., a condition observed in young children resembling spastic spinal paralysis; it is marked by hypotonia of the muscles of the trunk and hypertonia of the muscles of the extremities.

tubal i., a term descriptive of a corkscrew-like fallopian tube as seen in fetal life.

universal i., idiopathic i.

infarct (in'farkt) [L. *in-farcio,* pp. *-fartus* (*-ctus,* an incorrect form), to stuff into]. Infarction (2); an area of necrosis resulting from a sudden insufficiency of arterial or venous blood supply.

anemic i., white i. (1); pale i.; an i. in which little or no bleeding into tissue spaces occurs when the blood supply is obstructed.

bland i., an uninfected i.

bone i., an area of bone tissue that has become necrotic as a result of loss of its arterial blood supply.

Brewer's i.'s, dark-red, wedge-shaped areas resembling i.'s, seen on section of a kidney in pyelonephritis.

embolic i., an i. caused by an embolus.

hemorrhagic i., red i.; hemorrhagic gangrene (1); an i. red in color from infiltration of blood from collateral vessels into the necrotic area.

pale i., anemic i.

red i., hemorrhagic i.

septic i., an area of necrosis resulting from vascular obstruction due to emboli comprised of clumps of bacteria or infected material.

thrombotic i., an i. caused by a thrombus.

uric acid i., precipitates of uric acid distending renal collecting tubules in the newborn; since there is no necrosis, the term infarct is a misnomer.

white i., **(1)** anemic i.; **(2)** in the placenta, intervillous fibrin with ischemic necrosis of villi.

Zahn's i., a pseudoinfarct of the liver, consisting of an area of congestion with parenchymal atrophy but no necrosis; due to obstruction of a branch of the portal vein.

infarction (in-fark'shŭn). **1.** Sudden insufficiency of arterial or venous blood supply due to emboli, thrombi, vascular torsion, or pressure that produces a macroscopic area of necrosis; the heart, brain, spleen, kidney, intestine, lung, and testes are likely to be affected, as are tumors, especially of the ovary or uterus. **2.** Infarct.

anterior myocardial i., i. involving the anterior wall of the heart, and producing indicative electrocardiographic changes in the anterior chest leads.

anteroinferior myocardial i., i. involving both anterior and inferior walls of the heart simultaneously.

anterolateral myocardial i., extensive anterior i. producing indicative changes across the precordium as well as in leads I and aVL.

anteroseptal myocardial i., an anterior i. in which indicative electrocardiographic changes are confined to the right chest leads (V_1-V_4).

cardiac i., myocardial i.

diaphragmatic myocardial i., inferior myocardial i.

inferior myocardial i., diaphragmatic myocardial i.; i. in which the inferior or diaphragmatic wall of the heart is involved, produc-

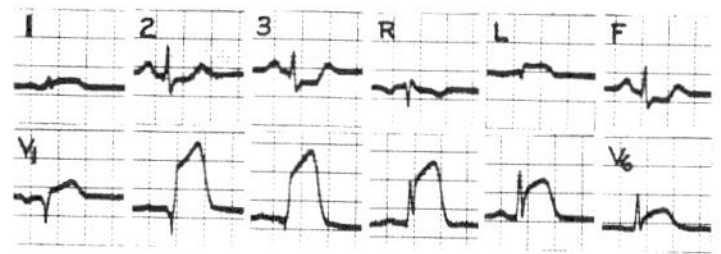

Acute Anterolateral Myocardial Infarction

ing indicative changes in leads II, III, and aVF in the electrocardiogram.
inferolateral myocardial i., i. involving the inferior and lateral surfaces of the heart and producing indicative changes in the electrocardiogram in leads II, III, aVF, V5, and V6.
lateral myocardial i., i. involving only the lateral wall of the heart, producing indicative electrocardiographic changes confined to leads I, aVL, V5, and V6.
myocardial i. (MI), cardiac i.; i. of an area of the heart muscle, usually as a result of occlusion of a coronary artery.
myocardial i. in H-form, i. involving the septum along with both inferior and anterior walls to make an H-shaped configuration.
nontransmural myocardial i. (NTMI), necrosis of heart muscle that fails to extend from the endocardium to the epicardium, often erroneously considered benign.
posterior myocardial i., i. involving the posterior wall of the heart; also formerly used of i.'s involving the inferior or diaphragmatic surface of the heart.
silent myocardial i., i. that produces none of the characteristic symptoms and signs of myocardial i.
subendocardial myocardial i., i. that involves only the layer of muscle subjacent to the endocardium.
through-and-through myocardial i., transmural myocardial i.
transmural myocardial i., through-and-through myocardial i.; i. that involves the whole thickness of the heart muscle from endocardium to epicardium.
watershed i., cortical i. in an area of blood supply between two major cerebral arteries.

infect (in-fekt') [L. *in- ficio,* pp. *-fectus,* to dip into, dye, corrupt, infect, fr. *in* + *facio,* to make]. **1.** To enter, invade, or inhabit another organism, causing infection or contamination. **2.** To dwell internally, endoparasitically, as opposed to externally (infest).

infection (in-fek'shŭn). Endoparasitism; multiplication of parasitic organisms within the body; multiplication of "normal" bacterial flora of the intestinal tract is not usually viewed as i.
agonal i., terminal i.
apical i., implantation of microorganisms at the apex of a tooth, usually the result of the migration of microorganisms from the pulp canal through the apical foramen.
cross i., i. spread from one source to another, person to person, animal to person, person to animal, animal to animal.
cryptogenic i., bacterial, viral, or other i., the source of which is unknown.
droplet i., i. acquired through the inhalation of droplets or aerosols of saliva or sputum containing virus or other microorganisms expelled by another person during sneezing, coughing, laughing, or talking.
endogenous i., i. caused by an infectious agent already present in the body, the previous i. having been inapparent.
focal i., an old term which distinguishes local i.'s (focal) from generalized i.'s (sepsis).
latent i., an asymptomatic i. capable of manifesting symptoms under particular circumstances or if activated.
mass i., i. resulting from the entrance of a large number of pathogens into the circulation or tissues.
mixed i., i. by more than one variety of pathogenic microorganisms.
pyogenic i., i. characterized by severe local inflammation, usually with pus formation, generally caused by one of the pyogenic bacteria.
scalp i., an i. external to the galea; *e.g.,* folliculitis or cellulitis.
secondary i., an i., usually septic, occurring in a person or animal already suffering from an i. of another nature.
terminal i., agonal i.; an acute i., commonly pneumonic or septic, occurring toward the end of any disease (usually chronic), and often the cause of death.
Vincent's i., necrotizing ulcerative *gingivitis.*
zoonotic i., an i. shared in nature by man with other species of vertebrate animals.

infection-immunity. See under immunity.

infectiosity (in-fek-shē-os'i-tē). Infectiousness.

infectious (in-fek'shŭs). **1.** Capable of being transmitted by infection, with or without actual contact. **2.** Infective. **3.** Denoting a disease due to the action of a microorganism.

infectiousness (in-fek'shŭs-nes). Infectivity; infectiosity; the state or quality of being infectious.

infective (in-fek'tiv). Infectious (2); producing or relating to an infection.

infectivity (in-fek-tiv'i-tē). Infectiousness.

infecundity (in-fē-kŭn'di-tē) [L. *infecunditas,* barrenness]. Female *sterility.*

inferior (in-fē'rē-ōr) [L. lower]. **1.** Situated below or directed downward. **2** [NA]. In human anatomy, situated nearer the soles of the feet in relation to a specific reference point; opposite of superior. **3.** Less useful or of poorer quality.

inferiority (in-fēr-ē-ōr'i-tē). The condition or state of being or feeling inadequate or inferior, especially to others similarly situated.

infertility (in-fer-til'i-tē) [L. *in-* neg. + *fertilis,* fruitful]. Relative sterility; diminished or absent fertility; does not imply (either in the male or the female) the existence of as positive or irreversible a condition as sterility.

infest (in-fest') [L. *infesto,* pp. *-atus,* to attack]. To occupy a site and dwell ectoparasitically on external surface tissue, as opposed to internally (infect).

infestation (in-fes-tā'shŭn). Ectoparasitism; the act or process of infesting.

infiltrate (in-fil'trāt) [L. *in* + Mediev. L. *filtro,* pp. *-atus,* to strain through felt, fr. *filtrum,* felt]. **1.** To perform or undergo infiltration. **2.** Infiltration (2).
Assmann's tuberculous i., infraclavicular i.
infraclavicular i., Assmann's tuberculous i.; an incipient lesion of tuberculous infection.

infiltration (in'fil-trā'shŭn). **1.** The act of permeating or penetrating into a substance, cell, or tissue; said of gases, fluids, or matter held in solution. **2.** Infiltrate (2); the gas, fluid, or dissolved matter that has entered any substance, cell, or tissue. **3.** Injection of solution into tissues, as in infiltration anesthesia. **4.** Extravasation of solutions intended for intravascular injection.
adipose i., growth of normal adult fat cells in sites where they are not usually present.
calcareous i., calcification.
cellular i., migration of cells from their sources of origin, or direct extension of cells as a result of unusual growth and multiplication, thereby resulting in fairly well-defined foci, irregular accumulations, or diffusely distributed individual cells in the connective tissue and interstices of various organs and tissues; used especially with reference to such changes associated with inflammations and certain types of malignant neoplasms.
epituberculous i., an i. superimposed upon a tuberculous lesion.
fatty i., abnormal accumulation of fat droplets in the cytoplasm of cells, particularly of fat derived from outside the cells. See also

fatty *degeneration.*
gelatinous i., gray i.
gray i., gelatinous i.; a term sometimes used for the relatively rapidly formed, semisolid, gray or gray-white exudate (chiefly necrotic cells and remnants of tissue, and macrophages) resulting from unusually acute, overwhelming, diffuse tuberculous infection in the lung.
lipomatous i., lipomatous hypertrophy; nonencapsulated adipose tissue forming a lipoma-like mass, usually in the cardiac interatrial septum where it may cause arrythmia and sudden death.
paraneural i., i. adjacent to or along a nerve.
perineural i., i. about a nerve.

infinity (in-fin'i-tē). Infinite *distance.*

infirm (in-ferm') [L. *in-firmus,* fr. *in-* neg. + *firmus,* strong]. Weak or feeble because of old age or disease.

infirmary (in-fer'mă-rē) [L. *infirmarium;* see infirm]. A clinic or small hospital, especially in a school or college.

infirmity (in-fer'mi-tē) [see infirm]. A weakness; an abnormal, more or less disabling, condition of mind or body.

inflammable (in-flam'ă-bl) [L. *in-,* intensive, + flamma, flame]. Flammable.

inflammation (in-flă-mā'shŭn) [L. *inflammo,* pp. *-atus,* fr. *in,* in, + *flamma,* flame]. A fundamental pathologic process consisting of a dynamic complex of cytologic and histologic reactions that occur in the affected blood vessels and adjacent tissues in response to an injury or abnormal stimulation caused by a physical, chemical, or biologic agent, including: 1) the local reactions and resulting morphologic changes, 2) the destruction or removal of the injurious material, 3) the responses that lead to repair and healing. The so-called "cardinal signs" of i. are: *rubor,* redness; *calor,* heat (or warmth); *tumor,* swelling; and *dolor,* pain; a fifth sign, *functio laesa,* inhibited or lost function, is sometimes added. All of the signs may be observed in certain instances, but no one of them is necessarily always present.
acute i., any i. that has a fairly rapid onset, quickly becomes severe, and has a relatively clear and distinct termination; usually manifested for only a few days, but may persist for several days or even a few weeks.
adhesive i., i. in which the amount of fibrin in the exudate is sufficient to result in a slight or moderate degree of adherence of adjacent tissues, as in healing by first intention.
allergic i., see allergic *reaction.*
alterative i., degenerative i.; a local reaction to injury, occasionally observed in the walls of blood vessels and in parenchymal cells of various organs in reacting to certain chemicals, viruses, and other intracellular agents; the response is characterized by degenerative changes in the cytoplasm and nucleus, frequently resulting in necrosis, but exudation (if any) is ordinarily observed only in the wall of the affected vessel, or in the interstices immediately adjacent to the affected vessel or parenchymal cells.
atrophic i., fibroid i.; a form of chronic i. or repeated episodes of acute i. in which the continued or recurrent proliferation of fibroblasts results in the formation of fibrous tissue that eventually contracts and leads to compression and atrophy of parenchymal tissue.
catarrhal i., an inflammatory process that is most frequent in the respiratory tract, but may occur in any mucous membrane, and is characterized by hyperemia of the mucosal vessels, edema of the interstitial tissue, enlargement of the secretory epithelial cells (which proliferate and form conspicuous globules of mucus), and an irregular layer of viscous, mucinous material on the surface; as exudation progresses, variable numbers of neutrophils migrate into the affected tissue and are included in the exudate, along with fragments of degenerated and necrotic epithelial cells; such an i. may frequently become mucopurulent.
chronic i., an i. that may begin with a relatively rapid onset or in a slow, insidious, and even unnoticed manner, tends to persist for several weeks, months or years, and has a vague and indefinite termination; results when the injuring agent (or products resulting from its presence) persists in the lesion, and the host's tissues respond in a manner (or to a degree) that is not sufficient to overcome completely the continuing effects of the injuring agent.
croupous i., an acute fibrinous i. in which a fairly tenacious pseudomembrane is formed in the larynx and frequently extends into the trachea and bronchi; the coagulated exudate may interfere with the passage of air and with the proper oxygenation of blood. See also pseudomembranous i.
degenerative i., alterative i.
exudative i., i. in which the conspicuous or distinguishing feature is an exudate, which may be chiefly serous, serofibrinous, fibrinous, or mucous (*i.e.,* relatively few cells are present), or may be characterized by relatively large numbers of neutrophils, eosinophils, lymphocytes, monocytes, or plasma cells, frequently with one or two types being predominant; it occurs not only as a separate and distinct pathologic process, but also frequently as a part of certain granulomatous i.'s.
fibrinopurulent i., a purulent i. in which the exudate contains an unusually large amount of fibrin; also, a fibrinous or serofibrinous i. in which the accumulation of large numbers of polymorphonuclear leukocytes results in liquefactive necrosis of tissue and the formation of pus with a relatively large quantity of fibrin.
fibrinous i., an exudative i. in which there is a disproportionately large amount of fibrin.
fibroid i., atrophic i.
granulomatous i., a form of proliferative i. See also granuloma.
hyperplastic i., proliferative i.
immune i., see allergic *reaction.*
interstitial i., i. in which the inflammatory reaction occurs chiefly in the supportive fibrous connective tissue or stroma of an organ.
necrotic i., necrotizing i., usually an acute inflammatory reaction in which the predominant histologic change is fairly rapid necrosis that occurs diffusely or extensively in relatively large foci throughout the affected tissue, frequently with only little or no evidence of cells in the exudate.
productive i., a vague term ordinarily used with reference to proliferative i., with or without an exudate; also sometimes used to indicate any i. in which grossly visible exudate is formed.
proliferative i., hyperplastic i.; an inflammatory reaction in which the distinguishing feature is an actual increase in the number of tissue cells, especially the reticuloendothelial macrophages, in contrast to cells exuded from blood vessels; in addition, exudates of various types are likely to be observed in granulomas and other forms of proliferative i., but the latter may occur without an exudate being formed (as in certain infections caused by virus).
pseudomembranous i., a form of exudative i. that involves mucous and serous membranes; relatively large quantities of fibrin in the exudate result in a rather tenacious membrane-like covering that is fairly adherent to the underlying acutely inflamed tissue; the pseudomembrane usually contains (in addition to the dense network of fibrin) varying quantities of plasma protein, degenerated and necrotic elements from the affected tissue, polymorphonuclear leukocytes, bacteria, etc.
purulent i., suppurative i.; an acute exudative i. in which the accumulation of polymorphonuclear leukocytes is sufficiently great that their enzymes cause liquefaction of the affected tissues, focally or diffusely; the purulent exudate is frequently termed pus, and consists of plasma and its constituents, end products of the enzymatic digestion of tissue, degenerated and necrotic cells and their debris, polymorphonuclear leukocytes and other white blood cells, the causal agent of the i., etc.
sclerosing i., i. leading to extensive formation of fibrous and scar tissue.

serofibrinous i., i. in which the exudate consists chiefly of serous fluid with an unusually large proportion of fibrin.

serous i., an exudative i. in which the exudate is predominantly fluid (*i.e.*, exuded from the blood vessels), with the protein, electrolytes, and other material contained therein; relatively few (if any) cells are observed.

subacute i., an i. that is intermediate in duration between that of an acute i. and that of a chronic i., usually persisting longer than 3 or 4 weeks.

suppurative i., purulent i.

inflammatory (in-flam'ă-tōr-ē). Pertaining to, characterized by, resulting from, or becoming affected by inflammation.

inflation (in-flā'shŭn) [L. *inflatio,* fr. *in-flo,* pp. *-flatus,* to blow into, inflate]. Vesiculation (2); distention by a fluid or gas.

inflator (in-flā'ter, -tŏr). An instrument for injecting air.

inflection, inflexion (in-flek'shŭn) [L. *in-flecto,* pp. *-flexus,* to bend]. **1.** An inward bending. **2.** Obsolete term for diffraction.

influenza (in-flū-en'ză) [It. fr. L. *in-fluo,* pr. p. *influens*] Grippe; grip; flu; an acute infectious respiratory disease, caused by orthomyxoviruses, in which the inhaled virus attacks the respiratory epithelial cells of susceptible persons and produces a catarrhal inflammation; characterized by sudden onset, chills, fever of short duration (3 days), severe prostration, headache, muscle aches, and a cough which is usually dry until secondary infection occurs. The disease commonly occurs in epidemics, sometimes in pandemics, which develop quickly and spread rapidly; mortality rate is normally low, but may be high in cases with secondary bacterial pneumonia, particularly in the elderly and those with underlying debilitating diseases; strain-specific immunity develops, but mutations in the virus are frequent and the immunity usually does not affect new, antigenically different strains.

i. A, i. caused by strains of influenza virus type A; the infections occur in epidemics which vary in size and severity; perhaps the most important of the three types of i. (A, B, and C).

Asian i., a worldwide i., apparently originating in China in the summer of 1957, which produces a much milder disease than that of the pandemic of 1917–1919.

avian i., fowl *plague.*

i. B, i. caused by strains of influenza virus type B; outbreaks are usually more limited than those due to influenza virus type A, although infections by the two types are clinically indistinguishable; occasionally associated with Reye's syndrome.

i. C, i. caused by strains of type C influenza virus; the disease is milder than that caused by types A and B, and has become uncommon in recent years.

endemic i., i. nostras; i., usually of a less severe type, occurring with some degree of regularity during the cold season, especially in the larger cities of the world.

equine i., a highly contagious upper respiratory infection of horses and other equids caused by equine strains of influenza virus type A; characterized by fever and respiratory signs similar to but more severe than those of equine rhinopneumonitis; edema of the lower trunk and limbs (epizootic cellulitis) may occur; the disease is frequently fatal when secondary bacterial pneumonia intervenes.

Hong Kong i., influenza caused by a serotype of influenza virus type A and first identified in Hong Kong.

i. nos'tras, endemic i.

Spanish i., i. which caused several waves of pandemic in 1918–1919, resulting in over 20 million deaths worldwide; it was particularly severe in Spain (hence the name), but now is thought to have originated in the U.S. as a form of swine i.

swine i., an acute respiratory disease of swine caused by strains of influenza virus type A; it is believed to have become adapted to swine in the United States during the great human pandemic in 1918; fatal cases, as in such cases of pandemic i. in man, are commonly associated with secondary bacterial pneumonia.

influenzal (in-flū-en'zăl). Relating to, marked by, or resulting from, influenza.

Influenzavirus (in-flū-en'ză-vī-rŭs). The genus of Orthomyxoviridae that comprises the influenza viruses types A and B. Each type of virus has a stable nucleoprotein group antigen common to all strains of the type, but distinct from that of the other type; each also has a mosaic of surface antigens (hemagglutinin and neuraminidase) which characterize the strains and which are subject to variations of two kinds: 1) a rather continual shift that occurs independently within the groups of hemagglutinin and neuraminidase antigens; 2) after a period of years, a sudden shift (notably in type A virus of human origin) to a different group of hemagglutinin and neuraminidase antigens. The sudden major shifts are the basis of subdivisions of type A virus of human origin. Strain notations indicate type, geographic origin, year of isolation, and, in the case of type A strains, the characterizing subtypes of hemagglutinin and neuraminidase antigens (*e.g.,* A/Hong Kong/1/68 (H_3 N_2); B/Hong Kong/5/72).

infold (in-fōld'). To inclose within a fold, as in "infolding" an ulcer of the stomach, in which the walls on either side of the lesion are brought together and sutured.

informed consent. A form of agreement, usually in writing, by a patient or his legal representative to a course of medical or surgical management suggested by a physician or surgeon; based upon a full and complete discussion between patient and physician or surgeon of the potential benefits, risks, and complications of the proposed course of management, as well as a discussion of alternative courses of management.

informosomes (in-fōr'mō-sōmz). Name suggested for the bodies composed of messenger (informational) RNA and protein that are found in the cytoplasm of animal cells.

infra- [L. below]. Prefix denoting a position below the part denoted by the word to which it is joined.

infra-axillary (in'fră-ak'si-lār-ē). Subaxillary.

infrabulge (in'fră-bŭlj). **1.** That portion of the crown of a tooth gingival to the height of contour. **2.** That area of a tooth where the retentive portion of a clasp of a removable partial denture is placed.

infracardiac (in'fră-kar'dē-ak). Beneath the heart; below the level of the heart.

infracerebral (in'fră-ser'e-brăl). Pertaining to that portion of the nervous system below the level of the cerebrum.

infraclavicular (in'fră-kla-vik'yū-lăr). Subclavian (1).

infraclusion (in-fră-klū'zhŭn). Infraocclusion; infraversion (3); the state wherein a tooth has failed to erupt to the maxillomandibular plane of interdigitation.

infracortical (in-fră-kōr'ti-kăl). Beneath the cortex of an organ, mainly the brain or kidney. See subcortical.

infracostal (in-fră-kos'tăl). Subcostal (1).

infracotyloid (in-fră-kot'i-loyd). Below the acetabulum or cotyloid cavity.

infracristal (in-fră-kris'tăl) [infra- + L. *crista,* crest]. Below the supraventricular crest; usually used in reference to ventricular septal defect.

infraction (in-frak'shŭn) [L. *infractio,* a breaking, fr. *infringere,* to break]. Infracture; a fracture; especially one without displacement.

infracture (in-frak'chūr). Infraction.

infradentale (in'fră-den-tă'lē). Lower alveolar point; in craniometrics, the apex of the septum between the mandibular central incisors.

infradian (in-frā'dē-ăn) [infra- + L. *dies,* day]. Relating to biologic variations or rhythms occurring in cycles less frequent than every 24 hours. *Cf.* circadian; ultradian.

infradiaphragmatic (in'fră-dī'ă-frag-mat'ik). Subdiaphragmatic.

infraduction (in-fră-dŭk'shŭn). Deorsumduction.

infraglenoid (in'fră-glē'noyd). Subglenoid, inferior to the glenoid cavity of the scapula.

infraglottic (in-fră-glot'ik). Subglottic; inferior to the glottis.

infrahepatic (in-fră-he-pat'ik). Subhepatic.

infrahyoid (in'fră-hī'oyd). Subhyoid; subhyoidean; below the hyoid bone; denoting especially a group of muscles: the sternohyoideus, sternothyroideus, thyrohyoideus, and omohyoideus.

inframammary (in-fră-mam'ă-rē). Submammary (2); inferior to the mammary gland.

inframamillary (in-fră-mam'ĭ-lăr-ē). Relating to that which is situated below a nipple.

inframandibular (in-fră-man-dib'yū-lăr). Submandibular.

inframarginal (in-fră-mar'ji-năl). Below any margin or edge.

inframaxillary (in-fră-mak'si-lă-rē). Mandibular.

infranatant (in'fră-nā'tănt) [infra- + L. *natare*, to swim]. See infranatant *fluid*.

infraocclusion (in'fră-ō-klū'zhŭn). Infraclusion.

infraorbital (in'fră-ōr'bi-tăl). Suborbital; below or beneath the orbit.

infrapatellar (in-fră-pa-tel'ăr). Subpatellar (2); inferior to the patella; denoting especially a bursa, a pad of fat, or a synovial fold.

infrapsychic (in-fră-sī'kik). Denoting ideas or actions originating below the level of consciousness.

infrared (in'fră-red). That portion of the electromagnetic spectrum with wavelengths between 770 and 1000 nm.

infrascapular (in-fră-skap'yū-lăr). Subscapular (2); inferior to the scapula.

infrasonic (in'fră-son'ik) [infra- + L. *sonus*, sound]. Denoting those frequencies that lie below the range of human hearing.

infraspinatus (in-fră-spī-nā'tŭs). See under musculus.

infraspinous (in-fră-spī'nŭs). Subspinous; below a spine or spinous process; specifically, the fossa infraspinata.

infrasplenic (in'fră-splen'ik, -sple'nik). Beneath or below the spleen.

infrasternal (in-fră-ster'năl). Substernal (2); inferior to the sternum.

infrasubspecific (in'fră-sŭb-spe-si'fik). Denoting a category of organisms of rank lower than subspecies.

infratemporal (in-fră-tem'pō-răl). Below the temporal fossa.

infrathoracic (in'fră-thō-ras'ik). Below or at the lower portion of the thorax.

infratonsillar (in-fră-ton'si-lăr). Below the palatine tonsil or cerebellar tonsil.

infratrochlear (in'fră-trok'lē-ăr). Inferior to the trochlea or pulley of the superior oblique muscle of the eye.

infraumbilical (in'fră-ŭm-bil'i-kăl). Subumbilical; inferior to the umbilicus.

infraversion (in'fră-ver'shŭn). **1.** A turning (version) downward. **2.** In physiological optics, rotation of both eyes downward. **3.** Infraclusion.

infriction (in-frik'shŭn) [L. *in*, on, + *frictio*, a rubbing]. The application of liniments or ointments combined with friction.

infundibula (in-fŭn-dib'yū-lă). Plural of infundibulum.

infundibular (in-fŭn-dib'yū-lăr). Relating to an infundibulum.

infundibulectomy (in'fŭn-dib'yū-lek'tō-mē) [infundibulum + G. *ektomē*, excision]. Excision of the infundibulum, especially of hypertrophied myocardium encroaching on the ventricular outflow tract.

infundibuliform (in-fŭn-dib'yū-li-fōrm) [L. *infundibulum*, funnel, + *forma*, form]. Choanoid.

infundibulin (in-fŭn-dib'yū-lin). A 20% solution of an extract of the posterior lobe of the hypophysis cerebri.

infundibulofolliculitis (in-fŭn-dib'yū-lō-fo-lik'yū-lī'tis). Inflammation of the follicular infundibulum, the superficial part of the hair follicle above the opening of the sebaceous gland.

disseminated recurrent i., a pruritic papular follicular eruption of the trunk and proximal extremities; usually occurs in blacks.

infundibuloma (in-fŭn-dib'yū-lō'mă) [infundibulum + G. *-oma*, tumor]. A piloid astrocytoma arising in tissues adjacent to the third ventricle of the cerebrum.

infundibulo-ovarian (in-fŭn-dib'yū-lō-ō-vā'rē-an). Relating to the fimbriated extremity of a uterine tube and the ovary.

infundibulopelvic (in-fŭn-dib'yū-lō-pel'vik). Relating to any two structures called infundibulum and pelvis, such as the expanded portion of a calyx and the pelvis of the kidney, or the fimbriated extremity of the uterine tube and the pelvis.

infundibulum, pl. **infundibula** (in-fŭn-dib'yū-lŭm, -yū-lă) [L. a funnel]. **1** [NA]. A funnel or funnel-shaped structure or passage. **2.** I. tubae uterinae. **3.** The expanding portion of a calix as it opens into the pelvis of the kidney. **4** [NA]. Official alternative name for *conus* arteriosus. **5.** Termination of a bronchiole in the alveolus. **6.** Termination of the cochlear canal beneath the cupola. **7** [NA]. The funnel-shaped, unpaired prominence of the base of the hypothalamus behind the optic chiasm, enclosing the infundibular recess of the third ventricle and continuous below with the stalk of the hypophysis. **8.** Mark (2); i. of teeth; the contact surface indentation in the incisor and cheek teeth of a horse.

ethmoid i., i. ethmoidale.

i. ethmoida'le [NA], ethmoid i.; a passage from the middle meatus of the nose communicating with the anterior ethmoidal cells and frontal sinus.

i. hypothal'ami [NA], hypothalamic i.; the apical portion of the tuber cinereum extending into the stalk of the hypophysis.

hypothalamic i., i. hypothalami.

i. of lungs, in the embryo, one of the expanded extremities of the subdivisions of the lung buds; in later development minute pouches (the air sacs) appear in its wall.

i. of teeth, i. (8).

i. tu'bae uteri'nae [NA], i. of the uterine tube; infundibulum (2); the funnel-like expansion of the abdominal extremity of the uterine (fallopian) tube.

i. of uterine tube, i. tubae uterinae.

infusible (in-fū'zi-bl). **1.** Incapable of being melted or fused. **2.** Capable of being made into an infusion.

infusion (in-fyū'zhŭn) [L. *infusio*, fr. *in-fundo*, pp. *-fusus*, to pour in]. **1.** The process of steeping a substance in water, either cold or hot (below the boiling point), in order to extract its soluble principles. **2.** A medicinal preparation obtained by steeping the crude drug in water. **3.** The introduction of fluid other than blood, *e.g.*, saline solution, into a vein.

infusodecoction (in-fyū'zō-dē-kok'shŭn). **1.** Infusion followed by decoction. **2.** A medicinal preparation made by steeping the crude drug first in cold water and then in boiling water.

Infusoria (in-fyūsō'rē-ă) [a Mod. L. use of the pl. of L. *infusorium*, a vessel for lamp oil, fr. *in-fundo*, to pour in]. Archaic term for Ciliaphora.

infusorian (in-fyū-sō'rē-an). Archaic term for a member of the class Infusoria, now the phylum Ciliophora.

ingesta (in-jes'tă) [pl. of L. *ingestum*, ntr. pp. of *in- gero*, *-gestus*, to carry in]. Solid or liquid nutrients taken into the body.

ingestion (in-jes'chŭn) [L. *ingestio*, a pouring in]. **1.** Introduction of food and drink into the stomach. **2.** Incorporation of particles into the cytoplasm of a phagocytic cell by invagination of a portion of the cell membrane as a vacuole.

ingestive (in-jes'tiv). Relating to ingestion.

Ingrassia, Giovanni F., Italian anatomist, 1510–1580. See I.'s *apophysis, wing.*

ingravescent (in-gră-ves'ent) [L. *ingravesco,* to grow heavier, fr. *gravis,* heavy]. Increasing in severity.

inguen (ing'gwen) [L.]. *Regio* inguinalis.

inguinal (ing'gwi-năl). Relating to the groin.

inguinocrural (ing'gwi-nō-krū'răl). Relating to the groin and the thigh.

inguinodynia (ing'gwi-nō-din'ē-ă) [L. *inguen (inguin-),* groin, + G. *odynē,* pain]. Pain in the groin.

inguinolabial (ing'gwi-nō-lā'bē-ăl). Relating to the groin and the labium.

inguinoperitoneal (ing'gwi-nō-per'i-tō-nē'ăl). Relating to the groin and the peritoneum.

inguinoscrotal (ing'gwi-nō-skrō'tăl). Relating to the groin and the scrotum.

inhalant (in-hā'lant) [see inhalation]. **1.** That which is inhaled; a remedy given by inhalation. **2.** A drug (or combination of drugs) with high vapor pressure, carried by an air current into the nasal passage, where it produces its effect. **3.** Insufflation (2); group of products consisting of finely powdered or liquid drugs that are carried to the respiratory passages by the use of special devices such as low pressure aerosol containers. See also inhalation; aerosol.

inhalation (in-hă-lā'shŭn) [L. *in-halo,* pp. *-halatus,* to breathe at or in]. **1.** Inspiration; the act of drawing in the breath. **2.** Drawing a medicated vapor in with the breath. **3.** A solution of a drug or combination of drugs for administration as a nebulized mist intended to reach the respiratory tree.

solvent i., i. of volatile organic solvents used in glue, nail polish remover, lacquer thinners, cleaning fluid, lighter fluid, and gasoline, for the purpose of self-intoxication. See also glue-sniffing.

inhale (in-hāl'). Inspire; to draw in the breath.

inhaler (in-hāl'er). **1.** Respirator (1). **2.** An apparatus for administering pharmacologically active agents by inhalation.

inherent (in-her'ent) [L. *inhaerens,* sticking to, adhering]. Occurring as a natural part or consequence.

inheritance (in-her'i-tans) [L. *heredito,* inherit, fr. *heres (hered-),* an heir]. **1.** Characters or qualities that are transmitted from parent to offspring. **2.** That which is inherited. **3.** The act of inheriting.

alternative i., **(1)** mendelian i. **(2)** Galton's term for an assumed form in which all the characters are derived from one parent.

blending i., Galton's term for that form in which the maternal and paternal characters appear to blend in the offspring.

codominant i., i. in which two alleles are individually expressed in the presence of the other; there may be other alleles at the locus that may or may not exhibit codominance.

collateral i., the appearance of characters in collateral members of a family group, as when an uncle and a niece show the same character inherited from a common ancestor; it occurs with recessive characters appearing irregularly, in contrast to dominant characters transmitted directly from one generation to the next.

cytoplasmic i., extranuclear i.; transmission of characters dependent on self-perpetuating elements not nuclear in origin.

dominant i., see *dominance* of genes.

extrachromosomal i., transmission of characters dependent on some factor not connected with the chromosomes.

extranuclear i., cytoplasmic i.

galtonian i., polygenic i.; i. in accordance with the principles of Galton's law and galtonian genetics.

holandric i., Y-linked i.

hologynic i., transmission of a trait from mother to all daughters and no sons, attributed to attached (partially fused) X chromosomes, to cytoplasmic i., or to sex limitation with abnormal segregation.

homochronous i., i. of characters that appear in the offspring at the same age as they appeared in the parent.

maternal i., transmission of characters that are dependent on peculiarities of the egg cytoplasm produced, in turn, by nuclear genes.

mendelian i., alternative i.; i. in which some characters are derived from one parent, others from the other parent; controlled entirely or overwhelmingly by a single genetic locus. See Mendel's law (*law* of segregation; *law* of independent assortment).

mosaic i., i. in which the paternal influence is dominant in one group of cells and the maternal in another.

multifactorial i., i. involving many factors, of which at least one is genetic but none is of overwhelming importance, as in the causation of a disease by multiple genetic and environmental factors.

polygenic i., galtonian i.

recessive i., see *dominance of genes.*

sex-influenced i., i. that is autosomal but has a different intensity of expression in the two sexes, *e.g.,* male pattern baldness.

sex-limited i., i. of a trait that can be expressed in one sex only, *e.g.,* hemophilia A.

sex-linked i., the pattern of inheritance that may result from a mutant gene located on either the X or Y chromosome.

X-linked i., the pattern of i. that may result from a mutant gene located on an X chromosome.

Y-linked i., holandric i.; the pattern of i. that may result from a mutant gene located on a Y chromosome.

inherited (in-her'it-ed). Inborn.

inhibin (in-hib'in). Name proposed for a postulated nonsteroidal polar substance of testicular origin that depresses the gonadotropic activity of the pituitary gland.

inhibit (in-hib'it). To curb or restrain.

inhibitine (in-hib'i-tēn). Carnosine.

inhibition (in-hi-bish'ŭn) [L. *in-hibeo,* pp. *-hibitus,* to keep back, fr. *habeo,* to have]. **1.** Depression or arrest of a function. **2.** In psychoanalysis, the restraining of instinctual or unconscious drives or tendencies, especially if they conflict with one's conscience or with societal demands. **3.** In psychology, a generic term for a variety of processes associated with the gradual attenuation, masking, and extinction of a previously conditioned response.

allogeneic i., i. of allogeneic cells that occurs when they are cultured after having been mixed together with added phytohemagglutinin (which causes the cells to adhere to each other); plaques develop in which cell growth is inhibited, seemingly because allogeneic cells in contact cause death of each other.

central i., suppression or diminution of outgoing impulses from a reflex center.

competitive i., selective i.; blocking of the action of an enzyme on its substrate by replacing the latter with a similar but inactive compound, one capable of combining with the active site of the enzyme but not being acted upon or split by it.

contact i., cessation of replication of dividing cells which come into contact, as in the center of a healing wound.

feedback i., i. of activity by an end product of the action; *e.g.,* thyroliberin stimulates thyroglobulin production, and thyroglobulin decreases thyrotropin formation.

hapten i. of precipitation, i. of precipitation that occurs when the precipitin has combined with hapten of the same specificity as the subsequently added antigen.

hemagglutination i., i. of nonimmune hemagglutination by antibody specific for the nonspecific hemagglutinin; *e.g.,* viral hemagglutination will not occur if antibody specific for the virus is added before addition of red blood cells. The i. is specific and is widely used for virus identification and for antibody determination.

noncompetitive i., a type of enzyme i. in which the inhibiting compound does not compete with the natural substrate for the active site on the enzyme, but inhibits reaction by combining with the enzyme-substrate complex, once the latter has been formed.
potassium i., arrest of the heart in the fully relaxed state as a result of potassium intoxication.
proactive i., a type of interference or negative transfer, observed in memory experiments and other learning situations, when something learned previously interferes with present learning or recall. *Cf.* retroactive i.
reciprocal i., **(1)** reciprocal *innervation;* **(2)** systematic *desensitization.*
reflex i., a situation in which sensory stimuli decrease reflex activity.
residual i., the i. or suppression of tinnitus by use of a sound-generating device (residual inhibitor) which masks the sounds of tinnitus and produces residual sound-inhibiting effect when the device is turned off.
retroactive i., the partial or complete obliteration of memory by a more recent event, particularly new learning. *Cf.* proactive i.
selective i., competitive i.
Wedensky i., i. of muscle response resulting from application of a series of rapidly repeated stimuli to the motor nerve where slower frequency of stimulation results in muscle response.

inhibitor (in-hib'i-ter, -tōr). **1.** An agent that restrains or retards physiologic, chemical, or enzymatic action. **2.** A nerve, stimulation of which represses activity.
angiotensin converting enzyme i. (ACEI), a class of drugs used in the treatment of hypertension; they produce a reduction of peripheral arterial resistance, although the exact mechanism of action has not been fully determined.
C1 esterase i., an α_2-neuraminoglycoprotein that inhibits the enzymatic activity of C̄1 esterase, the activated first component of complement.
carbonate dehydratase i., carbonic anhydrase i.; an agent, usually chemically related to the sulfonamides, that inhibits the activity of carbonate dehydratase, producing a general decrease in the formation of H_2CO_3 in the tissues. See also acetazolamide; dichlorphenamide.
carbonic anhydrase i., carbonate dehydratase i.
cholinesterase i., a drug, such as neostigmine, which, by inhibiting biodegradation of acetylcholine, restores myoneural function in myasthenia gravis or after nondepolarizing neuromuscular relaxants have been administered.
human α_1 proteinase i. (α_1PI), α-1-*antitrypsin.*
monoamine oxidase i. (MAOI), any of the hydrazine ($-NHNH_2$) and hydrazide ($-CONHNH_2$) derivatives that inhibit several enzymes and raise the brain norepinephrine and 5-hydroxytryptamine levels; used as antidepressant and hypotensive agents.
residual i., a sound-generating device, worn in the ear, which inhibits or suppresses the sounds of tinnitus by masking, with residual inhibitory effect when the device is turned off.
trypsin i., **(1)** a peptide hydrolyzed off trypsinogen under the catalytic influence of enteropeptidase, with trypsin produced as a result; so called because the peptide masks or inhibits the active site of the trypsin molecule; **(2)** one of the polypeptides, from various sources (*e.g.,* human and bovine colostrum, soybeans, egg white), that inhibit the action of trypsin.
α_1-trypsin i., α-1-*antitrypsin.*

inhibitory (in-hib'i-tōr-ē). Restraining; tending to inhibit.

iniac (in'ē-ak). Inial; relating to the inion.

iniad (in'ē-ad) [L. *ad,* to]. In a direction toward the inion.

inial (in'ē-ăl). Iniac.

iniencephaly (in'ē-en-sef'ă-lē) [G. *inion,* back of the head, + *enkephalos,* brain]. Malformation consisting of a cranial defect at the occiput, with the brain exposed; often in combination with a cervical rachischisis and retroflexion.

inion (in'ē-on) [G. nape of the neck] [NA]. A point located on the external occipital protuberance at the intersection of the midline with a line drawn tangent to the uppermost convexity of the right and left superior nuchal lines.

iniopagus (in'ē-op'ă-gŭs) [inion + G. *pagos,* fixed]. *Craniopagus* occipitalis.

iniops (in'ē-ops) [inion + G. *ōps,* eye, face]. *Janiceps* asymmetrus.

initiation (i-ni-shē-ā'shŭn). The first stage of tumor induction by a carcinogen; subtle alteration of cells by exposure to a carcinogenic agent so that they are likely to form a tumor upon subsequent exposure to a promoting agent (promotion).

initis (in-ī'tis) [G. *is* (*in-*), fiber, + *-itis* , inflammation]. **1.** Inflammation of fibrous tissue. **2.** Myositis.

inject (in-jekt') [L. *injicio,* to throw in]. To introduce into the body; denoting a fluid forced into one of the cavities, beneath the skin, or into a blood vessel. See also injection.

injectable (in-jek'tă-bl). **1.** Capable of being injected into anything. **2.** Capable of receiving an injection.

injected (in-jek'ted). **1.** Denoting a fluid introduced into the body. **2.** Denoting blood vessels visibly distended with blood.

injection (in-jek'shŭn) [L. *injicio,* pp. *-jectus,* to throw]. **1.** Introduction of a medicinal substance or nutrient material into the subcutaneous cellular tissue (subcutaneous or hypodermic i.), the muscular tissue (intramuscular i.), a vein (intravenous i.), an artery (intraarterial i.), the rectum (rectal i. or enema), the vagina (vaginal i., or douche), the urethra, or other canals or cavities of the body. **2.** An injectable pharmaceutical preparation. **3.** Congestion or hyperemia.
depot i., an i. of a substance in a vehicle which tends to keep it at the site of i. so that absorption occurs over a prolonged period.
hypodermic i., hypodermic (2); the administration of a remedy in liquid form by i. into the subcutaneous connective tissues.
insulin i., regular insulin i.; a preparation that may contain 20, 40, 80, 100, or 500 USP insulin units per ml, although the trend is toward standardizing all insulin preparations at 100 units per ml; it is administered subcutaneously, occasionally intravenously, and has a rapid onset of action, has a brief duration (5 to 7 hours), and is compatible for mixing with long-acting insulin preparations; used in the treatment of diabetic acidosis and insulin coma.
intrathecal i., introduction of material for diffusion throughout the subarachnoid space by means of lumbar puncture.
intraventricular i., the introduction of materials for diffusion throughout the ventricular and subarachnoid space by means of ventricular puncture.
jet i., hypodermic i. of drugs by a jet injector.
lactated Ringer's i., a sterile solution of calcium chloride, potassium chloride, sodium chloride, and sodium lactate in water for injection; used intravenously as a systemic alkalizer and a fluid and electrolyte replenisher.
regular insulin i., insulin i.
Ringer's i., a sterile solution of sodium chloride, potassium chloride, and calcium chloride, containing in each 100 ml between 820 and 900 mg of sodium chloride, between 25 and 35 mg of potassium chloride, and between 30 and 37 mg of calcium chloride; used intravenously as a fluid and electrolyte replenisher.
sensitizing i., an i. that sensitizes a person so that subsequent exposure to the antigen (allergen) evokes an allergic response.
Z-tract i., a technique in which the skin and subcutaneous tissue are displaced laterally before inserting the needle intramuscularly; used to prevent leakage along the track of the needle and consequent tissue irritation.

injector (in-jek'ter). A device for making injections.
jet i., an i. that utilizes high pressure to force a liquid through a

small orifice at a velocity sufficient to penetrate skin or mucous membrane without the use of a needle.

injure (in'jer). To wound, hurt, or harm.

injury (in'jer-ē) [L. *injuria,* fr. *in-* neg. + *jus (jur-),* right]. The damage or wound of trauma.
blast i., tearing of lung tissue or rupture of abdominal viscera without external i., as by the force of an explosion.
closed head i., a head i. in which continuity of the scalp and mucous membranes is maintained.
contrecoup i. of brain, an i. occurring beneath the skull opposite to the area of impact.
coup i. of brain, an i. occurring directly beneath the skull at the area of impact.
current of i., see under current.
degloving i., avulsion of the skin of the hand (or foot) in which the part is skeletonized by removal of most or all of the skin and subcutaneous tissue.
egg-white i., egg-white *syndrome.*
hyperextension-hyperflexion i., violence to the body causing the unsupported head to hyperextend and hyperflex the neck rapidly; does not imply any specific resultant trauma or pathology.
i. of intervertebral disk, see traumatic cervical *discopathy.*
open head i., a head i. in which there is a loss of continuity of scalp or mucous membranes; the term is sometimes used to indicate a communication between the exterior and the intracranial cavity. See also penetrating *wound.*
pneumatic tire i., separation of the skin and subcutaneous tissue from the underlying fascia occurring when an extremity is crushed and rolled over by the tire of a vehicle; may occur particularly in cases of obesity.
whiplash i., popular term for hyperextension-hyperflexion i.

inlay (in'lā). **1.** In dentistry, a prefabricated restoration sealed in the cavity with cement. **2.** A graft of bone into a bone cavity. **3.** A graft of skin into a wound cavity for epithelialization. **4.** In orthopedics, an orthomechanical device inserted into a shoe; commonly called an "arch support."
epithelial i., inlay *graft.*
gold i., a gold restoration fabricated by casting in a mold made from a wax pattern; the restoration is sealed in the prepared cavity with dental cement.
porcelain i., a fused porcelain restoration luted in a cavity prepared in a tooth.

in'let. A passage leading into a cavity.
pelvic i., *apertura* pelvis superior.

innate (i'nāt, i-nāt') [L. *in-nascor,* pp. *-natus,* to be born in, pp. as adj. inborn, innate]. Inborn.

innervation (in'er-vā'shŭn) [L. *in,* in, + *nervus,* nerve]. The supply of nerve fibers functionally connected with a part.
reciprocal i., reciprocal inhibition (1); contraction in a muscle is accompanied by a loss of tone or by relaxation in the antagonistic muscle.

innidiation (i-nid-ē-ā'shŭn) [L. *in,* in, + *nidus,* nest]. Colonization (1); indenization; the growth and multiplication of abnormal cells in another location to which they have been transported by means of lymph or the blood stream, or both. See also metastasis.

innocent (in'ō-sent) [L. *innocens (-ent-),* fr. *in,* neg., + *noceo,* to injure]. **1.** Not apparently harmful. **2.** Free from moral wrong.

innocuous (i-nok'yū-ŭs) [L. *innocuus*]. Innoxious; harmless.

innominatal (i-nom'i-nā-tăl). Relating to the hip bone.

innominate (i-nom'i-nāt) [L. *innominatus,* fr. *in-* neg. + *nomen (nomin-),* name]. Without a name; used to describe anatomic structures, *e.g.,* innominate artery or vein and, particularly, the innominate bone.

innoxious (i-nok'shŭs) [L. *in-noxius,* fr. *in,* neg. + *noceo,* to injure]. Innocuous.

Ino Symbol for inosine.

ino-, in- [G. *is (in-),* fiber]. Obsolete combining forms relating to fiber, or meaning fibrous; replaced in most terms by fibro-.

inoculability (i-nok'yū-lă-bil'i-tē). The quality of being inoculable.

inoculable (i-nok'yū-lă-bl). **1.** Transmissible by inoculation. **2.** Susceptible to a disease transmissible by inoculation.

inoculate (i-nok'yū-lāt) [L. *inoculo,* pp. *-atus,* to ingraft]. **1.** To introduce the agent of a disease or other antigenic material into the subcutaneous tissue or a blood vessel, or through an abraded or absorbing surface for preventive, curative, or experimental purposes. **2.** To implant microorganisms or infectious material into or upon culture media. **3.** To communicate a disease by transferring its virus.

inoculation (i-nok-yū-lā'shŭn). Introduction into the body of the causative organism of a disease.
stress i., in clinical psychology, an approach intended to provide patients with cognitive and attitudinal skills that they can use to cope with stress.

inoculum (i-nok'yū-lŭm). The microorganism or other material introduced by inoculation.

Inocybe (i-nō'sī-bē). A genus of mushrooms containing several species that have a high yield of muscarine.

inopectic (in-ō-pek'tik). Relating to inopexia.

inoperable (in-op'er-ă-bl). Denoting that which cannot be operated upon, or cannot be corrected or removed by an operation.

inorganic (in-ōr-gan'ik). **1.** Not organic; not formed by living organisms. **2.** See inorganic *compound.*

inosamine (in-ōs'ă-mēn). An inositol in which an —OH group is replaced by an $-NH_2$ group.

inoscopy (in-os'kō-pē) [ino- + G. *skopeō,* to look at]. The microscopic examination of biologic materials (*e.g.,* tissue, sputum, clotted blood, and so on) after dissecting or chemically digesting the fibrillary elements and strands of fibrin.

inosculate (in-os'kyū-lāt) [L. *in,* in, + *osculum,* dim. of *os,* mouth]. Anastomose.

inosculation (in'os-kyū-lā'shŭn). Anastomosis.

inose (in'ōs). Inositol.

inosemia (in-ō-sē'mē-ă) [inose + G. *haima,* blood]. **1.** The presence of inositol in the circulating blood. **2.** Fibremia.

inosinate (in-ō'si-nāt). A salt or ester of inosinic acid.

inosine (Ino) (in'ō-sēn). 9-β-D-Ribosylhypoxanthine; a nucleoside formed by the deamination of adenosine.

inosine pranobex (in'ō-sēn pran'ō-beks). A 1:3 molar complex of 1-dimethylamino-propan-2-ol-4-acetamidobenzoate and inosine, used as an antiviral agent.

inosinic acid (in-ō-sin'ik). Inosine phosphate; a mononucleotide found in muscle and other tissues.

inosinyl (in-ō'si-nil). The radical of inosinic acid.

inosite (in'ō-sīt). Inositol.

inositide (in-ō'si-tīd). Term sometimes used for phosphatidylinositol.

inositol (in-ō'si-tōl, -tol). Cyclohexitol; inose; inosite; lipositol; antialopecia or mouse antialopecia factor; hexahydroxycyclohexane; a member of the vitamin B complex necessary for growth of yeast and of mice; absence from the diet causes alopecia and dermatitis in mice and "spectacle eyes" in rats. It occurs in a number of stereoisomeric forms: *cis-, epi-, allo-. neo-, myo-, muco-, chiro-,* and *scyllo-* inositols; the most abundant naturally occurring one is *myo*-inositol (usually meant when "inositol" occurs alone).
i. niacinate, hexanicotinoyl inositol; a peripheral vasodilator.

***meso*-inositol.** **1.** Generic term for any isomer of i. in which the hydroxyl groups are so arranged that the molecule as a whole possesses a plane of symmetry and is optically inactive. **2.** Former name for *myo*-inositol.

***myo*-inositol.** 1,2,3,5/4,6-Inositol; a constituent of various phosphatidylinositols and the most widely distributed form of i. found in microorganisms, higher plants, and animals. In plants, it is found as phytic acid and as phytin; partially phosphorylated and free forms occur throughout nature, and in many tissues.

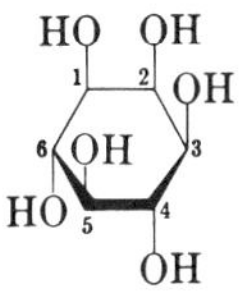

***myo*-Inositol**

inosituria (in′ō-sī-tū′rē-ă) [inositol + G. *ouron,* urine]. Inosuria (1); the excretion of inositol in the urine.

inosose (in′ōs-ōs). 2,3,4,5,6-Pentahydroxycyclohexanone; inositol in which the C-1 is a ketone rather than an alcohol.

inosuria (in-ō-sū′rē-a). **1.** Inosituria. **2.** The occurrence of fibrin in the urine.

inotropic (in-ō-trop′ik) [ino- + G. *tropos,* a turning]. Influencing the contractility of muscular tissue.

negatively i., weakening muscular action.

positively i., strengthening muscular action.

Inoviridae (i-nō-vir′i-dē). Provisional name for a family of filamentous bacterial viruses with a genome of single-stranded DNA (molecular weight 1.9 to 2.7 $\times$ 10^6). Coliphage fd, the type species of the fd phage group genus, adsorbs to the tips of pili of male enterobacteria and, after multiplication, particles are released without causing lysis of the host bacterium.

in phase. Moving in the same direction at the same time; a possible characteristic of two simultaneous oscillations of similar frequency.

inquest (in′kwest) [L. *in,* in, + *quaero,* pp. *quaisitus,* to seek]. A legal inquiry into the cause of sudden, violent, or mysterious death.

inquiline (in′kwi-līn, -lin) [L. *inquilinus,* an inhabitant of a place that is not his own, fr. *in,* in, + *colo,* to inhabit]. An animal that lives habitually in the abode of some other species (an oyster crab within the shell of an oyster) causing little or no inconvenience to the host. See also commensal.

insalivate (in-sal′i-vāt). To mix the food with saliva during mastication.

insalivation (in-sal-i-vā′shŭn). The mixing of the food with saliva.

insalubrious (in-să-lū′brē-ŭs) [L. *in-salubris,* unwholesome]. Unwholesome; unhealthful; usually in reference to climate.

insane (in-sān′) [L. *in-* neg. + *sanus,* sound, sane]. **1.** Of unsound mind; deranged; crazy. **2.** Relating to insanity.

insanitary (in-san′i-tār-ē) [L. *in-* neg. + *sanus,* sound]. Unsanitary; injurious to health, usually in reference to an unclean or contaminated environment.

insanity (in-san′i-tē) [L. *in-* neg. + *sanus,* sound]. **1.** An outmoded term comparable to severe mental illness or psychosis. **2.** In law, that degree of mental illness which negates the individual's legal responsibility or capacity.

basedowian i., obsolete term for a bipolar affective disorder of psychotic intensity occurring in thyrotoxicosis.

criminal i., in forensic psychiatry, a term that is defined by such legal precedents as the American Law Institute rule, Durham rule, M'Naghten rule, and New Hampshire rule (*q.v.* under rule).

inscriptio (in-skrip′shē-ō) [L. fr. *in-scribo,* pp. *-scriptus,* to write on]. Inscription.

i. tendin′ea, *intersectio* tendinea.

inscription (in-skrip′shŭn) [L. *inscriptio*]. Inscriptio. **1.** The main part of a prescription; that which indicates the drugs and the quantity of each to be used in the mixture. **2.** A mark, band, or line.

tendinous i., *intersectio* tendinea.

Insecta (in-sek′tă) [L. pl. of *insectus,* insect, fr. *in- seco,* pp. *-sectus,* to cut into]. Hexapoda; the insects, the largest class of the phylum Arthropoda and the largest major grouping of living things, chiefly characterized by flight, great adaptability, vast speciation in terrestrial and freshwater environments, and possession of three pairs of jointed legs and, usually, two pairs of wings. Some are parasitic, others serve as intermediate hosts for parasites, including those that cause many human diseases. Some are wingless; others, such as the Diptera, have only one pair of wings. Respiration is by tracheoles, cuticle-lined air tubes that pass air directly to the tissues. Development in higher forms is holometabolous and passes through distinctive egg, larval, pupal, and adult stages.

insectarium (in-sek-tā′rē-ŭm) [L.]. Place for keeping and breeding insects for scientific purposes.

insecticide (in-sek′ti-sīd) [insect + L. *caedō,* to kill]. An agent that kills insects.

insectifuge (in-sek′ti-fūj) [insect + L. *fugo,* to put to flight]. A substance that drives off insects.

Insectivora (in-sek-tiv′ō-ră) [insect + L. *voro,* to devour]. An order of small, plantigrade, placental mammals that are extremely active and often highly predaceous; they feed mostly on insects and small rodents, although the jes or potomogale of Africa feeds on fish. Eight living families include the solenodons of Cuba and Haiti, tenrecs of Madagascar, hedgehog of Europe and Asia, and shrews and moles of the U.S., Africa, and Asia.

insectivorous (in-sek-tiv′ō-rŭs) [insect + L. *voro,* to devour]. Insect-eating.

insecurity (in-sē-kyūr′i-tē). A feeling of unprotectedness and helplessness.

insemination (in-sem-i-nā′shŭn) [L. *in-semino,* pp. *-atus,* to sow or plant in, fr. *semen,* seed]. Semination; deposit of seminal fluid within the vagina, normally during coitus.

artificial i., the introduction of semen into the vagina other than by coitus.

heterologous i. (AID), artificial i. with semen from a donor who is not the woman's husband.

homologous i. (AIH), artificial i. with the husband's semen.

insenescence (in-sē-nes′ens) [L. *insenesco,* to begin to grow old]. The process of growing old.

insensible (in-sen′si-bl) [L. *in-sensibilis,* fr. *in,* neg. + *sentio,* pp. *sensus,* to feel]. **1.** Unconscious. **2.** Not appreciable by the senses.

insertion (in-ser′shŭn) [L. *insertio,* a planting in, fr. *inserto, -sertus,* to plant in]. **1.** A putting in. **2.** The attachment of a muscle to the more movable part of the skeleton, as distinguished from origin. **3.** In dentistry, the intraoral placing of a dental prosthesis. **4.** Intrusion of fragments of any size from molecular to cytogenetic into the normal genome.

parasol i., velamentous i.

velamentous i., parasol i.; a form of i. of the fetal blood vessels into the placenta, in which the vessels separate before reaching the placenta and develop toward it in a fold of amnion, somewhat like the ribs of an open parasol.

insheathed (in-shēthd′). Enclosed in a sheath or capsule.

insidious (in-sid′ē-ŭs) [L. *insidiosus,* cunning, fr. *insidioe* (pl.), an ambush]. Treacherous; stealthy; denoting a disease that progresses gradually with inapparent symptoms.

insight (in′sīt). Self-understanding as to the motives and reasons behind one's actions.

in situ (in sī'tū) [L. *in,* in, + *situs,* site]. In position, not extending beyond the focus or level of origin.

insolation (in-sō-lā'shŭn) [L. *insolare,* to place in the sun]. **1.** Exposure to the sun's rays. **2.** Sunstroke.

insoluble (in-sol'yū-bl). Not soluble.

insomnia (in-som'nē-ă) [L. fr. *in-* priv. + *somnus,* sleep]. Inability to sleep, in the absence of external impediments, such as noise, a bright light, etc., during the period when sleep should normally occur; may vary in degree from restlessness or disturbed slumber to a curtailment of the normal length of sleep or to absolute wakefulness.

insomniac (in-som'nē-ak). **1.** A sufferer from insomnia. **2.** Exhibiting, tending toward, or producing insomnia.

insorption (in-sōrp'shŭn) [L. *in,* in, + *sorbēre,* to suck]. Movement of substances from the lumen of the gut into the blood.

inspectionism (in-spek'shŭn-izm). Sexual pleasure from looking at genitals.

inspersion (in-sper'shŭn, -zhŭn) [L. *inspersio,* fr. *in-spergo,* pp. *-spersus,* to scatter upon, fr. *spargo,* to scatter]. Sprinkling with a fluid or a powder.

inspiration (in-spi-rā'shŭn) [L. *inspiratio,* fr. *in-spiro,* pp. *-atus,* to breathe in]. Inhalation (1).

crowing i., noisy breathing associated with respiratory obstruction, usually at the larynx.

inspiratory (in-spī'ră-tō-rē). Relating to or timed during inhalation.

inspire (in-spīr'). Inhale.

inspirometer (in-spiī-rom'ĕ-ter) [L. *in-spiro,* to breathe in, + G. *metron,* measure]. An instrument for measuring the force, frequency, or volume of inspirations.

inspissate (in-spis'āt). To perform or undergo inspissation.

inspissation (in-spi-sā'shŭn) [L. *in,* intensive, + *spisso,* pp. *-atus,* to thicken]. **1.** The act of thickening or condensing, as by evaporation or absorption of fluid. **2.** An increased thickening or diminished fluidity.

inspissator (in-spis'ă-tōr). An apparatus for evaporating fluids.

instability (in-stă-bil'i-tē). The state of being unstable, or lacking stability.

vertebral cervical i., excessive mobility of cervical vertebrae due to damage to ligaments. See also vertebral cervical *subluxation.*

instar (in'stahr) [L. form]. Any of the successive nymphal stages in the metamorphosis of hemimetabolous insects (simple or incomplete metamorphosis), or the stages of larval change by successive molts that characterize the holometabolous insects (complex or complete metamorphosis).

in'step. The arch, or highest part of the dorsum of the foot. See also tarsus.

instillation (in-sti-lā'shŭn) [L. *instillatio,* fr. *in-stillo,* pp. *-atus,* to pour in by drops, fr. *stilla,* a drop]. Dropping of a liquid on or into a part.

instillator (in'sti-lā-ter). Dropper; a device for performing instillation.

instinct (in'stinkt) [L. *instinctus,* impulse]. **1.** An enduring disposition or tendency of an organism to act in an organized and biologically adaptive manner characteristic of its species. **2.** The unreasoning impulse to perform some purposive action without an immediate consciousness of the end to which that action may lead. **3.** In psychoanalytic theory, the forces assumed to exist behind the tension caused by the needs of the id.

aggressive i., death i.

death i., aggressive i.; the i. of all living creatures toward self-destruction, death, or a return to the inorganic lifelessness from which they arose.

ego i.'s, self-preservative needs and self-love, as opposed to object love; drives that are primarily erotic.

herd i., social i.; tendency or inclination to band together with and share the customs of others of a group, and to conform to the opinions and adopt the views of the group.

life i., sexual i.; the i. of self-preservation and sexual procreation; the basic urge toward preservation of the species.

sexual i., life i.

social i., herd i.

instinctive, instinctual (in-stink'tiv, -stink'chū-ăl). Relating to instinct.

instrument (in'strū-ment) [L. *instrumentum*]. A tool or implement.

diamond cutting i.'s, in dentistry, cylinders, disks, and other cutting i.'s to which numerous small diamond pyramids have been held by a plating of metal.

Krueger i. stop, a mechanical device limiting the insertion of a root canal i. into a canal.

plugging i., plugger.

purse-string i., an intestinal clamp with jaws at an angle to the handle; when closed across the bowel, large grooved interdigitating serrations allow passage of a straight needle and suture through each side to form a purse-string suture, after which the clamp is removed.

Sabouraud-Noiré i., an obsolete device for measuring the quantity of x-rays by means of the change in color of a disk of barium platinocyanide which exposure to them produces; the unit used in this method is called teinte B, or tint B = erythema dose.

stereotactic i., stereotaxic i., an apparatus attached to the head, used to localize precisely an area in the brain by means of coordinates related to intracerebral structures.

test handle i., a root canal i. the handle of which is similar to a collet chuck and which can be secured in position on the root canal i. to adjust its effective length.

instrumentarium (in'strū-men-tār'ē-ŭm). A collection of instruments and other equipment for an operation or for a medical procedure.

instrumentation (in'strū-men-tā'shŭn). **1.** The use of instruments. **2.** In dentistry, the application of armamentarium in a restorative procedure.

insuccation (in'sŭ-kā'shŭn) [L. *insuco,* pp. *-atus,* to soak in, fr. *in,* in, + sucus, juice, sap (improp. *succ-*)]. Maceration or soaking, especially of a crude drug to prepare it for further pharmaceutical operation.

insudate (in'sū-dāt) [L. *in,* in, + *sudo,* pp. *-atus,* to sweat]. Fluid swelling within an arterial wall (ordinarily serous), differing from an exudate in that it does not come to lie extramurally.

insufficiency (in-sŭ-fish'en-sē) [L. *in-,* neg. + *sufficientia,* to suffice]. **1.** Lack of completeness of function or of power. **2.** Incompetence (1).

acute adrenocortical i., addisonian or adrenal crisis; Bernard-Sergent syndrome; severe adrenocortical i. when an intercurrent illness or trauma causes an increased demand for adrenocortical hormones in a patient with adrenal insufficiency due to disease or use of relatively large amounts of similar hormones as therapy; characterized by nausea, vomiting, hypotension, and frequently hyperthemia, hyponatremia, hyperkalemia, and hypoglycemia.

adrenocortical i., hypocorticoidism; loss, to varying degrees, of adrenocortical function.

aortic i., see valvular i.

cardiac i., heart *failure* (1).

chronic adrenocortical i., Addison's disease; adrenocortical i. usually as the result of idiopathic atrophy or destruction of both adrenal glands by tuberculosis, an autoimmune process, or other diseases; characterized by fatigue, decreased blood pressure, weight loss, increased melanin pigmentation of the skin and mucous membranes, anorexia, and nausea or vomiting; without appropriate replacement therapy, it can progress to acute adrenocortical i.

convergence i., that condition in which an esophoria or esotropia is more marked for far vision than for near vision.

coronary i., inadequate coronary circulation leading to anginal pain.

divergence i., that condition in which an exophoria or extropia is more marked for near vision than for far vision.

i. of eyelids, a condition in which the eyelids are closed only by conscious effort, and are not fully closed during sleep.

hepatic i., defective functional activity of the liver cells.

latent adrenocortical i., adrenocortical i. not clinically evident but which can become severe if a sudden stress, such as an intercurrent acute illness, develops.

mitral i., see valvular i.

muscular i., failure of any muscle to contract with its normal force, especially such failure of any of the eye muscles.

myocardial i., heart *failure* (1).

parathyroid i., hypoparathyroidism.

partial adrenocortical i., normal basal adrenocortical function with failure of adrenocortical reserve to respond to ACTH stimulation.

primary adrenocortical i., adrenocortical i. caused by disease, destruction, or surgical removal of the adrenal cortices.

pulmonary i., see valvular i.

pyloric i., patulousness of the pyloric outlet of the stomach, allowing regurgitation of duodenal contents into the stomach.

renal i., defective function of the kidneys, with accumulation of waste products (particularly nitrogenous) in the blood.

respiratory i., failure to adequately provide oxygen to the cells of the body and to remove excess carbon dioxide from them.

secondary adrenocortical i., adrenocortical i. caused by failure of ACTH secretion resulting from anterior pituitary disease, or by ACTH inhibition resulting from exogenous steroid therapy.

tricuspid i., see valvular i.

uterine i., atony of the uterine musculature.

valvular i., failure of the cardiac valves to close perfectly, thus allowing regurgitation of blood past the closed valve; named, according to the valve involved, aortic, mitral, pulmonary, or tricuspid i.

velopharyngeal i., anatomical or functional deficiency in the soft palate or superior constrictor muscle, resulting in the inability to achieve velopharyngeal closure.

venous i., inadequate drainage of venous blood from a part, resulting in edema or dermatosis.

insufflate (in-sŭf′lāt) [L. *in-sufflo,* to blow on or into]. To blow into; to blow a powder, aerosol, or vapor into a body cavity or into an airway.

insufflation (in-sŭf-lā′shŭn). **1.** The act or process of insufflating. **2.** Inhalant (3).

perirenal i., injection of air or carbon dioxide about the kidneys for roentgenographic visualization of the adrenal glands.

tubal i., Rubin *test.*

insufflator (in′sŭf-lā-ter). An instrument used in insufflation.

insula, gen. and pl. **insulae** (in′sū-lă, -lē) [L. island]. **1** [NA]. Insular cortex or area; island of Reil; an oval region of the cerebral cortex overlying the capsula extrema, lateral to the lenticular nucleus, buried in the depth of the fissura lateralis cerebri (sylvian fissure). **2.** Island. **3.** Any circumscribed body or patch on the skin.

Haller's i., Haller's annulus; a doubling of the thoracic duct for part of its course through the thorax.

insular (in′sū-lăr). Relating to any insula, especially the island of Reil.

insulate (in′sŭ-lāt) [L. *insulatus,* made like an island]. To prevent the passage of electric or radiant energy by the interposition of a nonconducting substance.

insulation (in-sŭ-lā′shŭn). **1.** The act of insulating. **2.** The nonconducting substance so used. **3.** The state of being insulated.

insulator (in′sŭ-lā-ter). A nonconducting substance used as insulation.

insulin (in′sŭ-lin). A peptide hormone, secreted by beta cells in the islets of Langerhans, that promotes glucose utilization, protein synthesis, and the formation and storage of neutral lipids; obtained from various animals and available in a variety of preparations, i. is used parenterally in the treatment of diabetes mellitus.

atypical i., an insulin-like material whose biological effects are not inhibited by i. antiserum; present in large amounts in the plasma of obese adult diabetics, but in low concentrations in juvenile and nonobese adult diabetics.

biphasic i., the specific antidiabetic principle of the pancreas of the ox in a solution of that from the pancreas of the pig.

globin zinc i., a sterile solution of i. modified by the addition of zinc chloride and globin; it contains 40 or 80 units per ml; duration of action is about 18 hours.

human i., a protein that has the normal structure of i. produced by the human pancreas, but is prepared by recombinant DNA techniques and by semisynthetic processes.

immunoreactive i. (IRI), that portion of i. in blood measured by immunochemical methods for the hormone; presumed to represent the free (unbound) and biologically active fraction of total blood i.

isophane i., NPH i.; a modified form of i. composed of i., protamine, and zinc; an intermediately acting preparation used for the treatment of diabetes mellitus.

lente i., insulin zinc *suspension.*

NPH i. [*N*eutral *P*rotamine *H*agedorn], isophane i.

protamine zinc i., i. modified by the addition of protamine and zinc chloride; it contains 40 or 80 units per ml.

semilente i., prompt insulin zinc *suspension.*

ultralente i., extended insulin zinc *suspension.*

insulinemia (in′sŭ-li-nē′mē-ă) [insulin + G. *haima,* blood]. Literally, insulin in the circulating blood; usually connotes abnormally large concentrations of insulin in the circulating blood.

insulinogenesis (in′sŭ-lin-ō-jen′ĕ-sis) [insulin + G. *genesis,* production]. Production of insulin.

insulinogenic, insulogenic (in′sŭ-lin-ō-jen′ik, in′sŭ-lō-jen′ik). Relating to insulinogenesis.

insulinoma (in′sŭ-li-nō′mă). Insuloma; an islet cell adenoma that secretes insulin.

insulitis (in′sŭ-lī′tis) [L. *insula,* island, + *-itis,* inflammation]. Inflammation of the islands of Langerhans, with lymphocytic infiltration which may result from viral infection and be the initial lesion of insulin-dependent diabetes mellitus.

insuloma (in-sŭ-lō′mă) [L. *insula,* island, + *-oma,* tumor]. Insulinoma.

insult (in′sŭlt) [LL. *insultus,* fr L. *insulto,* to spring upon] An injury, attack, or trauma.

insusceptibility (in′sŭ-sep′ti-bil′i-tē) [L. *suscipio,* pp. *-ceptus,* to take upon one, fr. *sub,* under, + *capio,* to take]. Immunity.

int. cib. Abbreviation for L. *inter cibos,* between meals.

integration (in-tĕ-grā′shŭn) [L. *integro,* pp. *-atus,* to make whole, fr. *integer,* whole]. **1.** The state of being combined, or the process of combining, into a complete and harmonious whole. **2.** In physiology, the process of building up, as by accretion, anabolism, etc. **3.** In mathematics, the process of ascertaining a function from its differential. **4.** In molecular biology, a recombination event in which a genetic element is inserted.

personality i., the useful organization of old and new experience, data, and emotional capacities into the personality; the harmonious organization of the personality.

integrity (in-teg'ri-tē). Soundness or completeness of structure; a sound or unimpaired condition.

marginal i. of amalgam, the ability of a dental amalgam restoration to maintain its original marginal form at the cavosurface margins.

integument (in-teg'yū-ment) [L. *integumentum,* a covering, fr. *intego,* to cover]. **1.** *Integumentum* commune. **2.** The rind, capsule, or covering of any body or part.

integumentary (in-teg-yū-men'tă-rē). Relating to the integument. See also cutaneous; dermal.

integumentum commune (in-teg-yū-men'tŭm ko-myūn') [NA]. Integument (1); the enveloping membrane of the body; includes, in addition to the epidermis and dermis, all of the derivatives of the epidermis, *i.e.,* hairs, nails, sudoriferous and sebaceous glands, and mammary glands.

intellectualization (in-te-lek'chū-ăl-i-zā'shŭn) [L. *intellectus,* perception, discernment]. An unconscious defense mechanism in which reasoning, logic, or attention to intellectual minutiae is used in an attempt to avoid confrontation with an objectionable impulse, affect, or interpersonal situation.

intelligence (in-tel'i-jens) [L. *intelligentia*]. **1.** An individual's aggregate capacity to act purposefully, think rationally, and deal effectively with his environment, especially in relation to the extent of his perceived effectiveness in meeting challenges. **2.** In psychology, an individual's relative standing on two quantitative indices, measured i. and effectiveness of adaptive behavior; a quantitative score or similar index on both indices constitutes the operational definition of i.

abstract i., the capacity to understand and manage abstract ideas and symbols.

measured i., that i. which can be ranked relative to an age or peer group quantitative index through scores on i. tests.

mechanical i., the capacity to understand and manage technical mechanisms.

social i., the capacity to understand and manage human relations and social affairs.

intemperance (in-tem'per-ăns) [L. *intemperantia,* fr. *in-,* neg. + *temperantia,* moderation]. Lack of proper self-control, usually in reference to the use of alcoholic beverages. *Cf.* incontinence (2).

intensimeter (in-ten-sim'ĕ-ter). An instrument for measuring intensity of radiation.

intensity (in-ten'si-tē) [L. *in- tendo,* pp. *-tensus,* to stretch out]. Marked tension; great activity; strength; often used simply to denote a measure of the degree or amount of some quality.

luminous i. (I), candle-power; the luminous flux per unit solid angle in a given direction.

i. of sound, the objective measurement of the amplitude of vibration of a sound wave.

intensive (in-ten'siv). Relating to or marked by intensity; denoting a form of treatment by means of very large doses or of substances possessing great strength or activity.

intention (in-ten'shŭn) [L. *intentio,* a stretching out; intention]. **1.** An objective. **2.** In surgery, a process or operation.

inter- [L. *inter,* between]. Prefix conveying the meaning of between, among.

interacinar (in-ter-as'i-nar). Interacinous.

interacinous (in-ter-as'i-nŭs). Interacinar; between the acini of a gland.

interalveolar (in'ter-al-vē'ō-lăr). Between any alveoli, especially the alveoli of the lungs.

interannular (in-ter-an'yū-lăr) [inter- + L. *anulus,* ring]. Between any two ringlike structures or constrictions.

interarch (in'ter-arch). See interarch *distance.*

interarticular (in-ter-ar-tik'yū-lăr) [inter- + L. *articulus,* joint]. **1.** Between two joints. **2.** Between two joint surfaces.

interarytenoid (in'ter-ăr'i-tē'noyd). Between the arytenoid cartilages.

interasteric (in-ter-ă-stē'rik). Between the two asteria. See asterion.

interatrial (in-ter-ā'trē-ăl). Interauricular (1); between the atria of the heart.

interauricular (in'ter-aw-rik'yū-lăr). **1.** Interatrial. **2.** Between the auricles or pinnae.

interbody (in'ter-bod'ē). Between the bodies of two adjacent vertebrae.

intercadence (in-ter-kā'dens) [inter- + L. *cado,* pr. p. *cadens* (*-ent-*), to fall]. The occurrence of an extra beat between the two regular pulse beats.

intercadent (in-ter-kā'dent). Irregular in rhythm; characterized by intercadence.

intercalary (in-ter'kă-ler-ē, in-ter-kal'er-ē) [L. *intercalarius,* concerning an insertion]. **1.** Occurring between two others; as in a pulse tracing, an upstroke interposed between two normal pulse beats. **2.** In fungi, located in a hypha or between hyphal segments, not at a hyphal terminus.

intercalated (in-ter'kă-lā-ted) [L. *intercalatus*]. Interposed; inserted between two others.

intercanalicular (in-ter-kan-ă-lik'yū-lăr). Between canaliculi.

intercapillary (in-ter-kap'i-lā-rē). Between or among capillary vessels.

intercarotic, intercarotid (in-ter-ka-rot'ik, -id). Between the internal and external carotid arteries.

intercarpal (in-ter-kar'păl). Between the carpal bones.

intercartilaginous (in'ter-kar-ti-laj'i-nŭs). Interchondral; between or connecting cartilages.

intercavernous (in'ter-kav'er-nŭs). Between two cavities.

intercellular (in-ter-sel'yū-lăr). Between or among cells.

intercentral (in-ter-sen'trăl). Connecting or lying between two or more centers.

intercentrum, pl. **intercentra** (in-ter-sen'trŭm, -tră). In veterinary anatomy, an intervertebral disk between vertebrae, and the hemal arch beneath vertebrae of some reptiles, birds, and mammals. See also hemal *arch.*

intercerebral (in'ter-ser'ē-brăl). Between the cerebral hemispheres.

interchondral (in-ter-kon'drăl) [inter- + L. *chondros,* cartilage]. Intercartilaginous.

intercilium (in-ter-sil'ē-ŭm) [inter- + L. *cilium,* eyelid]. Glabella.

interclavicular (in-ter-kla-vik'yū-lăr). Between or connecting the clavicles.

intercoccygeal (in'ter-kok-sij'ē-ăl). Situated between unfused segments of the coccyx.

intercolumnar (in-ter-kō-lŭm'nar). Between any two columns, as the columns or crura of the superficial inguinal ring.

intercondylar, intercondylic, intercondyloid (in-ter-kon'di-lăr, -kon-dil'ik, -kon'di-loyd). Between two condyles.

intercostal (in-ter-kos'tăl) [inter- + L. *costa,* rib]. Between the ribs.

intercostohumeral (in'ter-kos'tō-hyū'mer-ăl). Relating to an intercostal space and the arm. See *nervi* intercostobrachiales.

intercostohumeralis (in-ter-kos'tō-hyū-mer-ā'lis). See *nervi* intercostobrachiales.

intercourse (in'ter-kōrs) [L. *intercursus,* a running between]. Communication or dealings between or among people.

sexual i., coitus.

intercricothyrotomy (in-ter-krī'kō-thī-rot'ō-mē). Cricothyrotomy.

intercristal (in-ter-kris'tăl). Between two crests, as between the crests of the ilia, applied to one of the pelvic measurements.

intercross (in'ter-kros). A mating between two individuals both heterozygous at a specified locus or loci.

intercrural (in-ter-krū'răl). Between two crura; *e.g.,* the cerebral peduncles of the brain, the superficial inguinal ring, etc.

intercurrent (in-ter-ker'ent) [inter- + L. *curro,* pr. p. *currens* (*-ent-*), to run]. Intervening; said of a disease attacking a person already ill of another malady.

intercuspation (in'ter-kŭs-pā'shŭn). Intercusping. **1.** The cusp-to-fossa relation of the maxillary and mandibular posterior teeth to each other. **2.** Interdigitation (4); the interlocking or fitting together of the cusps of opposing teeth.

intercusping (in-ter-kŭs'ping) [L. *inter,* among, mutually, + cusp]. Intercuspation.

intercutaneomucous (in'ter-kyū-tā'nē-ō-mū'kŭs). Between skin and mucous membrane, as in the cheek or lip or at the mucocutaneous border of the lips or anus.

interdeferential (in-ter-def-er-en'shăl). Between the deferent ducts.

interdental (in-ter-den'tăl) [inter- + L. *dens,* tooth]. **1.** Between the teeth. **2.** Denoting the relationship between the proximal surfaces of the teeth of the same arch.

interdentium (in-ter-den'shē-ŭm). The interval between any two contiguous teeth.

interdigit (in-ter-dij'it). That part of the sloping extremity of the hand or foot lying between any two adjacent fingers or toes.

interdigital (in-ter-dij'i-tăl). Between the fingers or toes.

interdigitation (in'ter-dij-i-tā'shŭn) [inter- + L. *digitus,* finger]. **1.** The mutual interlocking of toothed or tonguelike processes. **2.** The processes thus interlocked. **3.** Infoldings or plicae of adjacent cell or plasma membranes. **4.** Intercuspation (2).

interdisciplinary (in-ter-dis'i-pli-năr-ē) [inter- + L. *disciplina,* knowledge]. Denoting the overlapping interests of different fields of medicine and science.

interface (in'ter-fās). A surface that forms a common boundary of two bodies.

crystalline i., in dentistry, a boundary between adjacent crystals.

dermoepidermal i., the line of meeting of the dermis and epidermis.

metal i., in dentistry, a boundary between metal and nonsolvent solder, or between metal and surface oxide.

structural i., in dentistry, a boundary between tooth and restorative material.

interfacial (in-ter-fā'shăl). Relating to an interface.

interfascicular (in'ter-fă-sik'yū-lăr). Between fasciculi.

interfemoral (in-ter-fem'ŏ-răl). Between the thighs.

interference (in-ter-fēr'ens) [inter- + L. *ferio,* to strike]. **1.** The coming together of waves in various media in such a way that the crests of one series correspond to the hollows of the other, the two thus neutralizing each other; or so that the crests of the two series correspond, thus increasing the excursions of the waves. **2.** Collision within the myocardium of two waves of excitation, as is seen in fusion beats. **3.** In A-V dissociation, the disturbance of the regular rhythm of the ventricles by a conducted impulse from the atria, *i.e.,* by a ventricular capture. **4.** The condition in which infection of a cell by one virus prevents superinfection by another virus, or in which superinfection prevents effects which would result from infection by either virus alone, even though both viruses persist.

bacterial i., the condition in which colonization by one bacterial strain prevents colonization by another strain.

cuspal i., deflective occlusal *contact.*

interferometer (in'ter-fe-rom'ĕ-ter). An instrument for measuring minute distances or movements through the interference of light waves thereby produced.

electron i., an i. that employs an electron beam in place of a light beam.

interferometry (in'ter-fe-rom'ĕ-trē). Measurement of minute distances or movements by interaction of waves of electromagnetic energy.

electron i., i. in which a beam of electrons is used instead of a beam of light.

interferon (INF) (in-ter-fēr'on). A class of small (MW 26,000–38,000) glycoproteins that exert antiviral activity at least in homologous cells through cellular metabolic processes involving synthesis of double-stranded RNA, which is an intermediate in replication of RNA viruses. INF is classified into three groups, alpha, beta, and gamma, based on their cells of origin and method of induction; Arabic numerals and letters are appended to the Greek letter to delineate subcategories.

i. alpha, leukocyte i.; i. elaborated by leukocytes in response to viral infection or stimulation with double-stranded RNA; INF-α-2A and -2B are protein products made by recombinant DNA techniques and are used as antineoplastic agents.

antigen i., i. gamma.

i. beta, fibroblast i.; i. elaborated by fibroblasts in response to the same stimuli as i. alpha.

fibroblast i., i. beta.

i. gamma, immune or antigen i.; i. elaborated by lymphocytes in response to mitogenic stimulation.

immune i., i. gamma.

leukocyte i., i. alpha.

interfibrillar, interfibrillary (in'ter-fī'bri-lăr, -fī-bril'ăr, -fī'bri-lăr-ē). Between fibrils.

interfibrous (in-ter-fī'brŭs). Between fibers.

interfilamentous (in'ter-fil-ă-men'tŭs). Between filaments.

interfrontal (in-ter-fron'tăl). Between the unfused halves of the frontal bone; denoting a suture there present.

interganglionic (in'ter-gang'lē-on'ik). Between or among or connecting ganglia.

intergemmal (in'ter-jem'ăl) [inter- + L. *gemma,* bud]. Between any two or more budlike or bulblike bodies such as the taste buds; denoting especially a nerve termination between two end bulbs.

interglobular (in-ter-glob'yū-lăr). Between globules.

intergluteal (in-ter-glū'tē-ăl) [inter- + G. *gloutos,* buttock]. Between the buttocks.

intergonial (in-ter-gō'nē-ăl) [inter- + G. *gōnia,* angle]. Between the two gonia. See gonion.

intergyral (in-ter-jī'răl). Between the gyri or convolutions of the brain.

interhemicerebral (in'ter-hem'ē-ser'ē-brăl). Intercerebral; between the cerebral hemispheres.

interictal (in-ter-ik'tăl) [inter- + L. *ictus,* stroke]. Denoting the interval between convulsions.

interior (in-tēr'ē-ōr). Relating to the inside; situated within.

interischiadic (in-ter-is-kē-ad'ik). Intersciatic; between the two ischia; especially, between the two tuberosities of the ischia.

interkinesis (in'ter-ki-nē'sis) [inter- + G. *kinēsis,* movement]. Interphase.

interlamellar (in'ter-lă-mel'ăr, -lam'ĕ- lăr). Between lamellae.

interleukin-1 (IL-1) (in-ter-lū'kin). A lymphokine and polypeptide hormine that is synthesized by monocytes, and that acts on the hypothalamus to induce fever and directly on skeletal muscle to promote protein catabolism.

interleukin-2 (IL-2). A lymphokine and polypeptide hormone that is produced by both T helper and suppressor lymphocytes and that functions to govern clonal expansion and reactivity of T lymphocytes.

interlobar (in-ter-lō'bar). Between the lobes of an organ or other structure.

interlobitis (in'ter-lō-bī'tis). Inflammation of the pleura separating two pulmonary lobes.

interlobular (in-ter-lob'yū-lăr). Between the lobules of an organ.

intermalleolar (in-ter-mal-ē'ō-lăr). Between the malleoli.

intermammary (in-ter-mam'ă-rē) [inter- + L. *mamma*, breast]. Between the breasts.

intermammillary (in-ter-mam'i-lā-rē) [inter- + L. *mammilla*, breast, nipple]. Between the breasts; between the nipples; denoting a line drawn between the two nipples.

intermarriage (in-ter-mar'ij). **1.** Marriage of relatives. **2.** Marriage of persons of different races or cultures.

intermaxilla (in-ter-maks-il'ă). *Os* incisivum.

intermaxillary (in-ter-mak'si-lā-rē). Between the maxillae, or upper jaw bones.

intermediary (in'ter-mē'dē-ār-ē) [L. *intermedius*, lying between, fr. *medius*, middle]. Occurring between.

intermediate (in'ter-mē'dē-it). **1.** Between two extremes; interposed; intervening. **2.** A substance formed in the course of chemical reactions which then proceeds to participate rapidly in further reactions, so that at any given moment it is present in minute concentrations only; such substances, when appearing in the course of the reactions involved in metabolism, are metabolic i.'s. **3.** In dentistry, a cement base. **4.** Intermedius.

intermedin (in-ter-mē'din). Melanotropin.

intermediolateral (in-ter-mē'dē-ō-lat'er-ăl). Intermediate, and to one side, not central.

intermedius (in-ter-mē'dē-ŭs) [L.] [NA]. Intermediate (4); an element or organ between right and left (or lateral and medial) structures.

intermembranous (in-ter-mem'bră-nŭs). Between membranes.

intermeningeal (in'ter-me-nin'jē-ăl). Between the meninges.

intermenstrual (in-ter-men'strū-ăl). Between two consecutive menstrual periods.

intermetacarpal (in-ter-met'ă-kar'păl). Between the metacarpal bones.

intermetameric (in'ter-met'ă-mer'ik). Between two metameres; denoting especially the intervertebral disks.

intermetatarsal (in-ter-met'ă-tar'săl). Between the metatarsal bones.

intermetatarseum (in-ter-met'ă-tar'sē-ŭm). *Os* intermetatarseum.

intermission (in-ter-mish'ŭn) [L. *intermissio*, fr. *intermitto*, to leave off, intermit, fr. *mitto*, to send]. **1.** A temporary cessation of symptoms or of any action. **2.** An interval between two paroxysms of a disease such as malaria.

intermit'. To cease for a time.

intermittence, intermittency (in-ter-mit'ens, -en-sē). **1.** A condition marked by intermissions or interruptions in the course of a disease or other process or state or in any continued action; denoting especially a loss of one or more pulse beats. **2.** Complete cessation of symptoms between two periods of activity of a disease.

intermittent (in-ter-mit'ent). Marked by intervals of complete quietude between two periods of activity.

intermuscular (in-ter-mŭs'kyū-lăr). Between the muscles.

in'tern [F. *interne*, inside]. An advanced student or recent graduate undertaking further education by assisting in the medical or surgical care of hospital patients, with supervision and instruction; formerly, one who resided within the institution.

internal (in-ter'năl) [L. *internus*]. Interior; away from the surface; often incorrectly used to mean medial.

internalization (in-ter'năl-i-zā'shŭn). Adopting as one's own the standards and values of another person or society.

internarial (in-ter-nā'rē-ăl). Internasal; between the nares or nostrils.

internasal (in-ter-nā'săl). Internarial.

International Committee of the Red Cross. A neutral Swiss organization serving as an intermediary between nations in armed conflict and in civil war or internal strife, to help victims receive protection and other humanitarian assistance under the Geneva Conventions in accordance with the fundamental principles of the Red Cross.

International System of Units (SI) [Fr. *Système International d'Unités*]. A system of measurements, based on the metric system, adopted at the 11th General Conference on Weights and Measures of the International Organization for Standardization (1960) to cover both the coherent units (basic, supplementary, and derived units) and the decimal multiples and submultiples of these units formed by use of prefixes proposed for general international scientific and technological use. SI proposes seven basic units: meter (m), kilogram (kg), second (s), ampere (A), Kelvin (K), candela (cd), and mole (mol) for the basic quantities of length, mass, time, electric current, temperature, luminous intensity, and amount of substance; supplementary units proposed are radian (rad) for plane angle and steradian (sr) for solid angle; derived units (*e.g.*, force, power, frequency) are stated in terms of the basic units (*e.g.*, velocity is in meters per second, m/s^{-1}). Multiples (prefixes) in descending order are: exa- (E, 10^{18}), peta- (P, 10^{15}), tera- (T, 10^{12}), giga- (G, 10^{9}), mega- (M, 10^{6}), kilo- (k, 10^{3}), hecto- (h, 10^{2}), deca- (da, 10^{1}), deci- (d, 10^{-1}), centi- (c, 10^{-2}), milli- (m, 10^{-3}), micro- (μ, 10^{-6}), nano- (n, 10^{-9}), pico- (p, 10^{-12}), femto- (f, 10^{-15}), atto- (a, 10^{-18}). Those involving a multiple of 10^3 are recommended; compounds of these are not recommended (*e.g.*, mμ for n).

interneuromeric (in'ter-nūr-ō-mer'ik). Between the neuromeres.

interneurons (in'ter-nū'ronz). Combinations or groups of neurons between sensory and motor neurons which govern coordinated activity.

internist (in-ter'nist, in'ter-nist). A physician trained in internal medicine.

internodal (in-ter-nō'dăl). Between two nodes; relating to an internode.

internode (in'ter-nōd). Internodal *segment.*

internuclear (in-ter-nū'klē-ăr). Between nerve cell groups in the brain or retina.

internuncial (in-ter-nun'sē-ăl) [L. *inter-nuntius* (or *-nuncius*), a messenger between two parties, fr. *inter*, between, + *nuncius*, a messenger]. **1.** Indicating a neuron functionally interposed between two or more other neurons. **2.** Acting as a medium of communication between two organs.

internus (in-ter'nŭs) [L.] [NA]. Internal.

interocclusal (in'ter-ō-klū'săl). Between the occlusal surfaces of opposing teeth.

interoceptive (in'ter-ō-sep'tiv) [inter- + L. *capio*, to take]. Relating to the sensory nerve cells innervating the viscera (thoracic, abdominal and pelvic organs, and the cardiovascular system), their sensory end organs, or the information they convey to the spinal cord and the brain.

interoceptor (in'ter-ō-sep'ter) [inter- + L. *capio*, to take]. One of the various forms of small sensory end organs (receptors) situated within the walls of the respiratory and gastrointestinal tracts or in other viscera.

interolivary (in-ter-ol'i-vār-ē). Between the left and right inferior olive of the medulla oblongata.

interorbital (in-ter-ōr'bi-tăl). Between the orbits.

interosseal (in-ter-os'ē-ăl). Interosseous.

interossei (in-ter-os'ē-ī). Plural of interosseus.

interosseous (in'ter-os'ē-ŭs) [inter- + L. *os,* bone]. Interosseal; lying between or connecting bones; denoting certain muscles and ligaments.

interosseus, pl. **interossei** (in'ter-os'ē-ŭs, -os'e-ī). See entries under musculus.

interpalpebral (in-ter-pal'pe-brăl). Between the eyelids.

interparietal (in'ter-pă-rī'ĕ-tăl) [inter- + L. *paries,* wall]. Between the walls of a part, or between the parietal bones.

interparoxysmal (in'ter-par-ok-siz'măl). Occurring between successive paroxysms of a disease.

interpediculate (in-ter-pe-dik'yū-lāt). Between vertebral pedicles.

interpeduncular (in-ter-pe-dŭnk'yū-lăr). Between any two peduncles.

interpersonal (in-ter-per'sŏn-ăl). Pertaining to relations and social exchanges between persons.

interphalangeal (in'ter-fă-lan'jē-ăl). Between two phalanges; denoting the finger or toe joints.

interphase (in'ter-fāz). Interkinesis; karyostasis; the stage between two successive divisions of a cell nucleus in which the biochemical and physiologic functions of the cell are performed, and during which replication of chromatin occurs.

interphyletic (in'ter-fī-let'ik) [inter- + G. *phylē,* tribe]. Denoting the transitional forms between two kinds of cells during the course of metaplasia.

in'terplant. The material transferred from donor to host in interplanting.

interplant'ing. In experimental embryology, the transferring of a primordial cell mass from one embryo to an indifferent environment in another embryo, as in chorioallantoic grafts or intraocular transplants.

interpretation (in-ter-pre-tā'shŭn). **1.** In psychoanalysis, the characteristic therapeutic intervention of the analyst. **2.** In clinical psychology, drawing inferences and formulating the meaning in terms of the psychological dynamics inherent in an individual's responses to psychological tests.

interproximal (in-ter-prok'si-măl). Between adjoining surfaces.

interpubic (in-ter-pyū'bik). Between the two pubic bones.

interpupillary (in-ter-pyū'pi-lār-ē). Between the pupils.

interradial (in-ter-rā'dē-ăl). Situated between radii or rays.

interrenal (in-ter-rē'năl). Between the two kidneys.

interscapular (in-ter-skap'yū-lăr). Between the scapulae.

interscapulum (in-ter-skap'yū-lŭm). The part of the back between the shoulders, or that between the scapulae.

intersciatic (in-ter-sī-at'ik). Interischiadic.

intersectio, pl. **intersectiones** (in'ter-sek'shē-ō, -sek-shē-ō'nēz) [L.] [NA]. Intersection; the site of crossing of two structures.

i. tendin'ea [NA], tendinous intersection or inscription; inscriptio tendinea; a tendinous band or partition running across a muscle.

intersection (in'ter-sek-shŭn). Intersectio.

tendinous i., *intersectio* tendinea.

intersectiones (in-ter-sek-shē-ō'nēz). Plural of intersectio.

intersegmental (in-ter-seg-men'tăl). Between two segments, such as metameres or myotomes.

interseptal (in-ter-sep'tăl). Lying between two septa.

interseptovalvular (in'ter-sep-tō-val'vyū-lăr). Between the embryonic septum primum and septum spurium.

interseptum (in-ter-sep'tŭm) [L]. Diaphragma.

intersexual (in-ter-seks'yū-ăl). Relating to or characterized by intersexuality.

intersexuality (in'ter-seks-yū-al'i-tē). The condition of having both male and female characteristics; being intermediate between the sexes.

interspace (in'ter-spās). Any space between two similar objects, such as a costal i. or interval between two ribs.

interspinal (in-ter-spī'năl). Interspinous; between two spines, such as the spinous processes of the vertebrae.

interspinalis (in-ter-spī-nā'lis). See entries under musculus.

interspinous (in-ter-spī'nŭs). Interspinal.

interstice, pl. **interstices** (in-ter'stis, -sti-sēz) [L. *interstitium,* fr. *sisto,* to stand]. Interstitium.

interstitial (in-ter-stish'ăl). **1.** Relating to spaces or interstices in any structure. **2.** Relating to spaces within a tissue or organ, but excluding such spaces as body cavities or potential space. *Cf.* intracavitary.

interstitium (in-ter-stish'ē-ŭm) [L.]. Interstice; a small area, space, or gap in the substance of an organ or tissue. See also connective *tissue.*

intersystole (in'ter-sis'tō-lē). Intersystolic period; atriocarotid interval; the period intervening between the systole of the atrium and that of the ventricle of the heart.

intertarsal (in-ter-tar'săl). Between the tarsal bones.

interthalamic (in-ter-thal'ă-mik). Between the thalami.

intertransversalis (in-ter-trans-ver-sā'lis). Intertransversarius; see entries under musculus.

intertransverse (in'ter-trans'vers). Between the transverse processes of the vertebrae.

intertriginous (in-ter-trij'i-nŭs). Characterized by or related to intertrigo.

intertrigo (in-ter-trī'gō) [L. a galling of the skin, fr. *inter,* between, + *tero,* to rub]. Dermatitis occurring between folds or juxtaposed surfaces of the skin, as between the buttocks, between the scrotum and the thigh, beneath pendulous breasts, etc.; caused by sweat retention, moisture, warmth, and concomitant overgrowth of resident microorganisms.

intertrochanteric (in'ter-trō-kan-tār'ik). Between the two trochanters of the femur.

intertubular (in-ter-tū'byū-lăr). Between or among tubules.

interureteral (in'ter-yū-rē'ter-ăl). Interureteric; between the two ureters.

interureteric (in-ter-yū-rē-tār'ik). Interureteral.

interval (in'ter-văl) [L. *inter-vallum,* space between breastworks in a camp, an interval, fr. *vallum,* a rampart, wall]. A time or space between two periods or objects; a break in continuity.

A-H i., the time from the initial rapid deflection of the wave to the initial rapid deflection of the His bundle (H) potential; it approximates the conduction time through the A-V node (normally 50-120 msec).

A-N i., the time between onset of the atrial deflection and the nodal potential (normally 40-100 msec).

atriocarotid (a-c) i., intersystolic period; intersystole; the time between the beginning of the atrial and that of the carotid waves in a tracing of the jugular pulse.

A-V i., the time from the beginning of atrial systole to the beginning of ventricular systole as measured from pressure pulses or car-

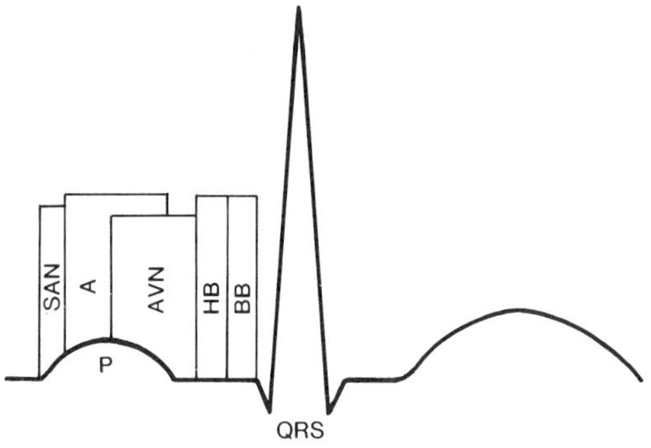

Interval

Diagram of activation sequence of the functional regions in the P-QRS interval in a conventional electrocardiogram. *SAN*, sinoatrial node; A, atrium; *AVN*, atrioventricular node; *HB*, His bundle; *BB*, bundle branches.

diac volume curves in animals, or from the electrocardiogram in man.

BH i., the time of His bundle deflection (normally 15-20 msec).

cardioarterial (c-a) i., the time between the apex beat of the heart and the radial pulse beat.

coupling i., the i., usually expressed in hundredths of a second, between a normal sinus beat and the ensuing premature beat.

escape i., the time between the patient's own depolarization (ectopic or sinus beat) and the initial pacemaker impulse (a preset i. in the circuitry); it may be either a shorter or a longer time period than the pulse i.

focal i., the distance between the anterior and posterior focal points of the eye.

H-V i., the time from the initial deflection of the His bundle (H) potential and the onset of ventricular activity (normally 35-45 msec).

interectopic i., the distance between consecutive ectopic complexes in the electrocardiogram.

isometric i., presphygmic i.

lucid i., in psychoses or delirium, a rational period appearing in the course of the mental disorder.

P-A i., the time from onset of the P wave to the initial rapid deflection of the A wave in the His bundle electrogram (normally 25-45 msec); it represents the intra-atrial conduction time.

passive i., the period of rest of the heart.

P-J i., the time elapsing from the beginning of the P wave to the end of the QRS complex (J for junction between QRS and S-T segment) in the electrocardiogram.

postsphygmic i., a period of isometric relaxation; the interval in the cardiac cycle following the sphygmic period, *i.e.,* from the closure of the semilunar valves to the opening of the atrioventricular valves.

P-P i., the distance between consecutive P waves in the electrocardiogram.

P-Q i., P-R i.

P-R i., P-Q i.; in the electrocardiogram, the time elapsing between the beginning of the P wave and the beginning of the QRS complex; it corresponds to the a-c interval of the venous pulse and is normally 0.12-0.20 sec.

presphygmic i., isometric period or i.; the brief period at the beginning of the ventricular systole during which the pressure rises before the semilunar valves open.

Q-R i., the time elapsing from the onset of the QRS complex to the peak of the R wave; measures the time of onset of the intrinsicoid deflection.

Q-RB i., the time between the onset of the Q wave of the QRS complex and the right bundle-branch potential (normally 15-20 msec).

QRS i., the duration of the QRS complex in the electrocardiogram.

Q-S_2 i., electromechanical *systole.*

Q-T i., in the electrocardiogram, the time elapsing from the beginning of the QRS complex to the end of the T wave; it represents the total duration of electrical activity of the ventricles.

R-R i., the time elapsing between two consecutive QRS complexes in the electrocardiogram.

sphygmic i., ejection period; the period in the cardiac cycle when the semilunar valves are open and blood is being ejected from the ventricles into the arterial system.

Sturm's i., the distance between the anterior and posterior focal lines in a spherocylindrical lens combination.

systolic time i.'s, see electromechanical *systole;* left ventricular ejection *time;* preejection *period.*

intervascular (in-ter-vas'kyū-lăr). Between blood or lymph vessels.

intervention (in-ter-ven'shŭn). An action or ministration that produces an effect or that is intended to alter the course of a pathologic process.

crisis i., a psychotherapeutic technique directed at counseling at the time of an acute life crisis and limited in aim to helping resolve the crisis.

interventricular (in-ter-ven-trik'yū-lăr). Between the ventricles.

intervertebral (in-ter-ver'te-brăl). Between two vertebrae.

intervillous (in-ter-vil'ŭs). Between or among villi.

intestinal (in-tes'ti-năl). Relating to the intestine.

intestine (in-tes'tin) [L. *intestinum*]. Intestinum (1).

large i., *intestinum* crassum.

small i., *intestinum* tenue.

intestinotoxin (in-tes'ti-nō-tok'sin). Enterotoxin.

intestinum, pl. **intestina** (in-tes-tī'nŭm, -nă) [L. *intestinus,* internal, ntr. as noun, the entrails, fr. *intus,* within] **1** [NA]. Intestine; gut (1); bowel; the digestive tube passing from the stomach to the anus. It is divided primarily into the i. tenue (small intestine) and the i. crassum (large intestine). **2** [neuter of *intestinus].* Inward; inner.

i. ce'cum, blind gut. See cecum.

i. cras'sum [NA], large intestine; the portion of the digestive tube extending from the ileocecal valve to the anus; it comprises the cecum, colon, rectum, and anal canal.

i. il'eum, twisted intestine. See ileum.

i. jeju'num, empty intestine. See jejunum.

i. rec'tum, straight intestine. See rectum.

i. ten'ue [NA], small intestine; the portion of the digestive tube between the stomach and the cecum or beginning of the large intestine; it consists of three portions: duodenum, jejunum, and ileum.

i. ten'ue mesenteria'le, the freely movable portion of the small intestine supplied with a mesentery, comprising the jejunum and ileum.

intima (in'ti-mă) [L. fem. of *intimus,* inmost]. Innermost. See *tunica* intima.

intimal (in'ti-măl). Relating to the intima or inner coat of a vessel.

intimitis (in-ti-mī'tis) [intima + G. *-itis,* inflammation]. Inflammation of an intima, as in endangiitis.

proliferative i., eruption characterized by dusky erythema and small ulcers due to proliferative changes in capillary bed.

intoe (in'tō). *Metatarsus* varus.

intolerance (in-tol'er-ăns). Abnormal metabolism, excretion, or other disposition of a given substance; term often used to indicate impaired disposal of dietary constituents.

hereditary fructose i., a metabolic error due to deficiency of hepatic fructose 1-phosphate aldolase, the second enzyme in the specific fructose pathway; vomiting and hypoglycemia follow ingestion of fructose; prolonged fructose ingestion in young children results in their failure to thrive and in jaundice, hepatomegaly, albuminuria, aminoaciduria, and sometimes cachexia and death; autosomal recessive inheritance in most families.

lactose i., a disorder characterized by abdominal cramps and diarrhea after consumption of food containing lactose (*e.g.*, milk, ice cream); believed to reflect a deficiency of intestinal lactase and may appear first in young adults who have previously tolerated milk well as infants.

intorsion (in-tōr'shŭn) [L. *in- torqueo,* pp. *tortus,* to twist]. Conjugate rotation of the upper poles of each cornea inward.

intortor (in-tōr'tōr). Medial rotator; a muscle that turns a part medialward. See also invertor.

intoxation (in-tok-sā'shŭn) [see intoxication]. Poisoning, especially by the toxic products of bacteria or poisonous animals, other than alcohol.

intoxicant (in-tok'si-kant). **1.** Having the power to intoxicate. **2.** An intoxicating agent, such as alcohol.

intoxication (in-tok-si-kā'shŭn) [L. *in,* in, + G. *toxicon,* poison]. **1.** Poisoning. **2.** Acute *alcoholism.*

acid i., poisoning by acid products (β-oxybutyric acid, diacetic acid, or acetone), formed as a result of faulty metabolism, or by acids introduced from without; marked by epigastric pain, headache, loss of appetite, constipation, restlessness, and an odor of acetone in the breath, followed by air hunger, coma, and collapse.

anaphylactic i., i. following an anaphylactic reaction.

citrate i., a toxic condition that may develop during massive replacement therapy with transfused blood that contains citrate as an anticoagulant; the citrate combines with calcium ions and may result in tetany.

intestinal i., autointoxication.

septic i., septicemia.

water i., severe overhydration resulting, through diuresis, in salt depletion with salivation, nausea and vomiting, restlessness, weakness, ataxia, tremors, and sometimes convulsions and death.

intra- [L. within]. Prefix meaning within. See also endo-, ento-.

intra-abdominal (in'tră-ab-dom'i-năl). Within the abdomen.

intra-acinous (in-tră-as'i-nŭs). Within an acinus.

intra-adenoidal (in'tră-ad-ĕ-noy'dăl). Within the adenoids.

intra-arterial (in'tră-ar-tēr'ē-ăl). Within an artery or the arteries.

intra-articular (in'tră-ar-tik'yūlăr) [intra- + L. *articulus,* joint]. Within the cavity of a joint.

intra-atrial (in'tră-ā-trē-ăl). Within one or both of the atria of the heart.

intra-aural (in'tră-aw'răl) [intra- + L. *auris,* ear]. Within the ear.

intra-auricular (in'tră-aw-rik'yū-lăr). **1.** Within an auricle (*e.g.*, of the ear). **2.** Obsolete term for intra-atrial.

intrabronchial (in-tră-brong'kē-ăl). Endobronchial; within the bronchi or bronchial tubes.

intrabuccal (in'tră-bŭk'ăl) [intra- + L. *bucca,* cheek]. **1.** Within the mouth. **2.** Within the substance of the cheek.

intracanalicular (in'tră-kan-ă-lik'yū-lăr). Within a canaliculus or canaliculi.

intracapsular (in'tră-kap'sū-lăr). Within a capsule, especially the capsule of a joint.

intracardiac (in'tră-kar'dē-ak) [intra- + G. *kardia,* heart]. Endocardiac, endocardial (1); intracordial; within one of the chambers of the heart.

intracarpal (in-tră-kar'păl). Within the carpus; among the carpal bones.

intracartilaginous (in'tră-kar-ti-laj'i-nŭs). Enchondral; endochondral; within a cartilage or cartilaginous tissue.

intracatheter (in'tră-kath'e-ter). A plastic tube, usually attached to the puncturing needle, inserted into a blood vessel for infusion, injection, or pressure monitoring.

intracavitary (in'tră-cav'i-tār-ē). Within an organ or body cavity.

intracelial (in'tră-sē'lē-ăl) [intra- + G. *koilia,* cavity]. Endoceliac; within any of the body cavities, especially within one of the ventricles of the brain.

intracellular (in-tră-sel'yū-lăr). Within a cell or cells.

intracerebellar (in'tră-ser-ĕ-bel'ăr). Within the cerebellum.

intracerebral (in'tră-ser'ē-brăl). Within the cerebrum.

intracervical (in'tră-ser'vi-kăl). Endocervical (1).

intracisternal (in'tră-sis-ter'năl). Within one of the subarachnoid cisternae; usually refers to the introduction of a cannula into the cisterna cerebellomedullaris for aspiration of cerebrospinal fluid or the injection of air into the ventricles of the brain.

intracolic (in'tră-kol'ik). Within the colon.

intracordal (in'tră-kōr'dăl) [intra- + L. *cor,* heart]. Intracardiac.

intracoronal (in'tră-kōr'ō-năl). Within the crown portion of a tooth.

intracorporeal (in'tră-kōr-po'rē-ăl) [intra- + L. *corpus,* body]. **1.** Within the body. **2.** Within any structure anatomically styled a corpus.

intracorpuscular (in'tră-kōr-pŭs'kyū-lăr). Intraglobular (2); within a corpuscle, especially a red blood corpuscle.

intracostal (in'tră-kos'tăl). On the inner surface of the ribs.

intracranial (in'tră-krā'nē-ăl). Within the skull.

intractable (in'trak'tă-bl) [L. *in-tractabilis,* fr. *in-* neg. + *tracto,* to draw, haul]. **1.** Refractory (1). **2.** Obstinate (1).

intracutaneous (in'tră-kū-tā'nē-ŭs) [intra- + L. *cutis,* skin]. Intradermal; intradermic; within the substance of the skin, particularly the dermis.

intracystic (in'tră-sis'tik). Within a cyst or the urinary bladder.

in'trad. Toward the inner part.

intradermal, intradermic (in'tră-der'măl, -der'mik) [intra- + G. *derma,* skin]. Intracutaneous.

intraduct (in'tră-dŭkt). Within the duct or ducts of a gland.

intradural (in'tră-dū'răl). Within or enclosed by the dura mater.

intraembryonic (in'tră-em-brē-on'ik). Within the embryonic body, *e.g.*, the portion of the umbilical vein within the embryo (in contrast to the portion in the umbilical cord which is discarded at birth). *Cf.* extraembryonic.

intraepidermal (in'tră-ep-i-der'măl). Within the epidermis.

intraepiphysial (in'tră-ep-i-fiz'ē-ăl). Within the epiphysis of a long bone.

intraepithelial (in'tră-ep-i-thē'lē-ăl). Within or among the epithelial cells.

intrafaradization (in'tră-fa-ră-di-zā'shŭn). Application of a faradic cauterizing current to the inner surface of a cavity or hollow organ.

intrafascicular (in'tră-fă-sik'yū-lăr). Within the fasciculi of a tissue or structure (*e.g.*, fasciculus intrafasciculus).

intrafebrile (in'tră-fē'bril, -feb'ril). Intrapyretic; occurring during the febrile stage of a disease.

intrafilar (in'tră-fī'lăr) [intra- + L. *filum,* thread]. Lying within the meshes of a network.

intrafusal (in'tră-fyū'săl). Applied to structures within the muscle spindle.

intragalvanization (in'tră-gal-van-i-zā'shŭn). Application of a galvanic cauterizing current to the interior of a cavity or hollow organ.

intragastric (in'tră-gas'trik). Within the stomach.

intragemmal (in'tră-jem'ăl) [intra- + L. *gemma,* bud]. Within any budlike or bulblike body; denoting especially a nerve termination within an end bulb or taste bud.

intraglandular (in'tră-glan'dū-lăr). Within a gland or glandular tissue.

intraglobular (in'tră-glob'yū-lăr). **1.** Within a globule in any sense. **2.** Intracorpuscular.

intragyral (in'tră-jī'răl). Within a gyrus or convolution of the brain.

intrahepatic (in'tră-he-pat'ik). Within the liver.

intrahyoid (in'tră-hī'oyd). Within the hyoid bone; denoting certain accessory thyroid glands that lie in the hollow or within the substance of the hyoid bone.

intralaryngeal (in'tră-lă-rin'jē-ăl). Within the larynx.

intraligamentous (in'tră-lig-ă-men'tŭs). Within a ligament, especially the broad ligament of the uterus.

intralobar (in'tră-lō'bar). Within a lobe of any organ or other structure.

intralobular (in'tră-lob'yū-lăr). Within a lobule.

intralocular (in-tră-lok'yū-lăr). Within the loculi of any structure or part.

intraluminal (in-tră-lū'mi-năl). Intratubal.

intramedullary (in'tră-med'yū-lăr-ē). **1.** Within the bone marrow; **2.** Within the spinal cord; **3.** Within the medulla oblongata.

intramembranous (in'tră-mem'bră-nŭs). **1.** Within, or between the layers of, a membrane. **2.** Denoting a method of bone formation directly from mesenchymal cells without an intervening cartilage stage, as distinguished from intracartilaginous bone formation.

intrameningeal (in'tră-mē-nin'jē-ăl). Within or enclosed by the meninges of the brain or spinal cord.

intramolecular (in'tră-mō-lek'yū-lăr). Referring to situations and events within a molecule.

intramural (in'tră-myū'răl). Intraparietal (1); within the substance of the wall of any cavity or hollow organ.

intramuscular (I.M., i.m.) (in'tră-mŭs'kyū-lăr). Within the substance of a muscle.

intramyocardial (in'tră-mī'ō-kar'dē-ăl). Within the myocardium.

intramyometrial (in'tră-mī'ō-mē'trē-ăl). Within the muscular coat of the uterus.

intranasal (in'tră-nā'săl). Within the nasal cavity.

intranatal (in'tră-nā'tăl) [intra- + L. *natalis,* relating to birth]. During or at the time of birth.

intraneural (in'tră-nū'răl) [intra- + G. *neuron,* nerve]. Within a nerve.

intranuclear (in'tră-nū'klē-ăr). Within the nucleus of a cell.

intraocular (in'tră-ok'yū-lăr). Within the eyeball.

intraoral (in'tră-ō'răl) [intra- + L. *os,* mouth]. Within the mouth.

intraorbital (in'tră-ōr'bi-tăl). Within the orbit.

intraosseous (in'tră-os'ē-ŭs) [intra- + L. *os,* bone]. Intraosteal; within bone.

intraosteal (in'tră-os'tēăl). Intraosseous.

intraovarian (in'tră-ō-vā'rē-an). Within the ovary.

intraovular (in'tră-ov'yū-lăr). Within the ovum.

intraparietal (in'tră-pă-rī'ē-tăl). **1.** Intramural. **2.** Denoting the intraparietal sulcus.

intrapartum (in'tră-par'tŭm) [intra- + L. *partus,* childbirth]. During labor and delivery or childbirth. *Cf.* antepartum; postpartum.

intrapelvic (in'tră-pel'vik). Within the pelvis.

intrapericardiac, intrapericardial (in'tră-per'ē-kar'dē-ak, -kar'dē-ăl). Endopericardiac; within the pericardial cavity.

intraperitoneal (I.P., i.p.) (in'tră-per'i-tō-nē'ăl). Within the peritoneal cavity.

intrapersonal (in'tră-per'sŏn-ăl). Intrapsychic.

intrapial (in'tră-pī'ăl). Within the pia mater.

intrapleural (in'tră-plū'răl). Within the pleura or the pleural cavity.

intrapontine (in'tră-pon'tīn). Within the pons of the brainstem.

intraprostatic (in'tră-pros-tat'ik). Within the prostate gland.

intraprotoplasmic (in'tră-prō-tō-plas'mik). Within the protoplasm of a cell.

intrapsychic (in'tră-sī'kik). Intrapersonal; denoting the psychological dynamics that occur inside the mind without reference to the individual's exchanges with other persons or events.

intrapulmonary (in'tră-pul'mo-nār-ē). Within the lungs.

intrapyretic (in'tră-pī-ret'ik) [intra- + L. *pyretos,* fever]. Intrafebrile.

intrarectal (in'tră-rek'tăl). Within the rectum.

intrarenal (in'tră-rē'năl) [intra- + L. *ren,* kidney]. Within the kidney.

intraretinal (in'tră-ret'i-năl). Within the retina.

intrarrhachidian, intrarachidian, (in'tră-ră-kid'ē-an) [intra- + G. *rachis,* spine]. Intraspinal.

intrascrotal (in'tră-skrō'tăl). Within the scrotum.

intraspinal (in'tră-spī'năl). Intrarrhachidian; intrarachidian; within the vertebral canal or spinal cord.

intrasplenic (in'tră-splen'ik). Within the spleen.

intrastromal (in'tră-strō'măl). Within the stroma or foundation substance of any organ or part.

intrasynovial (in'tră-si-nō'vē-ăl). Within the synovial sac of a joint or a synovial tendon sheath.

intratarsal (in'tră-tar'săl). Within the tarsus; among the tarsal bones.

intrathecal (in'tră-thē'kăl). **1.** Within a sheath. **2.** Within either the subarachnoid or the subdural space.

intrathoracic (in'tră-thō-ras'ik). Within the cavity of the chest.

intratonsillar (in'tră-ton-si-lăr). Within the substance of a tonsil.

intratubal (in'tră-tū'băl). Intraluminal; within any tube.

intratubular (in'tră-tū'byū-lăr). Within any tubule.

intratympanic (in'tră-tim-pan'ik). Within the middle ear or tympanic cavity.

intrauterine (in'tră-yū'ter-in). Within the uterus.

intravasation (in'trav-ă-sā'shŭn) [intra- + L. *vas,* vessel]. Entrance of foreign matter into a blood vessel.

intravascular (in'tră-vas'kyū-lăr). Within the blood vessels or lymphatics.

intravenation (in'tră-ven-ā'shŭn). Entrance of foreign matter into vein.

intravenous (I.V., i.v.) (in'tră-vē'nŭs). Endovenous; within a vein or veins.

intraventric'ular (I-V) (in'tră-ven-trik'yū-lăr). Within a ventricle of the brain or heart.

intravesical (in'tră-ves'i-kăl). Within a bladder, especially the urinary bladder.

intra vitam (in'tră vī'tăm) [L. *vita,* life]. During life.

intravitelline (in'tră-vi-tel'in, -ēn). Within the vitellus or yolk.

intravitreous (in'tră-vit'rē-ŭs). Within the vitreous body.

intrinsic (in-trin'sik) [L. *intrinsecus,* on the inside]. **1.** Inherent; belonging entirely to a part. **2.** In anatomy, denoting those muscles of the limbs whose origin and insertion are both in the same limb or segment of a limb, distinguished from the extrinsic muscles which have their origin in some part of the trunk outside of the pelvic or shoulder girdle; applied also to the ciliary muscle as distinguished from the recti and other orbital muscles which are on the eyeball.

intro- [L. *intro,* into]. Prefix meaning in or into.

introducer (in-trō-dūs'er) [L. *intro-duco,* to lead into, introduce]. Intubator; an instrument, such as a catheter, needle, or endotracheal tube, for introduction of a flexible device.

introflection, introflexion (in'trō-flek'shŭn) [intro- + L. *flecto,* pp. *flectus,* to bend]. A bending inward.

introgastric (in-trō-gas'trik) [intro- + G. *gastēr,* belly, stomach]. Leading or passed into the stomach.

introitus (in-trō'i-tŭs) [L. entrance, fr. *intro-eo,* to go into]. The entrance into a canal or hollow organ, as the vagina.

introjection (in-trō-jek'shŭn) [intro- + L. *jacto,* to throw]. A psychological defense mechanism involving appropriation of an external happening and its assimilation by the personality, making it a part of the self.

intromission (in-trō-mish'ŭn) [intro- + L. *mitto,* to send]. The insertion or introduction of one part into another.

intromittent (in-trō-mit'ent). Conveying or sending into a body or cavity.

intron (in'tron). Intervening sequence; a portion of DNA that lies between two exons, is transcribed into RNA as usual, but does not appear in that RNA after maturation, and so is not expressed (as protein) in protein synthesis.

introspection (in-trō-spek'shŭn) [intro- + L. *specto,* to look at, inspect]. Looking inward; self-scrutinizing; contemplating one's own mental processes.

introspective (in-trō-spek'tiv). Relating to introspection.

introsusception (in'trō-sŭs-sep'shŭn). Intussusception.

introversion (in-trō-ver'zhŭn) [intro- + L. *verto,* pp. *versus,* to turn]. **1.** The turning of a structure into itself. See also intussusception, invagination. **2.** A trait of preoccupation with oneself, as practiced by an introvert. *Cf.* extraversion.

introvert **1** (in'trō-vert). One who tends to be introspective, self-centered, and takes small interest in the affairs of others. *Cf.* extrovert. **2** (in-trō-vert'). To turn a structure into itself.

intubate (in'tū-bāt). To perform intubation.

intubation (in-tū-bā'shŭn) [L. *in,* in, + *tuba,* tube]. Insertion of a tubular device into a canal, hollow organ, or cavity; specifically, passage of an oro- or nasotracheal tube for anesthesia or for control of pulmonary ventilation.
altercursive i., diversion of secretion intermittently to the exterior from its normal destination, *e.g.,* of the bile from the intestine.
aqueductal i., insertion of a tube in the sylvian aqueduct to relieve atresia or narrowing of the aqueduct.
blind nasotracheal i., passage of an endotracheal tube through the nose and into the larynx without using a laryngoscope.
endotracheal i., intratracheal i.; passage of a tube through the nose or mouth into the trachea for maintenance of the airway during anesthesia or for maintenance of an imperiled airway.
intratracheal i., endotracheal i.
nasotracheal i., endotracheal i. through the nose.
orotracheal i., endotracheal i. through the mouth.

intubator (in'tū-bā-tōr). Introducer.

intumesce (in-tū-mes') [L. *in- tumesco,* to swell up, fr. *tumeo,* to swell]. To swell up; to enlarge.

intumescence (in-tū-mes'ens). **1.** Intumescentia. **2.** The process of enlarging or swelling; used to describe the spinal enlargements.
tympanic i., *intumescentia* tympanica.

intumescent (in-tū-mes'ent). Enlarging; swelling; becoming enlarged or swollen.

intumescentia (in-tū-mes-sen'shē-ă) [Mod. L.] [NA]. Intumescence (1); an anatomical swelling, enlargement, or prominence.
i. cervica'lis [NA], cervical enlargement of the spinal cord; a spindle-shaped swelling of the spinal cord extending from the third cervical to the second thoracic vertebra, with maximum thickness opposite the fifth or sixth cervical vertebra.
i. gangliofor'mis, *ganglion* geniculi.
i. lumba'lis [NA], lumbar enlargement of spinal cord; a spindle-shaped swelling of the spinal cord beginning at the level of the tenth thoracic vertebra and tapering into the conus medullaris, with maximum thickness opposite the last thoracic vertebra.
i. tympan'ica, tympanic intumescence; a swelling, not ganglionic, on the tympanic branch of the glossopharyngeus nerve; it is regarded as possibly similar to the carotid glomus.

intussusception (in'tŭs-sŭ-sep'shŭn) [L. *intus,* within, + *sus- cipio,* to take up, fr. *sub* + *capio,* to take]. Introsusception; the taking up or receiving of one part within another, especially the infolding of one segment of the intestine within another. See also introversion; invagination.
colic i., the ensheathing of one portion of the colon into another.
double i., a second i. that involves the bowel above the first; the first i. is followed by contraction of the bowel wall around it, and the solid mass so formed is enveloped by the proximal portion of the bowel and is thus the cause of the second i.
ileal i., i. in which one portion of the ileum is ensheathed in another portion of the same division of the bowel.

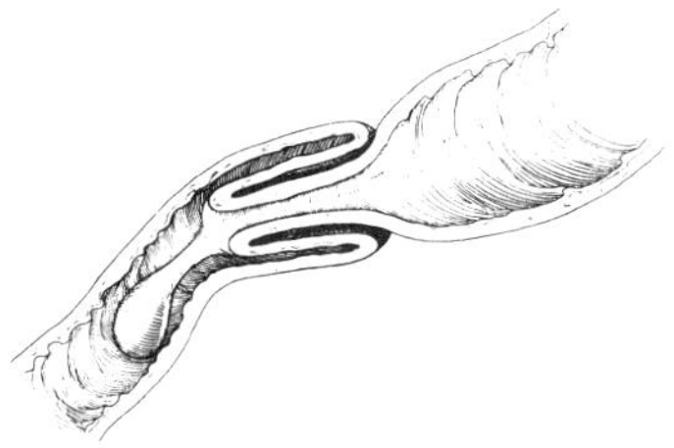

Ileal Intussusception with Pedunculated Tumor

ileocecal i., i. in which the lower segment of the ileum passes through the valve of the colon into the cecum.
ileocolic i., i. in which the lower portion of the ileum with the valve of the cecum passes into the ascending colon.
jejunogastric i., a rare complication following gastrojejunostomy in which the afferent or the efferent loop of bowel invaginates into the stomach.
retrograde i., the invagination of a lower segment of the bowel into one just above.

intussusceptive (in'tŭs-sŭ-sep'tiv). Relating to or characterized by intussusception.

intussusceptum (in'tŭs-sŭ-sep'tŭm). The inner segment in an intussusception; that part of the bowel which is received within the other part.

intussuscipiens (in'tŭs-sŭ-sip'ē-enz) [L. *intus,* within, + *suscipiens,* pr. p. of *suscipio,* to take up]. The portion of the bowel, in intussusception, which receives the other portion.

inulase (in'yū-lās). Inulinase.

inulin (in'yū-lin). Dahlin; alant starch; alantin; a fructose polysaccharide from the rhizome of *Inula helenium* or *elecampane* (family Compositae) and other plants; a hygroscopic powder used by intravenous injection to determine the rate of glomerular filtration. *Cf.* i. *clearance.* Also used in bread for diabetics.

inulinase (in'yū-lin-ās) [EC 3.2.1.7]. Inulase; an enzyme acting upon 2,1-β-D-fructoside links in inulin, releasing fructose.

inulol (in'yū-lol). Alantol.

inunction (in-ŭngk'shŭn) [L. *inunctio,* an anointing, fr. *inunguo,* pp.

-unctus, to smear on]. Administration of a drug in ointment form by rubbing to cause absorption of the active ingredient.

in utero (in yū'ter-ō) [L.]. Within the womb; not yet born.

invaccination (in-vak-si-nā'shŭn). Accidental inoculation of some disease, *e.g.*, syphilis, during vaccination.

in vacuo (in vak'yū-ō) [L.]. In a vacuum, *i.e.*, under reduced pressure.

invaginate (in-vaj'i-nāt) [L. *in*, in, + *vagina*, a sheath]. To ensheathe, infold, or insert a structure within itself or another.

invagination (in-vaj'i-nā'shŭn). **1.** The ensheathing, infolding, or insertion of a structure within itself or another. **2.** The state of being invaginated. See also introversion; intussusception.
basilar i., platybasia.

invaginator (in-vag'i-nā-ter, -tōr). An instrument for pushing inward any tissue.

invalid (in'vă-lid) [L. *in-* neg. + *validus*, strong]. **1.** Weak; sick. **2.** A person in a disabling but not necessarily completely incapacitating condition.

invalidism (in'vă-lid-izm). The condition of being an invalid.

invasin (in-vā'sin). Hyaluronidase (1).

invasion (in-vā'zhŭn) [L. *invasio*, fr. *in- vado*, pp. *-vasus*, to go into, attack]. **1.** The beginning or incursion of a disease. **2.** Local spread of a malignant neoplasm by infiltration or destruction of adjacent tissue; for epithelial neoplasms, i. signifies infiltration beneath the epithelial basement membrane.

invasive (in-vā'siv). **1.** Denoting or characterized by invasion. **2.** Denoting a procedure requiring insertion of an instrument or device into the body through the skin or a body orifice for diagnosis or treatment.

inventory (in'ven-tōr-ē). A detailed, often descriptive, list of items.
personality i., a psychological test for evaluation of habitual modes of behavior, thinking, and feeling relevant to one's peer group.

invermination (in-ver-mi-nā'shŭn) [L. *in*, in, + *vermis* (*vermin-*), worm]. Helminthiasis.

inversion (in-ver'zhŭn) [L. *inverto*, pp. *-versus*, to turn upside down, to turn about]. **1.** A turning inward, upside down, or in any direction contrary to the existing one. **2.** Conversion of a disaccharide or polysaccharide by hydrolysis into a monosaccharide; specifically, the hydrolysis of sucrose to glucose and fructose; so called because of the change in optical activity. **3.** Alteration of a DNA molecule made by removing a fragment, reversing its orientation, and putting it back into place. **4.** Heat-induced transition of silica, in which the quartz tridymite or cristobalite changes its physical properties as to thermal expansion.
i. of chromosomes, a chromosome aberration resulting from a double break in a segment of the chromosome, with end for end rotation of the fragment between the fracture lines, and refusion of the fragments; this results in reversal of the order of genes in the segment.
paracentric i., i. in a chromosome of a single segment in which the centromere is not included.
pericentric i., i. in a chromosome of a single segment that includes the centromere.
i. of the uterus, a turning of the uterus inside out, usually following childbirth.
visceral i., *situs* inversus.

invert (in'vert) [see inversion]. **1.** In chemistry, subjected to inversion, *e.g.*, invert sugar. **2.** Rarely used term for a homosexual.

invertase (in'ver-tās). β-Fructofuranosidase.

Invertebrata (in-ver-tĕ-brā'tă). A general category of the kingdom Animalia (multicellular animals) including those phyla whose members lack a notochord; *i.e.*, all animals except vertebrates in the phylum Chordata.

invertebrate (in-ver'tĕ-brāt). **1.** Not possessed of a spinal or vertebral column. **2.** Any animal except the craniate members of the phylum Chordata.

invertin (in'ver-tin). β-Fructofuranosidase.

invertor (in-ver'ter, -tōr) [see inversion]. A muscle that inverts or causes inversion or turns a part, such as the foot, inward.

invest'ing. 1. In dentistry, covering or enveloping wholly or in part an object such as a denture, tooth, wax form, crown, etc., with a refractory investment material before curing, soldering, or casting. **2.** In psychoanalysis, charging an object with psychic energy or cathexis.
vacuum i., the i. of a pattern within a vacuum.

invest'ment. 1. In dentistry, any material used in investing. **2.** In psychoanalysis, the psychic charge or cathexis invested in an object.
refractory i., an i. material which can withstand the high temperatures used in soldering or casting.

inveterate (in-vet'er-āt) [L. *in-vetero*, pp. *-atus*, to render old, fr. *vetus*, old]. Chronic; long seated; firmly established; said of a disease or of confirmed habits.

inviscation (in-vis-kā'shŭn) [L. *in*, in, on, + *viscum*, birdlime]. **1.** Smearing with mucilaginous matter. **2.** The mixing of the food, during mastication, with the buccal secretions.

in vitro (in vē'trō) [L. in glass]. In an artificial environment, referring to a process or reaction occurring therein, as in a test tube or culture media. *Cf.* in vivo.

in vivo (in vē'vō) [L. in the living being]. In the living body, referring to a process or reaction occurring therein. *Cf.* in vitro.

involucre (in'vō-lū-ker). Involucrum.

involucrin (in-vō-lū'krin) [fr. L. *involucrum*, a wrapper]. A nonkeratin soluble precursor of the highly cross-linked protein known as the corneocyte envelope.

involucrum, pl. **involucra** (in-vō-lū'krŭm, -lū'kră) [L. a wrapper, fr. *in-volvo*, to roll up]. Involucre. **1.** An enveloping membrane, *e.g.*, a sheath or sac. **2.** The sheath of new bone that forms around a sequestrum.

involuntary (in-vol'ŭn-tār-ē) [L. *in-* neg. + *voluntarius*, willing, fr. *volo*, to wish]. **1.** Independent of the will; not volitional. **2.** Contrary to the will.

involution (in-vō-lū'shŭn) [L. *in-volvo*, pp. *-volutus*, to roll up]. Catagenesis. **1.** Return of an enlarged organ to normal size. **2.** Turning inward of the edges of a part. **3.** In psychiatry, mental decline associated with advanced age.
senile i., the retrogression of vital organs and processes incident to aging.
i. of the uterus, the process of reduction of the uterus to its normal nonpregnant size and state following childbirth.

involutional (in-vō-lū'shŭn-ăl). Relating to involution.

iobenzamic acid (ī-ō-ben-zam'ik). *N*- (3-Amino-2,4,6-triiodobenzoyl)-*N*- phenyl-β-alanine; a radiographic contrast medium.

iocetamic acid (ī'ō-sē-tam'ik). *N*-Acetyl-*N*-(3-amino-2,4,6-triiodophenyl)-2-methyl-β-alanine; a radiopaque contrast medium.

iodamide (ī-ō'dă-mīd). Ametriodinic acid; α,5-diacetamide-2,4,6-triiodo-*m*-toluic acid; a radiopaque contrast medium.

Iodamoeba (ī-od-ă-mē'bă). A genus of parasitic amebae in the superclass Rhizopoda, order Amoebida.
I. bütsch'lii, a parasitic ameba in the large intestine of man; trophozoites are usually 9 to 14 μm in diameter; the cysts are usually 8 to 10 μm in diameter, uninucleate and somewhat irregular in shape, with a thick wall and a large compact mass of glycogen that stains deeply with a solution of iodine; clinically recognizable amebiasis caused by this organism is rare, but probably occurs, with

symptoms resembling those of chronic disease caused by *Entamoeba histolytica;* it is also found in other primates and is the commonest ameba of pigs.

iodate (ī'ō-dāt). A salt of iodic acid.

iodic (ī-od'ik). **1.** Relating to, or caused by, iodine or an iodide. **2.** Denoting a compound of iodine in its pentavalent state.

iodic acid. HIO_3; crystalline powder, soluble in water; used as an astringent, caustic, disinfectant, deodorant, and intestinal antiseptic.

iodide (ī'ō-dīd). The negative ion of iodine, I^-.

i. peroxidase [EC 1.11.1.8], iodotyrosine deiodase; iodinase; an oxidoreductase catalyzing reactions between iodine and water to yield iodide and H_2O_2; also catalyzes iodination and deiodination of tyrosine compounds.

iodimetry (ī-ō-dim'ĕ-trē) [iodine + G. *metron,* measure]. Iodometry.

iodinase (ī'ō-din-ās). *Iodide* peroxidase.

iodinate (ī'ō-di-nāt). To treat or combine with iodine.

iodine (ī'ō-dīn, -dēn) [G. *iōdēs,* violet-like, fr. *ion,* a violet, + *eidos,* form]. Iodum; a nonmetallic chemical element, symbol I, atomic no. 53, atomic weight 126.91; used in the manufacture of i. compounds and as a catalyst, reagent, tracer, topical antiseptic, therapy in thyroid disease, antidote for alkaloidal poisons, and in certain stains and solutions.

butanol-extractable i. (BEI), i. that can be separated from plasma proteins by butanol or other extractable solvents; used to measure thyroid function.

Gram's i., a solution containing i. and potassium iodide, used in Gram's stain.

protein-bound i. (PBI), thyroid hormone in its circulating form, consisting of one or more of the iodothyronines bound to one or more of the serum proteins.

radioactive i., the i. radioisotopes ^{131}I, ^{125}I, or ^{123}I used as tracers in biology and medicine.

tamed i., iodophor.

iodine-123 (^{123}I). A radioisotope of iodine with a pure gamma emission and a physical half-life of 13.1 hr, used for studies of thyroid disease.

iodine-125 (^{125}I). Radioactive iodine isotope that decays by K-capture (internal conversion) with a half-life of 60 days; used as a tracer in thyroid studies and as a label in immunoassay.

iodine-127 (^{127}I). Stable, nonradioactive iodine; it is the most abundant iodide isotope found in nature.

iodine-131 (^{131}I). A radioactive iodine isotope; beta emitter with a half-life of 8.05 days; used as a tracer in thyroid studies, as therapy in hyperthyroidism and thyroid cancer, and as a label in immunoassay.

iodine-132 (^{132}I). A gamma-emitting radioisotope of iodine with a physical half-life of 2.4 hr, usually obtained from a tellurium-132 radionuclide generator; its clinical use has been supplanted by ^{131}I and ^{123}I.

iodine-fast. Denoting hyperthyroidism unresponsive to iodine therapy, which develops frequently in most cases so treated.

iodinophil, iodinophile (ī-ō-din'ō-fil, -fīl) [iodine + G. *philos,* fond]. **1.** Iodinophilous; staining readily with iodine. **2.** Any histologic element that stains readily with iodine.

iodinophilous (ī-ō-din-of'i-lŭs). Iodinophil (1).

iodipamide (ī-ō-dip'ă-mīd). Adipiodone; 3,3′- (adipoyldiimino) bis[2,4,6-triiodobenzoic acid]; a radiographic contrast medium for the biliary system.

i. sodium, sodium salt of i., for injection.

iodism (ī'ō-dizm). Poisoning by iodine, a condition marked by severe coryza, an acneform eruption, weakness, salivation, and foul breath; caused by the continuous administration of iodine or one of the iodides.

iodize (ī'ō-dīz). To treat or impregnate with iodine.

iodized oil (ī'ō-dīzd). An iodine addition product of vegetable oils, containing not less than 38% and not more than 42% of organically combined iodine; a radiopaque medium.

iodoacetamide (ī-ō'dō-ă-sē'tă-mīd). ICH_2-$CONH_2$; a chemical reacting readily with sulfhydryl groups and therefore a strong inhibitor of many enzymes.

iodoalphionic acid (ī-ō'dō-al-fē-on'ik). β-(4-Hydroxy-3,5-diiodophenyl)-α-phenylpropionic acid; a rarely used radiographic contrast medium.

iodocasein (ī-ō-dō-kā'sēn). A compound of iodine with casein, in which the iodine is attached to tyrosine molecules; possesses thyroxine activity.

iodochlorhydroxyquin, iodochlorohydroxyquinoline (ī'ō-dō-klōr'hī-drok'si-kwin, -klōr'ō-hī-drok'si-kwin'ō-lēn). Chloriodoquin; clioquinol; 5-chloro-7-iodo-8-quinolinol; 5-chloro-8-hydroxy-7-iodoquinoline; used topically as a local anti-infective and in a wide range of dermatoses, intravaginally in *Trichomonas vaginalis* vaginitis, and internally for the treatment of mild or asymptomatic intestinal amebiasis.

iodochlorol (ī'ō-dō-klōr'ol). Chloriodized oil.

iododerma (ī-ō'dō-der'mă). An eruption of follicular papules and pustules, or a granulomatous lesion, caused by iodine toxicity or sensitivity.

iodoform (ī-ō'dō-fōrm). Triiodomethane; CHI_3; a topical antiseptic.

iodoglobulin (ī-ō'dō-glob'yū-lin). Thyroglobulin (1).

iodogorgoic acid (ī-ō'dō-gōr-gō'ik). 3,5-Diiodotyrosine; a precursor of thyroxine.

iodohippurate sodium (ī-ō'dō-hip'pū-rāt). Sodium *o*-iodohippurate; a radiopaque compound used intravenously, orally, or for retrograde urography. When tagged with iodine-131, it is used to measure renal function externally in radioisotopic renography.

iodomethamate sodium (ī-ō'dō-meth'ă-māt). Disodium *N*-methyl-3,5-diiodo-4-pyridone-2,6-dicarboxylate; an organic iodine radiopaque compound formerly used in intravenous urography or retrograde pyelography.

iodometric (ī-ō'dō-met'rik). Relating to iodometry.

iodometry (ī-ō-dom'ĕ-trē) [iodine + G. *metron,* measure]. Iodimetry; analytical techniques involving titrations in which iodine is either formed or consumed, the sudden appearance or disappearance of iodine marking the end point.

iodopanoic acid (ī-ō'dō-pa-nō'ik). Iopanoic acid.

iodophendylate (ī-ō'dō-fen'dil-āt). Iophendylate.

iodophilia (ī-ō'dō-fil'ē-ă) [iodine + G. *phileō,* to love]. An affinity for iodine, as manifested by some leukocytes in certain conditions. When treated with a solution of iodine and potassium iodide, normal polymorphonuclear leukocytes stain a fairly bright yellow; in certain pathologic conditions, the polymorphonuclear leukocytes frequently stain diffusely brown or yellow-brown; the reaction may be intracellular (as described) or extracellular, affecting the particles in the immediate vicinity of the leukocytes.

iodophor (ī-ō'dō-fōr) [iodine + G. *phora,* a carrying]. Tamed iodine; a combination of iodine with a surfactant carrier, usually polyvinylpyrrolidone. Commercial preparations generally contain 1% "available" iodine, which is slowly released to take effect against microorganisms; used as skin disinfectants, particularly for surgical scrubs.

iodophthalein (ī-ō'dō-thal'ēn, -dof-thal'e-in). Tetraiodophenolphthalein sodium; the disodium salt has been used in x-ray examination of the gallbladder.

iodoproteins (ī-ō'dō-prō'tēnz). Proteins containing iodine bound to tyrosine groups.

iodopsin (ī-ō-dop'sin). Visual violet; a visual pigment, composed of 11-*cis*-retinal bound to an opsin, found in the cones of the retina.

iodopyracet (ī-ō'dō-pī'ră-set). Diodone; diethanolamine acetate; 3,5-diiodo-4-pyridone-*N*- acetate; a radiopaque medium used intravenously in urography; also used to determine the renal plasma flow and the renal tubular excretory mass.

iodotherapy (ī'ō-dō-thār'ă-pē). Treatment with iodine.

iodothyronines (ī-ō'dō-thī'rō-nēnz). Iodinated derivatives of thyronine.

iodotyrosine (ī-ō'dō-tī'rō-sēn). An iodinated tyrosine.
i. deiodase, *iodide* peroxidase.

iodoxamate meglumine (ī-ō-doks'ă-māt). 3,3'-[Ethylenebis(oxyethylene-oxyethylenecarbonylimino)]bis-[2,4,6-triiodobenzoic acid] compound with 1-deoxy-1-(methylamino)-D-glucitol (1:2); a radiopaque medium used primarily for cholecystography.

iodum (ī'ō-dŭm) [L.]. Iodine.

ioduria (ī-ō-dū'rē-ă). Urinary excretion of iodine.

ioglycamic acid (ī'ō-glī-kam'ik). 3,3'-(Diglycoloyldiimino) bis(2,4,6-triiodobenzoic acid); radiographic contrast medium for the biliary system.

iohexol (ī-ō-heks'ol). $C_{19}H_{26}I_3N_3O_9$; a diagnostic radiopaque medium used intrathecally and intravascularly.

iometer (ī-om'ĕ-ter) [ion + G. *metron,* measure]. An apparatus for measuring ionization.

ion (ī'on) [G. *iōn,* going]. An atom or group of atoms carrying an electric charge by virtue of having gained or lost one or more valence electrons. I.'s charged with negative electricity (anions) travel toward a positive pole (anode); those charged with positive electricity (cations) travel toward a negative pole (cathode). I.'s may exist in solid, liquid, or gaseous environments, although those in liquid (electrolytes) are more common and familiar.
aquo-i., see *aquo-ion.*
dipolar i.'s, zwitterions; i.'s possessing both a negative charge and a positive charge, each localized at a different point in the molecule which thus has both positive and negative "poles"; amino acids are the most notable dipolar i.'s, containing a positively charged NH_3^+ group and a negatively charged COO^- group attached to carbon-2 (the α-carbon atom).
gram-i., see *gram-ion.*
hydride i., the H^- i., transferred to acceptor molecules in some biological oxidations.
hydrogen i. (H^+), a hydrogen atom minus its electron and therefore carrying a unit positive charge; in water, it combines with a water molecule to form hydronium i., H_3O^+.
hydronium i., oxonium i.; the hydrated proton, H_3O^+, the form in which hydrogen i. exists in aqueous solutions.
oxonium i., hydronium i.
sulfonium i., a compound in which a sulfur atom has three single covalent bonds and therefore has a positive charge analogous to the nitrogen of an ammonium compound; *e.g., S-* adenosylmethionine.

Ionescu. See Jonnesco.

ion exchange (ī'on eks-chanj'). See anion exchange; cation exchange.

ion exchanger (ī'on eks-chanj'er). See anion exchanger; cation exchanger.

ionic (ī-on'ik). Relating to an ion.

ionium (ī-ō'nē-ŭm) [G. *iōn,* going]. Former term for thorium-230.

ionization (ī'on-i-zā'shŭn). **1.** Dissociation into ions, occurring when an electrolyte is dissolved in water or certain liquids, or when molecules are subjected to electrical discharge or ionizing radiation. **2.** Production of ions as a result of interaction of radiation with matter. **3.** Iontophoresis.

ionize (ī'on-īz). To separate into ions; to dissociate atoms or molecules into electrically charged atoms or radicals.

ionogram (ī'on-ō-gram). Electropherogram.

ionone (ī'ō-nōn). A cyclic ketone with an odor of violets, the α and B varieties of which differ in the location of the double bond in the ring: provitamins A and vitamin A have i. configuration in the ring portion; α-carotene contains one α- and one β-ionone, β-carotene contains two β-ionones, and γ-carotene contains one β-ionone.

ionopherogram (ī'on-ō-fer'ō-gram). Electropherogram.

ionophore (ī-on'ō-fōr) [ion + G. *phore,* a bearer]. A compound or substance that forms a complex with an ion and transports it across a membrane; Na^+, Ca^{2+}.

ionophoresis (ī-on'ō-fōr-ē'sis) [ion + G. *phorēsis,* a carrying]. Electrophoresis.

ionophoretic (ī-on'ō-fōr-et'ik). Electrophoretic.

iontophoresis (ī-on'tō-fōr-ē'sis) [ion + G. *phorēsis,* a carrying]. Iontotherapy; ionization (2); ionic medication; the introduction into the tissues, by means of an electric current, of the ions of a chosen medicament.

iontophoretic (ī-on'tō-fōr-et'ik). Relating to iontophoresis.

iontoquantimeter (ī-on'tō-kwon-tim'ĕ-ter) [ion + L. *quantus,* how much, + G. *metron,* measure]. An obsolete device for determining the quantity of x-rays by measuring the resulting ionization.

iontotherapy (ī-on'tō-thār'ă-pē). Iontophoresis.

iopamidol (ī-ō-pam'i-dol). $C_{17}H_{22}I_3N_3O_8$; a diagnostic radiopaque medium used in myelography, arteriography, urography and ventriculography.

iopanoic acid (ī'ō-pa-nō'ik). Iodopanoic acid; 3-amino-α-ethyl-2,4,6-triiodohydrocinnamic acid; a creamy, organic, radiopaque iodine compound, insoluble in water; used as a contrast medium in cholecystography.

iophendylate (ī-ō-fen'dil-āt). Iodophendylate; ethyl 10-(*p*-iodophenyl)undecylate; a mixture of isomers of ethyl iodophenylundecylate, an absorbable iodized fatty acid of low viscosity; used for roentgenography of the spinal cord, biliary tree, sinuses, and body cavities.

iophenoxic acid (ī'ō-fen-oks'ik). α-Ethyl-3-hydroxy-2,4,6-triiodohydrocinnamic acid; a radiographic contrast medium.

iophobia (ī-ō-fō'bē-ă) [G. *ios,* poison, + *phobos,* fear]. Morbid fear of poisons.

iotacism (ī-ō'tă-sizm) [G. *iōta,* the letter i]. A speech defect marked by the frequent substitution of a long *e* sound (that of the Greek iota) for other vowels.

iothalamate sodium (ī-ō-thal'ă-māt). Sodium salt of iothalamic acid; used as a radiopaque medium.

iothalamic acid (ī'ō-thă-lam'ik). 5-Acetamido-2,4,6-triiodo-*N*-methylisophthalamic acid; an x-ray contrast medium.

iothiouracil sodium (ī'ō-thī-ō-yūr'ă-sil). The sodium salt of 5-iodo-2-thiouracil; an organic iodine derivative of thiouracil with the thyroid-involuting action of iodine and the capability inhibiting thyroxine production.

ioxaglate (ī-oks-ag'lāt). A diagnostic radiopaque medium, usually a combination of i. meglumine ($C_{24}H_{21}I_6N_5O_8 \cdot C_7H_{17}NO_5$), and i. sodium ($C_{24}H_{20}I_6N_5NaO_8$). used in angiography, aortography, arteriography, venography, and urography.

I.P., i.p. Abbreviation for intraperitoneal, or intraperitoneally.

ipecac (ip'ē-kak). Ipecacuanha.
powdered i., a form of i. used in the preparation of ipecac syrup.

ipecacuanha (ip-ē-kak-yū-an′ă) [native Brazilian word]. Ipecac; the dried root of *Uragoga (Cephaelis) ipecacuanha* (family Rubiaceae), a shrub of Brazil and other parts of South America; contains emetine, cephaeline, emetamine, ipecacuanhic acid, psychotrine, and methylpsychotrine; has expectorant, emetic, and antidysenteric properties.

de-emetinized i., i. from which the emetic principle has been extracted; has been used as an antidysenteric agent.

prepared i., a fine powder to contain 2% of the total alkaloids of i., calculated as emetine.

ipodate sodium (ī′pō-dāt). Sodium 3-[(dimethylaminomethylene)amino]-2,4,6-triiodohydracinnamate; a radiopaque medium.

ipomea (ī-pō-mē′ă) [G. *ips (ip-)*, a worm, + *homoios*, like]. Orizaba jalap root; Mexican scammony root; the dried root of *Ipomoea orizabensis* (family Convolvulaceae). See also ipomea *resin.*

Ipomoea (ī-pō-mē′ă) [L. ipomea]. A plant genus of the family Convolvulaceae.

I. rubrocoeru′lea var. **prae′cox,** ololiuqui; morning glory (1); the seeds contain lysergic acid amide, isolysergic acid amide, chanoclavine, elymoclavine, and other ergot (indole) alkaloids; ingestion of the seeds produces hallucinatory and euphoric effects.

I. versico′lor, *I. tricolor; I. violacea;* pearly gates; the seeds contain hallucinogenic ergot (indole) alkaloids.

IPPB Abbreviation for intermittent positive pressure *breathing.*

IPPV Abbreviation for intermittent positive pressure *ventilation.*

ipratropium (i-pră-trō′pē-ŭm). (8*r*)-3α-Hydroxy-8-isopropyl-1α*H*,-5α*H*-tropanium bromide(±)-tropate monohydrate; a synthetic quaternary ammonium compound, chemically related to atropine, that has anticholinergic activity and is used as an inhalant in the treatment of bronchospasm.

iproniazid (ī-prō-nī′ă-zid). 1-Isonicotinoyl-2-isopropylhydrazine; an antituberculous and antidepressant agent similar to isoniazid, but more toxic and rarely used; it inhibits monoamine oxidase.

ipronidazole (ī-prō-nī′dă-zōl). 2-Isopropyl-1-methyl-5-nitroimidazole; an antiprotozoal agent.

iproveratril (ī-prō-ver′ă-tril). Verapamil.

iPrSGal Abbreviation for isopropylthiogalactoside.

Ips Abbreviation for pipsyl.

ipsefact (ip′se-fakt) [L. *ipse*, self, + *factum*, a thing done]. All parts or aspects of the environment that an individual, colony, population, or species of animal has modified chemically or physically by its own behavior (*e.g.*, a nest or home, rodent or deer runs, excrement, pheromones).

ipsilateral (ip-si-lat′er-ăl) [L. *ipse*, same, + *latus (later-)*, side]. Homolateral; on the same side, with reference to a given point, *e.g.*, a dilated pupil on the same side as an extradural hematoma with contralateral limbs being paretic.

IPSP Abbreviation for inhibitory postsynaptic *potential.*

IPTG Abbreviation for isopropylthiogalactoside.

IPV Abbreviation for inactivated poliovirus vaccine. See poliovirus *vaccines.*

IQ Abbreviation for intelligence *quotient.*

Ir Symbol for iridium.

IRI Abbreviation for immunoreactive *insulin.*

irid-. See irido-.

iridal (ī′ri-dăl, ir′i-dăl). Iridial; iridian; iridic; relating to the iris.

iridectomy (ir′i-dek′tō-mē) [irido- + G. *ektomē*, excision]. Excision of a portion of the iris.

buttonhole i., peripheral i.

optical i., i. performed for the purpose of improving vision by making an artificial pupil.

peripheral i., stenopeic i.; buttonhole i.; in narrow-angle glaucoma, the surgical removal of a minute portion of the iris at its root; in intracapsular extraction of cataract, removal of one or more minute sections near the peripheral border, leaving the pupillary margin intact.

sector i., an i. in which a portion of the pupillary margin is excised.

stenopeic i., peripheral i.

therapeutic i., an i. performed for the prevention or cure of disease, *e.g.*, angle-closure glaucoma.

iridectropium (ir′i-dek-trō′pē-ŭm) [irido- + G. *ektropion*, everted eyelid]. *Ectropion* uveae.

iridencleisis (ir′i-den-klī′sis) [irido- + G. *enkleiō*, to shut in]. Holth's operation; the incarceration of a portion of the iris by corneoscleral incision in glaucoma to effect filtration between the anterior chamber and subconjunctival space.

iridentropium (ir′i-den-trō′pē-ŭm) [irido- + G. *entropia*, a turning toward]. *Entropion* uveae.

irideremia (ir′i-der-ē′mē′ă, ī′rid-) [irido- + G. *erēmia*, absence]. Condition wherein the iris is so rudimentary as to appear to be absent. *Cf.* aniridia.

irides (ir′i-dēz) [G.]. Plural of iris.

iridescent (ir-i-des′ent) [G. *iris*, rainbow]. Presenting multiple bright refractile colors, typically as a result of optical interference when incident white light is broken into its spectral components when reflected back through several thin-layered films.

iridesis (i-rid′ē-sis, ī-ri-dē′sis) [irido- + G. *desis*, a binding together]. Iridodesis; ligature of a portion of the iris brought out through an incision in the cornea.

iridial, iridian, iridic (ī-rid′ē-al, ī-rid′ē-an, ī-rid′ik; i-rid′-). Iridal.

iridin (ir′i-din). **1.** Irigenin 7-glucoside from orris root, *Iris florentina.* **2.** Irisin; a resinoid from blue flag, *Iris versicolor;* used as a cholagogue and cathartic.

iridium (i-rid′ē-ŭm). A white, silvery metallic element, symbol Ir, atomic no. 77, atomic weight 192.2.

irido-, irid- [G. *iris (irid-)*, rainbow]. Combining forms relating to the iris.

iridoavulsion (ir′i-dō-ă-vŭl′shŭn). Avulsion, or tearing away, of the iris.

iridocele (ir′i-dō-sēl) [irido- + G. *kēlē*, hernia]. Herniation of a portion of the iris through a corneal defect.

iridochoroiditis (ir′i-dō-kō-roy-dī′tis). Inflammation of both iris and choroid.

iridocoloboma (ir′i-dō-ko-lō-bō′mă) [irido- + G. *kolobōma*, coloboma]. A coloboma or congenital defect of the iris.

iridocorneal (ir′i-dō-kōr′nē-ăl). Relating to the iris and the cornea.

iridocyclectomy (ir′i-dō-sī-klek′tō-mē) [irido- + G. *kyklos*, circle (ciliary body), + *ektomē*, excision]. Removal of the iris and ciliary body for excision of a tumor.

iridocyclitis (ir′i-dō-sī-klī′tis) [irido- + G. *kyklos*, circle (ciliary body), + *-itis*, inflammation]. Inflammation of both iris and ciliary body. See also iritis; uveitis.

hypertensive i., secondary glaucoma due to vasodilation of the iris or obstruction of intraocular circulation with inflammatory cells.

i. sep′tica, Behçet's *syndrome.*

iridocyclochoroiditis (ir′i-dō-sī′klō-kō-royd-ī′tis). Inflammation of the iris, involving the ciliary body and the choroid.

iridocystectomy (ir′i-dō-sis-tek′tō-mē) [irido- + G. *kystis*, bladder (capsule), + *ektomē*, excision]. An operation for making an artificial pupil when posterior synechiae follow extracapsular extraction of cataract; the border of the iris and a portion of the capsule of the lens are drawn out through an incision in the cornea and cut off.

iridodesis (ir-i-dod'ĕ-sis). Obsolete term for iridesis.

iridodiagnosis (ir'i-dō-dī-ag-nō'sis). Diagnosis of systemic affections through observation of changes in form and color of the iris.

iridodialysis (ir'i-dō-dī-al'i-sis) [irido- + G. *dialysis,* loosening]. A colobomatous defect of the iris caused by its separation from the scleral spur.

iridodiastasis (ir'i-dō-dī-as'tă-sis) [irido- + G. *diastasis,* a separation]. A colobomatous defect affecting the peripheral border of the iris with an intact pupil.

iridodilator (ir'i-dō-dī-lā'ter). Causing dilation of the pupil; applied to the musculus dilator pupillae.

iridodonesis (ir'i-dō-dō-nē'sis) [irido- + G. *doneō,* to shake to and fro]. Tremulous iris; agitated motion of the iris.

iridokinesis, iridokinesia (ir'i-dō-ki-nē'sis, -ki-nē'zē-ă) [irido- + G. *kinēsis,* movement]. Movement of the iris in contracting and dilating the pupil.

iridokinetic (ir'i-dō-ki-net'ik). Iridomotor; relating to the movements of the iris.

iridology (ir-i-dol'ō-jē) [irido- + G. *logos,* study]. A system of medicine based on an examination of the iris, utilizing a chart on which certain areas of the iris are diagnostically specific for particular organs, systems, and structures.

iridomalacia (ir'i-dō-mă-lā'shē-ă) [irido- + G. *malakia,* softness]. Degenerative softening of the iris.

iridomesodialysis (ir'i-dō-mes'ō-dī-al'i-sis) [irido- + G. *mesos,* middle, + *dialysis,* loosening]. Separation of adhesions around the inner margin of the iris.

iridomotor (ir'i-dō-mō'tŏr). Iridokinetic.

iridoncosis (ir'i-dong-kō'sis) [irido- + G. *onkos,* mass, + *-ōsis,* condition]. Thickening of the iris.

iridoncus (ir-i-dong'kŭs) [irido- + G. *onkos,* mass]. A tumefaction of the iris.

iridoparalysis (ir'i-dō-pă-ral'i-sis). Iridoplegia.

iridopathy (ir-i-dop'ă-thē). Pathologic lesions in the iris.

iridoplegia (ir'i-dō-plē'jē-ă) [irido- + G. *plēgē,* stroke]. Iridoparalysis; paralysis of the musculus sphincter pupillae.
complete i., paralysis of both the dilator and sphincter muscles of the iris.
reflex i., absence of the pupillary light reflex, as in the Argyll Robertson pupil.
sympathetic i., i. due to the paralysis of the sympathetically innervated dilator pupillae muscle.

iridoptosis (ir'i-dop-tō'sis) [irido- + G. *ptosis,* a falling]. Prolapse of the iris.

iridorrhexis (ir'i-dō-rek'sis) [irido- + G. *rhēxis,* rupture]. Tearing the iris from the scleral spur in order to increase the breadth of a coloboma.

iridoschisis (ir-i-dos'ki-sis) [irido- + G. *schisma,* cleft]. Separation of the anterior layer of the iris from the posterior layer; ruptured anterior fibers float in the aqueous.

iridoschisma (ir'i-dō-skiz'mă) [irido- + G. *schisma,* a cleft]. Simple coloboma of the iris.

iridosclerotomy (ir'i-dō-skle-rot'ō-mē) [irido- + sclera, + G. *tomē,* incision]. An incision involving both sclera and iris.

iridosteresis (ir'i-dō-ste-rē'sis) [irido- + G. *sterēsis,* a loss]. Loss or absence of all or part of the iris.

iridotasis (ir'i-dot'ă-sis) [irido- + G. *tasis,* a stretching]. An operation consisting of stretching the iris and incarcerating it in the limbal incision; a substitute for iridencleisis in glaucoma.

iridotomy (ir-i-dot'ō-mē) [irido- + G. *tomē,* incision]. Corotomy; iritomy; irotomy; transverse division of some of the fibers of the iris, forming an artificial pupil.

Iridoviridae (ir'i-do-vir'i-dē). A family of viruses including iridescent viruses of insects (*Iridovirus*), the virions of which are nonenveloped, and, probably, also viruses of vertebrates (perhaps including African swine fever virus), the virions of which have envelopes containing 15% lipid. In general, the virus has large icosahedral virions (130 to 300 nm in diameter), the capsids of which contain about 1500 capsomeres. The genome is a single molecule of double stranded DNA with molecular weight of 130 to 160 $\times$ 10^6.

Iridovirus (ir'i-dō-vī'rŭs). A genus of viruses (family Iridoviridae) comprised of the iridescent insect viruses of which the type species is the tipular iridescent virus.

irigenin (i-ri-jen'in). A trihydroxy trimethoxy isoflavone component of iridin.

iris, pl. irides (ī'ris, ir'i-dēz) [G. rainbow. The iris of the eye] [NA]. The anterior division of the vascular tunic of the eye, a diaphragm, perforated in the center (the pupil), attached peripherally to the scleral spur; it is composed of stroma and a double layer of pigmented retinal epithelium from which are derived the sphincter and dilator muscles of the pupil.
i. bombé, a condition occurring in posterior annular synechia, in which an increase of fluid in the posterior chamber causes a forward bulging of the peripheral i.
plateau i., in angle-closure glaucoma, a flat appearance of the i. rather than a forward convexity.
tremulous i., iridodonesis.

iris frill. Collarette.

irisin (ī'ri-sin). Iridin (2).

irisopsia (ī-ri-sop'sē-ă) [G. *iris,* rainbow, + *opsis,* appearance]. The appearance of rainbow colors about objects.

iritic (ī-rit'ik). Relating to iritis.

iritides (ī-rit'i-dēz). Alternate plural of iritis.

iritis (ī-rī'tis). Inflammation of the iris. See also iridocyclitis and uveitis.
i. blenorrhagique à rechutes (blen-ō-rah'jēk ah rā-shūt'), i. recidivans staphylococco-allergica; i. with recurrent hypopyon.
i. catamenia'lis, i. recurring at the menstrual periods.
Doyne's guttate i., accumulation of cellular and fibrinous inflammatory cells, mainly of epithelial and hystiocytic mononuclear phagocytes, on the surface of the iris.
fibrinous i., acute inflammation of the iris, with profuse exudate occurring in uveitis of tertiary syphillis.
follicular i., chronic i. with glassy nodules situated deep down between the anterior and posterior layers of the iris.
i. glaucomato'sa, an outpouring of exudate and cells after control of angle-closure glaucoma.
hemorrhagic i., i. with such severe hyperemia that hyphema occurs.
nodular i., i. with aggregations of round cells in the iris.
i. ob'turans, chronic i. accompanying tuberculous uveitis.
plastic i., i. with a fibrinous exudation.
quiet i., i. without inflammatory signs such as redness or edema of the cornea.
i. recid'ivans staph'ylococco-aller'gica, i. blenorrhagique à rechutes.
serous i., inflammation of the iris, with a serous exudate in the anterior chamber.
spongy i., i. with a fibrinous coagulum in the anterior chamber of the eye.
sympathetic i., i. consecutive to a similar condition in the other eye.

iritomy (ī-rit'ō-mē). Iridotomy.

iron (ī'ern, ī'rŭn) [A.S. *iren*]. A metallic element, symbol Fe, atomic no. 26, atomic weight 55.85, that occurs in the heme of hemoglobin, myoglobin, transferrin, ferritin, and iron-containing porphyrins, and is an essential component of enzymes such as catalase, peroxidase, and the various cytochromes; its salts are used medicinally. For individual salts not listed below, see ferric and ferrous entries.

albuminized i., i. albuminate, a compound of i. oxide and albumin; rendered soluble by the presence of sodium citrate; occurs as reddish brown, lustrous granules, odorless or nearly so; used in anemia.

i. alum, ferric ammonium sulfate.

i. dextrin, a complex of dextrin with ferric hydroxide; used intravenously in the treatment of iron deficiency.

peptonized i., peptonate of i.; a compound of i. oxide and peptone, rendered soluble by the presence of sodium citrate; used in the treatment of iron deficiency anemia.

i. protoporphyrin, a protoporphyrin to which an i. atom is complexed; *e.g.,* heme.

i. pyri'tes, native sulfide of i.

i. sorbitex, i. sorbitol; a complex of iron, sorbitol, and citric acid in stable solution for intramuscular administration in the treatment of iron deficiency anemia in patients who are unable to take sufficient amounts of iron by the oral route.

i. sorbitol, i. sorbitex.

iron-52 (**^{52}Fe**). A radioactive iron isotope; a cyclotron-produced positron emitter with a half-life of 8.2 hr, used to study iron metabolism.

iron-55 (**^{55}Fe**). An iron isotope; a positron emitter with half-life of 2.7 years; used (less often than Fe^{59}) as tracer in study of iron metabolism.

iron-59 (**^{59}Fe**). An iron isotope; a beta emitter with half-life of 45.1 days; used as tracer in study of iron metabolism.

irotomy (ī-rot'ō-mē). Iridotomy.

irradiate (i-rā'dē-āt) [see irradiation]. To apply radiation from a source to a structure or organism.

irradiation (i-rā-dē-ā'shŭn) [L. *ir-radio, (in-r),* pp. *-radi-atus,* to beam forth]. **1.** The subjective enlargement of a bright object seen against a dark background. **2.** Exposure to the action of electromagnetic radiation (*e.g.,* heat, light, radium). **3.** The spreading of nervous impulses from one area in the brain or cord, or from a tract, to another tract. See also radiation.

irrational (i-rash'ŭn-ăl) [L. *irrationalis,* without reason]. Not rational; unreasonable (contrary to reason) or unreasoning (not exercising reason).

irreducible (ir-rē-dū'si-bl, i-rē-). **1.** Not reducible; incapable of being made smaller. **2.** In chemistry, incapable of being made simpler, or of being replaced, hydrogenated, or reduced in positive charge.

irrespirable (ir-rē-spīr'ă-bl). **1.** Incapable of being inhaled because of irritation to the airway, resulting in breath-holding. **2.** Denoting a gas or vapor either poisonous or containing insufficient oxygen. **3.** Denoting an aerosol composed of particles with aerodynamic size larger than 10 μ.

irresponsibility (ir'rē-spons-i-bil'i-tē). The state of not being responsible, for conscious or unconscious reasons,

criminal i., the state, usually attributed to mental defect or disease, that renders a person not responsbile for his criminal conduct.

irresuscitable (ir'rē-sŭs'i-tă-bl). Incapable of being revived.

irreversible (ir-rē-ver'si-bl) [L. *in-* (*ir-*) neg. + *re- verto,* pp. *-versus,* to turn back]. Incapable of being reversed; permanent.

irrigate (ir'i-gāt) [L. *ir-rigo,* pp. *-atus,* to irrigate, fr. *in,* on, + *rigo,* to water]. To perform irrigation.

irrigation (ir-i-gā'shŭn) [see irrigate]. The washing out of a cavity or wound with a fluid.

drip-suck i., infusion-aspiration *drainage.*

irrigator (ir'i-gā-ter). An appliance used in irrigation.

irritability (ir'i-tă-bil'i-tē) [L. *irritabilitas,* fr. *irrito,* pp. *-atus,* to excite]. The property inherent in protoplasm of reacting to a stimulus.

electric i., the response of a nerve or muscle to the passage of a current of electricity; in cases of degeneration in nerve or muscle this i. is altered or lost. See modal, qualitative, and quantitative *alteration.*

myotatic i., the ability of a muscle to contract in response to the stimulus produced by a sudden stretching.

irritable (ir'i-tă-bl). **1.** Capable of reacting to a stimulus. **2.** Tending to react immoderately to a stimulus. *Cf.* excitable.

irritant (ir'i-tant). **1.** Irritating; causing irritation. **2.** Any agent with this action.

primary i., a substance that causes inflammation and other evidence of irritation, particularly of the skin, on first contact or exposure; a reaction of irritation not dependent on a mechanism of sensitization.

irritation (ir-i-tā'shŭn) [L. *irritatio*]. **1.** Extreme incipient inflammatory reaction of the tissues to an injury. **2.** The normal response of nerve or muscle to a stimulus. **3.** The evocation of a normal or exaggerated reaction in the tissues by the application of a stimulus.

irritative (ir-i-tā'tiv). Causing irritation.

irrumation (ir'ū-mā'shŭn) [L. *irrumo,* pp. *-atus,* to give suck]. Fellatio.

irruption (i-rŭp'shŭn) [L. *irruptio,* fr. *irrumpo,* to break in]. Act or process of breaking through to a surface.

irruptive (i-rŭp'tiv). Relating to or characterized by irruption.

IRV Abbreviation for inspiratory reserve *volume.*

Irvine, A. Ray, Jr., U.S. ophthalmologist, *1917. See I.-Gass *syndrome.*

Isamine blue (is'ă-mēn, ī'să-). Pyrrol blue.

isauxesis (ī-sawk-zē'sis) [G. *isos,* even, + *auxēsis,* increase]. Growth of parts at the same rate as growth of the whole.

ischemia (is-kē'mē-ă) [G. *ischō,* to keep back, + *haima,* blood]. Local anemia due to mechanical obstruction (mainly arterial narrowing) of the blood supply.

myocardial i., inadequate circulation of blood to the myocardium, usually as a result of coronary artery disease. See also *angina* pectoris; myocardial *infarction.*

postural i., the reduced blood pressure and flow induced in a part, *e.g.,* the leg or foot, by raising it above the heart level; used to reduce bleeding during surgical operations on the extremities.

i. ret'inae, diminished blood supply in the retina due to failure of the arterial circulation; it may occur as a result of arterial embolism or spasm; poisoning, as by quinine; or exsanguination from recurring profuse hemorrhages (*e.g.,* in parturition, gastric and duodenal ulcers, and pulmonary tuberculosis); bilateral transitory or permanent blindness may result.

silent i., myocardial i. without accompanying signs or symptoms of angina pectoris. See also silent myocardial *infarction.*

ischemic (is-kē'mik). Relating to or affected by ischemia.

ischesis (is-kē'sis) [G. *ischō,* to hold back]. Suppression of any discharge, especially of a normal one.

ischia (is'kē-ă). Plural of ischium.

ischiadic (is-kē-ad'ik). Sciatic (1).

ischiadicus (is-kē-ad'i-kŭs) [L.] [NA]. Ischial or sciatic.

ischial (is'kē-ăl). Sciatic (1).

ischialgia (is-kē-al'jē-ă) [G. *ischion,* hip, + *algos,* pain]. **1.** Ischiodynia; ischioneuralgia; pain in the hip; specifically, the ischium. **2.** Rarely used term for sciatica.

ischiatic (is-kē-at'ik). Sciatic (1).

ischidrosis (is-ki-drō'sis) [G. *ischō,* to hold back, + *hidrōsis,* perspiration]. Anhidrosis.

ischio- [G. *ischion,* hip-joint, haunch (ischium)]. Combining form relating to the ischium.

ischioanal (is-kē-ō-ā'năl). Relating to the ischium and the anus.

ischiobulbar (is-kē-ō-bŭl'bar). Relating to the ischium and the bulb of the penis.

ischiocapsular (is-kē-ō-kap'sū-lăr). Relating to the ischium and the capsule of the hip joint; denoting that part of the capsule which is attached to the ischium.

ischiocavernosus (is'kē-ō-kav-er-nō'sŭs). See under musculus.

ischiocavernous (is-kē-ō-kav'er-nŭs). Relating to the ischium and the corpus cavernosum.

ischiocele (is'kē-ō-sēl) [ischio- + G. *kēlē,* hernia]. Sciatic *hernia.*

ischiococcygeal (is-kē-ō-kok-sij'ē-ăl). Relating to the ischium and the coccyx.

ischiococcygeus (is-kē-ō-kok-sij'ē-ŭs). See under musculus.

ischiodynia (is'kē-ō-din'ē-ă) [ischio- + G. *odynē,* pain]. Ischialgia (1).

ischiofemoral (is-kē-ō-fem'ō-răl). Relating to the ischium, or hip bone, and the femur, or thigh bone.

ischiofibular (is'kē-ō-fib'yū-lăr). Relating to or connecting the ischium and the fibula.

ischiomelus (is-ki-om'ĕ-lŭs) [ischio- + G. *melos,* limb]. Unequal conjoined twins in which the parasite, often only an arm or a leg, arises from the pelvic region of the autosite.

ischioneuralgia (is-kē-ō-nū-ral'jē-ă). Ischialgia.

ischionitis (is'kē-ō-nī'tis). Inflammation of the ischium.

ischiopagus (is-kē-op'ă-gŭs) [ischio- + G. *pagos,* fixed]. Conjoined twins united in their ischial region.

ischioperineal (is'kē-ō-per-i-nē'ăl). Relating to the ischium and the perineum.

ischiopubic (is'kē-ō-pū'bik). Relating to both ischium and pubis.

ischiorectal (is'kē-ō-rek'tăl). Relating to the ischium and the rectum.

ischiosacral (is'kē-ō-sā'krăl). Relating to the ischium and the sacrum.

ischiothoracopagus (is'kē-ō-thōr-ă-kop'ă-gŭs). Iliothoracopagus.

ischiotibial (is'kē-ō-tib'ē-ăl). Relating to or connecting the ischium and the tibia.

ischiovaginal (is-kē-ō-vaj'i-năl). Relating to the ischium and the vagina.

ischiovertebral (is-kē-ō-ver'tĕ-brăl). Relating to the ischium and the vertebral column.

ischium, gen. **ischii,** pl. **ischia** (is'kē-ŭm, is'kē-ă) [Mod. L. fr. G. *ischion,* hip]. *Os* ischii.

ischochymia (is-kō-kī'mē-ă) [G. *ischō,* to keep back, + *chymos,* juice]. Retention of food in the stomach due to dilation of that organ.

ischuretic (is-kū-ret'ik). **1.** Relating to or relieving ischuria. **2.** An agent that relieves retention or suppression of urine.

ischuria (is-kū'rē-ă) [G. *ischō,* to keep back, + *ouron,* urine]. Retention or suppression of urine.

isethionate (ī-sĕ-thī'ō-nāt). A salt or ester of isethionic acid.

isethionic acid (ī'sĕ-thī-on'ik). 2-Hydroxyethanesulfonic acid; $HOCH_2CH_2SO_3H$; a colorless viscous liquid, miscible with water and alcohols, that forms crystalline salts with organic acids.

Ishak. See Luna-I. *stain.*

Ishihara, Shinobu, Japanese ophthalmologist, 1879–1963. See I.'s *test.*

isinglass (ī'zing-glas) [Old Ger. *huysenblas,* sturgeon's bladder]. Ichthyocolla.

island (ī'land) [A.S. *īgland*]. Insula (2); in anatomy, any isolated part, separated from the surrounding tissues by a groove, or marked by difference in structure.

blood i., blood islet; an aggregation of splanchnic mesodermal cells on the embryonic yolk sac, with the potentiality of forming vascular endothelium and primitive blood cells.

bone i., a macroscopic cluster of cortical bone cells in medullary bone, frequently seen in roentgenograms of the bony pelvis and upper femora.

i.'s of Calleja, dense clusters of very small nerve cells (granule cells) characteristic of the olfactory tubercle at the base of the forebrain.

Langerhans' i.'s, *islets* of Langerhans.

pancreatic i.'s, islets of Langerhans.

i. of Reil, insula (1).

islet (ī'let). A small island.

blood i., blood *island.*

i.'s of Langerhans, Langerhans' islands; pancreatic i.'s or islands; i. tissue; cellular masses varying from a few to hundreds of cells lying in the interstitial tissue of the pancreas; they are composed of different cell types which comprise the endocrine portion of the pancreas and are the source of insulin and glucagon.

pancreatic i.'s, i.'s of Langerhans.

principal i.'s, separate globular aggregates made up mostly of endocrine pancreatic tissue; present in some fishes and snakes.

-ism [G. *-isma, -ismos,* noun-forming suffix]. **1.** Denoting a medical condition or a disease resulting from or involving some specified thing. **2.** Denoting a practice or doctrine. *Cf.* -ia.

-ismus [L. fr. G. *-ismos,* suffix forming nouns of action]. L. for -ism; customarily used to imply spasm, contraction.

iso- [G. *isos,* equal] **1.** Prefix meaning equal, like. **2.** In chemistry, prefix indicating "isomer of" (isomerism); *e.g.,* isocyanate vs. cyanate. **3.** In immunology, prefix designating sameness with respect to species; in recent years, the meaning has shifted to sameness with respect to genetic constitution of individuals.

isoagglutination (ī'sō-ă-glū-ti-nā'shŭn) [iso- + L. *ad,* to, + *gluten,* glue]. Isohemagglutination; agglutination of red blood cells as a result of the reaction between an isoagglutinin and specific antigen in or on the cells.

isoagglutinin (ī'sō-ă-glū'ti-nin). Isohemagglutinin; an isoantibody that causes agglutination of cells.

isoagglutinogen (ī'sō-ă-glū-tin'ō-jen). An isoantigen that induces agglutination of the cells to which it is attached upon exposure to its specific isoantibody.

isoallele (ī'sō-ă-lēl'). One of a number of alleles that can be mutually distinguished only by special analyses.

isoalloxazine (ī'sō-ă-loks'ă-zēn). The heterocyclic compound of riboflavin and other flavins.

isoamidone (ī-sō-am'i-dōn). Isomethadone.

isoaminile (ī-sō-am'i-nīl). 4-(Dimethylamino)-2-isopropyl-2-phenylvaleronitrile; an antitussive agent.

isoamyl (ī-sō-am'il). See amyl.

isoamylase (ī-sō-am'il-ās) [EC 3.2.1.68]. A hydrolase that cleaves 1,6-α-D-glucosidic branch linkages in glycogen, amylopectin, and their β-limit dextrins; part of the complex known as debranching enzyme.

isoamylhydrocupreine (ī-sō-am'il-hī-drō-kū'prē-ēn). A topical anesthetic and dental antiseptic.

isoandrosterone (ī'sō-an-dros'ter-ōn). Epiandrosterone.

isoantibody (ī′sō-an′ti-bod-ē) [G. *isos,* equal]. **1.** An antibody that occurs only in some individuals of a species and reacts specifically with the corresponding isoantigen; the latter does not occur naturally in the cells of the same individual who has the antibody. For specific i.'s of blood groups, see Blood Groups appendix. **2.** Sometimes used as a synonym of alloantibody.

isoantigen (ī′sō-an′ti-jen). **1.** An antigenic substance that occurs only in some individuals of a species, such as the blood group antigens of man. For specific i.'s of blood groups, see Blood Groups appendix. **2.** Sometimes used as a synonym of alloantigen.

isobar (ī′sō-bar) [iso- + G. *baros,* weight]. **1.** One of two or more nuclides having the same total number of protons plus neutrons, but with different distribution; *e.g.,* argon-40 with 18 protons and 22 neutrons, potassium-40 with 19 protons and 21 neutrons, calcium-40 with 20 protons and 20 neutrons. The product of a β-disintegration is an i. of its parent. **2.** The line on a map connecting points of equal barometric pressure.

isobaric (ī-sō-bar′ik). **1.** Having equal weights or pressures. **2.** With respect to solutions, having the same density as the diluent or medium; *e.g.,* in spinal anesthesia, an i. solution has the same specific gravity as has spinal fluid.

isobestic (ī-sō-bes′tik). Erroneous spelling of isosbestic.

isobornyl thiocyanoacetate (ī-sō-bōr′nil thī-ō-sī′ă-nō-as′ĕ-tāt). $C_{13}H_{19}NO_2S$; a pediculicide.

isobucaine hydrochloride (ī-sō-byū′kān). 2-(Isobutylamino)-2-methylpropyl benzoate hydrochloride; a local anesthetic used in dentistry.

isobuteine (ī-sō-byū′tē-ēn). *S*- (2-Carboxypropyl)cysteine; a sulfur-containing compound in urine.

isobutyl alcohol (ī-sō-byū′til). See *butyl* alcohol.

isobutyl nitrite. A liquid present in commercial amyl nitrite, with similar antispasmodic and vasodilator properties.

isobutyric acid (ī′sō-byū-tir′ik). See butyric acid.

isobuzole (ī-sō-byū′zōl). Glysobuzole; *N*-(5-isobutyl-1,3,4-thiadiazol-2-yl)-*p*-methoxybenzenesulfonamide; an oral hypoglycemic agent for the treatment of diabetes mellitus.

isocapnia (ī-sō-kap′nē-ă) [iso- + G. *kapnos,* vapor]. A state in which the arterial carbon dioxide pressure remains constant or unchanged.

isocarboxazid (ī′sō-kar-bok′să-zid). 1-Benzyl-2-(5-methyl-3-isoxazolylcarbonyl)hydrazine; a monoamine oxidase inhibitor used in the treatment of depressive disorders.

isocellular (ī′sō-sel′yū-lăr) [iso- + L. *cellula,* dim, of *cella,* a storeroom]. Composed of cells of equal size or of similar character.

isochoric (iī′sō-kōr′ik) [iso- + G. *chōra,* space]. Isovolumic.

isochromatic (ī-sō-krō-mat′ik) [iso- + G. *chrōma,* color]. **1.** Isochroous; of uniform color. **2.** Denoting two objects of the same color.

isochromatophil, isochromatophile (ī′sō-krō-mat′ō-fil, fīl) [iso- + G. *chrōma,* color, + *philos,* fond]. Having an equal affinity for the same dye; said of cells or tissues.

isochromosome (ī′sō-krō′mō-sōm). A chromosomal aberration that arises as a result of transverse rather than longitudinal division of the centromere during meiosis; two daughter chromosomes are formed, each lacking one chromosome arm but with the other doubled.

isochronia (ī-sō-krō′nē-ă) [iso- + G. *chronos,* time]. **1.** The state of having the same chronaxie. **2.** Agreement, with respect to time, rate, or frequency, between processes.

isochronous (ī-sok′rō-nŭs). Occurring during the same time.

isochroous (ī-sok′rō-ŭs). Isochromatic (1).

isocitrase, isocitratase (ī-sō-sit′rās, -sit′ră-tās). Isocitrate lyase.

isocitrate dehydrogenase (ī-sō-sit′rāt). Isocitric acid dehydrogenase; oxalosuccinic carboxylase; one of two enzymes (EC 1.1.1.41 and .42) that catalyze the conversion of *threo*-D_S-isocitrate, the product of the action of isocitrate lyase, to α-ketoglutarate (2-oxoglutarate); one of the reactions of the tricarboxylic acid cycle.

isocitrate lyase [EC 4.1.3.1]. Isocitratase; isocitritase; isocitrase; an enzyme that catalyzes the aldol condensation of glyoxylate and succinate, forming *threo*-D_S-isocitrate.

isocitric acid (ī-sō-sit′rik). $HOOCCH_2CH(COOH)CH(OH)$-$COOH$; an intermediate in the tricarboxylic acid cycle.

i. a. dehydrogenase, isocitrate dehydrogenase.

isocitritase (ī-sō-sit′ri-tās). Isocitrate lyase.

isocline (ī′sō-klīn) [iso- + G. *klinein,* to slope]. A line in a geographical region that joins points at which in a population there are constant expected frequencies for the various alleles at a genetic locus. See also cline.

isocoria (ī-sō-kō′rē-ă) [iso- + G. *korē,* pupil]. Equality in the size of the two pupils.

isocortex (ī-sō-kōr′teks). Homotypic cortex; neocortex; neopallium; O. and C. Vogt's term for the larger part of the mammalian cerebral cortex, distinguished from the allocortex by being composed of a larger number of nerve cells arranged in six layers. See also *cortex* cerebri.

isocyanate (ī-sō-sī′ă-nāt). The radical $-N=C=O$ from isocyanic acid.

isocyanic acid (ī-sō-sī′ă-nik). HNCO; a highly reactive chemical.

isocyanide (ī-sō-sī′ă-nīd). The radical –NC; organic i.'s are called isonitriles.

isocytolysin (ī′sō-sī-tol′i-sin). A cytolysin that reacts with the cells of certain other animals of the same species, but not with the cells of the individual that formed the i.

isodactylism (ī-sō-dak′ti-lizm) [iso- + G. *daktylos,* finger]. Condition in which each of the fingers or toes are approximately of equal length.

isodense (ī′sō-dens). Denoting a tissue having a radiopacity (radiodensity) similar to that of another or adjacent tissue.

isodulcit (ī-sō-dŭl′sit). L-Rhamnose.

isodynamic (ī′sō-dī-nam′ik) [iso- + G. *dynamis,* force]. **1.** Of equal force or strength. **2.** Relating to foods or other materials that liberate the same amount of energy on combustion.

isodynamogenic (ī′sō-dī-nă-mō-jen′ik, -dī-nam′ō-) [iso- + G. *dynamis,* force, + *-gen,* producing]. **1.** Isoenergetic. **2.** Producing equal nerve force.

isoelectric (ī′sō-ē-lek′trik). Isopotential; of equal electrical potential. *Cf.* isoelectric *point.*

isoenergetic (ī′sō-en-er-jet′ik). Isodynamogenic (1); exerting equal force; equally active.

isoenzyme (ī-sō-en′zīm). Isozyme; one of a group of enzymes that are very similar in catalytic properties but may be differentiated by variations in physical properties, such as isoelectric point or electrophoretic mobility; *e.g.,* lactate dehydrogenase, a tetramer composed of varying amounts of α and β subunits (*i.e.,* 4α; 3α + 1β; 2α + 2β; 1α + 3β; and 4β).

isoerythrolysis (ī′sō-ĕ-rith-rol′i-sis). Destruction of erythrocytes by isoantibodies.

neonatal i., **(1)** i. in the newborn animal; **(2)** hemolytic icterus of the newborn.

isoetharine (ī-sō-eth′ă-rēn). α-(1-Isopropylaminopropyl)-protocatechuyl alcohol; a bronchodilator for the treatment of bronchial asthma.

isofluorphate (ī-sō-flūr′fāt). Diisopropyl fluorophosphate;

$[(CH_3)_2CH–O]_2P(O)F$; a toxic cholinergic agent that acts by irreversible inhibition of cholinesterase; an ophthalmic cholinergic agent; also used in biochemical research as an enzyme inhibitor.

isoflurane (ī-sō-flūr'ăn). 1-Chloro-2,2,2-trifluoro-ethyl difluoromethyl ether; a nonflammable, nonexplosive, halogenated ether with potent anesthetic action; an isomer of enflurane.

isogamete (ī-sō-gam'ēt) [iso- + G. *gametēs* or *gametē,* husband or wife]. **1.** One of two or more similar cells by the conjugation or fusion of which, with subsequent division, reproduction occurs. **2.** A gamete of the same size as the gamete with which it unites.

isogamy (ī-sog'ă-mē) [iso- + G. *gamos,* marriage]. Conjugation between two equal gametes, or two individual cells alike in all respects.

isogeneic, isogenic (ī'sō-jĕ-nē'ik, -jen'ik). Syngeneic.

isogenesis (ī-sō-jen'ĕ-sis) [iso- + G. *genesis,* production]. Identity of morphologic development.

isogenous (ī-soj'ĕ-nŭs) [iso- + G. *genos,* family, kind]. Of the same origin, as in development from the same tissue or cell.

isogentiobiose (ī'sō-jen-shi-ō-bī'ōs). Isomaltose.

isoglutamine (ī-sō-glū'tă-mēn). $H_2NCO–CH(NH_2)CH_2CH_2$-COOH; a glutamic amide.

isognathous (ī-sog'nă-thŭs) [iso- + G. *gnathos,* jaw]. Having jaws of approximately the same width.

isograft (ī'sō-graft). Synograft.

isohemagglutination (ī'sō-hē'mă-glū'ti-nā'shŭn) [iso- + G. *haima,* blood, + L. *ad,* to, + *gluten,* glue]. Isoagglutination.

isohemagglutinin (ī'sō-hē'mă-glū'ti-nin). Isoagglutinin.

isohemolysin (ī'sō-hē-mol'i-sin). An isolysin that reacts with red blood cells.

isohemolysis (ī'sō-hē-mol'i-sis) [iso- + G. *haima,* blood, + *lysis,* dissolution]. A form of isolysis in which there is dissolution of red blood cells as a result of the reaction between an isolysin (isohemolysin) and specific antigen in or on the cells.

isohydric (ī-sō-hī'drik). Denoting two substances possessing the same pH.

isohydruria (ī'sō-hī-drū'rē-ă) [iso- + hydruria]. Fixation of the pH of the urine without the usual variation.

isohypercytosis (ī'sō-hī-per-sī-tō'sis) [iso- + G. *hyper,* above, + *kytos,* cell, + *-osis,* condition]. Obsolete term for a condition in which the number of leukocytes in the circulating blood is increased, but the relative proportions of the various types (especially the granulocytes) are within the usual range.

isohypocytosis (ī'sō-hī-pō-sī-tō'sis) [iso- + G. *hypo,* below, + *kytos,* cell, + *-osis,* condition]. Obsolete term for a condition in which there is an abnormally small number of leukocytes in the circulating blood, but the relative proportions of the various types (especially the granulocytes) are within the usual range.

isoiconia (ī'sō-ī-kō'nē-ă) [iso- + G. *eikōn,* image, + *-ia,* condition]. Equality of the two retinal images.

isoiconic (ī'sō-ī-kon'ik). Marked by or relating to isoiconia.

isoimmunization (ī'sō-im'yū-nī-zā'shŭn). Development of a significant titer of specific antibody as a result of antigenic stimulation with material contained on or in the red blood cells of another individual of the same species; *e.g.,* i. is likely to occur when an Rh-negative person is treated with a transfusion of Rh-positive blood from another human being, or an Rh-negative woman has a pregnancy in which the fetus inherits Rh-positive red blood cells.

isolate (ī'sō-lāt) [It. *isolare;* Mediev. L. *insulo,* pp. *-atus,* to insulate, fr. L. *insula,* island]. **1.** To separate, to set apart others; that which is so treated. **2.** To free from chemical contaminants. **3.** In psychoanalysis, to separate experiences or memories from the affects pertaining to them. **4.** Viable organisms separated on a single occasion from a field sample in experimental hosts, culture systems, or stabilates.

genetic i., a group that, for social, religious, geographical, or other reasons, behaves as a deme.

mating i., a population separated from its neighbors by any means (cultural, geographic, etc.) so that all or most matings occur within the population group.

isolation (ī-sō-lā'shŭn). Separation from others, as of an individual from a community because of communicable disease.

isolecithal (ī-sō-les'i-thăl). Denoting an ovum in which there is a moderate amount of uniformly distributed yolk.

isoleucine (Ile) (ī-sō-lū'sēn). 2-Amino-3-methylvaleric acid; $CH_3CH_2CH(CH_3)CH(NH_2)COOH$; an amino acid found in almost all proteins; an isomer of leucine and, like it, a dietary essential.

isoleucyl (Ile) (ī-sō-lū'sil). The acyl radical of isoleucine.

isoleukoagglutinin (ī'sō-lū'kō-ă-glū'ti-nin). Naturally occurring abnormal antibody in the blood of some persons with certain conditions, capable of agglutinating human leukocytes.

isologous (lī-sol'ō-gŭs) [iso- + G. *logos,* ratio]. Syngeneic.

isolysin (ī-sol'i-sin). An antibody that combines with, sensitizes, and results in complement-fixation and dissolution of cells that contain the specific isoantigen; i.'s occur in the blood of some members of a species and they react with the cells of that species, but not with the cells of the individual (or the same type) in which the i.'s are naturally formed.

isolysis (ī-sol'i-sis) [iso- + G. *lysis,* dissolution]. Lysis or dissolution of cells as a result of the reaction between an isolysin and specific antigen in or on the cells. See also isohemolysis.

isolytic (ī-sō-lit'ik). Pertaining to, characterized by, or causing isolysis.

isomaltase (ī-sō-mal'tās). Oligo-1,6-glucosidase.

isomaltose (ī-sō-mal'tōs). Isogentiobiose; a disaccharide in which two glucose molecules are attached by an α-1,6 link, rather than an α-1,4 link as in maltose.

isomastigote (ī-sō-mas'ti-gōt) [iso- + G. *mastix,* whip]. Denoting a protozoan having two or four flagella of equal length at one extremity.

isomer (ī'sō-mer) [iso- + G. *meros,* part]. **1.** One of two or more substances displaying isomerism; *e.g.,* L-glucose and D-glucose. **2.** One of two or more nuclides having the same atomic and mass numbers but differing in energy states for a finite period of time; *e.g.,* ^{99m}Tc and ^{99}Tc.

isomerase (ī-som'er-ās). A class of enzymes (EC class 5) catalyzing the conversion of a substance to an isomeric form; *e.g.,* glucose-phosphate isomerase (EC 5.3.1.9).

isomeric (ī-sō-măr'ik). Isomerous; relating to or characterized by isomerism.

isomerism (ī-som'er-izm). The existence of a chemical compound in two or more forms that are identical with respect to percentage composition but differ as to the positions of one or more atoms within the molecules, and also in physical and chemical properties.

geometric i., a form of i. displayed by unsaturated or ring compounds where free rotation about a carbon bond is restricted; *e.g.,* the i. of a *cis-* or *trans-*compound.

optical i., stereoisomerism involving the arrangement of substituents about an asymmetric carbon atom or atoms so that there is a difference in the behavior of the various isomers with regard to the extent of their rotation of the plane of polarized light.

stereochemical i., stereoisomerism.

structural i., i. involving the same atoms in different arrangements; *e.g.,* butyric acids, leucine and isoleucine, glucose and fructose.

isomerization (ī-som′er-ī-zā′shŭn). A process in which one isomer is formed from another, as in the action of isomerases.

isomerous (ī-som′er-ŭs). Isomeric.

isomethadone (ī-sō-meth′ă-dōn). Isoamidone; 6-(dimethylamino)-5-methyl-4,4-diphenyl-3-hexanone; a narcotic analgesic.

isometheptene (ī′sō-meth-ep′ten). *N*,1,5-Trimethyl-4-hexenylamine; an unsaturated aliphatic sympathomimetic amine with antispasmodic and vasoconstrictor actions.

isometric (ī-sō-met′rik) [iso- + G. *metron*, measure]. **1.** Of equal dimensions. **2.** In physiology, denoting the condition when the ends of a contracting muscle are held fixed so that contraction produces increased tension at constant overall length. *Cf.* auxotonic; isotonic (3); isovolumic.

isometropia (ī′sō-me-trō′pē-ă) [iso- + G. *metron*, measure, + *ōps* (*ōp*-), eye]. Equality in refraction in the two eyes.

isomorphic (ī-sō-mōr′fik). Isomorphous.

isomorphism (ī-sō-mōr′fizm) [iso- + G. *morphē*, shape]. Similarity of form between two or more organisms or between parts of the body.

isomorphous (ī-sō-mōr′fŭs). Isomorphic; having the same form or shape, or being morphologically equal.

isonaphthol (ī-sō-naf′thol). β-Naphthol.

isoncotic (ī-son-kot′ik). Of equal oncotic pressure.

isoniazid (ī-sō-nī′ă-zid). Isonicotinic acid hydrazide; $C_6H_7N_3O$; a compound effective in the treatment of tuberculosis.

isonicotinic acid (ī-sō-nik-ō-tin′ik). 4-Pyridinecarboxylic acid; its hydrazide is isoniazid.

isonitrile (ī-sō-nī′tril). An organic isocyanide.

isonitrosoacetone (ī′sō-nī-trō-sō-as′ĕ-tōn). Monoisonitrosoacetone; pyruvaldoxine; propanone 1-oxine; $CH_3CO{-}CH{=}NOH$; a cholinesterase reactivator that can penetrate the blood-brain barrier readily and cause significant reactivation of phosphorylated acetylcholinesterase in the central nervous system; used to protect human beings and animals against otherwise lethal poisoning with organophosphorous anticholinesterase agents.

isonormocytosis (ī′sō-nōr-mō-sī-tō′sis) [iso- + L. *norma*, rule, + G. *kytos*, cell, + *-osis*, condition]. Dinormocytosis; obsolete term for a condition in which the actual number and the relative proportions of the various types of leukocytes in the circulating blood are within normal range.

iso-osmotic (ī′sō-os-mot′ik). Isosmotic.

isopathy (ī-sop′ă-thē) [iso- + G. *pathos*, suffering]. Treatment of disease by means of the causal agent or a product of the same disease, or of a diseased organ by an extract of a similar organ from a healthy animal. See also homeopathy.

isopentyl (ī-sō-pen′til). See amyl.

isopentylhydrocupreine (ī-sō-pen′til-hī-drō-kū′prē-ēn). Euprocin hydrochloride.

isophagy (ī-sof′ă-jē) [iso- + G. *phagein*, to eat]. Autolysis.

isophoria (ī-sō-fō′rē-ă) [iso- + G. *phora*, movement]. A condition in which a muscular imbalance remains constant with changes of direction of gaze.

isopia (ī-sō′pē-ă) [iso- + G. *ōps* (*ōp*-), eye]. Equality in all respects of the two eyes, and of vision.

isoplassonts (ī-sō-plas′onts) [iso- + G. *plassō*, to form]. Like-formed entities having certain features in common.

isoplastic (ī-sō-plas′tik) [iso- + G. *plassō*, to form]. Syngeneic.

isopleth (ī′sō-pleth). A line on a Cartesian nomogram consisting of all points that represent a particular value of a variable; *e.g.*, an isobar is an i. for a particular pressure.

isopotential (ī′sō-pō-ten′chŭl). Isoelectric.

isoprecipitin (ī′sō-prē-sip′i-tin) [iso- + precipitin]. An antibody that combines with and precipitates soluble antigenic material in the plasma or serum, or in an extract of the cells, from another member, but not all members, of the same species.

isoprenaline hydrochloride (ī-sō-pren′ă-lēn). Isoproterenol hydrochloride.

isoprenaline sulphate. Isoproterenol sulfate.

isoprene (ī′sō-prēn). Hemiterpene; 2-methyl-1,3-butadiene; $CH_2{=}CH{-}C(CH_3){=}CH_2$; an unsaturated five-carbon hydrocarbon with a branched chain, which in the plant kingdom is used as the basis for the formation of isoprenoids; *e.g.*, terpenes, carotenoids, and related pigments, rubber. Fat-soluble vitamins either are isoprenoid or have isoprenoid side chains; steroids are synthesized via isoprenoid intermediates.

isoprenoids (ī-sō-prēn′oydz). Polymers whose carbon skeletons consist in whole or in large part of isoprene units joined end to end; *e.g.*, carotene, lycopene, vitamin A. Vitamins K and E and the coenzymes Q have isoprenoid side chains.

isopropamide iodide (ī-sō-prō′pă-mīd). (3-Carbamoyl-3,3-diphenylpropyl) diisopropylmethylammonium iodide; an anticholinergic agent.

isopropanol (ī-sō-prō′pă-nol). Isopropyl alcohol.

isoprophenamine hydrochloride (ī′sō-prō-fen′ă-mēn). Clorprenaline hydrochloride.

isopropyl alcohol (ī-sō-prō′pil). Isopropanol; dimethylcarbinol; $(CH_3)_2CHOH$; an isomer of propyl alcohol and a homologue of ethyl alcohol, similar in its properties, when used externally, to the latter, but more toxic when taken internally; used as an ingredient of various cosmetics and of medicinal preparations for external use; also available as isopropyl rubbing alcohol, which contains 68 to 72% of isopropyl alcohol (by volume) in water; used as a rubefacient.

isopropylarterenol hydrochloride (ī-sō-prō′pil-ar-ter′ĕ-nol). Isoproterenol hydrochloride.

isopropylcarbinol (ī′sō-prō-pil-kar′bin-ol). See *butyl* alcohol.

isopropyl myristate (ī-sō-prō′pil). A pharmaceutic aid used in topical medicinal preparations to promote absorption through the skin.

isopropylthiogalactoside (IPTG, iPrSGal) (ī-sō-pro′pil-thī′ō-gă-lak′tō-sīd). An artificial galactoside capable of inducing β-galactosidase in *Escherichia coli* without being split, as are the natural substrates such as lactose.

isoproterenol hydrochloride (ī′sō-prō-ter′ĕ-nol). Isopropylarterenol hydrochloride; isoprenaline hydrochloride; 3,4-dihydroxy-α-[(isopropylamino)methyl]-benzyl alcohol hydrochloride; a sympathomimetic β-receptor stimulant possessing the inhibitory properties and the cardiac excitatory, but not the vasoconstrictor, actions of epinephrine. Chemically it differs from epinephrine in having an isopropyl group replacing the methyl group attached to the nitrogen atom; used in the treatment of bronchial asthma and heart block, including Adams-Stokes attacks.

isoproterenol sulfate. Isoprenaline sulphate; used for inhalation as an aerosol in the treatment of acute asthmatic attacks and chronic pulmonary emphysema.

isopter (ī-sop′ter) [iso- + G. *optēr*, observer]. A curve of equal retinal sensitivity in the visual field designated by a fraction, the numerator being the diameter of a test object, and the denominator, the testing distance.

isopyrocalciferol (ī-sō-pī′rō-cal-sif′er-ol). 9β-Ergosterol; a thermal decomposition product of calciferol; a stereoisomer of pyrocalciferol and ergosterol.

isoquinoline (ī-sō-kwin′ō-lēn). Benzo[*c*]pyridine; ring structure characteristic of the group of opium alkaloids represented by papaverine. See fig. on p. 808.

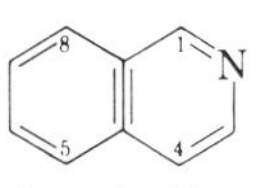

Isoquinoline

isoriboflavin (ī′sō-rī′bō-flā-vin). 8-Demethyl-6-methylriboflavin; a riboflavin antimetabolite, differing from riboflavin in that the methyl groups on the isoalloxazine nucleus are in the 6,7 positions rather than the 7,8.

isorrhea (ī-sō-rē′ă) [iso- + G. *rhoia*, a flow]. Equality of intake and output of water; maintenance of water equilibrium.

isosbestic (ī-sos-bes′tik) [Ger. *isosbestisch*, fr. G. *isos*, equal, + *sbestos*, extinguished]. Denoting the wavelength of light at which two related compounds have identical extinction coefficients; *e.g.*, the wavelength at which the absorption spectra of hemoglobin and oxyhemoglobin cross is their i. point. Spectrophotometry at that wavelength measures total concentration of hemoglobin, regardless of the extent to which it might be oxygenated.

isosensitize (ī-sō-sen′si-tīz). Autosensitize.

isosexual (ī-sō-sek′shū-ăl). **1.** Relating to the existence of characteristics or feelings of both sexes in one person. **2.** Descriptive of somatic characteristics possessed by, or of processes occurring within, an individual that are consonant with the sex of that individual.

isosmotic (ī′sos-mot′ik). Iso-osmotic; having the same total osmotic pressure or osmolality as another fluid (ordinarily intracellular fluid); such a fluid is not isotonic if it includes solutes that freely permeate cell membranes.

isosorbide dinitrate (ī-sō-sōr′bīd dī-nī′trāt). 1,4:3,6-Dianhydro-D-glucitol dinitrate; a coronary vasodilator; large doses may produce headache, flushing of the face, palpitation, fainting, and methemoglobinemia.

Isospora (ī-sos′pō-ră) [iso- + G. *sporos*, seed]. A genus of coccidia (family Eimeriidae, class sporozoea), with species chiefly in mammals; the ripe oocysts contain two sporocysts, each of which contains four sporozoites. This genus is now known to be closely related to *Toxoplasma* and *Sarcocystis*, with a similar sexual phase in the life cycle and a similar apical complex.

I. bel′li, a relatively rare species occurring in the small intestine of man, most common in the tropics but probably of worldwide distribution; most infections are subclinical, but sometimes they may cause mucous diarrhea.

I. bigem′ina, a species that occurs in the small intestine of the dog, cat, fox, mink, and possibly other carnivores; the most pathogenic coccidium in dogs and cats, causing enteritis and diarrhea; the oocysts are usually sporulated when passed in the feces, but are indistinguishable from those of *Toxoplasma gondii*, so considerable question remains as to the status of these parasites.

I. ca′nis, a species of worldwide distribution that is mildly pathogenic in dogs and is not infective in cats.

I. fe′lis, a species found in the small intestine and sometimes the cecum and colon of cats, lions, and other felids; it is only slightly, if at all, pathogenic in cats and is not infective in dogs.

I. rivol′ta, a species that occurs in the small intestine of dogs, cats, dingos, and probably other wild carnivores; pathogenic capabilities are similar to those of *I. bigemina*.

I. su′is, a species that affects the small intestine of the pig, producing mild diarrhea.

isospore (ī′sō-spōr). See anisospore.

isosporiasis (ī-sos-pō-rī′ă-sis). Disease caused by infection with a species of Isospora, such as *I. belli* of humans; human disease usually is mild except in cases of immunosuppression, as in AIDS, where it may cause an intractable diarrhea.

isostere (ī′sō-stēr) [iso- + G. *stereos*, solid]. One of two or more atoms or molecules having the same electron arrangement; *e.g.*, N_2 and CO.

isosthenuria (ī-sos′thē-nū′rē-ă, ī′sō-sthē-) [iso- + G. *sthenos*, strength, + *ouron*, urine]. A state in chronic renal disease in which the kidney cannot form urine with a higher or a lower specific gravity than that of protein-free plasma; specific gravity of the urine becomes fixed around 1.010, irrespective of the fluid intake.

isosuccinic acid (ī′sō-sŭk-sin′ik). Methylmalonic acid.

isosulfamerazine (ī′sō-sŭl-fă-mer′ă-zēn). Sulfaperin.

isosulfan blue (ī-sō-sŭl′fan). $C_{27}H_{31}N_2NaO_6S_2$; a dye used as a radiographic adjunct to mark lymphatic vessels during lymphography.

isothermal (ī-sō-ther′măl) [iso- + G. *thermē*, heat]. Having the same temperature.

isothiocyanate (ī′sō-thī-ō-sī′ă-nāt). The radical of isothiocyanic acid, $-N{=}C{=}S$.

isothipendyl (ī′sō-thī-pen′dil). 10-(2-Dimethylamino-2-methylethyl)-10*H*-pyrido[3,2-*b*][1,4]benzothiazine; an antihistaminic.

isotone (ī′sō-tōn). One of several nuclides having the same number of neutrons in their nuclei; *e.g.*, ${}^{39}_{19}K$ and ${}^{40}_{20}Ca$ with 20 each, ${}^{56}_{26}Fe$ and ${}^{58}_{28}Ni$ with 30 each.

isotonia (ī-sō-tō′nē-ă) [iso- + G. *tonos*, tension]. A condition of tonic equality in which tension or osmotic pressure in two substances or solutions is the same.

isotonic (ī-sō-ton′ik). **1.** Relating to isotonicity or isotonia. **2.** Having equal tension; denoting solutions possessing the same osmotic pressure; more specifically, limited to solutions in which cells neither swell nor shrink. Thus, a solution that is isosmotic with intracellular fluid will not be i. if it includes solute, such as urea, that freely permeates cell membranes. **3.** In physiology, denoting the condition when a contracting muscle shortens against a constant load, as when lifting a weight. *Cf.* auxotonic; isometric (2).

isotonicity (ī-sō-tō-nis′i-tē). **1.** The quality of possessing and maintaining a uniform tone or tension. **2.** The property of a solution in being isotonic.

isotope (ī′sō-tōp) [iso- + G. *topos*, part, place]. One of two or more nuclides that are chemically identical yet differ in mass number, since their nuclei contain different numbers of neutrons; individual i.'s are named with the inclusion of their mass number in superior position (${}^{12}C$) and the atomic number (nuclear protons) in inferior position (${}_{6}C$).

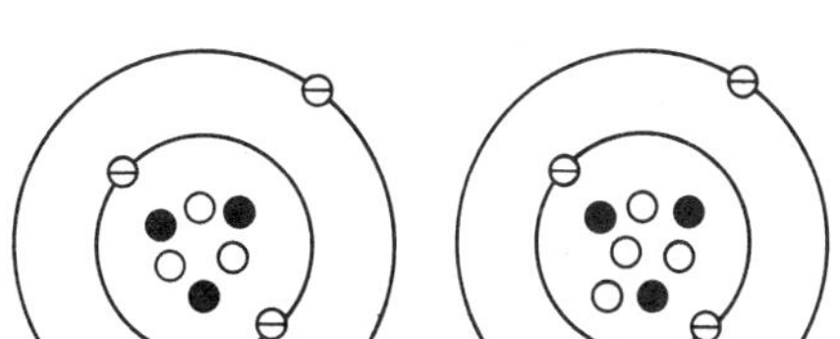

Lithium-6 (${}_{3}Li^{6}$) Lithium-7 (${}_{3}Li^{7}$)

Isotopes of Lithium
Proton, ●; neutron, ○; electron, ⊖

radioactive i., an i. with an unstable nuclear composition; such nuclei decompose spontaneously by emission of a nuclear electron (*β*-particle) or helium nucleus (*α*-particle and radiation (*γ*-rays), thus achieving a stable nuclear composition; used as tracers, and as radiation and energy sources.

stable i., a nonradioactive nuclide; an i. that shows no tendency to undergo radioactive decomposition.

isotopic (ī-sō-top'ik). Of identical chemical composition but differing in some physical property, such as atomic weight.

isotransplantation (ī'sō-tranz-plan-tā'shŭn). Transfer of an isograft (syngraft).

isotretinoin (ī-sō-tret'i-noyn). 13-*cis*-Retinoic acid; a retinoid used for treatment of severe recalcitrant cystic acne.

isotropic, isotropous (ī-sō-trop'ik, ī-sot'rō-pŭs) [iso- + G. *tropē,* a turn]. Having properties which are the same in all directions.

isotype (ī'sō-tīp). An antigenic determinant (marker) that occurs in all members of a subclass of an immunoglobulin class. Whereas a given allotypic marker or determinant is thought to occur in only one subclass, an antigenic marker which is isotypic in one subclass may also occur as an allotypic marker in another subclass.

isotypic (ī-sō-tip'ik). Pertaining to an isotype.

isovaleric acid (ī'so-vă-lār'ik, -lēr'ik). 3-Methylbutyric acid; $(CH_3)_2CHCH_2COOH$; a metabolic intermediate in oxidative processes.

isovalericacidemia (ī'sō-vă-lār'ik-as-i-dē'mē-ă). A disorder of leucine metabolism characterized by the excessive production of isovaleric acid upon protein ingestion or during infectious episodes; severe metabolic acidosis results from the large quantities of acid formed; autosomal recessive inheritance.

isovalthine (ī-sō-val'thēn). *S*- (1-Carboxy-2-methylpropyl)cysteine; $(CH_3)_2CHCH(COOH)\text{–}S\text{–}CH_2CH(NH_2)COOH$; a sulfur-containing compound found in urine.

isovolume (ī-sō-vol'yūm). At the same or equal volume. See also isovolumic.

isovolumetric (ī'sō-vol-yū-met'rik). Isovolumic.

isovolumic (ī'sō-vol-yū'mik). Isovolumetric; isochoric; occurring without an associated alteration in volume, as when, in early ventricular systole, the muscle fibers initially increase their tension without shortening so that ventricular volume remains unaltered. See also isometric.

isoxsuprine hydrochloride (ī-soks'sū-prēn). 1-(*p*-Hydroxyphenyl)-2-[(1'-methyl-2'-phenoxy)ethylamino]-1-propanol hydrochloride; a sympathomimetic amine with potent inhibitory effects on vascular, uterine, and other smooth muscles; used as a vasodilator in various vascular diseases and as a uterine relaxant.

isozyme (ī'sō-zīm). Isoenzyme.

issue (ish'ū) [Fr. a going out]. **1.** A suppurating or discharging sore, acting as a counterirritant, sometimes maintained by the presence of a foreign body in the tissues; once regarded as a means of escape for peccant humors. **2.** A discharge of pus, blood, or other matter. **3.** A point in question or a matter of dispute.

nature-nurture i., a controversy concerning the relative importance of heredity (nature) and environment (nurture) in various aspects of individual development, such as intelligence.

isthmectomy (is-mek'tō-mē) [G. *isthmos,* isthmus, + *ektomē,* excision]. Excision of the midportion of the thyroid.

isthmic, isthmian (is'mik, is'mē-an). Denoting an anatomical isthmus.

isthmoparalysis (is'mō-pă-ral'i-sis) [G. *isthmos,* isthmus, + paralysis]. Isthmoplegia; faucial paralysis; paralysis of the velum pendulum palati and the muscles forming the anterior pillars of the fauces.

isthmoplegia (is'mō-plē'jē-ă) [G. *isthmos,* isthmus, + *plēgē,* stroke]. Isthmoparalysis.

isthmus, pl. **isthmi, isthmuses** (is'mŭs, -mī, -mŭs-ez) [G. *isthmos*]. **1.** A constriction connecting two larger parts of an organ or other anatomical structure. **2.** A narrow passage connecting two larger cavities. **3.** The narrowest portion of the brainstem at the junction between midbrain and hindbrain.

i. of aorta, i. aortae.

i. aor'tae [NA], i. of aorta; a slight constriction of the aorta immediately distal to the left subclavian artery at the point of attachment of the ductus arteriosus.

i. of auditory tube, i. tubae auditivae.

i. of cartilage of ear, i. cartilaginis auris.

i. cartilag'inis au'ris [NA], i. of cartilage of ear; a narrow bridge connecting the cartilage of the external acoustic meatus and the lamina tragica with the main portion of the cartilage of the auricle.

i. of cingular gyrus, i. gyri cinguli.

i. of eustachian tube, i. tubae auditivae.

i. of external acoustic meatus, i. meatus acustici externi.

i. of fauces, i. faucium.

i. fau'cium [NA], i. of fauces; the constricted and short space which establishes the connection between the cavity of the mouth and the oral part of the pharynx.

i. glan'dulae thyroid'eae [NA], i. of thyroid; the central part of the thyroid gland joining the two lateral lobes.

Guyon's i., i. uteri.

i. gy'ri cin'guli [NA], i. of the cingular gyrus; i. of the gyrus fornicatus or limbic lobe; the narrowing of the gyrus cinguli, at its transition with the hippocampal gyrus behind and below the splenium of the corpus callosum, caused by the anterior extension of the conjoined parieto-occipital and calcarine sulci.

i. of gyrus fornicatus, i. gyri cinguli.

i. of His, i. rhombencephali.

Krönig's i., the narrow straplike portion of the resonant field which extends over the shoulder, connecting the larger areas of resonance over the pulmonary apex in front and behind.

i. of limbic lobe, i. gyri cinguli.

i. mea'tus acus'tici exter'ni, i. of external acoustic meatus; the narrowest portion of this canal near its deep termination.

pharyngeal i., choana.

i. pharyngonasa'lis, choana.

i. pros'tatae [NA], i. of prostate; the narrow middle part of the prostate anterior to the urethra.

i. of prostate, i. prostatae.

i. rhombenceph'ali [NA], rhombencephalic i.; i. of His; **(1)** a constriction in the embryonic neural tube delineating the mesencephalon from the rhombencephalon; **(2)** the anterior portion of the rhombencephalon connecting with the mesencephalon.

rhombencephalic i., i. rhombencephali.

i. of thyroid, i. glandulae thyroideae.

i. tu'bae auditi'vae [NA], i. of auditory or eustachian tube; the narrowest portion of the auditory tube at the junction of the cartilaginous and bony portions.

i. tu'bae uteri'nae [NA], i. of uterine tube; the narrow portion of the uterine tube adjoining the uterus.

i. u'teri [NA], i. of the uterus; Guyon's i.; ostium uteri internum; os uteri internum; orificium internum uteri; an elongated constriction at the junction of the body and cervix of the uterus.

i. of uterine tube, i. tubae uterinae.

i. of uterus, i. uteri.

Vieussens' i., *limbus* fossae ovalis.

itaconic acid (it'ă-kon'ik). Methylenesuccinic acid. $CH_2{=}C(COOH)CH_2COOH$; the decarboxylation product of *cis*-aconitic acid.

itch [A.S. *gikkan*]. **1.** A peculiar irritating sensation in the skin that arouses the desire to scratch. **2.** Common name for scabies. **3.** Pruritus (2).

azo i., itching that occurs among workers in azo dyes.

baker's i., an eruption on the hands and arms of bakers due to an allergic reaction to flour or other substances handled.

barber's i., *tinea* barbae.

bath i., bath *pruritus.*
coolie i., cutaneous *ancylostomiasis.*
copra i., a dermatitis occurring in workers in copra mills, caused by the presence of a mite, *Tyrophagus putrescentiae.*
Cuban i., alastrim.
dew i., cutaneous *ancylostomiasis.*
dhobie i., *tinea* cruris.
frost i., *dermatitis* hiemalis.
grain i., a cutaneous eruption occasionally noted in farmers and grain handlers, caused by the action of the mite *Pyemotes tritici.*
grocer's i., a vesicular dermatitis seen in grocers and bakers who handle sugar or flour; caused by a mite of the genus *Glycophagus.*
ground i., cutaneous *ancylostomiasis.*
jock i., *tinea* cruris.
kabure i., *schistosomiasis* japonica.
lumberman's i., *dermatitis* hiemalis.
mad i., pseudorabies.
Malabar i., *tinea* imbricata.
Norway i., Norwegian *scabies.*
poultryman's i., eruption due to infestation with the mite, *Dermanyssus gallinae.*
prairie i., pruritus of varied origin, affecting farm laborers.
rice i., cutaneous schistosomiasis japonica.
Saint Ignatius' i., pellagra.
straw i., straw-bed i., dermatitis pediculoides ventricosus; an urticarial eruption caused by the mite, *Pyemotes tritici* (*Pediculoides ventricosus*), which can infest straw used in mattresses.
summer i., *pruritus* aestivalis.
swamp i., cutaneous *ancylostomiasis.*
swimmer's i., **(1)** cutaneous *ancylostomiasis;* **(2)** schistosome *dermatitis.*
toe i., cutaneous *ancylostomiasis.*
warehouseman's i., eczema of the hands from handling irritating substances.
washerwoman's i., an eczematous eruption of the hands and arms of washerwomen, dishwashers, and others whose hands are excessively immersed in water.
water i., **(1)** cutaneous *ancylostomiasis;* **(2)** schistosome *dermatitis.*
winter i., *dermatitis* hiemalis.

itch'ing. Pruritus (1); an uncomfortable sensation of irritation of the skin or mucous membranes which causes scratching or rubbing of the affected parts.

-ite [G. *-itēs,* fem. *-itis*]. **1.** Suffix denoting of the nature of, resembling. **2.** In chemistry, denoting a salt of an acid that has the termination -ous. **3.** In comparative anatomy, a suffix denoting an essential portion of the part to the name of which it is attached. See also - ites.

iter (ī'ter) [L. *iter* (*itiner-*), a way, journey]. A passage leading from one anatomical part to another.
i. a ter'tio ad quar' tum ventric'ulum [L. path from the third to the fourth ventricle], *aqueductus* cerebri.
i. chor'dae ante'rius, Huguier's or Civinini's canal; a canal in the petrotympanic or glaserian fissure, near its posterior edge, through which the chorda tympani nerve issues from the skull.
i. chor'dae poste'rius, *canaliculus* chordae tympani.
i. den'tis, den'tium, the route or routes by which one or more teeth erupt.

iteral (ī'ter-ăl). Relating to an iter.

-ites [G. *itēs,* m., or *-ites,* n.]. Adjectival suffix to nouns, corresponding to L. *-alis, -ale,* or *-inus, -inum,* or E. -y, -like, or the hyphenated nouns; the adjective so formed is used without the qualified noun. The feminine form, *-itis* (agreeing with *nosos,* disease), is so often associated with inflammatory disease that it has acquired in most cases the significance of inflammation. Thus, tympanites is *ho tympanites oidēma,* the drumlike swelling of the abdomen, but tympanitis is *hē tympanitis nosos,* the inflammation of the tympanum. See also -ite.

ithykyphosis, ithycyphosis (ith'ĭ-kī-fō'sis, ith'ĭ-sī-) [G. *ithys,* straight, + *kyphos,* a hump]. Obsolete term for pure kyphosis without lateral displacement of the spine.

ithylordosis (ith'ē-lōr-dō'sis) [G. *ithys,* straight, + *lordōsis,* a forward curvature of the spine, fr. *lordos,* bent backward (opp. of *kyphos,* humped]. Obsolete term for a pure lordosis without lateral curvature of the spine.

-itides. Plural of -itis.

-itis [G. fem. of *-ites*]. See -ites.

Ito, Hayozo, Japanese physician, *1865. See I.-Reenstierna *test.*

Ito, Minor, 20th century Japanese dermatologist. See I.'s *nevus; hypomelanosis* of I.

Ito, T., 20th century Japanese physician. See I. *cells.*

ITP Abbreviation for idiopathic thrombocytopenic *purpura;* inosine 5'-triphosphate.

itramin tosylate (ī'tră-min). 2-Aminoethyl nitrate *p-* toluene sulfonate; a vasodilator.

IU Abbreviation for international *unit.*

IUCD Abbreviation for intrauterine contraceptive *device.*

IUD Abbreviation for intrauterine *device.*

IV, iv Abbreviation for intravenous, or intravenously.

I-V Abbreviation for intraventricular.

Ivemark, Biörn I., Swedish pathologist, *1925. See I.'s *syndrome.*

ivermectin (ī-ver-mek'tin). A 22,23-dihydro derivative of avermectin B_1, a macrocyclic lactone produced by the actinomycete *Streptomyces avermitilis;* active at extremely low dosages against a wide variety of nematode and arthropod parasites, and commercially used for treatment and control of parasites in cattle, horses, and sheep.

ivory (ī'vō-rē) [L. ebur]. A term applied to the tusks of the elephant, walrus, narwhal, hippopotamus, and warthog, and to all of the teeth of the sperm whale; the material is dentinum, the inner layer of the tooth derived from the mesoderm. In all of these animals, as well as in several others, the hard enamel layer fails to develop, or develops incompletely, leaving the softer dentinum core exposed.

IVP Abbreviation for intravenous pyelogram.

Ivy, Robert H., U.S. oral and plastic surgeon, 1881–1974. See I. loop *wiring.*

Iwanoff, Alexander, Russian ophthalmologist, 1836–1880. See I.'s *cysts.*

Ixodes (ik-sō'dēz) [G. *ixōdēs,* sticky, like bird-lime, fr. *ixos,* mistletoe, + *eidos,* form]. A genus of hard ticks (family Ixodidae), many species of which are parasitic on man and animals; severe reactions frequently follow their bites; they are characterized by an anal groove surrounding the anus anteriorly, absence of eyes and festoons, and marked sexual dimorphism; about 40 species have been described from North America.
I. bicor'nis, a species, found in Mexico, whose bite causes fever and extreme malaise.
I. cook'ei, a species that is a vector of Powassan virus in Canada.
I. damm'ini, a species that is a vector of Lyme disease and human babesiosis in the U.S.
I. holocyc'lus, a species in Australia that infests the kangaroo and transmits a paralytic disease to young cattle.
I. pacif'icus, the California black-legged tick, a species that is the vector of Lyme disease in the western U.S.
I. persulca'tus, a species that is a vector for Russian spring-summer encephalitis, and is associated with the taiga forest of the USSR.
I. pilo'sus, the paralysis tick, a species that infests sheep in South

Africa and causes paralysis.

I. rici'nus, the castor bean tick, a species that infests cattle, sheep, and wild animals, and transmits the virus of louping ill, the piroplasm *Babesia bovis,* and the Central European tick-borne encephalitis virus.

I. scapula'ris, the black-legged or shoulder tick, a species found on animals in the southern and eastern U.S.; capable of inflicting a painful bite to man.

I. spinipal'pis, a species parasitic on wild rodents in British Columbia and the vector of Powassan virus in mice of the genus *Peromyscus.*

ixodiasis (ik-sō-dī'ă-sis). **1.** Skin lesions caused by the bites of certain ixodid ticks; in some cases the tick burrows under the skin, causing some degree of irritation, but in most cases an urticarioid eruption is the only result. **2.** Any disease, such as Rocky Mountain spotted fever or Lyme disease, that is transmitted by ticks.

ixodic (ik-sod'ik). Relating to or caused by ticks.

ixodid (ik'sō-did). Common name for members of the family Ixodidae.

Ixodidae (ik-sod'i-dē) [G. *ixōdēs,* sticky]. A family of ticks (order Acarina, suborder Ixodides), the so-called "hard" ticks, characterized by rigid body form, presence of a dorsal shield, and an anteriorly projecting capitulum. It includes the genera *Ixodes, Hyalomma, Amblyomma, Boophilus, Margaropus, Dermacentor, Haemaphysalis,* and *Rhipicephalus,* species of which transmit many important human and animal diseases and cause tick paralysis; they occasionally attack man, a few habitually so.

Ixodoidea (ik'sō-dō-id'ē-ă) [G. *ixōdēs,* sticky]. Superfamily of the order Acarina that includes the families Ixodidae and Argasidae.

ixomyelitis (iks-ō-mī-ĕ-lī'tis) [G. *ixys,* small of the back]. Inflammation of the lumbar spinal cord.

J

J Symbol for joule; Joule's *equivalent.*

J Symbol for flux (4).

jaagziekte (yahg'zēk-tē) [Afrikaans, *drive sickness*]. Pulmonary *adenomatosis* of sheep.

Jaboulay, Mathieu, French surgeon, 1860–1913. See J. *pyloroplasty;* J.'s *amputation, method.*

Jaccoud, Sigismond, French physician, 1830–1913. See J.'s *arthritis, arthropathy.*

jacket (jak'et). **1.** A fixed bandage applied around the body in order to immobilize the spine. **2.** In dentistry, a term commonly used in reference to an artificial crown composed of fired porcelain or acrylic resin.

Minerva j., a plaster of Paris body cast incorporating the head and trunk for fracture of the cervical spine.

Sayre's j., a plaster of Paris j. applied while the patient is suspended by the head and axillae.

straight j., see under S.

jackscrew (jak'skrū). A threaded device used in appliances for the separation of approximated teeth or jaws.

Jackson, Jabez N., U.S. surgeon, 1868–1935. See J.'s *membrane, veil.*

Jackson, John Hughlings, British neurologist, 1835–1911. See jacksonian *epilepsy;* J.'s *law, rule, sign, syndrome.*

jacksonian (jak-sō'nē-an). Described by John Hughlings Jackson. See jacksonian *epilepsy.*

Jacobaeus, Hans C., Swedish surgeon, 1879–1937. See J. *operation.*

Jacobson, Ludwig L., Danish anatomist, 1783–1843. See J.'s *anastomosis, canal, cartilage, nerve, organ, plexus, reflex.*

Jacod's syndrome. See under syndrome.

Jacquart, Henri, 19th century French physician. See J.'s facial *angle.*

Jacquemet, Marcel, French anatomist, 1872–1908. See J.'s *recess.*

Jacquemin, Emile, 19th century French chemist. See under *test.*

Jacquemin's test. See under test.

Jacques, Paul, 19th century French physician. See J. *plexus.*

Jacquet, Leonard L., French dermatologist, 1860–1914. See J.'s *erythema.*

jactitation (jak-ti-tā'shŭn) [L. *jactatio,* a tossing, fr. *jacto,* pp. *-atus,* to throw]. Extreme restlessness or tossing about from side to side.

Jadassohn, Josef, German dermatologist in Switzerland, 1863–1936. See J.'s *nevus;* Borst-J. type intraepidermal *epithelioma;* J.-Pellizzari *anetoderma;* J.-Tièche *nevus;* J.-Lewandowski *syndrome.*

Jaeger, Eduard, Ritter von Jaxthal, Austrian ophthalmologist, 1818–1884. See J.'s *test-types.*

Jaffe, Henry L., U.S. pathologist, *1907. See J.-Lichtenstein *disease.*

Jaffe, Max, German biochemist, 1841–1911. See J. *reaction;* J.'s *test.*

Jahnke's syndrome. See under syndrome.

Jakob, Alfons M., German neuropsychiatrist, 1884–1931. See Creutzfeldt-J. or J.-Creutzfeldt *disease.*

jal'ap [*Jalapa* or *Xalapa,* a Mexican city whence the drug was exported]. The tuberous root of *Exogonium purga* or *Ipomoea purga* (family Convolvulaceae); used as a cathartic.

James, George C.W., 20th century British radiologist. See Swyer-J. *syndrome.*

James, T.N., U.S. cardiologist and physiologist, *1925. See J. *fibers, tract.*

James, William, U.S. psychologist, 1842–1910. See J.-Lange *theory.*

Janet, Pierre M.F., French neurologist, 1859–1947. See J.'s *test.*

Janeway, Edward G., U.S. physician, 1841–1911. See J. *lesion.*

janiceps (jan'i-seps) [L. *Janus,* a Roman diety having two faces, + *caput,* head]. Conjoined twins having their two heads fused together, with the faces looking in opposite directions. See also craniopagus; syncephalus.

j. asym'metrus, iniops; syncephalus asymmetros; a j. with one very small and imperfectly developed face.

j. parasit'icus, a j. in which one of the twins is a small and incompletely formed parasite attached to the more fully formed autosite.

Jansen, Albert, German otologist, 1859–1933. See J.'s *operation.*

Jansky, Jan, Prague physician, 1873–1921. See J.-Bielschowsky *disease,* J.'s *classification.*

Janus green B [C.I. 11050]. Diethylsafraninazodimethylaniline chloride, $C_{30}H_{31}N_6Cl$; a basic dye used in histology and to stain mitochondria supravitally.

jar. 1. To jolt or shake. **2.** A jolting or shaking.

heel j., the patient standing on tiptoe feels pain on suddenly bringing the heels to the ground: **(1)** in the spine in Pott's disease or disk space infection; **(2)** in one lumbar region in renal calculus.

jargon (jar'gŏn) [Fr. gibberish]. **1.** Language or terminology peculiar to a specific field, profession, or group. **2.** Paraphasia.

Jarisch, Adolf, Austrian dermatologist, 1850–1902. See J.-Herxheimer *reaction;* Bezold-J. *reflex.*

Jarjavay, Jean F., French anatomist and surgeon, 1815–1868. See J.'s *ligament.*

Jatropha (jat'rō-fă) [G. *iatros,* physician, + *trophē,* nourishment]. A genus of plants of the family Euphorbiaceae; a poisonous plant found in eastern Africa and the West Indies.

J. cur'cas, *J. glandulifera;* Barbados nut or physic-nut, the seed of which furnishes a purgative oil similar to croton oil.

J. glandulif'era, *J. curcas.*

J. u'rens, a species of South America; the macerated fresh leaves are used as a rubefacient and stimulating poultice; the seeds fu nish a purgative oil.

jaundice (jawn'dis) [Fr. *jaune,* yellow]. Icterus; a yellowish staining of the integument, sclerae, and deeper tissues and the excretions with bile pigments, which are increased in the plasma.

acholuric j., j. with excessive amounts of unconjugated bilirubin in the plasma and without bile pigments in the urine.

black j., **(1)** obsolete term for *icterus* neonatorum; **(2)** obsolete term for *icterus* melas.

catarrhal j., obsolete term for viral *hepatitis* type A.

cholestatic j., j. produced by inspissated bile or bile plugs in small biliary passages in the liver.

chronic acholuric j., hereditary *spherocytosis.*

chronic familial j., hereditary *spherocytosis.*

chronic idiopathic j., Dubin-Johnson *syndrome.*

congenital hemolytic j., hereditary *spherocytosis.*

familial nonhemolytic j., constitutional hepatic dysfunction; benign familial icterus; Gilbert's disease or syndrome; Hebra's disease (2); mild j. due to increased amounts of unconjugated bilirubin in the plasma without evidence of liver damage, biliary obstruction, or hemolysis; thought to be due to an inborn error of metabolism in which the excretion of bilirubin by the liver is defective, ascribed to decreased conjugation of bilirubin as a glucuronide.

hematogenous j., hemolytic j.

hemolytic j., hematogenous or toxemic j.; j. resulting from increased production of bilirubin from hemoglobin as a result of any process (toxic, congenital, or immune) causing increased destruction of erythrocytes.
hepatocellular j., j. resulting from diffuse injury or inflammation or failure of function of the liver cells, usually referring to viral or toxic hepatitis.
hepatogenous j., j. resulting from disease of the liver, as distinguished from that due to blood changes.
homologous serum j., obsolete term for viral *hepatitis* type B.
infectious j., **(1)** Weil's *disease;* **(2)** sometimes used in referring to infectious (viral) *hepatitis.*
leptospiral j., j. associated with infection by various species of *Leptospira.*
malignant j., *icterus* gravis.
mechanical j., obstructive j.
j. of the newborn, *icterus* neonatorum.
nonobstructive j., any j. in which the main biliary passages are not obstructed, *e.g.*, hemolytic j. or j. due to hepatitis.
nuclear j., kernicterus.
obstructive j., mechanical j.; j. resulting from obstruction to the flow of bile into the duodenum, whether intra- or extrahepatic.
painless j., j. not associated with abdominal pain; usually used for obstructive j. resulting from obstruction of the common bile duct at the head of the pancreas by a tumor or impaction of a stone.
physiologic j., physiologic *icterus.*
regurgitation j., j. due to biliary obstruction, the bile pigment having been conjugated and secreted by the hepatic cells and then reabsorbed into the bloodstream.
retention j., j. due to insufficiency of liver function or to an excess of bile pigment production; the bilirubin is unconjugated since it has not passed through the liver cells; van den Bergh test is indirect.
spherocytic j., hemolytic j. associated with spherocytosis.
toxemic j., hemolytic j.

jaundice root. Hydrastis.

jaw [A.S. *ceōwan,* to chew]. **1.** One of the two bony structures, in which the teeth are set, forming the framework of the mouth. **2.** Common name for either the maxillae or the mandible.
crackling j., chronic subluxation with clicking on motion.
Hapsburg j. and lip, prognathism and pouting lower lip, characteristic of the Hispano-Austrian imperial dynasty.
lock-j., trismus.
lower j., mandibula.
lumpy j., actinomycosis.
parrot j., a condition caused by protrusion of incisor teeth.
upper j., maxilla.

Jaworski, Walery, Polish physician, 1849–1924. See J.'s *bodies.*

Jeanselme, A. Edouard, French dermatologist, 1858–1935. See J.'s *nodules.*

jecur, gen. **jecoris** (jek'ŭr, -ōr-is) [L.]. Obsolete term for the liver.

Jeghers, Harald J., U.S. physician, *1904. See Peutz-J. *syndrome;* J. Peutz syndrome.

jejun-. See jejuno-.

jejunal (je-jū'năl). Relating to the jejunum.

jejunectomy (je-jū-nek'tō-mē) [jejunum + G. *ektomē,* excision]. Excision of all or a part of the jejunum.

jejunitis (je-jū-nī'tis). Inflammation of the jejunum.

jejuno-, jejun- [L. *jejunus,* empty]. Combining forms relating to the jejunum.

jejunocolostomy (je-jū-nō-kō-los'tō-mē) [jejuno- + colon + G. *stoma,* mouth]. Establishment of a communication between the jejunum and the colon.

jejunoileal (je-jū'nō-il'ē-ăl). Relating to the jejunum and the ileum.

jejunoileitis (je-jū'nō-il-ē-ī'tis). Inflammation of the jejunum and ileum.

jejunoileostomy (je-jū'nō-il-ē-os'tō-mē) [jejuno- + ileum + G. *stoma,* mouth]. Establishment of a new communication between the jejunum and the ileum.

jejunojejunostomy (je-jū'nō-jĕ-jū-nos'tō-mē) [jejuno- + jejuno- + G. *stoma,* mouth]. An anastomosis between two portions of jejunum.

jejunoplasty (je-jū'nō-plas-tē) [jejuno- + G. *plastos,* molded]. A corrective surgical procedure on the jejunum.

jejunostomy (je-jū-nos'tō-mē) [jejuno- + G. *stoma,* mouth]. Operative establishment of an opening from the abdominal wall into the jejunum, usually with creation of a stoma on the abdominal wall.

jejunotomy (je-jū-not'ō-mē) [jejuno- + G. *tomē,* incision]. Incision into the jejunum.

jejunum (jĕ-jū'nŭm) [L. *jejunus,* empty]. [NA]. The portion of small intestine, about 8 feet in length, between the duodenum and the ileum.

Jellinek, Stefan, Austrian physician, *1871. See J.'s *sign.*

jelly (jel'ē) [L. *gelo,* to freeze]. A semisolid tremulous compound usually containing some form of gelatin in solution.
cardiac j., term introduced by C.L. Davis for the gelatinous, noncellular material between the endothelial lining and the myocardial layer of the heart in very young embryos; later in development it serves as a substratum for cardiac mesenchyme.
interlaminar j., term introduced by B.M. Patten for the gelatinous material between ectoderm and endoderm that serves as the substrate on which mesenchymal cells migrate.
Wharton's j., the mucous connective tissue of the umbilical cord.

jellyfish (jel'ē-fish). Marine coelenterates (class Hydrozoa) including some poisonous species, notably *Physalia,* the Portuguese man-of-war; toxin is injected into the skin by nematocysts on the tentacles, causing linear wheals.

Jendrassik, Ernö, Hungarian physician, 1858–1936. See J.'s *maneuver.*

Jenner, Harley D., Canadian physician, *1907. See J.-Kay *unit.*

Jenner, Louis, British physician, 1866–1904. See J.'s *stain.*

Jensen, Carl O., Danish veterinary surgeon and pathologist, 1864–1934. See J.'s *sarcoma.*

Jensen, Edmund Z., Danish ophthalmologist, 1861–1950. See J.'s *disease.*

jerk. 1. A sudden pull. **2.** Deep *reflex.*
ankle j., Achilles *reflex.*
chin j., jaw *reflex.*
crossed j., crossed *reflex.*
crossed adductor j., crossed adductor *reflex.*
crossed knee j., crossed knee *reflex.*
elbow j., triceps *reflex.*
jaw j., jaw *reflex.*
knee j., patellar *reflex.*
supinator j., brachioradial *reflex.*

jerks (pl.). Chorea or any form of tic.

Jervell, Anton, 20th century Norwegian cardiologist. See J. and Lange-Nielsen *syndrome.*

Jesuits' bark. Cinchona.

jet lag. An imbalance of the normal circadian rhythm resulting from subsonic or supersonic travel through a varied number of time zones and leading to fatigue, irritability, and various constitutional disturbances.

Jeune, M., 20th century French pediatrician. See J.'s *syndrome.*

Jewett, Hugh J., U.S. urologist, *1903. See J. *sound.*

Jewett and Strong staging. See under staging.

jig'ger. Common name for *Tunga penetrans.* See also chigoe.

jim'son weed. *Datura stramonium.*

jird (jerd). A rodent of the genus *Meriones;* distinct from the gerbil, with which it is frequently confused.

Jk blood group. See Kidd blood group, Blood Groups appendix.

JNA Abbreviation for *Jena Nomina Anatomica,* 1935. See *Nomina Anatomica.*

Jobert de Lamballe, Antoine J., French surgeon, 1799–1867. See J. de L.'s *fossa, suture.*

Jod-Basedow, jodbasedow (yod-bas'ĕ-dō) [Ger. *Jod,* iodine, + K.A. von *Basedow*]. See Jod-Basedow *phenomenon.*

Joest, Ernst, German veterinary pathologist, 1873–1926. See J. *bodies.*

Joffroy, Alexis, French physician, 1844–1908. See J.'s *reflex, sign.*

Johne, H. Albert, German physician, 1839–1910. See johnin; J.'s *bacillus, disease.*

johnin (yō'nin) [A. *Johne*]. A product used as a diagnostic agent, analogous to tuberculin but made from *Mycobacterium paratuberculosis* (the causative organism of Johne's disease) grown in a broth medium containing *M. phlei* (timothy hay bacillus); used as an allergen to provoke reactions in infected animals.

Johnson, Frank B., U.S. pathologist, *1919. See Dubin-J. *syndrome.*

Johnson, Frank C., U.S. pediatrician, 1894–1934. See Stevens-J. *syndrome.*

Johnson, Harry B., U.S. dentist. See J.'s *method.*

Johnson, Treat Baldwin, U.S. chemist, 1875–1947. See under Wheeler-J. *test.*

JOINT

joint (joynt) [L. *junctura;* fr. *jungo,* pp. *junctus,* to join]. Articulatio.

acromioclavicular j., *articulatio* acromioclavicularis.

ankle j., *articulatio* talocruralis.

anterior intraoccipital j., *synchondrosis* intraoccipitalis anterior.

arthrodial j., *articulatio* plana.

atlanto-occipital j., *articulatio* atlanto-occipitalis.

ball-and-socket j., *articulatio* spheroidea.

biaxial j., one in which there are two principal axes of movement situated at right angles to each other; *e.g.,* saddle j.'s.

bicondylar j., *articulatio* bicondylaris.

bilocular j., one in which the intra-articular disk is complete, dividing the j. into two distinct cavities.

Budin's obstetrical j., *synchondrosis* intraoccipitalis posterior.

calcaneocuboid j., *articulatio* calcaneocuboidea.

capitular j., *articulatio* capitis costae.

carpal j.'s, *articulationes* intercarpeae.

carpometacarpal j.'s, *articulationes* carpometacarpeae.

carpometacarpal j. of thumb, *articulatio* carpometacarpea pollicis.

cartilaginous j., *articulatio* cartilaginis.

Charcot's j., neuropathic j.

Chopart's j., *articulatio* tarsi transversa.

Clutton's j.'s, symmetrical arthrosis in cases of congenital syphilis.

coccygeal j., *articulatio* sacrococcygea.

cochlear j., spiral or screw j.; a variety of hinge j. in which the elevation and depression, respectively, on the opposing articular surfaces form part of a spiral, flexion being then accompanied by a certain amount of lateral deviation.

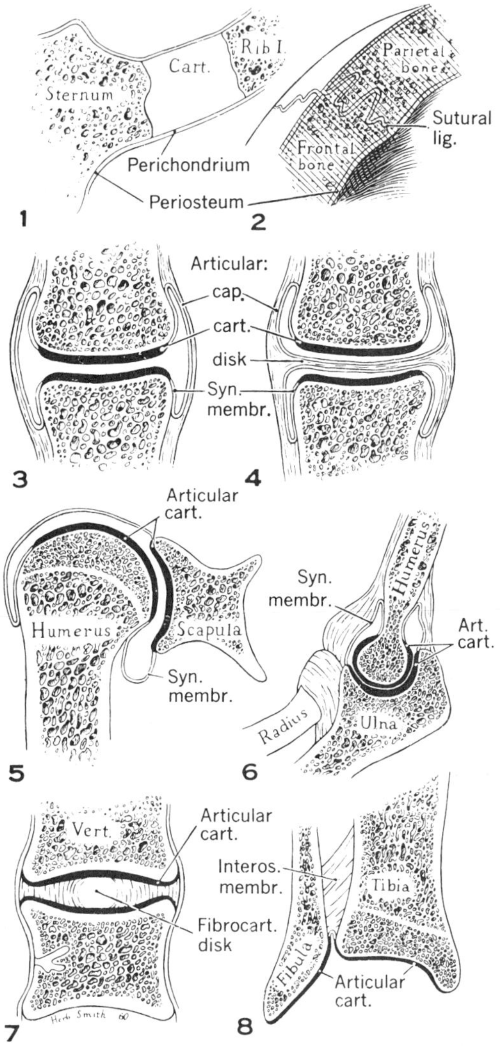

Types of Joint

1, Cartilaginous, synchondrosis; *2,* fibrous, suture; *3,* synovial, simple; *4,* synovial, with articular disk; *5,* synovial, spheroid (ball and socket); *6,* synovial, ginglymus (hinge); *7,* cartilaginous, symphysis; *8,* fibrous, syndesmosis.

coffin j., the distal interphalangeal articulation of the horse, a compound synovial j. between the middle and distal phalanges and also with the distal sesamoid or navicular bone on the caudal side.

compound j., *articulatio* composita.

condylar j., *articulatio* ellipsoidea.

costochondral j., *articulatio* costochondralis.

costotransverse j., *articulatio* costotransversaria.

costovertebral j.'s, *articulationes* costovertebrales.

cotyloid j., *articulatio* spheroidea.

cricoarytenoid j., *articulatio* cricoarytenoidea.

cricothyroid j., *articulatio* cricothyroidea.

Cruveilhier's j., *articulatio* atlantoaxialis mediana.

cubital j., *articulatio* cubiti.

cuboideonavicular j., a fibrous j. between adjacent parts of the cuboid and navicular bones; occasionally a synovial cavity is found here as an extension of the cuneonavicular j.

cuneocuboid j., the synovial articulation between the lateral surface of the lateral cuneiform and the anterior two-thirds of the medial surface of the cuboid.
cuneometatarsal j.'s, *articulationes* tarsometatarseae.
cuneonavicular j., *articulatio* cuneonavicularis.
dentoalveolar j., gomphosis.
diarthrodial j., *articulatio* synovialis.
digital j.'s, *articulationes* interphalangeae.
DIP j.'s, distal interphalangeal j.'s.
distal interphalangeal j.'s, DIP j.'s; the synovial j.'s between the middle and distal phalanges of the fingers and of the toes.
j.'s of ear bones, *articulationes* ossiculorum auditis.
elbow j., *articulatio* cubiti.
ellipsoidal j., *articulatio* ellipsoidea.
enarthrodial j., *articulatio* spheroidea.
false j., pseudarthrosis.
femoropatellar j., the articulation of the facets on the articular surface of the patella with corresponding surfaces on the femoral condyles.
fibrous j., *articulatio* fibrosa.
flail j., a j. with loss of function caused by loss of the power to stabilize the j. in any plane within its normal range of motion.
j.'s of free inferior limb, *articulationes* membri inferioris liberi.
j.'s of free superior limb, *articulationes* membri superioris liberi.
ginglymoid j., ginglymus.
gliding j., *articulatio* plana.
gompholic j., gomphosis.
j. of head of rib, *articulatio* capitis costae.
hemophilic j., chronic arthroplasty due to repeated hemarthrosis in a hemophiliac.
hinge j., ginglymus.
hip j., *articulatio* coxae.
humeroradial j., *articulatio* humeroradialis.
humeroulnar j., *articulatio* humeroulnaris.
hysterical j., a simulation of j. disease, with symptoms of pain, possibly swelling, and impairment of motion.
immovable j., *articulatio* fibrosa.
incudomalleolar j., *articulatio* incudomallearis.
incudostapedial j., *articulatio* incudostapedia.
j.'s of inferior limb girdle, *articulationes* cinguli membri inferioris.
inferior radioulnar j., *articulatio* radioulnaris distalis.
inferior tibiofibular j., *syndesmosis* tibiofibularis.
interarticular j.'s, *articulationes* zygapophyseales.
intercarpal j.'s, *articulationes* intercarpeae.
interchondral j.'s, *articulationes* interchondrales.
intercuneiform j.'s, the articulations between contiguous surfaces of the cuneiform bones.
intermetacarpal j.'s, *articulationes* intermetacarpeae.
intermetatarsal j.'s, *articulationes* intermetatarseae.
interphalangeal j.'s, *articulationes* interphalangeae.
intersternebral j.'s, *synchondroses* intersternebrales.
intertarsal j.'s, *articulationes* intertarseae.
jaw j., *articulatio* temporomandibularis.
knee j., *articulatio* genus.
lateral atlantoaxial j., *articulatio* atlantoaxialis lateralis.
lateral atlantoepistrophic j., *articulatio* atlantoaxialis lateralis.
Lisfranc's j.'s, *articulationes* tarsometatarseae.
lumbosacral j., *articulatio* lumbosacralis.
Luschka's j.'s, uncovertebral j.'s; small synovial j.'s between adjacent lateral lips of the bodies of the lower cervical vertebrae.
mandibular j., *articulatio* temporomandibularis.
manubriosternal j., *synchondrosis* manubriosternalis.
median atlantoaxial j., *articulatio* atlantoaxialis mediana.
metacarpophalangeal j.'s, *articulationes* metacarpophalangeae.
metatarsophalangeal j.'s, *articulationes* metatarsophalangeae.
middle atlantoepistrophic j., *articulatio* atlantoaxialis mediana.
middle carpal j., *articulatio* mediocarpea.
midtarsal j., *articulatio* tarsi transversa.
mortise j., *articulatio* talocruralis.
movable j., *articulatio* synovialis.
MP j.'s, (1) *articulationes* metacarpophalangeae; **(2)** *articulationes* metatarsophalangeae.
multiaxial j., polyaxial j.; one in which movement occurs in a number of axes. See *articulatio* spheroidea.
neurocentral j., neurocentral *synchondrosis.*
neuropathic j., neuropathic arthritis or arthropathy; tabetic arthropathy; Charcot's joint; destructive j. disease caused by diminished proprioceptive sensation, with gradual destruction of the j. by repeated subliminal injury, commonly associated with tabes dorsalis or diabetic neuropathy.
peg-and-socket j., gomphosis.
petro-occipital j., *synchondrosis* petro-occipitalis.
phalangeal j.'s, *articulationes* interphalangeae.
PIP j.'s, proximal interphalangeal j.'s.
pisotriquetral j., *articulatio* ossis pisiformis.
pivot j., *articulatio* trochoidea.
plane j., *articulatio* plana.
polyaxial j., multiaxial j.
posterior intraoccipital j., *synchondrosis* intraoccipitalis posterior.
proximal interphalangeal j.'s, PIP j.'s; the synovial j.'s between the proximal and middle phalanges of the fingers and of the toes.
radiocarpal j., *articulatio* radiocarpea.
rotary j., rotatory j., *articulatio* trochoidea.
sacrococcygeal j., *articulatio* sacrococcygea.
sacroiliac j., *articulatio* sacroiliaca.
saddle j., *articulatio* sellaris.
schindyletic j., schindylesis.
screw j., cochlear j.
shoulder j., *articulatio* humeri.
simple j., *articulatio* simplex.
socket j., *articulatio* spheroidea.
spheno-occipital j., *synchondrosis* spheno-occipitalis.
spheroid j., *articulatio* spheroidea.
spiral j., cochlear j.
sternal j.'s, *synchondroses* sternales.
sternoclavicular j., *articulatio* sternoclavicularis.
sternocostal j.'s, *articulationes* sternocostales.
stifle j., stifle; the femorotibial articulation in the hind leg of the horse and other quadrupeds; it corresponds to the knee in man.
subtalar j., *articulatio* subtalaris.
j.'s of superior limb girdle, *articulationes* cinguli membri superioris.
superior radioulnar j., *articulatio* radioulnaris proximalis.
superior tibiofibular j., *articulatio* tibiofibularis.
suture j., sutura.
synarthrodial j., (1) *articulatio* fibrosa; **(2)** *articulatio* cartilaginis.
synchondrodial j., synchondrosis.
syndesmodial j., syndesmotic j., syndesmosis.
synovial j., *articulatio* synovialis.
talocalcaneal j., *articulatio* subtalaris.
talocalcaneonavicular j., *articulatio* talocalcaneonavicularis.
tarsal j.'s, *articulationes* intertarseae.
tarsometatarsal j.'s, *articulationes* tarsometatarseae.
temporomandibular j., *articulatio* temporomandibularis.
thigh j., *articulatio* coxae.
tibiofibular j., inferior, *syndesmosis* tibiofibularis.
tibiofibular j., superior, *articulatio* tibiofibularis.
transverse tarsal j., *articulatio* tarsi transversa.
trochoid j., *articulatio* trochoidea.
uncovertebral j.'s, Luschka's j.'s.
uniaxial j., one in which movement is around one axis only.
unilocular j., one in which an intra-articular disk is incomplete or

absent, the j. having but a single cavity.
wedge-and-groove j., schindylesis.
wrist j., *articulatio* radiocarpea.
xiphisternal j., *synchondrosis* xiphosternalis.
zygapophysial j.'s, *articulatio* zygapophyseales.

joint mice. Small fibrous, cartilaginous, or bony loose bodies in the synovial cavity of a joint.

Jolles, Adolf, Austrian chemist, *1863. See J.'s *test.*

Jolly, Friedrich, German neurologist, 1844–1904. See J.'s *reaction.*

Jolly, Justin, French histologist, 1870–1953. See J. *bodies;* Howell-J. *bodies.*

Jones, Ernest, British psychiatrist, 1879–1958. See Ross-J. *test.*

Jones, Henry Bence. See Bence Jones, Henry.

Jonnesco (Ionescu), Thomas, Bucharest surgeon, 1860–1926. See J.'s *fossa.*

Jonston, Johns, Scottish physician in Poland, 1603–1675. See J.'s *alopecia, area.*

Joseph, Jacques, German surgeon, 1865–1934. See J. *rhinoplasty.*

Joubert, M., 20th century Canadian neurologist. See J.'s *syndrome.*

Joule, James P., British physicist, 1818–1889. See joule; J.'s *equivalent.*

joule (J) (jūl, jowl) [J.P. *Joule*]. A unit of energy; the heat generated, or energy expended, by an ampere flowing through an ohm for 1 second; equal to 10^7 ergs, and to a newton-meter. It is an approved multiple of the SI fundamental unit of energy, the erg, and is intended to replace the calorie (4.187 J).

juccuya (ū-kū'yă). Cutaneous *leishmaniasis.*

Judkins, Melvin P., U.S. radiologist, *1922. See J. *technique.*

juga (jū'gă). Plural of jugum.

jugal (jū'găl) [L. *jugalis,* yoked together, fr. *jugum,* a yoke]. **1.** Connecting; yoked. **2.** Relating to the zygomatic bone.

jugale (jū-gā'lē). Jugal point; a craniometric point at the union of the temporal and frontal processes of the zygomatic bone.

jugomaxillary (jū'gō-mak'si-lār-ē). Relating to the zygomatic bone and the maxilla.

jugular (jŭg'yū-lar) [L. *jugulum,* throat]. **1.** Relating to the throat or neck. **2.** Relating to the j. veins. **3.** A j. vein.

jugulum (jŭg'yū-lŭm). Throat (2).

jugum, pl. **juga** (jū'gŭm, -gă) [L. a yoke]. **1.** Yoke; a ridge or furrow connecting two points. **2.** A type of forceps.
j. alveola're, pl. **ju'ga alveola'ria** [NA], alveolar yoke; one of the eminences on the outer surface of the alveolar process of the maxilla or mandible, formed by the roots of the incisor teeth.
j. sphenoida'le [NA], planum sphenoidale; a plane surface on the sphenoid bone, in front of the sella turcica, connecting the two lesser wings, and forming part of the anterior cranial fossa.

juice (jūs) [L. *jus,* broth]. **1.** The interstitial fluid of a plant or animal. **2.** A digestive secretion.
appetite j., gastric j. secreted upon the sight or smell of food and at the time of eating, influenced by the attractiveness of the food and delight in the food ingested; a conditioned reflex.
cancer j., turbid, white to yellow-white or gray-white fluid (chiefly plasma) that may be expressed from certain forms of malignant neoplastic tissue, and is likely to contain neoplastic cells and debris; formed especially in relatively large, degenerating, partly necrotic foci of rapidly growing neoplastic tissue.
gastric j., the digestive fluid secreted by the glands of the stomach; a thin colorless liquid of acid reaction containing primarily hydrochloric acid, chymosin, pepsinogen, and intrinsic factor plus mucus.
intestinal j., an alkaline straw-colored fluid secreted by the intestinal glands; its enzymes (peptidases, saccharases, nucleases, lecithinases, phosphatases, lipases) complete the hydrolysis of carbohydrates, proteins, and lipids.
pancreatic j., the external secretion of the pancreas; a clear alkaline fluid containing several enzymes: α-amylase, nucleases, trypsinogen, chymotrypsinogen, and triacylglycerol lipase.

junction (jŭngk'shŭn). Junctura (2).
amelodental j., amelodentinal j., rarely used terms for dentinoenamel j.
amnioembryonic j., the line of amniotic attachment to the periphery of the embryonic disk.
anorectal j., the site of transition from rectum to anus.
cementodentinal j., dentinocemental j.; the surface at which the cementum and dentin of the root of a tooth are joined.
cementoenamel j., the surface at which the enamel of the crown and the cementum of the root of a tooth are joined. See also cervical *line.*
choledochoduodenal j., that part of the duodenal wall traversed by the ductus choledochus, ductus pancreaticus, and ampulla.
dentinocemental j., cementodentinal j.
dentinoenamel j., the surface at which the enamel and the dentin of the crown of a tooth are joined.
electrotonic j., gap j.
esophagogastric j., the line at the cardiac orifice of the stomach where there is a transition from the stratified squamous epithelium of the esophagus to the simple columnar epithelium of the stomach.
gap j., macula communicans; nexus; electrotonic j. or synapse; an intercellular j. formerly considered to be a tight, membrane-to-membrane j. (macula occludens) but now shown to have a 2 nm gap between apposed cell membranes; the gap is not blank but contains subunits in the form of polygonal lattices; it occurs in epithelia, between certain nerve cells, and in smooth and cardiac muscle; it is believed to mediate electrotonic coupling which allows ionic currents to pass from one cell to another. See also synapse.
intercellular j.'s, specializations of the cellular margins which contribute to the adhesion or allow for communication between cells; they include the macula adherens (desmosome), zonula adherens, zonula occludens, and nexus (gap junction).
intermediate j., *zonula* adherens.
j. of lips, *commissura* labiorum.
mucocutaneous j., the site of transition from epidermis to the epithelium of a mucous membrane.
muscle-tendon j., muscle-tendon *attachment.*
myoneural j., neuromuscular j.; the synaptic connection of the axon of the motor neuron with a muscle fiber. See motor *endplate.*
neuroectodermal j., neurosomatic j.; the margin of the embryonic neural plate separating it from the embryonic ectoderm; cells from this region form the neural crest.
neuromuscular j., myoneural j.
neurosomatic j., neuroectodermal j.
sacrococcygeal j., *articulatio* sacrococcygea.
sclerocorneal j., *limbus* corneae.
squamocolumnar j., the site of transition from stratified squamous epithelium to columnar epithelium, usually characterized by stratified columnar epithelium.
ST j., J *point.*
tight j., an intercellular j. between epithelial cells in which the outer leaflet of lateral cell membranes fuse to form a variable number of parallel interweaving strands that greatly reduce transepithelial permeability to macromolecules, solutes, and water via the paracellular route.
tympanostapedial j., *syndesmosis* tympanostapedia.

junctura, pl. **juncturae** (jŭngk-tū'ră, -rē) [L. a joining]. **1.** Articulatio. **2.** Juncture; junction; the point, line, or surface of union of two parts, mainly bones or cartilages.

j. cartilag'inea, *articulatio* cartilaginis.

junctu'rae cin'guli mem'bri superio'ris, *articulationes* cinguli membri superioris.

j. fibro'sa, *articulatio* fibrosa.

j. lumbosacra'lis, *articulatio* lumbosacralis.

junctu'rae mem'bri inferio'ris li'beri, *articulationes* membri inferioris liberi.

junctu'rae mem'bri superio'ris li'beri, *articulationes* membri superioris liberi.

junctu'rae os'sium, alternative name for articulationes. See articulatio.

j. sacrococcyge'a, *articulatio* sacrococcygea.

j. synovia'lis, *articulatio* synovialis.

junctu'rae ten'dinum, *connexus* intertendineus.

junctu'rae zygapophysea'les, *articulationes* zygapophyseales.

juncture (jŭngk'chūr). Junctura (2).

Jung, Carl Gustav, Swiss psychiatrist and psychologist, 1875–1961. See jungian *psychoanalysis.*

Jung, Karl G., Swiss anatomist, 1793–1864. See J.'s *muscle.*

jungian (yung'ē-an). Attributed to or described by Carl Gustav Jung.

Jüngling, Adolph O., German surgeon, 1884–1944. See J.'s *disease.*

juniper (jū'ni-per) [L. the juniper-tree]. Juniper berries; the dried ripe fruit of *Juniperus communis* (family Pinaceae).

j. berry oil, a volatile oil distilled from the fruit of *Juniperus communis;* a diuretic.

j. tar, cade oil; the empyreumatic volatile oil obtained from the woody portion of *Juniperus oxycedrus;* used externally for skin diseases.

Junius, Paul, Ger. ophthalmologist, *1871. See Kuhnt-J. *degeneration, disease.*

Junod, Victor T., French physician, 1809–1881. See J.'s *boot.*

jurisprudence (jūr-is-prū'dens) [L. *juris prudentia,* knowledge of law]. The science of law, its principles and concepts.

dental j., forensic *dentistry.*

medical j., forensic *medicine.*

justo major (jus'tō mā'jer). See *pelvis* justo major.

justo minor (jus'tō mī'ner). See *pelvis* justo minor.

juxtaepiphysial (jŭks'tă-ep-i-fiz'ē-ăl). Close to or adjoining an epiphysis.

juxtaglomerular (jŭks'tă-glō-mer'yū-lăr). Close to or adjoining a renal glomerulus.

juxtallocortex (jŭks'tă-lō-kōr'teks). O. Vogt's collective term for several regions of the cerebral cortex which occupy an intermediate position between the isocortex and the allocortex.

juxtaposition (jŭks-tă-pō-zish'ŭn) [L. *juxta,* near to, + *positio,* a placing, fr. *pono,* pp. *positus,* to place]. A position side by side. See also apposition; contiguity.

K

K 1. Symbol for potassium; phylloquinone; kelvin. **2.** In optics, the coefficient of scleral rigidity. **3.** In contact lens fitting, the radius of curvature of the flattest meridian of the apical cornea.

K Symbol for dissociation constant. Thus, K_a is the symbol for the dissociation constant of an acid; K_b, of a base; K_i, of an enzyme-inhibitor complex; K_m, of the Michaelis-Menten constant; K_w, of water.

k Symbol for kilo-.

k Symbol for rate or velocity constant.

K and k blood groups. See Kell blood group, Blood Groups appendix.

Ka Abbreviation for kathode or kathodal.

kabure (kah-bū'rē). *Schistosomiasis* japonica.

Kaes, Theodor, German neurologist, 1852–1913. See *line* of K.; *band* of K.-Bechterew.

kafindo (kă-fin'dō). Onyalai.

Kaiserling, Karl, German pathologist, 1869–1942. See K.'s *fixative.*

kak-, kako-. See caco-.

kakké (kahk'kā) [Jap.]. Beriberi.

kal-, kali- [L. *kalium,* potassium]. Combining forms relating to potassium; sometimes improperly written as *kalio-.*

kala azar (kah'lah ah-zahr') [Hind. *kala,* black, + *azar,* poison]. Visceral *leishmaniasis.*

kalemia (kă-lē'mē-ă). The presence of potassium in the blood.

kaliopenia (kā'lē-ō-pē'nē-ă) [Mod. L. *kalium,* potassium, + G. *penia,* poverty]. Insufficiency of potassium in the body.

kaliopenic (kā'lē-ō-pē'nik). Relating to kaliopenia.

Kalischer, Siegfried, German physician, *1862. See Sturge-K.-Weber *syndrome.*

kalium (kā'lē-ŭm) [Mod. L. fr. Ar. *quali,* potash]. Potassium.

kaliuresis (kā'lē-yū-rē'sis). Kaluresis.

kaliuretic (kā'lē-yū-ret'ik). Kaluretic.

kallak (kah-lak') [Eskimo word meaning skin disease]. A peculiar pustular dermatitis observed among the Eskimos.

kallidin (kal'i-din). Bradykininogen; kallidin I or 10; lysylbradykinin; bradykinin with a lysyl group attached to the amino terminus; this group can be removed by an aminopeptidase in the blood to yield bradykinin; a decapeptide vasodilator.
- **k. I,** bradykinin.
- **k. II,** kallidin.
- **k. 9,** bradykinin.
- **k. 10,** kallidin.

kallikrein (kal-i-krē'in). Kininogenase; kininogenin; a group of enzymes (*e.g.,* plasma, tissue, pancreatic, urinary, submandibular k.) that can convert kininogen by proteolysis to bradykinin or kallidin; trypsin and plasmin can also effect the conversion.

Kallmann, Franz Josef, U.S. medical geneticist and psychiatrist, 1897–1965. See K.'s *syndrome.*

kaluresis (kal-yū-rē'sis) [Mod. L. *kalium,* potassium, + G. *ouresis,* urination]. Kaliuresis; the increased urinary excretion of potassium.

kaluretic (kal-yū-ret'ik). Kaliuretic; relating to, causing, or characterized by kaluresis.

kanamycin sulfate (kan-ă-mī'sin). An antibiotic substance derived from strains of *Streptomyces kanamycetius;* a thermostable, water-soluble, polybasic substance consisting of two amino sugars glycosidally linked to deoxystreptamine. The antibacterial activity *in vitro* is nearly identical with that of neomycin and is active against many aerobic Gram-positive and Gram-negative bacteria (*Aerobacter, Escherichia coli, Proteus, Klebsiella, Neisseria, Shigella,* and *Salmonella*). Excessive doses and prolonged administration may result in irreversible damage to the auditory portion of the eighth cranial nerve; disturbances of equilibrium may also occur.

Kandori, Fumio, Japanese ophthalmologist, *1904. See fleck *retina* (of K.).

Kanner, Leo, Austrian psychiatrist in U. S., *1894. See K.'s *syndrome.*

kanyemba (kan-yem'bă). Chiufa.

kaolin (kā'ō-lin) [Ch. *kao lin,* High Ridge, name of a locality in China where the substance is found in abundance]. Aluminum silicate; powdered and freed from gritty particles by elutriation; used as a demulcent and adsorbent; in dentistry, used to add toughness and opacity to porcelain teeth.

kaolinosis (kā'ō-lin-ō'sis). Pneumonoconiosis caused by the inhalation of clay dust.

Kaposi, Moritz K., Austrian dermatologist, 1837–1902. See K.'s varicelliform *eruption, sarcoma.*

kappacism (kap'ă-sizm) [G. *kappa,* the letter k]. Faulty pronunciation of the "k" sound.

Karmen, Albert, U.S. internist and pathologist, *1930. See K. *unit.*

Karmen cannula. See under cannula.

Karnofsky, D.A., 20th century U.S. physician. See K. *scale.*

Kartagener, Manes, Swiss physician, *1897. See K.'s *syndrome, triad.*

karyo- [G. *karyon,* nucleus]. Combining form denoting nucleus.

karyochrome (kar'ē-ō-krōm) [karyo- + G. *chroma,* color]. A nerve cell body having little or no Nissl substance visible but a nucleus which stains intensely.

karyoclasis (kar-ē-ok'lă-sis) [karyo- + G. *klasis,* a breaking]. Karyorrhexis.

karyocyte (kar'ē-ō-sīt) [karyo- + G. *kytos,* cell]. A young, immature normoblast.

karyogamic (kar-ē-ō-gam'ik). Relating to or marked by karyogamy.

karyogamy (kar-ē-og'ă-mē) [karyo- + G. *gamos,* marriage]. Fusion of the nuclei of two cells, as occurs in fertilization or true conjugation.

karyogenesis (kar-ē-ō-jen'ĕ-sis) [karyo- + G. *genesis,* production]. Formation of the nucleus of a cell.

karyogenic (kar-ē-ō-jen'ik). Relating to karyogenesis; forming the nucleus.

karyogonad (kar'ē-ō-gō'nad) [karyo- + G. *gone,* generation, descent]. Micronucleus (2).

karyogram (kar'ē-ō-gram). Karyotype.

karyokinesis (kar'ē-ō-ki-nē'sis) [karyo- + G. *kinesis,* movement]. Mitosis.

karyokinetic (kar'ē-ō-ki-net'ik). Mitotic.

karyolymph (kar'ē-ō-limf) [karyo- + L. *lympha,* clear water]. Nuclear hyaloplasm or sap; nucleochylema; nucleochyme; the presumably fluid substance or gel of the nucleus in which stainable elements were believed to be suspended; much that was formerly considered to be k. is now known to be euchromatin.

karyolysis (kar-ē-ol'i-sis) [karyo- + G. *lysis,* dissolution]. Apparent destruction of the nucleus of a cell by swelling and the loss of affinity of its chromatin for basic dyes.

karyolytic (kar'ē-ō-lit'ik). Relating to karyolysis.

karyomicrosome (kar-ē-ō-mī'krō-sōm) [karyo- + G. *mikros,* small, + *soma,* body]. Nucleomicrosome; one of the minute particles or granules making up the substance of the cell nucleus.

karyomitosis (kar'ē-ō-mī-tō'sis). Mitosis.

karyomitotic (kar'ē-ō-mī-tot'ik). Mitotic.

karyomorphism (kar'ē-ō-mōr'fizm) [karyo- + G. *morphē,* form]. **1.** Development of the nucleus of a cell. **2.** Denoting the nuclear shapes of the cells, especially of the leukocytes.

karyon (kar'ē-on) [G. *karyon,* a nut, kernel]. Nucleus (1).

karyophage (kar'ē-ō-fāj) [karyo- + G. *phagein,* to devour]. An intracellular parasite that feeds on the host nucleus.

karyoplasm (kar'ē-ō-plazm). Rarely used term for nucleoplasm.

karyoplasmolysis (kar'ē-ō-plaz-mol'i-sis). Achromatolysis.

karyoplast (kar'ē-ō-plast) [karyo- + G. *plastos,* formed]. A cell nucleus surrounded by a narrow band of cytoplasm and a plasma membrane.

karyopyknosis (kar'ē-ō-pik-nō'sis) [karyo- + G. *pyknos,* thick, crowded, + *-osis,* condition]. Cytologic characteristics of the superficial or cornified cells of stratified squamous epithelium in which there is shrinkage of the nuclei and condensation of the chromatin into structureless masses.

karyorrhexis (kar-ē-ō-rak'sis) [karyo- + G. *rhexis,* rupture]. Karyoclasis; fragmentation of the nucleus whereby its chromatin is distributed irregularly throughout the cytoplasm; a stage of necrosis usually followed by karyolysis.

karyosome (kar'ē-ō-sōm) [karyo- + G. *sōma,* body]. Chromocenter; chromatin or false nucleolus; net knot; a mass of chromatin often found in the interphase cell nucleus representing a more condensed zone of chromatin filaments.

karyostasis (kar-ē-os'tă-sis) [karyo- + G. *stasis,* a standing still]. Interphase.

karyotheca (kar'ē-ō-thē'kă) [karyo- + G. *thēkē,* box, sheath]. Nuclear *envelope.*

karyotype (kar'ē-ō-tīp). Idiogram (1); karyogram; the chromosome characteristics of an individual or of a cell line, usually presented as a systematized array of metaphase chromosomes from a photomicrograph of a single cell nucleus arranged in pairs in descending order of size and according to the position of the centromere.

karyozoic (kar'ē-ō-zō'ik) [karyo- + G. *zōon,* animal]. Denoting a parasite inhabiting the cell nucleus of its host.

Kasabach, Haig H. See K.-Merritt *syndrome.*

Kasai, Morio, 20th century Japanese surgeon. See K. *operation.*

kasai (kă-sī'). Belgian Congo anemia; a form of anemia occurring in natives of the area formerly known as the Belgian Congo, with associated edema of subcutaneous tissues, depigmented regions in the skin, and various gastrointestinal disturbances; thought to result from deficiencies in nutrition.

Kashin, Nikolai I., Russian orthopedist, 1825–1872. See K.-Bek *disease.*

Kasten, Frederick H., U.S. histochemist and cell biologist, *1927. See K.'s fluorescent Schiff *reagents,* fluorescent Feulgen *stain,* fluorescent PAS *stain.*

kat Abbreviation for katal.

kata- [G. *kata,* down]. Alternative spelling for cata-, combining form meaning down.

katal (kat) (kat'ăl). Unit of catalytic activity equal to one mole per second, as of the amount of enzyme that catalyzes transformation of one mole of substrate per second.

katathermometer (kat'ă-ther-mom'ĕ-ter). An alcohol-filled thermometer of specified design which is heated above ambient temperature and then allowed to cool; the time taken to cool between specified temperatures is a measure of the heat content of the environment that takes into account air movement as well as temperature. The bulb may be silvered to minimize radiation effects or blackened to maximize them.

Katayama, Kunika, Japanese physician, 1856–1931. See K.'s *test.*

kathodal, kathode (Ka) (kath'ō-dăl, kath'ōd). Obsolete spelling of cathodal, cathode.

kation (kat'ī-on). Obsolete spelling of cation.

Katz, Bernard, British neurophysiologist and Nobel laureate, *1911. See Goldman-Hodgkin-K. *equation.*

kava (kah'vah) [Hawaiian name]. **1.** Methysticum. **2.** Yaqona.

Kawasaki, Tomisaku, 20th century Japanese pediatrician. See K. *disease.*

Kay, Herbert D., British biochemist, *1893. See Jenner-K. *unit.*

Kayser, Bernhard, German physician, 1869–1954. See K.-Fleischer *ring.*

Kazanjian, Varaztad H., Armenian otorhinolaryngologist in the U.S., *1879. See K.'s *operation.*

kb Abbreviation for kilobase.

kc Abbreviation for kilocycle.

kcal Abbreviation for kilogram *calorie;* kilocalorie.

Kearns, Thomas P., U.S. ophthalmologist, *1922. See K.-Sayre *syndrome.*

Keating-Hart, Walter V., French physician, 1870–1922. See K.-H.'s *method.*

ked. *Melophagus ovinus.*

keel (kēl). Paratyphoid or salmonellosis of ducklings.

Keen, William W., U.S. surgeon, 1837–1932. See K.'s *operation, sign.*

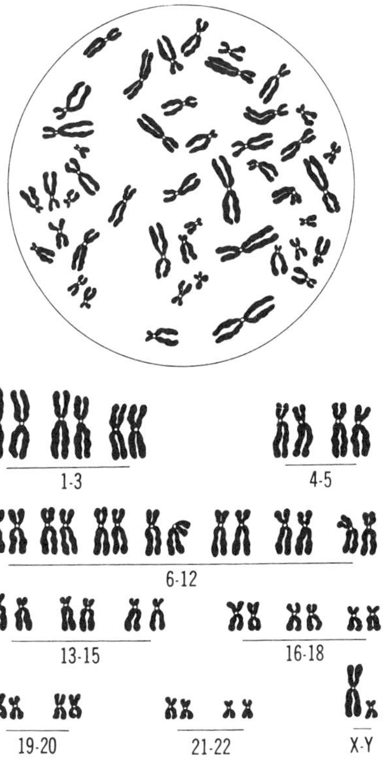

Karyotype of a Normal Human Cell

Kegel, A.H., 20th century U.S. gynecologist. See K.'s *exercises.*

Kehr, Hans, German surgeon, 1862–1916. See K.'s *incision, sign.*

keirospasm (kī'rō-spazm) [G. *keirō,* to shear]. Shaving *cramp.*

Keith, Sir Arthur, British anatomist, 1866–1955. See K.'s *bundle, node;* K. and Flack *node.*

K-el Abbreviation for phyllochromenol.

kelectome (kē'lek-tōm) [G. *kēlē,* tumor, + *ektomē,* excision]. An instrument used, like the harpoon, to remove a specimen of tumor substance for examination.

kelis (kē'lis) [G. *kēlis,* a stain, spot, blemish]. **1.** Obsolete term for morphea. **2.** Obsolete term for keloid.

Kell blood group. See Blood Groups appendix.

Keller, William Lordan, U.S. surgeon, *1874. See K. *bunionectomy.*

Kellie, George, 18th century Scottish anatomist. See Monro-K. *doctrine.*

Kelly, Adam B., British otolaryngologist, 1865–1941. See Paterson-K. *syndrome.*

Kelly, Howard A., U.S. gynecologist, 1858–1943. See K. *clamp;* K.'s *operation,* rectal *speculum.*

keloid (kē'loyd) [G. *kēlē,* a tumor (or *kēlis,* a spot), + *eidos,* appearance]. Cheloid; a nodular, frequently lobulated, firm, movable, nonencapsulated, often linear mass of hyperplastic scar tissue, consisting of wide irregularly distributed bands of collagenous fibrous tissue; occurs in the dermis and adjacent subcutaneous tissue, usually after trauma, surgery, a burn, or severe cutaneous disease such as cystic acne, and is more common in non-Causcasians.

acne k., a chronic eruption of fibrous papules which develop at the site of follicular lesions, usually on the back of the neck at the hairline. Also called dermatitis papillaris capillitii; folliculitis keloidalis; sycosis frambesiformis.

keloidosis (kē'loy-dō'sis). Multiple keloids.

keloplasty (kē'lō-plas-tē) [keloid + G. *plastos,* formed]. Operative removal of a scar or keloid.

kelosomia (kē-lō-sō'mē-ă). Celosomia.

Kelvin, Lord William Thomson, British physicist, 1824–1907. See kelvin; K. *scale.*

kelvin [W. T. *Kelvin*]. A unit of thermodynamic temperature. See Kelvin *scale.*

Kendall. See Abell-K. *method.*

Kendall, Edward C. U.S. biochemist and Nobel laureate, 1886–1972. See K.'s *compounds.*

Kennedy, Edward, U.S. dentist, *1883. See K. *classification.*

Kennedy, Robert Foster, U.S. neurologist, 1884–1952. See K.'s *syndrome;* Foster K. *syndrome.*

Kenny, Sister Elizabeth, Australian nurse, 1886–1952. See K.'s *treatment.*

keno- [G. *kenos,* empty]. See ceno- (3).

Kent, Albert F.S., British physiologist, 1863–1958. See K.'s *bundle;* K.-His *bundle.*

kephalin (kef'ă-lin). Cephalin.

Kerandel, Jean F., French physician, 1873–1934. See K.'s *symptom.*

keraphyllocele (ker-ă-fil'ō-sēl) [G. *keras,* horn, + *phyllon,* leaf, + *kēlē,* hernia, tumor]. A horny tumor on the internal face of the wall of a horse's foot.

kerasin (ker'ă-sin). Cerasin; obsolete term for glucocerebroside.

kerat-. See kerato-.

keratan sulfate (ker'ă-tan). Keratosulfate; a type of sulfated mucopolysaccharide containing D-galactose in place of the uronic acid of hyaluronic acid or chondroitin; found in cartilage, bone, connective tissue, and the cornea.

keratectasia (ker-ă-tek-tā'zē-ă) [kerato- + G. *ektasis,* extrusion]. Keratoectasia; herniation of the cornea.

keratectomy (ker-ă-tek'tō-mē) [kerato- + G. *ektomē,* excision]. Excision of a portion of the cornea.

keratein (ker'ă-tē-in). The easily digested reduction product of keratin, in which the disulfide links are reduced to SH groups, the individual peptide chains being separated.

keratiasis (ker-ă-tī'ă-sis). Keratosis.

keratic (ke-rat'ik) [G. *keras* (*kerat-*), horn]. Horny.

keratin (ker'ă-tin). Ceratin; a scleroprotein or albuminoid present largely in cuticular structures (*e.g.,* hair, nails, horns); it contains a relatively large amount of sulfur, is insoluble in the gastric juices, and is sometimes used for coating enteric pills that are intended to be dissolved only in the intestine. α-Keratin has a folded configuration; β-keratin has an extended configuration.

keratinases (ker'ă-tin-ās-ez). Hydrolases [EC 3.4.99.11 and 3.4.24.10] catalyzing the hydrolysis of keratin.

keratinization (ker'ă-tin-i-zā'shŭn). Cornification; hornification; keratin formation or development of a horny layer; may also apply to premature formation of keratin.

keratinized (ker'ă-ti-nīzd). Cornified; having become horny.

keratinocyte (ke-rat'i-nō-sīt). A cell of the living epidermis and certain oral epithelium that produces keratin in the process of differentiating into the dead and fully keratinized cells of the stratum corneum.

keratinosome (ke-rat'i-nō-sōm). Membrane-coating granule; lamellar granule; Odland body; a membrane-bound granule, 100 to 500 nm in diameter, located in the upper layers of the stratum spinosum of certain stratified squamous epithelia.

keratinous (ke-rat'i-nŭs). **1.** Relating to keratin. **2.** Horny.

keratitis (ker-ă-tī'tis) [kerato- + G. *-itis,* inflammation]. Inflammation of the cornea. See also keratopathy.

actinic k., a reaction of the cornea to ultraviolet light.

alphabetical k., letter-shaped k.; folds in Bowman's membrane with severe corneal inflammation.

deep punctate k., sharply defined opacities in an otherwise clear cornea, occurring in syphilitic iritis.

dendriform k., dendritic k., a form of herpetic k.

diffuse deep k., k. profunda.

Dimmer's k., k. nummularis.

k. discifor'mis, disk-shaped infiltration of the corneal stroma seen in virus infections, particularly herpetic, and after trauma.

exposure k., lagophthalmic k.

fascicular k., a phlyctenular k. followed by the formation of a band or fascicle of blood vessels extending from the margin toward the center.

k. filamento'sa, a condition characterized by the formation of epithelial filaments of varying size and length on the corneal surface.

geographic k., k. with coalescence of superficial lesions in herpes keratitis.

herpetic k., herpes corneae; herpetic keratoconjunctivitis; inflammation of the cornea (or cornea and conjunctiva) due to herpesvirus type 1.

hypopyon k., purulent k. with ulcer resulting in the accumulation of pus in the anterior chamber.

infectious bovine k., pinkeye (2); a highly contagious keratoconjunctivitis that occurs in range or pastured cattle during the summer months, is transmitted most commonly by contact with infectious discharges, and is caused by *Moraxella bovis.*

interstitial k., parenchymatous k.; a chronic inflammation of the corneal stroma, often with neovascularization.

lagophthalmic k., exposure k.; inflammation of the cornea resulting from irritation caused by inability to close the eyelids.

letter-shaped k., alphabetical k.
k. linea'ris mi'grans, inflammatory opacity in parenchymatous k.
marginal k., phlyctenular conjunctivitis occurring at the sclerocorneal junction.
metaherpetic k., postinfectious corneal inflammation in herpetic k. as a result of structural damage to the cornea; not due to virus replication.
mycotic k., an infection of the cornea of the eye caused by a fungus.
necrogranulomatous k., k. characterized by the formation of necrotizing granulomas; an occasional complication of rheumatoid arthritis or Wegener's granulomatosis.
neuroparalytic k., inflammation of the cornea occurring after corneal anesthesia.
k. nummula'ris, Dimmer's k.; coin-shaped or round, discrete, grayish areas 0.5 to 1.5 mm in diameter scattered throughout the various layers of the cornea.
parenchymatous k., interstitial k.; a chronic inflammation, with cellular infiltration of the middle and posterior layers of the cornea.
k. period'ica fu'gax, labile, bilateral, deep corneal inflammation, causing scarring.
phlyctenular k., scrofulous k.; an inflammation of the corneal conjunctiva with the formation of small red nodules of lymphoid tissue (phlyctenulae) near the corneoscleral limbus.
polymorphic superficial k., epithelial degeneration occurring in starvation.
k. profun'da, diffuse deep k.; a deep-seated inflammation of the cornea, accompanied more or less by opacity; probably a hypersensitivity reaction to a chronic infection.
punctate k., k. puncta'ta, keratic *precipitates.*
sclerosing k., inflammation of the cornea complicating scleritis; characterized by opacification of the corneal stroma.
scrofulous k., phlyctenular k.
serpiginous k., hypopyon ulcer (3); pneumococcus or serpent ulcer of cornea; ulcus serpens corneae; a severe, creeping, central, suppurative ulcer often due to pneumococci.
k. sic'ca, *keratoconjunctivitis* sicca.
superficial linear k., spontaneous, painful k. with epithelial erosion and folds in Bowman's membrane.
superficial punctate k., Thygeson's disease; epithelial punctate k. associated with viral conjunctivitis; occasionally may follow exposure to ultraviolet light.
trachomatous k., vascular k. at upper corneoscleral limbus, resulting in pannus.
vascular k., superficial cellular infiltration of the cornea and neovascularization between Bowman's membrane and the epithelium.
vesicular k., k. with coalescence of areas of epithelial corneal edema.
xerotic k., keratomalacia.

kerato-, kerat- [G. *keras,* horn]. Combining forms denoting: **1.** The cornea. **2.** Horny tissue or cells. See also cerat-, cerato-.

keratoacanthoma (ker'ă-tō-ak'an-thō'mă). A rapidly growing tumor which may be umbilicated, usually occurring on exposed areas of the skin, which invades the dermis but remains localized and usually resolves spontaneously if untreated; microscopically, the nodule is composed of well-differentiated squamous epithelium with a central keratin mass that opens on the skin surface.

keratoangioma (ker'ă-tō-an-jē-ō'mă). Angiokeratoma.

keratoatrophoderma (ker'ă-tō-at'rō-fō-der'mă) [kerato- + G. *atrophia,* atrophy, + *derma,* skin]. Porokeratosis.

keratocele (ker'ă-tō-sēl) [kerato- + G. *kēlē,* hernia]. Hernia of Descemet's membrane through a defect in the outer layer of the cornea.

keratoconjunctivitis (ker'ă-tō-kon-jŭngk'ti-vī'tis). Inflammation of the conjunctiva and of the cornea; phlyctenular hypersensitivity reaction of corneal and conjunctival epithelium to endogenous toxin.
atopic k., inflammation of the conjunctiva and cornea, secondary to atopic eczema.
epidemic k., virus k.; follicular conjunctivitis followed by subepithelial corneal infiltrates; often caused by adenovirus type 8, less commonly by other types.
flash k., ultraviolet k.
herpetic k., herpetic *keratitis.*
k. sic'ca, keratitis sicca; dry eye syndrome; k. associated with decreased tears. See also Sjögren's (H.S.C.) *syndrome.*
superior limbic k., inflammatory edema of the superior corneoscleral limbus.
ultraviolet k., actinic, arc-flash, snow, or welder's conjunctivitis; flash k.; electric ophthalmia; ophthalmia nivalis; acute k. resulting from exposure to intense ultraviolet irradiation.
vernal k., vernal *conjunctivitis.*
virus k., epidemic k.

keratoconus (ker'ă-tō-kō'nŭs) [kerato- + G. *kōnos,* cone]. Conical cornea; a conical protrusion of the cornea caused by thinning of the stroma; usually bilateral. See also Fleischer's *ring;* Munson's *sign.*

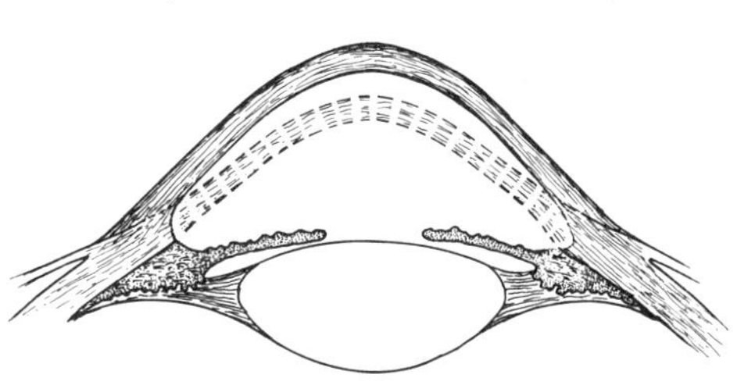

Keratoconus

keratocricoid (ker'ă-tō-krī'koyd). Ceratocricoid.

keratocyst (ker'ă-tō-sist). Odontogenic cyst derived from remnants of the dental lamina and appearing as a unilocular or multilocular radiolucency which may produce jaw expansion; epithelial lining is characterized microscopically by a uniform thickness, a corrugated superficial layer of paraperatin, and a prominent basal layer composed of palisaded columnar cells.

keratocyte (ker'ă-tō-sīt). The fibroblastic stromal cell of the cornea.

keratoderma (ker'ă-tō-der'mă) [kerato- + G. *derma,* skin]. **1.** Any horny superficial growth. **2.** A generalized thickening of the horny layer of the epidermis.
k. blennorrhag'ica, *keratosis* blennorrhagica.
k. eccen'trica, porokeratosis.
lymphedematous k., mossy *foot.*
mutilating k., keratoma hereditaria mutilans; Vohwinkel syndrome; diffuse k. of the extremities, with the development during childhood of constricting fibrous bands around the middle phalanx of the fingers or toes which may lead to spontaneous amputation; autosomal dominant inheritance.
k. palma'ris et planta'ris, palmoplantar k.
palmoplantar k., k., keratosis, ichthyosis, or tylosis palmaris et plantaris; k. symmetrica; keratoma plantare sulcatum; the occurrence of symmetrical diffuse or patchy areas of hypertrophy of the horny layer of the epidermis on the palms and soles; a group of ectodermal dysplasias of considerable variety, and either autosomal dominant or recessive inheritance.
k. planta're sulca'tum, cracked heel; hyperkeratosis and fissure formation on the soles.
punctate k., keratoma disseminatum; keratosis punctata; horny papules over the palms, soles, and digits which may develop central craters; autosomal dominant inheritance.
senile k., solar *keratosis.*
k. symmet'rica, palmoplantar k.

keratodermatitis (ker'ă-tō-der-mă-tī'tis) [kerato- + G. *derma,* skin, + *-itis,* inflammation]. Inflammation with proliferation of the horny layer of the skin.

keratoectasia (ker'ă-tō-ek-tā'zē-ă). Keratectasia.

keratoepithelioplasty (ker'ă-tō-ep-i-thē'lē-ō-plas-tē). Keratoplasty with transplantation of corneal epithelium and minimal supporting tissue.

keratogenesis (ker'ă-tō-jen'ĕ-sis) [kerato- + G. *genesis,* production]. Production or origin of horny cells or tissue.

keratogenetic (ker'ă-tō-jĕ-net'ik). Relating to keratogenesis.

keratogenous (ker-ă-toj'ĕ-nŭs). Causing a growth of cells that produce keratin and result in the formation of horny tissue, such as fingernails, scales, feathers, etc.

keratoglobus (ker-ă-tō-glō'bŭs) [kerato- + L. *globus,* ball]. Anterior *megalophthalmus.*

keratoglossus (ker'ă-tō-glos'sŭs). *Musculus* chondroglossus.

keratohyal (ker'ă-tō-hī'ăl). Ceratohyal.

keratohyalin (ker'ă-tō-hī'ă-lin) [kerato- + hyalin]. The substance in the large basophilic granules of the stratum granulosum of the epidermis.

keratoid (ker'ă-toyd) [kerato- + G. *eidos,* resemblance]. **1.** Horny. **2.** Resembling corneal tissue.

keratoleptynsis (ker'ă-tō-lep-tin'sis) [kerato- + G. *leptynsis,* a making thin]. **1.** Gutter *dystrophy* of cornea. **2.** An operation for removing the surface of the cornea and replacement by bulbar conjunctiva for cosmetic reasons.

keratoleukoma (ker'ă-tō-lū-kō'mă) [kerato- + G. *leukos,* white, + *-ōma,* growth]. A white corneal opacity.

keratolysis (ker-ă-tol'i-sis) [kerato- + G. *lysis,* loosening]. **1.** Separation or loosening of the horny layer of the epidermis. **2.** Deciduous skin; specifically, a disease characterized by a shedding of the epidermis recurring at more or less regular intervals.
k. exfoliati'va, erythema or erythroderma exfoliativa; familial continual skin peeling characterized by a separation of stratum corneum in leaflike flakes occurring everywhere except on the palms and soles; the cause is unknown.
pitted k., noninflammatory bacterial infection of the plantar, and (occasionally) the palmar surfaces producing small depressions in the stratum corneum, usually at the weight-bearing sites.

keratolytic (ker'ă-tō-lit'ik). Relating to keratolysis.

keratoma (ker-ă-tō'mă) [kerato- + G. *-oma,* tumor]. **1.** Callosity. **2.** A horny tumor.
k. dissemina'tum, punctate *keratoderma.*
k. heredita'ria mu'tilans, mutilating *keratoderma.*
k. malig'num, congenital ichthyosiform *erythroderma.*
k. planta're sulca'tum, palmoplantar *keratoderma.*
senile k., solar *keratosis.*

keratomalacia (ker'ă-tō-mă-lā'shē-ă) [kerato- + G. *malakia,* softness]. Xerotic keratitis; Brazilian ophthalmia; dryness with ulceration and perforation of the cornea, with absence of inflammatory reactions, occurring in cachectic children; results from severe vitamin A deficiency.

keratome (ker'ă-tōm). Keratotome; a knife used for incising the cornea.

keratometer (ker-ă-tom'ĕ-ter) [kerato- + G. *metron,* measure]. Ophthalmometer; an instrument for measuring the curvature of the anterior corneal surface.

keratometry (ker-ă-tom'ĕ-trē). Measurement of the radii of corneal curvature.

keratomileusis (ker'ă-tō-mī-lū'sis) [coinage, prob. fr. G. *keras* (*kerat-*), horn, cornea, + *smileusis,* carving]. Alteration of the refraction of the cornea by removal of a deep corneal lamella, freezing it, grinding a new curvature on a lathe, and then replacing it in the bed from which it was removed.

keratomycosis (ker-ă-tō-mī-kō'sis). Fungal infection of the cornea.

keratonosis (ker'ă-tō-nō'sis) [kerato- + G. *-osis,* condition]. Any abnormal noninflammatory, usually hypertrophic, affection of the horny layer of the skin.

keratopachyderma (ker'ă-tō-pak-i-der'mă) [kerato- + G. *pachys,* thick, + *derma,* skin]. A syndrome of congenital deafness with development of hyperkeratosis of the skin of the palms, soles, elbows, and knees in childhood, and with bandlike constrictions of the fingers; autosomal dominant inheritance.

keratopathy (ker-ă-top'ă-thē) [kerato- + G. *pathos,* suffering, disease]. A noninflammatory disorder of the cornea.
band-shaped k., a horizontal, gray, interpalpebral opacity of the cornea that begins at the periphery and progresses centrally; occurs in hypercalcemia, chronic iridocyclitis, and Still's disease.
bullous k., edema of the corneal stroma and epithelium; occurs in Fuchs' epithelial dystrophy, advanced glaucoma and iridocyclitis, and sometimes after intraocular lens implantation.
climatic k., Labrador k.; a bilateral, symmetrical corneal dystrophy caused by prolonged exposure to extremes of heat or cold; nodular opacities are limited to the interpalpebral area and vision is only mildly affected.
filamentary k., formation of fine elongations of corneal epithelium in inflammation, edema, and degenerative states.
Labrador k., climatic k.
lipid k., occurrence of fats in an area of corneal vascularization.
striate k., corneal stromal edema with formation of criss-cross tracts.
vesicular k., corneal epithelial edema with formation of vacuoles.

keratophakia (ker'ă-tō-fak'ē-ă) [kerato- + G. *phakos,* lens]. Keratophakic keratoplasty; implantation of a donor cornea or plastic lens within the corneal stroma to modify refractive error.

keratoplasty (ker'ă-tō-plas-tē) [kerato- + G. *plassō,* to form]. Transplantation or trepanation of cornea; corneal transplantation or trepanation; corneal graft; the removal of a portion of the cornea containing an opacity and the insertion in its place of a piece of cornea of the same size and shape removed from elsewhere.
allopathic k., corneal transplant with donor material of glass, plastic, or other inert material.
autogenous k., corneal transplant with donor material from the same individual.
epikeratophakic k., epikeratophakia.
heterogenous k., corneal transplant with donor material from another species.
homogenous k., corneal transplant with donor material from another individual of the same species.
keratophakic k., keratophakia.
lamellar k., layered k., nonpenetrating k.
nonpenetrating k., lamellar or layered k.; k. in which only the anterior layer of the cornea is used (not a tectonic k.).
optical k., transplantation of transparent corneal tissue to replace a leukoma or scar that impairs vision.
penetrating k., perforating k.; corneal transplant with replacement of all layers of the cornea, but retaining the peripheral cornea.
perforating k., penetrating k.
tectonic k., grafting to replace lost corneal tissue.
total k., corneal transplant in which the entire cornea is removed and replaced.

keratoprosthesis (ker'ă-tō-pros-thē'sis) [kerato- + G. *prosthesis,* addition]. Replacement of the central area of an opacified cornea by plastic.

keratorhexis, keratorrhexis (ker'ă-tō-rek'sis) [kerato- + G. *rhexis,* a bursting]. Rupture of the cornea, due to trauma or perforating ulcer.

keratorus (ker-a-tō'rŭs) [kerat- + L. *torus,* swelling, knot, bulge]. Vault-like corneal herniation with severe regular myopic astigmatism.

keratoscleritis (ker'ă-tō-skle-rī'tis). Inflammation of both cornea and sclera.

keratoscope (ker'ă-tō-skōp) [kerato- + G. *skopeō,* to examine]. Placido's disk; an instrument marked with lines or circles by means of which the corneal reflex can be observed.

keratoscopy (ker-ă-tos'kō-pē) [kerato- + G. *skopeō,* to examine]. **1.** Examination of the reflections from the anterior surface of the cornea in order to determine the character and amount of corneal astigmatism. **2.** A term first applied by Cuignet to his method of retinoscopy.

keratose (ker'ă-tōs). Relating to or marked by keratosis.

keratosis, pl. **keratoses** (ker-ă-tō'sis, -sēz) [kerato- + G. *-osis,* condition]. Keratiasis; any lesion on the epidermis marked by the presence of circumscribed overgrowths of the horny layer.
actinic k., solar k.
arsenical k., multiple keratoses, most commonly of the palms and soles but also of the fingers and proximal portions of the extremities, resulting from long-term arsenic ingestion; they may become malignant.
k. blennorrhag'ica, keratoderma blennorrhagica; pustules and crusts associated with Reiter's disease; at one time incorrectly believed to be due to gonorrhea.
k. diffu'sa feta'lis, *ichthyosis* vulgaris.
k. follicula'ris, Darier's disease; k. vegetans; a familial eruption, beginning usually in childhood, in which keratotic papules originating from both follicles and intrafollicular epidermis of the trunk, face, scalp, and axillae become crusted and verrucous; the papules are often intensely pruritic.
k. follicula'ris contagio'sa, Brooke's disease (2); a rare condition simulating k. follicularis.
inverted follicular k., a solitary benign epithelial tumor of hair follicle origin, consisting of a lobulated epidermal downgrowth of keratinizing squamous cells with a pattern of eddies or whorls.
k. labia'lis, thickening of stratum corneum on the lips.
lichenoid k., a solitary benign papule or plaque, with microscopic features resembling lichen planus, occurring on sun-exposed or unexposed skin.
k. ni'gricans, *acanthosis* nigricans.
k. obtu'rans, laminated epithelial plug; an accretion of epithelia in the external auditory canal.
k. palma'ris et planta'ris, palmoplantar *keratoderma.*
k. pilo'ris atroph'icans fa'ciei, erythema and horny plugs of outer portions of the eyebrows and destruction of follicles; onset in early infancy.
k. puncta'ta, punctate *keratoderma.*
k. ru'bra figura'ta, *erythrokeratoderma* variabilis.
seborrheic k., k. seborrhe'ica, basal cell papilloma; seborrheic wart or verruca; superficial, benign, verrucous lesions consisting of proliferating epidermal cells, especially of basal type, enclosing horn cysts; they usually occur after the third decade.
senile k., k. seni'lis, solar k.
solar k., a premalignant warty lesion occurring on the sun-exposed skin of the face or hands in aged light-skinned persons; hyperkeratosis may form a cutaneous horn, and squamous cell carcinoma of low-grade malignancy may develop. Also called actinic k.; senile k., keratoderma, keratoma, or wart; k. senilis; verruca senilis or plana senilis.
tar k., warty lesions of the face and hands resulting from repeated, prolonged exposure to tar and pitch; also occurs as keratoacanthoma-like lesions that can become malignant, particularly on the scrotum.
k. veg'etans, k. follicularis.

keratosulfate (ker'ă-tō-sŭl-fāt). Keratan sulfate.

keratotome (ker'ă-tō-tōm). Keratome.

keratotomy (ker'ă-tot'ō-mē) [kerato- + G. *tomē,* incision]. Incision through the cornea.
delimiting k., Gifford's operation; incision in the cornea along the margin of an advancing ulcer.
radial k., modification of refractive error by multiple symmetrical partial thickness corneal incisions extending peripherally from the margin of the central uncut clear zone.
refractive k., modification of corneal curvature by means of corneal incisions to minimize hyperopia, myopia, or astigmatism.

keraunophobia (kē-raw'nō-fō'bē-ă) [G. *keraunos,* thunderbolt, + *phobos,* fear]. Morbid fear of thunder and lightning.

Kerckring (Kerckringius), Theodor, Dutch anatomist, 1640–1693. See K.'s *center, folds, ossicle, valves.*

kerion (kē'rē-on) [G. *kērion,* honeycomb; a skin disease, fr. *kēros,* beeswax]. A granulomatous secondarily infected lesion complicating fungal infection of the hair; typically, a raised boggy lesion.
Celsus k., *tinea* kerion.

Kerley, Peter J., British radiologist, *1900. See K. B *lines.*

kernicterus (ker-nik'ter-ŭs) [Ger. *Kern,* kernel (nucleus), + *Ikterous,* jaundice]. Nuclear jaundice; a grave form of icterus neonatorum associated with high levels of unconjugated bilirubin, a breakdown product of hemoglobin, or, in very low birth weight infants, with modest degrees of bilirubinemia; yellow staining and degenerative lesions are found in the lenticular nucleus, subthalamus, Ammon's horn, and other areas of intracranial gray matter; occurrence in the newborn from accelerated destruction of red blood cells in erythroblastosis fetalis is associated with Rh incompatibility. Characterized clinically by opisthotonus, high-pitched cry, abnormal or absent Moro reflex, and abnormal eye movements.

Kernig, Vladimir, Russian physician, 1840–1917. See K.'s *sign.*

Kernohan, J.W., U.S. pathologist, *1897. See K.'s *notch.*

keroid (ker'oyd) [G. *keroeidēs,* horn-like]. Horny.

kerosene (ker'ō-sēn). A mixture of petroleum hydrocarbons, chiefly of the methane series; the fifth fraction in the distillation of petroleum, used as fuel for lamps and stoves, as a degreaser and cleaner, and in insecticides. Contact on human skin can lead to irritation and infection; inhalation may cause headache, drowsiness, coma; swallowing causes irritation, vomiting, and diarrhea. Vomiting should not be induced, as aspiration of vomitus causes pneumonitis.

kerotherapy (ker-ō-thār'ă-pē) [G. *kēros,* wax, + *therapeia,* treatment]. Treatment of burns and denuded surfaces with wax or paraffin preparations.

Kerr, Harry Hyland, U.S. surgeon, *1881. See Parker-K. *suture.*

Kestenbaum's sign. See under sign.

ketal (kē'tăl). $R_2C(OR')_2$; a hydrated ketone in which both hydroxyl groups are esterified with alcohols.

ketamine (kēt'ă-mēn). DL-2-(*o*-Chlorophenyl)-2-(methylamino)cyclohexanone; a parenterally administered anesthetic that produces catatonia, profound analgesia, increased sympathetic activity, and little relaxation of skeletal muscles; side effects include sialorrhea and occasional pronounced dysphoria, especially in adults.

ketene (kē'tēn). $CH_2{=}C{=}O$; a very reactive acetylating agent, used in chemical syntheses.

keto-. Combining form denoting a compound containing a ketone group; replaced by oxo- in systematic nomenclature.

keto acid (kē'tō). Oxo acid; an acid containing a ketone group (–CO–) in addition to the acid group(s).

3-ketoacid-CoA transferase. 3-Oxoacid-CoA transferase.

ketoacidosis (kē′tō-as-i-dō′sis). Acidosis, as in diabetes or starvation, caused by the enhanced production of ketone bodies.

ketoaciduria (kē′tō-as-i-dū′rē-ă). Excretion of urine having an elevated content of ketonic acids.
branched chain k., maple syrup urine *disease.*

β-ketoacyl-ACP reductase (kē-tō-as′il). 3-Oxoacyl-ACP reductase.

β-ketoacyl-ACP synthase. 3-Oxoacyl-ACP synthase.

3-ketoacyl-CoA thiolase. Acetyl-CoA acyltransferase.

ketobemidone (kē-tō-bem′i-dōn). 1-[4-(*m*-Hydroxyphenyl)-1-methyl-4-piperidyl]-1-propanone; an analgesic with narcotic properties.

ketoconazole (kē-tō-kō′nă-zōl). (±)-*cis*-1-Acetyl-4-[*p*-[2-(2,4-dichlorophenyl)-2-(imidazol-1-ylmethyl)1,3-dioxolan-4-yl]methoxy]phenyl]piperazine; a broad spectrum antifungal agent used to treat systemic and topical fungal infections.

α-ketodecarboxylase (kē′tō-dē-kar-boks′i-lās). Formerly, the enzyme system converting pyruvate (a 2-oxoacid) to acetyl-CoA and CO_2, with reduction of NAD^+ to NADH and the participation of lipoamide and thiamin pyrophosphate; now known to involve at least three enzymes in succession: pyruvate dehydrogenase, dihydrolipoamide acetyltransferase, and dihydrolipoamide dehydrogenase.

ketogenesis (kē-tō-jen′ĕ-sis). Metabolic production of ketones.

ketogenic (kē-tō-jen′ik). Giving rise to ketones in metabolism.

α-ketoglutaric dehydrogenase (kē′tō-glū-tar′ik). 2-Oxoglutarate dehydrogenase.

ketoheptose (kē-tō-hep′tōs). Heptulose; a seven-carbon sugar possessing a ketone group.

ketohexose (kē-tō-heks′ōs). Hexulose; a six-carbon sugar possessing a ketone group; *e.g.,* fructose.

β-ketohydrogenase (kē-tō-hī′drō-jen-ās). 3-Hydroxyacyl-CoA dehydrogenase.

ketohydroxyestrin (kē′tō-hī-drok-sē-es′trin). Estrone.

ketol (kē′tol). A ketone that has an OH group near the CO group. In an α-k., the OH is attached to a carbon atom that is attached to the CO carbon atom; in a β-k., one carbon atom intervenes.

ketole (kē′tōl). Indole.

ketole group. Carbon 1 and 2 of a 2-ketose ($HOCH_2CO$–); transketolation from D-xylose 5′-phosphate to C-1 of aldoses is important in various metabolic pathways involving carbohydrates (*e.g.,* photosynthesis, Dickens shunt); the two-carbon unit is transferred as α,β-dihydroxyethyl thiamin pyrophosphate.

ketolytic (kē-tō-lit′ik). Causing the dissolution of ketone or acetone substances, referring usually to oxidation products of glucose and allied substances.

ketone (kē′tōn). A substance with the carbonyl group $-\overset{\mathrm{O}}{\overset{\|}{\mathrm{C}}}-$ linking two carbon atoms; the most important in medicine and the simplest in chemistry is dimethyl k. (acetone).

ketone alcohol. A compound containing a carbonyl or ketone group as well as a hydroxyl group; *e.g.,* dihydroxyacetone (glycerone).

ketone-aldehyde mutase. Lactoylglutathione lyase.

ketonemia (kē-tō-nē′mē-ă) [ketone + G. *haima,* blood]. The presence of recognizable concentrations of ketone bodies in the plasma.

ketonic (kē-tōn′ik). Pertaining to, or possessing the characteristics of, a ketone.

ketonization (kē-tō-ni-zā′shŭn). Conversion into a ketone.

ketonuria (kē-tō-nū′rē-ă). Enhanced urinary excretion of ketone bodies.
branched chain k., maple syrup urine *disease.*

ketopantoic acid (kē′tō-pan-tō′ik). Oxidized precursor of pantoic acid, intermediate on the synthetic pathway between α-ketoisovaleric acid and pantothenic acid.

ketopentose (kē-tō-pen′tōs). A five-carbon sugar in which carbons 2, 3, or 4 make up part of a carbonyl group; *e.g.,* ribulose.

ketoprofen (kē-tō-prō′fen). *m*-Benzoylhydratropic acid; a nonsteroidal anti-inflammatory analgesic.

β-ketoreductase (kē′tō-rē-dŭk′tās). 3-Hydroxyacyl-CoA dehydrogenase.

ketose (kē′tōs). A carbohydrate containing the characteristic carbonyl group of the ketones; *e.g.,* fructose, ribulose, sedoheptulose.

ketose-1-phosphate aldolase. Fructose bisphosphate aldolase.

ketose reductase. D-Sorbitol-6-phosphate dehydrogenase.

ketosis (kē-tō′sis) [ketone + *-osis,* condition]. A condition characterized by the enhanced production of ketone bodies, as in diabetes mellitus or starvation.
bovine k., a common metabolic disease of cows which appears as a rule within a few weeks after parturition; characterized by hypoglycemia, ketonuria, loss of appetite, lethargy, loss of milk production, and rapid emaciation.

17-ketosteroids (17-KS) (kē-tō-stēr′oydz). 17-Oxosteroids; nominally, any steroid with a ketone group on C-17; commonly used to designate urinary C_{19} steroidal metabolites of androgenic and adrenocortical hormones that possess this structural feature.

α-ketosuccinamic acid (kē′tō-sŭk-si-nam′ik). NH_2-CO-CH_2-CO-COOH; the transamination product of asparagine.

ketosuccinic acid (kē-tō-sŭk′si-nik). Oxaloacetic acid.

β-ketothiolase (kē-tō-thī′ō-lās). Acetyl-CoA acyltransferase.

Key, Ernst A.H., Swedish anatomist and physician, 1832–1901. See K.-Retzius *corpuscles, foramen; sheath* of K. and Retzius.

keyway (kē′wā). The female portion of a precision attachment.

kg Abbreviation for kilogram.

khat (kot). The tender fresh parts of *Catha edulis.*

khellin (kel′in) [Ar. *khella*]. Dimethoxymethylfuranochromone; the active principle in extracts of *Ammi visnaga,* an umbelliferous plant growing in the Near East; used in angina pectoris and asthma.

KHN Abbreviation for Knoop hardness *number.*

kick (kik). A brisk mechanical stimulus.
atrial k., the increased efficiency of ventricular ejection resulting from the priming force contributed by atrial contraction immediately before ventricular ejection and thus still contributing an influence as the ventricular ejection begins.
idioventricular k., the increased contractility of the initially contracting ventricular fibers which, by stretching the later contracting fibers, increases their force of contraction.

Kidd blood group. See Blood Groups appendix.

kidney (kid′nē) [A.S. *cwith,* womb, belly, + *neere,* kidney]. One of the two organs (L. *ren,* G. *nephros*) that excrete the urine. The k.'s are bean-shaped organs (about 11 cm long, 5 cm wide, and 3 cm thick) lying on either side of the vertebral column, posterior to the peritoneum, about opposite the twelfth thoracic and first three lumbar vertebrae.
amyloid k., waxy k.; a k. in which amyloidosis has occurred, usually in association with some chronic illness such as multiple myeloma, tuberculosis, osteomyelitis, or other chronic suppurative inflammation; such k.'s are moderately enlarged and grossly manifest a waxy appearance, with amyloid deposited beneath the endothelium in the glomerular loops and in the arterioles, apparently beginning as foci of thickening of the basement membranes.

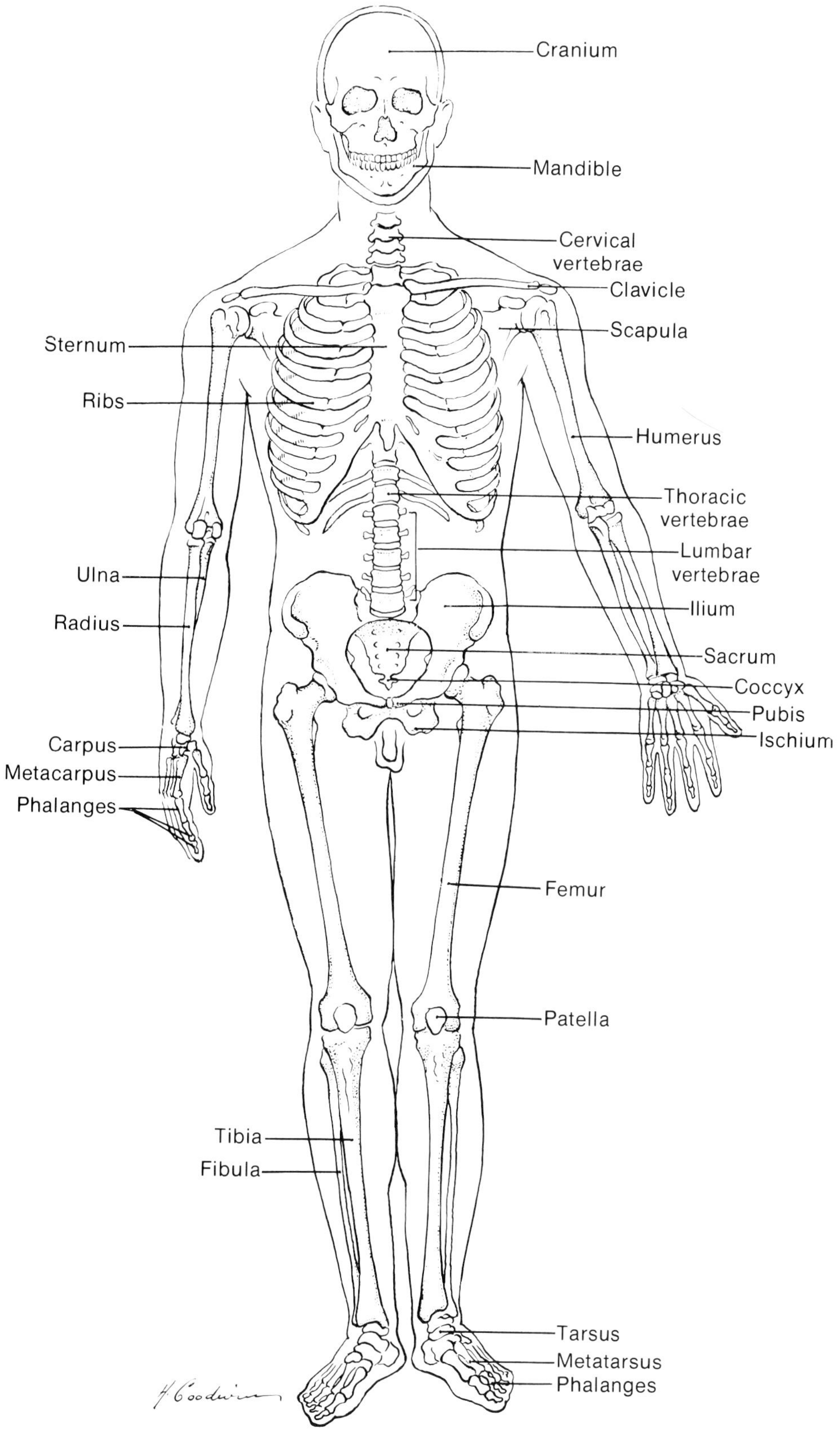

PLATE 1

Human Skeleton, Anterior View

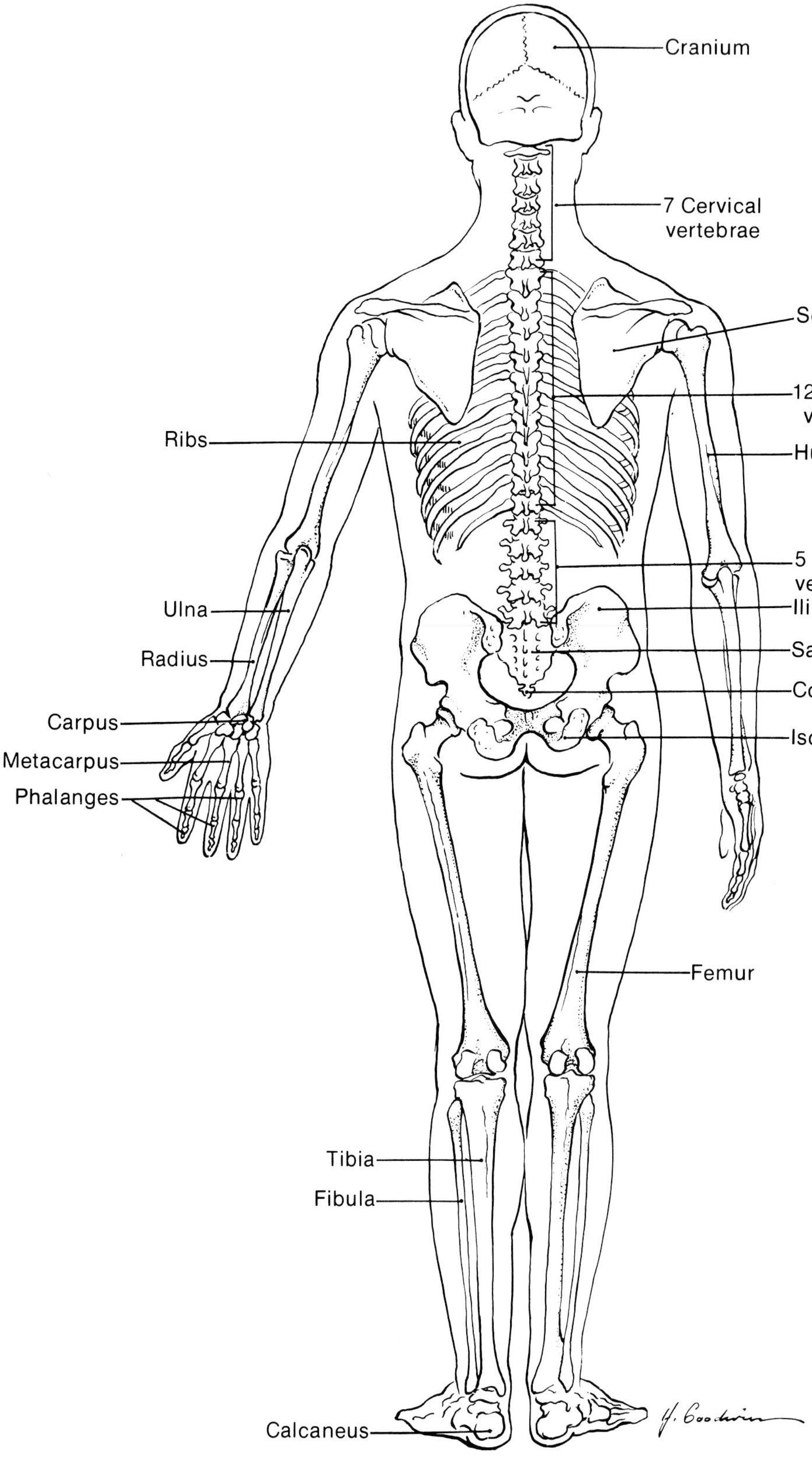

PLATE 2

Human Skeleton, Posterior View

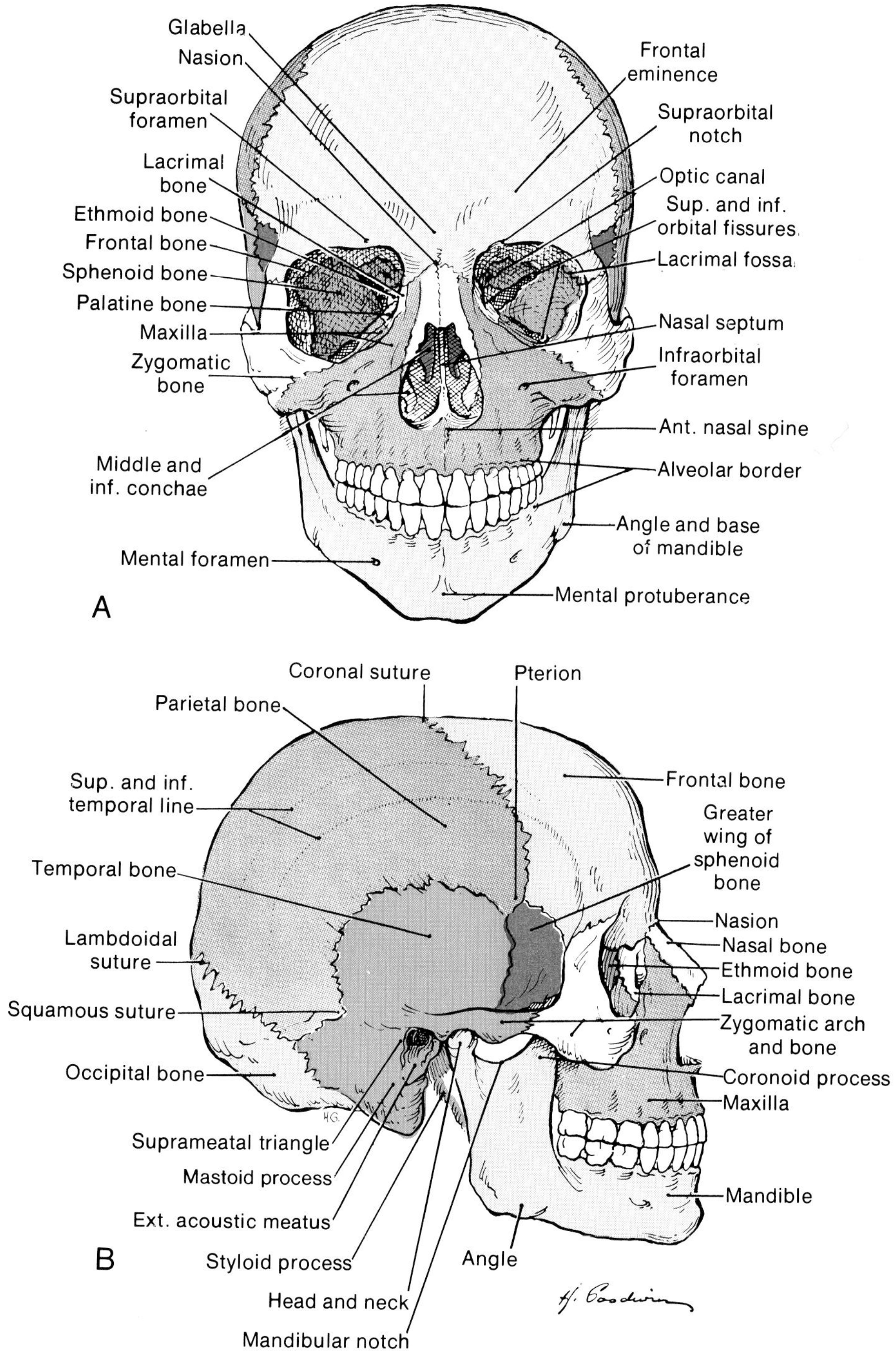
Glabella
Nasion
Supraorbital foramen
Lacrimal bone
Ethmoid bone
Frontal bone
Sphenoid bone
Palatine bone
Maxilla
Zygomatic bone
Middle and inf. conchae
Mental foramen
A
Frontal eminence
Supraorbital notch
Optic canal
Sup. and inf. orbital fissures
Lacrimal fossa
Nasal septum
Infraorbital foramen
Ant. nasal spine
Alveolar border
Angle and base of mandible
Mental protuberance
Coronal suture
Pterion
Parietal bone
Sup. and inf. temporal line
Temporal bone
Lambdoidal suture
Squamous suture
Occipital bone
Suprameatal triangle
Mastoid process
Ext. acoustic meatus
B
Styloid process
Head and neck
Mandibular notch
Angle
Frontal bone
Greater wing of sphenoid bone
Nasion
Nasal bone
Ethmoid bone
Lacrimal bone
Zygomatic arch and bone
Coronoid process
Maxilla
Mandible

PLATE 3

The Skull: A, Anterior View (Norma Facialis); B, Lateral View (Norma Lateralis)

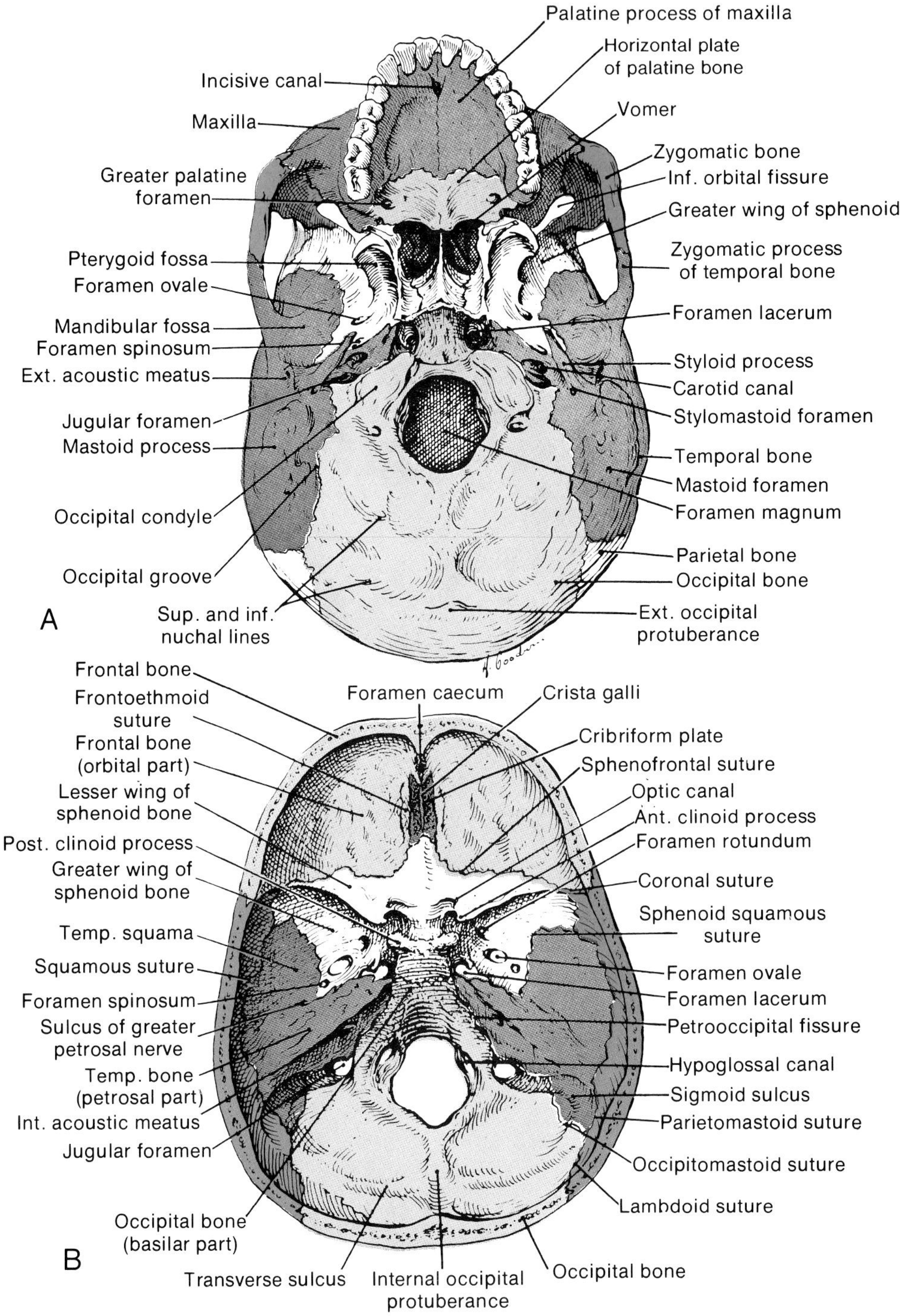
Palatine process of maxilla
Horizontal plate of palatine bone
Incisive canal
Maxilla
Vomer
Zygomatic bone
Greater palatine foramen
Inf. orbital fissure
Greater wing of sphenoid
Pterygoid fossa
Zygomatic process of temporal bone
Foramen ovale
Mandibular fossa
Foramen lacerum
Foramen spinosum
Styloid process
Ext. acoustic meatus
Carotid canal
Jugular foramen
Stylomastoid foramen
Mastoid process
Temporal bone
Mastoid foramen
Occipital condyle
Foramen magnum
Parietal bone
Occipital groove
Occipital bone
A
Sup. and inf. nuchal lines
Ext. occipital protuberance
Frontal bone
Foramen caecum
Crista galli
Frontoethmoid suture
Cribriform plate
Frontal bone (orbital part)
Sphenofrontal suture
Lesser wing of sphenoid bone
Optic canal
Ant. clinoid process
Post. clinoid process
Foramen rotundum
Greater wing of sphenoid bone
Coronal suture
Sphenoid squamous suture
Temp. squama
Squamous suture
Foramen ovale
Foramen spinosum
Foramen lacerum
Sulcus of greater petrosal nerve
Petrooccipital fissure
Temp. bone (petrosal part)
Hypoglossal canal
Sigmoid sulcus
Int. acoustic meatus
Parietomastoid suture
Jugular foramen
Occipitomastoid suture
Lambdoid suture
Occipital bone (basilar part)
B
Transverse sulcus
Internal occipital protuberance
Occipital bone

PLATE 4

The Skull: A, External View of the Base (Norma Basilaris); B, Internal View of the Base

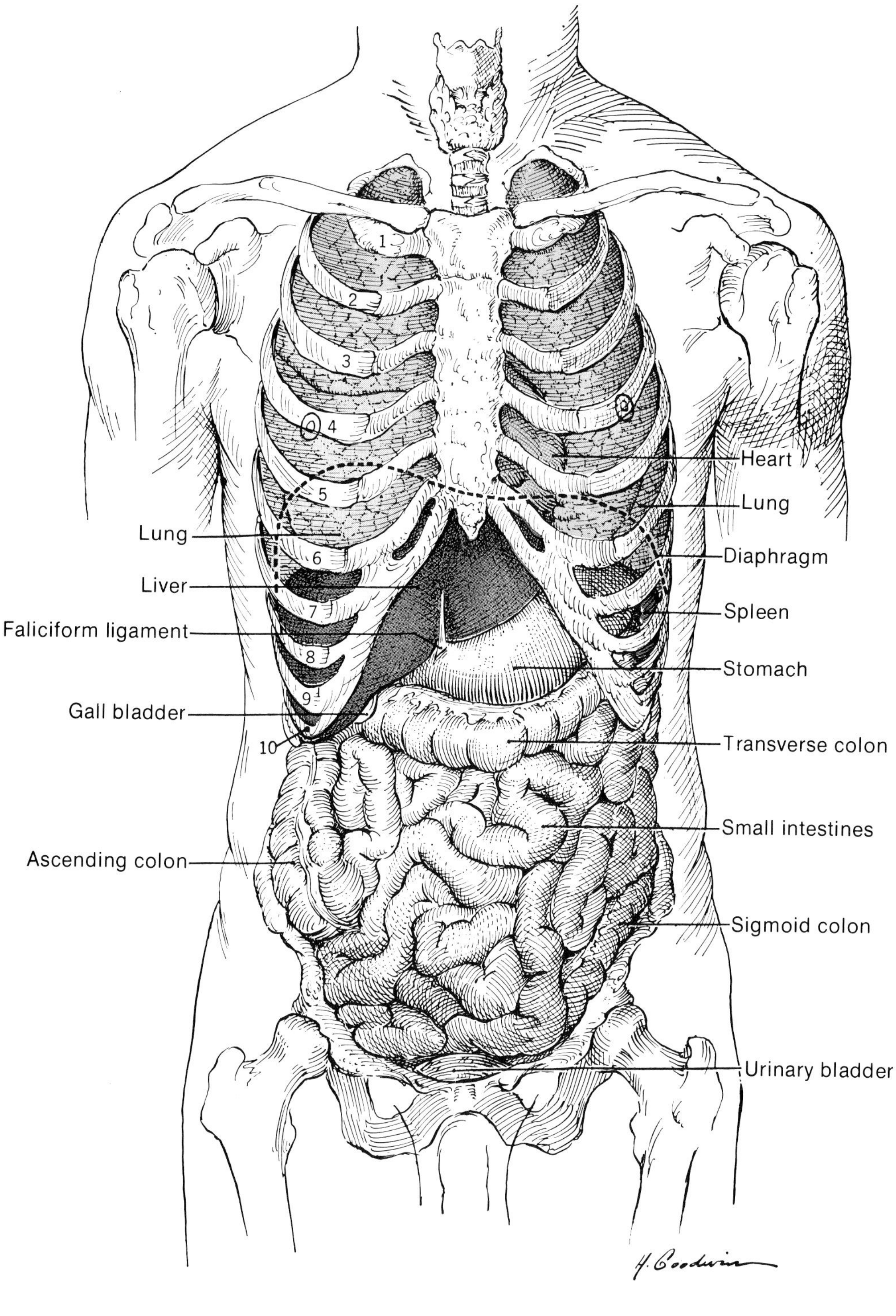

PLATE 5

Abdominal and Thoracic Viscera, Anterior View (After Pernkopf)

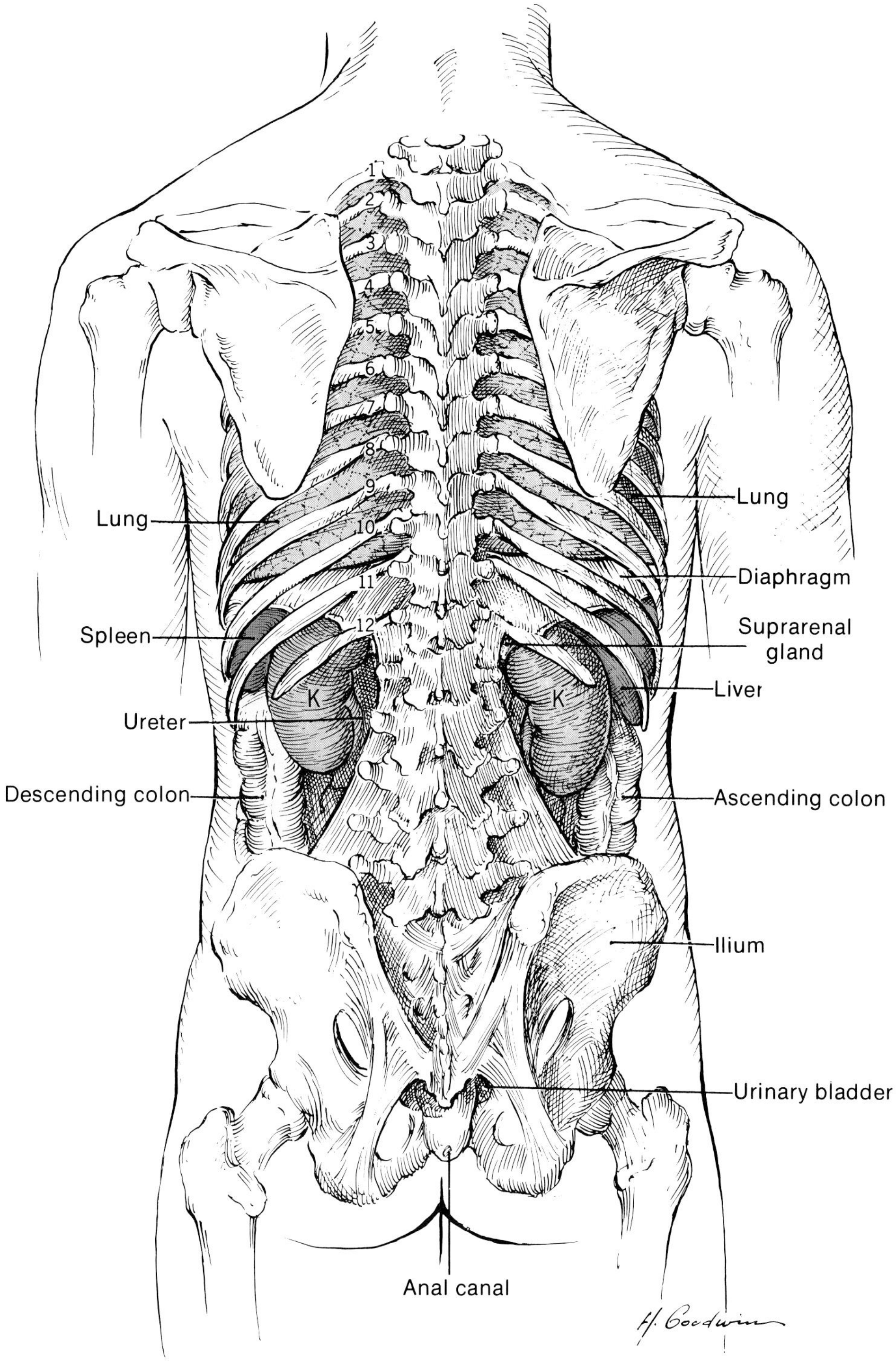

PLATE 6

Abdominal and Thoracic Viscera, Posterior View (After Pernkopf)

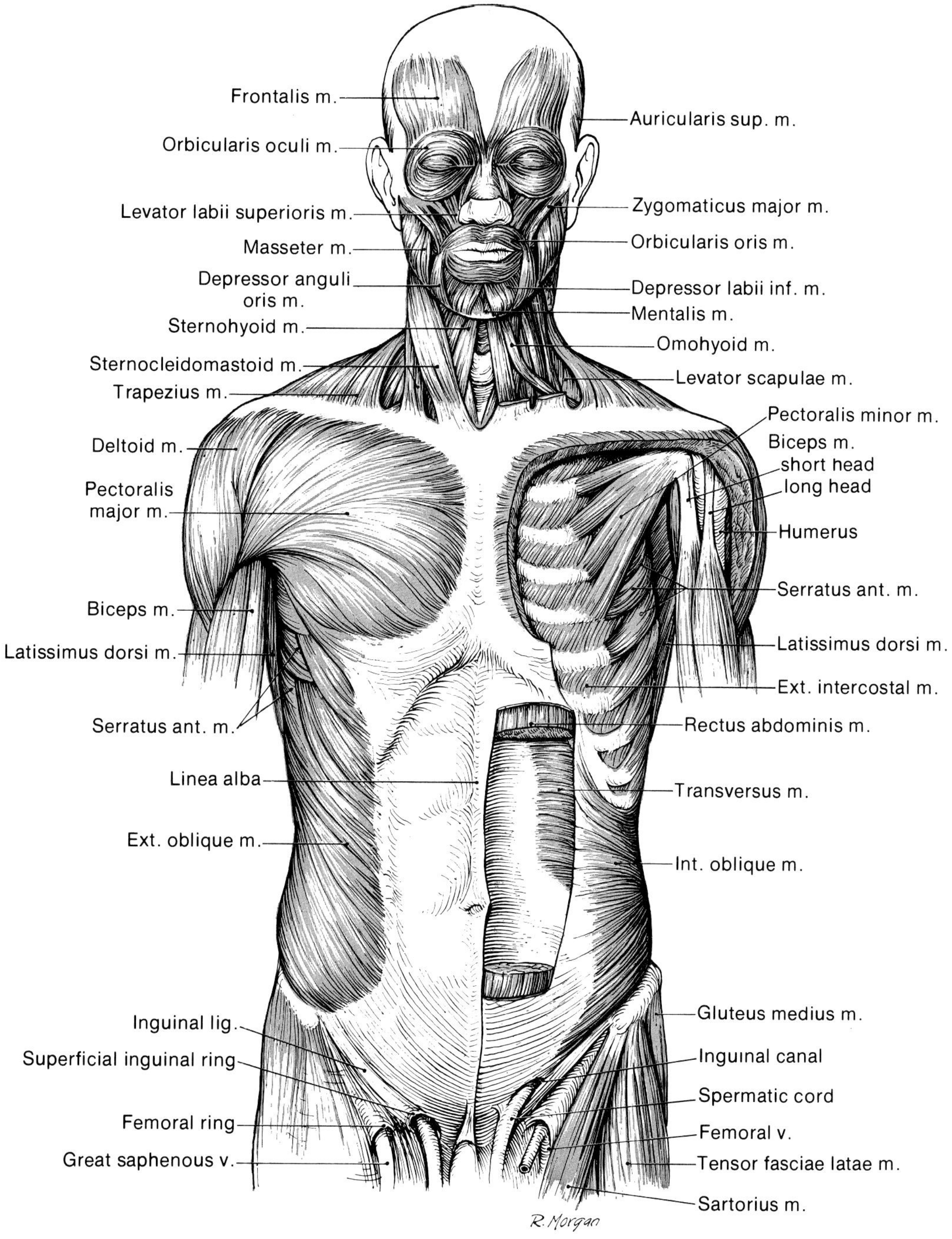
Frontalis m.
Auricularis sup. m.
Orbicularis oculi m.
Levator labii superioris m.
Zygomaticus major m.
Masseter m.
Orbicularis oris m.
Depressor anguli oris m.
Depressor labii inf. m.
Mentalis m.
Sternohyoid m.
Omohyoid m.
Sternocleidomastoid m.
Levator scapulae m.
Trapezius m.
Pectoralis minor m.
Deltoid m.
Biceps m.
short head
long head
Pectoralis major m.
Humerus
Serratus ant. m.
Biceps m.
Latissimus dorsi m.
Latissimus dorsi m.
Ext. intercostal m.
Serratus ant. m.
Rectus abdominis m.
Linea alba
Transversus m.
Ext. oblique m.
Int. oblique m.
Gluteus medius m.
Inguinal lig.
Superficial inguinal ring
Inguinal canal
Spermatic cord
Femoral ring
Femoral v.
Great saphenous v.
Tensor fasciae latae m.
Sartorius m.
R. Morgan

PLATE 7

Muscles of Head, Neck, and Torso, Anterior View

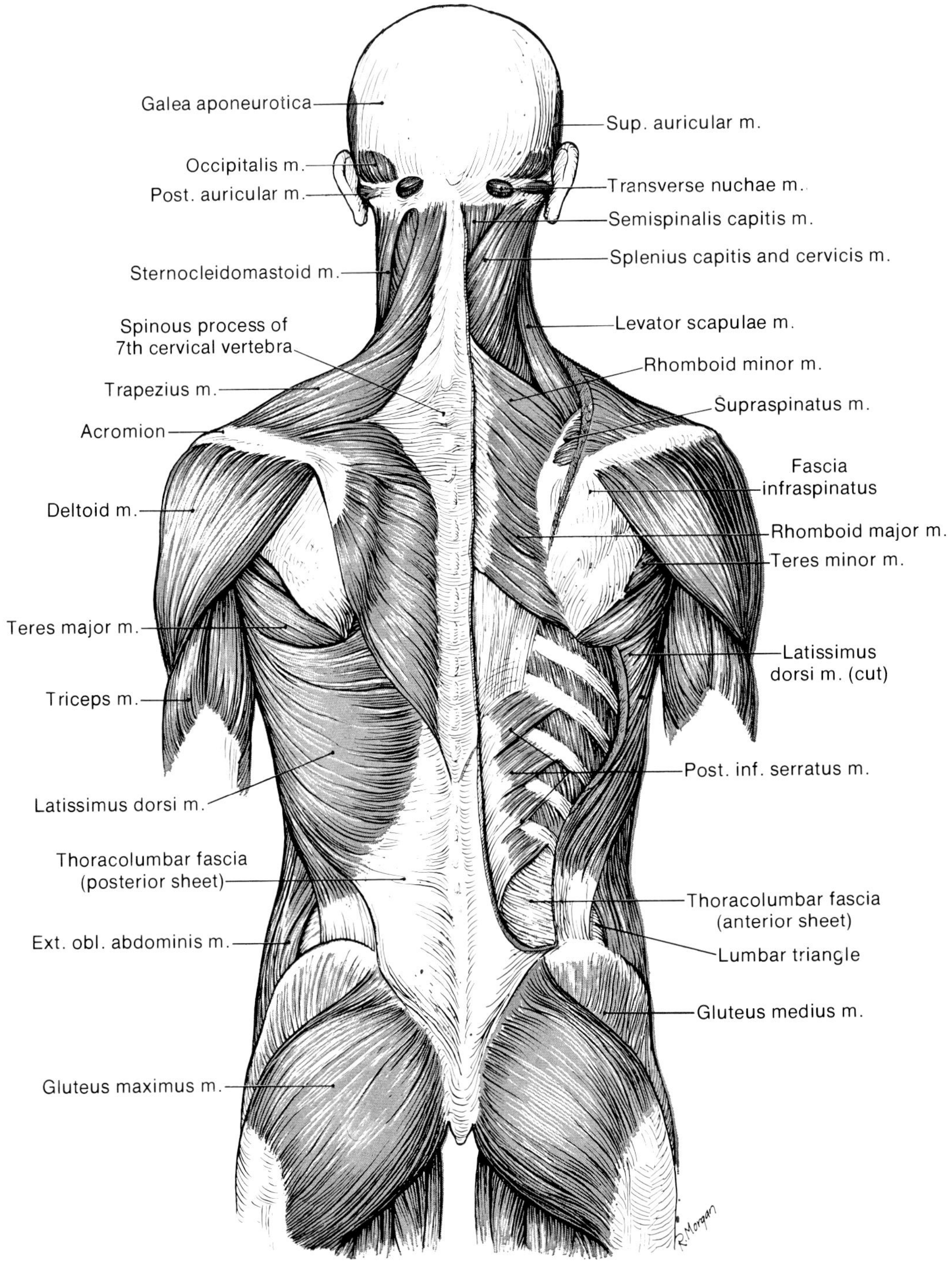

Galea aponeurotica
Sup. auricular m.
Occipitalis m.
Post. auricular m.
Transverse nuchae m.
Semispinalis capitis m.
Splenius capitis and cervicis m.
Sternocleidomastoid m.
Levator scapulae m.
Spinous process of 7th cervical vertebra
Rhomboid minor m.
Trapezius m.
Supraspinatus m.
Acromion
Fascia infraspinatus
Deltoid m.
Rhomboid major m.
Teres minor m.
Teres major m.
Latissimus dorsi m. (cut)
Triceps m.
Post. inf. serratus m.
Latissimus dorsi m.
Thoracolumbar fascia (posterior sheet)
Thoracolumbar fascia (anterior sheet)
Ext. obl. abdominis m.
Lumbar triangle
Gluteus medius m.
Gluteus maximus m.
R. Morgan

PLATE 8

Muscles of Trunk, Posterior View

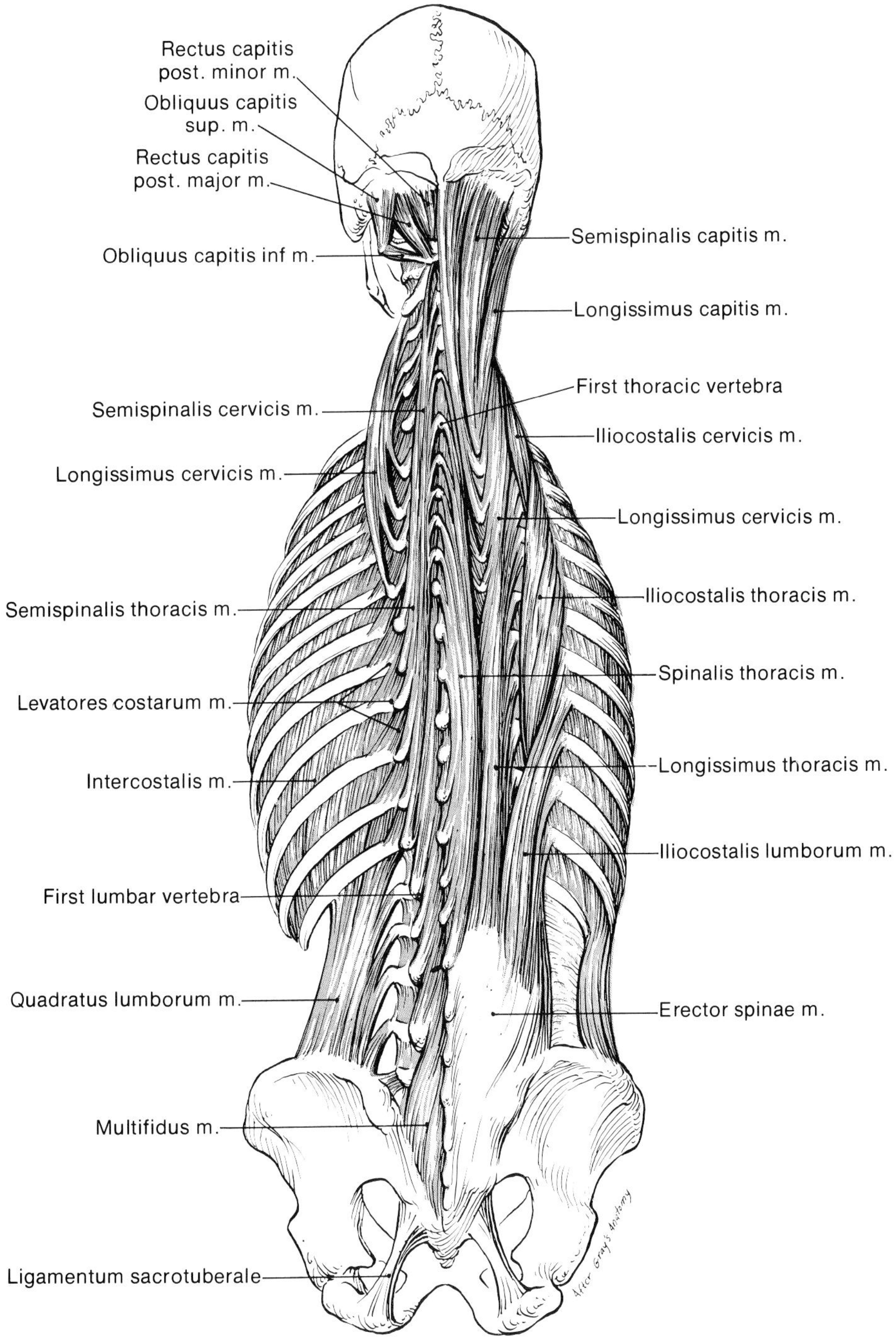
Rectus capitis post. minor m.
Obliquus capitis sup. m.
Rectus capitis post. major m.
Obliquus capitis inf m.
Semispinalis capitis m.
Longissimus capitis m.
First thoracic vertebra
Semispinalis cervicis m.
Iliocostalis cervicis m.
Longissimus cervicis m.
Longissimus cervicis m.
Iliocostalis thoracis m.
Semispinalis thoracis m.
Spinalis thoracis m.
Levatores costarum m.
Longissimus thoracis m.
Intercostalis m.
Iliocostalis lumborum m.
First lumbar vertebra
Quadratus lumborum m.
Erector spinae m.
Multifidus m.
Ligamentum sacrotuberale
After Gray's Anatomy

PLATE 9

Muscles of Back, Deep Dissection

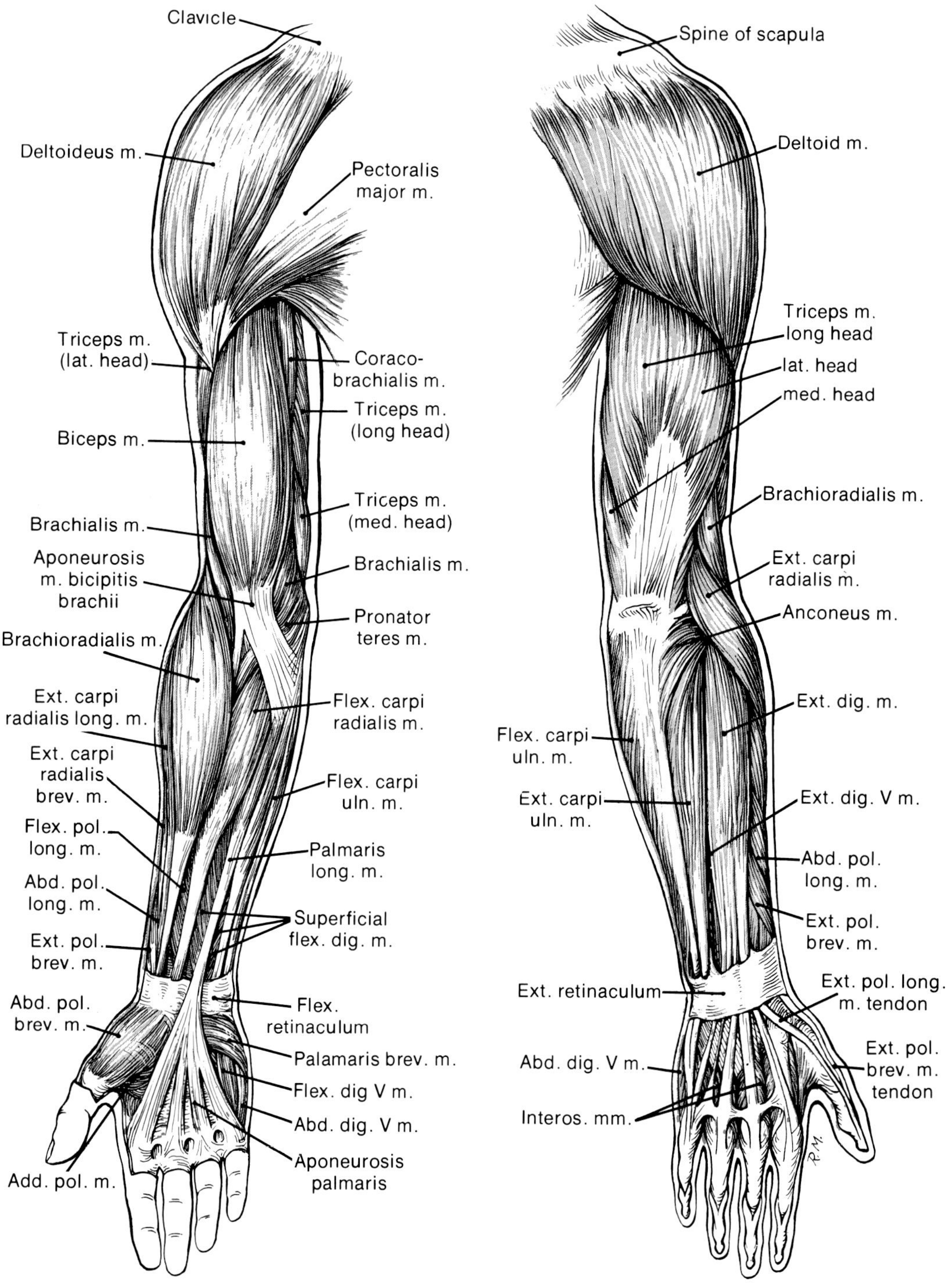

PLATE 10

Superficial Muscles of Right Upper Limb

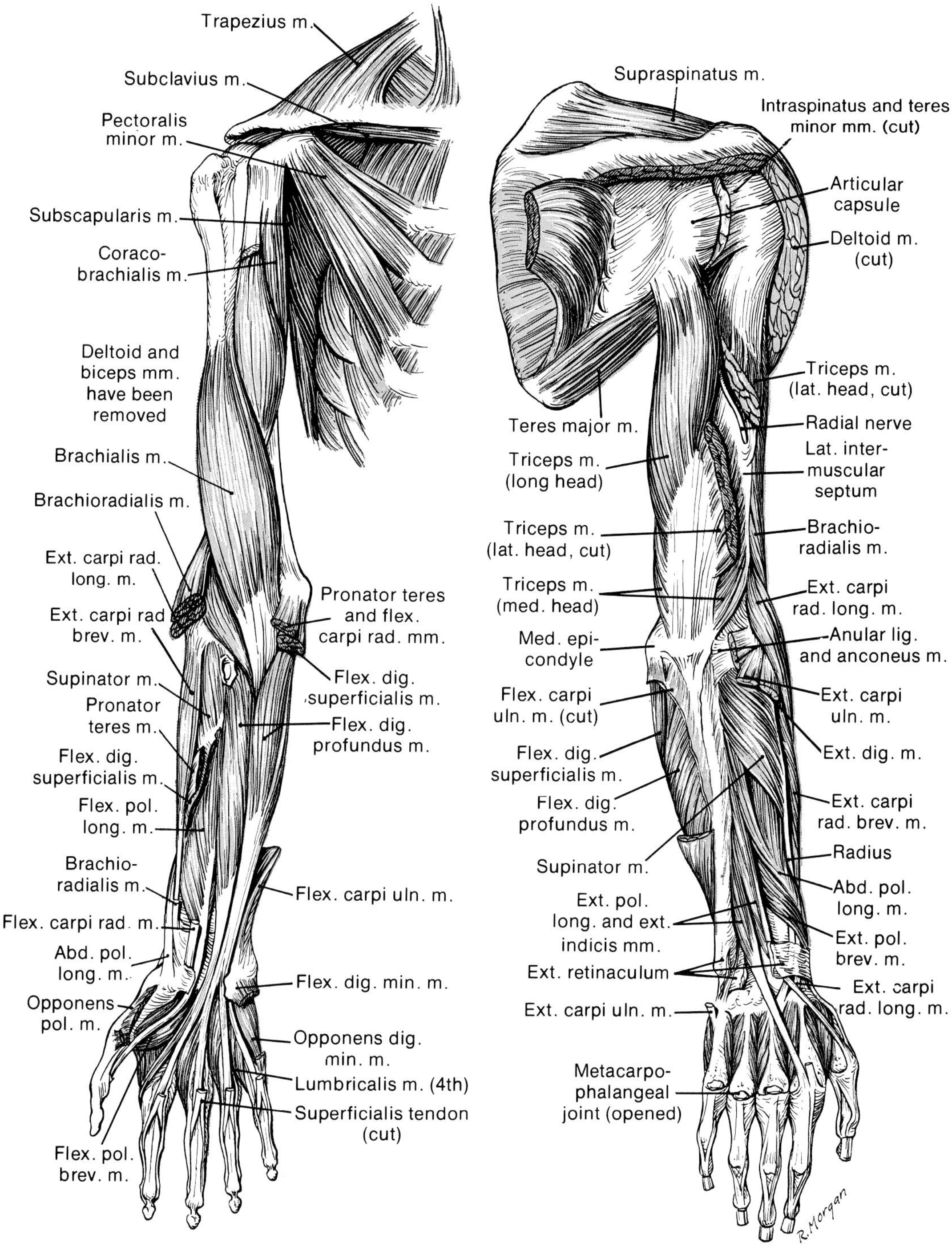
Trapezius m.
Subclavius m.
Pectoralis minor m.
Subscapularis m.
Coraco-brachialis m.
Deltoid and biceps mm. have been removed
Brachialis m.
Brachioradialis m.
Ext. carpi rad. long. m.
Ext. carpi rad brev. m.
Supinator m.
Pronator teres m.
Flex. dig. superficialis m.
Flex. pol. long. m.
Brachio-radialis m.
Flex. carpi rad. m.
Abd. pol. long. m.
Opponens pol. m.
Flex. pol. brev. m.
Pronator teres and flex. carpi rad. mm.
Flex. dig. superficialis m.
Flex. dig. profundus m.
Flex. carpi uln. m.
Flex. dig. min. m.
Opponens dig. min. m.
Lumbricalis m. (4th)
Superficialis tendon (cut)
Supraspinatus m.
Intraspinatus and teres minor mm. (cut)
Articular capsule
Deltoid m. (cut)
Teres major m.
Triceps m. (lat. head, cut)
Radial nerve
Triceps m. (long head)
Lat. inter-muscular septum
Triceps m. (lat. head, cut)
Brachio-radialis m.
Triceps m. (med. head)
Ext. carpi rad. long. m.
Med. epi-condyle
Anular lig. and anconeus m.
Flex. carpi uln. m. (cut)
Ext. carpi uln. m.
Ext. dig. m.
Flex. dig. superficialis m.
Flex. dig. profundus m.
Ext. carpi rad. brev. m.
Supinator m.
Radius
Abd. pol. long. m.
Ext. pol. long. and ext. indicis mm.
Ext. pol. brev. m.
Ext. retinaculum
Ext. carpi rad. long. m.
Ext. carpi uln. m.
Metacarpo-phalangeal joint (opened)
R. Morgan

PLATE 11

Muscles of Right Upper Limb, Deep Dissection

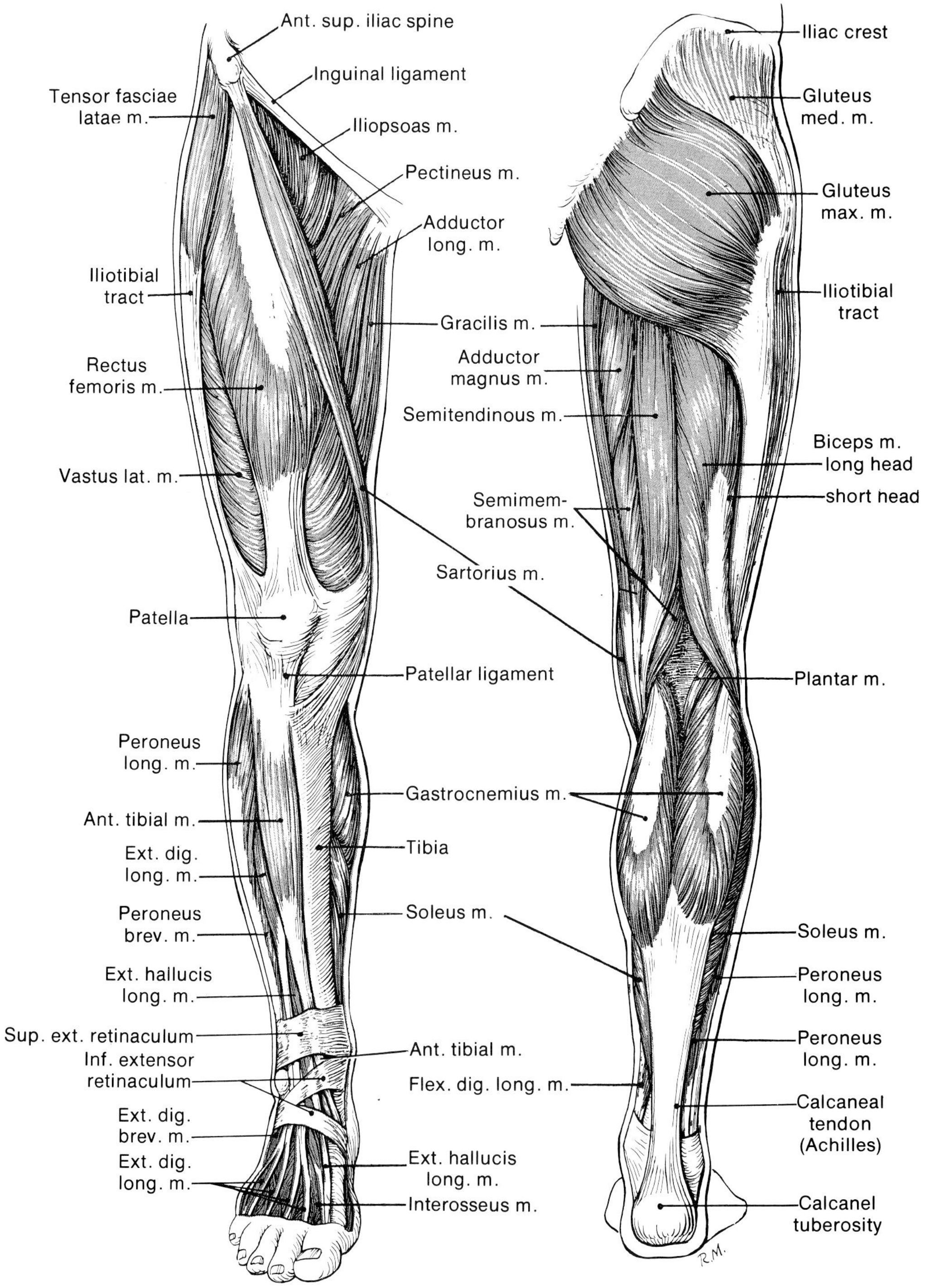
Ant. sup. iliac spine
Inguinal ligament
Tensor fasciae latae m.
Iliopsoas m.
Pectineus m.
Adductor long. m.
Iliotibial tract
Gracilis m.
Rectus femoris m.
Vastus lat. m.
Sartorius m.
Patella
Patellar ligament
Peroneus long. m.
Gastrocnemius m.
Ant. tibial m.
Tibia
Ext. dig. long. m.
Soleus m.
Peroneus brev. m.
Ext. hallucis long. m.
Sup. ext. retinaculum
Ant. tibial m.
Inf. extensor retinaculum
Flex. dig. long. m.
Ext. dig. brev. m.
Ext. dig. long. m.
Ext. hallucis long. m.
Interosseus m.
Iliac crest
Gluteus med. m.
Gluteus max. m.
Iliotibial tract
Adductor magnus m.
Semitendinous m.
Biceps m.
long head
short head
Semimem-branosus m.
Plantar m.
Soleus m.
Peroneus long. m.
Peroneus long. m.
Calcaneal tendon (Achilles)
Calcanel tuberosity
R.M.

PLATE 12

Superficial Muscles of Right Lower Limb

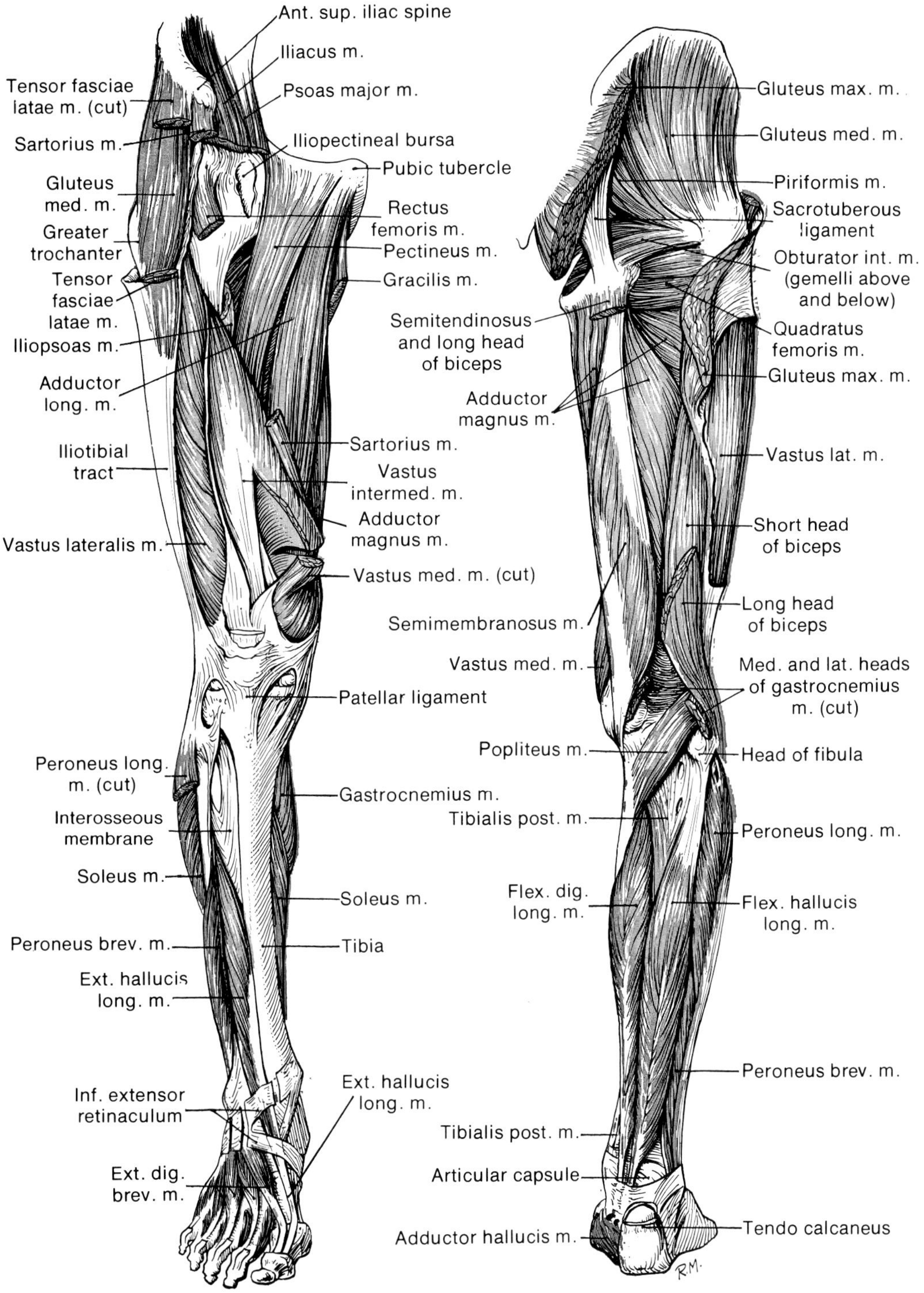
Ant. sup. iliac spine
Iliacus m.
Psoas major m.
Tensor fasciae latae m. (cut)
Sartorius m.
Iliopectineal bursa
Pubic tubercle
Gluteus med. m.
Rectus femoris m.
Greater trochanter
Pectineus m.
Tensor fasciae latae m.
Gracilis m.
Iliopsoas m.
Adductor long. m.
Iliotibial tract
Sartorius m.
Vastus intermed. m.
Adductor magnus m.
Vastus lateralis m.
Vastus med. m. (cut)
Patellar ligament
Peroneus long. m. (cut)
Gastrocnemius m.
Interosseous membrane
Soleus m.
Soleus m.
Peroneus brev. m.
Tibia
Ext. hallucis long. m.
Inf. extensor retinaculum
Ext. hallucis long. m.
Ext. dig. brev. m.
Gluteus max. m.
Gluteus med. m.
Piriformis m.
Sacrotuberous ligament
Obturator int. m. (gemelli above and below)
Semitendinosus and long head of biceps
Quadratus femoris m.
Gluteus max. m.
Adductor magnus m.
Vastus lat. m.
Short head of biceps
Long head of biceps
Semimembranosus m.
Vastus med. m.
Med. and lat. heads of gastrocnemius m. (cut)
Popliteus m.
Head of fibula
Tibialis post. m.
Peroneus long. m.
Flex. dig. long. m.
Flex. hallucis long. m.
Peroneus brev. m.
Tibialis post. m.
Articular capsule
Adductor hallucis m.
Tendo calcaneus
R.M.

PLATE 13

Muscles of Right Lower Limb, Deep Dissection

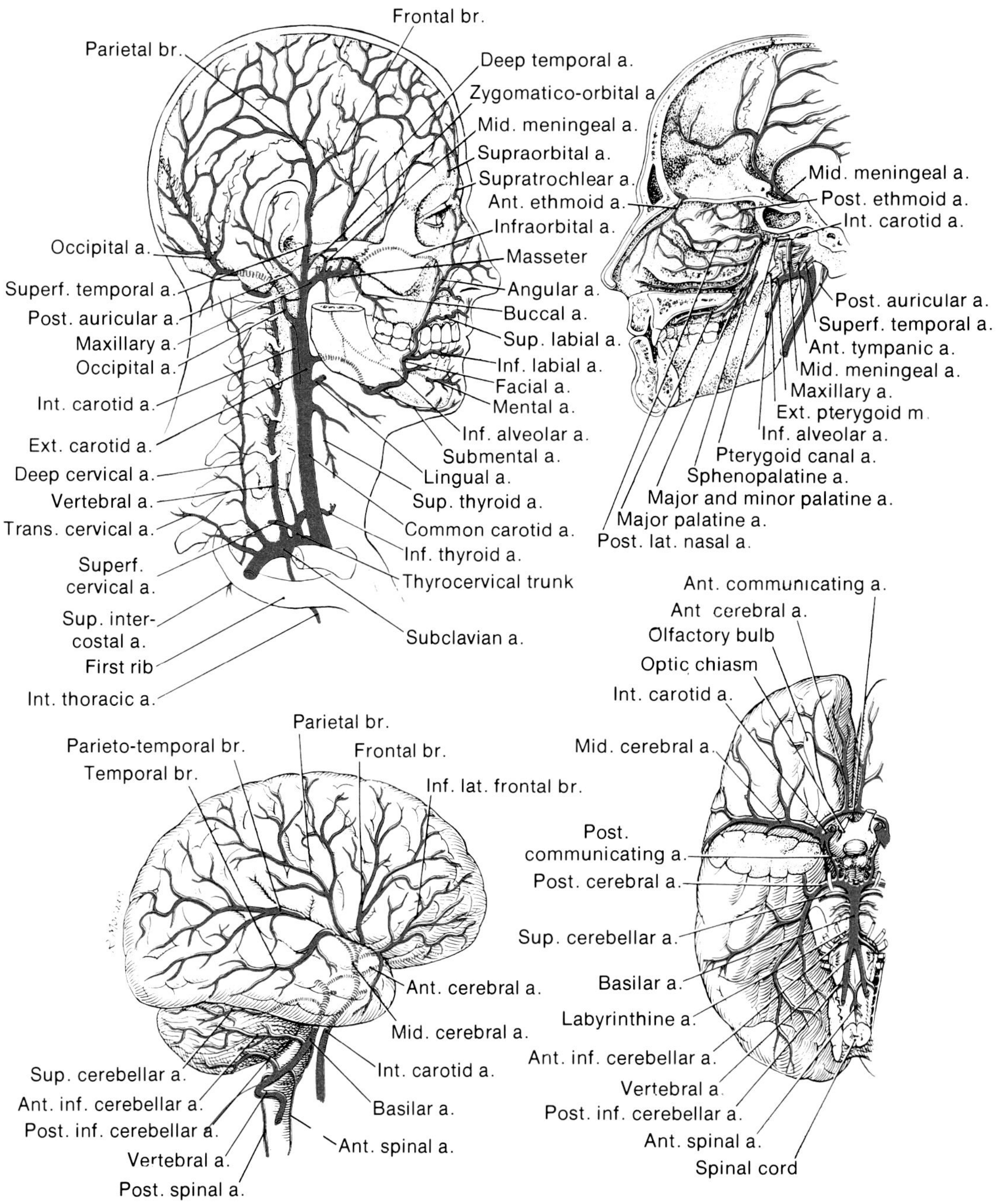
Frontal br.
Parietal br.
Deep temporal a.
Zygomatico-orbital a.
Mid. meningeal a.
Supraorbital a.
Supratrochlear a.
Ant. ethmoid a.
Infraorbital a.
Occipital a.
Masseter
Superf. temporal a.
Angular a.
Post. auricular a.
Buccal a.
Maxillary a.
Sup. labial a.
Occipital a.
Inf. labial a.
Facial a.
Int. carotid a.
Mental a.
Inf. alveolar a.
Ext. carotid a.
Submental a.
Deep cervical a.
Lingual a.
Vertebral a.
Sup. thyroid a.
Trans. cervical a.
Common carotid a.
Superf. cervical a.
Inf. thyroid a.
Thyrocervical trunk
Sup. intercostal a.
Subclavian a.
First rib
Int. thoracic a.
Mid. meningeal a.
Post. ethmoid a.
Int. carotid a.
Post. auricular a.
Superf. temporal a.
Ant. tympanic a.
Mid. meningeal a.
Maxillary a.
Ext. pterygoid m.
Inf. alveolar a.
Pterygoid canal a.
Sphenopalatine a.
Major and minor palatine a.
Major palatine a.
Post. lat. nasal a.
Ant. communicating a.
Ant cerebral a.
Olfactory bulb
Optic chiasm
Int. carotid a.
Mid. cerebral a.
Post. communicating a.
Post. cerebral a.
Sup. cerebellar a.
Basilar a.
Labyrinthine a.
Ant. inf. cerebellar a.
Vertebral a.
Post. inf. cerebellar a.
Ant. spinal a.
Spinal cord
Parietal br.
Parieto-temporal br.
Frontal br.
Temporal br.
Inf. lat. frontal br.
Ant. cerebral a.
Mid. cerebral a.
Int. carotid a.
Sup. cerebellar a.
Ant. inf. cerebellar a.
Basilar a.
Post. inf. cerebellar a.
Ant. spinal a.
Vertebral a.
Post. spinal a.

PLATE 14

Arteries of Head and Brain

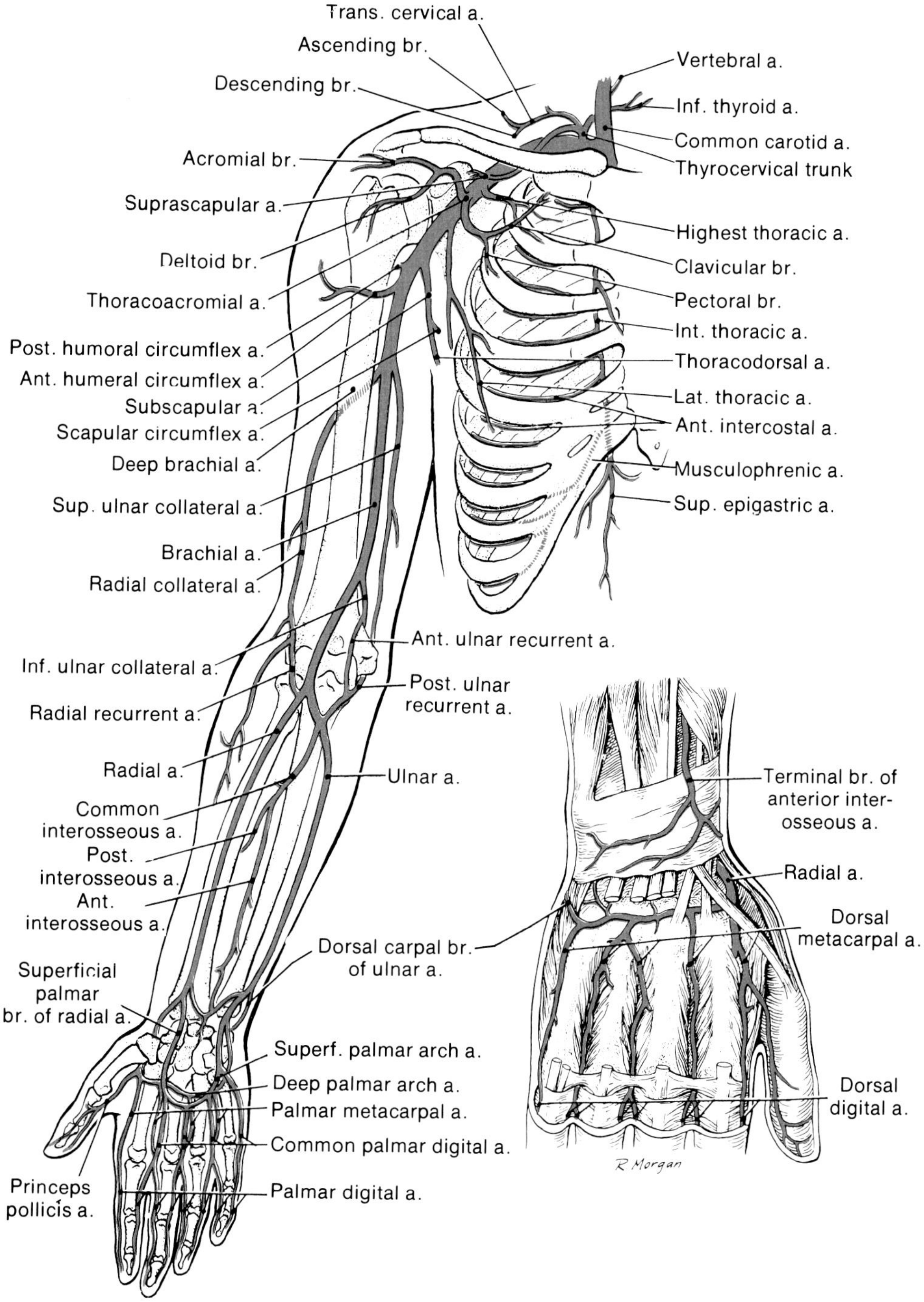
Trans. cervical a.
Ascending br.
Descending br.
Acromial br.
Suprascapular a.
Deltoid br.
Thoracoacromial a.
Post. humoral circumflex a.
Ant. humeral circumflex a.
Subscapular a.
Scapular circumflex a.
Deep brachial a.
Sup. ulnar collateral a.
Brachial a.
Radial collateral a.
Inf. ulnar collateral a.
Radial recurrent a.
Radial a.
Common interosseous a.
Post. interosseous a.
Ant. interosseous a.
Superficial palmar br. of radial a.
Princeps pollicis a.
Vertebral a.
Inf. thyroid a.
Common carotid a.
Thyrocervical trunk
Highest thoracic a.
Clavicular br.
Pectoral br.
Int. thoracic a.
Thoracodorsal a.
Lat. thoracic a.
Ant. intercostal a.
Musculophrenic a.
Sup. epigastric a.
Ant. ulnar recurrent a.
Post. ulnar recurrent a.
Ulnar a.
Dorsal carpal br. of ulnar a.
Superf. palmar arch a.
Deep palmar arch a.
Palmar metacarpal a.
Common palmar digital a.
Palmar digital a.
Terminal br. of anterior interosseous a.
Radial a.
Dorsal metacarpal a.
Dorsal digital a.
R Morgan

PLATE 15

Arteries of Upper Limb and Chest

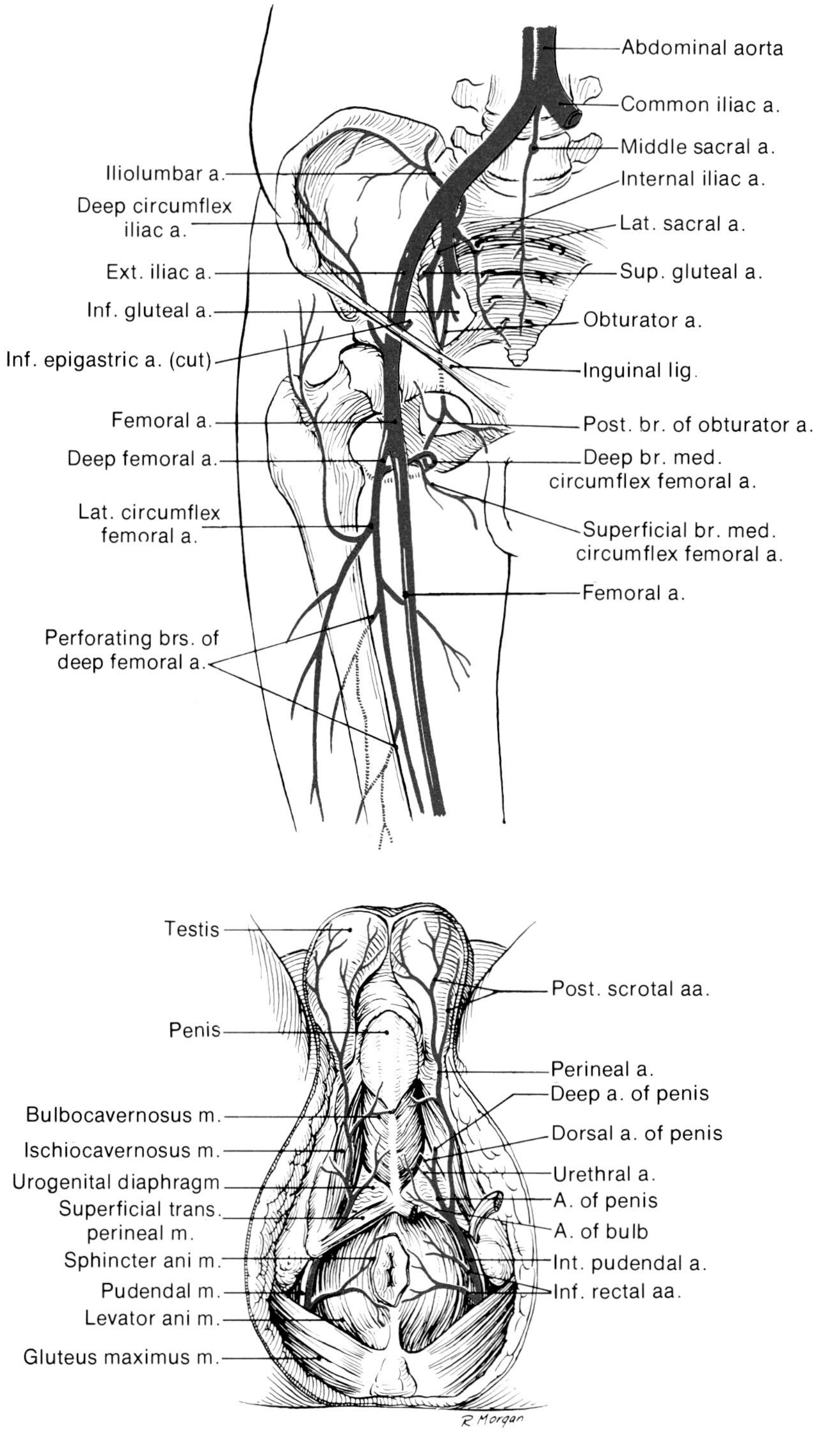
Abdominal aorta
Common iliac a.
Middle sacral a.
Internal iliac a.
Lat. sacral a.
Sup. gluteal a.
Obturator a.
Inguinal lig.
Post. br. of obturator a.
Deep br. med. circumflex femoral a.
Superficial br. med. circumflex femoral a.
Femoral a.
Iliolumbar a.
Deep circumflex iliac a.
Ext. iliac a.
Inf. gluteal a.
Inf. epigastric a. (cut)
Femoral a.
Deep femoral a.
Lat. circumflex femoral a.
Perforating brs. of deep femoral a.
Testis
Penis
Bulbocavernosus m.
Ischiocavernosus m.
Urogenital diaphragm
Superficial trans. perineal m.
Sphincter ani m.
Pudendal m.
Levator ani m.
Gluteus maximus m.
Post. scrotal aa.
Perineal a.
Deep a. of penis
Dorsal a. of penis
Urethral a.
A. of penis
A. of bulb
Int. pudendal a.
Inf. rectal aa.
R Morgan

PLATE 16

Arteries of Thigh and Perineum

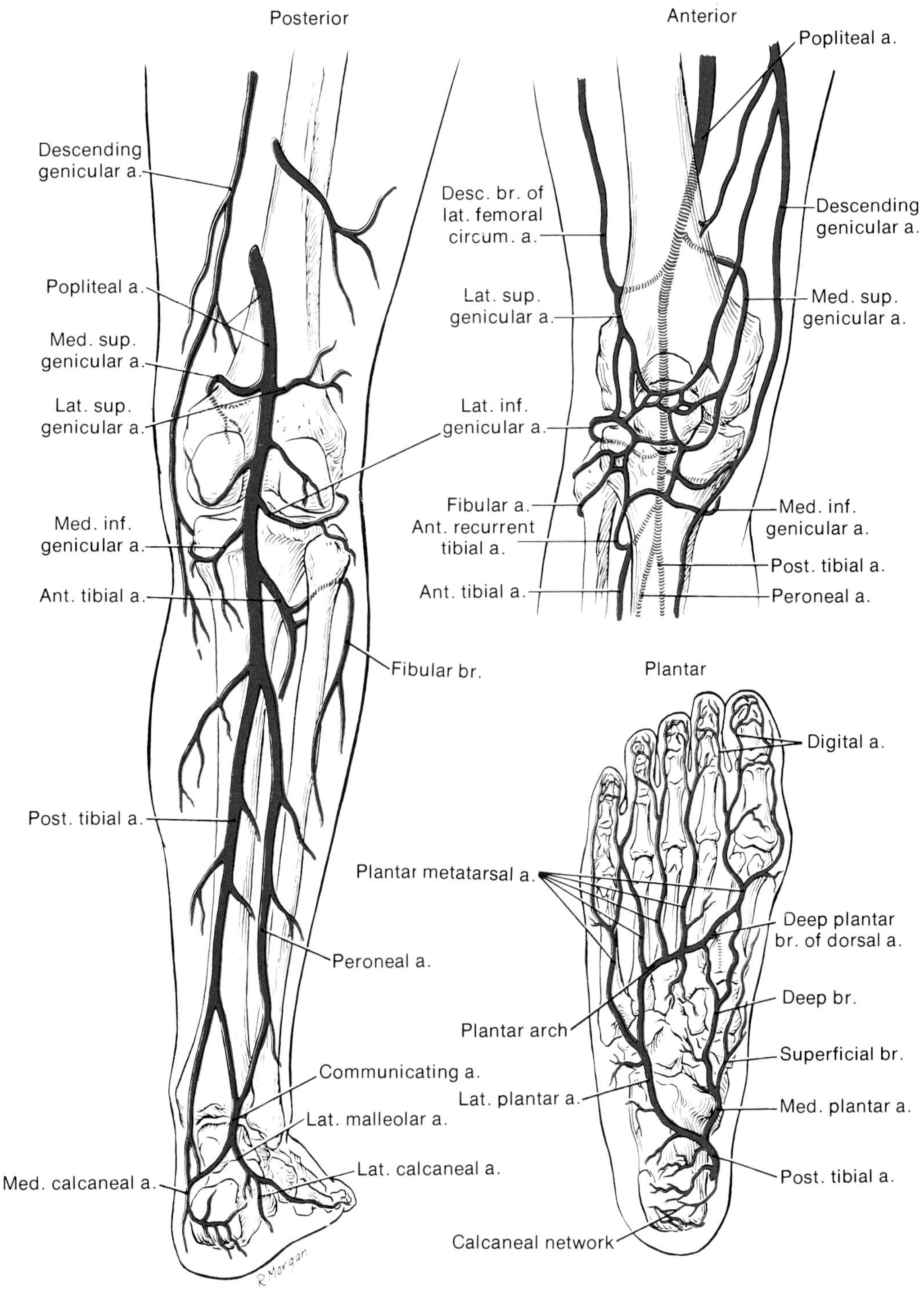

Posterior
Descending genicular a.
Popliteal a.
Med. sup. genicular a.
Lat. sup. genicular a.
Med. inf. genicular a.
Ant. tibial a.
Fibular br.
Post. tibial a.
Peroneal a.
Communicating a.
Lat. malleolar a.
Lat. calcaneal a.
Med. calcaneal a.
R. Morgan
Anterior
Popliteal a.
Desc. br. of lat. femoral circum. a.
Descending genicular a.
Lat. sup. genicular a.
Med. sup. genicular a.
Lat. inf. genicular a.
Fibular a.
Ant. recurrent tibial a.
Med. inf. genicular a.
Post. tibial a.
Ant. tibial a.
Peroneal a.
Plantar
Digital a.
Plantar metatarsal a.
Deep plantar br. of dorsal a.
Deep br.
Plantar arch
Superficial br.
Lat. plantar a.
Med. plantar a.
Post. tibial a.
Calcaneal network

PLATE 17

Arteries of Right Lower Limb in Relation to Bones

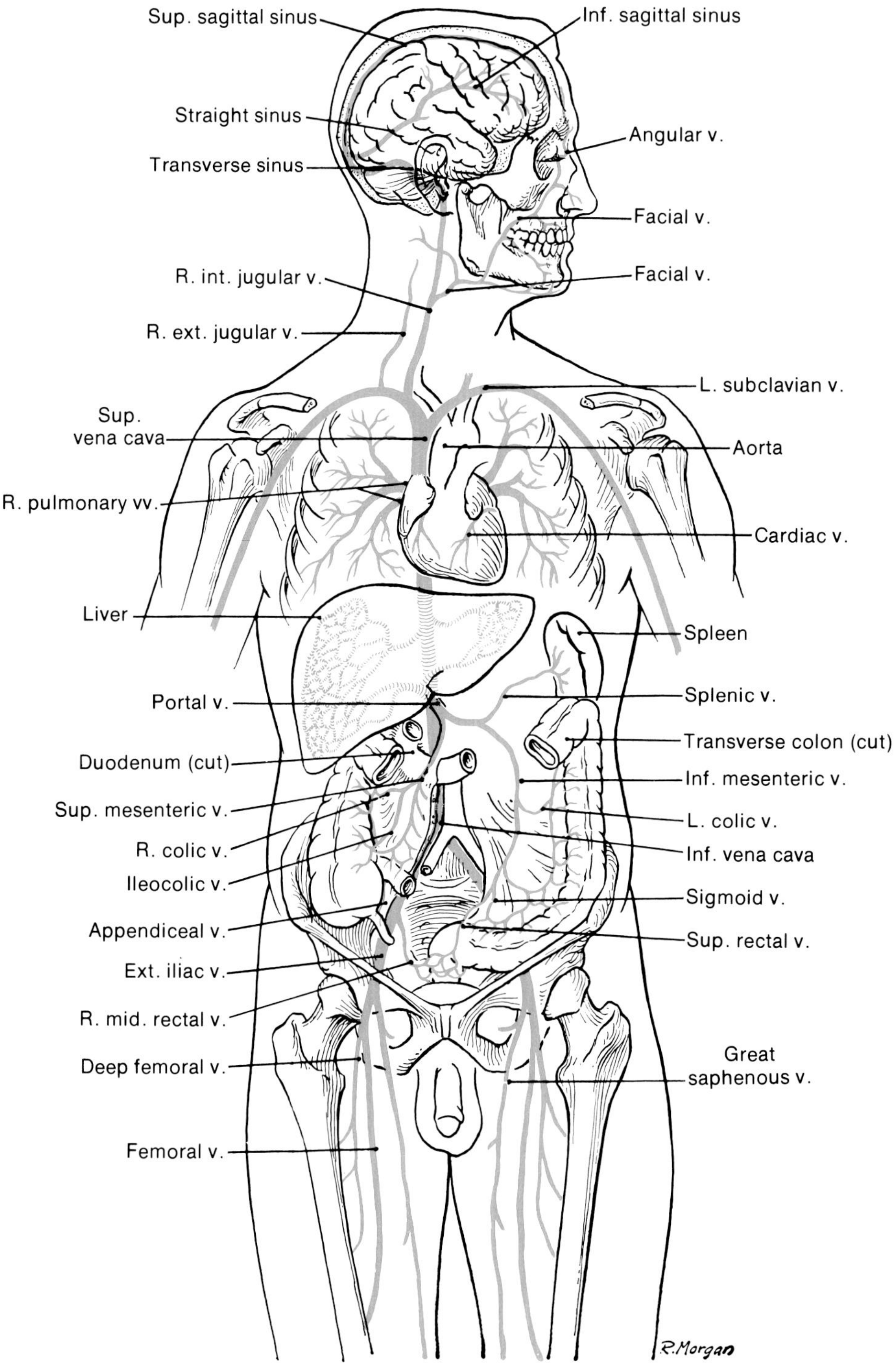
Sup. sagittal sinus
Inf. sagittal sinus
Straight sinus
Angular v.
Transverse sinus
Facial v.
R. int. jugular v.
Facial v.
R. ext. jugular v.
L. subclavian v.
Sup. vena cava
Aorta
R. pulmonary vv.
Cardiac v.
Liver
Spleen
Portal v.
Splenic v.
Transverse colon (cut)
Duodenum (cut)
Inf. mesenteric v.
Sup. mesenteric v.
L. colic v.
R. colic v.
Inf. vena cava
Ileocolic v.
Sigmoid v.
Appendiceal v.
Sup. rectal v.
Ext. iliac v.
R. mid. rectal v.
Great saphenous v.
Deep femoral v.
Femoral v.
R.Morgan

PLATE 18

Veins, Anterior View, Viscera Exposed

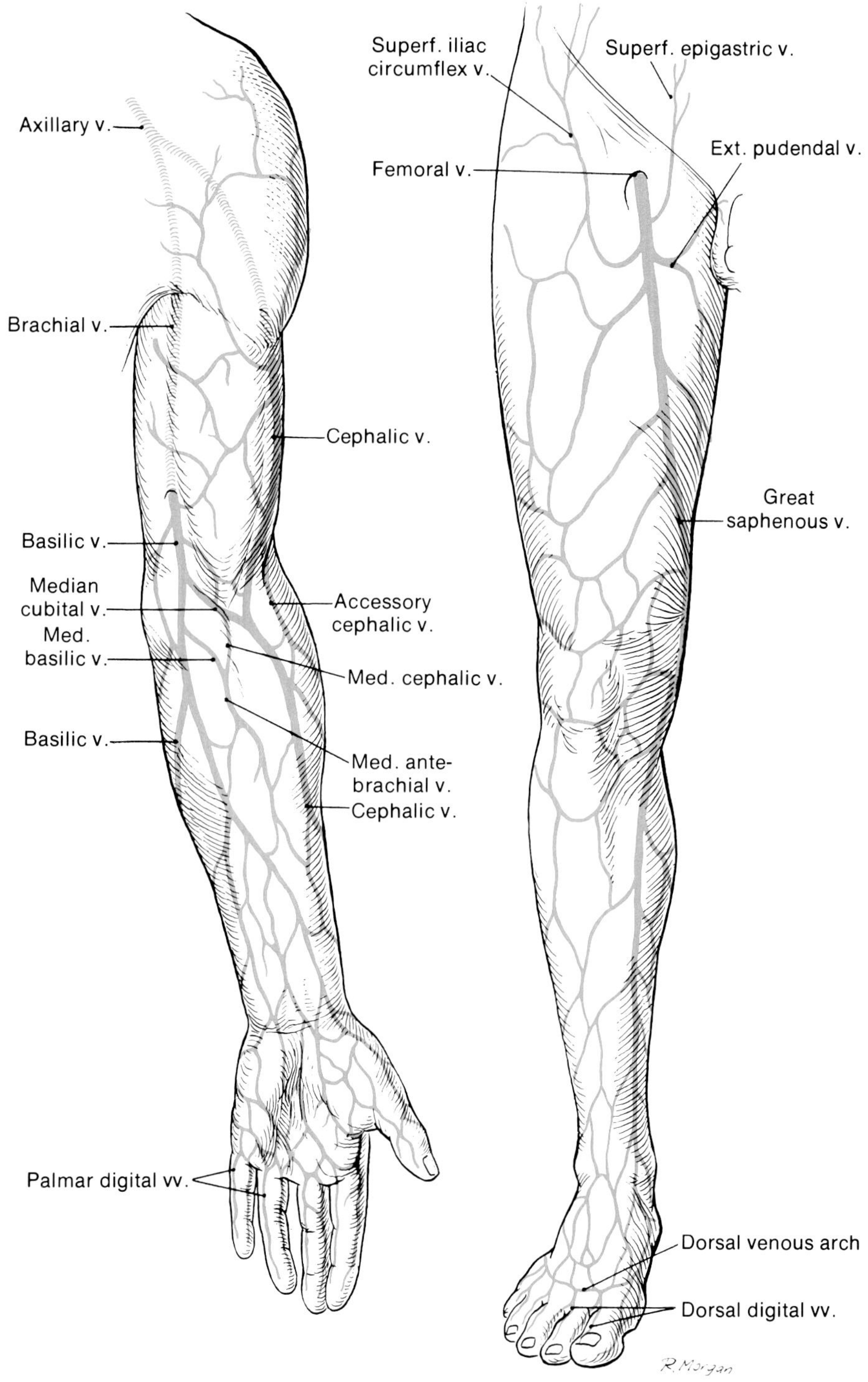
Axillary v.
Brachial v.
Cephalic v.
Basilic v.
Median cubital v.
Accessory cephalic v.
Med. basilic v.
Med. cephalic v.
Basilic v.
Med. ante-brachial v.
Cephalic v.
Palmar digital vv.
Superf. iliac circumflex v.
Superf. epigastric v.
Ext. pudendal v.
Femoral v.
Great saphenous v.
Dorsal venous arch
Dorsal digital vv.
R. Morgan

PLATE 19

Veins of Limbs

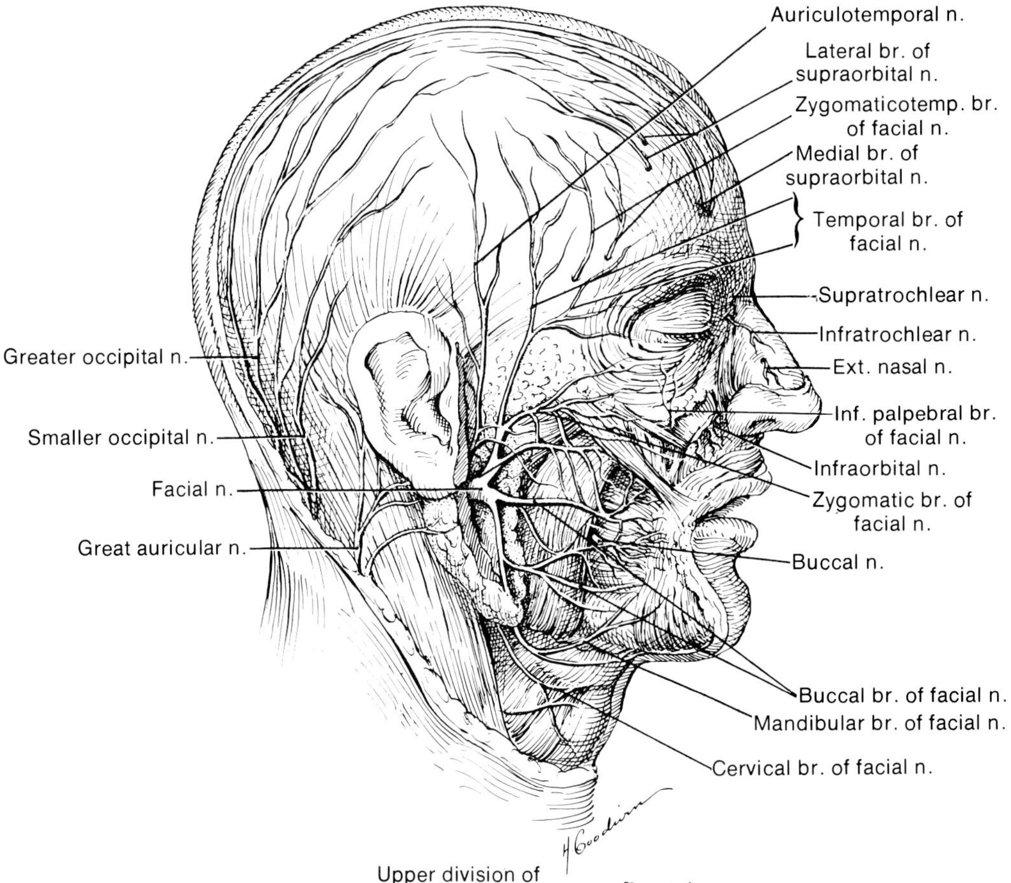

Auriculotemporal n.
Lateral br. of supraorbital n.
Zygomaticotemp. br. of facial n.
Medial br. of supraorbital n.
Temporal br. of facial n.
Supratrochlear n.
Infratrochlear n.
Ext. nasal n.
Inf. palpebral br. of facial n.
Infraorbital n.
Zygomatic br. of facial n.
Buccal n.
Buccal br. of facial n.
Mandibular br. of facial n.
Cervical br. of facial n.
Greater occipital n.
Smaller occipital n.
Facial n.
Great auricular n.

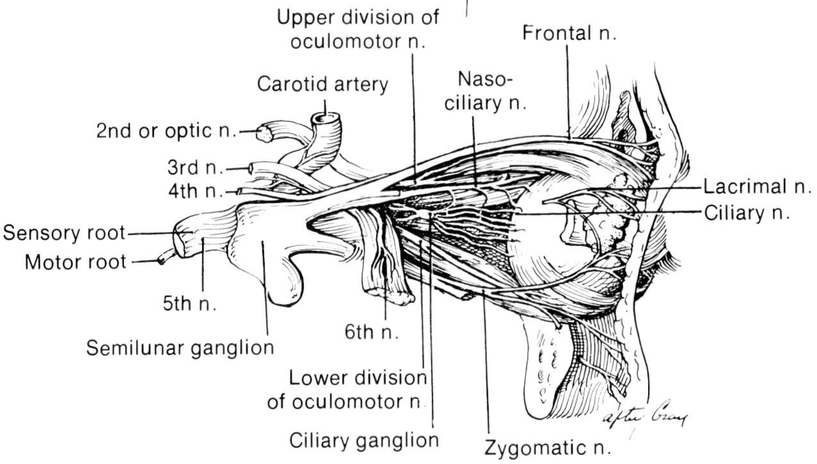

Upper division of oculomotor n.
Frontal n.
Carotid artery
Naso-ciliary n.
2nd or optic n.
3rd n.
4th n.
Lacrimal n.
Ciliary n.
Sensory root
Motor root
5th n.
6th n.
Semilunar ganglion
Lower division of oculomotor n.
Ciliary ganglion
Zygomatic n.

PLATE 20

Nerves of Head and Orbit

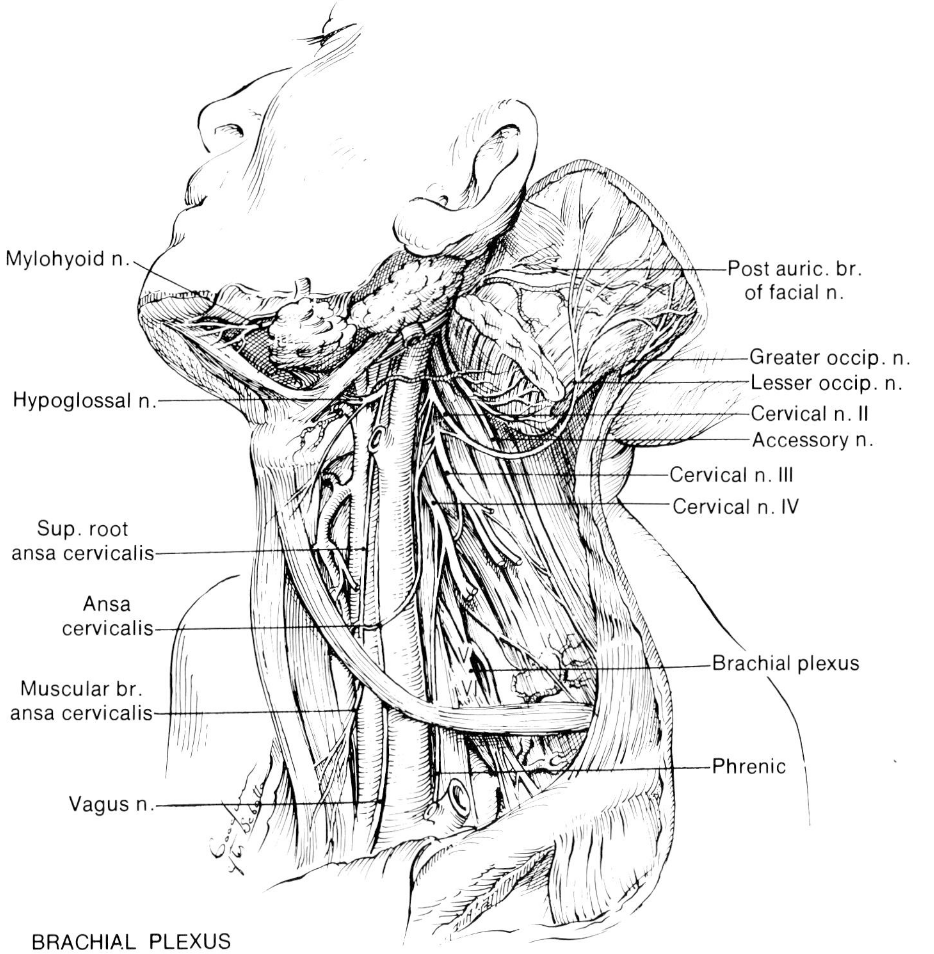

Mylohyoid n.
Hypoglossal n.
Sup. root ansa cervicalis
Ansa cervicalis
Muscular br. ansa cervicalis
Vagus n.
Post auric. br. of facial n.
Greater occip. n.
Lesser occip. n.
Cervical n. II
Accessory n.
Cervical n. III
Cervical n. IV
Brachial plexus
Phrenic

BRACHIAL PLEXUS

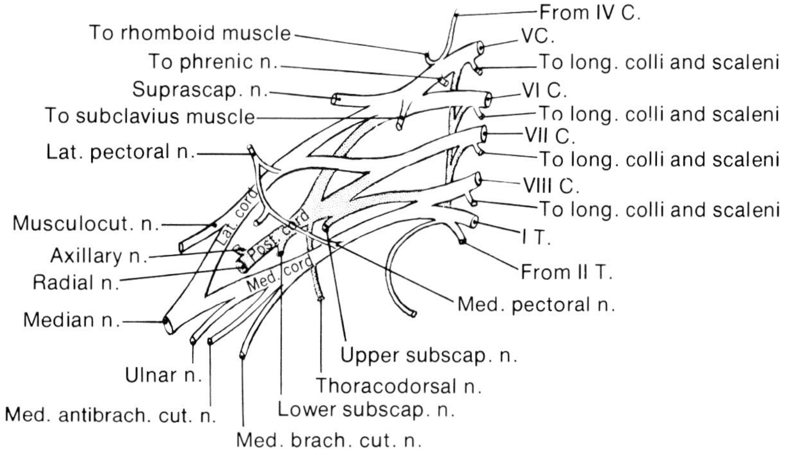

To rhomboid muscle
To phrenic n.
Suprascap. n.
To subclavius muscle
Lat. pectoral n.
Musculocut. n.
Axillary n.
Radial n.
Median n.
Ulnar n.
Med. antibrach. cut. n.
Med. brach. cut. n.
Lower subscap. n.
Thoracodorsal n.
Upper subscap. n.
Med. pectoral n.
From IV C.
VC.
To long. colli and scaleni
VI C.
To long. colli and scaleni
VII C.
To long. colli and scaleni
VIII C.
To long. colli and scaleni
I T.
From II T.
Lat. cord
Post. cord
Med. cord

PLATE 21

Nerves of Neck and Axilla

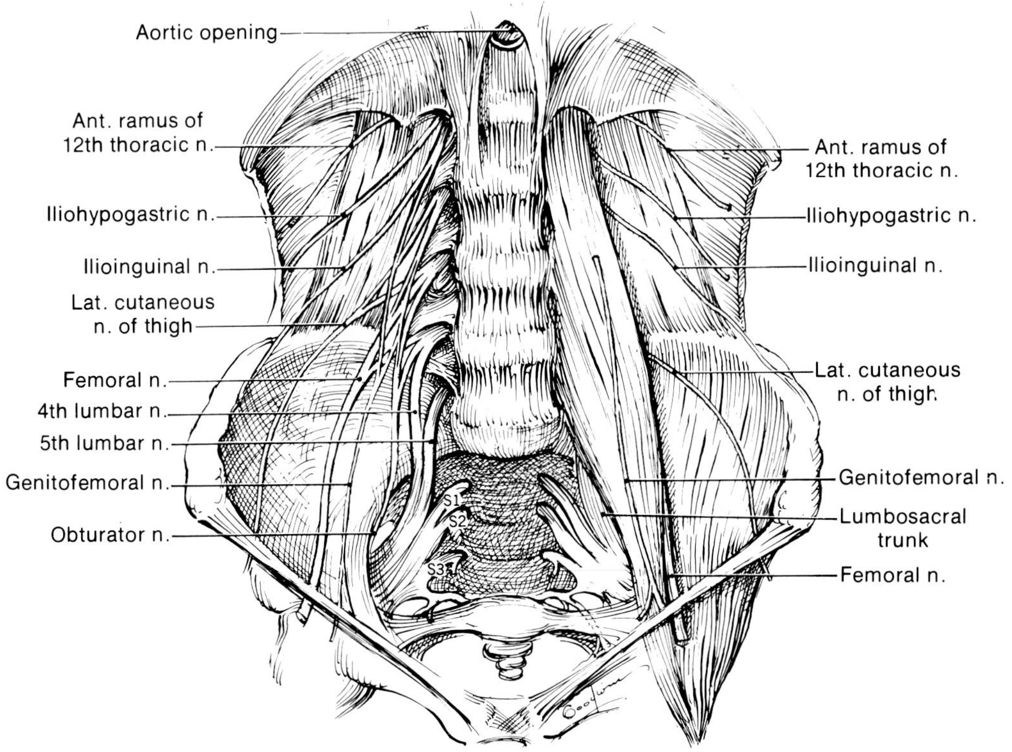
Aortic opening
Ant. ramus of 12th thoracic n.
Iliohypogastric n.
Ilioinguinal n.
Lat. cutaneous n. of thigh
Femoral n.
4th lumbar n.
5th lumbar n.
Genitofemoral n.
Obturator n.
S1
S2
S3
Ant. ramus of 12th thoracic n.
Iliohypogastric n.
Ilioinguinal n.
Lat. cutaneous n. of thigh
Genitofemoral n.
Lumbosacral trunk
Femoral n.

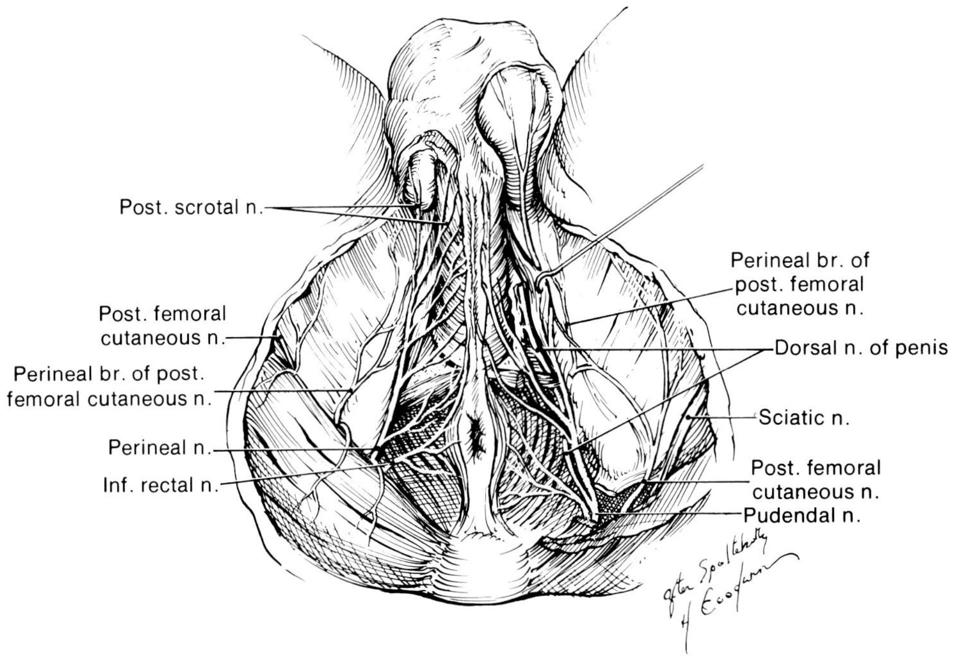
Post. scrotal n.
Post. femoral cutaneous n.
Perineal br. of post. femoral cutaneous n.
Perineal n.
Inf. rectal n.
Perineal br. of post. femoral cutaneous n.
Dorsal n. of penis
Sciatic n.
Post. femoral cutaneous n.
Pudendal n.

PLATE 22

Nerves of Lumbar and Sacral Plexuses

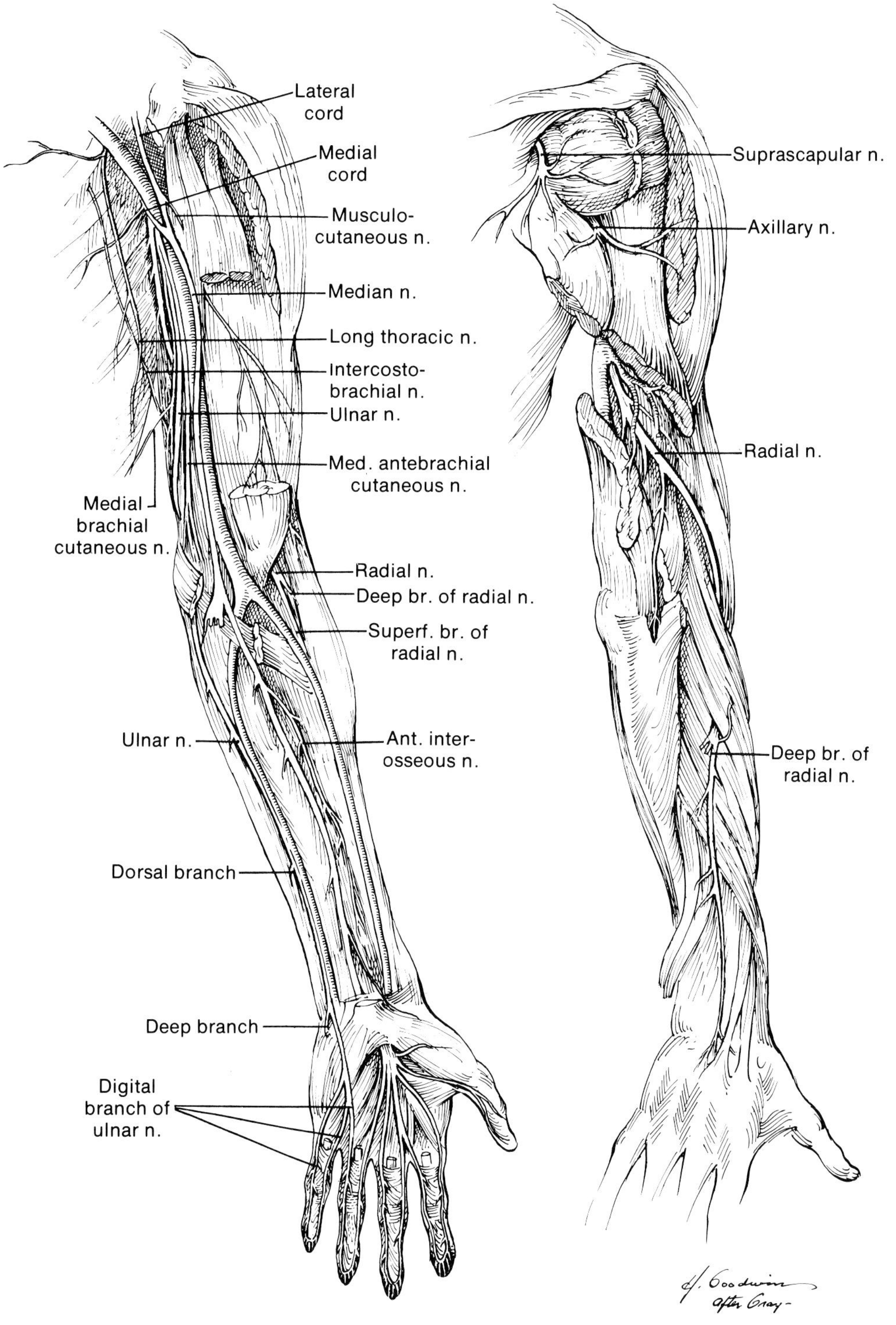
Lateral
cord
Medial
cord
Musculo-
cutaneous n.
Median n.
Long thoracic n.
Intercosto-
brachial n.
Ulnar n.
Med. antebrachial
cutaneous n.
Medial
brachial
cutaneous n.
Radial n.
Deep br. of radial n.
Superf. br. of
radial n.
Ulnar n.
Ant. inter-
osseous n.
Dorsal branch
Deep branch
Digital
branch of
ulnar n.
Suprascapular n.
Axillary n.
Radial n.
Deep br. of
radial n.

PLATE 23

Nerves of Upper Limb

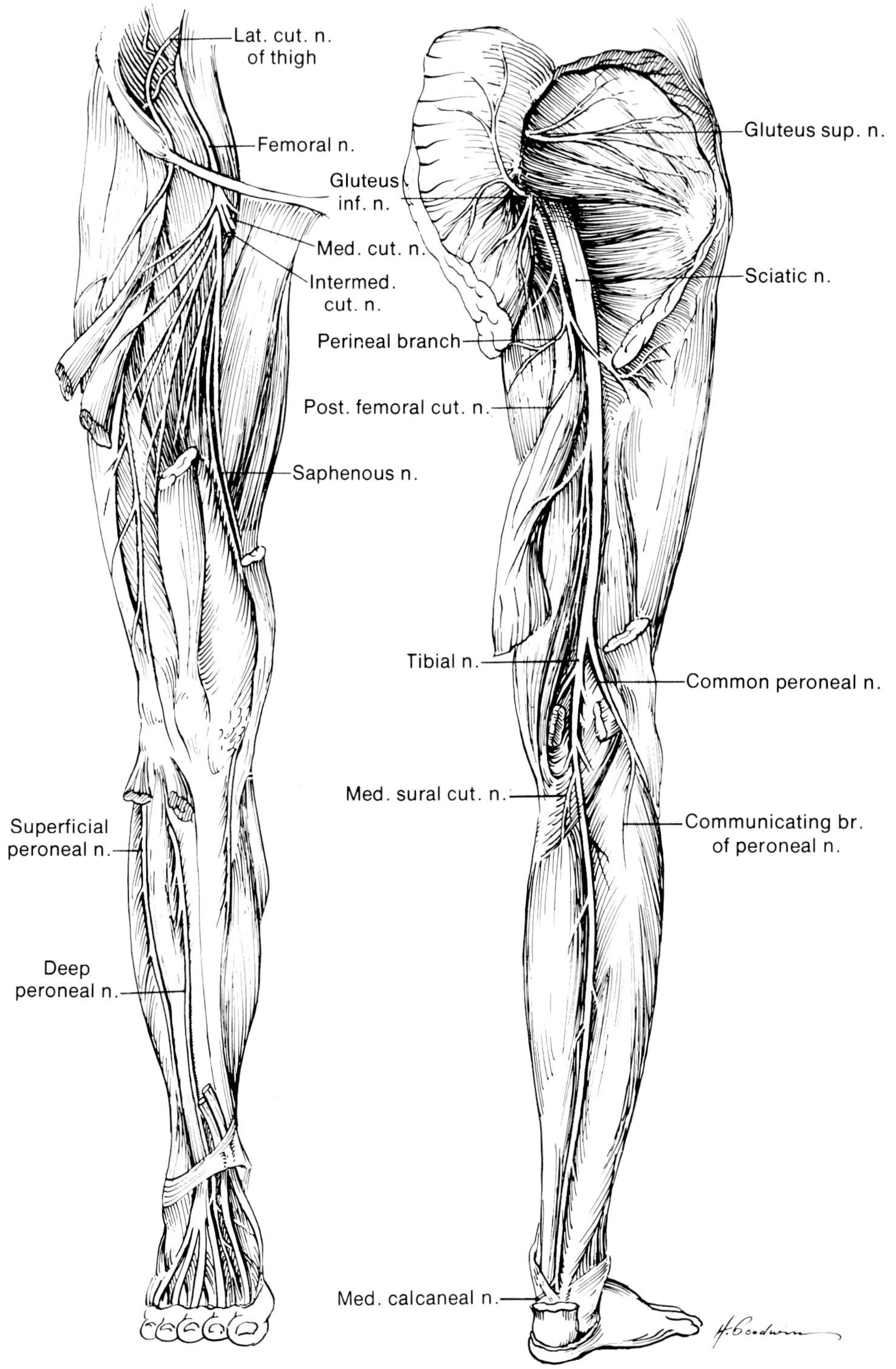
Lat. cut. n.
of thigh
Femoral n.
Gluteus
inf. n.
Med. cut. n.
Intermed.
cut. n.
Perineal branch
Post. femoral cut. n.
Saphenous n.
Superficial
peroneal n.
Deep
peroneal n.
Gluteus sup. n.
Sciatic n.
Tibial n.
Common peroneal n.
Med. sural cut. n.
Communicating br.
of peroneal n.
Med. calcaneal n.
H. Goodwin

PLATE 24

Nerves of Lower Limb

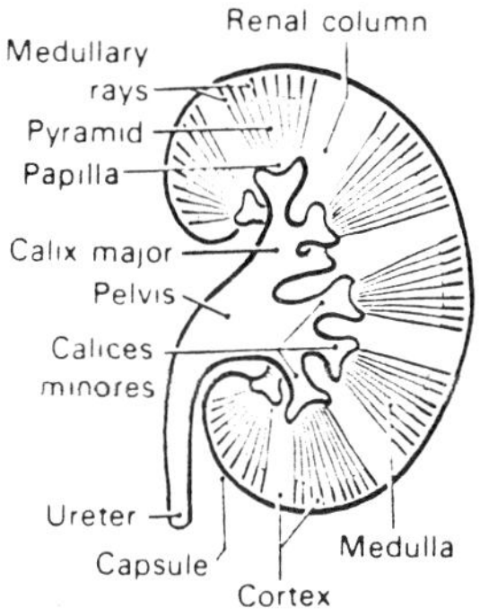

Kidney
Diagram of macroscopic structure, as seen on longitudinal section.

Armanni-Ebstein k., Armanni-Ebstein change; glycogen vacuolization of the loops of Henle, seen in diabetics before the introduction of insulin.
arteriolosclerotic k., a k. in which there is sclerosis of the arterioles, *i.e.,* arteriolar nephrosclerosis resulting from long-standing benign hypertension. Such k.'s tend to be pale red-brown or relatively gray, moderately reduced in size, and firmer than normal organs; the capsular surfaces are uniformly finely granular. Most of the arterioles are thickened and hyalinized, thereby resulting in varying degrees of narrowing of the lumens, ischemia, and fibrosis in the interstitial tissue, leading to uniform contraction of the cortex.
arteriosclerotic k., a k. in which there is sclerosis of arterial vessels larger than arterioles. Such k.'s are usually not significantly reduced in size, but are likely to be paler than usual; the capsular surface may be marked by a few, possibly several, conical, relatively deep V-shaped scars that result from fibrosis and ischemic atrophy of the region supplied by the affected vessel.
artificial k., hemodialyzer.
Ask-Upmark k., true renal hypoplasia with decreased lobules and deep transverse grooving of the cortical surfaces of the kidney.
atrophic k., a k. that is diminished in size because of inadequate circulation and/or loss of nephrons.
cake k., a solid irregularly lobed organ of bizarre shape, usually situated in the pelvis toward the midline, produced by fusion of the renal anlagen.
contracted k., a diffusely scarred k. in which the relatively large amount of abnormal fibrous tissue and ischemic atrophy leads to a moderate or great reduction in the size of the organ, as in arteriolar nephrosclerosis and chronic glomerulonephritis.
cow k., a k. containing an abnormally large number of minor calices, resembling normal bovine renal anatomy.
crush k., acute oliguric renal failure following crushing injuries of muscle; k.'s show the changes of hypoxic tubular damage, but pigment casts in renal tubules contain myoglobin.
cystic k., a general term used to indicate a k. that contains one or more cysts, including polycystic disease, solitary cyst, multiple simple cysts, and retention cysts (associated with parenchymal scarring).
disk k., pancake k.
duplex k., a k. in which two pelviocaliceal systems are present.
fatty k., a k. in which there is fatty metamorphosis of the parenchymal cells, especially fatty degeneration.
flea-bitten k., the k. seen at autopsy in some cases of bacterial endocarditis, the appearance being caused by diffuse petechial hemorrhages resulting from focal glomerulonephritis.
floating k., movable or wandering k.; the abnormally mobile k. in nephroptosia.
Formad's k., an enlarged and deformed k. sometimes seen in chronic alcoholism.
fused k., a single anomalous organ produced by fusion of the renal anlagen.
Goldblatt k., a k. whose arterial blood supply has been compromised, as a consequence of which arterial (renovascular) hypertension develops.
granular k., sclerotic k.; a k. in which fairly uniform, diffusely and evenly situated foci of scarring of the interstitial tissue of the cortex (and sometimes scarring of glomeruli), and the associated slight degree of bulging of groups of dilated tubules, leads to the development of a minutely bosselated surface; such k.'s are seen in arteriolar nephrosclerosis or chronic glomerulonephritis.
head k., pronephros (1).
hind k., metanephros.
horseshoe k., union of the lower or occasionally the upper extremities of the two k.'s by a band of tissue extending across the vertebral column.

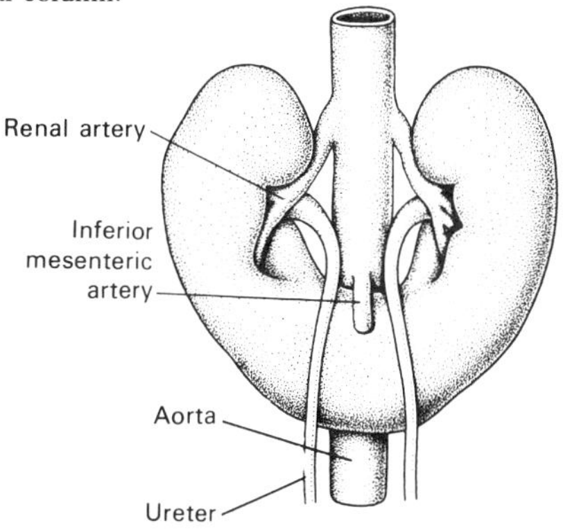

Horseshoe Kidney

medullary sponge k., cystic disease of the renal pyramids associated with calculus formation and hematuria; differs from cystic disease of the renal medulla in that renal failure does not usually develop.
middle k., mesonephros.
mortar k., putty k.
movable k., floating k.
pancake k., disk k.; a disk-shaped organ produced by fusion of both poles of the contralateral k. anlagen.
pelvic k., k. that has been displaced into the pelvis.
polycystic k., polycystic disease of the kidneys; a progressive disease characterized by formation of multiple cysts of varying size scattered diffusely throughout both k.'s, resulting in compression and destruction of k. parenchyma, usually with hypertension, gross hematuria, and uremia; there are two major types: 1) with onset in infancy or early childhood, usually with autosomal recessive inheritance; 2) with onset in adulthood, with autosomal dominant inheritance.
primordial k., pronephros.
putty k., mortar k.; a k. containing caseous material trapped by stricture of the ureter due to tuberculous granulations in renal tuberculosis.
pyelonephritic k., a k. deformed by multiple scars as a result of chronic or recurrent renal infection.
Rose-Bradford k., a form of fibrotic k. of inflammatory origin found in young persons.
sclerotic k., granular k.
supernumerary k., a k., in addition to the two usually present, developed from the splitting of the nephrogenic blastema, or from separate metanephric blastemas, into which partially or completely reduplicated ureteral stalks enter to form separate capsulated k.'s; in some cases, the separation of the reduplicated organ is incomplete.

wandering k., floating k.
waxy k., amyloid k.

Kiel classification. See under classification.

Kielland. See Kjelland.

Kien, Alphonse M.J., 19th century German physician. See Kussmaul-K. *respiration.*

Kienböck, Robert, Austrian roentgenologist, 1871–1953. See K.'s *atrophy, disease, dislocation, unit.*

Kiernan, Francis, British physician, 1800–1874. See K.'s *space.*

Kiesselbach, Wilhelm, German laryngologist, 1839–1902. See K.'s *area.*

Kilian, Hermann F., German gynecologist, 1800–1863. See K.'s *line.*

Killian, Gustav, German laryngologist, 1860–1921. See K.'s *bundle, operation.*

kilo- (k) [G. *chilioi,* one thousand] Prefix used in the SI and metric systems to signify one thousand (10^3).

kilobase (kb) (kil'ō-bās). Unit used in designating the length of a nucleic acid sequence; 1 kb equals a sequence of 1000 purine or pyramidine bases.

kilocalorie (kcal) (kil'ō-kal-ō-rē). Large *calorie.*

kilocycle (kc) (kil'ō-sī-kl). One thousand cycles per second.

kilogram (kg) (kil'ō-gram). The SI unit of mass, 1000 g or 1 cubic decimeter of water; equivalent to 15,432 gr, 2.205 lb. avoirdupois, or 2.68 lb. troy.

kilogram-meter. The energy exerted, or work done, when a mass of 1 kg is raised a height of 1 m; equal to 9.806 J in the SI system.

kiloroentgen (kil-ō-rent'gen). Term used to denote an exposure of 1000 roentgens.

kilovolt (kv) (kil'ō-vōlt). One thousand volts.

kilovoltmeter (kil'ō-vōlt-mē'ter). An instrument designed to measure electromotive force in kilovolts.

Kimmelstiel, Paul, German pathologist in the U.S., 1900–1970. See K.-Wilson *disease, syndrome.*

Kimura, T., 20th century Japanese pathologist. See K.'s *disease.*

kin-, kine- [G. *kinēsis,* movement]. Prefixes denoting movement. See also cine-.

kinanesthesia (kin-an-es-thē'zē-ă) [G. *kinēsis,* motion, + *an-* priv. + *aisthēsis,* sensation]. Cinanesthesia; a disturbance of deep sensibility in which there is inability to perceive either direction or extent of movement, the result being ataxia.

kinase (kī'nās). **1.** An enzyme catalyzing the conversion of a proenzyme to an active enzyme; *e.g.,* enteropeptidase (enterokinase). **2.** An enzyme catalyzing the transfer of phosphate groups to form triphosphates (ATP). For individual k.'s, see specific name.

kinase II. Peptidyl dipeptidase A.

kind'ling. Long-lasting epileptogenic changes induced by daily subthreshold electrical brain stimulation without apparent neuronal damage.

kin'dred. An aggregate of genetically related persons; distinguished from pedigree, which is a stylized representation of a k.

kinematics (kin-ĕ-mat'iks) [G. *kinēmatica,* things that move]. Cinematics; in physiology, the science concerned with movements of the parts of the body.

kinemometer (kin-ĕ-mom'ĕ-ter) [G. *kinēsis,* movement, + *metron,* measure]. An electromagnetic device, similar in principle to the velocity ballistocardiograph, used to measure the contraction and relaxation elicited in a tendon reflex.

kineplastics (kin'ĕ-plas-tiks). Cineplastic *amputation.*

kinesalgia (kin-ĕ-sal'jē-ă) [G. *kinēsis,* motion, + *algos,* pain]. Kinesialgia; pain caused by muscular movement.

kinescope (kin'ĕ-skōp) [G. *kinēsis,* motion, + *skopeō,* to examine]. Obsolete instrument for determining the refraction of the eyes; the subject observes the apparent "with" or "against" movement of the test object through a stenopeic slit moved across the front of the eye.

kinesi-, kinesio-, kineso- [G. *kinēsis,* motion]. Combining forms relating to motion.

kinesia (ki-nē'sē-ă, -nē'zē-) [G. *kinēsis,* movement]. Motion *sickness.*

kinesialgia (ki-nē-sē-al'jē-ă). Kinesalgia.

kinesiatrics (ki-nē'sē-at'riks) [G. *kinēsis,* movement, + *iatrikos,* relating to medicine]. Kinesitherapy.

kinesics (ki-nē'siks). The study of nonverbal, bodily motion in communication.

kinesimeter (kin-ĕ-sim'ĕ-ter) [G. *kinēsis,* movement, + *metron,* measure]. Kinesiometer; an instrument for measuring the extent of a movement.

kinesio-. See kinesi-.

kinesiology (ki-nē-sē-ol'ō-jē) [G. *kinēsis,* movement, + *-logos,* study]. The science or the study of movement, and the active and passive structures involved.

kinesiometer (ki-nē-sē-om'ĕ-ter). Kinesimeter.

kinesioneurosis (ki-nē'sē-ō-nū-rō'sis) [G. *kinēsis,* movement]. Rarely used term for a neurosis, or functional nervous disease, marked by tics, spasms, or other motor disorders.

kinesipathist (kin-ĕ-sip'ă-thist). A nonmedical person who treats disease by movements of various kinds.

kinesipathy (kin-ĕ-sip'ă-thē) [G. *kinēsis,* movement, + *pathos,* suffering]. **1.** An affection marked by motor disturbances. **2.** Kinesitherapy.

kinesis (ki-nē'sis) [G.]. Motion. As a termination, used to denote movement or activation, particularly the kind induced by a stimulus.

kinesitherapy (ki-nē-si-thār'ă-pē). Kinesipathy (2); kinesiatrics; treatment by means of a movement regimen. See subentries under movement.

kineso-. See kinesi-.

kinesophobia (ki-nē-sō-fō'bē-ă) [G. *kinēsis,* movement, + *phobos,* fear]. Morbid fear of movement.

kinesthesia (kin'es-thē'zē-ă) [G. *kinēsis,* motion, + *aisthēsis,* sensation]. **1.** The sense perception of movement; the muscular sense. **2.** An illusion of moving in space.

kinesthesiometer (kin'es-thē'zē-om'ĕ-ter) [kinesthesia, + G. *metron,* measure]. An instrument for determining the degree of muscular sensation.

kinesthetic (kin-es-thet'ik). Relating to kinesthesia.

kinetic (ki-net'ik) [G. *kinētikos,* of motion, fr. *kinētos,* moving]. Relating to motion or movement.

kinetics (ki-net'iks). The study of motion, acceleration, or rate of change.
chemical k., the study of the rates of chemical reactions.

kineto- [G. *kinētos,* moving, movable]. Combining form relating to motion.

kinetocardiogram (ki-nē'tō-kar'dē-ō-gram, ki-net'ō-). Graphic recording of the vibrations of the chest wall produced by cardiac activity.

kinetocardiograph (ki-nē'tō-kar'dē-ō-graf, ki-net'ō-). A device for recording precordial impulses due to cardiac movement; the absolute displacement of a point on the chest wall is recorded relative to a fixed reference point above the recumbent patient.

kinetochore (ki-nē'tō-kōr, ki-net'ō-) [kineto- + G. *chōra,* space]. Centromere (1).

kinetogenic (ki-nē-tō-jen'ik, ki-net-ō-). Causing or producing motion.

kinetoplasm (ki-nē'tō-plazm) [kineto- + G. *plasma,* a thing formed]. Cinetoplasm; cinetoplasma; kinoplasm. **1.** The most contractile part of a cell. **2.** The cytoplasm of the droplet which covers the sperm head during maturation.

kinetoplast (ki-nē'tō-plast, ki-net'ō-) [kineto- + G. *plastos,* formed]. An intensely staining rod-, disc-, or spherical-shaped extranuclear DNA structure found in parasitic flagellates (family Trypanosomatidae) near the base of the flagellum, posterior to the blepharoplast, and often at right angles to the nucleus. Electron micrographs show it to be part of a single giant mitochondrion filling most of the cytoplasm of amastigote flagellates, the k. portion being visible by light microscopy. DNA of the k. is termed kDNA to distinguish it from nuclear DNA, or nDNA. The k. divides independently, along with the basal body, prior to nuclear division. The term k. formerly included parabasal body and blepharoplast in a locomotory apparatus, but is now recognized as a distinct organelle of most trypanosomatids. See also parabasal *body.*

kinetoscope (kĭ-ne'to-skōp) [kineto- + G. *skopeō,* to examine]. An apparatus for taking serial photographs to record movement.

kinetosome (ki-nē'tō-sōm, ki-net'ō-) [kineto- + G. *sōma,* body]. Basal *body.*

King, Earl J., Canadian biochemist, *1901. See K. *unit;* K.-Armstrong *unit.*

Kingsley, N.W., U.S. dentist, 1829–1913. See K. *splint.*

kinic acid (kin'ik). Quinic acid.

kinin (kī'nin). One of a number of widely differing substances having pronounced and dramatic physiological effects. Some (*e.g.,* kallidin and bradykinin) are polypeptides, formed in blood by proteolysis secondary to some pathological process, that stimulate visceral smooth muscle but relax vascular smooth muscle, thus producing vasodilation; others (*e.g.,* kinetin) are plant growth regulators.

kininogen (ki-nin'ō-jen). The globulin precursor of a (plasma) kinin.

kininogenase (ki-nin'ō-jĕ-nās). Kallikrein.

kininogenin (ki-nin'ō-jen-in). Kallikrein.

kink. An angulation, bend, or twist.
Lane's k., Lane's *band.*

kino- [G. *kineō,* to move]. Combining form relating to movement.

kinocentrum (kin-ō-sen'trŭm) [kino- + G. *kentron,* center]. Cytocentrum.

kinocilium (kī-nō-sil'ē-ŭm) [kino- + cilium]. A cilium, usually motile, having nine peripheral double microtubules and two single central ones.

kinohapt (kin'ō-hapt) [kino- + G. *haptein,* to touch]. An esthesiometer for applying several stimuli to the skin at different distances and frequencies.

kinomometer (kin-ō-mom'ĕ-ter) [kino- + G. *metron,* measure]. An instrument for measuring degree of motion.

kinoplasm (kin'ō-plazm, kī'nō). Kinetoplasm.

kinoplasmic (kin-ō-plas'mik, kī-nō-) Relating to kinoplasm (kinetoplasm).

kin'ship. The state of being genetically related.

Kinyoun, J.J., early 20th century U.S. physician. See K. *stain.*

kion (kī'on) [G. *kiōn,* pillar, the uvula]. Obsolete term for uvula.

kion-, kiono- [G. *kiōn,* uvula]. Obsolete combining forms relating to the uvula. See uvul-, uvulo-.

Kirk, Norman Thomas, U.S. Army surgeon, 1888–1960. See K.'s *amputation.*

Kirkland, Olin, U.S. periodontist, 1876–1969. See K. *knife.*

Kirschner, Martin, German surgeon, 1879–1942. See K.'s *apparatus, wire.*

Kisch, Bruno, German physiologist, 1890–1966. See K.'s *reflex.*

Kitasato, Shibasaburo, Baron, Japanese bacteriologist, 1852–1931. See K.'s *bacillus.*

Kittrich, Miroslav. See K.'s *stain.*

Kjeldahl, Johan G.C., Danish chemist, 1849–1900. See K. *apparatus, method;* macro-K. *method;* micro-K. *method.*

Kjelland (Kielland), Christian, Norwegian obstetrician, 1871–1941. See K.'s *forceps.*

Klapp, Rudolph, German surgeon, 1873–1949. See K.'s *method.*

Klebs, Theodor Albrecht Edwin, German physician, 1834–1913. See *Klebsiella;* K-Loeffler *bacillus.*

Klebsiella (kleb-sē-el'ă) [E. *Klebs*]. A genus of aerobic, facultatively anaerobic, nonmotile, nonsporeforming bacteria (family Enterobacteriaceae) containing Gram-negative, encapsulated rods which occur singly, in pairs, or in short chains. These organisms produce acetylmethylcarbinol and lysine decarboxylase or ornithine decarboxylase. They do not usually liquefy gelatin. Citrate and glucose are ordinarily used as sole carbon sources. These organisms may or may not be pathogenic. They occur in the respiratory, intestinal, and urogenital tracts of man as well as in soil, water, and grain. The type species is *K. pneumoniae.*
K. ozae'nae, Abel's bacillus; a species which occurs in cases of ozena and other chronic diseases of the respiratory tract.
K. pneumo'niae, Friedländer's bacillus; pneumobacillus; a species which occurs in soil and water, on grain, and in the intestinal tract of man and other animals; it also occurs in association with several pathologic conditions, urinary tract infections, sputum, feces, and metritis in mares; capsular types 1, 2, and 3 of this organism may be causative agents in pneumonia; organisms previously identified as nonmotile strains of *Aerobacter aerogenes* are now placed in this species; it is the type species of *K.*
K. rhinosclero'matis, a species found in cases of rhinoscleroma.

kleeblattschädel (klā-blat-she'dl) [Ger.]. Cloverleaf skull. See cloverleaf skull *syndrome.*

Kleffner. See Landau-K. *syndrome.*

Kleihauer. See K.'s stain; Betke-K. *test.*

Klein, Edward E., Hungarian histologist, 1844–1925. See K.'s *muscle;* K. Gumprecht *nuclei.*

Kleine, Willi, 20th century German neuropsychiatrist. See K.-Levin *syndrome.*

kleptolagnia (klep-tō-lag'nē-ă) [G. *kleptō,* to steal, + *lagneia,* lust, coition]. Erotic feelings induced by stealing.

kleptomania (klep-tō-mā'nē-ă) [G. *kleptō,* to steal, + *mania,* insanity]. A disorder of impulse control characterized by a morbid tendency to steal.

kleptomaniac (klep-tō-mā'nē-ak). A person exhibiting kleptomania.

kleptophobia (klep-tō-fō'bē-ă) [G. *kleptō,* to steal, + *phobos,* fear]. Morbid fear of stealing or of becoming a thief.

Klinefelter, Harry F., Jr., U.S. physician, *1912. See K.'s *syndrome.*

Klinger-Ludwig acid-thionin stain for sex chromatin. See under stain.

Klippel, Maurice, French neurologist, 1858–1942. See K.'s *disease;* K.-Feil *syndrome;* K.-Trenaunay-Weber *syndrome.*

Klumpke, Augusta Dejerine-K., French neurologist, 1859–1927. See K.'s *paralysis;* K.-Déjérine *syndrome.*

Klüver, Heinrich, German-born U.S. neurologist, *1897. See K.-Barrera Luxol fast blue *stain;* K.-Bucy *syndrome.*

Knapp, Herman J., U.S. ophthalmologist, 1832–1911. See K.'s *streaks, striae.*

Knaus, Hermann, Austrian gynecologist, *1892. See Ogino-K. *rule.*

knee (nē) [A.S. *cneōw*]. **1.** Genu. **2.** See *articulatio* genus. **3.** Any recurved structure resembling a semiflexed knee. See genu (3), and geniculum.
Brodie's k., Brodie's disease (1); chronic hypertrophic synovitis of the k.
capped k., swelling of the bursa of the extensor metacarpi magnus muscle in cattle, usually caused by injury to the carpus in getting up and down on hard floors; *Brucella abortus* has been isolated from many of these cases.
housemaid's k., an adventitious occupational bursitis occurring over the tibial tuberosity, the area of contact when kneeling; not to be confused with prepatellar bursitis.
locked k., a condition in which the k. lacks full extension and flexion because of internal derangement, usually the result of a torn medial meniscus.

kneecap (nē'kap). Patella.

Knemidokoptes (nē'mi-dō-kop'tēz) [G. *knēmē,* leg, + *coptō,* to cut]. A genus of microscopic burrowing sarcoptid mites that infect fowl and caged birds; species include *K. laevis* var. *gallinae,* the depluming mite, and *K. mutans,* the scaly leg mite.

Knies, Max, German ophthalmologist, 1851–1917. See K.'s *sign.*

Kniest, Wilhelm, 20th century German pediatrician. See K. *syndrome.*

knife, pl. knives (nīf, nīvz). A cutting instrument used in surgery and dissection.

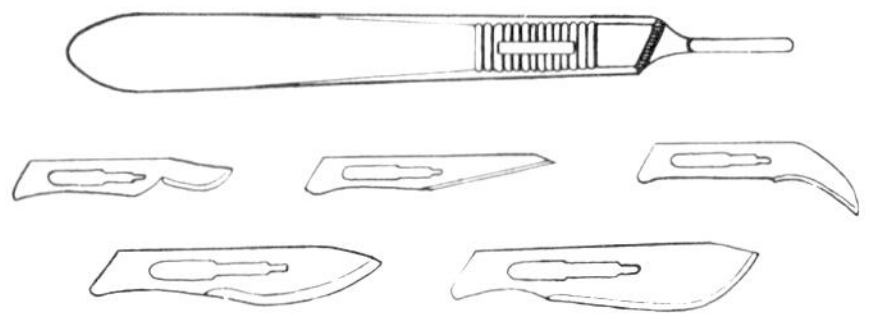

Knife
Bard-Parker handle with various blades

Beer's k., a triangular k. with a sharp point and one sharp edge, formerly used for incision for cataract.
cartilage k., chondrotome.
cautery k., a k. that sears while cutting, to diminish bleeding.
chemical k., term sometimes used for restriction *endonuclease.*
electrode k., a blade-shaped electrical instrument used to cut tissues by means of a high-frequency electrical current.
fistula k., fistulatome.
free-hand k., a manually operated k. or blade usually used to take split-thickness skin grafts; *e.g.,* Blair-Brown k., Humby k., Theirsh k.
Goldman-Fox knives, a set of knives used in periodontal surgery.
Graefe's k., a narrow-bladed k. used in making a section of the cornea.
hernia k., herniotome; a slender bladed k., with short cutting edge, for dividing the constricting tissues at the mouth of the hernial sac.
Kirkland k., a heart-shaped k. used in gingival surgery.
lenticular k., a scraper resembling a sharp spoon.
Liston's knives, long-bladed knives of various sizes used in amputations.
Merrifield k., a long, narrow, triangularly shaped k. used in gingival surgery.
valvotomy k., a k. used in mitral valvotomy.

knismogenic (nis'mō-jen'ik) [G. *knismos,* tickling, + *-gen,* production]. Causing a tickling sensation.

knismolagnia (nis-mō-lag'nē-ă) [G. *knismos,* tickling, + *lagneia,* lust]. Sexual gratification from the act of tickling.

knitting (nit'ing). Nonmedical term denoting the process of union of the fragments of a broken bone or of the edges of a wound.

knob (nob). A protuberance; a mass; a nodule.
Engelmann's basal k.'s, obsolete eponym for blepharoplast.
malarial k.'s, rounded protrusions of a red blood cell infected with *Plasmodium falciparum,* responsible for the adhesion of infected red cells to one another and to the endothelium of the blood vessels containing these infected cells; results in capillary blockage responsible for much of the pathology of malignant tertian malaria.

knock (nok). **1.** Colloquialism for a blow, especially a blow to the head. **2.** A sound simulating that of a blow or rap.
pericardial k., an early diastolic sound analogous to the normal third heart sound, but occurring somewhat earlier, due to rapid ventricular filling being abruptly halted by the restricting pericardium.

knock-knee (nok'nē). *Genu* valgum.

Knoll, Philipp, Bohemian physiologist, 1841–1900. See K.'s *glands.*

Knoop, Hedwig, German physician, *1908. See K.'s *theory.*

Knoop hardness number. See under number.

knot (not) [A.S. *cnotta*]. **1.** An intertwining of the ends of two cords, tapes, sutures, etc. in such a way that they cannot spontaneously become separated; or a similar twining or infolding of a cord in its continuity. **2.** In anatomy or pathology, a node, ganglion, or circumscribed swelling suggestive of a k.
false k.'s (of umbilical cord), local increases in length or varicosity of the umbilical vein, causing markedly apparent twisting of the cord.
Hensen's k., primitive *node.*
Hubrecht's protochordal k., primitive *node.*
net k., karyosome.
primitive k., primitive *node.*
protochordal k., primitive *node.*
syncytial k., syncytial bud or sprout; a localized aggregation of syncytiotrophoblastic nuclei in the villi of the placenta during early pregnancy.
true k. (of umbilical cord), actual intertwining of a segment of umbilical cord; circulation is usually not obstructed.
vital k., *noeud* vital.

knuckle (nŭk'l). **1.** A joint of a finger when the fist is closed, especially a metacarpophalangeal joint. **2.** A kink or loop of intestine, as in a hernia.
cervical aortic k., an anomalous aortic arch in which the aorta extends into the neck and forms an anteroposterior arch, which may be as high as the hyoid bone; the common carotid artery of one side is given off from the summit of the arch, and the common carotid of the other side arises from the more proximal part of the aorta; the pulsating arch may be mistaken for an aneurysm, but the radial pulses are equal.

knuckling (nŭk'ling). Talipes in the horse, caused by a contraction of the posterior fetlock tendons.

Kobelt, Georg L., German physician, 1804–1857. See K.'s *tubules.*

Kober, Philip A., U.S. chemist, *1884. See K. *test.*

Kober test. See under test.

Köbner, H., German dermatologist, 1838–1904. See K.'s *phenomenon.*

Koch, Robert, German bacteriologist and Nobel laureate, 1843–1910. See K.'s *bacilli,* blue *bodies, law,* old *tuberculin, phenomenon, postulates;* K.-Weeks *bacillus, conjunctivitis.*

Koch, Walter, German surgeon, *1880. See K.'s *node, triangle.*

Kocher, E. Theodor, Swiss surgeon and Nobel laureate, 1841–1917. See K. *clamp;* K.'s *incision, sign.*

Kock, Nils G., 20th century Swedish surgeon. See K. *pouch.*

Koenen's tumor. See under tumor.

Koenig, Franz, German surgeon, 1832–1910. See K.'s *syndrome.*

Koerber-Salus-Elschnig syndrome. See under syndrome.

Koerte, Werner, German surgeon, 1853–1937. See K.-Ballance *operation.*

Koettstorfer number. See under number.

Kogoj, Franz, Yugoslavian physician, *1894. See spongiform *pustule* of K.

Köhler, Alban, German roentgenologist, 1874–1947. See K.'s *disease.*

Köhler, August, German microscopist, 1866–1948. See K. *illumination.*

Köhlmeier, W., 20th century German physician. See K-Degos *disease.*

Kohlrausch, Otto L.B., German physician, 1811–1854. See K.'s *muscle, valves.*

Kohn, Hans N., German pathologist, *1866. See K.'s *pores.*

Kohnstamm, Oskar, German physician, 1871–1917. See K.'s *phenomenon.*

koilocyte (koy'lō-sīt) [G. *koilos,* hollow, + *kytos,* cell]. A squamous cell, often binucleated, showing a perinuclear hole; characteristic of condyloma acuminatum.

koilocytosis (koy'lō-sī-tō'sis) [G. *koilos,* hollow, + *kytos,* cell, + *-osis,* condition]. Perinuclear vacuolation. See also koilocyte.

koilonychia (koy-lō-nik'ē-ă) [G. *koilos,* hollow, + *onyx* (*onych-*), nail]. Celonychia; spoon nail; a malformation of the nails in which the outer surface is concave; often associated with hypochromic anemia, with rare occurrence as a familial trait.

koilosternia (koy-lō-ster'nē-ă) [G. *koilos,* hollow, + *sternon,* chest (sternum)]. *Pectus* excavatum.

Kojewnikoff (Kozhevnikov), Aleksei Y., Russian neurologist, 1836–1902. See K.'s *epilepsy.*

kojic acid (kō'jik). 5-Hydroxy-2-(hydroxymethyl)-4-pyranone; an antibiotic product of glucose catabolism in some molds; can be converted into flavor enhancers.

kola (kō'lă). Cola; the dried cotyledons of *Cola nitida* or other species of *Cola* (family Sterculiaceae) which contains caffeine, theobromine, and a soluble principle, colatin; used as a cardiac and central nervous system stimulant.

Kölliker, Rudolph A. von, Swiss histologist, 1817–1905. See K.'s *layer, reticulum.*

Kollmann, Arthur, 19th century German urologist. See K.'s *dilator.*

Kolmer, John A., U.S. pathologist, 1886–1962. See K. *test.*

Kolopp, P., 20th century French dermatologist. See Woringer-K. *disease.*

kolp-. See colp-.

kolytic (kō-lit'ik) [G. *kolyō,* to hinder]. Denoting an inhibitory action.

Kondoleon, Emmanuel, Greek surgeon, 1879–1939. See K. *operation.*

koniocortex (kō'nē-ō-kōr'teks) [G. *konis,* dust, + L. *cortex,* bark]. Regions of the cerebal cortex characterized by a particularly well developed inner granular layer (layer 4); this type of cerebral cortex is represented by the primary sensory areas 17 of the visual cortex, areas 1 to 3 of the somatic sensory cortex, and area 41 of the auditory cortex. See also *cortex* cerebri.

Koplik, Henry, U.S. physician, 1858–1927. See K.'s *spots, stigma* of degeneration.

kopophobia (kop-ō-fō'bē-ă) [G. *kopos,* fatigue, + *phobos,* fear]. Morbid fear of fatigue.

kopro-. See copro-.

Korányi, Baron F. von, Hungarian physician, 1828–1913. See K.'s *method.*

Korff, Karl von, 20th century German anatomist and histologist. See K.'s *fibers.*

Kornzweig, Abraham L. See Bassen-K. *syndrome.*

koro (kō'rō). Shook jong; an acute delusional state occurring in Macassars, natives of the Celebes and other parts of the East, in which the subject experiences a sensation that his penis is shriveling or is being drawn into the abdomen.

koronion (kŏ-rō'nē-on). Coronion.

Korotkoff, Nikolai S., Russian physician, 1874–1920. See K.'s *sounds, test.*

Korsakoff, Sergei S., Russian neurologist, 1853–1900. See K.'s *psychosis, syndrome;* Wernicke-K. *encephalopathy, syndrome.*

Koyanagi, Yosizo, Japanese ophthalmologist, 1880–1954. See Vogt-K. *syndrome.*

Koyter. See Coiter.

Kr Symbol for krypton.

Krabbe, Knud H., Danish neurologist, 1885–1961. See K.'s *disease, syndrome;* Christensen-K. *disease.*

krait (krīt). Elapid snakes of the genus *Bungaris,* found in northern India, whose bite is associated with generalized anesthetic and paralytic effects, as opposed to local pain, discoloration, or edema; neurotoxic symptoms are similar to those induced by cobra venom.

kra-kra. Craw-craw.

Krantz, Kermit E., U.S. obstetrician-gynecologist, *1923. See Marshall-Marchetti-K. *operation.*

Kraske, Paul, German surgeon, 1851–1930. See K.'s *operation.*

kraurosis vulvae (kraw-rō'sis vŭl'vē) [G. *krauros,* dry, brittle]. Leukokraurosis; atrophy and shrinkage of the epithelium of the vagina and vulva, often accompanied by a chronic inflammatory reaction in the deeper tissues, as in lichen sclerosus et atrophicus.

Krause, Arlington C., U.S. ophthalmologist, *1896. See K.'s *syndrome.*

Krause, Fedor, German surgeon, 1857–1937. See K. *graft;* K.'s *method;* Wolfe-K. *graft.*

Krause, Karl F.T., German anatomist, 1797–1868. See K.'s *glands, muscle.*

Krause, Wilhelm J.F., German anatomist, 1833–1910. See K.'s *bone,* end *bulbs,* respiratory *bundle, valve.*

Krebs, Sir Hans Adolph, German biochemist in England and Nobel laureate, 1900–1981. See K. *cycle;* K.-Henseleit *cycle;* K.-Ringer *solution.*

Kretschmann, Friederich, German otologist, 1858–1934. See K.'s *space.*

Kreysig, Friedrich L., German physician, 1770–1839. See K.'s *sign;* Heim-K. *sign.*

Krogh, August, Danish physiologist and Nobel laureate, 1874–1949. See K. *spirometer.*

Kromayer, Ernst L. F., German dermatologist, 1862–1933. See K.'s *lamp.*

Kronecker, Karl H., Swiss physiologist, 1839–1914. See K.'s *stain.*

Krönig, Georg, Berlin physician, 1856–1911. See K.'s *isthmus, steps.*

Krönlein, Rudolf U., surgeon, 1847–1910. See K. *operation;* K.'s *hernia.*

Krueger instrument stop. See under instrument.

Krukenberg, Adolph, German anatomist, 1816–1877. See K.'s *veins.*

Krukenberg, Friedrich, German pathologist, 1871–1946. See K.'s *amputation, spindle, tumor.*

Kruse, Walther, German bacteriologist, 1864–1943. See K.'s *brush;* Shiga-K. *bacillus.*

krymo-, kryo-. See crymo-, cryo-.

krypton (krip'ton) [G. *kryptos,* concealed]. One of the inert gases, present in small amount in the atmosphere; symbol Kr, atomic no. 36, atomic weight 83.80.

17-KS Abbreviation for 17-ketosteroids.

kubisagari, kubisagaru (kū-bi-sah-gah'rē, kū-bi-sah-gah'rū) [Jap. *kubi,* head, neck, + *sagaru,* to hang down]. Epidemic *vertigo.*

Kufs, H., German psychiatrist, 1871–1955. See K.'s *disease.*

Kugel's artery. See under artery.

Kugelberg, E., Swedish neurologist, *1913. See K.-Welander *disease;* Wohlfart-K.-Welander *disease.*

Kühne, Wilhelm (Willy) F., German physiologist and histologist, 1837–1900. See K.'s *fiber, methylene* blue, *phenomenon, plate, spindle.*

Kuhnt, Hermann, German ophthalmologist, 1850–1925. See K.'s *operation, spaces;* K.-Junius *degeneration, disease.*

Kulchitsky, Nicholas, Russian histologist, 1856–1925. See K. *cells.*

Külz, Rudolph E., German physician, 1845–1895. See K.'s *cylinder.*

Kümmell, Hermann, German surgeon, 1852–1937. See K.'s *spondylitis.*

Küntscher, Gerhard, German surgeon, 1902–1972. See K. *nail.*

Kupffer, Karl W. von, German anatomist, 1829–1902. See K. *cells.*

kurchi bark (ker'chē). Conessi.

Kurloff, Mikhail G., Russian physician, 1859–1932. See K.'s *bodies.*

Kürsteiner (Kuersteiner), W., 19th century German anatomist. See K.'s *canals.*

kuru (kū'rū) [native dialect, to shiver from fear or cold]. A progressive, fatal form of spongiform encephalopathy endemic to certain Melanesian tribes in the highlands of New Guinea, and due to a slow virus.

Kurzrok-Ratner test. See under test.

Kussmaul, Adolph, German physician, 1822–1902. See K. *respiration;* K.'s *aphasia, coma, disease,* paradoxical *pulse, sign, symptom;* K.-Kien *respiration;* K.-Landry *paralysis.*

Küster, Herman, 20th century German gynecologist. See Mayer-Rokitansky-K.-Hauser *syndrome;* Rokitansky-K.-Hauser *syndrome.*

Küstner, Heinz, German gynecologist, *1897. See Prausnitz-K. *antibody, reaction;* reversed Prausnitz-K. *reaction.*

kv Abbreviation for kilovolt.

Kveim, Morton A., Norwegian physician, *1892. See K. *antigen, test;* K.-Stilzbach *antigen, test;* Nickerson-K. *test.*

kwashiorkor (kwah-shē-ōr'kōr) [Native, red boy or displaced child]. Infantile pellagra; malignant malnutrition; a disease seen in African natives, particularly children one to three years old, due to dietary deficiency, particularly of protein; characterized by marked hypoalbuminemia, anemia, edema, pot belly, depigmentation of the skin, loss of hair or change in hair color to red, and bulky stools containing undigested food; fatty changes in the cells of the liver, atrophy of the acinar cells of the pancreas, and hyalinization of the renal glomeruli are found postmortem.

ky-. For words beginning thus and not found below, see cy-.

kyllosis (kil-ō'sis) [G. *kyllōsis,* a crippling]. Obsolete term for talipes.

kymatism (kī'mă-tizm) [G. *kyma,* wave]. Myokymia.

kymogram (kī'mō-gram). The graphic curve made by a kymograph.

kymograph (kī'mō-graf) [G. *kyma,* wave, + *graphō,* to record]. An instrument for recording wavelike motions or modulation, especially for recording variations in blood pressure; it consists of a drum usually revolved by clockwork and covered with smoked paper upon which the curve is inscribed by a stylet or other writing point.

kymography (kī-mog'ră-fē). Use of the kymograph.

kymoscope (kī'mō-skōp) [G. *kyma,* wave, + *skopeō,* to regard]. An apparatus for measuring the pulse waves, or the variation in blood pressure.

kynurenic acid (kin-yū-rē'nik, -ren'ik). 4-Hydroxyquinoline-2-carboxylic acid; a product of the metabolism of tryptophan; appears in human urine probably only in states of marked pyridoxine deficiency.

kynureninase (kī-nū-ren'i-nās) [EC 3.7.1.3]. A liver enzyme catalyzing the hydrolysis of the kynurenine side chain, with the formation of anthranilic acid and alanine, in tryptophan metabolism.

kynurenine (kī-nū'rē-nēn, -nin). 3-Anthraniloylalanine; a product of the metabolism of tryptophan, excreted in the urine in small amounts.

kynurenine formamidase. Formamidase.

kynurenine 3-hydroxylase. Kynurenine 3-monooxygenase.

kynurenine 3-monooxygenase [EC 1.14.13.9]. Kynurenine 3-hydroxylase; an enzyme catalyzing addition of a 3-OH to L-kynurenine, with the aid of NADPH and O_2.

kyphos (kī'fos) [G.]. A hump.

kyphoscoliosis (kī'fō-skō-lē-ō'sis). Kyphosis combined with scoliosis; severe, congestive heart failure is not infrequently a complication.

kyphosis (kī-fō'sis) [G. *kyphōsis,* hump-back, fr. *kyphos,* bent, hump-backed]. Cyphosis; a deformity of the spine characterized by extensive flexion.

juvenile k., Scheuermann's *disease.*

kyphotic (kī-fot'ik). Relating to or suffering from kyphosis.

kyphotone (kī'fō-tōn) [G. *kyphos,* hump, + *tonos,* brace]. A brace for use in tuberculosis of the spine.

Kyrle, J., 19th–20th century German dermatologist. See K.'s *disease.*

kyto-. See cyto-.

L

λ **1.** The 11th letter of the Greek alphabet. **2.** Symbol for wavelength; radioactive *constant;* Ostwald's solubility *coefficient.*

L **1.** Abbreviation for left (*e.g.,* left eye); lumbar vertebra (L1 to L5). **2.** Symbol for inductance; liter. **3.** Abbreviation for *limes;* used with a lower case letter, plus sign, subscript letter, or subscript plus sign as a symbol for various doses of toxin. See entries under dose.

L Prefix indicating a chemical compound to be structurally (sterically) related to L-glyceraldehyde. *Cf.* D-.

l Symbol for liter.

l- Prefix indicating a chemical compound to be levorotatory. *Cf. d-.*

La Symbol for lanthanum.

Laband, Peter F., U.S. dentist, *1900. See L.'s *syndrome.*

Labbé, Ernest M., French physician, 1870–1939. See L.'s neurocirculatory *syndrome.*

Labbé, Leon, French surgeon, 1832–1916. See L.'s *triangle, vein.*

label (lā'bĕl). Tag (1,2).

la belle indifference (lah bel an-dif-er-ahns') [Fr.]. A naive, inappropriate lack of emotion or concern for the implications of one's disability, typically seen in persons with conversion hysteria.

labetalol hydrochloride (la-bet'ă-lol). 5-[1-Hydroxy-2-[(1-methyl-3-phenylpropyl)amino]ethyl]salicyamide monohydrochloride; an α-adrenergic and β-adrenergic blocking agent used in the treatment of hypertension.

labia (lā'bē-ă). Plural of labium.

labial (lā'bē-ăl) [L. *labium,* lip]. **1.** Relating to the lips or any labium. **2.** Toward a lip. **3.** One of the letters formed by means of the lips.

labialism (lā'bē-ăl-izm). A form of stammering in which there is confusion in the use of the labial consonants.

labially (lā'bē-ăl-ē). Toward the lips.

labile (lā'bīl, -bil) [L. *labilis,* liable to slip, fr. *labor,* pp. *lapsus,* to slip]. Unstable; unsteady, not fixed; denoting: **1.** An adaptability to alteration or modification, *i.e.,* relatively easily changed or rearranged. **2.** Certain constituents of serum affected by increases in heat. **3.** An electrode that is kept moving over the surface during the passage of an electric current. **4.** In psychology or psychiatry, denoting free and uncontrolled expression of the emotions.

lability (lă-bil'i-tē). The state of being labile.

labio- [L. *labium,* lip]. Combining form relating to the lips. See also cheilo-.

labiocervical (lā'bē-ō-ser'vi-kăl) [labio- + L. *cervix,* neck]. Relating to a lip and a neck; specifically, to the labial or buccal surface of the neck of a tooth.

labiochorea (lā-bē-ō-kōr-ē'ă) [labio- + G. *choreia,* dance]. A chronic spasm of the lips, interfering with speech.

labioclination (lā'bē-ō-kli-nā'shŭn). Inclination of position more toward the lips than is normal; said of a tooth.

labiodental (lā-bē-ō-den'tăl) [labio- + L. *dens,* tooth]. Relating to the lips and the teeth; denoting certain letters the sound of which is formed by both lips and teeth.

labiogingival (lā'bē-ō-jin'ji-văl). Relating to the point of junction of the labial border and the gingival line on the distal or mesial surface of an incisor tooth.

labioglossolaryngeal (lā'bē-ō-glos'ō-lă-rin'jē-ăl) [labio- + G. *glōssa,* tongue, + larynx]. Relating to the lips, tongue, and larynx; describing bulbar paralysis in which these parts are involved.

labioglossopharyngeal (lā'bē-ō-glos'ō-fă-rin'jē-ăl) [labio- + G. *glōssa,* tongue, + pharynx]. Relating to the lips, tongue, and pharynx; describing bulbar paralysis involving these parts.

labiograph (lā'bē-ō-graf) [labio- + G. *graphō,* to record]. An instrument for recording the movements of the lips in speaking.

labiomental (lā'bē-ō-men'tăl) [labio- + L. *mentum,* chin]. Relating to the lower lip and the chin.

labiomycosis (lā'bē-ō-mī-kō'sis) [labio- + G. *mykēs,* fungus, + *-osis,* condition]. Rarely used term denoting any disease of the lips due to the presence of a fungus.

labionasal (lā'bē-ō-nā'săl). **1.** Relating to the upper lip and the nose, or to both lips and the nose. **2.** Denoting a letter which is both labial and nasal in the production of its sound.

labiopalatine (lā'bē-ō-pal'ă-tīn). Relating to the lips and the palate.

labioplacement (lā'bē-ō-plās'ment). Positioning (*e.g.,* of a tooth) more toward the lips than normal.

labioplasty (lā'bē-ō-plas-tē) [labio- + G. *plastos,* formed]. Plastic surgery of a lip.

labioversion (lā'bē-ō-ver-zhŭn). Malposition of an anterior tooth from the normal line of occlusion toward the lips.

labitome (lab'i-tōm) [G. *labis,* pincers, + *tomē,* an incision]. Cutting forceps; a forceps with sharp blades.

labium, gen. **labii,** pl. **labia** (lā'bē-ŭm, -bē-ē, -bē-ă) [L.] [NA]. **1.** Lip. **2.** Any lip-shaped structure.

l. ante'rius [NA], anterior lip; the portion of the vaginal part of the uterine cervix that bounds the ostium anteriorly. It is slightly shorter than l. posterius.

l. exter'num cris'tae ili'acae [NA], external lip of iliac crest; the roughened outer margin of the crest that gives attachment to the external oblique and latissimus dorsi muscles above and to the fasciae latae and the tensor fasciae latae muscle below.

l. infe'rius o'ris [NA], lower lip; the muscular fold bounding the opening of the mouth inferiorly.

l. inter'num cris'tae ili'acae [NA], internal lip of iliac crest; the roughened inner margin of the crest that gives attachment to parts of the transversus abdominis, quadratus lumborum, and erector spinae muscles.

l. later'le lin'eae as'perae [NA], lateral lip of linea aspera; the lateral margin of the linea aspera of the femur that gives attachment to the lateral intermuscular septum and the short head of the biceps femoris muscles.

l. lim'bi tympan'icum [NA], tympanic lip of limbus; the lower, long periosteal extension of the limbus laminae spiralis osseae that rests on the basilar lamina of the spiral organ (of Corti).

l. lim'bi vestibula're [NA], vestibular lip of limbus; lamina dentata; the upper, short periosteal extension of the limbus laminae spiralis osseae which provides the central attachment for the tectorial membrane.

l. ma'jus puden'di, pl. **la'bia majo'ra** [NA], large pudendal lip; one of two rounded folds of integument forming the lateral boundaries of the rima pudendi.

l. media'le lin'eae as'perae [NA], medial lip of the linea aspera; the medial margin of the linea aspera of the femur that provides attachment for part of the vastus medialis muscle.

l. mi'nus puden'di, pl. **la'bia mino'ra** [NA], small pudendal lip; nympha; one of two narrow longitudinal folds of mucous membrane enclosed in the cleft within the labia majora; posteriorly they gradually merge into the labia majora and join to form the fourchette, or frenulum labiorum pudendi; anteriorly each l. divides into two portions which unite with those of the opposite side in front of the glans clitoridis to form the prepuce.

la'bia o'ris [NA], lips of the mouth. See lip (1).

l. poste'rius [NA], posterior lip; the portion of the uterine cervix that bounds the ostium posteriorly. It is slightly longer than l. anterius.
l. supe'rius o'ris [NA], upper lip of mouth; the muscular fold forming the superior border of the mouth.
l. ure'thrae, one of the two lateral margins of the ostium urethrae externum.
la'bia u'teri, see l. anterius; l. posterius.
l. voca'le, pl. **la'bia voca'lia,** *plica* vocalis.

labor (lā'bŏr) [L. toil, suffering]. The process of expulsion of the fetus and the placenta from the uterus. The **stages of l.** include: **first s.,** beginning with the onset of uterine contractions through the period of dilation of the os uteri; **second s.,** the period of expulsive effort, beginning with complete dilation of the cervix and ending with expulsion of the infant; **third s.** or **placental s.,** the period beginning at the expulsion of the infant and ending with the completed expulsion of the placenta and membranes.
dry l., xerotocia; 1. after spontaneous loss of the amniotic fluid.
missed l., brief uterine contractions which do not lead to labor and expulsion of the infant, but which cease, resulting in the indefinite retension of the fetus (usually lifeless) either *in utero* or extrauterine, *e.g.,* in the abdominal cavity.
precipitate l., l. ending in rapid expulsion of the fetus.
premature l., onset of labor before the 37th completed week of pregnancy dated from the last normal menstrual period.

laboratorian (lab'ŏ-ră-tōr'ē-an). One who works in a laboratory; in the medical and allied health professions, one who examines or performs tests (or supervises such procedures) with various types of chemical and biologic materials, chiefly as an aid in the diagnosis, treatment, and control of disease, or as a basis for health and sanitation practices.

laboratory (lab'ŏ-ră-tō-rē, lab'ră-) [Mediev. L. *laboratorium,* a workplace, fr. L. *laboro,* pp. *-atus,* to labor]. A place equipped for the performance of tests, experiments, and investigative procedures and for the preparation of reagents, therapeutic chemical materials, and so on.
personal growth l., a sensitivity training area in which the primary emphasis is on each participant's potentialities for creativity, empathy, and leadership. See also sensitivity training *group.*

labra (lā'bră) [L.]. Plural of labrum.

labrale inferius (lă-bră'lē in-fē'rē-ŭs). A point where the boundary of the vermilion border of the lower lip and the skin is intersected by the median plane.

labrale superius (lă-bră'lē sū-pē'rē-ŭs). The point on the upper lip lying in the median sagittal plane on a line drawn across the boundary of the vermilion border and skin.

labrocyte (lab'rō-sīt). Mast *cell.*

labrum, pl. **labra** (lā'brŭm, lā'bră) [L.] [NA]. **1.** A lip. **2.** A lip-shaped structure.
l. acetabula're [NA], acetabular lip; circumferential cartilage (1); cotyloid ligament; ligamentum cotyloideum; a fibrocartilaginous rim attached to the margin of the acetabulum of the os coxae.
l. articula're [NA], articular lip; a fibrocartilaginous lip around the margin of the concave portion of some joints. See l. acetabulare; l. glenoidale.
l. glenoida'le [NA], glenoidal lip; glenoid ligament (1); articular margin; circumferential cartilage (2); ligamentum glenoidale; a ring of fibrocartilage attached to the margin of the glenoid cavity of the scapula to increase its depth.

labyrinth (lab'i-rinth). **1.** Labyrinthus. **2.** A group of upright test tubes terminating below in a base of communicating, alternately ∪ -shaped and ∩ -shaped tubes, used for isolating motile from nonmotile organisms in culture, or a motile from a less motile organism (as the typhoid from the colon bacillus), the former traveling faster and farther through the tubes than the latter.
bony l., *labyrinthus* osseus.
cochlear l., labyrinthus cochlearis.
ethmoidal l., *labyrinthus* ethmoidalis.
Ludwig's l., *pars* convoluta lobuli corticalis renis.
membranous l., *labyrinthus* membranaceus.
osseous l., *labyrinthus* osseus.
renal l., *pars* convoluta lobuli corticalis renis.
Santorini's l., *plexus* venosus prostaticus.
vestibular l., *labyrinthus* vestibularis.

labyrinthectomy (lab-ĭ-rin-thek'tō-mē) [labyrinth + G. *ektomē,* excision]. Excision of the labyrinth; a destructive operation to destroy labyrinthine function.

labyrinthine (lab-ĭ-rin'thin). Relating to any labyrinth.

labyrinthitis (lab'ĭ-rin-thī'tis). Otitis interna, intima, or labyrinthica; inflammation of the labyrinth (the internal ear), sometimes accompanied by vertigo.

labyrinthotomy (lab-ĭ-rin-thot'ō-mē) [labyrinth + G. *tomē,* incision]. Incision into the labyrinth.

labyrinthus (lab-i-rin'thŭs) [L. fr. G. *labyrinthos,* labyrinth] [NA]. Labyrinth (1); any of several anatomical structures with numerous intercommunicating cells or canals. **1.** The internal or inner ear, composed of the semicircular ducts, vestibule, and cochlea. **2.** Any group of communicating cavities, as in each lateral mass of the ethmoid bone, l. ethmoidalis. **3.** *Pars* convoluta lobuli corticalis renis.
l. cochlea'ris [NA], cochlear labyrinth; organ of hearing; the portion of the membranous labyrinth containing the spiral organ (of Corti). It is located in the cochlea surrounded by perilymph.
l. ethmoida'lis [NA], ethmoidal labyrinth; lateral mass of the ethmoid bone; a mass of air cells with thin bony walls forming part of the lateral wall of the nasal cavity; the cells are arranged in three groups, anterior, middle, and posterior, and are closed laterally by the orbital plate which forms part of the wall of the orbit.
l. membrana'ceus [NA], membranous labyrinth; an arrangement of communicating membranous sacs, filled with endolymph and surrounded by perilymph, lying within the cavity of the osseous labyrinth; its chief divisions are the cochlear labyrinth and the vestibular labyrinth.

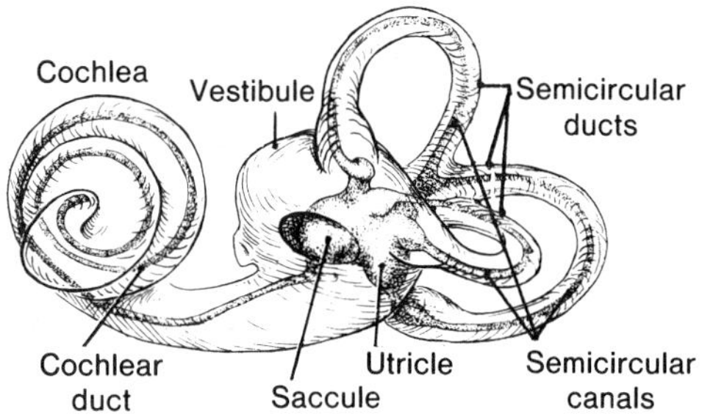

Labyrinthus Membranaceus (Membranous Labyrinth)
Left membranous labyrinth shown lying within the osseous labyrinth (labyrinthus osseus) of the otic capsule (lateral view).

l. os'seus [NA], osseous labyrinth; bony labyrinth; a series of cavities (cochlea, vestibule, and semicircular canals) in the petrous portion of the temporal bone which lodge the membranous labyrinth.
l. vestibula'ris [NA], vestibular labyrinth; the portion of the membranous labyrinth located within the semicircular canals and the vestibule of the osseous labyrinth. It is surrounded with perilymph and involved with vestibular functions.

lac, gen. **lactis** (lak, lak'tis) [L. milk] [NA]. **1.** Milk (1). **2.** Any whitish, milklike liquid.
l. sul'furis, precipitated sulfur.

l. vacci'num, cow's milk.

lacca (lak'ă). Shellac.

laccase (lak'ās) [EC 1.10.3.2]. Phenolase; polyphenol or urushiol oxidase; an enzyme oxidizing benzenediols to semiquinones with O_2.

lacerable (las'er-ă-bl) [L. *lacero*, to tear to pieces, fr. *lacer*, mangled]. Capable of being, or liable to be, torn.

lacerated (las'er-āted) [L. *lacero*, pp. *-atus*, to tear to pieces]. Torn; rent; having a ragged edge.

laceration (las-er-ā'shŭn) [L. *lacero*, pp. *-atus*, to tear to pieces]. **1.** A torn or jagged wound, or an accidental cut wound. **2.** The process or act of tearing the tissues.
brain l., gross tearing of neural tissue.
scalp l., a tear of the dermis or underlying tissues and galea aponeurotica of the scalp.
vaginal l., colporrhexis.

lacertus (lă-ser'tŭs) [L.]. **1.** Originally the muscular part of the upper limb from shoulder to elbow. **2** [NA]. A fibrous band or arm related to a muscle.
l. cor'dis, one of the trabeculae carneae.
l. fibro'sus, *aponeurosis* musculi bicipitis brachii.
l. of lateral rectus muscle, l. musculi recti lateralis.
l. me'dius, *ligamentum* longitudinale anterius.
l. mus'culi rec'ti latera'lis [NA], l. of lateral rectus muscle; the part of the tendon of origin of the lateral rectus muscle attaching to the greater wing of the sphenoid bone, lateral to the common tendinous ring; often incorrectly equated to the lateral check ligament of the eyeball.

lachrymal (lak'ri-măl). Lacrimal.

laciniae tubae (la-sin'ē-ē tū'bē) [L. *lacinia*, fringe]. *Fimbriae* tubae uterinae.

lacrimal (lak'ri-măl) [L. *lacrima*, a tear]. Lachrymal; relating to the tears, their secretion, the secretory glands, and the drainage apparatus.

lacrimation (lak'ri-mā'shŭn) [L. *lacrimatio*]. The secretion of tears, especially in excess.

lacrimator (lak'ri-mā-ter) [L. *lacrima*, tear]. An agent (such as tear gas) that irritates the eyes and produces tears.

lacrimatory (lak'ri-mă-tō-rē). Causing lacrimation.

lacrimotome (lak'ri-mō-tōm). A fine-bladed knife for use in lacrimotomy.

lacrimotomy (lak-ri-mot'ō-mē) [L. *lacrima*, tear, + G. *tomē*, incision]. The operation of incising the lacrimal duct or sac.

lact-, lacti-, lacto- [L. *lac, lactis*, milk]. Combining forms denoting milk.

lactacidemia (lak-tas-i-dē'mē-ă). Lacticacidemia.

lactacidosis (lak-tas-i-dō'sis). Acidosis due to increased lactic acid.

lactalbumin (lak-tal-byū'min). The albumin fraction of milk. It contains two proteins: α- and β-l.; the former, minor l., interacts with galactosyl transferase to form lactose synthase which synthesizes lactose from glucose and UDP-galactose in milk production.

lactam, lactim (lak'tam, -tim). Contractions of "lactoneamine" and "lactoneimine," and applied to the tautomeric forms –NH–CO– and –N=C(OH)–, respectively, observed in many purines, pyrimidines, and other substances; the latter form accounts for the acidic properties of uric acid.

β-lactam. A class of broad spectrum antibiotics that are structurally and pharmacologically related to the penicillins and cephalosporins.

β-lactamase (lak'tă-mās) [EC 3.5.2.6]. Penicillinase (1); cephalosporinase; an enzyme that brings about the hydrolysis of a β-lactam (as penicillin to penicilloic acid); found in most staphylococcus strains that are naturally resistant to penicillin.

lactase (lak'tās). β-D-Galactosidase.

lactate (lak'tāt). **1.** A salt or ester of lactic acid. **2.** To produce milk in the mammary glands.
l. dehydrogenase (LDH), lactic acid dehydrogenase; name for four enzymes: L-lactate (cytochrome, EC 1.1.2.3), D-lactate (cytochrome, EC 1.1.2.4), L-lactate (EC 1.1.1.27), and D-lactate (EC 1.1.1.2.8). The first of each pair transfers H to ferricytochrome *c* (EC 1.1.2.3 is cytochrome b_2), the second to NAD^+, in catalyzing the oxidation of lactate to pyruvate.
excess l., the increase in l. concentration beyond what would be expected from the increase in pyruvate concentration resulting from a change in redox potential; used as an index of anaerobic carbohydrate metabolism.

lactate 2-mono-oxygenase [EC 1.13.12.4]. Lactic acid oxidative decarboxylase; a flavoprotein oxidoreductase catalyzing oxidation (with O_2) of L-lactate to acetate plus CO_2.

lactation (lak-tā'shŭn) [L. *lactatio*, suckle]. **1.** Production of milk. **2.** Period following birth during which milk is secreted in the breasts.

lactational (lak-tā'shŭn-ăl). Relating to lactation.

lacteal (lak'tē-ăl). **1.** Relating to or resembling milk; milky. **2.** Chyle or lacteal vessel; a lymphatic vessel that conveys chyle from the intestine.
central l., the blindly ending lymphatic capillary in the center of an intestinal villus.

lactenin (lak'tĕ-nin). An antibacterial agent active against streptococci isolated from cow's milk.

lactescent (lak-tes'ent). Resembling milk; milky.

lacti-. See lact-.

lactic (lak'tik) [L. *lac* (*lact-*), milk]. Relating to milk.

lactic acid. 2-Hydroxypropionic acid; CH_3–CHOH–COOH; a normal intermediate in the fermentation (oxidation, metabolism) of sugar. In pure form, a syrupy, odorless, and colorless liquid obtained by the action of the l. a. bacillus on milk or milk sugar; in concentrated form, a caustic used internally to prevent gastrointestinal fermentation. A culture of the bacillus, or milk containing it, is usually given in place of the acid.

lactic acid dehydrogenase. *Lactate* dehydrogenase.

lacticacidemia (lak'tik-as-i-dē'mē-ă) [lactic acid + G. *haima*, blood]. Lactacidemia; the presence of dextrorotatory lactic acid in the circulating blood.

lactic acid oxidative decarboxylase. Lactate 2-mono-oxygenase.

lactiferous (lak-tif'er-ŭs) [lacti- + L. *fero*, to bear]. Lactigerous; yielding milk.

lactifugal (lak-tif'yū-găl). Lactifuge (1).

lactifuge (lak'ti-fyūj) [lacti- + L. *fugo*, to drive away]. Phygogalactic. **1.** Lactifugal; causing arrest of the secretion of milk. **2.** An agent having such an effect.

lactigenous (lak-tij'ĕ-nŭs) [lacti- + *-gen*, producing]. Producing milk.

lactigerous (lak-tij'er-ŭs) [lacti- + L. *gero*, to carry]. Lactiferous.

lactim (lak'tim). See lactam.

lactimorbus (lak-ti-mōr'bŭs) [lacti- + L. *morbus*, disease]. Milk *sickness*.

lactinated (lak'ti-nā-ted). Prepared with or containing milk sugar.

lacto-. See lact-.

Lactobacillaceae (lak'tō-bas'i-lā'sē-ē). A family of anaerobic to facultatively anaerobic, ordinarily nonmotile bacteria (order Eubacteriales) containing straight or curved, Gram-positive rods which usually occur singly or in chains; motile cells are peritrichous. These organisms have complex organic nutritional requirements; they produce lactic acid from carbohydrates. They are found in fermenting animal and plant products where carbohydrates are available; they are also found in the mouth, vagina, and intestinal tract of various warm-blooded animals including man. Only a few species are pathogenic. The type genus is *Lactobacillus.*

lactobacilli (lak-tō-bă-sil'ī). Plural of lactobacillus.

lactobacillic acid (lak'tō-bă-sil'ik). (1*R-cis*)- 2-Hexycyclopropanedecanoic acid;

$$CH_3(CH_2)_4CH_2—\overset{\overset{CH_2}{/\quad\backslash}}{CH — CH}—CH_2)_9COOH;$$

a major constituent of the lipids of lactobacilli; notable for the presence of a cyclopropane ring in the molecule.

Lactobacillus (lak-tō-bă-sil'ŭs) [lacto- + bacillus]. A genus of microaerophilic or anaerobic, nonsporeforming, ordinarily nonmotile bacteria (family Lactobacillaceae) containing Gram-positive rods which vary from long and slender cells to short coccobacilli; chains are commonly produced, especially in the later part of the logarithmic phase of growth. These organisms possess complex nutritional requirements, generally characteristic for each species; metabolism is fermentative and at least half of the end product is lactic acid. They are found in dairy products and effluents to grain and meat products, water, sewage, beer, wine, fruits and fruit juices, pickled vegetables, and in sour dough and mash, and are part of the normal flora of the mouth, intestinal tract, and vagina of many warm-blooded animals, including man; rarely are they pathogenic. The type species is *L. delbrueckii.*

L. acidoph'ilus, a species found in the feces of milk-fed infants and also in the feces of older persons on a high milk-, lactose-, or dextrin-containing diet.

L. bi'fidus, *Bifidobacterium bifidum.*

L. bi'fidus subsp. **pennsylva'nicus,** a bacterium present in human colostrum and milk, in the milk of other mammals, and in the feces of breast-fed infants; associated with a growth factor belonging to a group of N-containing polysaccharides with a high hexosamine content and known as bifidus factor.

L. bre'vis, a species widely distributed in nature, especially in plant and animal products; it is also found in the mouth and intestinal tract of humans and rats.

L. buch'neri, a species widely distributed in fermenting substances.

L. bulgar'icus, a species used in the production of yogurt.

L. ca'sei, a species found in milk and cheese.

L. catenafor'me, *Catenabacterium catenaforme;* an anaerobic species found in the intestines and pulmonary cavities of humans.

L. cellobio'sus, a species found in the mouth of man.

L. coproph'ilus, a species found in cow dung.

L. corynifor'mis, a species found primarily in silage but also in cow dung and dairybarn air.

L. curva'tus, a species found in cow dung, dairybarn air, silage, milk, and in a case of endocarditis.

L. delbrueck'ii, a species found in fermenting vegetables and grain mashes; it is the type species of the genus *L.*

L. desidio'sus, a species found in kefir grains.

L. fermen'ti, *L. fermentum.*

L. fermen'tum, *L. fermenti;* a species found widely distributed in nature, especially in fermenting plant and animal products.

L. fructiv'orans, a species isolated from spoiled mayonnaise and salad dressings.

L. helvet'icus, a species found in sour milk and Swiss cheese.

L. heterohio'chi, a species found in spoiled sake.

L. hilgar'dii, a species isolated from California table wines.

L. homohio'chi, a species found in spoiled sake.

L. jensen'ii, a species isolated from human sources such as vaginal discharge and blood clot.

L. lac'tis, a species found in milk and cheese; not pathogenic.

L. leichman'nii, a species found in dairy and plant products.

L. pastoria'nus, a species found in sour beer and distillery yeast.

L. planta'rum, a species found in dairy products and environments, fermenting plants, silage, sauerkraut, pickled vegetables, spoiled tomato products, sour dough, cow dung, and the human mouth, intestinal tract, and stools.

L. saliva'rius, a species found in the mouth and intestinal tract of the hamster, the mouth of man, and the intestinal tract of the hen.

L. thermoph'ilus, a thermophilic species so far found only in pasteurized milk.

L. tricho'des, a species found in wines containing 20% ethanol and in lees in California, Australia, France, and Spain; in California this organism is commonly referred to as the hair bacillus, cottony bacillus, cottony mold, or Fresno mold.

L. virides'cens, a species found in discolored cured meat products such as sausage and bologna.

lactobacillus (lak-tō-bă-sil'ŭs). A vernacular term used to refer to any member of the genus *Lactobacillus.*

lactobutyrometer (lak'tō-byū-ti-rom'ĕ-ter) [lacto- + G. *boutyron,* butter, + *metron,* measure]. A type of lactocrit.

lactocele (lak'tō-sēl) [lacto- + G. *kēlē,* tumor]. Galactocele.

lactochrome (lak'tō-krōm). Lactoflavin (1).

lactocrit (lak'tō-krit) [lacto- + G. *krinō,* to separate]. An instrument used to estimate the amount of butterfat in milk.

lactodensimeter (lak'tō-den-sim'ĕ-ter) [lacto- + L. *densus,* thick, + G. *metron,* measure]. A type of galactometer.

lactoferrin (lak'tō-făr-in). A transferrin found in the milk of several mammalian species and thought to be involved in the transport of iron to erythrocytes.

lactoflavin (lak'tō-flā-vin). **1.** Lactochrome; the flavin in milk. **2.** Riboflavin.

lactogen (lak'tō-jen) [lacto- + G. *-gen,* producing]. An agent that stimulates milk production or secretion.

human placental l. (HPL), l. isolated from human placentas and structurally similar to somatotropin; its biological activity weakly mimics that of somatotropin and prolactin. Also called chorionic "growth hormone-prolactin"; human chorionic somatomammotropic hormone; human chorionic somatomammotropin; purified placental protein; placenta protein, placental growth hormone.

lactogenesis (lak-tō-jen'ĕ-sis) [lacto- + G. *genesis,* production]. Milk production.

lactogenic (lak-tō-jen'ik). Pertaining to lactogenesis.

lactoglobulin (lak-tō-glob'yū-lin). The globulin present in milk, comprising 50 to 60% of bovine whey protein.

lactometer (lak-tom'ĕ-ter) [lacto- + G. *metron,* measure]. Galactometer.

lactonase (lak'tō-nās). Gluconolactonase.

lactone (lak'tōn). An organic anhydride formed from a hydroxyacid by the loss of water between an –OH and a –COOH group.

lactoperoxidase (lak'tō-per-oks'i-dās). A peroxidase obtained from milk.

lactoprotein (lak-tō-prō'tēn). Any protein normally present in milk.

lactorrhea (lak-tō-rē'ă) [lacto- + G. *rhoia,* a flow]. Galactorrhea.

lactoscope (lak'tō-skōp) [lacto- + G. *skopeō,* to view]. Galactoscope.

lactose (lak'tōs). Milk sugar; saccharum lactis; 4-(β-D-galactosido)-D-glucose; a disaccharide present in mammalian milk, occurring naturally as α- and β-lactose; obtained from cow's milk and used in modified milk preparations, in food for infants and convalescents, and in pharmaceutical preparations; large doses act as an osmotic diuretic and as a laxative.

lactosuria (lak'tō-sū'rē-ă) [lacto- + G. *ouron,* urine]. Excretion of lactose (milk sugar) in the urine; a common finding during pregnancy and lactation, and in the newborn, especially premature babies.

lactotherapy (lak-tō-thăr'ă-pē). Galactotherapy.

lactotropin (lak-tō-trō'pin). Prolactin.

lactovegetarian (lak'tō-vej-ĕ-tā'rē-ăn). One who lives on a mixed diet of milk and milk products, eggs, and vegetables, but eschews meat.

lactoylglutathione lyase (lak'tō-il-glū-tă-thī'ōn) [EC 4.4.1.5]. Glyoxalase I; aldoketomutase; ketone-aldehyde mutase; methylglyoxalase; a lyase cleaving lactoylglutathione to glutathione and methylglyoxal.

lactulose (lak'tū-lōs). 4-O-β-D-Galactopyranosyl-D-fructose; a synthetic disaccharide used to treat hepatic encephalopathy and chronic constipation.

lacuna, pl. lacunae (lă-kū'nă, -kū'nē) [L. a pit, dim. of *lacus,* a hollow, a lake]. **1** [NA]. A small space, cavity, or depression. **2.** A gap or defect. **3.** An abnormal space between strata or between the cellular elements of the epidermis. **4.** Corneal *space.*

cartilage l., cartilage space; a cavity within the matrix of cartilage, occupied by a chondrocyte.

l. cer'ebri, a small circumscribed loss of brain tissue surrounding one of the small arteries; rupture of the vessel is apt to occur into the cavity so produced.

Howship's lacunae, resorption lacunae; tiny depressions, pits, or irregular grooves in bone that is being resorbed by osteoclasts.

intervillous l., one of the blood spaces in the placenta into which the chorionic villi project.

lacunae latera'les [NA], parasinoidal sinuses; lateral lakes; lateral expansions of the sinus sagittalis superior of the dura mater, often increasing in width with advancing age until, in the very old, they may extend two centimeters lateral to the midline; the endothelium-lined lumen of the lacunae are usually reduced to a spongelike labyrinth by numerous arachnoid granulations and dural trabeculae.

l. mag'na, a recess on the roof of the fossa navicularis of the penis, formed by a fold of mucous membrane, the valve of the navicular fossa.

Morgagni's l., l. urethralis.

muscular l., l. musculorum.

l. musculo'rum [NA], muscular l.; the lateral compartment beneath the inguinal (Poupart's) ligament, for the passage of the iliopsoas muscle and femoral nerve; it is separated by the iliopectineal arch from the l. vasorum.

osseous l., a cavity in bony tissue occupied by an osteocyte.

l. pharyn'gis, a depression near the pharyngeal opening of the auditory (eustachian) tube.

resorption lacunae, Howship's lacunae.

trophoblastic l., one of the spaces in the early syncytiotrophoblastic layer of the chorion before the formation of villi; in human embryos maternal blood enters these spaces by the 10th day; with the differentiation of the chorionic villi they become intervillous spaces, sometimes called intervillous lacunae.

urethral l., l. urethralis.

l. urethra'lis, pl. lacu'nae urethra'les [NA], urethral l.; Morgagni's l.; one of a number of little recesses in the mucous membrane of the pars spongiosa urethrae into which empty the ducts of the urethral glands.

vascular l., l. vasorum.

l. vaso'rum [NA], vascular l.; the medial compartment beneath the inguinal ligament, for the passage to the femoral vessels; it is separated from the l. musculorum by the iliopectineal arch.

lacunar (lă-kū'năr). Relating to a lacuna.

lacunule (lă-kū'nūl) [Mod. L. *lacunula,* dim. of L. *lacuna*]. A very small lacuna.

lacus, pl. lacus (lā'kŭs) [L. lake]. Lake (1); a small collection of fluid.

l. lacrima'lis [NA], lacrimal lake or bay; the small cistern-like area of the conjunctiva at the medial angle of the eye, in which the tears collect after bathing the anterior surface of the eyeball and the conjunctival sac.

l. semina'lis, seminal lake; the vault of the vagina after insemination.

Ladd, William E., U.S. pediatric surgeon, 1880–1967. See L.'s *band, operation.*

Ladd-Franklin, Christine, U.S. psychologist, 1847–1930. See L.-F. *theory.*

Laelaps echidninus (lē'laps ē-kid-nī'nŭs). The spiny rat mite, a common worldwide ectoparasite of the wild Norway rat and occasionally found on the house mouse, cotton rat, and other rodents; it is the natural vector of *Hepatozoon muris* and can transmit the agent of tularemia experimentally. Junin virus has been isolated from this species in South America.

Laënnec, René T.H., French physician, 1781–1826. See L.'s *cirrhosis, pearls, thrombus.*

laetrile (lā'ĕ-tril). An allegedly antineoplastic drug consisting chiefly of amygdalin derived from apricot pits; its antitumor effect is unproven.

laev-. For words so beginning see levo-.

Lafora, Gonzalo Rodriguez, Spanish neurologist, 1887–1971. See L. *body;* L.'s *disease.*

lag. 1. To move or progress more slowly than normal; to fall behind. **2.** The act or condition of falling behind. **3.** The time interval between a change in one variable and a consequent change in another variable.

anaphase l., slow movement or no movement of one or more chromosomes during anaphase, resulting in such chromosomes being excluded from one of the daughter cells.

lagena, pl. lagenae (lă-jē'nă, -jē-nē) [L. flask]. One of the three parts of the membranous labyrinth of the inner ear of lower vertebrates; in mammals, l. becomes the cochlea.

lag'ging. Retarded or diminished ventilatory movement of the affected side of the chest due to pleural disease with muscle splinting or collapse of a lung.

lagomorph (lā'gō-mōrf). A member of the order Lagomorpha.

Lagomorpha (lā-gō-mōr'fă) [G. *lagōs,* hare, + *morphē,* form]. An order of herbivorous mammals (class Eutheria) resembling rodents (order Rodentia) but having two pairs of upper incisors one behind the other; it includes the rabbits, hares, and pikas.

lagophthalmia, lagophthalmos (lag-of-thal'mē-ă, -of-thal'mōs) [G. *lagōs,* hare, + *ophthalmos,* eye]. Hare's eye; a condition in which complete closure of the eyelids over the eyeball is difficult or impossible.

Lagrange, Pierre F., French ophthalmologist, 1857–1928. See L.'s *operation.*

Lahey, Frank H., U.S. surgeon, 1880–1935. See L. *forceps.*

lake (lāk) [A.S. *lacu,* fr. L. *lacus,* lake]. **1.** Lacus. **2.** To cause blood plasma to become red as a result of the release of hemoglobin from the erythrocytes, as when the latter are suspended in water.

capillary l., the total mass of blood contained in capillary vessels.

lacrimal l., *lacus* lacrimalis.

lateral l.'s, *lacunae* laterales.

seminal l., *lacus* seminalis.

subchorial l., subchorial *space.*

venous l.'s, (1) thin-walled collections of blood, resembling blood blisters, found commonly in the ears and less often on the lips and on the face and neck of elderly persons; **(2)** discontinuous venous cavities or channels. *Cf.* marginal *sinus* of placenta.

Laki-Lorand factor. See under factor.

laky (lā′kē). Pertaining to the transparent bright red appearance of blood serum or plasma, developing as a result of hemoglobin being released from destroyed red blood cells.

laliatry (lă-lī′ă-trē) [G. *lalia,* speech, chatter, + *iatria,* cure]. The study and treatment of speech disorders.

laliophobia (lal′ē-ō-fō′bē-ă) [G. *lalia,* speech, + *phobos,* fear]. Morbid fear of speaking or stuttering.

Lallemand, Claude F., French surgeon, 1790–1853. See L.'s *bodies;* Trousseau-L. *bodies.*

lalling (lal′ing) [G. *laleō,* to chatter]. A form of stammering in which the speech is almost unintelligible.

Lallouette, Pierre, French physician, 1711–1792. See L.'s *pyramid.*

lalochezia (lal-ō-kē′zē-ă) [G. *lalia,* speech, + *chezo,* to relieve oneself]. Emotional discharge gained by uttering indecent or filthy words.

lalognosis (lal′og-nō′sis) [G. *lalia,* speech, + *gnosis,* knowledge]. Understanding and knowledge of speech.

laloplegia (la-lō-plē′jē-ă) [G. *lalia,* speech, + *plēgē,* a stroke]. Paralysis of the muscles concerned in the mechanism of speech.

Lamarck, Jean-Baptiste P.A., French botanist, zoologist, and biological philosopher, 1744–1829. See lamarckian *theory.*

Lamaze, Fernand, French obstetrician, 1890–1957. See L. *method.*

LAMB Acronym for *l*entigines, *a*trial myxoma, *m*ucocutaneous myxomas, and *b*lue nevi. See LAMB *syndrome.*

lambda (lam′dă). **1.** The 11th letter of the Greek alphabet, λ. **2.** The craniometric point at the junction of the sagittal and lambdoid sutures.

lambdacism (lam′dă-sizm) [G. *lambda,* the letter L]. **1.** Mispronunciation or disarticulation of the letter *l.* **2.** Substitution of the letter *l* for the letter *r.*

lambdoid (lam′doyd) [lambda + G. *eidos,* resemblance]. Resembling the Greek letter lambda.

Lambert, Edward H., U.S. physician, *1915. See L.-Eaton, Eaton-L. *syndrome.*

lam′bert [J.H. *Lambert,* German physicist and mathematician, 1728–1777]. A unit of brightness; the brightness of a perfectly diffusing surface emitting or reflecting a total luminous flux of 1 lumen per sq cm of surface.

Lamblia intestinalis (lam′blē-ă in-tes-ti-nā′lis). Old term for *Giardia lamblia,* though still frequently used, especially by Soviet protozoologists.

lambliasis (lam-blī′ă-sis). Giardiasis.

lambo lambo (lam′bō-lam′bō). *Myositis* purulenta tropica.

lamella, pl. lamellae (lă-mel′ă, -mel′ē) [L. dim. of *lamina,* plate, leaf]. **1.** A thin sheet or layer, such as occurs in compact bone. **2.** Disk (3); a preparation in the form of a medicated gelatin disk, used as a means of making local applications to the conjunctiva in place of solutions.

annulate lamellae, several pairs of parallel, smooth membranes, each pair containing regularly spaced pores resembling those of the nuclear envelope; they occur in germ cells, embryonic cells, and neoplastic cells.

articular l., the compact layer of bone on its articular surface that is firmly attached to the overlying articular cartilage.

l. of bone, a concentric, circumferential, or interstitial l.

circumferential l., a bony l. that encircles the outer or inner surface of a bone.

concentric l., haversian l.; one of the tubular layers of bone surrounding the central canal in an osteon.

cornoid l., a narrow vertical column of parakeratosis in the epidermal stratum corneum; characteristic of porokeratosis.

elastic l., a thin sheet or membrane composed of elastic fibers; distinguished from elastic membrane, which usually refers to a condensed mass of fibers, as in an artery, whereas an elastic l. may be a looser elastic layer such as found in a vein or the respiratory tract.

enamel l., an organic defect in enamel; a thin, leaflike structure that extends from the enamel surface toward the dentinoenamel junction.

glandulopreputial l., a layer of embryonic epithelial tissue that gives rise to the prepuce.

ground l., interstitial l.

haversian l., concentric l.

intermediate l., interstitial l.

interstitial l., intermediate or ground l.; intermediary system; one of the lamellae of partially resorbed osteons occurring between newer, complete osteons.

triangular l., *tela* choroidea ventriculi tertii.

vitreous l., *lamina* basalis choroideae.

lamellar (lam′ĕ-lăr, lă-mel′ăr) **1.** Lamellate; lamellated; arranged in thin plates or scales. **2.** Relating to lamellae.

lamellate, lamellated (lam′ĕ-lāt, -ed). Lamellar (1).

lamellipodium, pl. **lamellipodia** (lă-mel-i-pō′dē-ŭm, -ă). A cytoplasmic veil produced on all sides of migrating polymorphonuclear leukocytes.

La Mer, Victor K. See L. *generator.*

LAMINA

lamina, pl. **laminae** (lam′i-nă, lam′i-nē) [L] [NA]. layer; thin plate or flat layer. See also layer; stratum.

l. affix′a [NA], that part of the medial ependymal wall of the lateral ventricle of the embryonic brain that in later development becomes adherent to the superior surface of the thalamus and thus comes to form the floor of the pars centralis of the lateral ventricle; it covers the thalamostriate and choroidal veins.

alar l. of neural tube, l. alaris.

l. ala′ris [NA], alar l. of the neural tube; alar or dorsal plate of the neural tube; l. dorsalis; wing plate; the dorsal division of the lateral walls of the neural tube in the embryo; it gives rise to neurons relaying afferent impulses to higher centers; in the adult such neurons compose the sensory nuclei of the spinal cord and brainstem.

lam′inae al′bae cerebel′li [NA], laminae medullares cerebelli; layers of white substance seen on section of the cerebellum.

l. ante′rior vagi′na mus′culi rec′ti abdo′minis [NA], anterior layer of the rectus abdominis sheath; the portion of the sheath of the rectus abdominis muscle that lies anterior to the muscle.

l. ar′cus ver′tebrae [NA], l. of vertebral arch; neurapophysis; the flattened posterior portion of the vertebral arch from which the spinous process extends.

basal l., **(1)** basement *membrane;* **(2)** *lamina* densa.

basal l. of choroid, l. basalis choroideae.

basal l. of neural tube, l. basalis.

l. basa′lis [NA], basal l. of the neural tube; basal or ventral plate of the neural tube; l. ventralis; the ventral division of the lateral walls of the neural tube in the embryo; it contains neuroblasts giving rise to somatic and visceral motor neurons.

l. basa′lis choroi′deae [NA], basal l. or layer of the choroid; l. vitrea; vitreous lamella; vitreous membrane (3); Bruch's or Henle's membrane; the transparent, nearly structureless inner layer of the choroid in contact with the pigmented layer of the retina.

l. basa′lis cor′poris cilia′ris [NA], basal layer of the ciliary body; the inner layer of the ciliary body, continuous with the basal layer of the choroid.

basement l., basement *membrane.*
basilar l., l. basilaris cochleae.

l. basila'ris coch'leae [NA], basilar l.; basilar membrane; membrana basilaris; the membrane extending from the osseous spiral l. to the basilar crest of the cochlea; it forms the greater part of the floor of the cochlear duct and supports the organ of Corti.
l. cartilag'inis cricoi'deae [NA], l. of cricoid cartilage; a quadrate plate forming the posterior part of the cricoid cartilage. It resembles the shield of a signet ring, the arch of the cricoid representing the remainder of the ring.

l. cartilag'inis latera'lis [NA], official alternative term for l. lateralis.
l. cartilag'inis media'lis [NA], official alternative term for l. medialis.
l. cartilag'inis thyroi'deae [NA], l. of thyroid cartilage; one of the paired (dextra et sinistra) quadrilateral plates of the thyroid cartilage that are joined anteriorly and form an open angle posteriorly.
l. choriocapilla'ris, l. choroidocapillaris.
l. choroi'dea, l. epithelialis.
l. choroi'dea epithelia'lis, l. epithelialis.

l. choroidocapilla'ris [NA], choriocapillary layer; l. choriocapillaris; membrana choriocapillaris; Ruysch's membrane; entochoroidea; the internal layer of the choroidea of the eye, composed of a very close capillary network.

l. cine'rea, l. terminalis cerebri.
l. cribro'sa os'sis ethmoida'lis [NA], cribriform plate of ethmoid bone; cribrum; sieve bone or plate; a horizontal l. from which are suspended the labyrinth, on either side, and the l. perpendicularis in the center; it fits into the ethmoidal notch of the frontal bone and supports the olfactory lobes of the cerebrum, being pierced with numerous openings for the passage of the olfactory nerves.
l. cribro'sa scle'rae, perforated layer of sclera; the portion of the sclera through which pass the fibers of the optic nerve.
l. of cricoid cartilage, l. cartilaginis cricoideae.
l. den'sa, basal lamina (2); the electron-dense central layer of the renal glomerulus, as seen in the electron microscope; on either side of this layer is a relatively electron-lucent layer, the l. rara.
dental l., dental *ledge.*
l. denta'ta, *labium* limbi vestibulare.
dentogingival l., dental *ledge.*
l. dex'tra cartilag'inis thyroi'dea [NA], right plate of thyroid cartilage; the thin quadrilateral plate of cartilage forming the right half of the thyroid cartilage.
l. dorsa'lis, l. alaris.
l. du'ra, the hard layer lining the dental alveoli.
l. elas'tica ante'rior, l. limitans anterior corneae.
l. elas'tica poste'rior, l. limitans posterior corneae.
elastic laminae of arteries, elastic layers of arteries; Henle's fenestrated elastic membrane; 1) external: the layer of elastic connective tissue lying immediately outside the smooth muscle of the tunica media; 2) internal: a fenestrated layer of elastic tissue of the tunica intima.
episcleral l., l. episcleralis.
l. episclera'lis [NA], episcleral l.; the layer of loose connective tissue on the external surface of the sclera.
epithelial l., l. epithelialis.
l. epithelia'lis [NA], epithelial l.; epithelial choroid layer; l. choroidea; l. choroidea epithelialis; the layer of modified ependymal cells that forms the inner layer of the tela choroidea, facing the ventricle.
l. exter'na cra'nii [NA], outer table of the skull; the outer compact layer of the cranial bones.
l. fibrocartilagin'ea interpu'bica, *discus* interpubicus.
l. fibroreticula'ris, a layer of the basement membrane in continuity with associated connective tissue; it is often discontinuous and may be lacking entirely in some cases.

l. fus'ca scle'rae [NA], brown layer; membrana fusca; a thin layer of loose, pigmented connective tissue on the inner surface of the sclera, connecting it with the choroid.
hepatic laminae, the plates of liver cells that radiate from the center of the liver lobule.
l. horizonta'lis os'sis palati'ni [NA], horizontal plate of palatine bone; the part of the palatine bone that forms the posterior part of the bony palate.
l. inter'na cra'nii [NA], inner table of skull; the inner compact layer of the cranial bones.
labiogingival l., a band of ectodermal epithelial cells growing into the mesenchyme of the embryonic jaws between the developing lip and the growing gingival elevation; it later opens to form the labiogingival groove.
l. latera'lis [NA], lateral layer; l. cartilaginis lateralis; lateral cartilaginous layer; the narrow lateral portion of the cartilaginous part of the auditory tube.
l. latera'lis proces'sus pterygoid'ei [NA], lateral plate of pterygoid process; the larger and more lateral of the two bony plates extending downward from the point of union of the body and greater wing of the sphenoid bone on either side.
lateral medullary l. of corpus striatum, l. medullaris lateralis corporis striati.
l. of lens, one of a series of concentric layers composed of the lens fibers that make up the substance of the lens.
l. lim'itans ante'rior cor'neae [NA], anterior limiting layer of cornea; l. elastica anterior; anterior elastic layer; Bowman's membrane; a transparent homogeneous acellular layer, 6 to 9 μm thick, lying between the basal l. of the outer layer of stratified epithelium and the substantia propria of the cornea; considered to be a basement membrane.
l. lim'itans poste'rior cor'neae [NA], posterior limiting layer of the cornea; l. elastica posterior; posterior elastic layer; entocornea; Duddell's or Descemet's membrane; vitreous membrane (1); a transparent homogeneous acellular layer between the substantia propria and the endothelial layer of the cornea; considered to be a highly developed basement membrane.
l. lu'cida, the lightly-staining layer of the basement membrane in contact with the plasmalemma of epithelial cells or other cells having an investment of basement membrane.
l. media'lis [NA], medial layer; l. cartilaginis medialis; medial cartilaginous layer; the broad medial portion of the cartilaginous part of the auditory tube.
l. media'lis proces'sus pterygoi'dei [NA], medial plate of pterygoid process; the smaller and more medial of the two bony plates extending downward from the point of union of the body and greater wing of the sphenoid bone on either side.
medial medullary l. of corpus striatum, l. medullaris medialis corporis striati.
lam'inae medulla'res cerebel'li, laminae albae cerebelli.
lam'inae medulla'res thal'ami [NA], medullary layers of thalamus; layers of myelinated fibers that appear on transverse sections of the thalamus; the l. medullaris externa marks the ventral and lateral borders of the thalamus and delimits it from the subthalamus and nucleus reticularis thalami; the l. medullaris interna is interposed between the mediodorsal and ventral nuclei of the thalamus and encloses the intralaminar nuclei (nuclei centromedianus, paracentralis, and centralis lateralis).
l. medulla'ris latera'lis cor'poris stria'ti [NA], lateral medullary l. of the corpus striatum; a thin, sharply defined layer of fibers separating the putamen from the globus pallidus.
l. medulla'ris media'lis cor'poris stria'ti [NA], medial medullary l. of the corpus striatum; a fiber layer separating the medial and lateral segments of the globus pallidus.
l. membrana'cea [NA], membranous layer; the connective tissue membrane that, with the l. lateralis, completes the lateral and inferior walls of the cartilaginous part of the auditory tube.

l. modi'oli [NA], plate of modiolus; a bony plate, the continuation of the modiolus and of the septum between the convolutions of the spiral canal of the cochlea extending upward toward the cupola, forming with the hamulus the helicotrema.
l. muscula'ris muco'sae [NA], muscular layer of the mucosa; muscularis mucosae; the thin layer of smooth muscle found in most parts of the digestive tube located outside the l. propria mucosae and adjacent to the tela submucosa.
orbital l. of ethmoid bone, l. orbitalis ossis ethmoidalis.
l. orbita'lis os'sis ethmoida'lis [NA], orbital l. or layer of ethmoid bone; l. papyracea; orbital, paper, or papyraceous plate; a thin plate of bone that forms a part of the medial wall of the orbit and bounds the ethmoidal labyrinth laterally.
osseous spiral l., l. spiralis ossea.
l. papyra'cea, l. orbitalis ossis ethmoidalis.
l. parieta'lis [NA], parietal layer; **l. p. pericar'dii,** the outer part of the serous pericardium supported by the fibrous pericardium; **l. p. tu'nicae vagina'lis tes'tis,** the outer part of the tunica vaginalis testis supported by the internal spermatic fascia.
periclaustral l., *capsula* externa.
l. perpendicula'ris [NA], perpendicular or vertical plate; pars perpendicularis; **(1)** a thin plate of bone projecting downward from the cribriform plate of the ethmoid; it forms part of the nasal septum; **(2)** the part of the palatine bone that extends vertically upward from the horizontal lamina; it forms part of the lateral wall of the nasal cavity.
l. poste'rior vagi'nae mus'culi rec'ti abdo'minis [NA], posterior layer of the rectus abdominis sheath; the portion of the sheath of the rectus abdominis muscle that lies posterior to the muscle; its free inferior margin forms the arcuate line.
l. pretrachea'lis [NA], pretracheal layer; pretracheal fascia; middle cervical fascia; Porter's fascia; the layer of fascia investing the infrahyoid muscles and contributing to the formation of the carotid sheath.
l. prevertebra'lis [NA], prevertebral layer; prevertebral fascia; the part of the cervical fascia which covers the bodies of the cervical vertebrae and the muscles attaching to them and to the anterior parts of their transverse processes.
primary dental l., dental *ledge.*
l. profun'da [NA], deep layer; **l. p. fas'ciae tempora'lis,** the deep part of the temporal fascia attaching to the medial surface of the zygomatic arch; **l. p. mus'culi levato'ris palpe'brae superio'ris,** the deeper fibers of the levator muscle of the superior eyelid which are inserted into the superior tarsal plate.
l. pro'pria muco'sae [NA], the layer of connective tissue underlying the epithelium of a mucous membrane.
pterygoid laminae, see l. lateralis processus pterygoidei and l. medialis processus pterygoidei.
l. quadrigem'ina, l. tecti mesencephali.
l. ra'ra, the relatively electron-lucent layer on either side of the l. densa.
reticular l., a major component of the basement membrane, as seen by light microscopy; it consists largely of reticular fibers and ground substances.
Rexed l., a cytoarchitectonic mapping of the layers of the spinal gray matter with Rexed 1 being the peripheral layer; Rexed 2, the substantia gelatinosa Rolandi; and Rexed 10, the glial layer around the central canal.
rostral l., l. rostralis.
l. rostra'lis, rostral l. or layer; teniola corporis callosi; a whitish line appearing on perfectly median sections of the brain as a thin bridge connecting the rostrum of the corpus callosum with the lamina terminalis; the l. rostralis contains no commissural fibers; instead, it corresponds to the line along which the pia mater reflects from the medial surface of one hemisphere to that of the other.
l. sep'ti pellu'cidi [NA], l. of the septum pellucidum; one of the two thin layers of the septum pellucidum, which extend from the corpus callosum to the fornix; often separated from each other by a space, the cavum septi pellucidi.
l. of septum pellucidum, l. septi pellucidi.
l. sinis'tra cartilag'inis thyroi'dea [NA], left plate of thyroid cartilage; the thin quadrilateral plate of the thyroid cartilage forming the left half of the thyroid cartilage.
l. spira'lis os'sea [NA], osseous spiral l.; spiral plate; a double plate of bone winding spirally around the modiolus dividing the spiral canal of the cochlea incompletely into two, scala tympani and scala vestibuli; between the two plates of this l. the fibers of the cochlear nerve reach the spiral organ (of Corti).
l. spira'lis secunda'ria [NA], secondary spiral plate; a ridge on the outer wall of the first turn of the cochlea opposite the spiral l.
l. superficia'lis [NA], superficial layer; **l. s. fas'ciae cervica'lis,** the part of the cervical fascia investing the sternocleidomastoid and trapezius muscles and completely encircling the neck; **l. s. fas'ciae tempora'lis,** the superficial part of the temporal fascia attaching to the lateral surface of the zygomatic arch; **l. s. mus'culi levato'ris palpe'brae superio'ris,** the superficial fibers of the levator muscle of the superior eyelid which are inserted into the skin of the superior eyelid.
l. suprachoroi'dea [NA], suprachoroid layer; ectochoroidea; a layer of loose, pigmented connective tissue on the outer surface of the choroid, resembling and attached to the l. fusca sclerae.
l. supraneuropor'ica, that part of the choroid membrane of the third ventricle that forms the roof of the foramen of Monro.
l. tec'ti mesenceph'ali [NA], tectum mesencephali; quadrigeminal plate; lamina quadrigemina; the roofplate of the mesencephalon formed by the corpora quadrigemina.
l. termina'lis cer'ebri [NA], terminal plate; velum terminale; l. cinerea; a thin plate passing upward from the optic chiasm and forming the rostral boundary of the third ventricle; membrane closing the rostral neuropore.
l. of thyroid cartilage, l. cartilaginis thyroideae.
l. tra'gi [NA], l. of tragus; a longitudinal curved plate of cartilage, the beginning of the cartilaginous portion of the external acoustic meatus.
l. of tragus, l. tragi.
l. vasculo'sa choroi'deae [NA], vascular layer of choroid coat of eye; Haller's vascular tissue; vascular layer; the outer portion of the choroid of the eye containing the largest blood vessels.
l. ventra'lis, l. basalis.
l. of vertebral arch, l. arcus vertebrae.
l. viscera'lis [NA], visceral layer; **l. v. pericar'dii,** epicardium; the inner part of the serous pericardium applied directly on the heart; **l. v. tu'nicae vagina'lis tes'tis,** the inner part of the tunica vaginalis testis applied directly to the testis and epididymis.
l. vit'rea, l. basalis choroideae.

laminagram (lam'i-nă-gram). A film taken by a laminagraph.
laminagraph (lam'i-nă-graf). Technique whereby tissues above and below the level of a suspected lesion are blurred out to emphasize a specific area.
laminagraphy (lam'i-nahg'ră-fē) [lamina + G. *graphē,* a writing]. Tomography.
laminar (lam'i-nar). **1.** Laminated; arranged in plates or laminae. **2.** Relating to any lamina.
laminaria (lam-i-nā'rē-ă) [L. *lamina,* a blade]. Sterile applicator made of kelp which, when placed in the cervical canal, absorbs moisture, swells, and gradually dilates the cervix.
laminarin (lam-i-nar'in). An algal polysaccharide, made up chiefly of β-D-glucose residues, obtained from *Laminaria* species (family Laminariaceae); variable proportions of the glucose chains contain at the potential reducing end a molecule of mannitol that can be sulfated.

l. sulfate, l. sulfated to varying degrees; two sulfate groups per glucose unit results in maximum stability and anticoagulant activity similar to that of heparin; l. with fewer sulfate groups has only antilipemic activity.

laminated (lam'i-nāt-ed). Laminar (1).

lamination (lam-i-nā'shŭn). **1.** An arrangement in the form of plates or laminae. **2.** Embryotomy by removing the fetal head in slices.

laminectomy (lam'i-nek'tō-mē) [L. *lamina,* layer, + G. *ektomē,* excision]. Rachiotomy; rachitomy; spondylotomy; excision of a vertebral lamina; commonly used to denote removal of the posterior arch.

laminin (lam'i-nin). A large polypeptide glycoprotein component of the basement membrane; particularly its unstained laminae.

laminitis (lam-i-nī'tis). **1.** Inflammation of any lamina. **2.** Founder (2); a painful inflammation of the sensitive lamina to which the hoof of the horse is attached.

laminotomy (lam'i-not'ō-mē) [L. *lamina,* layer, + G. *tomē,* incision]. An operation on one or more vertebral laminae.

lamins (lam'inz). Fibrous network associated with the inner membranes of cell nuclei, composed of polypeptides of varying molecular weights (60,000–80,000) and classified as A, B, C, etc. on the basis of physical properties.

lamp. Illuminating device; source of light. See also light.

annealing l., an alcohol l. with a soot-free flame used in dentistry to drive off the protective NH_3 gas coating from the surface of cohesive gold foil.

Edridge-Green l., a lantern used to test recognition of colored signals; it displays a single light with color filters in rotating disks that can be modified to simulate conditions of weather and atmosphere.

heat l., thermolamp; a l. that emits infrared light and produces heat; used to apply topical heat to the skin.

Kromayer's l., a U-shaped quartz l. of mercury vapor, giving out actinic rays; used in the treatment of skin diseases.

mignon l., a minute electric light used in various endoscopic instruments.

spirit l., a l., used mainly for heating in laboratory work, in which alcohol is burned.

ultraviolet l., a l. that emits rays in the ultraviolet band of the spectrum. See also ultraviolet.

uviol l., an electric l. with uviol glass, furnishing especially violet rays; used in phototherapy.

Wood's l., an ultraviolet l. with a nickel oxide filter that only passes light with a maximal wavelength of about 3660 Å; used to detect by fluorescence hairs infected with *Microsporum audouinii, M. canis, M. distortum,* or *M. ferrugineum,* producing greenish-yellow fluorescence.

Lamy, Maurice. See Maroteaux-L. *syndrome.*

lana, gen. and pl. **lanae** (lan'ă, lan'ē) [L.]. Wool.

lanatosides A, B, and **C** (lă-nat'ō-sīdz). Digilanides A, B, and C; the cardioactive precursor glycosides obtained from *Digitalis lanata.* Removal of the acetyl group yields desacetyllanatosides A, B, and C (purpurea glycosides A, B, and C, respectively); removal of the glucose from lanatosides A, B, and C yields acetyl digitoxin, acetylgitoxin, and acetyldigoxin, respectively; removal of glucose and the acetyl group yields digitoxin, gitoxin, and digoxin, respectively. See also purpurea glycosides.

lanatoside D (lă-nat'ō-sīd). A glycoside from the leaves of *Digitalis lanata,* yielding the genin diginatigenin (12-hydroxygitoxigenin; 16-hydroxydigoxigenin).

lance (lans) [L. *lancea,* a slender spear]. **1.** To incise a part, as an abscess or boil. **2.** A lancet.

Lancefield, Rebecca Craighill, U.S. bacteriologist, *1895. See L. *classification.*

lancet (lan'set) [Fr. *lancette*]. A surgical knife with a short, wide, sharp-pointed, two-edged blade.

gum l., a l. used for incising the gum over the crown of an erupting tooth.

spring l., a l. with a handle containing a blade that is activated by a spring.

thumb l., a l. with short flat blade which folds back, when closed, between two plates of the handle.

lancinating (lan'si-nāt'ing) [L. *lancino,* pp. *-atus,* to tear]. Denoting a sharp cutting or tearing pain.

Lancisi, Giovanni M., Italian physician, 1654–1720. See L.'s *sign, striae* lancisi.

Landau. See L.-Kleffner *syndrome.*

Landau-Kleffner syndrome. See under syndrome.

Landolfi's sign. See under sign.

Landolt, Edmund, French ophthalmologist, 1846–1926. See L.'s *bodies.*

Landouzy, Louis T.J., French neurologist, 1845–1917. See L.-Déjérine *dystrophy;* L.-Grasset *law.*

Landry, Jean B.O., French physician, 1826–1865. See L.'s *paralysis, syndrome;* Kussmaul-L. *paralysis;* L.-Guillain *syndrome.*

Landschutz tumor. See under tumor.

Landsteiner, Karl, Austrian-U.S. pathologist and Nobel laureate, 1868–1943. See L.-Donath *test;* Donath-L. cold *autoantibody, phenomenon.*

Landström, John, Swedish surgeon, 1869–1910. See L.'s *muscle.*

Landzert, T., 19th century German anatomist. See L.'s *fossa;* Grüber-L. *fossa.*

Lane, Sir W. Arbuthnot, British surgeon, 1856–1943. See L.'s *band, disease, plates.*

Lang, Basil T., British ophthalmologist, 1880–1928. See Frost-L. *operation.*

Lange, Carl F.A., German biochemist, *1883. See L.'s *solution, test.*

Lange, Carl G., Danish psychologist, 1834–1900. See James-L. *theory.*

Lange, Cornelia de. See De Lange, Cornelia.

Langenbeck, Bernhard R.K. von, German surgeon, 1810–1887. See L.'s *incision, triangle.*

Langendorff, Oscar, German physiologist, 1853–1908. See L.'s *method.*

Lange-Nielsen, F., 20th century Norwegian cardiologist. See Jervell and L.-N. *syndrome.*

Langer, Carl (Ritter von Edenberg) Austrian anatomist, 1819–1887. See L.'s *arch, lines, muscle.*

Langerhans, Paul, German anatomist, 1847–1888. See L.'s *cells, granule, islands; islets* of L.

Langhans, Theodor, German pathologist, 1839–1915. See L.'s *cells,* -type giant *cells, layer, stria.*

Langley, John N., British physiologist, 1852–1925. See L.'s *granules.*

Langmuir, Irving, U.S. chemist, 1881–1957. See L. *trough.*

language (lang'gwij) [L. *lingua*]. Any means or form, vocal or other, of expression or communication.

body l., **(1)** communication by means of bodily signs, *e.g.,* through the symptoms of hysterical conversion; **(2)** the expression of thoughts and feelings by means of nonverbal bodily movements, *e.g.,* gestures.

laniary (lan'i-ār-ē) [L. *laniarius,* to tear to pieces]. Adapted for tearing; in anatomy, sometimes applied to canine teeth, as l. teeth.

Lannelongue, Odilon M., French surgeon and pathologist, 1840–1911. See L.'s *foramina, ligaments.*

lanolin (lan'ō-lin) [L. *lana,* wool, + *oleum,* oil]. Hydrous wool fat; the purified fatlike substance from the wool of sheep, *Ovis aries* (family Bovidae); it contains not less than 25% and not more than 30% of water; used as a water-adsorbable ointment base. See also wool fat.

anhydrous l., wool fat; l. that contains not more than 0.25% of water; used as a water-adsorbable ointment base.

Lanterman, A.J., 19th century U.S. anatomist in Strasbourg. See L.'s *incisures, segments;* Schmidt-L. *clefts, incisures.*

lanthanic (lan'thă-nik) [G. *lanthanein,* to lie hidden]. Rarely used term denoting a disease process that produces no symptoms or clinical evidence of illness.

lanthanides (lan'thă-nīdz) [*lanthanum,* first element of the series]. Rare earth elements; those elements with atomic numbers 57–71 which closely resemble one another chemically and were once difficult to separate from one another.

lanthanum (lan'thă-nŭm) [G. *lanthanein,* to lie hidden]. A metallic element, symbol La, atomic no. 57, atomic weight 138.91; first of the rare earth elements (lanthanides).

l. nitrate, $La(NO_3)_3$; used in electron microscopy as a stain for extracellular mucopolysaccharides.

lanthionine (lan-thī'ō-nēn). 3,3'-Thiodialanine; $S(CH_2\text{-}CHNH_2\text{-}COOH)_2$; an amino acid obtained from wood which resembles cystine but has only one sulfur atom in the molecule rather than two.

lanuginous (lă-nū'ji-nŭs). Covered with lanugo.

lanugo (lă-nū'gō) [L. down, wooliness, from *lana,* wool] [NA]. Lanugo hair; fine, soft, unmedullated fetal or embryonic hair with minute shafts and large papillae; it appears toward the end of the third month of gestation.

Lanz, Otto, Swiss surgeon in Amsterdam, 1865–1935. See L.'s *line.*

LAP Abbreviation for leukocyte alkaline phosphatase. See alkaline *phosphatase.*

laparectomy (lap'ă-rek'tō-mē) [laparo- + G. *ektomē,* excision]. Excision of strips or gores from the abdominal wall and suture of the edges of the wounds, in cases of abnormal laxity of the abdominal muscles.

laparo- [G. *lapara,* flank, loins]. Combining form denoting the loins or, less properly, the abdomen in general.

laparocele (lap'ă-rō-sēl) [laparo- + G. *kēlē,* hernia]. Abdominal *hernia.*

laparogastroscopy (lap'ă-rō-gas-tros'kō-pē) [laparo- + G. *gastēr,* stomach, + *skopeō,* to view]. Inspection of interior of the stomach after a gastrotomy.

laparohysterectomy (lap'ă-rō-his-ter-ek'tō-mē). Abdominal *hysterectomy.*

laparohystero-oophorectomy (lap'ă-rō-his'ter-ō-ō-of'ō-rek'tō-mē) [laparo- + G. *hystera,* uterus, + oophorectomy]. Removal of the uterus and ovaries through an incision in the abdominal wall.

laparohysteropexy (lap'ă-rō-his'ter-ō-pek-sē) [laparo- + G. *hystera,* uterus, + *pēxis,* fixation]. Abdominal *hysteropexy.*

laparohysterosalpingo-oophorectomy (lap'ă-rō-his'ter-ō-sal'pin-gō-ō'of-ōr-ek'tō-mē). Removal of uterus and adnexa (tubes and ovaries) through an abdominal incision.

laparohysterotomy (lap'ă-rō-his-te-rot'ō-mē) [laparo- + G. *hystera,* uterus, + *tomē,* incision]. Abdominal *hysterotomy.*

laparomyomectomy (lap'ă-rō-mī-ō-mek'tō-mē). Abdominal *myomectomy.*

laparomyositis (lap'ă-rō-mī'ō-sī'tis) [laparo- + G. *mys,* muscle, + *-itis,* inflammation]. Inflammation of the lateral abdominal muscles.

laparorrhaphy (lap'ă-rōr'ă-fē). Celiorrhaphy.

laparosalpingectomy (lap'ă-rō-sal-pin-jek'tō-mē). Abdominal *salpingectomy.*

laparosalpingo-oophorectomy (lap'ă-rō-sal'ping-gō-ō-of'ō-rek'tō-mē). Abdominal salpingo-oophorectomy; removal of the fallopian tube and ovary through an abdominal incision.

laparosalpingotomy (lap'ă-rō-sal-ping-got'ō-mē). Abdominal *salpingotomy.*

laparoscope (lap'ă-rō-skōp) [laparo- + G. *skopeō,* to view]. Peritoneoscope.

laparoscopy (lap-ă-ros'kō-pē). Peritoneoscopy.

laparotomy (lap'ă-rot'ō-mē) [laparo- + G. *tomē,* incision]. **1.** Incision into the loin. **2.** Celiotomy.

laparotrachelotomy (lap'ă-rō-trak-ē-lot'ō-mē) [laparo- + G. *trachēlos,* neck, + *tomē,* incision]. A low cervical cesarean section.

laparouterotomy (lap'ă-rō-yū-ter-ot'ō-mē) [laparo- + uterus + G. *tomē,* incision]. Abdominal *hysterotomy.*

Lapicque, Louis, French physiologist, 1866–1952. See L.'s *law.*

lapinization (lap'i-ni-zā'shŭn) [Fr. *lapin,* rabbit]. Serial passage of a vaccine in rabbits.

lapinized (lap'i-nīzd) [Fr. *lapin,* rabbit]. Denoting viruses which have been adapted to develop in rabbits by serial transfers in this species.

Laplace, Ernest, U.S. surgeon, 1861–1924. See L.'s *forceps.*

Laplace, Pierre S. de, French mathematician, 1749–1827. See L.'s *law.*

Laquer, Ernst, German physiologist, *1910. See L.'s *stain* for alcoholic hyalin.

lar'bish. A form of creeping eruption observed in Senegal.

lard [L. *lardum*]. Adeps (2).

larkspur (lark'sper). *Delphinium ajacis.*

Laron, Zvi, Israeli pediatric endocrinologist, *1927. See L. type *dwarfism.*

Laroyenne, Lucien, French surgeon, 1831–1902. See L.'s *operation.*

Larrey, Baron Dominique Jean de, French surgeon, 1766–1842. See L.'s *amputation, cleft, ligation;* L.-Weil *disease.*

Larsen, Loren J., U.S. orthopedic surgeon, *1914. See L.'s *syndrome.*

Larsson, Tage. See Sjögren-L. *syndrome.*

larva, pl. larvae (lar'vă, lar'vē) [L. a mask]. **1.** The wormlike developmental stage or stages of an insect or helminth that are markedly different from the adult and undergo subsequent metamorphosis; a grub, maggot, or caterpillar. **2.** The second stage in the life cycle of a tick; the stage which hatches from the egg and, following engorgement, molts in the nymph. **3.** The young of fishes or amphibians which often differ in appearance from the adult.

filariform l., infective third-stage l. of the hookworm, *Ascaris,* and other nematodes with penetrating larvae or with larvae that migrate through the body to reach the intestine.

l. mi'grans, see *larva migrans.*

larvaceous (lar-vā'shŭs). Larvate.

larva currens (lar'vă kŭr'enz) [L. *larva,* mask + *currens,* racing]. Cutaneous larva migrans caused by rapidly moving larvae of *Strongyloides stercoralis* (up to 10 cm/hr), typically extending from the anal area down the upper thighs and observed as a rapidly progressing linear urticarial trail; may also be caused by zoonotic species of *Strongyloides.*

larval (lar'văl). **1.** Relating to larvae. **2.** Larvate.

larva migrans (lar'vă mī'granz) [L. *larva,* mask, + *migrare,* to transfer, migrate]. A larval worm, typically a nematode, that wanders for a period in the host tissues but does not develop to the adult stage; this usually occurs in abnormal hosts that inhibit normal development of the parasite.

cutaneous l. m., creeping eruption; dermatitis linearis migrans (1); myiasis linearis; an advancing serpiginous or netlike tunneling in the skin, with marked pruritus, caused by wandering hookworm larvae not adapted to intestinal maturation in man; especially common in the eastern and southern coastal U.S. and other tropical and subtropical coastal areas; various hookworms of dogs and cats have been implicated, chiefly *Ancylostoma braziliense* in the U.S., but also *A. caninum* of dogs, *Uncinaria stenocephala,* the European dog hookworm, and *Bunostomum phlebotomum,* the cattle hookworm; *Strongyloides* species of animal origin may also contribute to human cutaneous l. m.

ocular l. m., visceral l. m. involving the eyes, primarily of older children; clinical symptoms include decreased visual acuity and strabismus.

spiruroid l. m., extraintestinal migration by nematode larvae of the order Spiruroidea, not adapted to maturation in the human intestine; caused chiefly by species of *Gnathostoma spinigerum* and *G. hispidum* in Japan and Thailand, following ingestion of uncooked fish infected with encapsulated third-stage infective larvae, and possibly by ingestion of infected copepods (the first intermediate host) in contaminated drinking water; the anteriorly spined larvae produce serpiginous tunnels in the skin or may cause subcutaneous or pulmonary abscess, or may invade the eye or brain.

visceral l. m., a disease, chiefly of children, caused by ingestion of infective ova of *Toxocara canis,* less commonly by other ascarid nematodes not adapted to man, whose larvae hatch in the intestine, penetrate the gut wall, and wander in the viscera (chiefly the liver) for periods of up to 18 or 24 months; may be asymptomatic or may be marked by hepatomegaly (with granulomatous lesions caused by encapsulated larvae on the enlarged liver), pulmonary infiltration, fever, cough, hyperglobulinemia, and sustained high eosinophilia.

larvate (lar'vāt) [L. *larva,* mask]. Larvaceous; larval (2); masked or concealed; applied to a disease with undeveloped, absent, or atypical symptoms.

larvicidal (lar-vi-sī'dăl). Destructive to larvae.

larvicide (lar'vi-sīd) [larva + L. *caedo,* to kill]. An agent that kills larvae.

larviparous (lar-vip'ă-rŭs) [larva + L. *pario,* to bear]. Larvae-bearing; denoting passage of larvae, rather than eggs, from the body of the female, as in certain nematodes and insects.

larviphagic (lar'vi-fā'jik) [larva + G. *phagein,* to eat]. Consuming larvae; certain l. fish are used in mosquito control.

laryng-. See laryngo-.

laryngeal (lă-rin'jē-ăl). Relating in any way to the larynx.

laryngectomy (lar'in-jek'tō-mē) [laryngo- + G. *ektomē,* excision]. Excision of the larynx.

laryngemphraxis (lar'in-jem-frak'sis) [G. *emphraxis,* a stoppage]. Laryngeal obstruction from any cause.

larynges (lă-rin'jēz) [L.]. Plural of larynx.

laryngismus (lar-in-jiz'mŭs) [L. fr. G. *larynx,* + *-ismos,* -ism]. A spasmodic narrowing or closure of the rima glottidis.

l. strid'ulus, spasmus glottidis; pseudocroup; a spasmodic closure of the glottis, lasting a few seconds, followed by a noisy inspiration. *Cf. laryngitis* stridulosa.

laryngitic (lar-in-jit'ik). Relating to or caused by laryngitis.

laryngitis (lar-in-jī'tis) [laryngo- + G. *-itis,* inflammation]. Inflammation of the mucous membrane of the larynx.

chronic subglottic l., *chorditis* vocalis inferior.

croupous l., inflammation of the larynx associated with respiratory infection and croupy or noisy breathing.

membranous l., a form in which there is a pseudomembranous exudate on the vocal cords.

spasmodic l., l. stridulosa.

l. stridulo'sa, spasmodic l.; catarrhal inflammation of the larynx in children, accompanied by night attacks of spasmodic closure of the glottis, causing inspiratory stridor.

laryngo-, laryng- [G. *larynx*]. Combining forms relating to the larynx.

laryngocele (lă-ring'gō-sēl) [laryngo- + G. *kēle,* hernia]. An air sac communicating with the larynx through the ventricle, often bulging outward into the tissue of the neck, especially during coughing.

laryngofissure (lă-ring'gō-fish'er). Thyrofissure; thyroidotomy; thyrotomy (2); thyrochondrotomy; operative opening into the larynx, generally through the midline, commonly done for the excision of early carcinoma or the correction of laryngostenosis.

laryngograph (lă-ring'gō-graf) [laryngo- + G. *graphō,* to write]. An instrument for making a tracing of the movements of the larynx.

laryngology (lar'ing-gol'ō-jē) [laryngo- + G. *logos,* study]. The branch of medical science concerned with the larynx; the specialty of diseases of the larynx.

laryngomalacia (lă-ring'gō-mă-lā'shē-ă) [laryngo- + G. *malakia,* a softness]. *Chondromalacia* of the larynx.

laryngoparalysis (lă-ring'gō-pă-ral'i-sis). Laryngoplegia; paralysis of the laryngeal muscles.

laryngopathy (lar'ing-gop'ă-thē) [laryngo- + G. *pathos,* suffering]. Any disease of the larynx.

laryngophantom (lă-ring'gō-fan'tŭm) [laryngo- + G. *phantasma,* image]. A model of the larynx for use in the study of the anatomy or for practice in laryngoscopy.

laryngopharyngeal (lă-ring'gō-fă-rin'jē-ăl). Relating to both larynx and pharynx or to the laryngopharynx.

laryngopharyngectomy (lă-ring'gō-far'in-jek'tō-mē). Resection or excision of both larynx and pharynx.

laryngopharyngeus (lă-ring'gō-făr'in-jē'ŭs) [L.]. *Musculus* constrictor pharyngeus inferior.

laryngopharyngitis (lă-ring'gō-far-in-jī'tis). Inflammation of the larynx and pharynx.

laryngopharynx (lă-ring'gō-far-ingks). *Pars* laryngea pharyngis.

laryngophony (lar-ing-gof'ō-nē) [laryngo- + G. *phōnē,* voice]. The voice sounds heard in auscultation of the larynx.

laryngophthisis (lă-ring'gō-thī'sis) [laryngo- + G. *phthisis,* a wasting]. Tuberculosis of the larynx.

laryngoplasty (lă-ring'gō-plas-tē) [laryngo- + G. *plassō,* to form]. Reparative or plastic surgery of the larynx.

laryngoplegia (lă-ring'gō-plē'jē-ă) [laryngo- + G. *plēgē,* stroke]. Laryngoparalysis.

laryngoptosis (lă-ring-gō-tō'sis) [laryngo- + G. *ptōsis,* a falling]. An abnormally low position of the larynx at birth, which may be congenital or acquired; does not impair the health of the neonate. Some degree of l. occurs with aging.

laryngorhinology (lă-ring'gō-rī-nol'ō-jē) [laryngo- + G. *rhis,* nose, + *logos,* study]. The branch of medical science that has to do with affections of the larynx and of the nose.

laryngoscope (lă-ring'gō-skōp) [laryngo- + G. *skopeō,* to inspect]. Any of several types of hollow tubes, equipped with electrical lighting, used in examining or operating upon the interior of the larynx through the mouth.

laryngoscopic (lă-ring'gō-skop'ik). Relating to laryngoscopy.

laryngoscopist (lar'ing-gos'kō-pist). A person skilled in the use of the laryngoscope.

laryngoscopy (lar′ing-gos′kō-pē). Inspection of the larynx by means of the laryngoscope.
suspension l., support of the laryngoscope by leverage from the anterior chest wall or other supportive structure to provide maximum exposure of the pharyngeal cavity and larynx.

laryngospasm (lă-ring′gō-spazm). Glottidospasm; laryngospastic reflex; spasmodic closure of the glottic aperture.

laryngostenosis (lă-ring′gō-stĕ-nō′sis) [laryngo- + G. *stenōsis,* a narrowing]. Stricture or narrowing of the lumen of the larynx.

laryngostomy (lar′ing-gos′tō-mē) [laryngo- + G. *stoma,* mouth]. The establishment of a permanent opening from the neck into the larynx.

laryngostroboscope (lă-ring′gō-strō′bō-skōp, -strob′ō-skōp). Stroboscopic apparatus for observing the motion of the vocal cords during phonation.

laryngotome (lă-ring′gō-tōm). An instrument for use in laryngotomy.
dilating l., an instrument with almond-shaped extremity, in which is concealed a knife, used for the intralaryngeal division of strictures and cicatricial bands.

laryngotomy (lar-ing-got′ō-mē) [laryngo- + G. *tomē,* incision]. A surgical incision of the larynx.
inferior l., cricothyrotomy.
median l., laryngofissure.
superior l., incision through the thyrohyoid membrane.

laryngotracheal (lă-ring′gō-trā′kē-ăl). Relating to both larynx and trachea.

laryngotracheitis (lă-ring′gō-trā-kē-ī′tis). Inflammation of both larynx and trachea.
avian infectious l., a severe, specific, infectious disease of chickens and other birds, caused by a herpesvirus (family Herpetoviridae); manifested by severe hemorrhagic inflammation of the trachea and upper air passages.

laryngotracheobronchitis (lă-ring′gō-trā′kē-ō-brong-kī′tis). An acute respiratory infection involving the larynx, trachea, and bronchi. See croup.

laryngotracheotomy (lă-ring′gō-trā-kē-ot′ō-mē) [laryngo- + trachea + G. *tomē,* incision]. An incision through the cricoid cartilage and the upper tracheal rings.

laryngoxerosis (lă-ring′gō-zē-rō′sis) [laryngo- + G. *xērōsis,* a drying up]. An abnormal dryness of the laryngeal mucous membrane.

larynx, pl. larynges (lar′ingks, lă-rin′jēz) [Mod. L. fr. G.] [NA]. The organ of voice production; the part of the respiratory tract between the pharynx and the trachea; it consists of a framework of cartilages and elastic membranes housing the vocal folds and the muscles which control the position and tension of these elements.

lase (lāz). To cut, divide, or dissolve a substance, or to treat an anatomical structure, with a laser beam.

Lasègue, Ernest C., French physician, 1816–1883. See L.'s *disease, sign, syndrome.*

laser (lā′zer) [acronym coined from *l*ight *a*mplification by *s*timulated *e*mission of *r*adiation]. A device that concentrates high energies into an intense narrow beam of nondivergent monochromatic electromagnetic radiation; used in microsurgery, cauterization, and for a variety of diagnostic purposes. L.'s using ruby, argon, krypton, neodymium, helium-neon, or carbon dioxide are available.

Lash, Abraham Fae, U.S. obstetrician-gynecologist, *1898. See L.'s *operation.*

lash. An eyelash.

lasing (lā′zing). The use of a laser beam to cut, divide, or dissolve a substance, or to treat an anatomical structure.

Lasiohelea (las′ē-ō-hē′lē-ă). A genus of small bloodsucking gnats.

lassitude (las′i-tūd) [L. *lassitudo,* fr. *lassus,* weary]. A sense of weariness.

latah (lah′tah) [Malay, ticklish]. A nervous affection characterized by an exaggerated physical response to being startled or to unexpected suggestion, the subjects involuntarily uttering cries or executing movements in response to command or in imitation of what they hear or see in others. See also jumper *disease.*

Latarget, André, French anatomist, 1877–1947. See L.'s *nerve, vein.*

latebra (lat′ē-bră) [L. hiding place]. A flask-shaped region in large-yolked eggs extending from the animal pole to a dilated terminal portion near the center of the yolk; it contains the main bulk of the white yolk.

latency (lā′ten-sē). **1.** The state of being latent. **2.** In conditioning, the period of apparent inactivity between the time the stimulus is presented and the moment a response occurs. **3.** In psychoanalysis, the period of time from approximately age five to puberty.

latent (lā′tent) [L. *lateo,* pres. p. *latens (-ent-),* to lie hidden]. Not manifest, but potentially discernible.

laterad (lat′er-ad) [L. *latus,* side, + *ad,* to]. Toward the side.

lateral (lat′er-ăl) [L. *lateralis,* lateral, fr. *latus,* side]. **1.** On the side. **2.** Farther from the median or midsagittal plane. **3.** In dentistry, a position either right or left of the midsagittal plane.

lateralis (lat-er-ā′lis) [L.] [NA]. Lateral (1, 2).

laterality (lat-er-al′i-tē). Referring to a side of the body or of a structure; specifically, the dominance of one side of the brain or the body.
crossed l., right dominance of some members, *e.g.,* arm or leg, and left dominance of other members.

lateriflexion, lateriflection (lat-er-i-flek′shŭn). Lateroflexion.

latero- [L. *lateralis,* lateral, fr. *latus,* side]. Combining form meaning lateral, to one side, or relating to a side.

lateroabdominal (lat′er-ō-ab-dom′i-năl). Relating to the sides of the abdomen, to the loins or flanks.

laterodeviation (lat′er-ō-dē-vē-ā′shŭn) [latero- + L. *devio,* to turn aside, fr. *via,* a way]. A bending or a displacement to one side.

lateroduction (lat′er-ō-dŭk′shŭn) [latero- + L. *duco,* pp. *ductus,* to lead]. A drawing to one side; denoting a movement of a limb or rotation of the eyeball.

lateroflexion, lateroflection (lat′er-ō-flek′shŭn) [latero- + L. *flecto,* pp. *flexus,* to bend]. Lateriflexion; lateriflection; a bending or curvature to one side.

lateroposition (lat′er-ō-pō-zish′ŭn). A shift to one side.

lateropulsion (lat′er-ō-pŭl′shŭn) [latero- + L. *pello,* pp. *pulsus,* to push, drive]. An involuntary sidewise movement occurring in certain nervous affections.

laterotorsion (lat′er-ō-tōr′shŭn) [latero- + L. *torsio,* a twisting]. A twisting to one side; denoting rotation of the eyeball around its anteroposterior axis.

laterotrusion (lat′er-ō-trū′zhŭn) [latero- + L. *trudo,* pp. *trusus,* to thrust]. The outward thrust given by the muscles of mastication to the rotating mandibular condyle during movement of the mandible.

lateroversion (lat′er-ō-ver′shŭn) [latero- + L. *verto,* pp. *versus,* to turn]. Version to one side or the other, denoting especially a malposition of the uterus.

lathe (lādh). A motor-driven machine with a rotating shaft that can be fitted with various types of cutting instruments, grinding stones and polishing wheels; used in finishing and polishing dental appliances.

lathyrism (lath′i-rizm) [L. *lathyrus,* vetch]. Lupinosis. **1.** A disease occurring in Abyssinia, Algeria, and India, characterized by various nervous manifestations, tremors, spastic paraplegia, and parasthesias; prevalent in districts where vetches, khasari (*Lathyrus sativus*), and allied species form the main food. **2.** Poisoning of horses from eating certain varieties of peas, particularly *Lathyrus sativus*, a plant introduced into Europe from India; manifested by paralytic symptoms. See also githagism.

lathyrogen (lath'ĭ-rō-jen). An agent or drug, occurring naturally or used experimentally, that induces lathyrism.

Latrodectus (lat-rō-dek'tŭs) [L. *latro*, servant, robber, + G. *dēktēs*, a biter]. A genus of relatively small spiders, the widow spiders, capable of inflicting highly poisonous, neurotoxic, painful bites; they are responsible, along with *Loxosceles* (the brown spider), for most of the severe reactions from spider envenomation. Medically important species are known from Australia, North and South America, South Africa, and New Zealand. Some venomous species, in addition to *L. mactans* (the black widow spider), are *L. bishopi* (the red-legged widow spider), *L. euracaviensis*, *L. geometricus*, and *L. tredecimguttatus*.

L. mac'tans, the black widow spider, a venomous jet-black spider found in protected dark places; it is especially common in the southern U.S.; the full grown female (slightly more than 1 cm long) has a brilliant red dumbbell- or hourglass-shaped mark on the ventral aspect of the abdomen, and her bite may be extremely painful, producing a syndrome mimicking an acute abdominal crisis; some deaths, though rare, have been reported, particularly in small children; the male spider lacks the hourglass mark and is not venomous.

LATS Abbreviation for long-acting thyroid *stimulator.*

lattice (lat'is). A regular arrangement of units into an array such that a plane passing through two units of a particular type or in a particular interrelationship will pass through an indefinite number of such units; *e.g.*, the atom arrangement in a crystal.

latus (lā'tŭs) [L.]. Broad.

latus, gen. **lateris,** pl. **latera** (lā'tŭs, lat'er-is, lat'er-ă) [L.]. Flank; the side of the body between the pelvis and the ribs.

Latzko, Wilhelm, Austrian obstetrician, 1863–1945. See L.'s cesarean *section.*

laudable (law'dă-bl) [L. *laudabilis*, praiseworthy]. A term formerly used to describe pus, under the notion that suppuration in a wound favored healing.

laudanine (law'dă-nēn). $C_{20}H_{25}NO_4$; an isoquinoline alkaloid derived from the mother liquor of morphine; it causes tetanoid convulsions, with action similar to that of strychnine.

laudanosine (law'dă-nō-sēn). $C_{21}H_{27}NO_4$; an isoquinoline alkaloid obtained from the mother liquor of morphine; it causes tetanic convulsions.

laudanum (law'dă-nŭm) [G. *lēdanon*, a resinous gum]. A tincture containing opium.

Laugier, Stanislas, French surgeon, 1799–1872. See L.'s *hernia, sign.*

Laumonier, Jean B. P. N. R., French surgeon, 1749–1818. See L.'s *ganglion.*

Launois, Pierre E., French physician, 1856–1914. See L.-Cléret *syndrome;* L.-Bensaude *syndrome.*

Laurence, John Zachariah, British ophthalmologist, 1830–1874. See L.-Biedl *syndrome;* L.-Moon *syndrome;* L.-Moon-Bardet-Biedl *syndrome.*

Laurer, Johann F., German pharmacologist, 1798–1873. See L.'s *canal.*

lauric acid (law'rik). Dodecanoic acid; $CH_3(CH_2)_{10}COOH$; a fatty acid occurring in spermaceti, in milk, and in laurel, coconut, and palm oils.

Lauth, Ernst A., Strasbourg physician, 1803–1837. See L.'s *canal.*

Lauth, Thomas, German anatomist and surgeon, 1758–1826. See L.'s *ligament.*

Lauth's violet [Charles *Lauth*, English chemist, 1836–1913]. Thionine.

LAV Abbreviation for lymphadenopathy-associated *virus.*

lavage (lă-vahzh') [Fr. from L. *lavo*, to wash]. The washing out of a hollow cavity or organ by copious injections and rejections of fluid.

Lavdovsky, Michail D., Russian histologist, 1846–1902. See L.'s *nucleoid.*

Laverania (lav-er-ā'nē-ă) [C. *Laveran*, Fr. protozoologist and Nobel laureate, 1845–1922]. Old generic name for malaria-causing and other hematozoan protozoa. *L. falciparum* is a distinctive generic name for *Plasmodium falciparum*, and is preferred by some who believe that crescentic gametocytes should be the basis for classifying the causal agent of falciparum malaria in a separate genus. See *Plasmodium; Haemoproteus.*

laveur (lă-vŭr') [Fr.]. An instrument for irrigation or lavage.

LAW

law [A.S. *lagu*] **1.** A principle or rule. **2.** A statement of a sequence or relation of phenomena that is invariable under the given conditions. See also principle; rule; theorem.

all or none l., Bowditch's l.

Ambard's l.'s, obsolete l.'s for output of urea: 1) with the urinary urea concentration constant, urea output varies directly as the square of the concentration of the blood urea; 2) with the blood urea concentration constant, urea output varies inversely as the square root of its urinary concentration.

Ångström's l., a substance absorbs light of the same wavelength as it emits when luminous.

Arndt's l., a law stating that weak stimuli excite physiologic activity, moderately strong ones favor it, strong ones retard it, and very strong ones arrest it.

Arrhenius l., Arrhenius *doctrine.*

l.'s of association, principles formulated by Aristotle to account for the functional relationships between ideas; the l. of contiguity (association) proved most useful to experimental psychologists, culminating in modern studies of respondent conditioning.

l. of average localization, visceral pain is most accurately localized in the least mobile viscera and least accurately in the most mobile.

Avogadro's l., Avogadro's hypothesis or postulate; Ampère's postulate; equal volumes of gases contain equal numbers of molecules, the conditions of pressure and temperature being the same.

Baer's l., general organ characteristics appear earlier during embryogenesis than do special organ characteristics.

Baruch's l., the effect of any hydriatric procedure is in direct proportion to the difference between the temperature of the water and that of the skin; when the temperature of the water is above or below that of the skin the effect is stimulating; when the two temperatures are the same the effect is sedative.

Beer's l., the intensity of a color or of a light ray is inversely proportional to the depth of liquid through which it is transmitted; it is concluded that the absorption is dependent upon the number of molecules in the path of the ray.

Behring's l., parenteral administration of serum from an immunized person provides a relative, passive immunity to that disease (*i.e.*, prevents it, or favorably modifies its course) in a previously susceptible person.

Bell's l., Bell-Magendie l.; Magendie l.; the ventral spinal roots are motor, the dorsal are sensory.

Bell-Magendie l., Bell's l.

Bernoulli's l., Bernoulli's principle or theorem; when friction is negligible, the velocity of flow of a gas or fluid through a tube is inversely related to its pressure against the side of the tube; *i.e.,* velocity is greatest and pressure lowest at a point of constriction.

Berthollet's l., salts in solution will always react with each other so as to form a less soluble salt, if possible.

biogenetic l., l. of biogenesis, recapitulation *theory.*

Blagden's l., the depression of the freezing point of dilute solutions is proportional to the amount of the dissolved substance.

Bowditch's l., all or none l.; any stimulus, however feeble, capable of exciting a cardiac contraction will produce as powerful a contraction as the strongest stimulus; "minimal stimuli cause maximal pulsations."

Boyle's l., Mariotte's l.; at constant temperature, the volume of a given quantity of gas varies inversely with its absolute pressure.

Broadbent's l., lesions of the upper segment of the motor tract cause less marked paralysis of muscles that habitually produce bilateral movements than of those that commonly act independently of the opposite side.

Bunsen-Roscoe l., reciprocity l.; Roscoe-Bunsen l.; in two photochemical reactions, *e.g.,* the darkening of a photographic plate or film, if the product of the intensity of illumination and the time of exposure are equal, the quantities of chemical material undergoing change will be equal; the retina for short periods of exposure obeys this l.

Charles l., Gay-Lussac's l.; all gases expand equally on heating, namely, $^1/_{273}$ of their volume at 0°C for every degree Celsius.

l. of constant numbers in ovulation, the number of ova discharged at each ovulation is nearly constant for any given species.

l. of contiguity, when two ideas or psychologically perceived events have once occurred in close association they are likely to so occur again, the subsequent occurrence of one tending to elicit the other; this l. figures prominently in modern theories of conditioning and learning.

l. of contrary innervation, Meltzer's l.

Coppet's l., solutions having the same freezing point have equal concentrations of dissolved substances.

Courvoisier's l., Courvoisier's sign; enlargement of the gallbladder with jaundice is likely to result from carcinoma of the head of the pancreas and not from a stone in the common duct, because then the gallbladder is usually scarred from infection and does not distend.

Dale-Feldberg l., an identical chemical transmitter is liberated at all the functional terminals of a single neuron.

Dalton's l., l. of partial pressures; each gas in a mixture of gases exerts a pressure proportionately to the percentage of the gas and independently of the presence of the other gases present.

Dalton-Henry l., in dissolving a mixture of gases, a liquid will absorb as much of each gas in the mixture as if that were the only gas dissolved.

l. of definite proportions, Proust's l.; the relative weights of the several elements forming a chemical compound are invariable.

l. of denervation, when a structure is denervated, its irritability to certain chemical agents is increased; *e.g.,* the greater sensitivity of the pupil to acetylcholine after section and degeneration of the third nerve, and of the nictitating membrane to adrenaline after excision of the superior cervical ganglion.

Descartes' l., l. of refraction.

Donders' l., the rotation of the eyeball is determined by the distance of the object from the median plane and the line of the horizon.

Draper's l., a chemical change is produced in a photochemical substance only by those light rays that are absorbed by that substance.

Du Bois-Reymond's l., l. of excitation.

Dulong-Petit l., the heat capacity of the atoms of all simple solid bodies is the same.

Einthoven's l., Einthoven's equation; in the electrocardiogram the potential of any wave or complex in lead II is equal to the sum of the potentials of leads I and III.

Elliott's l., adrenaline acts upon those structures innervated by sympathetic nerve fibers.

l. of excitation, Du Bois-Reymond l.; a motor nerve responds, not to the absolute value, but to the alteration of value from moment to moment, of the electric current; *i.e.,* rate of change of intensity of the current is a factor in determining its effectiveness.

Faraday's l.'s, (1) the amount of an electrolyte decomposed by an electric current is proportional to the amount of the current; **(2)** when the same current is passed through several electrolytes, the amounts of the different substances decomposed are proportional to their chemical equivalents.

Farr's l., the curve of cases of an epidemic rises rapidly at first, then climbs slowly to a peak from which the fall is steeper than the previous rise.

Fechner-Weber l., Weber-Fechner l.

Ferry-Porter l., the critical fusion is directly proportional to the logarithm of the light intensity.

Flatau's l., a l. concerning the excentric position of the long spinal tracts; the greater the distance the nerve fibers run lengthwise in the cord, the more they tend to be situated toward its periphery.

Galton's l., l. of regression to mean; in a population mating at random, the progeny of a parent with extreme values for a measurable phenotype will tend on average to be nearer the population mean than to the extreme parent.

Gay-Lussac's l., Charles' l.

Gerhardt-Semon l., obsolete l. formerly used to account for the position of affected vocal cord or cords after injury to the recurrent laryngeal nerve or nerves.

Godélier's l., tuberculosis of the peritoneum is always associated with tuberculosis of the pleura on one or both sides.

Graham's l., the relative rapidity of diffusion of two gases varies inversely as the square root of their densities, *i.e.,* their molecular weights.

Grasset's l., Landouzy-Grasset l.

l. of gravitation, Newton's l.

Guldberg-Waage l., l. of mass action.

Haeckel's l., recapitulation *theory.*

Halsted's l., transplanted tissue will grow only if there is a lack of that tissue in the host.

Hamburger's l., albumins and phosphates pass from red corpuscles to serum and chlorides pass from serum to cells when blood is acid; the reverse occurs when blood is alkaline.

Hardy-Weinberg l., if mating occurs at random with respect to any one autosomal locus in a population in which the gene frequencies are equal in the two sexes, and the factors tending to change gene frequencies (mutation, differential selection, migration) are either absent or negligible, then in one generation the probabilities of all possible genotypes will on average equal the same proportions as if the genes were assembled at random. The l. does not apply to two or more loci jointly, nor to X-linked traits where the initial gene frequencies differ in the two sexes.

l. of the heart, Starling's l.; the energy liberated by the heart when it contracts is a function of the length of its muscle fibers at the end of diastole.

Heidenhain's l., glandular secretion is always accompanied by an alteration in the structure of the gland.

Hellin's l., twins occur once in 89 births, triplets once in 89^2, and quadruplets once in 89^3.

Henry's l., at equilibrium, the amount of gas dissolved in a given volume of liquid is directly proportional to the partial pressure of that gas in the gas phase.

Hilton's l., the nerve supplying a joint supplies also the muscles which move the joint and the skin covering the articular insertion of those muscles.

Hooke's l., the stress applied to stretch or compress a body is proportional to the strain, or change in length thus produced, so long as the limit of elasticity of the body is not exceeded.

l. of independent assortment, Mendel's second l.: different hereditary factors are assorted independently when the gametes are formed; must be modified by the restriction that linked genes do not assort independently.

l. of initial value, Wilder's l. of initial value.

l. of intestine, myenteric *reflex.*

l. of inverse square, as applied to point surfaces, the intensity of radiation is inversely proportional to the square of the distance from the source.

l. of isochronism, a nerve and the muscle which it innervates have the same chronaxie values.

isodynamic l., for energy purposes, the different foodstuffs may replace one another in accordance with their caloric values when burned in a calorimeter.

Jackson's l., loss of mental functions due to disease retraces in reverse order its evolutionary development.

Koch's l., Koch's *postulates.*

Landouzy-Grasset l., Grasset's l.; in lesions of one hemisphere, the patient's head is turned to the side of the affected muscles if there is spasticity and to that of the cerebral lesion if there is paralysis.

Lapicque's l., the chronaxie is inversely proportional to the diameter of an axon.

Laplace's l., the equilibrium relationship between transmural pressure difference (ΔP), wall tension (T), and radius of curvature (R) in a concave surface; for a sphere: $\Delta P = 2\ T/R$; for a cylinder: $\Delta P = T/R$.

Le Chatelier's l., Le Chatelier's principle; if external factors such as temperature and pressure disturb a system in equilibrium, adjustment occurs in such a way that the effect of the disturbing factors is reduced to a minimum.

Listing's l., when the eye leaves one object and fixes upon another, it revolves about an axis perpendicular to a plane cutting both the former and the present lines of vision.

Louis' l., **(1)** pulmonary tuberculosis usually begins in the left lung; **(2)** tuberculosis in any organ is accompanied by lesions in the lung.

Magendie's l., Bell's l.

Marey's l., the pulse rate varies inversely with the blood pressure; *i.e.,* the pulse is slow when the pressure is high; an expression of baroreceptor reflex influences on heart rate.

Marfan's l., the healing of localized tuberculosis protects against subsequent development of pulmonary tuberculosis.

Mariotte's l., Boyle's l.

l. of mass action, mass l., Guldberg-Waage l.; the rate of a chemical reaction is proportional to the concentrations of the reacting substances.

Meltzer's l., l. of contrary innervation; "all living functions are continually controlled by two opposite forces: augmentation or action on the one hand, and inhibition on the other."

Mendel's l.'s, **(1)** M.'s first l.: see l. of segregation; **(2)** M.'s second l.: see l. of independent assortment.

Mendeléeff's l., periodic l.; the properties of elements are periodical functions of their atomic weights; *i.e.,* if the elements are arranged in the order of their atomic weights, every element in the series will be related in respect to its properties to the eighth in order before or after it.

l. of the minimum, growth and development of plants and animals are determined by the availability of that essential nutrient which is present in the smallest amount.

Müller's l., l. of specific nerve energies; each type of sensory nerve ending, however stimulated (electrically, mechanically, etc.) gives rise to its own specific sensation; moreover, each type of sensation depends not upon any special character of the different nerves but upon the part of the brain in which their fibers terminate.

l. of multiple proportions, l. of reciprocal proportions.

Nasse's l., an early statement of the pattern of X-linked recessive inheritance: hemophilia affects only boys but is transmitted through mothers and sisters.

Neumann's l., in compounds of analogous chemical constitution, the molecular heat, or the product of the specific heat by the atomic weight, is always the same.

Newton's l., l. of gravitation; the attractive force between any two bodies is proportional to the product of their masses, and inversely proportional to the square of the distance between their centers.

Nysten's l., rigor mortis affects first the muscles of the head and spreads toward the feet.

Ochoa's l., the content of the X-chromosome tends to be phylogenetically conserved.

Ohm's l., in an electric current passing through a wire, the intensity of the current (I) in amperes equals the electromotive force (E) in volts divided by the resistance (R) in ohms: $I = (E/R)$.

l. of partial pressures, Dalton's l.

Pascal's l., fluids at rest transmit pressure equally in every direction.

periodic l., Mendeléeff's l.

Pflüger's l., l. of polar excitation.

Plateau-Talbot l., when successive light stimuli follow each other sufficiently rapidly to become fused, their apparent brightness is diminished.

Poiseuille's l., in laminar flow, the volume of a homogeneous fluid passing per unit time through a capillary tube is directly proportional to the pressure difference between its ends and to the fourth power of its internal radius, and inversely proportional to its length and to the viscosity of the fluid.

l. of polar excitation, Pflüger's l.; a given segment of a nerve is irritated by the development of catelectrotonus and the disappearance of anelectrotonus, but the reverse does not hold; *i.e.,* excitation occurs at the cathode when the circuit is closed and at the anode when it is opened.

l. of priority, use of the earliest published name (senior synonym) of two or more names of an organism as the correct name.

Profeta's l., the subject of congenital syphilis is immune against the acquired disease.

Proust's l., l. of definite proportions.

Raoult's l., the vapor pressure of a solution is that of the pure solvent multiplied by the mole-fraction of the solvent in the solution.

l. of recapitulation, recapitulation *theory.*

l. of reciprocal proportions, l. of multiple proportions; the relative weights in which two substances form a chemical union singly with a third are the same as, or simple multiples of, those in which they unite with each other; a corollary of the law of definite proportions.

reciprocity l., Bunsen-Roscoe l.

l. of referred pain, pain arises only from irritation of nerves which are sensitive to those stimuli that produce pain when applied to the surface of the body.

l. of refraction, Snell's or Descartes' l.; for two given media, the sine of the angle of incidence bears a constant relation to the sine of the angle of refraction.

l. of regression to mean, Galton's l.

Riccò's l., for small images, light intensity × area = constant for the threshold.

Ritter's l., a nerve is stimulated at both the opening and the closing of an electrical current. See l. of polar excitation.

Roscoe-Bunsen l., Bunsen-Roscoe l.

Rosenbach's l., **(1)** in affections of the nerve trunks or nerve centers, paralysis of the flexor muscles appears later than that of the extensors; **(2)** in cases of abnormal stimulation of organs with rhythmical functional periodicity, there is often a grouping of the

individual acts with corresponding lengthening of the pauses, in such a way that the proportion of total rest and activity remains nearly the same.
Rubner's l.'s of growth, **(1)** the l. of constant energy consumption: the rapidity of growth is proportional to the intensity of the metabolic processes; **(2)** the l. of the constant growth quotient: in most young mammals 24% of the entire food energy, or calories, is utilized for growth, in man only 5% is utilized.
Schütz' l., Schütz' *rule.*
second l. of thermodynamics, the entropy of the universe moves toward a maximum; similarly, the entropy of any isolated microcosm (*e.g.,* a chemical reaction) proceeds spontaneously only in that direction that yields an increase in entropy, entropy being maximal at equilibrium. To quote G.N. Lewis: Every process that occurs spontaneously is capable of doing work; to reverse any such process requires the expenditure of work from the outside.
l. of segregation, Mendel's first l.: factors which affect development retain their individuality from generation to generation, do not become contaminated when mixed in a hybrid, and become sorted out from one another when the gametes are formed.
Semon's l., an obsolete l. stating that injury to the recurrent laryngeal nerve results in paralysis of the abductor muscle of the vocal cords before paralysis of the adductor muscles.
Sherrington's l., every dorsal spinal nerve root supplies a particular area of the skin, the dermatome(3), which is, however, invaded above and below by fibers from the adjacent spinal segments.
l. of similars, see *similia similibus curantur.*
Snell's l., l. of refraction.
Spallanzani's l., the younger the individual the greater is the regenerative power of its cells.
Starling's l., l. of the heart.
Stokes' l., a muscle lying above an inflamed mucous or serous membrane is frequently the seat of paralysis.
Tait's l., an obsolete dictum that an exploratory laparotomy should be performed in every case of obscure pelvic or abdominal disease that threatens health or life.
Thoma's l.'s, the development of blood vessels is governed by dynamic forces acting on their walls as follows: an increase in velocity of blood flow causes dilation of the lumen; an increase in lateral pressure on the vessel wall causes it to thicken; an increase in end-pressure causes the formation of new capillaries.
van der Kolk's l., in a mixed nerve, the sensory fibers are distributed to the parts moved by the muscles controlled by the motor fibers.
van't Hoff's l., **(1)** in stereochemistry, all optically active substances have one or more multivalent atoms united to four different atoms or radicals so as to form in space an unsymmetrical arrangement; **(2)** the osmotic pressure exerted by any substance in very dilute solution is the same that it would exert if present as gas in the same volume as that of the solution; or, at constant temperature, the osmotic pressure of dilute solutions is proportional to the concentration (number of molecules) of the dissolved substance; **(3)** the rate of chemical reactions increases between two- and threefold for each 10°C rise in temperature.
Virchow's l., there is no special or distinctive neoplastic cell, inasmuch as the component cells of neoplasms originate from preexisting forms.
Vogel's l., when a phenotype may be transmitted by various modes of mendelian inheritance, the dominant will have the least deleterious phenotype, the recessive the most, and the X-linked intermediate between the two.
wallerian l., after section of the posterior root of a spinal nerve between the root ganglion and the spinal cord, the central portion degenerates; after division of the anterior root, the peripheral portion degenerates; the trophic center of the posterior root is therefore the ganglion, that of the anterior root the spinal cord.
Weber's l., Weber-Fechner law.
Weber-Fechner l., Fechner-Weber l.; Weber's l.; the intensity of a sensation varies by a series of equal increments (arithmetically) as the strength of the stimulus is increased geometrically; if a series of stimuli is applied and so adjusted in strength that each stimulus causes a just perceptible change in intensity of the sensation, then the strength of each stimulus differs from the preceding one by a constant fraction; thus, if a just perceptible change in a visual sensation is produced by the addition of 1 candle to an original illumination of 100 candles, 10 candles will be required to produce any change in sensation when the original illumination was one of 1000 candles.
Weigert's l., overproduction theory; the loss or destruction of a part or element in the organic world is likely to result in compensatory replacement and overproduction of tissue during the process of regeneration or repair (or both), as in the formation of callus when a fractured bone heals.
Wilder's l. of initial value, l. of initial value; the direction of response of a body function to any agent depends to a large degree on the initial level of that function.
Williston's l., as the vertebrate scale is ascended, the number of bones in the skull is reduced.
Wolff's l., every change in the form and the function of a bone, or in its function alone, is followed by certain definite changes in its internal architecture and secondary alterations in its external conformation.

Lawford's syndrome. See under syndrome.

Lawless' stain. See under stain.

Lawrence, R.D., 20th century British physician. See L.-Seip *syndrome.*

lawrencium (law-ren'sē-ŭm) [E.O. *Lawrence,* U.S. physicist and Nobel laureate, 1901–1958]. An artificial transplutonium element; symbol Lr, atomic number 103.

laxation (lak-sā'shŭn) [see laxative]. Bowel movement, with or without laxatives.

laxative (lak'să-tiv) [L. *laxativus,* fr. *laxo,* pp. *-atus,* to slacken, relax]. **1.** Mildly cathartic; having the action of loosening the bowels. **2.** A mild cathartic; a remedy that moves the bowels slightly without pain or violent action.

laxator tympani (lak-sā'tor tim'pan-ī) [Mod. L.]. One of two supposed muscles, probably ligaments of the malleus.

LAYER

layer (lā'er). A sheet of one substance lying upon another, and distinguished from it by a difference in texture or color, or by not being continuous with it. See also stratum; lamina.
ameloblastic l., enamel l.; the internal l. of the enamel organ.
anterior elastic l., *lamina* limitans anterior corneae.
anterior limiting l. of cornea, *lamina* limitans anterior corneae.
anterior l. of rectus abdominis sheath, *lamina* anterior vagina musculi recti abdominis.
bacillary l., l. of rods and cones.
basal l., *stratum* basale.
basal cell l., *stratum* basale epidermidis.
basal l. of choroid, *lamina* basalis choroideae.
basal l. of ciliary body, *lamina* basalis corporis ciliaris.
l. of Bechterew, *band* of Kaes-Bechterew.
blastodermic l.'s, the primordial cell l.'s on the yolk surface of a telolecithal egg; in earliest stages protoderm, later differentiating into ectoderm, endoderm, and mesoderm.

brown l., *lamina* fusca sclerae.
cambium l., **(1)** the inner osteogenic l. of the periosteum; **(2)** a highly cellular zone immediately beneath the epithelium covering a botryoid sarcoma.
l.'s of cerebellar cortex, see *cortex* cerebelli.
l.'s of cerebral cortex, see *cortex* cerebri.
cerebral l. of retina, *stratum* cerebrale retinae.
Chievitz' l., in the developing retina of an embryo, a transitory zone between the inner and outer neuroblastic l.'s that is devoid of nuclei.
choriocapillary l., *lamina* choroidocapillaris.
circular l.'s of muscular tunics, see *stratum* circulare tunicae muscularis coli, intestini tenuis, recti, and ventriculi.
circular l. of tympanic membrane, *stratum* circulare membranae tympani.
claustral l., the l. of subcortical gray matter between the external capsule and the white matter of the insula or extreme capsule.
clear l. of epidermis, *stratum* lucidum.
columnar l., *stratum* basale epidermidis.
conjunctival l. of bulb, *tunica* conjunctiva bulbi.
conjunctival l. of eyelids, *tunica* conjunctiva palpebrarum.
corneal l. of epidermis, *stratum* corneum epidermidis.
cornified l. of nail, *stratum* corneum unguis.
cutaneous l. of tympanic membrane, *stratum* cutaneum membranae tympani.
deep l., *lamina* profunda.
elastic l.'s of arteries, elastic *laminae* of arteries.
elastic l.'s of cornea, see *lamina* limitans anterior corneae and *lamina* limitans posterior corneae.
enamel l., ameloblastic l.
ependymal l., ventricular l.; ependymal zone; an inner epithelial l. of cells bordering the lumen of the embryonic neural tube and brain, formed during the latter's stratification, and persisting in modified form throughout life.
epithelial l.'s, see epithelium.
epithelial choroid l., *lamina* epithelialis.
epitrichial l., the superficial flattened-cell l. of the epidermis of a young embryo before the definitive stratification has developed.
fibrous l., the outer dense connective tissue l. of the periosteum.
fillet l., *stratum* lemnisci.
fusiform l., multiform, polymorphous, or spindle-celled l.; layer 6 of the cortex cerebri.
ganglionic l. of cerebellar cortex, *stratum* neuronorum piriformium.
ganglionic l. of cerebral cortex, layer 5 of the cortex cerebri.
ganglionic l. of optic nerve, *stratum* ganglionare nervi optici.
ganglionic l. of retina, *stratum* ganglionare retinae.
germ l., one of the three primordial cell l.'s (ectoderm, endoderm, mesoderm) established in an embryo during gastrulation and the immediately following stages.

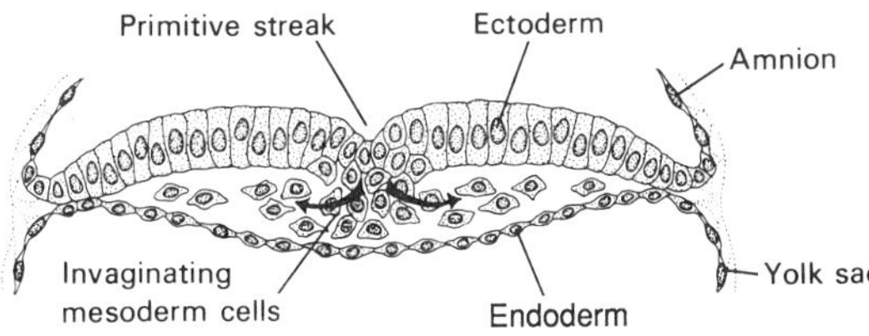

Embryonic Germ Layers
Transverse section through the region of the primitive streak of a 16-day presomite human embryo.

germinative l., *stratum* basale epidermidis.
germinative l. of nail, *stratum* germinativum unguis.
glomerular l. of olfactory bulb, a l. composed of spherical bodies, called glomeruli, formed by the synapses of mitral cells with the olfactory nerve fibers derived from the cells of the olfactory epithelium.
granular l. of cerebellar cortex, *stratum* granulosum cerebelli.
granular l.'s of cerebral cortex, layers 2 (outer) and 4 (inner) of the cortex cerebri.
granular l. of epidermis, *stratum* granulosum epidermidis.
granular l.'s of retina, nuclear l.'s of the retina.
granular l. of a vesicular ovarian follicle, *stratum* granulosum folliculi ovarici vesiculosi.
gray l. of superior colliculus, *stratum* griseum colliculi superioris.
half-value l. (HVL), the thickness of an absorber necessary to reduce the intensity of a beam of radiation to one-half its initial density.
Henle's l., the outer l. cells of the inner root sheath of the hair follicle.
Henle's fiber l., the l. of inner cone fibers in the central area of the retina.
Henle's nervous l., entoretina.
horny l. of epidermis, *stratum* corneum epidermidis.
horny l. of nail, *stratum* corneum unguis.
Huxley's l., Huxley's membrane or sheath; a l. of cells interposed between Henle's membrane and the cuticle of the inner root sheath of the hair follicle.
infragranular l., the cellular band deep to the inner granular l. of the human cerebral cortex which differentiates into the ganglionic l. and multiform l. by the sixth fetal month.
intermediate l., mantle l.
Kölliker's l., the l. of connective tissue in the iris.
Langhans' l., cytotrophoblast.
lateral l., *lamina* lateralis.
lateral cartilaginous l., *lamina* lateralis.
latticed l., a cortical cell l. in the hippocampus.
limiting l.'s of cornea, *lamina* limitans anterior corneae and posterior corneae.
longitudinal l.'s of muscular tunics, see *stratum* longitudinale tunicae muscularis coli, intestini tenuis, recti, and ventriculi.
malpighian l., malpighian *stratum.*
mantle l., intermediate l.; mantle zone (1); the nuclear zone of the developing neural tube between the marginal l. and the ependymal l.
marginal l., marginal zone; the outer, nonnuclear l. of the embryonic neural tube; into its fibrous network grow the longitudinal nerve fibers which eventually become the white matter of the cord and brain stem.
medial l., *lamina* medialis.
medial cartilaginous l., *lamina* medialis.
medullary l.'s of thalamus, *laminae* medullares thalami.
membranous l., *lamina* membranacea.
Meynert's l., pyramidal cell l.
molecular l., *stratum* moleculare.
molecular l. of cerebellar cortex, *stratum* moleculare cerebelli.
molecular l. of cerebral cortex, plexiform l. of cerebral cortex; layer 1 of the cortex cerebri.
molecular l.'s of olfactory bulb, the l.'s, composed mainly of nerve fibers, on the outer and inner sides of the l. of mitral cells of the bulb.
molecular l. of retina, *stratum* moleculare retinae.
multiform l., fusiform l.
muscular l. of mucosa, *lamina* muscularis mucosae.
neural l. of retina, *stratum* cerebrale retinae.
neuroepithelial l. of retina, *stratum* neuroepitheliale retinae.
Nitabuch's l., Nitabuch's *membrane.*
nuclear l.'s of retina, granular l.'s of the retina; stratum nucleare externum et internum retinae; the outer nuclear layer, layer 4, of the retina, *stratum* neuroepitheliale retinae, and the inner layer, layer 6, of the retina, *stratum* ganglionare retinae.
odontoblastic l., a l. of connective tissue cells at the periphery of

the dental pulp of the tooth.
optic l., *stratum* opticum.
orbital l. of ethmoid bone, *lamina* orbitalis ossis ethmoidalis.
osteogenetic l., the inner bone-forming l. of the periosteum.
palisade l., *stratum* basale epidermidis.
papillary l., *stratum* papillare corii.
parietal l., *lamina* parietalis.
perforated l. of sclera, *lamina* cribrosa sclerae.
pigmented l. of ciliary body, *stratum* pigmenti corporis ciliaris.
pigmented l. of iris, *stratum* pigmenti iridis.
pigmented l. of retina, *stratum* pigmenti retinae.
l. of piriform neurons, *stratum* neuronorum piriformium.
plasma l., still l.
plexiform l., *stratum* moleculare.
plexiform l. of cerebral cortex, molecular l. of cerebral cortex.
plexiform l.'s of retina, *stratum* plexiforme externum et internum retinae; l.'s of the retina where synapses occur; in the external l., processes of rods and cones synapse with bipolar neuron dendrites; in the internal l., axon terminals of bipolar cells synapse with ganglion cell dendrites. See retina.
polymorphous l., fusiform l.
posterior elastic l., *lamina* limitans posterior corneae.
posterior limiting l. of cornea, *lamina* limitans posterior corneae.
posterior l. of rectus abdominis sheath, *lamina* posterior vaginae musculi recti abdominis.
pretracheal l., *lamina* pretrachealis.
prevertebral l., *lamina* prevertebralis.
prickle cell l., *stratum* spinosum epidermidis.
Purkinje's l., *stratum* neuronorum piriformium.
pyramidal cell l., Meynert's l.; layer 3 of the cortex cerebri.
radiate l. of tympanic membrane, *stratum* radiatum membranae tympani.
Rauber's l., the thinned out trophoblastic membrane over the embryonic disk in developing carnivores and ungulates.
reticular l. of corium, *stratum* reticulare corii.
l.'s of retina, see retina.
l. of rods and cones, bacillary l.; the l. of the retina next to the pigment l. and containing the visual receptors; see also retina; granular l.'s of the retina; *stratum* neuroepitheliale retinae.
rostral l., *lamina* rostralis.
Sattler's elastic l., the middle l. of the choroid.
l.'s of skin, see epidermis; corium.
sluggish l., still l.
somatic l., the external l. of the lateral mesoderm of the embryo, lying adjacent to the ectoderm and together with it constituting the somatopleure.
spindle-celled l., fusiform l.
spinous l., *stratum* spinosum epidermidis.
splanchnic l., the internal l. of the lateral mesoderm, lying adjacent to the endoderm and together with it forming the splanchnopleure.
still l., sluggish or plasma l.; Poiseuille's space; the l. of the bloodstream in the capillary vessels, next to the wall of the vessel, that flows slowly and transports the white blood cells along the l. wall, while in the center the flow is rapid and transports the red blood cells.
subendocardial l., the loose connective tissue l. that joins the endocardium and myocardium; in the ventricles, it contains branches of the conducting system of the heart.
subendothelial l., the thin l. of connective tissue lying between the endothelium and elastic lamina in the intima of blood vessels.
subpapillary l., the vascular l. of the corium.
superficial l., *lamina* superficialis.
suprachoroid l., *lamina* suprachoroidea.
Tomes' granular l., a thin l. of dentin adjacent to the cementum, appearing granular in ground sections; the granules are small uncalcified spaces.
vascular l., *lamina* vasculosa choroideae.
vascular l. of choroid coat of eye, *lamina* vasculosa choroideae.
ventricular l., ependymal l.
visceral l., *lamina* visceralis.
Waldeyer's zonal l., *fasciculus* dorsolateralis.
Weil's basal l., Weil's basal zone; the l. beneath the odontoblasts of the tooth; it contains reticular fibers but few if any cells.
zonular l., *stratum* zonale.

lazaret, lazaretto (laz'ă-ret, -ret'ō) [It. *lazzaretto,* fr. *lazzaro,* a leper]. Obsolete term for: **1.** Leprosarium. **2.** A hospital for the treatment of contagious diseases. **3.** A place of detention for persons in quarantine.

LBF Abbreviation for *Lactobacillus bulgaricus* factor.

LBT Abbreviation for lupus band *test.*

LD Abbreviation for lethal *dose.*

LDH Abbreviation for *lactate* dehydrogenase.

LDL Abbreviation for low density lipoprotein. See lipoprotein.

LE, L.E. Abbreviation for left eye; *lupus* erythematosus.

leaching (lēch'ing) [A.S. *leccan,* to wet]. Lixiviation; removal of the soluble constituents of a substance by running water through it.

lead (led). Plumbum; a metallic element, symbol Pb, atomic no. 82, atomic weight 207.21; occurs in nature as an oxide or one of the salts, but chiefly as the sulfide, or galena.
l. acetate, sugar of l.; has been used as an astringent in diarrhea, and in aqueous solution as a wet dressing in certain dermatoses.
black l., graphite.
l. carbonate, white l.; ceruse; a heavy white powder that is insoluble in water; occasionally, it is used to relieve irritation in dermatitis, but it is used largely in the manufacture of paint and in the arts and is thus productive of l. poisoning.
l. chromate, chrome yellow.
l. monoxide, l. oxide; l. oxide (yellow); massicot; litharge; has been used as an ingredient in external applications such as l. plaster.
l. oxide (yellow), l. monoxide.
red l., l. tetroxide.
red oxide of l., l. tetroxide.
l. sulfide, PbS; galena; the native form in which l. is chiefly found.
l. tetraethyl, tetraethyllead.
l. tetroxide, red l.; red oxide of l.; a bright orange-red powder that turns black when heated; used in ointments and plasters.
white l., l. carbonate.

lead (lēd). The electrical connection for taking records by means of the electrocardiograph.
ABC l.'s, the l.'s for recording a vectorcardiogram utilizing the Arrighi triangle.
bipolar l., a record obtained with two electrodes placed on different regions of the body, each electrode contributing significantly to the record; *e.g.,* a standard limb l.
CB l., a chest l. with the indifferent electrode placed upon the subject's back.
CF l., a chest l. with the indifferent electrode placed on the subject's left leg.
chest l.'s, precordial l.'s; semidirect l.'s; those in which the exploring electrode is on the chest overlying the heart or its vicinity.
CL l., a chest l. with the indifferent electrode placed on the subject's left arm.
CR l., a chest l. with the indifferent electrode placed on the subject's right arm.
direct l., in electrocardiography, a l. recorded with the exploring electrode placed directly on the surface of the exposed heart.
esophageal l., a record obtained with the exploring electrode lying within the lumen of the esophagus; of particular value in obtaining

sizable atrial deflections and therefore helpful in the recognition of arrhythmias.

indirect l., standard l.

intracardiac l., the record obtained when the exploring electrode is placed within one of the heart's chambers, usually by means of cardiac catheterization.

limb l., one of the three standard l.'s or one of the unipolar limb l.'s (aVR, aVL, aVF).

precordial l.'s, chest l.'s.

semidirect l.'s, chest l.'s.

standard l., indirect l.; one of the three original bipolar limb l.'s of the clinical electrocardiogram, designated I, II and III: l. I records the potential difference between the right and left arms; l. II the difference between right arm and left leg; and l. III the difference between left arm and left leg.

unipolar l.'s, those in which the exploring electrode is on the chest in the vicinity of the heart or on one of the limbs, while the other or indifferent electrode is the central terminal.

V l., a chest l. with the central terminal as the indifferent electrode.

League of Red Cross Societies. The international federation of national Red Cross and similar societies.

learned helplessness. A laboratory model of depression involving both classical (respondent) and instrumental (operant) conditioning techniques; application of unavoidable shock is followed by failure to cope in situations where coping might otherwise be possible.

learning (lern'ing). Generic term for the relatively permanent change in behavior that occurs as a result of practice. See also conditioning, forgetting, memory.

incidental l., passive l.; l. without a direct attempt.

latent l., that l. which is not evident to the observer at the time it occurs, but which is inferred from later performance in which l. is more rapid than would be expected without the earlier experience.

passive l., incidental l.

rote l., the l. of arbitrary relationships, usually by repetition of the l. procedure through memorization and without an understanding of the relationships.

state-dependent l., l. during a specific state of sleep or wakefulness, or during a chemically altered state, where retrieval of learned information (*e.g.,* as measured by performance of a learned response) cannot be demonstrated unless the subject is restored to the state that originally existed during l.

Le Bel, Joseph Achille, French chemist, 1847–1930. See L. B.-van't Hoff *rule.*

Leber, Theodor, German ophthalmologist, 1840–1917. See L.'s hereditary optic *atrophy, plexus,* idiopathic stellate *retinopathy; amaurosis* congenita of L.

Le Chatelier, Henri L., French physical chemist, 1850–1936. See L. C.'s *law, principle.*

lecithal (les'i-thăl) [G. *lekithos,* egg yolk]. Having a yolk or pertaining to the yolk of any egg; used especially as a suffix.

lecithin (les'i-thin) [G. *lekithos,* egg yolk]. Traditional term for 1,2-diacyl-*sn*-glycero-3-phosphocolines or 3-*sn*-phosphatidylcholines, phospholipids that on hydrolysis yield two fatty acid molecules and a molecule each of glycerophosphoric acid and choline. In some varieties of l., both fatty acids are saturated, others contain only unsaturated acids (*e.g.,* oleic, linoleic, or arachidonic acid); in others again, one fatty acid is saturated, the other unsaturated. L.'s are yellowish or brown waxy substances, readily miscible in water in which they appear under the microscope as irregular elongated particles known as "myelin forms," and are found in nervous tissue, especially in the myelin sheaths, in egg yolk, and as essential constituents of animal and vegetable cells.

l. acyltransferase, lecithin-cholesterol acyltransferase.

lecithinase (les'i-thi-nās). Phospholipase.

l. A, phospholipase A_2.

l. B, lysophospholipase.

l. C, phospholipase C.

l. D, phospholipase D.

lecithin-cholesterol acyltransferase [EC 2.3.1.43]. Lecithin acyltransferase; an enzyme that transfers an acyl residue from a lecithin to cholesterol, forming a 1-acylglycerophosphocholine (a lysolecithin) and a cholesterol ester.

lecithoblast (les'i-thō-blast) [G. *lekithos,* egg yolk, + *blastos,* germ]. One of the cells proliferating to form the yolk-sac endoderm.

lecithoprotein (les'i-thō-prō'tēn). A conjugated protein, with lecithin as the prosthetic group.

Leclef. See Denys-Leclef *phenomenon.*

lectin (lek'tin). A protein of plant (usually seed) or animal origin that effects agglutination, precipitation, or other phenomena resembling the action of specific antibody, but that is not an antibody in that it was not evoked by an antigenic stimulus; l.'s include plant agglutinins (phytoagglutinins, phytohemagglutinins), plant precipitins, and perhaps certain animal proteins; some have mitogenic properties.

Lederer, Max, U.S. pathologist, 1885–1952. See L.'s *anemia.*

ledge (lej). In anatomy, a structure resembling a ledge. See also shelf; lamina.

dental l., a band of ectodermal cells growing from the epithelium of the embryonic jaws into the underlying mesenchyme; local buds from the l. give rise to the primordia of the enamel organs of the teeth. Also called enamel l.; dental shelf; dental, primary dental, or dentogingival lamina.

enamel l., dental l.

Lee, Robert, British physician, 1793–1877. See L.'s *ganglion.*

Lee, Roger I., U.S. physician, *1881. See L.-White *method.*

leech (lēch) [A.S. *laece,* a physician; a leech, because of its therapeutic use]. **1.** A bloodsucking aquatic annelid worm (genus *Hirudo,* class Hirudinea) formerly used in medicine for local withdrawal of blood. For various l. species, see *Hirudo.* **2.** To treat medically by applying leeches.

Leede, Carl S., U.S. physician, *1882. See Rumpel-L. *sign, test.*

Leeuwenhoek, Anton van, Dutch microscopist, 1632–1723. See L.'s *canals.*

Lefèvre, Paul, 20th century French dermatologist. See Papillon-L. *syndrome.*

Le Fort, Léon C., French surgeon and gynecologist, 1829–1893. See L. *sound;* L.'s *amputation, fracture.*

left-eyed. Sinistrocular.

left-footed. Sinistropedal.

left-handed. Sinistromanual; denoting the habitual or more skillful use of the left hand for writing and for most manual operations.

left-sidedness. The normal left-sided location of certain unpaired organs, such as the spleen and most of the stomach.

bilateral l., polysplenia syndrome; a syndrome in which normally unpaired organs develop more symmetrically in mirror image; two spleens, one on each side, are usually present, and cardiovascular anomalies are common.

leg. The segment of the inferior limb between the knee and the ankle; commonly used to mean the entire inferior limb.

l. of antihelix, *crus* anthelicis.

Barbados l., elephantiasis.

bow-l., bowleg. See *genu* varum.

elephant l., elephantiasis.

milk l., *phlegmasia* alba dolens.

restless l.'s, restless legs *syndrome.*

rider's l., a strain of the adductor muscles of the thigh.
scaly l., a thickened, encrusted condition of the legs of fowls caused by the mite, *Knemidokoptes mutans*.
tennis l., a rupture of the gastrocnemius muscle at the musculotendinous junction, resulting from forcible contractions of the calf muscles; commonly seen in tennis players.
white l., *phlegmasia* alba dolens.

Legal, Emmo, German physician, 1859–1922. See L.'s *test*.

Legendre, Gaston L.J., French physician, *1887. See L.'s *sign*.

Legg, Arthur T., U.S. surgeon, 1874–1939. See L.-Calvé-Perthes *disease*.

-legia [L. *legere*, to read]. Suffix, that properly relates to reading, as distinguished from the G. derivatives, *-lexis* and *-lexy*, which signify speech.

Legionella (lē-jŭ-nel'lă). A genus of aerobic, motile, non acid-fast, non-encapsulated, Gram-negative bacilli (family Legionellaceae) that have a nonfermentative metabolism and require L-cysteine-HCl and iron salts for growth; they are water-dwelling and airborne spread, and are pathogenic for man. The type species is *L. pneumophila*.
L. bozeman'ii, a species that causes human pneumonia.
L. micda'dei, Pittsburgh pneumonia agent; a species that causes Pittsburgh pneumonia, a variant of Legionnaires' disease.
L. pneumo'phila, a species that is the etiologic agent of Legionnaires' disease; it is the type species of the genus *L.*

legionellosis (lē-jŭ-nel-ō'sis). Legionnaires' *disease*.

legumin (lĕ-gū'min, leg'ū-min). Avenin.

leguminivorous (le-gū-mi-niv'ō-rŭs). Feeding on beans, peas, and other legumes.

Lehmann, J.O. Orla, Swedish physician, *1927. See Börjeson-Forssman-L. *syndrome*.

Leichtenstern, Otto, German physician, 1845–1900. See L.'s *phenomenon, sign*.

Leigh, Denis, British psychiatrist, *1915. See L.'s *disease*.

Leiner, Karl, Austrian pediatrician, 1871–1930. See L.'s *disease*.

leio- [G. *leios*, smooth]. Combining form meaning smooth. See also lio-.

leiodermia (lī-ō-der'mē-ă) [leio- + G. *derma*, skin]. Smooth, glossy skin.

leiomyofibroma (lī-ō-mī'ō-fī-brō'mă). Fibroleiomyoma.

leiomyoma (lī'ō-mī-ō'mă) [leio- + G. *mys*, muscle, + *-oma*, tumor]. A benign neoplasm derived from smooth (nonstriated) muscle.
l. cu'tis, dermatomyoma; cutaneous eruption of small painful nodules composed of smooth muscle fibers.
parasitic l., a uterine l. which has become detached from the uterus and adherent to another peritoneal surface from which it derives a blood supply.
vascular l., angioleiomyoma; angiomyofibroma; angiomyoma; a markedly vascular l., apparently arising from the smooth muscle of blood vessels.

leiomyomatosis (lī'ō-mī'ō-mă-tō'sis). The state of having multiple leiomyomas throughout the body.

leiomyosarcoma (lī'ō-mī'ō-sar-kō'mă) [leio- + myosarcoma]. A malignant neoplasm derived from smooth (nonstriated) muscle.

leiotrichous (lī-ot'ri-kŭs) [leio- + G. *thrix*, hair]. Having straight hair.

leipo-. For words so beginning see lipo-.

Leipzig yellow [C.I. 77600]. *Chrome* yellow.

Leishman, Sir William B., British surgeon, 1865–1926. See *Leishmania*; L.'s chrome *cells, stain*; L.-Donovan *body*.

Leishmania (lēsh-man'ē-ă) [W. B. *Leishman*]. A genus of digenetic, asexual, protozoan flagellates (family Trypanosomatidae) that occur as amastigotes in the macrophages of vertebrate hosts, and as promastigotes in invertebrate hosts and in cultures. Species are largely indistinguishable morphologically, but may be separated by clinical manifestations, geographic distribution and epidemiology, developmental patterns of promastigotes in their sandfly hosts, virulence testing of clones *in vivo*, the effect of test sera on growth in culture, cross-immunity tests, and serotyping with promastigote excreted factors; strains also can be distinguished by various biochemical analyses. Such procedures have identified all of the recognized groups and confirmed the separation of New World leishmaniasis agents into two species complexes, *L. mexicana* and *L. braziliensis*.
L. aethio'pica, a recently discovered African species of *L.* responsible for human cutaneous leishmaniasis in Ethiopia, with a reservoir of human infection in the rock hyraxes, *Procavia capensis* and *Heterohyrax brucei*, and in Kenya, with reservoirs in the tree hyrax, *Dendrohyrax arboreus*, and the giant rat, *Cricetomys gambianus;* vectors are the sandflies *Phlebotomus longpipes* and *P. pedifer*. It causes a cutaneous leishmaniasis of three types: classical oriental sore, mucocutaneous leishmaniasis, and diffuse cutaneous leishmaniasis; ulceration is late or absent and healing takes one to three years.
L. brazilien'sis, a species that is the causal agent of mucocutaneous leishmaniasis, endemic in southern Mexico and Central and South America, and transmitted by various species of *Lutzomyia* (New World sandflies); forest rodents and other neotropical arboreal animals serve as reservoir hosts. *L. braziliensis* is currently divided into three clinically, epidemiologically, and biochemically distinct strains or subspecies: *L. b. braziliensis, L. b. guyanensis,* and *L. b. panamensis*.
L. brazilien'sis brazilien'sis, the type subspecies of *L. braziliensis* and the agent of mucocutaneous leishmaniasis. A natural reservoir of infection remains unknown, but the proven vector in Brazil is *Lutzomyia (Psychodopygus) wellcomei;* other sandflies may also transmit the infection.
L. brazilien'sis guyanen'sis, a subspecies within the *L. braziliensis* complex from Brazil and Guyana, and the cause of the cutaneous leishmaniasis condition locally known as "pian bois"; the reservoir host in Brazil is the sloth *Choloepus hoffmani* and the vector is the sandfly *Lutzomyia umbratilis*.
L. brazilien'sis panamen'sis, a subspecies of *L. braziliensis* found in Panama, Colombia, and neighboring regions; it causes ulcerating lesions of cutaneous leishmaniasis which do not heal spontaneously and often involve nearby lymphatic tissues, but nasopharyngeal involvement is rare. The sloth *Choloepus hoffmani* is the reservoir in Panama and Costa Rica; the sandfly *Lutzomyia trapidoi* has been proven to be a vector.
L. donova'ni, a species that is the causal agent of visceral leishmaniasis in Mediterranean and adjacent countries, the south central USSR, eastern India, northern China, Kenya, Ethiopia, and the Sudan; also found in Brazil, Argentina, Colombia, and Venezuela; in the Old World, it is transmitted by various species of *Phlebotomus;* New World vectors are presumed to be species of *Lutzomyia;* dogs and other carnivores are known as reservoir hosts in some areas. The intracellular amastigote form multiplies in macrophages and produces a reticuloendothelial hyperplasia grossly affecting the spleen and liver, with other lymphoid tissues being involved as well, resulting in severe hepatosplenomegaly which usually is fatal if untreated.
L. donova'ni archibal'di, see *L. donovani donovani*.
L. donova'ni chaga'si, a subspecies of *L.* found in South America, chiefly in Brazil, producing visceral leishmaniasis; infections have been found in domestic dogs and in foxes, though the primary reservoir host is unclear. The vector remains undiscovered, and the taxonomic status of this subspecies is uncertain.
L. donova'ni donova'ni, the type subspecies and agent of visceral leishmaniasis in Asia, Africa, and the Indian subcontinent; a few

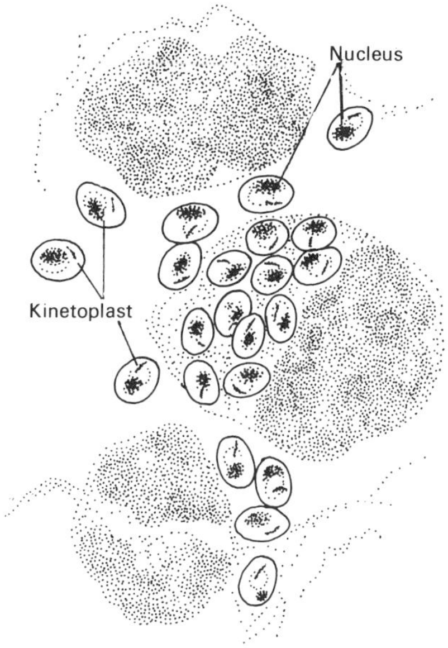

Leishmania donovani
Leishmanial forms of parasite in bone marrow smear (×2000).

cases occur in the south central USSR, and in Iran, Iraq, and possibly Yemen; the dog and jackal are animal reservoirs. The form in Africa may be this subspecies, though the name *L. donovani archibaldi* is also used.
L. donova'ni infan'tum, a strain or subspecies of *L. donovani* that causes visceral leishmaniasis in young children in Mediterranean countries; the reservoir is the domestic dog.
L. furunculo'sa, former name for *L. tropica.*
L. ma'jor, *L. tropica major;* a species responsible for zoonotic cutaneous leishmaniasis in a large area of the Mediterranean region and Asia Minor. The animal reservoirs are usually ground squirrels, such as *Rhombomys opimus* in the USSR and elsewhere in south central Asia, and other rodents in northwest India, the Middle East, and northern Africa; proven sandfly vectors include *Phlebotomous papatasi, P. duboscqi,* and *P. salehi.*
L. mexica'na, *L. tropica mexicana;* the agent of many forms of cutaneous leishmaniasis, now considered a complex of several subspecies or possibly species, each with distinctive DNA and enzyme characteristics, distribution, and vector-reservoir host association, resulting in distinct manifestations of human leishmaniasis; reservoir hosts are extremely diverse and include a wide array of arboreal rodents as well as marsupials, primates, and small carnivores. Typical disease forms caused by this species are chiclero's ulcer and diffuse cutaneous leishmaniasis, in contrast with mucocutaneous leishmaniasis, more characteristic of *L. braziliensis* infection.
L. mexica'na amazonen'sis, a particularly widespread form of *L. mexicana* in the Amazon basin (Bolivia, Brazil, Colombia, Ecuador, and southern Venezuela), where it infects a variety of forest rodents, the reservoirs of human infection. The disease is rare in man, but the single or multiple lesions, when induced, rarely heal spontaneously; the disseminated form is common, but nasopharyngeal involvement does not occur. The vector is the sandfly *Lutzomyia flaviscutellata.*
L. mexica'na garnha'mi, a recently described subspecies of *L. mexicana,* found in western Venezuela, causing single or multiple lesions in man that heal spontaneously in about six months; the probable sandfly vector is *Lutzomyia townsendi.*
L. mexica'na mexica'na, a species described from Mexico, Guatemala, and Belize; agent of a form of New World cutaneous leishmaniasis called chiclero's ulcer, associated with chicle gum and mahogany forest workers. The New World sandfly, *Lutzomyia olmcca,* is a proven vector of this subspecies.
L. mexica'na pifa'noi, *L. pifanoi;* a strain of *L. mexicana* accorded species status by those who consider it responsible for the diffuse or disseminated form of cutaneous leishmaniasis. It is responsible for this condition in Venezuela, where it was described, but it is now recognized that several species and subspecies of *L.* cause similar disseminated forms of leishmaniasis in widely separated regions (*L. mexicana amazonensis, L. aethiopica*); absence or suppression of the cell-mediated immune response in the host is also an important factor in induction of diffuse cutaneous leishmaniasis.
L. mexica'na venezuelen'sis, a recently described subspecies of *L. mexicana* from Venezuela that causes indolent, nodular, single lesions of cutaneous leishmaniasis to develop, sometimes with curable disseminated cutaneous leishmaniasis; infection has also been found in equines.
L. peruvia'na, species of *L.* found infecting man in the high Andean valleys of Peru and Bolivia; cause of a distinct form of New World cutaneous leishmaniasis called uta.
L. pifa'noi, *L. mexicana pifanoi.*
L. trop'ica, species that is the causal agent of anthroponotic cutaneous leishmaniasis; formerly endemic throughout the Mediterranean basin, the Middle East, parts of the southern USSR and elsewhere in Asia, and also reported from western Africa: it is transmitted by *Phlebotomus papatasii, P. sergenti,* and related species of sandflies; small rodents such as various ground squirrels serve as reservoir hosts.
L. trop'ica ma'jor, *L. major.*
L. trop'ica mexica'na, *L. mexicana.*

leishmaniasis (lēsh'mă-nī'ă-sis). Leishmaniosis; infection with a species of *Leishmania* resulting in a clinically ill-defined group of diseases traditionally divided into four major types: 1) visceral l. (kala azar); 2) Old World cutaneous l.; 3) New World cutaneous l.; 4) mucocutaneous l. Each is clinically and geographically distinct and each has in recent years been further subdivided into clinical and epidemiological subdivisions to give a more natural breakdown. Transmission is by various sandfly species of the genus *Phlebotomus* or *Lutzomyia.*
acute cutaneous l., zoonotic cutaneous l.
American l., l. america'na, mucocutaneous l.
anergic l., diffuse cutaneous l.
anthroponotic cutaneous l., urban, chronic, or dry cutaneous l.; a form of Old World cutaneous l. confined to urban areas in Syria, Iran, Iraq, Israel, Kuwait, Afghanistan, Greece, and possibly Turkey, Pakistan, and the USSR, where it formerly was more common and widespread. No animal reservoir host has been found, but proven vector sandflies are *Phlebotomous papatasi* and *P. sergenti.* The lesion tends to be a painless, chronic, dry ulceration that develops two to eight months after the bite, healing spontaneously in about a year, and often leaving a characteristic disfiguring indented scar.
canine l., a mild infection of dogs, usually confined to the muzzle or ears, produced by human disease-causing species of *Leishmania;* dogs therefore are important reservoirs of human infection, such as with visceral l. in the Mediterranean region.
chronic cutaneous l., anthroponotic cutaneous l.
cutaneous l., Old World l.; juccuya; infection with promastigotes (leptomonads) of *Leishmania tropica* and of *L. major* inoculated into the skin by the bite of an infected sandfly, *Phlebotomus* (commonly *P. papatasi*); it is endemic in parts of Asia Minor, northern Africa, and India, and is known by innumerable names, each indicating its locality (*e.g.,* Aleppo, Bagdad, Delhi, or Jericho boil; Aden ulcer; Biskra button); the ulcer begins as a papule that enlarges to a nodule and then breaks down into an ulcer. Two distinctive clinical and epidemiological diseases are recognized, the more

common and widespread zoonotic rural disease with a moist acute form, caused by *L. major,* with reservoir rodent hosts; and an urban, anthroponotic, dry, chronic form of l. caused by *L. tropica,* without a reservoir host, and now largely controlled. See zoonotic cutaneous l.; anthroponotic cutaneous l.
diffuse l., diffuse cutaneous l.
diffuse cutaneous l., diffuse, pseudolepromatous, or anergic l.; disseminated cutaneous l.; l. tegumentaria diffusa; l. caused by several New and Old World species and strains of *Leishmania* (*L. mexicana amazonensis, L. m. pifanoi,* possibly *L. m. garnhami* and *L. m. venezuelensis;* in Ethiopia, *L. aethiopica,* and unidentified leishmanial agents in Namibia and Tanzania). The condition is associated with a suppressed cell-mediated immune response, so that the non-ulcerating, non-necrotizing cutaneous lesions can spread widely over the body; great numbers of parasite-filled macrophages are found in the dermal lesions. Healing does not appear to occur unless an acquired cellular hypersensitivity can develop.
disseminated cutaneous l., diffuse cutaneous l.
dry cutaneous l., anthroponotic cutaneous l.
infantile l., visceral l. in infants, from *Leishmania donovani infantum.*
lupoid l., l. recidivans.
mucocutaneous l., New World, American, or nasopharyngeal l.; l. americana; a grave disease caused by *Leishmania braziliensis braziliensis,* endemic in southern Mexico and Central and South America, except for the equatorial region of Chile; the organism does not invade the viscera, and the disease is limited to the skin and mucous membranes, the lesions resembling the sores of cutaneous l. caused by *L. mexicana* or *L. tropica;* the chancrous sores heal after a time, but some months or years later, fungating and eroding forms of ulceration may appear on the tongue and buccal or nasal mucosa; many variants of the disease exist, marked by differences in distribution, vector, epidemiology, and pathology, which suggest that it may in fact be caused by a number of closely related etiological agents. See also espundia.
nasopharyngeal l., mucocutaneous l.
New World l., mucocutaneous l.
Old World l., cutaneous l.
pseudolepromatous l., diffuse cutaneous l.
l. recid'ivans, lupoid l.; a partially healing leishmanial lesion caused by *Leishmania tropica* and characterized by an extreme form of cellular immune response, intense granuloma production, fibrinoid necrosis without caseation, and frequent development of satellite lesions that continue the production of granulomatous tissue without healing, sometimes over a period of many years; organisms are difficult to demonstrate but can be cultured.
rural cutaneous l., zoonotic cutaneous l.
l. tegumenta'ria diffu'sa, diffuse cutaneous l.
urban cutaneous l., anthroponotic cutaneous l.
visceral l., kala azar; tropical splenomegaly; black sickness; Assam, Burdwan, cachectic, or Dumdum fever; a chronic disease, occurring in India, Assam, China, the USSR, Kenya, Sudan, and various parts of South America (chiefly Brazil), caused by *Leishmania donovani* and transmitted by the bite of an appropriate species of sandfly of the genus *Phlebotomus* or *Lutzomyia;* the organisms grow and multiply in macrophages, eventually causing them to burst and liberate amastigote parasites which then invade other macrophages; proliferation of macrophages in the bone marrow causes crowding out of erythroid and myeloid elements, resulting in leukopenia, and anemia, splenomegaly, and hepatomegaly which are characteristic, along with enlargement of lymph nodes; fever, fatigue, malaise, and secondary infections also occur.
wet cutaneous l., zoonotic cutaneous l.
zoonotic cutaneous l., rural, wet, or acute cutaneous l.; a form of cutaneous l. characterized by rural distribution of human cases near infected rodents, particularly communal ground squirrels; characterized by acute rapidly developing dermal lesions that become severely inflamed, with moist necrotizing sores or ulcers that heal in two to eight months after a two to four month incubation period; among nonimmune immigrants, multiple lesions may develop, which heal more slowly and leave disabling or disfiguring scars. A strong delayed hypersensitivity and involvement of immune complexes play a role in necrosis, which is part of the healing process and of the strong specific immunity that follows.

leishmaniosis (lēsh'man-ē-ō'sis). Leishmaniasis.

leishmanoid (lēsh'mă-noyd). A condition resembling leishmaniasis.
dermal l., post-kala azar dermal l.
post-kala azar dermal l., dermal l.; a chronic, progressive, granulomatous, nonulcerating hypopigmented nodular cutaneous outbreak that may appear 6 months to 5 years after spontaneous or drug cure of visceral leishmaniasis (kala azar); this condition was first described in India and is most characteristic of kala azar in that country.

Leiter, Russell G., U.S. psychologist, *1901. See L. International Performance *Scale.*

Lejeune, Jerôme J.L.M., French cytogeneticist, *1926. See L. *syndrome.*

lema (lē'mă) [G. *lēmē,* a humor, gum, rheum]. Sebum palpebrale; secretions from a meibomian gland, collected at the inner canthus.

Lembert, Antoine, French surgeon, 1802–1851. See L.'s *suture,* Czerny-L. *suture.*

lemic (lē'mik) [G. *loimos,* plague]. Relating to plague or any epidemic disease.

Lemli, Luc. See Smith-L.-Opitz *syndrome.*

lemmoblast (lem'ō-blast) [G. *lemma,* husk, + *blastos,* germ]. In an embryo, a cell of neural crest origin capable of forming a cell of the neurolemma sheath.

lemmocyte (lem'ō-sīt) [G. *lemma,* husk, + *kytos,* cell]. One of the cells of the neurolemma.

lemniscus, pl. **lemnisci** (lem-nis'kŭs, -nis'ī) [L. from G. *lēmniskos,* ribbon or fillet] [NA]. Fillet (1); a bundle of nerve fibers ascending from sensory relay nuclei to the thalamus.
acoustic l., l. lateralis.
auditory l., l. lateralis.
gustatory l., the uncrossed secondary-sensory fiber system ascending from the rhombencephalic gustatory nucleus to the parabrachial nuclei (rostral pontine level) and directly to the thalamic gustatory nucleus (ventral postero-medial nucleus, pars parvicellularis).
l. latera'lis [NA], acoustic l.; auditory l. or tract; lateral fillet; a bundle of ascending fibers that originate from the cochlear and auditory relay nuclei of the rhombencephalon, enter the corpus trapezoideum, a transverse fiber stratum in which about half their number decussate, and from here turn rostrally along the lateral side of the spinothalamic tract; in the midbrain, it arches dorsally and enters the inferior colliculus in which all of its fibers terminate; the auditory pathway is transsynaptically extended from here by the brachium of the inferior colliculus to the medial geniculate body of the thalamus, from which in turn the auditory radiation leads to the auditory cortex; intercalated in the trapezoid body and along the ascending trajectory of the l. are several cell groups in which part of the fibers synapse.
medial l., l. medialis.
l. media'lis [NA], medial fillet or l.; Reil's ribbon or band (2); a band of white fibers originating from the gracile and nuclei and decussating in the lower medulla; thence it passes upward through the center of the medulla oblongata, close to the median raphe; on entering the pons it spreads out laterally to form a flat band ascending over the dorsal border of the pontine nuclei; in the mesencephalon it passes over the dorsal border of the substantia nigra and is displaced laterally by the red nucleus; passing medial to the

medial geniculate body, the bundle enters and terminates in the nucleus ventralis posterior of the thalamus. Throughout their course, the fibers retain a somatotopic order such that those originating from the nucleus gracilis and representing the lower extremity lie lateral to those originating in the nucleus cuneatus and representing the arm. The l. medialis conveys somatic-sensory information involved in tactile discrimination (two-point discrimination), position sense, and vibration sense.
l. spina'lis [NA], *tractus* spinothalamicus.
trigeminal l., l. trigeminalis.
l. trigemina'lis [NA], trigeminal l.; collective term denoting the fibers ascending from the sensory nucleus of the trigeminus; one such fiber system originates from the main sensory nucleus, largely decussates, and joins the medial l. with which it enters the nucleus ventralis posterior thalami, terminating in the mediodorsal region of that nucleus; a second, uncrossed, fiber group follows an ascending course through central parts of the mesencephalic tegmentum ("dorsal trigeminal l."). The l. trigeminalis conveys tactile, pain, and temperature impulses from the skin of the face, the mucous membranes of the nasal and oral cavities, and the eye, as well as proprioceptive information from the facial and masticatory muscles.

lemon (lem'ŏn) [L. *limon*]. The fruit of *Citrus limon* (family Rutaceae); a source of citric and ascorbic acid; the freshly expressed juice of the ripe fruit is used as a refrigerant diuretic in fever, in the form of lemonade.

lemon yellow. *Chrome* yellow.

Lendrum, A.C., 20th century Scottish pathologist. See L.'s phloxine-tartrazine *stain;* Fraser-L. *stain* for fibrin.

Lenègre, Jean, 20th century French cardiologist. See L.'s *disease, syndrome.*

length. Linear distance between two points.
arch l., the amount of space required for the permanent teeth as measured from the mesial aspect of the first molar on one side to the mesial aspect of the first molar on the opposite side, as measured through the contact points along an imaginary line of the dental arch.
available arch l., the amount of space available for the permanent teeth around the dental arch from first permanent molar to first permanent molar.
crown-heel l., l. of an outstretched embryo or fetus from skull vertex to heel.
crown-rump l. (CR, CRL), a measurement from the skull vertex to the midpoint between the apices of the buttocks of an embryo or fetus, that permits approximation of embryonic or fetal age.
required arch l., the sum of the mesiodistal widths of the permanent teeth from first permanent molar to first permanent molar.

Lenhossék, Michael (Mihály) von, Hungarian anatomist, 1863–1937. See L.'s *processes.*

lenitive (len'i-tiv) [L. *lenio,* pp. *lenitus,* to soften, fr. *lenis,* mild]. **1.** Soothing; relieving discomfort or pain. **2.** Rarely used term for a demulcent.

Lennert, K. See L.'s *lymphoma;* L. *classification.*

Lennox, William G., U.S. neurologist, *1884. See L. *syndrome;* L.-Gastaut *syndrome.*

Lenoir, Camille A.H., French anatomist, *1867. See L.'s *facet.*

lens (lenz) [L. a lentil]. **1.** A transparent material with one or both surfaces having a concave or convex curve; acts upon electromagnetic energy to cause convergence or divergence of light rays. **2** [NA]. Crystalline l.; the transparent biconvex cellular refractive structure lying between the iris and the vitreous, consisting of a soft outer part (cortex) with a denser part (nucleus), and surrounded by a basement membrane (capsule); the anterior surface has a cuboidal epithelium, and at the equator the cells elongate to become lens fibers.

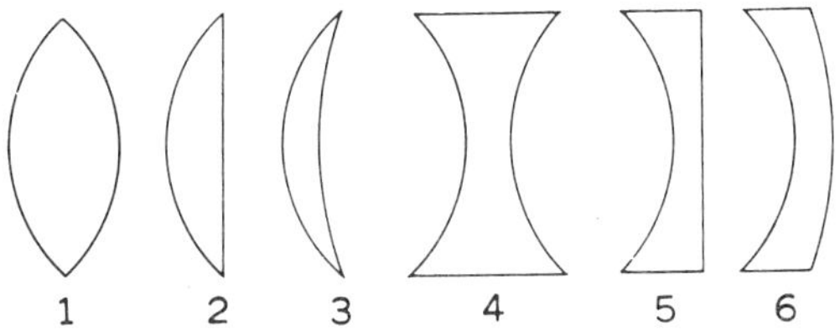

Types of Lens
1, Biconvex; *2,* planoconvex; *3,* concavoconvex, converging meniscus; *4,* biconcave; *5,* planoconcave; *6,* convexoconcave, diverging meniscus.

achromatic l., a compound l. made of two or more l.'s having different indices of refraction, so correlated as to minimize chromatic aberration.
aplanatic l., periscopic meniscus; a l. designed to correct spherical aberration and coma.
apochromatic l., a compound l. designed to correct both spherical and chromatic aberrations.
aspheric l., a l. with a paraboloidal surface that eliminates spherical aberration.
astigmatic l., cylindrical l.
biconcave l., concavoconcave or double concave l.; a l. that is concave on two opposing surfaces.
biconvex l., convexoconvex or double convex l.; a l. with both surfaces convex.
bifocal l., a l. used in cases of presbyopia, in which one portion is suited for distant vision, the other for reading and close work in general; the reading addition may be cemented to the l., fused to the front surface, or ground in one-piece form; other bifocal l.'s are the flat-top Franklin type, or blended invisible.
cataract l., any l. prescribed for aphakia.
compound l., an optical system of two or more lenses.
concave l., minus l.; a diverging minus power lens.
concavoconcave l., biconcave l.
concavoconvex l., a converging meniscus l. that is concave on one surface and convex on the opposite surface.
contact l., a l. that fits over the cornea and sclera or cornea only; used to correct refractive errors.
convex l., plus l.; a converging l.
convexoconcave l., a minus power l. having one surface convex and the opposite surface concave, with the latter having the greater curvature.
convexoconvex l., biconvex l.
corneal l., contact l. of plastic without scleral portions.
crystalline l., lens (2).
cylindrical l. (C, cyl.), astigmatic l.; a l. in which one of the surfaces is curved in one meridian and less curved in the opposite meridian.
decentered l., a l. so mounted that the visual axis does not pass through the axis of the l.
double concave l., biconcave l.
double convex l., biconvex l.
eye l., ocular l.; the upper of the two planoconvex l.'s of Huygens' ocular.
field l., the lower of the two planoconvex l.'s of Huygens' ocular.
Fresnel l., a l. with a surface consisting of a concentric series of zones that duplicate the power of a l. or prism but with less thickness.
immersion l., an objective (for a microscope) constructed in such a manner that the lower l. may be moved downward into direct contact with a fluid which is placed on the object being examined; by using a fluid with a refractive index closely similar to that of glass, the loss of light is minimized.

meniscus l., meniscus; a l. having a spherical concave curve on one side and a spherical convex curve on the other. See also relevant subentries under meniscus.
minus l., concave l.
multifocal l., a l. with segments providing two or more powers; commonly, a trifocal l.
ocular l., eye l.
omnifocal l., a l. for near and distant vision in which the reading portion is a continuously variable curve.
orthoscopic l., a spectacle l. corrected for distortion and curvature of the periphery.
periscopic l., a lens with 1.25 D base curve.
photochromic l., a light-sensitive spectacle l. that reduces light transmission in sunlight and increases transmission in reduced light.
planoconcave l., a l. that is flat on one side and concave on the other.
planoconvex l., a l. that is flat on one side and convex on the other.
plus l., convex l.
safety l., a l. that meets government specifications of impact resistance; the increased impact resistance required for safety l.'s is obtained by tempering, by an ion-exchange process, or by using laminated or plastic lenses.
slab-off l., a spectacle l. with a base-up prism below; used in unequal myopia to equalize image displacement when reading.
spherical l. (S or sph.), a l. in which all refracting surfaces are spherical.
spherocylindrical l., spherocylinder; a combined spherical and cylindrical l., one surface being spherical, the other cylindrical.
toric l., a lens in which both meridians are curved but not to the same degree.
trial l.'s, a series of cylindrical and spherical l.'s used in testing vision.
trifocal l., a l. with segments of three focal powers: distant, intermediate, and near.

lensectomy (len-sek'tō-mē) [lens + G. *ektomē*, excision]. Removal of the lens of the eye by an infusion-aspiration cutter; often done by puncture incision through the pars plana in the course of vitrectomy.

lensometer (len-zom'ĕ-ter) [lens + G. *metron*, measure]. Focimeter; vertometer; an instrument to measure spectacle power.

lensopathy (lenz-op'ă-thē) [lens + G. *pathos*, suffering]. The process by which tear proteins are deposited on a contact lens.

lenticonus (len-ti-kō'nŭs) [lens + L. *conus*, cone]. Conical projection of the anterior or posterior surface of the lens of the eye, occurring as a developmental anomaly.

lenticula (len-tik'yū-lă) [L. dim. of *lens*]. **1.** *Nucleus* lentiformis. **2.** Lentigo.

lenticular (len-tik'yū'lăr) [L. *lenticula*, a lentil]. **1.** Relating to or resembling a lens of any kind. **2.** Of the shape of a lentil.

lenticulo-optic (len-tik'yū-lō-op'tik). Relating to the lentiform nucleus and the optic tract; specifically refers to branches of the middle cerebral artery considered to supply these structures.

lenticulopapular (len-tik'yū-lō-pap'yū-lăr). Indicating an eruption with dome-shaped or lens-shaped papules.

lenticulostriate (len-tik'yū-lō-strī'āt). Relating to the nucleus lentiformis and the nucleus caudatus; specifically refers to branches of the middle cerebral artery supplying these gray masses.

lenticulothalamic (len-tik'yū-lō-tha-lam'ik). Pertaining to the lentiform (lenticular) nucleus and the thalamus.

lenticulus, pl. lenticuli (len-tik'yū-lŭs, -lī) [L. dim. of *lens, lentis*, a little lens]. Prosthetophacos; pseudophacos; an intraocular lens prosthesis placed in the anterior or posterior chamber of the eye, or attached to the iris after cataract extraction.

lentiform (len'ti-fōrm). Lens-shaped.

lentigines (len-tij'i-nēz) [L.]. Plural of lentigo.

lentiginosis (len-tij-i-nō'sis). Presence of lentigenes in very large numbers or in a distinctive configuration.
centrofacial l., uncommon autosomal dominant syndrome of small hyperpigmented macules appearing in a horizontal band across the center of the face at one year, increasing in number up to ten years, and associated with other defects.
generalized l., lentigines occurring singly or in groups from infancy onward.
periorificial l., Peutz-Jeghers *syndrome*.

lentiglobus (len-ti-glō'bŭs) [lens + L. *globus*, sphere]. Rare congenital anomaly with a spheroid elevation on the posterior surface of the lens of the eye.

lentigo, pl. lentigines (len-tī'gō, len-tij'i-nēz) [L. fr. *lens (lent-)*, a lentil]. Lenticula (2); a brown macule resembling a freckle except that the border is usually regular, and microscopic proliferation of rete ridges is present; scattered solitary nevus cells are seen in the basal cell layer. See also junction *nevus*.
malignant l., melanosis circumscripta precancerosa; precancerous melanosis of Dubreuilh; Hutchinson's or melanotic freckle; a brown or black mottled, irregularly outlined, slowly enlarging lesion resembling a lentigo in which there are increased numbers of scattered, frequently atypical, melanocytes in the epidermis, usually occurring on the face of older persons; malignant change is frequent, but the resulting melanomas are not highly malignant; development of a dark papule or nodule indicates an invasion of the dermis.
senile l., liver spot; a variably pigmented l. occurring on exposed skin of older Caucasians.

lentigomelanosis (len-tī'gō-mel'ă-nō'sis). Malignant lesions originating in lentigines.

Lentivirinae (len'ti-vir'i-nē) [L. *lentus*, sluggish, slow]. A subfamily of viruses (family Retroviridae) that includes the slow viruses of sheep (Visna virus and maedi virus) and human T-cell lymphotropic viruses; the viruses resemble the C-type RNA tumor viruses (Oncovirinae) in many ways, including production of reverse transcriptase.

lentivirus (len'ti-vī-rŭs). Any virus of the subfamily Lentivirinae.

lentogenic (len-tō-jen'ik) [L. *lentus*, sluggish, inactive, + G. *-gen*, producing]. Denoting the virulence of a virus capable of inducing lethal infection in embryonic hosts after a long incubation period and an inapparent infection in immature and adult hosts; the term is used in characterizing Newcastle disease virus, particularly strains used as vaccines administered in water or as sprays.

lentula, lentulo (len'tyū-lă, -lō) [L. *lentus*, pliant, flexible]. A motorized, flexible, spiral wire instrument used in dentistry to apply paste filling material into the root canal(s) of a tooth.

leontiasis (lē-on-tī'ă-sis) [G. *leōn (leont-)*, lion]. Leonine facies; the ridges and furrows on the forehead and cheeks of patients with advanced lepromatous leprosy, giving a leonine appearance.
l. os'sea, Virchow's disease (2); an overgrowth of the bones of the face, and sometimes of the cranium, causing a general enlargement of all the features.

LEOPARD Acronym for *l*entigines (multiple), *e*lectrocardiographic abnormalities, *o*cular hypertelorism, *p*ulmonary stenosis, *a*bnormalities of genitalia, *r*etardation of growth, and *d*eafness (sensorineural).

leopard's bane. Arnica.

Leopold, Christian G., German physician, 1846–1911. See L.'s *maneuvers*.

Lepehne, Georg, German physician, *1887. See L.-Pickworth *stain*.

leper (lep′er) [G. *lepra*]. A person who has leprosy.

lepidic (lĕ-pid′ik) [G. *lepis (lepid-)*, scale, rind]. Relating to scales or a scaly covering layer.

Lepidoptera (lep-i-dop′ter-ă) [G. *lepis*, scale, + *pteron*, wing]. An order of insects comprised of the moths and butterflies, characterized by wings covered with delicate scales.

lepidosis (lep-i-dō′sis) [G. *lepis*, scale, rind, + *-osis*, condition]. Any scaly or desquamating eruption.

Leporipoxvirus (lep′ō-ri-poks′vī-rŭs) [L. *leporis*, gen. of *lepus*, a hare, + virus]. The genus of viruses (family Poxviridae) that comprises the fibroma and myxoma viruses of rabbits; unlike the orthopoxviruses, they are ether-sensitive.

lepothrix (lep′ō-thriks) [G. *lepos*, rind, husk, + *thrix*, hair]. *Trichomycosis* axillaris.

lepra (lep′ră) [G. leprosy]. Obsolete term for leprosy.

leprechaunism (lep′rĕ-kawn-izm) [Irish *leprechaun*, elf]. Donohue's disease; a congenital form of dwarfism characterized by extreme growth retardation, endocrine disorders, and emaciation, with elfin facies and large low-set ears; autosomal recessive inheritance.

lep′rid [G. *lepra*, leprosy, + *-id* (1)]. Early cutaneous lesion of leprosy.

leprologist (lĕ-prol′ō-jist). A physician who specializes in the study of leprosy.

leprology (lĕ-prol′ō-jē) [G. *lepra*, leprosy, + *logos*, study]. The science and study of leprosy.

leproma (lĕ-prō′mă) [G. *lepros*, scaly, + *-oma*, tumor]. A fairly well circumscribed discrete focus of granulomatous inflammation, caused by *Mycobacterium leprae*, which consists chiefly of an accumulation of large mononuclear phagocytic cells in which the cytoplasm seems finely vacuolated (*i.e.*, foam cells); the foamlike character of the macrophages is related to the engulfing of numerous acid-fast organisms.

lepromatous (lep-rō′mă-tŭs). Pertaining to, or characterized by, the features of a leproma.

lepromin (lep′rō-min). An extract of tissue infected with *Mycobacterium leprae* used in skin tests to classify the stage of leprosy. See also l. *reaction*, *test*.

leprosarium (lep′rō-sar′ē-ŭm). A hospital especially designed for the care of those suffering from leprosy, especially those who need expert care.

leprose (lep′rōs). Leprous.

leprosery (lep′rō-ser-ē). A leper home or colony.

leprostatic (lep-rō-stat′ik). **1.** Inhibiting to the growth of *Mycobacterium leprae*. **2.** An agent having this action.

leprosy (lep′rō-sē) [G. *lepra*, from *lepros*, scaly]. **1.** A name given in Biblical times to various cutaneous diseases, especially those of a chronic or contagious nature, which probably included psoriasis and leukoderma. **2.** Hansen's disease; chronic granulomatous infection caused by *Mycobacterium leprae* (Hansen's bacillus) and affecting cooler parts of the body such as the skin.

anesthetic l., a form of l. chiefly affecting the nerves, marked by hyperesthesia succeeded by anesthesia, and by paralysis, ulceration, and various trophic disturbances, terminating in gangrene and mutilation. Also called Danielssen's or Danielssen-Boeck disease; dry or trophoneurotic l.

articular l., mutilating l.; a late stage of anesthetic l.

borderline l., dimorphous l.; a form of l. that is very unstable immunologically; the cutaneous nerves frequently present bacilli, but the lepromin test is usually negative; cutaneous lesions are comprised of flat bands or plaques.

cutaneous l., tuberculoid l.

dimorphous l., borderline l.

dry l., anesthetic l.

histoid l., a form of lepromatous l. with lesions resembling dermatofibromas or neurofibromas.

indeterminate l., a transitory form of l. in which the immunologic status is not yet formed, and the histologic and clinical features are not yet characteristic of any of the major types of l.

lazarine l. [*Lazarus*, Biblical character], Lucio's l.

lepromatous l., a form of l. in which nodular cutaneous lesions are infiltrated, have ill-defined borders, and are bacteriologically positive; the lepromin test is negative, *i.e.*, the immunologic mechanism of the patient is not responsive to the *Mycobacterium leprae* infection.

Lucio's l., Lucio's l. phenomenon; lazarine l.; an acute form occurring in pure diffuse lepromatous l. presenting irregularly shaped, intensely erythematous, tender plaques, especially of the legs, with tendency to ulceration and scarring.

macular l., a form of tuberculoid l. in which the lesions are small, hairless, and dry, and are erythematous in light skin and hypopigmented or copper-colored in dark skin.

Malabar l., elephantiasis.

mouse l., murine l., rat l.

mutilating l., articular l.

nodular l., tuberculoid l.

rat l., mouse or murine l.; a slowly but progressively fatal form of l. occurring in rats, caused by *Mycobacterium lepraemurium;* it appears in two forms, glandular and musculocutaneous; causes induration, alopecia, and eventually ulceration.

smooth l., tuberculoid l.

trophoneurotic l., anesthetic l.

tuberculoid l., cutaneous, smooth, or nodular l.; a benign, stable, and resistant form of the disease in which the lepromin reaction is strongly positive and in which the lesions are erythematous, insensitive, infiltrated plaques with clear-cut edges.

leprotic (lep-rot′ik). Leprous.

leprous (lep′rŭs). Leprose; leprotic; relating to or suffering from leprosy.

-lepsis, -lepsy [G. *lēpsis*, seizure]. Combining forms denoting seizure.

lepto- [G. *leptos*, slender, delicate, weak]. Combining form meaning light, slender, thin, or frail.

leptocephalous (lep-tō-sef′ă-lŭs) [lepto- + G. *kephalē*, head]. Having an abnormally narrow cranium.

leptocephaly (lep-tō-sef′ă-lē) [lepto- + G. *kephalē*, head]. A malformation characterized by an abnormally narrow cranium.

leptochroa (lep-tō-krō′ă) [lepto- + G. *chrōa*, skin]. Abnormally delicate skin.

leptochromatic (lep′tō-krō-mat′ik). Having a very fine chromatin network.

leptocyte (lep′tō-sīt) [lepto- + G. *kytos*, cell]. A target or Mexican hat cell, *i.e.*, an unusually thin or flattened red blood cell in which there is a central rounded area of pigmented material, a middle clear zone that contains no pigment, and an outer pigmented rim at the edge of the cell. L.'s are thought to be erythrocytes in which the cellular envelope or membrane is unusually large in proportion to its contents.

leptocytosis (lep′tō-sī-tō′sis). The presence of leptocytes in the circulating blood, as in thalassemia, some instances of jaundice (even in the absence of anemia), occasional examples of hepatic disease (in the absence of jaundice), and some patients who have had the spleen removed.

leptodactylous (lep-tō-dak′ti-lŭs) [lepto- + G. *daktylos*, finger]. Having slender fingers.

leptodermic (lep-tō-der′mik) [lepto- + G. *derma*, skin]. Thin-skinned.

leptomeningeal (lep′tō-me-nin′jē-ăl). Pertaining to the leptomeninges.

leptomeninges (lep-tō-me-nin'jēz) [lepto- + G. *mēninx,* pl. *mēninges,* membrane]. Piarachnoid; pia-arachnoid; meninx tenuis; collective term denoting the soft membranes enveloping brain and spinal cord: pia mater and arachnoidea mater, as distinguished from dura mater, the pachymeninx.

leptomeningitis (lep'tō-men-in-jī'tis). Pia-arachnitis; inflammation of leptomeninges. See also arachnoiditis.
basilar l., inflammation of the arachnoid at the base of the brain; often found in chronic meningitis of tuberculous, luetic, or mycotic origin.

leptomeninx (lep'tō-mē'ninks). Singular of leptomeninges.

leptomere (lep'tō-mēr) [lepto- + G. *meros,* part]. A very minute particle of living matter; Asclepiades believed the body was composed of an aggregation of vast numbers of l.'s.

leptomonad (lep'tō-mō'nad, lep-tom'ō-nad). **1.** Common name for a member of the genus *Leptomonas.* **2.** See promastigote.

Leptomonas (lep'tō-mō'nas, lep-tom'ō-nŭs) [lepto- + G. *monas,* unit]. A genus of asexual, monogenetic, parasitic flagellates (family Trypanosomatidae) commonly found in the hindgut of insects.

leptonema (lep-tō-nē'mă) [lepto- + G. *nēma,* thread]. Leptotene.

leptophonia (lep'tō-fō'nē-ă) [lepto- + G. *phōnē,* sound, voice]. Hypophonia.

leptophonic (lep'tō-fon'ik). Weak-voiced.

leptopodia (lep-tō-pō'dē-ă) [lepto- + G. *pous,* foot]. The condition of having slender feet.

leptoprosopia (lep'tō-prō-sō'pē-ă) [lepto- + G. *prosōpon,* face]. Narrowness of the face.

leptoprosopic (lep'tō-prō-sō'pik). Having a thin, narrow face.

leptorrhine (lep'tō-rīn) [lepto- + G. *rhis,* nose]. Having a thin nose. Applied to a skull with a nasal index below 47 (Frankfort agreement) or 48 (Broca).

leptoscope (lep'tō-skōp). An apparatus for measuring cell membranes.

leptosomatic, leptosomic (lep'tō-sō-mat'ik, -tō-sō'mik) [lepto- + G. *sōma,* body]. Having a slender, light, or thin body.

Leptospira (lep'tō-spī'ră) [lepto- + G. *speira,* a coil]. A genus of aerobic bacteria (order Spirochaetales) containing thin, tightly coiled organisms 6 to 20 μm in length. They possess an axial filament, and one or both ends may be bent into a semicircular hook. They stain with difficulty except with Giemsa's stain or silver impregnation. The type species is *L. interrogans.*
L. inter'rogans, a species containing more than one hundred named parasitic or pathogenic serovars. It is the type species of the genus *L.*

leptospire (lep'tō-spīr). Common name for any organism belonging to the genus *Leptospira.*

leptospirosis (lep'tō-spī-rō'sis). Infection with species of *Leptospira.*

leptospiruria (lep'tō-spī-rū'rē-ă). Presence of species of the genus *Leptospira* in the urine, as a result of leptospirosis in the renal tubules.

leptotene (lep'tō-tēn) [lepto- + G. *tainia,* band, tape]. Leptonema; early stage of prophase in meiosis in which the chromosomes contract and become visible as long filaments well separated from each other.

leptothricosis (lep'tō-thri-kō'sis). Obsolete term for any disease caused by the now invalid genus *Leptothrix.*

Leptothrix (lep'tō-thriks). Invalid name for a genus of organisms that would probably now be classified as actinomycetes, nocardiae, or corynebacteria.

Leptotrichia (lep-tō-trik'ē-ă) [lepto- + G. *thrix,* hair]. A genus of anaerobic, nonmotile bacteria containing Gram-negative, straight or slightly curved rods, 5 to 15 μm in length, with one or both ends rounded, often pointed. Granules are distributed evenly along the long axis, and one or more large granules may localize near the end of the cell. Branched or clubbed forms do not occur. Two or more cells join together and form septate filaments of varying length; in older cultures, filaments up to 200 μm may form and twist around each other; large, coccoid bodies may be found within a filament as a cell lyses. Carbon dioxide is essential for optimal growth. Lactic acid is produced from glucose. These organisms occur in the oral cavity of man. The type species is *L. buccalis.*
L. bucca'lis, a species found in the human mouth; it is the type species of the genus *L.*

Leptotrombidium (lep'tō-trom-bid'ē-ŭm). An important genus of trombiculid mites, formerly considered a subgenus of the genus *Trombicula,* which includes all of the vectors of scrub typhus (tsutsugamushi disease). Members of *L.* that serve as vectors of scrub typhus are within the *L. deliense* group: *L. akamushi* is the classical vector in Japan; *L. deliense* is the primary vector, extending from New Guinea, Australia, the Philippines, China, and Southeast Asia to western Pakistan; *L. fletcheri* is found in Malaysia, New Guinea, and the Philippines. Some eight other species have also been implicated in scrub typhus transmission in more limited areas.
L. akamu'shi, *Trombicula akamushi;* one of two species, the other being *L. deliensis* (*T. deliensis*), implicated in the transmission of *Rickettsia tsutsugamushi,* agent of tsutsugamushi disease in Japan and elsewhere in the Orient; the larvae of these species are characteristic parasites of rodents, which therefore are reservoirs of human infections, although the mites themselves are also reservoirs, as their rickettsial parasites are transovarially transmitted from generation to generation (a requirement for transmission to man as only larval mites feed parasitically and then only once in their lifetimes).

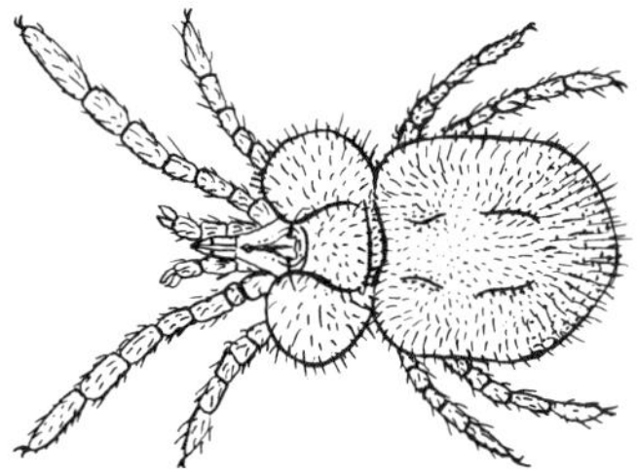

Leptotrombidium akamushi
Adult (×20)

Leri, André, French orthopedic surgeon, 1875–1930. See L.'s *pleonosteosis, sign;* L.-Weill *disease, syndrome.*

Leriche, René, French surgeon, 1879–1955. See L.'s *operation, syndrome.*

Lermoyez, Marcel, French otolaryngologist, 1858–1929. See L.'s *syndrome.*

Lerner, I.M., U.S. population geneticist, 1910–1967. See L. *homeostasis.*

Leroy, Edgar August, French physician, *1883. See Fiessinger-L.-Reiter *syndrome.*

lesbian (lez'bē-ăn). **1.** One who practices lesbianism. **2.** Pertaining to or characteristic of lesbianism.

lesbianism (lez'bē-ăn-izm) [G. *lesbios,* relating to the island of Lesbos]. Sapphism; tribadism; homosexuality between women.

Lesch, Michael, U.S. pediatrician, *1939. See L.-Nyhan *syndrome.*

Leser, Edmund, German surgeon, 1828–1916. See L.-Trélat *sign.*

lesion (lē'zhŭn) [L. *laedo,* pp. *laesus,* to injure]. **1.** A wound or injury. **2.** A pathologic change in the tissues. **3.** One of the individual points or patches of a multifocal disease.

Baehr-Lohlein l., Lohlein-Baehr l.

benign lymphoepithelial l., benign tumor-like masses of lymphoid tissue in the parotid gland, containing scattered small, mainly solid islands of epithelial cells.

Bracht-Wachter l., a focal collection of lymphocytes and mononuclear cells within the myocardium in bacterial endocarditis.

caviar l., a dilated vein or varicule existing in the venous collecting system under the tongue.

coin l.'s of lungs, solitary, round, circumscribed shadows found in the lungs in x-ray examinations; some common causes are tuberculosis, carcinoma, cysts, infarcts, or vascular anomalies.

Councilman's l., Councilman *body.*

Duret's l., small hemorrhage(s) in the floor of the fourth ventricle or beneath the aqueduct of Sylvius.

Ghon's primary l., Ghon's *tubercle.*

gross l., a l. plainly visible to the naked eye.

Hill-Sachs l., an irregularity seen in the head of the humerus following dislocation of the shoulder; caused by impaction of the head of the humerus against the edge of the glenoid.

Janeway l., a small erythematous or hemorrhagic l. seen in some cases of bacterial endocarditis, usually on the palm or sole.

Lennert's l., Lennert's *lymphoma.*

Lohlein-Baehr l., Baehr-Lohlein l.; focal embolic glomerulonephritis occurring in bacterial endocarditis.

Mallory-Weiss l., Mallory-Weiss tear; laceration of the gastric cardia, as seen in the Mallory-Weiss syndrome.

precancerous l., a noncancerous l. with a predictable likelihood of becoming malignant; *e.g.,* actinic keratosis or keratosis senilis.

radial sclerosing l., radial scar; a variant of sclerosing adenosis of the breast with central scar formation and radiating hyperplastic ducts.

ring-wall l., a small ring hemorrhage in the brain that stimulates proliferation of a glial ring.

supranuclear l., upper motor neuron l.; injury to cerebral (corticonuclear) fibers between the cerebral cortex and brainstem or spinal motor nerve nucleus.

upper motor neuron l., supranuclear l.

wire-loop l., thickening of the basement membrane, with fibrinoid staining, of scattered peripheral capillaries in renal glomeruli; characteristic of renal involvement in systemic lupus erythematosus; the appearance of an affected capillary wall resembles a loop used in microbiology.

Lesser's triangle. See under triangle.

Lesshaft, Pjotr F., Russian physician, 1836–1909. See L.'s *triangle.*

lethal (lē'thăl) [L. *letalis,* fr. *letum,* death]. Pertaining to or causing death; denoting especially the causal agent.

clinical l., a disorder that culminates in death.

genetic l., a disorder that prevents effective reproduction by those affected; *e.g.,* Klinefelter syndrome.

lethality (lē-thal'i-tē). The quality or state of being lethal.

lethargy (leth'ar-jē) [G. *lēthargis,* drowsiness]. A state of deep and prolonged unconsciousness, resembling profound slumber, from which one can be aroused but into which one immediately relapses.

LETS Acronym for *l*arge, *e*xternal *t*ransformation-*s*ensitive fibronectin. See fibronectin.

Letterer, Erich, German pathologist, *1895. See L.-Siwe *disease.*

Leu Symbol for leucine radical.

leuc-, leuco- [G. *leukos,* white]. For terms beginning thus and not found here, see leuk-, leuko-.

leucin (lū'sin). Leukin.

leucine (lū'sēn). 2-Amino-4-methylvaleric acid; $(CH_3)_2CHCH_2CH(NH_2)COOH$; one of the amino acids of proteins; an essential amino acid.

leucine aminopeptidase. Aminopeptidase (cytosol).

leucinosis (lū'si-nō'sis). A condition in which there is an abnormally large proportion of leucine in the tissues and body fluids.

leucinuria (lū-si-nū'rē-ă). The excretion of leucine in the urine.

leucitis (lū-sī'tis). Scleritis.

Leucocytozoon (lū'kō-sī-tō-zō'on) [G. *leukos,* white, + *kytos,* cell, + *zōon,* animal]. *Leukocytozoon;* a genus of sporozoan parasites (family Plasmodiidae, suborder Haemosporina) that attack the immature red blood cells of birds and are capable of causing acute outbreaks of disease, particularly in turkeys and ducks; vectors are black flies, *Simulium* species, and the bloodsucking gnat *Culicoides.*

L. marchou'xi, a species of unknown pathogenicity, but fairly common in wild doves and pigeons.

L. sabraze'si, a species that is a cause of leucocytozoonosis of chickens, particularly in Indochina, Malaysia, India, Sumatra, and Java.

L. simon'di, a species that causes disease in domestic and wild ducks, geese, and related waterfowl in the northern U.S. and Canada; it is severely pathogenic, especially in young birds.

L. smith'i, a species that causes disease in domestic turkeys.

leucocytozoonosis (lū'kō-sī'tō-zo-ō-nō'sis). Leukocytozoonosis; infection of ducks, turkeys, chickens, pigeons, and doves with species of *Leucocytozoon.* The disease is most acute and damaging in young turkeys and ducks, and is characterized by enlargement of the spleen and liver, anemia, listlessness, weakness, and frequently death.

leucoharmine (lū-kō-har'mēn). Harmine.

leucoline (lū'kō-lēn). Quinoline.

leucomethylene blue (lu'kō-meth'i-lēn). Methylene white; the reduced and colorless form of methylene blue.

Leuconostoc (lū-kō-nos'tok) [G. *leukos,* white, + *nostoc,* a genus of algae (a word coined by Paracelsus)]. A genus of microaerophilic to facultatively anaerobic bacteria (family Lactobacillaceae) containing Gram-positive, spherical cells which may, under certain conditions, lengthen and become pointed and even form rods. Lactic and acetic acids are produced by these organisms. They are found in plant juices and in milk. The type species is *L. mesenteroides.*

L. citrovo'rum, a species found in milk and dairy products; growth of these organisms is stimulated by a hemopoietic factor resembling folic acid.

L. mesenteroi'des, a species found in fermenting vegetables and other plant materials and in prepared meat products; it is an active slime (dextran) producer, the dextran commonly used as a plasma expander; it is the type species of the genus *L.*

leuco patent blue (lū'kō pat'ent) [C.I. 42051]. Patent blue V; a sulfonated triphenylmethane dye reduced and decolorized with zinc and acetic acid to produce a stable solution; used to demonstrate hemoglobin peroxidase.

leucovorin (lū'kō-vōr-in). Folinic acid.

l. calcium, calcium folinate; the calcium salt of leucovorin (folinic acid); used to counteract toxic effects of folic acid antagonists, for the treatment of megaloblastic anemias, and as an adjunct to cyanocobalamin in pernicious anemia.

Leudet, Théodor E., French physician, 1825–1887. See L.'s *tinnitus.*

leuenkephalin (lū-en-kef'ă-lin). See enkephalins.

leuk-. See leuko-.

leukanemia (lū-kă-nē'mē-ă) [leukemia + anemia]. Former term for erythroleukemia.

leukapheresis (lū'kă-fē-rē'sis) [leuko- + G. *aphairesis,* a withdrawal]. A procedure, analogous to plasmapheresis, in which leukocytes are removed from the withdrawn blood and the remainder is retransfused into the donor.

leukasmus (lū-kaz'mŭs) [G. *leukasmos,* a growing white]. Vitiligo.

leukemia (lū-kē'mē-ă) [leuko- + G. *haima,* blood]. Leukocytic sarcoma; progressive proliferation of abnormal leukocytes found in hemopoietic tissues, other organs, and usually in the blood in increased numbers. L. is classified by the dominant cell type, and by duration from onset to death. This occurs in *acute l.* within a few months in most cases, and is associated with symptoms that suggest acute infection, with severe anemia, hemorrhages, and slight enlargement of lymph nodes or the spleen. The duration of *chronic l.* exceeds one year, with a gradual onset of symptoms of anemia or marked enlargement of spleen, liver, or lymph nodes.

acute promyelocytic l., l. presenting as a severe bleeding disorder, with infiltration of the bone marrow by abnormal promyelocytes and myelocytes, a low plasma fibrinogen, and defective coagulation.

adult T-cell l. (ATL), adult T-cell *lymphoma.*

aleukemic l., l. in which abnormal (or leukemic) cells are absent in the peripheral blood.

basophilic l., basophilocytic l., mast cell l.; a form of granulocytic l. in which there are unusually great numbers of basophilic granulocytes in the tissues and circulating blood; in some instances, the immature and mature basophilic forms may represent from 40 to 80% of the total numbers of white blood cells.

l. cu'tis, yellow-brown, red, blue-red, or purple, sometimes nodular lesions associated with diffuse infiltrations or massive accumulations of leukemic cells in the skin; the involvement may be diffuse and generalized, *i.e.,* so-called universal l. cutis, or it may be localized.

embryonal l., stem cell l.

eosinophilic l., eosinophilocytic l., a form of granulocytic l. in which there are conspicuous numbers of eosinophilic granulocytes in the tissues and circulating blood, or in which such cells are predominant; in chronic disease of this type, the total white blood cell count may be as high as 200,000 to 250,000 per cu mm, with as many as 80 or 90% being eosinophils, chiefly adult forms.

feline l., a leukemic disorder of cats caused by feline l. virus and characterized by depression and mild fever, and by the presence of tumors in the mediastinal and mesenteric lymph nodes, followed by multiple tumor formation throughout the body; during the terminal stages of the disease lymphoblasts may appear in the peripheral blood.

l. of fowls, avian *leukosis.*

granulocytic l., myelocytic, myeloid, myelogenic, or myelogenous l.; leukemic myelosis (1); a form of l. characterized by an uncontrolled proliferation of myelopoietic cells in the bone marrow and in extramedullary sites, and the presence of large numbers of immature and mature granulocytic forms in various tissues (and organs) and in the circulating blood; the total count may range from 1000 (aleukemic variety) to several hundred thousand per cu mm. The predominant cell is usually of the neutrophilic series, but, in a few instances, eosinophilic or basophilic granulocytes, or even megakaryocytes, may represent the chief form; early in granulocytic l., the circulating blood may contain excessive numbers of all of the granulocytic forms.

hairy cell l., leukemic reticuloendotheliosis; a rare, usually chronic disorder characterized by proliferation of hairy cells in reticuloendothelial organs and blood.

leukemic l., a redundant term sometimes used to emphasize the occurrence of abundant numbers of leukemic cells in the circulating blood; this classic form of l. is usually termed simply *leukemia.*

leukopenic l., a form of lymphocytic, granulocytic, or monocytic l. in which the total number of white blood cells in the circulating blood is in the normal range, or may be diminished to various levels that are significantly less than normal.

lymphatic l., lymphocytic l.

lymphoblastic l., acute lymphocytic l. in which the abnormal cells are chiefly (or almost totally) blast forms of the lymphocytic series, or in which unusually large numbers of the immature forms occur in association with adult lymphocytes.

lymphocytic l., lymphoid or lymphatic l.; a variety of l. characterized by an uncontrolled proliferation and conspicuous enlargement of lymphoid tissue in various sites (*e.g.,* lymph nodes, spleen, bone marrow, lungs), and the occurrence of increased numbers of cells of the lymphocytic series in the circulating blood and in various tissues and organs; in chronic disease, the cells are adult lymphocytes, whereas conspicuous numbers of lymphoblasts are observed in the more acute syndromes.

lymphoid l., lymphocytic l.

mast cell l., basophilic l.

mature cell l., chronic granulocytic l.

megakaryocytic l., an unusual form of myelopoietic disease that is characterized by a seemingly uncontrolled proliferation of megakaryocytes in the bone marrow, and sometimes by the presence of a considerable number of megakaryocytes in the circulating blood. When bone marrow is examined at various intervals in some instances of chronic myelocytic l., the proliferation of megakaryocytes is more prominent than that of the granulocytes; at such times, the circulating blood may contain megakaryocytes or fragments of megakaryocytic nuclei and cytoplasm, or both, amounting to as much as 5 or 6% of the total number of leukocytes.

meningeal l., infiltration of the meninges by leukemic cells, a common occurrence in relapse following systemic administration of chemotherapeutic agents to leukemia patients.

micromyeloblastic l., a form of myelocytic l. in which relatively large proportions of micromyeloblasts are found in the circulating blood and in bone marrow and other tissues.

mixed l., mixed cell l., term infrequently used as a designation for granulocytic l., thereby emphasizing the occurrence of different types of cells in the myeloid series (*i.e.,* neutrophilic, eosinophilic, and basophilic granulocytes), in contrast to the comparatively monotonous pattern observed in lymphocytic and monocytic l.

monocytic l., leukemic reticulosis; a form of l. characterized by large numbers of cells that can be definitely identified as monocytes, in addition to larger, apparently related cells formed from the uncontrolled proliferation of the reticuloendothelial tissue; l. in which these two types of cells seem to "overrun" the usual sites of the reticuloendothelial system, and occur in conspicuous numbers in the circulating blood, is frequently referred to as the Schilling type of monocytic l., or sometimes as true monocytic l. The disease runs an acute or subacute course in older persons, and is characterized by swelling of gums, oral ulceration, bleeding in skin or mucous membranes, secondary infection, and splenomegaly.

myeloblastic l., leukemic myelosis (2); a form granulocytic l. in which there are large numbers of myeloblasts in various tissues (and organs) and in the circulating blood; the immature forms may amount to 30 to 60% (or even a greater proportion) of the increased total number of white blood cells. Used synonymously for acute granulocytic l., although myeloblastic l. may be a terminal event in the course of chronic granulocytic l.

myelocytic, myelogenic, myelogenous, or **myeloid l.,** granulocytic l.

myelomonocytic l., Naegeli type of monocytic l.; a variant of granulocytic l. with monocytosis in the peripheral blood.

Naegeli type of monocytic l., myelomonocytic l.

neutrophilic l., an unusual form of chronic granulocytic l. in which the greatly increased number of leukocytes in the circulating blood are mature polymorphonuclear neutrophils, with virtually no young or immature granulocytes being observed.

plasma cell l., an unusual disease characterized by leukocytosis and other signs and symptoms that are suggestive of l., in association with diffuse infiltrations and aggregates of plasma cells in the spleen, liver, bone marrow, and lymph nodes, and the presence of considerable numbers of plasma cells in the circulating blood; the total number of leukocytes in the latter may range from normal levels to 80,000 or 90,000 per cu mm, and 5 to 90% may be plasma cells; multiple myelomas are observed in some examples of plasma cell l., but discrete nodules are not formed in bone. Although there are other clinicopathologic differences in the two conditions, they may be phases of the same basic process.

polymorphocytic l., granulocytic l., especially any variety in which the predominant cells are mature, segmented granulocytes.

Rieder cell l., a special form of acute granulocytic l. in which the affected tissues and the circulating blood contain relatively large numbers of atypical myeloblasts (*i.e.,* Rieder cells) that have the usual, faintly granular, immature type of cytoplasm, and a bizarre, comparatively mature nucleus with several wide and deep indentations (suggestive of lobulation).

Schilling type of monocytic l., see monocytic l.

splenic l., a form of l. in which there is an unusually great degree of enlargement of the spleen, as observed frequently in chronic granulocytic l.

stem cell l., embryonal l.; a form of l. in which the abnormal cells are thought to be the precursors of lymphoblasts, myeloblasts, or monoblasts.

subleukemic l., leukopenic or subleukemic myelosis; hypoleukemia; subleukemia; a form of l. in which abnormal cells are present in the peripheral blood, but the total leukocyte count is not elevated.

leukemic (lū-kē'mik). Pertaining to, or having the characteristics of, any form of leukemia.

leukemid (lū-kem'id) [leuko- + G. *haima,* blood, + *id* (1)]. Any nonspecific type of cutaneous lesion that is frequently associated with leukemia (as a feature of the syndrome), but is not a localized accumulation of leukemic cells, although, occasionally, the nonspecific lesions present specific leukemic cells in the infiltrate; *e.g.,* petechiae, vesicles, wheals, bullae, hematomas, pustules, papules, and the lesions of exfoliative dermatitis and herpes zoster.

leukemogen (lū-kē'mō-jen). Any substance or entity (*e.g.,* benzene, ionizing radiation) considered to be a causal factor in the occurrence of leukemia.

leukemogenesis (lū-kē-mō-jen'ē-sis) [leukemia + G. *genesis,* production]. The causation (or induction), development, and progression of a leukemic disease.

leukemogenic (lū-kē-mō-jen'ik). Pertaining to the causation, induction, and development of leukemia; manifesting the ability to cause leukemia.

leukemoid (lū-kē'moyd) [leukemia + G. *eidos,* resemblance]. Resembling leukemia in various signs and symptoms, especially with reference to changes in the circulating blood. See also *leukemoid reaction.*

leukemoid reaction. A moderate, advanced, or sometimes extreme degree of leukocytosis in the circulating blood, closely similar or possibly identical to that occurring in various forms of leukemia, but not the result of leukemic disease; usually, there is a disproportionate increase in the number of forms (including immature stages) in one series of leukocytes, and various examples of myelocytic, lymphocytic, monocytic, or plasmocytic l. r. may be also indistinguishable from leukocytosis that is associated with certain forms of leukemia. L. r.'s are sometimes observed as a feature of: 1) infectious disease caused by certain bacteria and other biologic agents, *e.g.,* tuberculosis, diphtheria, chickenpox, and others; 2) intoxication of various types, *e.g.,* eclampsia, serious burns, mustard gas poisoning, and others; 3) malignant neoplasms, *e.g.,* carcinoma of the colon, of the lung, of the kidney, or of other organs; 4) acute hemorrhage or hemolysis.

lymphocytic l. r., leukocytosis of varying degree, with adult lymphocytes and immature forms amounting to 40% (or more) of the total number of white blood cells in the circulating blood; may be observed in association with pertussis, infectious mononucleosis, gonorrhea, chickenpox, and sarcoidosis.

monocytic l. r., leukocytosis of varying degree, *e.g.,* 30,000 to 40,000/cu mm, with adult monocytes and immature forms amounting to 30% (or more) of the total number of white blood cells in the circulating blood; may be observed in association with tuberculosis, especially the first infection, miliary type.

myelocytic l. r., leukocytosis of at least moderate degree, *e.g.,* 50,000 or more per cu mm, with a few immature forms, *e.g.,* 1 or 2% myelocytes, but chiefly mature polymorphonuclear leukocytes in the circulating blood; may be observed in association with tuberculosis, chronic osteomyelitis, various types of empyema, malaria, pneumococcal pneumonia, meningococcal meningitis, Hodgkin's disease, and metastases of carcinoma in the bone marrow.

plasmocytic l. r., the presence of unusual numbers of plasma cells, *i.e.,* plasmocytosis, in the bone marrow; may be observed in association with sarcoidosis, rheumatoid arthritis, cirrhosis, Hodgkin's disease, and certain of the so-called collagen diseases.

leukin (lū'kin). Leucin; a thermostable bactericidal substance extracted from leukocytes.

leuko-, leuk- [G. *leukos,* white]. Combining forms meaning white. For some words beginning thus, see leuc- and leuco-.

leukoagglutinin (lū'kō-ă-glū'ti-nin). An antibody that agglutinates white blood cells.

leukobilin (lū-kō-bil'in) [leuko- + L. *bilis,* bile]. An older term designating the relatively clear, almost colorless, viscid fluid that occurs in the gallbladder, intestines, or both as a result of obstruction of the bile ducts in various sites; this so-called white bile is actually the secretion of the mucous membrane, without the usual color resulting from bile pigments.

leukoblast (lū'kō-blast) [leuko- + G. *blastos,* germ]. Proleukocyte; an immature white blood cell that is transitional between the lymphoidocyte (or the myeloblast of Naegeli and Downey) and the promyelocyte; the cytoplasm is polychromatophilic or slightly acidophilic and, as compared with the lymphoidocyte, the nuclear network of chromatin is thicker and the nucleoli less distinct.

granular l., promyelocyte.

leukoblastosis (lū'kō-blas-tō'sis). A general term for the abnormal proliferation of leukocytes, especially that occurring in myelocytic and lymphocytic leukemia.

leukochloroma (lū'kō-klō-rō'mă) [leuko- + G. *chlorōs,* green, + -*oma,* tumor]. Myelocytomatosis (1).

leukocidin (lū-kos'i-din, lū-kō-sī'din) [leukocyte + L. *caedo,* to kill]. A heat-labile substance that is elaborated by many strains of *Staphylococcus aureus, Streptococcus pyogenes,* and pneumococci and manifests a destructive action on leukocytes, with or without lysis of the cells.

leukocoria (lū-kō-kō'rē-ă) [leuko- + G. *korē,* pupil]. Leukokoria; white pupillary reflex; reflection from a white mass within the eye giving the appearance of a white pupil.

leukocytactic (lū'kō-sī-tak'tik). Leukocytotactic.

leukocytal (lū-kō-sī'tăl). Leukocytic.

leukocytaxia, leukocytaxis (lū'kō-sī-tak'sē-ă, -tak'sis). Leukocytotaxia.

leukocyte (lū'kō-sīt) [leuko- + G. *kytos,* cell]. White blood cell; a type of cell formed in the myelopoietic, lymphoid, and reticular portions of the reticuloendothelial system in various parts of the body, and normally present in those sites and in the circulating blood (rarely in other tissues). Under various abnormal conditions, the total numbers or proportions, or both, may be characteristically increased, decreased, or not altered, and they may be present in other tissues and organs. L.'s represent three lines of development from primitive elements: myeloid, lymphoid, and monocytic series. On the basis of features observed with various methods of staining with polychromatic dyes (*e.g.,* Wright's stain, and others), cells of the myeloid series are frequently termed granular l.'s, or granulocytes; cells of the lymphoid and monocytic series also have granules in the cytoplasm but, owing to their tiny inconspicuous size and different properties (frequently not clearly visualized with routine methods), lymphocytes and monocytes are sometimes termed nongranular or agranular l.'s. Granulocytes are commonly known as polymorphonuclear l.'s (also polynuclear or multinuclear l.'s), inasmuch as the mature nucleus is divided into two to five rounded or ovoid lobes that are connected with thin strands or small bands of chromatin; they consist of three distinct types: neutrophils, eosinophils, and basophils, named on the basis of the staining reactions of the cytoplasmic granules. Cells of the lymphocytic series occur as two, somewhat arbitrary, normal varieties: small and large lymphocytes; the former represent the ordinary forms and are conspicuously more numerous in the circulating blood and normal lymphoid tissue; the latter may be found in normal circulating blood, but are more easily observed in lymphoid tissue. The small lymphocytes have nuclei that are deeply or densely stained (the chromatin is coarse and bulky) and almost fill the cells, with only a slight rim of cytoplasm around the nuclei; the large lymphocytes have nuclei that are approximately the same size as, or only slightly larger than, those of the small forms, but there is a broader, easily visualized band of cytoplasm around the nuclei. Cells of the monocytic series are usually larger than the other l.'s, and are characterized by a relatively abundant, slightly opaque, pale blue or blue-gray cytoplasm that contains myriads of extremely fine reddish-blue granules. Monocytes are usually indented, reniform, or shaped similarly to a horseshoe, but are sometimes rounded or ovoid; their nuclei are usually large and centrally placed and, even when eccentrically located, are completely surrounded by at least a small band of cytoplasm.

acidophilic l., eosinophilic l.

agranular l., nongranular l.

basophilic l., basocyte; basophilocyte; mast l.; a polymorphonuclear l. characterized by many large, coarse, metachromatic granules (dark purple or blue-black when treated with Wright's or similar stains) which usually fill the cytoplasm and may almost mask the nucleus; these l.'s are unique in that they usually do not occur in increased numbers as the result of acute infectious disease, and their phagocytic qualities are probably not significant; the granules, which contain heparin and histamine, may degranulate in response to hypersensitivity reactions and can be of significance in general inflammation.

cystinotic l., a l. having an enhanced content of cystine, found in patients with disorders characterized by the storage of cystine; within the l., the cystine, largely in noncrystalline form, is associated with dense lysosomal particles.

endothelial l., endotheliocyte; old term for a monocyte, a type of l. thought to be derived from reticuloendothelial tissue.

eosinophilic l., eosinophil; eosinocyte; acidocyte; acidophilic or oxyphilic l.; oxyphil (2); a polymorphonuclear l. characterized by many large or prominent, refractile, cytoplasmic granules that are fairly uniform in size and bright yellow-red or orange when treated with Wright's or similar stains; the nuclei are usually larger than those of neutrophils, do not stain as deeply, and characteristically have two lobes (a third lobe is sometimes interposed on the connecting strand of chromatin); these l.'s are motile phagocytes with distinctive antiparasitic functions.

filament polymorphonuclear l., any mature polymorphonuclear l., especially a neutrophilic l., in which the lobes of the nucleus are interconnected with a thin strand or filament of chromatin.

globular l., a type of wandering cell with a small, round nucleus found in the epithelium and lamina propria of the intestinal mucosa of many animals; its cytoplasm contains large eosinophilic globules or droplets.

granular l., any one of the polymorphonuclear l.'s, especially a neutrophilic l. See also granulocyte; basophilic l.; eosinophilic l.

hyaline l., old term for a monocyte, and for a mononuclear macrophage in various lesions.

mast l., basophilic l.

motile l., any l. that manifests active ameboid movement, especially a mature granulocytic l. (eosinophils are less motile than neutrophils or basophils); monocytes manifest a slow, but persistent, wavelike movement.

multinuclear l., polymorphonuclear l.

neutrophilic l., a neutrophilic granulocyte, the most frequent of the polymorphonuclear l.'s, and also the most active phagocyte among the various types of white blood cells; when treated with Wright's stain (or similar preparations), the fairly abundant cytoplasm is faintly pink, and numerous tiny, slightly refractile, relatively bright pink or violet-pink, diffusely scattered granules are recognizable in the cytoplasm; the deeply stained blue or purple-blue nucleus is sharply distinguished from the cytoplasm and is distinctly lobated, with thin strands of chromatin connecting the three to five lobes.

nonfilament polymorphonuclear l., a neutrophil, basophil, or eosinophil that is not completely matured, *i.e.,* the lobes of the nuclei remain connected with bands of chromatin, in contrast to the thin strands observed in mature cells.

nongranular l., agranular l.; a general, nonspecific term frequently used with reference to lymphocytes, monocytes, and plasma cells; although the cytoplasm of a lymphocyte or monocyte contains tiny granules, it is "nongranular" in comparison with that of a neutrophil, basophil, or eosinophil. See also l.

nonmotile l., a term sometimes used with reference to lymphocytes, monocytes, and plasma cells; although such forms actually have some degree of motility, they are "nonmotile" in comparison with the actively ameboid, neutrophilic, basophilic, and eosinophilic l.'s.

oxyphilic l., eosinophilic l.

polymorphonuclear l., polynuclear l., multinuclear l.; common term for granulocyte or granulocytic l.; the term includes basophilic, eosinophilic, and neutrophilic l.'s, but is usually used especially with reference to the neutrophilic l.'s.

segmented l., any mature polymorphonuclear l., especially a neutrophilic l.

transitional l., old term for a monocyte.

Türk's l., Türk *cell.*

leukocythemia (lū'kō-sī-thē'mē-ă) [leukocyte + G. *haima,* blood]. An undesirable term for leukemia.

leukocytic (lū-kō-sit'ik). Leukocytal; pertaining to or characterized by leukocytes.

leukocytoblast (lū-kō-sī'tō-blast) [leukocyte + G. *blastos,* germ]. A nonspecific term for any immature cell from which a leukocyte develops, including lymphoblast, myeloblast, and the like.

leukocytoclasis (lū'kō-sī-tok'lă-sis) [leuko- + G. *kytos,* cell, + *klasia,* a breaking]. Karyorrhexis of leukocytes.

leukocytogenesis (lū'kō-sī-tō-jen'ĕ-sis) [leukocyte + G. *genesis,* production]. The formation and development of leukocytes.

leukocytoid (lū'kō-sī-toyd) [leukocyte + G. *eidos,* resemblance]. Resembling a leukocyte.

leukocytolysin (lū'kō-sī-tol'i-sin). Leukolysin; any substance (including lytic antibody) that causes dissolution of leukocytes.

leukocytolysis (lū'kō-sī-tol'i-sis) [leukocyte + G. *lysis,* dissolution]. Leukolysis; dissolution or lysis of leukocytes.

leukocytolytic (lū'kō-sī-tō-lit'ik). Leukolytic; pertaining to, causing, or manifesting leukocytolysis.

leukocytoma (lū'kō-sī-tō'mă) [leukocyte + G. *-oma,* tumor]. A fairly well circumscribed, nodular, dense accumulation of leukocytes.

leukocytometer (lū'kō-sī-tom'ĕ-ter) [leukocyte + G. *metron,* measure]. A standarized glass slide that is suitably ruled for counting the leukocytes in a measured volume of accurately diluted blood (or other specimens).

leukocytopenia (lū'kō-sī-tō-pē'nē-ă). Leukopenia.

leukocytoplania (lū'kō-sī-tō-plā'nē-ă) [leukocyte + G. *planē,* a wandering]. Movement of leukocytes from the lumens of blood vessels, through serous membranes, or in the tissues.

leukocytopoiesis (lū'kō-sī-tō-poy-ē'sis) [leukocyte + G. *poiēsis,* a making]. Leukopoiesis.

leukocytosis (lū'kō-sī-tō'sis) [leukocyte + G. *-osis,* condition]. An abnormally large number of leukocytes, as observed in acute infections. A white blood cell count of 10,000 or more per cu mm usually indicates l. Most examples of l. represent a disproportionate increase in the number of cells in the neutrophilic series, and the term is frequently used synonymously with the designation neutrophilia. L. of 15,000 to 25,000 per cu mm is frequently observed in various pathologic conditions, and values as high as 40,000 are not unusual; occasionally, as in some examples of leukemoid reactions, white blood cell counts may range up to 100,000 per cu mm.
absolute l., an actual increase in the total number of leukocytes in the circulating blood, as distinguished from a relative increase (such as that observed in dehydration).
agonal l., terminal l.
basophilic l., basocytosis; the presence of an abnormally large number of basophilic granulocytes in the blood.
digestive l., l. occurring normally after ingestion of food.
distribution l., an abnormally large proportion of one or more types of leukocytes.
emotional l., an abnormally high white blood cell count that is thought to be related only to an emotional disturbance.
eosinophilic l., eosinophilia; a form of relative l. in which the greatest proportionate increase is in the eosinophils.
lymphocytic l., lymphocytosis.
monocytic l., monocytosis.
neutrophilic l., neutrophilia.
l. of the newborn, an apparently "physiologic" l. usually observed in newborn infants, in whom the white blood cell counts are usually greater than 10,000 per cu mm, and sometimes range to 45,000 per cu mm, resulting chiefly from increased numbers of neutrophils (especially single and bilobed forms). On the third or fourth day of life, the count generally decreases rapidly, and then fluctuates for several days; beginning about the fourth week of life, a relative lymphocytosis is observed, and this normally continues for a few years.
physiologic l., any form of l. that is associated with apparently normal situations and that is not directly related to a pathologic condition; *e.g.,* the temporary increase in the total number of white blood cells that may occur during a single day, or from day to day, as well as in the newborn period, during childhood, after strenuous exercise, during attacks of paroxysmal tachycardia, and in association with various other situations.
relative l., an increased proportion of one or more types of leukocytes in the circulating blood, without an actual increase in the total number of white blood cells.
terminal l., agonal l.; one that occurs in a person just prior to death, especially in one who has a "slow death."

leukocytotactic (lū'kō-sī-tō-tak'tik). Leukocytactic; leukotactic; pertaining to, characterized by, or causing leukocytotaxia.

leukocytotaxia (lū-kō-sī-tō-tak'sē-ă) [leukocyte + G. *taxis,* arrangement]. Leukocytaxia; leukocytaxis; leukotaxia; leukotaxis. **1.** The active ameboid movement of leukocytes, especially the neutrophilic granulocytes, either toward (**positive l.**) or away from (**negative l.**) certain microorganisms as well as various substances frequently formed in inflamed tissue. **2.** The property of attracting or repelling leukocytes.

leukocytotoxin (lū'kō-sī-tō-tok'sin) [leukocyte + G. *toxikon,* poison]. Leukotoxin; any substance that causes degeneration and necrosis of leukocytes, including leukolysin and leukocidin.

Leukocytozoon (lū'kō-sī-tō-zō'on). *Leucocytozoon.*

leukocytozoonosis (lū'kō-sī'tō-zō-ō-nō'sis). Leucocytozoonosis.

leukocyturia (lū'kō-sī-tū'rē-ă) [leukocyte + G. *ouron,* urine]. The presence of leukocytes in urine that is recently voided or collected by means of a catheter.

leukoderma (lū-kō-der'mă). Achromoderma; alphodermia; hypomelanosis; leukopathia; leukopathy; an absence of pigment, partial or total, in the skin.
acquired l., vitiligo.
l. acquisi'tum centrifu'gum, halo *nevus.*
l. col'li, syphilitic l.
congenital l., albinism.
syphilitic l., l. or melanoleukoderma colli; a fading of the roseola of secondary syphilis, leaving reticulated depigmented and hyperpigmented areas located chiefly on the sides of the neck.

leukodermatous (lū-kō-der'mă-tŭs). Relating to or resembling leukoderma.

leukodontia (lū-kō-don'shē-ă) [leuko- + G. *odous,* tooth]. The condition of having white teeth.

leukodystrophia (lū-kō-dis-trō'fē-ă). Leukodystrophy.
l. cer'ebri progres'siva, leukodystrophy.

leukodystrophy (lū-kō-dis'trō-fē) [leuko- + G. *dys,* bad, + *trophē,* nourishment]. Leukodystrophia; leukodystrophia cerebri progressiva; leukoencephalopathy; sclerosis of the white matter; generic term for a group of white matter diseases, some familial, characterized by progressive cerebral deterioration in early life and pathologically by primary absence or degeneration of the myelin of the central and peripheral nervous systems with glial reaction; probably related to a defect in lipid metabolism. See also spongy *degeneration.*
globoid cell l., diffuse infantile familial sclerosis; a metabolic encephalopathy of infancy with rapidly progressive cerebral degeneration, massive loss of myelin, severe astrocytic gliosis, and infiltration of the white matter with characteristic multinucleate globoid cells; metabolically there is gross deficiency of cerebrosidase (galactosylceramide β-galactosidase); autosomal recessive inheritance.
metachromatic l., sulfatide lipidosis; sulfatidosis; a metabolic disorder characterized by myelin loss, accumulation of metachromatic lipids (galactosyl sulfatidates) in the white matter of the central and peripheral nervous systems, a marked excess of sulfatidate in the white matter and in urine, progressive paralysis, and mental retardation; psychosis and dementia are seen in adults; autosomal recessive inheritance.

leukoedema (lū'kō-e-dē'mă). A bluish-white opalescence of the buccal mucosa which becomes the normal mucosal color on stretching the tissue; most commonly observed in blacks and may be considered a normal anatomic variation.

leukoencephalitis (lū'kō-en-sef-ă-lī'tis). Encephalitis restricted to the white matter.
acute epidemic l., Strumpell's disease (2); acute primary hemorrhagic meningoencephalitis; a disease characterized by acute onset of fever, followed by convulsions, delirium, and coma, and associated with perivascular demyelination and hemorrhagic foci in the central nervous system.
subacute sclerosing l., inclusion body *encephalitis.*

leukoencephalopathy (lū'kō-en-sef-ă-lop'ă-thē) [leuko- + G. *enkephalos,* brain, + *pathos,* suffering]. Leukodystrophy.

progressive multifocal l., a rare, subacute, afebrile disease characterized by areas of demyelinization surrounded by markedly altered neuroglia, including inclusion bodies in glial cells; it occurs usually in individuals with leukemia, lymphoma, or other debilitating diseases, or in those who have been receiving immunosuppressive treatment.

leukoerythroblastosis (lū'kō-ĕ-rith'rō-blas-tō'sis). Myelophthisic, myelopathic, osteosclerotic, or leukoerythroblastic anemia; any anemic condition resulting from space-occupying lesions in the bone marrow; the circulating blood contains immature cells of the granulocytic series and nucleated red blood cells, frequently in numbers that are disproportionately large in relation to the degree of anemia.

leukokeratosis (lū'kō-ker-ă-tō'sis). Rarely used term for leukoplakia.

leukokoria (lū-kō-kō'rē-ă). Leukocoria.

leukokraurosis (lū'kō-kraw-rō'sis). *Kraurosis* vulvae.

leukolymphosarcoma (lū'kō-lim'fō-sar-kō'mă). Leukosarcoma.

leukolysin (lū-kol'i-sin). Leukocytolysin.

leukolysis (lū-kol'i-sis). Leukocytolysis.

leukolytic (lū-kō-lit'ik). Leukocytolytic.

leukoma (lū-kō'mă) [G. whiteness, a white spot in the eye, fr. *leukos*, white]. Albugo; a dense, opaque, white opacity of the cornea.

adherent l., a cicatrix of the cornea to which a portion of the iris is attached.

leukomatous (lū-kō'mă-tŭs). Denoting leukoma.

leukomyelopathy (lū'kō-mī'ĕ-lop'ă-thē) [leuko- + G. *myelos*, marrow, + *pathos*, suffering]. Any systemic disease involving the white matter or the conducting tracts of the spinal cord.

leukon (lū'kon). The total mass of circulating leukocytes as well as the cells and leukopoietic cells from which it originates.

leukonecrosis (lū'kō-ne-krō'sis) [leuko- + G. *nekrōsis*, deadness]. White *gangrene*.

leukonychia (lū-kō-nik'ē-ă) [leuko- + G. *onyx* (*onych-*), nail]. Leukopathia unguis; achromia or canities unguium; the occurrence of white spots or patches under the nails, due to the presence of air bubbles between the nail and its bed; the decoloration may be total or in the form of lines (striate l.) or dots (punctate l.).

leukopathia, leukopathy (lū-kō-path'ē-ă, lū-kop'ă-thē) [leuko- + G. *pathos*, disease]. Leukoderma.

acquired l., vitiligo.

congenital l., albinism.

l. un'guis, leukonychia.

leukopedesis (lū'kō-pē-dē'sis) [leuko- + G. *pēdēsis*, a leaping]. The movement of white blood cells (especially polymorphonuclear leukocytes) through the walls of capillaries and into the tissues.

leukopenia (lū-kō-pē'nē-ă) [leuko(cyte) + G. *penia*, poverty]. Leukocytopenia; the antithesis of leukocytosis; any situation in which the total number of leukocytes in the circulating blood is less than normal, the lower limit of which is generally regarded as 5000/cu mm.

basophilic l., basocytopenia; basopenia; a decrease in the number of basophilic granulocytes normally present in the circulating blood (difficult to evaluate, owing to the small and variable number normally present).

eosinophilic l., a decrease in the number of eosinophilic granulocytes normally present in the circulating blood.

lymphocytic l., lymphopenia.

monocytic l., monocytopenia.

neutrophilic l., neutropenia.

leukopenic (lū-kō-pē'nik). Pertaining to leukopenia.

leukophlegmasia (lū-kō-fleg-mā'zē-ă) [leuko- + phlegmasia]. Lymphatic *edema*.

l. do'lens, *phlegmasia* alba dolens.

leukoplakia (lū-kō-plā'kē-ă) [leuko- + G. *plax*, plate]. A white patch of oral mucous membrane which cannot be wiped off and cannot be diagnosed clinically as any specific disease entity; in current usage, a clinical term without histologic or premalignant connotation.

hairy l., a white lesion appearing on the tongue, occasionally on the buccal mucosa, of patients with AIDS; the lesion appears raised, with a corrugated or "hairy" surface due to keratin projections.

l. vul'vae, leukoplakic vulvitis; an atrophic thickening and keratinization of the vulvar epithelium, often associated with papillary hypertrophy; the lesion has a patchy white appearance.

leukopoiesis (lū'kō-poy-ē'sis) [leuko- + G. *poiēsis*, a making]. Leukocytopoiesis; formation and development of the various types of white blood cells.

leukopoietic (lū'kō-poy-et'ik). Pertaining to or characterized by leukopoiesis, as manifested by portions of the bone marrow and reticuloendothelial and lymphoid tissues, which form (respectively) the granulocytes, monocytes, and lymphocytes.

leukoprotease (lū-kō-prō'tē-ās). An ill-defined proteolytic enzyme product of polynuclear leukocytes, formed in an area of inflammation, that causes liquefaction of dead tissue.

leukoriboflavin (lū-kō-rī'bō-flā-vin). The colorless nonfluorescing dihydro compound formed by the reduction of riboflavin.

leukorrhagia (lū-kō-rā'jē-ă) [leuko- + G. *rhēgnymi*, to burst forth]. Leukorrhea.

leukorrhea (lū-kō-rē'ă) [leuko- + G. *rhoia*, flow]. Leukorrhagia; discharge from the vagina of a white or yellowish viscid fluid containing mucus and pus cells.

menstrual l., intermittent l. recurring at or just before each menstrual period.

leukorrheal (lū-kō-rē'ăl). Relating to or characterized by leukorrhea.

leukosarcoma (lū'kō-sar-kō'mă). Leukolymphosarcoma; leukemia developing in a person with preexisting lymphosarcoma involving the lymph nodes and various other tissues and organs.

leukosarcomatosis (lū'kō-sar-kō-mă-tō'sis). A condition characterized initially by numerous widespread nodules or masses of lymphosarcoma, and the subsequent presence of similar cells in the circulating blood as in leukosarcoma.

leukosis (lū-kō'sis). Abnormal proliferation of one or more of the leukopoietic tissues; the term includes myelosis, certain forms of reticuloendotheliosis, and lymphadenosis.

avian l., fowl, leukemia of fowls; a group of conditions (*e.g.*, lymphoid, erythroid, or myeloid l.) that occur chiefly in chickens and are characterized by an abnormal proliferation of myelopoietic, erythropoietic, or lymphoid tissues; etiologic agents are a group of closely related viruses, and the conditions are transmissible. See also avian leukosis-sarcoma *complex*.

enzootic bovine l., a fatal infectious disease of cattle older than 3 years caused by the bovine leukemia virus; characterized clinically by enlargement of peripheral lymph nodes, anorexia, weight loss, and decreased milk production, and pathologically by development of lymphosarcoma in various tissues and organs.

sporadic bovine l., a rare disease of cattle less than 3 years of age, of unknown cause, characterized by the development of lymphosarcoma; three clinicopathological forms are recognized: calf or juvenile form, thymic form, and cutaneous form.

leukotactic (lū-kō-tak'tik). Leukocytotactic.

leukotaxia (lū-kō-tak'sē-ă). Leukocytotaxia.

leukotaxine (lū-kō-tak'sēn). A cell-free nitrogenous material prepared from injured, acutely degenerating tissue and from inflammatory exudates.

leukotaxis (lū-kō-tak'sis). Leukocytotaxia.

leukotic (lū-kot'ik). Pertaining to, characterized by, or manifesting leukosis.

leukotome (lū'kō-tōm). An instrument for performing leukotomy.

leukotomy (lū-kot'ō-mē) [leuko- + G. *tomē,* a cutting]. Incision into the white matter of the frontal lobe of the brain.
prefrontal l., prefrontal *lobotomy.*
transorbital l., transorbital *lobotomy.*

leukotoxin (lū-kō-tok'sin). Leukocytotoxin.

leukotrichia (lū-kō-trik'ē-ă) [leuko- + G. *thrix,* hair]. Whiteness of the hair.
l. annula'ris, ringed *hair.*

leukotrichous (lū-kot'ri-kŭs). Having white hair.

leukotrienes (lū-kō-trī'ēnz). Products of arachidonic acid metabolism with postulated physiologic activity such as mediators of inflammation and roles in allergic reactions; differ from the related prostaglandins and thromboxanes by not having a central ring. So named because discovered in association with leukocytes and of three double bonds in the first leukotriene discovered (most have four); letters A through E identify the five metabolites thus far isolated, with subscript numbers to indicate the number of double bonds (*e.g.,* leukotriene C_4).

Leukovirus (lū'kō-vī'rŭs). A former genus composed of the RNA tumor viruses now included in the family Retroviridae.

leuprolide acetate (lū'prō-līd). A synthetic nonapeptide analog of naturally occurring gonadotropin-releasing hormone; used in the palliative treatment of advanced prostatic cancer.

Lev, Maurice, U.S. pathologist, *1908. See L.'s *disease, syndrome.*

Levaditi, Constantin, Roumanian bacteriologist in Paris, 1874–1928. See L. *stain.*

levallorphan tartrate (lev-ă-lōr'fan). 1-*N*-Allyl-3-hydroxymorphinan tartrate; the *N*-allyl analogue of levorphanol, antagonistic to the actions of narcotic analgesics; used in the treatment of respiratory depression due to overdosage of narcotics.

lev'an. Fructosan.

levansucrase (lev-an-sū'krās) [EC 2.4.1.10]. An enzyme catalyzing transfer of the fructose moiety of sucrose to polyfructose (a levan), leaving the glucose moiety free.

levarterenol (lev-ar-tēr'ē-nol). Norepinephrine.
l. bitartrate, *norepinephrine* bitartrate.

levator (le-vā'ter, tōr) [L. a lifter, fr. *levo,* pp. *-atus,* to lift, fr. *levis,* light]. **1.** A surgical instrument for prying up the depressed part in a fracture of the skull. **2.** One of several muscles whose action is to raise the part into which it is inserted.

LeVeen, Harry H., U.S. surgeon, *1914. See L. *shunt.*

lev'el. Any rank, position, or status in a graded scale of values.
acoustic reference l., the biological reference l. for sound measurements. When the term decibel is used to indicate the noise l., a reference quantity is implied; this reference value is usually expressed as a sound pressure of 20 micronewtons per square meter. The reference l. is referred to as 0 decibels, the baseline of the scale of noise l.'s; this baseline is considered the weakest sound that can be heard by a person with very good hearing in an extremely quiet location. Other equivalent reference l.'s still being used include 0.0002 microbar and 0.0002 dyne per square centimeter.
l. of aspiration, in clinical psychology, the degree or quality of performance which an individual desires to attain or feels he can achieve.
Clark's l., the l. of invasion of primary malignant melanoma of the skin from the epidermis: I, into the underlying papillary dermis; II, to the junction of the papillary and reticular dermis; III, into the reticular dermis; IV, into the subcutaneous fat. The prognosis is worse with each successive deeper l. of invasion.
hearing l., the measure of the status of hearing as read directly on the hearing loss scale of an audiometer; described in decibels as a deviation from a standard value for zero on the audiometer.
sound pressure l. (SPL), a measure of sound energy relative to 0.0002 dynes/cm^2, expressed in decibels.
window l., the CT number that is the midpoint of a given window width, varying from +500 to −500 (or +1000 to −1000, depending on the type of machine).

Leventhal, Michael L., U.S. obstetrician-gynecologist, 1901–1971. See Stein-L. *syndrome.*

lever (lev'er, lē'ver) [Fr. *lever,* to lift]. An instrument used to lift or pry.
dental l., elevator (2).

leverage (lē'ver-ij). **1.** The actual lift or elevating direction of lever or elevator. **2.** The mechanical advantage gained thereby.

Lévi, E. Leopold, French endocrinologist, 1868–1933. See dominantly inherited L.'s *disease;* Lorain-L. *dwarfism, infantilism, syndrome.*

Levin, Abraham L., U.S. physician, 1880–1940. See L. *tube.*

Levin, Max, U.S. neurologist, *1901. See Kleine-L. *syndrome.*

Levine, Samuel A., U.S. cardiologist, 1891–1966. See Lown-Ganong-L. *syndrome.*

Levinea (lĕ-vin'ē-ă) [Max *Levine,* U.S. bacteriologist, *1889]. A former genus of bacteria (famiy Enterobacteriaceae) whose species are now assigned to the genus *Citrobacter.*
L. amalona'tica, *Citrobacter amalonaticus.*
L. malona'tica, *Citrobacter diversus.*

levitation (lev-i-tā'shŭn) [L. *levitas,* lightness]. Support of the patient on a cushion of air.

Leviviridae (lĕ-vi-vir'i-dē) [L. *levis,* light (not heavy)]. Provisional name for a family of small, nonenveloped, isometric bacterial viruses with genomes of single-stranded RNA (MW 1×10^6). Virions adsorb to the sides of bacterial pili, and crystalline arrays are formed in infected bacteria. The type species is coliphage R17.

levo- [L. *laevus,* left]. Prefix denoting left, toward or on the left side.

levobunolol hydrochloride (lē-vō-byū'nō-lol). (−)-5-[3-(*tert*-Butylamino)-2-hydroxy-propoxy]-3,4-dihydro-1(2*H*)-naphthalenone hydrochloride; a *β*-adrenergic blocking agent used primarily as an eyedrop in the treatment of chronic open-angle glaucoma and ocular hypertension.

levocardia (lē-vō-kar'dē-ă) [levo- + G. *kardia,* heart]. Situs inversus of the other viscera but with the heart normally situated on the left; congenital cardiac lesions are commonly associated.

levocardiogram (lē-vō-kar'dē-ō-gram). That part of the bicardiogram, or normal curve, that is the effect of the left ventricle.

levoclination (lē'vō-kli-nā'shŭn) [levo- + L. *clino,* pp. *-atus,* to bend]. Levotorsion (2).

levocycloduction (lē'vō-sī-klō-dŭk'shŭn) [levo- + cyclo- + L. *duco,* pp. *ductus,* to lead]. Rotation of the upper pole of one cornea to the left.

levodopa (lē-vō-dō'pă). L-Dopa; the biologically active form of dopa; an antiparkinsonian agent.

levoduction (lē-vō-dŭk'shŭn) [levo- + L. *duco,* pp. *ductus,* to lead]. Rotation of one eye to the left.

levoform (lē'vō-fōrm). Denoting the structure of a substance that rotates the plane of polarized light counterclockwise (left).

levoglucose (lē-vō-glū'kōs). Fructose.

levogram (lē'vō-gram). Electrocardiographic record in an experimental animal representing spread of impulse through the left ventricle alone.

levogyrate, levogyrous (lē-vō-jī'rāt, -jī'rŭs) [levo- + L. *gyro,* to turn in a circle]. Levorotatory.

levonordefrin (lē′vō-nōr-def′rin). α-(1-Aminoethyl)-3,4-dihydroxybenzyl alcohol; used as a nasal decongestant and as a vasoconstrictor given with infiltration anesthetics.

levophacetoperane (lē′vō-fa-sē-top′er′ān). α-Phenyl-2-piperidinemethanol acetate; an antidepressant with anorexigenic properties.

levophobia (lev′ō-fō′bē-ă). Fear of objects to the left.

levopropoxyphene napsylate (lē′vō-prō-pok′si-fēn). α-4-(Dimethylamino)-3-methyl-1,2-diphenyl-2-butanol propionate 2-naphthalenesulfonate; an antitussive.

levorotation (lē-vō-rō-tā′shŭn) [levo- + L. *rotare,* to turn]. **1.** A turning or twisting to the left; in particular, the counterclockwise twist given the plane of plane-polarized light by solutions of certain optically active substances. *Cf.* dextrorotation. **2.** Sinistrotorsion.

levorotatory (lē-vō-rō′tă-tōr-ē). Levogyrate; levogyrous; denoting levorotation, or certain crystals or solutions capable of doing so; as a chemical prefix, usually abbreviated *l*-. *Cf.* dextrorotatory.

levorphanol tartrate (lev-ōrf′ă-nol). L-3-Hydroxy-*N*-methylmorphinan tartrate dihydrate; an analgesic similar in action to morphine.

levotorsion (lē-vō-tōr′shŭn) [levo- + L. *torsio,* a twisting]. **1.** Sinistrotorsion. **2.** Levoclination; rotation of the upper pole of the cornea to the left.

levoversion (lē′vō-ver′zhŭn) [levo- + L. *verto,* pp. *versus,* to turn]. **1.** Version toward the left. **2.** Conjugate rotation of both eyes to the left.

Levret, André, French obstetrician, 1703–1780. See L.'s *forceps;* Mauriceau-L. *maneuver.*

levulan (lev′yū-lan). Fructosan.

levulic acid (lev′yū-lik). Levulinic acid.

levulin (lev′yū-lin). Fructosan.

levulinate (lev′yū-lin-āt). A salt or ester of levulinic acid.

levulinic acid (lev-yū-lin′ik). Levulic acid; 4-oxopentanoic acid; $CH_3COCH_2CH_2COOH$, formed by the action of hot, strong acids on hexoses. See also δ-aminolevulinic acid.

levulosan (lev′yū-lō-san). Fructosan.

levulose (lev′yū-lōs). Fructose.

levulosemia (lev′yū-lō-sē′mē-ă). Fructosemia.

levulosuria (lev′yū-lō-sū′rē-ă). Fructosuria.

Lévy, Gabrielle, French neurologist, 1886–1935. See Roussy-L. *disease, syndrome.*

Lewandowski, Felix, German dermatologist, 1879–1921. See L.-Lutz *disease;* Jadassohn-L. *syndrome; nevus* elasticus of L.

Lewis (Le) blood group. See Blood Groups appendix.

lewisite (lū′i-sīt) [W. Lee *Lewis,* Chicago chemist 1898–1943]. Dichloro(2-chlorovinyl)arsine; β-chlorovinyldichloroarsine; $C_2H_2AsCl_3$; a war gas. It is a vesicant, a lung irritant like mustard gas, a systemic poison entering the circulation through the lungs or skin, and a mitotic poison arresting mitosis in the metaphase; dimercaprol is the antidote.

Lewy (Lewey), Frederic H., German neurologist in the U.S., 1885–1950. See L. *bodies.*

-lexis, -lexy [G. *-lex-* fr. *legein, lexai,* to speak]. Suffixes that properly relate to speech, although often confused with -legia (Latin *-legis*) and thus erroneously employed to relate to reading.

Leyden, Ernst V. von, German physician, 1832–1910. See L.'s *ataxia, crystals, neuritis;* L.-Möbius muscular *dystrophy.*

Leydig, Franz von, German anatomist, 1821–1908. See L.'s *cells;* L. cell *adenoma.*

leydigarche (lī′dig-ar-kē) [Leydig (see Leydig cells), + G. *arche,* beginning]. Obsolete term for the beginning of gonadal function in the male, *i.e.,* male puberty.

Lf, L_f See under dose.

LFA Abbreviation for left frontoanterior *position.*

LFP Abbreviation for left frontoposterior *position.*

LFT Abbreviation for left frontotransverse *position.*

LH Abbreviation for luteinizing *hormone.*

Lhermitte, Jean, French neurologist, 1877–1959. See L.'s *sign;* L.-Duclos *disease.*

LH/FSH-RF Abbreviation for luteinizing hormone/follicle-stimulating hormone-releasing *factor.*

LH-RF Abbreviation for luteinizing hormone-releasing *factor.*

LH-RH Abbreviation for luteinizing hormone-releasing *hormone.*

Li Symbol for lithium.

Li, Frederick P., 20th century epidemiologist. See L.-Fraumeni cancer *syndrome.*

liberator (lib′er-ā-ter, tōr). An agent that stimulates or activates a physiological chemical or an enzymatic action.

histamine l.'s, substances that cause the release of histamine from mast cells or basophils.

liberomotor (lib′er-ō-mō′ter) [L. *liber,* free, + *motor,* mover]. Relating to voluntary movements.

libidinization (li-bid′i-ni-zā′shŭn). Erotization.

libidinous (li-bid′i-nŭs) [L. *libidinosus,* fr. *libido* (*libidin-*), pleasure, desire]. Lascivious; erotic; invested with or arousing sexual desire or energy.

libido (li-bē′dō, -bī′dō) [L. lust]. **1.** Conscious or unconscious sexual desire. **2.** Any passionate interest or form of life force. **3.** In Jungian psychology, synonymous with psychic *energy.*

object l., l. invested in the object, in contradistinction to that invested in the ego.

Libman, Emanuel, U.S. physician, 1872–1946. See L.-Sacks *endocarditis, syndrome.*

Liborius, Paul, 19th century Kronstadt bacteriologist. See L.'s *method.*

lice (līs). Plural of louse.

lichen (lī′ken) [G. *leichēn,* lichen; a lichen-like eruption]. A discrete flat papule or an aggregate of papules giving a patterned configuration resembling lichens growing on rocks.

l. acumina′tus, l. planus.

l. a′grius, Celsus' papules; acute papular eczema of severe type.

l. al′bus, chronic lichenoid dermatitis with depigmentation.

l. annula′ris, *granuloma* annulare.

l. hemorrhag′icus, a papular eruption due to hemorrhage into the hair follicles.

l. infan′tum, *miliaria* rubra.

l. i′ris, ringworm with concentric rings of erythematous papules.

l. myxedemato′sus, papular mucinosis; a lichenoid eruption of papules or plaques of mucinous edema due to deposit of acid mucopolysaccharides in the skin, in the absence of endocrine disease.

l. niti′dus, small minute asymptomatic whitish or pinkish papules; lesions, which are flat-topped, may coexist with l. planus and may involve male genitalia.

l. nu′chae, l. simplex of the neck, usually in women.

l. obtu′sus, a form in which the papules are large and rounded instead of flattened.

oral (erosive) l. planus, oral manifestations of l. planus characterized by white striae (Wickham's striae) of the oral mucous membrane and sometimes associated with ulceration; patients may or may not exhibit a history of cutaneous l. planus.

oral (nonerosive) l. planus, an oral disease characterized clinically by lesions appearing as a network of fine or thick, violaceous, inter-

lacing lines (Wickham's striae) forming a wide variety of patterns on the oral mucosa.
l. planopila'ris, l. planus et acuminatus atrophicans; Graham Little syndrome; follicular hyperkeratosis of the scalp with l. planus elsewhere.
l. pla'nus, l. acuminatus; l. ruber planus; Wilson's l.; eruption of flat-topped, shiny, violaceous papules on flexor surfaces, male genitalia, and buccal mucosa; may form linear groups; individual lesions may be angular or umbilicated; hypertrophic lesions may form on legs.
l. pla'nus et acumina'tus atro'phicans, l. planopilaris.
l. pla'nus annula'ris, a form in which the papules are grouped in ring figures.
l. pla'nus follicula'ris, l. planus of the hair follicles, usually of the scalp.
l. pla'nus hypertro'phicus, l. planus verrucosus; l. ruber verrucosus; verrucoid or warty lesions occurring on legs and thighs in association with l. planus elsewhere.
l. pla'nus verruco'sus, l. planus hypertrophicus.
l. ru'ber, old term for l. planus.
l. ru'ber monilifor'mis, a rare dermatosis consisting of small reddish papules arranged in narrow beaded bands and covering large areas of the body.
l. ru'ber pla'nus, l. planus.
l. ru'ber verruco'sus, l. planus hypertrophicus.
l. sclero'sus et atro'phicus, an eruption consisting of white atrophic papules which may be discrete or confluent and may contain a central depression or a black keratotic plug microscopically showing epidermal hyperkeratosis and atrophy, superficial dermal edema and homogenization, and mid-dermal inflammation; often associated with kraurosis vulvae.
l. scrofuloso'rum, papular *tuberculid.*
l. sim'plex, Vidal's disease; a small, intensely pruritic, lichenified area in post-adolescence, on almost any part of the body, in single or multiple sites.
l. spinulo'sus, eruption of conical papules, of unknown cause, which have an adherent scaly surface; may be related to l. planus.
l. stria'tus, a self-limited papular eruption occurring primarily in children (more commonly in females); the lesions are arranged in linear groups and usually occur on one extremity.
l. strophulo'sus, *miliaria* rubra.
l. syphilit'icus, follicular *syphilid.*
tropical l., l. trop'icus, *miliaria* rubra.
l. urtica'tus, prurigo infantilis; papular urticaria; urticaria papulosa; a type of urticaria occurring in children, in which the lesions are papules, or small papules and vesicles.
l. variega'tus, maculopapular *erythroderma.*
Wilson's l., l. planus.

lichenification (lī'ken-i-fi-kā'shŭn) [lichen + L. *facio,* to make]. Lichenization; leathery induration and thickening of the skin with hyperkeratosis, due to a chronic inflammation caused by scratching or long-continued irritation.

lichenin (lī'ken-in). Moss starch; a variety of starch obtained from Iceland moss; used as a demulcent.

lichenization (lī'ken-i-zā'shŭn). Lichenification.

lichenoid (lī'kĕ-noyd). **1.** Resembling lichen. **2.** Accentuation of normal skin markings observed in cases of chronic eczema. **3.** Microscopically resembling lichen planus.

Lichtenstein, Louis, U.S. physician, *1906. See Jaffe-L. *disease.*

Lichtheim, Ludwig, German physician, 1845–1928. See L.'s *sign;* Dejerine-L. *phenomenon.*

licorice (lik'ŏ-ris). Glycyrrhiza.

lid [A.S. *hlid*]. See eyelid.
granular l.'s, trachoma.

Liddell, Edward G.T., British neurophysiologist, 1895–1981. See L.-Sherrington *reflex.*

lidocaine hydrochloride (lī'dō-kān). Diethylamino-2,6-acetoxylidide hydrochloride; a local anesthetic with pronounced antiarrhythmic and anticonvulsant properties.

lidoflazine (lī-dō-flā'zēn). 4-[4,4-Bis(*p*-fluorophenyl)butyl]-1-piperazineaceto-2',6'-xylidide; a coronary vasodilator.

lie (lī). Relationship of the long axis of the fetus to that of the mother.
longitudinal l., that relationship in which the long axis of the fetus is longitudinal and roughly parallel to the long axis of the mother; the presenting part may be either the head or the breech.
oblique l., that relationship in which the long axis of the fetus crosses the maternal axis at an angle other than a right angle.
transverse l., that relationship in which the long axis of the fetus is transverse or at right angles to that of the mother.

Lieberkühn, Johann N., German anatomist, 1711–1756. See L.'s *crypts, follicles, glands.*

lieberkühn (lē'ber-kūn) [J.N. *Lieberkühn*]. A concave reflector around the objective of a microscope, for the purpose of directing a concentrated beam of light on the material being examined.

Liebermann, Leo von S., Hungarian physician, 1852–1926. See Burchard-L. *reaction;* L.-Burchard *test.*

Liebermeister, Carl von, German physician, 1833–1901. See L.'s *rule.*

Liebig, Baron Justus von, German chemist, 1803–1873. See L.'s *theory.*

lie detector. Polygraph (2).

lien-, lieno- [L. *lien,* spleen]. Combining forms relating to the spleen; most terms beginning thus are obsolete or obsolescent. See splen- and spleno-.

lien (lī'en) [L.] [NA]. Official alternative term for splen.
l. accesso'rius, *splen* accessorius.
l. mo'bilis, floating *spleen.*
l. succenturia'tus, *splen* accessorius.

lienal (lī'ĕ-năl). Splenic.

lienculus (lī-en'kyū-lŭs) [Mod. L. dim. of L. *lien,* spleen]. *Splen* accessorius.

lienectomy (lī'ĕ-nek'tō-mē). Obsolete term for splenectomy.

lienomedullary (lī'ĕ-nō-med'yū-lār-ē) [lieno- + G. *medulla,* marrow]. Splenomyelogenous.

lienomyelogenous (lī'ĕ-nō-mī-ĕ-loj'ĕ-nŭs). Splenomyelogenous.

lienopancreatic (lī'ĕ-nō-pan'krē-at'ik). Splenopancreatic.

lienorenal (lī'ĕ-nō-rē'năl) [lieno- + L. *ren,* kidney]. Splenonephric; splenorenal; relating to the spleen and the kidney.

lienteric (lī-en-ter'ik). Relating to, or marked by, lientery.

lientery (lī'en-ter-ē) [G. *leienteria,* fr. *leios,* smooth, + *enteron,* intestine]. Passage of undigested food in the stools.

lienunculus (lī'ĕ-nun'kyū-lŭs) [Mod. L. dim. of L. *lien,* spleen]. *Splen* accessorius.

Liesegang, Ralph E., German chemist, 1869–1947. See L. *rings.*

Lieutaud, Joseph, French anatomist and pathologist, 1703–1780. See L.'s *body, triangle, trigone, uvula.*

life (līf) [A.S. *lif*]. **1.** Vitality, the essential condition of being alive; the state of existence characterized by active metabolism. **2.** The existence of animals and plants.
half-l., see half-life.
postnatal l., that interval of l. after birth; in man, usually divided into periods: neonatal, infancy, childhood, adolescence, and adulthood.
prenatal l., that interval of l. between conception and birth; in humans, usually divided into embryonic and fetal periods.

sexual l., in psychiatry and psychoanalysis, the specifically erotic or sexual interests, fantasies, inclinations, and conduct of the patient.
vegetative l., the simple metabolic and reproductive activity of man or animals, apart from the exercise of conscious mental or psychic processes.

life events. Occurrences in one's daily life that act as stressors.

life-span. **1.** The duration of existence of an individual. **2.** The normal or average duration of existence of a given species. See also longevity.

life-style. The general behavior pattern of an individual as expressed by his/her attitudes, motives, manner of coping, and other factors.

LIGAMENT

ligament (lig′ă-ment) [L. *ligamentum,* a band, bandage]. Ligamentum.
accessory l.'s, l.'s about a joint that are in addition to the articular capsule. They may lie within, or on the outside of the latter.
accessory plantar l.'s, *ligamenta* plantaria.
accessory volar l.'s, *ligamenta* palmaria.
acromioclavicular l., *ligamentum* acromioclaviculare.
alar l.'s, **(1)** *ligamenta* alaria; **(2)** *plicae* alares.
alveolodental l., periodontal l.
annular l., orbicular l.; ligamentum annulare; one of a number of l.'s encircling various parts; the principal annular l.'s are those of the stapes, radius, and trachea. See *ligamentum* annulare bulbi, digitorum, radii, stapedis; *ligamenta* annularia trachealia.
annular l. of the radius, *ligamentum* annulare radii.
annular l. of the stapes, *ligamentum* annulare stapedis.
annular l.'s of the trachea, *ligamenta* annularia trachealia.
anococcygeal l., *ligamentum* anococcygeum.
anterior costotransverse l., *ligamentum* costotransversarium superius.
anterior cruciate l., *ligamentum* cruciatum anterius.
anterior l. of head of fibula, *ligamentum* capitis fibulae anterius.
anterior longitudinal l., *ligamentum* longitudinale anterius.
anterior l. of malleus, *ligamentum* mallei anterius.
anterior meniscofemoral l., *ligamentum* meniscofemorale anterius.
anterior sacrococcygeal l., *ligamentum* sacrococcygeum anterius.
anterior sacroiliac l.'s, *ligamenta* sacroiliaca anteriora.
anterior sacrosciatic l., *ligamentum* sacrospinale.
anterior sternoclavicular l., *ligamentum* sternoclaviculare (1).
anterior talofibular l., *ligamentum* talofibulare anterius.
anterior talotibial l., *pars* tibiotalaris anterior. See also *ligamentum* deltoideum.
anterior tibiofibular l., *ligamentum* tibiofibulare anterius.
apical l. of dens, *ligamentum* apicis dentis.
Arantius' l., *ligamentum* venosum.
arcuate popliteal l., *ligamentum* popliteum arcuatum.
arcuate pubic l., *ligamentum* arcuatum pubis.
arterial l., *ligamentum* arteriosum.
l.'s of auditory ossicles, *ligamenta* ossiculorum auditus.
auricular l.'s, *ligamenta* auricularia.
axis l. of malleus, Helmholtz' axis l.
Bardinet's l., the posterior band of the ulnar collateral l. of the elbow.
Barkow's l., the l.'s on the anterior and posterior aspects of the elbow joint.
Bellini's l., a fasciculus of the articular capsule l. of the hip extending to the great trochanter.
Berry's l., the lateral l.'s of the thyroid gland.
Bertin's l., *ligamentum* iliofemorale.
Bichat's l., the lower fasciculus of the posterior sacroiliac l.
bifurcated l., *ligamentum* bifurcatum.
Bigelow's l., *ligamentum* iliofemorale.
Botallo's l., *ligamentum* arteriosum.
Bourgery's l., *ligamentum* popliteum obliquum.
broad l. of the uterus, *ligamentum* latum uteri.
Brodie's l., transverse humeral l.
Burns' l., *cornu* superius (2).
calcaneocuboid l., *ligamentum* calcaneocuboideum.
calcaneofibular l., *ligamentum* calcaneofibulare.
calcaneonavicular l., *ligamentum* calcaneonaviculare.
calcaneotibial l., *pars* tibiocalcanea. See also *ligamentum* deltoideum.
Caldani's l., *ligamentum* coracoclaviculare.
Campbell's l., suspensory l. of axilla.
Camper's l., *membrana* perinei.
capsular l., ligamentum capsulare; thickened portions of the fibrous membrane of an articular capsule.
cardinal l., cervical l. of the uterus.
caroticoclinoid l., the l. that connects the anterior to the middle clinoid process of the sphenoid bone.
carpometacarpal l.'s, *ligamenta* carpometacarpalia.
caudal l., *retinaculum* caudale.
ceratocricoid l., *ligamentum* ceratocricoideum.
cervical l. of uterus, Mackenrodt's l.; cardinal l.; ligamentum transversalis colli; a fibrous band attached to the uterine cervix and the vault of the lateral fornix of the vagina; continuous with the tissue ensheathing the pelvic vessels.
check l.'s of eyeball, medial and lateral, Mauchart's l.'s; expansions of the sheaths of the medial and lateral rectus muscles of the eyeball which are attached, respectively, to the lacrimal bone and to the orbital (Whitnall's) tubercle of the zygomatic bone; they serve to prevent overaction of these muscles.
check l.'s of odontoid, *ligamenta* alaria.
chondroxiphoid l., *ligamentum* costoxiphoideum.
ciliary l., *musculus* ciliaris.
Civinini's l., *ligamentum* pterygospinale.
Clado's l., a mesenteric fold running from the broad l. on the right side to the appendix.
collateral l., *ligamentum* collaterale.
Colles' l., *ligamentum* reflexum.
conjugate l., ligamentum conjugale; a l. in some mammals which is the homologue of the intra-articular l. present in the joints between the heads of the ribs and the vertebrae.
conoid l., *ligamentum* conoideum.
Cooper's l.'s, **(1)** *ligamenta* suspensoria mammae; **(2)** *ligamentum* pectineale; **(3)** transverse l. of elbow.
coracoacromial l., *ligamentum* coracoacromiale.
coracoclavicular l., *ligamentum* coracoclaviculare.
coracohumeral l., *ligamentum* coracohumerale.
corniculopharyngeal l., ligamentum cricopharyngeum.
coronary l. of knee, portions of the articular capsule of the knee joint which connect the circumference of a semilunar cartilage with the margins of the condyles of the tibia.
coronary l. of liver, *ligamentum* coronarium hepatis.
costoclavicular l., *ligamentum* costoclaviculare.
costocolic l., *ligamentum* phrenicocolicum.
costotransverse l., *ligamentum* costotransversarium.
costoxiphoid l., *ligamentum* costoxiphoideum.
cotyloid l., *labrum* acetabulare.
Cowper's l., the part of the fascia lata which is anterior to and provides origin for fibers of the pectineus muscle.
cricopharyngeal l., *ligamentum* cricopharyngeum.
cricosantorinian l., ligamentum cricopharyngeum.

cricothyroid l., *ligamentum* cricothyroideum.
cricotracheal l., *ligamentum* cricotracheale.
crucial l., **(1)** see *retinaculum* musculorum extensorum inferius and superius; **(2)** *ligamenta* cruciata genus; **(3)** *ligamentum* cruciforme atlantis; **(4)** *pars* cruciformis vaginae fibrosae.
cruciate l. of the atlas, *ligamentum* cruciforme atlantis.
cruciate l.'s of knee, *ligamenta* cruciata genus.
cruciate l. of leg, *retinaculum* musculorum extensorum inferius.
cruciform l. of atlas, *ligamentum* cruciforme atlantis.
Cruveilhier's l.'s, *ligamenta* plantaria.
cuboideonavicular l., *ligamentum* cuboideonaviculare.
cuneocuboid l., *ligamentum* cuneocuboideum.
cuneonavicular l.'s, *ligamenta* cuneonavicularia.
cystoduodenal l., a peritoneal fold that sometimes passes from the gallbladder to the first part of the duodenum.
deep dorsal sacrococcygeal l., *ligamentum* sacrococcygeum posterius profundum.
deep posterior sacrococcygeal l., ligamentum sacrococcygeum posterius profundum.
deep transverse metacarpal l., *ligamentum* metacarpale transversum profundum.
deep transverse metatarsal l., *ligamentum* metatarsale transversum profundum.
deltoid l., *ligamentum* deltoideum.
Denonvilliers' l., *ligamentum* puboprostaticum.
denticulate l., *ligamentum* denticulatum.
Denucé's l., *ligamentum* quadratum.
diaphragmatic l. of the mesonephros, urogenital mesentery; that segment of the urogenital ridge which extends from the mesonephros to the diaphragm.
dorsal carpal l., *retinaculum* extensorum.
dorsal carpometacarpal l.'s, *ligamenta* carpometacarpalia dorsalia.
dorsal cuboideonavicular l., ligamentum cuboideonaviculare dorsale.
dorsal cuneocuboid l., *ligamentum* cuneocuboideum dorsale.
dorsal cuneonavicular l.'s, *ligamenta* cuneonavicularis dorsalia.
dorsal metacarpal l.'s, *ligamenta* metacarpalia dorsalia.
dorsal metatarsal l.'s, *ligamenta* metarsalia dorsalia.
dorsal radiocarpal l., *ligamentum* radiocarpale dorsale.
dorsal sacroiliac l.'s, *ligamenta* sacroiliaca posteriora.
duodenorenal l., ligamentum duodenorenale; a fold of peritoneum occasionally passing from the termination of the hepatoduodenal l. to the front of the right kidney.
l. of epididymis, *ligamentum* epididymidis.
epihyal l., *ligamentum* stylohyoideum.
external collateral l. of wrist, *ligamentum* collaterale carpi radiale.
extracapsular l.'s, *ligamenta* extracapsularia.
falciform l., *processus* falciformis.
falciform l. of liver, *ligamentum* falciforme hepatis.
fallopian l., *ligamentum* inguinale.
Ferrein's l., *ligamentum* laterale articulationis temporomandibularis.
fibular collateral l., *ligamentum* collaterale fibulare.
Flood's l., a band of the ligamentum coracohumerale, attached to the lower part of the lesser tuberosity of the humerus.
fundiform l. of foot, Retzius' l.
fundiform l. of penis, *ligamentum* fundiforme penis.
gastrocolic l., *ligamentum* gastrocolicum.
gastrodiaphragmatic l., *ligamentum* gastrophrenicum.
gastrolienal l., *ligamentum* gastrosplenicum.
gastrophrenic l., *ligamentum* gastrophrenicum.
gastrosplenic l., *ligamentum* gastrosplenicum.
genital l., suspensory l. of the gonad; an embryonic mesenchymatous band providing support for the internal genitalia.
genitoinguinal l., *ligamentum* genitoinguinale.
Gerdy's l., suspensory l. of axilla.
Gillette's suspensory l., *tendo* cricoesophageus.
Gimbernat's l., *ligamentum* lacunare.
gingivodental l., periodontal l.
glenohumeral l.'s, *ligamenta* glenohumeralia.
glenoid l., **(1)** *labrum* glenoidale; **(2)** *ligamenta* plantaria.
glossoepiglottic l., an elastic ligamentous band passing from the base of the tongue to the epiglottis in the middle glossoepiglottic fold.
Günz' l., a portion of the superficial layer of the obturator membrane.
hammock l., the part of the periodontium below the growing end of the root of the tooth.
l. of head of femur, *ligamentum* capitis femoris.
l.'s of head of fibula, *ligamenta* capitis fibulae.
Helmholtz' axis l., axis l. of malleus; a l. forming the axis about which the malleus rotates; it consists of two portions extending from the anterior and the posterior border, respectively, of the tympanic notch to the malleus.
Hensing's l., the left superior colic l.; a small serous horizontal or oblique fold sometimes found extending between the upper end of the descending colon and the abdominal wall.
hepatocolic l., *ligamentum* hepatocolicum.
hepatoduodenal l., *ligamentum* hepatoduodenale.
hepatoesophageal l., ligamentum hepatoesophageum; the part of the lesser omentum that extends between the liver and the abdominal part of the esophagus.
hepatogastric l., *ligamentum* hepatogastricum.
hepatorenal l., *ligamentum* hepatorenale.
Hesselbach's l., *ligamentum* interfoveolare.
Hey's l., *cornu* superius marginis falciformis.
Holl's l., l. joining the corpora cavernosa clitoridis in front of the urinary meatus.
Hueck's l., *reticulum* trabeculare.
Humphry's l., *ligamentum* meniscofemorale posterius.
Hunter's l., *ligamentum* teres uteri.
hyalocapsular l., ligamentum hyaloideo-capsulario; attachment of the vitreous body to the posterior surface of the lens of the eye.
hyoepiglottic l., *ligamentum* hyoepiglotticum.
hypsiloid l., *ligamentum* iliofemorale.
iliofemoral l., *ligamentum* iliofemorale.
iliolumbar l., *ligamentum* iliolumbale.
iliopectineal l., *arcus* iliopectineus.
iliotrochanteric l., the lateral strong band of the Y-shaped iliofemoral l.; it is attached below to the tubercle at the upper part of the intertrochanteric line.
l. of incus, *ligamentum* incudis.
inferior calcaneonavicular l., *ligamentum* calcaneonaviculare plantare.
inferior l. of epididymis, *ligamentum* epididymidis inferius.
inferior pubic l., *ligamentum* arcuatum pubis.
inferior transverse scapular l., *ligamentum* transversum scapulae inferius.
infundibulo-ovarian l., *fimbria* ovarica.
infundibulopelvic l., *ligamentum* suspensorium ovarii.
inguinal l., *ligamentum* inguinale.
inguinal l. of the kidney, the segment of the mesonephros extending to the inguinal region.
intercapital l., *ligamentum* intercapitale.
intercarpal l.'s, *ligamenta* intercarpalia.
interclavicular l., *ligamentum* interclaviculare.
interclinoid l., a band of dura mater connecting the anterior and posterior clinoid processes of the sphenoid bone.
intercornual l., *ligamentum* sacrococcygeum laterale.
intercostal l.'s, *membranae* intercostalia.
intercuneiform l.'s, *ligamenta* intercuneiformia.
interfoveolar l., *ligamentum* interfoveolare.

intermetacarpal l.'s, *ligamenta* metacarpalia.
intermetatarsal l.'s, *ligamenta* metatarsalia.
internal collateral l. of the wrist, *ligamentum* collaterale carpi ulnare.
interosseous cuneocuboid l., *ligamentum* cuneocuboideum interosseum.
interosseous cuneometatarsal l.'s, *ligamenta* cuneometatarsalia interossea.
interosseous metacarpal l.'s, *ligamenta* metacarpalia interossea.
interosseous metatarsal l.'s, *ligamenta* metatarsalia interossea.
interosseous sacroiliac l.'s, *ligamenta* sacroiliaca interossea.
interosseous talocalcaneal l., *ligamentum* talocalcaneare interosseum.
interspinous l., *ligamentum* interspinale.
intertransverse l., *ligamentum* intertransversarium.
intra-articular l. of costal head, *ligamentum* capitis costae intraarticulare.
intra-articular sternocostal l., *ligamentum* sternocostale intraarticulare.
intracapsular l.'s, *ligamenta* intracapsularia.
ischiocapsular l., *ligamentum* ischiofemorale.
ischiofemoral l., *ligamentum* ischiofemorale.
Jarjavay's l., *plica* rectouterina.
jugal l., *ligamentum* cricopharygeum.
Krause's l., *ligamentum* transversum perinei.
laciniate l., *retinaculum* musculorum flexorum.
lacunar l., *ligamentum* lacunare.
Lannelongue's l.'s, *ligamenta* sternopericardiaca.
lateral l. of ankle, the ligamentum calcaneofibulare, ligamentum talofibulare anterius, and ligamentum talofibulare posterius.
lateral arcuate l., *ligamentum* arcuatum laterale.
lateral l.'s of the bladder, condensations of fibroareolar tissue which pass one from each side of the bladder to blend with the pelvic fascia; smooth muscle is usually present in this tissue and is referred to as the musculus rectovesicalis.
lateral costotransverse l., *ligamentum* costotransversarium laterale.
lateral l. of elbow, *ligamentum* collaterale radiale.
lateral l. of knee, *ligamentum* collaterale fibulare.
lateral malleolar l., see *ligamentum* tibiofibulare anterius; *ligamentum* tibiofibulare posterius.
lateral l. of malleus, *ligamentum* mallei laterale.
lateral palpebral l., *ligamentum* palpebrale laterale.
lateral puboprostatic l., *ligamentum* puboprostaticum laterale.
lateral sacrococcygeal l., *ligamentum* sacrococcygeum laterale.
lateral talocalcaneal l., *ligamentum* talocalcaneare laterale.
lateral l. of temporomandibular joint, *ligamentum* laterale articulationis temporomandibularis.
lateral thyrohyoid l., *ligamentum* thyrohyoideum laterale.
lateral umbilical l., *ligamentum* umbilicale laterale.
lateral l. of wrist, *ligamentum* collaterale carpi radiale.
Lauth's l., *ligamentum* transversum atlantis.
l. of left superior vena cava, ligamentum venae cavae sinistrae; the obliterated left common cardinal vein that extends from the left brachiocephalic vein to the oblique vein of the left atrium.
left triangular l., *ligamentum* triangulare sinistrum.
lienophrenic l., *ligamentum* splenorenale.
lienorenal l., *ligamentum* splenorenale.
Lisfranc's l.'s, *ligamenta* cuneometatarsalia interossea.
Lockwood's l., suspensory l. of eyeball.
longitudinal l., *ligamentum* longitudinale.
long plantar l., *ligamentum* plantare longum.
lumbocostal l., *ligamentum* lumbocostale.
Luschka's l.'s, *ligamenta* sternopericardiaca.
Mackenrodt's l., cervical l. of the uterus.
l.'s of malleus, see *ligamentum* mallei anterius, laterale, and superius.
Mauchart's l.'s, see check l.'s of the eyeball, medial and lateral.
Meckel's l., Meckel's *band.*
medial l., **(1)** *ligamentum* deltoideum; **(2)** *ligamentum* mediale.
medial arcuate l., *ligamentum* arcuatum mediale.
medial calcaneocuboid l., *ligamentum* bifurcatum.
medial l. of elbow, *ligamentum* collaterale ulnare.
medial l. of knee, *ligamentum* collaterale tibiale.
medial palpebral l., *ligamentum* palpebrale mediale.
medial puboprostatic l., *ligamentum* puboprostaticum mediale.
medial talocalcaneal l., *ligamentum* talocalcaneare mediale.
medial umbilical l., *ligamentum* umbilicale mediale.
medial l. of wrist, *ligamentum* collaterale carpi ulnare.
median arcuate l., *ligamentum* arcuatum medianum.
median thyrohyoid l., *ligamentum* thyrohyoideum medianum.
meniscofemoral l.'s, see *ligamentum* meniscofemorale anterius; *ligamentum* meniscofemorale posterius.
metacarpal l.'s, *ligamenta* metacarpalia.
metatarsal l.'s, *ligamenta* metatarsalia.
middle costotransverse l., *ligamentum* costotransversarium.
middle umbilical l., *ligamentum* umbilicale medianum.
nuchal l., *ligamentum* nuchae.
oblique l. of elbow joint, *chorda* obliqua.
oblique popliteal l., *ligamentum* popliteum obliquum.
occipitoaxial l.'s, l.'s connecting the axis with the occipital bone. See *ligamenta* alaria and *ligamentum* apicis dentis.
odontoid l., *ligamenta* alaria.
orbicular l., annular l.
orbicular l. of radius, *ligamentum* annulare radii.
ovarian l., *ligamentum* ovarii proprium.
palmar l.'s, *ligamenta* palmaria.
palmar carpometacarpal l.'s, *ligamenta* carpometacarpalia palmaria.
palmar metacarpal l.'s, ligamenta metacarpalia palmaria.
palmar radiocarpal l., *ligamentum* radiocarpale palmare.
palmar ulnocarpal l., *ligamentum* ulnocarpale palmare.
patellar l., *ligamentum* patellae.
pectinate l. of iridocorneal angle, *reticulum* trabeculare.
pectinate l. of iris, *reticulum* trabeculare.
pectineal l., *ligamentum* pectineale.
peridental l., periodontal l.
periodontal l., alveolodental, gingivodental, or peridental l.; periodontal membrane; tapetum alveoli; the connective tissue that surrounds the tooth root and attaches it to its bony socket; it consists of fibers anchored in the cementum and extending into the alveolar bone.
Petit's l., *plica* rectouterina.
phrenicocolic l., *ligamentum* phrenicocolicum.
phrenicolienal l., *ligamentum* splenorenale.
phrenicosplenic l., *ligamentum* splenorenale.
phrenogastric l., *ligamentum* gastrophrenicum.
phrenosplenic l., *ligamentum* splenorenale.
pisohamate l., *ligamentum* pisohamatum.
pisometacarpal l., *ligamentum* pisometacarpeum.
pisounciform l., *ligamentum* pisohamatum.
pisouncinate l., *ligamentum* pisohamatum.
plantar l.'s, *ligamenta* plantaria.
plantar calcaneocuboid l., *ligamentum* calcaneocuboideum plantare.
plantar calcaneonavicular l., *ligamentum* calcaneonaviculare plantare.
plantar cuboideonavicular l., *ligamentum* cuboideonaviculare plantare.
plantar cuneocuboid l., *ligamentum* cuneocuboideum plantare.
plantar cuneonavicular l.'s, *ligamenta* cuneonavicularia plantaria.
plantar metatarsal l.'s, *ligamenta* metatarsalia plantaria.
posterior costotransverse l., *ligamentum* costotransversarium

laterale.
posterior cricoarytenoid l., *ligamentum* cricoarytenoideum posterius.
posterior cruciate l., *ligamentum* cruciatum posterius.
posterior l. of head of fibula, *ligamentum* capitis fibulae posterius.
posterior l. of incus, *ligamentum* incudis posterius.
posterior l. of knee, *ligamentum* popliteum arcuatum.
posterior longitudinal l., *ligamentum* longitudinale posterius.
posterior meniscofemoral l., *ligamentum* meniscofemorale posterius.
posterior occipitoaxial l., *membrana* tectoria.
posterior sacroiliac l.'s, *ligamenta* sacroiliaca posteriora.
posterior sacrosciatic l., *ligamentum* sacrotuberale.
posterior sternoclavicular l., *ligamentum* sternoclaviculare posterius.
posterior talofibular l., *ligamentum* talofibulare posterius.
posterior talotibial l., *pars* tibiotalaris posterior. See also *ligamentum* deltoideum.
posterior tibiofibular l., *ligamentum* tibiofibulare posterius.
Poupart's l., *ligamentum* inguinale.
proper l. of ovary, *ligamentum* ovarii proprium.
pterygomandibular l., *raphe* pterygomandibularis.
pterygospinal l., *ligamentum* pterygospinale.
pterygospinous l., *ligamentum* pterygospinale.
pubocapsular l., *ligamentum* pubofemorale.
pubofemoral l., *ligamentum* pubofemorale.
puboprostatic l., *ligamentum* puboprostaticum.
pubovesical l., *ligamentum* pubovesicale.
pulmonary l., *ligamentum* pulmonale.
quadrate l., *ligamentum* quadratum.
radial collateral l., *ligamentum* collaterale radiale.
radial collateral l. of wrist, *ligamentum* collaterale carpi radiale.
radiate l. of rib, *ligamentum* capitis costae radiatum.
radiate sternocostal l.'s, *ligamenta* sternocostalia radiata.
radiate l. of wrist, *ligamentum* carpi radiatum.
reflex l., *ligamentum* reflexum.
Retzius' l., fundiform l. of foot; the deep attachment of the inferior extensor retinaculum in the sinus tarsi; it acts as a sling for the extensor tendons of the toes.
rhomboid l., *ligamentum* costoclaviculare.
right triangular l., *ligamentum* triangulare dextrum.
ring l., *zona* orbicularis.
round l. of elbow joint, *chorda* obliqua.
round l. of femur, *ligamentum* capitis femoris.
round l. of liver, *ligamentum* teres hepatis.
round l. of uterus, *ligamentum* teres uteri.
sacrodural l., ligamentum sacrodurale; a longitudinal bundle of fibrous filaments running from the midline of the inferior part of the dural sac to the posterior longitudinal ligament of the sacrum.
sacrospinous l., *ligamentum* sacrospinale.
sacrotuberous l., *ligamentum* sacrotuberale.
serous l., ligamentum serosum; one of a number of peritoneal folds attaching certain of the viscera to the abdominal wall or to each other.
sheath l.'s, see *vaginae* fibrosae digitorum manus and pedis; *vagina* fibrosa tendinis.
Simonart's l.'s, amniotic *bands.*
Soemmering's l., small fibers attaching the lacrimal gland to the periorbita.
sphenomandibular l., *ligamentum* sphenomandibulare.
spinoglenoid l., *ligamentum* transversum scapulae inferius.
spiral l. of cochlea, *crista* spiralis.
splenorenal l., *ligamentum* splenorenale.
spring l., *ligamentum* calcaneonaviculare plantare.
Stanley's cervical l.'s, fibers of the capsule of the hip joint reflected onto the neck of the femur.
stellate l., *ligamentum* capitis costae radiatum.
sternoclavicular l., *ligamentum* sternoclaviculare.
sternopericardial l., *ligamentum* sternopericardiaca.
stylohyoid l., *ligamentum* stylohyoideum.
stylomandibular l., *ligamentum* stylomandibulare.
stylomaxillary l., *ligamentum* stylomandibulare.
superficial dorsal sacrococcygeal l., *ligamentum* sacrococcygeum posterius superficiale.
superficial posterior sacrococcygeal l., *ligamentum* sacrococcygeum posterius superficiale.
superficial transverse metacarpal l., *ligamentum* metacarpale transversum superficiale.
superficial transverse metatarsal l., *ligamentum* metatarsale transversum superficiale.
superior costotransverse l., *ligamentum* costotransversarium superius.
superior l. of epididymis, *ligamentum* epididymidis superius.
superior l. of incus, *ligamentum* incudis superius.
superior l. of malleus, *ligamentum* mallei superius.
superior pubic l., *ligamentum* pubicum superius.
superior transverse scapular l., *ligamentum* transversum scapulae superius.
suprascapular l., *ligamentum* transversum scapulae superius.
supraspinous l., *ligamentum* supraspinale.
suspensory l. of axilla, Campbell's or Gerdy's l.; the continuation of the clavipectoral fascia downward to attach to the axillary fascia; it maintains the characteristic hollow of the armpit.
suspensory l.'s of breast, *ligamenta* suspensoria mammae.
suspensory l. of clitoris, *ligamentum* suspensorium clitoridis.
suspensory l.'s of Cooper, *ligamenta* suspensoria mammae.
suspensory l. of esophagus, *tendo* cricoesophageus.
suspensory l. of eyeball, Lockwood's l.; a thickening of the inferior part of the bulbar sheath which supports the eye within the orbit; it extends between the lateral and medial orbital margins and includes the medial and lateral cheek l.'s.
suspensory l. of gonad, genital l.
suspensory l. of lens, *zonula* ciliaris.
suspensory l. of ovary, *ligamentum* suspensorium ovarii.
suspensory l. of penis, *ligamentum* suspensorium penis.
suspensory l. of testis, the cranial atrophic portion of the urogenital ridge attached to the cranial pole of the intra-abdominal embryonic testis.
suspensory l. of thyroid gland, one of several fibrous bands which pass from the sheath of the thyroid gland to the thyroid and cricoid cartilages.
sutural l., a delicate membrane binding the bones at the cranial sutures.
synovial l., one of the large synovial folds in a joint.
talocalcaneal l., *ligamentum* talocalcaneare.
talonavicular l., *ligamentum* talonaviculare.
tarsal l.'s, *ligamenta* tarsi.
tarsometatarsal l.'s, *ligamenta* tarsometatarsalia.
temporomandibular l., *ligamentum* laterale articulationis temporomandibularis.
Teutleben's l., *ligamentum* pulmonale.
thyroepiglottic l., thyroepiglottidean l., *ligamentum* thyroepiglotticum.
tibial collateral l., *ligamentum* collaterale tibiale.
tibiofibular l., see *ligamentum* tibiofibulare anterius, medium, and posterius.
tibionavicular l., *pars* tibionavicularis. See also *ligamentum* deltoideum.
transverse l. of acetabulum, *ligamentum* transversum acetabuli.
transverse l. of atlas, see *ligamentum* cruciforme atlantis.
transverse carpal l., *retinaculum* flexorum.
transverse crural l., *retinaculum* musculorum extensorum superius.
transverse l. of elbow, Cooper's l. (3); a bundle of fibers running

from the olecranon to the coronoid process in association with the ulnar collateral l.
transverse humeral l., Brodie's l.; a fibrous band running more or less obliquely from the greater to the lesser tuberosity of the humerus, bridging over the bicipital groove.
transverse l. of knee, *ligamentum* transversum genus.
transverse l. of leg, *retinaculum* musculorum extensorum superius.
transverse metacarpal l., *ligamentum* metacarpale transversum profundum.
transverse metatarsal l., *ligamentum* metatarsale transversum profundum.
transverse l. of pelvis, *ligamentum* transversum perinei.
transverse l. of perineum, *ligamentum* transversum perinei.
transverse tibiofibular l., the distal continuation of the interosseous membrane forming a strong l. that unites the distal end of the tibia and fibula; it lies deep to the posterior tibiofibular l.
trapezoid l., *ligamentum* trapezoideum.
Treitz' l., *musculus* suspensorius duodeni.
triangular l., *membrana* perinei.
triangular l.'s of liver, see *ligamentum* triangulare dextrum and *ligamentum* triangulare sinistrum.
ulnar collateral l., *ligamentum* collaterale ulnare.
ulnar collateral l. of wrist, *ligamentum* collaterale carpi ulnare.
urachal l., *ligamentum* umbilicale medianum.
uterosacral l., *plica* rectouterina.
Valsalva's l.'s, *ligamenta* auricularia.
venous l., *ligamentum* venosum.
ventral sacrococcygeal l., *ligamentum* sacrococcygeum anterius.
ventral sacroiliac l.'s, *ligamenta* sacroiliaca anteriora.
ventricular l., *ligamentum* vestibulare.
vertebropelvic l.'s, see *ligamenta* iliolumbale, sacrospinale, and sacrotuberale.
vesicoumbilical l., one of the ligaments between the urinary bladder and the umbilicus. See *ligamentum* umbilicale medianum and *ligamentum* umbilicale mediale.
vesicouterine l., uterovesical fold; plica uterovesicalis; plica vesicouterina; a peritoneal fold extending from the uterus to the posterior portion of the bladder.
vestibular l., *ligamentum* vestibulare.
vocal l., *ligamentum* vocale.
volar carpal l., *retinaculum* flexorum.
Weitbrecht's l., *chorda* obliqua.
Winslow's l., *ligamentum* collaterale fibulare.
Wrisberg's l., *ligamentum* meniscofemorale posterius.
Y-shaped l., *ligamentum* iliofemorale.
yellow l., *ligamentum* flavum.
Zaglas' l., a short thick fibrous band extending from the posterior superior spine of the ilium to the second transverse tubercle of the sacrum.
Zinn's l., *annulus* tendineus communis.

---

ligamenta (lig'ă-men'tă) [L.]. Plural of ligamentum.

ligamentopexis, ligamentopexy (lig'ă-men-tō-pek'sis, -pek'sē) [ligament + G. *pēxis,* fixation]. Shortening of any ligament of the uterus.

ligamentous (lig'ă-men'tŭs). Relating to or of the form or structure of a ligament.

LIGAMENTUM

---

ligamentum, pl. **ligamenta** (lig'ă-men'tŭm, -men'tă) [L. a band, tie, fr. *ligo,* to bind] [NA]. Ligament. **1.** A band or sheet of fibrous tissue connecting two or more bones, cartilages, or other structures, or serving as support for fasciae or muscles. **2.** A fold of peritoneum supporting any of the abdominal viscera. **3.** Any structure resembling a l. though not performing the function of such. **4.** The cordlike remains of a fetal vessel or other structure that has lost its original lumen.
l. acromioclavicula're [NA], acromioclavicular ligament; a fibrous band extending from the acromion of the scapula to the clavicle.
ligamen'ta ala'ria [NA], alar ligaments (1); odontoid ligaments; check ligaments of odontoid; one of a pair of short stout bands that extends from the side of the dens of the axis to the tubercle on the medial aspect of the occipital condyle.
l. annula're, annular *ligament.*
l. annula're bul'bi, *reticulum* trabeculare.
l. annula're digito'rum, *pars* annularis vaginae fibrosae.
l. annula're ra'dii [NA], annular ligament of radius; l. orbiculare radii; the ligament that holds the head of the radius in the radial notch of the ulna.
l. annula're stape'dis [NA], annular ligament of stapes; a ring of elastic fibers that attaches the base of the stapes to the margin of the fenestra vestibuli.
ligamen'ta annula'ria trachea'lia [NA], annular ligaments of trachea; ligamenta trachealia; the fibrous membranes that connect adjacent tracheal cartilages.
l. anococcy'geum [NA], anococcygeal ligament; anococcygeal body; Symington's anococcygeal body; raphe anococcygea; a musculofibrous band that passes between the anus and the coccyx.
l. ap'icis den'tis [NA], apical ligament of dens; a ligament that extends from the apex of the dens of the axis to the anterior margin of the foramen magnum.
l. arcua'tum latera'le [NA], lateral arcuate ligament; lateral lumbocostal arch; arcus lumbocostalis lateralis; one of Haller's arches; a thickening of the fascia of the quadratus lumborum muscle between the transverse process of the first lumbar vertebra and the twelfth rib on either side that gives attachment to a portion of the diaphragm.
l. arcua'tum media'le [NA], medial arcuate ligament; medial lumbocostal arch; arcus lumbocostalis medialis; one of Haller's arches; a tendinous thickening of the psoas fascia that extends from the body of the first lumbar vertebra to its transverse process on either side. A portion of the diaphragm arises from it.
l. arcua'tum media'num [NA], median arcuate ligament; a tendinous connection between the crura of the diaphragm that arches in front on the aorta.
l. arcua'tum pu'bis [NA], arcuate pubic ligament; inferior pubic ligament; the ligament that arches across the inferior aspect of the pubic symphysis.
l. arterio'sum [NA], arterial ligament; Botallo's ligament; the remains of the ductus arteriosus.
ligamen'ta auricula'ria [NA], auricular ligaments; Valsalva's ligaments; the three ligaments that attach the auricle to the side of the head: **l. auricula're ante'rius,** which extends from the root of the zygomatic process to the spine of the helix; **l. auricula're poste'rius,** which extends from the mastoid process to the conchal eminence; **l. auricula're supe'rius,** which extends from the superior margin of the osseous external acoustic meatus to the spine of the helix.
ligamen'ta ba'sium, see ligamenta metacarpalia ligamenta metatarsalia.
l. bifurca'tum [NA], bifurcated ligament; medial calcaneocuboid ligament; a strong V-shaped ligament on the dorsum of the foot that passes from the calcaneus distal to the tarsal sinus and attaches to cuboid and navicular bones; it is divided into the l. calcaneocuboideum and the l. cascaneonaviculare.
l. calcaneocuboi'deum [NA], calcaneocuboid ligament; the lateral

part of the l. bifurcatum.
l. calcaneocuboi'deum planta're [NA], plantar calcaneocuboid ligament; a strong band that passes forward and medially from the plantar surface of the calcaneus to the cuboid bone.
l. calcaneofibula're [NA], calcaneofibular ligament; the middle of the three fascicles that reinforce the lateral side of the ankle joint, the remaining two being the anterior and posterior talofibular ligaments.
l. calcaneonavicula're [NA], calcaneonavicular ligament; the medial part of the l. bifurcatum.
l. calcaneonavicula're planta're [NA], plantar calcaneonavicular ligament; inferior calcaneonavicular ligament; spring ligament; a dense fibroelastic ligament that extends from the sustentaculum tali to the plantar surface of the navicular bone; it supports the head of the talus.
l. calcaneotibia'le, *pars* tibiocalcanea. See also l. deltoideum.
l. cap'itis cos'tae intra-articula're [NA], intra-articular ligament of costal head; transverse fibers extending within the capsule from the ridge between the two facets on the head of the rib to the intervertebral disk.
l. cap'itis cos'tae radia'tum [NA], radiate ligament of rib; stellate ligament; l. radiatum; the radiate, stellate, or anterior costovertebral ligament connecting the head of each rib to the bodies of the two vertebrae with which it articulates.
l. cap'itis femo'ris [NA], ligament of head of femur; round ligament of the femur; l. teres femoris; a flattened ligament that passes from the fovea in the head of the femur to the borders of the acetabular notch; an artery often passes to the head of the femur with the ligament.
l. cap'itis fib'ulae [NA], ligament of head of fibula; **l. c. f. ante'rius,** anterior ligament of head of fibula; a ligament uniting the anterior part of the head of the fibula to the tibia; **l. c. f. poste'rius,** posterior ligament of head of fibula; a ligament uniting the posterior part of the head of the fibula to the tibia.
ligamen'ta capitulo'rum transver'sa, see l. metacarpeum transversum profundum; l. metatarseum transversum profundum.
l. capsula're, capsular *ligament.*
l. car'pi dorsa'le, *retinaculum* extensorum.
l. car'pi radia'tum [NA], radiate ligament of wrist; the ligament that extends from the capitate bone to the scaphoid, lunate, and triquetrum on the palmar side of the wrist.
l. car'pi transver'sum, *retinaculum* flexorum.
l. car'pi vola're, *retinaculum* flexorum.
ligamen'ta carpometacarpa'lia [NA], carpometacarpal ligaments; the ligaments uniting the metacarpal and carpal bones; **l. c. dorsa'lia** [NA], dorsal carpometacarpal ligaments; fibrous bands that connect the dorsal surfaces of the carpal and metacarpal bones; **l. c. palma'ria** [NA], palmar carpometacarpal ligaments; fibrous bands that connect the palmar surfaces of the carpal and metacarpal bones.
l. cauda'le, *retinaculum* caudale.
l. ceratocricoid'eum, ceratocricoid *ligament;* one of three ligaments (anterior, posterior, and lateral) reinforcing the capsule of the cricothyroid articulation on either side.
l. collatera'le, pl. **ligamen'ta collatera'lia** [NA], collateral ligament; one of a number of ligaments on either side of, and serving as a radius of movement of, the joint having a hingelike movement; they occur at the following joints: elbow, knee, wrist, and the metacarpo- or metatarsophalangeal, proximal interphalangeal, and distal interphalangeal joints of the hands and feet.
l. collatera'le car'pi radia'le [NA], radial collateral ligament of wrist; external collateral or lateral ligament of wrist; the ligament that extends distally from the styloid process of the radius to the carpal bones.
l. collatera'le car'pi ulna're [NA], ulnar collateral ligament of wrist; internal collateral or medial ligament of wrist; a ligament that passes from the styloid process of the ulna to the pisiform and triquetrum.
l. collatera'le fibula're [NA], fibular collateral ligament; lateral ligament of knee; Winslow's ligament; the cordlike ligament that passes from the lateral epicondyle of the femur to the head of the fibula.
l. collatera'le radia'le [NA], radial collateral ligament; lateral ligament of elbow; the ligament that connects the lateral epicondyle of the humerus with the annular ligament of the radius.
l. collatera'le tibia'le [NA], tibial collateral ligament; medial ligament of knee; the broad fibrous band that passes from the medial epicondyle of the femur to the medial margin and medial surface of the tibia; the medial meniscus is attached to its deep surface.
l. collatera'le ulna're [NA], ulnar collateral ligament; medial ligament of elbow; the triangular ligament extending from the medial epicondyle of the humerus to the medial side of the coronoid process and olecranon of the ulna.
l. col'li cos'tae, l. costotransversarium.
l. conjuga'le, conjugate *ligament.*
l. conoid'eum [NA], conoid ligament; the medial part of the coracoclavicular ligament that attaches to the conoid tubercle of the clavicle.
l. coracoacromia'le [NA], coracoacromial ligament; the heavy arched fibrous band that passes between the coracoid process and the acromion above the shoulder joint.
l. coracoclavicula're [NA], coracoclavicular ligament; Caldani's ligament; the strong ligament that unites the clavicle to the coracoid process; it is subdivided into the l. conoideum and the l. trapezoideum.
l. coracohumera'le [NA], coracohumeral ligament; the ligament that passes from the base of the coracoid process to the greater tubercle of the humerus.
l. corniculopharynge'um, l. cricopharyngeum.
l. corona'rium hep'atis [NA], coronary ligament of liver; peritoneal reflections from the liver to the diaphragm at the margins of the bare area of the liver.
l. costoclavicula're [NA], costoclavicular ligament; rhomboid ligament; the ligament that connects the first rib and the clavicle near its sternal end.
l. costotransversa'rium [NA], costotransverse ligament; middle costotransverse ligament; l. colli costae; the ligament that connects the dorsal aspect of the neck of a rib to the ventral aspect of the corresponding transverse process.
l. costotransversa'rium ante'rius, l. costotransversarium superius.
l. costotransversa'rium latera'le [NA], lateral costotransverse ligament; posterior costotransverse ligament; l. costotransversarium posterius; l. tuberculi costae; the short quadrangular ligament that passes across behind the costotransverse joint from the tip of the transverse process to the posterior surface of the neck of the rib.
l. costotransversa'rium poste'rius, l. costotransversarium laterale.
l. costotransversa'rium supe'rius [NA], superior costotransverse ligament; anterior costotransverse ligament; l. costotransversarium anterius; the fibrous band that extends upward from the neck of a rib to the transverse process of the next higher vertebra.
l. costoxiphoi'deum [NA], costoxiphoid ligament; chondroxiphoid ligament; the ligament that connects the xiphoid process to the seventh, and often to the sixth, costal cartilages.
l. cotyloid'eum, *labrum* acetabulare.
l. cricoarytenoi'deum poste'rius [NA], posterior cricoarytenoid ligament; the ligament that passes downward from the posterior border of the arytenoid cartilage to the lamina of the cricoid cartilage.
l. cricopharynge'um [NA], cricopharyngeal ligament; ligamentum corniculopharyngeum; corniculopharyngeal ligament; ligamentum jugale; jugal or cricosantorinian ligament; an elastic band connecting the tip of the corniculate (Santorini's) cartilage and the lamina of the cricoid cartilage and continuing into the pharyngeal mucosa covering the cricoid lamina.

l. cricothyroi'deum [NA], cricothyroid ligament; the strong band that connects the cricoid and thyroid cartilages in the midline anteriorly; it is continuous posteriorly with the conus elasticus.
l. cricotrachea'le [NA], cricotracheal ligament; cricotracheal membrane; a fibrous band connecting the cricoid cartilage with the first ring of the trachea.
ligamen'ta crucia'ta digito'rum, *pars* cruciformis vaginae fibrosae.
ligamen'ta crucia'ta ge'nus [NA], cruciate ligaments of the knee; crucial ligament (2); the two ligaments which pass from the intercondylar area of the tibia to the intercondylar fossa of the femur.
l. crucia'tum ante'rius [NA], anterior cruciate ligament; the ligament that extends from the anterior intercondylar area of the tibia to the posterior part of the medial surface of the lateral condyle of the femur.
l. crucia'tum atlan'tis, l. cruciforme atlantis.
l. crucia'tum cru'ris, *retinaculum* musculorum extensorum inferius.
l. crucia'tum poste'rius [NA], posterior cruciate ligament; the strong fibrous cord that extends from the posterior intercondylar area of the tibia to the anterior part of the lateral surface of the medial condyle of the femur.
l. crucia'tum ter'tium ge'nus, l. meniscofemorale posterius.
l. crucifor'me atlan'tis [NA], cruciform or cruciate ligament of atlas; crucial ligament (3); l. cruciatum atlantis, the strong ligament that lies posterior to the dens of the axis; it consists of the transverse ligament of the atlas (l. transversum atlantis or Lauth's ligament) and longitudinal fibers (fasciculi longitudinales).
l. cuboideonavicula're [NA], cuboideonavicular ligament; **l. c. dorsa'le,** dorsal cuboideonavicular ligament; the ligament that unites the dorsal surfaces of the cuboid and navicular bones of the tarsus; **l. c. planta're,** plantar cuboideonavicular ligament; the ligament that unites the plantar surfaces of the cuboid and navicular bones of the tarsus.
l. cuneocuboid'eum [NA], cuneocuboid ligament; **l. c. dorsa'le,** dorsal cuneocuboid ligament; the fibrous band that unites the dorsal margins of the lateral cuneiform and cuboid bones; **l. c. interos' seum,** the fibrous band that unites adjacent margins of the distal end of the lateral cuneiform and cuboid bones; **l. c. planta're,** plantar cuneocuboid ligament; the fibrous band that unites the apex of the lateral cuneiform with the medial margin of plantar suface of the cuboid.
ligamen'ta cuneometatara'lia interos'sea [NA], interosseous cuneometatarsal ligaments; Lisfranc's ligaments; ligaments that pass from the cuneiform bones to the metatarsals, the one from the first cuneiform to the second metatarsal being the strongest.
ligamen'ta cuneonavicula'ria [NA], cuneonavicular ligaments; ligamenta navicularicuneiformia; **l. c. dorsa'lia,** dorsal cuneonavicular ligaments; several ligaments connecting the dorsal surface of the navicular with the three cuneiform bones; **l. c. planta'ria,** plantar cuneonavicular ligaments; several ligaments connecting the plantar surface of the navicular with the three cuneiform bones.
l. deltoi'deum [NA], deltoid ligament; l. mediale (1); medial ligament (1); a ligament consisting of four parts which pass downward from the medial malleolus of the tibia to the tarsal bones: pars tibionavicularis, pars tibiocalcanea, pars tibiotalaris anterior and pars tibiotalaris posterior.
l. denticula'tum [NA], denticulate ligament; a serrated, shelflike extension of the spinal pia mater projecting in a frontal plane from either side of the cervical and thoracic spinal cord; its 21 pointed processes fuse laterally with the arachnoid and dura mater midway between the exits of the roots of adjacent spinal nerves.
l. duc'tus veno'si, l. venosum.
l. duodenorena'le, duodenorenal *ligament.*
l. epididym'idis [NA], ligament of the epididymis; one of two folds of the tunica vaginalis between the epididymis and the testis; **l. e. infe'rius,** inferior ligament of epididymis; the fold between the body of the epididymis and the testis; **l. e. supe'rius,** superior ligament of the epididymis; the fold between the head of the epididymis and the testis.
ligamen'ta extracapsula'ria [NA], extracapsular ligaments; ligaments associated with a synovial joint but separate from and external to its articular capsule.
l. falcifor'me, *processus* falciformis.
l. falcifor'me hep'atis [NA], falciform ligament of liver; a crescentic fold of peritoneum extending to the surface of the liver from the diaphragm and anterior abdominal wall; the round ligament lies in its free inferior border.
l. fla'vum [NA], yellow ligament; one of the paired ligaments of yellow elastic fibrous tissue, which bind together the laminae of adjoining vertebrae.
l. fundifor'me pe'nis [NA], fundiform ligament of penis; a band of elastic fibers that extends from the linea alba above the pubic symphysis splitting to surround the penis before attaching to the fascia of the penis.
l. gastrocol'icum [NA], gastrocolic ligament; the portion of the greater omentum that extends between the stomach and the transverse colon.
l. gastroliena'le [NA], official alternate term for *ligamenta* gastrosplenicum.
l. gastrophren'icum [NA], gastrophrenic, gastrodiaphragmatic, or phrenogastric ligament; the portion of the greater omentum that extends from the greater curvature of the stomach to the inferior surface of the diaphragm.
l. gastrosple'nicum [NA], gastrolienal or gastrosplenic ligament; gastrosplenic omentum; the portion of the greater omentum that lies between the greater curvature of the stomach and the hilum of the spleen.
l. genitoinguina'le [NA], genitoinguinal ligament; plica gubernatrix; in the fetus, a fold of the mesorchium containing the gubernaculum testis.
ligamen'ta glenohumera'lia [NA], glenohumeral ligaments; three fibrous bands that reinforce the anterior part of the articular capsule of the shoulder joint; they are attached to the margin of the glenoid cavity of the scapula and to the anatomic neck of the humerus.
l. glenoida'le, *labrum* glenoidale.
l. hepatocol'icum [NA], hepatocolic ligament; an inconstant extension of the hepatoduodenal ligament to the transverse colon.
l. hepatoduodena'le [NA], hepatoduodenal ligament; the portion of the lesser omentum that connects the liver and duodenum.
l. hepatoesopha'geum, hepatoesophageal *ligament.*
l. hepatogas'tricum [NA], hepatogastric ligament; the part of the lesser omentum that extends between the liver and lesser curvature of the stomach.
l. hepatorena'le [NA], hepatorenal ligament; a prolongation of the coronary ligament downward over the right kidney.
l. hyaloi'deo-capsula'rio, hyalocapsular *ligament.*
l. hyoepiglot'ticum [NA], hyoepiglottic ligament; a short elastic band that unites the epiglottis to the upper border of the hyoid bone.
l. hyothyroi'deum latera'le, l. thyrohyoideum laterale.
l. hyothyroi'deum me'dium, l. thyrohyoideum medianum.
l. iliofemora'le [NA], iliofemoral ligament; hypsiloid or Y-shaped ligament; Bertin's or Bigelow's ligament; a triangular ligament attached by its apex to the anterior inferior spine of the ilium and rim of the acetabulum, and by its base to the anterior intertrochanteric line of the femur; the strong medial band is attached to the lower part of the intertrochanteric line; the strong lateral part is fixed to the tubercle at the upper part of this line; the bands diverge, forming a Y-like figure with a weak area between.
l. iliolumba'le [NA], iliolumbar ligament; the strong ligament that connects the fourth and fifth lumbar vertebrae with the ilium.
l. iliopectinea'le, *arcus* iliopectineus.

l. in'cudis [NA], ligament of the incus; **l. i. poste'rius,** a ligament attaching the short process of the incus to the fossa incudis; **l. i. supe'rius,** a thin ligament running from the body of the incus to the roof of the epitympanic recess.
l. inguina'le [NA], inguinal ligament; Poupart's ligament; crural, femoral, or fallopian arch; arcus inguinalis; fallopian ligament; a fibrous band formed by the inferior border of the aponeurosis of the external oblique that extends from the anterior superior spine of the ilium to the pubic tubercle.
l. intercapita'le, intercapital ligament; a part of the l. capitis costae intraarticulare; which connects the heads of opposite ribs by passing over the intervertebral fibrocartilage, and thus holds the ribs in their articular sockets; not present in man but well developed in the dog and cat.
ligamen'ta intercarpa'lia [NA], intercarpal ligaments; three sets of short fibrous bands that bind together the two rows of carpal bones; according to their location they are named **l. i. dorsa'lia, l. i. interos'sea,** and **l. i. palma'ria.**
l. interclavicula're [NA], interclavicular ligament; a strong ligament that connects the two sternoclavicular joints across the upper border of the manubrium.
ligamen'ta intercosta'lia, *membranae* intercostalia.
ligamen'ta intercuneifor'mia [NA], intercuneiform ligaments; fibrous bands that unite the cuneiform bones; they are arranged in three sets: **l. i. dorsa'lia, l. i. interos'sea,** and **l. i. planta'ria.**
l. interfoveola're [NA], interfoveolar ligament; Hesselbach's ligament; fibrous or muscular strands that lie medial to the deep inguinal ring, extending from the lower border of the transversus muscle to the lacunar ligament and pectineal fascia.
l. interspina'le [NA], interspinous ligament; bands of fibrous tissue that connect the spinous processes of adjacent vertebrae.
l. intertransversa'rium [NA], intertransverse ligament; one of the ligaments that connect the transverse processes of adjacent vertebrae.
ligamen'ta intracapsula'ria [NA], intracapsular ligaments; ligaments located within and separate from the articular capsule of a synovial joint.
l. ischiocapsula're, l. ischiofemorale.
l. ischiofemora'le [NA], ischiofemoral ligament; ischiocapsular ligament; ligamentum ischiocapsulare; the thickened part of the capsule of the hip joint that passes from the ischium upward and laterally over the femoral neck; some of its fibers continue into the zona orbicularis.
l. juga'le, l. cricopharyngeum.
l. lacinia'tum, *retinaculum* musculorum flexorum.
l. lacuna're [NA], lacunar ligament; Gimbernat's ligament; a curved fibrous band that passes horizontally backward from the medial end of the inguinal ligament to the pectineal line; it forms the medial boundary of the femoral ring.
l. latera'le articulatio'nis temporomandibula'ris [NA], lateral ligament of temporomandibular joint; Ferrein's ligament; temporomandibular ligament; l. temporomandibulare; the capsular ligament that passes obliquely down and backward across the lateral surface of temporomandibular joint.
l. la'tum pulmo'nis, l. pulmonale.
l. la'tum u'teri [NA], broad ligament of uterus; the peritoneal fold passing from the lateral margin of the uterus to the wall of the pelvis on either side.
l. lienorena'le [NA], l. splenorenale.
l. longitudin'ale [NA], longitudinal ligament; one of two extensive fibrous bands running the length of the vertebral column: **l. l. ante'rius,** anterior longitudinal ligament; lacertus medius; the wide fibrous band interconnecting the anterior surfaces of the vertebral bodies; **l. l. poste'rius,** posterior longitudinal ligament; the wide fibrous band interconnecting the posterior surfaces of the vertebral bodies.
l. lumbocosta'le [NA], lumbocostal ligament; a strong band that unites the twelfth rib with the tips of the transverse processes of the first and second lumbar vertebrae.
l. mal'lei ante'rius [NA], anterior ligament of malleus; consists of two portions: Meckel's band, passing from the base of the anterior process to the spine of the sphenoid through the petrotympanic fissure; and the anterior ligament of Helmholtz, extending from the anterior aspect of the neck of the malleus to the anterior boundary of the tympanic notch.
l. mal'lei latera'le [NA], lateral ligament of malleus; a short fan-shaped ligament converging from the posterior half of the tympanic notch to the neck of the malleus.
l. mal'lei supe'rius [NA], superior ligament of malleus; a ligament extending from the head of the malleus to the roof of the epitympanic recess.
l. malle'oli latera'lis, see l. tibiofibulare anterius and posterius.
l. media'le [NA], medial ligament (2); **(1)** l. deltoideum; **(2)** the bundle of fibers strengthening the medial part of the articular capsule of the temporomandibular joint.
l. menis'ci latera'lis, l. meniscofemorale posterius.
l. meniscofemora'le [NA], meniscofemoral ligament; one of two ligaments that extend from the posterior part of the lateral meniscus to the lateral surface of the medial meniscus: **l. m. ante'rius,** anterior meniscofemoral ligament; Humphry's ligament; the band that passes anterior to the posterior cruciate ligament; **l. m. poste'rius,** posterior meniscofemoral ligament; Wrisberg's ligament; the band that passes posterior to the posterior cruciate ligament.
l. metacarpa'le transver'sum profun'dum [NA], deep transverse metacarpal ligament; transverse metacarpal ligament; the ligament that interconnects the heads of the second to fifth metacarpals; it lies in the plane of the palmar interosseous fascia.
l. metacarpa'le transver'sum superficia'le [NA], superficial transverse metacarpal ligament; Gerdy's fibers; a thickening of the superficial fascia in the most distal part of the palm.
ligamen'ta metacarpa'lia [NA], metacarpal ligaments; intermetacarpal ligaments; **l. m. dorsa'lia,** dorsal metacarpal ligaments; fibrous bands connecting the dorsal aspects of the bases of metacarpals two to five; **l. m. interos'sea,** interosseous metacarpal ligaments; fibrous bands connecting the bases of metacarpals two to five; they extend between the dorsal and palmar metacarpal ligaments; **l. m. palma'ria,** palmar metacarpal ligaments; fibrous bands connecting the palmar aspects of the bases of metacarpals two to five.
l. metatarsa'le transver'sum profun'dum [NA], deep transverse metatarsal ligament; transverse metatarsal ligament; the ligament that interconnects the heads of the metatarsals.
l. metatarsa'le transver'sum superficia'le [NA], superficial transverse metatarsal ligament; l. natatorium; a thickening of the superficial fascia under the heads of the metatarsal bones.
ligamen'ta metatarsa'lia [NA], metatarsal ligaments; intermetatarsal ligaments; **l. m. dorsa'lia,** dorsal metatarsal ligaments; fibrous bands that connect the dorsal aspects of the bases of the metatarsals; **l. m. interos'sea,** interosseous metatarsal ligaments; fibrous bands that connect the bases of the metatarsals, they extend between the dorsal and plantar metatarsal ligaments; **l. m. planta'ria,** plantar metatarsal ligaments; fibrous bands connecting the plantar aspects of the bases of the metatarsals.
l. natato'rium, l. metacarpeum transversum superficiale.
ligamen'ta navicularicuneifor'mia, ligamenta cuneonavicularia.
l. nu'chae [NA], nuchal ligament; apparatus ligamentosus colli; a sagittal ligamentous band at the back of the neck, formed of thickened supraspinous ligaments; it extends from the external occipital protuberance to the posterior border of the foramen magnum, cranially, to the seventh cervical spinous process, caudally.
l. orbicula're ra'dii, l. annulare radii.
ligamen'ta ossiculo'rum au'ditus [NA], ligaments of auditory ossicles; the ligaments connecting the ear bones with one another and with the walls of the tympanic cavity.

l. ova'rii pro'prium [NA], proper ligament of ovary; ovarian ligament; a cordlike bundle of fibers passing to the side of the uterus from the lower end of the ovary, between the folds of the broad ligament.
ligamen'ta palma'ria [NA], palmar ligaments; accessory volar ligaments; the fibrocartilaginous plates, one located on the anterior aspect of each metacarpophalangeal and interphalangeal joint, that are firmly attached to the bases of the phalanges and articulate with the heads of the next proximal bones.
l. palpebra'le exter'num, l. palpebrale laterale.
l. palpebra'le latera'le [NA], lateral palpebral ligament; l. palpebrale externum; l. tarsale externum; the band that attaches the tarsal plates to the orbital eminence of the zygomatic bone.
l. palpebra'le media'le [NA], medial palpebral ligament; l. tarsale internum; tendo oculi; tendo palpebrarum; the fibrous band that attaches the medial ends of the tarsal plates to the maxilla at the medial orbital margin.
l. patel'lae [NA], patellar ligament; a strong flattened fibrous band passing from the apex and adjoining margins of the patella to the tuberosity of the tibia.
l. pectina'tum [NA], *reticulum* trabeculare.
l. pectina'tum an'guli iridocornea'lis, *reticulum* trabeculare.
l. pectina'tum ir'idis, *reticulum* trabeculare.
l. pectinea'le [NA], pectineal ligament; Cooper's ligament (2); a thick, strong fibrous band that passes laterally from the lacunar ligament along the pectineal line of the pubis.
l. phrenicocol'icum [NA], phrenicocolic ligament; sustenaculum lienis; costocolic ligament; a triangular fold of peritoneum attached to the left flexure of the colon and to the diaphragm, on which rests the inferior pole or extremity of the spleen.
l. phrenicoliena'le [NA], *ligamentum* splenorenale.
l. phrenicosple'nicum [NA], l. splenorenale.
l. pisohama'tum [NA], pisohamate ligament; pisounciform or pisouncinate ligament; a strong fibrous band that extends from the pisiform bone to the hook of the hamate.
l. pisometacarpe'um [NA], pisometacarpal ligament; a strong fibrous band extending from the pisiform bone to the base of the fifth metacarpal bone; this ligament, together with the pisohamate ligament, forms the insertion of the flexor carpi ulnaris.
l. planta're lon'gum [NA], long plantar ligament; a strong ligament that extends from the calcaneus to the cuboid and lateral metatarsals on the plantar aspect of the foot.
ligamen'ta planta'ria [NA], plantar ligaments; glenoid ligaments (2); accessory plantar ligaments; Cruveilhier's ligaments; the counterparts in the foot of the ligamenta palmaria, in the hand.
l. poplite'um arcua'tum [NA], arcuate popliteal ligament; posterior ligament of knee; a broad fibrous band attached above to the lateral condyle of the femur and passing medially and downward in the posterior part of the capsule of the knee joint, arching over the tendon of the popliteus muscle.
l. poplite'um obli'quum [NA], oblique popliteal ligament; Bourgery's ligament; a fibrous band that extends across the back of the knee from the insertion of the semimembranosus on the medial condyle of the tibia to the lateral condyle of the femur.
l. pterygospina'le [NA], pterygospinal or pterygospinous ligament; Civinini's ligament; a membranous ligament extending from the spine of the sphenoid to the upper part of the posterior border of the lateral pterygoid lamina.
l. pu'bicum supe'rius [NA], superior pubic ligament; fibers that pass transversely above the pubic symphysis.
l. pubocapsula're, l. pubofemorale.
l. pubofemora'le [NA], pubofemoral ligament; pubocapsular ligament; l. pubocapsulare; a thickened part of the capsule of the hip joint that extends from the superior ramus of the pubis to the intertrochanteric line of the femur.
l. puboprostat'icum [NA], puboprostatic ligament; Denonvillier's ligament; the localized thickening of the superior fascia of the pelvic diaphragm anteriorly that anchors the prostate and neck of the bladder to the pubis on each side. It is composed of medial and lateral parts and usually contains smooth muscle.
l. puboprostat'icum latera'le, lateral puboprostatic ligament. See l. puboprostaticum.
l. puboprostat'icum media'le, medial puboprostatic ligament. See l. puboprostaticum.
l. pubovesica'le [NA], pubovesical ligament; in the female the fascial thickening comparable to the l. puboprostaticum.
l. pulmona'le [NA], pulmonary ligament; Teutleben's ligament; l. latum pulmonis; the reflection of pleura from the mediastinum to the lung which continues as a two-layered fold below the root of the lung.
l. quadra'tum [NA], quadrate ligament; Denucé's ligament; fibers that pass from the distal margin of the radial notch of the ulna to the neck of the radius.
l. radia'tum, l. capitis costae radiatum.
l. radiocarpa'le dorsa'le [NA], dorsal radiocarpal ligament; the ligament that extends from the distal end of the radius posteriorly to the proximal row of carpal bones.
l. radiocarpa'le palma're [NA], palmar radiocarpal ligament; a strong ligament that passes from the distal end of the radius to the proximal row of carpal bones on the anterior surface of the wrist joint.
l. reflex'um [NA], reflex ligament; Colles' ligament; fascia triangularis abdominis; triangular fascia; a triangular fibrous band extending from the aponeurosis of the external oblique to the pubic tubercle of the opposite side.
l. sacrococcyg'eum ante'rius [NA], anterior or ventral sacrococcygeal ligament, the continuation of the anterior longitudinal ligament uniting the sacrum and coccyx.
l. sacrococcyg'eum latera'le [NA], lateral sacrococcygeal ligament; intercornual ligament; a ligament that extends from the lateral inferior margin of the sacrum to the transverse process of the first coccygeal vertebra.
l. sacrococcyg'eum poste'rius profun'dum [NA], deep posterior sacrococcygeal ligament; the continuation of the posterior longitudinal ligament uniting the sacrum and coccyx.
l. sacrococcyg'eum poste'rius superficia'le [NA], superficial posterior or dorsal sacrococcygeal ligament; the continuation of the supraspinal ligament from the sacrum to the coccyx.
l. sacrodura'le, sacrodural *ligament.*
ligamen'ta sacroili'aca ante'riora [NA], anterior or ventral sacroiliac ligaments; the strong fibrous bands that reinforce the sacroiliac joint anteriorly.
ligamen'ta sacroili'aca interos'sea [NA], interosseous sacroiliac ligaments; short obliquely directed fibrous bands that pass between the sacrum and ilium in the narrow cleft behind the auricular surfaces of these bones.
ligamen'ta sacroil'aca poste'riora [NA], posterior or dorsal sacroiliac ligaments; the heavy fibrous bands that pass from the ilium to the sacrum posterior to the sacroilac joint.
l. sacroili'acum poste'rius, l. sacroiliaca posteriora.
l. sacrospina'le [NA], sacrospinous ligament; anterior sacrosciatic ligament; l. sacrospinosum; the fibrous band that passes from the ischial spine to the sacrum and coccyx.
l. sacrospino'sum, l. sacrospinale.
l. sacrotubera'le [NA], sacrotuberous ligament; posterior sacrosciatic ligament; l. sacrotuberosum; the ligament that passes from the ischial tuberosity to the ilium, sacrum, and coccyx.
l. sacrotubero'sum, l. sacrotuberale.
l. sero'sum, serous *ligament.*
l. sphenomandibula're [NA], sphenomandibular ligament; the fibrous band that passes from the spine of the sphenoid bone to the lingula of the mandible.
l. spira'le coch'leae [NA], official alternative term for *crista* spiralis.

l. sple'norenale [NA], splenorenal ligament; lienorenal ligament; lienophrenic ligament; phrenicosplenic, phrenosplenic, or phrenicolienal ligament; l. lienoreale; l. phrenicosplenicum or phrenicolienale l.; the portion of the greater omentum which extends from the spleen to the diaphragm near the left kidney.

l. sternoclavicula're [NA], sternoclavicular ligament; **l. s. ante'rius,** anterior sternoclavicular ligament; a fibrous band that reinforces the sternoclavicular anteriorly; **l. s. poste'rius,** posterior sternoclavicular ligament; a fibrous band that reinforces the sternoclavicular joint posteriorly.

l. sternocosta'le intra-articula're [NA], intra-articular sternocostal ligament; a ligament within the articular capsule between a costal cartilage and the sternum; especially well developed at second costal cartilage.

ligamen'ta sternocosta'lia radia'ta [NA], radiate sternocostal ligaments; fibers of the articular capsule that radiate from the costal cartilages to the anterior surface of the sternum.

ligamen'ta sternoper'icardi'aca [NA], sternopericardial ligaments; Lannelongue's or Luschka's ligaments; fibrous bands that pass from the pericardium to the sternum.

l. stylohyoi'deum [NA], stylohyoid ligament; epihyal ligament; a fibrous cord that passes from the tip of the styloid process to the lesser cornu of the hyoid bone; it is occasionally ossified.

l. stylomandibula're [NA], stylomandibular ligament; stylomaxillary ligament; a condensation of the deep cervical fascia extending from the tip of the styloid process of the temporal bone to the posterior border of the angle of the jaw.

l. supraspina'le [NA], supraspinous ligament; the longitudinal fibrous band attached to the tips of the spinous processes of the vertebrae: in the cervical region it is altered to form the ligamentum nuchae.

ligamen'ta suspenso'ria mam'mae [NA], suspensory ligaments of breast; suspensory ligaments of Cooper; Cooper's ligaments (1); well developed retinacula cutis that extend from the overlying skin to the fibrous stroma of the mammary gland.

l. suspenso'rium clitor'idis [NA], suspensory ligament of clitoris; a fibrous band that extends from the pubic symphysis to the fascia of the clitoris.

l. suspenso'rium ova'rii [NA], suspensory ligament of ovary; infundibulopelvic ligament; a band of peritoneum that extends upward from the upper pole of the ovary; it contains the ovarian vessels and ovarian plexus of nerves.

l. suspenso'rium pe'nis [NA], suspensory ligament of penis; a fibrous band that extends from the pubic symphysis to the deep fascia of the penis.

l. talocalcanea're [NA], talocalcaneal ligament; any of three ligaments uniting the talus and calcaneus: **l. t. interos'seum,** interosseous talocalcaneal ligament; a strong fibrous band occupying the tarsal sinus; **l. t. latera'le,** lateral talocalcaneal ligament; a ligament extending from the trochlea of the talus to the lateral surface of the calcaneus; **l. t. media'le,** medial talocalcaneal ligament; a ligament extending from the medial tuberosity of the posterior talar process and the sustentaculum tali.

l. talofibula're ante'rius [NA], anterior talofibular ligament; the band of fibers that extends from the lateral malleolus to the neck of the talus.

l. talofibula're poste'rius [NA], posterior talofibular ligament; the nearly horizontal fibrous band that extends from the posterior border of the talus to the malleolar fossa.

l. talonavicula're [NA], talonavicular ligament; the broad band that passes from the dorsal side of the neck of the talus to the dorsal surface of the navicular bone.

l. talotibia'le ante'rius, *pars* tibiotalaris anterior. See also l. deltoideum.

l. talotibia'le poste'rius, *pars* tibiotalaris posterior. See also l. deltoideum.

l. tarsa'le exter'num, l. palpebrale laterale.

l. tarsa'le inter'num, l. palpebrale mediale.

ligamen'ta tar'si [NA], tarsal ligaments; the ligaments that interconnect the tarsal bones; they are grouped into three sets: **l. t. dorsa'lia, l. t. interos'sea,** and **l. t. planta'ria,** and are individually named according to their attachments.

ligamen'ta tarsometatarsa'lia [NA], tarsometatarsal ligaments; the ligaments that unite tarsal and metatarsal bones; they are arranged in dorsal, interosseous, and plantar sets.

l. temporomandibula're, l. laterale articulationis temporomandibularis.

l. te'res fem'oris, l. capitis femoris.

l. te'res hep'atis [NA], round ligament of liver, the remains of the umbilical vein.

l. te'res u'teri [NA], round ligament of the uterus; Hunter's ligament; a fibromuscular band that is attached to the uterus on either side in front of and below the opening of the uterine tube; it passes through the inguinal canal to the labium majus.

l. tes'tis, the caudal portion of the embryonic urogenital ridge; the upper third of the gubernaculum testis.

l. thyroepiglot'ticum [NA], thyroepiglottic or thyroepiglottidean ligament; an elastic band that connects the petiole of the epiglottis to the interior of the thyroid cartilage near the superior thyroid notch.

l. thyrohyoi'deum latera'le [NA], lateral thyrohyoid ligament; l. hyothyroideum laterale; a band that extends from the superior cornu of the thyroid cartilage to the tip of the greater cornu of the hyoid bone.

l. thyrohyoi'deum media'num [NA], median thyrohyoid ligament; l. hyothyroideum medium; the central thickened portion of the thyrohyoid membrane.

l. tibiofibula're ante'rius [NA], anterior tibiofibular ligament; the ligament that binds the anterior aspect of the tibiofibular syndesmosis.

l. tibiofibula're me'dium, *membrana* interossea cruris.

l. tibiofibula're poste'rius [NA], posterior tibiofibular ligament; the fibrous band that crosses the posterior aspect of the tibiofibular syndesmosis.

l. tibionavicula're, *pars* tibionaviculare. See also l. deltoideum.

ligamen'ta trachea'lia [NA], ligamenta anularia trachealia.

l. transversa'lis col'li, cervical *ligament* of uterus.

l. transver'sum acetab'uli [NA], transverse ligament of acetabulum; the ligament that passes across the acetabular notch.

l. transver'sum atlan'tis [NA], Lauth's ligament; it forms the transversal part of the cruciforme atlantis.

l. transver'sum cru'ris, *retinaculum* musculorum extensorum superius.

l. transver'sum ge'nus [NA], transverse ligament of knee; a transverse band that passes between the lateral and medial menisci in the anterior part of the knee joint.

l. transver'sum pel'vis, l. transversum perinei.

l. transver'sum perine'i [NA], l. transversum pelvis; transverse ligament of perineum; transverse ligament of pelvis; Krause's ligament; the thickened anterior border of the urogenital diaphragm, formed by the fusion of its two fascial layers.

l. transver'sum scap'ulae infe'rius [NA], inferior transverse scapular ligament; spinoglenoid ligament; an inconstant fibrous band that passes from the lateral border of the spine of the scapula to the posterior margin of the glenoid cavity.

l. transver'sum scap'ulae supe'rius [NA], superior transverse scapular ligament; suprascapular ligament; the strong fibrous band that bridges the scapular notch.

l. trapezoi'deum [NA], trapezoid ligament; the lateral part of the coracoclavicular ligament that attaches to the trapezoid line of the clavicle.

l. triangula're, *membrana* perinei.

l. triangula're dex'trum [NA], right triangular ligament; a triangular fold of peritoneum that passes from the right lobe of the liver to the diaphragm; it is continuous with the coronary ligament.

l. triangula're sinis'trum [NA], left triangular ligament; a triangular fold of peritoneum that extends from the left lobe of the liver to the diaphragm.

l. tuber'culi cos'tae, l. costotransversarium laterale.

l. ulnocarpa'le palma're [NA], palmar ulnocarpal ligament; the fibrous band that passes from the ulnar styloid process to the carpal bones.

l. umbilica'le latera'le, lateral umbilical ligament; an old name for l. umbilicale mediale.

l. umbilica'le media'le [NA], medial umbilical ligament; the obliterated umbilical artery that persists as a fibrous cord passing upward alongside the bladder to the umbilicus.

l. umbilica'le media'num [NA], middle umbilical ligament; urachal ligament; the remnant of the urachus, contained in the plica umbilicalis mediana; it persists as a midline fibrous cord between the apex of the bladder and the umbilicus.

l. ve'nae ca'vae sinis'trae, ligament of left superior vena cava; the obliterated left common cardinal vein; it extends from the left brachiocephalic vein to the oblique vein of the left atrium.

l. veno'sum [NA], venous ligament; Arantius' ligament; a thin fibrous cord, lying in the fissura ligamenti venosi, the remains of the ductus venosus of the fetus.

l. ventricula're, l. vestibulare.

l. vestibula're [NA], vestibular ligament; ventricular ligament; l. ventriculare; the thin fibrous layer that lies in the ventricular fold of the larynx.

l. voca'le [NA], vocal ligament; the band that extends on either side from the thyroid cartilage to the vocal process of the arytenoid cartilage; it is the upper border of the conus elasticus of the larynx.

---

ligand (lig'and, lī'gand) [L. *ligo,* to bind]. **1.** An organic molecule attached to a central metal ion by multiple coordination bonds; *e.g.,* the porphyrin portion of heme, the corrin nucleus of the B_{12} vitamins. **2.** An organic molecule attached to a tracer element; *e.g.,* a radioisotope.

ligase (lī'gās). Generic term for enzymes (EC class 6) catalyzing the joining of two molecules coupled with the breakdown of a pyrophosphate bond in ATP or a similar compound. See also synthetase.

ligate (lī'gāt) [L. *ligo,* pp. *-atus,* to bind]. To apply a ligature.

ligation (lī-gā'shŭn) [L. *ligatio,* fr. *ligo,* to bind]. Application of a ligature.

Larrey's l., a l. of the femoral artery immediately below the inguinal ligament.

pole l., a l. at root of an organ to shut off or to diminish blood supply.

surgical l., in dentistry, the surgical exposure of an unerupted tooth so that a metal ligature can be placed around its cervix and fastened to an orthodontic appliance to facilitate eruption.

tooth l., the binding together of teeth with wire for stabilization and immobilization following traumatic injury or orthognathic surgery, or during periodontal therapy.

tubal l., interruption of the continuity of the oviducts by cutting, cautery, or by a plastic or metal device to prevent future conception.

ligator (lī'gā-ter, -tōr). An instrument used in the ligation of vessels in deep and nearly inaccessible parts.

ligature (lig'ă-chūr) [L. *ligatura,* a band or tie, fr. *ligo,* to tie]. **1.** A thread, wire, fillet, or the like, tied tightly around a blood vessel, the pedicle of a tumor, or other structure to constrict it. **2.** In orthodontics, a wire or other material used to secure an orthodontic attachment or tooth to an archwire.

Desault's l., a l. of the femoral artery in the adductor muscle, for treatment of popliteal aneurysm.

elastic l., **(1)** a rubber l. that slowly constricts; **(2)** in orthodontics, a stretchable threadlike material that may be tied from a tooth to an archwire or from tooth to tooth to gain movement of these units.

intravascular l., balloon occlusion of the feeding vessels of a cerebral arteriovenous malformation.

nonabsorbable l., a permanent l. of inert material, such as silk, wire, or synthetic fiber, that does not undergo dissolution in human tissues.

occluding l., a l. to shut off completely the distal blood supply.

provisional l., a l. applied to an artery in continuity at the beginning of an operation to prevent hemorrhage, but removed when the operation is completed.

soluble l., a temporary l. that of material that can be absorbed by human tissues.

Stannius l., a l. placed either around the junction between the sinus venosus and atrium of the frog or turtle heart (first Stannius l.) or around the atrioventricular junction (second Stannius l.); demonstrates that the cardiac impulse is conducted from sinus venosus to atria to ventricle, but that successive chambers possess automaticity since each may continue to beat, but the atria now have a slower rate than the sinus venosus and the ventricle either does not contract or beats at a slower rate than the atria.

suboccluding l., a l. to diminish blood supply and encourage collateral circulation.

suture l., a l. applied by passing a needle with attached thread through or around a structure to more firmly secure the l.

light (līt) [A.S. *leōht*]. That portion of electromagnetic radiation to which the retina is sensitive. See also subentries under lamp.

cold l., **(1)** bioluminescence; **(2)** fluorescent l. as opposed to incandescent l.

Finsen l., the violet and ultraviolet rays of the spectrum filtered out of the sunlight by a hollow planoconvex lens filled with an ammoniacal solution of copper sulfate; usually, instead of the filtered sunlight, the carbon electric arc is used, the rays being made parallel by two planoconvex lenses. It was formerly used in the treatment of cutaneous tuberculosis.

infrared l., see infrared.

minimum l., see visual *threshold.*

polarized l., l. in which, as a result of reflection or transmission through certain media, the vibrations are all in one plane, transverse to the ray, instead of in all planes.

reflected l., l. directed backward from a mirror.

refracted l., bent rays of l. changed in passage from one transparent medium to another of unequal density. See also refraction.

Simpson l., a lamp emitting ultraviolet rays, produced by an electric arc between two electrodes, one of tungstate of iron and the other of manganese.

transmitted l., l. passed through a transparent medium.

Wood's l., ultraviolet l. produced by Wood's lamp.

lightening (līt'en-ing). Sensation of decreased abdominal distention during the later weeks of pregnancy following the descent of the fetal head into the pelvic inlet.

light green SF yellowish [C.I. 42095]. An acid arylmethane dye, used as a cytoplasmic stain in plant and animal histology; fades badly in bright light.

Lignac, G.O.E., Dutch pediatrician. See L.-Fanconi *syndrome.*

lig'nin [L. *lignum,* wood]. A polymer of coniferyl alcohol accompanying cellulose and present in vegetable fiber and wood cells; a source of vanillin (by oxidation of l.).

lignoceric acid (lig-nō-sār'ik, -sēr'ik). Tetracosanoic acid; $CH_3(CH_2)_{22}COOH$; an acid present in one type of sphingomyelin.

Lillie, Ralph D., U.S. pathologist, 1896–1979. See L.'s *stains,* Glenner-L. *stain* for pituitary.

Lilly, John C., U.S. physiologist, *1915. See Silverman-L. *pneumotachograph.*

limb (lim) [A.S. *lim*]. **1.** An extremity; a member; an arm or leg. **2.** A segment of any jointed structure. See also crus.

ampullary l.'s of semicircular ducts, *crura* membranacea ampullaria.
anacrotic l., the ascending l. of an arterial pulse tracing.
anterior l. of internal capsule, *crus* anterius capsulae internae.
anterior l. of stapes, *crus* anterius stapedis.
l.'s of bony semicircular canals, *crura* ossea canales semicirculares.
common l. of membranous semicircular ducts, *crus* membranaceum commune ductus semicircularis.
l. of helix, *crus* helicis.
inferior l., *membrum* inferius.
lateral l., *crus* laterale.
medial l., *crus* mediale.
pelvic l., *membrum* inferius.
phantom l., stump hallucination; pseudesthesia (3); the sensation that an amputated l. is still present, often associated with painful paresthesia.
posterior l. of internal capsule, *crus* posterius capsulae internae.
posterior l. of stapes, *crus* posterius stapedis.
retrolenticular l. of internal capsule, *pars* retrolentiformis capsulae internae.
simple membranous l. of semicircular duct, *crus* membranaceum simplex ductus semicircularis.
sublenticular l. of internal capsule, *pars* sublentiformis capsulae internae.
superior l., *membrum* superius.
thoracic l., *membrum* superius.

limbic (lim'bik). **1.** Relating to a limbus. **2.** Relating to the limbic *system.*

limbus, pl. **limbi** (lim'bŭs, lim'bī) [L. a border] [NA]. The edge, border, or fringe of a part.

l. acetab'uli [NA], margin of the acetabulum; the rim of bone around the acetabulum to which is attached the labrum acetabulare.
l. alveola'ris, (1) *arcus* alveolaris mandibulae; **(2)** *arcus* alveolaris maxillae.
l. cor'neae [NA], corneal margin; sclerocorneal junction; the margin of the cornea overlapped by the sclera.
l. fos'sae ova'lis [NA], margin of the fossa ovalis; annulus ovalis; Vieussens' annulus, isthmus, limbus, or ring; a muscular ring surrounding the fossa ovalis in the wall of the right atrium of the heart.
l. lam'inae spira'lis os'seae [NA], the border of the spiral lamina; the thickened periosteum covering the upper plate of the lamina spiralis ossea of the cochlea.
l. membra'nae tym'pani, margin of the tympanic membrane attaching to the tympanic sulcus.
lim'bi palpebra'les [NA], borders of eyelids; **l. p. anterio'res,** anterior border of the eyelids; the margin of the eyelids near the skin; **l. p. posterio'res,** posterior border of the eyelids; the margin of the eyelids near the conjunctiva.
l. penicilla'tus, brush *border.*
l. stria'tus, striated *border.*
Vieussens' l., l. fossae ovalis.

lime (līm). **1.** Calx (1); calcium oxide; CaO; an alkaline earth oxide occurring in grayish white masses (quicklime); on exposure to the atmosphere it becomes converted into calcium hydrate and calcium carbonate (air-slaked l.); direct addition of water to calcium oxide produces calcium hydrate (slaked l.). **2.** Fruit of the l. tree, *Citrus medica* (family Rutaceae), which is a source of ascorbic acid and acts as an antiscorbutic agent.

air-slaked l., see lime (1).
chlorinated l., bleaching powder; obtained by the action of chlorine on calcium hydroxide; used to prepare surgical chlorinated soda solution and as a disinfectant and deodorant.
slaked l., see lime (1).
sulfurated l., crude *calcium* sulfide.

limen, pl. **limina** (li'men, lim'i-nă) [L.] [NA]. Threshold (3); entrance; the external opening of a canal or space, such as l. insulae.

l. in'sulae [NA], threshold of the island of Reil; the band of transition between the anterior portion of the gray matter of the insula and the anterior perforated substance; it is formed by a narrow strip of olfactory cortex along the lateral side of the lateral olfactory stria.
l. na'si [NA], threshold of the nose; a ridge marking the boundary between the nasal cavity proper and the vestibule.

limes (L) (lī'mēz) [L.]. A boundary, limit, or threshold. See also L *doses.*

liminal (lim'i-năl) [L. *limen* (*limin-*), a threshold]. **1.** Pertaining to a threshold. **2.** Pertaining to a stimulus just strong enough to excite a tissue, *e.g.,* nerve or muscle.

liminometer (lim-i-nom'ĕ-ter) [L. *limen,* threshold, + G. *metron,* measure]. An instrument for measuring the strength of a stimulus which is barely sufficient to produce a reflex response.

lim'it [L. *limes,* boundary]. A boundary or end.

elastic l., the greatest stress to which a material may be subjected and still be capable of returning to its original dimensions when the forces are released.
Hayflick's l., the l. of human cell division in subcultures; such cells will divide only about 50 times before dying out.
proportional l., the greatest stress that a material is capable of sustaining without any deviation from proportionality of stress to strain (Hooke's law).
quantum l., the shortest wavelength found in an x-ray spectrum.
short-term exposure l. (STEL), the maximum concentration of a chemical to which workers may be exposed continuously for up to 15 minutes without danger to health or work efficiency and safety.

Limnatis nilotica (lim-nā'tis nī-lot'i-kă) [G. *limnē,* pool]. The horse leech; a species of land-leech of southern Europe and northern Africa which may infest the nostrils or gullet and, attaching itself to the mucous membrane, may cause hemorrhages and anemia in horses and other animals drinking leech-infested water.

limnemia (lim-nē'mē-ă) [G. *limnē,* marsh, + *haima,* blood]. Chronic *malaria.*

limnemic (lim-nē'mik). Suffering from chronic malaria.

limnology (lim-nol'ō-jē) [G. *limnē,* pool, + *logos,* study]. Study of the physical, chemical, meteorological, and biological conditions in fresh water; a branch of ecology.

limon, gen. **limonis** (lī'mon, li-mō'nis) [L.]. Lemon.

limophoitas (lī'mō-foy'tas) [G. *limos,* hunger, + *phoitas,* frenzy]. Rarely used term for a psychosis induced by starvation.

limophthisis (lī-mof'thī-sis) [G. *limos,* hunger, + *phthisis,* wasting]. Rarely used term for emaciation from lack of sufficient nourishment.

limosis (lī-mō'sis) [G. *limos,* hunger]. Hunger, especially abnormal or inordinate hunger.

limp. A lame walk with a yielding step. See also claudication.

lincomycin (lin-kō-mī'sin). An antibacterial substance, composed of substituted pyrrolidine and octapyranose moities, produced by *Streptomyces lincolnensis;* active against Gram-positive organisms; used medicinally as l. hydrochloride.

lincture, linctus (link'chūr, link'tŭs) [L. *lingo,* pp. *linctus,* to lick]. An electuary or a confection; originally a medical preparation taken by licking.

lindane (lin'dān). Gamma-benzene hexachloride; 1,2,3,4,5,6-hexachlorocyclohexane; used as scabicide, pediculocide, and insecticide

(10 times more toxic for house flies than DDT).

Lindau, Arvid, Swedish pathologist, 1892–1958. See L.'s *disease, tumor;* von Hippel-L. *disease, syndrome.*

Lindbergh, Charles A., U.S. aviator, 1902–1974. See Carrel-L. *pump.*

Lindemann, Edward E., U.S. surgeon, 1879–1919. See L.'s *cannula.*

Lindner, Karl, Austrian ophthalmologist, 1883–1961. See L.'s *bodies, operation.*

Lindqvist, Johan Torsten, Swedish physician, *1906. See Fahraeus-L. *effect.*

LINE

line (līn) [L. *linea,* a linen thread, a string, line, fr. *linum,* flax]. **1.** A mark, strip, or streak. See also linea. **2.** A unit of measurement used by histologists in the 19th century; it varied in different countries from $^1/_{10}$ to $^1/_{12}$ of an English inch, but the most widely used unit was the Paris l. **3.** A laboratory derivative of a stock of organisms maintained under defined physical conditions. **4.** A section of tubing supplying fluid or conducting impulses for monitoring equipment; *e.g.,* intravenous l., arterial l.

absorption l.'s, the dark l.'s in the solar spectrum due to absorption by the solar and the earth's atmosphere; the phenomenon occurs because rays passing from an incandescent body through a colder medium are absorbed by elements in that medium.

accretion l.'s., l.'s seen in microscopic sections of the enamel, marking successive layers of added material.

alveolonasal l., a l. connecting the alveolar point and the nasion.

Amberg's lateral sinus l., a l. dividing the angle formed by the anterior edge of the mastoid process and the temporal l.

anocutaneous l., *linea* anocutanea.

anterior axillary l., *linea* axillaris anterior.

anterior median l., *linea* mediana anterior.

arcuate l., *linea* arcuata.

arterial l., an intra-arterial catheter.

axillary l., see *linea* axillaris anterior, media, and posterior.

azygos venous l., medial sympathetic l.; in the embryo, a longitudinal venous channel lying dorsolateral to the aorta and medial to the sympathetic trunk; the right side forms the azygos vein, the left side the hemiazygos vein.

Baillarger's l.'s, Baillarger's bands; two laminae of white fibers that course parallel to the surface of the cerebral cortex and are visible as outer and inner l.'s in sections cut perpendicular to the surface; the l. of Gennari in the calcarine cortex represents the outer of these lines.

base l., a l. corresponding to the base of the skull, passing from the infraorbital ridge to the midline of the occiput, cutting the external auditory meatus.

basinasal l., nasobasilar l.; a l. connecting the basion and the nasion.

Beau's l.'s, transverse depressions on the fingernails and intermittent thinning of the hair shaft following severe febrile disease, malnutrition, trauma, coronary occlusion, etc.

l. of Bechterew, band of Kaes-Bechterew.

bismuth l., a black zone on the gingiva, often the first sign of poisoning from prolonged parenteral administration of bismuth.

black l., *linea* nigra.

blue l., a bluish l. along the free border of the gingiva, occurring in chronic heavy metal poisoning.

Bolton-nasion l., Bolton *plane.*

Brödel's bloodless l., l. in section of the kidney demarcating the areas of distribution of the anterior and posterior branches of the renal artery.

Burton's l., a bluish l. on the free border of the gingiva, occurring in lead poisoning.

calcification l.'s of Retzius, l.'s of Retzius; incremental l.'s of rhythmic deposition of successive layers of enamel matrix during development.

Camper's l., the l. running from the inferior border of the ala of the nose to the superior border of the tragus of the ear.

cell l., in tissue culture, the cells growing in the first or later subculture from a primary culture. See also established cell l.

cement l., the refractile boundary of an osteon or interstitial lamellar system in compact bone.

cervical l., a continuous anatomical irregular curved l. marking the cervical end of the crown of a tooth and the cementoenamel junction.

Chamberlain's l., a l. drawn from the posterior margin of the hard palate to the dorsum of the foramen magnum; in basilar impression, the odontoid process rises above this l.

Chaussier's l., the anteroposterior l. of the corpus callosum as appearing on median section of the brain.

Clapton's l., a greenish discoloration of the marginal gingiva in cases of chronic copper poisoning.

cleavage l.'s, Langer's l.'s; linear openings made when a pin is driven into the skin of a cadaver, resulting from the principle axis of orientation of the subcutaneous connective tissue fibers and varying in direction with the region of the body surface.

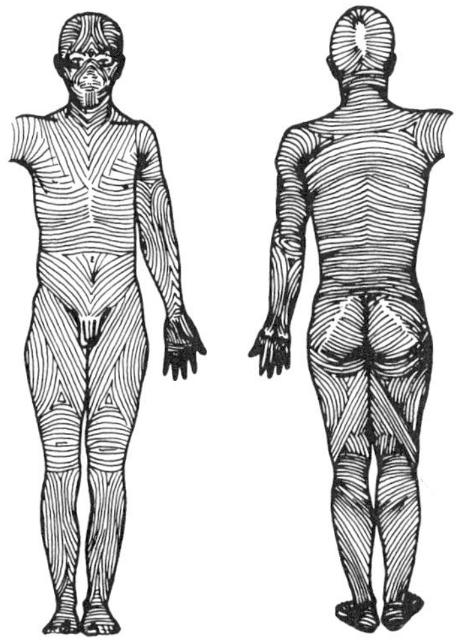

Cleavage Lines of the Skin
(After Langer)

Conradi's l., a l. extending from the base of the ensiform cartilage to the apex beat of the heart, corresponding approximately to the lower edge of the cardiac area.

contour l.'s of Owen, Owen's l.'s.

Correra's l., a l. between lungs and thoracic cage, seen on x-ray visualization.

costoclavicular l., *linea* parasternalis.

costophrenic septal l.'s, Kerley-B l.'s.

Crampton's l., a l. from the apex of the cartilage of the last rib downward and forward nearly to the crest of the ilium, then forward parallel with it to a little below the anterior superior spine; a guide to the common iliac artery.

Daubenton's l., the l. passing between the opisthion and the basion. See also Daubenton's *angle,* Daubenton's *plane.*

l. of demarcation, a zone of inflammatory reaction separating a

gangrenous area from healthy tissue.
demarcation l. of retina, junction of avascular and vascular retina in retinopathy of prematurity.
Dennie's l., Dennie's fold; an accentuated line or fold below the margin of the lower eyelid; characteristic in atopic dermatitis.
dentate l., *linea* anocutanea.
developmental l.'s, developmental *grooves.*
Douglas' l., *linea* arcuata vaginae musculi recti abdominis.
Eberth's l.'s, l.'s appearing between the cells of the myocardium when stained with silver nitrate.
Egger's l., the circular l. of adhesion between the vitreous and posterior lens.
Ehrlich-Türk l., the vertical, thin deposition of material on the posterior surface of the cornea in uveitis.
epiphysial l., *linea* epiphysialis.
established cell l., cells growing in culture after at least 70 subcultures at intervals of 3 days.
Farre's l., a whitish l. marking the insertion of the mesovarium on the ovary.
Feiss l., a l. running from the medial malleolus to the plantar aspect of the first metatarsophalangeal joint.
l. of fixation, a l. joining the object (or point of fixation) with the fovea.
Fleischner l.'s, linear shadows on the roentgenogram of the chest, indicating foci of lobular atelectasis.
Fraunhofer's l.'s, a number of the most prominent of the absorption l.'s of the solar spectrum.
fulcrum l., rotational axis; an imaginary l. around which a removable partial denture tends to rotate.
Futcher's l., a dorso-ventral line of pigmentation occurring symmetrically and bilaterally for about 10 cm along the lateral edge of the biceps muscle, seen in blacks.
l. of Gennari, Gennari's band, stripe; stria of Gennari; a prominent white line appearing in perpendicular sections of the visual cortex (Brodmann's area 17) at about mid-thickness of the cortical gray matter, corresponding to the particularly well developed outer line of Baillarger of that cortical area, and composed largely of tangentially disposed intracortical association fibers.
germ l., a collection of haploid cells derived from the specialized cells of the primitive gonad.
gluteal l., *linea* glutea.
Granger's l., in x-ray demonstration of the skull, a l. produced by the groove of the optic nerve.
growth l.'s, Harris l.'s; dense, transverse l.'s seen in radiographs of long bones, representing regrowth after temporary cessation of longitudinal growth.
Gubler's l., the level of the superficial origin of the trigeminus on the pons, a lesion below which causes Gubler's paralysis.
gum l., the position of the margin of the gingiva in relation to the teeth in the dental arch.
Haller's l., *linea* splendens.
Hampton l., a radiolucent region indicating mucosal edema, contrasted against the radiopaque barium in benign gastric ulcerations.
Harris' l.'s, growth l.'s.
Head's l.'s, Head's zones; tender l.'s or zones; bands of cutaneous hyperesthesia associated with acute or chronic inflammation of the viscera.
Hensen's l., H *band.*
highest nuchal l., *linea* nuchae suprema.
high lip l., the greatest height to which the lip is raised in normal function or during the act of smiling broadly.
Hilton's white l., white l. of anal canal.
His' l., a l. extending from the tip of the anterior nasal spine (acanthion) to the hindmost point on the posterior margin of the foramen magnum (opisthion), dividing the face into an upper and a lower, or dental part.
Holden's l., the crease or furrow of the skin of the groin caused by flexion of the thigh.
Hudson's l., Hudson-Stähli l.; Stahl's l.; a brown, horizontal l. across the lower third of the cornea, occasionally seen in the aged and also in association with corneal opacities.
Hudson-Stähli l., Hudson's l.
Hunter's l., *linea* alba.
Hunter-Schreger l.'s, Hunter-Schreger *bands.*
iliopectineal l., *linea* terminalis.
imbrication l.'s of von Ebner, incremental l.'s of von Ebner, incremental l.'s in the dentin of the tooth that reflect variations in mineralization during dentin formation; the distance between the l.'s corresponds to the daily rate of dentin formation.
incremental l.'s, (**1**) in the enamel, calcification l.'s of Retzius; (**2**) in the dentin, imbrication or incremental l.'s of von Ebner, and Owen's l.'s.
inferior nuchal l., *linea* nuchae inferior.
inferior temporal l., *linea* temporalis inferior.
infracostal l., *planum* subcostale.
intercondylar l., *linea* intercondylaris.
intermediate l. of iliac crest, *linea* intermedia cristae iliacae.
internal oblique l., *linea* mylohyoidea.
interspinal l., *planum* interspinale.
intertrochanteric l., *linea* intertrochanterica.
intertubercular l., *planum* intertuberculare.
isoelectric l., the base l. of the electrocardiogram.
l. of Kaes, *band* of Kaes-Bechterew.
Kerley B l.'s, costophrenic septal l.'s; fine horizontal l.'s a few centimeters above the costophrenic angle in the chest x-ray; thought to be due to distention of interlobular lymphatics with edema fluid.
Kilian's l., a transverse l. marking the promontory of the pelvis.
Langer's l.'s, cleavage l.'s.
Lanz's l., *planum* interspinale.
lateral l., see lateral line *system.*
lateral sympathetic l., thoracolumbar venous l.
lead l., deposits of lead sulfide in the gingiva in areas of chronic inflammation.
low lip l., (**1**) the lowest position of the lower lip during the act of smiling or voluntary retraction; (**2**) the lowest position of the upper lip at rest.
M l., M band; mesophragma; a fine l. in the center of the A band of the sarcomere of striated muscle myofibrils.
mamillary l., *linea* mamillaris.
mammary l., a transverse l. drawn between the two nipples.
McKee's l., a l. drawn from the tip of the cartilage of the eleventh rib to a point 3.5 cm medial to the anterior superior spine, then curved downward, forward, and inward to just above the deep inguinal ring; a guide to the common iliac artery.
medial sympathetic l., azygos venous l.
median l., see *linea* mediana anterior; *linea* mediana posterior.
Mees' l.'s, Mees' stripes; horizontal white bands of the nails seen in chronic arsenical poisoning, and occasionally in leprosy.
mercurial l., a bluish brown pigmentation seen at the gingival margin and associated with mercury poisoning (mercurial stomatitis).
Meyer's l., a l. through the axis of the big toe and passing the midpoint of the heel in a normal foot.
midaxillary l., *linea* axillaris media.
midclavicular l., *linea* medioclavicularis.
middle axillary l., *linea* axillaris media.
milk l., mammary *ridge.*
Monro's l., Monro-Richter l.
Monro-Richter l., Monro's l.; Richter-Monro l.; a l. passing from the umbilicus to the anterior superior iliac spine.
Muehrcke's l.'s, white l.'s, parallel with the lanula and separated from each other by normal pink areas; associated with hypoalbu-

minemia; the l.'s do not move forward with nail growth, but disappear when the serum albumen returns to normal.
mylohyoid l., *linea* mylohyoidea.
nasobasilar l., basinasal l.
Nélaton's l., Roser-Nélaton l.; a l. drawn from the anterior superior iliac spine to the tuberosity of the ischium; normally the great trochanter lies in this l., but in cases of iliac dislocation of the hip or fracture of the neck of the femur the trochanter is felt above the l.
neonatal l., neonatal ring; in deciduous teeth, a l. of demarcation between prenatal and postnatal enamel.
nipple l., *linea* mamillaris.
Obersteiner-Redlich l., Obersteiner-Redlich *zone.*
oblique l., *linea* obliqua.
l. of occlusion, the alignment of the occluding surfaces of the teeth in the horizontal plane. See also occlusal *plane.*
Ogston's l., a l. drawn from the adductor tubercle of the femur to the intercondylar notch; a guide to resection of the medial condyle for knock-knee.
Ohngren's l., a theoretical plane passing between the medial canthus of the eye and the angle of the mandible; used as an arbitrary dividing l. in classifying localized tumors of the maxillary sinus; tumors above the l. invade vital structures early and have a poorer prognosis, whereas those below the l. have a more favorable prognosis.
Owen's l.'s, contour l.'s of Owen; accentuated incremental l.'s in the dentin thought to be due to disturbances in the mineralization process.
parasternal l., *linea* parasternalis.
paravertebral l., *linea* paravertebralis.
Paris l., a unit of microscopic measurement as used in Kölliker's *Mikroskopische Anatomie;* it was equal to 0.0888138 of an inch.
pectinate l., *linea* anocutanea.
pectineal l., *linea* pectinea.
pectineal l. of pubis, *pecten* ossis pubis.
pleuroesophageal l., a boundary l. seen normally in an x-ray of the chest.
Poirier's l., a l. extending from the nasion to the lambda.
popliteal l., *linea* musculi solei.
postaxillary l., *linea* axillaris posterior.
posterior axillary l., *linea* axillaris posterior.
posterior median l., *linea* mediana posterior.
Poupart's l., a perpendicular l. passing through the center of the inguinal ligament on either side; it marks off the hypochondriac, lumbar, and iliac from the epigastric, umbilical, and hypogastric regions, respectively.
preaxillary l., *linea* axillaris anterior.
pure l., isogenic *strain.*
Reid's base l., a l. drawn from the inferior margin of the orbit to the auricular point (center of the aperture of the external auditory canal) and extending backward to the center of the occipital bone. Used as the zero plane in computed tomography.
retentive fulcrum l., **(1)** an imaginary l. connecting the retentive points of clasp arms on retaining teeth adjacent to mucosa-borne denture bases; **(2)** an imaginary l. connecting the retentive points of clasp arms, around which l. the denture tends to rotate when subjected to forces such as the pull of sticky foods.
l.'s of Retzius, calcification l.'s of Retzius.
Richter-Monro l., Monro-Richter l.
Roser-Nélaton l., Nélaton's l.
sagittal l., any anteroposterior l.
Salter's incremental l.'s, transverse l.'s sometimes seen in dentin, due to improper calcification.
S-BP l., a l. connecting the sella with the Bolton point; it indicates the posterior portion of the cranial base in cephalometrics.
scapular l., *linea* scapularis.
Schreger's l.'s, Hunter-Schreger *bands.*
semicircular l., *linea* arcuata vaginae musculi recti abdominis.
semilunar l., *linea* semilunaris.
Sergent's white l., white l.
Shenton's l., a curved l. formed by the top of the obturator foramen and the inner side of the neck of the femur, seen in a radiograph of the normal joint; it is disturbed in many lesions of the hip joint, such as congenital dislocation or hip fracture.
S-N l., a l. connecting a point (S) representing the center of the sella turcica with the frontonasal junction (N); it denotes the anterior portion of the cranial base in cephalometrics.
soleal l., *linea* musculi solei.
l. for soleus muscle, *linea* musculi solei.
Spigelius' l., *linea* semilunaris.
spiral l., *linea* intertrochanterica.
stabilizing fulcrum l., an imaginary l. connecting occlusal rests, around which l. the denture tends to rotate under masticatory force.
Stahl's l., Hudson's l.
sternal l., *linea* sternalis.
Stocker's l., a fine l. of pigment in the corneal epithelium near the head of a pterygium.
subcostal l., *planum* subcostale.
superior nuchal l., *linea* nuchae superior.
superior temporal l., *linea* temporalis superior.
supracrestal l., *planum* supracristale.
survey l., clasp guideline; Cummer's guideline; **(1)** a l. scribed on an abutment tooth of a dental cast by means of a dental surveyor indicating the height of contour of the tooth according to a specific path of insertion; **(2)** a l. which serves as a guide in the proper location of various parts of a clasp assembly for a removable partial denture.
Sydney l., Sydney *crease.*
sylvian l., the l. of the posterior limb of the lateral sulcus (sylvian fissure) of the cerebral cortex.
temporal l., see *linea* temporalis inferior; *linea* temporalis superior.
tender l.'s, Head's l.'s.
terminal l., *linea* terminalis.
thoracolumbar venous l., lateral sympathetic l.; a longitudinal venous channel lying dorsolateral to the aorta and lateral to the sympathetic trunk in the embryo; thought to be equivalent to the supracardinal veins in lower mammals.
Topinard's l., a l. running between the glabella and the mental point.
transverse l., *linea* transversa.
trapezoid l., *linea* trapezoidea.
Ullmann's l., the l. of displacement in spondylolisthesis.
Vesling's l., *raphe* scroti.
vibrating l., the imaginary l. across the posterior part of the palate, marking the division between the movable and immovable tissues.
l. of vision, visual *axis.*
Voigt's l.'s, boundaries on a skin area innervated by a main cutaneous nerve.
Wegner's l., a narrow, whitish, slightly curved l. representing an area of preliminary calcification at the junction of the epiphysis and diaphysis of a long bone, related to syphilitic epiphysitis.
white l., **(1)** linea alba; **(2)** Sergent's white l.; a pale streak appearing within 30 to 60 seconds after stroking the skin with a fingernail, and lasting for several minutes; regarded as a sign of diminished arterial tension.
white l. of anal canal, Hilton's white l.; a bluish pink, narrow, wavy zone in the mucosa of the anal canal below the pectinate l. at the level of the interval between the subcutaneous part of the external sphincter and the lower border of the internal sphincter.
Z l., Z band or disk; intermediate disk; a cross striation bisecting the I band of striated muscle myofibrils and serving as the anchoring point of actin filaments at either end of the sarcomere.

l.'s of Zahn, striae of Zahn; riblike markings seen by the naked eye on the surface of antemortem thrombi; they consist of a branching framework of platelets and fibrin separating the coagulated blood cells.

Zöllner's l.'s, figures devised to show the possibility of optical illusions; a common one consists of two parallel l.'s which are met by numerous short lines obliquely placed; the parallel lines then seeming to converge or diverge.

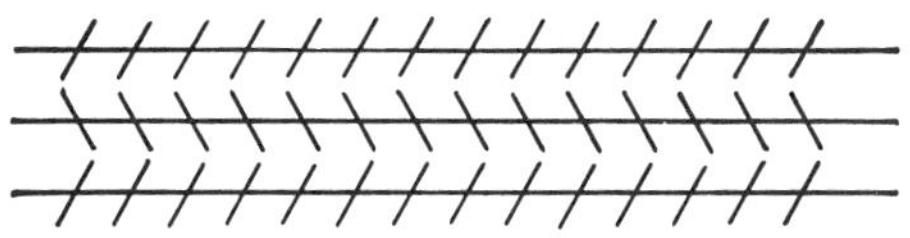

Zöllner's Lines

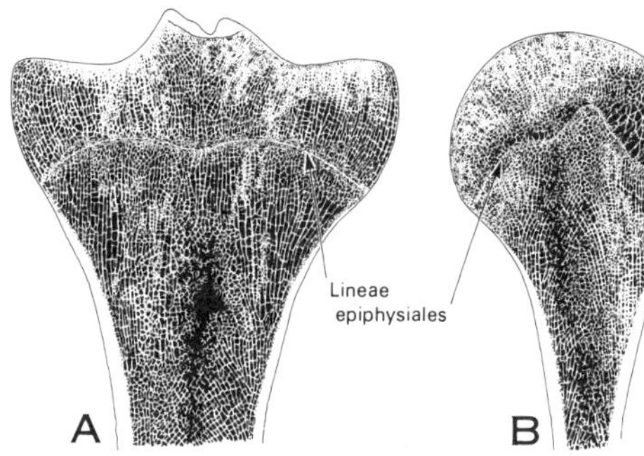

Lineae Epiphysiales

Epiphysial lines of (*A*) proximal end of tibia and (*B*) proximal end of humerus.

LINEA

linea, gen. and pl. **lineae** (lin'ē-ă, -ē-ē) [L.] [NA]. Line; in anatomy, a long narrow mark, strip, or streak distinguished from the adjacent tissues by color, texture, or elevation.

l. adminic'ulum, see *adminiculum* lineae albae.

l. al'ba [NA], white line (1); Hunter's line; a fibrous band running vertically the entire length of the center of the anterior abdominal wall, receiving the attachments of the oblique and transverse abdominal muscles.

lin'eae albican'tes, *striae* cutis distensae.

l. anocuta'nea [NA], anocutaneous line; dentate or pectinate line; the line between the simple columnar epithelium of the rectum and the stratified epithelium of the anal canal.

l. arcua'ta [NA], arcuate line; **l. a. os'sis il'ii,** the iliac portion of the terminal line of the pelvis; **l. a. vagi'nae mus'culi rec'ti abdom'inis,** semicircular line; l. semicircularis; Douglas' line; a crescentic line, not always clearly defined, which marks the lower limit of the posterior layer of the sheath of the rectus abdominis muscle.

l. as'pera [NA], rough line; a rough ridge with two pronounced lips running down the posterior surface of the shaft of the femur; the lateral lip (labium laterale) is a continuation of the crista glutea, the medial lip (labium mediale) of the linea intertrochanterica; it affords attachment to the vastus medialis, adductor longus, adductor magnus, adductor brevis, the short head of the biceps, and the vastus lateralis muscles.

lin'eae atroph'icae, *striae* cutis distensae.

l. axilla'ris ante'rior [NA], anterior axillary line; preaxillary line; l. preaxillaris; a vertical line extending inferiorly from the anterior axillary fold.

l. axilla'ris me'dia [NA], middle axillary line; midaxillary line; l. medio-axillaris; a vertical line midway between the anterior and posterior axillary folds.

l. axilla'ris poste'rior [NA], posterior axillary line; postaxillary line; l. postaxillaris; a vertical line extending inferiorly from the posterior axillary fold.

l. cor'neae seni'lis, *arcus* cornealis.

l. epiphysia'lis [NA], epiphysial line; synchondrosis epiphyseos; the line of junction of the epiphysis and diaphysis of a long bone where growth in length occurs.

l. glu'tea [NA], gluteal line; one of three rough curved lines on the outer surface of the ala of the ilium: **l. g. ante'rior** (or middle), **infe'rior,** and **poste'rior;** the two areas bounded by these give attachment to the gluteus minimus muscle below and gluteus medius above.

l. intercondyla'ris [NA], intercondylar line; a faint transverse ridge separating the floor of the intercondylar fossa from the popliteal surface of the femur; it affords attachment to the posterior portion of the articular capsule of the knee.

l. interme'dia cris'tae ili'acae [NA], intermediate line of the iliac crest; the line on the crest of the ilium between the outer and inner lips.

l. interspina'lis [NA], alternate term for *planum* interspinale.

l. intertrochanter'ica [NA], intertrochanteric line; spiral line; l. spiralis; a rough line that separates the neck and shaft of the femur anteriorly; it passes downward and medially from the greater trochanter and continues into the medial lip of the linea aspera.

l. intertubercula'ris [NA], alternate term for *planum* intertuberculare.

l. mamilla'ris [NA], mamillary line; nipple line; a perpendicular line passing through the nipple on either side.

l. media'na ante'rior [NA], anterior median line; the line of intersection of the midsagittal plane with the anterior surface of the body.

l. media'na poste'rior [NA], posterior median line; the line of intersection of the midsagittal plane with the posterior surface of the body.

l. medio-axilla'ris [NA], an alternate term for l. axillaris media.

l. medioclavicula'ris [NA], midclavicular line; a vertical line passing through the midpoint of the clavicle.

l. mus'culi sol'ei [NA], line for the soleus muscle; soleal or popliteal line; l. poplitea; a ridge which extends obliquely downward and medially across the back of the tibia from the fibular articular facet; it gives origin to the soleus muscle.

l. mylohyoi'dea [NA], mylohyoid line or ridge; internal oblique line; a ridge on the inner surface of the mandible running from a point inferior to the mental spine upward and backward to the ramus behind the last molar tooth; it gives attachment to the mylohyoid muscle and superior constrictor of the pharynx.

l. ni'gra, black line; the l. alba in pregnancy, which then becomes pigmented.

l. nu'chae infe'rior [NA], inferior nuchal line; a ridge that extends laterally from the external occipital crest toward the jugular process of the occipital bone.

l. nu'chae media'na, *crista* occipitalis externa.

l. nu'chae supe'rior [NA], superior nuchal line; the ridge that extends laterally from the external occipital protuberance toward the lateral angle of the occipital bone; it gives attachment to the trapezius, sternocleidomastoid, and splenius capitis muscles.

l. nu'chae supre'ma [NA], highest nuchal line; a line above and parallel to the superior nuchal line on the external surface of the occipital bone; it gives attachment to the epicranial aponeurosis and occipitalis muscle.

l. obli'qua [NA], oblique line; **l. o. cartilag'inis thyroi'dea,** a ridge on the outer surface of the thyroid cartilage that gives attachment to the sternothyroid and thyrohyoid muscles; **l. o. mandib'ulae,** the line on the external surface of the mandible that extends from the mental tubercle to the ramus and separates the alveolar and basilar parts of the bone.

l. parasterna'lis [NA], parasternal line; costoclavicular line; a vertical line equidistant from the sternal and midclavicular lines.

l. paravertebra'lis [NA], paravertebral line; a vertical line corresponding to the tips of the transverse processes of the vertebrae.

l. pectine'a [NA], pectineal line; a ridge running down the posterior surface of the shaft of the femur from the lesser trochanter to which the pectineus muscle attaches.

l. poplite'a, l. musculi solei.

l. postaxilla'ris [NA], an alternate term for l. axillaris posterior.

l. preaxilla'ris [NA], an alternate term for l. axillaris anterior.

l. scapula'ris [NA], scapular line; a vertical line passing through the inferior angle of the scapula.

l. semicircula'ris, l. arcuata vaginae musculi recti abdominis.

l. semiluna'ris [NA], semilunar line; Spigelius' line; the slight groove in the external abdominal wall parallel to the lateral edge of the rectus sheath.

l. spira'lis, l. intertrochanterica.

l. splen'dens, Haller's line; a thickened band of pia mater along the midline of the anterior surface of the spinal cord.

l. sterna'lis [NA], sternal line; a vertical line corresponding to the lateral margin of the sternum.

l. subcosta'lis [NA], an alternate term for *planum* subcostalis.

l. supracrista'lis [NA], alternate term for *planum* supracristalis.

l. tempora'lis infe'rior [NA], inferior temporal line; the lower of two curved lines on the parietal bone; it marks the limit of attachment of the temporal muscle.

l. tempora'lis supe'rior [NA], superior temporal line; the upper of two curved lines on the parietal bone; the temporal fascia is attached to it.

l. termina'lis [NA], terminal line; iliopectineal line; an oblique ridge on the inner surface of the ilium and continued on the pubis, which forms the lower boundary of the iliac fossa; it separates the true from the false pelvis.

l. transver'sa [NA], transverse line; one of four ridges that cross the pelvic surface of the sacrum; these mark the positions of the intervertebral disks between the bodies of the five sacral vertebrae in the immature bone.

l. trapezoi'dea [NA], trapezoid line or ridge; the area on the inferior surface of the clavicle near its lateral extremity on which the trapezoid ligament attaches.

---

linear (lin'ē-ăr). Pertaining to or resembling a line.

line'breeding. A practice of successive inbreeding of closely related individuals with the object of concentrating the genetic characteristics of some individual, or group.

liner (lī'ner). A layer of protective material.

asbestos l., a layer of asbestos used to line a dental casting ring so that during the heating and expansion of the investment the compression of the l. will free the investment from the restraint of the ring.

cavity l., varnish.

Lineweaver, Hans, U.S. physical chemist, *1907. See L.-Burk *equation.*

Ling, Per Henrik, Swedish hygienist, 1776–1839. See L.'s *method.*

Lingelsheimia (ling'el-shī'mē-ă) [W. von *Lingelsheim*]. *Acinetobacter.*

L. anitra'ta, *Acinetobacter calcoaceticus.*

lingism (ling'izm). Ling's *method.*

lingua, gen. and pl. linguae (ling'gwă, ling'gwē) [L. tongue] [NA]. **1.** Glossa; tongue; a mobile mass of muscular tissue covered with mucous membrane, occupying the cavity of the mouth and forming part of its floor, constituting also by its posterior portion the anterior wall of the pharnyx. It bears the organ of taste and assists in mastication, deglutition, and articulation. **2.** One of a number of tongue-like anatomical structures.

l. cerebel'li, *lingula* cerebelli.

l. dissec'ta, geographic *tongue.*

l. fissura'ta, fissured *tongue.*

l. frena'ta, a tongue with a very short frenum constituting tongue-tie.

l. geograph'ica, geographic *tongue.*

l. ni'gra, black *tongue.*

l. plica'ta, fissured *tongue.*

lingual (ling'gwăl). **1.** Glossal; relating to the tongue or any tongue-like part. **2.** Next to or toward the tongue.

Linguatula (ling-gwat'yū-lă) [L. *linguatulus,* tongued]. A genus of endoparasitic bloodsucking arthropods (family Linguatulidae, class Pentastomida), commonly known as tongue worms; once thought to be degenerate Acarina, but now generally considered to be a small but distinctive early offshoot of the Arthropoda. Adult worms are found in lungs or air passages of various hosts (*e.g.,* reptiles, birds, carnivores); young worms are found in a great variety of hosts, including man, but chiefly in animals that serve as prey.

L. rhina'ria, *L. serrata.*

L. serra'ta, *L. rhinaria;* a species most common in Europe, but also found in the United States, South America, and probably elsewhere; the adult is a whitish, soft, flattened, annulated worm equipped with hooks by which it attaches itself to the nasal mucosa of dogs and other canids; the larvae develop in the liver and lymph nodes of rodents, swine, cattle, and sometimes man and other primates.

linguatuliasis (ling-gwat-yū-lī'ă-sis). Infection with *Linguatula.* See also halzoun.

Linguatulidae (ling-gwat'yū-li-dē). One of the families of Pentastomida of medical interest, the other being the Porocephalidae. L. have flattened bodies; adults inhabit the nasal cavities of various carnivores, such as the dog and cat, and larval forms are found in tissues of rodents, herbivores, and other animals; both larvae and adults have been reported from man.

linguiform (ling'gwi-fōrm). Tongue-shaped.

lingula, pl. lingulae (ling'gyū-lă, -lē) [L. dim. of *lingua,* tongue] [NA]. **1.** A term applied to several tongue-shaped processes. **2.** When not qualified, the l. cerebelli.

l. cerebel'li [NA], lingula (2); lingua cerebelli; tongue of the cerebellum; a tongue-shaped sequence of flattened cerebellar folia forming the anterior (or superior) extreme of the cerebellar vermis, extending forward on the surface of the velum medullare superius between the two emerging superior cerebellar peduncles.

l. of left lung, l. pulmonis sinistri.

l. mandib'ulae [NA], l. of mandible; mandibular tongue; Spix's spine; a pointed tongue of bone overlapping the mandibular foramen, giving attachment to the sphenomandibular ligament.

l. of mandible, l. mandibulae.

l. pulmo'nis sinis'tri [NA], lingula of left lung; a projection from the upper lobe of the left lung which bounds the cardiac notch inferiorly.

l. sphenoida'lis [NA], l. of sphenoid; a slender process projecting posteriorly between the body and greater wing of the sphenoid bone, on either side, forming the lateral margin of the carotid groove.

lingular (ling'gyū-lăr). Pertaining to any lingula.

lingulectomy (ling'gyū-lek'tō-mē). **1.** Glossectomy. **2.** Excision of the lingular portion of the left upper lobe of the lung.

linguo- [L. *lingua,* tongue]. Combining form relating to the tongue.

linguoclination (ling'gwō-kli-nā'shŭn). Axial inclination of a tooth when the crown is inclined toward the tongue more than is normal.

linguoclusion (ling-gwō-klū'zhŭn). Lingual occlusion (1); displacement of a tooth toward the interior of the dental arch, or toward the tongue. See also lingual *occlusion* (2).

linguodistal (ling-gwō-dis'tăl). Relating to the lingual and distal part of the tooth, *e.g.,* the l. cusp. See also distolingual.

linguogingival (ling-gwō-jin'ji-văl). **1.** Relating to the gingival third of the lingual surface of a tooth. **2.** Relating to the angle or point of junction of the lingual border and gingival line on the distal or mesial surface of an incisor tooth.

linguo-occlusal (ling'gwō-ŏ-klū'săl). Relating to the line of junction of the lingual and occlusal surfaces of a tooth.

linguopapillitis (ling'gwō-pap'i-lī'tis). Small painful ulcers involving the papillae on the tongue margins.

linguoplate (ling'gwō-plāt). Lingual plate; a partial denture major connector formed as a lingual bar extended to cover the cingula of the lower anterior teeth.

linguoversion (ling'gwō-ver-zhŭn). Malposition of a tooth lingual to the normal position.

liniment (lin'i-ment) [L., fr. *lino,* to smear]. A liquid preparation for external application or application to the gums; they may be clear dispersions, suspensions, or emulsions, and are frequently applied by friction to the skin; used as counterirritants, rubefacients, anodynes, or cleansing agents.

linin (lī'nin) [L. *linum,* fr. G. *linon,* flax]. **1.** A bitter glycoside obtained from *Linum catharticum* (family Linaceae). **2.** A protein in linseed. **3.** Obsolete term for the threadlike, nonstaining (achromatic) substance of the cell nucleus, on which chromatin granules were thought to be suspended.

lining (līn'ing). A coating applied to the pulpal wall(s) of a restorative dental preparation to protect the pulp from thermal or chemical irritation; usually a vehicle containing a varnish, resin, and/or calcium hydroxide.

linitis (li-nī'tis, lī-nī'tis) [G. *linon,* flax, linen cloth, + *-itis,* inflammation]. Inflammation of cellular tissue, specifically of the perivascular tissue of the stomach.

l. plas'tica, originally believed to be an inflammatory condition, but now recognized to be due to infiltrating scirrhous carcinoma causing extensive thickening of the wall of the stomach; often called leather-bottle stomach.

linkage (lingk'ij). **1.** A chemical covalent bond. **2.** The relationship between syntenic loci sufficiently close so that the respective alleles are not inherited independently by the offspring; a characteristic of loci, not genes.

genetic l., see l. (2).

medical record l., the assemblage of lifetime or long term individual medical histories from vital and medical data derived from multiple sources.

sex l., a form of inheritance related to sex as a result of the gene concerned being carried on the X chromosome. A man receives all his sex-linked genes from his mother and transmits them to his daughters but not to his sons; a recessive sex-linked character is much more likely to be expressed in the male. See also sex *chromosome;* sex-linked *gene.*

linkage map. An abstract mathematical representation of genetic loci that conserves order of loci which are spaced in such a way that the distances are algebraically additive; conventionally, a map is scaled so that as distances between loci become smaller the ratio of the map distance to the value of the recombination fraction approaches 1.

linked. Said of two genetic loci that exhibit linkage.

link'er. A fragment of synthetic DNA containing a restriction site that may be used for splicing of genes.

Linognathus (li-nog'nă-thŭs) [G. *linon,* flax, thread, + *gnathos,* jaw]. A genus of sucking lice (order Anoplura, family Linognathidae) that includes the species *L. africanus,* the African blue louse of sheep and goats; *L. ovillus,* the sheep body louse; *L. pedalis,* the foot louse of sheep; *L. setosus,* the sucking louse of the dog and other canids; *L. stenopsis,* the sucking louse of goats; and *L. vituli,* the "long-nosed" sucking louse, ox louse, or blue louse of cattle.

linoleate (li-nō'lē-āt). Salt of linoleic acid.

linoleic acid (lin-ō-lē'ik) [L. *linum,* flax, + *oleum,* oil]. Linolic acid; 9,12-octadecadienoic acid; $CH_3(CH_2)_3(CH_2CH{=}CH)_2(CH_2)_7COOH$; a doubly unsaturated fatty acid, occurring widely in plant glycerides, that is essential in nutrition.

linolenic acid (lin-ō-len'ik). 9,12,15-Octadecatrienoic acid; $CH_3(CH_2CH{=}CH)_3(CH_2)_7COOH$; an unsaturated fatty acid that is essential in nutrition.

linolic acid (lin-ōl'ik). Linoleic acid.

linseed (lin'sēd) [G. *linon,* flax]. Flaxseed; the dried ripe seed of *Linum usitatissimum* (family Linaceae), flax, the fiber of which is used in the manufacture of linen; an infusion is used as a demulcent in catarrhal affections of the respiratory and urogenital tracts, and the ground seeds are used in making poultices.

l. oil, flaxseed oil; a fatty oil expressed from the ripe seeds of *Linum usitatissimum;* used in the preparation of lime liniment.

lint [O.E. *lin,* flax]. A soft, absorbent material used in surgical dressings, usually in the form of a thick, loosely woven material (sheet or patent l.).

lio-. See leio.

liothyronine (lī-ō-thī'rō-nēn). 3,5,3'-Triiodothyronine.

l. sodium, see under sodium.

liotrix (lī'ō-triks). A mixture of liothyronine sodium and levothyroxine sodium; used as a thyroid hormone.

lip-. See lipo-.

lip [A.S. *lippa*]. **1.** Labium oris; one of the two muscular folds with an outer mucosa having a stratified squamous epithelial surface layer which bound the mouth anteriorly. **2.** Any liplike structure bounding a cavity or groove. See also entries under labium; labrum.

acetabular l., *labrum* acetabulare.

anterior l., *labium* anterius.

articular l., *labrum* articulare.

cleft l., harelip; cheiloschisis; chiloschisis; a congenital facial deformity of the l. (usually the upper l.) due to failure of mesodermal penetration of the ectodermal grooves at the line of fusion of the medial and lateral nasal processes and the maxillary process; frequently but not necessarily associated with cleft alveolus and cleft palate.

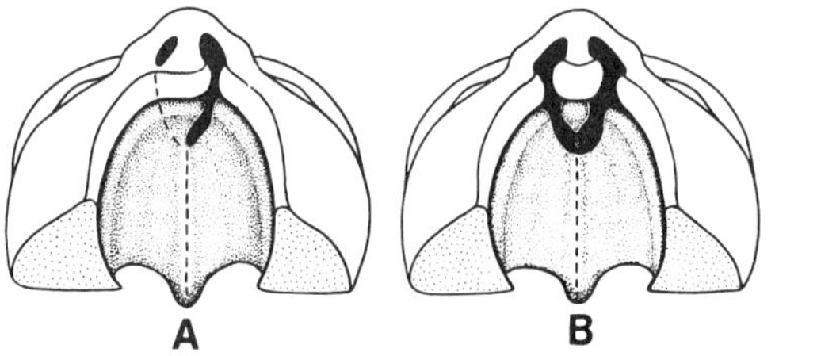

Cleft Lip
A, unilateral; *B,* bilateral.

external l. of iliac crest, *labium* externum cristae iliacae.

glenoidal l., *labrum* glenoidale.

Hapsburg l., see Hapsburg *jaw.*

internal l. of iliac crest, *labium* internum cristae iliacae.

large pudendal l., *labium* majus pudendi.

lateral l. of linea aspera, *labium* laterale lineae asperae.
lower l., *labium* inferius oris.
medial l. of linea aspera, *labium* mediale lineae asperae.
lips of mouth, *labia* oris.
posterior l., *labium* posterius.
rhombic l., the thickened alar plate of the embryonic rhombencephalon.
small pudendal l., *labium* minus pudendi.
tympanic l., *labium* limbi tympanicum.
upper l., *labium* superius oris.
vestibular l., *labium* limbi vestibulare.

lipancreatin (li-pan'krē-ă-tin, -krē'ă-tin). Pancrelipase.

liparocele (lip'ă-rō-sēl) [G. *liparos,* fatty, + *kēlē,* tumor, hernia]. An omental hernia.

lipase (lip'ās). In general, any fat-splitting or lipolytic enzyme; *e.g.,* triacylglycerol lipase, phospholipase A_2, lipoprotein lipase.

lipectomy (lip-ek'tō-mē) [lipo- + G. *ektomē,* excision]. Surgical removal of fatty tissue, as in cases of adiposity.

lipedema (lip'e-dē'mă) [lipo- + G. *oidēma,* swelling]. Chronic swelling, usually of the lower extremities, particularly in middle-aged women, caused by the widespread even distribution of subcutaneous fat and fluid.

lipemia (lip-ē'mē-ă) [lipid + G. *haima,* blood]. The presence of an abnormally large amount of lipids in the circulating blood. Also called hyperlipemia; hyperlipidemia; hyperlipoidemia; lipidemia; lipoidemia.
alimentary l., postprandial l.; relatively transient l. occurring after the ingestion of foods with a large content of fat.
diabetic l., development of lactescent plasma upon ingestion of dietary lipids; a rare manifestation of uncontrolled diabetes mellitus caused by defective metabolism of dietary lipids and abolished by the administration of insulin.
postprandial l., alimentary l.
l. retina'lis, a creamy appearance of the retinal blood vessels that occurs when the lipids of the blood exceed 5%.

lipemic (li-pē'mik). Relating to lipemia.

lip'id [G. *lipos,* fat]. "Fat-soluble," an operational term describing a solubility characteristic, not a chemical substance, *i.e.,* denoting substances extracted from animal or vegetable cells by nonpolar or "fat" solvents; included in the heterogeneous collection of materials thus extractable are fatty acids, glycerides and glyceryl ethers, phospholipids, sphingolipids, alcohols and waxes, terpenes, steroids, and "fat-soluble" vitamins A, D, and E.
anisotropic l., a l. in the form of doubly refractive droplets.
brain l., impure cephalin possessing marked hemostatic action when locally applied.
compound l.'s, heterolipids.
isotropic l., a l. occurring in the form of singly refractive droplets.
simple l.'s, homolipids.

lipidemia (lip'i-dē'mē-ă). Lipemia.

lipidosis, pl. **lipidoses** (lip-i-dō'sis, -sēz) [lipid + G. *-ōsis,* condition]. Inborn or acquired disorder of lipid metabolism.
cerebral l., cerebral *sphingolipidosis.*
cerebroside l., Gaucher's *disease.*
ganglioside l., gangliosidosis.
glycolipid l., Fabry's *disease.*
sphingomyelin l., Niemann-Pick *disease.*
sulfatide l., metachromatic *leukodystrophy.*

lip'in. Former term for lipid.

Lipmann, Fritz A., German biochemist in the U.S. and Nobel laureate, *1899. See Warburg-L.-Dickens *shunt.*

lipo-, lip- [G. *lipos,* fat]. Combining forms relating to fat or lipid.

lipoamide (lip-ō-am'īd, -am'id). See lipoic acid.

lipoamide dehydrogenase. Dihydrolipoamide dehydrogenase.

lipoamide disulfide. Oxidized lipoic acid in amide combination with the ϵ-amino group of a lysine of pyruvic acid dehydrogenase.

lipoamide reductase (NADH). Dihydrolipoamide dehydrogenase.

lipoarthritis (lip'ō-ar-thrī'tis) [lipo- + arthritis]. Inflammation of the periarticular fatty tissues of the knee.

lipoate (lip'ō-āt). A salt or ester of lipoic acid.

lipoate acetyltransferase. Dihydrolipoamide acetyltransferase.

lipoatrophia (lip'ō-ă-trō'fē-ă). Lipoatrophy.
l. annula'ris, a rare condition of unknown cause characterized by localized panatrophy, a depressed area encircling the arm with sclerosis and atrophy of fat.
l. circumscrip'ta, localized fat atrophy.

lipoatrophy (lip-ō-at'rō-fē) [G. *lipos,* fat, + *a-,* priv. + *trophē,* nourishment]. Lipoatrophia; lipoatrophic diabetes; Lawrence-Seip syndrome; loss of subcutaneous fat which may be total, congenital, and associated with hepatomegaly, excessive bone growth, and insulin-resistant diabetes.
insulin l., insulin *lipodystrophy.*
partial l., progressive *lipodystrophy.*

lipoblast lip'ō-blast) [lipo- + G. *blastos,* germ]. An embryonic fat cell.

lipoblastoma (lip'ō-blas-tō'mă). **1.** Liposarcoma. **2.** A benign subcutaneous tumor composed of embryonal fat cells separated into distinct lobules, occurring usually in infants.

lipoblastomatosis (lip'ō-blas-tō-mă-tō'sis). A diffuse form of lipoblastoma that infiltrates locally but does not metastasize.

lipocardiac (lip'ō-kar'dē-ak) [lipo- + G. *kardia,* heart]. **1.** Relating to fatty heart. **2.** Denoting a person suffering from fatty degeneration of the heart.

lipocatabolic (lip'ō-kat-ă-bol'ik). Relating to the breakdown (catabolism) of fat.

lipocele (lip'ō-sēl) [lipo- + G. *kēlē,* tumor]. Adipocele; presence of fatty tissue, without intestine, in a hernia sac.

lipoceratous (lip-ō-ser'ă-tŭs). Adipoceratous.

lipocere (lip'ō-sēr) [lipo- + L. *cera,* wax]. Adipocere.

lipochondrodystrophy (lip'ō-kon-drō-dis'trō-fē). Hurler's *syndrome.*

lipochrome (lip'ō-krōm) [lipo- + G. *chroma,* color]. **1.** Chromolipid; a pigmented lipid, *e.g.,* lutein, carotene. **2.** A term sometimes used to designate the wear-and-tear pigments, *e.g.,* lipofuscin, hemofuscin, ceroid. More precisely, l.'s are yellow pigments that seem to be identical to carotene and xanthophyll and are frequently found in the serum, skin, adrenal cortex, corpus luteum, and arteriosclerotic plaques, as well as in the liver, spleen, and adipose tissue; l.'s do not stain with the ordinary dyes for fat. **3.** The pigment produced by certain bacteria.

lipoclasis (li-pok'lă-sis) [lipo- + G. *klasis,* a breaking]. Lipolysis.

lipoclastic (lip-ō-klas'tik). Lipolytic.

lipocrit (lip'ō-krit) [lipo- + G. *krinō,* to separate]. An apparatus and procedure for separating and volumetrically analyzing the amount of lipid in blood or other body fluid.

lipocyte (lip'ō-sīt) [lipo- + G. *kytos,* cell]. Fat-storing *cell.*

lipodermoid (lip-ō-der'moyd) [lipo- + dermoid]. Congenital, yellowish-white, fatty, benign tumor located subconjunctivally.

lipodieresis (lip'ō-dī-er'ĕ-sis) [lipo- + G. *dieresis,* division]. Lipolysis.

lipodystrophia (lip'ō-dis-trō'fē-ă). Lipodystrophy.
l. intestina'lis, Whipple's *disease.*
l. progessi'va supe'rior, progressive *lipodystrophy.*

lipodystrophy (lip-ō-dis'trō-fē) [lipo- + G. *dys-,* bad, difficult, + *trophē,* nourishment]. Lipodystrophia; defective metabolism of fat.
congenital total l., l. characterized by almost complete lack of subcutaneous fat, accelerated rate of growth and skeletal development during the first 3 to 4 years of life, muscular hypertrophy, cardiac enlargement, hepatosplenomegaly, hypertrichosis, renal enlargement, hyperlipemia, and hypermetabolism; probably autosomal recessive inheritance.
insulin l., insulin lipoatrophy; dystrophic atrophy of subcutaneous tissues in diabetics at the site of frequent injections of insulin.
intestinal l., Whipple's *disease.*
membranous l., a rare metabolic disease in which bone marrow fat cells are transformed into thick convoluted PAS-staining membranes enclosing weakly osmophilic material; leads to progressive cystic resorption of limb bones, and dementia with sudanophilic leukodystrophy.
progressive l., lipodystrophia progressiva superior; partial lipoatrophy; Barraquer's or Simons' disease; a condition characterized by a complete loss of the subcutaneous fat of the upper part of the torso, the arms, neck, and face, sometimes with an increase of fat in the tissues about and below the pelvis.

lipoedema (lip'ō-e-dē'mă). Cellulite (2); edema of subcutaneous fat, causing painful swellings, especially of the legs in women.

lipoferous (lip-of'er-ŭs) [lipo- + L. *fero,* to carry]. Transporting fat.

lipofibroma (lip'ō-fī-brō'mă). A benign neoplasm of fibrous connective tissue, with conspicuous numbers of adipose cells.

lipofuscin (lip-ō-fyūs'in). Brown pigment granules representing lipid-containing residues of lysosomal digestion and considered one of the aging or "wear and tear" pigments; found in liver, kidney, heart muscle, adrenal, and ganglion cells.

lipofuscinosis (lip'ō-fyūs-i-nō'sis). Abnormal storage of any one of a group of fatty pigments.
ceroid l., cerebral *sphingolipidosis,* late juvenile type.

lipogenesis (lip-ō-jen'ĕ-sis) [lipo- + G. *genesis,* production]. Adipogenesis; the production of fat, either fatty degeneration or fatty infiltration; also applied to the normal deposition of fat or to the conversion of carbohydrate or protein to fat.

lipogenic (lip-ō-jen'ik). Adipogenic; adipogenous; lipogenous; relating to lipogenesis.

lipogenous (li-poj'ĕ-nŭs). Lipogenic.

lipogranuloma (lip'ō-gran-yū-lō'mă). Oleoma; oleogranuloma; eleoma; oil tumor; a nodule or focus of granulomatous inflammation (usually of the foreign-body type) in association with lipid material deposited in tissues, *e.g.,* after the injection of certain oils. See also paraffinoma.

lipogranulomatosis (lip'ō-gran'yū-lō-mă-tō'sis). **1.** Presence of lipogranulomas. **2.** Local inflammatory reaction to necrosis of adipose tissue.
disseminated l., Farber's disease or syndrome; a form of mucolipodosis, developing soon after birth and due to deficiency of ceramidase; characterized by swollen joints, subcutaneous nodules, lymphadenopathy, and accumulation in lysosomes of affected cells of PAS-positive lipid consisting of ceramide.

lipohemia (lip-ō-hē'mē-ă). Obsolete term for lipemia.

lipoic acid (li-pō'ik). Thioctic acid; ovoprotogen; protogen; protogen A; acetate-replacement or pyruvate oxidation factor; factor II (2); 6,8-dimercapto-octanoic acid; functions as the amide (lipoamide) in the oxidized (–S–S–) form in the transfer of "active aldehyde" (acetyl), the two-carbon fragment resulting from decarboxylation of pyruvate, from α-hydroxyethylthiamin pyrophosphate to acetyl-CoA, itself being reduced (to the –SH HS– form) in the process; present in yeast and liver extracts, and may be useful in the treatment of mushroom poisoning.

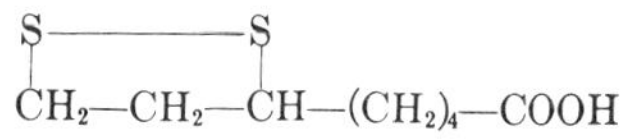

Lipoic acid (oxidized form)

lipoid (lip'oyd) [lipo- + G. *eidos,* appearance]. Adipoid. **1.** Resembling fat. **2.** Former term for lipid.

lipoidemia (lip-oy-dē'mē-ă). Lipemia.

lipoidosis (lip-oy-do'sis). Presence of anisotropic lipoids in the cells.
l. cor'neae, *arcus* cornealis.
l. cu'tis et muco'sae, lipid *proteinosis.*

lipolipoidosis (lip'ō-lip-oy-dō'sis). Fatty infiltration, both neutral fats and anisotropic lipoids being present in the cells. See also liposis (2).

lipolysis (li-pol'i-sis) [lipo- + G. *lysis,* dissolution]. Lipoclasis; lipodieresis; the splitting up (hydrolysis), or chemical decomposition, of fat.

lipolytic (lip-ō-lit'ik). Lipoclastic; relating to or causing lipolysis.

lipoma (li-pō'mă) [lipo- + G. *-oma,* tumor]. Adipose tumor; pimeloma; a benign neoplasm of adipose tissue, comprised of mature fat cells.
l. annula're col'li, an encircling growth of l. (or coalescent l.'s) in the neck, resulting in a collar-like enlargement. See also Madelung's neck.
l. arbores'cens, an irregularly shaped l. involving the synovial membrane of a joint, resulting in fingerlike or treelike hyperplastic folds in the villi.
atypical l., pleomorphic l.; subcutaneous l., occurring primarily in older men on the posterior neck, shoulders, and back, which is benign but microscopically atypical, containing multinucleated giant cells.
l. capsula're, a well circumscribed mass resulting from a greatly increased amount of adipose tissue adjacent to the breast.
l. caverno'sum, angiolipoma.
l. fibro'sum, fibrolipoma.
infiltrating l., liposarcoma.
lipoblastic l., liposarcoma.
l. myxomato' des, myxolipoma.
l. ossif'icans, a l. in which metaplasia occurs and small foci of bone are formed.
l. petrif'icans, a l. in which degeneration and necrosis results in a considerable amount of dystrophic calcification.
pleomorphic l., atypical l.
l. sarcomato'des, l. sarcomato'sum, liposarcoma.
spindle cell l., a microscopically distinctive form of l. in which adipose tissue is infiltrated by fibroblasts and collagen.
telangiectatic l., angiolipoma.

lipomatoid (li-pō'mă-toyd). Resembling a lipoma, frequently said of accumulations of adipose tissue that is not thought to be neoplastic.

lipomatosis (lip'ō-mă-tō'sis). Adiposis.
encephalocraniocutaneous l., a rare syndrome of multiple fibrolipomas or angiofibroma of the face, scalp, and neck present at birth, sometimes with symptomatic intracranial lipomas.
multiple symmetric l., symmetric adenolipomatosis; Launois-Bensaude syndrome; Madelung's disease; accumulation and progressive enlargement of collections of adipose tissue in the subcutaneous tissue of the head, neck, upper trunk, and upper portions of the upper extremities; seen primarily in adult males and of unknown cause.
l. neurot'ica, *adiposis* dolorosa.

lipomatous (li-pō'mă-tŭs). Pertaining to or manifesting the features of lipoma, or characterized by the presence of a lipoma (or lipomas).

lipomeningocele (lip'ō-mē-ning'gō-sēl) [lipo- + G. *mēninx,* membrane, + *kēlē,* tumor]. An intraspinal cauda equinal lipoma associated with a spina bifida.

lipomucopolysaccharidosis (lip'ō-myū'ko-pol-ē-sak'ă-ri-dō'sis). *Mucolipidosis* I.

liponucleoproteins (lip'ō-nū'klē-ō-prō'tēnz). Associations or complexes containing lipids, nucleic acids, and proteins.

Liponyssus (lip-ō-nis'ŭs) [lipo- + G. *nyssō,* to prick]. Former name for *Ornithonyssus.*

lipopenia (lip-ō-pē'nē-ă) [lipo- + G. *penia,* poverty]. An abnormally small amount, or a deficiency, of lipids in the body.

lipopenic (lip-ō-pē'nik). **1.** Relating to or characterized by lipopenia. **2.** An agent or drug that produces a reduction in the concentration of lipids in the blood.

lipopeptid (lip-ō-pep'tid). A compound or complex of lipid and amino acids.

lipophage (lip'ō-fāj) [G. *lipos,* fat, + *phagein,* to eat]. A cell that ingests fat.

lipophagia (lip-ō-fā'jē-ă). Lipophagy.
l. granulomato'sis, Whipple's *disease.*

lipophagic (lip-ō-fā'jik). Relating to lipophagy.

lipophagy (lip-of'ă-jē) [lipo- + G. *phagein,* to eat]. Lipophagia; ingestion of fat by a lipophage.

lipophanerosis (lip'ō-fan-er-ō'sis) [lipo- + G. *phaneros,* visible, + *-osis,* condition]. A change in certain cells whereby previously invisible fat becomes demonstrable as small sudanophilic droplets. See fatty *degeneration.*

lipophil (lip'ō-fil) [lipo- + G. *philos,* fond of]. A substance with lipophilic (hydrophobic) properties.

lipophilic (lip-ō-fil'ik). Capable of dissolving, of being dissolved in, or of absorbing lipids.

lipophosphodiesterase I (lip'ō-fos'-fō-dī-es'ter-ās). *Phospholipase* C.

lipophosphodiesterase II. *Phospholipase* D.

lipopolysaccharide (lip'ō-pol'ē-sak'ă-rīd). A compound or complex of lipid and carbohydrate.

lipoprotein (lip-ō-prō'tēn). Complexes or compounds containing lipid and protein. Almost all the lipids in plasma are present as l.'s and are therefore transported as such. Plasma l.'s migrate electrophoretically with the α- and β-globulins, but are presently characterized by their flotation constants (densities) as follows: chylomicra, $< 1{,}006$; very low density (VLDL), 1.006-1.019; low density (LDL), 1.019-1.063; high density (HDL), 1.063-1.21; very high density (VHDL), > 1.21. They range in molecular weight from 200,000 to 10,000,000 and from 4 to 95% lipid (the higher the density, the lower the lipid content). The very low- and low-density fractions appear in the β_1-globulin fraction and are particularly rich in triacylglycerols and cholesterol esters, respectively; the high-density and very high-density fractions appear in the α_1-globulin fraction.

α_1-lipoprotein. A lipoprotein fraction of relatively low molecular weight, high density, rich in phospholipids, and found in the α_1-globulin fraction of human plasma.

β_1-lipoprotein. A lipoprotein fraction of relatively high molecular weight, low density, rich in cholesterol, and found in the β-globulin fraction of human plasma.

lipoprotein lipase [EC 3.1.1.34]. Diacylglycerol or diglyceride lipase; an enzyme that cleaves one fatty acid from a triacylglycerol; its activity is enhanced by heparin and inactivated by heparinase. See also clearing *factors.*

lipoprotein-X. An abnormal lipoprotein found in patients with obstructive jaundice.

liposarcoma (lip'ō-sar-kō'mă) [lipo- + *sarx,* flesh, + *-oma,* tumor]. A malignant neoplasm of adults that occurs especially in the retroperitoneal tissues and the thigh, usually deep in the intermuscular or periarticular planes; histologically, l.'s are large tumors that may be composed of well differentiated fat cells or may be dedifferentiated, either myxoid, round celled, or pleomorphic, usually in association with a rich network of capillaries; recurrences are common, and dedifferentiated l.'s metastasize to the lungs or serosal surfaces. Also called lipoblastoma (1); infiltrating or lipoblastic lipoma; lipoma sarcomatodes or sarcomatosum.

liposis (li-pō'sis) [lipo- + G. *-osis,* condition]. **1.** Adiposis. **2.** Fatty infiltration, neutral fats being present in the cells. See also lipolipoidosis.

lipositol (lip-os'i-tol). Inositol.

liposoluble (lip-ō-sol'yū-bl). Fat-soluble.

liposome (lip'ō-sōm) [lipo- + G. *sōma,* body]. A spherical particle of lipid substance suspended in an aqueous medium within a tissue.

liposuctioning (lip'ō-sŭk'shŭn-ing). Removal of fat by high vacuum pressure; used in body contouring.

lipothiamide pyrophosphate (lip-ō-thī'am-īd). Name once given to the coenzymes of the multi-enzyme complex catalyzing the formation of acetyl-CoA from pyruvate and involving lipoamide and diphosphothiamin, on the assumption that the lipoamide and thiamin pyrophosphate are a single compound. See lipoic acid.

lipotrophic (lip-ō-trof'ik). Relating to lipotrophy.

lipotrophy (li-pot'rō-fē) [lipo- + G. *trophē,* nourishment]. An increase of fat in the body.

lipotropic (lip-ō-trop'ik). **1.** Pertaining to substances preventing or correcting the fatty liver of choline deficiency. **2.** Relating to lipotropy.

lipotropin (li-pō-trō'pin). Lipotropic or pituitary lipotropic hormone; lipid-mobilizing hormone; a pituitary hormone mobilizing fat from adipose tissue. β-Lipotropin is a single-chain peptide of about 90 residues that contains the sequences of endorphins and metenkephalin, and may be a precursor of β-melanotropin and β-endorphin; γ-lipotropin is shorter and is identical in sequence to the first 58 residues of β-lipotropin; both contain sequences common to ACTH and β-melanotropin.

lipotropy (li-pot'rō-pē) [lipo- + G. *tropē,* turning]. **1.** Affinity of basic dyes for fatty tissue. **2.** Prevention of accumulation of fat in the liver. **3.** Affinity of nonpolar substances for each other.

lipovaccine (lip'ō-vak-sēn). A vaccine having a vegetable oil as a menstruum. See adjuvant *vaccine.*

lipovitellin (lip'ō-vi-tel'in). Vitellin.

lipoxenous (li-pok'sĕ-nŭs). Pertaining to lipoxeny.

lipoxeny (li-pok'sĕ-nē, lī-) [G. *leipō,* to leave, + *xenos,* host]. Desertion of the host by a parasite when the development of the latter is complete.

lipoxidase (li-poks'i-dās). Lipoxygenase.

lipoxygenase (li-poks'ē-jĕ-nās) [EC 1.13.11.12]. Lipoxidase; carotene oxidase; an enzyme that catalyzes the oxidation of unsaturated fatty acids with O_2 to yield peroxides of the fatty acids.

lipoyl (lip'ō-il). The acyl radical of lipoic acid.

lipoyl dehydrogenase. Dihydrolipoamide dehydrogenase.

lipping (lip'ing). The formation of a liplike structure, as at the articular end of a bone in osteoarthritis.

lippitude, lippitudo (lip'i-tūd, lip-i-tū'dō) [L., fr. *lippus,* blear-eyed]. Blear *eye.*

Lipschütz, Benjamin, Austrian physician, 1878–1931. See L. *cell;* L.'s *ulcer.*

lipuria (li-pū'rē-ă) [lipo- + G. *ouron,* urine]. Adiposuria; presence of lipids in the urine.

lipuric (li-pū'rik). Pertaining to lipuria.

liquefacient (lik'we-fā'shent) [L. *lique-facio*, pres. p. *-faciens*, to make fluid, fr. ligueo, to be liquid]. **1.** Making liquid; causing a solid to become liquid. **2.** Denoting a resolvant supposed to cause the resolution of a solid tumor by liquefying its contents.

liquefaction (lik-wĕ-fak'shŭn) [see liquefacient]. The act of becoming liquid; change from a solid to a liquid form.

liquefactive (lik-wĕ-fak'tiv). Relating to liquefaction.

liquescent (li-kwes'ent) [L. *liquesco*, to become liquid]. Becoming or tending to become liquid.

liqueur (li-ker') [Fr.]. A cordial; a spirit containing sugar and aromatics.

liquid (lik'wid) [L. *liquidus*]. **1.** An inelastic substance, like water, that is neither solid nor gaseous. **2.** Flowing like water.

Cotunnius' l., perilympha.

liquor, gen. **liquoris,** pl. **liquores** (lik'er, lik'wōr; -wōr-is, -wō'rēs) [L.]. **1.** Any liquid or fluid. **2.** A term used for certain body fluids. **3.** The pharmacopeial term for any aqueous solution (not a decoction or infusion) of a nonvolatile substance and for aqueous solutions of gases. See also solution.

l. am'nii, amniotic *fluid.*

l. cerebrospina'lis [NA], cerebrospinal fluid (CSF); neurolymph; a fluid largely secreted by the choroid plexuses of the ventricles of the brain, filling the ventricles and the subarachnoid cavities of the brain and spinal cord.

l. cotun'nii, perilympha.

l. enter'icus, intestinal secretions.

l. follic'uli, the fluid within the antrum of the ovarian follicle.

malt l., a beverage brewed from malt, such as beer or ale.

Morgagni's l., Morgagni's humor; a fluid found postmortem between the epithelium and the fibers of the lens, resulting from the liquefaction of a semifluid material existing there during life.

mother l., the saturated solution remaining after a crystallization or precipitation.

Scarpa's l., endolympha.

spirituous l., a strong alcoholic l. obtained by distillation, such as whiskey.

vinous l., wine (1).

liquorice (lik'ŏ-ris). Glycyrrhiza.

liquorrhea (lik-ŏ-rē'ă) [L. *liquor*, fluid, + G. *rhoia*, flow]. The flow of liquid.

Lisch, Karl, Austrian ophthalmologist, *1907. See L. *nodule.*

Lisfranc (de St. Martin), Jacques, French surgeon, 1790–1847. See L.'s *amputation, joints, ligament, operation;* scalene *tubercle* of L.

lisinopril (līs-in'ō-pril). 1-[N^2-[(S)-1-Carboxy-3-phenylpropyl]-L-lysyl]-L-proline dihydrate; an angiotensin-converting enzyme inhibitor used in the treatment of hypertension.

Lison, Lucien, Belgian scientist, *1907. See L.-Dunn *stain.*

lisp'ing. Parasigmatism; sigmatism; mispronunciation of the sibilants *s* and *z.*

lissamine rhodamine B 200 (lis'să-mēn rō'dă-mēn). Sulforhodamine B.

Lissauer, Heinrich, German neurologist, 1861–1891. See L.'s *bundle, fasciculus, tract,* marginal *zone.*

lissencephalia (lis'en-sĕ-fā'lē-ă) [G. *lissos*, smooth, + *enkephalos*, brain]. Agyria.

lissencephalic (lis'en-sĕ-fal'ik). Pertaining to, or characterized by, lissencephalia.

lissencephaly (lis-en-sef'ă-lē) [G. *lissos*, smooth, + *enkephalos*, brain]. Agyria.

lissive (lis'iv) [G. *lissos*, smooth]. Having the property of relieving muscle spasm without causing flaccidity.

lissosphincter (lis'ō-sfingk'ter) [G. *lissos*, smooth, + sphincter]. Smooth muscular sphincter; a sphincter of smooth musculature.

lissotrichic, lissotrichous (lis-ō-trik'ik, -trik'ŭs) [G. *lissos*, smooth, + *thrix (trich-)*, hair]. Having straight hair.

Lister, Joseph (Lord Lister), British surgeon, 1827–1912. See *Listerella, Listeria,* listerism; L.'s *dressing, method, tubercle.*

Listerella (lis'ter-el'ă) [Joseph *Lister*]. In bacteriology, a rejected generic name sometimes cited as a synonym of *Listeria.* The type species is *L. hepatolytica.*

Listeria (lis-tēr-ē-ă) [Joseph *Lister*]. A genus of aerobic to microaerophilic, motile, peritrichous bacteria (family Corynebacteriaceae) containing small, coccoid, Gram-positive rods; these organisms tend to produce chains of three to five cells and, in the rough state, elongated and filamentous forms. Cells 18 to 24 hours old may show a palisade arrangement with a few V or Y forms; the bacteria produce acid but no gas from glucose and are found in the feces of man and other animals, on vegetation, and in silage and are parasitic on poikilothermic and warm-blooded animals, including man. The type species is *L. monocytogenes.*

L. denitrif'icans, a species found in cooked blood of beef; pathogenic to rats and mice when injected intraperitoneally.

L. gra'yi, a species found in the feces of chinchillas.

L. monocytog'enes, a species causing meningitis, encephalitis, septicemia, endocarditis, abortion, abscesses, and local purulent lesions; it is often fatal; it is found in healthy ferrets, insects, and the feces of chinchillas, ruminants, and man, as well as in sewage, decaying vegetation, silage, soil, and fertilizer.

listeriosis (lis-tēr'ē-ō'sis) [fr. organism *Listeria*]. Listeria meningitis; a sporadic disease of animals and occasionally man caused by the bacterium, *Listeria monocytogenes.* The infection in sheep and cattle frequently involves the central nervous system, causing various neurologic signs; in monogastric animals and fowl, the chief manifestations are septicemia and necrosis of the liver.

listerism (lis'ter-izm). Lister's *method.*

Listing, Johann B., German physiologist, 1808–1882. See L.'s reduced *eye, law.*

Liston, Robert, British surgeon, 1794–1847. See L.'s *knives, shears, splint.*

lisuride (lī'sūr-īd). A soluble ergot derivative with endocrine effects similar to those of bromocriptine; a serotonin inhibitor.

liter (L, l) (lē'ter) [Fr., fr. G. *litra*, a pound]. A measure of capacity of 1000 cubic centimeters or 1 cubic decimeter; equivalent to 1.0567 quarts.

lith-. See litho-.

lithagogue (lith'ă-gog) [litho- + G. *agōgos*, drawing forth]. Causing the dislodgment or expulsion of calculi, especially urinary calculi.

litharge (lith'arj) [litho- + G. *argyros*, silver]. Lead monoxide.

lithectomy (li-thek'tō-mē) [litho- + G. *ektomē*, excision]. Lithotomy.

lithiasis (li-thī'ă-sis) [litho- + G. *-iasis*, condition]. Formation of calculi of any kind, especially of biliary or urinary calculi.

l. conjuncti'vae, deposits of cellular degeneration into hard masses in Henle's glands.

pancreatic l., the formation of stones in the pancreas, usually associated with chronic inflammation and obstruction of the pancreatic ducts.

lithic acid (lith'ik). *Uric* acid.

lithium (lith'ē-ŭm) [Mod. L. fr. G. *lithos*, a stone]. An element of the alkali metal group, symbol Li, atomic no. 3, atomic weight 6.940.

l. bromide, LiBr; a white deliquescent powder, used as a sedative and hypnotic.

l. carbonate, Li_2CO_3; an antirheumatic and antilithic agent, also used in the treatment and prophylaxis of depressive, hypomanic, and manic phases of bipolar affective disorders.

l. citrate, $Li_3C_6H_5O_7 \cdot 4H_2O$; a diuretic and antirheumatic, also used in the treatment of manic psychosis.

effervescent l. citrate, a preparation containing l. citrate, sodium bicarbonate, tartaric acid, and citric acid; same use as potassium or sodium citrate.

l. tungstate, used in electron microscopy as a negative stain.

litho-, lith- [G. *lithos,* stone]. Combining forms relating to a stone or calculus, or to calcification.

Lithobius (li-thō'bē-ŭs) [litho- + G. *bios,* life]. A genus of centipedes characterized by 15 pairs of legs. Species common in the U.S. include *L. multidentatus* and *L. forficatus.*

lithocholic acid (lith-ō-kō'lik). 3α-Hydroxy-5β-cholan-24-oic acid; one of the acids isolated from human bile.

lithoclast (lith'ō-klast) [litho- + G. *klastos,* broken]. Lithotrite.

lithocystotomy (lith'ō-sis-tot'ō-mē) [litho- + G. *kystis,* bladder, + *tomē,* incision]. Vesical lithotomy.

lithodialysis (lith'ō-dī-al'i-sis) [litho- + G. *dialysis,* a breaking up]. Fragmentation or solution of a calculus.

lithogenesis, lithogeny (lith-ō-jen'ĕ-sis, lith-oj'ĕ-nē) [litho- + G. *genesis,* production]. Formation of calculi.

lithogenic (lith-ō-jen'ik). Promoting the formation of calculi.

lithogenous (lith-oj'ĕ-nŭs). Calculus-forming.

lithoid (lith'oyd) [litho- + G. *eidos,* resemblance]. Resembling a calculus or stone.

lithokelyphopedion, lithokelyphopedium (lith-ō-kel'ĕ-fō-pē'dē-on, -ŭm) [litho- + G. *kelyphos,* husk, shell, + *paidion,* child]. A lithopedion in which the fetal parts in contact with the surrounding membranes, as well as the membranes, are calcified.

lithokelyphos (lith-ō-kel'ĕ-fos) [litho- + G. *kelyphos,* rind, shell]. A type of lithopedion in which the fetal membranes alone undergo calcification.

litholabe (lith'ō-lāb) [litho- + G. *lambanein, labein,* to grasp]. Obsolete instrument for holding a bladder calculus during its removal.

litholapaxy (li-thol'ă-pak-sē) [litho- + G. *lapaxis,* an emptying out]. The operation of crushing a stone in the bladder and washing out the fragments through a catheter.

litholysis (li-thol'i-sis) [litho- + G. *lysis,* dissolution]. The dissolution of urinary calculi.

litholyte (lith'ō-līt). An instrument for injecting calculary solvents.

litholytic (li-thō-lit'ik) [litho- + G. *lysis,* dissolution]. **1.** Tending to dissolve calculi. **2.** An agent having such properties.

lithometer (li-thom'ĕ-ter) [litho- + G. *metron,* measure]. An instrument for measuring the size of a vesical calculus.

lithomyl (lith'ō-mil) [litho- + G. *mylē,* mill]. An instrument for pulverizing a stone in the bladder.

lithonephritis (lith'ō-ne-frī'tis). Interstitial nephritis associated with calculus formation.

lithopedion, lithopedium (lith-ō-pē'dē-on, -ŭm) [litho- + G. *paidion,* small child]. A retained fetus, usually extrauterine, which has become calcified.

lithophone (lith'ō-fōn) [litho- + G. *phōnē,* sound]. An instrument that emits a sound on contact with a stone in the bladder.

lithoscope (lith'ō-skōp) [litho- + G. *skopeō,* to view]. Obsolete term for cystoscope.

lithotome (lith'ō-tōm). A knife used in lithotomy.

lithotomist (li-thot'ō-mist). A person skilled in lithotomy.

lithotomy (li-thot'ō-mē) [litho- + G. *tomē,* incision]. Lithectomy; cutting for stone; a cutting operation for the removal of a calculus, especially a vesical calculus.

bilateral l., obsolete term for a l. in which the perineal incision is made transversely across the median raphe.

high l., suprapubic l.

lateral l., l. in which the perineum is incised to one side of the median line.

marian l. [L. *mas* (*mar-*), male], median l.

median l., marian l.; l. in which the perineal incision is made in the median raphe.

perineal l., l. in which the bladder is approached by an incision in the perineum.

prerectal l., l. by an incision in midline of perineum anterior to anus.

suprapubic l., high l.; l. in which the bladder is entered by an incision immediately above the symphysis pubis.

vaginal l., l. in which the bladder is entered through an incision in the vagina.

vesical l., lithocystotomy; removal of stones from the bladder by an open operation.

lithotresis (lith-ō-trē'sis) [litho- + G. *trēsis,* a boring]. The boring of holes in a calculus to facilitate its crushing.

ultrasonic l., the demolition of calculi by high frequency sound waves.

lithotripsy (lith'ō-trip-sē) [litho- + G. *tripsis,* a rubbing]. Lithotrity; the crushing of a stone in the bladder or urethra.

lithotriptic (lith-ō-trip'tik). **1.** Relating to lithotripsy. **2.** An agent that effects the dissolution of a calculus.

lithotriptor (lith-ō-trip'tŏr). A device used to crush a urinary calculus in lithotripsy.

lithotriptoscope (lith-ō-trip'tō-skōp). An endoscope used with a lithotrite.

lithotriptoscopy (lith'ō-trip-tos'kŏ-pē) [litho- + G. *tribō,* to rub, crush, + *skopeō,* to view]. Crushing of a stone in the bladder under direct vision.

lithotrite (lith'ō-trīt) [litho- + G. *tero,* pp. *tritus,* to rub]. Lithoclast; a mechanical instrument used to crush a urinary calculus in lithotripsy.

lithotrity (li-thot'ri-tē). Lithotripsy.

lithotroph (lith'ō-trof). An organism whose carbon needs are satisfied by carbon dioxide.

lithuresis (lith'yū-rē'sis) [litho- + G. *ourēsis,* urination]. The passage of gravel in the urine.

lithureteria (lith'yū-rē-tē'rē-ă) [litho- + G. *ourētēr,* ureter]. Ureterolithiasis.

lithuria (li-thū'rē-ă) [lithic (acid) + G. *ouron,* urine]. Excretion of uric acid or urates in large amount in the urine.

litmus (lit'mŭs) [a corruption of *lacmus,* fr. deu *lacmus,* fr. Dutch *lakmoes*] [old C.I. 1242]. A blue coloring matter obtained from *Roccella tinctoria* and other species of lichens, the principal component of which is azolitmin; used as an indicator (reddened by acids and turned blue again by alkalies).

Litten, Moritz, German physician, 1845–1907. See L.'s *phenomenon.*

litter (lit'er) [Fr. *litière;* fr. *lit,* bed]. **1.** A stretcher or portable couch for moving the sick or injured. **2.** Brood (1); a group of animals of the same parents, born at the same time.

Little, James L., U.S. surgeon, 1836–1885. See L.'s *area.*

Little, William J., British surgeon, 1810–1894. See L.'s *disease.*

Littré, Alexis, French anatomist, 1658–1726. See L.'s *glands, hernia.*

littritis (li-trī'tis). Inflammation of Littré's glands.

Litzmann, Karl K.T., German gynecologist, 1815–1890. See L.'s *obliquity.*

livebirth, live birth (līv'berth). The birth of an infant who shows evidence of life after birth. See also liveborn *infant.*

livedo (li-vē'dō) [L. lividness, fr. *liveo,* to be black and blue]. A bluish discoloration of the skin, either in limited patches or general.
postmortem l., postmortem hypostasis, lividity, or suggillation; a purple coloration of dependent parts, except in areas of contact pressure, appearing within one half to two hours after death, as a result of gravitational movement of blood within the vessels.
l. racemo'sa, l. reticularis.
l. reticula'ris, l. racemosa; dermatopathia pigmentosa reticularis; angiitis livedo reticularis; a purplish network-patterned discoloration of the skin caused by dilation of capillaries and venules due to alteration of a site or changes in underlying blood vessels including hyalinizing vasculation; rarely appears as a developmental defect.
l. reticula'ris idiopath'ica, an extensive and permanent form of l. reticularis; in rare instances associated with central arterial disease.
l. reticula'ris symptomat'ica, a discoloration or mottling of the skin due to some demonstrable cause, such as seen in erythema ab igne, in certain tuberculids, or as a reaction to exposure to cold.
l. telangiectat'ica, a permanent mottling of the skin due to an anomaly, probably congenital, of the cutaneous capillaries; a form of l. reticularis.

livedoid (liv'ĕ-doyd). Pertaining to or resembling livedo.

liv'er [A.S. *lifer*]. Hepar; the largest gland of the body, lying beneath the diaphragm in the right hypochondrium and upper part of the epigastrium; it is of irregular shape and weighs from 1 to 2 kg, or about $^1/_{40}$ the weight of the body. It secretes the bile and is also of great importance in both carbohydrate and protein metabolism.
cardiac l., cardiac *cirrhosis.*
desiccated l., a dried undefatted powder prepared from mammalian l.'s used as human food; contains riboflavin, nicotinic acid, and choline; used in the treatment of macrocytic anemias and as a nutritional supplement.
fatty l., hepatic steatosis; yellow discoloration of the l. due to fatty degeneration of l. parenchymal cells.
frosted l., hyaloserositis of the liver. Also called zuckergussleber; icing or sugar-icing l.; Curschmann's disease.
hobnail l., in Laënnec's cirrhosis, the contraction of scar tissue and hepatic cellular regeneration which causes a nodular appearance of the l.'s surface.
icing l., frosted l.
lardaceous l., waxy l.
nutmeg l., chronic passive congestion of the l., causing accentuation of the lobular pattern with red central and yellow or tan periportal zones.
polycystic l., polycystic liver disease; gradual cystic dilation of intralobular bile ducts (Meyenburg's complexes) that fail to involute in embryologic development of the l.; frequently associated with bilateral congenital polycystic kidneys and occasionally with cystic involvement of the pancreas, lungs, and other organs.
sugar-icing l., frosted l.
wandering l., hepatoptosis.
waxy l., lardaceous l.; amyloid degeneration of the l.

livetin (liv'ĕ-tin). Any of the three major water-soluble proteins in egg yolk: α-**livetin,** serum albumin; β-**livetin,** α-glycoprotein; γ-**livetin,** serum γ-globulin.

liv'id [L. *lividus,* being black and blue]. Having a black and blue or a leaden or ashy gray color, as in discoloration from a contusion, congestion, or cyanosis.

lividity (li-vid'i-tē). The state of being livid.
postmortem l., postmortem *livedo.*

livor (lī'vōr) [L. a black and blue spot]. The livid discoloration of the skin on the dependent parts of a corpse.

lixiviation (lik-siv-ē-ā'shŭn) [L. *lixivius,* made into lye, fr. *lix,* lye]. Leaching.

lixivium (lik-siv'ē-ŭm) [L. ntr. of *lixivius,* made into lye]. Lye.

LLL Abbreviation for left lower lobe (of lung).

Lloyd's reagent. See under reagent.

LLQ Abbreviation for left lower quadrant (of abdomen).

L.M. Abbreviation for licentiate in midwifery.

LMA Abbreviation for left mentoanterior *position.*

LMP Abbreviation for left mentoposterior *position.*

LMT Abbreviation for left mentotransverse *position.*

LNPF Abbreviation for lymph node permeability *factor.*

Lo, L_0 See under dose.

LOA Abbreviation for left occipitoanterior *position.*

load (lōd). A departure from normal body content, as of water, salt, or heat; positive l.'s are quantities in excess of the normal; negative l.'s are quantities in deficit.
electronic pacemaker l., the impedance to the output, the standard l. being 500 ohms resistance ± 1%.
genetic l., the aggregate of more or less harmful genes that are carried, mostly hidden, in the genome that may be transmitted to descendants and cause morbidity and disease; in classical genetic dynamics, genetic l. may be seen as undischarged genetic debts that result from previous mutations, each of which is supposed to exact an average number of lethal equivalents dependent only on the pattern of inheritance, regardless of how mild or severe the phenotype may be.

loading (lōd'ing). Administration of a substance for the purpose of testing metabolic function.
salt l., the administration of 2 g of sodium chloride (with a regular diet) 3 times a day for 4 days; a diagnostic test in primary aldosteronism, in which the salt l. produces the typical plasma electrolyte pattern.

Loa loa (lō'ă lō'ă). The African eye worm, a species of the family Onchocercidae (superfamily Filarioidea) that is indigenous to the western part of equatorial Africa, especially in the region of the Congo River, and is the causal agent of loiasis. Adult worms are white or gray-white, cylindroid, and threadlike, the males averaging 25 to 35 by 0.3 to 0.4 mm (with a curved tail) and the females ranging from 50 to 60 by 0.4 to 0.6 mm; microfilariae are ensheathed, with nuclei extending to the tip of the tail. The life cycle is somewhat similar to that of *Wuchereria* species; man is the only known definitive host, and parasites are transmitted by *Chrysops* flies (family Tabanidae); infective larvae from the latter require 3 years or more to mature in man, and the adult forms may persist in man for as long as 17 years. See also loiasis.

lobar (lō'bar). Relating to any lobe.

lobate (lō'bāt). Lobose; lobous. **1.** Divided into lobes. **2.** Lobe-shaped; denoting a bacterial colony with a deeply undulate margin.

lobe (lōb) [G. *lobos,* lobe]. **1.** Lobus. **2.** A rounded projecting part, as the l. of the ear. See also lobule; lobulus. **3.** One of the larger divisions of the crown of a tooth, formed from a distinct point of calcification.
anterior l. of hypophysis, official alternative name for adenohypophysis. See also hypophysis.
caudate l., *lobus* caudatus.
l.'s of cerebrum, *lobi* cerebri.
cuneiform l., *lobulus* biventer.
ear l., *lobulus* auriculae.
falciform l., *gyrus* cinguli.
flocculonodular l., the small posterior and inferior subdivision of the cerebellar cortex that borders the line of attachment of the choroid roof of the rhomboid fossa, and consists of the left and right flocculus together with the unpaired nodulus (the most posterior of the folia composing the vermis cerebelli). Its major afferent connections come from the vestibular nuclei and directly from the ves-

tibular nerve; it projects largely to the vestibular nuclei, directly and by way of the nucleus fastigii.
frontal l., *lobus* frontalis cerebri.
Home's l., the enlarged middle l. of the prostate gland.
inferior l. of lung, *lobus* inferior pulmonis.
left l., *lobus* sinister.
left l. of liver, *lobus* hepatis sinister.
limbic l., as originally defined by P. Broca: the nearly closed ring of the brain structures surrounding the hilus, or margin, of the cerebral hemisphere of mammals; it is composed of the gyrus fornicatus (gyrus cinguli and gyrus parahippocampalis), the hippocampus, and the amygdala. See limbic *system.*
lingual l., *cingulum* dentis.
lower l. of lung, *lobus* inferior pulmonis.
l.'s of mammary gland, *lobi* glandulae mammariae.
middle l. of prostate, *lobus* medius prostatae.
middle l. of right lung, *lobus* medius pulmonis dextri.
nervous l., *lobus* nervosus.
occipital l., *lobus* occipitalis cerebri.
parietal l., *lobus* parietalis cerebri.
placental l., Cotyledons of the human placenta, viewed on the maternal surface as irregularly shaped elevations or l.'s.
posterior l. of hypophysis, neurohypophysis.
l. of prostate, *lobus* prostatae.
pyramidal l. of thyroid gland, *lobus* pyramidalis glandulae thyroideae.
quadrate l., **(1)** *lobus* quadratus; **(2)** *lobulus* quadrangularis; **(3)** precuneus.
renal l., *lobus* renalis.
Riedel's l., lobus linguiformis; lobus appendicularis; an occasional tongue-like process extending downward from the right l. of the liver lateral to the gallbladder; a similar process may, though rarely, extend from the left lobe.
right l., *lobus* dexter.
right l. of liver, *lobus* hepatis dexter.
Spigelius' l., *lobus* caudatus.
superior l. of lung, *lobus* superior pulmonis.
supplemental l., in dental anatomy, an extra l.; one that is not included in the typical formation of a tooth.
temporal l., *lobus* temporalis.
l.'s of thyroid gland, *lobi* glandulae thyroideae.
upper l. of lung, *lobus* superior pulmonis.

lobectomy (lō-bek'tō-mē) [G. *lobos,* lobe, + *ektomē,* excision]. Excision of a lobe of any organ or gland.

lobelia (lō-bē'lē-ă). Asthma-weed (1); wild tobacco; the dried leaves and tops of *Lobelia inflata* (family Lobeliaceae); it contains several alkaloids: lobeline, lobelamine, lobelanidine, lobelanine, norlobelanine, norlobelanidine, and isolobelanine. The fluidextract and the tincture have been used as an expectorant in asthma and chronic bronchitis.

lobeline (lō'bĕ-lēn, lob'ĕ-lēn, -lin). A piperidylacetophenone; an alkaloid of lobelia with the same actions as nicotine, but with less potency.
l. sulfate, a form of l. occurring in yellow friable masses, soluble in water; used in whooping cough and asthma; it has been suggested as a smoking deterrent.

lobi (lō'bī) [L.]. Plural of lobus.

lobitis (lō-bī'tis). Inflammation of a lobe.

Lobo, Jorge, 20th century Brazilian physician. See L.'s *disease.*

Loboa loboi (lō-bō'ă lō-bō'ē). A species of fungus causing lobomycosis. The organism is still classified by some as *Paracoccidioides brasiliensis,* which causes paracoccidioidomycosis.

lobomycosis (lō-bō-mī-kō'sis). Lobo's disease; a chronic localized mycosis of the skin resulting in fibrous nodules or keloids that contain budding, thick-walled cells, *i.e.,* the tissue form of *Loboa loboi,* the causative fungus, which has never been cultured and has not infected laboratory animals.

lobopodium, pl. **lobopodia** (lō'bō-pō'dē-ŭm, -dē-ă) [G. *lobos,* lobe, + *pous,* foot]. A thick lobose pseudopodium.

lobose, lobous (lō'bōs, lō'bŭs). Lobate.

lobotomy (lō-bot'ō-mē) [G. *lobos,* lobe, + *tomē,* a cutting]. **1.** Incision into a lobe. **2.** Division of one or more nerve tracts in a lobe of the cerebrum.
prefrontal l., prefrontal leukotomy; division of one or more nerve tracts in the prefrontal area of the brain for surgical treatment of pain and emotional disorder.
transorbital l., transorbital leukotomy; l. by an approach through the roof of the orbit, behind the frontal sinus.

Lobry de Bruyn, Cornelius A., Dutch chemist, 1857–1904. See L. d. B.-van Ekenstein *transformation.*

Lobstein, Johann F.G., German pathologist, 1777–1835. See L.'s *ganglion, syndrome.*

lobular (lob'yū-lăr). Relating to a lobule.

lobulate, lobulated (lob'yū-lāt, -ed). Divided into lobules.

lobule (lob'yūl). Lobulus.
ansiform l., comprises the greater part of the hemisphere of the cerebellum; its superior and inferior surfaces are separated by the horizontal fissure into major parts known as crus I (lobulus semilunaris superior) and crus II (lobulus semilunaris inferior).
anterior lunate l., *lobulus* semilunaris superior.
l. of auricle, *lobulus* auriculae.
biventral l., *lobulus* biventer.
central l., *lobulus* centralis cerebelli.
crescentic l.'s of the cerebellum, *lobulus* semilunaris inferior and *lobulus* semilunaris superior.
l.'s of epididymis, *lobuli* epididymidis.
hepatic l., *lobulus* hepatis.
inferior parietal l., *lobulus* parietalis inferior.
inferior semilunar l., *lobulus* semilunaris inferior.
l.'s of mammary gland, *lobuli* glandulae mammariae.
paracentral l., *lobulus* paracentralis.
portal l. of liver, a conceptual unit of the liver, emphasizing its exocrine function in bile secretion, which comprises a roughly triangular shaped cross-sectional area with a portal canal at its center and three or more venae centrales hepatis at its periphery.
posterior lunate l., *lobulus* semilunaris inferior.
primary pulmonary l., pulmonary *acinus.*
quadrangular l., *lobulus* quadrangularis.
quadrate l., **(1)** *lobulus* quadrangularis; **(2)** precuneus.
renal cortical l., *lobulus* corticalis renalis.
respiratory l., pulmonary *acinus.*
secondary pulmonary l., a pyramidal mass of lung tissue whose sides are bounded by the incomplete interlobular connective tissue septa and whose base, which is 1 to 2 cm in diameter, usually faces the pleural surface of the lung; l.'s which occupy a more central position in the lung are not well defined and are considered to consist of three to five pulmonary acini with proximate terminal bronchioles.
simple l., *lobulus* simplex.
slender l., *lobulus* gracilis.
superior parietal l., *lobulus* parietalis superior.
superior semilunar l., *lobulus* semilunaris superior.
l.'s of testis, *lobuli* testis.
l.'s of thymus, *lobuli* thymi.
l.'s of thyroid gland, *lobuli* glandulae thyroideae.

lobulet, lobulette (lob'yū-let'). A very small lobule or one of the smaller subdivisions of a lobule.

lobulus, gen. and pl. **lobuli** (lob'yū-lŭs, yū-lī) [Mod. L. dim. of *lobus,* lobe] [NA]. Lobule; a small lobe or subdivision of a lobe.
l. auric'ulae [NA], lobule of the auricle; ear lobe; the lowest part

of the auricle; it consists of fat and fibrous tissue not reinforced by the auricular cartilage.

l. biven'ter [NA], biventral lobule; cuneiform lobe; l. biventralis; l. cuneiformis; a lobule on the undersurface of each cerebellar hemisphere, divided by a curved sulcus into a lateral and medial portion; it corresponds to the pyramid of the vermis.

l. biventra'lis, l. biventer.

l. centra'lis cerebel'li [NA], central lobule; a division of the superior vermis of the cerebellum between the lingula and the monticulus.

l. cli'vi, declive.

l. cortica'lis rena'lis [NA], renal cortical lobule; reniculus (1); one of the subdivisions of the kidney, consisting of a pars radiata or medullary ray and that portion of the pars convoluta (renal corpuscles and convoluted tubules) associated with its collecting duties.

l. cul'minis, culmen.

l. cune'iform'is, l. biventer.

lob'uli epididym'idis [NA], lobules of the epididymis; coni epididymidis or vasculosi; vascular cones; Haller's cones; the coiled portion of the efferent ductules that constitute the head of the epididymis; these join the ductus epididymidis.

l. fo'lii, the part of the superior vermis of the cerebellum lying immediately behind the posterior superior fissure and caudal to the l. clivi.

l. fusifor'mis, *gyrus* fusiformis.

lob'uli glan'dulae mamma'riae [NA], lobules of the mammary gland; subdivisions of the lobes of the mammary gland.

lob'uli glan'dulae thyroi'deae [NA], lobules of the thyroid gland; the subdivisions of the lobes, consisting of incompletely separated, irregular groups of thyroid follicles (20 to 40 in number) bound together by delicate connective tissue.

l. grac'ilis, slender lobule; the anterior portion of the posterioinferior lobule of the cerebellum, the posterior portion being the l. semilunaris inferior; the two correspond to the tuber of the vermis.

l. hep'atis [NA], hepatic lobule; the polygonal histologic unit of the liver consisting of masses of liver cells arranged around a central vein, a terminal branch of one of the hepatic veins; at the periphery are located preterminal and terminal branches of the portal vein, hepatic artery, and bile duct.

l. paracentra'lis [NA], paracentral lobule; a division of the medial aspect of the pallium, lying above the sulcus cinguli and bounded by the precentral sulcus in front and the pars marginalis of the sulcus cinguli behind.

l. parieta'lis infe'rior [NA], inferior parietal lobule; inferior parietal gyrus; the area of the parietal lobe of the cerebrum lying below the interparietal sulcus; it contains the angular and the supramarginal gyri.

l. parieta'lis supe'rior [NA], superior parietal lobule; superior parietal gyrus; the area of the convex surface of the parietal lobe of the cerebrum lying between the longitudinal fissure and the interparietal sulcus behind the posterior central gyrus; it is continuous with the precuneus on the medial aspect of the hemisphere.

l. quadrangula'ris [NA], quadrate lobe (2); quadrangular lobe; quadrate or quadrangular lobule; l. quadratus (1); the main portion of the superior part of each hemisphere of the cerebellum, corresponding to the monticulus of the vermis; it is divided into two portions, the anterior and the posterior crescentic lobules, corresponding to the culmen and the declive of the vermis.

l. quadra'tus, **(1)** l. quadrangularis; **(2)** precuneus.

l. semiluna'ris infe'rior [NA], inferior semilunar lobule; posterior lunate lobule; crus II; the part of the superior surface of the cerebellar hemisphere lying behind the fissura horizontalis.

l. semiluna'ris supe'rior [NA], superior semilunar lobule; anterior lunate lobule; crus I; the part of the superior surface of the cerebellar hemisphere lying rostral to the fissura horizontalis, and adjoining the folium of the vermis.

l. sim'plex [NA], simple lobule; the smaller anterior part of the posterior lobe of the cerebellum, demarcated by fissura prima from the anterior lobe rostrally and from the large caudal subdivision of the posterior lobe caudally.

lob'uli tes'tis [NA], lobules of the testis; the subdivisions of the parenchyma of the testis formed by delicate fibrous septa that pass inward from the tunica albuginea to converge at the mediastinum testis.

lobuli thy'mi [NA], lobules of the thymus; areas of thymic tissue 0.5 to 2 mm in diameter with a cortex and medulla.

lo'bus, gen. and pl. **lo'bi** (lō'bŭs, lō'bī) [LL. fr. G. *lobos*] [NA]. Lobe (1); one of the subdivisions of an organ or other part, bounded by fissures, connective tissue, septa, or other structural demarcations.

l. ante'rior hypophys'eos [NA], adenohypophysis.

l. appendicula'ris, Riedel's *lobe.*

l. az'ygos, a small accessory lobe sometimes found on the upper part of the right lung; separated from the rest of the upper lobe by a deep groove lodging the azygos vein.

l. cauda'tus [NA], caudate lobe; Spigelius' lobe; a small lobe of the liver situated posteriorly between the sulcus for the vena cava and the fissure for the ligamentum venosum.

lobi cer'ebri [NA], lobes of the cerebrum; the major divisions of the cerebral hemisphere; they include the frontal, parietal, temporal, and occipital lobes, named for the overlying bones of the skull.

l. cli'vi, the clivus monticuli and the posterior crescentic lobules of the cerebellum considered as one lobe.

l. dex'ter [NA], right lobe; the right subdivision of several glands, *e.g.,* prostate, thyroid, thymus.

l. falcifor'mis, *gyrus* cinguli.

l. fronta'lis cer'ebri [NA], frontal lobe; the portion of each cerebral hemisphere anterior to the central sulcus.

lo'bi glan'dulae mamma'riae [NA], lobes of the mammary gland; the 15 to 20 separate portions of the mammary gland that comprise the corpus mammae; each is drained by a single lactiferous duct.

lo'bi glan'dulae thyroi'deae [NA], lobes of the thyroid gland; the two major divisions of the gland lying on the right (l. dexter) and left (l. sinistra) side of the trachea and connected by the isthmus. A smaller pyramidal lobe is frequently present as an upward extension from the isthmus.

l. glandula'ris hypophys'eos, l. anterior hypophyseos.

l. hep'atis dex'ter [NA], right lobe of the liver; the largest lobe of the liver, separated from the left lobe above and in front by the falciform ligament and from the caudate and quadrate lobes by the sulcus for the vena cava and the fossa for the gallbladder; it contains two segments, anterior and posterior.

l. hep'atis sinis'ter [NA], left lobe of the liver; it is separated from the right lobe above and in front by the falciform ligament, and from the quadrate and caudate lobes by the fissure for the ligamentum teres and the fissure for the ligamentum venosum; the distribution of the portal vein, hepatic artery, and bile ducts does not correspond to the gross lobar divisions of the liver. It contains two segments, medial and lateral.

l. infe'rior pulmo'nis [NA], inferior or lower lobe of the lung; it is located below and behind the oblique fissure and contains five bronchopulmonary segments, superior, medial basal, anterior basal, lateral basal and posterior basal.

l. linguifor'mis, Riedel's *lobe.*

l. me'dius prosta'tae [NA], middle lobe of prostate; Morgagni's caruncle; the portion of the prostate lying between the urethra and the ejaculatory ducts; indistinct unless hypertrophied.

l. me'dius pulmo'nis dex'tri [NA], middle lobe of the right lung; it is located anteriorly between the horizontal and oblique fissures and includes lateral and medial bronchopulmonary segments.

l. nervo'sus, nervous lobe; the bulbous part of the neurohypophysis attached to the hypothalamus by the infundibulum. It is composed of pituicytes, blood vessels, and terminals of nerve fibers from the supraoptic and paraventricular nuclei.

l. occipita'lis cer'ebri [NA], occipital lobe; the posterior, somewhat pyramid-shaped part of each cerebral hemisphere, demarcated by no distinct surface markings on the lateral convexity of the hemisphere from the parietal and temporal lobes, but sharply delineated from the parietal lobe by the parieto-occipital sulcus on the medial surface.

l. parieta'lis cer'ebri [NA], parietal lobe; the middle portion of each cerebral hemisphere, separated from the frontal lobe by the central sulcus, from the temporal lobe by the lateral sulcus in front and an imaginary line projected posteriorly, and from the occipital lobe only partially by the parieto-occipital sulcus on its medial aspect.

l. poste'rior hypophys'eos [NA], official alternative name for neurohypophysis. See also hypophysis.

l. prosta'tae [NA], lobe of prostate; one of the lateral lobes (right or left) or the middle lobe or isthmus of the prostate; in the adult the lobes are ill-defined.

l. pyramida'lis glan'dulae thyroi'deae [NA], pyramidal lobe of thyroid gland; Morgagni's appendix; Lalouette's pyramid; pyramid of thyroid; an inconstant narrow lobe of the thyroid gland that arises from the upper border of the isthmus and extends upward, sometimes as far as the hyoid bone; it marks the point of continuity with the ductus thyroglossus.

l. quadra'tus [NA], quadrate lobe (1); a lobe on the inferior surface of the liver located between the fossa for the gallbladder and the fissure for the ligamentum teres.

l. rena'lis [NA], renal lobe; one of the subdivisions of the kidney, consisting of a renal pyramid and the cortical tissue associated with it.

l. sinis'ter [NA], left lobe; the left subdivision of several glands, *e.g.,* prostate, thyroid, thymus.

l. supe'rior pulmo'nis [NA], superior or upper lobe of the lung; the lobe of the right lung that lies above the oblique and horizontal fissures and includes the apical, posterior and anterior bronchopulmonary segments; in the left lung, the lobe lies above the oblique fissure and contains the apicoposterior, anterior, superior lingular and inferior lingular segments.

l. tempora'lis [NA], temporal cortex or lobe; a long lobe, the lowest of the major subdivisions of the cortical mantle, forming the posterior two-thirds of the ventral surface of the cerebral hemisphere, separated from the frontal and parietal lobes above it by the lateral sulcus arbitrarily delineated by an imaginary plane from the occipital lobe with which it is continuous posteriorly. The temporal lobe has a heterogeneous composition: in addition to a large neocortical component consisting of the superior, middle, and inferior temporal gyri and the lateral and medial occipitotemporal gyri, it includes the largely juxtallocortical parahippocampal gyrus with its paleocortical (olfactory) uncus and, beneath the latter, the amygdala.

local (lō'kăl) [L. *localis,* fr. *locus,* place]. Having reference or confined to a limited part; not general or systemic.

localization (lō'kăl-i-zā'shŭn). **1.** Limitation to a definite area. **2.** The reference of a sensation to its point of origin. **3.** The determination of the location of a morbid process.

auditory l., in sensory psychology, the naming or pointing to directions from which sounds emanate.

cerebral l., the mapping of the cerebral cortex into areas and the correlation of the various areas with cerebral function, or the diagnosis of the situation in the cerebrum of a brain lesion based on the signs and symptoms manifested by the patient or on radiographic studies.

germinal l., determination in very young embryos of the presumptive areas for specific organs or structures.

pneumotaxic l., l. on a grid of basal structures in the brain outlined by ventriculography.

spatial l., the reference of a visual sensation to a definite locality in space.

sterotaxic l., l. of intracerebral nuclei by coordinates with reference to anatomical landmarks in the brain.

localized (lō'kăl-īzd). Restricted or limited to a definite part.

locant (lō'kant). A number or letter preceding a substituent name in the name of a complex chemical that specifies the position (location) of the substituent on the parent molecule; *e.g.,* 5 in 5-methyluridine; *S* in *S*- adenosylmethionine.

locator (lō'kā-ter, tōr). An instrument or apparatus for finding the position of a foreign object in tissue.

lochia (lō'kē-ă) [G. neut. pl. of *lochios,* relating to childbirth, fr. *lochos,* childbirth]. Dicharges from the vagina of mucus, blood, and tissue debris, following childbirth.

l. al'ba, l. purulenta; the last discharge no longer tinged with blood.

l. cruen'ta, l. rubra; the initial discharge stained with blood.

l. purulen'ta, l. alba.

l. ru'bra, l. cruenta.

l. sanguinolen'ta, thick, dark red vaginal discharge seen a few days after delivery.

l. sero'sa, a thin and watery l.

lochial (lō'kē-ăl). Relating to the lochia.

lochiometra (lō-kē-ō-mē'tră) [G. *mētra,* womb]. Distention of the uterus with retained lochia.

lochiometritis (lō-kē-ō-mē-trī'tis). Puerperal metritis.

lochioperitonitis (lō'kē-ō-per'i-tō-nī'tis). Puerperal peritonitis.

lochiorrhagia (lō-kē-ō-rā'jē-ă) [lochia + G. *rhēgnymi,* to burst forth]. Lochiorrhea.

lochiorrhea (lō-kē-ō-rē'ă) [lochia + G. *rhoia,* a flow]. Lochiorrhagia; profuse flow of the lochia.

loci (lō'sī). Plural of locus.

Locke, Frank S., British physiologist, 1871–1949. See L.'s *solutions,* L.-Ringer *solution.*

lockjaw (lok'jaw). Trismus.

Lockwood, Charles B., British anatomist and surgeon, 1858–1914. See L.'s *ligament.*

loco (lō'kō) [Sp. crack-brained]. Locoweed disease; a disease affecting cattle on the great plains of the western U.S. caused by eating the locoweed; characterized by paresis, incoordination, dullness, and a tendency to become solitary in habit.

locomotive (lō-kō-mō'tiv). Locomotor.

locomotor (lō-kō-mō'ter) [L. *locus,* place, + L. *moveo,* pp. *motus,* to move]. Locomotive; locomotory; relating to locomotion, or movement from one place to another.

locomoto'rial. Relating to the locomotorium.

locomotorium (lō'kō-mō-tō'rē-um) [L. *locus,* place, + *motorius,* moving]. The locomotor apparatus of the body.

locomotory (lō-kō-mō'tō-rē). Locomotor.

locular (lok'yū-lăr). Relating to a loculus.

loculate (lok'yū-lāt). Containing numerous loculi.

loculation (lok-yū-lā'shŭn). **1.** A loculate region in an organ or tissue, or a loculate structure formed between surfaces of organs, mucous or serous membranes, and so on. **2.** The process that results in the formation of a loculus or loculi.

loculus, pl. loculi (lok'yū-lŭs, -lī) [L. dim. of *locus,* place]. A small cavity or chamber.

locus, pl. loci (lō'kŭs, lō'sī) [L.]. A place; usually, a specific site.

l. ceru'leus [NA], substantia ferruginea; l. cinereus or ferrugineus; a shallow depression, of a blue color in the fresh brain, lying laterally in the most rostral portion of the rhomboidal fossa near the cerebral aqueduct; it lies near the lateral wall of the fourth ventricle of about 20,000 melanin-pigmented neuronal cell bodies whose norepinephrine-containing axons have a remarkably wide distribution in the cerebellum as well as in the hypothalamus and cerebral cortex.

l. cine'reus, l. ceruleus.

complex l., a collection of closely linked genetic loci, as in the major histocompatibility complex l.

l. of control, a theoretical construct designed to assess a person's perceived control over his/her own behavior; classified as *internal* if the person feels in control of events, *external* if others are perceived to have that control.

l. ferrugin'eus, l. ceruleus.

genetic l., any of the homologous parts of a pair of chromosomes that may be occupied by allelic genes; the concept of a l. is somewhat idealized, not taking into account accidents that may occur in meiosis such as duplication of loci as a result of unequal crossing-over, translocations, inversions, etc.

l. ni'ger, *substantia* nigra.

l. perfora'tus anti'cus, *substantia* perforata anterior.

l. perfora'tus posti'cus, *substantia* perforata posterior.

sex-linked l., any l. that in normal karyotypes is borne on a heterosome; usually applied to an X-linked l.

X-linked l., any l. that in normal karyotypes is borne on the X chromosome.

Y-linked l., any (haploid) l. that in normal karyotypes is borne on the Y chromosome.

Loeb, Leo, U.S. pathologist, 1869–1959. See L.'s *deciduoma.*

Loeffler, Friedrich A. J., German bacteriologist and surgeon, 1852–1915. See L.'s *bacillus,* blood culture *medium, stains, methylene* blue; Klebs-L. *bacillus.*

Loevit, Moritz, Austrian pathologist, 1851–1918. See L.'s *cells.*

Loewenthal, Wilhelm, German physician, 1850–1894. See L.'s *bundle, reaction, tract.*

Loewi, Otto, German pharmacologist in New York and Nobel laureate, 1873–1961. See L.'s *sign.*

lofentanil (lō-fen'tă-nil). $C_{25}H_{32}N_2O_3$; a potent, longlasting narcotic and analgesic that is chemically related to fentanyl.

Löffler, Wilhelm, Swiss physician, *1887. See L.'s *disease, endocarditis, syndrome.*

log-. See logo-.

logagnosia (log-ag-nō'sē-ă) [logo- + G. *agnosia,* ignorance]. Aphasia.

logagraphia (log-ă-graf'ē-ă) [logo- + G. *a-* priv. + *graphō,* to write]. Agraphia.

logamnesia (log-am-nē'zē-ă) [logo- + G. *amnēsia,* forgetfulness]. Aphasia.

Logan, William H.G., early 20th century U.S. plastic surgeon. See L.'s *bow.*

logaphasia (log-ă-fā'zē-ă) [logo- + G. *aphasia,* speechlessness]. Aphasia of articulation.

logasthenia (log-as-thē'nē-ă) [logo- + G. *astheneia,* weakness]. Aphasia.

logetronography (lō-jet'ron-og'ră-fē). A method of printing in which special details are emphasized by purely electronic means in a very dense or very thin low contrast area in a manner that allows the desired emphasis to be obtained. Used especially in emphasizing details of x-ray films.

-logia. **1** [G. *logos,* discourse, treatise]. Suffix expressing in a general way the study of the subject noted in the body of the word, or a treatise on the same; the Eng. equivalent is -logy, or, with a connecting vowel, -ology. **2** [G. *legō,* to collect]. Suffix signifying collecting or picking.

logo-, log- [G. *logos,* word, discourse]. Combining forms relating to speech, or words.

logopathy (log-op'ă-thē) [logo- + G. *pathos,* suffering]. Any speech disorder.

logopedia (log-ō-pē'dē-ă). Logopedics.

logopedics (log'ō-pē'diks) [logo- + G. *pais (paid-),* child]. Logopedia; a branch of science concerned with the physiology and pathology of the organs of speech and with the correction of speech defects.

logoplegia (log-ō-plē'jē-ă) [logo- + G. *plēgē,* stroke]. Paralysis of the organs of speech.

logorrhea (log-ō-rē'ă) [logo- + G. *rhoia,* a flow]. Rarely used term for abnormal or pathologic garrulousness.

logospasm (log'ō-spazm) [logo- + G. *spasmos,* spasm]. **1.** Stuttering. **2.** Explosive *speech.*

logotherapy (log'ō-thār'ă-pē) [logo- + G. *therapeia,* cure]. A form of psychotherapy which places special emphasis on the patient's spiritual life and on the physician as "medical minister."

-logy [G. *logos,* treatis, discourse]. See -logia.

Lohlein-Baehr lesion. See under lesion.

Lohnstein, Theodor, German physician, 1866–1918. See L.'s *saccharimeter.*

loiasis (lō-ī'ă-sis). A chronic disease caused by *Loa loa,* with symptoms and signs first occurring approximately three to four years after a bite by an infected tabanid fly. When the infective larvae mature, the adult worms move about in an irregular course through the connective tissue of the body (as rapidly as 1 cm per minute), frequently becoming visible beneath the skin and mucous membranes; *e.g.,* in the back, scalp, chest, inner surface of the lip, and especially on the conjunctiva. The worms provoke hyperemia and exudation of fluid, often a host response to the worm products, a Calabar or fugitive swelling which causes no serious damage and subsides as the parasites move on; the patient is annoyed by the "creeping" in the tissues and intense itching, as well as occasional pain, especially when the swelling is in the region of tendons and joints. Most patients have an eosinophilia of 10 to 30 or 40% in the circulating blood.

loin (loyn) [Fr. *longe;* E. *lumbus*]. Lumbus.

Lok. See Luer-L. *syringe.*

loliism (lō'li-izm) [L. *lolium,* darnel, tares]. Poisoning by the seeds of a grass, *Lolium temulentum* (in the form of flour made into bread), characterized by giddiness, tremor, green vision, dilated pupils, prostration, and sometimes vomiting.

Lombard, Etienne, French physician, 1868–1920. See L. voice-reflex *test.*

lomustine (lō-mŭs'tēn). 1-(2-Chloroethyl)-3-cyclohexyl-1-nitrosourea; CCNU; an antineoplastic agent.

London, Fritz, German-U.S. physicist, 1900–1954. See L. *forces.*

Long, John H., U.S. physician, 1856–1927. See L.'s *coefficient, formula.*

long-chain fatty acid–CoA ligase [EC 6.2.1.3]. Acyl-CoA synthetase(2); fatty acid thiokinase (long chain); acyl-activating enzyme (1); a ligase forming acyl-CoA's from long chain fatty acids at the expense of ATP.

longevity (lon-jev'i-tē). Macrobiosis; duration of a particular life beyond the norm for the species. See also life-span.

longitudinal (lon'ji-tū'di-năl) [L. *longitudo,* length]. Running lengthwise; in the direction of the long axis of the body or any of its parts.

longitudinalis (lon'ji-tū'di-nā'lis) [NA]. Longitudinal.

longitype (lon'ji-tīp). Ectomorph.

Longmire, William P., Jr., U.S. surgeon, *1913. See L.'s *operation.*

Looney, Joseph M., U.S. biochemist, *1896. See Folin-L. *test.*

loop (lūp) [M.E. *loupe*]. **1.** A sharp curve or complete bend in a vessel, cord, or other cylindrical body, forming an oval or circular ring. **2.** A wire (usually of platinum or nichrome) fixed into a handle at one end and bent into a circle at the other, rendered sterile by flaming, and used to transfer microorganisms.

Biebl l., a continuous l. of small intestine brought through the abdominal wall to a subcutaneous location, for observation of motility.

bulboventricular l., the portion of the early somite embryonic cardiac tube which evolves into the ventricle and bulbus cordis.

capillary l.'s, small blood vessels in the dermal papillae.

cervical l., *ansa* cervicalis.

gamma l., Granit's l.; gamma motor system; the reflex arc consisting of small anterior horn cells and neuroma, their small fibers projecting to the intrafusal bundle producing its contraction, which initiates the afferent impulses that pass through the posterior root to the anterior horn cells, inducing a stretch reflex.

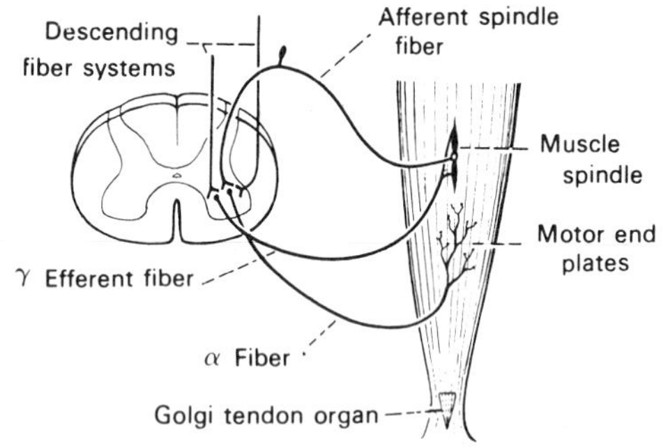

Schematic Diagram of the Gamma Loop

Gerdy's interatrial l., a muscular fasciculus in the interatrial septum of the heart, passing backward from the atrioventricular groove.

Granit's l., gamma l.

Henle's l., nephronic l.

Hyrtl's l., Hyrtl's anastomosis; a communicating l. between the right and left hypoglossal nerves, lying between the geniohyoid and genioglossus muscles or in the substance of the geniohyoid; it is found in about one in ten persons.

lenticular l., *ansa* lenticularis.

memory l., an electronic device for retrieving data that had been displayed upon the oscilloscope at an earlier time; used for reviewing electrical events immediately preceding a specific disturbance.

Meyer-Archambault l., the fibers of the visual radiation that loop around the tip of the temporal horn.

nephronic l., Henle's l. or ansa; the U-shaped part of the nephron extending from the proximal to the distal convoluted tubules, consisting of descending and ascending limbs, located in the medulla renalis and medullary ray.

peduncular l., *ansa* peduncularis.

l.'s of spinal nerves, *ansae* nervorum spinalium.

subclavian l., *ansa* subclavia.

vector l., an irregularly elliptical curve representing the average direction and magnitude of the heart's action from moment to moment throughout the cardiac cycle. See also vector (2), and vectorcardiogram.

ventricular l., the l. in the bulboventricular region of the embryonic heart.

Vieussens' l., *ansa* subclavia.

loosening of association. A manifestation of a severe thought disorder characterized by the lack of an obvious connection between one thought or phrase and the next, or with the response to a question.

Looser, Emil, Swiss physician, 1877–1936. See L.'s *zones.*

LOP Abbreviation for left occipitoposterior *position.*

lop-ear (lop'ēr). Congenital deformity of the external ear, with poor development of helix and anthelix.

loperamide hydrochloride (lō-per'ă-mīd). 4-(*p*-Chlorophenyl)-4-hydroxy-*N,N*-dimethyl-α,α-diphenyl-1-piperidinebutyramide monohydrochloride; an antiperistaltic agent used to treat diarrhea.

lophodont (lof'ō-dont) [G. *lophos,* ridge, + *odous,* tooth]. Having the crowns of the molar teeth formed in transverse or longitudinal crests or ridges, in contrast to bunodont.

Lophophora williamsii (lō-fof'ō-ră wil-yăm'sē-ī). *Anhalonium lewinii* (family Cactaceae); the botanical origin of peyote (mescal button); it contains over a dozen alkaloids, of which mescaline is the most important; others are pellotine, anhalomine, anhalonidine, anhalamine, anhalinine, anhalidine, and lophophorine.

lophotrichate (lō-fot'ri-kāt). Lophotrichous.

lophotrichous (lō-fot'ri-kŭs) [G. *lophos,* crest, + *thrix,* hair]. Lophotrichate; referring to a bacterial cell with two or more flagella at one or both poles.

lopremone (lō'pre-mōn). Former name for protirelin.

Lorain, Paul, French physician, 1827–1875. See L.'s *disease;* L.-Lévi *dwarfism, infantilism, syndrome.*

lorazepam (lō-ră'zē-pam). 7-Chloro-5-(*o*-chlorophenyl)-1,3-dihydro-3-hydroxy-2*H*-1,4-benzodiazepin-2-one; an antianxiety drug.

lordoscoliosis (lōr'dō-skō-lē-ō'sis) [G. *lordos,* bent back, + *skoliōsis,* crookedness, fr. *skolios,* bent, aslant]. Combined backward and lateral curvature of the spine.

lordosis (lōr-dō'sis) [G. *lordōsis,* a bending backward]. Hollow or saddle back; an abnormal extension deformity: backward curvature; anteroposterior curvature of the spine, generally lumbar with the convexity looking anteriorly.

lordotic (lōr-dot'ik). Pertaining to or marked by lordosis.

Lorenz, Adolf, Austrian surgeon, 1854–1946. See L.'s *sign.*

Loschmidt, Joseph (Johann), Czechoslovakian chemist and physicist, 1821–1895. See L.'s *number.*

LOT Abbreviation for left occipitotransverse *position.*

lotion (lō'shŭn) [L. *lotio,* a washing, fr. *lavo,* to wash]. A class of pharmacopeial preparations that are liquid suspensions or dispersions intended for external application; some consist of finely powdered, insoluble solids held in more or less permanent suspension by suspending agents or surface-active agents, or both; others are oil-in-water emulsions stabilized by surface-active agents.

Louis, Pierre C.A., French physician, 1787–1872. See L.'s *angle, law.*

Louis-Bar, Denise. See L.-B. *syndrome.*

loupe (lūp) [Fr.]. A magnifying lens.

binocular l., a magnifying device, attached to spectacles or a headband, worn as a visual aid when performing operations on small structures.

louse, pl. **lice** (lows, līs) [A.S. *lūs*]. Common name for members of the ectoparasitic insect orders Anoplura (sucking lice) and Mallophaga (biting lice). Important species are *Felicola subrostrata* (cat l.), *Goniocotes gallinae* (fluff l.), *Goniodes dissimilis* (brown chicken l.), *Haemodipsus ventricosus* (rabbit l.), *Lipeurus caponis* (wing l.), *Menacanthus stramineus* (chicken body l.), *Phthirus pubis* (crab or pubic l.), and *Polyplax serratus* (mouse l.).

biting l., chewing l., feather l., ectoparasites (order Mallophaga) chiefly found on birds, where they feed on feathers, hair, epidermal debris, and (less commonly) on blood; they possess nipper-like, heavily sclerotized mandibles and a characteristic broad head;

many species are host-specific.
sucking l., bloodsucking mammalian ectoparasites (order Anoplura), characterized by a narrow head with piercing and sucking mouthparts that lie in a sac concealed in the head.

lousiness (low'zē-nes). Pediculosis.

lousy (low'sē). Pediculous.

lovastatin (lō-vă-stat'in). Mevinolin; a cholesterol-lowering agent, isolated from a strain of *Aspergillus terreus,* that reduces both normal and elevated serum cholesterol.

Lovén, Otto C., Swedish physician, 1835–1904. See L. *reflex.*

Lovibond's angle, Lovibond's profile sign. See under angle; sign.

Low, George C., British physician, 1872–1952. See Castellani-L. *sign.*

Lowe, Charles U., U.S. pediatrician, *1921. See L.'s *syndrome,* L.-Terrey-MacLachlan *syndrome.*

Löwe, Karl F., German optician, 1874–1955. See L.'s *ring.*

Löwenberg, Benjamin B., French laryngologist, 1836–1905. See L.'s *canal, forceps, scala.*

Löwenstein, L.W. See Buschke-L. *tumor.*

Lower, Richard, British anatomist and physiologist, 1631–1691. See L.'s *ring, tubercle.*

Lown, Bernard, U.S. cardiologist, *1921. See L.-Ganong-Levine *syndrome.*

Lowry, Brian, 20th century Canadian medical geneticist. See Coffin-L. *syndrome.*

Lowsley, Oswald S., U.S. urologist, *1884. See L. *tractor.*

loxapine (lok'să-pēn). 2-Chloro-11-(4-methyl-1-piperazinyl)dibenz[*b.f*][1,4]-oxazepine; an antianxiety agent used as the succinate and hydrochloride salts.

loxia (lok'sē-ă) [G. *loxos,* oblique, slanting]. Torticollis.

loxophthalmus (loks'of-thal'mŭs) [G. *loxos,* slanting, + *ophthalmos,* eye]. Obsolete term for strabismus.

Loxosceles (lok-sos'ĕ-lēz) [G. *loxos,* oblique, + *skelos,* leg]. A genus of venomous spiders, the brown spiders, marked by a fiddle-shaped pattern on the cephalothorax, and found chiefly in South America. They inflict a highly ulcerative, spreading dermal lesion at the site of the bite (loxoscelism). Important species include *L. laeta,* the Chilean brown spider; *L. reclusus,* the brown spider of North America; and *L. rufipes,* the Peruvian brown spider.

loxoscelism (lok-sos'ĕ-lizm). A clinical illness produced by the brown recluse spider, *Loxosceles reclusus,* of North America; characterized by gangrenous slough at the site of the bite, nausea, malaise, fever, hemolysis, and thrombocytopenia.

Loxotrema ovatum (lok-sō-trē'mă ō-vā'tŭm) [G. *loxos,* slanting, + *trēma,* a hole; L. *ovatus,* egg-shaped]. Former name for *Metagonimus yokogawai.*

lozenge (loz'enj) [Fr. *losange,* fr. *lozangé,* rhombic]. Troche.

LPH Abbreviation for lipotropic *hormone.*

L.P.N. Abbreviation for licensed practical *nurse.*

Lr Symbol for lawrentium.

Lr, L_r See under dose.

L.R.C.P. Abbreviation for Licentiate of the Royal College of Physicians (of England).

L.R.C.P.(E) Abbreviation for Licentiate of the Royal College of Physicians (Edinburgh).

L.R.C.P.(I) Abbreviation for Licentiate of the Royal College of Physicians (Ireland).

L.R.C.S. Abbreviation for Licentiate of the Royal College of Surgeons (of England).

L.R.C.S.(E) Abbreviation for Licentiate of the Royal College of Surgeons (Edinburgh).

L.R.C.S.(I) Abbreviation for Licentiate of the Royal College of Surgeons (Ireland).

LRF Abbreviation for luteinizing hormone-releasing *factor.*

L.R.F.P.S. Abbreviation for Licentiate of the Royal Faculty of Physicians and Surgeons, a Scottish institution.

LRH Abbreviation for luteinizing hormone-releasing *hormone.*

LSA Abbreviation for left sacroanterior *position.*

LSD Abbreviation for *lysergic acid* diethylamide.

LSP Abbreviation for left sacroposterior *position.*

LST Abbreviation for left sacrotransverse *position.*

LTH Abbreviation for luteotropic *hormone.*

LTM Abbreviation for long term *memory.*

Lu Symbol for lutetium.

Lubarsch, Otto, German pathologist, 1860– 1933. See L.'s *crystals.*

Luc, Henri, French laryngologist, 1855–1925. See L.'s *operation,* Caldwell-L. *operation,* Ogston-L. *operation.*

lucanthone hydrochloride (lū-kan'thōn). 1,2'-Diethylaminoethylamino-4-methylthiaxanthone hydrochloride; used in the treatment of urinary schistosomiasis (*Schistosoma haematobium*) and intestinal schistosomiasis (*S. mansoni*).

Lucas, Richard C., British anatomist and surgeon, 1846–1915. See L.'s *groove.*

lucensomycin (lū-sen-sō-mī'sin). Lucimycin; an antibiotic isolated from cultures of *Streptomyces lucensis;* an antifungal agent.

lucent (lū'sent) [L. *lucere,* to shine]. Bright; clear; translucent.

Lucibacterium (lū'si-bak-tēr-ē-ŭm) [L. *lucere,* to shine, + bacterium]. A genus of aerobic to facultatively anaerobic, motile, peritrichous bacteria containing Gram-negative rods. Their metabolism is fermentative, and they are usually luminescent. They occur on the surface of dead fish and in sea water. The type species is *L. harveyi.*
L. harveyi, *Photobacterium harveyi;* a species of luminescent bacteria found in sea water; it is the type species of the genus *L.*

lucid (lū'sid) [L. *lucidus,* clear]. Clear, not obscured or confused, as in a l. moment or spoken expression.

lucidification (lū-sid'i-fi-kā'shŭn) [L. *lucidus,* clear, + *facere,* to make]. Clarification.

lucidity (lū-sid'i-tē). The quality or state of being lucid.

luciferases (lū-sif'er-ās-ĕz) [L. *lux,* light + *fero,* to bear]. Enzymes present in certain luminous organisms that act to bring about the oxidation of luciferins; energy produced in the process is liberated as bioluminescence.

luciferins (lū-sif'er-inz). Chemical substances present in certain luminous organisms that, when acted upon by luciferases, produce bioluminescence.

lucifugal (lū-sif'yū-găl) [L. *lux,* light, + *fugio,* to flee from]. Avoiding light.

Lucilia (lū-sil'ē-ă). A genus of scavenging blowflies (family Calliphoridae), commonly called bluebottle or greenbottle flies, whose larvae feed on carrion or excrement; they occasionally cause wound infestation or myiasis.
L. cae'sar, a species whose larvae formerly were used in the treatment of septic wounds.
L. cupri'na, the most important cause of blowfly strike of sheep in Australia and South Africa.
L. illus'tris, a metallic blue-green blowfly widely distributed in North America; the eggs are deposited chiefly on animal carcasses.
L. serica'ta, *Phaenicia sericata.*

lucimycin (lū-si-mī'sin). Lucensomycin.

Lucio, R., Mexican physician, 1819–1866. See L's *leprosy,* leprosy *phenomenon.*

lucipetal (lū-sip'i-tăl) [L. *lux,* light, + *peto,* to seek]. Seeking light.

Lucké, Balduin, U.S. pathologist, 1889–1954. See L. *carcinoma;* L.'s *adenocarcinoma, virus.*

Lücke, George A., German surgeon, 1829–1894. See L.'s *test.*

Lückenschädel (luk-en-shā'dl) [Ger. *Lücke,* gap + *Schädel,* skull]. Craniolacunia.

lucotherapy (lū'kō-thār-ă-pē) [L. *lux,* light, + G. *therapeia,* therapy]. Phototherapy.

ludic (lū'dik) [G. *ludus,* game]. Playlike; playfully pretending.

Ludloff, Karl, Breslau surgeon, 1864–1945. See L.'s *sign.*

Ludwig, Daniel, German anatomist, 1625–1680. See L.'s *angle.*

Ludwig, Karl F.W., German anatomist and physiologist, 1816–1895. See depressor *nerve* of L.; L.'s *ganglion, labyrinth, nerve, stromuhr.*

Ludwig, Kurt, German anatomist, *1922. See Klinger-L. acid-thionin *stain.*

Ludwig, Wilhelm Friedrich von, German surgeon, 1790–1865. See L.'s *angina.*

Luebering, J. See Rapoport-L. *shunt.*

Luer, German instrument maker, †1883. See L. *syringe;* L.-Lok *syringe.*

lues (lū'ēz) [L. pestilence]. A plague or pestilence; specifically, syphilis.
l. vene'rea, syphilis.

luetic (lū-et'ik). Syphilitic.

Luft, John H., U.S. histologist, *1927. See L.'s potassium permanganate *fixative.*

Luft, Rolf. See L.'s *disease.*

Lugol, Jean G.A., French physician, 1786–1851. See L.'s iodine *solution.*

Lukes-Collins classification. See under classification.

LUL Abbreviation for left upper lobe (of lung).

luliberin (lū-lib'er-in). Luteinizing hormone-releasing hormone; a decapeptide hormone from the hypothalamus that stimulates the anterior pituitary to release both follicle-stimulating hormone and luteinizing hormone.

lumbago (lŭm-bā'gō) [L. fr. *lumbus,* loin]. Lumbar rheumatism; pain in mid and lower back; a descriptive term not specifying cause.
ischemic l., an intermittent claudication of the back; a vascular form of backache characterized by a painful cramp of the muscles in the lumbar region excited by the exertion of walking or standing and promptly relieved by rest.

lumbar (lŭm'bar) [L. *lumbus,* a loin]. Relating to the loins, or the part of the back and sides between the ribs and the pelvis.

lumbarization (lŭm'bar-i-zā'shŭn). A congenital anomaly of the lumbosacral junction characterized by lumbar development of the first sacral vertebra; there are six lumbar vertebrae instead of five.

lumbi (lŭm'bī) [L.]. Plural of lumbus.

lumboabdominal (lŭm'bō-ab-dom'i-năl). Relating to the sides and front of the abdomen.

lumbocolostomy (lŭm'bō-kō-los'tō-mē) [L. *lumbus,* loin, + G. *kolon,* colon, + *stoma,* mouth]. Formation of a permanent opening into the colon via an incision through the lumbar region.

lumbocolotomy (lŭm'bō-kō-lot'ō-mē) [L. *lumbus,* loin, + G. *kolon,* colon, + *tomē,* incision]. Incision into the colon through the lumbar region.

lumbocostal (lŭm'bō-kos'tăl) [L. *lumbus,* loin, + *costa,* rib]. **1.** Relating to the lumbar and the hypochondriac regions. **2.** Relating to the lumbar vertebrae and the ribs; denoting a ligament connecting the first lumbar vertebra with the neck of the twelfth rib.

lumboiliac (lŭm-bō-il'ē-ak). Lumboinguinal.

lumboinguinal (lŭm'bō-ing'gwi-năl) [L. *lumbus,* loin, + *inguen* (*inguin-*), groin]. Lumboiliac; relating to the lumbar and the inguinal regions.

lumbo-ovarian (lŭm-bō-ō-vā'rē-an). Relating to the ovary and the lumbar regions.

lumbosacral (lŭm'bō-sā'krăl). Sacrolumbar; relating to the lumbar vertebrae and the sacrum.

lumbrical (lŭm'bri-kăl) [L. *lumbricus,* earthworm]. Lumbricoid (1).

lumbricalis (lŭm-bri-kā'lis) [L. *lumbricus,* an earthworm]. See entries under *musculus* lumbricalis.

lumbricidal (lŭm-bri-sī'dăl). Destructive to lumbricoid (intestinal) worms.

lumbricide (lŭm'bri-sīd) [L. *lumbricus,* worm, + *caedo,* to kill]. An agent that kills lumbricoid (intestinal) worms.

lumbricoid (lŭm'bri-koyd) [L. *lumbricus,* earthworm, + G. *eidos,* resemblance]. **1.** Lumbricus (1); lumbrical; denoting or resembling a roundworm, especially *Ascaris lumbricoides.* See also scolecoid (2); vermiform. **2.** Obsolete common name for *Ascaris lumbricoides.*

lumbricosis (lŭm'bri-kō'sis). Infection with lumbricoids or round intestinal worms.

lumbricus (lŭm'bri-kŭs) [L. earthworm]. **1.** Lumbricoid (1). **2.** Obsolete name for *Ascaris lumbricoides.*

lumbus, gen. and pl. **lumbi** (lŭm'bŭs, -bī) [L.] [NA]. Loin; the part of the side and back between the ribs and the pelvis.

lumen, pl. **lumina, lumens** (lū'men, -min-ă, -menz) [L. light, window]. **1.** The space in the interior of a tubular structure, such as an artery or the intestine. **2.** The unit of luminous flux; the luminous flux emitted in a solid angle of 1 steradian by a uniform point source of light having a luminous intensity of 1 candela.
residual l., residual *cleft.*

lumichrome (lū'mi-krōm). 7,8-Dimethylalloxazine; riboflavin minus its ribityl side chain; produced by ultraviolet irradiation of riboflavin in acid solution.

lumiflavin (lū'mi-flā-vin). 7,8,10-Trimethylisoalloxazine; a yellow photoderivative of riboflavin, bearing a methyl group in place of the ribityl; produced by ultraviolet irradiation of riboflavin in alkaline solution.

lumina (lū'mi-nă) [L.]. Plural of lumen.

luminal (lū'mi-năl). Relating to the lumen of a blood vessel or other tubular structure.

luminescence (lū-mi-nes'ens) [L. *lumen,* light]. Emission of light from a body as a result of a chemical reaction. See bioluminescence.

luminiferous (lū-mi-nif'er-ŭs) [L. *lumen,* light, + *fero,* to carry]. Producing or conveying light.

luminophore (lū'mi-nō-fōr) [L. *lumen,* light, + G. *phoros,* bearing]. An atom or atomic grouping in an organic compound that increases its ability to emit light.

luminous (lū'mi-nŭs) [L. *lumen,* light]. Emitting light, with or without accompanying heat.

lumirhodopsin (lū'mi-rō-dop'sin). An intermediate between rhodopsin and all-*trans-* retinal plus opsin during bleaching of rhodopsin by light.

lumpectomy (lŭm-pek'tō-mē). A tylectomy, especially of a malignant lesion from the breast with preservation of essential anatomy of the breast.

Luna, Lee G., 20th century U.S. medical technologist. See L.-Ishak *stain.*

lunacy (lū'nă-sē) [L. *luna,* moon]. **1.** Formerly, a form of insanity characterized by alternating lucid and insane periods, believed to be influenced by phases of the moon. **2.** Any form of insanity. **3.** Insanity as defined variously by law.

lunar (lū'ner) [L. *luna,* moon]. **1.** Relating to the moon or to a month. **2.** Lunate (1); semilunar; resembling the moon in shape, especially a half moon. See also crescentic. **3.** Relating to silver (the moon was the symbol of silver in alchemy).

lunare (lū-nā'rē). *Os* lunatum.

lunate (lū'nāt). **1.** Lunar (2). **2.** Relating to the lunate bone (os lunatum).

lunatic (lū'nă-tik) [see lunacy]. Obsolete term for a mentally ill person.

lunatomalacia (lū-nā'tō-mă-lā'shē-ă). Kienböck's *disease.*

lung (lŭng) [A.S. *lungen*]. Pulmo; one of a pair of viscera occupying the cavity of the thorax, the organs of respiration in which aeration of the blood takes place. As a rule, the right l. is slightly larger than the left and is divided into three lobes (an upper, a middle, and a lower or basal), while the left has but two lobes (an upper and a lower or basal). Each l. is irregularly conical in shape, presenting a blunt upper extremity (the apex), a concave base following the curve of the diaphragm, an outer convex surface (facies costalis), an inner or mediastinal surface (facies mediastinalis), a thin and sharp anterior border (margo anterior), and a thick and rounded posterior border (margo posterior).

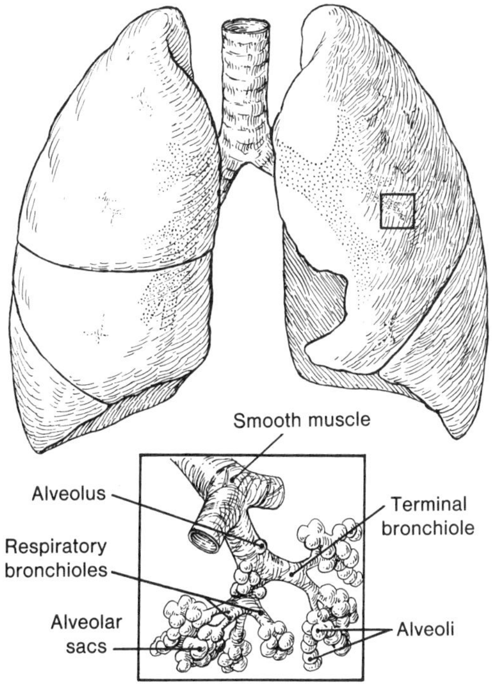

Lungs and Terminal Respiratory Units of Bronchial Tree

air-conditioner l., an extrinsic allergic alveolitis caused by forced air contaminated by thermophilic actinomycetes and other organisms.

bird-breeder's l., bird-fancier's l., bird-breeder's disease; extrinsic allergic alveolitis caused by inhalation of particulate avian emanations; sometimes specified by avian species, *e.g.,* pigeon-breeder's l., budgerigar-breeder's l.

black l., a form of pneumoconiosis, common in coal miners, characterized by deposit of carbon particles in the l.

butterfly l., hemorrhagic markings appearing on an animal's l. after inoculation with *Leptospira interrogans* (*L. icterohaemorrhagiae*).

cardiac l., disturbance in pulmonary anatomy and physiology secondary to valvular disease of the heart or to other disturbances of circulation incident to cardiac disease.

cheese worker's l., extrinsic allergic alveolitis caused by inhalation of spores of *Penicillium casei* from moldy cheese.

collier's l., anthracosis.

farmer's l., thresher's l.; a hypersensitivity pneumonitis characterized by fever and dyspnea, caused by inhalation of organic dust from moldy hay containing spores of actinomycetes such as *Micromonospora vulgaris, M. faeni, Thermopolyspora polyspora,* and certain true fungi, which thrive in the elevated temperatures of hay lofts and silos; repeated exposure may result in alveolar sensitization and, ultimately, granulomatous lung disease with severe l. disability.

fibroid l., chronic interstitial pneumonia in a l.

honeycomb l., the radiological and gross appearance of the l.'s resulting from diffuse fibrosis and cystic dilation of bronchioles; of unknown cause or a sequel of any of several diseases, including eosinophilic granuloma and sarcoidosis.

hyperlucent l., the radiographic finding that one l. is less dense than the other normal l., as from infection, bronchial foreign body, etc.

iron l., Drinker *respirator.*

malt-worker's l., extrinsic allergic alveolitis caused by inhalation of spores of *Aspergillus clavatus* and *A. fumigatus* from contaminated barley during the manufacture of beer.

mason's l., silicosis occurring in stone masons.

miner's l., anthracosis.

mushroom-worker's l., extrinsic allergic alveolitis caused by inhalation of spores of the mold *Thermopolyspora polyspora* or *Micromonospora vulgaris* from contaminated mushrooms under cultivation.

postperfusion l., a condition in which abnormal pulmonary function develops in patients who have undergone cardiac surgery involving the use of an extracorporeal circulation.

pump l., shock l.

quiet l., the collapse of a l. during thoracic operations undertaken to facilitate surgical procedure through absence of l. movement.

shock l., wet, white, or pump l.; in shock, the development of edema, impaired perfusion, and reduction in alveolar space so that the alveoli collapse.

thresher's l., farmer's l.

trench l., a psychogenic hyperventilation marked by paroxysmal attacks of rapid breathing, without any signs of organic disease, observed in stressful situations such as battle.

uremic l., uremic pneumonia (1); uremic pneumonitis; perihilar edema of the l. associated with renal failure and hypertension; the peripheral parts of the l. remain clear.

vanishing l., see vanishing lung *syndrome.*

welder's l., relatively benign form of pneumoconiosis, associated with welding, resulting from deposition of fine metallic particles in the l.

wet l., white l., shock l.

lungworms (lŭng'wermz). Nematodes that inhabit the air passages of animals, chiefly in the family Metastrongylidae (or Protostrongylidae). See *Dictyocaulus; Metastrongylus; Protostrogylus; Muellerius; Aelurostrongylus; Crenosoma.*

lunula, pl. **lunulae** (lū'nū-lă, -lē) [L. dim. of *luna,* moon]. **1** [NA]. Half-moon; selene unguium; the pale arched area at the proximal portion of the nail plate. **2.** A small semilunar structure.

azure l. of nails, bluish nonblanching discoloration of the lunulae of all the fingernails in hepatolenticular degeneration.
l. val'vulae semiluna'ris [NA], l. of the semilunar valve; the free border of a semilunar valve at each side of the nodulus valvulae semilunaris.

lupiform (lū'pi-fōrm). Lupoid.

lupinidine (lū-pin'i-dēn). Sparteine.

lupinosis (lū-pi-nō'sis) [L. *lupinus,* lupine, fr. *lupus,* wolf]. Lathyrism.

lupoid (lū'poyd) [L. *lupus* + G. *eidos,* resemblance]. Lupiform; resembling lupus.

lupous (lū'pŭs). Relating to lupus.

lupulin (lū'pū-lin). Humulin; a sticky, yellowish, granular material consisting of entire multicellular glandular hairs (trichomes) from the fruit and bracts of the hop vine, *Humulus lupulus;* the essential oils and resins of these glandular hairs are responsible for the characteristic bitter taste of beer or medicinals made from hops; has been used as an antispasmodic and sedative.

lupus (lū'pŭs) [L. wolf]. A term originally used to depict erosion (as if gnawed) of the skin, now used with modifying terms designating the various diseases listed below.
chronic discoid l. erythemato'sus, discoid l. erythematosus.
discoid l. erythemato'sus, chronic discoid l. erythematosus; a form of l. erythematosus in which only cutaneous lesions are present; these commonly appear on the face and are atrophic plaques with erythema, hyperkeratosis, follicular plugging, and telangiectasia; in some instances systemic l. erythematosis may develop.
disseminated l. erythemato'sus, systemic l. erythematosus.
l. erythemato'des, l. erythematosus.
l. erythemato'sus (LE), l. erythematodes or superficialis; an illness which may be chronic (characterized by skin lesions alone), subacute (characterized by recurring superficial nonscarring skin lesions that are more disseminate and present more acute features both clinically and histologically than those seen in the chronic discoid phase), or systemic or disseminated (in which the LE cell test may be positive and in which there is almost always involvement of vital structures. See also discoid l. erythematosus; systemic l. erythematosus.
l. erythemato'sus profun'dus, a subcutaneous panniculitis with marked lymphocyte infiltration of fat lobules giving rise to deep-seated, firm, rubbery nodules that sometimes become ulcerated, usually of the face; may occur in SLE with or without overlying skin lesions.
l. hypertroph'icus, l. tumidus; a form of l. vulgaris in which the tubercles are grouped into prominent hypertrophic nodules with deep-seated scarring, usually on the chin.
l. livi'do, persistent cyanotic lesions on the extremities, associated with the cutaneous manifestations of Raynaud's disease.
l. lymphat'icus, *lymphangioma* circumscriptum.
l. milia'ris dissemina'tus fa'ciei, a millet-like papular eruption of the face, associated with a positive anergy to tuberculin and (histopathologically) with tuberculoid structure.
l. mu'tilans, cutaneous tuberculosis with extensive destruction of tissue; *e.g.,* amputation of fingers, erosion of the skin or cartilage of the nose.
l. papillomato'sus, *tuberculosis* cutis verrucosa.
l. per'nio, sarcoid lesions, resembling those of frostbite, involving ears, cheeks, nose, hands, and fingers.
l. psori'asis, a form of l. vulgaris in which scaling predominates and simulates psoriasis.
l. sclero'sus, a permanent thickening of the skin due to excessive connective tissue formation in l. vulgaris lesions.
l. seba'ceus, l. erythematosus with lesions on the face in butterfly areas.
l. serpigino'sus, a cutaneous tuberculous lesion that spreads peripherally, healing centrally with scar formation.
l. superficia'lis, l. erythematosus.
systemic l. erythemato'sus (SLE), disseminated l. erythematosus; an inflammatory connective tissue disease with variable features, frequently including fever, weakness and fatigability, joint pains or arthritis resembling rheumatoid arthritis, diffuse erythematous skin lesions on the face, neck, or upper extremities, with liquefaction degeneration of the basal layer and epidermal atrophy, lymphadenopathy, pleurisy or pericarditis, glomerular lesions, anemia, hyperglobulinemia, and a positive LE cell test, with serum antinuclear antibodies.
l. tuberculo'sus, l. vulgaris.
l. tu'midus, l. hypertrophicus.
l. verruco'sus, *tuberculosis* cutis verrucosa.
l. vulga'ris, tuberculosis cutis luposa; l. tuberculosus; cutaneous tuberculosis with characteristic nodular lesions on the face, particularly about the nose and ears.
l. vulga'ris erythematoi'des, a form of cutaneous tuberculosis having a superficial resemblance to l. erythematosus.

LUQ Abbreviation for left upper quadrant (of abdomen).

lura (lū'ră) [L. the mouth of a bottle]. The contracted termination of the infundibulum of the brain.

lural (lū'răl). Pertaining to the lura.

Luschka, Hubert, German anatomist, 1820–1875. See L.'s *bursa, cartilage, ducts, gland,* cystic *glands, joints, ligaments, sinus, tonsil; foramen* of L.

Luse, Sarah A., 20th century U.S. physician. See L. *bodies.*

lusus naturae (lū'sŭs na-tū'rē) [L. a sport of nature]. A conspicuous congenital abnormality.

lute (lūt) [L. *lutum,* mud]. To seal or fasten with wax or cement.

luteal (lū'tē-ăl) [L. *luteus,* saffron-yellow]. Relating to the corpus luteum; l. cells, l. hormone, etc.

lutecium (lū-tē'sē-ŭm). Lutetium.

lutein (lū'tē-in) [L. *luteus,* saffron-yellow]. **1.** The yellow pigment in the corpus luteum, in the yolk of eggs, or any lipochrome. **2.** Xanthophyll. **3.** The dried powdered corpora lutea of the hog, formerly used as a progesterone source.

luteinization (lū'tē-in-i-zā'shŭn). Transformation of the mature ovarian follicle and its theca interna into a corpus luteum after ovulation; formation of luteal tissue.

luteinize (lū'tē-ī-nīz). To form luteal tissue.

luteinoma (lū'tē-i-nō'mă). Luteoma.

Lutembacher, René, French cardiologist, 1884–1916. See L.'s *syndrome.*

luteogenic (lū'tē-ō-jen'ik). Luteinizing; inducing the production or growth of corpora lutea.

luteohormone (lū'tē-ō-hōr'mōn). Progesterone.

luteol, luteole (lū'tē-ol, -ōl). Xanthophyll.

luteolin (lū-tē-ō'lin). Cyanidenon; 3′,4′,5,7-tetrahydroxyflavone; the aglycon of galuteolin and cynaroside.

luteolysin (lū-tē-ol'i-sin) [L. *luteus,* saffron-yellow, + G. *lysis,* dissolution]. Any agent, natural or compounded, that destroys the function of the corpus luteum.

luteolysis (lū-tē-ol'i-sis). Degeneration or destruction of ovarian luteinized tissue.

luteolytic (lū-tē-ō-lit'ik). Promoting or characteristic of luteolysis.

luteoma (lū-tē-ō'mă). Luteinoma; an ovarian tumor of granulosa or theca-lutein cell origin, producing progesterone effects on the uterine mucosa.
pregnancy l., a benign lutein cell tumor of the ovary.

luteotropic, luteotrophic (lū'tē-ō-trop'ik, -trof'ik). Having a stimulating action on the development and function of the corpus luteum.

luteotropin (lū'tē-ō-trō'pin). Luteotropic hormone; an anterior pituitary hormone whose action maintains the function of the corpus luteum.

lutetium (lū-tē'shē-ŭm) [L. *Lutetia,* Paris]. Lutecium; a rare earth element; symbol Lu, atomic no. 71, atomic weight 174.99.

luteus (lū-tē'ŭs) [L.] [NA]. Luteal.

Lutheran (Lu) blood group. See Blood Groups appendix.

lutropin (lū'trō-pin). Luteinizing hormone or principle; interstitial cell-stimulating h.; a glycoprotein h. that stimulates the final ripening of the follicles and the secretion of progesterone by them, their rupture to release the egg, and the conversion of the ruptured follicle into the corpus luteum.

lututrin (lū'tū-trin). A water-soluble protein-like fraction extracted from the corpus luteum of sows' ovaries, resembling relaxin; it causes uterine relaxation and is used in dysmenorrhea.

Lutz, Alfredo, 20th century Brazilian physician. See Lewandowski-L. *disease;* L.-Splendore-Almeida *disease.*

Lutzomyia (lūt-zō-mī'ă). A genus of New World sandflies or blood-sucking midges (family Psychodidae) that serve as vectors of leishmaniasis and Oroyo fever; formerly combined with the Old World sandfly genus *Phlebotomus.*

L. flaviscutella'ta, *Phlebotomus flaviscutellatus;* a sandfly species that is a vector of *Leishmania mexicana,* the agent of chiclero's ulcer.

L. interme'dius, one of a group of sandfly species that are vectors of *Leishmania braziliensis,* the agent of espundia.

L. longipal'pis, *Phlebotomus longipalpis.*

L. peruen'sis, a sandfly species that is a vector of *Leishmania peruviana,* the agent of uta.

lux (lŭks) [L. light]. Meter-candle; candle-meter; a unit of light or illumination; the reception of a luminous flux of 1 lumen per square meter of surface.

luxatio (lŭk-sā'shē-ō) [L. *luxo,* pp. *-atus,* to dislocate]. Luxation.

l. erec'ta, subglenoid dislocation of the head of the humerus; the arm is raised and abducted and cannot be lowered.

l. perinea'lis, a condition in which the head of the femur is dislocated to the perineum.

luxation (lŭk-sā'shŭn) [L. *luxatio*]. Luxatio. **1.** Dislocation. **2.** In dentistry, the dislocation or displacement of the condyle in the temporomandibular fossa, or of a tooth from the alveolus.

Malgaigne's l., nursemaid's *elbow.*

Luxol fast blue. Name for a group of closely related copper phthalocyanin dyes used as stains (with PAS, PTAH, hematoxylin, silver nitrate, etc.) for myelin in nerve fibers.

luxus (lŭks'ŭs) [L. extravagance, luxury]. Excess of any sort.

Luys, Jules B., French physician, 1828–1897. See L.'s *body; centre* médian de L.; *corpus* luysii; *nucleus* of L.

LVET Abbreviation for left ventricular ejection *time.*

L.V.N. Abbreviation for licensed vocational *nurse.*

Lw Former symbol for lawrencium.

lyase (lī'ās). Class name for those enzymes removing groups nonhydrolytically (EC class 4); prefixes such as "hydro-," "ammonia-," etc., are used to indicate the type of reaction. Trivial names for lyases include synthases, decarboxylases, aldolases, dehydratases. *Cf.* synthase; synthetase.

lycanthropy (lī-kan'thrō-pē) [G. *lykos,* wolf, + *anthropos,* man]. The morbid delusion that one is a wolf, possibly a mental atavism of the werewolf superstition.

lycoctonine (lī-kok'tō-nēn). An alkaloid, $C_{25}H_{41}NO_7$, obtained from *Aconitum lycoctonum,* an exceedingly poisonous species of aconite; it also occurs in other species of *Aconitum* and *Delphinium.*

lycopene (lī'kō-pēn). ψ,ψ-Carotene; the red pigment of the tomato that may be considered chemically as the parent substance from which all natural carotenoid pigments are derived; an unsaturated hydrocarbon made up of 8 isoprene units, two of them hydrogenated, with 11 conjugated double bonds.

lycopenemia (lī'kō-pē-nē'mē-ă) [lycopene + G. *haima,* blood]. A condition in which there is a high concentration of lycopene in the blood, producing carotenoid-like yellowish pigmentation of the skin; found in people who consume excessive amounts of tomatoes or tomato juice, or lycopene-containing fruits and berries.

Lycoperdon (līkō-per'don) [G. *lykos,* wolf, + *perdesthai,* to break wind]. Puffball; a genus of fungi (family Lycoperdaceae), some species of which have been used medicinally, *e.g.,* in folk medicine, by nasal inhalation to treat epistaxis. The spores of *L. bovista* (*L. gemmatum, L. caelatum*) and of *L. pyriforme* may rarely produce lycoperdonosis.

lycoperdonosis (lī'kō-per-don-ō'sis). A persisting pneumonitis following inhalation of spores of the puffballs *Lycoperdon pyriforme* and *L. bovista.*

lycophora (lī-kof'ō-ră). The 10-hooked larva of primitive tapeworms of the subclass Cestodaria.

lycopodium (lī-kō-pō'dē-ŭm) [G. *lykos,* wolf, + *pous,* foot]. Vegetable sulfur; club moss; the spores of *Lycopodium clavatum* (family Lycopodiaceae) and other species of *L.;* a yellow, tasteless, and odorless powder, used as a dusting powder and in pharmacy to prevent the agglutination of pills in a box.

lye (lī) [A.S. *leáh*] Lixivium; the liquid obtained by leaching wood ashes. See *potassium* hydroxide; *sodium* hydroxide.

Lyell, Aian. See L.'s *disease, syndrome.*

lygophilia (lī-gō-fil'ē-ă) [G. *lygē,* twilight, + *phileō,* to love]. Morbid preference for dark places.

lymecycline (lī-mē-sī'klēn). Tetracycline-methylene lysine; an antimicrobial agent.

Lymnaea (lim-nē'ă) [G. *limnē,* marsh]. A genus of snails, species of which are invertebrate hosts for the liver or sheep liver fluke, *Fasciola hepatica,* and other trematodes.

lymph-. See lympho-.

lymph (limf) [L. *lympha,* clear spring water]. Lympha; a clear, transparent, sometimes faintly yellow and slightly opalescent fluid that is collected from the tissues throughout the body, flows in the lymphatic vessels (through the lymph nodes), and is eventually added to the venous blood circulation. L. consists of a clear liquid portion, varying numbers of white blood cells (chiefly lymphocytes), and a few red blood cells.

aplastic l., corpuscular l.; l. containing a relatively large number of leukocytes, but comparatively little fibrinogen; such l. does not form a good clot and manifests only a slight tendency to become organized.

blood l., l. exuded from the blood vessels and not derived from the fluid in the tissue spaces.

corpuscular l., aplastic l.

croupous l., a form of inflammatory l. with an unusually large content of fibrinogen; as a result of the fibrin that is formed in relatively dense mats, a pseudomembrane is likely to be produced.

dental l., dentinal *fluid.*

euplastic l., l. that contains relatively few leukocytes, but a comparatively high concentration of fibrinogen; such l. clots fairly well and tends to become organized with fibrous tissue.

fibrinous l., a euplastic or croupous l.

inflammatory l., plastic l.; a faintly yellow, usually coagulable fluid (*i.e.,* euplastic l.) that collects on the surface of an acutely inflamed membrane or cutaneous wound.

intercellular l., the fluid in the potential spaces between cells in

the various organs and tissues.
intravascular l., l. within the lymphatic vessels, in contrast to intercellular l. and l. that has exuded from the vessels.
plastic l., inflammatory l.
tissue l., true l., *i.e.*, l. derived chiefly from fluid in tissue spaces (in contrast to blood l.).
vaccine l., vaccinia l., that collected from the vesicles of vaccinia infection, and used for active immunization against smallpox.

lympha (lim'fă) [L.] [NA]. Lymph.

lymphaden-. See lymphadeno-.

lymphaden (limf'ă-den) [lymph- + G. *adēn*, gland]. Lymphonodus.

lymphadenectomy (lim-fad-ĕ-nek'tō-mē) [lymphadeno- + G. *ektomē*, excision]. Excision of lymph nodes.

lymphadenitis (lim'-fad'ĕ-nī'tis) [lymphadeno- + G. *-itis*, inflammation]. Inflammation of a lymph node or lymph nodes.
caseous l., a specific disease of sheep caused by *Corynebacterium pseudotuberculosis* and characterized by slowly progressing caseation necrosis of the lymph nodes, particularly those of the thorax.
dermatopathic l., dermatopathic *lymphadenopathy.*
paratuberculous l., chronic inflammation of certain lymph nodes, not specifically tuberculous (*i.e.*, tubercle bacilli are not demonstrable), but associated with proved tuberculous inflammation in another part or organ of the body.
regional granulomatous l., cat-scratch *disease.*
tuberculous l., l. resulting from infection by *Mycobacterium tuberculosis.*

lymphadeno-, lymphaden- [L. *lympha*, spring water, + G. *adēn*, gland]. Combining forms relating to the lymph nodes.

lymphadenography (lim-fad'ĕ-nog'ră-fē) [lymphadeno- + G. *graphō*, to write]. X-ray visualization of lymph nodes after injection of a contrast medium; a type of lymphography.

lymphadenoid (lim-fad'ĕ-noyd) [lymphadeno- + G. *eidos*, resemblance]. Relating to, or resembling, or derived from a lymph node.

lymphadenoma (lim-fad'ĕ-nō'mă) [lymphadeno- + G. *-ōma*, tumor]. Lymphoadenoma. Obsolete term for: **1.** An enlarged lymph node. **2.** Hodgkin's disease.

lymphadenomatosis (lim-fad'ĕ-nō-mă-tō'sis). Obsolete term for a condition characterized by the presence of several to numerous enlarged lymph nodes, as in lymphosarcoma or Hodgkin's disease.

lymphadenopathy (lim-fad-ĕ-nop'ă-thē) [lymphadeno- + G. *pathos*, suffering]. Any disease process affecting a lymph node or lymph nodes.
angioimmunoblastic l., immunoblastic l.; acute or subacute generalized l. in older persons associated with polyclonal hypergammaglobulinemia, anemia, hepatosplenomegaly, fever, weight loss, and occasionally a rash, not responding to chemotherapy; the enlarged nodes show proliferation of immunoblasts, plasma cells, and capillaries surrounded by PAS-positive material; death may result from infection or subsequent development of lymphoma.
dermatopathic l., lipomelanic reticulosis; dermatopathic lymphadenitis; enlargement of lymph nodes, with proliferation of pale-staining interdigitating reticulum cells and macrophages containing fat and melanin; secondary to various forms of dermatitis, particularly with pruritus or exfoliation.
immunoblastic l., angioimmunoblastic l.

lymphadenosis (lim-fad'ĕ-nō'sis) [lymphadeno- + G. *-osis*, condition]. The basic underlying proliferative process that results in enlargement of lymph nodes, as in lymphocytic leukemia and certain inflammations.
benign l., infectious *mononucleosis.*
malignant l., obsolete term for malignant *lymphoma.*

lymphadenovarix (lim-fad'ĕ-nō-vā'riks) [lymphadeno- + L. *varix*]. Varicose deformity of a lymph node associated with lymphangiectasis.

lymphagogue (limf'ă-gog) [lymph + G. *agōgos*, drawing forth]. An agent that increases the formation and flow of lymph.

lymphangeitis (lim-fan'jē-ī'tis). Lymphangitis.

lymphangi-. See lymphangio-.

lymphangial (lim-fan'jē-ăl). Relating to a lymphatic vessel.

lymphangiectasis, lymphangiectasia (lim-fan'jē-ek'tă-sis, -ek-tā'zē-a) [lymphangio- + G. *ektasis*, a stretching]. Lymphectasia; telangiectasia lymphatica; dilation of the lymphatic vessels, the basic process that may result in the formation of a lymphangioma.
cavernous l., *lymphangioma* cavernosum.
cystic l., *lymphangioma* cysticum.
intestinal l., familial l. with intestinal loss of lymph causing lymphocytopenia and hypogammaglobulinemia.
simple l., *lymphangioma* simplex.

lymphangiectatic (lim-fan'jē-ek-tat'ik). Relating to or characterized by lymphangiectasis.

lymphangiectodes (lim-fan'jē-ek-tō'dēz) [lymphangio- + G. *ektasis*, a stretching, + *eidos*, appearance]. *Lymphangioma* circumscriptum.

lymphangiectomy (lim-fan'jē-ek'tō-mē) [lymphangio- + G. *ektomē*, excision]. Excision of a lymph channel.

lymphangiitis (lim-fan'jē-ī'tis). Lymphangitis.

lymphangio-, lymphangi- [L. *lympha*, spring water, + G. *angeion*, vessel]. Combining forms relating to the lymphatic vessels.

lymphangioendothelioma (lim-fan'jē-ō-en'dō-thē-lē-ō'mă). A neoplasm consisting of irregular groups or small masses of endothelial cells, as well as congeries of tubate structures that are thought to be derived from lymphatic vessels.

lymphangiography (lim-fan'jē-og'ră-fē) [lymphangio- + G. *graphō*, to write]. X-ray visualization of lymphatics and lymph nodes following the injection of a contrast medium; a type of lymphography.

lymphangiology (lim-fan-jē-ol'ō-jē) [lymphangio- + G. *logos*, study]. Lymphology; the branch of medical science concerned with the lymphatic vessels.

lymphangioma (lim-fan'jē-ō'mă) [lymphangio- + G. *-oma*, tumor]. Angioma lymphaticum; a fairly well circumscribed nodule or mass of lymphatic vessels or channels that vary in size, are usually greatly dilated, and are lined with normal endothelial cells; lymphoid tissue is usually present in the peripheral portions of the lesions, which are present at birth, or shortly thereafter, and probably represent anomalous development of lymphatic vessels (rather than true neoplasms); they occur most frequently in the neck and axilla, but may also develop in the arm, mesentery, retroperitoneum, and other sites.
l. capilla're varico'sum, l. circumscriptum.
l. caverno'sum, cavernous lymphangiectasia; a condition of conspicuous dilation of lymphatic vessels in a fairly circumscribed region, frequently with the formation of cavities or "lakes" filled with lymph.
l. circumscrip'tum, l. superficium simplex or capillare varicosum; lymphangiectodes; lupus lymphaticus; a congenital nevoid lesion consisting of a circumscribed group of tense lymph vesicles; the surface may be verrucous due to a thickened keratin layer over the vesicles.
l. cys'ticum, cystic lymphangiectasis; a condition characterized by a fairly well circumscribed group of several or numerous, cyst-like, dilated vessels or spaces lined with endothelium and filled with lymph.
l. sim'plex, simple lymphangiectasis; a circumbscribed region or focus of several to numerous lymphatic vessels that are moderately dilated.
l. superfic'ium sim'plex, l. circumscriptum.
l. tubero'sum mul'tiplex, a cutaneous lesion characterized by mul-

tiple, slightly red, cystlike nodules (located chiefly on the trunk), resulting from fairly large lymphatic vessels and spaces, and groups of proliferating endothelial cells; the lesion has some gross resemblance to spiradenoma, except for the characteristic location.

l. xanthelasmoid'eum, a capillary l. with colloid degeneration of the elastic tissues of the skin, characterized by yellow-brown or gray-brown plaques that may be only slightly raised above the surface of the skin.

lymphangiomatous (lim-fan'jē-ō'mă-tŭs). Pertaining to, characterized by, or containing lymphangioma.

lymphangion (lim-fan'jē-on) [L. *lympha,* lymph, + G. *angeion,* vessel]. A lymphatic vessel. See *vasa* lymphatica.

lymphangiophlebitis (lim-fan'jē-ō-flĕ-bī'tis). Inflammation of the lymphatic vessels and veins.

lymphangioplasty (lim-fan'jē-ō-plas-tē) [lymphangio- + G. *plastos,* formed]. Lymphoplasty; surgical alteration of lymphatic vessels.

lymphangiosarcoma (lim-fan'jē-ō-sar-kō'mă). A malignant neoplasm derived from vascular tissue, *i.e.*, an angiosarcoma, in which the neoplastic cells originate from the endothelial cells of lymphatic vessels, usually developing in the arm several years after radical mastectomy.

lymphangiotomy (lim-fan'jē-ot'ō-mē) [lymphangio- + G. *tomē,* incision]. Incision of lymphatic vessels.

lymphangitis (lim-fan-jī'tis) [lymphangio- + G. *-itis,* inflammation]. Lymphangeitis; lymphangiitis; inflammation of the lymphatic vessels.

l. carcinomato'sa, extensive lymphatic permeation by tumor cells, with surrounding fibrosis, producing visible or palpable cords, especially in pleura or skin overlying a carcinoma.

epizootic l., l. epizoot'ica, l. primarily involving the lymph channels of the skin of the legs and chest of horses and mules in Europe, Asia, and Africa; the causative agent is *Histoplasma capsulatum* var. *farciminosum.*

lymphapheresis (lim'fă-fĕ-rē'sis). Lymphocytapheresis.

lymphatic (lim-fat'ik) [L. *lymphaticus,* frenzied; Mod. L. use, of or for lymph]. **1.** Pertaining to lymph, a vascular channel that transports lymph, or a lymph node. **2.** Sometimes used to pertain to a sluggish or phlegmatic characteristic.

afferent l., *vas* afferens (3).

efferent l., *vas* efferens (3).

lymphaticostomy (lim-fat-i-kos'tō-mē) [lymphatic + G. *stoma,* mouth]. Making an opening into a lymphatic duct.

lymphatitis (lim-fă-tī'tis) [lymphatic + G. *-itis,* inflammation]. Inflammation of the lymphatic vessels or lymph nodes.

lymphatology (lim-fă-tol'ō-jē) [lymphatic + G. *logos,* study]. The study of the lymphatic system.

lymphatolysis (lim'fă-tol'i-sis) [lymphatic + G. *lysis,* dissolution]. Destruction of the lymphatic vessels or lymphoid tissue, or both.

lymphatolytic (lim'fă-tō-lit'ik). Pertaining to or characterized by lymphatolysis.

lymphectasia (lim-fek-tā'zē-ă) [lymph + G. *ektasis,* a stretching]. Lymphangiectasis.

lymphedema (limf'e-dē'mă) [lymph + G. *oidēma,* a swelling]. Swelling (especially in subcutaneous tissues) as a result of obstruction of lymphatic vessels or lymph nodes and the accumulation of large amounts of lymph in the affected region.

congenital l., see hereditary l.

hereditary l., trophedema; permanent pitting edema usually confined to the lower extremities; two types, congenital (Milroy's disease), or with onset at about the age of puberty (Meige's disease); autosomal dominant inheritance.

l. pre'cox, primary l.

primary l., l. precox; a form of l. observed chiefly in young women and girls, characterized by diffuse swelling of the lower extremities.

lymphemia (lim-fē'mē-ă) [lymph(ocyte) + G. *haima,* blood]. The presence of unusually large numbers of lymphocytes or their precursors, or both, in the circulating blood.

lymphization (lim-fi-zā'shŭn). The formation of lymph.

lympho-, lymph- [L. *lympha,* spring water]. Combining forms relating to lymph.

lymphoadenoma (lim'fō-ad'ĕ-nō'mă). Lymphadenoma.

lymphoblast (lim'fō-blast) [lympho- + G. *blastos,* germ]. Lymphocytoblast; a young immature cell that matures into a lymphocyte and is characterized by more abundant cytoplasm, a nucleus in which the chromatin is finer than that in a lymphocyte (but coarser than that in the myeloblast), and one or two rather prominent nucleoli.

lymphoblastic (lim-fō-blas'tik). Pertaining to the production of lymphocytes.

lymphoblastoma (lim-fō-blas-tō'mă) [lymphoblast + G. *-oma,* tumor]. A form of malignant lymphoma in which the chief cells are lymphoblasts.

giant follicular l., nodular *lymphoma.*

lymphoblastosis (lim'fō-blas-tō'sis) [lymphoblast + G. *-osis,* condition]. The presence of lymphoblasts in the peripheral blood; sometimes used as a synonym for acute lymphocytic leukemia.

lymphocele (lim'fō-sēl) [lympho- + G. *kēlē,* tumor]. Lymphocyst; a cystic mass that contains lymph, usually from diseased or injured lymphatic channels.

lymphocerastism (lim-fō-ser'as-tizm) [lympho- + G. *kerastos,* mixed, mingled]. The process of formation of cells in the lymphocytic series.

lymphocinesis, lymphocinesia (lim'fō-si-nē'sis, nē-zē-ă). Lymphokinesis.

lymphocyst (lim'fō-sist) [lympho- + G. *kystis,* bladder]. Lymphocele.

lymphocytapheresis (lim'fō-sī-tă-fĕ-rē'sis) [lymphocyte + G. *aphairesis,* a withdrawal]. Lymphapheresis; separation and removal of lymphocytes from the withdrawn blood, with the remainder of the blood retransfused into the donor.

lymphocyte (lim'fō-sīt) [lympho- + G. *kytos,* call]. Lymph cell; lympholeukocyte; a white blood cell formed in lymphatic tissue throughout the body (*e.g.,* lymph nodes, spleen, thymus, tonsils, Peyer's patches, and sometimes in bone marrow) and in normal adults comprising approximately 22 to 28% of the total number of leukocytes in the circulating blood. L.'s are generally small (7 to 8 μm), but larger forms are frequent (10 to 20 μm); with Wright's (or a similar) stain, the nucleus is deeply colored (purple-blue), and is composed of dense aggregates of chromatin within a sharply defined nuclear membrane; the nucleus is usually round, but may be slightly indented, and is eccentrically situated within a relatively small amount of light blue cytoplasm that ordinarily contains no granules; especially in larger forms, the cytoplasm may be fairly abundant and include several bright red-violet fine granules; in contrast to granules of the myeloid series of cells, those in l.'s do not yield a positive oxidase or peroxidase reaction.

B l., B cell (2); an immunologically important l. that is not thymus-dependent, is of short life, and resembles the bursa-derived l. of birds in that it is responsible for the production of immunoglobulins, *i.e.,* it is the precursor of the plasma cell and does not play a role in cell-mediated immunity. See also T l.

Rieder's l., an abnormal form of l. that has a greatly indented (or lobed), slightly twisted nucleus; such cells are usually observed in certain examples of chronic lymphocytic leukemia.

T l., T cell; a thymocyte-derived l. of immunological importance that is long-lived (months to years) and is responsible for cell-me-

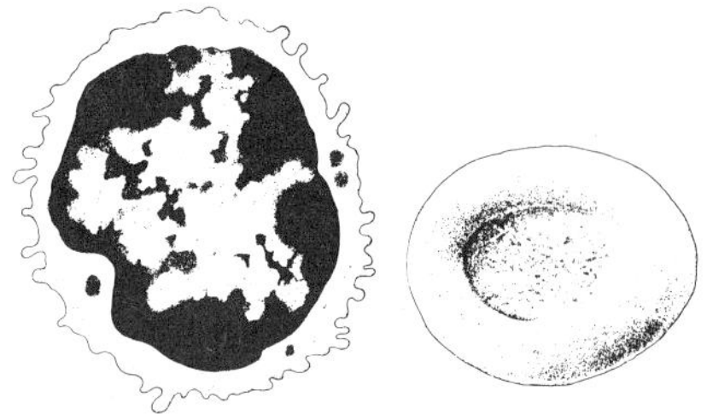

Human Lymphocyte
As seen under the electron microscope, with erythrocyte (right), to show comparative sizes.

diated immunity. T l.'s form rosettes with sheep erythrocytes and, in the presence of transforming agents (mitogens), differentiate and divide. See also B l.

transformed l., see lymphocyte *transformation.*

lymphocythemia (lim'fō-sī-thē'mē-ă). Lymphocytosis.

lymphocytic (lim-fō-sit'ik). Pertaining to or characterized by lymphocytes.

lymphocytoblast (lim-fō-sī'tō-blast) [lymphocyte, + G. *blastos,* germ]. Lymphoblast.

lymphocytoma (lim'fō-sī-tō'mă) [lymphocyte + G. *-oma,* tumor]. A circumscribed nodule or mass of mature lymphocytes, grossly resembling a neoplasm.

benign l. cutis, Spiegler-Fendt pseudolymphoma or sarcoid; a skin nodule caused by dense infiltration of the dermis by lymphocytes and histiocytes, often forming lymphoid follicles, separated from the epidermis by a narrow noninfiltrating layer.

lymphocytopenia (lim'fō-sī-tō-pē'nē-ă). Lymphopenia.

lymphocytopoiesis (lim'fō-sī-tō-poy-ē'sis) [lymphocyte + G. *poiēsis,* a making]. The formation of lymphocytes.

lymphocytosis (lim'fō-sī-tō'sis). Lymphocytic leukocytosis; lymphocythemia; a form of actual or relative leukocytosis in which there is an increase in the number of lymphocytes.

lymphoderma (lim'fō-der'mă) [lympho- + G. *derma,* skin]. A condition resulting from any disease of the cutaneous lymphatic vessels.

l. pernicio'sa, obsolete term for *leukemia* cutis.

lymphoduct (lim'fō-dŭkt) [lympho- + L. *ductus,* a leading]. A lymphatic vessel. See *vasa* lymphatica.

lymphoepithelioma (lim'fō-ep-i-thē-lē-ō'mă). A poorly differentiated radiosensitive squamous cell carcinoma involving lymphoid tissue in the region of the tonsils and nasopharynx; composed of irregular sheets, or small groups, of neoplastic epithelial cells (squamous or undifferentiated), with a slight to moderate amount of fibrous stroma that contains numerous lymphocytes; metastasizes at an early stage to cervical lymph nodes.

lymphogenesis (lim-fō-gen'ē-sis) [lympho- + G. *genesis,* production]. Lymph production.

lymphogenic (lim-fō-jen'ik). Lymphogenous (1).

lymphogenous (lim-foj'ē-nŭs). **1.** Lymphogenic; originating from lymph or the lymphatic system. **2.** Producing lymph.

lymphoglandula (lim-fō-glan'dū-lă). Lymphonodus.

lymphogranuloma (lim'fō-gran-yū-lō'mă). **1.** Old nonspecific term used with reference to a few basically dissimilar diseases in which the pathologic processes result in granulomas or granuloma-like lesions, especially in various groups of lymph nodes (which then become conspicuously enlarged). **2.** Old term for Hodgkin's disease.

l. benig'num, old term for sarcoidosis.

l. inguina'le, venereal l.

l. malig'num, old term for Hodgkin's disease.

Schaumann's l., old eponym for sarcoidosis.

venereal l., l. vene'reum, a venereal infection usually caused by *Chlamydia trachomatis,* and characterized by a transient genital ulcer and inguinal adenopathy in the male; in the female, perirectal lymph nodes are involved and rectal stricture is a common occurrence. Also called l. inguinale; lymphopathia venereum; climatic or tropical bubo; sixth veneral disease; Nicolas-Favre disease.

lymphogranulomatosis (lim-fō-gran'yū-lō-mă-tō'sis). Any condition characterized by the occurrence of multiple and widely distributed lymphogranulomas.

lymphography (lim-fog'ră-fē) [lympho- + *graphō,* to write]. Visualization of lymphatics (lymphangiography), lymph nodes (lymphadenography), or both by roentgenography following the injection of a contrast medium.

lymphohistiocytosis (lim'fō-his'tē-ō-sī-tō'sis). Proliferation or infiltration of lymphocytes and histiocytes.

lymphoid (lim'foyd) [lympho- + G. *eidos,* appearance]. **1.** Resembling lymph or lymphatic tissue, or pertaining to the lymphatic system. **2.** Adenoid (1).

lymphoidectomy (lim-foy-dek'tō-mē) [lymphoid + G. *ektomē,* excision]. Excision of lymphoid tissue.

lymphoidocyte (lim-foy'dō-sīt). A primitive mesenchymal cell believed to be capable of differentiating into all types of lymphoid cells, including lymphocytes, littoral cells, and reticular cells of lymph nodes.

lymphokines (lim'fō-kīnz). Soluble substances, released by sensitized lymphocytes on contact with specific antigen, which help effect cellular immunity by stimulating activity of monocytes and macrophages; these include, among others, chemotactic, mitogenic (blastogenic), migration-inhibitory, and transfer factors, lymphotoxin, and interleukin-2.

lymphokinesis (lim'fō-ki-nē'sis) [lympho- + G. *kinēsis,* movement]. Lymphocinesia; lymphocinesis. **1.** Circulation of lymph in the lymphatic vessels and through the lymph nodes. **2.** Movement of endolymph in the semicircular canals of the inner ear.

lympholeukocyte (lim'fō-lū'kō-sīt). Lymphocyte.

lymphology (lim-fol'ō-jē) [lympho- + G. *logos,* study]. Lymphangiology.

lymphoma (lim-fō'mă) [lympho- + G. *-oma,* tumor]. Malignant l.; general term for ordinarily malignant neoplasms of lymphoid and reticuloendothelial tissues which present as apparently circumscribed solid tumors composed of cells that appear primitive or resemble lymphocytes, plasma cells, or histiocytes. L.'s appear most frequently in lymph nodes, spleen, or other normal sites of lymphoreticular cells; when disseminated, l.'s, especially of the lymphocytic type, may invade the peripheral blood and manifest as leukemia. L.'s are classified by cell type, degrees of differentiation, and nodular or diffuse pattern; Hodgkin's disease and Burkitt's l. are special forms.

adult T cell l. (ATL), adult T-cell leukemia; an acute or subacute disease associated with a human T-cell virus, with lymphadenopathy, hepatosplenomegaly, skin lesions, peripheral blood involvement, and hypercalcemia.

benign l. of the rectum, lymphoid polyp; a rectal polyp composed of lymphoid tissue with follicle formation, covered by mucosa.

Burkitt's l., a form of malignant l. reported in African children, frequently involving facial bones, ovaries, and abdominal lymph nodes, which are infiltrated by undifferentiated stem cells with scattered pale macrophages containing nuclear debris; undifferentiated cells show numerous mitoses from lymphoid germinal center B-cells. Geographical distribution of Burkitt's l. suggests that it may be transmitted by biting insects and caused by Epstein-Barr virus; occasional cases of l. with similar features have been reported in the United States.

diffuse small cleaved cell l., diffuse poorly differentiated lymphocytic l.; follicular center cell l.'s that lack a follicular pattern; malignancy is of intermediate grade.

follicular l., nodular l.

follicular predominantly large cell l., nodular histiocytic l.; a B-cell l. of intermediate malignancy.

follicular predominantly small cleaved cell l., poorly differentiated lymphocytic l.

histiocytic l., reticulum cell sarcoma; a malignant tumor of reticular tissue composed predominantly of neoplastic histiocytes. See also large cell l.

immunoblastic l., immunoblastic sarcoma; a monomorphous proliferation of immunoblasts involving the lymph nodes; it may develop in some patients with angioimmunoblastic lymphadenopathy.

large cell l., l. composed of large mononuclear cells of undetermined type. Many l.'s formerly classified as histiocytic have in recent years been shown to consist of large lymphocytes.

Lennert's l., Lennert's lesion; malignant l. with a high proportion of diffusely scattered epitheliod cells. tonsillar involvement, and an unpredictable course.

lymphoblastic l., a diffuse l. in children, with supradiaphragmatic distribution and T-lymphocytes having convoluted nuclei; many patients develop acute lymphoblastic leukemia.

malignant l., lymphoma.

Mediterranean l., immunoproliferative small intestine *disease.*

nodular l., follicular l.; giant follicular lymphoblastoma; Brill-Symmers disease; malignant l. arising from lymphoid follicular B cells which may be small or large, growing in a nodular pattern.

nodular histiocytic l., follicular predominantly large cell l.

non-Hodgkin's l., a l. other than Hodgkin's disease, classified by Rappaport into a nodular or diffuse tumor pattern and by cell type; a working or international formulation separates such l.'s into low, intermediate, and high grade malignancy and into cytologic subtypes reflecting follicular center cell or other origin.

poorly differentiated lymphocytic l. (PDLL), follicular predominantly small, cleaved cell l.; a B-cell l. with nodular or diffuse lymph node or bone marrow involvement by large lymphoid cells.

small lymphocytic l., well differentiated lymphocytic l.

well differentiated lymphocytic l. (WDLL), small lymphocytic l.; essentially the same disease as chronic lymphocytic leukemia, except that lymphocytes are not increased in the peripheral blood; lymph nodes are enlarged and other lymphoid tissue or bone marrow is infiltrated by small lymphocytes.

lymphomatoid (lim-fō'mă-toyd). Resembling a lymphoma.

lymphomatosis (lim'fō-mă-to'sis). Any condition characterized by the occurrence of multiple, widely distributed sites of involvement with lymphoma.

avian l., fowl l.; a group of virus-induced transmissible diseases of chickens and some other birds in which there is lymphoid cell infiltration or formation of lymphomatous tumors in various tissues and organs; the two principal diseases are: 1) the avian leukosis-sarcoma complex-induced lymphoid leukosis, involving the bursa fabricii and various visceral organs; 2) Marek's disease, caused by the avian lymphomatosis virus and involving primarily the peripheral nerves and gonads and, to a lesser and more variable extent, other visceral organs, skin, muscle, and the eye. Variability of lesion site prompted other names for avian l., such as big liver disease, ocular l., visceral l. neurolymphomatosis gallinarum, and fowl paralysis.

fowl l., avian l.

ocular l., see avian l.

visceral l., see avian l.

lymphomatous (lim-fō'mă-tŭs). Pertaining to or characterized by lymphoma.

lymphomyeloma (lim'fō-mī'ĕ-lō'mă) [lympho- + G. *myelos,* marrow, + *-oma,* tumor]. A medullary neoplasm that consists of uninuclear, relatively small cells with morphologic features resembling those of lymphocytic forms.

lymphomyxoma (lim'fō-mik-sō'mă) [lympho- + G. *myxa,* mucus, + *-oma,* tumor]. A soft nonmalignant neoplasm that contains lymphoid tissue in a matrix of loose, areolar connective tissue.

LYMPHONODUS

lymphonodus, pl. **lymphonodi** (lim'fō-nō'dŭs, -nō'dī) [lympho- + L. *nodus,* node] [NA]. Lymph node or gland; nodus lymphaticus; lymphoglandula; lymphaden; one of numerous round, oval, or bean-shaped bodies located along the course of lymphatic vessels, varying greatly in size (1 to 25 mm in diameter) and usually presenting a depressed area, the hilum, on one side through which blood vessels enter and efferent lymphatic vessels emerge. The structure consists of a fibrous capsule and internal trabeculae supporting lymphoid tissue and lymph sinuses; lymphoid tissue is arranged in nodules in the cortex and cords in the medulla of a node, with afferent vessels entering at many points of the periphery.

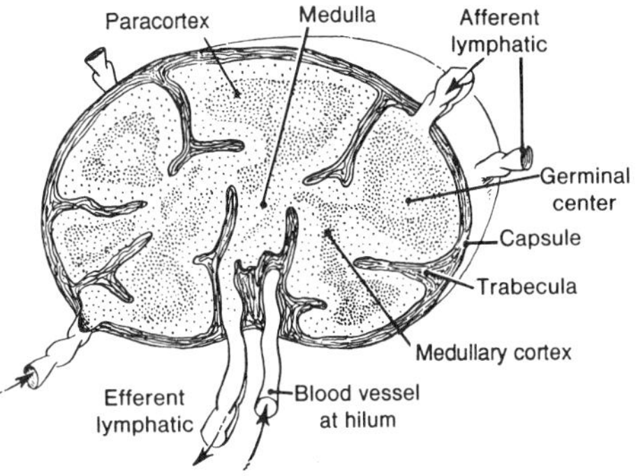

Lymphonodus (cross section)

lymphono'di abdom'inis viscera'les [NA], visceral abdominal lymph nodes; the numerous lymph nodes associated with the visceral branches of the aorta.

lymphono'di anorecta'les [NA], alternate term for lymphonodi pararectales.

lymphono'di appendicula'res [NA], appendicular lymph nodes; nodes along the appendicular artery; they receive afferent vessels from the vermiform appendix and send efferent vessels to the ileocolic lymph nodes.

l. ar'cus ve'na az'ygos [NA], lymph node of azygos arch; a lymph node of the posterior mediastinal group located adjacent to the arch of the azygos vein.

lymphono'di axilla'res [NA], axillary lymph nodes; axillary glands; numerous nodes around the axillary veins which receive the lymphatic drainage from the upper limb, shoulder girdle, and mammary gland; they drain into the subclavian trunk.

lymphono'di brachia'les [NA], brachial lymph nodes; lateral axillary lymph nodes; lymph nodes along the brachial vein that receive lymph drainage from most of the free superior limb and send efferent vessels to the axillary lymph nodes.

lymphono'di bronchopulmona'les, bronchopulmonary lymph nodes.

lymphono'di cervica'les anterio'res [NA], anterior cervical lymph nodes; the group of lymph nodes located in the anterior region of the neck, divided into superficial and deep groups: **l. c. anterio'res**

superficia'les, superficial anterior cervical lymph nodes; the lymph nodes in the subcutaneous tissue of the anterior region of the neck; **l. c. anterio'res profun'di,** deep anterior cervical lymph nodes; the lymph nodes near the larynx, trachea, and thyroid gland.

lymphono'di cervica'les latera'les profun'di [NA], deep lateral cervical lymph nodes; the lymph nodes located in the posterior triangle of the neck beneath the deep cervical fascia; they empty into the jugular trunk on the right or left side; the group is subdivided into four smaller chains: lymphonodi jugulares anteriores; lymphonodi jugulares laterales; lymphonodi comitantes nervi accessorii; and lymphonodi supraclaviculares.

lymphono'di cervica'les latera'les superficia'les [NA], superficial lateral cervical lymph nodes; one to four nodes lying along the external jugular vein; they drain the skin and superficial structures over the region of the sternocleidomastoid muscle and send efferent vessels to the deep lateral cervical lymph nodes.

lymphono'di coeli'aci [NA], celiac lymph nodes; celiac glands; nodes located along the celiac trunk which drain lymph from the stomach, duodenum, pancreas, spleen, and biliary tract.

lymphono'di col'ici dex'tri [NA], right colic lymph nodes; nodes located along the right colic artery that drain the upper part of the ascending colon.

lymphono'di col'ici me'dii [NA], middle colic lymph nodes; nodes along the middle colic artery and its branches that drain the right colic flexure and most of the transverse colon.

lymphono'di col'ici sinis'tri [NA], left colic lymph nodes; small nodes along the left colic artery and its branches that drain the left flexure and upper part of the descending colon; efferent vessels pass to the inferior mesenteric nodes.

lymphono'di comitan'tes ner'vi accesso'rii, companion lymph nodes of accessory nerve; accessory nerve lymph nodes; the nodes of the deep lateral cervical group that are located along the accessory nerve; their efferent vessels pass to the supraclavicular lymph nodes.

lymphono'di cubita'les [NA], cubital lymph nodes; lymph nodes of elbow; epitrochlear nodes; two groups of nodes, superficial and deep, lying along the basilic vein above the medial epicondyle; they receive afferents from the ulnar side of the forearm and hand, and send efferents to the brachial nodes.

lymphono'di epigas'trici inferio'res [NA], inferior epigastric lymph nodes; three or four nodes placed along the inferior epigastric vessels; they receive afferents from the lower abdominal wall and empty into the external iliac nodes.

lymphono'di facia'les [NA], facial lymph nodes; a chain of lymph nodes lying along the facial artery that receive afferent vessels from the eyelids, nose, cheek, lip, and gums, and send efferent vessels to the submandibular nodes.

lymphono'di gas'trici dex'tri [NA], right gastric lymph nodes; small nodes along the course of the right gastric artery that drain part of the lesser curvature of the stomach.

lymphono'di gas'trici sinis'tri [NA], left gastric lymph nodes; superior gastric lymph nodes; nodes located along the left gastric artery and its branches; they are divided into paracardial, upper and lower groups.

lymphono'di gastro-omenta'les dex'tri [NA], right gastro-omental or gastroepiploic lymph nodes; inferior gastric lymph nodes; nodes located in the greater omentum along the right gastroepiploic artery that drain part of the greater curvature of the stomach and the greater omentum.

lymphono'di gastro-omenta'les sinis'tri [NA], left gastro-omental or gastroepiploic lymph nodes; nodes located in the greater omentum along the left gastroepiploic artery that drain part of the greater curvature of the stomach and greater omentum.

lymphono'di glutea'les [NA], gluteal lymph nodes; nodes of the internal iliac group; They are subdivided into two groups: **l. g. inferio'res,** located along the inferior gluteal artery; **l. g. superio'res,** located along the superior gluteal artery.

lymphono'di hepat'ici [NA], hepatic lymph nodes; nodes located along the hepatic artery as far as the porta hepatis; they drain the liver, gallbladder, stomach, duodenum, and pancreas, and send efferents to the celiac nodes.

lymphono'di ileocol'ici [NA], ileocolic lymph nodes; nodes located along the ileocolic artery that drain lymph from the ascending colon to the superior mesenteric nodes.

lymphono'di ili'aci commu'nes [NA], common iliac lymph nodes; nodes located in association with the common iliac artery; they are subdivided into five groups: **l. i. c. interme'dii,** between the artery and the common iliac vein; **l. i. c. latera'les,** lateral to the artery; **l. i. c. media'les,** medial to the artery; **l. i. c. promonto'rii,** at the sacral promontory; and **l. i. c. subaor'tici,** at the bifurcation of the aorta; they all receive afferent vessels from the external and internal iliac nodes and send efferent vessels to the lumbar nodes.

lymphono'di ili'aci exter'ni [NA], external iliac lymph nodes; nodes located in association with the external iliac artery; they are subdivided into three groups: **l. i. e. interme'dii,** between the artery and the external iliac vein; **l. i. e. latera'les,** lateral to the artery; and **l. i. e. media'les,** medial to the artery; they all receive afferent vessels from the inguinal nodes, lower abdominal wall, and pelvic viscera, and send efferent vessels to the common iliac nodes.

lymphono'di ili'aci inter'ni [NA], internal iliac lymph nodes; nodes that lie along the internal iliac artery and its branches; they receive lymph from the pelvic viscera, the gluteal region, and the deep parts of the perineum, and send efferent vessels to the common iliac nodes.

lymphono'di inguina'les profun'di [NA], deep inguinal lymph nodes; several small nodes deep to the fascia lata and medial to the femoral vein; they receive lymph from the deep structures of the lower limb, from the glans penis and from superficial inguinal nodes; efferents pass to the external iliac nodes.

lymphono'di inguina'les superficia'les [NA], superficial inguinal lymph nodes; a group of 12 to 20 nodes that lie in the subcutaneous tissue below the inguinal ligament and along the terminal part of the great saphenous vein; they drain the skin and subcutaneous tissue of the lower abdominal wall, perineum, buttock, external genitalia, and lower limb; they are subdivided into three groups: **l. i. inferio'res,** located inferior to the saphenous opening; **l. i. superolatera'les,** located lateral to the saphenous opening; and **l. i. superomedia'les,** located medial to the saphenous opening.

lymphono'di intercosta'les [NA], intercostal lymph nodes; one or two small nodes located posteriorly in each intercostal space; they receive lymph from the parietal pleura, intercostal space, and posterior body wall; the nodes in the upper spaces empty into the thoracic duct; the nodes in the lower spaces form a descending intercostal trunk that opens into the cisterna chyli.

lymphono'di interili'aci [NA], interiliac lymph nodes; several lymph nodes located between the external and internal iliac arteries and the obturator artery; these nodes are considered by some to be part of the medial external iliac nodes.

lymphono'di interpectora'les [NA], interpectoral or pectoral lymph nodes; small lymph nodes located between the pectoralis major and minor muscles; they receive lymph from the muscles and the mammary gland, and deliver lymph to the axillary lymphatic plexus.

lymphono'di jugula'res anterio'res [NA], anterior jugular lymph nodes; nodes of the deep lateral cervical group located anterior to the internal jugular vein; two nodes are specifically named: n. jugulodigastricus and n. jugulo-omohyoideus.

lymphono'di jugula'res latera'les [NA], lateral jugular lymph nodes; nodes of the deep lateral cervical group lying lateral to the internal jugular vein; they usually empty into the jugular trunk.

lymphono'di jux'ta-esophagea'les pulmona'les [NA], juxta-esophageal pulmonary lymph nodes; juxta-esophageal lymph n.'s; several nodes of the posterior mediastinal group located along either side of the esophagus; they receive lymph from both the esophagus and the lungs.

lymphono'di juxta-intestina'les [NA], juxta-intestinal lymph nodes; the mesenteric lymph nodes located in immediate proximity to the jejunum or ileum.

lymphono'di liena'les [NA], alternate term for *nodi* lymphatici splenici.

lymphono'di lumba'les dex'tri [NA], right lumbar lymph nodes; the chain of lymph nodes associated with the inferior vena cava; it is divided into three groups: **lymphono'di cava'les latera'les** on the right of the inferior vena cava; **lymphono'di precava'les,** in front of the inferior vena cava; **lymphono'di postcava'les,** behind the inferior vena cava.

lymphono'di lumba'les interme'dii [NA], intermediate lumbar lymph nodes; the chain of lymph nodes located between the aorta and the inferior vena cava.

lymphono'di lumba'les sinis'tri [NA], left lumbar lymph nodes; the chain of lymph nodes associated with the aorta in the abdomen; it is divided into three groups: **lymphono'di aor'tici latera'les,** on the left of the aorta; **lymphono'di preaor'tici,** in front of the aorta; **lymphono'di postaor'tici,** behind the aorta.

lymphono'di mastoi'dei [NA], mastoid or retroauricular lymph nodes; two or three nodes that lie posterior to the mastoid process; they receive afferent lymphatic vessels from the scalp and auricle and send efferent vessels to the deep anterior cervical nodes.

lymphono'di mediastina'les anterio'res [NA], anterior mediastinal lymph nodes; located in the superior mediastinum in relation to the great vessels, these nodes receive lymph from the thymus, pericardium and right side of the heart; their efferent vessels join those of the tracheal nodes to form the bronchomediastinal trunks.

lymphono'di mediastina'les posterio'res [NA], posterior mediastinal lymph nodes; nodes located along the thoracic aorta; they receive vessels from the esophagus, diaphragm, liver and pericardium and send efferents to the thoracic duct and inferior tracheobronchial nodes.

lymphono'di mesenter'ici [NA], mesenteric lymph nodes; nodes located in the mesentery; they are of two classes: lymphonodi juxta-intestinales; lymphonodi superiores or centrales.

lymphono'di mesocol'ici [NA], mesocolic lymph nodes; nodes located in the mesocolon; they are of two classes: **lymphono'di paracol'ici,** located in immediate proximity to the colon; **lymphono'di col'ici,** located along the arteries supplying the colon.

lymphono'di obturato'rii [NA], obturator lymph nodes; nodes of the internal iliac group located along the obturator artery.

lymphono'di occipita'les [NA], occipital lymph nodes; one or two small nodes along the occipital vessels close to the trapezius muscle that receive afferents from the posterior scalp and drain into the deep cervical nodes.

lymphono'di pancreat'ici [NA], pancreatic lymph nodes; nodes draining the body and tail of the pancreas; they are subdivided into two groups: **l. p. inferio'res,** located along the inferior pancreatic artery; **l. p. superio'res,** located along the splenic artery near the origin of its pancreatic branches.

lymphono'di pancreat'icoduodena'les [NA], pancreaticoduodenal lymph nodes; nodes along the superior and inferior pancreaticoduodenal arteries.

lymphono'di pancreat'icoliena'les, lymphonodi pancreatici superiores.

lymphono'di paramamma'rii [NA], paramammary lymph nodes; several lymph nodes on the lateral side of the mammary gland that receive afferents from the mammary gland and send efferents to the axillary lymph nodes.

lymphono'di pararecta'les [NA], pararectal or anorectal lymph nodes; lymphonodi anorectales; nodes located on either side of the rectum; they send efferents to the middle rectal and superior rectal nodes.

lymphono'di parasterna'les [NA], parasternal lymph nodes; a number of small nodes that lie along the course of the internal thoracic vessels; lymph enters these nodes from the anterior intercostal spaces, pericardium, diaphragm, liver and mammary gland; the efferent vessels pass upward to join the bronchomediastinal trunk of the same side.

lymphono'di paratrachea'les [NA], paratracheal or tracheal lymph nodes; nodes along the sides of the trachea in the neck and in the posterior mediastinum.

lymphono'di parauteri'ni [NA], parauterine lymph nodes; nodes on either side of the uterus draining lymph to the internal iliac nodes and to the lumbar nodes via lymphatic vessels following the ovarian arteries.

lymphono'di paravagina'les [NA], paravaginal lymph nodes; lymph nodes in association with the vagina; they drain to the internal iliac nodes.

lymphono'di paravesicula'res [NA], paravesical lymph nodes; the lymph nodes located around the urinary bladder and, in the male, the prostate; there are three groups: **lymphono'di prevesicula'res,** in front of the bladder; **lymphono'di vesica'les latera'les,** on the right and left sides; **lymphono'di postvesicula'res,** behind the bladder.

lymphono'di parotid'ei intraglandula'res [NA], intraglandular parotid lymph nodes; small lymph nodes of the deep parotid group lying within the parotid gland.

lymphono'di parotid'ei profun'di [NA], deep parotid lymph nodes; the group of lymph nodes associated with the parotid gland lying deep to the parotid masseteric fascia.

lymphono'di parotid'ei subfascia'les infra-auricula'res [NA], infra-auricular subfascial parotid lymph nodes; small lymph nodes located deep to the parotid fascia and below the ear.

lymphono'di parotid'ei subfascia'les praeauricula'res [NA], preauricular subfascial parotid lymph nodes; small lymph nodes located deep to the parotid fascia and in front of the ear.

lymphono'di parotid'ei superficia'les [NA], superficial parotid lymph nodes; several small lymph nodes located in the subcutaneous tissue in the parotid region.

lymphono'di pericardia'les latera'les [NA], small lymph nodes located along the pericardiacophrenic artery; they drain the pericardium.

lymphono'di phren'ici inferio'res [NA], inferior phrenic lymph nodes; small lymph nodes associated with the inferior phrenic vessels.

lymphono'di phren'ici superio'res [NA], superior phrenic lymph nodes; diaphragmatic nodes; three groups of small nodes, anterior, middle, and posterior, on the upper surface of the diaphragm; they receive afferents from the liver, diaphragm, and intercostal spaces and send efferents to parasternal and posterior mediastinal nodes.

lymphono'di poplitea'les [NA], popliteal lymph nodes; two groups of nodes located in the popliteal fossa: the superficial popliteal lymph nodes, located around the termination of the small saphenous vein, that drain the skin of the back of the leg and lateral side of the foot; and the deep popliteal lymph nodes, located around the popliteal vessels, that drain the superficial group, the deep structures of the leg, and the knee joint.

lymphono'di prececa'les [NA], prececal lymph nodes; nodes located in front of the cecum draining lymph to the ileocolic nodes.

lymphono'di prelarynge'ales [NA], prelaryngeal lymph nodes; lymph nodes of the deep anterior cervical group that lie in front of the larynx; they drain into the deep lateral cervical nodes.

lymphono'di prepericardia'les [NA], prepericardiac lymph nodes; several small lymph nodes located between the pericardium and the sternum.

lymphono'di pretrachea'les [NA], pretracheal lymph nodes; lymph nodes of the deep anterior cervical group that lie in front of the trachea; they drain into the deep lateral cervical group or into the anterior mediastinal group.

lymphono'di prevertebra'les [NA], prevertebral lymph nodes; lymph nodes posterior to the thoracic aorta.

lymphono'di promonto'rii [NA], promontory lymph nodes; nodes of the common iliac group located at the promontory of the sacrum.

lymphono'di pulmona'les, pulmonary lymph *nodes.*

lymphono'di pylo'rici [NA], pyloric or gastroduodenal lymph nodes; a group of nodes surrounding the pylorus, draining lymph into the right gastric or the right gastro-omental lymph nodes; it is divided into three smaller groups: nodus suprapylo'ricus, above the pylorus; no'di subpylo'rici, subpyloric nodes; below the pylorus; no'di retropylo'rici, retropyloric nodes; behind the pylorus.

lymphono'di recta'les superio'res [NA], superior rectal lymph nodes; nodes of the inferior mesenteric group, located along the superior rectal artery.

lymphono'di retroceca'les [NA], retrocecal lymph nodes; nodes located behind the cecum draining lymph into the ileocolic nodes.

lymphono'di retropharyngea'les [NA], retropharyngeal lymph nodes; the three groups of lymph nodes, one median and two lateral, located between the pharynx and the prevertebral fascia; they receive lymph from the nasopharynx, the auditory tube, and the atlanto-occipital and atlantoaxial joints.

lymphono'di sacra'les [NA], sacral lymph nodes; nodes in the concavity of the sacrum that drain the rectum and posterior pelvic wall.

lymphono'di sigmoi'dei [NA], sigmoid lymph nodes; nodes of the inferior mesenteric group, located along the sigmoid arteries.

lymphono'di sple'nici [NA], splenic lymph nodes; nodes near the hilum of the spleen; they receive afferents from the spleen and stomach, and send efferents to the pancreatic nodes.

lymphono'di subaor'tici [NA], subaortic lymph nodes; nodes of the common iliac group located at the bifurcation of the aorta.

lymphono'di submandibula'res [NA], submandibular lymph nodes; four or five nodes that lie between the mandible and the submandibular gland; they receive vessels from the face below the eye and from the tongue and drain into the deep cervical nodes; particularly the jugulodigastric node.

lymphono'di submenta'les [NA], submental lymph nodes; small nodes that lie superficial to the mylohyoid muscle; they receive afferents from the lower lip, chin, and the tip of the tongue, and send efferents to the deep lateral cervical nodes.

lymphono'di superio'res centra'les [NA], the mesenteric lymph nodes located along the intestinal branches of the superior mesenteric artery.

lymphono'di supraclavicula'res [NA], supraclavicular lymph nodes; the portion of the deep lateral cervical group located between the inferior belly of the omohyoid muscle and the clavicle; afferent vessels come from adjacent regions including the mediastinum; efferent vessels terminate in the subclavian trunk.

lymphono'di thyroi'dei [NA], thyroid lymph nodes; nodes of the deep anterior cervical group located around the thyroid gland; they drain into the deep lateral cervical group.

lymphono'di tracheobronchia'les inferio'res [NA], inferior tracheobronchial lymph nodes; bifurcation lymph nodes; several large lymph nodes inferior to the tracheal bifurcation; they receive afferents from the bronchopulmonary nodes and the heart; and send efferents to the superior tracheobronchial and tracheal nodes.

lymphono'di tracheobronchia'les superio'res [NA], superior tracheobronchial lymph nodes; several large lymph nodes of the posterior mediastinal group located superior to the bronchi at their union with the trachea.

---

lymphopathia (lim-fō-path'ē-ă). Lymphopathy.

l. vene'reum, seldom used term for *lymphogranuloma* venereum.

lymphopathy (lim-fop'ă-thē) [lympho- + G. *pathos,* suffering]. Lymphopathia; any disease of the lymphatic vessels or lymph nodes.

lymphopenia (lim-fō-pē'nē-ă) [lympho- + G. *penia,* poverty]. Lymphocytopenia; lymphocytic leukopenia; a reduction, relative or absolute, in the number of lymphocytes in the circulating blood.

lymphoplasmapheresis (lim'fō-plaz'mă-fĕ-rē'sis) [lymphocyte + plasma + G. *aphairesis,* a withdrawal]. Separation and removal of lymphocytes and plasma from the withdrawn blood, with the remainder of the blood retransfused into the donor.

lymphoplasty (lim'fō-plas-tē). Lymphangioplasty.

lymphopoiesis (lim-fō-poy-ē'sis) [lympho- + G. *poiēsis,* a making]. The formation of lymphocytes.

lymphopoietic (lim-fō-poy-et'ik). Pertaining to or characterized by lymphopoiesis.

lymphoreticulosis (lim'fō-rĕ-tik-yū-lō'sis). Proliferation of the reticuloendothelial cells (macrophages) of the lymph glands.

benign inoculation l., cat-scratch *disease.*

lymphorrhagia (lim-fō-rā'jē-ă) [lympho- + G. *rhēgnymi,* to burst forth]. Lymphorrhea.

lymphorrhea (lim-fō-rē'ă) [lympho- + G. *rhoia,* a flow]. Lymphorrhagia; an escape of lymph on the surface from ruptured, torn, or cut lymphatic vessels.

lymphorrhoid (lim'fō-royd). A dilation of a lymph channel, resembling a hemorrhoid.

lymphosarcoma (lim'fō-sar-kō'mă) [lympho- + G. *sarkōma,* sarcoma]. Lymphatic sarcoma; a diffuse lymphocytic lymphoma.

bovine l., a systemic malignancy of the lymphoreticular system of cattle which is seen in two etiologically and clinically distinct forms, enzootic bovine *leukosis* and sporadic bovine *leukosis.*

lymphosarcomatosis (lim'fō-sar-kō'mă-tō'sis). A condition characterized by the presence of multiple, widely distributed masses of lymphosarcoma.

lymphosis (lim-fō'sis). Undesirable term for lymphocytic *leukemia.*

lymphostasis (lim-fos'tă-sis) [lympho- + G. *stasis,* a standing still]. Obstruction of the normal flow of lymph.

lymphotaxis (lim-fō-tak'sis) [lympho- + G. *taxis,* orderly arrangement]. The exertion of an effect that attracts or repels lymphocytes.

lymphotoxicity (lim'fō-tok-sis'i-tē). The potential of an antibody in the serum of an allograft recipient to react directly with the lymphocytes or other cells of an allograft donor to produce a hyperacute type of graft rejection.

lymphotoxin (lim'fō-tok-sin). A lymphokine that lyses or damages many cell types.

lymphotrophy (lim-fot'rō-fē) [lympho- + G. *trophē,* nourishment]. Nourishment of the tissues by lymph in parts devoid of blood vessels.

lymphuria (lim-fū'rē-ă) [lympho- + G. *ouron,* urine]. Discharge of lymph in the urine.

lynestrenol (lin-es'tren-ol). Ethinylestrenol; 17α-ethynylestr-4-en-17β-ol; 3-desoxynorlutin; a progestational agent, used with mestranol as an oral contraceptive.

lyo- [G. *lyō,* to loosen, dissolve] Combining form relating to dissolution. See also lyso-.

lyoenzyme (lī-ō-en'zīm). Extracellular *enzyme.*

lyolysis (lī-ol'i-sis). Rarely used term for solvolysis.

Lyon, B. B. Vincent, U.S. physician, 1880–1953. See Meltzer-L. *test.*

Lyon, Mary F., British cytogeneticist, *1925. See L. *hypothesis; lyonization.*

lyonization (lī'on-i-zā'shŭn) [M. *Lyon*]. X-inactivation; the phenomenon, common but not universal, for X-linked loci whereby in each cell one or another of the genes is inactivated apparently at random and has no phenotypic expression; its randomness explains the variable expressivity of X-linked traits in women. See also dosage *compensation;* Lyon *hypothesis.*

lyophil, lyophile (lī'ō-fil, -fīl). A substance that is lyophilic.

lyophilic (lī-ō-fil'ik) [lyo- + G. *phileō,* to love]. Lyotropic; in colloid chemistry, denoting a dispersed phase having a pronounced affinity for the dispersion medium; when the dispersed phase is l., the colloid is usually a reversible one.

lyophilization (lī-of'i-li-zā'shŭn). Freeze-drying; the process of isolating a solid substance from solution by freezing the solution and evaporating the ice under vacuum.

lyophobe (lī'ō-fōb). A substance that is lyophobic.

lyophobic (lī-ō-fo'bik) [lyo- + G. *phobos,* fear]. In colloid chemistry, denoting a dispersed phase having but slight affinity for the dispersion medium; when the dispersed phase is l., the colloid is usually an irreversible one.

lyosorption (lī-ō-sōrp'shŭn). Adsorption of a liquid on a solid surface.

lyotropic (lī-ō-trop'ik) [lyo- + G. *tropē,* a turning]. Lyophilic.

lypressin (lī'pres-in). 8-Lysine vasopressin; [Lys[8]]vasopressin; vasopressin containing lysine in position 8; an antidiuretic and vasopressor hormone.

lyra (lī'ră) [L. and G. lyre]. A lyre-shaped structure.
l. davidis, lyre of David, obsolete terms for *commissura* fornicis.
l. uteri'na, *plicae* palmatae.

Lys Symbol for lysine, or its radicals in peptides.

lys- See lyso-.

lysate (lī'sāt). Material produced by the destructive process of lysis.

lyse (līz). Lyze; to break up, to disintegrate, to effect lysis.

lysemia (lī-sē'mē-ă) [lyso- + G. *haima,* blood]. Disintegration or dissolution of red blood cells and the occurrence of hemoglobin in the circulating plasma and in the urine.

lysergamide (lī-serj'ă-mīd). *Lysergic acid* amide.

lysergic acid (lī-ser'jik). D-Lysergic acid; a cleavage product of alkaline hydrolysis of ergot alkaloids, with mol wt 268.3; occurs as shiny crystals, slightly soluble in water.

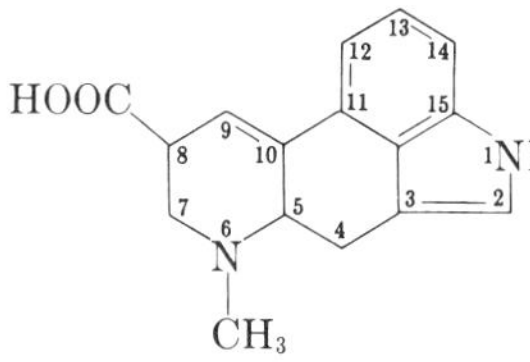

Lysergic acid

l. a. amide, lysergamide; ergine; a psychotomimetic agent present in *Rivea corymbosa* and *Ipomoea tricolor;* possesses less hallucinogenic potency than does l. a. diethylamide.
l. a. diethylamide (LSD), lysergide; peripherally, a serotonin antagonist; 1 to 2 μg per kg induces hallucinatory states of a visual rather than auditory nature; its use may precipitate psychoses; it is occasionally used in the treatment of chronic alcoholism and psychotic disorders.
l. a. monoethylamide, a psychotomimetic agent present in *Rivea corymbosa* and *Ipomoea tricolor;* possesses less hallucinatory potency than does l. a. diethylamide.

lysergide (lī-ser'jīd). *Lysergic acid* diethylamide.

lysin (lī'sin). **1.** A specific complement-fixing antibody that acts destructively on cells and tissues; the various types are designated in accordance with the form of antigen that stimulates the production of the l., *e.g.,* hemolysin, bacteriolysin. **2.** Any substance that causes lysis.

lysine (Lys) (lī'sēn). 2,6-Diaminohexanoic acid; $NH_2(CH_2)_4CH(NH_2)COOH$; an essential α-amino acid found in many proteins; distinguished by an ε-amino group.
l. decarboxylase [EC 4.1.1.18], an enzyme that catalyzes the decarboxylation of l., with the production of cadaverine.

8-lysine vasopressin. Lypressin.

lysinemia (lī-si-nē'mē-ă). Increased concentration of lysine in the blood, associated with mental and physical retardation.

lysinogen (lī-sin'ō-jen). An antigen that stimulates the formation of a specific lysin.

lysinogenic (lī'si-nō-jen'ik). Having the property of a lysinogen.

lysinuria (lī-si-nū'rē-ă). The presence of lysine in the urine.

lysis (lī'sis) [G. dissolution or loosening]. **1.** Gradual subsidence of the symptoms of an acute disease, a form of the curative process, as distinguished from crisis. **2.** Destruction of red blood cells, bacteria, and other structures by a specific lysin, usually referred to by the structure destroyed (*e.g.,* hemolysis, bacteriolysis, nephrolysis); may be a direct toxin or act by an immune mechanism, such as antibody reacting with antigen on the surface of a target cell, usually by binding an activation of a series of proteins in the blood with enzymatic activity (complement system).

lyso-, lys- [G. *lysis,* a loosening or dissolution] Combining forms relating to lysis, or dissolution. See also lyo-.

lysocephalin (lī-sō-sef'ă-lin). A lysophosphatidic acid esterified with serine or ethanolamine, *i.e.,* a lysophosphatidylserine or -ethanolamine; analogous to lysolecithin.

lysogen (lī'sō-jen) [lysin + G. *-gen,* producing]. **1.** That which is capable of inducing lysis. **2.** A bacterium in the state of lysogeny.

lysogenesis (lī-sō-jen'ĕ-sis). The production of lysins.

lysogenic (lī-sō-jen'ik). **1.** Causing or having the power to cause lysis, as the action of certain antibodies and chemical substances. **2.** Pertaining to bacteria in the state of lysogeny.

lysogenicity (lī'sō-jĕ-nis'i-tē). The property of being lysogenic.

lysogenization (lī'sō-jĕ-ni-zā'shŭn, lī-soj'ĕ-ni-zā'shŭn). The process by which a bacterium becomes lysogenic.

lysogeny (lī-soj'ĕ-nē). The phenomenon of a culture of a bacterial strain being capable of inducing, by means of its contained bacteriophage, general lysis in a culture of another bacterial strain without itself undergoing obvious lysis; in such lysogenic cultures, probacteriophage is associated with the genome of all the bacteria, rendering the bacteria immune to infection by the free bacteriophage always present in the culture due to constant dissociation, at a slow rate, of probacteriophage and freeing of infectious particles. Genes of some prophages may determine new host properties (*e.g.,* toxins of diphtheria and scarlet fever).

lysokinase (lī-sō-kī'nās). Term proposed for activator agents (*e.g.,* streptokinase, urokinase, staphylokinase) that produce plasmin by indirect or multiple-stage action on plasminogen.

lysolecithin lī-sō-les'i-thin). Lysophosphatidylcholine; a lysophosphatic acid that contains choline; capable of lysing erythrocytes.

lysolecithinase (lī-sō-les'i-thin-ās). Lysophospholipase.

lysophosphatidic acid (lī'sō-fos'fă-tid'ik). A phosphatidic acid in which only one of the two hydroxyl groups of the glycerophosphate is esterified.

lysophosphatidylcholine (lī'sō-fos'fă-tī'dil-kō'lēn). Lysolecithin.

lysophosphatidylserine (lī'sō-fos'fă-tī'dil-ser'ēn). Phosphatidylserine from which one fatty acid residue has been removed from the glycerol moiety. *Cf.* lysophosphatidic acid.

lysophospholipase (lī'sō-fos'fō-lip'ās) [EC 3.1.1.5]. Phospholipase B; lecithinase B, lysolecithinase; a hydrolase removing the single acyl group from a lysolecithin, leaving glycerophosphocholine.

lysosome (lī'sō-sōm) [lyso- + G. *soma,* body]. A cytoplasmic membrane-bound vesicle measuring 5-8 nm (primary l.) and containing a wide variety of glycoprotein hydrolytic enzymes active at an acid pH; serves to digest exogenous material, such as bacteria, as well as effete organelles of the cells.

definitive l.'s, secondary l.'s.

primary l.'s, l.'s produced at the Golgi apparatus where hydrolytic enzymes are incorporated; they fuse with phagosomes or pinosomes to become secondary l.'s.

secondary l.'s, definitive l.'s; l.'s in which lysis takes place, owing to the activity of hydrolytic enzymes; they are believed to eventually become residual bodies.

lysozyme (lī'sō-zīm) [EC 3.2.1.17]. Muramidase; mucopeptide glycohydrolase; an enzyme hydrolyzing 1,4-β links between *N*-acetylmuramic acid and *N*-acetylglucosamine, and thus destructive to cell walls of certain bacteria; present in tears and some other body fluids, in egg white, and in some plant tissues.

lyssa (lis'ă) [G. *madness*]. **1.** Worm (2); a cartilage in the tongue of the dog. **2.** Old term for rabies.

Lyssavirus (lis'ă-vī-rŭs). A genus of viruses (family Rhabdoviridae) that includes the rabies virus group.

lysyl (lī'sil). The univalent radical of lysine.

lysyl-bradykinin (lī'sil-brad-ē-kī'nin). Kallidin.

lytic (lit'ik). Pertaining to lysis.

lytta (lit'ă). Old term for rabies.

lyxitol (lik'si-tol). A pentitol (reduced lyxose) occurring in lyxoflavin.

lyxoflavin (lik-sō-flā'vin). A compound similar to riboflavin except that D-lyxitol is present in place of the D-ribitol group; present in small quantity in cardiac muscle.

lyxose (lik'sōs). An aldopentose isomeric with ribose.

lyxulose (liks'yū-lōs). The 2-keto derivative of lyxose.

lyze (līz). Lyse.

M

μ [mu, 12th letter of the G. alphabet] Symbol for micro-(2); micron; dynamic *viscosity.*

$\mu\mu$ Symbol for micromicro-.

μ**m** Symbol for micrometer.

M **1.** Symbol for mega-; morgan; moles per liter (also written *M* or M); myopia or myopic. **2.** Symbol for a blood factor. See MNSs blood group, Blood Groups appendix.

M. Abbreviation for L. *misce,* mix.

M_r Symbol for molecular weight *ratio.*

M Symbol for moles per liter (also written M or *M*).

m Symbol for meter; milli-; minim.

m- Abbreviation for *meta-* (3).

mμ Symbol for millimicron.

MA Abbreviation for mental *age.*

ma Abbreviation for milliampere.

MAA Abbreviation for macroaggregated *albumin.*

MAC Abbreviation for minimal alveolar (anesthetic) *concentration.*

Mac-. For proper names beginning thus, see also Mc-.

Macaca (mă-kah'kă) [Pg. *macaco,* monkey]. A large genus of Old World monkeys (family Cercopithecidae) that includes the macaque and rhesus monkeys, and the barbary apes. *M. mulatta,* the rhesus monkey, is used as a research animal.

macaque (mă-kahk') [Fr.]. See *Macaca.*

Macchiavello's stain. See under stain.

MacConkey, Alfred T., British bacteriologist, 1861–1931. See M. *agar.*

Mace, MACE Acronym for *m*ethylchloroform 2-chlor*ace*tophenone (the classical lacrimator) in a light petroleum dispersant and a pressurized propellant.

macerate (mas'er-āt) [see maceration]. To soften by steeping or soaking.

maceration (mas-er-ā'shŭn) [L. *macero,* pp. *-atus,* to soften by soaking]. **1.** Softening by the action of a liquid. **2.** Softening of tissues after death by nonputrefactive (sterile) autolysis; seen especially in the stillborn, with bullous separation of the epidermis.

Macewen, Sir William, Scottish surgeon, 1848–1924. See M.'s *sign, symptom, triangle.*

Mach, Ernst, Austrian scientist, 1838–1916. See M.'s *band,* M. *number.*

Machado-Guerreiro test. See under test.

Machado-Joseph disease. Surnames of two families studied in major descriptions of the disease. See under disease.

Mache, Heinrich, Austrian physicist, *1876. See M. *unit.*

machine (mă-shēn') [L. *machina,* contrivance]. Any mechanical apparatus or device.

anesthesia m., equipment used for inhalation anesthesia, including flowmeters, vaporizers, and sources of compressed gases, but not including the anesthetic circuit or mechanisms for elimination of carbon dioxide.

heart-lung m., a device incorporating a blood pump (artificial heart) and a blood oxygenator (artificial lung) to provide extracorporeal circulation and oxygenation of the blood during cardiac surgery.

panoramic rotating m., an x-ray machine using a reciprocating motion of the tube and extraoral film to produce radiographs of all the teeth and surrounding structures.

Macintosh, Charles, Scottish chemist, 1766–1843. See M. *blockers.*

Mackay, R. Stuart, U.S. physicist, *1924. See M.-Marg *tonometer.*

Mackenrodt, Alwin K., German gynecologist, 1859–1925. See M.'s *incision, ligaments.*

Mackenzie, Sir James, Scottish physician practicing in London, 1853–1925. See M.'s *polygraph.*

Mackenzie, Richard J., Scottish surgeon, 1821–1854. See M.'s *amputation.*

MacLachlan, E.A. See Lowe-Terrey-M. *syndrome.*

Macleod, Roderick, Scottish physician, 1795–1852. See M.'s *rheumatism.*

Macleod, William Mathieson, British physician, 1911–1977. See M.'s *syndrome.*

maclurin (mă-klūr'in) [C.I. 75240]. A natural dye associated with morin and derived from fustic; used to dye fabrics with various metal mordants. It turns deep green on addition of ferric chloride.

MacNeal, Ward J., U.S. bacteriologist, 1881–1946. See M.'s tetrachrome blood *stain.* Novy and M.'s blood *agar.*

macr-. See macro-.

Macracanthorhynchus (mak'ră-kan-thō-ring'kŭs) [macro- + G. *akantha,* thorn, + *rhynchos,* snout]. A genus of giant thorny-headed worms (class Acanthocephala).

M. hirudina'ceus, the giant thorny-headed worm of the pig, approximately the size of the giant roundworm (*Ascaris*); it inhabits the intestinal tract where nodules develop at the site of penetration of the spiny proboscis of each worm; it has occasionally been reported in man; transmission is by ingestion of infected insects, frequently dung beetles or cockroaches that have fed on feces of infected pigs containing viable eggs and have developed the cystacanth stage infective to the vertebrate host, including man.

macrencephaly, macrencephalia (mak'ren-sef'ă-lē, -sĕ-fā'lē-ă) [macro- + G. *enkephalos,* brain]. Hypertrophy of the brain; the condition of having a large brain.

macro-, macr- [G. *makros,* large]. Combining form meaning large, long. See also mega-, megalo-.

macroadenoma (mak'rō-ad-ĕ-nō'mă). A pituitary adenoma larger than 10 mm in diameter.

macroamylase (mak-rō-am'i-lās). Descriptive term applied to a form of serum amylase in which the enzyme is present as a complex joined to a globulin; the molecular weight of the enzyme alone is 50,000, whereas that of the complex probably exceeds 160,000; hence, renal excretion of the complex is not appreciable.

macroamylasemia (mak'rō-am'i-lā-sē'mē-ă) [macroamylase + G. *haima,* blood]. A form of hyperamylasemia, in which a portion of serum amylase exists as macroamylase.

macrobacterium (mak'rō-bak-tēr'ē-ŭm). Megabacterium.

macrobiosis (mak'rō-bī-ō'sis) [macro- + G. *bios,* life]. Longevity.

macrobiote (mak-rō-bī'ōt) [macro- + G. *bios,* life]. An organism that is long-lived.

macrobiotic (mak'rō-bī-ot'ik). **1.** Long-lived. **2.** Tending to prolong life.

macrobiotics (mak'rō-bī-ot'iks). The study of the prolongation of life.

macroblast (mak'rō-blast) [macro- + G. *blastos,* germ]. A large erythroblast.

macroblepharia (mak'rō-ble-fār'ē-ă) [macro- + G. *blepharon,* eyelid]. A condition characterized by abnormally large eyelids.

macrobrachia (mak-rō-brā'kē-ă) [macro- + G. *brachiōn,* arm]. Condition of having abnormally thick or long arms.

macrocardia (mak-rō-kar'dē-ă). Cardiomegaly.

macrocephalic, macrocephalous (mak'rō-se-fal'ik, -sef'ă-lŭs) [macro- + G. *kephalē,* head]. Megacephalic.

macrocephaly, macrocephalia (mak-rō-sef'ă-lē, -sĕ-fā'lē-ă) [macro- + G. *kephalē,* head]. Megacephaly.

macrocheilia, macrochilia (mak-rō-kī'lē-ă) [macro- + G. *cheilos,* lip]. **1.** Macrolabia; abnormally enlarged lips. **2.** Cavernous lymphangioma of the lip, a condition of permanent swelling of the lip resulting from the presence of greatly distended lymphatic spaces.

macrocheiria, macrochiria (mak-rō-kī'rē-ă) [macro- + G. *cheir,* hand]. Cheiromegaly; chiromegaly; megalocheiria; megalochiria; a condition characterized by abnormally large hands.

macrochemistry (mak-rō-kem'is-trē). The use of chemical procedures, the reactions of which (color change, effervescence, etc.) are visible to the unaided eye. *Cf.* microchemistry.

macrochilia (mak-rō-kī'lē-ă). Macrocheilia.

macrochiria (mak-rō-kī'rē-ă). Macrocheiria.

macrochylomicron (mak'rō-kī-lō-mī'kron). An unusually large chylomicron.

macrocnemia (mak-rō-nē'mē-ă) [macro- + G. *knēmē,* leg]. A condition characterized by enlargement of the shins.

macrococcus (mak'rō-kok'ŭs). Megacoccus.

macrocolon (mak'rō-kō'lon). A sigmoid colon of unusual length; a variety of megacolon.

macroconidium, pl. **macroconidia** (mak'rō-kō-nid'ē-ŭm, -ă) [macro- + Mod. L. dim. fr. G. *Konis,* dust]. **1.** A conidium, or exospore, of large size. **2.** In fungi, the larger of two distinctively different-sized types of conidia in a single species, thick- or thin-walled and composed of 2 to 10 cells; characteristic of most dermatophytes.

macrocornea (mak-rō-kōr'nē-ă). Megalocornea; an abnormally large cornea.

macrocranium (mak-rō-krā'nē-ŭm). An enlarged skull, especially the bones containing the brain, as seen in hydrocephalus; the face appears relatively small in comparison.

macrocryoglobulin (mak-rō-krī-ō-glob'yū-lin). A macroglobulin that has the properties of a cryoglobulin.

macrocryoglobulinemia (mak'rō-krī-ō-glob'yū-lin-ē'mē-ă). The presence of cold-precipitating macroglobulins in the peripheral blood; such macrocryoglobulins are often called cold hemagglutinins.

macrocyst (mak'rō-sist). A cyst of macroscopic proportions.

macrocytase (mak-rō-sī'tās). According to Metchnikoff, a cytase or complement, formed by the large uninuclear leukocytes, which is effective in the destruction of tissue cells, blood cells, etc.

macrocyte (mak'rō-sīt) [macro- + G. *kytos,* a hollow (cell)]. Macroerythrocyte; a large erythrocyte, such as those observed in pernicious anemia.

macrocythemia (mak'rō-sī-thē'mē-ă) [macrocyte + G. *haima,* blood]. Macrocytosis; megalocythemia; megalocytosis; the occurrence of unusually large numbers of macrocytes in the circulating blood.

hyperchromatic m., an inexact term frequently used for macrocytes that contain an unusually large amount of hemoglobin, but are actually normochromic; although the total mass of hemoglobin is greater than normal (owing to the large cells), the percentage of hemoglobin in the cells is not greater than normal.

macrocytosis (mak'rō-sī-tō'sis) [macrocyte + G. *-osis,* condition]. Macrocythemia.

macrodactylia, macrodactylism, macrodactyly (mak-rō-dak-til'ē-ă, -dak'til-izm, dak'ti-lē). Megadactyly.

macrodont (mak'rō-dont) [macro- + G. *odous* (*odont-*), tooth]. Megadont; megalodont. **1.** A tooth of abnormally large and frequently distorted proportions, either localized or generalized. **2.** Denoting a skull with a dental index above 44.

macrodontia, macrodontism (mak-rō-don'shē-ă, -don'tizm). Megalodontia; megadontism; the state of having abnormally large teeth.

macrodystrophia lipomatosa (mak'rō-dis-trō'fē-ă lip-ō-mă-tō'să). A rare nonfamilial disease characterized by enlargement of the fingers by lipomas, with painful degenerative arthropathy of the metacarpophalangeal and interphalangeal joints.

macroencephalon (mak'rō-en-sef'ă-lon) [macro- + G. *enkephalos,* brain]. Megaloencephalon.

macroerythroblast (mak'rō-ĕ-rith'rō-blast). Macronormochromoblast; a large erythroblast.

macroerythrocyte (mak'rō-ĕ-rith'rō-sīt). Macrocyte.

macroesthesia (mak'rō-es-thē'zē-ă) [macro- + G. *aisthēsis,* sensation]. A subjective sensation that all objects are larger than they are.

macrogamete (mak-rō-gam'ēt) [macro- + G. *gametē,* wife]. Megagamete; the female element in anisogamy; it is the larger of the two sex cells, with more reserve material, and usually nonmotile.

macrogametocyte (mak'rō-gă-mē'tō-sīt). Macrogamont; the female gametocyte or mother cell producing the female or macrogamete among fungi or protozoa that undergo anisogamy.

macrogamont (mak-rō-gam'ont). Macrogametocyte.

macrogamy (mă-krog'ă-mē) [macro- + G. *gamos,* marriage]. Conjugation of two adult cells or gametes.

macrogastria (mak-rō-gas'trē-ă). Megalogastria.

macrogenitosomia (mak'rō-jen'i-tō-sō'mē-ă) [macro- + L. *genitalis,* genital, + G. *sōma,* body]. Excessive bodily and genital development.

m. pre'cox, Pellizzi's syndrome; a disorder in which gonadal maturation (puberty) and the adolescent growth spurt in bodily height occur in the first decade of life; often associated with a pineal tumor or lesions in hypothalamic areas known to regulate gonadotrophin secretion.

m. pre'cox su'prarena'lis, precocious somatic growth and isosexual maturation of secondary sexual characteristics, as the consequence of an adrenocortical tumor.

macroglia (ma-krog'lē-ă) [macro- + G. *glia,* glue]. Astrocyte.

macroglobulin (mak-rō-glob'yū-lin). Plasma globulin of unusually large molecular weight, *e.g.,* as much as 1,000,000.

macroglobulinemia (mak'rō-glob'yū-li-nē'mē-ă). The presence of macroglobulins in the circulating blood, as in some patients with multiple myeloma.

Waldenström's m., Waldenström's syndrome or purpura; hyperglobulinemic purpura; m. occurring in elderly persons, especially women, characterized by proliferation of cells resembling lymphocytes or plasma cells in the bone marrow, anemia, increased sedimentation rate, and hyperglobulinemia with a narrow peak in γ-globulin or β_2-globulin at about 19 S units. The spleen, liver, or lymph nodes are often enlarged and there is frequently purpura or mucosal bleeding.

macroglossia (mak-rō-glos'ē-ă) [macro- + G. *glōssa,* tongue]. Megaloglossia; enlargement of the tongue, either developmental in origin or secondary to a neoplasm or vascular hamartoma.

macrognathia (mak-rō-nā'thē-ă) [macro- + G. *gnathos,* jaw]. Megagnathia; enlargement or elongation of the jaw.

macrography (mă-krog'ră-fē) [macro- + G. *graphō,* to write]. Megalographia; writing with very large letters.

macrogyria (mak-rō-jī'rē-ă) [macro- + G. *gyros,* circle (gyrus)]. Congenitally larger than normal convolutions of the cerebral cortex.

macrolabia (mak'rō-lā'bē-ă) [macro- + L. *labium,* lip]. Macrocheilia (1).

macroleukoblast (mak-rō-lū'kō-blast). An unusually large leukoblast.

macrolides (mak'rō-līdz). A class of antibiotics discovered in streptomycetes, characterized by molecules made up of large-ring lactones; *e.g.* erythromycin.

macromania (mak-rō-mā'nē-ă) [macro- + G. *mania,* frenzy]. Rarely used term for: **1.** Megalomania. **2.** A delusion that all objects surrounding the subject, or the subject himself or his body parts, are of immense size.

macromastia, macromazia (mak-rō-mas'tē-a, -mā'zē-ă) [macro- + G. *mastos,* breast]. Abnormally large breasts. See also hypermastia (2).

macromelanosome (mak-rō-mel'ă-nō-sōm). Giant *melanosome.*

macromelia (mak-rō-mē'lē-ă) [macro- + G. *melos,* limb]. Megalomelia; abnormal size of one or more of the extremities.

macromere (mak'rō-mēr) [macro- + G. *meros,* part]. A blastomere of large size, as in amphibians.

macromerozoite (mak'rō-mer-ō-zō'īt) [macro- + G. *mēros,* part, + *zōon,* animal]. Megamerozoite; a large merozoite.

macromolecule (mak-rō-mol'ĕ-kyūl). A molecule of colloidal size; *e.g.,* proteins, nucleic acids, polysaccharides.

macromonocyte (mak-rō-mon'ō-sīt). An unusually large monocyte.

macromyeloblast (mak-rō-mī'ĕ-lō-blast). An abnormally large myeloblast.

macronormoblast (mak-rō-nōr'mō-blast). **1.** A large normoblast. **2.** A large, incompletely hemoglobiniferous, nucleated red blood cell with a "cart-wheel" nucleus.

macronormochromoblast (mak'rō-nōr-mō-krō'mō-blast). Macroerythroblast.

macronucleus (mak-rō-nū'klē-ŭs). **1.** Meganucleus; a nucleus that occupies a relatively large portion of the cell, or the larger nucleus where two or more are present in a cell. **2.** Trophonucleus; somatic or trophic nucleus; the larger of the two nuclei in ciliates, which governs vegetative metabolic functions and not reproduction. See also micronucleus (2).

macronutrients (mak-rō-nū'trē-ents). Nutrients required in the greatest amount; *e.g.,* carbohydrates, protein, fats.

macronychia (mak-rō-nik'ē-ă) [macro- + G. *onyx,* nail]. Megalonychosis; abnormally large fingernails or toenails.

macroparasite (mak-rō-par'ă-sīt). A parasite, such as a louse or an intestinal worm, that is visible to the naked eye.

macropathology (mak'rō-pa-thol'ō-jē). The phase of pathology that pertains to the gross anatomical changes in disease.

macropenis (mak-rō-pē'nis). Macrophallus; megalopenis; megalophallus; an abnormally large penis.

macrophage (mak'rō-fāj) [macro- + G. *phagein,* to eat]. Clasmatocyte; macrophagocyte; rhagiocrine cell; any mononuclear, actively phagocytic cell arising from monocytic stem cells in the bone marrow; these cells are widely distributed in the body and vary in morphology and motility, though most are large, long-lived cells with a nearly round nucleus and have abundant endocytic vacuoles, lysosomes, and phagolysosomes. Phagocytic activity is typically mediated by serum recognition factors, including certain immunoglobulins and components of the complement system, but also may be nonspecific for some inert materials and bacteria, as in the case of alveolar m.'s; m.'s also are involved in both the production of antibodies and in cell-mediated immune responses, participate in presenting antigens to lymphocytes, and secrete a variety of immunoregulatory molecules.

alveolar m., dust cell; coniophage; a vigorously phagocytic m. on the epithelial surface of lung alveoli where it ingests inhaled particulate matter.

fixed m., resting wandering c.; a relatively immotile m. found in connective tissue, lymph nodes, spleen, and bone marrow.

free m., an actively motile m. typically found in sites of inflammation.

Hansemann m., large histiocytes with abundant cytoplasm that may contain Michaelis-Gutmann bodies and one or several nuclei; described in lesions of malacoplakia.

macrophagocyte (mak-rō-fag'ō-sīt). Macrophage.

macrophallus (mak-rō-fal'lŭs) [macro- + G. *phallos,* penis]. Macropenis.

macrophthalmia (mak-rof-thal'mē-ă) [macro- + G. *ophthalmos,* eye]. Megalophthalmus.

macropodia (mak-rō-pō'dē-ă) [macro- + G. *pous,* foot]. Megalopodia; pes gigas; abnormally large feet.

macropolycyte (mak-rō-pol'ē-sīt) [macro- + G. *polys,* many, + *kytos,* cell]. An unusually large polymorphonuclear neutrophilic leukocyte that contains a multisegmented nucleus *e.g.,* 8, 10, or more lobes); the arrangement of chromatin is less compact than in the normal neutrophil, and the cytoplasmic granules tend to be larger and more acidophilic. Such changes frequently precede significant alterations in the red blood cells, *e.g.,* as in pernicious anemia and certain other forms of anemia.

macropromyelocyte (mak'rō-prō-mī'ĕ-lō-sīt). An unusually large promyelocyte.

macroprosopia (mak'rō-prō-sō'pē-ă) [macro- + G. *prosōpon,* face]. Megaprosopia; a condition in which the face is too large in proportion to the size of the cranial vault.

macroprosopous (mak-rō-prō'sō-pŭs, -prō-sō'pŭs). Megaprosopous; relating to or exhibiting macroprosopia.

macropsia (mă-krop'sē-ă) [macro- + G. *opsis,* vision]. Megalopsia; megalopia; perception of objects as larger than they are.

macrorhinia (mak-rō-rin'ē-ă) [macro- + G. *rhis* (*rhin-*), nose]. Excessive size of the nose, either congenital or pathologic.

macroscelia (mak-rō-sē'lē-ă) [macro- + G. *skelos,* leg]. Abnormally increased length or thickness of the legs.

macroscopic (mak-rō-skop'ik). **1.** Of a size visible with the naked eye or without the use of a microscope. **2.** Relating to macroscopy.

macroscopy (mă-kros'kō-pē) [macro- + G. *skopeō,* to view]. Examination of objects with the naked eye.

macrosigmoid (mak-rō-sig'moyd). Megasigmoid; enlargement or dilation of the sigmoid colon.

macrosis (mă-krō'sis) [G.]. Increase in length or volume.

macrosmatic (mak'roz-mat'ik) [macro- + G. *osmē,* smell]. Denoting an abnormally keen olfactory sense.

macrosomia (mak-rō-sō'mē-ă) [macro- + G. *sōma,* body]. Megasomia; abnormally large size of the body.

macrosplanchnic (mak-rō-splangk'nik). Megalosplanchnic.

macrospore (mak'rō-spōr) [macro- + G. *sporos,* seed]. Megaspore; megalospore; the larger of two spore types of certain protozoans or fungi.

macrostereognosis (mak'rō-ster-ē-og-nō'sis) [macro- + G. *stereos,* solid, + *gnōsis,* recognition]. An error of perception in which objects appear larger than they are.

macrostomia (mak-rō-stō'mē-ă) [macro- + G. *stoma,* mouth]. Abnormally large size of the mouth.

macrotia (mak-rō'shē-ă) [macro- + G. *ous,* ear]. Congenital excessive enlargement of the auricle.

macrotome (mak'rō-tōm) [macro- + G. *tomē,* cutting]. An instrument for making gross anatomical sections.

macula, pl. **maculae** (mak'yū-lă, -yū-lē) [L. a spot]. Spot (1); macule. **1** [NA]. A small spot, perceptibly different in color from the surrounding tissue. **2.** A small, discolored patch or spot on the skin, neither elevated above nor depressed below the skin's surface. See also subentries under spot.

mac'ulae acus'ticae, see m. sacculi and m. utriculi.

m. adher'ens, desmosome.

m. al'bida, pl. **mac'ulae al'bidae,** m. lactea or tendinea; tendinous or white spot; tache blanche; tache laiteuse (2); gray-white or white, rounded or irregularly shaped, slightly opaque patches or spots that are sometimes observed postmortem in the epicardium, especially in middle-aged or older persons; they result from fibrous thickening, and sometimes hyalinization, of the epicardium; Similar lesions may also occur in the visceral layer of the peritoneum.

m. atroph'ica, an atrophic glistening white spot on the skin.

m. ceru'lea, blue spot (1); tache bleuâtre; a bluish stain on the skin caused by the bites (saliva) of fleas or lice.

m. commu'nicans, gap *junction.*

m. commu'nis, the thickened area in the medial wall of the auditory vesicle that later subdivides, forming the maculae of both the sacculus and utriculus as well as the cristae of the ampullae of the semicircular ducts.

m. cor'neae, corneal spot; a moderately dense opacity of the cornea.

m. cribro'sa, pl. **mac'ulae cribro'sae,** [NA], one of three areas on the wall of the vestibule of the labyrinth, marked by numerous foramina giving passage to nerve filaments supplying portions of the membranous labyrinth; **m.c. infe'rior,** located in the posterior osseous ampulla for passage of posterior ampullary nerve fibers; **m.c. me'dia,** area near the base of the cochlea through which the saccular nerve fibers pass; **m.c. supe'rior,** perforated area above the elliptical recess for passage of the utriculoampullary nerve fibers; **m.c. quar'ta,** a name sometimes applied to the opening for the cochlear nerve.

m. den'sa, a closely packed group of densely staining cells in the distal tubular epithelium of a nephron, in direct apposition to the juxtaglomerular cells; they may function as either chemoreceptors or as baroreceptors feeding information to the juxtaglomerular cells.

false m., an extrafoveal point of fixation.

m. fla'va, a yellowish spot at the anterior extremity of the rima glottidis where the two vocal folds join.

m. germinati'va, archaic term for the nucleolus in the nucleus of an ovum.

m. gonorrho'ica, Saenger's m.; a spot of red brighter than the surrounding membrane, at the congested orifice of the duct of Bartholin's gland, sometimes seen in gonorrhea.

honeycomb m., cystoid macular degeneration; edema of the macular region of the retina.

m. lac'tea, m. albida.

m. lu'tea, m. retinae.

mongolian m., mongolian *spot.*

m. pellu'cida, follicular *stigma.*

m. ret'inae [NA], m. lutea; yellow spot; area centralis; punctum luteum; macular area; Soemmering's spot; an oval area of the sensory retina, 3 by 5 mm, temporal to the optic disk corresponding to the posterior pole of the eye; at its center is the fovea centralis, which contains only retinal cones.

m. sac'culi [NA], saccular spot; the oval neuroepithelial sensory receptor in the anterior wall of the saccule; hair cells of the neuroepithelium support the membrana statoconiorum and have terminal arborizations of vestibular nerve fibers around their bodies.

Saenger's m., m. gonorrhoica.

m. tendin'ea, m. albida.

m. utric'uli [NA], utricular spot; the neuroepithelial sensory receptor in the inferolateral wall of the utricle; hair cells of the neuroepithelium support the membrana statoconiorum and have terminal arborizations of vestibular nerve fibers around their bodies; sensitive to linear acceleration in the longitudinal axis of the body and to gravitational influences.

macular, maculate (mak'yū-lăr, -lāt). **1.** Relating to or marked by macules. **2.** Denoting the central retina, especially the macula retinae.

maculation (mak-yū-lā'shŭn). The formation or the presence of macules.

macule (mak'yūl) [L. *macula,* spot]. Macula.

maculocerebral (mak'yū-lō-ser'ĕ-brăl). Relating to the macula lutea and the brain; denoting a type of nervous disease marked by degenerative lesions in both the retina and the brain.

maculoerythematous (mak'yū-lō-er-i-thē'mă-tŭs). Denoting lesions that are erythematous and macular, covering wide areas.

maculopapule (mak'yū-lō-pap'yūl). A lesion with a sessile base that slopes from a papule in the center.

maculopathy (mak-yū-lop'ă-thē). Macular retinopathy; any pathological condition of the macula lutea.

bull's-eye m., an ocular condition in which edema or degeneration of the sensory retina at the posterior pole of the eye causes alternating areas of light and dark, as in a target; seen in toxic, inflammatory, and hereditary conditions.

cystoid m., cystic degeneration of the central retina; it may occur after cataract extraction, in senile macular degeneration, and in other retinal abnormalities.

familial pseudoinflammatory m., familial macular degeneration resembling inflammatory changes.

nicotinic acid m., m. observed in persons taking 3000 mg or more of nicotinic acid daily; normal vision returns after this medication is discontinued.

mad [A.S. *gemād*]. Colloquialism for: **1.** Rabid. **2.** Mentally ill; insane.

madarosis (mad-ă-rō'sis) [G. a falling off of the eyelashes, fr. *madaō,* to fall off (of hair)]. Milphosis.

madder (mad'er) [A.S. *maedere*]. Turkey red; the dried and powdered root of *Rubia tinctorum* (family Rubiaceae); it contains several glycosides which upon fermentation give the red dyes, alizarin and purpurin. When m. (or alizarin) is fed to young animals, the calcium in newly deposited bone salt, hydroxyapatite, is stained red.

Maddox, Ernest E., British ophthalmologist, 1860–1933. See M.'s *rod.*

Madelung, Otto W., German surgeon, 1846–1926. See M.'s *deformity, disease, neck.*

madescent (mă-des'ent) [L. *madesco,* to become moist]. Becoming moist; slightly moist.

madidans (mad'i-danz) [L. *madido,* pres. p. *-ans,* to moisten]. Moist; denoting certain skin lesions.

Madlener, Max, German surgeon, 1868–1951. See M. *operation.*

madness (mad'nes). The state of being mad.

Madsen, Thorvald J.M., *1870. See Arrhenius-M. *theory.*

Madurella (mad'yū-rel'ă) [*Madura,* India]. A genus of fungi including a number of species, such as *M. grisea* and *M. mycetomi,* that cause mycetoma.

maduromycosis (mad'yū-rō-mī-kō'sis) [*Madura,* India, + mycosis]. Mycetoma (1).

maedi (mā'dē) [Icelandic, dyspnea]. A chronic, progressive, contagious interstitial pneumonitis of sheep caused by a slow virus (subfamily Lentivirinae); it is now believed that maedi and visna are two histopathological and clinical manifestations of the same viral infection.

mafenide (mā′fe-nīd). 4-Homosulfanilamide hydrochloride; α-amino-*p*-toluenesulfonamide hydrochloride; a topical antibacterial agent active against anaerobic pathogens. M. acetate is the preferred salt for ointment; m. hydrochloride is the preferred salt for solution.

Maffucci, Angelo, Italian physician, 1847–1903. See M.'s *syndrome.*

magaldrate (mag′al-drāt). A chemical combination of aluminum hydroxide and magnesium hydroxide, used as an antacid.

Magendie, François, French physiologist, 1783–1855. See M.'s *foramen, law, spaces;* M.-Hertwig *sign, syndrome.*

magenstrasse (mag′en-stras′e) [Ger. *Magen,* stomach, + *Strasse,* road]. The name sometimes applied to the passageway which food takes after it passes through the cardia, namely along the lesser curvature into the gastroduodenal junction.

maggot (mag′ot). A fly larva or grub.
cheese m., *Philopia casei.*
surgical m., an obsolete therapy of wound debridement and removal of abscessed tissues by the use of sterilized botfly m.'s of the species *Phaenicia sericata, Lucilia caesar,* and *Phormia regina.*
wool m., fleece worm; the larva of one of several species of blowflies which deposit eggs on sheep, causing myiasis.

magistral (maj′is-trăl) [L. *magister,* master]. Denoting a preparation compounded according to a physician's prescription, in contrast to officinal (derived from a pharmacist's stock).

magma (mag′mă) [G. a soft mass or salve, fr. *massō,* to knead]. **1.** A soft mass left after extraction of the active principles. **2.** A salve or thick paste.
m. reticula′re, delicate noncellular strands running between the yolk-sac and the outer wall of the blastocyst.

Magnan, Valentin J.J., Paris psychiatrist, 1835–1916. See M.'s trombone *movement, sign.*

magnesia (mag-nē′zhŭh) [see magnesium]. *Magnesium* oxide.
calcined m., *magnesium* oxide.
m. magma, *milk* of magnesia.

magnesium (mag-nē′zē-ŭm) [Mod. L. fr. G. *Magnēsia,* a region in Thessaly]. An alkaline earth element, symbol Mg, atomic no. 12, atomic weight 24.31, that oxidizes to magnesia.
m. aluminum silicate, aluminum m. silicate; m. aluminosilicate dihydrate; an antacid.
m. bacteriopheophytinate, see bacteriochlorophyll.
m. benzoate, has been used in gout and rheumatoid arthritis.
m. carbonate, used in gastric and intestinal acidity and as a laxative.
m. chloride, $MgCl_2 \cdot 6H_2O$; has been used as a laxative.
m. citrate, $Mg_3(C_6H_5O_7)_2 \cdot 14H_2O$; a laxative.
dried m. sulfate, exsiccated m. sulfate; dried Epsom salts.
effervescent m. citrate, m. carbonate, citric acid, sodium bicarbonate, and sugar, moistened with alcohol, passed through a sieve, and dried to a coarse granular powder; used as a laxative.
effervescent m. sulfate, effervescent Epsom salt; m. sulfate, sodium bicarbonate, tartaric acid, and citric acid, moistened, passed through a sieve, and dried to a coarse granular powder; a purgative.
m. hydroxide, $Mg(OH)_2$; an antacid and laxative.
m. lactate, a laxative.
m. oxide, magnesia; calcined magnesia; used as an antacid and laxative.
m. peroxide, decomposes in water to hydrogen peroxide; used as an ingredient in dentifrices and in antiseptic dusting powder.
m. phytinates, chlorophyll *α* and *β*.
m. salicylate, a sodium-free salicylate derivative with anti-inflammatory, analgesic, and antipyretic actions; used for relief of mild to moderate pain.
m. stearate, a compound of m. with variable proportions of stearic and palmitic acids; used in the preparation of tablets, as a lubricant, and as an ingredient in some baby powders.
m. sulfate, Epsom salt; active ingredient of most natural laxative waters; used as a promptly acting cathartic in certain poisonings, in the treatment of increased intracranial pressure and edema, as an anticonvulsant in eclampsia (when administered intravenously), and as an anti-inflammatory (when applied locally).
tribasic m. phosphate, tertiary m. phosphate, $Mg_3(PO_4)_2 \cdot 5H_2O$; it is used as an antacid but it does not produce systemic alkalization; 1 g is equivalent in neutralizing power to about 0.46 g of sodium bicarbonate.
m. trisilicate, $2MgO \cdot 3SiO_2 \cdot n\ H_2O$; a compound of m. oxide and silicon dioxide with varying proportions of water; occurs in nature as meerschaum, pararepiolite, and repiolite; a gastric antacid.

mag′net [G. *magnēs*]. **1.** A body that has the property of attracting particles of iron, cobalt, nickel, or any of various metallic alloys and that when freely suspended tends to assume a definite direction between the magnetic poles of the earth (magnetic polarity). **2.** A bar or horseshoe-shaped piece of iron or steel that has been made magnetic by contact with another m. or, as in an electromagnet, by passage of electric current around a metallic (iron) core.
Haab's m., a powerful electric m. used for removing intraocular chips of iron or steel.

magnet′ic. 1. Relating to or characteristic of a magnet. **2.** Possessing magnetism.

magnetism (mag′nĕ-tizm). The property of mutual attraction or repulsion possessed by magnets.

magnetocardiography (mag′nĕ-tō-kar-dē-og′ră-fē). Measurement of the magnetic field of the heart, produced by the same ionic currents that generate the electrocardiogram, and showing the characteristic P, QRS, T, and U waves.

magnetoencephalogram (MEG) (mag-nē′tō-en-sef′ă-lō-gram). A gauss-time record of the magnetic field of the brain.

magnetoencephalography (mag-nē′tō-en-sef-ă-log′ră-fē). The process of recording the brain's magnetic field.

magnetometer (mag-nĕ-tom′ĕ-ter). An instrument for detecting and measuring the magnetic field.

magneton (mag′nĕ-ton). A unit of measurement of the magnetic moment of a particle (*e.g.,* atom or subatomic particle).
Bohr m., electron m.; a constant in the equation relating the difference in energies between parallel and antiparallel spin alignments of electrons in a magnetic field; the net magnetic moment of one unpaired electron; used in electron spin resonance spectrometry for detection and estimation of free radicals.
electron m., Bohr m.
nuclear m., a constant in the equation relating the difference in energies between parallel and antiparallel spin alignments of atomic nuclei in a magnetic field; used in nuclear magnetic resonance spectrometry.

magnetotherapy (mag-nē′tō-thār′ă-pē). Attempted treatment of disease by application of magnets.

magnification (mag′ni-fi-kā′shŭn) [L. *magnifico,* pp. *-atus,* to magnify]. **1.** The seeming increase in size of an object viewed under the microscope; when noted, this increased size is expressed by a figure preceded by ×, indicating the number of times its diameter is enlarged. **2.** The increased amplitude of a tracing, as of a muscular contraction, caused by the use of a lever with a long writing arm, *i.e.,* one in which the fulcrum is placed nearer to the muscle than to the writing point.

magnitude (mag′ni-tūd). Size or extent.
average pulse m., the amplitude of pulse averaged throughout its duration; identical with peak amplitude for a square wave or pulse without droop.

peak m., the greatest pulse amplitude.

magnocellular (mag'nō-sel'yū-lăr) [L. *magnus,* large, + cellular]. Composed of cells of large size.

magnum (mag'nŭm) [L. *magnus,* large]. *Os* capitatum.

Magnus, Rudolph, German physiologist, 1873–1927. See M.'s *sign* of death.

magnus (mag'nŭs) [L.]. Large; great; denoting a structure of large size.

Mahaim, I. See M. *fibers.*

Ma-huang (mah-hwahng) [Chinese]. *Ephedra equisetina.*

maidenhead (mā'den-hed). Infrequently used term for the intact hymen of a virgin.

maidism (mā'dizm) [*Zea mays,* maize]. Pellagra.

Maier, Rudolf, German physician, 1824–1888. See M.'s *sinus.*

maim (mām). To disable or cripple by an injury.

main (man) [Fr.]. Hand.
m. d'accoucheur, accoucheur's *hand.*
m. en crochet, a permanent flexure of the fourth and fifth fingers, resembling the hand of a woman crocheting with three fingers bent to guide the thread.
m. en griffe, clawhand.
m. en lorgnette, opera-glass *hand.*
m. fourché (fōr-shā), cleft *hand.*

mainstreaming (mān'strēm-ing). Deinstitutionalization; providing the least restrictive environment (socially, physically, and educationally) for chronically disabled individuals by introducing them into the natural environment rather than segregating them into homogeneous groups living in sheltered environments under constant supervision.

maintainer (mān-tā'ner). A device utilized to hold or keep teeth in a given position.
space m., space retainer; an orthodontic appliance used to prevent the loss of space or the shifting of teeth following extraction or premature loss of teeth.

maise oil (māz). Corn oil.

maintenance (mān'ten-ans). The extent to which the patient continues good health practices without supervision, incorporating them into a general life-style. *Cf.* compliance (1); adherence (2).

Maissiat, Jacques H., French anatomist, 1805–1878. See M.'s *band.*

Majocchi, Domenico, Italian dermatologist, 1849–1929. See M. *granulomas;* M.'s *disease.*

major (mā'jōr) [L. comparative of *magnus,* great]. Larger or greater in size of two similar structures.

Makeham, William Matthew, 19th century British actuary. See M.'s *hypothesis.*

Maklakov, Aleksey Nikolaevich, Russian ophthalmologist, 1837–1895. See M. applanation *tonometer.*

mal- [L. *malus,* bad]. Combining form meaning ill or bad.

mal (mahl) [Fr. fr. L. *malum,* an evil]. A disease or disorder.
m. de caderas, a disease of horses in some South American countries caused by *Trypanosoma equinum* and manifested by emaciation, remittent fever, weakness (especially of the hind quarters, from which the disease gets its name), and eventually death; the trypanosome has a reservoir in the giant rodent, the capybara; cattle, sheep, and goats are only mildly affected; man is not susceptible.
m. de Cayenne, elephantiasis.
m. de la rosa, m. rosso, pellagra.
m. de los pintos, pinta.
m. de Meleda, endemic symmetrical keratoderma of the extremities occurring on the island of Meleda off the coast of Dalmatia.
m. de mer, seasickness.
m. de San Lazaro, elephantiasis.
grand m. (grahn), generalized tonic-clonic *epilepsy.*
m. morado, onchocerciasis.
m. perforant, perforating *ulcer* of foot.
petit m. (pĕ-tē') [Fr. small], absence.

mala (mā'lă) [L. cheek bone]. **1.** Cheek. **2.** *Os* zygomaticum.

malabsorption (mal-ab-sōrp'shŭn). Imperfect, inadequate, or otherwise disordered gastrointestinal absorption.

Malacarne, Michele V.G., Italian surgeon, 1744–1816. See M.'s *pyramid, space.*

malachite green (mal'ă-kīt) [G. *malachē,* a mallow] [C.I. 42000]. Tetramethyl-di-*p*- aminotriphenylcarbinol; a dye that has been used as a wound antiseptic, as a treatment of mycotic skin infections, and in biological staining of tissues and bacteria.

malacia (mă-lā'shē-ă) [G. *malakia,* a softness]. Malacosis; mollities (2); a softening or loss of consistency and contiguity in any of the organs or tissues. Also used as combining form in suffix position.

malacic (mă-lā'sik). Malacotic.

malaco- [G. *malakos,* soft; *malakia,* a softness]. Combining form meaning soft or softening.

malacoplakia (mal'ă-kō-plā'kē-ă) [malaco- + G. *plax,* plate, plaque]. Rare lesion in the mucosa of the urinary bladder, more frequently in women, characterized by numerous mottled yellow and gray soft plaques and nodules that consist of numerous macrophages and calcospherites (Michaelis-Guttmann bodies) which may form around intracellular bacteria.

malacosis (mal'ă-kō'sis). Malacia.

malacotic (mal'ă-kot'ik). Malacic; pertaining to or characterized by malacia.

malacotomy (mal'ă-kot'ō-mē) [malaco- + G. *tomē,* incision]. Obsolete term for incision of soft parts, especially of the abdominal wall.

malactic (mă-lak'tik) [G. *malaktikos,* softening]. Emollient.

maladie (mal'ă-dē') [Fr.]. Malady.
m. de Roger [Fr.], Roger's *disease.*

maladjustment (mal-ad-jŭst'ment). In the mental health professions, an inability to cope with the problems and challenges of everyday living.
social m., m. without manifest psychiatric disorder, as that occasioned by an inability to cope with social situations.

malady (mal'ă-dē) [Fr. *maladie,* illness]. A disease or illness, especially a chronic, usually fatal, one.

malagma (mă-lag'mă) [G. a poultice]. A cataplasm or emollient.

malaise (mă-lāz') [Fr. discomfort]. A feeling of general discomfort or uneasiness, an out-of-sorts feeling, often the first indication of an infection or other disease.

malalignment (mal-ă-līn'ment). Displacement of a tooth or teeth from a normal position in the dental arch.

malar (mā'lăr). Relating to the mala, the cheek or cheek bones.

malaria (mă-lār'ē-ă) [It. *malo* (fem. *mala,* bad, + *aria,* air, referring to the old theory of the miasmatic origin of the disease]. Marsh, paludal, or jungle fever; swamp fever (2); a disease caused by the presence of the sporozoan *Plasmodium* in human or other vertebrate red blood cells and is transmitted to humans by the bite of an infected female mosquito of the genus *Anopheles,* which previously sucked the blood from a person with m; human infection begins with the exoerythrocytic cycle in liver parenchyma cells, followed by a series of erythrocytic schizogenous cycles repeated at regular intervals; production of gametocytes in other red cells provides future gametes for another mosquito infection. See also *Plasmodium* and species subentries.

acute m., a form of m. that may be intermittent or remittent, consisting of a chill accompanied and followed by fever with its attendant general symptoms, and terminating in a sweating stage; the paroxysms, caused by release of merozoites from infected cells, recur every 48 hours in tertian (vivax or ovale) m., every 72 hours in quartan (malariae) m., and at indefinite but frequent intervals, usually about 48 hours, in malignant tertian (falciparum) m.
algid m., a form of falciparum m. chiefly involving the gut and other abdominal viscera; **gastric a. m.** is characterized by persistent vomiting; **dysenteric a. m.** is characterized by bloody diarrheic stools in which enormous numbers of infected red blood cells are found.
autochthonous m., disease acquired by mosquito transmission in an area where m. regularly occurs.
avian m., plasmodial infections of domestic and wild birds, transmitted chiefly by culicine mosquitoes.
benign tertian m., vivax m.
bilious remittent m., a form of falciparum m. characterized by bilious vomiting, bilious diarrhea, etc.
cerebral m., a form of falciparum m. characterized by cerebral involvement, with extreme hyperthermia and headache, and a case fatality rate of about 50%.
chronic m., malarial cachexia; limnemia; m. that develops after frequently repeated attacks of one of the acute forms, usually falciparum m.; it is characterized by profound anemia, enlargement of the spleen, emaciation, mental depression, sallow complexion, edema of ankles, feeble digestion, and muscular weakness.
m. comato'sa, falciparum m. complicated by coma.
double tertian m., see quotidian m.
falciparum m., pernicious m.; malignant tertian m. or fever; aestivoautumnal or falciparum fever; m. caused by *Plasmodium falciparum* and characterized by 48-hour malarial paroxysms of severe form that occur with acute cerebral, renal, or gastrointestinal manifestations in severe cases, chiefly caused by the large number of red blood cells affected and the tendency for infected red cells to become sticky and clump, thus blocking capillaries. See also malarial *knobs.*
induced m., m. acquired by artificial means, *e.g.,* via blood transfusion, common syringes, or malariotherapy.
intermittent m., a malarial fever, usually of the tertian or quartan type, in which there is complete apyrexia, with absence of the other symptoms, in the intervals between the paroxysms.
malariae m., quartan m. or fever; a malarial fever with paroxysms that recur every 72 hours or every fourth day, reckoning the day of the paroxysm as the first; due to the schizogony and invasion of new red blood corpuscles by *Plasmodium malariae.*
malignant tertian m., falciparum m.
monkey m., simian m.
nonan m., a malarial fever with paroxysms that occur every ninth day, *i.e.,* every eighth day following the preceding paroxysm, the day of each paroxysm being included in the computation.
ovale m., ovale tertian m., m. caused by *Plasmodium ovale.*
pernicious m., falciparum m.
quartan m., malariae m.
quotidian m., quotidian fever; m. in which the paroxysms occur daily; usually a double tertian m., in which there is an infection by two distinct groups of *Plasmodium vivax* parasites sporulating alternately every 48 hours, but may also be an infection by the pernicious form of malarial parasite, *P. falciparum,* combined with *P. vivax,* or infection by two distinct *P. falciparum* generations; which mature on different days; may also develop from infection with *P. knowlesi.*
relapsing m., renewal of clinical activity at some interval after the primary attack.
remittent m., a malarial fever, usually of the severe falciparum type, in which the temperature falls but not to the normal level during the interval between two pronounced paroxysms.
simian m., monkey m.; plasmodial infection of monkeys and apes, as with human m., transmitted chiefly by anopheline mosquitoes; a number of *Plasmodium* species are responsible, with Southeast Asia and Africa being the apparent centers of evolution; among the 20 plasmodial agents described from nonhuman primates, some resemble and induce a malarial infection similar to those caused by the four species of *Plasmodium* from man, from which the agents of human m. appear to be derived.
tertian m., vivax m.
therapeutic m., intentionally induced m., formerly used against neurosyphilis and certain other paralytic diseases; the mechanism is thought to be immunological, with *Plasmodium* antibodies cross-reacting against the spirochetes or other agents.
vivax m., tertian or benign tertian m.; tertian or vivax fever; a malarial fever with paroxysms that recur every 48 hours or every other day (every third day, reckoning the day of the paroxysm as the first); the fever is induced by release of merozoites and their invasion of new red blood corpuscles.

malarial (mă-lār'ē-ăl). Pertaining to or affected with malaria.

malariology (mă-lār-ē-ol'ō-jē). A study of malaria in all aspects, with particular reference to epidemiology and control.

malarious (mă-lār'ē-ŭs) Relating to or characterized by the prevalence of malaria.

Malassez, Louis C., French physiologist, 1842–1910. See *Malassezia;* M.'s epithelial *rests.*

Malassezia (mal-ă-sā'zē-ă) [L. C. *Malassez*]. A genus of fungi (family Cryptococcaceae) of low pathogenicity that lack the ability to synthesize medium-chain and long-chain fatty acids, and require an exogenous supply of these lipids for growth as can be found in the skin.
M. fur'fur, *Pityrosporum orbiculare;* a fungus species which causes tinea versicolor.
M. ova'lis, *Pityrosporum ovale;* a species of yeast found in superficial epidermal scales and hair follicles on oily skin, of borderline pathogenicity; once thought to be the cause of dandruff.

malassimilation (mal'ă-sim-i-lā'shŭn). Incomplete or faulty assimilation.

malate (mal'āt). A salt or ester of malic acid.

malate dehydrogenase. An enzyme that catalyzes, through NAD or NADP, the dehydrogenation of malate to oxaloacetate or its decarboxylation to pyruvate. At least six are known (EC 1.1.1.37–.40, 1.1.1.82–.83), distinguished by their products, use of NAD or NADP, and specificity of substrate. Also called malic acid dehydrogenase; malic dehydrogenase; malic enzyme; pyruvic-malic carboxylase.

malate synthase [EC 4.1.3.2]. Malate-condensing enzyme; glyoxylate transacetylase; an enzyme catalyzing the condensation of acetyl-CoA with glyoxylate to form malate.

malathion (mal-ă-thī'on, mă-lă'thi-on). *S*-(1,2-Dicarboxyethyl)*O,O*-dimethyldithiophosphate; an organophosphorous compound used as an insecticide and veterinary ectoparasiticide; considered to be less toxic than parathion.

malaxation (mal'ak-sā'shŭn) [L. *malaxo,* pp. *-atus,* to soften]. **1.** Formation of ingredients into a mass for pills and plasters. **2.** A kneading process in massage.

maldigestion (mal-dī-jes'chŭn). Imperfect digestion.

Maldonado-San Jose stain. See under stain.

male (māl) [L. *masculus,* fr. *mas,* male]. **1.** In zoology, denoting the sex to which those belong that produce spermatozoa; an individual of that sex. **2.** Masculine.
genetic m., (1) an individual with a karyotype containing a Y chromosome; **(2)** an individual whose cell nuclei do not contain Barr sex chromatin bodies, which are normally present in females and absent in m.'s; patients with ambiguous sexual development

and those with Turner's syndrome are classed as genetic m.'s or genetic females by absence or presence of Barr bodies even though their sex chromosome complement may be abnormal.

XX m., a clear male phenotype in the presence of a 46,XX karyotype; presumably the vital parts of the Y chromosome, at least in some of these persons, are located elsewhere in the genome as a result of translocation.

XXY m., see Klinefelter's *syndrome.*

XYY m., see XYY *syndrome.*

Malecot, Achille-Etienne, French surgeon, *1852. See M. *catheter.*

maleic acid (mă-lē'ik). Toxilic acid; (*Z*)-butenedioic acid; HOOC-CH=CH-COOH; the *cis* isomer of fumaric acid; used for preparing maleate salts of antihistaminics and similar drugs.

malemission (mal-ē-mish'ŭn) [mal- + L. *e-mitto,* pp. *missus,* to send out]. Failure of semen to be ejected from the penis in coitus.

maleruption (mal-ē-rŭp'shŭn). Faulty eruption of teeth.

malformation (mal-fōr-mā'shŭn). Failure of proper or normal development; more specifically, a primary structural defect that results from a localized error of morphogenesis; *e.g.,* cleft lip. *Cf.* deformation.

Arnold-Chiari m., Arnold-Chiari *deformity.*

malfunction (mal-fŭnk'shŭn). Disordered, inadequate, or abnormal function.

Malgaigne, Joseph F., French surgeon, 1806–1865. See M.'s *amputation, fossa, hernia, luxation, triangle.*

Malherbe, A. See M.'s *disease,* calcifying *epithelioma.*

malic acid (mal'ik, mā'lik). Hydroxysuccinic acid; HOOC-CH_2-CHOH-COOH; an acid found in apples and various other tart fruits; an intermediate in the tricarboxylic acid cycle.

malic acid dehydrogenase. Malate dehydrogenase.

malic dehydrogenase. Malate dehydrogenase.

malignancy (mă-lig'nan-sē). The property or condition of being malignant.

malignant (mă-lig'nănt) [L. *maligno,* pres. p. *-ans (ant-),* to do anything maliciously]. **1.** Resistant to treatment; occurring in severe form, and frequently fatal; tending to become worse and lead to an ingravescent course. **2.** In reference to a neoplasm, having the property of locally invasive and destructive growth and metastasis.

malinger (mă-ling'ger). To engage in malingering.

malingerer (mă-ling'ger-er). One who engages in malingering.

malingering (mă-ling'ger-ing) [Fr. *malingre,* poor, weakly]. Feigning illness or disability to escape work, excite sympathy, or gain compensation.

malinterdigitation (mal'in-ter-dij'i-tā'shŭn). Faulty intercuspation of teeth.

Mall, Franklin P., U.S. anatomist and embryologist, 1862–1917. See M.'s *formula, ridges,* periportal *space* of M.

malleable (mal'ē-ă-bl) [L. *malleus,* a hammer]. Capable of being shaped by being beaten or by pressure; a property of certain metals such as gold and silver.

malleation (mal-ē-ā'shŭn) [L. *malleus,* a hammer]. A form of tic, in which the hands twitch in a hammering motion against the thighs.

mallebrin (mal'e-brin). *Aluminum* chlorate nonahydrate.

mallein (mal'ē-in). An allergin, analogous to tuberculin, made from the growth products of *Pseudomonas mallei,* the causative agent of glanders; used as a diagnostic agent to provoke reactions in animals affected with glanders.

malleinization (mal'ē-in-i-zā'shŭn). Inoculation with mallein.

malleoincudal (mal'ē-ō-ing'kū-dăl). Relating to the malleus and the incus in the tympanum.

malleolar (mă-lē'ō-lăr). Relating to one or both malleoli.

malleolus, pl. **malleoli** (ma-lē'ō-lŭs, -lī) [L. dim. of *malleus,* hammer] [NA]. A rounded bony prominence such as those on either side of the ankle joint.

external m., m. lateralis.

inner m., m. medialis.

internal m., m. medialis.

lateral m., m. lateralis.

m. latera'lis [NA], lateral m.; extramalleolus; external or outer m.; the process at the lateral side of the lower end of the fibula, forming the projection of the lateral part of the ankle.

medial m., m. medialis.

m. media'lis [NA], medial m.; internal or inner m.; the process at the medial side of the lower end of the tibia, forming the projection of the medial side of the ankle.

outer m., m. lateralis.

malleotomy (mal'ē-ot'ō-mē). **1** [malleus + G. *tomē,* incision]. Division of the malleus. **2** [malleolus + G. *tomē,* incision]. Division of the ligaments holding the malleoli in apposition in order to permit their separation in certain cases of clubfoot.

malleus, gen. and pl. **mallei** (mal'ē-ŭs, mal'ē-ī) [L. a hammer] [NA]. Hammer; the largest of the three auditory ossicles, resembling a club rather than a hammer; it is regarded as having a head or caput, below which is the neck or collum, and from this diverge the handle or manubrium, and the slender, anterior process; from the base of the manubrium the short lateral process arises. The manubrium and lateral process are firmly attached to the tympanic membrane, and the head articulates with a saddle-shaped surface on the body of the incus.

Mallophaga (mă-lof'ă-gă) [G. *mallos,* wool, + *phagein,* to eat]. An order of biting lice that cause irritation by feeding on hair, feathers, and skin, and on blood and exudates when present; most species are found on birds, but some are found on common domestic animals. The genera *Menacanthus* and *Menopon* (family Menoponidae) attack domestic fowl, as do *Columbicola, Chelopistes, Lipeurus,* and other genera of the family Philopteridae, while *Bovicola, Felicola,* and *Trichodectes* (family Trichodectidae) infest domestic mammals.

Mallory, Frank B., U.S. pathologist, 1862–1941. See M. *bodies;* M.'s *stains;* picro-M. trichrome *stain.*

Mallory, G. Kenneth, U.S. pathologist, *1926. See M.-Weiss *lesion, syndrome, tear.*

malnutrition (mal-nū-trish'ŭn). Faulty nutrition resulting from malassimilation, poor diet, or overeating.

malignant m., kwashiorkor.

malocclusion (mal-ō-klū'zhŭn). **1.** Any deviation from a physiologically acceptable contact of opposing dentitions. **2.** Any deviation from a normal occlusion.

Maloney bougies. See under bougie.

malonic acid (mălō'nik, -lon'ik). Propanedioic acid; HOOC–CH_2–COOH; a dicarboxylic acid of importance in intermediary metabolism.

malonyl (mal'ō-nil). The divalent radical derived from malonic acid.

m. transacylase, ACP-malonyltransferase.

malonyl-CoA. Malonylcoenzyme A; the condensation product of malonic acid and coenzyme A, an intermediate in fatty acid synthesis.

malonylcoenzyme A (mal'ō-nil-kō-en'zīm). Malonyl-CoA.

malonylurea (mal'ō-nil-yū-rē'ă). Barbituric acid.

Malpighi, Marcello, Italian anatomist, histologist, and embryologist, 1628–1694. See malpighian *bodies, capsules, cell, corpuscles, glands, glomerulus, layer, nodules, pyramid, rete, stigmas, stratum, tubules, tuft, vesicles.*

malpighian (mahl-pig'ē-an). Described by or attributed to Marcello Malpighi.

malposition (mal-pō-zish'ŭn). Dystopia.

malpractice (mal-prak'tis). Mistreatment of a patient through ignorance, carelessness, neglect, or criminal intent.

malpresentation (mal'prē-sen-tā'shŭn). Faulty presentation of the fetus; presentation of any part other than the occiput.

malrotation (mal-rō-tā'shŭn). Failure during embryonic development of normal rotation of all or part of an organ or system such as gut tube, kidney, or spinal cord.

malt (mawlt) [A.S. *mealt*]. The seed of barley or other grain, artificially germinated and dried, containing dextrin, maltose, small amounts of glucose, and amylolytic enzymes. Used in the form of an extract as a digestive and flavoring agent.

maltase (mawl-tās). α-D-Glucosidase.
acid m., exo-1,4-α-D-glucosidase.

maltobiose (mawl-tō-bī'ōs). Maltose.

maltose (mawl-tōs). Maltobiose; malt sugar; 4-(α-D-glucosido)-D-glucose; a disaccharide formed in the hydrolysis of starch and consisting of two glucose residues bound by a 1,4-α-glycoside link.

maltotetrose (mawl-tō-tet'rōs). A saccharide comprised of four glucose units in the α-1,4 linkage.

malum (mā'lŭm) [L. an evil]. A disease.
m. artic'ulorum seni'lis, arthritis in the aged.
m. cor'dis, heart disease.
m. cox'ae, disease of the hip joint.
m. cox'ae seni'le, senile hip disease; deformity of the head of the femur caused by ischemic damage.
m. per'forans pe'dis, perforating ulcer of the foot occurring in certain neuropathies.
m. vene'reum, syphilis.
m. vertebra'le suboccipita'le, Rust's *disease*.

malunion (mal-yūn'yŭn). Incomplete union, or union in a faulty position, after fracture or a wound of the soft parts.

Maly, Richard L., Austrian physiological chemist, 1839–1894. See M.'s *test*.

mamanpian (mă-mon-pē-on') [Fr. *maman*, mother + *pian*, yaw]. Mother *yaw*.

mamelon (mam'ĕ-lon) [Fr. nipple]. One of the rounded prominences, three in number, on the cutting edge of an incisor tooth when it first pierces the gum.

mamelonated (mam'ĕ-lon-āt-ed) [Fr. *mamelon*, nipple]. Having rounded, teatlike elevations; nodulated.

mamelonation (mam'ĕ-lō-nā'shŭn). The formation of rounded projections or nodules on bony and other structures.

mamil-, mamilli- [L. *mamilla*, nipple]. Combining forms relating to the mamillae. See also mammil-, mammilli-.

mamilla, pl. mamillae (mă-mil'ă, mă-mil'ē) [L. nipple]. **1.** A small rounded elevation resembling the female breast. **2.** *Papilla* mammae.

mamillare (mam-i-lā'rē) [L.]. Mamillary.

mamillaria (mam-i-lā'rē-ă). See *corpus* mamillare.

mamillary (mam'i-lăr-ē). Relating to or shaped like a nipple.

mamillate, mamillated (mam'i-lāt, -lāt'ed). Studded with nipple-like projections.

mamillation (mam-i-lā'shŭn). **1.** A nipple-like projection. **2.** The condition of being mamillated.

mamilliform (mă-mil'i-fōrm) [L. *mamilla*, nipple, + *forma*, form]. Nipple-shaped.

mamma, gen. and pl. mammae (mam'ă, mam'ē) [L.] [NA]. Breast (2); the organ of milk secretion; one of two hemispheric projections of variable size situated in the subcutaneous layer over the pectoralis major muscle on either side of the chest; it is rudimentary in the male. See *glandula* mammaria.
m. accesso'ria [NA], accessory breast; supernumerary m.; a milk-secreting gland located elsewhere than at the normal place on the chest and existing in addition to the two usual mammae.
m. errat'ica, a supernumerary breast aberrantly located, *i.e.*, in some part other than the milk line.
m. masculi'na [NA], male breast; m. virilis; one of the two, usually rudimentary, mammary glands in the male.
supernumerary m., m. accessoria.
m. viri'lis, m. masculina.

mammal (mam'ăl). An animal of the class Mammalia.

mammalgia (mă-mal'jē-ă) [L. *mamma*, breast, + G. *algos*, pain]. Mastodynia.

Mammalia (mă-mā'lē-ă) [L. *mamma*, breast]. The highest class of living organisms; it includes all the vertebrate animals (monotremes, marsupials, and placentals) that suckle their young, possess hair, and (except for the egg-laying monotremes) bring forth living young rather than eggs.

mammaplasty (mam'ă-plas-tē) [L. *mamma*, breast, + G. *plastos*, formed]. Mammoplasty; mastoplasty; plastic surgery of the breast to alter its shape, size, or position, or all of these.
augmentation m., plastic surgery to enlarge the breast, often by insertion of an implant.
reconstructive m., the making of a simulated breast by plastic surgery, to replace the appearance of one that has been removed.
reduction m., plastic surgery of the breast to reduce its size and (frequently) to improve its shape and position.

mammary (mam'ă-rē). Relating to the breasts.

mammectomy (ma-mek'tō-mē) [L. *mamma*, breast, + *ektomē*, excision]. Mastectomy.

mammiform (mam'i-fōrm) [L. *mamma*, breast, + *forma*, form]. Mammose (1); resembling a breast; breast-shaped.

mammil-, mammilli- [L. *mammilla (mamilla)*, nipple]. Combining forms relating to the mamillae. See also mamil-, mamilli-.

mammillaplasty (ma-mil'ă-plas-tē) [L. *mammilla*, nipple, + G. *plastos*, formed]. Theleplasty; plastic surgery of the nipple and areola.

mammillitis (mam-i-lī'tis) [L., *mamilla*, nipple, + G. *-itis*, inflammation]. Inflammation of the nipple.
bovine herpes m., bovine ulcerative m.; an ulcerative disease of the skin of the bovine teat caused by bovine herpesvirus type 2.
bovine ulcerative m., bovine herpes m.
bovine vaccinia m., a poxlike disease of the skin of the bovine teat caused by vaccinia virus.

mammitis (ma-mī'tis) [L. *mamma*, breast, + G. *-itis*, inflammation]. Mastitis.

mammo- [L. *mamma*, breast]. Combining form relating to the breasts.

mammogram (mam'ō-gram). The record produced by mammography.

mammography (ma-mog'ră-fē) [mammo- + G. *graphō*, to write]. Roentgenographic examination of the breast by means of x-rays, ultrasound, nuclear magnetic resonance, etc.

mammoplasty (mam'ō-plas-tē) [mammo- + G. *plastos*, formed]. Mammaplasty.

mammose (mam'mōs). **1.** Mammiform. **2.** Having large breasts.

mammotomy (ma-mot'ō-mē) [mammo- + G. *tomē*, incision]. Mastotomy.

mammotroph (mam'ō-trof). Prolactin cell; an acidophilic cell of the adenohypophysis that produces prolactin.

mammosomatotroph (mam'ō-sō-mat'ō-trof). A cell of the adenohypophysis that produces prolacting and somatotropin.

mammotropic, mammotrophic (mam-ō-trop'ik, -trof'ik) [mammo- + G. *tropos,* a turning]. Having a stimulating effect upon the development, growth, or function of the mammary glands.

mammotropin, mammotrophin (mam-ō-trō'pin, -trō'fin). Obsolete terms for prolactin.

Man Symbol for mannose or its radicals in polysaccharides.

manchette (man-shet') [Fr.]. A circular band formed mainly of microtubules at the caudal pole of the nucleus of a developing spermatozoon.

mandelate (man'de-lāt). A salt or ester of mandelic acid.

mandelic acid (man-del'ik). Phenylglycolic or hydroxytoluic acid; $C_6H_5CHOHCOOH$; a urinary antibacterial agent (both bactericidal and bacteriostatic).

Mandelin's reagent. See under reagent.

mandelytropine (man-de-lit'rō-pēn). Homatropine.

mandible (man'di-bl). Mandibula.

mandibula, pl. **mandibulae** (man-dib'yū-lă, -lē) [L. a jaw, fr. *mando,* pp. *mansus,* to chew] [NA]. Mandible; mandibulum; jaw bone; lower jaw; submaxilla; a U-shaped bone, forming the lower jaw, articulating by its upturned extremities with the temporal bone on either side.

mandibular (man-dib'yū-lăr). Inframaxillary; submaxillary (1); relating to the lower jaw.

mandibulectomy (man-dib-yū-lek'tō-mē) [mandibula + G. *ektomē,* excision]. Excision of the lower jaw.

mandibulofacial (man-dib'yū-lō-fā'shăl). Relating to the mandible and the face.

mandibulo-oculofacial (man-dib'yū-lō-ok'yū-lō-fā'shăl). Relating to the mandible and the orbital part of the face.

mandibulopharyngeal (man-dib'yū-lō-fa-rin'jē-ăl). Relating to the mandible and the pharynx; denoting the region between the pharynx and the ramus of the mandible, in which are found the internal carotid artery, the internal jugular vein, and the vagus, glossopharyngeal, accessory, and hypoglossal nerves.

mandibulum (man-dib'yū-lŭm). Mandibula.

mandragora (man-drag'ō-rā) [G. *mandragoras*]. The European mandrake, *Mandragora officinalis,* or *Atropa mandragora* (family Solanaceae), the mandrake of the Bible; its properties are similar to those of stramonium, hyoscyamus, and belladonna.

mandrake (man'drāk) [thr. L., fr. G. *mandragoras*]. **1.** See mandragora. **2.** See podophyllum.

man'drel, man'dril [G. *mandra,* a stable; the bed in which a ring's stone is set]. **1.** The shaft or spindle to which a tool is attached and by means of which it is rotated. **2.** Mandrin. **3.** In dentistry, an instrument used in a handpiece to hold a disk, stone, or cup used for grinding, smoothing, or finishing.

man'drill. Common name for a species of monkey of the genus *Cynocephalus,* with a short tail and doglike head.

man'drin [Fr. *mandrin,* mandrel]. Mandrel (2); a stiff wire or stylet inserted in the lumen of a soft catheter to give it shape and firmness while passing through a hollow tubular structure.

maneuver (mă-nū'ver) [Fr. *manoeuvre,* fr. L. *manu operari,* to work by hand]. A planned movement or procedure.

Adson m., Adson's *test.*

Bill's m., forceps rotation of the fetal head at mid-pelvis before extraction of the head.

Bracht m., delivery of a fetus in breech position by extension of the legs and trunk of the fetus over the symphysis pubis and abdomen of the mother; the fetal head is born spontaneously as the legs and trunk are lifted above the maternal pelvis, and as the body of the infant is extended by the operator.

Brandt-Andrews m., the expression of the placenta by grasping the umbilical cord with one hand and placing the other hand on the abdomen, with the fingers over the anterior surface of the uterus at the junction of the lower uterine segment and the corpus uteri.

Buzzard's m., testing the patellar reflex while the sitting patient makes firm pressure on the floor with the toes.

Credé's m.'s, Credé's *methods.*

DeLee's m., key-in-lock m.

Ejrup m., demonstration of collateral circulation by reduction in the prominence of activity of the greater arteries and reduced pulse volume following muscular activity.

Hampton m., rolling a supine patient on his right and then left side to obtain an air contrast x-ray film of the antrum and duodenum in gastrointestinal fluoroscopy.

Heimlich m., a planned action designed to expel an obstructing bolus of food from the throat by placing a fist on the abdomen between the navel and the costal margin, grasping the fist with the other hand, and forcefully thrusting it inward and upward so as to force air up the trachea and dislodge the obstruction.

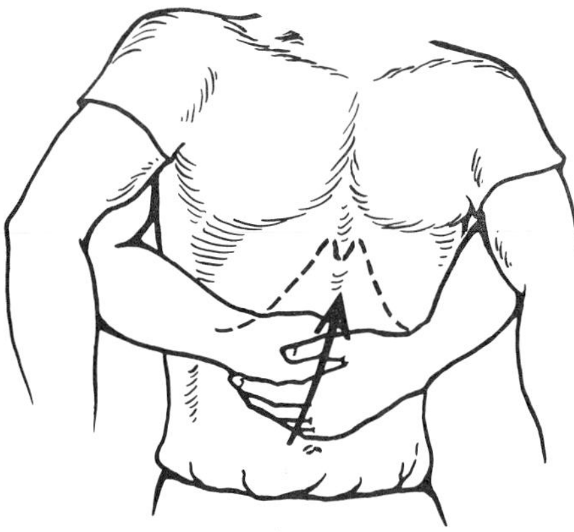

Heimlich Maneuver

Hillis-Müller m., manual pressure on the term fundus while a finger in the rectum determines the descent of the head into the pelvis engagement.

Hueter's m., pressing the patient's tongue downward and forward with the left forefinger in passing a stomach tube.

Jendrassik's m., a method of emphasizing the patellar reflex: the subject hooks his hands together by the flexed fingers and pulls against them with all his strength.

key-in-lock m., DeLee's m.; a method by which obstetrical forceps are used to rotate the fetal head.

Leopold's m.'s, four m.'s employed to determine fetal position: 1) determination of what is in the fundus; 2) evaluation of the fetal back and extremities; 3) palpation of the presenting part above the symphysis; 4) determination of the direction and degree of flexion of the head.

Mauriceau's m., Mauriceau-Levret m.; a method of assisted breech delivery in which the infant's body is astraddle the right forearm, and the middle finger of the right hand is in the fetal mouth to maintain flexion while traction is made upon the shoulders by the other hand.

Mauriceau-Levret m., Mauriceau's m.

McDonald's m., measurement of uterus from the upper border of the symphysis to a line tangential to the fundus over the abdomen with a tape to determine the height of the uterus; this figure divided by 3.5 gives the approximate age of the fetus in lunar months.

Müller's m., after a forced expiration, an attempt at inspiration is made with closed mouth and nose or closed glottis, whereby the negative pressure in the chest and lungs is made very subatmospheric; the reverse of Valsalva *maneuver.*

Pajot's m., traction downward on the forceps lock with one hand while traction is applied with the other hand to bring the fetal head down in the axis of the birth canal.
Pinard's m., in management of a frank breech presentation, pressure on the popliteal space is made by the index finger while the other three fingers flex the leg while sliding it along the other thigh as the foot of the flexed leg is brought down and out.
Prague m., a technique for delivery of the fetus in breech position when the fetal occiput is posterior; one hand of the operator delivers the shoulders, while making pressure over the symphysis pubis with the other hand.
Ritgen's m., delivery of a child's head by pressure on the perineum while controlling the speed of delivery by pressure with the other hand on the head.
Scanzoni's m., forceps rotation and traction in a spiral course, with reapplication of forceps for delivery.
Sellick's m., pressure applied to the cricoid cartilage, to prevent regurgitation during endotracheal intubation in the anesthetized patient.
Valsalva m., (1) forced expiratory effort with closed nose and mouth to inflate the eustachian tubes and middle ears; *e.g.,* as used by persons descending from high altitudes; **(2)** any forced expiratory effort against a closed airway, whether at the nose and mouth or at the glottis, the reverse of Müller's *maneuver;* because high intrathoracic pressure impedes venous return to the right atrium, this m. is used to study cardiovascular effects of raised peripheral venous pressure and decreased cardiac filling and cardiac output.
Wigand m., an assisted breech delivery with pressure above the symphysis while the fetus lies astraddle the operator's other arm.

manganese (mang'gă-nēz) [Mod. L. *manganesium, manganum,* an altered form of *magnesium*]. Manganum; a metallic element resembling and often associated, in ores, with iron; symbol Mn, atomic no. 25, atomic weight 54.94; manganous salts are sometimes used in medicine.

manganic (mang-gan'ik). Denoting the trivalent cation of manganese, Mn^{3+}.

manganous (mang'gă-nŭs). Denoting the divalent cation of manganese, Mn^{2+}.

manganum (man'gă-nŭm) [L.]. Manganese.

mange (mānj) [Fr. *manger,* to eat]. A cutaneous disease of domestic and wild animals caused by any one of several genera of skin-burrowing mites; in man, mite infestations are usually referred to as scabies or itch.
chorioptic m., m. caused by mites of the genus *Chorioptes;* in many cases it involves the skin of much of the body.
demodectic m., follicular m.; an infection of the hair follicles and sebaceous glands with mites of the genus *Demodex;* they occur in man and a number of domesticated animals; although they cause a benign disease in most species, these mites can cause severe and extensive dermatitis ("red mange") in dogs.
ear m., otodectic m.
follicular m., demodectic m.
notoedric m., m. of cats caused by the mite, *Notoedres cati.*
otodectic m., ear m.; disease resulting from heavy infestation with *Otodectes cynotis* in the ears of dogs, cats, foxes, and other carnivores and manifested by head shaking, continual ear scratching, and ear droop; observed in severe cases are torticollis, circling, epileptoid fits with purulent inflammation and discharge of the external ear, and possible perforation of the tympanic membrane. See also otoacariasis.
psoroptic m., hair loss or m. caused by infestation with *Psoroptes.*
red m., demodectic m. in dogs.
sarcoptic m., a cutaneous disease of domestic animals caused by subspecies *Sarcoptes scabiei* or other species of the genus *Sarcoptes.*

-mania [G. frenzy]. Combining form, used in the suffix position, usually referring to an abnormal love for, or morbid impulse toward, some specific object, place, or action.

mania (mā'nē-ă) [G. frenzy]. An emotional disorder characterized by euphoria, increased psychomotor activity, rapid speech, flight of ideas, decreased need for sleep, distractibility, grandiosity, and poor judgment; usually occurs in bipolar disorder.

maniac (mā'nē-ak). **1.** One suffering from mania. **2.** Obsolete term for a mentally ill or disturbed person.

maniacal (mă-nī'ă-kăl). Manic; relating to or characterized by mania.

manic (man'ik, mā'nik). Maniacal.

manic-depressive. 1. Pertaining to a manic-depressive psychosis (bipolar *disorder*). **2.** One suffering from such a disorder.

manicy (man'i-sē). Behavior characteristic of the manic phase of bipolar disorder.

manifestation (man'i-fes-tā'shŭn). The display or disclosure of characteristic signs or symptoms of an illness.
behavioral m., a m. characterized by defects in personality structure with minimal anxiety and little or no sense of distress, indicative of a psychiatric disorder; occasionally encephalitis or head injury will produce the clinical picture which is properly diagnosed as chronic brain disorder with behavioral m.'s.
neurotic m., a m. characterized by such defenses as conversion, dissociation, displacement, phobia formation, or repetitive thoughts and acts being utilized to handle anxiety; in contrast to psychotic m.'s, gross distortion or falsification of reality is not exhibited, and gross disintegration of the personality is not usually observed.
psychophysiologic m., a m. characterized by the visceral expression of affect, the symptoms due to a chronic and exaggerated state of the physiologic expression of emotion with the feeling repressed; such m.'s are commonly characteristic of psychosomatic disorders.
psychotic m., a m. characterized by a varying degree of personality disintegration and distortion or falsification of reality in various spheres; persons exhibiting such a m. fail in effective relationships to other people or to their work.

manikin (man'i-kin) [dim. of *man*]. A model, especially one with removable pieces, of the human body or any of its parts. See also phantom (2).

maniphalanx (man'i-fā'langks) [L. *manus,* hand, + *phalanx*]. A phalanx of the hand; a bony segment of a finger; distinguished from pediphalanx.

Mann, Frank C., U.S. surgeon, 1887–1962. See M.-Bollman *fistula;* M.-Williamson *operation, ulcer.*

Mann's methyl blue-eosin stain. See under stain.

manna (man'ă) [L., fr. G. *manna,* fr. Heb. *mān*]. A saccharine exudation from *Fraxinus ornus,* flowering ash, a tree of the Mediterranean shores, used as a laxative, especially for children. It is available as **m. cannellata,** a flake m.; **m. in lacrimis,** m. in tears or small flakes; and **m. communis** or **m. in sortis,** m. in sorts.

mannans (man'anz). Mannosans; polysaccharides of mannose, found in various legumes and in the ivory nut.

mannerism (man'er-izm). A peculiar or unusual characteristic mode of movement, action, or speech.

mannite (man'īt). Mannitol.

mannitol (man'i-tol). Mannite; manna sugar; the hexahydric alcohol, widespread in plants, derived by reduction of fructose; used in renal function testing to measure glomerular filtration, and intravenously as an osmotic diuretic.
m. hexanitrate, nitromannitol; an explosive compound formed by the nitration of m.; when diluted with carbohydrate substances (one part of m. hexanitrate to nine or more parts of carbohydrate)

it is not explosive, and is used as a vasodilator and hypotensive agent; it is slower in action than nitroglycerin.

Mannkopf, Emil W., German physician, 1836–1918. See M.'s *sign.*

mannoheptulose (man-ō-hep'tū-lōs). See D-*manno-* -heptulose.

mannomustine (man-ō-mŭs'tēn). 1-6-Bis(2-chloroethylamino)-1,6-dideoxy-D-mannitol dihydrochloride; mannitol nitrogen mustard; an antineoplastic agent.

mannosans (man'o-sanz). Mannans.

mannose (Man) (man'ōs). Carubinose; seminose; an aldohexose obtained from various plant sources (*i.e.,* from mannans).

mannose-1-phosphate guanylyltransferase(GDP) [EC 2.7.7.22]. GDPmannose phosphorylase; a transferase that catalyzes the transfer of GDP to the mannose of mannose 1-phosphate.

mannoside (man'ō-sīd). A glycoside of mannose.

mannosidosis (man'ō-si-dō'sis). Congenital deficiency of α-mannosidase; associated with mental retardation, kyphosis, enlarged tongue, and vacuolated lymphocytes, with accumulation of mannose in tissues; autosomal recessive inheritance.

mannuronic acid (man-yū-ron'ik). Uronic acid derived from the oxidation of mannose.

manometer (mă-nom'ĕ-ter) [G. *manos,* thin, scanty, + *metron,* measure]. An instrument for indicating the pressure of any fluid or the difference in pressure between two fluids, whether gas or liquid.
aneroid m., dial m.; a m. in which the pressure is indicated by a revolving pointer moved by a diaphragm or Bourdon tube exposed to the pressure.
dial m., aneroid m.
differential m., any device that indicates the difference in pressure between two fluids, regardless of any changes in their absolute pressures.
mercurial m., an m. in which the varying pressures are shown by differences of elevation in a column of mercury.

manometric (man-ō-met'rik). Relating to a manometer.

manometry (mă-nom'ĕ-trē) [see manometer]. Manoscopy; measurement of the pressure of gases by means of a manometer.
esophageal m., measurement of intra-esophageal pressures at one or more sites by intraluminal pressure-sensitive instruments.

manoscopy (mă-nos'kō-pē). Manometry.

man. pr. Abbreviation for L. *mane primo,* early morning, first thing in the morning.

Manson, Sir Patrick, British authority on tropical medicine, 1844–1922. See *Mansonella, Mansonia;* M.'s *disease, pyosis, schistosomiasis,* eye *worm.*

Mansonella (man-sō-nel'ă). A genus of filaria, widely distributed in tropical Africa and South America, that infects the peritoneal cavity, serous surfaces, or skin with unsheathed microfilariae in the skin or blood of man and other primates. The important human parasites *M. perstans* and *M. streptocerca* formerly were placed in the genera *Dipetalonema, Acanthocheilonema,* and *Tetrapetalonema.*
M. demarqua'yi, *M. ozzardi.*
M. ozzar'di, *M. demarquayi; M. tucumana;* a filarial parasite occurring in Yucatan, Panama, Colombia, northern Argentina, Guyana, French Guiana, and the islands of St. Vincent and Dominica, causing mansonelliasis; the microfilariae are not ensheathed, and there are no nuclei in the pointed tail; the life cycle is similar to that of *Wuchereria bancrofti;* man is the only known definitive host, and the intermediate hosts are biting midges, *Culicoides furens* and possibly *c. paraensis.*
M. per'stans, the "persistent filaria," a species widely prevalent in tropical Africa and northern South America where it infects human peritoneal and other body cavities, but is non- or mildly pathogenic; characteristic subperiodic microfilariae occur in peripheral blood. It is transmitted in Africa by the biting midges *Culicoides austeni* and *C. grahami.*
M. streptocer'ca, a filarial species in man that produces nonperiodic sheathless microfilariae found in the circulating blood; may cause a lichenoid condition or edema of the skin; commonly found in the corium of the skin of west African residents and transmitted by the biting midge, *Culicoides grahami.*
M. tucuma'na, *M. ozzardi.*

mansonelliasis (man'sō-nel-ī'ă-sis). Infection with a species of *Mansonella,* transmitted to man by biting midges of the genus *Culicoides;* adult worms live in the serous cavities, especially the peritoneal cavity, in mesenteric and perivisceral adipose tissue, and in the skin.

Mansonia (man-sō'nē-ă) [P. *Manson*]. A genus of brown or black medium-sized mosquitoes (tribe Culicini), often having banded abdomen and legs; larvae and pupae have modified breathing tubes enabling them to pierce aquatic plants to obtain air. *M.* mosquitoes are distributed worldwide and, in tropical areas, are important vectors of *Brugia malayi;* in some areas they also transmit *Wuchereria bancrofti.*

Mansonoides (man-sō-noy'dēz). A subgenus of *Mansonia.*

mantle (man'tl). **1.** A covering layer. **2.** Pallium.
brain m., pallium.
myoepicardial m., the dorsal wall of the primitive pericardium which in the early somite embryo becomes both the epicardium and the myocardium.

Mantoux, Charles, French physician, 1877–1947. See M. *pit, test.*

manubrium, pl. **manubria** (mă-nū'brē-ŭm, -ă) [L. handle] [NA]. The portion of the sternum or of the malleus that represents the handle.
m. mal'lei [NA], the handle of the malleus; the portion that extends downward, inward, and backward from the neck of the malleus; it is embedded throughout its length in the tympanic membrane.
m. ster'ni [NA], episternum; presternum; the upper segment of the sternum, a flattened, roughly triangular bone, occasionally fused with the body of the sternum, forming with it a slight angle, the sternal angle.

manudynamometer (man'yū-dī-nă-mom'ĕ-ter) [L. *manus,* hand, + G. *dynamis,* force, + *metron,* measure]. In dentistry, a device for measuring the force exerted by the thrust of an instrument.

manus, gen. and pl. **manus** (mā'nŭs) [L.] [NA]. Hand; the distal portion of the superior limb, comprised of the carpus, metacarpus, and digits.

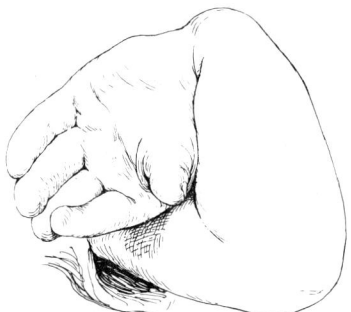

Manus Vara
Clubhand with radial deviation.

m. ca'va, a condition of extreme concavity of the palm of the hand.
m. exten'sa, m. superextensa; clubhand with deviation backward.
m. flex'a, clubhand with forward deviation.

m. pla'na, flat hand; loss of normal arches of the hand.
m. superexten'sa, m. extensa.
m. val'ga, clubhand with deviation to the ulnar side.
m. va'ra, clubhand with deviation to the radial side.

MAO Abbreviation for monoamine oxidase.

MAOI Abbreviation for monoamine oxidase *inhibitor.*

map distance. The degree of separation of two loci on a linkage map, measured in morgans or centimorgans.

mappine (map'ēn). Bufotenine.

mapping function. In linkage analysis, a formula that converts the recombination fraction (on the probability scale) into map distance (in morgans).

maprotiline (ma-prō'ti-lēn). *N*- Methyl-9,10-ethanoanthracene-9(10*H*)-propylamine; a tricyclic antidepressant used in the treatment of various depressive illnesses, and for relief of anxiety associated with depression.

Marañón, Gregorio, Spanish endocrinologist, 1887–1960. See M.'s *sign, syndrome.*

marantic (mă-ran'tik) [G. *marantikos,* wasting]. Marasmic.

marasmic (mă-raz'mik). Marantic; relating to or suffering from marasmus.

marasmoid (mă-raz'moyd) [G. *marasmos,* withering, + eidos, resemblance]. Resembling marasmus.

marasmus (mă-raz'mŭs) [G. *marasmos,* withering]. Marantic atrophy; Parrot's disease (3); pedatrophia; pedatrophy; cachexia, especially in young children, primarily due to prolonged dietary deficiency of protein and calories.

marc (mark) [Fr. fr. *marcher,* to trample]. The residue remaining after percolation of a drug.

Marcacci, Arturo, Italian physiologist, 1854–1915. See M.'s *muscle.*

Marchand, Felix, German pathologist, 1846–1928. See M.'s *adrenals, rest,* wandering *cell.*

Marchant, Gérard T.J., French surgeon, 1850–1903. See M.'s *zone.*

Marchesani, Oswald, 1900–1952. See M. *syndrome;* Weill-M. *syndrome.*

Marchetti, Andrew A., U.S. obstetrician and gynecologist, 1901–1970. See Marshall-M.-Krantz *operation.*

Marchi, Vittorio, Italian physician, 1851–1908. See M.'s *fixative, reaction, stain, tract.*

Marchiafava, Ettore, Italian pathologist, 1847–1935. See M.-Bignami *disease;* M.-Micheli *anemia, syndrome.*

marcid (mar'sid) [L. *marcidus;* fr. *marceo,* to wither]. Emaciating; tabid; wasting away.

Marcille, Maurice, 1871–1941. See M.'s *triangle.*

marcor (mar'kōr) [L. fr. *marceo,* to wither]. Obsolete term for marasmus.

Marcus Gunn, Robert. See *Gunn,* Robert Marcus.

Marek, Josef, Hungarian veterinarian and pathologist, 1867–1952. See M.'s *disease;* disease *virus.*

Marey, Ettienne J., French physiologist, 1830– 1904. See M.'s *law.*

Marfan, Antoine Bernard-Jean, French pediatrician, 1858–1942. See M.'s *disease, law, syndrome.*

marfanoid (mar'fan-oyd). Resembling the phenotype of Marfan's syndrome.

Marg, Elwin, U.S. physicist, *1918. See Mackay-M. *tonometer.*

Margaropus (mar-gar'ō-pŭs) [G. *margaros,* pearl oyster, + *pous,* foot]. A genus of ixodid ticks closely resembling *Boophilus,* but not having festoons or ornamentations; they are characterized by greatly enlarged posterior legs and a prolonged median plate.
M. winthe'mi, the one-host South American winter horse tick; it also sometimes attacks cattle and sheep.

margin (mar'jin) [L. *margo,* border, edge]. Margo; a boundary, edge, or border, as of a surface or structure. See also border, edge.
m. of acetabulum, *limbus* acetabuli.
anterior m., *margo* anterior.
articular m., *labrum* glenoidale.
cavity m., the periphery of a filling, the line of junction between a restoration and the external surface of a tooth.
cervical m., **(1)** gingival m.; **(2)** termination of a restoration in the gingival area.
ciliary m., **(1)** *margo* ciliaris iridis; **(2)** the tarsal border of an eyelid.
corneal m., *limbus* corneae.
m. of eyelid, *margo* palpebrae.
falciform m., *margo* falciformis.
fibular m. of foot, *margo* lateralis pedis.
m. of fossa ovalis, *limbus* fossa ovalis.
free m., *margo* liber.
frontal m., *margo* frontalis.
gingival m., cervical m. (1); gingival crest; **(1)** the most coronal portion of the gingiva surrounding the tooth; **(2)** the edge of the free gingiva.
incisal m., *margo* incisalis.
inferior m., *margo* inferior.
inferolateral m., *margo* inferior cerebri.
inferomedial m., *margo* medialis cerebri.
infraorbital m., *margo* infraorbitalis.
interosseous m., *margo* interosseus.
lacrimal m., *margo* lacrimalis.
lambdoid m., *margo* lambdoideus.
lateral m., *margo* lateralis.
mastoid m., *margo* mastoideus.
medial m., *margo* medialis.
mesovarian m., *margo* mesovaricus.
nasal m., *margo* nasalis.
occipital m., *margo* occipitalis.
parietal m., *margo* parietalis.
posterior m., *margo* posterior.
pupillary m., *margo* pupillaris iridis.
right m. of heart, *margo* dexter cordis.
m. of safety, the m. between the therapeutic dose and the toxic dose of a drug.
squamous m., *margo* squamosus.
superior m., *margo* superior.
superomedial m., *margo* superior cerebri.
supraorbital m., *margo* supraorbitalis.
m. of the tongue, *margo* linguae.
ulnar m., *margo* medialis antebrachii.
zygomatic m., *margo* zygomaticus.

marginal (mar'ji-năl). Relating to a margin.

Marginal Line Calculus Index (MLC). An index which scores supragingival calculus found in cervical areas paralleling marginal gingiva.

margination (mar'ji-nā'shŭn). A phenomenon that occurs during the relatively early phases of inflammation; as a result of dilation of capillaries and slowing of the bloodstream, leukocytes tend to occupy the periphery of the cross-sectional lumen and adhere to the endothelial cells that line the vessels.
m. of placenta, see *placenta* marginata.

margines (mar'ji-nēz) [L.]. Plural of margo.

marginoplasty (mar'ji-nō-plas-tē). Plastic surgery of the tarsal border of an eyelid.

margo, gen. marginis, pl. margines (mar'gō, mar'ji-nis, -nēz) [L.] [NA]. Margin.

m. ante'rior [NA], anterior margin; anterior border; **m. a. fib'ulae,** a ridge on the shaft of the fibula to which is attached the anterior intermuscular septum of the leg; **m. a. pancrea'tis,** the sharp margin between the anterior and inferior surfaces of the pancreas; **m. a. pulmo'nis,** the sharp margin separating the costal and mediastinal surfaces of the lung; **m. a. ra'dii,** the ridge on the shaft of the radius extending from the radial tuberosity to the anterior part of the styloid process; **m. a. tes'tis,** the rounded, free, anterior portion of the testis; **m. a. tib'iae,** tibial crest; the subcutaneous ridge of the tibia that extends from the tuberosity to the anterior part of the medial malleolus; **m. a. ul'nae,** the ridge on the body of the ulna that extends from the tuberosity to the anterior part of the styloid process.

m. cilia'ris i'ridis [NA], ciliary margin of the iris; the peripheral border of the iris attached to the ciliary body.

m. dex'ter cor'dis [NA], right margin of the heart; the border between the sternocostal and diaphragmatic surfaces of the heart; it is fairly well defined in fixed hearts but is rounded and indefinite in the living heart.

m. falcifor'mis [NA], falciform margin; the sharply curved, free margin of the saphenous opening in the fascia lata; medially, it ends in a superior and an inferior horn.

m. fibula'ris pedis [NA], an alternate term for m. lateralis pedis.

m. fronta'lis [NA], frontal margin; **m. f. os'sis parieta'lis,** the margin of the parietal bone that articulates with the frontal bone; **m. f. os'sis sphenoida'lis,** the margin of the greater wing of the sphenoid bone that articulates with the frontal bone.

m. incisa'lis [NA], incisal edge, margin, or surface; cutting edge (2); shearing edge; the part of an anterior tooth farthest from the apex of the root.

m. infe'rior [NA], inferior margin or border; **m. i. cer'ebri,** m. inferolateralis; inferolateral margin; the irregular, discontinuous margin of the cerebral hemisphere at the junction of the inferior and superolateral surfaces; **m. i. hep'atis,** the sharp border of the liver that separates the diaphragmatic and visceral surfaces; **m. i. lie'nis,** the border of the spleen separating the renal and diaphragmatic surfaces; **m. i. pancrea'tis,** the border of the pancreas separating the inferior and posterior surfaces; **m. i. pulmo'nis,** the sharp border of the lung that separates the diaphragmatic surface from the costal and mediastinal surfaces.

m. inferolatera'lis [NA], an alternate term for m. inferior cerebri.

m. inferomedia'lis [NA], an alternate term for m. medialis cerebri.

m. infraorbita'lis [NA], infraorbital margin; the lower border of the entrance to the orbit, formed by the maxilla medially and the zygomatic bone laterally.

m. interos'seus [NA], interosseous margin; interosseous crest; **m. i. fib'ulae,** the ridge along the medial border of the fibula to which is attached the interosseous membrane; **m. i. ra'dii,** the ridge along the medial side of the radius to which is attached the interosseous membrane; **m. i. tib'iae,** the ridge along the lateral border of the tibia to which is attached the interosseous membrane; **m. i. ul'nae,** the ridge along the lateral side of the body of the ulna to which is attached the interosseous membrane.

m. lacrima'lis [NA], lacrimal margin; the margin of the nasal surface of the maxilla that articulates with the lacrimal bone.

m. lambdoid'eus [NA], lambdoid margin; the margin of the occipital squama that articulates with the parietal bones in the lambdoid suture.

m. latera'lis [NA], lateral margin; **m. l. antebra'chii,** m. radialis; radial border; the radial or lateral border of the forearm; **m. l. pe'dis,** m. fibularis pedis; fibular margin of the foot; the border of the foot between the small toe and the heel; **m. l. humer'ii,** the ridge on the humerus that extends from the greater tubercle to the lateral epicondyle; **m. l. re'nis,** the convex lateral border of the kidney; **m. l. scap'ulae,** the border of the scapula extending from the glenoid fossa to the inferior angle; **m. l. un'guis,** the sides of the nail extending from the concealed to the free borders.

m. li'ber [NA], free margin; **m. l. ova'rii,** the posterior margin of the ovary; **m. l. un'guis,** the distal border of the nail that overhangs the tip of the digit.

m. lin'guae [NA], margin of the tongue; the lateral border that separates the dorsum from the inferior surface of the tongue on each side, the two borders meeting anteriorly at the apex.

m. mastoi'deus [NA], mastoid margin; the margin of the occipital squama that articulates with the temporal bone.

m. media'lis [NA], medial margin; **m. m. antebra'chii,** m. ulnaris; ulnar margin; the ulnar or medial border of the forearm; **m. m. cer'ebri,** m. inferomedialis; inferomedial margin; the irregular border of the cerebral hemisphere at the junction of the inferior and medial surfaces; **m. m. glan'dulae suprarena'lis,** the paravertebral border of the suprarenal gland; **m. m. humer'ii,** the ridge on the humerus that extends from the crest of the lesser tubercle to the medial epicondyle; **m. m. pe'dis,** m. tibialis; tibial border; the border of the foot from the great toe to the heel; **m. m. re'nis,** the concave border of the kidney; **m. m. scap'ulae,** the border of the scapula that extends from the superior angle to the inferior angle; **m. m. tib'iae,** the rounded border of the tibia that separates the posterior and medial surfaces.

m. mesova'ricus [NA], mesovarian margin; the border of the ovary to which the mesovarium is attached.

m. nasa'lis [NA], nasal margin; the border of the frontal bone that articulates with the nasal bones.

m. occipita'lis [NA], occipital margin; **m. o. os'sis parieta'lis,** the posterior margin of the parietal bone that articulates with the occipital squama; **m. o. os'sis tempora'lis,** that part of the temporal bone that articulates with the occipital squama.

m. occul'tus un'guis [NA], occult border of the nail; the proximal border of the nail entirely covered by the nail wall.

m. palpe'brae, margin of eyelid.

m. parieta'lis [NA], parietal margin; **m. p. os'sis fronta'lis,** the margin of the frontal bone that articulates with the parietal bone; **m. p. os'sis sphenoida'lis,** the margin of the greater wing of the sphenoid that articulates with the parietal bone; **m. p. os'sis tempora'lis,** the border of the squamous part of the temporal bone that articulates with the parietal bone.

m. poste'rior [NA], posterior margin; **m. p. fib'ulae,** the ridge on the posterior aspect of the fibula extending from the head to the medial aspect of the peroneal groove; **m. p. par'tis petro'sae os'sis tempora'lis,** posterior border of petrous part of temporal bone; the margin of the petrous part of the temporal bone that extends from the apex to the jugular notch; it articulates with the basal and jugular portions of the occipital bone. **m. p. ra'dii,** the ridge on the radius that extends from the tuberosity to the tubercle on the posterior aspect of the distal extremity; **m. p. tes'tis,** the rounded posterior portion of the testis into which the vessels enter; **m. p. ul'nae,** the sinuous ridge on the posterior aspect of the ulna that extends from near the olecranon to the styloid process.

m. pupilla'ris ir'idis [NA], pupillary margin of the iris; the inner border of the iris that forms the edge of the pupil.

m. radia'lis [NA], m. lateralis antebrachii.

m. sagitta'lis [NA], sagittal border; the medial border of the parietal bone entering into the sagittal suture.

m. sphenoida'lis [NA], sphenoidal border; the part of the border of the squamous part of the temporal bone that articulates with the greater wing of the sphenoid.

m. squamo'sus [NA], squamous margin; **m. s. os'sis parieta'lis,** the lateral border of the parietal bone that articulates with the squamous part of the temporal bone; **m. s. os'sis sphenoida'lis,** the margin of the greater wing of the sphenoid bone that articulates with the squamous part of the temporal bone.

m. supe'rior [NA], superior margin; **m. s. cer'ebri,** m. superomedialis; superomedial margin; the curved margin of the cerebral hemisphere at the junction of the superolateral and medial surfaces; **m. s. glan'dulae suprarena'lis,** the border of the suprarenal gland at the superior junction of the anterior and posterior surfaces; **m. s. lie'nis,** the notched border of the spleen that separates the gastric and disphragmatic surfaces; **m. s. pancrea'tis,** the border of the body of the pancreas that separates the anterior and posterior surfaces; **m. par'tis petro'sae os'sis tempora'lis,** superior border of petrous part of temporal bone; the margin that separates the anterior and posterior surfaces of the petrous part of the temporal bone; **m. s. scap'ulae,** the border of the scapula that extends from the glenoid fossa to the superior angle.

m. superomedia'lis [NA], m. superior cerebri.

m. supraorbita'lis [NA], supraorbital margin; supraorbital arch or ridge; the curved superior border of the entrance to the orbit.

m. tibia'lis [NA], m. medialis pedis.

m. ulna'ris [NA], m. medialis antebrachii.

m. u'teri [NA], border of the uterus; the right or left margin of the utcrus along which thc broad ligamcnt is attachcd. Thc utcrinc tube and round ligament attach to the uterus at the upper part of the border.

m. zygomat'icus [NA], zygomatic margin; the border of the greater wing of the sphenoid that articulates with the zygomatic bone.

Marie, Pierre, French neurologist, 1853–1940. See M.'s *ataxia, disease;* Charcot-M.-Tooth *disease,* Bamberger-M. *disease, syndrome;* M.-Strümpell *disease;* Strümpell-M. *disease;* Brissaud-M. *syndrome.*

marihuana (mar-i-wah'nă) [fr. Sp. *Maria- Juana,* Mary-Jane]. Popular name for the dried flowering leaves of *Cannabis sativa,* which are smoked as cigarettes, "joints," or "reefers." In the U.S. m. includes any part of, or any extracts from, the female plant. Alternative spellings are mariguana, marijuana. See also cannabis.

Marinesco, Georges, Rumanian neurologist, 1863–1938. See M.'s succulent *hand;* M.-Garland *syndrome,* M.-Sjögren *syndrome.*

marinobufotoxin (mar'i-nō-bū'fō-toks-in). A poison produced by the parotid gland of *Bufo marinus* (family Bufonidae), a large toad native to Central and South America; used in tropical countries for insect control.

Marion, Georges, French urologist, 1869–1932. See M.'s *disease.*

Mariotte, Edmé, French physicist, 1620–1684. See M.'s *bottle, experiment, law,* blind *spot.*

mariposia (mār-i-pō'zē-ă) [L. *mare,* the sea, + G. *posis,* drinking]. Thallasoposia; abnormal consumption of sea water as a result of psychogenic factors.

Marjolin, Jean N., French physician, 1780–1850. See M.'s *ulcer.*

marjoram (mar'jō-ram). Sweet, leaf, or garden m.; the leaves, with and without a small portion of the flowering tops of *Majorana hortensis* (*Origanum majorana*) (family Labiatae), are used as seasoning and medicinally as a stimulant, carminative, and emmenagogue.

mark [A.S. *mearc*]. **1.** Any spot, line, or other figure on the cutaneous or mucocutaneous surface, visible through difference in color, elevation, or other peculiarity. **2.** Infundibulum (8).

alignment m., m.'s made in tracings while the kymograph or other recording apparatus is at rest in order to indicate the time relations between two tracings inscribed one above the other, *e.g.,* jugular and radial pulses.

dhobie m., dhobie mark *dermatitis.*

port-wine m., *nevus* flammeus.

strawberry m., strawberry *nevus.*

Unna's m., nape *nevus.*

washerman's m., dhobie mark *dermatitis.*

mark'er. 1. A device used to make a mark or to indicate measurement. **2.** A characteristic or factor by which a cell or molecule can be recognized or identified.

allotypic m., allotype.

Amsler's m., obsolete term for a caliper compass, used in eye surgery.

cell m., an identifying characteristic of a cell; *e.g.,* formation of rosettes with sheep erythrocytes as a m. of T lymphocytes, or the presence of surface immunoglobulin as a m. of B lymphocytes.

genetic m., genetic *determinant.*

linkage m., a locus at which there is a high probability of heterozygotes (indispensible state for linkage analysis).

oncofetal m., a tumor m. produced by tumor tissue and by fetal tissue of the same type as the tumor, but not by normal adult tissue from which the tumor arises.

time m., an instrument that marks the time, usually in seconds or fractions of seconds, on a kymograph record in physiologic experiments.

tumor m., a substance, released into the circulation by tumor tissue, whose detection in the serum indicates the presence and specific type of tumor.

Marme's reagent. See under reagent.

marmorated (mar'mō-rā-ted) [L. *marmoratus,* marbled]. Denoting a condition in which the appearance of the skin is streaked like marble. See also *cutis* marmorata.

mar'mot [Fr. *marmotte*]. A woodchuck or groundhog; a hibernating rodent that may serve as reservoir host of plague bacillus in North America.

Maroteaux, Pierre. See M.-Lamy *syndrome.*

Marquis' reagent. See under reagent.

marrow (mar'ō) [A.S. *mearh*]. **1.** A highly cellular hematopoietic connective tissue filling the medullary cavities and spony epiphyses of bones which becomes predominantly fatty with age, particularly in the long bones of the limbs. **2.** Any soft gelatinous or fatty material resembling the m. of bone. See also medulla.

bone m., *medulla* ossium.

red bone m., *medulla* ossium rubra.

spinal m., *medulla* spinalis.

yellow bone m., *medulla* ossium flava.

Marsh, Hadleigh, U.S. veterinary pathologist, 1888–1971. See M.'s ovine progressive *pneumonia.*

Marshall, Don, U.S. ophthalmologist, *1905. See M. *syndrome.*

Marshall, Eli K., U.S. pharmacologist, 1889–1966. See M.'s *method.*

Marshall, John, English anatomist, 1818–1891. See M.'s vestigial *fold,* oblique *vein.*

Marshall, Victor F., U.S. urologist, *1913. See M.-Marchetti-Krantz *operation.*

Marshallagia marshalli (mar-sha-lā'jē-ă mar-shal'ī). One of the medium stomach worms of the nematode family Trichostrongylidae, found in the abomasum of sheep, goats, camels, and various wild ruminants.

marshmallow root (marsh'mal-ō). Althea.

marsupial (mar-sū'pē-ăl) [L. *marsupium,* a pouch]. **1.** A member of the order Marsupalia which includes such mammals as kangaroos, wombats, bandicoots, and opossums, the female of which has an abdominal pouch for carrying the young. **2.** Of or pertaining to marsupials.

marsupialization (mar-sū'pē-ăl-i-zā'shŭn) [L. *marsupium,* pouch]. Exteriorization of a cyst or other such enclosed cavity by resecting the anterior wall and suturing the cut edges of the remaining wall to adjacent edges of the skin, thereby creating a pouch.

marsupium (mar-sū'pē-ŭm) [L. pouch]. **1.** Scrotum. **2.** A pouch or sac; *e.g.,* in marsupials.

Martegiani, J., 19th century Italian anatomist. See M.'s *area, funnel.*

Martin, August E., German gynecologist, 1847–1933. See M.'s *tube.*

Martin, Henry A., U.S. surgeon, 1824–1884. See M.'s *bandage, disease.*

Martin, J.E. See Thayer-M. *medium.*

Martinotti, Giovanni, Italian physician, 1857–1928. See M.'s *cell.*

martius yellow (marsh'ē-ŭs) [Karl A. *Martius,* Ger. chemist, *1920] [C.I. 10315]. 2,4-Dinitro-α-naphthol; $C_{10}H_6N_2O_5$; an acid dye used as a plasma stain in plant and animal histlogy, and as a light filter for photomicrography.

Martorell, Fernando *Martorell* Otzet, 20th century Spanish cardiologist. See M.'s *syndrome.*

Maryland coma scale. See coma *scale.*

mas Abbreviation for milliampere-second.

maschaladenitis (mas'kăl-ad'ē-nī'tis) [G. *maschalē,* axilla, + *adēn,* gland, + *-itis,* inflammation]. Inflammation of the axillary glands.

maschale (mas'kăl-ē) [G.]. *Fossa* axillaris.

maschalephidrosis (mas'kăl-ef-i-drō'sis) [G. *maschalē,* axilla, + *ephidrōsis,* perspiration]. Sweating in the axillae.

maschaloncus (mas-kăl-ong'kŭs) [G. *maschalē,* axilla, + *onkos,* mass]. A neoplasm in the axilla.

maschalyperidrosis (mas'kăl-i-per-i-drō'sis) [G. *maschalē,* axilla, + *hyper,* over, + *hidrōs,* sweat]. Excessive sweating in the axillae.

masculine (mas'kyū-lin) [L. *masculus,* male, fr. *mas,* male]. Male (2); relating to or marked by the characteristics of the male sex or gender.

masculine protest. Adler's term to describe the movement of individuals from passive to active roles in a desire to escape from the feminine role.

masculinity (mas-kyū-lin'i-tē). The qualities and characteristics of a male.

masculinization (mas'kyū-lin-i-zā'shŭn) [L. *masculus,* male]. The condition marked by the attainment of male characteristics, such as facial hair.

masculinize (mas'kyū-li-nīz). To confer the qualities or characteristics peculiar to the male.

masculinovoblastoma (mas'kyū-lin-ō'vō-blas-tō'mă). An ovarian neoplasm that causes varying degrees of masculinization, *e.g.,* distribution of hair, change in voice, hypertrophy of the clitoris; m. consists of cords or anastomosing columns of cells with vesicular nuclei and indistinct cytoplasm, and is usually well vascularized; m.'s are thought by some to be derived from rests of adrenal cortical tissue, and they are morphologically similar to certain types of arrhenoblastoma.

masculinus (mas-kyū-lī'nŭs) [L.] [NA]. Masculine.

Masini, Giulio, Italian physician, 1874–1937. See M.'s *sign.*

mask. 1. Any of a variety of disease states producing alteration or discoloration of the skin of the face. **2.** The expressionless appearance seen in certain diseases; *e.g.,* Parkinson's facies. **3.** A facial bandage. **4.** A shield designed to cover the mouth and nose for maintenance of antiseptic conditions. **5.** A device designed to cover the mouth and nose for administration of inhalation anesthetics, oxygen, or other gases.

ecchymotic m., a dusky discoloration of the head and neck occurring when the trunk has been subjected to sudden and extreme compression, as in traumatic asphyxia.

Hutchinson's m., the sensation in tabes dorsalis as if the face were covered with a m. or with cobwebs.

luetic m., a dirty brownish yellow pigmentation, blotchy in character, resembling that of chloasma, occurring on the forehead, temples, and sometimes the cheeks in patients with tertiary syphilis.

m. of pregnancy, melasma.

nonrebreathing m., a m. fitted with both an inhalation valve and an exhalation valve so that all exhaled gas is vented to the external atmosphere and inhaled gas comes only from a reservoir connected to the m.

tropical m., *chloasma* bronzinum.

masked (maskt). Concealed.

mask'ing. 1. The use of noise of any kind to interfere with the audibility of another sound. For any given intensity, low pitched tones have a greater m. effect than those of a high pitch. **2.** In audiology, the use of a noise applied to one ear while testing the hearing acuity of the other ear. **3.** The hiding of smaller rhythms in the brain wave record by larger and slower ones whose wave form they distort. **4.** In dentistry, an opaque covering used to camouflage the metal parts of a prosthesis.

Maslow, Abraham H., U. S. psychologist, 1908–1970. See M.'s *hierarchy.*

masochism (mas'ō-kizm, maz'ō-) [Leopold von Sacher-*Masoch,* Austrian novelist, 1836–1895]. **1.** Passive algolagnia; a form of perversion, often sexual in nature, in which a person experiences pleasure in being abused and maltreated. *Cf.* sadism. **2.** A general orientation in life that personal suffering relieves guilt and leads to a reward.

masochist (mas'ō-kist). The passive party in the practice of masochism.

Mason, Edward E., U.S. surgeon, *1920. See M. *operation.*

masque biliaire (mask bil-ē-ār') [Fr.]. Periocular hyperpigmentation in middle-aged women, unrelated to any systemic disease.

mass [L. *massa,* a dough-like mass]. **1.** Massa. **2.** In pharmacy, a soft solid preparation containing an active medicinal agent, of such consistency that it can be divided into small pieces and rolled into pills. **3.** One of the seven fundamental quantities of the SI system; its unit is the kilogram, defined as the m. of the international prototype of the kilogram, which is made of platinum-iridium and kept at the International Bureau of Weights and Measures.

apperceptive m., the already existing knowledge base in a similar or related area with which the new perceptual material is articulated.

filar m., reticular *substance* (1).

injection m., colored solutions or suspensions injected into the vascular system to render vessels and their walls prominent; useful for gross preparations and for study under low magnification after clearing; most fluids contain warm gelatin and the coloring materials are carmine, Berlin blue, or carbon.

inner cell m., embryoblast.

lateral m. of atlas, *massa* lateralis atlantis.

lateral m. of ethmoid bone, *labyrinthus* ethmoidalis.

pilular m., any soft solid drug m. that is of the proper consistency to be made into pills.

sclerotic cemental m., florid osseous or cemental dysplasia; gigantiform cementoma; benign fibro-osseous jaw lesions of unknown etiology, occurring predominantly in middle-aged black females, which present as large painless radiopaque masses usually involving several quadrants of the jaw.

tubular excretory m., the m. of functioning excretory tubules of the kidney determined from the excretion of iodopyracet, or other compounds processed in the kidney primarily by tubular secretion, when large doses are used.

massa, gen. and pl. **massae** (mas'să, mas'sē) [L.] [NA]. Mass (1); a lump or aggregation of coherent material.

m. interme'dia, *adhesio* interthalamica.

m. latera'lis atlan'tis [NA], lateral mass of the atlas; the thick lateral part of the atlas on each side that articulates above with the occipital condyle and below with the axis.

massage (mă-sahzh') [Fr. from G. *massō,* to knead]. Tripsis (2); a method of manipulation of the body by rubbing, pinching, kneading, tapping, etc.

cardiac m., manual rhythmic compression of the ventricles to maintain the circulation.
closed chest m., external cardiac m.; rhythmic compression of the heart between sternum and spine by depressing the lower sternum backward with heels of hands, the patient lying supine.
external cardiac m., closed chest m.
gingival m., mechanical stimulation of the gingiva by rubbing or pressure.
nerve-point m., gelotripsy.
open chest m., rhythmic manual compression of the ventricles of the heart with the hand inside the thoracic cavity.
prostatic m., **(1)** manual expression of prostatic secretions by digital rectal technique; **(2)** the emptying of prostatic sini and ducts by repeated downward compression maneuvers, used in the treatment of various congestive and inflammatory prostatic conditions.
vibratory m., seismotherapy; sismotherapy; vibrotherapeutics; very rapid tapping of the surface effected by means of an instrument, usually with elastic tip.

Masselon, M. Julián, Paris physician, 1844–1917. See M.'s *spectacles.*

masseter (mă-sē′ter) [G. *masētēr,* masticator]. See *musculus* masseter.

masseur (mă-ser′) [Fr. see *massage*]. **1.** A man who massages. **2.** An instrument used in mechanical massage.

masseuse (mă-sūz′). A woman who massages.

massicot (mas′i-kot). *Lead* monoxide.

Masson, C.L. Pierre, Canadian pathologist, 1880–1959. See M.'s *pseudoangiosarcoma; stains;* M.-Fontana ammoniacal silver *stain.*

massotherapy (mas-ō-thăr′ă-pē) [G. *massō,* to knead, + *therapeia,* treatment]. The therapeutic use of massage.

mast-. See masto-.

mastadenitis (mast′ad-ĕ-nī′tis) [masto- + G. *adēn,* gland, + *-itis,* inflammation]. Mastitis.

mastadenoma (mast′ad-ĕ-nō′mă) [masto- + G. *adēn,* gland, + *-ōma,* tumor]. An adenoma of the breast.

Mastadenovirus (mast-ad′ĕ-nō-vī′rŭs). A genus of the family Adenoviridae, including adenoviruses that infect mammals, with at least 37 antigenic types (species) being infective for man. They cause minor respiratory infections in children, epidemic acute respiratory disease in military recruits, acute follicular conjunctivitis in adults, and epidemic keratoconjunctivitis; many infections are inapparent.

mastalgia (mas-tal′jē-ă) [masto- + G. *algos,* pain]. Mastodynia.

mastatrophy, mastatrophia (mas-tat′rō-fē, mast-ă-trō′fē-ă) [masto- + atrophy]. Atrophy or wasting of the breasts.

mastauxe (mas-tawk′sē) [masto- + G. *auxē,* increase]. Hypertrophy of the breast.

mastectomy (mas-tek′tō-mē) [masto- + G. *ektomē,* excision]. Mammectomy; excision of the breast.
extended radical m., excision of the entire breast including the nipple, areola, and overlying skin, as well as the pectoral muscles and the lymphatic-bearing tissues of the axilla and chest wall.
modified radical m., excision of the entire breast including the nipple, areola, and overlying skin, as well as the lymphatic-bearing tissue in the axilla.
radical m., Halsted's o. (2); excision of the entire breast including the nipple, areola, and overlying skin, as well as the pectoral muscles, lymphatic-bearing tissue in the axilla, and various other neighboring tissues.
simple m., total m.; excision of the breast including the nipple, areola, and most of the overlying skin.
subcutaneous m., excision of the breast tissues, but sparing the skin, nipple, and areola; usually followed by implantation of a prosthesis.
total m., simple m.

Master, Arthur M., U.S. physician, *1895. See M.'s *test,* two-step exercise *test.*

Masters, William H., U.S. gynecologist, *1915. See Allen-M. *syndrome.*

mastic (mas′tik) [G. *mastichē,* the resin of the mastich tree]. Mastich; mastiche; a resinous exudate from *Pistacia lentiscus* (family Anacardiaceae), a small tree of the Mediterranean shores; used in chewing gum, as an enteric coating, and as a temporary filling material in dentistry.

masticate (mas′ti-kāt). To chew; to perform mastication.

mastication (mas-ti-kā′shŭn) [L. *mastico,* pp. *-atus,* to chew]. The process of chewing food in preparation for deglutition and digestion; the act of grinding or comminuting with the teeth.

masticatory (mas′ti-kă-tō-rē). Relating to mastication.

mastich, mastiche (mas′tik, mas′ti-kē). Mastic.

Mastigophora (mas′ti-gof′ō-ră) [G. *mastix* (*mastig-*), a whip, + *phoros,* bearing]. The flagellates, a subphylum of Protozoa having one or more locomotory flagella, a single vesicular nucleus, and symmetric binary fission; sexual reproduction is unknown in many groups (*e.g., Volvox, Trypanosoma, Euglena*). It consists of two classes: Phytomastigophorea (to which *Euglena* belongs), which contains chlorophyll and is therefore photosynthetic and holophytic (although this has secondarily been lost in some groups), and Zoomastigophorea (including *Trypanosoma* and *Leishmania*), which lacks chromatophores and is heterotrophic.

mastigote (mas′ti-gōt) [G. *mastix,* a whip]. An individual flagellate.

mastitis (mas-tī′tis) [masto- + G. *-itis,* inflammation]. Mammitis; mastadenitis; inflammation of the breast.
bovine m., a disease complex which occurs in acute, gangrenous, chronic, and subclinical forms of inflammation of the bovine udder, and is due to a variety of infectious agents; animal care, hygiene, and management are important factors in this dairy cow disease of great economic import.
chronic cystic m., fibrocystic *disease* of the breast.
gargantuan m., obsolete term for chronic inflammation of the breast with great enlargement of the gland.
glandular m., parenchymatous m.
granulomatous m., a rare granulomatous inflammation of lobular breast tissue, with multinucleated giant cells; sarcoidosis is excluded by the frequent presence of neutrophils and absence of involvement of other tissues.
interstitial m., inflammation of the connective tissue of the mammary gland.
lactational m., puerperal m.
m. neonator′um, m. in the secreting breast tissue of the newborn, usually staphylococcal.
ovine m., bluebag; an acute inflammation of the sheep udder, usually gangrenous.
parenchymatous m., glandular m.; inflammation of the secreting tissue of the breast.
phlegmonous m., abscess or cellulitis of the breast.
plasma cell m., a condition of the breasts characterized by tumorlike indurated masses containing numerous plasma cells, usually resulting from mammary duct ectasia; although clinically resembling malignant disease (attachment to skin and enlargement of axillary lymph nodes), it is not neoplastic.
puerperal m., lactational m.; m., usually suppurative, occurring in the later part of the puerperium.
retromammary m., submammary m.
stagnation m., caked breast; painful distention of the breast occurring during the latter days of pregnancy and the first days of lactation.

submammary m., retromammary m.; inflammation of the tissues lying deep to the mammary gland.
suppurative m., inflammation of the breast due to infection with pyogenic bacteria.

masto-, mast- [G. *mastos,* breast]. Combining forms relating to the breast.

mastoccipital (mast'ok-sip'-i-tăl). Masto-occipital.

mastocyte (mas'tō-sīt). Mast *cell.*

mastocytogenesis (mas'tō-sī'tō-jen'ĕ-sis). Formation and development of mast cells.

mastocytoma (mas'tō-sī-tō'mă) [mastocyte + G. *-oma,* tumor]. A fairly well-circumscribed accumulation or nodular focus of mast cells, grossly resembling a neoplasm.

mastocytosis (mas'tō-sī-tō'sis) [mastocyte + G. *-osis,* condition]. Abnormal proliferation of mast cells in a variety of tissues; may be systemic, involving a variety of organs, or cutaneous (urticaria pigmentosa).

mastodynia (mas-tō-din'ē-ă) [masto- + G. *odynē,* pain]. Mastalgia; mazodynia; mammalgia; pain in the breast. See also mammary *neuralgia.*

mastoid (mas'toyd) [masto- + G. *eidos,* resemblance]. **1.** Resembling a mamma; breast-shaped. **2.** Mastoidal; relating to the m. process, antrum, cells, etc.

mastoidal (mas-toy'dăl). Mastoid (2).

mastoidale (mas-toy-dā'lē). The lowest point on the contour of the mastoid process.

mastoidectomy (mas'toy-dek'tō-mē) [mastoid (process) + G. *ektomē,* excision]. Hollowing out of the mastoid process by curetting, gouging, drilling, or otherwise removing the bony partitions forming the mastoid cells.
radical m., typanomeatomastoidectomy; an operation to exteriorize and join the mastoid air cells, the middle ear space, and the external meatus, often for extensive cholesteatoma.

mastoideocentesis (mas-toyd'ē-ō-sen-tē'sis) [mastoid + G. *kentēsis,* puncture]. The operation of drilling or chiseling into the mastoid cells and antrum.

mastoiditis (mas-toy-dī'tis). Mastoid empyema; inflammation of any part of the mastoid process.
Bezold's m., m. with perforation medially into the digastric groove and forming a deep neck abscess.
sclerosing m., a chronic m. in which the trabeculae are greatly thickened, almost or entirely obliterating the cells.

mastoidotomy (mas'toy-dot'ō-mē) [mastoid (process) + G. *tomē,* cutting]. Incision into the subperiosteum or the mastoid process of the temporal bone.

mastoncus (mas-tong'kŭs) [masto- + G. *onkos,* mass]. A tumor or swelling of the breasts.

masto-occipital (mas'tō-ok-sip'i-tăl). Mastoccipital; relating to the mastoid portion of the temporal bone and to the occipital bone, denoting the suture uniting them.

mastoparietal (mas'tō-pa-rī'ĕ-tăl). Relating to the mastoid portion of the temporal bone and to the parietal bone, denoting the suture uniting them.

mastopathy (mas-top'ă-thē) [masto- + G. *pathos,* suffering]. Mazopathy (2); any disease of the breasts.

mastopexy (mas'tō-pek-sē) [masto- + G. *pēxis,* fixation]. Plastic surgery to affix sagging breasts in a more elevated and normal position, often with some improvement in shape.

mastoplasia (mas-tō-plā'zē-ă) [masto- + G. *plasis,* a molding]. Mazoplasia; enlargement of the breast.

mastoplasty (mas'tō-plas-tē) [masto- + G. *plastos,* formed]. Mammaplasty.

mastoptosis (mas-top-tō'sis) [masto- + G. *ptōsis,* a falling]. Ptosis or sagging of the breast.

mastorrhagia (mas-tō-rā'jē-ă) [masto- + G. *rhēgnymi,* to burst forth]. Hemorrhage from a breast.

mastoscirrhus (mas-tō-skir'ŭs, -sir'ŭs). Obsolete term for a scirrhous carcinoma of the breast.

mastosquamous (mas'tō-skwā'mŭs). Relating to the mastoid and the squamous portions of the temporal bone.

mastosyrinx (mas'tō-sir'ingks) [masto- + G. *syrinx,* tube]. A fistula of the mammary gland.

mastotomy (mas-tot'ō-mē) [masto- + G. *tomē,* incision]. Mammotomy; incision of the breast.

masturbate (mas'ter-bāt) [L. *masturbari,* pp. *masturbatus*]. To practice masturbation.

masturbation (mas-ter-bā'shŭn) [L. *masturbatio*]. Erotic stimulation of the genitals, usually resulting in orgasm, achieved by means other than sexual intercourse.
false m., peotillomania.

Masugi, Matazo. See M.'s *nephritis.*

Matas, Rudolph, U.S. surgeon, 1860–1957. See M.'s *operation.*

match'ing. The process of making a study group and a comparison group in an epidemiological study comparable with respect to extraneous or confounding factors such as age, sex, or breed.

maté (mah-tā') [Sp. *maté,* a vessel in which the leaves are prepared]. Paraguay tea; the dried leaves of *Ilex paraguayensis* and other species of *Ilex* (family Aquifoliaceae), shrubs growing in Paraguay and Brazil, which contain caffeine and tannin; used in South American countries as a beverage and medicinally as a diuretic and diaphoretic, and for the relief of headache.

materia (mă-tē'rē-ă) [L. substance]. Substance or matter.
m. al'ba [L. white matter], accumulation or aggregation of microorganisms, desquamated epithelial cells, blood cells and food debris loosely adherent to surfaces of plaques, teeth, gingiva or dental appliances.
m. med'ica [L. medical matter], old term for: **(1)** that aspect of medical science concerned with the origin and preparation of drugs, their doses, and their mode of administration; **(2)** any agent used therapeutically. See also pharmacognosy; pharmacology.

material (mă-tēr'ē-ăl) [L. *materialis,* fr. *materia,* substance]. That of which something is made or composed; the constituent element of a substance.
base m., any substance from which a denture base may be made, such as shellac, acrylic resin, vulcanite, polystyrene, metal, etc.
cross-reacting m. (CRM), a biological chemical substance sufficiently different from a reference substance (R) to have a perceptibly different function from R but sufficiently similar to R that it reacts with anti-R antibodies; *e.g.,* mutant factor VIII may be defective or even inert in coagulation and yet be immunologically identified as factor VIII.
dental m., any m. used in dentistry.
impression m., any substance or combination of substances used for making a negative reproduction or impression.
plastic restoration m., in dentistry, any m. that may be shaped directly to the tooth cavity, such as amalgam, cement, or resin.
restorative dental m.'s, m.'s used to replace oral tissues in dentistry; *e.g.,* amalgam, gold alloys, cements, procelain, plastics, and denture m.'s.

materies morbi (mă-tē'rē-ēz mōr'bī) [L. the matter of disease]. The substance acting as the immediate cause of a disease.

maternal (mă-ter'năl) [L. *maternus,* fr. *mater,* mother]. Relating to or derived from the mother.

maternity (mă-ter'ni-tē) [see maternal]. Motherhood.

mating (māt'ing). The pairing of male and female for the purpose of reproduction.

assortative m., a practice of m. in a population in which at some specified locus persons mate preferentially according to phenotype or genotype; may be positive, as when similar persons tend to choose each other, or negative.
cross m., see subentries under cross.
random m., panmixis; a practice of m. in a population in which at some specified locus m. occurs with an expected frequency predicted by the product of the frequencies in the population.

matrass (mat'răs) [Fr. *matras*]. A long-necked glass vessel used for heating dry substances in chemical manipulations.

matrical (mat'ri-kăl). Matricial; relating to any matrix.

matricaria (mat-ri-kā'rē-ă) [L. *matrix,* womb]. German or wild chamomile; the flowers of *Matricaria chamomilla* (family Compositae); used internally as a tonic and externally as a counterirritant. See also chamomile.

matrices (mā'tri-sēz, mat'rĭ-sēz) [L.]. Plural of matrix.

matricial (mă-trish'ăl). Matrical.

matricide (mat'ri-sīd) [L. *mater,* mother, + *caedo,* to kill]. **1.** The killing of one's mother. **2.** One who commits such an act.

matrilineal (mat-ri-lin'ē-ăl) [L. *mater,* mother, + *linea,* line]. Denoting descent through the female line.

matrix, pl. **matrices** (mā'triks, mat'riks; mā'tri-sēz, mat'ri-sēz) [L. womb; female breeding animal]. **1** [NA]. The formative portion of a tooth or a nail. **2.** The intercellular substance of a tissue. **3.** A mold in which anything is cast or swaged; a counterdie; a specially shaped instrument, plastic material, or metal strip used for holding and shaping the material used in filling a tooth cavity.
amalgam m., a device used during placement of the amalgam mass within a compound cavity preparation, facilitating proper condensation and contour thereof by providing a confining wall.
bone m., the intercellular substance of bone tissue consisting of collagen fibers, ground substance, and inorganic bone salts.
cartilage m., the intercellular substance of cartilage consisting of fibers and ground substance.
cell m., cytoplasmic m.
cytoplasmic m., cell m.; cytomatrix; a fluid cytoplasmic substance filling the interstices of the cytoskeleton.
mitochondrial m., m. mitochondrialis.
m. mitochondria'lis, mitochondrial m.; the substance occupying the space enclosed by the inner membrane of a mitochondrium; it contains enzymes, filaments of DNA, ribosomes, granules, and inclusions of protein crystals, glycogen, and lipid.
nail m., m. unguis.
territorial m., cartilage *capsule.*
m. un'guis [NA], nail m.; nail bed; keratogenous membrane; onychostroma; the area of the corium on which the nail rests; it is extremely sensitive and presents numerous longitudinal ridges on its surface. According to some anatomists, the nail bed is the portion covered by the body of the nail, the nail m. being only the part on which the root of the nail rests.

mat'ter [L. *materies,* substance]. Substance. See also substantia.
gray m., *substantia* grisea.
pontine gray m., *nuclei* pontis.
white m., *substantia* alba.

maturate (mat'yū-rāt) [L. *maturo,* pp. *-atus,* to make ripe, fr. *maturus,* ripe]. To suppurate.

maturation (mat-yū-rā'shŭn) [L. *maturatio,* a ripening, fr. *maturus,* ripe]. **1.** Achievement of full development or growth. **2.** Developmental changes that lead to maturity.

mature (mă-chūr, -tūr) [L. *maturus,* ripe]. **1.** Ripe; fully developed. **2.** To ripen; to become fully developed.

maturity (mă-chūr'i-tē). A state of full development or completed growth.

Mauchart (Mauchard), Burkhard D., German anatomist, 1696–1751. See M.'s *ligaments.*

Maurer, Georg, German physician in Sumatra, *1909. See M.'s *clefts, dots.*

Mauriac, Pierre, 20th century French physician. See M.'s *syndrome.*

Mauriceau, François, French obstetrician, 1637–1709. See M.'s *maneuver;* M-Levret *maneuver.*

Mauthner, Ludwig, Austrian ophthalmologist, 1840–1894. See M.'s *cell, sheath, test.*

maxilla, gen. and pl. **maxillae** (mak-sil'ă, mak-sil'ē) [L. jawbone] [NA]. Upper jaw bone; upper jaw; an irregularly shaped bone, supporting the superior teeth and taking part in the formation of the orbit, hard palate, and nasal cavity.

maxillary (mak'si-lār-ē). Relating to the maxilla, or upper jaw.

maxillectomy (mak-sil-ek'tō-mē) [maxilla + G. *ektomē,* excision]. Excision of the maxilla.

maxillitis (mak'si-lī'tis). Inflammation of the maxilla.

maxillodental (mak-sil'ō-den'tăl). Relating to the upper jaw and its associated teeth.

maxillofacial (mak-sil'ō-fā'shăl). Pertaining to the jaws and face, particularly with reference to specialized surgery of this region.

maxillojugal (mak-sil'ō-jū'găl). Relating to the maxilla and the zygomatic bone.

maxillomandibular (mak-sil'ō-man-dib'yū-lăr). Relating to the upper and lower jaws.

maxillopalatine (mak-sil'ō-pal'ă-tīn). Relating to the maxilla and the palatine bone.

maxillotomy (mak-si-lot'ō-mē) [maxilla + G. *tomē,* incision]. Surgical sectioning of the maxilla to allow movement of all or a part of the maxilla into the desired portion.

maxilloturbinal (mak-sil'lō-ter'bi-năl). Relating to the inferior nasal concha.

Maximow, Alexander A., Russian physician in U.S., 1874–1928. See M.'s *stain* for bone marrow.

maximum (mak'si-mŭm) [L. neuter of *maximus,* greatest]. The greatest amount, value, or degree attained or attainable.
glucose transport m., the maximal rate of reabsorption of glucose from the glomerular filtrate; it amounts to approximately 320 mg/min in man.
transport m., tubular m. (Tm), the maximal rate of secretion or reabsorption of a substance by the renal tubules.

Maxwell, Alice F., U.S. obstetrician-gynecologist, 1890–1961. See Goldberg-M. *syndrome.*

Maxwell, James Clerk, British physicist, 1831–1879. See M.'s *spot.*

Maxwell, Patrick W., Irish ophthalmologist, 1856–1917. See M.'s *ring.*

May, Richard, German physician. See M.-Hegglin *anomaly.*

May apple. Podophyllum.

May-Grünwald stain. See under stain.

Mayer, Karl, Austrian neurologist, 1862–1932. See M.'s *reflex.*

Mayer, Karl, W., German gynecologist, 1795–1868. See M.'s *pessary.*

Mayer, Paul, German histologist, 1848–1923. See M.'s hemalum *stain;* mucicarmine *stain.*

Mayer-Rokitansky-Küster-Hauser syndrome. See under *syndrome.*

mayidism (mā'id-izm) [*Zea mays,* maize]. Pellagra.

Mayo, Charles H., U.S. surgeon, 1865–1939. See M. *bunionectomy.*

Mayo, William J., U.S. surgeon, 1861–1939. See M.'s *operation, vein.*

Mayo-Robson, Sir Arthur W., British surgeon, 1853–1933. See M.-R.'s *point, position.*

Mayou, Marmaduke Stephen, British ophthalmologist, 1876–1934. See Batten-M. *disease.*

mazamorra (maz-ă-mōr'ă). Name given in Puerto Rico to a dermatitis caused by penetration of the skin by ancylostome larvae.

maze (māz) [M.E. *masen,* to confuse]. A labyrinth; frequently used to study higher functions of the nervous system in rats.

mazindol (mā'zin-dol). An isoindole anorexiant that is distinctive in not having the phenethylamine chain common to sympathomimetic amines.

mazo-. [G. *mazos,* breast]. Combining form relating to the breast. See also masto-.

mazodynia (mā-zō-din'ē-ă) [mazo- + G. *odynē,* pain]. Mastodynia.

mazolysis (mā-zol'i-sis) [G. *maza,* placenta, + *lysis,* a loosening]. Detachment of the placenta.

mazopathy, mazopathia (mā-zop'ă-thē, mā-zō-path'ē-ă). **1** [G. *maza,* a barley cake (placenta), + *pathos,* suffering]. Any disease of the placenta. **2** [G. *mazos,* breast]. Mastopathy.

mazopexy (mā'zō-pek-sē). [mazo- + G. *pēxis,* fixation]. Rarely used term for mastopexy.

mazoplasia (mā-zō-plā'zē-ă). [mazo- + G. *plasia,* a moulding]. Mastoplasia.

Mazzoni, Vittorio, Italian physician, 1880–1940. See M.'s *corpuscle,* Golgi-M. *corpuscle.*

Mazzotti reaction or **test.** See under reaction, test.

Mb, MbCO, MbO_2 Symbols for myoglobin and its combinations with CO and O_2.

MBC Abbreviation for maximum breathing *capacity.*

M.C. Abbreviation for *Magister Chirurgiae,* Master of Surgery; Medical Corps.

mc Former abbreviation for millicurie.

MCH Abbreviation for mean corpuscular *hemoglobin.*

M.Ch. Abbreviation for *Magister Chirurgiae,* Master of Surgery.

MCHC Abbreviation for mean corpuscular hemoglobin *concentration.*

mCi Abbreviation for millicurie.

MCR Abbreviation for steroid metabolic clearance *rate.*

MCV Abbreviation for mean corpuscular *volume.*

McArdle, Brian, 20th century British neurologist. See M.'s *disease;* M.-Schmid-Pearson *disease.*

McBurney, Charles, U.S. surgeon, 1845–1913. See M.'s *incision, point.*

McCarthy, Daniel J., U.S. neurologist, 1874–1958. See M.'s *reflexes.*

McCrea, Lowrain E., U.S. urologist, *1896. See M. *sound.*

McCune, Donovan J., U.S. pediatrician, *1902. See M.-Albright *syndrome.*

McDonald, Ellice, U.S. gynecologist, 1876–1955. See M.'s *maneuver.*

McGoon, Dwight C., U.S. surgeon, *1925. See McG.'s *technique.*

McIndoe, Sir Archibald H., British surgeon, 1900–1960. See M.'s *operation.*

McKee, George Kenneth, British orthopedic surgeon, *1930. See M.'s *line.*

McLean, Malcolm, U.S. obstetrician, 1848–1924. See Tucker-M. *forceps.*

McMurray, Thomas P., British surgeon, *1889. See M. *test.*

McPhail, M.K., Canadian physiologist, *1907. See M. *test.*

McReynolds, John O., U.S. ophthalmologist, 1865–1942. See M.'s *operation.*

McVay, Chester B., U.S. surgeon, *1911. See M.'s *operation.*

M.D. Abbreviation of *Medicinae Doctor,* Doctor of Medicine.

Md Symbol for mendelevium.

MDF Myocardial depressant *factor.*

M'Dowel, Benjamin G., Irish anatomist, 1829–1885. See *frenulum* of M.

M.D.S. Abbreviation of Master of Dental Surgery.

Me Symbol for methyl.

Meadows, William Robert, U.S. cardiologist, *1919. See M.'s *syndrome.*

meal (mēl). The food consumed at regular intervals or at a specified time.

Boyden m., a m. consisting of three or four egg yolks, beaten up in milk and seasoned with sugar, port wine, etc., used to test the evacuation time of the gallbladder; $^2/_3$ to $^3/_4$ of the contents will be normally evacuated within 40 minutes.

test m., toast and tea, or crackers and tea, or gruel or other bland food, given to stimulate gastric secretion before withdrawing gastric contents for analysis.

mean (mēn). A statistical measurement of central tendency or average of a set of values, usually assumed to be the arithmetic m. unless otherwise specified.

arithmetic m., the m. calculated by adding a set of values and then dividing the sum by the number of values.

geometric m., the m. calculated as the antilogarithm of the arithmetic mean of the logarithms of the individual values; it can also be calculated as the nth root of the product of n values.

harmonic m., the m. calculated as the number of values being averaged, divided by the sum of their reciprocals.

standard error of the m., a statistical index of the probability that a given sample m. is representative of the m. of the population from which the sample was drawn.

Means, James H., U.S. physician, 1885–1967. See M.'s *sign.*

measle (mē'zl). **1.** The larva (*Cysticercus cellulosae*) of *Taenia solium,* the pork tapeworm. **2.** The larva (*Cysticercus bovis*) of *Taenia saginata,* the beef tapeworm.

measles (mē'zlz) [D. *maselen*]. **1.** Morbilli; an acute exanthematous disease, caused by m. virus and marked by fever and other constitutional disturbances, a catarrhal inflammation of the respiratory mucous membranes, and a generalized maculopapular eruption of a dusky red color; the eruption occurs early on the buccal mucous membrane in the form of Koplik's spots, a manifestation utilized in early diagnosis; average incubation period is from 10 to 12 days. **2.** A disease of swine caused by the presence of *Cysticercus cellulosae,* the measle or larva of *Taenia solium,* the pork tapeworm. **3.** A disease of cattle caused by the presence of *Cysticercus bovis,* the measle or larva of *Taenia saginata,* the beef tapeworm of man.

atypical m., the rather severe, unusual clinical manifestations of natural m. virus infection in persons with waning vaccination immunity, particularly in those who had received formaldehyde-inactivated vaccine; an accelerated allergic reaction apparently resulting from an anamnestic antibody response, characterized by high fever, absence of Koplik's spots, a shortened prodromal period, atypical rash, and pneumonia.

black m., **(1)** hemorrhagic m.; **(2)** Rocky Mountain spotted *fever.*

German m., rubella.

hemorrhagic m., black m. (1); a severe form in which the eruption is dark in color due to effusion of blood into affected areas of the skin.

three-day m., rubella.

tropical m., a disease of uncertain character, somewhat resembling rubella, occurring in southern China.

measly (mē'zlē). Pertaining to pork or beef infected with the cysticerci of *Taenia solium* or *T. saginata,* respectively.

measurement (mezh'ŭr-ment). Determination of a dimension or quantity.
end-point m., analytical m. at the end of a chemical reaction, as opposed to making the m. while the reaction proceeds.
kinetic m., continuous or frequent monitoring of the readings in a chemical reaction to determine its rate.
nasion-pogonion m., facial *plane.*

meatal (mē-ā'tăl). Relating to a meatus.

meato- [L. *meatus*]. Combining form relating to a meatus.

meatomastoidectomy (mē'ă-tō-mas-toy-dek'tō-mē). A modified mastoidectomy to exteriorize mastoid air cells into the external auditory meatus, preserving the tympanic cavity and ossicles.

meatometer (mē-ă-tom'ĕ-ter) [meato- + G. *metron,* measure]. An instrument for measuring the size of a meatus, especially the meatus of the urethra.

meatoplasty (mē'ă-tō-plas-tē). Plastic surgery of a meatus or canal, *e.g.,* the external auditory meatus or the urethral meatus.

meatorrhaphy (mē-ă-tōr'ă-fē) [meato- + G. *rhaphē,* suture]. Closing by suture of the wound made by performing a meatomy.

meatoscope (mē-at'ō-skōp) [meato- + G. *skopeō,* to view]. A form of speculum for examining a meatus, especially the meatus of the urethra.

meatoscopy (mē-ă-tos'kŏ-pē) [meato- + G. *skopeō,* to view]. Inspection, usually instrumental, of any meatus, especially of the meatus of the urethra.

meatotome (mē-at'ō-tōm). A knife with short cutting edge for use in meatotomy.

meatotomy (mē-ă-tot'ō-mē) [meato- + G. *tomē,* incision]. Porotomy; an incision made to enlarge a meatus, *e.g.,* of the urethra or ureter.

meatus, pl. **meatus** (mē-ā'tŭs) [L. a going, a passage, fr. *meo,* pp. *meatus,* to go, pass] [NA]. A passage or channel, especially the external opening of a canal.
m. acus'ticus exter'nus [NA], external acoustic m.; external auditory m.; antrum auris; auditory canal; the passage leading inward through the tympanic portion of the temporal bone, from the auricle to the membrana tympani; it consists of an osseous (internal) portion and a fibrocartilaginous (external) portion, the **m. acus'ticus exter'nus cartilagin'eus.**
m. acus'ticus inter'nus [NA], internal acoustic or internal auditory m.; a canal running from the internal acoustic pore, through the petrous portion of the temporal bone, ending at the fundus where a thin plate of bone separates it from the vestibule; it gives passage to the facial and vestibulocochlear nerves together with the labyrinthine artery and veins.
external acoustic m., m. acusticus externus.
external auditory m., m. acusticus externus.
fish-mouth m., a red and swollen condition of the orifice of the urethra (urinary m.) in gonorrhea.
internal acoustic m., m. acusticus internus.
internal auditory m., m. acusticus internus.
m. na'si [NA], any of three passages in the nasal cavity formed by the projection of the conchae: **m. n. infe'rior,** lies below the inferior concha; **m. n. me'dius,** lies between the middle and inferior conchae; **m. n. supe'rior,** lies between the superior and middle conchae.
m. nasopharyn'geus [NA], nasopharyngeal passage; the posterior part of the nasal cavity from the posterior limits of the conchae to the choanae.
ureteral m., *ostium* ureteris.
m. urina'rius, *ostium* urethrae externum.

mebanazine (mē-ban'ă-zēn). (1-Phenylethyl)methylbenzyl)hydrazine; an antidepressant with inhibitory effect on monoamine oxidase.

mebendazole (mē-ben'dă-zōl). Methyl 5-benzoylbenzimidazole-2-carbamate; an effective broad-spectrum nematicidal agent against intestinal nematodes such as pinworm, hookworm, whipworm, and *Ascaris.*

mebeverine hydrochloride (mĕ-bev'er-ēn). 4-[Ethyl(*p*-methoxy-*α*-methylphenethyl)amino] butyl veratrate hydrochloride; an intestinal antispasmodic.

mebhydroline (meb-hī'drō-lēn). 5-Benzyl-2,3,4,5-tetrahydro-2-methyl-1*H*-pyrido[4,3-*b*]indole; an antihistaminic.

mebrophenhydramine (mĕ-brō-fen-hī'dră-mēn). 2-(*p*-Bromo-*α*-methyl-*α*-phenylbenzyloxy)-*N,N*-dimethylethylamine; an antihistaminic.

mebutamate (mĕ-byū'tă-māt). Carbamic acid 2-sec-butyl-2-methyltrimethylene ester; chemically, it differs only slightly from meprobamate, and possesses similar CNS-depressant properties.

mecamylamine hydrochloride (mek'ă-mil'ă-mēn). 3-Methylaminoisocamphane hydrochloride; a secondary amine that blocks transmission of impulses at autonomic ganglia (similar to but more effective than hexamethonium); used in the management of severe hypertension.

mechanical (mĕ-kan'i-kăl) [G. *meckanikos,* relating to a machine, fr. *mēchanē,* a contrivance, machine]. **1.** Performed by means of some apparatus, not manually. **2.** Explaining phenomena in terms of mechanics. **3.** Automatic.

mechanicoreceptor (mĕ-kan'i-kō-rē-sep'ter, tōr). Mechanoreceptor.

mechanics (mĕ-kan'iks) [see mechanical]. The science of the action of forces in promoting motion or equilibrium.
body m., the study of the action of muscles in producing motion or posture of the body.

mechanism (mek'ă-nizm) [G. *mēchanē,* a contrivance]. **1.** An arrangement or grouping of the parts of anything that has a definite action. **2.** The means by which an effect is obtained.
association m., the cerebral m. whereby the memory of past sensations may be compared or associated with present ones.
countercurrent m., see countercurrent exchanger; countercurrent multiplier.
defense m., **(1)** a psychological means of coping with conflict or anxiety, *e.g.,* conversion, denial, dissociation, rationalization, repression, sublimation; **(2)** the psychic structure underlying a coping strategy; **(3)** immunological m.
Douglas m., m. of spontaneous evolution in transverse lie; extreme lateral flexion of the vertebral column with birth of the lateral aspect of thorax before the buttocks.
Duncan's m., passage of the placenta from the uterus with the rough side foremost.
gating m., **1.** occurrence of the maximum refractory period among cardiac conducting cells approximately 2 mm proximal to the terminal Purkinje fibers in the ventricular muscle, beyond which the refractory period is shortened through a sequence of Purkinje cells, transitional cells, and muscular cells; gating m. may be a cause of ventricular aberration, bidirectional tachycardia, and concealed extrasystoles. *Cf.* gate *theory;* **(2)** a m. by which painful impulses may be blocked from entering the spinal cord.
immunological m., defense m. (3); the groups of cells (chiefly lymphocytes and cells of the reticuloendothelial system) that function in establishing active acquired immunity (induced sensitivity, allergy).
ping-pong m., a special bi-bi reaction in which an enzyme reacts with one substrate to form a product and a modified enzyme, the latter then reacting with a second substrate to form a second, final product, and regenerating the original enzyme. See fig. on p. 930.
pressoreceptive m., the pressoreceptor system, especially of the carotid sinuses and aortic arch.

$$E + S_1 \rightarrow EM + P_1$$
$$EM + S_2 \rightarrow E + P_2$$
$$\text{Sum: } S_1 + S_2 \rightarrow P_1 + P_2$$

Ping-Pong Mechanism

proprioceptive m., the m. of sense of position and movement, by which muscular movements can be adjusted to a great degree of accuracy and equilibrium be maintained.

Schultze's m., expulsion of the placenta with the fetal surface foremost.

mechanocardiography (mek'ă-nō-kar-dē-og'ră-fē). Use of graphic tracings reflecting the mechanical effects of the heart beat, such as the carotid pulse tracing or apexcardiogram.

mechanocyte (mek'ă-nō-sīt). An *in vitro* tissue culture fibroblast.

mechanophobia (mek'ă-nō-fō'bē-ă) [G. *mēchanē,* machine, + *phobos,* fear]. Morbid fear of machinery.

mechanoreceptor (mek'ă-nō-rē-sep'tōr). Mechanicoreceptor; a receptor which responds to mechanical pressure or distortion; *e.g.,* receptors in the carotid sinuses, touch receptors in the skin.

mechanoreflex (mek'ă-nō-rē'fleks). A reflex triggered by stimulation of a mechanoreceptor.

mechanotherapy (mek'ă-nō-thār'ă-pē) [G. *mēchanē,* machine, + *therapeia,* treatment]. Treatment of disease by means of apparatus or mechanical appliances of any kind.

mèche (māsh) [Fr. wick]. A strip of gauze or other material used as a tent or drain.

mechlorethamine hydrochloride (mek'lōr-eth'ă-mēn). Mustine hydrochloride; 2,2'-dichloro-*N*-methyldiethylamine hydrochloride; methyl-bis(beta-chloroethyl)amine hydrochloride; nitrogen mustard hydrochloride; HN2; it is cytotoxic for all cells, but with a special affinity for bone marrow, lymphatic tissues, and rapidly proliferating cells of certain neoplasms. Used for the palliative treatment of Hodgkin's disease, lymphosarcoma, and certain chronic leukemias.

mecillinam (me-sil'i-nam). Amdinocillin.

mecism (mē'sizm) [G. *mēkos,* length, *-ismos,* condition]. Abnormal elongation of the body or one or more of its parts.

Mecistocirrus (mē-sis-tō-sir'ŭs) [G. *mēkistos,* very long, + L. *cirrus,* curl, the protruding male organ of a nematode]. A monotypic genus of trichostrongylid nematodes (subfamily Mecistocirrinae), with the single species, *M. digitatus;* it is not grossly distinguished from *Haemonchus contortus* and has about the same effect on the host. *M.* is distributed chiefly in Asia in cattle, sheep, buffalo, bison, the stomach of pigs, and occasionally in man.

Mecke's reagent. See under reagent.

Meckel, Johann F., the elder, German anatomist and obstetrician, 1714–1774. See M.'s *band, cavity, ganglion, ligament, space.*

Meckel, Johann F., the younger, German comparative anatomist and embryologist, 1781–1833. See M. *scan, syndrome;* M.'s *cartilage, diverticulum, plane;* M.-Gruber *syndrome.*

meclastine (mĕ-klas'tēn). Clemastine.

meclizine hydrochloride (mek'li-zēn). Meclozine hydrochloride; 1-(*p*-chlorobenzhydryl)-4-(*m*-methylbenzyl) piperazine dihydrochloride; an antihistaminic useful in the prevention and relief of motion sickness and symptoms caused by vestibular disorders.

meclofenamate sodium (mek-lō-fen'ă-māt). Monosodium *N*- (2,6-dichloro-*m*- tolyl)anthranilate monohydrate; a nonsteroidal anti-inflammatory agent with analgesic and antipyretic actions.

meclofenoxate (mek'lō-fen-ok'sāt). 2-(Dimethylamino)ethyl (4-chlorophenoxy)acetate; an analeptic.

mecloqualone (mek-lō-kwah'lōn). 3-(2-Chlorophenyl)-2-methyl-4(3*H*)-quinazolinone; a sedative and hypnotic.

meclozine hydrochloride (mek'lō-zēn). Meclizine hydrochloride.

mecometer (mē-kom'ĕ-ter) [G. *mēkos,* length, + *metron,* measure]. An instrument, like calipers with a scale attachment, for measurement of newborn infants.

meconate (mek'ō-nāt) [G. *mēkōn,* poppy]. A salt or ester of meconic acid.

meconic acid (me-kon'ik). 3-Hydroxy-4-oxy-4*H*-pyran-2,6-dicarboxylic acid; obtained from opium; it forms soluble salts (meconates) with many of the alkaloids of opium.

meconin (mek'ō-nin). Opianyl; $C_{10}H_{10}O_4$; the lactone of meconic acid, found also in *Hydrastis canadensis;* a hypnotic.

meconiorrhea (mē-kō'nē-ō-rē'ă) [meconium + G. *rhoia,* flow]. Passage, by the newborn infant, of an abnormally large amount of meconium.

meconism (mē'kō-nizm) [G. *mēkōn,* poppy]. Opium addiction or poisoning.

meconium (mē-kō'nē-ŭm) [L., fr. G. *mēkōnion,* dim. of *mēkōn,* poppy]. **1.** The first intestinal discharges of the newborn infant, greenish in color and consisting of epithelial cells, mucus, and bile. **2.** Opium.

medazepam hydrochloride (mĕ-daz'ĕ-pam). 7-Chloro-2,3-dihydro-1-methyl-5-phenyl-1*H*-1,4-benzodiazepine monohydrochloride; an antianxiety agent.

medfalan (med'fal-an). Medphalan.

media (mē'dē-ă) [L. fem. of *medius,* middle]. **1.** *Tunica* media. **2.** Plural of medium.

mediad (mē'dē-ad). Toward the middle line.

medial (mē'dē-ăl) [L. *medialis,* middle]. Relating to the middle or center; nearer to the median or midsagittal plane.

medialecithal (mē'dē-ă-les'i-thăl) [L. *medialis,* medial, + G. *lekithos,* egg yolk]. Denoting an egg with a moderate amount of yolk, as in amphibians.

medialis (mē-dē-ā'lis) [L.] [NA]. Medial.

median (mē'dē-an) [L. *medianus,* middle]. **1.** Central; middle; lying in the midline. **2.** The middle value in a set of measurements; like the mean, a measure of central tendency.

medianus (mē-dē-ā'nŭs) [L.] [NA]. Median (1).

mediastinal (mē'dē-as-tī'năl). Relating to the mediastinum.

mediastinitis (mē'dē-as-ti-nī'tis). Inflammation of the cellular tissue of the mediastinum.

idiopathic fibrous m., mediastinal *fibrosis.*

mediastinography (mē'dē-as-ti-nog'ră-fē). [mediastinum + G. *graphō,* to write]. X-ray examination of the mediastinum.

gaseous m., x-ray examination of mediastinum after injection of air (artificial pneumomediastinum).

mediastinopericarditis (me'dē-as'tin-ō-per'i-kar-dī'tis). Inflammation of the pericardium and of the surrounding mediastinal cellular tissue.

mediastinoscope (mē-dē-as'tin'-ō-skōp). An endoscope for inspection of mediastinum through a suprasternal incision.

mediastinoscopy (mē'dē-as-ti-nos'kō-pē) [mediastinum + G. *skopeō,* to view]. Exploration of the mediastinum through a suprasternal incision, for biopsy of paratracheal lymph nodes.

mediastinotomy (mē'dē-as-ti-not'ō-mē) [mediastinum + G. *tomē,* incision]. Incision into the mediastinum.

mediastinum (me'dē-as-tī'nŭm) [Mod. L. a middle septum, fr. Mediev. L. *mediastinus,* medial, fr. L. *mediastinus,* a lower servant, fr. *medius,* middle] [NA]. **1.** A septum between two parts of an organ or a cavity. **2.** Interpulmonary septum; septum mediastinale; interpleural or mediastinal space; the median partition of the thoracic cavity, covered by the mediastinal pleura and containing all the thoracic viscera and structures except the lungs. It is divided arbitrarily into four parts: **m. supe'rius,** superior m.; that part lying above the pericardium; it contains the arch of the aorta and the vessels arising from it, the brachiocephalic veins, and upper portion of the superior vena cava, the trachea, the esophagus, the thoracic duct, the thymus, and the phrenic, vagus, cardiac, and left recurrent laryngeal nerves. The region below is the **m. infe'rius,** inferior m.; subdivided into three regions, middle, anterior, and posterior; **m. me'dium,** middle m.; contains the pericardium and its contents and the phrenic nerves and accompanying vessels; **m. ante'rius,** anterior m.; the narrow region between the pericardium and the sternum containing some lymph nodes and vessels and branches of the internal thoracic artery; **m. poste'rius,** posterior m.; postmediastinum m.; lies between the pericardium and the vertebral column, below the level of the fourth thoracic vertebra; it contains the descending aorta, thoracic duct, esophagus, azygos veins, and vagus nerves.

m. tes'tis [NA], septum of the testis; corpus highmori; corpus highmorianum; Highmore's body; a mass of fibrous tissue continuous with the tunica albuginea, projecting into the testis from its posterior border.

mediate [L. *mediatus,* fr. *medio,* pp. *-atus,* to divide in the middle]. **1.** (mē'dē-it). Situated between; intermediate. **2.** (mē'dē-āt). To effect something by means of an intermediary substance, as in complement-mediated phagocytosis.

mediation (mē-dē-ā'shŭn). The action of an intermediary substance (mediator).

mediator (mē'dē-ā-ter, -tōr). An intermediary substance or thing.

pharmacologic m.'s of anaphylaxis, substances released from mast (and other) cells by the reaction of antigen and specific homocytotropic antibody on their surfaces; they include histamine, slow-reacting substance of anaphylaxis (SRS-A), bradykinin, and (in some species of animals) serotonin.

medicable (med'i-kă-bl). Treatable, with hope of a cure.

medical (med'i-kăl) [L. *medicalis,* fr *medicus,* physician]. **1.** Medicinal (2); relating to medicine or the practice of medicine. **2.** Medicinal (1).

medical transcriptionist. An individual who performs machine transcription of physician-dictated medical reports concerning a patient's health care which become part of the patient's permanent medical record; a certified m. t. (CMT) has satisfied the requirements for certification by the American Association of Medical Transcription.

medicament (me-dik'ă-ment, med'i-kă-ment) [L. *medicamentum,* medicine]. A medicine, medicinal application, or remedy.

medicamentosus (med'i-kă-men-tō'sŭs) [L.]. Relating to a drug; denoting a drug eruption.

medicate (med'i-kāt) [L. *medico,* pp. *-atus,* to heal]. **1.** To treat disease by the giving of drugs. **2.** To impregnate with a medicinal substance.

medicated (med'i-kāt-ed). Impregnated with a medicinal substance.

medication (med-i-kā'shŭn). **1.** The act of medicating. **2.** A medicinal substance, or medicament.

arrhenic m., treatment of disease by means of the organic preparations of arsenic, the cacodylates, and methylarsinates.

ionic m., iontophoresis.

preanesthetic m., drugs administered prior to an anesthetic to decrease anxiety and to obtain a smoother induction to, maintenance of, and emergence from anesthesia.

medicator (med'i-kā-ter, -tōr). **1.** An instrument for use in making therapeutic applications to the deeper parts of the body. **2.** One who gives medicaments for the relief of disease; sometimes applied in derision to one who prescribes drugs for minor ailments.

medicephalic (mē'dē-se-fal'ik). Median cephalic; denoting the communicating vessel between the median and the cephalic veins of the forearm.

medicinal (mĕ-dis'i-năl). **1.** Medical (2); relating to medicine having curative properties. **2.** Medical (1).

medicinal scarlet red. Scarlet red.

medicine (med'i-sin) [L. *medicina,* fr. *medicus,* physician (see medicus)]. **1.** A drug. **2.** The art of preventing or curing disease; the science concerned with disease in all its relations. **3.** The study and treatment of general diseases or those affecting the internal parts of the body.

adolescent m., ephebiatrics; hebiatrics; the branch of medicine concerned with the treatment of youth in the approximate age range of 13 to 21 years.

aerospace m., a branch of m. combining the areas of concern of both aviation and space m.

aviation m., aeromedicine; the study and practice of m. as it applies to physiologic problems peculiar to aviation.

behavioral m., an interdisciplinary field concerned with the development and integration of behavioral and biomedical science, knowledge, and techniques relevant to health and illness, and to its application to prevention, diagnosis, treatment, and rehabilitation.

clinical m., the study and practice of m. in relation to the actual patient; the art of m. as distinguished from laboratory science.

defensive m., diagnostic or therapeutic measures conducted primarily as a safeguard against possible subsequent malpractice liability.

experimental m., the scientific investigation of medical problems by experimentation upon animals or by clinical research.

family m., the medical specialty concerned with providing continuous, comprehensive care to all age groups, from first patient contact to terminal care, with special emphasis on care of the family as a unit.

fetal m., fetology; study of the growth, development, care, and treatment of the fetus, and of environmental factors harmful to the fetus.

folk m., treatment of ailments in the home by remedies and simple measures based upon experience and knowledge handed on from generation to generation.

forensic m., legal m.; medical jurisprudence; **(1)** the relation and application of medical facts to legal matters; **(2)** the law in its bearing on the practice of medicine.

holistic m., an approach to medical care that emphasizes the study of all aspects of a person's health, especially that a person should be considered as a unit, including psychological as well as social and economic influences on health status.

internal m., the branch of m. concerned with nonsurgical diseases in adults, but not including diseases limited to the skin or to the nervous system.

legal m., forensic m.

military m., the practice of m. as applied to the special circumstances associated with military life.

neonatal m., neonatology.

nuclear m., the clinical discipline concerned with the diagnostic, therapeutic, and investigative uses of radionuclides, excluding the therapeutic use of sealed radiation sources.

osteopathic m., osteopathy (2).

patent m., a m., usually of secret composition or patented, advertised to the public.

perinatal m., perinatology.

physical m., physiatry; the study and treatment of disease mainly by mechanical and other physical methods.

podiatric m., podiatry.

preventive m., the branch of medical science concerned with the prevention of disease and with promotion of physical and mental health, through study of the etiology and epidemiology of disease processes.

proprietary m., a medicinal compound the formula and mode of manufacture of which are the property of the maker.
psychosomatic m., the study and treatment of diseases, disorders, or abnormal states in which psychological processes and reactions are believed to play a prominent role.
quack m., a compound advertised falsely as curative of a certain disease or diseases.
socialized m., the organization and control of medical practice by a government agency, the practitioners being employed by the organization from which they receive standardized compensation for their services, and to which the public contributes usually in the form of taxation.
space m., the field of m. concerned with physiologic diseases or disturbances resulting from the unique conditions of space travel.
sports m., a field of m. that uses a holistic, comprehensive, and multidisciplinary approach to health care for those engaged in a sporting or recreational activity.
tropical m., the branch of m. concerned with diseases, mainly of parasitic origin, in areas having a tropical climate.
veterinary m., the field concerned with the diseases and health of all animal species other than man.

medico- [L. *medicus,* physician]. Combining form meaning medical.

medicobiologic, medicobiological (med′i-kō-bī-ō-loj′ik, -loj′i-kăl). Pertaining to the biologic aspects of medicine.

medicochirurgical (med′i-kō-kī-rŭr′ji-kăl) [medico- G. *cheirourgia,* surgery]. Relating to both medicine and surgery, or to both physicians and surgeons.

medicolegal (med′i-kō-lē′găl) [medico- + L. *legalis,* legal]. Relating to both medicine and the law. See also forensic *medicine.*

medicomechanical (med′i-kō-mĕ-kan′i-kăl). Relating to both medicinal and mechanical measures in therapeutics.

medicophysical (med′i-kō-fiz′i-kăl). Relating to disease and the condition of the body in general; *e.g.,* a m. examination, in which a person is examined in order to determine the presence or absence of disease as well as to note the general physical condition.

medicopsychology (med′i-kō-sī-kol′ō-jē). Psychology in its relation to medicine.

medio-, medi- [L. *medius,* middle]. Combining forms meaning middle, or median.

mediocarpal (mē′dē-ō-kar′păl). Mesocarpal; midcarpal. **1.** Relating to the central part of the carpus. **2.** Carpocarpal; denoting the articulation between the two rows of carpal bones.

medioccipital (mē′dē-ok-sip′i-tăl). Midoccipital.

mediodens (mē′dē-ō-dens) [medio- + L. *dens,* tooth]. A supernumerary tooth located between the two maxillary central incisors.

mediodorsal (mē′dē-ō-dōr′săl). Relating to the median plane and the dorsal plane.

mediolateral (mē′dē-ō-lat′er-ăl). Relating to the median plane and a side.

medionecrosis (mē′dē-ō-ne-krō′sis). Necrosis of a tunica media.
m. of the aorta, cystic medial *necrosis.*
m. aor′tae idiopath′ica cys′tica, cystic medial *necrosis.*

mediotarsal (mē′dē-ō-tar′săl). Midtarsal; mesotarsal; tarsotarsal; relating to the middle of the tarsus; denoting the articulations of the tarsal bones with each other.

mediotrusion (mē′dē-ō-trū′zhŭn) [medio- + L. *trudo,* pp. *trusus,* to thrust]. A thrusting of the mandibular condyle toward the midline during movement of the mandible.

mediotype (mē′dē-ō-tīp). Mesomorph.

medisect (mē′di-sekt) [L. *medius,* middle, + *seco,* pp. *sectus,* to cut]. To incise in the median line.

medium, pl. **media** (mē′dē-ŭm, -ă) [L. neuter of *medius,* middle]. **1.** A means; that through which an action is performed. **2.** A substance through which impulses or impressions are transmitted. **3.** Culture m. **4.** The liquid holding a substance in solution or suspension.
clearing m., a m. used in histology for making specimens translucent or transparent.
complete m., a m. for an *in vitro* culture that contains the supplemental nutrients as well as the basic nutrients to support fastidious or mutant growth requirements.
contrast m., any material relatively opaque to the x-rays, such as barium, used in roentgenography to visualize the stomach, intestine, or other organ; occasionally refers to air.
culture m., m. (3); a substance, either solid or liquid, used for the cultivation, isolation, identification, or storage of microorganisms; blood and chocolate agar are used routinely for isolation; the addition of several chemical substances serves to identify various organisms, and maintenance of growth requires media to be tailored to the metabolic requirements of the particular organism.
Czapek-Dox m., Czapek's solution *agar.*
dispersion m., external *phase.*
Dorset's culture egg m., a m. for cultivating *Mycobacterium tuberculosis;* it consists of the whites and yolks of four fresh eggs and a solution of sodium chloride.
Eagle's basal m., a solution of various salts containing 13 naturally occurring amino acids, several vitamins, two antibiotics, and phenol red; used as a tissue culture medium.
Eagle's minimum essential m. (MEM), a tissue culture m. similar to Eagle's basal medium but with different amounts and a few exclusions (*e.g.,* antibiotics and phenol red).
Endo's m., Endo *agar.*
external m., external *phase.*
Loeffler's blood culture m., a culture m. consisting of beef blood serum, sheep blood serum, and beef bouillon containing peptone, glucose, and sodium chloride; used for the isolation of *Corynebacterium diphtheriae.*
motility test m., a culture m. with a concentration of agar that produces a less solid consistency than usual and allows motile organisms to grow away from the line of inoculation; used to differentiate species of bacteria.
mounting m., a substance, usually resinous, used for mounting a cover glass on histologic suspensions.
passive m., a m. that produces no change in the specimens placed in it.
selective m., a culture m. containing ingredients that inhibit growth of contaminants or microorganisms other than that desired.
separating m., **(1)** any coating which serves to prevent one surface from adhering to another; **(2)** in dentistry, a material usually applied to a cast to facilitate separation from the resin denture base after curing; a coating on impressions to facilitate removal of the cast.
Simmons' citrate m., a diagnostic m. used in the differentiation of species of Enterobacteriaceae, based on their ability to utilize sodium citrate as the sole source of carbon.
support m., the material in which separation takes place, as in separation of components in electrophoresis.
Thayer-Martin m., a modified chocolate agar (plate or slant) containing antibiotics (vancomycin, colistin, nystatin) and enriched with chemical and vitamin supplements; widely used for cultivation of *Neisseria gonorrhoeae* and *N. meningitidis.*
transport m., a m. for transporting clinical specimens to the laboratory for examination.

medius (mē′dē-ŭs) [L.] [NA]. Middle; denoting an anatomical structure that is between two other similar structures or that is midway in position.

MEDLARS Abbreviation for Medical Literature Analysis and

Retrieval System, a computerized index system of the U.S. National Library of Medicine.

MEDLINE [MEDLARS-on-line] A telephone linkage between a number of medical libraries in the United States and MEDLARS for rapid provision of medical bibliographies.

medorrhea (mē-dōr-rē'ă) [G. *mēdos* (sing.), the bladder, *medea* (pl.), the genitals, + *rhoia,* flow]. Gleet.

medphalan (med'fă-lan). Medfalan; D-phenylalanine mustard; D-sarcolysine; D-3-[*p* -[*bis* -(2-chloroethyl)amino]-phenyl]-alanine; an antineoplastic agent.

medrogestone (med-rō-jes'tōn). 6,17α-Dimethyl-4,6-pregnadiene-3,20-dione; an oral progestin.

medroxyprogesterone acetate (med-rok'sē-prō-jes'ter-ōn). 17α-Hydroxy-6α-methylprogesterone; a progestational agent that is active orally as well as parenterally, and more potent than progesterone; used, in combination with ethynyl estradiol, as an oral contraceptive.

medrylamine (med-ril'ă-mēn). 2-(*p*-Methoxy-α-phenylbenzyloxy-*N,N*-dimethylethylamine; an antihistaminic.

medrysone (med'ri-sōn). 11β-hydroxy-6α-methylpregn-4-ene-3,20-dione; a glucocorticoid used topically as an anti-inflammatory agent, usually on the eye.

medulla, pl. **medullae** (me-dŭl'ă, me-dŭl'ē) [L. marrow, fr. *medius,* middle] [NA]. Substantia medullaris (1); any soft marrow-like structure, especially in the center of a part.

m. of adrenal gland, m. glandulae suprarenalis.

m. glan'dulae suprarena'lis, m. of adrenal gland; it is composed principally of anastomosing cords of cells in the core of the gland; the cells display a chromaffin reaction because of the presence of epinephrine and norepinephrine in their granules.

m. of hair shaft, the central axis of some hairs, containing a column of large vacuolated and keratinized cells; the medullary portion is surrounded by the cortex.

m. of kidney, m. renalis.

m. of lymph node, m. nodi lymphatici.

m. no'di lymphat'ici, m. of a lymph node; the central portion of a node consisting of cordlike masses of lymphocytes, plasma cells, and macrophages in a stroma of reticular fibers separated by lymph sinuses; it reaches the surface of the node at the hilum.

m. oblonga'ta [NA], myelencephalon; the most caudal subdivision of the brainstem, immediately continuous with the spinal cord, extending from the lower border of the decussation of the pyramid to the pons; its ventral surface resembles that of the spinal cord except for the bilateral prominence of the inferior olive; the dorsal surface of its upper half forms part of the floor of the fourth ventricle. Motor nuclei of the m. oblongata include the hypoglossal nucleus, the dorsal motor nucleus, and the nucleus ambiguus of the vagus; sensory nuclei include the nuclei of the posterior column (gracilis and cuneatus), the cochlear and vestibular nuclei, the mid-portion of the spinal nucleus of the trigeminus, and the nucleus of the solitary tract.

m. os'sium [NA], bone marrow; the tissue filling the cavities of bones, having a stroma of reticular fibers and cells; **m. o. fla'va,** yellow bone marrow, bone marrow in which the meshes of the reticular network are filled with fat; **m. o. ru'bra,** red bone marrow, bone marrow in which the meshes contain the developmental stages of erythrocytes, leukocytes, and megakaryocytes.

m. rena'lis, [NA], m. of the kidney; the inner, darker portion of the kidney parenchyma consisting of the renal pyramids.

m. spina'lis [NA], spinal marrow; spinal cord; the elongated cylindrical portion of the cerebrospinal axis, or central nervous system, which is contained in the spinal or vertebral canal.

medullar (med-yŭl'ăr). Medullary.

medullary (med'ŭ-lăr-ē, mē-dul'er-ē, med'yū-lăr-ē). Medullar; relating to the medulla or marrow.

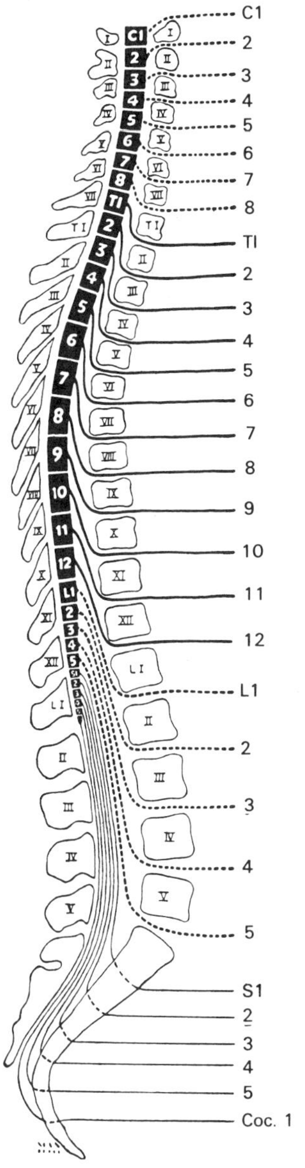

Segments of Spinal Cord (Medulla Spinalis)
Diagram of the position of the spinal cord segments with reference to the bodies and spinous processes of the vertebrae. Note also the place of origin of the nerve roots from the spinal cord and their emergence from the corresponding intervertebral foramina (Haymaker and Woodhall).

medullated (med'ŭ-lā-ted, med'yū-). **1.** Having a medulla or medullary substance. **2.** Myelinated.

medullation (med'ŭ-lā'shŭn, med'yū-). **1.** Acquiring, or the act of formation of, marrow or medulla. **2.** Myelination.

medullectomy (med-ū-lek'tō-mē, med-yū-) [medulla + G. *ektomē,* excision]. Excision of any medullary substance.

medullization (med'ŭ-li-zā'shŭn, med'yū-). Enlargement of the medullary spaces in rarefying osteitis.

medullo- [L. *medulla*]. Combining form meaning medulla.

medulloarthritis (med-ŭ-lō-ar-thrī′tis). Inflammation of the cancellous articular extremity of a long bone.

medulloblastoma (med′ŭ-lō-blas-tō′mă). A glioma consisting of neoplastic cells that resemble the undifferentiated cells of the primitive medullary tube; m.'s are usually located in the vermis of the cerebellum, and may be implanted discretely or coalescently on the surfaces of the cerebellum, brainstem, and spinal cord; they comprise approximately 3% of all intracranial neoplasms, and occur approximately twice as frequently in boys as in girls; the neoplastic cells are compactly arranged, rounded or ovoid, with hyperchromatic nuclei in relatively scant cytoplasm, and lie in small and poorly defined groups, or, occasionally, in a pseudorosette pattern.

medullocell (med′ŭ-lō-sel; med′yū-). Myelocyte (2).

medulloepithelioma (me′dŭ-lō-ep′ĭ-thē-lē-ō′mă). A rare, primitive, rapidly growing intracranial neoplasm thought to originate from the cells of the embryonic medullary canal and hence included with ependymoblastomas by some neuropathologists; ganglion cells and astrocyte maturation has also been reported. Tumors that occur in the ciliary body are referred to as embryonal m.'s.
adult m., malignant ciliary *epithelioma.*
embryonal m., dictyoma; embryonal tumor of ciliary body; an epitheliomatous tumor of the nonpigmented layer of the ciliary epithelium.

medullomyoblastoma (med′ŭ-lō-mī′ō-blas-tō′mă, med′yū-). A rare histologic variant of medulloblastoma with scattered smooth and striated muscle cells incorporated into the neoplasm.

Meeh, K., 19th century German physiologist. See M. *formula,* M.-DuBois *formula.*

Mees' lines or **stripes.** See under lines, stripes.

Meesman, A., 20th century German ophthalmologist. See M. *dystrophy.*

mefenamic acid (me-fĕ-nam′ik). *N*-(2,3-Xylyl)anthranilic acid; an analgesic with anti-inflammatory properties.

mefenorex hydrochloride (me-fen′ō-reks). *N*-(3-Chloropropyl)-α-methylphenethylamine hydrochloride; a sympathomimetic drug with anorexic activity.

mefexamide (mĕ-fek′ă-mīd). *N*-[2-Diethylamino)ethyl]-2-(*p*-methoxyphenoxy)acetamide; an antidepressant.

MEG Abbreviation for magnetoencephalogram.

mega- [G. *megas,* big] **1.** Combining form meaning large, oversize. See also macro-; megalo-. **2. (M).** Prefix used in the SI and metric systems to signify one million (10^6).

megabacterium (meg′ă-bak-tēr′ē-ŭm). Macrobacterium; a bacterium of unusually large size.

megabladder (meg′ă-blad-er). Megacystis.

megacardia (meg-ă-kar′dē-ă). Cardiomegaly.

megacaryoblast (meg-ă-kar′ē-ō-blast). Megakaryoblast.

megacaryocyte (meg-ă-kar′ē-ō-sīt). Megakaryocyte.

megacephalia (meg-ă-se-fā′lē-ă). Megacephaly.

megacephalic (meg′ă-se-fal′ik). Macrocephalic; macrocephalous; megacephalous; relating to or characterized by megacephaly.

megacephalous (meg-ă-sef′ă-lŭs). Megacephalic.

megacephaly (meg-ă-sef′ă-lē) [mega- + G. *kephalē,* head]. Megacephalia; macrocephalia; macrocephaly; megalocephaly; megalocephalia; a condition, either congenital or acquired, in which the head is abnormally large; usually applied to an adult skull with a capacity of over 1450 cc.

megacins (meg′ă-sinz). Antibacterial proteins produced by strains of *Bacillus megaterium.*

megacoccus, pl. **megacocci** (meg′ă-kok′ŭs, -kok′sī). Macrococcus; a coccus of unusually large size.

megacolon (meg′ă-kō′lon). Giant colon; a condition of extreme dilation and hypertrophy of the colon.
congenital m., m. congen′itum, Hirschsprung's disease; congenital dilation and hypertrophy of the colon due to absence (aganglionosis) or marked reduction (hypoganglionosis) in the number of ganglion cells of the myenteric plexus of the rectum and a varying but continuous length of gut above the rectum; also seen in dogs.

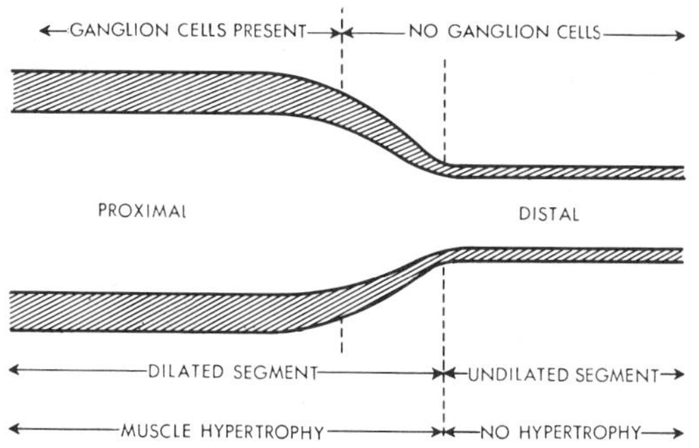

Congenital Megacolon
(After Bodian, Stephens, and Ward.)

idiopathic m., m., found in children or adults, without distal obstruction or absence of ganglion cells; the muscle of the dilated colon is thin.
toxic m., acute nonobstructive dilation of the colon, seen in fulminating ulcerative colitis.

megacycle (meg′ă-sī-kl). One million cycles per second.

megacystis (meg′ă-sis-tis) [mega- + *kystis,* bladder]. Megabladder; megalocystis; pathologically large bladder in children.

megadactyly, megadactylia, megadactylism (meg-ă-dak′ti-lē, -dak-til′ē-ă -dak′til-izm) [mega- + G. *daktylos,* digit]. Condition characterized by enlargement of one or more digits (fingers or toes). Also called megalodactylia; megalodactylism; megalodactyly; macrodactylia; macrodactylism; macrodactyly; dactylomegaly.

megadolichocolon (meg′ă-dol′i-kō-kō′lon) [mega- + G. *dolichos,* long, + *kolon,* colon]. Excessive length and dilation of colon.

megadont (meg′ă-dont) [mega- + G. *odous (odont-),* tooth]. Macrodont.

megadontism (meg-ă-don′tizm). Macrodontia.

megadyne (meg′ă-dīn). One million dynes.

megaesophagus (meg′ă-ē-sof′ă-gŭs, meg′ă-e-sof′). Great enlargement of the lower portion of the esophagus, as seen in patients with achalasia and Chagas' disease.

megagamete (meg-ă-gam′ēt). Macrogamete.

megagnathia (meg-ă-nā′thē-ă). Macrognathia.

megahertz (MHz) (meg′ă-hertz). One million hertz.

megakaryoblast (meg-ă-kar′ē-ō-blast). Megacaryoblast; the precursor of a megakaryocyte.

megakaryocyte (meg-ă-kar′ē-ō-sīt) [mega- + G. *karyon,* nut (nucleus), + *kytos,* hollow vessel (cell)]. Megacaryocyte; megalokaryocyte; thromboblast; a large cell (as much as 100 μm in diameter) with a polyploid nucleus that is usually multilobed; n.'s are normally present in bone marrow, not in the circulating blood, and give rise to blood platelets.

megal- See megalo-.

megalecithal (meg-ă-les′i-thăl) [mega- + G. *lekithos,* yolk]. Denoting an egg rich in yolk, as in bony fishes, reptiles, and birds.

megalgia (meg-al′jē-ă) [megal- + G. *algos,* pain]. Very severe pain.

megalo-, megal- [G. *megas (megal-),* large]. Combining forms meaning large. See also macro-, mega-.

megaloblast (meg'ă-lō-blast) [megalo- + G. *blastos,* + germ, sprout]. A large, nucleated, embryonic type of cell that is a precursor of erythrocytes in an abnormal erythropoietic process observed almost exclusively in pernicious anemia; an m.'s four stages of development are as follows: 1) promegaloblast, 2) basophilic m., 3) polychromatic m., 4) orthochromatic m. See also erythroblast.

megalocardia (meg'ă-lō-kar'dē-ă) [megalo- + G. *kardia,* heart]. Cardiomegaly.

megalocephaly, megalocephalia (meg'ă-lō-sef'ă-lē, -sĕ-fā'lē-ă). Megacephaly.

megalocheiria, megalochiria (meg'ă-lō-kī'rē-ă) [megalo- + G. *cheir,* hand]. Macrocheiria.

megalocornea (meg'ă-lō-kōr'nē-ă). Macrocornea.

megalocystis (meg'ă-lō-sis'tis) [megalo- + G. *kystis,* bladder]. Megacystis.

megalocyte (meg'ă-lō-sīt) [megalo- + G. *kytos,* cell]. A large (10 to 20 μm) nonnucleated red blood cell.

megalocythemia (meg'ă-lō-sī-thē'mē-ă). Macrocythemia.

megalocytosis (meg'ă-lō-sī-tō'sis). Macrocythemia.

megalodactylia, megalodactylism, megalodactyly (meg'ă-lō-dak-til'ē-ă, -dak'til-izm, -dak'ti-lē). Megadactyly.

megalodont (meg'ă-lō-dont). Macrodont.

megalodontia (meg'ă-lō-don'shē-ă). Macrodontia.

megaloencephalic (meg'ă-lō-en'sĕ-fal'ik). Denoting an abnormally large brain.

megaloencephalon (meg'ă-lō-en-sef'ă-lon) [megalo- + G. *enkephalos,* brain]. Macroencephalon; an abnormally large brain.

megaloencephaly (meg'ă-lō-en-sef'ă-lē) [megalo- + G. *enkephalon,* brain]. Abnormal largeness of the brain.

megaloenteron (meg'ă-lō-en'ter-on) [megalo- + G. *enteron,* intestine]. Enteromegalia; enteromegaly; abnormal largeness of the intestine.

megalogastria (meg'ă-lō-gas'trē-ă) [megalo- + G. *gastēr,* stomach]. Macrogastria; abnormally large size of the stomach.

megaloglossia (meg'ă-lō-glos'sē-ă) [megalo- + G. *glōssa,* tongue]. Macroglossia.

megalographia (meg'ă-lō-graf'ē-ă). Macrography.

megalohepatia (meg'ă-lo-he-pat'ē-ă). Hepatomegaly.

megalokaryocyte (meg'ă-lō-kar'ē-ō-sīt). Megakaryocyte.

megalomania (meg'ă-lō-mā'nē-ă) [megalo- + G. *mania,* frenzy]. Morbid verbalized overevaluation of oneself or of some aspect of oneself.

megalomaniac (meg'ă-lō-mā'nē-ak). A person exhibiting megalomania.

megalomelia (meg'ă-lō-mē'lē-ă). Macromelia.

megalonychosis (meg'ă-lon-i-kō'sis) [megalo- + G. *onyx,* nail, *-osis,* condition]. Macronychia.

megalopenis (meg'ă-lō-pē'nis). Macropenis.

megalophallus (meg'ă-lō-fal'ŭs). Macropenis.

megalophthalmus (meg'ă-lof-thal'mŭs) [megalo- + G. *ophthalmos,* eye]. Macrophthalmia; megophthalmus; abnormally large eyes.

anterior m., keratoglobus; m. affecting the anterior segment of the eyeball, with associated changes in the zonular ligament and the lens.

megalopia (meg-ă-lō'pē-ă) Macropsia.

megalopodia (meg'ă-lō-pō'dē-ă) [megalo- + G. *pous,* foot]. Macropodia.

megalopsia (meg-ă-lop'sē-ă). Macropsia.

megalosplanchnic (meg'ă-lō-splangk'nik) [megalo- + G. *splanchnon,* viscus]. Macrosplanchnic; having abnormally large viscera.

megalosplenia (meg'ă-lō-splē'nē-ă). Splenomegaly.

megalospore (meg'ă-lō-spōr). Macrospore.

megalosyndactyly, megalosyndactylia (meg'ă-lō-sin-dak'ti-lē, -dak-til'ē-ă) [megalo- + G. *syn,* together, + *daktylos,* finger]. Condition of webbed or fused fingers or toes of large size.

megaloureter (meg'ă-lō-yū-rē'ter). Megaureter; a congenitally enlarged ureter without evidence of obstruction or infection.

megalourethra (meg'ă-lō-yū-rē'thră). Megaurethra; congenital dilation of the urethra.

megamerozoite (meg'ă-mer-ō-zō'īt). Macromerozoite.

meganucleus (meg-ă-nū'klē-ŭs). Macronucleus (1).

megaprosopia (meg'ă-prō-sō'pē-ă) [mega- + G. *prosopon,* face]. Macroprosopia.

megaprosopous (meg-ă-pros'ō-pŭs). Macroprosopous.

megarectum (meg-ă-rek'tŭm). Extreme dilation of the rectum.

megaseme (meg'ă-sēm) [mega- + G. *sēma,* sign]. Denoting an orbital aperture with an index above 89.

megasigmoid (meg-ă-sig'moyd). Macrosigmoid.

-megaly [G. *megas (megal-),* large]. Suffix meaning large.

megasomia (meg-ă-sō'mē-ă). Macrosomia.

megaspore (meg'ă-spōr). Macrospore.

megathrombocyte (meg-ă-throm'bō-sīt) [mega- + G. *thrombos,* clot, + *kytos,* cell]. A large blood platelet, especially a young one recently released from the bone marrow.

megaureter (meg'ă-yū-rē'ter). Megaloureter.

megaurethra (meg'ă-yū-rē'thră). Megalourethra.

megavolt (meg'ă-vōlt). One million volts.

megavoltage (meg'ă-vol'tij). In radiation therapy, a vague term for voltage above one million volts.

megestrol acetate (me-jes'trōl). 17α-Hydroxy-6-methylpregna-4,6-diene-3,20-dione acetate; a synthetic progestin with progestational effects similar to those of progesterone; used in threatened and habitual abortion, endometriosis, and menstrual disorders; claimed to be superior to 19-nor compounds as an antifertility agent because it has less effect on the endometrium and vagina; in combination with ethynyl estradiol, it acts as an oral contraceptive.

meglumine (meg'lū-mēn). USAN-approved contraction for *N*-methylglucamine.

m. acetrizoate, a radiographic contrast medium.

m. diatrizoate, methylglucamine diatrizoate; *N*-methylglucamine salt of 3,5-diacetamido-2,4,6-triiodobenzoic acid; a water-soluble organic iodine compound used for excretory urography for contrast visualization of the cardiovascular system, and orally for roentgenography of the gastrointestinal tract.

m. iothalamate, *N*-methylglucamine salt of iothalmic acid (60% solution); a diagnostic radiopaque medium for intravascular use in angiography and urography.

megohm (meg'ōm). One million ohms.

megophthalmus (meg-of-thal'mŭs). Megalophthalmus.

megoxycyte (meg-oks'ē-sīt). Megoxyphil.

megoxyphil, megoxyphile (meg-oks'ē-fil, fīl) [mega- + G. *oxys,* acid, + *phileō,* to like]. Megoxycyte; an eosinophilic leukocyte containing coarse granules.

megrim (mē'grim). Obsolete term for migraine.

Meibom (Meibomius), Hendrik (Heinrich), German anatomist, 1638–1700. See meibomian *conjunctivitis, cyst, glands, sty.*

meibomian (mī-bō'mē-an). Attributed to or described by Meibom.

meibomitis, meibomianitis (mī'bō-mī'tis, mī-bō'mē-ă-nī'tis). Inflammation of the meibomian glands.

Meier, Georg, German serologist, *1875. See Porges-M. *test.*

Meige, Henri, French physician, 1866–1940. See M.'s *disease.*

Meigs, Joe V., U.S. gynecologist, 1892–1963. See M.'s *syndrome.*

Meinicke, Ernst, German physician, 1878–1945. See M. *test.*

meio-. For words beginning thus and not found here, see mio-.

meiosis (mī-ō'sis) [G. *meiōsis,* a lessening]. Meiotic division; the special process of cell division that results in the formation of gametes, consisting of two nuclear divisions in rapid succession that result in the formation of four gametocytes, each containing half the number of chromosomes found in somatic cells.

meiotic (mī-ot'ik). Pertaining to meiosis.

Meissel. See Wachstein-M. *stain* for calcium-magnesium-ATPase.

Meissner, Georg, German histologist, 1829–1905. See M.'s *corpuscle, plexus.*

mel-, melo-. **1** [G. *melos,* limb]. Combining form indicating limb. **2** [G. *mēlon,* cheek]. Combining form indicating cheek. **3** [L. *mel, mellis,* honey; G. *meli, melitos,* honey]. Combining form relating to honey or sugar. See also meli-. **4** [G. *mēlon,* sheep]. Combining form relating to sheep.

mel. **1.** Honey. **2.** Unit of pitch; a pitch of 1000 mels results from a simple tone of frequency 1000 Hz, 40 dB above the normal threshold of audibility.

melagra (mĕ-lag'ră) [G. *melos,* limb, + *agra,* seizure]. Rheumatic or myalgic pains in the arms or legs.

melalgia (mĕ-lal'jē-ă) [G. *melos,* a limb, + *algos,* pain]. Pain in a limb; specifically, burning pain in the feet extending up the leg and even to the thigh, and thickening of the walls of the blood vessels with obliteration of the vascular lumina; thought to be indicative of a vitamin deficiency disease.

melamine formaldehyde (mel'ă-mēn). Melamine *resin.*

melan-, melano- [G. *melas,* black]. Combining forms meaning black or extreme darkness of hue.

melancholia (mel-an-kō'lē-ă) [melan- + G. *cholē,* bile. See humoral *doctrine*]. Melancholy. **1.** A severe form of depression marked by anhedonia, insomnia, psychomotor changes, and guilt. **2.** A symptom occurring in other conditions, marked by depression of spirits and by a sluggish and painful process of thought.

hypochondriacal m., m. with many associated physical complaints, often with little basis in fact.

involutional m., a depressive disorder of middle life, commonly associated with the climacteric.

melancholic (mel-an-kol'ik). **1.** Relating to or characteristic of melancholia. **2.** Formerly, denoting a temperament characterized by irritability and a pessimistic outlook.

melancholy (mel'an-kol-ē). Melancholia.

melanedema (mel'an-e-dē'mă) [melan- + G. *oidēma,* swelling]. Anthracosis.

melanemia (mel-ă-nē'mē-ă) [melan- + G. *haima,* blood]. The presence of dark brown, almost black, or black granules of insoluble pigment (melanin) in the circulating blood.

melanidrosis (mel'an-i-drō'sis). See chromidrosis; pseudochromhidrosis.

melaniferous (mel-ă-nif'er-ŭs) [melan- (melanin) + L. *ferro,* to carry]. Containing melanin or other black pigment.

melanin (mel'ă-nin) [G. *melas* (*melan-*), black]. Melanotic pigment; any of the dark brown to black polymers of indole 5,6-quinone and/or 5,6-dihydroxyindole 2-carboxylic acid that normally occur in the skin, hair, pigmented coat of the retina, and inconstantly in the medulla and zona reticularis of the adrenal gland. M. may be formed *in vitro* or biologically by oxidation of tyrosine or tryptophan, the usual mechanism being the enzymatic oxidation of tyrosine to 3,4-dihydroxyphenylalanine (dopa) and dopaquinone by monophenol monooxygenase, and the further oxidation (probably spontaneous) of this intermediate to m.

artificial m., factitious m., melanoid.

melanism (mel'ă-nizm). Unusually marked, diffuse, melanin pigmentation of body hair and skin, (usually not affecting the iris); autosomal dominant inheritance. See also melanosis.

melano-. See melan-.

melanoameloblastoma (mel'ă-nō-am'ē-lō-blas-tō'mă). Melanotic neuroectodermal *tumor.*

melanoblast (mel'ă-nō-blast) [melano- + G. *blastos,* germ, sprout]. A cell derived from the neural crest; it migrates to various parts of the body during the relatively early phases of embryonic life, and then becomes a mature melanocyte capable of forming melanin.

melanoblastoma (mel'ă-nō-blas-tō'mă) [melano- + G. *blastos,* germ, sprout, + *-ōma,* tumor]. Melanoma.

melanocarcinoma (mel'ă-nō-kar-si-nō'mă). Melanoma.

melanocomous (mel-ă-nok'ō-mŭs) [melano- + G. *komē,* hair of the head]. Melanotrichous.

melanocyte (mel'ă-nō-sīt) [melano- + G. *kytos,* cell]. Pigment cell of the skin; melanodendrocyte; a cell located in the basal layer of the epidermis with branching processes by means of which melanosomes are transferred to epidermal cells, resulting in pigmentation.

melanocytoma (mel'ă-nō-sī-tō'mă) [megalo- + cyto- + G. *-oma;* tumor]. **1.** A pigmented tumor of the uveal stroma. **2.** Usually benign melanoma of the optic disk, appearing in markedly pigmented individuals as a small deeply pigmented tumor at the edge of the disk, sometimes extending into the retina and choroid; malignant metaplasia is rare.

melanodendrocyte (mel'ă-nō-den'drō-sīt) [melano- + G. *dendron,* tree, + *kytos,* a hollow (cell)]. Melanocyte.

melanoderma (mel'ă-nō-der'mă) [melano- + G. *derma,* skin]. An abnormal darkening of the skin by deposition of excess melanin, or of metallic substances such as silver and iron.

m. cachectico'rum, m. of the cachectic, occurring in certain chronic diseases, such as malaria and tuberculosis.

m. chloas'ma, melasma.

parasitic m., vagabond's, vagrant's, or Greenhow's disease; excoriations and m. caused by scratching the bites of the body louse, *Pediculus corporis.*

racial m., the normally dark skin of blacks and certain other races.

senile m., melasma universale; cutaneous pigmentation occurring in the aged.

melanodermatitis (mel'ă-nō-der-mă-tī'tis). Excessive deposit of melanin in an area of dermatitis.

melanodermic (mel'ă-nō-der'mik). Relating to or marked by melanoderma.

melanogen (mĕ-lan'ō-jen, mel'ă-nō-jen) [melanin + G. *-gen,* producing]. A colorless substance that may be converted into melanin; *e.g.,* some patients with widespread metastases of melanoma excrete m. in their urine, and melanin is formed when the urine is exposed to air (*i.e.,* oxidized) for a few hours.

melanogenemia (mel'ă-nō-jĕ-nē'mē-ă) [melanogen + G. *haima,* blood]. The presence of melanin precursors in the blood; may occur in malignant melanoma with metastasis.

melanogenesis (mel'ă-nō-jen'ĕ-sis) [melanin + G. *genesis,* production]. Formation of melanin.

melanoglossia (mel'ă-nō-glos'ē-ă) [melano- + G. *glōssa,* tongue]. Black *tongue.*

melanoid (mel'ă-noyd). Artificial or factitious melanin; a dark pigment, resembling melanin, formed from glucosamines in chitin.

melanokeratosis (mel'ă-nō-ker-ă-tō'sis) [melano- + kerato- + G. *-osis,* condition]. Migration of conjunctival melanoblasts into the cornea.

melanoleukoderma (mel'ă-nō-lū-kō-der'mă) [melano- + G. *leukos,* white, + *derma,* skin]. Marbled, or marmorated, skin.
m. col'li, syphilitic *leukoderma.*

melanoma (mel'ă-nō'mă) [melano- + G. *-ōma,* tumor]. Melanotic carcinoma; melanocarcinoma; melanoblastoma; malignant m.; a malignant neoplasm, derived from cells that are capable of forming melanin, which may occur in the skin of any part of the body, in the eye, or, rarely, in the mucous membranes of the genitalia, anus, oral cavity, or other sites; occurs mostly in adults and may originate *de novo* or from a pigmented nevus or malignant lentigo. In the early phases, the cutaneous form is characterized by proliferation of cells at the dermal-epidermal junction which soon invade adjacent tissue extensively. The cells vary in amount and pigmentation of cytoplasm; the nuclei are relatively large and frequently bizarre in shape, with prominent acidophilic nucleoli; and mitotic figures tend to be numerous. M.'s frequently metastasize widely, and the regional lymph nodes, liver, lungs, and brain are likely to be involved.
acral lentiginous m., a form of malignant lentigo m. that occurs in areas not excessively exposed to sunlight and where hair follicles are absent.
amelanotic m., an anaplastic m. consisting of cells derived from melanoblasts but not forming melanin.
benign juvenile m., spindle or epithelioid cell nevus; Spitz nevus; a benign, slightly pigmented or red superficial small skin tumor composed of spindle-shaped, epithelioid, and multinucleated cells; most common in children but also appearing in adults.
Cloudman m., a transplantable m. that arose spontaneously in a mouse of DBA strain, and which grows and metastasizes in mice of related strains.
halo m., a rare condition in which a m. is surrounded by an irregular area of depigmentation.
Harding-Passey m., a melanin-forming tumor that arose spontaneously in a non-inbred mouse, and that is transplantable to mice of many strains but does not ordinarily metastasize.
malignant m., melanoma.
malignant m. in situ, a m. limited to the epidermis and composed of nests and single upper epidermal atypical melanocytes that may be round with abundant cytoplasm (pagetoid cells); local excision is curative. Malignant lentigo may be considered a special type of malignant m. in situ.
malignant lentigo m., a m. arising from a malignant lentigo.
minimal deviation m., a m. showing less cytologic atypia than is usual in m. cells invading the dermis.
nodular m., primary cutaneous m. characterized by dermal invasion extending to the lateral margins of epidermal involvement or ulceration.
subungual m., melanotic whitlow; a m. beginning in the skin at the border of or beneath the nail.
superficial spreading m., primary cutaneous m. characterized by intraepidermal growth extending laterally beyond the site of dermal invasion.

melanomatosis (mel'ă-nō-mă-tō'sis) [melanoma + G. *-osis,* condition]. A condition characterized by numerous, widespread lesions of melanoma.

melanonychia (mel'ă-nō-nik'ē-ă) [melano- + G. *onyx* (*onych-*), nail]. Black pigmentation of the nails.

melanopathy (mel'ă-nop'ă-thē) [melano- + G. *pathos,* suffering]. Any disease marked by abnormal pigmentation of the skin.

melanophage (mel'ă-nō-fāj, mĕ-lan'ō-fāj) [melano- + G. *phagein,* to eat]. A histiocyte that has phagocytized melanin.

melanophore (mel'ă-nō-fōr, mĕ-lan'ō-fōr) [melano- + G. *phoros,* bearing]. A dermal pigment cell that does not secrete its pigment granules; it is well developed in fish, amphibians, and reptiles, but largely confined to the choroid of the eye and the mongolian spots in humans.

melanoplakia (mel'ă-nō-plā'kē-ă) [melano- + G. *plax,* plate, plaque]. The occurrence of pigmented patches on the tongue and buccal mucous membrane.

melanoprotein (mel'ă-nō-prō'tēn). A protein complex containing melanin.

melanorrhagia (mel'ă-nō-rā'jē-ă) [melano- + G. *rhēgnymi,* to burst forth]. Melena.

melanorrhea (mel'ă-nō-rē'ă) [melano- + G. *rhoia,* a flow]. Melena.

melanosis (mel-ă-nō'sis) [melano- + G. *-osis,* condition]. **1.** Abnormal dark brown or brown-black pigmentation of various tissues or organs, as the result of melanins or, in some situations, other substances that resemble melanin to varying degrees; *e.g.,* m. of the skin may occur in sunburn, during pregnancy, and as a result of various diseases, infections, and neoplasms. **2.** Cachexia resulting from widespread metastases of melanoma.
m. circumscrip'ta precancero'sa, malignant *lentigo.*
m. co'li, m. of the large intestinal mucosa due to accumulation of pigment of uncertain composition within macrophages in the lamina propria.
m. cori'i degenerati'va, a congenital abnormality in which pigment is deposited in whorls and streaks; vesicles occasionally occur, and it may be associated with cardiac or neurologic disorders.
neurocutaneous m., cutaneous giant pigmented nevi associated with m. of the leptomeninges; malignant melanomas may develop in the skin or meninges.
oculodermal m., Ota's nevus; pigmentation of the conjunctiva and skin around the eye, usually unilateral; seen especially in women of Oriental races.
precancerous m. of Dubreuilh, malignant *lentigo.*
Riehl's m., a brown pigmentary condition of the exposed portions of the skin of the neck and face with melanin pigment in dermal macrophages, thought to result from materials, such as oil, encountered in various occupations.

melanosity (mel-ă-nos'i-tē). Darkness of complexion.

melanosome (mel'ă-nō-sōm) [melano- + G. *sōma,* body]. The generally oval pigment granule (0.2 by 0.6 μm) produced by melanocytes.
giant m., melanin macroglobule; macromelanosome; a large spherical m. (1 to 6 μ in diameter) formed in the cytoplasm of melanocytes in café-au-lait spots and other melanocytic disorders.

melanotic (mel'ă-not'ik). **1.** Pertaining to the presence, normal or pathologic, of melanin. **2.** Relating to or characterized by melanosis.

melanotrichous (mel-ă-not'ri-kŭs) [melano- + G. *thrix* (*trich-*), hair]. Melanocomous; having black hair.

melanotroph (mel'ă-nō-trōf) [melano- + G. *trophē,* nourishment]. A cell of the intermediate lobe of the hypophysis that produces melanotropin.

melanotropin (mel'ă-nō-trōp-in). Melanocyte-stimulating hormone; intermedin; melanophore-expanding principle; a peptide hormone secreted by the intermediate lobe of the hypophysis which causes dispersion of melanin by melanophores, resulting in darkening of the skin, presumably by promoting melanin synthesis; this effect is readily demonstated in some lower vertebrates, such as frogs and fish.

melanuria (mel-ă-nū'rē-ă) [melano- + G. *ouron,* urine]. The excretion of urine of a dark color, resulting from the presence of melanin or other pigments or from the action of phenol, creosote, resorcin, and other coal tar derivatives.

melanuric (mel-ă-nū'rik). Pertaining to or characterized by melanuria.

melarsoprol (me-lar'sō-prol). 2-*p*-(4,6-Diamino-1,3,5-triazine-2-ylamino)phenyl-4-hydroxymethyl-1,3,2-dithioarsolan; used in the treatment of the meningoencephalitic stages of trypanosomiasis; may produce a fatal reactive encephalopathy.

melasma (mĕ-laz'mă) [G. a black color, a black spot]. Melanoderma chloasma; mask of pregnancy; a patchy or generalized pigmentation of the skin. See also chloasma.
m. gravida'rum, chloasma occurring in pregnancy.
m. universa'le, senile *melanoderma.*

melatonin (mel-ă-tōn'in). *N*-Acetyl-5-methoxytryptamine; a substance formed by the mammalian pineal gland that appears to depress gonadal function in mammals and causes contraction of amphibian melanophores.

Melchior. See Dyggve-M.-Clausen *syndrome.*

melena (me-lē'nă) [G. *melaina,* fem. of *melas,* black]. Melanorrhea; melanorrhagia; passage of dark colored, tarry stools, due to the presence of blood altered by the intestinal juices. *Cf.* hematochezia.
m. neonato'rum, m. of the newborn, a form occurring in young infants.
m. spu'ria, passage in the stool of blood which has been swallowed, especially that swallowed by nurslings from a fissured nipple.
m. ve'ra, true m. as distinguished from m. spuria.

melenemesis (mel-ĕ-nem'ĕ-sis) [G. *melas,* black, + *emesis,* vomiting]. Vomiting of dark colored or blackish material. See also black *vomit.*

Meleney, Frank L., U.S. surgeon, 1889–1963. See M.'s synergistic *gangrene, ulcer.*

melengestrol acetate (mel-en-jes'trōl). 17α-Acetoxy-6-methyl-16-methylene-4,6-pregnadiene-3,20-dione; a progestational agent.

meletin (mel'ĕ-tin). Quercetin.

meli- [G. *meli,* honey]. Combining form relating to honey or sugar. See also mel- (3).

melibiase (mel-i-bī'ās). α-D-Galactosidase. -D-Galactosidase.

melibiose (mel-i-bī'ōs). 6-*O*-α-D-Galactopyranosyl-D-glucose; a disaccharide formed by the hydrolysis of raffinose by β-fructofuranosidase.

melicera, meliceris (mel-i-sē'ră, mel-i-sē'ris) [G. *meli- kēris,* a tumor, fr. *melikēron,* honeycomb, fr. *meli,* honey, + *kēros,* wax]. A hygroma or other type of cyst that contains a relatively thick, tenacious, semifluid material.

melioidosis (mel'ē-oy-dō'sis) [G. *mēlis,* a distemper of asses, + *eidos,* resemblance, + *-osis,* condition]. Pseudoglanders; an infectious disease of rodents in India and Southeast Asia that is caused by *Pseudomonas pseudomallei* and is communicable to man. The characteristic lesion is a small caseous nodule, found generally throughout the body, which breaks down into an abscess; symptoms vary according to the tracts or organs involved.

melissa (me-lis'ă) [G. a bee]. Sweet balm; lemon lobelia; sweet Mary; the leaves from the tops of *Melissa officinalis* (family Labiatae), a plant of southern Europe; a diaphoretic.

melissophobia (mĕ-lis'ō-fō'bē-ă) [G. *melissa,* bee, + *phobos,* fear]. Apiphobia.

melitis (mē-lī'tis) [G. *mēlon,* cheek, + *-itis,* inflammation]. Inflammation of the cheek.

melitose (mel'i-tōs). Raffinose.

melitracen hydrochloride (mel-i-trā'sen). 9,10,Dihydro-10,10-dimethyl-9-(3-dimethylaminopropylidene)anthracene hydrochloride; an antidepressant.

melitriose (mel-i-trī'ōs). Raffinose.

melituria (mel-i-tū'rē-ă) [G. *meli,* honey, + *ouron,* urine]. Obsolete term for glycosuria.

Melkersson, Ernst G., Swedish physician, 1898–1932. See M.-Rosenthal *syndrome.*

mellitum, gen. **melliti,** pl. **mellita** (me-lī'tŭm, -tī, tă) [L. neut. of *mellitus,* honeyed]. A pharmaceutical preparation with honey as an excipient.

Melnick, John C., U.S. radiologist, *1928. See M.-Needles *syndrome.*

melo-. See mel-.

melocervicoplasty (mel-ō-ser'vi-kō-plas-tē) [melo- + L. *cervix,* neck, + G. *plastos,* formed]. Plastic surgery of the cheek and neck.

melomania (mel-ō-mā'nē-ă) [G. *melos,* song + *mania,* frenzy]. An abnormal fascination with or devotion to music.

melomelia (mel-ō-mē'lē-ă) [G. *melos* + *melos,* limb]. A malformation in which the fetus has normal and rudimentary accessory limbs. *Cf.* micromelia.

melonoplasty (mē'lon-ō-plas-tē) [G. *mēlon,* cheek, + *plastos,* formed]. Obsolete spelling for meloplasty.

Melophagus (mē-lof'ă-gŭs) [G. *mēlon,* sheep, + *phagein,* to eat]. A genus of louse flies (family Hippoboscidae) that includes the ectoparasite of sheep, *M. ovinus.* See also *Hippobosca.*
M. ovi'nus, ked; a wingless, flattened, hairy, leathery parasitic fly found in the wool of sheep and on goats; it is cosmopolitan in sheep, in which it sucks blood and causes much skin irritation.

meloplasty (mel'ō-plas-tē) [melo- + G. *plastos,* formed]. Plastic surgery of the cheek.

melorheostosis (mel'ō-rē-os-tō'sis) [G. *melos,* limb, + *rheos,* stream, + *osteon,* bone, + *-ōsis*]. Osteosis eburnisans monomelica; rheostosis confined to the long bones.

melosalgia (mel-ō-sal'jē-ă) [G. *melos,* limb, + *algos,* pain]. Pain in the lower limbs.

meloschisis (me-los'ki-sis) [G. *mēlon,* cheek, + *schisis,* a cleaving]. Congenital cleft in the cheek.

melotia (me-lō'shē-ă) [G. *mēlon,* cheek, + *ous,* ear]. Congenital displacement of the auricle.

melphalan (mel'fă-lan). L-Phenylalanine mustard; L-sarcolysine; L-3-[*p*- [*bis* (2-chloroethyl)- amino]- phenyl]alanine; a phenylalanine derivative of nitrogen mustard; an alkalylating antineoplastic agent.

Meltzer, Samuel J., U.S. physiologist, 1851–1920. See M.'s *law;* M.-Lyon *test.*

mem'ber [L. *membrum*]. A limb.
virile m., penis.

membra (mem'bră) [L.] [NA]. Plural of membrum.

MEMBRANA

membrana, gen. and pl. **membranae** (mem-brā'nă, -brā'nē) [L.] [NA]. Membrane; a thin sheet or layer of pliable tissue, serving as a covering or envelope of a part, the lining of a cavity, as a partition or septum, or to connect two structures.
m. abdom'inis, peritoneum.
m. adamanti'na, *cuticula* dentis.
m. adventi'tia, **(1)** *tunica* adventitia; **(2)** *decidua* capsularis.
m. atlanto-occipita'lis ante'rior [NA], anterior atlanto-occipital membrane; the fibrous layer that extends from the anterior arch of the atlas to the anterior margin of the foramen magnum.
m. atlanto-occipita'lis poste'rior [NA], posterior atlanto-occipital membrane; the fibrous membrane that attaches between the poste-

rior arch of the atlas and the posterior margin of the foramen magnum.
m. basa'lis duc'tus semicircula'ris [NA], the basal membrane underlying the epithelium of the semicircular duct.
m. basila'ris, *lamina* basilaris cochleae.
m. capsula'ris, the hyaloid vascular network around the posterior pole of the lens in the embryo.
m. capsulopupilla'ris, the lateral portion of the vascular tunic of the lens of the eye in the embryo.
m. carno'sa, *tunica* dartos.
m. cer'ebri, any one of the cerebral meninges.
m. choriocapilla'ris, *lamina* choroidocapillaris.
m. cor'dis, pericardium.
m. cricothyroi'dea, *conus* elasticus.
m. decid'ua [NA], deciduous membrane; decidua; Hunter's membrane; caduca; the mucous membrane of the pregnant uterus which has already undergone certain changes, under the influence of the ovulation cycle, to fit it for the implantation and nutrition of the ovum; so-called because the m. is cast off after labor. See also subentries under decidua.
m. e'boris, ivory membrane; the lining membrane of the pulp cavity of a tooth, consisting of the odontoblastic layer.
m. fibroelas'tica laryn'gis [NA], a layer of elastic fibers, taking the place in the larynx of the submucosa.
m. fibro'sa [NA], fibrous membrane; fibrous articular capsule; stratum fibrosum; the outer fibrous part of the capsule of a synovial joint which may in places be thickened to form capsular ligaments.
m. flac'cida, *pars* flaccida membranae tympani.
m. fus'ca, *lamina* fusca sclerae.
m. germinati'va, blastoderm.
m. granulo'sa, *stratum* granulosum folliculi ovarici vesiculosi.
m. hyaloi'dea, m. vitrea.
m. hyothyroi'dea, m. thyrohyoidea.
membran'nae intercosta'lia [NA], intercostal membranes or ligaments; ligamenta intercostalia; the membranous layers between ribs; **m. intercosta'lis exter'na,** the membrane that replaces the external intercostal muscle anteriorly; **m. intercosta'lis inter'na,** the membrane that replaces the internal intercostal muscle posteriorly.
m. interos'sea antebra'chii [NA], interosseous membrane of the forearm; the dense membrane that connects the interosseous margins of the radius and ulna.
m. interos'sea cru'ris [NA], interosseous membrane of the leg; ligamentum tibiofibulare medium; the dense fibrous layer that connects the interosseous margins of the tibia and fibula.
m. lim'itans, limiting *membrane* of retina.
m. lim'itans gli'ae, a dense, resilient membrane forming the true capsule of the brain and spinal cord, composed of the processes of astrocytes (macroglia cells) and covered throughout by the pia mater which firmly adheres to it; the two membranes are collectively called the pial-glial membrane.
m. muco'sa, *tunica* mucosa.
m. nic'titans, *plica* semilunaris conjunctivae (2).
m. obturato'ria [NA], obturator membrane; the thin membrane of strong interlacing fibers filling the obturator foramen.
m. perine'i [NA], perineal membrane; fascia diaphragmatis urogenitalis inferior; inferior fascia of the urogenital diaphragm; Camper's ligament; ligamentum triangulare; triangular ligament; the layer of fascia extending between the ischiopubic rami inferior to the sphincter urethrae and the deep transverse perineal muscles.
m. pituito'sa, *tunica* mucosa nasi.
m. preformati'va, the thickened m. formed by fusion of Korff's fibers and the basement membrane of the ameloblasts in a developing tooth.
m. pro'pria duc'tus semicircula'ris [NA], the meshwork of connective tissue fibers between the semicircular duct and the bony semicircular canal; it encloses the perilymph in its spaces.

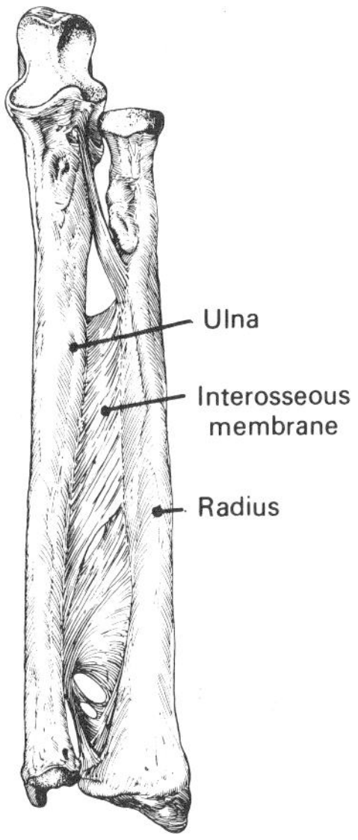

Membrana Interossea (Interosseous Membrane) of the Forearm

m. pupilla'ris [NA], pupillary membrane; Wachendorf's membrane; the thin, central portion of the iridopupillary lamina occluding the pupil in fetal life (the membrane normally atrophies about the seventh prenatal month but strands may persist); failure to regress may cause congenital blindness.
m. quadrangula'ris [NA], quadrangular membrane; Tourtual's membrane; the elastic membrane that extends from the ventricular fold of the larynx upward to the aryepiglottic fold; it attaches anteriorly to the epiglottis.
m. reticula'ris [NA], reticular membrane; the membrane formed by cuticular plates of the cells of the spiral organ of Corti; it appears netlike when viewed from above.
m. sero'sa, (1) *tunica* serosa; **(2)** serosa (2).
m. seroti'na, obsolete synonym of *decidua* basalis.
m. spira'lis [NA], alternate term for *paries* tympanicus ductus cochlearis.
m. stape'dis [NA], stapedial membrane; the delicate mucosal layer that bridges the space between the crura and base of the stapes.
m. statoconio'rum [NA], statoconial membrane; otolithic membrane; a gelatinous membrane supported by the hairs of the hair cells of the maculae of the saccule and utriculus of the inner ear; adhering to the surface are numerous crystalline particles called statoconia.
m. ster'ni [NA], sternal membrane; interlacing fibers from the anterior costosternal ligaments covering the anterior surface of the sternum.
m. stria'ta, *zona* striata.
m. succin'gens [L. *succingere,* to surround], pleura.
m. suprapleura'lis [NA], suprapleural membrane; Sibson's fascia; Sibson's aponeurosis; the thickened portion of endothoracic fascia extending over the cupola of the pleura and reinforcing it; it attaches to the inner border of the first rib and to the transverse process of the seventh cervical vertebra.
m. synovia'lis [NA], synovial membrane; stratum synoviale; synovium; the connective tissue membrane that lines the cavity of a synovial joint and produces the synovial fluid; it does not cover the articular cartilage of the bones.
m. tecto'ria [NA], tectorial membrane; apparatus ligamentosus

weitbrechti; posterior occipitoaxial ligament; the upper continuation of the anterior part of the posterior longitudinal ligament attached to the upper surface of the basilar portion of the occipital bone and the bodies of the second and third cervical vertebrae.
m. tecto'ria duc'tus cochlea'ris [NA], tectorial membrane of the cochlear duct; Corti's membrane; tectorium (2); a gelatinous membrane that overlies the spiral organ (Corti) in the inner ear.
m. ten'sa, *pars* tensa membranae tympani.
m. thyrohyoi'dea [NA], thyrohyoid membrane; m. hyothyroidea; a thin, fibrous, membranous sheet filling the gap between the hyoid bone and the thyroid cartilage.
m. tym'pani [NA], tympanic or drum membrane; membrane of tympanum; eardrum; drum; drumhead; myringa; myrinx; a thin tense membrane forming the greater part of the lateral wall of the tympanic cavity and separating it from the external acoustic meatus; it constitutes the boundary between the external and middle ear, is covered on both surfaces with epithelium, and in the pars tensa has an intermediate layer of outer radial and inner circular collagen fibers.

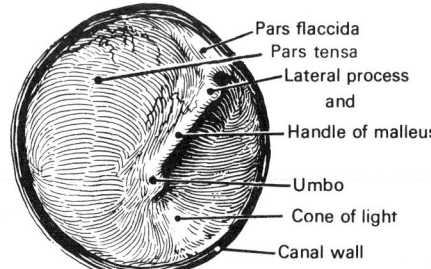

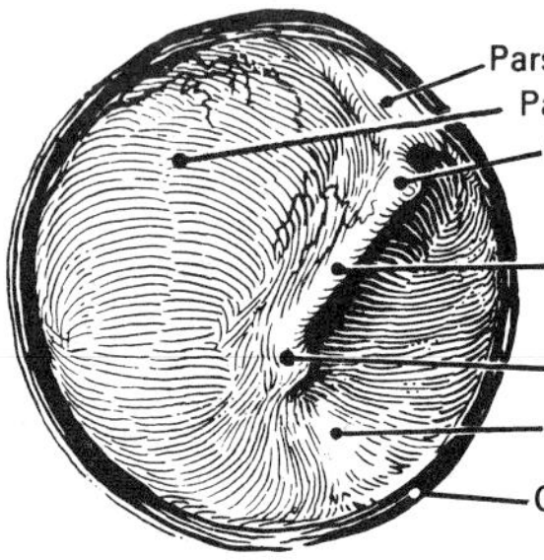

Right Membrana Tympani
As seen through an aural speculum

m. tym'pani secunda'ria [NA], secondary tympanic membrane; Scarpa's membrane; the membrane closing the fenestra cochleae or rotunda.
m. versic'olor, tapetum (2).
m. vestibula'ris [NA], *paries* vestibularis ductus cochlearis.
m. vi'brans, *pars* tensa membranae tympani.
m. vitelli'na, yolk membrane; **(1)** vitelline or ovular membrane; the membrane enveloping the yolk; specifically, the thickened cell membrane of large-yolked ova; **(2)** sometimes used to designate the zona pellucida of a mammalian ovum.
m. vit'rea [NA], vitreous membrane (2); m. hyaloidea; hyaloid membrane; tunica vitrea; a condensation of fine collagen fibers in places in the cortex of the vitreous body; formerly thought to form a membrane or capsule at its periphery.

membranaceous (mem-brā-nā'shŭs). Membranous.
membranate (mem'brā-nāt). Of the nature of a membrane.

MEMBRANE

membrane (mem'brān) [L. *membrana*, a skin or membrane that covers parts of the body, fr. *membrum*, a member]. Membrana.
adamantine m., *cuticula* dentis.
allantoid m., allantois.
alveolodental m., periodontium.
anal m., the dorsal portion of the embryonic cloacal m. after its division by the urorectal septum.
anterior atlanto-occipital m., *membrana* atlanto-occipitalis anterior.
arachnoid m., arachnoidea.
atlanto-occipital m., *membrana* atlanto-occipitalis.
basement m., basal lamina (1); basement lamina; basilemma; an amorphous extracellular layer closely applied to the basal surface of epithelium and also investing muscle cells, fat cells, and Schwann cells; thought to be a selective filter and to serve both structural and morphogenetic functions. It is composed of three successive layers (lamina lucida, lamina densa, and lamina fibroreticularis), a matrix of collagen (of which type IV is unique to this membrane), and several glycoproteins.
basilar m., *lamina* basilaris cochleae.
Bichat's m., the inner elastic m. of arteries.
Bogros' serous m., a m. of the episcleral space (of Tenon).
Bowman's m., *lamina* limitans anterior corneae.
Bruch's m., *lamina* basalis choroideae.
Brunn's m., the epithelium of the olfactory region of the nose.
bucconasal m., oronasal m.; a thin, transient epithelial sheet separating the primitive nasal cavity from the stomodeum in the seven-week-old human embryo.
buccopharyngeal m., oral or oropharyngeal m.; a bilaminar (ectoderm and endoderm) m. derived from the prochordal plate; after the embryonic head fold has evolved it lies at the caudal limit of the stomodeum.
cell m., cytolemma; cytomembrane; plasmalemma; plasmolemma; plasma m.; the protoplasmic boundary of all cells which controls permeability and may serve other functions through surface specializations; *e.g.,* active ion transport absorption by formation of pinocytotic vesicles; receptor-mediated antigen recognition, etc.; in structure, it is trilaminar and consists of the electron-dense lamina externa and lamina interna with an electron-lucent lamina intermedia.
chorioallantoic m., extraembryonic m. formed by fusion of chorion and allantois.
cloacal m., a transitory m. in the caudal area of the ventral wall of the embryo, separting the endodermal from the ectodermal cloaca; it is divided into anal and genitourinary m.'s that break down during the eighth to ninth week to establish the external opening for the alimentary and genitourinary tracts.
closing m.'s, pharyngeal m.'s; thin sheets, composed of ectoderm externally and endoderm internally, which separate the pharyngeal pouches from overlying branchial clefts in the early embryo.
Corti's m., *membrana* tectoria ductus cochlearis.
cricothyroid m., *conus* elasticus.
cricotracheal m., *ligamentum* cricotracheale.
cricovocal m., *conus* elasticus.
croupous m., false m.
deciduous m., *membrana* decidua.
Descemet's m., *lamina* limitans posterior corneae.
diphtheritic m., the false m. forming on the mucous surfaces in diphtheria.
drum m., *membrana* tympani.
Duddell's m., *lamina* limitans posterior corneae.
dysmenorrheal m., a m., resembling the decidua, cast off in cases of membranous dysmenorrhea.
egg m., the investing envelope of the ovum; **primary e. m.** is produced from ovarian cytoplasm; **secondary e. m.** is the product of the ovarian follicle; **tertiary e. m.** is secreted by the lining of the oviduct.
elastic m., a m. formed of elastic connective tissue, present as fenestrated lamellae in the coats of the arteries and elsewhere.
embryonic m., fetal m.
enamel m., the internal layer of the enamel organ formed by the enamel cells.
epipapillary m., **(1)** a congenital m. covering the optic disk; **(2)** the glial remnants of Bergmeister's *papilla.*
epiretinal m., a m., usually acquired, covering a portion of the

retina and composed of fibrous tissue from metaplasia of retinal pigment epithelial cells or glia.
exocelomic m., Heuser's m.; a layer of cells delaminated from the inner surface of the blastocystic cytotrophoblast and from the envelope of the primary yolk sac during the second week of embryonic life.
false m., pseudomembrane; croupous m.; neomembrane; plica (2); a thick, tough fibrinous exudate on the surface of a mucous m. or the skin.
fenestrated m., an elastic m., as in elastic laminae of arteries.
fertilization m., a viscous m. formed on the inner surface of the vitelline m. from the cytoplasm of the egg cell after entry of the sperm, preventing the entry of additional sperm.
fetal m., embryonic m.; a structure or tissue that develops from the fertilized ovum but does not form part of the embryo proper.
fibrous m., *membrana* fibrosa.
Fielding's m., tapetum (2).
flaccid m., *pars* flaccida membranae tympani.
germ m., germinal m., blastoderm.
glassy m., **(1)** the basement m. present between the stratum granulosum and the theca interna of a vesicular ovarian follicle; it becomes very prominent in large atretic follicles; **(2)** hyaline m. (2); the basement m. and associated connective tissue of the hair follicle.
Henle's m., *lamina* basalis choroideae.
Henle's fenestrated elastic m., elastic *laminae* of arteries.
Heuser's m., exocelomic m.
Hunter's m., *membrana* decidua.
Huxley's m., Huxley's *layer.*
hyaline m., **(1)** the thin, clear basement m. beneath certain epithelia; **(2)** glassy m. (2).
hyaloid m., *membrana* vitrea.
hyoglossal m., a delicate fibrous m. that extends between the hyoid bone and the tongue.
intercostal m.'s, *membranae* intercostalia.
interosseous m. of forearm, *membrana* interossea antebrachii.
interosseous m. of leg, *membrana* interossea cruris.
ivory m., *membrana* eboris.
Jackson's m., Jackson's veil; a thin vascular m. or veil-like adhesion, covering the anterior surface of the ascending colon from the cecum to the right flexure; it may cause obstruction by kinking of the bowel.
keratogenous m., *matrix* unguis.
limiting m. of neural tube, the inner and outer aspects of the developing neural tube, formed from footplates of the cytoplasmic processes of ependymal cells passing centripetally and centrifugally, respectively.
limiting m. of retina, membrana limitans; one of two layers of the retina: **internal l. m.,** formed by the expanded inner ends of Müller's fibers; **outer l. m.,** not a membrane but a row of junctional complexes.
medullary m., endosteum.
mucous m.'s, see entries under *tunica* mucosa.
Nasmyth's m., *cuticula* dentis.
nictitating m., *plica* semilunaris conjunctivae (2).
Nitabuch's m., Nitabuch's layer or stria; a layer of fibrin between the boundary zone of compact endometrium and the cytotrophoblastic shell in the placenta.
nuclear m., nuclear *envelope.*
obturator m., *membrana* obturatoria.
olfactory m., that part of the nasal mucosa having olfactory receptor cells and glands of Bowman.
oral m., buccopharyngeal m.
oronasal m., bucconasal m.
oropharyngeal m., buccopharyngeal m.
otolithic m., *membrana* statoconiorum.
ovular m., *membrana* vitellina (1).
Payr's m., a fold of peritoneum that crosses over the left flexure of the colon.
pericardiopleural m., pleuropericardial m.
peridental m., periodontium.
perineal m., *membrana* perinei.
periodontal m., periodontal *ligament.*
periorbital m., periorbita.
pharyngeal m.'s, closing m.'s.
pial-glial m., the dual outer lining of the brain and spinal cord, composed of the membrana limitans gliae and the pia mater.
pituitary m., *tunica* mucosa nasi.
placental m., placental barrier; the semipermeable layer of fetal tissue separating the maternal from the fetal blood in the placenta; composed of: 1) endothelium of the fetal vessels in the chorionic villi, 2) stromata of the villi, 3) cytotrophoblast (negligible after the fifth month of gestation), and 4) syncytial trophoblast covering the villi; placental m. acts as a selective m. regulating passage of substances from the maternal to the fetal blood.
plasma m., cell m.
pleuropericardial m., pericardiopleural m.; a tissue fold jutting into the embryonic pericardioperitoneal canals; it separates the developing pericardium from the pleural cavity.
pleuroperitoneal m., pleuroperitoneal fold; a tissue fold jutting into the caudal portion of the embryonic pericardioperitoneal canal; it develops into the dorsal portion of the definitive diaphragm.
posterior atlanto-occipital m., *membrana* atlanto-occipitalis posterior.
postsynaptic m., that part of the plasma m. of a neuron or muscle fiber with which an axon terminal forms a synaptic junction; in many instances, at least part of such a small postsynaptic m. patch shows characteristic morphological modifications such as greater thickness and higher electron-density, believed to correspond to the transmitter-sensitive receptor site of such synapses.
presynaptic m., that part of the plasma m. of an axon terminal that faces the plasma m. of the neuron or muscle fiber with which the axon terminal establishes a synpatic junction; many synaptic junctions exhibit structural presynaptic characteristics, such as conical, electron-dense internal protrusions, that distinguish it from the remainder of the axon's plasma m. See also synapse.
primary egg m., see egg m.
proligerous m., *cumulus* oophorus.
prophylactic m., pyogenic m.
pupillary m., *membrana* pupillaris.
pyogenic m., prophylactic m.; a layer of pus cells lining an abscess cavity which have not yet autolyzed.
quadrangular m., *membrana* quadrangularis.
Reissner's m., *paries* vestibularis ductus cochlearis.
reticular m., *membrana* reticularis.
Rivinus' m., *pars* flaccida membrane tympani.
Ruysch's m., *lamina* choroidocapillaris.
Scarpa's m., *membrana* tympani secundaria.
schneiderian m. [Schneider, C.V. Ger. anatomist, 1614–1680], *tunica* mucosa nasi.
Schultze's m., *regio* olfactoria tunicae mucosae nasi.
secondary egg m., see egg m.
secondary tympanic m., *membrana* tympani secundaria.
semipermeable m., a m. that is relatively permeable to the solvent but relatively impermeable to all or at least some of the solutes in either or both of the solutions separated by the m.
serous m., *tunica* serosa.
Shrapnell's m., *pars* flaccida membranae tympani.
spiral m., *paries* tympanicus ductus cochlearis.
stapedial m., *membrana* stapedis.
statoconial m., *membrana* statoconiorum.
sternal m., *membrana* sterni.
striated m., *zona* striata.
suprapleural m., *membrana* suprapleuralis.

synovial m., *membrana* synovialis.
tectorial m., *membrana* tectoria.
tectorial m. of cochlear duct, *membrana* tectoria ductus cochlearis.
tertiary egg m., see egg m.
thyrohyoid m., *membrana* thyrohyoidea.
Toldt's m., the anterior layer of the renal fascia.
Tourtual's m., *membrana* quadrangularis.
tympanic m., *membrana* tympani.
m. of tympanum, *membrana* tympani.
undulating m., undulatory m., a locomotory organelle of certain flagellate (trypanosome and trichomonad) parasites, consisting of a finlike extension of the limiting m. with the flagellar sheath; wavelike rippling of the undulating m. produces a characteristic movement.
unit m., the trilaminar structure of the plasmalemma and other intercellular membranes, when seen in cross-section with the electron microscope, composed of two electron-dense laminae approximately 20 Å thick separated by a less dense lamina 35 Å thick.
urogenital m., the ventral portion of the embryonic cloacal m. after its division by the urorectal septum.
urorectal m., in the embryo, urorectal septum separating the cloaca into urogenital sinus and rectum.
uteroepichorial m., rarely used term for *decidua* parietalis.
vaginal synovial m., *vagina* synovialis tendinis.
vestibular m., *paries* vestibularis ductus cochlearis.
virginal m., hymen.
vitelline m., *membrana* vitellina (1).
vitreous m., **(1)** *lamina* limitans posterior corneae; **(2)** *membrana* vitrea; **(3)** *lamina* basalis choroideae.
Wachendorf's m., *membrana* pupillaris.
yolk m., *membrana* vitellina.
Zinn's m., the anterior layer of the iris.

---

membranectomy (mem-bră-nek'tō-mē) [membrane + G. *ektomē,* excision]. Removal of the membranes of a subdural hematoma.

membranelle (mem-bră-nel'). A minute membrane formed of fused cilia, found in certain ciliate protozoa.

membraniform (mem-brā'ni-fōrm). Membranoid; of the appearance or character of a membrane.

membranocartilaginous (mem'bră-nō-kar-ti-laj'i-nŭs). **1.** Partly membranous and partly cartilaginous. **2.** Derived from both membrane and cartilage; denoting certain bones.

membranoid (mem'bră-noyd). Membraniform.

membranous (mem'bră-nŭs). Hymenoid (1); membranaceous; relating to or of the form of a membrane.

membrum, pl. **membra** (mem'brŭm, mem'bră) [L. member] [NA]. A limb; a member.
m. infe'rius [NA], inferior limb; pelvic limb; lower extremity; the hip, thigh, leg, ankle, and foot.
m. mulieb're, clitoris.
m. supe'rius [NA], superior limb; thoracic limb; upper extremity; the shoulder, arm, forearm, wrist, and hand.
m. vir'ile, penis.

memory (mem'ō-rē) [L. *memoria*]. **1.** General term for the recollection of that which was once experienced or learned. **2.** The mental information processing system that receives (registers), modifies, stores, and retrieves informational stimuli; composed of three stages: encoding, storage, and retrieval.
affect m., the emotional element recurring whenever a significant experience is recalled.
anterograde m., m. for that which occurred after an event such as a brain injury.
long-term m. (LTM), that phase of the m. process considered the permanent storehouse of information which has been registered, encoded, passed into the short-term m., coded, rehearsed, and finally transferred and stored for future retrieval; material and information retained in LTM underlies cognitive abilities.
remote m., m. for events of long ago as opposed to recent events.
retrograde m., m. for that which occurred before an event such as a brain injury.
screen m., in psychoanalysis, a consciously tolerable m. that unwittingly serves as a cover for another associated m. which would be emotionally painful if recalled.
selective m., reception or retrieval of only some of the events in an experience.
senile m., m. that is good for remote events, often in contrast to current events; characteristically seen in aged persons.
short-term m. (STM), that phase of the m. process in which stimuli that have been recognized and registered are stored briefly; decay occurs rapidly, typically within seconds, but may be held indefinitely by using rehearsal as a holding process by which to recycle material over and over through STM.
subconscious m., information not immediately available for recall.

memotine hydrochloride (mem'ō-tēn). 3,4-Dihydro-1-[(*p*-methoxyphenoxy)methyl]isoquinoline hydrochloride; an antiviral drug.

menacme (me-nak'mē) [G. *mēn,* month, + *akmē,* prime]. The period of menstrual activity in a woman's life.

menadiol diacetate (men-ă-dī'ol). Vitamin K_4; acetomenaphthone; 2-methyl-1,4-naphthohydroquinone diacetate; menadiol acetylated at both OH's; a prothrombogenic vitamin.

menadiol sodium diphosphate. Tetrasodium 2-methyl-1,4-naphthalenediol-*bis* (dihydrogen phosphate); a dihydro derivative of menadione, with similar vitamin K activity.

menadione (men-ă-dī'ōn) Menaphthone; menaquinone; 2-methyl-1,4-naphthoquinone; the root of compounds that are 3-multiprenyl derivatives of m. and known as the menaquinones or vitamins K_2.

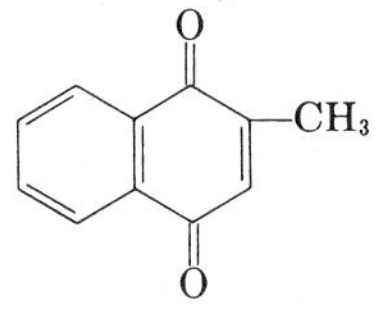

Menadione

m. reductase, NAD(P)H dehydrogenase (quinone).
m. sodium bisulfite, menaphthone sodium bisulfite; it possesses the same action and is used for the same purposes as m. or vitamin K; it differs, however, from m. in being water-soluble.

menaphthone (men-ă-naf'thōn). Menadione.

menaquinone (MK) (men'ă-kwin'ōn, -kwī'nōn). Menadione.

menaquinone-6 (MK-6). Vitamin K_2 or K_2(30); hexaprenylmenaquinone; prenylmenaquinone-6; 2-methyl-3-hexaprenyl-1,4-naphthoquinone; isolated from putrified fish meal; potency is about 60% of that of phylloquinone (vitamin K_1).

menaquinone-7 (MK-7). Vitamin K_2(35); menaquinone-6 with a 3-heptaprenyl side-chain.

menarche (me-nar'kē) [G. *mēn,* month, + *archē,* beginning]. Establishment of the menstrual function; the time of the first menstrual period.

menarcheal, menarchial (me-nar'kē-ăl). Pertaining to the menarche.

Mendel, Gregor J., Austrian geneticist, 1822–1884. See mendelian *character, inheritance, ratio;* M.'s *laws.*

Mendel, Kurt, German neurologist, 1874–1946. See M.'s instep *reflex;* Bechterew-M. *reflex.*

Mendeléeff (Mendeleev), Dimitri (Dmitri) I., Russian chemist, 1834–1907. See mendelevium, M.'s *law.*

mendelevium (men-dĕ-lē'vē-ŭm) [*D. Mendeléeff*]. An element, atomic no. 101, symbol Md, prepared in 1955 by bombardment of einsteinium with alpha particles.

mendelian (men-dē'lē-ăn). Attributed to or described by Gregor Mendel; usually referring to the behavior and the mechanism of the genetic transmission of single-locus traits.

mendelism (men'del-izm). The hereditary principles derived from Mendel's laws.

mendelizing (men'del-īz-ing). Denoting a pattern of inheritance of a trait that corresponds phenotypically to the segregation of known or putative genes at one predominating genetic locus.

Mendelson, Curtis L., U.S. physician, *1913. See M.'s *syndrome.*

Ménétrièr, Pierre E., French physician, 1859–1935. See M.'s *disease, syndrome.*

Menge, Karl, German gynecologist, 1864–1945. See M.'s *pessary.*

Ménière, Prosper, French physician, 1799–1862. See M.'s *disease, syndrome.*

mening-. See meningo-.

meningeal (mĕ-nin'jē-ăl, men'in-jē'ăl). Relating to the meninges.

meningeocortical (mĕ-nin'jē-ō-kōr'ti-kăl). Meningocortical.

meningeorrhaphy (mĕ-nin'jē-ōr'ă-fē) [G. *mēninx* (*mēning-*), membrane, + *rhaphē,* suture]. Suture of the cranial or spinal meninges or of any membrane.

meninges (mĕ-nin'jēz). Plural of meninx.

meningioma (mĕ-nin'jē-ō'mă) [mening- + G. *-oma,* tumor]. A benign, encapsulated neoplasm of arachnoidal origin, occurring in adults; most frequent form consists of elongated, fusiform cells in whorls and pseudolobules with psammoma bodies frequently present; m.'s tend to occur along the superior sagittal sinus, along the sphenoid ridge, or in the vicinity of the optic chiasm; in addition to meningothelial m., angiomatous, chondromatous, osteomatous, lipomatous, melanotic, and fibrosarcomatous varieties are recognized.

cutaneous m., a lesion in the skin and subcutis composed of meningoepithelial cells; occurs as a developmental error in children or as an extension of an aggressive intracranial m. in adults.

psammomatous m., psammoma.

meningiomatosis (mĕ-nin'jē-ō-mă-tō'sis). The presence of multiple meningiomas, sometimes seen in von Recklinghausen's disease.

meningism (men'in-jizm, mĕ-nin'jizm). Pseudomeningitis; a condition of irritation of the brain or spinal cord in which the symptoms simulate a meningitis, but in which no actual inflammation of these membranes is present.

meningitic (men'in-jit'ik). Relating to or characterized by meningitis.

meningitis pl. **meningitides** (men-in-jī'tis, -jit'i-dēz) [mening- + G. *itis,* inflammation]. Inflammation of the membranes of the brain or spinal cord. See also arachnoiditis; leptomeningitis.

basilar m., m. at the base of the brain, due usually to tuberculosis, syphilis, or any low-grade chronic granulomatous process; may result in an internal hydrocephalus.

cerebrospinal m., meningococcal m.

eosinophilic m., angiostrongylosis.

epidemic cerebrospinal m., meningococcal m.

epidural m., *pachymeningitis* externa.

external m., *pachymeningitis* externa.

internal m., *pachymeningitis* interna.

listeria m., listeriosis.

meningococcal m., cerebrospinal m. or fever; epidemic cerebrospinal m.; an acute infectious disease affecting children and young adults, caused by *Neisseria meningitidis;* characterized by nasopharyngeal catarrh, headache, vomiting, convulsions, stiffness in the neck (nuchal rigidity), photophobia, constipation, cutaneous hyperesthesia, a purpuric or herpetic eruption, and the presence of Kernig's sign.

neoplastic m., neoplastic arachnoiditis; infiltration of subarachnoid space by neoplastic cells, typically medulloblastoma or metastatic carcinoma.

occlusive m., leptomeningitis causing occlusion of the spinal fluid pathways.

otitic m., infection of the meninges secondary to mastoiditis or otitis media.

serous m., acute m. with secondary external hydrocephalus.

tuberculous m., cerebral tuberculosis (1); inflammation of the cerebral leptomeninges marked by the presence of granulomatous inflammation; it is usually confined to the base of the brain (basilar m., internal hydrocephalus) and is accompanied in children by an accumulation of spinal fluid in the ventricles (acute hydrocephalus).

meningo-, mening- [G. *mēninx,* membrane]. Combining forms relating to meninges.

meningocele (mĕ-ning'gō-sēl) [meningo- + G. *kēlē,* tumor]. Protrusion of the membranes of the brain or spinal cord through a defect in the skull or spinal column.

spurious m., traumatic m.; an extracranial or extraspinal accumulation of cerebrospinal fluid, due to meningeal tear.

traumatic m., spurious m.

meningococcemia (mĕ-ning'gō-kok-sē'mē-ă). Presence of meningococci (*Neisseria meningitidis*) in the circulating blood.

meningococcus, pl. **meningococci** (mĕ-ning'gō-kok'ŭs, -kok'sī) [meningo- + G. *kokkos,* berry]. *Neisseria meningitidis.*

meningocortical (mĕ-ning'gō-kōr'ti-kăl). Meningeocortical; relating to the meninges and the cortex of the brain.

meningocyte (mĕ-ning'gō-sīt) [meningo- + G. *kytos,* cell]. A mesenchymal epithelial cell of the subarachnoid space; it may become a macrophage.

meningoencephalitis (mĕ-ning'gō-en-sef'ăl-ī'tis) [meningo- + G. *enkephalos,* brain, + *-itis,* inflammation]. Cerebromeningitis; encephalomeningitis; an inflammation of the brain and its membranes.

acute primary hemorrhagic m., acute epidemic *leukoencephalitis.*

biundulant m., tick-borne *encephalitis* (Central European subtype).

eosinophilic m., a disease caused by infection with the rat lungworm, *Angiostrongylus cantonensis,* whose larvae, ingested with infected slugs or land snails (or some unidentified transport host), migrate from intestine to the meninges of the brain where the disease is produced; it is usually mild, of short duration, and characterized by fever, eosinophilia, and white blood cells (rarely nematode larvae) in the spinal fluid.

herpetic m., a severe form of m. caused by herpesvirus type 1 and associated with a high mortality rate; definite diagnosis depends upon isolation of the virus or demonstration of viral antigens.

mumps m., a usually benign nervous system infection arising during the active phase of clinical mumps parotiditis.

primary amebic m., an invasive, rapidly fatal cerebral infection by soil amebae, chiefly *Naegleria fowleri,* found in man and other primates and experimentally in rodents; the disease is characterized by a high fever, neck rigidity, and symptoms associated with upper respiratory infection such as cough and nausea; although organisms have been cultured from various organs, the brain is the primary focus, especially the olfactory lobes and cerebral cortex, which are first attacked by the amebae that enter from nasal mucosa through the cribiform plate; death usually occurs two to three days after onset of symptoms.

syphilitic m., a secondary or tertiary stage manifestation of syphilis; rarely fatal.

meningoencephalocele (mĕ-ning′gō-en-sef′ă-lō-sēl) [meningo- + G. *enkephalos,* brain, + *kēlē,* hernia]. Encephalomeningocele; a protrusion of the meninges and brain through a congenital defect in the cranium, usually in the frontal or occipital region.

meningoencephalomyelitis (mĕ-ning′gō-en-sef′ă-lō-mī-ĕ-lī′tis) [meningo + G. *enkephalos,* brain, + *myelos,* marrow, + *-itis,* inflammation]. Inflammation of the brain and spinal cord together with their membranes.

meningoencephalopathy (mĕ-ning′gō-en-sef-ă-lop′ă-thē) [meningo- + G. *enkephalos,* brain, + *pathos,* suffering]. Encephalomeningopathy; disorder affecting the meninges and the brain.

meningomyelitis (mĕ-ning′gō-mī′ĕ-lī′tis) [meningo- + G. *myelos,* marrow, + *-itis,* inflammation]. Inflammation of the spinal cord and of its enveloping arachnoid and pia mater, and less commonly also of the dura mater.

meningomyelocele (mĕ-ning-gō-mī′ĕ-lō-sēl) [meningo- + G. *myelos,* marrow, + *kēlē,* tumor]. Myelomeningocele; myelocystomeningocele; protrusion of the membranes and cord through a defect in the vertebral column.

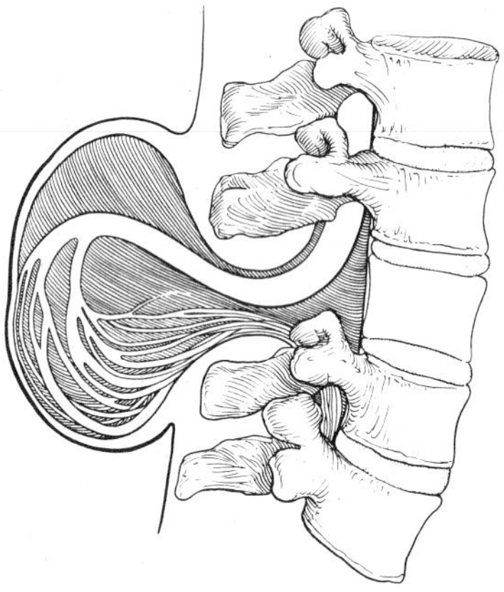

Meningomyelocele

meningo-osteophlebitis (mĕ-ning′gō′os-tē-ō-flĕ-bī′tis). Inflammation of the veins of the periosteum.

meningoradicular (mĕ-ning′gō-ra-dik′yū-lăr) [meningo- + L. *radix,* root]. Relating to the meninges covering cranial or spinal nerve roots.

meningoradiculitis (mĕ-ning′gō-ra-dik-yū-lī′tis). Inflammation of the meninges and roots of the nerves.

meningorrhachidian (mĕ-ning′gō-ra-kid′ē-an) [meningo- + G. *rhachis,* spine]. Relating to the spinal cord and its membranes.

meningorrhagia (mĕ-ning′gō-rā′jē-ă) [meningo- + G. *rhēgnymi,* to burst forth]. Hemorrhage into or beneath the cerebral or spinal meninges.

meningosis (men′ing-gō′sis) [meningo- + G. *-ōsis,* condition]. Membranous union of bones, as in the skull of the newborn.

meningovascular (mĕ-ning′gō-vas′kyū-lăr). Concerning the blood vessels in the meninges; or the meninges and blood vessels.

meninguria (men-ing-gū′rē-ă) [meningo- + G. *ouron,* urine]. The passage of membraniform shreds in the urine.

meninx, gen. **meningis,** pl. **meninges** (mē′ningks, men′ingks, mĕ-nin′jes, -jēz) [Mod. L. fr. G. *mēninx,* membrane]. Any membrane; specifically, one of the membranous coverings of the brain and spinal cord. See also arachnoidea, dura mater, pia mater.

m. fibro′sa, rarely used term for dura mater.

m. primiti′va, the embryonic loose mesenchymatous tissue surrounding the brain and spinal cord; from it the three definite meninges (arachnoidea, dura mater, and pia mater) are derived.

m. sero′sa, arachnoidea.

m. ten′uis, the leptomeninges.

m. vasculo′sa, rarely used term for pia mater.

meniscectomy (men′i-sek′tō-mē) [G. *mēniskos,* crescent (meniscus) + *ektomē,* excision]. Excision of a meniscus, usually from the knee joint.

menisci (mĕ-nis′sī). Plural of meniscus.

meniscitis (men′i-sī′tis) [G. *mēniskos,* crescent (meniscus), + *-itis,* inflammation]. Inflammation of a fibrocartilaginous meniscus.

meniscocyte (mĕ-nis′kō-sīt) [G. *mēniskos,* a crescent, + *kytos,* a hollow (cell)]. Sickle *cell.*

meniscocytosis (mĕ-nis′kō-sī-tō′sis) [meniscocyte + G. *-osis,* condition]. Obsolete term for sickle cell *anemia.*

meniscopexy (mĕ-nis′kō-pek-sē). Meniscorrhaphy; surgical procedure anchoring the medial meniscus to its former attachment.

meniscorrhaphy (men-is-kōr′ă-fē). Meniscopexy.

meniscotome (mĕ-nis′kō-tōm) [G. *mēniskos,* crescent (meniscus) + *tomē,* incision]. An instrument used in the removal of a meniscus.

meniscus, pl. **menisci,** (mĕ-nis′kŭs, mĕ-nis′sī) [G. *mēniskos,* crescent]. **1.** Meniscus *lens.* **2** [NA]. A crescent-shaped structure. **3.** A crescent-shaped fibrocartilaginous structure of the knee, the acromio- and sterno-clavicular and the temporo-mandibular joints.

articular m., m. articularis.

m. articula′ris [NA], articular m.; articular crescent; a crescent-shaped intra-articular fibrocartilage found in certain joints.

converging m., positive m.; a m. in which the convexity exceeds the concavity.

diverging m., negative m.; a convexoconcave lens in which the concavity has a greater radius than does the convexity.

lateral m., m. lateralis.

m. latera′lis [NA], lateral m.; external semilunar fibrocartilage; attached to the lateral border of the upper articular surface of the tibia.

medial m., m. medialis.

m. media′lis [NA], medial m.; falciform cartilage; internal semilunar fibrocartilage of knee joint; attached to the medial border of the upper articular surface of the tibia.

negative m., diverging m.

periscopic m., aplanatic *lens.*

positive m., converging m.

tactile m., m. tactus.

m. tac′tus [NA], tactile m.; tactile disk; Merkel's tactile cell or disk; Merkel's corpuscle; a specialized tactile sensory nerve ending in the epidermis, characterized by a terminal cuplike expansion of

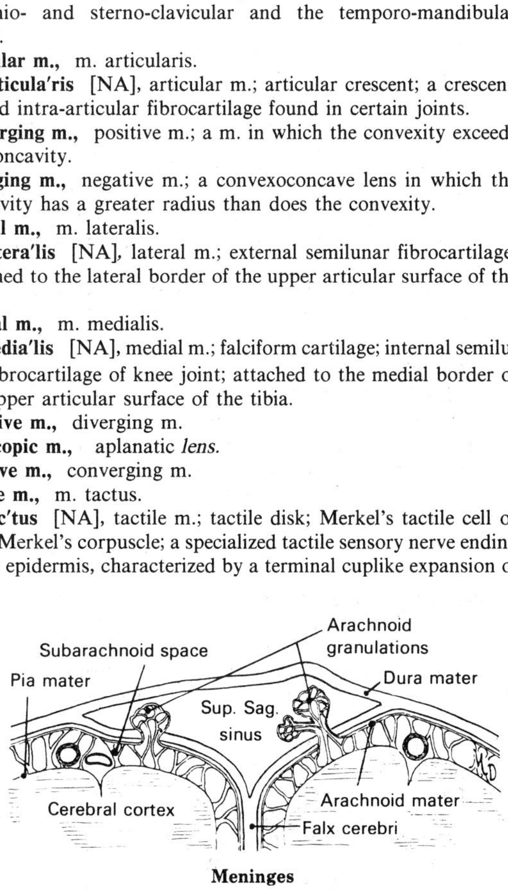

Meninges

Coronal section to show the cerebral meninges in relation to the brain.

an intraepidermal axon in contact with the base of a single modified keratinocyte.

Menkes, John H., U.S. neurologist, *1928. See M.'s *syndrome.*

meno- [G. *mēn,* month]. Combining form denoting relationship to the menses.

menocelis (men-ō-sē'lis) [meno- + G. *kēlis,* spot]. A dark macular or petechial eruption sometimes occurring in cases of amenorrhea.

menometrorrhagia (men'ō-mē-trō-rā'jē-ă) [meno- + G. *mētra,* uterus, + *rhēgnymi,* to burst forth]. Irregular or excessive bleeding during menstruation and between menstrual periods.

menopausal (men'ō-paw-zăl). Associated with or occasioned by the menopause.

menopause (men'ō-pawz) [meno- + G. *pausis,* cessation]. Permanent cessation of the menses; termination of the menstrual life.

menophania (men-ō-fā'nē-ă) [meno- + G. *phainō,* to show]. First sign of the menses at puberty.

Menopon (men'ō-pon). A genus of biting lice (family Menoponidae, order Mallophaga) found on birds; it includes important pests that infect domestic fowl, such as *M. gallinae* (*M. pallidum*). the shaft louse of poultry, a light yellow louse about 1.7 to 2.0 mm long, found on barnyard fowl, ducks, and pigeons.

menorrhagia (men-ō-rā'jē-ă) [meno- + G. *rhēgnymi,* to burst forth]. Hypermenorrhea.

menorrhalgia (men-ō-ral'jē-ă) [meno- + G. *algos,* pain]. Dysmenorrhea.

menoschesis (me-nos'ke-sis, men-ō-skē'sis) [meno- + G. *schesis,* retention]. Suppression of menstruation.

menostasis, menostasia (mē-nos'tă-sis, men-ō-stā'zē-ă) [meno- + G. *stasis,* a standing]. Rarely used term for amenorrhea.

menostaxis (men-ō-stak'sis) [meno- + G. *staxis,* a dripping]. Hypermenorrhea.

menotropins (men-ō-trō'pinz). Extract of postmenopausal urine containing primarily the follicle-stimulating hormone. See also human menopausal *gonadotropin.*

menouria (men-ō-yū'rē-ă) [meno- + G. *ouron,* urine, + *-ia,* condition]. Menstruation occurring through the urinary bladder as a result of vesicouterine fistula.

menoxenia (men-ō-zē'nē-ă, men'ok-sē'nē-ă) [meno- + G. *xenos,* strange]. Any abnormality of menstruation.

menses (men'sēz) [L. pl. of *mensis,* month]. Menstrual period; catamenia; emmenia; a periodic physiologic hemorrhage, occurring at approximately 4-week intervals, and having its source from the uterine mucous membrane; under normal circumstances, the bleeding is preceded by ovulation and predecidual changes in the endometrium. See also menstrual *cycle.*

menstrual (men'strū-ăl) [L. *menstrualis*]. Catamenial; emmenic; relating to the menses.

menstruant (men'strū-ant). Menstruating.

menstruate (men'strū-āt) [L. *menstruo,* pp. *-atus,* to be menstruant]. To undergo menstruation.

menstruation (men-strū-ā'shŭn) [see menstruate]. Cyclic endometrial shedding and discharge of a bloody fluid from the uterus during the menstrual cycle.

anovular m., anovulational or nonovulational m.; menstrual bleeding without the discharge of an ovum; also occurs in subhuman primates.

anovulational m., anovular m.

nonovulational m., anovular m.

retained m., hematocolpos.

retrograde m., a flow of menstrual blood back through the fallopian tubes; it sometimes carries with it endometrial cells, giving rise to endometriosis.

supplementary m., bleeding from the navel or urinary tract due to endometriosis occurring at the time of m.

suppressed m., nonappearance of menstrual bleeding from whatever cause.

vicarious m., bleeding from any surface other than the mucous membrane of the uterine cavity, occurring periodically at the time when the normal m. should take place.

menstruum, pl. **menstrua** (men'strū-ŭm, -strū-ă) [Mediev. L. menstrual fluid, thought to possess certain solvent properties, ntr. of L. *menstruus,* monthly]. Old term for solvent.

mensual (men'sū-ăl, -shū-ăl) [L. *mensis,* month]. Monthly.

mensuration (men-sū-rā'shŭn) [L. *mensuratio,* fr. *mensuro,* to measure]. The act or process of measuring.

mentagra (men-tag'ră) [L. tetter on the chin, fr. *mentum,* chin, + G. *agra,* a seizure]. Sycosis.

men'tal. 1 [L. *mens (ment-),* mind]. Relating to the mind. **2** [L. *mentum,* chin]. Genial; genian; relating to the chin.

mentalis (men-tā'lis) [L.]. See under musculus.

mentality (men-tal'i-tē). The functional attributes of the mind; mental activity.

mentation (men-tā'shŭn). The process of reasoning and thinking.

Menten, Maud L., Canadian pathologist in U.S., 1879–1960. See Michaelis-M. *constant, hypothesis.*

Mentha (men'thă) [L.]. Mint; a genus of plants of the family Labiatae. M. piperita is peppermint; M. pulegium, pennyroyal; M. viridis, spearmint.

menthane (men'thān) 1-Isopropyl-4-methylcyclohexane; the cyclic terpene parent of alcohols such as menthol, terpin.

men'thol. Peppermint camphor; *p* -menthan-3-ol; an alcohol obtained from peppermint oil or other mint oils, or prepared synthetically; used as an antipruritic and topical anesthetic, in nasal sprays and inhalers, and as a flavoring agent.

camphorated m., a liquid obtained by triturating equal parts of camphor and m.; used locally as a counterirritant and (diluted) as a spray in rhinitis and pharyngitis.

mentolabialis (men'tō-lā-bē-ā'lis) [L.]. The mentalis and depressor labii inferioris considered as one muscle.

men'ton [L. *mentum,* chin]. In cephalometrics, the lowermost point in the symphysial shadow as seen on a lateral jaw projection.

mentoplasty (men'tō-plas-tē) [L. *mentum,* chin, + G. *plastos,* formed]. Genioplasty; plastic surgery of the chin, whereby its shape or size is altered.

mentum, gen. **menti** (men'tŭm, -tī) [L.] [NA]. The chin.

menyanthes (men-yan'thēz). Buckbean.

mepacrine hydrochloride (mep'ă-krēn). Quinacrine hydrochloride.

meparfynol (me-par'fin-ol). 3-Methyl-1-pentyn-3-ol; a hypnotic and sedative.

mepazine acetate (mep'ă-zēne). 10-[(1-Methyl-3-piperidyl) methyl]phenothiazine acetate; a phenothiazine derivative with actions and uses similar to those of chlorpromazine. Also available as m. hydrochloride.

mepenzolate bromide (me-pen'zō-lāt). *N*-Methyl-3-piperidyl benzilate methyl bromide; an anticholinergic drug.

meperidine hydrochloride (me-per'i-dēn). Ethyl 1-methyl-4-phenylisonipecotate hydrochloride; a narcotic analgesic.

mephenesin (me-fen'ĕ-sin). 3-*o* -Toloxy-1,2-propanediol; a skeletal muscle relaxant; also available as m. carbamate.

mephenoxalone (me-fen-ok'să-lōn). 5-[(*o*-Methoxyphenoxy)-methyl]-2-oxazolidinone; a mild tranquilizer and muscle relaxant.

mephentermine (me-fen'ter-mēn). *N*-α,α-trimethylphenethylamine; a sympathomimetic amine.
m. sulfate, used topically as a nasal decongestant and systemically for its pressor effects in acute hypotensive states.

mephenytoin (mĕ-fen'i-tō-in). Methoin; 5-ethyl-3-methyl-5-phenylhydantoin; an anticonvulsant.

mephitic (me-fit'ik) [L. *mephitis,* a noxious exhalation]. Foul, poisonous, or noxious.

mephobarbital (mef-ō-bar'bi-tawl). 5-Ethyl-1-methyl-5-phenylbarbituric acid; used as a sedative and long-acting hypnotic, and as an anticonvulsant in the management of epilepsy.

mepivacaine hydrochloride (me-piv'ă-kān). *d*-1-*N*-Methylpipecolic acid 2,6-dimethylanilide hydrochloride; a local anesthetic agent.

meprednisone (me-pred'ni-sōn). 17,21-Dihydroxy-16β-methylpregna-1,4-diene-3,11,20-trione; a glucocorticoid for oral use.

meprobamate (me-prō'bă-māt). 2-Methyl-2-*n*- propyl-1,3-propanediol dicarbamate; a skeletal muscle relaxant with action similar to that produced by mephenesin but of longer duration; used in the management of certain disorders associated with abnormal motor activity, as a mild hypnotic, and as an antianxiety agent.

mepyramine maleate (me-pir'ă-mēn). Pyrilamine maleate.

mepyrapone (me-pir'ă-pōn). Metyrapone.

mEq, meq Abbreviation for milliequivalent.

-mer. **1.** Suffix attached to a prefix such as mono-, di-, poly-, tri-, etc., to indicate the smallest unit of a repeating structure; *e.g.,* polymer. **2.** Suffix denoting a member of a particular group; *e.g.,* isomer, enantiomer.

meralgia (me-ral'jē-ă) [G. *mēros,* thigh, + *algos,* pain]. Pain in the thigh; specifically, m. paresthetica.
m. paraesthet'ica, tingling, formication, itching, and other forms of paresthesia in the outer side of the lower part of the thigh in the area of distribution of the lateral femoral cutaneous nerve; there may be pain, but the skin is usually hypesthetic to the touch. Also called Bernhardt's or Roth's disease; Roth-Bernhardt disease; Bernhardt-Roth syndrome.

meralluride (mer-al'yū-rīd). *N*-[[2-Methoxy-3-[(1,2,3,6-tetrahydro-1,3-dimethyl-2,6-dioxopurin-7-yl) mercuri]propyl]carbamoyl]succinamic acid; a mercurial diuretic.

merbromin (mer-brō'min). The disodium salt of 2,7-dibromo-4-hydroxymercurifluorescein; an organic mercurial antiseptic compound that also has staining properties similar to those of eosin and phloxine, with strong affinity for cytoplasmic structures; also used histochemically to stain protein-bound sulfhydryl and disulfide groups for bright-field and fluorescence microscopy.

mercaptal (mer-kap'tăl). A substance derived from an aldehyde by the replacement of the bivalent oxygen by two thioalkyl (–SR) groups.

mercaptan (mer-kap'tan). **1.** Thioalcohol; a class of substances in which the oxygen of an alcohol has been replaced by sulfur. **2.** In dentistry, a class of elastic impression compounds sometimes referred to as rubber base materials.
methyl m., methanethiol; CH_3SH; formed in the intestines by bacterial action on sulfur-containing proteins and appears in urine after ingestion of asparagus (contributing to the characteristic odor); also used in the manufacture of various organic sulfur-containing pesticides and fungicides.

mercapto-. Prefix indicating the presence of a thiol group, –SH.

mercaptoacetic acid (mer-kap'tō-ă-sē'tik). Thioglycolic acid.

mercaptol (mer-kap'tol). A substance derived from a ketone by the replacement of the bivalent oxygen by two thioalkyl (–SR) groups.

mercaptomerin sodium (mer-kap-tom'ĕ-rin, mer-kap-tō-mer'in). *N*-(γ-Carboxymethylmercaptomercuri-β-methoxy)propylcamphoramic acid disodium salt; a mercurial diuretic.

mercaptopurine (mer-kap-tō-pūr'ēn). 6-Purinethiol; an analogue of hypoxanthine and of adenine; an antineoplastic agent.

mercapturic acid (mer-kap-tyūr'ik). A condensation product of cysteine with aromatic compounds, such as bromobenzene; formed biologically via glutathione in the liver and excreted in the urine.

Mercier, Louis A., French urologist, 1811– 1882. See M.'s *bar, sound, valve;* median *bar* of M.

mercocresols (mer-kō-krē'solz). A mixture consisting of equal parts by weight of *sec*-amyltricresol and *o*-hydroxyphenylmercuric chloride; it possesses fungicidal, germicidal, and bacteriostatic action.

mercumatilin (mer'kyū-mă-til'in, -mat'i-lin). 8-(2'-Methoxy-3'-hydroxymercuripropyl) coumarin-3-carboxylic acid (mercumallylic acid) and theophylline; a mercurial diuretic; also available as m. sodium.

mercuramide (mer-kū'ră-mīd). Mersalyl.

mercurial (mer-kyū'rē-ăl). **1.** Relating to mercury. **2.** Any salt of mercury used medicinally.

mercurialentis (mer-kyū'rē-ă-len'tis). A brown discoloration of the anterior capsule of the lens caused by mercury; early sign of mercurial poisoning.

mercurialism (mer-kyū'rē-ă-lizm). Mercury *poisoning.*

***p*-mercuribenzoate** (mer-kyūr-i-ben'zō-āt). A commonly used enzyme inhibitor because of its reaction with sulfhydryl groups; usually *p*-chloromercuribenzoate or *p*-hydroxymercuribenzoate is used.

mercuric (mer-kyū'rik). Denoting a salt of mercury in which the ion of the metal is bivalent, as in corrosive sublimate, mercuric chloride, $HgCl_2$; the mercurous chloride is calomel, HgCl.

mercuric chloride. Mercury bichloride or perchloride; corrosive mercury chloride; corrosive sublimate; $HgCl_2$; a topical antiseptic and disinfectant for inanimate objects.
ammoniated m. chloride, ammoniated *mercury.*

mercuric iodide, red. Mercury biniodide or deutoiodide; HgI_2; has been used as an antiseptic and as a disinfectant for inanimate objects.

mercuric oleate. An ointment-like preparation used in parasitic skin diseases.

mercuric oxide, red. Red precipitate; the red precipitate of HgO; it has been used externally as an antiseptic in chronic skin diseases and fungus infections.

mercuric oxide, yellow. Yellow precipitate; the yellow precipitate of HgO; used externally as an antiseptic in the treatment of inflammatory conditions of the eyelids and the conjunctivae.

mercuric salicylate. Mercury subsalicylate; a powder used externally in the treatment of parasitic and fungus skin diseases.

mercurophen (mer-kyū'-rō-fen). Sodium hydroxymercury-*o*-nitrophenolate; a local antiseptic.

mercurophylline sodium (mer-kyūr-of'i-lēn). The sodium salt of β-methoxy-γ-hydroxymercuripropylamide of trimethylcyclopentanedicarboxylic acid, and theophylline; a mercurial diuretic.

mercurous (mer-kyū'rūs, mer'kyū-rūs). Denoting a salt of mercury in which the ion of the metal is univalent, as in calomel, mercurous chloride, HgCl; the mercuric chloride is corrosive sublimate, $HgCl_2$.

mercurous chloride. Calomel.

mercurous iodide. Yellow mercury iodide; mercury protoiodide; HgI; used externally as an ointment in eye diseases.

mercury (mer'kyū-rē) [L. *Mercurius,* Mercury, the god of trade, messenger of the gods; in Mediev. L., quicksilver, mercury]. Quicksilver; hydrargyrum; a liquid metallic element, symbol Hg, atomic no. 80, atomic weight 200.59; used in thermometers, barometers, manometers, and other scientific instruments; some salts and organic mercurials are used medicinally.

ammoniated m., ammoniated mercuric chloride; white mercuric precipitate; $HgNH_2Cl$; used in ointment for the treatment of skin diseases.

m. bichloride, m. perchloride, corrosive m. chloride, mercuric chloride.

m. biniodide, mercuric iodide, red.

m. deutoiodide, mercuric iodide, red.

m. protoiodide, mercurous iodide.

m. subsalicylate, mercuric salicylate.

yellow m. iodide, mercurous iodide.

mere-, mero- [G. *mĕros,* part]. Combining forms meaning part; also indicating one of a series of similar parts. See also -mer.

Merendino, K. Alvin, U.S. surgeon, *1914. See M.'s *technique.*

mereprine (mer'ĕ-prēn). Doxylamine succinate.

merethoxylline procaine (mer-ĕ-thok'si-lēn). Dehydro-2-[*N*-(3'-hydroxymercuri-2'-methoxyethoxy)propylcarbamoyl]phenoxyacetic acid (merethoxylline), 2-diethylaminoethyl *p*-aminobenzoate (procaine), and theophylline; a mixture of the procaine salt of merethoxylline and anhydrous theophylline; used as a mercurial diuretic.

meridian (mĕ-rid'-ē-an) [L. *meridianus,* pertaining to midday, on the south side, southern]. **1.** A line encircling a globular body at right angles to its equator and touching both poles, or the half of such a circle extending from pole to pole. **2.** In acupuncture, the lines connecting different anatomical sites.

m. of cornea, any line bisecting the cornea through its apex.

m.'s of eye, *meridiani* bulbi oculi.

meridiani (mĕ-rid-ē-ā'nī). Plural of meridianus.

meridianus, pl. **meridiani** (mĕ-rid'ē-ā'nŭs, -nī) [L.] [NA]. Meridian.

meridiani bul'bi oc'uli [NA], meridians of eye; lines surrounding the surface of the eyeball passing through both anterior and posterior poles.

meridional (mĕ-rid'ē-ō-năl). Relating to a meridian.

merispore (mer'i-spōr) [G. *meros,* a part, + *sporos,* seed]. A secondary spore, one resulting from the segmentation of another (compound or septate) spore.

meristematic (mer'is-tē-mat'ik) [G. *merizein,* to divide]. Pertaining (in fungi) to an area (meristem) of the hyphae or of other specialized structures from which new growth occurs.

meristic (mĕ-ris'tik) [G. *meristikos,* suitable for dividing]. Symmetrical; that which can be divided evenly; denoting bilateral or longitudinal symmetry in the arrangement of parts in one organism.

Merkel, Friedrich S., German anatomist and physiologist, 1845–1919. See M.'s *corpuscle,* tactile *cell,* tactile *disk.*

Merkel, Karl L., German anatomist and laryngologist, 1812–1876. See M.'s *filtrum* ventriculi, *fossa, muscle.*

mero-. See mere-.

meroacrania (mer'ō-ă-krā'nē-ă) [mero- + G. *a-* priv. + *kranion,* skull]. Congenital lack of a part of the cranium other than the occipital bone.

meroanencephaly (mer'ō-an-en-sef'ă-lē) [mero- + G. *an-* priv. + *enkephalos,* brain]. A type of anencephaly in which the brain and cranium are present in rudimentary form.

merocele (mēr'ō-sēl) [G. *mēros,* thigh, + *kele,* hernia]. Femoral *hernia.*

merocrine (mer'ō-krin, -krīn, -krēn) [mero- + G. *krinō,* to separate]. See under gland.

merodiastolic (mer'ō-dī-ă-stol'ik) [mero- + diastole]. Partially diastolic; relating to a part of the diastole of the heart.

merogenesis (mer-ō-jen'ĕ-sis) [mero- + G. *genesis,* origin]. Reproduction by segmentation.

merogenetic, merogenic (mer-ō-jĕ-net'ik, -ō-jen'ik). Relating to merogenesis.

merogony (mĕ-rog'ō-nē) [mero- + G. *gonē,* generation]. **1.** The incomplete development of an ovum which has been disorganized. **2.** A form of asexual schizogony, typical of sporozoan protozoa, in which the nucleus divides several times before the cytoplasm divides; the schizont divides to form merozoites in this asexual phase of the life cycle.

meromelia (mer-ō-mē'lē-ă) [mero- + G. *melos,* a limb]. Partial absence of a free limb (exclusive of girdle).

meromicrosomia (mer'ō-mī'krō-sō'mē-ă) [mero- + G. *mikros,* small, + *sōma,* body]. Abnormal smallness of some portion of the body; local dwarfism.

meromyosin (mer-ō-mī'ō-sin). A subunit of the tryptic digestion of myosin; two types are produced, H-m. and L-m.

H-m. [H for "heavy"], one of the relatively heavy products (molecular weight about 232,000) of the action of trypsin on myosin; it carries the ATPase activity of myosin.

L-m. [L for "light"], the relatively low-molecular-weight product (molecular weight about 96,000) of the tryptic digestion of myosin.

meront (mer'ont). A stage in the life cycle of sporozoans in which multiple asexual fission (schizogony) occurs, resulting in production of merozoites. See also schizont.

merorachischisis, merorrhachischisis (mer'ō-rā-kis'ki-sis) [mero- + G. *rhachis,* spine, + *schisis,* fissure]. Mesorrhachischis; rachischisis partialis; fissure of a portion of the spinal cord.

merosmia (me-roz'mē-ă) [mero- + G. *osmē,* smell]. A condition in which the perception of certain odors is wanting; analogous to color blindness.

merosystolic (mer'ō-sis-tol'ik) [mero- + systole]. Partially systolic; relating to a portion of the systole of the heart.

merotomy (me-rot'ō-mē) [mero- + G. *tomē,* incision]. The procedure of cutting into parts, as the cutting of a cell into separate parts to study their capacity for survival and development.

merozoite (mer-ō-zō'īt) [mero- + G. *zōon,* animal]. Endodyocyte (2); schizozoite; the motile infective stage of sporozoan protozoa that results from schizogony or a similar type of asexual reproduction; *e.g.,* endodyogeny or endopolygeny. M.'s form at the surface of schizonts, blastophores, or invaginations into schizonts, and are responsible for the vast reproductive powers of sporozoan parasites; this is seen in human malaria, where the cyclic production of m.'s produces the typical fever and chill syndrome.

merozygote (mĕ-rō-zī'gōt) [mero- + *zygōtos,* yoked]. In microbial genetics, an organism that, in addition to its own original genome (endogenote), contains a fragment (exogenote) of a genome from another organism; the relatively small size of the exogenote permits a diploid condition for only a limited region of the endogenote.

merphalan (mer'fă-lan). Sarcolysine; the racemic mixture of melphalan and medphalan; an antineoplastic agent.

Merrifield knife. See under knife.

Merritt, Katharine K., U.S. pediatrician, *1886. See Kasabach-M. *syndrome.*

mersalyl (mer'să-lil). Mercuramide; sodium salt of (3-hydroxymercuric-2-methoxypropyl)salicylamide-*O*-acetic acid; a mercurial diuretic.

m. acid, a mixture of *o*-carboxymethylsalicyl-(3-hydroxymercuric-2-methoxypropyl)-amide and its anhydrides; same use as m.

m. theophylline, m. plus theophylline added to inhibit decomposition of m.

Méry, Jean, French anatomist, 1645–1722. See M.'s *gland.*

Merzbacher, Ludwig, German physician in Argentina, *1875. See M.-Pelizaeus *disease.*

mes-. See meso-.

mesad (mē'zad, mē'sad) [G. *mesos,* middle, + L. *ad,* to]. Mesiad; passing or extending toward the median plane of the body or of a part.

mesal (mē'zăl, mē'săl) [G. *mesos,* middle]. Rarely used term referring to the median plane of the body or a part.

mesalamine (me-sal'ă-mēn). 5-Aminosalicyclic acid; a salicylate used in the treatment of active mild to moderate distal ulcerative colitis, proctosigmoiditis, and proctitis.

mesameboid (mez-ă-mē'boyd) [mes- + G. *amoibē,* change (ameba), + *eidos,* resemblance]. Minot's term for a primitive, "wandering" cell derived from mesoderm, probably a hemocytoblast.

mesangial (mes-an'jē-ăl). Referring to the mesangium.

mesangium (mes-an'jē-ŭm) [mes- + G. *angeion,* vessel]. A central part of the renal glomerulus between capillaries; mesangial cells are phagocytic and for the most part separated from capillary lumina by endothelial cells.
extraglomerular m., Polkissen of Zimmerman; mesangial cells which fill the triangular space between the macula densa and the afferent and efferent arterioles of the juxtaglomerular apparatus.

mesaortitis (mes-ā-ōr-tī'tis) [mes- + aortitis]. Inflammation of the middle or muscular coat of the aorta.

mesareic, mesaraic (mes-ă-rā'ik) [G. *mesaraion,* mesentery, fr. *mesos,* middle, + *araia,* flank, belly]. Mesenteric.

mesarteritis (mes-ar-ter-ī'tis) [mes- + arteritis]. Inflammation of the middle (muscular) coat of an artery.

mesaticephalic (mē-sat'i-se-fal'ik) [G. *mesatos,* midmost, + *kephalē,* head]. Mesocephalic.

mesatipellic, mesatipelvic (mē-sat'i-pel'ik, -pel'vik) [G. *mestatos,* midmost, + *pellis,* a bowl (pelvis)]. Denoting an individual with a pelvic index between 90 and 95; the superior strait has a round appearance, with the transverse diameter longer than the anteroposterior by 1 cm or less.

mesaxon (mez-ak'son, mes-). The plasma membrane of the neurolemma which is folded in to surround a nerve axon. In electron micrographs this double layer resembles a mesentery in appearance.

mescal buttons (mes'kal). The dried slices of the cactus *Lophophora williamsii,* containing mescaline and related alkaloids.

mescaline (mes'kă-lēn). 3,4,5-Trimethoxyphenethylamine; the most active alkaloid present in the buttons of a small cactus, *Lophophora williamsii.* M. produces psychotomimetic effects similar to those produced by LSD: alteration in mood, changes in perception, reveries, visual hallucinations, delusions, depersonalization, mydriasis, hippus, and increases in body temperature and blood pressure; psychic dependence, tolerance, and cross tolerance to LSD and psilocybin develop.

mesectic (me-sek'tik) [mes- + G. *echō,* to have]. Obsolete term denoting a specimen of blood that has a normal percentage saturation of oxygen at any given pressure.

mesectoderm (mez-ek'tō-derm) [mes- + ectoderm]. **1.** Cells in the area around the dorsal lip of the blastopore where mesoderm and ectoderm undergo a process of separation. **2.** Ectomesenchyme; that part of the mesenchyme derived from ectoderm, especially from the neural crest in the cephalic region in very young embryos.

mesencephalic (mez-en'se-fal'ik). Relating to the mesencephalon.

mesencephalitis (mez'en-sef'ă-lī'tis). Inflammation of the midbrain (mesencephalon); sometimes noted in *Listeria* infection of the nervous system.

mesencephalon (mez-en-sef'ă-lon) [mes- + G. *enkephalos,* brain] [NA]. Midbrain; midbrain vesicle; that part of the brainstem developing from the middle of the three primary cerebral vesicles of the embryo (the caudal of these being the rhombencephalon or hindbrain, the rostral the prosencephalon or forebrain). In the adult, the m. is characterized by the unique conformation of its roof plate, the lamina tecti mesencephali, composed of the bilaterally paired superior and inferior colliculus, and by the massive paired prominence of the crus cerebri at its ventral surface. On transverse section, its patent central canal, the aqueductus cerebri, is surrounded by a prominent ring of gray matter poor in myelinated fibers; the periaqueductal gray is ventrally and laterally adjoined by the myelin-rich tegmentum mesencephali, and covered dorsally by the lamina tecti mesencephali. Prominent cell groups of the m. include the motor nuclei of the trochlear and oculomotor nerves, the red nucleus, and the substantia nigra.

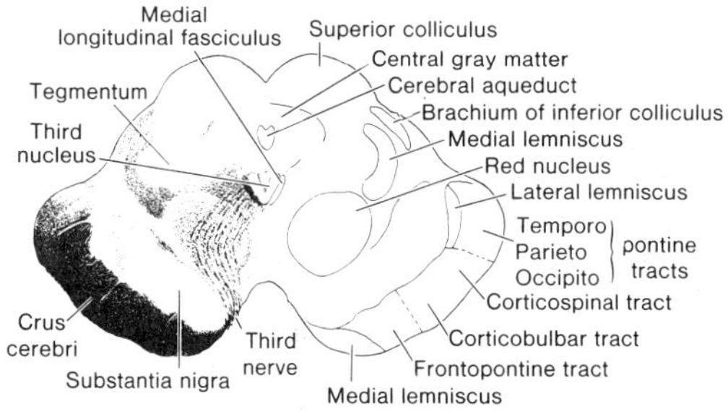

Mesencephalon
Schematic transverse section through upper portion of midbrain.

mesencephalotomy (mez'en-sef'ă-lot'ōmē) [mesencephalon + G. *tomē,* incision]. **1.** The sectioning of any structure in the midbrain, especially of the spinothalamic tracts for the relief of unbearable pain or the cerebral peduncle for dyskinesias. **2.** Spinothalamic *tractotomy,* mesencephalic.

mesenchyma (mē-seng'ki-mă, mē-zeng'). Mesenchyme.

mesenchymal (mē-seng'ki-măl, mez-eng-kī'măl). Relating to the mesenchyme.

mesenchyme (mez'en-kīm) [mes- + G. *enkyma,* infusion]. Mesenchyma. **1.** An aggregation of mesenchymal cells. **2.** Primordial embryonic tissue consisting of mesenchymal cells, usually stellate in form, supported in interlaminar jelly.
interzonal m., an area of avascular m. between adjacent skeletal elements in the embryo; it denotes the region of future joints.
synovial m., vascular m. surrounding the interzonal m.; it develops into the synovial membrane of a joint.

mesenchymoma (mez'en-kī-mō'mă). A neoplasm in which there is a mixture of mesenchymal derivatives, other than fibrous tissue. A **benign m.** may contain foci of vascular, muscular, adipose, osteoid, osseous, and cartilaginous tissue; such neoplasms are sometimes classed under a compounded name, *e.g.*, angioleiomyolipoma, and the like, but the broader term may be preferred. A **malignant m.** may also occur as a similar mixture of two or more types of mesenchymal cells that are malignant (other than fibrous tissue cells).

mesenteric (mez-en-ter'ik). Mesareic; mesaraic; relating to the mesentery.

mesenteriolum (mez-en-ter-ē'ō-lŭm) [Mod. L. dim. of *mesenterium,* mesentery]. Mesoenteriolum; a small mesentery, as one of an intestinal diverticulum.
m. proces'sus vermifor'mis, mesoappendix.

mesenteriopexy (mes'en-ter-ē-ō-pek'sē) [mesentery + G. *pēxis,* fixation]. Mesopexy; fixation or attachment of a torn or incised mesentery.

mesenteriorrhaphy (mez'en-ter-ē-ōr'ă-fe]) [mesentery + G. *rhaphē,* suture]. Mesorrhaphy; suture of the mesentery.

mesenteriplication (mez'en-ter-i-pli-kā'shŭn) [mesentery + L. *plico,* pp. *-atus,* to fold]. Reducing redundancy of a mesentery by making one or more tucks in it.

mesenteritis (mez'en-ter-ī'tis). Inflammation of the mesentery.

mesenterium (mez'en-ter'ē-ŭm) [Mod. L.] [NA]. Mesentery.
m. dorsa'le com'mune, mesentery (2).

mesenteron (mez-en'ter-on) [mes- + G. *enteron,* intestine]. The midportion of the insect alimentary canal and site of digestion; the m. may possess anterior finger-like projections, the gastric ceca, and a tubular anterior midgut, followed posteriorly by the saccular ventriculus, or stomach.

mesentery (mes'en-ter-ē) [Mod. L. *mesenterium,* fr. G. *mesenterion,* fr. G. *mesos,* middle, + *enteron,* intestine]. Mesenterium. **1.** A double layer of peritoneum attached to the abdominal wall and enclosing in its fold a portion or all of one of the abdominal viscera, conveying to it its vessels and nerves. **2.** Mesenterium dorsale commune; mesostenium; the fan-shaped fold of peritoneum encircling the greater part of the small intestines (jejunum and ileum) and attaching it to the posterior abdominal wall.
m. of appendix, mesoappendix.
urogenital m., diaphragmatic *ligament* of the mesonephros.

mesh'work. See network.
trabecular m., *reticulum* trabeculare.

mesiad (mē'zē-ad, mes'ē-ad). Mesad.

mesial (mē'zē-ăl, mes'ē-ăl) [G. *mesos,* middle]. Proximal (2); toward the median plane following the curvature of the dental arch, in contrast to distal (2).

mesio- [G. *mesos,* middle]. Combining form (especially in dentistry) meaning mesial.

mesiobuccal (mē'zē-ō-bŭk'ăl). Relating to the mesial and buccal surfaces of a tooth; denoting especially the angle formed by the junction of these two surfaces.

mesiobucco-occlusal (mē'zē-ō-bŭk'ō-ō-klū'săl). Relating to the angle formed by the junction of the mesial, buccal, and occlusal surfaces of a bicuspid or molar tooth.

mesiobuccopulpal (mē'zē-ō-bŭk'ō-pŭl'păl). Relating to the angle denoting the junction of mesial, buccal and pulpal surfaces in a tooth cavity preparation.

mesiocervical (mē'zē-ō-ser'vi-kăl). **1.** Relating to the line angle of a cavity preparation at the junction of the mesial and cervical walls. **2.** Pertaining to the area of a tooth at the junction of the mesial surface and the cervical region.

mesioclusion (mē'zē-ō-klū'zhŭn). Mesial occlusion (2); a malocclusion in which the mandibular arch articulates with the maxillary arch in a position mesial to normal; in Angle's classification, a Class III malocclusion.

mesiodens (mē'zē-ō-denz) [mesio- + L. *dens,* tooth]. A supernumerary tooth located in the midline of the anterior maxillae, between the maxillary central incisor teeth.

mesiodistal (mē'zē-ō-dis'tăl). Denoting the plane or diameter of a tooth cutting its mesial and distal surfaces.

mesiodistocclusal (MOD) (mē'zē-ō-dist'ō-klū'săl, -zăl). Denoting three-surface cavity or cavity preparation or restoration (class 2, Black classification) in the premolars (bicuspids) and molars.

mesiogingival (mē'zē-ō-jin'ji-văl). Relating to the angle formed by the junction of the mesial surface with the gingival line of a tooth.

mesiognathic (mē'zē-ō-nath'ik). Denoting malposition of one or both jaws forward from their normal position.

mesioincisal (mē'zē-ō-in-sī'săl, -zăl). Relating to the mesial and incisal surfaces of a tooth; denoting the angle formed by their junction.

mesiolabial (mē'zē-ō-lā'bē-ăl). Relating to the mesial and labial surfaces of a tooth; denoting especially the angle formed by their junction.

mesiolingual (mē'zē-ō-ling'gwăl). Relating to the mesial and lingual surfaces of a tooth; denoting especially the angle formed by their junction.

mesiolinguo-occlusal (mē'zē-ō-ling'gwō-ō-klū'săl, -zăl). Denoting the angle formed by the junction of the mesial, lingual, and occlusal surfaces of a bicuspid or molar tooth.

mesiolinguopulpal (mē'zē-ō-ling'gwō-pŭl'păl). Relating to the angle denoting the junction of the mesial, lingual, and pulpal surfaces in a tooth cavity preparation.

mesion (mē'zē-on, mes'i-on). Meson.

mesio-occlusal (mē'zē-ō-ō-klū'săl, -zăl). Denoting the angle formed by the junction of the mesial and occlusal surfaces of a bicuspid or molar tooth.

mesio-occlusion (mē'zē-ō-ō-klū'zhŭn). Mesial *occlusion* (1).

mesioplacement (mē'zē-ō-plās'ment). Mesioversion.

mesiopulpal (mē'zē-ō-pŭl'păl). Pertaining to the inner wall or floor of a cavity preparation on the mesial side of a tooth.

mesioversion (mē'zē-ō-ver-zhŭn). Mesioplacement; malposition of a tooth distal to normal, in a posterior direction following the curvature of the dental arch.

mesmerism (mes'mer-izm) [F.A. *Mesmer,* Austrian physician, 1733–1815]. A system of therapeutics from which were developed hypnotism and therapeutic suggestion.

mesmerize (mes'mer-īz) [see mesmerism]. Obsolete term for hypnotize.

meso-, mes- [G. *mesos,* middle]. **1.** Prefix meaning middle, or mean, or used to give an indication of intermediacy. **2.** Prefix designating a mesentery or mesentery-like structure.

mesoappendix (mez'ō-ă-pen'diks) [NA]. Mesentery of the appendix; mesenteriolum processus vermiformis; the short mesentery of the appendix lying behind the terminal ileum.

mesoarium (mez-ō-ār'ē-ŭm). Mesovarium.

mesobilane (mez-ō-bī'lān). Mesobilirubinogen; urobilinogen IX-α; a reduced mesobilirubin with no double bonds between the pyrrole rings and, consequently, colorless. See also bilirubinoids.

mesobilene, mesobilene-β (mez-ō-bī'lēn). Urobilin IX-α; a bilirubinoid.

mesobilirubin (mez'ō-bil-i-rū'bin). A compound differing from bilirubin only in that the vinyl groups of bilirubin are reduced to ethyl groups. See also bilirubinoids.

mesobilirubinogen (mez'ō-bil-i-rū-bin'ō-jen). Mesobilane.

mesobiliviolin (mez'ō-bil-i-vī-ō'lin). A bilirubinoid.

mesoblast (mez'ō-blast) [meso- + G. *blastos,* germ]. Mesoderm.

mesoblastema (mez'ō-blas-tē'mă) [meso- + G. *blastēma,* a sprout]. All the cells collectively which constitute the early undifferentiated mesoderm.

mesoblastemic (mez'ō-blas-tē'mik). Relating to or derived from the mesoblastema.

mesoblastic (mez'ō-blas'tik). Relating to or derived from the mesoderm.

mesocardia (mez'ō-kar'dē-ă) [meso- + G. *kardia,* heart]. **1.** Atypical position of the heart in a central position in the chest, as in early embryonic life. **2.** Plural of mesocardium.

mesocardium, pl. **mes'ocar'dia** (mez-ō-kar'dē-ŭm) [meso- + G. *kardia,* heart]. The double layer of splanchnic mesoderm supporting the embryonic heart in the pericardial cavity.
dorsal m., the part of the m. dorsal to the embryonic heart.
ventral m., the part of the m. ventral to the embryonic cardiac tube; transitory in all vertebrates; in the higher mammals, it breaks through as soon as its component layers of epicardium make contact with each other.

mesocarpal (mez'ō-kar'păl). Mediocarpal.

mesocecal (mez'ō-sē'kăl). Relating to the mesocecum.

mesocecum (mez'ō-sē'kŭm) [meso- + cecum]. Part of the mesocolon, supporting the cecum, that occasionally persists when the ascending colon becomes retroperitoneal during fetal life.

mesocephalic (mez'ō-se-fal'ik) [meso- + G. *kephalē,* head]. Mesocephalous; mesaticephalic; normocephalic; having a head of medium length; denoting a skull with a cephalic index between 75 and 80 and with a capacity of 1350 to 1450 ml, or an individual with such a skull.

mesocephalous (mez'ō-sef'ă-lŭs). Mesocephalic.

mesocolic (mez'ō-kol'ik). Relating to the mesocolon.

mesocolon (mez'ō-kō'lon) [meso- + *kolon,* colon] [NA]. The fold of peritoneum attaching the colon to the posterior abdominal wall; **m. ascen'dens,** ascending, **m. transver'sum,** transverse, **m. descen' dens,** descending, and **m. sigmoi'deum,** sigmoid or pelvic, correspond to the respective divisions of the colon; the ascending and descending portions are usually more or less deficient or absent.

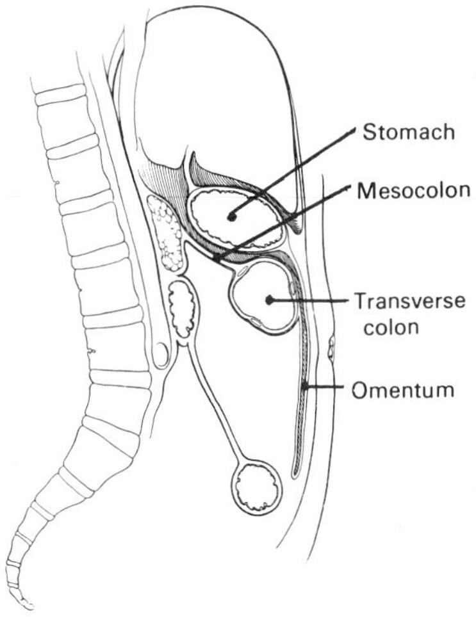

Mesocolon

mesocolopexy. (mez'ō-kō'lō-pek-sē) [meso- + G. *kolon,* colon, + *pēxis,* fixation]. Mesocoloplication; an operation for shortening the mesocolon, for correction of undue mobility and ptosis.

mesocoloplication (mes'ō-kō'lō-pli-kā'shŭn) [meso- + G. *kolon,* colon, + L. *plico,* pp. *-atus,* to fold]. Mesocolopexy.

mesocord (mez'ō-kōrd). A fold of amnion that sometimes binds a segment of the umbilical cord to the placenta.

mesocuneiform (mez-ō-kū'nē-i-fōrm). *Os* cuneiforme intermedium.

mesoderm (mez'ō-derm) [meso- + G. *derma,* skin]. Mesoblast; the middle of the three primary germ layers of the embryo (the others being ectoderm and endoderm); m. is the origin of all connective tissues, all body musculature, blood, cardiovascular and lymphatic systems, most of the urogenital system, and the lining of the pericardial, pleural, and peritoneal cavities.

branchial m., m. surrounding the primitive stomodeum and pharynx; it develops into the pharyngeal arches.

extraembryonic m., primary m.; cells or tissues which, though derived from the zygote, are not part of the embryo proper but form the fetal membranes.

gastral m., m. in lower vertebrates formed by constriction from the roof of the archenteron or yolk sac.

intermediate m., a continuous band of m. between the segmented paraxial m. medially and the lateral plate m. laterally; from it develops the nephrogenic cord.

intraembryonic m., secondary m.; m. derived from the primitive streak and lying between the ectoderm and endoderm.

lateral m., lateral plate m.

lateral plate m., lateral m.; the peripheral thinned out portion of intraembryonic m. which is continuous with the extraembryonic m. beyond the margins of the embryonic disk; in it develops the intraembryonic celom.

paraxial m., a thickened mass lying at either side of the midline embryonic notochord; on segmentation, it forms the paired somites.

primary m., extraembryonic m.

prostomial m., m. that arises in lower vertebrates by continued proliferation at the lateral lips of the blastopore.

secondary m., intraembryonic m.

somatic m., the m. adjacent to the ectoderm in the early embryo, after foundation of the intraembryonic celom.

somitic m., muscle derived from cells situated in or derived from somites.

splanchnic m., the layer of lateral plate m. adjacent to the endoderm.

visceral m., the splanchnic m. or the branchial m.

mesodermic (mez-ō-der'mik). Relating to the mesoderm.

mesodiastolic (mez-ō-dī-ă-stol'ik). Middiastolic.

mesodont (mez'ō-dont) [meso- + G. *odous,* tooth]. Having teeth of medium size; denoting a skull with a dental index between 42 and 43.9.

mesoduodenal (mez'ō-dū-ō-dē'năl). Relating to the mesoduodenum.

mesoduodenum (mez'ō-dū'ō-dē'nŭm, -dū-od'ē-nŭm). The mesentery of the duodenum.

mesoenteriolum (mes'ō-en-ter-ē'ō-lŭm). Mesenteriolum.

mesoepididymis (mez-ō-ep-i-did'i-mis) [meso- + epididymis]. An occasional fold of the tunica vaginalis binding the epididymis to the testis.

mesogaster (mez-ō-gas'ter). Mesogastrium.

mesogastric (mez-ō-gas'trik). Relating to the mesogastrium.

mesogastrium (mez-ō-gas'trē-ŭm) [meso- + G. *gastēr* stomach]. Mesogaster; in the embryo, the mesentery in relation to the dilated portion of the enteric canal which is the future stomach.

mesogenic (mez-ō-jen'ik) [meso- + G. *-gen,* producing]. Denoting the virulence of a virus capable of inducing lethal infection in embryonic hosts, after a short incubation period, and an inapparent infection in immature and adult hosts; used in characterizing Newcastle disease virus, particularly strains used in parenteral vaccination of chickens.

mesogenitale (mez'ō-jen-i-tā'lē). The embryonic mesentery by which the genital ridge is connected to the mesonephros.

mesoglia (me-sog'lē-ă) [meso- + G. *glia,* glue]. Mesoglial cells; neuroglial cells of mesodermal origin. See also microglia.

mesogluteal (mez'ō-glū'tē-ăl). Relating to the musculus gluteus medius.

mesogluteus (mez'ō-glū-tē'ŭs). *Musculus* gluteus medius.

mesognathic (mez-ō-nath'ik, -og-nath'ik). **1.** Relating to the mesognathion. **2.** Mesognathous.

mesognathion (mez'ō-nā'thēon, -og-nā'thē-on, nath'ē-on) [meso- + G. *gnathos,* jaw]. The lateral segment of the premaxillary or incisive bone external to the endognathion.

mesognathous (me-zog'nă-thŭs). Mesognathic (2); having a face with slightly projecting jaw, one with a gnathic index from 98 to 103.

mesoileum (mez-ō-il'ē-ŭm). The mesentery of the ileum.

mesojejunum (mez'ō-je-jū'nŭm). The mesentery of the jejunum.

mesolepidoma (mes'ō-lep'i-dō'mă) [meso- + G. *lepis,* rind, + *-oma,* tumor]. A neoplasm derived from the persistent embryonic mesothelium.

mesolobus (me-sol'ō-bŭs) [meso- + L. *lobus,* lobe]. Obsolete term for *corpus* callosum.

mesolymphocyte (mez-ō-lim'fō-sīt) [meso- + lymphocyte]. A mononuclear leukocyte of medium size, probably a lymphocyte, with a deeply staining nucleus of large size but relatively smaller than that in most lymphocytes.

mesomelia (mez-ō-mē'lē-ă) [meso- + G. *melos,* limb]. The condition of having abnormally short forearms and lower legs.

mesomelic (mez-ō-mē'lik). Pertaining to the middle segment of a limb.

mesomere (mez'ō-mēr) [meso- + G. *meros,* part]. A blastomere of a size intermediate between a macromere and a micromere.

mesomeric (mez-ō-mer'ik). Pertaining to mesomerism.

mesomerism (mĕ-som'er-izm). Displacement of electrons within a molecule in such a way as to create fractional charges on different parts of the molecule.

mesometritis (mez'ō-mē-trī'tis) [meso- + G. *mētra,* uterus, + *-itis,* inflammation]. Myometritis.

mesometrium (mez'ō-mē'trē-ŭm) [meso- + G. *mētra,* uterus] [NA]. The broad ligament of the uterus, below the mesosalpinx.

mesomorph (mez'ō-mōrf) [meso- + G. *morphē,* form]. Mediotype; a constitutional body type or build (biotype or somatotype) in which tissues that originate from the mesoderm prevail; from the morphological standpoint, there is a balance between trunk and limbs. See also hypermorph, hypomorph, ectomorph, endomorph.

mesomorphic (mez-ō-mōrf'ik). Relating to mesomorphs.

meson (mez'on, mē'zon, mes'on) [G. neuter of *mesos,* middle]. Mesion; an elementary particle having a rest mass intermediate in value between the mass of an electron and that of a proton.

mesonephric (mez-ō-nef'rik). Relating to the mesonephros.

mesonephroi (mez'ō-nef'roy). Plural of mesonephros.

mesonephroma (mez'ō-ne-frō'mă) Wolffian duct or mesometanephric carcinoma; mesonephric adenocarcinoma; clear cell adenocarcinoma (2); mesonephroid tumor; a relatively rare malignant neoplasm of the ovary and corpus uteri, thought to originate in mesonephric structures that become misplaced in ovarian tissue during embryonic development; characterized by a tubular pattern, with focal proliferation of epithelial cells with clear cytoplasm or of the hob-nail type; so-called glomeruloid structures are reported, *i.e.,* small convolutions or tufts of tiny tubate formations with capillaries extending into the spaces.

mesonephros, pl. mesonephroi (mez'ō-nef'ros, -roy) [meso- + G. *nephros,* kidney] [NA]. Wolffian body; middle kidney; one of three excretory organs appearing in the evolution of vertebrates; in life forms with a metanephros, the m. is located between the regressing pronephros and the metanephros, cephalic to the latter. In young mammalian embryos, the m. is well developed and briefly functional until establishment of the metanephros, the definitive kidney; in older embryos, the m. undergoes regression as an excretory organ, but its duct system is retained in the male as the epididymis and ductus deferens.

mesoneuritis (mez'ō-nū-rī'tis). Inflammation of a nerve or of its connective tissue without involvement of its sheath.

nodular m., inflammation of the connective tissue beneath the nerve sheath, with the formation of circumscribed fibrous thickenings.

meso-ontomorph (mez-ō-on'tō-mōrf) [meso- + G. *ōn,* being, + *morphē,* form]. A broad, stocky individual.

mesopexy (mez'ō-pek-sē). Mesenteriopexy.

mesophil, mesophile (mez'ō-fil, -fīl) [meso- + G. *philos,* fond]. A microorganism with an optimum temperature between 25°C and 40°C, but growing within the limits of 10°C and 45°C.

mesophilic (mez'ō-fil'ik). Pertaining to a mesophil.

mesophlebitis (mez'ō-flĕ-bī'tis) [meso- + phlebitis]. Inflammation of the middle coat of a vein.

mesophragma (mez-ō-frag'mă) [meso- + G. *phragma,* a fence]. M *line.*

mesophryon (mez-of'ri-on) [meso- + Gr. *ophrys,* eyebrow]. Glabella (2).

mesopic (me-zō'pik) [meso- + G. *opsis,* vision]. Pertaining to illumination between the photopic and scotopic ranges.

mesoporphyrins (mez-ō-pōr'fi-rinz). Porphyrin compounds resembling the protoporphyrins except that the vinyl side chains of the latter are reduced to ethyl side chains; *e.g.,* mesobilane.

mesoprosopic (mez'ō-prō-sop'ik) [meso- + G. *prosōpon,* face]. Having a face of moderate width, *i.e.,* with a facial index of about 90.

mesopulmonum (mez-ō-pŭl'mon-ŭm) [meso- + L. *pulmo,* lung]. The mesentery of the embryonic lung.

mesorchial (mez-ōr'kē-ăl). Relating to the mesorchium.

mesorchium (mez-ōr'kē-ŭm) [meso- + G. *orchis,* testis]. **1.** In the fetus, a fold of tunica vaginalis testis supporting the mesonephros and the developing testis. **2.** In the adult, a fold of tunica vaginalis testis between the testis and epididymis.

mesorectum (mez'ō-rek'tŭm). The peritoneal investment of the rectum, covering the upper part only.

mesoridazine besylate (mez-ō-rid'ă-zēn). 10-[2-(1-Methyl-2-piperidyl)ethyl]-2-(methylsulfinyl)phenothiazone; a biotransformation product of thioridazine; an antipsychotic.

mesorrhachischisis (mez'ō-rā-kis'ki-sis). Merorrhachischisis.

mesorrhaphy (mez-ōr'ă-fē). Mesenteriorrhaphy.

mesorrhine (mez'ō-rin) [meso- + G. *rhis* (*rhin-*), nose]. Having a nose of moderate width. Denoting a skull with a nasal index from 47 to 51 (Frankfort agreement) or 48 to 53 (Broca).

mesosalpinx (mez'ō-sal'pinks) [meso- + G. *salpinx,* trumpet] [NA]. The part of the broad ligament investing the uterine (fallopian) tube.

mesoscope (mez'ō-skōp) [meso- + G. *skopeō,* to view]. An instrument for viewing objects that are larger than microscopic but cannot be seen distinctly with the naked eye.

mesoseme (mez'ō-sēm) [meso- + G. *sēma,* sign]. Denoting an orbital aperture with an index between 84 and 89; characteristic of the white race.

mesosigmoid (mez'ō-sig'moyd). The mesocolon of the sigmoid colon.

mesosigmoiditis (mes'ō-sig-moy-dī'tis). Inflammation of the mesosigmoid.

mesosigmoidopexy (mez-ō-sig-moy'dō-pek-sē). Surgical fixation of the mesosigmoid.

mesosomatous (mez'ō-so'mă-tŭs). Denoting a person of medium height.

mesosomia (mez'ō-sō'mē-ă) [meso- + G. *sōma,* body]. Medium height.

mesostenium (mez'ō-stē'nē-ŭm). Mesentery (2).

mesosternum (mez'ō-ster'nŭm) [meso- + G. *sternon,* chest]. *Corpus* sterni.

mesosyphilis (mez-ō-sif'i-lis). Secondary *syphilis.*

mesosystolic (mez'ō-sis-tol'ik). Midsystolic.

mesotarsal (mez'ō-tar'săl). Mediotarsal.

mesotendineum (mez'ō-ten-din'ē-ŭm) [NA]. Mesotendon; the synovial layers that pass from a tendon to the wall of a tendon sheath in certain places where tendons lie within osteofibrous canals.

mesotendon (mez'ō-ten'don). Mesotendineum.

mesothelia (mez-ō-thē'lē-ă). Plural of mesothelium.

mesothelial (mez-ō-thē'lē-ăl). Relating to the mesothelium.

mesothelioma (mez'ō-thē-lē-ō'mă) [mesothelium + G. *-oma,* tumor]. A rare neoplasm derived from the lining cells of the pleura and peritoneum which grows as a thick sheet covering the viscera, and is composed of spindle cells or fibrous tissue which may enclose glandlike spaces lined by cuboidal cells.
benign m. of genital tract, adenomatoid *tumor.*

mesothelium, pl. **mesothelia** (mez-ō-thē'lē-ŭm, -lē-ă) [meso- + epithelium]. A single layer of flattened cells forming an epithelium that lines serous cavities; *e.g.,* peritoneum, pleura, pericardium.

mesothorium (mez'ō-thōr'ē-ŭm). The first two disintegration products of thorium; mesothorium 1 is ^{228}Ra, a beta emitter with a half-life of 6.7 years, decaying into mesothorium 2, which is ^{228}Ac, a beta emitter with a half-life of 6.13 hr, which disintegrates to radiothorium (^{228}Th).

mesotropic (mez'ō-trop'ik) [meso- + G. *tropē,* a turning]. Turned toward the median plane.

mesouranic (mes'ō-yū-ran'ik) [meso- + G. *ouranos,* palate]. Mesuranic; having a palatal index between 110 and 115.

mesovarium, pl. **mesovaria** (mez'ō-vā'rē-ŭm, -ă) [meso- + L. *ovarium,* ovary] [NA]. Mesoarium; a short peritoneal fold connecting the anterior border of the ovary with the posterior layer of the broad ligament of the uterus.

Mesozoa (mez-ō-zō'ă) [meso- + G. *zōon,* animal]. A small phylum of about 50 species of parasites of marine invertebrates with complex life cycles. M. are classified with the Metazoa, but they are regarded by some observers as intermediate between unicellular and multicellular animals; others consider them a degenerate group of flatworms. M. are divided into two very distinct orders, the Orthonectida and Dicyemida; the latter are nephridial parasites of squids, octopods, and cuttlefish.

messenger (mes'en-jer). **1.** That which carries a message. **2.** Having message-carrying properties.
first m., a hormone that has a transaction with adenosine 3',5'-cyclic phosphate (second m.) at or near the cell membrane.
second m., see adenosine 3',5'-cyclic phosphate.

messenger RNA. See under ribonucleic acid.

mestanolone (mes-tan'ō-lōn). 17β-Hydroxy-17-methyl-5α-androstan-3-one; an androgenic steroid with anabolic properties.

mestenediol (mes-tēn'dī-ol). Methandriol.

mestranol (mes'tră-nōl). 3-Methoxy-19-nor-17α-pregna-1,3,5(10)-trien-20-yn-17-ol; the 3 methyl ether of ethynyl estradiol; an estrogen used in many oral contraceptive preparations.

mesulphen (mĕ-sŭl'fen). 2-7-Dimethylthianthrene; a topical scabicide with antipruritic properties.

mesuranic (mez'yū-ran'ik). Mesouranic.

MET Abbreviation for metabolic *equivalent.*

Met Symbol for methionine or its radicals in peptides.

meta- [G. after, between, over] **1.** In medicine and biology, a prefix denoting the concept of after, subsequent to, behind, or hindmost; corresponds to L. *post-.* **2.** Prefix denoting joint, action sharing. **3** (*m-*). In chemistry, an italicized prefix denoting a compound formed by two substitutions in the benzene ring separated by one carbon atom, *i.e.,* linked to the first and third, second and fourth, etc., carbon atoms of the ring. For terms beginning with *meta-,* or *m-,* see the specific name.

metabasis (mĕ-tab'ă-sis) [G. a passing over, change, fr. *metabainō,* to pass over]. A change of any kind in symptoms or course of a disease.

metabiosis (met'ă-bī-ō'sis) [meta- + G. *biōsis,* way of life]. Dependence of one organism on another for its existence. *Cf.* commensalism; mutualism; parasitism.

metabolic (met-ă-bol'ik). Relating to metabolism.

metabolimeter (met'ă-bŏ-lim'ĕ-ter). A modified calorimeter for measuring the rate of basal metabolism.

metabolin (mĕ-tab'ō-lin). Metabolite.

metabolism (mĕ-tab'ō-lizm) [G. *metabolē,* change]. The sum of the chemical changes occurring in tissue, consisting of anabolism, those reactions that convert small molecules into large, and catabolism, those reactions that convert large molecules into small, including both endogenous large molecules as well as biodegradation of xenobiotics.
basal m., basal metabolic rate; oxygen utilization of an individual during minimal physiologic activity while awake; determined by measuring oxygen consumption of a fasting subject at complete bodily and mental rest and a room temperature of 20°C.
carbohydrate m., oxidation, breakdown, and synthesis of carbohydrates in the tissues.
electrolyte m., the chemical changes that various essential minerals (*e.g.,* sodium, potassium, calcium, magnesium) undergo in the tissues.
fat m., oxidation, decomposition, and synthesis of fats in the tissues.
protein m., proteometabolism; decomposition and synthesis of protein in the tissues.
respiratory m., the exchange of respiratory gases in the lungs, oxidation of foodstuffs in the tissues, and production of carbon dioxide and water.

metabolite (mĕ-tab'ō-līt). Metabolin; any product (foodstuff, intermediate, waste product) of metabolism, especially of catabolism.

metabolize (mĕ-tab'ō-līz). To undergo the chemical changes of metabolism.

metabutethamine hydrochloride (met'ă-byūt-eth'ă-mēn). 2-(Isobutylamino)ethanol *m*-aminobenzoate monohydrochloride; a local anesthetic.

metabutoxycaine hydrochloride (met'ă-byū-tok'si-kān). 3-Amino-2-butoxy-benzoic acid β-diethylaminoethyl ester hydrochloride; a local anesthetic.

metacarpal (met'ă-kar'păl). Relating to the metacarpus.

metacarpectomy (met'ă-kar-pek'tō-mē) [metacarpus + G. *ektomē,* excision]. Excision of one or all of the metacarpals.

metacarpophalangeal (met'ă-kar'pō-fă-lan'jē-ăl). Relating to the metacarpus and the phalanges; denoting the articulations between them.

metacarpus, pl. **metacarpi** (met'ă-kar'pŭs, -kar'pī) [meta- + G. *karpos,* wrist] [NA]. The five bones of the hand between the carpus and the phalanges.

metacentric (met-ă-sen'trik) [meta- + G. *kentron,* circle]. Having the centromere about equidistant from the extremities, said of a chromosome.

metacercaria, pl. **metacercariae** (met'ă-ser-kar'ē-ă, -ē) [meta- + G. *kerkos,* tail]. The post-cercarial encysted stage in the life history of a fluke, prior to transfer to the definitive host. Some cercariae attach themselves to grass or other vegetation, form m., and later are ingested by herbivores, as in *Fasciola* and similar forms; others encyst in muscles of fish, as in *Clonorchis,* or in crayfish, as in *Paragonimus.*

metacestode (met-ă-ses'tōd). The larval stages of a tapeworm, including the metamorphosis of the oncosphere to the first evidence of sexuality in the adult worm, differentiation of the scolex, and beginning of proglottid formation; it includes the procercoid and plerocercoid stages of pseudophyllid cestodes, and the cysticercus, cysticercoid, coenurus, and hydatid stages of cyclophyllidean cestodes.

metachloral (met-ă-klō'răl). *m-* Chloral.

metachromasia (met'ă-krō-mā'zē-ă) [meta- + G. *chrōma*, color]. **1.** Metachromatism (2); the condition in which a cell or tissue component takes on a color different from the dye solution with which it is stained. **2.** A change in the characteristic color of certain basic thyazine dyes, such as toluidine blue, when the dye molecules are bound in proximate array to tissue polyanionic polymers, such as glycoaminoglycans.

metachromatic (met'ă-krō-mat'ik). Metachromophil; metachromophile; denoting cells or dyes which exhibit metachromasia.

metachromatism (met-ă-krō'mă-tizm) [meta- + G. *chrōma*, color]. **1.** Any color change, whether natural or produced by basic aniline dyes. **2.** Metachromasia (1).

metachroming (met'ă-krō'ming). The process of mixing a metal mordant with a dye before applying the dye to a tissue or fabric.

metachromophil, metachromophile (met-ă-krō'mō-fil, -fīl) [meta- + G. *chrōma*, color, + *philos*, fond]. Metachromatic.

metachronous (mĕ-tak'rō-nŭs) [meta- + G. *chronos*, time]. Not synchronous; multiple separate occurrences, such as multiple primary cancers developing at intervals.

metachrosis (met-ă-krō'sis) [meta- + G. *chrōsis*, a coloring]. A change of color, such as occurs in certain animals, *e.g.*, the chameleon, by expansion and contraction of chromatophores.

metacone (met'ă-kōn) [meta- + G. *kōnos*, cone]. The distobuccal cusp of an upper molar tooth.

metaconid (met-ă-kon'id, -kō'nid). The mesolingual cusp of a lower molar tooth.

metacontrast (met-ă-kon'trast). Inhibition of the brightness of illumination when an adjacent visual field is illuminated.

metaconule (met-ă-kon'yūl) [meta- + G. *kōnos*, a cone]. The distal intermediate cusp of an upper molar tooth.

metacresol (met-ă-krē'sol). *m*-Cresol.

metacryptozoite (met'ă-krip-tō-zō'īt) [meta- + G. *kryptos*, hidden, + *zōon*, animal]. The exoerythrocytic stage that develops from merozoites formed by the first, or cryptozoite, generation; the cryptozoite and metacryptozoite generations comprise the primary exoerythrocytic stages of malaria development (prepatent period) prior to infection of red blood cells.

metacyesis (met-ă-sī-ē'sis) [meta- + G. *kyesis*, pregnancy]. Ectopic *pregnancy*.

metadysentery (met-ă-dis'en-tār-ē). Old term for bacillary *dysentery*.

metagenesis (met-ă-jen'ĕ-sis) [meta- + G. *genesis*, production]. *Alternation* of generations.

Metagonimus (met-ă-gon'i-mŭs) [meta- + G. *gonimos*, productive]. A genus of flukes (superfamily Heterophyoidea) that encyst on fish and infect various fish-eating animals, including man. *M. yokogawai*, an intestinal fluke widely distributed in the Far East and Balkan states and one of the smallest (1–2.5 mm) flukes infecting humans, is passed from *Semisulcospira* snails to cyprinoid fish and then to man and other fish-eating mammals and birds.

metaicteric (met-ă-ik'ter-ik) [meta- + G. *ikterikos*, jaundiced]. Occurring as a sequel of jaundice.

metainfective (met'ă-in-fek'tiv). Occurring subsequent to an infection; denoting specifically a febrile condition that is sometimes observed during convalescence from an infectious disease.

metakinesis, metakinesia (met'ă-ki-nē'sis, -ki-nē'sē-ă) [meta- + G. *kinēsis*, movement]. Moving apart; the separation of the two chromatids of each chromosome and their movement to opposite poles in the anaphase of mitosis.

metal (met'ăl) [L. *metallum*, a mine, a mineral, fr. G. *metallon*, a mine, pit]. One of the electropositive elements, either amphoteric or basic, usually characterized by properties such as luster, malleability, ductility, the ability to conduct electricity, and the tendency to lose rather than gain electrons in chemicals.

alkali m., an alkali of the family Li, Na, K, Rb, Cs, and Fr, all of which have highly ionized hydroxides.

alkali earth m., see alkaline earth *elements*.

Babbitt m., an alloy of antimony, copper, and tin; used occasionally in dentistry.

base m., basic m., a m. that is readily oxidized; *e.g.*, iron, copper.

colloidal m., electrosol; a colloidal solution of a m. obtained by passing electric sparks between terminals of the m. in distilled water.

d'Arcet's m., an alloy of lead, bismuth, and tin; used in dentistry.

fusible m., a m. with a low melting point.

light m., a m. with a specific gravity of less than 4.

noble m., noble element; a m. that cannot be oxidized by heat alone, nor readily dissolved by acid; *e.g.*, gold, platinum.

rare earth m., see lanthanides.

respiratory m., a m. present in certain respiratory pigments; *e.g.*, iron, manganese, copper, vanadium.

metaldehyde (met-al'dĕ-hīd) [meta- + aldehyde]. A polymer of acetaldehyde.

metallic (mĕ-tal'ik). Relating to, composed of, or resembling metal.

metallo- [see metal]. Combining form relating to metal, or meaning metallic.

metallocyanide (mĕ-tal-ō-sī'ă-nīd). A compound of cyanogen with a metal forming an ionic radical that combines with a basic element to form a salt; *e.g.*, potassium ferricyanide, $K_3Fe(CN)_6$.

metalloenzyme (mĕ-tal-ō-en'zīm). An enzyme containing a metal (ion) as an integral part of its active structure; *e.g.*, cytochromes (Fe, Cu), aldehyde oxidase (Mo), catechol oxidase (Cu), carbonic anhydrase (Zn).

metalloflavodehydrogenase (mĕ-tal'ō-flā'vō-dē-hī'drō-jen-ās). An oxidizing enzyme, containing one of the flavin nucleotides as coenzyme, plus a metal ion that is also necessary to the action; the metal may be Fe (as in succinate dehydrogenase), Cu (as in urate oxidase), or Mo (as in xanthine oxidase).

metalloid (met'ă-loyd) [metal + G. *eidos*, resemblance]. Resembling a metal in at least one amphoteric form; *e.g.*, silicon and germanium as semiconductors.

metallophilia (mĕ-tal'ō-fil'ē-ă) [metallo- + G. *philos*, fond]. Affinity for metal salts; *e.g.*, the affinity of the cytoplasm of cells of the reticuloendothelial system for silver carbonate stain and salts of gold and iron.

metallophobia (mĕ-tal-ō-fō'bē-ă) [G. *metallon*, metal, + *phobos*, fear]. Morbid fear of metal objects.

metalloporphyrin (mĕ-tal-ō-pōr'fi-rin). A combination of a porphyrin with a metal, *e.g.*, Fe (hematin), Mg (as in chlorophyll), Cu (in hemocyanin), Zn.

metalloprotein (mĕ-tal-ō-prō'tēn). A protein with a tightly bound metal ion or ions; *e.g.*, hemoglobin.

metalloscopy (met-ă-los'kō-pē) [metallo- + G. *skopeō*, to examine]. Testing the action of various metals applied to the surface of the body.

metallothionein (mĕ-tal-ō-thī'ō-nēn). Name proposed for a small protein, rich in sulfur-containing amino acids, that is synthesized in the liver and kidney in response to the presence of divalent ions (zinc, mercury, cadmium, copper, etc.) and that binds these ions tightly; of importance in ion transport and detoxification.

metaluetic (met′ă-lū-et′ik) [meta- + L. *lues,* pestilence]. Metasyphilitic.

metamer (met′ă-mer) [meta- + -mer]. An entity that is similar to, but ultimately differentiable from, another entity.

metamere (met′ă-mēr) [meta- + G. *meros,* part]. One of a series of homologous segments in the body. See also somite.

metameric (met-ă-mer′ik). Relating to or showing metamerism, or occurring in a metamere.

metamerism (me-tam′er-izm). **1.** A type of anatomic structure exhibiting serially homologous metameres; in primitive forms, such as the annelids, the metameres are almost alike in structure; in vertebrates, specialization in the cephalic region masks the underlying m. which is still clearly evident in serially repeated vertebrae, ribs, intercostal muscles, and spinal nerves, and in young vertebrate embryos. **2.** In chemistry, rarely used synonym for isomerism.

metamorphopsia (met′ă-mōr-fop′sē-ă) [meta- + G. *morphē,* shape, + *opsis,* vision]. Distortion of visual images.

metamorphosis (met-ă-mōr′fō-sis, -mōr-fō′sis) [G. *metamorphasis,* transformation fr. *meta,* beyond, over, + *morphē,* form]. Allaxis; transformation (1); a change in form, structure, or function.

complete m., holometabolous m.; insect development from egg, through successive larval instars, pupa, and adult; the latter is distinct from the first two forms of the insect, permitting specialization of feeding (larval) and reproductive-flying functions (adult); characteristic of the higher insect orders, such as Coleoptera (beetles), Hymenoptera (bees, wasps, ants), Diptera (two-winged flies), and Siphonaptera (fleas).

fatty m., fatty change; the appearance of microscopically visible droplets of fat in the cytoplasm of cells. See also fatty *degeneration.*

heterometabolous m., incomplete m.

holometabolous m., complete m.

incomplete m., heterometabolous m.; the development of a nymph into the imago which in many respects resembles the former; characteristic of more primitive insect orders, such as Heteroptera (true bugs), Orthoptera (locusts, grasshoppers), and Blatterria (roaches).

retrograde m., cataplasia.

metamorphotic (met′ă-mōr-fot′ik). Relating to or marked by metamorphosis.

metamyelocyte (met-ă-mī′el-ō-sīt) [meta- + G. *myelos,* marrow, + *kytos,* cell]. Juvenile cell; a transitional form of myelocyte with nuclear construction that is intermediate between the mature myelocyte (myelocyte C of Sabin) and the two-lobed granular leukocyte.

metanephric (met-ă-nef′rik). Of or pertaining to the metanephron.

metanephrine (met-ă-nef′rin). 3-*O*-Methylepinephrine; a catabolite of epinephrine found, together with normetanephrine, in the urine and in some tissues, resulting from the action of catechol-*O*-methyltransferase on epinephrine; has no sympathomimetic actions.

metanephrogenic, metanephrogenous (met′ă-nef-rō-jen′ik, -nĕ-froj′ĕ-nŭs) [meta- + G. *nephros,* kidney, + *-gen,* producing]. Applied to the more caudal part of the intermediate mesoderm which, under the inductive action of the metanephric diverticulum, has the potency to form metanephric tubules.

metanephros, pl. **metanephroi** (met-ă-nef′ros, -roy) [meta- + G. *nephros,* kidney]. Hind kidney; the most caudally located of the three excretory organs appearing in the evolution of the vertebrates (the others being the pronephros and the metanephros); in mammalian embryos, the m. develops caudal to the mesonephros during its regression, becoming the permanent kidney.

metaneutrophil, metaneutrophile (met-ă-nū′trō-fil, -fīl) [meta- + L. *neuter,* neither, + G. *philos,* fond]. Not staining true with neutral dyes.

metanil yellow (mĕt′ă-nil) [C.I. 13065]. A monoazo acid dye, $C_{18}H_{14}N_3O_3SNa$, used as a cytoplasmic and connective tissue stain.

metaphase (met′ă-fās) [meta- + G. *phasis,* an appearance]. The stage of mitosis or meiosis in which the chromosomes become aligned on the equatorial plate of the cell with the centromeres mutually repelling each other. In mitosis and in the second meiotic division, the centromeres of each chromosome divide and the two daughter centromeres are directed toward opposite poles of the cell; in the first division of meiosis, the centromeres do not divide but the centromeres of each pair of homologous chromosomes become directed toward opposite poles.

metaphosphoric acid (met′ă-fos-fōr′ik). Glacial phosphoric acid.

metaphysial, metaphyseal (met-ă-fiz′ē-ăl). Relating to a metaphysis.

metaphysis, pl. **metaphyses** (mĕ-taf′i-sis, -sēz) [meta- + G. *physis,* growth] [NA]. Growth zone between the epiphysis and diaphysis during development of a bone.

metaphysitis (mĕ-taf′i-sī′tis). Inflammation of the metaphysis.

metaplasia (met-ă-plā′zē-ă) [G. *metaplasis,* transformation]. Metaplasis (2); abnormal transformation of an adult, fully differentiated tissue of one kind into a differentiated tissue of another kind; an acquired condition, in contrast to heteroplasia.

agnogenic myeloid m., primary myeloid m.

apocrine m., alteration of acinar epithelium of breast tissue to resemble apocrine sweat glands; seen commonly in fibrocystic disease of the breasts.

autoparenchymatous m., m. occurring in the parenchymal cells proper to the tissue.

intestinal m., the transformation of mucosa, particularly in the stomach, into glandular mucosa resembling that of the intestines, although usually lacking villi.

myeloid m., a syndrome characterized by anemia, enlargement of the spleen, nucleated red blood cells and immature granulocytes in the circulating blood, and conspicuous foci of extramedullary hemopoiesis in the spleen and liver; may develop in the course of polycythemia rubra vera and there is a high incidence of development of myeloid leukemia.

primary myeloid m., agnogenic myeloid m.; myeloid m. occurring as the primary condition, often in association with myelofibrosis.

secondary myeloid m., symptomatic myeloid m.; myeloid m. occurring in individuals with another disease.

squamous m., epidermalization; the transformation of glandular or mucosal epithelium into stratified squamous epithelium.

squamous m. of amnion, *amnion* nodosum.

symptomatic myeloid m., secondary myeloid m.

metaplasis (mĕ-tap′lă-sis) [G. a transformation]. **1.** E.H. Haeckel's term for the stage of completed growth or development of the individual. **2.** Metaplasia.

metaplasm (met′ă-plazm) [meta- + G. *plasma,* something formed]. Cell *inclusions* (1).

metaplastic (met-ă-plas′tik). Pertaining to metaplasia or metaplasis.

metaplexus (met′ă-plek′sŭs) [meta- + L. *plexus,* an interweaving]. The choroid plexus in the fourth ventricle of the brain.

metapophysis (met′ă-pof′i-sis) [meta- + G. *apophysis,* a process]. *Processus* mamillaris.

metapore (met′ă-pōr) [meta- + G. *poros,* pore]. *Apertura* mediana ventriculi quarti.

metaprotein (met-ă-prō′tēn). Nondescript term for a derived protein obtained by the action of acids or alkalies, soluble in weak acids or alkalies but insoluble in neutral solutions; *e.g.,* albuminate.

metaproterenol sulfate (met′ă-prō-ter′ĕ-nol). Orciprenaline sulphate; 3,5-dihydroxy-α-[(isopropylamino)methyl]benzyl alcohol sulfate; a sympathomimetic bronchodilator used for the treatment of bronchial asthma.

metapsychology (met'ă-sī-kol'ō-jē) [G. *meta,* beyond, transcending, + psychology]. **1.** A systematic attempt to discern and describe what lies beyond the empirical facts and laws of psychology, such as the relations between body and mind, or concerning the place of the mind in the universe. **2.** In psychoanalysis, or psychoanalytic m., psychology concerning the fundamental assumptions of the freudian theory of the mind, which entail five points of view: 1) dynamic, concerning psychologic forces; 2) economic, concerning psychologic energy; 3) structural, concerning psychologic configurations; 4) genetic, concerning psychologic origins; 5) adaptive, concerning psychologic relations with the environment.

metapyretic (met'ă-pī-ret'ik) [meta- + G. *pyretos,* fever]. Postfebrile.

metapyrocatechase (met'ă-pī-rō-kat'ĕ-kās). Catechol 3,4-dioxygenase.

metaraminol bitartrate (met-ă-ram'i-nol). *l*-α-(1-Aminoethyl)-*m*-hydroxybenzyl alcohol hydrogen *d*-tartrate; a potent sympathomimetic amine used for the elevation and maintenance of blood pressure in acute hypotensive states and topically as a nasal decongestant.

metarteriole (met'ar-tēr'ē-ōl) [meta- + arteriole]. One of the small peripheral blood vessels between the arterioles and the true capillaries that contain scattered groups of smooth muscle fibers in their walls.

metarubricyte (met-ă-rū'bri-sīt). Orthochromatic normoblast. See discussion under erythroblast.

pernicious anemia type m., orthochromatic megaloblast. See discussion under erythroblast.

metastable (met'ă-stā-bl) [meta- + L. *stabilis,* stable]. **1.** Of uncertain stability; in a condition to pass into another phase when slightly disturbed; *e.g.,* water, when cooled below the freezing point may remain liquid but will at once congeal if a piece of ice is added. **2.** Denoting the excited condition of the nucleus of a radionuclide isomer that reaches a lower energy state by the process of isomeric transition decay without changing its atomic number or weight; *e.g.,* ${}^{99m}_{43}Tc \rightarrow {}^{99}_{43}Tc + \gamma$.

metastasis, pl. **metastases** (mĕ-tas'tă-sis, -sēz) [G. a removing, fr. *meta,* in the midst of, + *stasis,* a placing]. **1.** The shifting of a disease, or its local manifestations, from one part of the body to another, as in mumps when the symptoms referable to the parotid gland subside and the testis becomes affected. **2.** The spread of a disease process from one part of the body to another, as in the appearance of neoplasms in parts of the body remote from the site of the primary tumor; results from dissemination of tumor cells by the lymphatics or blood vessels, or by direct extension through serous cavities or subarachnoid or other spaces. **3.** Transportation of bacteria from one part of the body to another, through the bloodstreams (**hematogenous m.**) or through lymph channels (**lymphogenous m.**).

biochemical m., the transportation and induction of abnormal immunochemical specificities in apparently normal organs.

calcareous m., the deposit of calcareous material in remote tissues in the event of extensive resorption of osseous tissue in caries, malignant neoplasms, and so on.

pulsating metastases, metastases to bone, usually from hypernephromas, but occasionally from thyroid tumors; may have expansile pulsation and a continuous bruit.

satellite m., m. within the immediate vicinity of a primary malignant neoplasm; *e.g.,* skin adjacent to a melanoma.

metastasize (mĕ-tas'tă-sīz). To pass into or invade by metastasis.

metastatic (met-ă-stat'ik). Relating to metastasis.

metasternum (met'ă-ster'nŭm). *Processus* xiphoideus.

metastrongyle (met-ă-stron'jīl). Common name for members of the genus *Metastrongylus* or of the family Metastrongylidae.

Metastrongylus (met-ă-stron'jĭ-lŭs) [meta- + G. *strongylos,* round]. A genus of nematode lungworms (family Metastrongylidae), the only genus in its subfamily (Metastrongylinae). The four known species are found only in pigs; transmission is by earthworm intermediate hosts.

M. a'pri, a common lungworm species that occurs in larger bronchi of wild and domestic pigs, where it is highly pathogenic, causing verminous pneumonia, consolidation of lungs, emphysema, loss of condition, and reduced growth.

M. elonga'tus, *M. salmi.*

M. pudendotec'tus, a lungworm species, considerably smaller than *M. apri,* found in domestic and wild pigs.

M. sal'mi, *M. elongatus;* a species that occurs in the trachea, bronchi, and bronchioles of domestic and wild pigs.

metasyphilis (met-ă-sif'i-lis). **1.** The constitutional state due to congenital syphilis without local lesions. **2.** Parasyphilis.

metasyphilitic (met'ă-sif-i-lit'ik). Metaluetic. **1.** Relating to metasyphilis. **2.** Following or occurring as a sequel of syphilis. **3.** Parasyphilitic.

metatarsal (met'ă-tar'săl). Relating to the metatarsus or to one of the metatarsal bones.

metatarsalgia (met'ă-tar-sal'jē-ă) [meta- + G. *algos,* pain]. Pain in the forefoot in the region of the heads of the metatarsals.

metatarsectomy (met'ă-tar-sek'tō-mē) [metarsus + G. *ektomē,* excision]. Excision of the metatarsus.

metatarsophalangeal (met'ă-tar'sō-fă-lan'jē-ăl). Relating to the metatarsal bones and the phalanges; denoting the articulations between them.

metatarsus, pl. **metatarsi** (met'ă-tar'sŭs, -sī) [meta- + G. *tarsos,* tarsus] [NA]. The distal portion of the foot between the instep and the toes, having as its skeleton the five long bones (metatarsal bones) articulating posteriorly with the cuboid and cuneiform bones and distally with the phalanges.

m. adductova'rus, fixed deformity of the foot in which both adductus and varus vectors contribute to the resultant foot posture.

m. adduc'tus, a fixed deformity of the foot in which the forepart of the foot is angled away from the main longitudinal axis of the foot toward the midline; usually congenital in origin.

m. atav'icus, abnormal shortness of the first metatarsal bone as compared with the second.

m. la'tus, talipes transversoplanus; deformity caused by sinking down of the transverse arch of the foot.

m. va'rus, intoe; fixed deformity of the foot in which the forepart of the foot is rotated on the long axis of the foot, so that the plantar surface faces the midline of the body.

metathalamus (met'ă-thal'ă-mŭs) [meta- + G. *thalamos,* thalamus] [NA]. The most caudal and ventral part of the thalamus, composed of the medial and lateral geniculate bodies.

metathesis (me-tath'ĕ-sis) [meta- + G. *thesis,* a placing]. **1.** Transfer of a pathologic product (*e.g.,* a calculus) from one place to another where it causes less inconvenience or injury, when it is not possible or expedient to remove it from the body. **2.** In chemistry, a double decomposition, wherein a compound, A-B, reacts with another compound, C-D, to yield A-C + B-D, or A-D + B-C.

metatroph (met'ă-trof). An organism that requires complex organic sources of carbon and nitrogen for growth.

metatrophic (met-ă-trof'ik) [meta- + G. *trophē,* nourishment]. Denoting the ability to undertake anabolism or to obtain nourishment from varied sources, *i.e.,* both nitrogenous and carbonaceous organic matter.

metatropic (met-ă-trop'ik) [meta- + G. *tropē,* a turning]. Denoting a reversion to a previous state.

metatypical (met-ă-tip'i-kăl). Pertaining to tissue that is formed of elements identical to those occurring in that site under normal conditions, but the various elements are not arranged in the usual normal pattern.

metaxalone (mĕ-tak'să-lōn). 5-[(3,5-Xylyloxy)methyl]-2-oxazolidinone; 5-(3,5-dimethylphenoxymethyl)-2-oxazolidinone; a centrally acting skeletal muscle relaxant.

Metazoa (met-ă-zō'ă) [meta- + G. *zōon,* animal]. A subkingdom of the kingdom Animalia, including all multicellular animal organisms in which the cells are differentiated and form tissues; distinguished from the subkingdom Protozoa, or unicellular animal organisms.

metazoonosis (met'ă-zō-ō-nō'sis) [meta- + G. *zōon,* animal, + *nosos,* disease]. A zoonosis that requires both a vertebrate and an invertebrate host for completion of its life cycle; *e.g.,* the arbovirus, infections of man and other vertebrates.

Metchnikoff, Elie, Russian biologist in Paris and Nobel laureate, 1845–1916. See M.'s *theory.*

metencephalic (met'en-se-fal'ik). Relating to the metencephalon.

metencephalon (met'en-sef'ă-lon) [meta- + G. *enkephalos,* brain] [NA]. The anterior of the two major subdivisions of the rhombencephalon (the posterior being the myelencephalon or medulla oblongata), composed of the pons and the cerebellum.

Metenier's sign. See under sign.

metenkephalin (met-en-kef'ă-lin). See enkephalins.

meteorism (mē'tē-ō-rizm) [G. *meteōrismos,* a lifting up]. Tympanites.

meteoropathy (mē'tē-ōr-op'ă-thē) [G. *meteōra,* things high in the air, + *pathos,* suffering]. Rarely used term for ill health due to climatic conditions.

meteorotropic (mē'tē-ōr-ō-trop'ik) [G. *meteora,* things high in the air, + G. *tropos,* a turning]. Denoting diseases affected in their incidence by the weather.

meter (m) (mē'ter) [Fr. *metre;* G. *metron,* measure]. **1.** The fundamental unit of length in the SI and metric systems, equivalent to 39.37 inches. **2.** A device for measuring the quantity of that which passes through it.

atom m., Ångstrom *unit.*

rate m., a device that continuously displays the magnitude of events averaged over varying time intervals.

ventilation m., a m. used to measure tidal and minute ventilatory volumes.

Venturi m., a device for measuring flow of a fluid in terms of the drop in pressure when the fluid flows into the constriction of a Venturi tube.

meter-candle (mē'ter-kan'dl). Lux.

metergasia (met-er-gā'zē-ă) [G. *meta,* denoting change, + *ergasia,* work]. Change of function.

metestrus, metestrum (met-es'trŭs, -trŭm) [meta- + estrus]. The period between estrus and diestrus in the estrous cycle.

metformin (met-fōr'min). 1,1-Dimethylbiguanide; an oral hypoglycemic agent.

meth-, metho-. Chemical prefixes usually denoting a methyl or methoxy group.

methacholine chloride (meth'ă-kō-lēn). Acetyl-β-methylcholine chloride; a derivative of acetylcholine; a parasympathomimetic agent used as a vasodilator in peripheral vascular disease, and for inducing hyperemia in arthritis, its action being brought about locally by iontophoresis; also available as m. bromide.

methacrylate resin (meth-ak'ri-lāt). See under resin.

methacrylic acid (meth'ă-kril'ik). Methylacrylic acid; occurs in oil from Roman camomile; used in the manufacture of methacrylate resins and plastics.

methacycline hydrochloride (meth-ă-sī'klēn). 6-Methylene-5-hydroxytetracycline hydrochloride; an antimicrobial agent.

methadone hydrochloride (meth'ă-dōn). 6-Dimethylamino-4,4-diphenyl-3-heptanone hydrochloride; a synthetic narcotic drug; an orally effective analgesic similar in action to morphine but with slightly greater potency and longer duration. It produces psychic and physical dependence, but withdrawal symptoms are relatively mild; used as a replacement (oral route) for morphine and heroin; also used during withdrawal treatment in morphine and heroin addiction.

methallenestril (meth'ă-len-es'tril). α,α-Dimethyl-β-ethyl-6-methoxy-2-naphthalene propionic acid; an orally effective, nonsteroid estrogenic compound.

methamphetamine hydrochloride (meth-am-fet'ă-mēn). Methylamphetamine hydrochloride; *d*-desoxyephedrine hydrochloride; *d-N,*α-dimethylphenethylamine hydrochloride; a sympathomimetic agent that exerts greater stimulating effects upon the central nervous system than does amphetamine; widely used by drug abusers via the oral and intravenous ("mainlining") routes; strong psychic dependence may develop.

methampyrone (meth-am-pī'rōn). Dipyrone.

methandienone (meth-an-dī'ĕ-nōn). Methandrostenolone.

methandriol (meth-an'drē-ol). Mestenediol; 17-methyl-5-androstene-3β,17β-diol; the methyl derivative of androstenediol, with similar actions and uses.

methandrostenolone (meth-an-drō-sten'ō-lōn). Methandienone; 17β-hydroxy-17α-methyl-1,4-androstadiene-3-one; a methylated dehydrotestosterone; an orally effective anabolic steroid that may promote nitrogen retention when combined with an adequate diet; in addition, it can exert typically androgenic effects.

methane (meth'ān). Marsh gas; CH_4; an odorless gas produced by the decomposition of organic matter; explosive when mixed with 7 or 8 volumes of air, constituting then the firedamp in coal mines.

Methanobacteriaceae (meth'ă-nō-bak-tēr-ē-ā'sē-ē). A family of bacteria containing Gram-negative and Gram-positive, motile or nonmotile, strictly anaerobic rods and cocci, which obtain energy either by the reduction of carbon dioxide to form methane or by the fermentation of compounds such as acetate and methanol with the production of methane and carbon dioxide; they are found in anaerobic habitats such as sediments of natural waters, soil, anaerobic sewage digestors, and the gastrointestinal tract of animals.

methanogen (meth-an'ō-jen). Any methane-producing bacterium of the family Methanobacteriaceae.

methanol (meth'ă-nol). *Methyl* alcohol.

methantheline bromide (meth-an'thĕ-lēn). β-Diethylaminoethyl-9-xanthenecarboxylate methobromide; C_{21}-$H_{26}BrNO_3$; an anticholinergic drug.

methapyrilene (meth-ă-pir'i-lēn). 2-[(2-Dimethylaminoethyl)-2-thenylamino]pyridine; an antihistamine. M. fumarate is administered topically on the skin; m. hydrochloride is the preferred salt for oral or parenteral use.

methaqualone (meth-ă-kwā'lōn). 2-Methyl-3-*o*-tolyl-4(3*H*)-quinazolinone; a sedative and hypnotic, also a drug of abuse; available as the hydrochloride.

metharbital (meth-ar'bi-tahl). 5,5-Diethyl-1-methylbarbituric acid; an *N*-methylated derivative of barbital with anticonvulsant properties similar to those of phenobarbital.

methargen (meth'ar-jen). 2,2'-Dinaphthylmethane-3,3'-disulfonic acid disilver salt; a topical antiseptic agent.

methazolamide (meth-ă-zol'ă-mīd). *N*-(4-Methyl-2-sulfamoyl-Δ^2-1,3,4-thiadiazolin-5-ylidene)acetamide; a carbonic anhydrase inhibitor with uses similar to those of acetazolamide.

metHb Abbreviation for methemoglobin.

methdilazine hydrochloride (meth-dil'ă-zēn). 10-(1-Methyl-3-pyrrolidylmethyl)phenothiazine hydrochloride; a phenothiazine compound with antihistaminic activity; used in the treatment of various dermatoses to relieve pruritus.

methemalbumin (met'hēm-al-bū'min, -hem-al'bū-min). An abnormal compound formed in the blood as a result of heme combining with plasma albumin.

methemalbuminemia (met'hēm-al-bū-min-ē'mē-ă). The presence of methemalbumin in the circulating blood, indicative of hemoglobin breakdown; found in some patients with blackwater fever or paroxysmal nocturnal hemoglobinuria; described as a means of differentiating severe (hemorrhagic) from mild (edematous) pancreatitis, and also has been described in other acute conditions such as strangulation obstruction and mesenteric artery occlusion.

methemoglobin (metHb) (met-hē-mō-glō'bin). Ferrihemoglobin; a transformation product of oxyhemoglobin because of the oxidation of the normal Fe^{2+} to Fe^{3+}, thus converting ferroprotoporphyrin to ferriprotoporphyrin; it contains oxygen in firm union with ferric iron, thus being chemically different from oxyhemoglobin and useless for respiration; found in sanguineous effusions and in the circulating blood after poisoning with acetanilid, potassium chlorate, and other substance.

m. reductase, a flavoenzyme catalyzing the reduction of m. to hemoglobin in the red blood cell.

methemoglobinemia (met-hē'mō-glō-bi-nē'mē-ă, meth'ĕ-mō-) [methemoglobin + G. *haima,* blood]. The presence of methemoglobin in the circulating blood.

acquired m., enterogenous or secondary m.; m. caused by various chemical agents, such as nitrites.

congenital m., primary or hereditary m.; hereditary methemoglobinemic cyanosis; **(1)** m. due to formation of any one of a group of abnormal hemoglobins collectively known as hemoglobin M; slate-gray cyanosis occurs in early infancy, without pulmonary or cardiac disease, and is resistant to ascorbic acid or methylene blue therapy; autosomal dominant inheritance; **(2)** m. due to deficiency of cytochrome b_5 reductase, the enzyme responsible for reduction of intraerythrocyte methemoglobin; cyanosis is improved by ascorbic acid or methylene blue; autosomal recessive inheritance.

enterogenous m., acquired m.

hereditary m., congenital m.

primary m., congenital m.

secondary m., acquired m.

methemoglobinuria (met-hē'mō-glō-bi-nū'rē-ă, meth'ĕ-mō-) [methemoglobin + G. *ouron,* urine]. The presence of methemoglobin in the urine.

methenamine (me-then'ă-mēn). Hexamine; hexamethylenamine; hexamethylenetetramine; ammonioformaldehyde; $C_6H_{12}N_4$; a condensation product obtained by the action of ammonia upon formaldehyde; a urinary antiseptic.

m. hippurate, hexamethylenetetramine hippurate; a urinary antiseptic.

m. mandelate, $C_{14}H_{20}N_4O_3$; a urinary antiseptic.

m. salicylate, hexamethylenetetramine salicylate; a uric acid solvent and urinary antiseptic.

methenamine-silver. A hexamethylenetetramine-silver complex prepared by adding silver nitrate to methenamine; a white precipitate appears in the solution which dissolves upon shaking and is stable under refrigeration; used in various histological and histochemical staining methods. See also Gomori's methenamine-silver *stains.*

methene (meth'ēn). Methylene.

methicillin sodium (meth-i-sil'in). Sodium methicillin; sodium 2,6-dimethoxyphenylpenicillin monohydrate; a semisynthetic penicillin salt for parenteral administration; restriction of its use to infections caused by penicillin G-resistant staphylococci is recommended; it is less effective than penicillin G in infections caused by hemolytic streptococci, pneumococci, gonococci, and penicillin G-sensitive staphylococci.

methimazole (me-thim'ă-zōl). 1-Methylimidazole-2-thiol; an antithyroid drug similar in action to propylthiouracil.

methiodal sodium (meth-ī'ō-dăl). An iodine-containing radiopaque medium, formerly used for examination of the urinary tract.

methionine (Met) (me-thī'ō-nēn). 2-Amino-4-(methylthio)butyric acid; $CH_3S\text{–}CH_2CH_2CHNH_2\text{–}COOH$; an essential amino acid and the most important natural source of "active methyl" groups in the body, hence usually involved in methylations *in vivo;* the DL-form is used as an adjunct in the treatment of liver diseases.

active m., *S*-adenosylmethionine.

m. adenosyltransferase [EC 2.5.1.6], methionine-activating enzyme; an enzyme catalyzing the condensation of methionine and ATP, forming *S*-adenosylmethionine.

m. sulfoxime, a toxic derivative of m. formed when proteins containing it are treated with nitrogen chloride to give $\text{–}SO(NH)CH_3$ in place of $\text{–}SCH_3$.

methisazone (mĕ-this'ă-zōn). *N*-Methylisatin 3-semicarbazone; 1- methylindole-2,3-dione 3-thiosemicarbazone; an antiviral agent.

methixene hydrochloride (me-thik'sēn). 1-Methyl-3-(thioxanthen-9-ylmethyl)piperidine hydrochloride; an anticholinergic agent.

metho-. See meth-.

methocarbamol (meth-ō-kar'bă-mol). 2-Hydroxy-3-*o*- methoxyphenoxypropyl carbamate; a centrally acting skeletal muscle relaxant, chemically related to mephenesin carbamate; it is slower in onset of action but of longer duration, and may be administered intravenously, intramuscularly, or orally.

METHOD

method (meth'ŏd) [G. *methodos;* fr. *meta,* after, + *hodos,* way]. The mode or manner or orderly sequence of events of a process or procedure. See also entries under fixative; operation; procedure; stain; technique.

Abbott's m., a m. of treatment of scoliosis by use of a series of plaster jackets applied after partial correction of the curvature by external force.

Abell-Kendall m., a standard m. for estimation of total serum cholesterol involving saponification of cholesterol ester by hydroxide, extraction with petroleum ether, and color development with acetic anhydride-sulfuric acid; the m. avoids interference by bilirubin, protein, and hemoglobin.

activated sludge m., a m. of sewage disposal in which the sewage is treated with 15% bacterially active, liquid sludge, which is produced by repeated vigorous aeration of fresh sewage to form floccules or sediment; when this flocculation process is complete, the resulting activated sludge contains large numbers of bacteria, together with yeasts, molds, and protozoa, which actively effect the oxidation of organic compounds; this mixture is piped to a sedimentation tank, the effluent from which is completely treated sewage.

Altmann-Gersh m., the m. of rapidly freezing a tissue and dehydrating it in a vacuum.

Anel's m., ligation of an artery immediately above (on the proximal side of) an aneurysm.

Antyllus' m., ligature of the artery above and below an aneurysm, followed by incision into and emptying of the sac.

aristotelian m., a m. of study that stresses the relation between a general category and a particular object.
Ashby m., a differential agglutination m. for estimating erythrocyte life span; compatible blood possessing a group factor that the recipient lacks is transferred to the recipient; after the transfusion, sera with potent agglutinins for the recipient's red cells are added to samples of the recipient's blood, and the unagglutinated red cells are counted; using this technique the red cell life span in normal persons is found to be 110 to 120 days.
auxanographic m., diffusion m.; a m. for the study of bacterial enzymes in which agar is mixed with the material (*e.g.,* starch or milk) which is to serve as an indicator of the enzyme action and is inoculated and plated; if the bacteria produce enzymes digesting the admixed material, there will be a zone of clearing in the medium about each colony.
Barraquer's m., zonulolysis.
Beck's m., a permanent opening into the stomach made from its greater curvature.
Bier's m., **(1)** intravenous regional *anesthesia;* **(2)** treatment of various surgical conditions by reactive hyperemia.
Born m. of wax plate reconstruction, the making of three-dimensional models of structures from serial sections; it depends on the building up of a series of wax plates, cut out to scaled enlargements of the individual sections involved in the region to be reconstructed.
Brasdor's m., treatment of aneurysm by ligation of the artery immediately below (on the distal side of) the tumor.
broad marginal confrontation m., Jaboulay's m.
Callahan's m., chloropercha m.
Carpue's m., Indian *rhinoplasty.*
Charters' m., a method of toothbrushing utilizing a restricted circular motion with the bristles inclined coronally at a 45 degree angle.
Chayes' m., a m. of replacing lost teeth utilizing a mechanical device for the fixation and stabilization of the dental prosthesis which allows "movement in function" of the abutment teeth.
chloropercha m., Callahan's or Johnson's m.; a m. of filling the root canals of teeth by dissolving gutta-percha cones in a chloroform-rosin medium within the root canal.
closed circuit m., a m. for measuring oxygen consumption in which the subject rebreathes an initial quantity of oxygen through a carbon dioxide absorber and the decrease in the volume of oxygen being rebreathed is noted.
confrontation m., a m. of perimetry; the examiner compares the visual fields of the patient with his own by facing the patient who has one eye covered and the other fixed upon the corresponding (confronting) eye of the examiner. The examiner then holds his finger midway between the patient and himself and moves it slowly in different directions until the patient fails to see it. In each instance the finger is moved again toward the original position until it is just seen by the subject.
cooled-knife m., the cutting of frozen sections with a knife cooled to a few degrees below the freezing point.
copper sulfate m., a m. for the determination of specific gravity of blood or plasma in which the blood or plasma is delivered by drops into solutions of copper sulfate graded in specific gravity by increments of 0.004, each of bottles of solution being within the expected range of the blood or plasma sample; the specific gravity of the copper sulfate solution in which the drop of blood or plasma remains suspended indefinitely indicates the specific gravity of the sample.
correlational m., a statistical m., most often used in clinical and other applied areas of psychology, to study the relationship which exists between one characteristic and another in an individual.
Credé's m.'s, Credé's maneuvers; **(1)** instillation of one drop of a 2% solution of silver nitrate into each eye of the newborn infant, to prevent ophthalmia neonatorum; **(2)** resting the hand on the fundus uteri from the moment of the expulsion of the fetus, and gently rubbing in case of hemorrhage or failing contraction; then, when the afterbirth is loosened it is expelled by firm compression or squeezing of the fundus by the hand; **(3)** use of manual pressure on bladder, particularly a paralyzed bladder, to express urine.
cross-sectional m., in developmental psychology, the study of the life span involving comparison of groups of individuals at different age levels. *Cf.* longitudinal m.
definitive m., an analytical procedure for the measurement of a specified analyte in a specified material which is known to give essentially the true value for the concentration of the analyte.
Dick m., Dick *test.*
Dieffenbach's m., a plastic operation for covering a defect by sliding a flap with broad pedicle.
diffusion m., auxanographic m.
direct m. for making inlays, direct technique; in dentistry, an inlay technique in which the wax pattern is made directly in the prepared cavity in the tooth.
disk sensitivity m., a procedure for testing the relative effectiveness of various antibiotics; small disks of paper (or other suitable material) are impregnated with known, appropriate amounts of antibiotic, and then placed on the surface of semisolid medium that has been previously inoculated with the organism being tested; after suitable periods of incubation at 37°C, the lack of growth in zones about the various disks indicates the relative effectiveness of the antibiotic.
double antibody m., double antibody *precipitation.*
Edman m., see phenylisothiocyanate.
Eggleston m., rapid digitalization by means of large doses of digitalis leaf or tincture frequently repeated.
Eicken's m., facilitation of hypopharyngoscopy by means of forward traction on the cricoid cartilage by a laryngeal probe.
experimental m., in experimental psychology, control of environmental, physiological, or attitudinal factors to observe dependent changes in aspects of experience and behavior.
flash m., sterilization of milk by raising it rapidly to a temperature of 178°F, holding it there for a short time, and reducing it rapidly to 40°F.
flotation m., any of several procedures for concentrating helminth eggs for more reliable results when eggs are difficult to find in direct examination; the flotation m.'s depend on flotation of helminth eggs on the surface of a liquid of sufficiently high specific gravity, approximately 1.180; 1 part feces mixed in about 10 parts saturated saline will float most protozoan cysts and nonpercolated helminth eggs. See also zinc sulfate flotation centrifugation m.
Gärtner's m., a m. of measuring venous pressure, based upon Gärtner's vein phenomenon; with the patient sitting erect a vein is selected on the back of the hand which is held horizontal a little below the level of the right atrium, and then is raised slowly; when the vein is observed to collapse, the distance between its level and that of the atrium is measured with a millimeter rule; this distance gives the venous pressure in millimeters of blood; thus the vein itself is used as a manometer communicating with the right atrium.
Gerota's m., injection of the lymphatics with a dye that is soluble in chloroform or ether but not in water; alkanin, red sulfide of mercury, and Prussian blue are said to be suitable for this purpose.
glucose oxidase m., a highly specific m. for measurement of glucose in serum or plasma by reaction with glucose oxidase, in which gluconic acid and hydrogen peroxide are formed.
Gräupner's m., a test of the sufficiency of the heart muscle; if a normal subject takes a measured amount of exercise, the pulse rate rises, and after it has begun to fall the systolic blood pressure begins to rise, reaching its maximum a few minutes after the pulse rate; in the case of a weakened heart, the rise in blood pressure is delayed and the amount of increase diminished; in seriously weakened hearts, a fall in blood pressure occurs.
Gruber's m., a modification of the Politzer m. in which the patient

does not swallow, but says "hoc" at the instant of compression of the bag.

Hammerschlag's m., a hydrometric m. of determining the specific gravity of the blood by allowing a drop of blood to fall into each of a series of tubes containing mixtures of chloroform and benzene of known graded specific gravities; the specific gravity of that mixture in which the drop remains exactly suspended, neither rising nor falling, corresponds to the specific gravity of the blood sample.

hexokinase m., the most specific m. for measuring glucose in serum or plasma, wherein hexokinase plus ATP transforms glucose to glucose 6-phosphate plus ADP; glucose 6-phosphate is then reacted with NADP and glucose 6-phosphate dehydrogenase to form NADP which is measured spectrophotometrically.

Hilton's m., division of the nerves supplying a part, for the relief of pain in ulcers.

Hirschberg's m., a m. of measuring the amount of deviation of a strabismic eye, by observing the reflection of a light fixated by the straight eye on the cornea of the deviating eye.

Holmgren m., Holmgren's *test.*

Hung's m., Wilson's m.

immunofluorescence m., any m. in which a fluorescent-labeled antibody is used to detect the presence or determine the location of the corresponding antigen.

impedance m., a m. for localizing brain structures by measuring impedance of electric current.

Indian m., Indian *rhinoplasty.*

indirect m. for making inlays, indirect technique; a method whereby the inlay is constructed entirely on a model made from an impression of the prepared tooth or teeth in the mouth.

indophenol m., a m. of determining quantitatively the amount of vitamin C in plant and animal tissue based on the rapid reduction of a standardized indophenol solution to a colorless compound by vitamin C in acid solution.

introspective m., in functionalism, the systematic study of mental phenomena by contemplating the processes in one's own conscious experiences.

Italian m., Italian *rhinoplasty.*

Jaboulay's m., broad marginal confrontation m.; anastomosis of arteries by splitting the cut ends a short distance and then suturing the flaps together, applying intima to intima.

Johnson's m., chloropercha m.

Keating-Hart's m., fulguration in the treatment of external cancer or of the field of operation after the removal of a malignant growth.

Kjeldahl m., see macro- and micro-Kjeldahl m.'s.

Klapp's m., treatment of scoliosis by a series of systematic crawling movements whereby the spine is bent laterally and made more flexible.

Krause's m., see Krause *graft.*

Lamaze m., a technique of psychoprophylactic preparation for childbirth, designed to minimize the pain of labor.

Langendorff's m., perfusion of the isolated mammalian heart by carrying fluid under pressure into the sectioned aorta, and thus into the coronary system.

Lee-White m., a m. for determining coagulation time of venous blood in tubes of standard bore at body temperature.

Liborius' m., a m. for culturing anaerobic bacteria; a stab culture is made in the appropriate agar medium, then more of the same medium is liquefied and poured into the test tube on top of the stab culture, effectually sealing it from the air.

Ling's m., lingism; gymnastic exercises (as in Swedish movements) without the use of apparatus.

Lister's m., listerism; antiseptic surgery, as first advocated by Lister in 1867; the operation was performed under a cloud of diluted carbolic acid spray, the instruments were dipped in a carbolic solution before use, and the wound was dressed with a thick layer of carbolized gauze; from this was developed the present practice of aseptic surgery.

lod m. [logarithm of the odds], a method of linkage analysis using an examination of the common logarithm of the ratio of the likelihood for a particular value of the recombination fraction to that if the recombination fraction is 0.5 (*i.e.,* no linkage); thus, a lod score of 3 for a recombination fraction of 0.2 means that the data are 1000 times more readily explained by supposing that recombination fraction than by supposing the loci are unlinked.

longitudinal m., in developmental psychology, the study of the life span of one individual involving comparisons of different age levels. *Cf.* cross-sectional m.

macro-Kjeldahl m., a procedure for analyzing the content of nitrogenous compounds in urine, serum, or other specimens, usually to determine relatively large amounts of nitrogen (*e.g.,* 20 to 100 mg); the specimen is treated with a digestion mixture (copper sulfate and sulfuric acid), heated thoroughly, and made alkaline with a solution of sodium hydroxide; ammonia is then distilled from the mixture, trapped in a boric acid-indicator solution, and titrated with standard hydrochloric or sulfuric acid.

Marshall's m., a quantitative procedure for estimating free and conjugated sulfanilamide in body fluids.

micro-Astrup m., an interpolation technique for acid-base measurement, based on pH and the use of the Siggaard-Andersen nomogram to determine the base deficit as an expression of metabolic acidosis and the arterial P_{CO_2} as an expression of respiratory acidosis or alkalosis.

micro-Kjeldahl m., a modification of the macro-Kjeldahl m. designed for the analysis of nitrogenous compounds in relatively small quantities, *e.g.,* specimens in which the total content of nitrogen is in the range of 1 to a few mg.

Moore's m., treatment of aneurysm by the introduction of silver or zinc wire into the sac to induce fibrin deposition.

Müller's m., obsolete term for resection of the sclera for detachment of the retina.

Needles' split cast m., split cast m.

Nikiforoff's m., the fixing of blood films by immersion for 5 to 15 minutes in absolute alcohol, a mixture of equal parts of alcohol and ether, or pure ether.

Ochsner's m., an obsolete treatment of appendicitis, when surgery is not advisable, by peristaltic rest.

Ollier's m., see Ollier *graft.*

open circuit m., a m. for measuring oxygen consumption and carbon dioxide production by collecting the expired gas over a known period of time and measuring its volume and composition.

Orsi-Grocco m., palpatory percussion of the heart.

Pachon's m., cardiography, carried out with the patient lying on the left side.

paracelsian m., the use of chemical agents only in the treatment of disease.

parallax m., localization of a foreign body by observation of dense areas on the fluoroscopic screen while the tube is moving at determined distances from the body.

Pavlov m., the m. of studying conditioned reflex activity by the observation of a motor indicator, such as the salivary or electroencephalographic response.

Politzer m., inflation of the eustachian tube and tympanum by forcing air into the nasal cavity at the instant the patient swallows.

Porges m., a m. of destroying the capsule of bacteria by heating with N/4 hydrochloric acid and neutralizing with NaOH.

Purmann's m., treatment of aneurysm by extirpation of the sac.

Quick's m., prothrombin *test.*

reference m., an analytical procedure sufficiently free of random or systematic error to make it useful for validating proposed new analytical procedures for the same analyte.

Rehfuss m., fractional m. of gastric activity: a fine tube with fenestrated metal tip is left in the stomach after a test meal, and small quantities (6 or 8 ml) of the stomach contents are removed at 15-minute intervals and examined.

Reverdin's m., see Reverdin *graft.*
rhythm m., rhythm (2); a natural contraceptive m. that spaces human sexual intercourse to avoid the fertile period of the menstrual cycle.
Rideal-Walker m., see Rideal-Walker *coefficient.*
Roux's m., division of the inferior maxilla in the median line, to facilitate the operation of ablation of the tongue.
Scarpa's m., cure of aneurysm by ligation of the artery at some distance above the sac.
Schäfer's m., an obsolete m. of resuscitation in cases of drowning or asphyxia; the patient is laid face downward and natural breathing is imitated by gentle intermittent pressure over the lower part of the thorax at the rate of about 15 times a minute.
Schede's m., supplying the defect in bone, after removal of a sequestrum or scraping away carious material, by allowing the cavity to fill with blood which may become organized (Schede's clot).
Schick m., Schick *test.*
Schmidt-Thannhauser m., a m. for fractionation of nucleic acid, based upon the fact that RNA but not DNA is hydrolyzed to nucleotides by alkali; RNA can be hydrolyzed in about 2 hours in 0.75 N NaOH, but 18 hours and 0.3 N NaOH usually are used.
Shaffer-Hartman m., an obsolete m. for the quantitative determination of glucose in biological fluids, based on the reduction of copper by the reducing group of the sugar.
Somogyi m., see Somogyi *unit.*
split cast m., Needles' split cast m.; **(1)** a procedure for placing indexed casts on an articulator to facilitate their removal and replacement on the instrument; **(2)** the procedure of checking the ability of an articulator to receive or be adjusted to a maxillomandibular relation record.
Stas-Otto m., a m. of extraction of alkaloids from plants and animal bodies: the substance is digested in alcohol and tartaric acid, the fatty and resinous matters are precipitated with water, the fluid is made alkaline, and the alkaloids are extracted with ether or chloroform.
Stroganoff's m., treatment of eclampsia by morphine, chloral hydrate, shielding the patient from all external sources of irritation, and rapid delivery.
Thane's m., a m. for indicating the position of the central sulcus (Rolando's fissure) of the brain; the upper end of the sulcus corresponds to the midpoint of a line drawn from the glabella to the inion.
Theden's m., treatment of aneurysms or of large sanguineous effusions by compression of the entire limb with a roller bandage.
Thiersch's m., see Thiersch *graft.*
thiochrome m., a m. for the determination of thiamin based upon the production of thiochrome when the vitamin is oxidized by alkaline ferricyanide to yield the fluorescent compound, thiochrome.
ultropaque m., a rapid m. for examining thick (1 to 3 mm) sections of fresh tissue with the ultramicroscope, making use of an objective built in an illuminator so that the light is reflected down upon the tissue.
Wardrop's m., treatment of aneurysm by ligation of the artery at some distance beyond the sac, leaving one or more branches of the artery between the sac and the ligature.
Westergren m., a procedure for estimating the sedimentation rate of red blood cells in fluid blood by mixing venous blood with an aqueous solution of sodium citrate and allowing it to stand in an upright standard pipet filled to the zero mark; the fall of the red blood cells, in millimeters, is then observed in 1 hr; the normal rate for men is 0 to 15 mm (average, 4 mm), and for women 0 to 20 mm (average, 5mm).
Wheeler m., a surgical procedure for correction of cicatricial ectropion.
Wilson's m., Hung's m.; a simple saline flotation m. for concentrating helminth eggs in the feces. See flotation m.
Wolfe's m., see Wolfe *graft.*
zinc sulfate flotation centrifugation m., a flotation m. in which the fecal specimen is suspended in tap water, strained through wet gauze, centrifuged, resuspended in tap water, washed and recentrifuged several times, and then suspended in 33% solution of zinc sulfate and centrifuged at top speed for 45 to 60 sec; a bacteriologic loop may be used to pick up the surface layer, which contains protozoan cysts and helminth eggs.

methodism (meth'ŏd-izm). Solidism.

methohexital sodium (meth-ō-heks'i-tawl). Sodium α-*dl*-methyl-5-allyl-5-(1-methyl-2-pentynyl) barbiturate; an ultrashort-acting barbiturate used intravenously for induction and for general anesthesia of short duration.

methoin (meth'ō-in). Mephenytoin.

methonium compounds (me-thō'nē-ŭm). See under compound.

methophenazine (me-thō-fen'ă-zēn). 3,4,5-Trimethoxybenzoic acid 2-{4-[3-(2-chlorophenothiazin-10-yl)propyl]-1-piperazinyl}ethyl ester; an antipsychotic.

methopholine (me-thō-fō'lēn). 1-(*p*-Chlorophenethyl)-1,2,3,4-tetrahydro-6,7-dimethoxy-2-methylisoquinoline; an analgesic.

methopterin (meth-op'ter-in). 10-Methylfolic acid; 10-methylpteroylglutamic acid; a folic acid antagonist.

methorphinan (meth-ōr'fi-nan). 3-Hydroxy-*N*-methylmorphinan; $C_{17}H_{23}NOHBr$. See dextromethorphan; levorphanol.

methoserpidine (meth-ō-ser'pi-dēn). 10-Methoxydeserpidine; an antihypertensive agent similar in its actions to reserpine.

methotrexate (meth-ō-trek'sāt). Amethopterin; methylaminopterin; 4-amino-10-methylfolic acid; a folic acid antagonist used as an antineoplastic agent.

methotrimeprazine (meth'ō-trī-mep'ră-zēn). 10-[3-(Dimethylamino)-2-methylpropyl]-2-methoxyphenothiazine; a phenothiazine analgesic.

methoxamine hydrochloride (me-thok'să-mēn). α-(1-Aminoethyl)-2,5-dimethoxybenzyl alcohol; β-hydroxy-β-(2,5-dimethoxyphenyl) isopropylamine hydrochloride; a sympathomimetic amine.

methoxsalen (me-thok'să-len). δ-Lactone of 3-(6-hydroxy-7-methoxybenzofuranyl) acrylic acid; a methoxypsoralen derivative that increases melanin production in the skin when exposed to ultraviolet light; used orally and topically in the treatment of idiopathic vitiligo, and also as a suntan accelerator and sun protectant.

methoxy-. Chemical prefix denoting substitution of a methoxyl group.

4-methoxybenzoic acid (meth-ok'sē-ben-zō'ik). Anisic acid.

methoxyflurane (me-thok-sē-flūr'ān). 2,2-Dichloro-1,1-difluoroethyl methyl ether; a potent, nonflammable, nonexplosive inhalation anesthetic; low vapor pressure makes induction of anesthesia slow; very high lipid solubility may prolong recovery; adverse side effects include high output renal failure due to increased plasma concentrations of inorganic fluoride, a metabolic breakdown product of m.

methoxyl (me-thok'sil). The group, $-OCH_3$.

methoxyphenamine hydrochloride (me-thok-sē-fen'ă-mēn). β-(*o*-Methoxyphenyl)isopropylmethylamine hydrochloride; a sympathomimetic amine.

methscopolamine bromide (meth-skō-pol'ă-mēn). Epoxytropine tropate methylbromide; a parasympatholytic drug similar to atropine; the methyl nitrate has the same action and uses.

methsuximide (meth-sŭk'si-mīd). *N*,2-Dimethyl-2-phenylsuccinimide; an antiepileptic effective against petit mal and psychomotor epilepsy.

methyclothiazide (meth'i-klō-thī'ă-zīd). 6-Chloro-3-(chloro-methyl)-3,4-dihydro-2-methyl-2*H*-1,2,4-benzothiadiazine-7-sulfonamide-1,1-dioxide; an orally effective diuretic and antihypertensive agent of the thiazide group.

methyl (Me) (meth'il) [G. *methy,* wine, + *hylē,* wood]. The radical, $-CH_3$.

active m., a m. group attached to a quaternary ammonium ion or a tertiary sulfonium ion that can take part in transmethylation reactions; *e.g.,* m. groups in choline and in *S*-adenosylmethionine, which are thus m. donors.

m. alcohol, wood alcohol; methanol; carbinol; wood naphtha; wood spirit; pyroxylic spirit; pyroligneous alcohol or spirit; CH_3OH; a flammable, toxic, mobile liquid, used as an industrial solvent, antifreeze, and in chemical manufacture; ingestion may result in severe acidosis, visual impairment, and other effects on the central nervous system.

m. aldehyde, formaldehyde.

angular m., a m. group attached to carbon 10 (between rings A and B) or to carbon 13 (between rings C and D) of the steroid nucleus.

m. chloride, chloromethane.

m. cysteine hydrochloride, mecysteine hydrochloride; the methyl ester of cysteine hydrochloride; a mucolytic agent.

m. hydroxybenzoate, methylparaben.

m. isobutyl ketone, 4-methyl-2-pentanone, an alcohol denaturant; in high concentrations it has narcotic action; in relatively low concentrations it may be irritating to the eyes and mucous membranes.

m. methacrylate, a thermoplastic material used for denture bases.

m. nicotinate, nicotinic acid methyl ester; used as rubefacient.

m. salicylate, the methyl ester of salicylic acid, produced synthetically or distilled from *Gaultheria procumbens* (family Ericaceae) or from *Betula lenta* (family Betulaceae); used externally and internally for the treatment of various forms of rheumatism.

methylacrylic acid (meth'il-ă-kril'ik). Methacrylic acid.

methylamphetamine hydrochloride (meth'il-am-fet'ă-mēn). Methamphetamine hydrochloride.

methylate (meth'i-lāt). **1.** To mix with methyl alcohol. **2.** To introduce a methyl group. **3.** A compound in which a metal ion methyl replaces the alcoholic hydrogen of alcohol.

methylation (meth-i-lā'shŭn). Addition of methyl groups; in histochemistry, used to esterify carboxyl groups and remove sulfate groups by treating tissue sections with hot methanol in the presence of hydrochloric acid; the net effect being to reduce tissue basophilia and abolish metachromasia.

methylatropine bromide (meth-il-at'rō-pēn, -pin). Atropine methylbromide; a cycloplegic.

methylbenzene (meth-il-ben'zēn). Toluene.

methylbenzethonium chloride (meth'il-ben-zĕ-thō'nē-ŭm). Benzyldimethyl {2-[2-(*p*-1,1,3,3-tetramethylbutylcresoxy)ethoxy]-ethyl}ammonium chloride; a quaternary ammonium compound having a surface action like that of other cationic detergents; generally germicidal and bacteriostatic; used to rinse infant diapers and bed linen in the prevention of ammonia dermatitis.

methyl blue [C.I. 42780]. A sulfonated triphenylrosaniline dye used as a stain for cytoplasm, collagen, and Negri bodies, and as an antiseptic.

methylcarnosine (meth-il-kar'nō-sēn). Anserine.

methylcellulose (meth-il-sel'yū-lōs). A methyl ester of cellulose that forms a colorless liquid when dissolved in water, alcohol, or ether; used to increase bulk of the intestinal contents, to relieve constipation, or of the gastric contents, to reduce appetite in obesity; also used dissolved in water as a spray to cover burned areas.

methylchloroform (meth-il-chlōr'ō-fōrm). Trichloroethane.

3 (or 20)-**methylcholanthrene** (meth'il-kōl-an'thrēn). A highly carcinogenic hydrocarbon that can be formed chemically from deoxycholic or cholic acids, or from cholesterol; the choice between 3- or 20- for the methyl group depends upon whether hydrocarbon (inner) or steroid (outer) numbering is chosen; in the latter case, the formal relationship to the cholic acids and cholesterol is clear.

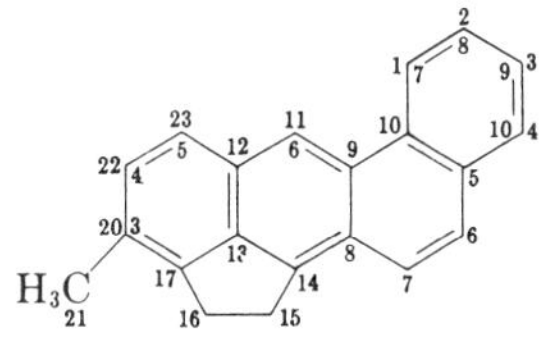

3 (or 20)-Methylcholanthrene

methylcysteine synthase (meth-il-sis'tē-ēn). Cystathionine β-synthase.

methyldihydromorphinone hydrochloride (meth'il-dī-hī'drō-mōr'fi-nōn). Metopon hydrochloride.

methyldopa (meth-il-dō'pă). (L)-3-(3,4-Dihydroxyphenyl)-2-methylalanine; an antihypertensive agent, also used as the ethyl ester hydrochloride, with the same action and uses.

methylene (meth'i-lēn). Methene; the radical, $-CH_2-$.

methylene azure. *Azure* I.

methylene blue [C.I. 52015]. 3,7-bis(Dimethylamino)phenazathionium chloride; tetramethylthionine chloride; a basic dye easily oxidized to azure, with dye mixtures; used in histology and microbiology, to stain intestinal protozoa in wet mount preparations, to track RNA and RNase in electrophoresis, and as an antidote for methemoglobinemia; its redox indicator properties are useful in milk bacteriology.

Kühne's m. b., m. b. in absolute alcohol and phenol solution.

Loeffler's m. b., a stain for diphtheria organisms that contains m. b. in dilute ethanol plus a slight amount of potassium hydroxide; dye solution gives best results when aged to a polychrome state.

new m. b. [C.I. 52030], a basic thiazin dye, $C_{18}H_{22}N_3SCl$, used for supravital staining of reticulocytes in blood smears.

polychrome m. b., an alkaline solution of m. b. which undergoes progressive oxidative demethylation with aging (ripening) to produce a mixture of m. b., azures, and m. violet; boiling with sodium carbonate or other oxidizing agents accomplishes this result quickly, although it is not as highly regarded.

methylenesuccinic acid (meth'il-ēn-sŭk'sin-ik). Itaconic acid.

methylene white. Leucomethylene blue.

methylenophil, methylenophile (meth-i-lēn'ō-fil, -fīl) [methylene + G. *philos,* fond]. Methylenophilic; methylenophilous; staining readily with methylene blue; denoting certain cells and histologic structures.

methylenophilic, methylenophilous (meth'i-lē-nō-fil'ik, meth'il-ĕ-nof'i-lŭs). Methylenophil.

methylergometrine maleate (meth'il-er-gō-met'rēn). Methylergonovine maleate.

methylergonovine maleate (meth'il-er-gō-nō'vēn). Methylergometrine maleate; *d*-lysergic acid-*dl*-hydroxybutylamide-2-maleate; a partially synthesized derivative of lysergic acid with oxytocic action, used to prevent or treat postpartum uterine atony and hemorrhage.

methylglucamine (meth-il-glū'kă-mēn). Meglumine.

m. diatrizoate, *meglumine* diatrizoate.

m. iodipamide, bis-*N*-methylglucamine salt of iodipamide; a water-soluble organic iodine compound used for intravenous cholangiography and cholecystography.

methylglyoxal (meth'il-glī-ok'săl). Pyruvaldehyde; pyruvic aldehyde; CH_3-CO_3-CHO; the aldehyde of pyruvic acid.

m. bis(guanylhydrazone), 1,1′-[(methylethanediylidene)dinitrilo] diguanidine; an antineoplastic agent.

methylglyoxalase (meth′il-glī-oks′ă-lās). Lactoylglutathione lyase.

methyl green [C.I. 42585]. A basic triphenylmethane dye used as a chromatin stain and, in combination with pyronin, for differential staining of RNA (red) and DNA (green); also used as a tracking dye for DNA in electrophoresis.

methylhexaneamine (meth′il-hek-sān′ă-mēn, -min). 4-Methyl-2-hexylamine; a volatile sympathetic amine base, used as an inhalant nasal decongestant.

methylkinase (meth′il-kī′nās). Methyltransferase.

methylmalonic acid (meth′il-mă-lon′ik). 2-Methylpropanedioic acid, an important intermediate in fatty acid metabolism.

methylmalonic acidemia. A heterogeneous group of disorders characterized by accumulation of methylmalonic acid in the blood, cerebrospinal fluid, and urine. See methylmalonic aciduria.

methylmalonic aciduria. Excretion of excessive amounts of methylmalonic acid in urine due to deficiency of activity of methylmalonyl-CoA mutase or a deficiency of cobalamin reductase. Two types occur: 1) congenital, a metabolic error resulting in severe ketoacidosis developing shortly after birth, with urine that also contains long chain ketones; autosomal recessive inheritance; 2) acquired, a type developing in vitamin B_{12} deficiency.

methylmalonyl-CoA mutase (meth-il-mal′on-il) [EC 5.4.99.2]. An enzyme that interchanges methylmalonyl-CoA and succinyl-CoA.

methylmorphine (meth-il-mōr′fēn). Codeine.

methylnortestosterone (meth′il-nōr-tes-tos′ter-ōn). Normethandrone.

methylol (meth′i-lol). Hydroxymethyl; the radical, $-CH_2OH$.

methyl orange [C.I. 13025]. Helianthin; $C_{14}H_{14}N_3O_3SNa$; a weakly acid dye used as a pH indicator (red at 3.0, yellow at 4.4).

methylose (meth′i-lōs). A sugar in which the carbon atom farthest from the carbonyl group is a methyl (CH_3).

methylparaben (meth-il-par′ă-ben). Methyl hydroxybenzoate; methyl *p*-hydroxybenzoate; an antifungal preservative.

methylpentose (meth-il-pen′tōs). A hexose (a 6-deoxyhexose) in which carbon-6 is part of a methyl group; *e.g.,* rhamnose, fucose.

methylphenidate hydrochloride (meth-il-fen′i-dāt). Methyl α-phenyl-2-piperidineacetate hydrochloride; a central nervous system stimulant used to produce mild cortical stimulation in various types of depressions; commonly used in the treatment of hyperkinetic or hyperactive children.

methylprednisolone (meth′il-pred-nis′ŏ-lōn). 6-α-Methylprednisolone; an anti-inflammatory glucocorticoid.

m. acetate, 6-methylprednisolone-21-acetate; has the same actions and uses as m.; aqueous suspensions are suitable for intrasynovial and soft tissue injection.

sodium m. succinate, sodium 6-methylprednisolone-21-succinate; it has the same metabolic and anti-inflammatory actions as the parent compound, m.; because of its solubility it can be administered in small volumes.

methyl red [C.I. 13020]. $C_{15}H_{15}N_30_2$; a weakly acid dye used as a pH indicator (red at 4.4, yellow at 6.2); easily reduced with loss of color, and pH readings must be made rapidly.

5-methylresorcinol (meth′il-rē-sōr′sin-ol). Orcinol.

methylrosaniline chloride (meth′il-rō-zan′i-lēn, -lin). Crystal violet.

methyltestosterone (meth′il-tes-tos′ter-ōn). A methyl derivative of testosterone, with the same actions and uses, except that it is active when given orally or sublingually.

methylthioadenosine (meth′il-thī′ō-ă-den′ō-sēn). Thiomethyladenosine; adenosine carrying an $-SCH_3$ group in place of OH at position 5′; the $-SCH_3$ group is transferred to α-aminobutyric acid to form methionine in some bacteria. M. is formed from *S*-adenosylmethionine in the course of spermidine synthesis by loss of the alanine group.

methylthiouracil (meth′il-thī-ō-yū′ră-sil). 6-Methyl-2-thiouracil; an antithyroid compound with the same action as thiouracil, but with a smaller dose required.

methyltocol (meth-il-tō′kol). A methylated tocol; *e.g.,* tocotrienol, the tocopherols.

methyltransferase (meth-il-trans′fer-ās) [EC 2.1.1.]. Transmethylase; methylkinase; demethylase; any enzyme transferring methyl groups from one compound to another.

methyl violet [C.I. 42535]. Mixtures of tetra-, penta-, or pararosanilin which vary in shade of violet depending on the extent of methylation (designated R for reddish shades, B for bluish shades); the hexamethyl compound is known as crystal violet, the pentamenthyl compound as methyl violet 6B. As stains, m. v. has many bacteriological, histological, and cytological applications.

methyl yellow. Butter yellow.

methyprylon(e) (meth-i-prī′lon, -lōn). 3,3-Diethyl-2,4-dioxo-5-methylpiperidine; a sedative and hypnotic.

methysergide maleate (meth-i-ser′jīd). N-[1-(Hydroxymethyl)propyl]-1-methyl-D-lysergamide bimaleate; a serotonin antagonist, weakly adrenolytic, chemically related to methylergonovine; used in the prophylactic treatment of vascular headache (migraine); untoward effects are common.

methysticum (mĕ-this′ti-kŭm). Kava (1); the root of *Piper methysticum* (family Piperaceae), a plant of the Pacific islands, used by the natives as an intoxicant. It has been used in diarrhea and in inflammatory affection of the urogenital tract.

metMb Abbreviation for metmyoglobin.

metmyoglobin (metMb) (met′mī-ō-glō′bin). Myoglobin in which the ferrous ion of the heme prosthetic group is oxidized to ferric ion.

metoclopramide hydrochloride (met′ō-klō-pram′īd). 4-Amino-5-chloro-*N*-[2-(diethylamino)-ethyl]-*o*-anisamide hydrochloride; an antiemetic agent.

metocurine iodide (met-ō-kyūr′ēn). Dimethyl tubocurarine iodide; dimethyl *d*-tubocurarine; (+)-*O,O*′-dimethylchondrocurarine diiodide; a nondepolarizing neuromuscular blocking agent used to provide relaxation during surgical operations.

metolazone (me-tol′ă-zōn). 7-Chloro-1,2,3,4-tetrahydro-2-methyl-4-oxo-3-*o*-tolyl-6-quinazolinesulfonamide; a diuretic with antihypertensive activity.

metonymy (mĕ-ton′i-mē) [meta- + G. *ōnyma,* name]. Imprecise or circumscribed labeling of objects or events, said to be characteristic of the language disturbance of schizophrenics; *e.g.,* the patient speaks of having had a "menu" rather than a "meal."

metopagus (mĕ-top′ă-gŭs) [G. *metōpon,* forehead, + *pagos,* something fixed]. Conjoined twins united at the forehead.

metopic (me-tō′pik, me-top′ik) [G. *metōpon,* forehead]. Relating to the forehead or anterior portion of the cranium.

metopion (mĕ-tō′pē-on) [G. *metōpon,* forehead]. Metopic point; a craniometric point midway between the frontal eminences.

metopism (met′ō-pizm) [G. *metōpon,* forehead]. Persistence of the frontal suture in the adult.

metopon hydrochloride (met′ō-pon). Methyldihydromorphinone hydrochloride; a derivative of morphine with similar pharmacologic actions.

metopoplasty (met′ō-pō-plas-tē, me-top′ō-plas-tē) [G. *metōpon,* forehead, + *plastos,* formed]. Plastic surgery of the skin or bone of the forehead.

metoposcopy (met'ō-pos'kō-pē) [G. *metōpon,* forehead, + *skopeō,* to view]. The study of physiognomy.

metoprolol tartrate (me-tō'prō-lol). 1-Isopropylamino-3-[*p*-(2-methoxyethyl)phenoxy]-2-propanol (2:1) dextrotartrate salt; a *β*-adrenergic blocking agent used in the treatment of hypertension.

Metorchis (met-ōr'kis) [G. *meta,* behind, + *orchis,* testicle]. A genus of opisthorchid fish-borne flukes parasitic in the gallbladder of fish-eating mammals and birds, common in north temperate regions. *M. conjunctus* is a species that occurs in dogs and cats, and occasionally in man, in North America.

metoxenous (me-tok'sĕ-nŭs) [G. *meta,* beyond, + *xenos,* host]. Heterecious.

metoxeny (me-tok'sĕ-nē) [G. *meta,* beyond, + *xenos,* host]. **1.** Heterecism. **2.** Change of host by a parasite.

metr-, metra-, metro- [G. *mētra,* uterus]. Combining forms denoting the uterus. See also hystero- (1), utero-.

metra (mē'tră) [G. uterus]. Uterus.

metratonia (mē-tră-tō'nē-ă). [metra- + G. *a-* priv. + *tonos,* tension]. Atony of the uterine walls after childbirth.

metratrophy, metratrophia (mē-trat'rō-fē, mē-tră-trō'fē-ă) [metra- atrophy]. Uterine atrophy.

metria (mē'trē-ă) [G. *mētra,* uterus]. Pelvic cellulitis or other inflammatory affection in the puerperal period.

metric (met'rik) [G. *metrikos,* fr. *metron,* measure]. Quantitative; relating to measurement. See metric *system.*

metrifonate (me-trī'fō-nāt). Trichlorfon.

metriocephalic (met'rē-ō-se-fal'ik) [G. *metrios,* moderate, fr. *metron,* measure, + *kephalē,* head]. Having a head well proportioned to height; denoting a skull with an index between 72 and 77. See also orthocephalic.

metritis (mē-trī'tis) [G. *mētra,* uterus, + *-itis,* inflammation]. Uteritis; inflammation of the uterus.

contagious equine m., a highly contagious venereal disease of horses and other Equidae caused by a Gram-negative non-motile coccobacillus that produces an endometritis, cervicitis, and vaginitis, affecting breeding and fertility.

metrizamide (me-triz'ă-mīd). Metrizoate sodium.

metrizoate sodium (met-ri-zō'āt). Metrizamide; sodium 3-acetamido-5-(*N*-methylacetamido)-2,4,6-triiodobenzoate; a diagnostic radiopaque medium.

metro- [G. *metra,* uterus]. See metr-.

metrocyte (mē'trō-sīt) [G. *mētēr,* mother, + *kytos,* a hollow (cell)]. Mother *cell.*

metrodynamometer (mē-trō-dī'nă-mom'ĕ-ter) [metro- + G. *dynamis,* power, + *metron,* measure]. Instrument for measuring the force of uterine contractions.

metrodynia (mē-trō-dī'ē-ă) [metro- + G. *odynē,* pain]. Hysteralgia.

metrofibroma (mē'trō-fī-brō'mă). A fibroma of the uterus.

metrography (mē-trog'ră-fē) [metro- + G. *graphō,* to write]. Hysterography.

metrolymphangitis (mē'trō-lim-fan-jī'tis) [metro- + lymphangitis]. Inflammation of the uterine lymphatics.

metromalacia (mē'trō-mă-lā'shē-ă) [metro- + G. *malakia,* softness]. Metromalacoma; metromalacosis; pathologic softening of the uterine tissues.

metromalacoma, metromalacosis (mē'trō-mal-ă-kō'mă, -kō'sis). Metromalacia.

metromania (met-rō-mā'nē-ă) [G. *metron,* measure, + *mania,* frenzy]. Rarely used term for an incessant writing of verses.

metronidazole (met-rō-ni'dă-zōl). 2-Methyl-5-nitroimidazole-1-ethanol; an orally effective trichomonicide used in the treatment of infections caused by *Trichomonas vaginalis* and *Entamoeba histolytica.*

metronoscope (mĕ-tron'ō-skōp) [G. *metron,* measure, + *skopeō,* to view]. A tachistoscopic apparatus that exposes for timed intervals short selections of printed matter for reading; used in testing and developing reading speed.

metroparalysis (mē'trō-pă-ral'i-sis) [metro- + paralysis]. Flaccidity or paralysis of the uterine muscle during or immediately after childbirth.

metropathia (mē-trō-path'ē-ă) [L.]. Metropathy.

m. hemorrhag'ica, abnormal, excessive, often continuous uterine bleeding due to persistence and exaggeration of the follicular phase of the menstrual cycle; the endometrium is the seat of glandular hyperplasia with cyst formation (see Swiss cheese *endometrium*).

metropathic (mē-trō-path'ik). Relating to or caused by uterine disease.

metropathy (mē-trop'ă-thē) [metro- + G. *pathos,* suffering]. Metropathia; any disease of the uterus, especially of the myometrium.

metroperitonitis (mē'trō-per-i-tō-nī'tis) [metro- + peritonitis]. Perimetritis; inflammation of the uterus involving the peritoneal covering.

metrophlebitis (mē'trō-flĕ-bī'tis) [metro- + G. *phleps,* vein, + *-itis,* inflammation]. Inflammation of the uterine veins usually following childbirth.

metroplasty (met'trō-plas-tē, mē'trō-). Uteroplasty.

metrorrhagia (mē-trō-rā'jē-ă) [metro- + G. *rhēgnymi,* to burst forth]. Any irregular, acyclic bleeding from the uterus between periods.

m. myopath'ica, postpartum hemorrhage due to flaccidity of the uterine muscle.

metrorrhea (mē'trō-rē'ă) [metro- + G. *rhoia,* a flow]. Discharge of mucus or pus from the uterus.

metrorrhexis (mē'trō-rek'sis) [metro- + G. *rhēxis,* rupture]. Hysterorrhexis.

metrosalpingitis (mē'trō-sal-pin-jī'tis) [metro- + G. *salpinx,* trumpet (oviduct), + *-itis,* inflammation]. Inflammation of the uterus and of one or both fallopian tubes.

metrosalpingography (mē'trō-sal-pin-gog'ră-fē) [metro- + G. *salpinx,* tube, + *graphō,* to write]. Hysterosalpingography.

metroscope (mē'trō-skōp) [metro- + G. *skōpeō,* to view]. Hysteroscope.

metrostaxis (mē-trō-stak'sis) [metro- + G. *staxis,* a dripping]. Small but continuous hemorrhage of the uterine mucous membrane.

metrostenosis (mē'trō-ste-nō'sis) [metro- + G. a *stenosis,* narrowing]. A narrowing of the uterine cavity.

metrotomy (mē-trot'ō-mē) [metro- + G. *tomē,* incision]. Hysterotomy.

metyrapone (mĕ-tir'ă-pōn). Mepyrapone; 2-methyl-1,2-di-3-pyridyl-1-propanone; an inhibitor of adrenocortical steroid C-11*β* hydroxylation, administered orally or intravenously to determine the ability of the pituitary gland to increase its secretion of corticotropin; because 11-deoxycorticosteroids, as a consequence of m. administration, only weakly inhibit pituitary corticotropin secretion, the normal pituitary gland will appreciably increase its output of this hormone.

metyrosine (mĕ-tī'rō-sin, -sēn). *α*-Methyl-*p*-tyrosine, an inhibitor of tyrosine hydroxylase and therefore a powerful inhibitor of catecholamine synthesis; used for controlling the manifestations of pheochromocytoma, in preoperative preparation, or in instances where surgical resection is contraindicated or incomplete.

Mev Symbol for 1 million electron-volts.

mevalonic acid (mev-ă-lon′ik). Hiochic acid; 3,5-dihydroxy-3-methylpentanoic acid; precursor of squalene and steroids.

mevinolin (me-vin′ō-lin). Lovastatin.

mexenone (mek′sĕ-nōn). 2-Hydroxy-4-methoxy-4′-methylbenzophenone; a sun-screening agent.

Meyenburg, H. von. See M.'s *complex, disease;* M.-Altherr-Uehlinger *syndrome.*

Meyer, Adolf, U.S. psychiatrist, 1866–1950. See M.-Archambault *loop.*

Meyer, Edmund V., German laryngologist, 1864–1931. See M.'s *cartilages.*

Meyer, Georg H., Swiss anatomist, 1815–1892. See M.'s *disease, line, sinus.*

Meyer, Hans H., German pharmacologist, 1853–1939. See M.-Overton *theory* of narcosis.

Meyer, Willy, U.S. surgeon, 1854–1932. See M.'s *reagent.*

Meyer-Betz, Friedrich, 20th century German physician. See M.-B. *syndrome.*

Meyerhof, Otto F., German biochemist and Nobel laureate, 1884–1951. See Embden-M. *pathway;* Embden-M.-Parnas *pathway.*

Meyer-Schwickerath, Gerhard Rudolph Edmund, German ophthalmologist, *1920. See M.-S. *operation;* M.-S. and Weyers *syndrome.*

Meynert, Theodor H., Vienna neurologist, 1833–1892. See M.'s retroflex *bundle, cells, commissures, decussation, fasciculus, layer.*

mexiletin hydrochloride (meks-il′ĕ-tēn). 1-(2,6-Dimethylphenoxy)-2-propanamine; an orally active antiarrhythmic agent used to suppress symptomatic ventricular arrhythmias.

mezlocillin sodium (mez-lō-sil′in). $C_{21}H_{24}NaN_5O_8S_2$; an extended spectrum penicillin antibiotic used intravenously and intramuscularly.

Mg Symbol for magnesium.

mg Symbol for milligram.

MHC Abbreviation for major histocompatilibity *complex.*

mho (mō) [*ohm* reversed]. Siemens.

MHz Symbol for megahertz.

MI Abbreviation for myocardial *infarction.*

mianserin hydrochloride (mē-an′ser-in). 1,2,3,4,10,14b-Hexahydro-2-methyldibenzo[*c,f*] pyrazino-[1,2-*a*]azepine monohydrochloride; an antihistaminic with antiserotonin activity.

Mibelli, Vittorio, Italian dermatologist, 1860–1910. See M.'s *angiokeratoma, disease.*

MIC Abbreviation for minimal inhibitory *concentration.*

micellar (mī-sel′er, mi-). Having the properties of an assemblage of micelles, *i.e.,* of a gel.

micelle (mi-sel′, mī-sel′) [L. *micella,* small morsel, dim. of *mica,* morsel, grain]. Nägeli's term for elongated sub(light)microscopic particles, detected in hydrogels, of supramolecular character and crystalline structure; now defined as one of two classes of colloidal particle: those consisting of many molecules, the other class being single macromolecules light- or sub-microscopic in size. A m. is thus a structural unit of the disperse phase in a gel, a unit whose repetition in three dimensions constitutes the micellar structure of the gel; it does not denote the individual particles in free suspension or solution, or the unit structure of a crystal.

Michaelis, Leonor, U.S. chemist, 1875–1949. See M.-Gutmann *body;* M.-Menten *constant, hypothesis.*

Michel's spur. See under spur.

Micheli, Ferdinando, Italian physician, 1872–1936. See Marchiafava-M. *anemia, syndrome.*

miconazole nitrate (mī-kon′ă-zōl). 1-[2,4-Dichloro-β-[(2,4-dichlorobenzyl)oxy]phenethyl]imidazole mononitrate; an antifungal agent.

micr-. See micro-.

micracoustic (mī′kră-kū′stik) [micro- + G. *akoustikos,* relating to hearing, fr. *akouō,* to hear]. Micrococustic. **1.** Relating to faint sounds. **2.** Magnifying very faint sounds so as to make them audible.

micrencephalia (mī′kren-se-fā′lē-ă). Micrencephaly.

micrencephalous (mī-kren-sef′ă-lŭs). Having a small brain.

micrencephaly (mī-kren-sef′ă-lē) [micro- + G. *enkephalos,* brain]. Micrencephalia; microencephaly; abnormal smallness of the brain.

micro-, micr- [G. *mikros,* small] **1.** Prefixes denoting smallness. **2.** Prefix used in the SI and metric systems to signify one-millionth (10^{-6}) of such unit. **3.** In chemistry, prefix to terms denoting chemical examination, methods, etc. that utilize minimal quantities of the substance to be examined; *e.g.,* a drop or two in place of one or more milliliters. **4.** Combining forms meaning microscopic.

microabscess (mī′krō-ab′ses). A very small circumscribed collection of leukocytes in solid tissues.

Munro's m., Munro's abscess; a microscopic collection of polymorphonuclear leukocytes found in the stratum corneum in psoriasis.

Pautrier's m., Pautrier's abscess; a microscopic lesion in the epidermis, seen in mycosis fungoides; it is composed of the same type of mononuclear cells as those that form the infiltrate in the corium.

microadenoma (mī′krō-ad-ĕ-nō′mă). A pituitary adenoma less than 10 mm in diameter; may cause hypersecretion syndromes.

microaerobion (mī′krō-ā-rō′bī-on). A microaerophilic microorganism.

microaerophil, microaerophile (mī-krō-ār′ō-fil, -fīl) [micro- + G. *aēr,* air, + *philos,* fond]. **1.** An aerobic bacterium that requires oxygen, but less than is present in the air, and grows best under modified atmospheric conditions. **2.** Microaerophilic; microaerophilous; relating to such an organism.

microaerophilic (mī′krō-ār-ō-fil′ik). Microaerophil (2).

microaerophilous (mī′krō-ār-ŏf′i-lŭs). Microaerophil (2).

microaerosol (mī-krō-ār′ō-sol). A suspension in air of particles that are submicronic or, more frequently, from 1 to 10 μ in diameter.

microanalysis (mī′krō-ă-nal′i-sis). Analytic techniques involving unusually small samples.

microanastomosis (mī′krō-ă-nas-tō-mō′sis). Anastomosis of minute structures performed under a surgical microscope.

microanatomist (mī′krō-ă-nat′ō-mist). Histologist.

microanatomy (mī′krō-ă-nat′ō-mē). Histology.

microaneurysm (mī′krō-an′yū-rizm). Focal dilation of retinal capillaries occurring in diabetes mellitus, retinal vein obstruction, and absolute glaucoma, or of arteriolocapillary junctions in many organs in thrombotic thrombocytopenic purpura.

microangiography (mī′krō-an-jē-og′ră-fē). Microarteriography; the radiography of the finer vessels of an organ after the injection of a contrast medium and enlarging the resulting radiograph.

microangiopathy (mī′krō-an-jē-op′ă-thē). Capillaropathy.

thrombotic m., thrombosis within small blood vessels, as in thrombotic thrombocytopenic purpura.

microangioscopy (mī′krō-an-jē-os′kŏ-pē). Capillarioscopy.

microarteriography (mī′krō-ar-tēr-ē-og′ră-fē). Microangiography.

microbalance (mī′krō-bal-ans). A balance designed for use in weighing unusually small samples of materials.

microbe (mī′krōb) [Fr., fr. G. *mikros,* small, + *bios,* life]. Any very minute organism. As originated, the word was intended as a collective term for the large variety of microorganisms then known in the 19th century; modern usage has retained the original collective meaning but expanded it to include both microscopic and ultramicroscopic organisms (spirochetes, bacteria, rickettsiae, and viruses). These organisms are considered to form a biologically distinctive group, in that the genetic material is not surrounded by a nuclear membrane, and mitosis does not occur during replication.

microbial (mī-krō'bē-ăl). Microbic; microbiotic (2); relating to a microbe or to microbes.

Microbial associates (mī-krō'bē-ăl ă-sō'shē-ăts). Flora (2).

microbic (mī-krō'bik). Microbial.

microbicidal (mī-krō'bi-sī'dăl). Microbicide (1); destructive to microbes.

microbicide (mī-krō'bi-sīd) [microbe + L. *caedo,* to kill]. **1.** Microbicidal. **2.** An agent destructive to microbes; a germicide; an antiseptic.

microbid (mī-krō'bid) [micro- + G. *bios,* life, + *eidēs,* resembling]. Cutaneous allergic response to superficial bacterial infection.

microbiologic (mī'krō-bī-ō-loj'ik). Relating to microbiology.

microbiologist (mī'krō-bī-ol'ō-jist). Protistologist, one who specializes in the science of microbiology.

microbiology (mī'krō-bī-ol'ō-jē) [Fr. *microbiologie*]. Protistology; the science concerned with microscopic and ultramicroscopic organisms.

microbiotic (mī'krō-bī-ot'ik). **1.** Short-lived. **2.** Microbial.

microbism (mī'krō-bizm). Infection with microbes.

latent m., the presence of pathogenic microorganisms in the body that elicit no symptoms; the condition of a pathogen carrier.

microblast (mī'krō-blast) [micro- + G. *blastos,* sprout, germ]. A small, nucleated, red blood cell.

microblepharia, microblepharism, microblepharon (mī'krō-ble-far'ē-ă, -blef'ăr-izm, -blef'ă-ron) [micro- + G. *blepharon,* eyelid, + *-ia,* condition]. Eyelids with abnormal vertical shortness.

microbody (mī'krō-bod-ē). Peroxisome.

microbrachia (mī-krō-brā'kē-ă) [micro- + G. *brachiōn,* arm]. Abnormal smallness of the arms.

microbrenner (mī-krō-bren'er) [micro- + Ger. *Brenner,* burner]. An electric cautery with needle point.

microcardia (mī-krō-kar'dē-ă) [micro- + G. *kardia,* heart]. Abnormal smallness of the heart.

microcentrum (mī-krō-sen'trŭm) [micro- + G. *kentron,* center]. Cytocentrum.

microcephalia (mī-krō-se-fā'lē-ă). Microcephaly.

microcephalic (mī'krō-sĕ-fal'ik). Microcephalous; nanocephalic; nanocephalous; having a small head.

microcephalism (mī-krō-sef'ă-lizm). Microcephaly.

microcephalous (mī-krō-sef'ă-lŭs). Microcephalic.

microcephaly (mī-krō-sef'ă-lē) [micro- + G. *kephalē,* head]. Microcephalia; microcephalism; nanocephalia; nanocephaly; abnormal smallness of the head; applied to a skull with a capacity below 1350 cc.

encephaloclastic m., complex growth disturbances in the brain as a result of regressive changes in fetal life.

schizencephalic m., dysgenic process resulting in focal cerebral defects.

microcheilia, microchilia (mī-krō-kī'lē-ă) [micro- + G. *cheilos,* lip]. Smallness of the lips.

microcheiria, microchiria (mī-krō-kī'rē-ă) [micro- + G. *cheir,* hand]. Smallness of the hands.

microchemistry (mī-krō-kem'is-trē). The use of chemical procedures involving minute quantities or reactions not visible to the unaided eye. *Cf.* macrochemistry.

microchilia (mī-krō-kī'lē-ă). Microcheilia.

microchiria (mī-krō-kī'rē-ă). Microcheiria.

microcide (mī'krō-sīd). *Glucose* oxidase.

microcinematography (mī'kro-sin-ĕ-mă-tog'ră-fē) [micro- + G. *kinēma,* movement, + *graphō,* to write]. The application of moving pictures taken through magnifying lenses to the study of an organ or system in motion; *e.g.,* the circulation in living embryos.

microcirculation (mī'krō-sir-kyū-lā'shŭn). Passage of blood in the smallest vessels, namely arterioles, capillaries, and venules.

Micrococcaceae (mī'krō-kok-ā'sē-ē). A family of bacteria (order Eubacteriales) containing Gram-positive spherical cells which occur singly or in pairs, tetrads, packets, irregular masses, or even chains. Rarely are these organisms motile. Free living, saprophytic, parasitic, and pathogenic species occur. The type genus is *Micrococcus.*

micrococci (mī'krō-kok'sī). Plural of micrococcus.

Micrococcus (mī'krō-kok-ŭs) [micro- + G. *kokkos,* berry]. A genus of bacteria (family Micrococcaceae) containing Gram-positive, spherical cells that occur in irregular masses, never in packets. Some species are motile or produce motile mutants. These organisms are saprophytic, facultatively parasitic, or parasitic but are not truly pathogenic. The type species is *M. luteus.* It is the type genus of the family Micrococcaceae.

M. can'didus, a species found in skin secretions, milk, and dairy products.

M. conglomera'tus, a species found in infections, milk, dairy products, dairy utensils, and water.

M. cryoph'ilus, a species found in frozen meat products.

M. fla'vus, a species found in skin gland secretions, milk, dairy products, and dairy utensils.

M. lu'teus, a saphrophytic species found in milk and dairy products and on dust particles; it is the type species of the genus *M.*

M. morrhu'a, a species found in sea-water brine, sea salt, and salt lakes; also found in association with a red discoloration of salted fish.

M. ure'ae, a species found in stale urine or in soil containing urine.

M. var'ians, a species found in body secretions, dairy products, dairy utensils, dust, and fresh and salt water.

micrococcus, pl. **micrococci** (mī'krō-kok'ŭs, -kok'sī). A vernacular term used to refer to any member of the genus *Micrococcus.*

microcolitis (mī'krō-kō-lī'tis). Colitis which is not seen by endoscopy, but in which microscopic examination of biopsies shows nonspecific mucosal inflammation.

microcolon (mī'krō-kō-lon). A small colon, often arising from a decreased functional state.

microconidium, pl. **microconidia** (mī'krō-kō-nid'ē-ŭm, -ă). In fungi, the smaller of two distinctively different-sized types of conidia in a single species, usually single-celled and spherical, ovoid, pyriform, or clavate.

microcoria (mī-krō-kō'rē-ă) [micro- + G. *korē,* pupil]. A congenitally small pupil with an inability to dilate.

microcornea (mī'krō-kōr'nē-ă). An abnormally small cornea.

microcoulomb (mī-krō-kū'lom). One-millionth of a coulomb.

microcoustic (mī'krō-kū'stik). Micracoustic.

microcrystalline (mī'krō-krys'tă-lin). Occurring in minute crystals.

microcurie (μ**Ci**) (mī'krō-kyū'rē). A measure of radium emanation, one-millionth of a curie; 3.7×10^4 disintegrations per second.

microcyst (mī'krō-sist). A tiny cyst, frequently of such dimensions that a magnifying lens or microscope is required for observation.

microcyte (mī'krō-sīt) [micro- + G. *kytos,* cell]. Microerythrocyte; a small (5 μm or less) non-nucleated red blood cell.

microcythemia (mī'krō-sī-thē'mē-ă) [microcyte + G. *haima,* blood]. Microcytosis; the presence of many microcytes in the circulating blood.

microcytosis (mī'krō-sī-tō'sis) [microcyte + G. *-osis,* condition]. Microcythemia.

microdactylia (mī'krō-dak-til'ē-ă). Microdactyly.

microdactylous (mī-krō-dak'ti-lŭs). Relating to or characterized by microdactyly.

microdactyly (mī-krō-dak'ti-lē) [micro- + G. *dactylos,* finger, toe]. Microdactylia; smallness or shortness of the fingers or toes.

microdissection (mī'krō-di-sek'shŭn). Dissection of tissues under a microscope or magnifying glass, usually done by teasing the tissues apart by means of needles.

microdont (mī'krō-dont) [micro- + G. *odous (odont-),* tooth]. Having small teeth; denoting a skull with a dental index below 41.9.

microdontia, microdontism (mī-krō-don'shē-ă, -don'tizm) [micro- + G. *odous,* tooth]. A condition in which a single tooth, or pairs of teeth, or the whole dentition, may be disproportionately small.

microdose (mī'krō-dōs). A very small dose.

microdrepanocytosis (mī'krō-drep'ă-nō-sī-tō'sis) [microcytosis + drepanocytosis]. A chronic hemolytic anemia resulting from interaction of the genes for sickle cell anemia and thalassemia.

microdysgenesia (mī'krō-dis-ge-nē'sē-ă). Increase in partially distopic neurons in the stratum zonale, white matter, hippocampus and cerebellar cortex, producing an indistinct border between cortex and subcortical white matter and a columnar arrangement of cortical neurons; seen in patients with primary generalized epilepsy.

microelectrode (mī'krō-ē-lek'trōd). An electrode of very fine caliber consisting usually of a fine wire or a glass tube of capillary diameter (10 μm to 1 mm) drawn to a fine point and filled with saline or a metal such as gallium or indium (while melted); used in physiologic experiments to stimulate or to record action currents of extracellular or intracellular origin.

microencephaly (mī'krō-en-sef'ă-lē). Micrencephaly.

microerythrocyte (mī'krō-ĕ-rith'rō-sīt). Microcyte.

microevolution (mī'krō-ev-ŏ-lū'shŭn). The evolution of bacteria and other microorganisms through mutations.

microfibril (mi-kro-fi'bril). A very small fibril having an average diameter of 130 Å; it may be a bundle of still smaller elements, the microfilaments.

microfilament (mī-krō-fil'ă-ment). The finest filamentous element of the cytoskeleton, having a diameter of about 5 nm and consisting primarily of actin. See also actin filament.

microfilaremia (mī'krō-fil-ă-rē'mē-ă). Infection of the blood with microfilariae. M. caused by *Wuchereria bancrofti* is characterized by sharp nocturnal periodicity, apparently tied to the nocturnal habits of the vector mosquitoes; in geographic areas where mosquitoes are not strictly night-biters (as in parts of Polynesia), the microfilarial periodicity is modified or absent. See also periodic *filariasis.*

microfilaria, pl. **microfilariae** (mī'krō-fi-lar'ē-ă, -ē). Term for embryos of filarial nematodes in the family Onchocercidae. See *Filaria.* In the past this term has been used as a generic designation (e.g., *Microfilaria bancrofti, M. malaya*).

microgamete (mī-krō-gam'ēt) [micro- + G. *gametēs,* husband]. The male element in anisogamy, or conjugation of cells of unequal size; it is the smaller of the two cells and actively motile.

microgametocyte (mī-krō-gam'ĕ-tō-sīt). Microgamont; the mother cell producing the microgametes, or male elements of sexual reproduction in sporozoan protozoans and fungi.

microgamont (mī-krō-gam'ont). Microgametocyte.

microgamy (mī-krog'ă-mē) [micro- + G. *gamos,* marriage]. Conjugation between two young cells, the recent product of sporulation or some other form of reproduction.

microgastria (mī-krō-gas'trē-ă) [micro- + G. *gastēr,* stomach]. Smallness of the stomach.

microgenia (mī-krō-jēn'ē-ă) [micro- + G. *geneion,* chin]. Abnormal smallness of the chin.

microgenitalism (mī-krō-jen'i-tal-izm). Abnormal smallness of the external genital organs.

microglia (mī-krog'lē-ă) [micro- + G. *glia,* glue]. Microglia or microglial cells; Hortega cells; small neuroglial cells, possibly of mesodermal origin, which may become phagocytic, in areas of neural damage or inflammation.

microgliacyte (mī-krōg'lē-ă-sīt) [micro- + G. *glia,* glue, + *kytos,* cell]. A cell, especially an embryonic cell, of the microglia.

microglioma (mī-krog'lē-ō'mă) [microglia + G. *-oma,* tumor]. An intracranial neoplasm of microglial cell origin that is structurally similar to reticulum cell sarcoma.

microgliomatosis (mī'krō-glē-ō-mă-tō'sis). A condition characterized by the presence of multiple microgliomas.

microgliosis (mī-krog'lē-ō'sis) [microglia + G. *-osis,* condition]. Presence of microglia in nervous tissue secondary to injury.

microglossia (mī-krō-glos'ē-ă) [micro- + G. *glōssa,* tongue]. Smallness of the tongue.

micrognathia (mī-krō-nā'thē-ă, mī-krog-nath'ē-ă) [micro- + G. *gnathos,* jaw]. Abnormal smallness of the jaws, especially of the mandible.

m. with peromelia, Hanhart's syndrome; hypoplasia of the mandible with malformed and missing teeth, birdlike face, and severe deformities of the hands and forearms and sometimes of feet and legs.

microgram (μg) (mī'krō-gram). One-millionth of a gram.

micrograph (mī'krō-graf) [micro- + G. *graphō,* to write]. **1.** An instrument that magnifies the microscopic movements of a diaphragm by means of light interference and records them on a moving photographic film; may be used for recording various pulse curves, sound waves, and any forms of motion that may be communicated through the air to a diaphragm. **2.** Photomicrograph.

electron m., the image produced by the electron beam of an electron microscope, recorded on an electron-sensitive plate or film.

micrography (mī-krog'ră-fē) [micro- + G. *graphō,* to write]. **1.** Writing with very minute letters, sometimes observed in psychoses and in paralysis agitans. **2.** A description of objects seen with a microscope. **3.** Photomicrography.

microgyria (mī-krō-jī'rē-ă) [micro- + G. *gyros,* convolution]. Abnormal narrowness of the cerebral convolutions.

microhepatia (mī-krō-he-pat'ē-ă) [micro- + G. *hepar (hepat-),* liver]. Abnormal smallness of the liver.

microhm (mī'krōm). Micro-ohm; one-millionth of an ohm.

microincineration (mī'krō-in-sin'ĕ-rā'shŭn). Spodography; combustion, in a furnace, of organic constituents in a tissue section so that the remaining mineral ash can be examined microscopically.

microincision (mī-krō-in-sizh'ŭn). An incision made with the aid of a microscope.

microinvasion (mī'krō-in-vā'zhŭn). Invasion of tissue immediately adjacent to a carcinoma in situ, the earliest stage of malignant neoplastic invasion.

microkymatotherapy (mī'krō-kī-mat'ō-thār'ă-pē) [micro- + G. *kyma,* a wave, + *therapeia,* treatment]. Microwave therapy; treatment with high frequency radiations of 3,000,000,000 Hz (3000

MHz), at a wavelength of 10 cm.

microleukoblast (mī-krō-lū'kō-blast). Micromyeloblast.

microliter (uL,μl) (mī'krō-lē-ter). One-millionth of a liter.

microlith (mī'krō-lith) [micro- + G. *lithos,* stone]. A minute calculus, usually multiple and constituting a coarse sand called gravel.

microlithiasis (mī-krō-li-thī'ă-sis). The formation, presence, or discharge of minute concretions, or gravel.

pulmonary alveolar m., microscopic granules of calcium or bone disseminated throughout the lungs.

micrology (mī-krol'ō-jē) [micro- + G. *logos,* study]. The science concerned with microscopic objects, of which histology is a branch.

micromania (mī-krō-mā'nē-ă) [micro- + G. *mania,* frenzy]. A delusion of self-depreciation, or that one's own body is of minute size.

micromanipulation (mī'krō-mă-nip'yū-lā'shŭn). Dissection, teasing, stimulation, etc., under the microscope, of minute structures; *e.g.,* tissue cells or unicellular organisms.

micromanipulator (mī'krō-mă-nip'yū-lā'ter, -tōr). An instrument used in micromanipulation, whereby microdissection, microinjection, and other maneuvers are performed, usually with the aid of a microscope.

micromazia (mī-krō-mā'zē-ă) [micro- + G. *mazos,* breast]. Condition in which the breasts are rudimentary and functionless.

micromelia (mī-krō-mē'lē-ă) [micro- + G. *melos,* limb]. Nanomelia; condition of having disproportionately short or small limbs. See also achondroplasia.

micromere (mī'krō-mēr) [micro- + G. *meros,* a part]. A blastomere of small size.

micromerozoite (mī'krō-mer-ō-zō'īt). A small merozoite.

micrometastasis (mī'krō-mĕ-tas'tă-sis). A stage of metastasis when the secondary tumors are too small to be clinically detected, as in micrometastatic disease.

micrometastatic (mī'krō-met-ă-stat'ik). Denoting or characterized by micrometastasis, as in m. disease.

micrometer (μm) (mī'krō-mē-ter). One-millionth of a meter.

micrometer (mī-krom'ĕ-ter) [micro- + G. *metron,* measure]. A device for measuring various types of objects in an accurate and precise manner; in medicine and biology, the term is usually used with reference to a glass slide or lens that is accurately marked for measuring microscopic forms.

caliper m., a gauge with a calibrated m. screw for the measurement of thin objects such as microscope cover glasses and slides.

filar m., an ocular micrometer with a line moved by a ruled drum such that a movement of the line of 0.005 mm or less may be made in relation to fixed parallel lines.

ocular m., a glass disk that fits in a microscope eyepiece and that has a ruled scale; when calibrated with a slide m., direct measurements of a microscopic object can be made.

slide m., a scale made on a microscope slide with lines ruled in divisions, usually, of 0.01 mm.

micrometry (mī-krom'ĕ-trē). Measurement of objects with some type of micrometer and a microscope.

micromicro- (μμ). Prefix formerly used to signify one-trillionth (10^{-12}); now pico-.

micromicrogram (μμg) (mī'krō-mī'krō-gram). Former term for picogram.

micromicron (μμ) (mī-kro-mī'kron). Former term for picometer.

micromolar (mī-krō-mō'lar). Denoting a concentration of 10^{-6} mole per liter (10^{-6} M or 1 μM).

micromole (μmol) (mī'krō-mōl). One-millionth of a mole.

micromotoscope (mī'krō-mō'tō-skōp) [micro- + L. *motus,* motion, + G. *skopeō,* to view]. A cinematoscope for representing the movements of amebas and other motile microscopic objects.

micromyelia (mī'krō-mī-ē'lē-ă) [micro- + G. *myelos,* marrow]. Abnormal smallness or shortness of the spinal cord.

micromyeloblast (mī-krō-mī'el-ō-blast). Microleukoblast; a small myeloblast, often the predominating cell in myeloblastic leukemia.

micron (μ) (mī'kron). Former term for micrometer.

microneedle (mī'krō-nē'dl). A small glass needle used in micrurgical manipulation.

microneme (mī'krō-nēm) [micro- + G. *nema,* thread]. Sarconeme; a small, osmiophilic, cordlike twisted organelle found in the anterior region of many sporozoans; one of the characteristics that helps to define the subphylum Apicomplexa.

micronic (mī-kron'ik). Of the size of 1 micron (micrometer).

micronodular (mī'krō-nod'yū-lăr) [G. *mikros,* small]. Characterized by the presence of minute nodules; denoting a somewhat coarser appearance than that of a granular tissue or substance.

micronucleus (mī-krō-nū'klē-ŭs). **1.** A small nucleus in a large cell, or the smaller nuclei in cells that have two or more such structures. **2.** Gametic, germ, gonad, or reproductive nucleus; karyogonad; the smaller of the two nuclei in ciliates dividing mitotically and bearing specific inheritable material. See also macronucleus (2).

micronutrients (mī-krō-nū'trē-ents). Essential food factors required in only small quantities by the body; *e.g.,* vitamins, trace minerals.

micronychia (mī-krō-nik'ē-ă) [micro- + G. *onyx,* nail]. Abnormal smallness of nails.

micronystagmus (mī'krō-nis-tag'mŭs) [micro- + G. *nystagmos,* a nodding]. Minimal amplitude nystagmus; nystagmus of so small an amplitude that it is not detected by the usual clinical tests.

micro-ohm (mī'krō-ōm). Microhm.

microorganism (mī'krō-ōr'gan-izm). A microscopic organism (plant or animal).

microparasite (mī-krō-par'ă-sīt). A parasitic microorganism.

micropathology (mī'krō-pa-thol'ō-jē) [micro- + G. *pathos,* suffering, + *logos,* study]. The microscopic study of disease changes.

micropenis (mī-krō-pē'nis). Microphallus; abnormally small penis.

microphage (mī'krō-fāj) [micro- + phag(ocyte)]. Microphagocyte; a polymorphonuclear leukocyte that is phagocytic. See also phagocyte.

microphagocyte (mī-krō-fāj'ō-sīt). Microphage.

microphallus (mī-krō-fal'ŭs). Micropenis.

microphobia (mī-krō-fō'bē-ă) [micro- + G. *phobos,* fear]. Fear of minute objects, microorganisms, germs, etc.

microphone (mī'krō-fōn) [micro- + G. *phōnē,* sound]. An instrument for magnifying sounds or for converting sounds to electrical impulses.

microphonia, microphony (mī-krō-fō'nē-ă, mī-krof'ō-nē) [micro- + G. *phōnē,* voice]. Hypophonia.

microphonoscope (mī-krō-fō'nō-skōp). A stethoscope with a diaphragm attachment for magnifying the sound.

microphotograph (mī-krō-fō'tō-graf). A minute photograph of any object, as distinguished from a photomicrograph.

microphthalmia, microphthalmos (mī'krof-thal'mē-ă, -thal'mos) [micro- + G. *ophthalmos,* eye]. Nanophthalmia; nanophthalmos; abnormal smallness of one or both eyeballs.

micropipette, micropipet (mī'krō-pi-pet', -pī-pet'). A pipette designed for the measurement of very small volumes.

microplania (mī-krō-plā'nē-ă) [micro- + L. *planus,* flat]. Decreased horizontal diameter of erythrocytes.

microplasia (mī-krō-plā'zē-ă) [micro- + G. *plasis,* a shaping, forming]. Stunted growth, as in dwarfism.

microplethysmography (mī'krō-pleth-iz-mog'ră-fē). The technique of measuring minute changes in the volume of a part as a result of blood flow into or out of it.

micropodia (mī-krō-pō'dē-ă) [micro- + G. *pous*, foot]. Abnormal smallness of the feet.

micropore (mī'krō-pōr) [micro- + G. *poros*, pore]. An organelle formed by the pellicle of all stages of sporozoan protozoa of the subphylum Apicomplexa and also found in developmental stages that may lack the inner pellicle layer; it is composed of two concentric rings (in transverse section), the inner of which corresponds with an invagination of the outer pellicle membrane. M.'s thus far observed seem to serve as feeding organelles; their role in nonfeeding developmental forms is unknown.

micropromyelocyte (mī'krō-prō-mī'el-ō-sīt). A cell derived from a promyelocyte.

microprosopia (mī'krō-prō-sō'pē-ă) [micro- + G. *prosōpon*, face]. A condition characterized by an abnormally small or imperfectly developed face.

micropsia (mī-krop'sē-ă) [micro- + G. *opsis*, sight]. Perception of objects as smaller than they are.

micropuncture (mī'krō-pŭnk-chūr). A puncture made with the aid of a microscope.

micropyle (mī'krō-pīl) [micro- + G. *pylē*, gate]. **1.** Minute opening believed to exist in the investing membrane of certain ova as a point of entrance for the spermatozoon. **2.** Former name for micropore.

microradiography (mī'krō-rā-dē-og'ră-fē). Making radiographs that can be enlarged.

microrefractometer (mī'krō-rē-frak-tom'ĕ-ter). A refractometer used in the study of blood cells.

microrespirometer (mī'krō-res-pi-rom'ĕ-ter). An apparatus for measuring the utilization of oxygen by small particles of isolated tissues or cells or particles of cells.

microsaccades (mī'krō-să-kādz') [micro- + Fr. *saccade*, sudden check (of a horse)]. Minute to and fro movements of the eyes.

microscintigraphy (mī'krō-sin-tig'ră-fē). Imaging of small anatomic structures by use of a radionuclide in conjunction with a special collimator which "magnifies" the image; specifically, the use of technetium-99m in conjunction with a pinhole collimator to image the lacrimal drainage.

microscope (mī'krō-skōp) [micro- + G. *skopeō*, to view]. An instrument that gives an enlarged image of an object or substance that is minute or not visible with the naked eye; usually the term denotes a compound m.; for low magnifications the term simple m., or magnifying glass, is used.

binocular m., a m. having two eyepieces; it may be a compound m. or a stereoscopic m.

color-contrast m., a type of m. in which the condenser stop is of one color and the annulus is a complement of it so that unstained objects are observed in one color on a field of the other.

comparator m., a device constructed with one or more m.'s having micrometer eyepieces used to measure dimensional changes during setting or temperature changes.

compound m., a m. having two or more lenses.

dark-field m., a m. that has a special condenser and objective with a diaphragm or stop such that light is scattered from the object observed, with the result that the object appears bright on a dark background.

electron m., a visual and photographic m. in which electron beams with wavelengths thousands of times shorter than visible light are utilized in place of light, thereby allowing much greater resolution and magnification; in this technique, the electrons are transmitted through a very thin section of an embedded dehydrated specimen maintained in a vacuum.

fluorescence m., see fluorescence *microscopy*.

flying spot m., a m. in which a moving spot of light is imaged in the object plane, the energy transmitted by the specimen being detected with a photoelectric cell; the light source may be a cathode ray tube, a scanning disk or drum, or an oscillating mirror.

Greenough m., stereoscopic m.

infrared m., a m. that is equipped with infrared transmitting optics and that measures the infrared absorption of minute samples with the aid of photoelectric cells; images may be observed with image converters or television.

interference m., a specially constructed m. in which the entering light is split into two beams which pass through the specimen and are recombined in the image plane where interference effects make transparent (invisible) refractile object details become visible as intensity differences; permits measurements of light retardation, index of refraction, and thickness and mass of specimen, and is useful in the examination of living or unstained cells.

laser m., a m. in which a laser beam is focused on a microscopic field, causing it to vaporize; the emitted radiation is analyzed by means of a microspectrophotometer; at a low intensity the laser is employed as the light source in an interference m.

opaque m., epimicroscope.

operating m., surgical m.

phase m., phase-contrast m., a specially constructed m. that has a special condenser and objective containing a phase-shifting ring whereby small differences in index of refraction are made visible as intensity or contrast differences in the image; particularly useful for examining structural details in transparent specimens such as living or unstained cells and tissues.

polarizing m., a m. equipped with a polarizing filter below and above the specimen which forms an image by the influence of specimen birefringence on polarized light; the polarizing direction of the two filters is typically adjustable which, together with a graduated rotating stage, permits measurement of the angular value of different refractive indices in either biological or chemical specimens.

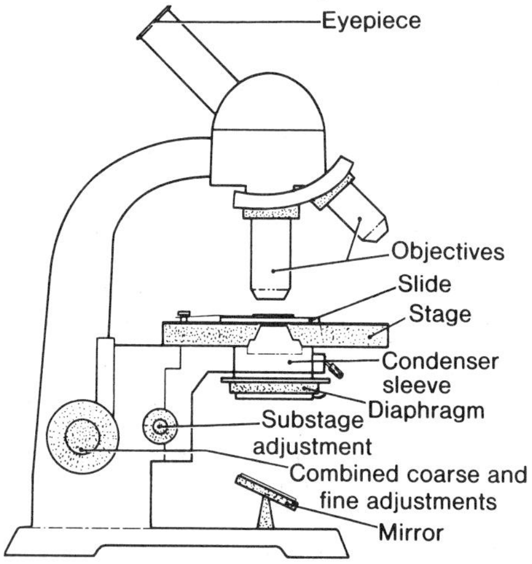

Compound Light Microscope

Rheinberg m., a modified form of dark-field m. in which the central opaque stop in the condenser is replaced by a colored filter, producing a background of contrasting color against which the specimen is illuminated.

scanning electron m., a m. in which the object in a vacuum is scanned in a wide pattern by a slender electron beam, generating reflected and secondary electrons from the specimen surface which are used to modulate the image on a synchronously scanned cathode ray tube; with this method a three-dimensional image is obtained, with both high resolution and great depth of focus.

simple m., single m., a m. that has a single magnifying lens.

stereoscopic m., Greenough m.; a m. having double eyepieces and objectives and thus independent light paths, giving a three-dimensional image.

stroboscopic m., a m. which has a light source that flashes at a constant rate so that an analysis of the motility of an object may be made; it may be used for high speed or low speed (time-lapse) cinephotomicrography.

surgical m., operating m.; a binocular m. used to obtain good visualization of fine structures in the operating field; in the standing type of m., a motorized zoom lens system operated by hand or foot controls provides an adjustable working distance; in headborne models, interchangeable oculars provide the magnification needed.

television m., a m. in which the image is observed by a television camera which produces a television display; it is used for quantitative studies, display to a large audience, or examinations in ultraviolet and infrared regions of the spectrum.

ultra-m., see ultramicroscope.

ultrasonic m., a m. that has lenses designed to use acoustic energy so that the ultrasonic wavelengths may be utilized; by means of transducers, the information is translated to a form that may be visualized or recorded.

ultraviolet m., a m. having optics of quartz and fluorite which allow transmission of light waves shorter than those of the visible spectrum, *i.e.,* below 400 nm; the image is made visible by photography, fluorescence of special glasses, or television; in a scanning instrument the receptor is a multiplier phototube.

x-ray m., a m. in which images are obtained by using x-rays as an energy source which are recorded on a very fine-grained film, or the image is enlarged by projection; if film is used, it may be examined with the light m. at fairly high magnifications.

microscopic, microscopical (mī-krō-skop'ik, -i-kăl). **1.** Of minute size; visible only with the aid of the microscope. **2.** Relating to a microscope.

microscopy (mī-kros'kō-pē). Investigation of minute objects by means of a microscope.

electron m., examination of minute objects by use of an electron microscope.

fluorescence m., a procedure based on the fact that fluorescent materials emit visible light when they are irradiated with ultraviolet or violet-blue visible rays; some materials manifest this property naturally, whereas others may be treated with fluorescent solutions (somewhat analogous to staining); when the absorption of the specimen is in the relatively long ultraviolet range, a filter that transmits these radiations is used, and a yellow filter is placed on or in the ocular; the background field is then dark, and any yellow or red fluorescence becomes visible.

immersion m., see immersion (3).

immune electron m., electron m. of biological specimens to which specific antibody has been bound.

immunofluorescence m., see immunofluorescence.

microseme (mī'krō-sēm) [micro- + G. *sēma,* sign]. Denoting a skull with an orbital index below 84.

microsides (mī'krō-sīdz). Fatty acid esters of trehalose and mannose isolated from diphtheria bacilli.

microsmatic (mī'kroz-mat'ik) [micro- + G. *osmē,* sense of smell]. Having a weakly developed sense of smell.

microsome (mī'krō-sōm) [micro- + G. *sōma,* body]. One of the small spherical vesicles derived from the endoplasmic reticulum after disruption of cells and ultracentrifugation.

microsomia (mī-krō-sō'mē-ă) [micro- + G. *sōma,* body]. Nanocormia; abnormal smallness of body, as in dwarfism.

microspectrophotometry (mī'krō-spek-trō-fō-tom'ĕ-trē). A technique for characterizing and quantitating nucleoproteins in single cells or cell organelles by their natural absorption spectra (ultraviolet) or after binding stoichiometrically in selective cytochemical staining reactions, as in the Feulgen stain for DNA. See also cytophotometry.

microspectroscope (mī-krō-spek'trō-skōp). An instrument for observing the optical spectrum of microscopic objects.

microspherocytosis (mī'krō-sfēr'ō-sī-tō'sis). A condition of the blood seen in hemolytic icterus in which small spherocytes are predominant; the red blood cells are smaller and more globular than normal.

microsphygmy (mī'krō-sfig'mē) [micro- + G. *sphygmos,* pulse]. Microsphyxia; smallness of the pulse.

microsphyxia (mī-krō-sfik'sē-ă) [micro- + G. *sphyxis,* pulse]. Microsphygmy.

microsplanchnic (mī-krō-splangk'nik) [micro- + G. *splanchna,* viscera]. Referring to smallness of the abdominal viscera.

microsplenia (mī-krō-sple'nē-ă). Abnormal smallness of the spleen.

Microspora (mī-krō-spōr'ă) [micro- + G. *sporos,* seed]. Cnidospora; a protozoan phylum that includes the genus *Nosema* and *Encephalitozoon,* and is characterized by the presence of unicellular spores with an imperforate wall and an extrusion apparatus having a polar tube and a polar cap; mitochondria are absent. They are intracellular parasites of invertebrates and lower vertebrates, with rare examples in higher vertebrates.

Microsporasida (mī'krō-spōr-as'i-dă). Microsporida.

Microsporida (mī-krō-spō'ri-dă). Microsporasida; Cnidosporidia; an order of the protozoan class Microsporea and phylum Microspora, characterized by minute spores with a single long, coiled, tubular filament enclosing the infective cell or sporoplasm. They are typically parasites of invertebrates and lower vertebrates, although fish and higher vertebrates (including man) have been infected. The order includes genera such as *Encephalitozoon* and *Nosema.*

Microsporum (mī-kros'pŏ-rŭm, mī-krō-spō'rŭm) [micro- + G. *sporos,* seed]. A genus of pathogenic fungi causing dermatophytosis. In appropriate culture media, characteristic macroconidia are seen; microconidia are rare in most species.

M. audoui'nii, an anthrophilic species that used to cause epidemic tinea capitis in children.

M. ca'nis, the principal cause of ringworm in dogs and cats and a zoophilic species causing sporadic dermatophytosis in man.

M. distor'tum, a zoophilic species that causes dermatophytosis in man and animals; seen among laboratory animal handlers.

M. ferrugin'eum, an anthropophilic species that causes dermatophytosis, primarily in Japan and the Far East.

M. ful'vum, a geophilic species that causes dermatophytosis in man and is a member of the *M. gypseum* complex whose ascomycetous state elevates it to the rank of a specific species.

M. gal'linae, a species that causes dermatophytosis in fowl and, occasionally, in man; due to its broadly clavate macroconidia, it was until recently erroneously classified as a species of *Trichophyton.*

M. gyp'seum, a cause of ringworm in dogs and horses and occasionally other animal species; a geophilic complex of species causing sporadic dermatophytosis in man.

M. na'num, a geophilic species that is the principal cause of ringworm in pigs; rarely causes dermatophytosis in man.

M. persic'olor, a geophilic species that causes dermatophytosis in voles, field voles, and, occasionally, man; its ascomycetous state is *Nannizzia persicolor.*

M. vanbreusegh'emi, a zoophilic species that causes dermatophytosis in dogs and squirrels, and occasionally in man.

microstethophone (mī-krō-steth'ō-fōn) [micro- + G. *stēthos,* chest, + *phōnē,* sound]. Microstethoscope.

microstethoscope (mī-krō-steth′ō-skōp). Microstethophone; a stethoscope that amplifies the sounds heard.

microstomia (mī-krō-stō′mē-ă) [micro- + G. *stoma*, mouth]. Smallness of the oral aperture.

microsurgery (mī-krō-ser′jer-ē). Surgical procedures performed under the magnification of a surgical microscope.

microsuture (mī-krō-sū′chūr). Tiny caliber suture material, often 9-0 or 10-0, with an attached needle of corresponding size, for use in microsurgery.

microsyringe (mī′krō-si-rinj′). A hypodermic syringe having a micrometer screw attached to the piston, whereby accurately measured minute quantities of fluid may be injected.

microthelia (mī-krō-thē′lē-ă) [micro- + G. *thēlē*, nipple]. Smallness of the nipples.

microtia (mī-krō′shē-ă) [micro- + G. *ous*, ear]. Smallness of the auricle or pinna of the ear.

microtome (mī′krō-tōm). Histotome; an instrument for making sections of biological tissue for examination under the microscope. See also ultramicrotome.

microtomy (mī-krot′ō-mē) [micro- + G. *tomē*, incision]. Histotomy; the making of thin sections of tissues for examination under the microscope.

microtonometer (mī′krō-tō-nom′ĕ-ter) [micro- + G. *tonos*, tone, + *metron*, measure]. A small tonometer invented by Krogh, originally intended for animals but later adapted to man, for determining the tensions of oxygen and carbon dioxide in arterial blood; it provides the means of bringing a small bubble of air into gaseous equilibrium with a sample of blood obtained by arterial puncture.

Microtrombidium (mī′krō-trom-bid′ē-ŭm) [micro- + Mod. L. *trombidium*, a timid one]. A genus of chigger or harvest mites that cause severe itching from the presence of the larval stage (chigger) in the skin.

microtropia (mī-krō-trō′pē-ă) [micro- + G. *tropē*, a turn, turning]. Strabismus of less than four degrees, associated with amblyopia, eccentric fixation, or anomalous retinal correspondence.

microtubule (mī-krō-tū′byūl). A cylindrical cytoplasmic element, 200 to 270 Å in diameter and of variable length, that occurs widely in the cytoskeleton of plant and animal cells; m.'s increase in number during mitosis and meiosis, where they may be related to movement of the chromosomes or chromatids on the nuclear spindle during nuclear division.

subpellicular m., subpellicular fibril; a m. lying beneath the unit membrane (pellicle) of many protozoans, often as a palisade of longitudinally arranged fibrils connected by fine lateral bridges that support the external cell form; in certain sporozoan stages a fixed number of m.'s are found, extending longitudinally from the polar ring.

microvesicle (mī-krō-ves′i-kl). A space formed within the epidermis that is too small to be recognized as a blister.

microvillus, pl. **microvilli** (mī-krō-vil′ŭs, -vil′ī). One of the minute projections of cell membranes greatly increasing surface area; microvilli form the striated or brush borders of certain cells.

Microviridae (mī-krō-vir′i-dē). Provisional name for a family of small, spherical, bacterial viruses with a genome of single-stranded DNA (MW 1.7 × 10^6); includes the genus *Morulavirus*.

microvolt (μV) (mī′krō-vōlt). One-millionth of a volt.

microwaves (mī′krō-wāvz). Microelectric waves; that portion of the radio wave spectrum of shortest wavelength, including the region with wavelengths of 1 mm to 30 cm (1000 to 300,000 megacycles per second).

microwelding (mī-krō-weld′ing). A method of fastening or joining stainless steel sutures or such sutures to needles.

microxyphil (mī-krok′si-fil) [micro- + G. *oxys*, acid, + *philos*, fond]. A multinuclear oxyphil leukocyte.

microzoon (mī-krō-zō′on) [micro- + G. *zōon*, animal]. A microscopic form of the animal kingdom; a protozoon.

micrurgical (mī-krer′ji-kăl) [micro- + G. *ergon*, work]. Relating to procedures performed on minute structures under a microscope.

miction (mik′shŭn). Urination.

micturate (mik′chū-rāt) [see micturition]. Urinate.

micturition (mik-chū-rish′ŭn) [L. *micturio*, to desire to make water]. **1.** Urination. **2.** The desire to urinate. **3.** Frequency of urination.

M.I.D. Abbreviation for minimal infecting *dose*.

mid- [A.S. *mid, midd*]. Combining form meaning middle.

midazolam (mi-daz′ō-lam). $C_{18}H_{13}ClFN_3$; a benzodiazepine with sedative and anxiolytic properties; used as an intravenous anesthetic.

midazolam hydrochloride. 8-Chloro-6-(6-fluorophenyl)-1-methyl-4*H*- imidazo[1,5-*a*][1,4]benzodiazepine monohydrochloride; a short-acting injectable benzodiazapine central nervous system depressant used for preoperative sedation.

midbody (mid′bod′ē). intermediate body of Flemming; a dense stalk of residual interzonal spindle fibers (microtubules) and actin-containing filaments that connects daughter cells during telophase.

midbrain (mid′brān). Mesencephalon.

midcarpal (mid′kar-păl). Mediocarpal.

midgracile (mid-gras′il). Denoting an occasional fissure dividing the gracile lobe of the cerebellum into two parts.

midgut (mid′gŭt). **1.** The central portion of the digestive tube; the small intestine. **2.** The portion of the embryonic gut tract between the foregut and the hindgut.

midmenstrual (mid′men′strū-ăl). Denoting the period about midway between two menstrual periods.

midoccipital (mid′ok-sip′i-tăl). Medioccipital; relating to the central portion of the occiput.

midpain (mid′pān). Intermenstrual *pain* (1).

midplane (mid′plān). Pelvic *plane* of least dimensions.

midriff (mid′rif) [A.S. *mid*, middle, + *hrif*, belly]. Diaphragma (2).

midsection (mid′sek-shŭn). A cut or section through the middle of an organ.

midsternum (mid′ster′nŭm). *Corpus* sterni.

midtarsal (mid′tar′săl). Mediotarsal.

midwife (mid′wīf) [A.S. *mid*, with, + *wif*, wife]. A person qualified to practice midwifery, having specialized training in obstetrics and child care with the training to carry out emergency measures in the absence of medical help.

midwifery (mid′wīf′rē, mid′wif′ĕ-rē). Independent care of essentially normal, healthy women and infants by a midwife, antepartally, intrapartally, postpartally, and/or obstetrically in a hospital, birth center, or home setting, and including normal delivery of the infant, with medical consultation, collaborative management, and referral of cases in which abnormalities develop; strong emphasis is placed on educational preparation of parents for childbearing and childrearing, with an orientation toward childbirth as a normal physiological process requiring minimal intervention.

Miescher, Johann F., Swiss pathologist, 1811–1887. See M.'s *elastoma, granulomatosis, tubes.*

migraine (mī′grān, mi-grān′) [through O. Fr., fr. G. *hēmi- krania*, pain on one side of the head, fr. *hēmi-*, half, + *kranion*, skull]. Sick, bilious, blind, or vascular headache; hemicrania (1); megrim; a symptom complex occurring periodically and characterized by pain in the head (usually unilateral), vertigo, nausea and vomiting, photophobia, and scintillating appearances of light. Classified as classic m., common m., cluster headache, hemiplegic m., ophthalmoplegic m., and ophthalmic m.

abdominal m., paroxysmal abdominal pain without apparent cause, perhaps a form of epilepsy.

classic m., m. with visual or other prodromes.

common m., m. without prodromes.

fulgurating m., m. characterized by its abrupt commencement and the severity of the episode.

Harris' m., periodic migrainous *neuralgia.*

hemiplegic m., a form associated with transient hemiplegia.

ophthalmic m., a form of m. accompanied by marked disturbances of vision.

ophthalmoplegic m., a form of m. associated with paralysis of the eye muscles.

migration (mī-grā'shŭn) [L. *migro,* pp. *-atus,* to move from place to place]. **1.** Passing from one part to another, said of certain morbid processes or symptoms. **2.** Diapedesis. **3.** Movement of a tooth or teeth out of normal position. **4.** Movement of molecules during electrophoresis.

epithelial m., apical shift of epithelial attachment, exposing more of the tooth crown.

m. of ovum, the transperitoneal passage of an ovum from the ovarian follicle into the uterine tube (oviduct).

Mikity, Victor G., U.S. radiologist, *1919. See Wilson-M. *syndrome.*

Mikulicz, Johannes von M.-Radecki, Polish surgeon in Breslau, 1850–1905. See M.'s *aphthae, cells, clamp, disease, drain, operation, syndrome;* M.-Vladimiroff or Vladimiroff-M. *amputation;* Heineke-M. *pyloroplasty.*

Miles, William E., British surgeon, 1869–1947. See M.'s *operation, resection.*

milia (mil'ē-ă). Plural of milium.

Milian, Gaston, French dermatologist, 1871–1945. See M.'s *disease, erythema.*

miliaria (mil-ē-ā'rē-ă) [L. *miliarius,* relating to millet, fr. *milium,* millet]. Miliary fever (2); an eruption of minute vesicles and papules due to retention of fluid at the orifices of sweat glands.

m. al'ba, m. with vesicles containing a milky fluid.

apocrine m., Fox-Fordyce *disease.*

m. crystalli'na, crystal rash; sudamina (2); a noninflammatory form of m. in which the vesicles are filled with clear fluid.

m. profun'da, pale firm papules, most commonly on the trunk; it is asymptomatic and results from severe damage to the sweat ducts after repeated episodes of m. rubra or from experimental injury.

pustular m., an eruption of pustules that occurs usually in very hot weather and mostly on the flexor aspects of the limbs, the groins, and the axillae; the lesions are situated at the orifices of sweat glands.

m. ru'bra, an eruption of papules and vesicles at the orifices of sweat glands, accompanied by redness and inflammatory reaction of the skin. Also called strophulus; lichen infantum, strophulosus, or tropicus; tropical lichen; heat, summer, or wildfire rash; prickly heat.

miliary (mil'ē-ā-rē, mil'yă-rē) [see miliaria]. **1.** Resembling a millet seed in size (about 2 mm). **2.** Marked by the presence of nodules of millet seed size on any surface.

milieu (mēl-yū') [Fr. *mi,* fr. L. *medius,* middle, + *leiu,* fr. L. *locus,* place]. **1.** Surroundings; environment. **2.** In psychiatry, the social setting of the mental patient, *e.g.,* the hospital.

m. intérieur, m. inter'ne, the internal environment; the fluids bathing the tissue cells of multicellular animals.

milium, pl. milia (mil'ē-ŭm, -ē-ă) [L. millet]. Pearly or sebaceous tubercle; tuberculum sebaceum; whitehead (1); a small subepidermal keratin cyst, usually multiple and therefore commonly referred to in the plural.

colloid m., *elastosis* colloidalis conglomerata.

milk [A.S. *meolc*]. **1.** Lac (1); a white liquid, containing proteins, sugar, and lipids, secreted by the mammary glands, and designed for the nourishment of the young. **2.** Any whitish milky fluid; *e.g.,* the juice of the coconut or a suspension of various metallic oxides. **3.** A pharmacopeial preparation that is a suspension of insoluble drugs in a water medium; distinguished from gels mainly in that the suspended particles of m. are larger. **4.** Strip (1).

acidophilus m., m. inoculated with a culture of *Bacillus acidophilus.*

m. of bismuth, a suspension of bismuth hydroxide and bismuth subcarbonate in water; used in gastrointestinal disorders as a protective agent.

buddeized m., see Budde *process.*

certified m., cow's m. that does not have more than the maximal permissible limit of 10,000 bacteria per ml at any time prior to delivery to the consumer, and that must be cooled to 10°C or less and maintained at that temperature until delivery.

certified pasteurized m., cow's m. in which the maximum permissible limit for bacteria should not be more than 10,000 bacteria per ml before pasteurization and not more than 500 bacteria per ml after pasteurization; it must be cooled to 7.2°C or less and maintained at that temperature until delivery.

condensed m., a thick liquid prepared by the partial evaporation of cow's m., with or without the addition of sugar.

crop m., pigeon's m.

fortified vitamin D m., m. produced through direct addition of vitamin D; standardized at 400 USP units per quart.

irradiated vitamin D m., cow's m. exposed in a thin film to ultraviolet light and standardized to contain 400 USP units of vitamin D per quart.

lactobacillary m., m. inoculated with a culture of *Bacillus acidophilus, B. bulgaricus,* or other lactic acid-forming microorganism.

m. of magnesia, magnesia magma; mixture of magnesium hydroxide; an aqueous solution of magnesium hydroxide, used as an antacid and laxative.

metabolized vitamin D m., m. produced by feeding irradiated yeast to cows; standardized to contain not less than 400 USP units per quart.

modified m., cow's m. altered, by increasing the fat and reducing the amount of protein, to resemble human m. in composition.

perhydrase m., m. treated by the addition of hydrogen peroxide. See Budde *process.*

pigeon's m., crop m.; a secretion formed by glands in the mucosa of the pigeon's crop with which the young are fed; it is increased under the influence of prolactin.

skim m., skimmed m., the aqueous (noncream) part of m. from which casein is isolated.

m. of sulfur, precipitated *sulfur.*

uterine m., a whitish fluid secretion between the villi of the placenta, which nourishes the implanting ovum.

vitamin D m., cow's m. to which vitamin D has been added, to contain 400 USP units of vitamin D per quart.

witch's m., a secretion of colostrum-like m. sometimes occurring in the glands of newborn infants of either sex 3 to 4 days after birth and lasting a week or two; due to endocrine stimulation from the mother before birth.

Milkman, Louis A., U.S. roentgenologist, 1895–1951. See M.'s *syndrome.*

milkpox (milk'poks). Alastrim.

Millard, Auguste L.J., French physician, 1830–1915. See M.-Gubler *syndrome.*

Miller, Thomas Grier, U.S. physician, *1886. See M.-Abbott *tube.*

Miller, Willoughby D., U.S. dentist, 1853–1907. See M.'s chemicoparasitic *theory.*

Milles' syndrome. See under syndrome.

millet seed (mil'et). The seed of a grass, *Panicum miliaceum,* used as a rough designation of size of cutaneous and other lesions; it is the equivalent of about 2 mm, or $^1/_{12}$ inch, in diameter.

milli- (m) [L. *mille,* one thousand] Prefix used in the SI and metric systems to signify one-thousandth (10^{-3}).

milliampere (ma) (mil'ē-am'pēr). One thousandth of an ampere.

millibar (mil'i-bar). One-thousandth of a bar; 100 newtons/sq m; 0.75006 mm Hg; standard atmospheric pressure is 1013 millibars.

millicurie (mCi) (mil'i-kyū'rē). A unit of radioactivity equivalent to 3.7×10^7 disintegrations per second.

milliequivalent (mEq, meq) (mil'i-ē-kwiv'ă-lent). One-thousandth equivalent; 10^{-3} mole divided by valence.

milligram (mg) (mil'i-gram). One-thousandth of a gram.

milligramage (mil'i-gram-āj). Milligram hour.

milligram hour. Milligramage; a unit of exposure in radium therapy, *i.e.,* the application of 1 milligram of radium during 1 hour.

millilambert (mil-i-lam'bert). One thousandth of a lambert; a unit of brightness equal to 0.929 lumen per square foot (roughly, 1 equivalent footcandle).

milliliter (mL, ml) (mil'i-lē-ter). One-thousandth of a liter.

millimeter (mm) (mil'i-mē-ter). One-thousandth of a meter.

millimicro-. Prefix formerly used to signify one-billionth (10^{-9}); now nano-.

millimicron (mμ) (mil'i-mī-kron). Former term for nanometer.

millimole (mmol) (mil'i-mōl). One-thousandth of a gram-molecule.

milling-in (mil'ing-in). Refining the occlusion of teeth by the use of abrasives between their occluding surfaces while the dentures are rubbed together in the mouth or on the articulator.

milliosmole (mil'i-oz-mōl). One-thousandth of an osmole.

millipede (mil'i-pēd) [milli- + L. *pes, pedis,* foot]. A venomous nonpredaceous arthropod of the order Diplopoda, characterized by two pairs of legs per leg-bearing segment. The venom is purely defensive, oozed or squirted from pores along the body, producing irritation to the skin or severe inflammation if it reaches the eyes.

millisecond (ms, msec) (mil'i-sek'ŏnd). One-thousandth of a second.

millivolt (mV, mv) (mil'i-vōlt). One thousandth of a volt.

Millon, Auguste N.E., French chemist, 1812–1867. See M. *reaction;* M.'s *reagent;* M.-Nasse *test.*

milphosis (mil-fō'sis) [G. *milphōsis*]. Madarosis; loss of eyelashes.

Milroy, William F., U.S. physician, 1855–1942. See M.'s *disease.*

Milton, John L., British dermatologist, 1820–1898. See M.'s *disease.*

mimesis (mi-mē'sis, mī-) [G. *mimēsis,* imitation, fr. *mimeomai,* to mimic]. **1.** Hysterical simulation of organic disease. **2.** The symptomatic imitation of one organic disease by another.

mimetic (mi-met'ik, mī-) [G. *mimētikos,* imitative]. Relating to mimesis.

mimic (mim'ik) [G. *mimikos,* imitating, fr. *mimos,* a mimic]. To imitate or simulate.

mimmation (mi-mā'shŭn) [Ar. *mim,* the letter m]. A form of stammering in which the m-sound is given to various letters.

mind [A.S. *gemynd*]. **1.** The organ or seat of consciousness and higher functions of the human brain, such as cognition, reasoning, and willing. **2.** The organized totality of all mental processes and psychic activities, with emphasis on the relatedness of the phenomena.

prelogical m., prelogical *thinking.*
subconscious m., subliminal *self.*

mind-reading. Telepathy.

mineral (min'er-ăl) [L. *mineralis,* pertaining to mines, fr. *mino,* to mine]. Any homogeneous inorganic material usually found in the earth's crust.

mineralocoid (min-er-al'ō-koyd). Mineralocorticoid.

mineralocorticoid (min'er-al-ō-kōr'ti-koyd). Mineralocoid; one of the steroids of the adrenal cortex that influences salt (sodium and potassium) metabolism.

mineral oil. Heavy liquid petrolatum; liquid paraffin or petroleum; a mixture of liquid hydrocarbons obtained from petroleum, used as a vehicle in pharmaceutical preparations.

minilaparotomy (min'ē-lap-ă-rot'ō-mē). Technique for sterilization by surgical ligation of the fallopian tubes, performed through a small suprapubic incision.

min'im [L. *minimus,* least]. **1 (m).** A fluid measure, $^1/_{60}$ of a fluidrachm; in the case of water about one drop. **2.** Smallest; least; the smallest of several similar structures.

minocycline (min-ō-sī'klēn). A substituted naphthacenecarboxamide; an antibacterial drug related to tetracycline.

minor (mī'ner) [L.]. Smaller; lesser; denoting the smaller of two similar structures.

minoxidil (mi-nok'si-dil). 2,4-Diamino-6-piperidinopyrimidine 3-oxide; an antihypertensive agent.

mint [G. *mintha*]. Mentha.

mio- [G. *meiōn,* less]. Combining form meaning less.

miocardia (mī-ō-kar'dē-ă) [mio- + G. *kardia,* heart]. Systole.

miodidymus, miodymus (mī-ō-did'i-mŭs, mī-od'i-mŭs) [mio- + G. *didymos,* twin]. Unequal conjoined twins with the smaller head fused to the larger in the occipital region.

miolecithal (mī-ō-les'i-thal) [mio- + G. *lekithos,* egg yolk]. Denoting an egg with little yolk which is uniformly dispersed throughout the egg.

mionectic (mī-ō-nek'tik) [mio- + G. *echō,* to have]. An obsolete term denoting less than the normal; used especially with reference to blood that has an abnormally low percentage of saturation with oxygen at a certain pressure.

miopragia (mī-ō-prā'jē-ă) [mio- + G. *prassō,* to do]. Diminished functional activity in a part.

miopus (mī-ō'pŭs) [mio- + *ōps,* eye]. Unequal conjoined twins with heads united in such a manner that one face is rudimentary.

miosis (mī-ō'sis) [G. *meiosis,* a lessening]. **1.** Contraction of the pupil. **2.** Rarely used term for the period of decline of a disease in which the intensity of the symptoms begins to diminish. **3.** Incorrect alternative spelling for meiosis.

paralytic m., m. due to paralysis of the dilator muscle of the pupil.
spastic m., m. due to spasmodic contraction of the sphincter muscle of the pupil.

miosphygmia (mī'ō-sfig'mē-ă) [mio- + G. *sphygmos,* pulse]. Microsphygmy; condition in which pulse beats are fewer than heart beats.

miotic (mī-ot'ik). **1.** Relating to or characterized by contraction of the pupil. **2.** An agent that causes the pupil to contract.

miracidium, pl. **miracidia** (mī-ră-sid'ē-ŭm, -ă) [G. *meirakidion,* boy]. The ciliated first-stage larva of a trematode that emerges from the egg and must penetrate into the tissues of an appropriate intermediate host snail if it is to continue its life cycle; followed by development into a mother sporocyst and by production of a number of offspring of successive larval generations. See also sporocyst (1).

Mirchamp's sign. See under sign.

mire (mēr) [L. *miror,* pp. *-atus,* to wonder at]. One of the test objects in the ophthalmometer; its image is measured to determine the radii of curvature of the cornea.

Mirizzi, P.L., 20th century Argentinian physician. See M.'s *syndrome.*

mirror (mir'ŏr) [Fr. *miroir,* fr. L. *miror,* to wonder at]. A polished surface reflecting the rays of light from objects in front of it.
concave m., a spherical reflecting surface that constitutes a segment of the interior of a sphere.
convex m., a spherical reflecting surface that constitutes a segment of the exterior of a sphere.
head m., a circular concave m. attached to a head band, used to project a beam of light into a cavity, such as the nose or larynx, for purposes of examination and permitting binocular vision.
mouth m., a small m. on a handle used to facilitate visualization in the examination of the teeth.
van Helmont's m., obsolete term for *centrum* tendineum.

mirror-writing (mir'ŏr-rīt-ing). Retrography; writing backward, from right to left, the letters appearing like ordinary writing seen in a mirror.

miryachit (mir-yach'it). Myriachit; a nervous affection observed in Siberia. See jumper *disease.*

misandry (mis'an-drē) [G. *miseō,* to hate, + *anēr, andros,* male]. Aversion to or hatred of men.

misanthropy (mis-an'thrō-pē) [G. *miseō,* to hate, + *anthrōpos,* man]. Aversion to people; hatred of mankind.

miscarriage (mis-kar'ij). Spontaneous expulsion of the products of pregnancy before the middle of the second trimester.

miscarry (mis-kar'ē). To have a miscarriage.

miscegenation (mis'e-jĕ-nā'shŭn) [L. *misceo,* to mix, + *genus,* descent, race]. Marriage or interbreeding of individuals of different races.

miscible (mis'i-bl) [L. *misceo,* to mix]. Capable of being mixed and remaining so after the mixing process ceases.

misdiagnosis (mis'dī-ag-nō'sis). A wrong or mistaken diagnosis.

miserotia (mis-ĕ-rō'shi-ă) [G. *miseō,* to hate, + *eros,* physical love]. Dislike of or aversion to physical love.

misogamy (mi-sog'ă-mē) [G. *miseō,* to hate, + *gamos,* marriage]. Aversion to marriage.

misogyny (mi-soj'i-nē) [G. *miseō,* to hate, + *gynē,* woman]. Aversion to or hatred of women.

misologia (mis-ō-lō'jē-ă) [G. *miseō,* to hate, + *logos,* reasoning, discussion]. Aversion to talking or to mental activity.

misoneism (mis-ō-nē'izm) [G. *miseō,* to hate, + *neos,* new]. Dislike of and disinclination to accept new ideas.

misopedia, misopedy (mis-ō-pē'dē-ă, -op'ĕ-dē) [G. *miseō,* to hate, + *pais* (*paid-*), child]. Aversion to or hatred of children.

mistletoe (mis'l-tō). Viscum (1).

Mitchell, Silas Weir, U.S. neurologist, poet, and novelist, 1829–1914. See M.'s *disease, treatment.*

mite (mīt) [A.S.]. A minute arthropod of the order Acarina, a vast assemblage of parasitic and (primarily) free-living organisms. Most are still undescribed, and only a relatively small number are of medical or veterinary importance as vectors or intermediate hosts of pathogenic agents, by directly causing dermatitis or tissue damage, or by causing blood or tissue fluid loss. The six-legged larvae of trombiculid m.'s, the chigger m.'s (*Tromicula*), are parasitic of man and many mammals and birds, and are important as vectors of scrub typhus (tsutsugamushi disease) and other rickettsial agents. Some other important m.'s are *Acarus hordei* (barley m.), *Demodex folliculorum* (follicular or mange m.), *Dermanyssus gallinae* (red hen-m.), *Ornithonyssus bacoti* (tropical rat m.), *O. bursa* (tropical fowl m.), *O. sylviarum* (northern fowl m.), *Pyemotes tritici* (straw or grain itch m.), and *Sarcoptes scabei* (itch m.).

mitella (mī-tel'ă) [L. dim. of *mitra,* a bandage, band]. A sling for the arm.

mithramycin (mith-ră-mī'sin). Aureolic acid; mitramycin; an antibiotic produced by *Streptomyces argillaceus* and *S. tanashiensis;* possesses antineoplastic activity.

mithridatism (mith'ri-dā'tizm, mith-rid'ă-tizm) [*Mithridates,* King of Pontus (132–63 B.C.), supposedly an unsuccessful suicide (by poison) because of repeated small doses taken to become invulnerable to assassination by poison]. Immunity against the action of a poison produced by small and gradually increasing doses of the same.

miticidal (mī-ti-sī'dăl). Destructive to mites.

miticide (mī'ti-sīd) [mite + L. *caedo,* to kill]. An agent destructive to mites.

mitigate (mit'i-gāt) [L. *mitigo,* pp. *-atus,* to make mild or gentle, fr. *mitis,* mild, + *ago,* to do, make]. Palliate.

mitis (mī'tis) [L.]. Mild.

mitochondria (mī-tō-kon'drē-ă). Plural of mitochondrion.

mitochondrial (mī-tō-kon'drē-ăl). Relating to mitochondria.

mitochondrion, pl. mitochondria (mī-tō-kon'drē-on, -kon'drē-ă) [G. *mitos,* thread, + *chondros,* granule, grits]. Altmann's granule (2); an organelle of the cell cytoplasm consisting of two sets of membranes, a smooth continuous outer coat and an inner membrane arranged in tubules or more often in folds that form platelike double membranes called cristae; mitochondria are the principal energy source of the cell and contain the cytochrome enzymes of terminal electron transport and the enzymes of the citric acid cycle, fatty acid oxidation, and oxidative phosphorylation.
m. of hemoflagellates, the "mother m.," from which smaller mitochondria appear to arise.

mitogen (mī'tō-jen) [mitosis + G. *-gen,* producing]. Transforming agent; a substance that stimulates mitosis and lymphocyte transformation; includes not only the substances associated with lectins, but also substances from streptococci (associated with streptolysin S) and from strains of α-toxin-producing staphylococci.
pokeweed m. (PWM), a m. from *Phytolacca americana* (pokeweed) which stimulates chiefly B lymphocytes.

mitogenesis (mī-tō-jen'ĕ-sis) [mitosis + G. *genesis,* origin]. The process of induction of mitosis in a cell.

mitogenetic (mī'tō-jĕ-net'ik). Pertaining to the factor or factors causing cell mitosis.

mitogenic (mī-tō-jen'ik). Pertaining to a mitogen.

mitomycin (mī-tō-mī'sin). Antibiotic produced by *Streptomyces caespitosus,* variants of which are designated m. A, m. B, etc.; m. C is an antineoplastic agent.

mitosis, pl. mitoses (mī-tō'sis, -sēz) [G. *mitos,* threat]. Karyokinesis; karyomitosis; mitotic or indirect nuclear division; the usual process of cell reproduction consisting of a sequence of modifications of the nucleus (prophase, prometaphase, metaphase, anaphase, telophase) that result in the formation of two daughter cells with exactly the same chromosome and DNA content as that of the original cell. See also cell *cycle.*
heterotype m., a variety of m. in which the halved chromosomes are united at their ends forming ring-like figures.
multipolar m., a pathologic form in which the spindle has three or more poles resulting in the formation of a corresponding number of nuclei.
somatic m., the ordinary process of m. as it occurs in the somatic or body cells, characterized by the formation of a definite number of chromosomes, varying according to the species (in humans the number is 46).

mitotane (mī'tō-tān). 1,1-Dichloro-2-(*o*-chlorophenyl)-2-(*p*-chlorophenyl)ethane; an antineoplastic agent.

mitotic (mī-tot′ik). Karyokinetic; karyomitotic; relating to or marked by mitosis.

mitoxantrone hydrochloride (mī-tō-zan′trōn). 1,4-Dihydro-5,8-bis[[2-[2-hydroxyethyl)-amino]ethyl]anthraquinone dihydrochloride; a synthetic anti-neoplastic used intravenously in the initial therapy for acute nonlymphocytic leukemia in adults.

mitral (mī′trăl) [L. *mitra,* a coif or turban]. **1.** Relating to the mitral or bicuspid valve. **2.** Shaped like a bishop's miter; denoting a structure resembling the shape of a headband or turban.

mitralization (mī′tră-li-zā′shŭn). Straightening of the left heart border in the chest roentgenogram due to increased prominence of the left atrial appendage and/or the pulmonary salient; an unreliable criterion.

mitramycin (mit-ră-mī′sin). Mithramycin.

Mitsuda, Kensuke, Japanese physician, *1876. See M. *antigen, reaction.*

mittelschmerz (mit′el-schmārts) [Ger. Mittelschmerz, middle + pain]. Intermenstrual pain (2); middle pain; abdominal pain occurring at the time of ovulation, resulting from irritation of the peritoneum by bleeding from the ovulation site.

Mitzuo, Gentaro, Japanese ophthalmologist, 1876–1913. See M.'s *phenomenon.*

mixing (mik′sing). The mingling or blending of particles or components, especially of different kinds.
phenotypic m., the condition in which bacteriophage particles released from a bacterium with a mixed infection have components from both the infecting phages.

mixture (miks′chŭr) [L. *mixtura* or *mistura*]. **1.** A mutual incorporation of two or more substances, without chemical union, the physical characteristics of each of the components being retained. A **mechanical m.** is a m. of particles or masses distinguishable as such under the microscope or in other ways; a **physical m.** is a more intimate m. of molecules, as in the case of gases and many solutions. **2.** In chemistry, a mingling together of two or more substances without the occurrence of a reaction by which they would lose their individual properties, *i.e.,* without permanent gain or loss of electrons. **3.** In pharmacy, a preparation, consisting of a liquid holding an insoluble medicinal substance in suspension by means of acacia, sugar, or some other viscid material.
Bordeaux m., a plant fungicidal m., comprising copper sulfate (5 parts) and calcium oxide (5 parts) in water (400 parts) freshly mixed; the CaO is added to the $CuSO_4$ solution.
extemporaneous m., a m. prepared at the time ordered, according to the directions of a prescription, as distinguished from a stock preparation.

Miyagawa, Yoneji, Japanese bacteriologist, 1885–1959. See *Miyagawanella;* M. *bodies.*

Miyagawanella (mē′yă-gah′wă-nel′ă) [Y. *Miyagawa*]. Formerly considered a genus of Chlamydiaceae, but now synonymous with *Chlamydia.*

MK, MK-6, MK-7 Abbreviation for menaquinone, menaquinone-6, and menaquinone-7, respectively.

MKS, mks Abbreviation for meter-kilogram-second. See under system; unit.

mL, ml Abbreviation for milliliter.

MLC Abbreviation for Marginal Line Calculus Index.

MLD, mld Abbreviation for minimal lethal *dose.*

mm Abbreviation for millimeter.

M-mode. TM-mode; a diagnostic ultrasound presentation of the temporal changes in echoes in which the depth of echo-producing interfaces is displayed along one axis and time (T) is displayed along the second axis, recording motion (M) of the interfaces toward and away from the transducer; a one-dimensional study of the target time movement is produced.

mmol Abbreviation for millimole.

MMPI Abbreviation for Minnesota multiphasic personality inventory *test.*

MMR Abbreviation for measles, mumps, and rubella *vaccine.*

Mn Symbol for manganese.

M'Naghten, Daniel, British criminal, tried in March, 1843. See M. *rule.*

mneme (nē′mē) [G. *mnēmē,* memory]. **1.** Term coined by Richard Semon to denote the ability to remember which he believed all living cells possessed. **2.** The enduring quality in the mind that accounts for the facts of memory; the engram of a specific experience.

mnemenic, mnemic (nē-men′ik, nē′mik). Relating to memory.

mnemism (nē′mizm) [G. *mnēmē,* memory]. Mnemic *hypothesis.*

mnemonic (nē-mon′ik). Anamnestic(1).

mnemonics (nē-mon′iks) [G. *mnēmonikos,* mnemonic, pertaining to memory]. The art of improving the memory; a system for aiding the memory.

MNSs blood group. See Blood Groups appendix.

M.O. Abbreviation for Medical Officer.

Mo Symbol for molybdenum.

mobilization (mō′bi-li-zā′shŭn) [see mobilize]. **1.** Making movable; restoring the power of motion in a joint. **2.** The act or the result of the act of mobilizing; exciting a hitherto quiescent process into physiologic activity.
stapes m., an operation to remobilize the footplate of the stapes to relieve conductive hearing impairment caused by its immobilization through otosclerosis or middle ear disease.

mobilize (mō′bi-līz) [Fr. *mobiliser,* to liberate, make ready, fr. L. *mobilis,* movable]. **1.** To liberate material stored in the body; more specifically, to move a substance from tissue stores into the bloodstream. **2.** To excite quiescent material to physiologic activity.

Mobitz, Woldemar, German cardiologist, *1889. See M. types of atrioventricular *block.*

Möbius, Paul J., German physician, 1853–1907. See M.'s *disease, sign, syndrome;* Leyden-M. muscular *dystrophy.*

MOD Abbreviation for mesiodistocclusal.

modality (mō-dal′i-tē) [Mediev. L. *modalitas,* fr. L. *modus,* a mode]. **1.** A form of application or employment of a therapeutic agent or regimen. **2.** Various forms of sensation, *e.g.,* touch, vision, etc.

mode (mōd) [L. *modus,* a measure, quantity]. In a set of measurements, that value which appears most frequently.

model (mod′ĕl). **1.** A representation of something, often idealized or modified to make it conceptually easier to understand. **2.** Something to be imitated. **3.** In dentistry, a cast.
animal m., in comparative or experimental medicine, the analog in some other animal species of a disease of man, whether spontaneous or induced.
Bingham m., a m. representing the flow behavior of a Bingham plastic, in the idealized case.
computer m., computer simulation; a mathematical representation of the functioning of a system, presented in the form of a computer program.
medical m., a set of assumptions that views behavioral abnormalities in the same framework as physical disease or abnormalities.

modeling (mod′ĕl-ing). **1.** In learning theory, the acquiring and learning of a new skill by observing and imitating that behavior being performed by another individual. **2.** In behavior modification, a treatment procedure whereby the therapist or another significant person presents (models) the target behavior which the learner is to imitate and make part of his repertoire. **3.** A continuous process by which a bone is altered in size and shape during its growth by resorption and formation of bone at different sites and rates.

modification (mod'i-fi-kā'shŭn). A nonhereditary change in an organism; *e.g.*, one that is acquired from its own activity or environment.

behavior m., the systematic use of principles of conditioning and learning, especially operant or instrumental conditioning, to teach certain skills or to extinguish undesirable behaviors, attitudes, or phobias.

modiolus, pl. **modi'oli** (mō-dī'ō-lŭs, -ō-lī) [L., the nave of a wheel]. **1** [NA]. Columella cochleae; the central cone-shaped core of spongy bone about which turns the spiral canal of the cochlea. **2.** M. labii.

m. la'bii, a point near the corner of the mouth where several muscles of facial expression converge.

modulation (mod-yū-lā'shŭn) [L. *modulari,* to measure off properly]. **1.** The functional and morphologic fluctuation of cells in response to changing environmental conditions. **2.** Systematic variation in a characteristic (*e.g.*, frequency, amplitude) of a sustained oscillation to code additional information.

modulus (moj'yū-lŭs, mod'yū-) [L. dim. of *modus,* a measure, quantity]. A coefficient expressing the magnitude of a physical property by a numerical value.

bulk m., m. of volume elasticity.

m. of elasticity, a coefficient expressing the ratio between stress per unit area acting to deform a body and the amount of deformation that results from it.

m. of volume elasticity, bulk m.; a coefficient expressing the ratio between pressure acting to change the volume of a substance and the amount of change that results from it.

Young's m., a type of m. of elasticity which specifies the force applied to a body in one direction, per unit cross-sectional area of the body perpendicular to that direction, divided by the fractional change in length of the body in that direction.

Moeller, Alfred, German bacteriologist, *1868. See M.'s grass *bacillus*.

Moeller, Julius O.L., German surgeon, 1819–1887. See M.'s *glossitis*.

mofebutazone (mof-ĕ-byū'tă-zōn). 4-Butyl-1-phenyl-3,5-pyrazolidinedione; an anti-inflammatory agent used for the treatment of arthritis.

mogiarthria (moj-i-ar'thrē-ă) [G. *mogis,* with difficulty, + *arthroun,* to articulate]. Speech defect due to muscular incoordination.

mogigraphia (moj-i-graf'ē-ă) [G. *mogis,* with difficulty, + *graphē,* writing]. Writer's *cramp*.

mogilalia (moj-i-lā'lē-ă) [G. *mogis,* with difficulty, + *lalia,* speech]. Molilalia; stuttering stammering, or any speech defect.

mogiphonia (moj-i-fō'nē-ă) [G. *mogis,* with difficulty, + *phōnē,* voice]. Laryngeal spasm occurring in public speakers as a result of overuse of the voice.

Mohrenheim, Joseph J. Freiherr von, Austrian-Russian surgeon, 1755–1799. See M.'s *fossa, space*.

Mohs, Frederick E., U.S. surgeon, *1910. See M. fresh tissue chemosurgery *technique*.

Mohs, Friedrich, German mineralogist, 1773–1839. See M. *scale*.

moiety (moy'i-tē) [M.E. *moite,* a half]. Originally, a half; now, loosely, a portion of something.

mol Abbreviation for mole (3).

molal (mō'lăl). Denoting one mole of solute dissolved in 1000 grams of solvent; such solutions provide a definite ratio of solute to solvent molecules. *Cf.* molar (4).

molality (mō-lal'i-tē). Moles of solute per kilogram of solvent. *Cf.* molarity (4).

molar (mō'lăr). **1** [L. *molaris,* relating to a mill, millstone]. Denoting a grinding, abrading, or wearing away. **2.** *Dens* molaris. **3** [L. *moles,* mass]. Massive; relating to a mass; not molecular. **4.** Denoting a concentration of 1 gram-molecular weight (1 mole) of solute per liter of solution, the common unit of concentration in chemistry. *Cf.* molal. **5.** Denoting specific quantity, *e.g.*, molar volume (volume of 1 mole).

first (permanent) m., sixth permanent tooth or fourth deciduous tooth in the maxilla and mandible on either side of the midsagittal plane of the head following the arch form.

Moon's m.'s, small dome-shaped first m. teeth occurring in congenital syphilis.

mulberry m., a m. tooth with alternating nonanatomical depressions and rounded enamel nodules on its crown surface, usually associated with congenital syphilis.

second m., seventh permanent or fifth deciduous tooth in the maxilla and mandible on either side of the midsagittal plane of the head following the arch form.

sixth-year m., the first permanent m. tooth.

third m., eighth permanent tooth in the maxilla and mandible on either side of the midsagittal plane of the head following the arch form.

twelfth-year m., the second permanent m. tooth.

molariform (mō-lar'i-fōrm) [molar (tooth) + L. *forma,* form]. Having the form of a molar tooth.

molarity (mō-lar'i-tē). Moles per liter of solution (mol/L). *Cf.* molality.

mold (mōld). Mould. **1.** A filamentous fungus, generally a circular colony that may be cottony, wooly, etc., or glabrous, but with filaments not organized into large fruiting bodies, such as mushrooms. **2.** A shaped receptacle into which wax is pressed or fluid plaster is poured in making a cast. **3.** To shape a mass of plastic material according to a definite pattern. **4.** To change in shape; denoting especially the adaptation of the fetal head to the pelvic canal. **5.** The term used to specify the shape of an artificial tooth (or teeth).

molding (mōld'ing). Shaping by means of a mold.

border m., tissue m.; tissue-trimming; muscle-trimming; the shaping of an impression material by the manipulation or action of the tissues adjacent to the borders of an impression.

compression m., **(1)** the act of pressing or squeezing together to form a shape in a mold; **(2)** the adaptation of a plastic material to the negative form of a split mold by pressure. See also injection m.

injection m., the adaptation of a plastic material to the negative form of a closed mold by forcing the material into the mold through appropriate gateways. See also compression m. (2).

tissue m., border m.

mole (mōl). **1** [A.S. *māēl* (L. *macula*), a spot]. *Nevus* pigmentosus. **2** [L. *moles,* mass]. An intrauterine mass formed by the degeneration of the partly developed products of conception. **3 (mol).** In the SI system, the unit of amount of substance, defined as that amount of a substance containing as many "elementary entities" as there are atoms in 0.0120 kg of carbon-12; "elementary entities" may be atoms, molecules, ions, or any describable entity or defined mixture of entities; in practical terms, the mole is 6.0225×10^{23} "elementary entities." See also Avogadro's *number*.

blood m., fleshy m.

Breus m., an aborted ovum in which the fetal surface of the placenta presents numerous hematomata with an absence of blood vessels in the chorion and an ovum much smaller in size than normal in relation to the duration of the pregnancy.

carneous m., fleshy m.

cystic m., hydatidiform m.

false m., an intrauterine polypus.

fleshy m., blood or carneous m.; a shapeless fetal mass.

grape m., hydatidiform m.
hairy m., *nevus* pilosus.
hydatidiform m., hydatid m., cystic, grape, or vesicular m.; a vesicular or polycystic mass resulting from the proliferation of the trophoblast, with hydropic degeneration and avascularity of the chorionic villi.
invasive m., *chorioadenoma* destruens.
spider m., arterial *spider.*
vesicular m., hydatidiform m.

molecular (mō-lek'yū-lăr). Relating to molecules.

molecule (mol'ĕ-kyūl) [Mod. L. *molecula,* dim. of L. *moles,* mass]. The smallest possible quantity of a di-, tri-, or polyatomic substance that retains the chemical properties of the substance.

molilalia (mol'i-lā'lē-ă) [G. *molis,* with difficulty (a later form of *mogis*), + *lalia,* talking]. Mogilalia.

molimen, pl. **molimina** (mō-lī'men, -lim'i-nă) [L. an endeavor]. An effort; laborious performance of a normal function.
m. climacte'reium vir'ile, a condition resembling neurasthenia, occurring in men of 45 to 55 years of age; may be psychosomatic or due to alteration in testicular androgen secretion.
menstrual molimina, premenstrual *syndrome.*

molindone hydrochloride (mō-lin'dōn). 3-Ethyl-6,7-dihydro-2-methyl-5-(morpholinomethyl)indol-4(5*H*)-one monohydrochloride; an antipsychotic.

Molisch, Hans, Austrian chemist, 1856–1937. See M.'s *test.*

Moll, Jacob A., Dutch oculist, 1832–1914. See M.'s *glands; adenocarcinoma* of M.

mollities (mō-lish'i-ēz) [L. *mollis,* soft]. **1.** Characterized by a soft consistency. **2.** Malacia (1).

mollusc (mol'ŭsk). Mollusk.

Mollusca (mo-lŭs'kă) [L. *mollusca,* a nut with a thin shell, fr. *mollis,* soft]. A phylum of the subkingdom Metazoa with soft, unsegmented bodies, consisting of an anterior head, a dorsal visceral mass and a ventral foot. Most forms are enclosed in a protective calcareous shell. M. includes the classes Gastropoda (snails, whelks, slugs), Pelecypoda (oysters, clams, mussels), Cephalopoda (squids, octopuses), Amphineura (chitons), Scaphopoda (tooth shells), and the class of primitive metameric mollusks, Monoplacophora.

molluscous (mo-lŭs'kŭs). Relating to or resembling molluscum.

molluscum (mo-lŭs'kŭm) [L. *molluscus,* soft]. A disease marked by the occurrence of soft rounded tumors of the skin.
m. contagio'sum, m. verrucosum; an infectious disease of the skin caused by a virus of the family Poxviridae and characterized by the appearance of few to numerous small, pearly, umbilicated papular epithelial lesions that contain numerous inclusion bodies (m. bodies); occurs in anthropoid apes as well as in man.
m. fibro'sum, old term for neurofibromatosis.
m. fibro'sum gravida'rum, *fibroma* molle gravidarum.
m. verruco'sum, m. contagiosum.

mollusk (mol'ŭsk). Mollusc; common name for members of the phylum Mollusca, although usually restricted to the gastropods and bivalves.

Moloney, John B., 20th century U.S. oncologist. See M.'s *virus.*

Moloney, Paul J., Canadian physician, 1870–1939. See M. *test.*

Moloy, Howard C., U.S. obstetrician, 1903–1953. See Caldwell-M. *classification.*

molt (mōlt) [L. *muto,* to change]. Moult; to cast off feathers, hair, or cuticle; to undergo ecdysis. See also desquamate.

mol wt Abbreviation for molecular *weight.*

molybdate (mō-lib'dāt). A salt of molybdic acid.

molybdenic, molybdenous (mō-lib'den-ik, -den-ŭs). Relating to molybdenum.

molybdenum (mō-lib'dĕ-nŭm) [G. *molybdaina,* a piece of lead; a metal, prob. galena, fr. *molybdos,* lead]. A silvery white metallic element, symbol Mo, atomic no. 42, atomic weight 95.94.

molybdenum-99 (^{99}Mo). A reactor-produced radioisotope of molybdenum with a half-life of 68.3 hr, used in the manufacture of radionuclide generators for the production of technetium-99m.

molybdic (mō-lib'dik). Denoting molybdenum in the 6+ state, as in MoO_3.

molybdic acid. MoO_3,H_2O; a yellowish crystalline acid, forming molybdates.

molybdous (mō-lib'dŭs). Denoting molybdenum in the 4+ state, as in MoO_2.

molysmophobia (mŏ-liz-mō-fō'bē-ă) [G. *molysma,* filth, infection, + *phobos,* fear]. Morbid fear of infection.

momism (mom'izm). Excessive or overbearing mothering, especially as attributed to American cultural stereotypes.

mon-. See mono-.

monad (mō'nad, mon'ad) [G. *monas,* the number one, unity]. **1.** A univalent element or radical. **2.** A unicellular organism. **3.** In meiosis, the single chromosome derived from a tetrad after the first and second maturation divisions.

Monakow, Constantin von, Swiss histologist, 1853–1930. See M.'s *bundle, nucleus, syndrome, tract.*

monamide (mon-am'id). Monoamide.

monamine (mon-am'in). Monoamine.

monaminuria (mon'am-i-nū'rē-ă). Monoaminuria.

monangle (mon'ang-gl). Having only one angle, denoting a dental instrument that has only one angle between the handle or shaft and the working portion (blade or nib).

monarda (mon-ar'dă). The leaves of *Monarda punctata* (family Labiatae), American horsemint, a labiate plant of the U.S. east of the Mississippi; the main commercial source of natural thymol; used as a carminative in colic.

monarthric (mon-ar'thrik). Monarticular.

monarthritis (mon-ar-thrī'tis). Arthritis of a single joint.

monarticular (mon-ar-tik'yū-lăr). Uniarticular; monarthric; relating to a single joint.

monaster (mon-as'ter) [mono- + G. *astēr,* star]. Mother star; the single star figure at the end of prophase in mitosis.

monathetosis (mon-ath-ĕ-tō'sis). Athetosis affecting one hand or foot.

monatomic (mon-ă-tom'ik). **1.** Relating to or containing a single atom. **2.** Monovalent (1).

monaural (mon-aw'răl) [mono- + L. *auris,* ear]. Pertaining to one ear.

monaxonic (mon-aks-on'ik) [mono- + G. *axōn,* axle]. **1.** Having but one axis, being therefore elongated and slender. **2.** Having one axon.

Mönckeberg, Johann G., German pathologist, 1877–1925. See M.'s *arteriosclerosis, calcification, degeneration, disease.*

Mondini. See M. *deafness, dysplasia.*

Mondonesi, Filippo, Italian physician. See M.'s *reflex.*

Mondor, Henri, French surgeon, 1885–1962. See M.'s *disease.*

moner (mō'ner) [G. *monērēs,* solitary, fr. *monos,* alone]. Obsolete designation for a non-nucleated mass of protoplasm.

Monera (mō-nē'ră) [pl. of Mod. L. *moneron,* fr. G. *monērēs,* solitary]. The prokaryotes, a kingdom of primitive microbial organisms characterized by having no defined nucleus or chromosomes; DNA that is not membrane-bound; and absence of centrioles, mitotic spindle, microtubules, and mitochondria; division of the ill-defined nuclear zone (nucleoid) is by separation of two masses attached to parts of the cell membrane, then growing apart (a form of amitosis). M. includes the blue-green algae and bacteria; viruses, which lack a true cell, may have originated as "escaped nucleic acids" or "wild genes" from eukaryotic cells and are not included.

moneran (mō-nē'ran). A member of the prokaryote kingdom Monera.

monesthetic (mon-es-thet'ik) [mono- + G. *aisthēsis,* sense perception]. Relating to a single sense or sensation.

monestrous (mon-es'trŭs). Having but one estrous cycle in a mating season.

Monge Medrano, Carlos, Peruvian professor of medicine and high altitude specialist, 1884–1970. See M.M's *disease.*

mongol (mon'gōl). Obsolete term for an individual with Down's syndrome.

mongolian (mon-gō'lē-ăn). **1.** Mongoloid (1). **2.** Relating to a member of the Mongolian race.

mongolism (mon'gō-lizm) [*Mongol,* member of the major ethnic group native to Asia, + ism]. Obsolete term for Down's *syndrome.*
translocation m., a condition in which, as a result of translocation of a large part of chromosome 21 to another chromosome, an individual has virtually the genetic content of three chromosomes 21 and thus has the phenotype of Down's syndrome but with the normal number of chromosomes.

mongoloid (mon'gō-loyd). **1.** Mongolian (1); relating to or characterized by features associated with Down's syndrome. **2.** An individual with Down's syndrome.

Moniezia expansa (mon-i-ē'zē-ă ek-span'să). The broad tapeworm (family Anoplocephalidae) of sheep and cattle, occurring in the small intestine and reaching a length of 12 to 15 feet; infections are usually benign. Cysticercoids develop in soil-dwelling oribatid mites commonly ingested with grass by herbivores.

monilated (mon'i-lāt-ed). Moniliform.

monilethrix (mō-nil'ē-thriks) [L. *monile,* necklace, + G. *thrix,* hair]. Aplasia pilorum propia; beaded or moniliform hair; a developmental ectodermal defect in which brittle hairs show a series of constrictions, giving the appearance of a string of fusiform beads; probably due to an underlying metabolic disorder.

Monilia (mo-nil'ē-ă) [L. *monile,* necklace]. Generic term for a group of fungi that are commonly known as fruit molds; the sexual state is *Neurospora.* A few closely related pathogenic organisms formerly classified in this genus are now properly termed *Candida.*

Moniliaceae (mō-nil-ē-ā'sē-ē). A family of Fungi Imperfecti (order Moniliales) which includes *Sporothrix schenckii,* the causative agent of sporotrichosis.

monilial (mō-nil'ē-ăl). Precisely, pertaining to the *Monilia,* but, in medicine, frequently used incorrectly with reference to the genus *Candida.*

moniliasis (mō-ni-lī'ă-sis). Candidiasis.

moniliform (mō-nil'i-fōrm) [L. *monile,* necklace, + *forma,* appearance]. Monilated; shaped like a string of beads or beaded necklace.

Moniliformis (mō-nil-i-fōr'mis) [L. *monile,* necklace, + *forma,* appearance]. A genus of the class (or phylum) Acanthocephala, the thorny-headed worms. *M. dubius,* the common spiny-headed worm of house rats, is transmitted by infected cockroaches, *Periplaneta americana;* a few infections in man have been reported. *M. moniliformis* is a species normally found in rodents and a rare parasite of man.

moniliid (mō-nil'ē-id). Minute macular or papular lesions occurring as an allergic reaction to monilial infection.

monism (mō'nizm) [G. *monos,* single]. A metaphysical system in which all of reality is conceived as a unified whole.

monistic (mo-nis'tik). Pertaining to monism.

monitor (mon'i-ter, -tōr). A device that records specified data for a given series of events, operations, or circumstances.
cardiac m., an electronic m. which, when connected to the patient, signals each heart beat with a flashing light, an electrocardiographic curve, or an audible signal.
electronic fetal m., an apparatus for continuous monitoring of the fetal heart before or during labor.
Holter m., a technique for long-term recording of electrocardiographic signals continuously on magnetic tape, and replaying it at rapid speed, for scanning and selection of significant but fleeting changes that might otherwise escape notice.

monkey-paw (mong'kē-paw). A contracture of the hand resulting from median nerve palsy; the thumb cannot be opposed to the tips of the fingers.

monkeypox (mŏng'kē-poks). A disease of monkeys and rarely man caused by the monkeypox virus; human disease clinically resembles smallpox.

monkshood (monks'hud). See aconite.

mono-, mon- [G. *monos,* single]. Prefixes denoting the participation or involvement of a single element or part; corresponds to L. *uni-.*

mono-amelia (mon-ō-ă-mē'lē-ă). Absence of one limb.

monoamide (mon-ō-am'īd, -id). Monamide; a molecule containing one amide group.

monoamine (mon-ō-am'īn, -in). Monamine; a molecule containing one amine group.

monoamine oxidase (MAO). *Amine* oxidase (flavin-containing).

monoaminergic (mon'ō-am-i-ner'jik) [monoamine + G. *ergon,* work]. Referring to nerve cells or fibers that transmit nervous impulses by the medium of a catecholamine or indolamine.

monoaminuria (mon'ō-am-i-nū'rē-ă). Monaminuria; the excretion of any monoamine in the urine.

monoamniotic (mon'ō-am-nē-ot'ik). Denoting two or more progeny of a multiple pregnancy that have shared a common amniotic sac.

monoassociated (mon'ō-ă-sō'shē-ā-tĕd). Denoting a germ-free organism that becomes colonized by a single microbial species.

monobactam (mon-ō-bak'tam). A class of antibiotic that has a monocyclic beta-lactam nucleus and are structurally different from other beta-lactams; *e.g.,* aztreonam.

monobasic (mon-ō-bā'sik). Denoting an acid with only one replaceable hydrogen atom, or only one replaced hydrogen atom.

monobenzone (mon-ō-ben'zōn). *p*-Benzyloxyphenol; a melanin-pigment inhibiting agent; used topically for the treatment of hyperpigmentation caused by formation of melanin.

monoblast (mon'ō-blast) [mono- + G. *blastos,* germ]. An immature cell that develops into a monocyte.

monobrachius (mon-ō-brā'kē-ŭs) [mono- + G. *brachiōn,* arm]. The condition of being one-armed.

monobromated, monobrominated (mon-ō-brō'māt-ed, -brō'min-āt-ed). Denoting a chemical compound with one atom of bromine per molecule.

monocardian (mon-ō-kar'dē-an). Having a heart with a single atrium and ventricle.

monocephalus (mon-ō-sef'ă-lŭs). Syncephalus.

monochlorphenamide (mon'ō-klōr-fen'ă-mīd). Clofenamide.

monochord (mon'ō-kōrd). An instrument used in hearing tests.

monochorea (mon'ō-kō-rē'ă). Chorea affecting the head alone or only one extremity.

monochorial (mon-ō-kō-rē'ăl). Monochorionic.

monochorionic (mon'ō-kōr-ē-on'ik). Monochorial; relating to or having a single chorion; denoting monovular twins.

monochroic (mon-ō-krō'ik). Monochromatic.

monochromasia (mon'ō-krō-mā'zē-ă). Achromatopsia.

monochromasy (mon-ō-krō'mă-sē). Achromatopsia.
blue cone m., see incomplete *achromatopsia.*
pi cone m., see incomplete achromatopsia.
rod m., complete *achromatopsia.*

monochromatic (mon'ō-krō-mat'ik). **1.** Monochroic; monochromic; having but one color. **2.** Indicating a light of a single wavelength. **3.** Relating to or characterized by monochromatism.

monochromatism (mon-ō-krō'mă-tizm) [mono- + G. *chrōma,* color]. **1.** The state of having or exhibiting only one color. **2.** Achromatopsia.

monochromatophil, monochromatophile (mon'ō-krō-mat'ō-fil, -fīl) [mono- + G. *chrōma,* color, + *philos,* fond]. Monochromophil; monochromophile. **1.** Taking only one stain. **2.** A cell or any histologic element staining with only one kind of dye.

monochromator (mon-ō-krō'mă-ter, -tōr). A prism or diffraction grating used in spectrophotometry to isolate a narrow spectral range.

monochromic (mon-ō-krō'mik). Monochromatic.

monochromophil, monochromophile (mon-ō-krō'mō-fil, -fīl). Monochromatophil.

monocle (mon'ŏ-kl). A lens used for one eye, usually in the correction of presbyopia.

monoclinic (mon-ō-klin'ik) [mono- + G. *klinein,* to incline]. Relating to crystals with a single oblique inclination.

monoclonal (mon-ō-klō'năl). In immunochemistry, pertaining to a protein from a single clone of cells, all molecules, of which are the same; *e.g.,* in the case of Bence Jones protein, the chains are all κ or λ.

monoclonal peak. A narrow band visible on electrophoresis or an abnormal arc seen on immunoelectrophoresis, thought to represent immunoglobulin of one cell clone.

monocranius (mon-ō-krā'nē-ŭs) [mono- + G. *kranion,* cranium]. Syncephalus.

monocrotaline (mon-ō-crō'tă-lin). Crotaline; an alkaloid in the seeds, leaves, and stems of *Crotalaria spectabilis* (family Leguminosae), a plant poisonous to livestock and poultry in the southern U.S.

monocrotic (mon'ō-krot'ik) [mono- + G. *krotos,* a beat]. Denoting a pulse the curve of which presents no notch in the downward line.

monocrotism (mon-ok'rō-tizm) [mono- + G. *krotos,* a beat]. The state in which the pulse is monocrotic.

monocular (mon-ok'yū-lăr) [mono- + L. *oculus,* eye]. Relating to, affecting, or visible by one eye only.

monoculus (mon-ok'yū-lŭs) [L. a one-eyed man, a hybrid word fr. G. *monos,* single, + L. *oculus,* eye]. **1.** Cyclops. **2.** A bandage applied to one eye only.

monocyte (mon'ō-sīt) [mono- + G. *kytos,* cell]. A relatively large mononuclear leukocyte (16 to 22 μm in diameter), that normally constitutes 3 to 7% of the leukocytes of the circulating blood, and is normally found in lymph nodes, spleen, bone marrow, and loose connective tissue. When treated with the usual dyes, m.'s manifest an abundant pale blue or blue-gray cytoplasm that contains numerous, fine, dustlike, red-blue granules; vacuoles are frequently present; the nucleus is usually indented, or slightly folded, and has a stringy chromatin structure that seems more condensed where the delicate strands are in contact. See also monocytoid *cell,* endothelial *leukocyte.*

monocytopenia (mon'ō-sī-tō-pē'nē-ă) [mono- + G. *kytos,* cell, + *penia,* poverty]. Monocytic leukopenia; monopenia; diminution in the number of monocytes in the circulating blood.

monocytosis (mon'ō-sī-tō'sis). Monocytic leukocytosis; an abnormal increase in the number of monocytes in the circulating blood.
avian m., bluecomb *disease* of chickens.

monodactyly, monodactylism (mon-ō-dak'ti-lē, -dak'-ti-lizm) [mono- + G. *daktylos,* digit]. The presence of a single finger on the hand, or a single toe on the foot.

monodermoma (mon'ō-der-mō'mă) [mono- + G. *derma,* skin, + *-ōma,* tumor]. A neoplasm composed of tissues from a single germinal layer.

monodiplopia (mon'ō-di-plō'pē-ă). Monocular *diplopia.*

monodisperse (mon'ō-dis-pers). Of relatively uniform size; said of aerosol suspensions with size variation of less than $\pm 20\%$.

monoethanolamine (mon'ō-eth-ă-nol'ă-mēn). 2-Aminoethanol; a surfactant; the oleate is used as a sclerosing agent in the treatment of varicose veins.

monogametic (mon'ō-gă-met'ik). Homogametic.

monogamy (mon-og'ă-mē) [mono- + G. *gamos,* marriage]. The marriage or mating system in which each partner has but one mate.

monogenesis (mon-ō-jen'ĕ-sis) [mono- + G. *genesis,* origin, production]. **1.** The production of similar organisms in each generation. See also *alternation* of generations. **2.** The production of young by a single parent as in nonsexual generation and parthenogenesis. **3.** The process of parasitizing a single host, in which the life cycle of the parasite is passed; *e.g., Boophilus annulatus,* the one-host cattle tick, or certain trematodes of the order Monogenea.

monogenetic (mon'ō-jĕ-net'ik). Monoxenous; relating to monogenesis.

monogenic (mon-ō-jen'ik). Relating to a hereditary disease or syndrome, or to an inherited characteristic, controlled by alleles at a single genetic locus.

monogenous (mō-noj'ĕ-nŭs). Asexually produced, as by fission, gemmation, or sporulation.

monogerminal (mon-ō-jer'mi-năl). Unigerminal.

monograph (mon'ō-graf) [mono- + G. *graphē,* a writing]. A treatise on a particular subject or specific aspect of a subject.

monohydrated (mon-ō-hī'drā-ted). Containing or united with a single molecule of water per molecule of substance.

monohydric (mon-ō-hī'drik). Having but one hydrogen atom in the molecule.

monoideism (mon'ō-ī-dē'izm) [mono- + G. *idea,* form, idea]. A marked preoccupation with one idea or subject; a slight degree of monomania.

monoinfection (mon'ō-in-fek'shŭn). Simple infection with a single variety of microorganism.

monoisonitrosoacetone (mon'ō-ī'sō-nī-trō'sō-as'ĕ-tōn). Isonitrosoacetone.

monolayers (mon-ō-lā'erz). **1.** Films, one molecule thick, formed on water by certain substances, such as proteins and fatty acids, characterized by molecules containing some atom groupings that are soluble in water and other atom groupings that are insoluble in water. **2.** A confluent sheet of cells, one cell deep, growing on a surface in a cell culture.

monolocular (mon-ō-lok'yū-lăr) [mono- + L. *loculus,* a small place]. Unicameral; unicamerate; having one cavity or chamber.

monomania (mon-ō-mā'nē-ă) [mono- + G. *mania,* frenzy]. An obsession or abnormally extreme enthusiasm for a single idea or subject; a psychosis marked by the limitation of the symptoms rather strictly to a certain group, as the delusion in paranoia.

monomaniac (mon-ō-mā'nē-ak). **1.** One exhibiting monomania. **2.** Characterized by or relating to monomania.

monomastigote (mon-ō-mas′ti-gōt) [mono- + G. *mastix, a whip*]. A mastigote having only one flagellum.

monomelic (mon-ō-mel′ik) [mono- + G. *melos*, limb]. Relating to one limb.

monomer (mon′ō-mer) [mono- + -mer]. **1.** The molecular unit that, by repetition, constitutes a large structure or polymer; *e.g.*, ethylene, $CH_2{=}CH_2$, is the monomer of polyethylene, $H(CH_2)_nH$. **2.** The protein structural unit of a virion capsid. See virion. **3.** The protein subunit of a protein composed of several loosely associated such units.

monomeric (mon-ō-mer′ik) [mono- + G. *meros*, part]. **1.** Consisting of a single part. **2.** In genetics, relating to a hereditary disease or characteristic controlled by genes at a single locus. **3.** Consisting of monomers.

monometallic (mon′ō-mĕ-tal′ik). Containing one atom of a metal per molecule.

monomicrobic (mon′ō-mī-krō′bik). Denoting a monoinfection.

monomolecular (mon′ō-mō-lek′yū-lăr). Unimolecular; denoting a single molecule.

monomorphic (mon-ō-mōr′fik) [mono- + G. *morphē*, shape]. Of one shape; unchangeable in shape.

monomphalus (mon-om′fă-lŭs) [mono- + G. *omphalos*, umbilicus]. Omphalopagus.

monomyoplegia (mon′ō-mī′ō-plē′jē-ă) [mono- + G. *mys*, muscle, + *plēgē*, a stroke]. Paralysis limited to one muscle.

monomyositis (mon′ō-mī-ō-sī′tis). Inflammation of a single muscle.

mononeme (mon′ō-nēm). An unpaired helix of nucleic acid, as occurs in a chromatid.

mononeural, mononeuric (mon′ō-nū′răl, -nū′rik). **1.** Having only one neuron. **2.** Supplied by a single nerve.

mononeuralgia (mon′ō-nū-ral′jă). Pain along the course of one nerve.

mononeuritis (mon′ō-nū-rī′tis). Inflammation of a single nerve.
m. mul′tiplex, inflammation of several nerves in unrelated portions of the body.

mononeuropathy (mon′ō-nū-rop′ă-thē). Disease involving a single nerve.
m. mul′tiplex, involvement of several individual nerves.

mononoea (mon-ō-nē′ă) [mono- + G. *noēsis*, idea]. Fixation of the mind on one subject.

mononuclear (mon-ō-nū′klē-ăr). Having only one nucleus; used especially in reference to blood cells.

mononucleosis (mon′ō-nū-klē-ō′sis). Presence of abnormally large numbers of mononuclear leukocytes in the circulating blood, especially with reference to forms that are not normal.
infectious m., benign lymphadenosis; glandular fever; an acute febrile illness caused by the Epstein-Barr virus; characterized by fever, sore throat, enlargement of lymph nodes and spleen, and leukopenia that changes to lymphocytosis during the second week; the circulating blood usually contains abnormal, large lymphocytes that have a resemblance to monocytes, and there is heterophil antibody that may be completely adsorbed on beef erythrocytes, but not on guinea pig kidney antigen. Collections of the characteristic abnormal lymphocytes may be present not only in the lymph nodes and spleen, but in various other sites, such as the meninges, brain, and myocardium.

mononucleotide (mon-ō-nū′klē-ō-tīd). Nucleotide.

monooctanoin (mon-ok-tan′ō-in). A semisynthetic esterfied glycerol used as a solubilizing agent for radiolucent gallstones retained in the biliary tract following cholecystectomy.

monooxygenases (mon-ō-ok′si-jĕ-nā-sez). Oxidoreductases that induce the incorporation of one atom of oxygen from O_2 into the substance being oxidized.

monoparesis (mon′o-pa-rē′sis, -par′ĕ-sis). Paresis affecting a single extremity or part of an extremity.

monoparesthesia (mon′ō-par-es-thē′zē-ă). Paresthesia affecting a single region only.

monopathic (mon-ō-path′ik). Relating to a monopathy.

monopathy (mon-op′ă-thē) [mono- + G. *pathos*, suffering]. **1.** A single uncomplicated disease. **2.** A local disease affecting only one organ or part.

monopenia (mon-ō-pē′nē-ă). Monocytopenia.

monophagism (mō-nof′ă-jizm) [mono- + G. *phagein*, to eat]. Habitual eating of but one kind of food or but one meal a day.

monophasia (mon-ō-fā′zē-ă) [mono- + G. *phasis*, speech]. Inability to speak other than a single word or sentence.

monophasic (mon-ō-fā′zik). **1.** Marked by monophasia. **2.** Occurring in or characterized by only one phase or stage. **3.** Fluctuating from the baseline in one direction only.

monophenol monooxygenase (mon-ō-fē′nol) [EC 1.14.18.1]. Monophenol oxidase; tyrosinase; cresolase; a copper-containing oxidoreductase that catalyzes the oxidation of *o*-diphenols to *o*-quinones by O_2, with the incorporation of one of the two oxygen atoms in the product; it also catalyzes the oxidation of monophenols, such as tyrosine, to dihydroxyphenylalanine (dopa), a precursor of melanin and epinephrine (catecholamines), and can act as a catechol oxidase.

monophenol oxidase. Monophenol monooxygenase.

monophobia (mon-ō-fō′bē-ă) [mono- + G. *phobos*, fear]. Morbid fear of solitude or of being left alone.

monophthalmos (mon-of-thal′mos) [mono- + G. *ophthalmos*, eye]. Failure of outgrowth of a primary optic vesicle with absence of ocular tissues; the remaining eye is often maldeveloped.

monophthalmus (mon′of-thal′mŭs) [mono- + G. *ophthalmos*, eye]. Cyclops.

monophyletic (mon′ō-fī-let′ik) [mono- + G. *phylē*, tribe]. **1.** Having a single source of origin; derived from one line of descent, in contrast to polyphyletic. **2.** In hematology, relating to monophyletism.

monophyletism (mon-ō-fī′lĕ-tizm) [mono- + G. *phylē*, tribe]. Monophyletic theory; in hematology, the theory that all the blood cells are derived from one common stem cell or histioblast.

monophyodont (mon-ō-fī′ō-dont) [mono- + G. *phyō*, to grow, + *odous* (*odont-*), tooth]. Having one set of teeth only; without deciduous dentition.

monoplasmatic (mon′ō-plas-mat′ik) [mono- + G. *plasma*, thing formed]. Formed of but one tissue.

monoplast (mon′ō-plast) [mono- + G. *plastos*, formed]. A unicellular organism that retains the same structure or form throughout its existence.

monoplastic (mon-ō-plas′tik). Undergoing no change in structure; relating to a monoplast.

monoplegia (mon-ō-plē′jē-ă) [mono- + G. *plēgē*, a stroke]. Paralysis of one limb.
m. masticato′ria, unilateral paralysis of the muscles of mastication (masseter, temporal, pterygoid).

monoploid (mon′ō-ployd). [mono- + G. *ploides*, in form]. Haploid.

monopodia (mon-ō-pō′dē-ă) [mono- + G. *pous*, foot]. Malformation in which only one foot is externally recognizable.

monops (mon′ops) [mono- + G. *ōps*, eye]. Cyclops.

monoptychial (mon-ō-tī′kē-ăl) [mono- + G. *ptychē*, fold]. Arranged in a single but folded layer, as the cells in the epithelium of the gallbladder or certain glands.

monorchia (mon-ōr′kē-ă). Monorchism.

monorchidic, monorchid (mon-ōr-kid′ik, mon-ōr′kid). **1.** Having but one testis. **2.** Having apparently but one testis, the other being undescended.

monorchidism (mon-ōr′ki-dizm). Monorchism.

monorchism (mon′ōr-kizm) [mono- + G. *orchis,* testis]. Monorchia; monorchidism; a condition in which only one testis is apparent, the other being absent or undescended.

monorecidive (mon-o-res′i-dēv) [mono- + L. *recidivus,* relapsing]. Denoting a late or tertiary manifestation of syphilis which takes the form of an ulcerated papule located at the site of the original chancre.

monorhinic (mon-ō-rin′ik) [mono- + G. *rhis* (*rhin-*), nose]. Single-nosed; used to characterize conjoined twins in which cephalic fusion has left only a single nose evident.

monosaccharide (mon-ō-sak′ă-rīd). Monose; a carbohydrate that cannot form any simpler sugar by simple hydrolysis; *e.g.,* pentoses, hexoses.

monoscelous (mon-ō-sel′ŭs, -skel′ŭs) [mono- + G. *skelos,* leg]. Having only one leg.

monoscenism (mon-ō-sē′nizm) [mono- + G. *skēnē,* tent (stage drop)]. Morbid concentration on some past experience.

monose (mon′ōs). Monosaccharide.

monosodium glutamate (MSG) (mon-ō-sō′dē-ŭm glū′tă-māt). $C_5H_8NNaO_4 \cdot H_2O$; the monosodium salt of the naturally occurring L form of glutamic acid; used as a flavor enhancer which is a cause or contributing factor to "Chinese restaurant" syndrome; also used intravenously as an adjunct in treatment of encephalopathies associated with hepatic disease.

monosome (mon′ō-sōm) [mono- + chromosome]. Accessory *chromosome.*

monosomia (mon-ō-sō′mē-ă) [mono- + G. *sōma,* body]. In conjoined twins, a condition in which the trunks are completely merged although the heads remain separate.

monosomic (mon-ō-sō′mik). Relating to monosomy.

monosomous (mon-ō-sō′mŭs). Characterized by or pertaining to monosomia.

monosomy (mon′ō-sō-mē) [see monosome]. Absence of one chromosome of a pair of homologous chromosomes. See also chromosomal *deletion.*

monospasm (mon′ō-spazm). Spasm affecting only one muscle or group of muscles, or a single extremity.

monospermy (mon′ō-sper-mē) [mono- + G. *sperma,* seed]. Fertilization by the entrance of only one spermatozoon into the egg.

Monosporium apiospermum (mon-ō-spō′rē-ŭm ap′ē-ō-sper′mŭm). *Scedosporium apiospermum.*

Monostoma (mō-nos′tō-mă, mon-ō-stō′mă) [mono- + G. *stoma,* mouth]. Archaic name for a genus of trematodes, based on the presence of a single sucker.

monostome (mon′ō-stōm) [mono- + G. *stoma,* mouth]. Common name for digenetic trematodes that possess a single sucker, oral or ventral, rather than both. See also *Monostoma.*

monostotic (mon-os-tot′ik) [mono- + G. *osteon,* bone]. Involving only one bone.

monostratal (mon-ō-strā′tăl) [mono- + L. *stratum,* layer]. Composed of a single layer.

monosubstituted (mon-ō-sŭb′sti-tū-tĕd). In chemistry, denoting an element or radical, only one atom or unit of which is found in each molecule of a substitution compound.

monosymptomatic (mon′ō-simp-tō-mat′ik). Denoting a disease or morbid condition manifested by only one marked symptom.

monosynaptic (mon′ō-si-nap′tik). Referring to direct neural connections (those not involving an intermediary neuron); *e.g.,* the direct connection between primary sensory nerve cells and motor neurons characterizing the monosynaptic reflex arc.

monosyphilide (mon-o-sif′i-lid). Marked by the occurrence of a single syphilitic lesion.

monoterpenes (mon-ō-ter′pēnz). Hydrocarbons or their derivatives formed by the condensation of two isoprene units, and therefore containing 10 carbon atoms; *e.g.,* camphor.

monothermia (mon-ō-ther′mē-ă) [mono- + G. *thermē,* heat]. Evenness of bodily temperature; absence of an evening rise in body temperature.

monothioglycerol (mon′ō-thī-ō-glis′er-ol). α-Monothioglycerol; thioglycerol; 3-mercapto-1,2-propanediol; used to promote wound healing.

monotocous (mō-not′ō-kŭs) [mono- + G. *tokos,* birth]. Producing a single offspring at a birth.

Monotremata (mon-ō-trē′mă-tă) [mono- + G. *trēma,* a hole]. An order of egg-laying mammals that have a cloaca or common chamber which receives digestive, urinary, and reproductive products; only Australia has such forms, the duck-billed platypus (*Ornithorhynchus*) and the echidna (*Tachyglossus*).

monotreme (mon′ō-trēm). A member of the order Monotremata.

monotrichate (mō-not′ri-kāt) Monotrichous.

monotrichous (mō-not′ri-kŭs). Monotrichate; uniflagellate; denoting a microorganism possessing a single flagellum or cilium.

monovalence, monovalency (mon-ō-vā′lens, -vā′len-sē). Univalence; univalency; a combining power (valence) equal to that of a hydrogen atom.

monovalent (mon-ō-vā′lent). **1.** Monatomic; univalent; having the combining power (valence) of a hydrogen atom. **2.** Pertaining to a monovalent (specific) antiserum.

monoxenous (mon-oks′ĕ-nŭs) [mono- + G. *xenos,* stranger]. Monogenetic.

monoxide (mon-ok′sīd). Any oxide having only one atom of oxygen; *e.g.,* CO.

monozoic (mon-ō-zō′ik). Unisegmented, as in cestodarian tapeworms. See polyzoic.

monozygotic, monozygous (mon-ō-zī-got′ik, -zī′gŭs) [mono- + G. *zygōtos,* yoked]. Denoting twins derived from a single fertilized ovum. See under twin.

Monro, Alexander Sr., Scottish anatomist and surgeon, 1697–1767. See *bursa* of M.

Monro, Alexander, Jr., Scottish anatomist, 1733–1817. See M.'s *doctrine, foramen, line, sulcus;* M.-Kellie *doctrine;* M.-Richter *line;* Richter-M. *line.*

mons, gen. **montis,** pl. **montes** (monz, mon′tis, mon′tēz) [L. a mountain] [NA]. An anatomical prominence or slight elevation above the general level of the surface.

m. pu′bis [NA], pubic mound; m. veneris; pubis (3); the prominence caused by a pad of fatty tissue over the symphysis pubis in the female.

m. ure′teris, a pinkish prominence on the wall of the bladder marking each ureteral orifice.

m. ven′eris [L. *Venus*], m. pubis.

Monson, George S., U.S. dentist, 1869–1933. See M. *curve;* anti-Monson *curve.*

mon′ster [L. *monstrum,* an evil omen, a prodigy, a wonder]. Outmoded term for malformed embryos, fetuses, or individuals. See teras; terato- entries.

Monteggia, Giovanni B., Italian surgeon, 1762–1815. See M.'s *fracture.*

Montgomery, William F., Irish obstetrician, 1797–1859. See M.'s *follicles, glands, tubercles.*

monticulus, pl. **monticuli** (mon-tik'yū-lŭs, -lī) [L. dim. of *mons,* mountain]. **1.** Any slight rounded projection above a surface. **2.** The central portion of the superior vermis forming a projection on the surface of the cerebellum; its anterior and most prominent portion is called the culmen, its posterior sloping portion, the declive.

mood (mūd). The emotional state of an individual.

mood swing. Oscillation of a person's emotional feeling tone between periods of euphoria and depression.

Moon, Henry, British surgeon, 1845–1892. See M.'s *molars.*

Moon, Robert C., U.S. ophthalmologist, 1844–1914. See Laurence-M. *syndrome;* Laurence-M.-Bardet-Biedl *syndrome.*

Moore, Charles H., British surgeon, 1821–1870. See M.'s *method.*

Moore, Robert Foster, British ophthalmologist, 1878–1963. See M.'s lightning *streaks.*

Mooren, Albert, German ophthalmologist, 1828–1899. See M.'s *ulcer.*

Mooser, Hermann, Swiss pathologist in Mexico, *1891. See M. *bodies.*

MOPP Acronym for *m*echlorethamine, *O*ncovin (vincristine), *p*rocarbazine, and *p*rednisone, a chemotherapy regimen used in the treatment of Hodgkin's disease.

Morand, Sauveur F., French surgeon, 1697–1773. See M.'s *foot, spur.*

Morat, Pierre, French physiologist, 1846–1920. See Dastre-M. *law.*

Morax, Victor, French ophthalmologist, 1866–1935. See *Moraxella;* M.-Axenfeld *conjunctivitis, diplobacillus.*

Moraxella (mōr'ak-sel'ă) [V. *Morax*]. A genus of obligately aerobic nonmotile bacteria (family Neisseriaceae) containing Gram-negative coccoids or short rods which usually occur in pairs. They do not produce acid from carbohydrates, are oxidase-positive and penicillin-susceptible, and are parasitic on the mucous membranes of man and other mammals. The type species is *M. lacunata.*

M. bo'vis, a species causing pinkeye in cattle.

M. lacuna'ta, Morax-Axenfeld diplobacillus; a species causing conjunctivitis in man; it is the type species of the genus *M.*

M. nonliquefa'ciens, a species found in the respiratory tract of man, especially in the nose; usually not pathogenic, but occasionally causes sinusitis.

M. osloen'sis, a species found in the genitourinary tract, blood, spinal and chest fluids, and nose; rarely found in the respiratory tract; usually not pathogenic, although some strains have been isolated from serious pathologic conditions in man.

M. phenylpyru'vica, a species of unknown pathogenicity found in the genitourinary tract, blood, cerebrospinal fluid, and in pus from various lesions.

morbid (mōr'bid) [L. *morbidus,* ill, fr. *morbus,* disease]. **1.** Diseased or pathologic. **2.** In psychology, abnormal or deviant.

morbidity (mōr-bid'i-tē). **1.** A diseased state. **2.** Morbility; the ratio of sick to well in a community. See also morbidity *rate.* **3.** The frequency of the appearance of complications following a surgical procedure or other treatment.

puerperal m., illness arising during the first 10 days of the post-partum period, *i.e.,* a temperature of 38°C (100.4°F) or more on any two days of the first 10, excluding the first 24 hours.

morbific (mōr-bif'ik) [L. *morbus,* disease, + *facio,* to make]. Pathogenic.

morbigenous (mor-bij'ĕ-nŭs) [L. *morbus,* disease, + G. *-gen,* producing]. Pathogenic.

morbility (mōr-bil'i-tē). Morbidity (2).

morbilli (mōr-bil'ī) [Mediev. L. *morbillus,* dim. of L. *morbus,* disease]. Measles (1).

morbilliform (mōr-bil'i-fōrm) [see morbilli]. Resembling measles (1).

Morbillivirus (mōr-bil'i-vī'rŭs). A genus of the family Paramyxoviridae, including measles, canine distemper, and bovine rinderpest viruses, all of which seem to lack neuraminidase activity.

morbilous (mōr-bil'ŭs) [see morbilli]. Relating to measles (1).

morbus (mōr'bŭs) [L. disease]. Disease (1).

morcel (mōr-sel') [Fr. *morceler,* to subdivide]. To remove piecemeal.

morcellation (mōr-se-lā'shŭn) [Fr. *morceler,* to subdivide]. Morcellment; division into and removal of small pieces, as of a tumor.

morcellement (mōr-sel-maw') [Fr.]. Morcellation.

mordant (mōr'dant) [L. *mordeo,* to bite]. **1.** A substance capable of combining with a dye and the material to be dyed, thereby increasing the affinity or binding of the dye; *e.g.,* a m. commonly used to promote staining with hematoxylin is alum. **2.** To treat with a m.

mor. dict. Abbreviation for L. *moro dicto,* as directed.

Morel, Benedict A., French psychiatrist, 1809–1873. See M.'s *ear;* Stewart-M. *syndrome.*

Morerastrongylus costaricensis (mōr'er-ă-stron'ji-lŭs kos'tar-i-sen'sis). *Angiostrongylus costaricensis.*

Morgagni, Giovanni B., Italian anatomist and pathologist, 1682–1771. See morgagnian *cyst;* M.'s *appendix, cartilage, caruncle, cataract, columns, concha, crypts, cyst, disease, foramen, fossa, fovea, frenum, globules, humor, hydatid, lacuna, liquor, nodule, prolapse, retinaculum, sinus, spheres, syndrome, tubercle, valves, ventricle;* M.-Adams-Stokes *syndrome; frenulum* of M.

Morgan, Harry de R., British physician, 1863–1931. See M.'s *bacillus.*

morgan (M) (mōr'găn) [T.H. *Morgan,* U.S. geneticist, 1866–1945]. The standard unit of genetic distance on the genetic map: the distance between two loci such that on average one crossing over will occur per miosis; for working purposes, the centimorgan (.001 M) is used.

Morgan's fold. See under fold.

morgue (mōrg) [Fr.]. Mortuary (2). **1.** A building where unidentified dead are kept pending identification before burial. **2.** A building or room in a hospital where the dead are kept pending autopsy, burial, or cremation.

moria (mōr'ē-ă) [G. *mōria,* folly, fr. *mōros,* stupid, dull]. **1.** Hebetude; rarely used term denoting foolishness or dullness of comprehension. **2.** Rarely used term for a mental state marked by frivolity, joviality, an inveterate tendency to jest, and inability to take anything seriously.

moribund (mōr'i-bŭnd) [L. *moribundus,* dying, fr. *morior,* to die]. Dying; at the point of death.

morin (mōr'in) [C.I. 75660]. 2',3,4',5,7-Pentahydroxyflavone; a natural yellow dye obtained from fustic and often associated with the dye maclurin; used as a fluorochrome for detection of metals, particularly aluminum. Fluorescent morinates are also formed with beryllium, gallium, indium, scandium, thorium, titanium, and zirconium.

Morison, James R., British surgeon, 1853–1939. See M.'s *pouch.*

Mörner, Karl A.H., Swedish chemist, 1855–1917. See M.'s *test.*

morning glory (mōr'ning glō'rē). **1.** *Ipomoea rubrocoerulea.* **2.** *Rivea corymbosa.*

Moro, Ernst, German physician, 1874–1951. See M. *reflex.*

moron (mōr'on) [G. *mōros,* stupid]. An obsolete term for a subclass of mental retardation or the individual classified therein.

moroxydine (mō-rok'si-dēn). Abitilguanide; 4-morpholinecarboximidoylguanidine; an antiviral agent.

morph-. See morpho-.

morphazinamide hydrochloride (mōr-fă-zin′ă-mīd). Morinamide hydrochloride; *N*-(morpholinomethyl)pyrazinecarboxamide hydrochloride; an antituberculous agent.

morphea (mōr-fē′ă) [G. *morphē,* form, figure]. Localized scleroderma; cutaneous lesion(s) characterized by indurated, slightly depressed plaques of thickened dermal fibrous tissue, of a whitish or yellowish white color surrounded by a pinkish or purplish halo.
m. acroter′ica, m. confined chiefly to the extremities.
m. al′ba, m. in which there is reduction or absence of normal skin pigmentation.
m. gutta′ta, white spot disease; small discrete, white, waxy, indurated lesions due to localized degenerative changes in the fibrous tissue.
m. herpetifor′mis, m. distributed along the course of distribution of a nerve, similar to the distribution of the lesions of herpes zoster.
m. linea′ris, m. in which lesions are arranged in bands.
m. pigmento′sa, localized scleroderma in which there is an increase in pigmentation.

morpheme (mōr′fēm) [morph- + G. *phēmē,* voice]. The smallest linguistic unit with a meaning.

morphine (mōr′fēn, mōr-fēn′) [L. *Morpheus,* god of dreams or of sleep]. $C_{17}H_{19}NO_3$; the major phenanthrene alkaloid of opium; contains 9 to 14% of anhydrous m. It produces a combination of depression and excitation in the central nervous system and some peripheral tissues; predominance of either central stimulation or depression depends upon the species and dose; repeated administration leads to the development of tolerance, physical dependence, and (if abused) psychic dependence. Used as an analgesic, sedative, and anxiolytic.
m. hydrochloride, white acicular or cubical crystals of bitter taste, soluble in about 25 parts of water.
m. sulfate, a narcotic analgesic consisting of feathery, silky crystals or a white crystalline powder of bitter taste; when exposed to the air it gradually loses water of crystallization.

morpho-, morph- [G. *morphē,* form, shape]. Combining forms relating to form, shape, or structure.

morphogenesis (mōr-fō-jen′ĕ-sis) [morpho- + G. *genesis,* production]. Differentiation of cells and tissues in the early embryo which establishes the form and structure of the various organs and parts of the body.

morphogenetic (mōr′fō-jĕ-net′ik). Relating to morphogenesis.

morphologic (mōr-fō-loj′ik). Relating to morphology.

morphology (mōr-fol′ō-jē) [morpho- + G. *logos,* study]. The science concerned with the configuration or the structure of animals and plants.

morphometric (mōr′fō-met′rik). Pertaining to morphometry.

morphometry (mōr-fom′ĕ-trē) [morpho- + G. *metron,* measure]. The measurement of the form of organisms or their parts.

morphon (mōr′fon) [G. *morphē,* form]. Any one of the individual structures entering into the formation of an organism; a morphologic element, such as a cell.

morphosis (mōr-fō′sis) [G. formation, act of forming]. Mode of development of a part.

morphosynthesis (mōr-fō-sin′thĕ-sis) [morpho- + synthesis]. An awareness of space and of body schema represented in the parietal lobes of the cerebral cortex.

morphotype (mōr′fō-tīp) [morpho- + G. *typos,* stamp, model]. An infrasubspecific group of bacterial strains distinguishable from other strains of the same species on the basis of morphologic characters which may or may not be associated with a change in serologic state.

Morquio, Louis, Uruguayan physician, 1867–1935. See M.'s *disease, syndrome;* M.-Ullrich *disease;* Brailsford-M. *disease.*

morrhuate sodium (mōr′rū-āt) [fr. *Gadus morrhua,* cod]. The sodium salts of the fatty acids of cod liver oil; a sclerosing agent used in the treatment of varicose veins, mixed with a local anesthetic.

Morris, John McL., U.S. surgeon, *1914. See M. *syndrome.*

Morrison, Ashton B., Irish pathologist in the U.S., *1922. See Verner-M. *syndrome.*

mors, gen. **mortis** (mōrz, mōr′tis) [L.]. Death.
m. thy′mica, old term for sudden death in young children, usually the result of infection; formerly erroneously attributed to an enlarged thymus. See also sudden infant death *syndrome.*

mor. sol. Abbreviation for L. *moro solito,* as usual, as customary.

morsulus (mōr′sū-lŭs) [Mod. L. dim. of L. *morsus,* a bite]. Troche.

mortal (mōr′tăl) [L. *mortalis,* fr. *mors,* death]. **1.** Pertaining to, or causing death. **2.** Destined to die.

mortality (mōr-tal′i-tē) [L. *mortalitus,* fr. *mors* (*mort-*), death]. **1.** The state of being mortal. **2.** Mortality *rate.* **3.** A fatal outcome.

mortar (mōr′tăr) [L. *mortarium*]. A vessel with rounded interior in which crude drugs and other substances are crushed or bruised by means of a pestle.

Mortierella (mōr′tē-ĕ-rel′ă). A genus of saprophytic fungi (class Zygomycetes, family Mucoraceae) commonly found in nature and occasionally causing zygomycosis in man.

mortification (mōr′ti-fi-kā′shŭn) [L. *mors* (*mort-*), death, + *facio,* to make]. Gangrene.

mortified (mōr′ti-fīd). Gangrenous.

mortise (mōr′tēs). The seating for the talus formed by the union of the fibula and the tibia at the ankle joint.

Morton, Dudley J., U.S. orthopedist, 1884–1960. See M.'s *syndrome.*

Morton, Samuel G., U.S. physician, 1799–1851. See M.'s *plane.*

Morton, Thomas G., U.S. physician, 1835–1903. See M.'s *neuralgia.*

mortuary (mōr′tyū-ăr-ē) [L. *mortuus,* dead, part. adj. fr. *morior,* pp. *mortuus,* to die]. **1.** Relating to death or to burial. **2.** Morgue.

morula (mōr′ū-lă, mōr′yū-) [Mod. L. dim. of L. *morus,* mulberry]. The mass of blastomeres resulting from the early cleavage divisions of the zygote. In ova with little yolk, the m. is a spheroidal mass of cells; in forms with considerable yolk, the configuration of the m. stage is greatly modified.

morulation (mōr-ū-lā′shŭn, mōr-yū-). Formation of the morula.

Morulavirus (mōr′ū-lă-vī′rŭs, mōr′yū-) [Mod. L. *morula,* dim. of L. *morum,* mulberry]. Provisional name for a genus of viruses (family Microviridae) that includes the $\phi\ \chi$ phage group of bacterial viruses.

moruloid (mōr′ū-loyd, mōr′yū-). Resembling a morula.

Morvan, Augustin M., French physician, 1819–1897. See M.'s *chorea, disease.*

mosaic (mō-zā′ik) [Mod. L. *mosaicus, musaicus,* pertaining to the Muses, artistic]. **1.** Inlaid; resembling inlaid work. **2.** The juxtaposition in an organism of genetically different tissues, resulting from somatic mutation (gene mosaicism), an anomaly of chromosome division resulting in two or more types of cells containing different numbers of chromosomes (chromosome mosaicism), or chimerism (cellular mosaicism).

mosaicism (mō-zā′i-sizm). Condition of being mosaic (2).
cellular m., a chimerism in which a tissue contains cells from different zygotes; *e.g.,* in man, involving erythrocytes.
chromosome m., see mosaic (2).
gene m., see mosaic (2).
germinal m., gonadal m., a state in which cells in a sector of a go-

nad are of a form not present in either parent, due to mutation in an intermediate progenitor of that sector.

Moschcowitz, Eli, U.S. physician, 1879–1964. See M.'s *disease.*

moschus (mos'kŭs) [G. *moschos,* musk]. Musk.

Mosler, Karl F., German physician, 1831–1911. See M.'s *diabetes.*

mosquito, pl. **mosquitoes** (mŭs-kē'tō, -tōs) [Sp. dim. of *mosca,* fly, fr. L. *musca,* a fly]. A blood-sucking dipterous insect of the family Culicidae. *Aedes, Anopheles, Culex, Mansonia,* and *Stegomyia* are the genera containing most of the species involved in the transmission of protozoan and other disease-producing parasites.

Moss, Gerald, U.S. physician, *1931. See M. *tube.*

Moss, Melvin L., U.S. oral pathologist, *1923. See Gorlin-Chaudhry-M. *syndrome.*

moss [A.S. *meōs*]. **1.** Any low growing, delicate cryptogamous plant of the class Musci. **2.** Popularly, any one of a number of lichens and seaweeds.
Ceylon m., a source of agar-agar.
club m., lycopodium.
Iceland m., cetraria.
Irish m., chondrus (2).
muskeag m., sphagnum m.
pearl m., chondrus (2).
peat m., sphagnum m.
sphagnum m., muskeag or peat m.; a highly absorbent m. used as a substitute for absorbent cotton or gauze in surgical dressing and sanitary napkins.

Mosso, Angelo, Italian physiologist, 1846–1910. See M.'s *ergograph, sphygmomanometer.*

Moszkowicz, Ludwig, Austrian surgeon, 1873–1945. See M.'s *test.*

Motais, Ernst, French ophthalmologist, 1845–1913. See M.'s *operation.*

mote (mōt) [A.S. *mot*]. A small particle; a speck.
blood m.'s, hemoconia.

mother (mŭth'er) [A.S. *mōdor*] **1.** The female parent. **2.** Any cell or other structure from which other similar bodies are formed.
surrogate m., a female whose ovum is fertilized by donor-contributed sperm and whose pregnancy is then carried normally to term with the intention of giving the infant up for adoption to the couple whose male partner has contributed the sperm.

mother of vinegar [A.S. *modder,* mud]. In vinegar, the fungus of acetous fermentation appearing as a stringy sediment.

motile (mō'til) [see motion]. **1.** Having the power of spontaneous movement. **2.** Denoting the type of mental imagery in which one learns and recalls most readily that which has been felt. *Cf.* audile; visile. **3.** A person having such mental imagery.

motilin (mō-til'in). A 22-amino acid polypeptide occurring in duodenal mucosa as a controller of normal gastrointestinal motor activity; in minute (ng) doses, it induces powerful motor activity increases in the fundic gland area and antral pouches of the stomach, with an increase in pepsin output from the former.

motility (mō-til'i-tē). The power of spontaneous movement.

motion (mō'shŭn) [L. *motio,* movement, fr. *moveo,* pp. *motus,* to move]. **1.** A change of place or position. *Cf.* movement (1). **2.** Defecation. **3.** Stool.
brownian m., brownian *movement.*
continuous passive m. (CPM), a technique in which a joint, usually the knee, is moved constantly in a mechanical splint to prevent stiffness and to increase the range of motion.

motivation (mō-ti-vā'shŭn) [ML. *motivus,* moving]. In psychology, the aggregate of all the individual motives and drives operative in an individual at any given moment which influence will and cause behavior.
extrinsic m., the search for satisfaction, or to avoid dissatisfaction, through non-task aspects of the environment such as seeking comfort, safety, and security from others or through the efforts of others.
intrinsic m., derivation of personal satisfaction through self-initiated achievement and behavior.
personal m., an individual's predispositions and expectations that give meaning and direction to personality functioning.

motive (mō'tiv) [L. *moveo,* to move, to set in motion]. **1.** Learned drive; a predisposition, need, or specific state of tension within an individual which arouses, maintains, and directs behavior toward a goal. **2.** The reason attributed to or given by an individual for a behavioral act.
achievement m., a chronic need to succeed in the face of recognizable obstacles; its strength is usually diagnosed from recurring themes in stories told by the individual while taking a thematic apperception test or from other assessment instruments used by clinical psychologists.
mastery m., the need to be assertive, to stand out in a crowd, to be dominant.

motofacient (mō-tō-fā'shent) [L. *motus,* motion, + *facio,* to make]. Causing motion; denoting the second phase of muscular activity in which actual movement is produced.

motoneuron (mō'tō-nū'ron). Motor *neuron.*

motor (mō'ter) [L. a mover, fr. *movere,* to move]. That which imparts movement. As applied to living organisms, alteration in muscle tone. **1.** In anatomy and physiology, denoting those neural structures which by the impulses generated and transmitted by them cause muscle fibers or pigment cells to contract, or glands to secrete. See also motor *cortex;* motor *endplate;* motor *neuron.* **2.** In psychology, denoting the organism's overt reaction to a stimulus (motor response).
m. oc'uli, *nervus* oculomotorius.
plastic m., an artificial point of attachment on an amputation stump to which is fastened the cord or extensor by which movement is transmitted to an artificial limb; used in cinematization.

motorial (mō-tōr'ē-ăl). Relating to motion, to a motor nerve or the motor nucleus.

motormeter (mō'ter-mē'ter). A device for determining the amount, force, and rapidity of movement.

mottling (mot'ling) [E. *motley,* variegated in color]. An area of skin comprised of macular lesions of varying shades or colors.

Motulsky dye reduction test. See under test.

moulage (mū-lazh') [F. a molding]. A reproduction in wax of a skin lesion, tumor, or other pathologic state.

mould (mōld). Mold.

moult (mōlt). Molt.

mounding (mownd'ing). Myoedema.

Mounier-Kuhn, P., 20th century French physician. See M.-K. *syndrome.*

mount (mownt). **1.** To prepare for microscopic examination. **2.** To climb on for purposes of copulation.

mounting (mownt'ing). In dentistry, the laboratory procedure of attaching the maxillary and/or mandibular cast to an articulator.
split cast m., **(1)** a cast with key grooves on its base, mounted on an articulator for the purpose of easy removal and accurate replacement; split remounting metal plates may be used instead of grooves in casts; **(2)** a means for testing the accuracy of articulator adjustment.

mourn (mōrn). To express grief or sorrow as a result of loss. In psychoanalysis, mourning is the frequently unexpressed process of responding to loss of a cathectic object which, in contrast to melancholia, usually does not involve loss of self-esteem.

mouse (mows). A small rodent belonging to the genus *Mus.*

multimammate m., an African rodent, *Praomys natalensis,* widely used in cancer research.
New Zealand mice, inbred strains of mice, either black (NZB) or white (NZW), unique among strains used in experimental immunology because of their proclivity to spontaneous immunologic abnormalities and disorders ranging from autoallergy (autoimmunity) to B lymphocyte tumors.
nude m., a hairless mutant m. with thymic hypoplasia, lacking T cells.

mousepox (mows'poks). Ectromelia (2).

mouth (mowth) [A.S. *mūth*]. **1.** *Cavitas* oris. **2.** The opening, usually the external opening, of a cavity or canal. See os (2); ostium; orifice.
carp m., a m. like that of the carp, with downturning of the corners; observed in Cornelia de Lange syndrome and Silver-Russel dwarfism.
denture sore m., mucosal erythema underlying a denture base, usually representing inflammation caused by ill-fitting dentures, poor oral hygiene, or *Candida albicans.*
parrot m., a condition of the horse in which the upper jaw is relatively longer than the lower, resulting in elongation of the upper incisors.
sore m., see soremouth.
tapir m., bouche de tapir; protrusion of the lips due to weakness of the oral muscle in certain forms of juvenile muscular dystrophy.
trench m., necrotizing ulcerative *gingivitis.*
m. of the womb, *ostium* uteri.

mouth guard. A pliable plastic device, adapted to cover the maxillary teeth, which is worn to reduce potential injury to oral structures during participation in contact sports.

mouth stick. A prosthesis which is held by the teeth and utilized by handicapped persons to perform such actions as typing, painting, and lifting small objects.

mouth'wash. Collutorium; collutory; a medicated liquid used for cleaning the mouth and treating diseased states of its mucous membranes.

movement (mūv'ment) [L. *moveo,* pp. *motus,* to move]. **1.** The act of motion; said of the entire body or of one or more of its numbers or parts. **2.** Stool. **3.** Defecation.
active m., m. effected by the organism itself, unaided by external influences.
adversive m., a rotation of the eyes, head, or trunk about the long axis of the body.
after-m., Kohnstamm's *phenomenon.*
ameboid m., the m. characteristic of leukocytes and protozoan organisms of the superclass Rhizopoda. See also streaming m.; filopodium; lobopodium.
assistive m., in massage, a m. which the partially paralyzed muscle of the patient would be unable to perform unaided but which is effected with the graduated assistance of the operator.
associated m., involuntary m. in a limb corresponding to one voluntarily executed in its fellow.
Bennett m., the bodily lateral m. or lateral shift of the mandible during a laterotrusive m.
border m.'s, any extreme compass of mandibular m. limited by bone, ligaments, or soft tissues; usually applied to horizontal mandibular m.'s.
border tissue m.'s, the action of the muscles and other tissues adjacent to the borders of a denture.
brownian m., brownian motion, brownian-Zsigmondy m.; molecular m.; pedesis; erratic, nondirectional, zigzag m. observed by ultramicroscope in certain colloidal solutions and by microscope in suspensions of light particulate matter that results from the jostling or bumping of the larger particles by the molecules in the suspending medium which are regarded as being in continuous motion.
brownian-Zsigmondy m., brownian m.
cardinal ocular m.'s, eye rotations to the right and left, upward to the right and left, and downward to the right and left, to diagnose positions of gaze.
choreic m., an involuntary spasmodic twitching or jerking in groups of muscles not associated in the production of definite purposeful m.'s.
ciliary m., the rhythmic, sweeping m. of epithelial cell cilia, of ciliate protozoans, or the sculling m. of flagella, effected possibly by the alternate contraction and relaxation of contractile threads (myoids) on one side of the cilium or flagellum.
circus m., circus rhythm; a contraction or excitation wave traveling continuously in circular fashion around a ring of muscle or through the wall of the heart.
cogwheel ocular m.'s, loose, jerky ocular rotations replacing smooth following rotations.
conjugate m. of eyes, rotation of the two eyes in the same direction. See also version (4).
decomposition of m., a manifestation of cerebellar disease in which a muscular movement is not carried out smoothly but in a series of component motions.
disjugate m. of eyes, rotation of the two eyes in opposite directions, as in convergence or divergence.
drift m.'s, drifts.
fetal m., the m. characteristic of the fetus *in utero;* usually commences between the sixteenth and eighteenth weeks of pregnancy. See also quickening.
fixational ocular m., rotation of the eyes during voluntary fixation on an object; tremors, flicks, and drifts occur.
flick m.'s, flicks.
free mandibular m.'s, **(1)** any mandibular m.'s made without tooth interference; **(2)** any uninhibited m.'s of the mandible.
functional mandibular m.'s, all natural, proper, or characteristic m.'s of the mandible made during speech, mastication, yawning, swallowing, and other associated m.'s.
fusional m., a reflex m. that tends to move the visual axes to the object of fixation so that stereoscopic vision is possible.
hinge m., an opening or closing m. of the mandible on the hinge axis.
intermediary m.'s, in dentistry, all m.'s between the extremes of mandibular excursions.
jaw m.'s, mandibular m.'s.
lateral m., in dentistry, m. of the mandible to the side.
lightning eye m.'s, ocular *myoclonus.*
Magnan's trombone m., an involuntary forward and back m. of the tongue when it is drawn out of the mouth; may be seen in several basal ganglia disorders.
mandibular m., jaw m.'s; **(1)** m.'s of the lower jaw; **(2)** all changes in position of which the mandible is capable.
mass m., mass *peristalsis.*
molecular m., brownian m.
morphogenetic m., the streaming of cells in the early embryo to form tissues or organs.
muscular m., m. caused by the contraction of the myofibrils of the muscle cells.
neurobiotactic m., the streaming of nerve cells toward the area from which they receive the most stimuli.
non-rapid eye m. (NREM), slow oscillation of the eyes during sleep.
opening m., in dentistry, m. of the mandible executed during jaw separation.
paradoxical m. of eyelids, spontaneous, involuntary elevation or lowering of the eyelids, associated with m. of extraocular muscles or muscles of mastication (external pterygoids).
passive m., allokinesis (1); m. imparted to an organism or any of its parts by external agency; m. of any joint effected by the hand of another person, or by mechanical means, without participation of

the subject himself.

pendular m., a to-and-fro m. of the intestine, without any propelling or peristaltic action, whereby the contents are churned and thoroughly mixed with the intestinal ferments.

perverted ocular m., a condition in which attempts to move eyes affected by partial ophthalmoplegia excite a m. in another direction.

protoplasmic m., m. produced by the inherent power of contraction and relaxation of protoplasm; such m.'s are of three kinds: muscular, streaming, and ciliary.

rapid eye m.'s (REM), symmetrical quick scanning m.'s of the eyes occurring many times during sleep in clusters for 5 to 60 minutes; associated with dreaming.

reflex m., allokinesis (2); an involuntary m. resulting from a sensory stimulus.

resistive m., in massage, a m. made by the patient against the efforts of the operator, or one forced by the operator against the resistance of the patient.

saccadic m., **(1)** a quick rotation of the eyes from one fixation point to another as in reading; **(2)** the rapid correction m. of a jerky nystagmus, as in labyrinthine and optokinetic nystagmus.

streaming m., the form of m. characteristic of the protoplasm of leukocytes, amebae, and other unicellular organisms; it involves the massing of the protoplasm at a point where surface pressure is least and its extrusion in the form of a pseudopod; the protoplasm may return to the body of the cell, resulting in the retraction of the pseudopod, or the entire mass may flow into the latter and thereby result in locomotion of the cell.

Swedish m.'s, Swedish gymnastics; a form of kinesitherapy in which certain systematized m.'s of the body and limbs are regulated by resistance made by an attendant.

translatory m., the motion of the body at any instant when all points within the body are moving at the same velocity and in the same direction.

vermicular m., peristalsis.

Mowry's colloidal iron stain. See under stain.

moxa (mok'să) [Jap. *moe kusa,* burning herb]. A cone or cylinder of cotton wool or other combustible material, placed on the skin and ignited in order to produce counterirritation. See also moxibustion.

moxalactam disodium (moks-ă-lak'tam). $C_{20}H_{18}N_6Na_2O_9S$; a broad spectrum β-lactam antibiotic related to the penicillins and cephalosporins.

moxibustion (mok-sĭ-bŭs'chŭn). Burning of herbal agents, such as moxa, on the skin as a counterirritant in the treatment of disease; a component of traditional Chinese and Japanese medicine.

moxisylyte (mok-sĭ'si-līt). Thymoxamine; 5-(2-dimethylaminoethoxy)carvacrol acetate; used as an α-adrenergic blocking agent for treatment of peripheral vascular disease.

MPD Abbreviation for maximal permissible *dose.*

MPS Abbreviation for mononuclear phagocyte *system.*

MQ Former abbreviation for menaquinone; now MK.

M.R.C.P. Abbreviation for Member of the Royal College of Physicians (of England).

M.R.C.P.(E) Abbreviation for Member of the Royal College of Physicians (Edinburgh).

M.R.C.P.(I) Abbreviation for Member of the Royal College of Physicians (Ireland).

M.R.C.S. Abbreviation for Member of the Royal College of Surgeons (England).

M.R.C.S.(E) Abbreviation for Member of the Royal College of Surgeons (Edinburgh).

M.R.C.S.(I) Abbreviation for Member of the Royal College of Surgeons (Ireland).

M.R.C.V.S. Abbreviation for Member of the Royal College of Veterinary Surgeons (of the United Kingdom).

MRD, mrd Abbreviation for minimal reacting *dose.*

MRI Abbreviation for magnetic resonance *imaging.*

mRNA Abbreviation for messenger *ribonucleic acid.*

MS Abbreviation for multiple *sclerosis.*

ms Abbreviation for millisecond.

M.S.D. Abbreviation for Master of Science in Dentistry.

msec Abbreviation for millisecond.

MSG Abbreviation for monosodium glutamate.

MSH Abbreviation for melanocyte-stimulating *hormone.*

MTF Abbreviation for modulation transfer *function.*

M.u. Abbreviation for Mache *unit.*

m.u. Abbreviation for mouse *unit.*

mu (myū). Twelfth letter of the Greek alphabet, μ(*q.v.*).

mucase (myū'kās). Mucinase.

Much, Hans C. R., German physician, 1880–1932. See M.'s *bacillus.*

Mucha, Victor, Austrian dermatologist, 1877–1919. See M.-Habermann *disease, syndrome.*

muci- [L. *mucus*]. Combining form for mucus, mucous, or mucin. See also muco-, myxo-.

mucicarmine (myū-si-kar'mīn). A red stain containing aluminum chloride and carmine; used to detect epithelial mucins and mucin-secreting adenocarcinomas; also used to demonstrate the capsule of *Cryptococcus* neoformans and other fungi.

mucid (myū'sid). Muciparous.

muciferous (myū-sif'er-ŭs). Muciparous.

mucification (myū'si-fi-kā'shŭn) [L. *mucus* + *facio,* to make]. A change produced in the vaginal mucosa of spayed experimental animals following stimulation with estrogen; characterized by the formation of tall columnar cells secreting mucus.

muciform (myū'si-fōrm). Blennoid; mucoid (2); myxoid; resembling mucus.

mucigenous (myū-sij'ĕ-nŭs). Muciparous.

mucihematein (myū-si-hē'mă-tē-in). A violet-blue staining fluid containing aluminum chloride and hematein; used to detect connective tissue mucins.

mucilage (myū'si-lij) [L. *mucilago*]. A pharmacopeial preparation consisting of a solution in water of the mucilaginous principles of vegetable substances; used as a soothing application to the mucous membranes and in the preparation of official and extemporaneous mixtures.

mucilaginous (myū-sĭ-laj'i-nŭs). **1.** Resembling mucilage; *i.e.,* adhesive, viscid, sticky. **2.** Muciparous.

mucin (myū'sin). A secretion containing carbohydrate-rich glycoproteins such as that from the goblet cells of the intestine, the submaxillary glands, and other mucous glandular cells; it is also present in the ground substance of connective tissue, especially mucous connective tissue, is soluble in alkaline water, and is precipitated by acetic acid.

gastric m., a white or yellowish powder which forms a viscous opalescent fluid with water, prepared from mucosa of hog's stomach by pepsin-hydrochloric acid digestion and precipitation of the supernatant fluid with 60% alcohol; used in peptic ulcer for its protective and lubricating action.

mucinase (myū'si-nās). Mucase; mucopolysaccharidase; a term specifically applied to hyaluronate lyase, hyaluronoglucosaminidase, and hyaluronoglucuronidase (hyaluronidases), but more loosely to any enzyme that hydrolyzes mucopolysaccharide substances (mucins).

mucinemia (myū-si-nē'mē-ă) [mucin + G. *haima,* blood]. Myxemia; the presence of mucin in the circulating blood.

mucinogen (myū'sin-ō-jen) [mucin + G. *-gen,* producing]. A glycoprotein that forms mucin through the imbibition of water.

mucinoid (myū'si-noyd). **1.** Mucoid (1). **2.** Resembling mucin.

mucinolytic (myū'si-nō-lit'ik). Capable of bringing about the hydrolysis of mucin, as by a mucinase.

mucinosis (myū-si-nō'sis) [mucin + G. *-osis,* condition]. A condition in which mucin is present in the skin in excessive amounts, or in abnormal distribution; classified as: **metabolic m.,** diffuse or pretibial myxedema, lichen myxedematosus, gargoylism; **secondary m.,** degeneration in tumors; **localized m.,** follicular, papular, plaque-like, focal, and myxoid or synovial cyst.
follicular m., a relatively uncommon benign eruption of discrete lesions on the face or scalp, usually in young people, in which there are cystic mucinous changes in the pilosebaceous units in the involved area; may also develop in mycosis fungoides.
papular m., *lichen* myxedematosus.
reticular erythematous m. (REM), REM *syndrome.*

mucinous (myū'si-nŭs). Mucoid (3); relating to or containing mucin.

mucinuria (myū-si-nū'rē-ă) [mucin + G. *ouron,* urine]. The presence of mucin in the urine.

muciparous (myū-sip'ă-rŭs) [mucin + L. *pario,* to bring forth, bear]. Producing or secreting mucus. Also called mucid; muciferous; mucigenous; mucilaginous (2); blennogenic; blennogenous.

mucitis (myū-sī'tis). Inflammation of a mucous membrane.

Muckle, T.J. See M.-Wells *syndrome.*

muco- [L. *mucus*]. Combining form for mucus, mucous, mucosa (mucous membrane). See also muci-, myxo-.

mucocele (myū'kō-sēl) [muco- + G. *kēlē,* tumor, hernia]. **1.** Mucous *cyst.* **2.** A mucous polypus. **3.** A retention cyst of the lacrimal sac, paranasal sinuses, appendix, or gallbladder.

mucoclasis (myū-kok'lă-sis) [muco- + G. *klasis,* a breaking off]. Denudation of any mucous surface.

mucocolitis (myū'kō-kō-lī'tis). Mucous *colitis.*

mucocolpos (myū-kō-kol'pos) [muco- + G. *kolpos,* vagina]. Presence of mucus in the vagina.

mucocutaneous (myū'kō-kyū-tā'nē-ŭs). Cutaneomucosal; relating to mucous membrane and skin; denoting the line of junction of the two at the nasal, oral, vaginal, and anal orifices.

mucoenteritis (myū'kō-en-ter-ī'tis). **1.** Inflammation of the intestinal mucous membrane. **2.** Mucomembranous *enteritis.*

mucoepidermoid (myū'kō-ep-i-der'moyd). Denoting a mixture of mucus-secreting and epithelial cells, as in m. carcinoma.

mucoglobulin (myū-kō-glob'yū-lin). A glycoprotein or mucoprotein in which the protein component is a globulin.

mucoid (myū'koyd) [mucus + G. *eidos,* appearance]. **1.** Mucinoid (1); general term for a mucin, mucoprotein, or glycoprotein. **2.** Muciform. **3.** Mucinous.

mucolipidosis, pl. **mucolipidoses** (myū'kō-lip-i-dō'sis, -sēz). Any of a group of lysosomal storage diseases in which symptoms of visceral and mesenchymal mucopolysaccharide, glycoprotein, oligosaccharide, and/or glycolipid storage are present; clinically, they bear a superficial resemblance to the mucopolysaccharidoses; autosomal recessive inheritance.
m. I, lipomucopolysaccharidosis; m. with mild Hurler-like symptoms, mild dysostosis multiplex, and moderate mental retardation.
m. II, I-cell or inclusion cell disease; m. of early onset and with severe Hurler-like symptoms, but with normal urinary mucopolysaccharides, vacuolated lymphocytes, and inclusion bodies in cultured fibroblasts (I-cells); lysosomal enzymes are increased in serum, spinal fluid, and urine.
m. III, pseudopolydystrophy; m. with mild Hurler-like symptoms, restricted joint mobility, short stature, mild mental retardation, and dysplastic skeletal changes, especially of the hip; aortic and mitral valve disease are often present.
m. IV, psychomotor retardation with cloudy corneas and retinal degeneration, with inclusion cells in cultured fibroblasts; may be due to a deficiency of neuramidase.

mucolysis (myū-kol'i-sis) [muco- + G. *lysis,* dissolution]. The solution, digestion, or liquefaction of mucus.

mucolytic (myū-kō-lit'ik). Capable of dissolving, digesting, or liquefying mucus.

mucomembranous (myū'kō-mem'bră-nŭs). Relating to a mucous membrane.

mucopeptide (myū-kō-pep'tīd). A peptide found in combination with polysaccharides containing muramic or sialic acids.
m. glycohydrolase, lysozyme.

mucoperiosteal (myū'kō-per-ē-os'tē-ăl). Relating to mucoperiosteum.

mucoperiosteum (myū'kō-per-ē-os'tē-ŭm). Mucous membrane and periosteum so intimately united as to form practically a single membrane, as that covering the hard palate.

mucopolysaccharidase (myū'kō-pol-ē-sak'ă-ri-dās). Mucinase.

mucopolysaccharide (myū'kō-pol-ē-sak'ă-rīd). General term for a protein-polysaccharide complex obtained from proteoglycans and containing as much as 95% polysaccharide; m.'s include the blood group substances. A more modern term is glycosaminoglycan, as all of the known six classes contain major amounts of glucosamine and galactosamine.

mucopolysaccharidosis, mucopolysaccharidoses (myū'kō-pol-ē-sak'ă-ri-dō'sis, -sēz). Any of a group of lysosomal storage diseases that have in common a disorder in metabolism of mucopolysaccharides, as evidenced by excretion of various mucopolysaccharides in urine and infiltration of these substances into connective tissue, with resulting various defects of bone, cartilage, and connective tissue.
type I m., Hurler's *syndrome.*
type IS m., Scheie's *syndrome.*
type II m., Hunter's *syndrome.*
type III m., Sanfilippo's *syndrome.*
type IV m., Morquio's *syndrome.*
type V m., former designation for Scheie's *syndrome.*
type VI m., Maroteaux-Lamy *syndrome.*
type VII m., m. due to β-glucuronidase deficiency.

mucopolysacchariduria (myū'kō-pol-ē-sak'ă-ri-dū'rē-ă). The excretion of mucopolysaccharides in the urine.

mucoprotein (myū-kō-prō'tēn). General term for a protein-polysaccharide complex, usually implying that the protein component is the major part of the complex, in contradistinction to mucopolysaccharide; m.'s include the α_1- and α_2-globulins of serum (and others). Sometimes called glycoproteins, although this term usually refers to those m.'s containing less than 4% carbohydrate.
Tamm-Horsfall m., the matrix of urinary casts derived from the secretion of renal tubular cells.

mucopurulent (myū-kō-pū'rū-lent). Puromucous; pertaining to an exudate that is chiefly purulent (pus), but containing relatively conspicuous proportions of mucous material.

mucopus (myū'kō-pŭs). Mycopus; a mucopurulent discharge; a mixture of mucous material and pus.

Mucor (myū'kōr). A genus of fungi (class Zygomycetes, family Mucoraceae), most species of which are saprobic; several are pathogenic and may cause zygomycosis in man.

Mucoraceae (myū'kōr-a'sē-ē) [L. *mucor,* mold]. A family of fungi (class Zygomycetes) comprised of terrestrial, aquatic, and sometimes parasitic organisms; includes the genera *Mucor, Absidia, Rhizopus,* and *Mortierella.* Although the various species of the four genera are ordinarily saprobic, free-living forms, some of them cause zygomycosis (mucormycosis) in man.

mucormycosis (myū'kōr-mī-kō'sis). Zygomycosis.

mucosa (myū-kō'să) [L. fem. of *mucosus,* mucous]. See *tunica* mucosa.
alveolar m., the mucous membrane apical to the attached gingiva.
gingival m., that portion of the oral mucous membrane that covers and is attached to the necks of the teeth and the alveolar process of the jaws; it is demarcated from lining m. on the facial aspect by a clearly defined line which marks the mucogingival junction, and, in contrast to the lining m., is keratinized and lighter in color; on the palatal surface, the gingiva blends imperceptibly with the palatal m.
olfactory m., *regio* olfactoria tunicae mucosae nasi.
respiratory m., *regio* respiratoria tunicae mucosae nasi.

mucosal (myū-kō'săl). Relating to the mucosa or mucous membrane.

mucosanguineous, mucosanguinolent (myū'kō-sang-gwin'ē-ŭs, -ō-lent) [muco- + L. *sanguis,* blood]. Pertaining to an exudate or other fluid material that has a relatively high content of blood and mucus.

mucosectomy (myū-kō-sek'tō-me). Excision of the mucosa, usually of the rectum prior to ileoanal anastomosis for treatment of ulcerative colitis.

mucoserous (myū-kō-sē'rŭs). Pertaining to an exudate or secretion that consists of both mucus and serum or a watery component.

mucostatic (myū-kō-stat'ik) [muco- + G. *stasis,* a standing]. **1.** Denoting the normal relaxed condition of mucosal tissues covering the jaws. **2.** Arresting the secretion of mucus.

mucosulfatidosis (myū'kō-sŭl-fă-ti-dō'sis). A combination of metachromatic leukodystrophy and mucopolysaccharidosis caused by deficiency of sulfatase enzymes such as arylsulfatases A, B, and C, and steroid sulfatases; characterized by coarse facial features, ichthyosis, hepatosplenomegaly, and skeletal abnormalities, with increased urinary excretion of dermatan and heparan sulfates.

mucous (myū'kŭs) [L. *mucosus,* mucous, fr. *mucus*] Relating to mucus or a m. membrane.

mucoviscidosis (myū'kō-vis-i-dō'sis). Cystic *fibrosis.*

mucro, pl. **mucrones** (myū'krō, myū-krō'nēz) [L. point, sword]. A term applied to the pointed extremity of a structure.
m. cor'dis, *apex* cordis.
m. ster'ni, *processus* xiphoideus.

mucron (myū'kron). Attachment organelle of aseptate gregarines, similar to an epimerite; the latter is set off from the rest of the gregarine body by a septum.

mucronate (myū'krō-nāt) [L. *mucronatus,* pointed]. Xiphoid.

mucus (myū'kŭs) [L.]. The clear viscid secretion of the mucous membranes, consisting of mucin, epithelial cells, leukocytes, and various inorganic salts suspended in water.
glairy m., pituita.

Muehrcke, Robert C. See Muehrcke's *lines.*

Mueller. U.S. manufacturer of surgical instruments. See M. electronic *tonometer.*

Muellerius capillaris (myū-ler'ē-ŭs kap-i-lā'ris). One of the most common species of hair lungworms (subfamily Protostrongylinae) of sheep, goats, and deer. It is smaller than *Dictyocaulus,* inhabits the smaller bronchi and lung parenchyma, and is relatively nonpathogenic to its host.

muffle (mŭf'l). A refractory core that is wound with resistant wire for electrical heating, or a similar core for gas, etc., usually in conjunction with a furnace.

Muir-Torre syndrome. See under syndrome.

Mules, Philip H., British ophthalmologist, 1843–1905. See M.'s *operation.*

muliebria (mū'lē-ē'brē-ă) [L. neut pl. of *muliebris,* relating to *mulier,* a woman]. The female genital organs.

Müller, Friedrich von, German physician, 1858–1941. See M.'s *sign.*

Müller, Heinrich, German anatomist, 1820–1864. See M.'s radial *cells, fibers, muscle, trigone.*

Müller, Hermann F., German histologist, 1866–1898. See formol-M. *fixative;* M.'s *fixative.*

Müller, Johannes P., German anatomist, physiologist, and pathologist, 1801–1858. See M.'s or müllerian *capsule, duct, experiment, law, maneuver, tubercle.*

Müller, Leopold, Czechoslovakian ophthalmologist, 1862–1936. See M.'s *method.*

Müller, Peter, German obstetrician, 1836–1922. See Hillis-M. *maneuver.*

Müller, Walther, 20th century German physicist. See Geiger-M. *counter, tube.*

müllerian (myū-ler'ē-an). Attributed to or described by Johannes Müller.

mulling (mŭl'ing). In dentistry, the final step of mixing dental amalgam, when the triturated mass is kneaded to complete the amalgamation.

multangular (mŭl-tang'gyū-lăr). Having many angles.

multi- [L. *multus,* much, many]. Prefix denoting many, properly joined only to words of L. derivation; corresponds to G. *poly-.* See also *pluri-.*

multiarticular (mŭl'tē-ar-tik'yū-lăr) [multi- + L. *articulus,* joint]. Polyarthric; polyarticular; relating to or involving many joints.

multibacillary (mŭl-tē-bas'i-lăr-ē). Made up of, or denoting the presence of, many bacilli.

multicapsular (mŭl-tē-kap'sū-lăr). Having numerous capsules.

multicellular (mŭl-tē-sel'yū-lăr). Composed of many cells.

Multiceps (mŭl'ti-seps) [multi- + L. *caput,* head]. A genus of taeniid tapeworms in which the larval forms in herbivores occur in the form of a coenurus (multiple scoleces invaginated within a single cyst).
M. mul'ticeps, a species the mature form of which occurs in the intestines of dogs; the coenurus develops in the brains of herbivorous animals, especially sheep; the cyst is often called *Coenurus cerebralis.*
M. seria'lis, a species the mature form of which is found in the intestine of dogs; the coenurus is found in the subcutaneous tissues of rabbits.

multicuspid (mŭl-tē-kŭs'pid). Multicuspidate (2).

multicuspidate (mŭl-tē-kŭs'pi-dāt). **1.** Having more than two cusps. **2.** Multicuspid; a molar tooth with three or more cusps or projections on the crown.

multifetation (mŭl-tē-fe-tā'shŭn). Superfetation.

multifid (mŭl'tē-fid) [L. *multifidus,* fr. *multus,* much, + *findo,* to cleave]. Divided into many clefts or segments.

multifidus (mŭl-tif'i-dŭs) [L.]. **1.** Multifid. **2.** See *musculus* multifidus.

multifocal (mŭl-tē-fō'kăl). Relating to or arising from many foci.

multiform (mŭl'ti-fōrm). Polymorphic.

multiglandular (mŭl-tē-glan'dyū-lăr). Pluriglandular.

multigravida (mŭl-tē-grav'i-dă) [multi- + L. *gravida,* pregnant]. A pregnant woman who has been pregnant one or more times previously.

multi-infection (mŭl'tē-in-fek'shŭn). Mixed infection with two or more varieties of microorganisms developing simultaneously.

multilobar, multilobate, multilobed (mŭl-tē-lō'bar, -lō'bāt, -lōbd'). Having several lobes.

multilobular (mŭl-tē-lob'yū-lăr). Having many lobules.

multilocal (mŭl-tē-lō'kăl). Denoting traits with an etiology comprising effects of multiple genetic loci operating together and simultaneously.

multilocular (mŭl-tē-lok'yū-lăr). Plurilocular; many-celled; having many compartments or loculi.

multimammae (mŭl-tē-mam'ē) [multi- + L. *mamma*, breast]. Polymastia.

multinodal (mŭl-tē-nō'dăl). Having many nodes.

multinodular, multinodulate (mŭl-tē-nod'yū-lăr, -yū-lāt). Having many nodules.

multinuclear, multinucleate (mŭl-tē-nū'klē-ăr, -āt). Polynuclear; polynucleate; plurinuclear; having two or more nuclei.

multinucleosis (mŭl'tē-nūk-lē-ō'sis). Polynucleosis.

multipara (mŭl-tip'ă-ră) [multi- + L. *pario*, to bring forth, to bear]. A woman who has given birth at least two times to an infant, liveborn or not weighing 500 g or more, or having an estimated length of gestation of at least 20 weeks.

grand m., a m. who has given birth seven or more times.

multiparity (mŭl-tē-păr'i-tē). Condition of being a multipara.

multiparous (mŭl-tip'ă-rŭs). Relating to a multipara.

multipartial (mŭl'tē-par'shăl). Polyvalent, with respect to an antiserum.

multiple (mŭl'ti-pl) [L. *multiplex*, fr. *multus*, many, + *plico*, pp. -*atus*, to fold]. Manifold; repeated several times; occurring in several parts at the same time, as m. arthritis, m. neuritis.

multipolar (mŭl-tē-pō'lăr). Having more than two poles; denoting a nerve cell in which the branches project from several points.

multirooted (mŭl-tē-rūt'ed). Having more than two roots.

multirotation (mŭl'tē-rō-tā'shŭn). Mutarotation.

multisynaptic (mŭl'tē-si-nap'tik). Polysynaptic.

multivalence, multivalency (mŭl-tē-vā'lens, -vā'len-sē). The state of being multivalent.

multivalent (mŭl-tē-vā'lent). Polyvalent (1). **1.** In chemistry, having a combining power (valence) of more than one hydrogen atom. **2.** Efficacious in more than one direction.

mummification (mŭm'i-fi-kā'shŭn) [mummy + L. *facio*, to make]. **1.** Dry *gangrene*. **2.** Shrivelling of a dead, retained fetus. **3.** In dentistry, treatment of inflamed dental pulp with fixative drugs (usually formaldehyde derivatives) in order to retain teeth so treated for relatively short periods; generally acceptable only for primary (deciduous) teeth.

mumps (mŭmpz) [dialectic Eng. *mump*, a lump or bump]. Epidemic *parotiditis*.

metastatic m., m. complicated by involvement of the testis or the breast.

Münchhausen, Baron Karl F.H. von, German nobleman, soldier, and raconteur, 1720–1797. See M. *syndrome*.

Munro, John C., U.S. surgeon, 1858–1910. See M.'s *point*.

Munro, William J., 19th century Australian dermatologist. See M.'s *abscess*, *microabscess*.

Munsell, Albert H., U.S. artist, 1858–1918. See Farnsworth-M. color *test*.

Munsell, Hazel E., U.S. chemist, *1891. See Sherman-M. *unit*.

Munson's sign. See under sign.

Münzer, Egmont, Austrian physician, 1865–1924. See *tract* of M. and Wiener.

mural (myū'răl) [L. *muralis;* fr. *murus*, wall]. Relating to the wall of any cavity.

muramic acid (myū-ram'ik). 2-Amino-3-*O*-(1-carboxyethyl)-2-deoxy-D-glucose; glucosamine and lactate in ether linkage between the 3 and 2 positions, respectively; a constituent of the mureins in bacterial cell walls.

muramidase (myū-ram'i-dās). Lysozyme.

mureins (myūr'ēnz). Peptidoglycans composing the sacculus or cell casing of bacteria, consisting of linear polysaccharides of alternating *N*-acetylglucosamine and *N*-acetylmuramic acid units, to the lactate side chains of which are linked oligopeptides; independent chains are cross-linked in three dimensions via the peptides or the 6-OH groups (the latter may be linked via phosphate to a teichoic acid).

Muret, Paul-Louis, French physician, *1878. See Quénu-M. *sign*.

murexide (myū-rek'sīd, -sid). The ammonium salt of purpuric acid, formerly used as a dye but superseded by the aniline colors.

muriate (myū'rē-āt) [L. *muria*, brine]. Former term for chloride.

muriatic (myū-rē-at'ik) [L. *muriaticus*, pickled in brine, fr. *muria*, brine]. Hydrochloric; relating to brine.

muriatic acid. Hydrochloric acid.

Muridae (myū'ri-dē) [L. *mus* (*mur-*), a mouse]. The largest family of Rodentia and of mammals, embracing the Old World mice and rats.

muriform (myūr'i-fōrm) [L. *murus*, wall]. Denoting an aggregation of cells fitting together like stones in a stone wall.

murine (myū'rīn, -rin, -rēn) [L. *murinus*, relating to mice, fr. *mus* (*mur-*), a mouse]. Relating to animals of the family Muridae.

murmur (mer'mer) [L.]. **1.** Susurrus; a soft sound, like that made by a somewhat forcible expiration with the mouth open, heard on auscultation of the heart, lungs, or blood vessels. **2.** An other-than-soft sound, which may be loud, harsh, frictional, etc. *e.g.*, organic cardiac m.'s are generally loud and harsh; pericardial m.'s are frictional.

accidental m., an evanescent cardiac m. not due to valvular lesion.

anemic m., a nonvalvular m. heard on auscultation of the heart and large blood vessels in cases of profound anemia.

aortic m., a m. produced at the aortic orifice, either obstructive or regurgitant.

arterial m., a m. heard on auscultating an artery.

atriosystolic m., presystolic m.

Austin Flint m., Flint's m.

bellows m., a blowing m.

brain m., sounds produced by intracranial aneurysms or arterial venous aneurysms in congenital dysplastic angiomatosis.

Cabot-Locke m., an early diastolic m., like that of aortic insufficiency, heard best at the left lower sternal border in severe anemia.

cardiac m., a m. produced within the heart, at one of its orifices.

cardiopulmonary m., cardiorespiratory m.; an innocent extracardiac m., synchronous with the heart's beat but disappearing when the breath is held, believed due to movement of air in a segment of lung compressed by the contracting heart.

cardiorespiratory m., cardiopulmonary m.

Carey Coombs m., Coombs m.; a blubbering apical middiastolic m. occurring in the acute stage of rheumatic mitral valvulitis and disappearing as the valvulitis subsides.

Cole-Cecil m., the diastolic m. of aortic insufficiency when well or predominantly heard in the left axilla.

continuous m., a m. that is heard without interruption throughout systole and into diastole.

Coombs m., Carey Coombs m.

crescendo m., a m. that increases in intensity and suddenly ceases; the presystolic m. of mitral stenosis.

Cruveilhier-Baumgarten m., a venous m. heard over collateral

veins, connecting portal and caval venous systems, on the abdominal wall. See also Cruveilhier-Baumgarten *sign.*
diamond-shaped m., a crescendo-decrescendo m., from the shape of the frequency intensity curve of the phonocardiogram.
diastolic m., a m. heard during diastole.
Duroziez' m., Duroziez' *symptom.*
dynamic m., a heart m. due to anemia or to any cause other than a valvular lesion.
early diastolic m., a m. that begins with the second heart sound, as the m. of aortic insufficiency.
ejection m., a diamond-shaped systolic m. ending before the second heart sound and produced by the ejection of blood into aorta or pulmonary artery.
endocardial m., a m. arising, from any cause, within the heart.
exocardial m., a pericardial friction m.
extracardiac m., a m. heard over the precordium but originating from structures other than the heart; the term includes pericardial friction rubs and cardiopulmonary m.'s.
Flint's m., Austin Flint m.; a diastolic m., similar to that of mitral stenosis, heard at the cardiac apex in some cases of free aortic insufficiency; it is thought to be caused by the turbulent regurgitating stream from the aorta mixing into the stream simultaneously entering from the left atrium through the mitral valve, and perhaps by the posterior movement of the anterior leaflet of the mitral valve in that turbulence.

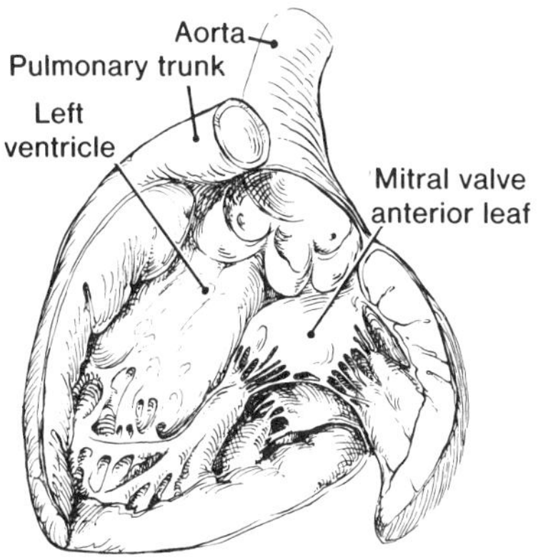

Flint's Murmur
Mechanism of production

Fräntzel's m., m. of mitral stenosis when louder at its beginning and end than in its midportion.
functional m., innocent m.; inorganic m.; a cardiac m. not associated with a heart lesion.
Gibson m., the typical continuous "machinery-like" m. of patent ductus arteriosus.
Graham Steell's m., Steell's m.; an early diastolic m. of pulmonic insufficiency secondary to pulmonary hypertension, as in mitral stenosis.
hemic m., a cardiac or vascular m. heard in anemic persons who have no valvular lesion, probably due to the increased blood velocity that characterizes anemia.
Hodgkin-Key m., a musical diastolic m. associated with retroversion of an aortic cusp.
holosystolic m., pansystolic m.
hourglass m., one in which there are two areas of maximum loudness decreasing to a point midway between the two.
innocent m., functional m.
inorganic m., functional m.
late apical systolic m., a m. ordinarily considered benign, or even extracardiac, with a possible relationship to pericardial disease; it often represents mitral insufficiency, often localized and of moderate severity but with propensity for developing bacterial endocarditis, and is frequently associated with systolic click and Barlow syndrome; a balloon or billowing mitral valve leaflet can produce either a click, murmur, or both, as it prolapses during systole into the left atrium.
late diastolic m., presystolic m.
machinery m., the long "continuous" rumbling m. of patent ductus arteriosus.
middiastolic m., a m. beginning after the A-V valves have opened in diastole, *i.e.,* an appreciable time after the second heart sound, as the m. of mitral stenosis.
mill wheel m., water wheel m.; churning cardiac m. produced by air embolism to the heart.
mitral m., a m. produced at the mitral valve, either obstructive or regurgitant.
muscular m., the sound produced by contracting muscular tissue.
musical m., a cardiac m. having a musical character.
nun's m., venous *hum.*
obstructive m., a m. caused by narrowing of one of the valvular orifices.
organic m., a m. caused by an organic lesion.
pansystolic m., holosystolic m.; a m. occupying the entire systolic interval, from first to second sound.
pericardial m., a friction sound, synchronous with the heart movements, heard in certain cases of pericarditis.
pleuropericardial m., a pleural friction sound over the pericardial region, synchronous with the heart's action, and simulating a pericardial m.
presystolic m., atriosystolic m.; late diastolic m.; a m. heard at the end of ventricular diastole (during atrial systole), usually due to obstruction at one of the atrioventricular orifices.
pulmonary m., pulmonic m., a m. produced at the pulmonary orifice of the heart, either obstructive or regurgitant.
regurgitant m., a m. due to leakage or backward flow at one of the valvular orifices of the heart.
respiratory m., vesicular *respiration.*
Roger's m., bruit de Roger; a loud pansystolic m. maximal at the left sternal border, caused by a small ventricular septal defect.
sea gull m., a musical m. supposed to imitate the sea gull's cry.
seesaw m., to-and-fro m.
Steell's m., Graham Steell's m.
stenosal m., an arterial m. due to narrowing of the vessel from pressure or organic change.
Still's m., an innocent musical m. resembling the noise produced by a twanging string.
systolic m., a m. heard during ventricular systole.
to-and-fro m., see-saw m.; m. heard in both systole and diastole of the heart, as in aortic stenosis and insufficiency.
tricuspid m., a m. produced at the tricuspid orifice, either obstructive or regurgitant.
vascular m., a m. originating in a blood vessel.
venous m., a m. heard over a vein.
vesicular m., vesicular *respiration.*
water wheel m., mill wheel m.

muromonab-CD3 (myū-rō-mō'nab). A murine monoclonal antibody to the T3 (CD3) antigen of human T lymphocytes, used as an immunosuppressant in the treatment of acute allograft rejection following renal transplantation.

Murphy, John B., U.S. surgeon, 1857–1916. See M. *drip;* M.'s *button.*

murrina (mū-rē'nă) [Fr. *morine;* Sp. *morriña,* cattle plague, prob. fr. L. *morior,* to die]. A disease of horses, mules, and burros in Panama caused by *Trypanosoma evansi* and characterized by emaciation, weakness, anemia, edema, ecchymotic conjunctivitis, fever, and paralysis of the hind legs.

Mus (mŭs) [L. *mus (mur-),* a mouse]. A genus of the family Muridae that includes about 16 species of mice; domesticated strains are numerous and genetically well defined, the most popular being the albino and piebald strains.

Musca (mŭs'kă) [L. fly]. A genus of flies (family Muscidae, order Diptera) that includes the common housefly, *M. domestica,* a species universally associated with humans, particularly under unsanitary conditions; it breeds in filth and organic waste, and is involved in the mechanical transfer of numerous pathogens.

muscae volitantes (mŭs'sē, mŭs'kē vol-i-tan'tēs) [L. pl. of *musca,* fly; pres. p. pl. of *volito,* to fly to and fro]. Floaters; appearance of moving spots before the eyes, arising from remnants of the embryologic hyaloid vascular system in the vitreous humor.

muscarine (mŭs'kă-rēn, -rin). A toxin with neurologic effects, first isolated from *Amanita muscaria* (fly agaric and also present in some species of *Hebeloma* and *Inoccybe.* The quaternary trimethylammonium salt of 2-methyl-3-hydroxy-5-(aminomethyl)-tetrahydrofuran, it is a cholinergic substance whose pharmacologic effects resemble those of acetylcholine and post ganglionic parasympathetic stimulation (cardiac inhibition, vasodilation, salivation, lacrimation, bronchoconstriction, gastrointestinal stimulation).

muscarinic (mŭs-kă-rin'ik). **1.** Having a muscarine-like action, *i.e.,* producing effects that resemble postganglionic parasympathetic stimulation. **2.** An agent that stimulates the postganglionic parasympathetic receptor. See also muscarine; nicotinic.

muscarinism (mŭs'kă-rin-ism). Mycetism.

Musci (mŭs'sī) [L. pl. of *muscus,* moss]. The class of plants that includes the mosses.

muscicide (mŭs'i-sīd) [L. *musca,* fly, + *caedo,* to kill]. An agent destructive to flies.

Muscidae (mŭs'i-dē) [L. *musca,* fly]. The family of flies (order Diptera) that includes the houseflies (*Musca*) and stable flies (*Stomoxys*).

MUSCLE

muscle (mŭs'ĕl) [L. *musculus*]. A primary tissue, consisting predominantly of highly specialized contractile cells, which may be classified as skeletal m., cardiac m., or smooth m.; microscopically, the latter is lacking in transverse striations characteristic of the other two types. For gross anatomical description, see musculus.

m.'s of abdomen, *musculi* abdominis.

abdominal external oblique m., *musculus* obliquus externus abdominis.

abdominal internal oblique m., *musculus* obliquus internus abdominis.

abductor m. of great toe, *musculus* abductor hallucis.

abductor m. of little finger, *musculus* abductor digiti minimi manus.

abductor m. of little toe, *musculus* abductor digiti minimi pedis.

adductor m. of great toe, *musculus* adductor hallucis.

adductor m. of thumb, *musculus* adductor pollicis.

Aeby's m., *musculus* cutaneomucosus.

Albinus' m., **(1)** *musculus* risorius; **(2)** *musculus* scalenus minimus.

anconeus m., *musculus* anconeus.

antagonistic m.'s, those having an opposite function, the contraction of one neutralizing that of the other.

anterior auricular m., *musculus* auricularis anterior.

anterior cervical intertransverse m.'s, *musculi* intertransversarii anteriores cervicis.

anterior rectus m. of head, *musculus* rectus capitis anterior.

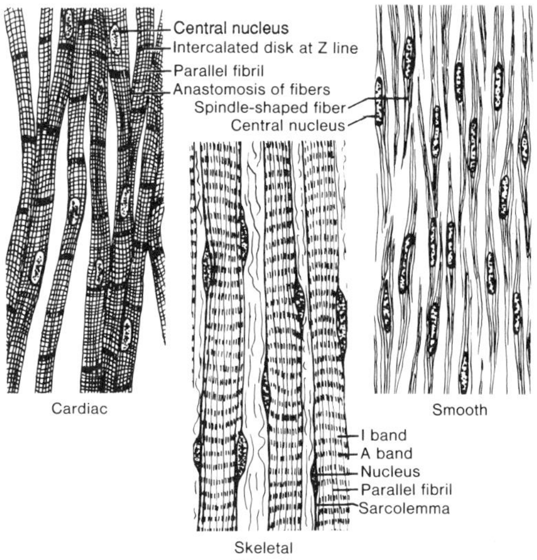

Muscle

anterior scalene m., *musculus* scalenus anterior.

anterior serratus m., *musculus* serratus anterior.

anterior tibial m., *musculus* tibialis anterior.

antigravity m.'s, the m.'s that maintain the posture characteristic of a given animal species. In most mammals they are the extensor m.'s.

m. of antitragus, *musculus* antitragicus.

appendicular m., one of the skeletal m.'s of the limbs.

articular m., *musculus* articularis.

articular m. of elbow, *musculus* articularis cubiti.

articular m. of knee, *musculus* articularis genus.

aryepiglottic m., *musculus* aryepiglotticus.

m.'s of auditory ossicles, *musculi* ossiculorum auditus.

axial m., one of the skeletal m.'s of the trunk or head.

Bell's m., a band of muscular fibers, forming a slight fold in the wall of the bladder, running from the uvula to the opening of the ureter on either side, bounding the trigonum.

biceps m. of arm, *musculus* biceps brachii.

biceps m. of thigh, *musculus* biceps femoris.

bipennate m., *musculus* bipennatus.

Bochdalek's m., *musculus* triticeoglossus.

Bovero's m., *musculus* cutaneomucosus.

Bowman's m., *musculus* ciliaris.

brachial m., *musculus* brachialis.

brachiocephalic m., *musculus* brachiocephalicus.

brachioradial m., *musculus* brachioradialis.

branchiomeric m.'s, the m.'s derived from branchial arch mesoderm that provide a large portion of the musculature for the face and neck.

Braune's m., *musculus* puborectalis.

broadest m. of back, *musculus* latissimus dorsi.

bronchoesophageal m., *musculus* bronchoesophageus.

Brücke's m., Crampton's m.; the part of the ciliary m. formed by the meridional fibers.

cardiac m., m. of heart; the muscle comprising the myocardium, consisting of anastomosing transversely striated m. fibers formed of cells united at intercalated disks; the one or two nuclei of each cell are centrally located and the longitudinally arranged myofibrils have considerable sarcoplasm around them; connective tissue is limited to reticular and fine collagenous fibers.

Casser's perforated m., *musculus* coracobrachialis.

cervical iliocostal m., *musculus* iliocostalis cervicis.
cervical interspinal m., *musculus* interspinalis cervicis.
cervical longissimus m., *musculus* longissimus cervicis.
cervical rotator m.'s, *musculi* rotatores cervicis.
cheek m., *musculus* buccinator.
chin m., *musculus* mentalis.
ciliary m., *musculus* ciliaris.
coccygeal m., *musculus* coccygeus.
m.'s of coccyx, *musculi* coccygei.
Coiter's m., *musculus* corrugator supercilii.
compressor m. of lips, *musculus* cutaneomucosus.
coracobrachial m., *musculus* coracobrachialis.
corrugator m., *musculus* corrugator supercilii.
cowl m., *musculus* trapezius.
Crampton's m., Brücke's m.
cremaster m., *musculus* cremaster.
cricothyroid m., *musculus* cricothyroideus.
cruciate m., *musculus* cruciatus.
cutaneomucous m., *musculus* cutaneomucosus.
cutaneous m., *musculus* cutaneus.
dartos m., *tunica* dartos.
deep flexor m. of fingers, *musculus* flexor digitorum profundus.
deep transverse m. of perineum, *musculus* transversus perinei profundus.
deltoid m., *musculus* deltoideus.
depressor m. of epiglottis, *musculus* thyroepiglotticus.
depressor m. of eyebrow, *musculus* depressor supercilii.
depressor m. of lower lip, *musculus* depressor labii inferioris.
depressor m. of septum, *musculus* depressor septi.
digastric m., **(1)** a m. with two fleshy bellies separated by a fibrous insertion; **(2)** *musculus* digastricus.
dilator m., *musculus* dilator.
dorsal m.'s, *musculi* dorsi.
dorsal interosseous m. of foot, *musculus* interosseus dorsalis pedis.
dorsal interosseous m. of hand, *musculus* interosseus dorsalis manus.
dorsal sacrococcygeal m., *musculus* sacrococcygeus dorsalis.
Dupré's m., *musculus* articularis genus.
Duverney's m., *musculus* orbicularis oculi pars lacrimalis.
elevator m. of anus, *musculus* levator ani.
elevator m. of prostate, *musculus* levator prostatae.
elevator m. of rib, *musculus* levator costae.
elevator m. of scapula, *musculus* levator scapulae.
elevator m. of soft palate, *musculus* levator veli palatini.
elevator m. of thyroid gland, *musculus* levator glandulae thyroideae.
elevator m. of upper eyelid, *musculus* levator palpebrae superioris.
elevator m. of upper lip, *musculus* levator labii superioris.
elevator m. of upper lip and wing of nose, *musculus* levator labii superioris alaeque nasi.
epicranial m., *musculus* epicranius.
erector m.'s of the hairs, *musculi* arrectores pilorum.
erector m. of spine, *musculus* erector spinae.
extensor m. of fingers, *musculus* extensor digitorum.
extensor m. of little finger, *musculus* extensor digiti minimi.
external intercostal m., *musculus* intercostalis externus.
external obturator m., *musculus* obturator externus.
external pterygoid m., *musculus* pterygoideus lateralis.
external sphincter m. of anus, *musculus* sphincter ani externus.
m.'s of eyeball, *musculi* bulbi.
facial m.'s, *musculi* faciales.
m.'s of facial expression, *musculi* faciales.
femoral m., *musculus* vastus intermedius.
fixator m., a m. that acts as a stabilizer of one part of the body during movement of another part.
fusiform m., *musculus* fusiformis.
Gantzer's m., an accessory m. extending from the superficial flexor of the digits to the deep flexor of the digits.
gastrocnemius m., *musculus* gastrocnemius.
Gavard's m., oblique fibers in the muscular coat of the stomach.
genioglossal m., *musculus* genioglossus.
geniohyoid m., *musculus* geniohyoideus.
gluteus maximus m., *musculus* gluteus maximus.
gluteus medius m., *musculus* gluteus medius.
gluteus minimus m., *musculus* gluteus minimus.
gracilis m., *musculus* gracilis.
great adductor m., *musculus* adductor magnus.
greater pectoral m., *musculus* pectoralis major.
greater posterior rectus m. of head, *musculus* rectus capitis posterior major.
greater psoas m., *musculus* psoas major.
greater rhomboid m., *musculus* rhomboideus major.
greater zygomatic m., *musculus* zygomaticus major.
Guthrie's m., *musculus* sphincter urethrae.
hamstring m.'s, the m.'s at the back of the thigh, comprising the biceps, the semitendinosus, and the semimembranosus.
m.'s of head, *musculi* capitis.
m. of heart, cardiac m.
Horner's m., *musculus* orbicularis oculi pars lacrimalis.
Houston's m., *compressor* venae dorsalis penis.
hyoglossal m., *musculus* hyoglossus.
iliac m., *musculus* iliacus.
iliococcygeal m., *musculus* iliococcygeus.
iliocostal m., *musculus* iliocostalis.
iliopsoas m., *musculus* iliopsoas.
index extensor m., *musculus* extensor indicis.
inferior constrictor m. of pharynx, *musculus* constrictor pharyngis inferior.
inferior gemellus m., *musculus* gemellus inferior.
inferior lingual m., *musculus* longitudinalis inferior.
inferior oblique m., *musculus* obliquus inferior.
inferior oblique m. of head, *musculus* obliquus capitis inferior.
inferior posterior serratus m., *musculus* serratus posterior inferior.
inferior rectus m., *musculus* rectus inferior.
inferior tarsal m., *musculus* tarsalis inferior.
infrahyoid m.'s, *musculi* infrahyoidei.
infraspinatus m., *musculus* infraspinatus.
innermost intercostal m., *musculus* intercostalis intimus.
intermediate great m., *musculus* vastus intermedius.
intermediate vastus m., *musculus* vastus intermedius.
internal intercostal m., *musculus* intercostalis internus.
internal obturator m., *musculus* obturator internus.
internal pterygoid m., *musculus* pterygoideus medialis.
internal sphincter m. of anus, *musculus* sphincter ani internus.
interspinal m.'s, *musculi* interspinales.
intertransverse m.'s, *musculi* intertransversarii.
involuntary m.'s, m.'s not ordinarily under control of the will; except in the case of the heart, they are smooth (nonstriated) m.'s.
ischiocavernous m., *musculus* ischiocavernosus.
Jung's m., *musculus* pyramidalis auriculae.
Klein's m., *musculus* cutaneomucosus.
Kohlrausch's m., the longitudinal m.'s of the rectal wall.
Krause's m., *musculus* cutaneomucosus.
Landström's m., microscopic m. fibers in the fascia behind and about the eyeball, attached anteriorly to the lids and anterior orbital fascia; its action is to draw the eyeball forward and the lids backward, resisting the pull of the four orbital m.'s.
Langer's m., axillary *arch.*
large m. of helix, *musculus* helicis major.
m.'s of larynx, *musculi* laryngis.
lateral cricoarytenoid m., *musculus* cricoarytenoideus lateralis.

lateral great m., *musculus* vastus lateralis.
lateral lumbar intertransverse m.'s, *musculi* intertransversarii laterales lumborum.
lateral pterygoid m., *musculus* pterygoideus lateralis.
lateral rectus m., *musculus* rectus lateralis.
lateral rectus m. of the head, *musculus* rectus capitis lateralis.
lateral vastus m., *musculus* vastus lateralis.
lesser rhomboid m., *musculus* rhomboideus minor.
lesser zygomatic m., *musculus* zygomaticus minor.
long abductor m. of thumb, *musculus* abductor pollicis longus.
long adductor m., *musculus* adductor longus.
long extensor m. of great toe, *musculus* extensor hallucis longus.
long extensor m. of thumb, *musculus* extensor pollicis longus.
long extensor m. of toes, *musculus* extensor digitorum longus.
long fibular m., *musculus* peroneus longus.
long flexor m. of great toe, *musculus* flexor hallucis longus.
long flexor m. of thumb, *musculus* flexor pollicis longus.
long flexor m. of toes, *musculus* flexor digitorum longus.
long m. of head, *musculus* longus capitis.
longissimus capitis m., *musculus* longissimus capitis.
long m. of neck, *musculus* longus colli.
long palmar m., *musculus* palmaris longus.
long peroneal m., *musculus* peroneus longus.
long radial extensor m. of wrist, *musculus* extensor carpi radialis longus.
lumbar iliocostal m., *musculus* iliocostalis lumborum.
lumbar interspinal m., *musculus* interspinalis lumborum.
lumbar quadrate muscle, *musculus* quadratus lumborum.
lumbar rotator m.'s, *musculi* rotatores lumborum.
lumbrical m. of foot, *musculus* lumbricalis pedis.
lumbrical m. of hand, *musculus* lumbricalis manus.
Marcacci's m., a sheet of smooth m. fibers underlying the areola and nipple of the mammary gland.
m.'s of mastication, see *musculus* masseter, temporalis, pterygoideus lateralis, and pterygoideus medialis.
medial great m., *musculus* vastus medialis.
medial lumbar intertransverse m.'s, *musculi* intertransversarii mediales lumborum.
medial pterygoid m., *musculus* pterygoideus medialis.
medial rectus m., *musculus* rectus medialis.
medial vastus m., *musculus* vastus medialis.
Merkel's m., *musculus* ceratocricoideus.
middle constrictor m. of pharynx, *musculus* constrictor pharyngis medius.
middle scalene m., *musculus* scalenus medius.
mimetic m.'s, *musculi* faciales.
mucocutaneous m., *musculus* cutaneomucosus.
Müller's m., (1) *musculus* orbitalis; **(2)** *fibrae* circulares; **(3)** *musculus* tarsalis superior.
multipennate m., *musculus* multipennatus.
mylohyoid m., *musculus* mylohyoideus.
nasal m., *musculus* nasalis.
m.'s of neck, *musculi* colli.
m. of notch of helix, *musculus* incisurae helicis.
oblique arytenoid m., *musculus* arytenoideus obliquus.
oblique m. of auricle, *musculus* obliquus auriculae.
occipitofrontal m., *musculus* occipitofrontalis.
ocular m.'s, see appropriate entries under *musculus* rectus and *musculus* obliquus.
Oehl's m.'s, strands of m. fibers in the chordae tendineae of the left atrioventricular valve.
omohyoid m., *musculus* omohyoideus.
opposer m. of little finger, *musculus* opponens digiti minimi.
opposer m. of thumb, *musculus* opponens pollicis.
orbicular m., *musculus* orbicularis.
orbicular m. of eye, *musculus* orbicularis oculi.
orbicular m. of mouth, *musculus* orbicularis oris.

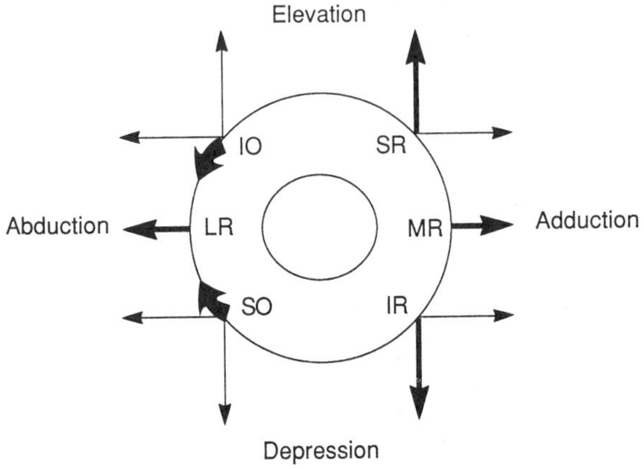

Ocular Muscles

Diagram showing actions in the right eye: clockwise arrows indicate intorsion; counterclockwise arrows indicate extorsion; heavy arrows indicate primary action; light arrows indicate secondary action. *IO*, inferior oblique; *SR*, superior rectus; *MR*, medial rectus; *IR*, inferior rectus; *SO*, superior rectus; *LR*, lateral rectus.

orbital m., *musculus* orbitalis.
palatoglossus m., *musculus* palatoglossus.
palatopharyngeal m., *musculus* palatopharyngeus.
palatouvularis m., *musculus* uvulae.
palmar interosseous m., *musculus* interosseous palmaris.
panniculus carnosus m., (1) a sheet of m., lying beneath the skin, by which the skin can be made to shiver; it is especially well developed in the horse; **(2)** in man, platysma.
papillary m., *musculus* papillaris.
pectinate m.'s, *musculi* pectinati.
pectineal m., *musculus* pectineus.
pennate m., see *musculus* bipennatus and *musculus* unipennatus.
perineal m.'s, *musculi* perinei.
piriform m., *musculus* piriformis.
plantar m., *musculus* plantaris.
plantar interosseous m., *musculus* interosseous plantaris.
plantar quadrate m., *musculus* quadratus plantae.
pleuroesophageal m., *musculus* pleuroesophageus.
popliteal m., *musculus* popliteus.
posterior auricular m., *musculus* auricularis posterior.
posterior cervical intertransverse m.'s, *musculi* intertransversarii posteriores cervicis.
posterior cricoarytenoid m., *musculus* cricoarytenoideus posterior.
posterior scalene m., *musculus* scalenus posterior.
posterior tibial m., *musculus* tibialis posterior.
Pozzi's m., *musculus* extensor digitorum brevis manus.
procerus m., *musculus* procerus.
pubococcygeal m., *musculus* pubococcygeus.
puboprostatic m., *musculus* puboprostaticus.
puborectal m., *musculus* puborectalis.
pubovaginal m., *musculus* pubovaginalis.
pubovesical m., *musculus* pubovesicalis.
pyramidal m., *musculus* pyramidalis.
pyramidal m. of auricle, *musculus* pyramidalis auriculae.
quadrate m., *musculus* quadratus.
quadrate m. of loins, *musculus* quadratus lumborum.
quadrate pronator m., *musculus* pronator quadratus.
quadrate m. of sole, *musculus* quadratus plantae.
quadrate m. of thigh, *musculus* quadratus femoris.

quadrate m. of upper lip, *musculus* quadratus labii superioris.
quadriceps m. of thigh, *musculus* quadriceps femoris.
radial flexor m. of wrist, *musculus* flexor carpi radialis.
rectococcygeal m., *musculus* rectococcygeus.
rectourethral m., *musculus* rectourethralis.
rectovesical m., *musculus* rectovesicalis.
rectus m. of abdomen, *musculus* rectus abdominis.
rectus m. of thigh, *musculus* rectus femoris.
red m., a m. in which small dark fibers predominate; myoglobin is abundant and great numbers of mitochondria occur.
Reisseisen's m.'s, microscopic smooth m. fibers in the smallest bronchial tubes.
rider's m.'s, the adductor m.'s of the thigh, which come into play especially in horseback riding.
Riolan's m., **(1)** marginal fibers of the palpebral part of the musculus orbicularis oculi; **(2)** *musculus* cremaster.
risorius m., *musculus* risorius.
rotator m.'s, *musculi* rotatores.
Rouget's m., *fibrae* circulares.
round pronator m., *musculus* pronator teres.
Ruysch's m., the muscular tissue of the fundus uteri.
salpingopharyngeal m., *musculus* salpingopharyngeus.
Santorini's m., *musculus* risorius.
scalp m., *musculus* epicranius.
Sebileau's m., deep fibers of the dartos tunic which pass into the scrotal septum.
second tibial m., *musculus* tibialis secundus.
semimembranosus m., *musculus* semimembranosus.
semispinal m., *musculus* semispinalis.
semispinal m. of head, *musculus* semispinalis capitis.
semispinal m. of neck, *musculus* semispinalis cervicis.
semispinal m. of thorax, *musculus* semispinalis thoracis.
semitendinous m., semitendinosus m., *musculus* semitendinosus.
shawl m., obsolete term for *musculus* trapezius.
short abductor m. of thumb, *musculus* abductor pollicis brevis.
short adductor m., *musculus* adductor brevis.
short extensor m. of great toe, *musculus* extensor hallucis brevis.
short extensor m. of thumb, *musculus* extensor pollicis brevis.
short extensor m. of toes, *musculus* extensor digitorum brevis.
short fibular m., *musculus* peroneus brevis.
short flexor m. of great toe, *musculus* flexor hallucis brevis.
short flexor m. of little finger, *musculus* flexor digiti minimi brevis manus.
short flexor m. of little toe, *musculus* flexor digiti minimi brevis pedis.
short flexor m. of thumb, *musculus* flexor pollicis brevis.
short flexor m. of toes, *musculus* flexor digitorum brevis.
short palmar m., *musculus* palmaris brevis.
short peroneal m., *musculus* peroneus brevis.
short radial extensor m. of wrist, *musculus* extensor carpi radialis brevis.
Sibson's m., *musculus* scalenus minimus.
skeletal m., musculus skeleti; grossly, a collection of striated muscle fibers connected at either or both extremities with the bony framework of the body; it may be an appendicular or an axial muscle; histologically, a m. consisting of elongated, multinucleated, transversely striated skeletal muscle fibers together with connective tissues, blood vessels, and nerves; individual m. fibers are surrounded by fine reticular and collagen fibers (endomysium); bundles (fascicles) of m. fibers are surrounded by irregular connective tissue (perimysium); the entire m. is surrounded, except at the m. tendon junction, by a dense connective tissue (epimysium).
smaller m. of helix, *musculus* helicis minor.
smaller pectoral m., *musculus* pectoralis minor.
smaller posterior rectus m. of head, *musculus* rectus capitis posterior minor.
smaller psoas m., *musculus* psoas minor.
smallest scalene m., *musculus* scalenus minimus.
smooth m., unstriated or unstriped m.; one of the m.'s of the internal organs, blood vessels, hair follicles, etc.; contractile elements are elongated, usually spindle-shaped cells with centrally located nuclei and a length from 20 to 200 μm, or even longer in the pregnant uterus; although transverse striations are lacking, both thick and thin myofibrils occur; smooth m. fibers are bound together into sheets or bundles by reticular fibers, and frequently elastic fiber nets are also abundant. See also involuntary m.'s.
Soemmering's m., *musculus* levator glandulae thyroideae.
soleus m., *musculus* soleus.
sphincter m., *musculus* sphincter.
sphincter m. of common bile duct, *musculus* sphincter ductus choledochi.
sphincter m. of pancreatic duct, *musculus* sphincter ductus pancreatici.
sphincter m. of pupil, *musculus* sphincter pupillae.
sphincter m. of pylorus, *musculus* sphincter pylori.
sphincter m. of urethra, *musculus* sphincter urethrae.
sphincter m. of urinary bladder, *musculus* sphincter vesicae.
spinal m., *musculus* spinalis.
spinal m. of head, *musculus* spinalis capitis.
spinal m. of neck, *musculus* spinalis cervicis.
spinal m. of thorax, *musculus* spinalis thoracis.
spindle-shaped m., *musculus* fusiformis.
splenius m. of head, *musculus* splenius capitis.
splenius m. of neck, *musculus* splenius cervicis.
stapedius m., *musculus* stapedius.
sternal m., *musculus* sternalis.
sternochondroscapular m., *musculus* sternochondroscapularis.
sternoclavicular m., *musculus* sternoclavicularis.
sternocleidomastoid m., *musculus* sternocleidomastoideus.
sternohyoid m., *musculus* sternohyoideus.
sternomastoid m., *musculus* sternocleidomastoideus.
sternothyroid m., *musculus* sternothyroideus.
strap m.'s, *musculi* infrahyoidei.
striated m., skeletal or cardiac m. in which cross striations occur in the fibers as a result of regular overlapping of thick and thin myofilaments.
styloauricular m., *musculus* styloauricularis.
styloglossus m., *musculus* styloglossus.
stylohyoid m., *musculus* stylohyoideus.
stylopharyngeal m., *musculus* stylopharyngeus.
subanconeus m., *musculus* articularis cubiti.
subclavian m., *musculus* subclavius.
subcostal m., *musculus* subcostalis.
subcrural m., *musculus* articularis genus.
suboccipital m.'s, *musculi* suboccipitales.
subquadricipital m., *musculus* articularis genus.
subscapular m., *musculus* subscapularis.
superficial flexor m. of fingers, *musculus* flexor digitorum superficialis.
superficial lingual m., *musculus* longitudinalis superior.
superficial transverse m. of perineum, *musculus* transversus perinei superficialis.
superior auricular m., *musculus* auricularis superior.
superior constrictor m. of pharynx, *musculus* constrictor pharyngis superior.
superior gemellus m., *musculus* gemellus superior.
superior oblique m., *musculus* obliquus superior.
superior oblique m. of head, *musculus* obliquus capitis superior.
superior posterior serratus m., *musculus* serratus posterior superior.
superior rectus m., *musculus* rectus superior.
superior tarsal m., *musculus* tarsalis superior.
supinator m., *musculus* supinator.
supraclavicular m., *musculus* supraclavicularis.

suprahyoid m.'s, *musculi* suprahyoidei.
supraspinous m., *musculus* supraspinatus.
suspensory m. of duodenum, *musculus* suspensorius duodeni.
synergistic m.'s, m.'s having a similar and mutually helpful function or action.
tailor's m., *musculus* sartorius.
temporal m., *musculus* temporalis.
temporoparietal m., *musculus* temporoparietalis.
tensor m. of fascia lata, *musculus* tensor fasciae latae.
tensor m. of soft palate, *musculus* tensor veli palatini.
tensor tarsi m., *musculus* orbicularis oculi pars lacrimalis.
tensor m. of tympanic membrane, *musculus* tensor tympani.
teres major m., *musculus* teres major.
teres minor m., *musculus* teres minor.
Theile's m., *musculus* transversus perinei superficialis.
third peroneal m., *musculus* peroneus tertius.
thoracic interspinal m., *musculus* interspinalis thoracis.
thoracic intertransverse m.'s, *musculi* intertransversarii thoracis.
thoracic longissimus m., *musculus* longissimus thoracis.
thoracic rotator m.'s, *musculi* rotatores thoracis.
m.'s of thorax, *musculi* thoracis.
thyroarytenoid m., *musculus* thyroarytenoideus.
thyroepiglottic m., thyroepiglottidean m., *musculus* thyroepiglotticus.
thyrohyoid m., *musculus* thyrohyoideus.
Tod's m., *musculus* obliquus auriculae.
m.'s of tongue, *musculi* linguae.
Toynbee's m., *musculus* tensor tympani.
tracheloclavicular m., *musculus* tracheloclavicularis.
m. of tragus, *musculus* tragicus.
transverse m. of abdomen, *musculus* transversus abdominis.
transverse arytenoid m., *musculus* arytenoideus transversus.
transverse m. of auricle, *musculus* transversus auriculae.
transverse m. of chin, *musculus* transversus menti.
transverse m. of nape, *musculus* transversus nuchae.
transverse m. of thorax, *musculus* transversus thoracis.
transverse m. of tongue, *musculus* transversus linguae.
transversospinal m., *musculus* transversospinalis.
trapezius m., *musculus* trapezius.
Treitz' m., *musculus* suspensorius duodeni.
triangular m., **(1)** *musculus* triangularis; **(2)** *musculus* depressor anguli oris.
triceps m. of arm, *musculus* triceps brachii.
triceps m. of calf, *musculus* triceps surae.
two-bellied m., *musculus* digastricus.
ulnar extensor m. of wrist, *musculus* extensor carpi ulnaris.
ulnar flexor m. of wrist, *musculus* flexor carpi ulnaris.
unipennate m., *musculus* unipennatus.
unstriated m., unstriped m., smooth m.
m. of uvula, *musculus* uvulae.
Valsalva's m., *musculus* tragicus.
ventral sacrococcygeal m., *musculus* sacrococcygeus ventralis.
vertical m. of tongue, *musculus* verticalis linguae.
vestigial m., an imperfect structure in man corresponding to a functioning m. in the lower animals.
vocal m., *musculus* vocalis.
voluntary m., one whose action is under the control of the will; all the striated m.'s, except the heart, are voluntary m.'s.
white m., a m. in which pale large fibers predominate; mitochondria and myoglobin are relatively sparse compared to red m.
Wilson's m., **(1)** *musculus* sphincter urethrae; **(2)** certain fibers of the levator ani.
wrinkler m. of eyebrow, *musculus* corrugator supercilii.

muscle-bound (mŭs'ĕl-bownd). Denoting a condition in which individual muscles are overdeveloped but dysynergic in concerted action.

muscle-trimming. Border *molding.*

muscone (mŭs'kōn). Muskone.

musculamine (mŭs'kyūl-ă-mēn). Spermine.

muscular (mŭs'kyū-lăr). **1.** Relating to a muscle or the muscles. **2.** Having well developed musculature.

muscularis (mŭs-kyū-lā'ris) [Mod. L. muscular]. The muscular coat of a hollow organ or tubular structure.
m. muco'sae, *lamina* muscularis mucosae.

muscularity (mŭs'kyū-lar'i-tē). The state or condition of having well developed muscles.

musculature (mŭs'kyū-lă-chūr). The arrangement of the muscles in a part or in the body as a whole.

musculoaponeurotic (mŭs'kyū-lō-ap'ō-nū-rot'ik). Relating to muscular tissue and an aponeurosis of origin or insertion.

musculocutaneous (mŭs'kyū-lō-kyū-tā'nē-ŭs). Myocutaneous; myodermal; relating to both muscle and skin.

musculomembranous (mŭs'kyū-lō-mem'bră-nŭs). Relating to both muscular tissue and membrane; denoting certain muscles, such as the occipitofrontalis, that are largely membranous.

musculophrenic (mŭs'kyū-lō-fren'ik). Relating to the muscular portion of the diaphragm; denoting an artery supplying this part.

musculoskeletal (mŭs'kyū-lō-skel'ĕ-tăl). Relating to muscles and to the skeleton, as, for example, the m. system.

musculospiral (mŭs'kyū-lō-spī'răl). Denoting the musculospiral nerve. See *nervus* radialis.

musculotendinous (mŭs'kyū-lō-ten'di-nŭs). Relating to both muscular and tendinous tissues.

musculotropic (mŭs'kyū-lō-trop'ik). Affecting, acting upon, or attracted to muscular tissue.

MUSCULUS

musculus, gen. and pl. **musculi** (mŭs'kyū-lŭs, -kyū-lī) [L. a little mouse, a muscle, fr. *mus (mur-)*, a mouse]. [NA]. Muscle; one of the contractile organs of the body by which movements of the various organs and parts are effected; typical m. is a mass of m. fibers (venter or belly), attached at each extremity, by means of a tendon, to a bone or other structure; the more proximal or more fixed attachment is called the *origin,* the more distal or more movable attachment is the *insertion;* the narrowing part of the belly which is attached to the tendon of origin is called the caput or head. For histologic description, see muscle.
mus'culi abdom'inis [NA], muscles of abdomen; muscles forming the wall of the abdomen including rectus abdominis, external and internal oblique muscles, transversus abdominis, and quadratus abdominis.
m. abduc'tor dig'iti min'imi ma'nus [NA], abductor muscle of little finger; m. abductor digiti quinti (1); *origin,* pisiform bone and pisohamate ligament; *insertion,* medial side of base of proximal phalanx of the little finger; *action,* abducts and flexes little finger; *nerve supply,* ulnar.
m. abduc'tor dig'iti min'imi pe'dis [NA], abductor muscle of little toe; m. abductor digiti quinti (2); *origin,* lateral and medial processes of calcanean tuberosity; *insertion,* lateral side of proximal phalanx of fifth toe; *action,* abducts and flexes little toe; *nerve supply,* lateral plantar nerve.
m. abduc'tor dig'iti quin'ti, **(1)** m. abductor digiti minimi manus; **(2)** m. abductor digiti minimi pedis.

m. abduc'tor hal'lucis [NA], abductor muscle of great toe; *origin,* medial process of tuber calcanei, flexor retinaculum, and plantar aponeurosis; *insertion,* medial side of proximal phalanx of great toe; *action,* abducts great toe; *nerve supply,* medial plantar.

m. abduc'tor pol'licis bre'vis [NA], short abductor muscle of thumb; *origin,* tubercle of trapezium and flexor retinaculum; *insertion,* lateral side of proximal phalanx of thumb; *action,* abducts thumb; *nerve supply,* median.

m. abduc'tor pol'licis lon'gus [NA], long abductor muscle of thumb; m. extensor ossis metacarpi pollicis; *origin,* interosseous membrane and posterior surfaces of radius and ulna; *insertion,* lateral side of base of first metacarpal bone; *action,* abducts and assists in extending thumb; *nerve supply,* radial.

m. accesso'rius glu'teus min'imus, m. scansorius.

m. adduc'tor bre'vis [NA], short adductor muscle; *origin,* superior ramus of pubis; *insertion,* upper third of medial lip of linea aspera; *action,* adducts thigh; *nerve supply,* obturator.

m. adduc'tor hal'lucis [NA], adductor muscle of great toe; *origin,* by two heads, the caput transversum from the capsules of the lateral four metatarsophalangeal joints and the caput obliquum from the lateral cuneiform and bases of the third and fourth metatarsal bones; *insertion,* lateral side of base of proximal phalanx of great toe; *action,* adducts great toe; *nerve supply,* lateral plantar.

m. adduc'tor lon'gus [NA], long adductor muscle; *origin,* symphysis and crest of pubis; *insertion,* middle third of medial lip of linea aspera; *action,* adducts thigh; *nerve supply,* obtutator.

m. adduc'tor mag'nus [NA], great adductor muscle; *origin,* ischial tuberosity and ischiopubic ramus; *insertion,* linea aspera and adductor tubercle of femur; *action,* adducts and extends thigh; *nerve supply,* obturator and sciatic.

m. adduc'tor min'imus, a small flat muscle constituting the upper portion of the adductor magnus, *insertion,* the space above linea aspera.

m. adduc'tor pol'licis [NA], adductor muscle of thumb; *origin,* by two heads, the caput transversum from the shaft of the third metacarpal and the caput obliquum from the front of the base of the second metacarpal, the trapezoid and capitate bones; *insertion,* medial side of base of proximal phalanx of thumb; *action,* adducts thumb; *nerve supply,* ulnar.

m. ancone'us [NA], anconeus muscle; anconeus (2); *origin,* back of lateral condyle of humerus; *insertion,* olecranon process and posterior surface of ulna; *action,* extends forearm and abducts ulna in pronation of wrist; *nerve supply,* radial.

m. antitrag'icus [NA], muscle of antitragus; a band of transverse muscular fibers on the outer surface of the antitragus, arising from the border of the intertragic notch and inserted into the anthelix and cauda helicis.

mus'culi arrecto'res pilo'rum [NA], erector muscles of hairs; bundles of smooth muscle fibers, attached to the deep part of the hair follicles, passing outward alongside the sebaceous glands to the papillary layer of the corium; they act to pull the hairs erect.

m. articula'ris [NA], articular muscle; a muscle that inserts directly onto the capsule of a joint, acting to retract the capsule in certain movements.

m. articula'ris cu'biti [NA], articular muscle of elbow; subanconeus muscle; the name applied to a small slip of the medial head of the triceps that inserts into the capsule of the elbow joint.

m. articula'ris ge'nus [NA], articular muscle of the knee; Dupré's muscle; subcrural or subquadricipital muscle; m. subcrureus; *origin,* lower fourth of anterior surface of shaft of femur; *insertion,* capsule of knee joint; *action,* retracts suprapatellar bursa; *nerve supply,* femoral.

m. aryepiglot'ticus [NA], aryepiglottic muscle; the fibers of the oblique arytenoid muscle that extend from the summit of the arytenoid cartilage to the side of the epiglottis; *action,* constricts the laryngeal aperture.

m. arytenoi'deus obli'quus [NA], oblique arytenoid muscle; *origin,* muscular process of arytenoid cartilage; *insertion,* summit of arytenoid cartilage of opposite side and the aryepiglottic fold as far as the epiglottis; *action,* narrows rima glottidis; *nerve supply,* recurrent laryngeal.

m. arytenoi'deus transver'sus [NA], transverse arytenoid muscle; a band of muscular fibers passing between the two arytenoid cartilages posteriorly; *action,* narrows the rima glottidis; *nerve supply,* recurrent laryngeal.

m. aryvoca'lis, a number of the deeper fibers of the vocalis muscle attached directly to the outer side of the true vocal cord.

m. attol'lens au'rem, m. attol'lens auric'ulam, m. auricularis superior.

m. a'ttrahens au'rem, m. a'ttrahens auric'ulam, m. auricularis anterior.

m. auricula'ris ante'rior [NA], anterior auricular muscle; m. attrahens aurem or auriculam; *origin,* galea aponeurotica; *insertion,* cartilage of auricle; *action,* draws pinna of ear upward and forward; *nerve supply,* facial. Considered by some to be the anterior part of the m. temporoparietalis.

m. auricula'ris poste'rior [NA], posterior auricular muscle; m. retrahens aurem or auriculam; *origin,* mastoid process; *insertion,* posterior portion of root of auricle; *action,* draws back the pinna; *nerve supply,* facial.

m. auricula'ris supe'rior [NA], superior auricular muscle; m. attollens aurem or auriculam; attollens aurem, auriculam; *origin,* galea aponeurotica; *insertion,* cartilage of auricle; *action,* draws pinna of ear upward and backward; *nerve supply,* facial. Considered by some to be the posterior part of the m. temporoparietalis.

m. az'ygos u'vu'lae, m. uvulae.

m. bi'ceps bra'chii [NA], biceps muscle of arm; *origin,* long head (caput longum) from supraglenoidal tuberosity of scapula, short head (caput breve) from coracoid process; *insertion,* tuberosity of radius; *action,* flexes and supinates forearm; *nerve supply,* musculocutaneous.

m. bi'ceps fem'oris [NA], biceps muscle of thigh; m. biceps flexor cruris; *origin,* long head (caput longum) from tuberosity of ischium, short head (caput breve) from lower half of lateral lip of linea aspera; *insertion,* head of fibula; *nerve supply,* long *action,* flexes knee and rotates leg laterally; *nerve supply,* long head, tibial, short head, peroneal.

m. bi'ceps flex'or cru'ris, m. biceps femoris.

m. bipenna'tus [NA], bipennate muscle; a muscle with a central tendon toward which the fibers converge on either side like the barbs of a feather.

m. biven'ter mandib'ulae, m. digastricus.

m. brachia'lis [NA], brachial muscle; *origin,* lower two-thirds of anterior surface of humerus; *insertion,* coronoid process of ulna; *action,* flexes forearm; *nerve supply,* musculocutaneous and (usually) radial.

m. brachicephal'icus, brachiocephalic muscle; in animals, a compound muscle passing from the brachium or humerus to the head and the dorsal cervical raphe; the clavicular insertion or clavicle subdivides the muscle.

m. brachioradia'lis [NA], brachioradial muscle; m. supinator longus; *origin,* lateral supracondylar ridge of humerus; *insertion,* front of base of styloid process of radius; *action,* flexes forearm and assists slightly in supination; *nerve supply,* radial.

m. bronchoesopha'geus [NA], bronchoesophageal muscle; muscular fascicles, arising from the wall of the left bronchus, which reinforce the musculature of the esophagus.

m. buccina'tor [NA], cheek muscle; *origin,* posterior portion of alveolar portion of maxilla and mandible and pterygomandibular ligament or raphe; *insertion,* orbicularis oris at angle of mouth; *action,* flattens cheek, retracts angle of mouth; *nerve supply,* facial.

m. buccopharyn'geus, see m. constrictor pharyngis superior.

mus'culi bul'bi [NA], muscles of eyeball; the muscles within the orbit including the four rectus muscles; two oblique muscles, and the levator of the superior eyelid.

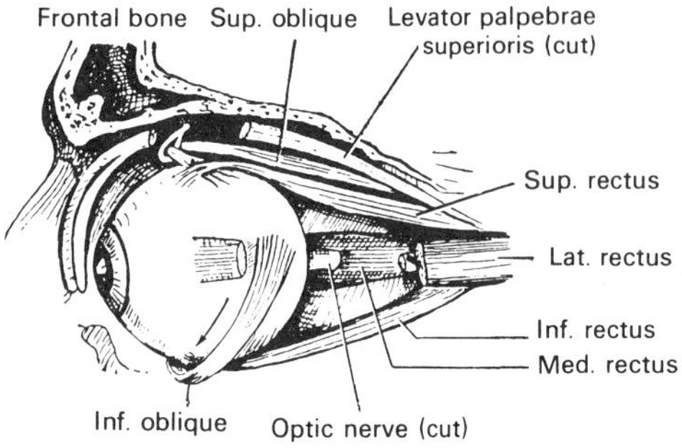

Musculi Bulbi (Muscles of the Eyeball)

m. bulbocaverno'sus, m. bulbospongiosus.
m. bulbospongio'sus [NA], sphincter vaginae; m. ejaculator seminis; m. bulbocavernosus; m. sphincter vaginae. In the male: *origin,* the perineal membrane fascia on the dorsum of the bulb of the penis; *insertion,* central tendon of the perineum and the median raphe on the free surface of the bulb; *action,* constricts bulbous urethra. In the female: *origin,* the dorsum of the clitoris, the corpus cavernosum, and the perineal membrane; *insertion,* central tendon of the perineum; *action,* acts as a weak sphincter of the vagina; *nerve supply,* pudendal.
m. cani'nus, m. levator anguli oris.
mus'culi cap'itis [NA], muscles of head; the muscles of expression, of mastication, and the suboccipital muscles in general.
m. cephalopharyn'geus, m. constrictor pharyngis superior.
m. ceratocricoi'deus [NA], Merkel's muscle; a fasciculus from the m. cricoarytenoideus posterior inserted into the inferior cornu of the thyroid cartilage.
m. ceratopharyn'geus, see m. constrictor pharyngis medius.
m. cervica'lis ascen'dens, m. iliocostalis cervicis.
m. chondroglos'sus [NA], ceratoglossus; keratoglossus; muscular fibers occasionally separated from the hyoglossus, but usually forming part of it.
m. chondropharyn'geus, see m. constrictor pharyngis medius.
m. cilia'ris [NA], ciliary muscle or ligament; Bowman's muscle; the smooth muscle of the ciliary body; it consists of circular fibers (fibrae circulares, or Müller's muscle) and radiating fibers (fibrae meridionales, or Brücke's muscle); *action,* it changes the shape of the lens in the process of accommodation.
m. cleidoepitrochlea'ris, the anterior portion of the deltoid, arising from the clavicle.
m. cleidomastoi'deus, the portion of the sternocleidomastoid muscle passing between the clavicle and the mastoid process.
m. cleido-occipita'lis, the portion of the sternocleidomastoid muscle between the clavicle and the superior nuchal line.
mus'culi coccyg'ei [NA], muscles of coccyx; the muscles of the coccyx considered as a group, including the m. coccygeus and the inconstant m. sacrococcygeus ventralis and dorsalis.
m. coccyg'eus [NA], coccygeal muscle; m. ischiococcygeus; *origin,* spine of ischium and sacrospinous ligament; *insertion,* sides of lower part of sacrum and upper part of coccyx; *action,* assists in raising and supporting pelvic floor; *nerve supply,* third and fourth sacral.
mus'culi col'li [NA], muscles of neck; the anterolateral muscles of the neck including the platysma, sternocleidomastoid, suprahyoid muscles, infrahyoid muscles, longus colli and scalene muscles.
m. complex'us, m. semispinalis capitis.
m. complex'us mi'nor, m. longissimus capitis.
m. compres'sor na'ris, see m. nasalis.
m. compres'sor ure'thrae, m. sphincter urethrae.
m. constric'tor pharyn'gis infe'rior [NA], inferior constrictor muscle of pharynx; m. laryngopharyngeus; *origin,* outer surfaces of thyroid (pars thyropharyngea) and cricoid (pars cricopharyngea) cartilages; *insertion,* pharyngeal raphe in the posterior portion of wall of pharynx; *action,* narrows lower part of pharynx in swallowing; *nerve supply,* pharyngeal plexus.
m. constric'tor pharyn'gis me'dius [NA], middle constrictor muscle of pharynx; *origin,* stylohyoid ligament, lesser cornu of the hyoid bone (pars chondropharyngeus) and greater cornu of the hyoid bone (pars ceratopharyngeus); *insertion,* pharyngeal raphe in the posterior wall of the pharynx; *action,* narrows pharynx in the act of swallowing; *nerve supply,* pharyngeal plexus.
m. constric'tor pharyn'gis supe'rior [NA], superior constrictor muscle of pharynx; m. cephalopharyngeus; *origin,* medial pterygoid plate (pars pterygopharyngea), pterygomandibular raphe (pars buccopharyngea), mylohyoid line of mandible (pars mylopharyngea), and the mucous membrane of the floor of the mouth and the side of the tongue (pars glossopharyngea); *insertion,* pharyngeal raphe in the posterior wall of the pharynx; *action,* narrows pharynx; *nerve supply,* pharyngeal plexus.
m. constric'tor ure'thrae, m. sphincter urethrae.
m. coracobrachia'lis [NA], coracobrachial muscle; Casser's perforated muscle; *origin,* coracoid process of scapula; *insertion,* middle of medial border of humerus; *action,* adducts and flexes the arm; *nerve supply,* musculocutaneous.
m. corruga'tor cu'tis a'ni, smooth muscle fibers radiating from the anal opening superficial to the external sphincter.
m. corruga'tor supercil'ii [NA], corrugator muscle; wrinkler muscle of eyebrow; Coiter's muscle; *origin,* from orbital portion of m. orbicularis oculi and nasal prominence; *insertion,* skin of eyebrow; *action,* draws medial end of eyebrow downward and wrinkles forehead vertically; *nerve supply,* facial.
m. cremas'ter [NA], cremaster muscle; Riolan's muscle (2); *origin,* from m. obliquus internus and inguinal ligament; *insertion,* cremasteric fascia and pubic tubercle; *action,* raises testicle; *nerve supply,* genitofemoral; in the male the muscle envelops the spermatic cord and testis, in the female, the round ligament of the uterus.
m. cricoarytenoi'deus latera'lis [NA], lateral cricoarytenoid muscle; *origin,* upper margin of arch of cricoid cartilage; *insertion,* muscular process of arytenoid; *action,* narrows rima glottidis; *nerve supply,* recurrent laryngeal.
m. cricoarytenoi'deus poste'rior [NA], posterior cricoarytenoid muscle; *origin,* depression on posterior surface of lamina of cricoid; *insertion,* muscular process of arytenoid; *action,* widens rima glottidis; *nerve supply,* recurrent laryngeal.
m. cricopharyn'geus, see m. constrictor pharyngis inferior.
m. cricothyroi'deus [NA], cricothyroid muscle; *origin,* anterior surface of arch of cricoid; *insertion,* pars recta, the anterior or straight part, passes upward to ala of thyroid; pars obliqua, the posterior or oblique part, passes more outward to inferior cornu of thyroid; *action,* makes vocal folds tense; *nerve supply,* superior laryngeal.
m. crucia'tus [NA], cruciate muscle; a general type of muscle in which the muscles or bundles of muscle fibers cross in a X-shaped configuration; *e.g.,* the oblique arytenoid muscles.
m. cutaneomuco'sus, cutaneomucous or mucocutaneous muscle; compressor muscle of the lips; Aeby's, Bovero's, Klein's, or Krause's muscle; "sucking muscle;" a labial muscle formed by sagittal fibers running from the skin to the mucous membrane.
m. cuta'neus [NA], cutaneous muscle; a muscle that lies in the subcutaneous tissue and attaches to the skin; it may or may not have a bony attachment. The muscles of expression are the chief examples of cutaneous muscles in the human.
m. deltoi'deus [NA], deltoid muscle; deltoid (2); *origin,* lateral third of clavicle, lateral border of acromion process, lower border of spine of scapula; *insertion,* lateral side of shaft of humerus a little above its middle; *action,* abduction, flexion, extension, and rota-

tion of arm; *nerve supply,* axillary from fifth and sixth cervical through brachial plexus.
m. depres'sor an'guli o'ris [NA], triangular muscle (2); m. triangularis (2); m. triangularis labii inferiores; *origin,* lower border of mandible anteriorly; *insertion,* blends with other muscles in lower lip near angle of mouth; *action,* pulls down corners of mouth; *nerve supply,* facial.
m. depres'sor la'bii inferio'ris [NA], depressor muscle of lower lip; m. quadratus labii inferioris; m. quadratus menti; *origin,* anterior portion of lower border of mandible; *insertion,* m. orbicularis oris and skin of lower lip; *action,* depresses lower lip; *nerve supply,* facial.
m. depres'sor sep'ti [NA], depressor muscle of septum; a vertical fasciculus from the m. orbicularis oris passing upward along the median line of the upper lip, and inserted into the cartilaginous septum of the nose; *action,* depresses septum; *nerve supply,* facial.
m. depres'sor supercil'ii [NA], depressor muscle of eyebrow; fibers of the orbital part of the m. orbicularis oculi which insert in the eyebrow; *action,* depresses eyebrow; *nerve supply,* facial.
m. detru'sor uri'nae, dutrusor urinae; the muscular coat of the bladder.
m. diaphrag'ma, see diaphragma.
m. digas'tricus [NA], digastric muscle (2); two-bellied muscle; m. biventer mandibulae; biventer mandibulae; consists of two bellies united by a central tendon which is connected to the body of the hyoid bone; *origin,* by posterior belly (venter posterior) from digastric groove medial to the mastoid process; *insertion,* by anterior belly (venter anterior) into lower border of mandible near midline; *action,* elevates the hyoid when mandible is fixed; depresses the mandible when hyoid is fixed; *nerve supply,* posterior belly from facial, anterior belly by mylohyoid from mandibular division of trigeminal.
m. dilata'tor, m. dilator.
m. dila'tor, dilator muscle; m. dilatator; a muscle which opens an orifice or dilates the lumen of an organ; it is the dilating or opening component of a pylorus (the other component is the m. sphincter).
m. dila'tor i'ridis, m. dilator pupillae.
m. dila'tor na'ris, see m. nasalis.
m. dila'tor pupil'lae [NA], dilator of pupil; dilator iridis; m. dilator iridis; the radial muscular fibers extending from the sphincter pupillae to the ciliary margin; some anatomists regard them as elastic, not muscular, in man.
m. dila'tor pylo'ri gastroduodena'lis, the longitudinal muscular fibers that open the gastroduodenal junction.
m. dila'tor pylo'ri ilea'lis, the longitudinal muscular fibers that open the ileal orifice at the level of the cecocolic junction.
m. dila'tor tu'bae, that portion of m. tensor veli palatini that attaches to the mucous membrane of the auditory tube; formerly described as a separate muscle.
mus'culi dor'si [NA], dorsal muscles; the muscles of the back in general, including those attaching the shoulder girdle to the trunk posteriorly, the posterior serratus muscles, and the erector spinae.
m. ejacula'tor sem'inis, m. bulbospongiosus.
m. epicra'nius [NA], epicranial muscle; scalp muscle; composed of the galea aponeurotica and the muscles inserting into it, *i.e.,* the m. occipitofrontalis and m. temporoparietalis.
m. epitrochleoancone'us, an occasional muscle *origin,* from the back of the medial condyle of the humerus, and *insertion* into the medial side of the olecranon process.
m. erec'tor clitor'idis, m. ischiocavernosus.
m. erec'tor pe'nis, m. ischiocavernosus.
m. erec'tor spi'nae [NA], erector muscle of spine; sacrospinalis; m. sacrospinalis; *origin,* from sacrum, ilium, and spines of lumbar vertebrae; it divides into three columns, m. iliocostalis, m. longissimus, and m. spinalis, which insert into ribs and vertebrae with additional muscle slips joining the columns at successively higher levels; *action,* extends vertebral column; *nerve supply,* posterior branches of spinal nerves.
m. exten'sor bre'vis digito'rum, m. extensor digitorum brevis.
m. exten'sor bre'vis pol'licis, m. extensor pollicis brevis.
m. exten'sor car'pi radia'lis bre'vis [NA], short radial extensor muscle of wrist; *origin,* lateral epicondyle of humerus; *insertion,* base of third metacarpal bone; *action,* extends and abducts wrist radialward; *nerve supply* radial.
m. exten'sor car'pi radia'lis lon'gus [NA], long radial extensor muscle of wrist; *origin,* lateral supracondylar ridge of humerus; *insertion,* back of base of second metacarpal bone; *action,* extends and deviates wrist radialward; *nerve supply,* radial.
m. exten'sor car'pi ulna'ris [NA], ulnar extensor muscle of wrist; *origin,* lateral epicondyle of humerus (caput humerale) and oblique line and posterior border of ulna (caput ulnare); *insertion,* base of fifth metacarpal bone; *action,* extends and abducts wrist ulnarward; *nerve supply,* radial (posterior interosseous).
m. exten'sor coccyg'is, m. sacrococcygeus dorsalis.
m. exten'sor dig'iti min'imi [NA], extensor muscle of little finger; m. extensor digiti quinti proprius; m. extensor minimi digiti; *origin,* lateral epicondyle of humerus; *insertion,* dorsum of proximal, middle, and distal phalanges of little finger; *action,* extends fingers; *nerve supply,* radial (posterior interosseous).
m. exten'sor dig'iti quin'ti pro'prius, m. extensor digiti minimi.
m. exten'sor digito'rum [NA], extensor muscle of fingers; m. extensor digitorum communis; *origin,* lateral epicondyle of humerus; *insertion,* by four tendons into the base of the proximal and middle and base of the distal phalanges; *action,* extends fingers; *nerve supply,* radial (posterior interosseous).
m. exten'sor digito'rum bre'vis [NA], short extensor muscle of toes; m. extensor brevis digitorum; *origin,* dorsal surface of calcaneus; *insertion,* by four tendons fusing with those of the extensor digitorum longus, and by a slip attached independently to the base of the proximal phalanx of the great toe; *action,* extends toes; *nerve supply,* deep peroneal.
m. exten'sor digito'rum bre'vis ma'nus, Pozzi's muscle; a short extensor muscle of the fingers of rare occurrence, and comparable to the short extensor of the toes.
m. exten'sor digito'rum commu'nis, m. extensor digitorum.
m. exten'sor digito'rum lon'gus [NA], long extensor muscle of toes; m. extensor longus digitorum; *origin,* lateral condyle of tibia, upper two-thirds of anterior margin of fibula; *insertion,* by four tendons to the dorsal surfaces of the bases of the proximal, middle, and distal phalanges of the second to fifth toes; *action,* extends the four lateral toes; *nerve supply,* deep branch of peroneal.
m. exten'sor hal'lucis bre'vis [NA], short extensor muscle of great toe; the medial belly of m. extensor digitorum brevis, the tendon of which is inserted into the base of the proximal phalanx of the great toe.
m. exten'sor hal'lucis lon'gus [NA], long extensor muscle of great toe; *origin,* lateral surface of tibia and interosseous membrane; *insertion,* base of distal phalanx of great toe; *action,* extends the great toe; *nerve supply,* anterior tibial.
m. exten'sor in'dicis [NA], index extensor muscle; m. extensor indicis proprius; *origin,* dorsal surface of ulna; *insertion,* dorsal extensor aponeurosis of index finger; *action,* assists in extending the forefinger; *nerve supply,* radial.
m. exten'sor in'dicis pro'prius, m. extensor indicis.
m. exten'sor lon'gus digito'rum, m. extensor digitorum longus.
m. exten'sor lon'gus pol'licis, m. extensor pollicis longus.
m. exten'sor min'imi dig'iti, m. extensor digiti minimi.
m. exten'sor os'sis metacar'pi pol'licis, m. abductor pollicis longus.
m. exten'sor pol'licis bre'vis [NA], short extensor muscle of thumb; m. extensor brevis pollicis; *origin,* dorsal surface of radius; *insertion,* base of proximal phalanx of thumb; *action,* extends and abducts the thumb; *nerve supply,* radial.
m. exten'sor pol'licis lon'gus [NA], long extensor muscle of

thumb; m. extensor longus pollicis; *origin,* posterior surface of ulna; *insertion,* base of distal phalanx of thumb; *action,* extends distal phalanx of thumb; *nerve supply,* radial.

mus'culi facia'les [NA], facial muscles; muscles of facial expression; mimetic muscles; the numerous muscles supplied by the facial nerve that are attached to and move the skin of the face. The NA also includes some masticatory muscles in this group.

m. fibula'ris brev'is [NA], m. peroneus brevis.

m. fibula'ris long'us [NA], m. peroneus longus.

m. fibula'ris ter'tius [NA], m. peroneus tertius.

m. flex'or accesso'rius [NA], m. quadratus plantae.

m. flex'or bre'vis digito'rum, m. flexor digitorum brevis.

m. flex'or bre'vis hal'lucis, m. flexor hallucis brevis.

m. flex'or car'pi radia'lis [NA], radial flexor muscle of wrist; *origin,* medial condyle of humerus; *insertion,* anterior surface of bases of second and third metacarpal bones; *action,* flexes and abducts wrist radialward; *nerve supply,* median.

m. flex'or car'pi ulna'ris [NA], ulnar flexor muscle of wrist; *origin,* humeral head (caput humerale) from medial condyle of humerus, ulnar head (caput ulnare) from olecranon and upper three-fifths of posterior border of ulna; *insertion,* pisiform bone; *action,* flexes and abducts wrist ulnarward; *nerve supply,* ulnar.

m. flex'or dig'iti min'imi brev'is ma'nus [NA], short flexor muscle of little finger; *origin,* hamulus of hamate bone; *insertion,* medial side of proximal phalanx of little finger; *action,* flexes proximal phalanx of little finger; *nerve supply,* ulnar.

m. flex'or dig'iti min'imi brev'is pe'dis [NA], short flexor muscle of little toe; *origin,* base of metatarsal bone of the little toe and sheath of m. peroneus longus; *insertion,* lateral surface of base of proximal phalanx of little toe; *action,* flexes the proximal phalanx of the little toe; *nerve supply,* lateral plantar.

m. flex'or digito'rum bre'vis [NA], short flexor muscle of toes; m. flexor brevis digitorum; *origin,* medial tubercle of calcaneus and central portion of plantar fascia; *insertion,* middle phalanges of four lateral toes by tendons perforated by those of the flexor longus; *action,* flexes lateral four toes; *nerve supply,* medial plantar.

m. flex'or digito'rum lon'gus [NA], long flexor muscle of toes; m. flexor longus digitorum; *origin,* middle third of posterior surface of tibia; *insertion,* by four tendons, perforating those of the flexor brevis, into bases of distal phalanges of four lateral toes; *action,* flexes second to fifth toes; *nerve supply,* tibial nerve.

m. flex'or digito'rum profun'dus [NA], deep flexor muscle of fingers; m. flexor profundus; *origin,* anterior surface of upper third of ulna; *insertion,* by four tendons, piercing those of the superficialis, into base of distal phalanx of each finger; *action,* flexes distal phalanges of fingers; *nerve supply,* ulnar and median (anterior interosseous muscle).

m. flex'or digito'rum subli'mis, m. flexor digitorum superficialis.

m. flex'or digito'rum superficia'lis [NA], superficial flexor muscle of fingers; m. flexor digitorum sublimis; m. flexor sublimis; *origin,* humeroulnar head (caput humeroulnare) from the medial epicondyle of the humerus, the medial border of the coronoid process, and a tendinous arch between these points, radial head (caput radiale) from the oblique line and middle third of the lateral border of the radius; *insertion,* by four split tendons, passing to either side of the profundus tendons, into sides of middle phalanx of each finger; *action,* flexes middle phalanges of the fingers; *nerve supply,* median.

m. flex'or hal'lucis bre'vis [NA], short flexor muscle of great toe; m. flexor brevis hallucis; *origin,* medial surface of cuboid and middle and lateral cuneiform bones; *insertion,* by two tendons, embracing that of the flexor longus hallucis, into the sides of the base of the proximal phalanx of the great toe; *action,* flexes great toe; *nerve supply,* medial and lateral plantar.

m. flex'or hal'lucis lon'gus [NA], long flexor muscle of great toe; m. flexor longus hallucis; *origin,* lower two-thirds of posterior surface of fibula; *insertion,* base of distal phalanx of great toe; *action,* flexes great toe; *nerve supply,* medial plantar.

m. flex'or lon'gus digito'rum, m. flexor digitorum longus.

m. flex'or lon'gus hal'lucis, m. flexor hallucis longus.

m. flex'or lon'gus pol'licis, m. flexor pollicis longus.

m. flex'or pol'licis bre'vis [NA], short flexor muscle of thumb; *origin,* superficial portion from flexor retinaculum of wrist, deep portion from ulnar side of first metacarpal bone; *insertion,* base of proximal phalanx of thumb; *action,* flexes proximal phalanx of thumb; *nerve supply,* median and ulnar.

m. flex'or pol'licis lon'gus [NA], long flexor longus muscle of thumb; m. flexor pollicis; *origin,* anterior surface of middle third of radius; *insertion,* distal phalanx of thumb; *action,* flexes distal phalanx of thumb; *nerve supply,* median palmar interosseous.

m. flex'or profun'dus, m. flexor digitorum profundus.

m. flex'or subli'mis, m. flexor digitorum superficialis.

m. fronta'lis, see m. occipitofrontalis.

m. fusifor'mis [NA], fusiform muscle; spindle-shaped muscle; one that has a fleshy belly, tapering at either extremity.

m. gastrocne'mius [NA], gastrocnemius muscle; gastrocnemius; *origin,* by two heads (caput laterale and caput mediale) from the lateral and medial condyles of the femur; *insertion,* with soleus by tendo calcaneus (achillis) into lower half of posterior surface of calcaneus; *action,* plantar flexion of foot; *nerve supply,* tibial.

m. gemel'lus infe'rior [NA], inferior gemellus muscle; origin, tuberosity of ischium; *insertion,* tendon of m. obturator internus; *action,* rotates thigh laterally; *nerve supply,* sacral plexus.

m. gemel'lus supe'rior [NA], superior gemellus muscle; *origin,* ischial spine and margin of lesser sciatic notch; *insertion,* tendon of m. obturator internus; *action* rotates thigh laterally; *nerve supply,* sacral plexus.

m. genioglos'sus [NA], genioglossal muscle; m. geniohyoglossus; one of the paired lingual muscles; *origin,* mental spine of the mandible; *insertion,* lingual fascia beneath the mucous membrane and epiglottis; *action,* depresses and protrudes the tongue; *nerve supply,* hypoglossal.

m. geniohyoglos'sus, m. genioglossus.

m. geniohyoi'deus [NA], geniohyoid m.; geniohyoid; geniohyoideus; *origin,* mental spine of mandible; *insertion,* body of hyoid bone; *action,* draws hyoid forward, or depresses jaw when hyoid is fixed; *nerve supply,* fibers from first and second cervical accompanying hypoglossal.

m. glossopalati'nus, m. palatoglossus.

m. glossopharyn'geus, see m. constrictor pharyngis superior.

m. glu'teus max'imus [NA], gluteus maximus muscle; *origin,* ilium behind posterior gluteal line, posterior surface of sacrum and coccyx, and sacrotuberous ligament; *insertion,* iliotibial band of fascia lata and gluteal ridge of femur; *action,* extends thigh; *nerve supply,* inferior gluteal.

m. glu'teus me'dius [NA], gluteus medius muscle; mesogluteus; *origin,* ilium between anterior and posterior gluteal lines; *insertion,* lateral surface of great trochanter; *action,* abducts and rotates thigh; *nerve supply,* superior gluteal.

m. glu'teus min'imus [NA], gluteus minimus muscle; *origin,* ilium between anterior and inferior gluteal lines; *insertion,* great trochanter of femur; *action,* abducts thigh; *nerve supply,* superior gluteal.

m. glu'teus quar'tus, m. scansorius.

m. grac'ilis [NA], gracilis muscle; *origin,* ramus of pubis near symphysis; *insertion,* shaft of tibia below medial tuberosity; *action,* adducts thigh, flexes knee, rotates leg medially; *nerve supply,* obturator.

m. hel'icis ma'jor [NA], large muscle of helix; a narrow band of muscular fibers on the anterior border of the helix arising from the spine and inserted at the point where the helix becomes transverse.

m. hel'icis mi'nor [NA], smaller muscle of helix; a band of oblique fibers covering the crus helicis.

m. hyoglos'sus [NA], hyoglossal muscle; *origin,* body and greater horn of hyoid bone; *insertion,* side of the tongue; *action,* retracts and pulls down side of tongue; *nerve supply,* motor by hypoglossal, sensory by lingual.

m. hypopharyn'geus, see m. constrictor pharyngis medius.

m. ili'acus [NA], iliac muscle; *origin,* iliac fossa; *insertion,* tendon of psoas, anterior surface of lesser trochanter, and capsule of hip joint; *action,* flexes thigh and rotates it medially; *nerve supply,* lumbar plexus.

m. ili'acus mi'nor, m. iliocapsularis; the fibers of the iliacus arising from the anterior inferior iliac spine and inserted into the iliofemoral ligament, sometimes distinctly separate from the rest of the muscle.

m. iliocapsula'ris, m. iliacus minor.

m. il'iococcyg'eus [NA], iliococcygeal muscle; the posterior part of the levator ani arising from the tendinous arch of the levator ani muscle and inserting on the anococcygeal ligament and coccyx.

m. iliocosta'lis [NA], iliocostal muscle; the lateral division of the erector spinae, having three subdivisions: m. iliocostalis lumborum, m. iliocostalis thoracis, and m. iliocostalis cervicis.

m. iliocosta'lis cer'vicis [NA], cervical iliocostal muscle; m. cervicalis ascendens; cervicalis ascendens (1); *origin,* angles of upper six ribs; *insertion,* transverse processes of middle cervical vertebrae; *action,* extends, abducts, and rotates cervical vertebrae; *nerve supply,* dorsal branches of upper thoracic nerves.

m. iliocosta'lis dor'si, m. iliocostalis thoracis.

m. iliocosta'lis lumbo'rum [NA], lumbariliocostal muscle; m. sacrolumbalis; *origin,* with erector spinae; *insertion,* the angles of lower six ribs; *action,* extends, abducts, and rotates lumbar vertebrae; *nerve supply,* dorsal branches of thoracic and lumbar nerves.

m. iliocosta'lis thora'cis [NA], thoracic iliocostal muscle; m. iliocostalis dorsi; *origin,* medial side of angles of lower six ribs; *insertion,* angles of upper six ribs; *action,* extends, abducts, and rotates thoracic vertebrae; *nerve supply,* dorsal branches of thoracic nerves.

m. iliopso'as [NA], iliopsoas muscle; a compound muscle, consisting of the m. iliacus and m. psoas major.

m. incisi'vus la'bii inferior'is, inferior incisive bundle of origin of m. orbicularis oris.

m. incisi'vus la'bii superior'is, superior incisive bundle of origin of m. orbicularis oris.

m. incisu'rae hel'icis [NA], muscle of notch of helix; Santorini's muscle; m. intertragicus; an occasional muscle on the cranial surface of the auricle spanning the antitragohelicine fissure.

m. infracosta'lis, pl. **infracosta'les,** m. subcostalis.

mus'culi infrahyoi'dei [NA], infrahyoid muscles; strap muscles; the small, flat muscles inferior to the hyoid bone including the sternohyoideus, omohyoideus, sternothyroideus, thyrohyoideus and levator glandulae thyroideae.

m. infraspina'tus [NA], infraspinatus muscle; *origin,* infraspinous fossa of scapula; *insertion,* middle facet of great tubercle of humerus; *action,* extends arm and rotates it laterally; *nerve supply,* suprascapular from fifth to sixth cervical.

m. intercosta'lis exter'nus, pl. **intercosta'les exter'ni** [NA], external intercostal muscle; each arises from lower border of one rib and passes obliquely downward and forward to be inserted into the upper border of rib below; *action,* contract during inspiration, also maintain tension in the intercostal spaces to resist mediolateral movement; *nerve supply,* intercostal.

m. intercosta'lis inter'nus, pl. **intercosta'les inter'ni** [NA], internal intercostal muscle; each arises from lower border of rib and passes obliquely downward and backward to be inserted into upper border of rib below; *action,* contract during expiration, also maintain tension in the intercostal spaces to resist mediolateral movement; *nerve supply,* intercostal.

m. intercosta'lis in'timus pl. **intercosta'les in'timi** [NA], innermost intercostal muscle; a layer parallel to the internal intercostal muscle but separated from it by the intercostal vessels and nerves.

m. interos'seus dorsa'lis ma'nus, pl. **interos'sei dorsa'les ma'nus** [NA], dorsal interosseous muscle of hand; four muscles in the hand; *origin,* sides of adjacent metacarpal bones; *insertion,* proximal phalanges and extensor expansion, first on radial side of index, second on radial side of middle finger, third on ulnar side of middle finger, fourth on ulnar side of ring finger; *action,* abducts index, abducts or adducts middle finger, abducts ring finger; *nerve supply,* ulnar.

m. interos'seus dorsa'lis pe'dis, pl. **interos'sei dorsa'les pe'dis** [NA], dorsal interosseous muscle of foot; four muscles in the foot; *origin,* from sides of adjacent metatarsal bones; *insertion,* first into medial, second into lateral side of proximal phalanx of second toe, third and fourth into lateral side of proximal phalanx of third and fourth toes; *action,* first adducts second toe; second, third, and fourth abduct second, third, and fourth toes; *nerve supply,* lateral plantar.

m. interos'seus palma'ris, pl. **interos'sei palma'res** [NA], palmar interosseous muscle; m. interosseus volaris; three muscles in the hand; *origin,* first from ulnar side of second metacarpal, second and third from radial sides of fourth and fifth metacarpals; *insertion,* first into ulnar side of index, second and third into radial sides of ring and little fingers; *action,* adducts fingers toward axis of middle finger; *nerve supply,* ulnar.

m. interos'seus planta'ris, pl. **interos'sei planta'res** [NA], plantar interosseous muscle; three muscles; *origin,* the medial side of the third, fourth, and fifth metatarsal bones; *insertion,* corresponding side of proximal phalanx of the same toes; *action,* adducts three lateral toes; *nerve supply,* lateral plantar.

m. interos'seus vola'ris, m. interosseus palmaris.

mus'culi interspina'les [NA], interspinal muscles; the paired muscles between spinous processes of adjacent vertebrae; subdivided into cervical, thoracic, and lumbar muscles.

m. interspina'lis cer'vicis [NA], cervical interspinal muscle; *origin,* tubercle of spinous process of cervical vertebra; *insertion,* tubercle of spinous process of next superior vertebra; *action,* extends the neck; *nerve supply,* dorsal branches of cervical nerves.

m. interspina'lis lumbo'rum [NA], lumbar interspinal muscle; *origin,* superior margin of lumbar spinous process; *insertion,* inferior margin of next superior spinous process; *action,* extends lumbar vertebrae; *nerve supply,* dorsal branches of lumbar nerves.

m. interspina'lis thora'cis [NA], thoracic interspinal muscle; often poorly developed or absent muscles between spinous process of thoracic vertebrae; *action,* extends thoracic vertebrae; *nerve supply,* dorsal branches of thoracic nerves.

m. intertra'gicus, m. incisurae helicis.

mus'culi intertransversa'rii [NA], intertransverse muscles; the paired muscles between transverse processes of adjacent vertebrae; there are anterior and posterior muscles in the cervical region; lateral and medial muscles in the lumbar region; and single muscles in the thoracic region.

mus'culi intertransversa'rii anterio'res cer'vicis [NA], anterior cervical intertransverse muscles; *origin,* anterior tubercle of cervical transverse process; *insertion,* anterior tubercle of next superior transverse process; *action,* abducts cervical vertebrae; *nerve supply,* ventral branch of cervical nerves.

mus'culi intertransversa'rii latera'les lumbo'rum [NA], lateral lumbar intertransverse muscles; *origin,* transverse processes of lumbar vertebrae; *insertion,* next superior transverse process; *action,* abducts lumbar vertebrae; *nerve supply,* ventral branches of lumbar nerves.

mus'culi intertransversa'rii media'les lumbo'rum [NA], medial lumbar intertransverse muscles; *origin,* accessory and mamillary processes of lumbar vertebrae; *insertion,* corresponding processes of next superior vertebra; *action,* abducts lumbar vertebrae; *nerve supply,* dorsal branches of lumbar nerves.

mus'culi intertransversa'rii posterio'res cer'vicis [NA], posterior cervical intertransverse muscles; *origin,* pars lateralis, posterior tubercle of cervical transverse process; pars medialis; transverse process; *insertion,* corresponding parts of next superior transverse process; *action,* abducts cervical vertebrae; *nerve supply,* pars lateralis; ventral branches of cervical nerves; pars medialis, dorsal branches of cervical nerves.

mus'culi intertransversa'rii thora'cis [NA], thoracic intertransverse muscles; *origin,* transverse processes of thoracic vertebrae; *insertion,* next superior transverse process; *action,* abducts thoracic vertebrae; *nerve supply,* dorsal branches of thoracic nerves.

m. ischiocaverno'sus [NA], ischiocavernous muscle; m. erector penis or clitoridis; *origin,* ramus of ischium; *insertion,* corpus cavernosum penis (or clitoridis); *action* compresses the crus of the penis (or clitoris) forcing blood in its sinuses into the distal part of the corpus cavernosum; *nerve supply,* perineal.

m. ischiococcyg'eus, m. coccygeus.

m. keratopharyn'geus, see m. constrictor pharyngis medius.

mus'culi laryn'gis [NA], muscles of larynx; the intrinsic muscles that regulate the length, position and tension of the vocal cords and adjust the size of the openings between the aryepiglottic folds, the ventricular folds and the vocal folds.

m. laryngopharyn'geus, m. constrictor pharyngis inferior.

m. latis'simus dor'si [NA], broadest muscle of back; *origin,* spinous processes of lower five or six thoracic and the lumbar vertebrae, median ridge of sacrum, and outer lip of iliac crest; *insertion,* with teres major into posterior lip of bicipital groove of humerus; *action,* adducts arm, rotates it medially, and extends it; *nerve supply,* thoracodorsal.

m. leva'tor a'lae na'si, alar insertion of m. levator labii superioris alaeque nasi.

m. leva'tor an'guli o'ris [NA], m. triangularis labii superioris; m. caninus; *origin,* canine fossa of maxilla; *insertion,* orbicularis oris and skin at angle of mouth; *action,* raises angle of mouth; *nerve supply,* facial.

m. leva'tor an'guli scap'ulae, m. levator scapulae.

m. leva'tor a'ni [NA], elevator muscle of anus; formed by m. puborectalis, m. levator prostatae (m. pubovaginalis), m. pubococcygeus, and m. iliococcygeus; *origin,* back of pubis, tendinous arch of the levator ani, and spine of ischium; *insertion,* anococcygeal ligament, sides of the lower part of the sacrum and of coccyx; *action,* draws the anus upward in defecation; supports the pelvic viscera; *nerve supply,* fourth sacral.

m. leva'tor cos'tae, pl. **levato'res costa'rum** [NA], elevator muscle of rib; **musculi levatores costarum breves,** *origin,* the transverse processes of last cervical and eleven thoracic vertebrae; *insertion* ribs immediately below, between angle and tubercle; **musculi levatores costarum longi,** *insertion,* the second rib below their origin; *action,* raise ribs; *nerve supply,* intercostal.

m. leva'tor glan'dulae thyroi'deae [NA], elevator muscle of thyroid gland; Soemmering's muscle; a fasciculus occasionally passing from the thyrohyoid muscle to the isthmus of the thyroid gland.

m. leva'tor la'bii inferio'ris, m. mentalis.

m. leva'tor la'bii superio'ris [NA], elevator muscle of the upper lip; caput infraorbitale quadrati labii superioris; *origin,* maxilla below infraorbital foramen; *insertion,* orbicularis oris of upper lip; *action,* elevates upper lip; *nerve supply,* facial.

m. leva'tor la'bii superio'ris alae'que na'si [NA], elevator muscle of upper lip and wing of nose; caput angulare quadrati labii superioris; *origin,* root of nasal process of maxilla; *insertion,* ala of nose and m. orbicularis oris of upper lip; *action,* elevates upper lip and wing of nose; *nerve supply,* facial.

m. leva'tor pala'ti, m. levator veli palatini.

m. leva'tor palpe'brae superio'ris [NA], elevator muscle of upper eyelid; m. orbitopalpebralis; *origin,* orbital surface of the lesser wing of the sphenoid, above and anterior to the optic canal; *insertion,* skin of eyelid, tarsal plate, and orbital walls, by medial and lateral expansions of the aponeurosis of insertion; *action,* raises the upper eyelid; *nerve supply,* oculomotor.

m. leva'tor prosta'tae [NA], elevator muscle of prostate; in the male, the most medial fibers of the levator ani muscle that extend from the pubis into the fascia of the prostate.

m. leva'tor scap'ulae [NA], elevator muscle of scapula; m. levator anguli scapulae; *origin,* from posterior tubercles of transverse processes of four upper cervical vertebrae; *insertion,* into superior angle of scapula; *action,* raises the scapula; *nerve supply,* dorsal nerve of scapula.

m. leva'tor ve'li palati'ni [NA], elevator muscle of soft palate; m. levator palati; m. petrostaphylinus; *origin,* apex of petrous portion of temporal bone and lower part of cartilaginous auditory (eustachian) tube; *insertion,* aponeurosis of soft palate; *action,* raises soft palate; *nerve supply,* pharyngeal plexus.

mus'culi lin'guae [NA], muscles of tongue; the extrinsic muscles include the genioglossus, hyoglossus, chondroglossus, styloglossus and glossopalatinus; the intrinsic muscles are the vertical, transverse and the superior and inferior longitudinal.

m. longis'simus [NA], the intermediate division of the erector spinae muscle having three subdivisions, m. longissimus capitis, m. longissimus cervicis, and m. longissimus thoracis.

m. longis'simus cap'itis [NA], longissimus capitis muscle; m. trachelomastoideus; m. transversalis capitis; m. complexus minor; *origin,* from transverse processes of upper thoracic and transverse and articular processes of lower and middle cervical vertebrae; *insertion,* into mastoid process; *action,* keeps head erect, draws it backward or to one side; *nerve supply,* dorsal branches of cervical nerves.

m. longis'simus cer'vicis [NA], cervical longissimus muscle; m. transversalis cervicis or colli; *origin,* transverse processes of upper thoracic vertebrae; *insertion,* transverse processes of middle and upper cervical vertebrae; *action,* extends cervical vertebrae; *nerve supply,* dorsal branches of lower cervical and upper thoracic nerves.

m. longis'simus dor'si, m. longissimus thoracis.

m. longis'simus thora'cis [NA], thoracic longissimus muscle; m. longissimus dorsi; *origin,* with iliocostalis and from transverse processes of lower thoracic vertebrae; *insertion,* by lateral slips into most or all of the ribs between angles and tubercles and into tips of transverse processes of upper lumbar vertebrae, and by medial slips into accessory processes of upper lumbar and transverse processes of thoracic vertebrae; *action,* extends vertebral column; *nerve supply,* dorsal branches of thoracic and lumbar nerves.

m. longitudina'lis infe'rior [NA], inferior lingual muscle; an intrinsic muscle of the tongue, cylindrical in shape, occupying the underpart on either side; *action,* shortens the lower part of the tongue; *nerve supply,* motor by hypoglossal, sensory by lingual.

m. longitudina'lis supe'rior [NA], superficial lingual muscle; an intrinsic muscle of the tongue, running from base to tip on the dorsum just beneath the mucous membrane; *action,* shortens the upper part of the tongue; *nerve supply,* motor by hypoglossal, sensory by lingual.

m. lon'gus cap'itis [NA], long muscle of head; m. rectus capitis anticus major; *origin,* anterior tubercles of transverse processes of third to sixth cervical vertebrae; *insertion,* basilar process of occipital bone; *action,* twists or bends neck forward; *nerve supply,* cervical plexus.

m. lon'gus col'li [NA], long muscle of neck; medial, *origin,* the bodies of the third thoracic to the fifth cervical vertebrae; *insertion,* the bodies of the second to fourth cervical vertebrae; superolateral, *origin,* the anterior tubercles of the transverse processes of the third to fifth cervical vertebrae and is inserted into the anterior tubercle of the atlas; inferolateral, *origin,* the bodies of the first to third thoracic vertebrae; *insertion,* the anterior tubercles of the transverse processes of the fifth and sixth cervical vertebrae; *action,* for all three parts, twist neck and bend neck forward; *nerve supply,* for all three parts, ventral branches of cervical.

m. lumbrica'lis ma'nus, pl. **lumbrica'les ma'nus** [NA], lumbrical muscle of the hand; four muscles in the hand; *origin,* the two lateral, from the radial side of the tendons of the flexor digitorum profundus going to the index and middle fingers, the two medial, from the adjacent sides of the second and third, and third and fourth tendons; *insertion,* radial side of extensor tendon on dorsum of each of the four fingers; *action,* flexes and proximal and extends the middle and distal phalanges; *nerve supply,* the two radial by the median, the two ulnar by the ulnar.

m. lumbrica'lis pe'dis, pl. **lumbrica'les pe'dis** [NA], lumbricales muscle of foot; four muscles in the foot; *origin,* first from tibial side of tendon to second toe of flexor digitorum longus, second, third, and fourth, from adjacent sides of all four tendons of this m.; *insertion,* tibial side of extensor tendon on dorsum of each of the four lateral toes; *action,* flex the proximal and extend the middle and distal phlanges; *nerve supply,* lateral and medial plantar.

m. masse'ter [NA], *origin,* pars superficialis, inferior border of the anterior two-thirds of the zygomatic arch; pars profunda, inferior border and medial surface of the zygomatic arch; *insertion,* lateral surface of ramus and coronoid process of the mandible; *action,* closes jaw; *nerve supply,* masseteric from mandibular division of trigeminal.

m. menta'lis [NA], chin muscle; m. levator labii inferioris; *origin,* incisor fossa of mandible; *insertion,* skin of chin; *action,* raises and wrinkles skin of chin, thus elevating the lower lip; *nerve supply,* facial.

m. multif'idus [NA], m. multifidus spinae; *origin,* from the sacrum, sacroiliac ligament, mammillary processes of the lumbar vertebrae, transverse processes of thoracic vertebrae, and articular processes of last four cervical vertebrae; *insertion,* into the spinous processes of all the vertebrae up to and including the axis; *action,* rotates vertebral column; *nerve supply,* dorsal branches of spinal nerve.

m. multif'idus spi'nae, m. multifidus.

m. multipenna'tus [NA], multipennate muscle; a muscle with several central tendons toward which the muscle fibers converge like the barbs of feathers.

m. mylohyoi'deus [NA], mylohyoid muscle; *origin,* mylohyoid line of mandible; *insertion,* upper border of hyoid bone and raphe separating muscle from its fellow; *action,* elevates floor of mouth and the tongue, depresses jaw when hyoid is fixed; *nerve supply,* mylohyoid from mandibular division of trigeminal.

m. mylopharyn'geus, see m. constrictor pharyngis superior.

m. nasa'lis [NA], nasal muscle; consists of the pars transversa, arising from the maxilla on each side and passing across the bridge of the nose, and the pars alaris, arising from the maxilla and attaching to the ala of the nose; the pars alaris dilates the nostrils; *nerve supply,* facial.

m. obli'quus auric'ulae [NA], oblique muscle of auricle; Tod's muscle; a thin band of oblique muscular fibers extending from the upper part of the eminence of the concha to the convexity of the helix, running across the groove corresponding to the crus anthelicis inferior.

m. obli'quus cap'itis infe'rior [NA], inferior oblique muscle of head; *origin,* spinous process of axis; *insertion,* transverse process of the atlas; *action,* rotates head; *nerve supply,* suboccipital.

m. obli'quus cap'itis supe'rior [NA], superior oblique muscle of head; *origin,* transverse process of atlas; *insertion,* lateral third of inferior nuchal line; *action,* rotates head; *nerve supply,* suboccipital.

m. obli'quus exter'nus abdom'inis [NA], abdominal external oblique muscle; *origin,* fifth to twelfth ribs; *insertion,* anterior half of lateral lip of iliac crest, inguinal ligament, and anterior layer of the sheath of the rectus; *action,* diminishes capacity of abdomen, draws thorax downward; *nerve supply,* ventral branches of lower thoracic nerves.

m. obli'quus infe'rior [NA], inferior oblique muscle; *origin,* orbital plate of maxilla lateral to the lacrimal groove; *insertion,* sclera between the superior and lateral recti; *action,* primary, extorsion; secondary, elevation and abduction; *nerve supply,* oculomotor.

m. obli'quus inter'nus abdom'inis [NA], abdominal internal oblique muscle; *origin,* iliac fascia deep to lateral part of inguinal ligament, anterior half of crest of ilium, and lumbar fascia; *insertion,* tenth to twelfth ribs and sheath of rectus; some of the fibers from inguinal ligament terminate in the falx inguinalis; *action,* diminishes capacity of abdomen, bends thorax forward; *nerve supply,* lower thoracic.

m. obli'quus supe'rior [NA], superior oblique muscle; *origin,* above the medial margin of the optic canal; *insertion,* by a tendon passing through the trochlea, or pulley, and then reflected backward, downward, and laterally to the sclera between the superior and lateral recti; *action,* primary, intorsion; secondary, depression and abduction; *nerve supply,* trochlear nerve.

m. obturato'r exter'nus [NA], external obturator muscle; *origin,* lower half of margin of obturator foramen and adjacent part of external surface of obturator membrane; *insertion,* trochanteric fossa of greater trochanter; *action,* rotates thigh laterally; *nerve supply,* obturator.

m. obturato'r inter'nus [NA], internal obturator muscle; *origin,* pelvic surface of obturator membrane and margin of obturator foramen; *insertion,* medial surface of greater trochanter; *action,* rotates thigh laterally; *nerve supply,* sacral plexus.

m. occipita'lis, see m. occipitofrontalis.

m. occipitofronta'lis, [NA], occipitofrontal muscle; it is a part of m. epicranius; the occipital belly (venter occipitalis) arises from the occipital bone and inserts into the galea aponeurotica; the frontal belly (venter frontalis) arises from the galea and inserts into the skin of the eyebrow and nose; *action,* to move the scalp; *nerve supply,* facial.

m. omohyoi'deus [NA], omohyoid muscle; omohyoid; formed of two bellies attached to intermediate tendon; *origin,* by inferior belly from upper border of scapula between superior angle and notch; *insertion,* by superior belly into hyoid bone; *action,* depresses hyoid; *nerve supply,* upper cervical through ansa cervicalis.

m. oppo'nens dig'iti min'imi [NA], opposer muscle of little finger; m. opponens digiti quinti; m. opponens minimi digiti; *origin,* hamulus of the hamate bone and flexor retinaculum; *insertion,* shaft of fifth metacarpal; *action,* draws ulnar side of hand toward center of palm; *nerve supply,* ulnar.

m. oppo'nens dig'iti quin'ti, m. opponens digiti minimi.

m. oppo'nens min'imi dig'iti, m. opponens digiti minimi.

m. oppo'nens pol'licis [NA], opposer muscle of thumb; *origin,* ridge of trapezium and flexor retinaculum; *insertion,* anterior surface of first metacarpal bone; *action,* opposes thumb to other fingers; *nerve supply,* median.

m. orbicula'ris [NA], orbicular muscle; a sphincter-like sheet of muscle that encircles an orifice such as the mouth or the palpebral fissures.

m. orbicula'ris oc'uli [NA], sphincter oculi or oris; orbicular muscle of eye; m. orbicularis palpebrarum; consists of three portions: pars orbitalis, or external portion, arises from frontal process of maxilla and nasal process of frontal bone, encircles aperture of orbit, and is inserted near origin; pars palpebralis, or internal portion, arises from medial palpebral ligament, passes through each eyelid, and is inserted into lateral palpebral raphe; pars lacrimalis (tensor tarsi muscle, Duverney's or Horner's muscle) arises from posterior lacrimal crest and passes across lacrimal sac to join palpebral portion; *action,* closes eye, wrinkles forehead vertically; *nerve supply,* facial.

m. orbicula'ris o'ris [NA], orbicular muscle of mouth; m. sphincter oris; *origin,* by nasolabial band from septum of the nose, by superior incisive bundle from incisor fossa of maxilla, by inferior incisive bundle from lower jaw each side of symphysis; *insertion,* fibers surround mouth between skin and mucous membrane of lips and cheeks, and are blended with other muscles; *action,* closes lips; *nerve supply,* facial.

m. orbicula'ris palpebra'rum, m. orbicularis oculi.
m. orbita'lis [NA], orbital muscle; Müller's muscle (1); a rudimentary nonstriated muscle, crossing the infraorbital groove and sphenomaxillary fissure, intimately united with the periosteum of the orbit.
m. orbitopalpebra'lis, m. levator palpebrae superioris.
mus'culi ossiculo'rum audi'tus [NA], muscles of auditory ossicles; the m. stapedius and m. tensor tympani.
m. palatoglos'sus [NA], palatoglossus muscle; m. glossopalatinus; forms anterior pillar of fauces; *origin,* oral surface of soft palate; *insertion,* side of tongue; *action,* raises back of tongue and narrows fauces; *nerve supply,* pharyngeal plexus.
m. palatopharyn'geus [NA], palatopharyngeal muscle; m. pharyngopalatinus; forms the posterior pillar of the fauces; *origin,* soft palate; *insertion,* posterior border of thyroid cartilage and aponeurosis of pharynx; *action,* narrows fauces, depresses soft palate, elevates pharynx and larynx; *nerve supply,* pharyngeal plexus.
m. palatosalpin'geus, m. tensor veli palatini.
m. palatostaphyli'nus, a bundle of muscular fibers from the tensor veli palatini joining the m. uvulae.
m. palma'ris bre'vis [NA], short palmar muscle; *origin,* ulnar side of central portion of the palmar aponeurosis; *insertion,* skin of ulnar side of hand; *action,* wrinkles skin on medial side of palm; *nerve supply,* ulnar.
m. palma'ris lon'gus [NA], long palmar muscle; *origin,* medial epicondyle of humerus; *insertion,* flexor retinaculum of wrist and palmar fascia; *action,* makes palmar fascia tense and flexes the hand and forearm; is occasionally absent; *nerve supply,* median.
m. papilla'ris [NA], papillary muscle; one of the group of myocardial bundles which terminate in the chordae tendineae which attach to the cusps of the atrioventricular valves; each has an anterior and a posterior papillary muscle; the right ventricle sometimes has a septal papillary muscle.
mus'culi pectina'ti [NA], pectinate muscles or fibers; prominent ridges of atrial myocardium located on the inner surface of much of the right atrium and both auricles.
m. pectin'eus [NA], pectineal muscle; *origin,* crest of pubis; *insertion,* pectineal line of femur; *action,* adducts thigh and assists in flexion; *nerve supply,* obturator and femoral.
m. pectora'lis ma'jor [NA], greater pectoral muscle; *origin,* pars clavicularis, medial half of clavicle; pars sternocostalis, anterior surface of manubrium and body of sternum and cartilages of first to sixth ribs; pars abdominalis, aponeurosis of obliquus externus; *insertion,* crest of greater tubercle of humerus; *action,* adducts and medially rotates arm; *nerve supply,* anterior thoracic.
m. pectora'lis mi'nor [NA], smaller pectoral muscle; *origin,* third to fifth ribs at the costochondral articulations; *insertion,* tip of coracoid process of scapula; *action,* draws down scapula or raises ribs; *nerve supply,* anterior thoracic.
mus'culi perine'i [NA], perineal muscles; the muscles located in the perineal region; these are m. sphincter ani externus, m. transversus perinei superficialis, m. ischiocavernosus, m. bulbospongiosus, m. transversus perinei profundus, and m. sphincter urethrae.
m. peroneocalca'neus, an occasional muscle arising from the shaft of the fibula and inserted into the calcaneus.
m. perone'us bre'vis [NA], short peroneal or fibular muscle; m. fibularis brevis; *origin,* lower two-thirds of lateral surface of fibula; *insertion,* base of fifth metatarsal bone; *action,* everts foot; *nerve supply,* peroneal.
m. perone'us lon'gus [NA], long peroneal or fibular muscle; m. fibularis longus; *origin,* upper two-thirds of outer surface of fibula and lateral condyle of tibia; *insertion,* by tendon passing behind lateral malleolus and across sole of foot to medial cuneiform and base of first metatarsal; *action,* plantar flexes and everts foot; *nerve supply,* peroneal.
m. perone'us ter'tius [NA], third peroneal or fibular muscle; m. fibularis tertius; *origin,* in common with m. extensor digitorum longus; *insertion,* dorsum of base of fifth metatarsal bone; *nerve supply,* deep branch of peroneal; *action,* assists in dorsal flexion of foot.
m. petropharyn'geus, an occasional accessory levator muscle of the pharynx, arising from the undersurface of the petrous portion of the temporal bone and inserted into the pharynx.
m. petrostaphyli'nus, m. levator veli palatini.
m. pharyngopalati'nus, m. palatopharyngeus.
m. pirifor'mis [NA], piriform muscle; m. pyriformis; *origin,* margins of pelvic sacral foramina and greater sciatic notch of ilium; *insertion,* upper border of great trochanter; *action,* rotates thigh laterally; *nerve supply,* sciatic plexus.
m. planta'ris [NA], plantar muscle; m. tibialis gracilis; *origin,* lateral supracondylar ridge; *insertion,* medial margin of tendo achillis and deep fascia of ankle; *action,* plantar flexion of foot; *nerve supply,* tibial nerve.
m. platys'ma, platysma.
m. platys'ma myoi'des, platysma.
m. pleuroesopha'geus [NA], pleuroesophageal muscle; muscular fasciculi, arising from the mediastinal pleura, which reinforce musculature of esophagus.
m. poplite'us [NA], popliteal muscle; popliteus; *origin,* lateral condyle of femur; *insertion,* posterior surface of tibia above oblique line; *action,* flexes leg and rotates it medially; *nerve supply,* tibial.
m. proce'rus [NA], procerus muscle; procerus; m. pyramidalis nasi; *origin,* from membrane covering bridge of nose; *insertion,* into frontalis; *action,* assists frontalis; *nerve supply,* branch of facial.
m. prona'tor pe'dis, m. quadratus plantae.
m. prona'tor quadra'tus [NA], quadrate pronator muscle; *origin,* distal fourth of anterior surface of ulna; *insertion,* distal fourth of anterior surface of radius; *action,* pronates forearm; *nerve supply,* anterior interosseous.
m. prona'tor ra'dii te'res, m. pronator teres.
m. prona'tor te'res [NA], round pronator muscle; m. pronator radii teres; *origin,* superficial head (caput humerale) from the medial epicondyle of the humerus, deep head (caput ulnare) from the medial side of the coronoid process of the ulna; *insertion,* middle of the lateral surface of the radius; *action,* pronates forearm; *nerve supply,* median.
m. prostat'icus, *substantia* muscularis prostatae.
m. pso'as ma'jor [NA], greater psoas muscle; *origin,* bodies of vertebrae and intervertebral disks from the twelfth thoracic to the fifth lumbar, and transverse processes of the lumbar vertebrae; *insertion,* lesser trochanter of femur; *action,* flexes thigh; *nerve supply,* lumbar plexus.
m. pso'as mi'nor [NA], smaller psoas muscle; an inconstant muscle, absent in about 40%; *origin,* bodies of twelfth thoracic and first lumbar vertebrae and disk between them; *insertion,* iliopubic eminence with iliac fascia; *action,* assists in flexion of lumbar spine; *nerve supply,* lumbar plexus.
m. pterygoi'deus exter'nus, m. pterygoideus lateralis.
m. pterygoi'deus inter'nus, m. pterygoideus medialis.
m. pterygoi'deus latera'lis [NA], lateral pterygoid muscle; external pterygoid muscle; m. pterygoideus externus; *origin,* inferior head from lateral lamina of pterygoid process; superior head from infratemporal crest and adjacent greater wing of the sphenoid; *insertion,* into pterygoid pit of mandible and articular disk; *action,* brings jaw forward, opens jaw; *nerve supply,* nerve to lateral pterygoid from mandibular division of trigeminal.
m. pterygoi'deus media'lis [NA], medial pterygoid muscle; internal pterygoid muscle; m. pterygoideus internus; *origin,* pterygoid fossa of sphenoid and tuberosity of maxilla; *insertion,* medial surface of mandible between angle and mylohyoid groove; *action,* raises mandible closing jaw; *nerve supply,* nerve to medial pterygoid from mandibular division of trigeminal.
m. pterygopharyn'geus, see m. constrictor pharyngis superior.

m. pterygospino'sus, a muscular slip, occasionally present, passing between the spine of the sphenoid bone and the posterior margin of the lateral pterygoid plate.
m. pubococcyg'eus [NA], pubococcygeal muscle; fibers of the levator ani, arising from the pelvic surface of the body of the pubis, attaching to the coccyx.
m. puboprostat'icus [NA], puboprostatic muscle; smooth muscle fibers within the puboprostatic ligament.
m. puborecta'lis [NA], puborectal muscle; Braune's muscle; the part of the m. levator ani that passes from the body of the pubis around the anus to form a muscular sling at the level of the anorectal junction; it relaxes during defecation.
m. pubovagina'lis [NA], pubovaginal muscle; in the female, the most medial fibers of the levator ani muscle that extend from the pubis into the lateral walls of the vagina.
m. pubovesica'lis [NA], pubovesical muscle; smooth muscle fibers within the pubovesical ligament in the female.
m. pyramida'lis [NA], pyramidal muscle; *origin,* crest of pubis; *insertion,* lower portion of linea alba; *action,* makes linea alba tense; *nerve supply,* last thoracic.
m. pyramida'lis auric'ulae [NA], pyramidal muscle of auricle; Jung's muscle; an occasional prolongation of the fibers of the tragicus to the spina helicis.
m. pyramida'lis na'si, m. procerus.
m. pyrifor'mis, m. piriformis.
m. quadra'tus [NA], quadrate muscle; a muscle that is more or less square in shape.
m. quadra'tus fem'oris [NA], quadrate muscle of the thigh; *origin,* lateral border of tuberosity of ischium; *insertion,* intertrochanteric ridge; *action,* rotates thigh laterally; *nerve supply,* sacral plexus.
m. quadra'tus la'bii inferio'ris, m. depressor labii inferioris.
m. quadra'tus la'bii superior'is, quadrate muscle of upper lip; composed of three heads usually described as three muscles; they are the caput angulare or m. levator labii superioris alaeque nasi; caput infraorbitale or m. levator labii superioris; caput zygomaticum or m. zygomaticus minor. See also entries under caput.
m. quadra'tus lumbo'rum [NA], lumbar quadrate muscle; quadrate muscle of loins, *origin,* iliac crest, iliolumbar ligament, and transverse processes of lower lumbar vertebrae; *insertion,* twelfth rib and transverse processes of upper lumbar vertebrae; *action,* abducts trunk; *nerve supply,* upper lumbar.
m. quadra'tus men'ti, m. depressor labii inferioris.
m. quadra'tus plan'tae [NA], plantar quadrate muscle; quadrate muscle of sole; m. flexor accessorius; m. pronator pedis; caro quadrata sylvii; *origin,* by two heads from the lateral and medial borders of the inferior surface of the calcaneus; *insertion,* tendons of flexor digitorum longus; *action,* assists long flexor; *nerve supply,* lateral plantar.
m. quad'riceps exten'sor fem'oris, m. quadriceps femoris.
m. quad'riceps fem'oris [NA], quadriceps muscle of thigh; m. quadriceps extensor femoris; *origin,* by four heads: rectus femoris, vastus lateralis, vastus intermedius, and vastus medialis; *insertion,* patella, and thence by ligamentum patellae to tuberosity of tibia; *action,* extends leg; flexes thigh by action of rectus femoris; *nerve supply,* femoral.
m. rectococcyg'eus [NA], rectococcygeal muscle; a band of smooth muscle fibers passing from the posterior surface of the rectum to the anterior surface of second or third coccygeal segment.
m. rectourethra'lis [NA], rectourethral muscle; smooth muscle fibers that pass forward from the longitudinal muscle layer of the rectum to the membranous urethra in the male.
m. rectouteri'nus [NA], a band of fibrous tissue and smooth muscle fibers passing between the cervix uteri and the rectum in the rectouterine fold, on either side.
m. rectovesica'lis [NA], rectovesical muscle; smooth muscle fibers in the sacrogenital fold in the male; they correspond to m. rectouterinus.
m. rec'tus abdom'inis [NA], rectus muscle of abdomen; *origin,* crest and symphysis of the pubis; *insertion,* xiphoid process and fifth to seventh costal cartilages; *action,* flexes vertebral column, draws thorax downward; *nerve supply,* branches of lower thoracic.
m. rec'tus cap'itis ante'rior [NA], anterior straight muscle of head; m. rectus capitis anticus minor; *origin,* transverse process and lateral mass of atlas; *insertion,* basilar process of occipital bone; *action,* turns and inclines head forward; *nerve supply,* first and second cervical.
m. rec'tus cap'itis an'ticus ma'jor, m. longus capitis.
m. rectus cap'itis an'ticus mi'nor, m. rectus capitis anterior.
m. rec'tus cap'itis latera'lis [NA], lateral rectus muscle of head; *origin,* transverse process of atlas; *insertion,* jugular process of occipital bone; *action,* inclines head to one side; *nerve supply,* ventral branch of first cervical (suboccipital).
m. rec'tus cap'itis poste'rior ma'jor [NA], greater posterior rectus muscle of head; m. rectus capitis posticus major; *origin,* spinous process of axis; *insertion,* middle of inferior nuchal line of occipital bone; *action,* rotates and draws head backward; *nerve supply,* dorsal branch of first cervical (suboccipital).
m. rec'tus cap'itis poste'rior mi'nor [NA], smaller posterior rectus muscle of head; m. rectus capitis posticus minor; *origin,* from posterior tubercle of atlas; *insertion,* medial third of inferior nuchal line of occipital bone; *action,* rotates head and draws it backward; *nerve supply,* dorsal branch of first cervical (suboccipital).
m. rec'tus cap'itis pos'ticus ma'jor, m. rectus capitis posterior major.
m. rec'tus cap'itis pos'ticus mi'nor, m. rectus capitis posterior minor.
m. rec'tus exter'nus, m. rectus lateralis.
m. rec'tus fem'oris [NA], rectus muscle of thigh; *origin,* anterior inferior spine of ilium and upper margin of acetabulum; *insertion,* common tendon of quadriceps femoris.
m. rec'tus infe'rior [NA], inferior rectus muscle; *origin,* inferior part of the anulus tendineus communis (ligament of Zinn); *insertion,* inferior part of sclera of the eye; *action,* primary, depression; secondary, adduction and extorsion. *nerve supply,* oculomotor.
m. rec'tus inter'nus, m. rectus medialis.
m. rec'tus latera'lis [NA], lateral rectus muscle; abducens oculi; m. rectus externus; *origin,* lateral part of the anulus tendineus communis that bridges superior orbital fissure; *insertion,* lateral part of sclera of eye; *action,* abduction; *nerve supply,* abducens.
m. rec'tus media'lis [NA], medial rectus muscle; m. rectus internus; *origin,* medial part of the anulus tendineus communis; *insertion,* medial part of sclera of the eye; *action,* adduction; *nerve supply,* oculomotor.
m. rec'tus supe'rior [NA], superior rectus muscle; attollens oculi; *origin,* superior part of annulus tendineus communis (ligament of Zinn); *insertion,* superior part of sclera of the eye; *action,* primary, elevation; secondary, adduction and intorsion; *nerve supply,* oculomotor.
m. rec'tus thora'cis, m. sternalis.
m. ret'rahens au'rem or **auric'ulam,** m. auricularis posterior.
m. rhomboatloi'deus, an occasional muscle arising with the rhomboids from the cervical and thoracic vertebrae and inserted into the atlas.
m. rhomboi'deus ma'jor [NA], greater rhomboid muscle; *origin,* spinous processes and corresponding supraspinous ligaments of first four thoracic vertebrae; *insertion,* medial border of scapula below spine; *action,* draws scapula toward vertebral column; *nerve supply,* dorsal nerve of scapula.
m. rhomboi'deus mi'nor [NA], lesser rhomboid muscle; *origin,* spinous processes of sixth and seventh cervical vertebrae; *insertion,* medial margin of scapula above spine; *action,* draws scapula toward vertebral column and slightly upward; *nerve supply,* dorsal nerve of scapula.

m. riso'rius [NA], risorius muscle; Albinus' muscle (1); Santorini's muscle; *origin,* from platysma and fascia of masseter; *insertion,* orbicularis oris and skin at corner of mouth; *action,* draws out angle of mouth; *nerve supply,* facial.

mus'culi rotato'res [NA], rotator muscles; a number of short transversospinal muscles chiefly developed in the thoracic region; they arise from the transverse process of one vertebra and are inserted into the root of the spinous process of the next two or three vertebrae above; *action,* rotate the vertebral column; *nerve supply,* dorsal branches of the spinal.

mus'culi rotato'res cer'vicis [NA], cervical rotator muscles; the rotator muscles attached to the cervical vertebrae.

mus'culi rotato'res lumbo'rum [NA], lumbar rotator muscles; the rotator muscles of the lumbar vertebrae.

mus'culi rotato'res thora'cis [NA], thoracic rotator muscles; the rotators of the thoracic vertebrae.

m. sacrococcyg'eus ante'rior, m. sacrococcygeus ventralis.

m. sacrococcyg'eus dorsa'lis [NA], dorsal sacrococcygeal muscle; m. extensor coccygis; m. sacrococcygeus posterior; an inconstant and poorly developed muscle on the dorsal surfaces of the sacrum and coccyx, the remains of a portion of the caudal musculature of lower animals.

m. sacrococcyg'eus poste'rior, m. sacrococcygeus dorsalis.

m. sacrococcyg'eus ventra'lis [NA], ventral sacrococcygeal muscle; m. sacrococcygeus anterior; an inconstant muscle on the pelvic surfaces of the sacrum and coccyx, the remains of a portion of the caudal musculature of lower animals.

m. sacrolumba'lis, m. iliocostalis lumborum.

m. sacrospina'lis, m. erector spinae.

m. salpingopharyn'geus [NA], salpingopharyngeal muscle; *origin,* medial lamina of cartilaginous part of auditory tube; *insertion,* muscular layer of pharynx in association with m. palatopharyngeus; *action,* assists in elevating pharynx and, according to some, assists in opening the auditory tube during swallowing; *nerve supply,* pharyngeal plexus.

m. sarto'rius [NA], tailor's muscle; *origin,* anterior superior spine of ilium; *insertion,* medial border of tuberosity of tibia; *action,* flexes thigh and leg, rotates leg medially and thigh laterally; *nerve supply,* femoral.

m. scale'nus ante'rior [NA], anterior scalene muscle; m. scalenus anticus; *origin,* anterior tubercles of transverse processes of third to sixth cervical vertebrae; *insertion,* scalene tubercle of first rib; *action,* raises first rib; *nerve supply,* cervical plexus.

m. scale'nus an'ticus, m. scalenus anterior.

m. scale'nus me'dius [NA], middle scalene muscle; *origin,* costotransverse lamellae of transverse processes of second to sixth cervical vertebrae; *insertion,* first rib posterior to subclavian artery; *action,* raises first rib; *nerve supply,* cervical plexus.

m. scale'nus min'imus [NA], smallest scalene muscle; Albinus' muscle (2); Sibson's muscle; an occasional independent muscular fasciculus between the scalenus anterior and medius, and having the same action and innervation.

m. scale'nus poste'rior [NA], posterior scalene muscle; m. scalenus posticus; *origin,* posterior tubercles of transverse processes of fourth to sixth cervical vertebrae; *insertion,* lateral surface of second rib; *action,* elevates second rib; *nerve supply,* cervical and brachial plexuses.

m. scale'nus pos'ticus, m. scalenus posterior.

m. scanso'rius, m. accessorius gluteus minimus; m. gluteus quartus; anterior fibers of the gluteus minimus (according to some anatomists the piriformis) which are sometimes distinct from the main portion of the muscle.

m. semimembrano'sus [NA], semimembranosus muscle; *origin,* tuberosity of ischium; *insertion,* medial condyle of tibia and by membrane to tibial collateral ligament of knee joint, popliteal fascia, and lateral condyle of femur; *action,* flexes leg and rotates it medially, and makes capsule of knee joint tense; *nerve supply,* tibial.

m. semispina'lis [NA], semispinal muscle; the superficial part of the transverospinal muscle; comprised of m. semispinalis capitis, m. semispinalis cervicis, and m. semispinalis thoracis.

m. semispina'lis cap'itis [NA], semispinal muscle of head; m. complexus; *origin,* transverse processes of five or six upper thoracic and articular processes of four lower cervical vertebrae; *insertion,* occipital bone between superior and inferior nuchal lines; *action,* rotates head and draws it backward; *nerve supply,* dorsal branches of cervical.

m. semispina'lis cer'vicis [NA], semispinal muscle of neck; m. semispinalis colli; continuous with m. semispinalis thoracis; *origin,* transverse processes of second to fifth thoracic vertebrae; *insertion,* spinous processes of axis and third to fifth cervical vertebrae; *action,* extends cervical spine; *nerve supply,* dorsal branches of cervical and thoracic.

m. semispina'lis col'li, m. semispinalis cervicis.

m. semispina'lis dor'si, m. semispinalis thoracis.

m. semispina'lis thora'cis [NA], semispinal muscle of thorax; *origin,* transverse processes of fifth to eleventh thoracic vertebrae; *insertion,* spinous processes of first four thoracic and fifth and seventh cervical vertebrae; *action,* extends vertebral column; *nerve supply,* dorsal branches of cervical and thoracic.

m. semitendino'sus [NA], semitendinous muscle; semitendinosus muscle; *origin,* ischial tuberosity; *insertion,* medial surface of upper fourth of shaft of tibia; *action,* extends thigh, flexes leg and rotates it medially; *nerve supply,* tibial.

m. serra'tus ante'rior [NA], anterior serratus muscle; m. serratus magnus; costoscapularis; *origin,* from center of lateral aspect of first eight to nine ribs; *insertion,* superior and inferior angles and intervening medial margin of scapula; *action,* rotates scapula and pulls it forward, elevates ribs; *nerve supply,* long thoracic from brachial plexus.

m. serra'tus mag'nus, m. serratus anterior.

m. serra'tus poste'rior infe'rior [NA], inferior posterior serratus muscle; *origin,* with latissimus dorsi, from spinous processes of two lower thoracic and two upper lumbar vertebrae; *insertion,* into lower borders of last four ribs; *action,* draws lower ribs backward and downward; *nerve supply,* ninth to twelfth intercostal.

m. serra'tus poste'rior supe'rior [NA], superior posterior serratus muscle; *origin,* from spinous processes of two lower cervical and two upper thoracic vertebrae; *insertion,* into lateral side of angles of second to fifth ribs; *nerve supply,* first to fourth intercostals.

m. skel'eti, skeletal *muscle.*

m. sol'eus [NA], soleus muscle; *origin,* posterior surface of head and upper third of shaft of fibula, oblique line and middle third of medial margin of tibia, and a tendinous arch passing between tibia and fibula over the popliteal vessels; *insertion,* with gastrocnemius by tendo calcaneus (achillis) into tuberosity of calcaneus; *action,* plantar flexion of foot; *nerve supply,* tibial.

m. sphenosalpingostaphyli'nus, m. tensor veli palatini.

m. sphinc'ter [NA], sphincter muscle; sphincter; a muscle that encircles a duct, tube or orifice in such a way that its contraction constricts the lumen or orifice; it is the closing component of a pylorus (the outer component is the m. dilator).

m. sphincter ampullae hepatopancreat'icae [NA], Glisson's sphincter; Oddi's sphincter; the smooth muscle sphincter of the hepatopancreatic ampulla within the duodenal papilla.

m. sphinc'ter a'ni exter'nus [NA], external sphincter muscle of the anus; a fusiform ring of striated muscular fibers surrounding the anus, attached posteriorly to the coccyx and anteriorly to the central tendon of the perineum; it is subdivided into a pars subcutanea, pars superficialis, and pars profunda.

m. sphinc'ter a'ni inter'nus [NA], internal sphincter muscle of anus; a smooth muscle ring, formed by an increase of the circular fibers of the rectum, situated at the upper end of the anal canal.

m. sphinc'ter duc'tus choledo'chi [NA], choledochal sphincter;

Boyden's sphincter; sphincter or sphincter muscle of common bile duct; smooth muscle sphincter of the common bile duct immediately proximal to the hepatopancreatic ampulla.
m. sphinc'ter duc'tus pancreat'ici, sphincter muscle of the pancreatic duct; smooth muscle sphincter of the main pancreatic duct immediately proximal to the hepatoduodenal, ampulla.
m. sphinc'ter o'ris, m. orbicularis oris.
m. sphinc'ter pupil'lae [NA], sphincter muscle of pupil; sphincter pupillae; a ring of smooth muscle fibers surrounding the pupillary border of the iris.
m. sphinc'ter pylo'ri [NA], sphincter muscle of pylorus; pyloric sphincter; a thickening of the circular layer of the gastric musculature encircling the gastroduodenal junction.
m. sphinc'ter ure'thrae [NA], sphincter urethrae; m. compressor urethrae; m. constrictor urethrae; m. sphincter urethrae membranaceae; sphincter muscle of urethra; Guthrie's muscle; Wilson's muscle (1); *origin,* ramus of pubis; *insertion,* with fellow in median raphe behind and in front of urethra; *action,* constricts membranous urethra; *nerve supply,* pudendal.
m. sphinc'ter ure'thrae membrana'ceae, m. sphincter urethrae.
m. sphinc'ter vagi'nae, m. bulbospongiosus.
m. sphinc'ter vesi'cae, sphincter vesicae; sphincter muscle of urinary bladder; annulus urethralis; traditionally recognized as a vesical sphincter made up of a thickening of the middle muscular layer of the bladder around the urethral opening; although no annular sphincter exists, a sphincteric action is attributed to the bundle of muscles in the region of the neck of the urinary bladder.
m. spina'lis [NA], spinal muscle; the medial component of the erector spinae muscle; it is comprised of m. spinalis capitis, m. spinalis cervicis, and m. spinalis thoracis.
m. spina'lis cap'itis [NA], spinal muscle of head; biventer cervicis; an inconstant extension of spinalis cervicis to the occipital bone, sometimes fusing with semispinalis capitis.
m. spina'lis cer'vicis [NA], spinal muscle of neck; m. spinalis colli; an inconstant or rudimentary muscle; *origin,* spinous processes of sixth and seventh cervical; *insertion,* spinous processes of axis and third cervical vertebra; *action,* extends cervical spine; *nerve supply,* dorsal branches of cervical.
m. spina'lis col'li, m. spinalis cervicis.
m. spina'lis dor'si, m. spinalis thoracis.
m. spina'lis thora'cis [NA], spinal muscle of thorax; m. spinalis dorsi; *origin,* spinous processes of upper lumbar and two lower thoracic vertebrae; *insertion,* spinous processes of middle and upper thoracic vertebrae; *action,* supports and extends vertebral column; *nerve supply,* dorsal branches of thoracic and upper lumbar.
m. sple'nius cap'itis [NA], splenius muscle of head; *origin,* from ligamentum nuchae of last four cervical vertebrae and supraspinous ligament of first and second thoracic vertebrae; *insertion,* lateral half of superior nuchal line and mastoid process; *action,* rotates head and extends neck; *nerve supply,* dorsal branches of second to sixth cervical.
m. sple'nius cer'vicis [NA], splenius muscle of neck; m. splenius colli; *origin,* from supraspinous ligament and spinous processes of third to fifth thoracic vertebrae; *insertion,* posterior tubercles of transverse processes of first and second (sometimes third) cervical vertebrae; *action,* rotates and extends neck; *nerve supply,* dorsal branches of fourth to eighth cervical.
m. sple'nius col'li, m. splenius cervicis.
m. stape'dius [NA], stapedius muscle; stapedius; *origin,* internal walls of pyramidal eminence in tympanic cavity; *insertion,* neck of the stapes; *action,* draws head of stapes backward; *nerve supply,* facial.
m. sterna'lis [NA], sternal muscle; m. rectus thoracis; an inconstant muscle, running parallel to the sternum across the costosternal origin of the pectoralis major, and usually connected with the sternocleidomastoid and rectus abdominis muscles.
m. sternochondroscapula'ris, sternochondroscapular muscle; an occasional muscle arising from the manubrium sterni and first costal cartilage and passing lateralward and backward to be inserted into the upper border of the scapula.
m. sternoclavicula'ris, sternoclavicular muscle; an occasional muscle, a slip from the subclavius muscle, passing from the upper part of the sternum to the clavicle beneath the pectoralis major.
m. sternocleidomastoi'deus [NA], sternocleidomastoid muscle; sternomastoid muscle; *origin,* by two heads from anterior surface of manubrium sterni and sternal end of clavicle; *insertion,* mastoid process and lateral half of superior nuchal line; *action,* turns head obliquely to opposite side; when acting together, flex the neck and extend the head; *nerve supply,* motor by accessory, sensory by cervical plexus.
m. sternofascia'lis, an occasional muscular slip arising from the manubrium sterni and inserted into the fascia of the neck.
m. sternohyoi'deus [NA], sternohyoid muscle; *origin,* posterior surface of manubrium sterni and first costal cartilage; *insertion,* body of hyoid bone; *action,* depresses hyoid bone; *nerve supply,* upper cervical through ansa cervicalis.
m. sternothyroi'deus [NA], sternothyroid muscle; *origin,* posterior surface of manubrium sterni and first or second costal cartilage; *insertion,* oblique line of thyroid cartilage; *action,* depresses larynx; *nerve supply,* upper cervical through the ansa cervicalis.
m. styloauricula'ris, styloauricular muscle; an occasional small muscle extending from the root of the styloid process to the cartilage of the meatus of the ear.
m. styloglos'sus [NA], styloglossus muscle; *origin,* lower end of styloid process; *insertion,* side and undersurface of tongue; *action,* retracts tongue; *nerve supply,* hypoglossal.
m. stylohyoi'deus [NA], stylohyoid muscle; *origin,* styloid process of temporal bone; *insertion,* hyoid bone by two slips on either side of intermediate tendon of digastric; *action,* elevates hyoid bone; *nerve supply,* facial.
m. stylolaryn'geus, that part of the stylopharyngeus which is inserted into the thyroid cartilage.
m. stylopharyn'geus [NA], stylopharyngeal muscle; *origin,* root of styloid process; *insertion,* thyroid cartilage and wall of pharynx; *action,* elevates pharynx and larynx; *nerve supply,* glossopharyngeal.
m. subcla'vius [NA], subclavian muscle; *origin,* first costal cartilage; *insertion,* inferior surface of acromial end of clavicle; *action,* fixes clavicle or elevates first rib; *nerve supply,* subclavian from brachial plexus.
m. subcosta'lis, pl. **subcosta'les** [NA], subcostal muscle; m. infracostalis; one of a number of inconstant muscles having the same direction as the intercostales interni, but passing deep to one or more ribs.
m. subcuta'neus col'li, platysma.
mus'culi suboccipita'les [NA], suboccipital muscles; a group of muscles located immediately below the occipital bone; they are: m. rectus capitis anterior, m. rectus capitis posterior major and minor, m. rectus capitis lateralis, m. obliquus capitis superior and inferior.
m. subscapula'ris [NA], subscapular muscle; *origin,* subscapular fossa; *insertion,* lesser tuberosity of humerus; *action,* rotates arm medially; *nerve supply,* upper and lower subscapular from fifth and sixth cervical.
m. supina'tor [NA], supinator muscle; m. supinator radii brevis; *origin,* lateral epicondyle of humerus and supinator ridge of ulna; *insertion,* anterior and lateral surface of radius; *action,* supinates the forearm; *nerve supply,* radial (posterior interosseous).
m. supina'tor lon'gus, m. brachioradialis.
m. supina'tor ra'dii brev'is, m. supinator.
m. supraclavicula'ris, supraclavicular muscle; an anomalous muscular slip running from the upper edge of the manubrium sterni lateralward to about the middle of the upper surface of the clavicle.
mus'culi suprahyoi'dei [NA], suprahyoid muscles; the group of muscles attached to the upper part of the hyoid bone including the

digastricus, stylohyoideus, mylohyoideus, and geniohyoideus.
m. supraspina'lis, one of a number of muscular bands passing between the tips of the spinous processes of the cervical vertebrae.
m. supraspina'tus [NA], supraspinous muscle; *origin,* supraspinous fossa of scapula; *insertion,* great tuberosity of humerus; *action,* abducts arm; *nerve supply,* suprascapular from fifth and sixth cervical.
m. suspenso'rius duode'ni [NA], suspensory muscle of duodenum; Treitz' muscle or ligament; a broad flat band of smooth muscle and fibrous tissue attached to the right crus of the diaphragm and to the duodenum at its junction with the jejunum.

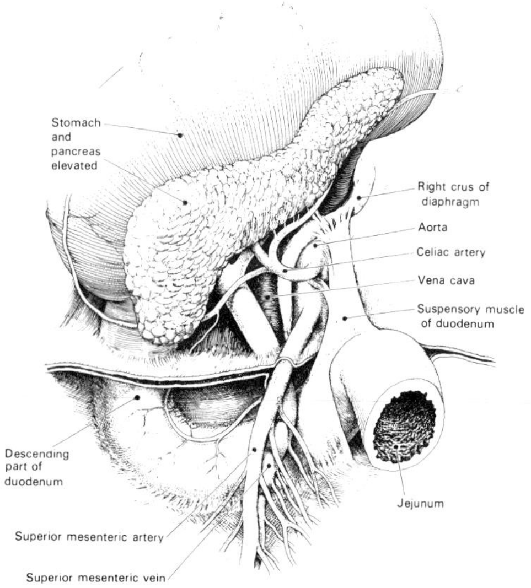

Musculus Suspensorius Duodeni

m. tarsa'lis infe'rior [NA], inferior tarsal muscle; poorly developed smooth muscle in the lower eyelid that acts to widen the palpebral fissure.
m. tarsa'lis supe'rior [NA], superior tarsal muscle; Müller's muscle (3); a well defined layer of smooth muscle that extends from the aponeurosis of the m. levator palpebrae superioris to the superior tarsus; it is innervated by sympathetic nerves and acts to hold the upper lid in an elevated position.
m. tempora'lis [NA], temporal muscle; *origin,* temporal fossa; *insertion,* coronoid process of mandible and anterior border of ramus; *action,* closes jaw; *nerve supply,* deep temporal branches of mandibular division of trigeminal.
m. temporoparieta'lis [NA], temporoparietal muscle; the part of m. epicranius that arises from the lateral part of the galea aponeurotica and inserts in the cartilage of the auricle. See also m. auricularis anterior and m. auricularis superior.
m. ten'sor fas'ciae fem'oris, m. tensor fasciae latae.
m. ten'sor fas'ciae la'tae [NA], tensor muscle of the fascia lata; m. tensor fasciae femoris; *origin,* anterior superior spine and adjacent lateral surface of the ilium; *insertion,* iliotibial band of fascia lata; *action,* tenses fascia lata; flexes, abducts and medially rotates thigh; *nerve supply,* superior gluteal.
m. ten'sor pala'ti, m. tensor veli palatini.
m. ten'sor tar'si, m. orbicularis oculi pars lacrimalis.
m. ten'sor tym'pani [NA], tensor muscle of the tympanic membrane; Toynbee's muscle; *origin,* the cartilaginous part of the auditory (eustachian) tube and the walls of its canal just above the bony portion of the auditory tube; *insertion,* handle of malleus; *action,* draws the handle of the malleus medialward and tenses the tympanic membrane; *nerve supply,* branches of trigeminal through the otic ganglion.
m. ten'sor ve'li palati'ni [NA], tensor muscle of soft palate m. tensor palati; m. palatosalpingeus; m. sphenosalpingostaphylinus; dilator tubae; *origin,* scaphoid fossa of sphenoid, cartilaginous and membranous part of auditory (eustachian) tube and spine of sphenoid; *insertion,* posterior border of hard palate and aponeurosis of soft palate; *action,* tenses the soft palate; opens auditory tube; *nerve supply,* branches of trigeminal nerve through the otic ganglion.
m. te'res ma'jor [NA], teres major muscle; *origin,* inferior angle and lower third of border of scapula; *insertion,* medial border of intertubercular groove of humerus; *action,* adducts and extends arm and rotates it medially; *nerve supply,* lower subscapular from fifth and sixth cervical.
m. te'res mi'nor [NA], teres minor muscle; *origin,* upper two-thirds of the lateral border of scapula; *insertion,* lower facet of great tuberosity of humerus; *action,* adducts arm and rotates it laterally; *nerve supply,* axillary from fifth and sixth cervical.
m. tetrago'nus, platysma.
mus'culi thora'cis [NA], muscles of thorax; the muscles attaching to the rib cage including the pectoral muscles, serratus anterior, subclavius, levator muscles, intercostal muscles, transverse thoracic muscle, subcostal muscles, and diaphragm.
m. thyroarytenoi'deus [NA], thyroarytenoid muscle; m. thyroarytenoideus externus; *origin,* inner surface of thyroid cartilage; *insertion,* muscular process and outer surface of arytenoid; *action,* shortens vocal cords; *nerve supply,* recurrent laryngeal.
m. thyroarytenoi'deus exter'nus, m. thyroarytenoideus.
m. thyroarytenoi'deus inter'nus, m. vocalis.
m. thyroepiglot'ticus [NA], thyroepiglottic or thyroepiglottidean muscle; depressor muscle of the epiglottis; *origin,* inner surface of thyroid cartilage in common with m. thyroarytenoideus; *insertion,* aryepiglottic fold and margin of epiglottis; *action,* depresses base of epiglottis; *nerve supply,* recurrent laryngeal.
m. thyrohyoi'deus [NA], thyrohyoid muscle; apparently a continuation of the sternothyroid; *origin,* oblique line of thyroid cartilage; *insertion,* body of hyoid bone; *action,* approximates hyoid bone to the larynx; *nerve supply,* upper cervical passing with hypoglossal.
m. thyropharyn'geus, see m. constrictor pharyngis inferior pars thyropharyngea.
m. tibia'lis ante'rior [NA], anterior tibial muscle; m. tibialis anticus; *origin,* upper two-thirds of lateral surface of tibia, interosseous membrane, and intermuscular septum; *insertion,* medial cuneiform and base of first metatarsal; *action,* dorsiflexion and inversion of foot; *nerve supply,* deep peroneal.
m. tibia'lis an'ticus, m. tibialis anterior.
m. tibia'lis gra'cilis, m. plantaris.
m. tibia'lis poste'rior [NA], posterior tibial muscle; m. tibialis posticus; *origin,* soleal line and posterior surface of tibia, the head and shaft of the fibula between the medial crest and interosseous border, and the posterior surface of interosseous membrane; *insertion,* navicular, three cuneiform, cuboid, and second, third, and fourth metatarsal bones; *action,* plantar flexion and inversion of foot; *nerve supply,* tibial.
m. tibia'lis pos'ticus, m. tibialis posterior.
m. tibia'lis secun'dus, second tibial muscle; an inconstant muscle, of small size, arising from the back of the tibia and inserted into the articular capsule of the ankle joint.
m. tibiofascia'lis ante'rior, m. tibiofascia'lis anticus, separate fibers of the tibialis anterior inserted into the fascia of the dorsum of the foot.
m. trachea'lis [NA], the band of smooth muscular fibers in the fibrous membrane connecting posteriorly the ends of the tracheal rings.
m. tracheloclavicula'ris, tracheloclavicular muscle; an anomalous muscle occasionally arising from the cervical vertebrae and in-

serted into the lateral end of the clavicle.
m. trachelomastoi'deus, m. longissimus capitis.
m. tra'gicus [NA], muscle of the tragus; Valsalva's muscle; a band of vertical muscular fibers on the outer surface of the tragus of the ear.
m. transversa'lis abdom'inis, m. transversus abdominis.
m. transversa'lis cap'itis, m. longissimus capitis.
m. transversa'lis cer'viscis, m. transversa'lis col'li, m. longissimus cervicis.
m. transversa'lis na'si, see m. nasalis, pars transversa.
m. transversospina'lis [NA], transversospinal muscle; the group of muscles that originate from transverse processes of vertebrae and pass to spinous processes of higher vertebrae; they act as rotators and include the semispinalis (capitis, cervicis, thoracis), multifidus, and rotatores (cervicis, thoracis, lumborum).
m. transver'sus abdom'inis [NA], transverse muscle of the abdomen; m. transversalis abdominis; *origin,* seventh to twelfth costal cartilages, lumbar fascia, iliac crest, and inguinal (Poupart's) ligament; *insertion,* xiphoid cartilage and linea alba and, through falx inguinalis, pubic tubercle and pecten; *action,* compresses abdominal contents; *nerve supply,* lower thoracic.
m. transver'sus auric'ulae [NA], transverse muscle of auricle; a band of sparse muscular fibers on the cranial surface of the auricle, extending from the eminence of the concha to the eminence of the scapha.
m. transver'sus lin'guae [NA], transverse muscle of tongue; an intrinsic muscle of the tongue, the fibers of which arise from the septum and radiate to the dorsum and sides; *action,* decreases lateral dimension of the tongue; *nerve supply,* hypoglossal for motor, lingual for sensory.
m. transver'sus men'ti [NA], transverse muscle of chin; inconstant fibers of the m. depresser anguli oris which continue into the neck and cross to the opposite side inferior to the chin.
m. transver'sus nu'chae [NA], transverse muscle of nape; an occasional muscle passing between the tendons of the trapezius and sternocleidomastoid, possibly a fasciculus of the auricularis posterior.
m. transver'sus perine'i profun'dus [NA], deep transverse muscle of perineum; *origin,* ramus of ischium; *insertion,* with its fellow in a median raphe; *action,* assists sphincter urethrae; *nerve supply,* pudendal.
m. transver'sus perine'i superficia'lis [NA], superficial transverse muscle of perineum; Theile's muscle; an inconstant muscle; *origin,* ramus of ischium; *insertion,* central tendon of perineum; *action,* draws back and fixes the central tendon of the perineum; *nerve supply,* pudendal.
m. transver'sus thora'cis [NA], transverse muscle of thorax; m. triangularis sterni; *origin,* dorsal surface of xiphoid cartilage and lower portion of dorsal surface of body of sternum; *insertion,* second to sixth costal cartilages; *action,* narrows chest; *nerve supply,* intercostal.
m. trape'zius [NA], trapezius muscle; cowl muscle; *origin,* medial third of superior nuchal line, external occipital protuberance, ligamentum nuchae, spinous processes of seventh cervical and the thoracic vertebrae and corresponding supraspinous ligaments; *insertion,* lateral third of posterior surface of clavicle, medial side of acromion, and upper border of the spine of the scapula; *action,* draws head to one side or backward, rotates scapula; *nerve supply,* motor by accessory, sensory by cervical plexus.
m. triangula'ris, triangular muscle; **(1)** [NA], a muscle that is triangular in shape; **(2)** m. depressor anguli oris.
m. triangula'ris la'bii inferior'is, m. depressor anguli oris.
m. triangula'ris la'bii superior'is, m. levator anguli oris.
m. triangula'ris ster'ni, m. transversus thoracis.
m. tri'ceps bra'chii [NA], triceps muscle of arm; *origin,* long or scapular head (caput longum) lateral border of scapula below glenoid fossa, lateral head (caput laterale) lateral and posterior surface of humerus below greater tubercle, medial head (caput mediale) posterior surface of humerus below radial groove; *insertion,* olecranon of ulna; *action,* extends forearm; *nerve supply,* radial.
m. tri'ceps su'rae [NA], triceps muscle of calf; the gastrocnemius and soleus considered as one muscle.
m. triticeoglos'sus, Bochdalek's muscle; an occasional thin band of muscular fibers passing between the root of the tongue and the cartilago triticea.
m. unipenna'tus [NA], unipennate muscle; a muscle with a lateral tendon to which the fibers are attached obliquely, like one half of a feather.
m. u'vulae [NA], muscle of uvula; m. azygos uvulae; palatouvularis muscle; *origin,* posterior nasal spine; *insertion,* forms chief bulk of the uvula; *action,* raises the uvula; *nerve supply,* pharyngeal plexus.
m. vas'tus exter'nus, m. vastus lateralis.
m. vas'tus interme'dius [NA], intermediate vastus muscle; intermediate great muscle; femoral muscle; crureus; *origin,* upper three-fourths of anterior surface of shaft of femur; *insertion,* tibial tuberosity by way of common tendon of quadriceps femoris and ligamentum patellae; *action,* extends leg; *nerve supply,* femoral.
m. vas'tus inter'nus, m. vastus medialis.
m. vas'tus latera'lis [NA], lateral vastus muscle; lateral great muscle; m. vastus externus; *origin,* lateral lip of linea aspera as far as great trochanter; *insertion,* tibial tuberosity by way of common tendon of quadriceps femoris and ligamentum patellae; *action,* extends leg; *nerve supply,* femoral.
m. vas'tus media'lis [NA], medial vastus muscle; medial great muscle; m. vastus internus; *origin,* medial lip of linea aspera; *insertion,* tibial tuberosity by way of common tendon of quadriceps femoris and ligamentum patellae; *action,* extends leg; *nerve supply,* femoral.
m. ventricula'ris, fibers of the thyroarytenoid which pass into the false vocal cord.
m. vertica'lis lin'guae [NA], vertical muscle of tongue; an intrinsic muscle of the tongue, consisting of fibers that pass from the aponeurosis of the dorsum to the aponeurosis of the inferior surface; *action,* decreases the superior to inferior dimension of the tongue; *nerve supply,* hypoglossal for motor, lingual for sensory.
m. voca'lis [NA], vocal muscle; m. thyroarytenoideus internus; *origin,* depression between the two laminae of thyroid cartilage; *insertion,* vocal process of arytenoid; *action,* shortens and relaxes vocal cords; *nerve supply,* recurrent laryngeal.
m. zygomat'icus, m. zygomaticus major.
m. zygomat'icus ma'jor [NA], greater zygomatic muscle; m. zygomaticus; *origin,* zygomatic bone anterior to temporozygomatic suture; *insertion,* muscles at angle of mouth; *action,* draws upper lip upward and laterally; *nerve supply,* facial.
m. zygomat'icus mi'nor [NA], lesser zygomatic muscle; caput zygomaticum quadrati labii superioris; *origin,* zygomatic bone posterior to zygomaticomaxillary suture; *insertion,* orbicularis oris of upper lip; *action,* draws upper lip upward and outward; *nerve supply,* facial.

mushbite (mŭsh'bīt). A maxillomandibular record made by introducing a mass of soft wax into the patient's mouth and instructing the patient to bite into it to the desired degree; not a generally accepted procedure.

musicotherapy (myū'sik-ō-thăr'ă-pē). Treatment of mental disorders by means of music.

Musset, L.C. Alfred de, French poet, 1810–1857; person in whom M.'s *sign* was studied.

mussitation (mŭs-i-tā'shŭn) [L. *mussito,* to murmur constantly, fr. *musso,* pp. *-atus,* to mutter]. Movements of the lips as if speaking, but without sound; observed in delirium and in semicoma.

Mussy. See Guéneau de Mussy.

must (mŭst) [L. *mustum,* new wine, ntr. of *mustus,* fresh]. Unfermented juice of the grape or other fruits.

Mustard, W.T., Canadian thoracic surgeon, *1914. See M. *operation, procedure.*

mustard (mŭs'tard) [O. Fr. *moustarde,* fr. L. *mustum,* must]. The dried ripe seeds of *Brassica alba* (white m.) and *B. nigra* (black m.) (family Cruciferae).

black m., the dried ripe seed of *Brassica nigra* or of *B. juncea;* it is the source of allyl isothiocyanate; it contains sinigrin (potassium myronate); myrosin; sinapine sulfocyanate; erucic, behenic, and synapolic acids; and fixed oil; a prompt emetic, a rubefacient, and a condiment.

m. chlorohydrin, hemisulfur m.

hemisulfur m., m. chlorohydrin; semisulfur m.; 2-(2-chloroethylthio)ethanol; an antineoplastic agent.

nitrogen m.'s, compounds of the general formula R—$N(CH_2CH_2Cl)$; the prototype is HN2 nitrogen m., mechlorethamine, in which R is CH_3. Some have been used therapeutically for their destructive action upon lymphoid tissue in lymphosarcoma, leukemia, Hodgkin's disease, and certain other cancers. See also mechlorethamine hydrochloride.

semisulfur m., hemisulfur m.

sulfur m., mustard *gas.*

uracil m., see under uracil.

white m., the ripe seeds of *Brassica* (*Sinapsis*) *alba;* less pungent than black m., but with the same constituents and uses.

mustard oil. Term applied to any of the organic isothiocyanates in general, but more specifically to allyl isothiocyanate; such oils are metabolically convertible to thiocyanates and may thus lead to goiter.

expressed m. o., the fixed oil expressed from the seeds of *Brassica alba* and *B. nigra;* it contains the glycerides of oleic, arachidic, and other fatty acids; used as salad oil and in the manufacture of oleomargarine.

volatile m. o., *allyl* isothiocyanate.

mustine hydrochloride (mŭs'tēn). Mechlorethamine hydrochloride.

mutacism (myū'tă-sizm). Mytacism.

mutagen (myū'tă-jen) [L. *muto,* to change, + G. *-gen,* producing]. Any agent that can cause a mutation, *e.g.,* radioactive substances, x-rays, or certain chemicals.

frame-shift m., a m., such as an acridine derivative, that causes a reading-frame-shift mutation.

mutagenesis (myū-tă-jen'ĕ-sis). Production of a mutation.

insertional m., mutation caused by insertion of new genetic material into a normal gene, particularly of retroviruses into chromosomal DNA.

mutagenic (myū-tă-jen'ik). Having the power to cause mutations.

mutant (myu'tant). **1.** A phenotype in which a mutation is manifested. **2.** A gene that is rare and usually harmful, in contrast to a wild-type gene.

active m., a m. with overt phenotypic expression.

conditionally lethal m., conditional-lethal m., a viral m. that can replicate under some (permissive) conditions but not under other (restrictive or nonpermissive) conditions, the parent ("wild" type) strain being able to replicate under both conditions. See suppressor-sensitive m.; temperature-sensitive m.

inactive m., silent m.; a m. that is not phenotypically manifest.

silent m., inactive m.

suppressor-sensitive m., a conditionally lethal, host range, bacteriophage m. that is productive of nonsense codons and can replicate only in a host bacterium able to effect "translation" of the nonsense codon in a "meaningful" way; the mutation effects are lethal (*i.e.,* prevent replication of the virus) in a bacterium without such a suppressor mechanism.

temperature-sensitive m., a viral m. that is able to replicate at one portion of a temperature range but not at another, the parent ("wild" type) strain being able to replicate over the whole temperature range.

mutarotase (myū'tă-rō-tās). Aldose 1-epimerase.

mutarotation (myū'tă-rō-tā'shŭn). Birotation; multirotation; the process of changing specific rotation; *e.g.,* a solution of α-D-glucose recrystallized from its solution in acetic acid and freshly dissolved in water gives a rotation of $[\alpha]_D^{20} = +112.2°$, but when recrystallized from a boiling aqueous solution (as the β-form) it shows an initial rotation of $[\alpha]_D^{20} = +18.7°$; either solution upon standing slowly changes its specific rotation to a value of $[\alpha]_D^{20} = +52.7°$, indicating a mixture of the two.

mutase (myū'tās). Any enzyme that catalyzes the apparent migration of groups within one molecule, *e.g.,* phosphoglycerate phosphomutase; sometimes the transfer is from one molecule to another, *e.g.,* phosphoglucomutase, phosphoglyceromutase (both phosphotransferases).

mutation (myū-tā'shŭn) [L. *muto,* pp. *-atus,* to change]. **1.** A change in the character of a gene that is perpetuated in subsequent divisions of the cell in which it occurs; a change in the sequence of base pairs in the chromosomal molecule. **2.** De Vries' term for the sudden production of a species, as distinguished from variation.

addition-deletion m., reading-frame-shift m.

amber m., a m. that results in the formation of termination codon UAG, which results in the premature termination of a polypeptide chain; named from the appearance of the *Escherichia coli* culture plate when the m. was first observed.

back m., reverse m.; reversion of a gene to an ancestral form due to further m. to the original codon or one coding for the same amino acid.

frame-shift m., reading-frame-shift m.

induced m., a m. caused by exposure to a mutagen.

lethal m., a mutant trait that leads to a phenotype incompatible with effective reproduction.

missense m. [L. *mitto,* to send away], a m. in which a base change or substitution results in a codon that causes insertion of a different amino acid into the growing polypeptide chain, giving rise to an altered protein.

natural m., spontaneous m.

neutral m., a m. with a negligible impact on genetic fitness.

new m., redundant term for a heritable trait present in the offspring but in neither parent.

nonsense m., suppressor m.

ochre m., a m. yielding the termination codon UAA, resulting in premature termination of a polypeptide chain; named from the appearance of the *Escherichia coli* culture plate when the m. was the first observed.

point m., a m. that involves a single nucleotide; it may consist of loss of a nucleotide, substitution of one nucleotide for another, or the insertion of an additional nucleotide.

reading-frame-shift m., addition-deletion or frame-shift m.; a m. that results from a nucleotide insertion into, or deletion from, the normal DNA sequence; since the genetic code is read three nucleotides at a time, all nucleotide triplets distal to the mutation will be out of phase and misread.

reverse m., back m.

silent m., the form of a genetic trait distinguishable at the genotypic level but not at the level of arbitrary phenotype (*e.g.,* clinical, immunological, or electrophoretic).

somatic m., a m. occurring in the general body cells (as opposed to the germ cells).

spontaneous m., natural m.; a m. that arises naturally and not as a

result of exposure to mutagens.
suppressor m., nonsense m.; a m. that alters the anticodon in a tRNA so that it is complementary to a termination codon, thus suppressing termination of the amino acid chain.
transition m., a point m. involving substitution of one base-pair for another, *i.e.,* replacement of one purine for another and of one pyrimidine for another pyrimidine without change in the purine-pyrimidine orientation.
transversion m., a point m. involving base substitution in which the orientation of purine and pyrimidine is reversed, in contradistinction to transition m.

mute (myūt) [L. *mutus*]. **1.** Unable or unwilling to speak. **2.** A person who has not the faculty of speech.

mutein (myū'tēn). General term for a protein arising as a result of a mutation.

mutilation (myū-ti-lā'shŭn) [L. *mutilatio,* fr. *mutilo,* pp. *-atus,* to maim]. Disfigurement or injury by removal or destruction of any conspicuous or essential part of the body.

mutism (myū'tism) [L. *mutus,* mute]. **1.** The state of being silent. **2.** Organic or functional absence of the faculty of speech.
akinetic m., a syndrome characterized by m., loss of voluntary and emotional movement, and apparent loss of emotional feeling; related to lesions of the upper brainstem.
elective m., voluntary m.; m. due to hysteria, abnormal inhibition, or emotional causes.
voluntary m., elective m.

muton (myū'ton). In genetics, the smallest unit of a chromosome in which alteration can be effective in causing a mutation.

mutualism (myū'tyū-ăl-izm). Symbiotic relationship in which both species derive benefit. *Cf.* commensalism; metabiosis; parasitism.

mutualist (myū'tyū-ăl-ist) [L. *mutuus,* in return, mutual]. Symbion.

muzzle (mŭz'l). The snout of an animal.

Mv Former symbol for mendelevium.

mV, mv Abbreviation for millivolt.

MVV Abbreviation for maximum voluntary *ventilation.*

MW Abbreviation for molecular *weight.*

my. Abbreviation of myopia.

myalgia (mī-al'jē-ă) [G. *mys,* muscle, + *algos,* pain]. Myodynia; myoneuralgia; myosalgia; muscular pain.
epidemic m., epidemic *pleurodynia.*
m. ther'mica, heat *cramps.*

myasthenia (mī-as-thē'nē-ă) [G. *mys,* muscle, + *astheneia,* weakness]. Muscular weakness.
m. angiosclerot'ica, intermittent *claudication.*
m. cor'dis, amyocardia.
m. gra'vis, Goldflam or Hoppe-Goldflam disease; a chronic progressive muscular weakness, beginning usually in the face and throat, unaccompanied by atrophy; due to a defect in myoneural conduction.

myasthenic (mī'as-then'ik). Relating to myasthenia.

myatonia, myatony (mī-ă-tō'nē-ă, mī-at'ō-nē) [G. *mys,* muscle, + *a* priv. + *tonos,* tone]. Amyotonia; abnormal extensibility of a muscle.
m. congen'ita, *amyotonia* congenita.

myatrophy (mī-at'rō-fē). Myoatrophy.

mycelia (mī-sē'lē-ă). Plural of mycelium.

mycelian (mī-sē'lē-an). Pertaining to a mycelium.

mycelioid (mī-sē'lē-oyd) [mycelium + G. *eidos,* resemblance]. Resembling a mycelium.

mycelium, pl. **mycelia** (mī-sē'lē-ŭm, -ă) [G. *mykēs,* fungus, + *hēlos,* nail, wart, excrescence on animal or plant]. The mass of hyphae making up a colony of fungi.
aerial m., the portion of m. that grows upward or outward from the surface of the substrate, and from which propagative spores develop in or on characteristic structures that are distinctive for various generic groups.
nonseptate m., one in which there are no septa, or "cross-walls," in the hyphae; inasmuch as the latter are not divided into numerous individual cells, the multinucleated protoplasm may flow throughout the tubelike structures.
septate m., one in which septa, or "cross-walls," divide the hyphae into numerous uninucleated or multinucleated cells.

mycet-, myceto- [G. *mykēs,* fungus]. Combining forms relating to fungus. See also myco-.

mycete (mī'sēt) [G. *mykēs,* fungus]. A fungus.

mycetism, mycetis'mus (mī'sē-tizm, -tiz'mŭs) [G. *mykēs,* fungus]. Muscarinism; poisoning by certain species of mushrooms.
m. cerebra'lis, a condition characterized by transient hallucinogenic symptoms following ingestion of mushrooms such as *Psilocybe* and *Panaeolus.*
m. cholifor'mis, a severe and occasionally fatal illness due to the consumption of *Amanita phalloides* and other poisonous mushroom species.
m. gastrointestina'lis, a relatively mild type of mushroom poisoning characterized by nausea, vomiting, and diarrhea, caused by eating certain species of *Boletus, Lactarius, Entoloma,* and *Lepiota.*
m. nervo'sa, mushroom poisoning that involves the parasympathetic nervous system and causes gastrointestinal distress, after consumption of species such as *Amanita, Inocybe,* and *Clitocybe.*
m. sanguina'reus, a transient hemoglobinuria and jaundice caused by eating the mushroom *Helvella esculenta,* both raw and cooked.

mycetogenetic, mycetogenic (mī-sē'tō-jĕ-net'ik, -jen'ik; mī'sē-tō-) [G. *mykēs,* fungus, + *gennētos,* begotten]. Mycetogenous; caused by fungi.

mycetogenous (mī-sē-toj'ĕ-nŭs). Mycetogenetic.

mycetoma (mī-sē-tō'mă). **1.** Madura boil; Bouffardi's black mycetoma; Madura or fungous foot; maduromycosis; a chronic infection usually involving the feet (and rarely the hands and other sites), and characterized by the formation of localized lesions with tumefactions and multiple draining sinuses. The exudate contains granules that may be yellow, white, red, brown, or black, depending upon the causative agent. M. is caused by two principal groups of microorganisms: 1) actinomycotic m. is caused by actinomycetes, including species of *Streptomyces,* and *Nocardia,* 2) eumycotic mycetoma is caused by true fungi, including species of *Madurella, Exophiala, Pseudallescheria, Curvularia, Neotestudina, Pyrenochaeta, Aspergillus,* and *Acremonium.* **2.** Any tumor produced by filamentous fungi.
Bouffardi's black m., mycetoma (1).
Bouffardi's white m., a form common in India and found occasionally in Somaliland, caused by the organism *Streptomyces somaliensis;* in this variety, the muscles, tendons, and bones of the foot are destroyed by the disease process; numerous draining sinuses discharge yellowish grains, clustered like fish roe.
Brumpt's white m., m. caused by *Pseudallescheria boydii,* occurring in temperate and subtropical areas in India; small, white to yellow, hard to soft granules are discharged through the draining sinuses.
Carter's black m., m. caused by *Madurella mycetomi* which is prevalent in Italy, parts of Africa, and India; the exuded granules are black.
Nicolle's white m., m. caused by a species of *Aspergillus,* and producing relatively large granules, about the size of a pea; infection occurs from barley grain.
Vincent's white m., m. caused by *Nocardia madurae* and occur-

ring in North Africa, India, the Argentine, and Cuba.

mycid (mī'sid) [G. *mykēs,* fungus, + -id]. An allergic reaction to a remote focus of mycotic infection.

myco- [G. *mykēs,* fungus]. Combining form relating to fungus. See also mycet-.

mycobacteria (mī'kō-bak-tē'rē-ă). Organisms belonging to the genus *Mycobacterium.*

group I m., photochromogens; m. that produce a bright yellow color when grown in the presence of light. Organisms placed in this group appear to belong to the species *Mycobacterium kansasii.*

group II m., scotochromogens; m. that produce a yellow pigment even when grown in the dark; when grown in the light, the pigment is orange. These organisms behave as do saprophytes in man and are nonpathogenic to laboratory animals.

group III m., nonchromogens; m. that are either colorless or that slowly produce a light yellow pigment when grown in the presence of light. Organisms placed in this group belong to the species *Mycobacterium intracellulare.*

group IV m., m. that grow rapidly and that do not produce pigment. Organisms placed in this group belong to such species as *Mycobacterium ulcerans* and *M. marinum.*

Mycobacteriaceae (mī'kō-bak-tēr-ē-ā'sē-ē). A family of aerobic bacteria (order Actinomycetales) containing Gram-positive, spherical to rod-shaped cells. Branching does not occur under ordinary cultural conditions. They may or may not be acid-fast. They occur in soil and dairy products and as parasites on man and other animals. The type genus is *Mycobacterium.*

mycobacteriosis (mī'kō-bak-tēr'ē-ō'sis). Infection with mycobacteria.

Mycobacterium (mī'kō-bak-tēr'ē-ŭm) [myco- + bacterium]. A genus of aerobic, nonmotile bacteria (family Mycobacteriaceae) containing Gram-positive, acid-fast, slender, straight or slightly curved rods; slender filaments occasionally occur, but branched forms rarely are produced. Parasitic and saprophytic species occur. The type species is *M. tuberculosis.* It is the type genus of the family Mycobacteriaceae.

M. absces'sus, a species orginally found in a traumatic infection of the human knee.

M. a'vium, tubercle bacillus (3); a species causing tuberculosis in fowl and other birds.

M. bal'nei, a later, subjective synonym of *M. marinum.*

M. bo'vis, *M. tuberculosis* subsp. *bovis;* tubercle bacillus (2); a species which is the primary cause of tuberculosis in cattle; transmissible to man and other animals, causing tuberculosis.

M. fortu'itum, a saprophytic species found in soil and in infections of humans, cattle, and cold-blooded animals.

M. intracellula're, Battey bacillus; a species found in lung lesions and sputum of man; may cause bone and tendon-sheath lesions in rabbits; some strains are pathogenic for mice.

M. kansas'ii, a species causing a tuberculosis-like pulmonary disease; also found to cause infections (and usually lesions) in spinal fluid, spleen, liver, pancreas, testes, hip joint, knee joint, finger, wrist, and lymph nodes.

M. lep'rae, Hansen's bacillus; leprosy bacillus; a species that causes Hansen's disease; recently identified from wild leprous armadillos (*Dasypus novemcinctus*) in Texas.

M. lepraemu'rium, a species which causes rat leprosy.

M. maria'num, a subjective synonym of *M. scrofulaceum.*

M. mari'num, a species causing spontaneous tuberculosis in salt water fish; it also occurs in other cold-blooded animals, in some swimming pools, irrigation canals and ditches, and ocean beaches. *M. balnei* is a later, subjective synonym of *M. marinum.*

M. micro'ti, a species causing generalized tuberculosis in voles; transmissible to guinea pigs, rabbits, and calves, causing localized infections.

M. paratuberculo'sis, Johne's bacillus; a species causing Johne's disease, a chronic enteritis in cattle.

M. phle'i, timothy hay bacillus; Moeller's grass bacillus; a species found in soil and dust and on plants.

M. platypoeci'lus, a species found in skin ulcers, liver, spleen, gills, and kidneys of diseased platyfish.

M. scrofula'ceum, a species frequently associated with cervical adenitis in children; also found in a skin lesion of a leprosy patient. A subjective synonym is *M. marianum.*

M. smeg'matis, mist bacillus; a saprophytic species of bacteria found in smegma from the genitalia of man and many of the lower animals; it is also found in soil, dust, and water.

M. thamno'pheos, a species found as a parasite in the garter snake and other cold-blooded vertebrates; experimentally it causes tuberculosis in snakes, frogs, lizards, and fish; it is not pathogenic for guinea pigs, rabbits, or fowl.

M. tuberculo'sis, Koch's bacillus (1); tubercle bacillus (human); a species which causes tuberculosis in man; it is the type species of the genus *M.*

M. tuberculo'sis subsp. **bo'vis,** *M. bovis.*

M. ul'cerans, a species causing Buruli ulcers in man; transmissible from soil, usually after an injury, and possibly by an insect vector.

M. xen'opi, M. xen'opei, a species found in a skin lesion of a cold-blooded animal, *Xenopus laevis;* a rare cause of nosocomial human pulmonary tuberculosis.

mycobactin (mī'kō-bak'tin). A complex lipid factor reported to be required for the growth of *Mycobacterium tuberculosis* in human plasma; appears to be identical with the lipid factor extracted from *M. phlei* and essential for the growth of *M. johnei.*

mycocide (mī'kō-sīd) [myco- + L. *caedo,* to kill]. Fungicide.

Mycoderma (mī-kō-der'mă) [myco- + G. *derma,* skin]. Obsolete genus of fungi now classified as *Blastomyces, Candida,* and *Paragcoccidioides.*

mycodermatitis (mī'kō-der-mă-tī'tis). A nonspecific term used to designate an eruption of mycotic (fungus, yeast, mold) origin.

mycogastritis (mī'kō-gas-trī'tis) [myco- + G. *gastēr,* stomach, + *-itis,* inflammation]. Inflammation of the stomach due to the presence of a fungus.

mycolic acids (mī-kol'ik). Mykol; long-chain cyclopropanecarboxylic acids (C_{19}–C_{21}), further substituted by long-chain (C_{24}–C_{30}) alkanes containing free hydroxyl groups, found in certain bacteria; these waxy substances appear to be responsible for the acid-fastness of the bacteria that contain them.

mycologist (mī-kol'ō-jist). A person specializing in mycology.

mycology (mī-kol'ō-jē) [myco- + G. *logos,* study]. The study of fungi: their classification, edibility, cultivation, and biology.

medical m., the study of fungi that produce disease in man and other mammalians, and of the diseases they produce, their ecology, and their epidemiology.

mycomyringitis (mī'kō-mir-in-jī'tis) [myco- + Mod. L. *myringa,* drum-membrane, + G. *-itis,* inflammation]. Myringomycosis; an obsolete term denoting an inflammation of the membrana tympani caused by the presence of *Aspergillus* or other fungus.

mycophage (mī'kō-fāj) [myco- + G. *phagein,* to eat]. A virus the host of which is a fungus, in contradistinction to a bacteriophage, the host of which is a bacterium. See also mycovirus.

Mycoplasma (mī'kō-plaz-mă) [myco- + G. *plasma,* something formed (plasm)]. *Asterococcus;* a genus of aerobic to facultatively anaerobic bacteria (family Mycoplasmataceae) containing Gram-negative cells which do not possess a true cell wall but are bounded by a three-layered membrane; they do not revert to bacteria containing cell walls or cell wall fragments. The minimal reproductive units of these organisms are 0.2 to 0.3 μm in diameter. The cells are pleomorphic, and in liquid media appear as coccoid bodies, rings, or filaments. Colonies usually consist of a central core, growing down into the medium, surrounded by superficial peripheral growth. They require sterol for growth. They also require enrichment with serum or ascitic fluid. These organisms are found in humans and other animals and are parasitic to pathogenic. The type species is *M. mycoides.*

M. agalact'iae, a species causing contagious agalactia of sheep and goats, a common disease in the Mediterranean region.

M. bucca'le, *M. orale 2;* a species which is an infrequent parasitic inhabitant of the human oropharynx; it is the predominant mycoplasma in the oropharynx of nonhuman primates.

M. conjuncti'vae subsp. **o'vis,** a subspecies associated with pinkeye of sheep.

M. fau'cium, *M. orale 3;* a species which is a rare member of the normal flora of the human oropharynx; it is occasionally found in the oropharynx of nonhuman primates.

M. fermen'tans, a species found in ulcerative genital lesions associated with fusiform bacteria and spirilla and also on the apparently normal genital mucosa of humans.

M. gallisep'ticum, a species causing chronic respiratory disease of chickens and infectious sinusitis of turkeys.

M. granula'rum, *Acholeplasma granularum.*

M. hom'inis, a species found in the genital tract and anal canal of humans; also found in the blood of a patient with puerperal septicemia and in pus of a bronchopleural fistula.

M. hyorhi'nis, a species found in the nasal cavity of swine; associated with arthritis and polyserositis in domestic pigs.

M. hyosyno'viae, a species found in the joints and respiratory tract of swine, and associated with arthritis and polyserositis in domestic pigs.

M. hypopneumo'niae, a species causing mycoplasma pneumonia of pigs.

M. laidla'wii, *Acholeplasma laidlawii.*

M. meleag'ridis, a species causing air sacculitis in turkeys.

M. mycoi'des, a species containing two subspecies: *M. mycoides* subsp. *mycoides,* the type subspecies, and *M. mycoides* subsp. *capri;* the former causes contagious bovine pleuropneumonia in cattle; the latter causes contagious pleuropneumonia in sheep and goats; it is the type species of the genus *M.*

M. neuroly'ticum, a species found in normal and diseased mice; causes "rolling disease."

M. ora'le 1, *M. pharyngis.*

M. ora'le 2, *M. buccale.*

M. ora'le 3, *M. faucium.*

M. pharyn'gis, *M. orale 1;* a species occurring as a commensal in the human oropharynx.

M. pneumo'niae, Eaton agent; a species causing primary atypical pneumonia in man.

M. saliva'rium, a species found in human saliva.

M. syno'viae, a species found in the hock joint of a fowl; causes infectious synovitis in chickens.

mycoplasma, pl. **mycoplasmata** (mī-kō-plaz'mă, -plaz'mah-tă). A vernacular term used only to refer to any member of the genus *Mycoplasma.*

Mycoplasmatales (mī'kō-plaz'mă-tā'lēz). An order of Gram-negative bacteria containing cells which are bounded by a three-layered membrane but which do not possess a true cell wall. The minimal reproductive units are 0.2 to 0.3 μm in diameter. Pathogenic and saprophytic species occur. These organisms reproduce through the breaking up of branched filaments into coccoid, filterable elementary bodies. The order includes the so-called pleuropneumonia-like *organisms* (PPLO).

mycopus (mī'kō-pŭs). Mucopus.

mycose (mī'kōs). Trehalose.

mycosis, pl. **mycoses** (mī-kō'sis, -sēz) [myco- + G. *-osis,* condition]. Any disease caused by a fungus or yeast.

m. cu'tis chron'ica, a chronic dermatomycosis caused by a fungus.

m. framboesioi'des, yaws.

m. fungoi'des, a chronic progressive lymphoma arising in the skin which initially simulates eczema or other inflammatory dermatoses; the appearance of plaques is associated with acanthosis and bandlike infiltration of the upper dermis by a pleomorphic infiltrate including atypical T lymphocytes which also collect in clear spaces in the lower epidermis (Pautrier's microabscesses); in advanced cases, ulcerated tumors and infiltrations of lymph nodes may occur.

Gilchrist's m., obsolete term for blastomycosis.

m. intestina'lis, gastroenteric form of anthrax, the symptoms of which are those of gastroenteritis followed by toxemia and general depression.

mycostatic (mī-kō-stat'ik). Fungistatic.

mycosterols (mī-kos'ter-olz). Sterols obtained from fungi.

mycotic (mī-kot'ik). Relating to or caused by a fungus.

mycotoxicosis (mī'kō-tok-si-kō'sis). Poisoning due to the ingestion of preformed substances produced by the action of certain fungi on particular foodstuffs, or ingestion of the fungi themselves.

mycotoxins (mī'kō-tok-sinz). Toxic compounds produced by certain fungi, some of which are used for medicinal purposes; *e.g.,* muscarine, psilocybin.

mycovirus (mī'kō-vī-rŭs). A virus that infects fungi.

mydaleine (mī-dā'lē-ēn) [G. *mydaleos,* moldy, fr. *mydos,* dampness]. A poisonous ptomaine formed in putrefying liver and other viscera; it acts specifically upon the heart, causing arrest of its action in diastole.

mydatoxin (mī-dă-tok'sin) [G. *mydos,* dampness, decay, + *toxikon,* poison]. A ptomaine from putrefying viscera and flesh.

mydriasis (mi-drī'ă-sis) [G.]. Dilation of the pupil.

alternating m., m. alternately affecting each eye because of alternating Horner's syndrome or anisocoria.

amaurotic m., a m. of both eyes, resulting from impaired visual input from one or both eyes.

paralytic m., pupillary dilation due to paralysis of the sphincter muscle of the pupil induced by anticholinergic drugs given topically or systemically, or resulting from lesions of the oculomotor nucleus or nerve, contusion of the eyeball, or glaucoma.

spasmodic m., spastic m.

spastic m., spasmodic m.; pupillary dilation due to contraction of the dilator muscle of the pupil induced by adrenergic drugs or by stimulation of the sympathetic pathway.

springing m., sudden and temporary m. from any cause.

mydriatic (mi-drē-at'ik). **1.** Causing mydriasis or dilation of the pupil. **2.** An agent that dilates the pupil.

myectomy (mī-ek'tō-mē) [G. *mys,* muscle, + *ektomē,* excision]. Exsection of a portion of a muscle.

myectopy, myectopia (mī-ek'tō-pē, mī-ek-tō'pē-ă) [G. *mys,* muscle, + *ektopos,* out of place]. Dislocation of a muscle.

myel-, myelo- [G. *myelos,* medulla, marrow]. Combining forms denoting relationship to: **1.** The bone marrow. **2.** The spinal cord and medulla oblongata. **3.** The myelin sheath of nerve fibers.

myelapoplexy (mī'el-ap'ō-plek'sē) [myel- + G. *apoplēxia,* apoplexy]. Hematomyelia.

myelatelia (mī'el-ă-tē'lē-ă) [myel- + G. *ateleia,* incompleteness]. Developmental defect of the spinal cord.

myelauxe (mī-el-awk'sē) [myel- + G. *auxē,* increase]. Hypertrophy of the spinal cord.

myelemia (mī-ĕ-lē'mē-ă) [myel- + G. *haima,* blood]. Myelocytosis.

myelencephalon (mī'el-en-sef'ă-lon) [myel- + G. *enkephalos,* brain] [NA]. *Medulla* oblongata.

myelic (mī-el'ik). Relating to (1) the spinal cord, or (2) bone marrow.

myelin (mī'ĕ-lin). **1.** The lipoproteinaceous material, composed of regularly alternating membrana of lipid lamellae (cholesterol, phospholipids, sphingolipids, phosphatidates) and protein, of the myelin sheath. **2.** Droplets of lipid formed during autolysis and postmortem decomposition.

myelinated (mī'ĕ-li-nāt-ed). Medullated (2); having a myelin sheath.

myelination (mī'ĕ-li-nā'shŭn). Myelinization; myelinogenesis; medullation (2) the acquisition, development, or formation of a myelin sheath around a nerve fiber.

myelinic (mī'ĕ-lin'ik). Relating to myelin.

myelinization (mī'ĕ-li-nī-zā'shŭn). Myelination.

myelinoclasis (mī'ĕ-li-nok'lă-sis) [myelin + G. *klasis,* a breaking]. Destruction of myelin. See also demyelination, dysmyelination.

myelinogenesis (mī'ĕ-lin-ō-jen'ĕ-sis) [myelin + G. *genesis,* production]. Myelination.

myelinolysis (mī'ĕ-li-nol'i-sis) [myelin + G. *lysis,* dissolution]. Dissolution of the myelin sheaths of nerve fibers.

central pontine m., localized loss of myelin within the midbase of the pons; related to malnutrition and often to alcoholism.

myelitic (mī-ĕ-lit'ik). Relating to or affected by myelitis.

myelitis (mī-ĕ-lī'tis) [myel- + G. *-itis,* inflammation]. **1.** Inflammation of the spinal cord. **2.** Inflammation of the bone marrow.

acute transverse m., acute inflammation and softening of the spinal cord; involves the entire thickness of the spinal cord but is limited in length.

ascending m., progressive inflammation involving successively higher areas of the spinal cord.

bulbar m., inflammation of the medulla oblongata.

concussion m., traumatic myelopathy.

Foix-Alajouanine m., subacute necrotizing m.

funicular m., **(1)** inflammation involving any of the columns of the spinal cord; **(2)** subacute combined *degeneration* of the spinal cord.

subacute necrotizing m., Foix-Alajouanine m.; angiodysgenetic myelomalacia; a disorder of the lower spinal cord resulting in progressive paraplegia.

systemic m., inflammation confined to special tracts of the spinal cord.

transverse m., inflammation involving the entire thickness of the spinal cord, but of limited longitudinal extent.

myelo-. See myel-.

myeloarchitectonics (mī'ĕ-lō-ar'ki-tek-ton'iks). The pattern of myelinated nerve fibers in the brain, as distinguished from cytoarchitectonics.

myeloblast (mī'ĕ-lō-blast) [myelo- + G. *blastos,* germ]. Premyelocyte; an immature cell (10 to 18 μm in diameter) in the granulocytic series, occurring normally in bone marrow, but not in the circulating blood (except in certain diseases). When stained with the usual dyes, the cytoplasm is light blue, nongranular, and variable in amount, sometimes being only a thin rim around the nucleus; the latter is deep purple-blue with finely divided, punctate, threadlike chromatin that is somewhat condensed at the periphery. A few light blue nucleoli are usually present in the nucleus, and these generally disappear as the m. matures into a promyelocyte and then a myelocyte. M.'s ordinarily yield a negative reaction with peroxidase.

myeloblastemia (mī'ĕ-lō-blas-tē'mē-ă) [myeloblast + G. *haima,* blood]. The presence of myeloblasts in the circulating blood.

myeloblastoma (mī'ĕ-lō-blas-tō'mă) [myeloblast + G. *-oma,* tumor]. A nodular focus or fairly well circumscribed accumulation of myeloblasts, as sometimes observed in acute myeloblastic leukemia and chlorosis.

myeloblastosis (mī'ĕ-lō-blas-tō'sis). The presence of unusually large numbers of myeloblasts in the circulating blood, or tissues, or both (as in acute leukemia).

avian m., fowl m., disease caused by the avian leukosis-sarcoma virus, characterized by progressive anemia, enormous numbers of myeloblasts in the blood, weakness, and death.

myelocele (mī'ĕ-lō-sēl). **1** [myelo- + G. *kēle,* hernia]. Protrusion of the spinal cord in spina bifida. **2** [G. *myelos,* marrow, + *koilia,* a hollow]. The central canal of the spinal cord.

myelocyst (mī'ĕ-lō-sist) [myelo- + G. *kystis,* bladder]. Any cyst (usually lined with columnar or cuboidal cells) that develops from a rudimentary medullary canal in the central nervous system.

myelocystic (mī'ĕ-lō-sist'ik). Pertaining to or characterized by the presence of a myelocyst.

myelocystocele (mī'ĕ-lō-sis'tō-sēl) [myelo- + G. *kystis,* bladder, + *kēlē,* tumor]. Spina bifida containing spinal cord substance.

myelocystomeningocele (mī'ĕ-lō-sis'tō-mĕ-ning'gō-sēl) [myelo- + G. *kystis,* bladder, + *mēninx* (*mēning-*), membrane, + *kēlē,* hernia]. Meningomyelocele.

myelocyte (mī'ĕ-lō-sīt) [myelo- + G. *kytos,* cell]. **1.** Myelomonocyte; a young cell of the granulocytic series, occurring normally in bone marrow, but not in circulating blood (except in certain diseases). When stained with the usual dyes, the cytoplasm is distinctly basophilic and relatively more abundant than in myeloblasts or promyelocytes, even though m.'s are smaller cells; numerous cytoplasmic granules (*i.e.,* neutrophilic, eosinophilic, or basophilic) are present in the more mature forms of m.'s, and the first two types are peroxidase-positive. The nuclear chromatin is coarser than that observed in myeloblasts, but it is relatively faintly stained and lacks a well defined membrane; the nucleus is fairly regular in contour (*i.e.,* not indented), and seems to be "buried" beneath the numerous cytoplasmic granules. **2.** Medullocell; a nerve cell of the gray matter of the brain or spinal cord.

m. A, the youngest form of m., characterized by only a few (not more than ten) cytoplasmic granules, which are most reliably demonstrated by means of staining with neutral red; the mitochondria are numerous, and resemble those of the myeloblast.

m. B, the intermediate form of m., characterized by approximately 30 to 100 (or more) cytoplasmic granules scattered among the mitochondria; the latter are less numerous than in m.'s of the A stage, and they are frequently displaced toward the periphery of the cell.

m. C, the most mature of the m.'s characterized by numerous cytoplasmic granules that are recognizable as neutrophilic, eosinophilic, and basophilic; with neutral red these are stained, respectively, red, bright yellow, and deep maroon; C m.'s are frequently larger than earlier forms; if the nucleus is indented, the m. is maturing into a metamyelocyte.

myelocythemia (mī'ĕ-lō-sī-thē'mē-ă) [myelocyte + G. *haima,* blood]. The presence of myelocytes in the circulating blood, especially in persistently large numbers (as in myelocytic leukemia).

myelocytic (mī'ĕ-lō-sit'ik). Pertaining to or characterized by myelocytes.

myelocytoma (mī'ĕ-lō-sī-tō'mă) [myelocyte + G. *-oma,* tumor]. A nodular focus or fairly well circumscribed, relatively dense accumulation of myelocytes, as in certain tissues of persons with myelocytic leukemia.

myelocytomatosis (mī'ĕ-lō-sī'tō-mă-tō'sis). **1.** Leukochloroma; a form of tumor involving chiefly the myelocytes. **2.** A rare leukosis of fowl marked by the presence of white tumors composed of myeloid cells, located principally along the sternum and in the liver.

myelocytosis (mī'ĕ-lō-sī-tō'sis) [myelocyte + G. *-osis,* condition]. Myelemia; the occurrence of abnormally large numbers of myelocytes in the circulating blood, or tissues, or both.

myelodiastasis (mī'ĕ-lō-dī-as'tă-sis) [myelo- + G. *diastasis,* separation]. Softening and destruction of the spinal cord.

myelodysplasia (mī'ĕ-lō-dis-plā'zē-ă) [myelo- + G. *dys-,* difficult, + *plasis,* a molding]. **1.** An abnormality in development of the spinal cord. **2.** Inappropriate term for spina bifida occulta.

myelofibrosis (mī'ĕ-lō-fī-brō'sis). Myelosclerosis; osteomyelofibrotic syndrome; fibrosis of the bone marrow, especially generalized, associated with myeloid metaplasia of the spleen and other organs, leukoerythroblastic anemia, and thrombocytopenia, although the bone marrow often contains many megakaryocytes.

myelogenesis (mī'ĕ-lō-jen'ĕ-sis). Development of bone marrow.

myelogenetic, myelogenic (mī'ĕ-lō-jĕ-net'ik, -jen'ik). **1.** Relating to myelogenesis. **2.** Myelogenous; produced by or orginating in the bone marrow.

myelogenous (mī-ĕ-loj'ĕ-nŭs). Myelogenetic (2).

myelogone, myelogonium (mī'ĕ-lō-gōn, -gō'nē-ŭm) [myelo- + G. *gonē,* seed]. An immature white blood cell of the myeloid series that is characterized by a relatively large, fairly deeply stained, finely reticulated nucleus that contains palely stained nucleoli, and a scant amount of rimlike, nongranular, moderately basophilic cytoplasm. M.'s are difficult to distinguish from lymphoblasts and monoblasts, unless one evaluates them in relation to the more mature forms usually associated with the younger cells.

myelogram (mī-el'ō-gram). Roentgenographic study of the spinal cord.

myelography (mī'ĕ-log'ră-fē) [myelo- + G. *graphē,* a drawing]. X-ray visualization of the spinal cord or its extension after the injection of a radiopaque substance into the spinal subarachnoid space.

myeloic (mī-ĕ-lō'ik). Pertaining to the tissue and precursor cells from which neutrophils, eosinophils, and basophils are derived.

myeloid (mī'ĕ-loyd). **1.** Pertaining to, derived from, or manifesting certain features of the bone marrow. **2.** Sometimes used with reference to the spinal cord. **3.** Pertaining to certain characteristics of myelocytic forms, but not necessarily implying origin in the bone marrow.

myeloidosis (mī'ĕ-loy-dō'sis). General hyperplasia of myeloid tissue.

myeloleukemia (mī'ĕ-lō-lū-kē'mē-ă). A form of leukemia in which the abnormal cells are derived from myelopoietic tissue.

myelolipoma (mī'ĕ-lō-li-pō'mă). A misnomer for certain nodular foci that are not neoplasms, but probably represent accumulations of cells derived from localized proliferation of reticuloendothelial tissue in the blood sinuses of the adrenal glands; grossly, the nodules may seem to be adipose tissue, but actually are foci of bone marrow containing erythropoietic or myeloid cells.

myelolymphocyte (mī'ĕ-lō-lim'fō-sīt). An abnormal form of the lymphocytic series in the bone marrow, and presumed to be formed in that tissue.

myelolysis (mī-ĕ-lol'i-sis). Decomposition of myelin.

myeloma (mī-ĕ-lō'mă) [myelo- + G. *-oma,* tumor]. **1.** A tumor composed of cells derived from hemopoietic tissues of the bone marrow. **2.** A plasma cell tumor.

Bence Jones m., L-chain m. or disease; multiple m. in which the malignant plasma cells excrete only light chains of one type (either κ or λ); lytic bone lesions occur in about 60% of the cases, and light chains (Bence Jones protein) occur in the urine; amyloidosis and severe renal failure are more common than in multiple m.

endothelial m., Ewing's *tumor.*

giant cell m., giant cell *tumor* of bone.

L-chain m., Bence Jones m.

multiple m., m. mul'tiplex, multiple myelomatosis; myelomatosis multiplex; an uncommon disease that occurs more frequently in men than in women and is associated with anemia, hemmorrhages, recurrent infections, and weakness. Ordinarily, it is regarded as a malignant neoplasm that originates in bone marrow and involves chiefly the skeleton, with clinical features attributable to the sites of involvement and to abnormalities in formation of plasma protein; characterized by numerous diffuse foci or nodular accumulations of abnormal or malignant plasma cells in the marrow of various bones (especially the skull), causing palpable swellings of the bones, and occasionally in extraskeletal sites; radiologically, the bone lesions have a characteristic punched-out appearance. The myeloma cells produce abnormal proteins in the serum and urine; those formed in any one example of multiple m. are different from other m. proteins, as well as from normal serum proteins, the most frequent abnormalities in the metabolism of protein being: 1) the occurrence of Bence Jones proteinuria, 2) a great increase in monodonal γ-globulin in the plasma, 3) the occasional formation of cryoglobulin, and 4) a form of primary amyloidosis. The Bence Jones protein is not a derivative of abnormal serum protein, but seems to be formed *de novo* from amino acid precursors. See also plasma cell m.

nonsecretory m., multiple m. in which there is no detectable paraproteinemia or paraproteinuria.

plasma cell m., **(1)** multiple m.; **(2)** plasmacytoma of bone, which is usually a solitary lesion and not associated with the occurrence of Bence Jones protein or other disturbances in the metabolism of protein (as observed in multiple m.). Some observers emphasize that the solitary lesion probably represents an early phase of classic multiple m., or an example of the latter in which only one focus is recognized.

myelomalacia (mī'ĕ-lō-ma-lā'shē-ă). [myelo- + G. *malakia,* a softness]. Softening of the spinal cord.

angiodysgenetic m., subacute necrotizing *myelitis.*

myelomatosis (mī'ĕ-lō-mă-tō'sis). A disease characterized by the occurrence of myelomas in various sites.

multiple m., m. mul'tiplex, multiple *myeloma.*

myelomeningocele (mī'ĕ-lō-mĕ-ning'gō-sēl) [myelo- + G. *mēninx,* membrane, + *kēlē,* hernia]. Meningomyelocele.

myelomere (mī'ĕ-lō-mēr) [myelo- + G. *meros,* part]. Neuromere of the spinal cord.

myelomonocyte (mī'ĕ-lō-mon'ō-sīt). Myelocyte (1).

myeloneuritis (mī'ĕ-lō-nū-rī'tis). Neuromyelitis.

myelonic (mī-ĕ-lon'ik) [G. *myelon,* fr. *myelos,* marrow]. Relating to the spinal cord.

myeloparalysis (mī'ĕ-lō-pă-ral'i-sis). Spinal *paralysis.*

myelopathic (mī'ĕ-lō-path'ik). Relating to myelopathy.

myelopathy (mī-ĕ-lop'ă-thē) [myelo- + G. *pathos,* suffering]. **1.** Disturbance or disease of the spinal cord. **2.** A disease of the myelopoietic tissues.

carcinomatous m., paracarcinomatous m.; degeneration or necrosis of the spinal cord associated with a carcinoma.

compressive m., destruction of spinal cord tissue caused by pressure from neoplasms, hematomas, or other masses.

diabetic m., degenerative changes in spinal cord tissue occurring as a complication of diabetes mellitus.

paracarcinomatous m., carcinomatous m.

radiation m., damage (planned or unplanned) to the spinal cord from exposure to x-rays or similar radiation.

myeloperoxidase (mī'el-ō-per-oks'i-dās). A peroxidase occurring in phagocytic cells that can oxidize halogen ions (*e.g.,* I^-) to the free halogen.

myelopetal (mī-ĕ-lop'ĕ-tăl) [myelo- + L. *peto,* to seek]. Proceeding in a direction toward the spinal cord; said of different nerve impulses.

myelophthisic (mī'ĕ-lō-tiz'ik, -thiz'ik). Relating to or suffering from myelophthisis.

myelophthisis (mī'ĕ-lof'thi-sis, mī'ĕ-lō-tī'sis, -tē'sis) [myelo- + G. *phthisis,* a wasting away]. **1.** Wasting or atrophy of the spinal cord as in tabes dorsalis. **2.** Panmyelophthisis; replacement of hemopoietic tissue in the bone marrow by abnormal tissue, usually fibrous tissue or malignant tumors which are most commonly metastatic carcinomas.

myeloplast (mī'ĕ-lō-plast) [myelo- + G. *plastos,* formed]. Any of the leukocytic series of cells in the bone marrow, especially young forms.

myeloplegia (mī'ĕ-lō-plē'jē-ă) [myelo- + G. *plēgē,* a stroke]. Spinal *paralysis.*

myelopoiesis (mī'ĕ-lō-poy-ē'sis) [myelo- + G. *poiēsis,* a making]. Formation of the tissue elements of bone marrow, or any of the types of blood cells derived from bone marrow, or both processes.

myelopoietic (mī'ĕ-lō-poy-et'ik). Relating to myelopoiesis.

myeloproliferative (mī'ĕ-lō-prō-lif'er-ă-tiv). Pertaining to or characterized by unusual proliferation of myelopoietic tissue.

myeloradiculitis (mī'ĕ-lō-ra-dik-yū-lī'tis) [myelo- + L. *radicula,* root, + G. *-itis,* inflammation]. Inflammation of the spinal cord and nerve roots.

myeloradiculodysplasia (mī'ĕ-lō-ra-dik'yū-lō-dis-plā-zē-ă) [myelo- + L. *radicula,* root, + dysplasia]. Congenital maldevelopment of the spinal cord and spinal nerve roots.

myeloradiculopathy (mī'ĕ-lō-ră-dik'yū-lop'ă-thē) [myelo- + L. *radicula,* root, + G. *pathos,* disease]. Radiculomyelopathy; disease involving the spinal cord and nerve roots.

myeloradiculopolyneuronitis (mī'ĕ-lō-ra-dik'yū-lō-pol'ē-nū-ron-ī'tis). Acute idiopathic *polyneuritis.*

myelorrhagia (mī'ĕ-lō-rā'jē-ă) [myelo- + G. *rhēgnymi,* to burst forth]. Hematomyelia.

myelorrhaphy (mī-ĕ-lōr'ă-fē) [myelo- + G. *rhaphē,* a seam]. Suture of a wound of the spinal cord.

myelosarcoma (mī'ĕ-lō-sar-kō'mă) [myelo- + G. *sarx,* flesh, + *-ōma,* tumor]. A malignant neoplasm derived from bone marrow or one of its cellular elements.

myelosarcomatosis (mī'ĕ-lō-sar-ko-mă-tō'sis). Widespread myelosarcomas.

myeloschisis (mī-ĕ-los'ki-sis) [myelo- + G. *schisis,* a cleaving]. Cleft spinal cord resulting from failure of the neural folds to close normally in the formation of the neural tube; inevitably spina bifida is a sequel.

myelosclerosis (mī'ĕ-lō-skle-rō'sis) [myelo- + G. *sklērōsis,* induration]. Myelofibrosis.

myelosis (mī-ĕ-lō'sis). **1.** A condition characterized by abnormal proliferation of tissue or cellular elements of bone marrow, *e.g.,* multiple myeloma, myelocytic leukemia, myelofibrosis. **2.** A condition in which there is abnormal proliferation of medullary tissue in the spinal cord, as in a glioma.

aleukemic m., m. with absence of abnormal cellular elements in peripheral blood.

chronic nonleukemic m., a condition in which there is abnormal proliferation of leukopoietic tissue that results in immature white blood cells in the circulating blood, but the total count is within the normal range.

erythremic m., a neoplastic process involving the erythropoietic tissue, characterized by anemia, irregular fever, splenomegaly, hepatomegaly, hemorrhagic disorders, and numerous erythroblasts in all stages of maturation (with disproportionately large numbers of less mature forms) in the circulating blood; postmortem studies reveal primitive erythroblasts and reticuloendothelial cells, not only in hemopoietic organs, but also in the kidneys, adrenal glands, and other sites. Acute and chronic forms are recognized, but in the latter there is less prominence of the immature cells; the former is also called Di Guglielmo's disease and acute erythremia.

funicular m., subacute combined *degeneration* of the spinal cord.

leukemic m., **(1)** granulocytic *leukemia;* **(2)** myeloblastic *leukemia.*

leukopenic m., subleukemic m., subleukemic *leukemia.*

myelospongium (mī'ĕ-lō-spŭn'jē-ŭm) [myelo- + G. *spongos,* sponge]. The fibrocellular meshwork in the spinal cord of the embryo, from which the neuroglia is developed.

myelosyphilis (mī'ĕ-lō-sif'i-lis). Syphilis of the spinal cord.

myelosyringosis (mī'ĕ-lō-si-rin-gō'sis). Syringomyelia.

myelotome (mī'ĕ-lō-tōm) [myelo- + G. *tomos,* cutting]. An instrument used in making serial sections of the spinal cord or for incising the spinal cord.

myelotomography (mī'ĕ-lō-tō-mog'ră-fē). Tomographic depiction of the spinal subarachnoid space filled with contrast media.

myelotomy (mī-ĕ-lot'ō-mē) [myelo- + G. *tomē,* incision]. Incision of the spinal cord.

Bischof's m., longitudinal incision of the spinal cord through the lateral column for spasticity.

commissural m., midline m.

midline m., commissural m., commissurotomy (2); section of the midline transverse fibers of the spinal cord.

T m., midline m. with lateral cuts into the anterior horns.

myelotoxic (mī'ĕ-lō-tok'sik). **1.** Inhibitory, depressant, or destructive to one or more of the components of bone marrow. **2.** Pertaining to, derived from, or manifesting the features of diseased bone marrow.

myenteric (mī-en-ter'ik). Relating to the myenteron.

myenteron (mī-en'ter-on) [G. *mys,* muscle, + *enteron,* intestine]. The muscular coat, or muscularis, of the intestine.

myesthesia (mī-es-thē'zē-ă) [G. *mys,* muscle, + *aisthēsis,* sensation]. Kinesthetic or muscular sense; deep or mesoblastic sensibility; myoesthesis; myoesthesia; the sensation felt in muscle when it is contracting; awareness of movement or activity in muscles or joints; sense of position or movement mediated in large part by the posterior columns and medial lemniscus. See also bathyesthesia.

myiasis (mī-ī'ă-sis) [G. *myia,* a fly]. Any infection due to invasion of tissues or cavities of the body by larvae of dipterous insects.

African furuncular m., cordylobiasis.

aural m., invasion of the external, middle, or inner ear by larvae of dipterous insects.

creeping m., m. causing suppurating cutaneous sinuses which may be mistaken for the creeping eruption of cutaneous larva migrans.

human botfly m., dermatobiasis.

intestinal m., presence of larvae of certain dipterous insects in the gastrointestinal tract, as of *Musca domestica* (domestic housefly), the cheese mite, and *Fannia canicularis* (lesser housefly).

m. linea'ris, cutaneous *larva migrans.*

nasal m., fly larva invasion of the nasal passages, due most commonly in the U.S. to primary screw-worms, the larvae of *Cochliomyia hominivorax,* which develop in the nasal or aural cavity.

ocular m., ophthalmomyiasis; invasion of the conjunctival sac or eyeball by larvae of flies, *e.g., Hypoderma bovis, H. lineata, Sarcophaga,* or *Gasterophilus intestinalis.*

m. oestruo'sa, m. due to a species of the family Oestridae, the gadflies or botflies.

subcutaneous m., invasion of subcutaneous tissues by the larvae of dipterous insects.

tumbu dermal m., cordylobiasis.

wound m., traumatic m., the infestation of a surface wound or other open lesion by fly larvae.

myitis (mī-ī'tis) [G. *mys,* muscle, + *-itis,* inflammation]. Myositis.

mykol (mī'kol). Mycolic acids.

mylabris (mil'ă-bris) [G. a cockroach found in mills and bakehouses, fr. *mylē,* mill]. The dried beetle, *Mylabris phalerata;* a vesicant similar to cantharis.

mylohyoid (mī'lō-hī'oyd) [G. *mylē,* a mill, in pl. *mylai,* molar teeth]. Relating to the molar teeth, or posterior portion of the lower jaw, and to the hyoid bone; denoting various structures. See entries under nerve, muscle, region, and sulcus.

mylohyoideus (mī-lō-hī-oy'dē-ŭs). *Musculus* mylohyoideus.

myo- [G. *mys,* muscle]. Combining form relating to muscle.

myoalbumin (mī'ō-al-byū'min). Albumin in muscle tissue, possibly the same as serum albumin.

myoarchitectonic (mī'ō-ar'ki-tek-ton'ik) [myo- + G. *architektonikos,* relating to construction]. Relating to the structural arrangement of muscle or of fibers in general.

myoatrophy (mī-ō-at'rō-fē). Myatrophy; muscular atrophy.

myoblast (mī'ō-blast) [myo- + G. *blastos,* germ]. Sarcogenic cell; sarcoblast; a primitive muscle cell with the potentiality of developing into a muscle fiber.

myoblastic (mī-ō-blas'tik). Relating to a myoblast or to the mode of formation of muscle cells.

myoblastoma (mī'ō-blas-tō'mă) [myo- + G. *blastos,* germ, + *-oma,* tumor]. A tumor of immature muscle cells.
granular cell m., granular cell *tumor.*

myobradia (mī-ō-brā'dē-ă) [myo- + G. *bradys,* slow]. Sluggish reaction of muscle following stimulation.

myocardia (mī-ō-kar'dē-ă). Plural of myocardium.

myocardial (mī-ō-kar'dē-ăl). Relating to the myocardium.

myocardiograph (mī'ō-kar'dē-ō-graf) [myo- + G. *kardia,* heart, + *graphō,* to record]. An instrument composed of a tambour with recording lever attachment, by means of which a tracing is made of the movements of the heart muscle.

myocardiopathy (mī'ō-kar-dē-op'ă-thē) [myocardium + G. *pathos,* suffering]. Cardiomyopathy.

myocardiorraphy (mī'ō-kar-dē-ōr'ă-fē) [myocardium + G. *raphē,* suture]. Suture of the myocardium.

myocarditis (mī'ō-kar-dī'tis). Inflammation of the muscular walls of the heart.
acute isolated m., Fiedler's m.; an acute interstitial m. of unknown cause, the endocardium and pericardium being unaffected.
Fiedler's m., acute isolated m.
fragmentation m., fragmentation of the myocardium as the result of inflammation.
giant cell m., acute isolated m. characterized by infiltration by granulomas containing giant cells.
indurative m., chronic m. leading to hardening of the muscular wall of the heart.

myocardium, pl. **myocardia** (mī-ō-kar'dē-ŭm, -kar'dē-ă) [myo- + G. *kardia,* heart] [NA]. The middle layer of the heart, consisting of cardiac muscle.

myocardosis (mī'ō-kar-dō'sis). **1.** A condition marked by symptomatic signs of cardiac trouble without any discoverable pathologic lesion. **2.** Any degenerative condition of the heart muscle except myofibrosis.

myocele (mī'ō-sēl). **1** [myo- + G. *kēlē,* hernia]. Protrusion of muscle substance through a rent in its sheath. **2** [myo- + G. *koilia,* a cavity]. Somite cavity; the small cavity that appears in somites.

myocelialgia (mī'ō-sē-lē-al'jē-ă) [myo- + G. *koilia,* the belly, + *algos,* pain]. Obsolete term for celiomyalgia.

myocelitis (mī'ō-sē-lī'tis) [myo- + G. *koilia,* belly, + *-itis,* inflammation]. Inflammation of the abdominal muscles.

myocellulitis (mī'ō-sel-yū-lī'tis) [myo- + Mod. L. *cellularis,* cellular (tissue), + G. *-itis,* inflammation]. Inflammation of muscle and cellular tissue.

myocerosis (mī'ō-sē-rō'sis) [myo- + G. *kēros,* wax]. Myokerosis; waxy degeneration of the muscles.

myochrome (mī'ō-krōm). Rarely used term for cytochrome found in muscle tissue.

myochronoscope (mī-ō-kron'ō-skōp) [myo- + G. *chronos,* time, + *skopeō,* to examine]. An instrument for timing a muscular impulse, *i.e.,* the interval between the application of the stimulus and the muscular movement in response.

myocinesimeter (mī'ō-sin-ĕ-sim'ĕ-ter). Myokinesimeter.

myoclonia (mī'ō-klō'nē-ă) [myo- + G. *klonos,* a tumult]. Any disorder characterized by myoclonus.
fibrillary m., tetanilla (1); the twitching of a limited part or group of fibers of a muscle.

myoclonic (mī-ō-klon'ik). Showing myoclonus.

myoclonus (mī-ok'lō-nŭs, mī-ō-klo'nŭs) [myo- + G. *klonus,* tumult]. Clonic spasm or twitching of a muscle or group of muscles.
m. mul'tiplex, a disorder marked by rapid contractions occurring simultaneously or consecutively in various unrelated muscles. Also called Friedreich's disease; polyclonia; polymyoclonus; paramyoclonus.
nocturnal m., frequently repeated muscular jerks occurring at the moment of dropping off to sleep.
ocular m., lightning eye movements; rapid bursts of small ocular saccadic movements that usually follow gaze toward the paretic or ataxic side of the body.
palatal m., rhythmic contractions of the soft palate, the facial muscles, and the diaphragm, related to lesions of the olivocerebellar pathways. See also palatal *nystagmus.*
stimulus sensitive m., m. induced by a variety of stimuli, *e.g.,* talking, calculation, loud noises, tapping, etc.

myocolpitis (mī-ō-kol-pī'tis) [myo- + G. *kolpos,* bosom (vagina), + *-itis,* inflammation]. Inflammation of the muscular tissue of the vagina.

myocomma, pl. **myocommata** (mī-ō-kom'ă, -kom'ă-tă) [myo- + G. *komma,* a coin or the stamp of a coin]. Myoseptum; the connective tissue septum separating adjacent myotomes.

myocrismus (mī-ō-kris'mŭs) [myo- + G. *krizō,* to squeak]. A creaking sound sometimes heard on auscultation of a contracting muscle.

myocutaneous (mī-ō-kyū-tā'nē-ŭs) [myo- + L. *cutis,* skin]. Musculocutaneous.

myocyte (mī'ō-sīt) [myo- + G. *kytos,* cell]. A muscle cell.
Anitschkow m., cardiac *histiocyte.*

myocytolysis (mī-ō-sī-tol'i-sis) [myo- + G. *kytos,* cell, + *lysis,* a loosening]. Dissolution of muscle fiber.
m. of heart, local loss of myocardial syncytium as a result of a metabolic imbalance, insufficient in intensity or duration (or both) to cause stromal injury or to elicit any reactive exudation.

myocytoma (mī'ō-sī-tō'mă). A benign neoplasm derived from muscle.

myodegeneration (mī'ō-dē-jen-ĕ-rā'shŭn). Muscular degeneration.

myodemia (mī-ō-dē'mē-ă) [myo- + G. *dēmos,* tallow]. Fatty degeneration of muscle.

myodermal (mī-ō-der'mal) [myo- + G. *derma,* skin]. Musculocutaneous.

myodiastasis (mī'ō-dī-as'tă-sis) [myo- + G. *diastasis,* separation]. Separation of muscle.

myodynamia (mī'ō-dī-nā'mē-ă) [myo- + G. *dynamis,* power]. Muscular strength.

myodynamics (mī'ō-dī-nam'iks). The dynamics of muscular action.

myodynamometer (mī'ō-dī-nă-mom'ĕ-ter) [myo- + G. *dynamis,* force, + *metron,* measure]. An instrument for determining muscular strength.

myodynia (mī'ō-din'ē-ă) [myo- + G. *odynē,* pain]. Myalgia.

myodystony (mī-ō-dis'tō-nē) [myo- + G. *dys-,* difficult, + *tonos,* tone, tension]. A condition of slow relaxation, interrupted by a succession of slight contractions, following electrical stimulation of a muscle.

myodystrophy, myodystrophia (mī-ō-dis'trō-fē, mī'-ō-dis-trō'fē-ă) [myo- + G. *dys-,* difficult, poor, + *trophē,* nourishment]. Muscular *dystrophy.*

myoedema (mī'ō-e-dē'mă) [myo- + G. *oidēma,* swelling]. Idiomuscular contraction; mounding; myoidema; a localized contraction of a degenerating muscle, occurring at the point of a sharp blow, independent of the nerve supply.

myoelastic (mī'ō-e-las'tik). Pertaining to closely associated smooth muscle fibers and elastic connective tissue.

myoelectric (mī'ō-ē-lek'trik). Relating to the electrical properties of muscle.

myoendocarditis (mī-ō-en'dō-kar-dī'tis) [myo- + G. *endon,* within, + *kardia,* heart, + *-itis,* inflammation]. Inflammation of the muscular wall and lining membrane of the heart.

myoepithelial (mī'ō-ep-i-thē'lē-ăl). Relating to myoepithelium.

myoepithelioma (mī'ō-ep-i-thē-lē-ō'mă) [myo- + epithelium, + G. *-ōma,* tumor]. A benign tumor of myoepithelial cells.

myoepithelium (mī'ō-ep-i-thē'lē-ŭm) [myo- + epithelium]. Muscle epithelium; spindle-shaped, contractile, smooth muscle-like cells of epithelial origin which are arranged longitudinally or obliquely around sweat glands and the secretory alveoli of the mammary gland; stellate myoepithelial cells occur around lacrimal and some salivary gland secretory units.

myoesthesis, myoesthesia (mī'ō-es-thē'sis, -thē'zē-ă). Myesthesia.

myofascial (mī-ō-fash'ē-ăl). Of or relating to the fascia surrounding and separating muscle tissue.

myofascitis (mī'ō-fă-sī'tis). *Myositis* fibrosa.

myofibril (mī-ō-fī'bril) [myo- + Mod. L. *fibrilla,* fibril]. Myofibrilla; muscular fibril; one of the fine longitudinal fibrils occurring in a skeletal or cardiac muscle fiber comprising many regularly overlapped ultramicroscopic thick and thin myofilaments.

myofibrilla, pl. **myofibrillae** (mī'ō-fī-bril'ă, -bril'ē). Myofibril.

myofibroblast (mī-ō-fī'brō-blast). A cell thought to be responsible for contracture of wounds; such cells have some characteristics of smooth muscle, such as contractile properties and fibrils, and are also believed to produce, temporarily, type III collagen.

myofibroma (mī'ō-fī-brō'mă). A benign neoplasm that consists chiefly of fibrous connective tissue, with variable numbers of muscle cells forming portions of the neoplasm.

myofibrosis (mī'ō-fī-brō'sis). Chronic myositis with diffuse hyperplasia of the interstitial connective tissue pressing upon and causing atrophy of the muscular tissue.
m. cor'dis, m. of the heart walls.

myofibrositis (mī'ō-fī-brō-sī'tis). Inflammation of the perimysium.

myofilaments (mī-ō-fil'ă-ments). The ultramicroscopic threads of filamentous proteins making up myofibrils in striated muscle. Thick ones contain myosin and thin ones actin; thick and thin m.'s also occur in smooth muscle fibers but are not regularly arranged in discrete myofibrils and thus do not impart a striated appearance to these cells.

myofunctional (mī'ō-fŭnk'shŭn-ăl). **1.** Relating to function of muscles. **2.** In dentistry, relating to the role of muscle function in the etiology or correction of orthodontic problems.

myogen (mī'ō-jen) [myo- + G. *-gen,* producing]. Myosinogen; proteins extracted from muscle with cold water, largely the enzymes promoting glycolysis; from the residue, alkaline 0.6 M KCl extracts actin and myosin as actomyosin, with myosin further separable into two meromyosins by proteinase treatment.

myogenesis (mī-ō-jen'ĕ-sis) [myo- + G. *genesis,* origin]. Formation of muscle cells or fibers.

myogenetic, myogenic (mī-ō-jĕ-net'ik, -jen'ik). Myogenous. **1.** Originating in or starting from muscle. **2.** Relating to the origin of muscle cells or fibers.

myogenous (mī-oj'ĕ-nŭs). Myogenetic.

myoglobin (Mb) (mī-ō-glō'bin). Myohemoglobin; muscle hemoglobin; the oxygen-transporting protein of muscle, resembling blood hemoglobin in function but containing only one heme as part of the molecule (rather than the four of hemoglobin), and with a molecular weight one-quarter that of hemoglobin.

myoglobinuria (mī'ō-glō-bi-nū'rē-ă). Idiopathic paroxysmal rhabdomyolysis; Meyer-Betz syndrome; excretion of myoglobin in the urine; occurs as a result of muscle degeneration which releases myoglobin into the blood, certain types of trauma (crush syndrome), advanced or protracted ischemia of muscle, or as a paroxysmal process of unknown etiology.
paralytic m., *azoturia* of horses.

myoglobulin (mī-ō-glob'yū-lin). Globulin present in muscle tissue.

myoglobulinuria (mī'ō-glob'yū-li-nū'rē-ă). The excretion of myoglobulin in the urine.

myognathus (mī-og'nă-thŭs, mī-ō-nāth'ŭs) [myo- + G. *gnathos,* jaw]. An unequal conjoined twin in which the rudimentary head of the parasite is attached to the lower jaw of the autosite by muscle and skin only.

myogram (mī'ō-gram) [myo- + G. *gramma,* a drawing]. Muscle curve; the tracing made by a myograph.

myograph (mī'ō-graf) [myo- + G. *graphō,* to write]. A recording instrument by which tracings are made of muscular contractions.
palate m., palatograph.

myographic (mī-ō-graf'ik). Relating to a myogram, or the record of a myograph.

myography (mī-og'ră-fē). **1.** The recording of muscular movements by the myograph. **2.** Descriptive myology; a description of or treatise on the muscles.

myohemoglobin (mī'ō-hēm-ō-glō'bin). Myoglobin.

myoid (mī'oyd) [myo- + G. *eidos,* appearance]. **1.** Resembling muscle. **2.** One of the fine, contractile, threadlike protoplasmic elements found in certain epithelial cells in lower animals. **3.** A contractile part of retinal cones in certain fish and amphibia. In mammals, the m. is the inner part of the inner segment of rods and cones; it contains microtubules, the Golgi apparatus, endoplasmic reticulum, and ribosomes, but no myofibrils.

myoidema (mī-oy-dē'mă) [myo- + G. *oidēma,* swelling]. Myoedema.

myoischemia (mī'ō-is-kē'mē-ă). A condition of localized deficiency or absence of blood supply in muscular tissue.

myokerosis (mī'ō-kē-rō'sis). Myocerosis.

myokinase (mī-ō-kī'nās). *Adenylate* kinase.

myokinesimeter (mī'ō-kin-ē-sim'ĕ-ter) [myo- + G. *kinesis,* movement, + *metron,* measure]. Myocinesimeter; a device for registering the exact time and extent of contraction of the larger muscles of the lower extremity in response to electric stimulation.

myokymia (mī-ō-kī'mē-ă) [myo- + G. *kyma,* wave]. Kymatism; a benign condition, often familial, characterized by an irregular twitching of most of the muscles.

hereditary m., a syndrome consisting of m., hypoglycemia, and disturbed thyroid function.

myolemma (mī-ō-lem'ă). Sarcolemma.

myolipoma (mī'ō-li-pō'mă). A benign neoplasm that consists chiefly of fat cells (adipose tissue), with variable numbers of muscle cells forming portions of the neoplasm.

myologia (mī'ō-lō'jē-ă) [NA]. Myology.

myologist (mī-ol'ō-jist). One learned in the knowledge of muscles.

myology (mī-ol'ō-jē) [myo- + G. *logos,* study]. Myologia; sarcology (1); the branch of science concerned with the muscles and their accessory parts, tendons, aponeuroses, bursae, and fasciae.

descriptive m., myography (2).

myolysis (mī-ol'i-sis) [myo- + G. *lysis,* dissolution]. Dissolution or liquefaction of muscular tissue, frequently preceded by degenerative changes such as infiltration of fat, atrophy, and fatty degeneration.

cardiotoxic m., cardiomalacia occurring in fever and various systemic infections.

myoma (mī-ō'mă) [myo- + G. *-oma,* tumor]. A benign neoplasm of muscular tissue. See also leiomyoma; rhabdomyoma.

myomalacia (mī'ō-mă-lā'shē-ă) [myo- + G. *malakia,* softness]. Pathologic softening of muscular tissue.

myomatous (mī-ō'mă-tŭs). Pertaining to or characterized by the features of a myoma.

myomectomy (mī-ō-mek'tō-mē) [myoma + G. *ektomē,* excision]. Operative removal of a myoma, specifically of a uterine myoma.

abdominal m., celiomyomectomy; laparomyomectomy; removal of a myoma of the uterus through an abdominal incision.

vaginal m., colpomyomectomy; removal of a myoma of the uterus through the vagina.

myomelanosis (mī'ō-melă-nō'sis) [myo- + G. *melanōsis,* becoming black]. Abnormal dark pigmentation of muscular tissue. See also melanosis.

myomere (mī'ō-mēr) [myo- + G. *meros,* a part]. Muscular segment within a metamere.

myometer (mī-om'ĕ-ter) [myo- + G. *metron,* measure]. An instrument for measuring the extent of a muscular contraction.

myometrial (mī-ō-mē'trē-ăl). Relating to the myometrium.

myometritis (mī'ō-mē-trī'tis) [myo- + G. *mētra,* uterus, + *-itis,* inflammation]. Mesometritis; inflammation of the muscular wall of the uterus.

myometrium (mī'ō-mē'trē-ŭm) [myo- + G. *mētra,* uterus] [NA]. The muscular wall of the uterus.

myomitochondrion, pl. **myomitochondria** (mī'ō-mī'tō-kon'drē-on, -drē-ă). Sarcosome (2); a mitochondrion of a muscle fiber.

myomotomy (mī-ō-mot'ō-mē) [myoma + G. *tomē,* incision]. Incision of a myoma.

myon (mī'on) [G. *mys,* muscle]. An individual muscle unit.

myonecrosis (mī'ō-nĕ-krō'sis). Necrosis of muscle.

clostridial m., gas *gangrene.*

myoneme (mī'ō-nēm) [myo- + G. *nēma,* thread]. **1.** A muscle fibril. **2.** One of the contractile fibrils of certain protozoans; thought to function in an analogous fashion to metazoan muscle fibers.

myoneural (mī-ō-nū'răl) [myo- + G. *neuron,* nerve]. Relating to both muscle and nerve; denoting specifically the synapse of the motor neuron with striated muscle fibers: myoneural junction or motor endplate. See also neuromuscular.

myoneuralgia (mī'ō-nū-ral'jē-ă) [myo- + G. *neuron,* nerve, + *algos,* pain]. Myalgia.

postural m., muscle pain associated with cramped position, stress of standing with improper posture, etc.

myoneurasthenia (mī'ō-nū-ras-thē'nē-ă). Muscular weakness associated with neurasthenia.

myoneuroma (mī'ō-nū-rō'mă) [myo- + G. *neuron,* nerve, + *-oma,* tumor]. A tumefaction consisting chiefly of abnormally proliferating Schwann cells, with variable numbers of muscle cells forming portions of the mass; m.'s are probably malformations, rather than true neoplasms.

myonosus (mī-on'ō-sŭs) [myo- + G. *nosos,* disease]. Myopathy.

myonymy (mī-on'i-mē) [myo- + G. *onyma* or *onoma,* name]. Nomenclature of the muscles.

myopachynsis (mī'ō-pă-kin'sis) [myo- + G. *pachynsis,* a thickening]. Muscular hypertrophy.

myopalmus (mī-ō-pal'mŭs) [myo- + G. *palmos,* a quivering]. Muscle twitching.

myoparalysis (mī-ō-pă-ral'i-sis). Muscular paralysis.

myoparesis (mī'ō-pă-rē'sis, -par'ē-sis). Slight muscular paralysis.

myopathic (mī-ō-path'ik). Denoting a disorder involving muscular tissue.

myopathy (mī-op'ă-thē) [myo- + G. *pathos,* suffering]. Myonosus; any abnormal condition or disease of the muscular tissues; commonly designates a disorder involving skeletal muscle.

carcinomatous m., Lambert-Eaton *syndrome.*

centronuclear m., myotubular m.; slowly progressive generalized muscle weakness and atrophy beginning in childhood; on biopsy of skeletal muscle, the nuclei of most muscle fibers are seen to be located near the center of a small fiber (the normal position for a 10-week embryo) rather than at the periphery of the fiber; familial incidence.

distal m., m. affecting predominantly the distal portions of the limbs; onset is usually after age 40, with weakness and wasting of small muscles of the hands; autosomal dominant inheritance.

mitochondrial m., weakness and hypotonia of muscles, primarily those of the neck, shoulder, and pelvic girdles, with onset in infancy or childhood; on biopsy, giant, bizarre mitochondria are seen located between muscle fibrils just beneath the sarcolemma.

myotubular m., centronuclear m.

nemaline m., rod m.; congenital, nonprogressive muscle weakness that is most evident in the proximal muscles; named after the characteristic nemaline (threadlike) rods seen in the muscle cells composed of Z-band material.

ocular m., a specific type of progressive muscular dystrophy that begins with the gradual onset of ptosis and sequential involvement of the other extraocular muscles.

rod m., nemaline m.

thyrotoxic m., extreme muscular weakness in severe thyrotoxicosis affecting muscles of limbs and trunk as well as those used in speech and swallowing.

myopericarditis (mī'ō-per-i-kar-dī'tis) [myo- + pericarditis]. Inflammation of the muscular wall of the heart and of the enveloping pericardium.

myoperitonitis (mī'ō-per-i-tō-nī'tis). Inflammation of the parietal peritoneum with myositis of the abdominal wall.

myophone (mī'ō-fōn) [myo- + G. *phōnē,* sound]. An instrument to enable one to hear the murmur of muscular contractions.

myopia (M or **my.),** (mī-ō'pē-ă) [G. fr. *myo,* to shut, + *ōps,* eye]. Shortsightedness; nearsightedness; near or short sight; that optical condition in which only rays a finite distance from the eye focus on the retina.

axial m., m. due to elongation of the globe of the eye.

curvature m., m. due to refractive errors resulting from excessive corneal curvature.

degenerative m., pathologic m.

index m., m. arising from increased refractivity of the lens, as in nuclear sclerosis.

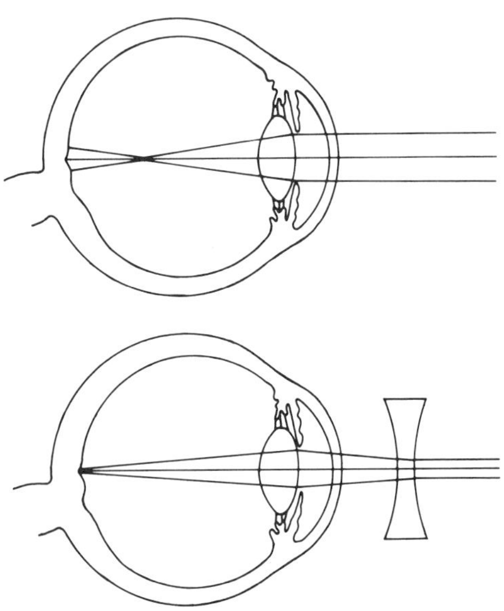

Myopia
Top, light rays in unaided myopia; *bottom,* after correction by concave lens.

malignant m., pathologic m.
night m., m. occurring in a normally emmetropic eye because long light rays focus in front of the retina.
pathologic m., degenerative or malignant m.; progressive m. marked by fundus changes, posterior staphyloma, and subnormal corrected acuity.
prematurity m., m. observed in infants of low birth weight or in association with retrolental fibroplasia.
senile lenticular m., second *sight.*
simple m., m. arising from failure of correlation of the refractive power of the anterior segment and the length of the eyeball.
space m., a type of m. arising when no contour is imaged on the retina.
transient m., m. observed in accommodative spasm secondary to iridocyclitis or ocular contusion.

myopic (mī-op'ik, -ō'pik). Relating to or suffering from myopia.

myoplasm (mī'ō-plazm) [myo- + G. *plasma,* a thing formed]. The contractile portion of the muscle cell, as distinguished from the sarcoplasm.

myoplastic (mī-ō-plas'tik). Relating to the plastic surgery of the muscles, or to the use of muscular tissue in correcting defects.

myoplasty (mī'ō-plas-tē) [myo- + G. *plastos,* formed]. Plastic surgery of muscular tissue.

myopolar (mī-ō-pō'lăr). Relating to muscular polarity, or to the portion of muscle between two electrodes.

myoprotein (mī-ō-prō'tēn). Protein occurring in muscle.

myorhythmia (mī'ō-ridh'mē-ă) [myo- + G. *rhythmos,* rhythm]. A form of hyperkinesia in which the tremor rate (2 to 4 per second) is irregular and slower than in alternating tremor, with greater frequency and higher voltage of the associated spike potentials in the electromyogram.

myorrhaphy (mī-ōr'ă-fē) [myo- + G. *raphē,* seam]. Suture of a muscle.

myorrhexis (mī-ō-rek'sis) [myo- + G. *rhēxis,* a rupture]. Tearing of a muscle.

myosalgia (mī-ō-sal'jē-ă). Myalgia.

myosalpingitis (mī'ō-sal-pin-jī'tis) [myosalpinx + G. *-itis* inflammation]. Inflammation of the muscular tissue of the uterine tube.

myosalpinx (mī'ō-sal'pingks) [myo- + salpinx]. The muscular tunic of the uterine tube.

myosarcoma (mī'ō-sar-kō'mă). A general term for a malignant neoplasm derived from muscular tissue. See also leiomyosarcoma, rhabdomyosarcoma.

myosclerosis (mī'ō-skle-rō'sis). Chronic myositis with hyperplasia of the interstitial connective tissue.

myoseism (mī'ō-sīzm) [myo- + G. *seismos,* a shaking, shock, fr. *seiō,* fut. *seisō,* to shake]. Nonrhythmic spasmodic muscular contractions.

myoseptum (mī-ō-sep'tŭm) [myo- + L. *saeptum,* a barrier]. Myocomma.

myosin (mī'ō-sin). A globulin present in muscle; in combination with actin, it forms actomyosin.

myosinogen (mī-ō-sin'ō-jen). Myogen.

myosinose (mī'ō-si-nōs). A proteose formed by the partial hydrolysis of myosin.

myosis (mī-ō'sis). Obsolete alternative spelling for miosis (2).

myositic (mī-ō-sit'ik). Relating to myositis.

myositis (mī-ō-sī'tis) [myo- + G. *-itis,* inflammation]. Myitis; initis (2); inflammation of a muscle.
acute disseminated m., multiple m.
cervical m., see posttraumatic neck *syndrome.*
epidemic m., m. epidem'ica acu'ta, epidemic *pleurodynia.*
m. fibro'sa, myofascitis; interstitial m.; Froriep's induration; induration of a muscle through an interstitial growth of fibrous tissue.
infectious m., inflammation of the voluntary muscles, marked by swelling and pain, affecting usually the shoulders and arms, though almost the entire body may be involved.
interstitial m., m. fibrosa.
multiple m., acute disseminated m.; pseudotrichiniasis; pseudotrichinosis; the occurrence of multiple foci of acute inflammation in the muscular tissue and overlying skin in various parts of the body, accompanied by fever and other signs of systemic infection. See also dermatomyositis.
m. ossif'icans, ossification or deposit of bone in muscle with fibrosis, causing pain and swelling in muscles.
m. ossif'icans circumscrip'ta, local deposit of bone in a muscle, usually following prolonged trauma; *e.g.,* riders' bone.
m. ossif'icans progressi'va, a rare and frequently fatal mutation, beginning in early life, characterized by progressive ossification of the muscles; it is not strictly a m., but a noninflammatory ossification.
proliferative m., a rapidly growing benign infiltrating fibrous nodule in skeletal muscle, containing characteristic giant cells resembling ganglion cells.
m. purulen'ta trop'ica, tropical m. or pyomyositis; lambo lambo; bungpagga; a disease observed in Samoa and in tropical Africa, marked by pains in the extremities, fever of a remittent or intermittent type, and abscesses in the muscles in various parts of the body (may result in death from sepsis); causative organisms are *Staphylococcus aureus* and *Streptococcus pyogenes,* but the disease is usually associated with parasitic infections.
tropical m., m. purulenta tropica.

myospasm, myospasmus (mī'ō-spazm, mī-ō-spaz'mŭs). Spasmodic muscular contraction.
cervical m., see posttraumatic neck *syndrome.*

myospherulosis (mī'ō-sfēr-ū-lō'sis) [myo- + L. *sphaerula,* small sphere, + G. *-osis,* condition]. A chronic granulomatous reaction to undetermined spherical structures frequently contained within a microscopic cyst; first reported in cystic lesions in skeletal muscle from eastern Africa and subsequently in nasal infections in the U.S.

myosthenometer (mī'ō-sthĕ-nom'ĕ-ter) [myo- + G. *sthenos*, strength, + *metron*, measure]. An instrument for measuring the power of muscle groups.

myostroma (mī-ō-strō'mă) [myo- + G. *strōma*, mattres]. The supporting connective tissue or framework of muscular tissue.

myostromin (mī-ō-strō'min). A protein found in muscle stroma.

myotactic (mī-ō-tak'tik) [myo- + L. *tactus*, a touching]. Relating to the muscular sense.

myotasis (mī-ot'ă-sis) [myo- + G. *tasis*, a stretching]. Stretching of a muscle.

myotatic (mī-ō-tat'ik). Relating to myotasis.

myotenositis (mī'ō-te-nō-sī'tis) [myo- + G. *tenōn*, tendon, + *-itis*, inflammation]. Inflammation of a muscle with its tendon.

myotenotomy (mī'ō-te-not'ō-mē) [myo- + G. *tenōn*, tendon, + *tomē*, incision]. Tenontomyotomy; tenomyotomy; cutting through the principal tendon of a muscle, with division of the muscle itself in whole or in part.

myothermic (mī-ō-ther'mik) [myo- + G. *thermē*, heat]. Relating to the increased temperature in muscular tissue resulting from its contraction.

myotome (mī'ō-tōm) [myo- + G. *tomos*, a cut]. **1.** A knife for dividing muscle. **2.** Muscle plate; in embryos, that part of the somite that develops into skeletal muscle. **3.** All muscles derived from one somite and innervated by one segmental spinal nerve. **4.** In primitive vertebrates, the muscular part of a metamere.

myotomy (mī-ot'ō-mē) [myo- + G. *tomē*, excision]. **1.** Anatomy or dissection of the muscles. **2.** Surgical division of a muscle.

myotone (mī'ō-tōn). Myotony.

myotonia (mī-ō-tō'nē-ă) [myo- + G. *tonos*, tension, stretching]. Delayed relaxation of a muscle after a strong contraction, or prolonged contraction after mechanical stimulation (as by percussion) or brief electrical stimulation.

m. acquis'ita, Talma's disease; acquired m. following injury or disease.

m. atroph'ica, myotonic *dystrophy*.

m. congen'ita, Thomsen's disease; a hereditary disease marked by momentary tonic spasms occurring when a voluntary movement is attempted.

m. dystroph'ica, myotonic *dystrophy*.

m. neonato'rum, neonatal *tetany*.

myotonic (mī-ō-ton'ik). Pertaining to or exhibiting myotonia.

myotonoid (mī-ot'ŏ-noyd) [myo- + G. *tonos*, tone, tension, + *eidos*, resemblance]. Denoting a muscular reaction, naturally or electrically excited, characterized by slow contraction and, especially, slow relaxation.

myotonus (mī-ot'ŏ-nŭs) [myo- + G. *tonos*, tension, stretching]. A tonic spasm or temporary rigidity of a muscle or group of muscles.

myotony (mī-ot'ŏ-nē) [myo- + G. *tonos*, tension]. Myotone; muscular tonus or tension.

myotrophy (mī-ot'rō-fē) [myo- + G. *trophē*, nourishment]. Nutrition of muscular tissue.

myotube (mī'ō-tūb). A skeletal muscle fiber formed by the fusion of myoblasts during a developmental stage; a few myofibrils occur at the periphery with the central core occupied by nuclei and sarcoplasm so that the fiber has a tubular appearance.

myotubule (mī-ō-tū'būl). Former term for myotube.

Myoviridae (mī-ō-vir'i-dē). Provisional name for a family of relatively large bacterial viruses with complex contractile tails, heads that are usually elongated but are isometric in some species, and a double-stranded DNA genome (MW 21 to 190 $\times$ 10^6). It includes the T-even phage group and probably other genera.

myriachit (mir-yah'chit) [Kalmuk?]. Miryachit.

myrica (mir'i-kă). Bayberry bark; the bark of *Myrica cerifera* (family Myricaceae); used in diarrhea and icterus, and externally in sore throat.

myricin (mir'i-sin). Myricyl palmitate, a white, almost odorless solid that is the chief constituent of beeswax.

myring-. See myringo-.

myringa (mi-ring'gă) [Mod. L. drum membrane]. *Membrana* tympani.

myringectomy (mir-in-jek'tō-mē) [myring- + G. *ektomē*, excision]. Myringodectomy; excision of the tympanic membrane.

myringitis (mir-in-jī'tis) [myring- + G. *-itis*, inflammation]. Tympanitis; inflammation of the tympanic membrane.

m. bulbo'sa, myringodermatitis.

bullous m., painful inflammation of the tympanic membrane accompanied by bullae, probably of viral etiology.

myringo-, myring- [Mod. L. *myringa*]. Combining forms denoting the membrana tympani.

myringodectomy (mi-ring'gō-dek'tō-mē). Myringectomy.

myringodermatitis (mi-ring'gō-der-mă-tī'tis). Myringitis bulbosa; inflammation of the meatal or outer surface of the drum membrane and the adjoining skin of the external auditory canal.

myringomycosis (mi-ring'gō-mī-kō'sis). Mycomyringitis.

myringoplasty (mi-ring'gō-plas'tē) [myringo- + G. *plassō*, to form]. Operative repair of a damaged tympanic membrane.

myringostapediopexy (mi-ring'gō-stā-pē'dē-ō-pek'sē) [*myringo-* + L. *stapes*, stirrup (stapes), + G. *pēxis*, fixation]. A technique of tympanoplasty in which the drum membrane or grafted drum membrane is brought into functional connection with the stapes.

myringotome (mi-ring'gō-tōm) [myringo- + G. *tomē*, excision]. A knife used for paracentesis of the tympanic membrane.

myringotomy (mir-ing-got'ō-mē) [myringo- + G. *tomē*, excision]. Tympanotomy; tympanostomy; paracentesis of the tympanic membrane.

myrinx (mī'ringks, mir'ringks) [Mod. L. *myringa, drum membrane*]. *Membrana* tympani.

myristica (mi-ris'ti-kă) [G. *myrizō*, to anoint, fr. *myron*, an unguent]. Nutmeg.

m. oil, nutmeg oil.

myristic acid (mi-ris'tik). Tetradecanoic acid; $CH_3(CH_2)_{12}$COOH; a saturated fatty acid present as an acylglycerol in milk, vegetable fats, and cod liver oil.

myristicin (mī-ris'ti-sin). A constituent of nutmeg thought to be responsible, at least in part, for the bizarre central nervous system symptoms produced by the ingestion of large amounts of nutmeg.

myristoleic acid (mi-ris-tō-lē'ik). 9-Tetradecenoic acid; a 14-carbon unsaturated fatty acid with a double bond between carbons 9 and 10; the 14-carbon analog of oleic acid.

myrmecia (mĭr-mē'shē-ă) [G. *murmex*, ant]. A form of viral wart in which the lesion has a domed surface (*i.e.*, an ant hill configuration) and is associated with eosinophilic intranuclear and intracytoplasmic inclusion bodies in the epidermal cells.

myrosinase (mī-rō'si-nās). Thioglucosidase.

myrrh (mer) [G. *myrrha*]. A gum resin from *Commiphora molmol* and *C. phora abyssinica* (family Burseraceae) and other species of *C.*, a shrub of Arabia and eastern Africa; used as an astringent, tonic, and stimulant, and locally for diseases of the oral cavity and in mouthwashes.

mysophilia (mī-sō-fil'ē-ă) [G. *mysos*, defilement, + *philos*, fond]. Sexual interest in excretions.

mysophobia (mī-sō-fō'bē-ă) [G. *mysos*, defilement, + *phobos*, fear].

Morbid fear of dirt or defilement from touching familiar objects.

mytacism (mī'tă-sizm) [G. *my*, the letter μ]. Mutacism; a form of stammering in which the letter *m* is frequently substituted for other consonants.

myurous (mī-yū'rŭs) [G. *mys*, mouse, + *ouros*, tail]. Gradually decreasing, as a mouse's tail, in thickness; rarely used term denoting certain symptoms in process of cessation, or the heartbeat in certain cases in which it grows feebler and feebler for a while and then strengthens.

myx-. See myxo-.
m. labia'lis, *cheilitis* glandularis.

myxadenoma (mik-sad-ĕ-nō'mă). A benign neoplasm derived from glandular epithelial tissue, *i.e.*, an adenoma, in which the loose connective tissue of the stroma resembles relatively primitive mesenchymal tissue.

myxasthenia (mik-sas-thē'nē-ă) [myx- + G. *astheneia*, weakness]. Faulty secretion of mucus.

myxedema (mik-se-dē'mă) [myx- + G. *oidema*, swelling]. Hypothyroidism characterized by a relatively hard edema of subcutaneous tissue, with increased content of proteoglycans in the fluid; characterized by somnolence, slow mentation, dryness and loss of hair, increased fluid in body cavities such as the pericardial sac, subnormal temperature, hoarseness, muscle weakness, and slow return of a muscle to the neutral position after a tendon jerk; usually caused by removal or loss of functioning thyroid tissue.
circumscribed m., pretibial m.; nodules and plaques of mucoid edema of the skin, usually in the pretibial region, occurring in some patients with hyperthyroidism.
congenital m., cretinism.
infantile m., m. beginning during infancy in consequence of some acquired injury of the thyroid gland or of the presence of cretinism.
operative m., m. developing after thyroidectomy.
pituitary m., m. resulting from inadequate secretion of the thyrotropic hormone; commonly occurs in association with inadequate secretion of other anterior pituitary hormones.
pretibial m., circumscribed m.

myxedematoid (mik-sĕ-dem'ă-toyd). Resembling myxedema.

myxedematous (mik-sĕ-dem'ă-tŭs). Relating to myxedema.

myxemia (mik-sē'mē-ă) [myx- + G. *haima*, blood]. Mucinemia.

myxo-, myx- [G. *myxa*, mucus]. Combining forms relating to mucus. See also muci-, muco-.

myxochondrofibrosarcoma (mik'sō-kon'drō-fī'brō-sar-kō'mă) [myxo- + G. *chondros*, cartilage, + L. *fibra*, fiber, + G. *sarx*, flesh, + *-ōma*, tumor]. A malignant neoplasm derived from fibrous connective tissue, *i.e.*, a fibrosarcoma, in which there are intimately associated foci of cartilaginous and myxomatous tissue.

myxochondroma (mik'sō-kon-drō'mă) [myxo- + G. *chondros*, cartilage, + *-ōma*, tumor]. Myxoma enchondromatosum; a benign neoplasm of cartilaginous tissue, *i.e.*, a chondroma, in which the stroma resembles relatively primitive mesenchymal tissue.

Myxococcidium stegomyiae (mik'sō-kok-sid'ē-ŭm steg-ō-mī'ē-ē). A protozoon once found in the body of the mosquito, *Stegomyia calopus*, that had fed on the blood of a patient with yellow fever; the organism was then postulated, incorrectly, to be the causal agent of yellow fever.

myxocyte (mik'sō-sīt) [myxo- + G. *kytos*, cell]. One of the stellate or polyhedral cells present in mucous tissue.

myxofibroma (mik'sō-fī-brō'mă) [myxo- + L. *fibra*, fiber, + G. *-ōma*, tumor]. Fibroma myxomatodes; myxoma fibrosum; a benign neoplasm of fibrous connective tissue that resembles primitive mesenchymal tissue.

myxofibrosarcoma (mik'sō-fī'brō-sar-kō'mă) [myxo- + L. *fibra*, fiber, + G. *sarx*, flesh, + *-ōma*, tumor]. A malignant fibrous histiocytoma with a predominance of myxoid areas that resemble primitive mesenchymal tissue.

myxoid (mik'soyd) [myxo- + G. *eidos*, resemblance]. Mucoid; resembling mucus.

myxolipoma (mik'sō-li-pō'mă) [myxo- + G. *lipos*, fat, + *-ōma*, tumor]. Lipoma myxomatodes; myxoma lipomatosum; a benign neoplasm of adipose tissue in which portions of the tumor resemble mucoid mesenchymal tissue.

myxoma (mik-sō'mă) [myxo- + G. *-ōma*, tumor]. A benign neoplasm derived from connective tissue, consisting chiefly of polyhedral and stellate cells that are loosely embedded in a soft mucoid matrix, thereby resembling primitive mesenchymal tissue; occur frequently intramuscularly (where may be mistaken for a sarcoma), also in the jaw bones, and encysted in the skin (focal mucinosis and dorsal wrist ganglion).
atrial m., a primary cardiac neoplasm arising most commonly in the left atrium as a soft polypoid mass attached by a stalk to the septum; it may resemble an organized mural thrombus, and the symptoms may include cardiac murmurs, which change with alteration of body position, and signs of mitral stenosis or insufficiency.
m. enchondromato'sum, myxochondroma.
m. fibro'sum, myxofibroma.
m. lipomato'sum, myxolipoma.
odontogenic m., a benign, expansile, multilocular radiolucent neoplasm of the jaws consisting of myxomatous fibrous connective tissue; presumably derived from the mesenchymal components of the odontogenic apparatus.
m. sarcomato'sum, myxosarcoma.

myxomatosis (mik'sō-mă-tō'sis). **1.** A fatal disease of European rabbits (*Oryctolagus cuniculus*) marked by purulent conjunctivitis and the development of myxomatous growths in the skin; caused by rabbit myxoma virus and transmitted mechanically by mosquitoes; natural hosts are rabbits of the genus *Sylvilagus* in California and Brazil, in which the infection is not fatal and causes only local swelling. **2.** Mucoid *degeneration*. **3.** Multiple myxomas.

myxomatous (mik-sō'mă-tŭs). **1.** Pertaining to or characterized by the features of a myxoma. **2.** Said of tissue that resembles primitive mesenchymal tissue.

myxomycete (mik'sō-mī-sēt). A member of the class Myxomycetes.

Myxomycetes (mik'sō-mī-sē'tēz) [myxo- + G. *mykēs*, fungus]. A class of fungi containing the slime molds, which occur on rotting vegetation but are not pathogenic for man.

myxoneuroma (mik'sō-nū-rō'mă) [myxo- + G. *neuron*, nerve, + *-ōma*, tumor]. **1.** A tumefaction resulting from abnormal proliferation of Schwann cells, in which focal or diffuse degenerative changes result in portions that resemble primitive mesenchymal tissue. **2.** Obsolete term for a neurilemoma, meningioma, or glioma in which the stroma is myxomatous in nature.

myxopapilloma (mik'sō-pap-i-lō'mă) [myxo- + L. *papilla*, a nipple, + G. *-ōma*, tumor]. A benign neoplasm of epithelial tissue in which the stroma resembles primitive mesenchymal tissue.

myxopoiesis (mik'sō-poy-ē'sis) [myxo- + G. *poiēsis*, a making]. Mucus production.

myxorrhea (mik-sō-rē'ă) [myxo- + G. *rhoia*, a flow]. Blennorrhea.
m. gas'trica, gastromyxorrhea.

myxosarcoma (mik'sō-sar-kō'mă) [myxo- + G. *sarx*, flesh, + *-ōma*, tumor]. Myxoma sarcomatosum; a sarcoma, usually a liposarcoma or malignant fibrous histiocytoma, with an abundant component of myxoid tissue resembling primitive mesenchyme containing connective tissue mucin.

Myxospora (mik-sō-spō'ră) [myxo- + G. *sporos*, seed]. A subphylum of the phylum Protozoa, characterized by the presence of spores of multicellular origin, usually with two or three valves, two or more polar filaments, and an ameboid sporoplasm; parasitic in lower vertebrates, especially common in fishes. Important genera include *Ceratomyxa, Hanneguya, Leptotheca, Myxidium,* and *Myxobolus.*

myxospore (mik'sō-spōr) [myxo- + G. *sporos,* seed]. Obsolete term for the spore of a myxomycete.

Myxosporea (mik'sō-spō-rē'ă). A class of Myxozoa with spores containing one to six (usually two) polar capsules, each containing a coiled polar filament; parasitic in the celom or tissues of cold-blooded vertebrates, especially fishes. Important genera include *Ceratomyxa, Hanneguya, Leptotheca, Myxidium,* and *Myxobolus.*

myxovirus (mik'sō-vī'rŭs). Term formerly used for viruses with an affinity for mucins, now included in the families Orthomyxoviridae and Paramyxoviridae. The m.'s included influenza virus, parainfluenza virus, respiratory syncytial virus, measles virus, and mumps virus.

Myxozoa (mik-sō-zō'ă) [myxo- + G. *zoa,* animal]. A phylum of the subkingdom Protozoa, characterized by spores of multicellular origin (usually with two or three valves), one to six polar capsules or nematocysts (each with a coiled hollow filament), and a one- to many-nucleated ameboid sporoplasm; parasitic in annelids and other invertebrates (class Actinosporea; subclass Actinomyxa) and in lower vertebrates (class Myxosporea).

N

ν **1.** Thirteenth letter of the Greek alphabet, nu. **2.** Symbol for kinematic *viscosity.*

N 1. Symbol for newton; nitrogen. **2.** Designation for an inherited blood factor. See MNSs blood group, Blood Groups appendix.

N. Symbol for normal concentration. See normal (3).

n Symbol for nano-(2); refractive *index.*

N.A. Abbreviation for numerical *aperture.*

NA Abbreviation for *Nomina Anatomica.*

Na Symbol for sodium (natrium).

nabilone (nab'i-lōn). (±)-3-(1,1-Dimethylheptyl-6-6a*β*,7,8,10,-10a*α*-hexahydro-1-hydroxy-6,6-dimethyl-9*H*- dibenzo[*b,d*]pyran-9-one; a synthetic cannabinoid used in the treatment of nausea and vomiting associated with cancer chemotherapy.

Naboth, Martin, German anatomist and physician, 1675–1721. See nabothian *cyst, follicle.*

nacreous (nā'krē-ŭs) [Fr. *nacre,* mother-of-pearl]. Lustrous, like mother-of-pearl.

N.A.D. Abbreviation for no appreciable disease; nothing abnormal detected (British).

NAD Abbreviation for nicotinamide adenine dinucleotide.

NAD$^+$ Abbreviation for nicotinamide adenine dinucleotide (oxidized form).

NADase. NAD$^+$ nucleosidase.

NADH Abbreviation for nicotinamide adenine dinucleotide (reduced form).

NADH dehydrogenase [EC 1.6.99.3]. Cytochrome *c* reductase; an iron-containing flavoprotein oxidizing NADH to NAD$^+$.

NADH dehydrogenase (quinone) [EC 1.6.99.5]. An enzyme oxidizing NADH with quinones (*e.g.,* menaquinone) as acceptors.

NADH-hydroxylamine reductase [EC 1.6.6.11]. An enzyme reducing hydroxylamine to ammonia with NADH as hydrogen donor.

Nadi reaction. See under reaction.

nadide (nā'dīd). 3-Carbamoyl-1-*β*- D-ribofuranosylpyridinium hydroxide; a nicotinamide adenine dinucleotide compound used as an antogonist to alcohol and narcotics.

NAD$^+$ nucleosidase [EC 3.2.2.5]. NADase; DPNase; an enzyme cleaving NAD to nicotinamide and adenosinediphosphoribose.

nadolol (nā'dō-lol). 1-(*tert*-Butylamino)-3-[(5,6,7,8-tetrahydro-*cis*-6,7-dihydroxy-1-naphthyl)oxy]-2-propanol; a *β*-adrenergic blocking agent with actions similar to those of propanolol.

NADP Abbreviation for nicotinamide adenine dinucleotide phosphate.

NADP$^+$ Abbreviation for nicotinamide adenine dinucleotide phosphate (oxidized form).

NADPH Abbreviation for nicotinamide adenine dinucleotide phosphate (reduced form).

NADPH-cytochrome c_2 reductase [EC 1.6.2.5]. Cytochrome c_2 reductase; an enzyme catalyzing the reduction of ferricytochrome c_2 to ferrocytochrome c_2 at the expense of NADPH.

NADPH dehydrogenase [EC 1.6.99.1]. NADPH diaphorase; old yellow or Warburg's old yellow enzyme; a flavoprotein oxidizing NADPH to NADP$^+$.

NADPH dehydrogenase (quinone) [EC 1.6.99.6]. A flavoprotein similar to NADH dehydrogenase (quinone), but oxidizing NADPH.

NAD(P)H dehydrogenase (quinone) [EC 1.6.99.2]. Menadione, quinone, or phylloquinone reductase; DT-diaphorase; a flavoprotein oxidizing NADH or NADPH to NAD$^+$ or NADP$^+$ with quinones (*e.g.,* menadione) as hydrogen acceptors.

NADPH diaphorase. NADPH dehydrogenase.

NADPH-ferrihemoprotein reductase (fer'ī-hē-mō-prō'tēn, fer'ē) [EC 1.6.2.4]. Cytochrome reductase; an enzyme catalyzing the reduction of a ferricytochrome by NADPH to a ferrocytochrome.

NAD(P)$^+$ nucleosidase [EC 3.2.2.6]. An enzyme hydrolyzing NAD(P) to release free nicotinamide and adenosinediphosphoribose (phosphate).

Naegeli, Oskar, 20th century Swiss physician. See N. *syndrome.*

Naegeli, Otto, Swiss physician, 1871–1938. See N. type of monocytic *leukemia.*

Naegleria (nā-glē'rē-ă). A genus of free-living soil, water, and sewage ameba (order Schizopyrenida, family Vahlkampfiidae) one species of which, *N. fowleri,* has been implicated as the causative agent of the rapidly fatal primary amebic meningoencephalitis. Infection has been traced to swimming pools (including indoor chlorinated pools); entry is by the nasal mucosa, from which the amebae reach the meninges and brain through the cribriform plate and olfactory nerves. Other soil amebae that have been implicated, although of far less epidemiological significance, include the genera *Acanthamoeba* and *Hartmanella,* the latter being a suspected but unproved causative agent.

nafcillin (naf'sil'in). 6-(2-Ethoxy-1-naphthamido)penicillin; a semisynthetic penicillin derived from 6-aminopenicillanic acid; resistant to penicillinase, and effective against *Staphylococcus aureus.*
n. sodium, a penicillinase-resistant penicillin.

Naffziger, Howard C., U.S. surgeon, 1884–1961. See N. *operation, syndrome.*

nafronyl oxalate (naf'rō-nil). 2-(Diethylamino)ethyl tetrahydro-*α*-(1-naphthylmethyl)-2-furanpropionate oxalate; a vasodilator drug.

naftifine hydrochloride (naf'ti-fēn). (*E*)-*N*- Cinnamyl-*N*- methyl-1-naphthalenemethylamine hydrochloride; a broad spectrum antifungal agent used in the topical treatment of tinea infections.

nagana (nah-gah'nah). An acute or chronic disease of cattle, dogs, pigs, horses, sheep, and goats in sub-Saharan Africa; marked by fever, anemia, and cachexia, varying in severity with the parasite and the host. A collective term for diseases caused by *Trypanosome brucei brucei, T. congolense,* and *T. vivax.*

Nagel, Willibald, A., German ophthalmologist and physiologist, 1870–1911. See N.'s *test.*

Nägele, Franz K., German obstetrician, 1777–1851. See N.'s *obliquity, pelvis, rule.*

Nageotte, Jean, French histologist, 1866–1948. See N. *cells.*

nail (nāl) [A.S. *naegel*]. **1.** Unguis. **2.** A slender rod of metal, bone, or other solid substance, used in operations to fasten together the divided extremities of a broken bone.
egg shell n., hapalonychia.
half and half n., division of the n. by a transverse line into a proximal dull white part and a distal pink or brown part; seen in uremia.
hippocratic n.'s, the coarse curved n.'s capping clubbed digits (hippocratic fingers).
ingrown n., acronyx; onychocryptosis; onyxis; unguis aduncus; unguis incarnatus; a toenail, one edge of which is overgrown by the nailfold, producing a pyogenic granuloma; due to faulty trimming of the toenails or pressure from a tight shoe.
Küntscher n., an intramedullary n. used for internal fixation of a fracture.

parrot-beak n., a markedly curved fingernail.
pincer n., transverse overcurvature of the n. that increases distally, causing the lateral borders of the n. to pinch the soft tissue with resulting tenderness; may result from a developmental anomaly or subungual exostosis.
racket n., a broad flat thumbnail resulting from a congenital shorter and wider distal phalanx of the thumb.
reedy n., a n. marked by longitudinal ridges and furrows.
shell n., bronchiectasis with excessive longitudinal curvature of the nail plate and atrophy of the nail bed and underlying bone.
Smith-Petersen n., a flanged n. for pinning a fracture of the neck of the femur.
spoon n., koilonychia.
Terry's n.'s, a white, ground-glass-like opacity of the n.'s with a zone of normal pink at the distal edge of the n.'s; associated with liver disease (most commonly, cirrhosis of the liver).
yellow n., the complete or almost complete cessation of all nail growth, with thickening of the nails, increase in the convexity, loss of cuticles, and yellowing; the resulting onycholysis can cause loss of some of the nails, usually permanent, although the nails can occasionally become normal; the condition may be caused by lymphedema and is often associated with chronic bronchitis or bronchiectasis.

nailing (nāl'ing). Act of inserting or driving a nail into the ends of a fractured bone.

Najjar, Victor A., U.S. physician and biochemist, *1914. See Crigler-N. *syndrome.*

Nakanishi, K., Japanese physician. See N.'s *stain.*

nalbuphine hydrochloride (nal-byū'fēn). 17-(Cyclobutylmethyl)-4,5α-epoxymorphinan-3,6α, 14-triol hydrochloride; a synthetic opioid analgesic chemically related to oxymorphone, a narcotic, and to naloxone, a narcotic antagonist, with both agonist and antagonist narcotic properties.

nalidixic acid (nal-i-dik'sik). 1-Ethyl-1,4-dihydro-7-methyl-4-oxo-1,8-naphthyridine-3-carboxylic acid; an orally effective antibacterial agent used in the treatment of genitourinary tract infections.

nalorphine (nal-ōr'fēn). *N*- Allylnormorphine; $C_{19}H_{21}NO_3$; an antagonist of most of the depressant and stimulatory effects of morphine and related narcotic analgesics; precipitates severe withdrawal symptoms in morphine addicts, is used in the diagnosis of suspected morphine addiction, and counteracts the respiratory depression produced by morphine and related compounds; when administered in the absence of narcotics, n. has mild analgesic and respiratory depressant effects in nonaddicts.

naloxone hydrochloride (nal-ok'sōn). 1-*N*-Allyl-7,8-dihydro-14-hydroxymorphinone hydrochloride; a potent antagonist of endorphins and narcotics, including pentazocine; devoid of pharmacologic action when administered without narcotics.

naltrexone (nal-treks'ōn). 17-(Cyclopropylmethyl)-4,5-epoxy-3,14-dihydroxymorphinan-6-one; an endorphin and narcotic antagonist; devoid of pharmacologic action when administered in the absence of narcotics.

NAME Acronym for *n*evi, *a*trial myxoma, *m*yxoid neurofibromas, and *e*philides. See NAME *syndrome.*

nandrolone (nan'drō-lōn). 17β-Hydroxy-4-estrene-3-one; a semi-synthetic, parenterally administered, anabolic, androgenic steroid.
n. decanoate, an anabolic androgen.
n. phenpropionate, n. phenylpropionate; a moderately long-acting synthetic anabolic androgen.
n. phenylpropionate, n. phenpropionate.

nanism (nan'izm) [G. *nanos;* L. *nanus,* dwarf]. Dwarfism.

Nannizzia (nă-niz'ē-ă). A genus of ascomycetous fungi comprised of *Microsporum* species in their perfect state.

nano- [G. *nānos,* dwarf] **1.** Combining form relating to dwarfism (nanism). **2 (n).** Prefix used in the SI and metric systems to signify one-billionth (10^{-9}).

nanocephalia (nan'ō-se-fā'lē-ă). Microcephaly.

nanocephalous, nanocephalic (nan-ō-sef'ă-lŭs, -se-fal'ik). Microcephalic.

nanocephaly (nan-ō-sef'ă-lē) [nano- + G. *kephale,* head]. Microcephaly.

nanocormia (nan-ō-kōr'mē-ă) [nano- + G. *kormos,* trunk]. Microsomia.

nanogram (ng) (nan'ō-gram). One-billionth of a gram.

nanoid (nan'oyd) [nano- + G. *eidos,* resemblance]. Dwarflike.

nanomelia (nan-ō-mē'lē-ă) [nano- + G. *melos,* limb]. Micromelia.

nanometer (nm) (năn-om'ĕ-ter). One-billionth of a meter.

nanophthalmia, nanophthalmos (nan-of-thal'mē-ă, -mos) [nano- + G. *ophthalmos,* eye]. Microphthalmia.

Nanophyetus salmincola (na-nō'fī-ĕ-tŭs sal-min'kō-lă). *Troglotrema salmincola;* a digenetic fish-borne fluke (family Nanophyetidae) of dogs and other fish-eating mammals; the vector of *Neorickettsia helmintheca,* the agent of salmon poisoning.

nanous (nā'nŭs). Dwarfish.

Nanta. See Gandy-N. *disease.*

nanukayami (nă-nū-kă-yah'mē). Nanukayami *fever.*

nanus (nā'nŭs) [L.; G. *nanos*]. Dwarf.

NAP Abbreviation for *Nomina Anatomica Parisiensia.*

nape (nāp). Nucha.

napex (nā'peks). The area of the scalp just below the occipital protuberence.

naphazoline hydrochloride (nă-faz'ō-lēn, naf-az'-). Naphthazoline hydrochloride; 2-(1-naphthylmethyl)-2-imidazoline hydrochloride; a sympathomimetic amine, used as a topical vasoconstrictor; available as n. nitrate, with the same uses.

naphtha (naf'thă) [G.]. *Petroleum* benzin.
coal tar n., benzene.
wood n., *methyl* alcohol.

naphthalene (naf'thă-lēn). Tar camphor; naphthalin; a carcinogenic and toxic hydrocarbon obtained from coal tar; used for many syntheses in industry and in some moth repellents.

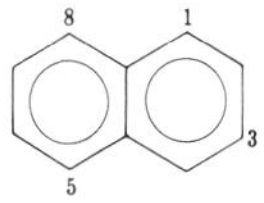

Naphthalene

naphthalenol (naf-thal'ĕ-nol). Naphthol.

naphthalin (naf'thă-lin). Naphthalene.

naphthazoline hydrochloride (naf-thaz'ō-lēn). Naphazoline hydrochloride.

naphthol (naf'thol). Naphthalenol; $C_{10}H_7OH$; a phenol of naphthalene, occurring in two forms: **α-n.,** a dye intermediate used in cytochemistry for arginine localization; **β-n.,** isonaphthol, used as an anthelmintic and antiseptic. Both forms are also used in the manufacture of dyes, organic chemicals, and rubber products.

naphthol yellow S [C.I. 10316]. 8-Hydroxy-5,7-dinitro-2-naphthalene sulfonic acid; an acid dye used as a stain for basic proteins in microspectro-photometry.

naphtholate (naf'thō-lāt). A compound of naphthol in which the hydrogen in the hydroxyl radical is substituted by a base.

naphthoquinone (naf-thō-kwin'ōn). A quinone derivative of naphthalene, reducible to naphthohydroquinone; 1,4-naphthoquinone derivatives have vitamin K activity *e.g.,* (menaquinone).

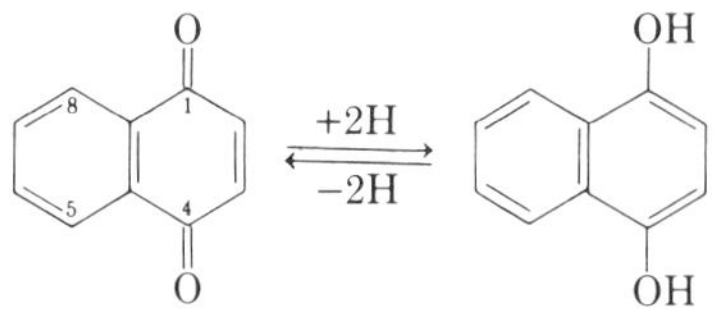

1,4-Naphthoquinone

naphthyl (naf'thil). The radical of naphthalene, $C_{10}H_7$–.

α-naphthylthiourea (ANTU) (naf'thil-thī'ō-yū-rē'ă). 1-(1-Naphthyl)-2-thiourea; a derivative of thiourea; a highly toxic antithyroid agent, especially to small mammals, causing pulmonary edema, fatty degeneration of the liver, and low body temperature; used as a rat poison.

napier (nā'pē-er) [John *Napier,* Scottish mathematician, 1550–1617]. Neper.

naprapathy (nă-prap'ă-thē) [Bohemian *napravit,* to correct, + G. *pathos,* suffering]. A system of therapeutic manipulation based on the theory that morbid symptoms are dependent upon strained or contracted ligaments in the spine, thorax, or pelvis.

naproxen (nă-prok'sēn). (+)-6-Methoxy-α-methyl-2-naphthaleneacetic acid; an anti-inflammatory analgesic agent used in the treatment of rheumatoid conditions.

napsylate (nap'si-lāt). USAN-approved contraction for 2-naphthalenesulfonate.

Narath, Albert, Dutch surgeon, 1864–1924. See N.'s *operation.*

narceine (nar'sē-ēn). An alkaloid of opium; $C_{23}H_{27}NO_8$. Ethylnarceine is a narcotic, analgesic, and antitussive.

narcissism (nar-sis'izm, nar'si-sizm) [*Narkissos,* G. myth. char.]. **1.** Self-love; autosexualism (2); autophilia; sexual attraction toward one's own person. **2.** A state in which the individual regards everything in relation to himself and not to other persons or things.
primary n., in psychoanalysis, the original psychic energy embodied or invested in the ego.
secondary n., in psychoanalysis, the psychic energy once attached to external objects, but now withdrawn from those objects and reinvested in the ego.

narco- [G. *narkoun,* to benumb, deaden]. Combining form relating to stupor or narcosis.

narcoanalysis (nar'kō-ă-nal'i-sis). Narcosynthesis; psychotherapeutic treatment under light anesthesia, originally used in acute combat cases during World War II. See also narcotherapy.

narcohypnia (nar-kō-hip'nē-ă) [narco- + G. *hypnos,* sleep]. A general numbness sometimes experienced at the moment of waking.

narcohypnosis (nar'kō-hip-nō'sis) [narco- + G. *hypnos,* sleep]. Stupor or deep sleep induced by hypnosis.

narcolepsy (nar'kō-lep-sē) [narco- + G. *lēpsis,* seizure]. Paroxysmal sleep; hypnolepsy; Friedmann's disease; Gélineau's syndrome; a sudden uncontrollable disposition to sleep occurring at irregular intervals, with or without obvious predisposing or exciting cause, usually involving an abnormality in sleep-stage sequencing.

narcosis (nar-kō'sis) [G. a benumbing]. General and nonspecific reversible depression of neuronal excitability, produced by a number of physical and chemical agents, usually resulting in stupor rather than in anesthesia (with which n. was once synonymous).
nitrogen n., **(1)** n. produced by nitrogenous materials such as occurs in certain forms of uremia and hepatic coma; **(2)** the stuporous condition characterized by disorientation and by loss of judgment and skill, attributed to an increased pressure of nitrogen as occurs with divers breathing air during underwater operations. Commonly referred to as "rapture of the deep."

narcosynthesis (nar-kō-sin'thĕ-sis). Narcoanalysis.

narcotherapy (nar-kō-thār'ă-pē). Psychotherapy conducted with the patient under the influence of a sedative or narcotic.

narcotic (nar-kot'ik) [G. *narkōtikos,* benumbing]. **1.** Any substance producing stupor associated with analgesia. **2.** Specifically, a drug derived from opium or opium-like compounds, with potent analgesic effects associated with significant alteration of mood and behavior, and with the potential for dependence and tolerance following repeated administration. **3.** Capable of inducing a state of stuporous analgesia.

***dl*-narcotine** (nar'kō-tēn). Gnoscopine.

***l*-α-narcotine.** Noscapine.

narcotism (nar'kō-tizm). **1.** Stuporous analgesia induced by a narcotic. **2.** Addiction to a narcotic.

naris, pl. **nares** (nā'ris, -rē-ŭm, -res) [L.] [NA]. Nostril; prenaris; anterior opening on either side of the nasal cavity.
anterior n., n.
posterior n., choana.

nasal (nā'zăl) [L. *nasus,* nose]. Rhinal; relating to the nose.

nascent (nas'ent, nā'sent) [L. *nascor,* pres. p. *nascens,* to be born]. **1.** Beginning; being born or produced. **2.** Denoting the state of a chemical element at the moment it is set free from one of its compounds.

nasioiniac (nā'zē-ō-in'ē-ak). Relating to the nasion and inion; denoting the distance in a straight line between the frontonasal suture and the external occipital protuberance.

nasion (nā'zē-on) [L. *nasus,* nose] [NA]. Nasal point; a point on the skull corresponding to the middle of the nasofrontal suture.

Nasmyth, Alexander, London dentist, †1847. See N.'s *cuticle, membrane.*

naso- [L. *nasus,* nose]. Combining form relating to the nose.

nasoantral (nā'zō-an'trăl). Relating to the nose and the maxillary sinus.

nasociliary (nā'zō-sil'ē-ār-ē). See *nervus* nasociliaris.

nasofrontal (nā-zō-frŭn'tăl). Relating to the nose and forehead, or to the nasal cavity and frontal sinuses.

nasogastric (nā-zō-gas'trik). Pertaining to or involving the nasal passages and the stomach, as in n. intubation.

nasolabial (nā-zō-lā'bē-ăl) [naso- + G. *labium,* lip]. Relating to the nose and upper lip.

nasolacrimal (nā-zō-lak'ri-măl). Relating to the nasal and the lacrimal bones, or to the nasal cavity and the lacrimal ducts.

naso-oral (nā-zō-ō'răl). Relating to the nose and mouth.

nasopalatine (nā'zō-pal'ă-tēn, -tin). Relating to the nose and the palate.

nasopharyngeal (nā'zō-fă-rin'jē-ăl). Rhinopharyngeal (1). **1.** Relating to the nose or nasal cavity and the pharynx. **2.** *Pars* nasalis pharyngis.

nasopharyngitis (nā'zō-far-in-jī'tis). Rhinopharyngitis.

nasopharyngolaryngoscope (nā'zō-fa-ring'gō-lā-ring'gō-skōp). An instrument, often of fiberoptic type, used to visualize the upper airways and pharynx.

nasopharyngoscope (nā'zō-fa-ring'gō-skōp). Telescopic instrument, electrically lighted, for examination of the nasal passages and the nasopharynx.

nasopharyngoscopy (nā'zō-fa-ring-gos'kō-pē) [nasopharynx + G. *skopeō,* to view]. Examination of the nasopharynx by flexible or rigid optical instruments, or with a mirror.

nasopharynx (nā'zō-far'ingks). *Pars* nasalis pharyngis.

nasorostral (nā'zō-ros'trăl). Relating to the nasal cavity and the rostrum of the sphenoid bone.

nasoscope (nā'zō-skōp). Rhinoscope.

nasosinusitis (nā'zō-sī-nŭ-sī'tis). Inflammation of the nasal cavities and of the accessory sinuses.

Nasse's law. See under law.

nasus (nā'sŭs) [L.] [NA]. Nose. **1.** N. externus. **2.** That portion of the respiratory pathway above the hard palate; includes both the n. externus and the cavum nasi.
n. exter'nus [NA], external nose; nasus (1); the visible portion of the nose which forms a prominent feature of the face; it consists of a root, dorsum and apex from above downward and is perforated inferiorly by two nostrils separated by a septum.

natal (nā'tăl). 1 [L. *natalis,* fr. *nascor,* pp. *natus,* to be born]. Relating to birth. 2 [L. *nates,* buttocks]. Relating to the buttocks or nates.

natality (nā-tal'i-tē) [see natal (1)]. The birth rate; the ratio of births to the general population.

natamycin (nā-tă-mī'sin). Pimaricin.

nates (nā'tēz) [L. pl. of *natis*] [NA]. The buttocks; breech; clunes; the prominence formed by the gluteal muscles on either side.

natimortality (nā'ti-mōr-tal'i-tē) [L. *natus,* birth, + *mortalitus,* fr. *mors,* death]. The perinatal death rate; the proportion of fetal and neonatal deaths to the general natality.

National Formulary (NF). An official compendium formerly issued by the American Pharmaceutical Association but now published by the United States Pharmacopeia Convention for the purpose of providing standards and specifications which can be used to evaluate the quality of pharmaceuticals and therapeutic agents.

natremia, natriemia (nā-trē'mē-ă, nā'trē-ē'mē-ă) [natrium, sodium, + G. *haima,* blood]. The presence of sodium in the blood.

natrexone hydrochloride (nă-treks'on). 17-(Cyclopropylmethyl)4,5α-epoxy-3,14-dihydroxymorphinan-6-one hydrochloride; a narcotic antagonist used in maintenance therapy of detoxified, formerly opiod-dependent, patients.

natriferic (nā-trif'er-ik) [natrium + L. *ferro,* to carry]. Tending to increase sodium transport.

natrium (nā'trē-ŭm) [Ar. *natrūm,* fr. G. *nitron,* carbonate of soda]. Sodium.

natriuresis (nā'trē-yū-rē'sis) [natrium + G. *ouron,* urine]. Urinary excretion of sodium; commonly designates enhanced sodium excretion, which may occur in certain diseases or as a result of the administration of diuretic drugs.

natriuretic (nā'trē-yū-ret'ik). **1.** Pertaining to or characterized by natriuresis. **2.** A substance that increases urinary excretion of sodium, usually as a result of decreased tubular reabsorption of sodium ions from glomerular filbrate.

naturopath (nā'chūr-ō-path). One who practices naturopathy.

naturopathic (nā'chūr-ō-path'ik). Relating to or by means of naturopathy.

naturopathy (nā-chūr-op'ă-thē). A system of therapeutics in which neither surgical nor medicinal agents are used, dependence being placed only on natural (nonmedicinal) forces.

naupathia (naw-path'ē-ă) [G. *naus,* ship, + *pathos,* suffering]. Seasickness.

nausea (naw'zē-ă, -zhă) [L. fr. G. *nausia,* seasickness, fr. *naus,* ship]. Symptoms resulting from an inclination to vomit.
epidemic n., epidemic *vomiting.*
n. gravida'rum, morning *sickness.*

nauseant (naw'zē-ănt). **1.** Nauseating; causing nausea. **2.** An agent that causes nausea.

nauseate (naw'zē-āt). To cause an inclination to vomit.

nauseated (naw'zē-ā-ted). Affected with nausea.

nauseous (naw'zē-ŭs, naw'shŭs). Causing nausea.

Nauta, Walle J.H., U.S. neuroscientist, *1916. See N.'s *stain.*

navel (nā'vel) [A.S. *nafela*]. Umbilicus.

navicula (nă-vik'yū-lă) [L. dim of *navis,* ship]. A small boat-shaped structure.

navicular (nă-vik'yū-lăr) [L. *navicularis,* relating to shipping]. Scaphoid.

navicularthritis (nă-vik'yū-lar-thrī'tis) [navicular + arthritis]. Navicular *disease.*

Nb Symbol for niobium.

NBT Abbreviation for nitro blue *tetrazolium.*

Nd Symbol for neodymium.

Ne Symbol for neon.

nealbarbital (nē-al-bar'bi-tahl). 5-Allyl-5-neopentylbarbituric acid; a sedative and hypnotic.

nearsightedness (nēr'sīt-ed-nes). Myopia.

nearthrosis (nē-ar-thrō'sis) [G. *neos,* new, + *arthrōsis,* a jointing]. A new joint; *e.g.,* a pseudarthrosis arising in an ununited fracture, or an artificial joint resulting from a total joint replacement operation.

nebramycin (neb-ră-mī'sin). A complex of substances produced by *Streptomyces tenebrarius;* an antibacterial agent.

nebula, pl. neb'ulae (neb'yū-lă, -lē) [L. fog, cloud, mist]. **1.** A translucent foglike opacity of the cornea. **2.** A class of oily preparations, intended for application by atomization. See spray.

nebularine (neb-yū-lăr'in). Ribosylpurine; purine ribonucleoside; a slightly toxic nucleoside isolated from the mushroom *Agaricus nebularis.*

nebulization (neb'yū-li-zā'shŭn) [L. *nebula,* mist]. Spraying or vaporization.

nebulize (neb'yū-līz) [L. *nebula,* mist]. To break up a liquid into a fine spray or vapor; to vaporize.

nebulizer (neb'yū-līz-er). A device used to reduce liquid medication to extremely fine cloudlike particles; useful in delivering medication to deeper parts of the respiratory tract. See also atomizer; vaporizer.
jet n., an atomizer that uses a gas stream to change a liquid into small particles.
spinning disk n., a n. in which water is changed into small particles as it is thrown by centrifugal force from a spinning disk.
ultrasonic n., a humidifier using high-frequency electricity to power a transducer that vibrates 1,350,000 times per second and changes water up into particles 0.5 to 3 μm in size in its nebulizing chamber; used in inhalation therapy.

Necator (nē-kā'tŏr) [L. a murderer]. A genus of nematode hookworms (family Ancylostomatidae, subfamily Necatorinae) distinguished by two chitinous cutting plates in the buccal cavity and fused male copulatory spicules. Species include *N. americanus,* the so-called New World hookworm (although it is also prevalent in the tropics of Africa, southern Asia, and Polynesia); the adults of this species attach to villi in the small intestine and suck blood, causing abdominal discomfort, diarrhea (usually with melena) and cramps, anorexia, loss of weight, and hypochromic microcytic anemia, which may occur in advanced disease. See also *Ancylostoma.* See fig. on p. 1026.

necatoriasis (nē-kă-tō-rī'ă-sis). Hookworm disease caused by *Necator,* the resulting anemia being usually less severe than that from ancylostomiasis.

neck (nek) [A.S. *hnecca*]. **1.** Collum. **2.** In anatomy, any constricted portion having a fancied resemblance to the n. of an animal. **3.** The germinative portion of an adult tapeworm which develops the segments or proglottids; the region of cestode segmentation behind the scolex.

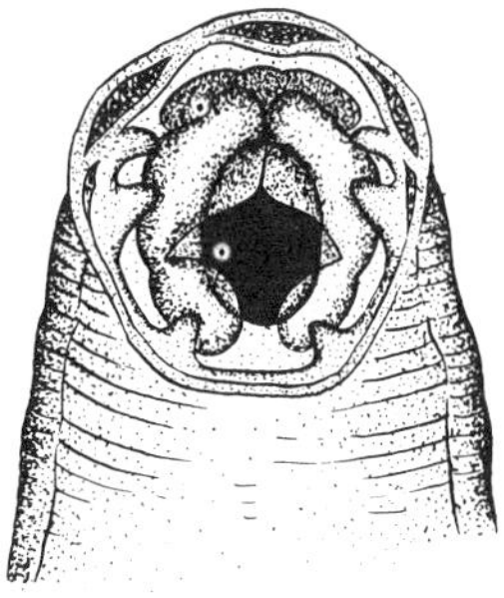

Necator americanus
Mouth and buccal cavity.

anatomical n. of humerus, *collum* anatomicum humeri.
buffalo n., combination of moderate kyphosis with thick heavy fat pad on the n., seen especially in persons with Cushing's disease or syndrome.
bull n., a heavy thick n. caused by hypertrophied muscles or enlarged cervical lymph nodes.
dental n., *cervix* dentis.
n. of femur, *collum* ossis femoris.
n. of fibula, *collum* fibulae.
n. of gallbladder, *collum* vesicae biliaris.
n. of glans penis, *collum* glandis penis.
n. of hair follicle, *collum* folliculi pili.
n. of humerus, *collum* humeri.
Madelung's n., multiple symmetric lipomatosis (Madelung's disease) confined to the n.
n. of malleus, *collum* mallei.
n. of mandible, *collum* mandibulae.
n. of radius, *collum* radii.
n. of rib, *collum* costae.
n. of scapula, *collum* scapulae.
stiff n., torticollis.
surgical n. of humerus, *collum* chirurgicum humeri.
n. of talus, *collum* tali.
n. of thigh bone, *collum* ossis femoris.
n. of tooth, *cervix* dentis.
n. of urinary bladder, *cervix* vesicae urinariae.
n. of uterus, *cervix* uteri.
webbed n., the broad n. due to lateral folds of skin extending from the clavicle to the head; occurs in Turner's syndrome and in Noonan's syndrome.
n. of womb, *cervix* uteri.
wry n., torticollis.

necklace (nek'lās). Term used to describe a skin rash that encircles the neck.
Casal's n., a dermatitis partly or completely encircling the lower part of the neck in pellagra.
n. of Venus, obsolete term for syphilitic *leukoderma.*

necr-. See necro-.

necrectomy (ne-krek'tō-mē) [necr- + G. *ektomē,* excision]. Operative removal of any necrosed tissue.

necro-, necr- [G. *nekros,* corpse]. Combining forms relating to death or to necrosis.

necrobiosis (nek'rō-bī-ō'sis) [necro- + G. *biōs,* life]. Bionecrosis. **1.** Physiologic or normal death of cells or tissues as a result of changes associated with development, aging, or use. **2.** Necrosis of a small area of tissue.
n. lipoid'ica, n. lipoid'ica diabetico'rum, a condition, sometimes associated with diabetes, in which one or more yellow, atrophic, shiny lesions develop on the legs (typically pretibial); characterized histologically by n. in the cutis.

necrobiotic (nek'rō-bī-ot'ik). Pertaining to or characterized by necrobiosis.

necrocytosis (nek'rō-sī-tō'sis) [necro- + G. *kytos,* cell, + *-osis,* condition]. A process that results in, or a condition that is characterized by, the abnormal or pathologic death of cells.

necrogenic (nek-rō-jen'ik) [necro- + G. *genesis,* origin]. Necrogenous; relating to, living in, or having origin in dead matter.

necrogenous (nĕ-kroj'ĕ-nŭs). Necrogenic.

necrogranulomatous (nek'rō-gran-yū-lō'mă-tŭs). Having the characteristics of a granuloma with central necrosis.

necrologist (nĕ-krol'ō-jist). A student of, or a specialist in, necrology.

necrology (nĕ-krol'ō-jē) [necro- + G. *logos,* study]. The science of the collection, classification, and interpretation of mortality statistics.

necrolysis (nĕ-krol'i-sis) [necro- + G. *lysis,* loosening]. Necrosis and loosening of tissue.
toxic epidermal n. (TEN), a syndrome in which a large portion of the skin becomes intensely erythematous and peels off in the manner of a second-degree burn, often simultaneous with the formation of flaccid bullae, resulting from drug sensitivity or of unknown cause; the level of separation is subepidermal, unlike staphylococcal scalded skin syndrome in which there is subcorneal change.

necromania (nek-rō-mā'nē-ă) [necro- + G. *mania,* frenzy]. **1.** A morbid tendency to dwell with longing on death. **2.** A morbid attraction to dead bodies.

necrometer (nĕ-krom'ĕ-ter) [necro- + G. *metron,* measure]. An instrument for measuring a dead body or any of its parts or organs.

necroparasite (nek-rō-par'ă-sīt). Saprophyte.

necropathy (nĕ-krop'ă-thē) [necro- + G. *pathos,* disease]. A tendency to tissue death or gangrene.

necrophagous (nĕ-krof'ă-gŭs) [necro- + G. *phagein,* to eat]. **1.** Living on carrion. **2.** Necrophilous.

necrophilia, necrophilism (nek-rō-fil'ē-ă, nĕ-krof'i-lizm) [necro- + G. *phileō,* to love]. **1.** A morbid fondness for being in the presence of dead bodies. **2.** The impulse to have sexual contact, or the act of such contact, with a dead body, usually of males with female corpses.

necrophilous (nĕ-krof'i-lŭs) [necro- + G. *philos,* fond]. Necrophagous (2); having a preference for dead tissue; denoting certain bacteria.

necrophobia (nek-rō-fō'bē-ă) [necro- + G. *phobos,* fear]. Morbid fear of corpses.

necropsy (nek'rop-sē) [necro- + G. *opsis,* view]. Autopsy (1).

necrosadism (nek-rō-săd'izm) [necro- + sadism]. Sexual gratification derived by mutilating corpses.

necroscopy (nĕ-kros'kŏ-pē) [necro- + G. *skopeō,* to examine]. Autopsy (1).

necrose (nĕ-krōz'). **1.** To cause necrosis. **2.** To become the site of necrosis.

necrosis (nĕ-krō'sis) [G. *nekrōsis,* death, fr. *nekroō,* to make dead]. Pathologic death of one or more cells, or of a portion of tissue or organ, resulting from irreversible damage; earliest irreversible changes are mitochondrial, consisting of swelling and granular calcium deposits seen by electron microscopy; most frequent visible alterations are nuclear: pyknosis, shrunken and abnormally dark basophilic staining; karyolysis, swollen and abnormally pale basophilic staining; or karyorrhexis, rupture and fragmentation of the nucleus. After such changes, the outlines of individual cells are indistinct, and affected cells may become merged, sometimes form-

ing a focus of coarsely granular, amorphous, or hyaline material.
aseptic n., n. occurring in the absence of infection.
avascular n., n. due to deficient blood supply.
bridging hepatic n., area of liver n. which bridge adjacent portal areas and central veins; subsequent post-necrotic collapse and fibrosis is likely to result in cirrhosis.
caseous n., caseation n., caseous degeneration; n. characteristic of certain inflammations (*e.g.,* tuberculosis, histoplasmosis), which represents n. with loss of separate structures of the various cellular and histologic elements; affected tissue manifests the friable, crumbly consistency and dull, opaque quality observed in cheese.
central n., n. involving the deeper or inner portions of a tissue, or an organ or its units.
coagulation n., a type of n. in which the affected cells or tissue are converted into a dry, dull, fairly homogeneous eosinophilic mass without nuclear staining, as a result of the coagulation of protein as occurs in an infarct; microscopically, the necrotic process involves chiefly the cells, and remnants of histologic elements (*e.g.,* elastin, collagen, muscle fibers) may be recognizable, as well as "ghosts" of cells and portions of cell membranes; may be caused by heat, ischemia, and other agents that destroy tissue, including enzymes that would continue to alter the devitalized cellular substance.
colliquative n., liquefactive n.
cystic medial n., medionecrosis of the aorta; medionecrosis aortae idiopathica cystica; mucoid medial degeneration; Erdheim disease; loss of elastic and muscle fibers in the aortic media, with accumulation of mucopolysaccharide, sometimes in cystlike spaces between the fibers; a disease of unknown cause, which may be inherited and which predisposes to dissecting aneurysms.
epiphysial aseptic n., aseptic n. of bony epiphyses, probably due to ischemia; it may affect the upper end of the femur (Legg-Calvé-Perthes disease), the tibial tubercle (Osgood-Schlatter disease), the tarsal navicular bone or the patella (Köhler's disease), the second metatarsal head (Freiberg's disease), vertebral bodies (Scheuermann's disease), or the capitellum of the humerus (Panner's disease).
fat n., steatonecrosis; the death of adipose tissue, characterized by the formation of small (1 to 4 mm), dull, chalky, gray or white foci; these represent small quantities of calcium soaps formed in the affected tissue when fat is hydrolyzed into glycerol and fatty acids.
fibrinoid n., n. in which the necrotic tissue has some staining reactions resembling fibrin and becomes deeply eosinophilic, homogenous, and refractile.
focal n., occurrence of numerous, relatively small or tiny, fairly well circumscribed, usually spheroidal portions of tissue that manifest coagulative, caseous, or gummatous n. and are characteristically associated with agents that are hematogenously disseminated; frequently observed only in histologic sections, but the foci may be as large as 1 to 3 mm and macroscopically visible; arbitrarily, foci larger than that are usually not termed focal n.
ischemic n., n. caused by hypoxia resulting from local deprivation of blood supply, as by infarction.
laminar cortical n., the breaking down of a definite cell layer in the cerebral cortex, encountered typically after temporary cardiac arrest or perinatal hypoxia.
liquefactive n., colliquative n.; a type of n. characterized by a fairly well circumscribed, microscopically or macroscopically visible lesion that consists of the dull, opaque or turbid, gray-white to yellow-gray, soft or boggy, partly or completely fluid remains of tissue that became necrotic and was digested by enzymes, especially proteolytic enzymes liberated from disintegrating leukocytes; it is classically observed in abscesses, and frequently in infarcts of the brain.
mummification n., dry *gangrene.*
progressive emphysematous n., gas *gangrene.*
renal papillary n., necrotizing papillitis; n. of renal papillae, occurring in acute pyelonephritis, especially in diabetics, or in analgesic nephropathy; renal failure may result.
simple n., a stage of coagulation n.; the occurrence of a coarsely granular or hyaline change in the cytoplasm, and the lack of a recognizable nucleus, with the general configuration of the dead cells being relatively unchanged.
subcutaneous fat n. of newborn, *sclerema* neonatorum.
suppurative n., liquefactive n. with pus formation.
total n., **(1)** complete n. of the cytologic and histologic elements in a portion of tissue, as in caseous n.; **(2)** death of an entire organ or part.
Zenker's n., Zenker's *degeneration.*
zonal n., n. predominantly affecting or limited to an anatomical zone, especially parts of the hepatic lobules defined according to proximity to either the portal tracts or central (hepatic) veins.

necrospermia (nek-rō-sper'mē-ă) [necro- + G. *sperma,* seed]. A condition in which there are dead or immobile spermatozoa in the semen.

necrosteon, necrosteosis (nĕ-kros'tē-on, nĕ-kros-tē-ō'sis) [necro- + G. *osteon,* bone]. Gangrene of bone.

necrotic (nĕ-krot'ik). Pertaining to or affected by necrosis.

necrotomy (ne-krot'ō-mē) [necro- + G. *tomē,* cutting]. **1.** Dissection. **2.** Operation for the removal of a necrosed portion of bone (sequestrum).
osteoplastic n., removal of a bone sequestrum through a hinged window of bone which is then replaced.

needle (nē'dl). **1.** A slender, usually sharp-pointed, instrument used for puncturing tissues, suturing, or passing a ligature around an artery. **2.** A hollow n. used for injection, aspiration, biopsy, or to guide introduction of a catheter into a vessel or other space. **3.** To separate the tissues by means of one or two n.'s, in the dissection of small parts. **4.** To perform discission of a cataract by means of a knife n.
aneurysm n., artery n., a blunt-pointed, curved n., set in a handle, with the eye at the point, used for passing a ligature around an artery.
aspirating n., a hollow n. used for withdrawing fluid from a cavity, when combined with an aspirator tube attached to one end.
atraumatic n., an eyeless surgical n. with the suture permanently fastened into a hollow end.
biopsy n., a hollow n. used to obtain a core of tissue for histologic study.
cataract n., knife n.
couching n., an obsolete instrument used in couching.
Deschamps n., a n. with a long shaft for passing sutures in the deep tissues.
Emmet's n., a strong n. with the eye in the point, having a wide curve, and set in a handle, used to pass a ligature around an undissected structure.
exploring n., a strong n. with a longitudinal groove, which is thrust into a tumor or cavity to determine the presence of fluid, the latter escaping externally along the groove.
Francke's n., a small lancet-shaped spring-activated n., used to evacuate a small effusion of blood.
Frazier's n., a n. for draining lateral ventricles of brain.
Gillmore n., a device for obtaining the setting time of dental cement.
Hagedorn n., a curved surgical n. flattened on the sides.
hypodermic n., a hollow n., similar to but smaller than an aspirating n., attached to a syringe; used primarily for injection.
knife n., cataract n.; a very narrow, needle-pointed knife used in discission of a cataract.
lumbar puncture n., a n., provided with a stylet, for entering the spinal canal or cisterna magna, with a bore of at least 1 mm and 40 mm or more in length.
Salah's sternal puncture n., a wide-bore n. for obtaining samples of red marrow from the sternum.

spatula n., a minute n. with a flat (non-cutting) concave surface, used by eye surgeons.

stop-n., a surgical n., with the eye at the tip, the shank of which has a projecting shelf to arrest the n. when it has passed the desired distance through the tissues.

Tuohy n., a n. with a lateral opening at the distal end, designed to cause a catheter passing through the n.'s lumen to exit laterally at a 45° angle; used to place catheters into the subarachnoid or epidural space.

Vicat n., a device for obtaining the setting time of plaster and other materials.

needle-holder, needle-carrier, needle-driver. Needle forceps; an instrument for grasping a needle in suturing.

Needles, Carl F., U.S. pediatrician, *1935. See Melnick-N. *syndrome.*

Needles, J.W., U.S. dentist. See N.'s split cast *method.*

needling (nēd'ling). Discission of a soft or secondary cataract.

Neelsen, Friedrich K.A., German pathologist, 1854–1894. See Ziehl-N. *stain.*

neencephalon (nē-en-sef'ă-lon) [G. *neos,* new, + *enkephalos,* brain]. Neoencephalon; Edinger's term for the higher levels of the central nervous system superimposed upon the metameric or propriospinal system (paleencephalon).

NEEP Abbreviation for negative end-expiratory *pressure.*

nefopam hydrochloride (nef'ō-pam). 3,4,5,6-Tetrahydro-5-methyl-1-phenyl-1*H*-2,5-benzoxazocine hydrochloride; an analgesic agent.

Neftel, William B., U.S. neurologist, 1830–1906. See N.'s *disease.*

negation (nĕ-gā'shŭn). Denial.

negative (−) (neg'ă-tiv) [L. *negativus,* fr. *nego,* to deny]. **1.** Not affirmative; refutative; not positive; not abnormal. **2.** Denoting failure of response, absence of a reaction, or absence of an entity or condition in question.

false n., a n. test result in a subject which possesses the attribute for which the test is being conducted.

negative G. Gravity in a foot-to-head direction in flying, or in standing on one's head; opposite of positive G.

negative S. Flotation *constant.*

negativism (neg'ă-tiv-izm). A tendency to do the opposite of what one is requested to do, or to stubbornly resist for no apparent reason; seen in catatonic states.

negatron (neg'ă-tron). Term used for an electron to emphasize its negative charge in contradistinction to the positive charge carried by the otherwise similar positron.

Negri, Adelchi, Italian physician, 1876–1912. See N. *bodies, corpuscles.*

Negro, Camillo, Italian neurologist, 1861–1927. See N.'s *phenomenon.*

Neisser, Albert L.S., Breslau physician, 1855–1916. See *Neisseria;* N.'s *coccus, syringe.*

Neisser, Max, German bacteriologist, 1869–1938. See N.'s *stain.*

Neisseria (nī-sē'rē-ă) [A. *Neisser*]. A genus of aerobic to facultatively anaerobic bacteria (family Neisseriaceae) containing Gram-negative cocci which occur in pairs with the adjacent sides flattened. These organisms are parasites of animals. The type species is *N. gonorrhoeae.*

N. ca'viae, a species found in the pharyngeal region of guinea pigs and perhaps of other animals.

N. fla'va, a species found in the mucous membranes of the human respiratory tract.

N. flaves'cens, a species found in cerebrospinal fluid in cases of meningitis; probably occurs in the mucous membranes of the human respiratory tract.

N. gonorrhoe'ae, gonococcus; Neisser's coccus; a species that causes gonorrhea and other infections in man; the type species of the genus *N.*

N. haemol'ysans, a species found in the mucous membranes of the human respiratory tract.

N. meningi'tidis, meningococcus; Weichselbaum's coccus; a species found in the nasopharynx of man but not in other animals; the causative agent of meningococcal meningitis; virulent organisms are strongly Gram-negative and occur singly or in pairs; in the latter case the cocci are elongated and are arranged with long axes parallel and facing sides kidney-shaped; groups characterized by serologically specific capsular polysaccharides are designated by capital letters (the main serogroups being A, B, C, and D).

N. sic'ca, a species found in the mucous membranes of the human respiratory tract.

N. subfla'va, a species found in the mucous membranes of the human respiratory tract; easily confused with *N. meningitidis.*

neisseria, pl. **neisseriae** (nī-sē'rē-ă, nī-sē'rē-ē). A vernacular term used to refer to any member of the genus *Neisseria.*

Nélaton, Auguste, French surgeon, 1807–1873. See N.'s *catheter, dislocation, fibers, line, sphincter;* Roser-N. *line.*

Nelson, Don H., U.S. internist, *1925. See N. *syndrome, tumor.*

Nelson, R.S. See Sprinz-N. *syndrome.*

nem [Ger. *Nahrungs Einheit Milch,* milk nutrition unit]. A nutritional unit defined as 1 gram breast milk of specific nutritional components having a caloric value equivalent to $^2/_3$ calorie.

nema-, nemat-, nemato- [G. *nēma,* thread]. Combining forms meaning thread, threadlike.

nemathelminth (nem-ă-thel'minth). A member of the former phylum Nemathelminthes.

Nemathelminthes (nem'ă-thel-min'thēz) [nemat- + G. *helmins, helminthos,* worm]. Aschelminthes; formerly considered a phylum to incorporate the pseudocelomate organisms, which now are divided into the distinct phyla Acanthocephala, Entoprocta, Rotifera, Gastrotricha, Kinorhyncha, Nematoda, and Nematomorpha.

nematocidal (nem'ă-tō-sī'dăl). Destructive to nematode worms.

nematocide (nĕ-mat'ō-sīd) [nematode + L. *caedo,* to kill]. An agent that kills nematodes.

nematocyst (nem'ă-tō-sist) [nemato- + G. kystis, bladder]. Cnida; cnidocyst; a stinging cell of coelenterates consisting of a poison sac and a coiled barbed sting capable of being ejected and penetrating the skin of an animal on contact; of considerable consequence in large jellyfish and in the Portuguese man-of-war whose large numbers of these stinging cells can cause great pain and even death.

Nematoda (nem-ă-tō'dă) [nemat- + G. *eidos,* form]. The roundworms, a large phylum that includes many of the helminths parasitic in man and a far greater number of plant-parasitic and free-living soil and aquatic nonparasitic species. For practical purposes, the parasitic nematodes may be placed in two groups, based on their adult habitat in the human body: 1) the intestinal roundworms (*e.g.,* the genera *Ascaris, Trichuris, Ancylostoma, Necator, Strongyloides, Enterobius,* and *Trichinella*); and 2) the filarial roundworms of the blood, lymphatic tissues, and viscera (*e.g.,* the genera *Wuchereria, Mansonella, Loa, Onchocerca,* and il Dracunculus).

nematode (nem'ă-tōd). A common name for any roundworm of the phylum Nematoda.

nematodiasis (nem'ă-tō-dī'ă-sis). Infection with nematode parasites.

cerebrospinal n., invasion of the central nervous system by wandering nematode larvae; *e.g., Setaria* species in horses, *Angiostrongylus cantonensis* in rats and humans.

Nematodirella longispiculata (nē′mă-tō-di-rel′ă lon′gi-spik-yū-lā′tă). One of the thread-necked trichostrongyle nematodes in the small intestine of sheep, goats, reindeer, moose, musk ox, and pronghorn.

Nematodirus (nem-ă-tō′di-rŭs). The genus of thread-necked or thin-necked trichostrongyles; slender, relatively elongated nematodes occurring in herbivorous animals, usually in the small intestine. Generally, they are not believed to be highly pathogenic except in poorly fed, heavily infected animals. Species include *N. abnormalis,* common in the U.S. and occurring in sheep, goats, camels, and mule deer; *N. filicollis,* occurring worldwide in sheep, goats, oxen, and various wild ruminants; *N. helvetianus,* in cattle, sheep, goats, and camels in Europe, Asia, and the Americas; *N. lanceolatus,* in sheep and pronghorns in the Americas; *N. leporis,* in domestic rabbits and wild cottontail rabbits in North America; and *N. spathiger,* the most common, widespread, and abundant species, in sheep, cattle, camels, and other ruminants.

nematoid (nem′ă-toyd). Relating to nematodes.

nematologist (nem-ă-tol′ō-jist). A specialist in nematology.

nematology (nem-ă-tol′ō-jē) [nematode + G. *logos,* study]. The science concerned with all aspects of nematodes, their biology, and their importance to man.

nematospermia (nem′ă-tō-sper′mē-ă) [nemat- + G. *sperma,* seed]. Spermatozoa with an elongated tail, as in humans, in contrast to spherospermia.

neo- [G. *neos,* new]. Prefix meaning new or recent.

neoantigens (nē-ō-an′ti-jenz). Tumor *antigens.*

neoarsphenamine (nē′ō-ar-sfen′ă-mēn). Sodium arsphenamine methylenesulfoxylate; formerly used as an antisyphilitc agent.

neoarthrosis (nē-ō-ar-thrō′sis). Nearthrosis.

Neoascaris vitulorum (nē-ō-as′kă-ris vit-yū-lō′rŭm). The large roundworm occurring in the small intestine of cattle, water buffalo, and (rarely) sheep; although uncommon in the U.S., it is a serious cattle parasite in many other areas. Experimental infection has been produced in rodents and man.

neobiogenesis (nē′ō-bī-ō-jen′ĕ-sis) [neo- + G. *bios,* life, + *genesis,* origin]. The theory that life can originate from nonliving matter.

neoblastic (nē-ō-blas′tik) [neo- + G. *blastos,* germ, offspring]. Developing in or characteristic of new tissue.

neocerebellum (nē′ō-ser-ĕ-bel′ŭm) [NA]. Corticocerebellum; phylogenetic term referring to the larger lateral portion of the cerebellar hemisphere receiving its dominant input from the pontine nuclei which, in turn, are dominated by afferent nerves originating from all parts of the cerebral cortex; phylogenetically, of more recent origin than the archicerebellum and paleocerebellum, n. reaches its largest development in man and other primates.

neochymotrypsinogen (nē-ō-kī′mō-trip-sin′ō-jen). An intermediate in the conversion of chymotrypsin to α-chymotrypsin by chymotrypsin cleavage.

neocinchophen (nē-ō-sin′kō-fen). The ethyl ester of 6-methyl-2-phenylquinolin-4-carboxylic acid; its action and uses are similar to those of cinchophen.

neocortex (nē-ō-kōr′teks). Isocortex.

neocystostomy (nē′ō-sis-tos′tō-mē) [neo- + G. *kystis,* bladder, + *stoma,* mouth]. An operation in which the ureter or a segment of the ileum is implanted into the bladder.

neodymium (nē-ō-dim′ē-ŭm) [neo- + G. *didymos,* twin (of lanthanum)]. One of the rare earth elements; symbol Nd, atomic no. 60, atomic weight 144.24.

neoencephalon (nē-ō-en-sef′ă-lon). Neencephalon.

neofetal (nē-ō-fē′tăl). Relating to the neofetus.

neofetus (nē-ō-fē′tŭs). The intrauterine organism at about 8 weeks in the transition period between embryo and fetus.

neoformation (nē′ō-fōr-mā′shŭn). **1.** Formation of neoplasia, or a neoplasm. **2.** Sometimes used to indicate the process of regeneration, or a regenerated tissue or part.

neogala (nē-og′ă-lă) [neo- + G. *gala,* milk]. The first milk formed in the breasts after childbirth.

neogenesis (nē-ō-jen′ĕ-sis) [neo- + G. *genesis,* origin]. Regeneration (1).

neogenetic (nē′ō-je-net′ik). Pertaining to or characterized by neogenesis.

neokinetic (nē′ō-ki-net′ik) [neo- + G. *kinētikos,* relating to movement]. Denoting one of the divisions of the motor system, the function of which is the transmission of isolated synergic movements of voluntary origin; it represents a more highly specialized form of movement than the paleokinetic function.

neolallism (nē-ō-lal′izm) [neo- + G. *laleō,* to chatter]. Abnormal use of neologisms in speech.

neologism (nē-ol′ō-jizm) [neo- + G. *logos,* word]. A new word or phrase, or an existing word used in a new sense; in psychiatry, such usages may have meaning only to the patient or be indicative of his condition.

neomembrane (nē-ō-mem′brān). False *membrane.*

neomorph, neomorphism (nē′ō-mōrf, nē′ō-mōr′fizm) [neo- + G. *morphē,* form]. A new formation; a structure found in higher organisms, only slight or no traces of which exist in lower orders.

neomycin sulfate (nē-ō-mī′sin). The sulfate of an antibacterial substance produced by the growth of *Streptomyces fradiae,* active against a variety of Gram-positive and Gram-negative bacteria.

neon (nē′on) [G. *neos,* new]. An inert gaseous element in the atmosphere, separated from argon by Ramsay in 1898; symbol Ne, atomic no. 10, atomic weight 20.183.

neonatal (nē-ō-nā′tăl) [neo- + L. *natalis,* relating to birth]. Newborn; relating to the period immediately succeeding birth and continuing through the first 28 days of life.

neonate (nē′ō-nāt) [L. *neonatus,* newborn]. A neonatal infant.

neonatologist (nē′ō-nā-tol′ō-jist). One who specializes in neonatology.

neonatology (nē′ō-nā-tol′ō-jē) [neo- + L. *natus,* pp. born, + G. *logos,* theory]. The medical specialty concerned with disorders of the neonate.

neopallium (nē-ō-pal′ē-ŭm). Isocortex.

neopathy (nē-op′ă-thē) [neo- + G. *pathos,* disease]. A new lesion or pathologic process.

neophobia (nē-ō-fō′bē-ă) [neo- + G. *phobos,* fear]. Morbid aversion to, or dread of, novelty or the unknown.

neophrenia (nē-ō-frē′nē-ă) [neo- + G. *phrēn,* mind]. Any major mental disorder (psychosis) occurring in childhood.

neoplasia (nē-ō-plā′zē-ă) [neo- + G. *plasis,* a molding]. The pathologic process that results in the formation and growth of a neoplasm.

cervical intraepithelial n., dysplastic changes beginning at the squamocolumnar junction in the uterine cervix which may be precursors of squamous cell carcinoma: grade 1, mild dysplasia involving the lower one-third or less of the epithelial thickness; grade 2, moderate dysplasia with one-third to two-thirds involvement; grade 3, severe dysplasia or carcinoma in situ, with two-thirds to full-thickness involvement.

multiple endocrine n., type 1, familial endocrine *adenomatosis,* type 1.

multiple endocrine n., type 2, familial endocrine *adenomatosis,* type 2.

neoplasm (nē′ō-plazm) [neo- + G. *plasma,* thing formed]. New growth; tumor (2); an abnormal tissue that grows by cellular proliferation more rapidly than normal and continues to grow after the stimuli that initiated the new growth cease. N.'s show partial or complete lack of structural organization and functional coordination with the normal tissue, and usually form a distinct mass of tissue which may be either benign (benign *tumor*) or malignant (cancer).

histoid n., a n. characterized by a cytohistologic pattern that closely resembles the tissue from which the neoplastic cells are derived.

neoplastic (nē-ō-plas'tik). Pertaining to or characterized by neoplasia, or containing a neoplasm.

neopterin (nē-op'ter-in). A pteridine present in body fluids; elevated levels result from immune system activation, malignant disease, allograft rejection, and viral infections (especially as in AIDS).

neopyrithiamin (nē'ō-pir-i-thī'ă-min). Pyrithiamin.

neoretinene B (nē-ō-ret'i-nēn). 11-*cis*-Retinol.

Neorickettsia helmintheca (nē'ō-ri-ket'sē-ă hel-min'thē-kă). A rickettsial organism that is the agent of salmon disease of dogs and is transmitted by the heterophyid fluke, *Nanophytes salmincola.*

neostigmine (nē-ō-stig'min). $C_{12}H_{19}BrN_2O_2$; a synthetic compound, closely similar in action to physostigmine (eserine); a reversible cholinesterase inhibitor, used as the bromide or methylsulfate salts in the treatment of myasthenia gravis, postoperative distention, urinary retention, overdose of tubocurarine, and as a pregnancy test.

neostomy (nē-os'tō-mē) [neo- + G. *stoma,* mouth]. Surgical construction of a new or artificial opening.

neostriatum (nē-ō-strī-ā'tŭm). The caudate nucleus and putamen considered as one and distinguished from the globus pallidus (paleostriatum).

neostrophingic (nē'ō-strō-fin'jik) [neo- + G. *strophē,* turning, + hinge]. A "new turning," describing surgical mobilization of the mitral valve by extension of the arcuate line in valve closure a little past the normal limits at both ends, thus rehinging the septal leaflet and making it more flexible.

neoteny (nē-ot'ĕ-nē) [neo- + G. *tenō,* to stretch]. Prolongation of the larval state, as in the Mexican tiger salamander or axolotl, or in certain termite castes held in the larval stage as future replacements of the queen. *Cf.* pedogenesis.

Neotestudina rosati (nē'ō-tes-tū-dī'nă rō-sā'tī). A species of fungus which causes white grain mycetoma in Somalia and elsewhere in Africa.

neothalamus (nē-ō-thal'ă-mŭs). The portion of the thalamus projecting to the neocortex.

neotyrosine (nē-ō-tī'rō-sēn). Dimethyltyrosine; a tyrosine antimetabolite.

neovascularization (nē'ō-vas'kyū-lar-i-zā'shŭn). Proliferation of blood vessels in tissue not normally containing them, or proliferation of blood vessels of a different kind than usual in tissue.

nep'er (Np) [fr. *neperus,* latinized form of (John) *Napier*]. Napier; a unit for comparing the magnitude of two powers, usually in electricity or acoustics; it is one half of the natural logarithm of the ratio of the two powers.

nephelometer (nef-ĕ-lom'ĕ-ter) [G. *nephelē,* cloud, + *metron,* measure]. An instrument used in nephelometry.

nephelometry (nef-ĕ-lom'ĕ-trē). A technique for estimation of the number and size of particles in a suspension by measurement of light scattered from a beam of light passed through the solution.

nephr-. See nephro-.

nephradenoma (nef'rad-ĕ-nō'mă) [nephr- + adenoma]. Adenoma of the kidney.

nephralgia (ne-fral'jē-ă) [nephr- + G. *algos,* pain]. Pain in the kidney.

nephralgic (ne-fral'jik). Relating to nephralgia.

nephrasthenia (nef-ras-thē'nē-ă) [nephr- + G. *asthenia,* weakness]. Obsolete term for a mild nephrosis, a condition of imperfect functioning of the kidney, giving rise to slight urinary signs, but without actual disease of the renal tubules.

nephratonia, nephratony (nef-ră-tō'nē-ă, -frat'ō-nē) [nephr- + G. *a-* priv. + *tonos,* tension]. Obsolete term for diminished functional activity of the kidneys.

nephrectasis, nephrectasia (ne-frek'tă-sis, ne-frek-tā'zē-ă) [nephr- + G. *ektasis,* a stretching]. Obsolete term for dilation or distention of the pelvis of the kidney.

nephrectomy (ne-frek'tō-mē) [nephr- + G. *ektomē,* excision]. Removal of a kidney.

abdominal n., anterior n.; removal of the kidney by an incision through the anterior abdominal wall; performed by either a transperitoneal or extraperitoneal technique.

anterior n., abdominal n.

lumbar n., n. through an incision in the flank or loin, usually with the patient in the lateral position.

paraperitoneal n., n. performed by an extraperitoneal incision.

posterior n., retroperitoneal removal of a kidney through an incision in the posterior lumbar muscles, usually with the patient in a prone position.

nephredema (nef-re-dē'mă) [nephr- + G. *oidēma,* swelling]. Edema caused by renal disease; rarely, edema of the kidney.

nephrelcosis (nef-rel-kō'sis) [nephr- + G. *helkōsis,* ulceration]. Ulceration of the mucous membrane of the pelvis or calices of the kidney.

nephric (nef'rik). Renal; relating to the kidney.

nephridium, pl. **nephridia** (ne-frid'ē-ŭm, -ă) [G. *nephridios,* relating to the kidney]. One of the paired, segmentally arranged excretory tubules of invertebrates such as the annelids.

nephritic (ne-frit'ik). Relating to or suffering from nephritis.

nephritis, pl. **nephritides** (ne-frī'tis, -frit'i-dēz) [nephr- + G. *-itis,* inflammation]. Inflammation of the kidneys.

acute n., acute *glomerulonephritis.*

acute interstitial n., interstitial n. with variable tubular damage and infiltration by numerous neutrophils, due to bacterial infection, urinary tract obstruction, or other causes (including drugs) which may be hypersensitivity reactions; accompanied by renal failure, fever, blood or tissue eosinophilia, and rash.

analgesic n., analgesic nephropathy; chronic interstitial n. with renal papillary necrosis, occurring in patients with a long history of excessive consumption of analgesics, especially those containing phenacetin.

anti-basement membrane n., glomerulonephritis produced by autologous or heterologous antibodies to the glomerular capillary basement membranes, the latter known as anti-kidney serum n.

anti-kidney serum n., experimental glomerulonephritis produced by injection of antiserum to kidney.

chronic n., chronic *glomerulonephritis.*

Ellis types 1 and 2 n., Ellis types 1 and 2 *glomerulonephritis.*

focal n., focal *glomerulonephritis.*

glomerular n., glomerulonephritis.

n. gravida'rum, n. developing in pregnancy.

hemorrhagic n., acute glomerulonephritis accompanied by hematuria.

hereditary n., familial renal disease progressing to chronic renal failure, especially in males; associated with nerve deafness.

immune complex n., an immune complex disease resulting from glomerular deposits, as in systemic lupus erythematosus.

interstitial n., a form of n. in which the interstitial connective tissue is chiefly affected.

lupus n., glomerulonephritis occurring in some patients with systemic lupus erythematosus, characterized by hematuria and a progressive course culminating in renal failure, often without hypertension; sometimes also applied to the nephrotic syndrome in patients with systemic lupus. Renal biopsies in patients with a progressive course show diffuse proliferative glomerulonephritis; in milder cases, there are focal proliferative glomerular lesions or mesangial nephritis.

Masugi's n., glomerulonephritis produced by injecting into rats a rabbit antiserum prepared against rat kidney tissue suspensions.
mesangial n., glomerulonephritis with an increase in glomerular mesangial cells or matrix, or mesangial deposits.

salt-losing n., Thorn's syndrome; a rare disorder resulting from renal tubular damage of unknown etiology; mimics adrenocortical insufficiency in that abnormal renal loss of sodium chloride occurs, accompanied by hyponatremia, azotemia, acidosis, dehydration, and vascular collapse.
scarlatinal n., acute glomerulonephritis occurring as a complication of scarlet fever.
serum n., glomerulonephritis occurring in serum sickness or in animals injected with foreign serum protein.
subacute n., subacute *glomerulonephritis.*
suppurative n., focal glomerulonephritis with abscess formation in the kidney.
syphilitic n., a rare complication of congenital and secondary syphilis, with the nephrotic syndrome, resulting from glomerular immune-complex deposits.
transfusion n., renal failure and tubular damage resulting from the transfusion of incompatible blood; the hemoglobin of the hemolyzed red cells is deposited as casts in the renal tubules.
trench n., obsolete term for glomerulonephritis occurring in soldiers subjected to cold and damp conditions in trenches.
tuberculous n., n., mainly interstitial, due to the tubercle bacillus.
tubulointerstitial n., n. affecting renal tubules and interstitial tissue, with infiltration by plasma cells and mononuclear cells; seen in lupus n., allograft rejection, and methicillin sensitization.
uranium n., an experimental n. produced by the administration of uranium nitrate.

nephritogenic (nef'ri-tō-jen'ik) [nephritis + G. *genesis,* production]. Causing nephritis; said of conditions or agents.

nephro-, nephr- [G. *nephros,* kidney]. Combining forms denoting the kidney. See also reno-.

nephroblastema (nef'rō-blas-tē'mă) [nephro- + G. *blastema,* a sprout]. Nephric *blastema.*

nephroblastoma (nef'rō-blas-tō'mă). Wilms' *tumor.*

nephrocalcinosis (nef'rō-kal-si-nō'sis) [nephro- + calcinosis]. A form of renal lithiasis characterized by diffusely scattered foci of calcification in the kidneys; deposits of calcium phosphate, calcium oxalate monohydrate, and similar compounds are usually demonstrable radiologically.

nephrocapsectomy (nef'rō-kap-sek'tō-mē) [nephro- + L. *capsula,* a small box, + G. *ektomē,* excision]. Obsolete operation for decortication, or decapsulation, of the kidney.

nephrocardiac (nef'rō-kar'dē-ak) [nephro- + G. *kardia,* heart]. Cardiorenal.

nephrocele (nef'rō-sēl). **1** [nephro- + G. *kēlē,* hernia]. Hernial displacement of a kidney. **2** [nephro- + G. *koilōma,* a hollow (celom)]. Nephrotomic cavity; nephrocelom; in lower vertebrates, the developmental cavity connecting the myocele with the celom.

nephrocelom (nef-rō-sē'lom) [nephro- + G. *koilōma,* a hollow (celom)]. Nephrocele (2).

nephrocystosis (nef'rō-sis-tō'sis) [nephro- + G. *kystis,* cyst, + *-osis,* condition]. Formation of renal cysts.

nephrogenetic, nephrogenic (nef'rō-jĕ-net'ik, -jen'ik) [nephro- + G. *genēsis,* origin]. Developing into kidney tissue.

nephrogenous (ne-froj'ĕ-nŭs). Developing from kidney tissue.

nephrogram (nef'rō-gram). Examination of the kidney parenchyma by x-ray after the intravenous injection of a radiopaque substance.

nephrography (ne-frog'ră-fē) [nephro- + G. *graphō,* to write]. Radiography of the kidney.

nephrohydrosis (nef'rō-hī-drō'sis). Hydronephrosis.

nephroid (nef'royd) [nephro- + G. *eidos,* resemblance]. Reniform; kidney-shaped; resembling a kidney.

nephrolith (nef'rō-lith) [nephro- + G. *lithos,* stone]. Renal *calculus.*

nephrolithiasis (nef'rō-li-thī'ă-sis). Presence of renal calculi.

nephrolithotomy (nef'rō-li-thot'ō-mē) [nephro- + G. *lithos,* stone, + *tomē,* incision]. Incision into the kidney for the removal of a renal calculus.

nephrology (ne-frol'ō-jē) [nephro- + G. *logos,* study]. The branch of medical science concerned with medical diseases of the kidneys.

nephrolysin (ne-frol'i-sin). An antibody that causes destruction of the cells of the kidneys, formed in response to the injection of an emulsion of renal substance; it is specific for the species from which the antigen was prepared.

nephrolysis (ne-frol'i-sis) [nephro- + G. *lysis,* dissolution]. **1.** Freeing of the kidney from inflammatory adhesions, with preservation of the capsule. **2.** Destruction of renal cells.

nephrolytic (nef-rō-lit'ik) Nephrotoxic (2); pertaining to, characterized by, or causing nephrolysis.

nephroma (ne-frō'mă) [nephro- + G. *-oma,* tumor]. A tumor arising from renal tissue.
mesoblastic n., Wilms' *tumor.*

nephromalacia (nef'rō-mă-lā'shē-ă) [nephro- + G. *malakia,* softness]. Softening of the kidneys.

nephromegaly (nef-rō-meg'ă-lē) [nephro- + G. *megas,* great]. Extreme hypertrophy of one or both kidneys.

nephromere (nef'rō-mēr) [nephro- + G. *meros,* a part]. That portion of the intermediate mesoderm from which segmented kidney tubules develop.

nephron (nef'ron) [G. *nephros,* kidney]. A long convoluted tubular structure in the kidney, consisting of the renal corpuscle, the proximal convoluted tubule, the nephronic loop, and the distal convoluted tubule. See also uriniferous *tubule.*

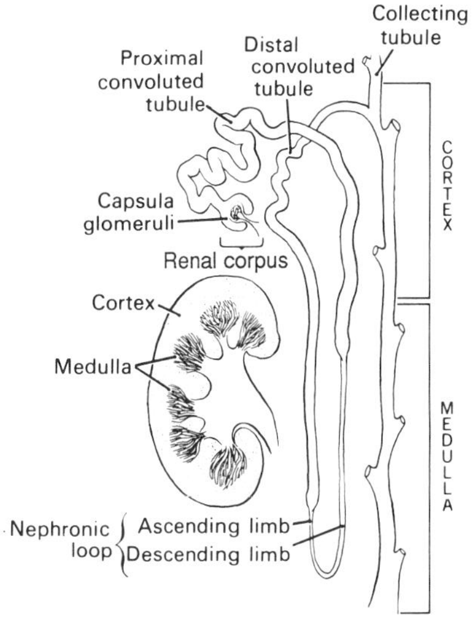

Diagram of the Nephron

nephropathia epidemica (nef-rō-path'ē-ă ep-i-dem'i-kă). A generally benign form of epidemic hemorrhagic fever reported in Scandinavia.

nephropathy (ne-frop'ă-thē) [nephro- + G. *pathos,* suffering]. Nephrosis (1); renopathy; any disease of the kidney.
analgesic n., analgesic *nephritis.*
Balkan n., Danubian endemic familial n.; interstitial chronic nephritis of unknown etiology, originally described as a disease endemic in the Balkans, characterized by insidious onset, scanty urinary findings, anemia, and acidosis.
Danubian endemic familial n., Balkan n.
hypokalemic n., vacuolar nephrosis; vacuolation of the epithelial cytoplasm of renal convoluted tubules in patients seriously depleted of potassium; vacuoles do not contain fat or glycogen, concentrating ability is impaired, polyuria and polydipsia are common, and pyelonephritis may develop.
IgA n., focal *glomerulonephritis.*
IgM n., mesangial proliferative *glomerulonephritis.*

nephropexy (nef'rō-pek-sē) [nephro- + G. *pēxis,* fixation]. Operative fixation of a floating or mobile kidney.

nephrophthisis (nef-rof'thĭ-sis, -tĭ-sis) [nephro- + G. *phthisis,* a wasting]. **1.** Suppurative nephritis with wasting of the substance of the organ. **2.** Tuberculosis of the kidney.
familial juvenile n., cystic *disease* of renal medulla, autosomal recessive type.

nephroptosis, nephroptosia (nef-rop-tō'sis, -tō'sē-ă) [nephro- + G. *ptōsis,* a falling]. Prolapse of the kidney.

nephropyelitis (nef'rō-pī-ĕ-lī'tis). Pyelonephritis.

nephropyeloplasty (nef-rō-pī'el-ō-plas-tē) [nephro- + G. *pyelos,* trough (pelvis), + *plastos,* formed]. Plastic or reparative surgery of the kidney and renal pelvis.

nephropyosis (nef'rō-pī-ō'sis) [nephro- + G. *pyōsis,* suppuration]. Pyonephrosis.

nephrorrhaphy (nef-rōr'ă-fē) [nephro- + G. *raphē,* a suture]. Nephropexy by suturing the kidney.

nephrosclerosis (nef'rō-skle-rō'sis) [nephro- + G. *sklērosis,* hardening]. Induration of the kidney from overgrowth and contraction of the interstitial connective tissue.
arterial n., arterionephrosclerosis; senile n.; patchy atrophic scarring of the kidney due to arteriosclerotic narrowing of the lumens of large branches of the renal artery, occurring in old or hypertensive persons and occasionally causing hypertension.
arteriolar n., arteriolonephrosclerosis; benign n.; renal scarring due to arteriolar sclerosis resulting from longstanding hypertension; the kidneys are finely granular and mildly or moderately contracted, with hyaline thickening of the walls of afferent glomerular arterioles and hyaline scarring of scattered glomeruli; chronic renal failure develops infrequently.
benign n., arteriolar n.
malignant n., the renal changes in malignant hypertension; subcapsular petechiae, necrosis in the walls of scattered afferent glomerular arterioles, and red blood cells and casts in the urine, with uremia as a common termination.
senile n., arterial n.

nephrosclerotic (nef'rō-skle-rot'ik). Pertaining to or causing nephrosclerosis.

nephrosis (ne-frō'sis) [nephro- + G. *-osis,* condition]. **1.** Nephropathy. **2.** Degeneration of renal tubular epithelium. **3.** Nephrotic *syndrome.*
acute n., acute oliguric renal failure, especially that caused by certain poisons.
amyloid n., **(1)** renal *amyloidosis;* **(2)** the nephrotic syndrome due to deposition of amyloid in the kidney.
cholemic n., obsolete term for the occurrence of acute renal failure in jaundiced patients; the kidneys contain tubular casts of bile and may show tubular necrosis, but there is little evidence that jaundice or bile casts directly damage the kidneys.
familial n., the nephrotic syndrome appearing in siblings in infancy, without nerve deafness.
hemoglobinuric n., acute oliguric renal failure associated with hemoglobinuria, due to massive intravascular hemolysis, *e.g.,* following an incompatible blood transfusion; the kidneys show the morphologic changes of hypoxic n.
hypoxic n., acute oliguric renal failure following hemorrhage, burns, shock, or other causes of hypovolemia and reduced renal blood flow; frequently associated with patchy tubular necrosis, tubulorrhexis, and distal tubular casts of hemoglobin.
lipoid n., minimal-change disease; nil disease; idiopathic nephrotic syndrome occurring most commonly in children, in which glomeruli show minimal changes with no thickening of the basement membranes, fat vacuoles in the tubular epithelium, and fusion of glomerular foot processes.
lower nephron n., obsolete term for acute tubular necrosis.
osmotic n., swelling of renal tubular epithelium associated with glomerular filtration of sugars and dextrose; the swelling is due to formation of cytoplasmic vesicles by pinocytosis, and is reversible, probably with no dysfunction, when produced by glucose or mannitol.
toxic n., acute oliguric renal failure due to chemical poisons, septicemia, or bacterial toxemia; frequently associated with extensive necrosis of proximal convoluted tubules.
vacuolar n., hypokalemic *nephropathy.*

nephrospasia, nephrospasis (nef-rō-spā'sē-ă, nef-ros'pă-sis) [nephro- + G. *spasis,* a pulling]. Obsolete term for floating kidney in which the organ is attached only by the blood vessels entering at the hilus.

nephrostogram (ne-fros'tō-gram). A radiograph of the kidney after opacification of the renal pelvis by a contrast agent administered by a nephrostomy tube.

nephrostoma, nephrostome (ne-fros'tō-mă, nef'rō-stōm) [nephro- + G. *stoma,* mouth]. One of the ciliated funnel-shaped openings by which pronephric and some primitive mesonephric tubules communicate with the celom.

nephrostomy (ne-fros'tō-mē) [nephro- + G. *stoma,* mouth]. Establishment of an opening between the pelvis of the kidney through its cortex to the exterior of the body.

nephrotic (nef-rot'ik). Relating to, caused by, or similar to nephrosis.

nephrotome (nef'rō-tōm) [nephro- + G. *tomē,* a cutting]. The intermediate mesoderm, sometimes so designated because it evolves into nephric primordia.

nephrotomic (nef-rō-tom'ik). Relating to the nephrotome.

nephrotomogram (nef-rō-tō'mō-gram). A sectional x-ray examination of the kidneys following the intravenous administration of water-soluble iodinated contrast material for the purpose of improving visualization of renal parenchymal abnormalities.

nephrotomography (nef'rō-tō-mog'ră-fē). X-ray examination of the kidney by tomography.

nephrotomy (ne-frot'ō-mē) [nephro- + G. *tomē,* incision]. Incision into the kidney.
anatrophic n., Smith-Boyce operation; an incision into the posterolateral renal parenchyma, gaining access to the calyceal system through an avascular plane between anterior and posterior branches of the renal artery; used for removal of calyceal and branched renal calculi, with maximum exposure yet minimal bleeding or parenchymal damage.

nephrotoxic (nef-rō-tok′sik) **1.** Pertaining to nephrotoxin; toxic to renal cells. **2.** Nephrolytic.

nephrotoxicity (nef′rō-tok-sis′i-tē). The quality or state of being toxic to kidney cells.

nephrotoxin (nef-rō-tok′sin). A cytotoxin that is specific for cells of the kidney.

nephrotrophic (nef-rō-trof′ik). Renotrophic.

nephrotropic (nef-rō-trop′ik). Renotrophic.

nephrotuberculosis (nef′rō-tū-ber-kyū-lō′sis). Tuberculosis of the kidney.

nephroureterectomy (nef′rō-yū-rē′ter-ek′tō-mē) [nephro- + ureter + G. *ektomē*, excision]. Surgical removal of a kidney and its ureter.

nephroureterocystectomy (nef′rō-yū-rē′ter-ō-sis-tek′tō-mē) [nephro- + ureter + G. *kystis*, bladder, + *ektomē*, excision]. Removal of kidney, ureter, and part or all of the bladder.

nepiology (nep-ē-ol′ō-jē) [G. *nepios* (adj.), infant, + *logos*, study]. Obsolete term for neonatology.

neptunium (nep-tū′nē-ŭm) [planet, *Neptune*]. A radioactive element; symbol Np, atomic no. 93; first element of the transuranian series (not found in nature).

Néri's sign. See under sign.

neriine (nē′ri-ēn). Conessine.

Nernst, Walther, Berlin physicist, 1864–1941. See N.'s *equation, theory.*

NERVE

nerve (nerv) [L. nervus]. A cordlike structure composed of one or more fascicles of myelinated or unmyelinated n. fibers, or more often mixtures of both, together with connective tissue within the fascicle and around the neurolemma of individual n. fibers (endoneurium), around each fascicle (perineurium), and around the entire n. and its nourishing blood vessels (epineurium). For gross anatomical description, see nervus.

abducent n., *nervus* abducens.
accelerator n.'s, the slender n.'s establishing the sympathetic innervation of the heart; originating from ganglion cells of the superior, middle, and inferior cervical ganglion of the sympathetic trunk, hence unmyelinated, the efferent fibers of the accelerator n.'s upon stimulation increase the heart rate.
accessory n., *nervus* accessorius.
accessory phrenic n.'s, *nervi* phrenici accessorii.
acoustic n., *nervus* vestibulocochlearis.
afferent n., centripetal or esodic n.; a n. conveying impulses from the periphery to the central nervous system.
Andersch's n., *nervus* tympanicus.
anococcygeal n.'s, *nervi* anococcygei.
anterior ampullar n., *nervus* ampullaris anterior.
anterior antebrachial n., *nervus* interosseus anterior.
anterior auricular n.'s, *nervi* auriculares anteriores.
anterior crural n., *nervus* femoralis.
anterior ethmoidal n., *nervus* ethmoidalis anterior.
anterior interosseous n., *nervus* interosseus anterior.
anterior labial n.'s, *nervi* labiales anteriores.
anterior scrotal n.'s, *nervi* scrotales anteriores.
anterior supraclavicular n., *nervus* supraclavicularis medialis.
anterior tibial n., *nervus* peroneus profundus.
aortic n., depressor n. of Ludwig; Cyon's n.; Ludwig's n.; a branch of the vagus which ends in the aortic arch and base of the heart; composed entirely of afferent fibers; its stimulation elicits a brainstem reflex which causes slowing of the heart, dilation of the peripheral vessels, and a fall in blood pressure.
Arnold's n., *ramus* auricularis vagi.
articular n., *nervus* articularis.
auditory n., *nervus* cochlearis.
augmentor n.'s, accelerator n.'s, called augmentor because their action is to increase the force as well as the rate of the heart beat.
auriculotemporal n., *nervus* auriculotemporalis.
autonomic n., a bundle of nerve fibers belonging or relating to the autonomic nervous system.
axillary n., *nervus* axillaris.
baroreceptor n., pressoreceptor n.
Bell's respiratory n., *nervus* thoracicus longus.
Bock's n., *ramus* pharyngeus.
buccal n., *nervus* buccalis.
buccinator n., *nervus* buccalis.
caroticotympanic n., *nervus* caroticotympanicus.
carotid sinus n., *ramus* sinus carotici.
cavernous n.'s of clitoris, *nervi* cavernosi clitoridis.
cavernous n.'s of penis, *nervi* cavernosi penis.
centrifugal n., efferent n.
centripetal n., afferent n.
cervical n.'s, *nervi* cervicales.
circumflex n., *nervus* axillaris.
coccygeal n., *nervus* coccygeus.
cochlear n., *nervus* cochlearis.
common fibular n., *nervus* peroneus communis.
common palmar digital n.'s, *nervi* digitales palmares communes.
common peroneal n., *nervus* peroneus communis.
common plantar digital n.'s, *nervi* digitales plantares communes.
cranial n.'s, *nervi* craniales.
cubital n., *nervus* ulnaris.
cutaneous n., *nervus* cutaneus.
cutaneous cervical n., *nervus* transversus colli.
Cyon's n., aortic n.
dead n., misnomer for nonvital dental pulp.
deep fibular n., *nervus* peroneus profundus.
deep peroneal n., *nervus* peroneus profundus.
deep petrosal n., *nervus* petrosus profundus.
deep temporal n.'s, *nervi* temporales profundi.
dental n., **(1)** layman's term for a dental pulp; **(2)** see *nervus* alveolaris inferior, *nervi* alveolares superiores.
depressor n. of Ludwig, aortic n.
dorsal n. of clitoris, *nervus* dorsalis clitoridis.
dorsal digital n.'s, *nervi* digitales dorsales.
dorsal digital n.'s of foot, *nervi* digitales dorsales pedis.
dorsal interosseous n., *nervus* interosseus posterior.
dorsal lateral cutaneous n., *nervus* cutaneus dorsalis lateralis.
dorsal medial cutaneous n., *nervus* cutaneus dorsalis medialis.
dorsal n. of penis, *nervus* dorsalis penis.
dorsal n. of scapula, *nervus* dorsalis scapulae.
dorsal n.'s of toes, *nervi* digitales dorsales pedis.
efferent n., centrifugal or exodic n.; a n. conveying impulses from the central nervous system to the periphery.
eighth cranial n., *nervus* vestibulocochlearis.
eleventh cranial n., *nervus* accessorius.
esodic n., afferent n.
excitor n., a n. conducting impulses that stimulate to increased function.
excitoreflex n., a visceral n. the special function of which is to cause reflex action.
exodic n., efferent n.
n. of external acoustic meatus, *nervus* meatus acustici externi.
external carotid n.'s, *nervi* carotici externi.
external respiratory n. of Bell, *nervus* thoracicus longus.
external saphenous n., *nervus* suralis.

facial n., *nervus* facialis.
femoral n., *nervus* femoralis.
fifth cranial n., *nervus* trigeminus.
first cranial n., *nervi* olfactorii.
fourth cranial n., *nervus* trochlearis.
fourth lumbar n., furcal n.
frontal n., *nervus* frontalis.
furcal n., nervus furcalis; fourth lumbar nerve; the ventral branch of the n. is forked to enter into the formation of both lumbar and sacral plexuses.
Galen's n., Galen's *anastomosis.*
gangliated n., a sympathetic n.
Gaskell's n.'s, rarely used eponym for the accelerator n.'s of the heart.
genitocrural n., *nervus* genitofemoralis.
genitofemoral n., *nervus* genitofemoralis.
glossopharyngeal n., *nervus* glossopharyngeus.
great auricular n., *nervus* auricularis magnus.
great sciatic n., *nervus* ischiadicus.
greater occipital n., *nervus* occipitalis major.
greater palatine n., *nervus* palatinus major.
greater petrosal n., *nervus* petrosus major.
greater splanchnic n., *nervus* splanchnicus major.
greater superficial petrosal n., *nervus* petrosus major.
hemorrhoidal n.'s, see *plexus* rectalis superior; *plexus* rectalis medii; *nervi* rectales inferiores.
Hering's sinus n., *ramus* sinus carotici.
hypogastric n., *nervus* hypogastricus.
hypoglossal n., *nervus* hypoglossus.
iliohypogastric n., *nervus* iliohypogastricus.
ilioinguinal n., *nervus* ilioinguinalis.
inferior alveolar n., *nervus* alveolaris inferior.
inferior cervical cardiac n., *nervus* cardiacus cervicalis inferior.
inferior cluneal n.'s, *nervi* clunium inferiores.
inferior dental n., *nervus* alveolaris inferior.
inferior gluteal n., *nervus* gluteus inferior.
inferior hemorrhoidal n.'s, *nervi* rectales inferiores.
inferior laryngeal n., *nervus* laryngeus inferior.
inferior maxillary n., *nervus* mandibularis.
inferior rectal n.'s, *nervi* rectales inferiores.
inferior vesical n.'s, several small n.'s passing from the pudendal plexus to the bladder.
infraorbital n., *nervus* infraorbitalis.
infratrochlear n., *nervus* infratrochlearis.
inhibitory n., a n. conveying impulses that diminish functional activity in a part.
intercostal n.'s, *nervi* intercostales.
intercostobrachial n.'s, *nervi* intercostobrachiales.
intercostohumeral n.'s, *nervi* intercostobrachiales.
intermediary n., *nervus* intermedius.
intermediate n., *nervus* intermedius.
intermediate dorsal cutaneous n., *nervus* cutaneus dorsalis intermedius.
intermediate supraclavicular n., *nervus* supraclavicularis intermedius.
internal carotid n., *nervus* caroticus internus.
internal saphenous n., *nervus* saphenus.
interosseous n. of leg, *nervus* interosseus cruris.
Jacobson's n., *nervus* tympanicus.
jugular n., *nervus* jugularis.
lacrimal n., *nervus* lacrimalis.
Latarget's n., *plexus* hypogastricus superior.
lateral ampullar n., *nervus* ampullaris lateralis.
lateral anterior thoracic n., *nervus* pectoralis lateralis.
lateral cutaneous n. of calf, *nervus* cutaneus surae lateralis.
lateral cutaneous n. of forearm, *nervus* cutaneus antebrachii lateralis.
lateral cutaneous n. of thigh, *nervus* cutaneus femoris lateralis.
lateral pectoral n., *nervus* pectoralis lateralis.
lateral plantar n., *nervus* plantaris lateralis.
lateral popliteal n., *nervus* peroneus communis.
lateral supraclavicular n., *nervus* supraclavicularis lateralis.
lesser internal cutaneous n., *nervus* cutaneus brachii medialis.
lesser occipital n., *nervus* occipitalis minor.
lesser palatine n.'s, *nervi* palatini minores.
lesser petrosal n., *nervus* petrosus minor.
lesser splanchnic n., *nervus* splanchnicus minor.
lesser superficial petrosal n., *nervus* petrosus minor.
lingual n., *nervus* lingualis.
long buccal n., *nervus* buccalis.
long ciliary n., *nervus* ciliaris longus.
long saphenous n., *nervus* saphenus.
long subscapular n., *nervus* thoracodorsalis.
long thoracic n., *nervus* thoracicus longus.
lower lateral cutaneous n. of arm, *nervus* cutaneus brachii lateralis inferior.
lowest splanchnic n., *nervus* splanchnicus imus.
Ludwig's n., aortic n.
lumbar n.'s, *nervi* lumbales.
lumbar splanchnic n.'s, *nervi* splanchnici lumbales.
lumboinguinal n., femoral branch of genitofemoral n. See *nervus* genitofemoralis.
mandibular n., *nervus* mandibularis.
masseteric n., *nervus* massetericus.
masticator n., *radix* motoria nervi trigemini.
maxillary n., *nervus* maxillaris.
medial anterior thoracic n., *nervus* pectoralis medialis.
medial cutaneous n. of arm, *nervus* cutaneus brachii medialis.
medial cutaneous n. of forearm, *nervus* cutaneus antebrachii medialis.
medial cutaneous n. of leg, *nervus* cutaneus surae medialis.
medial pectoral n., *nervus* pectoralis medialis.
medial plantar n., *nervus* plantaris medialis.
medial popliteal n., *nervus* tibialis.
medial supraclavicular n., *nervus* supraclavicularis medialis.
median n., *nervus* medianus.
mental n., *nervus* mentalis.
middle cervical cardiac n., *nervus* cardiacus cervicalis medius.
middle cluneal n.'s, *nervi* clunium medii.
middle meningeal n., *ramus* meningeus medius nervi maxillaris.
middle supraclavicular n., *nervus* supraclavicularis intermedius.
mixed n., a n. containing both afferent and efferent fibers.
motor n., an efferent n. conveying an impulse that excites muscular contraction.
motor n. of face, *nervus* facialis.
musculocutaneous n., *nervus* musculocutaneus.
musculocutaneous n. of leg, *nervus* peroneus superficialis.
musculospiral n., *nervus* radialis.
mylohyoid n., *nervus* mylohyoideus.
nasal n., *nervus* nasociliaris.
nasociliary n., *nervus* nasociliaris.
nasopalatine n., *nervus* nasopalatinus.
ninth cranial n., *nervus* glossopharyngeus.
obturator n., *nervus* obturatorius.
oculomotor n., *nervus* oculomotorius.
olfactory n., *nervi* olfactorii.
ophthalmic n., *nervus* ophthalmicus.
optic n., *nervus* opticus.
orbital n., *nervus* zygomaticus.
parasympathetic n., one of the n.'s of the parasympathetic nervous system.
pathetic n., *nervus* trochlearis.
pelvic splanchnic n.'s, *nervi* splanchnici pelvini.
perineal n.'s, *nervi* perineales.

peroneal communicating n., *ramus* communicans peroneus.
phrenic n., *nervus* phrenicus.
pneumogastric n., *nervus* vagus.
popliteal communicating n., *nervus* cutaneus surae medialis.
posterior ampullar n., *nervus* ampullaris posterior.
posterior antebrachial n., *nervus* interosseus posterior.
posterior auricular n., *nervus* auricularis posterior.
posterior cutaneous n. of arm, *nervus* cutaneus brachii posterior.
posterior cutaneous n. of forearm, *nervus* cutaneus antebrachii posterior.
posterior cutaneous n. of thigh, *nervus* cutaneus femoris posterior.
posterior ethmoidal n., *nervus* ethmoidalis posterior.
posterior interosseous n., *nervus* interosseus posterior.
posterior labial n.'s, *nervi* labiales posteriores.
posterior scapular n., *nervus* dorsalis scapulae.
posterior scrotal n.'s, *nervi* scrotales posteriores.
posterior supraclavicular n., *nervus* supraclavicularis lateralis.
posterior thoracic n., *nervus* thoracicus longus.
presacral n., *plexus* hypogastrica superior.
pressor n., an afferent n., stimulation of which excites a reflex vasoconstriction, thereby raising the blood pressure.
pressoreceptor n., baroreceptor n.; a n. composed of afferent fibers the endings of which are sensitive to increases in mechanical pressure; the term specifically refers to sensory n.'s innervating the walls of hollow organs.
proper palmar digital n.'s, *nervi* digitales palmares proprii.
proper plantar digital n.'s, *nervi* digitales plantares proprii.
pterygoid n., *nervus* pterygoideus.
n. of pterygoid canal, *nervus* canalis pterygoidei.
pterygopalatine n.'s, *rami* ganglionares.
pudendal n., *nervus* pudendus.
pudic n., *nervus* pudendus.
radial n., *nervus* radialis.
recurrent n., *nervus* laryngeus recurrens.
recurrent laryngeal n., *nervus* laryngeus recurrens.
recurrent meningeal n., *ramus* meningeus medius nervi maxillaris.
n. to rhomboid, *nervus* dorsalis scapulae.
saccular n., *nervus* saccularis.
sacral n.'s, *nervi* sacrales.
sacral splanchnic n.'s, *nervi* splanchnici sacrales.
saphenous n., *nervus* saphenus.
sciatic n., *nervus* ischiadicus.
second cranial n., *nervus* opticus.
secretory n., a n. conveying impulses that excite functional activity in a gland.
sensory n., an afferent n. conveying impulses that are processed by the central nervous system so as to become part of the organism's perception of self and its environment.
seventh cranial n., *nervus* facialis.
short ciliary n., *nervus* ciliaris brevis.
short saphenous n., *nervus* suralis.
sinus n. of Hering, *ramus* sinus carotici.
sinuvertebral n., *ramus* meningeus nervorum spinalium.
sixth cranial n., *nervus* abducens.
small deep petrosal n., *nervus* caroticotympanicus.
smallest splanchnic n., *nervus* splanchnicus imus.
small sciatic n., *nervus* cutaneus femoris posterior.
n. of smell, *nervi* olfactorii.
somatic n., one of the n.'s of sensation or motion, as distinguished from the trophic and secretory n.'s.
space n., one of the branches of the vestibulocochlear n. distributed to the semicircular canals.
spinal n.'s, *nervi* spinales.
spinal accessory n., *nervus* accessorius.
splanchnic n., one of the n.'s supplying the viscera. See *nervus* splanchnicus imus, major, and minor; *nervi* splanchnici lumbales, pelvini, and sacrales.
n. to stapedius muscle, *nervus* stapedius.
subclavian n., *nervus* subclavius.
subcostal n., *nervus* subcostalis.
sublingual n., *nervus* sublingualis.
suboccipital n., *nervus* suboccipitalis.
subscapular n., *nervus* subscapularis.
superficial cervical n., *nervus* transversus colli.
superficial fibular n., *nervus* peroneus superficialis.
superficial peroneal n., *nervus* peroneus superficialis.
superior alveolar n.'s, *nervi* alveolares superiores.
superior cervical cardiac n., *nervus* cardiacus cervicalis superior.
superior cluneal n.'s, *nervi* clunium superiores.
superior dental n.'s, *nervi* alveolares superiores.
superior gluteal n., *nervus* gluteus superior.
superior laryngeal n., *nervus* laryngeus superior.
superior maxillary n., *nervus* maxillaris.
supraorbital n., *nervus* supraorbitalis.
suprascapular n., *nervus* suprascapularis.
supratrochlear n., *nervus* supratrochlearis.
sural n., *nervus* suralis.
sympathetic n., one of the n.'s of the sympathetic nervous system.
temporomandibular n., *nervus* zygomaticus.
n. of tensor tympani muscle, *nervus* tensoris tympani.
n. of tensor veli palatini muscle, *nervus* tensoris veli palatini.
tenth cranial n., *nervus* vagus.
tentorial n., *ramus* tentorii.
terminal n.'s, *nervi* terminales.
third cranial n., *nervus* oculomotorius.
third occipital n., *nervus* occipitalis tertius.
thoracic n.'s, *nervi* thoracici.
thoracic cardiac n.'s, *nervi* cardiaci thoracici.
thoracodorsal n., *nervus* thoracodorsalis.
tibial n., *nervus* tibialis.
tibial communicating n., *nervus* cutaneus surae medialis.
Tiedemann's n., a sympathetic n. accompanying the central artery of the retina in the optic n.
transverse n. of neck, *nervus* transversus colli.
trifacial n., *nervus* trigeminus.
trigeminal n., *nervus* trigeminus.
trochlear n., *nervus* trochlearis.
twelfth cranial n., *nervus* hypoglossus.
tympanic n., *nervus* tympanicus.
n. of tympanic membrane, *ramus* membranae tympani.
ulnar n., *nervus* ulnaris.
upper lateral cutaneous n. of arm, *nervus* cutaneus brachii lateralis superior.
utricular n., *nervus* utricularis.
utriculoampullar n., *nervus* utriculoampullaris.
vaginal n.'s, *nervi* vaginales.
vagus n., *nervus* vagus.
Valentin's n., a n. that connects the pterygopalatine ganglion with the abducens n.
vascular n., *nervus* vascularis.
vasomotor n., a motor n. effecting dilation (vasodilator n.) or contraction (vasoconstrictor n.) of the blood vessels.
vertebral n., *nervus* vertebralis.
vestibular n., *nervus* vestibularis.
vestibulocochlear n., *nervus* vestibulocochlearis.
vidian n., *nervus* canalis pterygoidei.
volar interosseous n., *nervus* interosseus anterior.
Wrisberg's n., **(1)** *nervus* cutaneus brachii medialis; **(2)** *nervus* intermedius.
zygomatic n., *nervus* zygomaticus.

nervi (ner'vī) [L.] [NA]. Plural of nervus.

nervimotility (ner-vi-mō-til'i-tē). Neurimotility; capability of movement in response to a nervous stimulus.

nervimotion (ner-vi-mō'shŭn). Movement in response to a nervous stimulus.

nervimotor (ner-vi-mō'ter). Neurimotor; relating to a motor nerve.

nervine (ner'vīn). Acting therapeutically, especially as a sedative, upon the nervous system.

nervone (ner'vōn). A cerebroside containing nervonic acid.

nervonic acid (ner-von'-ik). *cis*-15-Tetracosanoic acid; a 24-carbon straight-chain fatty acid unsaturated between C-15 and C-16; occurs in cerebrosides such as nervone.

nervosism (ner'vō-sizm) [L. *nervosus*, nervous]. **1.** Neurasthenia (1). **2.** Hypothetical dependence of psychiatric conditions upon alterations of nerve force.

nervous (ner'vŭs) [L. *nervosus*]. **1.** Relating to a nerve or the nerves. **2.** Easily excited or agitated; suffering from mental or emotional instability; tense or anxious. **3.** Formerly, denoting a temperament characterized by excessive mental and physical alertness, rapid pulse, excitability, often volubility, but not always fixity of purpose.

nervous breakdown. Nonmedical term for an emotional or mental illness; often a euphemism for a psychiatric disorder.

nervousness (ner'vŭs-nes). A condition of being nervous (2).

NERVUS

nervus, gen. and pl. **nervi** (ner'vŭs, -vī) [L.] [NA]. Nerve; a whitish cord, made up of nerve fibers arranged in bundles (fascicles) held together by a connective tissue sheath, by which stimuli are transmitted from the central nervous system to a part of the body or the reverse. Nerve branches are given in the definition of the major nerve; many are also listed and defined under ramus. For a histological description, see nerve.

n. abdu'cens [NA], abducent nerve; sixth cranial nerve; a small motor nerve supplying the lateral rectus muscle of the eye; its origin is in the dorsal part of the tegmentum of the pons just below the surface of the rhomboid fossa, and it emerges from the brain in the fissure between the medulla oblongata and the posterior border of the pons; it passes through the cavernous sinus and enters the orbit through the superior orbital fissure.

n. accesso'rius [NA], accessory nerve; spinal accessory nerve; eleventh cranial nerve; accessorius willisii; arises by two sets of roots: cranial, emerging from the side of the medulla, and spinal, emerging from the ventrolateral part of the first five cervical segments of the spinal cord; these roots unite to form the accessory nerve trunk, which divides into two rami, internal and external; the internal ramus, carrying fibers of the cranial root, unites with the vagus in the jugular foramen and supplies the muscles of the pharynx, larynx, and soft palate; the external ramus continues independently through the jugular foramen to supply the sternocleidomastoid and trapezius muscles.

n. acu'sticus, n. vestibulocochlearis.

n. alveola'ris infe'rior [NA], inferior alveolar nerve; inferior dental nerve; one of the terminal branches of the mandibular, it enters the mandibular canal to be distributed to the lower teeth, periosteum, and gingiva of the mandible; a branch, the mental nerve, passes through the mental foramen to supply the skin of the lower lip and chin.

ner'vi alveola'res superio'res [NA], superior alveolar nerves; superior dental nerves; three branches (posterior, middle, and anterior) of the maxillary nerve that enter the maxilla to supply the upper teeth and gingiva.

n. ampulla'ris ante'rior [NA], anterior ampullar nerve; a branch of the utriculoampullar nerve that supplies the crista ampullaris of the anterior semicircular duct.

n. ampulla'ris latera'lis [NA], lateral ampullar nerve; a branch of the utriculoampullar nerve that supplies the crista ampullaris of the lateral semicircular duct.

n. ampulla'ris poste'rior [NA], posterior ampullar nerve; a branch of the vestibular part of the eighth nerve that supplies the crista ampullaris of the posterior semicircular duct.

ner'vi anococcyg'ei [NA], anococcygeal nerves; several small nerves arising from the coccygeal plexus, supplying the skin over the coccyx.

n. antebra'chii ante'ior [NA], official alternative term for n. interosseus anterior.

n. antebra'chii poste'rior [NA], official alternative term for n. interosseus posterior.

n. articula'ris [NA], articular nerve; a branch of a nerve supplying a joint.

ner'vi auricula'res anterio'res [NA], anterior auricular nerves; branches of the auriculotemporal nerve that supply the tragus and upper part of the auricle.

n. auricula'ris mag'nus [NA], great auricular nerve; arises from the second and third cervical, supplies the skin of part of the ear, adjacent portion of the scalp, cheek, and angle of the jaw.

n. auricula'ris poste'rior [NA], posterior auricular nerve; the first extracranial branch of the facial nerve; it passes behind the ear, supplying the auricularis posterior and intrinsic muscles of the auricle and, through its occipital branch, innervating the occipital belly of the occipitofrontal muscle.

n. auriculotempora'lis [NA], auriculotemporal nerve; a branch of the mandibular, usually by two roots embracing the middle meningeal artery; it passes through the parotid gland, terminating in the skin of the temple and scalp, and sends branches to the external acoustic meatus, tympanic membrane, parotid gland and auricle as well as a communicating branch to the facial nerve.

n. axilla'ris [NA], axillary nerve; circumflex nerve; arises from the posterior cord of the brachial plexus in the axilla, passes downward and laterally with the posterior circumflex artery, and winds round the surgical neck of the humerus supplying the deltoid and teres minor muscles.

n. bucca'lis [NA], buccal nerve; buccinator nerve; long buccal nerve; a sensory branch of the mandibular division of the trigeminal nerve; it passes downward and forward on the buccinator muscle to supply the buccal mucous membrane and skin of the cheek near the angle of the mouth.

n. cana'lis pterygoi'dei [NA], nerve of pterygoid canal; vidian nerve; radix facialis; facial root; the nerve constituting the motor and sympathetic roots of the pterygopalatine ganglion; it is formed in the foramen lacerum by the union of the greater petrosal and the deep petrosal nerves, and runs through the pterygoid canal to the pterygopalatine fossa.

ner'vi cardi'aci thora'cici [NA], thoracic cardiac nerves; branches from the second to fifth segments of the thoracic sympathetic trunk that pass forward to enter the cardiac plexus.

n. cardi'acus cervica'lis infe'rior [NA], inferior cervical cardiac nerve; a nerve passing from the cervicothoracic ganglion to the cardiac plexus.

n. cardi'acus cervica'lis me'dius [NA], middle cervical cardiac nerve; a bundle of fibers running downward, from the middle cervical ganglion along the subclavian artery (on the left) or the brachiocephalic (on the right side) to join the cardiac plexus.

n. cardi'acus cervica'lis supe'rior [NA], superior cervical cardiac nerve; a nerve which arises from the lower part of the superior cervical ganglion and passes down to form, with branches of the vagus, the cardiac plexus.

ner'vi carot'ici exter'ni [NA], external carotid nerves; a number of sympathetic nerve fibers extending upward from the superior cervical ganglion along the external carotid artery, forming the external carotid plexus.
n. caroticotympan'icus, pl. **ner'vi caroticotympan'ici** [NA], caroticotympanic nerve; small deep petrosal nerve; one of two sympathetic branches from the internal carotid plexus to the tympanic plexus.
n. carot'icus inter'nus [NA], internal carotid nerve; a sympathetic nerve extending upward from the superior cervical ganglion along the internal carotid artery, forming the internal carotid plexus.
ner'vi caverno'si clitor'idis [NA], cavernous nerves or plexus of clitoris; they correspond to the nervi cavernosi penis in the male.
ner'vi caverno'si pe'nis [NA], cavernous nerves or plexus of penis; two nerves, major and minor, derived from the inferior hypogastric plexus supplying sympathetic and parasympathetic fibers to the corpus cavernosum.
ner'vi cervica'les [NA], cervical nerves; nerves whose nuclei of origin are situated in the cervical spinal cord.
n. cervica'lis superficia'lis, n. transversus colli.
n. cilia'ris bre'vis, pl. **ner'vi cilia'res bre'ves** [NA], short ciliary nerve; one of a number of branches of the ciliary ganglion, supplying the ciliary muscles, iris, and tunics of the eyeball.
n. cilia'ris lon'gus, pl. **ner'vi cilia'res lon'gi** [NA], long ciliary nerve; one of two or three branches of the nasociliary nerve, supplying the ciliary muscles, iris, and cornea.
ner'vi clu'nium inferio'res [NA], inferior cluneal nerves, branches of the posterior femoral cutaneous nerve supplying the skin of the lower half of the gluteal region.
ner'vi clu'nium me'dii [NA], middle cluneal nerves; terminal branches of the dorsal rami of the sacral nerves, supplying the skin of the mid-gluteal region.
ner'vi clu'nium superio'res [NA], superior cluneal nerves; terminal branches of the dorsal rami of the lumbar nerves, supplying the skin of the upper half of the gluteal region.
n. coccyg'eus [NA], coccygeal nerve; a small nerve, the lowest of the spinal nerves, entering into the formation of the coccygeal plexus.
n. cochlea'ris [NA], cochlear nerve; pars cochlearis; inferior part of vestibulocochlear nerve; cochlear part of vestibulocochlear nerve; auditory nerve; the part of the vestibulocochlear nerve peripheral to the radix cochlearis; it is composed of the nerve processes which have their terminals on the four rows of neuroepithelial cells (hair cells) and the bipolar neurons of the spiral ganglion. See also *radix* cochlaris.
n. commu'nicans perone'us (fibula'ris), *ramus* communicans peroneus.
ner'vi crania'les [NA], cranial nerves; those nerves that emerge from, or enter, the brain, in contrast to the spinal nerves. The twelve paired cranial nerves are the olfactory, optic, oculomotor, trochlear, trigeminal, abducent, facial, vestibulocochlear, glossopharyngeal, vagal, accessory, and hypoglossal. (For definitions, see the corresponding Latin terms under nervus.)
n. cuta'neus [NA], cutaneous nerve; a mixed nerve supplying a region of the skin, including its blood vessels, smooth muscle and glands.
n. cuta'neus antebra'chii latera'lis [NA], lateral cutaneous nerve of forearm; the terminal cutaneous branch of the musculocutaneous nerve that supplies the skin of the radial side of the forearm.
n. cuta'neus antebra'chii media'lis [NA], medial cutaneous nerve of forearm; arises from the medial cord of the brachial plexus, passes downward in company with the brachial artery and then the basilic vein, and supplies the skin of the anterior and ulnar surfaces of the forearm.
n. cuta'neus antebra'chii poste'rior [NA], posterior cutaneous nerve of forearm; a branch of the radial nerve supplying the skin of the dorsal surface of the forearm.

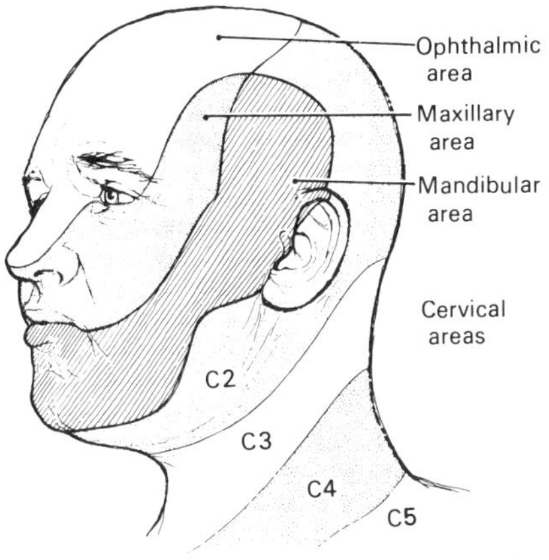

Cutaneous Nerve Supply of the Face

n. cuta'neus bra'chii latera'lis infe'rior [NA], lower lateral cutaneous nerve of arm; a branch of the radial nerve supplying the skin of the lower lateral aspect of the arm; it frequently is a branch of the posterior antebrachial nerve.
n. cuta'neus bra'chii latera'lis supe'rior [NA], upper lateral cutaneous nerve of arm; a branch of the axillary supplying the skin over the lower portion of the deltoid and for a distance below its insertion.
n. cuta'neus bra'chii media'lis [NA], medial cutaneous nerve of arm; lesser internal cutaneous nerve; Wrisberg's nerve (1); arises from the medial cord of the brachial plexus, unites in the axilla with the lateral cutaneous branch of the second intercostal nerve, and supplies the skin of the medial side of the arm.
n. cuta'neus bra'chii poste'rior [NA], posterior cutaneous nerve of arm; a branch of the radial nerve supplying the skin of the posterior surface of the arm.
n. cuta'neus dorsa'lis interme'dius [NA], intermediate dorsal cutaneous nerve; the lateral terminal branch of the superficial peroneal nerve, supplying the dorsum of the foot and dorsal nerves to the toes.
n. cuta'neus dorsa'lis latera'lis [NA], dorsal lateral cutaneous nerve; the continuation of the sural nerve in the foot, supplying the lateral margin and dorsum.
n. cuta'neus dorsa'lis media'lis [NA], dorsal medial cutaneous nerve; the medial terminal branch of the superficial peroneal nerve, supplying the dorsum of the foot and dorsal nerves to the toes.
n. cuta'neus femo'ris latera'lis [NA], lateral cutaneous nerve of thigh; arises from the second and third lumbar nerves, supplies the skin of the anterolateral and lateral surfaces of the thigh.
n. cuta'neus femo'ris poste'rior [NA], posterior cutaneous nerve of thigh; small sciatic nerve; arises from the first three sacral nerves, supplies the skin of the posterior surface of the thigh and of the popliteal region; it gives off a perineal branch that passes to the scrotum or labia majora.
n. cuta'neus su'rae latera'lis [NA], lateral cutaneous nerve of calf; it arises from the common peroneal in the popliteal space and is distributed to the skin of the inferolateral surface of the calf.
n. cuta'neus su'rae media'lis [NA], medial cutaneous nerve of leg; tibial or popliteal communicating nerve; arises from the tibial in the popliteal space, passes down the calf between the two heads of the gastrocnemius and unites in the middle of the leg with the communicating branch of the common peroneal to form the sural nerve, distributed to the skin of the distal and lateral surfaces of the leg and ankle.
ner'vi digita'les dorsa'les [NA], dorsal digital nerves; nerves of the hand supplying the skin of the dorsal surface of the fingers.

ner'vi digita'les dorsa'les pe'dis [NA], dorsal digital nerves of foot; dorsal nerves of toes; nerves of the foot supplying the skin of the proximal and middle phalanges.
ner'vi digita'les palma'res commu'nes [NA], common palmar digital nerves; four nerves in the palm that send branches (nervi digitales palmares proprii) to adjacent sides of two digits; three are branches of the median, one is from the ulnar.
ner'vi digita'les palma'res pro'prii [NA], proper palmar digital nerves; the palmar nerves of the digits of the hand derived from common palmar digital nerves; each nerve supplies a palmar quadrant of a digit and a part of the dorsal surface of the distal phalanx.
ner'vi digita'les planta'res commu'nes [NA], common plantar digital nerves; these include three nerves derived from the medial plantar and one from the lateral plantar that supply the skin of the ball of the foot and terminate as proper plantar digital nerves to the side of each toe.
ner'vi digita'les planta'res pro'prii [NA], proper plantar digital nerves; the ten nerves derived from the common plantar digital nerves; each nerve supplies a plantar quadrant of a toe and part of the dorsal surface of the distal phalanx.
n. dorsa'lis clitor'idis [NA], dorsal nerve of clitoris; the deep terminal branch of the pudendal, supplying especially the glans clitoridis.
n. dorsa'lis pe'nis [NA], dorsal nerve of penis; the deep terminal branch of the pudendal running along the dorsum of the penis, supplying the skin of the penis, the prepuce, and the glans.
n. dorsa'lis scap'ulae [NA], dorsal nerve of scapula; posterior scapular nerve; nerve to rhomboid; arises from the fifth to seventh cervical nerves and passes downward to supply the levator scapulae and the rhomboideus major and minor muscles.
ner'vi erigen'tes, [NA], *nervi* splanchnici pelvini.
n. ethmoida'lis ante'rior [NA], anterior ethmoidal nerve; a branch of the nasociliary nerve.
n. ethmoida'lis poste'rior [NA], posterior ethmoidal nerve; a branch of the nasociliary nerve.
n. facia'lis [NA], facial nerve; seventh cranial nerve; motor nerve of face; its origin is in the tegmentum of the lower portion of the pons, and it emerges from the brain at the posterior border of the pons; it leaves the cranial cavity through the internal acoustic meatus where it is joined by the n. intermedius, traverses the facial canal in the petrous portion of the temporal bone, and makes its exit through the stylomastoid foramen; it passes through the parotid gland and reaches the facial muscles through various branches.
n. femora'lis [NA], femoral nerve; anterior crural nerve; arises from the second, third, and fourth lumbar nerves in the substance of the psoas muscle and enters the thigh lateral to the femoral vessels; it supplies muscles and skin of the anterior region of the thigh.
n. fibula'ris commu'nis [NA], n. peroneus communis.
n. fibula'ris profun'dus [NA], n. peroneus profundus.
n. fibula'ris superficia'lis [NA], n. peroneus superficialis.
n. fronta'lis [NA], frontal nerve; a branch of the ophthalmic nerve which divides within the orbit into the supratrochlear and the supraorbital nerves.
n. furca'lis, furcal *nerve.*
n. genitofemora'lis [NA], genitofemoral nerve; genitocrural nerve; arises from the first and second lumbar nerves, passes distad along the anterior surface of psoas major muscle and divides into genital and femoral branches.
n. glossopharyn'geus [NA], glossopharyngeal nerve; ninth cranial nerve; it emerges from the rostral end of the medulla and passes through the jugular foramen to supply sensation to the pharynx and posterior third of the tongue; it also carries motor fibers to the stylopharyngeus muscle and the parasympathetic fibers to the otic ganglion.
n. glu'teus infe'rior [NA], inferior gluteal nerve; arises from the fifth lumbar and first and second sacral nerves, and supplies the gluteus maximus muscle.
n. glu'teus supe'rior [NA], superior gluteal nerve; arises from the fourth and fifth lumbar and first sacral nerves, and supplies the gluteus medius and minimus and tensor fasciae latae muscles.
n. hemorrhoida'lis, see *plexus* rectalis superior; *plexus* rectales medii; *plexus* rectales inferiores; *nervi* rectales inferiores.
n. hypogas'tricus [NA], hypogastric nerve; one of the two nerve trunks (right and left) which lead from the superior hypogastric plexus into the pelvis to join the inferior hypogastric plexuses.
n. hypoglos'sus [NA], hypoglossal nerve; twelfth cranial nerve; arises from an oblong nucleus in the medulla and emerges by several root filaments between the pyramid and the olive; it passes through the hypoglossal canal, then courses downward and forward to supply the intrinsic and extrinsic muscles of the tongue.
n. iliohypogas'tricus [NA], iliohypogastric nerve; arises from the first lumbar nerve; it supplies the abdominal muscles and the skin of the lower part of the anterior abdominal wall.
n. ilioinguina'lis [NA], ilioinguinal nerve; arises from the first lumbar nerve, passes through the superficial inguinal ring to supply the skin of the upper medial thigh and scrotum or labia majora.
n. im'par, *filum* terminale.
n. infraorbita'lis [NA], infraorbital nerve; the continuation of the maxillary nerve after it has entered the orbit, traversing the infraorbital canal to reach the face; it supplies the upper incisors, canine and premolars, the upper gums, the inferior eyelid and conjunctiva, part of the nose and the superior lip.
n. infratrochlea'ris [NA], infratrochlear nerve; a branch of the nasociliary nerve running beneath the pulley of the superior oblique muscle to the front of the orbit, and supplying the skin of the eyelids and root of the nose.
ner'vi intercosta'les [NA], intercostal nerves; ventral branches of the thoracic nerves.
ner'vi intercostobrachia'les [NA], intercostobrachial or intercostohumeral nerves; branches of the second and third intercostal nerves which pass to the skin of the medial side of the arm.
n. interme'dius [NA], intermediary or intermediate nerve; Wrisberg's nerve (2); pars intermedia (3); portio intermedia; a root of the facial nerve containing sensory fibers whose cell bodies are located in the geniculate ganglion and autonomic fibers whose cell bodies are located in the superior salivatory nucleus.
n. interos'seus ante'rior [NA], anterior interosseous or antebrachial nerve; n. antebrachii anterior; volar interosseous nerve; a branch of the median supplying the flexor pollicis longus, part of flexor digitorum profundus and the pronator quadratus muscles.
n. interos'seus cru'ris [NA], interosseous nerve of leg; a nerve given off from one of the muscular branches of the tibial nerve which passes down over the posterior surface of the interosseous membrane supplying it and the two bones of the leg.
n. interos'seus dorsa'lis, n. interosseus posterior.
n. interos'seus poste'rior [NA], posterior interosseous or antebrachial nerve; n. antebrachii posterior; n. interosseus dorsalis; dorsal interosseous nerve; the deep terminal branch of the radial nerve, supplying the supinator and all the extensor muscles in the forearm.
n. ischia'dicus [NA], sciatic nerve; great sciatic nerve; arises from the sacral plexus, passes through the greater sciatic foramen and down the thigh, at about the middle of which it divides into the common peroneal and tibial nerves.
n. jugula'ris [NA], jugular nerve; a communicating branch between the superior cervical ganglion of the sympathetic nerve, the superior ganglion of the vagus nerve, and the inferior ganglion of the glossopharyngeal nerve.
ner'vi labia'les anterio'res [NA], anterior labial nerves; branches of the ilioinguinal nerve distributed to the labia majora.
ner'vi labia'les posterio'res [NA], posterior labial nerves; terminal branches of the perineal nerve, supplying the skin of the posterior portion of the labia and the vestibule of the vagina, corresponding to the posterior scrotal nerves in the male.

n. lacrima'lis [NA], lacrimal nerve; a branch of the ophthalmic nerve supplying the upper eyelid, conjunctiva, and lacrimal gland.
n. laryn'geus infe'rior [NA], inferior laryngeal nerve; the terminal branch of the recurrent laryngeal nerve; it supplies all laryngeal muscles except the cricothyroid and the mucosa inferior to the vocal folds.
n. laryn'geus recur'rens [NA], recurrent laryngeal nerve; recurrent nerve; a branch of the vagus nerve curving upward, on the right side round the root of the subclavian artery, on the left side round the arch of the aorta, then passing up behind the common carotid artery and between the trachea and the esophagus to the larynx; it supplies cardiac, tracheal, and esophageal branches terminating as the inferior laryngeal nerve.
n. laryn'geus supe'rior [NA], superior laryngeal nerve; a branch of the vagus nerve at the inferior ganglion; at the thyroid cartilage it divides into two branches; the internal laryngeal nerve supplies the mucous membrane of the larynx superior to the vocal folds, and the external laryngeal nerve supplies the inferior pharyngeal constrictor and the cricothyroid muscle.
n. lingua'lis [NA], lingual nerve; one of the branches of the mandibular nerve, passing medial to the lateral pterygoid muscle, between the medial pterygoid and the mandible, and beneath the mucous membrane of the floor of the mouth to the side of the tongue over the anterior two-thirds of which it is distributed: it supplies also the mucous membrane of the floor of the mouth.
ner'vi lumba'les [NA], lumbar nerves; five nerves on each side, emerging from the lumbar portion of the spinal cord; the first four nerves enter into the formation of the lumbar plexus, the fourth and fifth into that of the sacral plexus.
n. mandibula'ris [NA], mandibular nerve; inferior maxillary nerve; the third division of the trigeminal nerve formed by the union of sensory fibers from the trigeminal (gasserian) ganglion and the motor root in the foramen ovale, through which the nerve emerges; its branches are: meningeal, masseteric, deep temporal, lateral and medial pterygoid, buccal, auriculotemporal, lingual, and inferior alveolar.
n. masseter'icus [NA], masseteric nerve; a muscular branch of the mandibular nerve passing to the medial surface of the masseter muscle which it supplies.
n. maxilla'ris [NA], maxillary nerve; superior maxillary nerve; the second division of the trigeminal nerve, passing from the trigeminal (gasserian) ganglion through the foramen rotundum into the pterygopalatine fossa, where it gives off ganglionic branches to the pterygopalatine ganglion and continues forward to give off the zygomatic nerve and enter the orbit, where it is named the infraorbital nerve.
n. mea'tus acus'tici exter'ni [NA], nerve of external acoustic meatus; a branch of the auriculotemporal nerve supplying the lining of the external acoustic meatus.
n. media'nus [NA], median nerve; formed by the union of medial and lateral roots from the medial and lateral cords of the brachial plexus, respectively; it supplies muscular branches in the anterior region of the forearm and muscular and cutaneous branches in the hand.
n. menta'lis [NA], mental nerve; a branch of the inferior alveolar nerve, arising in the mandibular canal and passing through the mental foramen to the chin and lower lip.
n. musculocuta'neus [NA], musculocutaneous nerve; arises from lateral cord of the brachial plexus, passes through the coracobrachialis muscle, and then downward between the brachialis and biceps, supplying these three muscles and being prolonged as the lateral cutaneous nerve of the forearm.
n. mylohyoi'deus [NA], mylohyoid nerve; a small branch of the inferior alveolar nerve given off just before the nerve enters the mandibular foramen, distributed to the anterior belly of the digastric muscle and to the mylohyoid muscle.
n. nasocilia'ris [NA], nasociliary nerve; nasal nerve; a branch of the ophthalmic nerve in the superior orbital fissure, passing through the orbit, entering the cranial cavity through the anterior ethmoidal foramen, and then the nasal cavity, through the nasal fissure; its branches are the communicating branch to the ciliary ganglion, the long ciliary nerves, the infratrochlear, and nasal branches, supplying the mucous membrane of nose, the skin of the tip of the nose, and the conjunctiva.
n. nasopalati'nus [NA], nasopalatine nerve; a branch from the pterygopalatine ganglion, passing through the sphenopalatine foramen, down the nasal septum, and through the incisive foramen to supply the mucous membrane of the hard palate.
ner'vi nervo'rum, nerves distributed to the sheaths of nerve trunks.
n. obturato'rius [NA], obturator nerve; arises from the second, third, and fourth lumbar nerves in the psoas muscle, crosses the brim of the pelvis, and enters the thigh through the obturator canal; it supplies muscles and skin on the medial side of the thigh.
n. occipita'lis ma'jor [NA], greater occipital nerve; medial branch of the dorsal ramus of the second cervical nerve; sends branches to the semispinalis capitis and multifidus cervicis, but is mainly cutaneous, supplying the back part of the scalp.
n. occipita'lis mi'nor [NA], lesser occipital nerve; arises from the ventral rami of the second and third cervical nerves; supplies the skin of the posterior surface of the pinna and the adjacent portion of the scalp.
n. occipita'lis ter'tius [NA], third occipital nerve; medial branch of the dorsal ramus of the third cervical nerve; this is usually joined with the greater occipital, but may exist as an independent nerve supplying cutaneous branches to the scalp and nucha.
n. octa'vus, n. vestibulocochlearis.
n. oculomoto'rius [NA], oculomotor nerve; oculomotorious; third cranial nerve; motor oculi; it supplies all the extrinsic muscles of the eye, except the lateral rectus and superior oblique; it also supplies the levator palpebrae superioris, the ciliary muscle, and the sphincter pupillae; its origin is in the midbrain below the cerebral aqueduct; it emerges from the brain in the interpeduncular fossa, pierces the dura mater to the side of the posterior clinoid process, passes in the lateral wall of the cavernous sinus and enters the orbit through the superior orbital fissure.
ner'vi olfacto'rii [NA], olfactory nerve; first cranial nerve; nerve of smell; fila olfactoria; collective term denoting the numerous olfactory filaments: slender fascicles each composed of the thin, unmyelinated axons of 8 to 12 of the bipolar olfactory receptor cells in the olfactory portion of the nasal mucosa; the olfactory filaments pass through the cribriform plate of the ethmoid bone and enter the olfactory bulb, where they terminate in synaptic contact with mitral cells, tufted cells, and granule cells. See also *tractus* olfactorius.
n. ophthal'micus [NA], ophthalmic nerve; a branch of the trigeminal nerve that passes forward from the trigeminal ganglion in the lateral wall of the cavernous sinus, entering the orbit through the superior orbital fissure; through its branches, frontal, lacrimal, and nasociliary, it supplies sensation to the orbit and its contents, the anterior part of the nasal cavity, and the skin of the nose and forehead.
n. op'ticus [NA], optic nerve; second cranial nerve; originating from the ganglion cells of the retina, it passes out of the orbit through the optic canal to the chiasm, where part of the fibers cross to the opposite side and pass through the optic tract to the geniculate bodies, superior colliculus, and the pretectum.
n. palati'nus ma'jor [NA], greater palatine nerve; a branch of the pterygopalatine ganglion that passes downward through the greater palatine canal to supply the mucosa and glands of the hard palate, and the anterior part of the soft palate.
ner'vi palati'ni mino'res [NA], lesser palatine nerves; usually two, these nerves emerge through the lesser palatine foramina and supply the mucosa and glands of the soft palate and uvula; they are

branches of the pterygopalatine ganglion and contain sensory fibers of the maxillary and facial nerves.
n. pectora'lis lateral'is [NA], lateral pectoral nerve; lateral anterior thoracic nerve; a nerve that arises from the lateral cord of the brachial plexus to supply the pectoral muscles.
n. pectoral'is medial'is [NA], medial pectoral nerve; medial anterior thoracic nerve; a nerve that arises from the medial cord of the brachial plexus to supply the pectoral muscles.
ner'vi perinea'les [NA], perineal nerves; the superficial terminal branches of the pudendal nerve, supplying most of the muscles of the perineum as well as the skin of that region.
n. perone'us commu'nis [NA], common peroneal or fibular nerve; lateral popliteal nerve; n. fibularis communis; one of the terminal divisions of the sciatic nerve, passing through the lateral portion of the popliteal space to opposite the head of the fibula where it divides into the superficial and deep peroneal nerves.
n. perone'us profun'dus [NA], deep peroneal or fibular nerve; anterior tibial nerve; n. fibularis profundus; one of the terminal branches of the common peroneal nerve, passing into the anterior compartment of the leg; it supplies the tibialis anterior, extensor hallucis longus, extensor digitorum longus, and peroneus tertius muscles, and also the skin of the great toe and medial surface of the second toe.
n. perone'us superficia'lis [NA], superficial peroneal or fibular nerve; musculocutaneous nerve of leg; n. fibularis superficialis; a branch of the common peroneal nerve which passes downward in front of the fibula to supply the long and short peroneal muscles and terminate in the skin of the dorsum of the foot and toes.
n. petro'sus ma'jor [NA], greater petrosal nerve; greater superficial petrosal nerve; the parasympathetic root of the pterygopalatine ganglion; a branch from the knee of the facial nerve running through a canal and groove on the anterior surface of the petrous part of the temporal bone beside the foramen lacerum through the pterygoid canal to reach the pterygopalatine ganglion.
n. petro'sus mi'nor [NA], lesser petrosal nerve; lesser superficial petrosal nerve; the parasympathetic root of the otic ganglion, derived from the tympanic plexus; it leaves the tympanic cavity through the canal for the lesser petrosal nerve and passes within the cranium to the sphenopetrosal fissure, or to the foramen ovale, or to the petrosal foramen through which it reaches the otic ganglion.
n. petro'sus profun'dus [NA], deep petrosal nerve; great deep petrosal branch of the carotid plexus; the sympathetic part of the nerve of the pterygoid canal; it arises from the internal carotid plexus and joins the greater petrosal nerve at the entrance of the pterygoid canal.
n. pharyn'geus, *ramus* pharyngeus.
ner'vi phren'ici accesso'rii [NA], accessory phrenic nerves; accessory nerve strands that arise from the fifth cervical nerve, often as branches of the nerve to the subclavius, passing downward to join the phrenic nerve.
n. phren'icus [NA], phrenic nerve; arises from the cervical plexus, chiefly from the fourth cervical nerve, passes downward in front of the anterior scalene muscle and enters the thorax between the subclavian artery and vein behind the sternoclavicular articulation; it then passes in front of the root of the lung to the diaphragm; it is mainly the motor nerve of the diaphragm but sends sensory fibers to the pericardium (ramus pericardiacus), and branches (rami phrenicoabdominales) that communicate with branches from the celiac plexus.
n. planta'ris latera'lis [NA], lateral plantar nerve; one of the two terminal branches of the tibial nerve; it courses along the lateral side of the sole, dividing into superficial and deep branches; it supplies the skin of the lateral aspect of the sole and the lateral one and one-half toes; it innervates the intrinsic muscles of the plantar part of the foot with the exception of the abductor hallucis and the flexor digitorum brevis.
n. planta'ris media'lis [NA], medial plantar nerve; one of the two terminal branches of the tibial nerve; it courses along the medial aspect of the sole to supply the abductor hallucis and flexor digitorum brevis and, by way of common and proper digital branches, to innervate the skin of the medial part of the foot and medial three and one-half toes.
n. presacra'lis [NA], official alternative name for *plexus* hypogastricus superior.
n. pterygoi'deus [NA], pterygoid nerve; one of two motor branches, lateral and medial, of the mandibular nerve, supplying the lateral and medial pterygoid muscles.
ner'vi pterygopalati'ni, *rami* ganglionares.
n. puden'dus [NA], pudendal nerve; pudic nerve; plexus pudendus nervosus; formed by fibers from the second, third, and fourth sacral nerves; it passes through the greater sciatic foramen and accompanies the internal pudendal artery, terminating as the dorsal nerve of the penis or of the clitoris.
n. radia'lis [NA], radial nerve; musculospiral nerve; arises from the posterior cord of the brachial plexus; it curves round the posterior surface of the humerus and passes down to the cubital fossa where it divides into its two terminal branches, the superficial ramus and the deep ramus; it supplies muscular and cutaneous branches to the dorsal aspect of the arm and forearm.
ner'vi recta'les inferio'res [NA], inferior rectal nerves; inferior hemorrhoidal nerves; several branches of the pudendal nerve that pass to the sphincter ani externus and the skin of the anal region.
n. saccula'ris [NA], saccular nerve; a branch of the vestibular nerve going to the macula sacculi.
ner'vi sacra'les [NA], sacral nerves; five nerves issuing from the sacral foramina on either side; the ventral branches of the first three enter into the formation of the sacral plexus, and the last two into the coccygeal plexus.
n. saphe'nus [NA], saphenous nerve; long or internal saphenous nerve; a branch of the femoral, extending from the femoral triangle to the foot, becoming subcutaneous on the medial side of the knee; it supplies cutaneous branches to the skin of the leg and foot, by way of infrapatellar and medial crural branches.
ner'vi scrota'les anterio'res [NA], anterior scrotal nerves; branches of the ilioinguinal nerve; distributed to the skin of the root of the penis, and the anterior surface of the scrotum.
ner'vi scrota'les posterio'res [NA], posterior scrotal nerves; several terminal branches of the perineal nerve supplying the skin of the posterior portion of the scrotum, corresponding to the posterior labial nerves in the female.
n. spermat'icus exter'nus, *ramus* genitalis.
ner'vi sphenopalati'ni, *rami* ganglionares.
ner'vi spina'les [NA], spinal nerves; the nerves emerging from the spinal cord; there are 31 pairs, each attached to the cord by two roots, anterior and posterior, or ventral and dorsal; the latter is provided with a circumscribed enlargement, the spinal ganglion; the two roots unite in the intervertebral foramen, and the nerve almost immediately divides again into ventral and dorsal rami, or anterior and posterior primary divisions, the former supplying the foreparts of the body and the limbs, the latter the muscles and skin of the back.
ner'vi splanch'nici lumba'les [NA], lumbar splanchnic nerves; branches from the lumbar sympathetic trunks that pass anteriorly to join the celiac, intermesenteric, aortic, and superior hypogastric plexuses.
ner'vi splanch'nici pelvi'ni [NA], pelvic splanchnic nerves; nervi erigentes; branches from the second, third, and fourth sacral nerves that join the inferior hypogastric plexus; they carry parasympathetic and sensory fibers.
ner'vi splanch'nici sacra'les [NA], sacral splanchnic nerves; branches from the sacral sympathetic trunk that pass to the inferior hypogastric plexus.
n. splanch'nicus i'mus [NA], lowest splanchnic nerve; smallest

splanchnic nerve; a nerve containing the sympathetic fibers for the renal plexus, usually contained in the lesser splanchnic nerve, but occasionally existing as an independent nerve.

n. splanch'nicus ma'jor [NA], greater splanchnic nerve; arises from the fifth or sixth to the ninth or tenth thoracic sympathetic ganglia and passes downward along the bodies of the thoracic vertebrae, to join the celiac plexus.

n. splanch'nicus mi'nor [NA], lesser splanchnic nerve; arises from the last two thoracic sympathetic ganglia and passes to the aorticorenal ganglion.

n. stape'dius [NA], nerve to stapedius muscle; a branch of the facial arising in the facial canal and innervating the stapedius muscle.

n. statoacus'ticus, n. vestibulocochlearis.

n. subcla'vius [NA], subclavian nerve; a branch from the superior trunk of the brachial plexus supplying the subclavius muscle.

n. subcosta'lis [NA], subcostal nerve; the ventral ramus of the twelfth thoracic nerve; it courses below the last rib, supplies parts of the abdominal muscles and gives off cutaneous branches to the skin of the lower abdominal wall and to the gluteal region.

n. sublingua'lis [NA], sublingual nerve; a branch of the lingual to the sublingual gland and mucous membrane of the floor of the mouth.

n. suboccipita'lis [NA], suboccipital nerve; dorsal ramus of the first cervical nerve, passing through the suboccipital triangle and sending branches to the rectus capitis posterior major and minor, obliquus capitis superior and inferior, rectus capitis lateralis, and semispinalis capitis.

n. subscapula'ris [NA], subscapular nerve; a branch of the posterior cord of the brachial plexus, supplying the subscapularis muscle.

n. supraclavicula'ris interme'dius [NA], middle supraclavicular nerve; intermediate supraclavicular nerve; one of several nerves arising from the cervical plexus which pass down across the clavicle to supply the skin, in the infraclavicular region.

n. supraclavicula'ris latera'lis [NA], lateral supraclavicular nerve; posterior supraclavicular nerve; one of several branches of the cervical plexus which descend to the skin over the acromion and deltoid region.

n. supraclavicula'ris media'lis [NA], medial supraclavicular nerve; anterior supraclavicular nerve; one of several nerves arising from the cervical plexus which supply the skin over the upper medial part of the thorax.

n. supraorbita'lis [NA], supraorbital nerve; a branch of the frontal leaving the orbit through the supraorbital foramen or notch and dividing into branches distributed to the forehead and scalp, upper eyelid, and frontal sinus.

n. suprascapula'ris [NA], suprascapular nerve; arises from the fifth and sixth cervical, passes downward parallel to the cords of the brachial plexus, then through the scapular notch, supplying the supraspinatus and infraspinatus muscles, and also sending branches to the shoulder joint.

n. supratrochlea'ris [NA], supratrochlear nerve; a branch of the frontal supplying the medial part of the upper eyelid, the central part of the skin of the forehead, and the root of the nose.

n. sura'lis [NA], sural nerve; short or external saphenous nerve; formed by the union of the medial sural cutaneous from the tibial and the peroneal communicating branch of the common peroneal nerve, about the middle of the calf; thence it accompanies the small saphenous vein around the lateral malleolus to the dorsum of the foot.

ner'vi tempora'les profun'di [NA], deep temporal nerves; two branches, anterior and posterior, from the mandibular nerve, supplying the temporal muscle.

n. tenso'ris tym'pani [NA], nerve of tensor tympani muscle; a branch of the mandibular nerve passing through the otic ganglion without synapse to supply the tensor tympani muscle.

n. tenso'ris ve'li palati'ni [NA], nerve of tensor veli palatini muscle; a branch of the mandibular nerve passing through the otic ganglion without synapse to supply the tensor veli palatini muscle.

n. tento'rii, *ramus* tentorii.

ner'vi termina'les [NA], terminal nerves; delicate plexiform nerve strands passing parallel and medial to the olfactory tracts, distributing peripherally with the olfactory nerves and passing centrally into the anterior perforated substance; they are considered to have an autonomic function but the exact nature of this is unknown.

ner'vi thora'cici [NA], thoracic nerves; twelve nerves on each side, mixed motor and sensory, supplying the muscles and skin of the thoracic and abdominal walls.

n. thora'cicus lon'gus [NA], long thoracic nerve; posterior thoracic nerve; external respiratory nerve of Bell; Bell's respiratory nerve; arises from the fifth, sixth, and seventh cervical nerves, descends the neck behind the brachial plexus, and is distributed to the serratus anterior muscle.

n. thoracodorsa'lis [NA], thoracodorsal nerve; long subscapular nerve; arises from the posterior cord of the brachial plexus; it contains fibers from the sixth, seventh, and eighth cervical nerves and supplies the latissimus dorsi muscle.

n. tibia'lis [NA], tibial nerve; medial popliteal nerve; one of the two major divisions of the sciatic nerve, it courses down the back of the leg to terminate as the medial and lateral plantar nerves in the foot; it supplies the hamstring muscles, the muscles of the back of the leg and the plantar aspect of the foot, as well as the skin on the back of the leg and sole of the foot.

n. transver'sus col'li [NA], transverse nerve of neck; superficial cervical nerve; cutaneous cervical nerve; n. cervicalis superficialis; a branch of the cervical plexus that supplies the skin over the anterior triangle of the neck.

n. trigem'inus [NA], trigeminal nerve; trifacial nerve; fifth cranial nerve; the chief sensory nerve of the face and the motor nerve of the muscles of mastication; its nuclei are in the mesencephalon and in the pons extending down into the cervical portion of the spinal cord; it emerges by two roots, sensory and motor, from the lateral portion of the surface of the pons, and enters a cavity of the dura mater, cavum trigeminale (of Meckel), at the apex of the petrous portion of the temporal bone, where the sensory root expands to form the trigeminal (gasserian) ganglion; from there the three divisions (ophthalmic, maxillary, and mandibular) arise.

n. trochlea'ris [NA], trochlear nerve; fourth cranial nerve; pathetic nerve; supplies the superior oblique muscle of the eye; its origin is in the midbrain below the cerebral aqueduct, its fibers decussate in the superior medullary velum, and emerge from the brain at the side of the frenulum; it passes in the lateral wall of the cavernous sinus to enter the orbit through the superior orbital fissure.

n. tympan'icus [NA], tympanic nerve; Andersch's or Jacobson's nerve; a nerve from the inferior ganglion of the glossopharyngeal nerve, passing to the tympanic cavity, forming there the tympanic plexus which supplies the mucous membrane of the tympanic cavity, mastoid cells, and auditory tube; parasympathetic fibers also pass through the tympanic nerve via the lesser petrosal nerve to the otic ganglion to supply the parotid gland.

n. ulna'ris [NA], ulnar nerve; cubital nerve; arises from the medial cord of the brachial plexus and passes down the arm, behind the medial epicondyle of the humerus, and down the ulnar side of the forearm to the hand; it gives off numerous muscular and cutaneous branches in the forearm and supplies intrinsic muscles of the hand and the skin of the medial side of the hand.

n. utricula'ris [NA], utricular nerve; a branch of the utriculoampullar nerve, supplying the macula of the utricle.

n. utriculoampulla'ris [NA], utriculoampullar nerve; a division of the vestibular part of the eighth cranial nerve; it gives off branches to the macula of the utricle (n. utricularis) and to the cristae of the ampullae of the anterior and lateral semicircular ducts (n. ampullaris anterior, n. ampullaris lateralis).

ner'vi vagina'les [NA], vaginal nerves; several nerves passing from the uterovaginal plexus to the vagina.

n. va'gus [NA], vagus nerve; pneumogastric nerve; tenth cranial nerve; a mixed nerve that arises by numerous small roots from the side of the medulla oblongata, between the glossopharyngeal above and the accessory below; it leaves the cranial cavity by the jugular foramen and passes down to supply the pharynx; larynx, lungs, heart, esophagus, stomach, and most of the abdominal viscera.

n. vascula'ris [NA], vascular nerve; a small nerve filament that supplies the wall of a blood vessel.

n. vertebra'lis [NA], vertebral nerve; a branch from the cervicothoracic ganglion that ascends along the vertebral artery to the level of the axis or atlas, giving branches to the cervical nerves and meninges.

n. vestibula'ris [NA], vestibular nerve; pars vestibularis; vestibular part of vestibulocochlear nerve; superior part of vestibulocochlear nerve; the part of the vestibulocochlear nerve peripheral to the radix vestibulochochlearis; it is composed of the nerve processes which have their terminals on the hair cells of hair cells in the ampullae of the semicircular ducts and the maculae of the saccule and utricle and the bipolar neurons of the vestibular ganglion. See also *radix* vestibulocochlearis.

n. vestibulocochlea'ris [NA], vestibulocochlear nerve; eighth cranial nerve; acoustic nerve; n. acusticus, octavus, or statoacusticus; octavus; a composite sensory nerve innervating the receptor cells of the membranous labyrinth; it consists of two major, anatomically and functionally distinct components each of which have different central connections: radix vestibularis and radix cochlearis. See under radix.

n. zygomat'icus [NA], zygomatic nerve; orbital or temporomandibular nerve; a branch of the maxillary in the inferior orbital fissure through which it passes; it divides into a ramus zygomaticotemporalis and a ramus zygomaticofacialis, which supply the skin of the temporal and zygomatic regions.

nesidiectomy (nē-sid'ē-ek'tō-mē) [G. *nēsidion,* islet, dim. of *nēsos,* island, + *ektomē,* excision]. Excision of islet tissue of the pancreas.

nesidioblast (nē-sid'ē-ō-blast) [G. *nēsidion,* dim. of *nēsos,* island, + *blastos,* germ]. A pancreatic islet-forming cell.

nesidioblastoma (nē-sid'ē-ō-blas-tō'mă) [nesidioblast + G. *-oma,* tumor]. Islet cell *adenoma.*

nesidioblastosis (ne-sid'ē-ō-blas-tō'sis) [nesidioblast + G. *-osis,* tumor]. Hyperplasia of the cells of the islets of Langerhans.

Nessler, A., German chemist, 1827–1905. See N.'s *reagent.*

nesslerize (nes'ler-īz). To treat with Nessler's reagent; used in the determination of urea nitrogen in the blood and in the urine.

nest [A.S.]. A group or collection of similar objects. See also nidus.

Brunn's n.'s, glandlike invaginations of surface transitional epithelium in the mucosa of the lower urinary tract.

cell n.'s, a small focus or accumulation of one type of cell that is different from the other cells in the tissue.

epithelial n., keratin *pearl.*

net. Network (1).

Chiari's n., abnormal fibrous or lacelike strands in the right atrium, extending from the margins of the coronary or caval valves and attaching to the atrial wall along the line of the crista terminalis; results when resorption of the septum spurium is markedly less than normal.

chromidial n., a reticulum of basophilic-staining material in the cytoplasm of certain cells.

Netherton, Earl W., U.S. dermatologist. See N.'s *syndrome.*

netilmicin sulfate (net-il-mī'sin). $(C_{21}H_{41}N_5O_7)_2{\cdot}5H_2SO_4$; a parenteral aminoglycoside antibiotic used for short-term treatment of serious or life-threatening bacterial infections.

nettle (net'l) [A.S. *netele*] Urtica.

network (net'werk). **1.** Net; a structure bearing a resemblance to a woven fabric. See also rete; reticulum. **2.** The persons in a patient's environment, especially as significant for the course of the illness.

acromial n., *rete* acromiale.

arterial n., *rete* arteriosum.

articular n. of elbow, *rete* articulare cubiti.

articular n. of knee, *rete* articulare genus.

articular vascular n., *rete* vasculosum articulare.

chromatin n., the appearance of basophilic material in the nuclei of many cells after fixation. See also chromatin.

dorsal carpal n., *rete* carpi dorsale.

dorsal venous n. of foot, *rete* venosum dorsale pedis.

dorsal venous n. of hand, *rete* venosum dorsale manus.

n. of heel, *rete* calcaneum.

lateral malleolar n., *rete* malleolare laterale.

linin n., see linin (3).

medial malleolar n., *rete* malleolare mediale.

patellar n., *rete* patellae.

peritarsal n., the lymphatic vessels along the margin of the eyelid.

plantar venous n., *rete* venosum plantare.

Purkinje's n., the n. formed by Purkinje's fibers beneath the endocardium.

subpapillary n., the capillary blood vessels in the deeper layers of the skin.

trabecular n., *reticulum* trabeculare.

Neubauer, Johann E., German anatomist, 1742–1777. See N.'s *artery.*

Neufeld, Fred, German bacteriologist, 1869–1945. See N. *reaction,* capsular *swelling.*

Neumann, Ernst F.C., German histologist, anatomist, and pathologist, 1834–1918. See N.'s *cells, sheath;* Rouget-N. *sheath.*

Neumann, Franz E., German physicist, 1798–1895. See N.'s *law.*

Neumann, Isidor Edler von Heilwart, Austrian dermatologist, 1832–1906. See N.'s *disease.*

neur-, neuri-, neuro- [G. *neuron,* nerve]. Combining forms denoting a nerve or relating to the nervous system.

neuragmia (nū-rag'mē-ă) [neur- + G. *agmos,* fracture]. Rupture or tearing asunder of a nerve.

neural (nūr'ăl) [G. *neuron,* nerve]. **1.** Relating to any structure composed of nerve cells or their processes, or that on further development will evolve into nerve cells. **2.** Referring to the dorsal side of the vertebral bodies or their precursors, where the spinal cord is located, as opposed to hemal (2).

neuralgia (nū-ral'jē-ă) [neur- + G. *algos,* pain]. Neurodynia; nerve pain; pain of a severe, throbbing, or stabbing character in the course or distribution of a nerve.

atypical facial n., atypical trigeminal n.

atypical trigeminal n., atypical facial n.; periodic pain in any region of the face, teeth, tongue, and occasionally in the occipital or shoulder area, which lasts several minutes to several days but has no trigger point and lacks the paroxysmal character of tic douloureux.

epileptiform n., trigeminal n.

facial n., trigeminal n.

n. facia'lis ve'ra, geniculate n.

Fothergill's n., trigeminal n.

geniculate n., n. facialis vera; Hunt's n.; geniculate otalgia; a severe paroxysmal lancinating pain deep in the ear, on the anterior wall of the external meatus, and on a small area just in front of the pinna.

glossopharyngeal n., glossopharyngeal tic; paroxysmal lancinating pain in the throat or palate.

hallucinatory n., reminiscent n.; an impression of local pain persisting after an attack of n. has ceased.

Hunt's n., geniculate n.
idiopathic n., nerve pain not due to any apparent cause.
intercostal n., pain in the chest wall due to n. of one or more of the intercostal nerves.
mammary n., n. of the intercostal nerve or nerves supplying the breast.
Morton's n., n. of an interdigital nerve, usually the anastomotic branch between the medial and lateral plantar nerves, resulting from compression of the nerve by the metatarsophalangeal joint.
occipital n., see posttraumatic neck *syndrome.*
periodic migrainous n., Harris' migraine; recurrent facial pain and headache, more common in men than in women.
red n., erythromelalgia.
reminiscent n., hallucinatory n.
sciatic n., sciatica.
Sluder's n., sphenopalatine n.
sphenopalatine n., Sluder's n.; n. of the lower half of the face, with pain referred to the root of the nose, upper teeth, eyes, ears, mastoid, and occiput, in association with nasal congestion and rhinorrhea occurring in infection of the nasal sinuses, and produced by lesions of the sphenopalatine ganglion; ocular hyperemia and excessive lacrimation may occur.
stump n., pain experienced as coming from an absent part, caused by irritation of neuromas in the scarred tissue of an amputation stump.
suboccipital n., see posttraumatic neck *syndrome.*
supraorbital n., n. of the supraorbital nerve.
symptomatic n., n. occurring as a symptom of some local or systemic disease not involving primarily nerve structures.
trifacial n., trigeminal n.
trigeminal n., severe, paroxysmal bursts of pain in one or more branches of the trigeminal nerve; often induced by touching trigger points in or about the mouth. Also called trifacial, facial, epileptiform, or Fothergill's n.; Fothergill's disease (1); tic douloureux; prosopalgia; prosoponeuralgia; trismus dolorificus.

neuralgic (nū-ral'jik). Relating to, resembling, or of the character of, neuralgia.

neuralgiform (nū-ral'ji-fōrm). Resembling or of the character of neuralgia.

neuramebimeter (nūr'am-ē-bim'ĕ-ter) [neur- + G. *amoibē,* exchange, return, answer, + *metron,* measure]. An instrument for measuring the rapidity of response of a nerve to any stimulus.

neuraminic acid (nūr'ă-min'ik). Prehemataminic acid; 5-amino-3,5-dideoxy-D-*glycero*-D-*galacto*-2-nonulopyranosonic acid; an aldol product of mannosamine and pyruvic acid, linking the C-1 of the former to the C-3 of the latter. The *N*- and *O*-acyl derivatives of n. are known as sialic acids and are constituents of gangliosides and of the polysaccharide components of muco- and glycoproteins from many tissues, secretions, and species.

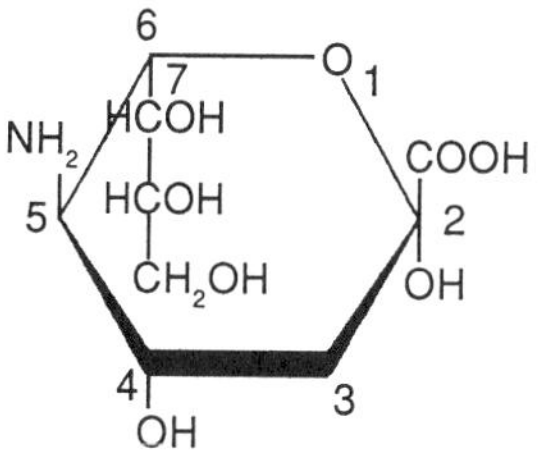

Neuraminic acid

neuraminidase (nūr-ă-min'i-dās). Sialidase.

α_2-neuraminoglycoprotein (nūr-ă-min'ō-glī-kō-prō'tēn). A glycoprotein that contains neuraminic acid and which during electrophoresis migrates with the α_2 portion of serum proteins. See also Cl-esterase *inhibitor.*

neuranagenesis (nūr'an-ă-jen'ĕ-sis) [neur- + G. *ana,* up, again, + *genesis,* origin]. Regeneration of a nerve.

neurapophysis (nūr-ă-pof'i-sis) [neur- + G. *apophysis,* offshoot]. *Lamina* arcus vertebrae.

neurapraxia (nūr-ă-prak'sē-ă) [neur- + G. a- priv. + *praxis,* action]. Loss of conduction in a nerve without structural degeneration, caused by a focal lesion and normally followed by a return of function.

neurarchy (nūr'ar-kē) [neur- + G. *archē,* dominion]. The dominant action of the nervous system over the physical processes of the body.

neurasthenia (nūr-as-thē'nē-ă) [neur- + G. *astheneia,* weakness]. Nervosism (1); an ill-defined condition, commonly accompanying or following depression, characterized by vague functional fatigue.
angiopathic n., angioparalytic n., pulsating n.; a form of mild n. in which the chief complaint is of a universal throbbing or sense of pulsation throughout the body.
gastric n., a condition marked by gastric atony and distention, dyspepsia, and mild neurasthenic symptoms.
n. gra'vis, a condition of extreme and lasting n.
n. pre'cox, primary n.; a form of nervous exhaustion appearing in the adolescent period.
primary n., n. precox.
pulsating n., angiopathic n.
sexual n., a form in which sexual erethism, weakness, or perversion is a marked symptom.
traumatic n., posttraumatic *syndrome.*

neurasthenic (nūr-as-then'ik). Relating to, or suffering from, neurasthenia.

neurasthenic helmet. A feeling of pressure over the entire cranium in certain cases of neurasthenia.

neuraxis (nū-rak'sis). The axial, unpaired part of the central nervous system: spinal cord, rhombencephalon, mesencephalon, and diencephalon, in contrast to the paired cerebral hemisphere or telencephalon.

neuraxon, neuraxone (nū-rak'son, -sōn) [neur- + G. *axōn,* axis]. Obsolete term for axon.

neurectasis, neurectasia, neurectasy (nū-rek'tă-sis, nūr-ek-tā'zē-ă, -ek'tă-sē) [neur- + G. *ektasis,* extension]. Neurotension; neurotony; the operation of stretching a nerve or nerve trunk.

neurectomy (nū-rek'tō-mē) [neur- + G. *ektomē,* excision]. Neuroectomy; excision of a segment of a nerve.
presacral n., presacral sympathectomy; Cotte's operation; removal of the presacral nerve to relieve severe dysmenorrhea.
retrogasserian n., trigeminal *rhizotomy.*

neurectopia, neurectopy (nūr-ek-tō'pē-ă, -ek'tō-pē) [neur- + G. *ektopos,* fr. *ek,* out of, + *topos,* place]. **1.** Dislocation of a nerve trunk. **2.** A condition in which a nerve follows an anomalous course.

neurepithelium (nūr'ep-i-thē'lē-ŭm). Neuroepithelium.

neurergic (nū-rer'jik) [neur- + G. *ergon,* work]. Relating to the activity of a nerve.

neurexeresis (nūr-ek-ser'ĕ-sis) [neur- + G. *exairesis,* a taking out, fr. *haireō,* to grasp, take]. Tearing out or evulsion of a nerve.

neuri-. See neur-.

neuriatria, neuriatry (nūr-ē-at'rē-ă, nū-rī'ă-trē) [neur- + G. *iatreia,* medical treatment]. Treatment of nervous diseases.

neuridine (nūr'i-dēn). Spermine.

neurilemma (nūr-i-lem'ă) [neuri + G. *lemma,* husk]. Neurolemma; sheath of Schwann; a cell that enfolds one or more axons of the peripheral nervous system; in myelinated fibers its plasma membrane forms the lamellae of myelin.

neurilemoma (nūr'i-lē-mō'mă) [neurilemma + G. *-oma,* tumor]. Neurinoma; neuroschwannoma; schwannoma (2); a benign, encapsulated neoplasm in which the fundamental component is structurally identical to a syncytium of Schwann cells; the neoplastic cells proliferate within the endoneurium, and the perineurium forms the capsule. The neoplasm may originate from a peripheral or sympathetic nerve, or from various cranial nerves, particularly the eighth nerve; when the nerve is small, it is usually found (if at all) in the capsule of the neoplasm; if the nerve is large, the n. may develop within the sheath of the nerve, the fibers of which may then spread over the surface of the capsule as the neoplasm enlarges. Microscopically, n.'s are composed of combinations of two cell types, Antoni types A and B (see below), either of which may be predominant in various examples of n.'s. See also neurofibroma.
acoustic n., acoustic *neurinoma.*
Antoni type A n., relatively solid or firm neoplastic tissue that consists of Schwann cells arranged in twisting bundles and associated with delicate reticulin fibers; the nuclei of the Schwann cells are frequently grouped in parallel rows (so-called palisades), and the nuclei and fibers sometimes form exaggerated tactile corpuscles, called Verocay bodies.
Antoni type B n., relatively soft neoplastic tissue that consists of Schwann cells in a haphazard or nondescript type of arrangement among reticulin fibers and tiny cystlike foci; fat-laden macrophages may be observed in some of the larger neoplasms.

neurility (nū-ril'i-tē). The property, inherent in nerves, of conducting stimuli.

neurimotility (nūr'i-mō-til'i-tē). Nervimotility.

neurimotor (nūr-i-mō'ter). Nervimotor.

neurine (nūr'ēn). Trimethylvinylammonium hydroxide; $CH_2{=}CH{-}N^+(CH_3)_3OH$; a toxic amine that is a product of decomposing animal matter (dehydration of choline) and a poisonous constituent of mushrooms.

neurinoma (nūr-i-nō'mă). Neurilemoma.
acoustic n., a benign neoplasm of the intracranial segment of the eighth cranial nerve, producing cerebellar, lower cranial nerve, and brainstem signs and symptoms. Also called acoustic neurilemoma, neuroma, or schwannoma; cerebellopontine angle tumor; eighth nerve tumor.

neurit, neurite (nūr'it, nūr'īt) [G. *neuritēs,* of a nerve]. Obsolete term for axon.

neuritic (nū-rit'ik). Relating to neuritis.

neuritis, pl. neuritides (nū-rī'tis, nū-rit'i-dēz) [neuri- + G. *-itis,* inflammation]. Inflammation of a nerve, associated with neuralgia, hyperesthesia, anesthesia, paresthesia, paralysis, muscular atrophy in the region supplied by the affected nerve, and with absence of the reflexes.
adventitial n., inflammation of the sheath of a nerve. See also perineuritis.
ascending n., inflammation progressing upward along a nerve trunk in a direction away from the periphery.
axial n., parenchymatous n.
brachial n., brachial plexus *neuropathy.*
central n., parenchymatous n.
descending n., inflammation progressing downward along a nerve trunk in a direction toward the periphery.
Eichhorst's n., interstitial n.
endemic n., beriberi.
fallopian n., facial *palsy.*
interstitial n., Eichhorst's n.; inflammation of the connective tissue framework of a nerve.
intraocular n., inflammation of the retinal portion of the optic nerve.
Leyden's n., fatty degeneration of the fibers of the affected nerve.
multiple n., polyneuritis.
occipital n., see posttraumatic neck *syndrome.*
optic n., retrobulbar n.; inflammation of the optic nerve. See also *neuromyelitis* optica.
parenchymatous n., axial or central n.; inflammation of the nervous substance proper, the axons, and myelin.
retrobulbar n., optic n.
sciatic n., inflammation of the sciatic nerve, causing sciatica.
segmental n., inflammation occurring at several points along the course of a nerve. See also segmental *neuropathy.*
suboccipital n., see posttraumatic neck *syndrome.*
toxic n., n. due to the action of alcohol, lead, arsenic, or some other poison.
traumatic n., inflammation of a nerve following an injury.

neuro-. See neur-.

neuroallergy (nūr-ō-al'er-jē). An allergic reaction in nervous tissue.

neuroanastomosis (nūr'ō-an-as-tō-mō'sis). Surgical formation of a junction between nerves.

neuroanatomy (nūr'ō-ă-nat'ō-mē). The anatomy of the nervous system.

neuroarthropathy (nūr'ō-ar-throp'ă-thē) [neuro- + G. *arthron,* joint, + *pathos,* suffering, disease]. A trophoneurosis affecting one or more joints.

neuroaugmentation (nūr'ō-awg-men-tā'shūn). Use of electrical stimulation to supplement activity of the nervous system.

neuroaugmentive (nūr'ō-awg-men'tiv). Related to neuroaugmentation.

neurobiotaxis (nūr'ō-bī-ō-tak'sis) [neuro- + G. *bios,* life, + *taxis,* arrangement]. Tendency of the nerve cells to move toward the area from which they receive the most stimuli.

neuroblast (nūr'ō-blast) [neuro- + G. *blastos,* germ]. An embryonic nerve cell.

neuroblastoma (nūr'ō-blas-tō'mă). A malignant neoplasm characterized by immature, only slightly differentiated nerve cells of embryonic type, *i.e.,* neuroblasts; typical cells are relatively small (10 to 15 μm in diameter) with disproportionately large, darkly staining, vesicular nuclei and scant, palely acidophilic cytoplasm; they may be arranged in sheets, irregular clumps, or cordlike groups, as well as occurring individually and in pseudorosettes (with nuclei arranged peripherally about the centrally directed cytoplasmic processes); ordinarily, the stroma is sparse, and foci of necrosis and hemorrhage are not unusual. N.'s occur frequently in infants and children in the mediastinal and retroperitoneal regions (approximately 30% associated with the adrenal glands); widespread metastases to the liver, lungs, lymph nodes, cranial cavity, and skeleton are very common.
olfactory n., olfactory esthesioneuroblastoma; a rare, often slowly growing malignant tumor of primitive nerve cells, usually arising in the olfactory area of the nasal cavity.

neurocardiac (nūr-ō-kar'dē-ak) [neuro- + G. *kardia,* heart]. **1.** Relating to the nerve supply of the heart. **2.** Relating to a cardiac neurosis.

neurocele (nūr'ō-sēl) [neuro- + G. *koilos,* hollow]. Rarely used collective term for the central cavity of the cerebrospinal axis; the combined ventricles of the brain and central canal of the spinal cord.

neurochemistry (nūr-ō-kem'is-trē). The science concerned with the chemical aspects of nervous system structure and function.

neurochitin (nūr-ō-kī'tin) [neuro- + G. *chitōn,* tunic]. Neurokeratin.

neurochorioretinitis (nūr-ō-kōr'ē-ō-ret-in-ī'tis). Inflammation of the choroid, the retina, and the optic nerve.

neurochoroiditis (nūr'ō-kō-roy-dī'tis). Inflammation of the choroid and the optic nerve.

neurocladism (nū-rok'lă-dizm) [neuro- + G. *klados,* a young branch]. Odogenesis; the outgrowth of axons from the central stump to bridge the gap in a cut nerve.

neurocranium (nūr-ō-krā'nē-ŭm) [neuro- + G. *kranion,* skull]. Those bones of the skull enclosing the brain, as distinguished from the bones of the face.

cartilaginous n., in the embryo, that part of the base of the skull first laid down in cartilage and then ossified.

membranous n., the vault of the embryonic skull which is ossified in membrane.

neurocristopathy (nūr'ō-kris-top'ă-thē) [neuro- + L. *crista,* crest, + G. *pathos,* suffering]. Developmental anomaly of the neural crest manifested by abnormal development and tumors of the neural axis.

neurocyte (nūr'o-sīt) [neuro- + G. *kytos,* cell]. Neuron.

neurocytolysis (nūr'ō-sī-tol'i-sis) [neuro- + G. *kytos,* cell, + *lysis,* dissolution]. Destruction of neurons.

neurocytoma (nūr'ō-sī-tō'mă) [neuro- + G. *kytos,* cell, + *-oma,* tumor]. Ganglioneuroma.

neurodendrite (nūr-ō-den'drīt). Dendrite (1).

neurodendron (nūr-ō-den'dron). Dendrite (1).

neurodermatitis (nūr'ō-der-mă-tī'tis) [neuro- + G. *derma,* skin, + *-itis,* inflammation]. Neurodermatosis; a chronic lichenified skin lesion, localized or disseminated; a term loosely applied to atopic dermatitis or chronic lichen simplex.

neurodermatosis (nūr'ō-der-mă-tō'sis). Neurodermatitis.

neurodynamic (nūr'ō-dī-nam'ik) [neuro- + G. *dynamis,* force]. Pertaining to nervous energy.

neurodynia (nūr-ō-din'ē-ă) [neuro- + G. *odynē,* pain]. Neuralgia.

neuroectoderm (nūr-ō-ek'tō-derm). That central region of the early embryonic ectoderm which on further development forms the brain and spinal cord, and also evolves into the nerve cells and neurolemma or Schwann cells of the peripheral nervous system.

neuroectodermal (nūr'ō-ek-tō-der'măl). Relating to the neuroectoderm.

neuroectomy (nūr-ō-ek'tō-mē). Neurectomy.

neuroencephalomyelopathy (nūr'ō-en-sef'ă-lō-mī-ĕ-lop'ă-thē). Disease of the brain, spinal cord, and nerves.

neuroendocrine (nūr-ō-en'dō-krin). **1.** Pertaining to the anatomical and functional relationships between the nervous system and the endocrine apparatus. **2.** Descriptive of cells that release a hormone into the circulating blood in response to a neural stimulus. Such cells may comprise a peripheral endocrine gland (*e.g.,* the insulin-secreting beta cells of the islets of Langerhans in the pancreas and the adrenaline-secreting chromaffin cells of the adrenal medulla); others are neurons in the brain (*e.g.,* the neurons of the supraoptic nucleus that release antidiuretic hormone from their axon terminals in the posterior lobe of the hypophysis).

neuroendocrinology (nūr-ō-en'dō-krin-ol'ō-jē). The specialty concerned with the anatomical and functional relationships between the nervous system and the endocrine apparatus.

neuroepithelial (nūr'ō-ep-i-thē'lē-ăl). Relating to the neuroepithelium.

neuroepithelium (nūr'ō-ep-i-thē'lē-ŭm) [NA]. Neuroepithelial cells; neurepithelium; epithelial cells specialized for the reception of external stimuli. Most neuroepithelial cells, notably the hair cells of the inner ear and the receptor cells of the taste buds, are not true neurons but transducer cells that stand in synaptic contact with the peripheral endings of sensory ganglion cells. The neuroepithelial receptor cells of the olfactory epithelium, by contrast, are true peripheral neurons whose extremely thin, unmyelinated axons compose the olfactory filaments that enter the olfactory bulb of the cerebral hemisphere. The NA also applies the term to the rods and cones of the retina.

n. of ampullary crest, n. cristae ampullaris.

n. cris'tae ampulla'ris [NA], n. of the ampullary crest; the specialized sensory hair cells in the ampullary crest of the ampulla of each semicircular duct.

n. of macula, n. maculae.

n. mac'ulae [NA], n. of the macula; the specialized sensory hair cells of the epithelium of the macula sacculi and macula utriculi.

neurofibril (nūr-ō-fī'bril). A filamentous structure seen with the light microscope in the nerve cell's body, dendrites, axon, and sometimes synaptic endings, as aggregations of much finer ultramicroscopic elements, the neurofilaments and microtubules; their functional significance remains to be established.

neurofibrillar (nūr-ō-fī'bri-lăr) Relating to neurofibrils.

neurofibroma (nūr'ō-fī-brō'mă). Schwannoma (1); fibroneuroma; a moderately firm, benign, encapsulated tumor resulting from proliferation of Schwann cells in a disorderly pattern that includes portions of nerve fibers; in neurofibromatosis, n.'s are multiple.

plexiform n., fibrillary or plexiform neuroma; a type of n., representing an anomaly rather than a true neoplasm, in which the proliferation of Schwann cells occurs from the inner aspect of the nerve sheath, thereby resulting in an irregularly thickened, distorted, tortuous structure; in some instances, the process extends along the course of the nerve and may eventually involve the spinal roots and the spinal cord.

storiform n., pigmented *dermatofibrosarcoma protuberans.*

neurofibromatosis (nūr'ō-fī-brō-mă-tō'sis). Two distinct disorders of autosomal dominant inheritance with marked clinical variability: **1.** (von) Recklinghausen's disease; n. characterized by café au lait spots, intertriginous freckling, iris hamartomas, and multiple skin neurofibromas; may be associated with optic gliomas, spinal and peripheral nerve neurofibromas, macrocephaly, neurologic or mental impairment, or bone abnormalities. **2.** Bilateral acoustic n.; n. characterized by bilateral acoustic neuromas manifested by loss of hearing and facial weakness, headache, and varying sensorineural impairment; café au lait spots, skin neurofibromas, and intertriginous freckling are less common.

abortive n., incomplete n.

incomplete n., abortive n.; multiple neurofibromas with minimal manifestations, perhaps limited to café-au-lait spots; individuals with minimal lesions may have offspring with severe involvement.

neurofilament (nūr-ō-fil'ă-ment). A class of intermediate filaments found in neurons.

neuroganglion (nūr-ō-gang'lē-on). Ganglion (1).

neurogastric (nūr-ō-gas'trik). Relating to the innervation of the stomach.

neurogenesis (nūr-ō-jen'ĕ-sis) [neuro- + G. *genesis,* production]. Formation of the nervous system.

neurogenic, neurogenetic (nūr-ō-jen'ik, -jĕ-net'ik). **1.** Neurogenous; originating in, starting from, or caused by, the nervous system or nerve impulses. **2.** Relating to neurogenesis.

neurogenous (nū-roj'ĕ-nŭs). Neurogenic (1).

neuroglia (nū-rog'lē-ă) [neuro- + G. *glia,* glue]. Glia; reticulum (2); Kölliker's reticulum; non-neuronal cellular elements of the central and peripheral nervous system; formerly believed to be merely supporting cells but now thought to have important metabolic functions, since they are invariably interposed between neurons and the blood vessels supplying the nervous system. In central nervous tissue they include oligodendroglia cells, astrocytes, ependymal cells, and microglia cells. The satellite cells of ganglia and the neurolemmal or Schwann cells around peripheral nerve fibers can be interpreted as the oligodendroglia cells of the peripheral nervous system.

neurogliacyte (nū-rog'lē-ă-sīt) [neuro- + G. *glia,* glue, + *kytos,* cell]. A neuroglia cell. See neuroglia.

neuroglial, neurogliar (nū-rog'lē-ăl, -lē-ăr). Relating to neuroglia.

neurogliomatosis (nū-rog'lē-ō-mă-tō'sis). Gliomatosis.

neurogram (nūr'ō-gram) [neuro- + G. *gramma,* something written]. The imprint on the brain substance theoretically remaining after every mental experience, *i.e.,* the engram or physical register of the mental experience, stimulation of which retrieves and reproduces the original experience, thereby producing memory.

neurography (nū-rog'ră-fē) [neuro- + G. *graphō,* to write]. A method of depicting the state of a peripheral nerve, such as electrical recording or radiographic visualization by contrast media.

neurohemal (nūr-ō-hē'măl) [neuro- + hemal, relating to blood vessels]. Descriptive of structures containing neurosecretory neurons, whose axons form no synapses with other neurons and whose axonal endings are modified to permit storage and release into the circulation of neurosecretory material.

neurohistology (nūr'ō-his-tol'ō-jē). Histoneurology; the microscopic anatomy of the nervous system.

neurohormone (nūr-ō-hōr'mōn). A hormone formed by neurosecretory cells and liberated by nerve impulses.

neurohumor (nūr-ō-hyū'mer). The active chemical substance liberated at nerve endings with exciting effect on adjacent structures.

neurohypophysial (nūr'ō-hī-pō-fiz'ē-ăl). Relating to the neurohypophysis.

neurohypophysis (nūr'ō-hī-pof'i-sis) [neuro- + hypophysis] [NA]. Lobus posterior hypophyseous; posterior lobe of hypophysis; pars nervosa hypophyseos; it is composed of the infundibulum and the lobus nervosus, *q.v.* See also hypophysis.

neuroid (nūr'oyd) [neuro- + G. *eidos,* resemblance]. Resembling a nerve; nervelike.

neurokeratin (nūr-ō-kār'ă-tin) [neuro- + G. *keras,* horn]. Neurochitin. **1.** The proteinaceous network that remains of the myelin sheath of axons following fixation and the removal of the fatty material; the reticular appearance is probably a fixation artifact. **2.** The insoluble protein matter of brain remaining after extraction with solvents following proteolytic digestion; it differs in composition from other keratins.

neurolemma (nūr-ō-lem'ă) [neuro- + G. *lemma,* husk]. Neurilemma.

neuroleptanalgesia (nūr'ō-lept-an-ăl-jē'zē-ă). An intense analgesic and amnesic state produced by administration of narcotic analgesics and neuroleptic drugs; unconsciousness may or may not occur, and cardiorespiratory function may be altered.

neuroleptanesthesia (nūr'ō-lept-an-es-thē'zē-ah). A technique of general anesthesia based upon intravenous administration of neuroleptic drugs, together with inhalation of a weak anesthetic with or without neuromuscular relaxants.

neuroleptic (nūr-ō-lep'tik) [neuro- + G. *lēpsis,* taking hold]. **1.** Neuroleptic *agent.* **2.** Denoting a condition similar to that produced by such an agent.

neurolinguistics (nur'ō-ling-gwis'tiks). The branch of medical science concerned with the neuroanatomical basis of speech and its disorders.

neurologist (nū-rol'ō-jist). A specialist in the diagnosis and treatment of nervous system diseases.

neurology (nū-rol'ō-jē) [neuro- + G. *logos,* study]. The branch of medical science concerned with the nervous system and its disorders.

neurolymph (nūr'ō-limf) [neuro- + L. *lympha,* clear water]. *Liquor* cerebrospinalis.

neurolymphomatosis (nūr'ō-lim-fō-mă-tō'sis). Lymphoblastic invasion of a nerve.

n. gallina'rum, see avian *lymphomatosis.*

neurolysin (nū-rol'i-sin). Neurotoxin; an antibody causing destruction of ganglion and cortical cells, obtained by the injection of brain substance.

neurolysis (nū-rol'i-sis) [neuro- + G. *lysis,* dissolution]. **1.** Destruction of nerve tissue. **2.** Freeing of a nerve from inflammatory adhesions.

neurolytic (nūr-ō-lit'ik). Relating to neurolysis.

neuroma (nū-ro'mă) [neuro- + G. *-oma,* tumor]. General term for any neoplasm derived from cells of the nervous system; on the basis of newer knowledge pertaining to cytologic and histologic characteristics, a variety of neoplasms, formerly placed in the general category of n., may now be classified in more specific categories, *e.g.,* ganglioneuroma, neurilemoma, pseudoneuroma, and others.

acoustic n., acoustic *neurinoma.*

amputation n., traumatic n.

n. cu'tis, neurofibroma of the skin.

false n., traumatic n.

fibrillary n., plexiform *neurofibroma.*

plexiform n., plexiform *neurofibroma.*

n. telangiecto'des, a neurofibroma with a conspicuous number of blood vessels, some of which have unusually large lumens (in proportion to the thickness of the walls).

traumatic n., amputation or false n.; pseudoneuroma; the proliferative mass non-neoplastic of Schwann cells and neurites that may develop at the proximal end of a severed or injured nerve.

Verneuil's n., a nodular enlargement of the cutaneous nerves.

neuromalacia (nūr'ō-mă-lā'shē-ă) [neuro- + G. *malakia,* softness]. Pathologic softening of nervous tissue.

neuromast (nūr'ō-mast). See lateral line sense *organ.*

neuromatosis (nūr'ō-mă-tō'sis). The presence of multiple neuromas, as in neurofibromatosis.

neuromelanin (nūr-ō-mel'ă-nin). A modified form of melanin pigment normally found in certain neurons of the nervous system, especially in the substantia nigra and locus ceruleus.

neuromere (nūr'ō-mēr) [neuro- + G. *meros,* part]. Rhombomere; neural segment; that part of the neural tube within a metamere.

neuromimesis (nūr'ō-mi-mē'sis) [neuro- + G. *mimēsis,* imitation]. Obsolete term for hysterical or neurotic simulation of disease.

neuromimetic (nūr'ō-mi-met'ik). Relating to the action of a drug that mimics the response of an effector organ to nerve impulses.

neuromuscular (nūr-ō-mŭs'kyū-lăr). Referring to the relationship between nerve and muscle, in particular to the motor innervation of skeletal muscles and its pathology (*e.g.,* neuromuscular disorders). See also myoneural.

neuromyasthenia (nūr'ō-mī-as-thē'nē-ă) [neuro- + G. *mys,* muscle, + *a-* priv. + *sthenos,* strength]. Muscular weakness, usually of emotional origin.

epidemic n., Akureyri or Iceland disease; benign or epidemic myalgic encephalomyelitis; an epidemic disease of unknown origin and, often, insidious onset, characterized by stiffness of the neck and back, headache, diarrhea, fever, and localized muscular weakness; restricted almost exclusively to adults, affecting women more than men.

neuromyelitis (nūr'ō-mī-el-ī'tis) [neuro- + G. *myelos,* marrow, + *-itis,* inflammation]. Myeloneuritis; neuritis combined with spinal cord inflammation.

n. op'tica, Devic's disease; a demyelinating disorder associated with transverse myelopathy and optic neuritis.

neuromyopathy (nūr'ō-mī-op'ă-thē) [neuro- + G. *mys,* muscle, + *pathos,* disease]. A disorder of muscle, anatomical or physiological, due to disease or disorder of its nerve supply.

carcinomatous n., n. associated with carcinoma, especially of the lung.

neuromyositis (nūr'ō-mī-ō-sī'tis) [neuro- + G. *mys,* muscle, + -*itis,* inflammation]. Neuritis with inflammation of the muscles with which the affected nerve or nerves are in relation.

neuron (nūr'on) [G. *neuron,* a nerve]. **1.** Neurone; nerve cell; neurocyte; the morphological and functional unit of the nervous system, consisting of the nerve cell body, the dendrites, and the axon. **2.** Obsolete term for axon.

autonomic motor n., see motor n.

bipolar n., a n. that has two processes arising from opposite poles of the cell body.

gamma motor n.'s, gamma *loop.*

ganglionic motor n., see motor n.

Golgi type I n., nerve cells whose long axons leave the gray matter of which they form a part.

Golgi type II n., nerve cells with short axons which ramify in the gray matter.

intercalary n., internuncial n.

internuncial n., intercalary n.; a n. interposed between and connecting two other n.'s.

lower motor n., clinical term used to indicate the final motor n.'s which innervate the skeletal muscles; distinguished from upper motor n.'s of the motor cortex that contribute to the pyramidal or corticospinal tract. See also motor n.

motor n., motoneuron; a nerve cell in the spinal cord, rhombencephalon, or mesencephalon characterized by having an axon that leaves the central nervous system to establish a functional connection with an effector (muscle or glandular) tissue; **somatic m. n.'s** directly synapse with striated muscle fibers by motor endplates; **visceral** or **autonomic m. n.'s** (preganglionic m. n.'s), by contrast, innervate smooth muscle fibers or glands only by the intermediary of a second, peripheral, n. (postganglionic or ganglionic m. n.) located in an autonomic ganglion. See also motor *endplate; systema* nervosum autonomicum.

multipolar n., a n. with several processes, usually an axon and three or more dendrites.

postganglionic motor n., see motor n.

preganglionic motor n., see motor n.

pseudounipolar n., unipolar n.

somatic motor n., see motor n.

unipolar n., pseudounipolar n.; pseudounipolar or unipolar cell; a n. whose cell body emits a single axonal process resulting from the fusion of two polar processes during development; at a variable distance from the cell body, the process divides into a peripheral axon branch extending outward as a peripheral afferent (sensory) nerve fiber, and a central axon branch that enters into synaptic

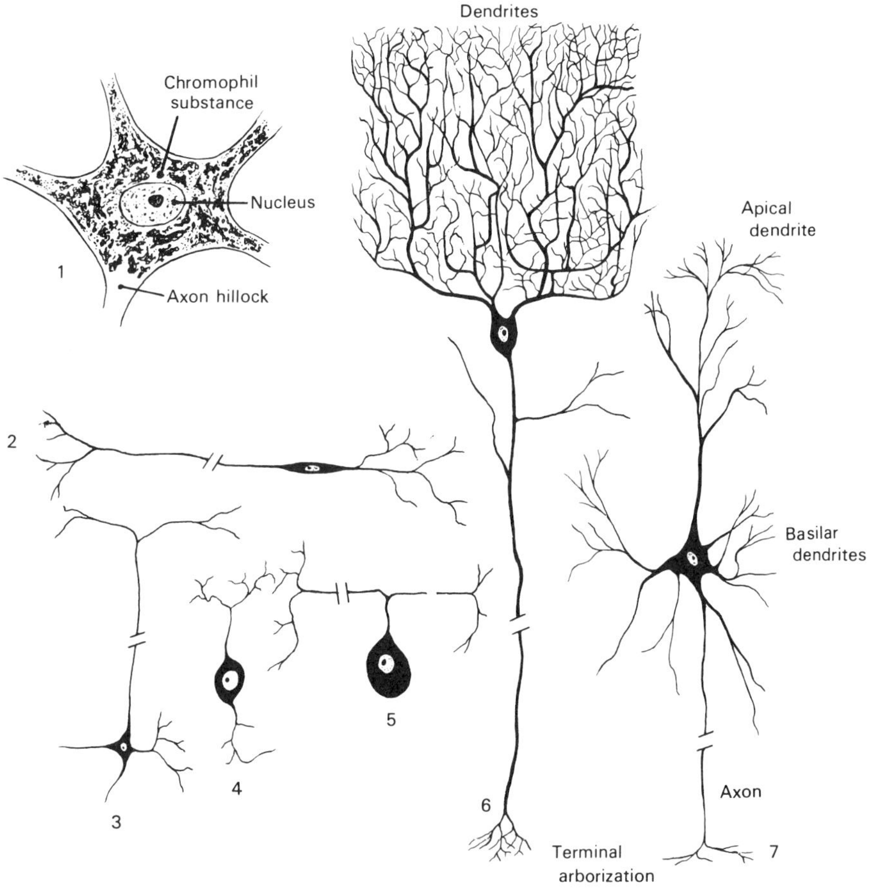

Some Types of Neuron

1, Typical nerve cell body showing internal structure; *2,* horizontal cell (of Cajal) from cerebral cortex; *3,* Martinotti's cell; *4,* bipolar cell; *5,* unipolar cell (posterior root ganglion); *6,* Purkinje cell; *7,* pyramidal cell of motor area of cerebral cortex. Sheaths are not shown.

contact with n.'s in the spinal cord or brainstem. With the single known exception of the n.'s composing the mesencephalic nucleus of the trigeminus, unipolar n.'s are the exclusive neural elements of the sensory ganglia. The lack of dendritic processes of these primary sensory n.'s is only apparent: the dendritic pole of the unipolar n. is represented by the unmyelinated terminal ramifications of the peripheral axon branch.

upper motor n., clinical term indicating those n.'s of the motor cortex that contribute to the formation of the pyramidal or corticospinal and corticobulbar tracts, as distinguished from the lower motor n.'s innervating the skeletal muscles. Although not motor n.'s in the strict sense, these cortical n.'s became colloquially classified as motor n.'s because their stimulation produces movement and their destruction causes severe disorders of movement. See also motor n.; motor *cortex.*

visceral motor n., see motor n.

neuronal (nūr'ō-năl, nū-rō'năl). Pertaining to a neuron.

neurone (nūr'ōn). Neuron (1).

neuronephric (nūr-ō-nef'rik) [neuro- + G. *nephros,* kidney]. Relating to the nerve supply of the kidney.

neuronevus (nūr-ō-nē'vŭs). A variety of intradermal nevus in which nests of atrophic nevus cells in the lower dermis are hyalinized and resemble nerve bundles.

neuronitis (nūr-ŏ-nī'tis). Degenerative inflammation of nerve cells.

neuronopathy (nūr-ō-nop'ă-thē). Disorder, often toxic, of the neuron (1).

sensory n., n. confined to dorsal root and gasserian ganglia.

neuronophage (nū-ron'ō-fāj) [neuron + G. *phagein,* to eat]. A phagocyte that ingests neuronal elements. See microglia.

neuronophagia, neuronophagy (nūr'on'ō-fā'jē-ă, nūr-ō-nof'ă-jē) [neuron + G. *phagein,* to eat]. Phagocytosis of nerve cells.

neuronyxis (nūr-ō-nik'sis) [neuro- + G. *nyxis,* pricking]. Acupuncture of a nerve.

neuro-oncology (nūr'ō-on-kol'ō-jē) [neuro- + onco- + G. *logos,* study]. The study of tumors of the nervous system.

neuro-ophthalmology (nūr'ō-of-thal-mol'ō-jē). Neurophthalmology; that branch of medical science concerned with the relationship of the eyes and their associated parts to the central nervous system, and their disorders.

neuro-otology (nūr'ō-ō-tol'ō-jē). The science concerned with labyrinthine affections and with those brain lesions complicating or related to disease of the ear.

neuropapillitis (nūr'ō-pap-i-lī'tis). Inflammation of the optic nerve within the eye.

neuroparalysis (nūr'ō-pă-ral'i-sis). Paralysis resulting from disease of the nerve supplying the affected part.

neuroparalytic (nūr'ō-pa-ră-lit'ik). Denoting or characterized by neuroparalysis.

neuropath (nūr'ō-path). One who suffers from or is predisposed to some disease of the nervous system.

neuropathic (nūr-ō-path'ik). Relating in any way to neuropathy.

neuropathogenesis (nūr'ō-path-ō-jen'ĕ-sis) [neuro- + G. *pathos,* suffering, + *genesis,* origin]. The origin or causation of a disease of the nervous system.

neuropathology (nūr'ō-pa-thol'ō-jē). **1.** Pathology of the nervous system. **2.** That branch of pathology concerned with the nervous system.

neuropathy (nū-rop'ă-thē) [neuro- + G. *pathos,* suffering]. **1.** A classical term for any disorder affecting any segment of the nervous system. **2.** In contemporary usage, a disease involving the cranial or spinal nerves.

asymmetric motor n., n. in which the loss of function is more marked in the extremities of one side of the body.

brachial plexus n., neuralgic amyotrophy; brachial neuritis; acute brachial radiculitis; shoulder girdle or shoulder-hand syndrome; an acute syndrome of unknown etiology characterized by pain in the shoulder girdle; followed by flaccid weakness of the muscles supplied by the brachial plexus and mild sensory loss in the affected dermatomes; EMG shows evidence of denervation but normal conduction velocities; usually, spontaneous recovery occurs within months.

diabetic n., a combined sensory and motor n., typically symmetric and segmental, and involving, as well, autonomic fibers; seen frequently in older diabetic persons.

diphtheritic n., a rapidly developing peripheral n. caused by a toxin elaborated by *Corynebacterium diphtheriae.*

entrapment n., a region of traumatic neuritis in which the nerve is maintained in an irritated state by external pressure created by encroachment or impingement from a nearby anatomical structure; *e.g.,* pressure on the median nerve by swollen tendons and their sheaths in the carpal tunnel producing the carpal tunnel syndrome.

familial amyloid n., familial amyloidosis; a disorder in which various peripheral nerves are infiltrated with amyloid and their functions disturbed; characteristically, it begins during mid-life and is found largely in persons of Portuguese descent; autosomal dominant inheritance. Other rare clinical types occur.

giant axonal n., a generalized disorder of neurofilaments with progressive peripheral neural degeneration in childhood.

hereditary hypertrophic n., Dejerine's or Dejerine-Sottas disease; a progressive chronic sensorimotor polyneuropathy associated with swelling and mucoid degeneration of peripheral nerves; autosomal dominant inheritance.

hereditary sensory radicular n., n. characterized by the occurrence of severe, relapsing foot ulcerations of neuropathic origin, destruction of terminal digits of feet and hands, and a loss of sensation; autosomal dominant inheritance.

hypertrophic interstitial n., onion bulb n.; sensorimotor neuropathy characterized pathologically by collections of Schwann cell processes arranged concentrically around one or more nerve fibers. For hereditary types, see hereditary hypertrophic n.

ischemic optic n., optic nerve n. secondary to arteriosclerosis (arteritic) or temporal arteritis.

isoniazid n., an axonal form of n. seen in some patients treated with isoniazid.

lead n., a progressive, often symmetric, segmental peripheral n. seen in chronic lead intoxication; characterized by wrist-drop.

leprous n., a slowly developing granulomatous n., commonly seen in leprosy, caused by *Mycobacterium leprae.*

motor dapsone n., a peripheral n. due to ingestion of 4,4-deaminodiphenylsulphone.

onion bulb n., hypertrophic interstitial n.

segmental n., demyelination of scattered segments of peripheral nerves, with relating sparing of axons; noted in diabetes, arsenic poisoning, lead poisoning, diphtheria, and leprosy.

symmetric distal n., n. in which the motor weakness is equal on both sides of the body.

vitamin B_{12} n., subacute combined *degeneration* of the spinal cord.

neuropeptide (nūr-ō-pep'tīd). Any of a variety of peptides found in neural tissue; *e.g.,* endorphins, enkephalins.

neuropharmacology (nūr'ō-far'mă-kol'ō-jē). The study of drugs that affect neuronal tissue.

neurophilic (nūr-ō-fil'ik) [neuro- + G. *philos,* fond]. Neurotropic.

neurophonia (nūr-ō-fō'nē-ă) [neuro- + G. *phōnē,* voice]. A spasm or tic of the muscles of phonation causing involuntary sounds or cries.

neurophthalmology (nūr'of-thal-mol'ō-jē). Neuro-ophthalmology.

neurophysins (nūr-ō-fiz'inz). A family of proteins synthesized in the hypothalamus as part of the large precursor protein that includes vasopressin and oxytocin in the neurosecretory granules; n. function as carriers in the transport and storage of neurohypophysial hormones.

neurophysiology (nūr'ō-fiz-ē-ol'ō-jē). Physiology of the nervous system.

neuropil, neuropile (nūr'ō-pil, -pīl) [neuro- + G. *pilos,* felt]. The complex, feltlike net of axonal, dendritic, and glial arborizations that forms the bulk of the central nervous system's gray matter, and in which the nerve cell bodies lie embedded.

neuroplasm (nūr'ō-plazm). The protoplasm of a nerve cell.

neuroplasty (nūr'ō-plas-tē) [neuro- + G. *plastos,* formed]. Plastic surgery of the nerves.

neuroplegic (nūr-ō-plē'jik) [neuro- + G. *plēgē,* a stroke]. Pertaining to paralysis due to nervous system disease.

neuropodia (nūr-ō-pō'dē-ă) [pl. of *neuropodium* or *neuropodion,* fr. neuro- + G. *podion,* little foot]. Axon *terminals.*

neuropore (nūr'ō-pōr) [neuro- + G. *poros,* pore]. An opening in the embryo leading from the central canal of the neural tube to the exterior of the tube.

caudal n., the temporary opening at the extreme caudal end of the neural tube in early embryos.

rostral n., the temporary opening at the extreme rostral (cephalic) end of the early embryonic forebrain.

neuropsychiatry (nūr'ō-sī-kī'ă-trē). The specialty dealing with both organic and psychic disorders of the nervous system.

neuropsychologic, neuropsychological (nūr'ō-sī-kō-loj'ik, -loj'i-kăl). Pertaining to neuropsychology.

neuropsychology (nūr'ō-sī-kol'ō-jē). A specialty of psychology concerned with the study of the relationships between the brain and behavior, including the use of psychological tests and assessment techniques to diagnose specific cognitive and behavioral deficits and to prescribe rehabilitation strategies for their remediation.

neuropsychopathic (nūr'ō-sī-kō-path'ik). Relating to neuropsychopathy.

neuropsychopathy (nūr'ō-sī-kop'ă-thē). An emotional illness of neurologic and/or functional origin.

neuropsychopharmacology (nūr'ō-sī'kō-far-mă-kol'ō-jē). Psychopharmacology.

neuroradiology (nūr'ō-rā-dē-ol'ō-jē). The study of the nervous system using x-ray examination and similar methods.

neurorecidive (nūr-ō-res'i-dēv) [neuro- + L. *recidivus,* recurring]. Neurorelapse.

neurorecurrence (nūr'ō-rē-ker'ens). Neurorelapse.

neurorelapse (nūr'ō-rē-laps'). Neurorecurrence; neurorecidive; the recurrence of neurological symptoms upon initiation of therapy, especially with antisyphilitic drugs.

neuroretinitis (nūr'ō-ret-i-nī'tis). Inflammation of the retina and optic nerve.

neurorrhaphy (nūr-ōr'ă-fē) [neuro- + G. *rhaphē,* suture]. Neurosuture; nerve suture; joining together, usually by suture, of the two parts of a divided nerve.

neurosarcocleisis (nūr'ō-sar-kō-klī'sis) [neuro- + G. *sarx,* flesh, + *kleisis,* closure]. An operation for the relief of neuralgia, consisting of resection of one of the walls of the osseous canal traversed by the nerve and transposition of the nerve into the soft tissues.

neurosarcoidosis (nūr'ō-sar-koy-dō'sis). A granulomatous disease of unknown etiology involving the central nervous system, usually with concomitant systemic involvement.

neuroschwannoma (nūr'ō-shwah-nō'mă). Neurilemoma.

neurosciences (nūr-ō-sī'en-sez). The scientific disciplines concerned with the development, structure, function, chemistry, pharmacology, clinical assessments, and pathology of the nervous system.

neurosecretion (nūr'ō-sē-krē'shŭn). The release of a secretory substance from the axon terminals of certain nerve cells in the brain into the circulating blood. The secretory product may be a true hormone, *e.g.,* the antidiuretic hormone released from the axon terminals of the neurons composing the supraoptic nucleus of the hypothalamus; in the case of the so-called releasing-factor neurons of the hypothalamus the cell product is not a systemic hormone in its own right but elicits the release of trophic hormones by the anterior lobe of the hypophysis, substances that in turn stimulate peripheral endocrine glands to release their systemically active hormones.

neurosecretory (nūr'ō-sē'krē-tōr-ē, -sē-krē'tōr-ē). Relating to neurosecretion.

neurosis, pl. **neuroses** (nū-rō'sis, -sēz) [neuro- + G. *-osis,* condition]. **1.** A psychological or behavioral disorder in which anxiety is the primary characteristic; defense mechanisms or any of the phobias are the adjustive techniques which an individual learns in order to cope with this underlying anxiety. In contrast to the psychoses, persons with a n. do not exhibit gross distortion of reality or disorganization of personality. **2.** A functional nervous disease, or one for which there is no evident lesion. **3.** A peculiar state of tension or irritability of the nervous system; any form of nervousness.

accident n., traumatic n.

anxiety n., anxiety state; chronic abnormal distress and worry to the point of panic, associated with overaction of the sympathetic nervous system.

association n., a n. in which association of ideas causes mental repetition of an experience.

battle n., war n.

cardiac n., cardioneurosis; anxiety concerning the state of the heart, as a result of palpitation, chest pain, or other symptoms not due to heart disease. See also neurocirculatory *asthenia.*

character n., a subclass of personality disorders.

compensation n., the development of symptoms of n. believed to be motivated by the desire for, and hope of, monetary gain.

compulsive n., obsessive-compulsive n.

conversion hysteria n., conversion *hysteria.*

expectation n., a condition in which anticipation of an event produces neurotic symptoms.

experimental n., a behavior disorder produced experimentally, as when an organism is required to make a discrimination of extreme difficulty and "breaks down" in the process.

military n., war n.

noogenic n., in existential psychiatry, the neurotic symptomatology resulting from existential frustration.

obsessive-compulsive n., compulsive n.; a disorder characterized by the persistent and repetitive intrusion of unwanted thoughts, urges, or actions that the individual is unable to prevent; the compulsive thoughts may consist of single words, ideas, or ruminations often perceived by the sufferer as nonsensical; the repetitive urges or actions vary from simple movements to complex rituals; anxiety or distress is the underlying emotion or drive state, and the ritualistic behavior is a learned method of reducing the anxiety.

occupational n., professional n., craft palsy; functional, occupational, or professional spasm; a functional disorder of a group of muscles used chiefly in one's occupation, marked by the occurrence of spasm, paresis, or incoordination on attempt to repeat the habitual movements; *e.g.,* writer's cramp.

oedipal n., continuation of the oedipus complex into adulthood.

pension n., a type of compensation n., motivated by the desire for premature retirement on pension.

postconcussion n., a type of traumatic n. following a cerebral concussion.

posttraumatic n., traumatic n.
n. tar'da, neurotic patterns developing in older people, related to organic cerebral lesions.
torsion n., *dysbasia* lordotica progressiva.
transference n., in psychoanalysis, the phenomenon of the patient's developing a strong emotional relationship with the analyst, symbolizing an emotional relationship with a family figure; analysis of this n. comprises an important part of psychoanalytic treatment.
traumatic n., accident or posttraumatic n.; any functional nervous disorder following an accident or injury.
war n., battle or military n.; a stress condition or mental disorder induced by conditions existing in warfare. See also battle *fatigue.*

neurospasm (nūr'ō-spazm). Muscular spasm or twitching caused by a disordered nerve supply.

neurosplanchnic (nūr-ō-splangk'nik) [neuro- + G. *splanchnon,* a viscus]. Neurovisceral.

neurospongium (nūr-ō-spon'jē-ŭm, -spŭn'jē-ŭm) [neuro- + G. *spongion,* small sponge]. **1.** Obsolete term for the plexus of neurofibrils within nerve cells. **2.** Obsolete designation for the reticular layer of the retina.

Neurospora (nū-ros'pōr-ă) [neuro- + G. *spora,* seed]. Pink bread mold; a genus of fungi (class Ascomycetes) grown in cultures and used in research in genetics and cellular biochemistry.

neurosthenia (nūr-ō-sthē'nē-ă) [neuro- + G. *sthenos,* force]. A condition in which the nerves respond with abnormal force or rapidity to slight stimuli.

neurostimulator (nūr-ō-stim'yū-lā-ter). A device for chronic electrical excitation of the central or peripheral nervous system.

neurosurgeon (nūr-ō-ser'jŭn). A surgeon specializing in operations on the nervous system.

neurosurgery (nūr-ō-ser'jer-ē). Surgery of the nervous system.
functional n., destruction or chronic excitation of a part of the brain to treat disordered behavior or function.

neurosuture (nūr-ō-sū'chūr). Neurorrhaphy.

neurosyphilis (nūr-ō-sif'i-lis). Nervous system manifestations of syphilis, including tabes dorsalis, general paresis, meningovascular syphilis.

neurotabes (nūr-ō-tā'bēz) [neuro- + L. *tabes,* a wasting away]. Déjérine's peripheral n.; polyneuritis with ataxic symptoms.
Dejerine's peripheral n., neurotabes.

neurotendinous (nūr-ō-ten'di-nŭs). Relating to both nerves and tendons.

neurotensin (nū-rō-ten'sin). A 13-amino acid peptide neurotransmitter found in synapsomes in the hypothalamus, amygdala, basal ganglia, and dorsal gray matter of the spinal cord; it plays a role in pain perception, but its analgesic effects are not blocked by opioid antagonists; it also affects pituitary hormone release and gastrointestinal function.

neurotension (nūr-ō-ten'shŭn). Neurectasia.

neurothekeoma (nūr-ō-thē'kē-ō-mă). A benign myxoma of cutaneous nerve sheath origin.

neurothele (nūr'ō-thēl) [neuro- + G. *thēlē,* nipple]. Nerve *papilla.*

neurotherapeutics, neurotherapy (nūr'ō-thār'ă-pyū'tiks, -thār'ă-pē). The treatment of nervous disorders.

neurothlipsis, neurothlipsia (nūr-ō-thlip'sis, -sē-ă) [neuro- + G. *thlipsis,* pressure]. Pressure on one or more nerves.

neurotic (nū-rot'ik). Relating to or suffering from a neurosis.

neuroticism (nū-rot'i-sizm). The condition or psychological trait of being neurotic.

neurotization (nūr'ō-ti-zā'shŭn). The acquisition of nervous substance; the regeneration of a nerve.

neurotize (nūr'ō-tīz). To provide with nerve substance.

neurotmesis (nūr-ot-mē'sis) [neuro- + G. *tmēsis,* a cutting]. A condition in which there is complete division of a nerve.

neurotology (nūr-ō-tol'ō-jē) [neuro- + G. *ous (ot-),* ear, + *logos,* study]. Neuro-otology.

neurotome (nūr'ō-tōm) [neuro- + G. *tomē,* a cutting]. A very slender knife or needle, used for teasing apart nerve fibers in microdissection.

neurotomy (nū-rot'ō-mē) [neuro- + G. *tomē,* a cutting]. Operative division of a nerve.
retrogasserian n., trigeminal *rhizotomy.*

neurotonic (nūr-ō-ton'ik). **1.** Relating to neurotony. **2.** Strengthening or stimulating impaired nervous action. **3.** An agent that improves the tone or force of the nervous system.

neurotony (nū-rot'ō-nē) [neuro- + G. *tonos,* tension]. Neurectasia.

neurotoxic (nūr-ō-tok'sik). Poisonous to nervous substance.

neurotoxin (nūr-ō-tok'sin). Neurolysin.

neurotransmission (nūr'ō-trans-mish'ŭn). Neurohumoral *transmission.*

neurotransmitter (nūr'ō-trans-mit'er) [neuro- + L. *transmitto,* to send across]. Any specific chemical agent released by a presynaptic cell, upon excitation, that crosses the synapse to stimulate or inhibit the postsynaptic cell.

neurotrauma (nūr-ō-traw'mă) [neuro- + G. *trauma,* injury]. **1.** Trauma of the nervous system. **2.** Neurotrosis; trauma or wounding of a nerve.

neurotripsy (nūr-ō-trip'sē) [neuro- + G. *tripsis,* a rubbing]. Operative crushing of a nerve.

neurotrophic (nūr-ō-trof'ik). Relating to neurotrophy.

neurotrophy (nū-rot'rō-fē) [neuro- + G. *trophē,* nourishment]. Nutrition and metabolism of tissues under nervous influence.

neurotropic (nūr-ō-trop'ik). Neurophilic; having an affinity for the nervous system.

neurotropy, neurotropism (nū-rot'rō-pē, -pizm) [neuro- + G. *tropē,* a turning]. **1.** Affinity of basic dyes for nervous tissue. **2.** The attraction of certain pathogenic microorganisms, poisons, and nutritive substances toward the nerve centers.

neurotrosis (nūr-ō-trō'sis) [neuro- + G. *trōsis,* a wounding]. Neurotrauma (2).

neurotubule (nūr'ō-tū-byūl). One of the microtubules, 10 to 20 nm in diameter, occurring in the cell body, dendrites, axon, and in some synaptic endings of neurons.

neurovaccine (nūr-ō-vak'sēn). A fixed or standardized vaccine virus of definite strength, obtained by continued passage through the brain of rabbits.

neurovaricosis, neurovaricosity (nūr'ō-var-i-kō'sis, -var-i-kos'i-tē) [neuro- + L. *varix,* varicosis]. A condition marked by multiple swellings along the course of a nerve.

neurovascular (nūr-ō-vas'kyū-lăr). Relating to both nervous and vascular systems; relating to the nerves supplying the walls of the blood vessels, the vasomotor nerves.

neurovegetative (nūr-ō-vej'ĕ-tā-tiv). Neurovisceral.

neurovirus (nūr-ō-vī'rŭs). Vaccine virus modified by means of passage into and growth in nervous tissue.

neurovisceral (nūr-ō-vis'er-ăl) [neuro- + L. *viscera,* the internal organs]. Neurovegetative; neurosplanchnic; referring to the innervation of the internal organs by the autonomic nervous system.

neurula, pl. neurulae (nūr'ū-lă, -lē) [neur- + L. *-ulus,* small one]. Stage in embryonic development in which the prominent processes are the formation of the neural plate and the plate's closure to form the neural tube.

neurulation (nūr-ū-lā'shŭn) [see neurula]. Processes involved in the formation of the neurula stage.

Neusser, Edmund von, Austrian physician, 1852–1912. See N.'s *granules.*

neutral (nū'trăl) [L. *neutralis,* fr. *neuter,* neither]. **1.** Exhibiting no positive properties; indifferent. **2.** In chemistry, neither acid nor alkaline.

neutralization (nū'trăl-i-zā'shŭn). **1.** The change in reaction of a solution from acid or alkaline to neutral by the addition of just a sufficient amount of an alkaline or of an acid substance, respectively. **2.** The rendering ineffective of any action, process, or potential.

neutralize (nū'tră-līz). To effect neutralization.

neutral red [C.I. 50040]. Toluylene red; N^8,N^8,3-trimethyl-2,8-phenazinediamine monohydrochloride; used as an indicator (red at pH 6.8, yellow at 8.0), as a vital dye to stain granules and vacuoles in living cells, in testing the secretion of acid by the stomach (given with a test meal), and in general histologic staining.

neutrino (nū-trē'nō) [neutron + It. dim. *-ino*]. A subatomic particle having zero rest mass and no charge, traveling always at the speed of light, and rarely interacting with matter.

neutro-, neutr- [L. *neutralis,* fr. *neuter,* neither]. Combining forms meaning neutral.

neutroclusion (nū-trō-klū'zhŭn) [neutro- + occlusion]. Neutral occlusion (2); a malocclusion in which there is a normal anteroposterior relationship between the maxilla and mandible; in Angle's classification, a Class I malocclusion.

neutron (nū'tron) [L. *neuter,* neither]. An electrically neutral particle in the nuclei of all atoms (except hydrogen-1) with a mass approximately that of a proton; in isolation, it breaks down to a proton and an electron with a half-life of about 12 minutes.
epithermal n., a n. having an energy in the range immediately above the thermal range, *i.e.,* having an energy between a few hundredths and approximately 100 ev.

neutropenia (nū-trō-pē'nē-ă) [neutrophil + G. *penia,* poverty]. Neutrophilic leukopenia; neutrophilopenia; the presence of abnormally small numbers of neutrophils in the circulating blood.
cyclic n., periodic n.
periodic n., cyclic n.; n. recurring at regular intervals (14 to 45 days), in association with various types of infectious diseases, *e.g.,* stomatitis, cutaneous ulcers, furuncles, arthritis, and others.

neutrophil, neutrophile (nū'trō-fil, -fīl) [neutro- + G. *philos,* fond]. **1.** A mature white blood cell in the granulocytic series, formed by myelopoietic tissue of the bone marrow (sometimes also in extramedullary sites), and released into the circulating blood, where they normally represent from 54% to 65% of the total number of leukocytes. When stained with the usual Romanovsky type of dyes, n.'s are characterized by: 1) a nucleus that is dark purple-blue, lobated (three to five distinct lobes joined by thin strands of chromatin), and has a rather coarse network of fairly dense chromatin; 2) a cytoplasm that is faintly pink (sharply contrasted with the nucleus) and contains numerous fine pink or violet-pink granules, *i.e.,* not acidophilic or basophilic (as in eosinophils or basophils). The precursors of n.'s, in order of increasing maturity, are: myeloblasts, myelocytes, and metamyelocytes or "juvenile" forms, including the "stabkernige" or staff cells (also known as stabs or band forms). Although the terms neutrophilic leukocytes and neutrophilic granulocytes include younger cells in which neutrophilic granules are recognized, the two expressions are frequently used as synonyms for n.'s, which are mature forms unless otherwise indicated by a modifying term, such as immature n. See also leukocyte, leukocytosis, and their subentries. **2.** Any cell or tissue that manifests no special affinity for acid or basic dyes, *i.e.,* the cytoplasm stains approximately equally with either type of dye.
band n., band *cell.*
hypersegmented n., an aged and degenerated n. in which there may be 6 to 10 lobes in the nucleus.
immature n., a young n.; the term is usually used with reference to stab n.'s (or other "juvenile" n.'s), neutrophilic granulocytes in which the nucleus is indented but not distinctly segmented.
juvenile n., any cell of the granulocytic series in which the neutrophilic granules are recognizable and the nucleus is indented (the first phase of segmentation).
mature n., segmented n.
segmented n., mature n.; a fully matured n. that has at least 2 (and as many as 5) distinct lobes in the nucleus and manifests active ameboid motion.
stab n., band *cell.*

neutrophilia (nū-trō-fil'ē-ă). Neutrophilic leukocytosis; an increase of neutrophilic leukocytes in blood or tissues; also frequently used synonymously with leukocytosis, inasmuch as the latter is generally the result of an increased number of neutrophilic granulocytes in the circulating blood (or in the tissues, or both). N. is usually absolute, *i.e.,* there is an increase in the total number of leukocytes as well as an increased percentage of neutrophils; in some instances, n. may be relative, *i.e.,* there is an increased percentage of neutrophils, but the total number of all types of leukocytes may be within the normal range.

neutrophilic (nū-trō-fil'ik). **1.** Pertaining to or characterized by neutrophils, such as an exudate in which the predominant cells are n. granulocytes. **2.** Neutrophilous; characterized by a lack of affinity for acid or basic dyes, *i.e.,* staining approximately equally with either type.

neutrophilopenia (nū'trō-fil-ō-pē'nē-ă) [neutrophil + G. *penia,* poverty]. Neutropenia.

neutrophilous (nū-trof'i-lŭs). Neutrophilic (2).

neutrotaxis (nū-trō-tak'sis) [neutrophil + G. *taxis,* arrangement]. A phenomenon in which neutrophilic leukocytes are stimulated by a substance in such a manner that they are either attracted, and move toward it (**positive n.**), or they are repelled, and move away from it (**negative n.**); in some instances, there is no effect (sometimes called **indifferent n.**).

nevi (nē'vī) [L.]. Plural of nevus.

nevocyte (nē'vō-sīt). Nevus *cell.*

nevoid (nē'voyd) [L. *naevus,* mole (nevus), + G. *eidos,* resemblance]. Nevose (2); nevous (2); resembling a nevus.

nevolipoma (nē'vō-li-pō'mă) [nevus + lipoma]. Nevus lipomatodes or lipomatosis; unsatisfactory terms for a lesion that is basically a nevus, with a stroma of fibrous and adipose elements.

nevose, nevous (nē'vōs, -vŭs) **1.** Marked with nevi. **2.** Nevoid.

nevoxanthoendothelioma (nē'vō-zan'thō-en'dō-thē-lē-ō'mă) [nevus + G. *xanthos,* yellow, + endothelioma]. Juvenile *xanthogranuloma.*

nevus, pl. **nevi** (nē'vŭs, -vī) [L. *naevus,* mole, birthmark]. Spiloma; spilus. **1.** Birthmark; a circumscribed malformation of the skin, especially if colored by hyperpigmentation or increased vascularity; a n. may be predominantly epidermal, adnexal, melanocytic, vascular, or mesodermal, or a compound overgrowth of these tissues. **2.** A benign localized overgrowth of melanin-forming cells of the skin present at birth or appearing early in life.
acquired n., a melanocytic n. that is not visible at birth, but appears in childhood or adult life.
n. ane'micus, a functional developmental defect characterized by pale, round or oval, flat lesions, indistinguishable from surrounding normal skin on diascopy.
n. angiecto'des, n. vascularis.
n. angiomato'des, a diffuse angiomatous formation in the subcutaneous connective tissue.

n. arachnoi'deus, n. ara'neus, arterial *spider.*
balloon cell n., a n. in which many of the cells are large, with clear cytoplasm.
basal cell n., a hereditary disease noted in infancy or adolescence, characterized by lesions of the eyelids, nose, cheeks, neck, and axillae, appearing as uneroded flesh-colored papules, some becoming pedunculated, and histologically indistinguishable from basal cell epithelioma; also noted are punctate keratotic lesions of the palms and soles; the lesions usually remain benign; ulceration and invasion are evidence of malignant changes; autosomal dominant inheritance with high penetrance.
bathing trunk n., giant pigmented n.; Tierfellnaevus; a large hairy congenital pigmented n. with a predilection for the entire lower trunk; malignant melanoma may develop in childhood.
Becker's n., pigmented hairy epidermal n.; a n. first seen as an irregular pigmentation of the shoulders, upper chest, or scapular area, gradually enlarging irregularly and becoming thickened and hairy.
blue n., Jadassohn-Tièche n.; a dark blue or blue-black n. covered by smooth skin and formed by spindle-shaped melanocytes in the dermis.
blue rubber-bleb nevi, a syndrome characterized by erectile, easily compressible, thin-walled hemangiomatous nodules, widely distributed in the skin and in the alimentary canal, and sometimes in other tissues; lesions in the gut may perforate or cause hemorrhage, and the patient may be anemic from continual bleeding.
capillary n., capillary hemangioma of the skin.
n. caverno'sus, cavernous *hemangioma.*
cellular blue n., a blue n. in which melanocytes are numerous, large, and closely packed, and which may extend deeply into the subcutis; malignant change is very rare.
n. comedon'icus, comedo n., n. follicularis keratosis; congenital linear keratinous cystic invaginations of the epidermis, with failure of development of normal pilosebaceous follicles.
compound n., a n. in which there are nests of n. cells in the epidermal-dermal junction and in the dermis.
congenital n., a melanocytic n. that is visible at birth, is often larger than an acquired n., and more frequently involves deeper dermal structures.
dysplastic n., see dysplastic nevus *syndrome.*
n. elas'ticus of Lewandowski, plaques of smooth or nodular papules, skin- or ivory-colored, occuring symmetrically on the trunk or extremities; now known to be a collagenous n.
epidermic-dermic n., junction n.
epithelioid cell n., benign juvenile *melanoma.*
faun tail n., a circumscribed growth of hair of the lumbosacral area, associated with diastematomyelia.
n. flam'meus, flame n., port-wine mark or stain; a large n. vascularis having a purplish color; it is usually found on the head and neck and persists throughout life.
n. follicula'ris kerato'sis, n. comedonicus.
giant pigmented n., bathing trunk n.
halo n., circumnevic vitiligo; leukoderma acquisitum centrifugum; Sutton's disease (1) or n.; a benign, sometimes multiple, melanocytic n. in which involution occurs with a central brown mole surrounded by a uniformly depigmented zone or halo.
intradermal n., a n. in which nests of melanocytes are found in the dermis, but not at the epidermal-dermal junction; benign pigmented nevi in adults are most commonly intradermal.
Ito's n., pigmentation of skin (mongolian spot) innervated by lateral branches of the supraclavicular nerve and the lateral cutaneous nerve of the arm, due to scattered melanocytes in the dermis.
Jadassohn's n., n. sebaceus.
Jadassohn-Tièche n., blue n.
junction n., epidermic-dermic n.; a n. consisting of nests of melanocytes in the basal cell zone, at the junction of the epidermis and dermis, appearing as a slightly raised, small, flat, nonhairy pigmented (brown or black) tumor.
n. lipomato'des, n. lipomato'sus, nevolipoma.
n. lu'pus, obsolete term for *angioma* serpiginosum.
n. lymphat'icus, a cutaneous lymphangioma.
nape n., Unna's mark; a pale vascular birthmark found on the nape of the neck in 25 to 50% of normal persons.
oral epithelial n., white sponge n.
organoid n., n. sebaceus.
Ota's n., oculodermal *melanosis.*
n. papillomato'sus, a prominent wartlike mole.
pigmented hair epidermal n., Becker's n.
n. pigmento'sus, mole (1); a benign pigmented melanocytic proliferation; raised or level with the skin, present at birth or arising early in life.
n. pilo'sus, hairy mole; a mole covered with an abundant growth of hair.
n. sanguin'eus, n. vascularis.
n. seba'ceus, Jadassohn's or organoid n.; congenital papillary acanthosis of the epidermis, with hypoplasia of sebaceous glands developing at puberty and presence of apocrine glands in non-apocrine areas of the skin (commonly the scalp).
spider n., arterial *spider.*
n. spi'lus, a flat mole.
spindle cell n., benign juvenile *melanoma.*
Spitz n., benign juvenile *melanoma.*
strawberry n., strawberry birthmark or mark; a small n. vascularis resembling a strawberry in size, shape, and color; it usually disappears spontaneously in early childhood.
Sutton's n., halo n.
n. syring'ocystad'enomato'sus papillif'erus, an organoid epithelial defect with apocrine structures predominating.
systematized n., a developmental dysplasia of the skin; extensive, patterned, and usually unilateral.
n. u'nius lat'eris, a congenital systematized linear n. limited to one side of the body or to portions of the extremities on one side; lesions are often extensive, forming wave-like bands on the trunk, and spiraling streaks on the extremities.
n. vascula'ris, n. vasculo'sus, capillary or superficial angioma; n. angiectodes or sanguineus; a congenital red discoloration of the skin, of irregular size and boundaries, caused by an overgrowth of the cutaneous capillaries; most of these capillary hemangiomas regress spontaneously; strawberry n. and n. flammeus are types of n. vascularis.
n. veno'sus, a n. formed of a patch of dilated venules.
verrucous n., a skin-colored or darker wartlike, often linear, lesion appearing at birth or early in childhood, and occurring in various sizes and locations, single or multiple.
white sponge n., familial white folded dysplasia; oral epithelial n.; a hereditary condition of the oral cavity characterized by soft, white or opalescent, thickened and corrugated folds of mucous membrane; other mucosal sites are occasionally involved simultaneously.
woolly-hair n., allotrichia circumscripta; a circumscribed congenital kinking or woolliness of scalp hair, appearing during infancy (or as late as age 19) in a previously normal hair site and enlarging for a period of 2 to 3 years.

newborn (nū'bōrn). Neonatal.

Newcastle disease. See under disease.

Newcomer's fixative. See under fixative.

New Hampshire rule. See under rule.

Newton, Sir Isaac, British physicist, 1642–1727. See newton; newtonian *aberration, constant* of gravitation, *flow, viscosity;* N.'s *disk, law.*

newton (N) (nū'tŏn) [I. *Newton*]. Derived unit of force in the SI system, expressed as meters-kilograms per second squared (m/kg/s^{-2}); equivalent to 10^5 dynes in the CGS system.

newton-meter. A unit of the MKS system, expressed as energy expended, or work done, by a force of 1 newton acting through a distance of 1 meter; equal to 1 joule (10^7 ergs).

nexus, pl. **nexus** (nek'sŭs) [L. interconnection]. Gap *junction.*

Nezelof, C., French pathologist, *1922. See N. *syndrome,* N. type of thymic *alymphoplasia.*

NF Abbreviation for *National Formulary.*

ng Abbreviation for nanogram.

NGF Abbreviation for nerve growth *factor.*

N.H.S. Abbreviation for National Health Service (England).

NH_2-terminal. Amino-terminal.

Ni Symbol for nickel.

niacin (nī'ă-sin). Nicotinic acid.

niacinamide (nī'ă-sin-am'īd). Nicotinamide.

nialamide (nī-al'ă-mīd). *N*-Benzyl-*β*-(isonicotinoylhydrazine) propionamide; a monoamine oxidase inhibitor used in the treatment of depressive disorders.

nib. In dentistry, the portion of a condensing instrument that comes into contact with the restorative material being condensed; its end, the face, is smooth or serrated.

niche (nitch, nēsh) [Fr.]. **1.** A space, site, or recess that can be suitably filled. **2.** In contrast radiography, an eroded or ulcerated area which can be detected when it fills with a contrast medium. **3.** An ecological term for the position occupied by a species in a biotic community, particularly its relationships to various other competitor, predator, prey, and parasite species.

enamel n., enamel *crypt.*

Haudek's n., archaic term for an apparent projection from the wall of the stomach sometimes seen in roentgenograms of gastric ulcer, due actually to the filling of the cavity of the ulcer with contrast medium.

nick (nik). In molecular biology, a hydrolytic cleavage of a phosphodiester bond in one strand of a double-stranded nucleic acid. *Cf.* cut.

nickel (nik'l) [abbrev. fr. Ger. *kupfer-nickel,* name of copper-colored ore from which nickel was first obtained; *nickel,* the Ger. word for a dwarfish imp]. A metallic element, symbol Ni, atomic no. 28, atomic weight 58.70, closely resembling cobalt and often associated with it.

Nickerson-Kveim test. See under test.

nicking (nik'ing). Localized constrictions in retinal blood vessels.

arteriovenous n., constriction of a retinal vein at an artery-vein crossing.

Nicklès, François J.J., French chemist, 1821–1869. See N.'s *test.*

niclosamide (ni-klō'să-mīd). *N*-(2'-Chloro-4'-nitrophenyl)-5-chlorosalicylamide; a teniacide effective against intestinal cestodes.

nicofuranose (ni-kō-fyū'ră-nōs). Fructose 1,3,4,6-tetranicotinate; a peripheral vasodilator.

Nicol, William, Edinburgh physicist, 1768–1851. See N. *prism.*

Nicolas, Joseph, French physician, *1868. See N.-Favre *disease.*

Nicolle, J.H., French microbiologist and Nobel laureate, 1866–1936. See N.'s white *mycetoma, stain* for capsules.

nicotinamide (nik-ō-tin'ă-mīd). Nicotinic acid amide; niacinamide; pyridine-3-carboxamide; the biologically active amide of nicotinic acid, used in the prevention and treatment of pellagra.

nicotinamide adenine dinucleotide (NAD). Ribosylnicotinamide 5'-phosphate (NMN) and adenosine 5'-phosphate (AMP) linked by pyrophosphate formation between the two phosphoric groups; attached as a prosthetic group to a protein, it serves as a respiratory enzyme (hydrogen acceptor and donor) through alternate oxidation and reduction ($NAD^+ \rightleftharpoons NADH$). See also entries under NAD and NADP.

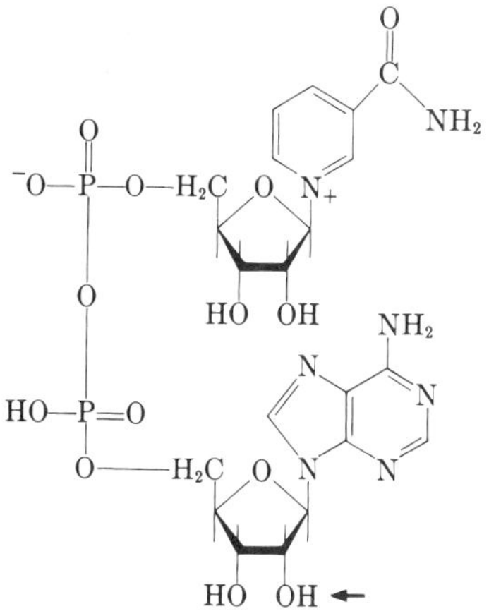

Oxidized NAD (NAD^+)
Arrow indicates location of the third phosphoric group in NADP.

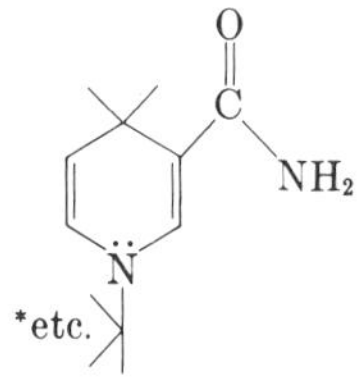

Reduced NAD (NADH) (Nicotinamide moiety)
* Denotes that remainder of NADH formula is identical with that shown for NAD^+.

nicotinamide adenine dinucleotide phosphate (NADP). A coenzyme of many oxidases (dehydrogenases), in which the reaction $NADP^+ + 2H \rightleftharpoons NADPH + H^+$ takes place; the third phosphoric group esterifies the 2'-hydroxyl of the adenosine moiety of NAD.

nicotinamide mononucleotide (NMN). A condensation product of nicotinamide and ribose 5-phosphate, linking the N of nicotinamide to the (*β*) C-1 of the ribose; in NAD, the ring is linked by the 5'-P to the 5'-P of AMP.

nicotinate (nik'ō-ti-nāt). Ester of nicotinic acid; some n.'s are used in ointments as rubefacients.

nicotine (nik'ō-tēn). 1-Methyl-2-(3-pyridyl)pyrrolidine; a poisonous volatile alkaloid derived from tobacco and responsible for many of the effects of tobacco; it first stimulates (small doses) then depresses (large doses) at autonomic ganglia and myoneural junctions. N. is an important tool in physiologic and pharmacologic investigation, is used as an insecticide and fumigant, and forms salts with most acids.

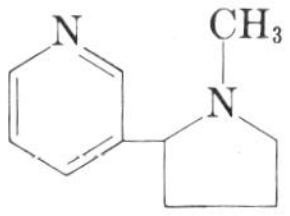

Nicotine

nicotinehydroxamic acid methiodide (nik'ō-tēn-hī'drok-sam'ik as'id mĕ-thī'ō-dīd). An effective cholinesterase reactivator, with actions that are most marked at the skeletal neuromuscular junction; antidotal effects are less striking at autonomic effector sites, and insignificant in the central nervous system.

nicotinic (nik-ō-tin'ik). Relating to the stimulating action of acetylcholine and other nicotine-like agents on autonomic ganglia, adrenal medulla, and the motor end-plate of striated muscle.

nicotinic acid. Niacin; anti-black tongue, anti-pellagra, or pellagra-preventing factor; pyridine-3-carboxylic acid; a part of the vitamin B complex; used in the prevention and treatment of pellagra, as a vasodilator, and as a cholesterol-lowering agent.

nicotinic acid amide. Nicotinamide.

nicotinic alcohol. Nicotinyl alcohol.

nicotinomimetic (nik-ō-tin'ō-mi-met'ik). Mimicking the action of nicotine.

nicotinyl alcohol (nik-ō-tin'il). Nicotinic alcohol; 3-pyridinemethanol; same action and use as nicotinyl tartrate.

nicotinyl tartrate. 3-Pyridinemethanol tartrate; a relatively weak peripheral vasodilator related to nicotinic acid; used in peripheral vascular disorders such as Raynaud's disease, acrocyanosis, and chilblains.

nicoumalone (ni-kū'mă-lōn). Acenocoumarol.

nictation (nik-tā'shŭn). Nictitation.

nictitate (nik'ti-tāt) [see nictitation]. To wink.

nictitation (nik-ti-tā'shŭn) [L. *nicto,* pp. *-atus,* to wink, fr. *nico,* to beckon]. Nictation; winking.

nidal (nī'dăl). Relating to a nidus, or nest.

nidation (nī-dā'shŭn) [L. *nidus,* nest]. Embedding of the early embryo in the uterine mucosa.

NIDDM Abbreviation for non-insulin dependent *diabetes* mellitus.

nidus, pl. nidi (nī'dŭs, nī'dī) [L. nest]. **1.** A nest. **2.** The nucleus or central point of origin of a nerve. **3.** A focus or point of lodgment and development of a pathogenic organism. **4.** The nucleus of a crystal; the coalescence of molecules or small particles that is the beginning of a crystal or similar solid deposit.

n. a'vis [L. bird's nest], a deep depression on each side of the inferior surface of the cerebellum, between the uvula and the biventral lobe, in which the tonsil rests.

n. hirun'dinis [L. swallow's nest], n. avis.

Nieden's syndrome. See under syndrome.

Niemann, Albert, German physician, 1880–1921. See N.-Pick *cell, disease.*

Niewenglowski, Gaston H., 19th century Paris scientist. See N. *rays.*

nifedipine (ni-fed'i-pēn). 1,4-Dihydro-2,6-dimethyl-4-(2-nitrophenyl)-3,5-pyridinedicarboxylic acid dimethyl ester; a calcium channel-blocking agent and coronary vasodilator.

nifenazone (ni-fen'ă-zōn). *N*-Antipyrinylnicotinamide; an analgesic and antipyretic.

nifuraldezone (nī-fyūr-al'dĕ-zōn). 5-Nitro-2-furaldehyde semioxamazone; an antibacterial agent.

nifuratel (nī-fyū'ră-tel). Methylmercadone; 5-[(methylthio)methyl]-3-[(5-nitrofurfurylidene)amino]-2-oxazolidinone; trichomonacide.

nifuroxime (nī-fyū-rok'sēm, -sim). *Anti*-5-nitro-2-furaldoxime; a furan derivative, principally effective against *Candida albicans.*

nigerose (nī'jĕ-rōs) [fr. *nigeran,* a polysaccharide synthesized by *Aspergillus niger*]. 3-*O*-α-D-Glucopyranosyl-D-glucose; a disaccharide obtained by the hydrolysis of amylopectins, consisting of two glucose residues bound in a 1–3 linkage.

nightguard (nīt'gard). A device used to stabilize the teeth and reduce the traumatic effects of bruxism.

nightmare (nīt'măr) [A.S. *nyht,* night, + *mara,* a demon]. Oneirodynia gravis; incubus (2); a terrifying dream, as in which one is unable to cry for help or to escape from a seemingly impending evil.

nightshade (nīt'shād). Any of a number of plants of the genus *Solanum* (family Solanaceae) and of some other genera of the family Solanaceae.

deadly n., belladonna.

night-terrors (nīt'tār-erz). Pavor nocturnus; a disorder allied to nightmare, occurring in children, in which the child awakes screaming with fright, the distress persisting for a time during a state of semiconsciousness.

nigra (nī'gră) [L. fr. *niger,* black]. In neuroanatomy, the *substantia* nigra.

nigricans (nī'gri-kanz) [L. fr. *niger,* black]. Blackish.

nigrities (nī-grish'i-ēz) [L. blackness, fr. *niger,* black]. A black pigmentation.

n. lin'guae, black *tongue.*

nigrosin, nigrosine (nī'grō-sin, -sēn) [C.I. 50420]. A variable mixture of blue-black aniline dyes; used as a histologic stain for nervous tissue and as a negative stain for studying bacteria and spirochetes; also used to discriminate between live and dead cells in dye-exclusion staining.

Nigrospora (nī-gros'pōr-ă). A genus of rapidly growing fungi that produces shiny, black conidia in cultures; it is a common contaminant in laboratory cultures and is nonpathogenic for man.

nigrostriatal (nī'grō-strī-ā'tăl). Referring to the efferent connection of the substantia nigra with the striatum. See *substantia* nigra.

NIH Abbreviation for National Institutes of Health (U.S. Public Health Service).

nihilism (nī'i-lizm, nī'hi-lizm) [L. *nihil,* nothing]. **1.** In psychiatry, the delusion of the nonexistence of everything, especially of the self or part of the self. **2.** Engagement in acts which are totally destructive to one's own purposes and those of one's group.

therapeutic n., a disbelief in the efficacy or value of therapy, as of drugs, psychotherapy, etc.

nikethamide (nī-keth'ă-mīd). *N,N*-Diethylpyridine-3-carboxamide; *N,N*-diethylnicotinamide; it acts mainly on the central nervous system, as a respiratory and cardiovascular stimulant.

Nikiforoff, Mikhail, Russian dermatologist, 1858–1915. See N.'s *method.*

Nikolsky, Pyotr V., Russian dermatologist, 1858–1940. See N.'s *sign.*

Nile blue A [C.I. 51180]. A basic oxazin dye, $C_{20}H_{20}N_3OCl$, used as a fat and vital stain, and in Kittrich's stain; as an indicator, it changes from blue to purplish red at pH 10 to 11.

ninhydrin (nin-hī'drin). 2,2-Dihydroxy-1,3-indanedione; reacts with free amino acids to yield CO_2, NH_3, and an aldehyde, the NH_3 produced yielding a colored product (diketohydrindylidene-diketohydrinamine, a bi-indanedione derivative). See also ninhydrin *reaction.*

niobium (nī-ō'bē-ŭm) [*Niobe,* G. myth.]. A rare metallic element, symbol Nb, atomic no. 41, atomic weight 92.91, usually found with tantalum.

nipple (nip'l) [dim. of A.S. *neb,* beak, nose (?)]. *Papilla* mammae.

niridazole (nī-rid'ă-zōl). 1-(5-Nitro-2-thiazolyl)-2-imidazolidinone; used for the treatment of schistosomiasis, amebiasis, and dracontiasis.

Nissen, Rudolf, Swiss surgeon, *1896. See N.'s *operation.*

Nissl, Franz, German neurologist, 1860–1919. See N. *bodies, degeneration, granules, substance;* N.'s *stain.*

nit [A.S. *knitu*]. **1.** The ovum of a body, head, or crab louse; it is attached to human hair or clothing by a layer of chitin. **2.** A unit of luminance; a luminous intensity of 1 candela per square meter of orthogonally projected surface.

Nitabuch, Raissa, 19th century German physician. See N.'s *layer, membrane, stria.*

niter (nī'ter) [G. *nitron,* soda, formerly not distinguished from potash]. *Potassium* nitrate.

cubic n., *sodium* nitrate.

niton (nī'ton). Archaic term for radon.

nitrate (nī'trāt). A salt of nitric acid.

nitrazepam (nī-trā'zĕ-pam). 1,3-Dihydro-7-nitro-5-phenyl-2*H*- 1,4-benzodiazepin-2-one; a hypnotic and sedative.

nitric acid (nī'trik). HNO_3; a strong acid oxidant.

fuming n. a. contains about 91% n. acid; used as a caustic.

nitric-oxide reductase [EC 1.7.99.2]. An enzyme oxidizing N_2 to NO, a first step in the fixing of atmospheric nitrogen by bacteria.

nitridation (nī-tri-dā'shŭn). Formation of nitrides; formation of nitrogen compounds through the action of ammonia (analogous to oxidation).

nitride (nī'trīd). A compound of nitrogen and one other element; *e.g.,* magnesium nitride, Mg_3N_2.

nitrification (nī'tri-fi-kā'shŭn). **1.** Bacterial conversion of nitrogenous matter into nitrates. **2.** Treatment of a material with nitric acid.

nitrile (nī'tril). An alkyl cyanide. Individual n.'s are named for the acid formed on hydrolysis; *e.g.,* CH_3CN is acetonitrile rather than methyl cyanide.

nitrilo-. Prefix indicating a tervalent nitrogen atom attached to three identical groups; *e.g.,* nitrilotriacetic acid, $N(CH_2COOH)_3$.

nitrimuriatic acid (nī'tri-myū-rē-at'ik). Nitrohydrochloric acid.

nitrite (nī'trīt). A salt of nitrous acid.

nitrituria (nī-tri-tū'rē-ă). The presence of nitrites in the urine, as a result of the action of *Escherichia coli, Proteus vulgaris,* and other microorganisms that may reduce nitrates.

nitro-. Prefix denoting the group $-NO_2$.

nitrocellulose (nī-trō-sel'yū-lōs). Pyroxylin.

nitrochloroform (nī-trō-klōr'ō-fōrm). Chloropicrin.

nitrofurans (nī-trō-fyū'ranz). Antimicrobials (*e.g.,* nitrofurazone) effective against Gram-positive and Gram-negative organisms.

nitrofurantoin (nī'trō-fyū-ran'tō-in). *N*-(5-Nitro-2-furfurylidene)-1-aminohydantoin; a urinary antibacterial agent with a wide range of activity against both Gram-positive and Gram-negative organisms; also available as n. sodium for injection.

nitrofurazone (nī-trō-fyū'ră-zōn). 5-Nitro-2-furaldehyde semicarbazone; a topical bacteriostatic and bactericidal agent.

nitrogen (nī'trō-jen) [L. *nitrum,* niter, + *-gen,* to produce]. **1.** A gaseous element, symbol N, atomic no. 7, atomic weight 14.007; forms about 77 parts by weight of the atmosphere. **2.** Pharmaceutical grade N_2, containing not less than 99.0% by volume of N_2; used as a diluent for medicinal gases, and for air replacement in pharmaceutical preparations.

blood urea n. (BUN), n., in the form of urea, in the blood; the most prevalent of nonprotein nitrogenous compounds in blood; ml. blood normally contains 10 to 15 mg of urea/100 ml. See also urea n.

filtrate n., nonprotein n. in various compounds that normally pass through the glomerular filtration, or through a filter in the laboratory (after proteins are precipitated).

heavy n., nitrogen-15.

n. monoxide, nitrous oxide.

nonprotein n. (NPN), rest n.; the n. content of other than protein bodies; *e.g.,* about one half the nonprotein n. in the blood is contained in urea.

n. pentoxide, nitric acid anhydride; N_2O_5; it forms nitric acid when dissolved in water.

rest n., nonprotein n.

undetermined n., the n. of blood, urine, etc., other than urea, uric acid, amino acids, etc., that can be directly estimated; in blood it amounts to about 25 mg per 100 ml.

urea n., the portion of n. in a biological sample, such as blood or urine, that derives from its content of urea. See also blood urea n.

urinary n., n. excreted as urea, amino acids, uric acid, etc., in the urine; 1 g of urinary n. indicates the breakdown in the body of 6.25 g of protein. See also n. *equivalent.*

nitrogen-13 (^{13}N). A cyclotron-produced, positron-emitting radioisotope of nitrogen with a physical half-life of 10 minutes; used in protein metabolism studies.

nitrogen-14 (^{14}N). The common nitrogen isotope, making up 99.635% of natural nitrogen.

nitrogen-15 (^{15}N). Heavy nitrogen; the less common stable nitrogen isotope, making up 0.365% of natural nitrogen.

nitrogenase (nī'trō-jĕ-nās). Formerly a general term used to describe enzyme systems that catalyze the reduction of molecular nitrogen to ammonia in nitrogen-fixing bacteria; now specifically applied to enzymes that carry out this reaction with reduced ferredoxin and ATP.

nitrogen distribution. Nitrogen partition.

nitrogen group. Five trivalent or quinquivalent elements whose hydrogen compounds are basic and whose oxyacids vary from monobasic to tetrabasic: nitrogen, phosphorus, arsenic, antimony, and bismuth.

nitrogen lag. The length of time after the ingestion of a given protein before the amount of nitrogen equal to that in the protein has been excreted in the urine.

nitrogen mustards. See under mustard.

nitrogenous (nī-troj'ĕ-nŭs). Relating to or containing nitrogen.

nitrogen partition. Nitrogen distribution; determination of the distribution of nitrogen in the urine among the various constituents.

nitroglycerin (nī-trō-glis'er-in). Glonoin; glyceryl trinitrate; trinitroglycerin; $C_3H_5(NO_3)_3$; an explosive yellowish oily fluid formed by the action of sulfuric and nitric acids on glycerin; used as a vasodilator, especially in angina pectoris.

nitrohydrochloric acid (nī'trō-hī-drō-klōr'ik). Aqua regia; nitrimuriatic acid; an extremely caustic mixture that contains 18 parts nitric acid and 82 parts hydrochloric acid.

nitromannitol (nī-trō-man'i-tol). *Mannitol* hexanitrate.

nitromersol (nī-trō-mer'sol). The anhydride of 4-nitro-3-hydroxymercuriorthocresol; a synthetic organic mercurial compound, used as an antiseptic for skin and mucous membranes.

nitrometer (nī-trom'ĕ-ter) [nitrogen + G. *metron,* measure]. A device for collecting and measuring the nitrogen set free in a chemical reaction.

nitron (nī'tron). 1,4-Diphenyl-3-phenylamino-1,2,4-triazolium hydroxide (inner salt); a reagent for the determination of nitric acid, perchlorate, and rhenium, as it is one of the few substances to form an insoluble nitrate.

nitrophenylsulfenyl (Nps) (nī'trō-fen'il-sŭl-fĕn'il). Nitrophenylthio; $O_2N{-}C_6H_4{-}S{-}$; a radical easily attached to NH_2 groups; used in peptide synthesis and protein chemistry.

nitroprusside (nī-trō-prŭs'īd). The anion $[Fe(CN)_5NO]^{=}$; as in sodium n.

nitrosamines (nī-trōs'am-ēnz). Amines substituted by a nitroso (NO) group, usually on a nitrogen atom, to yield *N*-nitrosamines ($R{-}NH{-}NO$ or $R_2N{-}NO$); can be formed by direct combination of an amine and nitrous acid (can be formed from nitrites in the acidic gastric juice); some are mutagenic and/or carcinogenic.

nitroso-. Prefix denoting a compound containing nitrosyl.

nitrosyl (nī'trō-sil). A univalent radical or atom group, –N=o, forming the nitroso compounds.

nitrous (nī'trŭs). Denoting a nitrogen compound containing one less atom of oxygen than the nitric compounds; one in which the nitrogen is present in its trivalent state.

nitrous acid. HNO_2; a standard biologic and clinical laboratory reagent.

nitrous oxide. Dinitrogen or nitrogen monoxide; laughing gas; N_2O; a nonflammable, nonexplosive gas that will support combustion; widely used as a rapidly acting, rapidly reversible, nondepressant, and nontoxic inhalation analgesic to supplement other anesthetics and analgesics; its anesthetic potency alone is inadequate to provide surgical anesthesia.

nitroxanthic acid (nī-trō-zan'thik). Picric acid.

nitroxoline (nī-trok'sō-lēn). 5-Nitro-8-quinolinol; an antibacterial agent.

nitroxy (nī-trok'sē) [contraction of nitryloxy]. The $-O-NO_2$ radical.

nitroxyl (nī-trok'sil). The nitrosyl hydride, HNO.

nitryl (nī'tril). The radical $-NO_2$ of the nitro compounds.

nizatidine (ni-zat'i-den). *N*-[2-[[[2-[(Dimethylamino)methyl]-4-thiazdyl]methyl]thio]ethyl]-*N*'-methyl-2-nitro-1,1-ethenediamine; a histamine H_2 antagonist used to treat active duodenal ulcers.

njovera (nyō-ver'ă) [Native]. A nonvenereal disease of children in Zimbabwe, indistinguishable from syphilis, due to an organism apparently identical with *Treponema pallidum;* probably the same as bejel.

N.K. Abbreviation for Nomenklatur Kommission.

nm Symbol for nanometer.

NMN Abbreviation for nicotinamide mononucleotide.

NMR Abbreviation for nuclear magnetic *resonance.*

No Symbol for nobelium.

nobelium (nō-bel'ē-ŭm) [*Nobel* Institute for Physics]. An unstable transuranium element, atomic no. 102, symbol No, prepared by bombardment of curium with carbon nuclei and similar heavy ions on other elements of the transuranium series.

Noble, Charles P., U.S. gynecologist, 1863–1935. See N.'s *position.*

Noble, Robert L., Canadian physiologist, *1910. See N.-Collip *procedure.*

Noble's stain. See under stain.

Nocard, Edmund I.E., French veterinarian, 1850–1903. See *Nocardia,* Nocardiaceae; Preisz-N. *bacillus.*

Nocardia (nō-kar'dē-ă) [E. *Nocard*]. A genus of aerobic nonmotile actinomycetes (family Nocardiaceae, order Actinomycetales), transitional between bacteria and fungi, containing variably acid-fast, slender rods or filaments, frequently swollen and occasionally branched, forming a mycelium. Coccus or bacillary forms are produced by these organisms, which are mainly saprophytic but may produce disease in man and other animals. The type species is *N. farcinica.*

N. africa'na, *Actinomadura pelletieri;* a species found in a case of mycetoma of the foot in South Africa.

N. asteroi'des, *N. leishmanii;* a species of aerobic, Gram-positive, partially acid-fast, branching organisms causing nocardiosis and possibly mycetoma in man.

N. brasilien'sis, a species that closely resembles *N. asteroides* and is a cause of mycetoma in man.

N. ca'viae, a species that causes mycetoma in man; it closely resembles *N. asteroides* but differs by its ability to decompose xanthine and by formation of acid from inositol and mannitol.

N. farci'nica, a species causing bovine farcy; it is the type species of the genus *N.*

N. gibso'nii, *Streptomyces gibsonii.*

N. leishma'nii, *N. asteroides.*

N. lu'rida, a species that produces ristocetin.

N. lu'tea, a species found in a case of actinomycosis of the lacrimal gland.

N. madu'rae, a species which causes actinomycotic mycetoma.

N. mediterra'nei, a species that produces rifamycin.

N. orienta'lis, a species that produces vancomycin.

nocardia, pl. **nocardiae** (nō-kar'dē-ă, nō-kar'dē-ē). A vernacular term used to refer to any member of the genus *Nocardia.*

Nocardiaceae (nō-kar-dē-ā'sē-ē) [E. *Nocard*]. A family of acid-fast, Gram-positive, aerobic bacteria (order Actinomycetales) that includes the genus *Nocardia.*

nocardiasis (nō-kar-dī'ă-sis). Nocardiosis.

nocardioform (nō-kar'dē-ō-fōrm). Denoting an organism that morphologically and culturally resembles members of the genus *Nocardia.*

nocardiosis (nō-kar-dē-ō'sis). Nocardiasis; a generalized disease in man caused by *Nocardia asteroides* (or occasionally by *N. farcinica*) and characterized by primary pulmonary lesions which may be subclinical or chronic with hematogenous spread, and usually with involvement of the central nervous system.

granulomatous n., a form of n. characterized by emaciation, abdominal distention, and replacement of lymphoid tissue in lymph nodes and spleen by granulomatous tissue.

noci- [L. *noceo,* to injure, hurt]. Combining form relating to hurt, pain, or injury.

nociceptive (nō-si-sep'tiv) [see nociceptor]. Capable of appreciation or transmission of pain.

nociceptor (nō-si-sep'ter, -tōr) [noci- + L. *capio,* to take]. A peripheral nerve organ or mechanism for the appreciation and transmission of painful or injurious stimuli.

nocifensor (nō-si-fen'ser) [noci- + L. *fendo* (only in compounds), to strike, ward off]. Denoting processes or mechanisms that act to protect the body from injury; specifically, a system of nerves in the skin and mucous membranes that react to adjacent injury by causing vasodilation.

noci-influence (nō'si-in'flū-ens). Injurious or harmful influence.

nociperception (nō'si-per-sep'shŭn) [noci- + perception]. The appreciation of injurious influences, referring to nerve centers.

noct- [L. *nox,* night]. Combining form meaning night, nocturnal. See also nycto-.

noctambulation (nok'tam-byū-lā'shŭn). Somnambulism (1).

noctambulism (nok-tam'byū-lizm). Somnambulism (1).

noct. maneq. Abbreviation for L. *nocte maneque,* at night and in the morning.

nocturia (nok-tū'rē-ă) [noct- + G. *ouron,* urine]. Nycturia; urinating at night, often because of increased nocturnal secretion of urine resulting from failure of suppression of urine flow during recumbency or from obstructive lesions in the lower urinary tract.

nocturnal (nok-ter'năl) [L. *nocturnus,* of the night]. Pertaining to the hours of darkness; opposite of diurnal (1).

nodal (nō'dăl). Relating to any node.

NODE

node (nōd) [L. *nodus,* a knot]. **1.** A knob or nodosity; a circumscribed swelling. **2.** A circumscribed mass of differentiated tissue. See nodus. **3.** A knuckle, or finger joint.

accessory nerve lymph n.'s, *lymphonodi* comitantes nervi accessorii; companion lymph nodes of accessory nerve; the nodes of the deep lateral cervical group that are located along the accessory nerve; their efferent vessels pass to the supraclavicular lymph nodes.
anorectal lymph n.'s, *lymphonodi* pararectales.
anterior cervical lymph n.'s, *lymphonodi* cervicales anteriores.
anterior jugular lymph n.'s, *lymphonodi* jugulares anteriores.
anterior mediastinal lymph n.'s, *lymphonodi* mediastinales anteriores.
anterior tibial n., *nodus* tibialis anterior.
apical lymph n.'s, the group of lymph n.'s located at the apex of the axillary fossa that receive lymphatic drainage from other groups of axillary n.'s.
appendicular lymph n.'s, *lymphonodi* appendiculares.
n. of Aschoff and Tawara, *nodus* atrioventricularis.
atrioventricular n., *nodus* atrioventricularis.
axillary lymph n.'s, *lymphonodi* axillares.
n. of azygos arch, *nodus* arcus vena azygos.
Babès' n.'s, collections of lymphocytes in the central nervous system found in rabies.
bifurcation lymph n.'s, *lymphonodi* tracheobronchiales inferiores.
brachial lymph n.'s, *lymphonodi* brachiales.
bronchopulmonary lymph n.'s, lymphonodi bronchopulmonales; lymph n.'s in the hilum of the lung that receive lymph from the pulmonary n.'s.
buccinator n., buccal n., *nodus* buccinatorius.
celiac lymph n.'s, *lymphonodi* coeliaci.
central lymph n.'s, **(1)** n.'s located around the midportion of the axillary artery; they receive afferent vessels from the brachial, paramammary, and interpectoral n.'s and send efferent vessels to the apical n.'s; **(2)** *nodi* lymphatici mesenteric superiores.
cervical paratracheal lymph n.'s, *lymphonodi* paratracheales cervicales.
n. of Cloquet, Rosenmüller's n. or gland; one of the deep inguinal lymph n.'s located in or adjacent to the femoral canal; sometimes mistaken for a femoral hernia when enlarged.
common iliac lymph n.'s, *lymphonodi* iliaci communes.
companion lymph n.'s of accessory nerve, accessory nerve lymph n.'s.
coronary n., the uppermost part of the atrioventricular n.
cubital lymph n.'s, *lymphonodi* cubitales.
cystic n., *nodus* cysticus.
deep anterior cervical lymph n.'s, *lymphonodi* cervicales anteriores profundi.
deep inguinal lymph n.'s, *lymphonodi* inguinales profundi.
deep lateral cervical lymph n.'s, *lymphonodi* cervicales laterales profundi.
deep parotid lymph n.'s, *lymphonodi* parotidei profundi.
delphian n. [fr. oracle of Delphi, Greece], a midline prelaryngeal lymph node, adjacent to the thyroid gland, enlargement of which is indicative of thyroid disease.
diaphragmatic n.'s, *lymphonodi* phrenici superiores.
Dürck's n.'s, a small cell infiltration of the perivascular lymphatic tissue, throughout the brain, cord, and meninges, occurring in human trypanosomiasis.
epitrochlear n.'s, *lymphonodi* cubitales.
external iliac lymph n.'s, *lymphonodi* iliaci externi.
facial lymph n.'s, *lymphonodi* faciales.
fibular n., *nodus* fibularis.
Flack's n., *nodus* sinuatrialis.
foraminal n., *nodus* foraminis.
gastroduodenal lymph n.'s, *lymphonodi* pylorici.
gluteal lymph n.'s, *lymphonodi* gluteales.
Haygarth's n.'s, Haygarth's nodosities; exostoses from the margins of the articular surfaces and from the periosteum and bone in the neighborhood of the joints of the fingers, leading to ankylosis and associated with lateral deflection of the fingers toward the ulnar side, which occur in rheumatoid arthritis.
Heberden's n.'s, Heberden's nodosities; Rosenbach's disease (1); tuberculum arthriticum (1); exostoses about the size of a pea or smaller, found on the terminal phalanges of the fingers in osteoarthritis, which are enlargements of the tubercles at the articular extremities of the distal phalanges.
hemal n., hemolymph n.; hemal, hemolymph, or vascular gland; a lymphoid structure in which the blood sinuses are present in place of lymph sinuses; hemal n.'s occur in ruminants and some other mammals, but their presence in man is questioned.
hemolymph n., hemal n.
Hensen's n., primitive n.
hepatic lymph n.'s, *lymphonodi* hepatici.
ileocolic lymph n.'s, *lymphonodi* ileocolici.
inferior epigastric lymph n.'s, *lymphonodi* epigastrici inferiores.
inferior mesenteric lymph n.'s, *nodi* lymphatici mesenterici inferiores.
inferior phrenic lymph n.'s, *lymphonodi* phrenici inferiores.
inferior tracheobronchial lymph n.'s, *lymphonodi* tracheobronchiales inferiores.
infra-auricular subfascial parotid lymph n.'s, *lymphonodi* parotidei subfasciales infra-auriculares.
intercostal lymph n.'s, *lymphonodi* intercostales.
interiliac lymph n.'s, *lymphonodi* interiliaci.
intermediate lacunar n., *nodus* lacunaris intermedius.
intermediate lumbar lymph n.'s, *lymphonodi* lumbales intermedii.
internal iliac lymph n.'s, *lymphonodi* iliaci interni.
interpectoral lymph n.'s, *lymphonodi* interpectorales.
intraglandular parotid lymph n.'s, *lymphonodi* parotidei intraglandulares.
jugulodigastric n., *nodus* jugulodigastricus.
jugulo-omohyoid n., *nodus* jugulo-omohyoideus.
juxta-esophageal pulmonary lymph n.'s, juxta-esophageal lymph n.'s, *lymphonodi* juxta-esophageales pulonares.
juxtaintestinal lymph n.'s, *lymphonodi* juxtaintestinales.
Keith's n., *nodus* sinuatrialis.
Keith and Flack n., *nodus* sinuatrialis.
Koch's n., *nodus* sinuatrialis.
lateral axillary lymph n.'s, *lymphonodi* brachiales.
lateral jugular lymph n.'s, *lymphonodi* jugulares laterales.
lateral lacunar n., *nodus* lacunaris lateralis.
lateral pericardiac lymph n.'s, *lymphonodi* pericardiales laterales.
left colic lymph n.'s, *lymphonodi* colici sinistri.
left gastric lymph n.'s, *lymphonodi* gastrici sinistri.
left gastroepiploic lymph n.'s, *lymphonodi* gastro-omentales sinistri.
left gastro-omental n.'s, *lymphonodi* gastro-omentales sinistri.
left lumbar lymph n.'s, *lymphonodi* lumbales sinistri.
n. of ligamentum arteriosum, *nodus* ligamentis arteriosi.
lumbar lymph n.'s, *lymphonodi* lumbales dextri, intermedii, and sinistri.
lymph n., lymphonodus.
lymph n.'s of elbow, *lymphonodi* cubitales.
malar n., *nodus* malaris.
mandibular n.'s, *nodus* mandibularis.
mastoid lymph n.'s, *nodi* lymphatici mastoidei.
medial lacunar n., *nodus* lacunaris medialis.
mesenteric lymph n.'s, *lymphonodi* mesenterici.
mesocolic lymph n.'s, *lymphonodi* mesocolici.
middle colic lymph n.'s, *lymphonodi* colici medii.
middle rectal n., *nodus* rectalis media; a node along the middle rectal artery that receives afferents from the pararectal nodes and sends efferents to the internal iliac nodes.

milkers' n.'s, pseudocowpox.
nasolabial n., *nodus* nasolabialis.
obturator lymph n.'s, *lymphonodi* obturatorii.
occipital lymph n.'s, *lymphonodi* occipitales.
Osler n., a tender cutaneous lesion characteristic of subacute bacterial endocarditis; small, raised, and discolored, these n.'s usually appear in the pads of fingers or toes.
pancreatic lymph n.'s, *lymphonodi* pancreatici.
pancreaticoduodenal lymph n.'s, *lymphonodi* pancreaticoduodenales.
pancreaticosplenic lymph n.'s, *lymphonodi* pancreaticolienales.
paramammary lymph n.'s, *lymphonodi* paramammarii.
pararectal lymph n.'s, *lymphonodi* pararectales.
parasternal lymph n.'s, *lymphonodi* parasternales.
paratracheal lymph n., *lymphonodi* paratracheales.
parauterine lymph n.'s, *lymphonodi* parauterini.
paravaginal lymph n.'s, *lymphonodi* paravaginales.
paravesical lymph n.'s, *lymphonodi* paravesicales.
parietal n.'s, *nodi* lymphatici parietales.
pectoral lymph n.'s, *lymphonodi* interpectorales.
peroneal n., *nodus* fibularis.
popliteal lymph n.'s, *lymphonodi* poplitei.
posterior mediastinal lymph n.'s, *lymphonodi* mediastinales posteriores.
posterior tibial n., *nodus* tibialis posterior.
preauricular subfascial parotid lymph n.'s, *lymphonodi* parotidei subfasciales praeauriculares.
prececal lymph n.'s, *lymphonodi* prececales.
prelaryngeal lymph n.'s, *lymphonodi* prelaryngei.
prepericardiac lymph n.'s, *lymphonodi* prepericardiaci.
pretracheal lymph n.'s, *lymphonodi* pretracheales.
prevertebral lymph n.'s, *lymphonodi* prevertebrales.
primitive n., primitive or protochordal knot; Hensen's n. or knot; Hubrecht's protochordal knot; a local thickening of the blastoderm at the cephalic end of the primitive streak of the embryo.
promontory lymph n.'s, *lymphonodi* promontorii.
pulmonary lymph n.'s, *lymphonodi* pulmonales; small nodes that occur along the bronchi within the lung; they receive the drainage from localized areas of the lung and send efferents to bronchopulmonary nodes.
pyloric lymph n.'s, *lymphonodi* pylorici.
Ranvier's n., a short interval in the myelin sheath of a nerve fiber, occurring between each two successive segments of the myelin sheath; at the n., the axon is invested only by short, finger-like cytoplasmic processes of the two neighboring Schwann cells or, in the central nervous system, oligodendroglia cells. See also myelin *sheath.*
retroauricular lymph n.'s, *lymphonodi* mastoidei.
retrocecal lymph n.'s, *lymphonodi* retrocecales.
retropharyngeal lymph n.'s, *lymphonodi* retropharyngeales.
retropyloric n.'s, *nodi* retropylorici.
right colic lymph n.'s, *lymphonodi* colici dextri.
right gastric lymph n.'s, *lymphonodi* gastrici dextri.
right gastroepiploic lymph n.'s, *lymphonodi* gastro-omentales dextri.
right gastro-omental lymph n.'s, *lymphonodi* gastro-omentales dextri.
right lumbar lymph n.'s, *lymphonodi* lumbales dextri.
Rosenmüller's n., n. of Cloquet.
n. of Rouviere, one of the lateral group of retropharyngeal lymph nodes. See *lymphonodi* retropharyngeales.
sacral lymph n.'s, *lymphonodi* sacrales.
sigmoid lymph n.'s, *lymphonodi* sigmoidei.
signal n., Virchow's n.; jugular gland; a firm supraclavicular lymph n., especially on the left side, sufficiently enlarged that it is palpable from the cutaneous surface; such a lymph n. is so termed because it may be the first recognized *presumptive* evidence of a malignant neoplasm in one of the viscera. A signal n. that is *known* to contain a metastasis from a malignant neoplasm is sometimes designated by an old eponym, Troisier's ganglion.
singer's n.'s, vocal cord *nodules.*
sinoatrial n., *nodus* sinuatrialis.
sinus n., *nodus* sinuatrialis.
splenic lymph n.'s, *lymphonodi* splenici.
subaortic lymph n.'s, *lymphonodi* subaortici.
subdigastric n., *nodus* jugulodigastricus.
submandibular lymph n.'s, *lymphonodi* submandibulares.
submental lymph n.'s, *lymphonodi* submentales.
subpyloric n., *nodi* subpylorici.
subscapular lymph n.'s, n.'s of the axillary region located along the subscapular artery and its branches; they receive afferent vessels from the dorsal surface of the thorax and scapular region, and send efferent vessels to the axillary lymphatic plexus.
superficial anterior cervical lymph n.'s, *lymphonodi* cerviacles anteriores superficiales.
superficial inguinal lymph n.'s, *lymphonodi* inguinales superficiales.
superficial lateral cervical lymph n.'s, *lymphonodi* cervicales laterales superficiales.
superficial parotid lymph n.'s, *lymphonodi* parotidei superficiales.
superior gastric lymph n.'s, *lymphonodi* gastrici sinistri.
superior mesenteric lymph n.'s, *nodi* lymphatici mesenterici superiores.
superior phrenic lymph n.'s, *lymphonodi* phrenici superiores.
superior rectal lymph n.'s, *lymphonodi* rectales superiores.
superior tracheobronchial lymph n.'s, *lymphonodi* tracheobronchiales superiores.
supraclavicular lymph n.'s, *lymphonodi* supraclaviculares.
suprapyloric n., *nodus* suprapylorious.
Tawara's n., *nodus* atrioventricularis.
teachers' n.'s, vocal cord *nodules.*
thyroid lymph n.'s, *lymphonodi* thyroidei.
tracheal lymph n.'s, *lymphonodi* paratracheales.
Troisier's n., Troisier's *ganglion.*
Virchow's n., signal n.
visceral n.'s, *nodi* viscerales.
vital n., *noeud* vital.

---

nodi (nō′dī) [L.]. Plural of nodus.

nodose (nō′dōs) [L. *nodosus*] Nodous; nodular; nodulous; nodulate; nodulated; having nodes or knotlike swellings.

nodositas (nō-dos′i-tas) [L. fr. *nodos,* a knot]. Nodosity.
n. crin′ium, *trichorrhexis* nodosa.

nodosity (nō-dos′i-tē) [L. *nodositas*] Nodositas. **1.** A node; a knoblike or knotty swelling. **2.** The condition of being nodose.
Haygarth's n.'s, Haygarth's *nodes.*
Heberden's n.'s, Heberden's *nodes.*

nodous, nodular, nodulate, nodulated (nō′dŭs, nod′yū-lăr, nod′yū-lāt, -lā′ted). Nodose.

nodulation (nod-yū-lā′shŭn). The formation or the presence of nodules.

nodule (nod′yūl) [L. *nodulus,* dim. of *nodus,* knot]. A small node. See also nodulus.
aggregated lymphatic n.'s, *folliculi* lymphatici aggregati.
Albini's n.'s, minute fibrous n.'s on the margins of the mitral and tricuspid valves of the heart, sometimes present in the neonate; described previously by Cruveilhier. *Cf. nodulus* valvulae semilunaris.
apple jelly n.'s, descriptive term for the papular lesions of lupus vulgaris, as they appear on diascopy.
Arantius' n., *nodulus* valvulae semilunaris.

Aschoff n.'s, Aschoff *bodies.*
Bianchi's n., *nodulus* valvulae semilunaris.
Bohn's n.'s, keratin-filled cysts of salivary gland origin located on the palate of newborn infants; also commonly but inappropriately applied to dental lamina cysts of the newborn.
Caplan's n.'s, Caplan's *syndrome.*
cold n., a thyroid n. with a much lower uptake of radioactive iodine than the surrounding parenchyma; about one in four prove to be malignant.
Dalen-Fuchs n.'s, collections of epithelial cells lying between Bruch's membrane and the retinal pigment epithelium in sympathetic ophthalmia and rarely in other granulomatous intraocular inflammations.
enamel n., enameloma.
Gamna-Gandy n.'s, Gamna-Gandy *bodies.*
Hoboken's n.'s, Hoboken's gemmules; gross dilations on the outer surface of the umbilical arteries. See also Hoboken's valves.
hot n., a thyroid n. with a much higher uptake of radioactive iodine than the surrounding parenchyma; usually benign but causing hyperthyroidism.
Jeanselme's n.'s, juxta-articular n.'s; a form of tertiary yaws that is characterized by the occurrence of n.'s on the arms and legs, situated usually near the joints.
juxta-articular n.'s, Jeanselme's n.'s.
Lisch n., iris hamartomas in segmental neurofibromatosis.
lymph n., *folliculus* lymphaticus.
malpighian n.'s, *folliculi* lymphatici lienales.
milkers' n.'s, pseudocowpox.
Morgagni's n., *nodulus* valvulae semilunaris.
primary n., a lymphatic n. having small lymphocytes and lacking a germinal center.
pulp n., pulp *stone.*
rheumatoid n.'s, subcutaneous n.'s, occurring most commonly over bony prominences, in some patients with rheumatoid arthritis; microscopically, the n.'s are foci of fibrinoid necrosis, surrounded by a palisade of fibroblasts.
Schmorl's n., prolapse of the nucleus pulposus into the spongiosa of a vertebra.
secondary n., a lymphatic n. having a germinal center.
n. of semilunar valve, *nodulus* valvulae semilunaris.
siderotic n.'s, Gamna-Gandy *bodies.*
singer's n.'s, vocal cord *nodules.*
Sister Joseph's n., a malignant intra-abdominal neoplasm metastatic to the umbilicus.
solitary n.'s of intestine, *folliculi* lymphatici solitarii.
splenic lymph n.'s, *folliculi* lymphatici lienales.
vocal cord n.'s, singer's or teacher's nodes; chorditis nodosa or tuberosa; small, circumscribed, beadlike enlargements on the vocal cords caused by overuse or abuse of the voice.

nodulous (nod'yū-lŭs). Nodose.

nodulus, pl. **noduli** (nod'yū-lŭs, -lī) [L. dim. of *nodus,*] [NA]. **1.** Nodule; a small node. **2.** The posterior extremity of the inferior vermis of the cerebellum, forming with the velum medullare posterius the central portion of the flocculonodular lobe.
n. carot'icus, *glomus* caroticum.
n. lymphat'icus, *folliculus* lymphaticus.
n. val'vulae semiluna'ris, pl. **nod'uli valvula'rum semiluna'rium** [NA], nodule of semilunar valve; corpus arantii; Arantius', Morgagni's, or Bianchi's nodule; a nodule at the center of the free border of each semilunar valve at the beginning of the pulmonary artery and aorta.

nodus, pl. **nodi** (nō'dŭs, -dī) [L. a knot] [NA]. Node; in anatomy, a circumscribed mass of tissue.
n. atrioventricula'ris [NA], atrioventricular node; node of Aschoff and Tawara; Tawara's node; a small node of specialized cardiac muscle fibers located near the ostium of the coronary sinus; it gives rise to the atrioventricular bundle of the conduction system of the heart.
n. buccinato'rius [NA], buccinator or buccal node; one of the chain of facial lymph nodes located superficial to the buccinator muscle.
n. cys'ticus [NA], cystic node; a lymph node at the neck of the gallbladder draining lymph into the hepatic nodes.
n. fibula'ris [NA], fibular or peroneal node; a small inconstant lymph node located along the course of the peroneal artery.
n. foram'inis [NA], foraminal node; one of the hepatic nodes located adjacent to the epiploic foramen.
n. jugulodigas'tricus [NA], jugulodigastric node; subdigastric node; a prominent lymph node in the deep lateral cervical group lying below the digastric muscle and anterior to the internal jugular vein; it receives lymphatic drainage from the pharynx, palatine tonsil, and tongue.
n. jugulo-omohyoi'deus [NA], jugulo-omohyoid node; a lymph node of the deep lateral cervical group that lies above the intermediate tendon of the omohyoid muscle and anterior to the internal jugular vein; it receives lymphatic drainage from the submental, submandibular, and deep anterior cervical nodes; its efferent vessels go to other deep lateral cervical nodes.
n. lacuna'ris interme'dius [NA], intermediate lacunar node; a lymph node of the external iliac group located between the external iliac artery and vein at the lacuna vasorum.
n. lacuna'ris latera'lis [NA], lateral lacunar node; a lymph node of the external iliac group located lateral to the external iliac artery at the lacuna vasorum.
n. lacuna'ris media'lis [NA], medial lacunar node; a lymph node of the external iliac group located medial to the external iliac vein at the lacuna vasorum.
n. ligamen'tis arterio'si [NA], node of ligamentum arteriosum; a lymph node of the anterior mediastinal group located adjacent to the ligamentum arteriosum.
nodi lymphat'ici centra'les, nodi lymphatici mesenterici superiores.
no'di lymphat'ici mesenter'ici inferio'res [NA], inferior mesenteric lymph nodes; nodes located along the inferior mesenteric artery and its branches that drain the upper part of the rectum, the sigmoid colon and descending colon.
no'di lymphat'ici mesenter'ici superio'res [NA], superior mesenteric lymph nodes; nodi lymphatici centrales; central lymph nodes (2); the numerous nodes located in the mesentery along the superior mesenteric artery and its branches to the jejunum and ileum, from which they receive lymph.
n. lymphat'icus, pl. **no'di lymphat'ici,** lymphonodus.
n. mala'ris [NA], malar node; one of the facial lymph nodes located near the zygomatic minor muscle.
n. mandibula'ris [NA], mandibular node; one of the facial lymph nodes located by the facial artery near the point it crosses the mandible.
n. nasolabia'lis [NA], nasolabial node; one of the facial lymph nodes located near the junction of the superior labial and facial arteries.
no'di parieta'les [NA], parietal nodes; the lymph nodes draining the walls of the abdomen or of the pelvis.
n. recta'lis me'dia, middle rectal *node.*
no'di retropylo'rici [NA], retropyloric nodes; a group of lymph nodes located behind the pylorus.
n. sinuatria'lis [NA], sinoatrial node; atrionector; S-A node; Flack's, Koch's, or Keith's node; Keith and Flack node; sinus node; the mass of specialized cardiac muscle fibers that normally acts as the "pacemaker" of the cardiac conduction system; it lies under the epicardium at the upper end of the sulcus terminalis.
no'di subpylo'rici [NA], subpyloric nodes; a group of lymph nodes located below the pylorus.
n. suprapylo'ricus [NA], suprapyloric node; a lymph node located above the pylorus.

n. tibia'lis ante'rior [NA], anterior tibial node; a small inconstant lymph node in front of the interosseous membrane along the upper part of the anterior tibial vessels.
n. tibia'lis poste'rior [NA], posterior tibial node; a small inconstant lymph node located along the course of the posterior tibial artery.
no'di viscera'les [NA], visceral nodes; the lymph nodes draining the viscera of the abdomen or of the pelvis.

noematic (nō-ē-mat'ik) [G. *noēma,* perception, a thought]. Noetic; relating to the mental processes.

noesis (nō-ē'sis) [G. *noēsis,* thought, intelligence]. Cognition, especially through direct and self-evident knowledge.

noetic (nō-et'ik). Noematic.

noeud vital (nū vē-tal') [Fr.]. Vital node or knot; a circumscript region in the lower part of the medulla oblongata, near the apex of the calamus scriptorius, interpreted by M. Flourens (1858) as a nerve center controlling respiration.

Noguchia (nō-gū'chē-ă) [Hideyo *Noguchi,* Japanese bacteriologist, 1876–1928]. A genus of aerobic to facultatively anaerobic, motile, peritrichous bacteria (family Brucellaceae) containing small, slender, Gram-negative, encapsulated rods. These organisms are present in the conjunctiva of man and other animals affected by a follicular type of disease. The type species is *N. granulosis.*
N. cunic'uli, a species which causes conjunctival folliculosis in rabbits.
N. granulo'sis, a species regarded by some as a cause of trachoma in man; it produces a granular conjunctivitis in monkeys and apes; it is the type species of the genus *N.*
N. sim'iae, a species which causes conjunctival folliculosis in monkeys (*Macacus rhesus*).

noise (noyz). Unwanted additions to a signal not arising at its source; *e.g.,* the 60-cycle frequency wave in an electrocardiogram.

noma (nō'mă) [G. *nomē,* a spreading (sore)]. Water canker; stomatonecrosis; stomatonoma; corrosive ulcer; a gangrenous stomatitis, usually beginning in the mucous membrane of the corner of the mouth or cheek, and then progressing fairly rapidly to involve the entire thickness of the lips or cheek (or both), with conspicuous necrosis and complete sloughing of tissue; usually observed in poorly nourished children and debilitated adults, especially in lower socioeconomic groups, and frequently preceded by another disease, *e.g.,* kala azar, dysentery, or scarlet fever. A similar process (n. pudendi, n. vulvae) may also involve the labia majora. Several organisms are usually found in the necrotic material, but fusiform bacilli, *Borrelia* organisms, staphylococci, and anaerobic streptococci are most frequently observed.

Nomarski, Georges, 20th century French optical inventor. See N. *optics.*

nomatophobia (nō'ma-tō-fō'bē-ă). Onomatophobia.

nomenclature (nō'men-klā-chūr, nō-men'klă-chūr). A set system of names used in any science, as of anatomic structures, organisms, etc.
binary n., binomial n., linnaean *system* of nomenclature.

Nomenklatur Kommission (N.K.). Committee on Nomenclature of the German Anatomical Society, appointed to revise or supplement the BNA (1895).

nomifensine maleate (nō-mi-fen'sēn). 8-Amino-1,2,3,4-tetrahydro-2-methyl-4-phenylisoquinoline maleate; an antidepressant.

Nomina Anatomica (NA) (nom'i-nă an-ă-tom'i-kă, nō'mi-nă an'ă-tō'mi-kă). Anatomical nomenclature; the modification of the Basle Nomina Anatomica or BNA system of anatomical terminology adopted in 1955 by the International Congress of Anatomists in Paris, France. The International Anatomical Nomenclature Committee is responsible for continued revisions of the NA which are reviewed and adopted by the International Congress of Anatomists meeting at five-year intervals since 1950.

nomogenesis (nō-mō-jen'ĕ-sis) [G. *nomos,* law, + *genesis,* origin]. A theory that evolution proceeds by predetermined law and cannot be modified by environment or chance events.

nomogram (nom'ō-gram) [G. *nomos,* law, + *gramma,* something written]. Nomograph (2); a series of scales arranged so that calculations can be performed graphically.
blood volume n., a n. used to predict blood volume on the basis of the individual's weight and height.
cartesian n., a n. based on rectangular coordinates, representing two variables, on which a family of isopleths is superimposed for each of the additional variables involved.
d'Ocagne n., an alignment chart consisting of an arrangement of three or more graduated lines (straight or curved), each constituting a scale of values of a variable, constructed so that any straight line crossing these scales connects the simultaneously compatible values; from values for any two variables, the values of all other variables can be determined.
Radford n., a n. used to predict necessary tidal volume for artificial respiration on the basis of respiratory rate, body weight, and sex; correction factors are supplied for activity, fever, altitude, metabolic acidosis, and alterations in dead space.
Siggaard-Andersen n., a n. used to predict acid-base composition of blood by the slope and position of a buffer line constructed when P_{CO_2} on a logarithmic scale is plotted against pH.

nomograph (nom'ō-graf) [G. *nomos,* law, + *graphō,* to write]. **1.** A graph consisting of three coplanar curves, usually parallel, each graduated for a different variable so that a straight line cutting all three curves intersects the related values of each variable. **2.** Nomogram.

nomothetic (nom-ō-thet'ik) [G. *nomos,* law, + *thesis,* a placing]. Denoting the generalizations pertaining to the behavior of groups of individuals as groups, as opposed to idiographic.

nomotopic (nō-mō-top'ik) [G. *nomos,* law, custom, + *topos,* place]. Relating to, or occurring at, the usual or normal place.

nonan (nō'nan) [L. *nonus,* ninth]. Occurring on the ninth day.

nonanedioic acid (nō-nān-dī'ō-ik). Azelaic acid.

***n*-nonanoic acid** (non-ă-nō'ik). Pelargonic acid.

nonbursate (non-ber'sāt) [L. *non,* not, + Mediev. L. *bursa,* purse]. Denoting a nontaxonomic division of Nematoda embracing those in which the male copulatory bursa is only a skin fold containing no fleshy ribs, as seen in the hookworms, and other bursate nematodes.

noncariogenic (non-kā'rē-ō-jen'ik). Not caries-producing.

noncellular (non-sel'yū-lăr). **1.** Subcellular; lacking cellular organization, as applied to viruses, which can only replicate within a cell, whether prokaryotic or eukaryotic. **2.** Acellular (1).

nonchromogens (non-krō'mō-jenz). Group III *mycobacteria.*

non compos mentis (non kom'pos men'tis) [L. *non,* not, + *compos,* participating, competent, + *mens,* gen. *mentis,* mind]. Not of sound mind; mentally incapable of managing one's affairs.

nondisease (non'dis-ēz). Absence of disease when a specific disease is suspected but not found.

nondisjunction (non-dis-jŭnk'shŭn). Failure of one or more pairs of chromosomes to separate at the meiotic stage of karyokinesis, with the result that both chromosomes are carried to one daughter cell and none to the other.
primary n., n. occurring in a previously normal cell.
secondary n., n. occurring in an aneuploid cell, which was the result of a primary n.

nonelectrolyte (non-ē-lek'trō-līt). A substance with molecules that do not, in solution, dissociate to ions, and, therefore, do not carry an electric current.

nonimmune (non-i-myūn'). Pertaining to an individual that is not immune or to a serum from such an individual.

nonimmunity (non-i-myūn'i-tē). Aphylaxis.

noninvasive (non-in-vā'siv). Denoting a procedure that does not require insertion of an instrument or device through the skin or a body orifice for diagnosis or treatment.

nonmedullated (non-med'yū-lāt-ed). Unmyelinated.

nonmyelinated (non-mī'ĕ-li-nāt'ed). Unmyelinated.

Nonne, Max, German physician, 1861–1959. See N.-Milroy *disease.*

non-neoplastic, nonneoplastic (non'nē-ō-plas'tik). Not neoplastic.

non-nucleated. (non-nū'klē-ā-ted). Having no nucleus.

nonocclusion (non-ŏ-klū'shŭn). Failure of a tooth to contact an opposing tooth.

nonose (non'ōs) [L. *nonus,* ninth]. A sugar with nine carbon atoms.

nonparous (non-par'ŭs). Nulliparous.

nonpenetrance (non-pen'ĕ-trans). **1.** The state in which a genetic trait, although present in the appropriate genotype (*i.e.,* homozygous, hemizygous, or heterozygous according to the state of dominance and mode of inheritance), fails to manifest itself in the phenotype. **2.** Obscuration of genetic traits by nongenetic mechanisms.

nonproprietary name (non-prō-prī'ĕ-tăr-ē). A short name (often called a generic name) of a chemical, drug, or other substance that is not subject to trademark (proprietary) rights but is, in contrast to a trivial name, recognized or recommended by government agencies (*e.g.,* Federal Food and Drug Administration) and by quasi-official organizations (*e.g.,* U.S. Adopted Names Council) for general public use. Like a proprietary name, it is almost always a coined designation derived without using set criteria. *Cf.* trivial name; proprietary name; semisystematic name; systematic name.

nonreset nodus sinuatrialis (non-rē'set nō'dŭs sī'nū-ā-trē-ā'lis). Nonreset of the sinoatrial node produced by a premature atrial depolarizaton when the sum of the duration of the premature cycle and the return cycle is fully compensatory, *i.e.,* twice the duration of the spontaneous cycle length. *Cf.* reset nodus sinuatrialis.

nonrotation (non-rō-tā'shŭn). Failure of normal rotation.
n. of intestine, a developmental anomaly resulting in the small intestine being on the right of the abdomen and the colon on the left.
n. of kidney, a developmental anomaly in which the hilum of the kidney retains its original position, facing ventrally.

nonsecretor (non-sē-krē'tŏr, -tōr). An individual whose saliva does not contain antigens of the ABO blood group. See also secretor.

nonunion (non'yūn-yŭn). Failure of normal healing of a fractured bone.

nonvalent (non-vā'lent). Having no valency; not capable of entering into chemical composition.

nonvascular (non-vas'kyū-lăr). Avascular.

nonverbal (non-ver'bl). Denoting communication without sounds or words; *e.g.,* by signs, symbols, facial expressions, gestures, posture.

nonviable (non-vī'ă-bl). **1.** Incapable of independent existence; often denoting a prematurely born fetus. **2.** Denoting a microorganism or parasite incapable of metabolic or reproductive activity.

Noonan, Jacqueline A., U.S. physician, *1921. See N.'s *syndrome.*

nor-. **1.** Chemical prefix denoting 1) elimination of one methylene group from a chain, the highest permissible locant being used; 2) contraction of a (steroid) ring by one CH_2 unit, the locant being the capital letter identifying the ring. Elimination of two methylene groups is denoted by the prefix dinor-; three groups, by trinor-, etc. **2.** Chemical prefix denoting "normal," *i.e.,* unbranched chain of carbon atoms in aliphatic compounds, as opposed to branched with the same number of carbon atoms; *e.g.,* norleucine, leucine.

noradrenaline (nor-ă-dren'ă-lin). Norepinephrine.
n. acid tartrate, *norepinephrine* bitartrate.
n. bitartrate, *norepinephrine* bitartrate.

nordefrin hydrochloride (nōr-def'rin). *dl*-α(1-Aminoethyl)-3,4-dihydrobenzyl alcohol hydrochloride; a sympathomimetic and vasoconstrictor.

norepinephrine (nōr'ep-i-nef'rin). Noradrenaline; levarterenol; *l*-α-(aminomethyl)-3,4-dihydroxybenzyl alcohol; a catecholamine hormone of which the natural form is D, although the L form has some activity; the base is considered to be the postganglionic adrenergic mediator. It is present in the adrenal medulla and in adult animals of most species in much smaller amounts than is epinephrine; possesses the excitatory actions of epinephrine, but has minimal inhibitory effects; has feeble effects on bronchial smooth muscle and metabolic processes; and differs from epinephrine in its cardiovascular action, chiefly vasoconstriction, exerting little effect upon the cardiac output. It is used medicinally as n. bitartrate.
n. bitartrate, levarterenol or noradrenaline bitartrate; noradrenaline acid tartrate; (−)-α-(aminomethyl)-3,4-dihydroxybenzyl alcohol tartrate. For actions and uses, see n.

norethandrolone (nōr-eth-an'drō-lōn). 17α-Ethyl-19-nortestosterone; 17α-ethyl-17-hydroxy-19-nor-androst-4-en-3-one; an androgenic steroid similar chemically and pharmacologically to testosterone.

norethindrone (nōr-eth'in-drōn). Norethisterone; 19-norethisterone; 19-nor-17α-ethinyltestosterone; 17α-ethynl-17β-hydroxy-4-estren-3-one; a potent orally effective progestational agent with some estrogenic and androgenic activity; used as a substitute for progesterone and, in combination with an estrogen, as an oral contraceptive.
n. acetate, 17-hydroxy-19-nor-17α-pregn-4-en-20-yn-3-one acetate; an orally active progestin with some estrogenic and androgenic activity, used to treat endometriosis and, with an estrogen, as an oral contraceptive.

norethisterone (nōr-eth-is'ter-ōn). Norethindrone.

norethynodrel (nōr-ĕ-thī'nō-drel). An orally active progestin with some estrogenic activity; used as a progestational agent and, in combination with mestranol, as an oral contraceptive.

norfloxacin (nōr-floks'ă-sin). 1-Ethyl-6-fluoro-1,4-dihydro-4-oxo-7-(1-piperazinyl)-3-quinolinecarboxylic acid; an oral broad spectrum quinoline antibacterial agent used in the treatment of urinary tract infections.

norgestrel (nōr-jes'trel). (±)-13-Ethyl-17-hydroxy-18,19-dinor-17α-pregn-4-en-20-yn-3-one; a progestin used in oral contraceptive products.

norleucine (nōr-lū'sin). Caprine; glycoleucine; α-amino-*n*-caproic acid; 2-aminohexanoic acid; an α-amino acid, isomer of leucine and isoleucine, but not found in proteins; a deamination product of lysine, to which it is linked in collagens.

norma, pl. normae (nōr'mă, nōr'mē) [L. a carpenter's square] [NA]. A line or pattern defining the contour of a part; extended to denote the outline of a surface, referring especially to the various aspects of the cranium.
n. ante'rior, n. facialis.
n. basila'ris [NA], basis cranii externa; n. ventralis; n. inferior; the outline of the inferior aspect of the skull.
n. facia'lis [NA], n. anterior; n. frontalis; the outline of the skull viewed from in front.
n. fronta'lis, n. facialis.
n. infe'rior, n. basilaris.
n. latera'lis [NA], n. temporalis; the profile of the skull; the outline of the skull viewed from either side.

n. occipita'lis [NA], n. posterior; the outline of the skull viewed from behind.
n. poste'rior, n. occipitalis.
n. sagitta'lis, the outline of a sagittal section through the skull.
n. supe'rior, n. verticalis.
n. tempora'lis, n. lateralis.
n. ventra'lis, n. basilaris.
n. vertica'lis [NA], n. superior; the outline of the surface of the skull viewed from above.

normal (nōr'măl) [L. *normalis,* according to pattern]. **1.** Typical; usual; healthy; according to the rule or standard. **2.** In bacteriology, nonimmune; untreated; denoting an animal, or the serum or substance contained therein, that has not been experimentally immunized against any microorganism or its products. **3.** (N). Denoting a solution containing 1 equivalent of replaceable hydrogen or hydroxyl per liter; *e.g.,* 1 M HCl is 1 N, but 1 M H_2SO_4 is 2 N. **4.** In psychiatry and psychology, denoting a state of effective function satisfactory to both the individual and his social milieu.

normalization (nōr'mal-i-zā'shŭn). **1.** Making normal or according to the standard. **2.** Reducing or strengthening of a solution to make it normal. **3.** Adjusting one curve to another by multiplication of the points of the one by some arbitrary factor.

normalize (nōr'măl-īz). To effect normalization.

normetanephrine (nōr-met'ă-nef'rin). 3-*O*-Methylnorepinephrine; a catabolite of norepinephrine found, together with metanephrine, in the urine and some tissues, resulting from the action of catechol-*O*-methyltransferase on norepinephrine; has no sympathomimetic actions.

normethadone (nōr-meth'ă-dōn). Desmethylmethadone; phenyldimazone; 6-dimethylamino-4,4-diphenyl-3-hexanone; an antitussive with narcotic properties.

normethandrone (nōr-meth'an-drōn). Methylnortestosterone; 17β-hydroxy-17-methylestr-4-en-3-one; an androgen.

normo- [L. *normalis,* normal, according to pattern]. Combining form meaning normal, usual.

normobaric (nōr-mō-bar'ik) [normo- + G. *baros,* weight]. Denoting a barometric pressure equivalent to sea level pressure.

normoblast (nōr'mō-blast) [normo- + G. *blastos,* sprout, germ]. A nucleated red blood cell, the immediate precursor of a normal erythrocyte in man. Its four stages of development are: 1) pronormoblast, 2) basophilic n., 3) polychromatic n., and 4) orthochromatic n. See discussion under erythroblast.

normocapnia (nōr-mō-kap'nē-ă) [normo- + G. *kapnos,* vapor]. A state in which the arterial carbon dioxide pressure is normal, about 40 mm Hg. See also eucapnia.

normocephalic (nōr'mō-se-fal'ik) [normo- + G. *kephalē,* head]. Mesocephalic.

normochromia (nōr-mō-krō'mē-ă) [normo- + G. *chrōma,* color]. Normal color; referring to blood in which the amount of hemoglobin in the red blood cells is normal.

normochromic (nōr-mō-krō'mik). Being normal in color; referring especially to red blood cells that possess the normal quantity of hemoglobin.

normocyte (nōr'mō-sīt) [normo- + G. *kytos,* cell]. Normoerythrocyte; a non-nucleated erythrocyte of normal size (average 7.5 μm); a normal, healthy red blood cell.

normocytosis (nōr'mō-sī-tō'sis). A normal state of the blood with regard to its component formed elements.

normoerythrocyte (nōr'mō-ĕ-rith'rō-sīt). Normocyte.

[illegible]lycemia (nōr'mō-glī-sē'mē-ă). Euglycemia.

[illegible]emic (nōr'mō-glī-sē'mik). Euglycemic.

[illegible]mia, normokaliemia (nōr'mō-kă-lē'mē-ă, -ka-lē-ē'mē-[illegible] [illegible]nal level of potassium in the blood.

normoplasia (nōr-mō-plā'zē-ă) [normo- + G. *plasis,* a forming]. A specific differentiation characteristic of a cell within normal limits.

normosthenuria (nōr'mō-sthĕ-nū'rē-ă) [normo- + G. *sthenos,* strength, + *ouron,* urine]. The excretion of normal urine in normal amount.

normotensive (nōr-mō-ten'siv). Normotonic (2); indicating a normal arterial blood pressure.

normothermia (nōr-mō-ther'mē-ă) [normo- + G. *thermē,* heat]. Environmental temperature that does not cause increased or depressed activity of body cells.

normotonic (nōr-mō-ton'ik). **1.** Eutonic; relating to or characterized by normal muscular tone. **2.** Normotensive.

normotopia (nōr-mō-tō'pē-ă) [normo- + G. *topos,* place]. The state of being in the normal place; used in reference to normal placement of an organ.

normotopic (nōr-mō-top'ik). Relating to normotopia; in the right place.

normovolemia (nōr'mō-vol-ē'mē-ă) [normo- + volume, + G. *haima,* blood]. A normal blood volume.

normoxia (nōr-mok'sē-ă) [normo- + oxygen]. A state in which the partial pressure of oxygen in the inspired gas is equal to that of air at sea level, about 150 mm Hg.

norophthalmic acid (nōr'of-thal-mik). *N*-[*N*-(γ-Glutamyl)alanyl]glycine; a tripeptide analogue of glutathione (cysteine replaced by alanine), found in the lens of the eye.

norpipanone (nōr-pip'ă-nōn). 4,4-Diphenyl-6-(1-piperidyl)-3-hexanone; an analgesic agent.

Norrie, Gordon, Danish ophthalmologist, 1855–1941. See N.'s *disease.*

Norris, Richard, British physiologist, 1831–1916. See N.'s *corpuscles.*

norsteroids (nōr-stēr'oydz). Steroids in which an angular methyl group is missing; most commonly, the group between the A and B rings (C-19).

norsympatol (nōr-sim'pă-tōl). Octopamine.

norsynephrine (nōr-si-nef'rin). Octopamine.

Norton, U.F., U.S. obstetrician. See N.'s *operation.*

nortriptyline hydrochloride (nōr-trip'ti-lēn). 10,11-Dihydro-*N*-methyl-5*H*-dibenzol[a,d]cycloheptene-Δ^5,γ-propylamine hydrochloride; an antidepressant.

norvaline (nōr-val'ēn, -vā'lēn). α-Aminovaleric acid; $CH_3(CH_2)_2CHNH_2COOH$; the straight chain analogue of valine; not found in proteins.

noscapine (nos'kă-pēn). Opianine; *l*-α-narcotine; 2-methyl-8-methoxy-6,7-methylenedioxy-1-(6,7-dimethoxy-3-phthalidyl)-1,2,3,4-tetrahydroisoguinoline; an isoquionoline alkaloid, occurring in opium, with papaverine-like action on smooth muscle; suppresses the cough reflex and is used as an antitussive; it appears to be without addiction liability.

nose (nōz) [A.S. *nosu*] Nasus.
brandy n., rhinophyma.
cleft n., a n. with a furrow where the bridge is normally present; due to failure of complete convergence of the paired primordia.
copper n., rhinophyma.
dog n., goundou.
external n., *nasus* externus.
hammer n., rhinophyma.
potato n., rhinophyma.
rum n., rhinophyma.
saddle n., a n. with markedly depressed bridge, seen in congenital syphilis or after injury from trauma or operation.
toper's n., rhinophyma.

nosebleed (nōs'blēd). Epistaxis.

Nosema (nō-sē'mă) [G. *nosēma*, plague, fr. *noseō*, to be sick, fr. *nosos*, disease]. A protozoan genus (family Nosematidae, order Microsporida, phylum Microspora) with species (*N. apis, N. bombycis*, and others) pathogenic for invertebrates of economic importance (bees, silkworms); others are being studied as possible agents of biological control of pest insects or other target invertebrates.

Nosematidae (nō-sē-mat'i-dē). A family of the class Microsporida that includes the genera *Encephalitozoon* and *Nosema*, containing several pathogenic and economically important species.

nosepiece (nōs'pēs). A microscope attachment, consisting of several objectives surrounding a central pivot.

nosetiology (nōs'ē-tē-ol'ō-jē) [G. *nosos*, disease, + *aitia*, cause, + *logos*, study]. Rarely used term for the study of the causes of disease.

noso- [G. *nosos*, disease]. Combining form relating to disease.

nosochthonography (nos'ok-thō-nog'ră-fē) [noso- + G. *chthōn*, the earth, + *graphē*, a description]. Geomedicine.

nosocomial (nos-ō-kō'mē-ăl) [G. *nosokomeian*, hospital, fr. *nosos*, disease, + *komeō*, to take care of]. **1.** Relating to a hospital. **2.** Denoting a new disorder (not the patient's original condition) associated with being treated in a hospital, such as a hospital-acquired infection.

nosogenesis, nosogeny (nos-ō-jen'ĕ-sis, no-soj'ĕ-nē) [noso- + G. *genesis*, production]. Rarely used terms for pathogenesis.

nosogenic (nos-ō-jen'ik). Pathogenic.

nosogeography (nos'ō-jē-og'ră-fē). Geomedicine.

nosographic (nos-ō-graf'ik). Relating to nosography, or the description of diseases.

nosography (nō-sog'ră-fē) [noso- + G. *graphē*, description]. A treatise on pathology or the practice of medicine.

nosologic (nos-ō-loj'ik). Relating to nosology.

nosology (nō-sol'ō-jē) [noso- + G. *logos*, study]. Nosonomy; nosotaxy; the science of classification of diseases.
psychiatric n., psychonosology.

nosomania (nos-ō-mā'nē-ă) [noso- + G. *mania*, insanity]. An unfounded morbid belief that one is suffering from some special disease.

nosometry (nō-som'ĕ-trē) [noso- + G. *metron*, measure]. Measurement of morbidity or of the sickness rate in occupations and social conditions.

nosomycosis (nos'ō-mī-kō'sis) [noso- + G. *mykēs*, fungus]. Any disease caused by a fungus.

nosonomy (nō-son'ō-mē) [noso- + G. *nomos*, law]. Nosology.

nosophilia (nos-ō-fil'ē-ă) [noso- + G. *phileō*, to love]. A morbid desire to be sick.

nosophobia (nos-ō-fō'bē-ă) [noso- + G. *phobos*, fear]. Pathophobia; an inordinate dread and fear of disease.

nosophyte (nos'ō-fīt) [noso- + G. *phyton*, plant]. A pathogenic microorganism of the plant kingdom.

nosopoietic (nos'ō-poy-et'ik) [noso- + G. *poiēsis*, a making]. Pathogenic.

Nosopsyllus (nos-ō-sil'ŭs) [noso- + G. *psylla*, flea]. A flea genus commonly found on rodents. *N. fasciatus*, the northern rat flea, is a species that infrequently transmits the plague bacillus to man.

nosotaxy (nos'ō-tak-sē) [noso- + G. *taxis*, arrangement]. Nosology.

nosotoxic (nos-ō-tok'sik). Relating to a nosotoxin or to nosotoxicosis.

nosotoxicosis (nos'ō-tok-si-kō'sis) [noso- + G. *toxicon*, poison]. A morbid state caused by a toxin. See also toxicosis.

nosotoxin (nos-ō-tok'sin). Rarely used term for any toxin associated with a disease.

nosotrophy (nos-ot'rō-fē) [noso- + G. *trophē*, nourishment]. Rarely used term for care of the sick.

nosotropic (nos-ō-trop'ik) [noso- + G. *tropē*, a turning]. Directed against the pathologic changes or symptoms of a disease.

nostalgia (nos-tal'jē-ă) [G. *nostos*, a return (home), + *algos*, pain]. The longing to return home, to a former time in one's life, or to familiar surroundings. *Cf.* apodemialgia.

nostomania (nos-tō-mā'nē-ă) [G. *nostos*, return, homecoming, + *mania*, frenzy]. An obsessive or abnormal interest in nostalgia, especially as an extreme manifestation of homesickness.

nostophobia (nos-tō-fō'bē-ă) [G. *nostos*, return, homecoming, + *phobos*, fear]. Morbid fear of returning home.

nos'tril. Naris.
internal n., secondary *choana*.

nostrum (nos'trŭm) [L. neuter of *noster*, our, "our own remedy"]. General term for a therapeutic agent, sometimes patented and usually of secret composition, offered to the general public as a specific remedy for any disease or class of diseases.

notal (nō'tăl) [G. *nōtos*, the back]. Relating to the back.

notalgia (nō-tal'jē-ă) [G. *nōtos*, the back, + *algos*, pain]. Obsolete term for dorsalgia.
n. paresthet'ica, localized pruritus in the oval-shaped area in the inferomedial border of the scapula, with no demonstrable changes in the skin except for what results from repeated and prolonged scratching; possibly X-linked dominant inherited trait.

notancephalia (nō'tan-se-fā'lē-ă) [G. *nōtos*, back, + *an-* priv. + *kephalē*, head]. Fetal malformation characterized by a bony deficiency, *i.e.*, absence of the occipital bone of the cranium.

notanencephalia (nō'tan-en-se-fā'lē-ă) [G. *nōtos*, back, + *an-* priv. + *enkephalos*, brain]. Fetal malformation characterized by a bony deficiency, *i.e.*, absence of the occipital bone of the cranium.

notatin (nō-tā'tin). *Glucose* oxidase.

NOTCH

notch. Incisura (2).
acetabular n., *incisura* acetabuli.
angular n., *incisura* angularis.
antegonial n., the highest point of the n. or concavity of the lower border of the ramus where it joins the body of the mandible.
anterior n. of cerebellum, *incisura* cerebelli anterior.
anterior n. of ear, *incisura* anterior auris.
aortic n., the slight n. in the sphygmographic tracing caused by the rebound at the closure of the aortic valves.
n. of apex of heart, *incisura* apicis cordis.
auricular n., **(1)** *incisura* anterior auris; **(2)** *incisura* terminalis auris.
cardiac n., *incisura* cardiaca.
cardiac n. of left lung, *incisura* cardiaca pulmonis sinistri.
n.'s in cartilage of external acoustic meatus, *incisurae* cartilaginis meatus acustici externi.
clavicular n., *incisura* clavicularis.
costal n., *incisura* costalis.
cotyloid n., *incisura* acetabuli.
craniofacial n., a defect in the osseous partition between the orbital and nasal cavities.
dicrotic n., the n. in a pulse tracing which precedes the second or dicrotic wave.
digastric n., *incisura* mastoidea.

ethmoidal n., *incisura* ethmoidalis.
fibular n., *incisura* fibularis.
frontal n., *incisura* frontalis.
greater sciatic n., *incisura* ischiadica major.
hamular n., pterygomaxillary n.
Hutchinson's crescentic n., the semilunar n. on the incisal edge of Hutchinson's teeth, encountered in congenital syphilis.
iliosciatic n., *incisura* ischiadica major.
inferior thyroid n., *incisura* thyroidea inferior.
interarytenoid n., *incisura* interarytenoidea.
interclavicular n., *incisura* jugularis sternalis.
intercondyloid n., *fossa* intercondylaris.
intertragic n., *incisura* intertragica.
intervertebral n., *incisura* vertebralis.
ischiatic n., see *incisura* ischiadica major; *incisura* ischiadica minor.
jugular n., *incisura* jugularis.
Kernohan's n., a n. in the cerebral peduncle due to displacement of the brainstem against the incisura of the tentorium by a transtentorial herniation.
lacrimal n., *incisura* lacrimalis.
lesser sciatic n., *incisura* ischiadica minor.
mandibular n., *incisura* mandibulae.
marsupial n., *incisura* cerebelli posterior.
mastoid n., *incisura* mastoidea.
nasal n., *incisura* nasalis.
pancreatic n., *incisura* pancreatis.
parietal n., *incisura* parietalis.
parotid n., the space between the ramus of the mandible and the mastoid process of the temporal bone.
popliteal n., *fossa* intercondylaris.
posterior n. of cerebellum, *incisura* cerebelli posterior.
preoccipital n., *incisura* preoccipitalis.
presternal n., *incisura* jugularis sternalis.
pterygoid n., *incisura* pterygoidea.
pterygomaxillary n., hamular n.; the n. or fissure between the tuberosity of the maxilla and the hamulus of the pterygoid process of the sphenoid bone.
radial n., *incisura* radialis.
Rivinus' n., *incisura* tympanica.
n. for round ligament of liver, *incisura* ligamenti teretis hepatis.
sacrosciatic n., *incisura* ischiadica major.
scapular n., *incisura* scapulae.
semilunar n., **(1)** *incisura* cerebelli anterior; **(2)** *incisura* trochlearis.
sigmoid n., *incisura* mandibulae.
sphenopalatine n., *incisura* sphenopalatina.
sternal n., *incisura* jugularis sternalis.
superior thyroid n., *incisura* thyroidea superior.
supraorbital n., *incisura* supraorbitalis.
suprascapular n., *incisura* scapulae.
suprasternal n., *incisura* jugularis sternalis.
n. of tentorium, *incisura* tentorii.
terminal n. of auricle, *incisura* terminalis auris.
trochlear n., *incisura* trochlearis.
tympanic n., *incisura* tympanica.
ulnar n., *incisura* ulnaris.
umbilical n., *incisura* ligamenti teretis.
vertebral n., *incisura* vertebralis.

notched. Emarginate.

notencephalocele (nō-ten-sef'ă-lō-sēl) [G. *nōtos,* back, + *enkephalos,* brain, + *kēlē,* hernia]. Malformation in the occipital portion of the cranium with protrusion of brain substance.

Nothnagel, C.W. Hermann, Austrian physician, 1841–1905. See N.'s *syndrome, test.*

notochord (nō'tō-kōrd) [G. *nōtos,* back, + *chordē,* cord, string]. **1.** In primitive vertebrates, the primary axial supporting structure of the body, derived from the notochordal or head process of the early embryo; an important organizer for determining the final form of the nervous system and related structures. **2.** Chorda dorsalis or vertebralis; in embryos, the axial fibrocellular cord about which the vertebral primordia develop; vestiges of it persist in the adult as the nuclei pulposi of the intervertebral disks.

notochordal (nō-tō-kōr'dăl). Relating to the notochord.

Notoedres cati (nō-tō-ed'rēz kā'tī). Sarcoptic mange mite of cats. Also called *Sarcoptes scabei minor.*

noumenal (nū'men-ăl) [G. *nooumenos,* perceived, fr. *noeō,* to perceive, think]. Intellectually, not sensuously, intuitional; relating to the object of pure thought divorced from all concepts of time or space.

nourishment (ner'ish-ment). A substance used to feed or to sustain life and growth of an organism.

nous (nūs, nows) [G. mind, reason]. A word originally used by Anaxagoras to mean an all-knowing, all-pervading spirit or force; in later Greek philosophy it came to mean simply mind, reason, or intellect.

novobiocin (nō-vō-bī'ō-sin). Streptonivicin; an antibacterial substance produced by fermentation from cultures of *Streptomyces niveus* or *S. spheroides,* effective against penicillin-resistant *Staphylococcus* and *Proteus;* also available as n. calcium and n. sodium.

Novy, Frederick G., U.S. bacteriologist, 1864–1957. See N. and MacNeal's blood *agar.*

noxa (nok'să) [L. injury, fr. *noceo,* to injure]. Anything that exerts a harmful influence, such as trauma, poison, etc.

noxious (nok'shŭs) [L. *noxius,* injurious, fr. *noceo,* to injure]. Injurious; harmful.

noxythiolin (nok-sē-thī'ō-lin). 1-(Hydroxymethyl)-3-methyl-2-thiourea; an antibacterial and antifungal agent.

Np **1.** Symbol for neptunium. **2.** Abbreviation for neper.

NPN Abbreviation for nonprotein *nitrogen.*

Nps Abbreviation for nitrophenylsulfenyl.

NREM Abbreviation for non-rapid eye *movement.*

nRNA Abbreviation for nuclear *ribonucleic acid.*

NSAID Abbreviation for nonsteroidal anti-inflammatory drug; *e.g.,* aspirin.

N-terminal. Amino-terminal.

NTMI Abbreviation for nontransmural myocardial *infarction.*

nu (nū). Thirteenth letter of the Greek alphabet, ν(*q.v.*).

nubecula (nū-bek'yū-lă) [L. dim. of *nubes,* cloud]. A faint cloud or cloudiness.

nucha (nū'kă) [Fr. *nuque*] [NA]. Nape; the back of the neck.

nuchal (nū'kăl). Relating to the nucha.

Nuck, Anton, Dutch anatomist, 1650–1692. See N.'s *diverticulum, hydrocele, canal* of N.

nucl-. See nucleo-.

nuclear (nū'klē-er). Relating to a nucleus, either cellular or atomic; in the latter sense, usually referring to radiation emanating from atomic nuclei (α, β, or γ) or to atomic fission.

nuclease (nū'klē-ās). General term for enzymes that catalyze the hydrolysis of nucleic acid into nucleotides or oligonucleotides by cleaving phosphodiester linkages. For n.'s not listed below, see the specific term.
Azotobacter n., Endonuclease (*Serratia marcescens*).
micrococcal n., micrococcal *endonuclease.*
mung bean n., Endonuclease S_1 (*Aspergillus*).

nucleate (nū'klē-āt). A salt of a nucleic acid.

nucleated (nū'klē-ā-ted). Provided with a nucleus, a characteristic of all true cells.

nucleation (nū-klē-ā'shŭn). Process of forming a nidus (4).
heterogeneous n., n. about a nidus composed of material other than that precipitating.
homogeneous n., n. about a nidus composed of material identical with that precipitating.

nuclei (nū'klē-ī). Plural of nucleus.

nucleic acid (nū-klē'ik, -klā'ik). A family of macromolecules, of molecular masses ranging upward from 25,000, found in the chromosomes, nucleoli, mitochondria, and cytoplasm of all cells, and in viruses; in complexes with proteins, they are called nucleoproteins. On hydrolysis they yield purines, pyrimidines, phosphoric acid, and a pentose, either D-ribose or D-deoxyribose; from the last, the n.a.'s derive their more specific names, ribonucleic acid and deoxyribonucleic acid. N.a.'s are linear (*i.e.,* unbranched) chains of nucleotides in which the 5′ phosphoric group of each one is esterified with the 3′ hydroxyl of the adjoining nucleotide.
infectious n. a., n. a. capable of effecting transfection.

nucleiform (nū'klē-i-fōrm). Nucleoid (1); shaped like or having the appearance of a nucleus.

nucleinase (nū'klē-in-ās). Obsolete term for nuclease.

nucleo-, nucl- [L. *nucleus*]. Combining forms for nucleus or nuclear.

nucleocapsid (nū'klē-ō-kap'sid). See virion.

nucleochylema (nū-klē-ō-kī-lē'mă) [nucleo- + G. *chylos,* juice]. Karyolymph.

nucleochyme (nū'klē-ō-kīm). Karyolymph.

nucleofugal (nū-klē-of'yū-găl) [nucleo- + L. *fugio,* to flee]. **1.** Moving within the cell body in a direction away from the nucleus. **2.** Moving in a direction away from a nerve nucleus; said of nerve transmission.

nucleohistone (nū'klē-ō-his'tōn). A complex of histone and deoxyribonucleic acid, the form in which the latter is usually found in the nuclei of cells; n. may be viewed as a salt between the basic protein and the acidic nucleic acid.

nucleoid (nū'klē-oyd) [nucleo- + G. *eidos,* resemblance]. **1.** Nucleiform. **2.** A nuclear inclusion body. **3.** Nucleus (2).
Lavdovsky's n., astrosphere.

nucleolar (nū-klē'ō-lăr). Relating to a nucleolus.

nucleoli (nū-klē'ō-lī). Plural of nucleolus.

nucleoliform (nū-klē'ō-lē-fōrm). Nucleoloid; resembling a nucleolus.

nucleoloid (nū-klē'ō-loyd) [nucleolus + G. *eidos,* resemblance]. Nucleoliform.

nucleolonema (nū-klē'ō-lō-nē'mă) [nucleolus + G. *nema,* thread]. The irregular network or rows of fine ribonucleoprotein granules or microfilaments forming most of the nucleolus.

nucleolus, pl. **nucleoli** (nū-klē'ō-lŭs, -lī) [L. dim of *nucleus,* a nut, kernel]. **1.** A small rounded mass within the cell nucleus where ribonucleoprotein is produced; it is usually single, but there may be several accessory nucleoli besides the principal one. The n. is composed of a meshwork (nucleolonema) of microfilaments and granules and the pars amorpha, now shown to have microfilaments also. **2.** A more or less central body in the vesicular nucleus of certain protozoa in which an endosome is lacking but one or more Feulgen-positive (DNA+) nucleoli are present; characteristic of certain sporozoans, flagellates, opalinids, dinoflagellates, and radiolarians among the Protozoa. The chromatin material is distributed throughout the nucleus rather than peripherally, as in the endosome type of nucleus of *Entamoeba.*
chromatin n., karyosome.
false n., karyosome.

nucleomicrosome (nū'klē-ō-mī'krō-sōm). Karyomicrosome.

nucleon (nū'klē-on). One of the subatomic particles of the atomic nucleus; *i.e.,* either a proton or a neutron.

nucleopetal (nū-klē-op'ĕ-tăl) [nucleo- + L. *peto,* to seek]. **1.** Moving in the cell body in a direction toward the nucleus. **2.** Moving in a direction toward a nerve nucleus; said of a nervous impulse.

Nucleophaga (nū-klē-of'ă-gă) [nucleo- + G. *phagein,* to eat]. A microsporan parasite of amebae which destroys the nucleus of its host.

nucleophil, nucleophile (nū'klē-ō-fil, -fīl) [nucleo- + G. *philos,* fond]. **1.** The electron donor atom in a chemical reaction in which a pair of electrons is picked up by an electrophil. **2.** Nucleophilic; relating to a nucleophil.

nucleophilic (nū'klē-ō-fil'ik). Nucleophil (2).

nucleophosphatases (nū'klē-ō-fos'fă-tās-ez). Nucleotidases.

nucleoplasm (nū'klē-ō-plazm). The protoplasm of the nucleus of a cell.

nucleoprotein (nū'klē-ō-prō'tēn). A complex of protein and nucleic acid, the form in which essentially all nucleic acids exist in nature; chromosomes and viruses are largely n.

nucleoreticulum (nū'klē-ō-rē-tik'yū-lŭm) [nucleo- + L. *reticulum,* dim. of *rete,* net]. The intranuclear network of chromatin or linin.

nucleorrhexis (nū'klē-ō-rek'sis) [nucleo- + G. *rhēxis,* rupture]. Fragmentation of a cell nucleus.

nucleosidases (nū'klē-ō-sī'dās-ez). Enzymes (EC subgroup 3.2.2) that catalyze the hydrolysis of nucleosides, releasing the purine or pyrimidine base.

nucleoside (nū'klē-ō-sīd). A compound of a sugar (usually ribose or deoxyribose) with a purine or pyrimidine base by way of an *N*-glycosyl link.
n. bisphosphate, a n. that carries two independent (*i.e.,* not linked to each other) phosphoric residues. *Cf.* n. diphosphate.
n. diphosphate, the pyrophosphoric ester of a n., *i.e.,* a n. in which the H of one of the ribose hydroxyls (usually the 5′) is replaced by a pyrophosphoric (diphosphoric) radical; *e.g.,* adenosine diphosphate. *Cf.* n. bisphosphate.
n. phosphate, a nucleotide, *e.g.,* AMP.
n. triphosphate, a n. in which the H of one of the ribose hydroxyls (usually the 5′) is replaced by a triphosphoric group, $-PO(OH)-O-PO(OH)-O-PO(OH)_2$; *e.g.,* adenosine triphosphate.

nucleosidediphosphate kinase (nū'klē-ō-sīd-dī-fos'fāt) [EC 2.7.4.6]. A phosphotransferase catalyzing transfer of one phosphate group from ATP to a nucleoside diphosphate to yield a nucleoside triphosphate and ADP.

nucleosidediphosphate sugars. Nucleoside diphosphates linked through the 5′-diphosphoric group with simple or complex carbohydrates; *e.g.,* GDP-mannose, UDP-glucose (UDPG), dTDP-glucosamine.

nucleosome (nū'klē-ō-sōm) [nucleo- + G. *sōma,* body]. A localized aggregation of histone and DNA that is evident when chromatin is in the uncondensed stage.

nucleospindle (nū'klē-ō-spin'dl). The fusiform body in mitosis.

nucleotidases (nū'klē-ō-tī-dās-ez). Nucleophosphatases; enzymes (EC class 3.1.3) that catalyze the hydrolysis of nucleotides into phosphoric acid and nucleosides; specificities are indicated by prefixes 3′- and 5′-.

nucleotide (nū'klē-ō-tīd). Mononucleotide; originally a combination of a (nucleic acid) purine or pyrimidine, one sugar (usually ribose or deoxyribose), and a phosphoric group; by extension, any compound containing a heterocyclic compound bound to a phosphorylated sugar by an *N*-glycosyl link (*e.g.,* adenosine phosphate, flavin mononucleotide). For individual n.'s see specific names.

nucleotidyltransferases (nū'klē-ō-tī'dil-trans'fer-ās-ez). Enzymes (EC class 2.7.7) transferring nucleotide residues (nucleotidyls) from nucleoside di- or triphosphates into dimer or polymer forms. Some n.'s bear specific names (*e.g.,* adenylyltransferases), or trivial names indicating the linkage hydrolyzed in the synthesis (pyrophosphorylases, phosphorylases), or names of the material synthesized (RNA or DNA polymerase).

nucleotoxin (nū'klē-ō-tok'sin). A toxin acting upon the cell nuclei.

NUCLEUS

nucleus, pl. **nuclei** (nū'klē-ŭs, nū'klē-ī) [L. a little nut, the kernel, stone of fruits, the inside of a thing, dim. of *nux,* nut]. **1.** Karyon; in cytology, typically a rounded or oval mass of protoplasm within the cytoplasm of a plant or animal cell; it is surrounded by a nuclear envelope, which encloses euchromatin, heterochromatin, and one or more nucleoli, and undergoes mitosis during cell division. **2.** Nucleoid (3); by extension, because of similar function, the genome of microorganisms (microbes) that is relatively simple in structure, lacks a nuclear membrane, and does not undergo mitosis during replication. See also virion. **3** [NA]. In neuroanatomy, a group of nerve cells in the brain or spinal cord that can be demarcated from neighboring groups on the basis of either differences in cell type or the presence of a surrounding zone of nerve fibers or cell-poor neuropil. **4.** Any substance, (*e.g.,* foreign body, mucus, crystal) around which a urinary or other calculus is formed. **5.** The central portion of an atom (composed of protons and neutrons) where most of the mass and all of the positive charge are concentrated.

abducens n., n. of abducent nerve, n. abducen'tis, n. nervi abducentis.

accessory cuneate n., n. cuneatus accessorius.

accessory olivary nuclei, see n. olivaris accessorius dorsalis and n. olivaris accessorius medialis.

n. accum'bens sep'ti, the region of fusion between the caput nuclei caudati and the putamen, covered on the ventral side by the olfactory tubercle. The name ("a nucleus leaning against the septum") refers to a medial, hook-shaped expansion of this anteroventral region of the striatum which curves under the floor of the frontal horn of the lateral ventricle and ascends for some distance into the ventral half of the septal region.

n. acu'sticus, see n. nervi vestibulocochlearis.

n. a'lae cine'reae, n. dorsalis nervi vagi.

almond n., *corpus* amygdaloideum.

ambiguous n., n. ambiguus.

n. ambig'uus [NA], ambiguous n.; a very slender, longitudinal column of motor neurons in the ventrolateral medulla oblongata; its efferent fibers leave with the vagus and glossopharyngeal nerve and innervate the striated muscle fibers of the pharynx (including the musculus levator veli palatini) and the vocal cord muscles of the larynx.

n. amyg'dalae, *corpus* amygdaloideum.

amygdaloid n., *corpus* amygdaloideum.

nu'clei anterio'res thal'ami [NA], anterior nuclei of the thalamus; collective term for three groups of nerve cells which together form the tuberculum anterius thalami: the n. anteroventralis, a relatively large n.; the n. anteromedialis; and the n. anterodorsalis, a small (but large-celled) n. The nuclei receive the mamillothalamic tract from the mamillary body, and additional afferents by way of the fornix; they project collectively to the cortex of the cingulate and parahippocampal gyrus.

anterior nuclei of thalamus, nuclei anteriores thalami.

n. anterodorsa'lis [NA], **anterodorsal thalamic n.,** see nuclei anteriores thalami.

n. anteromedia'lis [NA], **anteromedial thalamic n.,** see nuclei anteriores thalami.

n. anteroventra'lis [NA], **anteroventral thalamic n.,** see nuclei anteriores thalami.

arcuate n., n. arcuatus.

arcuate nuclei, nuclei arcuati.

nu'clei arcua'ti [NA], arcuate nuclei; a variable assembly of small cell groups, probably outlying components of the pontine nuclei, on the ventral and medial aspects of the pyramid in the medulla oblongata.

n. arcua'tus, arcuate n.; **(1)** n. arcuatus thalami. **(2)** posterior periventricular n.; a cell group in the hypothalamus, located in the lowest part of the infundibulum adjacent to the median eminence.

n. arcua'tus thal'ami, n. arcuatus (1); semilunar n. of Flechsig; thalamic gustatory n.; the small ventral region of the n. ventralis posteromedialis thalami in which the fibers of the gustatory lemniscus and secondary trigeminal tracts terminate; it projects to the lower part of the postcentral gyrus of the cerebral cortex.

auditory n., see n. nervi vestibulocochlearis.

n. basa'lis of Ganser, a large group of large cells in the substantia innominata, ventral to the lentiform n.

Bechterew's n., (1) n. vestibularis superior; see nuclei vestibulares; **(2)** n. centralis tegmenti superior; see nuclei raphes.

benzene n., the six carbon atoms of the benzene ring.

Blumenau's n., the lateral cuneate n. of the medulla oblongata.

branchiomotor nuclei, special visceral efferent (or motor) nuclei; collective term for those motoneuronal nuclei of the brainstem (n. ambiguus, facial motor n., motor n. of the trigeminus) that develop from the branchiomotor column of the embryo and innervate striated muscle fibers (muscles of mastication, facial musculature, pharynx and vocal cord muscles) developed from the mesenchyme of the branchial arches.

Burdach's n., n. cuneatus.

caudate n., n. caudatus.

n. cauda'tus [NA], caudate n.; caudatum; an elongated curved mass of gray matter, consisting of an anterior thick portion, the caput or head, which protrudes into the anterior horn of the lateral ventricle, a portion extending along the floor of the body of the lateral ventricle, known as the corpus, and an elongated curved thin portion, the cauda or tail, which curves downward, backward, and forward in the temporal lobe in the wall of the lateral ventricle.

n. centra'lis latera'lis thal'ami, the most lateral of the intralaminar nuclei of the thalamus.

n. centra'lis tegmen'ti supe'rior, Bechterew's n. (2); see nuclei raphes.

centromedian n., n. centromedianus.

n. centromedia'nus [NA], centromedian n.; centrum medianum; centre médian de Luys; a large, lentil-shaped cell group, the largest and most caudal of the intralaminar nuclei, located within the lamina medullaris interna of the thalamus between the mediodorsal n. and ventrobasal n.; so called by Luys because of its prominent appearance on frontal sections midway between anterior and posterior pole of the human thalamus. The n. receives numerous fibers from the internal segment of the globus pallidus by way of the fasciculus thalamicus of the ansa lenticularis, as well as from projections area 4 of the motor cortex; its major efferent connection is with the putamen although collaterals reach broad areas of the cerebral cortex.

Clarke's n., n. thoracicus.

cochlear nuclei, nuclei cochleares.

nu'clei cochlea'res [NA], cochlear nuclei; nuclei nervi cochlearis; the n. cochlearis dorsalis and n. cochlearis ventralis, located on the dorsal and lateral surface of the inferior cerebellar peduncle, in the floor of the lateral recess of the rhomboid fossa. They receive the incoming fibers of the cochlear part of the vestibulocochlear nerve and are the major source of origin of the lateral lemniscus or central auditory pathway.

n. collic'uli inferio'ris [NA], the nerve cell groups composing the colliculus inferior.
convergence n. of Perlia, Perlia's n.
n. cor'poris genicula'ti media'lis [NA], n. of the medial geniculate body; the nerve cell groups composing the medial geniculate body (corpus geniculatum mediale).
nu'clei cor'poris mamilla'ris [NA], n. of the mamillary body; a single large-celled lateral n. and a larger bipartite medial n. together comprising the corpus mamillare; present in the caudal hypothalamus.
nuclei of cranial nerves, nuclei nervorum cranialium.
cuneate n., n. cuneatus.
n. cunea'tus [NA], cuneate n.; n. funiculi cuneati; the larger Burdach's n.; of the three nuclei of the posterior column of the spinal cord; located near the dorsal surface of the medulla oblongata at and below the level of the obex, the n. receives posterior root fibers corresponding to the sensory innervation of the arm and hand of the same side; together with its medial companion, n. gracilis, it is the major source of origin of the medial lemniscus.
n. cunea'tus accesso'rius [NA], accessory, external, or lateral cuneate n.; Monakow's n.; a cell group lateral to the n. cuneatus which receives posterior-root fibers corresponding to the proprioceptive innervation of the arm and hand; it projects to the cerebellum by way of the cuneocerebellar tract, and can be considered the upper-extremity equivalent of n. thoracicus.
n. of Darkschewitsch, an ovoid cell group in the ventral central gray substance rostral to the oculomotor nucleus, receiving fibers from the vestibular nuclei by way of the medial longitudinal fasciculus; projections are not known, although some cross in the posterior commissure.
deep cerebellar nuclei, collective term for the nuclei dentatus, globosus, emboliformis, and tecti or fastigii of the cerebellum.
Deiters' n., n. vestibularis lateralis. See nuclei vestibulares.
dentate n. of cerebellum, n. dentatus cerebelli.
n. denta'tus cerebel'li [NA], dentate n. of the cerebellum; dentatum; corpus dentatum; the most lateral and largest of the deep cerebellar nuclei; it receives the axons of the Purkinje cells of the neocerebellum; together with the more medially located nuclei globosus and emboliformis it is the major source of fibers composing the massive superior cerebellar peduncle or brachium conjunctivum.

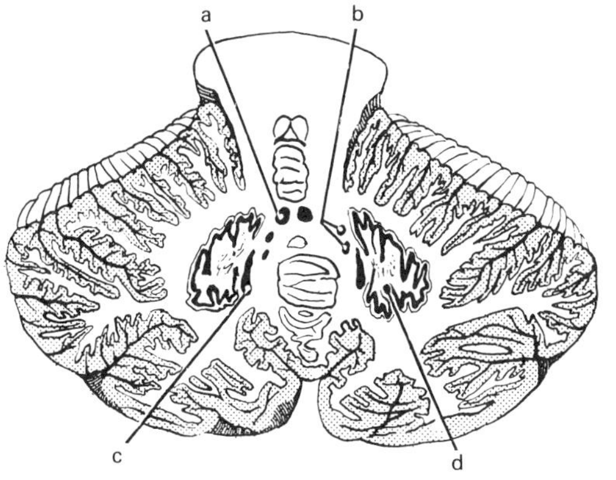

Cerebellar Nuclei
a, Nucleus fastigii; *b,* nucleus globosus; *c,* nucleus emboliformis; *d,* nucleus dentatus.

descending n. of the trigeminus, n. tractus spinalis nervi trigemini.
diploid n., a n. containing the diploid or normal double complement of chromosomes.
dorsal n., n. thoracicus.
dorsal accessory olivary n., n. olivaris accessorius dorsalis.
n. dorsa'lis, n. thoracicus.
n. dorsa'lis cor'poris trapezoi'dei [NA], oliva superior; superior olive; superior olivary n.; a circumscript, bipartite cell group located ventrolaterally in the lower pontine tegmentum, immediately dorsal to the trapezoid body; the n. receives fibers from both the ipsilateral and contralateral cochlear nuclei, and contributes fibers to the lateral (auditory) lemniscus of both sides. It is believed to be prominently involved in the function of spatial localization of sound.
n. dorsa'lis ner'vi va'gi [NA], dorsal n. of the vagus; dorsal motor n. of the vagus; n. alae cinereae; the visceral motor n. located in the vagal trigone (ala cinerea) of the floor of the fourth ventricle. It gives rise to the parasympathetic fibers of the vagus nerve innervating the heart muscle and the smooth musculature and glands of the respiratory and intestinal tracts.
dorsal motor n. of vagus, n. dorsalis nervi vagi.
dorsal n. of vagus, n. dorsalis nervi vagi.
dorsomedial n., n. medialis thalami.
dorsomedial hypothalamic n., n. dorsomedialis hypothalami.
n. dorsomedia'lis hypothal'ami [NA], dorsomedial hypothalamic n.; an oval cluster of cells located dorsal to the ventromedial hypothalamic n.
droplet nuclei, solid residues of evaporated droplets that are formed when expiratory droplets from infected hosts evaporate quickly in unsaturated atmospheres; these particles remain suspended in the air as a cloud, and can travel considerable distances in wind, thereby spreading some agents (*e.g.,* foot-and-mouth disease virus) between premises or even countries.
Edinger-Westphal n., a small group of preganglionic parasympathetic motor neurons in the midline near the rostral pole of the oculomotor n. of the midbrain; the axons of these motor neurons leave the brain with the oculomotor nerve and synapse on the cells of the ciliary ganglion which in turn innervate the sphincter muscle of the pupil and ciliary muscle. Destruction of this n. or its efferent fibers causes maximal paralytic dilation of the pupil; also demonstrated to project fibers to lower levels of the brainstem and all spinal levels.
emboliform n., n. emboliformis.
n. embolifor'mis [NA], emboliform n.; embolus (2); a small wedge-shaped mass of gray matter in the central white substance of the cerebellum just internal to the hilus of the dentate n.
external cuneate n., n. cuneatus accessorius.
n. facia'lis, n. nervi facialis.
facial motor n., n. nervi facialis.
n. fascic'uli gra'cilis, n. gracilis.
n. fasti'gii [NA], n. tecti; roof n.; fastigatum; the most medial of the deep cerebellar nuclei, lying medial to the n. interpositus, near the midline, in the white matter underneath the vermis of the cerebellar cortex. It receives the axons of Purkinje cells from all parts of the vermis. Its major projection is to the vestibular nuclei and medullary reticular formation.
n. fibro'sus lin'guae, *septum* linguae.
n. filifor'mis, n. paraventricularis.
n. funic'uli cunea'ti, n. cuneatus.
n. funic'uli gra'cilis, n. gracilis.
gametic n., micronucleus (2).
n. gelatino'sus, n. pulposus.
germ n., micronucleus (2).
n. gigantocellula'ris medul'lae oblonga'tae, one of the three nuclei of the reticular nuclei of the brainstem.
n. globo'sus [NA], spherical n.; a group of two or three small masses of gray substance in the white central core of the cerebellum, medial to the n. emboliformis.
n. of Goll, n. gracilis.

gonad n., micronucleus (2).
n. gra'cilis [NA], n. fasciculi gracilis; n. funiculi gracilis; n. of Goll; the medial one of the three nuclei of the dorsal column, the remaining two being the n. cuneatus and the n. cuneatus accessorius, which corresponds to the clava; it receives dorsal-root fibers conveying sensory innervation of the leg, and lower trunk, and projects, by way of the medial lemniscus, to the n. ventralis posterior of the thalamus.
Gudden's tegmental nuclei, nuclei tegmenti.
gustatory n., see rhombencephalic gustatory n., thalamic gustatory n.
n. haben'ulae [NA], habenular n.; ganglion habenulae; the gray matter of the habenula, composed of a small-celled medial and a larger-celled lateral habenular n.; both nuclei receive fibers from basal forebrain regions (septum, n. basalis, lateral preoptic n.); the lateral habenular n. receives an additional projection from the medial segment of the globus pallidus. Both nuclei project by way of the fasciculus retroflexus to the n. interpeduncularis and a medial zone of the midbrain tegmentum.
habenular n., n. habenulae.
hypoglossal n., n. nervi hypoglossi.
n. of hypoglossal nerve, n. nervi hypoglossi.
inferior olivary n., n. olivaris.
inferior salivary n., n. salivatorius inferior.
inferior vestibular n., n. vestibularis inferior; see nuclei vestibulares.
intercalated n., n. intercalatus.
n. intercala'tus [NA], intercalated n.; Staderini's n.; a small collection of nerve cells in the medulla oblongata lying lateral to the hypoglossal n.
intermediolateral n., n. intermediolateralis.
n. intermediolatera'lis, intermediolateral n.; intermediolateral cell column of spinal cord; the cell column that forms the lateral horn of the spinal cord's gray matter. Extending from the first thoracic through the second lumbar segment, the column contains the autonomic motor neurons that give rise to the preganglionic fibers of the sympathetic system.
intermediomedial n., n. intermediomedialis.
n. intermediomedia'lis, intermediomedial n.; a small group of scattered visceral motor neurons immediately ventral to the n. thoracicus in the thoracic and upper two lumbar segments of the spinal cord; considered to receive visceral afferent fibers at all spinal levels.
interpeduncular n., n. interpeduncularis.
n. interpeduncula'ris [NA], interpeduncular n. or ganglion; Gudden's ganglion; intercrural ganglion; ganglion isthmi; a median, unpaired, ovoid cell group at the base of the midbrain tegmentum between the cerebral peduncles; it receives the fasciculus retroflexus from the habenula, and projects to the raphe region (nuclei raphes) and periaqueductal gray substance of the midbrain.
n. interpos'itus, collective term denoting the nuclei globosus and emboliformis of the cerebellum.
interstitial n. of Cajal, n. interstitialis.
n. interstitia'lis [NA], interstitial n. of Cajal; a group of widely spaced, medium-sized neurons in the dorsomedial region of the upper mesencephalic tegmentum, immediately lateral to the n. of Darkschewitsch; together with the latter, the n. interstitialis is closely associated with the fasciculus longitudinalis medialis, via which it receives fibers from the vestibular nuclei and projects crossed fibers via the posterior commissure to the oculomotor n.; also projects fibers to all spinal levels. It is believed to be involved in the integration of head and eye movements, particularly eye movements of a vertical or oblique nature.
nu'clei intralamina'res thal'ami [NA], intralaminar nuclei of the thalamus; collective term denoting several cell groups embedded in the internal medullary lamina of the thalamus; n. centralis lateralis, n. paracentralis, and farthest caudally, the large n. centromedianus. The first two of these receive afferents from the cerebral cortex, brainstem, reticular formation, cerebellum, and spinal cord, and project more or less diffusely to large regions of the frontal and parietal cortex. See also n. centromedianus.
intralaminar nuclei of thalamus, nuclei intralaminares thalami.
Klein-Gumprecht shadow nuclei, shadow nuclei in degenerating lymphoidocytes and macrolymphocytes in leukemia.
lateral cuneate n., n. cuneatus accessorius.
n. latera'lis medul'lae oblonga'tae [NA], lateral n. of medulla oblongata; lateral reticular n.; a group of cells in the medulla oblongata, located between the inferior olive and the descending trigeminal n., receiving fibers from the spinal cord and motor cortex and projecting to the cerebellum.
n. latera'lis thal'ami [NA], lateral n. of the thalamus; the largest of the major subdivisions of the thalamus; the composite n. lateralis includes, from before backward, the n. lateralis anterior or dorsalis, n. lateralis intermedius, n. lateralis posterior, and pulvinar; together, these cell groups form most of the free dorsal surface of the posterior half of the thalamus and project to a very large region of parietal, occipitoparietal, and temporal cortex; its afferent connections are largely obscure, but the n. lateralis posterior and the pulvinar receive a projection from the superior colliculus.
n. of lateral lemniscus, n. lemnisci lateralis.
lateral n. of medulla oblongata, n. lateralis medullae oblongatae.
lateral preoptic n., n. preopticus lateralis.
lateral reticular n., n. lateralis medullae oblongatae.
lateral n. of thalamus, n. lateralis thalami.
lateral tuberal nuclei, nuclei tuberales.
lateral vestibular n., n. vestibularis lateralis; see nuclei vestibulares.
n. lemnis'ci latera'lis [NA], n. of the lateral lemniscus; a substantial cell mass embedded in the lateral lemniscus, immediately below the latter's entry into the inferior colliculus; the n. represents a synaptic way-station for part of the fibers of the lateral lemniscus.
n. of lens, n. lentis.
lenticular n., lentiform n., n. lentiformis.
n. lentifor'mis [NA], lentiform or lenticular n.; lenticula (1); the large cone-shaped mass of gray matter forming the central core of the cerebral hemisphere. The convex base of the cone, oriented laterally and rostrally, is formed by the putamen which together with the caudate nucleus composes the striatum; the apical part, oriented medially and caudally, consists of the two segments of the globus pallidus. The n. is ventral and lateral to the thalamus and caudate n., from which it is separated by the internal capsule, and together with the caudate n. composes the corpus striatum.
n. len'tis [NA], n. of lens; the core or inner dense portion of the lens of the eye.
n. of Luys, n. subthalamicus.
main sensory n. of the trigeminus, n. sensorius principalis nervi trigemini.
n. of the mamillary body, n. corporis mamillare.
masticatory n., n. masticato'rius, n. motorius nervi trigemini.
medial accessory olivary n., n. olivaris accessorius medialis.
medial central n. of thalamus, n. medialis centralis thalami.
n. of medial geniculate body, n. corporis geniculati medialis.
n. media'lis centra'lis thal'ami [NA], medial central n. of the thalamus; a small cell group in the massa intermedia of the thalamus, occupying the midline region of the internal medullary lamina, between the left and the right n. paracentralis.
n. media'lis thal'ami [NA], medial n. of the thalamus; mediodorsal or dorsomedial n.; a large, composite cell group in the dorsomedial region of the thalamus having reciprocal connections with the entire extent of the frontal cortex anterior to the motor cortex (area 4) and premotor cortex (area 6). The afferent connections of the n. medialis also include projections from the olfactory cortex and amygdala.
medial preoptic n., n. preopticus medialis.

medial n. of thalamus, n. medialis thalami.
medial vestibular n., n. vestibularis medialis. See nuclei vestibulares.
mediodorsal n., n. medialis thalami.
mesencephalic n. of the trigeminus, n. tractus mesencephali nervi trigemini.
Monakow's n., n. cuneatus accessorius.
motor nuclei, nuclei originis.
motor n. of facial nerve, n. nervi facialis.
n. moto'rius ner'vi trigem'ini [NA], masticatory n.; n. masticatorius; motor n. of the trigeminus; a group of motor neurons innervating the muscles of mastication (masseter, temporalis, internal and external pterygoid muscles) and the musculi tensor tympani and tensor veli palatini. The n. lies in the upper pontine tegmentum medial to the main sensory n. of the trigeminus; emerging root fibers form the portio minor of the trigeminal nerve.
motor n. of trigeminus, n. motorius nervi trigemini.
n. ner'vi abducen'tis [NA], n. of the abducent nerve; n. abducentis; abducens n.; a group of motor neurons in the lower part of the pons, innervating the lateral rectus muscle of the eye; unique among motor cranial nerve nuclei in that it consists of two distinct populations of neurons: neurons that give rise to fibers forming the abducens nerve root and those internuclear neurons whose processes cross the midline, ascend in the opposite medial longitudinal fasciculus, and terminate upon specific oculomotor neurons; considered a primary center for mechanisms controlling conjugate horizontal gaze.
nu'clei ner'vi cochlea'ris, nuclei cochleares.
n. ner'vi facia'lis [NA], facial motor n.; motor n. of the facial nerve; n. facialis; a group of motor neurons located in the ventrolateral region of the lower pontine tegmentum and innervating the facial muscles, the stapedius muscle in the middle ear, the posterior limb of the musculus digastricus, and the stylohyoid muscle.
n. ner'vi hypoglos'si [NA], n. of the hypoglossal nerve; hypoglossal n.; the motor n. innervating the intrinsic and extrinsic musculature of the tongue; it is located in the medulla oblongata near the midline, immediately beneath the floor of the inferior recess of the rhomboid fossa.
n. ner'vi oculomoto'rii [NA], n. of the oculomotor nerve; oculomotor n.; the composite group of motor neurons innervating all of the external eye muscles except the nusculus rectus lateralis and musculus obliquus superior, and including the musculus levator palpebrae superioris; the most rostral component of the n. is the Edinger-Westphal n. which innervates the musculi sphincter pupillae and ciliaris. The oculomotor n. lies in the rostral half of the midbrain, near the midline in the most ventral part of the central gray substance; fibers of the medial longitudinal fasciculus form its lateral borders.
n. ner'vi trochlea'ris [NA], n. of the trochlear nerve; trochlear n.; a group of motor neurons innervating the superior oblique muscle of the contralateral eye. The n. lies in the caudal half of the midbrain, behind the oculomotor n., in the most ventral part of the central gray substance, near the midline.
nu'clei ner'vi vestibulocochlea'ris [NA], the combined cochlear and vestibular nuclei in the brainstem that receive the incoming fibers of the eighth cranial nerve; see nuclei cochleares and nuclei vestibulares.
nu'clei nervo'rum crania'lium [NA], nuclei of the cranial nerves; groups of nerve cells associated with the cranial nerves either as motor nuclei (nuclei originis) or sensory nuclei (nuclei terminationis).
n. ni'ger, *substantia* nigra.
n. of oculomotor nerve, oculomotor n., n. nervi oculomotorii.
n. oliva'ris [NA], inferior olivary n.; a large aggregate of small densely packed nerve cells arranged in folded laminae shaped like a purse with the opening (hilum) directed medially. It corresponds in position to the oliva, projects to all parts of the contralateral half of the cerebellar cortex by way of the olivocerebellar tract, and is the major source of cerebellar climbing fibers. Its afferent connections include fibers from the spinal cord, the dentate nucleus and motor cortex, but its major input appears to be the central tegmental tract originating from multiple nuclei at midbrain levels.
n. oliva'ris accesso'rius dorsa'lis [NA], dorsal accessory olivary n.; a detached part of the n. olivaris dorsal to the latter's main body.
n. oliva'ris accesso'rius media'lis [NA], medial accessory olivary n.; a detached part of the n. olivaris medial to the latter's main body, against the lateral side of the medial lemniscus and pyramidal tract.
Onuf's n. [B. Onufrowicz], small somatic motor neurons in the ventral horn of the spinal cord at sacral 2 level which innervate the vesicorectal sphincters, that is, the external anal and the urethral sphincter; O.'s n. has been identified in the cat, dog, and man.
nuclei of origin, nuclei originis.
nu'clei ori'ginis [NA], nuclei of origin; motor nuclei; collections of motor neurons (forming a continuous column in the spinal cord, discontinuous in the medulla and pons) giving origin to the spinal and cranial motor nerves.
parabrachial nuclei, nuclei parabrachiales.
nuclei parabrachia'les, parabrachial nuclei; the cell groups flanking the brachium conjunctivum at levels immediately caudal to the inferior colliculus; they serve as way-stations in the pathways ascending from the n. tractus solitarii to the thalamus and hypothalamus, and receive afferent fibers from the hypothalamus and corpus amygdaloideum.
n. paracentra'lis thal'ami, paracentral n. of the rostral thalamus; one of the intralaminar nuclei of the thalamus, medial to the n. centralis lateralis.
paracentral n. of thalamus, n. paracentralis thalami.
paraventricular n., n. paraventricularis.
n. paraventricula'ris [NA], paraventricular n.; n. filiformis; a triangular group of large magnocellular neurons in the periventricular zone of the anterior half of the hypothalamus. The cells of the n. are similar to those of the supraoptic n.; the axons of about 20% of their number join in the formation of the supraopticohypophysial tract and are functionally associated with the posterior lobe of the hypophysis; they project fibers to the brainstem nuclei (dorsal motor n. and solitary n.) and to the intermediolateral cell column of the spinal cord at thoracic, lumbar, and spinal levels; similar descending autonomic fibers arise from the lateral and posterior hypothalamic nuclei.
Perlia's n., Spitzka's n.; convergence n. of Perlia; a small cell group located between the somatic cell columns of the oculomotor nuclei. Since it is placed between the groups of motor neurons innervating, respectively, the left and right medial rectus muscles, the n. is considered to possibly represent an integrating mechanism for ocular convergence.
phenanthrene n., misnomer for tetracyclic steroid n.
pontine nuclei, nuclei pontis.
nu'clei pon'tis [NA], pontine nuclei; pontine gray matter; the massive gray matter filling the basilar pons. The nuclei are of fairly homogeneous architecture and project to the cortex of the contralateral cerebellar hemisphere by way of the middle cerebellar peduncle. Their main afferents come from the entire extent of the cerebral neocortex by way of the longitudinal pontine bundles (corticopontine fibers); thus, the pontine nuclei form a major waystation in the impulse conduction from the cerebral cortex of one hemisphere to the posterior lobe of the opposite cerebellum.
n. poste'rior hypothal'ami [NA], posterior hypothalamic n.; a large, periventricular hypothalamic n. located dorsal to the mamillary body, continuous with the central gray substance of the mesencephalon.
posterior hypothalamic n., n. posterior hypothalami.
posterior periventricular n., n. arcuatus (2).

n. preop'ticus latera'lis [NA], lateral preoptic n.; a vaguely defined group of nerve cells in the lateral zone of the preoptic region.
n. preop'ticus media'lis [NA], medial preoptic n.; a group of nerve cells forming the medial zone of the preoptic region.
prerubral n., the gray matter of field H_2; see *fields* of Forel.
n. pulpo'sus [NA], n. gelatinosus; vertebral pulp; the soft fibrocartilage central portion of the intervertebral disk; regarded as a derivative of the notochord.

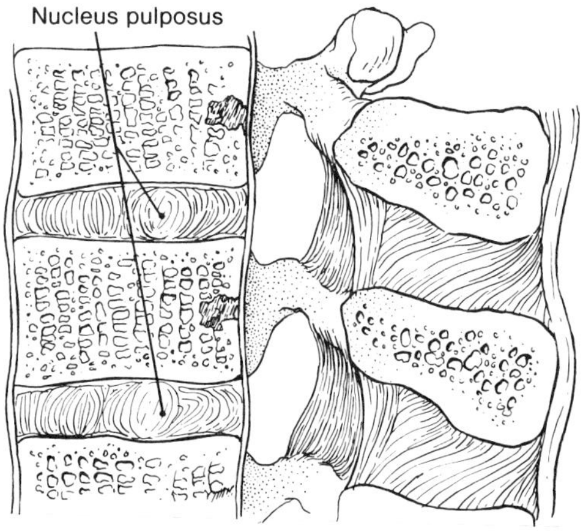

Nucleus Pulposus

n. pyramida'lis, obsolete term for n. olivaris accessorius medialis.
pyrrole n., of porphyrins, a cyclic tetrapyrrole; four pyrrole groups joined into a ring structure by way of –CH= (methylidyne) bridges between α (2) position of one pyrrole and α' (5) position of another pyrrole, the fourth pyrrole being joined to the first. See also porphin and porphyrin.
raphe nuclei, nuclei raphes.
nu'clei raph'es, raphe nuclei; collective term denoting a variety of unpaired nerve cell groups in and along the median plane of the mesencephalic and rhombencephalic tegmentum: the n. centralis tegmenti superior, and the n. raphis dorsalis, n. raphis pontis, n. raphis magnus, n. raphe pallidus, and n. raphe obscusis. These nuclei include neurons characterized by their containing the indolamine transmitter agent serotonin; their serotonin-carrying axons extend rostrally to the hypothalamus, septum, hippocampus, and cingulate gyrus and include projections to brainstem, cerebellum, and spinal cord.
red n., n. ruber.
reduction n., a n. that degenerates in the cell during the changes incident to fertilization.
reproductive n., micronucleus (2).
reticular nuclei of the brainstem, the vaguely delineated cell groups composing the gray matter of the reticular formation of the rhombencephalon and mesencephalon. In general, large-celled territories occupy the medial two-thirds of the reticular formation: n. gigantocellularis medullae oblongatae, nuclei tegmenti pontis caudalis and oralis. Smaller groups of reticular nuclei are found laterally and in paramedian locations; lateral nuclei receive sensory collaterals and project medially; paramedian reticular nuclei largely project to the cerebellum. See also *formatio* reticularis.
n. reticula'ris thal'ami [NA], reticular n. of the thalamus; a sheet of fairly large neurons covering the lateral, ventral, and rostral surfaces of the thalamus; its reticular appearance is caused by the numerous fascicles of the thalamic peduncles which traverse the n. The n. receives numerous fibers from the cerebral cortex but it has no cortical projection.
reticular n. of thalamus, n. reticularis thalami.
rhombencephalic gustatory n., the rostral one-third of the n. tractus solitarii, receiving afferents from the facial, glossopharyngeal, and vagus nerves conveying impulses originating from the receptor cells of the taste buds.
Roller's n., **(1)** lateral n. of the accessory nerve; **(2)** a small bulbar n. lying immediately anterior to the hypoglossal n., considered one of the perihypoglossal nuclei.
roof n., n. fastigii.
n. ru'ber [NA], red n.; a large, well defined, somewhat elongated cell mass, of reddish-gray hue in the fresh brain, located in the rostral mesencephalic tegmentum. The n. receives a massive projection from the contralateral half of the cerebellum by way of the superior cerebellar peduncle, and an additional projection from the ipsilateral motor cortex. Projections from the anterior interposed nucleus and motor cortex to the red nucleus are somatopically organized. Its efferent connections are with the contralateral rhombencephalic reticular formation and spinal cord by way of the rubrobulbar and rubrospinal tracts. Rubrospinal fibers have somatotopic origin.
n. salivato'rius infe'rior [NA], inferior salivary n.; a group of preganglionic parasympathetic motor neurons located in the reticular formation of the medulla oblongata dorsal to the n. ambiguus; its axons leave the brain with the glossopharyngeal nerve and govern secretion from the parotid gland by the intermediary of the ganglion oticum; cells of the inferior and superior n. are scattered and overlapping in lateral regions of the reticular formation.
n. salivato'rius supe'rior [NA], superior salivary n.; a group of preganglionic parasympathetic motor neurons situated rostrally and laterally to the inferior salivary n.; it governs secretion of the lacrimal, sublingual, and submaxillary glands by way of the facial nerve and the sphenopalatine and submandibular ganglia.
Schwalbe's n., n. vestibularis medialis. See nuclei vestibulares.
secondary sensory nuclei, nuclei terminationis.
segmentation n., the compound n. in the impregnated ovum, formed by conjugation of the nuclei of the germ cell and of the sperm cell, or of the female and the male pronucleus.
semilunar n. of Flechsig, n. arcuatus thalami.
n. senso'rius principa'lis ner'vi trigem'ini [NA], n. sensorius superior nervi trigemini; the main sensory n. of the trigeminal nerve.
n. senso'rius supe'rior ner'vi trigem'ini, n. sensorius principalis nervi trigemini.
shadow n., a n. that has lost its pigment and staining properties.
sole nuclei, an accumulation of skeletal muscle fiber nuclei at the myoneural junction.
n. of solitary tract, n. tractus solitarii.
somatic n., macronucleus (2).
somatic motor nuclei, collective term indicating the motor nuclei innervating the tongue musculature (n. nervi hypoglossi) and the extraocular eye muscles (n. nervi abducentis, n. nervi trochlearis, and n. nervi oculomotorii).
special visceral efferent (or **motor**) **nuclei,** branchiomotor nuclei.
sperm n., the head of the spermatozoon, which becomes spheroidal, after entering the ovum.
spherical n., n. globosus.
spinal n. of accessory nerve, n. spinalis nervi accessorii.
spinal n. of the trigeminus, n. tractus spinalis nervi trigemini.
n. spina'lis ner'vi accesso'rii [NA], spinal n. of the accessory nerve; a slender column of motor neurons extending longitudinally through the central part of the ventral horn of the upper five segments of the spinal cord, giving origin to the pars spinalis of the accessory nerve.
Spitzka's n., Perlia's n.
Staderini's n., n. intercalatus.
steroid n., tetracyclic steroid n.
Stilling's n., n. thoracicus.
subthalamic n., n. subthalamicus.
n. subthalam'icus [NA], subthalamic n.; n. or body of Luys; corpus luysi; a circumscript n., shaped like a biconvex lens, located in

the ventral part of the subthalamus on the dorsal surface of the peduncular part of the internal capsule immediately rostral to the substantia nigra. The n. receives a massive topographic projection from the lateral segment of the globus pallidus, and a somatopically organized projection from the ipsilateral motor cortex; a smaller bundle of afferents from the centromedian n. of the thalamus terminate in the rostral part of the n. The s. n. projects to both pallidal segments, to the pars reticulata of the substantia nigra, and in a small way to the ipsilateral pedunculopontine nucleus.
superior olivary n., n. dorsalis corporis trapezoidei.
superior salivary n., n. salivatorius superior.
superior vestibular n., n. vestibularis superior. See nuclei vestibulares.
supraoptic n., n. supraopticus hypothalami.
n. supraop'ticus hypothal'ami [NA], supraoptic n.; a large-celled neurosecretory n. in the hypothalamus, located over the lateral border of the optic tract, from which the supraopticohypophysial tract arises; its neurons produce and transport vasopressin released into the general circulation from the axon terminals in the supraopticohypophysial tract.
n. tec'ti, n. fastigii.
nu'clei tegmen'ti [NA], Gudden's tegmental nuclei; collective term for two small round cell groups in the caudal part of the midbrain (**n. t. pon'tis cauda'lis** and **n. t. pon'tis ora'lis**), associated with the mamillary body by way of the mamillary peduncle and mamillotegmental tract.
terminal nuclei, nuclei termina'les, nuclei terminationis.
nu'clei terminatio'nis [NA], nuclei terminales; terminal nuclei; secondary sensory nuclei; collective term indicating those nerve cell groups in the rhombencephalon and spinal cord in which the afferent fibers of the spinal and cranial nerves terminate.
tetracyclic steroid n., steroid n.; perhydrocyclopenta[*a*] phenanthrene; the group of four fused rings forming the framework or parent substance of the steroids.
thalamic gustatory n., n. arcuatus thalami.
thoracic n., n. thoracicus.
n. thorac'icus [NA], thoracic n.; dorsal n.; n. dorsalis; Clarke's n. or column; Stilling's n. or column; a column of large neurons located in the base of the posterior gray column of the spinal cord, extending from the first thoracic through the second lumbar segment; it gives rise to the dorsal spinocerebellar tract of the same side.
n. trac'tus mesenceph'ali ner'vi trigem'ini [NA], mesencephalic n. of the trigeminus; a long, narrow plate of unipolar neurons extending throughout the length of the midbrain, in and along the lateral angle of the central gray substance. The n. is the single known instance of primary sensory neurons enclosed in the central nervous system instead of in a peripheral sensory ganglion. Its peripheral axonal processes pass with the trigeminal nerve, give collaterals to the trigeminal motor n., and terminate in the muscles of mastication.
n. trac'tus solita'rii [NA], n. of solitary tract; a slender cell column extending sagittally through the dorsal part of the medulla oblongata, beneath the floor of the rhomboid fossa, immediately lateral to the sulcus limitans. It is the visceral sensory (visceral afferent) n. of the brainstem, receiving the afferent fibers of the vagus, glossopharyngeal, and facial nerves by way of the tractus solitarius. The caudal two-thirds of the n. process impulses originating in the pharynx, larynx, intestinal and respiratory tracts, and heart and large blood vessels; its rostral one-third receives impulses from the taste buds and is known as the rhombencephalic gustatory n.
n. trac'tus spina'lis ner'vi trigem'ini [NA], descending n. of the trigeminus; spinal n. of the trigeminus; the long sensory n. extending from the caudal border of the pontine sensory n. of the trigeminus down through the lateral region of the rhombencephalon into the upper three segments of the spinal cord's dorsal horn; it receives the fibers of the sensory root of the trigeminal nerve which descend along its lateral border as the tractus spinalis nervi trigemini.
trochlear n., n. of trochlear nerve, n. nervi trochlearis.
trophic n., macronucleus (2).
tuberal nuclei, nuclei tuberales.
nu'clei tubera'les [NA], tuberal nuclei; lateral tuberal nuclei; two or three small, encapsulated, round or ovoid clusters of cells in the lateral hypothalamic area along the surface of the tuber cinereum; their connections and functional significance are unknown.
ventral anterior n. of thalamus, n. ventralis anterior thalami.
ventral intermediate n. of thalamus, n. ventralis intermedius thalami.
n. ventra'lis ante'rior thal'ami, ventral anterior n. of the thalamus; the most rostral of the subdivisions of the ventral n., receiving projections from the globus pallidus and projecting to the premotor and frontal cortex.
n. ventra'lis cor'poris trapezoi'dei [NA], n. of trapezoid body; a cell group embedded among the fibers of the trapezoid body, the major decussation of the central auditory pathway, in the lower pons. The n. receives fibers from the contralateral cochlear nuclei and contributes fibers to the ascending auditory system or lateral lemniscus.
n. ventra'lis interme'dius thal'ami [NA], n. ventralis lateralis; ventral intermediate or ventral lateral n. of the thalamus; the composite middle third of the ventral n. receiving in its various parts distinctive projections from the contralateral half of the cerebellum (by way of the superior cerebellar peduncle) and the ipsilateral globus pallidus; nearly all parts of the n. projects to the motor cortex.
n. ventra'lis latera'lis, n. ventralis intermedius thalami.
n. ventra'lis poste'rior interme'dius thal'ami, ventral posterior intermediate n. of thalamus. See n. ventralis posterior thalami.
n. ventra'lis poste'rior thal'ami, ventrobasal n.; ventral posterior n. of thalamus; the large posterior part of the ventral n. of the thalamus receiving the somatic sensory lemnisci (medial lemniscus, spinothalamic tract, trigeminal lemniscus) and the ascending gustatory (taste) lemniscus, and projecting in turn by way of the internal capsule to the cortex of the postcentral gyrus. The n. is somatotopically organized and subdivided into a n. ventralis posterolateralis thalami representing the leg, a n. ventralis posterior intermedius thalami representing the arm, a n. ventralis posteromedialis thalami representing the face, and a n. arcuatus thalami receiving the gustatory lemniscus.
n. ventra'lis posterolatera'lis thal'ami [NA], ventral posterolateral or ventral posterior lateral n. of thalamus; lateral part of the ventrobasal nuclear complex. See n. ventralis posterior thalami.
n. ventra'lis posteromedia'lis thal'ami [NA], ventral posteromedial or ventral posterior medial n. of thalamus; medial part of the ventrobasal nuclear complex. See n. ventralis posterior thalami.
n. ventra'lis thal'ami [NA], ventral n. of the thalamus; a large, complex cell mass the external border of which forms the ventral and much of the lateral boundary, as well as the rostral border, of the thalamus; it can be subdivided into an anterior, intermediate, and posterior part.
ventral lateral n. of thalamus, n. ventralis intermedius thalami.
ventral posterior n. of thalamus, n. ventralis posterior thalami.
ventral posterior intermediate n. of thalamus, n. ventralis posterior intermedius thalami. See n. ventralis posterior thalami.
ventral posterolateral n. of thalamus, ventral posterior lateral n. of thalamus, n. ventralis posterolateralis thalami.
ventral posteromedial, posterior medial n. of thalamus, n. ventralis posteromedialis thalami.
ventral n. of thalamus, n. ventralis thalami.
ventral tier thalamic nuclei, collective term for nuclei in the ventral part of the lateral nuclear group, *e.g.*, n. ventralis anterior, lateralis, posterolateralis, and posteromedialis and the medial and lateral geniculate bodies. The basoventral nuclear complex consti-

tutes the caudal part of the ventral tier thalamic nuclei.
ventral n. of trapezoid body, n. ventralis corporis trapezoidei.
ventrobasal n., n. ventralis posterior thalami.
ventromedial n. of hypothalamus, n. ventromedialis hypothalami.
n. ventromedia'lis hypothal'ami [NA], ventromedial n. of the hypothalamus; a circumscript ovoid group of small neurons in the medial zone of the tuberal region of the hypothalamus. Bilateral destruction of this n. in the rat leads to severe obesity. It receives numerous fibers from the amygdala via the stria terminalis; its efferent connections are obscure.
vestibular nuclei, nuclei vestibulares.
nu'clei vestibula'res [NA], vestibular nuclei; a group of four main nuclei that include: the n. v. lateralis (Deiters' n.), n. v. medialis (Schwalbe's n.), n. v. superior (Bechterew's n.), and n. v. inferior, located in the lateral region of the hindbrain beneath the floor of the rhomboid fossa. They receive primary fibers of the vestibular nerve, are reciprocally connected with the flocculonodular lobe of the cerebellum, and project by way of the medial longitudinal fasciculus to the abducens, trochlear, and oculomotor nuclei and to the ventral horn of the spinal cord. The n. v. lateralis projects to the ipsilateral ventral horn of the spinal cord by the vestibulospinal tract.

---

nuclide (nū'klīd). A particular (atomic) nuclear species with defined atomic mass and number. See also isotope.

Nuel, Jean P., Belgian ophthalmologist and otologist, 1847–1920. See N.'s *space*.

NUG Abbreviation for necrotizing ulcerative *gingivitis*.

Nuhn, Anton, German anatomist, 1814–1889. See N.'s *gland*.

nulligravida (nŭl-i-grav'i-dă) [L. *nullus*, none, + *gravida*, pregnant]. A woman who has never conceived a child.

nullipara (nŭ-lip'ă-ră) [L. *nullus*, none, + *pario*, to bear]. A woman who has never borne children.

nulliparity (nŭl-i-par'i-tē). Condition of having borne no children.

nulliparous (nŭl-ip'ă-rŭs). Nonparous; never having borne children.

number (nŭm'ber). **1.** A symbol expressive of a certain value or of a specific quantity determined by count. **2.** The place of any unit in a series.
atomic n. (Z), charge n.; the n. of negatively charged electrons in an uncharged atom, or the number of protons in its nucleus; it indicates the position of the element in the periodic system.
Avogadro's n., Avogadro's constant; the n. of molecules in one gram-molecular weight (1 mole) of any compound; defined as the number of atoms in 0.0120 kg of pure carbon-12; equivalent to 6.0225×10^{23}.
Brinell hardness n. (BHN), a n. related to the size of the permanent impression made by a ball indenter of specified size (usually 10 mm in diameter) pressed into the surface of the material under a specified load:

$$\mathrm{BHN} = \frac{P}{\frac{\pi D}{2}\left(D - \sqrt{D^2 - d^2}\right)}$$

where P = applied load in kg, D = diameter of the ball in mm, and d = diameter of the impression in mm.
charge n., atomic n.
CT n., the n. used to designate the x-ray attenuation in each picture element (pixel) of the CT image.
electronic n., the n. of electrons in the outermost orbit (valence shell) of an element.
gold n., gold *equivalent*.
Hehner n., the weight of the nonvolatile fatty acids yielded by 5 g of a saponified fat or oil.
hydrogen n., the quantity of hydrogen that 1 g of fat will absorb; it is a measurement of the amount of unsaturated fatty acids in the fat. See also iodine n.
iodine n., iodine value; an indication of the quantity of unsaturated fatty acids present in a fat; it represents the number of grams of iodine absorbed by each 100 g of fat. See also hydrogen n.
Knoop hardness n. (KHN), a n. obtained by dividing the load in kg applied to a pyramid-shaped diamond of specific size divided by the projected area of the impression: KHN $= L/A$, where A = the projected area of the impression in mm^2 and L = the load in kg; used for measurements of hardness of any materials, especially very hard and brittle substances such as tooth dentin and enamel.
Koettstorfer n., saponification n.
Loschmidt's n., the n. of molecules in 1 ml of gas at 0°C and 1 atmosphere of presssure; Avogadro's n. divided by 22,400.
Mach n., a n. representing the ratio between the speed of an object moving through a fluid medium, such as air, and the speed of sound in the same medium.
mass n., the mass of the atom of a particular isotope relative to hydrogen-1 (or to $^1/_{12}$ the mass of carbon-12), generally very close to the whole number represented by the sum of the protons and neutrons in the atomic nucleus of the isotope (indicated in the name or symbol of the isotope; *e.g.*, oxygen-16, ^{16}O); not to be confused with the atomic weight of an element, which may include a number of isotopes in natural proportion.
Polenské n., the n. of milliliters of 0.1 N KOH required to neutralize the nonvolatile fatty acids obtained from 5 g of a saponified fat or oil.
Reichert-Meissl n., volatile fatty acid n.; an index of the volatile acid content of a fat; the n. of milliliters of 0.1 N KOH required to neutralize the soluble volatile fatty acids in 5 g of fat that has been saponified, acidified to liberate the fatty acids, and then steam-distilled.
saponification n., Koettstorfer n.; the n. of milliliters of KOH required to saponify 1 g of fat; an approximate measure of the average molecular weight of a fat, with which it varies inversely.
thiocyanogen n., thiocyanogen value; the n. of grams of thiocyanogen taken up by 100 g of fat; analogous to the iodine n., except that thiocyanogen will not add to all the double bonds in polyunsaturated fatty acids as will iodine.
transport n., the fraction of the total current carried through a solution by a particular type of ion present in that solution.
volatile fatty acid n., Reichert-Meissl n.
wave n., the n. of waves (of any wave form such as light or sound) per unit length.

numbness (nŭm'nes). Absence of perception of tactile, thermal, or noxious stimuli.
waking n., night palsy; a temporary n. and paresis of the extremities experienced on waking or after lying down for a long period.

nummiform (nŭm'i-fōrm). Nummular.

nummular (nŭm'yū-ler) [L. *nummus*, coin]. Nummiform. **1.** Discoid or coin-shaped; denoting the thick mucous or mucopurulent sputum in certain respiratory diseases, so called because of the disc shape assumed when it is flattened on the bottom of a sputum mug containing water or transparent disinfectant. **2.** Arranged like stacks of coins, denoting the lining up of the red blood cells into rouleaux formation.

nummulation (nŭm-yū-lā'shŭn). Formation of nummular masses.

nunnation (nŭ-nā'shŭn) [Ar. *nūn*, the letter n.]. A form of stammering in which the *n* sound is given to other consonants.

nurse (ners) [O. Fr. *nourice*, fr. L. *nutrix*, wet-nurse, nurse, fr. *nutrio*, to sucke, to tend]. **1.** To breast feed. **2.** To provide care of the sick. **3.** One who is trained in the scientific basis of nursing under defined standards of education and is concerned with the diagnosis and treatment of human responses to actual or potential health problems.

charge n., head n. (2); a n. in charge of a hospital patient-care unit.
clinical n. specialist, a n. with advanced degree, skill, and competence in a particular area of nursing practice such as in cardiology, oncology, or psychiatry.
community health n., public health n.
head n., **(1)** a n. supervising the nursing staff in a hospital; called "sister" in Great Britain; **(2)** charge n.
licensed practical n. (L.P.N.), licensed vocational n. (L.V.N.), a n. who has graduated from a program requiring fewer instructional hours than is required for a baccalaureate degree and who has passed a state examination for licensure.
private duty n., **(1)** a n. who is not a member of a hospital staff, but is called upon to take special care of an individual patient in a hospital or other setting; **(2)** a n. who specializes in the care of patients with diseases of a particular class, *e.g.,* surgical cases, tuberculosis, children's diseases.
public health n., community health n.; a n., working under the direction of a public health official, who acts as the connecting link between that official and the lay public, and whose duties are concerned with general health problems in the community.
registered n. (R.N.), a n. who has been registered and licensed to practice by a state authority.
scrub n., a n. who has scrubbed arms and hands, donned sterile gloves and, usually, a sterile gown, and assists an operating surgeon, primarily by passing instruments.
visiting n., a n. who is responsible for several sick persons, visiting each on a regular basis and performing the necessary nursing services.
wet n., a woman who breast-feeds a child not her own.

nurse anesthetist. A registered professional nurse with additional training in the administration of anesthetics, to function as an anesthetist under the direction of a physician.

nurse-midwife. A person formally educated in the two disciplines of nursing and midwifery, and who may be certified by the American College of Nurse-Midwives.

nurse practitioner (ners prak-tish'ŭ-ner). A registered nurse with special skills in assessing the physical and psychosocial status of patients, often as a colleague of a physician.

nursing (ner'sing). **1.** Feeding an infant at the breast; tending and taking care of a child. **2.** The scientific care of the sick by a professional nurse.

nursing home. A convalescent home or private facility for the care of individuals who do not require hospitalization and who cannot be cared for at home.

Nussbaum, Johann N. von, German surgeon, 1829–1890. See N.'s *bracelet.*

Nussbaum, Moritz, German histologist, 1850–1915. See N.'s *experiment.*

nutation (nū-tā'shŭn) [L. *annuere,* to nod]. The act of nodding, especially involuntary nodding.

nutgall (nŭt'gahl). Galla; gall (3); oak apple; an excrescence on the oak, *Quercus infectoria* (family Fagaceae) and other species of *Quercus,* caused by the deposit of the ova of a fly, *Cynips gallae tinctorae;* an astringent and styptic, by virtue of the tannin it contains.

nutmeg (nŭt'meg). Myristica; the dried ripe seed of *Myristica fragrans* (family Myristicaceae), deprived of its seed coat and arillode; an aromatic stimulant, carminative, condiment, and source of volatile and expressed nutmeg oils; it is consumed for its bizarre central nervous system effects. See also myristicin.

nutmeg oil. Myristica oil; the volatile oil distilled from the dried kernels of the ripe seeds of *Myristica fragrans;* used as a flavoring agent and a carminative; in large quantities, it may produce narcosis and delirium; the fixed oil expressed from *M. fragrans* is used as a rubefacient.

nutrient (nū'trē-ent) [L. *nutriens,* fr. *nutrio,* to nourish]. A constituent of food necessary for normal physiologic function.

nutrilites (nū'tri-līts) [L. *nutrio,* to suckle, nourish]. Essential nutritional factors.

nutrition (nū-trish'ŭn) [L. *nutritio,* fr. *nutrio,* to nourish]. **1.** Trophism (2); a function of living plants and animals, consisting in the taking in and metabolism of food material whereby tissue is built up and energy liberated. **2.** The study of the food and liquid requirements of human beings or animals for normal physiologic function, including need, maintenance, growth, activity, reproduction, and lactation.
total parenteral n. (TPN), n. maintained entirely by intravenous injection or other nongastrointestinal route.

nutritive (nū'tri-tiv). Alible. **1.** Pertaining to nutrition. **2.** Capable of nourishing.

nutriture (nū'tri-chūr) [L. *nutriture,* a nursing, fr. *nutrio,* to nourish]. State or condition of the nutrition of the body; state of the body with regard to nourishment.

Nuttallia (nŭ-tal'ē-ă) [G. H. F. *Nuttall,* U.S. biologist, 1862–1937]. Former name for *Babesia.*

nux vomica (nŭks vom'i-kă) [Mod. L. emetic nut, fr. L. *nux,* nut, + *vomo,* to vomit]. Strychnos seed; poison nut; Quaker button; the seed of *Strychnos nux-vomica* (family Logeniaceae), a tree of tropical Asia; it contains two alkaloids, strychnine and brucine; it has been used as a bitter tonic and central nervous system stimulant.

nyct-. See nycto-.

nyctalgia (nik-tal'jē-ă) [nyct- + G. *algos,* pain]. Night pain; denoting especially the osteocopic pains of syphilis occurring at night.

nyctalopia (nik-tă-lō'pē-ă) [nyct- + G. *alaos,* obscure, + *ōps,* eye]. Night blindness; nocturnal amblyopia; nyctanopia; day sight; decreased ability to see in reduced illumination.
n. with congenital myopia, an abnormality of X-linked inheritance characterized by low visual acuity, strabismus, or nystagmus.

nyctanopia (nik-tă-nō'pē-ă) [nyct- + G. *an-* priv. + *opsis,* sight]. Nyctalopia.

nycterine (nik'ter-īn, -in) [G. *nykterinos*]. **1.** By night. **2.** Dark or obscure.

nycterohemeral (nik'ter-ō-hē'mer-ăl) [G. *nykteros,* by night, nightly, + *hēmera,* day]. Nyctohemeral.

nycto-, nyct- [G. *nyx,* night]. Combining forms denoting night, nocturnal. See also noct-.

nyctohemeral (nik-tō-hē'mer-ăl) [nycto- + G. *hēmera,* day]. Nycterohemeral; both daily and nightly.

nyctophilia (nik-tō-fil'ē-ă) [nycto- + G. *philos,* fond]. Scotophilia; preference for the night or darkness.

nyctophobia (nik-tō-fō'bē-ă) [nycto- + G. *phobos,* fear]. Scotophobia; morbid fear of night or of the dark.

Nyctotherus (nik-tō-thē'rŭs) [G. *nyktothēras,* one who hunts by night, fr. *thēraō,* to hunt, fr. *thēr,* wild beast]. A genus of Ciliophora one species of which, *N. faba,* has been reported, though rarely, from the human intestine; it is generally found in amphibia.

nycturia (nik-tū'rē-ă). Nocturia.

Nyhan, William L. U.S. pediatrician, *1926. See Lesch-N. *syndrome.*

nylidrin hydrochloride (nī'li-drin, nil'). 1-(*p*-Hydroxyphenyl)-2-(1-methyl-3-phenylpropylamino) propanol hydrochloride; a sympathomimetic agent, similar to isoproterenol, that produces vasodilation of arterioles of skeletal muscles and increases muscle blood flow; used in the treatment of peripheral vascular diseases.

nymph (nimf) [G. *nymphē,* maiden]. **1.** The earliest series of stages in metamorphosis following hatching in the development of hemimetabolous insects (*e.g.,* locusts); the n. resembles the adult in many respects, but lacks full wing or genitalia development; it grows through successive instars without any intermediate or pupal stage into the imago or adult form. See also incomplete *metamorphosis;* complete *metamorphosis.* **2.** The third stage in the life cycle of a tick, between the larva and the adult.

nympha, pl. **nymphae** (nim'fă, nim'fē) [Mod. L., fr. G. *nymphē,* a bride]. One of the labia minora.

nymphal (nim'făl). **1.** Pertaining to a nymph. **2.** Pertaining to the labia minora (nymphae).

nymphectomy (nim-fek'tō-mē) [nympha + G. *ektomē,* excision]. Surgical removal of hypertrophied labia minora.

nymphitis (nim-fī'tis) [nympha + G. *-itis,* inflammation]. Inflammation of the labia minora.

nympho-, nymph- [L. *nympha*]. Combining forms denoting the nymphae (labia minora).

nympholabial (nim'fō-lā'bē-ăl). Relating to the labia minora (nymphae) and the labia majora; denoting a furrow between the two labia on each side.

nympholepsy (nim-fō-lep'sē) [nympho- + G. *lēpsis,* a seizure]. Ecstasy; transport, especially of an erotic nature.

nymphomania (nim-fō-mā'nē-ă) [nympho- + G. *mania,* frenzy]. Excessive eroticism or sexual behavior in a female; the counterpart of satyriasis in a male.

nymphomaniac (nim-fō-mā'nē-ak). A female exhibiting nymphomania.

nymphomaniacal (nim'fō-mă-nī'ă-kăl). Pertaining to, or exhibiting, nymphomania.

nymphoncus (nim-fong'kŭs) [nympho- + G. *onkos,* tumor]. Swelling or hypertrophy of one or both labia minora.

nymphotomy (nim-fot'ō-mē) [nympho- + G. *tomē,* incision]. Incision into the labia minora or the clitoris.

nystagmic (nis-tag'mik). Relating to or suffering from nystagmus.

nystagmiform (nis-tag'mi-fōrm). Nystagmoid.

nystagmogram (nis-tag'mō-gram). The tracing produced by a nystagmograph.

nystagmograph (nis-tag'mō-graf). An apparatus for measuring the amplitude, periodicity, and velocity of ocular movements in nystagmus, by measuring the change in the resting potential of the eye as the eye moves.

nystagmography (nis-tag-mog'ră-fē). The technique of recording nystagmus.

nystagmoid (nis-tag'moyd) [nystagmus + G. *eidos,* resemblance]. Nystagmiform; resembling nystagmus.

nystagmus (nis-tag'mŭs) [G. *nystagmos,* a nodding, fr. *nystazō,* to be sleepy, nod]. Ocular ataxia; rhythmical oscillation of the eyeballs, either pendular or jerky.

after-n., n. occurring after the abrupt cessation of rotation in the opposite direction of the rotatory n.

amaurotic n., ocular n.

ataxic n., unilateral n. with impairment of horizontal conjugate movement, most commonly due to multiple sclerosis.

caloric n., jerky n. induced by labyrinthine stimulation with hot or cold water in the ear. See also Bárány's *sign.*

central n., reflex from stimulation arising in the central nervous system.

cervical n., n. arising from a lesion of the proprioceptive mechanism of the neck.

Cheyne's n., a n. with a rhythm similar to that of Cheyne-Stokes respiration.

compressive n., a jerky n. resulting from unilateral changes of pressure in semicircular canals.

congenital n., **(1)** n. present at birth caused by lesions sustained *in utero* or at the time of birth; **(2)** inherited n., usually x-linked, without associated neurologic lesions and nonprogressive; **(3)** the n. associated with albinism, achromatopsia, and hypoplasia of the macula.

conjugate n., a n. in which the two eyes move simultaneously in the same direction.

deviational n., end-position n.

dissociated n., dysjunctive, incongruent, or irregular n.; a n. in which the movements of the two eyes are dissimilar in direction, amplitude, and periodicity.

downbeat n., a vertical n. with a rapid component downward, occurring in lesions of the lower part of the brainstem or cerebellum.

dysjunctive n., dissociated n.

end-position n., deviational n.; a jerky, physiologic n. occurring in a normal individual when attempts are made to fixate a point at the limits of the field of fixation.

fixation n., n. aggravated or induced by ocular fixation, arising as opticokinetic n., or resulting from midbrain lesions.

galvanic n., n. involving galvanic stimulation of the labyrinth.

gaze n., a n. occurring in partial gaze paralysis when an attempt is made to look in the direction of the palsy.

hysterical n., a n. with pendular oscillations of up to 1200 per minute, and with a prominent psychologic element.

incongruent n., dissociated n.

irregular n., dissociated n.

jerky n., n. in which there is a slow drift of the eyes in one direction, followed by a rapid recovery movement, always described in the direction of the recovery movement; it usually arises from labyrinthine or neurologic lesions or stimuli.

labyrinthine n., vestibular n.

latent n., jerky n. that is brought out by covering one eye.

lateral n., a form of n. in which the eyes oscillate from side to side.

miner's n., miner's disease (2); n. occurring in coal miners and related to lack of illumination as well as other factors.

minimal amplitude n., micronystagmus.

ocular n., amaurotic n.; the pendular or, rarely, jerky n. seen in severely reduced vision.

opticokinetic n., optokinetic n., railroad n.; n induced by looking at moving visual stimuli.

palatal n., a clonic spasm of the levator palati muscle, causing an audible click.

pendular n., a n. that, in most positions of gaze, has oscillations equal in speed and amplitude, usually arising from a visual disturbance.

perverted n., a vertical or oblique n. excited by caloric stimulation of horizontal semicircular canals.

positional n., n. occurring only when the head is in a particular position.

railroad n., opticokinetic n.

retraction n., Koerber-Salus-Elschnig syndrome; irregular, jerky n., either horizontal, vertical, or rotatory, with retraction of the eye into the orbit on attempt to change the direction of visual fixation.

rotational n., jerky n. arising from stimulation of the labyrinth by rotation of the head around any axis and induced by change of motion.

rotatory n., a movement of the eyes around the visual axis.

seesaw n., a n. in which one eye rotates upward as the other rotates downward, often combined with a torsional rotation.

strabismic n., n. associated with esotropia.

upbeat n., a vertical jerky n. with a rapid component upward, occurring with brainstem lesions.

vertical n., an up-and-down oscillation of the eyes.

vestibular n., labyrinthine n.; n. resulting from physiological stimuli to the labyrinth that may be rotatory, caloric, compressive, or galvanic, or due to labyrinthal lesions. See also Bárány's *sign.*

voluntary n., pendular n. in which the individual causes an extremely fine and rapid horizontal oscillation of the eyes.

nystatin (nī-stat′in, nis′tă-tin). Fungicidin; an antibiotic substance isolated from cultures of *Streptomyces noursei,* effective in the treatment of all forms of moniliasis, particularly monilial infections of the intestine, skin, and mucous membranes.

Nysten, Pierre H., French physician, 1771–1818. See N.'s *law.*

nyxis (nik′sis) [G.]. A pricking; puncture; paracentesis.

O

O **1.** Symbol for oxygen. **2.** Abbreviation for opening (in formulas for electrical reactions). **3.** Symbol for a blood group in the ABO system. See ABO blood group, Blood Groups appendix. **4.** An abbreviation derived from *ohne Hauch* (without a film), used as a designation for: 1) antigens that occur in the bacterial cell, in contrast to those in the flagella; 2) specific antibodies for such somatic antigens; 3) the agglutinative reaction between somatic antigen and its antibody.

o- In chemistry, abbreviation for ortho-(2).

oak apple. Nutgall.

oari-, oario- [G. *ōarion,* a small egg, dim. of *ōon,* egg]. Obsolete combining forms denoting ovary. See oo-, oophor-, ovario-.

oarium (ō-ar'ē-ŭm) [G. *ōarion,* a small egg]. Obsolete term for ovary.

oath (ōth). A solemn affirmation or attestation. See Hippocratic Oath; Veterinarian's Oath.

OB Abbreviation for obstetrics.

obdormition (ob-dōr-mish'ŭn) [L. *ob-dormio,* pp. *-itus,* to sleep]. Numbness of an extremity, due to pressure on the sensory nerve.

O'Beirne, James, Irish surgeon, 1786–1862. See O.'s *sphincter.*

obeliac (ō-bē'lē-ak). Relating to the obelion.

obeliad (ō-bē'lē-ad). Toward the obelion.

obelion (ō-bē'lē-on) [G. *obelos,* a spit]. A craniometric point on the sagittal suture between the parietal foramina near the lambdoid suture.

Obermayer, Friedrich, Austrian physician, 1861–1925. See O.'s *test.*

Obermeier, Otto H.F., German physician, 1843–1873. See O.'s *spirillum.*

Obersteiner, H., Austrian neurologist, 1847–1922. See O.-Redlich *line, zone.*

obese (ō-bēs') [L. *obesus,* fat, partic. adj., fr. *ob-edo,* pp. *-esus,* to eat away, devour]. Corpulent; excessively fat.

obesity (ō-bē'si-tē). Corpulence; adiposity (1); an abnormal increase of fat in the subcutaneous connective tissues.
hypothalamic o., o. caused by disease of the hypothalamus.
morbid o., o. sufficient to prevent normal activity or physiologic function, or to cause the onset of a pathologic condition.
simple o., o. resulting when caloric intake exceeds energy expenditure.

obex (ō'beks) [L. barrier] [NA]. The point on the midline of the dorsal surface of the medulla oblongata that marks the caudal angle of the rhomboid fossa or fourth ventricle. It corresponds to a small, transverse medullary fold overhanging the calamus scriptorius.

obfuscation (ob-fus-kā'shŭn) [L. *ob-fusco,* pp. *-atus,* to darken, fr. *fuscus,* dark, tawny]. **1.** A rendering dark or obscure. **2.** A deliberate attempt to confuse or to prevent understanding.

OB/GYN Abbreviation for obstetrics and gynecology.

object (ob'jekt). **1.** Anything to which thought or action is directed. **2.** In psychoanalysis, that through which an instinct can achieve its aim. **3.** In psychoanalysis, often used synonymously with person.
good o., in psychoanalysis, the good or supporting aspects of an important person in the patient's life, especially of a parent or parent-surrogate.
sex o., a person toward whom another is sexually attracted.
test o., **(1)** an o. having very fine surface markings, mounted on a slide, used to determine the defining power of the objective lens of a microscope; **(2)** the target in measurement of the visual field.

object choice. In psychoanalysis, the object (usually a person) upon which psychic energy is centered.

objective (ob-jek'tiv) [L. *ob- jicio,* pp. *-jectus,* to throw before]. **1.** Object glass; the lens or lenses in the lower end of the body tube of a microscope, by means of which the rays coming from the object examined are brought to a focus. **2.** Viewing events or phenomena as they exist in the external world, impersonally, or in an unprejudiced way; open to observation by oneself and by others. *Cf.* subjective.
achromatic o., an o. that is corrected for two colors chromatically, and one color spherically.
apochromatic o., an o. in which chromatic aberration is corrected for three colors and spherical abberation is corrected for two.
immersion o., a high power o. used with a drop of oil between the lens and the specimen on the slide, allowing a greater numerical aperture; similar lenses are available for use with water as the immersing liquid.

obligate (ob'li-gāt) [L. *ob-ligo,* pp. *-atus,* to bind to]. Without an alternative system or pathway.

oblique (ob-lēk') [L. *obliquus*] Slanting; deviating from the perpendicular or the horizontal.

obliquity (ob-lik'wi-tē). Asynclitism.
Litzmann o., posterior asynclitism; inclination of the fetal head so that the biparietal diameter is oblique in relation to the plane of the pelvic brim, the posterior parietal bone presenting to the parturient canal.
Nägele o., anterior asynclitism; inclination of the fetal head in cases of flat pelvis, so that the biparietal diameter is oblique in relation to the plane of the pelvic brim, the anterior parietal bone presenting to the parturient canal.

obliquus (ob-lī'kwŭs) [L. slanting, oblique]. Denoting a structure having an oblique course or direction; a name given, with further qualification, to several muscles. See entries under musculus.

obliteration (ob-lit-er-ā'shŭn) [L. *oblittero,* to blot out]. Blotting out, especially by filling of a natural space or lumen by fibrosis or inflammation.

oblongata (ob-long-gah'tă) [L. fem. of *oblongatus,* from *oblongus,* rather long]. *Medulla* oblongata.

OBS Organic brain *syndrome.*

observer (ob-zer'ver) [L. *observo,* to watch]. One who perceives, notices, or watches.
nonparticipant o., an investigator who studies a group of subjects engaged in certain activities but does not directly participate in these activities, presumably being able to study them more objectively.
participant o., an investigator who while studying the activities of a group of subjects also participates in their activities, presumably being able to gain more detailed, relevant information but with less objectivity.

obsession (ob-sesh'ŭn) [L. *obsideo,* pp. *-sessus,* to besiege, fr. *sedeo,* to sit]. A recurrent and persistent idea, thought, or impulse that is ego-dystonic, that is experienced as senseless or repugnant, and that the individual cannot voluntarily suppress.
impulsive o., an o. accompanied by action, sometimes becoming a mania.
inhibitory o., an o. involving an impediment to action, usually representing a phobia.

obsessive-compulsive. Having a tendency to perform certain repetitive acts or ritualistic behavior to relieve anxiety, as in obsessive-compulsive neurosis.

obsolescence (ob-sō-les'ens) [L. *obsolescere,* to grow out of use].

Falling into disuse; denoting the abolition of a function.

obstetric, obstetrical (ob-stet'rik, -ri-kăl). Relating to obstetrics.

obstetrician (ob-stĕ-trish'ŭn) [see obstetrics]. Accoucheur; a physician specializing in the medical care of women during pregnancy and childbirth.

obstetrics (OB) (ob-stet'riks) [L. *obstetrix,* a midwife, fr. *ob-sto,* to stand before, denoting the position formerly taken by the midwife]. Tocology; the specialty of medicine concerned with the care of women during pregnancy, parturition, and the puerperium.

obstinate (ob'sti-năt) [L. *obstinātus,* determined]. **1.** Intractable (2); refractory (2); firmly adhering to one's own purpose, opinion, etc.; not yielding to argument, persuasion, or entreaty. **2.** Refractory (1).

obstipation (ob-sti-pā'shŭn) [L. *ob,* against, + *stipo,* pp. *-atus,* to crowd]. Intestinal obstruction; severe constipation.

obstruction (ob-strŭk'shŭn) [L. *obstructio*]. Blockage or clogging, *e.g.,* by occlusion or stenosis.

closed-loop o., o. of a segment of intestine by rotation on a fixed point (volvulus); frequently impairs venous circulation of the affected bowel segment, resulting in strangulation and gangrene; the segment of intestine contained in a hernia can also become a closed-loop o. when sufficient compression occurs at the neck of the sac.

ureteropelvic o., a blocking or stenosis, usually congenital, at the junction of the renal pelvis and ureter, usually resulting in stasis, hydronephrosis, and calyceal clubbing.

ureterovesical o., o. of the lower ureter at its entrance into the bladder.

obstruent (ob'strū-ent) [L. *ob-struo,* to build against, obstruct]. **1.** Obstructing; blocking; clogging. **2.** An agent that obstructs or prevents a normal discharge, especially a discharge from the bowels.

obtund (ob-tŭnd') [L. *ob-tundo,* pp. *-tusus,* to beat against, blunt]. To dull or blunt, especially to blunt sensation or deaden pain.

obturation (ob-tū-rā'shŭn) [see obturator]. Obstruction or occlusion.

obturator (ob'tū-rā-tōr) [L. *obturo,* pp. *-atus,* to occlude or stop up]. **1.** Any structure that occludes an opening. **2.** Denoting the obturator foramen, the obturator membrane, or any of several parts in relation to this foramen. **3.** A prosthesis used to close an opening of the hard palate, usually a cleft palate. **4.** The stylus or removable plug used during the insertion of many tubular instruments.

obtuse (ob-tūs') [see obtund]. **1.** Dull in intellect; of slow understanding. **2.** Blunt; not acute.

obtusion (ob-tū'zhŭn). **1.** Dullness of sensibility. **2.** A dulling or deadening of sensibility.

occipital (ok-sip'i-tăl). Relating to the occiput.

occipitalis (ok'sip-i-tā'lis) [L.] [NA]. Occipital; referring to the occipital bone or to the back of the head.

occipitalization (ok'sip'i-tăl-i-zā'shŭn). Bony ankylosis between the atlas and occipital bone.

occipito- [L. *occiput*]. Combining form denoting the occiput or occipital structures.

occipitoatloid (ok-sip'i-tō-at'loyd). Relating to the occipital bone and the atlas; denoting the articulation between the two bones.

occipitoaxial, occipitoaxoid (ok-sip'i-tō-ak'sē-ăl, -ak'soyd). Relating to the occipital bone and the axis, or epistropheus.

occipitobregmatic (ok-sip'i-tō-breg-mat'ik). Relating to the occiput and the bregma; denoting a measurement in craniometry.

occipitofacial (ok-sip'i-tō-fā'shăl). Relating to the occiput and the face.

occipitofrontal (ok-sip'i-tō-frŭn'tăl). **1.** Relating to the occiput and the forehead. **2.** Relating to the occipital and frontal lobe of the cerebral cortex and association pathways that interconnect these regions.

occipitofrontalis (ok-sip'i-tō-frŭn-tā'lis) [L.]. See under musculus.

occipitomastoid (ok-sip'i-tō-mas'toyd). Relating to the occipital bone and the mastoid process.

occipitomental (ok-sip'i-tō-men'tăl). Relating to the occiput and the chin.

occipitoparietal (ok-sip'i-tō-pă-rī'ĕ-tăl). Relating to the occipital and the parietal bones.

occipitotemporal (ok-sip'i-tō-tem'pō-răl). Relating to the occiput and the temple, or the occipital and the temporal bones.

occipitothalamic (ok-sip'i-tō-tha-lam'ik). Relating to the nerve fibers leading from the occipital lobe of the cerebral cortex to the thalamus.

occiput, gen. occip'itis (ok'si-put, ok-sip'i-tis) [L.] [NA]. The back of the head.

occlude (ō-klūd) [see occlusion]. **1.** To close or bring together. **2.** To enclose, as in an occluded virus.

occluder (ō-klūd'er). In dentistry, a name given to some articulators.

occlusal (ō-klū'zăl). **1.** Pertaining to occlusion or closure. **2.** In dentistry, pertaining to the contacting surfaces of opposing occlusal units (teeth or occlusion rims), or the masticating surfaces of the posterior teeth.

occlusion (ō-klū'zhŭn) [L. *oc- cludo,* pp. *-clusus,* to shut up, fr. *ob.,* against, + *claudo,* to close]. **1.** The act of closing or the state of being closed. **2.** In chemistry, the absorption of a gas by a metal or the inclusion of one substance within another (as in a gelatinous precipitate). **3.** Any contact between the incising or masticating surfaces of the upper and lower teeth. **4.** The relationship between the occlusal surfaces of the maxillary and mandibular teeth when they are in contact.

abnormal o., an arrangement of the teeth which is not considered to be within the normal range of variation.

afunctional o., a malocclusion which does not permit normal function of the dentition.

anterior o., **(1)** the o. of anterior teeth; **(2)** mesial o. (1).

balanced o., balanced bite or articulation; the simultaneous contacting of the upper and lower teeth on the right and left and in the anterior and posterior occlusal areas in centric and eccentric positions within the functional range; used primarily in reference to the mouth, but also arranged and observed on articulators, developed to prevent a tipping or rotating of the denture bases in relation to the supporting structures.

bimaxillary protrusive o., an o. in which both the maxilla and mandible protrude, causing the long axes of the maxillary anterior teeth to be at an extremely acute angle to the mandibular teeth; may be secondary to a skeletal or dental deformity, or both; seen commonly in blacks.

buccal o., **(1)** malposition of a tooth toward the cheek; **(2)** the o. as seen from the buccal side of the teeth.

centric o., centric contact; **(1)** the relation of opposing occlusal surfaces which provides the maximum planned contact and/or intercuspation; **(2)** the o. of the teeth when the mandible is in centric relation to the maxillae.

coronary o., blockage of a coronary vessel, usually by thrombosis or atheroma, often leading to myocardial infarction.

distal o., **(1)** disto-occlusion; postnormal o.; retrusive o. (2); a tooth occluding in a position distal to normal; **(2)** distoclusion.

eccentric o., any o. other than centric.

edge-to-edge o., edge-to-edge bite; end-to-end bite or o.; an o. in which the anterior teeth of both jaws meet along their incisal edges when the teeth are in centric o.

end-to-end o., edge-to-edge o.

functional o., **(1)** any tooth contacts made within the functional range of the opposing teeth surfaces; **(2)** o. which occurs during function.
gliding o., dental *articulation.*
hyperfunctional o., occlusal stress of tooth or teeth exceeding normal physiologic demands.
labial o., **(1)** malposition of a tooth in a labial direction; **(2)** the o. as seen from the labial side of the arches.
lateral o., malposition of a tooth or an entire dental arch in a direction away from the midline.
lingual o., **(1)** linguoclusion; **(2)** interdigitation of the teeth as seen from the internal or lingual aspect.
mechanically balanced o., a balanced o. without reference to physiologic considerations, as on an articulator.
mesenteric artery o., obstruction of arterial flow in the mesenteric circulation by an embolus or thrombus; usually refers to o. of the superior mesenteric artery, although atherosclerotic narrowing may involve all three major splanchnic branches (celiac, superior, and inferior mesenteric).
mesial o., **(1)** mesio-occlusion; anterior o. (2); o. in which the mandibular teeth articulate with the maxillary teeth in a position anterior to normal; **(2)** mesioclusion.
neutral o., **(1)** normal o. (2); an arrangement of teeth such that the maxillary and mandibular first permanent molars are in normal anteroposterior relation; **(2)** neutroclusion.
normal o., **(1)** normal bite; that arrangement of teeth and their supporting structure which is usually found in health and which approaches an ideal or standard arrangement; **(2)** neutral o. (1).
pathogenic o., an occlusal relationship capable of producing pathologic changes in the supporting tissues.
physiologic o., o. in harmony with functions of the masticatory system.
physiologically balanced o., a balanced o. that is in harmony with the temporomandibular joints and the neuromuscular system.
posterior o., posteroclusion; the most effective contact of the molar and bicuspid teeth of both jaws which allows for all the natural movements of the jaws essential to normal mastication and closure.
postnormal o., distal o. (1).
protrusive o., o. which results when the mandible is protruded forward from centric position.
o. of pupil, the presence of an opaque membrane closing the pupillary area.
retrusive o., **(1)** a biting relationship in which the mandible is forcefully or habitually placed more distally than the patient's centric o.; **(2)** distal o. (1).
spherical form of o., an arrangement of teeth which places their occlusal surfaces on the surface of an imaginary sphere (usually 8 inches in diameter) with its center above the level of the teeth. See also Monson *curve.*
torsive o., torsiversion.
traumatic o., traumatogenic o.
traumatogenic o., traumatic o.; a malocclusion capable of producing injury to the teeth and/or associated structures.
working o., working *contacts.*

occlusive (ō-klū'siv). Serving to close; denoting a bandage or dressing that closes a wound and excludes it from the air.

occlusometer (ok-lū-som'ĕ-ter). Gnathodynamometer.

occult (ō-kŭlt', ok'ŭlt) [L. *oc-culo,* pp. *-cultus,* to cover, hide]. **1.** Hidden; concealed; not manifest. **2.** Denoting a concealed hemorrhage, the blood being so changed as not to be readily recognized. See occult *blood.* **3.** In oncology, a clinically unidentified primary tumor with recognized metastases.

Oceanospirillum (ō'shen-ō-spī-ril'ŭm) [L. *oceanus,* ocean, + *spirillum,* coil]. A genus of motile, nonsporeforming, aerobic bacteria (family Spirillaceae) containing Gram-negative, rigid, helical cells which are 0.3 to 1.2 μm in diameter. Motile cells contain bipolar fascicles of flagella. There is no growth anaerobically with nitrate. These organisms are chemoorganotrophic and possess a strictly respiratory metabolism; they neither oxidize nor ferment carbohydrates. These organisms are found in marine environments. There are at present five species in this genus, of which the type species is *O. linum.*

ocellus, pl. **ocelli** (ō-sel'ŭs, -lī) [L. dim. of *oculus,* eye]. **1.** Eyespot (2); the simple eye found in many invertebrates. **2.** Facet of the compound eye of an insect.

ochlophobia (ok-lō-fō'bē-ă) [G. *ochlos,* a crowd, + *phobos,* fear]. Morbid fear of crowds.

Ochoa's law. See under law.

ochrodermia (ō-krō-der'mē-ă) [G. *ōchros,* pale yellow, + *derma,* skin]. Yellow discoloration of the skin.

ochrometer (ō-krom'ĕ-ter) [G. *ōchros,* pale yellow, + *metron,* measure]. An instrument for determining the capillary blood pressure; one of two adjacent fingers is compressed by a rubber balloon until blanching of the skin occurs, after which the force necessary to accomplish this color change is read in millimeters of mercury.

ochronosis (o-kron-ō'sis) [G. *ōchros,* pale yellow, + *nosos,* disease]. A pathologic condition observed in certain persons with alkaptonuria, characterized by pigmentation of the cartilages and sometimes tissues such as muscle, epithelial cells, and dense connective tissue; may affect also the sclera, mucous membrane of the lips, and skin of the ears, face, and hands, and cause standing urine to be dark-colored and contain pigmented casts; pigmentation is thought to result from oxidized homogentisic acid, and cartilage degeneration results in osleoarthritis, particularly of the spine.
exogenous o., pigmentation of the cornea and of the skin of the face and hands from prolonged exposure to phenol or resinol.

ochronotic (ō-kron-ot'ik). Relating to or characterized by ochronosis.

Ochsner, Albert J., U.S. surgeon, 1858–1925. See O. *clamp;* O.'s *method.*

ocrylate (ok'ri-lāt). Octyl-2-cyanoacrylate; a tissue adhesive for surgery.

oct-, octa-, octi-, octo- [G. *oktō,* L. *octo,* eight]. Combining forms meaning eight.

octad (ok'tad) [L. *octo,* eight]. **1.** Octavalent. **2.** An octavalent element or radical.

octamethyl pyrophosphoramide (OMPA) (ok-tă-meth'il pī'rō-fos-fōr'ă-mīd). An anticholinesterase that is used as a plant insecticide.

octamylamine (ok-tă-mil'ă-mēn). *N*-Isopentyl-1,5-dimethylhexylamine; an anticholinergic agent.

octan (ok'tan) [L. *octo,* eight]. Applied to fever, the paroxysms of which recur every eighth day, the day of a paroxysm being counted as the first in the computation.

octanoate (ok'tă-nō-āt). Caprylate.

octanoic acid (ok'tă-nō-ik). Caprylic acid.

octapeptide (ok-tă-pep'tīd). A peptide made up of eight amino acid residues.

octaploidy (ok'tă-ploy'dē). See polyploidy.

octapressin (ok-tă-pres'in). Felypressin.

octavalent (ok'tă-vā'lent, ok-tav'ă-lent). Octad (1); denoting a chemical element or radical having a combining power (valency) of eight.

octavus (ok-tā'vŭs) [L.]. Eighth cranial nerve. See *nervus* vestibulocochlearis.

octi-. See oct-.

octo-. See oct-.

Octomitidae (ok-tō-mit'i-dē) [octo- + G. *mitos,* thread]. A family in the protozoan class Zoomastigophorea; flagellates with six to eight flagella arranged in pairs and a body that is bilaterally symmetric; it includes the common human intestinal parasite *G. lamblia.*

Octomitus hominis (ok-tom'i-tŭs hom'i-nis). *Pentatrichomonas hominis.*

octopamine (ok-tō'pă-mēn). Norsympatol; norsynephrine; α-(aminomethyl)-*p*-hydroxybenzyl alcohol; a sympathomimetic amine.

octose (ok'tōs). A sugar containing eight carbon atoms; synthetically prepared but not occurring as such in nature.

octoxynol (ok-tok'si-nol). Polyethylene glycol mono[*p*- (1,1,3,3,-tetramethylbutyl)phenyl]ether; a surfactant.

octulose (ok'tū-lōs). An eight-carbon monoketose.

octulosonic acid (ok'tū-lō-son'ik). The -onic acid formally formed by oxidation of carbon atom 1 of octulose to a carboxylic acid group; a condensation product of arabinose and phosphoenol-pyruvate analogous to neuraminic acid. It forms part of the repeating unit of the polysaccharides of the complex lipopolysaccharides of the Enterobacteriaceae constituting the characteristic somatic octose antigens.

octyl gallate (ok'til gal'āt). Octyl 3,4,5-trihydroxybenzoate; an antioxidant.

octylphenoxy polyethoxyethanol (ok'til-fe-nok'sē pol'ē-eth-ok'sē-eth'ă-nol). Mono-*p*- isooctyl phenyl ether of polyethylene glycol; a surface-active (wetting) agent.

ocular (ok'yū-lăr) [L. *oculus,* eye]. **1.** Ophthalmic. **2.** The eyepiece of a microscope, the lens or lenses at the observer end of a microscope, by means of which the image focused by the objective is viewed.

compensating o., an o. that compensates and corrects for the effects of chromatic aberration in the objective.

Huygens' o., the compound o. of a microscope, composed of two planoconvex lenses so arranged that the plane side of each is directed toward the observer.

Ramsden's o., an eyepiece of a microscope, consisting of two planoconvex lenses with convexities turned to each other.

wide field o., an o. that gives a larger than usual field of view and a high eyepoint.

ocularist (ok'yū-lăr-ist) [L. *oculus,* eye]. One skilled in the design, fabrication, and fitting of artificial eyes and the making of prostheses associated with the appearance or function of the eyes.

oculentum, pl. **oculenta** (ok-yū-len'tŭm, -tă) [Mod. L., fr. L. *oculus,* eye]. Ophthalmic *ointment.*

oculi (ok'yū-lī) [L.]. Plural of oculus.

oculist (ok'yū-list) [L. *oculus,* eye]. Ophthalmologist.

oculo- [L. *oculus,* eye]. Combining form denoting the eye, ocular. See also ophthalmo-.

oculoauriculovertebral (ok'yū-lō-aw-rik'yū-lō-ver'tē-brăl). Relating to the eyes, ears, and vertebrae.

oculocardiac (ok'yū-lō-kar'dē-ak). Relating to the eyes and heart.

oculocerebrorenal (ok'yū-lō-ser'ē-brō-rē'năl). Relating to the eyes, brain, and kidneys.

oculocutaneous (ok'yū-lō-kyū-tā'nē-ŭs). Relating to the eyes and the skin.

oculodentodigital (ok'yū-lō-den'tō-dij'i-tăl). Relating to the eyes, teeth, and fingers.

oculodermal (ok'yū-lō-der'măl). Relating to the eyes and skin.

oculofacial (ok-yū-lō-fā'shăl). Relating to the eyes and the face.

oculography (ok-yū-log'ră-fē) [oculo- + G. *graphē,* a writing]. A method of recording eye position and movements.

photosensor o., o. in which photocells are directed to the surface of the eye to record rotations.

oculogyria (ok'yū-lō-jī'rē-ă) [oculo- + G. *gyros,* circle]. The limits of rotation of the eyeballs.

oculogyric (ok'yū-lō-jī'rik). Referring to rotation of the eyeballs; characterized by oculogyria.

oculomandibulodyscephaly (ok'yū-lō-man-dib'yū-lō-dis-sef'ă-lē). *Dyscephalia* mandibulo-oculofacialis.

oculomotor (ok'yū-lō-mō'tōr) [L. *oculomotorius,* fr. oculo- + L. *motorius,* moving]. **1.** Relating to or causing movements of the eyeball. **2.** Pertaining to the o. cranial nerve.

oculomotorius (ok'yū-lō-mō-tō'rē-ŭs) [L.]. *Nervus* oculomotorius.

oculonasal (ok'yū-lō-nā'săl) [oculo- + L. *nasus,* nose]. Relating to the eyes and the nose.

oculopathy (ok-yū-lop'ă-thē). Ophthalmopathy.

oculoplethysmography (ok'yū-lō-pleth-iz-mog'ră-fē) [oculo- + G. *plēthymos,* increase, + *graphē,* to write]. Indirect measurement of the hemodynamic significance of internal carotid artery stenosis or occlusion by demonstration of an ipsilateral delay in the arrival of ocular pressure transmitted from branches of the ophthalmic artery.

oculopneumoplethysmography (ok'yū-lō-nū'mō-pleth-iz-mog'ră-fē). A method of bilateral measurement of ophthalmic artery pressure that reflects pressure and flow in the internal carotid artery. See oculoplethysmography.

oculopupillary (ok'yū-lō-pū'pi-lār-ē). Pertaining to the pupil of the eye.

oculovertebral (ok'yū-lō-ver'tē-brăl). Relating to the eyes and vertebrae.

oculozygomatic (ok'yū-lō-zī-gō-mat'ik). Relating to the orbit or its margin and the zygomatic bone.

oculus, gen. and pl. **oculi** (ok'yū-lŭs, -lī) [L.] [NA]. The eye, the organ of vision that consists of the eyeball and the optic nerve.

ocy- See oxy-.

ocytocin (ō-si-tō'sin) [G. *okytokos,* fast birth, prompt delivery]. Oxytocin.

OD Abbreviation for overdose.

O.D. Abbreviation for L. *oculus dexter,* right eye; Doctor of Optometry (see optometrist).

od [G. *hodos,* way]. A force assumed to be exerted upon the nervous system by magnets.

o.d. Abbreviation for L. *omni die,* every day.

odaxesmus (ō'dak-sez'mŭs) [G. *odaxēsmos,* an irritation, fr. *odax* (adv.), by biting.]. A biting sensation; a form of paresthesia.

odaxetic (ō'dak-set'ik) [G. *odaxēsmos,* an irritation]. **1.** Causing formication or itching. **2.** A substance or agent that causes formication or itching.

Oddi, Ruggero, 19th century Italian physician. See *sphincter of O.*

odditis (od-ī'tis). Inflammation of the junction of the duodenum and common bile duct at the sphincter of Oddi.

-odes [G. *eidos,* form, resemblance]. Suffix denoting having the form of, like, resembling.

Odland body. See under body.

odogenesis (ō-dō-jen'ē-sis) [G. *hodos,* path, + *genesis,* source]. Neurocladism.

odont-, odonto- [G. *odous* (*odont-*), tooth]. Combining forms, properly in words formed from G. roots, denoting a tooth or teeth.

odontagra (ō-don-tag'ră) [odonto- + G. *agra,* seizure]. Obsolescent term for toothache thought to be of gouty origin.

odontalgia (ō-don-tal'jē-ă) [odont- + G. *algos,* pain]. Toothache.

o. denta'lis, reflex pain in the ear due to dental disease, usually propagated along the auriculotemporal nerve.

odontalgic (ō-don-tal'jik). Relating to or marked by toothache.

odontectomy (ō-don-tek'tō-mē) [odont- + G. *ektomē,* excision]. Removal of teeth by the reflection of a mucoperiosteal flap and excision of bone from around the root or roots before the application of force to effect the tooth removal.

odonterism (ō-don'ter-izm) [odont- + G. *erismos,* quarrel]. Chattering of the teeth.

odontiasis (ō-don-tī'ă-sis). Teething.

odontinoid (ō-don'ti-noyd). **1.** Resembling dentin. **2.** A small excrescence from a tooth, most common on the root or neck. **3.** Toothlike.

odontitis (ō-don-tī'tis). Pulpitis.

odonto-. See odont-.

odontoameloblastoma (ō-don'tō-am'ĕ-lō-blas-tō'mă). Ameloblastic *odontoma.*

odontoblast (ō-don'tō-blast) [odonto- + G. *blastos,* sprout, germ]. Odontoplast; one of the dentin-forming cells, derived from mesenchyme (via neural crests), lining the pulp cavity of a tooth; o.'s are arranged in a layer peripherally in the dental pulp forming the dentinal matrix, with odontoblastic processes extending from each cell into a dentinal tubule; the cells generally are columnar in the coronal pulp, but are more cuboidal in the radicular area and adjacent to tertiary dentin.

odontoblastoma (ō-don'tō-blas-tō'mă) [odontoblast + G. *-oma,* tumor]. **1.** A tumor composed of neoplastic epithelial and mesenchymal cells that may differentiate into cells able to produce calcified tooth substances. **2.** An odontoma in its early formative stage.

odontoclast (ō-don'tō-klast) [odonto- + G. *klastos,* broken]. One of the cells believed to produce resorption of the roots of the deciduous teeth.

odontodynia (ō-don-tō-din'ē-ă) [odonto- + G. *odynē,* pain]. Toothache.

odontodysplasia (ō-don'tō-dis-plā'zē-ă). Odontogenic dysplasia; odontogenesis imperfecta; a developmental disturbance of one or of several adjacent teeth, of unknown etiology, characterized by deficient formation of enamel and dentin which results in an abnormally large pulp chamber and imparts a ghostlike radiographic image to the teeth; such teeth exhibit delayed eruption into the oral cavity.

odontogenesis (ō-don-tō-jen'ĕ-sis) [odonto- + G. *genesis,* production]. Odontogeny; odontosis; the process of development of the teeth.

o. imperfec'ta, odontodysplasia.

odontogeny (ō-don-toj'ĕ-nē). Odontogenesis.

odontoid (ō-don'toyd) [odont- + G. *eidos,* resemblance]. **1.** Dentoid; shaped like a tooth. **2.** Relating to the toothlike o. process of the second cervical vertebra.

odontology (ō-don-tol'ō-jē) [odonto- + G. *logos,* study]. Dentistry.

forensic o., forensic *dentistry.*

odontoloxia, odontoloxy (ō-don-tō-lok'sē-ă, ō-don-tol'ok-sē) [odonto- + G. *loxos,* slanting]. Odontoparallaxis.

odontolysis (ō-don-tol'i-sis) [odonto- + G. *lysis,* dissolution]. Erosion (3).

odontoma (ō-don-tō'mă) [odonto- + G. *-oma,* tumor]. **1.** A tumor of odontogenic origin. **2.** A hemartomatous odontogenic tumor comprised of enamel, dentin, cementum, and pulp tissue that may or may not be arranged in the form of a tooth.

ameloblastic o., odontoameloblastoma; a benign mixed odontogenic tumor comprised of an undifferentiated component histologically identical to an ameloblastoma and a well differentiated component identical to an odontoma; appears as a mixed radiolucent-radiopaque lesion and presents clinically as an ameloblastoma.

complex o., an o. in which the various odontogenic tissues are organized in a haphazard arrangement with no resemblance to teeth.

compound o., an o. in which the odontogenic tissues are organized and resemble anomalous teeth.

odontoneuralgia (ō-don'tō-nū-ral'jē-ă). Facial neuralgia caused by a carious tooth.

odontonomy (ō-don-ton'ō-mē). [odonto- + G. *onoma,* name]. Dental nomenclature.

odontonosology (ō-don'tō-nō-sol'ō-jē) [odonto- + G. *nosos,* disease, + *logos,* study]. Dentistry.

odontoparallaxis (ō-don'tō-par-ă-lak'sis) [odonto- + G. *parallax,* alternately]. Odontoloxia; odontoloxy; irregularity of the teeth.

odontopathy (ō-don-top'ă-thē) [odonto- + G. *pathos,* suffering]. Any disease of the teeth or of their sockets.

odontophobia (ō-don-tō-fō'bē-ă) [odonto- + G. *phobos,* fear]. Morbid fear of teeth.

odontoplast (ō-don'tō-plast) [odonto- + G. *plastos,* formed]. Rarely used term for odontoblast.

odontoplasty (ō-don'tō-plas-tē) [odonto- + G. *plassō,* to mold]. Surgical contouring of tooth surface to enhance plaque control and gingival morphology.

odontoprisis (ō-don-top'ri-sis) [odonto- + G. *prisis,* a sawing, a grinding]. Grinding together of the teeth.

odontoptosis (ō-don-top-tō'sis, -tō-tō'sis) [odonto- + G. *ptosis,* a falling]. Drooping downward of an upper tooth due to the loss of its lower antagonist(s).

odontorrhagia (ō-don-tō-rā'jē-ă) [odonto- + G. *rhēgnymi,* to burst forth]. Profuse bleeding from the socket after the extraction of a tooth.

odontoschism (ō-don'tō-skizm, -sizm) [odonto- + G. *schisma,* a cleft]. Fissure of a tooth.

odontoscope (ō-don'tō-skōp). An optical device, similar to a closed circuit television system, that projects the oral cavity onto a screen for multiple viewing.

odontoscopy (ō-don-tos'kō-pē) [odonto- + G. *skopeō,* to view]. **1.** Examination of the oral cavity by means of the odontoscope. **2.** Examination of the markings in prints of the cutting edges of the teeth; used, like fingerprints, as a method of personal identification.

odontosis (ō-don-tō'sis). Odontogenesis.

odontotherapy (ō-don-tō-thar'ă-pē). Treatment of diseases of the teeth.

odontotomy (ō-don-tot'ō-mē) [odonto- + G. *tomē,* incision]. Cutting into the crown of a tooth.

prophylactic o., a preventive operation in which imperfectly formed developmental grooves, pits, and fissures are opened up by means of a bur and filled in order to obviate future decay.

odor (ō'dŏr) [L.]. Scent; smell (3); emanation from any substance that stimulates the olfactory cells in the organ of smell.

odorant (ō'dŏr-ant). Odoriferous.

odoratism (ō-dŏr'ă-tizm) [fr. *Lathyrus odoratus,* sweet pea]. See lathyrism; osteolathyrism.

odoriferous (ō-dŏ-rif'er-ŭs) [odor + L. *fero,* to bear]. Odorant; odorous; having a scent, perfume, or odor.

odorimeter (ō'dŏ-rim'ĕ-ter). Instrument for performing odorimetry.

odorimetry (ō'dŏ-rim'ĕ-trē) [odor + G. *metron,* measure]. The determination of the comparative power of different substances in exciting olfactory sensations.

odorivection (ō-dŏr-i-vek'shŭn) [odor + L. *vector,* a carrier]. Conveying or bearing an odor, as on the air.

odorography (ō'dō-rog'ră-fē) [odor + G. *graphē,* a description]. Description of odors.

odorous (ō'dŏr-ŭs). Odoriferous.

O'Dwyer, Joseph P., U.S. physician, 1841–1898. See O'D.'s *tube.*

odyn-, odyno- [G. *odyne,* pain]. Combining forms meaning pain.

odynacusis (ō-din'ă-kū'sis) [odyn- + G. *akouō,* to hear]. Hypersensitiveness of the organ of hearing, so that noises cause actual pain.

odynometer (ō-di-nom'ĕ-ter) [odyno- + G. *metron,* measure]. Algesiometer.

odynophagia (ō-din-ō-fā'jē-ă) [odyno- + G. *phagein,* to eat]. Pain on swallowing.

odynophonia (ō-din-ō-fō'nē-ă) [odyno- + G. *phonē,* sound, voice]. Pain on using the voice.

Oe Symbol for oersted.

oe-. For words so beginning and not found here, see e-.

oedipism (ed'i-pizm) [*Oedipus,* G. myth. char.]. **1.** Self-infliction of injury to the eyes, usually an attempt at evulsion. **2.** Manifestation of the Oedipus complex.

Oehl, Eusebio, Italian anatomist, 1827–1903. See O.'s *muscles.*

Oehler, Johannes, German physician, *1879. See O.'s *symptom.*

oenanthal (ē-nan'thăl). Heptanal.

oersted (Oe) (er'sted) [Hans-Christian *Oersted* Danish physicist, 1777–1851]. A unit of magnetic field intensity; the magnetic field intensity that exerts a force of 1 dyne on unit magnetic pole; equal to $(1000/4\pi)$A/m.

oesophagostomiasis (ē-sof'ă-gō-stō-mī'ă-sis) [G. *oi-sophagos,* gullet (esophagus), + *stoma,* mouth, + *-iasis,* condition]. Esophagostomiasis; infection with nematode parasites of the genus *Oesophagostomum.*

Oesophagostomum (ē-sof-ă-gos'tō-mŭm) [G. *oisophagos,* gullet (esophagus), + *stoma,* mouth]. A genus of strongyle nematodes (subfamily Oesophagostominae) that encyst in the intestinal wall of herbivores and primates, causing nodular disease. Larvae appear to stimulate a host reaction in the intestinal wall, forming nodules in which the worms complete their development (unless the host is immune); they then leave the nodule and feed as adults in the lumen of the large intestine.

O. apios'tomum, a primate species that has been reported in northern Nigeria and central Africa to encyst under the submucosa of the human intestine and occasionally cause dysentery; a common parasite of monkeys and apes, both in captivity and in the wild.

O. brevicau'dum, a species that occurs in the cecum and colon of pigs in North America and India.

O. brump'ti, a species described from African monkeys and reported occasionally in man.

O. columbia'num, a species that occurs in sheep, goats, and wild African antelopes; except when present in large numbers, it does not appear to seriously affect the health of the host.

O. denta'tum, a species that affects the colon of swine; the lesions are similar to those in sheep.

O. georgia'num, a species that occurs in the cecum and colon of pigs in the U.S.

O. quadrispinula'tum, a species that occurs in the cecum and colon of pigs in the Americas, Europe, and Southeast Asia.

O. radia'tum, a species that occurs worldwide in cattle and water buffalo; the lesions are similar to those of sheep.

O. stephanos'tomum, a species occurring in chimpanzees, monkeys, and gorillas in Africa, but also reported from man and monkeys in Brazil.

O. venulo'sum, a species that occurs worldwide in the cecum and colon of cattle, sheep, goats, deer, and many other ruminants.

oestrids (est'ridz) [G. *oistros,* gadfly]. Common name for botflies of the family Oestridae, such as *Oestrus.*

oestrosis (es-trō'sis). Infection of small ruminants and rarely man with larvae of the fly *Oestrus ovis.*

Oestrus (es'tŭs) [G. *oistros,* gadfly]. A genus of tissue-invading flies that cause myiasis in sheep; the head botflies in the family Oestridae. *O. ovis* (a nose fly) is a grayish brown, robust, hairy, beelike botfly, imported from Europe, and now a serious pest in parts of the U.S.; larvae are deposited by the adult fly in the nostrils of sheep, and inch-long larvae develop in the paranasal sinuses, causing considerable mucous discharge and distress in old or weak sheep.

official (ŏ-fish'ăl) [L. *officialis,* fr. *officium,* a favor, service, fr. *opus,* work, + *facio,* to do]. Authoritative; denoting a drug or a chemical or pharmaceutical preparation recognized as standard in the pharmacopeia. *Cf.* officinal.

officinal (ŏ-fis'i-năl) [L. *officina,* shop]. Denoting a chemical or pharmaceutical preparation kept in stock, in contrast to magistral (prepared extemporaneously according to a physician's prescription); an o. preparation is often, though not necessarily, official.

Ogino, Kyusaka, 20th century Japanese physician. See O.-Knaus *rule.*

Ogston, Sir Alexander, Scottish surgeon, 1844–1929. See O.'s *line;* O.-Luc *operation.*

Oguchi, Chita, Japanese ophthalmologist, 1875–1945. See O.'s *disease.*

Ogura, Joseph H., U.S. otolaryngologist, *1915. See O. *operation.*

O'Hara, Michael, Jr., U.S. surgeon, 1869–1926. See O'H. *forceps.*

OHI Abbreviation for Oral Hygiene Index.

OHI-S Abbreviation for Simplified Oral Hygiene Index.

Ohm, Georg S., German physicist, 1787–1854. See ohm; O.'s *law.*

ohm (Ω) (ōm) [G. S. *Ohm*]. The practical unit of electrical resistance; the resistance of any conductor allowing 1 ampere of current to pass under the electromotive force of 1 volt.

ohmammeter (ōm-am'ĕ-ter). A combined ohmmeter and ammeter.

ohmmeter (ōm'ĕ-ter). An instrument for determining the resistance, in ohms, of a conductor.

ohne Hauch (ō'nă howch) [Ger. without breath]. Term used to designate the nonspreading growth of nonflagellated bacteria on agar media; also applied to somatic agglutination. See also O *antigen.*

Ohngren's line. See under line.

oi-. For words so beginning and not found here, see e-.

-oid [G. *eidos,* form, resemblance]. Suffix denoting resemblance to, joined properly to words formed from G. roots; equivalent to Eng. -form.

oidia (ō-id'ēă). Plural of oidium.

oidiomycin (ō-id'ē-ō-mī'sin). An antigen used to demonstrate cutaneous hypersensitivity in patients infected with one of the Candida species; one of a series of antigens used to demonstrate an immunocompromised patient's capacity to react to any cutaneous antigen.

oidium, pl. oidia (ō-id'ē-ŭm, ō-id'ē-ă) [Mod. L. dim. of G. *ōon,* egg]. Formerly used term for arthroconidium.

oil (oyl) [L. *oleum;* G. *elaion,* originally olive oil]. An inflammable liquid, of fatty consistence and unctuous feel, that is insoluble in water, soluble or insoluble in alcohol, and freely soluble in ether. O.'s are variously classified as animal, vegetable, and mineral o.'s according to their source (the mineral o.'s probably being of remote animal and vegetable origin); into fatty (fixed) and volatile o.'s; and into drying and nondrying (fatty) o.'s, the former becoming gradually thicker when exposed to the air and finally drying to a varnish, the latter not drying but liable to become rancid on exposure. Many of the o.'s, both fixed and volatile, are used in medicine. For individual o.'s, see the specific names.

essential o.'s, plant products, usually somewhat volatile, giving the odors and tastes characteristic of the particular plant, thus possessing the essence, *e.g.*, citral, pinene, camphor, menthane, terpenes. See also volatile o.

ethereal o., volatile o.

fatty o., fixed o.; an o. derived from both animals and plants; chemically, a glyceride of a fatty acid which, by substitution of the glycerine by an alkaline base, is converted into a soap; a fatty o., in contrast to a volatile o., is permanent, leaving a stain on an absorbent surface, and thus is not capable of distillation; it is obtained by expression or extraction; the consistency varies with the temperature, some being liquid (o.'s proper), others semisolid (fats), and others solid (tallows) at ordinary temperatures; both liquid and semisolid o.'s are congealed by cold and the solids are liquified by heat.

fixed o., fatty o.

joint o., synovia.

volatile o., ethereal o.; a substance of oily consistency and feel, derived from a plant and containing the principles to which the odor and taste of the plant are due (essential o.); in contrast to a fatty o., a volatile o. evaporates when exposed to the air and thus is capable of distillation; it may also be obtained by expression or extraction; many volatile o.'s, identical to or closely resembling the natural o.'s, can be made synthetically. Volatile o.'s are used in medicine as stimulants, stomachics, correctives, carminatives, and for purposes of flavoring.

oil red O [C.I. 26125]. 1-8-[4-(Dimethylphenylazo)dimethylphenylazo]-2-naphthalenol; a weakly acid diazo oil-soluble dye, used in histologic demonstration of neutral fats.

oil of vitriol. Sulfuric acid.

ointment (oynt'ment) [O. Fr. *oignement;* L. *unguo,* pp. *unctus,* to smear]. Salve; uncture; unguent; a semisolid preparation usually containing medicinal substances and intended for external application. O. bases used as vehicles fall into four general classes: 1) Hydrocarbon bases (oleaginous o. bases) keep medicaments in prolonged contact with the skin, act as occlusive dressings, and are used chiefly for emollient effects. 2) Absorption bases either permit the incorporation of aqueous solutions with the formation of a water-in-oil emulsion or are water-in-oil emulsions that permit the incorporation of additional quantities of aqueous solutions; such bases permit better absorption of some medicaments and are useful as emollients. 3) Water-removable bases (creams) are oil-in-water emulsions containing petrolatum, anhydrous lanolin, or waxes; they may be washed from the skin with water, and are thus more acceptable for cosmetic reasons; they favor absorption of serous discharges in dermatological conditions. 4) Water-soluble bases (greaseless ointment bases) contain only water-soluble substances. See also cerate.

eye o., ophthalmic o.

ophthalmic o., eye o.; oculentum; a special o. for application to the eye that must be free from particles and must be nonirritating to the eye.

-ol. Suffix denoting that a substance is an alcohol or a phenol.

olamine (ōl'ă-mēn). USAN-approved contraction for ethanolamine.

oleaginous (ō-lē-aj'i-nŭs) [L. *oleagineus,* pertaining to *olea,* the olive tree]. Oily or greasy.

oleander (ō-lē-an'der). The bark and leaves of *Nerium oleander* (family Apocynaceae), a shrub of the eastern Mediterranean; a diuretic and heart tonic.

oleandomycin phosphate (ō-lē-an-dō-mī'sin). An antibiotic substance produced by species of *Streptomyces antibioticus;* effective against staphylococci, streptococci, pneumococci, and some Gram-negative bacteria.

oleate (ō'lē-āt). **1.** A salt of oleic acid. **2.** A pharmacopeial preparation consisting of a combination or solution of an alkaloid or metallic base in oleic acid, used as an inunction.

olecranon (ō-lek'ră-non, ō'lē-krā'non) [G. the head or point of the elbow, fr. *ōlenē,* ulna, + *kranion,* skull, head] [NA]. Tip or point of elbow; o. process; the prominent curved proximal extremity of the ulna, the upper and posterior surface of which gives attachment to the tendon of the triceps muscle, the anterior surface entering into the formation of the trochlear notch.

olefin (ō'lē-fin). Any one of a group of hydrocarbons possessing one or more double bonds in the carbon chain; the simplest is ethylene.

oleic acid (ō-lē'ik) [L. *oleum,* oil]. 9-Octadecenoic acid; an unsaturated fatty acid that is the most widely distributed and abundant fatty acid in nature; used commercially in the preparation of oleates and lotions, and as a pharmaceutical solvent.

olein (ō'lē-in). Triolein; trioleoyl glycerol; glyceryl trioleate; found in fats and oils.

oleo- [L. *oleum,* oil]. Combining form relating to oil. See also eleo-.

oleogomenol (ō'lē-ō-gō'men-ol). Gomenol.

oleogranuloma (ō'lē-ō-gran-yū-lō-mă). Lipogranuloma.

oleoma (ō-lē-ō'mă). Lipogranuloma.

oleometer (ō-lē-om'ĕ-ter) [oleo- + G. *metron,* measure]. Eleometer; an instrument, similar to a hydrometer, for determining the specific gravity of oils.

oleopalmitate (ō'lē-ō-pal'mi-tāt). A double salt of oleic and palmitic acids.

oleoresin (ō'lē-ō-rez'in). **1.** A compound of an essential oil and resin, present in certain plants. **2.** A pharmaceutical preparation. See subentries under aspidium; capsicum; ginger.

oleosaccharum, pl. **oleosacchara** (ō'lē-ō-sak'ă-rŭm) [oleo- + G. *saccharon,* sugar]. Oil sugar; a class of preparations made by the trituration of a volatile oil (anise, fennel, lemon, etc.) with sugar; used as a diluent or corrigent of powerful or bad tasting drugs in powder form.

oleostearate (ō'lē-ō-stē'ă-rāt). A double salt of oleic and stearic acids.

oleosus (ō-lē-ō'sŭs) [L., fr. *oleum,* oil]. Greasy; relating to defects of the sebaceous apparatus.

oleotherapy (ō'lē-ō-thār'ă-pē) [oleo- + G. *therapeia,* therapy]. Eleotherapy; treatment of disease by an oil given internally or applied externally.

oleothorax (ō'lē-ō-thōr'aks) [oleo- + thorax]. Eleothorax; an obsolete form of treatment to compress the lung in pulmonary tuberculosis, for the relief of pyothorax, or to meet other indications, by the introduction of mineral oil or a mixture of gomenol and olive oil into the pleural cavity, either with or without artificial pneumothorax.

oleovitamin (ō'lē-ō-vī'tă-min). A solution of a vitamin in an edible oil.

o. A and D, a solution of vitamins A and D in fish liver oil or in an edible vegetable oil.

oleyl alcohol (ō-lē'il). A mixture of aliphatic alcohols consisting chiefly of $CH_3(CH_2)_7CH{=}CH(CH_2)_7CH_2OH$; used as an emulsifying aid and in the preparation of cold cream; found in fish oils.

olfactie, olfacty (ol-fak'tē) [see olfaction]. The unit of smell; the threshold of olfactory stimulation, or the point where the smell is just received in the olfactometer.

olfaction (ol-fak'shŭn) [L. *ol- facio,* pp. *-factus,* to smell]. Osmesis;

osphresis. **1.** Smell (2); the sense of smell. **2.** The act of smelling.

olfactology (ol′fak-tol′-ō-jē) [olfaction + G. *logos,* study]. Study of the sense of smell.

olfactometer (ol′fak-tom′ĕ-ter) [L. *olfactus,* smell, + G. *metron,* measure]. A device for estimating the keenness of the sense of smell.

olfactometry (ol′fak-tom′ĕ-trē). Determination of the degree of sensibility of the olfactory organ.

olfactophobia (ol-fak-tō-fō′bē-ă) [L. *olfactus,* smell, + G. *phobos,* fear]. Osmophobia; osphresiophobia; morbid fear of odors.

olfactory (ol-fak′tō-rē) [see olfaction]. Osmatic; osphretic; relating to the sense of smell.

olfacty (ol-fak′tē). Olfactie.

olibanum (ō-lib′ă-nŭm) [Ar. *al,* the, + *lubān,* frankincense]. Frankincense; thus; a gum resin from several trees of the genus *Boswellia* (family Burseraceae); has been used as a stimulant expectorant in bronchitis, for fumigations, and as incense.

olig-. See oligo-.

oligamnios (ol-i-gam′nē-os). Oligoamnios.

oligemia (ol-i-gē′mē-ă) [oligo- + G. *haima,* blood]. Olighemia; a deficiency in the amount of blood in the body.

oligemic (ol-i-gē′mik). Pertaining to or characterized by oligemia.

olighemia (ol-ig-hē′mē-ă). Oligemia.

olighidria, oligidria (ol-ig-hid′rē-ă, -id′rē-ă) [oligo- + G. *hidrōs,* sweat]. Scanty perspiration.

oligo-, olig- [G. *oligos,* few]. **1.** Combining forms denoting a few or a little. **2.** In chemistry, used in contrast to "poly-" in describing polymers; *e.g.,* oligosaccharide.

oligoamnios (ol′i-gō-am′nē-os) [oligo- + amnion]. Oligohydramnios; oligamnios; deficiency in the amount of the amniotic fluid.

oligocholia (ol′i-gō-kō′lē-ă) [oligo- + G. *cholē,* bile]. Hypocholia; a deficient secretion of bile.

oligochylia (ol′i-gō-kī′lē-ă) [oligo- + G. *chylos,* juice]. Hypochylia; a deficiency of gastric juice.

oligochymia (ol′i-gō-kī′mē-ă) [oligo- + G. *chymos,* juice]. A deficiency of chyme.

oligocystic (ol′i-gō-sis′tik) [oligo- + G. *kystis,* bladder, cyst]. Consisting of only a few cysts, as occasionally observed in certain examples of hydatidiform mole and other lesions that ordinarily have numerous cysts.

oligodactyly, oligodactylia (ol′i-gō-dak′ti-lē, -dak-til′ē-ă) [oligo- + G. *daktylos,* finger or toe]. Presence of fewer than five digits on one or more extremities.

oligodendria (ol′i-gō-den′drē-ă). Oligodendroglia.

oligodendroblast (ol′i-gō-den′drō-blast). A primitive glial cell that is the normal precursor cell of the oligodendrocyte.

oligodendroblastoma (ol′i-gō-den′drō-blas-tō′mă). A rare neoplasm of oligodendroblast origin and more rapid in growth than the oligodendroglioma.

oligodendrocyte (ol′i-gō-den′drō-sīt). A cell of the oligodendroglia.

oligodendroglia (ol′ī-gō-den-drog′lē-ă) [oligo- + G. *dendron,* tree, + *glia,* glue]. Oligodendria; one of the three types of glia cells (the other two being macroglia or astrocytes, and microglia) that, together with nerve cells, compose the tissue of the central nervous system. Oligodendroglia cells are characterized by variable numbers of veillike or sheetlike processes which are wrapped each around individual axons to form the myelin sheath of nerve fibers in the central nervous system (*cf.* Schwann cells in the peripheral nervous system); accordingly, they are more numerous in white matter than in gray matter.

oligodendroglioma (ol′i-gō-den′drō-glī-ō′mă). A relatively rare, moderately well differentiated, relatively slowly growing glioma that occurs most frequently in the cerebrum of adult persons; the neoplasm is grossly homogeneous, fairly well circumscribed, moderately firm, and somewhat gritty in consistency with interstitial calcification sufficiently dense so as to be detected by x-ray imaging of the skull. Microscopically, an o. is characterized by numerous, small, round, or ovoid, oligodendroglial cells with small, deeply stained nuclei (rarely observed in mitosis), and palely stained, indistinct cytoplasm; the neoplastic cells are rather uniformly distributed in a sparse, fibrillary stroma with scattered calcific bodies.

oligodipsia (ol′i-gō-dip′sē-ă) [oligo- + G. *dipsa,* thirst]. Abnormal lack of thirst. See also hypodipsia.

oligodontia (ol′i-gō-don′shē-ă) [oligo- + G. *odous,* tooth]. Hypodontia.

oligodynamic (ol′i-gō-dī-nam′ik) [oligo- + G. *dynamis,* power]. Active in very small quantity; *e.g.,* the germicidal effect of an exceedingly dilute solution (such as one to one hundred million) of copper in distilled water.

oligogalactia (ol′i-gō-gă-lak′tē-ă, -shē-ă) [oligo- + G. *gala,* milk]. Slight or scant secretion of milk.

oligoglucan-branching glycosyltransferase (ol′i-gō-glū′kan). 1,4-α-D-Glucan 6-α-D-glucosyltransferase.

oligo-1,6-glucosidase [EC 3.2.1.10]. Isomaltase; a glucanohydrolase cleaving α-1,6 links in isomaltose and dextrins produced from starch and glycogen by α-amylase.

oligohydramnios (ol′i-gō-hī-dram′nē-os) [oligo- + G. *hydōr,* water, + amnion]. Oligoamnios.

oligohydruria (ol′i-gō-hī-drū′rē-ă) [oligo- + G. *hydōr,* water, + *ouron,* urine]. Obsolete term for excretion of small quantities of urine, as seen in dehydration.

oligolecithal (ol′i-gō-les′i-thal) [oligo- + G. *lekithos,* yolk]. Having little yolk; denoting an egg in which there is only a little scattered deutoplasm.

oligomenorrhea (ol′i-gō-men-ō-rē′ă) [oligo- + menorrhea]. Scanty menstruation.

oligomer (ol′i-gō-mer). A polymer containing only a few repeating units, a "few" generally considered as less than 20.

oligomorphic (ol′-i-gō-mōr′fik) [oligo- + G. *morphē,* form]. Presenting few changes of form; not polymorphic.

oligonephronic (ol′i-gō-nef-ron′ik). Characterized by a reduced number of nephrons.

oligonucleotide (ol′i-gō-nū′klē-ō-tīd). A compound made up of the condensation of a small number of nucleotides. *Cf.* polynucleotide.

oligopepsia (ol′i-gō-pep′sē-ă). Hypopepsia.

oligoplastic (ol′i-gō-plas′tik) [oligo- + G. *plassō,* to form]. Deficient in reparative power.

oligopnea (ol′i-gop-nē′ă, -gop′nē-ă) [oligo- + G. *pnoē,* breath]. Hypopnea.

oligoptyalism (ol′i-gō-tī′ă-lizm, ol′i-gop-tī′) [oligo- + G. *ptyalon,* saliva]. Oligosialia; a scanty secretion of saliva.

oligoria (ol-i-gōr′ē-ă) [G. *oligōria,* negligence, slight esteem, fr. *oligos,* little, + *ōra,* care, regard]. An abnormal indifference toward or dislike of persons or things.

oligosaccharide (ol′i-gō-sak′ă-rīd). A compound made up of the condensation of a small number of monosaccharide units. *Cf.* polysaccharide.

oligosialia (ol′i-gō-sī-ă′lē-ă) [oligo- + G. *sialon,* saliva]. Oligoptyalism.

oligospermia, oligospermatism (ol-i-gō-sper′mē-ă, -mă-tizm). [oligo- + G. *sperma,* seed]. Oligozoospermatism; oligozoospermia; a subnormal concentration of spermatozoa in the penile ejaculate.

oligosymptomatic (ol′i-gō-simp-tō-mat′ik). Having few or minor symptoms.

oligosynaptic (ol′i-gō-si-nap′tik). Paucisynaptic; referring to neural conduction pathways that are interrupted by only a few synaptic junctions, *i.e.*, made up of a sequence of only few nerve cells, in contrast to polysynaptic pathways.

oligothymia (ol′i-gō-thī′mē-ă) [oligo- + -thymia]. Rarely used term for a poverty or loss of affect.

oligotrichia (ol′i-gō-trik′ē-ă). Hypotrichosis.

oligotrichosis (ol′i-gō-tri-kō′sis). Hypotrichosis.

oligotrophia, oligotrophy (ol′i-gō-trō′fē-ă, -got′rō-fē) [oligo- + G. *trophē*, nourishment]. Deficient nutrition.

oligozoospermatism, oligozoospermia (ol′i-gō-zō′ō-sper′mă-tizm, -sper′mē-ă) [oligo- + G. *zōon*, animal, + *sperma*, seed]. Oligospermia.

oliguresia, oliguresis (ol′i-gū-rē′sē-ă, -rē′sis) [oligo- + G. *ourēsis*, urination]. Oliguria.

oliguria (ol-i-gū′rē-ă) [oligo- + G. *ouron*, urine]. Oliguresia; scanty urination.

oliva, pl. **oli′vae** (ō-lī′vă) [L.] [NA]. Olive (1); inferior olive; olivary eminence or body; corpus olivare; a smooth oval prominence of the ventrolateral surface of the medulla oblongata lateral to the pyramidal tract, corresponding to the nucleus olivaris.
o. infe′rior, the oliva.
o. supe′rior, *nucleus* dorsalis corporis trapezoidei.

olivary (ol′i-vār-ē). **1.** Relating to the oliva. **2.** Relating to or shaped like an olive.

olive (ol′iv) [L. *oliva*]. **1.** Oliva. **2.** Common name for a tree of the genus *Olea* (family Oleaceae) or its fruit.
inferior o., oliva.
superior o., *nucleus* dorsalis corporis trapezoidei.

olive oil. The expressed oil of the fruit of *Olea europaea;* used as a cholagogue, laxative, and emollient, and in the preparation of liniments.

olivifugal (ol′i-vif′yū-găl) [oliva + L. *fugio*, to flee]. In a direction away from the olive.

olivipetal (ol′i-vip′ĕ-tăl) [oliva + L. *peto*, to seek]. In a direction toward the olive.

olivocochlear (ol′i-vō-kok′lē-ăr). See olivocochlear *bundle.*

olivopontocerebellar (ol′i-vō-pon′tō-sār-ĕ-bel′ar). Relating to the olivary nucleus, basis pontis, and cerebellum.

Ollendorf, H., German dermatologist. See Buschke-O. *syndrome.*

Ollier, Louis X.E.L., French surgeon, 1830–1900. See O. *graft; O.'s disease, method, theory;* O.-Thiersch *graft.*

-ology. See -logia.

ololiuqui (ō-lō-lyū′kē). A hallucinogen used in ceremonies by the Aztec Indians in Mexico. See also *Rivea corymbosa; Ipomoea rubrocoerulea.*

olophonia (ol′ō-fō′nē-ă) [G. *oloos*, destroyed, lost, + *phōnē*, voice]. Impaired speech due to an anatomical defect in the vocal organs.

Olszewski, Jerzy, Polish-Canadian neuropathologist, †1966. See Steele-Richardson-O. *disease, syndrome.*

-oma [G. *-ōma*]. Suffix, properly added only to words derived from G. roots, denoting a tumor or neoplasm.

omasitis (ō-mă-sī′tis). Inflammation of the omasum.

omasum (ō-mā′sŭm) [L. bullock's tripe]. Psalterium (2); the third stomach division of a ruminant.

-omata. Plural of -oma.

Ombrédanne, Louis, French surgeon, 1871–1956. See O. *operation.*

ombrophobia (om-brō-fō′bē-ă) [G. *ombros*, rainstorm, + *phobos*, fear]. Morbid fear of rain.

Omenn, Gilbert S., U.S. internist, *1941. See O's *syndrome.*

omental (ō-men′tăl). Epiploic; relating to the omentum.

omentectomy (ō-men-tek′tō-mē) [omentum + G. *ektomē*, excision]. Omentumectomy; resection or excision of the omentum.

omentitis (ō-men-tī′tis) [L. *omentum* + G. *-itis*, inflammation]. Peritonitis involving the omentum.

omento-, oment- [L. *omentum*]. Combining forms relating to the omentum. See also epiplo-.

omentofixation (ō-men′tō-fik-sā′shŭn). Omentopexy.

omentopexy (ō-men′tō-pek-sē) [omento- + G. *pēxis*, fixation]. Omentofixation. **1.** Suture of the great omentum to the abdominal wall to induce collateral portal circulation. **2.** Suture of the omentum to another organ to increase arterial circulation. See also omentoplasty.

omentoplasty (ō-men′tō-plas-tē) [omento- + G. *plastos*, formed]. Use of the greater omentum to cover or fill a defect, augment arterial or portal venous circulation, absorb effusions, or increase lymphatic drainage. See also omentopexy.

omentorrhaphy (ō-men-tōr′ă-fē) [omento- + G. *rhaphē*, suture]. Suture of an opening in the omentum.

omentovolvulus (ō-men-tō-vol′vyū-lŭs). Twisting of the omentum.

omentulum (ō-men′tyū-lŭm) [Mod. L. dim. of *omentum*]. *Omentum* minus.

omentum, pl. **omenta** (ō-men′tŭm, -tă) [L. the membrane that encloses the bowels] [NA]. A fold of peritoneum passing from the stomach to another abdominal organ.
gastrocolic o., o. majus.
gastrohepatic o., o. minus.
gastrosplenic o., *ligamentum* gastrosplenicum.
greater o., o. majus.
lesser o., o. minus.
o. ma′jus [NA], greater or gastrocolic o.; epiploon; caul (2); velum (3); a peritoneal fold passing from the greater curvature of the stomach to the transverse colon, hanging like an apron in front of the intestines.
o. mi′nus [NA], lesser or gastrohepatic o.; omentulum; Willis' pouch; a peritoneal fold passing from the margins of the porta hepatis and the bottom of the fissura ductus venosi to the lesser curvature of the stomach and to the upper border of the duodenum for a distance of about 2 cm beyond the gastroduodenal pylorus.

omentumectomy (ō-men-tŭ-mek′tō-mē). Omentectomy.

Ommaya, Ayub, 20th century U.S. neurosurgeon. See O. *reservoir.*

omn. hor. Abbreviation for L. *omni hora*, every hour.

omnipotence of thought (om-nip′ō-tens). A childish thought process whereby instantaneous realization of fantasies and wishes is expected.

omnivorous (om-niv′ŏ-rŭs) [L. *omnis*, all, + *voro*, to eat]. Living on food of all kinds, upon both animal and vegetable food.

omo- [G. *ōmos*, shoulder]. Combining form indicating relationship to the shoulder.

omoclavicular (ō′mō-kla-vik′yū-lăr). Relating to the shoulder and the clavicle; denoting an anomalous muscle attached to the coracoid process or upper edge of the scapula and to the clavicle.

omohyoid (ō-mō-hī′oyd). *Musculus* omohyoideus.

omophagia (ō-mō-fā′jē-ă) [G. *ōmos*, raw, + *phagein*, to eat]. The eating of raw food, especially of raw flesh.

omothyroid (ō-mō-thī′royd). Denoting a band of muscular fibers passing between the superior cornu of the thyroid cartilage and the omohyoid muscle.

OMP Abbreviation for orotidylic acid; orotidylate; oligo-*N*-methylmorpholinium propylene oxide.

OMPA Abbreviation for octamethyl pyrophosphoramide.

omphal-, omphalo- [G. *omphalos,* navel (umbilicus)]. Combining forms denoting relationship to the umbilicus.

omphalectomy (om-fă-lek'tō-mē) [omphal- + G. *ektomē,* excision]. Excision of the umbilicus or of a neoplasm connected with it.

omphalelcosis (om'fal-el-kō'sis) [omphal- + G. *helkōsis,* ulceration]. Ulceration at the umbilicus.

omphalic (om-fal'ik) [G. *omphalos,* umbilicus]. Umbilical.

omphalitis (om-fă-lī'tis). Inflammation of the umbilicus and surrounding parts.

omphalo-. See omphal-.

omphaloangiopagus (om'fă-lō-an-jē-op'ă-gŭs) [omphalo- + G. *angeion,* vessel, + *pagos,* something fixed]. Unequal conjoined twins in which the parasite derives its blood supply from the placenta of the autosite.

omphalocele (om'fal-ō-sēl, om'fă-lō-) [omphalo- + G. *kēlē,* hernia]. Exomphalos (3); congenital herniation of viscera into the base of the umbilical cord, with a covering membranous sac of peritoneum-amnion. The umbilical cord is inserted into the sac here, in contradistinction to its attachment in gastroschisis.

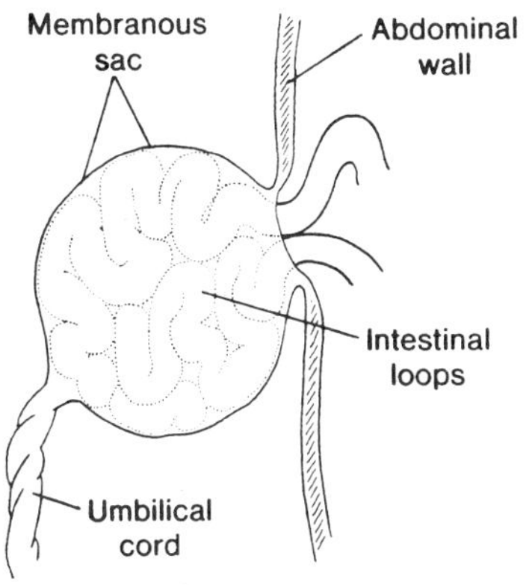

Omphalocele

omphaloenteric (om'fă-lō-en-tăr-ik). Relating to the umbilicus and the intestine.

omphalomesenteric (om'fă-lō-mez-en-tăr'ik). Obsolete term denoting relationship to the umbilicus and the mesentery or intestine.

omphalopagus (om'fă-lop'ă-gŭs) [omphalo- + G. *pagos,* something fixed]. Monomphalus; conjoined twins united at their umbilical regions.

omphalophlebitis (om'fă-lō-fle-bī'tis) [omphalo- + G. *phleps,* vein, + *-itis,* inflammation]. Inflammation of the umbilical veins.

omphalorrhagia (om'fă-lō-rā'jē-ă) [omphalo- + G. *rhēgnymi,* to burst forth]. Bleeding from the umbilicus.

omphalorrhea (om'fă-lō-rē'ă) [omphalo- + G. *rhoia,* flow]. A serous discharge from the umbilicus.

omphalorrhexis (om'fă-lō-rek'sis) [omphalo- + G. *rhēxis,* rupture]. Rupture of the umbilical cord during childbirth.

omphalos (om'fă-los) [G. navel]. Rarely used term for umbilicus.

omphalosite (om'fă-lō-sīt) [omphalo- + G. *sitos,* food]. Placental parasitic twin; the parasitic member of unequal monochorial twins which derives its blood supply from the placenta of the autosite and is incapable of independent existence after birth and separation from the placenta.

omphalospinous (om'fă-lō-spī'nŭs). Denoting a line connecting the umbilicus and the anterior superior spine of the ilium, on which lies McBurney's point.

omphalotomy (om-fă-lot'ō-mē) [omphalo- + G. *tomē,* incision]. Cutting of the umbilical cord at birth.

omphalotripsy (om'fă-lō-trip'sē) [omphalo- + G. *tripsis,* a rubbing]. Crushing, instead of cutting, the umbilical cord after childbirth.

omphalovesical (om'fă-lō-ves'i-kăl). Vesicoumbilical.

omphalus (om'fă-lŭs) [G. *omphalos,* navel]. Rarely used term for umbilicus.

OMS Organic mental *syndrome.*

onanism (ō'nan-izm) [*Onan,* son of Judah, who practiced it. Genesis 38:9]. **1.** Coitus interruptus; withdrawal of the penis before ejaculation, in order to prevent insemination and fecundation of the ovum. **2.** Incorrectly used as a synonym of masturbation.

oncho-. See onco-.

Onchocerca (ong-kō-ser'kă) [G. *onkos,* a barb, + *kerkos,* tail]. *Oncocerca;* a genus of elongated filariform nematodes (family Onchocercidae) that inhabit the connective tissue of their hosts, usually within firm nodules in which these parasites are coiled and entangled.

O. cervica'lis, a species common in the ligamentum nuchae of horses, mules, and asses, where it has been suspected of playing a role in fistulous withers and poll evil.

O. gibso'ni, a species that infects the subcutaneous tissues of cattle, buffalo, and sheep.

O. liena'lis, a species that inhabits the connective tissue around the ligamentum nuchae, tibiofemoral ligament, spleen capsule, and other sites in cattle and buffalo; although widely distributed, it is not common in the U.S.

O. vol'vulus, the blinding nodular worm, a species that causes onchocerciasis.

onchocerciasis (ong'kō-ser-kī'ă-sis). Oncocerciasis; onchocercosis; coast erysipelas; volvulosis; blinding disease; mal morado; infection with *Onchocerca* (especially *O. volvulus*), marked by nodular swellings forming a fibrous cyst enveloping the coiled parasites; microfilariae move freely out of the nodule and escape into the intercellular lymph in the dermis. Dermatological changes often develop, especially in Africa, resulting in intense pruritus, scaly or lichenoid skin, depigmentation, and destruction of elastic fibers. Most important are the ocular complications that may develop after a long chronic course, with blindness frequently occurring in advanced cases, probably as a result of the sensitization of the cornea to the microfilariae.

ocular o., Robles' disease; river blindness; ocular complications, such as keratitis, iridocyclitis, or retrobulbar neuritis, caused by the microfilariae of *Onchocerca volvulus.*

onchocercid (ong-kō-ser'kid). Common name for members of the family Onchocercidae.

Onchocercidae (ong-kō-ser'ki-dē). A family of nematode parasites (superfamily Filarioidea) characterized by production of microfilariae; it includes the genera *Onchocerca, Wuchereria, Brugia, Loa,* and *Mansonella.*

onchocercosis (ong'kō-ser-kō'sis). Onchocerciasis.

onco-, oncho- [G. *onkos,* bulk, mass]. Combining forms denoting a tumor or some relation to a tumor, or to bulk, volume.

Oncocerca (ong-kō-ser'kă). *Onchocerca.*

oncocerciasis (ong'kō-ser-kī'ă-sis). Onchocerciasis.

oncocyte (ong'kō-sīt) [onco- + G. *kytos,* cell]. A large, granular, acidophilic tumor cell containing numerous mitochondria; a neoplastic oxyphil cell.

oncocytoma (ong'kō-sī-tō'mă) [onco- + G. *kytos,* cell, + *-oma,* tumor]. Oxyphil adenoma; a glandular tumor composed of large cells with cytoplasm that is granular and eosionphilic due to the presence of abundant active mitochondria; occurs uncommonly in the kidney, salivary glands, and endocrine glands.

oncofetal (ong-kō-fē'tăl). Relating to tumor-associated substances present in fetal tissue, as o. antigens.

oncogene (ong'kō-jēn). Transforming gene; a viral gene, found in certain retroviruses, that may transform the host cell to a neoplastic phenotype but is not required for viral replication.

oncogenesis (ong-kō-jen'ĕ-sis) [onco- + G. *genesis,* production]. Origin and growth of a neoplasm.

oncogenic (ong-kō-jen'ik). Oncogenous.

oncogenous (ong-koj'ĕ-nŭs). Oncogenic; causing, inducing, or being suitable for the formation and development of a neoplasm.

oncograph (ong'kō-graf) [onco- + G. *graphē,* a record]. A recording oncometer, or the recording portion of an oncometer.

oncography (ong'kog'ră-fē). Graphic representation, by means of a special apparatus, of the size and configuration of an organ.

oncoides (ong-koy'dēz) (onco- + G. *eidos,* resemblance]. Intumescence or turgescence.

oncologist (ong-kol'ō-jist). A specialist in oncology.

oncology (ong-kol'ō-jē) [onco- + G. *logos,* study]. The study or science dealing with the physical, chemical, and biologic properties and features of neoplasms, including causation, pathogenesis, and treatment.

oncolysis (ong-kol'i-sis) [onco- + G. *lysis,* dissolution]. Destruction of a neoplasm; sometimes used with reference to the reduction of any swelling or mass.

oncolytic (ong-kō-lit'ik). Pertaining to, characterized by, or causing oncolysis.

oncoma (ong-kō'mă) [G. *onkos,* mass, + *-oma,* tumor]. Obsolescent term for neoplasm or tumor.

Oncomelania (ong'kō-mĕ-lā'nĭ-ă) [onco- + G. *melas (melan-),* black]. A medically important genus of amphibious freshwater operculate snails of the family Hydrobiidae (subfamily Hydrobiinae; subclass Prosobranchiata). In the Orient, several subspecies of *O. hupensis* serve as intermediate hosts of the oriental blood fluke, *Schistosoma japonicum.*

oncometer (ong-kom'ĕ-ter) [onco- + G. *metron,* measure]. **1.** An instrument for measuring the size and configuration of the kidneys and other organs. **2.** The measuring, as distinguished from the recording part of the oncograph.

oncometric (ong-kō-met'rik). Relating to oncometry.

oncometry (ong-kom'ĕ-trē). Measurement of the size of an organ.

oncornavruses (ong-kōr'nă-vī'rŭs-ez). Oncovirinae.

oncosis (ong-kō'sis) [G. *onkōsis,* swelling, fr. *onkos,* bulk, mass]. A condition characterized by the formation of one or more neoplasms or tumors.

oncosphere (ong'-kō-sfēr) [onco- + G. *sphaira,* sphere]. Hexacanth.

oncotherapy (ong-kō-thār'ă-pē). Treatment of tumors.

oncotic (ong-kot'ik). Relating to or caused by edema or any swelling (oncosis).

oncotomy (ong-kot'ō-mē) [onco- + G. *tomē,* incision]. Incision of an abscess, cyst, or other tumor.

oncotropic (ong'kō-trop'ik) [onco- + G. *tropē,* a turning]. Tumoraffin; manifesting a special affinity for neoplasms or neoplastic cells.

Oncovirinae (ong-kō-vir'i-nē). Oncornaviruses; a subfamily of viruses (family Retroviridae) composed of the RNA tumor viruses. Subgroups are based on antigenicity, host range, and kind of malignancy induced (avian, feline, hamster, or murine leukemia-sarcoma complex; murine mammary tumor virus; primate oncoviruses). Like other retroviruses, the oncoviruses contain RNA-dependent DNA polymerases (reverse transcriptases). Virions, on the basis of morphology and antigenicity, are of four types: 1) type A, found only within infected cells and seemingly immature in that there is no electron-dense nucleoid; 2) type B, having an eccentric electron-dense nucleoid and associated with the Bittner mammary tumor; 3) type C, having a centrally located, electron-dense nucleoid and associated with leukemia-sarcoma complexes of various species; 4) type D, having a central electron-dense nucleoid but differing in other respects from type C. An important aspect of these viruses seems to be utilization of viral reverse transcriptase to make DNA which can be integrated into the DNA of the host cell where it serves as a cellular gene.

oncovirus (ong'kō-vī'rŭs). Any virus of the subfamily Oncovirinae. See also oncogenic *virus.*

-one. Systematic suffix indicating a ketone (–CO–) group.

oneiric (ō-nī'rik) [G. *oneiros,* dream]. Oniric. **1.** Pertaining to dreams. **2.** Pertaining to the clinical state of oneirophrenia.

oneirism (ō-nī'rizm) [G. *oneiros,* dream]. A waking dream state.

oneirocritical (ō-nī-rō-krit'i-kăl) [G. *oneiros,* dream, + *kritikōs,* skilled in judgment]. Pertaining to the logic of dreams.

oneirodynia (ō-nī-rō-din'ē-ă) [G. *oneiros,* dream, + *odynē,* pain]. An unpleasant or painful dream.

o. acti'va, somnambulism (1).

o. gra'vis, nightmare.

oneirogmus (ō'nī-rog'mŭs) [G. *oneirōgmos,* an effusion of semen during sleep]. Nocturnal emission of semen, often related to erotic dreams. See also wet *dream.*

oneirology (ō-nī-rol'ō-jē) [G. *oneiros,* dream, + *logos,* study]. The study of dreams and their content.

oneirophrenia (ō-nī-rō-frē'nē-ă) [G. *oneiros,* dream, + *phrēn,* mind]. A state in which hallucinations occur, caused by such conditions as prolonged deprivation of sleep, sensory isolation, and a variety of drugs.

oneiroscopy (ō-nī-ros'kŏ-pē) [G. *oneiros,* dream, + *skopeō,* to examine]. Rarely used term for the diagnosis of a person's mental state by an analysis of his dreams.

oniomania (ō'nē-ō-mā'nē-ă) [G. *ōnios,* for sale, + *mania,* insanity]. Rarely used term for the morbidly exaggerated need or urge to buy beyond the realistic needs of the individual.

oniric (ō-nī'rik). Oneiric.

-onium. Suffix indicating a positively charged radical; *e.g.,* ammonium, NH_4^+.

onko-. See onco-.

onlay (on'lā). **1.** A metal (usually gold) cast restoration of the occlusal surface of a posterior tooth or the lingual surface of an anterior tooth, the entire surface of which is in dentin without side walls; retention in the anterior tooth is by pins and in the posterior by pins and/or boxes in retentive grooves in the buccal and lingual walls. **2.** A graft applied on the exterior of a bone.

onomatomania (on'ō-mat-ō-mā'nē-ă) [G. *onomo,* name, + *mania,* frenzy]. An abnormal impulse to dwell upon certain words and their supposed significance, or to frantically try to recall a particular word.

onomatophobia (on'ō-mat-ō-fō'bē-ă) [G. *onomo,* name, + *phobos,* fear]. Nomatophobia; abnormal dread of certain words or names because of their supposed significance.

onomatopoiesis (on'ō-mat'ō-poy-ē'sis) [G. *onoma,* name, + *poiēsis,* making]. The making of a name or word, especially to express or imitate a natural sound (*e.g.,* hiss, crash, boom); in psychiatry, the tendency to make new words of this type is said to characterize some persons with schizophrenia. See also neologism.

ontogenesis (on-tō-jen'ĕ-sis). Ontogeny.

ontogenetic, ontogenic (on'tō-jĕ-net'ik, -jen'ik). Relating to ontogeny.

ontogeny (on-toj'ĕ-nē) [G. *ōn,* being, + *genesis,* origin]. Ontogenesis; development of the individual, as distinguished from phylogeny, evolutionary development of the species.

Onufrowicz, B. See Onuf's *nucleus.*

onyalai (on-i-al'ā). Akembe; kafindo; an acute disease affecting natives of Central Africa, characterized by bloody vesicles of the mouth and other mucous surfaces, hematuria, and melena; defective nutrition may be the cause.

onych-. See onycho-.

onychalgia (on-i-kal'jē-ă) [onycho- + G. *algos,* pain]. Pain in the nails.

onychatrophia, onychatrophy (on'i-kă-trō'fē-ă, on-ik-at'rō-fē) [onycho- + G. *atrophia,* atrophy]. Atrophy of the nails.

onychauxis (on-i-kawk'sis) [onycho- + G. *auxē,* increase]. Marked overgrowth of the fingernails or toenails.

onychectomy (on-i-kek'tō-mē) [onycho- + G. *ectomē,* excision]. Ablation of a toenail or fingernail.

onychia (ō-nik'ē-ă) [onycho- + G. *-ia,* condition]. Onychitis; onyxitis; inflammation of the matrix of the nail.
o. latera'lis, paronychia.
o. malig'na, Wardrop's disease; acute o. occurring spontaneously in debilitated patients, or in response to slight trauma.
o. periungua'lis, paronychia.
o. sic'ca, a condition characterized by brittle nails.

onychitis (on-i-kī'tis). Onychia.

onycho-, onych- [G. *onyx,* nail]. Combining forms denoting nail.

onychoclasis (on-i-kok'lă-sis) [onycho- + G. *klasis,* breaking]. Breaking of the nails.

onychocryptosis (on'i-kō-krip-tō'sis) [onycho- + G. *kryptō,* to conceal]. Ingrown *nail.*

onychodystrophy (on'i-kō-dis'trō-fē) [onycho- + G. *dys-,* bad, + *trophē,* nourishment]. Dystrophic changes in the nails occurring as a congenital defect or due to any illness or injury that may cause a malformed nail.

onychograph (on'i-kō-graf) [onycho- + G. *graphō,* to write]. An instrument for recording the capillary blood pressure as shown by the circulation under the nail.

onychogryphosis (on'i-kō-gri-fō'sis). Onychogryposis.

onychogryposis (on'i-kō-gri-pō'sis) [onycho- + G. *grypōsis,* a curvature]. Onychogryphosis; gryposis unguium; enlargement with increased thickening and curvature of the fingernails or toenails.

onychoheterotopia (on'i-kō-het-er-ō-tō'pē-ă). Abnormal placement of nails.

onychoid (on'i-koyd) [onycho- + G. *eidos,* resemblance]. Resembling a fingernail in structure or form.

onychology (on-i-kol'ō-jē) [onycho- + G. *logos,* treatise]. Study of the nails.

onycholysis (on-i-kol'i-sis) [onycho- + G. *lysis,* loosening]. Loosening of the nails, beginning at the free border, and usually incomplete.

onychoma (on-i-kō'mă) [onycho- + G. *-ōma,* tumor]. A tumor arising from the nail bed.

onychomadesis (on'i-kō-mă-dē'sis) [onycho- + G. *madēsis,* a growing bald, fr. *madaō,* to be moist, (of hair) fall off]. Complete shedding of the nails, usually associated with systemic disease.

onychomalacia (on'i-kō-mă-lā'shē-ă) [onycho- + G. *malakia,* softness]. Abnormal softness of the nails.

onychomycosis (on'i-kō-mī-kō'sis) [onycho- + G. *mykes,* fungus, + *-ōsis,* condition]. Ringworm of nails; tinea unguium; a fungus infection of the nails, causing thickening, roughness, and splitting, usually caused by *Trichophyton rubrum* or *T. mentagrophytes.*

onychonosus (on-i-kon'ō-sŭs) [onycho- + G. *nosos,* disease]. Onychopathy.

onycho-osteodysplasia (on'i-kō-os'tē-ō-dis-plā'zē-ă). Nail-patella *syndrome.*

onychopathic (on'i-kō-path'ik). Relating to or suffering from any disease of the nails.

onychopathology (on'i-kō-pă-thol'ō-jē). Study of diseases of the nails.

onychopathy (on-i-kop'ă-thē) [onycho- + G. *pathos,* suffering]. Onychonosus; onychosis; any disease of the nails.

onychophagy, onychophagia (on-i-kof'ă-jē, on'i-kō-fā'jē-ă). [onycho- + G. *phagein,* to eat]. Habitual nailbiting.

onychophosis (on'i-kō-fō'sis) [onycho- + G. *phōs,* light, + *-osis,* condition]. A growth of horny epithelium in the nail bed.

onychophyma (on'i-kō-fī'mă) [onycho- + G. *phyma,* growth]. Swelling or hypertrophy of the nails.

onychoplasty (on'i-kō-plas-tē) [onycho- + G. *plastos,* formed, shaped]. A corrective or plastic operation on the nail matrix.

onychoptosis (on'i-kop-tō'sis) [onycho- + G. *ptōsis,* a falling]. Falling off of the nails.

onychorrhexis (on'i-kō-rek'sis) [onycho- + G. *rhēxis,* a breaking]. Abnormal brittleness of the nails with splitting of the free edge.

onychoschizia (on'i-kō-skiz'ē-ă) [onycho- + G. *schizein,* to divide, + *-ia,* condition]. Splitting of the nails in layers.

onychosis (on-i-kō'sis). Onychopathy.

onychostroma (on'i-kō-strō'mă) [onycho- + G. *strōma,* bedding]. *Matrix* unguis.

onychotillomania (on'i-kot'i-lō-mā'nē-ă) [onycho- + G. *tillein,* to pluck, + *mania,* insanity]. A tendency to pick at the nails.

onychotomy (on-i-kot'ō-mē) [onycho- + G. *tomē,* cutting]. Incision into a toenail or fingernail.

onychotrophy (on-i-kot'rō-fē) [onycho- + G. *trophē,* nourishment]. Nutrition of the nails.

onyx (on'iks) [G. nail]. Unguis.

onyxis (on-iks'is). Ingrown *nail.*

onyxitis (on-iks-ī'tis). Onychia.

oo- [G. *ōon,* egg. OO-]. Combining form denoting egg, ovary. See also oophor-, ovario-, ovi-, ovo-.

oocyesis (ō-ō-sī-ē'sis) [G. *ōon,* egg, + *kyēsis,* pregnancy]. Ovarian *pregnancy.*

oocyst (ō'ō-sist) [G. *ōon,* egg, + *kystis,* bladder]. The encysted form of the fertilized macrogamete, or zygote, in coccidian Sporozoea in which sporogonic multiplication occurs; results in the formation of sporozoites, infectious agents for the next stage of the sporozoan life cycle.

oocyte (ō'ō-sīt) [G. *ōon,* egg, + *kytos,* a hollow (cell)]. Ovocyte; the immature ovum. See fig. on p. 1088.
primary o., an o. during its growth phase and prior to completion of the first maturation division.
secondary o., an o. in which the first meiotic division is completed; the second meiotic division usually stops short of completion unless fertilization occurs.

oogenesis (ō-ō-jen'ĕ-sis) [G. *ōon,* egg, + *genesis,* origin]. Ovigenesis; ovogenesis; process of formation and development of the ovum.

oogenetic (ō-ō-jĕ-net'ik). Producing ova. Also called oogenic; oogenous; ovigenetic; ovigenic; ovigenous.

oogenic, oogenous (ō-ō-jen'ik, ō-oj'ĕ-nŭs). Oogenetic.

oogonium, pl. **oogonia** (ō-ō-gō'nē-ŭm, -ă) [G. *ōon,* egg, + *gonē,* generation]. **1.** The primitive egg mother cell, from which the oocytes are developed. **2.** In fungi, the female gametangium bearing one or more oospores.

ookinesis, ookinesia (ō'ō-ki-nē'sis, -zē-ă) [G. *ōon,* egg, + *kinēsis,* movement]. Chromosomal movements of the egg during maturation and fertilization.

ookinete (ō'ō-ki-ne't, -kī'ne't) [G. *ōon,* egg, + *kinētos,* motile]. Vermicule (2); the motile zygote of the malarial organism that penetrates the mosquito stomach to form an oocyst under the outer gut lining; the contents of the occyst subsequently divide to produce numerous sporozoites.

oolemma (ō-ō-lem'ă) [G. *ōon,* egg, + *lemma,* sheath]. Plasma membrane of the oocyte.

oomycosis (ō'ō-mī-kō'sis). A mycosis caused by fungi belonging to the class Oomycetes; *e.g.,* hyphomycosis, rhinosporidiosis.

oophagia, oophagy (ō-ō-fā'jē-ă, ō-of'ă-jē) [G. *ōon,* egg, + *phagein,* to eat]. The habitual eating of eggs; subsisting largely on eggs.

oophor-, oophoro- [Mod. L. *oophoron,* ovary, fr. G. *ōophoros,* egg-bearing]. Combining forms denoting the ovary. See also oo-, ovario-.

oophoralgia (ō-of-ōr-al'jē-ă) [oophor- + G. *algos,* pain]. Ovarialgia.

oophorectomy (ō-of-ōr-ek'tō-mē) [G. *ōon,* egg, + *phoros,* bearing, + *ectomē,* excision]. Ovariectomy.

oophoritis (ō-of-ōr-ī'tis) [G. *ōon,* egg, + *phoros,* a bearing, + *-itis,* inflammation]. Ovaritis; inflammation of an ovary.

oophoro-. See oophor-.

oophorocystectomy (ō-of'ōr-ō-sis-tek'tō-mē). Excision of an ovarian cyst.

oophorocystosis (ō-of'ōr-ō-sis-tō'sis). Ovarian cyst formation.

oophorohysterectomy (ō-of'ōr-ō-his-ter-ek'tō-mē). Ovariohysterectomy.

oophoroma (ō-of-ōr-ō'mă). Ovarioncus; an ovarian tumor.

oophoron (ō-of'ōr-on) [G. *ōon,* egg, + *phoros,* bearing]. Rarely used term for ovary.

oophoropathy (ō-of-ōr-op'ă-thē). Ovariopathy.

oophoropeliopexy (ō-of'ōr-ō-pel'i-ō-pek-sē) [oophoro- + G. *pellis,* pelvis, + *pēxis,* fixation]. Oophororrhaphy.

oophoropexy (ō-of'ōr-ō-pek-sē) [oophoro- + G. *pēxis,* fixation]. Surgical fixation or suspension of an ovary.

oophoroplasty (ō-of'ōr-ō-plas-tē) [oophoro- + G. *plastos,* formed, shaped]. Plastic operation upon an ovary.

oophororrhaphy (ō-of-ō-rōr'ă-fē) [oophoro- + G. *rhaphē,* suture]. Oophoropeliopexy; suspension of ovary by attachment to pelvic wall.

oophorosalpingectomy (ō-of'ōr-ō-sal-pin-jek'tō-mē). Ovariosalpingectomy.

oophorosalpingitis (ō-of'ōr-ō-sal-pin-jī'tis) [oophoro- + salpingitis]. Ovariosalpingitis.

oophorostomy (ō-of-ōr-os'tō-mē) [oophoro- + G. *stoma,* mouth]. Ovariostomy.

oophorotomy (ō-of-ōr-ot'ō-mē) [oophoro- + G. *tomē,* incision]. Ovariotomy.

oophorrhagia (ō-of-ōr-rā'jē-ă) [oophoro- + G. *rhēgnymi,* to burst forth]. Ovarian hemorrhage.

ooplasm (ō'ō-plazm) [G. *ōon,* egg, + *plasma,* a thing formed]. Protoplasmic portion of the ovum.

oosporangium (ō'ō-spō-ran'jē-ŭm) [oospore + G. *angeion,* vessel]. Obsolete term for oogonium (2).

oospore (ō'ō-spōr) [see *Oospora*]. A thick-walled fungus spore which develops from a female gamete either through fertilization or parthenogenesis in an oogonium.

oothec-, ootheco- [Mod. L. *ootheca*]. Obsolescent combining forms denoting the ovary. See oo-; oophor-; ovario-.

ootheca (ō-oth-ē'kă) [G. *ōon,* egg, + *thēkē,* box, case]. Rarely used term for ovary.

ootid (ō'ō-tid) [G. *ōotidion,* a diminutive egg. See -id (2)]. The nearly mature ovum after the first maturation has been completed and the second initiated; in most higher mammals, the second maturation division is not completed unless fertilization occurs.

ootype (ō'ō-tīp) [G. *ōon,* egg, + *typos,* stamp, print]. The central portion of the ovarian complex of trematodes and cestodes in which fertilization takes place and the vitellarian or eggshell materials are coated over the egg; this occurs in a rapid, stamping-mill sequence, after which eggs pass into the uterus for tanning of the shell, storage, and passage toward the genital pore.

opacification (ō-pas'i-fi-kā'shŭn) [L. *opacus,* shady]. **1.** The process of making opaque. **2.** The formation of opacities.

opacity (ō-pas'i-tē) [L. *opacitas,* shadiness]. **1.** A lack of transparency; an opaque or nontransparent area. **2.** Mental dullness.
snowball o., a spherical, white body seen in the vitreous in asteroid hyalosis.

opalescent (ō-pă-les'ent) [Fr. fr. L. *opalus,* opal]. Resembling an

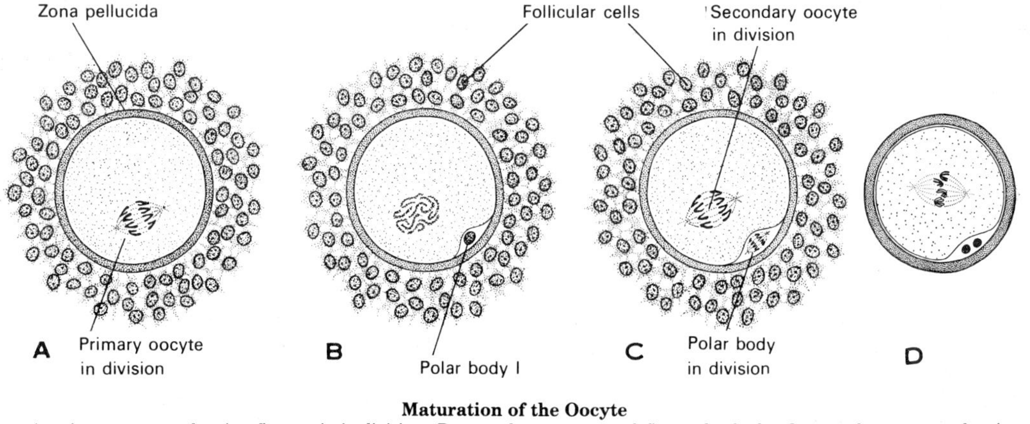

Maturation of the Oocyte
A, primary oocyte showing first meiotic division; *B,* secondary oocyte and first polar body; *C,* secondary oocyte showing second meiotic division immediately after ovulation; *D,* completion of secondary meiotic division with production of second polar body immediately after fertilization.

opal in the display of various colors; denoting certain bacterial cultures.

Opalski, Adam, Polish physician, 1897–1963. See O. *cell.*

opaque (ō-pāk′) [Fr. fr. L. *opacus,* shady]. Impervious to light; not translucent or only slightly so.

opeidoscope (op-ī′dō-skōp) [G. *ops* (*op-*), a voice, + *eidos,* appearance, + *skopeō,* to view]. An apparatus for study of voice vibrations by which the vibrations of a diaphragm, started by the voice, move a mirror by which a ray of light is reflected on a screen.

open (ō′pen) [A.S.]. **1.** Not closed; exposed, said of a wound. **2.** To enter or expose, as a wound or cavity.

opening (ō′pen-ing). Apertura. See also aperture; fossa; ostium; orifice.

access o., access.
aortic o., *hiatus* aorticus.
cardiac o., *ostium* cardiacum.
esophageal o., *hiatus* esophageus.
external urethral o., *ostium* urethrae externum.
femoral o., *hiatus* tendineus.
ileocecal o., *ostium* ileocecale.
o. of inferior vena cava, *ostium* venae cavae inferioris.
internal urethral o., *ostium* urethrae internum.
lacrimal o., *punctum* lacrimale.
pharyngeal o. of auditory tube, *ostium* pharyngeum tubae auditivae.
pharyngeal o. of eustachian tube, *ostium* pharyngeum tubae auditivae.
piriform o., *apertura* piriformis.
pulmonary o., *ostium* trunci pulmonalis.
o.'s of pulmonary veins, *ostia* venarum pulmonalium.
saphenous o., *hiatus* saphenus.
o. of superior vena cava, *ostium* venae cavae superioris.
tendinous o., *hiatus* tendineus.
tympanic o. of auditory tube, *ostium* tympanicum tubae auditivae.
tympanic o. of canal for chorda tympani, *apertura* tympanica canaliculi chordae tympani.
tympanic o. of eustachian tube, *ostium* tympanicum tubae auditivae.
ureteral o., *ostium* ureteris.
urethral o.'s, see *ostium* urethrae externum; *ostium* urethrae internum.
o. of uterus, *ostium* uteri.
vaginal o., *ostium* vaginae.
vertical o., vertical *dimension.*

operable (op′er-ă-bl). Denoting a patient or condition on which a surgical procedure can be performed with a reasonable expectation of cure or relief.

operant (op′er-ănt). Target behavior (1); target response; in conditioning, any behavior or specific response chosen by the experimenter; its frequency is intended to increase or decrease by the judicious pairing with it of a reinforcer when it occurs.

operate (op′er-āt) [L. *operor,* pp. *-atus,* to work, fr. *opus,* work]. **1.** To work upon the body by the hands or by means of cutting or other instruments to correct a surgical problem. **2.** To cause a movement of the bowels; said of a laxative or cathartic remedy.

OPERATION

operation (op-er-ā′shŭn). **1.** Any surgical procedure. **2.** The act, manner, or process of functioning. See also entries under method; procedure; technique.

Abbe o., use of an Abbe flap in plastic surgery of the lips.
Adams' o. for ectropion, excision of a wedge from the lateral margin of the eyelid in order to shorten it.
Ammon's o., blepharoplasty by transplantation from the cheek.
Anagnostakis' o., Hotz-Anagnostakis o.
Arlt's o., transplantation of the eyelashes back from the edge of the lid in trichiasis.
Baldy's o., Webster's o.; an obsolete o. for retrodisplacement of the uterus, consisting of bringing the round ligaments through the perforated broad ligaments and attaching them to each other and to the back of the uterus.
Ball's o., division of the sensory nerve trunks supplying the anus, for relief of pruritus ani.
Barkan's o., goniotomy for congenital glaucoma under direct observation of the anterior chamber angle.
Bassini's o., an o. for the radical cure of hernia; after reduction of the hernia, the sac is twisted, ligated, and cut off, then a new canal is made by uniting the edge of the internal oblique muscle to the inguinal ligament, placing on this the cord, and covering the latter by the external oblique muscle.
Baudelocque's o., an incision through the posterior cul-de-sac of the vagina for the removal of the ovum, in extrauterine pregnancy.
Beer's o., flap o. for cataract.
Belsey o., a transthoracic procedure for sliding hiatal hernia; the esophagus is intussuscepted into the stomach by two rows of interrupted sutures which pull and fold it into the subjacent gastric cardia, as well as attach it to the tendinous diaphragm; the posterior crural fibers are also approximated.
Billroth's o. I and II, (1) Billroth I anastomosis; excision of the pylorus with end-to-end anastomosis of stomach and duodenum; **(2)** Billroth II anastomosis; resection of the pylorus with the greater part of the lesser curvature of the stomach, closure of the cut ends of the duodenum and stomach, followed by a posterior gastrojejunostomy.
Blalock-Hanlon o., the creation of a large atrial septal defect as a palliative procedure for complete transposition of the great arteries.
Blalock-Taussig o., an o. for congenital malformations of the heart, in which an abnormally small volume of blood passes through the pulmonary circuit; blood from the systemic circulation is directed to the lungs by anastomosing the right or left subclavian artery to the right or left pulmonary artery.
Blaskovics' o., resection of the musculus levator palpebrae superioris for remedying blepharoptosis.
bloodless o., an o. performed with negligible loss of blood.
Bonnet's o., enucleation of the eyeball.
Bowman's o., (1) double-needle o. for dilaceration of a cataract, two lance-pointed needles being introduced through opposite sides of the cornea, the points meeting in the center of the lens and then being separated by moving the handles toward each other; **(2)** slitting the canaliculus for the relief of stenosis, to evacuate an abscess of the lacrimal sac, etc.
Bozeman's o., an o. for uterovaginal fistula, the cervix uteri being attached to the bladder and opening into its cavity.
Bricker o., an o. utilizing an isolated segment of ileum to collect urine from both ureters and conduct it to the skin surface.
Brock o., transventricular valvotomy for relief of pulmonic valvar stenosis.
Brunschwig's o., total pelvic *exenteration.*
Burow's o., an o. in which triangles of skin adjacent to a sliding flap are excised to facilitate movement of the flap.
Caldwell-Luc o., Luc's o.; intraoral antrostomy; an intraoral procedure for opening into the maxillary antrum through the supradental (canine) fossa above the maxillary premolar teeth.
capital o., obsolete term for an o. of such magnitude or involving vital organs to such an extent that it is *per se* dangerous to life.

Carmody-Batson o., reduction of fractures of the zygoma and zygomatic arch through an intraoral incision above the maxillary molar teeth.
Caslick's o., an o. for the correction of faulty conformation of the vulva of the mare, a frequent cause of low-grade vaginitis and infertility; consists of surgical closure of the dorsal portion of the vulva.
cesarean o., see cesarean *section* and cesarean *hysterectomy.*
commando o., commando *procedure.*
concrete o.'s, in the psychology of Piaget, a stage of development in thinking, occurring approximately between 7 and 11 years of age, during which a child becomes capable of reasoning about concrete situations.
Cotte's o., presacral *neurectomy.*
Dana's o., posterior *rhizotomy.*
Dandy o., **(1)** see third *ventriculostomy;* **(2)** see trigeminal *rhizotomy.*
Daviel's o., extracapsular cataract extraction.
debulking o., excision of a major part of a malignant tumor which cannot be completely removed, so as to enhance the effectiveness of subsequent radio- or chemotherapy.
decompression o.'s, see related subentries under decompression.
de Vincentiis o., goniotomy for congenital glaucoma.
Doyle's o., paracervical uterine denervation.
Dupuy-Dutemps o., a modified dacryocystorhinostomy for stenosis of the lacrimal duct.
Elliot's o., trephining of the eyeball at the corneoscleral margin to relieve tension in glaucoma.
Emmet's o., trachelorrhaphy.
Esser o., see inlay *graft.*
Estes o., an o. for sterility in which a portion of an ovary is implanted on one uterine cornu.
Estlander o., use of an Estlander flap in plastic surgery of the lips.
fenestration o., a rarely used surgical procedure producing an opening from the external auditory canal to the membranous labyrinth to improve hearing in hearing impairment of the conduction type.
Filatov's o., obsolete eponym for penetrating *keratoplasty.*
filtering o., a surgical procedure for creation of a fistula between the anterior chamber of the eye and the subconjunctival space in treatment of glaucoma.
Finney's o., gastroduodenostomy which creates, by the technique of closure, a large opening to insure free emptying from the stomach.
flap o., **(1)** flap *amputation* **(2)** in dental surgery, an o. in which a portion of the mucoperiosteal tissues is surgically detached from the underlying bone or impacted tooth for better access and visibility in exploring the area covered by the tissue. See also subentries under flap.
Foley o., Foley Y-plasty *pyelopasty.*
Fontan o., Fontan *procedure.*
formal o.'s, in the psychology of Piaget, a stage of development in thinking, occurring approximately between 11 and 15 years of age, during which a child becomes capable of reasoning about abstract situations; reasoning at this stage is comparable to that of normal adults but less sophisticated.
Fothergill's o., Manchester o.
Frazier-Spiller o., see trigeminal *rhizotomy.*
Fredet-Ramstedt o., pyloromyotomy.
Freund's o., **(1)** total abdominal hysterectomy for uterine cancer; **(2)** chondrotomy to relieve Freund's anomaly.
Frost-Lang o., insertion of a spherical prosthesis after the enucleation of the eyeball.
Gifford's o., delimiting *keratotomy.*
Gigli's o., pubiotomy.
Gilliam's o., an o. for retroversion of uterus by suturing round ligaments to abdominal wall fascia.
Gillies' o., a technique for reducing fractures of the zycoma and the zygomatic arch through an incision in the temporal region above the hairline.
Gil-Vernet o., extended *pyelotomy.*
Glenn's o., anastomosis between the superior vena cava and the right main pulmonary artery to increase pulmonary blood flow as a palliative correction for tricuspid atresia.
Graefe's o., **(1)** removal of cataract by a limbal incision with capsulotomy and iridectomy; **(2)** iridectomy for glaucoma.
Gritti's o., Gritti-Stokes *amputation.*
Halsted's o., **(1)** an o. for the radical correction of inguinal hernia; **(2)** radical *mastectomy.*
Hartmann's o., resection of the rectosigmoid colon beginning at or just above the peritoneal reflexion and extending proximally, with closure of the rectal stump and end-colostomy.
Heaney's o., technique for vaginal hysterectomy.
Heine's o., cyclodialysis.
Heller o., esophagomyotomy at the gastro-esophageal region.
Herbert's o., an o. for creating a filtering cicatrix in glaucoma by cutting and displacing, without removing, a wedge-shaped scleral flap.
Hill o., repair of hiatus hernia; narrowing the esophagogastric junction and attaching it to the right medial arcuate ligament.
Hoffa's o., in congenital dislocation of the hip, hollowing out the acetabulum and reduction of the head of the femur after severing the muscles inserted into the upper portion of the bone.
Hofmeister's o., partial gastrectomy with closure of a portion of the lesser curvature and retrocolic anastomosis of remainder to jejunum.
Holth's o., iridencleisis.
Hotz-Anagnostakis o., Anagnostakis' o.; an o. for the correction of entropion and trichiasis of cicatricial origin.
Huggins' o., orchidectomy performed for palliation or cure of cancer of prostate.
Hummelsheim's o., transplantation of a normal ocular rectus muscle, to substitute for a paralyzed muscle.
Hunter's o., ligation of the artery on the proximal side and at some distance from the sac, for correction of aneurysm.
Indian o., Indian *rhinoplasty.*
interval o., an o. performed during a period of quiescence or of intermission in the condition necessitating surgery.
Italian o., Italian *rhinoplasty.*
Jacobaeus o., pleurolysis.
Jansen's o., an o. for frontal sinus disease, the lower wall and lower portion of the anterior wall being removed and the mucous membrane curetted away.
Kasai o., portoenterostomy.
Kazanjian's o., surgical extension of the vestibular sulcus of edentulous ridges to increase their height and to improve denture retention. See also ridge *extension.*
Keen's o., removal of sections of the posterior branches of the spinal nerves to the affected muscles, and of the spinal accessory nerve, as a cure for torticollis.
Kelly's o., **(1)** correction of retroversion of the uterus by plication of uterosacral ligaments; **(2)** correction of urinary stress incontinence by vaginally placing sutures beneath the bladder neck.
Killian's o., an o. for frontal sinus disease in which the entire anterior wall is removed and the mucous membrane is curetted away; the ethmoid cells are scraped out through an opening in the nasal process of the maxillary bone, and the upper wall of the orbit is removed as well.
Koerte-Ballance o., operative anastomosis of the facial and hypoglossal nerves for the relief of facial paralysis.
Kondoleon o., excision of strips of subcutaneous connective tissue for the relief of elephantiasis.
Kraske's o., removal of the coccyx and excision of the left wing of the sacrum in order to afford approach for resection of the rectum for cancer or stenosis.

Krönlein o., orbital decompression through the anterior lateral wall of the orbit.
Kuhnt's o., conjunctival flap with a fornix base to cover a corneal laceration or corneascleral incision.
Ladd's o., division of Ladd's band to relieve duodenal obstruction in malrotation of the intestine.
Lagrange's o., a combined iridectomy and sclerectomy performed in glaucoma for the purpose of forming a filtering cicatrix.
Lambrinudi o., a form of triple arthrodesis done in such a manner as to prevent foot drop, usually as occurs in poliomyelitis.
Laroyenne's o., puncture of Douglas pouch to evacuate the pus and to secure drainage in cases of pelvic suppuration.
Lash's o., removal of a wedge of the internal cervical os with suturing of the internal os into a tighter canal structure.
Leriche's o., periarterial *sympathectomy.*
Lindner's o., posterior sclerectomy for relief of glaucoma.
Lisfranc's o., Lisfranc's *amputation.*
Longmire's o., intrahepatic cholangiojejunostomy with partial hepatectomy for biliary obstruction.
Luc's o., Caldwell-Luc o.
Madlener o., tubal sterilization by clamp and tie.
major o., an extensive, relatively difficult surgical procedure involving vital organs and/or in itself hazardous to life.
Manchester o. [*Manchester,* England], Fothergill's o.; a vaginal o. for prolapse of the uterus, consisting of cervical amputation and parametrial fixation (cardinal ligaments) anterior to the uterus.
Mann-Williamson o., an o. performed on experimental animals (dogs) in research on peptic ulcer, the duodenum with its alkaline secretions being transplanted into the ileum and the cut end of the jejunum anastomosed to the pylorus; the animals develop ulcers in the jejunum which directly receives the gastric juice.
morcellation o., vaginal hysterectomy in which the uterus is removed by lateral halves after being split.
Marshall-Marchetti-Krantz o., an o. for urinary stress incontinence, performed retropubically.
Mason o., gastric *bypass.*
Matas' o., aneurysmoplasty.
Mayo's o., an o. for the radical cure of umbilical hernia; the neck of the sac is exposed by two elliptical incisions, the gut is returned to the abdomen, the sac and adherent omentum are cut away, and the facial edges of the opening are overlapped with mattress sutures.
McReynolds' o., transplantation of the pterygium.
McVay's o., repair of inguinal and femoral hernias by suture of the the transversus abdominis muscle and its associated fasciae (transversus layer) to the pectineal ligament.
Meyer-Schwickerath o., photocoagulation of the retina or choroid.
mika o. [Australian native term], the establishment of a permanent fistula in the bulbous portions of the urethra in order to render the man incapable of procreating; said to be a practice among certain Australian aborigines.
Mikulicz' o., excision of bowel in two stages: 1) exteriorizing the diseased area, suturing efferent and afferent limbs together, and closing the abdomen around them, after which the diseased part is excised; 2) at a later time, cutting the spur with an enterotome and closing the stoma extraperitoneally.
Miles' o., Miles resection; combined abdominoperineal resection for carcinoma of the rectum.
minor o., a surgical procedure of relatively slight extent and not in itself hazardous to life.
Motais' o., transplantation of the middle third of the tendon of the superior rectus muscle of the eyeball into the upper lid, between the tarsus and skin, to supplement the action of the levator muscle in ptosis.
Mules' o., evisceration of the eyeball followed by the insertion within the sclera of a spherical prosthesis to support an artificial eye.
Mustard o., M. procedure; correction, at the atrial level, of hemodynamic abnormality due to transposition of the great arteries by an intraatrial baffle to direct pulmonary venous blood through the tricuspid orifice into the right ventricle and the systemic venous blood through the mitral valve into the left ventricle.
Naffziger o., orbital decompression for severe malignant exophthalmos by removal of the lateral and superior orbital walls.
Nissen's o., fundoplication.
Norton's o., extraperitoneal cesarean section by a paravesical approach.
Ogston-Luc o., an o. for frontal sinus disease; a skin incision is made from the inner third of the edge of the orbit toward the root of the nose or outward; the periosteum is pushed upward and outward, and the sinus is opened on the outer side of the median line; then a wide opening is made by curetting the nasofrontal duct, interior of the sinus, and anterior ethmoid cells.
Ogura o., orbital decompression by removal of the floor of the orbit through an opening made in the supradental (canine) fossa.
Ombrédanne o., transseptal orchiopexy; a technique whereby the mobilized testis is brought down into the scrotum and through the scrotal septum, to be affixed to the tissues in the contralateral scrotal pouch.
Payne o., a jejunoileal bypass for morbid obesity utilizing end-to-side anastomosis of the upper jejunum to the terminal ileum, with closure of the proximal end of the bypassed intestine.
plastic o., see plastic *surgery.*
Pólya's o., Pólya gastrectomy; partial gastrectomy with retrocolic anastomosis of the full width of stomach to jejunum.
Pomeroy's o., excision of a ligated portion of the fallopian tubes.
Porro o., cesarean *hysterectomy.*
Potts' o., Potts anastomosis; direct side-to-side anastomosis between aorta and pulmonary artery as a palliative procedure in congenital malformation of the heart.
Putti-Platt o., Putti-Platt procedure; a procedure for recurrent dislocation of shoulder joint.
radical o. for hernia, an o. by which the hernia is not only reduced, but the hernial defect is also repaired.
Ramstedt o., pyloromyotomy.
Récamier's o., curettage of the uterus.
Ridell's o., removal of the entire anterior and inferior walls of the frontal sinus, for chronic inflammation of that cavity.
Roux-en-Y o., Roux-en-Y anastomosis; anastomosis of the distal end of the divided upper jejunum to the stomach, esophagus, biliary tract, or other structure and anastomosis of the proximal end to the side of the jejunum a little further distal.
Saemisch's o., incision of the cornea to evacuate pus.
Saenger's o., cesarean section followed by careful closure of the uterine wound by three tiers of sutures.
Schauta vaginal o., an extensive extirpation of the uterus and the adnexa, using the vaginal approach facilitated by Schuchardt's o.
Schroeder's o., excision of diseased endocervical mucosa.
Schuchardt's o., a paravaginal rectal displacement incision, a surgical technique of making the upper vagina accessible for fistula closure or radical surgery via vaginam.
scleral buckling o., an o. performed in retinal detachment to indent the sclerochoroidal wall.
Scott o., a jejunoileal bypass for morbid obesity utilizing end-to-end anastomosis of the upper jejunum to the terminal ileum, with the bypassed intestine closed proximally and anastomosed distally to the colon.
second-look o., exploratory celiotomy within a year after apparently curative resection of intra-abdominal cancer, in patients with no sign or symptom of recurrence, to resect an occult tumor if present.
seton o., an o. for advanced glaucoma; passage of a suture or seton into the anterior chamber to act as a wick.

Shirodkar o., a cerclage procedure done by purse-string suturing of an incompetent cervical os with a nonabsorbent suture material.
Sistrunk o., excision of the thyroglossal cyst and duct including the midportion of the hyoid bone through, or near, which the duct traverses.
Smith's o., (Smith-Indian o.); a surgical technique for removal of cataract within the capsule.
Smith-Boyce o., anatrophic *nephrotomy.*
Smith-Indian o., Smith's o.
Smith-Robinson o., interbody spinal fusion through an anterior cervical approach.
Soave o., endorectal pull-through for treatment of congenital megacolon.
Spinelli o., an o. splitting the anterior wall of the prolapsed uterus and reversing the organ preliminary to reduction.
stapes mobilization o., now infrequently used o. involving fracture of tissue immobilizing the stapes to restore hearing; especially used in patients with otosclerosis.
Stoffel's o., division of certain motor nerves for the relief of spastic paralysis.
Stookey-Scarff o., see third *ventriculostomy.*
Sturmdorf's o., conical removal of the endocervix.
subcutaneous o., an o., as for the division of a tendon, performed without incising the skin other than by a minute opening made by the entering knife.
Syme's o., Syme's *amputation.*
tagliacotian o., Italian *rhinoplasty.*
talc o., poudrage (2); pericardial poudrage; an obsolescent o. in which magnesium silicate powder is applied to the epicardium to create a sterile granulomatous pericarditis and thus promote pericardial anastomoses with the coronary circulation.
TeLinde o., modified radical *hysterectomy.*
Torek o., a two-stage o. for bringing down an undescended testicle.
Trendelenburg's o., a pulmonary embolectomy.
Urban's o., extended radical mastectomy, including *en bloc* resection of internal mammary lymph nodes, part of the sternum, and costal cartilages.
Waters' o., an extraperitoneal cesarean section with a supravesical approach.
Webster's o., Baldy's o.
Weir's o., obsolete eponym for appendicostomy.
Wertheim's o., a radical o. for carcinoma of the uterus in which as much as possible of the vagina is excised and there is wide lymph node excision.
Wheelhouse's o., external *urethrotomy.*
Whipple's o., pancreatoduodenectomy.
Whitehead's o., excision of hemorrhoids by two circular incisions above and below involved veins, allowing normal mucosa to be pulled down and sutured to anal skin.
Ziegler's o., a V-shaped iridotomy for the formation of an artificial pupil.

operative (op'er-ă-tiv). **1.** Relating to, or effected by means of an operation. **2.** Active or effective.

operator (op'er-ā-ter). See operator *gene.*

opercular (ō-per'kyū-lăr). Relating to an operculum.

operculated (ō-per'kyū-lā-ted). Provided with a lid (operculum); denoting members of the mollusk class Gastropoda (the snails), subclass Prosobranchiata (operculate snails), and the eggs of certain parasitic worms such as the digenetic trematodes (except the schistosomes) and the broad fish tapeworm.

operculitis (ō-perk-yū-lī'tis) [operculum + G. *-itis,* inflammation]. Pericoronitis.

operculum, gen. **operculi,** pl. **opercula** (ō-per'kyū-lūm, -lī, -lă) [L. cover or lid, fr. *operio,* pp. *opertus,* to cover]. **1.** Anything resembling a lid or cover. **2** [NA]. In anatomy, the portions of the frontal, parietal, and temporal lobes bordering the lateral sulcus and covering the insula. **3.** Mucus sealing the endocervical canal of the uterus after conception has taken place. **4.** In parasitology, the lid or caplike cover of the shell opening of operculated freshwater snails in the subclass Prosobranchiata, and of the eggs of certain trematode and cestode parasites. **5.** The attached flap in the tear of retinal detachment. **6.** The mucosal flap partially or completely covering an unerupted tooth.
o. il'ei, Variolus' *sphincter.*
occipital o., a portion of the occipital lobe of the brain demarcated by the simian fissure when present in man.
trophoblastic o., the mushroom-shaped plug of fibrin that fills the aperture in the endometrium made by the implanting ovum.

operon (op'er-on). A genetic functional unit that controls production of a messenger RNA; it consists of an operator gene and two or more structural genes located in sequence in the cis position on one chromosome.

ophiasis (ō-fī'ă-sis) [G., fr. *ophis,* snake]. A form of alopecia areata in which the loss of hair occurs in bands partially or completely encircling the head.

Ophidia (ō-fid'ē-ă) [G. *ophidion,* dim. of *ophis,* a serpent]. The snakes, a suborder of the class Reptilia, including the families Colubridae, Crotalidae, Elapidae, Hydrophyidae, and Viperidae.

ophidiasis (ō'fi-dī'ă-sis) [G. *ophidion,* dim. of *ophis,* a serpent]. Ophidism; poisoning by a snake.

ophidiophobia (ō-fid'ē-ō-fō'bē-ă) [G. *ophidion,* a small snake, + *phobos,* fear]. Morbid fear of snakes.

ophidism (ō'fid-izm). Ophidiasis.

ophritis (of-rī'tis) [G. *ophrys,* eyebrow, + *-itis,* infammation]. Ophryitis; dermatitis in the region of the eyebrows.

ophryitis (of-rē-ī'tis). Ophritis.

ophryon (of'rē-on) [G. *ophrys,* eyebrow]. Supranasal or supraorbital point; the point on the midline of the forehead just above the glabella (1).

Ophryoscolecidae (of'rē-ō-skō-les'i-dē) [G. *ophrys,* eyebrow, + *scolex,* a worm]. A family of ciliate protozoa occurring in the rumen and reticulum of ruminant animals, characterized by having cilia arranged in spiral membranelles around the mouth (adoral) and in some genera also in a dorsal (metoral) position. The most important genera are *Entodinium, Diplodinium, Epidinium,* and *Ophryoscolex,* which are thought to contribute to ruminant nutrition by converting cellulose in plant material ingested by the ruminant into readily digestible animal protein of their own bodies.

ophryosis (of-rē-ō'sis) [G. *ophrys,* eyebrow, + *-osis,* condition]. Spasmodic twitching of the upper portion of the orbicularis palpebrarum muscle causing a wrinkling of the eyebrow.

ophthalm-. See ophthalmo-.

ophthalmalgia (of'thal-mal'jē-ă) [ophthalmo- + G. *algos,* pain]. Pain in the eyeball.

ophthalmia (of-thal'mē-ă) [G.]. Ophthalmitis. **1.** Severe, often purulent, conjunctivitis. **2.** Inflammation of the deeper structures of the eye.
Brazilian o., keratomalacia.
catarrhal o., mucous o.; a mild form of conjunctivitis with mucopurulent secretion.
caterpillar-hair o., o. nodosa.
o. eczemato'sa, phlyctenular *conjunctivitis.*
Egyptian o., trachoma.
electric o., ultraviolet *keratoconjunctivitis.*
gonorrheal o., blennophthalmia (2); blennorrhea conjunctivalis; acute purulent conjunctivitis excited by *Neisseria gonorrhoeae.*
granular o., trachoma.

o. hepa'tica, night blindness and degeneration of the retina and choroid after prolonged liver disease.
o. len'ta, subacute infective retinitis, usually secondary to subacute bacterial endocarditis.
metastatic o., **(1)** sympathetic o; **(2)** choroiditis in septicemia.
migratory o., sympathetic o.
mucous o., catarrhal o.
o. neonato'rum, blennorrhea neonatorum; infantile purulent conjunctivitis; a conjunctival inflammation occurring within the first 10 days of life; causes include *Neisseria gonorrhoeae, Staphylococcus, Streptococcus pneumoniae,* and *Chlamydia trachomatis.*
neuroparalytic o., corneal inflammation or ulceration following lesion of the ophthalmic branch of the trigeminal nerve.
o. niva'lis, ultraviolet *keratoconjunctivitis.*
o. nodo'sa, caterpillar-hair o.; pseudotuberculous o.; the presence of nodular swellings on the conjunctiva, due to penetration of ocular tissues by the hairs of caterpillars.
periodic o., moon blindness; an acute iridocyclitis of horses, involving one or both eyes; it subsides only to recur at intervals of varying length and usually ends in blindness; the cause is uncertain but some have associated it with leptospires; does not appear to be contagious.
phlyctenular o., phlyctenular *conjunctivitis.*
pseudotuberculous o., o. nodosa.
purulent o., purulent conjunctivitis, usually of gonorrheal origin.
reaper's o., vegetable o.
scrofulous o., phlyctenular *conjunctivitis.*
spring o., vernal *conjunctivitis.*
sympathetic o., migratory or transferred o.; metastic o. (1); a serous or plastic uveitis caused by a perforating wound of the uvea followed by a similar severe reaction in the other eye that may lead to bilateral blindness.
transferred o., sympathetic o.
vegetable o., reaper's o.; o. due to irritation from retention of plant constituents (such as grain, hops, hawthorn, thistles, burdock, and cotton or tobacco dust) within the conjunctival sac.

ophthalmic (of-thal'mik) [G. *ophthalmikos*]. Ocular (1); relating to the eye.

ophthalmic acid. A tripeptide occurring in calf lens, similar to glutathione but differing in the replacement of cysteine by α-amino-*n*-butyric acid (*i.e.,* in the replacement of –SH by $-CH_3$); a potent inhibitor of glyoxalase. *Cf.* norophthalmic acid.

ophthalmitis (of-thal-mī'tis). Ophthalmia.

ophthalmo-, ophthalm- [G. *ophthalmos,* eye]. Combining forms denoting relationship to the eye. See also oculo-.

ophthalmodiaphanoscope (of-thal'mō-dī-ă-fan'ō-skōp) [ophthalmo- + diaphanoscope]. An instrument for viewing the interior of the eye by transmitted light.

ophthalmodynamometer (of-thal'mō-dī-nă-mom'ĕ-ter) [ophthalmo- + G. *dynamis,* power, + *metron,* measure]. **1.** An instrument for determining the power of convergence of the eyes as regards the near point of vision. **2.** An instrument to measure the blood pressure in the retinal vessels.
Bailliart's o., an instrument used to measure the blood pressure of the central retinal artery; of value in diagnosing occlusion of the proximal carotid artery.
suction o., an o. with a suction disk which increases ocular pressure during ophthalmoscopic observation of the retinal artery.

ophthalmodynamometry (of-thal'mō-dī-nă-mom'ĕ-trē) [ophthalmo- + G. *dynamis,* power, + *metron,* measure]. **1.** The process of measuring the degree of power of the extraocular muscles. **2.** The measurement of blood pressure in the retinal vessels by means of an ophthalmodynamometer.

ophthalmogram (of-thal'mō-gram). The record made by an ophthalmograph, or the similar record made by electro-oculography.

ophthalmograph (of-thal'mō-graf). An instrument that records eye movements during reading by photographing a mark on the cornea or making a tracing of light reflexes.

ophthalmography (of-thal-mog'ră-fē) [ophthalmo- + G. *graphē,* a description]. Use of the ophthalmograph.

ophthalmolith (of-thal'mō-lith) [ophthalmo- + G. *lithos,* stone]. Dacryolith.

ophthalmologist (of-thal-mol'ō-jist). Oculist; a specialist in ophthalmology.

ophthalmology (of-thal-mol'ō-jē) [ophthalmo- + G. *logos,* study]. The medical specialty concerned with the eye, its diseases, and refractive errors.

ophthalmomalacia (of-thal'mō-mă-lā'shē-ă) [ophthalmo- + G. *malakia,* softness]. Abnormal softening of the eyeball.

ophthalmomelanosis (of-thal'mō-mel-ă-nō'sis). Melanotic discoloration of the conjunctiva and adjoining tissues.

ophthalmometer (of-thal-mom'ĕ-ter) [ophthalmo- + G. *metron,* measure]. Keratometer.

ophthalmomycosis (of-thal'mō-mī-kō'sis) [ophthalmo- + G. *mykēs,* fungus, + *-osis,* condition]. Any disease of the eye or its appendages caused by a fungus.

ophthalmomyiasis (of-thal'mō-mī-ī'ă-sis). Ocular *myiasis.*

ophthalmomyitis (of-thal'mō-mī-i'tis) [ophthalmo- + G. *mys,* muscle, + *-itis,* inflammation]. Inflammation of the extrinsic muscles of the eye.

ophthalmopathy (of-thal-mop'ă-thē) [ophthalmo- + G. *pathos,* suffering]. Oculopathy; any disease of the eyes.
endocrine o., exophthalmos caused by increased water content of retroocular orbital tissues; associated with thyroid disease, usually hyperthyroidism.
external o., any disease of the conjunctiva, cornea, or adnexa of the eye.
internal o., any disease of the internal structures of the eyeball.

ophthalmoplegia (of-thal-mō-plē'jē-ă) [ophthalmo- + G. *plēgē,* stroke]. Paralysis of one or more of the ocular muscles.
exophthalmic o., o. with protrusion of the eyeballs due to increased water content of orbital tissues incidental to thyroid disorders, usually hyperthyroidism.
o. exter'na, Ballet's disease; paralysis affecting one or more of the extrinsic eye muscles.
fascicular o., o. due to a lesion in the pons.
infectious o., transient or permanent nuclear paralysis of eye muscles, including the intraocular muscles, in encephalitis lethargica.
o. inter'na, paralysis affecting only the sphincter muscle of the pupil and the ciliary muscle.
o. internuclea'ris, o. in lesions of the medial longitudinal fasciculus, with failure of adduction in horizontal gaze but with retention of convergence.
nuclear o., o. due to a lesion of the nuclei of origin of the motor nerves of the eye.
orbital o., o. due to a lesion within the orbit.
Parinaud's o., Parinaud's *syndrome.*
o. partia'lis, incomplete o. involving only one or two of the extrinsic or intrinsic ocular muscles.
o. progressi'va, Graefe's disease; progressive upper bulbar palsy, due to degeneration of the nuclei of the motor nerves of the eye.
o. tota'lis, paralysis of both the extrinsic and intrinsic ocular muscles.

ophthalmoplegic (of-thal-mō-plē'jik). Relating to or marked by ophthalmoplegia.

ophthalmoscope (of-thal'mō-skōp) [ophthalmo- + G. *skopeō,* to examine]. Funduscope; a device for studying the interior of the eyeball through the pupil.
binocular o., an o. that provides a stereoscopic view of the fundus.

demonstration o., an o. by which the fundus may be seen simultaneously by more than one observer.
direct o., an instrument designed to visualize the interior of the eye, with the instrument relatively close to the subject's eye and the observer viewing an upright magnified image.
indirect o., an instrument designed to visualize the interior of the eye, with the instrument at arm's length from the subject's eye and the observer viewing an inverted image through a convex lens located between the instrument and the subject's eye.

ophthalmoscopic (of'thal-mō-skop'ik). Relating to examination of the interior of the eye.

ophthalmoscopy (of-thal-mos'kŏ-pē). Funduscopy; examination of the fundus of the eye by means of the ophthalmoscope.
direct o., o. performed with a direct ophthalmoscope.
indirect o., o. performed with an indirect ophthalmoscope.
o. with reflected light, examination of that part of the fundus adjacent to an area illuminated by a sharply focused light.

ophthalmotrope (of-thal'mō-trōp) [ophthalmo- + G. *tropos,* a turning]. A model of the two eyes, to each of which are attached weighted cords pulling in the direction of the six extrinsic eye muscles; used to demonstrate the action of the ocular muscles singly or in various combinations.

ophthalmovascular (of-thal'mō-vas'kyū-lăr). Relating to the blood vessels of the eye.

-opia [G. *ōps,* eye]. Suffix meaning vision.

opianine (ō-pī'ă-nēn). Noscapine.

opianyl (ō'pī-ă-nil). Meconin.

opiate (ō'pē-āt). Any preparation or derivative of opium.

opine (ō'pēn). A derivative of basic amino acids, produced by crown-gall tumors in plants.

opioid (ō'pē-oyd). Denoting synthetic narcotics that resemble opiates in action but are not derived from opium.

opiomelanocortin (ō'pē-ō-mel'ă-nō-kōr'tin). A linear polypeptide of the pituitary gland that contains in its sequence the sequences of endorphins, MSH, ACTH, and the like, which are split off enzymically; the nucleotide sequences coding have been determined for several species.

opipramol hydrochloride (ō-pip'ră-mōl). 4-[3-(5*H*-Dibenz[*b.f*]azepin-5-yl)propyl]-1-piperazineethanol dihydrochloride; an antidepressant agent.

opisthenar (ō-pis'thē-nar) [G. back of the hand, from *opisthen,* behind, + *thenar,* palm of the hand]. Dorsum of the hand.

opisthiobasial (ō-pis'thē-ō-bā'sē-ăl). Relating to both opisthion and basion; denoting a line connecting the two, or the distance between them.

opisthion (ō-pis'thē-on) [G. *opisthios,* posterior] [NA]. The middle point on the posterior margin of the foramen magnum, opposite the basion.

opisthionasial (ō-pis'thē-ō-nā'zē-ăl). Relating to the opisthion and the nasion; denoting the distance between the two points.

opistho- [G. *opisthen,* at the rear, behind]. Combining form denoting backward, behind, dorsal.

opisthocheilia, opisthochilia (op'is-thō-kī'lē-ă) [opistho- + G. *cheilos,* lip]. Recession of the lips.

opisthomastigote (ō-pis-thō-mas'ti-gōt) [opistho- + G. *mastix,* whip]. Term now used instead of herpetomonad for the stage of development of certain insect and plant parasitizing flagellates to avoid confusion between the stage and the genus *Herpetomonas.* In this stage the flagellum arises from the kinetoplast located behind the nucleus and emerges from the anterior end of the organism; an undulating membrane is absent.

opisthoporeia (ō-pis'thō-pō-rī'ă, -rē'ă) [opistho- + G. *poreia,* a walking, fr. *poreuō,* to go, walk]. Involuntary backward gait; frequently connected with parkinsonism.

opisthorchiasis (op'is-thōr-kī'ă-sis). Infection with the Asiatic liver fluke, *Opisthorchis viverrini,* or other opisthorchids.

opisthorchid (op-is-thōr'kid). Common name for members of the family Opisthorchiidae.

Opisthorchiidae (op'is-thōr-kē'i-dē). A family of trematodes that includes the genera *Opisthorchis* and *Clonorchis.*

Opisthorchis (op-is-thōr'kis) [opistho- + G. *orchis,* testis]. Genus of digenetic trematodes (family Opisthorchiidae) found in the bile ducts or gallbladder of fish-eating mammals, birds, and fish.
O. felin'eus, the cat liver fluke, a species frequently found as a parasite of man in Eastern Europe, Siberia, India, Japan, and Southeast Asia; adults are lancet-shaped, thin, relatively transparent, and hermaphroditic, with sizes ranging from 7 to 12 by 2 to 3 mm; ingested eggs hatch in *Bithynia* snails, and cercariae encyst on various species of freshwater fish; man acquires the infection by ingesting raw or inadequately cooked fish; the parasites sometimes cause no evidence of disease, but cholangitis, biliary cirrhosis, and chronic pancreatitis may occur.
O. sinen'sis, *Clonorchis sinensis.*
O. viverri'ni, a species closely related to O. *felineus,* very common in man in Thailand; causes opisthorchiasis.

opisthotic (op-is-thō'tik) [opistho- + G. *ous* (*ōt-*), ear]. Behind the ear.

opisthotonic (op-is-thot'ō-nik, ō-pis'thō-ton'ik). Relating to or characterized by opisthotonos.

opisthotonoid (op-is-thot'ō-noyd). Resembling opisthotonos.

opisthotonos, opisthotonus (op-is-thot'ō-nŭs) [opistho- + G. *tonos,* tension, stretching]. Tetanus dorsalis; tetanus posticus; a tetanic spasm in which the spine and extremities are bent with convexity forward, the body resting on the head and the heels.

Opitz, John M., U.S. pediatrician, *1935. See Smith-Lemli-O. *syndrome.*

opium (ō'pē-ŭm) [L. fr. G. *opion,* poppy-juice]. Gum opium; meconium (2); the air-dried milky exudation obtained by incising the unripe capsules of *Papaver somniferum* (family Papveraceae) or its variety, *P. album.* Contains some 20 alkaloids, including morphine, 9 to 16%; noscapine, 4 to 8%; codeine, 0.8 to 2.5%; papaverine, 0.5 to 2.5%; and thebaine, 0.5 to 2%. Used as an analgesic, hypnotic, and diaphoretic, and in diarrhea and spasmodic conditions.
Boston o., pudding o.; o. so diluted after importation as barely to meet the official requirements.
deodorized o., denarcotized o., powdered o. treated with purified petroleum benzine which removes certain nauseating and odorous constituents.
granulated o., o. dried and reduced to a coarse powder; it contains 10 to 10.5% anhydrous morphine.
powdered o., dried and finely powdered o. containing 10% morphine.
pudding o., Boston o.

opo- [G. *ōps,* face, eye]. Combining form relating to the face or eye.

opobalsamum (op-ō-bal'sa-mŭm) [G. *opobalsamon,* the juice of the balsam tree, fr. *opos,* juice, + *balsamon*] *Balm* of Gilead.

opodidymus (op-ō-did'i-mŭs) [G. *ōps,* eye, face, + *didymos,* twin]. Conjoined twins with a single body having two heads fused at the back with partially separated facial regions.

Oppenheim, Hermann, Berlin neurologist, 1858–1919. See O.'s *disease, gait, reflex, syndrome;* Ziehen-O. *disease.*

oppilation (op-i-lā'shŭn) [L. *oppilatio,* fr. *op-pilo* (*obp-*), pp. *-atus,* to stop up, fr. *pilo,* to ram down]. Obstruction or closing of the pores.

oppilative (op-i-lā'tiv). Obstructive to any secretion.

opponens (ŏ-pō′nens) [L. *op-pono* (*obp-*), pres. p. *-ens,* to place against, oppose]. A name given to several muscles of the fingers or toes, by the action of which these digits are opposed to the others.

opportunistic (op′ŏr-tū-nis′tik). **1.** Denoting an organism capable of causing disease only in a host whose resistance is lowered, *e.g.,* by other diseases or by drugs. **2.** Denoting a disease caused by such an organism.

op′sin. The protein portion of the rhodopsin molecule.

opsinogen (op-sin′ō-jen). Opsogen; a substance that stimulates the formation of opsonin, such as the antigen contained in a suspension of bacteria used for immunization.

opsiuria (op-sē-ū′rē-ă) [G. *opsi,* late, + *ouron,* urine]. A more rapid excretion of urine during fasting than after a full meal.

opsoclonus (op′sō-klō′nŭs) [G. *ōps, ōpos,* eye, + *klonos,* confused motion]. Rapid, irregular, nonrhythmic movements of the eye in horizontal and vertical directions.

opsogen (op′sō-jen). Opsinogen.

opsomania (op′sō-mā′nē-ă) [G. *opson,* seasoning, + *mania,* frenzy]. A longing for a particular article of diet, or for highly seasoned food.

opsonic (op-son′ik). Relating to opsonins or to their utilization.

opsonin (op′sō-nin) [G. *opsonein,* to cater, prepare food]. A substance that enhances phagocytosis.

common o., normal o.

immune o., specific o.

normal o., common or thermolabile o.; that normally present in the blood, *i.e.,* without stimulation by a known, specific antigen; it is relatively thermolabile and reacts with various organisms.

specific o., immune or thermostable o.; that formed in response to stimulation by a specific antigen, either as a result of an attack of a disease, or injections with a suitably prepared suspension of the specific microorganism; specific o. is more heat-stable than normal o., and reacts only with microorganisms that contain the specific antigens that stimulated formation of the antibody.

thermolabile o., normal o.

thermostable o., specific o.

opsonization (op′sō-nī-zā′shŭn). The process by which bacteria are altered in such a manner that they are more readily and more efficiently engulfed by phagocytes.

opsonocytophagic (op′sō-nō-sī′tō-fā′jik) [opsonin + G. *kytos,* a hollow (cell), + *phagein,* to eat]. Pertaining to the increased efficiency of phagocytic activity of the leukocytes in blood that contains specific opsonin.

opsonometry (op-sō-nom′ĕ-trē). Determination of the opsonic index or the opsonocytophagic activity.

opsonophilia (op-sō-nō-fil′ē-ă) [opsonin + G. *phileō,* to love]. The condition in which bacteria readily unite with opsonins, thereby sensitizing them for more effective phagocytosis.

opsonophilic (op-sō-nō-fil′ik). Pertaining to, characterized by, or resulting in opsonophilia.

optesthesia (op-tes-thē′zē-ă) [G. *optikos,* optical, + aisthēsis, sensation]. Visual sensibility to light stimuli.

optic, optical (op′tik, op′ti-kăl) [G. *optikos*]. Relating to the eye, vision, or optics.

optician (op-tish′an). One who practices opticianry.

opticianry (op-tish′an-rē). The professional practice of filling prescriptions for ophthalmic lenses, dispensing spectacles, and making and fitting contact lenses.

optico-. See opto-.

opticociliary (op′ti-kō-sil′ē-ăr-ē). Relating to the optic and ciliary nerves.

opticopupillary (op′ti-kō-pyū′pi-lăr-ē). Relating to the optic nerve and the pupil.

optics (op′tiks) [G. *optikos,* fr. *ōps,* eye]. The science concerned with the properties of light, its refraction and absorption, and the refracting media of the eye in that relation.

Nomarski o., an optical system for differential interference contrast microscopy.

optimism (op′ti-mizm) [L. *optimus,* best]. The tendency to look on the bright side of everything, to believe that there is good in everything.

therapeutic o., a belief in the efficacy of drugs and other therapeutic agents in the treatment of diseases.

optimum (op′ti-mŭm) [L. ntr. sing. of *optimus,* best]. The best or most suitable; *e.g.,* denoting the dose of a remedy likely to give most benefit with fewest side effects, the temperature at which an enzyme has maximal activity.

opto-, optico- [G. *optikos,* optical, from *ōps,* eye]. Combining forms meaning optical.

optokinetic (op′tō-ki-net′ik) [opto- + G. *kinēsis,* movement]. Pertaining to the occurrence of intermittent rotation of the eye when the subject looks at moving objects.

optomeninx (op′tō-mē′ninks) [opto- + G. *mēninx,* membrane]. Retina.

optometer (op-tom′ĕ-ter) [opto- + G. *metron,* measure]. An instrument for determining the refraction of the eye.

objective o., refractometer.

optometrist (op-tom′ĕ-trist). One who practices optometry.

optometry (op-tom′ĕ-trē). **1.** The profession concerned with the examination of the eyes and related structures to determine the presence of vision problems and eye disorders, and with the prescription and adaptation of lenses and other optical aids or the use of visual training for maximum visual efficiency. **2.** The use of an optometer.

optomyometer (op′tō-mī-om′ĕ-ter) [opto- + G. *mys,* muscle, + *metron,* measure]. An instrument for determining the relative power of the extrinsic muscles of the eye.

optotypes (op′tō-tīps) [opto- + G. *typos,* type]. Test letters. See *test types.*

OPV Abbreviation for oral poliovirus vaccine. See poliovirus *vaccines.*

ora (ō′ră) [L.]. Plural of L. *os,* the mouth.

ora, pl. **orae** (ō′ră, ō′rē) [L.] [NA]. An edge or a margin.

o. serra′ta [NA], the serrated extremity of the pars optica retinae, located a little behind the ciliary body and marking the limits of the percipient portion of the membrane.

orad (ōr′ad) [L. *os,* mouth, + *ad,* to]. **1.** In a direction toward the mouth. **2.** Situated nearer the mouth in relation to a specific reference point; opposite of aborad.

oral (ōr′ăl) [L. *os* (*or-*), mouth]. Relating to the mouth.

orale (ō-rā′lē) [Mod. L. punctum *orale,* oral point, fr. L. *os* (*or-*), mouth]. A point at the lingual side of the alveolar termination of the premaxillary suture.

Oral Hygiene Index (OHI). An index used in epidemiological studies of dental disease, to evaluate dental plaque and dental calculus separately.

orality (ōr-al′i-tē). In freudian psychology, a term used to denote the psychic organization derived from, and characteristic of, the oral period of psychosexual development.

Oram, S. See Holt-O. *syndrome.*

orange (ōr′enj) [O.F. *orenge,* fr. Ar. *nāranj,* the initial *n* being absorbed in Fr. article *une*]. **1.** The fruit of the orange tree, *Citrus aurantium* (family Rutaceae). **2.** A color between yellow and red in the spectrum. For individual orange dyes, see specific name.

bitter o. peel, the dried rind of the unripe but fully grown fruit; a flavoring agent.

bitter o. peel, dried, the dried outer part of the pericarp of the ripe, or nearly ripe, fruit; it contains not less than 2.5% v/w of volatile oil.

bitter o. peel, fresh, the outer part of the pericarp of the ripe, or nearly ripe, fruit; used to prepare the tincture and the syrup.

bitter o. peel oil, a volatile oil obtained by expression from the fresh peel of the bitter o.

orange G [C.I. 16230]. An azo dye, $C_{16}H_{10}N_2O_7S_2Na_2$, used as a cytoplasmic stain in histologic techniques.

orange wood. A soft wood used in dentistry for placement of bridges, crowns, etc. by biting pressure, also used as a burnishing point in the polishing of root surfaces.

Orbeli, Leon A., Russian physiologist, 1882–1958. See O. *effect.*

orbicular (or-bik'yū-lăr) [L. *orbiculus,* a small disk, dim. of *orbis,* circle]. Similar in form to an orb; circular in form.

orbiculare (ōr-bik-yū-lā'rē) [L., fr. *orbiculus,* a small disk]. *Processus* lenticularis incudis.

orbicularis (ōr-bik'yū-lā'ris) [L. fr. *orbiculus,* a small disk]. **1.** Circular; denoting a circular or disk-shaped structure. **2.** *Musculus* orbicularis.

orbiculus ciliaris (ōr-bik'yū-lŭs sil-ē-ār'is) [Mod. L.] [NA]. Ciliary disk or ring; annulus ciliaris; pars plana; the darkly pigmented posterior zone of the ciliary body continuous with the retina at the ora serrata.

orbit (ōr'bit). Orbita.

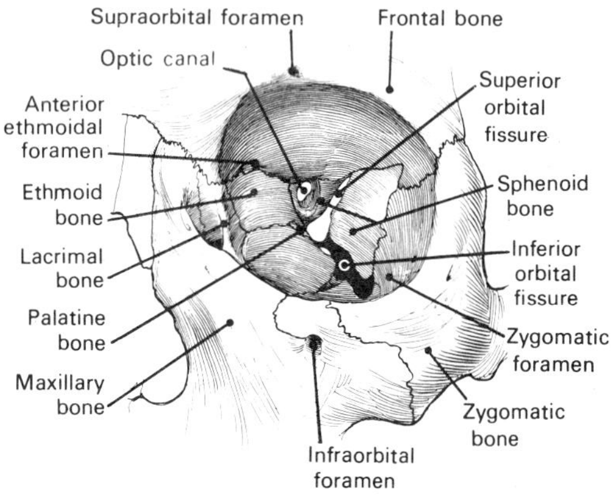

Orbit

orbita, gen. **orbita** (ōr'bi-tă, -tē) [L. a wheel-track, fr. *orbis,* circle] [NA]. Orbit; orbital cavity; eye socket; the bony cavity containing the eyeball and its adnexa; it is formed of parts of seven bones: the frontal, maxillary, sphenoid, lacrimal, zygomatic, ethmoid, and palatine bones.

orbital (ōr'bi-tăl). Relating to the orbits.

orbitale (ōr-bi-tā'lē) [L. of an orbit]. In cephalometrics, the lowermost point in the lower margin of the bony orbit that may be felt under the skin.

orbitography (ōr'bi-tog'ră-fē) [L. *orbita,* orbit, + G. *graphō,* to write]. A diagnostic technique for radiographic evaluation in suspected blow-out fracture of the orbit, using a water-soluble iodinated compound injected over the orbital floor.

orbitonasal (ōr'bi-tō-nā'săl). Relating to the orbit and the nose or nasal cavity.

orbitonometer (ōr'bi-tō-nom'ĕ-ter) [L. *orbita,* orbit, + G. *metron,* measure]. An instrument that measures the resistance offered to pressing the eyeball backwards into its socket.

orbitonometry (ōr'bi-tō-nom'ĕ-trē). Measurement by means of the orbitonometer.

orbitopagus (ōr-bi-top'ă-gŭs) [L. *orbita,* orbit, + G. *pagos,* something fixed]. Teratoma orbitae; unequal conjoined twins in which the parasite, usually very imperfectly developed, is attached at an orbit of the autosite.

orbitosphenoid (ōr'bi-tō-sfe'noyd). Relating to the orbit and the sphenoid bone.

orbitotomy (ōr-bi-tot'ō-mē) [L. *orbita,* orbit, + *tomas,* cut]. Surgical incision into the orbit.

Orbivirus (ōr'bi-vī-rŭs) [L. *orbis,* ring, + virus]. A genus of viruses of vertebrates (family Reoviridae) that multiply in insects, including certain viruses formerly included with the arboviruses. They are antigenically distinct from other groups of viruses and are characterized by an indistinct but rather large outer layer of capsomeres which give the appearance of rings (hence the name). The genus includes, among others, Colorado tick fever virus of man, bluetongue virus of sheep, and African horse sickness virus.

orcein (ōr'sē-in) [old C.I. 1242]. A natural dye derived from orcinol by treatment with air and ammonia, which as a purple dye complex is used in various histologic staining methods.

orchectomy (ōr-kek'tō-mē). Orchiectomy.

orchella (ōr-kel'ă) [old C.I. 1242]. Archil.

orcheo-. For words beginning thus, see orchio-.

orchi-, orchido-, orchio- [G. *orchis,* testis]. Combining forms denoting relationship to the testes.

orchialgia (ōr-kē-al'jē-ă) [orchi- + G. *algos,* pain]. Pain in the testis. Also called orchiodynia; orchioneuralgia; orchidalgia; testalgia.

orchiatrophy (ōr-kē-at'rō-fē). Atrophy or shrinking of the testis.

orchichorea (ōr'kē-kō-rē'ă) [orchi- + G. *choreia,* a dance]. Involuntary rising and falling movements of the testis.

orchidalgia (ōr-ki-dal'jē-ă) Orchialgia.

orchidectomy (ōr-ki-dek'tō-mē). Orchiectomy.

orchidic (ōr-kid'ik). Relating to the testis.

orchiditis (ōr-ki-dī'tis). Orchitis.

orchido-. See orchi-.

orchidometer (ōr-ki-dom'ĕ-ter) [orchido- + G. *metron,* measure]. **1.** A caliper device used to measure the size of testes. **2.** A set of sized models of testes for comparison of testicular development.

orchidoptosis (ōr'ki-dop-tō'sis) [orchido- + G. *ptosis,* a falling]. Ptosis of the male gonads.

orchidorraphy (ōr-ki-dōr'ă-fē). Orchiopexy.

orchiectomy (ōr-kē-ek'tō-mē) [orchi- + G. *ektomē,* excision]. Orchidectomy; orchectomy; testectomy; removal of one or both testes.

orchiepididymitis (ōr'kē-ep'i-did'i-mī'tis) [orchi- + epididymis, + G. *-itis,* inflammation]. Inflammation of the testis and epididymis.

orchil (ōr'kil) [old C.I. 1242]. Archil.

orchilytic (ōr-ki-lit'ik) [orchi- + G. *lytikos,* causing dissolution]. Destructive to the testis.

orchio-. See orchi-.

orchiocele (ōr'kē-ō-sēl) [orchio- + G. *kēlē,* hernia, tumor]. A testis retained in the inguinal canal.

orchiococcus (ōr'kē-ō-kok'ŭs) [orchio- + G. *kokkos,* berry (coccus)]. An old term for any Gram-negative diplococcus that resembles the gonococcus but is more easily cultivated on ordinary media; it is sometimes found in vaginal secretions. Such bacteria are now classified as species of *Neisseria,* along with *N. gonorrhoeae.*

orchiodynia (ōr'kē-ō-din'ē-ă) [orchi- + G. *odynē,* pain]. Orchialgia.

orchioncus (ōr-kē-ong′kŭs) [orchio- + G. *onkos,* bulk, mass]. A neoplasm of the testis.

orchioneuralgia (ōr′kē-ō-nū-ral′jē-ă) [orchio- + G. *neuron,* nerve, + *algos,* pain]. Orchialgia.

orchiopathy (ōr-kē-op′ă-thē) [orchio- + G. *pathos,* suffering]. Testopathy; disease of a testis.

orchiopexy (ōr′kē-ō-pek′sē) [orchio- + G. *pēxis,* fixation]. Orchiorrhaphy; orchidorrhaphy; cryptorchidopexy; surgical treatment of an undescended testicle by freeing it and implanting it into the scrotum.

transseptal o., Ombrédanne *operation.*

orchioplasty (ōr′kē-ō-plas-tē) [orchio- + G. *plastos,* formed]. Plastic surgery of the testis.

orchiorrhaphy (ōr-kē-ōr′ă-fē) [orchio- + G. *rhaphē,* a suture]. Orchiopexy.

orchiotherapy (ōr′kē-ō-thār′ă-pē). Treatment with testicular extracts.

orchiotomy (ōr-kē-ot′ō-mē) [orchio- + G. *tomē,* incision]. Orchotomy; incision into a testis.

orchis, pl. **orchises** (ōr′kis, ōr′ki-sēz) [G. testis, an orchid]. Testis.

orchitic (ōr-kit′ik). Denoting orchitis.

orchitis (ōr-kī′tis) [orchi- + G. *-itis,* inflammation]. Orchiditis; testitis; inflammation of the testis.

o. parotid′ea, o. associated with mumps.

traumatic o., simple inflammation of the testis caused by mechanical injury.

o. variolo′sa, o. complicating smallpox.

orchotomy (ōr-kot′ō-mē). Orchiotomy.

orcin (ōr′sin). Orcinol.

orcinol (ōr′sin-ol). Orcin; 5-methylresorcinol; 3,5-dihydroxytoluene; the parent substance of the natural dye orcein, obtained from certain colorless lichens (*Lecanora tinctoria, Rocella tinctoria*) by treatment with boiling water; used as an external antiseptic in various skin diseases and in chemistry as a reagent for pentoses.

orciprenaline sulfate (ōr-si-pren′ă-lēn). Metaproterenol sulfate.

ORD Abbreviation for optical rotatory *dispersion.*

Ord Symbol for orotidine.

ordeal bean (ōr′dē-ăl). Physostigma.

order (ōr′der) [L. *ordo,* regular arrangement]. In biological classification, the division just below the class (or subclass) and above the family.

pecking o., the establishment of a graded dominance in members of a group by the use of aggression.

orderly (ōr′der-lē). An attendant in a hospital unit who assists in the care of patients.

ordinate (ōr′di-nāt). In a plane cartesian coordinate system, the vertical axis (*y*). *Cf.* abscissa.

orectic (ō-rek′tik). Pertaining to or characterized by orexia.

orexia (ō-rek′sē-ă) [G. *orexis,* appetite]. **1.** The affective and conative aspects of an act, in contrast to the cognitive aspect. **2.** Appetite.

orexigenic (ō-rek-si-jen′ik). Appetite-stimulating.

orf. Contagious *ecthyma.*

organ (ōr′găn) [L. *organum,* fr. G. *organon,* a tool, instrument]. Organum; any part of the body exercising a specific function, as of respiration, secretion, digestion.

accessory o.'s, supernumerary o.'s.

accessory o.'s of eye, *organa* oculi accessoria.

annulospiral o., annulospiral *ending.*

Chievitz' o., a normal epithelial structure, possibly a neurotransmitter, found at the angle of the mandible with branches of the buccal nerve.

circumventricular o.'s, structures in or near the base of the brain that differ from other brain tissue in having capillaries lacking the usual blood-brain barrier, so that they are not isolated from many compounds in the blood; they are selectively stained by certain intravascular dyes.

Corti's o., *organum* spirale.

critical o., the o. or physiologic system that for a given method of administration would first be subjected to the legally defined maximum permissible radiation exposure as the dose of radioactive material is increased; *e.g.,* the kidney is the critical o. when ^{197}Hg-chlormerodrin is administered.

enamel o., a circumscribed mass of ectodermal cells budded off from the dental lamina; it becomes cup-shaped and develops on its internal face the ameloblast layer of cells which produce the enamel cap of a developing tooth.

end o., the special structure containing the terminal of a nerve fiber in peripheral tissue such as muscle, tissue, skin, mucous membrane, or glands. See also subentries under ending.

floating o., wandering o.

flower-spray o. of Ruffini, flower-spray *ending.*

genital o.'s. *organa* genitalia.

Golgi tendon o., neurotendinous o. or spindle; a proprioceptive sensory nerve ending embedded among the fibers of a tendon, often near the musculotendinous junction; it is compressed and activated by any increase of the tendon's tension, caused either by active contraction or passive stretch of the corresponding muscle.

gustatory o., *organum* gustus.

o. of hearing, *labyrinthus* cochlearis.

intromittent o., penis.

Jacobson's o., *organum* vomeronasale.

lateral line sense o., neuromast o.; a structure in fish consisting of a long groove or canal extending along each side of the trunk and tail and branching in the head region; the groove or tube is lined with neuroepithelial cells, some of which are in groups known as neuromasts; its function appears to be the detection of vibrations of low frequency.

neuromast o., lateral line sense o.

neurotendinous o., Golgi tendon o.

olfactory o., *organum* olfactus.

ptotic o., wandering o.

o. of Rosenmüller, epoophoron.

sense o.'s, *organa* sensuum.

o. of smell, *organum* olfactus.

spiral o., *organum* spirale.

subcommissural o., a microscopic organ, made up of columnar ciliated ependymal cells, located in the cerebral aqueduct beneath the posterior commissure of the brain; it is believed to have a neurosecretory function.

supernumerary o.'s, accessory o.'s; o.'s exceeding the normal number, which may develop from multiple foci of organization in an organ-formative field larger (originally) than that of the definitive main o.; such o.'s are aberrant but frequently not a cause of disease; illness may persist if they are left in the body after therapeutic removal of the main o.

target o., target (3); a tissue or o. upon which a hormone exerts its action; generally, a tissue or organ with appropriate receptors for a hormone.

o. of taste, *organum* gustus.

o. of touch, *organum* tactus.

urinary o.'s, *organa* urinaria.

vestibular o., collective term for the utricle, saccule, and semicircular ducts of the membranous labyrinth, each having a single patch of ciliated receptor epithelium innervated by the vestibular nerve: macula sacculi, macula utriculi, and cristae of the semicircular ducts.

vestibulocochlear o., *organum* vestibulocochleare.

vestigial o., a rudimentary structure in man corresponding to a

functional structure or o. in the lower animals.
o. of vision, *organum* visus.
vomeronasal o., *organum* vomeronasale.
wandering o., floating or ptotic o.; an o. with loose attachments, permitting its displacement.
Weber's o., *utriculus* prostaticus.
o.'s of Zuckerkandl, *corpora* paraaortica.

organa (ōr'gă-nă). Plural of organum.

organelle (or'gă-nel) [Mod. L. dim. of G. *organon,* organ]. Cell o.; organoid (3); one of the specialized parts of a protozoan or tissue cell; these subcellular units include mitochondria, the Golgi apparatus, nucleus and centrioles, granular and agranular endoplasmic reticulum, vacuoles, microsomes, lysosomes, plasma membrane, and certain fibrils, as well as plastids of plant cells.
cell o., organelle.
paired o.'s, rhoptries.

organic (ōr-gan'ik) [G. *organikos*] **1.** Relating to an organ. **2.** Relating to or formed by an organism. **3.** Organized; structural. **4.** See organic *compound.*

organicism (ōr-gan'i-sizm). A theory which attributes all diseases, in particular, all mental disorders, to organic lesions.

organicist (ōr-gan'i-sist). One who believes in, or subscribes to the views of, organicism.

organism (ōr'gă-nizm). Any living individual, whether plant or animal, considered as a whole.
calculated mean o. (CMO), a hypothetical o. whose characters are the means of both the positive and negative characters of the o.'s which belong to the same taxon as the CMO, as opposed to the hypothetical mean o.
fastidious o., a bacterial organism having complex nutritional requirements.
hypothetical mean o. (HMO), a hypothetical o. whose characters are the means of the positive characters of the organisms which belong to the same taxon as the HMO, as opposed to the calculated mean o.
pleuropneumonia-like o.'s (PPLO), the original name given to a group of bacteria which did not possess cell walls; these o.'s, isolated from man and other animals, soil, and sewage, are now assigned to the order Mycoplasmatales.

organization (ōr'gan-i-zā'shŭn). **1.** An arrangement of distinct but mutually dependent parts. **2.** The conversion of coagulated blood, exudate, or dead tissue into fibrous tissue.
pregenital o., in psychoanalysis, the o. or arrangement of the libido in the stages prior to that of genital primacy.

organize (ōr'gan-īz). To provide with, or to assume, a structure.

organizer (ōr'gan-ī-zer). H. Spemann's term originally applied to a group of cells on the dorsal lip of the blastopore inducing differentiation of cells in the embryo, and controlling growth and development of adjacent parts; now generally applied to any group of cells having such a controlling influence, the effects being brought about through the action of an evocator.
nucleolar o., nucleolar zone; the region of the satellites on the acrocentric chromosomes that is active in nucleolus formation.
primary o., the o. situated on the dorsal lip of the blastopore.
procentriole o., deuterosome.

organo- [G. *organon,* organ]. Combining form denoting organ or organic.

organoferric (ōr'gă-nō-făr'ik). Relating to an organic compound containing iron.

organogel (ōr-gan'ō-jel). A hydrogel with an organic liquid instead of water as the dispersion means.

organogenesis (ōr'gă-nō-jen'ĕ-sis) [organo- + G. *genesis,* origin]. Organogeny; formation of organs during development.

organogenetic, organogenic (ōr'gă-nō-jĕ-net'ik, -jen'ik). Relating to organogenesis.

organogeny (ōr-gan-oj'ĕ-nē). Organogenesis.

organography (ōr'gă-nog'ră-fē) [organo- + G. *graphē,* a writing]. A treatise on, or description of, the organs of the body.

organoid (ōr'gă-noyd) [organo- + G. *eidos,* resemblance]. **1.** Resembling in superficial appearance or in structure any of the organs or glands of the body. **2.** Composed of glandular or organic elements, and not of a single tissue; pertaining to certain neoplasms (*e.g.,* an adenoma) that contain cytologic and histologic elements arranged in a pattern that closely resembles or is virtually identical to a normal organ. See also histoid. **3.** Organelle.

organoleptic (ōr'gă-nō-lep'tik) [organo- + G. *lēptikos,* disposed to accept]. **1.** Stimulating any of the organs of sensation. **2.** Susceptible to a sensory stimulus.

organology (ōr-gă-nol'ō-jē) [organo- + G. *logos,* study]. Branch of science concerned with the anatomy, physiology, development, and functions of the various organs.

organoma (ōr-gă-nō'mă) [organo- + G. *-oma,* tumor]. A neoplasm that contains cytologic and histologic elements in such an arrangement that specific types of tissue, *e.g.,* thyroid glands, intestinal mucosa, ovarian stroma and follicles, may be identified in various parts. See also teratoma.

organomegaly (ōr'gă-nō-meg'ă-lē). Visceromegaly.

organomercurial (ōr-gan'ō-mer-kyū'rē-ăl). Any organic mercurial compound; *e.g.,* merbromin, thimerosal.

organometallic (ōr'gă-nō-me-tal'ik). Denoting an organic compound containing one or more metallic atoms in its structure.

organon, pl. **organa** (ōr'gă-non, ōr'gă-nă) [G. organ]. Organum.

organonomy (ōr-gă-non'ō-mē) [organo- + G. *nomos,* law]. The body of laws regulating the life processes of organized beings.

organonymy (ōr'gă-non'i-mē) [organo- + G. *onyma,* name]. The nomenclature of the organs of the body, as distinguished from toponymy.

organopathy (ōr-gă-nop'ă-thē) [organo- + G. *pathos,* suffering]. Any disease especially affecting one of the organs of the body.

organopexy, organopexia (ōr'gă-nō-pek-sē, -pek'sē-ă) [organo- + G. *pēxis,* fixation]. Fixation by suture or otherwise of a floating or ptotic organ.

organophilic (ōr'gă-nō-fil'ik). Pertaining to organophilicity.

organophilicity (ōr'gă-nō-fi-li'si-tē). Attraction of nonpolar substances (organic molecules) to each other.

organosol (ōr-gan'ō-sol). A hydrosol with an organic liquid instead of water as the dispersion means.

organotaxis (ōr'gă-nō-tak'sis) [organo- + G. *taxis,* orderly arrangement]. The tendency to migrate to a certain organ selectively.

organotherapy (ōr'gă-nō-thār'ă-pē). Treatment of disease by preparations made from animal organs; now frequently by synthetic preparations instead of extracts of a gland.

organotrophic (ōr'gă-nō-trof'ik) [organo- + G. *trophē,* nourishment]. Pertaining to the nourishment of an organ.

organotropic (ōr'gă-nō-trop'ik). Pertaining to or characterized by organotropism.

organotropism (ōr-gă-not'rō-pizm) [organo- + G. *tropē,* a turning]. Organotropy; the special affinity of particular drugs, pathogens, or metastatic tumors for particular organs or their component parts. *Cf.* parasitotropism.

organotropy (ōr-gă-not'rō-pē). Organotropism.

organ-specific. Denoting or pertaining to a serum produced by the injection of the cells of a certain organ or tissue that, when injected into another animal, destroys the cells of the corresponding organ.

organum, pl. **organa** (ōr'gă-nŭm, ōr'gă-nă) [L. tool, instrument].

[NA]. Organ.
o. au'ditus, o. vestibulocochleare.
or'gana genita'lia [NA], genital organs; genitalia; genitals; the organs of reproduction or generation, external and internal; **o. g. femini'na exter'na** [NA], external feminine genital organs; partes genitales femininae externae; the vulva and clitoris; **o. g. femini'na inter'na** [NA], internal feminine genital organs; the ovaries, uterine tubes, uterus, and vagina; **o. g. masculi'na exter'na** [NA], external masculine genital organs; partes genitales masculinae externae; the penis and scrotum; **o. g. masculi'na inter'na,** [NA], internal masculine genital organs; the testes, epididymides, deferent ducts, seminal vesicles, prostate, and bulbourethral glands.

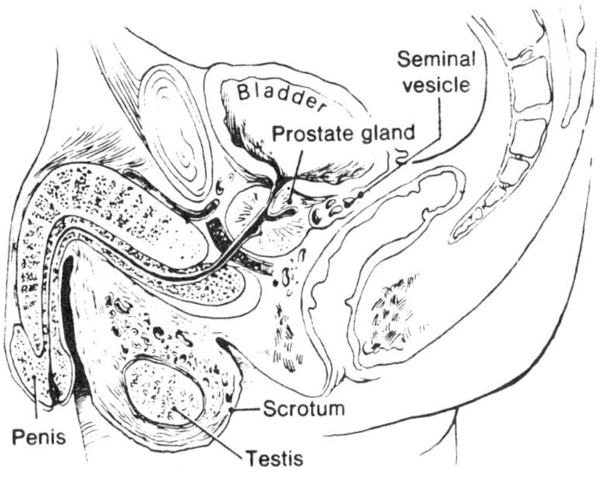

Male Genital Organs

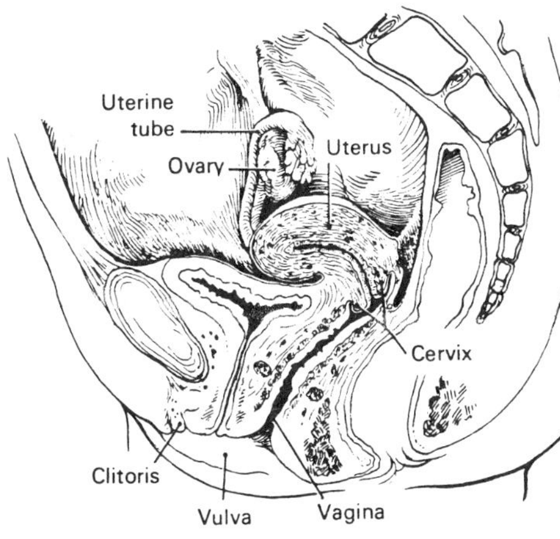

Female Genital Organs

o. gus'tus [NA], gustatory organ; organ of taste; located in the papillae of the mucous membrane of the tongue, chiefly in the vallate papillae.
or'gana oc'uli accesso'ria [NA], accessory organs of eye; the eyelids, lacrimal apparatus, and extrinsic muscles of the eyeball.
o. olfac'tus [NA], olfactory organ; organ of smell; the olfactory region in the superior portion of the nasal cavity.
or'gana sen'suum [NA], sense organs; the organs of special sense, including the eye, ear, olfactory organ, taste organs, and the accessory structures associated with these organs.
o. spira'le [NA], spiral organ; Corti's organ; acoustic papilla; a prominent ridge of highly specialized epithelium in the floor of the ductus cochlearis overlying the membrana basilaris, containing one inner row and three outer rows of hair cells, or cells of Corti (the auditory receptor cells innervated by the cochlear nerve) supported by various columnar cells: the pillars of Corti, cells of Hensen, and cells of Claudius; the o. spirale is partly overhung by an awning-like shelf, the membrana tectoria, the free marginal zone of which is covered by a gelatinous substance in which the stereocilia of the outer hair cells are embedded.
o. tac'tus, organ of touch; any one of the sensory end organs.
or'gana urina'ria [NA], urinary organs; organs involved with the formation, storage, and excretion of urine.
o. vestibulocochlea're [NA], vestibulocochlear organ; o. auditus; the external, middle, and internal ear.
o. vi'sus [NA], organ of vision; the eye and its adnexa.
o. vomeronasa'le [NA], vomeronasal organ; Jacobson's organ; a fine horizontal canal, ending in a blind pouch, in the mucous membrane of the nasal septum, beginning just behind and above the ductus incisivus.

orgasm (ōr'gazm) [G. *orgaō,* to swell, be excited]. Climax (2); the acme of the sexual act.

orgasmic, orgastic (ōr-gaz'mik, -gas'tik). Relating to, characteristic of, or tending to produce an orgasm.

orientation (ōr-ē-en-tā'shŭn) [Fr. *orienter,* to set toward the East, therefore in a definite position]. **1.** The recognition of one's temporal, spatial, and personal relationships and environment. **2.** The relative position of an atom with respect to one to which it is connected, *i.e.,* the direction of the bond connecting them.

orientomycin (or'ē-en-tō-mī'sin). Cycloserine.

orifice (or'i-fis) [L. *orificium*]. Orificium; any aperture or opening.
anal o., anus.
esophagogastric o., *ostium* cardiacum.
gastroduodenal o., *ostium* pyloricum.
golf-hole ureteral o., a retracted funnel-shaped condition of the ureteral o. in the wall of the bladder, due often to tuberculosis or a secondary sclerosis of the ureter.
mitral o., *ostium* atrioventriculare sinistrum.
pyloric o., *ostium* pyloricum.
root canal o., an opening in the pulp chamber leading to the root canal.
tricuspid o., *ostium* atrioventriculare dextrum.

orificial (ōr-i-fish'ăl). Relating to an orifice of any kind.

orificium, pl. **orificia** (ōr-i-fish'ē-ŭm, -ă) [L.] [NA]. Orifice.
o. exter'num u'teri, *ostium* uteri.
o. inter'num u'teri, *isthmus* uteri.
o. ure'teris, *ostium* ureteris.
o. ure'thrae exter'num, *ostium* urethrae externum.
o. vagi'nae, *ostium* vaginae.

origanum oil (ō-rig'ă-nŭm). The volatile oil (which contains carvacrol) obtained from various species of *Origanum* (family Labiatae); used as a rubefacient, as a constituent in veterinary liniments, and in microscopic techniques.

origin (ōr'i-jin) [L. *origo,* source, beginning, fr. *orior,* to rise]. **1.** The less movable of the two points of attachment of a muscle, that which is attached to the more fixed part of the skeleton. **2.** The starting point of a cranial or spinal nerve. The former have two o.'s: the **ental, deep,** or **real o.,** the cell group in the brain or medulla, whence the fibers of the nerve begin, and the **ectal, superficial,** or **apparent o.,** the point where the nerve emerges from the brain.

orizaba jalap root (ō-riz'ă-bă ja'lap). Ipomea.

Ormond, John K., U.S. urologist, *1886. See O.'s *disease.*

Orn Symbol for ornithine or its radical.

ornate (ōr'nāt) [L. *ornatus,* decorated]. A term that refers to the patterning of the scutum (gray or white markings on a dark background) in ixodid ticks.

ornithine (Orn) (ōr'ni-thēn, -thin). 2,5-Diaminovaleric acid; $NH_2(CH_2)_3CH(NH_2)COOH$; the amino acid formed when arginine is hydrolyzed by arginase; not a constituent of proteins, but an important intermediate in the urea cycle.

o. acetyltransferase, *glutamate* acetyltransferase.

o. carbamoyltransferase [EC 2.1.3.3], o. transcarbamoylase; an enzyme catalyzing formation of citrulline from o. and carbamoyl phosphate.

o. decarboxylase [EC 4.1.1.17], a bacterial enzyme catalyzing the decarboxylation of o. to putrescine.

o. transcarbamoylase, o. carbamoyltransferase.

ornithinemia (ōr'ni-thi-nē'mē-ă) [ornithine + G. *haima,* blood]. A toxic condition occasionally producing localized cerebral swelling, caused by abnormal amounts of ammonia in the blood.

ornithinuria (ōr'ni-thi-nū'rē-ă). Excretion of excessive amounts of ornithine in the urine.

Ornithodoros (ōr-ni-thod'ō-rŭs) [G. *ornis (ornith-),* bird, + *doros,* a leather bag]. A genus of soft ticks (family Argasidae) several species of which are vectors of pathogens of various relapsing fevers. They are characterized by a capitulum hidden below the hood and by disks and mamillae of the integument that are continuous from dorsal to ventral surfaces in a variety of patterns.

O. coria'ceus, pajaroello; a species common in the mountainous coastal areas of California; adults readily attack deer, cattle, and man, and have an irritating, painful, sometimes toxic bite.

O. errat'icus, a species the small variety of which is the vector of *Borrelia crocidurae* in Africa, the Near East, and central Asia; the large variety is the vector of *B. hispanica* in the Spanish peninsula and adjacent north Africa.

O. herm'si, a species that is a rodent parasite and vector of relapsing fever spirochetes, such as *Borrelia hermsii,* in the western U.S. and Canada.

O. lahoren'sis, a species that possibly transmits *Borrelia persica,* the agent of Persian relapsing fever.

O. mouba'ta complex, a group of four species in Africa; the taxonomy and ecology of this complex is of great significance because its members are vectors of relapsing fever spirochetes; members of the complex include *O. moubata* (various hosts), *O. compactus* (tortoises), *O. apertus* (porcupines), and *O. porcinus* (warthogs); a domestic subspecies of *O. porcinus,* in turn, forms three strains that feed chiefly on man, fowl, and swine.

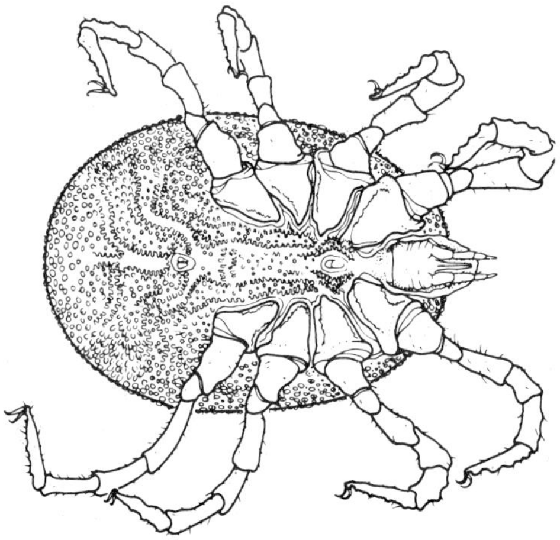

Ornithodoros moubata (×6)

O. pappil'ipes, the "Persian bug," a species found in the USSR and the Near East that transmits *Borrelia persica,* the pathogen in Iran of Persian relapsing fever.

O. par'keri, a species found in the western U.S. and a vector of *Borrelia parkeri.*

O. ru'dis, a species that is an important vector of relapsing fever spirochetes in Central and South America; possibly another complex similar to the *O. moubata* complex.

O. savi'gni, a species transmitting *Borrelia kochii,* an agent of relapsing fever of eastern Africa, southern Egypt, Ethiopia, and southwestern Asia.

O. talajé, a species found in Mexico and in Central and South America, where it feeds on wild rodents, domestic animals, and man; it delivers a painful, irritating bite and is a vector of *Borrelia mazzottii,* a cause of relapsing fever.

O. tholoza'ni, a species transmitting *Borrelia persica,* an agent of relapsing fever in the Middle East and central Asia.

O. turica'ta, a species that readily attacks man and other animals in the southern portion of the U.S. and Mexico; it is a vector of *Borrelia turicatae,* an agent of relapsing fever; the bite is painful and irritating.

O. venezuelen'sis, a species that is the vector of *Borrelia venezuelensis,* agent of relapsing fever in Colombia, Venezuela, and mountainous parts of South America.

O. verruco'sus, vector of *Borrelia caucasica.*

Ornithonyssus (ōr-ni-thon'i-sŭs) [G. *ornis (ornith-),* bird, + *nyssus,* to prick]. A genus of bird and rodent mites; species include *O. bacoti,* the tropical rat mite, a possible vector of murine typhus and a cause of human dermatitis; *O. bursa,* the tropical fowl mite; and *O. sylviarum,* the northern fowl mite.

ornithosis (ōr-ni-thō'sis) [G. *ornis (ornith-),* bird, + *-osis,* condition]. Originally, a disease in nonpsittacine birds (domestic fowls, ducks, pigeons, turkeys, and many wild birds) caused by *Chlamydia psittaci;* now, generally referred to as psittacosis.

Oro Symbol for orotic acid or orotate.

oro-. **1** [L. *os, oris,* mouth]. Combining form relating to the mouth. **2** [G. *orrhos,* whey, serum]. Obsolescent alternative spelling for orrho-. See sero-.

orodigitofacial (ōr'ō-dij'i-tō-fā'shăl). Relating to the mouth, fingers, and face.

orofacial (ōr-ō-fā'shăl). Relating to the mouth and face.

orolingual (ōr-ō-ling'gwăl). Relating to the mouth and tongue.

oronasal (ōr-ō-nā'săl). Relating to the mouth and nose.

oropharyngeal (ōr-ō-fă-rin'jē-ăl). Relating to the oropharynx.

oropharyngolaryngitis (ōr'ō-phă-rin'gō-la-rin'jī'tis). Inflammation of the mucosa of the upper respiratory-digestive tract, as from inhalation or ingestion of chemical or physical agents.

oropharynx (ōr'ō-far'ingks). [L. *os (or-),* mouth]. *Pars* oralis pharyngis.

orosomucoid (ōr'ō-sō-myū'koyd). α_1-acid glycoprotein; acid seromucoid; a subgroup of the α_1-globulin fraction of blood.

orotate (Oro) (ōr'ō-tāt). A salt or ester of orotic acid.

o. phosphoribosyltransferase [EC 2.4.2.10], orotidylic acid phosphorylase; a phosphoribosyltransferase synthesizing orotidylate from orotate and 5-phospho-α-D-ribosyl pyrophosphate.

orotic acid (oro) (ōr-ot'ik). 6-Carboxyuracil; uracil-6-carboxylic acid; an important intermediate in the formation of the pyrimidine nucleotides.

orotic aciduria [orotic acid + G. *ouron,* urine]. A rare disorder of pyrimidine metabolism characterized by hypochromic anemia with megaloblastic changes in bone marrow, leukopenia, retarded growth, and urinary excretion of orotic acid; autosomal recessive inheritance.

orotidine (Ord) (ō-rot'i-dēn). 1-Ribosylorotate; orotic acid ribonucleoside; uridine-6-carboxylic acid; an intermediate in the biosynthesis of the pyrimidine nucleosides (cytidine and uridine) that are found in nucleic acids.

orotidylate (OMP) (ō-rot-i-dil'āt). A salt or ester of orotidylic acid.

orotidylic acid (OMP) (ō-rot-i-dil′ik). Orotidine 5′-phosphate; an intermediate in the biosynthesis of the pyrimidine nucleosides (cytidine and uridine) that are found in nucleic acids.
o. a. phosphorylase, *orotate* phosphoribosyltransferase.

orphan (ōr′făn). See orphan *products.*

orphenadrine citrate (ōr-fen′ă-drēn). An antihistaminic that also has the same action and use as orphenadrine hydrochloride.

orphenadrine hydrochloride. *N,N*-Dimethyl-2(*o*-methyl-α-phenylbenzoyloxy)ethylamine hydrochloride; the *o*-methyl analogue of diphenhydramine hydrochloride; it reduces spasm of voluntary muscles, probably by action on the cerebral motor areas; used in the symptomatic treatment of paralysis agitans and drug-induced parkinsonism.

orrho- [G. *orrhos, oros,* whey, serum]. Obsolescent combining form denoting serum. See sero-.

orris (ōr′is). Iris (2).

orseillin BB (ōr-sil-in) [C.I. 26670]. A red disazo acid dye, $C_{24}H_{18}N_4O_7S_2Na_2$, used as a fungal and bacterial stain.

Orsi, Francesco, Italian physician, 1828–1890. See O.-Grocco *method.*

Orth, Johannes J., German pathologist, 1847–1923. See O.'s *fixative, stain.*

orth-. See ortho-.

orthergasia (ōrth-er-ga′zē-ă) [G. *orthos,* straight, correct, + *ergasia,* work]. Normal intellectual and emotional adjustment.

orthesis (ōr-thē′sis) [ortho- + *-esis,* process]. An orthopedic brace, splint, or appliance.

orthetics (ōr-thet′iks). Orthotics.

ortho-, orth- [Gr. *orthos,* correct, straight]. **1.** Prefix denoting straight, normal, or in proper order. **2 (*o*-).** In chemistry, italicized prefix denoting that a compound has two substitutions on adjacent carbon atoms in a benzene ring. For terms beginning *ortho-* or *o-,* see the specific name.

orthoacid (ōr′thō-as′id). An acid in which the number of hydroxyl groups equals the valence of the acid-forming element; *e.g.,* $C(OH)_4$, orthocarbonic acid. When there is no such acid, the one that most nearly approaches this condition is sometimes called an o.; *e.g.,* $PO(OH)_3$, orthophosphoric acid.

orthoarteriotony (ōr′thō-ar-tēr-ē-ot′ō-nē) [ortho- + G. *artēria,* artery, + *tonos,* tension]. Normal blood pressure.

orthobiosis (ōr′thō-bī-ō′sis) [ortho- + G. *biōsis,* life]. Correct living, both hygienically and morally.

orthocaine (ōr′thō-kān). The methyl ester of 3-amino-4-hydroxybenzoic acid; a surface anesthetic agent usually used in dusting powder form.

orthocephalic (ōr′thō-sĕ-fal′ik) [ortho- + G. *kephalē,* head]. Orthocephalous; having a head well proportioned to height; denoting a skull with a vertical index between 70 and 75. See also metriocephalic.

orthocephalous (ōr-thō-sef′ă-lŭs). Orthocephalic.

orthochorea (ōr′thō-kōr-ē′ă). A form of chorea in which the spasms occur only or chiefly when the patient is in the erect posture.

orthochromatic (ōr′thō-krō-mat′ic) [ortho- + G. *chrōma,* color]. Euchromatic (1); orthochromophil; orthochromophile; denoting any tissue or cell that stains the color of the dye used, *i.e.,* the same color as the dye solution with which it is stained.

orthochromophil, orthochromophile (ōr-thō-krō′mō-fil, -fīl) [ortho- + G. *chrōma,* color, + *philos,* fond]. Orthochromatic.

orthocrasia (ōr-thō-krā′sē-ă) [ortho- + G. *krasis,* a mixing, temperament]. Obsolete term for condition in which there is a normal reaction to drugs, articles of diet, etc.

orthocytosis (ōr′thō-sī-tō′sis) [ortho- + G. *kytos,* cell, + *-osis,* condition]. A condition in which all of the cellular elements in the circulating blood are mature forms, irrespective of the proportions of various types and total numbers.

orthodentin (ōr-thō-den′tin). Straight tubed dentin as seen in the teeth of mammals.

orthodigita (or-tho-dij′ī-tah) [ortho- + L. *digitus,* finger or toe]. Correction of malformations of fingers or toes.

orthodontia (ōr-thō-don′shē-ă). Orthodontics.

orthodontics (ōr-thō-don′tiks) [ortho- + G. *odous,* tooth]. Orthodontia; dental orthopedics; that branch of dentistry concerned with the correction and prevention of irregularities and malocclusion of the teeth.
surgical o., orthognathic surgery; the correction of occlusal abnormalities by the surgical repositioning of segments of the mandible or maxillae containing one to several teeth; or the bodily repositioning of entire jaws to improve function and esthetics.

or′thodont′ist. A dental specialist who practices orthodontics.

orthodromic (ōr-thō-drō′mik) [ortho- + G. *dromos,* course]. Dromic; denoting the propagation of an impulse along an axon in the normal direction. *Cf.* antidromic.

orthogenesis (ōr-thō-jen′ĕ-sis) [ortho- + G. *genesis,* origin]. The doctrine that evolution is governed by intrinsic factors, and occurs in definite directions.

orthogenic (ōr-thō-jen′ik). Relating to orthogenesis.

orthogenics (ōr-thō-jen′iks). The science concerned with the study and treatment of mental and physical defects that obstruct or retard normal development.

orthognathia (ōr-thō-nath′ē-ă) [ortho- + G. *gnathos,* jaw]. The study of the causes and treatment of conditions related to malposition of the bones of the jaws.

orthognathic, orthognathous (ōr-thō-nath′ik, ōr-thog′năthŭs) [ortho- + G. *gnathos,* jaw]. **1.** Relating to orthognathia. **2.** Having a face without projecting jaw, one with a gnathic index below 98.

orthograde (ōr′thō-grād) [ortho- + L. *gradior,* pp. *gressus,* to walk]. Walking or standing erect; denoting the posture of man; opposed to pronograde.

orthokeratology (ōr′thō-ker-ă-tol′ō-jē) [ortho- + G. *keras,* horn (cornea), + *logos,* science]. A method of molding the cornea with contact lenses to improve unaided vision.

orthokeratosis (ōr′thō-ker-ă-tō′sis) [ortho- + G. *keras,* horn, + *-osis,* condition]. Formation of an anuclear keratin layer.

orthokinetics (ōr-thō-ki-net′iks) [ortho- + G. *kinētikos,* movable, fr. *kineō,* to move]. A method advocated for the treatment of hypertrophic osteoarthritis in which an attempt is made to change muscular action from one group of muscles to another set of muscles to protect the diseased joint.

orthomechanical (ōr-thō-mĕ-kan′i-kăl) [ortho- + mechanical]. Pertaining to braces, prostheses, orthotic devices, and appliances.

orthomechanotherapy (ōr′thō-mĕ-kan-ō-thār′ă-pē) [ortho- + G. *mechane,* machine, + *therapeia,* medical treatment]. Treatment with braces, prostheses, orthotic devices, or appliances.

orthomelic (ōr-thō-mē′lik) [ortho- + G. *melos,* limb]. Correcting malformations of arms or legs.

orthometer (ōr-thom′ĕ-ter) [ortho- + G. *metron,* measure]. An instrument for determining the degree of protrusion or retraction of the eyeballs.

orthomolecular (ōr′thō-mō-lek′yū-lăr). Pauling's term denoting a therapeutic approach designed to provide an optimum molecular environment for body functions, with particular reference to the optimum concentrations of substances normally present in the human body, whether formed endogenously or ingested.

Orthomyxoviridae (ōr'thō-mik-sō-vir'i-dē). The family of viruses that comprises the three groups of influenza viruses, types A, B, and C. Virions are roughly spherical or filamentous, the former (the more common form) are 80 to 120 nm in diameter and ether-sensitive; envelopes are studded with surface projections; nucleocapsids are of helical symmetry, 6 to 9 nm in diameter, and contain single-stranded, segmented RNA. The nucleoprotein antigen of each type of virus is common to all strains of the type but distinct from those of the other two types; the mosaic of surface antigens varies from strain to strain. Nucleocapsids seem to be formed in the nuclei of infected cells, hemagglutinin and neuraminidase in the cytoplasm; virus maturation occurs during budding of the cell membrane. The only recognized genus is *Influenzavirus,* which comprises the strains of virus types A and B. Influenza virus type C differs from types A and B somewhat (*e.g.,* the "receptor-destroying enzyme" seems not to be a neuraminidase) and probably belongs to a separate genus. See also *Influenzavirus.*

orthopaedic, orthopedic (ōr-thō-pē'dik). Relating to orthopaedics.

orthopaedics, orthopedics (ōr-thō-pē'diks) [ortho- + G. *pais* (*paid-*), child]. The medical specialty concerned with the preservation, restoration, and development of form and function of the musculoskeletal system, extremities, spine, and associated structures by medical, surgical, and physical methods.

orthopaedist, orthopedist (ōr-thō-pē'dist). One who practices orthopaedics.

orthopedics (ōr-thō-pē'diks). Orthopaedics.

dental o., orthodontics.

functional jaw o., functional orthodontic therapy; utilization of muscle forces to effect changes in jaw position and tooth alignment by removable appliances.

orthopercussion (ōr'thō-per-kŭsh'ŭn). Very light percussion of the chest, made in a sagittal direction (*i.e.,* anteroposteriorly, and not perpendicularly to the wall of the chest); used to determine the size of the heart, the faint percussion sound disappearing when the heart is reached even though that may be overlapped by a layer of the lung.

orthophoria (ōr-thō-fōr'ē-ă) [ortho- + G. *phora,* motion]. Absence of heterophoria; the condition of binocular fixation in which the lines of sight meet at a distant or near point of reference in the absence of a fusion stimulus.

orthophoric (ōr-thō-fōr'ik). Pertaining to orthophoria.

orthophosphate (ōr-thō-fos'fāt). A salt or ester of orthophosphoric acid.

inorganic o. (P_i) any ion or salt form of phosphoric acid.

orthophosphoric acid (ōr'thō-fos-fōr'ik). Phosphoric acid, H_3PO_4, distinguished by ortho- from meta- and pyrophosphoric acids, $HPO_3)_n$ and $H_4P_2O_7$ respectively, which are anhydrides of H_3PO_4; the ultimate anhydride is phosphorus pentoxide, P_2O_5.

orthophrenia (ōr-thō-frē'nē-ă) [ortho- + G. *phrēn,* mind]. **1.** Soundness of mind. **2.** A condition of normal interpersonal relationships.

orthopnea (ōr-thop-nē'ă, ōr-thop'nē-ă) [ortho- + G. *pnoē,* a breathing]. Discomfort in breathing which is brought on or aggravated by lying flat. *Cf.* platypnea.

orthopneic (or'thop-ne'ik). Relating to or characterized by orthopnea.

Orthopoxvirus (ōr-thō-poks'vī-rŭs). The genus of the family Poxviridae which comprises the viruses of alastrim, vaccinia, variola, cowpox, ectromelia, monkeypox, and rabbitpox.

orthoprosthesis (ōr'thō-pros'thĕ-sis, -pros-thē'sis). An appliance used in the management of prosthetic problems related to alignment of teeth.

orthopsychiatry (ōr'thō-sī-kī'ă-trē). The science concerned with the study and treatment of disorders of behavior, especially in children.

Orthoptera (ōr-thop'ter-ă) [ortho- + G. *pteron,* a wing]. A large order of hemimetabolous insects that includes the locusts, grasshoppers, mantids, walking sticks, and related forms.

orthoptic (ōr-thop'tik). Relating to orthoptics.

orthoptics (ōr-thop'tiks) [ortho- + G. *optikos,* relating to sight]. The study and treatment of defective binocular vision, of defects in the action of the ocular muscles, or of faulty visual habits.

orthoptist (ōr-thop'tist). One skilled in orthoptics.

orthoscope (ōr'thō-skōp) [ortho- + G. *skopeō,* to view]. **1.** An instrument by means of which one is able to draw the outlines of the various normas of the skull. **2.** An instrument by which water is held in contact with the eye, thereby eliminating corneal refraction.

orthoscopic (ōr-thō-skop'ik). **1.** Relating to the orthoscope. **2.** Having normal vision. **3.** Denoting an object correctly observed by the eye.

orthoscopy (ōr-thos'kŏ-pē). Examination of the eye with the orthoscope.

orthosis, pl. **orthoses** (ōr-thō'sis, -sēz) [G. *orthōsis,* a making straight]. Straightening of a deformity, often by use of orthopedic appliances.

orthostatic (ōr-thō-stat'ik). Relating to an erect posture or position.

orthostereoscope (ōr'thō-ster'ē-ō-skōp). A rarely used instrument for stereoscopic x-ray.

orthosympathetic (ōr'thō-sim-pa-thet'ik). Referring to the sympathetic component of the autonomic nervous system, as distinguished from parasympathetic. See *systema* nervosum autonomicum.

orthothanasia (ōr'thō-thă-na'zē-ă) [ortho- + G. *thanatos,* death]. **1.** A normal or natural manner of death and dying. **2.** Sometimes used to denote the deliberate stopping of artificial or heroic means of maintaining life.

orthotics (ōr-thot'iks). Orthetics; the science concerned with the making and fitting of orthopaedic appliances.

orthotist (ōr'thō'tist). A maker and fitter of orthopaedic appliances.

orthotolidine (ōr-thō-tō'li-dēn). *o*-Tolidine; 3,3'-dimethylbenzidine; in the presence of peroxidase, o. (like benzidine) is oxidized to a blue color; since hemoglobin behaves like a peroxidase, o. has been used as an *in vitro* aid for the detection of occult blood in feces.

orthotonos, orthotonus (ōr-thot'ŏ-nos, -ō-nŭs) [ortho- + G. *tonos,* tension]. A form of tetanic spasm in which the neck, limbs, and body are held fixed in a straight line.

orthotopic (ōr-thō-top'ik) [ortho- + G. *topos,* place]. In the normal or usual position.

orthotropic (ōr-thō-trop'ik) [ortho- + G. *tropē,* a turn]. Extending or growing in a straight, especially a vertical, direction.

orthovoltage (ōr-thō-vōl'tij). In radiation therapy, a vague term for voltage between 400 and 600 kv.

Orton, S.T., U.S. neurologist, 1879–1975. See Wolf-O. *bodies.*

O.S. Abbreviation for L. *oculus sinster,* left eye.

Os Symbol for osmium.

os, gen. **o'ris,** pl. **o'ra** [L. mouth]. **1** [NA]. The mouth. **2.** Term applied sometimes to an opening into a hollow organ or canal, especially one with thick or fleshy edges.

incompetent cervical o., a defect in the muscular ring at the internal o. allowing premature dilation of the cervix.

Scanzoni's second o., pathologic retraction *ring.*

o. u'teri exter'num, *ostium* uteri.

o. u'teri inter'num, *isthmus* uteri.

OS

os, gen. **ossis,** pl. **ossa** (os, os'is, os'ă) [L. bone] [NA]. Bone; a portion of osseous tissue of definite shape and size, forming a part of the animal skeleton; in man there are 200 distinct ossa in the skeleton, not including the ossicula auditus of the tympanic cavity or the ossa sesamoidea other than the two patellae. Bone consists of a dense outer layer of compact substance or cortical substance covered by the periosteum, and an inner loose, spongy substance; the central portion of a long bone is filled with marrow. For histological description, see bone.

o. acromia'le, an acromion that is joined to the scapular spine by fibrous rather than by bony union.

o. basila're, basilar *bone.*

o. bre've [NA], short bone; one whose dimensions are approximately equal; it consists of a layer of cortical substance enclosing spongy substance and narrow. *Cf.* o. longum.

o. cal'cis, calcaneus.

o. capita'tum [NA], capitate (2); capitate bone; o. magnum; the largest of the carpal bones; located in the distal row.

os'sa car'pi [NA], carpal bones; see carpus (2) and the individual bones o. scaphoideum, o. lunatum, o. triquetrum, o. pisiforme, o. trapezium, o. trapezoideum, o. capitatum, o. hamatum.

o. centra'le [NA], central bone; a small bone occasionally found at the dorsal aspect of the wrist between the scaphoid, capitate, and trapezoid; it is developed as an independent cartilage in early fetal life but usually becomes fused with the scaphoid; it occurs normally in most monkeys.

o. centra'le tar'si, o. naviculare.

o. clito'ris, a small bone located in the clitoris of many carnivorous mammals. It is homologous with the o. penis of the male.

o. coc'cygis [NA], coccygeal bone; coccyx; tail bone; the small bone at the end of the vertebral column in man, formed by the fusion of four rudimentary vertebrae; it articulates above with the sacrum.

o. costa'le [NA], the bony part of a rib.

o. cox'ae [NA], coxal, hip, or innominate bone; coxa (1); o. innominatum; a large flat bone formed by the fusion of the ilium, ischium, and pubis (in the adult), constituting the lateral half of the pelvis; it articulates with its fellow anteriorly, with the sacrum posteriorly, and with the femur laterally.

ossa cra'nii [NA], cranial bones; the bones of the skull; they are the paired inferior nasal concha, lacrimal, maxilla, nasal, palatine, parietal, temporal, and zygomatic; and the unpaired ethmoid, frontal, occipital, sphenoid, and vomer.

o. cuboi'deum [NA], cuboid bone; the lateral bone of the distal row of the tarsus, articulating with the calcaneus, lateral cuneiform, navicular (occasionally), and fourth and fifth metatarsal bones.

o. cuneifor'me interme'dium [NA], intermediate, middle, or second cuneiform bone; mesocuneiform; wedge bone; a bone of the distal row of the tarsus; it articulates with the medial and lateral cuneiform, navicular, and second metatarsal bones.

o. cuneifor'me latera'le [NA], lateral cuneiform or third cuneiform bone; wedge bone; a bone of the distal row of the tarsus; it articulates with the intermediate cuneiform, cuboid, navicular, and second, third, and fourth metatarsal bones.

o. cuneifor'me media'le [NA], first or medial cuneiforme bone; wedge bone; the largest of the three cuneiform bones, the medial bone of the distal row of the tarsus, articulating with the intermediate cuneiform, navicular, and first and second metatarsal bones.

os'sa digito'rum [NA], bones of digits; the phalanges and sesamoid bones of the fingers and toes. See also phalanx (1).

o. ethmoida'le [NA], ethmoid bone; an irregularly shaped bone lying between the orbital plates of the frontal and anterior to the sphenoid bone; it consists of two lateral masses of thin plates enclosing air cells, attached above to a perforated horizontal lamina, the cribriform plate, from which descends a median vertical or perpendicular plate in the interval between the two lateral masses; the bone articulates with the sphenoid, frontal, maxillary, lacrimal, and palatine bones, the inferior nasal concha, and the vomer; it enters into the formation of the anterior cranial fossa, the orbits, and the nasal cavity.

os'sa fa'ciei, facial *bones.*

o. fem'oris [NA], thigh bone; femur (2); the long bone of the thigh, articulating with the hip bone proximally and the tibia and patella distally.

o. fronta'le [NA], frontal bone; coronale (1); the large single bone forming the forehead and the upper margin and roof of the orbit on either side; it articulates with the parietal, nasal, ethmoid, maxillary, and zygomatic bones, and with the lesser wings of the sphenoid.

o. hama'tum [NA], hamate, hooked, or unciform bone; hamatum; the bone on the medial (ulnar) side of the distal row of the carpus; it articulates with the fourth and fifth metacarpal, triquetral, lunate, and capitate.

o. hyoi'deum [NA], hyoid, lingual, or tongue bone; a U-shaped bone lying between the mandible and the larynx, suspended from the styloid processes by slender stylohyoid ligaments. See also *apparatus* hyoideus.

o. il'ium [NA], ilium; iliac or flank bone; the broad, flaring portion of the hip bone, distinct at birth but later becoming fused with the ischium and pubis; it consists of a body, which joins the pubis and ischium to form the acetabulum and a broad thin portion, called the ala or wing.

o. in'cae, o. interparietale.

o. incisi'vum [NA], incisive, intermaxillary, or premaxillary bone; o. intermaxillare or premaxillare; intermaxilla; premaxilla; Goethe's bone (2); the anterior and inner portion of the maxilla, which in the fetus and sometimes in the adult, is a separate bone; the incisive suture runs from the incisive canal between the lateral incisor and the canine tooth; according to K. Albrecht, the o. incisivum is further divided by a suture between the two incisor teeth on each side into two bones, the endognathion and the mesagnathion.

o. innomina'tum, o. coxae.

o. intermaxilla're, o. incisivum.

o. interme'dium, o. lunatum.

o. intermetatar'seum, a supernumerary bone at the base of the first metatarsal, or between the first and second metatarsal bones, usually fused with one or the other or with the medial cuneiform bone.

o. interparieta'le [NA], interparietal bone; incarial bone; o. incae; the upper part of the squama of the occipital bone, developed in membrane instead of in cartilage as is the rest of the occipital, and occasionally (especially in ancient Peruvian skulls) existing as a separate bone, separated from the remainder of the occipital by the sutura mendosa.

o. irregula're [NA], irregular bone; one of a group of bones having peculiar or complex forms, *e.g.,* vertebrae, many of the skull bones.

o. is'chii [NA], ischium; ischial bone; the lower and posterior part of the hip bone, distinct at birth but later becoming fused with the ilium and pubis; it consists of a body, where it joins the ilium and superior ramus of the pubis to form the acetabulum, and a ramus joining the inferior ramus of the pubis.

o. japon'icum, a bipartite or tripartite zygomatic bone, found with greater frequency in the Japanese than in other races.

o. lacrima'le [NA], lacrimal bone; o. unguis; an irregularly rectangular thin plate, forming part of the medial wall of the orbit be-

hind the frontal process of the maxilla; it articulates with the inferior nasal concha, ethmoid, frontal, and maxillary bones.
o. lon'gum [NA], long bone; pipe bone; one of the elongated bones of the extremities, consisting of a tubular shaft (diaphysis) and two extremities (epiphyses) usually wider than the shaft; the shaft is composed of compact bone surrounding a central medullary cavity. *Cf.* o. breve.
o. luna'tum [NA], lunate bone; semilunar bone; o. intermedium; lunare; one of the proximal row in the carpus between the scaphoid and triquetral; it articulates with the radius, scaphoid, triquetral, hamate, and capitate.
o. mag'num, o. capitatum.
o. mala're, o. zygomaticum.
os'sa mem'bri inferio'ris [NA], bones of inferior limb; these include the inferior limb girdle (hip bone) and the skeleton of the free inferior limb (femur, tibia, fibula, patella, tarsus, metatarsus, and bones of the toes).
os'sa mem'bri superio'ris [NA], bones of superior limb; these include the superior limb girdle (scapula and clavicle) and the skeleton of the free superior limb (humerus, radius, ulna, wrist bones, metacarpus, and bones of the fingers).
o. metacarpa'le, pl. **os'sa metacarpa'lia** [NA], one of the metacarpal bones, five long bones (numbered I to V, beginning with the bone on the radial or thumb side) forming the skeleton of the metacarpus or palm; they articulate with the bones of the distal row of the carpus and with the five proximal phalanges.
o. metatarsa'le, pl. **os'sa metatarsa'lia** [NA], one of the metatarsal bones; the five long bones numbered I to V beginning with the bone on the medial side forming the skeleton of the anterior portion of the foot, articulating posteriorly with the three cuneiform and the cuboid bones, anteriorly with the five proximal phalanges.
o. multan'gulum ma'jus, o. trapezium.
o. multan'gulum mi'nus, o. trapezoideum.
o. nasa'le [NA], nasal bone; an elongated rectangular bone which, with its fellow, forms the bridge of the nose; it articulates with the frontal bone superiorly, the ethmoid and the frontal process of the maxilla posteriorly, and its fellow medially.
o. navicula're [NA], navicular bone; o. centrale tarsi; central bone of ankle; a bone of the tarsus on the medial side of the foot articulating with the head of the talus, the three cuneiform bones, and occasionally the cuboid.
o. navicula're ma'nus, o. scaphoideum.
o. occipita'le [NA], occipital bone; a bone at the lower and posterior part of the skull, consisting of three parts (basilar, condylar, and squamous), enclosing a large oval hole, the foramen magnum; it articulates with the parietal and temporal bones on either side, the sphenoid anteriorly, and the atlas below.
o. odontoi'deum, the dens of the axis when anomalously not fused with the body of the axis.
o. orbicula're, *processus* lenticularis incudis.
o. palati'num [NA], palatine bone; an irregularly shaped bone posterior to the maxilla, which enters into the formation of the nasal cavity, the orbit, and the hard palate; it articulates with the maxilla, inferior nasal concha, sphenoid, and ethmoid bones, the vomer and its fellow of the opposite side.
o. parieta'le [NA], parietal bone; a flat, curved bone of irregular quadrangular shape, at either side of the vault of the cranium; it articulates, with its fellow medially, with the frontal anteriorly, the occipital posteriorly, and the temporal and sphenoid inferiorly.
o. pe'nis, baculum; penis bone; a bone of variable size and shape, located in the glans penis or glans clitoridis of all animals, except man, ungulates, elephants, whales, and a few others; it is particularly well developed in carnivora, and in the dog may reach a length of more than 10 cm; its size and shape are often a characteristic of a species.
o. pisifor'me [NA], pisiform bone; lentiform bone; a small bone resembling a pea in size and shape, in the proximal row of the carpus, lying on the anterior surface of the triquetral with which alone it articulates; it gives insertion to the tendon of the flexor carpi ulnaris muscle.
o. pla'num [NA], flat bone; a type of bone characterized by its thin, flattened shape, such as the scapula or certain of the cranial bones.
o. pneumat'icum [NA], pneumatic bone; hollow bone; a bone that is hollow or contains many air cells, such as the mastoid process of the temporal bone.
o. premaxilla're, o. incisivum.
o. pterygoi'deum, *processus* pterygoideus.
o. pu'bis [NA], pubic bone; pubis (1); the anteroinferior portion of the hip bone, distinct at birth but later becoming fused with the ilium and ischium; it is composed of a body which articulates with its fellow at the symphysis pubis, and two rami; the superior ramus enters into the formation of the acetabulum, the inferior ramus fuses with the ramus of the ischium.
o. pyramida'le, o. triquetrum.
o. sa'crum [NA], sacred bone; sacrum; vertebra magna; the segment of the vertebral column forming part of the pelvis; a broad, slightly curved, spade-shaped bone, thick above, thinner below, closing in the pelvic girdle posteriorly; it is formed by the fusion of five originally separate sacral vertebrae; it articulates with the last lumbar vertebra, the coccyx, and the hip bone on either side.
o. scaphoi'deum [NA], scaphoid bone; navicular bone of hand; o. naviculare manus; the largest bone of the proximal row of the carpus on the lateral (radial) side, articulating with the radius, lunate, capitate, trapezium, and trapezoid.
o. sesamoi'deum, pl. **os'sa sesamoi'dea** [NA], sesamoid bone; a bone formed in a tendon where it passes over a joint.
o. sphenoida'le [NA], sphenoid bone; a bone of most irregular shape occupying the base of the skull; it is described as consisting of a central portion, or body, and six processes: two greater wings, two lesser wings and two pterygoid processes; it articulates with the occipital, frontal, ethmoid, and vomer, and with the paired temporal, parietal, zygomatic, palatine and sphenoidal concha bones.
o. subtibia'le, an inconstant bone found very rarely in the distal articular end of the tibia.
o. suprasterna'le, pl. **os'sa suprasterna'lia** [NA], suprasternal bone; episternal bone; Breschet's bones; one of the small ossicles occasionally found in the ligaments of the sternoclavicular articulation.
os'sa sutura'rum [NA], sutural, epactal, or wormian bones; Andernach's ossicles; epactal ossicles; small irregular bones found along the sutures of the cranium, particularly related to the parietal bone.
o. syl'vii, *processus* lenticularis incudis.
os'sa tar'si [NA], tarsal bones. See tarsus (1).
o. tempora'le [NA], temporal bone; a large irregular bone situated in the base and side of the skull; it consists of three parts, squamous, tympanic and petrous, which are distinct at birth; the petrous part contains the vestibulocochlear organ; the bone articulates with the sphenoid, parietal, occipital, and zygomatic bones, and by a synovial joint with the mandible.
o. tibia'le poste'rius, o. tibia'le posti'cum, tibiale posticum; a sesamoid bone in the tendon of the tibialis posterior muscle, occasionally fused with the tuberosity of the navicular.
o. trape'zium [NA], trapezium bone; trapezium; o. multangulum majus; greater multangular bone; the lateral (radial) bone in the distal row of the carpus; it articulates with the first and second metacarpals, scaphoid, and trapezoid bones.
o. trapezoi'deum [NA], trapezoid bone; trapezoid (3); lesser multangular bone; o. multangulum minus; a bone in the distal row of the carpus; it articulates with the second metacarpal, trapezium, capitate, and scaphoid.
o. triangula're, **(1)** o. trigonum; **(2)** o. triquetrum.

o. tribasila're, the single bone resulting from the fusion in infancy of the occipital and temporal bones at the base of the cranial cavity.

o. trigo'num [NA], triangular bone; o. triangulare (1); an independent ossicle sometimes present in the tarsus; usually it forms part of the talus, constituting the lateral tubercle of the posterior process.

o. trique'trum [NA], triquetral bone; triquetrum; cubital, three-cornered, cuneiform, or pyramidal bone; o. pyramidale; o. triangulare (2); pyramidale; a bone on the medial (ulnar) side of the proximal row of the carpus, articulating with the lunate, pisiform, and hamate.

o. un'guis, o. lacrimale.

o. vesalia'num, Vesalius' bone; the tuberosity of the fifth metatarsal bone sometimes existing as a separate bone.

o. zygomat'icum [NA], zygomatic bone; yoke, jugal, or malar bone; cheek bone; o. malare; mala; zygoma (1); a quadrilateral bone which forms the prominence of the cheek; it articulates with the frontal, sphenoid, temporal, and maxillary bone.

---

osazone (ō'să-zōn). Dihydrazone; the compound formed by certain sugars (*e.g.,* glucose, galactose, fructose) with excess hydrazines, possessing two hydrazones on carbons 1 and 2 instead of only one at C-1, as in the ordinary hydrazone; o.'s formed with phenylhydrazine (phenylosazones) are used to characterize and identify certain sugars.

osche-, oscheo- [G. *oschē,* scrotum]. Combining forms denoting the scrotum.

oscheal (os'kē-ăl). Scrotal.

oscheitis (os-kē-ī'tis) [osche- + G. *-itis,* inflammation]. Inflammation of the scrotum.

oschelephantiasis (osk'el-ĕ-fan-tī'ă-sis) [osche- + elephantiasis]. An enlargement or elephantiasis of the scrotum.

oscheohydrocele (os-kē-ō-hī'drō-sēl) [oscheo- + G. *hydōr,* water, + *kēlē,* tumor]. Scrotal hydrocele.

oscheoplasty (os'kē-ō-plas-tē) [oscheo- + *plastos,* formed]. Scrotoplasty.

oscillation (os-i-lā'shŭn) [L. *oscillatio,* fr. *oscillo,* to swing]. **1.** A to-and-fro movement. **2.** A stage in the vascular changes in inflammation in which the accumulation of leukocytes in the small vessels arrests the passage of blood and there is simply a to-and-fro movement at each cardiac contraction.

oscillator (os'si-lā-ter). **1.** An apparatus somewhat like a vibrator, used to give a form of mechanical massage. **2.** An electric circuit designed to generate alternating current at a particular frequency. **3.** Any device that produces oscillation.

oscillograph (ŏ-sil'ō-graf). An instrument that records oscillations, usually electrical.

oscillography (os-i-log'ră-fē). The study of the records made by an oscillograph.

oscillometer (os-i-lom'ĕ-ter) [L. *oscillo,* to swing, + G. *metron,* measure]. An apparatus for measuring oscillations of any kind, especially those of the bloodstream in sphygmometry. See also sphygmo-oscillometer.

oscillometric (os'i-lō-met'rik). Relating to the oscillometer or the records made by its use.

oscillometry (os-i-lom'ĕ-trē). The measurement of oscillations of any kind with an oscillometer.

oscillopsia (os-i-lop'sē-ă) [L. *oscillo,* to swing, + G. *opsis,* vision]. Oscillating vision; the subjective sensation of oscillation of objects viewed.

oscilloscope (ŏ-sil'ō-skōp). An oscillograph in which the record of oscillations is continuously visible.

cathode ray o. (CRO), the common form of o., in which a varying electrical signal (*y*) vertically deflects an electron beam impinging on a fluorescent screen, while some other function (*x* or time) deflects the beam horizontally; the result is a visual graph of *y* plotted against *x* or time with negligible distortion by inertia.

storage o., a cathode ray o. in which the visual record of oscillations persists on the fluorescent screen until erased electrically.

oscitate (os'i-tāt) [L. *oscito,* fr. *os,* mouth, + *cieo,* to put in motion]. To yawn; to gape.

oscitation (os'i-tā'shŭn) [L. *oscitatio*]. Yawning.

osculum, pl. oscula (os'kyū-lŭm, -lă) [L. dim.of *os,* mouth]. A pore or minute opening.

-ose. 1. In chemistry, a termination usually indicating a carbohydrate. **2.** [L. *-osus,* full of, abounding]. Suffix appended to some L. roots, with significance of the more common -ous (2).

-oses. Plural of -osis.

Osgood, Robert B., U.S. orthopedic surgeon, 1873–1956. See O.-Schlatter *disease.*

OSHA Abbreviation for Occupational Safety and Health Administration of the U.S. Department of Labor, responsible for establishing and enforcing safety and health standards in the workplace.

-osis, pl. -oses [G.]. Suffix, properly added only to words formed from G. roots, meaning a process, condition, or state, usually abnormal or diseased. It denotes primarily any production or increase, physiologic or pathologic, and secondarily an invasion, and increase within the organism, of parasites; in the latter sense, it is similar to and often interchangeable with G. *-iasis,* as seen in trichinosis, trichiniasis.

Osler, Sir William, Canadian-American physician, 1849–1919. See O.'s *disease, node, sign;* Rendu-O.-Weber *disease, syndrome.*

osmate (os'māt). A salt of osmic acid.

osmatic (oz-mat'ik) [G. *osmē,* smell]. Olfactory.

osmesis (oz-mē'sis) [G. *osmēsis,* smelling]. Olfaction.

osmic acid (oz'mik). Osmium tetroxide; OsO_4; a volatile caustic and strong oxidizing agent; colorless crystals, poorly soluble in water, but soluble in organic solvents; the aqueous solution is a fat and myelin stain and a general fixative for electron microscopy.

osmicate (oz'mi-kāt). To stain or fix with osmic acid.

osmication, osmification (os'mi-kā'shŭn, os'mi-fi-kā'shŭn). The fixation of tissue with an osmic acid solution.

osmics (oz'miks) [G. *osmē,* smell]. The science of olfaction.

osmidrosis (oz-mi-drō'sis) [G. *osmē,* smell, + *hidrōs,* sweat]. Bromidrosis.

osmiophilic (oz'mi-ō-fil'ik) [osmium + G. *phileō,* to love]. Readily stained with osmic acid.

osmiophobic (oz'mi-ō-fō'bik) [osmium + G. *phobos,* fear]. Not readily stained with osmic acid.

osmium (oz'mē-ŭm) [G. *osmē,* smell, because of the strong odor of the tetroxide]. A metallic element of the platinum group, symbol Os, atomic no. 76, atomic weight 190.2.

o. tetroxide, osmic acid.

osmo-. 1 [G. *ōsmos,* impulsion]. Combining form denoting osmosis. **2** [G. *osmē,* smell]. Combining form denoting smell or odor.

osmoceptor (os-mō-sep'ter, tōr). Osmoreceptor.

osmodysphoria (oz'mō-dis-fōr'ē-ă) [G. *osmē,* smell, + *dys-,* bad, + *phora,* a carrying]. An abnormal dislike of certain odors.

osmogram (oz'mō-gram) [G. *osmē,* smell, + *gramma,* a drawing]. Electro-olfactogram.

osmolality (os-mō-lal'i-tē). Osmotic concentration, defined as the number of osmoles (Φn moles, where n is the number of particles or ions formed upon dissociation of a solute in solution; *e.g.,* $n = 2$ for sodium chloride and $n = 1$ for glucose) of a solute per kg of solvent (water); thus, o. is given by Φnc, where c is the molal concentration of solute. The o. of a given solution is numerically equal to the molality of an ideal solution of a nonelectrolyte having the same freezing point. It is approximated by the quotient of the freezing point depression of an aqueous solution below that of water (Δ°C) and the molal freezing point depression for water (*ca.* 1.86°C per mol of undissociated solute per kg of water); *i.e.*, o. = Δ/1.86.

calculated serum o., the calculation of serum o. from serum sodium, glucose, and urea nitrogen values by a variety of formulae, the most common of which is:

$1.86 \times [Na^{30}] + \text{glucose(mg/dl)}/18 + \text{BUN(mg/dl)}/2.8$

osmolar (os-mō'lăr). Osmotic.

osmolarity (os-mō-lăr'i-tē). The osmotic concentration of a solution expressed as osmoles of solute per liter of solution.

osmole (os'mōl). The molecular weight of a solute, in grams, divided by the number of ions or particles into which it dissociates in solution.

osmology (os-mol'ō-jē). **1.** Osphresiology; the study of odors, their production, and their effects. **2.** The study of osmosis.

osmometer (os-mom'ĕ-ter). An instrument for measuring osmolality by freezing point depression or vapor pressure elevation techniques.

osmometry (os-mom'ĕ-trē). Measurement of osmolality by use of an osmometer.

osmophil, osmophilic (os'mō-fil, -fil'ik) [osmo(sis) + G. *phileō*, to love]. Flourishing in a medium of high osmotic pressure.

osmophobia (oz-mō-fō'bē-ă) [G. *osmē*, smell, + phobia]. Olfactophobia.

osmophore (oz'mō-fōr) [G. *osmē*, smell, + *phonos*, bearing]. The group of atoms in the molecule of a compound that is responsible for the compound's characteristic odor.

osmoreceptor (os'mō-rē-sep'ter, -tōr). Osmoceptor. **1** [G. *osmos*, impulsion]. A receptor in the central nervous system (probably the hypothalamus) that responds to changes in the osmotic pressure of the blood. **2** [G. *osmē*, smell]. A receptor that receives olfactory stimuli.

osmoregulatory (os-mō-reg'yū-lă-tōr-ē). Influencing the degree and rapidity of osmosis.

osmose (os'mōs). **1.** To move through a membrane by osmosis. **2.** Obsolete term for osmosis.

osmosis (os-mō'sis) [G. *ōsmos*, a thrusting, an impulsion]. The process by which solvent tends to move through a semipermeable membrane from a solution of lower to a solution of higher osmolal concentration of the solutes to which the membrane is relatively impermeable.

reverse o., movement of solvent in the opposite direction from o., *i.e.*, pressure filtration of solvent through a semipermeable membrane that will hold back the solutes; commonly replaced by filtration or ultrafiltration when speaking of capillary membranes, as in the renal glomerulus.

osmosity (os-mos'i-tē). An indirect measure of the osmotic characteristics of a solution, in terms of a comparable sodium chloride solution, now rendered obsolete by the more precisely defined term osmolality.

osmotherapy (os'mō-thār'ă-pē) [osmosis + therapy]. Dehydration by means of intravenous injections of hypertonic solutions of sodium chloride, dextrose, urea, mannitol, or other osmotically active substances, or by oral administration of glycerine, isosorbide, glycine, etc.; used in the treatment of cerebral edema and increased intracranial pressure.

osmotic (os-mot'ik). Osmolar; relating to osmosis.

osphresio- [G. *osphrēsis*, smell]. Combining form denoting odor or the sense of smell.

osphresiolagnia (os-frē'zē-ō-lag'nē-ă) [osphresio- + G. *lagneia*, lust]. Sexual excitement produced by odors.

osphresiologic (os-frē-zē-ō-loj'ik). Relating to osphresiology.

osphresiology (os-frē'zē-ol'ō-jē) [osphresio- + G. *logos*, study]. Osmology (1).

osphresiophilia (os-frē'zē-ō-fil'ē-ă) [osphresio- + G. *phileō*, to love]. An unusual interest in odors.

osphresiophobia (os-frē'zē-ō-fō'bē-ă) [osphresio- + G. *phobos*, fear]. Olfactophobia.

osphresis (os-frē'sis) [G. *osphrēsis*, smell]. Olfaction.

osphretic (os-fret'ik). Olfactory.

ossa (os'ă) [L.]. Plural of L. *os*, bone.

ossein, osseine (os'ē-in) [L. *os*, bone]. Collagen.

osselet (os'ĕ-let) [L. dim. of *os*, bone]. A periostitis of the anterior margin of the third metacarpal bone or first phalanx near the fetlock, characterized first by a painful, soft swelling and later by exostosis; a cause of lameness in horses, particularly young race horses in training.

osseo- [L. *osseus*, bony]. Combining form denoting bony. See also ossi-, osteo-.

osseocartilaginous (os'ē-ō-kar-ti-laj'i-nŭs). Osteocartilaginous; osteochondrous; relating to, or composed of, both bone and cartilage.

osseomucin (os'ē-ō-myū'sin). The ground substance of bony tissue.

osseomucoid (os'ē-ō-myū'koyd). A mucoid derived from ossein.

osseous (os'ē-ŭs) [L. *osseus*] Osteal; bony, of bone-like consistency or structure.

ossi- [L. *os*, bone]. Combining form denoting bone. See also osseo-, osteo-.

ossicle (os'i-kl) [L. *ossiculum*, dim. of *os*, bone]. Ossiculum.

Andernach's o.'s, *ossa* suturarum.

auditory o.'s, *ossicula* auditus.

Bertin's o.'s, *conchae* sphenoidales.

epactal o.'s, *os* suturarum.

Kerckring's o., Kerckring's *center*.

ossicula (ō-sik'yū-lă) [L.]. Plural of ossiculum.

ossicular (ō-sik'yū-lăr). Pertaining to an ossicle.

ossiculectomy (os'i-kyū-lek'tō-mē) [L. *ossiculum*, ossicle, + G. *ektomē*, excision]. Removal of one or more of the ossicles of the middle ear.

ossiculotomy (os'i-kyū-lot'ō-mē) [L. *ossiculum*, ossicle, + G. *tomē*, incision]. Division of one of the processes of the ossicles of the middle ear, or of a fibrous band causing ankylosis between any two ossicles.

ossiculum, pl. **ossicula** (ō-sik'yū-lŭm, -lă) [L. dim. of *os*, bone] [NA]. Ossicle; bonelet; a small bone; specifically, one of the bones of the tympanic cavity or middle ear.

ossicula audi'tus [NA], auditory ossicles; ear bones; ossicular chain; the small bones of the middle ear; malleus, incus, and stapes; they are articulated to form a chain for the transmission of sound from the tympanic membrane to the oval window.

ossic'ula menta'lia, small nodules of bone that appear at the symphysis menti shortly before birth and fuse with the mandible after birth.

ossiferous (ō-sif'er-ŭs) [ossi- + L. *fero*, to bear]. Containing or producing bone.

ossific (o-sif'ik). Relating to a change into, or formation of, bone.

ossification (os'i-fi-kā'shŭn) [L. *ossificatio*, fr. *os*, bone, + *facio*, to make]. **1.** The formation of bone. **2.** A change into bone.

endochondral o., formation of osseous tissue in association with

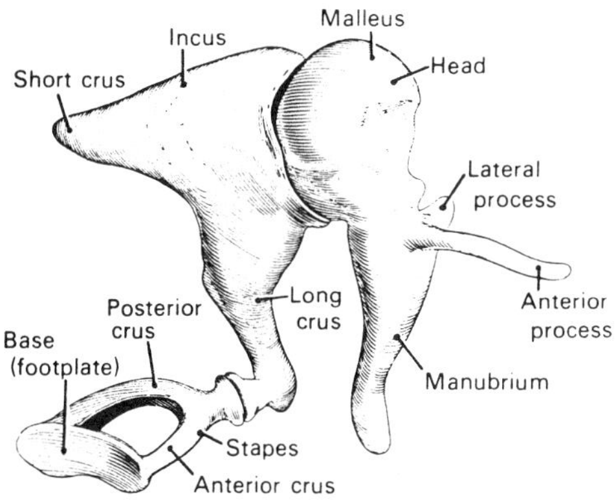

Ossicula Auditus

calcifying cartilage (the process by which bones grow in length); in long bones, endochondral o. is seen at the epiphysial cartilage plate by formation of bone trabeculae on a framework of calcified cartilage by the action of osteoblasts.
intramembranous o., membranous o.
membranous o., intramembranous o., development of osseous tissue within mesenchymal tissue without prior cartilage formation, such as occurs in the frontal and parietal bones.
metaplastic o., the formation of irregular foci of bone (sometimes including bone marrow) in various soft structures, such as the muscles, lungs, brain, and other sites where osseous tissue is abnormal.

ossiform (os'i-fōrm) [ossi- + L. *forma,* form]. Osteoid (1).

ossify (os'i-fī) [ossi- + L. *facio,* to make]. To form bone or convert into bone.

ost-, oste-. See osteo-.

osteal (os'tē-ăl) [G. *osteon,* bone]. Osseous.

ostealgia (os-tē-al'jē-ă) [osteo- + G. *algos,* pain]. Osteodynia; pain in a bone.

ostealgic (os-tē-al'jik). Relating to or marked by bone pain.

osteanagenesis (os'tē-an-ă-jen'ĕ-sis). Osteoanagenesis.

osteanaphysis (os'tē-ă-naf'i-sis) [osteo- + G. *anaphysis,* a growing again]. Osteoanagenesis.

ostectomy (os-tek'tō-mē) [osteo- + G. *ektomē,* excision]. Osteoectomy. **1.** Surgical removal of bone. **2.** In dentistry, resection of supporting osseous structure to eliminate periodontal pockets.

ostein, osteine (os'tē-in) [G. *osteon,* bone]. Collagen.

osteitic (os-tē-it'ik). Ostitic; relating to or affected by osteitis.

osteitis (os-tē-ī'tis) [osteo- + G. *-itis,* inflammation]. Ostitis; inflammation of bone.
alveolar o., alveoalgia.
caseous o., tuberculous caries in bone.
central o., **(1)** osteomyelitis; **(2)** endosteitis.
condensing o., sclerosing o.
cortical o., periostitis with involvement of the superficial layer of bone.
o. defor'mans, Paget's disease (1).
o. fibro'sa cir'cumscrip'ta, monostotic fibrous *dysplasia.*
o. fibro'sa cys'tica, Recklinghausen's disease of bone; parathyroid osteosis; increased osteoclastic resorption of calcified bone with replacement by fibrous tissue, due to primary hyperparathyroidism or other causes of the rapid mobilization of mineral salts.
o. fibro'sa disseminat'a, polyostotic fibrous *dysplasia.*
hematogenous o., any o. caused by infection carried in the bloodstream.
localized o. fibro'sa, monostotic fibrous *dysplasia.*
multifocal o. fibro'sa, polyostotic fibrous *dysplasia.*
renal o. fibro'sa, renal *rickets.*
sclerosing o., condensing o.; Garré's disease; fusiform thickening or increased density of bones, of unknown cause; it has been considered a form of chronic nonsuppurative osteomyelitis.
o. tuberculo'sa mul'tiplex cys'tica, Jüngling's disease; an o. of tuberculous origin, marked by numerous small cavities in the osseous substance.

ostembryon (os-tem'brē-on) [osteo- + G. *embryon,* embryo]. Archaic term for lithopedion.

ostemia (os-tē'mē-ă) [osteo- + G. *haima,* blood]. Congestion or hyperemia of a bone.

ostempyesis (os'tem-pī-ē'sis) [osteo- + G. *empyēsis,* suppuration]. Suppuration in bone.

osteo-, ost-, oste- [G. *osteon,* bone]. Combining forms denoting bone. See also osseo-, ossi-.

osteoanagenesis (os'tē-ō-an-ă-jen'ĕ-sis) [osteo- + G. *ana,* again, + *genesis,* generation]. Osteanagenesis; osteanaphysis; reproduction of bone.

osteoarthritis (os'tē-ō-ar-thrī'tis). Osteoarthrosis; degenerative or hypertrophic arthritis; degenerative joint disease; arthritis characterized by erosion of articular cartilage, either primary or secondary to trauma or other conditions, which becomes soft, frayed, and thinned with eburnation of subchondral bone and outgrowths of marginal osteophytes; pain and loss of function result; primary o., mainly affecting weight-bearing joints, is common in older persons.
hyperplastic o., hypertrophic pulmonary *osteoarthropathy.*

osteoarthropathy (os'tē-ō-ar-throp'ă-thē) [osteo- + G. *arthron,* joint, + *pathos,* suffering]. A disorder affecting bones and joints.
hypertrophic pulmonary o., Bamberger-Marie disease or syndrome; pneumogenic or pulmonary o., hyperplastic osteoarthritis; expansion of the distal ends, or the entire shafts, of the long bones, sometimes with erosions of the articular cartilages and thickening and villous proliferation of the synovial membranes, and frequently clubbing of fingers; the disorder occurs in chronic pulmonary disease, in heart disease, and occasionally in other acute and chronic disorders; also occurs in dogs as a result of *Spirocerca lupi* infection of the esophagus.
idiopathic hypertrophic o., o., not secondary to pulmonary or other progressive lesions, which may occur alone (acropathy) or as part of the syndrome of pachydermoperiostosis.
pneumogenic o., hypertrophic pulmonary o.
pulmonary o., hypertrophic pulmonary o.

osteoarthrosis (os'tē-ō-ar-thrō'sis) [osteo- + G. *arthron,* joint, + *-osis,* condition]. Osteoarthritis.

osteoblast (os'tē-ō-blast) [osteo- + G. *blastos,* germ]. Osteoplast; a bone-forming cell derived from mesenchyme forming an osseous matrix in which it becomes enclosed as an osteocyte.

osteoblastic (os'tē-ō-blas'tik). Relating to the osteoblasts.

osteoblastoma (os'tē-ō-blas-tō'mă). Giant osteoid osteoma; an uncommon benign tumor of osteoblasts with areas of osteoid and calcified tissue, occurring most frequently in the spine of a young person.

osteocarcinoma (os'tē-ō-kar'si-nō'mă). Undesirable nonspecific term for a metastasis of carcinoma in a bone, or a carcinoma that contains foci of osseous tissue (as a result of metaplasia).

osteocartilaginous (os'tē-ō-kar-ti-laj'i-nŭs). Osseocartilaginous.

osteochondritis (os'tē-ō-kon-drī'tis) [osteo- + G. *chondros,* cartilage, + *-itis,* inflammation]. Inflammation of a bone and its cartilage.
o. defor'mans juveni'lis, Legg-Calvé-Perthes *disease.*
o. defor'mans juveni'lis dor'si, Scheuermann's *disease.*
o. dis'secans, complete or incomplete separation of a portion of joint cartilage and underlying bone, usually involving the knee,

associated with epiphyseal aseptic necrosis.
syphilitic o., Wegner's disease; inflammation of the epiphysial line associated with congenital syphilis.

osteochondrodystrophia deformans (os'tē-ō-kon'drō-dis-trō'fē-ă dē-fōr'manz). Chondro-osteodystrophy.

osteochondrodystrophy (os'tē-ō-kon'drō-dis'trō-fē). Chondro-osteodystrophy.

osteochondroma (os'tē-ō-kon-drō'mă) [osteo- + G. *chondros,* cartilage, + *-oma,* tumor]. Solitary osteocartilaginous exostosis; a benign cartilaginous neoplasm that consists of a pedicle of normal bone (protruding from the cortex) covered with a rim of proliferating cartilage cells; may originate from any bone that is preformed in cartilage, but is most frequent near the ends of long bones, usually in patients who are 10 to 25 years of age; the lesion is frequently not noticed, unless it is traumatized or of large size; multiple o.'s are inherited and referred to as hereditary multiple exostoses.

osteochondromatosis (os'tē-ō-kon-drō-mă-tō'-sis). Hereditary multiple *exostoses.*
synovial o., synovial *chondromatosis.*

osteochondrosarcoma (os'tē-ō-kon'drō-sar-kō'-mă) [osteo- + G. *chondros,* cartilage, + *sarx,* flesh, + *-oma,* tumor]. Chondrosarcoma arising in bone. Sarcomas in bone containing foci of neoplastic cartilage as well as bone are classified as osteogenic sarcomas.

osteochondrosis (os'tē-ō-kon-drō'sis) [osteo- + G. *chondros,* cartilage, + *-osis,* condition]. Any of a group of disorders of one or more ossification centers in children, characterized by degeneration or aseptic necrosis followed by reossification; includes the various forms of epiphysial aseptic necrosis.

osteochondrous (os'tē-ō-kon'drŭs) [osteo- + G. *chondros,* cartilage]. Osseocartilaginous.

osteoclasis, osteoclasia (os'tē-ok'lă-sis, os'tē-ō-klā'zē-ă) [osteo- + G. *klasis,* fracture]. Diaclasis; diaclasia; intentional fracture of a bone in order to correct deformity.

osteoclast (os'tē-ō-klast) [osteo- + G. *klastos,* broken]. **1.** Osteophage; a large multinucleated cell, possibly of monocytic origin, with abundant acidophilic cytoplasm, functioning in the absorption and removal of osseous tissue. **2.** An instrument used to fracture a bone to correct a deformity.

osteoclastic (os'tē-ō-klas'tik). Pertaining to osteoclasts, especially with reference to their activity in the absorption and removal of osseous tissue.

osteoclastoma (os'tē-ō-klas-tō'mă). Giant cell *tumor* of bone.

osteocranium (os'tē-ō-krā'nē-ŭm) [osteo- + G. *kranion,* skull]. The cranium of the fetus after ossification of the membranous cranium has made it firm.

osteocystoma (os'tē-ō-sis-tō'mă). Solitary bone *cyst.*

osteocyte (os'tē-ō-sīt) [osteo- + G. *kytos,* cell]. Bone cell or corpuscle; osseous cell; a cell of osseous tissue which occupies a lacuna and has processes which extend into canaliculi and make contact by means of gap junctions with other processes.

osteodentin (os'tē-ō-den'tin) [osteo- + L. *dens,* tooth]. Rapidly formed tertiary dentin that contains entrapped odontoblasts and few dentinal tubules, thereby superficially resembling bone.

osteodermatopoikilosis (os'tē-ō-der'mă-tō-poy-ki-lō'sis). [osteo- + G. *derma,* skin, + *poikilos,* dappled, + *-osis,* condition]. Buschke-Ollendorf syndrome; osteopoikilosis with skin lesions, most commonly small fibrous nodules on the posterior aspects of the thighs and buttocks; autosomal dominant inheritance with incomplete penetrance.

osteodermatous (os'tē-ō-der'mă-tŭs). Pertaining to or characterized by osteodermia.

osteodermia (os'tē-ō-der'mē-ă) [osteo- + G. *derma,* skin]. *Osteosis* cutis.

osteodesmosis (os'tē-ō-dez-mō'sis) [osteo- + G. *desmos,* a band (tendon), + *-osis,* condition]. Transformation of tendon into bony tissue.

osteodiastasis (os'tē-ō-dī-as'tă-sis) [osteo- + G. *diastasis,* a separation]. Separation of two adjacent bones, as of the cranium.

osteodynia (os-tē-ō-din'ē-ă) [osteo- + G. *odynē,* pain]. Ostealgia.

osteodysplasty (os'tē-ō-dis'plas-tē). [osteo- + G. *dys-,* bad, + *plastos,* formed]. Melnick-Needles syndrome; a generalized skeletal dysplasia with prominent forehead and small mandible; radiographically, there are irregular ribbon-like constrictions of the ribs and tubular bones; probably autosomal dominant inheritance.

osteodystrophia (os'tē-ō-dis-trō'fē-ă). Osteodystrophy.

osteodystrophy (os'tē-ō-dis'trō-fē) [osteo- + G. *dys,* difficult, imperfect, + *trophē,* nourishment]. Osteodystrophia; defective formation of bone; common in dogs with chronic nephritis.
Albright's hereditary o., Albright's syndrome (2); an inherited form of hypoparathyroidism associated with skeletal defects.
renal o., generalized bone changes resembling osteomalacia and rickets or osteitis fibrosa, occurring in children or adults with chronic renal failure.

osteoectasia (os'tē-ō-ek-tā'zē-ă) [osteo- + G. *ektasis,* a stretching]. Bowing of bones, particularly of the legs.

osteoectomy (os-tē-ō-ek'tō-mē). Ostectomy.

osteoepiphysis (os'tē-ō-e-pif'i-sis). An epiphysis of a bone.

osteofibroma (os'tē-ō-fī-brō'mă). A benign lesion of bone, probably not a true neoplasm, consisting chiefly of fairly dense, moderately cellular, fibrous connective tissue in which there are small foci of osteogenesis. Most examples of this condition, especially in the maxilla and mandible, probably represent foci of fibrous dysplasia; a few examples of fibrous lesions with foci of osteogenesis, especially in vertebral bodies, may be neoplasms.

osteofibrosis (os'tē-ō-fī-brō'sis). Fibrosis of bone, mainly involving red bone marrow.
periapical o., periapical cemental *dysplasia.*

osteogen (os'tē-ō-jen) [osteo- + G. *-gen,* producing]. A bone matrix-producing tissue or layer.

osteogenesis (os'tē-ō-jen'ĕ-sis) [osteo- + G. *genesis,* production]. Osteogeny; osteosis (2); ostosis (2); the formation of bone.
o. imperfec'ta, brittle bones; a condition of abnormal fragility and plasticity of bone, with recurring fractures on minimal trauma; variable associated features include deformity of long bones, blueness of sclerae, laxity of ligaments, and otosclerosis; inheritance is autosomal dominant in most families, but a rare autosomal recessive type also exists. In **o. i. congenita,** a more severe form, the fractures occur before or at birth; in **o. i. tarda,** a less severe form, the fractures occur later in childhood.

osteogenic, osteogenetic (os'tē-ō-jen'ik, -jĕ-net'ik). Osteogenous; osteoplastic (1); relating to osteogenesis.

osteogenous (os-tē-oj'ĕ-nŭs). Osteogenic.

osteogeny (os-tē-oj'ĕ-nē). Osteogenesis.

osteography (os'tē-og'ră-fē) [osteo- + G. *graphē,* a writing]. A treatise on or description of the bones.

osteohalisteresis (os'tē-ō-hal'is-ter-ē'sis) [osteo- + G. *hals,* salt, + *sterēsis,* privation]. Softening of the bones through absorption or insufficient supply of the mineral portion.

osteohypertrophy (os'tē-ō-hī-per'trō-fē) [osteo- + G. *hyper-* over, + *trophē,* nourishment]. Condition characterized by overgrowth of bones.

osteoid (os'tē-oyd) [osteo- + G. *eidos,* resemblance]. **1.** Ossiform; relating to or resembling bone. **2.** Newly formed organic bone matrix prior to calcification.

osteolathyrism (os'tē-ō-lath'i-rizm) [osteo- + lathyrism]. An experimental disease in rats, swine, turkeys, and other animals fed the seeds of certain species of *Lathyrus* (*e.g., L. odoratus,* sweet pea), or such nitriles as aminoacetonitrile or β-aminopropionitrile; the chief pathologic changes occur in connective tissue structures, as follows: 1) fibroblastic, chondroblastic, and osteoblastic proliferative changes in the periosteum; 2) degeneration, necrosis, and atypical proliferation of epiphysial cartilages; 3) an increase in adipose tissue of the bone marrow; 4) sometimes proliferation of synovial membranes; 5) relatively large foci of extensive destruction of elastic fibers in the aorta, especially in the thoracic aorta.

osteolipochondroma (os'tē-ō-lip'ō-kon-drō'mă) [osteo- + G. *lipos,* fat, + *chondros,* cartilage, + *-oma,* tumor]. A benign neoplasm of cartilaginous tissue, in which metaplasia occurs and foci of adipose cells and osseous tissue are formed.

osteologia (os-tē-ō-lō'jē-ă) [L.] [NA]. Osteology.

osteologist (os'tē-ol'ō-jist). A specialist in osteology.

osteology (os'tē-ol'ō-jē) [osteo- + G. *logos,* study]. Osteologia; the anatomy of the bones; the science concerned with the bones and their structure.

osteolysis (os-tē-ol'i-sis) [osteo- + G. *lysis,* dissolution]. Softening, absorption, and destruction of bony tissue, a function of the osteoclasts.

osteolytic (os-tē-ō-lit'ik). Pertaining to, characterized by, or causing osteolysis.

osteoma (os-tē-ō'mă) [osteo- + G. *-oma,* tumor]. A benign slow-growing mass of mature, predominantly lamellar bone, usually arising from the skull or mandible.

o. cu'tis, see *osteosis* cutis.

dental o., an exostosis arising from the root of a tooth.

giant osteoid o., osteoblastoma.

o. medulla're, an o. containing spaces that are filled (or partly filled) with various elements of bone marrow.

osteoid o., a painful benign neoplasm that usually originates in one of the bones of the lower extremities, especially the femur or tibia of adolescent and young adult persons; characterized by a nidus (usually no larger than 1 cm in diameter) that consists of osteoid material, vascularized osteogenic stroma, and poorly formed bone; around the nidus there is a relatively large zone of reactive thickening of the cortex.

o. spongio'sum, an o. that consists chiefly of cancellous bone tissue.

osteomalacia (os'tē-ō-mă-lā'shē-ă) [osteo- + G. *malakia,* softness]. Adult rickets; a disease characterized by a gradual softening and bending of the bones with varying severity of pain; softening occurs because the bones contain osteoid tissue which has failed to calcify due to lack of vitamin D or renal tubular dysfunction; more common in women than in men, o. often begins during pregnancy.

infantile o., juvenile o., rickets.

senile o., osteoporosis in the aged.

X-linked hypophosphatemic o., vitamin D-resistant *rickets.*

osteomalacic (os'tē-ō-mă-lā'sik). Relating to, or suffering from, osteomalacia.

osteomatoid (os-tē-ō'mă-toyd) [osteoma + G. *eidos,* appearance, form]. An abnormal nodule or small mass of overgrowth of bone, usually occurring bilaterally and symmetrically, in juxtaepiphysial regions, especially in long bones of the lower extremities; lesions are not actually neoplasms, but represent anomalous developments in which there are outpouchings of the cortex (in contrast to a growth superimposed on the cortex), and are more properly termed exostoses.

osteomere (os'tē-ō-mēr) [osteo- + G. *meros,* a part]. One of the series of bone segments, such as the vertebrae.

osteometry (os-tē-om'ĕ-trē) [osteo- + G. *metron,* measurement]. The branch of anthropometry concerned with the relative size of the different parts of the skeleton.

osteomyelitis (os'tē-ō-mī-ĕ-lī'tis) [osteo- + G. *myelos,* marrow, + *-itis,* inflammation]. Central osteitis (1); inflammation of the bone marrow and adjacent bone.

osteomyelodysplasia (os'tē-ō-mī'ĕ-lō-dis-plā'-zē-ă) [osteo- + G. *myelos,* marrow, + dysplasia]. A disease characterized by enlargement of the marrow cavities of the bones, thinning of the osseous tissue, large, thin-walled vascular spaces, leukopenia, and irregular fever.

osteon, osteone (os'tē-on, -ōn) [G. *osteon,* bone]. Haversian system; a central canal and the concentric osseous lamellae around it occurring in compact bone.

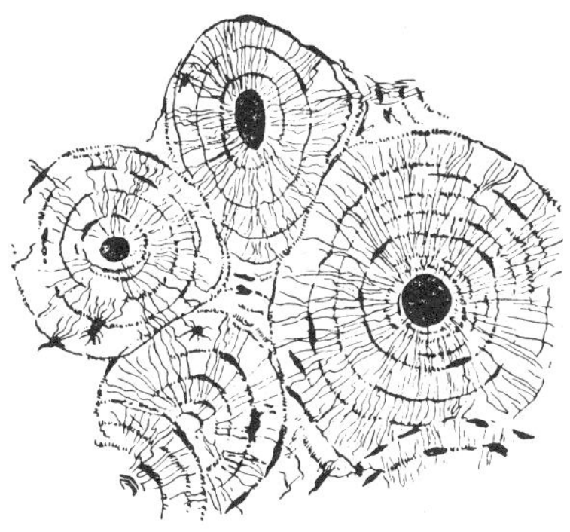

Osteons

Haversian systems and interstitial lamellae (cross section) of bone.

osteoncus (os-tē-ong'kŭs) [osteo- + G. *onkos,* bulk (swelling)]. An osteoma, sometimes used with reference to any neoplasm of a bone.

osteonecrosis (os'tē-ō-ne-krō'sis) [osteo- + G. *nekrōsis,* death]. The death of bone in mass, as distinguished from caries ("molecular death") or relatively small foci of necrosis in bone.

osteopath (os'tē-ō-path). Osteopathic *physician.*

osteopathia (os'tē-ō-path'ē-ă). Osteopathy (1).

o. conden'sans, osteopoikilosis.

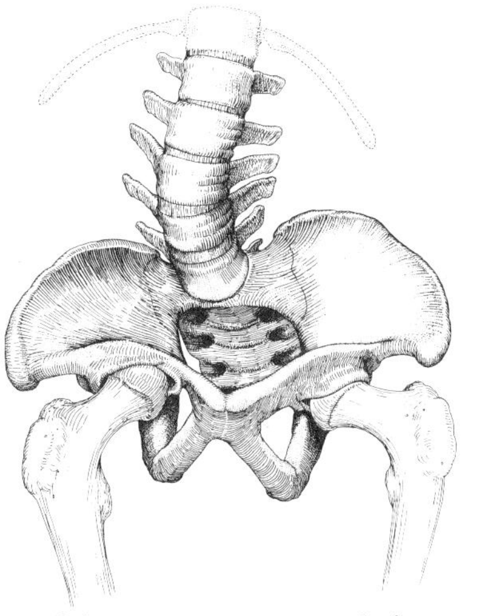

Spine and Pelvis in Osteomalacia

o. hemorrha'gica infan'tum, infantile *scurvy.*
o. stria'ta, Voorhoeve's disease; linear striations seen by x-ray visualization in the metaphyses of long bones and also flat bones; it may be a variant of osteopoikilosis.

osteopathic (os-tē-ō-path'ik). Relating to osteopathy.

osteopathology (os'tē-ō-pa-thol'ō-jē). Study of diseases of bone.

osteopathy (os-tē-op'ă-thē) [osteo- + G. *pathos,* suffering]. **1.** Osteopathia; any disease of bone. **2.** Osteopathic medicine; a school of medicine based upon a concept of the normal body as a vital machine capable, when in correct adjustment, of making its own remedies against infections and other toxic conditions; practitioners use the diagnostic and therapeutic measures of ordinary medicine in addition to manipulative measures.
alimentary o., bone disease due to dietary deficiency.

osteopedion (os'tē-ō-pē'dē-on) [osteo- + G. *paidion,* dim. of *pais,* a child]. Archaic term for lithopedion.

osteopenia (os'tē-ō-pē'nē-ă) [osteo- + G. *penia,* poverty]. **1.** Decreased calcification or density of bone; a descriptive term applicable to all skeletal systems in which such a condition is noted; carries no implication about causality. **2.** Reduced bone mass due to inadequate osteoid synthesis.

osteoperiostitis (os'tē-ō-per'ē-os-tī'tis). Inflammation of the periosteum and of the underlying bone.

osteopetrosis (os'tē-ō-pe-trō'sis) [osteo- + G. *petra,* stone, + *-osis,* condition]. Albers-Schönberg disease; marble bones; marble bone disease; excessive formation of dense trabecular bone and calcified cartilage, especially in long bones, leading to obliteration of marrow spaces and to anemia, with myeloid metroplasia and hepatosplenomegaly, beginning in infancy and with progressive deafness and blindness; autosomal recessive inheritance. A milder, autosomal dominant form has onset in childhood and no neurologic sequelae.
o. ac'ro-osteoly'tica, pyknodysostosis.
o. gallina'rum, a virus-induced bone tumor of chickens.

osteopetrotic (os'tē-ō-pe-trot'ik). Relating to osteopetrosis.

osteophage (os'tē-ō-fāj) [osteo- + G. *phagein,* to eat]. Osteoclast (1).

osteophagia (os'tē-ō-fā'jē-ă) [osteo- + G. *phagein,* to eat]. Eating of bones; perverted appetite seen in cattle suffering from mineral (phosphorus or calcium) deficiency.

osteophlebitis (os'tē-ō-fle-bī'tis) [osteo- + G. *phleps,* vein, + *-itis,* inflammation]. Inflammation of the veins of a bone.

osteophony (os'tē-of'ō-nē). Bone *conduction.*

osteophyma (os-tē-ō-fī'mă) [osteo- + G. *phyma,* tumor]. Osteophyte.

osteophyte (os'tē-ō-fīt) [osteo- + G. *phyton,* plant]. Osteophyma; a bony outgrowth or protuberance.

osteoplaque (os'tē-ō-plak) [osteo- + Fr. *plaque,* plate]. Any osseous layer.

osteoplast (os'tē-ō-plast) [osteo- + G. *plastos,* formed]. Osteoblast.

osteoplastic (os-tē-ō-plas'tik). **1.** Osteogenic. **2.** Relating to osteoplasty.

osteoplasty (os'tē-ō-plas-tē) [osteo- + G. *plastos,* formed]. **1.** Bone grafting; reparative or plastic surgery of the bones. **2.** In dentistry, resection of osseous structure to achieve acceptable gingival contour.

osteopoikilosis (os'tē-ō-poy-ki-lō'sis). [osteo- + G. *poikilos,* dappled, + *-osis,* condition]. Osteopathia condensans; mottled or spotted bones caused by widespread small foci of compact bone in the substantia spongiosa; autosomal dominant inheritance with incomplete penetrance. See also *osteopathia* striata.

osteoporosis (os'tē-ō-pō-rō'sis) [osteo- + G. poros, pore, + *-osis,* condition]. Reduction in the quantity of bone or atrophy of skeletal tissue; occurs in postmenopausal women and elderly men, resulting in bone trabeculae that are scanty, thin, and without osteoclastic resorption.
o. circumscrip'ta cra'nii, localized cranial o. often seen in Paget's disease.
juvenile o., idiopathic o. with onset before puberty, leading to pain or fractures, with spontaneous remission within a few years.
posttraumatic o., Sudeck's *atrophy.*

osteoporotic (os'tē-ō-pō-rot'ik). Pertaining to, characterized by, or causing a porous condition of the bones.

osteoradionecrosis (os'tē-ō-rā'dē-ō-ne-krō'sis). Necrosis of bone produced by ionizing radiation; may be planned or unplanned.

osteorrhaphy (os-tē-ōr'ă-fē) [osteo- + G. *rhaphē,* suture]. Osteosuture; wiring together the fragments of a broken bone.

osteosarcoma (os'tē-ō-sar-kō'mă). Osteogenic *sarcoma.*

osteosclerosis (os'tē-ō-skle-rō'sis) [osteo- + G. *sklērōsis,* hardness]. Abnormal hardening or eburnation of bone.
o. congen'ita, achondroplasia.

osteosclerotic (os'tē-ō-skle-rot'ik). Relating to, due to, or marked by hardening of bone substance.

osteoscope (os'tē-ō-skōp) [osteo- + G. *skopeō,* to view]. An obsolete apparatus enclosing certain bones of standard density and thickness, used for testing an x-ray machine.

osteosis (os-tē-ō'sis) [osteo- + G. *-osis,* condition]. **1.** Ostosis (1); a morbid process in bone. **2.** Osteogenesis.
o. cu'tis, dermostosis; osteodermia; bone formed in the skin by osseous metaplasia of calcium deposits. Also called osteoma cutis, although not neoplastic.
o. ebur'nisans monomel'ica, melorheostosis.
parathyroid o., *osteitis* fibrosa cystica.
renal fibrocystic o., renal *rickets.*

osteospongioma (os'tē-ō-spon'jē-ō'mă) [osteo- + G. *spongos,* sponge, + *-oma,* tumor]. General nonspecific term for a neoplasm in bone that results in thinning and fragmentation (thus, in softening) of the cortex.

osteosteatoma (os'tē-ō-stē'ă-tō'mă) [osteo- + G. *stear,* suet, fat, + *-oma,* tumor]. A benign mass, usually a lipoma or sebaceous cyst, in which small foci of bony elements are present.

osteosuture (os-tē-ō-sū'chūr). Osteorrhaphy.

osteosynthesis (os-tē-ō-sin'thē-sis). Internal fixation of a fracture by means of a mechanical device, such as a pin, screw, or plate.

osteothrombosis (os'tē-ō-throm-bō'sis). Thrombosis in one or more of the veins of a bone.

osteotome (os'tē-ō-tōm) [osteo- + G. *tomē,* incision]. An instrument for use in cutting bone.

osteotomy (os-tē-ot'ō-mē) [osteo- + G. *tomē,* incision]. Cutting a bone, usually by means of a saw or chisel.
"C" sliding o., an extraoral o. in the shape of a "C" performed bilaterally in the mandibular rami for the correction of retrognathia and/or apertognathia.
horizontal o., an o. performed intraorally for genioplasty; the inferior aspect of the anterior mandible is advanced or retruded by movement of the free segment.
sagittal split mandibular o., an intraoral surgical procedure for correction of retrognathism, apertognathia, and prognathism; the mandibular rami and posterior body are sectioned in the sagittal plane.
segmental alveolar o., an intraoral surgical procedure in which segments of alveolar bone containing teeth are sectioned between, and apically to, the teeth for the repositioning of the alveolus and teeth; it may be maxillary or mandibular, and may be combined with ostectomy.

sliding oblique o., an oral surgical procedure in which the mandibular ramus is cut vertically from the sigmoid notch to the angle to facilitate posterior repositioning of the mandible in correction of mandibular prognathism; it may be performed extraorally or intraorally, and is similar to vertical o.

vertical o., an oral surgical procedure similar to sliding oblique o.

osteotribe (os'tē-ō-trīb) [osteo- + G. *tribō,* to bruise, to grind down]. An instrument for crushing off bits of necrosed or carious bone.

osteotrite (os'tē-ō-trīt) [osteo- + L. *tritus,* a grinding, a wearing off]. An instrument with conical or olive-shaped tip having a cutting surface, resembling a dental burr, used for the removal of carious bone.

osteotrophy (os-tē-ot'rō-fē) [osteo- + G. *trophē,* nourishment]. Nutrition of osseous tissue.

osteotympanic (os'tē-ō-tim-pan'ik) [osteo- + G. *tympanon,* drum]. Otocranial.

Ostertagia (os-ter-tā'jē-ă) [R. von *Ostertag*]. The medium or brown stomach worm; a genus of small, slender, bloodsucking trichostrongyle nematodes found in the abomasum (rarely in the small intestine) of sheep, goats, cattle, and other ruminants. Species include *O. bisonis* in bison, cattle, and deer; *O. circumcincta,* the most economically important species found in sheep, which occurs worldwide in sheep, goats, camels, and wild ruminants; *O. lyrata* in cattle and wild ruminants; *O. occidentalis* in sheep, goats, pronghorn, mule deer, and other ruminants; *O. orloffi* in sheep, cattle, mule deer, and Barbary sheep in North America and the USSR; *O. ostertagi,* in cattle, sheep, and many wild ruminants; and *O. trifurcata* in sheep and goats, also reported from many wild ruminants.

ostia (os'tē-ă) [L.]. Plural of ostium.

ostial (os'tē-ăl). Relating to any orifice, or ostium.

ostitic (os-tī'tik). Osteitic.

ostitis (os-tī'tis). Osteitis.

ostium, pl. ostia (os'tē-ŭm, -ă) [L. door, entrance, mouth] [NA]. A small opening, especially one of entrance into a hollow organ or canal.

o. abdomina'le tu'bae uteri'na [NA], the fimbriated or ovarian extremity of an oviduct.

o. aor'tae [NA], aortic o.; o. arteriosum (2); the opening from the left ventricle into the ascending aorta; it is guarded by the aortic valve.

aortic o., o. aortae.

o. appen'dicis vermifor'mis [NA], the opening of the vermiform appendix into the lumen of the cecum.

o. arterio'sum, **(1)** o. trunci pulmonalis; **(2)** o. aortae.

os'tium atrioventricula're dex'tium [NA], tricuspid orifice; an atrioventricular opening which leads from the right atrium into the right ventricle of the heart.

o. atrioventricula're sinis'trum [NA], mitral orifice; an atrioventricular opening which leads from the left atrium into the left ventricle of the heart.

o. cardi'acum [NA], cardiac opening; esophagogastric orifice; the trumpet-shaped opening of the esophagus into the stomach.

o. ileoceca'le [NA], ileocecal opening; the opening of the terminal ileum into the large intestine at the transition between the cecum and the ascending colon.

o. inter'num, o. uterinum tubae.

o. pharyn'geum tu'bae auditi'vae [NA], pharyngeal opening of auditory or eustachian tube; an opening in the upper part of the nasopharynx about 1.2 cm behind the posterior extremity of the inferior concha on each side.

o. pri'mum, interatrial *foramen* primum.

o. pylor'icum [NA], pyloric orifice; gastroduodenal orifice; the opening between the stomach and the superior part of the duodenum.

o. secun'dum, interatrial *foramen* secundum.

o. trun'ci pulmona'lis [NA], pulmonary opening; o. arteriosum (1); the opening of the pulmonary trunk from the right ventricle, guarded by the pulmonary valve.

o. tympan'icum tu'bae auditi'vae [NA], tympanic opening of auditory or eustachian tube; an opening in the anterior part of the tympanic cavity below the canal for the tensor tympani muscle.

o. ure'teris [NA], ureteral opening or meatus; orificium ureteris; the opening of the ureter in the bladder, situated one at each lateral angle of the trigone; wide gaping of the o. usually indicates vesicoureteral reflux.

o. ure'thrae exter'num [NA], external urethral opening; meatus urinarius; orificium urethrae externum; **(1)** the slitlike opening of the urethra in the glans penis; **(2)** the external orifice of the urethra (in the female) in the vestibule, usually upon a slight elevation, the papilla urethrae.

o. ure'thrae inter'num [NA], internal urethral opening; the internal opening or orifice of the urethra, at the anterior and inferior angle of the trigone.

o. u'teri [NA], o. of uterus; o. uteri externum; os uteri externum; orificium externum uteri; mouth of womb; the vaginal opening of the uterus.

o. u'teri exter'num, o. uteri.

o. u'teri inter'num, *isthmus* uteri.

o. uteri'num tu'bae [NA], o. internum; the uterine opening of the oviduct.

o. vagi'nae [NA], vaginal opening; orificium vaginae; the narrowest portion of the canal, in the floor of the vestibule posterior to the urethral orifice.

o. ve'nae ca'vae inferio'ris [NA], opening of inferior vena cava; the orifice through which the inferior vena cava opens into the right atrium.

o. ve'nae ca'vae superio'ris [NA], opening of superior vena cava; the point of entry of the superior vena cava into the right atrium.

os'tia vena'rum pulmona'lium [NA], openings of pulmonary veins; the orifices of the pulmonary veins, usually two on each side, in the wall of the left atrium.

o. veno'sum, see ostium atrioventriculare dextrum; ostium atrioventriculare sinistrum.

ostomate (os'tō-māt) [L. *ostium,* mouth]. Undesirable term for one who has an ostomy.

-ostomy. See -stomy.

ostomy (os'tō-mē) [L. *ostium,* mouth]. **1.** An artificial stoma or opening into the urinary or gastrointestinal canal, or the trachea. **2.** Any operation by which an opening is created between two hollow organs or between a hollow viscus and the abdominal wall or neck externally, as in tracheostomy.

ostosis (os-tō'sis). **1.** Osteosis (1). **2.** Osteogenesis.

ostraceous (os-trā'shŭs) [*Ostraeacea,* group including the oysters]. Denoting the heaping up of scales seen in psoriasis, which resembles the stratification of oyster shells.

ostreotoxism (os'trē-ō-tok'sizm) [G. *ostreon,* oyster, + *toxikon, poison*] Poisoning from eating infected or contaminated oysters.

Ostwald, Friedrich Wilhelm, German physical chemist, 1853–1932. See O.'s solubility *coefficient.*

OT Abbreviation for occupational therapist or therapy; Koch's old *tuberculin.*

ot- [G. *ous,* ear]. Combining form denoting the ear. See also auri-.

Ota, Masao T., Japanese dermatopathologist, 1885–1945. See O.'s *nevus.*

otalgia (ō-tal'jē-ă) [ot- + G. *algos,* pain]. Earache.

geniculate o., geniculate *neuralgia.*

reflex o., pain referred to the ear from disease in another part, most commonly laryngeal, tonsillar, or nasopharyngeal.

otalgic (ō-tal'jik). **1.** Relating to otalgia, or earache. **2.** A remedy for earache.

OTC Abbreviation for *o*ver *t*he *c*ounter, pertaining to a drug available without a prescription.

othematoma (ōt-hē-mă-tō'mă, ō-thē') [ot- + G. *haima,* blood, + *-oma,* tumor]. Hematoma auris; a purplish, rounded, hard swelling of the external ear, resulting from an effusion of blood between the cartilage and perichondrium; it may be caused by trauma or self-inflicted injury in the mentally ill.

othemorrhagia (ōt-hem-ō-rā'jē-ă, ō-them'ō-) [ot- + G. *haima,* blood, + *rhēgnymi,* to burst forth]. Bleeding from the ear.

other-directed (odh'er-di-rek'ted). Pertaining to a person readily influenced by the attitudes of others.

otiatria, otiatrics (ō-tē-at'rē-ă, -tē-at'riks) [ot- + G. *iatreia,* treatment]. The treatment of diseases of the ear.

otic (ō'tik) [G. *otikos,* fr. *ous,* ear]. Relating to the ear.

Otis, Arthur Brooks, U.S. respiratory physiologist, *1913. See Rahn-O. *sample.*

otitic (ō-tit'ik). Relating to otitis.

otitis (ō-tī'tis) [ot- + G. *-itis,* inflammation]. Inflammation of the ear.

aviation o., *aerotitis* media.

o. desquamati'va, o. externa with a copious brawny desquamation.

o. diphtherit'ica, diphtheritic inflammation of the external auditory meatus.

o. exter'na, inflammation of the external auditory canal.

o. exter'na circumscrip'ta, o. furunculosa; furunculosis of the external auditory canal.

o. exter'na diffu'sa, inflammation of the entire extent of the external auditory meatus.

o. exter'na hemorrhag'ica, inflammation, marked by the presence of one or more vesicles filled with blood on the wall of the bony portion of the external auditory canal.

o. furunculo'sa, o. externa circumscripta.

o. inter'na, labyrinthitis.

o. in'tima, labyrinthitis.

o. labyrin'thica, labyrinthitis.

o. me'dia, inflammation of the middle ear, or tympanum.

o. me'dia catarrha'lis, serous o.

o. me'dia purulen'ta, o. media suppurativa.

o. me'dia suppurati'va, o. media purulenta; suppurative inflammation of the middle ear.

o. mycot'ica, a fungous growth in the external auditory meatus, often of *Aspergillus niger.*

parasitic o., otoacariasis.

reflux o. me'dia, o. media caused by passage of nasopharyngeal secretions through the eustachian tube.

secretory o. me'dia, serous o.

serous o., o. media catarrhalis; secretory o. media; inflammation of middle ear mucosa, often accompanied by accumulation of fluid, secondary to eustachian tube obstruction.

oto- [G. *ous,* ear]. Combining form denoting the ear. See also auri-.

otoacariasis (ō'tō-ak-ă-rī'ă-sis). Parasitic otitis; an infestation of the auditory canal of cats, dogs, foxes, and other animals by auricular mites, chiefly *Otodectes cynotis,* which infest the ears and cause considerable discomfort and tenderness; in extreme cases, they cause symptoms such as loss of appetite, wasting, and fits. See also otodectic *mange.*

otoantritis (ō-tō-an-trī'tis). Inflammation of the mastoid antrum.

otobiosis (ō'tō-bī-ō'sis). Presence of larvae and the characteristic spiny nymphs of *Otobius megnini* in the external auditory canal of cattle, horses, cats, dogs, deer, coyotes, and other domestic and wild animals; they may remain in the ear for several months before dropping out to pupate and mature. Several records of human infection are known.

Otobius (ō-tō'bē-ŭs). A genus of argasid ticks similar to *Ornithodoros* but characterized by a granulated integument, a hypostome that is vestigial in the adult but well developed in the spiny nymphs, and the absence of eyes and hood. Two species are recognized: *O. lagophilus* (the face tick of rabbits), and *O. megnini,* the spinose ear tick that causes otobiosis in horses, cattle, sheep, dogs, and some wild animals; it occurs in southwestern parts of the U.S., where it is an important pest, and is also distributed worldwide.

otocephaly (ō-tō-sef'ă-lē) [oto- + G. *kephalē,* head]. Malformation characterized by markedly defective development of the lower jaw (micrognathia or agnathia) and the union or close approach of the ears (synotia) on the front of the neck.

otocerebritis (ō-tō-ser-ē-brī'tis). Otoencephalitis.

otocleisis (ō-tō-klī'sis) [oto- + G. *kleisis,* closure]. **1.** Closure of the eustachian tube. **2.** Closure, by a new growth or accumulation of cerumen, of the external auditory meatus.

otoconia, sing. **otoconium** (ō-to-kō'nē-ă, -ŭm). Statoconia.

otocranial (ō-tō-krā'nē-ăl). Osteotympanic; relating to the otocranium.

otocranium (ō'tō-krā'nē-um) [oto- + G. *kranion,* cranium]. The bony case of the internal and middle ear, consisting of the petrous portion of the temporal bone.

otocyst (ō'tō-sist) [oto- + G. *kystis,* a bladder]. **1.** Embryonic auditory vesicle. **2.** A balancing organ, analogous to the utricle of mammals, possessed by certain invertebrates containing grains of calcareous material or of sand.

Otodectes (ō-tō-dek'tēz) [oto- + *dektēs,* beggar, receiver]. A genus of ear mites (family Psoroptidae) consisting of a single species, *O. cynotis,* the cause of otodectic mange in dogs, cats, and other carnivores; the entire lifespan of this mite is spent in the ears (rarely on the body) of the host, where it feeds on epidermal debris; it can be found in the encrusted material scraped from infected ears.

otodectic (ō-tō-dek'tik). Of, relating to, or caused by mites of the genus *Otodectes.*

otodynia (ō-tō-din'ē-ă) [oto- + G. *odynē,* pain]. Earache.

otoencephalitis (ō'tō-en-sef-ă-lī'tis) [oto- + G. *enkephalos,* brain, + *-itis,* inflammation]. Otocerebritis; inflammation of the brain by extension of the process from the middle ear and mastoid cells.

otoganglion (ō'tō-gang'glē-on). *Ganglion* oticum.

otogenic, otogenous (ō'tō-jen'ik, ō-toj'ĕ-nŭs) [oto- + G. *-gen,* producing]. Of otic origin; originating within the ear, especially from inflammation of the ear.

otography (ō-tog'ră-fē) [oto- + G. *graphē,* a writing]. A treatise on, or a description of the ear.

otolaryngologist (ō'tō-lar-ing-gol'ŏ-jist). A physician who specializes in otolaryngology.

otolaryngology (ō'tō-lar-ing-gol'ŏ-jē) [oto- + G. *larynx,* + *logos,* study]. The combined specialties of diseases of the ear and larynx, often including upper respiratory tract and many diseases of the head and neck, tracheobronchial tree, and esophagus.

otoliths, otolites (ō'tō-lith, ō'tō-līt) [oto- + G. *lithos,* stone]. **1.** Statoconia. **2.** Otosteon (2).

otologic (ō'tō-loj'ik). Relating to otology.

otologist (ō-tol'ŏ-jist). A specialist in otology.

otology (ō-tol'ŏ-jē) [oto- + G. *logos,* study]. The branch of medical science concerned with the study, diagnosis, and treatment of diseases of the ear and related structures.

otomassage (ō'tō-mă-sahzh). Systematic and regular movement imparted to the tympanic membrane and ossicles, by means of sound waves, rapid jets of air in the external auditory meatus, or vibratory tapping of the drum membrane.

otomucormycosis (ō-tō-myū'kōr-mī-kō'sis). Mucormycosis of the ear.

-otomy. See -tomy.

otomycosis (ō'tō-mī-kō'sis) [oto- + G. *mykēs,* fungus]. An infection due to a fungus in the external auditory canal, usually unilateral, with scaling, itching, and pain as the primary symptoms.

otoneuralgia (ō'tō-nū-ral'jē-ă) [oto- + G. *neuron,* nerve, + *algos,* pain]. Earache of neuralgic origin, not caused by inflammation.

otopalatodigital (ō'tō-pal'ă-tō-dij'i-tăl). Relating to the ears, palate, and fingers.

otopathy (ō-top'ă-thē) [oto- + G. *pathos,* suffering]. Any disease of the ear.

otopharyngeal (ō'tō-fa-rin'jē-ăl). Relating to the middle ear and the pharynx.

otoplasty (ō'tō-plas-tē) [oto- + G. *plastos,* formed]. Reparative or plastic surgery of the auricle of the ear.

otopolypus (ō'tō-pol'ē-pŭs) [oto- + L. *polypus,* polyp]. A polyp in the external auditory meatus, usually arising from the middle ear.

otopyorrhea (ō-tō-pī-ō-rē'ă) [oto- + G. *pyon,* pus, + *rhoia,* a flow]. Chronic otitis media with perforation of the drum membrane and a purulent discharge.

otorhinolaryngology (ō'tō-rī'nō-lar-ing -gol'ō-jē) [oto- + G. *rhis,* nose, + *larynx,* larynx, + *logos,* study]. The combined specialties of diseases of the ear, nose, and larynx; now includes diseases of related structures of the head and neck. See also otolaryngology.

otorhinology (ō'tō-rī-nol'ō-jē) [oto- + G. *rhis,* nose, + *logos,* study]. The study of disease of the ear and nose.

otorrhagia (ō-tō-rā'jē-ă) [oto- + G. *rhēgnymi,* to burst forth]. Bleeding from the ear.

otorrhea (ō-tō-rē'ă) [oto- + G. *rhoia,* flow]. A discharge from the ear.

cerebrospinal fluid o., discharge of cerebrospinal fluid through the external auditory meatus or through the eustachian tube into the nasopharynx.

otosalpinx (ō-tō-sal'pingks) [oto- + G. *salpinx,* trumpet]. *Tuba* auditiva.

otosclerosis (ō'tō-sklē-rō'sis) [oto- + G. *sklērosis,* hardening]. A new formation of spongy bone about the stapes and fenestra vestibuli (ovalis), resulting in progressively increasing deafness, without signs of disease in the eustachian tube or tympanic membrane. See also Bezold's *triad.*

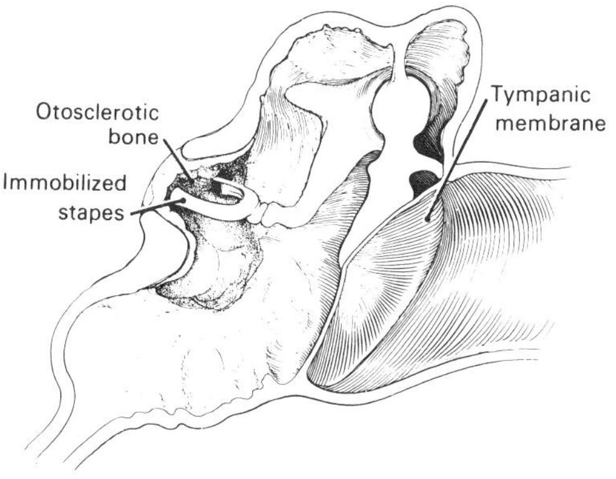

Otosclerosis

otoscope (ō'tō-skōp) [oto- + G. *skopeō,* to view]. Auriscope; an instrument for examining the drum membrane or auscultating the ear.

Siegle's o., an ear speculum with a bulb attachment by which the air pressure can be varied, thus imparting movement to the membrana tympani, if intact, while under inspection.

otoscopy (ō-tos'kō-pē) [oto- + G. *skopeō,* to view]. Inspection of the ear, especially of the drum membrane.

otosteal (ō-tos'tē-ăl) [oto- + G. *osteon,* bone]. Relating to the ossicles of the ear.

otosteon (ō-tos'tē-on) [oto- + G. *osteon,* bone]. **1.** One of the ossicles of the ear. **2.** Otolith or otolite (2); a concretion in the ear, larger than a statoconium.

ototomy (ō-tot'ō-mē) [oto- + G. *tomē,* incision]. Anatomy of the ear; dissection of the ear.

ototoxic (ō'tō-tok'sik) [oto- + G. *toxikon,* poison]. Having a toxic action upon the ear.

ototoxicity (ō-tō-tok-sis'i-te). The property of being ototoxic.

Otto, Adolph W., German surgeon, 1786–1845, See O. *pelvis;* O.'s *disease.*

Ottoson, David, 20th century Swedish physiologist. See O. *potential.*

O.U. Abbreviation for Latin *oculus uterque,* each eye or both eyes.

ouabain (wah'bān, wah'bah-in). G-strophanthin; acocantherin; $C_{29}H_{44}O_{12}8H_2O$; a glycoside and African arrow poison from ouabaio, obtained from the wood of *Acocanthera ouabaio* or from the seeds of *Strophanthus gratus;* its action is qualitatively identical to that of strophanthus and the digitalis glycosides; used for rapid digitalization.

Ouchterlony, Orjan, Swedish immunologist. See O. *test.*

oul-. For words beginning thus, see ulo-.

ounce (oz.) (owns) [L. *unica,* the twelfth part (of a pound or foot) hence also inch]. A weight containing 480 gr., or $^1/_{12}$ pound troy and apothecaries' weight, or $437^1/_2$ gr., $^1/_{16}$ pound avoirdupois. The apothecary oz. (used in the USP) contains 8 dr. and is equivalent to 31.10349 g; the avoirdupois oz. is equivalent to 28.35 g.

-ous. 1. Chemical suffix denoting that the element to the name of which it is attached is in one of its lower valencies. *Cf.* -ic (1). **2** [L. *-osus,* full of, abounding]. Suffix used to form an adjective from a noun.

outlet (owt'let). An exit or opening of a passageway.

pelvic o., *apertura* pelvis inferior.

out of phase. Not in phase, moving in opposite directions at the same time; 180° out of phase; a possible characteristic of two simultaneous oscillations of similar frequency.

outpatient (owt'pā'shent). A patient treated in a hospital dispensary or clinic instead of in a room or ward.

output (owt'put). The quantity produced, ejected, or excreted of a specific entity in a specified period of time or per unit time, *e.g.,* urinary sodium o.; the opposite of intake or input.

cardiac o., minute o.; the amount of blood ejected by the heart in a unit of time (*i.e.,* the minute volume), usually expressed in liters per minute.

minute o., cardiac o.

pacemaker o., electrical energy delivered into a standard load (500 ohms resistance).

stroke o., stroke *volume.*

ova (ō'vă) [L.]. Plural of ovum.

oval (ō'văl). **1.** Relating to an ovum. **2.** Egg-shaped, resembling in outline the longitudinal section of an egg.

ovalbumin (ō-văl-byū'min). Egg albumin; albumen; the chief protein occurring in the white of egg and resembling serum albumin.

ovalocyte (ō'văl-ō-sīt) [L. *ovalis,* oval, + G. *kytos,* cell]. Elliptocyte.

ovalocytosis (ō′vă-lō-sī-tō′sis). Elliptocytosis.

ovarialgia (ō-var-ē-al′jē-ă) [ovario- + G. *algos,* pain]. Oarialgia; oophoralgia; pain in an ovary.

ovarian (ō-var′ē-an). Relating to the ovary.

ovariectomy (ō-var-ē-ek′tō-mē) [ovario- + G. *ektomē,* excision]. Oophorectomy; ovariosteresis; excision of one or both ovaries.

ovario-, ovari- [L. *ovarium,* ovary]. Combining forms denoting ovary. See also oo-, oophor-, oophoro-.

ovariocele (ō-var′ē-ō-sēl) [ovario- + G. *kēlē,* hernia]. Hernia of an ovary.

ovariocentesis (ō-var′ē-ō-sen-tē′sis) [ovario- + G. *kentēsis,* puncture]. Puncture of an ovary or an ovarian cyst.

ovariocyesis (ō-var′ē-ō-sī-ē′sis) [ovario- + G. *kyēsis,* pregnancy]. Ovarian *pregnancy.*

ovariodysneuria (ō-var′ē-ō-dis-nū′rē-ă) [ovario- + G. *dys-,* bad, + *neuron,* nerve]. Ovarian pain or neuralgia.

ovariogenic (ō-var′ē-ō-jen′ik) [ovario- + G. *-gen,* producing]. Originating in the ovary.

ovariohysterectomy (ō-var′ē-ō-his-ter-ek′tō-mē) [ovario- + G. *hystera,* uterus, + *ektomē,* excision]. Oophorohysterectomy; removal of ovaries and uterus.

ovariolytic (ō-var′ē-ō-lit′ik) [ovario- + G. *lysis,* dissolution]. Destructive to the ovary.

ovarioncus (ō-var-ē-ong′kŭs) [ovario- + G. *onkos,* tumor]. Oophoroma.

ovariopathy (ō-var-ē-op′ă-thē) [ovario- + G. *pathos,* suffering]. Oophoropathy; any disease of the ovary.

ovariorrhexis (ō-var′ē-ō-rek′sis) [ovario- + G. *rhēxis,* rupture]. Rupture of an ovary.

ovariosalpingectomy (ō-var′ē-ō-sal-pin-jek′tō-mē) [ovario- + salpingectomy]. Oophorosalpingectomy; operative removal of an ovary and the corresponding oviduct.

ovariosalpingitis (ō-var′ē-ō-sal-pin-jī′tis) [ovario- + salpingitis]. Oophorosalpingitis; inflammation of ovary and oviduct.

ovariosteresis (ō-var′ē-ō-stĕ-rē′sis) [ovario- + G. *sterēsis,* deprivation, loss]. Ovariectomy.

ovariostomy (ō-var-ē-os′tō-mē) [ovario- + G. *stoma,* mouth]. Oophorostomy; establishment of a temporary fistula for drainage of a cyst of the ovary.

ovariotomy (ō-var-ē-ot′ō-mē) [ovario- + G. *tomē,* incision]. Oophorotomy; an incision into an ovary, *e.g.,* a biopsy or a wedge excision.

normal o., historically, removal of an apparently healthy ovary.

ovaritis (ō-vă-rī′tis). Oophoritis.

ovarium, pl. **ovaria** (ō-vār′ē-ŭm, -ă) [Mod. L. fr. *ovum,* egg] [NA]. Ovary.

o. biparti′tum, an ovary separated into two distinct parts.

o. disjunc′tum, an ovary partially or completely divided into two sections.

o. gyra′tum, an ovary showing curved or irregular grooves or furrows.

o. loba′tum, an ovary demarcated by deep furrows into two or more lobes.

o. masculi′num, *appendix* testis.

ovary (ō′vă-rē) [Mod. L. *ovarium,* fr. *ovum,* egg]. Ovarium; one of the paired female reproductive glands containing the ova or germ cells; the o.'s stroma is a vascular connective tissue containing numbers of ovarian follicles enclosing the ova; surrounding this stroma is a more condensed layer of stroma called the tunica albuginea.

mulberry o., the type of o. produced by the administration of an-

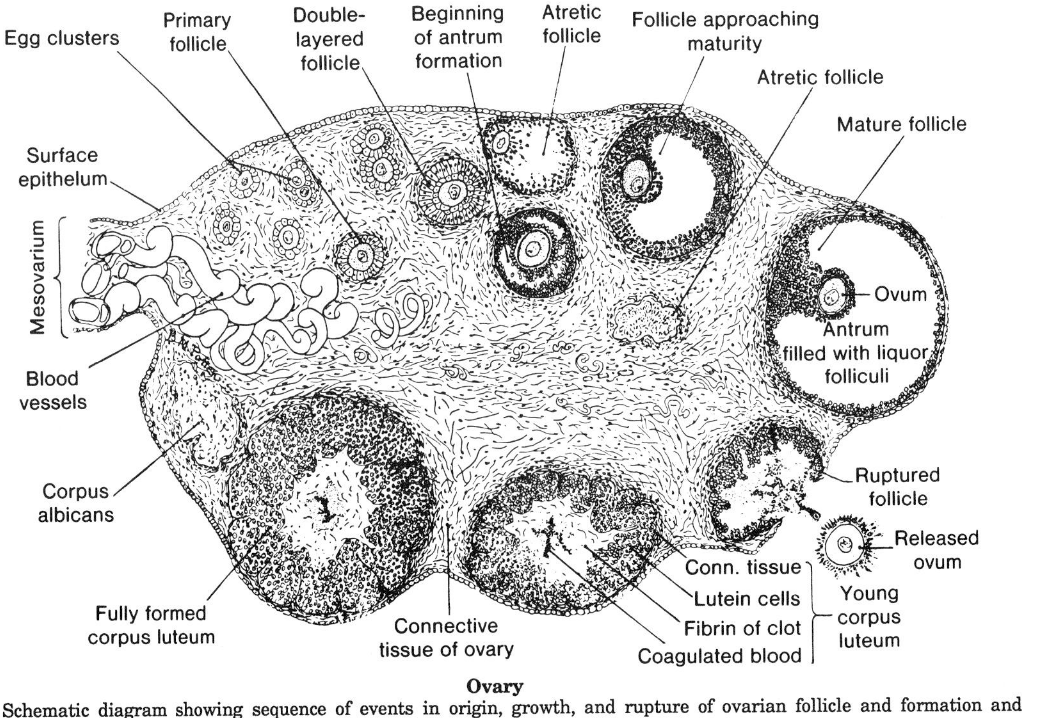

Ovary

Schematic diagram showing sequence of events in origin, growth, and rupture of ovarian follicle and formation and retrogression of corpus luteum. Follow clockwise around ovary, starting at mesovarium.

terior pituitary extracts to immature rats; such an o. contains many more follicles than normal, with the follicles in various stages of development and with prominent corpora lutea on their surfaces, thus the perceived resemblance to a mulberry.

polycystic o., enlarged cystic o.'s, pearl white in color, with thickened tunica albuginea, characteristic of the Stein-Leventhal syndrome; clinical features are abnormal menses, obesity, and evidence of masculinization, such as hirsutism and clitoromegaly.

third o., an accessory o.

overbite (ō'ver-bīt). Vertical *overlap.*

overclosure (ō'ver-klō-zher). A decrease in occlusal vertical dimension.

overcompensation (ō'ver-kom-pen-sā'shŭn). **1.** An exaggeration of personal capacity to overcome a real or imagined inferiority. **2.** The process in which a psychologic deficiency inspires exaggerated correction.

overcorrection (ō'ver-kō-rek'shŭn). In behavior modification treatment programs, especially those involving retardates, overlearning the desired target behavior beyond the set criterion to assure that the behavior will continue to meet the established criterion when the post-learning decrements and forgetting occur.

overdenture (ō-ver-den'chūr). Overlay *denture.*

overdetermination (o'ver-dē-ter'min-ā'shŭn). In psychoanalysis, the multiple causation of a single behavioral or emotional reaction, mental symptom, or dream.

overdominance (ō-ver-dom'i-năns). That state in which the heterozygote is more fit than the homozygous state for either of the alleles that it comprises.

overdominant (ō-ver-dom'i-nănt). Denoting heterogygous states that exhibit overdominance.

overeruption (ō'ver-ē-rŭp'shŭn). Occlusal projection of a tooth beyond the line of occlusion.

overextension (ō-ver-eks-ten'shŭn). Hyperextension.

overhang (ō'ver-hang). An excess of dental filling material beyond the cavity margin or normal tooth contour.

overhydration (ō'ver-hī-drā'shŭn). Hyperhydration.

overjet, overjut (ō'ver-jet, ō'ver-jŭt). Horizontal *overlap.*

overlap (ō'ver-lap). **1.** Suturing of one layer of tissue above or under another to gain strength. **2.** An extension or projection of one tissue over another.

horizontal o., overjet; overjut; the projection of the upper anterior and/or posterior teeth beyond their antagonists in a horizontal direction.

vertical o., overbite; **(1)** the extension of the upper teeth over the lower teeth in a vertical direction when the opposing posterior teeth are in contact in centric occlusion; **(2)** the distance that teeth lap over their antagonists vertically, especially for the distance that the upper incisal edges drop below the lower ones, but may also describe the vertical relations of opposing cusps; **(3)** the relationship of the maxillary incisors to the mandibular incisors when the incisal edges pass each other in centric occlusion.

overlay (ō'ver-lā). An addition to an already existing condition.

emotional o., the emotional component of an organic disability.

overlearning (ō'ver-lern'ing). In the psychology of memory, continuation of practice beyond the point where one is able to perform according to the specified criterion; typically, retention is longer after o. as compared with retention after practice only to the point of performance meeting the specified criterion.

overresponse (ō'ver-rē-spons'). An abnormally strong reaction to a stimulus.

overriding (ō'ver-rī'ding). **1.** Slippage of the lower fragment of a broken long bone upward and alongside the proximal portion. **2.** Denoting a fetal head which is palpable above the symphysis because of cephalopelvic disproportion.

overshoot (ō'ver-shūt). **1.** Generally, any initial change, in response to a sudden step change in some factor, that is greater than the steady-state response to the new level of that factor; common in systems in which inertia or a time lag in negative feedback outweighs any damping that may be present. Changes in a negative direction are sometimes distinguished by the term undershoot, and the two may alternate in an oscillatory fashion, as in the transient oscillations of a pendulum when released from an initial displacement. **2.** Momentary reversal of the membrane potential of a cell (inside becoming positive rather than negative relative to the outside) during an action potential; considered a form of o.(1) because, before discovery of o.(2), excitation was thought merely to depolarize the membrane to zero transmembrane potential.

Overton, Charles E., British biologist in Sweden, 1865–1933. See Meyer-O. *theory* of narcosis.

overtone (ō'ver-tōn). Any of the tones, other than the lowest or fundamental tone, of which a sound is composed.

psychic o., the mental associations related to any stimulus.

overventilation (ō'ver-ven-ti-lā'shŭn). Hyperventilation.

overwintering (ō'ver-win'ter-ing). Persistence of an infectious agent in its vector for extended periods, such as the cooler winter months, during which the vector has no opportunity to be reinfected or to infect another host.

ovi- [L. *ovum,* egg]. Combining form denoting egg. See also oo-, ovo-.

ovicidal (ō-vi-sī'dăl) [ovi- + L. *caedo,* to kill]. Causing death of the ovum.

oviducal (ō-vi-dū'kăl). Oviductal.

oviduct (ō'vi-dŭkt) [ovi- + L. *ductus,* a leading, fr. *duco,* pp. *ductus,* to lead]. *Tuba* uterina.

oviductal (ō-vi-dŭk'tăl). Oviducal; relating to a uterine tube.

oviferous (ō-vif'er-ŭs) [ovi- + L. *fero,* to carry]. Ovigerous; carrying or containing ova.

oviform (ō'vi-fōrm). Ovoid (2).

ovigenesis (ō-vi-jen'ĕ-sis). Oogenesis.

ovigenetic, ovigenic (ō-vi-jĕ-net'ik, -jen'ik). Oogenetic.

ovigenous (ō-vij'ĕ-nŭs). Oogenetic.

ovigerous (ō-vij'er-ŭs). Oviferous.

ovine (ō'vīn) [L. *ovinus,* relating to a sheep]. Relating to sheep; sheeplike.

ovinia (ō-vin'ē-ă) [L. *ovinus,* relating to a sheep]. Sheep-pox.

oviparity (ō-vi-par'i-tē) [ovi- + L. *pario,* to bear]. The quality of being oviparous.

oviparous (ō-vip'ă-rŭs) [L. *oviparus,* fr. *ovum,* egg, + *pario,* to bear]. Egg-laying; denoting those birds, fish, amphibians, reptiles, monotreme mammals, and invertebrates whose young develop in eggs outside of the maternal body.

oviposit (ō'vi-poz'it) [ovi- + L. *pono,* pp. *positus,* to place]. To lay eggs; applied especially to insects.

oviposition (ō'vi-pō-zish'ŭn). Act of laying or depositing eggs by insects.

ovipositor (ō-vi-poz'i-tŏr, -tōr). A specialized female organ especially well developed in insects for laying or depositing eggs.

ovist (ō'vist). A preformationist who believed that the female sex cell contained a miniature body susceptible to growth when stimulated by semen.

ovo- [L. *ovum,* egg]. Combining form denoting egg. See also oo-, ovi-.

ovocenter (ō'vō-sen'ter). Obsolete term for the centrosome of the impregnated ovum.

ovocyte (ō′vō-sīt) [ovo- + G. *kytos,* a hollow (cell)]. Oocyte.

ovoflavin (ō-vō-flā′vin). Riboflavin found in eggs.

ovogenesis (ō-vō-jen′ĕ-sis). Oogenesis.

ovoglobulin (ō-vō-glob′yū-lin). Globulin in the white of egg.

ovogonium (ō-vō-gō′nē-ŭm) [ovo- + G. *gonē,* generation]. Obsolete term for oogonium.

ovoid (ō′voyd) [ovo- + G. *eidos,* resemblance]. **1.** An oval or egg-shaped form. **2.** Oviform; resembling an egg.
fetal o., the form of the fetus *in utero;* its length is about one-half of the length of the extended fetus.
Manchester o. [University of *Manchester, England*], an egg-shaped radium applicator for placement in the lateral vaginal fornices.

ovolarviparous (ō′vō-lar-vip′ă-rŭs) [ovo- + L. *larva,* a mask, + *pario,* to bear]. Denoting certain nematodes and other invertebrates in which the eggs are hatched within the female, and the larvae developed or protected within the uterus until the correct time for their emergence.

ovomucin (ō-vō-myū′sin). A glycoprotein in the white of egg.

ovomucoid (ō-vō-myū′koyd). A mucoprotein obtained from the white of egg.

ovoplasm (ō′vō-plazm). Protoplasm of an unfertilized egg.

ovoprotogen (ō-vō-prō′tō-jen). Lipoic acid.

ovotestis (ō′vō-tes′tis). Gonad in which both testicular and ovarian components are present; a form of hermaphroditism.

ovotransferrin (ō′vō-trans-fār′in). Conalbumin.

ovovitellin (ō′vō-vī-tel′in). [ovo- + L. *vitellus,* yolk]. Vitellin.

ovoviviparous (ō′vō-vī-vip′ă-rŭs) [ovo- + L. *viviparus,* bringing forth alive, fr. *vivus,* alive, + *pario,* to bear]. Denoting those fish, amphibians, and reptiles that produce eggs which hatch within the body of the parent.

ovular (ov′yū-lăr, ō′vyū-). Relating to an ovule.

ovulation (ov′yū-lā′shŭn, ō′vyū-). Release of an ovum from the ovarian follicle.
anestrous o., discharge of ova occurring in animals without estrus.
paracyclic o., o. occurring in the menstrual cycle at any time other than the normally anticipated time; believed to be usually a psychogenic phenomenon.

ovulatory (ov′yū-lă-tō-rē, ō′vyū-). Relating to ovulation.

ovule (ov′yūl, ō′vyū-) [Mod. L. *ovulum,* dim. of L. *ovum,* egg]. Ovulum. **1.** The ovum of a mammal, especially while still in the ovarian follicle. **2.** A small beadlike structure bearing a fancied resemblance to an o.

ovulocyclic (ov′yū-lō-sī′klik, ō′vyū-). Denoting any recurrent phenomenon associated with and occurring at a certain time within the ovulatory cycle, as, for example, ovulocyclic porphyria.

ovulum, pl. **ovula** (ov′yū-lŭm, -lă, ō′vyū-). Ovule.

ovum, gen. **ovi,** pl. **ova** (ō′vŭm, -vī, -vă) [L. egg]. The female sex cell. When fertilized by a spermatozoon, an o. is capable of developing into a new individual of the same species; during maturation, the o., like spermatozoon, undergoes a halving of its chromosomal complement so that, at its union with the male gamete, the species number of chromosomes (46 in man) is maintained; yolk contained in the ova of different species varies greatly in amount and distribution, and influences the pattern of the cleavage division.
alecithal o., an o. in which the yolk is nearly absent, consisting of only a few particles.
blighted o., a fertilized o. whose development has ceased at an early stage.
centrolecithal o., one in which the yolk is mostly located near the center of the egg.
fertilized o., an o. impregnated by a spermatozoon.
isolecithal o., an o. in which there is only a small amount of evenly distributed yolk.
Peters' o., an o. with a presumptive fertilization age of about 13 days; for many years, one of very few young human embryos recovered in good condition and whose study furnished many facts regarding early embryonic changes.
telolecithal o., an o. in which there is a large amount of yolk massed at the vegetative pole, as in the eggs of birds and reptiles.

Owen, Sir Richard, British anatomist, 1804–1892. See O.'s *lines;* contour *lines* of O.; interglobular *space* of O.

Owren, Paul A., 20th century Norwegian physician. See O.'s *disease.*

oxa-. Combining form inserted in names of organic compounds to signify presence or addition of oxygen atom(s) in a chain or ring (as in ethers), not appended to either (as in ketones and aldehydes). See also hydroxy-; oxo-; oxy- (6).

oxacillin sodium (ok-să-sil′in). 5-Methyl-3-phenyl-4-isoxazolylpenicillin sodium; a semisynthetic penicillin used in the oral therapy of penicillin-resistant staphylococcal infections.

oxalaldehyde (ok-să-lal′dĕ-hīd). Glyoxal.

oxalate (ok′să-lāt). A salt of oxalic acid.

oxalemia (ok-să-lē′mē-ă) [oxalate + G. *haima,* blood]. The presence of an abnormally large amount of oxalates in the blood.

oxalic acid (ok-sal′ik). An acid, HOOC–COOH, found in many plants and vegetables, particularly in buckwheat (family Polygoniaceae) and *Oxalis* (family Oxalidaceae); used as a hemostatic in veterinary medicine, but toxic when ingested by man; also used in the removal of ink and other stains, and as a general reducing agent.

oxalo (ok′să-lō). The monoacyl radical, HOOC–CO– .

oxaloacetate transacetase (ok′să-lō-as′ĕ-tāt trans-as′ĕ-tās). *Citrate* synthase.

oxaloacetic acid (ok′să-lō-ă-sē′tik). Oxosuccinic acid; ketosuccinic acid; $HOOC–CO–CH_2COOH$; a ketodicarboxylic acid and important intermediate in the tricarboxylic acid cycle; the product formed when aspartic acid acts as amine donor in transamination reactions.

oxalosis (ok-să-lō′sis). Widespread deposition of calcium oxalate crystals in the kidneys, bones, arterial media, and myocardium, with increased urinary excretion of oxalate; may be an acquired disorder, as in oxalate poisoning, or represent one aspect of primary hyperoxaluria and o.

oxalosuccinic acid (ok′să-lō-sŭk-sin′ik). $HOOC–CO–CH(COOH)–CH_2–COOH$; the product of the dehydrogenation of isocitric acid under the catalytic influence of isocitrate dehydrogenase; an intermediate of the tricarboxylic acid cycle.

oxalosuccinic carboxylase. Isocitrate dehydrogenase.

oxalourea (ok′să-lō-yū-rē′ă). Oxalylurea.

oxaluria (ok-să-lū′rē-ă) [oxalate + G. *ouron,* urine]. Hyperoxaluria.

oxaluric acid (ok-să-lūr′ik). $NH_2CONHCOCOOH$; the ureide of oxalic acid, derived from uric acid or oxalylurea.

oxalyl (ok′să-lil). The diacyl radical, –CO–CO– .

oxalylurea (ok′să-lil-yū-rē′ă). Oxalourea; parabanic acid; the cyclic (end-to-end) amide anhydride of oxaluric acid; an oxidation product of uric acid.

oxamide (ok-sam′īd). The diamide of oxalic acid, $NH_2CO–CONH_2$.

oxammonium (ok-să-mō′nē-ŭm). Hydroxylamine.

oxamniquine (oks-am′ni-quin). $C_{14}H_{21}N_3O_3$; a tetrahydroquinoline derivative, similar to hycanthone and lucanthone, effective against *Schistosoma mansoni;* now largely superseded by the broad spectrum anthelmintic drug praziquantel.

oxanamide (ok-san'ă-mīd). 2-Ethyl-3-propylglycidamide; a sedative.

oxandrolone (ok-san'drō-lōn). 17β-Hydroxy-17α-methyl-2-oxa-5α-androstan-3-one (C-2 replaced by O in the androstane nucleus); an androgenic anabolic steroid.

oxaphenamide (ok-să-fen'ă-mīd). 4'-Hydroxysalicylanilide; a choleretic.

oxazepam (ok-sā'zĕ-pam). 7-Chloro-1,3-dihydro-3-hydroxy-5-phenyl-2*H*-1,4-benzodiazepin-2-one; a benzodiazepine chemically and pharmacologically related to chlordiazepoxide and diazepam; an antianxiety agent.

oxazin (ok'să-zin). Oxyiminodiphenylimine; $C_{12}H_{10}ON_2$; parent substance of a series of biological dyes, *e.g.*, gallocyanin, brilliant cresyl blue, cresyl violet acetate.

oxazole (ok'să-zōl). The fundamental ring system, C_3H_3ON.

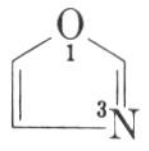

1,3-Oxazole

oxeladin (ok-sel'ă-din). 2-Ethyl-2-phenylbutyric acid 2-(2-diethylaminoethoxy)ethyl ester; an antitussive agent.

oxidant (ok'si-dant). The substance that is reduced and that, therefore, oxidizes the other component of an oxidation-reduction system.

oxidase (ok'si-dās). Oxydase; classically, one of a group of ensymes, now termed oxidoreductases (EC class 1), that bring about oxidation by the addition of oxygen to a metabolite or by the removal of hydrogen or of one or more electrons. O. is now used for those cases in which O_2 acts as an acceptor (of H or of electrons); those removing hydrogen are now termed dehydrogenases. For individual o.'s, see the specific names.
direct o., originally, an o. catalyzing the transfer of O_2 directly to other bodies; now termed oxygenase.
indirect o., originally, an o. that acts by reducing a peroxide; now termed peroxidase.

oxidasis (ok-si-dā'sis). Oxidation by an oxidase.

oxidation (ok-si-dā'shŭn). **1.** Oxidization; combination with oxygen; increasing the valence of an atom or ion by the loss from it of hydrogen or of one or more electrons thus rendering it more electropositive, as when iron is changed from the ferrous (2+) to the ferric (3+) state. **2.** In bacteriology, the aerobic dissimilation of substrates with the production of energy and water; in contrast to fermentation, the transfer of electrons in the o. process is accomplished via the respiratory chain, which utilizes oxygen as the final electron acceptor.
beta-o., o. of the β-carbon (carbon 3) of a fatty acid, forming the β-keto (β-oxo) acid analogue; of importance in fatty acid catabolism.
omega-o., o. at the carbon atom farthest removed (ω-carbon) from the carboxyl group (carbon 1).

oxidation-reduction. Any chemical oxidation or reduction reaction, which must, *in toto,* comprise both oxidation and reduction; the basis for calling all oxidative enzymes (formerly oxidases) oxidoreductases. Often shortened to "redox."

oxidative (ok-si-dā'tiv). Having the power to oxidize; denoting a process involving oxidation.

oxide (ok'sīd). A compound of oxygen with another element or a radical; *e.g.,* mercuric o., HgO.
acid o., an acid anhydride; an o. of an electronegative element or radical; it can combine with water to form an acid.
basic o., a base anhydride; an o. of an electropositive element or radical; it can combine with water to form a base.
indifferent o., neutral o.
neutral o., indifferent o.; an o. that is neither an acid nor a base; *e.g.,* water (hydrogen oxide, H_2O).

oxidization (ok'sid-i-zā'shŭn). Oxidation (1).

oxidize (ok'si-dīz). To combine or cause an element or radical to combine with oxygen or to lose electrons.

oxidoreductase (ok'si-dō-rē-dŭk'tās). An enzyme (EC class 1) catalyzing an oxidation-reduction reaction. Trivial names for o.'s include dehydrogenase, reductase, oxidase (where O_2 is the H acceptor), oxygenase (where O_2 is incorporated into the substrate), peroxidase (H_2O_2 is the acceptor; catalase is an exception), hydroxylase (coupled oxidation of two donors). See also oxidase.

oxime (ok'sēm). A compound resulting from the action of hydroxylamine, NH_2OH, on a ketone or an aldehyde to yield the group =N–OH attached to the former carbonyl carbon atom.
amide o.'s, amidoximes.

oximeter (ok-sim'ĕ-ter). An instrument for determining photoelectrically the oxygen saturation of a sample of blood.
cuvette o., an o. that reads the percentage of oxygen saturation of the blood as it passes through a cuvette outside the body.

oximetry (ok-sim'ĕ-trē). Measurement with an oximeter of the oxygen saturation of hemoglobin in a sample of blood.

oxo-. Prefix denoting addition of oxygen; used in place of keto- in systematic nomenclature. See also hydroxy-; oxa-; oxy-(6).

oxo acid (ok'sō). Keto acid.

3-oxoacid-CoA transferase [EC 2.8.3.5]. 3-Ketoacid-CoA transferase; acetoacetyl-succinic thiophorase; an enzyme catalyzing the conversion of acetoacetyl-CoA and succinate into succinyl-CoA and acetoacetate; malonyl-CoA can substitute for succinyl-CoA and other 3-oxo acids for the acetoacetate.

3-oxoacyl-ACP reductase (ok'sō-as'il). [EC 1.1.100]. β-Ketoacyl-ACP reductase; an enzyme oxidizing 3-hydroxyacyl-ACP to 3-oxoacyl-ACP, with $NADP^+$ as hydrogen acceptor; the reverse reaction is involved in the synthesis of fatty acids.

3-oxoacyl-ACP synthase [EC 2.3.1.41]. β-Ketoacyl-ACP synthase; acyl-malonyl-ACP synthase; an enzyme condensing malonyl-ACP and acyl-ACP to oxoacyl-ACP + ACP + CO_2, and similar reactions, as steps in fatty acid synthesis.

2-oxoglutarate dehydrogenase (ok'sō-glū-tar'āt) [EC 1.2.4.2]. β-Ketoglutarate dehydrogenase; an enzyme that catalyzes the oxidative decarboxylation of 2-ketoglutaric acid to succinyldihydrolipoate; the succinyl group is later transferred to CoA and the reduced lipoate is oxidized by NAD^+.

oxolamine (ok-sol'ă-mēn). 5-(2-Diethylaminoethyl)-3-phenyl-1,2,4-oxadiazole; used for treatment of bronchopulmonary infections.

oxolinic acid (ok-sō-lin'ik). 5-Ethyl-5,8-dihydro-8-oxo-1,3-dioxolo[4,5-*g*]quinoline-7-carboxylic acid; a quinolone antibacterial agent used in the treatment of urinary tract infections.

oxophenarsine hydrochloride (ok'sō-fen-ar'sēn). 3-Amino-4-hydroxyphenylarsineoxide hydrochloride; an antisyphilitic and antitrypanosomal agent.

17-oxosteroids (ok-sō-stēr'oydz). 17-Ketosteroids.

oxosuccinic acid (ok's-ō-sŭk-sin'ik). Oxaloacetic acid.

oxprenolol hydrochloride (oks-pren'ō-lol). 1-[*o*-(Allyloxy)-phenoxy]-3-(isopropylamino)-2-propanol hydrochloride; a β-receptor blocking agent with coronary vasodilator activity.

OXT Abbreviation for oxytocin.

oxtriphylline (oks-trī'fi-lin, oks'trī-fil'in). Choline theophyllinate; a true salt of theophylline; it has mild diuretic, myocardial stimulating vasodilator, and bronchodilator actions, with the same uses as theophylline, but is better absorbed and less irritating.

oxy- [G. *oxys,* keen]. **1.** Combining form denoting sharp, pointed; acid; acute; shrill; quick (incorrectly used for ocy-, from G. *ōkys,* swift). **2.** In chemistry, combining form denoting the presence of oxygen, either added or substituted, in a substance. See also hydroxy-; oxa-; oxo-.

oxyacoia, oxyakoia (ok'sē-ă-koy'ă) [G. *oxys,* acute, + *akoē,* hearing]. Increased sensitiveness to noises, occurring in facial paralysis, especially when the stapedius muscle is paralyzed.

oxyaphia (ok-sē-ā'fē-ă) [G. *oxys,* acute, + *haphē,* touch]. Hyperaphia.

oxybarbiturates (ok'sē-bar-bit'yūr-āts). Hypnotics of the barbiturate group in which the atom attached at the carbon-2 position is oxygen.

oxybenzone (ok-sē-ben'zōn). 2-Hydroxy-4-methoxybenzophenone; an ultraviolet screen for use in skin ointments and lotions.

oxybiotin (ok-sē-bī'ō-tin). An analogue and antimetabolite of biotin, in which the sulfur atom is replaced by oxygen.

oxybutynin chloride (ok-sē-byū'ti-nin). α-Phenylcyclohexaneglycolic acid 4-(diethylamino)-2-butynyl ester hydrochloride; an intestinal antispasmodic.

oxycalorimeter (ok'sē-kal-ō-rim'ĕ-ter). A calorimeter measuring energy content of substances in terms of oxygen consumed.

oxycellulose (ok-sē-sel'yū-lōs). Cellulose that has been oxidized by NO_2 or other oxidizing agents to the point where all or most of the glucose residues have been converted to glucuronic acid residues; used as an adsorbent in chromatography or other adsorption processes. See also oxidized *cellulose.*

oxycephalia (ok'sē-se-fā'lē-ă). Oxycephaly.

oxycephalic, oxycephalous (ok-sē-se-fal'ik, -sef'ă-lŭs). Acrocephalic; acrocephalous; hypsicephalic; relating to or characterized by oxycephaly.

oxycephaly (ok-sē-sef'ă-lē) [G. *oxys,* pointed, + *kephalē,* head]. Acrocephalia; acrocephaly; hypsicephaly; hypsocephaly; oxycephalia; turricephaly; steeple or tower skull; a type of craniosynostosis in which there is premature closure of the lambdoid and coronal sutures, resulting in an abnormally high, peaked, or conically shaped skull.

oxychloride (ok-sē-klōr'īd). A compound of oxygen with a metallic chloride; *e.g.,* a chlorate or perchlorate.

oxychromatic (ok'sē-krō-mat'ik) [G. *oxys,* sour, acid, + *chrōma,* color]. Acidophilic.

oxychromatin (ok-sē-krō'mă-tin). Oxyphil chromatin; chromatin that stains with acid dyes, as in interphase nuclei.

oxycodone (ok-sē-kō'dōn). 14-Hydroxydihydrocodeinone; a narcotic analgesic.

11-oxycorticoids (ok-sē-kōr'ti-koydz). Corticosteroids bearing an alcohol or ketonic group on carbon-11; *e.g.,* cortisone, cortisol.

oxydase (ok'sē-dās). Oxidase.

oxyesthesia (ok'sē-es-thē'zē-ă) [G. *oxys,* acute, + *aisthēsis,* sensation]. Hyperesthesia.

oxygen (ok'sē-jen). **1.** A gaseous element, symbol O, atomic no. 8, atomic weight 16.000+ on basis of $^{12}C = 12.0000$; the most abundant and widely distributed chemical element which combines with most of the other elements to form oxides and is essential to animal and plant life. **2.** A medicinal gas that contains not less than 99.0%, by volume, of O_2.

heavy o., oxygen-18.

hyperbaric o., high pressure o., o. at a pressure greater than 1 atmosphere. See also hyperbaric *oxygenation.*

singlet o., an excited or higher energy form of o. characterized by the spin of a pair of electrons in opposite directions, whereas electron spin is unidirectional in normal molecular o. Because of its great reactivity, singlet o. is a probable intermediate in most photooxidation reactions. Although it exists for no more than 0.1 sec, it may react with atmospheric pollutants to foster smog formation and may have harmful biological effects.

triplet o., the normal unexcited state of O_2 in the atmosphere, in which the unpaired pair of electrons are so displaced that their magnetic fields are oriented in the same direction, resulting in paramagnetism; each of the heat-generated spectral lines of such o. can be split by a magnetic field into a triplet. *Cf.* singlet o.

oxygen-15 (^{15}O). A cyclotron-produced, positron-emitting radioisotope of oxygen with a physical half-life of 2 minutes; used in studies of respiratory function.

oxygen-16 (^{16}O). The common o. isotope, making up 99.759% of natural o.; previously the standard nuclide for the mass numbers on the physical scale, its mass number being arbitrarily set equal to 16.000000. The standard is now ^{12}C, set equal to 12.000000.

oxygen-17 (^{17}O). The rarest of the stable o. isotopes, making up 0.037% of natural o.

oxygen-18 (^{18}O). Heavy o.; a stable o. isotope making up 0.204% of natural o.

oxygenase (ok'sē-jĕ-nās). Direct oxidase; one of a group of enzymes (EC subclass 1.13) catalyzing direct incorporation of O_2 into substrates; *e.g.,* tryptophan 2,3-dioxygenase (tryptophan pyrrolase) catalyzing reaction between O_2 and tryptophan to form formylkynurenine.

oxygenate (ok'sē-jĕ-nāt). To accomplish oxygenation.

oxygenation (ok'sē-jĕ-nā'shŭn). Addition of oxygen to any chemical or physical system.

apneic o., diffusion *respiration.*

hyperbaric o., an increased amount of oxygen in organs and tissues resulting from the administration of oxygen in a compression chamber at an ambient pressure greater than 1 atmosphere.

oxygenic (ok-sē-jen'ik). Pertaining to or containing oxygen.

oxygenize (ok'sē-jen-īz). To oxidize with oxygen.

oxygeusia (ok-sē-gū'sē-ă) [G. *oxys,* acute, + *geusis,* taste]. Hypergeusia.

oxyheme (ok'sē-hēm). Hematin.

oxyhemochromogen (ok'sē-hēm'ō-krō'mō-jen). Hematin.

oxyhemoglobin (HbO_2) (ok'sē-hē-mō-glō'bin). Oxygenated hemoglobin; hemoglobin in combination with oxygen, the form of hemoglobin present in arterial blood, scarlet or bright red when dissolved in water.

oxyiodide (ok-sē-ī'ō-dīd). A compound of oxygen with a metallic iodide, *e.g.,* an iodate or periodate.

oxykrinin (ok-sē-krin'in). Secretin.

oxylonprocaine hydrochloride (ok'sē-lon-prō'kān). Benoxinate hydrochloride.

oxymesterone (ok-sē-mes'te-rōn). 4,17β-Dihydroxy-17-methylandrost-4-en-3-one; an anabolic steroid.

oxymetazoline hydrochloride (ok'sē-mĕ-taz'ō-lēn). 6-Tert-butyl-3-(2-imidazolin-2-ylmethyl)-2,4-dimentylphenol hydrochloride; a vasoconstrictor used topically to reduce swelling and congestion of the nasal mucosa.

oxymetholone (ok-sē-meth'ō-lōn). 17β-Hydroxy-2- (hydroxymethylene)-17-methyl-5α-androstan-3-one; an androgenic anabolic steroid.

oxymorphone hydrochloride (ok-sē-mōr'fōn). 14-Hydroxydihydromorphinone hydrochloride; a semisynthetic narcotic analgesic closely related chemically to hydromorphone hydrochloride; its actions are similar to those of morphine, but more potent.

oxymyoglobin (ok'sē-mī-ō-glō'bin). Myoglobin in its oxygenated form, analogous in structure to oxyhemoglobin.

oxynervone (ok'sē-ner'vōn). Hydroxynervone.

oxyneurine (ok-sē-nūr'ēn). Betaine.

oxyntic (ok-sin'tik) [G. *oxynō,* to sharpen, make sour, acid]. Acid-forming, *e.g.,* the parietal cells of the gastric glands.

oxyosmia (ok-sē-oz'mē-ă) [G. *oxys,* acute + *osmē,* sense of smell]. Hyperosmia.

oxyosphresia (ok'sē-os-frē'zē-ă) [G. *oxys,* acute, + *osphrēsis,* smell]. Hyperosmia.

oxypertine (ok-sē-per'tēn). 5,6-Dimethoxy-2-methyl-3-[2-(4-phenyl-1-piperazinyl)ethyl]indole; an antianxiety agent; also available as the hydrochloride.

oxyphenbutazone (ok'sē-fen-bū'tă-zōn). 1-(p-Hydroxyphenyl)-2-phenyl-4-butyl-3,5-pyrazolidine-dione monohydrate; an orally effective analgesic and anti-inflammatory agent used (usually in short courses) for rheumatoid arthritis and gout.

oxyphencyclimine hydrochloride (ok'sē-fen-sī'klī-mēn). The hydrochloride of 1,4,5,6-tetrahydro-1-methylpyrimidin-2-ylmethyl-α-cyclohexyl-α-hydroxy-α-phenylacetate; an anticholinergic agent.

oxyphenisatin acetate (ok'sē-fe-nī'să-tin). Acetphenolisatin; endophenolphthalein; diacetyldiphenolisatin; 3,3-bis(*p*-acetoxyphenyl)oxindole; a cathartic with pharmacologic properties resembling those of phenolphthalein, except that it is not absorbed from the gastrointestinal tract.

oxyphenonium bromide (ok'sē-fe-nō'nē-ŭm). Diethyl(2-hydroxyethyl)methylammonium bromide α-phenyl-α-cyclohexylglycolate; a quaternary ammonium compound with anticholinergic action.

oxyphil, oxyphile (ok'sē-fil, -fīl) [G. *oxys,* sour, acid, + *philos,* fond]. **1.** Oxyphyl *cell.* **2.** Eosinophilic *leukocyte.* **3.** Oxyphilic.

oxyphilic (ok-sē-fil'ik). Oxyphil (3); having an affinity for acid dyes; denoting certain cell or tissue elements.

oxyphonia (ok-sē-fō'nē-ă) [G. *oxys,* sharp, + *phōnē,* voice]. Shrillness or high pitch of the voice.

oxypolygelatin (ok'sē-pol-ē-jel'ă-tin). A modified gelatin used as a plasma extender in transfusions.

oxypurine (ok-sē-pyūr'ēn). A purine containing oxygen; *e.g.,* hypoxanthine, xanthine, uric acid.

oxyrhine (ok'sē-rīn) [G. *oxys,* sharp, + *rhis* (*rhin-*), nose]. Having a sharp-pointed nose.

oxyrygmia (ok-sē-rig'mē-ă) [G. *oxys,* acid, + *erygmos,* eructation]. Obsolete term for eructation of acid fluid.

Oxyspirura mansoni (ok'-sē-spī-rū'ră man-sō'nī). Manson's eye worm; a widely distributed spiruroid nematode parasite found under the nictitating membrane in the eye of turkeys, chickens, peafowl, quail, and grouse; larvae develop to the infective stage in cockroaches.

oxytalan (ok-sit'ă-lan) [G. *oxys,* acid, + *talas,* suffering, resisting; coined term probably intended to mean "resistant to acid hydrolysis"]. A type of connective tissue fiber histochemically distinct from collagen or elastic fibers described in the periodontal membrane and gingivae.

oxytetracycline (ok'sē-tet-ră-sī'klīn). An antibiotic produced by the actinomycete, *Streptomyces rimosus,* present in the soil; its actions and uses are similar to those of tetracycline; available as the dihydrate, hydrochloride, and calcium.

oxythiamin (ok-sē-thī'ă-min). A molecule similar to that of thiamin but with a hydroxyl group replacing the amino group on the pyrimidine ring; a thiamin antagonist capable of inducing symptoms of thiamin deficiency on administration; increases thiamin excretion.

oxytocia (ok-sē-tō'sē-ă) [G. *okytokos,* swift birth]. Rapid parturition.

oxytocic (ok-sē-tō'sik). **1.** Hastening childbirth. **2.** Parturifacient (2).

oxytocin (OXT) (ok-sē-tō'sin) [G. *okytokos,* swift birth]. Ocytocin; α-hypophamine; a nonapeptide hormone of the neurohypophysis, differing from human vasopressin in having leucine at position 8 and isoleucine at position 3, that causes myometrial contractions at term and promotes milk release during lactation; used for the induction or stimulation of labor, in the management of postpartum hemorrhage and atony, and to relieve painful breast engorgement.
arginine o., o. with arginine at position 8 (identical with arginine vasotocin). See also arginine *vasopressin.*

oxyuriasis (ok-sē-yū-rī'ă-sis). Infection with nematode parasites of the genus *Oxyuris.*

oxyuricide (ok'sē-yū'ri-sīd) [oxyurid + L. *caedo,* to kill]. An agent that destroys pinworms.

oxyurid (ok-sē-yū'rid) [see *Oxyuris*]. Common name for members of the family Oxyuridae.

Oxyuridae (ok-sē-yū'ri-dē). A family of parasitic nematodes (superfamily Oxyuroidea) found in the large intestine or cecum of vertebrates and the intestine of invertebrates, especially insects and millipedes; it includes the genera *Aspiculurus, Enterobius, Oxyuris, Passalurus, Syphacia,* and *Thelandros.*

Oxyuris (ok'sē-yū'ris) [G. *oxys,* sharp, + *oura,* tail]. A genus of nematodes commonly called seatworms or pinworms (although the pinworm of man is the closely related form, *Enterobius vermicularis*). *O. equi,* the horse pinworm, is a common parasite of horses in all parts of the world, inhabiting the large intestine.

-oyl. Suffix denoting an acyl radical; -yl replaces -ic in acid names.

oz. Abbreviation for ounce.

ozena (ō-zē'nă) [G. *ozaina,* a fetid polypus, fr. *ozō,* to smell]. A disease characterized by intranasal crusting, atrophy, and fetid odor.

ozenous (ō'zē-nŭs). Relating to ozena.

ozocerite (ō-zō-sē'rīt). Ozokerite.

ozochrotia (ō-zō-krō'shē-ă) [G. *ozō,* to smell, + *chroa,* skin]. Bromidrosis.

ozokerite (ō-zō-kēr'īt). Ozocerite; a mixture of paraffinic and cycloparaffinic hydrocarbons occurring in nature; it has a higher melting point than synthetic paraffin, and is used as a substitute for beeswax.
purified o., ceresin.

ozonator (ō'zō-nā-ter, -tōr). An apparatus for generating ozone and diffusing it in the atmosphere of a room.

ozone (ō'zōn) [G. *ozō,* to smell]. O_3; a powerful oxidizing agent; air containing a perceptible amount of O_3 is formed by an electric discharge or by the slow combustion of phosphorus, and has an odor suggestive of CL_2 or SO_2.

ozonide (ō'zō-nīd). The unstable intermediate formed by the reaction of ozone with an unsaturated organic compound, especially with unsaturated fatty acids.

ozonolysis (ō-zō-nol'ĭ-sis) [ozone + G. *lysis,* dissolution]. The splitting of a double bond in a hydrocarbon chain upon treatment with ozone, with the formation of two aldehydes (an ozonide is the unstable intermediate); used to determine the structure of unsaturated fatty acids.

ozonometer (ō-zō-nom'ĕ-ter). A modified form of ozonoscope, in which by a series of test papers the amount of ozone in the atmosphere may be estimated.

ozonoscope (ō-zō'nō-skōp). Filter paper saturated with starch and potassium iodide or with litmus and potassium iodide; turns blue in the presence of ozone.

ozostomia (ō-zō-stō'mē-ă) [G. *ozō,* to smell, + *stoma,* mouth]. Halitosis.

P

P **1.** Symbol for peta-; phosphorus; pressure or partial *pressure,* frequently with subscripts indicating location and chemical species. **2.** Followed by a subscript, refers to the plasma concentration of the substance indicated by the subscript. **3.** A blood group designation. See P blood group, Blood Groups appendix.

P In nucleic acid terminology, symbol for phosphoric residue.

P_i Symbol for inorganic *orthophosphate.*

P_1 Abbreviation for parental *generation.*

P_{700} The pigment in chloroplasts bleached by light of wavelengths about 700 nm.

P_{870} The pigment in bacterial chromatophores bleached by light of wavelengths about 870 nm.

p **1.** Abbreviation for pupil; optic *papilla.* **2.** In polynucleotide symbolism, phosphoric ester or phosphate. **3.** Symbol for pico-(2). **4** [fr. Fr. *petit,* small]. In cytogenetics, symbol for the short arm of a chromosome.

***p*-** Abbreviation for *para-* (4).

P.A. Abbreviation for physician's assistant.

Pa Symbol for pascal; protactinium.

Paas, H.R., German physician. See P.'s *disease.*

PABA Abbreviation for *p*-aminobenzoic acid.

pablum (pab'lŭm). A precooked infant food, a mixture of wheat, oat, and corn meals, wheat embryo, alfalfa leaves, brewers' yeast, iron, and sodium chloride.

pabular (pab'yū-lăr). Relating to, or of the nature of, pabulum.

pabulum (pab'yū-lŭm) [L.]. Food or nutriment.

Pacchioni, Antonio, Italian anatomist, 1665–1726. See pacchionian *bodies, corpuscles, depressions, glands, granulations.*

pacchionian (pak-ē-ō'nē-an). Attributed to or described by Pacchioni.

pacefollower (pās'fawl-ō-er). Any cell in excitable tissue that responds to stimuli from a pacemaker.

pacemaker (pās'mā-ker) [L. *passus,* step, pace]. **1.** Biologically, any rhythmic center that establishes a pace of activity; **2.** An artificial regulator of rate activity. **3.** In chemistry, the substance whose rate of reaction sets the pace for a series of chain reactions; the rate-limiting reaction itself.

artificial p., any device that substitutes for the normal p. and controls the rhythm of the organ; especially an artificial cardiac p., which may be implanted in the chest, with electrodes attached to the external cardiac surface, or passed through the venous circulation into the right side of the heart (pervenous p.).

demand p., a form of artificial p. usually implanted into cardiac tissue because its output of electrical stimuli can be inhibited by endogenous cardiac electrical activity.

ectopic p., any p. other than the sinus node.

electric cardiac p., an electric device that can substitute for the normal cardiac p., controlling the heart's rhythm by artificial electric discharges.

external p., an artificial cardiac p. whose electrodes for delivering rhythmical electrical stimuli to the heart are placed on the chest wall.

fixed-rate p., an artificial p. that emits electrical stimuli at a constant frequency.

nuclear p., a nuclear-powered unit used to generate the electrical current for artificially pacing the heart.

pervenous p., an artificial p. passed through the venous circulation into the right side of the heart.

shifting p., wandering p.

subsidiary atrial p., secondary source for rhythmic control of the heart, available for controlling cardiac activity if the sinoatrial pacemaker fails; located within the crista terminalis and atrial free wall near the inferior vena cava.

wandering p., shifting p.; a disturbance of the normal cardiac rhythm in which the site of the controlling p. shifts from beat to beat, usually between the sinus and A-V nodes.

pachometer (pa-kom'ĕ-ter). Pachymeter.

Pachon, Michel V., French physiologist, 1867–1938. See P.'s *method, test.*

pachy- [G. *pachys,* thick]. Prefix to words formed from G. roots, denoting thick.

pachyblepharon (pak'ē-blef'ă-ron) [pachy- + G. *blepharon,* eyelid]. Tylosis ciliaris; thickening of the tarsal border of the eyelid.

pachycephalia (pak'ē-se-fā'lē-ă). Pachycephaly.

pachycephalic, pachycephalous (pak'ē-se-fal'ik, -sef'ă-lŭs). Relating to or marked by pachycephaly.

pachycephaly (pak-i-sef'ă-lē) [pachy- + G. *kephalē,* head]. Pachycephalia; abnormal thickness of the skull.

pachycheilia, pachychilia (pak-i-kī'lē-ă) [pachy- + G. *cheilos,* lip]. Swelling or abnormal thickness of the lips.

pachycholia (pak-i-kō'lē-ă) [pachy- + G. *cholē,* bile]. Inspissation of the bile.

pachychromatic (pak'ē-krō-mat'ik). Having a coarse chromatin reticulum.

pachychymia (pak-i-kī'mē-ă) [pachy- + G. *chymos,* juice]. Inspissation of the chyme.

pachydactylia (pak'ē-dak-til'ē-ă). Pachydactyly.

pachydactylous (pak-i-dak'ti-lŭs). Relating to or characterized by pachydactyly.

pachydactyly (pak-i-dak'ti-lē) [pachy- + G. *daktylos,* finger or toe]. Pachydactylia; enlargement of the fingers or toes, especially extremities; often see in neurofibromatosis.

pachyderma (pak-i-der'mă) [pachy- + G. *derma,* skin]. Pachydermatosis; pachydermia; abnormally thick skin. See also elephantiasis.

p. laryn'gis, a circumscribed connective tissue hyperplasia at the posterior commissure of the larynx.

p. lymphangiectat'ica, elephantiasis due to lymph stasis.

p. verruco'sa, chronic elephantiasis due to lymph stasis.

p. vesi'cae, elephantiasis with nodules comprised of lymph vesicles on skin surface.

pachydermatocele (pak'ē-der-mat'ō-sēl) [pachy- + G. *derma,* skin, + *kēlē,* tumor]. **1.** *Cutis* laxa. **2.** A huge neurofibroma.

pachydermatosis (pak'i-der'mă-tō'sis). Pachyderma.

pachydermatous (pak-i-der'mă-tŭs). Pachydermic; relating to pachyderma.

pachydermia (pak-i-der'mē-ă). Pachyderma.

pachydermic (pak-i-der'mik). Pachydermatous.

pachydermoperiostosis (pak-i-der'mō-per'ē-os-tō'sis) [pachy- + G. *derma,* skin, + periostosis]. A syndrome characterized by clubbing of the digits, periosteal new bone formation, especially over the distal ends of the long bones (idiopathic hypertrophic osteoarthropathy), and coarsening of the facial features with thickening, furrowing, and oiliness of the skin of the face and forehead (cutis verticis gyrata); there is seborrheic hyperplasia with open sebaceous pores filled with plugs of sebum; probably of autosomal dominant inheritance, usually more severe in males.

pachyglossia (pak-i-glos'ē-ă) [pachy- + G. *glōssa,* tongue]. An enlarged thick tongue.

pachygnathous (pă-kig'nath-ŭs) [pachy- + G. *gnathos,* jaw]. Characterized by a large or thick jaw.

pachygyria (pak-i-jī'rē-ă) [pachy- + G. *gyros,* circle]. Unusually thick convolutions of the cerebral cortex, related to defective development.

pachyhymenia (pak'ē-hī-me'nē-ă) [pachy- + G. *hymān,* membrane]. Pachymenia.

pachyhymenic (pak'ē-hī-men'ik). Pachymenic.

pachyleptomeningitis (pak'i-lep'tō-men-in-jī'tis) [G. *pachys,* thick, + *leptos,* thin, + *mēninx* (*mēning-*), membrane, + *-itis,* inflammation]. Inflammation of all the membranes of the brain or spinal cord.

pachylosis (pak-i-lō'sis) [G. *pachylos,* rather coarse]. A condition of roughness, dryness and thickening of the skin, usually on the lower extremities.

pachymenia (pak-i-mē'nē-ă) [pachy- + G. *hymēn,* a membrane]. Pachyhymenia; thickening of the skin or contiguous membranes.

pachymenic (pak-i-men'ik). Pachyhymenic; marked by or relating to pachymenia.

pachymeningitis (pak'i-men'in-jī'tis) [pachy- + G. *mēninx,* membrane, + *-itis,* inflammation]. Perimeningitis; inflammation of the dura mater.
p. exter'na, external or epidural meningitis; inflammation of the outer surface of the dura mater.
hemorrhagic p., subdural *hemorrhage.*
hypertrophic cervical p., a fibrotic and inflammatory thickening of spinal pachymeninges, particularly in the cervical region, resulting in spinal nerve radiculopathy; believed to be of syphilitic etiology.
p. inter'na, internal meningitis; inflammation of the inner surface of the dura mater.
pyogenic p., suppurative inflammation of the dura, often spreading from a neighboring osteomyelitis.

pachymeningopathy (pak'ē-mĕ-ning-gop'ă-thē) [pachy- + G. *mēninx* (*mēning-*), membrane, + *pathos,* disease]. Disease of the dura mater.

pachymeninx (pak'i-mē'ningks) [pachy- + G. *mēninx,* membrane]. The dura mater.

pachymeter (pă-kim'ĕ-ter) [pachy- + G. *metron,* measure]. Pachometer; an instrument for measuring the thickness of any object, especially of thin objects such as a plate of bone or a membrane.
optical p., a lens and/or mirror used to measure corneal thickness.

pachynema (pak-ē-nē'mă) [pachy- + G. *nēma,* thread]. Pachytene.

pachynsis (pă-kin'sis) [G. a thickening]. Any pathologic thickening.

pachyntic (pă-kin'tic). Relating to pachynsis.

pachyonychia (pak'ē-ō-nik'ē-ă) [pachy- + G. *onyx,* nail]. Abnormal thickness of the fingernails or toenails.
p. congen'ita, Jadassohn-Lewandowsky syndrome; a syndrome characterized by an abnormal thickness and elevation of nail plates with palmar and plantar hyperkeratosis; the tongue is whitish and glazed due to papillary atrophy; autosomal dominant inheritance.

pachyotia (pak-i-ō'shē-ă) [pachy- + G. *ous,* ear]. Thickness and coarseness of the auricles of the ears.

pachyperiostitis (pak'i-per'ē-ŏs-tī'tis) [pachy- + periostitis]. Proliferative thickening of the periosteum caused by inflammation.

pachyperitonitis (pak'i-per'i-tō-nī'tis) [pachy- + peritonitis]. Productive peritonitis; inflammation of the peritoneum with thickening of the membrane.

pachypleuritis (pak'ē-plū-rī'tis) [pachy- + pleura + G. *-itis,* inflammation]. Productive pleurisy; inflammation of the pleura with thickening of the membrane.

pachypodous (pă-kip'ō-dŭs) [pachy- + G. *pous,* foot]. Having large thick feet.

pachysalpingitis (pak'ē-sal-pin-jī'tis). Chronic interstitial salpingitis.

pachysalpingo-ovaritis (pak-i-sal'pin-gō-ō-va-rī'tis) [pachy- + salpinx + Mod. L. *ovarium,* ovary, + G. *-itis,* inflammation]. Chronic parenchymatous inflammation of the ovary and fallopian tube.

pachysomia (pak-i-sō'mē-ă) [pachy- + G. *sōma,* body]. Pathologic thickening of the soft parts of the body, notably in acromegaly.

pachytene (pak'i-tēn) [pachy- + G. *tainia,* band, tape]. Pachynema; the stage of prophase in meiosis in which pairing of homologous chromosomes is complete and the paired homologues may twine about each other as they continue to shorten; longitudinal cleavage occurs in each chromosome to form two sister chromatids so that each homologous chromosome pair becomes a set of four intertwined chromatids called a bivalent.

pachyvaginalitis (pak'i-vaj'i -năl-ī'tis) [pachy- + Mod. L. (tunica) *vaginalis,* + G. *-itis,* inflammation]. Chronic inflammation with thickening of the tunica vaginalis testis.

pachyvaginitis (pak'i-vaj'i-nī'tis) [pachy- + vagina + G. *-itis,* inflammation]. Chronic vaginitis with thickening and induration of the vaginal walls.
p. cys'tica, *vaginitis* emphysematosa.

Pacini, Filippo, Italian anatomist, 1812–1883. See pacinian *corpuscles,* Vater-P. *corpuscles.*

pacinian (pa-sin'ē-an, pa-chin'). Attributed to or described by Pacini.

pacinitis (pa-sin-ī'tis, pa-chin-). Inflammation of the pacinian corpuscles.

pack (pak). **1.** To fill, stuff, or tampon. **2.** To enwrap or envelop the body in a sheet, blanket, or other covering. **3.** To apply a dressing or covering to a surgical site. **4.** The items so used above.
cold p., a p. of cloth or other material wrung out of cold water or encasing ice.
dry p., a p. enveloping one in dry, warmed blankets in order to induce profuse perspiration.
hot p., a p. of cloth or other material wrung out of hot water, or producing moist heat by another means.
wet p., the usual form of p. using hot or cold moisture.

packer (pak'er). **1.** An instrument for tamponing. **2.** Plugger.

packing (pak'ing). **1.** Filling a natural cavity, a wound, or a mold with some material. **2.** The material so used. **3.** The application of a pack.
denture p., filling and compressing a denture base material into a mold in a flask.

pad. **1.** Soft material forming a cushion, used in applying or relieving pressure on a part, or in filling a depression so that dressings can fit snugly. **2.** A more or less encapsulated body of fat or some other tissue serving to fill a space or act as a cushion in the body.
abdominal p., laparotomy p.
dinner p., a p. of moderate thickness placed over the pit of the stomach before the application of a plaster jacket; after the plaster has set the p. is removed, leaving space for varying degrees of abdominal distention.
fat p., see *fat-pad.*
knuckle p.'s, **(1)** a congenital condition, an atavistic trait, in which thick p.'s of skin appear over the proximal phalangeal joints; occasionally associated with leukonychia and deafness; **(2)** a callus reaction in persons predisposed to producing callus and as the result of occupational or self-inflicted trauma.
laparotomy p., abdominal p.; a p. made from several layers of

gauze folded into a rectangular shape; used as a sponge, for packing off the viscera in abdominal operations, and in other ways.
Passavant's p., Passavant's *cushion*.
periarterial p., juxtaglomerular *body*.
pharyngoesophageal p.'s, pharyngoesophageal *cushions*.
retromolar p., pear-shaped area; a cushioned mass of tissue, frequently pear-shaped, located on the alveolar process of the mandible behind the area of the last natural molar tooth.
sucking p., suctorial p., *corpus* adiposum buccae.

Padykula-Herman stain for myosin ATPase. See under stain.

Paecilomyces (pē-sil-ō-mī'sēz). A genus of saprophytic imperfect fungi whose conidia-bearing hyphae superficially resemble the penicillus of *Penicillium;* isolated as contaminants.

paed-. For words so beginning see ped-.

PAF Abbreviation for platelet-aggregating (or -activating) *factor*.

Pagenstecher, Alexander, German ophthalmologist, 1828–1879. See P.'s *circle*.

Paget, Sir James, British surgeon, 1814–1899. See P.'s *cells, disease;* extramammary P. *disease;* P.-von Schrötter *syndrome*.

Paget-Eccleston stain. See under stain.

pagetic (pa-jet'ik). Relating to or suffering from Paget's disease.

pagetoid (paj'ĕ-toyd). Resembling or characteristic of Paget's disease.

pagophagia (pā-gō-fā'jē-ă) [G. *pagos,* frost, + *phagein,* to eat]. Compulsive and repeated ingestion of ice; sometimes associated with iron deficiency anemia.

-pagus [G. *pagos,* something fixed, fr. *pēgnymi,* to fasten together]. Termination denoting conjoined twins, the first element of the word denoting the parts fused. See also -didymus; -dymus.

PAH Abbreviation for *p*-aminohippuric acid.

paidology (pā-dol'ō-jē). Pedology.

pain (pān) [L. *poena,* a fine, a penalty]. **1.** An unpleasant sensation associated with actual or potential tissue damage, and mediated by specific nerve fibers to the brain where its conscious appreciation may be modified by various factors. **2.** Term used to denote a uterine contraction occurring in childbirth.
after-p.'s, see afterpains.
bearing-down p., a uterine contraction accompanied by straining and tenesmus; usually appearing in the second stage of labor.
dream p., hypnalgia.
expulsive p.'s, effective labor p.'s, associated with contraction of the uterine muscle.
false p.'s, ineffective uterine contractions, preceding and sometimes resembling true labor, but distinguishable from it by the lack of progressive effacement and dilation of the cervix.
girdle p., a painful sensation encircling the body like a belt, occurring in tabes dorsalis or other spinal cord disease.
growing p.'s, aching p.'s, frequently felt at night, in the limbs of growing children; attributed variously to growth, rheumatic state, faulty posture, fatigue, or ill-defined psychic causes.
heterotopic p., referred p.
homotopic p., p. felt at the point of injury.
hunger p., cramp in the epigastrium associated with hunger.
intermenstrual p., **(1)** midpain; pelvic discomfort occurring at midpoint of the menstrual cycle; **(2)** Mittelschmerz.
intractable p., p. resistant or refractory to ordinary analgesic agents.
labor p.'s, parodynia; rhythmical uterine contractions which under normal conditions increase in intensity frequency, and duration, culminating in vaginal delivery of the infant.
middle p., Mittelschmerz.
mind p., psychalgia (1).
nerve p., neuralgia.
night p., nyctalgia.
organic p., pain caused by an organic lesion.
phantom limb p., see phantom *limb*.
psychogenic p., psychalgia; (2); p. which is correlated with a psychological, emotional, or behavioral stimulus.
referred p., heterotopic p.; synalgia; telalgia; p. perceived as coming from an area or situation remote from its actual origin; *e.g.,* arm, elbow, or wrist p. felt in angina pectoris, or the p. above the clavicle in diaphragmatic pleurisy.
rest p., p. occurring usually in the extremities during rest in the sitting or lying position.
soul p., psychalgia (1).
tracheal p., trachealgia.

paint (pānt). A solution or suspension of one or more medicaments applied to the skin with a brush or large applicator; usually used in the treatment of widespread eruptions.
carbol-fuchsin p., Castellani's p.; a p. containing boric acid, phenol, resorcinol, fuchsin, acetone, and alcohol in water; used in the treatment of superficial mycotic infections.
Castellani's p., carbol-fuschin p.

pair (pār). Two objects considered together because of similarity, for a common purpose, or because of some attracting force between them.
base p., nucleoside or nucleotide p.; the complex of two heterocyclic nucleic acid bases, one a pyrimidine and the other a purine, brought about by hydrogen bonding between the 1 and 6 positions of the purine and the 3 and 4 positions of the pyrimidine; base pairing is the essential element in the structure of DNA proposed by Watson and Crick in 1953; usually guanine is paired with cytosine (G·C), and adenine with thymine (A·T) or uracil (A·U).
buffer p., an acid and its conjugate base (anion).
chromosome p., two chromosomes of the full diploid karyotype that are similar in form and function but that usually differ in content, one normally being inherited from each parent and one being transmitted to each progeny; in the heteromorphic sex (in humans, the male), one pair, the sex chromosomes, differs markedly in appearance, content, and function.
conjugate acid-base p., in prototonic solvents (*e.g.,* H_2O, NH_3, acetic acid), two molecular species differing only in the presence or absence of a hydrogen ion (*e.g.,* carbonic acid/bicarbonate ion or ammonium ion/ammonia); the basis of buffer action.
nucleoside p., nucleotide p., base p.

pajaroello (pah-har-wā'ō) [Am. Sp. *pajahuello,* fr. Sp. *paja,* straw, + *huello,* undersurface of hoof]. *Ornithodoros coriaceus.*

Pajot, Charles, French obstetrician, 1816–1896. See P.'s *maneuver*.

Palade, George E., Romanian-born electron microscopist and Nobel laureate, *1912. See P. *granule,* Weibel-P. *bodies*.

palatal (pal'ă-tăl). Palatine; relating to the palate or the palate bone.

palate (pal'ăt) [L. *palatum,* palate]. Palatum.
bony p., *palatum* osseum.
Byzantine arch p., incomplete fusion of the palatal process with the nasal spine.
cleft p., palatum fissum; palatoschisis; a congenital fissure in the median line of the p., often associated with cleft lip.

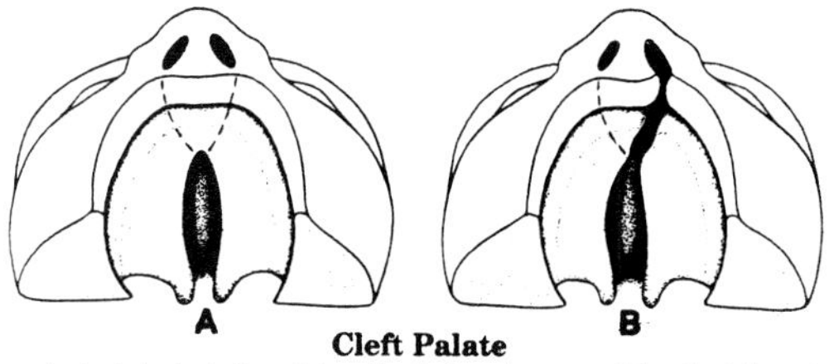

Cleft Palate
A, isolated cleft palate; *B*, cleft palate combined with unilateral anterior cleft.

falling p., uvuloptosis.
Gothic p., an abnormally highly arched p.
hard p., **(1)** *palatum* durum; **(2)** in cephalometrics, a line connecting the anterior and posterior nasal spines to represent the position of the bony p.
pendulous p., *uvula* palatina.
primary p., primitive p.; in the early embryo, the mesoderm-filled shelf that anteriorly separates the oral cavity below from the primitive nasal cavities above.
primitive p., primary p.
secondary p., the posterior portion of the embryonic p. from which develops the hard p. behind the incisive canal and the soft p.
soft p., *palatum* molle.

palatiform (pă-lat′i-fōrm). Palate-shaped; resembling the palate.

palatinase (pă-lat′i-nās). A maltase in the intestinal mucosa that hydrolyzes palatinose; probably oligo-1,6-glucosidase.

palatine (pal′ă-tīn). Palatal.

palatinose (pă-lat′i-nōs). A disaccharide consisting of glucose and fructose in α-1,6 linkage (sucrose is α-1,2).

palatitis (pal-ă-tī′tis). Uranisconitis; inflammation of the palate.

palato- [L. *palatum,* palate]. Combining form meaning palate.

palatoglossal (pal′ă-tō-glos′ăl). Relating to the palate and the tongue, or to the palatoglossus muscle.

palatoglossus (pal-ă-tō-glos′ŭs). *Musculus* palatoglossus.

palatognathous (pal′ă-tog′nă-thŭs) [palato- + G. *gnathos,* jaw]. Having a cleft palate.

palatogram (pal′ă-tō-gram). A registration of tongue action against the palate made by placing soft wax or powder on a baseplate.

palatograph (pal′ă-tō-graf) [palato- + G. *graphō,* to record]. Palate myograph; palatomyograph; an instrument used in recording the movements of the soft palate in speaking and during respiration.

palatomaxillary (pal′ă-tō-mak′si-lār-ē). Relating to the palate and the maxilla.

palatomyograph (pal′ă-tō-mī′ō-graf) [G. palato- + *mys,* muscle, + *graphō,* to record]. Palatograph.

palatonasal (pal-ă-tō-nā′sal). Relating to the palate and the nasal cavity.

palatopharyngeal (pal′ă-tō-fa-rin′jē-ăl). Relating to palate and pharynx.

palatopharyngeus (pal′ă-tō-far-in-jē′ŭs) [L.]. *Musculus* palatopharyngeus.

palatopharyngoplasty (pal′ă-tō-fa-rin′gō-plas-tē) [palato- + pharynx, + *plastos,* formed]. Uvulopalatoplasty; uvulopalatopharyngoplasty; surgical resection of unnecessary palatal and oropharyngeal tissue in selected cases of snoring, with or without sleep apnea.

palatopharyngorrhaphy (pal′ă-tō-far′in-gōr′ă-fē) [palato- + pharynx + G. *raphē,* suture]. Staphylopharyngorrhaphy.

palatoplasty (pal′ă-tō-plas-tē) [palato- + G. *plassō,* to form]. Staphyloplasty; uraniscoplasty; uranoplasty; surgery of the palate to restore form and function.

palatoplegia (pal′ă-tō-plē′jē-ă) [palato- + G. *plēgē,* stroke]. Staphyloplegia; paralysis of the muscles of the soft palate.

palatorrhaphy (pal-ă-tōr′ă-fē) [palato- + G. *rhaphē,* suture]. Staphylorrhaphy; uraniscorrhaphy; uranorrhaphy; velosynthesis; suture of a cleft palate.

palatosalpingeus (pal′ă-tō-sal-pin-jē′ŭs) [L.]. *Musculus* palatosalpingeus.

palatoschisis (pal-ă-tos′ki-sis) [palato- + G. *schisis,* fissure]. Cleft *palate.*

palatum, pl. **pala′ti** (pă-lā′tŭm) [L.] [NA]. Palate; uraniscus; roof of mouth; the bony and muscular partition between the oral and nasal cavities; popularly the uvula.
p. du′rum [NA], hard palate (1); the anterior part of the palate, consisting of the p. osseum covered above by the mucous membrane of the floor of the nasal cavity and below by the mucoperiosteum of the roof of the mouth which contains the palatine vessels, nerves, and mucous glands.
p. fis′sum, cleft *palate.*
p. mol′le [NA], soft palate; velum palatinum; velum pendulum palati; claustrum gutturis; claustrum oris; the posterior muscular portion of the palate, forming an incomplete septum between the mouth and the oropharynx, and between the oropharynx and the nasopharynx.
p. os′seum [NA], bony palate; a concave elliptical bony plate, constituting the roof of the oral cavity, formed of the palatine process of the maxilla and the horizontal plate of the palatine bone on either side.

paleencephalon (pā′lē-en-sef′ă-lon) [paleo- + G. *enkephalos,* brain]. L. Edinger's term for the metameric nervous *system.*

paleo-, pale- [G. *palaios,* old, ancient]. Combining forms denoting old, primitive, primary, early.

paleocerebellum (pā′lē-ō-ser′ĕ-bel′ŭm) [paleo- + L. *cerebellum*] [NA]. Phylogenetic term referring to all parts of the cerebellum comprising most of the vermis and the adjacent zones of the cerebellar hemisphere rostral to the primary fissure; p. is equated with the anterior lobe and corresponds to the zone of distribution of the spinocerebellar tracts and is sometimes called spinocerebellum; in phylogenetic age, it is thought to be intermediate between the archicerebellum and the neocerebellum.

paleocortex (pā′lē-ō-kōr′teks). The phylogenetically oldest part of the cortical mantle of the cerebral hemisphere represented by the olfactory cortex.

paleokinetic (pā′lē-ō-ki-net′ik) [paleo- + G. *kinētikos,* relating to movement]. Denoting the primitive motor mechanisms underlying muscular reflexes and automatic, stereotyped movements.

paleopathology (pā′lē-ō-pa-thol′ō-jē). [paleo- + pathology]. The science of disease in prehistoric terms as revealed in bones, mummies, and archaeologic artifacts.

paleostriatal (pā′lē-ō-strī-ā′tăl). Relating to the paleostriatum.

paleostriatum (pā′lē-ō-strī-ā′tŭm) [paleo- + L. *striatum*]. Term denoting the globus pallidus and expressing the hypothesis that this component of the corpus striatum developed earlier in evolution than the "neostriatum" or striatum (caudate nucleus and putamen) and is regarded as a diencephalic derivative.

paleothalamus (pā′lē-ō-thal′ă-mŭs). The intralaminar nuclei, believed to be the earliest components of the thalamus to evolve.

Palfyn (Palfin), Jean, Belgian surgeon and anatomist, 1650–1730. See P.'s *sinus.*

palikinesia, palicinesia (pal-i-ki-nē′zē-ă, -si-nē′zē-ă) [G. *palin,* again, + *kinēsis,* movement]. Involuntary repetition of movements.

palilalia (pal-i-lā′lē-ă) [G. *palin,* again, + *lalia,* a form of speech]. Paliphrasia.

palinal (pal′i-năl) [G. *palin,* backward]. Moving backward.

palindrome (pal′in-drōm) [G. *palindromos,* a running back]. In molecular biology, a self-complementary nucleic acid sequence; a sequence identical to its complementary strand, if both are "read" in the same 5′-to-3′ direction, or inverted repeating sequences running in opposite directions (but same 5′- to 3′- direction) on either side of an axis of symmetry; p.'s occur at sites of important reactions (*e.g.,* binding sites, sites cleaved by restriction enzymes).

palindromia (pal-in-drō′mē-ă) [G. *palindromos,* a running back, + *-ia,* condition]. A relapse or recurrence of a disease.

palindromic (pal-in-drom′ik). Relapsing; recurring.

palingenesis (pal-in-jen'ĕ-sis) [G. *palin*, again, + *genesis*, origin]. Production of characters typical of phylogenetically ancestral types. *Cf.* cenogenesis.

palinopsia (pal-i-nop'sē-ă) [G. *palin*, again, + *opsis*, vision]. Abnormal recurring visual hallucinations.

paliphrasia (pal-i-frā'zē-ă) [G. *palin*, again, + *phrasis*, speech]. Palilalia; in speech, involuntary repetition of words or sentences.

palisade (pal'i-săd) [Fr. *palissade*, fr. L. *palus*, a pale, stake]. In pathology, a row of elongated nuclei parallel to each other.

palladium (pă-lā'dē-ŭm) [fr. the asteroid, Pallas]. A metallic element resembling platinum, symbol Pd, atomic no. 46, atomic weight 106.4.

pallanesthesia (pal'an-es-thē'zē-ă) [G. *pallō*, to quiver, + *anaisthēsia*, insensibility]. Apallesthesia; absence of pallesthesia.

pallescense (pal-es'ens) [L. *palesco*, to become pale, fr. *palleo*, to be pale]. Pallor.

pallesthesia (pal'es-thē'zē-ă) [G. *pallō*, to quiver, + *aisthesis*, sensation]. Bone, pallesthetic, or vibratory sensibility; the appreciation of vibration, a form of pressure sense; most acute when a vibrating tuning fork is applied over a bony prominence.

pallesthetic (pal-es-thet'ik). Pertaining to pallesthesia.

pallial (pal'ē-ăl). Relating to the pallium.

palliate (pal'ē-āt) [L. *palliatus* (adj.), dressed in a *pallium*, cloaked]. Mitigate; to reduce the severity of; to relieve slightly.

palliative (pal-ē-ă-tiv). Mitigating; reducing the severity of; denoting the alleviation of symptoms without curing the underlying disease.

pallidal (pal'i-dăl). Relating to the pallidum.

pallidectomy (pal'i-dek'tō-mē) [pallidum + G. *ektomē*, excision]. Excision or destruction of the globus pallidus, usually by stereotaxy; a prefix may indicate the method used, *e.g.*, chemopallidectomy (destruction by a chemical agent), cryopallidectomy (destruction by cold).

pallidoamygdalotomy (pal'i-dō-ă-mig'dă-lot'ō-mē). Production of lesions in the globus pallidus and amygdaloid nuclei.

pallidoansotomy (pal'i-dō-an-sot'ō-mē). Production of lesions in the globus pallidus and ansa lenticularis.

pallidotomy (pal-i-dot'ō-mē) [pallidum + G. *tomē*, incision]. A destructive operation on the globus pallidus, done to relieve involuntary movements or muscular rigidity.

pallidum (pal'i-dŭm) [L. *pallidus*, pale]. *Globus* pallidus.

pallium (pal'ē-ŭm) [L. cloak] [NA]. Mantle (2); brain mantle; the cerebral cortex with the subjacent white substance.

pallor (pal'ŏr) [L.]. Pallescense; paleness, as of the skin.
cachectic p., achromasia (1).

palm (pahm, pawlm) [L. *palma*] Palma; palma manus; vola manus; the flat of the hand; the flexor or anterior surface of the hand, exclusive of the thumb and fingers; the opposite of the dorsum.
liver p., exaggerated erythema of the thenar and hypothenar eminences.

palma, pl. **palmae** (pawl'mă, pawl'mē) [L.] [NA]. Palm.
p. ma'nus [NA], palm of the hand. See palm.

palmar (pawl'măr) [L. *palmaris*, fr. *palma*]. Referring to the palm of the hand; volar.

palmaris (pawl-măr'is) [L.] [NA]. Palmar.

palmellin (pal'mel-in). A red coloring matter formed by an alga, *Palmella cruenta.*

Palmer, Walter L., U.S. physician, *1896. See P. acid *test* for peptic ulcer.

palmic (pal'mik). Beating; throbbing; relating to a palmus.

palmitaldehyde (pal-mi-tal'dĕ-hīd). Hexadecanal(dehyde); $CH_3(CH_2)_{14}CHO$; the 16-carbon aldehyde corresponding to palmitic acid; a constituent of plasmalogens.

palmitate (pal'mi-tāt). A salt of palmitic acid.

palmitic acid (pal-mit'ik). Hexadecanoic acid; $C_{16}H_{32}O_2$; a saturated fatty acid occurring in palm oil and other fats.

palmitin (pal'mi-tin). Tripalmitin; the triglyceride of palmitic acid occurring in palm oil.

palmitoleic acid (pal'mi-tō-lē'ik). 9-Hexadecenoic acid; a monounsaturated 16-carbon acid; one of the common constituents of the triacylglycerols of human adipose tissue.

palmityl alcohol (pal'mi-til). *Cetyl* alcohol.

palmodic (pal-mod'ik). Relating to palmus (1).

palmoscopy (pal-mos'kō-pē) [G. *palmos*, pulsation, + *skopeō*, to examine]. Examination of the cardiac pulsation.

palmus, pl. **palmi** (pal'mŭs, -mī) [G. *palmos*, pulsation, quivering]. **1.** Facial *tic.* **2.** Rhythmical fibrillary contractions in a muscle. See also jumper *disease.* **3.** The heart beat.

palpable (pal'pă-bl) [see palpation]. **1.** Perceptible to touch; capable of being palpated. **2.** Evident; plain.

palpate (pal'pāt). To examine by feeling and pressing with the palms of the hands and the fingers.

palpation (pal-pā'shŭn) [L. *palpatio*, fr. *palpo*, pp. *-atus*, to touch, stroke]. **1.** Examination with the hands, feeling for organs, masses, or infiltration of a part of the body, feeling the heart or pulse beat, vibrations in the chest, etc. **2.** Touching, feeling, or perceiving by the sense of touch.
light-touch p., a method of determining the outlines of organs or masses by lightly palpating the surface with the tip of a finger.

palpatopercussion (pal'pă-tō-per-kŭsh'ŭn). Examination by means of combined palpation and percussion.

palpebra, pl. **palpebrae** (pal-pē'bră, pē'brē) [L.] [NA]. Eyelid; blepharon; one of the two movable folds of skin (upper and lower eyelids) lined with conjunctiva in front of the eyeball.
p. III, *plica* semilunaris conjunctivae (2).
p. infe'rior [NA], lower eyelid.
p. supe'rior [NA], upper eyelid.
p. ter'tia, *plica* semilunaris conjunctivae (2).

palpebral (pal'pē-brăl). Relating to an eyelid or the eyelids.

palpebralis (pal'pē-brā'lis) [L.]. *Musculus* levator palpebrae superioris.

palpebrate (pal'pē-brāt) [L. *palpebra*, eyelid]. **1.** Having eyelids. **2.** To wink.

palpebration (pal-pē-brā'shŭn) [L. *palpebratio*]. Winking.

palpitatio cordis (pal-pi-tā'shē-ō kōr'dis). Palpitation of the heart.

palpitation (pal-pi-tā'shŭn) [L. *palpitatio*, to throb]. Trepidatio cordis; forcible pulsation of the heart, perceptible to the patient, usually with an increase in frequency or force, with or without irregularity in rhythm.

palsy (pawl'zē) [a corruption of O. Fr. fr. L. and G. *paralysis*]. Paralysis; often connotes partial paralysis or paresis.
Bell's p., facial p.
birth p., infantile diplegia or hemiplegia; obstetrical paralysis; paralysis, hemiplegia or diplegia, due to cerebral hemorrhage occurring at birth or to hypoxic injury of the fetal brain *in utero.*
brachial birth p., paralysis of the infant's arm due to injury received at birth; three types are recognized: 1) whole arm; 2) upper arm (Erb's p.); 3) forearm (Klumpke's paralysis).
bulbar p., progressive bulbar *paralysis.*
cerebral p., defect of motor power and coordination related to damage of the brain.
craft p., occupational *neurosis.*
creeping p., progressive muscular *atrophy.*

crutch p., crutch *paralysis.*
Erb's p., Duchenne-Erb or Erb's paralysis; a type of brachial birth p. in which there is paralysis of the muscles of the upper arm (deltoid, biceps, anterior brachial, and long supinator muscles) due to a lesion of the brachial plexus or of the roots of the fifth and sixth cervical nerves.
facial p., Bell's p.; facial paralysis; fallopian neuritis; facioplegia; prosopoplegia; a unilateral paralysis of the facial muscles supplied by the seventh nerve; probably due to a viral demyelinization of the facial nerve.
Féréol-Graux p., paralysis, nuclear in origin, of the lateral rectus muscle of one eye and the medial rectus muscle of the other eye because of a lesion in the fasciculus longitudinalis medialis.
lead p., lead paralysis; paralysis of the extensor muscles of the wrist causing wrist-drop; occurs in lead poisoning.
night p., waking *numbness.*
posticus p., paralysis of the cricoarytenoideus posticus muscle, resulting in the vocal cord being held in or near the midline.
pressure p., pressure *paralysis.*
progressive supranuclear p., a heterogeneous degeneration involving the brainstem, basal ganglia, and cerebellum, with nuchal dystonia and dementia.
scrivener's p., writer's *cramp.*
shaking p., trembling p., parkinsonism (1).
wasting p., progressive muscular *atrophy.*

Paltauf, Richard, Austrian pathologist, 1858–1924. See P.-Sternberg *disease.*

paludal (pal'ū-dăl) [L. *palus,* marsh]. Obsolete term for malarial.

pamabrom (pam'ă-brom). 8-Bromotheophylline compound with 2-amino-2-methyl-1-propanol; diuretic.

pamaquine (pam'ă-kwēn). An antimalarial agent, active against avian malaria and against the gametocytes of all malarial forms in man; it is more toxic than chloroquine or primaquine and has been replaced by primaquine.

pamoate (pam'ō-āt). USAN-approved contraction for 4,4'-methylenebis(3-hydroxy-2-naphthoate).

pampiniform (pam-pin'i-fōrm) [L. *pampinus,* a tendril, + *forma,* form]. Having the shape of a tendril; denoting a vinelike structure.

pampinocele (pam-pin'ō-sēl) [L. *pampinus,* tendril, + G. *kēlē,* tumor]. Varicocele.

Pan [G. myth. god of forest]. Genus of anthropoid apes including the gorilla and chimpanzee. *P. panisus* and *P. troglodytes* are chimpanzee species used in biologic experiments.

pan- [G. *pas,* all]. Prefix properly affixed to words derived from G. roots, denoting all, entire. See also pant-.

panacea (pan-ă-sē'ă) [G. *panakeia,* universal remedy, fr. Panacea, Aesculapius' daughter]. A cure-all; a remedy claimed to be curative of all diseases.

panagglutinable (pan-ă-glū'ti-nă-bl). Agglutinable with all types of human serum; denoting erythrocytes having this property.

panagglutinins (pan-ă-glū'ti-ninz). Agglutinins that react with all human erythrocytes.

panangiitis (pan'an-jē-ī'tis) [pan- + angiitis]. Inflammation involving all the coats of a blood vessel.

panarteritis (pan'ar-ter-ī'tis) [pan- + L. *arteria,* artery, + G. *-itis,* inflammation]. Endoperiarteritis; an inflammatory disorder of the arteries characterized by involvement of all structural layers of the vessels.

panarthritis (pan-ar-thrī'tis). **1.** Inflammation involving all the tissues of a joint. **2.** Inflammation of all the joints of the body.

panatrophy (pan-at'rō-fē). Pantatrophia; pantatrophy. **1.** Atrophy of all the parts of a structure. **2.** General atrophy of the body.

panblastic (pan-blas'tik) [pan- + G. *blastos,* germ]. Relating to all the primary germ layers.

pancarditis (pan-kar-dī'tis). Inflammation of all the structures of the heart.

Pancoast, Henry K., U.S. roentgenologist, 1875–1939. See P. *syndrome, tumor.*

Pancoast, Joseph, U.S. surgeon, 1805–1882. See P.'s *suture.*

pancolectomy (pan'kō-lek'tō-mē). Extirpation of the entire colon.

pancreas, pl. **pancreata** (pan'krē-as, pan-krē-ā'tă) [G. *pankreas,* the sweetbread, fr. *pas* (*pan*), all, + *kreas,* flesh] [NA]. Salivary gland of abdomen; an elongated lobulated gland, devoid of capsule, extending from the concavity of the duodenum to the spleen; it consists of a flattened head (caput) within the duodenal concavity, an elongated three-sided body (corpus) extending transversely across the abdomen, and a tail (cauda) in contact with the spleen. The gland secretes from the pars exocrina pancreatic juice which is discharged into the intestine and from the pars endocrina the internal secretions, insulin and glucagon.

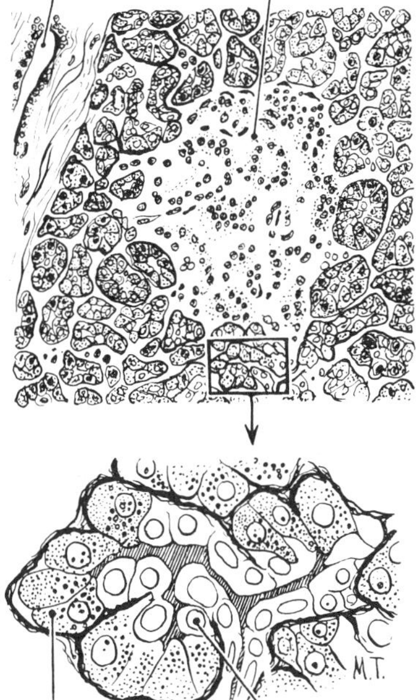

Pancreas (Cross Section)

p. accesso'rium [NA], a detached portion of pancreatic tissue sometimes found in the wall of the stomach or duodenum.
annular p., a ring of p. encircling the duodenum, caused by a failure of the embryologic ventral pancreas to migrate to the right of the duodenum.
Aselli's p., Aselli's *gland.*
p. divi'sum, a bifid, or divided, p. resulting from a congenital failure of the embryonic primordia to unite completely.
dorsal p., that portion of the pancreatic primordium of the embryo that arises as a dorsal bud from the foregut endoderm.
lesser p., *processus* uncinatus pancreatis.
p. mi'nus, *processus* uncinatus pancreatis.
small p., *processus* uncinatus pancreatis.
uncinate or **unciform p.,** *processus* uncinatus pancreatis.
ventral p., that portion of the primordium of the pancreas that

develops, together with the hepatic diverticulum, as a ventral bud from the foregut entoderm.

Willis' p., *processus* uncinatus pancreatis.

Winslow's p., *processus* uncinatus pancreatis.

pancreat-, pancreatico-, pancreato-, pancreo- [G. *pankreas*, pancreas]. Combining forms denoting the pancreas.

pancreatalgia (pan'krē-ă-tal'jē-ă) [pancreat- + G. *algos*, pain]. Pain arising from the pancreas, or felt in or near the region of the pancreas.

pancreatectomy (pan'krē-ă-tek'tō-mē) [pancreat- + G. *ektomē*, excision]. Pancreectomy; excision of the pancreas.

pancreatemphraxis (pan'krē-at-em-frak'sis) [pancreat- + G. *emphraxis*, a stoppage]. Obstruction in the pancreatic duct, causing swelling of the gland.

pancreatic (pan-krē-at'ik). Relating to the pancreas.

pancreatico-. See pancreat-.

pancreaticoduodenal (pan-krē-at'i-kō-dū'ō-dē'năl, -dū-od'ĕ-năl). Relating to the pancreas and the duodenum.

pancreatin (pan'krē-ă-tin). A mixture of the enzymes from the pancreas of the ox or hog, used internally as a digestive, and also as a peptonizing agent in preparing predigested foods; it contains the proteolytic trypsin, the amylolytic amylopsin, and the lipolytic steapsin.

pancreatitis (pan'krē-ă-tī'tis). Inflammation of the pancreas.

acute hemorrhagic p., an acute inflammation of the pancreas accompanied by the formation of necrotic areas and hemorrhages into the substance of the gland; clinically marked by sudden severe abdominal pain, nausea, fever, and leukocytosis; areas of fat necrosis are present on the surface of the pancreas and in the omentum due to the action of the escaped pancreatic enzyme (trypsin and lipase).

pancreato-. See pancreat-.

pancreatocholecystostomy (pan-krē-at'ō-kō-lē-sis-tos'tō-mē, pan'krē-ă-tō-). A surgical anastomosis between a pancreatic cyst or fistula and the gallbladder.

pancreatoduodenectomy (pan-krē-at'ō-dū-ō-dē-nek'tō-mē, pan'krē-ă-tō-). Whipple's operation; excision of all or part of the pancreas together with the duodenum.

pancreatoduodenostomy (pan-krē-at'ō-dū-ō-dē-nos'tō-mē, pan'krē-ă-tō-). Surgical anastomosis of a pancreatic duct, cyst, or fistula to the duodenum.

pancreatogastrostomy (pan-krē-at'ō-gas-tros'tō-mē, pan'krē-ă-tō-). Surgical anastomosis of a pancreatic cyst or fistula to the stomach.

pancreatogenic, pancreatogenous (pan'krē-ă-tō-jen'ik, -toj'ĕ-nŭs) [pancreato- + G. *genesis*, origin]. Of pancreatic origin; formed in the pancreas.

pancreatography (pan'krē-ă-tog'ră-fē) [pancreato- + G. *graphō*, to write]. Radiographic visualization of the pancreatic ducts, after injection of radiopaque material into the collecting system.

pancreatojejunostomy (pan-krē-at'ō-je-jū-nos'tō-mē, pan'krē-ă-tō-). Surgical anastomosis of a pancreatic duct, cyst, or fistula to the jejunum.

pancreatolith (pan-krē-at'ō-lith) [pancreato- + G. *lithos*, stone]. Pancreatic *calculus*.

pancreatolithectomy (pan-krē-at'ō-li-thek'tō-mē, pan'krē-ă-tō-) [pancreato- + G. *lithos*, stone, + *ektomē*, excision]. Pancreatolithotomy.

pancreatolithiasis (pan-krē-at'ō-li-thī'ă-sis, pan'krē-ă-tō-). Stones in the pancreas, usually found in the pancreatic duct system.

pancreatolithotomy (pan-krē-at'ō-li-thot'ō-mē, pan'krē-ă-tō-) [pancreato- + G. *lithos*, stone, + *tomē*, incision]. Pancreatolithectomy; removal of a pancreatic concretion.

pancreatolysis (pan'krē-ă-tol'i-sis) [pancreato- + G. *lysis*, dissolution]. Destruction of the pancreas.

pancreatolytic (pan'krē-ă-tō-lit'ik). Denoting pancreatolysis.

pancreatomegaly (pan'krē-ă-tō-meg'ă-lē) [pancreato- + G. *megas*, great]. Abnormal enlargement of the pancreas.

pancreatomy (pan'krē-at'ō-mē). Pancreatotomy.

pancreatopathy (pan'krē-ă-top'ă-thē) [pancreato- + G. *pathos*, suffering]. Pancreopathy; any disease of the pancreas.

pancreatopeptidase E (pan'krē-ă-tō-pep'ti-dās). See elastase.

pancreatotomy (pan'krē-ă-tot'ō-mē) [pancreato- + G. *tomē*, incision]. Pancreatomy; incision of the pancreas.

pancreatropic (pan'krē-ă-trop'ik) [pancreat- + G. *tropikas*, relating to a turning]. Exerting an action on the pancreas.

pancreectomy (pan-krē-ek'tō-mē). Pancreatectomy.

pancrelipase (pan-krē-lip'ās, -lī'pās). Lipancreatin; a concentrate of pancreatic enzymes standardized for lipase content; a lipolytic used for substitution therapy.

pancreo-. See pancreat-.

pancreolith (pan'krē-ō-lith) [pancreo- + G. *lithos*, stone]. Pancreatic *calculus*.

pancreopathy (pan-krē-op'ă-thē). Pancreatopathy.

pancreoprivic (pan'krē-ō-priv'ik) [pancreo- + L. *privus*, deprived of]. Without a pancreas.

pancreozymin (pan'krē-ō-zī'min). Cholecystokinin.

pancuronium bromide (pan-kyūr-ō'nē-ŭm). 2β,16β-Dipiperidino-5α-androstane-3α,17β-diol diacetate dimethobromide; a nondepolarizing steroidal neuromuscular blocking agent resembling curare but without its potential for ganglionic blockade, histamine release, or hypotension.

pancytopenia (pan'sī-tō-pē'nē-ă) [pan- + G. *kytos*, cell, + *penia*, poverty]. Pronounced reduction in the number of erythrocytes, all types of white blood cells, and the blood platelets in the circulating blood.

congenital p., Fanconi's p., Fanconi's *anemia*.

tropical canine p., canine *ehrlichiosis*.

pandemic (pan-dem'ik) [pan- + G. *dēmos*, the people]. Denoting a disease affecting or attacking the population of an extensive region; extensively epidemic.

pandemicity (pan-dĕ-mis'i-tē). The state or condition of being pandemic.

pandiculation (pan-dik-yū-lā'shŭn) [L. *pandiculor*, to stretch oneself, fr. *pando*, to spread out]. The act of stretching, as when awaking.

Pandy, Kalman, Hungarian neurologist, *1868. See P.'s *test, reaction*.

panencephalitis (pan'en-sef-ă-lī'tis). A diffuse inflammation of the brain.

nodular p., Pette-Döring disease; probably a form of subacute sclerosing p.

subacute sclerosing p., inclusion body *encephalitis*.

panendoscope (pan-en'dō-skōp) [pan- + G. *endon*, within, + *skopeō*, to view]. An illuminated instrument for inspection of the interior of the urethra as well as the bladder by means of a foroblique lens system.

panesthesia (pan-es-thē'zē-ă) [pan- + G. *aisthēsis*, sensation]. The sum of all the sensations experienced by a person at one time. See also cenesthesia.

Paneth, Josef, Austrian physician, 1857–1890. See P.'s granular *cells*.

pang. A sudden sharp, brief pain.

breast p., *angina* pectoris.

panglossia (pan-glos'ē-ă) [pan- + G. *glōssa,* tongue]. Abnormal or pathologic garrulousness.

panhidrosis (pan-hi-drō'sis). Panidrosis.

panhydrometer (pan-hī-drom'ĕ-ter) [pan- + G. *hydōr,* water, + *metron,* measure]. A hydrometer for determining the specific gravity of any liquid.

panhyperemia (pan'hī-per-ē'mē-ă) [pan- + G. *hyper,* over, + *haima,* blood]. Universal congestion or hyperemia.

panhypopituitarism (pan-hī'pō-pi-tū'i-tă-rizm). A state in which the secretion of all anterior pituitary hormones is inadequate or absent; caused by a variety of disorders that result in destruction or loss of function of substantially all of the anterior pituitary gland.

panic (pan'ik) [fr. G. myth. char., *Pan*]. Extreme and unreasoning anxiety and fear.

homosexual p., an acute, severe attack of anxiety based on unconscious conflicts regarding homosexuality.

panidrosis (pan-i-drō'sis) [pan- + G. *hidros,* sweat]. Panhidrosis; sweating of the entire surface of the body.

panimmunity (pan-i-myū'ni-tē). A general immunity to all infectious diseases.

panleukopenia (pan'lū-kō-pē'nē-ă). Feline infectious enteritis; feline distemper; feline agranulocytosis; a highly contagious and fatal disease of cats, particularly young cats, caused by feline panleukopenia virus and manifested by severe leukopenia, prostration, fever, vomiting and diarrhea.

panmixis (pan-mik'sis) [pan- + G. *mixis,* intercourse]. Random *mating.*

panmyelophthisis (pan'mī-ĕ-lof'thi-sis). Myelophthisis (2).

panmyelosis (pan'mī-ĕ-lō'sis) [pan- + G. *myelos,* marrow, + *-osis,* condition]. Myeloid metaplasia with abnormal immature blood cells in the spleen and liver, associated with myelofibrosis.

Panner, H.J., 20th century Danish radiologist. See P.'s *disease.*

panneuritis (pan-nū-rī'tis). Rarely used term meaning extreme polyneuritis.

p. endem'ica, beriberi.

panni (pan'ī). Plural of pannus.

panniculectomy (pa-nik-yū-lek'tō-mē). Surgical excision of redundant paniculus adiposus, usually of the abdomen.

panniculitis (pă-nik'yū-lī'tis) [panniculus + G. *-itis,* inflammation]. Inflammation of subcutaneous adipose tissue.

cytophagic p., chronic lobular p. with infiltration by histiocytes that have phagocytized red blood cells, leukocytes, and platelets; a hemorrhagic diathesis may result.

nodular nonsuppurative p., Weber-Christian disease; Christian's disease (2); a condition of unknown cause marked by recurring attacks of fever and the formation of tender red nodular indurated skin lesions; necrotic areas infiltrated by lipid macrophages are present in subcutaneous fat.

subacute migratory p., erythema nodosum migrans; nodular tender lesions of changing configuration on the lateral aspect of one or both legs, of many months duration; trauma may be the initiating factor.

panniculus, pl. **panniculi** (pă-nik'yū-lŭs, -lī) [L. dim. of *pannus,* cloth] [NA]. A sheet or layer of tissue.

p. adipo'sus [NA], the superficial fascia which contains a more or less fatty deposit in its areolar substance.

p. carno'sus, the skeletal muscle layer in the superficial fascia represented in man by the platysma muscle; it is much more extensive in lower mammals.

pannus, pl. **panni** (pan'ŭs, pan'ī) [L. cloth]. A membrane of granulation tissue covering a normal surface: **1.** the articular cartilages in rheumatoid arthritis and in chronic granulomatous diseases such as tuberculosis; **2.** the cornea in trachoma. See also corneal p.

corneal p., a fibrovascular connective tissue that proliferates in the anterior layers of the peripheral cornea in inflammatory corneal disease, particularly trachoma in which the p. involves the superior cornea. Three forms occur: **p. crassus** (thick), in which there are many blood vessels and the opacity is very dense; **p. siccus** (dry), p. with dry, glossy surface; **p. tenuis** (thin), in which there are few blood vessels and the opacity is slight.

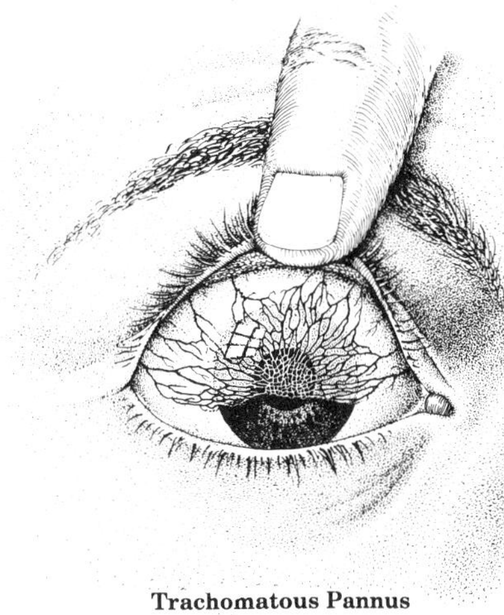

Trachomatous Pannus

phlyctenular p., p. occurring in phlyctenular conjunctivitis.

trachomatous p., p. of the superior cornea associated with trachoma.

panodic (pan-od'ik) [pan- + G. *hodos,* way]. Panthodic; pollodic; denoting a wide and extreme diffusion of a nerve impulse.

panophthalmia, panophthalmitis (pan'of-thal'mē-ă, -of'thal-mī'tis) [pan- + G. *ophthalmos,* eye]. Purulent inflammation of all parts of the eye.

panoptic (pan-op'tik) [pan- + G. *optikos,* relating to vision]. All-revealing, denoting the effect of multiple or differential staining.

panotitis (pan'ō-tī'tis) [pan- + G. *ous,* ear, + *-itis,* inflammation]. General inflammation of all parts of the ear; specifically, a disease which begins as an otitis interna, the inflammation subsequently extending to the middle ear and neighboring structures.

panphobia (pan-fō'bē-ă) [pan- + G. *phobos,* fear]. Fear of everything.

panplegia (pan-plē'jē-ă) [pan- + G. *plēgē,* stroke]. Paralysis of the four extremities.

Pansch, Adolf, German anatomist, 1841–1887. See P.'s *fissure.*

pansclerosis (pan-skle-rō'sis). Universal sclerosis of an organ or part.

pansinuitis (pan-sin-yū-ī'tis). Pansinusitis.

pansinusitis (pan-sī-nŭ-sī'tis). Pansinuitis; inflammation of all the accessory sinuses of the nose on one or both sides.

panspermia, panspermatism (pan-sper'mē-ă, -sper'mă-tizm) [pan- + G. *sperma,* seed]. The hypothetical doctrine of the omnipresence of minute forms and spores of animal and vegetable life, thus accounting for apparent spontaneous generation.

pansporoblast (pan-spō'rō-blast) [pan- + G. *sporos,* seed, + *blastos,* germ]. The reproductive sporoblast that gives rise to more than one spore in the order Myxosporida (class Myxosporea, phylum Myxozoa).

pansporoblastic (pan'spō-rō-blas'tik). Referring to a pansporoblast.

pansystolic (pan'sis-tol'ik). Holosystolic; lasting throughout systole, extending from first to second heart sound.

pant [Fr. *panteler,* to gasp]. To breathe rapidly and shallowly.

pant-, panto- [G. *pas,* all]. Prefixes properly affixed to words derived from G. roots, denoting all, entire. See also pan-.

pantachromatic (pan'tă-krō-mat'ik). Completely achromatic.

pantalgia (pan-tal'jē-ă) [pant- + G. *algos,* pain]. Pain involving the entire body.

pantamorphia (pan-tă-mōr'fē-ă) [pant- + G. *a-* priv. + *morphē,* shape]. Shapelessness; general or over-all malformation.

pantamorphic (pan-tă-mōr'fik). Relating to or characterized by pantamorphia.

pantanencephaly, pantanencephalia (pan'tan-en-sef'ă-lē, -se-fā'lē-ă) [pant- + G. *an-* priv. + *enkephalos,* brain]. Complete anencephaly.

pantankyloblepharon (pan'tan-kī-lō-blef'ă-ron). Blepharosynechia.

pantaphobia (pan-tă-fō'bē-ă) [pant- + G. *a-* priv. + *phobos,* fear]. Absolute fearlessness.

pantatrophia, pantatrophy (pan-tă-trō'fē-ă, pan-tat'rō-fē) [pant- + atrophy]. Panatrophy.

pantetheine (pan-tē-thē'in) *Lactobacillus bulgaricus* factor; the condensation product of pantothenic acid and aminoethanethiol, *N*-pantothenyl-2-aminoethanethiol, $HOCH_2C(CH_3)_2CHOH–CO–NH–CH_2CH_2CO–NH–CH_2CH_2SH$; an intermediate in biosynthesis of CoA via 4′-phosphopantetheine (phosphate on the terminal $–CH_2O$ group) and ATP.

p. kinase [EC 2.7.1.34], an enzyme that catalyzes the phosphorylation of pantetheine by ATP to pantetheine 4′-phosphate.

pantethine (pan'tĕ-thin). The disulfide formed from two pantetheines.

panthenol (pan'thĕ-nol). Dexpanthenol.

panthodic (pan-thod'ik). Panodic.

panto-. See pant-.

pantoate (pan'tō-āt). A salt or ester of pantoic acid.

pantograph (pan'tō-graf) [panto- + G. *graphō,* to record]. **1.** An instrument for reproducing drawings by a system of levers whereby a recording pencil is made to follow the movements of a stylet passing along the lines of the original. **2.** An instrument for reproducing graphically the contours of the chest. **3.** In dentistry, an instrument used to record mandibular border movements that may be transferred to make equivalent settings on an articulator.

pantoic acid (pan-tō'ik). 2,4-Dihydroxy-3,3-dimethylbutyric acid; $HOCH_2C(CH_3)_2CHOH–COOH$, the β-alanine amide of which is pantothenic acid.

pantomogram (pan'tō-mō-gram). A panoramic radiographic record of the maxillary and mandibular dental arches and their associated structures, obtained by a pantomograph.

pantomograph (pan'tō-mō-graf). A panoramic radiographic instrument that permits visualization of the entire dentition, alveolar bone, and contiguous structures on a single extraoral film.

pantomography (pan-tō-mog'ră-fē). A method of radiography by which a radiograph (pantomogram) of the maxillary and mandibular dental arches and their contiguous structures may be obtained on a single film.

pantomorphia (pan-to-mōr'fē-ă) [panto- + G. *morphē,* shape]. **1.** The condition of an organism, such as an ameba, that is capable of assuming all shapes. **2.** Perfect shapeliness or symmetry.

pantomorphic (pan-tō-mōr'fik). Capable of assuming all shapes.

pantonine (pan'tō-nēn). An amino acid identified in *Escherichia coli* which may be an intermediate in the biosynthesis of pantothenic acid by that organism, containing NH_2 in place of the α-OH group of pantothenic acid.

pantoscopic (pan-tō-skop'ik) [panto- + G. *skopeō,* to view]. Designed for observing objects at all distances; denoting bifocal lenses.

panothenate (pan-tō-then'āt). A salt or ester of pantothenic acid.

p. synthetase [EC 6.3.2.1], pantoate-activating enzyme; an enzyme that converts pantoate and β-alanine to pantothenate with cleavage of ATP to AMP and PP_i.

pantothenic acid (pan-tō-then'ik). *N*-(2,4-dihydroxy-3,3-dimethylbutyryl)-3-aminopropionic acid; $HOCH_2C(CH_3)_2CHOH–CO–NH–CH_2CH_2COOH$; the β-alanine amide of pantoic acid. A growth substance widely distributed in plant and animal tissues, and essential for growth of yeast and certain bacteria; deficiency in diet causes a dermatitis in chicks and rats and achromotrichia in the latter.

pantothenyl (pan-tō-then'il). The acyl radical of pantothenic acid.

p. alcohol, Dexpanthenol.

pantoyl (pan'tō-il). The acyl radical of pantoic acid.

pantoyltaurine (pan'tō-il-taw'rin, -rēn). Thiopanic acid; pantothenic acid in which the carboxyl group is replaced by a sulfonic acid group; analogous to pantothenic acid in structure, except that taurine replaces β-alanine in the molecule.

Panum, Peter L., Danish physiologist, 1820–1885. See P.'s *area.*

panzerherz (pahn'zer-härtz). [Ger. Panzerherz]. Armored *heart.*

PAP Abbreviation for *p*eroxidase *a*nti*p*eroxidase complex. See PAP *technique.*

pap. A food of soft consistency, like that of breadcrumbs soaked in milk or water.

papain, papainase (pa-pā'in, -ās) [EC 3.4.22.2]. Papayotin; a proteolytic enzyme, or a crude extract containing it, obtained from papaya latex. It has esterase, thiolase, transamidase, and transesterase activities, and is used as a protein digestant, meat tenderizer, and to prevent adhesions.

Papanicolaou, George N., Greek physician, anatomist, and cytologist, 1883–1962. See P. *examination, smear, stain.*

Papaver (pă-pā'ver, pă-pav'er) [L. poppy]. Poppy; a genus of plants, one species of which, *P. somniferum* (family Papaveraceae), furnishes opium.

papaveretum (pă-pav-er-ē'tŭm) [L. *papaver,* poppy]. A preparation of water soluble opium alkaloids, including 50% anhydrous morphine.

papaverine (pa-pav'er-ēn) [L. *papaver,* poppy]. A benzylisoquinoline alkaloid of opium that is not a narcotic but has mild analgesic action and is a powerful spasmolytic; does not evoke tolerance and has no addiction liability. Also available as p. hydrochloride.

papaw (pă-paw'). See papaya.

papaya (pă-pī'yah, pă-pā'yah) [Sp.]. Carica; the fruit of the papaw (pawpaw), *Carica papaya* (family Caricaceae), a tree of tropical America; it possesses a proteolytic action and is the source of papain.

papayotin (pap-ā'yō-tin). Papain.

paper (pā'per) [L. *papyrus;* G. *papyros,* a kind of rush, from which writing paper was made]. **1.** A square of p. folded over so as to form an envelope containing a dose of any medicinal powder. **2.** A piece of blotting p. or filter p. impregnated with a medicinal solution, dried, and burned; formerly, the fumes were inhaled in the treatment of asthma and other respiratory affections.

articulating p., occluding p.

Congo red p., p. impregnated with Congo red; used as a pH indicator, changing from blue-violet at 3.0 to red at 5.0.

filter p., an unsized p. used in pharmacy and chemistry for filtering solutions; many varieties are used for p. chromatography.

occluding p., articulating p.; an inked p. or ribbon interposed between natural or artificial teeth to determine tooth contacts.

Papez, J.W., U.S. anatomist, 1883–1958. See P. *circuit.*

PAPILLA

papilla, pl. **papillae** (pă-pil'ă, -pil'ē) [L. a nipple, dim. of *papula,* a pimple] [NA]. Any small nipple-like process.

acoustic p., *organum* spirale.

Bergmeister's p., a small mass of glial tissue that forms during fetal life a temporary conical investment of the hyaloid artery at its emergence into the vitreous chamber; vestiges of it may persist as a prepapillary membrane.

bile p., p. duodeni major.

p. of breast, p. mammae.

circumvallate p., p. vallata.

clavate papillae, papillae fungiformes.

conic papillae, papillae conicae.

papil'lae con'icae [NA], conic papillae; numerous projections on the dorsum of the tongue, scattered among the filiform papillae and similar to them, but shorter.

papil'lae co'rii [NA], papillae dermis.

papillae of corium, papillae dermis.

dentinal p., p. dentis.

p. den'tis [NA], dentinal p.; a projection of the mesenchymal tissue of the developing jaw into the cup of the enamel organ; its outer layer becomes specialized columnar cells, the odontoblasts, that form the dentin of the tooth.

dermal papillae, papillae dermis.

papil'lae der'mis [NA], dermal papillae; papillae of corium; papillae corii; the superficial projections of the corium or dermis that interdigitate with recesses in the overlying epidermis; they contain vascular loops and specialized nerve endings, and are arranged in ridgelike lines best developed in the hand and foot.

p. duod'eni ma'jor [NA], major duodenal p.; Santorini's major caruncle; bile p.; point of opening of the common bile duct and pancreatic duct into the duodenum; it is located posteriorly in the descending part of the duodenum.

p. duod'eni mi'nor [NA], minor duodenal p.; Santorini's minor caruncle; the site of the opening of the accessory pancreatic duct into the duodenum, located anterior to and slightly superior to the major p.

filiform papillae, papillae filiformes.

papil'lae filifor'mes [NA], filiform papillae; numerous elongated conical keratinized projections on the dorsum of the tongue.

papil'lae folia'tae [NA], foliate papillae; folia linguae; numerous projections arranged in several transverse folds upon the lateral margins of the tongue just in front of the palatoglossus muscle.

foliate papillae, papillae foliatae.

fungiform papillae, papillae fungiformes.

papil'lae fungifor'mes [NA], fungiform or clavate papillae; numerous minute elevations on the dorsum of the tongue, of a fancied mushroom shape, the tip being broader than the base; the epithelium of many of these papillae have taste buds.

hair p., p. pili.

p. inci'siva [NA], incisive or palatine p.; a slight elevation of the mucosa at the anterior extremity of the raphe of the palate.

incisive p., p. incisiva.

interdental p., interproximal p.; gingival septum; the gingiva that fills the interproximal space between two adjacent teeth.

interproximal p., interdental p.

lacrimal p., p. lacrimalis.

p. lacrima'lis [NA], lacrimal p.; a slight projection from the margin of each eyelid near the medial commisure, in the center of which is the punctum lacrimale or opening of the lacrimal duct.

lenticular papillae, *folliculi* linguales.

lingual p., **(1)** p. lingualis; **(2)** the lingual portion of the gingiva filling the interproximal space between adjacent teeth; in molar and premolar areas, there may be separate lingual and buccal papillae.

p. lingua'lis, pl. **papil'lae lingua'les** [NA], lingual p. (1); one of numerous variously shaped projections of the mucous membrane of the dorsum of the tongue.

major duodenal p., p. duodeni major.

p. mam'mae [NA], p. of the breast; nipple; mamilla (2); teat (1); thele; thelium (3); a wartlike projection at the apex of the mamma, on the surface of which the lactiferous ducts open; it is surrounded by a circular pigmented area, the areola.

minor duodenal p., p. duodeni minor.

nerve p., neurothele; one of the papillae in the skin containing a tactile corpuscle or other form of end organ.

p. ner'vi op'tici, *discus* nervi optici.

optic p., *discus* nervi optici.

palatine p., p. incisiva.

parotid p., p. parotidea.

p. paroti'dea [NA], parotid p.; the projection at the opening of the parotid duct into the vestibule of the mouth opposite the neck of the upper second molar tooth.

p. pi'li, hair p.; a knoblike indentation of the bottom of the hair follicle, upon which the hair bulb fits like a cap; it is derived from the corium and contains vascular loops for the nourishment of the hair root.

renal p., p. renalis.

p. rena'lis, pl. **papil'lae rena'les** [NA], renal p.; the apex of a renal pyramid which projects into a minor calyx; some 10 to 25 openings of papillary ducts occur on its tip, forming the area cribrosa.

retrocuspid p., a small tissue tag located on the mandibular gingiva lingual to the cuspid teeth; usually occurs bilaterally, is more commonly identified in children, and is considered a normal anatomic structure.

tactile p., one of the papillae of the skin containing a tactile cell or corpuscle.

urethral p., p. urethra'lis, the slight projection in the vestibule of the vagina marking the urethral orifice.

p. valla'ta, pl. **papil'lae valla'tae** [NA], vallate p.; circumvallate p.; one of eight or ten projections from the dorsum of the tongue forming a row anterior to and parallel with the sulcus terminalis; each p. is surrounded by a circular trench (fossa) having a slightly raised outer wall (vallum); on the sides of the vallate p. and the opposed margin of the vallum are numerous taste buds.

vallate p., p. vallata.

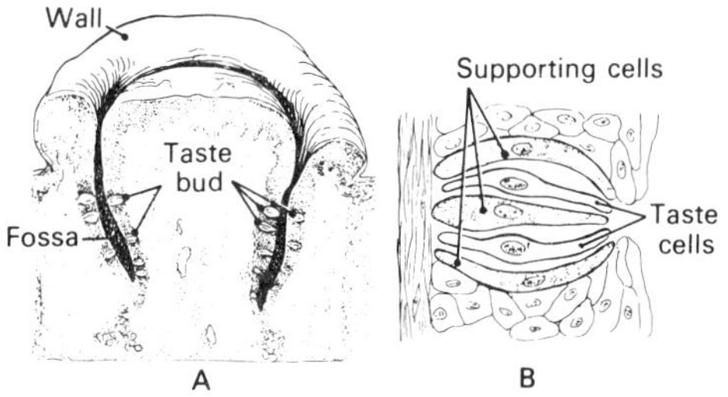

Papilla Vallata

A, microscopic section of papilla vallata of tongue; *B,* structure of taste bud.

vascular papillae, dermal papillae containing vascular loops.

papillary, papillate (pap'i-lār-ē, -i-lāt). Relating to, resembling, or provided with papillae.

papillectomy (pap-i-lek'tō-mē) [papilla + G. *ektomē,* excision]. Surgical removal of any papilla.

papilledema (pă-pil-e-dē'mă) [papilla + edema]. Choked disk; papillary stasis; edema of the optic disk; may be due to increased intracranial pressure, or part of a diffuse retinal edema, as in accelerated hypertension.

papilliferous (pap-i-lif'er-ŭs) [papilla + L. *fero,* to bear]. Provided with papillae.

papilliform (pă-pil'i-fōrm). Resembling or shaped like a papilla.

papillitis (pap-i-lī'tis) [papilla + G. *-itis,* inflammation]. **1.** Inflammation of the optic nerve at the level of the optic disk. **2.** Inflammation of the renal papilla.
necrotizing p., renal papillary *necrosis.*

papillo- [L. *papilla*]. Combining form denoting papilla, papillary.

papilloadenocystoma (pap'i-lō-ad'ĕ-nō-sis-tō'mă). A benign epithelial neoplasm characterized by glands or glandlike structures, formation of cysts, and finger-like projections of neoplastic cells covering a core of fibrous connective tissue.

papillocarcinoma (pap'i-lō-kar-si-nō'mă) [papilla + G. *karkinōma,* cancer]. **1.** A papilloma that has become malignant. **2.** A carcinoma that is characterized by papillary, finger-like projections of neoplastic cells in association with cores of fibrous stroma as a supporting structure.

papilloma (pap-i-lō'mă) [papilla + G. *-oma,* tumor]. Papillary tumor; villoma; a circumscribed benign epithelial tumor projecting from the surrounding surface; more precisely, a benign epithelial neoplasm consisting of villous or arborescent outgrowths of fibrovascular stroma covered by neoplastic cells.
p. acumina'tum, *condyloma* acuminatum.
basal cell p., seborrheic *keratosis.*
p. canalic'ulum, a papillomatous benign tumor arising within the duct of a gland.
canine oral p., warts affecting mucous membranes of young dogs; caused by a papillomavirus.
p. diffu'sum, widespread occurrence of p.'s.
duct p., intraductal p.
p. du'rum, hard p.; a wart, corn, or cutaneous horn.
fibroepithelial p., skin *tag.*
hard p., p. durum.
Hopmann's p., Hopmann's polyp; a papillomatous overgrowth of the nasal mucous membrane.
infectious p. of cattle, cattle warts; single or multiple rough nodules on the skin and mucous membranes caused by a papillomavirus; in young cattle, which are most susceptible, they are most numerous on the head, neck, and shoulders; in cows they usually affect the udder and teats.
p. inguina'le trop'icum, a cutaneous eruption, occurring in Colombia, characterized by numerous slender pink vegetations in the inguinal region.
intracystic p., a p. growing within a cystic adenoma, filling the cavity with a mass of branching epithelial processes.
intraductal p., duct p.; a small, often impalpable, benign p. arising in a lactiferous duct and frequently causing bleeding from the nipple.
inverted p., a mucosal tumor of the urinary bladder or nasal cavity in which proliferating epithelium is invaginated beneath the surface and is more smoothly rounded than in other p.'s.
p. mol'le, soft p.
p. neuropath'icum, p. neurot'icum, a papillomatous eruption or growth following the course of a nerve.
soft p., p. molle; **(1)** a p. with only a thin layer of horny epithelium; **(2)** any small soft growth; *e.g.,* a soft mole or nevus.
transitional cell p., a benign papillary tumor of transitional epithelium; in the urinary tract, called transitional cell carcinoma, grade 1, because of the likelihood of its recurrence.
p. vene'reum, *condyloma* acuminatum.
villous p., villous tumor; a p. composed of slender, finger-like excrescences occurring in the bladder or large intestine, or from the choroid plexus of the cerebral ventricles; villous p.'s of the colon are usually sessile and frequently become malignant.
zymotic p., yaws.

papillomatosis (pap'i-lō-mă-tō'sis). **1.** The development of numerous papillomas. **2.** Papillary projections of the epidermis forming a microscopically undulating surface.
confluent and reticulate p., Gougerot-Carteaud syndrome; a genodermatosis occurring predominantly in females with onset at puberty; characterized by discrete and confluent papules of the anterior and posterior mid-chest, spreading gradually.
florid oral p., diffuse involvement of the lips and oral mucosa with benign squamous papillomas; microscopically, it resembles verrucous carcinoma, but is not invasive or localized to a specific area of the oral mucosa.
juvenile p., a form of fibrocystic disease of the breast in young women, with florid and sclerosing adenosis that microscopically may suggest carcinoma.
laryngeal p., multiple squamous cell papillomas of the larynx, seen most commonly in young children, usually due to infection by the human papilloma virus which may be transmitted at birth from the maternal condylomata; recurrences are common, with remission after several years.
palatal p., inflammatory papillary *hyperplasia.*
subareolar duct p., adenoma of the nipple; erosive adenomatosis of the nipple; a benign tumor which may clinically resemble Paget's disease, but which is a papillary or solid growth of columnar and myoepithelial cells producing a florid pseudoinfiltrative pattern.

papillomatous (pap-i-lō'mă-tŭs). Relating to a papilloma.

Papillomavirus (pap-i-lō'mă-vī-rŭs). A genus of viruses (family Papovaviridae) containing DNA (MW 5×10^6), having virions about 55 nm in diameter, and including the papilloma and warts viruses of man and other animals.

Papillon, M.M. See P.-Lefèvre *syndrome.*

Papillon-Léage. See P. and Psaume *syndrome.*

papilloretinitis (pap'i-lō-ret-i-nī'tis). Papillitis with inflammation of adjacent parts of the retina.

papillotomy (pă-pi-lot'ō-mē) [papilla + G. *tome,* incision]. An incision into the major duodenal papilla.

papillula, pl. **papillulae** (pă-pil'yū-lă, -lē) [Mod. L. dim. of L. *papilla*]. A small papilla.

Papin, Denis, French physicist, 1647–1714. See P.'s *digester.*

Papovaviridae (pă-po'vă-vir'i-dē) [*pa*pilloma + *po*lyoma + *va*cuolating]. A family of small, antigenically distinct viruses that replicate in nuclei of infected cells; most have oncogenic properties. Virions are 45 to 55 nm in diameter, nonenveloped, and ether-resistant; capsids are icosahedral with 72 capsomeres, and they contain double-stranded DNA (MW 3 to 5×10^6). The family includes the genera *Papillomavirus* and *Polyomavirus.*

papovavirus (pă-pō'vă-vī'rŭs). Any virus of the family Papovaviridae.

PAPP Abbreviation for *p*-aminopropiophenone.

Pappenheim, Artur, German physician, 1870–1916. See P.'s *stain;* Unna-P. *stain.*

Pappenheimer bodies. See under body.

pappose, pappous (pap'pōs, pap'pŭs) [G. *pappos,* down]. Downy.

pappus (pap'ŭs) [G. *pappos,* down]. The first downy growth of beard.

PAPS Abbreviation for adenosine 3′-phosphate 5′-phosphosulfate.

papula, pl. **papulae** (pap'yū-lă, -lē) [L.]. Papule.

papular (pap'yū-lăr). Relating to papules.

papulation (pap-yū-lā'shŭn). The formation of papules.

papule (pap'yūl) [L. *papula,* pimple]. Papula; a small, circumscribed, solid elevation on the skin involving predominantly the epidermis or the dermis, depending on the type of pathological process.
 Celsus' p.'s, *lichen* agrius.
 follicular p., a papular lesion arising about a hair follicle; not specific for any condition.
 moist p., mucous p., *condyloma* latum.
 piezogenic pedal p., pressure-induced papules of the heel, occurring probably as a result of herniation of fat tissue resulting from degeneration of dermal collagen.
 split p.'s, p.'s at commissures of the mouth seen in some cases of secondary syphilis.

papuliferous (pap-yū-lif'er-ŭs) [papule + L. *fero,* to bear]. Having papules.

papulo- [L. *papula,* papule]. Combining form denoting papule.

papuloerythematous (pap'yū-lō-er-i-them'ă-tŭs, -thē'mă-tŭs). Denoting an eruption of papules on an erythematous surface.

papulopustular (pap'yū-lō-pŭs'tū-lăr). Denoting an eruption composed of papules and pustules.

papulopustule (pap'yū-lō-pŭs'tyūl). A small semisolid skin elevation which rapidly evolves into a pustule.

papulosis (pap-yū-lō'sis). The occurrence of numerous widespread papules.
 bowenoid p., a clinically benign form of intraepithelial neoplasia that microscopically resembles Bowes's disease or carcinoma in situ, occurring in young individuals of both sexes on the genital or perianal skin usually as multiple well demarcated pigmented warty papules.
 lymphomatoid p., a chronic papular and ulcerative variant of pityriasis lichenoides et varioliformis acuta characterized by dermal perivascular infiltration by atypical mononuclear cells suggestive of a lymphoma; it is usually benign, but occasional transformation to mycosis fungoides has been reported.
 malignant atrophic p., Degos' or Köhlmeier-Degos disease; Degos' syndrome; a cutaneovisceral syndrome characterized by pathognomonic umbilicated porcelain-white papules with elevated telangiectatic annular borders, followed by the development of intestinal ulcers which perforate, causing peritonitis; arterioles in the lesions are occluded by thrombosis and internal fibrosis, leading to progressive neurological disability and death.

papulosquamous (pap'yū-lō-skwā'mŭs) [papulo- + L. *squamosus,* scaly (squamous)]. Denoting an eruption composed of both papules and scales.

papulovesicle (pap'yū-lō-ves'i-kl). A small semisolid skin elevation which evolves into a blister.

papulovesicular (pap'yū-lō-ve-sik'yū-lăr). Denoting an eruption composed of papules and vesicles.

papyraceous (pap-i-rā'shŭs) [L. *papyraceus,* made of *papyrus*]. Like parchment or paper.

par [L. equal]. A pair; specifically a pair of cranial nerves, *e.g.,* p. nonum, ninth pair, glossopharyngeal; p. vagum, the vagus or tenth pair.

para- [G. alongside of, near]. **1.** Prefix denoting a departure from the normal. **2.** Prefix denoting involvement of two like parts or a pair. **3.** Prefix denoting adjacent, alongside, near, etc. **4 (*p*).** In chemistry, an italicized prefix designating two substitutions in the benzene ring arranged symmetrically, *i.e.,* linked to opposite carbon atoms in the ring. For words beginning with *para-* or *p-,* see the specific name.

para (par'ă) [L. *pario,* to bring forth]. A woman who has given birth to one or more infants. Para followed by a roman numeral or preceded by a Latin prefix (primi-, secundi-, terti-, quadri-, *etc.*) designates the number of times a pregnancy has culminated in a single or multiple birth; *e.g.,* **para I,** primipara; a woman who has given birth for the first time; **para II,** secundipara; a woman who has given birth for the second time to one or more infants. *Cf.* gravida.

para-appendicitis (par'ă-ă-pen-di-sī'tis). Periappendicitis.

paraballism (par-ă-bal'izm) [para- + G. *ballismos,* jumping about]. Severe jerking movements of both legs.

parabanic acid (par'ă-ban-ik). Oxalylurea.

parabiosis (par-ă-bī-ō'sis) [para- + G. *biōsis,* life]. **1.** Fusion of whole eggs or embryos, as occurs in conjoined twins. **2.** Surgical joining of the vascular systems of two organisms.

parabiotic (par-ă-bī-ot'ik). Relating to, or characterized by, parabiosis.

parablepsia (par-ă-blep'sē-ă) [para- + G. *blepsis,* sight]. Perverted vision, as in visual illusions or hallucination.

parabulia (par-ă-bū'lē-ă) [para- + G. *boulē,* will]. Perversion of volition or will in which one impulse is checked and replaced by another.

paracanthoma (par'ak-an-thō'mă) [para- + G. *akantha,* a thorn, + *-oma,* tumor]. A neoplasm arising from abnormal hyperplasia of the prickle cell layer of the skin.

paracanthosis (par'ak-an-thō'sis). **1.** The development of paracanthomas. **2.** A division of tumors that includes the cutaneous epitheliomas.

paracarmine (par'ă-kar'min, mēn). See under stain.

paracasein (par-ă-kā'sē-in). The compound produced by the action of rennin upon κ-casein (which liberates a glycoprotein), and that precipitates with calcium ion as the insoluble curd.

Paracelsus, Aureolus Theophrastus Bombastus von Hohenheim, Swiss physician, 1493–1541. See paracelsian *method.*

paracenesthesia (par'ă-sē-nes-thē'zē-ă) [para- + G. *koinos,* common, + *aisthestai,* to perceive]. Deterioration in one's sense of bodily well-being, *i.e.,* of the normal functioning of its organs.

paracentesis (par'ă-sen-tē'sis) [G. *parakentēsis,* a tapping for dropsy, fr. *para,* beside, + *kentēsis,* puncture]. Tapping (2); the passage into a cavity of a trocar and cannula, needle, or other hollow instrument for the purpose of removing fluid; variously designated according to the cavity punctured.

paracentetic (par-ă-sen-tet'ik). Relating to paracentesis.

paracentral (par-ă-sen'trăl). Close to or alongside the center or some structure designated "central."

paracervical (par-ă-ser'vi-kăl). Adjacent to the uterine cervix.

paracervix (par-ă-ser'viks) [NA]. The connective tissue of the pelvic floor extending from the fibrous subserous coat of the cervix of the uterus laterally between the layers of the broad ligament.

paracetaldehyde (par-as-ĕ-tal'dĕ-hīd). Paraldehyde.

paracetamol (par-ă-set'ă-mol). Acetaminophen.

parachlorophenol (par'ă-klōr-ō-fē'nol). *p*-Chlorophenol; a disinfectant effective against most Gram-negative organisms; also available as camphorated p.

paracholera (par-ă-kol'er-ă). A disease clinically resembling Asiatic cholera but due to a vibrio specifically different from *Vibrio cholerae.*

parachordal (par-ă-kōr'dăl) [para- + G. *chordē,* cord]. Alongside the anterior portion of the notochord in the embryo; designating the cartilaginous bars on either side which enter into the formation of the base of the skull.

parachroia (par-ă-kroy'ă) [para- + G. *chroia,* color]. Parachroma (1).

parachroma (par-ă-krō'mă) [para- + G. *chrōma,* color]. Parachroia (1); parachromatosis; abnormal coloration of the skin.

parachromatosis (par-ă-krō-mă-tō'sis). Parachroma (1).

parachymosin (par-ă-kī'mō-sin). An enzyme resembling chymosin.

paracinesia, paracinesis (par'ă-si-nē'zē-ă, -nē'sis). Parakenesia.

paracmasis (par-ak'mă-sis). Paracme.

paracmastic (par-ak-mas'tik). Relating to the paracme.

paracme (par-ak'mē) [G. the point at which the prime is past; fr. *para,* beyond, + *akmē,* highest point, prime]. Paracmasis. **1.** The stage of subsidence of a fever. **2.** The period of life beyond the prime; the decline or stage of involution of an organism.

Paracoccidioides brasiliensis (par'ă-kok-sid-ē-oy'dēz bră-sil-ē-en'sis). A dimorphic fungus that causes paracoccidioidomycosis. In tissues and on enriched culture medium at 37°C, it grows as large spherical or oval cells which bear single or several buds, and usually is identified by this characteristic; at lower temperatures, it grows slowly as a white mold with minimal sporulation and is non-characteristic.

paracoccidioidin (par'ă-kok-sid-ē-oy'din). A filtrate antigen prepared from the filamentous form of the pathogenic fungus, *Paracoccidioides brasiliensis;* used for demonstrating delayed type dermal hypersensitivity in populations and useful in demonstrating endemic areas in different geographic regions.

paracoccidioidomycosis (par'ă-kok-sid-ē-oy'dō-mī-kō'sis). South American blastomycosis; Almeida's or Lutz-Splendore-Almeida disease; paracoccidioidal granuloma; a chronic mycosis characterized by primary pulmonary lesions with dissemination to many visceral organs, conspicuous ulcerative granulomas of the buccal and nasal mucosa with extensions to the skin, and generalized lymphangitis; caused by *Paracoccidioides brasiliensis.*

paracolitis (par'ă-kō-lī'tis). Inflammation of the peritoneal coat of the colon.

paracolpitis (par'ă-kol-pī'tis) [para- + G. *kolpos,* vagina, + *-itis,* inflammation]. Paravaginitis.

paracolpium (par-ă-kol'pē-ŭm) [para- + G. *kolpos,* vagina]. The tissues alongside the vagina.

paracone (par'ă-kōn) [para- + G. *kōnos,* cone]. The mesiobuccal cusp of an upper molar tooth.

paraconid (par-ă-kon'id). The mesiobuccal cusp of a lower molar tooth.

paracortex (par-ă-kōr'teks). Deep or tertiary cortex; thymus-dependent zone; the area of a lymph node between the subcapsular cortex and the medullary cords; it contains mostly the long-lived lymphocytes derived from the thymus.

paracousis (par-ă-kū'sis). Paracusis.

paracrine (par'ă-krin). Referring to the release of locally acting substances from endocrine cells directly into the intercellular space of adjacent cells.

paracusis, paracusia (par'ă-kū'sis, -kū'sē-ă) [para- + G. *akousis,* hearing]. Paracousis. **1.** Impaired hearing. **2.** Auditory illusions or hallucinations.

false p., Willis' p.; the apparent increase in auditory acuity of a deaf person to conversation in noisy surroundings due to his companion unconsciously raising his voice.

p. loci, loss or diminution of the power of determining the direction of sound.

Willis' p., false p.

paracyesis (par-ă-sī-ē'sis) [para- + G. *kyēsis,* pregnancy]. Ectopic *pregnancy.*

paracystic (par-ă-sis'tik) [para- + G. *kystis,* bladder]. Paravesical; alongside or near a bladder, specifically the urinary bladder.

paracystitis (par'ă-sis-tī'tis) [para- + G. *kystis,* bladder, + *-itis,* inflammation]. Inflammation of the connective tissue and other structures about the urinary bladder.

paracystium (par-ă-sis'tē-ŭm) [para- + G. *kystis,* bladder]. The tissues adjacent to the urinary bladder.

paracytic (par-ă-sī'tik) [para- + G. *kytos,* cell]. **1.** Relating to cells other than those normal to the part where they are found. **2.** Between or among, but independent of, cells.

paradenitis (par'ad'ĕ-nī'tis) [para- + G. *adēn,* gland, + *-itis,* inflammation]. Inflammation of the tissues adjacent to a gland.

paradental (par-ă-den'tăl). Periodontal.

paradentium (par-ă-den'tē-ŭm). Periodontium.

paradidymal (par-ă-did'i-măl). **1.** Relating to the paradidymis. **2.** Alongside the testis.

paradidymis, pl. **paradidymides** (par'ă-did'i-mis, -di-dim'i-dēz) [para- + G. *didymos,* twin, in pl. *didymoi,* testes] [NA]. Parepididymis; a small body sometimes attached to the front of the lower part of the spermatic cord above the head of the epididymis; the remmants of tubules of the mesonephros.

paradipsia (par-ă-dip'sē-ă) [para- + G. *dipsa,* thirst]. A perverted appetite for fluids, ingested without relation to bodily need.

paradox (par'ă-doks) [G. *paradoxos,* incredible, beyond belief, fr. *doxa,* belief]. That which is apparently, though not actually, inconsistent with or opposed to the known facts in any case.

Weber's p., if a muscle is loaded beyond its power to contract it may elongate.

para-equilibrium (par'ă-ē'kwi-lib'rē-ŭm). Vertigo, often associated with nausea, nystagmus, and muscular weakness, due to irritation of the vestibular apparatus of the ear.

paraesthesia (par-es-thē'zē-ă). Paresthesia.

paraffin (par'ă-fin) [L. *parum,* little, + *affinis,* neighboring, akin, so called because of its slight tendency to chemical reaction]. **1.** One of the methane series of acyclic hydrocarbons. **2.** Hard p.

chlorinated p., a solvent for dichloramine-T.

hard p., p. (2); a purified mixture of solid hydrocarbons derived from petroleum.

liquid p., mineral oil.

white soft p., white *petrolatum.*

yellow soft p., petrolatum.

paraffinoma (par'ă-fi-nō'mă). Paraffin tumor; a tumefaction, usually a granuloma, caused by the prosthetic or therapeutic injection of paraffin into the tissues; sometimes used with reference to similar lesions resulting from the injection of any oil, wax, or the like. See also lipogranuloma.

Parafilaria multipapillosa (par'ă-fi-lā'rē-ă mul'ti-pap-i-lō'să). A common filarial parasite that causes dermatorrhagia parasitica.

paraflagella (par'ă-fla-jel'ă). Plural of paraflagellum.

paraflagellate (par-ă-flaj'ĕ-lāt). **1.** Having one or more paraflagella. **2.** Paramastigote.

paraflagellum, pl. **paraflagella** (par'ă-fla-jel'ŭm, -ă). A minute accessory flagellum sometimes present in addition to the ordinary flagellum of certain protozoans.

parafollicular (par-ă-fo-lik'yū-lăr). Associated spatially with a follicle.

paraformaldehyde (par-ă-fōr-mal'dĕ-hīd). Trioxymethylene; a polymer of formaldehyde, used as a disinfectant.

parafuchsin (par-ă-fuk'sin). Pararosanilin.

paragammacism (par'ă-gam'ă-sizm) [para- + G. *gamma,* the letter g]. Substitution of another letter sound for the g sound. See also gammacism.

paraganglia (par-ă-gang'glē-ă). Plural of paraganglion.

paraganglioma (par'ă-gang-glē-ō'mă). A neoplasm usually derived from the chromoreceptor tissue of a paraganglion, such as the carotid body, or the medulla of the adrenal gland; the latter is usually termed a chromaffinoma or pheochromocytoma.

nonchromaffin p., chemodectoma.

paraganglion, pl. **paraganglia** (par-ă-gang'glē-on, -ă). Chromaffin body; a small, roundish body containing chromaffin cells; a number of such bodies may be found retroperitoneally near the aorta and in organs such as the kidney, liver, heart, and gonads.

paragene (par'ă-jēn). Plasmid.

paragenital (par-ă-jen'i-tal). Alongside the gonads.

parageusia (par-ă-gyū'sē-ă, -jū'sē-ă) [para- + G. *geusis,* taste]. Disordered or perverted sense of taste.

parageusic (par-ă-gyū'sik). Relating to parageusia.

paragnathus (pa-rag'na-thŭs) [para- + G. *gnathos,* jaw]. **1.** An individual with an accessory lower jaw. **2.** A parasitic fetus attached to the jaw of the autosite.

paragnomen (par-ag-nō'men) [para- + G. *gnōmēn, gnōmē,* judgment]. An unexpected reaction.

paragonimiasis (par'ă-gon-i-mī'ă-sis). Pulmonary distomiasis; infection with a worm of the genus *Paragonimus,* especially *P. westermani.*

Paragonimus (par-ă-gon'i-mŭs) [para- + G. *gonimos,* with generative power]. A genus of lung flukes, parasitic in man and a wide variety of mammals, that feed upon crustacea carrying the metacercariae.

P. kellicot'ti, a species prevalent in certain wild animals, such as racoons, and occurring in dogs, in the Great Lakes region of the U.S.; it is morphologically similar to *P. westermani.*

P. rin'geri, *P. westermani.*

P. westerman'i, *P. ringeri;* the bronchial or lung fluke; a species that causes paragonimiasis, found chiefly in Japan, Korea, Taiwan, China, the Philippines, and Thailand; eggs are coughed up in sputum or swallowed and passed in the feces; miracidia invade *Melania* snails, and produce large numbers of stumpy-tailed cercariae that leave the snail and crawl into muscles and viscera of crayfish or crabs and encyst; in man the excysted worms invade the wall of the gut and migrate through the diaphragm into the lungs; the developing parasites cause an intense inflammatory reaction and eventually induce fibrous-walled nodules that usually contain a pair of adult worms, along with exudate, eggs, and remains of red blood cells; the fibroparasitic nodules may become contiguous and form multiloculated cystlike structures; in some instances, the flukes involve the brain, liver, peritoneum, intestine, or skin.

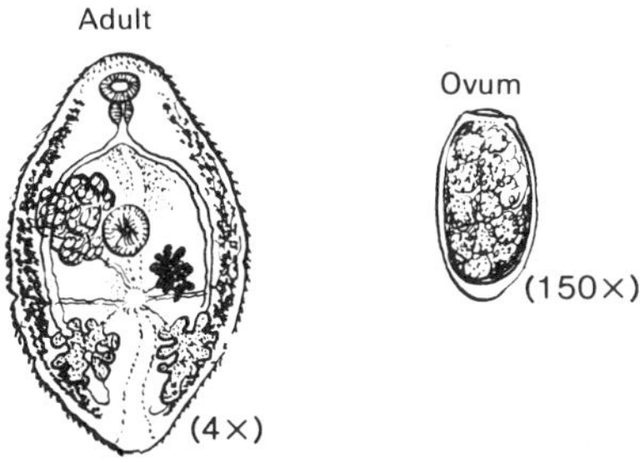

Paragonimus westermani
(After Jeffrey and Leach.)

paragonorrheal (par'ă-gon-ō-rē'ăl). Indirectly related to or consequent to gonorrhea.

paragrammatism (par-ă-gram'ă-tizm). Paraphasia.

paragraphia (par-ă-graf'ē-ă) [para- + G. *graphō,* to write]. **1.** Loss of the power of writing from dictation, although the words are heard and comprehended. **2.** Writing one word when another is intended.

parahemophilia (par'ă-hē-mō-fil'ē-ă). Owren's *disease.*

parahepatic (par-ă-he-pat'ik). Adjacent to the liver.

parahidrosis (par'ă-hi-drō'sis). Paridrosis.

parahormone (par-ă-hōr'mōn). A substance, product of ordinary metabolism, not produced for a specific purpose, that acts like a hormone in modifying the activity of some distant organ; *e.g.,* the action of carbon dioxide on the control of breathing.

parahypno'sis. (par'ă-hip-nō'sis). Disordered sleep, such as caused by nightmare or somnambulism.

parahypophysis (par'ă-hī-pof'i-sis). A small mass of pituitary tissue, or tissue resembling in structure the anterior lobe of the hypophysis, occasionally found in the dura mater lining of the sella turcica.

parakappacism (par'ă-kap'ă-sizm) [para- + G. *kappa,* the letter k]. Substitution of another letter sound for that of k. See also kappacism.

parakeratosis (par'ă-ker-ă-tō'sis). Retention of nuclei in the cells of the stratum corneum of the epidermis, observed in many scaly dermatoses such as psoriasis and exfoliative dermatitis.

p. ostra'cea, p. scutularis.

porcine p., a skin disease of young pigs characterized by a hard, scaly, proliferation of the surface layers of the skin. The extremities are commonly affected first, but it may involved the entire body.

p. psoriasifor'mis, an eruption marked by the presence of thick scales resembling those of psoriasis.

p. pustulo'sa, idiopathic subungual keratosis with nail deformity or pitting and with pustular or well demarcated scaling eczematous changes of the fingertips; usually seen in young girls.

p. scutula'ris, p. ostracea; a disease of the scalp marked by the formation of crusts that envelop the hairs.

p. variega'ta, *poikiloderma* atrophicans vasculare.

parakinesia, parakinesis (par'ă-ki-nē'zē-ă, -ki-nē'sis) [para- + G. *kinēsis,* movement]. Paracinesia; paracinesis; any motor abnormality.

paralalia (par-ă-lā'lē-ă) [para- + G. *lalia,* talking]. Any speech defect; especially one in which one letter is habitually substituted for another.

p. litera'lis, stammering.

paralambdacism (par-ă-lam'dă-sizm) [para- + G. *lambda,* letter l]. Mispronunciation of the letter l, or the substitution of some other letter for it. See also lambdacism.

paraldehyde (par-al'dĕ-hīd). Paracetaldehyde; $(CH_3CHO)_3$; a polymer of acetaldehyde; a safe potent hypnotic and sedative suitable for oral, rectal, intravenous, and intramuscular administration; its offensive odor limits its use.

paraleprosis (par-ă-lĕ-prō'sis). Presence of certain trophic or nerve changes suggesting an attenuated form of leprosy in regions where the disease has long prevailed.

paralepsy (par'ă-lep-sē) [G. para- + *lepsis,* seizure]. **1.** A temporary attack of mental inertia and hopelessness. **2.** A sudden alteration in mood or emotional tension.

paralexia (par-ă-lek'sē-ă) [para- + G. *lexis,* speech]. Misapprehension of written or printed words, other meaningless words being substituted for them in reading.

paralgesia (par-al-jē'zē-ă) [para- + G. *algēsis,* the sense of pain]. Painful paresthesia; any disorder or abnormality of the sense of pain.

paralgia (par-al'jē-ă) [para- + G. *algos,* pain]. Abnormal or unusual pain.

paralipophobia (par'ă-lip-ō-fō'bē-ă). Morbid fear of neglect or omission of some duty.

parallactic (par-ă-lak'tik). Relating to a parallax.

parallax (par'ă-laks) [G. alternately, fr. *par-allassō,* to make alternate, fr. *allos,* other]. **1.** The apparent displacement of an object that follows a change in the position from which it is viewed. **2.** See

phi *phenomenon.*
binocular p., stereoscopic p.; the difference in the angles formed by the lines of sight to two objects situated at different distances from the eyes; a factor in the visual perception of depth.
heteronymous p., the apparent movement of an object toward the closed eye; noted in exophoria.
homonymous p., the apparent movement of an object toward the open eye when one is closed; noted in esophoria.
stereoscopic p., binocular p.
vertical p., the relative vertical displacement of the image when each eye is closed in turn; seen in vertical diplopia, or heterophoria.

parallelism (par'ă-lel-izm) [para- + G. *allēlōn,* of one another, fr. *allos,* other]. **1.** The state of being structurally parallel. **2.** In psychology, the doctrine that for every conscious process there is a corresponding or parallel organic process, without asserting a causal interrelation between the two.

parallelometer (par'ă-lel-om'ĕ-ter). An apparatus used for paralleling the attachments and abutments for fixed or removable partial dentures.

parallergic (par-ă-ler'jik). Denoting an allergic state in which the body becomes predisposed to nonspecific stimuli following original sensitization with a specific allergen.

paralogia, paralogism, paralogy (par-ă-lō'jē-ă; pă-ral'ō-jizm, -ral'ō-jē) [G. *paralogia,* a fallacy, fr. *para,* beside, + *logos,* reason]. False reasoning, involving self-deception.
thematic p., false reasoning in relation chiefly to one theme or subject, upon which the mind dwells insistently.

paralysis, pl. **paralyses** (pă-ral'i-sis, -sēz) [G. fr. para- + *lysis,* a loosening]. **1.** Palsy; loss of power of voluntary movement in a muscle through injury to or disease of its nerve supply. **2.** Loss of any function, as sensation, secretion, or mental ability.
acute ascending p., Landry's p.; Kussmaul-Landry p.; a p. of rapid course beginning in the legs and involving progressively the trunk, arms, and neck, ending sometimes in death in from one to three weeks.
acute atrophic p., acute anterior *poliomyelitis.*
p. ag'itans, obsolete term for parkinsonism (1).
ascending p., p. that advances progressively from the periphery toward the nerve center, or from the lower toward the upper portions of the body.
Brown-Séquard's p., Brown-Séquard's *syndrome.*
bulbar p., progressive bulbar p.
central p., p. due to a lesion in the brain or spinal cord.
Chastek p., a disease of foxes and mink caused by feeding on raw fish of certain types which contain an enzyme destructive of thiamin; the thiamin deficiency causes loss of appetite, emaciation, and finally paralysis and death.
compression p., p. due to compression of a nerve, usually of the arm, due to prolonged pressure, *e.g.,* during sleep, or from the pressure of a crutch.
conjugate p., p. of one or more of the external muscles of the eye, resulting in loss of conjugate movement of the eyes.
crossed p., alternating *hemiplegia.*
crutch p., crutch palsy; a form of compression p. affecting the arm and caused by the pressure of the crosspiece of a crutch, usually involving the ulnar nerve.
decubitus p., a form of compression p. due to pressure on a nerve during sleep.
diphtheritic p., postdiphtheritic p.
diver's p., lay term for decompression *sickness.*
Duchenne's p., pseudohypertrophic muscular *dystrophy.*
Duchenne-Erb p., Erb's *palsy.*
Erb's p., Erb's *palsy.*
Erb's spinal p., chronic myelitis of syphilitic origin.
facial p., facial *palsy.*
familial periodic p., see hyperkalemic, hypokalemic, and normokalemic periodic p.
faucial p., isthmoparalysis.
fowl p., see avian *lymphomatosis.*
ginger p., jake p.
global p., p. of both whole sides of the body; survival is usually of short duration.
glossolabiolaryngeal p., glossolabiopharyngeal p., progressive bulbar p.
Gubler's p., Gubler's *syndrome.*
hyperkalemic periodic p., adynamia episodica hereditaria; a form of periodic p. in which the serum potassium level is elevated during attacks; onset occurs in infancy, attacks are frequent but relatively mild, and myotonia is often present; autosomal dominant inheritance.
hypokalemic periodic p., a form of periodic p. in which the serum potassium level is low during attacks; onset usually occurs between the ages of 7 and 21 years; attacks may be precipitated by exposure to cold, high carbohydrate meal, or alcohol, may last hours to days, and may cause respiratory p.; autosomal dominant inheritance with reduced penetrance in females.
immunological p., lack of specific antibody production after exposure to large doses of the antigen; immunological p. disappears when the antigen is eliminated.
infectious bulbar p., pseudorabies.
jake p., ginger p.; neuropathy produced by drinking synthetic Jamaican ginger (or "jake" in the vernacular) containing triorthocresylphosphate.
Klumpke's p., Klumpke-Dejerine syndrome; bracial plexus injury, often due to birth trauma, causing atrophic p. of the forearm and small muscles of the hand together with paralysis of the cervical sympathetic.
Kussmaul-Landry p., acute ascending p.
labial p., progressive bulbar p.
lambing p., pregnancy *disease* of sheep.
Landry's p., acute ascending p.
lead p., lead *palsy.*
mimetic p., p. of the facial muscles.
mixed p., combined motor and sensory p.
motor p., loss of the power of muscular contraction.
musculospiral p., p. of the muscles of the forearm due to injury of the radial (musculospiral) nerve.
myogenic p., acute anterior *poliomyelitis.*
normokalemic periodic p., sodium-responsive periodic p.; a form of periodic p. in which the serum potassium level is within normal limits during attacks; onset usually occurs between the ages of 2 and 5 years; there is often severe quadriplegia, usually improved by the administration of sodium salts; autosomal dominant inheritance.
obstetrical p., birth *palsy.*
ocular p., complete p. of extraocular and intraocular muscles.
parturient p., milk *fever* (2).
periodic p., term for a group of diseases characterized by recurring episodes of muscular weakness or flaccid p. without loss of consciousness, speech, or sensation; attacks begin when the patient is at rest, and there is apparent good health between attacks. See hyperkalemic periodic p.; hypokalemic periodic p.; normokalemic periodic p.
postdiphtheritic p., diphtheritic p.; p. affecting the uvula most frequently, but also any other muscle, due to toxic neuritis; usually appears in the second or third week following the beginning of the attack of diphtheria.
posti'cus p., p. of the posterior cricothyroid muscles.
Pott's p., Pott's *paraplegia.*
pressure p., pressure palsy; p. due to compression of a nerve, nerve trunk, or spinal cord.
progressive bulbar p., bulbar p. or palsy; labial, glossolabiolaryngeal, or glossolabiopharyngeal p.; Duchenne's disease (2); Erb's

disease; a progressive atrophy and p. of the muscles of the tongue, lips, palate, pharynx, and larynx, occurring in later life and due to atrophic degeneration of the neurons innervating these muscles.
pseudobulbar p., p. of the lips and tongue, simulating progressive bulbar p., due to cerebral lesions with bilateral involvement of the upper motor neurons; characterized by speech and swallowing difficulties, emotional instability, and spasmodic, mirthless laughter. Sometimes called laughing sickness.
pseudohypertrophic muscular p., pseudohypertrophic muscular *dystrophy.*
sensory p., loss of sensation; anesthesia.
sleep p., sleep dissociation; a condition in which the waking person is aware of the surroundings but is unable to move.
sodium-responsive periodic p., normokalemic periodic p.
spastic spinal p., spastic *diplegia.*
spinal p., myeloparalysis; myeloplegia; rachioplegia; loss of motor power due to a lesion of the spinal cord.
supranuclear p., p. due to lesions above the primary motor neurons.
tick p., an ascending p. caused by the continuing presence of *Dermacentor* and *Ixodes* attached in the occipital region or on the upper neck of humans, often hidden under long hair; reported from the western U.S., British Columbia, and other regions; occurs mainly in children, but also in dogs, calves, and sheep.
Todd's p., Todd's postepileptic p.; p. of temporary duration (normally not more than a few days) that occurs in the limb or limbs involved in jacksonian epilepsy after the seizure.
Todd's postepileptic p., Todd's p.
vasomotor p., vasoparesis.
wasting p., progressive muscular *atrophy.*
Zenker's p., paresthesia and p. in the area of the external popliteal nerve.

paralyssa (par'ă-lis'ă) [paralysis + G. *lyssa,* madness (rabies)]. A paralytic form of rabies caused by the bite of the vampire bat (*Desmodis*).

paralytic (par-ă-lit'ik). Relating to paralysis or to suffering from paralysis.

paralyzant (pă-ral'i-zant). **1.** Causing paralysis. **2.** Any agent, such as curare, that causes paralysis.

paralyze (par'ă-līz). To render incapable of movement.

paramagnetic (par'ă-mag-net'ik). Having the property of paramagnetism.

paramagnetism (par-ă-mag'nĕ-tizm). The property of being magnetic, as exhibited by assuming a position parallel with the lines of force between the two poles of a magnet; *e.g.,* molecules having an unpaired electron, such as Hb and O_2, exhibit a magnetic movement; combined, as in HbO_2, they are diamagnetic.

paramastigote (par-ă-mas'ti-gōt) [para- + G. *mastix,* whip]. Paraflagellate (2); a mastigote having two flagella, one long and one short.

paramastoid (par-ă-mas'toyd). Near the mastoid process.

Paramecium (par-ă-mē'shē-ŭm, -sē-ŭm) [G. *paramēkēs,* rather long, fr. *mēkos,* length]. An abundant genus of freshwater holotrichous ciliates, characteristically slipper-shaped and often large enough to be visible to the naked eye; commonly used for genetic and other studies.

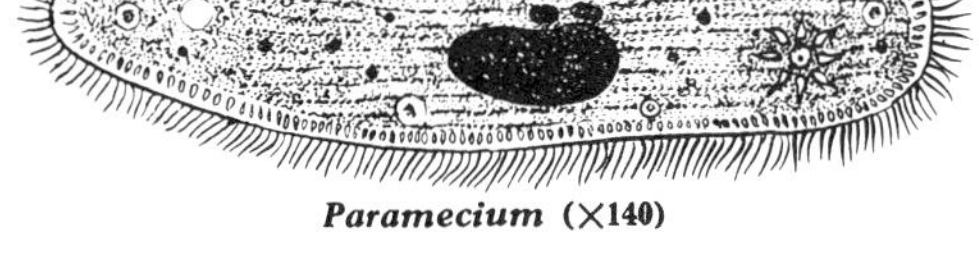

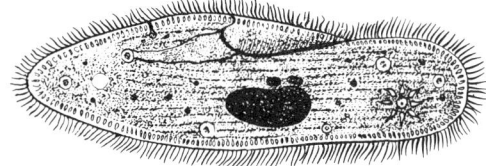

Paramecium **(×140)**

paramedian (par-ă-mē'dē-an). Paramesial; near the middle line.

paramedic (par-ă-med'ik). A person trained and certified to provide emergency medical care.

paramedical (par-ă-med'i-kăl). **1.** Related to the medical profession in an adjunctive capacity, *e.g.,* denoting allied health fields such as physical therapy, speech pathology, etc. **2.** Relating to a paramedic.

paramenia (par-ă-mē'nē-ă) [para- + G. *mēn,* month]. Any disorder or irregularity of menstruation.

paramesial (par-ă-mē'sē-ăl). Paramedian.

paramesonephric (par-ă-mes-ō-nef'rik). Close to or alongside the embryonic mesonephros.

parameter (pă-ram'ĕ-ter) [para- + G. *metron,* measure]. One of many ways of measuring or describing an object or evaluating a subject: **1.** In a mathematical expression, an arbitrary constant that can possess different values, each value defining other expressions, and can determine the specific form but not the general nature of the expression; *e.g.,* in the equation $y = a + bx$, a and b are parameters. **2.** In statistics, a term used to define a characteristic of a population, in contrast to a sample from that population; *e.g.,* the mean and standard deviation of a total population. **3.** In psychoanalysis, any tactic, other than interpretation, used by the analyst to further the patient's progress.

paramethadione (par'ă-meth-ă-dī'ōn). 3,5-Dimethyl-5-ethyloxazolidine-2,4-dione; an anticonvulsant used in petit mal epilepsy.

paramethasone (par-ă-meth'ă-sōn). 6α-Fluoro-11β,17,21-trihydroxy-16α-methyl-1,4-pregnadiene-3,20-dione; a glucocorticoid with anti-inflammatory effects and toxicity similar to those of prednisone.
p. acetate, acetic ester of p. at C-21; a glucocorticoid useful in the treatment of rheumatoid arthritis and other collagen diseases, allergic conditions, and certain hematologic disorders.

parametrial, (par-ă-mē'trē-ăl). Pertaining to the parametrium.

parametric (par-ă-met'rik). Relating to the parametrium, or structures immediately adjacent to the uterus.

parametrismus (par'ă-mĕ-triz'mŭs) [parametrium + G. *trismos,* a creaking]. Painful spasm of the muscular fibers in the broad ligaments.

parametritic (par'ă-me-trit'ik). Relating to parametritis.

parametritis (par'ă-me-trī'tis) [parametrium + G. *-itis,* inflammation]. Pelvic cellulitis; inflammation of the cellular tissue adjacent to the uterus.

parametrium, pl. **parametria** (par-ă-mē'trē-ŭm, -ă) [para- + G. *mētra,* uterus] [NA]. The connective tissue of the pelvic floor extending from the fibrous subserous coat of the supracervical portion of the uterus laterally between the layers of the broad ligament.

paramimia (par-ă-mim'ē-ă) [para- + G. *mimia,* imitation]. The use of gestures unsuited to the words which they accompany.

paramnesia (par-am-nē'zē-ă) [para- + G. *amnēsia,* forgetfulness]. False recollection, as of events that have never occurred.

Paramoeba (par-ă-mē'bă). *Entamoeba.*

paramolar (par-ă-mō-lăr). A supernumerary tooth lying between, lingual, or buccal to the maxillary or mandibular molars.

paramorphia (par-ă-mōr'fē-ă) [para- + G. *morphē,* shape]. Any abnormality in form or structure induced by environmental influences without any corresponding genetic change.

paramorphic (par-ă-mōr'fik). Relating to paramorphia.

paramorphine (par-ă-mōr'fēn). Thebaine.

Paramphistomatidae (par'am-fis-tō-mat'i-dē). A family of parasitic trematodes characterized by large fleshy bodies with a large posterior sucker; included are the genera *Paramphistomum, Gastrodiscoides,* and Watsonius.

paramphistomiasis (par'am-fis-tō-mī'ă-sis). Infection of animals and man with trematodes of the family Paramphistomatidae; human disease is caused by *Gastrodiscoides hominis* in Asia and *Watsonius watsoni* in Africa.

Paramphistomum (par-am-fis'tō-mŭm) [para- + G. *amphistomos,* having a double mouth, fr. *amphi,* two-sided, + *stoma,* mouth]. The rumen fluke, a genus of digenetic trematodes (family Paramphistomatidae) parasitic in the rumen or paunch of cattle; species include *P. microbothrioides, P. cervi,* and *P. liorchis.*

paramusia (par-ă-mū'zē-ă). Loss of the ability to read or to render music correctly.

paramyloidosis (pă-ram'i-loy-dō'sis). A variety of amyloid deposit seen in lymph nodes in some chronic nonspecific inflammations and in primary localized amyloidosis; histologic reactions are the same as in amyloidosis.

paramyoclonus (par'ă-mī-ok'lō-nŭs) [para- + G. *mys,* muscle, + *klonos,* a tumult]. *Myoclonus* multiplex.

paramyotonia (par'ă-mī-ō-tō'nē-ă). Paramyotonus; an atypical form of myotonia.

ataxic p., a disorder characterized by a tonic muscular spasm on attempted movement, associated with slight paresis and ataxia.

congenital p., p. congen'ita, Eulenburg's disease; a nonprogressive disease characterized by myotonia induced by exposure of muscles to cold; there are episodes of intermittent flaccid paralysis, but no atrophy or hypertrophy of muscles; autosomal dominant inheritance.

symptomatic p., a temporary rigidity of the muscles when first attempting to walk.

paramyotonus (par-ă-mī-ot'ō-nŭs). Paramyotonia.

Paramyxoviridae (par-ă-mik'sō-vir'i-dē). A family of RNA-containing viruses about twice the size of the influenza viruses (Orthomyxoviridae) but similar to them in morphology. Virions are 150 to 300 nm in diameter, enveloped, ether-sensitive, and contain RNA-dependent RNA polymerase. Nucleocapsids are helical, considerably larger than those of the influenza viruses, and contain single-stranded unsegmented RNA. Three genera are recognized: *Paramyxovirus, Morbillivirus,* and *Pneumovirus,* all of which cause cell fusion and produce cytoplasmic eosinophilic inclusions.

Paramyxovirus (par-ă-mik'sō-vī-rŭs). A genus of viruses (family Paramyxoviridae) that includes Newcastle disease, mumps, and parainfluenza viruses (types 1 to 5). They all have hemagglutinating and hemadsorbing activities, but only Newcastle disease and mumps viruses grow well in embryonated eggs.

paranalgesia (par-an-ăl-jē'zē-ă) [para- + analgesia]. Analgesia of the lower half of the body.

paranasal (par-ă-nā'săl). Alongside the nose.

paraneoplasia (par'ă-nē-ō-plā'zē-ă). Hormonal, neurological, hematological, and other clinical and biochemical disturbances associated with malignant neoplasms but not directly related to invasion by the primary tumor or its metastases.

paraneoplastic (par'ă-nē-ō-plas'tik). Relating to or characteristic of paraneoplasia.

paranephric (par-ă-nef'rik). **1.** Relating to the paranephros. **2.** Pararenal.

paranephros, pl. **paranephroi** (par-ă-nef'ros, -nef'roy) [para- + G. *nephros,* kidney]. *Glandula* suprarenalis.

paranesthesia (par-an-es-thē'zē-ă) [para- + anesthesia]. Anesthesia of the lower half of the body.

paraneural (par-ă-nūr'ăl) [para- + G. *neuron,* nerve]. Near or alongside a nerve.

paraneurone (par-ă-nūr'ōn). Neuroendocrine cell (2); a gland or aggregate of cells containing neurosecretory granules.

parangi (pă-rang'gē, -ran'jē). A disease similar to yaws, occurring in Sri Lanka.

paranoia (par-ă-noy'ă) [G. derangement, madness, fr. para- + *noeō,* to think]. A severe but rare mental disorder characterized by the presence of systematized delusions, often of a persecutory character, in an otherwise intact personality. See also paranoid *personality.*

acute hallucinatory p., a form in which there are interjected periods of hallucinations in addition to the systematized delusions.

litigious p., p. querulans.

p. origina'ria, a form occurring in children.

p. quer'ulans, litigious p.; a morbid state characterized by discontent and the disposition to complain of imaginary slights.

paranoiac (par-ă-noy'ak). **1.** Relating to or affected with paranoia. **2.** One who is suffering from paranoia.

paranoid (par'ă-noyd). **1.** Relating to or characterized by paranoia. **2.** Having delusions of persecution.

paranomia (par-ă-nō'mē-ă). [para- + G. *onoma,* name]. A form of aphasia in which objects are called by the wrong names.

paranuclear (par-ă-nū'klē-ăr). **1.** Paranucleate. **2.** Outside of, but near the nucleus.

paranucleate (par'ă-nū'klē-āt). Paranuclear (1); relating to or having a paranucleus.

paranucleolus (par'ă-nū-klē'ō-lŭs). See sex *chromatin.*

paranucleus (par-ă-nū'klē-ŭs). An accessory nucleus or small mass of chromatin lying outside of, though near, the nucleus.

paraomphalic (par'ă-om-fal'ik) [para- + G. *omphalos,* umbilicus]. Paraumbilical.

paraoperative (par-ă-op'er-ă-tiv). Perioperative.

paraoral (par-ă-ō'răl) [para- + L. *os* (*or-*), mouth]. Near or adjacent to the mouth.

paraovarian (par'ă-ō-var'ē-an). Parovarian (2).

paraoxon (par-ă-ok'son). Diethyl-4-nitrophenyl phosphate; an organophosphorous cholinesterase inhibitor used in insecticides; parathion is converted in the liver to p.

parapancreatic (par'ă-pan-krē-at'ik). Near or alongside of the pancreas.

paraparesis (par-ă-pă-rē'sis) [para- + paresis]. A slight degree of paralysis, affecting the lower extremities.

paraparetic (par'ă-pă-ret'ik). **1.** Relating to paraparesis. **2.** A person with paraparesis.

parapedesis (par'ă-pĕ-dē'sis) [para- + G. *pēdēsis,* a bending, deflection]. Excretion or secretion through an abnormal channel.

paraperitoneal (par'ă-per'i-tō-nē'ăl). Outside of or alongside the peritoneum.

parapestis (par-ă-pes'tis) [para- + G. *pestis,* plague]. Ambulant *plague.*

paraphasia (par-ă-fā'zē-ă) [para- + G. *phasis,* speech]. Paraphrasia; paragrammatism; pseudoagrammatism; jargon (2); a form of aphasia in which a person has lost the ability to speak correctly, substituting one word for another, and jumbling words and sentences unintelligibly.

thematic p., incoherent speech that wanders from the theme or subject under discussion.

paraphasic (par-ă-fā'sik). Relating to paraphasia.

paraphia (pa-rā'fē-ă) [para- + G. *haphē,* touch]. Parapsia; pseudaphia; pseudesthesia (1); any disorder of the sense of touch.

paraphilia (par-ă-fil'ē-ă) [para- + G. *philos,* fond]. Sexual *deviation.*

paraphimosis (par'ă-fī-mō'sis) [para- + G. phimosis]. **1.** Capistration; painful constriction of the glans penis by a phimotic foreskin, which has been retracted behind the corona. **2.** See p. palpebrae.

p. palpe'brae, total spastic eversion of the upper and lower eyelids.

paraphonia (par-ă-fō'nē-ă) [para- + G. *phōnē,* voice]. Any disorder of the voice, especially a change in its tone.

paraphora (pă-raf'ō-ră) [G. a going aside, derangement]. A slight emotional disturbance.

paraphrasia (par-ă-frā'zē-ă) [para- + G. *phrasis,* speech]. Paraphasia.

paraphysial, paraphyseal (par-ă-fiz'ē-ăl). Pertaining to the paraphysis.

paraphysis, pl. paraphyses (pă-raf'i-sis, -sēz) [G. an offshoot]. A median organ developing from the roofplate of the diencephalon in certain lower vertebrates.

parapineal (par-ă-pin'ē-ăl). Beside the pineal; denoting the visual or photoreceptive portion of the pineal body present, if not functioning, in certain lizards.

paraplasm (par'ă-plazm) [para- + G. *plasma,* a thing formed]. **1.** Obsolete term for hyaloplasm. **2.** Malformed or abnormal tissue.

paraplastic (par-ă-plas'tik). Relating to paraplasm.

paraplectic (par-ă-plek'tik) [G. *paraplēktikos,* paralyzed]. Paraplegic.

paraplegia (par-ă-plē'jē-ă) [para- + *plēgē,* a stroke]. Paralysis of both lower extremities and, generally, the lower trunk.

ataxic p., progressive ataxia and paresis of the leg muscles due to sclerosis of the lateral and posterior funiculi of the spinal cord.

congenital spastic p., infantile spastic p.; a spastic paralysis of the lower extremities occurring in the infant, due to meningeal hemorrhage following injury at birth; a form of obstetric paralysis or birth palsy.

p. doloro'sa, painful p.; paralysis of the lower extremities in which the affected parts, in spite of loss of motion and sensation, are the seat of excruciating pain; it occurs in certain cases of cancer of the spinal cord.

p. in extension, paralysis of the legs, maintained in an extended position by hypertonic extensor muscles.

p. in flexion, the fixation of the paralyzed legs in a flexed posture; usually in transection of the spinal cord.

infantile spastic p., congenital spastic p.

painful p., p. dolorosa.

Pott's p., Pott's paralysis; paralysis of the lower part of the body and the extremities, due to pressure on the spinal cord as the result of tuberculous spondylitis.

senile p., **(1)** simple weakness of the lower extremities, without atrophy or changes in the reflexes, occurring in the aged; **(2)** an acute p. due to hemorrhage or thrombosis of the spinal arteries; **(3)** a slowly developing paralysis of the lower, eventually of the upper, extremities, with involvement of the sphincters, due to softening of the anterior cornua of the spinal cord in the aged.

spastic p., tetanoid p.; paresis of the lower extremities with increased irritability and spasmodic contraction of the muscles.

superior p., paralysis of both arms.

tetanoid p., spastic p.

paraplegic (par-ă-plē'jik). Paraplectic; relating to or suffering from paraplegia.

parapoplexy (par-ap'ō-plek-sē). Pseudoapoplexy.

Parapoxvirus (par-ă-poks'vī-rŭs). The genus of viruses (family Poxviridae) that includes the contagious ecthyma of sheep, bovine papular stomatitis, and paravaccinia viruses. They possess the nucleoprotein antigen common to all viruses included in the family but differ from other poxviruses in morphology (*e.g.,* virions are smaller and have thicker external coats) and by not multiplying in embryonated eggs.

parapraxia (par-ă-prak'sē-ă) [para- + G. *praxis,* a doing]. A condition analogous to paraphasia and paragraphia in which there is a defective performance of purposive acts; *e.g.,* slips of the tongue, or mislaying of objects.

paraproctitis (par'ă-prok-tī'tis) [para- + G. *prōktos,* anus, + *-itis,* inflammation]. Inflammation of the cellular tissue surrounding the rectum.

paraproctium, pl. **paraproctia** (par'ă-prok'shē-um, -tē-ŭm; -ă) [para- + G. *prōktos,* anus]. The cellular tissue surrounding the rectum.

paraprostatitis (par'ă-pros-tă-tī'tis) [para- + L. *prostata,* prostate, + *-itis,* inflammation]. Inflammation of the tissue around the prostate gland.

paraprotein (par-ă-prō'tēn). **1.** An abnormal plasma protein, such as macroglobulin, cryoglobulin, and myeloma protein. **2.** Monoclonal *immunoglobulin.*

paraproteinemia (par'ă-prō-tēn-ē'mē-ă). The presence of abnormal proteins in the blood.

parapsia (pă-rap'sē-ă) [para- + G. *hapsis,* touch]. Paraphia.

parapsoriasis (par'ă-sō-rī'ă-sis). Xanthoerythrodermia perstans; a chronic dermatosis of unknown origin, with erythematous, papular, and scaling lesions appearing in persistent and often enlarging plaques, and resistant to treatment.

p. en plaque, a form of parapsoriasis which frequently develops into mycosis fungoides.

p. gutta'ta, asymptomatic finely scaling superficial erythematous papules on the trunk, thighs, and arms which may remit spontaneously.

p. lichenoi'des, *poikiloderma* atrophicans vasculare.

p. lichenoi'des et variolifor'mis acu'ta, *pityriasis* lichenoides et varioliformis acuta.

p. variolifor'mis, *pityriasis* lichenoides et varioliformis acuta.

parapsychology (par'ă-sī-kol'ō-jē). The study of extrasensory perception, such as thought transference (telepathy) and clairvoyance.

paraquat (par'ă-kwaht). 1,1'-Dimethyl-4,4'-dipyridilium; a weed-killer that produces delayed toxic effects on the liver, kidneys, and lungs when ingested; progressive interstitial pneumonia with proliferation of alveolar lining cells may develop.

pararama (par-ă-rā'mă). Painful or crippling disease of the fingers, first described in Brazilian rubber workers, produced by accidental contact with setae of the larva of the moth, *Premolis semirufa;* immediate pruritus, hyperemia, and local edema may be followed by chronic swelling and immobility that may lead to loss of one or more fingers, presenting a clinical picture corresponding to ankylosis.

pararectal (par-ă-rek'tăl). Near the rectum or rectus muscle.

parareflexia (par'ă-rē-flek'sē-ă). A condition characterized by abnormal reflexes.

pararenal (par-ă-rē'năl). Paranephric (2); near or adjacent to the kidneys.

pararhotacism (par'ă-rō'tă-sizm) [para- + G. *rho,* the letter r]. Substitution of another sound for that of r. See also rhotacism.

pararosanilin (par'ă-rō-san'i-lin) [C.I. 42500]. Parafuchsin; a tri(aminophenyl)methane hydrochloride; an important red biologic stain used in Schiff's reagent to detect cellular DNA (Feulgen stain), mucopolysaccharides (PAS stain), and proteins (ninhydrin-Schiff stain).

pararrhythmia (par-ă-ridh'mē-ă) [para- + G. *rhythmos,* rhythm]. A cardiac dysrhythmia in which two independent rhythms coexist, but not as a result of A-V block; p. thus includes parasystole and A-V dissociation (2), but not complete A-V block.

parasacral (par-ă-sā'krăl). Alongside the sacrum.

parasalpingitis (par'ă-sal-pin-jī'tis) [para- + salpinx + G. *-itis,* inflammation]. Inflammation of the tissues surrounding the fallopian or the eustachian tube.

Parascaris equorum (pa-ras'ka-ris ē-kwō'rŭm). *Ascaris equorum;* a large heavy-bodied ascarid nematode extremely common in the small intestine of horses and other equids. Larvae may develop in man or mice, but do not reach the adult stage.

parascarlatina (par'ă-skar-lă-tē'nă). Fourth *disease.*

parasecretion (par'ă-sē-krē'shŭn). Obsolete term for abnormal secretion.

parasexuality (par'ă-sek-shū-al'i-tē). Abnormal or perverted sexuality.

parasigmatism (par-ă-sig'mă-tizm) [para- + G. *sigma,* the letter s]. Lisping.

parasinoidal (par'ă-sī-noy'dăl). Near a sinus, particularly a cerebral sinus.

parasite (par'ă-sīt) [G. *parasitos,* a guest, fr. *para,* beside, + *sitos,* food]. **1.** An organism that lives on or in another and draws its nourishment therefrom. **2.** In the case of a fetal inclusion or conjoined twins, the usually incomplete twin that derives its support from the more nearly normal autosite.

autistic p., autochthonous p.; a p. descended from the tissues of the host.

autochthonous p., autistic p.

commensal p., see commensal (2).

euroxenous p., a p. with a broad or nonspecific host range.

facultative p., an organism that may either lead an independent existence or live as a p., in contrast to obligate p.

heterogenetic p., a p. whose life cycle involves an alternation of generations.

heteroxenous p., a p. that has more than one obligatory host in its life cycle.

incidental p., a p. that normally lives on a host other than its present host.

inquiline p., see inquiline.

malignant tertian malarial p., *Plasmodium falciparum.*

obligate p., a p. that cannot lead an independent nonparasitic existence, in contrast to facultative p.

quartan p., *Plasmodium malariae.*

specific p., a p. that habitually lives in its present host and is particularly adapted for the host species.

stenoxous p., a p. with a narrow or specific host range.

temporary p., an organism accidentally ingested that survives briefly in the intestine.

tertian p., *Plasmodium vivax.*

parasitemia (păr'ă-sī-tē'mē-ă). The presence of parasites in the circulating blood; used especially with reference to malarial and other protozoan forms, and microfilariae.

parasitic (par-ă-sit'ik). **1.** Relating to or of the nature of a parasite. **2.** Denoting organisms that normally grow only in or on the living body of a host.

parasiticidal (par'ă-sit-i-sī'dăl). Destructive to parasites.

parasiticide (par-ă-sit'i-sīd) [parasite + L. *caedo,* to kill]. An agent that destroys parasites.

parasitism (par'ă-si-tizm). A symbiotic relationship in which one species (the parasite) benefits at the expense of the other (the host). *Cf.* mutualism, commensalism.

multiple p., a condition in which parasites of different species parasitize a single host, in contrast to superparasitism (2) or hyperparasitism.

parasitize (par'ă-si-tīz). To invade as a parasite.

parasitocenose (par-ă-sī'tō-sē-nōz) [parasite + G. *koinos,* common, together]. Parasite-host ecosystem; complex of all parasite species and individuals associated with a specific host.

parasitogenesis (par'ă-sī-tō-jen'ĕ-sis). The evolution of relationships between parasite and host.

parasitogenic (par'-ă-sī-tō-jen'ik) [parasite + G. *-gen,* producing]. **1.** Caused by certain parasites. **2.** Favoring parasitism.

parasitoid (par-ă-sī'toyd) [parasite + G. *eidos,* appearance]. Denoting a feeding relationship intermediate between predation and parasitism, in which the p. eventually destroys its host; refers especially to parasitic wasps (order Hymenoptera) whose larvae feed on and finally destroy a grub or other arthropod host stung by the mother wasp prior to laying its egg(s) on the host.

parasitologist (par'ă-sī-tol'ō-jist). One who specializes in the science of parasitology.

parasitology (par'ă-sī-tol'ō-jē) [parasite + G. *logos,* study]. The branch of biology and of medicine concerned with all aspects of parasitism.

parasitome (par'ă-sī-tōm) [parasite + *-ome* (fr. G. *-ōma*), group, mass]. The total mass or number of individuals of all developmental stages of a single parasite species in one host.

parasitophobia (par'ă-sī-tō-fō'bē-ă) [parasite + G. *phobos,* fear]. Morbid fear of parasites.

parasitosis (par'ă-sī-tō'sis). Infestation or infection with parasites.

parasitotropic (par'ă-sī-tō-trop'ik). Pertaining to or characterized by parasitotropism.

parasitotropism (par'ă-sī-tot'rō-pizm) [parasite + G. *tropē,* a turning]. Parasitotropy; the special affinity of particular drugs or other agents for parasites rather than for their hosts, including microparasites that infect a larger parasite. *Cf.* organotropism.

parasitotropy (par'ă-sī-tot'rō-pē). Parasitotropism.

parasomnia (par-ă-som'nē-ă). Any dysfunction associated with sleep, *e.g.,* somnabulism, pavor nocturnus, enureseis, or nocturnal seizures.

paraspadia, paraspadias (par-ă-spā'dē-ă, -ŭs) [G. *para- spaō,* to draw aside]. An acquired condition in which there is an abnormal opening into the urethra to one side of the normal urethral lumen.

parastasis (par-ă-stā'sis) [G. standing shoulder to shoulder]. The relationship among causal mechanisms that can compensate for, or mask defects in, each other; in genetics, a relationship between non-alleles classified by some as a form of epistasis.

parasternal (par-ă-ster'năl). Alongside the sternum.

parastruma (par-ă-strū'mă) [para- + L. *struma,* a scrofulous tumor]. Obsolete term for a goitrous tumefaction resulting from enlargement of a parathyroid gland.

parasympathetic (par-ă-sim-pa-thet'ik) Pertaining to a division of the autonomic nervous system. See *systema* nervosum autonomicum.

parasympatholytic (par-ă-sim'pă-thō-lit'ik). Parasympathoparalytic; relating to an agent that annuls or antagonizes the effects of the parasympathetic nervous system; *e.g.,* atropine.

parasympathomimetic (par-ă-sim'pă-thō-mi-met'ik) [para- + G. *sympatheia,* sympathy, + *mimētikos,* imitative]. Relating to drugs or chemicals having an action resembling that caused by stimulation of the parasympathetic nervous system. See also cholinomimetic.

parasympathoparalytic (par-ă-sim'pă-thō-par-ă-lit'ik). Parasympatholytic.

parasympathotonia (par-ă-sim'pă-thō-tō'nē-ă). Vagotonia.

parasynanche (par'ă-si-nang'kē) [para- + cynanche]. Rheumatic inflammation of the muscles of the throat, or any angina, especially parotitis.

parasynapsis (par'ă-si-nap'sis) [para- + G. *synapsis,* a connection, junction]. Union of chromosomes side to side in the process of reduction.

parasynovitis (par'ă-si-nō-vī'tis) [para- + synovitis]. Inflammation of the tissues immediately adjacent to a joint.

parasyphilis (par-ă-sif'i-lis). Parasyphilosis; quaternary syphilis; metasyphilis (2); any condition indirectly due to syphilis.

parasyphilitic (par'ă-sif-i-lit'ik). Metasyphilitic (3); denoting certain diseases supposed to be indirectly due to syphilis but presenting none of the recognized lesions of that infection.

parasyphilosis (par'ă-sif-i-lō'sis). Parasyphilis.

parasystole (par-ă-sis'tō-lē) [para- + G. *systolē*, a contracting]. Parasystolic beat; a second automatic rhythm existing simultaneously with normal sinus rhythm, the parasystolic center being protected from the sinus impulses so that its rhythm is undisturbed.

parataxia (par-ă-tak'sē-ă). Parataxis.

parataxic (par-ă-tak'sik). Pertaining to parataxis.

parataxis (par-ă-tak'sis) [para- + G. *taxis*, orderly arrangement]. Parataxia; the psychological state or repository of attitudes, ideas, and experiences accumulated during personality development that are not effectively assimilated or integrated into the growing mass and residue of the other attitudes, ideas, and experiences of an individual's personality.

paratenesis (par-ă-te-nē'sis). Passage of an infective agent by one or a series of paratenic hosts in which the agent is transported between hosts but does not undergo further development.

paratenon (par-ă-ten'on) [para- + G. *tenōn*, tendon]. The tissue, fatty or synovial, between a tendon and its sheath.

paraterminal (par-ă-ter'mi-năl). Near or alongside any terminus.

parathion (par-ă-thī'on). Phosporothioic acid *O,O*- diethyl*O*- (4-nitrophenyl) ester; an organic phosphate insecticide, highly toxic to animals and man, that is an irreversible inhibitor of cholinesterases.

parathormone (par-ă-thōr'mōn). Parathyroid *hormone*.

parathymia (par-ă-thī'mē-ă) [para- + G. *thymos*, soul, mind]. Misdirection of the emotional faculties; disordered mood.

parathyrin (par-ă-thī'rin). Parathyroid *hormone*.

parathyroid (par-ă-thī'royd). **1.** Adjacent to the thyroid gland. **2.** *Glandula* parathyroidea.

parathyroidectomy (pa'ră-thī-roy-dek'to-mē) [parathyroid + G. *ektomē*, excision]. Excision of the parathyroid glands.

parathyrotropic, parathyrotrophic (par'ă-thī-rō-trop'ik, -trof'ik) [parathyroid + G. *tropē*, a turning; *trophē*, nourishment]. Influencing the growth or activity of the parathyroid glands.

paratrichosis (par'ă-tri-kō'sis) [para- + G. *trichōsis*, making or being hairy, fr. *thrix* (*trich-*), hair]. Any disorder in the growth of the hair, with particular reference to quantity.

paratripsis (par-ă-trip'sis) [G. friction, fr. *para*, beside, + *tripsis*, rubbing]. **1.** Chafing. **2.** Obsolete term for retardation of catabolism or of tissue waste.

paratriptic (par-ă-trip'tik). Causing or caused by chafing.

paratrophic (par-ă-trof'ik) [para- + G. *trophē*, nourishment]. Deriving sustenance from living organic material. See also metatrophic; prototrophic.

paratyphlitis (par'ă-tif-lī'tis) [para- + G. *typhlon*, cecum, + *-itis*, inflammation]. Inflammation of the connective tissue adjacent to the cecum.

paratyphoid (par-ă-tī'foyd). Paratyphoid *fever*.

paraumbilical (par'ă-ŭm-bil'i-kal). Paraomphalic; parumbilical; near the umbilicus.

paraurethral (par'ă-yū-rē'thrăl). Alongside the urethra.

paravaccinia (par'ă-vak-sin'ē-ă). Pseudocowpox.

paravaginal (par-ă-vaj'i-năl). Alongside the vagina.

paravaginitis (par'ă-vaj-i-nī'tis). Paracolpitis; inflammation of the connective tissue alongside the vagina.

paravalvular (par-ă-val'vyū-lăr). Alongside or in the vicinity of a valve.

paravenous (par'ă-vē'nŭs). Beside a vein.

paravertebral (par-ă-ver'tĕ-brăl). Alongside a vertebra or the vertebral column.

paravesical (par-ă-ves'i-kăl). Paracystic.

paraxial (par-ak'sē-ăl). By the side of the axis of any body or part.

paraxon (par-ak'son) [para- + G. *axōn*, axis]. A collateral branch of an axon.

Parazoa (par-ă-zō'ă). A subkingdom that includes the sponges (phylum Porifera), considered by many zoologists to be intermediate between the subkingdoms Protozoa and Metazoa.

parazoon (par-ă-zō'on) [para- + G. *zōon*, animal]. **1.** An animal parasite. **2.** A member of the subkingdom Parazoa.

parchment crackling (parch'ment krak'ling). The sensation as of the crackling of stiff paper or parchment, noted on palpation of the skull in cases of craniotabes.

Paré, Ambroïse, French surgeon, 1510–1590. See P.'s *suture*.

parectasis, parectasia (par-ek'tă-sis, -ek-tā'zē-ă) [G. *parektasis*, extrusion, fr. *para*, beside, + *ektasis*, extension]. Extreme distention of a cavity or other part.

parectropia (par-ek-trō'pē-ă) [G. *par-ektropē*, a turning aside]. Apraxia.

paregoric (par-ĕ-gōr'ik) [G. *parēgorkos*, soothing]. Camphorated opium tincture; an antiperistaltic agent containing powdered opium, anise oil, benzoic acid, camphor, glycerin, and diluted alcohol.

pareira (pă-rā'ē-ră) [Pg. *parreira*, vine trained against a wall]. Pareira brava, the root of *Chondodendron tomentosum* and other species of *Chondodendron* (family Menispermaceae), a vine of tropical America; one of the chief sources of *d*- tubocurarine; it has diuretic and urinary antiseptic properties.

parelectronomic (par'ĕ-lek-trō-nom'ik) [para- + G. *ēlektron*, amber (electricity), + *nomos*, law]. Not subject to the laws of electricity, *i.e.*, not excited by an electric stimulus.

parencephalia (par'en-se-fā'lē-ă) [para- + G. *enkephalos*, brain]. Condition of imperfect cerebral development.

parencephalitis (par'en-sef-ă-lī'tis) [parencephalon + G. *-itis*, inflammation]. Inflammation of the cerebellum.

parencephalocele (par-en-sef'ă-lō-sēl) [parencephalon + G. *kēle*, hernia]. Protrusion of the cerebellum through a defect in the cranium.

parencephalous (par-en-sef'ă-lŭs). Relating to parencephalia.

parenchyma (pă-reng'ki-mă) [G. anything poured in beside, fr. *parencheō*, to pour in beside]. **1.** The distinguishing or specific cells of a gland or organ, contained in and supported by the connective tissue framework, or stroma. **2.** The endoplasm of a protozoan cell. **p. tes'tis** [NA], the parenchyma of the testis, consisting of the seminiferous tubules located within the lobules.

parenchymal (pă-reng'ki-măl). Parenchymatous.

parenchymatitis (pă-reng'ki-mă-tī'tis). Inflammation of the parenchyma or differentiated substance of a gland or organ.

parenchymatous (par'eng-kim'ă-tŭs). Parenchymatous; relating to the parenchyma.

parenteral (pă-ren'ter-ăl) [para- + G. *enteron*, intestine]. By some other means than through the gastrointestinal tract; referring particularly to the introduction of substances into an organism by intravenous, subcutaneous, intramuscular, or intramedullary injection.

parepicele (par-ep'i-sēl) [para- + G. *epi,* upon, + *koilia,* a hollow]. The lateral recess of the fourth ventricle of the brain.

parepididymis (par'ep'i-did'i-mis). Paradidymis.

parepithymia (par'ep-i-thī'mē-ă) [para- + G. *epithymia,* desire]. A morbid longing; an abnormal desire or craving.

parerethisis (par-ĕ-rēth'i-sis) [para- + G. *erethizō,* to excite]. Abnormal or morbid excitement.

parergasia (par-er-gā'zē-ă) [para- + G. *ergasia,* work]. Obsolete term for schizophrenia.

paresis (pă-rē'sis, par'ĕ-sis) [G. a letting go, slackening, paralysis, fr. *paritēmi,* to let go]. **1.** Partial or incomplete paralysis. **2.** Dementia paralytica; paralytic dementia; Boyle's disease; a disease of the brain, syphilitic in origin, marked by progressive dementia, tremor, speech disturbances, and increasing muscular weakness; in a large proportion of cases there is a preliminary stage of irritability often followed by exaltation and delusions of grandeur.

parturient p., milk *fever* (2).

paresthesia (par-es-thē'zē-ă) [para- + G. *aisthēsis,* sensation]. Paraesthesia; an abnormal sensation, such as of burning, pricking, tickling, or tingling.

Berger's p., p. of the legs in young patients, especially at the beginning of a movement.

paresthetic (par-es-thet'ik). Relating to or marked by paresthesia; denoting numbness and tingling in an extremity which usually occurs on the resumption of the blood flow to a nerve following temporary pressure or mild injury.

paretic (pa-ret'ik). Relating to or suffering from paresis.

pareunia (par-yū'nē-ă) [G. *pareunos,* lying beside, fr. *para,* beside, + *eunē,* a bed]. Coitus.

pargyline hydrochloride (par'ji-lēn). *N*-Methyl-*N*-(2-propynyl)-benzylamine hydrochloride; a nonhydrazine monoamine oxidase inhibitor, used as an antihypertensive agent.

paridrosis (par-i-drō'sis) [para- + G. *hidrōsis,* sweating]. Parahidrosis; any derangement of perspiration.

paries, gen. **pari'etis,** pl. **parietes** (par'i-ēz, pā'rī-ēz; pă-rī'ĕ-tēz) [L. wall] [NA]. A wall, as of the chest, abdomen, or any hollow organ.

p. ante'rior vagi'nae [NA], anterior wall of vagina; it is somewhat shorter than the posterior wall and at its upper end is penetrated by the cervix uteri.

p. ante'rior ventric'uli [NA], anterior wall of stomach; the part of the gastric wall that faces the peritoneal cavity.

p. carot'icus ca'vi tym'pani [NA], anterior or carotid wall of middle ear; it contains the opening of the auditory (eustachian) tube.

p. exter'nus duc'tus cochlea'ris [NA], external wall of cochlear duct; the wall that faces the outer side of the cochlea.

p. infe'rior or'bitae [NA], inferior wall of orbit; the floor of the orbit; the shortest of the four walls of the orbit, sloping upward from the orbital margin; it is comprised of the maxilla and orbital process of the palatine bone.

p. jugula'ris ca'vi tym'pani [NA], jugular wall of middle ear; fundus tympani; inferior wall of the tympanic cavity; the floor of the tympanic cavity; a thin plate of bone separating the tympanic cavity from the jugular fossa.

p. labyrin'thicus ca'vi tym'pani [NA], labyrinthine or medial wall of middle ear; a bony layer separating the middle from the internal ear or labyrinth; it contains the fenestra vestibuli and the fenestra cochleae.

p. latera'lis or'bitae [NA], lateral wall of orbit; a triangular wall of the orbit formed by the zygomatic bone, the greater wing of the sphenoid bone, and a small part of the frontal bone; posteriorly it is bounded by the superior and inferior orbital fissures.

p. mastoi'deus ca'vi tym'pani [NA], mastoid or posterior wall of middle ear; it contains the opening into the mastoid antrum.

p. media'lis or'bitae [NA], medial wall of orbit; the thin, rectangular wall of the orbit formed by the orbital plate of the ethmoid, lacrimal, frontal and a small part of the sphenoid bones; the fossa for the lacrimal sac lies at its anterior limit.

p. membrana'ceus ca'vi tym'pani [NA], membranous or lateral wall of middle ear; the wall formed mainly by the membrana tympani.

p. membrana'ceus tra'cheae [NA], membranous wall of trachea; the part of the tracheal wall posteriorly that is not reinforced by tracheal cartilages.

p. poste'rior vagi'nae [NA], posterior wall of vagina; it is longer than the anterior wall and has a low ridge in the midline throughout most of its length.

p. posterior ventriculi [NA], posterior wall of stomach; that part of the gastric wall that faces the omental bursa.

p. supe'rior or'bitae [NA], superior wall of orbit; roof of orbit; formed by the orbital plate of the frontal bone and the lesser wing of the sphenoid bone, the optic canal opens at its posterior limit; an indentation, the fossa for the lacrimal gland, is located in the anterolateral part of the roof.

p. tegmenta'lis ca'vi tym'pani [NA], tegmental wall of middle ear; the superior wall, or roof, of the tympanic cavity, formed by the tegmen tympani of the temporal bone.

p. tympan'icus duc'tus cochlea'ris [NA], tympanic wall of cochlear duct; membrana spiralis; spiral membrane; the wall that separates the cochlear duct from the scala tympani; it consists of the osseous spiral lamina and the basilar membrane.

p. vestibula'ris duc'tus cochlea'ris [NA], vestibular wall of cochlear duct; membrana vestibularis; spiral or vestibular membrane; Reissner's membrane; the membrane separating the ductus cochlearis from the scala vestibuli; it consists of squamous epithelial cells with microvilli toward the ductus, a basement membrane, and a thin layer of connective tissue toward the scala.

parietal (pă-rī'ĕ-tăl). Relating to the wall of any cavity.

parietes (pă-rī'ĕ-tēz) [L.]. Plural of paries.

parieto- [L. *paries,* wall]. Combining form denoting relationship to a wall (paries).

parietofrontal (pa-rī'ĕ-tō-fron'tăl). Relating to the parietal and the frontal bones or the parts of the cerebral cortex corresponding thereto.

parietography (pa-rī'ĕ-tog'ră-fē) [parieto- + G. *graphē,* a writing]. A roentgenographic examination using a combination of pneumoperitoneum and air or barium in the stomach.

parietomastoid (pă-rī'ĕ-to-mas'toyd). Relating to the parietal bone and the mastoid portion of the temporal bone.

parieto-occipital (pă-rī'ĕ-tō-ok-sip'i-tăl). Relating to the parietal and occipital bones or to the parts of the cerebral cortex corresponding thereto.

parietosphenoid (pă-rī'ĕ-tō-sfē'noyd). Relating to the parietal and the sphenoid bones.

parietosplanchnic (pă-rī'ĕ-tō-splangk'nik). Parietovisceral.

parietosquamosal (pă-rī'ĕ-tō-skwā-mō'săl). Relating to the parietal bone and the squamous portion of the temporal bone.

parietotemporal (pă-rī'ĕ-tō-tem'pō-răl). Relating to the parietal and the temporal bones.

parietovisceral (pă-rī'ĕ-tō-vis'er-ăl). Parietosplanchnic; relating to the wall of a cavity and to the contained viscera.

Parinaud, Henri, French ophthalmologist, 1844–1905. See P.'s *conjunctivitis, ophthalmoplegia, syndrome,* oculoglandular *syndrome.*

Paris green. Cupric acetoarsenite, used as an insecticide and as a pigment.

Paris yellow [C.I. 77600]. *Chrome* yellow.

parity (par'ĭ-tē) [L. *pario,* to bear]. The condition of having given birth to an infant or infants, alive or dead; a multiple birth is considered as a single parous experience.

Park, Henry, British surgeon, 1744–1831. See P.'s *aneurysm.*

Park, William H., U.S. bacteriologist, 1863–1939. See P.-Williams *bacillus, fixative.*

Parker, Edward Mason, U.S. surgeon, 1860–1941. See P.-Kerr *suture.*

Parker, George H., U.S. zoologist, 1864–1955. See P.'s *fluid.*

Parker, Willard, U.S. surgeon, 1800–1884. See P.'s *incision.*

Parkinson, James, British physician, 1755–1824. See parkinsonism (1); P.'s *disease, facies.*

Parkinson, Sir John, British cardiologist, *1885. See Wolff-P.-White *syndrome.*

parkinsonian (par-kin-sō'nē-an). Relating to or the suffering from parkinsonism (1).

parkinsonism (par'kin-son-izm) [J. Parkinson]. **1.** Parkinson's disease; shaking or trembling palsy; spasmus agitans; a neurological syndrome usually resulting from deficiency of the neurotransmitter dopamine as the consequence of degenerative, vascular, or inflammatory changes in the basal ganglia; characterized by rhythmical muscular tremors, rigidity of movement, festination, droopy posture, and masklike facies. **2.** A syndrome similar to p. appearing as a side effect of certain antipsychotic drugs.

Parnas, Jakob Karol, Polish physiologic chemist, 1884–1955. See Embden-Meyerhof-P. *pathway.*

paroccipital (par'ok-sip'i-tăl) [para- + occipital]. Near or beside the occipital bone or the occiput.

parodontitis (par'ō-don-tī'tis). Obsolete term for periodontitis.

parodontium (par-ō-don'shē-ŭm) [para- + G. *odous,* tooth]. Periodontium.

parodynia (par-ō-din'ē-ă) [L. *pario,* to bear, + G. *odynē,* pain]. Labor *pains.*

parole (pă-rōl'). In psychiatry, term for conditional release of a formally committed patient from a mental hospital prior to formal discharge, so that the patient may be returned to the hospital if necessary without fresh legal action.

parolfactory (par-ol-fak'tōr-ē). Associated with or related to the olfactory system.

parolivary (par-ol'i-văr-ē) [para- + L. *oliva,* olive]. By the side of or near the oliva.

paromomycin sulfate (par'ō-mō-mī'sin). A broad spectrum antibiotic produced by *Streptomyces rimosus* forma *paromomycinus;* used in the treatment of bacterial enteritis and amebiasis, and for preoperative suppression of intestinal bacteria.

paromphalocele (par-om'fă-lō-sēl) [para- + G. *omphalos,* umbilicus, + *kēlē,* tumor, hernia]. **1.** A tumor near the umbilicus. **2.** A hernia through a defect in the abdominal wall near the umbilicus.

Parona, Francesco, 19th century Italian surgeon. See P.'s *space.*

paroneiria, paroniria (par-ō-nī'rē-ă) [para- + G. *oneiros,* dream]. Rarely used term for disagreeable or terrifying dreams.

p. sa'lax, rarely used term denoting restlessness in sleep, with lascivious dreams and nocturnal emissions.

paronychia (par-ō-nik'ē-ă) [para- + G. *onyx,* nail]. Onychia lateralis; onychia periungualis; inflammation of the nail fold with separation of the skin from the proximal portion of the nail; may be due to bacteria or fungi.

paronychial (par-ō-nik'ē-ăl). Relating to paronychia.

paroophoritis (par'ō-of'ō-rī'tis) [paroophoron + G. *-itis,* inflammation]. Inflammation of tissues adjacent to the ovaries.

paroöphoron (par-ō-of'ōr-on) [para- + oophoron, ovary] [NA]. Corpus pampiniforme; parovarium; remnants of the tubules and glomeruli of the lower part of the wolffian body appearing as a few scattered tubules in the broad ligament between the epoophoron and the uterus.

parophthalmia (par'of-thal'mē-ă) [para- + G. *ophthalmos,* eye]. Inflammation of the tissues around the eye.

paropsia, paropsis (par-op'sē-ă, par-op'sis) [para- + G. *opsis,* vision]. Disorientation of the perception of direction in hemianopia caused by occipital lesions.

parorchidium (par-ōr-kid'ē-ŭm) [para- + G. *orchis,* testis]. *Ectopia* testis.

parorchis (par-ōr'kis) [para- + G. *orchis,* testis]. Epididymis.

parorexia (par-ō-rek'sē-ă) [para- + G. *orexis,* appetite]. An abnormal or disordered appetite.

parosmia (par-oz'mē-ă) [para + G. *osmē,* sense of smell]. Parosphresia; any disorder of the sense of smell, especially subjective perception of nonexistent odors.

parosphresia (par-os-frē'zē-ă) [para- + G. *osphrēsis,* smell]. Parosmia.

parosteal (par-os'tē-ăl). Relating to the tissues immediately adjacent to the periosteum of a bone.

parosteitis (păr-os-tē-ī'tis) [para- + G. *osteon,* bone, + *-itis,* inflammation]. Parostitis; inflammation of the tissues immediately adjacent to a bone.

parosteosis, parostosis (par'os-tē-ō'sis, -os-tō'sis) [para- + G. *osteon,* bone, + *-osis,* condition]. **1.** Development of bone in an unusual location, as in the skin. **2.** Abnormal or defective ossification.

parostitis (par-os-tī'tis). Parosteitis.

parotic (pă-rot'ik) [para- + G. *ous,* ear]. Near or beside the ear.

parotid (pă-rot'id) [G. *parōtis* (*parōtid-*), the gland beside the ear, fr. *para,* beside, + *ous* (*ōt-*), ear]. Situated near the ear; denoting several structures in this neighborhood. Usually refers to the p. salivary gland.

parotidectomy (pă-rot'i-dek'tō-mē) [parotid + G. *ektomē,* excision]. Surgical removal of the parotid gland.

parotiditis (pă-rot-i-dī'tis). Parotitis; inflammation of the parotid gland.

epidemic p., mumps; an acute infectious and contagious disease caused by a Paramyxovirus and characterized by fever, inflammation and swelling of the parotid gland, sometimes of other salivary glands, and occasionally by inflammation of the testis, ovary, pancreas, or meninges.

postoperative p., an acute inflammation of the parotid gland occurring in the postoperative period, especially in debilitated or dehydrated patients; frequently results in abscess formation and rapidly spreading cellulitis that may become fatal.

punctate p., recurrent or chronic p. with terminal sialectasis, giving a punctate pattern on sialography; associated with epithelial hyperplasia of intralobular ducts, atrophy of acini, and lymphocytic infiltration.

parotidoauricularis (pă-rot'i-dō-aw-rik-yū-lā'ris). **1.** An occasional band of muscle fibers passing from the surface of the parotid gland to the auricle. **2.** Relating to the parotid gland and the external ear.

parotin (par'ō-tin). Salivary gland hormone; a globulin obtained from parotid glands, that causes hypocalcemia, has effects on mesenchymal tissues, produces first leukopenia and then leukocytosis, and promotes calcification of dentin.

parotitis (par-o-tī'tis). Parotiditis.

parous (par'ŭs) [L. *pario,* to bear]. Pertaining to parity.

parovarian (par-ō-var'ē-an). **1.** Relating to the paroophoron. **2.** Paraovarian; beside or in the neighborhood of the ovary.

parovariotomy (par'ō-var-ē-ot'ō-mē) [parovarium + G. *tomē,* incision]. Incision into or removal of a tumor of the parovarium.

parovaritis (par'ō-var-ī'tis). Inflammation of the parovarium.

parovarium (par-ō-var'ē-ŭm) [para- + L. *ovarium,* ovary]. Paroophoron.

paroxypropione (par-ok-si-prō'pē-ōn). *p*-Hydroxypropiophenone; an inhibitor of pituitary gonadotropic hormone.

paroxysm (par'ok-sizm) [G. *paroxysmos,* fr. *paroxynō,* to sharpen, irritate, fr. *oxys,* sharp]. **1.** A sharp spasm or convulsion. **2.** A sudden onset of a symptom or disease, especially one with recurrent manifestations such as the chills and rigor of malaria.

paroxysmal (par-ok-siz'măl). Relating to or occurring in paroxysms.

parricide (par'i-sīd) [L. *parricidium,* killing of close kin]. **1.** The killing of one's parent (patricide or matricide). **2.** One who commits such an act.

Parrot, Jules, French physician, 1829–1883. See P.'s *disease.*

Parry, Caleb H., British physician, 1755–1822. See P.'s *disease.*

PARS

pars, pl. **partes** (pars, par'tēz) [L. *pars* (*part-*) a part] [NA]. A part; a portion.

p. abdomina'lis [NA], abdominal part; **p. a. aor'tae** [NA], abdominal part of the aorta; aorta abdominalis; the part of the p. descendens aortae that supplies structures below the diaphragm. See also *ductus* thoracicus; **p. a. duc'tus thora'cicus** [NA], the part of the thoracic duct between the cisterna chyli and the aortic hiatus of the diaphragm; **p. a. esoph'agi** [NA], the part of the esophagus inferior to the diaphragm; **p. a. ure'teris** [NA], the part of the ureter between the renal pelvis and the brim of the pelvis.

p. ala'ris [NA], alar part. See *musculus* nasalis.

p. alveola'ris mandib'ulae [NA], alveolar part of mandible; the portion of the body of the mandible that surrounds and supports the lower teeth.

p. amor'pha, the part of the nucleolus which occupies irregular spaces in the nucleolonema and contains finely filamentous substance. See also p. granulosa.

p. annula'ris vagi'nae fibro'sae [NA], annulus of fibrous sheath; ligamentum annulare digitorum; one of the two circular fibrous bands of the fibrous sheaths of the fingers and toes attached to the shaft of the proximal and middle phalanges.

p. ante'rior [NA], anterior part; **p. a. commissu'rae anterio'ris** or **rostralis** [NA], the anterior part of the anterior or rostral commissure of the brain; **p. a. fa'cies diaphragma'tis** [NA], the part of the diaphragmatic surface of the liver deep to the costal arches and the xiphoid process; **p. a. for'nix vagi'nae** [NA], the portion of the fornix of the vagina anterior to the cervix uteri.

p. ascen'dens [NA], ascending part; **p. a. aor'tae** [NA], ascending part of the aorta; aorta ascendens; the part of the aorta from which arise the coronary arteries; **p. a. duode'ni** [NA], the terminal part of the duodenum, ascending from the horizontal part to the jejunum.

p. atlan'tica [NA], see *arteria* vertebralis.

p. autonom'ica [NA], autonomic part; systema nervosum autonomicum; autonomic, involuntary, vegetative, or visceral nervous system; that part of the nervous system which represents the motor innervation of smooth muscle, cardiac muscle, and gland cells. It consists of two physiologically and anatomically distinct, mutually antagonistic components: p. sympathetica and p. parasympathetica. In both of these parts the pathway of innervation consists of a synaptic sequence of two motor neurons, one of which lies in the spinal cord or brainstem as the preganglionic neuron, the thin but myelinated axon of which (preganglionic or B fiber) emerges with an outgoing spinal or cranial nerve and synapses with one or more of the postganglionic (or, more strictly, ganglionic) neurons composing the autonomic ganglia; the unmyelinated postganglionic fibers in turn innervate the smooth muscle, cardiac muscle, or gland cells. The preganglionic neurons of p. sympathetica lie in the columna lateralis of the thoracic and upper two lumbar segments of the spinal gray matter; those of p. parasympathetica compose the visceral motor (visceral efferent) nuclei of the brainstem as well as the columna lateralis of the second to fourth sacral segments of the spinal cord. The ganglia of the p. sympathetica are the paravertebral ganglia of the sympathetic trunk and the prevertebral or collateral ganglia; those of the p. parasympathetica lie either near the organ to be innervated or as intramural ganglia within the organ itself. Impulse transmission from preganglionic to the postganglionic neuron is mediated by acetylcholine in both the p. sympathetica and p. parasympathetica; transmission from the postganglionic fiber to the visceral effector tissues is classically said to be acetylcholine in p. parasympathetica and by noradrenalin in p. sympathetica; recent evidence suggests the existence of further non-cholinergic, non-adrenergic classes of postganglionic fibers.

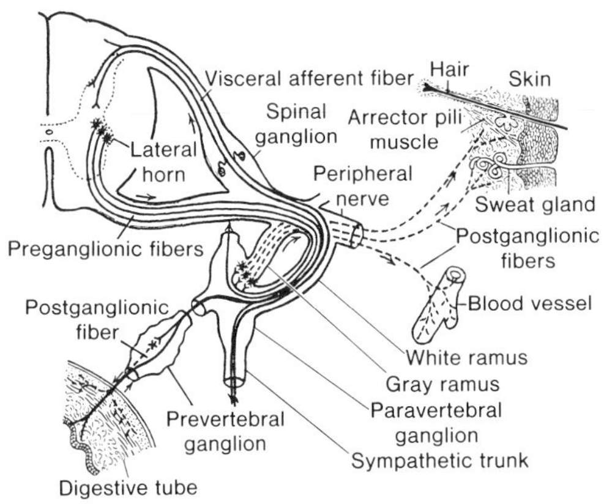

Pars Autonomica (Autonomic Nervous System)
Diagram of the neural reflex arcs of the sympathetic system.

p. basa'lis arte'riae pulmona'lis [NA], basal part of pulmonary artery; see *arteria* pulmonalis dextra; *arteria* pulmonalis sinistra.

p. basila'ris os'sis occipita'lis [NA], basal part of occipital bone; basilar apophysis; basilar process; the part of the occipital bone that lies anterior to the foramen magnum and joins with the body of the sphenoid bone.

p. basila'ris pon'tis, p. ventralis pontis.

p. buccopharyn'gea [NA], buccopharyngeal part. See *musculus* constrictor pharyngis superior.

p. cardi'aca ventric'uli [NA], cardiac part of stomach; cardia; the area of the stomach close to the esophageal opening (cardiac opening) which contains the cardiac glands.

p. cartilagin'ea sep'ti na'si, *cartilago* septi nasi.

p. cartilagin'ea tu'bae auditi'vae [NA], cartilaginous part of auditory tube; that portion of the auditory tube that is supported by cartilage; it continues anteromedially from the osseous part to open into the nasopharynx.

p. cartilagino'sa systema'tis skeleta'lis [NA], cartilaginous part of skeletal system; the part of the skeleton composed of cartilage.

p. cauda'lis [NA], caudal part; the lower part of the vestibular ganglion that receives fibers from the macula of the saccule and the ampulla of the posterior semicircular duct.

p. caverno'sa, p. spongiosa urethrae masculinae.

p. caverno'sa arte'riae carot'is inter'nae [NA], cavernous part of internal carotid artery; the tortuous portion of the internal carotid artery located within the cavernous sinus; it has numerous small branches.

p. ce'ca ret'inae, the embryological anterior part of the retina that evolves into the p. ciliaris retinae and p. iridica retinae.

p. centra'lis [NA], central part; systema nervosum centrale; central nervous system; the brain and the spinal cord.

p. centra'lis ventric'uli latera'lis [NA], cella media; the body of the lateral ventricle of the brain, extending from the interventricular foramen (of Monro) to the collateral trigone (*i.e.,* junction of posterior and inferior horns).

p. ceratopharyn'gea [NA], ceratopharyngeal part. See *musculus* constrictor pharyngis medius.

p. cerebra'lis arte'riae carot'is inter'nae [NA], cerebral part of internal carotid artery; the portion of the internal carotid artery that supplies the brain; its branches are: superior hypophyseal, clival, ophthalmic, anterior choroidal, anterior cerebral, and middle cerebral.

p. cervica'lis [NA], cervical part; **p. c. arte'riae carot'is inter'nae** [NA], cervical part of the internal carotid artery; the unbranched portion located in the neck; **p. c. duc'tus thora'cici** [NA], the portion of the thoracic duct above the first rib; **p. c. esoph'agi** [NA], cervical part of the esophagus; the part of the esophagus located in the neck; **p. c. medul'lae spina'lis** [NA], segmenta medullae spinalis cervicalia; cervical part or segments of the spinal cord; the part of the spinal cord that gives rise to the first eight pairs of spinal nerves.

p. chondropharyn'gea [NA], chondropharyngeal part. See *musculus* constrictor pharyngis medius.

p. cilia'ris ret'inae [NA], ciliary part of retina. See retina.

p. clavicula'ris [NA], clavicular part. See *musculus* pectoralis major.

p. coccyg'ea medul'lae spina'lis [NA], segmenta medullae spinalis coccygea; coccygeal part of spinal cord; segments of spinal cord; the terminal part of the spinal cord from which the three pairs of coccygeal nerves originate.

p. cochlea'ris [NA], *nervus* cochlearis.

p. convolu'ta lo'buli cortica'lis re'nis [NA], convoluted part of kidney lobule; labyrinthus (3); renal labyrinth; Ludwig's labyrinth; proximal and distal convoluted tubules and the associated renal corpuscles supplied by branches of the interlobular arteries.

p. corneosclera'lis [NA], corneoscleral part; the anterior part of the reticulum trabeculare, located between the venous sinus of the sclera, the scleral spur, and the posterior limiting membrane of the cornea.

par'tes corpo'ris huma'ni [NA], parts of human body; the head, neck, trunk, and limbs.

p. cortica'lis [NA], cortical part. See *arteria* cerebri media; *arteria* cerebri posterior.

p. costa'lis diaphragma'tis [NA], costal part of diaphragm; the part of the diaphragm that arises from the inner aspect of the lower six costal cartilages and the lower four ribs and inserts on the anterolateral part of the central tendon.

p. cricopharyn'gea [NA], cricopharyngeal part; Killian's bundle. See *musculus* constrictor pharyngis inferior.

p. crucifor'mis vagi'nae fibro'sae [NA], cruciform part of fibrous sheath; ligamenta cruciata digitorum; crucial ligament (4); the fibers of the fibrous sheath of the fingers and toes which form X-shaped patterns over the region of the interphalangeal joints.

p. cupula'ris [NA], cupular or cupulate part; the dome-shaped, highest portion of the epitympanic recess.

p. cys'tica, the smaller caudal division of the primitive embryonic hepatic bud, developing into the gallbladder and cystic duct.

p. descen'dens [NA], descending part; **p. d. aor'tae** [NA], descending part of the aorta; aorta descendens; a part of the aorta, further divided into the p. thoracica aortae and p. abdominalis aortae; **p. d. duode'ni** [NA], the second portion of the duodenum.

p. dex'tra [NA], right part; the part of the diaphragmatic surface of the liver deep to the bodies of the lower ribs on the right side.

p. dista'lis [NA], the larger part of the adenohypophysis composed of cords of epithelial cells individually specialized to secrete various tropic hormones which exert their effect on several target organs in the body. The secretory activity of these cells is under the control of either releasing or inhibiting factors elaborated by hypothalamic neurons and transported to the adenohypophysis by the hypothalamo-hypophysial portal system.

p. dorsa'lis pon'tis [NA], dorsal part of the pons; tegmentum of the pons; the part of the pons bounded laterally by the middle cerebellar peduncles and anteriorly by the p. ventralis pontis; it is continuous with the tegmentum of the mesencephalon and contains long tracts such as the medial and lateral lemnisci, cranial nerve nuclei, and reticular formation.

p. endocri'na pancrea'tis, see pancreas.

p. exocri'na pancrea'tis, see pancreas.

p. feta'lis placen'tae [NA], placenta fetalis; fetal placenta; the chorionic portion of the placenta, containing the fetal blood vessels, from which the funis develops; specifically, in humans, it develops from the chorion frondosum.

p. flac'cida membra'nae tym'pani [NA], membrana flaccida; flaccid membrane; Shrapnell's membrane; Rivinus' membrane; flaccid part of tympanic membrane.

p. fronta'lis corpo'ris callo'si, *forceps* minor.

par'tes genita'les femini'nae exter'nae, *organa* genitalia feminina externa.

par'tes genita'les masculi'nae exter'nae, *organa* genitalia masculina externa.

p. glossopharyn'gea [NA], glossopharyngeal part. See *musculus* constrictor pharyngis superior.

p. granulo'sa, the granular and filamentous part of the nucleolonema of the nucleolus.

p. hepat'ica, the larger cranial division of the primitive embryonic hepatic bud, developing into the liver proper.

p. horizonta'lis, horizontal part. See duodenum.

p. infe'rior [NA], inferior part; **p. i. duode'ni** [NA], the third part of the duodenum, **p. i. gang'lion vestibula'ris** [NA], the part of the vestibular ganglion that receives fibers from the macula of the saccule and the ampulla of the posterior semicircular duct; **p. i. ra'mus lingula'ris** [NA], the vein draining the inferior lingular bronchopulmonary segment of the left lung.

p. infraclavicula'ris plex'us brachia'lis [NA], infraclavicular part of brachial plexus; the part of the brachial plexus that extends from the level of the clavicle downward into the axilla; it includes the cords of the plexus and their branches.

p. infraloba'ris [NA], infralobar part; the vein draining the posterior segment of the right lung that emerges inferior to the superior lobe; tributary to the posterior branch of the right superior pulmonary vein.

p. infrasegmenta'lis [NA], p. intersegmentalis; infrasegmental or intersegmental part; a vein receiving blood from adjacent bronchopulmonary segments; it emerges from the inferior margin of a segment to become a tributary of a branch of a pulmonary vein.

p. infundibula'ris, p. tuberalis.

p. insula'ris [NA], insular part. See *arteria* cerebri media.

p. intercartilagin'ea ri'mae glot'tidis [NA], intercartilaginous part of glottic opening; glottis respiratoria; the opening between the vocal processes of the arytenoid cartilages.

p. interme'dia [NA], intermediate part; **p. i. lo'bi anterio'ris hypophys'eos** [NA], the part of the adenohypophysis located between the pars distalis and the nervous lobe; poorly developed in humans; **p. i. commissu'ra bulbo'rum** [NA], bulborum; *nervus* intermedius.

p. intermembrana'cea ri'mae glot'tidis [NA], intermembranous part of glottic opening; glottis vocalis; the portion of the opening anterior to the vocal processes of the arytenoid cartilages bounded by the vocal ligaments.

p. intersegmenta'lis [NA], official alternate term for p. infrasegmentalis.

p. intracanic'ulus ner'vi op'tici [NA], intracanicular part of optic nerve; the part of the optic nerve lying within the optic canal.

p. intracrania'lis [NA], intracranial part; **p. i. arte'riae vertebra'lis** [NA], see *arteria* vertebralis; **p. i. ner'vi op'tici** [NA], the part of the optic nerve between the optic canal and the optic chiasm.

p. intralamina'ris ner'vi op'tici [NA], intralaminar part of optic nerve; the portion of the optic nerve as it passes through the lamina cribrosa of the sclera.

p. intraloba'ris [NA], intralobar part; the vein draining the apical and posterior segments of the right lung; tributary to the posterior branch of the right superior pulmonary vein.

p. intraocula'ris ner'vi op'tici [NA], intraocular part of optic nerve; the part of the optic nerve within the eye; it is divided into intralaminar, postlaminar, and prelaminar parts.

p. intrasegmenta'lis [NA], intrasegmental part; a vein emerging from the bronchopulmonary segment it drains; a tributary to a branch of a pulmonary vein.

p. irid'ica ret'inae [NA], iridial part of retina. See retina.

p. labia'lis [NA], labial part; the major part of the obicularis oris muscle within the body of the lips.

p. lacrima'lis mus'culi orbicula'ris oc'uli [NA], see *musculus* orbicularis oculi.

p. laryn'gea pharyn'gis [NA], laryngeal part of pharynx; hypopharynx; laryngopharynx; laryngeal pharynx; the part of the pharynx lying below the aperture of the larynx and behind the larynx; it extends from the vestibule of the larynx to the esophagus at the level of the inferior border of the cricoid cartilage.

p. latera'lis [NA], lateral part; **p. l. ar'cus pe'dis longitudina'lis** [NA], see *arcus* pedis longitudinalis; **p. l. for'nix vagi'nae** [NA], see *fornix* vaginae; **p. l. mus'culi intertransversa'rii posterio'res cer'vicis** [NA], see *musculi* intertransversarii posteriores cervicis; **p. l. os'sis occipita'lis** [NA], exoccipital bone; the part of the occipital bone that lies on either side of the foramen magnum; **p. l. os'sis sa'cri** [NA], the lateral mass of the sacrum formed by the fused costal elements; **p. l. ve'nae pulmona'lis** [NA], the vein draining the lateral bronchopulmonary segment of the middle lobe of the right lung.

p. lumba'lis [NA], lumbar part; **p. l. diaphragma'tis** [NA], lumbar part of diaphragm; vertebral part of diaphragm; the portion of the diaphragm that arises from the upper lumbar vertebrae and from the medial and lateral arcuate ligaments. See *crus* dextrum, *crus* sinistrum, *ligamentum* arcuatum; **p. l. medul'lae spina'lis** [NA], segmenta medullae spinalis lumbalia; lumbar part or segments of the spinal cord; that part of the cord giving rise to the five pairs of lumbar nerves.

p. margina'lis [NA], marginal part; the part of the orbicularis oris muscle located in the margin of the lips, *i.e.,* the red area.

p. mastoi'dea, mastoid part; the portion of the petrous part of the temporal bone bearing the mastoid process.

p. media'lis [NA], medial part; **p. m. ar'cus pe'dis longitudina'lis** [NA], see *arcus* pedis longitudinalis; **p. m. mus'culi intertransversa'rii posterio'res cer'vicis** [NA], see *musculi* intertransversarii posteriores cervicis; **p. m. ve'nae pulmo'nis** [NA], the vein draining the medial bronchopulmonary segment of the middle lobe of the right lung.

p. mediastina'lis [NA], mediastinal part; the part of the medial surface of a lung in contact with the mediastinum.

p. membrana'cea [NA], membranous part; **p. m. sep'ti atrio'rum,** *septum* atrioventriculare; **p. m. sep'ti interventricula'ris** [NA], membranous septum (2); septum membranaceum ventriculorum; septum musculare ventriculorum; the membranous portion of the interventricular septum of the heart; **p. m. sep'ti na'si** [NA], membranous part of the nasal septum; membranous septum (1); the small portion of the nasal septum anterior to the portion supported by the cartilage of the nasal septum; **p. m. ure'thrae masculi'nae** [NA], membranous part of male urethra; membranous urethra; the portion of the male urethra, about 1 cm in length, extending from the prostate to the beginning of the urethra in the corpus spongiosum just beyond the bulb.

p. mo'bilis sep'ti na'si [NA], septum mobile nasi; the anterior movable part of the nasal septum formed by the medial crus of the greater alar cartilage on each side.

p. muscula'ris sep'ti interventricula'ris [NA], the muscular portion of the interventricular septum of the heart.

p. mylopharyn'gea [NA], mylopharyngeal part. See *musculus* constrictor pharyngis superior.

p. nasa'lis [NA], nasal part; **p. n. os'sis fronta'lis** [NA], nasal portion of the frontal bone which lies between the two orbital parts anteriorly and forms part of the roof of the nasal cavity; **p. n. pharyn'gis** [NA], nasal part of pharynx; nasal pharynx; pharyngonasal cavity; epipharynx; nasopharynx; rhinopharynx; the part of the pharynx that lies above the soft palate; anteriorly it opens into the nasal cavity.

p. nervo'sa hypophys'eos, neurohypophysis.

p. nervo'sa ret'inae [NA], see retina.

p. obli'qua, [NA], oblique part. See *musculus* cricothyroideus.

p. occipita'lis corpo'ris callo'si, *forceps* major.

p. opercula'ris, one of the three small cortical convolutions together forming a cover for the insular region. Opercular convolutions are frontal, temporal, and parietal.

p. op'tica ret'inae [NA], *stratum* cerebrale retinae.

p. ora'lis pharyn'gis [NA], oral part of pharynx; oropharynx; oral pharynx; the portion of the pharynx that lies posterior to the mouth; it is continuous above with the nasopharynx and below with the laryngopharynx.

p. orbita'lis, orbital part; **p. o. glan'dulae lacrima'lis** [NA], see *glandula* lacrimalis; **p. o. mus'culi orbicula'ris oc'uli** [NA], see *musculus* orbicularis oculi; **p. o. ner'vi op'tici** [NA], orbital part of optic nerve; the part of the optic nerve between the eye and the optic canal; **p. o. os'sis fronta'lis** [NA], the portion of the frontal bone that contributes to the formation of the orbits; the most rostral of three cortical convolutions that together form the inferior frontal gyrus.

p. os'sea sep'ti na'si [NA], bony part of nasal septum; the major portion of the nasal septum supported by the vomer and the perpendicular plate of the ethmoid.

p. os'sea systema'tis skeleta'lis [NA], osseous part of skeletal system; the part of the skeleton composed of bone.

p. os'sea tu'bae auditi'vae [NA], bony part of auditory tube; the portion of the auditory tube that passes from the tympanic cavity anteromedially through the semicanalis tubae auditivae.

p. palpebra'lis [NA], palpebral part; **p. p. glan'dulae lacrima'lis** [NA], see *glandula* lacrimalis; **p. p. mus'culi orbicula'ris oc'uli** [NA], see *musculus* orbicularis oculi.

p. parasympath'ica [NA], parasympathetic part; parasympathetic nervous *system;* bulbosacral or craniosacral system; the parasympathetic part of the autonomic nervous system. See p. autonomica.

p. pelvi'ca, pelvic part; **p. p. ure'teris** [NA], the part of the ureter between the brim of the pelvis and the urinary bladder; the upper pelvic portion of the embryologic urogenital sinus.

p. peripher'ica, peripheral part; systema nervosum periphericum; peripheral nervous system; the part of the nervous system external to the brain and spinal cord from their roots to their peripheral terminations. This includes the ganglia, both sensory and autonomic and any plexuses through which the nerve fibers run. See also p. autonomica.

p. perpendicula'ris, *lamina* perpendicularis.

p. petro'sa [NA], petrous part; **p. p. arte'riae carot'is inter'nae** [NA], petrous part of internal carotid artery; the part of the internal carotid artery in the carotid canal; its branches are carotidotympanic arteries and the artery of the pterygoid canal; **p. p. os'sis tempora'lis** [NA], petrous part of temporal bone; periotic, petrosal, or petrous bone; petrous pyramid; the part of the temporal bone that contains the structures of the inner ear and the second part of the internal carotid artery; in antenatal life it appears as a separate ossification center.

p. phal'lica, the lower portion of the urogenital sinus, related to the base of the genital tubercle.

p. pharyn'gea hypophys'eos, pharyngeal *hypophysis.*

p. pigmento'sa [NA], see retina.

p. pla'na, *orbiculus* ciliaris.

p. postcommunica'lis [NA], postcommunical part. See *arteria* cerebri anterior; *arteria* cerebri posterior.

p. poste'rior [NA], posterior part; **p. p. commissu'rae anterio'ris** [NA], the posterior portion of the anterior commissure of the brain; **p. p. fa'cies diaphragma'tis hep'atis** [NA], that portion of the diaphragmatic surface of the liver that includes the bare area and the caudate lobe; **p. p. for'nix vagi'nae** [NA], see *fornix* vaginae.

p. postlamina'ris ner'vi op'tici [NA], postlaminar part of optic nerve; the portion of the optic nerve posterior to the lamina cribrosa of the sclera.

p. postsulca'lis [NA], postsulcal part. See *dorsum* linguae.

p. precommunica'lis [NA], precommunical part. See *arteria* cerebri anterior; *arteria* cerebri posterior.

p. prelamina'ris ner'vi op'tici [NA], prelaminar part of optic nerve; the portion of the optic nerve anterior to the lamina cribrosa of the sclera.

p. presulca'lis [NA], presulcal part. See *dorsum* linguae.

p. profun'da [NA], deep part; **p. p. glan'dulae parotid'eae** [NA], see *glandula* parotidea; **p. p. mus'culi masse'teri** [NA], see *musculus* masseter; **p. p. mus'culi sphinc'teri a'ni exter'ni** [NA], see *musculus* sphincter ani externus.

p. prostat'ica ure'thrae [NA], prostatic urethra; the prostatic part of the male urethra, about 2.5 cm in length, that traverses the prostate.

p. pterygopharyn'gea [NA], pterygopharyngeal part. See *musculus* constrictor pharyngis superior.

p. pylo'rica ventric'uli [NA], pyloric part of the stomach; that portion of the stomach between the angular notch and the pylorus; its mucosa contains pyloric glands.

p. quadra'ta [NA], quadrate part; the part of the medial segment of the liver which includes the quadrate lobe.

p. radia'ta lo'buli cortica'lis re'nis [NA], medullary ray; Ferrein's pyramid; processus ferreini; the center of the renal lobule, which has the shape of a small, steep pyramid, consisting of straight tubular parts; these may be either ascending or descending limbs of the nephronic loop or collecting tubules.

p. rec'ta [NA], straight part. See *musculus* cricothyroideus.

p. retrolentifor'mis cap'sulae inter'nae [NA], retrolenticular limb of the internal capsule; that portion of the capsule caudal to the lentiform nucleus which contains large parts of the optic or geniculocalcarine radiation and other fiber systems.

p. rostra'lis [NA], rostral part; the superior part of the vestibular ganglion that receives fibers from the maculae of the utricle and the saccule and the ampullae of the anterior and lateral semicircular ducts.

p. sacra'lis medul'lae spina'lis [NA], segmenta medullae spinalis sacralis; sacral part or segments of the spinal cord; the part of the cord from which five pairs of sacral nerves originate.

p. sella'ris, *sella* turcica.

p. sphenoida'lis [NA], sphenoidal part. See *arteria* cerebri media.

p. spina'lis [NA], spinal part of accessory nerve; originates from the upper five or six cervical spinal segments, emerges from the lateral surface of the spinal cord and ascends through the foramen magnum to join the cranial root. See *radices* spinales.

p. spongio'sa ure'thrae masculi'nae [NA], spongiose part of male urethra; spongy or penile urethra; p. cavernosa; the portion of the male urethra, about 15 cm in length, which traverses the corpus spongiosum.

p. squamo'sa os'sis tempora'lis [NA], squama temporalis; the squamous portion of the temporal bone.

p. sterna'lis diaphragma'tis [NA], sternal part of diaphragm; the small slip on each side that arises from the inner surface of the xiphoid process and inserts on the central tendon.

p. sternocosta'lis [NA], sternocostal part. See *musculus* pectoralis major.

p. subcuta'nea [NA], subcutaneous part. See *musculus* sphincter ani externus.

p. sublentifor'mis cap'sulae inter'nae [NA], sublenticular limb of the internal capsule; the part of the internal capsule below the caudal third of the lentiform nucleus that contains the auditory radiation as well as that part of the optic radiation representing the upper part of the contralateral half of the binocular visual field.

p. superficia'lis [NA], superficial part; **p. s. glan'dulae parotid'eae** [NA], see *glandula* parotidea; **p. s. mus'culi masse'teri** [NA], see *musculus* masseter; **p. s. mus'culi sphinc'teri a'ni exter'ni** [NA], see *musculus* sphincter ani externus.

p. supe'rior [NA], superior part; **p. s. duode'ni** [NA], see duodenum; **p. s. fa'cies diaphragma'tis hep'atis** [NA], the convex superior portion of the diaphragmatic surface of the liver; **p. s. gang'lion vestibula'ris** [NA], the part of the vestibular ganglion that receives fibers from the maculae of the utricle and the saccule and the ampullae of the anterior and lateral semicircular ducts; **p. s. ra'mus lingula'ris** [NA], the vein that drains the superior lingular bronchopulmonary segment.

p. supraclavicula'ris plex'us brachia'lis [NA], supraclavicular part of brachial plexus; the part of the brachial plexus, including the roots, trunks, and divisions, that gives rise to the dorsal scapular, long thoracic, suprascapular and subclavian nerves.

p. sympath'ica [NA], sympathetic part; sympathetic nervous system (2); systema nervosum autonomicum; thoracolumbar system; the sympathetic part of the nervous system. See also p. autonomica.

p. tec'ta, hidden part; **p. t. duode'ni,** the part of duodenum covered by the root of the transverse mesocolon, the coalescence of the ascending mesocolon, and the root of the mesentery; **p. t. pancrea'tis,** hidden portion of the pancreas; part of the pancreas covered by the root of the transverse mesocolon, the coalescence of the ascending mesocolon, and the root of the mesentery; **p. t. rena'lis,** hidden portion of the kidney; part of the kidney covered by the root of the transverse mesocolon; **p. t. uretera'lis,** hidden portion of the ureter; part of the right ureter covered (crossed) by the root of the mesentery, and of the left ureter covered (crossed) by the root of the sigmoid mesocolon.

p. ten'sa membra'nae tym'pani [NA], tense part of tympanic membrane; membrana tensa; membrana vibrans; the greater portion of the membrana tympani which is tense and firm, contrasting with the small triangular pars flaccida.

p. termina'lis [NA], terminal part. See *arteria* cerebri media; *arteria* cerebri posterior.

p. thorac'ica, thoracic part; **p. t. aor'tae** [NA], thoracic part of aorta; aorta thoracica; the part of the p. descendens aortae that supplies structures as far down as the diaphragm; **p. t. duc'tus thorac'ici** [NA], see *ductus* thoracicus; **p. t. esoph'agi** [NA], thoracic part of the esophagus; the part of the esophagus between the thoracic inlet and the diaphragm; **p. t. medul'lae spina'lis** [NA], segmenta medullae spinalis thoracica; thoracic part or segments of the spinal cord; the part of the spinal cord from which the twelve pairs of thoracic nerves originate.

p. thyropharyn'gea [NA], thyropharyngeal part; see *musculus* constrictor pharyngis inferior.

p. tibiocalca'nea [NA], tibiocalcaneal part; calcaneotibial ligament; ligamentum calcaneotibiale; the part of the medial or deltoid ligament that extends from the medial malleolus to the sustentaculum tali of the calcaneus.

p. tibionavicula'ris [NA], tibionavicular part; tibionavicular ligament; ligamentum tibionaviculare; the part of the medial or deltoid liagment that extends from the medial malleolus to the navicular bone.

p. tibiotala'ris ante'rior [NA], anterior tibiotalar part; anterior talotibial ligament; ligamentum talotibiale anterius; the part of the medial or deltoid ligament that extends from the medial malleolus to the neck of the talus.

p. tibiotala'ris poste'rior [NA], posterior tibiotalar part; posterior talotibial ligament; ligamentum talotibiale posterius; the part of the medial or deltoid ligament that extends from the medial malleolus to the posterior process of the talus.

p. transver'sa [NA], transverse part; see *musculus* nasalis; the long unbranched part of the left branch of the portal vein.

p. transversa'ria [NA], see *arteria* vertebralis.

p. triangula'ris, the middle one of three small convolutions which together compose the inferior frontal gyrus of the cerebral cortex; the other two being the p. orbitalis and p. opercularis.

p. tubera'lis [NA], p. infundibularis; infundibular part; the upward extension of the anterior lobe that wraps around the infundibular stalk; its cells, mostly gonadotropic, are arranged in cords and clusters; it is supplied by the superior hypophyseal arteries and contains the first capillary bed and the venules of a portal system that carries neurosecretory factors from the hypothalamus to a second capillary bed in the adenohypophysis where they regulate the release of hormones. See also hypophysis.

p. tympan'ica os'sis tempora'lis [NA], tympanic part of temporal bone, that portion of the temporal bone forming the greater part of the wall of the external acoustic meatus.

p. umbilica'lis [NA], umbilical part; the highly branched part of the left branch of the portal vein; the round and venous ligaments attach to this part.

p. uteri'na [NA], uterine part; **p. u. placen'tae** [NA], maternal placenta; placenta uterina; the part of the placenta derived from the uterine tissue. See also placenta. **p. u. tu'bae uteri'nae** [NA], the part of the uterine tube located within the wall of the uterus.

p. uvea'lis [NA], uveal part; the posterior part of the reticulum trabeculare, located between the scleral spur, the ciliary body, and the anterior surface of the iris.

p. vaga'lis [NA], *radices* craniales.

p. ventra'lis pon'tis [NA], p. basilaris pontis; basilar or ventral part of the pons; the large ventral part of the pons occupied by the nuclei pontis, traversed longitudinally by corticopontine, corticobulbar, and corticospinal fibers, and transversally by pontocerebellar fibers. Pontocerebellar fibers converging laterally form the middle cerebellar peduncle or brachium pontis.

p. vertebra'lis [NA], vertebral part; the part of the medial surface of the lung in contact with the vertebral bodies.

p. vestibula'ris [NA], *nervus* vestibularis.

---

pars-planitis (parz'plā-nī'tis). A clinical syndrome consisting of inflammation of the peripheral retina and/or pars plana, exudation into the overlying vitreous base, and edema of the optic disk and adjacent retina.

part. See pars.

abdominal p., *pars* abdominalis.
alar p., *pars* alaris.
alveolar p. of mandible, *pars* alveolaris mandibulae.
anterior p., *pars* anterior.
anterior p. of pons, *pars* basilaris pontis.
anterior tibiotalar p., *pars* tibiotalaris anterior.
ascending p., *pars* ascendens.
ascending p. of aorta, *pars* ascendens aortae.
autonomic p., *pars* autonomica.
basal p. of occipital bone, *pars* basilaris ossis occipitalis.
basal p. of pulmonary artery, *pars* basalis arteriae pulmonalis.
basilar p. of pons, *pars* ventralis pontis.
bony p. of auditory tube, *pars* ossea tubae auditivae.
bony p. of nasal septum, *pars* ossea septi nasi.
buccopharyngeal p., *pars* buccopharyngea.
cardiac p. of stomach, *pars* cardiaca ventriculi.
cartilaginous p. of auditory tube, *pars* cartilaginea tubae auditivae.
cartilaginous p. of skeletal system, *pars* cartilaginosa systematis skeletalis.
cavernous p. of internal carotid artery, *pars* cavernosa arteriae carotis internae.
ceratopharyngeal p., *pars* ceratopharyngea.
cerebral p. of internal carotid artery, *pars* cerebralis arteriae carotis internae.
cervical p., *pars* cervicalis; **c. p. of esophagus,** *pars* cervicalis esophagi; **c. p. of internal carotid artery,** *pars* cervicalis arteriae carotis internae; **c. p. of spinal cord,** *pars* cervicalis medullae spinalis; **c. p. of thoracic duct,** see *ductus* thoracicus.
chondropharyngeal p., *pars* chondropharyngea.
ciliary p. of retina, *pars* ciliaris retinae.
clavicular p., *pars* clavicularis.
coccygeal p. of spinal cord, *pars* coccygea medullae spinalis.
cochlear p. of vestibulocochlear nerve, *nervus* cochlearis.
convoluted p. of kidney lobule, *pars* convoluta lobuli corticalis renis.
corneoscleral p., *pars* corneoscleralis.
cortical p., *pars* corticalis.
costal p. of diaphragm, *pars* costalis diaphragmatis.
cricopharyngeal p., *pars* cricopharyngea.
cruciform p. of fibrous sheath, *pars* cruciformis vaginae fibrosae.
cupular p., cupulate p., *pars* cupularis.
deep p., *pars* profunda.
descending p., *pars* descendens.
distal p. of anterior lobe of hypophysis, *pars* distalis lobi anterioris hypophyseos.
dorsal p. of pons, *pars* dorsalis pontis.
flaccid p. of tympanic membrane, *pars* flaccida membranae tympani.
glossopharyngeal p., *pars* glossopharyngea.
hidden p., *pars* tecta.
horizontal p., *pars* horizontalis.
p.'s of human body, *partes* corporis humani.
inferior p., *pars* inferior.
inferior p. of vestibulocochlear nerve, *nervus* cochlearis.
infraclavicular p. of brachial plexus, *pars* infraclavicularis plexus brachialis.
infralobar p., *pars* infralobaris.
infrasegmental p., *pars* infrasegmentalis.
infundibular p. of anterior lobe of hypophysis, *pars* infundibularis lobi anterioris hypophyseos.
insular p., *pars* insularis.
intercartilaginous p. of glottic opening, *pars* intercartilaginea rimae glottidis.
intermediate p., *pars* intermedia.
intermembranous p. of glottic opening, *pars* intermembranacea rimae glottidis.
intersegmental p., *pars* infrasegmentalis.
intracanicular p. of optic nerve, *pars* intracaniculus nervi optici.
intracranial p., *pars* intracranialis.
intralaminar p. of optic nerve, *pars* intralaminaris nervi optici.
intralobar p., *pars* intralobaris.
intraocular p. of optic nerve, *pars* intraocularis nervi optici.
intrasegmental p., *pars* intrasegmentalis.
iridial p. of retina, *pars* iridica retinae.
labial p., *pars* labialis.
laryngeal p. of pharynx, *pars* laryngea pharyngis.
lateral p., *pars* lateralis.
lumbar p., *pars* lumbalis; **l. p. of diaphragm,** *pars* lumbalis dia-

phragmatis; **l. p. of spinal cord,** *pars* lumbalis medullae spinalis.
marginal p., *pars* marginalis.
mastoid p., *pars* mastoidea.
medial p., *pars* medialis.
mediastinal p., *pars* mediastinalis.
membranous p., *pars* membranacea.
membranous p. of male urethra, *pars* membranacea urethrae masculinae.
membranous p. of nasal septum, *pars* membranacea septi nasi.
mylopharyngeal p., *pars* mylopharyngea.
nasal p., *pars* nasalis.
nasal p. of pharynx, *pars* nasalis pharyngis.
oblique p., *pars* obliqua.
optic p. of retina, *stratum* cerebrale retinae.
oral p. of pharynx, *pars* oralis pharyngis.
orbital p., *pars* orbitalis.
orbital p. of optic nerve, *pars* orbitalis nervi optici.
osseous p. of skeletal system, *pars* ossea systematis skeletalis.
palpebral p., *pars* palpebralis.
parasympathetic p., *pars* parasympathetica.
pelvic p., *pars* pelvica.
petrous p., *pars* petrosa; **p. p. of internal carotid artery,** *pars* petrosa arteriae carotis internae; **p. p. of temporal bone,** *pars* petrosa ossis temporalis.
postcommunical p., *pars* postcommunicalis.
posterior p., *pars* posterior.
posterior tibiotalar p., *pars* tibiotalaris posterior.
postlaminar p. of optic nerve, *pars* postlaminaris nervi optici.
postsulcal p., *pars* postsulcalis.
precommunical p., *pars* precommunicalis.
prelaminar p. of optic nerve, *pars* prelaminaris nervi optici.
presulcal p., *pars* presulcalis.
pterygopharyngeal p., *pars* pterygopharyngea.
pyloric p., of stomach, *pars* pylorica ventriculi.
quadrate p., *pars* quadrata.
right p., *pars* dextra.
sacral p. of spinal cord, *pars* sacralis medullae spinalis.
soft p.'s, the nonbony and noncartilaginous tissues of the body.
sphenoidal p., *pars* sphenoidalis.
spinal p. of accessory nerve, *pars* spinalis.
spongiose p. of the male urethra, *pars* spongiosa urethrae masculinae.
sternal p. of diaphragm, *pars* sternalis diaphragmatis.
sternocostal p., *pars* sternocostalis.
straight p., *pars* recta.
subcutaneous p., *pars* subcutanea.
superficial p., *pars* superficialis.
superior p., *pars* superior.
superior p. of vestibulocochlear nerve, *nervus* vestibularis.
supraclavicular p. of brachial plexus, *pars* supraclavicularis plexus brachialis.
sympathetic p., *pars* sympathica.
tense p. of the tympanic membrane, *pars* tensa membranae tympani.
terminal p., p. terminalis.
thoracic p., *pars* thoracica, **t. p. of aorta,** *pars* thoracica aortae; **t. p. of esophagus,** *pars* thoracica esophagi; **t. p. of spinal cord,** *pars* thoracica medullae spinalis; **t. p. of thoracic duct,** see *ductus* thoracicus.
thyropharyngeal p., *pars* thyropharyngea.
tibiocalcaneal p., *pars* tibiocalcanea.
tibionavicular p., *pars* tibionavicularis.
transverse p., *pars* transversa.
tympanic p. of temporal bone, *pars* tympanica ossis temporalis.
umbilical p., *pars* umbilicalis.
uterine p., *pars* uterina.
uveal p., *pars* uvealis.
vagal p. of accessory nerve, *radices* craniales.
ventral p. of the pons, *pars* ventralis pontis.
vertebral p., *pars* vertebralis.
vertebral p. of diaphragm, *pars* lumbalis diaphragmatis.
vestibular p. of vestibulocochlear nerve, *nervus* vestibularis.

part. aeq. Abbreviation for L. *partes aequales,* in equal parts (amounts).

partes (par'tēz). Plural of pars.

parthenogenesis (par'the-nō-jen'ĕ-sis) [G. *parthenos,* virgin, + *genesis,* product]. Apogamia; apogamy; apomixia; virgin generation; a form of nonsexual reproduction, or agamogenesis, in which the female reproduces its kind without fecundation by the male.

parthenophobia (par'the-nō-fō'bē-ă) [G. *parthenos,* virgin, + *phobos,* fear]. Morbid fear of girls.

particle (par'ti-kl) [L. *particula,* dim. of *pars,* part]. A very small piece or portion of anything.
alpha p., alpha ray; a p. consisting of two neutrons and two protons, and with a positive charge ($2e^+$), that is emitted energetically from the nuclei of unstable isotopes of high atomic number (elements of mass number from 82 up); its properties are identical to those of the helium nucleus.
beta p., beta ray; an electron, either positively (positron) or negatively (negatron) charged, emitted during beta decay of a radionuclide.
chromatin p.'s, fine bluish dots thought to represent remnants of the nucleus, occasionally seen in stained erythrocytes.
Dane p.'s, the larger spherical forms of hepatitis-associated antigens; they comprise the virion of hepatitis B virus, containing a 27-nm "core" in which DNA-dependent DNA polymerase and circular, double-stranded DNA have been found.
elementary p., **(1)** platelet; **(2)** one of the units occurring on the matrical surface of mitochondrial cristae; the head of the p., which measures about 90 Å, attaches to the membrane of the crista by a stalk 50 Å in length; the p.'s may be concerned with the electron transport system.
kappa p.'s, inheritable cytoplasmic symbionts, once thought to be p.'s mainly or exclusively of DNA, occurring in some strains of *Paramecium;* capable of producing a product lethal to other strains.
Zimmermann's elementary p., platelet.

particulate (par-tik'yū-lāt). Relating to or occurring in the form of fine particles.

particulates (par-tik'yū-lats). Formed elements, discrete bodies, as contrasted with the surrounding liquid or semiliquid material; *e.g.,* granules or mitochondria in cells.

parturient (par-tū'rē-ent) [L. *parturio,* to be in labor]. Relating to or in the process of childbirth.

parturifacient (par-tūr-ē-fā'shent) [L. *parturio,* to be in labor, + *facio,* to make]. Oxytocic. **1.** Inducing or accelerating labor. **2.** An agent that induces or accelerates labor.

parturiometer (par-tūr-ē-om'ĕ-ter) [L. *parturitio,* parturition, + G. *metron,* measure]. Device for determining the force of the uterine contractions in childbirth.

parturition (par-tūr-ish'ŭn) [L. *parturitio,* fr. *parturio,* to be in labor]. Childbirth.

part. vic. Abbreviation for L. *partes vicibus,* in divided doses.

parulis, pl. **parulides** (pă-rū'lis, -li-dēz) [G. *paroulis,* gumboil, fr. *para,* beside, + *oulon,* gum]. Gingival *abscess.*

parumbilical (par'ŭm-bil'i-kăl). Paraumbilical.

paruresis (par-yū-rē'sis). Inhibited micturition, especially in the presence of strangers.

parvalbumin (par-val-byū'min) [L. *parvus,* small, + albumin]. A small water-soluble calcium-binding protein distinct from calmodulin and other calcium-binding proteins; found in the brain, skeletal muscle, and retina, but not in the heart, liver, or spleen, of various species.

parvicellular (par-vi-sel′yū-lăr) [L. *parvus*, small, + Mod. L. *cellularis*, cellular]. Relating to or composed of cells of small size.

Parvobacteriaceae (par′vō-bak-tēr-ē-ā′sē-ē). A family name regarded as a former name for the bacterial family Brucellaceae. No type genus has ever been proposed for the family P.

parvoline (par′vō-lēn). A ptomaine, $C_9H_{13}N$, from decaying fish.

Parvoviridae (par-vō-vir′i-dē). A family of small viruses containing single-stranded DNA. Virions are 18 to 26 nm in diameter, are not enveloped, and are ether-resistant. Capsids are of cubic symmetry, with 32 capsomeres. Replication and assembly occur in the nucleus of infected cells. Three genera are recognized: *Parvovirus*, *Densovirus*, and an officially unnamed genus that includes the adeno-associated satellite virus.

Parvovirus (par′vō-vī-rŭs). A genus of viruses (family Parvoviridae) that replicate autonomously in suitable cells. The Kilham rat virus is the type species.

parvule (par′vūl) [L. *parvulus*, very small, fr. *parvus*, small]. A minute pill.

parvus (par′vŭs) [L.]. Small.

PAS Abbreviation for *p*- aminosalicylic acid; periodic acid-Schiff (stain).

PASA Abbreviation for *p*- aminosalicyclic acid.

Pascal, Blaise, French scientist, 1623–1662. See pascal; P.'s *law*.

pascal (Pa) (pas′kăl) [B. *Pascal*]. A derived unit of pressure in the SI system, expressed in newtons per square meter.

Pascheff (Pashev), Constantin (Konstantin), Bulgarian ophthalmologist, 1873–1961. See P.'s *conjunctivitis*.

Paschen, Enrique, German pathologist 1860– 1936. See P. *bodies*.

Pashev. See *Pascheff*, Constantin.

Pasini, Augustine, 20th century Argentine dermatologist. See *atrophoderma* of P. and Pierini.

pasiniazide (pas-i-nī′ă-zīd). Isoniazid 4-aminosalicylate; an antituberculostatic agent.

paspalism (pas′păl-izm) [G. *paspalos*, a kind of millet, fr. *pas*, all, + *palē*, meal]. Poisoning by seeds of a species of grass, *Paspalum scrobiculatum*.

passage (pas′ij) [Mediev. L. *passo*, to pass]. **1.** The act of passing. **2.** A discharge, as from the bowels or of urine. **3.** Inoculation of a series of animals with the same strain of a pathogenic microorganism whereby the virulence usually is increased, but is sometimes diminished. **4.** A channel, duct, pore, or opening.
nasopharyngeal p., *meatus* nasopharyngeus.

Passalurus ambiguus (pa-sal′yū-rŭs am-big′yū-ŭs). The rabbit pinworm, an oxyurid nematode found abundantly in the cecum and large intestine of rabbits.

Passavant, Philippas G., German physician, 1815–1893. See P.'s *bar, cushion, pad, ridge*.

Passey, R.D., 20th century British pathologist. See Harding-P. *melanoma*.

passiflora (pas-i-flō′ră) [L. *passio*, passion, + *flos* (*flor*-), flower]. The passion-flower, *Passiflora incarnata* (family Passifloraceae), a climbing herb of the southern U.S.; the dried flowering and fruiting top has been used in neuralgia, dysmenorrhea, and insomnia, and as an application to hemorrhoids and for burns.

passion (pash′ŭn) [L. *passio*, fr. *patior*, pp. *passus*, to suffer]. **1.** Intense emotion. **2.** Obsolete term for suffering or pain.

passive (pas′iv) [L. *passivus*, fr. *patior*, to endure]. Not active; submissive.

passivism (pas′iv-izm) [see passive]. **1.** An attitude of submission. **2.** A form of sexual perversion in which the subject, usually male, is submissive to the will of the partner, male or female, in sexual practices. See also pathic.

passivity (pas-iv′i-tē). **1.** The condition of a metal having formed a protective oxide coating; *e.g.*, rustless metals and aluminum become passive in air. **2.** In dentistry, the quality or condition of inactivity or rest assumed by the teeth, tissues, and denture when a removable partial denture is in place but not under masticatory pressure.

pasta, gen. and pl. **pastae** (pas′tă,-tē) [L.]. Paste.

paste (pāst) [L. *pasta*]. A soft semisolid of firmer consistency than pap, but soft enough to flow slowly and not to retain its shape.
dermatologic p., a class of preparations consisting of starch, dextrin, sulfur, calcium carbonate, or zinc oxide made into a p. with glycerin, soft soap, petrolatum, or some fat, with which is incorporated some medicinal substance.
desensitizing p., an ointment, usually caustic, coagulating or cytotoxic, formulated to be applied to the cervix of a tooth for the purpose of obtunding pain from sensitive, exposed cementum or dentin.

paster (pā′ster). The segment forming the part for near vision in two-piece bifocal lenses.

pas′tern [O. Fr. *pasturon*, pasture; because the shackle of a horse out at pasture is attached to this part of the leg]. The part of the leg of a horse and similar animals that lies between the fetlock joint and the hoof.

Pasteur, Louis, French chemist and bacteriologist, 1822–1895. See P. *vaccine*; P.'s *effect*.

Pasteurella (pas-ter-el′ă) [L. *Pasteur*] A genus of aerobic to facultatively anaerobic, nonmotile bacteria (family Brucellaceae) containing small, Gram-negative, ellipsoidal to elongated rods which, with special methods, show bipolar staining. These organisms are parasites of man and other animals, including birds. The type species is *P. multocida*.
P. anatipes′tifer, a species causing a respiratory disease in ducklings.
P. haemolyt′ica, a species associated with pneumonia in sheep, goats, and cattle, and causing mastitis in ewes.
P. multoci′da, a species which causes fowl cholera and hemorrhagic septicemia in warm-blooded animals and may infect dog or cat bites or scratches or cause septicema in humans with chronic disease. It is the type species of the genus *P.*
P. novici′da, a species pathogenic for white mice, guinea pigs, and hamsters; it produces lesions in experimental animals similar to those found in cases of tularemia; it is not known to infect man.
P. pes′tis, *Yersinia pestis*.
P. pfaf′fii, a species found in an epidemic of septicemia in canaries where it caused a necrotic enteritis; pathogenic for canaries, sparrows, pigeons, white mice, guinea pigs, and rabbits; not pathogenic for chickens.
P. pseudotuberculo′sis, *Yersinia pseudotuberculosis*.
P. septicae′miae, a species which causes fatal septicemia in young geese.
P. tularen′sis, *Francisella tularensis*.

pasteurella, pl. **pasteurellae** (pas-ter-el′ă, pas-ter-el′ē). A vernacular term used to refer to any member of the genus *Pasteurella*.

pasteurellosis (pas′ter-ĕ-lō′sis). Infection with bacteria of the genus *Pasteurella*.

pasteurization (pas′ter-i-zā′shŭn) [L. *Pasteur*]. The heating of milk, wines, fruit juices, etc., for about 30 minutes at 68°C (154.4°F) whereby living bacteria are destroyed, but the flavor or bouquet is preserved; the spores are unaffected, but are kept from developing by immediately cooling the liquid to 10°C (50°F) or lower. See also sterilization.

pasteurize (pas'ter-īz). To treat by pasteurization.

pasteurizer (pas'ter-ī-zer). An apparatus used in pasteurization.

Pastia, C., Roumanian physician. See P.'s *sign.*

pastil, pastille (pas'til, pas-tēl') [Fr. *pastille;* L. *pastillus,* a roll (of bread), dim. of *panis,* bread]. **1.** A small mass of benzoin and other aromatic substances to be burned for fumigation. **2.** Troche.
Sabouraud's p.'s, disks containing barium platinocyanide which undergo a color change when exposed to x-rays; previously used to indicate the administered dose.

past-pointing (past'poynt'ing). A test of the integrity of the vestibular apparatus of the ear and of cerebellar function: the patient, seated in a revolving chair, is rotated to the right ten times with eyes closed; then with the arm held horizontal, the right index finger is brought in touch with the tip of the examiner's finger; the arm is then raised vertically and the patient is instructed to touch the examiner's finger on bringing the arm once more to the horizontal; if the vestibular apparatus is normal, the finger will be brought down several inches to the right of the examiner's finger because the patient is still responding to the sensation of rotation to the left; the reverse is true on rotation to the left. In cerebellar disease, a patient attempting to reach a point with the finger will overshoot it. The test is also used in connection with caloric stimulation.

patagium, pl. **patagia** (pă-tā'jē-ŭm, -ă) [L. a gold edging on a woman's gown]. A winglike membrane.
cervical p., *pterygium* colli.

Patau, Klaus, 20th century U.S. cytogeneticist. See P.'s *syndrome.*

patch. A small circumscribed area differing in color or structure from the surrounding surface.
butterfly p., butterfly (2).
cotton-wool p.'s, cotton-wool spots; accumulations of cellular organelles in the retinal nerve fiber layer caused by damage to axons.
herald p., the initial oval-shaped papulosquamous lesion, heralding the widespread eruption of pityriasis rosea, and preceding the latter by several days to as long as 2 months.
Hutchinson's p., salmon p.
moth p., chloasma.
mucous p., an oval to round, yellow-gray to white, maturated lesion or lesions occurring on the mucous membranes; usually seen in secondary syphilis.
opaline p., a mucous p. of silver-gray appearance.
Peyer's p.'s, *folliculi* lymphatici aggregati.
salmon p., Hutchinson's p.; interstitial or parenchymatous keratitis giving rise to neovascularization of the cornea.
shagreen p., shagreen *skin.*
smoker's p.'s, obsolete term for leukoplakia.
soldier's p.'s, milk *spots* (1).

patefaction (pat-ĕ-fak'shŭn) [L. *pate-facio,* pp. *-factus,* to make lie open, fr. *pateo,* to lie open]. A laying open.

Patein, G., French physician, 1857–1928. See P.'s *albumin.*

patella, gen. and pl. **patellae** (pa-tel'ă, -ē) [L. a small plate, the kneecap, dim. of *patina,* a shallow disk, fr. *pateo,* to lie open] [NA]. Kneecap; the large sesamoid bone, in the combined tendon of the extensors of the leg, covering the anterior surface of the knee.
floating p., a p. riding high on effusion of the knee.
slipping p., spontaneous or easily provoked dislocation of the p.

patellalgia (pa-tĕ-lal'jē-ă). A painful condition involving the patella.

patellar (pa-tel'ăr). Relating to the patella.

patellectomy (pat'ĕ-lek'tō-mē) [patella + G. *ektomē,* excision]. Excision of the patella.

patelliform (pa-tel'i-fōrm). Of the shape of the patella.

patellometer (pat'ĕ-lom'ĕ-ter) [patella + G. *metron,* measure]. Instrument for measuring the patellar reflex.

patency (pā'ten-sē). The state of being freely open or exposed.
probe p. (of foramen ovale), a term introduced by B.M. Patten to cover incomplete fibrous adhesion of an adequate valvula foraminis ovalis in the postnatal closure of the foramen ovale.

patent (pa'tent, pā'tent) [L. *patens,* pres. p. of *pateo,* to lie open]. Patulous; open or exposed.

patent blue V. Leuco patent blue.

Paterson, Donald R., British otolaryngologist, 1863–1939. See P.-Kelly *syndrome.*

path-, patho-, -pathy, pathic [G. *pathos,* feeling, suffering, disease]. Combining forms meaning disease.

path [A.S. *paeth*] A road or way; the course taken by an electric current or by nervous impulses. See also pathway.
condyle p., the p. traveled by the mandibular condyle in the temporomandibular joint during the various mandibular movements.
generated occlusal p., a registration of the p.'s of movement of the occlusal surfaces of mandibular teeth on a plastic or abrasive surface attached to the maxillary arch. See also functional chew-in *record.*
incisal p., incisal *guidance.*
p. of insertion, the direction in which a dental prosthesis is placed upon or removed from the supporting tissues or abutment teeth.
milled-in p.'s, milled-in curves; **(1)** contours carved by various mandibular movements into the occluding surface of an occlusion rim, by teeth or studs placed in the opposing occlusion rim; the curves or contours may be carved into wax, modeling plastic, or plaster of Paris; **(2)** occlusal curves developed by masticatory or gliding movements of occlusion rims which are composed of materials including abrasives. See also functional chew-in *record.*
occlusal p., **(1)** a gliding occlusal contact; **(2)** the p. of movement of an occlusal surface.

pathema (pă-thē'mă) [G. *pathēma,* suffering]. Obsolete term for a disease or morbid condition.

pathergasia (path-er-gā'zē-ă) [G. *pathos,* disease, + *ergasia,* work]. Obsolete term for a physiologic or anatomical defect that limits normal emotional adjustment.

pathergy (path'er-jē) [G. *pathos,* disease, + *ergon,* work]. Those reactions resulting from a state of altered activity, both allergic (immune) and nonallergic.

pathetic (pă-thet'ik) [G. *pathētikos,* relating to the feelings]. **1.** Denoting the fourth cranial nerve (pathetic nerve), the nervus trochlearis. **2.** Denoting that which arouses sorrow or pity.

pathfinder (path'fīn-der). A filiform bougie for introduction through a narrow stricture end to serve as a guide for the passage of a larger sound or catheter.

pathic (path'ik) [G. *pathikos,* remaining passive]. A person who assumes the passive role in any abnormal sexual act. See also passivism.

patho-. See path-.

pathoamine (path-ō-am'ēn). A ptomaine; a toxic amine causing disease or resulting from a disease process.

pathobiology (path'ō-bī-ol'ō-jē). Pathology with emphasis more on the biological than on the medical aspects.

pathoclisis (path-ō-klis'is) [patho- + G. *klisis,* bending, proneness]. A specific tendency to sensitivity to special toxins; a tendency for toxins to attack certain organs.

pathocrinia (path-ō-krin'ē-ă) [patho- + G. *krinein,* to separate]. Obsolete term for any disorder of the endocrine glands.

pathodixia (path-ō-dik'sē-ă) [patho- + G. *deiknunai,* to show]. Rarely used term for a morbid desire to exhibit one's injured or diseased part.

pathodontia (path-ō-don'shē-ă) [patho- + G. *odous,* tooth]. The science concerned with diseases of the teeth.

pathoformic (path-ō-fōr′mik) [patho- + L. *formo,* to form]. Relating to the beginning of disease; denoting especially certain symptoms occurring in the transition period between a normal and a diseased state.

pathogen (path′ō-jen) [patho- + G. *-gen,* to produce]. Any virus, microorganism, or other substance causing disease.
behavioral p., the personal habits and lifestyle behaviors of an individual which are associated with an increased risk of physical illness and dysfunction. See also risk *factor.*
opportunistic p., an organism that is capable of causing disease only when the host's resistance is lowered, *e.g.,* by other diseases or drugs.

pathogenesis (path-ō-jen′ĕ-sis) [patho- + G. *genesis,* production]. The pathologic, physiologic, or biochemical mechanism resulting in the development of a disease or morbid process. *Cf.* etiology.
drug p., the production of morbid symptoms by drugs.

pathogenic, pathogenetic (path-ō-jen′ik, -jĕ-net′ik). Morbific; morbigenous; nosogenic; nosopoietic; causing disease or abnormality.

pathogenicity (path′ō-jĕ-nis′i-tē). The condition or quality of being pathogenic, or the ability to cause disease.

pathogeny (pă-thoj′ĕ-nē). Rarely used synonym for pathogenesis.

pathognomonic (path′og-nō-mon′ik) [see pathognomy]. Characteristic or indicative of a disease; denoting especially one or more typical symptoms, findings, or pattern of abnormalities specific for a given disease and not found in any other condition.

pathognomy (pă-thog′nō-mē) [patho- + G. *gnōmē,* a mark, a sign]. Diagnosis by means of a study of the typical symptoms of a disease, or of the subjective sensations of the patient.

pathognostic (path-og-nos′tik) [patho- + G. *gnōstikos,* pertaining to knowledge]. Rarely used synonym for pathognomonic.

pathography (pă-thog′ră-fē) [patho- + G. *graphē,* a description]. A treatise on or description of disease; a treatise on pathology.

patholesia (path-ō-lē′sē-ă) [path- + G. *lēsis,* choice, will]. Rarely used term for any impairment or abnormality of the will.

pathologic, pathological (path-ō-loj′ik, -i-kăl). **1.** Pertaining to pathology. **2.** Morbid or diseased; resulting from disease.

pathologist (pa-thol′ō-jist). A specialist in pathology; a physician who practices, evaluates, or supervises diagnostic tests, using materials removed from living or dead patients, and functions as a laboratory consultant to clinicians, or who conducts experiments or other investigations to determine the causes or nature of disease changes.

pathology (pa-thol′ō-jē) [patho- + G. *logos,* study, treatise]. The medical science, and specialty practice, concerned with all aspects of disease, but with special reference to the essential nature, causes, and development of abnormal conditions, as well as the structural and functional changes that result from the disease processes.
anatomical p., pathological anatomy; the subspecialty of p. that pertains to the gross and microscopic study of organs and tissues removed for biopsy or during postmortem examination, and also the interpretation of the results of such study.
cellular p., (1) the interpretation of diseases in terms of cellular alterations, *i.e.,* the ways in which cells fail to maintain homeostasis; **(2)** sometimes used as a synonym for cytopathology (1).
clinical p., (1) any part of the medical practice of p. as it pertains to the care of patients; **(2)** the subspecialty in p. concerned with the theoretical and technical aspects (*i.e.,* the methods or procedures) of chemistry, microbiology, parasitology, immunology, hematology, and other fields as they pertain to the diagnosis of disease and the care of patients, as well as to the prevention of disease.
comparative p., the p. of diseases of animals, especially in relation to human p.
dental p., oral p.
functional p., p. pertaining to abnormalities in function of a tissue, organ, or part, with or without associated changes in structure.
humoral p., the thesis that disorders in the fluids of the body, especially the blood, are the basic factors in disease.
medical p., p. pertaining to various diseases not suitable for treatment by surgery.
molecular p., the study of biochemical and biophysical cellular mechanisms as the basic factors in disease.
oral p., dental p.; the branch of dentistry concerned with the etiology, pathogenesis, and clinical, gross, and microscopic aspects of oral and paraoral disease, including oral soft tissues, the teeth, jaws, and salivary glands.
speech p., the science concerned with functional and organic speech defects and disorders.
surgical p., a field in anatomical p. concerned with examination of tissues removed from living patients for the purpose of diagnosis of disease and guidance in the care of patients.

pathometric (path-ō-met′rik). Relating to pathometry.

pathometry (pă-thom′ĕ-trē) [patho- + G. *metron,* measure]. Determination of the proportionate number of individuals affected with a certain disease at a given time, and of the conditions leading to an increase or decrease in this number.

pathomimesis (path′ō-mi-mē′sis) [patho- + G. *mimēsis,* imitation]. Pathomimicry; mimicry of a disease or dysfunction, whether intentional or unconscious.

pathomimicry (path-ō-mim′i-krē). Pathomimesis.

pathomiosis (path-ō-mī-ō′sis) [patho- + G. *meiōsis,* a lessening]. The attitude of a patient which leads him to minimize his disease.

pathomorphism (path-ō-mōr′fizm). Abnormal morphology.

pathonomia, pathonomy (path-ō-nō′mē-ă, pă-thon′ō-mē) [patho- + G. *nomos,* law]. The science of the laws of morbid changes.

pathophobia (path-ō-fō′bē-ă) [patho- + G. *phobos,* fear]. Nosophobia.

pathophysiology (path′ō-fiz-ē-ol′ō-jē). Derangement of function seen in disease; alteration in function as distinguished from structural defects.

pathopoiesis (path′ō-poy-ē′sis). [patho- + G. *poiēsis,* making]. Rarely used term for the mode of production of disease.

pathosis (pă-thō′sis) [patho- + G. *-osis,* condition]. A state of disease, diseased condition, or disease entity.

pathotropism (pa-thot′rō-pizm) [patho- + G. *tropos,* a turning]. Attraction of drugs toward diseased structures.

pathway (path′wā). **1.** A collection of axons establishing a conduction route for nerve impulses from one group of nerve cells to another group or to an effector organ composed of muscle or gland cells. **2.** Any sequence of chemical reactions leading from one compound to another; if taking place in living tissue, usually referred to as a **biochemical p.**
auditory p., neural paths and connections of the nervous system, including nuclei, beginning at the organ of Corti's hair cells, continuing along the eighth nerve, and terminating at the auditory cortex.
Embden-Meyerhof p., Embden-Meyerhof-Parnas p., the anaerobic glycolytic p. by which glucose (most notably in muscle) is converted to lactic acid.
pentose phosphate p., phosphogluconate p.; hexose monophosphate shunt; Dickens or Warburg-Lipmann-Dickens shunt; a secondary p. for the oxidation of glucose (not occurring in skeletal muscle), generating reducing power (NADPH) in the cytoplasm outside the mitochondria and synthesizing pentoses. It proceeds from glucose 6-phosphate to ribulose and ribose phosphates, thence (with xylulose 5-phosphate) to sedaneptulose 7-phosphate

and D-glyceraldehyde 3-phosphate; carbon dioxide is released in the gluconate-ribulose step. In plants, it participates in the formation of glucose from carbon dioxide in the dark reactions of photosynthesis.

phosphogluconate p., pentose phosphate p.

-pathy. See path-.

patient (pā'shent) [L. *patiens,* pres. p. of *patior,* to suffer]. One who is suffering from any disease and is under treatment for it. *Cf.* case (1).

target p., in psychoanalytic group therapy, the p. being analyzed in turn by another member p.

patricide (pat'ri-sīd) [L. *pater,* father, + *caedō,* to kill]. **1.** The killing of one's father. **2.** One who commits such an act.

Patrick, Hugh T., U.S. neurologist, 1860–1938. See P.'s *test.*

patrilineal (pat-ri-lin'ē-ăl) [L. *pater,* father, + *linea,* line]. Related to descent through the male line.

patten (pat'en) [Fr. *patin,* a clog]. A support placed under one shoe to equalize leg length when one leg is shorter than the other, or when one is artificially lengthened by a brace or splint.

pattern (pat'ern). **1.** A design. **2.** In dentistry, a form used in making a mold, as for an inlay or partial denture framework.

ballerina-foot p., a vigorous posteromedial contraction of the left ventricle coupled with convexity anteriorly, resulting from poor contraction of the opposing anterior wall; it is the most frequent dyssynergy observed in the prolapsed mitral valve leaflet syndrome, and produces a configuration of angiographic dye in the right anterior oblique projection resembling a ballerina's foot; sometimes called dancer's foot malformation.

hourglass p., a vigorous ringlike contraction observed angiographically in the left ventricular angiogram in the right anterior oblique projection, resembling an hourglass; it is seen in the prolapsed mitral valve leaflet syndrome.

juvenile p., a precordial T-wave inversion in an electrocardiogram, resembling that seen in normal children, which occurs as a normal variant in some adults, especially Blacks.

occlusal p., occlusal *form.*

wax p., wax form; a p. of wax of such shape that, when invested and burned out or otherwise eliminated, it will produce a mold in which a casting may be made.

patulin (pat'yū-lin). 4-Hydroxy-4*H*- furo[3,2-c]pyran-2(6*H*)-one; an antibiotic derived from metabolites of fungi, such as species of *Aspergillus, Penicillium,* and *Gymnoascus;* has carcinogenic activity.

patulous (pat'yū-lŭs) [L. *patulus,* fr. *pateo,* to lie open]. Patent.

paucibacillary (paw-sē-bas'i-lār-ē). Made up of, or denoting the presence of, few bacilli.

paucisynaptic (paw'sē-si-nap'tik) [L. *paucus,* few, + synapse]. Oligosynaptic.

Paul, Gustav, Austrian physician, 1859–1935. See P.'s *reaction, test.*

Pauli, Wolfgang, Austrian physicist, 1900–1958. See P.'s *principle.*

Pauling, Linus C., U.S. chemist and Nobel laureate, *1901. See P.'s *theory;* P.-Corey *helix.*

paunch (pawnch). Rumen.

pause (pawz) [G. *pausis,* cessation]. Temporary stop.

apneic p., cessation of air flow for more than 10 seconds. See sleep *apnea.*

compensatory p., the p. following an extrasystole, when the p. is long enough to compensate for the prematurity of the extrasystole; the short cycle ending with the extrasystole plus the p. following the extrasystole together equal two of the regular cycles.

postextrasystolic p., the somewhat prolonged cycle immediately following an extrasystole.

preautomatic p., a temporary p. in cardiac activity before an automatic pacemaker escapes. See also escape.

respiratory p., cessation of air flow for less than 10 seconds. See sleep *apnea.*

sinus p., a spontaneous interruption in the regular sinus rhythm, the p. lasting for a period that is not an exact multiple of the sinus cycle. See also sinus *arrest;* sinus *standstill.*

Pautrier, Lucien M.A., French dermatologist, 1876–1959. See P.'s *abscess, microabscess.*

Pauzat, Jean E., 19th century French physician. See P.'s *disease.*

pavex (pā'veks). An apparatus for producing passive vascular exercise in peripheral circulatory disorders by means of alternate positive and negative pressure.

Pavlov, Ivan P., Russian physiologist and Nobel laureate, 1849–1936. See pavlovian *conditioning;* P. *method, pouch, stomach; P.'s reflex.*

pavor nocturnus (pā'vōr nok-ter'nŭs) [L.]. Night-terrors.

Pavy, Frederick W., British physician, 1829–1911. See P.'s *disease.*

paw'paw. See papaya.

Paxton, Francis V., British physician, 1840–1924. See P.'s *disease.*

Payne, J. Howard, U.S. surgeon, *1916. See P. *operation.*

Payr, Erwin, German surgeon, 1871–1946. See P.'s *clamp, membrane, sign.*

P_B Symbol for barometric *pressure.*

Pb Symbol for lead (plumbum).

PBG Porphobilinogen.

PBI Abbreviation for protein-bound *iodine.*

p.c. Abbreviation for L. *post cibum,* after a meal.

PCB Polychlorinated *biphenyl.*

PCMB, *p* CMB Abbreviation for *p*-chloromercuribenzoic acid.

P_{CO_2}, pCO_2 Symbol for partial pressure (tension) of carbon dioxide. See partial *pressure.*

P-congenitale (kon-jen-i-tā'lē). The P-wave pattern in the electrocardiogram seen in some cases of congenital heart disease, consisting of tall peaked P waves in leads I, II, aVF, and aVL, with predominant positivity of diphasic waves in V1-2. See also Spannungs-P.

PCP Abbreviation for phencyclidine.

PCT Abbreviation for *porphyria* cutanea tarda.

Pd Symbol for palladium.

p.d. Abbreviation of prism *diopter.*

P-dextrocardiale (deks'trō-kar-dē-ā'lē). An electrocardiographic syndrome characteristic of overloading of the right atrium, often erroneously called P-pulmonale because the syndrome can result from any overloading of the right atrium (*e.g.,* tricuspid stenosis) and independently of cor pulmonale.

PDI Abbreviation for Periodontal Disease Index.

PDLL Abbreviation for poorly differentiated lymphocytic *lymphoma.*

peach kernel oil (pēch ker'nĕl). See persic oil.

peanut oil (pē'nŭt). Arachis oil; oil extracted from the kernels of one or more cultivated varieties of *Arachis hypogaea* (family Leguminosae); used as a solvent for intramuscular injections.

pearl (perl) **1.** A concretion formed around a grain of sand or other foreign body within the shell of certain mollusks. **2.** One of a number of small tough masses, such as mucus occurring in the sputum in asthma.

Elschnig p.'s, the proliferated anterior capsule of the lens of the eye after surgical capsulotomy or injury.

enamel p., enameloma.

epithelial p., keratin p.

Epstein's p.'s, multiple small white epithelial inclusion cysts found in the midline of the palate in newborn infants.
gouty p., a concretion of sodium urate on the cartilage of the ear, occurring in the gouty.
keratin p., squamous p.; epithelial p. or nest; a focus of central keratinization within concentric layers of abnormal squamous cells; seen in squamous cell carcinoma.
Laënnec's p.'s, obsolete term for small, round, translucent, tenacious bodies in the sputum of some persons with asthma; when floated in water, they become unfurled and are then recognizable as Curschmann's spirals.
squamous p., keratin p.

pearl-ash. Potash.

Pearson, Carl M. See McArdle-Schmid-P. *disease.*

Pearson, Karl, British mathematician, 1857–1936. See Poisson-P. *formula.*

peau d'orange (pō-dŏ-rahnj') [Fr. orange peel]. A swollen pitted skin surface overlying carcinoma of the breast in which there is both stromal infiltration and lymphatic obstruction with edema.

peccant (pek'ant) [L. *peccans (-ant-),* pres. p. of *pecco,* to sin]. Morbid; unhealthy; producing disease.

peccatiphobia (pek'kă-ti-fō'bē-ă) [L. *pecco,* to sin, + G. *phobos,* fear]. Morbid fear of sinning.

pecilo-. See poikilo-.

pecilocin (pĕ-sil'ō-sin). 1-(8-Hydroxy-6-methyl-1-oxo-2,4,6-dodecatrienyl)-2-pyrrolidinone; an antifungal agent.

Pecquet, Jean, French anatomist, 1622–1674. See P.'s *cistern, duct, receptaculum, reservoir.*

pectase (pek'tās) [EC 3.1.1.11]. Pectinesterase; an enzyme that converts pectin to galacturonic acid (pectic acid).

pecten (pek'ten) [L. comb]. **1** [NA]. A structure with comblike processes or projections. **2.** P. analis.
anal p., p. analis.
p. ana'lis [NA], anal p.; pecten (2); the middle third of the anal canal.
p. os'sis pu'bis [NA], p. pubis; pectineal line of pubis; the continuation on the superior ramus pubis of the terminal line, forming a sharp ridge.
p. pubis, p. ossis pubis.

pectenitis (pek-ten-ī'tis) [L. *pecten,* a comb, + G. *-itis,* inflammation]. Inflammation of the sphincter ani.

pectenosis (pek-ten-ō'sis). Exaggerated enlargement of the pecten band.

pectic (pek'tik) [G. *pēktos,* stiff, curdled]. Relating to any of the substances or materials now referred to as pectin.

pectic acid. Galacturonic acid.

pectin (pek'tin). Broad generic term for what are now called pectic substances or materials; specifically, a gelatinous substance, consisting largely of long chains of galacturonic acid units, that is extracted from fruits where it is presumed to exist as protopectin (pectose). Commercial p.'s are sometimes called pectinic acid and are used in the preparation of jams, jellies, and similar food products; therapeutically, they are used to control diarrhea (usually in conjunction with other agents), as a plasma expander, and as a protectant.

pectinase (pek'tin-ās). Polygalacturonase.

pectinate (pek'ti-nāt). **1.** Pectiniform; combed; comb-shaped. **2.** In fungi, used to describe a particular type of branching hyphae in cultures of dermatophytes.

pectineal (pek-tin'ē-ăl). Ridged; relating to the os pubis or to any comblike structure.

pectinesterase (pek-tin-es'ter-ās). Pectase.

pectineus (pek'ti-nē'ŭs) [L.]. **1.** Pectineal. **2.** See *musculus* pectineus.

pectinic acids (pek-tin'ik). Term sometimes used for commercial pectins.

pectiniform (pek-tin'i-fōrm). Pectinate (1).

pectization (pek-ti-zā'shŭn) [G. *pēktikos,* curdling]. In colloidal chemistry, coagulation.

pectoral (pek'tō-răl) [L. *pectoralis;* fr. *pectus,* breast bone]. Relating to the chest.

pectoralgia (pek-tō-ral'jē-ă) [L. *pectus (pector-),* chest, + G. *algos,* pain]. Pain in the chest.

pectoriloquy (pek-tō-ril'ō-kwē) [L. *pectus,* chest, + *loquor,* to speak]. Pectorophony; transmission of the voice sound through the pulmonary structures, so that it is clearly audible on auscultation of the chest; usually indicates consolidation of the underlying lung parenchyma.
aphonic p., Baccelli's *sign.*
whispered p., whispering p., whispered bronchophony; p. of whispered sounds in the same fashion as that of voice sounds.

pectorophony (pek-tō-rof'ō-nē) [L. *pectus,* chest, + G. *phōnē,* voice]. Pectoriloquy.

pectose (pek'tōs). Protopectin. See pectin.

pectous (pek'tŭs). **1.** Relating to or consisting of pectin or pectose. **2.** Denoting a firm coagulated condition sometimes assumed by a gel, which is permanent in that the substance cannot be made to reassume the gel form.

pectus, gen. **pectoris,** pl. **pectora** (pek'tŭs, pek'tō-ris, pek'tō-ră) [L.] [NA]. The anterior wall of the chest or thorax; the breast.
p. carina'tum, pigeon or chicken breast; keeled chest; flattening of the chest on either side with forward projection of the sternum resembling the keel of a boat.
p. excava'tum, a hollow at the lower part of the chest caused by a backward displacement of the xiphoid cartilage. Also called pectus recurvatum; funnel breast or chest; foveated chest; chonechondrosternon; koilosternia; trichterbrust.
p. recurva'tum, p. excavatum.

ped-, pedi-, pedo-. 1 [G. *pais,* child]. Combining forms denoting child. **2** [L. *pes,* foot]. Combining forms denoting feet.

pedal (ped'ăl) [L. *pedalis,* fr. *pes (ped-),* a foot]. Relating to the feet, or to any structure called pes.

pedatrophia, pedatrophy (ped-ă-trō'fē-ă, -at'rō-fē) [G. *pais (paid-),* child, + atrophy]. Marasmus.

pederast (ped'er-ast). One who practices pederasty.

pederasty (ped'er-as-tē) [G. *paiderastia;* fr. *pais (paid-),* boy, + *eraō,* to long for]. Homosexual anal intercourse, especially when practiced on boys.

Pedersen's speculum. See under speculum.

pedesis (pē-dē'sis) [G. *pēdēsis,* a leaping]. Brownian *movement.*

pedi-. See ped-.

pediatric (pē-dē-at'rik) [G. *pais (paid-),* child, + *iatrikos,* relating to medicine]. Relating to pediatrics.

pediatrician (pē'dē-ă-trish'ăn). Pediatrist; a specialist in pediatrics.

pediatrics (pē-dē-at'riks) [G. *pais (paid-),* child, + *iatreia,* medical treatment]. Pediatry; the medical specialty concerned with the study and treatment of children in health and disease during development from birth through aldolescence.

pediatrist (pē-dē-at'rist). Pediatrician.

pediatry (pē'dē-at-rē, pē-dī'ă-trē). Pediatrics.

pedicel (ped'i-sel) [Mod. L. *pedicellus,* dim. of L. *pes,* foot]. Foot process; footplate (2); the secondary process of a podocyte which helps form the visceral capsule of a renal corpuscle.

pedicellate (ped'i-sel-lāt). Pediculate.

pedicellation (ped'i-sĕ-lā'shŭn). Formation of a pedicle or peduncle.

pedicle (ped'ĭ-kl) [L. *pediculus,* dim. of *pes,* foot]. **1.** Pediculus (1). **2.** Peduncle (2); a stalk by which a nonsessile tumor is attached to normal tissue. **3.** A stalk through which a flap receives nourishment until its transfer to another site results in the nourishment coming from that site.
p. of arch of vertebra, *pediculus* arcus vertebrae.
Filatov-Gillies tubed p., tubed *flap.*

pedicterus (pē-dik'ter-ŭs) [G. *pais (paid-),* child, + *ikteros,* jaundice]. *Icterus* neonatorum.

pedicular (pĕ-dik'yū-lăr) [L. *pedicularis*]. Relating to pediculi, or lice.

pediculate (pĕ-dik'yū-lāt) [L. *pedicutatus*]. Pedicellate; pedunculate; not sessile, having a pedicle or peduncle.

pediculation (pĕ-dik'yū-lā'shŭn) [L. *pediculus,* louse]. Infestation with lice.

pediculi (pĕ-dik'yū-lī) [L.]. Plural of pediculus.

pediculicide (pĕ-dik'yū-li-sīd) [L. *pediculus,* louse, + *caedo,* to kill]. An agent used to destroy lice.

Pediculoides ventricosus (pĕ-dik-yū-loy'dēz ven-tri-kō'sŭs) [Mod. L., fr. L. *pediculus,* louse, + *venter,* belly]. *Pyemotes tritici.*

pediculophobia (pĕ-dik'yū-lō-fō'bē-ă) [L. *pediculus,* louse, + G. *phobos,* fear]. Phthiriophobia; morbid fear of infestation with lice.

pediculosis (pĕ-dik'yū-lō'sis) [L. *pediculus,* louse, + G. *-osis,* condition]. Lousiness; the state of being infested with lice.
p. cap'itis, pthiriasis capitis; the presence of lice on the hair of the head.
p. cor'poris, p. vestimenti or vestimentorum; pthiriasis corporis; the presence of body lice. See also parasitic *melanoderma.*
p. palpebra'rum, the presence of lice in the eyelashes.
p. pu'bis, pthiriasis.
p. vestimen'ti, p. vestimento'rum, p. corporis.

pediculous (pĕ-dik'yū-lŭs). Lousy; infested with lice.

Pediculus (pĕ-dik'yū-lŭs) [L.]. A genus of parasitic lice (family Pediculidae) that lives in the hair and feed periodically on blood. Important species include *P. humanus,* the species of louse infecting man; *P. humanus* var. *capitis,* the head louse of man; *P. humanus* var. *corporis* (also called *P. vestimenti* or *P. corporis*), the body louse or clothes louse, which lives and lays eggs (nits) in clothing and feeds on the human body; and *P. pubis* (see *Pthirus pubis*).

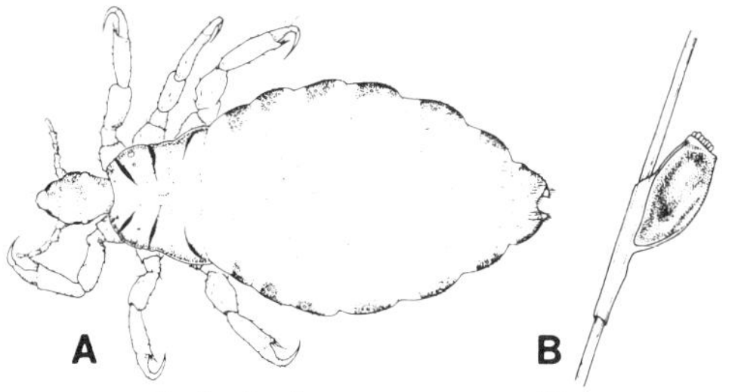

Pediculus humanus var. capitis
A, the female head louse (×17); *B,* egg or nit (×15), attached to hair.

pediculus, pl. **pediculi** (pĕ-dik'yū-lŭs, -lī) **1** [L. pedicle] [NA]. Pedicle (1); a constricted portion or stalk. **2** [L.]. A louse. See *Pediculus.*
p. ar'cus ver'tebrae [NA], pedicle of arch of vertebra; radix arcus vertebrae; the constricted portion of the arch on either side extending from the body to the lamina.

pedicure (ped'i-kyūr) [L. *pes (ped-),* foot, + *cura,* treatment]. Care and treatment of the feet.

pedigree (ped'i-grē) [M.E. *pedegra* fr. O.Fr. *pie de grue,* foot of crane]. Ancestral line of descent, especially as diagrammed on a chart to show ancestral history; used in genetics to analyze inheritance.

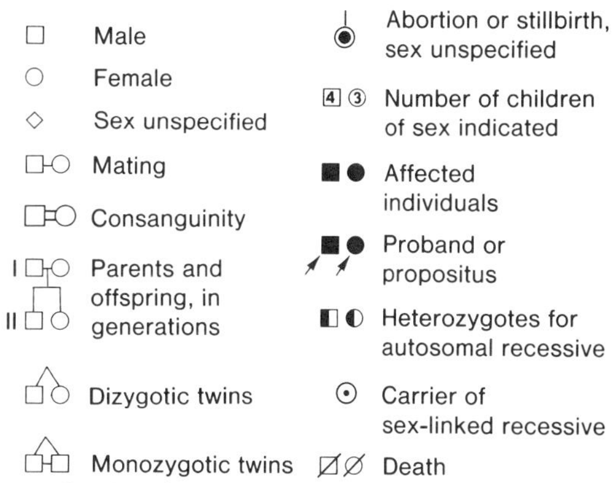

Symbols Commonly Used in Pedigree Charts

pediluvium (ped'i-lū'vē-ŭm) [L. *pes (ped-),* foot, + *luo,* to wash]. A foot bath.

pedionalgia (ped'ē-ō-nal'jē-ă) [G. *pedion,* a plain, sole of the foot, metatarsus, + *algos,* pain]. Pedioneuralgia; rarely used term for podalgia.

pedioneuralgia (ped'ē-ō-nū-ral'jē-ă). Pedionalgia.

pediophobia (pē'dē-ō-fō'bē-ă) [G. *paidion,* a little child, + *phobos,* fear]. Morbid fear aroused by the sight of a child or of a doll.

pediphalanx (ped'i-fā'langks) [L. *pes (ped-),* foot, + phalanx]. A phalanx of the foot, distinguished from maniphalanx.

pedo-. See ped-.

pedodontia (pē-dō-don'shē-ă). Pedodontics.

pedodontics (pē-dō-don'tiks) [G. *pais,* child, + *odous,* tooth]. Pediatric dentistry; pedodontia; the branch of dentistry concerned with the dental care and treatment of children.

pedodontist (pē-dō-don'tist). A dentist who practices pedodontics.

pedodynamometer (ped'ō-dī-nă-mom'ĕ-ter) [L. *pes (ped-),* foot, + G. *dynamis,* force, + G. *metron,* measure]. An instrument for measuring the strength of the leg muscles.

pedogenesis (pē-dō-jen'ĕ-sis) [G. *pais (paid-),* child, + *genesis,* origin]. Permanent larval stage with sexual development, as in certain gall midges (genus *Miastor*). *Cf.* neoteny.

pedogram (ped'ō-gram). A record made by the pedograph.

pedograph (ped'ō-graf) [L. *pes* (ped-), foot, + G. *graphō,* to write]. An instrument for recording and studying the gait.

pedography (pĕ-dog'ră-fē). Production of a record as made by a pedograph.

pedologist (pē-dol'ō-jist). A specialist in pedology.

pedology (pē-dol'ō-jē) [G. *pais (paid-),* child, + *logos,* study]. Paidology; the branch of biology and of sociology concerned with the child in his physical, mental, and social development.

pedometer (pĕ-dom-ĕ-ter) [L. *pes (ped-),* foot]. Podometer; an instrument for measuring the distance covered in walking.

pedomorphism (pē-dō-mōr'fizm) [G. *pais (paid),* child, + *morphē,* form]. Description of adult behavior in terms appropriate to child behavior.

pedophilia (pē-dō-fil'ē-ă) [G. *pais,* child, + *philos,* fond]. In psychiatry, an abnormal attraction to children by an adult for sexual purposes.

pedophilic (pē-dō-fil'ik). Relating to or exhibiting pedophilia.

Pedoviridae (ped-ō-vir'i-dē). Provisional name for a family of bacterial viruses with short tails and genomes of double-stranded DNA (MW 12 to 73 × 10^6); heads may be isometric or elongated. The family includes the T-7 phage group and probably other genera.

peduncle (pe-dŭng'kl, pē'dŭng-kl) [Mod. L. *pedunculus*, dim. of *pes*, foot]. **1.** Pedunculus. **2.** Pedicle (2).
cerebral p., see *pedunculus* cerebri and *crus* cerebri.
p. of corpus callosum, *gyrus* subcallosus.
p. of flocculus, *pedunculus* flocculi.
inferior cerebellar p., *pedunculus* cerebellaris inferior.
inferior thalamic p., *pedunculus* thalami inferior.
lateral thalamic p., *pedunculus* thalami lateralis.
p. of mamillary body, *pedunculus* corporis mamillaris.
middle cerebellar p., *pedunculus* cerebellaris medius.
olfactory p., *tractus* olfactorius.
superior cerebellar p., *pedunculus* cerebellaris superior.
ventral thalamic p., *pedunculus* thalami ventralis.

peduncular (pē-dŭng'kyū-lăr). Relating to a pedicle or peduncle.

pedunculate (pē-dŭng'kyū-lāt). Pediculate.

pedunculotomy (pe-dŭng'kyū-lot'ō-mē) [peduncle + G. *tomē*, incision]. **1.** A total or partial section of a cerebral peduncle. **2.** Pyramidal *tractotomy*, mesencephalic type.

pedunculus, pl. **pedunculi** (pe-dŭng'kyū-lŭs, -kyū-lī) [Mod. L. dim. of *pes*, foot] [NA]. Peduncle (1); a stalk or stem; in neuroanatomy, term loosely applied to a variety of stalklike connecting structures in the brain, composed either exclusively of white matter (*e.g.*, p. cerebellaris) or of white and gray matter (*e.g.*, p. cerebri).
p. cerebella'ris infe'rior [NA], inferior cerebellar peduncle; corpus restiforme; restiform body; large paired bundles of nerve fibers which develop on the dorsolateral surfaces of the upper medulla, extend under the lateral recesses of the rhomboid fossa and curve dorsally into the cerebellum medial to the middle cerebellar peduncle. Fibers forming this composite bundle originate from spinal neurons and medullary relay nuclei. The largest constituent is crossed fibers from the inferior olive; it also contains the dorsal spinocerebellar tract and cerebellar projections from the lateral reticular nucleus, the accessory cuneate nucleus, the paramedian reticular nuclei and the perihypoglossal nuclei. Vestibulocerebellar fibers are placed medially to the p. and are often separately identified as the juxtarestiform body.
p. cerebella'ris me'dius [NA], middle cerebellar peduncle; brachium pontis; the largest of three paired cerebellar peduncles, composed mainly of fibers that originate in the nuclei pontis, cross the midline in the pars basilaris pontis, and emerge on the opposite side as a massive bundle arching dorsally along the lateral side of the pontine tegmentum into the cerebellum; its fibers are distributed chiefly to the cortex of the cerebellar hemisphere.
p. cerebella'ris supe'rior [NA], superior cerebellar peduncle; brachium conjunctivum cerebelli; a large bundle of nerve fibers that originate from the nuclei dentatus and interpositus and emerges from the cerebellum in the rostral direction, along the lateral wall of the fourth ventricle. The bundle submerges from the dorsal surface of the brainstem into the mesencephalic tegmentum, where all of its fibers cross in the massive decussatio brachii conjunctivi. Part of the bundle terminates in the contralateral red nucleus; the bulk of the fibers continue rostrally to parts of the nuclei ventralis lateralis, ventralis posterolateralis, and centralis lateralis of the thalamus.
p. cer'ebri [NA], cerebral peduncle; originally denoting either of the two halves of the midbrain (a relatively narrow "neck" connecting the forebrain to the hindbrain), this term later came to refer to the crus cerebri together with the midbrain tegmentum, and is now even used occasionally to indicate the crus cerebri (basis pedunculi): the massive bundle of corticofugal fibers on either side at the ventral surface of the midbrain.
p. cor'poris callo'si [NA], *gyrus* subcallosus.
p. cor'poris mamilla'ris [NA], peduncle of mamillary body; fasciculus pedunculomamillaris; a fascicle of nerve fibers passing to the mamillary body along the ventral surface of the midbrain; it consists of fibers that originate from the dorsal and ventral tegmental nuclei.
p. floc'culi [NA], peduncle of flocculus; the bundle of afferent and efferent nerve fibers connecting the flocculus and the nodule of the cerebellum; part of its course is in the inferior medullary velum.
p. of pineal body, see habenula (2).
p. thal'ami infe'rior [NA], inferior thalamic peduncle; a large fiber bundle emerging from the anterior part of the thalamus in the ventral direction, in part joining the medial fibers of the internal capsule, in other part curving laterally around the medial margin of the capsule into the substantia innominata. Many of its fibers establish a reciprocal connection of the mediodorsal nucleus of the thalamus with the orbital gyri of the frontal lobe, but numerous other fibers constitute a conduction system from the amygdala and olfactory cortex to the mediodorsal nucleus. See also *ansa* peduncularis.
p. thal'ami latera'lis, lateral thalamic peduncle; the massive group of fibers that emerges from the laterodorsal side of the thalamus to join the corona radiata; it reciprocally connects the lateral nucleus and the geniculate bodies of the thalamus with the corresponding regions of the cerebral cortex.
p. thal'ami ventra'lis, ventral thalamic peduncle; the massive system of fiber bundles emerging through the ventral, lateral, and anterior borders of the thalamus to join the internal capsule and parts of the corona radiata; it contains the fibers reciprocally connecting the ventral thalamic nuclei with the precentral and postcentral gyri of the cerebral cortex.
p. vitelli'nus, yolk stalk.

peeling (pēl'ing) [M.E. *pelen*]. A stripping off or loss of epidermis, as in sunburn, postscarlatinal peeling, or toxic epidermal necrolysis.

peenash (pē'nash) [East Indian]. Rhinitis caused by insect larvae in the nasal passages.

PEEP Abbreviation for positive end-expiratory *pressure*.

peg. A cylindrical projection.
rete p.'s, rete *ridges*.

Peiffer, J. See Hirsch-P. *stain*.

pejorism (pē'jōr-izm) [L. *pejor*, worse]. A pessimistic attitude.

Pel, Pieter K., Dutch physician, 1852–1919. See P.-Ebstein *disease*, *fever*.

pelade (pē-lad', -lahd') [Fr. *peler*, to remove the hair from a hide]. Alopecia.

pelage (pel'ij) [Fr.]. The hairy covering of the body of animals; *e.g.*, the fur or coat.

pelargonic acid (pel-ar-gon'ik). *n*-Nonanoic acid; $CH_3(CH_2)_7COOH$; used in the manufacture of lacquers and plastics.

Pelger, Karel, Dutch physician, 1885–1931. See P.-Huët nuclear *anomaly*.

pelidnoma (pē-lid-nō'mă) [G. *pelidnos*, livid, + *-oma*, tumor]. Pelioma; a circumscribed, elevated, livid patch on the skin.

pelioma (pē-lē-ō'mă). Pelidnoma.

peliosis (pē-lē-ō'sis, pel-) [G. *peliōsis*, a livid spot, livor]. Purpura.
p. hep'atis, the presence throughout the liver of blood-filled cavities which may become lined by endothelium or become organized.

Pelizaeus, Friedrich, German neurologist, 1850–1917. See Merzbacher-P. *disease*.

pellagra (pĕ-lag′ră, pĕ-lā′gră) [It. *pelle,* skin, + *agro,* rough]. Saint Ignatius' itch; maidism; mal de la rosa; mal rosso; mayidism; psychoneurosis maidica; Alpine scurvy; an affection characterized by gastrointestinal disturbances, erythema (particularly of exposed areas) followed by desquamation, and nervous and mental disorders; may occur because of a poor diet, alcoholism, or some other disease causing impairment of nutrition; commonly seen when corn (maize) is a main nutrient in the diet, resulting in a deficiency of niacin.
infantile p., kwashiorkor.
secondary p., p. resulting from any morbid condition which impairs nutrition by increasing the requirement or reducing the available supply of vitamins.
p. sine p., p. without the characteristic skin lesions.

pellagroid (pĕ-lag′royd). Resembling pellagra.

pellagrous (pĕ-lag′rŭs). Relating to or suffering from pellagra.

Pellegrini, Augusto, 19th-20th century Italian surgeon. See P.'s or P.-Stieda *disease.*

pellet (pel′et) [Fr. *pelote;* L. *pila,* a ball]. **1.** A pilule, or minute pill. **2.** A small rod-shaped or ovoid dosage form that is sterile and is composed essentially of pure steroid hormones in compressed form, intended for subcutaneous implantation in body tissues; serves as a depot providing for the slow release of the hormone over an extended period of time.

pellicle (pel′i-kl) [L. *pellicula,* dim of *pellis,* skin]. **1.** Literally and nonspecifically, a thin skin. **2.** A film or scum on the surface of a liquid. **3.** Cell boundary of sporozoites and merozoites among members of the protozoan subphylum Apicomplexa (Sporozoa), consisting of an outer unit membrane and an inner layer of two unit membranes.
acquired p., acquired, acquired enamel, or posteruption cuticle; brown p.; a thin film (about 1 μm), derived mainly from salivary glycoproteins, which forms over the surface of a cleansed tooth crown when it is exposed to the saliva.
brown p., acquired p.

pellicular, pelliculous (pe-lik′yū-lăr, -lŭs). Relating to a pellicle.

Pellizzari, Pietro, Italian dermatologist, 1823–1892. See Jadassohn-P. *anetoderma.*

Pellizzi, G.B., 19th-20th century Italian physician. See P.'s *syndrome.*

pellote (pā-yō′tā) [Aztec, *peyotl*]. Peyote.

pellucid (pe-lū′sid) [L. *pellucidus*]. Allowing the passage of light.

pelma (pel′mă) [G.]. *Planta* pedis.

pelmatic (pel-mat′ik) [G. *pelma,* sole]. Relating to the sole of the foot.

pelmatogram (pel-mat′ō-gram) [G. *pelma* (*pelmat-*), sole of the foot, + *gramma,* a picture]. An imprint of the sole of the foot, made by resting the inked foot on a sheet of paper, or by pressing the greased foot on a plaster of Paris paste.

pelopathy (pē-lop′ă-thē) [G. *pēlos,* mud, + *pathos,* suffering]. Pelotherapy.

pelotherapy (pē′lō-thār-ă-pē) [G. *pēlos,* mud, + *therapeia,* treatment]. Pelopathy; application of peloids, such as mud, peat, or clay, to all or part of the body.

pelt. The hide of animals on which the hair, fur, or wool is left.

pelta (pel′tă) [L. a shield]. A crescentic, silver-staining, membranous organelle located anteriorly near the base of the flagella in certain flagellate protozoa, as in *Trichomonas.*

peltation (pel-tā′shŭn) [L. *pelta,* a light shield]. Protection provided by inoculation with an antiserum or with a vaccine.

pelvi-, pelvio-, pelvo- [L. *pelvis,* basin (pelvis)]. Combining forms relating to the pelvis.

pelvic (pel′vik). Relating to a pelvis.

pelvic direction (pel′vik dī-rek′shŭn). The direction of the axis of the pelvis.

pelvicephalography (pel′vi-sef-ă-log′ră-fē) [pelvi- + G. *kephalē,* head, + *graphō,* to write]. Cephalopelvimetry.

pelvicephalometry (pel′vi-sef-ă-lom′ĕ-trē) [pelvi- + G. *kephalē,* head, + *metron,* measure]. Measurement of the female pelvic diameters in relation to those of the fetal head.

pelvifixation (pel-vi-fik-sā′shŭn). Surgical attachment of a floating pelvic organ to the wall of the pelvic cavity.

pelvigraph (pel′vi-graf) [pelvi- + G. *graphō,* to write]. An instrument for drawing the contour and dimensions of the pelvis; may be drawn to scale.

pelvilithotomy (pel′vi-li-thot′ō-mē) [pelvi- + G. *lithos,* stone, + *tomē,* incision]. Pyelolithotomy.

pelvimeter (pel-vim′ĕ-ter). Instrument shaped like calipers for measuring the diameters of the pelvis.

pelvimetry (pel-vim′ĕ-trē) [pelvi- + G. *metron,* measure]. Measurement of the diameters of the pelvis.
manual p., measurement of the essential diameters of the bony pelvis using the hands.
planographic p., measurement of the bony pelvis through use of lateral and anterior x-ray films.
stereoscopic p., a seldom used measurement of the bony pelvis through use of stereoscopic imagery giving a three-dimensional picture of the pelvis.

pelvio-. See pelvi-.

pelviolithotomy (pel-vē-ō-li-thot′ō-mē). Pyelolithotomy.

pelvioperitonitis (pel′vē-ō-per-i-tō-nī′tis). Pelvic *peritonitis.*

pelvioplasty (pel′vē-ō-plas-tē) [pelvio- + G. *plastos,* formed]. **1.** Symphysiotomy or pubiotomy for enlargement of the female pelvic outlet. **2.** Pyeloplasty.

pelvioscopy (pel-vē-os′kō-pē) [pelvio- + G. *skopeō,* to view]. Pelvoscopy; examination of the pelvis for any purpose; *e.g.,* to determine its diameters.

pelviotomy, pelvitomy (pel′vē-ot′ō-mē) [pelvio- + G. *tomē,* incision]. **1.** Symphysiotomy. **2.** Pubiotomy. **3.** Pyelotomy.

pelviperitonitis (pel-vē-per-i-tō-nī′tis). Pelvic *peritonitis.*

PELVIS

pelvis, pl. **pelves** (pel′vis, pel′vēz) [L. basin] **1** [NA]. The massive cup-shaped ring of bone, with its ligaments, at the lower end of the trunk, formed of the os coxae (the pubic bone, ilium, and ischium) on either side and in front, and the sacrum, and coccyx posteriorly. **2.** Any basin-like or cup-shaped cavity, as the p. of the kidney.
android p., a masculine or funnel-shaped p.
anthropoid p., an apelike p., with a long anteroposterior diameter and a narrow transverse diameter.
assimilation p., a deformity in which the transverse processes of the last lumbar vertebra are fused with the sacrum, or the last sacral with the first coccygeal body.
beaked p., osteomalacic p.
brachypellic p., transverse oval p.; a p. in which the transverse diameter is more than 1 cm longer but less than 3 cm longer than the anteroposterior diameter.
caoutchouc p., rubber p.; in osteomalacia, a p. in which the bones are still soft.
contracted p., a p. with less than normal measurements in any diameter.

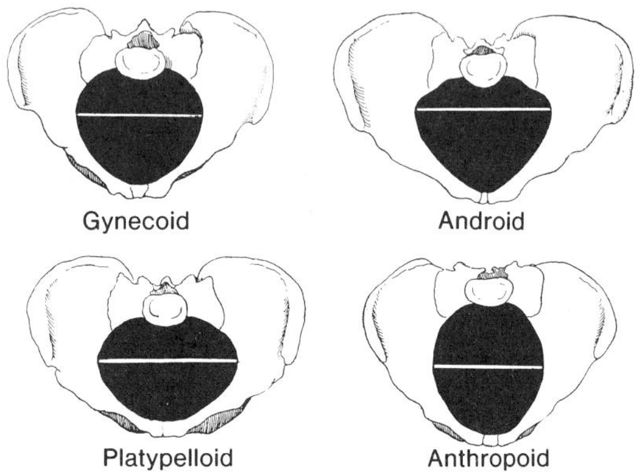

Types of Female Pelvis

cordate p., cordiform p., heart-shaped p.; a p. with sacrum projecting forward between the ilia, giving to the brim a heart shape.
Deventer's p., a p. with shortened anteroposterior diameter.
dolichopellic p., longitudinal oval p.; a p. in which the anteroposterior diameter is longer than the transverse.
dwarf p., p. nana; a very small p., in which the several bones are united by cartilage as in the infant.
false p., p. major.
flat p., p. plana; a p. in which the anteroposterior diameter is uniformly contracted, the sacrum being dislocated forward between the iliac bones.
frozen p., hardened p.; a condition in which the true p. is indurated throughout, especially by carcinoma.
funnel-shaped p., a p. in which the pelvic inlet dimensions are normal, but the outlet is contracted in the transverse or in both transverse and anteroposterior diameters.
p. of gallbladder, Hartmann's *pouch.*
gynecoid p., the normal female p.
hardened p., frozen p.
heart-shaped p., cordate p.
inverted p., split p. with separation at pubis.
p. jus'to ma'jor, a symmetrical p. with greater than normal measurements in all diameters.
p. jus'to mi'nor, a p. of the female type, but with all its diameters smaller than normal.
juvenile p., a p. justo minor in which the bones are slender.
kyphoscoliotic p., a p. with marked anteroposterior curvature of the spine combined with lateral spinal curvature, usually due to severe rickets.
kyphotic p., backward curvature of lumbar spine causing contraction of pelvic measurements.
large p., p. major.
longitudinal oval p., dolichopellic p.
lordotic p., a deformed p. associated with lordosis.
p. ma'jor [NA], large p.; false p.; p. spuria; the expanded portion of the p. above the brim.
masculine p., **(1)** a p. justo minor in which the bones are large and heavy; **(2)** a slight degree of funnel-shaped p. in the woman, in which the shape approximates that of the male p.
mesatipellic p., round p.; one in which the anteroposterior and transverse diameters are equal or the transverse diameter is not more than 1 cm longer than the anteroposterior diameter.
p. mi'nor [NA], small p.; true p.; p. vera; the cavity of the p. below the brim or superior aperture.
Nägele's p., an obliquely contracted or unilateral synostotic p., marked by arrest of development of one lateral half of the sacrum, usually ankylosis of the sacroiliac joint on that side, rotation of the sacrum toward the same side, and deviation of the symphysis pubis to the opposite side.
p. na'na, dwarf p.
p. obtec'ta, a form of kyphotic p. in which the angular curvature of the spine is low and extreme so that the spinal column projects horizontally across the inlet of the p.
osteomalacic p., beaked or rostrate p.; a pelvic deformity in osteomalacia; the pressure of the trunk on the sacrum and lateral pressure of the femoral heads produce a pelvic aperture that is three-cornered or has the shape of a heart or cloverleaf, while the pubic bone becomes beak-shaped.
Otto p., Otto's *disease.*
p. pla'na, flat p.
platypellic p., flat oval p., in which the transverse diameter is more than 3 cm longer than the anteroposterior diameter.
platypelloid p., simple flat p.
Prague p., spondylolisthetic p.
pseudo-osteomalacic p., an extreme degree of rachitic p., resembling the puerperal osteomalacic p., in which the pelvic canal is obstructed by a forward projection of the sacrum, and an approximation of the acetabula.
rachitic p., a contracted and deformed p., most commonly a flat p., occurring from rachitic softening of the bones in early life.
renal p., p. renalis.
p. rena'lis [NA], renal p.; a flattened funnel-shaped expansion of the upper end of the ureter receiving the calices, the apex being continuous with the ureter.
reniform p., a modified cordate p., with a long transverse diameter, giving the brim a kidney shape.
Robert's p., a p. which is narrowed transversely in consequence of the almost entire absence of the alae of the sacrum.
Rokitansky's p., spondylolisthetic p.
rostrate p., osteomalacic p.
round p., mesatipellic p.
rubber p., caoutchouc p.
scoliotic p., a deformed p. associated with lateral curvature of the spine.
small p., p. minor.
spider p., narrow calices of renal p.
split p., a p. in which the symphysis pubis is absent, the pelvic bones being separated by quite an interval; usually associated with exstrophy of the bladder.
spondylolisthetic p., Prague or Rokitansky's p.; a p. whose brim is more or less occluded by a forward dislocation of the body of the lower lumbar vertebra.
p. spu'ria, p. major.
transverse oval p., bracypellic p.
true p., p. minor.

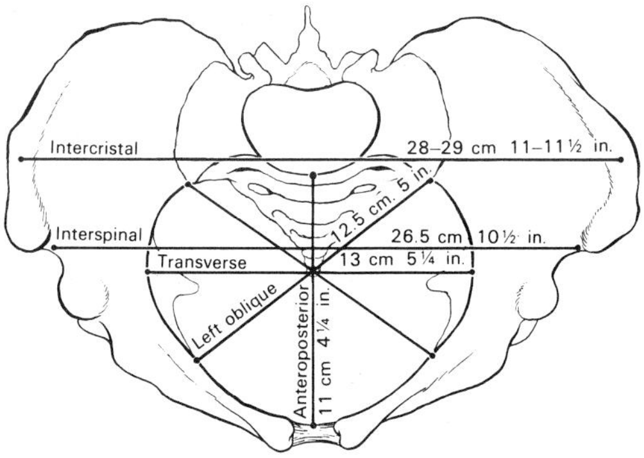

Diameters of Pelvis Major and Pelvic Brim

p. ve'ra, p. minor.

---

pelvisacral (pel-vi-sā'krăl). Relating to both the pelvis, or hip bones, and the sacrum.

pelviscope (pel'vi-skōp) [pelvi- + G. *skopeō,* to view]. Instrument for examining the interior of the pelvis.

pelvitherm (pel'vi-therm) [pelvi- + G. *thermē,* heat]. Instrument for applying heat to the pelvic organs.

pelvitomy (pel-vit'ō-mē). Pelviotomy.

pelviureterography (pel-vi-yū-rē-ter-og'ră-fē). Pyelography.

pelvo-. See pelvi-.

pelvocephalography (pel'vō-sef-ă-log'ră-fē). Cephalopelvimetry.

pelvoscopy (pel-vos'cō-pē). Pelvioscopy.

pelvospondylitis ossificans (pel'vō-spon-di-lī'tis os-if'i-kanz) [L. *pelvis,* basin, + G. *spondylos,* vertebra, + *-itis;* L. *os,* bone, + *facere,* to make]. Deposit of bony substance between the vertebrae of the sacrum.

pelyco- [G. *pelyx,* bowl (pelvis)]. Rarely used combining form denoting the pelvis. See pelvi-.

pemoline (pem'ō-lēn). 2-Imino-5-phenyl-4-oxazolidinone; a psychostimulant used in the treatment of minimal brain dysfunction in children.

pemphigoid (pem'fi-goyd) [G. *pemphix,* blister, + *eidos,* resemblance]. **1.** Resembling pemphigus. **2.** A disease resembling pemphigus but significantly distinguishable histologically (nonacantholytic) and clinically (generally benign course).

benign mucosal p., cicatricial p.; a chronic disease that produces adhesions and progressive cicatrization and shrinkage of the conjunctival, oral, and vaginal mucous membranes.

bullous p., a chronic, generally benign disease, most commonly of old age, characterized by tense nonacantholytic bullae in which serum antibodies are localized to the epidermal basement membrane, causing detachment of the entire epidermis.

cicatricial p., benign mucosal p.

ocular p., cicatricial *conjunctivitis.*

pemphigus (pem'fi-gŭs) [G. *pemphix,* a blister]. General term used to designate the chronic bullous diseases with acantholysis: p. foliaceous, p. erythematosus, or p. vegetans; also used with a modifying adjective to designate a variety of blistering skin diseases.

p. acu'tus, bullous fever; a pyogenic infection due to local trauma, that responds to antibiotic therapy; if untreated, the condition may become extensive and the patient seriously ill.

Brazilian p., fogo selvagem.

p. contagio'sus, Manson's pyosis; a superficial pyogenic infection.

p. croupo'sus, p. diptherit'icus, obsolete terms for the formation of a false membrane on the raw surface left after rupture of the bullae.

p. erythemato'sus, Senear-Usher disease or syndrome; an eruption involving the scalp, face, and trunk; the lesions are scaling erythematous macules and blebs, combining the clinical features of both lupus erythematosus and p. vulgaris; bullae are subcorneal; may be a variant of p. foliaceus.

familial benign chronic p., Hailey and Hailey disease; recurrent eruption of vesicles and bullae that become scaling and crusted lesions with vesicular borders, predominantly of the neck, groin, and axillary regions; irregular autosomal dominant inheritance.

p. folia'ceus, a generally chronic form of p. in which extensive exfoliative dermatitis, with no perceptible blistering, may be present in addition to the bullae; crusted acantholytic superficial epidermal lesions are usually present at the site of ruptured bullae.

p. gangreno'sus, **(1)** *dermatitis* gangrenosa infantum; **(2)** bullous *impetigo* of newborn.

p. lepro'sus, an eruption of bullae, occurring sometimes in the course of anesthetic leprosy.

p. veg'etans, **(1)** Neumann's disease; a form of p. vulgaris in which vegetations develop on the eroded surfaces left by ruptured bullae; new bullae continue to form; **(2)** Hallopeau's disease (2); a chronic benign vegetating form of p., with lesions commonly in the axillae and perineum; spontaneous remissions and occasionally permanent healing occur.

p. vulga'ris, a serious form of p., occurring in middle age, in which cutaneous flaccid acantholytic suprabasal bullae and oral mucosal erosions may be localized a few months before becoming generalized; blisters break easily and are slow to heal; results from the action of autoimmune antibodies that localize to intercellular sites of stratified squamous epithelium.

pempidine (pem'pi-dēn). Secondary amine of the mecamylamine group, effective as a ganglionic blocking agent; also available as p. tartrate, with the same uses.

pencil (pen'sil) [L. *penicillum,* a paint-brush]. **1.** A roll of material in the form of a cylinder. **2.** A stick, especially of caustic substances, pointed like a p. for local application. **3.** All the rays of light focused at a given point.

pendelluft (pen-del-lŭft') [Ger. *Pendel,* pendulum, + *Luft,* air]. Transient movement of gas out of some alveoli and into others when flow has just stopped at the end of inspiration, or such movement in the opposite direction just at the end of expiration; occurs when regions of the lung differ in compliance, airway resistance, or inertance so that the time constants of their filling (or emptying) in response to a change of transpulmonary pressure are not the same.

Pendred, Vaughan, British surgeon, 1869–1946. See P.'s *syndrome.*

penectomy (pē-nek'tō-mē) [L. *penis* + G. *ektomē,* excision]. Phallectomy.

penetrance (pen'ĕ-trans) [see penetration]. The frequency, expressed as a fraction or percentage, of individuals who are phenotypically affected, among persons of an appropriate genotype (*i.e.* homozygous or hemizygous for recessives, heterozygotes or homozygotes for dominants); factors affecting expression may be genetic, environmental, or due to purely random variation.

penetrate (pen'ĕ-trāt). To pierce; to pass into the deeper tissues or into a cavity.

penetration (pen-ĕ-trā'shŭn) [L. *penetratio,* fr. *penetro,* pp. *-atus,* to enter]. **1.** A piercing or entering. **2.** Mental acumen. **3.** Focal *depth.*

penetrometer (pen-ĕ-trom'ĕ-ter). An obsolete instrument for measuring the penetrating power of x-rays from any given source.

-penia [G. *penia,* poverty]. Combining form used in the suffix position to denote deficiency.

penial (pē'nē-ăl). Penile.

peniaphobia (pē'nē-ă-fō'bē-ă) [G. *penia,* poverty, + *phobos,* fear]. Morbid fear of poverty.

penicillamine (pen-i-sil'ă-mēn). *β,β*-Dimethylcysteine; *β*-thiovaline; a degradation product of penicillin; a chelating agent used in the treatment of lead poisoning, hepatolenticular degeneration, and cystinuria, and in the removal of excess copper in Wilson's disease; also available as p. hydrochloride.

penicillanate (pen-i-sil'ă-nāt). A salt of penicillanic acid.

penicillanic acid (pen-i-si-lan'ik). A penicillin without the characterizing R group (with H– replacing ROONH–) of penicillin.

penicillary (pen-i-sil'ă-rē). Denoting a penicillus (1).

penicillate (pen-i-sil'āt). **1.** Pertaining to a penicillus. **2.** Having a tuftlike structure.

penicillic acid (pen-i-sil'ik). An antibiotic produced by *Penicillium puberulum,* a mold found on maize, and from *P. cyclopium;* active against Gram-positive and Gram-negative bacteria but toxic to animal tissues. See fig. on p. 1158.

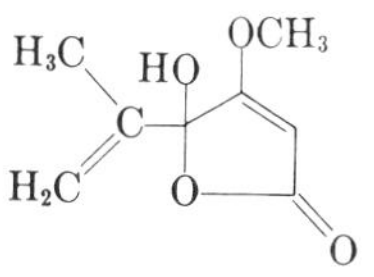

Penicillic acid

penicillin (pen-i-sil'in) [see penicillus]. **1.** Originally, an antibiotic substance obtained from cultures of the molds *Penicillium notatum* or *P. chrysogenum.* **2.** One of a family of natural or synthetic variants of penicillic acid. They are mainly bactericidal in action, are especially active against Gram-positive organisms, and show a particularly low toxic action on animal tissue.

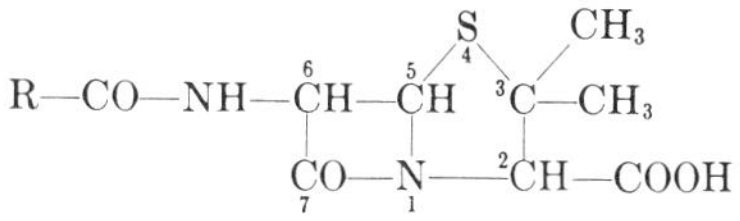

Penicillin

aluminum p., the trivalent aluminum salt of an antibiotic substance or substances produced by the growth of the molds *Penicillium notatum* or *P. chrysogenum;* used for oral or sublingual administration.

p. B, phenethicillin potassium.

buffered crystalline p. G, crystalline potassium p. G or crystalline sodium p. G buffered with not less than 4% and not more than 5% of sodium citrate.

chloroprocaine p. O, a crystalline salt of 2-chloroprocaine and p. O, insoluble in water; the level of the antibiotic in the blood persists for 24 hours; its antibacterial activity is similar to that of p. O and G.

p. G, benzylpenicillin; $R=C_6H_5CH_2$–; the most commonly used p. compound; it comprises 85% of the p. salts (sodium, potassium, aluminum, and procaine).

p. G benzathine, a benzylpenicillin compound with *N,N*- dibenzylethylenediamine (2:1); a relatively insoluble preparation that may remain in the body for 1 to 2 weeks.

p. G hydrabamine, a dipenicillin compound, a mixture of p. G salts consisting chiefly of the salt of the diacidic base *N,N'*-bis-(dehydroabietyl) ethylenediamine.

p. G potassium, potassium benzylpenicillin; the potassium salt of p. G, containing 85 to 90% p. G.

p. G procaine, procaine p; procaine benzylpenicillin; the procaine salt of p. G; it has a more prolonged action than p. G.

p. G sodium sodium benzylpenicillin; the sodium salt of p. G, containing not less than 85% p. G.

p. N, *cephalosporin* N.

p. O, allylmercaptomethylpenicillin; $R-=CH_2=CHCH_2SCH_2$–; produced by growing the mold in a medium containing allylmercaptomethylacetic acid; also available as the potassium and sodium salts.

p. phenoxymethyl, p. V.

p. V, p. phenoxymethyl; phenoxymethylpenicillin; $R=C_6H_5$-OCH_2–; obtained from *Penicillium chrysogenum* Q 176; a crystalline nonhydroscopic acid, very stable even in high humidity; it resists destruction by gastric juice; the potassium salt is used orally.

p. V benzathine, benzathine phenoxymethylpenicillin; p. for oral use.

p. V hydrabamine, hydrabamine phenoxymethylpenicillin; a compound with preparation and uses analogous to those of p. G hydrabamine.

penicillinase (pen-i-sil'i-nās). **1.** β-Lactamose. **2.** A purified enzyme preparation obtained from cultures of a strain of *Bacillus cereus;* formerly used in the treatment of slowly developing or delayed penicillin reactions.

penicillinate (pen-i-sil'i-nāt). A salt of a penicillic acid (*i.e.,* of a penicillin).

Penicillium (pen-i-sil'ē-ŭm) [see penicillus]. A genus of fungi (class Ascomycetes, order Aspergillales), species of which yield various antibiotic substances and biologicals; *e.g., P. citrinum* yields citrinin; *P. claviforme, P. expansum,* and *P. patulum* yield patulin; *P. chrysogenum* yields penicillin; *P. griseofulvin* yields griseofulvin; *P. notatum* yields penicillin and notatin; *P. cyclopium* and *P. puberulum* yield penicillic acid; *P. purpurogenum* and *P. rubrum* yield rubratoxin.

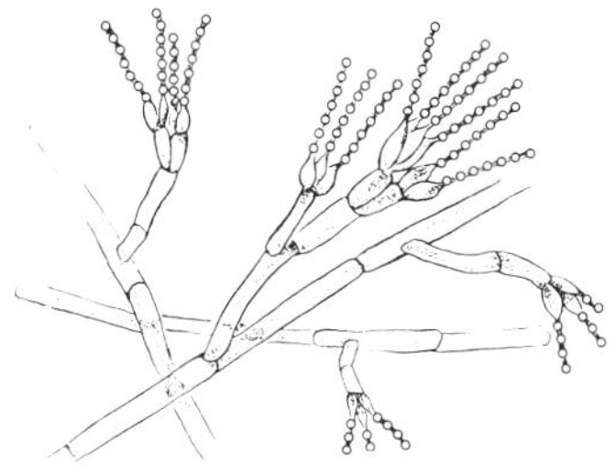

Penicillium

penicilloic acid (pen'i-si-lō'ik). Alkali and bacterial degradation product of a penicillin, resulting from hydrolysis of the 1,7 bond.

penicilloyl polylysine (pen-i-sil'ō-il). A preparation of polylysine and a penicillic acid, used intradermally in the diagnosis of penicillin sensitivity; sensitive persons may react with systemic manifestations, including generalized cutaneous eruptions.

penicillus, pl. **penicilli** (pen-i-sil'ŭs, -sil'ī) [L. paint brush]. **1** [NA]. One of the tufts formed by the repeated subdivision of the minute arterial twigs in the spleen. **2.** In fungi, one of the branched conidiophores bearing chains of conidia in *Penicillium* species.

penile (pē'nīl). Penial; relating to the penis.

penillic acids (pe-nil'ik). Acid degradation products of penicillins, produced by cleavage of the 1,7 bond, forming penicilloic acid, and formation of a bond between the exocyclic carbonyl carbon and N-1 with elimination of H_2O from those two and the exocyclic NH.

penin (pen'in). 6-Aminopenicillanic acid (NH_2 replacing RCONH– in penicillin); an intermediate in the synthesis of penicillins.

penis (pē'nis) [L. tail] [NA]. Coles; membrum virile; viral member; phallus; priapus; virga; intromittent organ; the organ of copulation in the male; it is formed of three columns of erectile tissue, two arranged laterally on the dorsum (corpora cavernosa p.) and one median below (corpus spongiosum); the urethra traverses the latter; the extremity (glans p.) is formed by an expansion of the corpus spongiosum, and is more or less completely covered by a free fold of skin (preputium).

bifid p., diphallus.

clubbed p., a deformity of the erect p. marked by a curve to one side or toward the scrotum.

double p., diphallus.

p. femin'eus, clitoris.

p. luna'tus, chordee (1).

p. mulie'bris, clitoris.

p. palma'tus, a p. enclosed by the scrotum.

webbed p., a p. whose undersurface is joined to the front of the scrotum by a fold of skin.

penischisis (pē-nis'ki-sis) [L. *penis* + G. *schisis,* fissure]. A fissure of the penis resulting in an abnormal opening into the urethra, either above (epispadia), below (hypospadia), or to one side (paraspadia).

penitis (pē-nī'tis). Phallitis; priapitis; obsolete term for inflammation of the penis.

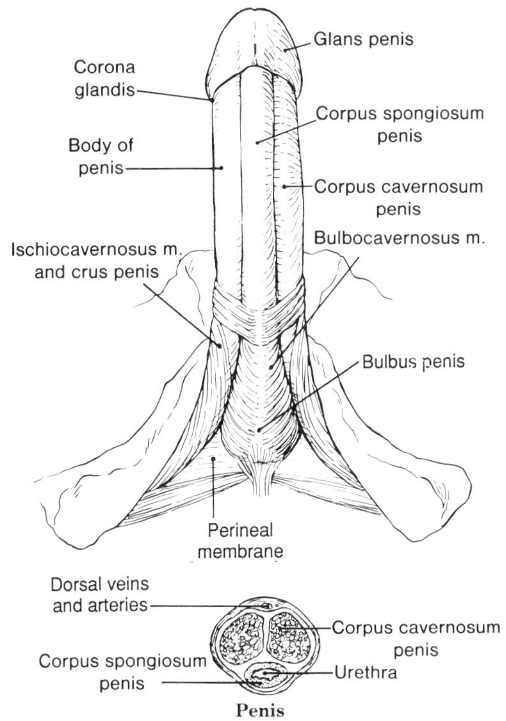

Penis
Top, skin and subcutaneous tissue removed in part to show structure of root of penis; *bottom,* transverse section of penis.

pennate (pen'āt) [L. *pennatus,* fr. *penna,* feather]. Penniform; feathered; resembling a feather.

penniform (pen'i-fōrm) [L. *penna,* feather, + *forma,* form]. Pennate.

pennyroyal (pen'ē-roy-ăl). A name in folk medicine given to *Mentha pulegium* (an aromatic p.), or to *Hedeoma pulegeoides* (American p.) (family Labiatae); an aromatic stimulant formerly used as an emmenagogue.

penoscrotal (pē'nō-skrō'tăl). Relating to both penis and scrotum.

penotomy (pē-not'o-mē) [L. *penis* + G. *tomē,* a cutting]. Phallotomy.

Penrose, Charles B., U.S. gynecologist, 1862–1925. See P. *drain.*

penta- [G. *pente,* five]. Combining form denoting five.

pentabasic (pen-tă-bā'sik) [penta- + G. *basis,* base]. Denoting an acid having five replaceable hydrogen atoms.

pen'tad [G. *pentas,* the number five]. **1.** A collection of five things in some way related. **2.** In chemistry, a pentavalent element.

pentadactyl, pentadactyle (pen-tă-dak'til) [penta- + G. *daktylos,* finger]. Quinquedigitate; having five fingers or toes on each hand or foot.

pentaerythritol (pen-tă-ē-rith'ri-tol). Tetrakis(hydroxymethyl)-methane; $C(CH_2OH)_4$; the tetranitrate is a coronary vasodilator with action similar to that of other slow acting organic nitrates.

pentagastrin (pen-tă-gas'trin). The substituted pentapeptide, Boc-Ala-Trp-Met-Asp-Phe(NH_2); a gastric acid stimulator.

pentalogy (pen-tal'ō-jē) [penta- + G. *logos,* treatise, word]. A combination of five elements, such as five concurrent symptoms.
p. of Fallot, Fallot's tetralogy with, in addition, a patent foramen ovale or atrial septal defect.

pentamer (pen'tă-mer) [penta- + G. *meros,* part]. See virion.

pentamethonium bromide (pen'tă-me-thō'nē-ŭm). Pentamethylene-*bis*[trimethylammonium bromide]; a ganglionic blocking agent with the same antihypertensive use as hexamethonium chloride.

pentamidine isethionate (pen-tam'i-dēn). *p,p'*-(Pentamethylenedioxy)dibenzamidinebis(*β*-hydroxyethanesulfonate); a toxic but effective drug used in the prophylaxis and treatment of early stages of both types of African sleeping sickness (Gambian and Rhodesian trypanosomiasis). It does not cross the blood-brain barrier and is not effective in the treatment of the advanced (neurological) stage of the disease. Also used to treat leishmaniasis that does not respond to therapy with pentavalent antimonials and in the treatment of pneumonia caused by *Pneumocystis carinii.*

pentanoic acid (pen-tă-nō'ik). Valeric acid.

pentapiperide fumarate (pen-tă-pip'er-īd). 3-Methyl-2-phenylvaleric acid 1-methyl-4-piperidyl ester fumarate; an intestinal antispasmodic.

pentapiperium methylsulfate (pen'tă-pī-per'ē-ŭm). 4-Hydroxy-1,1-dimethylpiperidinium methyl sulfate 3-methyl-2-phenylvalerate; an anticholinergic agent.

pentaquine (pen'tă-kwīn). 8-(5-Iso-propylamino)-6-methoxyquinoline; an antimalarial agent closely related chemically to pamaquine but less toxic and more effective; it is administered with quinine, the two drugs acting synergically; active against *Plasmodium vivax* infections.

Pentastoma (pen-tas'tō-mă) [penta- + G. *stoma,* mouth]. Older name for a genus of Pentastomida, now called *Linguatula.* The species described as *P. denticulatum* proved to be the larva of *Linguatula rhinaria,* sometimes parasitic in the nose of man and other mammals; adults are found in the lungs of reptiles.

pentastomiasis (pen'tă-stō-mī'ă-sis). Infection of herbivorous animals, swine, and man with larval Pentastomida; lesions occur principally in the lymph nodes of the digestive tract, where they often resemble those of tuberculosis.

Pentastomida (pen-tă-stom'i-dă) [see *Pentastoma*]. The tongue worms, a group of parasitic wormlike animals considered to form a distinct phylum thought to be descended from primitive arthropods, though they are modified by parasitism to form elongate, pseudosegmented, wormlike organisms with two to three pairs of budlike degenerate limbs in the larva and anterior, hollow, fanglike hooks in the adult. Adults are usually parasitic in the lungs or respiratory tract of vertebrates, usually in snakes and other reptiles, though one group parasitizes the air sacs of birds and one family (Linguatulidae) has become adapted to the lungs of mammal carnivores (families Felidae and Canidae). Larvae are found in the viscera of many hosts that serve as prey of the final hosts (insects, fish, amphibians, chiefly frogs, and mammals, chiefly rodents). Dogs may develop adult *Linguatula serrata* in their nasal passages from infective larvae (nymphs) in the viscera of sheep, cattle, or rabbits, which became infected from water or vegetation contaminated with eggs passed by infected dogs; humans also can develop a larval infection from this source. Human infection of liver, spleen, and lungs has been reported in Africa from *Armilifer armillatus* and in China by *A. moniliformis* from contaminated water or vegetation or from handling infected snakes.

pentatomic (pent'ă-tom-ik) [penta- + atomic]. Denoting five atoms per molecule.

Pentatrichomonas (pen'tă-trik-ō-mō'nas, pen'tă-trī-kom'ō-nas) [penta- + *Trichomonas*]. A genus of parasitic protozoan flagellates, formerly part of the genus *Trichomonas but now separated as a distinct genus by the presence of five anterior flagella and a granular parabasal body. The species P. hominis* lives as a commensal in the colon of man and other primates, dogs, cats, oxen, and various rodents.

pentavalent (pen-tă-vā′lent, pen-tav′ă-lent). Quinquevalent; having a combining power (valence) of five.

pentazocine (pen-taz′ō-sēn). 1,2,3,4,5,6-Hexahydro-6,11-dimethyl-3-(3-methyl-2-butenyl)-2,6-methano-3-benzazocin-8-ol; a potent analgesic with some addiction liability but only rare withdrawal syndrome and tolerance; available as the hydrochloride and lactate salts.

pentetate trisodium calcium (pen′tĕ-tāt). Calcium trisodium pentetate; the calcium trisodium salt of pentetic acid.

pentetic acid (pen-tet′ik). Diethylenetriamine pentaacetic acid; a pentaacetic acid triamine with affinity for heavy metals; used as the calcium sodium chelate in the treatment of iron-storage disease and poisoning from heavy metals and radioactive metals. See also ethylenediaminetetraacetic acid.

penthienate bromide (pen-thī′ĕ-nāt). 2-Diethylaminoethyl-α-cyclopentyl-2-thiopheneglycolate methylbromide; an anticholinergic agent.

pentifylline (pen-tif′i-lēn). 1-Hexyltheobromine; a vasodilator.

pentitol (pen′ti-tol). A reduced pentose; *e.g.*, ribitol, lyxitol.

pentobarbital (pen-tō-bar′bi-tahl). 5-(Ethyl-5-methylbutyl)barbituric acid; a sedative and short-acting hypnotic.

pentolinium tartrate (pen-tō-lin′ē-ŭm). Pentamethylene-1,1′-bis-(1-methylpyrrolidinium bitartrate; a quaternary ammonium compound with potent ganglionic blocking action; used in the management of severe and malignant hypertension and peripheral vasospastic diseases.

penton (pen′tōn). The pentagonal capsomere (p. base) along with the protruding fiber at each of the 12 vertices of the adenovirus capsid; antigenically, the p. base differs from the fiber, and both differ from the other (hexagonal) capsomeres.

pentosan (pen′tō-san). An oligosaccharide of a pentose.

pentose (pen′tōs). A monosaccharide containing five carbon atoms in the molecule; *e.g.*, arabinose, lyxose, ribose, xylose.

p. nucleotide, a nucleotide having a p. as the sugar component.

pentose nucleic acid. Older term for ribonucleic acid.

pentosuria (pen-tō-sū′rē-ă). The excretion of one or more pentoses in the urine.

alimentary p., the urinary excretion of L-arabinose and L-xylose, as the result of the excessive ingestion of fruits containing these pentoses.

essential p., primary p.; L-xylulosuria; a benign heritable disorder in which the urinary output of L-xylulose is 1 to 4 g per 24 hr; it occurs principally in Jewish people; autosomal recessive inheritance.

primary p., essential p.

pentoxide (pen-tok′sīd). An oxide containing five oxygen atoms; *e.g.*, phosphorus p., P_2O_5.

pentoxifylline (pen-toks-if′i-lēn). 1-(5-Oxohexyl)theobromine; a dimethylxanthine derivative that decreases blood viscosity and improves blood flow; used in the treatment of intermittent claudication.

pentulose (pen′tyū-lōs). A ketopentose; *e.g.*, ribulose.

pentyl (pen′til). Amyl.

pentylenetetrazol (pen′ti-lēn-tet′ră-zol). $C_6H_{10}N_4$; a powerful stimulant to the central nervous system; used to cause generalized convulsion in the shock treatment of emotional states and as a respiratory stimulant.

peotillomania (pē′ō-til-ō-mā′nē-ă) [G. *peos,* penis, + *tillō,* to pull out (of hair), + *mania,* frenzy]. False masturbation; pseudomasturbation; rarely used term for a nervous tic consisting of a constant pulling of the penis.

peplomer (pep′lō-mer) [see peplos]. A part or subunit of the peplos of a virion, the assemblage of which produces the complete peplos, produced from the peplos by detergent treatment.

peplos (pep′lōs) [G. an outer garment worn by women]. The coat or envelope of lipoprotein material that surrounds certain virions.

Pepper, William, Jr., U.S. physician, 1874–1947. See P. *syndrome.*

peppermint (pep′er-mint). The dried leaves and flowering tops of *Mentha piperita* (family Labiatae); a carminative and antiemetic.

p. camphor, menthol.

p. oil, the volatile oil distilled with steam from the fresh, overground parts of the flowering plant of *Mentha piperita,* rectified by distillation and neither partially nor wholly dementholized; a flavor.

pepsic (pep′sik). Peptic.

pepsin, pepsin A (pep′sin) [G. *pepsis,* digestion] [EC 3.4.23.1]. The principal digestive enzyme (protease) of gastric juice, formed from pepsinogen; it hydrolyzes peptide bonds at low pH values, preferably adjacent to phenylalanine and leucine residues, thus reducing proteins to smaller molecules (proteoses and peptones); p. B (EC 3.4.23.2) is similar to p. A, but formed from porcine pepsinogen B; p. C (EC 3.4.23.3) is also similar to p. A, and structurally related to it.

pepsinate (pep′si-nāt). To mix pepsin with.

pepsiniferous (pep-si-nif′er-ŭs). Pepsinogenous.

pepsinogen (pep-sin′ō-jen) [pepsin + G. *-gen,* producing]. Propepsin; a proenzyme formed and secreted by the chief cells of the gastric mucosa; the acidity of the gastric juice and pepsin itself remove 42 amino acid residues from p. to form active pepsin.

pepsinogenous (pep-sin-oj′ĕ-nŭs). Pepsiniferous; producing pepsin.

pepsinuria (pep-si-nū′rē-ă) [pepsin + G. *ouron,* urine]. Excretion of pepsin in the urine.

peptic (pep′tik) [G. *peptikos,* fr. *peptō,* to digest]. Pepsic; relating to the stomach, to gastric digestion, or to pepsin A.

peptidase (pep′ti-dās). Peptide hydrolase; any enzyme capable of hydrolyzing one of the peptide links of a peptide; *e.g.*, carboxypeptidases, aminopeptidases.

peptidase P. Peptidyl dipeptidase A.

peptide (pep′tīd). A compound of two or more amino acids in which the alpha carboxyl group of one is united with the alpha amino group of another, with the elimination of a molecule of water, thus forming a peptide bond, –CO–NH–.

adrenocorticotropic p., a p. with ACTH activity, isolated from pituitary extracts.

bradykinin-potentiating p., teprotide.

heteromeric p., a p. which, on hydrolysis, yields substances other than amino acids in addition to amino acids; *e.g.*, pteroylglutamic acid.

p. hydrolase [EC subclass 3.4], peptidase.

phenylthiocarbamoyl (PTC) p., the p. formed by combination of phenylisothiocyanate and an α-amino group of a peptide. See also phenylthiohydantoin.

S p., see S *protein.*

sigma p., a p. with one end bonded to a point within the chain, usually by means of the disulfide group of a cystine residue, so that only one end of the p. is free; so called since the p. chain has then the rough shape of the Greek letter sigma.

p. synthetase [EC sub-subclass 6.3.2], any enzyme that catalyzes the synthesis of peptide bonds, with the hydrolysis of a nucleoside triphosphate.

peptidergic (pep-ti-der′jik) [peptide + G. *ergon,* work]. Referring to nerve cells or fibers that are believed to employ small peptide molecules as their neurotransmitter.

peptidoglycan (pep′ti-dō-glī′kan). A compound containing amino acids (or peptides) linked to sugars, with the latter proponderant.

Cf. glycopeptide.

peptidoid (pep'ti-doyd). A condensation product of two amino acids involving at least one condensing group other than the α-carboxyl or α-amino group; *e.g.,* glutathione.

peptidolytic (pep'ti-dō-lit'ik) [peptide + G. *lytikos,* solvent]. Causing the cleavage or digestion of peptides.

peptidyl dipeptidase A (pep'ti-dil) [EC 3.4.15.1]. A hydrolase cleaving C-terminal dipeptides from a variety of substrates, including angiotensin I which is converted to angiotensin II. Also called dipeptidyl carboxypeptidase; angiotensin-converting enzyme; carboxycathepsin; kinase II; peptidase P.

peptization (pep-ti-zā'shŭn). In colloid chemistry, an increase in the degree of dispersion, tending toward a uniform distribution of the dispersed phase.

Peptococcaceae (pep'tō-kok-ā'sē-ē). A family of nonmotile, nonsporeforming, anaerobic bacteria (order Eubacteriales) containing Gram-positive (staining may be equivocal) cocci, 0.5 to 1.6 μm in diameter, which occur singly, in pairs, tetrads, and irregular masses but not in three-dimensional, cubic packets. These organisms are chemoorganotrophic and have complex nutritional requirements. Carbohydrates may or may not be fermented by these organisms, which produce gas, principally CO_2 and usually H_2, from amino acids, or carbohydrates, or both. They are found in the mouth and intestinal and respiratory tracts of man and other animals; they are frequently found in normal and pathologic human female urogenital tracts. The type genus is *Peptococcus.*

Peptococcus (pep'tō-kok'ŭs) [G. *peptō,* to digest, + *kokkos,* berry]. A genus of nonmotile, anaerobic, chemoorganotrophic bacteria (family Peptococcaceae) containing Gram-positive, spherical cells that occur singly, in pairs, tetrads, or irregular masses, rarely in short chains. They are frequently found in association with pathologic conditions. The type species is *P. niger.*

P. ac'tivus, a species found in cases of puerperal septicemia and in the female genital tract.

P. aerog'enes, a species found primarily on human mucous surfaces; also found in cases of puerperal fever, in the female genital tract, and in the tonsils and nose.

P. anaero'bius, a species found in appendices, the female genital tract, in cases of cystitis and draining sinus, and in tidal bay mud.

P. asaccharolyt'icus, a species found in the human large intestine, buccal cavity, pleura, uterus, and vagina.

P. constella'tus, a species found in tonsils, purulent pleurisy, appendix, the nose, throat, and gums, and infrequently on the skin and in the vagina.

P. ni'ger, a species found once, in the urine of an aged woman; type species of the genus *P.*

peptocrinine (pep-tō-krin'ēn). An extract of the intestinal mucosa resembling secretin.

peptogenic, peptogenous (pep-tō-jen'ik, pep-toj'ĕ-nŭs). **1.** Producing peptones. **2.** Promoting digestion.

peptolysis (pep-tol'i-sis). The hydrolysis of peptones.

peptolytic (pep-tō-lit'ik). **1.** Pertaining to peptolysis. **2.** Denoting an enzyme or other agent that hydrolyses peptones.

peptone (pep'tōn). Descriptive term applied to intermediate polypeptide products, formed in partial hydrolysis of proteins, that are soluble in water, diffusible, and not coagulable by heat; used in bacterial culture media.

peptonic (pep-ton'ik). Relating to or containing peptone.

peptonization (pep'ton-i-zā'shŭn). Conversion by enzymic action of native protein into soluble peptone.

Peptostreptococcus (pep'tō-strep-tō-kok'ŭs) [G. *peptō,* to digest, + *streptos,* curved, + *kokkos,* berry]. A genus of nonmotile, anaerobic, chemoorganotrophic bacteria (family Peptococcaceae) containing spherical to ovoid, Gram-positive cells which occur in pairs and short or long chains. These organisms are found in normal and pathologic female genital tracts and blood in puerperal fever, in respiratory and intestinal tracts of normal humans and other animals, in the oral cavity, and in pyogenic infections, putrefactive war wounds, and appendicitis; they may be pathogenic. The type species is *P. anaerobius.*

P. anaero'bius, a species found in the mouth, intestinal and respiratory tracts, and cavities, especially the vagina, of humans and other animals; it may be pathogenic; it is the type species of the genus *P.*

P. evolu'tus, a species found in the human respiratory tract, mouth, and vagina.

P. foeti'dus, a species found in abscesses, blood, the intestinal tract, vagina, and mouth of humans and other animals; it is sometimes fatal.

P. interme'dius, a species found in the human respiratory and digestive tracts, oral cavity, and vagina; it has been isolated from various pathologic conditions.

P. lanceola'tus, a species found in the human mouth, vagina, and intestinal tract; it has been isolated from putrid diarrhea, dental infection, vulvovaginitis, and arthritic and other abscesses.

P. mag'nus, a species found in putrefying butcher's meat and in a case of appendicitis.

P. mi'cros, a species found in natural cavities of man and other animals; it has been isolated from various pathologic conditions.

P. morbillo'rum, a species found in the nose, throat, eyes, ears, mucous secretions, and blood in cases of measles, being irrelevant, however, to the etiology of measles; probably present normally, developing as a secondary invader.

P. paleopneumo'niae, a species found in the buccal pharyngeal cavity and the upper respiratory tract of man.

P. par'vulus, a species isolated from the mouth and the respiratory tract.

P. plagarumbel'li, a species commonly found in septic war wounds.

P. produc'tus, a species found in natural cavities of man, especially respiratory cavities.

P. pu'tridus, a species found in the human mouth and intestinal tract but especially in the human vagina.

per- [L. through, throughout, extremely]. **1.** A prefix denoting through, conveying intensity. **2.** In chemistry, a prefix denoting either 1) more or most, with respect to the amount of a given element (usually oxygen, as in perchloric acid) or radical contained in a compound, or 2) the degree of substitution for hydrogen, as in peroxides, peroxy acids (*e.g.,* hydrogen peroxide, peroxyformic acid). See also peroxy-.

peracephalus (per-ă-sef'ă-lŭs) [per- + G. *a-* priv. + *kephalē,* head]. An omphalosite lacking head and arms, and with a defective thorax; typically, the body consists of little more than pelvis and legs.

peracetate (per-as'ĕ-tāt). A salt or ester of peracetic acid.

peracetic acid (per-ă-sē'tik). Peroxyacetic acid; acetyl hydroperoxide; a peroxide of acetic acid, $CH_3CO–O–OH$.

peracid (per-as'id). Peroxy acid; an acid containing a peroxide group (–O–OH); *e.g.,* peracetic acid.

peracute (per-ă-kyut') [L. *peracutus,* very sharply]. Very acute; said of a disease.

per anum (per ā'nŭm) [L.]. By or through the anus.

perarticulation (per'ar-tik'yū-lā'shŭn) [per- + L. *articulatio,* joint]. *Articulatio* synovialis.

peratodynia (per'ă-tō-din'ē-ă) [G. *peratos,* on the opposite side, + *odynē,* pain]. Obsolete term for pyrosis.

peraxillary (per-ak'si-lăr-ē). Through the axilla.

perazine (per'ă-zēn). 10-[3-(4-Methyl-1-piperazinyl)propyl]phenothiazine; an antipsychotic.

perboric acid (per-bōr'ik). Tetraboric acid.

percentile (per-sen'tīl). The rank position of an individual in a serial array of data, stated in terms of what percentage of the group he equals or exceeds.

percept (per'sept) [L. *perceptum,* a thing perceived]. **1.** That which is perceived; the complete mental image, formed by the process of perception, of an object present in space. **2.** In clinical psychology, a single unit of perceptual report, such as one of the responses to an inkblot in the Rorshach test.

perception (per-sep'shun). Esthesia (1); the mental process of becoming aware of or recognizing an object; primarily cognitive rather than affective or conative, although all three aspects are manifested.

conscious p., apperception (1).
depth p., the visual ability to judge depth or distance.
extrasensory p. (ESP), p. by means other than through the ordinary senses; *e.g.,* telepathy, clairvoyance, precognition.
facial p., the p. of objects through sensation in the skin of the face; supposedly present in the blind.
simultaneous p., a combination of two slightly dissimilar images into a single image.

perceptive (per-sep'tiv). Relating to or having the power of perception.

perceptivity (per-sep-tiv'i-tē). The power of perception.

perceptorium (per-sep-tōr'ē-ŭm). Sensorium (2).

perchloric acid (per-klōr'ik). $HClO_4$; the highest in oxygen content of the series of chlorine acids.

perchloride (per-klōr'īd). Hyperchloride; a chloride containing the highest possible amount of chlorine.

percolation (per-kō-lā'shŭn) [L. *percolatio,* fr. per- + *colare,* to strain]. **1.** Filtration. **2.** Extraction of the soluble portion of a solid mixture by passing a solvent liquid through it. **3.** Passage of saliva or other fluids into the interface between tooth structure and restoration; sometimes induced by thermal changes.

percolator (per'kō-lā-ter). A funnel-shaped vessel used for the process of percolation in pharmacy.

percomorph oil (per-kō-mōrf). A liver oil from fish of the order Percomorphi, with a standardized amount of vitamins A and D.

per contiguum (per kon-tig'yū-ŭm) [per- + L. *contiguus,* touching, fr. *tango,* to touch]. In contiguity; touching; denoting the mode by which an inflammation or other morbid process spreads into an adjacent contiguous structure.

per continuum (per kon-tin'yū-ŭm) [per- + L. *continuus,* holding together, continuous, fr. *teneo,* to hold]. In continuity; continuous; denoting the mode by which an inflammation or other morbid process spreads from one part to another through continuous tissue.

percuss (per-kŭs'). To perform percussion.

percussion (per-kŭsh'ŭn) [L. *percussio,* fr. *per-cutio,* pp. *-cussus,* to beat, fr. *quatio,* to shake, beat]. **1.** A diagnostic procedure designed to determine the density of a part by the sound produced by tapping the surface with the finger or a plessor; performed primarily over the chest to determine presence of normal air content in the lungs and over the abdomen to evaluate air in the loops of intestine. **2.** A form of massage, consisting of repeated blows or taps of varying force.

auscultatory p., auscultation of the chest or other part at the same time that p. is made, to aid in hearing the sound made by p.
bimanual p., immediate p. in which the finger of one hand taps the other hand.
clavicular p., p., usually direct, along the entire clavicle to demonstrate dullness, particularly in apical pulmonary tuberculosis.
deep p., heavy p. to obtain information about deeply situated organs or structures.
direct p., immediate p.
finger p., p. in which a finger of one hand is used as a plessimeter and one of the other hand as a plessor.
immediate p., direct p.; the striking of the part under examination directly with the finger or a plessor, without the intervention of another finger or plessimeter.
mediate p., p. effected by the intervention of a finger or a plessimeter between the striking finger or plessor and the part percussed.
palpatory p., plessesthesia; finger p. in which attention is focused upon the resistance and reverberation of the tissues under the finger as well as upon the sound elicited.
threshold p., p. effected by means of a glass rod as a plessimeter, the rod being inclined to the wall of the chest or abdomen and touching it only by one extremity.

percussor (per-kŭs'er). Plessor.

percutaneous (per-kyū-tā'nē-ŭs). Diadermic; transcutaneous; transdermic; denoting the passage of substances through unbroken skin, as in absorption by inunction.

perencephaly (per-en-sef'ă-lē) [G. *pēra,* a purse, a wallet, + *enkephalos,* brain]. A condition marked by one or more cerebral cysts.

Perez, Bernard, French physician, 1836–1903. See P. *reflex.*

Perez, George V., Spanish physician, †1920. See P, *sign.*

perfectionism (per-fek'shŭn-izm). A tendency to set rigid high standards of performance for oneself.

perflation (per-flā'shŭn) [L. *per-flo,* pp, *-flatus,* to blow through]. Blowing air into or through a cavity or canal in order to force apart its walls or to expel any contained material.

perforans (per'fō-rans) [L. perforating]. A term applied to several muscles and nerves which, in their course, perforate other structures.

perforated (per'fō-rāt-ed) [L. *perforatus,* fr. *per-foro,* pp. *-atus,* to bore through]. Pierced with one or more holes.

perforation (per-fō-rā'shŭn) [see perforated]. Tresis; abnormal opening in a hollow organ or viscus.

Bezold's p., p. on the inner surface of the mastoid portion of the temporal bone.

perforator (per'fōr-ā-ter). An instrument for perforation of cranium.

perforatorium (per-fōr-ă-tōr'ē-ŭm). A rod or fibrous cone located between the acrosome and the anterior pole of the nucleus in the spermatozoa of toads and birds; no corresponding structure evident in the subacrosomal space of mammalian spermatozoa.

performic acid (per-fōr'mik). Peroxyformic acid; H–CO–O–OH; an organic peracid used in cleaving disulfide links in peptides by oxidizing cystine to cysteic acid.

perfrigeration (per-frij-er-ā'shŭn) [L. *per-frigero,* pp. *-atus,* to make cold, fr. *frigus,* cold]. A minor degree of frostbite.

perfusate (per'fyū-sāt) [see perfuse]. The fluid used for perfusion; sometimes more broadly applied to fluid that has been forced through any more or less porous membrane or material.

perfuse (per-fyūs') [L. *perfusio,* fr. per- + *fusio,* a pouring]. To force blood or other fluid to flow from the artery through the vascular bed of a tissue or to flow through the lumen of a hollow structure (*e.g.,* an isolated renal tubule). *Cf.* perifuse; superfuse.

perfusion (per-fyū'zhŭn). **1.** The act of perfusing. **2.** The flow of blood or other perfusate per unit volume of tissue, as in ventilation/perfusion ratio.

regional p., p. of part of the body, especially a limb, and particularly with chemotherapeutic agents, for treatment of a malignant tumor, primary, recurrent, or metastatic.

pergolide mesylate (per'go-līd). 8β-[(Methylthio)methyl]-6-propylergoline monomethanesulfonate; an ergot derivative with dopaminergic properties.

perhexiline maleate (per-hek'si-lēn). 2-(2,2-Dicyclohexylethyl)piperidine maleate; a coronary vasodilator and diuretic.

perhydrocyclopenta[*a*]phenanthrene. Tetracyclic steroid *nucleus.*

peri- [G. around]. Prefix denoting around, about.

periacinal, periacinous (per-ē-as′i-năl, -i-nŭs). Surrounding an acinus.

periadenitis (per′ē-ad-ĕ-nī′tis) [peri- + G. *adēn,* gland, + *-itis,* inflammation]. Inflammation of the tissues surrounding a gland.
p. muco′sa necrot′ica recur′rens, *aphthae* major.

perianal (per-ē-ā′năl). Circumanal.

periangiocholitis (per′ē-an′jē-ō-kō-lī′tis) [peri- + G. *angeion,* vessel, + *cholē,* bile, + *-itis,* inflammation]. Pericholangitis.

periangitis (per′ē-an-jī′tis) [peri- + G. *angeion,* a vessel, + *-itis,* inflammation]. Perivasculitis; inflammation of the adventitia of a blood vessel or of the tissues surrounding it or a lymphatic vessel. See also periarteritis; periphlebitis; perilymphangitis.

periaortic (per′ē-ā-ōr′tik). Surrounding or adjacent to the aorta.

periaortitis (per′ē-ā-ōr-tī′tis). Inflammation of the adventitia of the aorta and of the tissues surrounding it.

periapex (per′ē-ā′peks) [peri- L. *apex,* tip]. The periapical structures, particularly periodontal membrane and adjacent bone.

periapical (per-ē-ap′i-kăl). **1.** At or around the apex of a root of a tooth. **2.** Denoting the periapex.

periappendicitis (per′ē-ă-pen-di-sī′tis). Para-appendicitis; inflammation of the tissue surrounding the vermiform appendix.
p. decidua′lis, the presence of decidual cells in the peritoneum of the vermiform appendix in cases of right tubal pregnancy with adhesions between the fallopian tube and the appendix.

periappendicular (per′ē-ap-en-dik′yū-lăr). Surrounding an appendix, especially the vermiform appendix.

periarterial (per′ē-ar-tē′rē-ăl). Surrounding an artery.

periarteritis (per′ē-ar-ter-ī′tis). Inflammation of the adventitia of an artery.
p. nodo′sa, *polyarteritis* nodosa.

periarthric (per′ē-ar′thrik). Circumarticular.

periarthritis (per′ē-ar-thrī′tis) [peri- + arthritis]. Exarteritis; inflammation of the parts surrounding a joint.

periarticular (per′ē-ar-tik′yū-lăr). Circumarticular.

periatrial (per′ē-ā′trē-ăl). Periauricular (1); surrounding the atrium of the heart.

periauricular (per′ē-aw-rik′yū-lăr). **1.** Periatrial. **2.** Periconchal. **3.** Around the external ear.

periaxial (per′ē-ak′sē-ăl). Surrounding an axis.

periaxillary (per′ē-ak′sē-lăr-ē). Circumaxillary.

periaxonal (per′ē-ak′sō-năl) [peri- + G. *axōn,* axis]. Surrounding the axon of a nerve.

periblast (per′i-blast) [peri- + G. *blastos,* germ]. A specialized region of yolk surface immediately peripheral to the blastoderm in telolecithal eggs.

peribronchial (per-i-brong′kē-ăl). Surrounding a bronchus or the bronchi.

peribronchiolar (per-i-brong′kē-ō′lăr). Surrounding the bronchioles.

peribronchiolitis (per′i-brong′kē-ō-lī′tis). Inflammation of the tissues surrounding the bronchioles.

peribronchitis (per′i-brong-kī′tis). Inflammation of the tissues surrounding the bronchi or bronchial tubes.

peribuccal (per′i-bŭk′ăl). Surrounding the cheek.

peribulbar (per-i-bŭl′băr). Circumbulbar; surrounding any bulb, especially the eyeball or the bulb of the urethra.

peribursal (per-i-ber′săl). Surrounding a bursa.

pericanalicular (per′i-kan-ă-lik′yū-lăr). Surrounding a canaliculus.

pericardectomy (per′i-kar-dek′tō-mē). Pericardiectomy.

pericardia (per-i-kar′dē-ă). Plural of pericardium.

pericardiac, pericardial (per-i-kar′dē-ak, -dē-ăl). **1.** Surrounding the heart. **2.** Relating to the pericardium.

pericardicentesis (per-i-kar′dē-sen-tē′sis). Pericardiocentesis.

pericardiectomy (per′i-kar-dē-ek′tō-mē) [pericardium + G. *ektomē,* excision]. Pericardectomy; excision of a portion of the pericardium.

pericardiocentesis (per-i-kar′dē-ō-sen-tē′sis) [peri- + G. *kardia,* heart, + *kentēsis,* puncture]. Pericardicentesis; paracentesis of the pericardium.

pericardioperitoneal (per-i-kar′dē-ō-per-i-tō-nē′ăl). Relating to the pericardial and peritoneal cavities.

pericardiophrenic (per-i-kar′dē-ō-fren′ik) [pericardium + G. *phrēn,* diaphragm]. Relating to the pericardium and the diaphragm.

pericardiopleural (per-i-kar′dē-ō-plūr′ăl). Relating to the pericardial and pleural cavities.

pericardiorrhaphy (per′i-kar-dē-ōr′ă-fē) [pericardium + G. *rhaphē,* suture]. Suture of the pericardium.

pericardiostomy (per′i-kar-dē-os′tō-mē) [pericardium + G. *stoma,* mouth]. Establishment of an opening into the pericardium.

pericardiotomy (per′i-kar-dē-ot′ō-mē) [pericardium + G. *tomē,* incision]. Pericardotomy; coleotomy; incision into the pericardium.

pericarditic (per′i-kar-dit′ik). Relating to pericarditis.

pericarditis (per′i-kar-dī′tis). Inflammation of the pericardium.
adhesive p., adherent pericardium; p. with adhesions between the two pericardial layers, between the pericardium and heart, or between the pericardium and neighboring structures.
chronic constrictive p., tuberculous or other infection of the pericardium, with thickening of the membrane and constriction of the cardiac chambers.
fibrinous p., acute p. with fibrinous exudate. Also known as hairy heart; p. sicca or villosa; shaggy pericardium. See also bread-and-butter *pericardium.*
internal adhesive p., concretio cordis.
p. oblit′erans, inflammation of the pericardium leading to adhesion of the two layers, obliterating the sac. See also adhesive p.
rheumatic p., fibrinous p. occurring in acute rheumatic fever.
p. sic′ca, fibrinous p.
uremic p., fibrinous p. seen in chronic renal failure.
p. villo′sa, fibrinous p.

pericardium, pl. **pericardia** (per-i-kar′dē-ŭm, -ă) [L. fr. G. *pericardion,* the membrane around the heart] [NA]. Capsula, membrana, or theca cordis; heart sac; the fibroserous membrane, consisting of mesothelium and submesothelial connective tissue, covering the heart and beginning of the great vessels. It is a closed sac having two layers: the visceral layer (epicardium), immediately surrounding the heart, and the outer parietal layer, forming the sac, composed of strong fibrous tissue, **p. fibrosum,** lined with serous membrane, **p. serosum.** The phrenic nerve divides the p. into antephrenic and retrophrenic portions; the pulmonary hilum divides both of these portions into suprahilar, hilar, and infrahilar portions.
adherent p., adhesive *pericarditis.*
bread-and-butter p., fibrinous pericarditis in which the visceral and parietal surfaces of the p. resemble those of two pieces of buttered bread that have been pressed together and then pulled apart.
p. fibro′sum [NA], fibrous p. See p.
p. sero′sum [NA], serous p. See p.

shaggy p., fibrinous *pericarditis.*

pericardotomy (per-i-kar-dot'ō-mē). Pericardiotomy.

pericecal (per'i-sē'kăl). Perityphlic; surrounding the cecum.

pericellular (per-i-sel'yū-lăr). Pericytial; surrounding a cell.

pericemental (per'i-sē-men'tăl). Periodontal.

pericementitis (per'i-sē-men-tī'tis). Obsolete term for periodontitis.

pericentral (per-i-sen'trăl). Surrounding the center.

perichareia (per'i-kă-rī'ă) [G. excessive joy, fr. *chairō,* to rejoice]. Rarely used term for delirious rejoicing.

pericholangitis (per'i-kō-lan-jī'tis) [peri- + G. *cholē,* bile, + *angeion,* vessel, + *-itis,* inflammation]. Periangiocholitis; inflammation of the tissues around the bile ducts.

perichondral, perichondrial (per-i-kon'drăl, -kon'drē-ăl). Relating to the perichondrium.

perichondritis (per'i-kon-drī'tis). Inflammation of the perichondrium.

peristernal p., Tietze's *syndrome.*

relapsing p., relapsing *polychondritis.*

perichondrium (per-i-kon'drē-ŭm) [peri- + G. *chondros,* cartilage] [NA]. The dense irregular connective tissue membrane around cartilage.

perichord (per'i-kōrd). Sheath of the notochord.

perichordal (per-i-kōr'dăl). Relating to the perichord.

perichoroidal (per-i-kō-roy'dăl). Surrounding the choroid coat of the eye.

perichrome (per'i-krōm) [peri- + G. *chrōma,* a color]. Denoting a nerve cell in which the chromophil substance, or stainable material, is scattered throughout the cytoplasm.

pericolic (per'i-kol'ik). Surrounding or encircling the colon.

pericolitis (per'i-kō-lī'tis). Pericolonitis; serocolitis; inflammation of the connective tissue or peritoneum surrounding the colon.

p. dex'tra, p. involving the ascending colon.

p. sinis'tra, perisigmoiditis.

pericolonitis (per'i-kō-lon-ī'tis). Pericolitis.

pericolpitis (per'i-kol-pī'tis) [peri- + G. *kolpos,* bosom (vagina), + *-itis,* inflammation]. Perivaginitis.

periconchal (per'i-kong'kăl). Periauricular (2); surrounding the concha of the auricle.

pericorneal (per-i-kōr'nē-ăl). Circumcorneal; perikeratic; surrounding the cornea.

pericoronal (per-i-kōr'ō-năl). Around the crown of a tooth.

pericoronitis (per-i-kōr-ō-nī'tis) [peri- + L. *corona,* crown, + G. *-itis,* inflammation]. Operculitis; inflammation around the crown of a tooth, usually one that is incompletely erupted into the oral cavity.

pericranial (per-i-krā'nē-ăl). Relating to the pericranium; surrounding the skull.

pericranitis (per'i-krā-nī'tis). Inflammation of the pericranium.

pericranium (per'i-krā'nē-ŭm) [peri- + G. *kranion,* skull] [NA]. Periosteum cranii, the periosteum of the skull.

pericyazine (per-i-sī'ă-zēn). 10-[3-(4-Hydroxypiperidinyl)propyl]-phenothiazine-2-carbonitrile; an antipsychotic.

pericystic (per'i-sis'tik) [peri- + G. *kystis,* bladder]. Perivesical. **1.** Surrounding the urinary bladder. **2.** Surrounding the gallbladder. **3.** Surrounding a cyst.

pericystitis (per'i-sis-tī'tis). Inflammation of the tissues surrounding a bladder, especially the urinary bladder.

pericystium (per-i-sis'tē-ŭm) [peri- + G. *kystis,* bladder, cyst]. **1.** The tissues surrounding the urinary bladder or gallbladder. **2.** A vascular investment of a cystic tumor.

pericyte (per'i-sīt) [peri- + G. *kytos,* cell]. Perithelial, pericapillary, or adventitial cell; one of the slender mesenchymal-like cells found in close association with the outside wall of postcapillary venules; it is relatively undifferentiated and may become a fibroblast, macrophage, or smooth muscle cell.

capillary p., Rouget *cell.*

pericytial (per'i-sish'ē-ăl, -sit'ē-ăl). Pericellular.

peridectomy (per-i-dek'tō-mē) [peri- + G. *ektomē,* excision]. Peritectomy.

peridens (per'i-denz) [peri- + L. *dens,* tooth]. A supernumerary tooth appearing elsewhere than the midline of the dental arch.

peridental (per-i-den'tăl). Periodontal.

peridentitis (per'i-den-tī'tis). Obsolete term for periodontitis.

peridentium (per'i-den'tē-ŭm). Periodontium.

periderm, periderma (per'i-derm, -i-der'mă) [peri- + G. *derma,* skin]. Epitrichium; the outermost layer of the epidermis of the embryo and fetus to the sixth month of intrauterine life; desquamated epitrichial cells are a considerable component of the vernix caseosa.

peridermal, peridermic (per-i-der'măl, -mik). Relating to the periderm.

peridesmic (per-i-dez'mik). **1.** Periligamentous; surrounding a ligament. **2.** Relating to the peridesmium.

peridesmitis (per'i-dez-mī'tis) [peri- + G. *desmos,* band, + *-itis,* inflammation]. Inflammation of the connective tissue surrounding a ligament.

peridesmium (per-i-dez'mē-ŭm) [peri- + G. *desmion (desmos),* band]. The connective tissue membrane surrounding a ligament.

perididymis (per-i-did'i-mis) [G. *didymos,* twin, pl. *didymoi,* testes]. *Tunica* albuginea testis.

perididymitis (per'i-did-i-mī'tis). Inflammation of the perididymis.

peridium (pe-rid'ē-ŭm) [G. *pēridion,* dim. of *pēra,* leather pouch]. In fungi, the hyphal structure which surrounds the asci.

peridiverticulitis (per'i-dī'ver-tik'yū-lī'tis). Inflammation of the tissues around an intestinal diverticulum.

periduodenitis (per'i-dū'ō-dē-nī'tis). Inflammation around the duodenum.

peridural (per-i-dū'răl). Epidural.

periencephalitis (per'ē-en-sef-ă-lī'tis) [peri- + G. *enkephalos,* brain]. Inflammation of the cerebral membranes, particularly leptomeningitis or inflammation of the pia mater.

perienteric (per-ē-en-ter'ik). Circumintestinal; surrounding the intestine.

perienteritis (per'ē-en-ter-ī'tis). Seroenteritis; inflammation of the peritoneal coat of the intestine.

periependymal (per'ē-e-pen'di-măl). Surrounding the ependyma.

periesophageal (per'ē-e-sof'ă-jē'ăl). Surrounding the esophagus.

periesophagitis (per'ē-e-sof'ă-jī'tis). Inflammation of the tissues surrounding the esophagus.

perifocal (per-i-fō'kăl). Surrounding a focus; denoting tissues, or the blood that they contain, in the vicinity of an infective focus.

perifollicular (per'i-fō-lik'yū-lăr). Surrounding a hair follicle; usually used to describe the histopathologic appearance of the infiltrate surrounding a hair follicle.

perifolliculitis (per'i-fō-lik'yū-lī'tis). The presence of an inflammatory infiltrate surrounding hair follicles; frequently occurs in conjunction with folliculitis.

p. absce'dens et suffo'diens, dissecting cellulitis; a chronic dissecting folliculitis of the scalp.

superficial pustular p., follicular *impetigo.*

perifuse (per'i-fyūs) [peri- + L. *fusio,* a pouring]. To flush a fresh supply of bathing fluid around all of the outside surfaces of a small piece of tissue immersed in it. *Cf.* perfuse; superfuse.

perifusion (per-i-fyū'shŭn). The act of perifusing.

periganglionic (per'i-gang-glē-on'ik). Surrounding a ganglion, especially a nerve ganglion.

perigastric (per-i-gas'trik) [peri- + G. *gastēr,* belly, stomach]. Surrounding the stomach.

perigastritis (per'i-gas-trī'tis). Inflammation of the peritoneal coat of the stomach.

perigemmal (per'i-jem'ăl) [peri- + L. *gemma,* bud]. Circumgemmal.

periglandulitis (per'i-glan-dū-lī'tis). Inflammation of the tissues surrounding a gland.

periglottic (per-i-glot'ik) [peri- + G. *glōssa* or *glōtta,* tongue]. Around the tongue, especially around the base of the tongue and the epiglottis, or around the glottis (laryngis), the rima glottidis.

periglottis (per-i-glot'is) [G. *periglōttis,* covering of the tongue]. The mucous membrane of the tongue.

perihepatic (per-i-he-pat'ik) [peri- + G. *hēpar,* liver]. Surrounding the liver.

perihepatitis (pĕr'i-hep-ă-tī'tis) [peri- + G. *hēpar,* liver, + *-itis,* inflammation]. Hepatic capsulitis; hepatitis externa; hepatoperitonitis; inflammation of the serous, or peritoneal, covering of the liver.

perihernial (per-i-her'nē-ăl). Surrounding a hernia.

peri-implantoclasia (per'ē-im-plan'tō-klā'zē-ă) [peri- + L. *im,* in, + *planto,* to plant, + G. *klasis,* breaking up]. In dentistry, a general term implying disease of the supporting bone involving an implant; the disease may be exfoliative, resorptive, traumatic, or ulcerative in nature.

perijejunitis (per'i-jĕ-jū-nī'tis). Inflammation around the jejunum.

perikaryon, pl. **perikarya** (per-i-kar'ē-on, -ă) [peri- + G. *karyon,* kernel]. **1.** The cytoplasm around the nucleus, such as that of the cell body of nerve cells. **2.** The body of the odontoblast, excluding the dentinal fiber. **3.** The cell body of the nerve cell, as distinguished from its axon and dendrites.

perikeratic (per-i-ke-rat'ik) [peri- + G. *keras,* horn]. Pericorneal.

perikymata, sing. **perikyma** (per-i-kī'mă-tă, -kī'mă) [peri- + G. *kyma,* wave]. The transverse ridges and grooves on the surface of tooth enamel.

perilabyrinthitis (per'i-lab'ĭ-rin-thī'tis). Inflammation of the parts about the labyrinth.

perilaryngeal (per'i-lă-rin'jē-ăl). Surrounding the larynx.

perilaryngitis (per'i-lar-in-jī'tis). Inflammation of the tissues around the larynx.

perilenticular (per-i-len-tik'yū-lăr). Circumlental; surrounding the lens of the eye.

periligamentous (per'i-lig-ă-men'tŭs). Peridesmic.

perilymph (per'i-limf). Perilympha.

perilympha (per'i-lim'fă) [peri- + L. *lympha,* a clear fluid (lymph)] [NA]. Perilymph; Cotunnius' liquid; liquor cotunnii; the fluid contained within the osseus labyrinth, surrounding and protecting the membranous labyrinth.

perilymphangial (per'i-lim-fan'jē-ăl). Surrounding a lymphatic vessel.

perilymphangitis (per'i-lim-fan-jī'tis). Inflammation of the tissues surrounding a lymphatic vessel.

perilymphatic (per'i-lim-fat'ik). **1.** Surrounding a lymphatic structure (node or vessel). **2.** The spaces and tissues surrounding the membranous labyrinth of the inner ear.

perimeningitis (per'i-men-in-jī'tis). Pachymeningitis.

perimeter (pe-rim'ĕ-ter) [G. *perimetros,* circumference, fr. *peri,* around, + *metron,* measure]. **1.** A circumference, edge, or border. **2.** An instrument, usually half a circle or sphere, used to measure the field of vision.

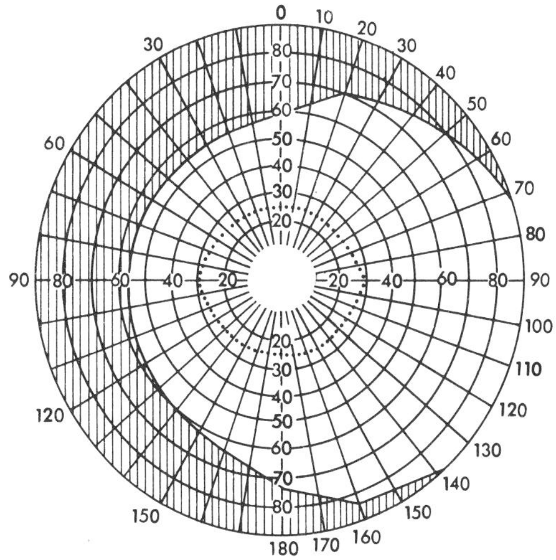

Perimeter Chart of Right Eye
The unshaded area is sensitive to light

arc p., a p. consisting of a semicircular frame at the center of which the patient looks while a white object is moving along the arc, the exact point where it becomes visible or invisible being noted and recorded on a chart.

Goldmann p., a projection p. that adds further precision by controlling the surrounding illumination.

projection p., a p. that uses as target a spot of light that can be adjusted rapidly as to size, brightness, and color, and moves silently at any desired speed.

Tübinger p. [*Tübingen,* German city], a static type of p. in which the stimulus is increased in intensity until it is detected.

perimetric (per-i-met'rik). **1** [G. *peri,* around, + *mētra,* uterus]. Periuterine; surrounding the uterus; relating to the perimetrium. **2** [G. *perimetros,* circumference]. Relating to the circumference of any part or area. **3.** Relating to perimetry.

perimetritic (per-i-me-trit'ik). Relating to or marked by perimetritis.

perimetritis (per'i-me-trī'tis) [perimetrium + G. *-itis,* inflammation]. Metroperitonitis.

perimetrium, pl. **perimetria** (per-i-mē'trē-ŭm, -ă) [peri- + G. *mētra,* uterus] [NA]. Tunica serosa uteri; the serous (peritoneal) coat of the uterus.

perimetry (pe-rim'ĕ-trē) [G. *perimetros,* circumference]. The determination of the limits of the visual field.

computed p., determination of the visual field by means of a programmed routine of stimulus and response.

flicker p., flicker fusion frequency technique; a technique of p. using the criterion of critical fusion frequency.

kinetic p., mapping of the visual field by using a moving test object.

mesopic p., exploration of the visual field in dim illumination.

objective p., determination of the visual field by pupillary constriction or electroencephalography.

quantitative p., a plotting of the visual field in isopters of equal retinal sensitivity.

scotopic p., p. of a dark-adapted eye.

static p., determination of the visual field by using test objects at fixed positions and gradually increasing luminance to the threshold of visibility.

perimyelis (per-i-mī'ĕ-lis) [peri- + G. *myelos,* marrow]. Endosteum.

perimyelitis (per'i-mī-ĕ-lī'tis). Endosteitis.

perimyoendocarditis (per-i-mī'ō-en-dō-kar-dī'tis). Endoperimyocarditis.

perimyositis (per'i-mī-ō-sī'tis). Perimysiitis (2); inflammation of the loose cellular tissue surrounding a muscle.

perimysial (per-i-mis'ē-ăl, -miz'ē-ăl). Relating to the perimysium; surrounding a muscle.

perimysiitis, perimysitis (per'i-mis-ē-ī'tis, -mī-sī'tis). **1.** Inflammation of the perimysium. **2.** Perimyositis.

perimysium, pl. **perimysia** (per-i-mis'ē-ŭm, -miz'ē-ŭm; -ē-ă) [peri- + G. *mys,* muscle] [NA]. The fibrous sheath enveloping each of the primary bundles of skeletal muscle fibers.

p. exter'num, epimysium.

p. inter'num, in the older literature, a term referring to the connective tissue around secondary and tertiary fascicles and individual fibers and also to the supporting framework of the myocardium.

perinatal (per-i-nā'tăl) [peri- + L. *natus,* pp. of *nascor,* to be born]. Occurring during, or pertaining to, the periods before, during, or after the time of birth; *i.e.,* before delivery from the 28th week of gestation through the first 7 days after delivery.

perinate (per'i-nāt). An infant in the perinatal period.

perinatologist (per-i-nā-tol'ō-jist). One who specializes in perinatology.

perinatology (per-i-nā-tol'ō-jē). A subspeciality of obstetrics concerned with care of the mother and fetus during pregnancy, labor, and delivery, particularly when the mother and/or fetus are ill or at risk of becoming ill.

perineal (per'i-nē'ăl). Relating to the perineum.

perineo- [L. fr. G. *perineos, perinaion*]. Combining form denoting the perineum.

perineocele (per-i-nē'ō-sēl) [perineo- + G. *kēlē,* hernia]. Perineal hernia; a hernia in the perineal region, either between the rectum and the vagina or the rectum and the bladder, or alongside the rectum.

perineometer (per'i-nē-om'ĕ-ter) [perineo- + G. *metron,* measure]. Instrument used to measure the strength of voluntary muscle contractions of the perineum.

perineoplasty (per-i-nē'ō-plas-tē). Plastic surgery of the perineum.

perineorrhaphy (per-i-nē-ōr'ă-fē). Suture of the perineum, performed in perineoplasty.

perineoscrotal (per-i-nē'ō-skrō'tăl). Relating to the perineum and the scrotum.

perineostomy (per-i-nē-os'tō-mē) [perineo- + G. *stoma,* mouth]. Urethrostomy through the perineum.

perineosynthesis (per'i-nē-ō-sin'thĕ-sis). Perineoplasty in a case of extensive laceration of the perineum.

perineotomy (per-i-nē-ot'ō-mē). Incision into the perineum as in external urethrotomy, lithotomy, etc., or to facilitate childbirth. See also episiotomy.

perineovaginal (per-i-nē'ō-vaj'i-năl). Relating to the perineum and the vagina.

perinephrial (per'i-nef'rē-ăl). Relating to the perinephrium.

perinephric (per'i-nef'rik). Perirenal; circumrenal; surrounding the kidney in whole or part.

perinephritis (per'i-ne-frī'tis). Inflammation of perinephric tissue.

perinephrium, pl. **perinephria** (per'i-nef'rē-ŭm, -nef'rē-ă) [peri- + G. *nephros,* kidney]. The connective tissue and fat surrounding the kidney.

perineum, pl. **perinea** (per'i-nē'ŭm, -nē'ă) [L. fr. G. *perineon, perinaion*] **1** [NA]. The area between the thighs extending from the coccyx to the pubis and lying below the pelvic diaphragm. **2.** The external surface of the central tendon of the perineum, lying between the vulva and the anus in the female and the scrotum and the anus in the male.

watering-can p., a p. riddled with fistulas resulting from urethral stricture.

perineural (per'i-nū'răl) [peri- + G. *neuron,* nerve]. Surrounding a nerve.

perineurial (per'i-nū'rē-ăl). Relating to the perineurium.

perineuritis (per'i-nū-rī'tis). Inflammation of the perineurium. See also adventitial *neuritis.*

perineurium, pl. **perineuria** (per-i-nū'rē-ŭm, -rē-ă) [L. fr. peri- + G. *neuron,* nerve]. The connective tissue sheath surrounding a fascicle of nerve fibers in a peripheral nerve; it consists of concentric layers of closely united flattened cells which alternate with layers of fine collagenous fibers having a predominantly longitudinal direction.

perinuclear (per-i-nū'klē-ăr). Circumnuclear; surrounding a nucleus.

periocular (per-i-ok'yū-lăr). Circumocular.

period (pēr'ē-ŏd) [G. *periodos,* a way round, a cycle, fr. *peri,* around, + *hodos,* way]. **1.** A certain duration or division of time. **2.** One of the stages of a disease, *e.g.,* p. of incubation, p. of convalescence. See also stage; phase. **3.** Colloquialism for menses.

absolute refractory p., the p. following excitation when no response is possible regardless of the intensity of the stimulus.

critical p., **(1)** in the first hours after birth, the p. of maximum imprintability; the period before and after which imprinting is difficult or impossible; **(2)** in animals, a p. when socialization is possible.

eclipse p., eclipse phase; the time between infection by (or induction of) a bacteriophage, or other virus, and the appearance of mature virus within the cell.

effective refractory p., the p. during which impulses may appear but are too weak to be conducted; the longest interval between adequate stimuli, falling just short of the time necessary to allow a propagated response to be evoked in a tissue by the second stimulus; it differs from the functional refractory p. in that it is a measure of stimulus interval rather than response interval of time.

ejection p., sphygmic *interval.*

extrinsic incubation p., the time interval between the acquisition of an infectious agent by a vector and the vector's ability to transmit the agent to other susceptible vertebrate hosts.

fertile p., the p. in a regularly menstruating woman's cycle, usually days 10 to 18 after the first day of the last menstrual cycle, during which conception is most likely.

functional refractory p., the minimum interval possible between successive responses to stimulation of a tissue.

Gap$_1$ p. (G$_1$ p.), the p. of the cell cycle after cell division when there is synthesis of RNA and protein; it may last for a few hours in rapidly growing tissue or a lifetime in non-renewing cells such as nerve cells.

Gap$_2$ p. (G$_2$ p.), the p. in the cell cycle when synthesis of DNA is completed but before mitosis begins.

incubation p., **(1)** latent p. (2); **(2)** incubative *stage.*

induction p., the interval between an initial injection of antigen and the appearance of demonstrable antibodies in the blood.

intersystolic p., atriocarotid *interval.*

intrapartum p., in obstetrics, the p. from the onset of labor to the end of the third stage of labor.

isoelectric p., the p. occurring in the electrocardiogram between the end of the S wave and the beginning of the T wave during which

electrical forces are acting in directions such as to neutralize each other so that there is no difference in potential under the two electrodes.
isometric p., presphygmic *interval.*
isometric p. of cardiac cycle, that p. in which the muscle fibers do not shorten although the cardiac muscle is excited and the pressure in the ventricles rises, extending from the closure of the atrioventricular valves to the opening of the semilunar valves.
latency p., latency *phase.*
latent p., **(1)** the p. elapsing between the application of a stimulus and the obvious response, *e.g.,* contraction of a muscle; **(2)** incubation p.; the p. of incubation of an infectious disease before the appearance of the prodromal symptoms.
masticatory silent p., a pause in electromyographic patterns associated with tooth contacts during chewing and biting; a part of the complex feedback mechanism of mandibular control involving receptors in the periodontal ligament and muscles.
menstrual p., menses.
missed p., the failure of menstruation to occur in any month at the expected time.
mitotic p. (M p.), the p. of the cell cycle when all phases of mitosis occur.
oedipal p., oedipal *phase.*
preejection p., the interval between onset of QRS complex and cardiac ejection; electromechanical systole minus ejection time.
prepatent p., the time interval between infection of an individual by a parasitic organism and first ability to detect a diagnostic stage of the organism from that host.
puerperal p., the p. elapsing between the termination of labor and the return of the generative tract to its normal condition; the 6 weeks following the completion of labor.
pulse p., the reciprocal of the repetition rate; *e.g.,* the interval between leading edges of successive pulses.
refractory p., **(1)** the p. following effective stimulation, during which excitable tissue such as heart muscle and nerve fails to respond to a stimulus of threshold intensity (*i.e.,* excitability is depressed); **(2)** a period of temporary psychophysiologic resistance to further sexual stimulation which occurs immediately following orgasm.
refractory p. of electronic pacemaker, the time required to restore full sensitivity after detecting cardiac activity or delivering a pacing impulse.
relative refractory p., the p. between the effective refractory p. and the end of the refractory p.; fibers then respond only to high intensity stimuli and the impulses conduct more slowly than normally.
safe p., the p. in the menstrual cycle when conception is least likely to occur, usually about 10 days before or after the onset of menstruation, since ovulation occurs about midway between two menstrual p.'s.
silent p., **(1)** the cessation of electrical responses from the contracting muscle during the experimental elicitation of a tendon jerk; **(2)** any pause in an otherwise continuous series of electrophysiologic events.
synthesis p. (S p.), the p. of the cell cycle when there is synthesis of DNA and histone; it occurs between Gap_1 and Gap_2.
total refractory p., the absolute refractory p. plus the relative refractory p.
vulnerable p. (of heart), a brief time during the cardiac cycle when stimuli are particularly likely to induce repetitive activity like tachycardia, flutter, or fibrillation which persists after the stimulus has ceased; for the ventricle, it occurs during the latter part of systole, during the relative refractory period coincident with the inscription of the T wave of the electrocardiogram.
Wenckebach p., a sequence of cardiac cycles in the electrocardiogram ending in a dropped beat due to A-V block, the preceding cycles showing progressively lengthening P-R intervals; the P-R interval following the dropped beat is again shortened.

periodate (per-ī'ō-dāt). A salt of periodic acid.

periodic (pēr-ē-od'ik). Recurring at regular intervals; denoting a disease with regularly recurring exacerbations or paroxysms.

periodic acid (per-ī'ō-dik). HIO_4, but existing in solution usually in hydrated form.

periodicity (pēr'ē-ō-dis'i-tē). Tendency to recurrence at regular intervals.
diurnal p., a circadian rhythm with primary expression of the p. during daylight hours, as in the release of microfilariae of *Loa loa* into the peripheral blood during the day, with far fewer released at night; associated with the day-biting habits of the vector, *Chrysops* species.
filarial p., the circadian rhythm observed in the appearance of filarial microfilariae in the peripheral blood. See also diurnal p.; nocturnal p.
lunar p., any rhythmic phenomenon that follows a lunar or monthly cycle.
malarial p., a clinical rhythmicity reflected in periodic fevers and chills recurring at approximately 48-hour intervals in tertian malaria (*Plasmodium vivax* or *P. ovale*) or at 72-hour intervals in quartan malaria (*P. malariae*); the rhythm of tertian or 48-hour cycles is frequently modified in malignant tertian or falciparum malaria (*P. falciparum*); associated with release of merozoites from red cells during erythrocytic schizogony, although the controlling mechanism for the synchronous release is unknown.
nocturnal p., a circadian rhythm with the p. expressed during nighttime hours, as in the night release of microfilariae of the human filaria *Wuchereria bancrofti* into the peripheral blood; this type of p. is found in regions where the vector mosquito is a night-biting species.
subperiodic p., a modified circadian rhythm in which the p. is not clearcut, as in certain zoonotic strains of Malayan filariasis caused by *Brugia malayi;* as in examples of strict filarial p., this response is correlated with the biting habits of the vector insect (mosquito), although the precise mechanism inducing this microfilarial response is not clearly established.

periodontal (per'ē-ō-don'tăl) [peri- + G. *odous,* tooth]. Pericemental; peridental; paradental; around a tooth.

Periodontal Disease Index (PDI). An index used for estimating the degree of periodontal disease based on the measurement of six representative teeth for gingival inflammation, pocket depth, calculus and plaque, attrition, mobility, and lack of contact.

Periodontal Index (PI). An index for the epidemiological classification of periodontal disease.

periodontia (per'ē-ō-don'shē-ă). **1.** Plural of periodontium. **2.** Periodontics.

periodontics (per'ē-ō-don'tiks) [peri- + G. *odous,* tooth]. Periodontia (2); the branch of dentistry concerned with the study of the normal tissues and the treatment of abnormal conditions of the tissues immediately about the teeth.

periodontist (per'ē-ō-don'tist). A dentist who specializes in periodontics.

periodontitis (per'ē-ō-don-tī'tis) [periodontium + G. *-itis,* inflammation]. **1.** Inflammation of the periodontium. **2.** A chronic inflammatory disease of the periodontium occurring in response to bacterial plaque on the adjacent teeth; characterized by gingivitis, destruction of the alveolar bone and periodontal ligament, apical migration of the epithelial attachment resulting in the formation of periodontal pockets, and ultimately loosening and exfoliation of the teeth.
apical p., inflammation of the periodontal ligament surrounding the root apex of a tooth; usually a consequence of pulpal inflammation or necrosis.

p. com'plex, vertical resorption of the alveolar process with pockets of uneven depth on adjacent teeth, and with traumatic occlusion as a factor.

juvenile p., periodontosis; a degenerative periodontal disease of adolescents in which the periodontal destruction is out of proportion to the local irritating factors present on the adjacent teeth; inflammatory changes become superimposed, and bone loss, migration, and extrusion are observed. Two forms are recognized: 1) localized, in which the destruction is limited to the incisors and first molars; 2) generalized, involving all of the teeth.

p. sim'plex, horizontal resorption of the alveolar process with pockets of even depth on adjacent teeth; traumatic occlusion is not a factor.

suppurative p., p. accompanied by purulent exudate.

periodontium, pl. **periodontia** (per'ē-ō-don'shē-ŭm, -shē-ă) [L. fr. peri- + G. *odous,* tooth] [NA]. Alveolodental or peridental membrane; paradentium; parodontium; peridentium; alveolar periosteum; periosteum alveolare; the tissues that surround and support the teeth, including the gingivae, cementum, periodontal ligament, and alveolar and supporting bone.

periodontoclasia (per'ē-ō-don-tō-klā'zē-ă) [periodontium + *klasis,* breaking]. Periodontolysis; destruction of periodontal tissues, gingiva, pericementum, alveolar bone, and cementum.

periodontolysis (per'ē-ō-don-tol'i-sis) [periodontium + G. *lysis,* dissolution]. Periodontoclasia.

periodontosis (per'ē-ō-don-tō'sis) [periodontium + G. *-osis,* condition]. Juvenile *periodontitis.*

periomphalic (per'ē-om-fal'ik) [peri- + G. *omphalos,* umbilicus]. Periumbilical.

perionychia (per-ē-ō-nik'ē-ă). Perionyxis; inflammation of the perionychium.

perionychium, pl. **perionychia** (per-ē-ō-nik'ē-ŭm, -nik'ē-ă) [peri- + G. *onyx,* nail]. Eponychium (2).

perionyx (per-ē-on'iks) [peri- + G. *onyx,* nail] [NA]. Remnant of the eponychium remaining in the narrow fold overlapping the proximal part of the lunula.

perionyxis (per'ē-ō-nik'sis). Perionychia.

perioophoritis (per'ē-ō-of'ō-rī'tis) [peri- + G. *oophoron,* ovary, + *-itis,* inflammation]. Periovaritis; inflammation of the peritoneal covering of the ovary.

perioophorosalpingitis (per'ē-ō-of'ō-rō-sal-pin-jī'tis) [peri- + G. *oophoron,* ovary, + salpingitis]. Perisalpingo-ovaritis; inflammation of the peritoneum and other tissues around the ovary and oviduct.

perioperative (per-ē-op'er-ă-tiv). Paraoperative; around the time of operation.

periophthalmic (per'ē-of-thal'mik) [peri- + G. *ophthalmos,* eye]. Circumocular.

periophthalmitis (per'ē-of-thal-mī'tis). Inflammation of the tissues surrounding the eye.

periople (per'ē-ō-pl) [G. *peri,* around, + *hoplon,* implement, shield]. Corium limbi; a region of the pododerm; the thin, hard, relatively impervious, outer layer of the horn wall of the hoof of an animal.

perioplic (per-ē-op'lik). Pertaining to the periople.

perioral (per-ē-ō'răl). Circumoral; peristomal; peristomatous; around the mouth.

periorbit (per-ē-ōr'bit). Periorbita.

periorbita (per'ē-ōr'bi-tă). [peri- + L. *orbita,* orbit] [NA]. Periorbit; orbital fascia; periorbital membrane; the periosteum of the orbit.

periorbital (per-ē-ōr'bi-tăl). **1.** Relating to the periorbita. **2.** Circumorbital.

periorchitis (per'ē-ōr-kī'tis) [peri- + G. *orchis,* testis, + *-itis,* inflammation]. Inflammation of the tunica vaginalis testis.

p. hemorrha'gica, chronic hematocele of the tunica vaginalis testis.

periost (per'ē-ost). Periosteum.

periostea (per-ē-os'tē-ă). Plural of periosteum.

periosteal (per-ē-os'tē-ăl). Periosteous; relating to the periosteum.

periosteitis (per'ē-os-tē-ī'tis). Periostitis.

periosteo- [Mod. L. *periosteum*]. Combining form denoting the periosteum.

periosteoma (per'ē-os'tē-ō'mă). Periostoma; periosteophyte; a neoplasm derived from the periosteum.

periosteomedullitis (per-ē-os'tē-ō-med-yū-lī'tis) [periosteo- + L. *medulla,* marrow, + G. *-itis,* inflammation]. Periosteomyelitis.

periosteomyelitis (per-ē-os'tē-ō-mī-ĕ-lī'tis) [periosteo- + G. *myelos,* marrow, + *-itis,* inflammation]. Periosteomedullitis; inflammation of the entire bone, with the periosteum and marrow.

periosteopathy (par'ē-os-tē-op'ă-thē). Any disease of the periosteum.

periosteophyte (per-ē-os'te-ō-fīt) [periosteo- + G. *phyton,* growth]. Periosteoma.

periosteosis (per'ē-os-tē-ō'sis). Periostosis; the formation of a periosteoma.

periosteotome (per'ē-os'tē-ō-tōm). Periostotome; a strong scapel-shaped knife, for cutting the periosteum.

periosteotomy (per'ē-os-tē-ot'ō-mē) [periosteo- + G. *tomē,* incision]. Periostotomy; the operation of cutting through the periosteum to the bone.

periosteous (per-ē-os'tē-ŭs). Periosteal.

periosteum, pl. **periostea** (per-ē-os'tē-ŭm, -ă) [Mod. L. fr. G. *periosteon,* ntr. of adj. *periosteos,* around the bones, fr. *peri,* around, + *osteon,* bone] [NA]. Periost; the thick fibrous membrane covering the entire surface of a bone except its articular cartilage. In young bones, it consists of two layers: an inner cellular layer which is osteogenic, forming new bone tissue, and an outer connective tissue layer conveying the blood vessels and nerves supplying the bone; in older bones, the osteogenic layer is reduced. See also perichondral *bone.*

alveolar p., p. alveola're, periodontium.

p. cra'nii, pericranium.

periostitis (per'ē-os-tī'tis). Periosteitis; inflammation of the periosteum.

orbital p., inflammation of periorbital soft tissues.

periostoma (per'ē-os-tō'mă). Periosteoma.

periostosis, pl. **periostoses** (per'ē-os-tō'sis, -sēz). Periosteosis.

periostosteitis (per-ē-os'tos-tē-ī'tis) [periosteum + G. *osteon,* bone, + *-itis,* inflammation]. Inflammation of a bone with involvement of the periosteum.

periostotome (per-ē-os'tō-tōm). Periosteotome.

periostotomy (per-ē-os-tot'ō-mē). Periosteotomy.

periotic (per'ē-ō'tik, -ot'ik) [peri- + G. *ous,* ear]. Surrounding the internal ear; referring to the petrous portion of the temporal bone, or the spaces and tissues in the bony labyrinth that surround the membranous labyrinth.

periovaritis (per'ē-ō-vă-rī'tis). Perioophoritis.

periovular (per'ē-ō'vyū-lăr). Surrounding the ovum.

peripachymeningitis (per'i-pak'ē-men-in-jī'tis) [peri- + pachymeninx (dura mater) + G. *-itis,* inflammation]. Inflammation of the parietal layer of the dura mater.

peripancreatitis (per'i-pan'krē-ă-tī'tis). Inflammation of the peritoneal coat of the pancreas.

peripapillary (per-i-pap'i-lăr-ē). Surrounding a papilla.

peripatetic (per'i-pă-tet'ik) [G. *peripatēsis,* a walking about]. Walking around; formerly used to describe a patient with "walking" typhoid fever.

peripenial (per-i-pē'nē-ăl). Surrounding the penis.

peripharyngeal (per'i-fă-rin'jē-ăl). Surrounding the pharynx.

peripherad (pĕ-rif'ĕ-rad) [G. *periphereia,* periphery, + L. *ad,* to]. In a direction toward the periphery.

peripheral (pĕ-rif'ĕ-răl). **1.** Relating to or situated at the periphery. **2.** Situated nearer the periphery of an organ or part of the body in relation to a specific reference point; opposite of central (centralis).

peripheralis (pĕ-rif-ĕ-rā'lis) [NA]. Peripheral.

peripherocentral (pĕ-rif'ĕ-rō-sen'trăl). Relating to both the periphery and the center of the body or any part.

periphery (pĕ-rif'ĕ-rē) [G. *periphereia,* fr. *peri,* around, + *pherō,* to carry]. **1.** The part of a body away from the center; the outer part or surface. **2.** Denture *border.*

periphlebitic (per'i-fle-bit'ik). Relating to periphlebitis.

periphlebitis (per'i-fle-bī'tis) [peri- + G. *phleps,* vein, + *-itis,* inflammation]. Inflammation of the outer coat of a vein or of the tissues surrounding it.

Periplaneta (per-i-pla-nē'tă) [peri- + G. *planētēs,* a roamer]. A genus of large cockroaches including several cosmopolitan household pests found wherever food is available, especially in moist protected areas. *P. americana* (American cockroach), a very large brownish-chestnut species, 30 to 40 mm long, is probably native to Africa but now universally distributed; *P. fulginosa* (the smoky-brown cockroach) is a common household pest in the eastern and southeastern U.S.

periplocin (pe-rip'lō-sin) [G. *peri-plokē,* a winding around, fr. *plekō,* to twine, plait]. Glucoperiplocymarin; a cardiotonic glycoside obtained from the bark and stems of *Periploca graeca* (family Asclepiadaceae), a plant of southern Europe.

peripolar (per-i-pō'lăr). Surrounding the pole or poles of any body, or any electric or magnetic poles.

peripolesis (per'i-pō-lē'sis) [peri- + G. *poleomai,* to wander]. Penetration of migrating cells between fixed tissue cells that are normally in close contact.

periporitis (per'i-pō-rī'tis) [peri- + G. *poros,* pore, + *-itis,* inflammation]. Miliary papules and papulovesicles with staphylococcic infection; most frequently on the face and in infants.

periportal (per-i-pōr'tăl). Peripylic; surrounding the portal vein.

periproctic (per'ē-prok'tik) [peri- + G. *prōktos,* anus]. Circumanal.

periproctitis (per'i-prok-tī'tis). Perirectitis; inflammation of the areolar tissue about the rectum.

periprostatic (per'i-pros-tat'ik). Surrounding the prostate.

periprostatitis (per'i-pros-tă-tī'tis). Inflammation of the tissues surrounding the prostate.

peripylephlebitis (per-i-pī'lē-fle-bī'tis) [peri- + G. *pylē,* gate, + *phleps,* vein, + *-itis,* inflammation]. Inflammation of the tissues around the portal vein.

peripylic (per-i-pī'lik) [peri- + G. *pylē,* portal, gate]. Periportal.

peripyloric (per'i-pī-lōr'ik, -pē-lōr'ik). Surrounding the pylorus.

perirectal (per'i-rek'tăl). Surrounding the rectum.

perirectitis (per'i-rek-tī'tis). Periproctitis.

perirenal (per'i-rē'năl) [peri- + L. *ren,* kidney]. Perinephric.

perirhinal (per'i-rī'năl) [peri- + G. *rhis,* nose]. Around the nose or nasal cavity.

perirhizoclasia (per'ē-rī-zō-klā'zē-ă) [peri- + G. *rhiza,* root, + *klasis,* destruction]. Inflammatory destruction of tissues immediately around the root of a tooth, *i.e.,* pericementum, cementum, and approximating layers of alveolar bone.

perisalpingitis (per-i-sal-pin-jī'tis) [peri- + G. *salpinx,* trumpet, + *-itis,* inflammation]. Inflammation of the peritoneum covering the fallopian tube.

perisalpingo-ovaritis (per'i-sal-ping'gō-ō-vă-rī'tis) [peri- + G. *salpinx,* trumpet, + ovary + G. *-itis,* inflammation]. Perioophorosalpingitis.

perisalpinx (per'i-sal'pingks) [peri- + G. *salpinx* (*salping-*), trumpet]. The peritoneal covering of the uterine tube.

periscopic (per'i-skop'ik) [peri- + G. *skopeō,* to view]. Denoting that which gives the ability to see objects to one side as well as in the direct axis of vision.

perisigmoiditis (per'i-sig-moy-dī'tis). Pericolitis sinistra; inflammation of the connective tissues surrounding the sigmoid flexure, giving rise to symptoms, referable to the left iliac fossa, similar to those of perityphlitis in the right iliac fossa.

perisinuous (per'i-sin'yū-ŭs). Surrounding a sinus, especially a sinus of the dura mater.

perispermatitis (per'i-sper-mă-tī'tis). Inflammation of the tissues around the spermatic cord.

p. sero'sa, hydrocele of the spermatic cord.

perisplanchnic (per'i-splangk'nik) [peri- + G. *splanchna,* viscera]. Perivisceral; surrounding any viscus or viscera.

perisplanchnitis (per'i-splangk-nī'tis) [peri- + G. *splanchna,* viscera, + *-itis,* inflammation]. Inflammation surrounding any viscus or viscera.

perisplenic (per-i-splen'ik). Around the spleen.

perisplenitis (per'i-sple-nī'tis). Inflammation of the peritoneum covering the spleen.

perispondylic (per-i-spon-dil'ik) [peri- + G. *spondylos,* vertebra]. Perivertebral.

perispondylitis (per-i-spon-di-lī'tis) [peri- + G. *spondylos,* vertebra, + *-itis,* inflammation]. Inflammation of the tissues about a vertebra.

perissodactyl, perissodactylous (pĕ-ris'ō-dak-til, -til-ŭs) [G. *perissos,* odd, + *daktylos,* finger or toe]. **1.** Imparidigitate; having an odd number of toes or digits on each foot or hand. **2.** Any mammal of the order *Perissodactyla,* comprising the odd-toed hoofed quadripeds, and including the tapirs, rhinoceros, and horses.

peristalsis (per-i-stal'sis) [peri- + G. *stalsis,* constriction]. Vermicular movement; the movement of the intestine or other tubular structure, characterized by waves of alternate circular contraction and relaxation of the tube by which the contents are propelled onward.

mass p., mass movement; forcible peristaltic movements of short duration, occurring only three or four times a day, which move the contents of the large intestine from one division to the next, as from the ascending to the transverse colon.

reversed p., antiperistalsis; a wave of intestinal contraction in a direction the reverse of normal, by which the contents of the intestine are forced backward.

peristaltic (per-i-stal'tik). Relating to peristalsis.

peristaphylitis (per'i-staf-i-lī'tis) [peri- + G. *staphylē,* uvula, + *-itis*]. Inflammation of the soft palate and parts about the uvula.

peristasis (pĕ-ris'tă-sis) [peri- + G. *stasis,* a standing still]. Peristatic hyperemia; phases of inactivity of vasoconstriction in inflammation.

peristole (pĕ-ris'tō-lē) [peri- + G. *stellō,* to contract]. The tonic activity of the walls of the stomach whereby the organ contracts about its contents; contrasting with the peristaltic waves passing from the cardia toward the pylorus (peristalsis).

peristolic (per-i-stol'ik). Relating to peristole.

peristoma (pe-ris'tō-mă, per-i-stō'mă). Peristome.

peristomal, peristomatous (per′i-stō′măl, -stō′mă-tŭs). Perioral.

peristome (per′i-stōm) [peri- + G. *stoma,* mouth]. Peristoma; a groove leading from the cytostome in ciliates and certain other forms of protozoa.

periston (per′i-ston). A plasma substitute consisting of fractionated polyvinyl pyrrolidone; mean molecular weight, 50,000.

peristrumous (per′i-strū′mŭs) [peri- + L. *struma,* goiter]. Situated about or near a goiter.

perisynovial (per′i-si-nō′vē-ăl). Around a synovial membrane.

perisystole (per-i-sis′tō-lē). Presystole.

perisystolic (per-i-sis-tol′ik). Presystolic.

peritectomy (per′i-tek′tō-mē) [peri- + G. *ektomē,* excision]. Peridectomy; peritomy (1); the removal of a paracorneal strip of the conjunctiva for the relief of corneal disease.

peritendineum, pl. **peritendinea** (per-i-ten-din′ē-ŭm, -ē-ŭ) [L. fr. peri- + G. *tenōn,* tendon] [NA]. One of the fibrous sheaths surrounding the primary bundles of fibers in a tendon.

peritendinitis (per′i-ten-di-nī′tis). Peritenontitis; inflammation of the sheath of a tendon.

p. calca′rea, a calcium (chalky) deposit around a tendon.

p. sero′sa, ganglion (2).

peritenon (per′i-ten-on) [peri- + G. *tenōn,* tendon]. *Vagina* tendinis.

peritenontitis (per′i-ten-on-tī′tis). Peritendinitis.

perithecium, pl. **perithecia** (per-i-thē′sē-ŭm, -sē-ă) [peri- + G. *thēkē,* flask]. In fungi, a flask-shaped ascocarp, one of the many shapes of structures which bear asci and ascospores; useful as an aid in identifying a fungus.

perithelioma (per′i-thē-lē-ō′mă). Hemangiopericytoma.

perithelium, pl. **perithelia** (per-i-thē′lē-ŭm, -ă) [peri- + G. *thēlē,* nipple]. The connective tissue that surrounds smaller vessels and capillaries.

Eberth's p., an incomplete layer of connective tissue cells encasing the blood capillaries.

perithoracic (per-i-thō-ras′ik). Surrounding or encircling the thorax.

perithyroiditis (per′i-thī-roy-dī′tis). Inflammation of the capsule or tissues surrounding the thyroid gland.

peritomist (pe-rit′ō-mist). One who performs circumcision.

peritomy (pe-rit′ō-mē) [G. *peritomē,* fr. *peri,* around, + *tomē,* incision]. **1.** Peritectomy. **2.** Circumcision (1).

peritoneal (per′i-tō-nē′ăl). Relating to the peritoneum.

peritonealgia (per′i-tō-nē-al′jē-ă) [peritoneum + G. *algos,* pain]. Pain in the peritoneum.

peritoneo- [L. *peritoneum*]. Combining form denoting the peritoneum.

peritoneocentesis (per′i-tō-nē′ō-sen-tē′sis) [peritoneum + G. *kentēsis,* puncture]. Paracentesis of the abdomen. Also called abdominocentesis; celiocentesis; celioparacentesis.

peritoneoclysis (per′i-tō-nē-ok′li-sis) [peritoneum, + G. *klysis,* a washing out]. Irrigation of the abdominal cavity.

peritoneopathy (per′i-tō-nē-op′ă-thē) [peritoneum, + *pathos,* suffering]. Inflammation or other disease of the peritoneum.

peritoneopericardial (per′i-tō-nē′ō-per′i-kar′dē-ăl). Relating to the peritoneum and the pericardium.

peritoneopexy (per′i-tō-nē′ō-pek-sē) [peritoneum + G. *pēxis,* fixation]. A suspension or fixation of the peritoneum.

peritoneoplasty (per′i-tō-nē′ō-plas-tē) [peritoneum + G. *plastos,* formed]. Loosening adhesions and covering the raw surfaces with peritoneum to prevent reformation.

peritoneoscope (per′i-tō-nē′ō-skōp) [peritoneum + G. *skopeō,* to view]. Laparoscope; an endoscope for examining the peritoneal cavity.

peritoneoscopy (per′i-tō-nē-os′kŏ-pē). Abdominoscopy; celioscopy; laparoscopy; ventroscopy; examination of the contents of the peritoneum with a peritoneoscope passed through the abdominal wall.

peritoneotomy (per′i-tō-nē-ot′ō-mē) [peritoneum + G. *tomē,* incision]. Incision of the peritoneum.

peritoneum, pl. **peritonea** (per′i-tō-nē′ŭm, -ă) [Mod. L. fr. G. *peritonaion,* fr. *periteino,* to stretch over] [NA]. Membrana abdominis; the serous sac, consisting of mesothelium and a thin layer of irregular connective tissue, that lines the abdominal cavity and covers most of the viscera contained therein; it forms two sacs: the peritoneal (or greater) sac and the omental bursa (lesser sac) connected by the foramen epiploicum.

p. parieta′le [NA], the layer of p. lining the abdominal walls.

p. viscera′le [NA], the layer of p. investing the abdominal organs.

peritonism (per′i-tō-nizm). **1.** A symptom complex marked by vomiting, pain, and shock associated with inflammation of any of the abdominal viscera in which the peritoneum is involved. **2.** Pseudoperitonitis; a neurosis in which the symptoms simulate those of peritonitis.

peritonitis (per′i-tō-nī′tis). Inflammation of the peritoneum.

adhesive p., a form of p. in which a fibrinous exudate occurs, matting together the intestines and various other organs.

benign paroxysmal p., familial paroxysmal *polyserositis.*

bile p., choleperitonitis; inflammation of the peritoneum caused by the escape of bile into the free peritoneal cavity.

chemical p., p. due to the escape of bile, contents of the gastrointestinal tract, or pancreatic juice into the peritoneal cavity; the contents of the fluid causes chemical injury, shock, and peritoneal exudation prior to occurrance of any associated infection.

chyle p., p. due to free chyle in the peritoneal cavity.

circumscribed p., localized p.

p. defor′mans, a chronic p. in which thickening of the membrane and contracting adhesions cause shortening of the mesentery and kinking and retraction of the intestines.

diaphragmatic p., p. affecting mainly the peritoneal surface of the diaphragm.

diffuse p., general p.

p. encap′sulans, a localized fibrous or adhesive p. remaining after a generalized p. has nearly disappeared; it is marked by pain, constipation, and a palpable tumor.

feline infectious p., a chronic progressive disease of domestic cats and other Felidae caused by a coronavirus and manifested by a variety of clinical syndromes with or without an effusive p.

fibrocaseous p., p. characterized by caseation and fibrosis, usually caused by the tubercle bacillus.

gas p., inflammation of the peritoneum accompanied by an intraperitoneal accumulation of gas.

general p., diffuse p.; p. throughout the peritoneal cavity.

localized p., circumscribed p.; p. confined to a demarcated region of the peritoneal cavity.

meconium p., p. caused by intestinal perforation in the fetus or newborn; associated with congenital obstruction or fibrocystic disease of the pancreas.

pelvic p., pelvioperitonitis; pelviperitonitis; localized inflammation of the peritoneum surrounding the uterus and fallopian tubes.

periodic p., familial paroxysmal *polyserositis.*

productive p., pachyperitonitis.

tuberculous p., p. caused by the tubercle bacillus.

peritonsillar (per′i-ton′si-lăr). Around a tonsil or the tonsils.

peritonsillitis (per′i-ton′si-lī′tis). Inflammation of the connective tissue above and behind the tonsil.

peritracheal (per-i-trā′kē-ăl). About the trachea.

peritrichal, peritrichate, peritrichic (pe-rit′ri-kăl, -rit′ri-kāt; per-i-trik′ik). Peritrichous (2).

Peritrichida (per-i-trik′i-dă) [peri- + G. *thrix*, hair]. An order of ciliates (subclass Peritrichia, phylum Ciliophora) characterized by a cylindrical shape with the cilia usually limited to the zone surrounding the mouth opening; includes the suborder Mobilina, whose members are all ecto- or endoparasites of aquatic invertebrates and vertebrates, of which the genus *Trichodina* includes economically important gill parasites of fish.

peritrichous (pe-rit′ri-kŭs) [peri- + G. *thrix*, hair]. **1.** Relating to cilia or other appendicular organs projecting from the periphery of a cell. **2.** Peritrichal; peritrichate; peritrichic; having flagella uniformly distributed over a cell; used especially with reference to bacteria.

peritrochanter′ic (per′i-trō′kan-ter′ik). Around a trochanter.

perityphlic (per′i-tif′lik) [peri- + G. *typhlon*, cecum]. Pericecal.

periumbilical (per′i-ŭm-bil′i-kăl). Periomphalic; around or near the umbilicus.

periungual (per′i-ŭng′gwăl) [peri- + L. *unguis*, nail]. Surrounding a nail; involving the nail folds.

periureteral, periureteric (per′i-yū-rē′ter-ăl, -yū′rē-ter′ik). Surrounding one or both ureters.

periureteritis (per′i-yū-rē′ter-ī′tis) [peri- + ureter + G. *-itis*, inflammation]. Inflammation of the tissues about a ureter.

p. plas′tica, idiopathic retroperitoneal *fibrosis*.

periurethral (per′i-yū-rē′thrăl). Surrounding the urethra.

periurethritis (per′i-yū-rē-thrī′tis) [peri- + urethra + G. *-itis*, inflammation]. Inflammation of the tissues about the urethra.

periuterine (per′i-yū′ter-in). Perimetric (1).

periuvular (per′i-yū′vyū-lăr). Around the uvula.

perivaginitis (per′i-vaj-i-nī′tis). Pericolpitis; inflammation of the connective tissue around the vagina.

perivascular (per′i-vas′kyū-lăr) [peri- + L. *vasculum*, vessel]. Circumvascular; surrounding a blood or lymph vessel.

perivasculitis (per′i-vas-kū-lī′tis). Periangitis.

perivenous (per-i-vē′nŭs). Surrounding a vein.

perivertebral (per-i-ver′te-brăl). Perispondylic; around a vertebra or vertebrae.

perivesical (per-i-ves′i-kăl) [peri- + L. *vesica*, bladder]. Pericystic.

perivisceral (per-ivis′er-ăl). Perisplanchnic.

perivisceritis (per′i-vis-er-ī′tis) [peri- + L. *viscera*, internal organs, + G. *-itis*, inflammation]. Inflammation surrounding any viscus or viscera.

perivitelline (per′i-vi-tel′in, -īn) [peri- + L. *vitellus*, yolk]. Surrounding the vitellus or yolk.

periwinkle (per′i-wing-kl). *Vinca rosea.*

perkinism (per′kin-izm) [Elisha *Perkins*, U.S. physician, 1741–1799]. A form of quackery purporting to treat disease by applying metals with magnetic and magic properties.

perlèche (per-lesh′) [Fr. *per*, intensive, + *lécher*, to lick]. Angular *cheilitis.*

Perlia, Richard, 19th century German ophthalmologist. See P.'s *nucleus*, convergence *nucleus* of P.

perlingual (per-ling′gwăl) [L. *per*, through, + *lingua*, tongue]. Through or by way of the tongue, denoting a method of medication.

Perls, Max, German pathologist, 1843–1881. See P.'s Prussian blue *stain, test.*

permanganate (per-mang′gă-nāt). A salt of permanganic acid.

permanganic acid (per-mang-gan′ik). An acid, $HMnO_4$, derived from manganese, forming permanganates with bases. See also *potassium* permanganate.

permeability (per′mē-ă-bil′i-tē). The property of being permeable.

permeable (per′mē-ă-bl) [L. *permeabilis* (see permeate)]. Pervious; permitting the passage of substances (*e.g.*, liquids, gases, heat), as through a membrane or other structure.

permeant (per′mē-ănt) [L. *permeabilis* (see permeate)]. Able to pass through a particular semipermeable membrane.

permease (per′mē-ās). Any of a group of membrane-bound carriers (enzymes) that effect the transport of solute through a semipermeable membrane.

permeate (per′mē-āt) [L. *permeo*, to pass through]. **1.** To pass through a membrane or other structure. **2.** That which can so pass.

permeation (per-mē-ā′shŭn) [L. *per-meo*, pp. *-meatus*, to pass through]. The process of spreading through or penetrating, as the extension of a malignant neoplasm by proliferation of the cells continuously along the blood vessels or lymphatics.

perniciosiform (per-nish′ē-o′si-fōrm). Rarely used term meaning apparently pernicious, denoting a condition or disease that appears to be pernicious or malignant.

pernicious (per-nish′ŭs) [L. *perniciosus*, destructive, fr. *pernicies*, destruction]. Destructive; harmful; denoting a disease of severe character and usually fatal without appropriate treatment.

perniosis (per-nē-ō′sis). [L. *pernio*, chilblain, + G. *-osis*, condition]. Chilblain.

pero- [G. *pēros*, maimed]. Combining form meaning maimed or malformed.

perobrachius (pē-rō-brā′kē-ŭs) [pero- + G. *brachiōn*, arm]. An individual with congenitally defective hands and forearms.

perocephalus (pē-rō-sef′ă-lŭs) [pero- + G. *kephalē*, head]. An individual with congenitally defective face and head.

perochirus (pē-rō-kī′rŭs) [pero- + G. *cheir*, hand]. An individual with congenitally defective hands.

perodactyly, perodactylia (pē-rō-dak′ti-lē, -dak-til′ē-ă) [pero- + G. *daktylos*, finger or toe]. Congenital condition characterized by deformed fingers or toes.

perogen (per′ō-jen). A preparation of sodium perborate that, when mixed with the accompanying catalyzer, liberates 10% of the oxygen in the salt.

peromelia, peromely (pē-rō-mē′lē-ă, pĕ-rom′ĕ-lē) [pero- + G. *melos*, limb]. Severe congenital malformations of extremities, including absence of hand or foot.

perone (per-ō′nē) [G. *peronē*, brooch, the small bone of the arm or leg, the fibula, fr. *peirō*, to pierce]. Fibula.

peroneal (per-ō-nē′ăl) [L. *peroneus*, fr. G. *peronē*, fibula]. Relating to the fibula, to the lateral side of the leg, or to the muscles there present.

peroneotibial (per′ō-nē′ō-tib′ē-ăl). Tibiofibular.

peropus (pē′rō-pŭs) [pero- + G. *pous*, foot]. A person with congenitally defective feet.

peroral (per-ō′răl) [L. *per*, through, + *os* (*or-*), mouth]. Through the mouth, denoting a method of medication or an approach.

per os [L.]. By or through the mouth, denoting a method of medication.

perosis (pē-rō′sis) [pero- + G. *-osis*, condition]. A nutritional disease of young birds (*e.g.*, chicks and turkeys) characterized by shortening and thickening of the limb bones and a deformity known as "slipped tendon," overcrowding, confinement, and wire floors without roosts are predisposing factors.

perosplanchnia (pē-rō-splank′nē-ă) [pero- + G. *splanchnon*, viscus]. Congenital malformation of the viscera.

perosseous (per-os'ē-ŭs) [L. *per,* through, + *os,* bone]. Through bone.

peroxi-. See peroxy-.

peroxidases (per-ok'si-dās-ez) [EC subclass 1.11]. Hydrogen peroxide reducing oxidoreductases; enzymes in animal and plant tissues that catalyze the dehydrogenation (oxidation) of various substances in the presence of hydrogen peroxide, which acts as hydrogen acceptor, being converted to water in the process; if the oxidized substance is iodide, yielding iodine, the enzyme may be termed iodide peroxidase (EC 1.11.1.8) and be involved in the iodination of tyrosine (as tyrosine iodinase or thyroid peroxidase).
horseradish p., an enzyme used in immunohistochemistry to label the antigen-antibody complex.

peroxide (per-ok'sīd). That oxide of any series that contains the greatest number of oxygen atoms; applied most correctly to compounds containing an –O–O–link, as in hydrogen peroxide (H–O–O–H).

peroxisome (per-ok'si-sōm) [peroxide + G. *sōma,* body]. Microbody; a membrane-bound organelle occurring in nearly all eukaryotic cells that often has an electron-dense crystalline inclusion containing catalase, urate oxidase, and other oxidative enzymes relating to the formation and degradation of H_2O_2; thought to be important in detoxifying various molecules and in catalyzing the breakdown of fatty acids to acetyl-CoA.

peroxy-. Prefix denoting the presence of an extra O atom, as in peroxides, peroxy acids (*e.g.,* hydrogen peroxide, peroxyformic acid). Often shortened to per-.

peroxyacetic acid (per-ok'sē-ă-sē'tik). Peracetic acid.

peroxyacetyl nitrate (per-ok-sē-ă-sē'til). The major pollutant responsible for eye and nose irritation in smog.

peroxy acid (per-ok'sē). Peracid.

peroxyformic acid (per-ok'sē-fōr'mik). Performic acid.

peroxyl (per-ok'sil). H–O–O; one of the free radicals presumed formed as a result of the bombardment of tissue by high energy radiation.

perphenazine (per-fen'ă-zēn). 2-Chloro-10-{3-[4-(2-hydroxyethyl)piperazinyl]propyl}phenothiazine; an antipsychotic.

per primam (intentionem) (per prī'mam in-ten-shē-ō'nem) [L.]. By first intention. See *healing* by first intention.

per rectum (per rek'tŭm) [L.]. By or through the rectum, denoting a method of medication.

persalt (per'sawlt). In chemistry, any salt that contains the greatest possible amount of the acid radical.

per saltum (per sal'tŭm) [L.]. At a leap; at one bound; not gradually or through different stages.

perseveration (per-sev-er-ā'shŭn). [L. *persevero,* to persist]. **1.** The constant repetition of a meaningless word or phrase. **2.** The duration of a mental impression, measured by the rapidity with which one impression follows another as determined by the revolving of a two-colored disk. **3.** In clinical psychology, the repetition of a previously appropriate or correct response, even though the repeated response has since become inappropriate or incorrect.

persic oil (per'sik). The fixed oil expressed from the kernels of varieties of *Prunus armeniaca* (apricot kernel oil) or *Prunus persica* (peach kernel oil); used as a vehicle.

persistence (per-sis'tens) [L. *persisto,* to abide, stand firm]. Obstinate continuation of characteristic behavior, or of existence in spite of opposition or adverse environmental conditions.
microbial p., the phenomenon of survival, in high concentration of an antimicrobial substance, of microbes that seem not to be resistant variants (mutants) since their progeny are fully susceptible.

persister (per-sis'ter). That which, or one who, is capable of persistence; especially a bacteria that exhibits microbial persistence.

persona (per-sō'nă) [L. *per,* through, + *sonare,* to sound: from the small megaphone in ancient dramatic masks, to aid in projecting the actor's voice]. In jungian psychology, the outer aspect of character, as opposed to anima (2); the assumed personality used to mask the true one.

personality (per-sŏn-al'i-tē). **1.** The unique self; the organized system of attitudes and behavioral predispositions by which one impresses and establishes relationships with others. **2.** An individual with a particular p. pattern.
allotropic p., see allotropic.
antisocial p., psychopathic p.; a p. disorder characterized by a continuous and persistent pattern of aggressive behavior in which the rights of others are violated.
authoritarian p., a cluster of p. traits reflecting a desire for security and order, *e.g.,* rigidity, highly conventional outlook, unquestioning obedience, scapegoating, desire for structured lines of authority.
avoidant p., a p. characterized by a hypersensitivity to potential rejection, humiliation, or shame, an unwillingness to enter into relationships without unusually strong guarantees of uncritical acceptance, social withdrawal in spite of a desire for affection and acceptance, and low self-esteem.
basic p., see basic personality *type.*
borderline p., see borderline p. *disorder.*
compulsive p., a p. characterized by rigidity, extreme inhibition, and excessive concern with conformity and adherence to standards of conscience either for the individual or for others.
cyclothymic p., a p. disorder in which a person experiences regularly alternating periods of elation and depression, usually not related to external circumstances.
dependent p., a p. in which a person passively allows others to assume responsibility for making decisions effecting him, characterized by a lack of self-confidence and an inability to function independently.
dual p., a mental disturbance in which a person assumes alternately two different identities without either p. being consciously aware of the other. See also multiple p.
histrionic p., hysterical p., a condition in which a person, typically immature, dependent, self-centered, and often vain, exhibits unstable, overreactive, and excitable behavior intended to gain attention even though he may not be aware of this intent.
inadequate p., a p. disorder, characterized by ineptness and emotional and physical instability, which renders the individual unable to cope with the normal vicissitudes of life.
masochistic p., a p. disorder in which the individual accepts exploitation and sacrifices self-interest while at the same time feeling morally superior, attempting to elicit sympathy, and inducing guilt in others.
multiple p., a dissociative disorder in which two or more distinct conscious p.'s alternately prevail in the same person, without any p. being aware of the other. See also dual p.
paranoid p., a p. disorder characterized by hypersensitivity, rigidity, unwarranted suspicion, jealousy, and a tendency to blame others and ascribe evil motives to them; though neither a neurosis or psychosis, it interferes with the individual's ability to maintain interpersonal relationships.
passive-aggressive p., a p. disorder in which aggressive feelings are manifested in passive ways, especially through mild obstructionism and stubbornness.
psychopathic p., antisocial p.
schizoid p., a disorder characterized by social withdrawal, emotional coldness or aloofness, and indifference to praise or criticism from others.
schizotypical p., a personality disorder characterized by eccentricities in thinking, appearance, and behavior; although not psychotic, individuals with such a disorder have unusual ideas and have difficulty relating to others.

shut-in p., a person who responds inadequately to contacts with other people.

syntonic p., a stable p., one characterized by even temperament.

type A p., type B p., see type A *behavior;* type B *behavior.*

person-years. The sum of the number of years that each member of a population has been afflicted by a certain condition; *e.g.,* years of treatment with a certain drug.

perspiration (pers-pi-rā'shŭn) [L. *per-spiro,* pp. *-atus,* to breathe everywhere]. **1.** Sweating; diaphoresis; sudation; the excretion of fluid by the sweat glands of the skin. **2.** All fluid loss through normal skin, whether by sweat gland secretion or by diffusion through other skin structures. **3.** Sweat (1); sudor; the fluid excreted by the sweat glands; it consists of water containing sodium chloride and phosphate, urea, ammonia, ethereal sulfates, creatinine, fats, and other waste products; the average daily quantity is estimated at about 1500 g. See also subentries under sweat.

insensible p., p. that evaporates before it is perceived as moisture on the skin; the term sometimes includes evaporation from the lungs.

sensible p., the p. excreted in large quantity, or when there is much humidity in the atmosphere, so that it appears as moisture on the skin.

perstillation (per-sti-lā'shŭn) [L. *per,* through, + *stillo,* to trickle, distil]. See pervaporation.

persuasion (per-swā'zhŭn). The act of influencing the mind of another, by authority, argument, or reason; an important element in most types of psychotherapy.

persulfate (per-sŭl'fāt). A salt of persulfuric acid.

persulfide (per-sŭl'fīd). **1.** That one of a series of sulfides that contains more atoms of sulfur than any other. **2.** The sulfur analogue of a peroxide.

persulfuric acid (per-sŭl-fyūr'ik). Peroxymonosulfuric acid, H_2SO_5; an oxidizing agent.

Perthes, Georg C., German surgeon, 1869–1927. See P. *disease, test;* Calvé-P. *disease;* Legg-Calvé-P. *disease.*

perthio-. Prefix denoting substitution of sulfur for every oxygen in a compound; *e.g.,* perthiocarbonic acid, H_2CS_3.

Pertik, Otto, Hungarian pathologist, 1852–1913. See P.'s *diverticulum.*

per tubam (per tū'băm) [L.]. Through a tube.

pertussis (per-tŭs'is) [L. *per,* very (intensive), + *tussis,* cough]. Whooping cough; an acute infectious inflammation of the larynx, trachea, and bronchi caused by *Bordetella pertussis;* characterized by recurrent bouts of spasmodic coughing which continues until the breath is exhausted, then ending in a noisy inspiratory stridor (the "whoop") caused by laryngeal spasm.

Peru'vian bark. Cinchona.

pervaporation (per'vap-ōr-ā'shŭn) [L. *per,* through, + *vapor,* steam]. The heating of a liquid within a dialyzing bag suspended over a hot plate, evaporation taking place rapidly through the membrane; any colloids in solution remain within the bag while crystalloids diffuse out and crystallize on the outer surface of the bag (perstillation).

perversion (per-ver'zhŭn) [L. *perversio,* fr. *per-verto,* pp. *-versus,* to turn about]. A deviation from the norm, especially concerning sexual interests or behavior.

polymorphous p., **(1)** in psychoanalytic theory, a child's variegated sexual activity and interests; **(2)** in general, the manifold p.'s shown by an adult.

sexual p., sexual *deviation.*

per'vert. One who practices perversions. See also deviant (2).

pervert'ed. Abnormal, deviant, or disordered.

per vias naturales (per vī'as nach'er-ā'lēz) [L.]. Through the natural passages; *e.g.,* denoting a normal delivery, as opposed to cesarean section, or the passage in stool of a foreign body instead of its surgical removal.

pervigilium (per-vi-jil'ē-ŭm) [L. a watching all night]. Wakefulness; sleeplessness.

pervious (per'vē-ŭs) [L. *pervius,* fr. *per,* through, + *via,* a way]. Permeable.

pes, gen. **pedis,** pl. **pedes** (pes, pē'dis, -dēz) [L.] **1** [NA]. Foot. **2.** Any footlike or basal structure or part. **3.** *Crus* cerebri. **4.** Talipes. In this sense, p. is always qualified by a word expressing the specific type.

p. abduc'tus. *talipes* valgus.

p. adduc'tus, *talipes* varus.

p. anseri'nus, **(1)** *plexus* intraparotideus; **(2)** the tendinous expansions of the sartorius, gracilis, and semitendinosus muscles at the medial border of the tuberosity of the tibia.

p. ca'vus, *talipes* cavus.

p. equi'noval'gus, *talipes* equinovalgus.

p. equi'nova'rus, *talipes* equinovarus.

p. febric'itans, elephantiasis.

p. gi'gas, macropodia.

p. hippocam'pi [NA], foot of the hippocampus; digitationes hippocampi; the anterior thickened extremity of the hippocampus.

p. pedun'culi, *crus* cerebri.

p. pla'nus, *talipes* planus.

p. prona'tus, *talipes* valgus.

p. val'gus, *talipes* valgus.

p. va'rus, *talipes* varus.

pessary (pes'ă-rē) [L. *pessarium, fr. G. pessos,* an oval stone used in certain games]. **1.** An appliance of varied form, introduced into the vagina to support the uterus or to correct any displacement. **2.** A medicated vaginal suppository.

diaphragm p., a ring with a covered opening, used as a platform to support uterus, bladder or rectum, or to prevent conception.

Dumontpallier's p., Mayer's p.; an elastic ring p.

Gariel's p., a hollow inflatable rubber p. made in the form of a ring or a pear.

Hodge's p., a double-curve oblong p. employed for the correction of retrodeviations of the uterus.

Mayer's p., Dumontpallier's p.

Menge's p., a ring p. with a central horizontal bar into which a detachable handle is inserted.

ring p., a ring of rubber, plastic, or metal in which the cervix rests; designed to support the uterus and to correct prolapse of that organ.

pessimism (pes'i-mizm) [L. *pessimus,* worst, irreg. superl. of *malus,* bad]. A tendency to see or anticipate the worst.

therapeutic p., a disbelief in the curative virtues of remedies in general and especially of drugs.

pest [L. *pestis*]. Plague (2).

fowl p., fowl *plague.*

swine p., hog *cholera.*

pesticemia (pes-ti-sē'mē-ă) [L. *pestis,* plague, + G. *haima,* blood]. Bacteremia due to *Yersinia pestis.*

pesticide (pes'ti-sīd). General term for an agent that destroys fungi, insects, rodents, or any other pest.

pestiferous (pes-tif'ĕ-rŭs). Pestilential.

pestilence (pes'ti-lens) [L. *pestilentia*]. **1.** Plague (2). **2.** An epidemic of any infectious disease.

pestilential (pes-ti-len'shăl). Pestiferous; relating to, or tending to produce, a pestilence.

pes'tis [L.]. Plague (2).

p. am'bulans, ambulant *plague.*

p. ful'minans, bubonic *plague.*

p. ma'jor, bubonic *plague.*
p. mi'nor, ambulant *plague.*
p. sid'erans, septicemic *plague.*

pestivirus (pes'ti-vī'rŭs). A genus of viruses (family Togaviridae) composed of the hog cholera virus and related viruses.

pestle (pes'l) [L. *pistillum,* fr. *pinso,* or *piso,* to pound]. An instrument in the shape of a rod with one rounded and weighted extremity, used for bruising, breaking, and triturating substances in a mortar.

PET Abbreviation for positron emission *tomography.*

peta- (P). Prefix used in the SI and metric systems to signify one quadrillion (10^{15}).

-petal [L. *peto,* to seek, strive for]. Suffix denoting movement toward the part indicated by the main portion of the word.

petechiae, sing. **petechia** (pe-tē'kē-ē, pe-tē'kē-ă; pē-tek'-) [Mod. L. form of It. *petecchie*]. Minute hemorrhagic spots, of pinpoint to pinhead size, in the skin which are not blanched by diascopy.
Tardieu's petechiae, Tardieu's *ecchymoses.*

petechial (pē-tē'kē-ăl, pē-tek'-). Relating to, accompanied by, or characterized by petechiae.

petechiasis (pe-te-kī'ă-sis). Formation of petechiae or purpura.

Peters, Albert, German physician, 1862–1938. See P.'s *anomaly.*

Peters, Hubert, Austrian obstetrician, 1859–1934. See P.'s *ovum.*

Petersen, C.F., Kiel surgeon, 1845–1908. See P.'s *bag.*

petiolate, petiolated (pet'ē-ō-lāt, -lāt-ed) [L. *petiolus*]. Petioled; having a stem or pedicle.

petiole (pet'ē-ōl). Petiolus.

petioled (pet'ē-ōld). Petiolate.

petiolus (pe-tī'ō-lŭs) [L. dim. of *pes* (foot), the stalk of a fruit]. Petiole; a stem or pedicle.
p. epiglot'tidis [NA], the lower end or pedicle of the cartilage of the epiglottis, attached to the superior notch of the thyroid cartilage.

Petit, Alexis T., French physician, 1791–1820. See Dulong-P. *law.*

Petit, Antoine, French surgeon and anatomist, 1718–1794. See P.'s *ligament.*

Petit, Francois P. du, French surgeon and anatomist, 1664–1741. See P.'s *canals, sinus.*

Petit, Jean L., Paris surgeon, 1674–1750. See P.'s *hernia, herniotomy,* lumbar *triangle.*

Petit, Paul, French anatomist, *1889. See P.'s *aponeurosis.*

petit mal (pĕ-tē'mal). Absence.

Petri, Julius, German bacteriologist, 1852–1921. See P. *dish.*

petrifaction (pet-ri-fak'shŭn) [L. *petra,* rock + *facio,* to make]. Fossilization, as in conversion into stone.

pétrissage (pā-trē-sazh') [Fr. kneading]. A manipulation in massage, consisting in a kneading of the muscles.

petro- [L. *petra,* rock; G. *petros,* stone]. Combining form denoting stone, stone-like hardness.

petroccipital (pet'rok-sip'i-tăl). Petro-occipital.

petrolatum (pet-rō-lā'tŭm). Petroleum jelly; yellow soft paraffin; a yellowish mixture of the softer members of the paraffin or methane series of hydrocarbons, obtained from petroleum as an intermediate product in its distillation; used as a soothing application to burns and abrasions of the skin, and as a base for ointments.
heavy liquid p., mineral oil.
hydrophilic p., p. composed of cholesterol 30 g, stearyl alcohol 30 g, white wax 80 g, and white p. 860 g, to make 1000 g.
light liquid p., light *mineral oil.*
white p., white soft paraffin; of the same composition as p. except that care is taken in its preparation to keep it colorless; used for the same purposes as p.

petroleum (pē-trō'lē-ŭm) [L. *petra,* rock, + *oleum,* oil]. Coal or rock oil; a mixture of liquid hydrocarbons found in the earth in various parts of the world and believed to be derived from fossilized animal and plant remains; the source of petrolatum, in addition to its use for lighting and heating purposes.
p. benzin, p. ether; benzin; benzine; naphtha; purified, low boiling fractions distilled from p. consisting of hydrocarbons, chiefly of the methane series; it is highly flammable, and its vapors, when mixed with air and ignited, may explode; used as a solvent.
p. ether, p. benzin.
liquid p., mineral oil.

petroleum jelly. Petrolatum.

petromastoid (pet'rō-mas'toyd). Petrosomastoid; relating to the petrous and the squamous portions of the temporal bone, which are usually united at birth by the petrosquamosal suture.

petro-occipital (pet'rō-ok-sip'i-tăl). Petroccipital; denoting the cranial suture between the occipital bone and the petrous portion of the temporal.

petropharyngeus (pet'rō-fă-rin-jē'ŭs). See under musculus.

petrosa, pl. **petrosae** (pe-trō'să,-sē) [L. fr. *petra,* rock]. The petrous portion of the temporal bone.

petrosal (pe-trō'săl). Petrous (2); relating to the petrosa.

petrosalpingostaphylinus (pet'rō-sal'pin-gō-staf-i-lī'nŭs) [petrosa + G. *salpinx,* trumpet, + *staphylē,* uvula]. Obsolete term for *musculus* levator veli palatini.

petrositis (pet-rō-sī'tis). Petrousitis; an inflammation involving the petrous portion of the temporal bone and its air cells.

petrosomastoid (pet-rō'sō-mas'toyd). Petromastoid.

petrosphenoid (pet'rō-sfē'noyd). Relating to the petrous portion of the temporal bone and to the sphenoid bone.

petrosquamosal, petrosquamous (pet'rō-skwā-mō'săl,-skwā'-mŭs). Squamopetrosal; relating to the petrous and the squamous portions of the temporal bone.

petrostaphylinus (pet'rō-staf-i-lī'nŭs) [G. *petra,* stone, + *staphylē,* uvula]. Obsolete term for *musculus* levator veli palatini.

petrous (pet'rŭs, pē'trŭs) [L. *petrosus,* fr. *petra,* a rock]. **1.** Of stony hardness. **2.** Petrosal.

petrousitis (pet-rū-sī'tis). Petrositis.

Pette, H.H. German neuropathologist, 1887–1964. See P.-Döring *disease.*

Pettit, Auguste, 19th century French physician. See Bachman-P. *test.*

Peutz, J.L.A. See P.-Jeghers *syndrome, Jeghers-P. syndrome.*

pexin (pek'sin). Chymosin.

pexinogen (pek-sin'ō-jen). Prochymosin.

pexis (pek'sis) [G. *pēxis,* fixation]. Fixation of substances in the tissues.

-pexy [G. *pēxis,* fixation]. Suffix meaning fixation, usually surgical.

Peyer, Johann K., Swiss anatomist, 1653–1712. See P.'s *glands, patches.*

peyote, peyotl (pā-yō'tē, pā-yō'tl) [Sp.] Pellote; Aztec name for *Lophophora williamsii.*

Peyronie, Francois de la, French surgeon, 1678–1747. See P.'s *disease.*

Peyrot, Jean J., French surgeon, 1843–1918. See P.'s *thorax.*

Pezzer, O. de, See de Pezzer.

Pfannenstiel, Hermann Johann, German gynecologist, 1862–1909. See P.'s *incision.*

Pfaundler, Meinhard von, German physician, 1872–1947. See P.-

Hurler *syndrome.*

Pfeiffer, R.A., 20th century German physician. See P. *syndrome.*

Pfeiffer, Richard F.J., German physician, 1858–1945. See *Pfeifferella;* P.'s blood *agar, bacillus, phenomenon.*

Pfeifferella (fī-fer-el'lă) [R. F. J. *Pfeiffer*] An obsolete genus of bacteria, the type species of which, *P. mallei,* formerly was placed in the genus *Actinobacillus* and presently is placed in the genus *Pseudomonas.*

PFFD Abbreviation for proximal femoral focal *deficiency.*

Pflüger, Eduard F. W., German anatomist and physiologist, 1829–1910. See P.'s *laws, tubules.*

Pfuhl, Eduard, German physician, 1852–1905. See P.'s *sign.*

pg Symbol for picogram.

PGA, PGB, PGC, PGD, etc. Abbreviations, with numerical subscripts according to structure, often used for prostaglandins. Letters A, B, etc. indicate the nature of the cyclopentane ring (substituents, double bonds, orientation); numerical subscripts indicate the number of double bonds in the alkyl chains.

PGR Abbreviation for psychogalvanic *response.*

P_2Gri Symbol for diphosphoglycerate.

Ph Symbol for phenyl.

pH [p (power) of H^+]. Symbol for the logarithm of the reciprocal of the H ion concentration; a solution with pH 7.00 is neutral, one with a pH of more than 7.0 is alkaline, one with a pH lower than 7.00 is acid.

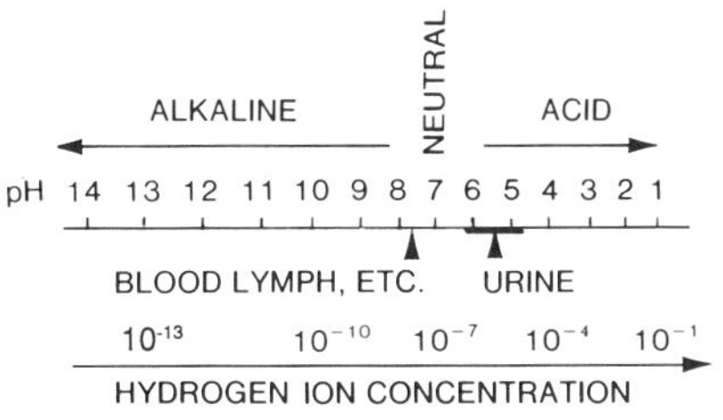

Diagram of pH Scale

critical pH, the pH range, about 5.5, at which saliva ceases to be saturated with respect to calcium and phosphate, and below which tooth mineral will dissolve.

optimum pH, the pH at which an enzymatic or any other reaction or process is most effective.

PHA Abbreviation for phytohemagglutinin.

phaco- [G. *phakos,* lentil (lens), anything shaped like a lentil]. Combining form meaning: **(1)** lens-shaped, or relating to a lens; **(2)** "mother-spot," as in phacomatosis.

phacoanaphylaxis (fak'ō-an-ă-fī-lak'sis). Hypersensitivity to protein of the lens of the eye.

phacocele (fak'ō-sēl) [phaco- + G. *kēlē,* hernia]. Hernia of the lens of the eye through the sclera.

phacocyst (fak'ō-sist) [phaco- + G. *kystis,* bladder]. *Capsula* lentis.

phacocystectomy (fak'ō-sis-tek'tō-mē) [phaco- + G. *kystis,* bladder, + *ektomē,* excision]. Surgical removal of a portion of the capsule of the lens of the eye.

phacodonesis (fak'ō-don-ē'sis) [phaco- + G. *doneo,* to shake to and fro]. Tremulousness of the lens of the eye.

phacoemulsification (fak'ō-ē-mŭl-si-fi-kā'shŭn). A method of emulsifying and aspirating a cataract with a low frequency ultrasonic needle.

phacoerysis (fak-ō-er'i-sis) [phaco- + G. *erysis,* pulling, drawing off]. Extraction of the lens of the eye by means of a suction cup called the erysophake.

phacofragmentation (fak'ō-frag'men-tā'shŭn). Rupture and aspiration of the lens.

phacoid (fak'oyd) [phaco- + G. *eidos,* resemblance]. Of lentil shape.

phacolysis (fă-kol'i-sis) [phaco- + G. *lysis,* dissolution]. Operative breaking down and removal of the lens.

phacolytic (fak-ō-lit'ik). Characterized by or referring to phacolysis.

phacoma (fa-kō'mă) [phaco- + G. *-oma,* tumor]. Phakoma; a hamartoma found in phacomatosis.

phacomalacia (fak'ō-mă-lā'shē-ă) [phaco- + G. *malakia,* softness]. Softening of the lens, as may occur in hypermature cataract.

phacomatosis (fak'ō-mă-tō'sis) [Van der Hoeve's coinage fr. G. *phakos,* mother-spot]. Phakomatosis; a generic term for a group of hereditary diseases characterized by hamartomas involving multiple tissues; *e.g.,* Lindau's disease, neurofibromatosis, Sturge-Weber syndrome, tuberous sclerosis.

phacometachoresis (fak'ō-met-ă-kō-rē'sis) [phaco- + G. *metachōrēsis,* change of place]. Obsolete term for luxation or subluxation of lens.

phacometer (fa-kom'ĕ-ter) [phaco- + G. *metron,* measure]. Obsolete term for lensometer.

phacoscope (fak'ō-skōp) [phaco- + G. *skopeō,* to view]. An instrument in the form of a dark chamber for observing the changes in the lens during accommodation.

Phaenicia sericata (fen-ī'sē-ă ser-i-kā'tă). *Lucilia sericata;* a common species of yellowish or metallic green blowfly (family Calliphoridae, order Diptera); an abundant scavenger feeding on carrion or excrement, and implicated in sheep strike and other forms of myiasis.

phaeo-. For terms beginning thus, see pheo-.

phaeohyphomycosis (fē'ō-hī'fō-mī-kō'sis) [G. *phaios,* dusky, + *hyphē,* web, + mycosis]. A group of superficial and deep infections caused by dematiaceous fungi that form hyphae and yeastlike cells in tissue, *i.e.,* dematiaceous fungal infections other than chromomycosis and mycetomas. In humans, cats, and horses, p. is caused by *Drechslera spicifera;* in chickens and turkeys by *Dactylaria gallopava.*

-phage, -phagia, -phagy [G. *phagein,* to eat]. Combining forms, used in the suffix position, meaning eating or devouring.

phage (fāj). Bacteriophage.

***β* p.,** *β corynebacteriophage.*

defective p., defective *bacteriophage.*

phagedena (faj-ĕ-dē'nă) [G. *phagedaina,* a canker]. An ulcer that rapidly spreads peripherally, destroying the tissues as it increases in size.

p. gangreno'sa, severe gangrene with sloughing.

p. nosocomia'lis, gangrene arising in a hospital from cross infection.

sloughing p., decubitus *ulcer.*

p. trop'ica, the tropical ulcer of Old World cutaneous leishmaniasis.

phagedenic (faj-ĕ-den'ik). Relating to or having the characteristics of phagedena.

phago- [G. *phagein,* to eat]. Combining form, used in the prefix position, denoting eating, devouring.

phagocyte (fag'ō-sīt) [phago- + G. *kytos,* cell]. Carrier or scavenger cell; a cell possessing the property of ingesting bacteria, foreign particles, and other cells. P.'s are divided into two general classes: 1) microphages, polymorphonuclear leukocytes which ingest chiefly bacteria; 2) macrophages, mononucleated cells (histiocytes and monocytes) which are largely scavengers, ingesting dead tissue and degenerated cells.

phagocytic (fag-ō-sit′ik). Relating to phagocytes or phagocytosis.

phagocytin (fag-ō-sī′tin). A very labile bactericidal substance that may be isolated from polymorphonuclear leukocytes.

phagocytize (fag′ō-si-tīz). Phagocytose.

phagocytoblast (fag-ō-sī′tō-blast) [phagocyte + G. *blastos,* germ]. A primitive cell developing into a phagocyte.

phagocytolysis (fag′ō-sī-tol′i-sis) [phagocyte + G. *lysis,* dissolution]. **1.** Phagolysis; destruction of phagocytes, or leukocytes, occurring in the process of blood coagulation or as the result of the introduction of certain antagonistic foreign substances into the body. **2.** A spontaneous breaking down of the phagocytes, preliminary (according to Metchnikoff) to the liberation of cytase, or complement.

phagocytolytic (fag′ō-sī-tō-lit′ik). Phagolytic; relating to phagocytolysis.

phagocytose (fag′ō-si-tōz). Phagocytize; to perform phagocytosis, denoting the action of phagocytic cells.

phagocytosis (fag′ō-sī-tō′sis) [phagocyte + G. *-osis,* condition]. The process of ingestion and digestion by cells of solid substances, *e.g.,* other cells, bacteria, bits of necrosed tissue, foreign particles.
induced p., p. occurring when bacteria subjected to the action of blood serum are brought in contact with leukocytes.
spontaneous p., p. occurring when a culture of bacteria is brought in contact with washed leukocytes in an indifferent medium, such as a physiologic salt solution.

phagodynamometer (fag′ō-dī-nă-mom′ĕ-ter) [phago- + G. *dynamis,* force, + *metron,* measure]. A device for measuring the force required to chew various foods.

phagolysis (fa-gol′i-sis). Phagocytolysis (1).

phagolysosome (fag-ō-lī′sō-sōm). A body formed by union of a phagosome or ingested particle with a lysosome having hydrolytic enzymes.

phagolytic (fag-ō-lit′ik). Phagocytolytic.

phagomania (fag-ō-mā′nē-ă) [phago- + G. *mania,* frenzy]. Rarely used term for a morbid desire to eat. See also bulimia.

phagophobia (fag-ō-fō′bē-ă) [phago- + G. *phobos,* fear]. Morbid fear of eating.

phagosome (fag′ō-sōm) [phago- + G. *soma,* body]. A vesicle that forms around a particle (bacterial or other) within the phagocyte that engulfed it, separates from the cell membrane, and then fuses with and receives the contents of cytoplasmic granules (lysosomes), thus forming a phagolysosome in which digestion of the engulfed particle occurs.

phagotype (fag′ō-tīp) [phago- + G. *typos,* type]. In microbiology, a subdivision of a species distinguished from other strains therein by sensitivity to a certain bacteriophage or set of bacteriophages.

-phagy. See -phage.

phako-. For words so beginning and not listed here, see phaco-.

phakoma (fa-kō′mă). Phacoma.

phakomatosis (fak′ō-mă-tō′sis). Phacomatosis.

phalacrosis (fal-ă-krō′sis) [G. *phalakrōsis,* fr. *phalos,* shining, white, fr. *phaō,* to shine]. Obsolete term for alopecia.

phalangeal (fă-lan′jē-ăl). Relating to a phalanx.

phalangectomy (fal-an-jek′tō-mē). Excision of one or more of the phalanges of hand or foot.

phalanges (fă-lan′jēz) [L.] [NA]. Plural of phalanx.

phalanx, gen. phalangis, pl. phalanges (fā′langks, fă-langks′, fă-lan′jis, -jēz) [L. fr. G. *phalanx (-ang-),* line of soldiers, bone between two joints of the fingers and toes]. **1** [NA]. One of the long bones of the digits, 14 in number for each hand or foot, two for the thumb or great toe, and three each for the other four digits; designated as proximal, middle, and distal, beginning from the metacarpus. **2.** One of a number of cuticular plates, arranged in several rows, on the surface of the spiral organ (of Corti), which are the heads of the outer row of pillar cells and of phalangeal cells; between them are the free ends of the hair cells.
tufted p., one of the terminal phalanges of the fingers in acromegaly; it has an expanded extremity resembling a sheaf of wheat.
ungual p., the distal p. of each of the digits; so called because of the flattened tuberosity at its termination which supports the nail.

phall-, phalli-, phallo- [G. *phallos,* penis]. Combining forms denoting the penis.

phallalgia (fal-al′jē-ă) [phall- + G. *algos,* pain]. Phallodynia.

phallectomy (fal-ek′tō-mē) [phall- + G. *ektomē,* excision]. Penectomy; surgical removal of the penis.

phallic (fal′ik) [G. *phallos,* penis]. **1.** Relating to the penis. **2.** In psychoanalysis, relating to the penis especially during the phases of infantile psychosexuality. See also phallic *phase.*

phallicism (fal′i-sizm). Phallism; worship of the male genitalia.

phalliform (fal′i-fōrm). Phalloid.

phallism (fal′i-sizm). Phallicism.

phallitis (fal-ī′tis). Penitis.

phallo-. See phall-.

phallocampsis (fal-ō-kamp′sis) [phallo- + G. *kampsis,* a bending]. Curvature of the erect penis. See also chordee.

phallocrypsis (fal-ō-krip′sis) [phallo- + G. *krypsis,* concealment]. Dislocation and retraction of the penis.

phallodynia (fal-ō-din′ē-ă) [phallo- + G. *odynē,* pain]. Phallalgia; pain in the penis.

phalloid (fal′oyd) [phallo- + G. *eidos,* resemblance]. Phalliform; resembling in shape a penis.

phalloidin (fă-loy′din). Best known of the toxic cyclic peptides produced by the poisonous mushroom, *Amanita phalloides;* closely related to amanitin.

phallolysin (fă-lol′i-sin). A glycoprotein that is the heat-sensitive (destroyed in cooking) toxin of the mushroom *Amanita phalloides.*

phalloncus (fal-ong′kŭs) [phallo- + G. *onkos,* mass]. A tumor or swelling of the penis.

phalloplasty (fal′ō-plas-tē) [phallo- + G. *plastos,* formed]. Plastic surgery of the penis.

phallorrhagia (fal-ō-rā′jē-ă) [phallo- + G. *rhēgnymi,* to burst forth]. Obsolete term for hemorrhage of the penis.

phallorrhea (fal-ō-rē′ă) [phallo- + G. *rhoia,* flow]. Discharge from the penis.

phallotomy (fal-ot′ō-mē) [phallo- + G. *tomē,* a cutting]. Penotomy; surgical incision into the penis.

phallus, pl. phalli (fal′ŭs, fal′ī) [L.; G. *phallos*]. Penis.

phanero- [G. *phaneros,* visible]. Combining form meaning visible, manifest.

phanerogenic (fan′er-ō-jen′ik) [phanero- + G. *genesis,* origin]. Denoting a disease the etiology of which is manifest. *Cf.* cryptogenic.

phaneromania (fan′er-ō-mā′nē-ă) [phanero- + G. *mania,* frenzy]. Constant preoccupation with some external part, as plucking the beard, pulling the lobe of the ear, picking at a pimple, etc.

phaneroscope (fan′er-ō-skōp) [phanero- + G. *skopeō,* to view]. A lens used to concentrate the light from a lamp upon the skin, to facilitate examination of lesions of the skin and subcutaneous tissues.

phanerosis (fan-er-ō′sis) [phanero- + G. *osis,* condition]. The act or process of becoming visible.
fatty p., presumed unmasking of previously invisible fat in the cytoplasm of cells; marked fatty metamorphosis is associated with

an absolute increase in the fat content of cells, so that the occurrence of p. is doubted.

phanerozoite (fan'er-ō-zō'īt) [phanero- + G. *zōon,* animal]. An exoerythrocytic tissue stage of malaria infection other than the primary exoerythrocytic stages (cryptozoite and metacryptozoite generations); consists chiefly of reinfection of the liver by merozoites produced by a blood infection (not found in falciparum malaria).

phanquone (fan'kwōn). 4,7-Phenanthroline-5,6-dione; an amebicide.

phantasia (fan-tā'zē-ă) [G. appearance]. Fantasy.

phantasm (fan'tazm) [G. *phantasma,* an appearance]. Phantom (1); the mental imagery produced by fantasy.

phantasmagoria (fan-taz-mă-gōr'ē-ă). A fantastic sequence of haphazardly associative imagery.

phantasmatomoria (fan-taz'mă-tō-mōr'ē-ă) [G. *phantasma,* an appearance, + *mōria,* folly]. Dementia with childish fantasies.

phantasmology (fan-tas-mol'ō-jē) [G. *phantasma,* an appearance, + *logos,* study]. The study of spiritualistic manifestations and of apparitions.

phantasmoscopia, phantasmoscopy (fan-taz-mō-skō'pē-ă, -mos'kō-pē) [G. *phantasma,* an appearance, + *skopeō,* to view]. The delusion of seeing phantoms.

phantom (fan'tŏm) [G. *phantasma,* an appearance]. **1.** Phantasm. **2.** A model, especially a transparent one, of the human body or any of its parts. See also manikin. **3.** In radiology, a mechanical or computer-originated model for predicting irradiation dosage deep in the body.
Schultze's p., a model of a female pelvis used in demonstrating the mechanism of childbirth and the application of forceps.

phantomize (fan'tŏm-īz). In psychiatry, to create mental imagery by fantasy.

pharmacal (far'mă-kăl). Pharmaceutic.

pharmaceutic, pharmaceutical (far-mă-sū'tik, sū'ti-kăl) [G. *pharmakeutikos,* relating to drugs]. Pharmacal; relating to pharmacy or to pharmaceutics.

pharmaceutics (far-mă-sū'tiks). **1.** Pharmacy (1). **2.** The science of pharmaceutical systems, *i.e.,* preparations, dosage forms, etc.

pharmaceutist (far-mă-sū'tist). Pharmacist.

pharmacist (far'mă-sist) [G. *pharmakon,* a drug]. Pharmaceutist; one who is licensed to prepare and dispense drugs and compounds and is knowledgable concerning their properties.

pharmaco- [G. *pharmakon,* drug, medicine]. Combining form relating to drugs.

pharmacochemistry (far'mă-kō-kem'is-trē). Pharmaceutical *chemistry.*

pharmacodiagnosis (far'mă-kō-dī-ag-nō'sis). Use of drugs in diagnosis.

pharmacodynamic (far'mă-kō-dī-nam'ik). Relating to drug action.

pharmacodynamics (far'mă-kō-dī-nam'iks) [pharmaco- + G. *dynamis,* force]. The study of uptake, movement, binding, and interactions of pharmacologically active molecules at their tissue site(s) of action.

pharmacoendocrinology (far'mă-kō-en'dō-krin-ol'ō-jē). The pharmacology of endocrine function.

pharmacogenetics (far'mă-kō-jĕ-net'iks). The study of genetically determined variations in responses to drugs in man or in laboratory organisms.

pharmacognosist (far-ma-kog'nō-sist). One skilled in pharmacognosy.

pharmacognosy (far-mă-kog'nō-sē) [pharmaco- + G. *gnōsis,* knowledge]. A branch of pharmacology concerned with the physical characteristics and botanical sources of crude drugs.

pharmacography (far-mă-kog'ră-fē) [pharmaco- + G. *graphē,* description]. A treatise on or description of drugs.

pharmacokinetic (far'mă-kō-ki-net'ik). Relating to the disposition of drugs in the body.

pharmacokinetics (far'mă-kō-ki-net'iks) [pharmaco- + G. *kinēsis,* movement]. Movements of drugs within biological systems, as affected by uptake, distribution, binding, elimination, and biotransformation; particularly the rates of such movements.

pharmacologic, pharmacological (far'mă-kō-loj'ik, -loj'i-kăl). **1.** Relating to pharmacology or to the composition, properties, and actions of drugs. **2.** Sometimes used in physiology to denote a dose (of a chemical agent that either is or mimics a hormone, neurotransmitter, or other naturally-occurring agent) that is so much larger or more potent than would occur naturally that it might have qualitatively different effects. *Cf.* homeopathic (2), physiologic (4), supraphysiologic.

pharmacologist (far-mă-kol'ō-jist). A specialist in pharmacology.
clinical p., a p. who has undergone training in basic pharmacology, clinical pharmacology, and one of several specialities of medical practice.

pharmacology (far-mă-kol'ō-jē) [pharmaco- + G. *logos,* study]. The science concerned with drugs, their sources, appearance, chemistry, actions, and uses.
biochemical p., a branch of p. concerned with the biochemical mechanisms responsible for the actions of drugs.
clinical p., the branch of p. concerned with the p. of therapeutic agents in the prevention, treatment, and control of disease in man.
marine p., a branch of p. concerned with pharmacologically active substances present in aquatic plants and animals; its objective is to find and develop new therapeutic agents.

pharmacomania (far'mă-kō-mā'nē-ă) [pharmaco- + G. *mania,* frenzy]. Morbid impulse to take drugs.

pharmacopedics, pharmacopedia (far'mă-kō-pē'diks, -pē'dē-ă) [pharmaco- + G. *paideia,* instruction, fr. *pais* (*paid-*), a child]. The teaching of pharmacy and pharmacodynamics.

Pharmacopeia, Pharmacopoeia (P) (far'mă-kō-pē'ă) [G. *pharmakopoiia,* fr. *pharmakon,* a medicine, + *poieo,* to make]. A work containing monographs of therapeutic agents, standards for their strength and purity, and their formulations. The various national pharmacopeias are referred to by abbreviations, of which the following are the most frequently encountered: *USP,* the Pharmacopeia of the United States of America (United States Pharmacopeia); *BP,* British Pharmacopoeia; *Codex medicamentarius,* the French Pharmacopeia; *I.C. Add.* (or *BA*), the Indian and Colonial Addendum to the BP; *IP,* International Pharmacopeia; *P. Austr.,* the Austrian Pharmacopeia; *Ph.G.,* the German Pharmacopeia (D.A.B.); *P. Helv.,* the Swiss Pharmacopeia. The first edition of the USP was compiled in 1820 and was made a legal standard by the terms of the National Food and Drugs Act in January, 1907.

pharmacopeial (far'mă-kō-pē'ăl). Relating to the Pharmacopeia; denoting a drug in the list of the Pharmacopeia. See also official.

pharmacophilia (far'mă-kō-fil'ē-ă) [pharmaco- + G. *phileō,* to love]. Morbid fondness for taking drugs.

pharmacophobia (far'mă-kō-fō'bē-ă) [pharmaco- + G. *phobos,* fear]. Morbid fear of taking drugs.

pharmacopsychosis (far'mă-kō-sī-kō'sis) [pharmaco- + psychosis]. Rarely used term for a psychosis causally related to taking a drug.

pharmacotherapy (far'mă-kō-thār'ă-pē) [pharmaco- + G. *therapeia,* therapy]. Treatment of disease by means of drugs. See also chemotherapy.

pharmacy (far'mă-sē) [G. *pharmakon,* drug]. **1.** Pharmaceutics (1); the practice of preparing and dispensing drugs. **2.** A drugstore.
clinical p., a branch of p. practice that emphasizes the therapeutic use of drugs rather than the preparation and dispensing of drugs.

Pharm. D. Abbreviation for Doctor of Pharmacy.

pharyng-. See pharyngo-.

pharyngalgia (far'ing-gal'jē-ă) [pharyng- + G. *algos,* pain]. Pharyngodynia; pain in the pharynx.

pharyngeal (fă-rin'jē-ăl) [Mod. L. *pharyngeus*]. Relating to the pharynx.

pharyngectomy (far'in-jek'tō-mē) [pharyng- + G. *ektomē,* excision]. Excision of a part of the pharynx.

pharyngemphraxis (far'in-jem-frak'sis) [pharyng- + G. *emphraxis,* a stoppage]. Pharyngeal obstruction.

pharynges (fă-rin'jēz). Plural of pharynx.

pharyngeus (far'in-jē'ŭs) [Mod. L.]. Pharyngeal.

pharyngismus (far-in-jiz'mŭs). Pharyngospasm; spasm of the muscles of the pharynx.

pharyngitic (far-in-jit'ik). Relating to pharyngitis.

pharyngitis (far-in-jī'tis) [pharyng- + G. *-itis,* inflammation]. Inflammation of the mucous membrane and underlying parts of the pharynx.
acute lymphonodular p., acute pharyngeal infection marked by reaction and hyperplasia in the lymph nodules on the posterior oropharyngeal wall, generally of bacterial etiology.
atrophic p., p. sicca; chronic p. accompanied by a varying degree of atrophy of the mucous glands and absence of their secretion.
croupous p., p. associated with an exudate resembling a membrane.
follicular p., granular p.
gangrenous p., putrid throat; gangrenous inflammation of the pharyngeal mucous membrane.
glandular p., granular p.
granular p., follicular or glandular p.; a form of p. in which the lymphoid follicles are enlarged, studding the mucous membrane as minute nodules or granules.
p. herpet'ica, p. characterized by vesicular eruption or shallow ulcers.
p. hypertroph'ica latera'lis, a form of chronic p. in which the glazed central portion is bounded on either side by a band of red, thickened mucous membrane.
membranous p., inflammation accompanied by a fibrinous exudate, forming a nondiphtheritic false membrane.
p. sic'ca, atrophic p.
ulcerative p., inflammation of the pharynx marked by ulceration of the mucosa; may have a viral etiology.
ulceromembranous p., inflammation of the pharyngeal mucosa with membranous debris overlaying the ulcerative lesions.

pharyngo-, pharyng- [Mod. L. fr. G. *pharynx*]. Combining forms denoting the pharynx.

pharyngocele (fă-ring'gō-sēl) [pharyngo- + G. *kēlē,* hernia]. A diverticulum from the pharynx.

pharyngodynia (fă-ring'gō-din'ē-ă) [pharyngo- + G. *odynē,* pain]. Pharyngalgia.

pharyngoepiglottic, pharyngoepiglottidean (fă-ring'gō-ep'i-glot'ik, -glo-tid'ē-an). Relating to the pharynx and the epiglottis.

pharyngoesophageal (fă-ring'gō-ē-sof'ă-jē'ăl). Relating to the pharynx and the esophagus.

pharyngoesophagoplasty (fă-ring'gō-ē-sof'ă-gō-plas-tē). Plastic surgery of the pharynx and esophagus.

pharyngoglossal (fă-ring'gō-glos'ăl). Relating to the pharynx and the tongue.

pharyngoglossus (fă-ring-gō-glos'ŭs). *Musculus* glossopharyngeus.

pharyngokeratosis (fă-ring'gō-ker-ă-tō'sis) [pharyngo- + G. *keras* (*kerat-*), horn]. Obsolete term for a thickening of the lining of the lymphoid follicles of the pharynx, with the formation of a tough, firmly adherent, pseudomembranous exudate.

pharyngolaryngeal (fă-ring'gō-lă-rin'jē-ăl). Relating to both the pharynx and the larynx.

pharyngolaryngitis (fă-ring'gō-lar-in-jī'tis). Inflammation of both the pharynx and the larynx.

pharyngolith (fă-ring'gō-lith) [pharyngo- + G. *lithos,* stone]. Pharyngeal calculus; a concretion in the pharynx.

pharyngology (făr'ing-gol'ō-jē) [pharyngo- + G. *logos,* study]. The medical science concerned with the study, diagnosis, and treatment of the pharynx.

pharyngomaxillary (fă-ring'gō-mak'si-lār-ē). Relating to the pharynx and the maxilla.

pharyngomycosis (fă-ring'gō-mī-kō'sis) [pharyngo- + G. *mykēs,* a fungus]. Invasion of the mucous membrane of the pharynx by fungi.

pharyngonasal (fă-ring'gō-nā'săl). Relating to the pharynx and the nasal cavity.

pharyngo-oral (fă-ring'gō-ō'răl) [pharyngo- + L. *os* (*or-*), mouth]. Relating to the pharynx and the mouth.

pharyngopalatine (fă-ring'gō-pal'ă-tīn). Relating to the pharynx and the palate.

pharyngopalatinus (fă-ring'gō-pal-ă-tī'nŭs) [L.]. *Musculus* palatopharyngeus.

pharyngopathy, pharyngopathia (far'ing-gop'ă-thē, fă-ring'gō-path'ē-ă) [pharyngo- + G. *pathos,* suffering]. Any disease of the pharynx.

pharyngoperistole (fă-ring'gō-pe-ris'tō-lē) [pharyngo- + G. *peristolē,* a drawing out]. Narrowing of the lumen of the pharynx.

pharyngoplasty (fă-ring'gō-plas-tē) [pharyngo- + G. *plastos,* formed]. Plastic surgery of the pharynx.

pharyngoplegia (fă-ring'gō-plē'jē-ă) [pharyngo- + G. *plēgē,* stroke]. Paralysis of the muscles of the pharynx.

pharyngorhinitis (fă-ring'gō-rī-nī'tis). Inflammation of the rhinopharynx, or of the mucous membrane of the pharynx and the nasal fossae.

pharyngorhinoscopy (fă-ring'gō-rī-nos'kŏ-pē) [pharyngo- + G. *rhis,* nose, + *skopeō,* to view]. Inspection of the rhinopharynx and posterior nares by means of the rhinoscopic mirror.

pharyngoscleroma (fă-ring'gō-skle-rō'mă) [pharyngo- + G. *sklērōma,* an induration]. A scleroma, or indurated patch, in the mucous membrane of the pharynx.

pharyngoscope (fă-ring'gō-skōp) [pharyngo- + G. *skopeō,* to view]. An instrument like a laryngoscope, used for inspection of the mucous membrane of the pharynx.

pharyngoscopy (far'ing-gos'kŏ-pē) [pharyngo- + G. *skopeō,* to view]. Inspection and examination of the pharynx.

pharyngospasm (fă-ring'gō-spazm). Pharyngismus.

pharyngostaphylinus (fă-ring'gō-staf-i-lī'nŭs) [L. fr. pharyngo- + G. *staphylē,* uvula]. *Musculus* palatopharyngeus.

pharyngostenosis (fă-ring'gō-ste-nō'sis) [pharyngo- + G. *stenōsis,* a narrowing]. Stricture of the pharynx.

pharyngotomy (far'ing-got'ō-mē) [pharyngo- + G. *tomē,* incision]. Any cutting operation upon the pharynx either from without or from within.

pharyngotonsillitis (fă-ring'gō-ton-si-lī'tis) [pharyngo- + tonsillitis]. Inflammation of the pharynx and tonsils.

pharyngotyphoid (fă-ring'gō-tī'foyd). Typhoid fever in which a sore throat is prominent among the initial symptoms.

pharyngoxerosis (fă-ring'gō-zē-rō'sis) [pharyngo- + G. *xerōsis,* a drying up]. Dryness of the pharyngeal mucous membrane.

pharynx, gen. **pharyngis,** pl. **pharynges** (far'ingks, fă-rin'jis, fă-rin'jēz) [Mod. L. fr. G. *pharynx* (*pharyng-*), the throat, the joint opening of the gullet and windpipe] [NA]. The upper expanded portion of the digestive tube, between the esophagus below and the mouth and nasal cavities above and in front.
laryngeal p., *pars* laryngea pharyngis.
nasal p., *pars* nasalis pharyngis.
oral p., *pars* oralis pharyngis.

phase (fāz) [G. *phasis,* an appearance]. **1.** A stage in the course of change or development. **2.** A homogeneous, physically distinct, and separable portion of a heterogeneous system; *e.g.,* oil, gum, and water are three p.'s of an emulsion. **3.** The time relationship between two or more events. **4.** A particular part of a recurring time-pattern or wave-form. See also stage; period.
anal p., in psychoanalytic personality theory, the stage of psychosexual development, occurring when a child is between 1 and 3 years, during which activities, interests, and concerns are centered around the anal zone.
aqueous p., the water portion of a system consisting of two liquid p.'s, one mainly water, the other a liquid immiscible with water (*e.g.,* benzene, ether).
cis p., see coupling p.
continuous p., external p.
coupling p., the physical relationship of two syntenic genes. If they are on the same chromosome, they are said to be "in coupling" or "in the cis p."; if on opposite members of a chromosome pair, "in repulsion" or "in the trans p."
discontinuous p., internal p.
dispersed p., internal p.
dispersion p., external p.
eclipse p., eclipse *period.*
eruptive p., that period in the tooth formation which includes the development of the roots, periodontal ligament, and dentogingival junction of the tooth.
external p., continuous or dispersion p.; dispersion or external medium; the medium or fluid in which a disperse is suspended.
genital p., in psychoanalytic personality theory, the final stage of psychosexual development, occurring during puberty, in which the individual's psychosexual development is so organized that sexual gratification can be achieved from genital-to-genital contact and the capacity exists for a mature affectionate relationship with an individual of the opposite sex.
internal p., dispersed or discontinous p.; the particles contained in a colloid solution.
lag p., a brief period in the course of the growth of a bacterial culture, especially at the beginning, during which the growth is very slow or scarcely appreciable.
latency p., latency period; in psychoanalytic personality theory, the period of psychosexual development in children, extending from about age 5 to the beginning of adolescence at age 12, during which the apparent cessation of sexual preoccupation during this period stems from a strong, aggressive blockade of libidinal and sexual impulses in an effort to avoid oedipal relationships; during this p., boys and girls are inclined to choose friends and join groups of their own sex.
logarithmic p., a period in the course of growth of a bacterial culture in which maximal multiplication is occurring by geometrical progression; thus, if the logarithms of their numbers are plotted against time, they will form a straight upward line.
luteal p., that portion of the menstrual cycle extending from the time of formation of the corpus luteum to the onset of menses, usually 14 days in length; **short l. p.,** a period of 10 days or less between ovulation and the onset of menses, frequently associated with infertility.
meiotic p., reduction p.; the stage of nuclear changes in the sexual cells during which reduction of the chromosomes takes place; it embraces the cell generations of the spermatocytes and oocytes.
negative p., the period during which the opsonic index is lowered following the injection of a vaccine.
oedipal p., oedipal period; in psychoanalysis, a stage in the psychosexual development of the child, characterized by erotic attachment to the parent of the opposite sex, repressed because of fear of the parent of the same sex; usually occurring between the ages of 3 and 6 years.
oral p., in psychoanalytic personality theory, the earliest stage in psychosexual development, lasting through the first 18 months of life, during which the oral zone is the center of the infant's needs, expression, gratification, and pleasurable erotic experiences; has a strong influence on the organization and development of the child's psyche.
phallic p., in psychoanalytic personality theory, the stage in psychosexual development, occurring when a child is between 2 and 6 years of age, during which interest, curiosity, and pleasurable experiences are centered around the penis in boys and the clitoris in girls.
positive p., the period following the negative p., during which the opsonic index rises.
postmeiotic p., postreduction p.; the stage following that of reduction of the chromosomes in the sexual cells, representing the mature forms of these cells, ending with the conjugation of the nuclei in the impregnated ovum.
postreduction p., postmeiotic p.
pregenital p., in psychoanalysis, the collective psychosexual development p.'s preceding the genital p.
premeiotic p., prereduction p.; the stage of nuclear changes in the sexual cells before the reduction of the chromosomes, embracing the cell generations up to that of the spermatogonia and oogonia.
pre-oedipal p., in psychoanalysis, the collective p.'s of psychosexual development preceding the oedipal p.
prereduction p., premeiotic p.
radial growth p., the early pattern of growth of cutaneous malignant melanoma, in which tumor cells spread laterally in the epidermis.
reduction p., meiotic p.
S p., a p. of DNA synthesis that follows gap 1 and precedes gap 2 in the mitotic cycle.
stationary p., the period in the course of growth of a bacterial culture during which the multiplication of the organisms becomes gradually less and finally ceases.
supernormal recovery p., a brief period during the recovery of cardiac muscle following excitation when the muscle is abnormally excitable; corresponds to the U wave in the electrocardiogram.
synaptic p., synapsis.
trans p., see coupling p.
vertical growth p., the late pattern of growth of cutaneous malignant melanoma in which epidermal tumor cells invade downward into the dermis.
vulnerable p., a period in the cardiac cycle during which an ectopic impulse may lead to repetitive activity such as flutter or fibrillation of the affected chamber.

phasmid (faz'mid). **1.** One of a pair of caudal chemoreceptors seen in nematodes of the class Secernentasida (Phasmidia). **2.** Common name for a member of the class Phasmidia, now Secernentasida.

Phasmidia (faz-mid'ē-ă) [G. *phasma,* appearance]. Secernentasida.

phasmophobia (fas-mō-fō'bē-ă) [G. *phasma,* apparition, + *phobos,* fear]. Morbid fear of ghosts.

phatnorrhagia (fat-nō-rā'jē-ă) [G. phatnōma, manger (alveolus), + G. *rhēgnymi,* to burst forth]. Hemorrhage from a dental alveolus.

Ph.D. Abbreviation for Doctor of Philosophy.

Phe Symbol for phenylalanine or its radical.

Phemister, Dallas B., American surgeon, 1882–1951. See P.'s *graft.*

phen-, pheno- [fr. G. *phainō,* to appear, show forth]. **1.** Combining form denoting appearance. **2.** In chemistry, combining form denoting derivation from benzene (phenyl-).

phenacaine hydrochloride (fen'ă-kān). Bis-(*p-* ethoxyphyenyl)acetamidine hydrochloride; a potent local surface anesthetic used in ophthalmology.

phenacemide (fe-nas'ĕ-mīd). Phenylacetylurea; an anticonvulsant used in the treatment of epilepsy.

phenacetin (fĕ-nas'ĕ-tin). Acetophenetidin; *p-* acetaminophenetide; *p-* acetphenetidine; $C_2H_5O–C_6H_4–NHCOCH_3$; an analgesic and antipyretic.

phenaceturic acid (fĕ-nas-ĕ-tūr'ik). Phenylaceturic acid; $C_6H_5CH_2CO–NH–CH_2COOH$; end product of the metabolism of phenylated fatty acids with even numbers of carbon atoms.

phenacridane chloride (fe-nas'ri-dān). 9-[*p-* (Hexyloxy)phenyl]-10-methylacridinium chloride; topical antiseptic.

phenacyclamine (fen-ă-sī'klă-mēn). Phenetamine.

phenadoxone hydrochloride (fen-ă-dok'sōn). Heptazone hydrochloride; 6-morpholino-4,4-diphenylheptan-3-one hydrochloride; an analgesic and hypnotic.

phenaglycodol (fen-ă-glī'kō-dol). 2-*p*-Chlorophenyl-3-methyl-2,3-butanediol; a central nervous system depressant used in the treatment of anxiety and simple neuroses.

phenanthrene (fĕ-nan'thrēn). $C_{14}H_{10}$; a compound isomeric with anthracene, derived from coal tar; a major component of steroids, as cyclopenta[α]-phenanthrene. Used as a basis for the synthesis of various dyes and drugs.

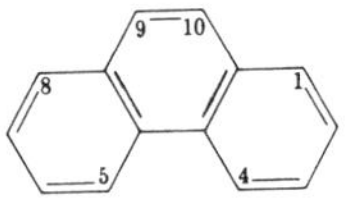

Phenanthrene

phenarsenamine (fen-ar-sen-am'ēn). Arsphenamine.

phenarsone sulfoxylate (fen-ar'sōn sŭl-fok'si-lāt). Sodium 3-amino-4-hydroxyphenylarsonate-*N-* methanolsulfoxylate; a pentavalent arsenical used in trichomonal vaginitis.

phenate (fē'nāt). Carbolate (1); a salt or ester of phenol (carbolic acid).

phenazacillin (fen-az-ă-sil'in). Hetacillin.

phenazocine (fen-ā'zō-sēn). 2'-Hydroxy-5,9-dimethyl-2-phenethyl-6,7-benzomorphan; a potent analgesic when given intramuscularly or intravenously, less effective orally.

phenazoline hydrochloride (fen-az'ō-lēn). Antazoline hydrochloride.

phenazopyridine hydrochloride (fen-ā-zō-pēr'i-dēn). 2,6-Diamino-3-(phenylazo)pyridine hydrochloride; a urinary antiseptic and anesthetic.

phencyclidine (PCP) (fen-sī'kli-dēn). 1-(1-Phenylcyclohexyl)piperidine; a substance of abuse, used for its hallucinogenic properties, which can produce profound psychological and behavioral disturbances; the hydrochloride has analgesic and anesthetic properties.

phendimetrazine tartrate (fen-di-met'ră-zēn). (*d*-3,4-Dimethyl-2-phenylmorpholine)-bitartrate; an anorexic agent.

phenelzine sulfate (fen'el-zēn). (2-Phenethyl) hydrazine sulfate; a monoamine oxidase inhibitor used as an antidepressant.

phenetamine (fĕ-net'ă-mēn). Phenacyclamine; 2-(Cyclohexylbenzyl)-*N,N,N',N'*-tetraethyl-1,3-propanediamine; an intestinal antispasmodic.

phenetharbital (fen-ĕ-thar'bi-tahl). *N-* Phenylbarbital; 5,5-diethyl-1-phenylbarbituric acid; an anticonvulsant agent.

phenethicillin potassium (fĕ-neth-i-sil'in). Penicillin B; α-phenoxyethylpenicillin potassium; a penicillin preparation that is stable in gastric acid and is rapidly but only partially absorbed from the gastrointestinal tract.

phenethyl alcohol (fĕ-neth'il). Phenylethyl alcohol.

phenetsal (fĕ-net'sal). Acetaminosalol.

pheneturide (fĕ-net'yū-rīd). Phenylethylacetylurea; (2-phenylbutyryl)urea; an antiepileptic similar in action to phenacemide.

phenformin hydrochloride (fen-fōr'min). 1-Phenylbiguanide monohydrochloride; an oral hypoglycemic agent no longer used in the U.S. because of the high incidence of fatal lactic acidosis associated with its use.

phenglutarimide hydrochloride (fen-glū-tar'i-mīd). The hydrochloride of α-2-diethylaminoethyl-α-phenylglutarimide; an antihistaminic used to decrease or prevent motion sickness, and to control Ménière's disease and vomiting.

phengophobia (fen-gō-fō'bē-ă) [G. *phengos,* daylight, + *phobos,* fear]. Morbid fear of daylight.

phenic acid (fē'nik). Phenol.

phenicarbazide (fen-i-kar'bă-zīd). 1-Phenylsemicarbazide; an antipyretic.

phenindamine tartrate (fĕ-nin'dă-mēn). 2-Methyl-9-phenyltetrahydro-1-pyridindene tartrate; an antihistaminic.

phenindione (fĕ-nin-dī'ōn). Phenylindanedione; 2-phenyl-1,3-indanedione: a synthetic anticoagulant with action and uses similar to those of bishydroxycoumarin.

pheniramine maleate (fĕ-nir'ă-mēn, -min). Prophenpyridamine maleate; 1-phenyl-1-(2-pyridyl)-3-dimethylaminopropane maleate; an antihistaminic.

phenmethylol (fen-meth'il-ol). *Benzyl* alcohol.

phenmetrazine hydrochloride (fen-met'ră-zēn). 2-Phenyl-3-methyltetrahydro-1,4-oxazine hydrochloride; an anorexic agent.

pheno-. See phen-.

phenobarbital (fē-nō-bar'bi-tahl). Phenylethylmalonylurea; phenylethylbarbituric acid; $CO(NHCO)_2C(C_2H_5)(C_6H_5)$; a long-acting oral or parenteral sedative and hypnotic; available as a sodium salt; also used in therapeutic management of epilepsy and induction of hepatic microsomal enzymes.

phenobutiodil (fen'ō-byū-tī'ō-dil). 2-(2,4,6-Triiodophenoxy)-butyric acid; a radiographic contrast medium for cholecystography.

phenocopy (fē'nō-kop'ē) [G. *phainein,* to display, + copy]. **1.** An individual with clinical or laboratory characteristics that would ordinarily assign him to a specific phenotype with respect to genetic abnormality, but whose characteristics are of environmental rather than genetic etiology. **2.** A condition of environmental etiology that mimics a condition usually of genetic etiology.

phenodeviant (fē-nō-dē'vē-ant). An individual with a phenotype significantly different from that of the population to which it belongs.

phenodin (fē'nō-din). Hematin.

phenol (fē'nol). Phenyl alcohol; phenic acid; carbolic acid; C_6H_5OH; an antiseptic and disinfectant; locally escharotic in concentrated form and neurolytic in 3 to 4% solutions; internally, a powerful escharotic poison.

camphorated p., camphorated carbolic acid, consisting of p., camphor, and liquid petrolatum; used as a local anesthetic and for the relief of toothache.

liquefied p., liquefied carbolic acid; p. liquefied by the addition of

10% of water.
p. oxidase, laccase.

phenolase (fē′nō-lās). Laccase.

phenolated (fē′nō-lāt-ed). Carbolated; impregnated or mixed with phenol.

phenolemia (fē-nol-ē′mē-ă) [phenol + G. *haima,* blood]. The presence of phenols in the blood.

phenology (fe-nol′ō-jē) [G. *phainō,* to appear, + *logos,* study]. The study of the biological rhythms of plants and animals, particularly those rhythms showing seasonal variation.

phenolphthalein (fē-nol-thal′ē-in, -thal′ēn). Obtained by the action of phenol on phthalic anhydride; used as a hydrogen ion indicator and as a laxative.

phenol red. Phenolsulfonphthalein.

phenolsulfonphthalein (PSP) (fē′nol-sŭl-fōn-thal′ē-in, -thal′ēn). Phenol red; occurs as a bright to dark red crystalline powder; widely used as an indicator in tissue culture media (yellow at pH 6.8, red at pH 8.4) and by parenteral injection as a test for renal function.

phenoluria (fē-nol-yū′rē-ă). The excretion of phenols in the urine.

phenomenology (fē-nom-ĕ-nol′ō-jē) [phenomenon, + G. *logos,* study]. **1.** The systematic description and classification of phenomena without attempt at explanation or interpretation. **2.** The study of human experiences, irrespective of objective-subjective distinctions. See also existential *psychology.*

PHENOMENON

phenomenon, pl. **phenomena** (fē-nom′ĕ-non, -nă) [G. *phainomenon,* fr. *phainō,* to cause to appear]. **1.** A symptom; an occurrence of any sort, whether ordinary or extraordinary, in relation to a disease. **2.** Any unusual fact or occurrence.

adhesion p., immune adherence p.; erythrocyte adherence p.; red cell adherence p.; a p. recognized in a variety of forms since the early years of the 20th century and manifested by the adherence of antigen-antibody-complement complex to "indicator cells" (microorganisms, platelets, leukocytes, or erythrocytes), the reaction being sensitive and specific for the antigen and antibody in the complex and requiring only the first four components of complement. When the antigen is a microorganism, adherence can be determined microscopically; when the antigen-antibody-complement complex is soluble, adherence causes agglutination of the indicator cells; when the antigen is on the surface of a cell (*e.g.,* leukocyte), the "target cell"-antibody-complement complex forms a rosette around the indicator cell.

AFORMED p. [*A*lternating, *f*ailure *o*f *r*esponse, *m*echanical, to *e*lectrical *d*epolarization], as pulsus alternans progresses to include inaudible alternating heart sounds, a state develops in which alternating heart depolarizations fail to eject any blood, thus allowing longer diastolic filling; the subsequent beat is then able to produce a significant ejection; at high rates the cardiac minute volume and blood pressure may appear normal.

Anrep p., homeometric autoregulation of the heart whereby cardiac performance improves as the afterload (aortic pressure) is increased.

aqueous influx p., Ascher's aqueous influx p.; the filling of the aqueous vein, which normally carries blood and aqueous, with aqueous, when the junction of the aqueous vein and the recipient vein is partially occluded.

Arias-Stella p., Arias-Stella effect or reaction; focal, unusual, decidual changes in endometrial epithelium, consisting of intraluminal budding, and nuclear enlargement and hyperchromatism with cytoplasmic swelling and vacuolation; may be associated with ectopic or uterine pregnancy.

arm p., Pool's p. (2).

Arthus p., Arthus reaction (1); a form of allergic inflammatory reaction observed in rabbits that become progressively more sensitive to an antigen (*e.g.,* horse serum) administered as a series of subcutaneous injections spaced at intervals of several days; the fifth or sixth dose is likely to result in a persistent swelling and firm indurated region that eventually becomes necrotic; the reaction is not confined to the region adjacent to the sites of previous injections, but is frequently observed at any site where the critical injection is made. A similar response may be observed when a cutaneous dose of antigen is administered to a rabbit sensitized 3 to 5 weeks previously by means of a series of 2 or 3 weekly intravenous doses of the same antigen. The reaction is caused by the inflammation that results from the deposition of antigen-antibody complexes in tissue spaces and in blood vessel walls, most of the damage seemingly being due to the polymorphonuclear leukocytes that phagocytize the deposits. The p., as described by Arthus, seems to be peculiar to rabbits, but similar reactions (Arthus-type reactions) are observed in guinea pigs, rats, and dogs, as well as in man, under appropriate conditions.

Ascher's aqueous influx p., aqueous influx p.

Aschner's p., oculocardiac *reflex.*

Ashley's p., oculocardiac *reflex.*

Ashman's p., aberrant ventricular conduction of a beat ending a short cycle that is preceded by a longer cycle during atrial fibrillation.

Aubert's p., a p. in which a bright perpendicular line appears to incline to one side when the observer turns the head to the opposite side in a dark room.

autoscopic p., the encountering of an image of oneself, the image being an illusion, a hallucination, or a vivid fantasy.

Babinski's p., Babinski's *sign* (1).

Bell's p., a patient with peripheral facial paralysis cannot close the eyelids of the affected side without at the same time moving the eyeball upward and outward.

Bombay p. [*Bombay,* India, where first reported], a rare recessive trait that is epistatic to the locus that regulates the phenotype at the ABO blood group; the Bombay locus manufactures H substance, which is the precursor from which the A and B phenotypes are elaborated; failure to produce H substance results in the Bombay trait and hence, no matter what the genotype at the ABO locus, the phenotype is O.

Bordet-Gengou p., the p. of complement fixation; when alexin (complement)-containing serum is added to a mixture of bacteria and specific antibody, the alexin is removed (fixed) and is not available to lyse subsequently added erythrocytes sensitized with specific antibody. See also Gengou p.

breakoff p., breakaway p., the occurrence, during high-altitude flight, of a sensation of being totally detached from the earth and one's fellow man.

Brücke-Bartley p., the sensation of glare in response to successive stimuli at frequencies just below the fusion point.

Capgras' p., Capgras' *syndrome.*

cervicolumbar p., a sense of weakness in the lower extremities on movement of the neck when a lesion is present in the upper portion of the spinal cord; or sensations referred to the neck when a lesion exists in the lower portion of the cord.

cogwheel p., Negro's p.; a sudden brief halt in usually smooth respiration or other motor activity.

constancy p., in perception, the tendency for brightness, color, size, or shape to remain relatively perceptually constant despite changes in any conditions of observation, *e.g.,* light or position.

crossed phrenic p., hemisection of the cord above the exit of the phrenic nerve paralyzes the ipsilateral half of the diaphragm; if the

contralateral phrenic nerve is then sectioned or blocked, contractions on the ipsilateral side are resumed.
Cushing p., Cushing effect or response; a rise in systemic blood pressure when the intracranial pressure acutely increases, usually in excess of 50% of the systolic arterial pressure.
Danysz p., reduction of the neutralizing effect of an antitoxin when toxin is mixed with it in divided portions, rather than adding the same total quantity of toxin in one step.
dawn p., abrupt increases in fasting levels of plasma glucose concentrations between 5 and 9 a.m., in the absence of antecedent hypoglycemia; occurs in diabetic patients receiving insulin therapy.
Debré p., in measles, the failure of the rash to develop at the site of immune serum injection.
declamping p., declamping shock; shock or hypotension following abrupt release of clamps from a large portion of the vascular bed, as from the aorta; apparently caused by transient pooling of blood in a previously ischemic area.
déjà vu p., the mental impression that a new experience (*e.g.,* a sight, sound, or action) has happened before; a common p. in normal persons that may occur more frequently or continuously in certain emotional or organic disorders. Also variously referred to as déjà entendu, déjà éprouvé, déjà fait, déjà pensé, déjà raconté, déjà vécu, or déjà voulu, depending on the experience or sense that is evoked.
Dejerine's hand p., Déjérine's reflex; clonic contractions of the flexors of the hand (wrist) on tapping the dorsum of the hand or the volar side of the forearm near the wrist; it occurs in normal persons but is exaggerated in pyramidal tract lesions.
Dejerine-Lichtheim p., Lichtheim's *sign.*
Denys-Leclef p., enhanced phagocytosis by leukocytes of microorganisms in the presence of immune serum.
d'Herelle p., Twort-d'Herelle p.
diaphragm p., Litten's or phrenic p.; phrenic wave; a lowering of the line of retraction on the side of the chest (marking the insertion of the diaphragm) during inspiration, and elevation of the same during expiration; the p. is absent in cases of distention of the pleural sac. See also paradoxical diaphragm p.
dip p., complete disappearance of ventricular excitability followed by progressive recovery within a few microseconds at the end of excitation; the muscle as a whole repolarizes somewhat inhomogeneously, so that this period is one of special sensitivity to exogenous or endogenous stimuli and reentry.
Donath-Landsteiner p., the hemolysis which results in a sample of blood of a subject of paroxysmal hemoglobinuria when the sample is cooled to around 5°C and then warmed again.
Doppler p., Doppler *effect.*
Duckworth's p., respiratory arrest before cardiac arrest as a result of intracranial disease.
Ehret's p., a sudden throb felt by the finger on the brachial artery, as the pressure in the cuff falls during a blood pressure estimation; said to indicate fairly accurately the diastolic pressure.
Ehrlich's p., the difference between the amount of diphtheria toxin that will exactly neutralize one unit of antitoxin and that which, added to one unit of antitoxin, will leave one lethal dose free is greater than one lethal dose of toxin; *i.e.,* it is necessary to add more than one lethal dose of toxin to a neutral mixture of toxin and antitoxin to make the mixture lethal (the basis of the L_+ dose).
erythrocyte adherence p., adhesion p.
escape p., failure of the pupil in an eye with optic neuritis to maintain constriction as both eyes are alternately stimulated with light.
facialis p., light rubbing of the skin or a tap on the zygoma causes a quick contraction of the lip and ala nasi; sometimes percussion above the zygoma causes contraction of the lip only; observed in tetany and sometimes in exophthalmic goiter.
finger p., Gordon's sign; a sign of organic hemiplegia; with the patient's elbow resting on a table, the patient's wrist is grasped by the examiner's hand, the thumb of which is used to exert pressure on the radial side of the patient's pisiform bone; if the hemiplegia is organic, some or all of the patient's fingers become extended and spread out in a fanlike form.
Friedreich's p., the tympanitic percussion sound over a pulmonary cavity is slightly raised in pitch on deep inspiration.
Galassi's pupillary p., orbicularis pupillary *reflex.*
Gallavardin's p., dissociation between the noisy and musical elements of the murmur of aortic stenosis, the musical element being better heard at the left sternal border and at the cardiac apex while the noisy element is better heard at the aortic area.
gap p., a short period in the cycle of the atrioventricular or intraventricular conduction allowing passage of an impulse which at other times would be blocked in transit.
Gärtner's vein p., fullness of the veins of the arm and hand held below heart level and collapse at a certain variable distance above that level.
generalized Shwartzman p., Sanarelli p.; Sanarelli-Shwartzman p.; when both the preparative injection of endotoxin-containing filtrate and the provocative injection are given intravenously 24 hours apart, the animal usually dies within 24 hours after the second inoculation; the characteristic lesions in the rabbit include widespread hemorrhages and bilateral cortical necrosis of the kidney; the p. is associated with a marked fall in the number of circulating leukocytes and platelets.
Gengou p., an extension of the Bordet-Gengou p.; noncellular antigens, when mixed with specific antibody, also fix alexin (complement).
gestalt p., see gestalt.
Goldblatt p., Goldblatt's hypertension; hypertension resulting from partial occlusion of a renal artery.
Grasset's p., Grasset-Gaussel p.; in organic paralysis of the lower extremity, the patient, lying on his back, can raise either limb separately, but not both together.
Grasset-Gaussel p., Grasset's p.
Gunn p., jaw-winking *syndrome.*
Hamburger's p., chloride *shift.*
Hill's p., Hill's *sign.*
hip p., Joffroy's *reflex.*
hip-flexion p., when a hemiplegic attempts to rise from a lying posture, the hip on the paralyzed side is flexed first; the same movement takes place on lying down.
Hoffmann's p., excessive irritability of the sensory nerves to electrical or mechanical stimuli in tetany.
Houssay p., see Houssay *animal.*
hunting p., hunting *reaction.*
Hunt's paradoxical p., in dystonia musculorum deformans, if an attempt is made at plantar flexion of the foot when the foot is in dorsal spasm the only response is an increase of the extensor, or dorsal, spasm; if, however, the patient is told to extend the foot which is already in a state of strong dorsal flexion, there will be a sudden movement of plantar flexion; the same p., *mutatis mutandis,* is observed when there is a condition of strong plantar flexion.
immune adherence p., adhesion p.
jaw-winking p., jaw-winking *syndrome.*
Jod-Basedow p., iodine-induced hyperthyroidism; induction of thyrotoxicosis in a previously euthyroid individual as a result of exposure to large quantities of iodine; occurs most often in areas of endemic iodine-deficient goiter and in patients with multinodular goiter; also can develop following use of iodine-containing agents for diagnostic studies.
knee p., patellar *reflex.*
Köbner's p., isomorphic response; an isomorphic reaction seen in response to trauma in previously uninvolved sites of patients with psoriasis, lichen planus, and verruca plana juvenilis.
Koch's p., **(1)** the p. of infection immunity; living tubercle bacilli (*Mycobacterium tuberculosis*) do not cause reinfection when inoculated into tuberculous guinea pigs (*i.e.,* the animals are "immune"

to reinfection) even though the original infections continue to develop and eventually cause death of the animals; **(2)** rise of temperature and increase of the local lesion, in a tuberculous subject, following an injection of tuberculin.
Kohnstamm's p., aftermovement; a slow, involuntary elevation of the arm after strong pressure against a firm object.
Kühne's p., when a constant current is passed through a muscle, an undulation is seen to pass from the positive to the negative pole.
LE p., the formation of LE cells in bone marrow or blood on adding serum from patients with disseminated lupus erythematosus.
leg p., Pool's p. (1).
Leichtenstern's p., Leichtenstern's *sign.*
Litten's p., diaphragm p.
Lucio's leprosy p., Lucio's *leprosy.*
Marcus Gunn p., jaw-winking *syndrome.*
misdirection p., aberrant *regeneration.*
Mitzuo's p., restoration of the normal color of the fundus with dark adaptation in Oguchi's disease.
Negro's p., cogwheel p.
no reflow p., absence of blood flow in a portion of the brain which has been damaged, usually by ischemia.
on-off p., a state in the treatment of Parkinson's disease by *l*-dopa, in which there is a rapid fluctuation of akinetic (off) and choreoathetotic (on) movements.
orbicularis p., constriction of the pupils when an effort is made to close eyelids forcibly held apart.
paradoxical diaphragm p., in pyopneumothorax, hydropneumothrax, and some cases of injury, the diaphragm on the affected side rises during inspiration and falls during expiration.
paradoxical pupillary p., paradoxical pupillary *reflex.*
peroneal p., tapping the peroneal nerve below the head of the fibula causes dorsal flexion and abduction of the foot.
Pfeiffer's p., the alteration and complete disintegration of cholera vibrios when introduced into the peritoneal cavity of an immunized guinea pig, or into that of a normal one if immune serum is injected at the same time; extended to include bacteriolysis in general.
phi p., an illusion of movement, which occurs by means of successive visual impressions at intervals of $^1/_{15}$ to $^1/_{20}$ sec; when an occluder is passed from one eye to the other while a small distant light is observed, the light seems to move with the occluder in exophoria, but in an opposite direction in esophoria.
phrenic p., diaphragm p.
Pool's p., **(1)** leg p.; Pool-Schlesinger sign; Schlesinger's sign; in tetany, spasm both of the extensor muscles of the knee and of the calf muscles when the extended leg is flexed at the hip; **(2)** arm p.; in tetany, contraction of the arm muscles following the stretching of the brachial plexus by elevation of the arm above the head with the forearm extended, resembles the contraction resulting from stimulation of the ulnar nerve.
pseudo-Graefe's p., retraction of the upper eyelid on downward movement of the eyes.
psi p., a p. that includes both psychokinesis and extrasensory perception.
Purkinje's p., Purkinje shift; in the light-adapted eye, the region of maximal brightness is in the yellow; in the dark-adapted eye, the region of maximal brightness is in the green.
quellung p., Neufeld capsular *swelling.*
radial p., dorsal flexion of the hand occurring involuntarily with palmar flexion of the fingers.
Raynaud's p., sensitivity of the hands and fingers to cold, as a result of spasm of the digital arteries, with blanching and numbness or pain of the fingers.
rebound p., **(1)** Stewart-Holmes *sign;* **(2)** generally, any p. in which a variable that has been displaced from its normal state by a disturbing influence temporarily deviates from normal in the opposite direction when the disturbing influence is suddenly removed, before finally stabilizing at its normal state, *i.e.,* a p. involving undershoot; *e.g.,* the subsequent hypoglycemia that may follow injection of glucose, because the initial hyperglycemia caused excessive secretion of insulin.
reclotting p., thixotropy.
red cell adherence p., adhesion p.
reentry p., see reentry.
release p., the increased tonus and hyperirritability of muscle-stretch reflexes which occur following damage of the upper portions of the extrapyramidal system.
Ritter-Rollet p., on equal electrical stimulation of motor nerve trunks, the flexor and abductor muscle groups react more readily than the extensors and adductors.
R-on-T p., a premature ventricular (QRS) complex in the electrocardiogram interrupting the T wave of the preceding beat.
Rust's p., in cancer or caries of the upper cervical vertebrae, the patient will always support the head by the hands when changing from the recumbent to the sitting posture or the reverse.
Sanarelli p., generalized Shwartzman p.
Sanarelli-Shwartzman p., generalized Shwartzman p.
Schellong-Strisower p., a reduction of the systolic blood pressure, accompanied sometimes by vertigo, on rising from the horizontal to the erect posture.
Schiff-Sherrington p., when the cord is transected in the mid-thoracic region or a little lower, the stretch and other postural reflexes of the upper extremity become exaggerated; if the transection is made in the sacral cord, a similar effect is observed in the lower limbs. The effect is regarded as a release p., *i.e.,* release from an inhibitory influence normally exerted by the spinal segments below the transection.
Schüller's p., in cases of functional hemiplegia the patient usually turns to the sound side in walking, but to the affected side in case of an organic lesion.
Schultz-Charlton p., Schultz-Charlton *reaction.*
Sherrington p., after the muscles of the leg have been deprived of their motor innervation by sectioning the ventral roots containing fibers for the sciatic nerve, and allowing time for the degeneration of the fibers to occur, stimulation of the sciatic nerve causes slow contraction of the muscles.
shot-silk p., shot-silk *retina.*
Shwartzman p., Shwartzman reaction; a rabbit is so prepared by the intradermal injection of a small quantity of a suspension or of a filtrate of a culture of *Salmonella typhi,* or certain other Gram-negative bacteria, that it will develop a hemorrhagic and necrotic lesion at the site of this preparatory inoculation following the intravenous injection, after a latent period (usually 24 hours); the active material which prepares the animal is endotoxin, a complex macromolecular phospholipid-polysaccharide which forms an integral part of the precipitates. See also generalized Shwartzman p.
Somogyi p., Somogyi effect; posthypoglycemic hyperglycemia; a rebound p. of reactive hyperglycemia following a period of relative hypoglycemia, which may be subclinical and difficult to detect; the hyperglycemia induces use of more insulin, thus aggravating the problem.
Soret's p., in a solution kept in a long, upright tube at room temperature, the upper part, being the warmer, is also the more concentrated.
Splendore-Hoeppli p., radiating or annular eosinophilic deposits of host-derived materials, and possibly of parasite antigens, which form around fungi, helminths, or bacterial colonies in tissue.
staircase p., treppe.
steal p., see steal.
Strassman's p., in the third stage of labor, failure of placental detachment indicated by transmission of pressure from the fundus uteri to the umbilical vein which becomes engorged.
Strümpell's p., tibial p.; dorsal flexion of the great toe, sometimes of the entire foot, in a paralyzed limb when the extremity is drawn up against the body, flexing both knee and hip.

symbiotic fermentation p., "two organisms, neither of which alone produces gas fermentation in certain carbohydrates, may do so when living in symbiosis or when artifically mixed" (Castellani).
Theobald Smith's p., a p. observed in guinea pigs that had survived use for diphtheria antitoxin standardization, the animals having been rendered highly susceptible to subsequent inoculation of horse serum.
tibial p., Strümpell's p.
toe p., Babinski's *sign* (1).
tongue p., Schultze's *sign.*
Tournay's p., Tournay's *sign.*
Twort p., Twort-d'Herelle p.
Twort-d'Herelle p., Twort p.; d.'Herelle p.; bacteriophagia; the lysis of bacteria by bacteriophage.
Tyndall p., the visibility of floating particles in gases or liquids when illuminated by a ray of sunlight and viewed at right angles to the illuminating ray.
Wenckebach p., progressive lengthening of A-V conduction time (P-R interval) until a beat is dropped; following the dropped beat the P-R interval is again shortened.
Westphal's p., Westphal's *sign.*
Westphal-Piltz p., Westphal's pupillary reflex; Piltz sign; pupillary constriction followed by dilation upon forcible closure of the eyelids.
Wever-Bray p., the action potentials in the acoustic nerve that correspond to auditory stimuli reaching the cochlea.

phenoperidine (fen-ō-per'i-dēn). 1-(3-Hydroxy-3-phenylpropyl)-4-phenylisonipecotic acid ethyl ester; an analgesic.

phenothiazine (fē-nō-thī'ă-zēn). Thiodiphenylamine; dibenzothiazine; a compound formerly used extensively for the treatment of intestinal nematodes in animals; without central nervous system depressant activity itself, it serves as the parent compound for synthesis of a large number of antipsychotic compounds, including chlorpromazine, thioridazine, perphenazine, and fluphenazine.

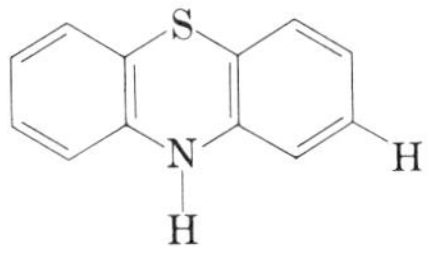

Phenothiazine

phenotype (fē'nō-tīp) [G. *phainein,* to display, + *typos,* model]. Manifestation of a genotype or the combined manifestation of several different genotypes. The discriminating power of the p. in identifying the genotype depends on its level of subtlety; thus special methods of carrier detection will distinguish them from normal subjects from whom they are inseparable on simple physical examination.

phenotypic (fē'nō-tip'ik, fen-ō-). Relating to phenotype.

phenoxazine (fe-nok'să-zēn). Phenothiazine in which S is replaced by O; as the 3-oxo derivative (phenoxazone), p. is the chromophore of actinomycins.

phenoxazone (fe-nok'să-zōn). See phenoxazine.

phenoxybenzamine hydrochloride (fē-nok'si-ben'ză-mēn). (2-Chloroethyl)-*N*-(1-methyl-2-phenoxyethyl benzylamine hydrochloride; a potent adrenergic (α-receptor) blocking agent of the β-haloalkylamines; selectively blocks the excitatory response of smooth muscle and exocrine glands to epinephrine; used in the treatment of peripheral vascular diseases.

2-phenoxyethanol (fē-nok-si-meth'ă-nol). 1-Hydroxy-2-phenoxyethane; an antibacterial agent used in the topical treatment of wound infections; it is active against Gram-negative bacteria that are resistant to most other antiseptics.

α-phenoxyethylpenicillin potassium (fē-nok'sē-eth'il-pen-i-sil'in). Phenethicillin potassium.

phenoxymethylpenicillin (fē-nok'si-meth'il-pen-i-sil'in). *Penicillin* V.

α-phenoxypropylpenicillin potassium (fē'nok-sē-prō'pil-pen-i-sil'in). Propicillin.

phenozygous (fē'nō-zī'gŭs, fe-noz'i-gŭs) [G. *phainō,* to show, + *zygon,* yoke]. Having a narrow cranium as compared with the width of the face, so that when the skull is viewed from above, the zygomatic arches are visible.

phenpentermine tartrate (fen-pen'ter-mēn). α,α,β-Trimethylphenethylamine; an anorexigenic agent.

phenprobamate (fen-prō'bă-māt). Proformiphen; 3-phenylpropyl carbamate; a skeletal muscle relaxant with antianxiety action.

phenprocoumon (fen-prō-kū'mon). 3-(1'-Phenylpropyl)-4-hydroxycoumarin; a long-acting orally effective anticoagulant.

phenpropionate (fen-prō'pē-ō-nāt). USAN-approved contraction for 3-phenylpropionate.

phensuximide (fen-sŭk'si-mīd). *N*-Methyl-2-phenylsuccinimide; an anticonvulsant drug used in the treatment of petit mal epilepsy.

phentermine (fen'ter-mēn). α,α-Dimethylphenethylamine; an anorexic agent; also available as the hydrochloride.

phentolamine hydrochloride (fen-tol'ă-mēn). 2-(*N'*-*p*- Tolyl-*N'*-*m*- hydroxyphenylaminomethyl)-imidazoline hydrochloride; an adrenergic (α-receptor) blocking agent.

phentolamine mesylate. Phentolamine methanesulfonate; the same actions as phentolamine hydrochloride, for intravenous use only.

phenyl (Ph) (fen'il). The univalent radical, C_6H_5–, of benzene.
p. alcohol, phenol.
p. aminosalicylate, *p*-aminosalicylic acid phenyl ester; an antituberculous drug.
p. salicylate, salol; the salicylic ester of phenol; the phenylic ester of salicylic acid; an intestinal analgesic and antipyretic; it has been used in the treatment of rheumatism, diarrhea, and pharyngitis, as an enteric coating for tablets, and in ointments for sunburn prevention.

phenylacetic acid (fen'il-ă-sē'tik). $C_6H_5CH_2COOH$; an abnormal product of phenylalanine catabolism, appearing in the urine in phenylketonuria.

phenylaceturic acid (fen'il-as-ĕ-tūr'ik). Phenaceturic acid.

phenylacetylurea (fen-il-as'ĕ-til-yū-rē'ă). Phenacemide.

phenylacrylic acid (fen'il-ă-kril'ik). Cinnamic acid.

phenylalaninase (fen-il-al'ă-nin-ās). Phenylalanine 4- monooxygenase.

phenylalanine (Phe) (fen-il-al'ă-nēn). 2-Amino-3-phenylpropionic acid; $C_6H_5CH_2CH(NH_2)COOH$; one of the common amino acids in proteins.

phenylalanine 4-hydroxylase. Phenylalanine 4-mono- oxygenase.

phenylalanine 4-monooxygenase [EC 1.14.16.1]. Phenylalaninase; phenylalanine 4-hydroxylase; an enzyme that catalyzes the oxidation of phenylalanine to tyrosine with O_2 and tetrahydropteridine (the latter forming the dihydro derivative) which is reduced by NADPH and a reductase to the active form.

phenylamine (fe-nil'ă-mēn). Aniline.

phenylbenzene (fen-il-ben'zēn). Biphenyl.

phenylbutazone (fen-il-byū'tă-zōn). 1,2-Diphenyl-4-butyl-3,5-pyrazolidinedione; a pyrazolone derivative; an analgesic, antipyretic, anti-inflammatory, and uricosuric agent.

phenylcarbinol (fen-il-kar'bi-nol). *Benzyl* alcohol.

phenylephrine hydrochloride (fen-il-ef′rin). (−)-*m*- Hydroxy-α-[(methylamino)methyl]benzyl alcohol hydrochloride; a sympathomimetic amine; a powerful vasoconstrictor, used as a nasal decongestant and mydriatic.

phenylethyl alcohol (fen-il-eth′il). Phenethyl alcohol; benzyl carbinol; 2-phenylethanol; $C_6H_5CH_2CH_2OH$; a natural constituent of some volatile oils (rose, geranium, neroli); used as an antibacterial agent in ophthalmic solutions.

phenylethylbarbituric acid (fen′il-eth′il-bar-bi-tyūr′ik). Phenobarbital.

phenylethylmalonylurea (fen′il-eth′il-mal′ō-nil-yū-rē′ă). Phenobarbital.

phenylglycolic acid (fen′il-glī-kol′ik). Mandelic acid.

phenylindanedione (fen′il-in-dān′dī-ōn). Phenindione.

phenylisothiocyanate (PhNCS, PITC) (fen′il-ī′sō-thī-ō-sī′ă-nāt). Edman's reagent; C_6H_5–N=C=S, a reagent that condenses with the free *N*-terminal amino group of a peptide chain to form a phenylthiohydantoin in the Edman method of identifying *N*-terminal amino acids.

phenylketonuria (PKU) (fen′il-kē′tō-nū′rē-ă) [phenyl + ketone + G. *ouron,* urine]. Folling's disease; congenital deficiency of phenylalanine 4-monooxygenase causing inadequate formation of tyrosine, elevation of serum phenylalanine, urinary excretion of phenylpyruvic acid, and accumulation of phenylalanine and its metabolites which can produce brain damage resulting in severe mental retardation, often with seizures, other neurologic abnormalities such as retarded myelination, and deficient melanin formation leading to hypopigmentation of the skin and eczema; autosomal recessive inheritance.

phenyllactic acid (fen-il-lak′tik). $C_6H_5CH_2CHOH–COOH$; a product of phenylalanine catabolism, appearing prominently in the urine in phenylketonuria.

phenylmercuric acetate (fen′il-mer-kyū′rik). Acetoxyphenylmercury; a bacteriostatic preservative, fungicide, and herbicide (especially for crabgrass).

phenylmercuric nitrate. Basic phenylmercuric nitrate; a mixture of phenylmercuric nitrate and phenylmercuric hydroxide; an antiseptic used for the prophylactic disinfection of the intact skin or of minor wounds.

phenylpiperone (fen-il-pip′er-ōn). Dipipanone.

phenylpropanolamine (fen′il-prō-pă-nol′ă-mēn). α-(1-Aminoethyl)-benzyl alcohol; a sympathomimetic amine, used as a nasal decongestant and bronchodilator.

phenylthiocarbamide (fen′il-thī-ō-kar′bă-mīd). Phenylthiourea.

phenylthiocarbamoyl (PTC) (fen′il-thī′ō-kar-bam′ō-il). See phenylthiocarbamoyl *peptide.*

phenylthiohydantoin (PTH) (fen′il-thī′ō-hī-dan′tō-in). The compound formed from an amino acid in the Edman method of protein degradation, in which phenylisothiocyanate reacts with the NH_2 of the N-terminal amino acid to form a phenylthiocarbamoyl peptide or protein, on which weak acids act to release the p. containing the N-terminal amino acid.

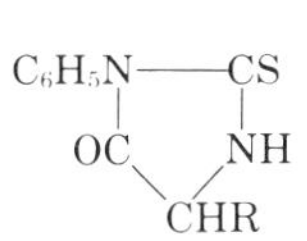

Phenylthiohydantoin

phenylthiourea (fen′il-thī′ō-yū-rē′ă). Phenylthiocarbamide; a substance that tastes bitter to some persons but is tasteless to others. The ability to taste it is inherited and dependent upon a single gene pair; "tasters" are either homozygous or heterozygous for the dominant allele. P. contains the N–C=S group upon which the taste peculiarity apparently depends, for goitrogenic or antithyroid substances (*e.g.,* thiourea and thiouracil), which also contain this group, possess the same property with respect to taste.

phenyltoloxamine (fen′il-tol-ok′să-mēn). *N,N*-dimethyl-2-(α-phenyl-*o*-tolyloxy)-ethylamine; an antihistaminic.

phenyltrimethylammonium (PTMA) (fen′il-trī-meth′il-ă-mō′nē-ŭm). A highly selective stimulant of the motor endplates of skeletal muscle.

phenyramidol hydrochloride (fen-i-ram′i-dol). α-(2-Pyridylaminomethyl)benzyl alcohol hydrochloride; an analgesic and a muscle relaxant.

phenytoin (fen′i-tō-in). 5,5-Diphenylhydantoin; an anticonvulsant used in the treatment of grand mal epilepsy. Also available as p. sodium, with the same uses as p.

pheo-. **1.** Prefix denoting the same substituents on a phorbin or phorbide (porphyrin) residue as are present in chlorophyll, excluding any ester residues and Mg. **2.** [G. *phaios,* dusky]. Combining form meaning dusky, gray, or dun.

pheochrome (fē′ō-krōm) [G. *phaios,* dusky, + *chrōma,* color]. **1.** Chromaffin. **2.** Staining darkly with chromic salts.

pheochromoblast (fē-ō-krō′mō-blast) [G. *phaios,* dusky, + *chrōma,* color, + *blastos,* germ]. A primitive chromaffin cell which, with sympathetoblasts, enters into the formation of the adrenal gland.

pheochromoblastoma (fē′ō-krō′mō-blas-tō′mă). Pheochromocytoma.

pheochromocyte (fē-ō-krō′mō-sīt) [pheochrome + G. *kytos,* cell]. Pheochrome cell (2); a chromaffin cell of a sympathetic paraganglion, medulla of an adrenal gland, or of a pheochromocytoma.

pheochromocytoma (fē′ō-krō′mō-sī-tō′mă). Pheochromoblastoma; a functional chromaffinoma, usually benign, derived from cells in the adrenal medullary tissue and characterized by the secretion of catecholamines, resulting in hypertension which may be paroxysmal and associated with attacks of palpitation, headache, nausea, dyspnea, anxiety, pallor, and profuse sweating. See also paraganglioma.

pheomelanin (fē-ō-mel′ă-nin) [G. *phaios,* dusky, + *melos (melan-),* black]. A type of melanin found in red hair.

pheomelanogenesis (fē′ō-mel′ă-nō-jen′ĕ-sis). The formation of pheomelanin by living cells.

pheomelanosome (fē-ō-mel′ă-nō-sōm). A spherical melanosome of pheomelanin in red hair.

pheophorbide (fē-ō-fōr′bīd). Phorbin with all the side-chains found in chlorophylls *a* and *b,* but lacking the phythyl group; termed p. *a* and p. *b* depending on the group (CH_3 or CHO) at C-7, respectively.

pheophorbin (fē-ō-fōr′bin). A chlorophyllide; that which remains of a chlorophyll molecule when the magnesium atom has been removed and the phytyl and methyl esters hydrolyzed to the free acids.

pheophytin (fē-ō-fī′tin). Pheophorbide with a phytyl ester on the C-17 propionic residue; chlorophyll less its magnesium atom.

pheresis (fe-rē′sis) [G. *aphairesis,* a withdrawal]. A procedure in which blood is removed from a donor, separated, and a portion retained, with the remainder returned to the donor. See also leukapheresis; plateletpheresis; plasmapheresis.

pheromones (fer′ō-mōnz) [G. *pherein,* to carry, + *horman,* to excite, stimulate]. A type of ectohormone secreted by an individual and perceived by a second individual of the same species, thereby producing a change in the sexual or social behavior of that individual.

Ph.G. **1.** Abbreviation for *Pharmacopoeia germanica;* German Pharmacopoeia. **2.** Abbreviation for Graduate in Pharmacy.

phial (fī'ăl) [G. *phialē,* a broad flat vessel]. Vial.

phialide (fī'ă-līd) [G. *phialē,* a broad, flat vessel]. In fungi, a conidiogenous cell in which the meristematic end remains unchanged as successive conidia are extruded out to form chains.

phialoconidium, pl. **phialoconidia** (fī'ă-lō-kon-id'ē-ŭm, -id'ē-ă). A conidium produced by a phialide.

Phialophora (fī-ă-lof'ō-ră) [G. *phialē,* a broad, flat vessel, + *phoreō,* to carry]. A genus of fungi of which at least two species, *P. verrucosa* and *P. dermatitidis,* cause chromoblastomycosis.

-phil, -phile, -philic, -philia [G. *philos,* fond, loving; *phileō,* to love]. Combining forms, used in the suffix position, to denote affinity for, or craving for. See also philo-.

philiater (fil'ē-ā'ter, fi-lī'ă-ter) [G. *philos,* fond, + *iatreia,* practice of medicine]. Rarely used term for one interested in the study of medicine.

Philip, Sir Robert W., Scottish physician, 1857–1939. See P.'s *glands.*

Philippe, Claudien, French pathologist, 1866–1903. See P.'s *triangle.*

Phillips, Charles, French urologist, 1809–1871. See P. *catheter.*

Phillipson's reflex. See under reflex.

philo- [G. *philos,* fond, loving; *phileō,* to love]. Combining form, used in the prefix position, to denote affinity or craving for. See also -phil.

philomimesia (fil'ō-mī-mē'sē-ă) [philo- + G. *mimēsis,* imitation]. Rarely used term for a morbid impulse to imitate or mimic.

Philopia casei (fil-ō'pē-ă kā'sē-ī). Cheese maggot; a species that may cause temporary intestinal myiasis.

philoprogenitive (fil'ō-prō-jen'i-tiv) [philo- + L. *progenies,* offspring, progeny]. **1.** Procreative, producing offspring. **2.** In psychiatry, manifesting an erotic or abnormal love for children.

philtrum, pl. **philtra** (fil'trŭm, -tră) [L., fr. G. *philtron,* a love-charm, depression on upper lip, fr. *phileo,* to love]. **1.** A philter or love potion. **2** [NA]. The infranasal depression; the groove in the midline of the upper lip.

phimosis, pl. **phimoses** (fī-mō'sis, -sēz) [G. a muzzling, fr. *phimos,* a muzzle]. Narrowness of the opening of the prepuce, preventing its being drawn back over the glans.

p. vagina'lis, narrowness of the vagina.

phimotic (fī-mot'ik). Pertaining to phimosis.

phleb-. See phlebo-.

phlebalgia (flĕ-bal'jē-ă) [phlebo- + G. *algos,* pain]. Pain originating in a vein.

phlebarteriectasia (fleb'ar-tēr-ē-ek-tā'zē-ă) [phlebo- + G. *arteria,* artery, + *ektasis,* a stretching]. Vasodilation.

phlebectasia (fleb-ek-tā'zē-ă) [phlebo- + G. *ektasis,* a stretching]. Venectasia; vasodilation of the veins.

phlebectomy (fle-bek'tō-mē) [phlebo- + G. *ektomē,* excision]. Venectomy; excision of a segment of a vein, performed sometimes for the cure of varicose veins. See also strip (2).

phlebectopia, phlebectopy (fleb-ek-tō'pēă, fle-bek'tō-pē) [phlebo- + G. *ektopos,* out of place]. Dislocation or abnormal course of a vein.

phlebemphraxis (fleb-em-frak'sis) [phlebo- + G. *emphraxis,* a stoppage]. A venous thrombosis.

phlebeurysm (fleb'yū-rizm) [phlebo- + G. *eurys,* wide]. Pathologic dilation (varix) of a vein.

phlebismus (fle-biz'mŭs) [phlebo- + G. *-ismos,* condition]. Venous congestion and phlebectasia.

phlebitic (fle-bit'ik). Relating to phlebitis.

phlebitis (fle-bī'tis) [phlebo- + G. *-itis,* inflammation]. Inflammation of a vein.

adhesive p., a form of p. in which the walls adhere, leading to obliteration of the vessel.

p. nodula'ris necroti'sans, obsolete term for p. in which tuberculous nodules are formed in the skin; the lesions spread peripherally and undergo central necrosis.

puerperal p., *phlegmasia* alba dolens.

septic p., inflammation of a vein due to bacterial infection.

sinus p., inflammation of a cerebral sinus.

phlebo-, phleb- [G. *phleps,* vein]. Combining forms denoting vein.

phleboclysis (flĕ-bok'li-sis) [phlebo- + G. *klysis,* a washing out]. Venoclysis; intravenous injection of an isotonic solution of dextrose or other substances in quantity.

drip p., intravenous injection of a liquid drop by drop, by the drip method.

phlebodynamics (fleb'ō-dī-nam'iks) [phlebo- + G. *dynamis,* force]. Laws and principles governing blood pressures and flow within the venous circulation.

phlebogram (fleb'ō-gram). [phlebo- + G. *gramma,* something written]. Venogram (2); a tracing of the jugular venous pulse.

phlebograph (fleb'ō-graf) [phlebo- + G. *graphō,* to write]. A venous sphygmograph; an instrument for making a tracing of the venous pulse.

phlebography (fle-bog'ră-fē) [phlebo- + G. *graphē,* a writing]. **1.** The recording of the venous pulse. **2.** Venography.

phleboid (fleb'oyd) [phlebo- + G. *eidos,* resemblance]. **1.** Resembling a vein. **2.** Venous. **3.** Containing many veins.

phlebolite (fleb'ō-līt). Phlebolith.

phlebolith (fleb'ō-lith) [phlebo- + G. *lithos,* stone]. Phlebolite; vein stone; a calcareous deposit in a venous wall or thrombus.

phlebolithiasis (fleb'ō-li-thī'ă-sis). The formation of phleboliths.

phlebology (flĕ-bol'ō-jē) [phlebo- + G. *logos,* study]. The branch of medical science concerned with the anatomy and diseases of the veins.

phlebomanometer (fleb'ō-mă-nom'ĕ-ter). A manometer for measuring venous blood pressure.

phlebometritis (fleb'ō-mē-trī'tis) [phlebo- + G. *metra,* uterus, + *-itis,* inflammation]. Inflammation of the uterine veins.

phlebomyomatosis (fleb'ō-mī-ō-mă-tō'sis) [phlebo- + myoma + G. *-osis,* condition]. Thickening of the walls of a vein by an overgrowth of muscular fibers arranged irregularly, intersecting each other without any definite relation to the axis of the vessel.

phlebophlebostomy (fleb'ō-fle-bos'tō-mē). Venovenostomy.

phleboplasty (fleb'ō-plas-tē) [phlebo- + G. *plastos,* formed]. Repair of a vein.

phleborrhagia (fleb-ō-rā'jē-ă) [phlebo- + G. *rhēgnymi,* to burst forth]. Venous hemorrhage.

phleborrhaphy (fle-bōr'ă-fē) [phlebo- + G. *rhaphē,* seam]. Suture of a vein.

phleborrhexis (fleb-ō-rek'sis) [phlebo- + G. *rhēxis,* rupture]. Rupture of a vein.

phlebosclerosis (fleb'ō-skle-rō'sis) [phlebo- + G. *sklērōsis,* hardening]. Venofibrosis; venosclerosis; fibrous hardening of the walls of the veins.

phlebostasis (fle-bos'tă-sis) [phlebo- + G. *stasis,* a standing still]. Venostasis. **1.** Abnormally slow motion of blood in veins, usually with venous distention. **2.** Bloodless phlebotomy; treatment of congestive heart failure by compressing proximal veins of the extremities with tourniquets.

phlebostenosis (fleb'ō-stē-nō'sis) [phlebo- + G. *stenōsis,* a narrowing]. Narrowing of the lumen of a vein from any cause.

phlebostrepsis (fleb-ō-strep'sis) [phlebo- + G. *strepsis,* a twisting].

Twisting the cut or torn end of a vein to arrest hemorrhage.

phlebothrombosis (fleb′ō-throm-bō′sis) [phlebo- + thrombosis]. Thrombosis, or clotting, in a vein without primary inflammation.

phlebotomine (flĕ-bot′ō-mēn). Relating to sand flies of the genus *Phlebotomus*.

phlebotomist (fle-bot′ō-mist). An individual trained and skilled in phlebotomy.

Phlebotomus (fle-bot′ō-mŭs) [phlebo- + G. *tomos*, cutting]. A genus of very small midges or bloodsucking sandflies of the family Psychodidae.

P. argen′tipes, the vector of kala azar in India.

P. chinen′sis, the vector of kala azar in China.

P. flaviscutel′latus, *Lutzomyia flaviscutellata*.

P. longipal′pis, *Lutzomyia longipalpis;* a vector of kala azar in South America.

P. ma′jor, a vector of kala azar in the Mediterranean region.

P. nogu′chi, the transmitter of *Bartonella* organisms, the causal agent of Oroya fever.

P. orienta′lis, a vector of kala azar in the Sudan.

P. papata′sii, transmitter of the virus of phlebotomus fever; also a vector of *Leishmania tropica* in the Mediterranean area.

P. pernicio′sus, a vector of kala azar in the Mediterranean region.

P. sergen′ti, a vector of *Leishmania tropica,* the cause of anthroponotic cutaneous leishmaniasis.

P. verruca′rum, a form found in Peru which transmits *Bartonella* organisms, the causal agent of Oroya fever.

phlebotomy (fle-bot′ō-mē) [phlebo- + G. *tomē*, incision]. Venesection; venotomy; incision into a vein for the purpose of drawing blood.

bloodless p., phlebostasis (2).

Phlebovirus (fleb′ō-vī-rŭs). A genus of virus (family Bunyaviridae) that contains at least 30 viruses which constitute a single serological group; transmitted by arthropods primarily of the genus *Phlebotomus*.

phlegm (flem) [G. *phlegma*, inflammation]. **1.** Abnormal amounts of mucus, especially as expectorated from the mouth. **2.** One of the four humors of the body, according to the humoral *doctrine*.

phlegmasia (fleg-mā′zē-ă) [G. fr. *phlegma*, inflammation]. Obsolete term for inflammation, especially when acute and severe.

p. al′ba do′lens, milk or white leg; leukophlegmasia dolens; puerperal phlebitis; thrombotic p.; an extreme edematous swelling of the leg following childbirth, due to thrombosis of the veins that drain the part.

cellulitic p., p. dolens; inflammatory swelling of the leg, following childbirth, due to septic inflammation of the connective tissue.

p. ceru′lea do′lens, thrombosis of the veins of a limb, with sudden severe pain with swelling, cyanosis, and edema of the part, followed by circulatory collapse and shock.

p. do′lens, cellulitic p.

p. malabar′ica, elephantiasis.

thrombotic p., p. alba dolens.

phlegmatic (fleg-mat′ik) [G. *phlegmatikos*, relating to phlegm]. Relating to the heavy one of the four humors (see phlegm), and therefore calm, apathetic, unexcitable.

phlegmon (fleg′mon) [G. *phlegmonē*, inflammation]. Obsolete term for an acute suppurative inflammation of the subcutaneous connective tissue.

diffuse p., a diffuse inflammation of the subcutaneous tissues accompanied by constitutional symptoms of sepsis.

emphysematous p., gas *gangrene*.

gas p., gas *gangrene*.

phlegmonous (fleg′mon-ŭs). Denoting phlegmon.

phlogiston (flō-jis′ton) [G. *phlogistos*, inflammable]. A hypothetical substance of negative mass that, according to the theory of Stahl was given off by a substance when it underwent combustion, thus accounting for the decrease in mass of the ash over the original substance; abandoned after the discoveries of Priestley and Lavoisier concerning oxygen.

phlogocyte (flō′gō-sīt) [G. *phlogōsis*, inflammation, + *kytos*, a hollow (cell)]. Obsolete term for one of a number of cells present in the tissues during the course of an inflammation.

phlogocytosis (flō′gō-sī-tō′sis). Obsolete term for a blood state in which there are many phlogocytes in the peripheral circulation.

phlogogenic, phlogogenous (flō-gō-jen′ik, flō-goj′ĕ-nŭs) [G. *phlox* (*phlog-*), flame, + *-gen*, producing]. Obsolete term for exciting inflammation.

phlogosin (flō′gō-sin) [G. *phlogōsis*, inflammation]. A substance, isolated from cultures of pus-producing cocci, injections of sterilized solutions of which will excite suppuration.

phlogotherapy (flō′gō-thār′ă-pē) [G. *phlogōsis*, inflammation, + therapy]. Nonspecific *therapy*.

phloroglucin, phloroglucinol, phloroglucol (flōr-ō-glū′sin, -glū′sin-ol, -glū′kol). 1,3,5- Trihydroxybenzene; an isomer of pyrogallol, obtained from resorcinol by fusion with caustic soda; used as a reagent with vanillin.

phloxine (flok-sēn, -sin) [C.I. 45405]. Dichloro- or tetrachlorotetrabromofluorescein; a red acid dye used as a cytoplasmic stain in histology.

phlyctena, pl. **phlyctenae** (flik-tē′nă, -nē) [G. *phlyktaina*, a blister made by a burn]. A small vesicle, especially one of a number of small blisters following a first degree burn.

phlyctenar (flik′tē-năr). Phlyctenous; relating to or marked by the presence of phlyctenae.

phlyctenoid (flik′tĕ-noyd) [G. *phlyktaina*, blister, + *eidos*, resemblance]. Resembling a phlyctena.

phlyctenosis (flik-tĕ-nō′sis). The occurrence of phlyctenae; a disease marked by a phlyctenar eruption.

phlyctenous (flik′tĕ-nŭs). Phlyctenar.

phlyctenula, pl. **phlyctenulae** (flik-ten′yū-lă) [Mod. L. dim. of G. *phlyktaina*, blister]. Phlyctenule; a small red nodule of lymphoid cells, with ulcerated apex, occurring in the conjunctiva.

phlyctenular (flik-ten′yū-lăr). Relating to a phlyctenula.

phlyctenule (flik′ten-yūl). Phlyctenula.

phlyctenulosis (flik-ten′yū-lō′sis). A nodular hypersensitive affection of corneal and conjunctival epithelium due to endogenous toxin.

PhNCS Symbol for phenylisothiocyanate.

phobanthropy (fō-ban′thrō-pē) [G. *phobos*, fear, + *anthrōpos*, man]. Anthropophobia.

PHOBIA

phobia (fō′bē-ă) [G. *phobos*, fear]. Any objectively unfounded morbid dread or fear. The word is used as a combining form in many terms expressing the object that inspires the fear.

school p., a young child's sudden aversion to or fear of attending school, usually considered a manifestation of separation anxiety.

alcoholism, alcoholophobia.

animals, zoophobia.

bees, apiphobia, melissophobia.

being beaten, rhabdophobia.

being buried alive, taphophobia.

being dirty, automysophobia.

being locked in, clithrophobia.
being stared at, scopophobia.
birth of malformed fetus, teratophobia.
blood or **bleeding,** hemophobia.
blushing, ereuthophobia.
cancer, cancerophobia, carcinophobia.
cats, ailurophobia.
childbirth, tocophobia.
children, pediophobia.
choking, pnigophobia.
climbing, climacophobia.
cold, psychrophobia.
colors, chromatophobia, chromophobia.
confinement, claustrophobia.
corpses, necrophobia.
crossing a bridge, gephyrophobia.
crowds, ochlophobia.
dampness, hygrophobia.
darkness, nyctophobia, scotophobia.
dawn, eosophobia.
daylight, phengophobia.
death, thanatophobia.
deep places, bathophobia.
deserted places, eremophobia.
dirt, mysophobia, rhypophobia.
disease, nosophobia, pathophobia.
disorder, ataxiophobia.
dogs, cynophobia.
dolls, pediophobia.
drafts, aerophobia, anemophobia.
drugs, pharmacophobia.
eating, phagophobia.
electricity, electrophobia.
enclosed space, claustrophobia.
error, harmatophobia.
everything, panphobia.
excrement, coprophobia.
fatigue, ponophobia, kopophobia.
fever, pyrexiophobia.
filth, rhypophobia.
fire, pyrophobia.
fish, ichthyophobia.
food, cibophobia.
forests, hylephobia.
fur, doraphobia.
germs, microphobia.
ghosts, phasmophobia.
girls, parthenophobia.
glare of light, photaugiaphobia.
glass, crystallophobia, hyalophobia.
God, theophobia.
hair, trichophobia, trichopathophobia.
heart disease, cardiophobia.
heat, thermophobia.
heights, acrophobia.
home, returning to, nostophobia.
human companionship, anthropophobia, phobanthropy.
ideas, ideophobia.
infection, molysmophobia.
insects, entomophobia.
itching, acarophobia.
jealousy, zelophobia.
lice, pediculophobia, phthiriophobia.
light, photophobia.
lightning, astrapophobia, keraunophobia.
machinery, mechanophobia.
malignancy, cancerophobia, carcinophobia.
many things, polyphobia.
marriage, gamophobia.
men (males), androphobia.
metal objects, metallophobia.
microorganisms, microphobia.
minute objects, microphobia.
mirrors, spectrophobia.
missiles, ballistophobia.
moisture, hygrophobia.
movements, kinesophobia.
nakedness, gymnophobia.
names, nomatophobia, onomatophobia.
neglect or **omission of duty,** paralipophobia.
night, nyctophobia.
novelty, neophobia.
odors, olfactophobia, osmophobia, osphresiophobia, bromidosiphobia.
open spaces, agoraphobia.
pain, algophobia.
parasites, parasitophobia.
phobias, phobophobia.
places, topophobia.
pleasure, hedonophobia.
pointed objects, aichmophobia.
poisoning, toxicophobia, iophobia.
poverty, peniaphobia.
precipices, cremnophobia.
pregnancy, maieusiophobia.
radiation, radiophobia.
rain, ombrophobia.
rectal disease, proctophobia, rectophobia.
religious or **sacred objects,** hierophobia.
responsibility, hypengyophobia.
rivers, potamophobia.
robbers, harpaxophobia.
sea, thalassophobia.
self, autophobia.
semen, loss of, spermatophobia.
sexual intercourse, coitophobia, cypridophobia.
sexual love, erotophobia.
sharp objects, belonephobia.
sin, hamartophobia.
sinning, pecattiphobia.
skin diseases, dermatophobia.
skin of animals, doraphobia.
sleep, hypnophobia.
snakes, ophidiophobia.
solitude, eremophobia, autophobia, monophobia.
sounds, acousticophobia, phonophobia.
speaking, laliophobia.
spiders, arachnephobia.
stairs, climacophobia.
stealing, kleptophobia.
strangers, xenophobia.
stuttering, laliophobia.
sun, heliophobia.
teeth, odontophobia.
thirteen, triskaidekaphobia.
thunder, keraunophobia, tonitrophobia, brontophobia.
time, chronophobia.
touching or **being touched,** aphephobia, haphephobia.
traveling, hodophobia.
trembling, tremophobia.
uncleanliness, automysophobia.
vaccination, vaccinophobia.
vehicles, amaxophobia, hamaxophobia.
venereal disease, cypridophobia, venereophobia.

voices, phonophobia.
walking, basiphobia.
water, aquaphobia.
wind, anemophobia.
women (females), gynephobia.
work, ergasiophobia.
worms, helminthophobia.
writing, graphophobia.

---

phobic (fō'bik). Pertaining to or characterized by phobia.

phobophobia (fō-bō-fō'bē-ă) [G. *phobos,* fear]. Morbid dread of developing some phobia.

phocomelia, phocomely (fō-kō-mē'lē-ă, fō-kom'ĕ-lē) [G. *phōkē,* a seal, + *melos,* extremity]. Defective development of arms or legs, or both, so that the hands and feet are attached close to the body, resembling the flippers of a seal.

pholcodine (fol'kō-dēn). 3-(2-Morpholinoethyl)morphine; a narcotic with little or no analgesic or europhorigenic activity, used mainly as an antitussive.

pholedrine (fōl'ĕ-drēn). *p*-[2-(Methylamino)propyl]phenol; a sympathomimetic agent for the treatment of shock; also an adrenergic and vasopressor.

Phoma (fō'mă). A genus of rapidly growing fungi that are common laboratory contaminants and common plant pathogens.

phon-. See phono-.

phonacoscope (fō-nak'ō-skōp) [phon- + G. *akouō,* to listen, + *skopeō,* to view]. An instrument for increasing the intensity of the percussion note or of the voice sounds, the examiner's ear or the stethoscope being placed on the opposite side of the chest.

phonacoscopy (fō-nă-kos'kŏ-pē). Examination of the chest by means of the phonacoscope.

phonal (fō'năl). [G. *phōnē,* voice]. Relating to sound or to the voice.

phonasthenia (fō-nas-thē'nē-ă) [phon- + G. *astheneia,* weakness]. Functional vocal fatigue; difficult or abnormal voice production, the enunciation being too high, too loud, or too hard.

phonation (fō-nā'shŭn) [G. *phōnē,* voice]. The utterance of sounds by means of vocal cords.

phonatory (fō'nă-tōr-ē). Relating to phonation.

phonautograph (fōn-aw'tō-graf) [phon- + G. *autos,* self, + *graphō,* to record]. An instrument for registering the vibrations of the voice or any other sound.

phoneme (fō'nēm) [G. *phōnēma,* a voice]. The smallest sound unit which, in terms of the phonetic sequences of sound, controls meaning.

phonemic (fō-nē'mik). Pertaining to or having the characteristics of a phoneme.

phonendoscope (fō-nen'dō-skōp) [phon- + G. *endon,* within, + *skopeō,* to view]. A stethoscope which intensifies the auscultatory sounds by means of two parallel resonating plates, one resting on the patient's chest or attached to a stethoscope tube, the other vibrating in unison with it.

phonetic (fō-net'ik) [G. *phōnētikos*]. Relating to speech or to the voice. See also phonic.

phonetics (fō-net'iks). Phonology; the science of speech and of pronunciation.

phoniatrics (fō-nē-at'riks) [phon- + G. *iatrikos,* of the healing art]. The study of speech habits; the science of speech.

phonic (fon'ik, fō'nik). Relating to sound or to the voice. See also phonetic.

phonism (fō'nizm). Auditory *synesthesia.*

phono-, phon- [G. *phōnē,* sound, voice]. Combining forms denoting sound, speech, or voice sounds.

phonoangiography (fō'nō-an-jē-og'ră-fē) [phono- + G. *angeion,* vessel, + *graphō,* to write]. Recording and analysis of the audible frequency-intensity components of the bruit of turbulent arterial blood flow through an atherosclerotic stenotic lesion.

phonocardiogram (fō-nō-kar'dē-ō-gram). A record of the heart sounds made by means of a phonocardiograph.

phonocardiograph (fō-nō-kar'dē-ō-graf). An instrument, utilizing a microphone, amplifier, and filter, for graphically recording the heart sounds, which are displayed on an oscilloscope or tracing.
linear p., a p. that records all chest wall vibrations resulting from cardiac activity with emphasis on low frequency vibrations.
logarithmic p., a p. that records only audible vibrations with emphasis on the higher frequencies.
spectral p., an instrument for recording the heart sounds in which the electrical changes created by the latter pass from a microphone through a series of filters, each of which is tuned to a particular frequency band; output from each filter is led to and activates a separate light which shines according to the intensity of the sound transmitted through the corresponding filter; the lights are arranged vertically in descending order of frequencies. A record is obtained by photographing the vertical row of lights.
stethoscopic p., a p. that records all sound vibrations, audible and inaudible, conveyed by the stethoscope; however, very slow vibrations are filtered out.

phonocardiography (fō'nō-kar-dē-og'ră-fē) [phono- + G. *kardia,* heart, + *graphō,* to record]. **1.** Recording of the heart sounds with a phonocardiograph. **2.** The science of interpreting phonocardiograms.

phonocatheter (fō-nō-kath'ĕ-ter). A cardiac catheter with diminutive microphone housed in its tip, for recording sounds and murmurs from within the heart and great vessels.

phonogram (fō'nō-gram) [phono- + G. *gramma,* diagram]. A graphic curve depicting the duration and intensity of a sound.

phonology (fō-nol'ō-jē) [phono- + G. *logos,* study]. Phonetics.

phonomania (fō-nō-mā'nē-ă) [G. *phonos,* murder, + *mania,* frenzy]. A homicidal mania.

phonometer (fō-nom'ĕ-ter) [phono- + G. *metron,* measure]. An instrument for measuring the pitch and intensity of sounds.

phonomyoclonus (fō'nō-mī-ok'lō-nŭs) [phono- + G. *mys,* muscle, + *klonos,* tumult]. A condition in which fibrillary muscular contractions are present, as evidenced by the sound heard on auscultation, even though not visible.

phonomyography (fō'nō-mī-og'ră-fē) [phono- + G. *mys,* muscle, + *graphē,* drawing]. The recording of the varying sounds made by contracting muscular tissue.

phonopathy (fō-nop'ă-thē) [phono- + G. *pathos,* suffering]. Any disease of the vocal organs affecting speech.

phonophobia (fō-nō-fō'bē-ă) [phono- + G. *phobos,* fear]. Morbid fear of one's own voice, or of any sound.

phonophore (fō'nō-fōr) [phono- + G. *phoros,* carrying]. A form of binaural stethoscope with a bell-shaped chest piece into which project the recurved extremities of the sound tubes.

phonophotography (fō'nō-fō-tog'ră-fē) [phono- + photography]. The recording on a moving photographic plate of the movements imparted to a diaphragm by sound waves.

phonopsia (fō-nop'sē-ă) [phono- + G. *opsis,* vision]. A condition in which the hearing of certain sounds gives rise to a subjective sensation of color.

phonoreceptor (fō'nō-rē-sep'ter). A receptor for sound stimuli.

phonorenogram (fō-nō-rē'nō-gram). A sound tracing of the renal arterial pulse recorded by means of a phonocatheter placed in the renal pelvis.

phonoscope (fō'nō-skōp) [phono- + G. *skopeō,* to view]. An instrument for recording ausculatory percussion; originally used for photographic recording of heart sounds.

phonoscopy (fō-nos'kō-pē). The recording made by a phonoscope.

phor-. See phoro-.

phorbide (fōr'bīd). Phorbin with the various side chains that are characteristic of the chlorophylls but lacking the phytyl ester; chlorin is the fundamental ring system of the p.'s.

phorbin (fōr'bin). The parent hydrocarbon of chlorophyll; differs from porphin (porphyrin) in the presence of an isocyclic ring formed by the addition of a two-carbon group bridging the 13 and 15 positions of porphin (porphyrin) and by saturation of the 17-18 double bond (with realignment of conjugated double bonds). Addition of hydrocarbon side-chains in specific locations yields p.'s characterized by prefixes; *e.g.,* pheophorbin.

phorbol (fōr'bol). The parent alcohol of the cocarcinogens, which are 12,13 (9,9a) diesters of p. found in croton oil; the hydrocarbon skeleton is a cyclopropa-benzazulene.

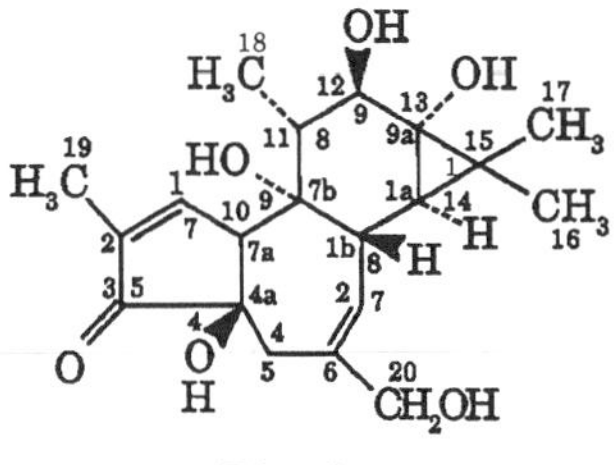

Phorbol

Outer numbers: phorbol numbering.
Inner numbers: cyclopropabenzazulene numbering.

phoresis (fōr'ĕ-sis, fō-rē'sis) [G. *phorēsis,* a being borne]. **1.** Electrophoresis. **2.** Epizoic commensalism; phoresy; a biological association in which one organism is transported by another, as in the attachment of the eggs of *Dermatobia hominis,* a human and cattle botfly, to the legs of a mosquito, which transports them to the human, cattle, or other host in which the botfly larvae can develop.

phoresy (for'ĕ-sē). Phoresis (2).

phoria (fōr'ē-ă) [G. *phora,* a carrying, motion]. The relative directions assumed by the eyes during binocular fixation of a given object in the absence of an adequate fusion stimulus. See anisophoria; cyclophoria; esophoria; exophoria; heterophoria; hyperphoria; hypophoria; orthophoria.

Phormia regina (fōr'mē-ă re-jī'nă). The black blowfly, the larvae of which were formerly used in the treatment of septic wounds because they secrete a proteolytic enzyme that aids in the removal of dead tissue; it is a frequent cause of maggot infestation of sheep, depositing eggs in the wool, and is a widely distributed cold weather species that lays its eggs on dead or decaying tissues.

phoro-, phor- [G. *phoros,* carrying, bearing]. Combining forms denoting carrying or bearing, a carrier or bearer, or phoria.

phorometer (fō-rom'ĕ-ter) [phoro- + G. *metron,* measure]. Originally, an apparatus to test oculomotor balance; now usually used as a synonym for phoro-optometer.

phoro-optometer (fō'rō-op-tom'ĕ-ter). An instrument for determining the oculomotor balance and refractive states of the eyes.

phoropter (fō-rop'ter). A device containing different lenses that is used for refraction of the eye.

phoroscope (fōr'ō-skōp) [phoro- + G. *skopeō,* to view]. An instrument for reproducing an image, as a photograph, from a distance.

phorozoon (fōr-ō-zō'on) [phoro- + G. *zōon,* animal]. The nonsexual stage in the life history of an animal that passes through several phases in its life cycle.

phos- [G. *phōs,* light]. Combined form denoting light.

phosgene (fos'jēn). Carbonyl chloride; $COCl_2$; a colorless liquid below 8°C, but an extremely poisonous gas at ordinary temperatures.

phosph-, phospho-, phosphor-, phosphoro- [G. *phōs,* light; *phoros,* carrying]. Prefixes indicating the presence of phosphorus in a compound. See phospho- for specific usage of that prefix.

phosphagen (fos'fă-jen). Phosphocreatine.

phosphagenic (fos-fă-jen'ik). Phosphate-producing.

phosphamic acid (fos-fam'ik). $R–NH–PO_3H_2$, one of the three types of high energy phosphates (the others being phosphophosphoric acids and phosphosulfuric acids).

phosphamidase (fos-fam'i-dās). Phosphoamidase.

phosphastat (fos'fă-stat) [phosphate + L. *status,* a standing]. A conceptual mechanism whereby the parathyroid hormone is increased when the levels of phosphorus rise to an above-normal level; there is as yet no satisfactory evidence for its existence.

phosphatase (fos'fă-tās). Any of a group of enzymes (EC sub-subclass 3.1.3) that liberate inorganic phosphate from phosphoric esters. See also phosphohydrolases.

acid p. [EC 3.1.3.2], a p. with an optimum pH of 5.4, notably present in the prostate gland; demonstrable in lysosomes with Gomori's nonspecific acid p. stain.

alkaline p. [EC 3.1.3.1], a p. with an optimum pH of 8.6, present ubiquitously; localized cytochemically in membranes by modifications of Gomori's nonspecific alkaline p. stain.

phosphate (fos'fāt). A salt or ester of phosphoric acid. For individual p.'s not listed here, see under the name of the base.

bone p., tribasic *calcium* phosphate.

cyclic p., Adenosine 3',5'-cyclic phosphate.

dihydrogen p., one-third-neutralized phosphoric acid; *e.g.,* NaH_2PO_4, KH_2PO_4.

disodium p., Na_2HPO_4.

energy-rich p.'s, high energy p.'s.

high energy p.'s, energy-rich p.'s; those p.'s that, on hydrolysis, yield an unusually large amount of energy; *e.g.,* nucleotide polyphosphates such as ATP, enol p.'s such as phospho*enol* pyruvate. See also high energy *compounds.*

monopotassium p., KH_2PO_4; a dihydrogen p. used as a reagent; commonly used in buffers.

monosodium p., NaH_2PO_4; a dihydrogen p. used as a reagent; commonly used in buffers.

normal p., a salt of phosphoric acid in which all the hydrogen atoms are displaced; *e.g.,* Na_3PO_4, $Na_4P_2O_7$.

organic p., an ester of phosphoric acid; *e.g.,* glycerol p., adenosine p., hexose p.

triple p., **(1)** magnesium ammonium p., $MgNH_4PO_4$; **(2)** a crude phosphate fertilizer product from phosphate rock and phosphoric acid.

phosphate acetyltransferase [EC 2.3.1.8]. Phosphotransacetylase; phosphoacylase; an enzyme catalyzing transfer of acetyl from acetyl-CoA to inorganic phosphate, forming acetyl phosphate.

phosphated (fos'fāt-ed). Containing phosphates.

phosphatemia (fos-fă-tē'mē-ă) [phosphate + G. *haima,* blood]. An abnormally high concentration of inorganic phosphates in the blood.

phosphatic (fos-fat'ik). Relating to or containing phosphates.

phosphatidal (fos-fă-tī'dăl). Older trivial name for alk-1-enylglycerophospholipid.

phosphatidase (fos-fă-tī'dās). Phospholipase A_2.

phosphatidate (fos-fă-tī'dāt). A salt or ester of a phosphatidic acid.

phosphatide (fos'fă-tīd). Former name for 1) phosphatidic acid and

2) phosphatidate.

phosphatidic acid (fos'fă-tid'ik). A derivative of glycerophosphoric acid in which the two remaining hydroxyl groups of the glycerol are esterified with fatty acids; *e.g.*, phosphatidic acids attached to choline are phosphatidylcholines (lecithins).

phosphatidolipase (fos'fă-tī-dō-lip'ās). Phospholipase A_2.

phosphatidyl (Ptd) (fos-fă-tī'dīl). The radical of a phosphatidic acid; *e.g.*, phosphatidylcholine.

phosphatidylcholine (PtdCho) (fos-fă-tī'dīl-kō'lēn). The condensation product of a phosphatidic acid and choline.

phosphatidylethanolamine (PtdEth) (fos-fă-tī'dīl-eth-ă-nol'ă-mēn). The condensation product of a phosphatidic acid and ethanolamine. See also cephalin.

phosphatidylglycerol (fos-fă-tī'dīl-glis'er-ol). A phosphatidic acid in which a second glycerol molecule replaces the usual choline, or ethanolamine or serine; a constituent in human amniotic fluid that denotes fetal lung maturity when present in the last trimester.

phosphatidylinositol (PtdIns) (fos-fă-tī'dīl-in-ō'si-tol). Phosphoinositide; a phosphatidic acid combined with inositol. Sometimes referred to as inositide.

phosphatidylserine (PtdSer) (fos-fă-tī'dīl-ser'ēn). The condensation product of phosphatidic acid and serine. See also cephalin.

phosphaturia (fos-fă-tū'rē-ă) [phosphate + G. *ouron*, urine]. Phosphoruria; phosphuria; excessive excretion of phosphates in the urine.

phosphene (fos'fēn) [G. *phōs*, light, + *phainō*, to show]. Sensation of light produced by mechanical or electrical stimulation of the peripheral or central optic pathway of the nervous system.

accommodation p., a p. occurring during accommodation, caused by sudden relaxation of the ciliary muscle.

phosphide (fos'fīd). A compound of phosphorus with valence −3; *e.g.*, sodium phosphide, Na_3P.

phosphine (fos'fēn, -fin). Hydrogen phosphide; phosphureted hydrogen; PH_3; a colorless poisonous war gas with a characteristic garlic-like odor; also the active agent in some rodenticides.

phosphinico-. Prefix indicating symmetrically doubly substituted phosphinic acid, $R_2P(O)OH$.

phosphite (fos'fīt). A salt of phosphorous acid.

phospho-. Prefix for *O*-phosphono-, which may replace the suffix phosphate; *e.g.*, glucose phosphate is *O*- phosphonoglucose or phosphoglucose. See also phosph-; phosphoryl-.

phosphoacylase (fos-fō-as'i-lās). Phosphate acetyltransferase.

phosphoamidase (fos-fō-am'i-dās) [EC 3.9.1.1]. Phosphamidase; an enzyme catalyzing the hydrolysis of phosphorus-nitrogen bonds, notably the hydrolysis of phosphocreatine to creatine and phosphoric acid.

phosphoamides (fos-fō-am'īdz). Amides of phosphoric acid (phosphoramidic acids) and their salts or esters (phosphoramidates), of the general formula $(HO)_2P(O){-}NH_2$; *e.g.*, creatine phosphate.

phosphoarginine (fos-fō-ar'gi-nēn). Arginine phosphate; a compound of arginine with phosphoric acid containing the phosphoamide bond; a source of energy in the contraction of muscle in invertebrates, corresponding to phosphocreatine in the muscles of vertebrates.

phosphocholine (fos-fō-kō'lēn). Phosphorylcholine; choline *O*-phosphate; $(CH_3)_3N^+{-}CH_2CH_2{-}OPO_3H^-$; important in choline metabolism, *e.g.*, as in cytidinediphosphocholine.

phosphocreatine (fos-fō-krē'ă-tēn). Creatine phosphate; phosphagen; a compound of creatine (through its NH_2 group) with phosphoric acid; a source of energy in the contraction of vertebrate muscle, its breakdown furnishing phosphate for the resynthesis of ATP from ADP by creatine kinase. *Cf.* phosphoarginine.

phosphodiester (fos'fō-dī-es'ter). A diesterified orthophosphoric acid, $RO{-}(PO_2H){-}OR'$, as in the nucleic acids.

p. hydrolases, phosphodiesterases.

phosphodiesterases (fos'fō-dī-es'ter-ās-ez). Phosphodiester hydrolases; enzymes (EC sub-subclass 3.1.4) cleaving phosphodiester bonds, such as those between nucleotides in nucleic acids, liberating smaller poly- or oligonucleotide units or mononucleotides but not inorganic phosphate.

spleen p., micrococcal *endonuclease.*

phosphodismutase (fos-fō-dis'myū-tās). Phosphomutase.

phosphoenolpyruvic acid (fos'fō-ē'nol-pī-rū'vik). $CH_2{=}C(OPO_3H_2){-}COOH$; the phosphoric ester of pyruvic acid in the latter's enol form; an intermediate in the conversion of glucose to pyruvic acid and an example of a high energy phosphate ester.

1-phosphofructaldolase (fos'-fō-frŭk-tal'dō-lās). Fructose-bisphosphate aldolase.

1-phosphofructokinase (fos'fō-frŭk-tō-kī'nās) [EC 2.7.1.56]. Fructose-1-phosphate kinase; an enzyme catalyzing phosphorylation of fructose 1-phosphate by ATP, etc., to fructose 1,6-bisphosphate.

6-phosphofructokinase [EC 2.7.1.11]. Phosphohexokinase; phosphofructokinase I; an enzyme that catalyzes the phosphorylation of fructose 6-phosphate by ATP or UTP, etc., to fructose 1,6-bisphosphate.

phosphogalactoisomerase (fos'fō-gă-lak'tō-ī-som'er-ās). UDP-glucose–hexose-l-phosphate uridylyltransferase.

phosphoglucokinase (fos'fō-glū-kō-kī'nās) [EC 2.7.1.10]. Glucose 1-phosphate kinase; an enzyme that, in the presence of ATP, catalyzes the phosphorylation of glucose 1-phosphate to glucose 1,6-bisphosphate; found in yeast and muscle.

phosphoglucomutase (fos'fō-glū-kō-myū'tās) [EC 5.4.2.2]. Glucose phosphomutase; an enzyme that catalyzes the reaction, glucose 1-phosphate→glucose 6-phosphate, with glucose 1,6-bisphosphate present.

phosphogluconate dehydrogenase (fos-fō-glū'kō-nāt) [EC 1.1.1.43]. 6-Phosphogluconic dehydrogenase; an enzyme catalyzing dehydrogenation (to NADP) of 6-phosphogluconate to 6-phospho-2-ketogluconate.

6-phosphogluconolactonase (fos'fō-glū'kō-nō-lak'tō-nās) [EC 3.1.1.31]. A hydrolase that catalyzes conversion of 6-phosphogluconolactone to 6-phosphogluconate.

phosphoglyceracetals (fos'fō-glis-er-as'ĕ-tālz). Plasmalogens.

phosphoglycerate kinase (fos-fō-glis'er-āt) [EC 2.7.2.3]. An enzyme catalyzing the formation of 3-phosphoglyceroyl phosphate from 3-phosphoglyceric acid and ATP.

phosphoglyceric acid (fos'fō-gli-ser'ik, -glis'er-ik). Glyceroyl phosphoric acid; glyceroyl phosphate; $CH_2OH{-}CHOH{-}CO{-}OPO_3H_2$; an acid anhydride between glyceric acid and phosphoric acid.

phosphoglycerides (fos-fō-glis'er-īdz). Acylglycerol and diacylglycerol phosphates; constituents of nerve tissue, and involved in fat transport and storage.

phosphoglyceromutase (fos'fō-glis'er-ō-myū'tās) [EC 5.4.2.1]. An isomerizing enzyme catalyzing the interconversion of 2-phosphoglyceric acid and 3-phosphoglyceric acid with 2,3-diphosphoglyceric acid present.

phosphohexokinase (fos'fō-hek-sō-kī'nās). 6-Phosphofructokinase.

phosphohexomutase (fos'fō-hek-sō-myū'tās). Glucosephosphate isomerase.

phosphohexose isomerase (fos-fō-hek'sōs). Glucosephosphate isomerase.

phosphohydrolases (fos-fō-hī'drō-lās-ez). Phosphoric monoester hydrolases; enzymes (EC sub-subclass 3.1.3) cleaving phosphoric acid (as orthophosphate) from its esters; trivial names usually end in phosphate.

phosphoinositide (fos'fō-in-ō'si-tīd). Phosphatidylinositol.

phosphokinase (fos-fō-kī'nās). A phosphotransferase or a kinase.

phospholipase (fos-fō-lip'ās). Lecithinase; an enzyme that catalyzes the hydrolysis of a phospholipid.

p. A_1 [EC 3.1.1.32], an enzyme converting a lecithin (1,2-diacylglycerophosphocholine) to a 2-acylglycerophosphocholine by splitting off the 1-acyl residue.

p. A_2 [EC 3.1.1.4], lecithinase A; phosphatidase; phosphatidolipase; an enzyme catalyzing conversion of a lecithin to a lysolecithin by removing the 2-acyl group; also acts on phosphatidylethanolamine, choline plasmalogen and phosphatidates by removing a fatty acid from the 2-position.

p. B, lysophospholipase.

p. C [EC 3.1.4.3], lipophosphodiesterase I; lecithinase C; *Clostridium welchii* α-toxin; *Clostridium oedematiens* β- and γ-toxins; an enzyme removing choline phosphate from a phosphatidylcholine; also acts on sphingomyelin.

p. D [EC 3.1.4.4], lipophosphodiesterase II; lecithinase D; choline phosphatase; an enzyme removing choline from a phosphatidylcholine; also acts on other phosphatidates.

phospholipid (fos-fō-lip'id). A lipid containing phosphorus, thus including the lecithins and other phosphatidic acids, sphingomyelin, and plasmalogens.

phosphomutase (fos-fō-myū'tās). Phosphodismutase; one of a number of enzymes (mutases) (EC sub-subclass 5.4.2) that apparently catalyze intramolecular transfer because the donor is regenerated (*e.g.,* phosphoglyceromutase, phosphoglucomutase).

phosphonecrosis (fos-fō-ne-krō'sis) [phosphorus + G. *nekrōsis,* death (necrosis)]. Necrosis of the osseous tissue of the jaw, as a result of poisoning by inhalation of phosphorus fumes, occurring especially in persons who work with the element.

phosphonium (fos-fō'nē-ŭm). The radical, $(PR_4)^+$.

***O*-phosphono-.** Prefix indicating a phosphonic acid radical ($-PO_3H_2$) attached through an oxygen atom, hence a phosphoric ester. See also phospho-.

phosphopentose isomerase (fos-fō-pen'tōs). Ribose-5-phosphate isomerase.

phosphoprotein (fos-fō-prō'tēn). A protein containing phosphoric groups attached directly to the side chains of some of its constituent amino acids, usually to the hydroxyl group of serine; *e.g.,* casein, vitellin.

phosphopyruvate hydratase (fos-fō-pī'rū-vāt). Enolase.

phosphor-, phosphoro-. See phosph-.

phosphor (fos'fōr) [G. *phōs,* light, + *phoros,* bearing]. A chemical substance that transforms incident electromagnetic or radioactive energy into light, as in scintillation radioactivity determinations.

phosphorated (fos'fōr-āt-ed). Forming a compound with phosphorus.

phosphorescence (fos-fō-res'ens) [G. *phōs,* light, + *phoros,* bearing]. The quality or property of emitting light without active combustion or the production of heat, generally as the result of prior exposure to radiation, which persists after the inciting cause is removed.

phosphorescent (fos'fō-res'ent). Having the property of phosphorescence.

phosphorhidrosis (fos'fōr-hī-drō'sis) [G. *phōs,* light, + *phoros,* bearing, + *hidrōsis,* sweating]. Phosphoridrosis; the excretion of luminous sweat.

phosphoriboisomerase (fos'fō-rī'bō-ī-som'er-ās). Ribose-5-phosphate isomerase.

phosphoribosylglycineamide synthetase (fos'fō-rī'bō-sil-gli-sin'ā-mīd) [EC 6.3.4.13]. Glycinamide ribonucleotide synthetase; an enzyme that adds glycine to ribosylamine 5-phosphate and cleaves ATP to ADP in the course of purine biosynthesis.

5-phospho-α-D-ribosyl pyrophosphate (PPRibP, PPRP, PRPP). 5-Phosphoribosyl diphosphate; ribose carrying a phosphate group on ribose carbon-5 and a pyrophosphate group on ribose carbon-1; an intermediate in the formation of the pyrimidine nucleotides.

phosphoribosyltransferase (fos'fō-rī'bō-sil-trans'fer-ās). One of a group of enzymes (EC sub-subclass 2.4.2, pentosyltransferases) that transfers ribose 5-phosphate from 5-phospho-α-D-ribosyl pyrophosphate to a purine, pyrimidine, or pyridine acceptor, forming a 5'-nucleotide and inorganic pyrophosphate, or ribose from ribosyl phosphate to a base, forming a nucleoside, or similar pentose transfers; important in nucleotide biosynthesis. Specific p.'s are preceded by the name of the acceptor base, *e.g.,* uracil phosphoribosyltransferase (EC 2.4.2.9).

phosphoribulokinase (fos'fō-rī'byū-lō-kī'nās) [EC 2.7.1.19]. An enzyme that, in the presence of ATP, catalyzes the phosphorylation of ribulose 5-phosphate to ribulose 1,5-bisphosphate, a reaction of importance in the carbon dioxide fixation cycle of photosynthesis.

phosphoribulose epimerase (fos-fō-rī'byū-lōs). Ribulose-phosphate 3-epimerase.

phosphoric acid (fos-fōr'ik). Orthophosphoric acid (*q.v.*); H_3PO_4; $PO(OH)_3$; a strong acid of industrial importance; dilute solutions have been used as urinary acidifiers and as dressings to remove necrotic debris. In dentistry, it comprises about 60% of the liquid used in zinc phosphate and silicate cements; solutions are used for conditioning enamel surfaces prior to applications of various types of resins.

cyclic p. a., **(1)** in general, a linear polymer of phosphoric acid residues in pyrophosphate linkage in which the α and ω residues are similarly linked to make one endless loop or cyclic compound; **(2)** specifically, a generic term applied to compounds in which one phosphoric acid residue is esterified to two hydroxyl groups of a single carbon chain, as in adenosine 3',5'-phosphoric acid, adenosine 2',3'-phosphoric acid, etc.

dilute p. a., a solvent containing 10% H_3PO_4.

glacial p. a., $(HPO_3)_n$; metaphosphoric acid; an anhydride of phosphoric acid used as a reagent, and in the manufacture of zinc oxyphosphate cement for dentistry.

phosphoridrosis (fos'fōr-i-drō'sis). Phosphorhidrosis.

phosphorism (fos'fōr-izm). Chronic poisoning with phosphorus.

phosphorized (fos'fōr-īzd). Containing phosphorus.

phosphorolysis (fos-fō-rol'i-sis). Phosphoroclastic cleavage; a reaction analogous to hydrolysis except that the elements of phosphoric acid, rather than of water, are added in the course of splitting a bond; *e.g.,* the conversion of glycogen to glucose 1-phosphate.

phosphorous (fos'fōr-ŭs, fos-fōr'ŭs). **1.** Relating to, containing, or resembling phosphorus. **2.** Referring to phosphorus in its lower (+3) valence state.

phosphorous acid. H_3PO_3; its salts are phosphites.

phosphoruria (fos-fō-rū'rē-ă). Phosphaturia.

phosphorus (fos'fōr-ŭs) [G. *phosphoros,* fr. *phōs,* light, + *phoros,* bearing]. A nonmetallic chemical element, symbol P, atomic no. 15, atomic weight 30.975, occurring extensively in nature always in combination as phosphates, phosphites, etc., and as the phosphate in every living cell; the elemental form is extremely poisonous, causing intense inflammation and fatty degeneration; repeated inhalation of p. fumes may cause necrosis of the jaw (phosphonecrosis).

amorphous p., red p., an allotropic form of p. formed by heating ordinary p., in the absence of oxygen, to 260°C; it occurs as an amorphous dark red mass or powder, nonpoisonous, and much less flammable than ordinary p.; it may be reconverted to the latter by heating to 454.4°C in nitrogen gas.

p. pentoxide, P_2O_5; the ultimate anhydride of orthophosphoric acid.

phosphorus-32. (^{32}P). Radioactive phosphorus isotope with atomic weight of 32; beta emitter with half-life of 14.3 days; used as tracer in metabolic studies and in the treatment of certain diseases of the osseous and hematopoietic systems.

phosphoryl-. Prefix incorrectly used to signify a phosphate (*e.g.,* phosphorylcholine) in place of the correct *O*- phosphono- or phospho-.

phosphoryl (fos'fō-ril). The radical, $PO^{\equiv}$, as in phosphoryl chloride, $POCl_3$.

phosphorylase (fos-fōr'i-lās) [EC 2.4.1.1]. An enzyme cleaving poly(1,4-α-D-glucosyl) to α-D-glucosyl phosphate with inorganic phosphate. Also known as P enzyme; p. *a;* amylophosphorylase; polyphosphorylase; glycogen p.; α-glucan p.

p. *a*, phosphorylase.

p. *b*, cleavage product of p. *a*. See p. phosphatase.

p. phosphatase [EC 3.1.3.17], phosphorylase-rupturing enzyme; PR enzyme (1); an enzyme catalyzing the conversion of one p. *a* into two p. *b* by splitting the former into halves, with release of four phosphates.

phosphorylases (fos-fōr'i-lās-ez). **1.** General term for enzymes transferring an inorganic phosphate group to some organic acceptor, hence belonging to the transferases. **2.** Specifically, enzymes that release a single glucose residue from a polyglucose as glucose 1-phosphate, the phosphate coming from inorganic orthophosphate; *e.g.,* phosphophorylase, sucrose p., cellobiose p.

nucleoside p., enzymes that catalyze the phosphorolysis of a nucleoside, forming the free purine of pyrimidine plus ribose (or deoxyribose 1-phosphate); *e.g.,* purine-nucleoside phosphorylases.

phosphorylation (fos'fōr-i-lā'shŭn). Addition of phosphate to an organic compound, such as glucose to produce glucose monophosphate, through the action of a phosphotransferase (phosphorylase) or kinase.

oxidative p., formation of high energy phosphoric bonds (*e.g.,* pyrophosphates) from the energy released by the dehydrogenation (*i.e.,* oxidation) of various substrates, most notably isocitric acid, α-ketoglutaric acid, succinic acid, and malic acid in the tricarboxylic acid cycle.

phosphorylcholine (fos'fōr-il-kō'lēn). Phosphocholine.

phosphorylethanolamine glyceridetransferase (fos'fōr-il-eth-ă-nol'ă-mēn). Ethanolaminephosphotransferase.

***O*^{3}-phosphoserine** (fos-fō-ser'ēn). $H_2O_3P—OCH_2CH(NH_2)$-COOH; the phosphoric ester of serine.

phosphosphingosides (fos-fō-sfing'gō-sīdz). Sphingomyelins.

phosphosugar (fos-fō-shug'er). A phosphorylated saccharide; any sugar containing an alcoholic group esterified with phosphoric acid.

phosphotransacetylase (fos'fō-trans-ă-set'i-lās). Phosphate acetyltransferase.

phosphotransferases (fos-fō-trans'fer-ās-ez). Transphosphatase; a subclass of transferases (EC subclass 2.7) transferring phosphorus-containing groups. P.'s include the "kinases" (2.7.1) transferring phosphate to alcohols, to carboxyl groups (2.7.2), to nitrogenous groups (2.7.3), or to another phosphate group (2.7.4). Phosphomutases (5.4.2) catalyze apparent intramolecular transfers; pyrophosphokinases (2.7.6) catalyze transfer of the pyrophosphate group; nucleotidyltransferases (2.7.7) catalyze transfer of the nucleotide (nucleotidyl) groups (including polyribonucleotide nucleotidyltransferase) and other similar groups (2.7.8).

phosphotriose isomerase (fos-fō-trī'ōs). Triosephosphate isomerase.

phosphotungstic acid (PTA) (fos-fō-tŭng'stik). A mixture of phosphoric and tungstic acids, approximately 24 WO_3, 2 H_3PO_4, 48 H_2O; a protein precipitant and reagent for arginine, lysine, histidine, and cystine; used with hematoxylin for nuclear and muscle staining; also used in electron microscopy as a stain for collagen and as a negative stain.

phosphuria (fos-fū'rē-ă). Phosphaturia.

phosvitin (fos-vī'tin). A phosphated protein constituting about 7% of the protein of egg yolk; it is about 60% serine, largely as phosphoserine, and has anticoagulant properties.

phot-. See photo-.

phot (fōt) [G. *phōs* (*phōt-*), light]. A unit of illumination; 1 p. equals 1 lumen/cm^2 of surface.

photalgia (fō-tal'jē-ă) [photo- + G. *algos,* pain]. Photodynia; pain caused by light; an extreme degree of photophobia.

photaugiaphobia (fō-taw'jē-ă-fō'bē-ă) [G. *phōtaugeia,* glare of light, + *phobos,* fear]. Morbid fear of, or overreaction to, a glare of light.

photechy (fō'tek-ē) [photo- + G. *ēchō,* echo]. The law that an irradiated body produces the same effects as the source of the radiation itself.

photerythrous (fō'tē-rith'rŭs) [photo- + G. *erythros,* red]. Deuteranopic.

photesthesia (fō-tes-thē'zē-ă) [photo- + G. *aisthēsis,* sensation]. Perception of light.

photic (fō'tik). Relating to light.

photism (fō'tizm). Pseudophotesthesia; production of a sensation of light or color by a stimulus to another sense organ, such as of hearing, taste, or touch.

photo-, phot- [G. *phōs* (*phōt-*), light]. Combining forms relating to light. In some old terms relating to x-rays, this element has been replaced by *radio-.*

photoactinic (fō'tō-ak-tin'ik) [photo- + G. *aktis,* ray]. Relating to radiation producing both luminous and chemical effects.

photoallergy (fō'tō-al'er-jē). See photosensitization.

photoautotroph (fō'tō-aw'tō-trōf) [photo- + G. *autos,* self, + *trophē,* nourishment]. An organism that depends on light for its energy and principally on carbon dioxide for its carbon.

photoautotrophic (fō-tō-aw'tō-trof'ik). Pertaining to a photoautotroph.

photobacteria (fō'tō-bak-tēr'ē-ă). Plural of photobacterium.

Photobacterium (fō'tō-bak-tēr'ē-ŭm). A genus of motile and nonmotile, aerobic to facultatively anaerobic bacteria (family Pseudomonadaceae) containing Gram-negative coccobacilli and occasional rods; under adverse conditions pleomorphic forms frequently occur. Motile cells have polar flagella. The metabolism of these organisms is fermentative. They are usually luminescent and occur symbiotically in tissues of luminous organs of cephalopods and deep-sea fishes and on the skin and in the intestines of some marine fish. The type species is *P. phosphoreum.*

P. harve'yi, *Lucibacterium harveyi.*

P. phospho'reum, a luminescent species found on dead fish and in sea water; it is the type species of the genus *P.*

photobacterium, pl. **photobacteria** (fō'tō-bak-tēr'ē-ŭm, -bak-tēr'ē-ă). A vernacular term used to refer to any member of the genus *Photobacterium.*

photobiology (fō'tō-bī-ol'ō-jē). The study of the effects of light upon plants and animals.

photobiotic (fō'tō-bī-ot'ik) [photo- + G. *bios,* life]. Living or flourishing only in the light.

photocatalyst (fō-tō-kat'ă-list) [photo- + G. *katalysis,* dissolution (catalysis)]. A substance that helps bring about a light-catalyzed reaction; *e.g.,* chlorophyll.

photoceptor (fō'tō-sep'ter, -tōr). Photoreceptor.

photochemical (fō-tō-kem'i-kăl). Denoting chemical changes caused by or involving light.

photochemistry (fō-tō-kem'is-trē). The branch of chemistry concerned with the chemical changes caused by or involving light.

photochemotherapy (fō'tō-kem-ō-ther'ă-pē, -kē-mō-). Photoradiation.

photochromogens (fō'tō-krō'mō-jenz) [photo- + G. *chrōma,* color, + *-gen,* producing]. Group I *mycobacteria.*

photocoagulation (fō'tō-kō-ag'yū-lā'shŭn) [photo- + L. *coagulo,* pp. *-atus,* to curdle]. A method by which a beam of electromagnetic energy is directed to a desired tissue under visual control; localized coagulation results from absorption of light energy and its conversion to heat or conversion of tissue to plasma (atoms stripped of electrons).

photocoagulator (fō'tō-kō-ag'yū-lā'ter, tōr). The apparatus used in photocoagulation.
laser p., a high-energy source of electromagnetic radiation. See laser.
xenon-arc p., a p. in which a xenon-arc bulb delivers radiation from the visible and near-infrared spectrum.

photodermatitis (fō'tō-der-mă-tī'tis) [photo- + G. *derma,* skin, + *-itis,* inflammation]. Dermatitis caused or elicited by exposure to ultraviolet light; may be phototoxic or photoallergic, and can result from topical application, ingestion, inhalation, or injection of mediating phototoxic or photoallergic material. See also photosensitization.

photodistribution (fō'tō-dis-tri-byū'shŭn). Areas on the skin that receive the greatest amount of exposure to sunlight, and which are involved in eruptions due to photosensitivity.

photodromy (fō-tod'rō-mē) [photo- + G. *dromos,* a running]. In the induced or spontaneous clarification of certain suspensions, the settlement of particles on the side nearest the light (**positive p.**) or on the dark side (**negative p.**).

photodynamic (fō'tō-dī-nam'ik) [photo- + G. *dynamis,* force]. Relating to the energy or force exerted by light.

photodynia (fō-tō-din'ē-ă) [photo- + G. *odynē,* pain]. Photalgia.

photodysphoria (fō'tō-dis-fōr'ē-ă) [photo- + G. *dysphoria,* extreme discomfort]. Extreme photophobia.

photoelectric (fō'tō-ē-lek'trik). Denoting electronic or electric effects produced by the action of light.

photoelectrometer (fō'tō-ē-lek-trom'ĕ-ter). A device employing a photoelectric cell for measuring the concentration of substances in solution.

photoelectron (fō'tō-ē-lek'tron). An electron freed by the action of light.

photoerythema (fō'tō-er-i-thē'mă) [photo- + G. *erythēma,* flush]. Erythema caused by exposure to light.

photoesthetic (fō'tō-es-thet'ik) [photo- + G. *aisthēsis,* sensation]. Sensitive to light.

photofluorography (fō'tō-flūr-og'ră-fē) [photo- + L. *fluor,* a flow, + G. *graphē,* a writing]. Fluorography; fluororoentgenography; recording of fluoroscopic views by conventional photography; used in mass roentgenographic examination of the lungs or the gastrointestinal tract.

photogastroscope (fō'tō-gas'trō-skōp) [photo- + G. *gastēr,* stomach, + *skopeō,* to view]. An instrument for taking photographs of the interior of the stomach.

photogen (fō'tō-jen) [photo- + G. *gen-,* producing]. A microorganism that produces luminescence.

photogenesis (fō-tō-jen'ĕ-sis) [photo- + G. *genesis,* production]. Production of light, as by bacteria, insects, or phosphorescence.

photogenic, photogenous (fō-tō-jen'ik, fō-toj'ĕ-nŭs). Denoting or capable of photogenesis.

photohemotachometer (fō'tō-hē'mō-tă-kom'ĕ-ter) [photo- + G. *haima,* blood, + *tachos,* speed, + *metron,* measure]. An appliance for recording photographically the rapidity of the blood current.

photoheterotroph (fō'tō-het'er-ō-trof, -trōf) [photo- + G. *heteros,* other, + *trophē,* nourishment]. An organism that depends on light for its energy and principally on organic compounds for its carbon.

photoheterotrophic (fō'tō-het'er-ō-trof'ik). Pertaining to a photoheterotroph.

photoinactivation (fō'tō-in-ak-ti-vā'shŭn). Inactivation by light; *e.g.,* as in the treatment of herpes simplex by local application of a photoactive dye followed by exposure to a fluorescent lamp.

photokinesis (fō'tō-ki-nē'sis) [photo- + G. *kinēsis,* movement]. Alteration of random movements of motile organisms in response to light.

photokinetic (fō'tō-ki-net'ik). **1.** Pertaining to photokinesis. **2.** Pertaining to photokinetics.

photokinetics (fō'tō-ki-net'iks) [photo- + G. *kinētikos,* relating to movement]. The changes in rate of a chemical reaction in response to light.

photokymograph (fō-tō-kī'mō-graf) [photo- + G. *kyma,* wave, + *graphō,* to record]. A device for moving film at a constant speed so that a continuous record of a physiologic event may be obtained, as by a beam of light shining on the film.

photology (fō-tol'ō-jē) [photo- + G. *logos,* study]. The science of light production and energy, especially in its therapeutic application.

photoluminescent (fō'tō-lū-mi-nes'ent) [photo- + L. *lumen,* light]. Having the ability to become luminescent upon exposure to visible light.

photolyase (fō-tō-lī'ās). See deoxyribodipyrimidine photolyase.

photolysis (fō-tol'i-sis) [photo- + G. *lysis,* dissolution]. Decomposition of a chemical compound by the action of light.

photolyte (fō'tō-līt). Any product of decomposition by light.

photolytic (fō-tō-lit'ik). Pertaining to photolysis.

photomacrography (fō'tō-mă-krog'ră-fē) [photo- + G. *makros,* large, + *graphō,* to write]. A technique for investigating and recording conditions and procedures involving small objects which ordinarily would be inspected through a loupe rather than a microscope.

photomania (fō-tō-mā'nē-ă) [photo- + G. *mania,* frenzy]. Morbid or exaggerated desire for light.

photometer (fō-tom'ĕ-ter) [photo- + G. *metron,* measure]. An instrument designed to measure the intensity of light or to determine the light threshold.
flame p., an instrument that uses flame emission spectrophotometry to measure the intensity and other properties of light.
flicker p., an instrument that compares two variable visual stimuli through control of the frequency of a flickering light.

photometry (fō-tom'ĕ-trē). The measurement of the intensity of light.

photomicrograph (fō'tō-mī'krō-graf) [photo- + G. *mikros,* small, + *graphē,* a record]. Micrograph (2); an enlarged photograph of an object viewed with a microscope, as distinguished from microphotograph.

photomicrography (fō'tō-mī-krog'ră-fē). Micrograph (3); the production of a photomicrograph.

photomyoclonus (fō'tō-mī-ok'lō-nŭs) [photo- + G. *mys,* muscle,

+ *klonos,* confused motion]. Clonic spasms of muscles in response to visual stimuli.
hereditary p., p. associated with diabetes mellitus, deafness, nephropathy, and cerebral dyfunction.

photon (fō'ton). **1.** Troland. **2.** In physics, a corpuscle of energy or particle of light; a quantum of light.

photoncia (fō-ton'sē-ă) [photo- + G. *onkos,* a mass (tumor)]. Any swelling resulting from the intense action of light.

photonosus (fō-ton'ō-sŭs) [photo- + G. *nosos,* disease]. Photopathy; any disease caused by excessive exposure to, or unusual intensity of, light, or resulting from phototoxicity or photoallergy.

photopathy (fō-top'ă-thē) [photo- + G. *pathos,* suffering]. Photonosus.

photoperceptive (fō'tō-per-sep'tiv). Capable of both receiving and perceiving light.

photoperiodism (fō'tō-pēr'ē-ō-dizm). The periodic (seasonal or diurnal) activities, behavior, or changes in plants or animals brought about by the action of light.

photophobia (fō-tō-fō'bē-ă) [photo- + G. *phobos,* fear]. **1.** Abnormal sensitivity to light, especially of the eyes. **2.** Morbid dread and avoidance of light.

photophobic (fō-tō-fō'bik). Relating to or suffering from photophobia.

photophore (fō'tō-fōr) [photo- + G. *phoros,* bearing]. **1.** A lamp with reflector used in laryngoscopy and in the examination of other internal parts of the body. **2.** In bacteriology, the organ producing intracellular bioluminescence in certain organisms.

photophosphorylation (fō-tō-fos'fōr-i-lā'shŭn). Formation of ATP as a result of absorption of light by chloroplast material.

photophthalmia (fō'tof-thal'mē-ă) [photo- + G. *ophthalmos,* eye]. Keratoconjunctivitis caused by ultraviolet energy, as in snow blindness, exposure to an ultraviolet lamp, arc welding, or the short circuit of a high-tension electric current. See also photoretinopathy.

photopia (fō-tō'pē-ă) [photo- + G. *opsis,* vision]. Photopic *vision.*

photopic (fō-top'ik). Pertaining to photopic vision.

photopsia (fō-top'sē-ă) [photo- + G. *opsis,* vision]. Photopsy; a subjective sensation of lights, sparks, or colors due to electrical or mechanical stimulation of the ocular system. See also Moore's lightning *streaks.*

photopsin (fō-top'sin). The protein moiety (opsin) of the pigment (iodopsin) in the cones of the retina.

photopsy (fō-top'sē). Photopsia.

photoptarmosis (fō'tō-tar-mō'sis) [photo- + G. *ptarmos,* a sneezing, + *-osis,* condition]. Reflex sneezing that occurs when bright light stimulates the retina.

photoptometry (fō'top-tom'ĕ-trē) [photo- + optometry]. Determination of the light threshold. See also photometry.

photoradiation (fō'tō-rā-dē-ā'shŭn). Photochemotherapy; photoradiation therapy; treatment of cancer by intravenous injection of a photosensitizing agent, such as hematoporphyrin, followed by exposure to visible light of superficial tumors or of deep tumors by a fiberoptic probe.

photoreaction (fō'tō-rē-ak'shŭn). A reaction caused or affected by light, *e.g.,* a photochemical reaction, photolysis, photosynthesis, phototropism, thymine dimer formation.

photoreactivation (fō'tō-rē-ak-ti-vā'shŭn). Activation by light of something or of some process previously inactive or inactivated.

photoreceptive (fō'tō-rē-sep'tiv). Functioning as a photoreceptor.

photoreceptor (fō'tō-rē-sep'ter, tōr) [photo- + L. *re-cipio,* pp. *-ceptus,* to receive, fr. *capio,* to take]. Photoceptor; a receptor that is sensitive to light, *e.g.,* a retinal rod or cone.

photoretinitis (fō'tō-ret'i-nī'tis). See photoretinopathy.

photoretinopathy (fō'tō-ret'i-nop'ă-thē) [photo- + retina, + G. *pathos,* suffering]. Electric or solar retinopathy; a macular burn from excessive exposure to sunlight or other intense light (*e.g.,* the flash of a short circuit); characterized subjectively by reduced visual acuity. See also eclipse *amblyopia.*

photoscan (fō'tō-skan). Scintiscan.

photosensitization (fō'tō-sen-si-ti-zā'shŭn). **1.** Sensitization of the skin to light, usually due to the action of certain drugs, plants, or other substances; may occur shortly after administration of the drug (phototoxic sensitivity), or may occur only after a latent period of from days to months (photoallergic sensitivity, or photoallergy). **2.** Photodynamic *sensitization.*

photosensor (fō'tō-sen'ser, sōr). A device designed to respond to light and to transmit resulting impulses for interpretation, movement, or operating control. See sensor.

photostable (fō'tō-stā-bl). Not subject to change upon exposure to light.

photostethoscope (fō-tō-steth'ō-skōp). Device that converts sound into flashes of light; used for continuous observation of the fetal heart.

photostress (fō'tō-stres). Exposure to intense illumination. See also p. *test.*

photosynthesis (fō-tō-sin'thĕ-sis) [photo- + G. *synthesis,* a putting together]. The compounding or building up of chemical substances under the influence of light; especially, the process by which green plants, using chlorophyll and the energy of sunlight, produce carbohydrates from water and carbon dioxide, liberating molecular oxygen in the process.

phototaxis (fō-tō-tak'sis) [photo- + G. *taxis,* orderly arrangement]. Reaction of living protoplasm to the stimulus of light, involving bodily motion of the whole organism toward (**positive p.**) or away from (**negative p.**) the stimulus. *Cf.* phototropism.

phototherapy (fō-tō-thār'ă-pē). Lucotherapy; light treatment; treatment of disease by means of light rays.

photothermal (fō-tō-ther'măl) [photo- + G. *thermē,* heat]. Relating to radiant heat.

phototonus (fō-tot'ō-nŭs) [photo- + G. *tonos,* tension]. Sensitivity to light.

phototoxic (fō-tō-tok'sik). Relating to, characterized by, or causing phototoxis.

phototoxis (fō-tō-tok'sis) [photo- + G. *toxikon,* poison]. The condition resulting from an overexposure to ultraviolet light, or from the combination of exposure to certain wavelengths of light and a phototoxic substance. See also photosensitization.

phototropism (fō-to'trō-pizm) [photo- + G. *tropē,* a turning]. Movement of a part of an organism toward (**positive p.**) or away from (**negative p.**) the stimulus of light. *Cf.* phototaxis.

photuria (fō-tū'rē-ă) [photo- + G. *ouron,* urine]. The passage of phosphorescent urine.

phragmoplast (frag'mō-plast) [G. *phragma,* hedge, enclosure, + *plassō,* to form]. Barrel-shaped enlargement of the spindle associated with formation of the new cell membrane during telophase in plant cells.

phren-. See phreno-.

phren (fren) [G. *phrēn,* the diaphragm, mind, heart (as seat of emotions)]. **1.** Diaphragma (2). **2.** The mind.

phrenalgia (fre-nal'jē-ă) [phren- + G. *algos,* pain]. **1.** Psychalgia (1). **2.** Pain in the diaphragm.

phrenectomy (fre-nek'tō-mē). Phrenicectomy.

phrenemphraxis (fren'em-frak'sis) [phren- + G. *emphraxis,* a stoppage]. Phreniclasia.

phrenetic (frĕ-net'ik) [G. *phrenitikos,* frenzied]. **1.** Frenzied; maniacal. **2.** An individual exhibiting such behavior.

phreni-, phrenico-. See phreno-.

-phrenia [G. *phrēn,* the diaphragm, mind, heart (as seat of emotions]. Suffix denoting diaphragm or mind.

phrenic (fren'ik). **1.** Relating to the diaphragm. **2.** Relating to the mind.

phrenicectomy (fren-i-sek'tō-mē) [phreni- + G. *ektomē,* excision]. Phrenectomy; phreniconeurectomy; phrenicoexeresis; exsection of a portion of the phrenic nerve, to prevent reunion such as may follow phrenicotomy.

phreniclasia (fren-i-klā'zē-ă) [phreni- + G. *klasis,* a breaking away]. Phrenemphraxis; phrenicotripsy; crushing of a section of the phrenic nerve to produce a temporary paralysis of the diaphragm.

phrenicoexeresis (fren'i-kō-ek-ser'ĕ-sis) [phrenico- + G. *exairesis,* a taking out, fr. *haireo,* to take, grasp]. Phrenicectomy.

phreniconeurectomy (fren'i-kō-nū-rek'tō-mē). Phrenicectomy.

phrenicotomy (fren-i-kot'ō-mē) [phrenico- + G. *tomē,* incision]. Section of the phrenic nerve in order to induce unilateral paralysis of the diaphragm, which is then pushed up by the abdominal viscera and exerts compression upon a diseased lung.

phrenicotripsy (fren'i-kō-trip'sē) [phrenico- + G. *tripsis,* a rubbing]. Phreniclasia.

phreno-, phren-, phreni-, phrenico- [G. *phrēn,* diaphragm, mind, heart (as seat of emotions)]. Combining forms denoting diaphragm, mind, or phrenic.

phrenocardia (fren-ō-kar'dē-ă) [phreno- + G. *kardia,* heart]. Cardiophrenia; precordial pain and dyspnea of psychogenic origin, often a symptom of anxiety neurosis.

phrenocolic (fren'ō-kol'ik) [phreno- + G. *kolon,* colon]. Relating to the diaphragm and the colon.

phrenocolopexy (fren-ō-kol'ō-pek-sē, -kō'lō-) [phreno- + G. *kolon,* colon, + *pēxis,* fixation]. Suture of a displaced or prolapsed transverse colon to the diaphragm.

phrenogastric (fren-ō-gas'trik) [phreno- + G. *gastēr,* stomach]. Relating to the diaphragm and the stomach.

phrenoglottic (fren-ō-glot'ik) [phreno- + G. *glōttis,* glottis]. Relating to the diaphragm and the glottis; denoting a spasm involving the diaphragm and the vocal cords.

phrenograph (fren'ō-graf) [phreno- + G. *graphō,* to record]. An instrument for recording graphically the movements of the diaphragm.

phrenohepatic (fren'ō-hĕ-pat'ik) [phreno- + G. *hepar,* liver]. Relating to the diaphragm and the liver.

phrenologist (frĕ-nol'ō-jist) [see phrenology]. One who claims to be able to diagnose mental and behavioral characteristics by a study of the external configuration of the skull.

phrenology (frĕ-nol'ō-jē) [phreno- + G. *logos,* study]. Craniognomy; Gall's craniology; an obsolete doctrine that each of the mental faculties is located in a definite part of the cerebral cortex, the size of which part varies in a direct ratio with the development of the corresponding faculty, this size being indicated by the external configuration of the skull.

phrenoplegia (fren-ō-plē'jē-ă) [phreno- + G. *plēgē,* stroke]. Paralysis of the diaphragm.

phrenoptosia (fren-op-tō'sē-ă) [phreno- + G. *ptōsis,* a falling]. An abnormal sinking down of the diaphragm.

phrenosin (fren'ō-sin). Cerebron; a cerebroside abundant in white matter of the brain, composed of cerebronic acid, galactose, and sphingosine.

phrenosinic acid (fren-ō-sin'ik). Cerebronic acid.

phrenospasm (fren'ō-spazm) [phreno- + G. *spasmos,* spasm]. Esophageal *achalasia.*

phrenosplenic (fren'ō-splen'ik) [phreno- + G. *splēn,* spleen]. Relating to the diaphragm and the spleen.

phrenotropic (fren-ō-trop'ik) [phreno- + G. *tropē,* a turning]. Affecting or working through the mind or brain.

phrictopathic (frik'tō-path'ik) [G. *phriktos,* causing a shudder, fr. *phrissō,* to bristle, shudder, + *pathos,* suffering]. Relating to a peculiar sensation, accompanied by shuddering, provoked by stimulation of a hysterical anesthetic area during the process of recovery.

phrynoderma (frin-ō-der'mă) [G. *phrynos,* toad, + *derma,* skin]. Toad skin; a follicular hyperkeratotic eruption thought to be due to deficiency of vitamin A.

phrynolysin (frī-nol'ĭ-sin) [G. *phrynos,* toad, + *lysis,* solution]. The poison of the fire-toad (*Bombinator igneus*).

PHS Abbreviation for Public Health Service.

pH-stat. A device for continuously sensing the pH of a solution and automatically adding acid or alkali as necessary to keep the pH constant; used to follow the time-course of reactions that liberate an acid or alkali.

phthalein (thal'ē-in). One of a group of highly colored compounds based on triphenylmethyl; *e.g.,* phenolphthalein.

phthalic acid (thal'ik). *o*-Benzenedicarboxylic acid; $C_6H_4(COOH)_2$.

phthaloyl (thal'ō-il). $-OC-C_6H_4-CO-$; the diacyl radical of phthalic acid.

phthalyl (thal'il). $-OC-C_6H_4-COOH$; the monoacyl radical of phthalic acid.

phthalylsulfacetamide (thal'il-sŭl-fă-set'ă-mīd). N^1-acetyl-N^4-phthalylsulfanilamide; a sulfonamide used in the treatment of enteric infections.

phthalylsulfathiazole (thal'il-sŭl-fă-thī'ă-zōl). 2-(N^4-Phthalylsulfanilamido)thiazole; a sulfonamide used in the treatment of enteric infections.

phthinoid (thin'oyd) [G. *phthinōdēs,* consumptive]. Obsolete term for wasting; consumptive; relating to or resembling phthisis.

phthiriophobia (thī'rē-ō-fō'bē-ă) [G. *phtheir,* louse, + *phobos,* fear]. Pediculophobia.

Phthirus (thī'rŭs) [L. *phthir;* G. *phtheir,* a louse]. See *Pthirus.*

phthisic, phthisical (tiz'ik, -i-kăl) [G. *phthisikos,* consumptive]. Obsolete terms relating to phthisis.

phthisio- [G. *phthisis,* a wasting]. Obsolete combining form pertaining to phthisis (tuberculosis).

phthisis (thī'sis, tī'sis) [G. a wasting]. **1.** Obsolete term for a wasting or atrophy, local or general. **2.** Obsolete term for consumption or, specifically, tuberculosis of the lungs.

aneurysmal p., the clinical picture of chest pain, cough with sputum, and hemoptysis sometimes produced by aortic aneurysm.

p. bul'bi, shrinkage of the eyeball after uveitis or other inflammatory disease.

essential p. bul'bi, a softening of the eyeball (ophthalmomalacia) and reduction in size, not due to inflammation.

marble cutters' p., obsolete term for calcicosis.

phyco- [G. *phykos,* seaweed]. Combining form denoting seaweed.

phycobilins (fī'kō-bil'inz, -bī'linz). Noncyclic tetrapyrroles, similar to bilirubin and urobilinogen, found in chloroplasts of certain algae; they function as light absorbers together with chlorophyll.

phycochrome (fī'kō-krōm) [phyco- + G. *chrōma,* color]. A bluish green coloring matter from certain algae; a phycobilin.

phycocyanin (fī-kō-sī'ă-nin) [phyco- + G. *kyanos,* blue]. A blue chromoprotein found in certain algae; the chromophore is a phycobilin.

phycoerythrin (fī'kō-ĕ-rith'rin) [phyco- + G. *erythros,* red]. A red chromoprotein found in red algae; the chromophore is a phycobilin.

Phycomycetes (fī'kō-mī-sē'tēz) [phyco- + G. *mykēs,* fungus]. Zygomycetes.

phycomycetosis (fī'kō-mī-sē-tō'sis). Zygomycosis.

phycomycosis (fī'kō-mī'kō-sis). Zygomycosis.

phygogalactic (fī-gō-gă-lak'tik) [G. *phygē,* flight, + *gala (galakt-),* milk]. Lactifuge.

phylacagogic (fī-lak-ă-goj'ik) [G. *phylaxis,* a guarding, protection, + *agogos,* leading]. Stimulating the production of protective antibodies.

phylaxis (fī-lak'sis) [G. a guarding, protection]. Protection against infection.

phyletic (fī-let'ik) [G. *phyletikos,* tribal, fr. *phylōn,* a tribe]. Denoting the mode of evolution characterized by sequential changes in a single line of descent without branching of lines; one species is transformed over a period of time to give rise to a single new species.

phyllo- [G. *phyllon,* leaf]. Combining form denoting leaf.

phyllochromanol (fil-ō-krō'mă-nol). The chroman form of reduced phylloquinone.

phyllochromenol (K-el) (fil-ō-krō'mĕ-nol). The chromenol form of phylloquinone.

phyllode (fil'ōd) [G. *phyllōdēs,* like leaves, fr. *phyllon,* leaf, + *eidos,* resemblance]. A flattened leaflike petiole; applied to any structure resembling a leaf, especially to a cross section of a neoplasm with a foliated structure, such as cystosarcoma phyllodes.

phylloerythrin (fil'ō-ĕ-rith'rin). Phytoporphyrin.

phylloporphyrin (fil-ō-pōr'fī-rin). 3,8-D-Ethyl-2,7,12,15,18-pentamethylporphyrin-17-propionic acid; a porphyrin derived from chlorophyll.

phyllopyrrole (fil-ō-pir'ōl). 3-Ethyl-2,4,5-trimethylpyrrole; a pyrrole derivative obtained by the reduction of chlorophyll.

phylloquinone, phylloquinone K (fil-ō-kwin'ōn, -kwī'nōn). Vitamin K_1 or $K_1(20)$; phytonadione; phytomenadione; 2-methyl-3-phytyl-1,4-naphthoquinone; 3-phytylmenaquinone; isolated from alfalfa; also prepared synthetically.
p. reductase, NAD(P)H dehydrogenase (quinone).

phylo- [G. *phylon,* tribe]. Combining form denoting tribe, race, or phylum.

phyloanalysis (fī'lō-ă-nal'i-sis) [phylo- + analysis]. **1.** The study of bioracial origins. **2.** A method of investigating individual and collective behavioral disorders putatively arising from impaired tensional processes.

phylogenesis (fī-lō-jen'ĕ-sis) [phylo- + G. *genesis,* origin]. Phylogeny.

phylogenetic, phylogenic (fī'lō-jĕ-net'ik, -jen'ik). Relating to phylogenesis.

phylogeny (fī-loj'ĕ-nē). Phylogenesis; the evolutionary development of a species, as distinguished from ontogeny, development of the individual.

phylum, pl. **phyla** (fī'lŭm, fī'lă) [Mod. L. fr. G. *phylon,* tribe]. A taxonomic division below the kingdom and above the class.

phyma (fī'mă) [G. a tumor]. A nodule or small rounded tumor of the skin.

phymatoid (fī'mă-toyd) [G. *phyma,* a tumor, + *eidos,* resemblance]. Resembling a neoplasm.

phymatorrhysin (fī'mă-tōr'i-sin) [G. *phyma (phymat-),* tumor, + *rhysis,* a flowing]. A variety of melanin obtained from certain melanotic neoplasms, and from hair and other heavily pigmented parts.

phymatosis (fī-mă-tō'sis). The growth or the presence of phymas or small nodules in the skin.

Physa (fī'să) [G. a pair of bellows; an air bubble; bladder]. Type genus of the freshwater pulmonate snails (family Physidae), which includes several common American species such as *P. parkeri, P. gyrina,* and *P. integra;* they are intermediate hosts of a number of bird and animal trematodes, including several that cause schistosome dermatitis in man.

physaliferous (fis-ă-lif'er-ŭs). Physaliphorous.

physaliform (fi-sal'i-fōrm) [G. *physallis,* bladder, bubble, + L. *forma,* form]. Like a bubble or small bleb.

physaliphore (fi-sal'i-fōr) [G. *physallis,* bladder, bubble, + *phoros,* bearing]. A mother cell, or giant cell containing a large vacuole, in a malignant growth.

physaliphorous (fis-ă-lif'ŏr-ŭs) [G. *physallis,* bladder, bubble, + *phoros,* bearing]. Physaliferous; having bubbles or vacuoles.

physalis (fis'ă-lis) [G. *physallis,* a bladder]. A vacuole in a giant cell found in certain malignant neoplasms, such as chordoma.

Physaloptera (fī'să-lop'ter-ă, fis-) [G. *physallis,* bladder, + *pteron,* wing]. A large genus of spiruroid roundworms parasitic in the stomach and duodenum of vertebrates, especially birds and mammals; they are transmitted via insect and annelid intermediate hosts and are frequently pathogenic, causing erosions and catarrhal gastritis. *P. caucasica* is a species reported in man in the southern USSR; *P. mordens* is a species from tropical Africa found only rarely in the esophagus, stomach, and intestine of man (probably cases of temporary infection from ingestion of infected insects).

physalopteriasis (fī'să-lop-ter-ī'ă-sis). Infection of animals and man with nematodes of the genus *Physaloptera.*

physeal (fiz'ē-ăl). Pertaining to the physis, or growth cartilage area, separating the metaphysis and the epiphysis.

physi-. See physio-.

physiatrics (fiz-ē-at'riks) [G. *physis,* nature, + *iatrikos,* healing]. **1.** Old term for physical *therapy.* **2.** Rehabilitation management.

physiatrist (fiz-ī'ă-trist). A physician who specializes in physical medicine.

physiatry (fi-zī'ă-trē). Physical *medicine.*

physic (fiz'ik) [G. *physikos,* natural, physical]. **1.** The art of medicine. **2.** A medicine; often a lay term for a cathartic.

physical (fiz'i-kăl) [Mod. L. *physicalis,* fr. G. *physikos*]. Relating to the body, as distinguished from the mind.

physician (fi-zish'ŭn) [Fr. *physicien,* a natural philosopher]. **1.** A doctor; a person who has been educated, trained, and licensed to practice the art and science of medicine. **2.** A practitioner of medicine, as contrasted with a surgeon.
osteopathic p., osteopath; a practitioner of osteopathy.

physician assistant (P.A.). A person who is trained, certified, and licensed to perform history taking, physical examination, diagnosis, and treatment of commonly encountered medical problems, and certain technical skills, under the supervision of a licensed physician, and who thereby extends the physician's capacity to provide medical care.

Physick, Philip Syng, U.S. surgeon, 1768–1837. See P.'s *pouches.*

physicochemical (fiz'i-kō-kem'i-kăl). Relating to the field of physical chemistry.

physics (fiz'iks) [see physic]. The branch of science concerned with the phenomena of matter, with the changes that matter undergoes without losing its chemical identity.

physio-, physi- [G. *physis,* nature]. Combining forms denoting physical (physiologic) or natural (relating to physics).

physiogenic (fiz'ē-ō-jen'ik) [physio- + G. *genesis*, origin]. Related to or caused by physiologic activity.

physiognomy (fiz-ē-og'nō-mē) [physio- + G. *gnōmōn*, a judge]. **1.** The countenance or habitus, especially regarded as an indication of character. **2.** Estimation of one's character and mental qualities by a study of the face and general bodily carriage.

physiognosis (fiz-ē-og-nō'sis) [physio- + G. *gnōsis*, knowledge]. Diagnosis of disease based upon a study of the facial appearance or bodily habitus.

physiologic, physiological (fiz-ē-ō-loj'ik, -loj'i-kăl). kō-sis). **1.** Relating to physiology. **2.** Normal, as opposed to pathologic; denoting the various vital processes. **3.** Denoting something that is apparent from its functional effects rather than from its anatomical structure; *e.g.*, a p. sphincter. **4.** Denoting a dose or the effects of such a dose (of a chemical agent that either is or mimics a hormone, neurotransmitter, or other naturally occurring agent) that is within the range of concentrations or potencies that would occur naturally. *Cf.* homeopathic(2); pharmocologic(2); supraphysiologic.

physiologicoanatomical (fiz'ē-ō-loj'i-kō-an-ă-tom'i-kăl). Relating to both physiology and anatomy.

physiologist (fiz-ē-ol'ō-jist). A specialist in physiology.

physiology (fiz-ē-ol'ō-jē) [L. or G. *physiologia*, fr. G. *physis*, nature, + *logos*, study]. The science concerned with the normal vital processes of animal and vegetable organisms, especially as to how things normally function in the living organism rather than to their anatomical structure, their biochemical composition, or how they are affected by drugs or disease.

comparative p., the science concerned with the differences in the vital processes in different species of organisms, particularly with a view to the adaptation of the processes to the specific needs of the species, to illuminating the evolutionary relationships among different species, or to establishing other interspecific generalizations and relationships.

developmental p., the study of physiologic processes in relation to embryonic development.

general p., the science of the functions or vital processes common to almost all living things, whether animal or plant, as opposed to aspects of p. peculiar to particular types of animals or plants, or to the application of p. to applied sciences such as medicine and agriculture.

hominal p., p. as applied to the elucidation of the normal functions of the human being.

pathologic p., physiopathology; that part of the science of disease concerned with disordered function, as distinguished from anatomical lesions.

physiomedical (fiz-ē-ō-med'i-kăl). Denoting the use of physical rather than medicinal measures in the treatment of disease.

physiopathologic (fiz'ē-ō-path-ō-loj'ik). Relating to pathologic physiology.

physiopathology (fiz'ē-ō-pă-thol'ō-jē). Pathologic *physiology.*

physiopsychic (fiz'ē-ō-sī'kik). Pertaining to both mind and body.

physiopyrexia (fiz'ē-ō-pī-rek'sē-ă) [physio- + G. *pyrexis*, feverishness]. Fever produced by a physical agent.

physiotherapeutic (fiz'ē-ō-ther-ă-pyū'tik). Pertaining to physical *therapy.*

physiotherapist (fiz'ē-ō-ther'ă-pist). A physical therapist. See physical *therapy* (2).

physiotherapy (fiz'ē-ō-ther'ă-pē) [physio- + G. *therapeia*, treatment]. Physical *therapy* (1).

oral p., the use of a toothbrush, interdental stimulator, floss, irrigating device, or other adjunctive aid to maintain oral health.

physique (fi-zēk') [Fr.]. Biotype; constitutional type; the physical or bodily structure; the "build."

physis (fī'sis) [G. growth]. A term sometimes used in referring to the *cartilago* epiphysialis.

physo- [G. *physaō*, to inflate, distend]. Combining form denoting: **1.** Tendency to swell or inflate. **2.** Relation to air or gas.

physocele (fī'sō-sēl) [physo- + G. *kelē*, tumor, hernia]. **1.** A circumscribed swelling due to the presence of gas. **2.** A hernial sac distended with gas.

Physocephalus sexalatus (fī'sō-sef'ă-lŭs sek'să-lā'tŭs) [G. *physa*, bellows, + *kephalē*, head]. A small species of spiruroid nematodes (family Spiruridae) found in the stomach of pigs, horses, camels, rabbits, and hares; worldwide in distribution, and especially prevalent in hogs.

physocephaly (fī-sō-sef'ă-lē) [physo- + G. *kephalē*, head]. Swelling of the head resulting from introduction of air into the subcutaneous tissues.

physometra (fī-sō-mē'tră) [physo- + G. *mētra*, uterus]. Uterine tympanites; distention of the uterine cavity with air or gas.

Physopsis (fī-sop'sis) [G. *physis*, growth, + *opseōs*, aspect, appearance]. A subgenus of the genus *Bulinus*, most species of which transmit the human blood fluke, *Schistosoma haematobium*, and some animal schistosomes in Africa south of the Sahara.

physopyosalpinx (fī'sō-pī-ō-sal'pingks) [physo- + G. *pyon*, pus, + *salpinx*, trumpet]. Pyosalpinx accompanied by a formation of gas in a fallopian tube.

physostigma (fī-sō-stig'mă) [G. *physa*, bellows, + *stigma*, a mark, spot; so called because of the shape of the stigma]. Calabar bean; ordeal bean; the dried seed of ***Physostigma venenosum*** (family Leguminosae), a vine of western Africa; it contains the alkaloids physostigmine (eserine), eseramine, eseridine (geneserine) and physovenine; in toxic doses it causes vomiting, colic, salivation, sweating, dyspnea, vertigo, slow pulse, and extreme prostration.

physostigmine (fī-sō-stig'mēn, -min). Eserine; an alkaloid of physostigma; it is a reversible inhibitor of the cholinesterases, and prevents destruction of acetylcholine; used as a cholinergic agent, and experimentally to enhance the action of acetylcholine at any of its sites of liberation.

p. salicylate, eserine salicylate; used by conjunctival instillation to reduce tension in glaucoma, in the treatment of postoperative intestinal atony and urinary retention, in the management of myasthenia gravis, and to counteract excessive doses of tubocurarine; also available as p. sulfate, with the same uses.

phyt-. See phyto-.

phytanate (fī'tan-āt). The anion of phytanic acid.

phytanate α-oxidase. An enzyme that oxidizes phytanic acid, removing the carboxyl group.

phytanic acid (fī-tan'ik). 3,7,11,15-Tetramethylhexadecanoic acid; an acid that accumulates in the serum and tissues of patients with Refsum's disease and is attributed to the hereditary absence of phytanate α-oxidase; arises from phytol and acts as an inhibitor of the α-oxidation of palmitic (hexadecanoic) acid.

6-phytase (fī'tās) [EC 3.1.3.26]. Phytate 6-phosphate; an enzyme hydrolyzing phytic acid, removing the 6-phosphoric group.

phytate (fī'tāt). A salt or ester of phytic acid.

phytic acid (fī'tik). The hexakisphosphoric ester of inositol; the mixed salt with magnesium and calcium is phytin.

phytin (fī'tin). The calcium magnesium salt of phytic acid; a dietary supplement used to provide calcium, organic phosphorus, and inositol.

phyto-, phyt- [G. *phyton*, a plant]. Combining forms denoting plants.

phytoagglutinin (fī'tō-ă-glū'ti-nin). A lectin that causes agglutination of erythrocytes or of leukocytes.

phytobezoar (fī-tō-bē'zōr) [phyto- + bezoar]. Food ball; a gastric concretion formed of vegetable fibers, with the seeds and skins of fruits, and sometimes starch granules and fat globules.

phytochemistry (fī-tō-kem'is-trē). The biochemical study of plants; concerned with the identification, biosynthesis, and metabolism of chemical constituents of plants.

phytocholesterol (fī'tō-kō-les'ter-ol). Phytosterol.

phytodermatitis (fī'tō-der-mă-tī'tis). Dermatitis caused by various mechanisms including mechanical and chemical injury, allergy, or photosensitization (phytophotodermatitis) at skin sites previously exposed to plants.

Phytoflagellata (fī'tō-flaj-ĕ-lā'tă) [phyto- + L. *flagellum,* a whip]. A subclass of Phytomastigophorea, the members of which have yellow or green chromatophores.

phytofluene (fī-tō-flū'ēn). Dodecahydrolycopene; 7,7',8,8',11,12-hexahydro-ψ,ψ-carotene; a possible colorless precursor of the plant carotenoids.

phytohemagglutinin (PHA) (fī'tō-hēm-ă-glū'ti-nin). Phytolectin; a phytomitogen from plants that agglutinates red blood cells. The term is commonly used specifically for the lectin obtained from the red kidney bean (*Phaseolus vulgaris*) which is also a mitogen that stimulates T lymphocytes more vigorously than B lymphocytes.

phytoid (fī'toyd) [G. *phytōdēs,* fr. *phyton,* plant, + *eidos,* resemblance]. Resembling a plant; denoting an animal having many of the biologic characteristics of a vegetable.

phytol (fī'tol). Phytyl alcohol; 3,7,11,15-tetramethyl-2-hexadecen-1-ol; an unsaturated primary alcohol derived from the hydrolysis of chlorophyll; a constituent of vitamins E and K_1.

phytolectin (fī-tō-lek'tin). Phytohemagglutinin.

Phytomastigina (fī'tō-mas-ti-jī'nă) [phyto- + G. *mastix,* whip]. Former term for plantlike flagellates, originally classified as a sub-order or order, raised to the class Phytomastigophorea (Phytomastigophorasida) in recent classifications.

Phytomastigophorasida (fī'tō-mas'ti-gō-fō-ras'i-dă). Phytomastigophorea.

Phytomastigophorea (fī'tō-mas'ti-gof-ō-rē'ă) [phyto- + G. *mastix,* whip, + *phoros,* bearing]. Phytomastigophorasida; a class of the subphylum Mastigophora (flagellates) within the phylum Sarcomastigophora (flagellate and ameboid protozoans), consisting mostly of free-living plantlike flagellates with or without chloroplasts, and usually with one or two flagella. *Cf.* Zoomastigophorea.

phytomenadione (fī'tō-men-ă-dī'ōn). Phylloquinone.

phytomitogen (fī-tō-mī'-tō-jen). A mitogenic lectin causing lymphocyte transformation accompanied by mitotic proliferation of the resulting blast cells identical to that produced by antigenic stimulation; *e.g.,* phytohemagglutinin, concanavalin A.

phytonadione (fī'tō-nā-dī'ōn). Phylloquinone.

phytonucleic acid (fī'tō-nū-klē'ik, -klā'ik). Obsolete term for ribonucleic acid.

phytophagous (fī-tof'ă-gŭs). [phyto- + G. *phagein,* to eat]. Plant-eating; vegetarian.

phytophlyctodermatitis (fī'tō-flik'tō-der-mă-ti'tis) [phyto- + G. *phlyktaina,* blister, + dermatitis]. Meadow *dermatitis.*

phytophotodermatitis (fī'tō-fō'tō-der-mă-tī'tis). Phytodermatitis resulting from photosensitization.

phytopneumoconiosis (fī'tō-nū'mō-kō-nē-ō'sis) [phyto- + pneumoconiosis]. A chronic fibrous reaction in the lungs due to the inhalation of dust particles of vegetable origin.

phytoporphyrin (fī-tō-pōr'fī-rin). Phylloerythrin; a porphyrin similar to the pheophorbide of the chlorophylls but with the vinyl group replaced by an ethyl group, with no methoxycarbonyl group, and minus two hydrogen atoms, producing one more double bond in ring D.

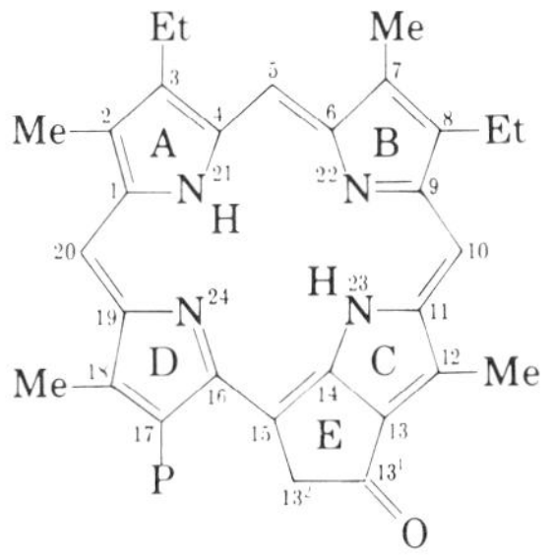

Phytoporphyrin
(Phylloerythrin in the Fischer system)

phytosphingosine (fī-tō-sfing'gō-sēn, -sin). 4*D*-hydroxysphinganine; 4-hydroxydihydrosphingosine; a sphingosine derivative isolated from various plants.

phytostearin (fī-tō-stē'ă-rin). Phytosterol.

phytosterin (fī-tō-stēr'in). Phytosterol.

phytosterol (fi-tō-stēr'ol). Phytocholesterol; phytostearin; phytosterin; generic term for the sterols of plants.

Phytotoxic (fī-tō-tok'sik). **1.** Poisonous to plant life. **2.** Pertaining to a phytotoxin.

phytotoxin (fī-tō-tok'sin) [phyto- + G. *toxikon,* poison]. Plant toxin; a substance similar in its properties to an extracellular bacterial toxin.

phytotrichobezoar (fī'tō-trik'ō-bē'zōr). Trichophytobezoar.

phytyl (fī'til). The radical, $-CH_2-CH{=}C(CH_3)-CH_2-[CH_2-CH_2-CH(CH_3)-CH_2-]_3H$, found in phylloquinone (vitamin K_1); a tetraprenyl radical, reduced in 3 of the 4 prenyl groups.

phytyl alcohol. Phytol.

PI Abbreviation for Periodontal Index.

pI The pH value for the isoelectric point of a given substance.

α_1PI Symbol for human α_1 proteinase *inhibitor.*

pia (pī'ă, pē'ă) [L. fem. of *pius,* tender]. Pia mater.

pia-arachnitis (pī'ă-ă-rak-nī'tis). Leptomeningitis.

pia-arachnoid (pī'ă-ă-rak'noyd, pē'ă-). Leptomeninges.

pial (pī'al, pē'al). Relating to the pia mater.

pia mater (pī'ă mā'ter, pē'ă mah'ter) [L. tender, affectionate mother]. Pia; a delicate vasculated fibrous membrane firmly adherent to the glial capsule of the brain (**p. m. enceph'ali** [NA]) and spinal cord (**p. m. spina'lis** [NA] or membrana limitans gliae); following exactly the outer markings of the cerebrum and also the ependymal lining circumference the choroid membranes and plexus, it invests the cerebellum but not so intimately as it does the cerebrum, not dipping down into all the smaller sulci. The p. m. and the arachnoid are collectively called leptomeninges, as distinguished from dura mater or pachymeninx.

pian (pē-an', pī'an). Yaws.

p. bois, bosch, bush, or forest yaws; a form of New World cutaneous leishmaniasis caused by *Leishmania braziliensis guyanensis* in the Amazon delta; a small proportion of cases are said to metastasize to the nasal mucosa with espundia-like involvement.

hemorrhagic p., *verruga* peruana.

piarachnoid (pī'ă-rak'noyd). Leptomeninges.

piblokto, pibloktog (pib-lok'tō) [Native]. A hysterical dissociative state, usually occurring in Eskimo women, in which the individual screams, tears off clothes, and runs out into the snow; afterward, there is no memory of the episode.

pica (pī'kă, pē'kă) [L. *pica,* magpie]. A perverted appetite for substances not fit as food or of no nutritional value; *e.g.,* clay, starch, ice.

Picchini's syndrome. See under syndrome.

Pick, Arnold, Prague psychiatrist, 1851–1924. See P.'s *atrophy, bundle, disease.*

Pick, Friedel, Prague physician, 1867–1926. See P.'s *bodies, disease, syndrome.*

Pick, Ludwig, German physician, 1868–1935. See P. *cell;* P.'s tubular *adenoma;* Niemann-P. *cell,* Niemann-P. *disease.*

pickling (pik'ling). In dentistry, the process of cleansing metallic surfaces of the products of oxidation and other impurities by immersion in acid.

Pickworth, F.A. See Lepehne-P. *stain.*

pico- [It. *piccolo,* small]. **1.** Combining form meaning small. **2 (p).** Bicro-; prefix used in the SI and metric systems to signify one-trillionth (10^{-12}).

picogram (pg) (pī'kō-gram). One-trillionth of a gram.

picolinic acid (pik-ō-lin'ik). Pyridine-4-carboxylic acid; an isomer of nicotinic acid.

picolinuric acid (pik-ō-li-nūr'ik). *N*-Picolinoylglycine; the amide, with glycine, of picolinic acid; hippuric acid analogue in which picolinic acid, rather than benzoic acid, is conjugated with glycine and excreted.

picometer (pm) (pī'kō-mē-ter). Bicron; one-trillionth of a meter.

Picornaviridae (pi-kōr-nă-vir'i-dē) [It. *piccolo,* very small, + RNA + -viridae]. A family of very small (20 to 30 nm) ether-resistant, nonenveloped viruses having a core of single-stranded RNA enclosed in a capsid of icosahedral symmetry with 32 capsomeres. Numerous species (including the polioviruses, coxsackieviruses, and echoviruses) are included in the family. There are four accepted genera: *Enterovirus, Rhinovirus, Cardiovirus,* and *Apthovirus.*

picornavirus (pi-kōr-nă-vī'rŭs). A virus of the family Picornaviridae.

picramic acid (pī-kram'ik). 2-Amino-4,6-dinitrophenol; red crystals sometimes found in the blood of persons poisoned with picric acid; formed as a result of partial reduction of the latter.

Picrasma (pi-kraz'mă) [L., fr. G. *pikrasmos,* bitterness]. See quassia.

picrate (pik'rāt). A salt of picric acid.

picric acid (pik'rik) [G. *pikros,* bitter]. 2,4,6-Trinitrophenol; nitroxanthic acid; carbazotic acid; $C_6H_2(NO_2)_3OH$; has been used as an application in burns, eczema, erysipelas, and pruritus.

picrocarmine (pik-rō-kar'min, -mēn). See under stain.

picroformol (pik'rō-fōr'mol). See under fixative.

picronigrosin (pik'rō-nī'grō-sin). See under stain.

picrotoxin (pik'rō-tok'sin) [G. *pikros,* bitter, + *toxicon,* poison]. Cocculin; a very bitter neutral principle derived from the fruit of *Anamirta cocculus* (family Menispermaceae); a central nervous system stimulant, used as an antidote for poisoning by barbiturates and certain other CNS-depressant drugs.

picrotoxinin (pik-rō-tok'si-nin). $C_{15}H_{16}O_6$; a lactone breakdown product of picrotoxin; pharmacological properties resemble those of picrotoxin.

picryl (pik'ril). 2,4,6-Trinitrophenyl; the organic radical derived from picric acid by removal of the hydroxyl group.

pictograph (pik'tō-graf). A vision test chart for illiterates.

PID Abbreviation for pelvic inflammatory *disease.*

piebaldism (pī'bawld-izm). Piebaldness.

piebaldness (pī'bawld-ness). Piebaldism; patchy absence of the pigment of scalp hair, giving a streaked appearance; patches of vitiligo may be present in other areas due to absence of melanocytes; often transmitted as an autosomal trait and may be associated with neurological defects (*e.g.,* Waardenburg syndrome).

piece (pēs). A part or portion.

end p., a part of the spermatozoon consisting of an axoneme surrounded only by the flagellar membrane.

Fab p., Fab *fragment.*

Fc p., Fc *fragment.*

middle p., a part of the spermatozoon characterized by an axoneme and by a sheath of mitochondria arranged in a tight helix.

principal p., the principal part of the spermatozoon which is about 45 μm long and has a characteristic fibrous sheath surrounding the axoneme.

piedra (pē-ā'dră) [Sp. a stone]. A fungus disease of the hair characterized by the hortae, of numerous waxy, small, hard, nodular masses. See also trichosporosis.

black p., p. involving the hairs of the scalp, caused by *Piedraia hortae* and characterized by firmly adherent black, hard, gritty nodules composed of an organized, firmly cemented mass of fungus cells; the fungal growth is always located above the level of the hair follicles; the disease occurs in humid tropical countries of the Americas, Africa, Southeast Asia, and Indonesia, and attacks chimpanzees and other primates as well as man.

p. nos'tras, a condition similar to p., but affecting the hair of the beard.

white p., p. of the beard, moustache, and genital areas, as well as the scalp, caused by *Trichosporon beigelii* and found in South America, Europe, and Japan; characterized by soft, mucilaginous, white to light brown nodules, within as well as on the hairs.

Piedraia (pī'ĕ-drī'ă) [see piedra]. A genus of fungi, based on *P. hortae,* which is probably the only species and which causes black piedra.

pieds terminaux (pē-e'ter-mē-nō') [Fr., end feet]. Axon *terminals.*

Pierini, Luigi, 20th century Argentine dermatologist. See *atrophoderma* of Pasini and P.

Pierre Robin. See Robin, Pierre.

piesesthesia (pī-ē-ses-thē'zē-ă) [G. *piesis,* pressure, + *aisthēsix,* sensation]. Pressure *sense.*

piesimeter, piesometer (pī-ĕ-sim'ĕ-ter, pī-ĕ-som'ĕ-ter) [G. *piesis,* pressure]. Piezometer; an instrument for measuring the pressure of a gas or a fluid.

Hales' p., a glass tube inserted into an artery at right angles to its axis, the pressure being shown by the height to which the blood ascends in the tube.

piesis (pī'ĕ-sis) [G. pressure]. Blood *pressure.*

piezochemistry (pī-ĕ-zō-kem'is-trē). The study of the effect of very high pressures on chemical reactions.

piezoelectric (pī'ĕ-zō-ĕ-lek'trik). Pertaining to piezoelectricity.

piezoelectricity (pī'ĕ-zō-ē-lek-tris'i-tē) [G. *piezō,* to press, squeeze, + electricity]. Electric currents generated by pressure upon certain crystals, *e.g.,* quartz, mica, calcite.

piezogenic (pī'ĕ-zō-jen'ik) [G. *piezo,* to press, squeeze, + *genesis,* origin]. Resulting from pressure.

piezometer (pī-ĕ-zom'ĕ-ter). Piesimeter.

PIF Abbreviation for prolactin inhibiting *factor.*

pig'bel. A type of necrotizing enteritis endemic in the Papua New Guinea highlands caused by the B toxin of *Clostridium perfringens* type C; occurs predominantly in children because of poor immunity to B toxin and a low level of intestinal proteases resulting from a diet low in protein and high in sweet potatoes.

pig'ment [L. *pigmentum,* paint]. **1.** Any coloring matter, as that of the red blood cells, hair, iris, etc., or the stains used in histologic or bacteriologic work, or that in paints. **2.** A medicinal preparation for external use, applied to the skin like paint.

bile p.'s, coloring matter in the bile derived from porphyrins by rupture of a methane bridge; *e.g.,* bilirubin, biliverdin.

formalin p., a p. formed when acid aqueous solutions of formaldehyde act on blood-rich tissues; characterized by rotation of the plane of polarized light, withstanding extraction in aqueous and lipid solvents, being bleached in acids and hydrogen peroxide; not formed when tissue is fixed with formaldehyde buffered to pH levels above 6.

hematogenous p., a p. derived from the hemoglobin of the red blood cells.

hepatogenous p., bile p. derived from the destruction of hemoglobin in the liver.

malarial p., a dark brown, granular p. which rotates the plane of polarized light and has other properties similar to formalin p.; occurs in parasites, such as *Plasmodium malariae,* around brain capillaries, and in fixed macrophages of spleen, liver, bone marrow, and lymph nodes. See malarial pigment *stain.*

melanotic p., melanin.

respiratory p.'s, the oxygen-carrying (colored) substances in blood and tissues (hemoglobin, myoglobin, hemocyanin, etc.).

visual p.'s, the photopigments in the retinal cones and rods that absorb light and initiate the visual process.

wear-and-tear p., lipofuscin that accumulates in aging or atrophic cells as a residue of lysosomal digestion.

pigmentary (pig'men-tār-ē). Relating to a pigment.

pigmentation (pig-men-tā'shŭn). Coloration, either normal or pathologic, of the skin or tissues resulting from a deposit of pigment.

arsenic p., generalized but spotty increased melanin p. of the skin in chronic arsenic poisoning.

exogenous p., discoloration of the skin or tissues by a pigment introduced from without.

pigmented (pig'men-ted). Colored as the result of a deposit of pigment.

pigmentolysin (pig-men-tol'i-sin) [L. *pigmentum,* pigment, + G. *lysis,* a loosening]. An antibody causing destruction of pigment.

pigmentum nigrum (pig-men'tŭm nī'grŭm). Melanin of the choroid coat of the eye.

pigmy (pig'mē). Pygmy.

Pignet, Maurice-C.J., French surgeon, *1871. See P.'s *formula.*

pilar, pilary (pī'lăr, pil'ă-rē) [L. *pilus,* hair]. Hairy.

pile (pīl). **1** [L. *pila,* pillar]. A series of plates of two different metals imposed alternately one on the other, separated by a sheet of material moistened with a dilute acid solution, used to produce a current of electricity. **2** [L. *pila,* ball]. An individual hemorrhoidal tumor. See hemorrhoids.

sentinel p., a circumscribed thickening of the mucous membrane at the lower end of a fissure of the anus.

thermoelectric p., thermopile.

pileous (pī'lē-ŭs) [L. *pilus,* hair]. Hairy.

piles (pīlz) [L. *pila,* a ball]. Hemorrhoids.

pileus (pī'lē-ŭs) [L. *pileum* or *pileus,* a felt cap]. A cap or shield; sometimes a caul.

pili (pī'lī) [L.] [NA]. Plural of pilus.

pilimiction (pī-li-mik'shŭn) [L. *pilus,* hair, + *mictio,* urination]. Passage of hairs in the urine, as in cases of dermoid tumors, or of threads of mucus in the urine.

pill [L. *pilula;* dim. of *pila,* ball]. A small globular mass of some coherent but soluble substance, containing a medicinal substance to be swallowed. See also tablet.

bread p., a placebo made of bread crumbs or other indifferent substances.

pep p.'s, colloquialism for tablets containing a central nervous system stimulant, especially amphetamine.

pillar (pil'ăr) [L. *pila*]. A structure or part having a resemblance to a column or pillar.

anterior p. of fauces, *arcus* palatoglossus.

anterior p. of fornix, *columna* fornicis.

Corti's p.'s, pillar *cells.*

p.'s of fauces, *arcus* palatini.

p.'s of fornix, the columna fornicis and crus fornicis.

p. of iris, *reticulum* trabeculare.

posterior p. of fauces, *arcus* palatopharyngeus.

posterior p. of fornix, *crus* fornicis.

pillet (pil'et). A small pill.

pill-rolling (pil'rōl'ing). A circular movement of the opposed tips of the thumb and the index finger appearing as a form of tremor in paralysis agitans.

pilo- [L. *pilus,* hair]. Combining form relating to hair.

pilobezoar (pī-lō-bē'zōr) [pilo- + bezoar]. Trichobezoar.

pilocarpine (pī-lō-kar'pēn) [G. *pilos,* a felt hat, + *karpos,* fruit]. An alkaloid obtained from the leaves of *Pilocarpus; Microphyllus* or *P. jaborandi* (family Rutaceae), shrubs of the West Indies and tropical America; a parasympathomimetic agent used as a diaphoretic, sialogogue, and stimulant of intestinal motility, and externally as a miotic and in the treatment of glaucoma; used as the hydrochloride and the nitrate salts.

pilocystic (pi'lō-sis'tik) [pilo- + G. *kystis,* bladder]. Denoting a dermoid cyst containing hair.

piloerection (pī'lō-ē-rek'shŭn). Erection of hair due to action of arrectores pilorum muscles.

piloid (pī'loyd) [pilo- + G. *eidos,* resemblance]. Hairlike; resembling hair.

pilojection (pī-lō-jek'shŭn) [pilo- + injection]. Process of shooting shafts of stiff mammalian hair into a saccular aneurysm in the brain in order to produce thrombosis.

pilomatrixoma (pī'lō-mā-trik-sō'mă) [pilo- + matrix + G. *-oma,* tumor]. Malherbe's calcifying epithelioma; Malherbe's disease; a benign tumor of the skin and subcutis, containing cells resembling basal cell carcinoma and areas of coagulation necrosis forming eosinophilic ghost cells with variable calcification and foreign body giant cell reaction in the fibrous stroma.

pilomotor (pī'lō-mō'ter) [pilo- + L. *motor,* mover]. Moving the hair; denoting the arrectores pilorum muscles of the skin and the postganglionic sympathetic nerve fibers innervating these small smooth muscles.

pilonidal (pī-lō-nī'dăl) [pilo- + L. *nidus,* nest]. Denoting a growth of hair in a dermoid cyst or in the deeper layers of the skin; in the latter instance, the misplaced hair may result from an ingrowth of cutaneous hair.

pilose (pī'lōs) [L. *pilosus*]. Hairy.

pilosebaceous (pī'lō-sē-bā'shŭs) [pilo- + L. *sebum,* suet]. Relating to the hair follicles and sebaceous glands.

pilosis (pī-lō'sis) [pilo- + G. *-osis,* condition]. Hirsutism.

Piltz, Jan, Polish neurologist, 1870–1931. See P. *sign;* Westphal-P. *phenomenon.*

pilula, gen. and pl. **pilulae** (pil'yū-lă, -lē) [L. dim. of *pila,* a ball]. A pill or pilule.

pilular (pil'yū-lăr). Relating to a pill.

pilule (pil'yūl) [L. *pilula*]. A small pill.

pilus, pl. **pili** (pī'lŭs, pī'lī) [L.]. **1** [NA]. Crinis; hair (1); one of the fine, filamentous epidermal growths covering the entire body except the palms and soles, and the flexor surfaces of the joints; the full length and texture of the hair varies markedly in different body sites. **2.** Fimbria (2); a fine filamentous appendage, somewhat analogous to the flagelium, that occurs on some bacteria. Pili consist only of protein and are shorter, straighter, much more numerous, and may be chemically similar to flagella; specialized pili (F pili, I pili, and other conjugative pili) seem to mediate bacterial conjugation. See also conjugative *plasmid*.

pi'li annula'ti, ringed *hair*.

pi'li cunicula'ti, ingrown *hairs*.

F pili, see pilus (2).

I pili, see pilus (2).

pi'li incarna'ti, ingrown *hairs*.

pi'li multigem'ini, the presence of several hairs in a single follicle.

R pili, specialized pili found on bacterial cells, similar to F pili and associated with R plasmids.

pi'li tor'ti, twisted hairs; a condition in which the hair shafts are twisted on the long axis, as a result of distortion of the follicles from a scarring inflammatory process, mechanical stress, or cicatrizing alopecia; the hair shafts resemble spangles in reflected light, are brittle, and break at varying lengths with many areas appearing bald with a dark stubble; as a developmental defect it can be manifested in such syndromes as Bjornstad's, Crandall's, and Menkes'.

pimaricin (pi-mar'i-sin). Natamycin; $C_{34}H_{49}NO_{14}$; an antifungal antibiotic for topical use, produced by *Streptomyces natalensis;* effective against *Aspergillus, Candida,* and *Mucor* species.

pimelic acid (pī-mel'ik). Heptanedioic acid; HOOC-$(CH_2)_5$COOH; an intermediate in the oxidation of oleic acid in some microorganisms; a precursor of biotin.

pimelo- [G. *pimelē,* soft fat, lard, fr. *piar,* fat]. Combining form denoting fat or fatty.

pimelopterygium (pim'ĕ-lō-tĕ-rij'i-ŭm) [pimelo- + pterygium]. A pterygium containing adipose tissue.

pimelorrhea (pim'ĕ-lō-rē'ă) [pimelo- + G. *rhoia,* a flux]. Fatty *diarrhea*.

pimelorthopnea (pim'ĕ-lōr-thop'nē-ă, -nē'ă) [pimelo- + G. *orthos,* straight, + *pnoē,* breath]. Piorthopnea; orthopnea, or difficulty in breathing in any but the erect posture, due to obesity.

pimenta, pimento (pi-men'tă, -tō) [Sp. fr. L. *pigmentum,* paint (Mediev. L. meaning, spice)]. Pimento; allspice; the dried fruit of *Pimenta officinalis* (family Myrtaceae), a tree native in Jamaica and other parts of tropical America, used as a carminative and aromatic spice; p. oil comprises 3 to 4% of the dried fruit.

p. oil, allspice oil; comprises 3 to 4.5% of the dried fruit.

piminodine (pi-min'ō-dēn). Ethyl-4-phenyl-1-[3-(phenylamino)-propyl]-piperidine-4-carboxylate; a potent narcotic analgesic chemically related to meperidine, with a duration of action shorter than that of morphine.

pimozide (pim'ō-zīd). 1-[1-[4,4-bis(*p*-Fluorophenyl)butyl]-4-piperidyl]-2-benzimidazolinone; a tranquilizing drug.

pimple (pim'pl). A papule or small pustule; usually meant to denote a lesion of acne.

pin. A metal rod used in surgical treatment of bone fractures. See also nail.

Steinmann p., a p. that is used to transfix bone for traction or fixation.

pinacyanol (pin-ă-sī'ă-nol) [old C.I. 808]. A basic dye, $C_{25}H_{25}N_2I$, used as a color sensitizer (violet red in water, blue in alcohol) in photography and for vital staining of leukocytes.

Pinard, Adolphe, French obstetrician, 1844–1934. See P.'s *maneuver*.

pincement (pans-mon') [Fr. pinching]. A pinching manipulation in massage.

Pindborg, Jens J., Danish oral pathologist, *1921. See P. *tumor*.

pindolol (pin'dō-lol). 1-(Indol-4-yloxy)-3-(isopropylamino)-2-propanol; a β-adrenergic blocking agent used in the treatment of hypertension.

pine (pīn) [L. *pinus,* a pine tree]. An evergreen coniferous tree of the genus *Pinus* (family Pinaceae), various species of which yield tar, turpentine, resin, and volatile oils.

p. oil, the volatile oil from the wood of *Pinus palustris* and other species of *Pinus;* used as a deodorant and disinfectant.

p.-needle oil, a volatile oil distilled with steam from the fresh leaf of *Pinus mugo;* has been used by inhalation and spray in catarrhal affections of the air passages, and locally in rheumatism; also used as a flavoring and in perfumery.

p. tar, liquid pitch; obtained by the destructive distillation of the wood of *Pinus palustris* and other species of *Pinus;* used internally as an expectorant, and externally in the treatment of skin diseases.

white p., the dried inner bark of *Pinus strobus,* used as an ingredient in cough syrups.

pineal (pin'ē-ăl) [L. *pineus,* relating to the pine, *pinus*] **1.** Piniform; shaped like a pine cone. **2.** Pertaining to the corpus pineale.

pinealectomy (pin'ē-ă-lek'tō-mē) [pineal + G. *ektomē,* excision]. Removal of the pineal body.

pinealocyte (pin-ē'al-ō-sīt) [pineal + G. *kytos,* cell]. Chief cell or parenchymatous cell of the corpus pineale; a cell of the pineal body with long processes ending in bulbous expansions. P.'s receive a direct innervation from sympathetic neurons which form recognizable synapses. The club-shaped endings of pinealocyte processes terminate in perivascular spaces surrounding capillaries.

pinealoma (pin'ē-ă-lō'mă) [pineal + G. *-oma,* tumor]. A relatively rare pineal neoplasm characterized by large, round, or polygonal, cells and small cells that resemble lymphocytes; a p. may cause hydrocephalus by pressure on the sylvian aqueduct; sometimes causes precocious puberty, as a result of hypothalamic involvement.

ectopic p., extrapineal p.; an undifferentiated neoplasm resembling a p., usually found near the pituitary gland; believed by some to be an undifferentiated teratoma.

extrapineal p., ectopic p.

pinealopathy (pin'ē-ă-lop'ă-thē) [pineal + G. *pathos,* disease]. Disease of the pineal gland.

pineapple (pīn'ap-ĕl). The fruit of *Ananas sativa* or *Bromelia ananas* (family Bromeliaceae); it contains a proteolytic and milk-clotting enzyme, bromelain.

Pinel, Philippe, French psychiatrist, 1745–1826. See P.'s *system*.

pineoblastoma (pin'ē-ō-blas-tō'mă) [pineal + G. *blastos,* germ, + *-oma,* tumor]. A poorly differentiated form of pinealoma.

pinguecula, pinguicula (ping-gwek'yū-lă) [L. *pinguiculus,* fattish, fr. *pinguis,* fat]. A yellowish accumulation of connective tissue that thickens the conjunctiva; occurs in the aged.

piniform (pin'i-fōrm, pī'ni-) [L. *pinus,* pine, + *forma,* form]. Pineal (1).

pinkeye (pink'ī). **1.** Acute contagious or acute epidemic *conjunctivitis*. **2.** Infectious bovine *keratitis*. **3.** In horses, a form of equine viral *enteritis*.

pinledge (pin'ledj). A cast metal dental restoration or technique that employs parallel pins as part of the casting to increase retention of the restoration.

pinna, pl. **pinnae** (pin'ă, pin'ē) [L. *pinna* or *penna,* a feather, in pl. a wing]. **1.** Auricula. **2.** A feather, wing, or fin.

p. na'si, *ala* nasi.

pinnal (pin'ăl). Relating to the pinna.

pinniped (pin'i-ped) [L. *pinna,* feather (wing), + *pes* (*ped-*), foot]. A member of the suborder Pinnipedia, aquatic carnivorous mammals with all four limbs modified into flippers (*e.g.,* seal, walrus).

pinocyte (pin'ō-sīt, pī'nō-) [G. *pineo,* to drink, + *kytos,* cell]. A cell that exhibits pinocytosis.

pinocytosis (pin'ō-sī-tō'sis, pī'nō-) [pinocyte + G. *-osis,* condition]. The cellular process of actively engulfing liquid, a phenomenon in which minute incuppings or invaginations are formed in the surface of the cell membrane and close to form fluid-filled vesicles; it resembles phagocytosis.

pinosome (pin'ō-sōm, pī'nō-) [G. *pineō,* to drink, + *sōma,* body]. A fluid-filled vacuole formed by pinocytosis.

Pins, Emil, Austrian physician, 1845–1913. See P.'s *sign, syndrome.*

pint (pīnt). A measure of quantity, containing 16 fluidounces, 28.875 cubic inches; 473.166 cc. An imperial p. contains 20 fluidounces, 34.659 cubic inches; 567.94 cc.

pinta (pin'tă, pēn'tă) [Sp. spot, blemish]. Azul; carate; spotted sickness; mal de los pintos; a disease caused by a spirochete, endemic in Mexico and Central America, and characterized by an eruption of patches of varying color that finally become white.

pin'tids [pinta + -id(1)]. Eruptions of plaque-like lesions in the secondary phase of pinta; the lesions, which vary in color (hypochromic, hyperchromic, and erythematosquamous), result in depigmentation.

pintoid (pin'toyd). Resembling pinta.

pinus (pī'nŭs) [L. a pine tree]. *Corpus* pineale.

pinworm (pin'werm). Seatworm; a member of the genus *Enterobius* or related genera of nematodes in the family Oxyuridae, abundant in a large variety of vertebrates, including such species as *Oxyuris equi* (the horse p.), *Enterobius vermicularis* (the human p.), *Syphacia* and *Aspiculuris* species (the mouse p.), *Passalurus ambiguus* (the rabbit p.), and *Syphacia muris* (the rat p.).

pioepithelium (pī'ō-ep-i-thē'lē-ŭm) [G. *piōn,* fat, + epithelium]. Fatty degenerated epithelium, or any epithelium containing fat globules.

Piophila casei (pī-of'i-lă kā'sē-ī) [L., fr. G. *piōn,* fat, + *philos,* fond; L. *caseus,* cheese]. The cheese fly, a species of muscoid flies whose eggs are deposited on exposed cheese, cured meats, and other foods and are thus ingested, sometimes giving rise to temporary intestinal myiasis, with diarrhea, colicky pains, and vomiting.

piorthopnea (pī-ōr-thop'nē-ă, -nē'ă) [G. *piōn,* fat, + *orthos,* straight, + *pnoē,* breath]. Pimelorthopnea.

pipamazine (pi-pam'ă-zēn). 1-[3-(2-Chlorophenothiazin-10-yl)propyl]isonipectoamide; a phenothiazine analogue with antiemetic and tranquilizing properties.

pipamperone (pi-pam'per-ōn). 1'-[3- (*p*-Fluorobenzoyl)propyl]-[1,4'-bipiperidine]-4'-carboxamide; an antipsychotic tranquilizer.

pipazethate (pi-paz'ĕ-thāt). 2-(2-Piperidinoethoxy)ethyl 10*H*-pyridol[3,2-*b*][1,4]benzothiazine-10-carboxylate; an antitussive agent.

pipecolic acid (pip'ĕ-kō'lik, -kol'ik). Pipecolinic acid; homoproline; dihydrobaikiaine; 2-piperidinecarboxylic acid; saturated picolinic acid; Δ^1 and Δ^6 dehydropipecolic acids are intermediates in the catabolism of lysine.

pipecolinic acid (pip-ĕ-kō-lin'ik, -kol'i-nik). Pipecolic acid.

pipenzolate methylbromide (pi-pen'zō-lāt). 1-Ethyl-3-piperidyl benzilate methylbromide; an anticholinergic drug.

Piper, E.B., U.S. obstetrician-gynecologist, 1881–1935. See P.'s *forceps.*

piper (pī'per) [L. pepper]. Black pepper, the dried unripe fruit of *Piper nigrum* (family Piperaceae), a climbing plant of the East Indies; used as a condiment, diaphoretic, stimulant, and carminative, and locally as a counterirritant.

piperacetazine (pi-per-ă-set'ă-zēn). 10-{3-[4-(2-Hydroxyethyl)-piperidino]-propyl} phenothiazin-2-yl methyl ketone; a tranquilizer.

piperazine (pi-per'ă-zēn, -zin). Diethylenediamine; pyrazine hexahydride; its former use in gout was based upon its property of dissolving uric acid *in vitro,* but it is ineffective in increasing uric acid excretion; its compounds are now used as anthelmintics in oxyuriasis and ascariasis.

p. adipate, a veterinary anthelmintic and filaricide.

p. calcium edetate, (ethylenedinitrilo)tetraacetic acid piperazine calcium salt; an anthelmintic.

p. citrate, a vermifuge for pinworms and roundworms.

p. estrone sulfate, a purified preparation of natural estrone sulfate; the p. acts as a buffer to increase the stability of estrone sulfate.

piperacillin sodium (pi-per'ă-sil'in). $C_{23}H_{26}N_5NaO_7S$; a semisynthetic extended spectrum penicillin active against a wide variety of Gram-positive and Gram-negative bacteria.

piperidine (pī'per-i-dēn). Hexahydropyridine; $C_5H_{11}N$; a compound from which are derived phenothiazine antipsychotics such as thioridazine hydrochloride and mesoridazine besylate.

piperidolate hydrochloride (pi-per'i-dō-lāt). 1-Ethyl-3-piperidyl diphenylacetate hydrochloride; an anticholinergic agent.

piperocaine hydrochloride (pip'er-ō-kān, pī'per-). 3-(2-Methyl-1-piperidyl)propyl benzoate hydrochloride; a rapidly acting local anesthetic for infiltration and nerve blocks.

piperoxan hydrochloride (pip-er-ok'san). Fourneau 933; 2-(1-piperidylmethyl)-1,4-benzodioxane hydrochloride; an adrenergic (α-receptor blocking agent of the Fourneau series of benzodioxanes); used as a diagnostic test for pheochromocytoma.

pipette, pipet (pī-pet', pi-pet') [Fr. dim. of *pipe,* pipe]. A graduated tube (marked in ml) used to transport a definite volume of a gas or liquid in laboratory work.

pipobroman (pip-ō-brō'man). 1,4-Bis(3-bromopropionyl)piperazine; an alkylating agent used in polycythemia vera and chronic granulocytic leukemia.

piposulfan (pi-pō-sŭl'fan). 1,4-Dihydracryloylpiperazine dimethanesulfonate; an antineoplastic agent.

pipradrol hydrochloride (pip'ră-drol). α-[2-Piperidyl]benzhydrol hydrochloride; a central nervous system stimulant.

piprinhydrinate (pip-rin-hī'dri-nāt). *N*-Methylpiperidyl 4-benzhydryl ether (diphenylpyralimine) 8-chlorotheophyllinate; an antihistaminic and antiemetic.

pipsyl (Ips) (pip'sil). *p*-Iodophenylsulfonyl, the radical of p. chloride that combines with the NH_2 groups of amino acids and proteins.

pirbuterol (pir-byū'ter-ol). α^6[(*tert*- Butylamino)methyl]-3-hydroxy-2,6-pyridine-dimethanol; a selective β_2-adrenergic bronchodilator used in the treatment of asthma.

Pirenella (pir-ĕ-nel'ă). A genus of marine and brackish water operculate (prosobranch) snails. *P. conica* is the initial intermediate host of *Heterophyes heterophyes,* the fish-borne fluke of humans and fish-eating birds and mammals along the Mediterranean and Red Sea coasts.

Pirie, George A., Scottish radiologist, 1864–1929. See P.'s *bone.*

piriform (pir'i-fōrm, pī'rē-) [L. *pirum,* pear, + *forma,* form]. Pyriform; pear-shaped.

pirinitramide (pir-i-nī'tră-mīd). Piritramide.

Pirogoff, Nikolai I., Moscow surgeon, 1810–1881. See P.'s *amputation, angle, triangle.*

piromen (pir'ō-men, pī'rō-). Pyromen; a sterile, nonprotein, nonanaphylactogenic extract of *Pseudomonas aeruginosa* and *Proteus vulgaris.* The active components are bacterial polysaccharides of low toxicity; used in the treatment of certain allergic, dermatologic, and ophthalmic disorders.

Piroplasma (pir'ō-plaz'mă, pī'rō-) [L. *pirum,* pear, + G. *plasma,* a thing formed]. Former name for *Babesia.*

Piroplasmida (pi'rō-plaz-mī'dă). An order of sporozoan protozoa (subclass Piroplasmia, class Sporozoea) consisting of the families Habesiidae, Theileriidae, and Dactylosomatidae; includes heteroxenous tick-borne blood parasites of vertebrates with reduced apical complex, lacking spores, and with asexual reproduction by binary fission or schizogony.

piroplasmosis (pir'ō-plas-mō'sis). Babesiosis.

piroxicam olamine (pir-oks'i-kam). 4-Hydroxy-2-methyl-*N*- 2-pyridyl-2*H*- 1,2-benzothiazine-3-carboxamide-1,1-dioxide; a nonsteroidal anti-inflammatory agent with analgesic and antipyretic actions.

pirprofen (pir-prō'fen). 3-Chloro-4-(3-pyrrolin-1-yl)hydratropic acid; an anti-inflammatory agent used in the treatment of rheumatoid arthritis.

Pirquet von Cesenatico, Clemens P., Austrian physician, 1874–1929. See P.'s *reaction, test.*

Pisces (pis'ēz, pī'sēz) [L. pl. of *piscis,* a fish]. A superclass of vertebrates, generally known as fish; the term is sometimes confined to the bony fishes.

pisiform (pis'i-fōrm) [L. *pisum,* pea, + *forma,* appearance]. Pea-shaped or pea-sized.

pit [L. *puteus*]. **1.** Any natural depression on the surface of the body, such as the axilla. *Cf.* dimple. **2.** One of the pinhead-sized depressed scars following the pustule of acne, chickenpox, or smallpox (pockmark). **3.** A sharp-pointed depression in the enamel surface of a tooth, due to faulty or incomplete calcification or formed at the confluent point of two or more lobes of enamel. **4.** To indent, as by pressure of the finger on the edematous skin; to become indented, said of the edematous tissues when pressure is made with the fingertip.

anal p., proctodeum (1).
articular p. of head of radius, *fovea* articularis capitis radii.
auditory p.'s, paired depressions, one on either side of the head of the embryo, marking the location of the future auditory vesicles.
buccal p., a structural depression found on the buccal enamel of molars.
central p., *fovea* centralis retinae.
costal p. of transverse process, *fovea* costalis processus transversus.
p. for dens of atlas, *fovea* dentis atlantis.
gastric p., *foveola* gastrica.
granular p.'s, *foveolae* granulares.
p. of head of femur, *fovea* capitis ossis femoris.
inferior articular p. of atlas, *facies* articularis inferior atlantis.
inferior costal p., *fovea* costalis inferior.
iris p.'s., colobomas affecting the stroma of the iris with pigment epithelium intact.
lens p.'s, the paired depressions formed in the superficial ectoderm of the embryonic head as the lens placodes sink in toward the optic cup; the external openings of the p.'s are closed as the lens vesicles are formed.
Mantoux p., tiny depressions of the palms and soles in basal cell nevus syndrome.
nail p.'s, small punctate depressions on the surface of the nail plate due to defective nail formation; seen in psoriasis and other disorders. See also geographic *stippling* of nails.
nasal p.'s, olfactory p.'s; the paired depressions formed when the nasal placodes come to lie below the general external contour of the developing face as a result of the rapid growth of the adjacent nasal elevations; the p.'s are the primordia of the rostral portions of the nasal chambers.
oblong p. of arytenoid cartilage, *fovea* oblonga cartilaginis arytenoideae.
olfactory p.'s, nasal p.'s.
postnatal p. of the newborn, *fovea* coccygis.
primitive p., a small depression extending beneath Hensen's node from the most cephalic part of the primitive groove.
pterygoid p., *fovea* pterygoidea.
p. of stomach, epigastric *fossa.*
sublingual p., *fovea* sublingualis.
superior articular p. of atlas, *facies* articularis superior atlantis.
superior costal p., *fovea* costalis superior.
suprameatal p., *foveola* suprameatica.
triangular p. of arytenoid cartilage, *fovea* triangularis cartilaginis arytenoideae.
trochlear p., *fovea* trochlearis.

PITC Abbreviation for phenylisothiocyanate.

pitch (pich) [L. *pix*]. A resinous substance obtained from tar after the volatile substances have been expelled by boiling.

Burgundy p., white p.; a resinous exudation from the spruce fir or Norway spruce, *Picea excelsa;* has been used as a counterirritant in the form of a plaster.
liquid p., *pine* tar.
white p., Burgundy p.

pitchblende (pich'blend). Uraninite; a mineral of pitchlike appearance, chiefly uranium dioxide, the main source of uranium and elements, such as radium, produced as a result of the radioactive breakdown of that element.

pith [A.S. *pitha*]. **1.** The center of a hair. **2.** The spinal cord and medulla oblongata. **3.** To pierce the medulla of an animal with a sharp instrument introduced at the base of the skull.

pithecoid (pith'ĕ-koyd) [G. *pithēkos,* ape, + *eidos,* resemblance]. Resembling an ape.

pithode (pith'ōd) [G. *pithōdēs,* like a jar, fr. *pithos,* earthenware wine-jar, + *eidos,* resemblance]. The nuclear spindle in karyokinesis.

Pitkin, George P., U.S. surgeon, 1885–1934. See P. *syringe.*

Pitot, Henri, French engineer, 1695–1771. See P. *tube.*

Pitres, Jean A., French physician, 1848–1927. See P.'s *area, sign.*

pit'ting. In dentistry, the formation of well defined, relatively deep depressions in a surface, usually used in describing defects in surfaces (often golds, solder joints, or amalgam). It may arise from a variety of causes, although the clinical occurrence is often associated with corrosion.

pituicyte (pi-tū'i-sīt) [pituitary + G. *kytos,* cell]. The primary cell of the posterior lobe of the pituitary gland, a fusiform cell closely related to neuroglia.

pituicytoma (pi-tū'i-sī-tō'mă) [pituicyte + G. *-oma,* tumor]. A rare gliogenous neoplasm derived from pituicytes, occurring in the posterior lobe of the pituitary gland and characterized by cells with relatively small, round or oval nuclei and long branching processes that form a complex network of cytoplasmic material, in which numerous small droplets of fat may be demonstrated by means of osmic acid (and certain other special stains).

pituita (pi-tū'i-tă) [L. phlegm or thick mucous secretion] [NA]. Glairy mucus; a thick nasal secretion.

pituitarism (pi-tū'i-tăr-izm). Pituitary dysfunction. See hyperpituitarism; hypopituitarism.

pituitarium (pi-tū-i-tā'rē-ŭm) [Mod. L.]. Pituitary.

pituitary (pi-tū'i-tăr-ē) [L. *pituita*]. Relating to the pituitary gland (hypophysis).

anterior p., the dried, partially defatted, and powdered anterior lobe of the p. gland of cattle, sheep, or swine; now rarely used therapeutically.
desiccated p., posterior p.
pharyngeal p., the embryonic remnant of the oral end of Rathke's pouch that is cut off from the adenohypophysis by the developing sphenoid bone; composed chiefly of chromophobes and, under

normal conditions, considered physiologically inactive.
posterior p., hypophysis sicca; desiccated p.; the cleaned, dried, and powdered posterior lobe obtained from the p. body of domestic animals used for food by man; an oxytocic, vasoconstrictor, antidiuretic, and a stimulant of intestinal motility.

pituitous (pi-tū'i-tŭs). Relating to pituita.

pityriasic (pit-i-rī'ă-sik). Relating to or suffering from pityriasis.

pityriasis (pit-i-rī'ă-sis) [G. fr. *pityron*, bran, dandruff]. A dermatosis marked by branny desquamation.
p. al'ba, patchy hypopigmentation of the skin resulting from mild dermatitis.
p. al'ba atroph'icans, a scaling condition of the skin followed by atrophy.
p. amianta'cea, *tinea* amiantacea.
p. cap'itis, dandruff.
p. circina'ta, p. rosea.
p. furfura'cea, obsolete synonym for dandruff.
p. lichenoi'des, maculopapular *erythroderma.*
p. lichenoi'des et variolifor'mis acu'ta, parapsoriasis lichenoides et varioliformis acuta; parapsoriasis varioliformis; Mucha-Habermann disease or syndrome; an acute dermatitis that runs a relatively mild course and is self-limited, although persistence of lesions and recurrence of attacks are not uncommon; vesicles, papules, and crusted lesions eventually produce smallpoxlike scars.
p. lin'guae, geographic *tongue.*
p. macula'ta, p. rosea.
p. ni'gra, *tinea* nigra.
p. ro'sea, p. cirrinata or maculata; a self-limited eruption of macules or papules involving the trunk and extremities and rarely the face; the lesions are usually oval and follow the lines of cleavage of the skin; the onset is frequently preceded by a single larger lesion known as the herald patch.
p. ru'bra, exfoliative *dermatitis.*
p. ru'bra pila'ris, a chronic eruption of the hair follicles, which become firm, red, surmounted with a horny plug, and often confluent to form scaly plaques; it is most conspicuously noted on the dorsa of the fingers and on the elbows and knees, and is associated with erythema, thickening of the palms and soles, and opaque thickening of the nails.
p. sic'ca, dandruff.
p. versic'olor, *tinea* versicolor.

pityroid (pit'i-royd) [G. *pityrōdēs*, branlike, fr. *pityron*, bran, + *eidos*, resemblance]. Furfuraceous.

Pityrosporum (pit-i-ros'pō-rŭm, pit'i-rō-spō'rŭm) [G. *pityron*, bran, + *sporos*, seed]. A genus of nonpathogenic fungi found in dandruff and seborrheic dermatitis.
p. orbicula're, *Malassezia furfur.*
P. ova'le, *Malassezia ovalis.*

pivalate (piv'ă-lāt). USAN-approved contraction for trimethylacetate, $(CH_3)_3C\text{–}CO_2^-$.

pivot (piv'ŏt). A post upon which something hinges or turns.
adjustable occlusal p., an occlusal p. which may be adjusted vertically by means of a screw or by other means.
occlusal p., an elevation contrived on the occlusal surface, usually in the molar region, designed to act as a fulcrum and to induce sagittal mandibular rotation.

pix, gen. picis (piks, pī'sis) [L]. Pitch.

pixel (pik'sel). A contraction for a picture element, which is a representation of a single volume element (voxel) of the display of the CT image.

PK Abbreviation for *pyruvate* kinase.

pK The negative logarithm of the ionization constant (K_a) of an acid; the pH at which equal concentrations of the acid and basic forms of a substance (usually a buffer) are present.

PKU Abbreviation for phenylketonuria.

placebo (plă-sē'bō) [L. I will please, future of *placeo*]. **1.** An inert substance given as a medicine for its suggestive effect. **2.** An inert compound identical in appearance with material being tested in experimental research, which may or may not be known to the physician and/or patient, administered to distinguish between drug action and suggestive effect of the material under study.

PLACENTA

placenta (plă-sen'tă) [L. a cake] [NA]. Organ of metabolic interchange between fetus and mother. It has a portion of embryonic origin, derived from a highly developed area of the outermost embryonic membrane (chorion frondosum), and a maternal portion formed by a modification of the part of the uterine mucosa (decidua basalis) in which the chorionic vesicle is implanted. Within the p., the chorionic villi, with their contained capillaries carrying blood of the embryonic circulation, are exposed to maternal blood in the intervillous spaces in which the villi lie; no direct mixing of fetal and maternal blood occurs, but the intervening tissue (the placental membrane) is sufficiently thin to permit the absorption of nutritive materials, oxygen, and some harmful substances, like viruses, into the fetal blood and the release of carbon dioxide and nitrogenous waste from it. At term, the human p. is disk-shaped, about 4 cm in thickness and 18 cm in diameter, and averages about $^1/_6$ to $^1/_7$ the weight of the fetus; its fetal face is smooth, being formed by the adherent amnion, with the umbilical cord normally attached near its center; the maternal face of a detached p. is rough because of the torn decidual tissue adhering to the chorion, and shows lobular elevations called cotyledons or lobes.

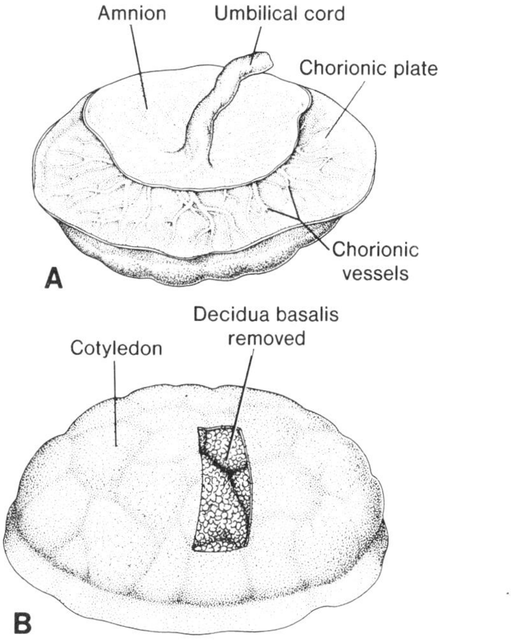

A Full Term Placenta
A, as seen from the fetal side; *B*, as seen from the maternal side.

accessory p., supernumerary or succenturiate p.; a mass of pla-

cental tissue distinct from the main p.
p. accre'ta, the abnormal adherence of the chorionic villi to the myometrium, associated with partial or complete absence of the decidua basalis and, in particular, the stratum spongiosum.
p. accre'ta ve'ra, the term applied when villi are in juxtaposition with the myometrium.
adherent p., a p. that fails to separate cleanly from the uterus after delivery.
annular p., zonary p.; a p. in the form of a band encircling the interior of the uterus.
battledore p., a p. in which the umbilical cord is attached at the border; so-called because of the fancied resemblance to the racquet (racket) used in battledore, a precursor to badminton.
bidiscoidal p., a p. with two separate disc-shaped portions attached to opposite walls of the uterus, normal for certain monkeys and shrews, and occasionally found in humans.
p. bilo'ba, p. bipartita; a p. duplex in which the two parts are separated by a constriction.
p. biparti'ta, p. biloba.
central p. previa, p. previa centralis.
chorioallantoic p., a p. (such as that of primates) in which the chorion is formed by the fusion of the allantoic mesoderm and vessels to the inner face of the serosa.
chorioamnionic p., a form of placentation in which the amnion is fused to the inside of the chorion, thus permitting interchange of water and electrolytes between mother and fetus.
choriovitelline p., a p. (seen in some lower animals) in which the chorion is formed by the fusion of yolk-sac mesoderm and vessels to the inner face of the serosa.
p. circumvalla'ta, a cup-shaped p. with raised edges, having a thick, round, white, opaque ring around its periphery; a portion of the decidua separates the margin of the p. from its chorionic plate; the remainder of the chorionic surface is normal in appearance, but the fetal vessels are limited in their course across the p. by the ring. See also p. marginata; p. reflexa.
cotyledonary p., a p. in which the substance is divided into lobes or cotyledons.
deciduate p., a p. in which the maternal decidua is cast off with the fetal p.
dichorionic diamniotic p., see twin p.
p. diffu'sa, p. membranaceae.
p. dimidia'ta, p. duplex.
disperse p., a p. in which the umbilical arteries divide dichotomously before entering the placental substance.
p. du'plex, p. dimidiata; a p. consisting of two parts, almost entirely detached, being united only at the point of attachment of the cord.
endotheliochorial p., a p. in which the chorionic tissue penetrates to the endothelium of the maternal blood vessels.
endothelio-endothelial p., a p. in which the endothelium of the maternal vessels comes in direct contact with the endothelium of the fetal vessels to form the placental barrier.
epitheliochorial p., a p. in which the chorion is merely in contact with, and does not erode, the endometrium.
p. extrachora'les, a p. in which the chorionic plate is limited by a thin membranous fold at the edge.
p. fenestra'ta, a p. in which there are areas of thinning, sometimes extending to entire absence of placental tissue.
fetal p., p. feta'lis, *pars* fetalis placentae.
hemochorial p., the type of p., as in man and some rodents, in which maternal blood is in direct contact with the chorion.
hemoendothelial p., the type of p., as in rabbits, in which the trophoblast becomes so attenuated that, by light microscopy, maternal blood appears to be separated from fetal blood only by the endothelium of the chorionic capillaries.
horseshoe p., an exaggerated p. reniformis curved in the form of a horseshoe.
incarcerated p., a p. held in the uterus by a contracted cervix.
p. incre'ta, a form of p. accreta in which the chorionic villi invade the myometrium.
labyrinthine p., a p. in which maternal blood circulates through channels within the fetal syncytiotrophoblast.
p. margina'ta, a p. with raised edges, less pronounced than the p. circumvallata. See also p. reflexa.
maternal p., *pars* uterina placentae.
p. membrana'cea, p. diffusa; an abnormally thin p. covering an unusually large area of the uterine lining.
monochorionic diamniotic p., see twin p.
monochorionic monoamniotic p., see twin p.
p. multilo'ba, a p. having more than three lobes separated from each other by simple constrictions, the fetus being single.
nondeciduous p., a p. in which the fetal p. is cast off, leaving the uterine mucosa intact (*e.g.,* an epitheliochorial p.).
p. pandurafor'mis, a form of p. dimidiata with the two halves placed side by side in a shape suggestive of a lutelike musical instrument (pandura).
p. percre'ta, the term applied when the villi have invaded the full thickness of myometrium to or through the serosa of the uterus, causing incomplete or complete uterine rupture, respectively.
p. pre'via, placental presentation; the condition in which the p. is implanted in the lower segment of the uterus, extending to the margin of the internal os of the cervix or partially or completely obstructing the os.
p. pre'via centra'lis, central or total p. previa; p. previa in which the p. entirely covers the internal os of the cervix.
p. pre'via margina'lis, p. previa in which the p. comes just to, but does not occlude, the internal os of the cervix.
p. pre'via partia'lis, p. previa in which the internal os of the cervix is partially covered by placental tissue.
p. reflex'a, an anomaly of the p. in which the margin is thickened so as to appear turned back upon itself. See also p. circumvallata and p. marginata.
p. renifor'mis, a kidney-shaped p.
retained p., incomplete separation of the p. and its failure to be expelled at the usual time after delivery of the child.
Schultze's p., a p. that appears at the vulva with the glistening fetal surface presenting.
p. spu'ria, a mass of placental tissue which has no vascular connection with the main p.
succenturiate p., accessory p.
supernumerary p., accessory p.
syndesmochorial p., in ruminant animals, a type of p. in which the chorion is attached to maternal connective tissue.
total p. pre'via, p. previa centralis.
p. tri'loba, p. tripartita.
p. triparti'ta, p. triplex; a p. consisting of three parts almost entirely separate, being joined together only by the blood vessels of the umbilical cord; the fetus is single.
p. tri'plex, p. tripartita.
twin p., the placenta(s) of a twin pregnancy; if dizygotic, the p.'s may be separate or fused, the latter retaining two amniotic and two chorionic sacs (**dichorionic diamniotic p.**); if monozygotic, the p. may be a **monochorionic monoamniotic** or **monochorionic diamniotic p.,** depending on the stage at which twinning took place; only if twinning occurs very early, may there be a fused p. with two chorionic and two amniotic membranes.
p. uteri'na, *pars* uterina placentae.
p. velamento'sa, a p. in which the umbilical cord is attached to the adjoining membranes, with the umbilical vessels spread out and entering the p. independently.
villous p., a p. in which the chorion forms villi.
zonary p., annular p.

placental (pla-sen'tăl). Relating to the placenta.

Placentalia (plas-en-tā'lē-ă) [L. *placenta*]. See *Eutheria.*

placentascan (pla-sen'tă-skan). Obsolete method of determining the location of the placenta by means of injected radioactive material and its localization and display by a scintillation detector.

placentation (plas-en-tā'shŭn). The structural organization and mode of attachment of fetal to maternal tissues in the formation of the placenta. Types of p. are defined under placenta.

placentitis (plas-en-tī'tis). Inflammation of the placenta.

placentography (plas-en-tog'ră-fē) [placenta + G. *graphō,* to write]. Roentgenography of the placenta following injection of a radiopaque substance.

indirect p., roentgenographic determination of the presence of placenta previa by estimating the distance between the presenting fetal part and the bladder filled with a radiopaque substance.

placentoma (plas-en-tō'mă). Deciduoma.

placentotherapy (plă-sen'tō-thār'ă-pē). Therapeutic use of an extract of placental tissue.

Placido da Costa, Antonio, Portuguese ophthalmologist, 1848–1916. See P.'s *disk.*

placode (plak'ōd) [G. *plakōdēs,* fr. *plax,* anything flat or broad, + *eidos,* like]. Local thickening in an embryonic epithelial layer; the cells of the p. ordinarily constitute a primordial group from which some organ or structure is later developed.

auditory p.'s, otic p.'s; paired ectodermal p.'s that sink below the general level of the superficial ectoderm to form the auditory vesicles.

epibranchial p.'s, ectodermal thickenings associated with the more dorsal parts of the embryonic branchial grooves; their cells are believed to contribute to formation of the cranial ganglia, especially those of nerves IX and X.

lens p.'s, optic p.'s; paired ectodermal p.'s that become invaginated to form the embryonic lens vesicles.

nasal p.'s, olfactory p.'s.

olfactory p.'s, nasal p.'s; paired ectodermal p.'s which come to lie in the bottom of the olfactory pits as the pits are deepened by the growth of the surrounding nasal processes.

optic p.'s, lens p.'s.

otic p.'s, auditory p.'s.

pladaroma, pladarosis (plad-ă-rō'mă,-rō'sis) [G. *pladaros,* wet, damp, flaccid, + *-oma,* tumor]. A soft wartlike growth on the eyelid.

plafond (plă-fon') [Fr. ceiling]. A ceiling, especially the ceiling of the ankle joint, *i.e.,* the articular surface of the distal end of the tibia.

plagio- [G. *plagios,* oblique]. Combining form denoting oblique, slanting.

plagiocephalic (plā'jē-ō-se-fal'ik). Plagiocephalous; relating to or marked by plagiocephaly.

plagiocephalism (plā'jē-ō-sef'ă-lizm). Plagiocephaly.

plagiocephalous (plā'jē-ō-sef'ă-lŭs). Plagiocephalic.

plagiocephaly (plā'jē-ō-sef'ă-lē) [G. *plagios,* oblique, + *kephalē,* head]. Plagiocephalism; an asymmetric craniostenosis due to premature closure of the lambdoid and coronal sutures on one side; characterized by an oblique deformity of the skull.

plague (plāg) [L. *plaga,* a stroke, injury]. **1.** Any disease of wide prevalence or of excessive mortality. **2.** Pest; pestis; pestilence (1); an acute infectious disease caused by *Yersinia pestis* and marked clinically by high fever, toxemia, prostration, a petechial eruption, lymph node enlargement, and pneumonia, or hemorrhage from the mucous membranes; primarily a disease of rodents, transmitted to man by fleas that have bitten infected animals. In man the disease takes one of four clinical forms: bubonic *p.,* septicemic *p.,* pneumonic *p.,* or ambulant *p.*

ambulant p., ambulatory p., parapestis; pestis ambulans; pestis minor; larval p.; a mild form of bubonic p. characterized by symptoms such as mild fever and lymphadenitis.

black p., see black *death.*

bubonic p., pestis fulminans; pestis major; glandular p.; polyadenitis maligna; the usual form of p. marked by inflammatory enlargement of the lymphatic glands in the groins, axillae, or other parts.

cattle p., rinderpest.

duck p., a viral enteritis of ducks and other waterfowl in Europe, Asia, and the U.S. caused by a herpesvirus; manifested by weakness, lethargy, and diarrhea accompanied by catarrhal hemorrhagic enteritis and echymotic hemorrhages in organs and muscles.

fowl p., fowl pest; avian influenza; a highly fatal and highly transmissible disease of gallinaceous and passerine birds, pigeons, ducks, and geese, caused by avian influenza virus type A; symptoms include dyspnea, edema of head and neck, cyanosis, diarrhea, and sometimes disturbances of the central nervous system.

glandular p., bubonic p.

hemorrhagic p., the hemorrhagic form of bubonic p.

larval p., ambulant p.

Pahvant Valley p., tularemia.

pneumonic p., plague pneumonia; a rapidly progressive and frequently fatal form of p. in which there are areas of pulmonary consolidation, with chill, pain in the side, bloody expectoration, and high fever.

rabbit p., rabbitpox.

septicemic p., pestis siderans; a generally fatal form of p. in which there is an intense bacteremia with symptoms of profound toxemia.

sylvatic p., bubonic p. in rats and other wild animals.

plakalbumin (plak-al-byū'min). The product of the action of subtilisin upon egg albumin, removing a hexapeptide.

plakins (plā'kinz). Bactericidal substances similar to leucins extracted from blood platelets.

plan-. See plano-.

plana (plā'nă) [L.]. Plural of planum.

planchet (plan'shet) [Fr. *planchette,* dim. of *planche,* plank]. A small, flat plate or dish used to support a sample for radioactivity determination; the sample is usually evaporated on (in) the p.

Planck, Max, German physicist, 1858–1947. See P.'s *constant, theory.*

PLANE

plane (plān) [L. *planus,* flat]. **1.** A flat surface. See planum. **2.** An imaginary surface formed by extension through any axis or two definite points in reference especially to craniometry and to pelvimetry.

Addison's clinical p.'s, a series of p.'s used as landmarks in thoracoabdominal topography; the trunk is divided vertically by a *median p.* from the upper border of the manubrium sterni to the symphysis pubis, by a *lateral p.* drawn vertically on either side through a point half way between the anterior superior iliac spine and the median p. at the interspinal p., and by an *interspinal p.* passing vertically through the anterior superior iliac spine on either side; transversely the trunk is divided by a *transthoracic p.* passing across the thorax 3.2 cm above the lower border of the corpus sterni, by a *transpyloric p.* midway between the jugular notch of the sternum and the pubic symphysis, corresponding to the disk between the first and second lumbar vertebrae, and by an *intertu-*

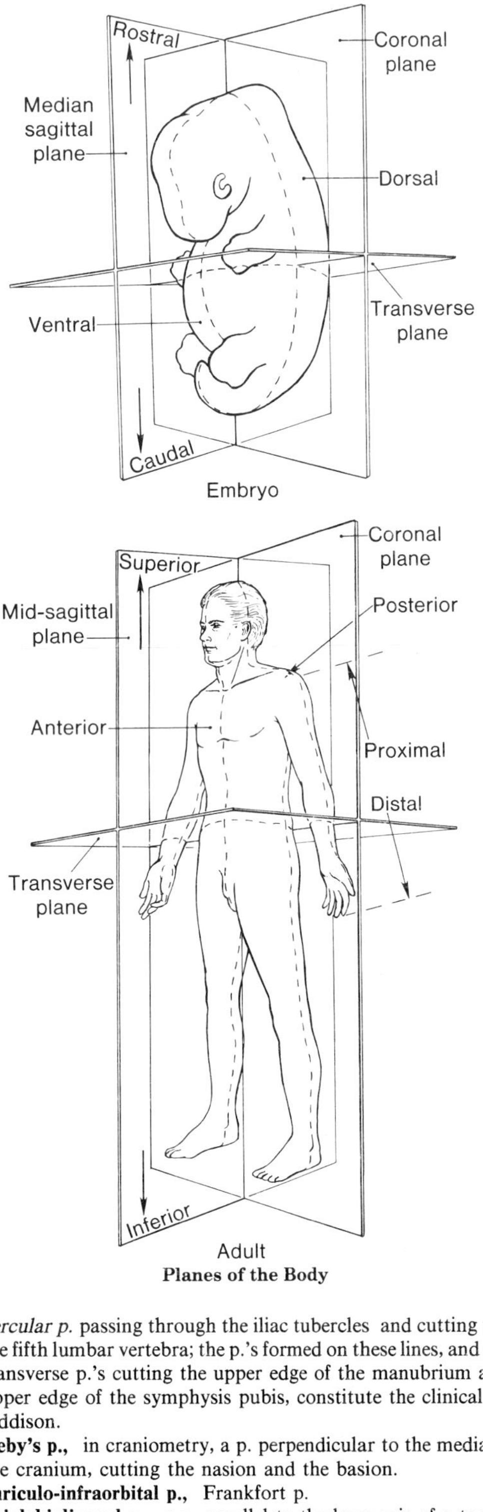

Planes of the Body

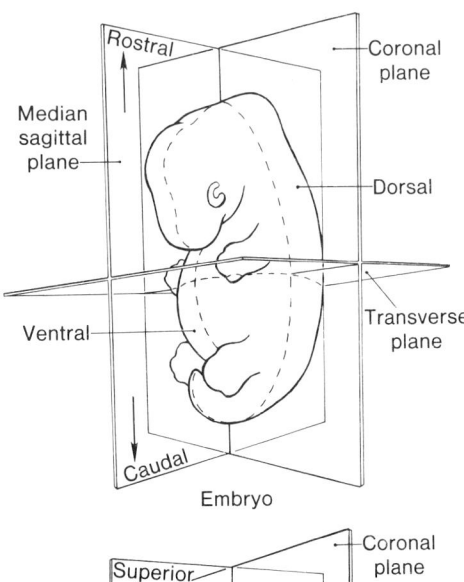

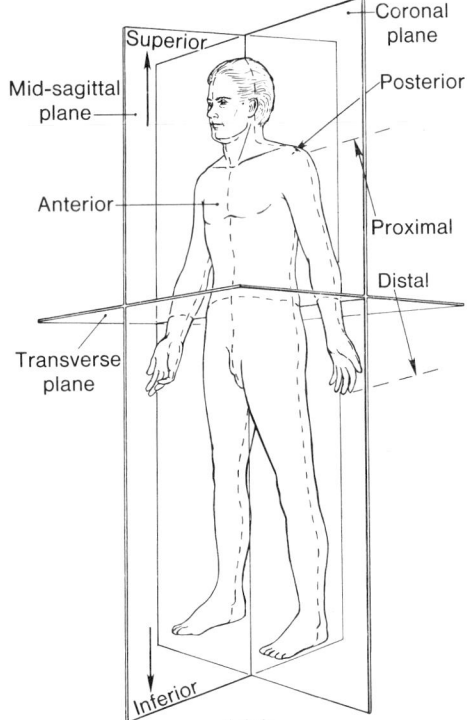

bercular p. passing through the iliac tubercles and cutting usually the fifth lumbar vertebra; the p.'s formed on these lines, and also on transverse p.'s cutting the upper edge of the manubrium and the upper edge of the symphysis pubis, constitute the clinical p.'s of Addison.
Aeby's p., in craniometry, a p. perpendicular to the median p. of the cranium, cutting the nasion and the basion.
auriculo-infraorbital p., Frankfort p.
axiolabiolingual p., a p. parallel to the long axis of a tooth and extending in a labiolingual direction.
axiomesiodistal p., a p. parallel to the long axes of the teeth and extending in a mesiodistal direction.
bite p., occlusal p.
Bolton p., Bolton-Broadbent p., Bolton-nasion p., Bolton-nasion line; a roentgenographic cephalometric p. extending from the Bolton point to nasion.
Broca's visual p., a p. drawn through the visual axes of each eye.
Camper's p., a p. running from the tip of the anterior nasal spine (acanthion) to the center of the bony external auditory meatus on the right and left sides.
canthomeatal p., a p. passing through the two lateral canthi and the center of the external acoustic meatus; this p. lies approximately midway between the Frankfort and the supraorbitmeatal p.'s.
coronal p., frontal p.; a vertical p. at right angles to a sagittal p., dividing the body into anterior and posterior portions.
datum p., an arbitrary p. used as a base from which to make craniometric measurements.
Daubenton's p., the p. of the foramen magnum. See also Daubenton's *angle,* Daubenton's *line.*
equatorial p., in metaphase of mitosis, the p. that contains all of the centromeres and their spindle attachments.
eye-ear p., Frankfort p.
facial p., nasion-pogonion measurement; a measurement of the bony profile of the face.
first parallel pelvic p., *apertura* pelvis superior.
fourth parallel pelvic p., *apertura* pelvis inferior.
Frankfort p., Frankfort horizontal p., eye-ear or auriculo-infraorbital p.; infraorbitomeatal p.; a standard craniometric reference p. passing through the right and left porion and the left orbitale; drawn on the profile radiograph or photograph from the superior margin of the acoustic meatus to the orbitale.
frontal p., coronal p.
guide p., a fixed or removable device used to displace a single tooth, an arch segment, or an entire arch toward an improved relationship.
horizontal p., transverse p.; a p. across the body at right angles to the coronal and sagittal p.'s.
p. of incidence, the p. perpendicular to a lens surface that contains the incident light ray.
infraorbitomeatal p., Frankfort p.
p. of inlet, *apertura* pelvis superior.
interspinal p., *planum* interspinale.
intertubercular p., *planum* intertuberculare.
labiolingual p., a p. parallel to the labial and lingual surfaces of the teeth.
p. of least pelvic dimensions, pelvic p. of least dimensions.
mean foundation p., the mean of the various irregularities in form and inclination of the basal seat; the ideal condition for denture stability exists when the mean foundation p. is most nearly at right angles to the direction of force.
Meckel's p., a craniometric p. cutting the alveolar and the auricular points.
median p., midsagittal p.; a vertical p. through the midline of the body that divides the body into right and left halves. See also Addison's clinical p.'s.
p. of midpelvis, pelvic p. of least dimensions.
midsagittal p., median p.
Morton's p., a p. passing through the summits of the parietal and occipital protuberances.
nasion-postcondylar p., a p. passing through the nasion anteriorly and to a point immediately behind each condylar process of the mandible, posteriorly.
nodal p., the p. corresponding to the optical center of a simple lens. See nodal *point.*
nuchal p., the external surface of the squamous part of the occipital bone below the superior nuchal line, giving attachment to the muscles of the back of the neck.
occipital p., planum occipitale; the external surface of the occipi-

tal bone above the superior nuchal line.
occlusal p., p. of occlusion, bite p.; an imaginary surface which is related anatomically to the cranium and which theoretically touches the incisal edges of the incisors and the tips of the occluding surfaces of the posterior teeth; it is not a p. in the true sense of the word but represents the mean of the curvature of the surface. See also *curve* of occlusion.
orbital p., planum orbitale; the orbital surface of the maxilla, lying perpendicular to the Frankfort p. at the orbitale.
p. of outlet, *apertura* pelvis inferior.
parasagittal p., any p. parallel to the sagittal p. or anteroposterior median p.
p. of pelvic canal, *axis* pelvis.
pelvic p. of greatest dimensions, second parallel pelvic p.; wide p.; the p. extending from the middle of the posterior surface of the pubic symphysis to the junction of the second and third sacral vertebrae, and laterally passing through the ischial bones over the middle of the acetabulum.

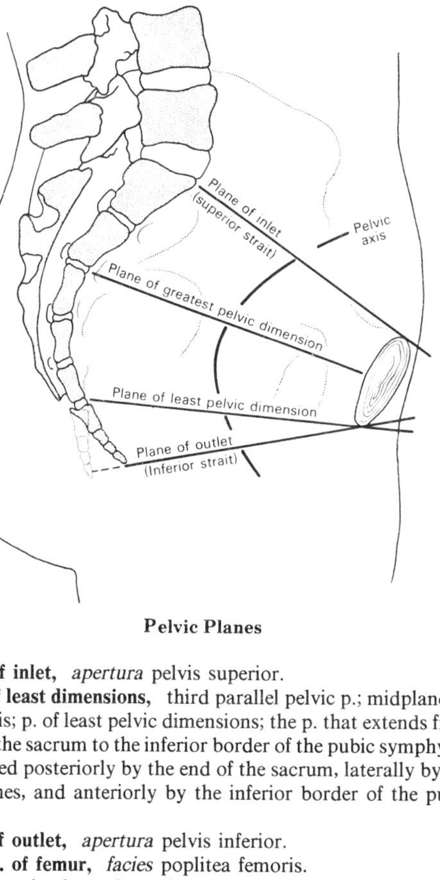

Pelvic Planes

pelvic p. of inlet, *apertura* pelvis superior.
pelvic p. of least dimensions, third parallel pelvic p.; midplane; p. of midpelvis; p. of least pelvic dimensions; the p. that extends from the end of the sacrum to the inferior border of the pubic symphysis; it is bounded posteriorly by the end of the sacrum, laterally by the ischial spines, and anteriorly by the inferior border of the pubic symphysis.
pelvic p. of outlet, *apertura* pelvis inferior.
popliteal p. of femur, *facies* poplitea femoris.
principal p., the theoretic p. of a compound lens system. See principal *point.*
p.'s of reference, p.'s which act as a guide to the location of other p.'s.
p. of regard, an imaginary p. through which the point of regard moves as the eyes are turned from side to side.
sagittal p., median p.; in a broad sense, s. p. is used for any p. parallel to the median.
second parallel pelvic p., pelvic p. of greatest dimensions.
spectacle p., the p. at which spectacles are worn.
sternal p., planum sternale; a p. indicated by the front surface of the sternum.
subcostal p., *planum* subcostale.
supracrestal p., *planum* supracristale.
supraorbitomeatal p., a p. passing the superior orbital margins and the superior margin of the external acoustic meatuses; it makes an angle of approximately 25 to 30 degrees with the Frankfort p. and is the p. in which routine CT (computed tomography) scans of the brain are made.
suprasternal p., a horizontal p. passing through the body at the level of the superior margin of the manubrium sterni.
temporal p., planum temporale; a slightly depressed area on the side of the cranium, below the inferior temporal line, formed by the temporal and parietal bones, the greater wing of the sphenoid, and a part of the frontal bone.
third parallel pelvic p., pelvic p. of least dimensions.
tooth p., any one of the imaginary p.'s of section of a tooth, such as the axial, horizontal, or vertical.
transpyloric p., *planum* transpyloricum.
transverse p., horizontal p.
wide p., pelvic p. of greatest dimensions.

plani-. See plano-.

planigraphy (pla-nig'ră-fē) [L. *planum,* plane, + G. *graphē,* a writing]. Tomography.

planimeter (plă-nim'ĕ-ter) [L. *planum,* plane, + G. *metron,* measure]. An instrument formed of jointed levers with a recording index, used for measuring the area of any surface, by tracing its boundaries.

planing (plān'ing). Dermabrasion.

planithorax (plan'i-thō'raks). A diagram of the chest showing the front and back in plane projection, after the manner of Mercator's projection of the earth's surface.

plankter (plangk'ter). Any type of plankton.

plankton (plangk'ton) [G. *planktos,* wandering]. A general term for many floating marine forms, mostly of microscopic or minute size, which are moved passively by winds, waves, tides, or currents; it includes diatoms, algae, copepods, and many protozoans, crustacea, mollusks, and worms.

planktonic (plangk-ton'ik). Relating to plankton; plankton-like.

plano-, plan-, plani-. 1 [L. *planum,* plane; *planus,* flat]. Combining forms relating to a plane, or meaning flat or level. **2** [G. *planos,* roaming, wandering]. Combining form meaning wandering.

planocellular (plā-nō-sel'yū-lăr) [L. *planus,* flat, + cellular]. Relating to or composed of flat cells.

planoconcave (plā'nō-kon'kāv). Flat on one side and concave on the other; denoting a lens of that shape.

planoconvex (plā'nō-kon'veks). Flat on one side and convex on the other; denoting a lens of that shape.

planography (pla-nog'ră-fē). Tomography.

planomania (plan-ō-mā'nē-ă) [G. *planos,* wandering, + *mania,* frenzy]. The morbid impulse to leave home and discard social restraints.

Planorbis (plan-ōr'bis) [G. *planos,* wandering, + L. *orbis,* circle, ring]. A European and North African genus of freshwater snails (family Planorbidae), including *P. planorbis,* intermediate host of the sheep and cattle fluke, *Paramphistoma cervi.*

planotopokinesia (plan'ō-top'ō-ki-nē'zē-ă) [G. *planos,* wandering, + *topos,* place, + *kinesis,* motion]. Loss of orientation in space.

planovalgus (plā-nō-val'gŭs) [plano- + L. *valgus,* turned outward]. A condition in which the longitudinal arch of the foot is flattened and everted.

planta, gen. and pl. **plantae** (plan'tă, plan'tē) [L.] [NA]. P. pedis.

p. pe'dis [NA], planta; pelma; the plantar surface or under part of the foot.

plantago (plan-tā'gō) [L. plantain]. The root and leaves of the common or large-leaved plantain, *Plantago major* (family Plantaginaceae).

p. ovata coating, the separated outer mucilaginous layers of *Plantago ovata* seeds; used in simple constipation associated with lack of sufficient bulk.

p. seed, plantain or psyllium seed, the dried ripe seed of *Plantago psyllium* or *P. arenaria* (*P. indica*) (Spanish or French psyllium seed), or of *P. ovata* (blond psyllium seed, or Indian plantago seed); light brown to chestnut brown ovate seeds, used as a laxative.

plantalgia (plan-tal'jē-ă) [L. *planta,* sole of foot, + G. *algos,* pain]. Pain on the plantar surface of the foot over the plantar fascia.

plantar (plan'tăr) [L. *plantaris*]. Relating to the sole of the foot.

plantaris (plan-tăr'is) [L.] [NA]. Plantar.

plantigrade (plan'ti-grād) [L. *planta,* sole, + *gradior,* to walk]. Walking with the entire sole and heel of the foot on the ground, as do man and bears. *Cf.* digitigrade.

planula, pl. **planulae** (plan'yū-lă, -lē) [L. dim. of *planum,* flat surface]. Name given by Lankester to a coelenterate embryo when it consists of the two primary germ layers only, the ectoderm and endoderm.

invaginate p., gastrula.

planum, pl. **plana** (plā'nŭm, plā'nă) [L. plane]. A plane or flat surface. See also plane.

p. interspina'le [NA], interspinal plane or line; linea interspinalis; Lanz's line; a horizontal plane passing through the anterior superior iliac spines; it marks the boundary between the lateral and umbilical regions superiorly and the inguinal and pubic regions inferiorly. See also Addison's clinical *planes.*

p. intertubercula're [NA], intertubercular plane or line; linea intertubercularis; a horizontal plane passing through the iliac tubercles. See also Addison's clinical *planes.*

p. occipita'le, occipital *plane.*

p. orbita'le, orbital *plane.*

p. poplite'um, *facies* poplitea femoris.

p. semiluna'tum, the area of epithelium bounding the sensory area of the crista ampullaris.

p. sphenoida'le, *jugum* sphenoidale.

p. sterna'le, sternal *plane.*

p. subcosta'le [NA], subcostal plane or line; linea subcostalis; infracostal line; a horizontal plane passing through the inferior limits of the costal margin, *i.e.,* the tenth costal cartilages; it marks the boundary between the hypochondriac and epigastric regions superiorly and the lateral and umbilical regions inferiorly.

p. supracrista'le [NA], supracrestal plane or line; linea supracristalis; a horizontal plane passing through the summits of the iliac crests; it usually passes through the fourth lumbar spinous process.

p. tempora'le, temporal *plane.*

p. transpylo'ricum [NA], transpyloric plane; a horizontal plane midway between the superior margins of the manubrium sterni and the symphysis pubis; the pyloris is not usually located on this plane. See Addison's clinical *planes.*

planuria (plă-nū'rē-ă) [G. *planos,* wandering, + *ouron,* urine]. **1.** Extravasation of urine. **2.** The voiding of urine from an abnormal opening.

plaque (plak) [Fr. a plate]. **1.** A patch or small differentiated area on a body surface (*e.g.,* skin, mucosa, or arterial endothelium) or on the cut surface of an organ such as the brain. **2.** An area of clearing in a flat confluent growth of bacteria or tissue cells, such as is caused by the lytic action of bacteriophage in an agar plate culture of bacteria, by the cytopathic effect of certain animal viruses in a sheet of cultured tissue cells, or by antibody (hemolysin) produced by lymphocytes cultured in the presence of erythrocytes and to which complement has been added. **3.** A sharply defined zone of demyelination characteristic of multiple sclerosis. **4.** See dental p.

atheromatous p., a well demarcated yellow area or swelling on the intimal surface of an artery; produced by intimal lipid deposit.

bacterial p., dental p. (2); mucous or mucinous p.; in dentistry, a mass of filamentous microorganisms and large variety of smaller forms attached to the surface of a tooth which, depending on bacterial activity and environmental factors, may give rise to caries, calculus, or inflammatory changes in adjacent tissue.

dental p., **(1)** the noncalcified accumulation mainly of oral microorganisms and their products, that adheres tenaciously to the teeth and is not readily dislodged; **(2)** bacterial p.

Hollenhorst p.'s, glittering, orange-yellow, atheromatous emboli in the retinal arterioles that contain cholesterin crystals and originate in the carotid artery.

mucous p., mucinous p., bacterial p.

neuritic p., senile p.

senile p., neuritic p.; a spherical mass of amyloid fibrils surrounded by distorted interwoven neuronal processes.

Plaque Index. An index for estimating the status of oral hygiene by measuring dental plaque which occurs in the areas adjacent to the gingival margin.

-plasia [G. *plassō,* to form]. Suffix meaning formation.

plasm (plazm). Plasma.

plasma-, plasmat-, plasmato-, plasmo- [G. *plasma,* something formed]. Combining forms denoting plasma.

plasma (plaz'mă) [G. something formed]. **1.** Blood p.; the fluid (noncellular) portion of the circulating blood, as distinguished from the serum obtained after coagulation. **2.** The fluid portion of the lymph. **3.** A "fourth state of matter" in which, owing to elevated temperature (*ca.* 10^6 degrees), atoms have broken down to form free electrons and more or less stripped nuclei; produced in the laboratory in connection with hydrogen fusion (thermonuclear) research.

antihemophilic p. (human), human p. in which the labile antihemophilic globulin component, present in fresh p., has been preserved; it is used to temporarily relieve dysfunction of the hemostatic mechanism in hemophilia.

blood p., plasma (1).

fresh frozen p. (FFP), separated p., frozen within 6 hours of collection, used in hypovolemia and coagulation factor deficiency.

p. hydrolysate, an artificial digest of protein derived from bovine blood p. prepared by a method of hydrolysis sufficient to provide more than half of the total nitrogen present in the form of α-amino nitrogen; used when high protein intake is indicated and cannot be accomplished through ordinary foods. See also *protein* hydrolysate.

p. mari'num, sea water diluted to make it isotonic with p.

muscle p., an alkaline fluid in muscle that is spontaneously coagulable, separating into myosin and muscle serum.

normal human p., citrated normal human p.; sterile p. obtained by pooling approximately equal amounts of the liquid portion of citrated whole blood from eight or more adult humans who have been certified as free from any disease which is tranmissible by transfusion, and treating it with ultraviolet irradiation to destroy possible bacterial and viral contaminants.

salted p., salted serum; the fluid portion of blood drawn from the vessels, which is prevented from coagulating by being drawn into a solution of sodium or magnesium sulfate.

plasmablast (plaz'mă-blast) [plasma + G. *blastos,* germ]. Plasmacytoblast; precursor of the plasma cell.

plasmacrit (plaz'mă-krit) [plasma + G. *krinō,* to separate]. A measure of the percentage of the volume of blood occupied by plasma, in contrast to a hematocrit.

plasmacyte (plaz'mă-sīt). Plasma *cell.*

plasmacytoblast (plas-mă-sī'tō-blast). Plasmablast.

plasmacytoma (plaz'mă-sī-tō'mă) [plasmacyte + G. *-oma,* tumor]. A discrete, presumably solitary mass of neoplastic plasma cells in bone or in one of various extramedullary sites; in man, such lesions are probably the initial phase of developing plasma cell myeloma.

plasmacytosis (plaz'mă-sī-tō'sis) [plasmacyte + G. *-osis,* condition]. **1.** Presence of plasma cells in the circulating blood. **2.** Presence of unusually large proportions of plasma cells in the tissues or exudates.

plasma expander (plaz'mă eks-pan'der). Plasma *substitute.*

plasmagene (plaz'mă-jēn) [plasma + gene]. Cytogene; a determinant of an inherited character located in the cytoplasm.

plasmals (plaz'mălz). Long chain aldehydes occurring in plasmalogens; *e.g.,* stearaldehyde, palmitaldehyde.

plasmalemma (plaz-mă-lem'ă) [plasma + G. *lemma,* husk]. Cell *membrane.*

plasmalogens (plaz-mal'ō-jenz). Phosphoglyceracetals; generic term for glycerophospholipids in which the glycerol moiety bears a 1-alkenyl ether group; e.g., alk-1-enylglycerophospholipid.

plasmapheresis (plaz'mă-fē-rē'sis) [plasma + G. *aphairesis,* a withdrawal]. Removal of whole blood from the body, separation of its cellular elements by centrifugation, and reinfusion of them suspended in saline or some other plasma substitute, thus depleting the body's own plasma without depleting its cells.

plasmapheretic (plaz'mă-fē-ret'ik). Relating to plasmapheresis.

plasmat-, plasmato-. See plasma-.

plasmatic (plaz-mat'ik). Plasmic; relating to plasma.

plasmatogamy (plaz-mă-tog'ă-mē). Plasmogamy.

plasmenic acid (plaz'men-ik). Proposed name for phosphatidates such as alk-1-enylglycerol (lipid).

plasmic (plaz'mik). Plasmatic.

plasmid (plaz'mid). Extra chromosomal element; extra chromosomal genetic element; paragene; a genetic particle that can stably function and replicate while physically separate from the chromosome of the host cell (chiefly bacterial) and that is not essential to the cell's basic functioning.

bacteriocinogenic p.'s, bacteriocinogens; bacteriocin factors; bacterial p.'s responsible for the elaboration of bacteriocins.

conjugative p., transmissible or infectious p.; a p. that can effect its own intercellular transfer by means of conjugation; this is accomplished by the bacterium being rendered a donor, a usual characteristic of which is the presence of specialized pili.

F p., F agent or factor; fertility agent or factor; sex factor; the prototype conjugative p. associated with conjugation in the K-12 strain of *Escherichia coli.*

F'p., F' agent or factor; F genote; a p. (episome) in which a segment of the bacterial chromosome has been included in an F p.

infectious p., conjugative p.

nonconjugative p., a p. that cannot effect conjugation and self-transfer to another bacterium (bacterial strain); transfer depends upon mediation of another (conjugative) p.

R p.'s, resistance p.'s

resistance p.'s, R p.'s or factors; resistance-transferring episomes; resistance factors; p.'s carrying genes responsible for antibiotic (or antibacterial drug) resistance among bacteria (notably Enterobacteriaceae); they may be conjugative or nonconjugative p.'s, the former possessing transfer genes (resistance transfer factor) lacking in the latter.

transmissible p., conjugative p.

plasmin (plaz'min) [EC 3.4.21.7]. Fibrinolysin; fibrinase (2); an enzyme hydrolyzing peptides and esters of arginine and lysine, and converting fibrin to soluble products; occurs in plasma as plasminogen (profibrinolysin) and is activated to plasmin by organic solvents, which remove an inhibitor, and by streptokinase, trypsin, and plasminogen activator, all cleaving a single arginyl-valyl bond.

plasminogen (plaz-min'ō-jen). See plasmin.

plasminokinase (plaz'min-ō-kī'nās). Streptokinase.

plasminoplastin (plaz'min-ō-plas'tin). Term proposed for activator agents that produce plasmin by direct action on plasminogen; *e.g.,* staphylokinase, plasminogen activator.

plasmo-. See plasma-.

plasmodia (plaz-mō'dē-ă) [L.]. Plural of plasmodium.

plasmodial (plaz-mō'dē-ăl). **1.** Relating to a plasmodium. **2.** Relating to any species of the genus *Plasmodium.*

plasmodiotrophoblast (plaz-mō'dē-ō-trō'fō-blast) [plasmodium + G. *trophē,* nourishment, + *blastos,* germ]. Syncytiotrophoblast.

Plasmodium (plaz-mō'dē-ŭm) [Mod. L. from G. *plasma,* something formed, + *eidos,* appearance]. A genus of the family Plasmodidae (suborder Haemosporina, subclass Coccidia), blood parasites of vertebrates, characterized by separate microgametes and macrogametes, a motile ookinete, sporogony in the invertebrate host, and merogony (schizogony) in the vertebrate host; includes the causal agents of malaria in man and other animals, with an asexual cycle occurring in liver and red blood cells of vertebrates and a sexual cycle in mosquitoes, the latter cycle resulting in the production of large numbers of infective sporozoites in the salivary glands of the vector which are transmitted when the mosquito bites and draws blood. Primate malaria is transmitted by various species of *Anopheles mosquitoes,* bird malaria by species of *Aedes, Culex, Anopheles,* and *Culiseta.*

P. aethio'picum, *P. falciparum.*

P. ber'ghei, a species that is the etiologic agent of rodent malaria from central Africa; an important source of experimental nonprimate mammal malaria.

P. brazilian'um, a species found in New World monkeys of the family Cebidae in northern South America and Panama which can cause mild malaria in man.

P. catheme'rium, a species that is the cause of a rapidly fatal, anemia-producing disease in canaries, also infecting sparrows and other passerine birds.

P. cynomol'gi, a species similar to *P. vivax* occurring naturally in the macaque, but infecting man both accidentally and experimentally; it produces a *P. vivax* type of malaria.

P. du'rae, a species that is the cause of an acute and often fatal malaria of young turkeys in Africa.

P. falcip'arum, *P. aethiopicum;* malignant tertian malarial parasite; *Laverania falciparum,* a species that is the causal agent of falciparum (malignant tertian) malaria; a young trophozoite is about one-fifth the size of an erythrocyte, but developing erythrocytic stages are rarely seen in circulating blood, as they render infected cells sticky and cause them to concentrate in pulmonary capillaries; a schizont occupies about one-half to two-thirds of the red blood cell and has fine sparse granules (observed in peripheral blood only from moribund patients); infected erythrocytes are normal or contracted in size and are likely to contain basophilic granules and red dots (Maurer's clefts or dots); multiple infection is extremely frequent and causes bouts of fever somewhat irregularly since the parasites' cycles of multiplication is usually asynchronous.

P. gallina'ceum, a species that is the cause of malaria in domestic chickens in southern Asia and Indonesia, sometimes with high mortality.

P. juxtanuclea're, a species that is a cause of chicken malaria in Mexico and South America, and in Sri Lanka and Malaysia.

P. knowles'i, a species from Southeast Asia that causes monkey malaria with a quotidian fever cycle; highly fatal in rhesus monkeys; naturally acquired by a human in Malayasia, and also transmitted to man experimentally.

P. ko'chi, a *P.* species now recognized as *Hepatocystis kochi.*

P. mala'riae, quartan parasite; a species that is the causal agent of quartan malaria; a ring-stage trophozoite is triangular, ovoid, or slightly bean-shaped, with fine or coarse black granules, approximately one-third the size of an eythrocyte; the schizont is oval or rounded, and nearly fills the red blood cell; infected erythrocytes are normal or slightly contracted in size, usually with no stippling (the two most important characteristics that distinguish it from *P. vivax*), although extremely fine Ziemann's dots may be observed; multiple infection is extremely rare, thus bouts of fever occur fairly regularly at 72-hour intervals; prolonged asymptomatic parasitemia is characteristic of the species and recrudescence of fever may occur 10 years or more after the initial episode.

P. ova'le, a species that is the agent of the least common form of human malaria; resembles *P. vivax* in its earlier stages, but often modifies the cell membrane, causing it to form a fimbriated outline, and often assume an oval shape; Schüffner's dots are abundant and appear early, host cells are normal or only slightly enlarged, and only about 8 to 10 grapelike merozoites are produced; fever is tertian and relapses are infrequent.

P. relic'tum, a species of worldwide distribution found in pigeons, doves, ducks, swans, and a great variety of other birds; it is highly pathogenic in pigeons, game birds, and others to which this strain is poorly adapted, causing anemia, weakness, and often death.

P. vi'vax, tertian parasite; a species that is the most common malarial parasite of man (except in west Africa, where lack of the Duffy antigen protects most of the resident populations, which has permitted *P. ovale* to replace *P. vivax*); the early trophozoite is irregular and ameboid in shape, one-fourth to one-third the size of a red blood cell, and contains several fine granules; the schizont is irregular in shape, fills the enlarged erythrocyte, and contains numerous yellow-brown pigment granules; affected red blood cells are pale, enlarged, and contain Schüffner's dots in the later stages of growth; multiple infection is common, causing bouts of fever fairly regularly at 48-hour intervals.

plasmodium, pl. **plasmodia** (plaz-mō'dē-ŭm, -dē-ă) [Mod. L. fr. G. *plasma,* something formed, + *eidos,* appearance]. A protoplasmic mass containing several nuclei, resulting from multiplication of the nucleus with cell division.

placental p., syncytiotrophoblast.

Plasmodromata (plaz-mō-drō'mă-tă) [plasmo- + G. *dromos,* a running, a course]. A former taxonomic category that included ameboid and flagellate Protozoa in which the nucleus is not separated into reproductive (micro-) and vegetative (macro-) portions; equivalent to the present phylum Sarcomastigophora.

plasmogamy (plaz-mog'ă-mē) [plasmo- + G. *gamos,* marriage]. Plasmatogamy; plastogamy; union of two or more cells with preservation of the individual nuclei; formation of a plasmodium.

plasmogen (plaz'mō-jen) [plasmo- + G. *-gen,* producing]. Protoplasm.

plasmokinin (plaz-mō-kī'nin). *Factor* VIII.

plasmolemma (plaz-mō-lem'ă). Cell *membrane.*

plasmolysis (plaz-mol'i-sis) [plasmo- + G. *lysis,* dissolution]. Protoplasmolysis. **1.** Dissolution of cellular components. **2.** Shrinking of plant cells by osmotic loss of cytoplasmic water.

plasmolytic (plaz-mō-lit'ik). Relating to plasmolysis.

plasmolyze (plaz'mō-līz). To cause the dissolution of the cellular constituents.

plasmon (plaz'mon). Plasmotype; the total of the genetic properties of the cell cytoplasm.

plasmorrhexis (plaz-mō-rek'sis). The splitting open of a cell from the pressure of the protoplasm.

plasmoschisis (plaz-mos'ki-sis) [plasmo- + G. *schisis,* a cleaving]. The splitting of protoplasm into fragments.

plasmosin (plaz'mō-sin). A highly viscous substance in cytoplasm containing discrete fibers of considerable length; a nucleoprotein regarded as the structural foundation of the cell.

plasmosome (plaz'mō-sōm) [plasmo- + G. *sōma,* body]. Obsolete term for nucleolus.

plasmotomy (plaz-mot'ō-mē) [plasmo- + G. *tomē,* incision]. A form of mitosis in multinuclear protozoan cells in which the cytoplasm divides into two or more masses, later reproducing, in some cases by sporulation.

plasmotropic (plaz-mō-trop'ik). Pertaining to or manifesting plasmotropism.

plasmotropism (plaz-mot'rō-pizm) [plasmo- + G. *tropē,* a turning]. A condition in which the bone marrow, spleen, and liver contain strongly hemolytic bodies that cause the destruction of the erythrocytes, although the latter are not affected while in the circulating blood.

plasmotype (plaz'mō-tīp). Plasmon.

plasmozyme (plaz'mō-zīm) [plasmo- + G. *zymē,* leaven]. Prothrombin.

plastein (plas'tē-in). Insoluble polypeptide formed through the random condensation of amino acid or peptides under the catalytic influence of a proteinaselike chymotrypsin; molecular weights as high as 500,000 are reported.

plas'ter [L. *emplastrum;* G. *emplastron,* plaster or mold]. **1.** A solid preparation which can be spread when heated, and which becomes adhesive at the temperature of the body; used to keep the edges of a wound in apposition, to protect raw surfaces, and, when medicated, to redden or blister the skin or to apply drugs to the surface to obtain their systemic effects. **2.** In dentistry, colloquialism for p. of Paris.

p. of Paris, exsiccated calcium sulfate from which the water of crystallization has been expelled by heat, but which, when mixed with water, will form a paste which subsequently sets.

plastic (plas'tik) [G. *plastikos,* relating to molding]. **1.** Capable of being formed or molded. **2.** A material that can be shaped by pressure or heat to the form of a cavity or mold.

Bingham p., a material that, in the idealized case, does not flow until a critical stress (yield stress) is exceeded, and then flows at a rate proportional to the excess of stress over the yield stress; real materials probably only approach this ideal model.

modeling p., modeling composition; impression or modeling compound; a thermoplastic material usually composed of gum damar and prepared chalk, used especially for making dental impressions.

plasticity (plas-tis'i-tē). The capability of being formed or molded; the quality of being plastic.

plastid (plas'tid) [G. *plastos,* formed, + -id]. **1.** Trophoplast; one of the differentiated structures in cytoplasm of plant cells where photosynthesis or other cellular processes are carried on. **2.** One of the granules of foreign or differentiated matter, food particles, fat, waste material, chromatophores, trichocysts, etc., in cells. **3.** A self-duplicating virus-like particle that multiplies within a host cell, such as kappa particles in certain paramecia.

blood p., any basic, morphologic unit in the biologic composition of blood, *e.g.,* an erythrocyte.

plastochromanol-3, plastochromanol E_3 (plas-tō-krō'man-ol). γ-Tocotrienol.

plastochromenol-8 (plas-tō-krō'men-ol). Solanochromene; the chromenol (isomeric) form of plastoquinone-9.

plastogamy (plas-tog'ă-mē). Plasmogamy.

plastoquinone (plas-tō-kwin'ōn, -kwī'nōn). 2,3-Dimethyl-1,4-benzoquinone with a multiprenyl side chain; a trivial name sometimes used for plastoquinone-9.

plastoquinone-9, plastoquinone E_9 (PQ-9). 2,3-Dimethyl-6-nonaprenyl-1,4-benzoquinone; one of a group of vitamins E and K and coenzymes Q; the isomeric form is plastochromenol-8.

plas'tron [Fr. a breastplate]. The sternum with costal cartilages attached.

-plasty [G. *plastos,* formed, shaped]. Suffix meaning molding or shaping or the result thereof, as of a surgical procedure.

plasty (plas'tē) [G. *plastos,* formed]. Surgical procedure for repair of a defect or restoration of form and/or function of a part.

plate (plāt) [O.Fr. *plat,* a flat object, fr. G. *platys,* flat, broad]. **1.** In anatomy, a thin, flat, structure, such as a lamina or lamella. **2.** A metal bar applied to a fractured bone in order to maintain the ends in apposition. **3.** The agar layer within a Petri dish or similar vessel. **4.** To form a very thin layer of a bacterial culture by streaking it on the surface of an agar p. (usually within a Petri dish) in order to isolate individual organisms from which a colonial clone will develop.

alar p. of neural tube, *lamina* alaris.
anal p., the anal portion of the cloacal p.
axial p., the primitive streak of an embryo.
basal p. of neural tube, *lamina* basalis.
base p., see baseplate.
blood p., platelet.
bone p., a metal bar with perforations for the insertion of screws; used to immobilize fractured segments.
buttress p., a metal p. used to support the internal fixation of a fracture.
cardiogenic p., the thickened layer of mesoderm from which the cardiopericardial primordia of very young embryos are derived.
chorionic p., that portion of the chorionic wall in the region of its uterine attachment; it consists of the mesoderm which lines the chorionic vesicle and is covered, on the maternal side, by the trophoblast which lines the intervillous spaces; in the last half of gestation, the mesodermal connective tissue is largely replaced by fibrinoid material, and the amniotic membrane is adherent to the fetal side of the plate.
cloacal p., a p., composed of a layer of cloacal endoderm in contact with a layer of proctodeal ectoderm, which subsequently ruptures, forming the anal and urogenital openings of the embryo.
cribriform p. of ethmoid bone, *lamina* cribrosa ossis ethmoidalis.
cutis p., dermatome (2).
dorsal p. of neural tube, *lamina* alaris.
end p., see endplate.
epiphysial p., *cartilago* epiphysialis.
equatorial p., the collected chromosomes at the equator of the spindle in the process of mitosis.
ethmovomerine p., the central portion of the ethmoid bone, forming a distinct element at birth.
flat p., a survey radiograph, usually of the abdomen without use of contrast media and with the patient recumbent; significant as an historic comparison to the characteristics of flexible film.
floor p., ventral p.; the thin ventral portion of the embryonic neural tube which merges on either side with the basal portion of the lateral p.'s.
foot p., see footplate.
frontal p., in the fetus, a cartilage p. between the lateral parts of ethmoid cartilage and the developing sphenoid bone.
horizontal p. of palatine bone, *lamina* horizontalis ossis palatini.
Kühne's p., the endplate of a motor nerve fiber in a muscle spindle.
Lane's p.'s, flattened, narrow, metal p.'s of various shapes and sizes, perforated for screws; used to hold the fragments of a fractured bone in apposition.
lateral p., a nonsegmented mass of mesoderm on the lateral periphery of the embryonic disk.
lateral p. of pterygoid process, *lamina* lateralis processus pterygoidei.
left p. of thyroid cartilage, *lamina* sinistra cartilaginis thyroidea.
lingual p., linguoplate.
medial p. of pterygoid process, *lamina* medialis processus pterygoidei.
medullary p., neural p.
p. of modiolus, *lamina* modioli.
motor p., a motor endplate.
muscle p., myotome (2).
nail p., unguis.
neural p., medullary p; the unpaired neuroectodermal region of the early embryo's dorsal surface which in later development is transformed into the neural tube and neural crest.
neutralization p., a metal p. used for the internal fixation of a long bone fracture to neutralize the forces producing displacement.
notochordal p., the sheet of notochordal cells that are intercalated in the endodermal roof of the primitive yolk sac.
oral p., a circumscribed area of fusion of foregut endoderm and stomodeal ectoderm in the embryo which breaks through early in development to establish the oral opening.
orbital p., *lamina* orbitalis ossis ethmoidalis.
palatal p., a partial denture major connector that has an anteroposterior width in excess of two maxillary premolars.
paper p., papyraceous p., *lamina* orbitalis ossis ethmoidalis.
parachordal p., the cartilage primordia of the base of the skull situated on either side of the cephalic part of the notochord.
parietal p., the outer of the two layers of the lateral mesoderm which becomes associated with the ectoderm; together they constitute the somatopleure.
perpendicular p., *lamina* perpendicularis.
polar p.'s, condensed platelike bodies at the ends of the spindle during mitosis of certain types of cells.
prechordal p., prochordal p.
prochordal p., prechordal p.; a small area immediately rostral to the cephalic tip of the notochord where ectoderm and endoderm are in contact; when turned under the growing head, it forms the oral p. in the floor of the stomodeum.
pterygoid p.'s, see *lamina* lateralis processus pterygoidei *lamina* medialis processus pterygoidei.
quadrigeminal p., *lamina* tecti mesencephali.
right p. of thyroid cartilage, *lamina* dextra cartilaginis thyroidea.
roof p., roofplate; the thin layer of the embryonic neural tube connecting the lateral p.'s dorsally.
secondary spiral p., *lamina* spiralis secundaria.
segmental p., segmental *zone.*
sieve p., *lamina* cribrosa ossis ethmoidalis.
sole p., obsolete term for sarcoplasm in which the ending of a motor nerve supposedly was embedded; now shown by electron microscopy that the nerve fiber does not penetrate the sarcolemma.
spiral p., *lamina* spiralis ossea.
suction p., in dentistry, a p. held in place by atmospheric pressure.
tarsal p.'s, see *tarsus* superior; *tarsus* inferior.
terminal p., *lamina* terminalis cerebri.
tympanic p., the bony p. between the anterior wall of the external acoustic meatus and the tympanic cavity and the posterior wall of the mandibular fossa.
urethral p., an epithelial p. located ventromedially in the developing genital tubercle of a young embryo; it later opens to form the lining of the penile urethra.
ventral p., floor p.
ventral p. of neural tube, *lamina* basalis.
vertical p., *lamina* perpendicularis.
visceral p., the inner of the two layers of the lateral mesoderm; the splanchnic mesoderm which becomes associated with the endoderm; together they constitute the splanchnopleure.
wing p., *lamina* alaris.

Plateau, Joseph Antoine Ferdinand, Belgian physicist, 1801–1883.

See P.-Talbot *law.*

plateau (plă-tō) [Fr.]. A flat elevated segment of a graphic record.
ventricular p., a level portion of the intraventricular blood pressure curve, representing graphically the maintenance of contraction of the ventricle.

platelet (plāt'let) [see plate]. An irregularly shaped disklike cytoplasmic fragment of a megakaryocyte which is shed in the marrow sinus and subsequently found in the peripheral blood where it functions in clotting. A p. contains granules in the central part (granulomere) and, peripherally, clear protoplasm (hyalomere), but no definite nucleus; is about one-third to one-half the size of an erythrocyte; and contains no hemoglobin. Also called blood p.; thrombocyte; thromboplastid (1); hemolamella; elementary particle(1) or body (2); Deetjen's bodies; Zimmermann's corpuscle, granule, or elementary particle; Hayem's hematoblast; blood disk or plate; Bizzozero's or third corpuscle.

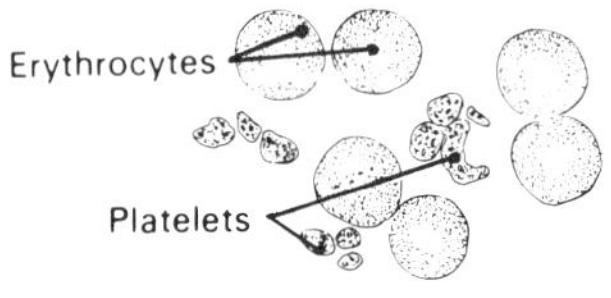

Blood Platelets
With erythrocytes for comparison of size (drawing taken from dry, stained smear of human blood).

plateletpheresis (plāt'let-fē-rē'sis) [platelet + G. *aphairesis,* a withdrawal]. Removal of blood from a donor with replacement of all blood components except platelets.

plating (plāt'ing). **1.** Sowing of bacteria on a solid medium in a Petri dish or similar container; the making of a plate culture. **2.** Application of a metal strip to keep the ends of a fractured bone in apposition. **3.** Electrolytic deposition of a metal.
compression p., a technique for internal fixation of fractures in which plates and screws are applied so as to produce compression of the line of fracture.

platinic (pla-tin'ik). Relating to platinum; denoting a compound containing platinum in its higher valency.

platinous (plat'i-nŭs). Relating to platinum; denoting a compound containing platinum in its lower valency.

platinum (plat'i-nŭm) [Mod. L., originally *platina,* fr. Sp. *plata,* silver]. A metallic element, symbol Pt, atomic No. 78, atomic weight 195.09, used for making small parts for chemical apparatus because of its resistance to acids; in powdered form **(p. black)** it is an important catalyst in hydrogenation. Some of its salts have been used in the treatment of syphilis.

platinum foil. Pure platinum rolled into extremely thin sheets; its high fusing point makes it suitable as a matrix for various soldering procedures in dentistry, and also suitable for providing internal form to porcelain restorations during their fabrication.

platinum group. A group of six amphoteric elements: iridium, osmium, palladium, platinum, rhodium, and ruthenium.

Platt, Sir Harry, British surgeon, *1886. See Putti-P. *operation, procedure.*

platy- [G. *platys,* flat, broad]. Combining form denoting width or flatness.

platybasia (plat-i-bā'sē-ă) [*platy-* + G. *basis,* ground]. Basilar invagination; a developmental anomaly of the skull or an acquired softening of the skull bones so that the floor of the posterior cranial fossa bulges upward in the region about the foramen magnum.

platycephaly (plat'i-sef'ă-lē) [platy- + G. *kephalē,* head]. Platycrania; flatness of the skull, a condition in which the vertical cranial index is below 70.

platycnemia (plat'ik-nē'mē-ă) [platy- + G. *knēmē,* leg]. Platycnemism; a condition in which the tibia is abnormally broad and flat.

platycnemic (plat'ik-nē'mik). Relating to or marked by platycnemia.

platycnemism (plat'ik-nē'mizm). Platycnemia.

platycrania (plat'i-krā'nē-ă) [platy- + G. *kranion,* skull]. Platycephaly.

platycyte (plat'i-sīt) [platy- + G. *kytos,* cell]. A relatively small giant cell sometimes formed in tubercles.

platyglossal (plat'i-glos'ăl) [platy- + G. *glōssa,* tongue]. Having a broad, flattened tongue.

platyhelminth (plat-i-hel'minth) [platy- + G. *helmins,* worm]. Common name for any flatworm of the phylum Platyhelminthes; any cestode (tapeworm) or trematode (fluke).

Platyhelminthes (plat'i-hel-min'thēz). A phylum of flatworms that are bilaterally symmetric, flattened, and acelomate. There is no digestive tract in some platyhelminths (Cestoda), or the gut may be incomplete (without an anus), as in the Trematoda; most of the forms are hermaphroditic. There are three major classes, but the parasitic species of medical and veterinary importance are in the subclass Cestoda (the true tapeworms) of the class Cestoidea, and in the subclass Digenea (the digenetic flukes) of the class Trematoda.

platyhieric (plat-i-hī-er'ik) [platy- + G. *heiron,* sacrum]. Having a broad sacrum.

platymeric (plat-i-mē'rik, -mer'ik) [platy- + G. *mēros,* thigh]. Having a broad femur.

platymorphia (plat'i-mōr'fē-ă) [platy- + G. *morphē,* shape]. Having a flat shape; denoting an eye with a short anteroposterior axis.

platyopia (plat'i-ō'pē-ă) [platy- + G. *ōps,* eye, face]. Broadness of the face; denoting a condition in which the orbitonasal index is less than 107.5.

platyopic (plat'i-op'ik, -ō'pik). Relating to or characterized by platyopia.

platypellic (plat-i-pel'ik) [platy- + G. *pellis,* bowl (pelvis)]. Platypelloid; having a broad pelvis, with an index below 90°. See platypellic *pelvis.*

platypelloid (plat-ē-pel'oyd). Platypellic.

platypnea (plă-tip'nē-ă) [platy- + G. *pnoē,* a breathing]. Difficulty in breathing when erect, relieved by recumbency. *Cf.* orthopnea.

platyrrhine (plat'i-rīn) [platy- + G. *rhis,* nose]. **1.** Characterized by a nose of large width in proportion to its length. **2.** Denoting a skull with a nasal index between 53 and 58.

platyrrhiny (plat'i-rī-nē). A condition in which the nose is wide in proportion to its length.

platysma, pl. **platysmas, platysmata** (plă-tiz'mă, -tiz'mă-tă) [G. *platysma,* a flatplate] [NA]. Musculus platysma; musculus platysma myoides; musculus subcutaneous colli; musculus tetragonus; panniculus carnosus muscle (2); tetragonus; *origin,* subcutaneous layer and fascia covering pectoralis major and deltoid at level of first or second rib; *insertion,* lower border of mandible, risorius and platysma of opposite side; *action,* depresses lower lip, wrinkles skin of neck and upper chest; *nerve supply,* cervical branch of facial.

platyspondylia, platyspondylisis (plat-i-spon-dil'ē-ă, plat'i-spon-dil'i-sis) [platy- + G. *spondylos,* vertebra]. Flatness of the bodies of the vertebrae.

platystencephaly (plă-tis'ten-sef'ă-lē) [G. *platystos,* widest, superl. of *platys,* wide, + *enkephalē,* brain]. Extreme width of the skull in the occipital region, with narrowing anteriorly and prognathism.

Plaut, Hugo K., German physician, 1858–1928. See P.'s *bacillus.*

Pleasure, Max A., U.S. dentist. See P. *curve.*

plectridium (plek-trid′ē-ŭm) [Mod. L. dim. of G. *plēktron,* an instrument to strike with]. A bacterial rod-shaped cell that contains a spore at one end, imparting a drumstick shape to the cell, such as the spore-containing cells in the organism causing tetanus, *Clostridium tetani.*

pledget (plej′et). A tuft of wool, cotton, or lint.

-plegia [G. *plēgē,* stroke]. Suffix denoting paralysis.

pleio-. Rarely used alternative spelling for pleo-.

pleiotropic (plī-ō-trop′ik). Polyphenic; denoting, or characterized by, pleiotropy.

pleiotropy, pleiotropia (plī-ot′rō-pē, plī′ō-trō′pē-ă) [pleio- + G. *tropos,* turning]. Production by a single mutant gene of apparently unrelated multiple effects at the clinical or phenotypic level; a pleiotropic gene produces a clinical syndrome.

pleo- [G. *pleiōn,* more]. Combining form denoting more.

pleochroic (plē-ō-krō′ik) [pleo- + G. *chroa,* color]. Pleochromatic.

pleochroism (plē-ok′rō-izm). Pleochromatism.

pleochromatic (plē-ō-krō-mat′ik). Pleochroic; relating to pleochromatism.

pleochromatism (plē-ō-krō′mă-tizm) [pleo- + G. *chrōma,* color]. Pleochroism; property of showing changes of color when illuminated along different axes, as certain crystals or liquids.

pleocytosis (ple′ō-sī-tō′sis) [pleo- + G. *kytos,* cell, + *-ōsis,* condition]. Presence of more cells than normal, often denoting leukocytosis and especially lymphocytosis or round cell infiltration; orginally applied to the lymphocytosis of the cerebrospinal fluid present in syphilis of the central nervous system.

pleomastia, pleomazia (plē-ō-mas′tē-ă, -mā′zē-ă) [pleo- + G. *mastos,* breast]. Polymastia.

pleomorphic (plē-ō-mōr′fik). **1.** Polymorphic. **2.** Among fungi, having two or more spore forms; also used to describe a sterile mutant dermatophyte resulting from degenerative changes in culture.

pleomorphism (plē-ō-mōr′fizm) [pleo- + G. *morphē,* form]. Polymorphism.

pleomorphous (plē-ō-mōr′fŭs). Polymorphic.

pleonasm (plē′ō-nazm) [G. *pleonasmos,* exaggeration, excessive, fr. *pleiōn,* more]. Excess in number or size of parts.

pleonectic (plē-ō-nek′tik). Obsolete term denoting specifically a blood that has a percentage saturation of oxygen above normal at any given pressure. See also mesectic; mionectic.

pleonexia (plē-ō-nek′sē-ă) [pleo- + G. *echō,* fut. *hexō,* to have]. Excessive greediness.

pleonosteosis (plē′on-os-tē-ō′sis) [pleo- + G. *osteon,* bone, + *-osis,* condition]. Superabundance of bone formation.

Leri's p., dyschondrosteosis.

pleoptics (plē-op′tiks) [pleo- + optics]. A term introduced by Bangerter to include all forms of treatment for amblyopia, particularly that associated with eccentric fixation.

pleoptophor (plē-op′tō-fōr) [pleo- + G. *optos,* visible, + *phoros,* bearing]. An instrument for the treatment of amblyopia.

plerocercoid (plē-rō-ser′koyd) [G. *plērēs,* full, complete, + *kerkos,* tail]. A stage in the development of a tapeworm following the procercoid stage, which develops in an animal serving as the second or subsequent intermediate host; a wormlike nonsegmented larva with an invaginated scolex at one end, usually unencysted in the flesh of various fishes, reptiles, or amphibians, the ingestion of which transmits the parasite to the final host. See also *Diphyllobothrium latum.*

plesio- [G. *plēsios,* close, near]. Combining form denoting nearness or similarity.

plesiomorphic (plē′sē-ō-mōr′fik). Plesiomorphous; similar in form.

plesiomorphism (plē′sē-ō-mōr′fizm) [plesio- + G. *morphē,* form]. Similarity in form.

plesiomorphous (plē′sē-ō-mōr′fŭs). Plesiomorphic.

pless-, plessi- [G. *plēssō,* to strike]. Combining forms denoting a striking, especially percussion.

plessesthesia (ples-es-thē′zē-ă) [G. *plēssō,* to strike, + *aisthēsis,* sensation]. Palpatory *percussion.*

plessimeter (ple-sim′ĕ-ter) [G. *plēssō,* to strike, + *metron,* measure]. Pleximeter; plexometer; an oblong flexible plate used in mediate percussion by being placed against the surface and struck with the plessor.

plessimetric (ples-i-met′rik). Relating to a plessimeter.

plessor (ples′er) [G. *plēssō,* to strike]. Plexor; percussor; a small hammer, usually with soft rubber head, used to tap the part directly, or with a plesssimeter, in percussion of the chest or other part.

plethora (pleth′ō-ră) [G. *plēthōrē,* fullness, fr. *plēthō,* to become full]. Repletion. **1.** Hypervolemia. **2.** An excess of any of the body fluids.

plethoric (ple-thōr′ik, pleth′ō-rik). Sanguine (1); sanguineous (2); relating to plethora.

plethysmograph (plĕ-thiz′mō-graf) [G. *plēthysmos,* increase, + *graphō,* to write]. A device for measuring and recording changes in volume of a part, organ, or whole body.

body p., a chamber apparatus surrounding the entire body, commonly used in studies of respiratory function.

pressure p., **(1)** a p. applied to part of the body, *e.g.,* a limb segment, and arranged so that volume is measured during temporary application of sufficient pressure to the part to empty its blood vessels; **(2)** a body p. in which changes of body volume are measured in terms of the consequent changes in air pressure in the body p.

volume-displacement p., a p., usually a body p., in which changes in volume displace a corresponding volume into or out of a very compliant measuring device, such as a Krogh spirometer or integrating flowmeter.

plethysmography (pleth-iz-mog′ră-fē) [G. *plēthysmos,* increase, + *graphē,* a writing]. Measuring and recording changes in volume of an organ or other part of the body by a plethysmograph.

impedance p., dielectrography; recording changes in electrical impedance between electrodes placed on opposite sides of a part of the body, as a measure of volume changes in the path of the current.

venous occlusion p., measurement of the rate of arterial inflow into an organ or limb segment by measuring its initial rate of increase in volume when its venous outflow is suddenly occluded.

plethysmometry (pleth-iz-mom′ĕ-trē) [G. *plēthysmos,* increase, + *metron,* measure]. Measuring the fullness of a hollow organ or vessel, as of the pulse.

pleur-, pleura-, pleuro- [G. *pleura;* a rib, the side]. Combining forms denoting rib, side, pleura.

pleura, gen. and pl. **pleurae** (plūr′ă, plūr′ē) [G. *pleura,* a rib, pl. the side] [NA]. Membrana succingens; the serous membrane enveloping the lungs and lining the walls of the pleural cavity.

cervical p., *cupula* pleurae.

p. costa′lis [NA], costal p.; the layer of parietal p. lining the chest walls.

diaphragmatic p., p. diaphragmatica.

p. diaphragmat′ica [NA], diaphragmatic p.; p. phrenica; the layer of parietal p. covering the upper surface of the diaphragm, except along its costal attachments and where it is covered with the pericardium.

p. mediastina′lis [NA], mediastinal p.; the continuation of the costal p. passing from the sternum to the vertebral column which covers the side of the mediastinum.

parietal p. p. parietalis.
p. parieta'lis [NA], parietal p.; that which lines the different parts of the wall of the pleural cavity; called costal, diaphragmatic, and mediastinal, according to the parts invested.
p. pericardi'aca, pericardial p., that portion of the mediastinal p. which is fused with the pericardium.
p. phren'ica, p. diaphragmatica.
p. pulmona'lis [NA], pulmonary p.; p. visceralis; the layer investing the lungs and dipping into the fissures between the several lobes.
visceral p., p. visceralis.
p. viscera'lis, p. pulmonalis.

pleuracentesis (plūr'ă-sen-tē'sis). Thoracentesis.

pleural (plūr'ăl). Relating to the pleura.

pleuralgia (plū-ral'jē-ă) [pleur- + G. *algos,* pain]. Rarely used synonym for pleurodynia (2).

pleurapophysis (plūr'ă-pof'i-sis) [pleur- + G. *apophysis,* process, offshoot]. A rib, or the process on a cervical or lumbar vertebra corresponding thereto. *Cf.* diapophysis.

pleurectomy (plū-rek'tō-mē) [pleur- + G. *ektomē,* excision]. Excision of pleura, usually parietal.

pleurisy (plūr'i-sē) [L. *pleurisis,* fr. G. *pleuritis*]. Pleuritis; inflammation of the pleura.
adhesive p., dry p.
benign dry p., epidemic *pleurodynia.*
costal p., inflammation of the pleura lining the thoracic walls.
diaphragmatic p., epidemic *pleurodynia.*
dry p., adhesive, fibrinous, or plastic p.; p. with a fibrinous exudation, without an effusion of serum, resulting in adhesion between the opposing surfaces of the pleura.
p. with effusion, serous or wet p.; p. accompanied by serous exudation.
encysted p., a form of serofibrinous p., in which adhesions occur at various points, circumscribing the serous effusion.
epidemic benign dry p., epidemic *pleurodynia.*
epidemic diaphragmatic p., epidemic *pleurodynia.*
fibrinous p., dry p.
hemorrhagic p., p. with an effusion of blood-stained serum.
interlobular p., inflammation limited to the pleura in the sulci between the pulmonary lobes.
plastic p., dry p.
productive p., pachypleuritis.
proliferating p., p. with a tendency for the proliferation of inflammatory exudate.
pulmonary p., visceral p.; inflammation of the pleura covering the lungs.
purulent p., suppurative p.; p. with empyema.
sacculated p., p. with the inflammatory exudate divided into separate regions by adhesions or inflammatory changes.
serofibrinous p., the more common form of p., characterized by a fibrinous exudate on the surface of the pleura and an extensive effusion of serous fluid into the pleural cavity.
serous p., p. with effusion.
suppurative p., purulent p.
typhoid p., obsolete term for acute or subacute p. with typhoid symptoms.
visceral p., pulmonary p.
wet p., p. with effusion.

pleuritic (plū-rit'ik). Pertaining to pleurisy.

pleuritis (plū-rī'tis) [G. fr. *pleura,* side, + *-itis,* inflammation]. Pleurisy.

pleuritogenous (plūr-i-toj'ĕ-nŭs) [G. *pleuritis,* pleurisy, + *genesis,* origin]. Tending to produce pleurisy.

pleuro-. See pleur-.

pleurocele (plūr'ō-sēl) [pleuro- + G. *kēlē,* hernia]. Pneumonocele.

pleurocentesis (plūr'ō-sen-tē'sis) [pleuro- + G. *kentēsis,* puncture]. Thoracentesis.

pleurocentrum (plūr'ō-sen'trŭm) [pleuro- + G. *kentron,* center]. One of the lateral halves of the body of a vertebra.

pleuroclysis (plūr-ok'li-sis) [pleuro- + G. *klysis,* a washing out]. Washing out of the pleural cavity.

pleurodesis (plūr-od'e-sis) [pleuro- + G. *desis,* a binding together]. The creation of a fibrous adhesion between the visceral and parietal layers of the pleura, thus obliterating the pleural cavity; it is performed surgically by the insertion of a sterile irritant into the pleural canal, and applied as treatment in cases of recurrent spontaneous pneumothorax, malignant pleural effusion, and chylothorax.

pleurodynia (plūr-ō-din'ē-ă) [pleuro- + G. *odynē,* pain]. Costalgia. **1.** Pleuritic pain in the chest. **2.** A painful rheumatic affection of the tendinous attachments of the thoracic muscles, usually of one side only.
epidemic p., an acute infectious disease usually occurring in epidemic form, characterized by paroxysms of pain, usually in the chest, and associated with strains of *Enterovirus* coxsackievirus type B. Also called Bornholm, Daae's, or Sylvest's disease; devil's grip; benign dry, diaphragmatic, epidemic benign dry, or epidemic diaphragmatic pleurisy; epidemic transient diaphragmatic spasm; epidemic myalgia or myositis.

pleurogenic (plūr-ō-jen'ik) [pleuro- + G. *-gen,* producing]. Pleurogenous (1); of pleural origin; beginning in the pleura.

pleurogenous (plūr-oj'ĕ-nŭs). **1.** Pleurogenic. **2.** In fungi, denoting spores or conidia developed on the sides of a conidiophore or hypha.

pleurography (plūr-og'ră-fē) [pleuro- + G. *graphō,* to write]. Roentgenography of the pleural cavity.

pleurohepatitis (plūr'ō-hep-ă-tī'tis) [pleuro- + G. *hēpar,* liver, + *-itis,* inflammation]. Hepatitis with extension of the inflammation to the neighboring portion of the pleura.

pleurolith (plūr'ō-lith) [pleuro- + G. *lithos,* stone]. Pleural calculus; a concretion in the pleural cavity.

pleurolysis (plūr-ol'i-sis) [pleuro- + G. *lysis,* dissolution]. Jacobaeus operation; locating pleural adhesions by the aid of an endoscope and then dividing them with the electric cautery.

pleuropericardial (plūr'ō-per-i-kar'dē-ăl). Relating to both pleura and pericardium.

pleuropericarditis (plūr'ō-per-i-kar-dī'tis) [pleuro- + pericardium + G. *-itis,* inflammation]. Combined inflammation of the pericardium and of the pleura.

pleuroperitoneal (plūr'ō-per-i-tō-nē'ăl). Relating to both pleura and peritoneum.

pleuropneumonia (plūr'ō-nū-mō'nē-ă). Specific infectious diseases in domestic ruminants, characterized by inflammation of the lungs and pleura; caused by *Mycoplasma mycoides* sp. *mycoides.*
contagious bovine p. (CBPP), a highly infectious disease of cattle caused by *Mycoplasma mycoides* sp. *mycoides* and occurring in acute, subacute, and chronic septicemic forms.
contagious caprine p., an acute disease of goats caused by *Mycoplasma mycoides* sp. *capri.*

pleuropulmonary (plūr-ō-pul'mō-ner-ē). Relating to the pleura and the lungs.

pleurorrhea (plūr-ō-rē'ă) [pleuro- + G. *rhoia,* a flow]. Hydrothorax.

pleurothotonos, pleurothotonus (plūr-ō-thot'ō-nŭs) [G. *pleurothen,* from the side, + *tonos,* tension]. Tetanus lateralis; lateral bending of the body; formerly seen as a common symptom of conversion hysteria.

pleurotomy (plū-rot'ō-mē) [pleuro- + G. *tomē,* incision]. Thoracotomy.

pleurotyphoid (plur-ō-tī'foyd). Typhoid fever in which the early stage is masked by the physical signs of pleurisy.

pleurovisceral (plūr'ō-vis'er-ăl). Visceropleural.

plexal (plek'săl). Relating to a plexus.

plexectomy (plek-sek'tō-mē) [plexus + G. *ektomē,* excision]. Surgical excision of a plexus.

plexiform (plek'si-fōrm) [plexus + L. *forma,* form]. Weblike, or resembling or forming a plexus.

pleximeter (plek-sim'i-ter) [G. *plēxis,* stroke]. Plessimeter.

plexitis (plek-sī'tis). Inflammation of a plexus.

plexogenic (plek'sō-jen-ik) [plexus + G. *-gen,* producing]. Giving rise to weblike or plexiform structures.

plexometer (plek-som'ĕ-ter). Plessimeter.

plexor (plek'ser) [G. *plēxis,* a stroke]. Plessor.

PLEXUS

plexus, pl. (L.) **plexus,** (Eng.) **plexuses** (plek'sŭs, -sŭs-ez) [L. a braid] [NA]. A network or interjoining of nerves and blood vessels or of lymphatic vessels.

abdominal aortic p., p. aorticus abdominalis.

annular p., p. annularis; a nerve p. near the corneoscleral junction from which myelinated and unmyelinated nerves pass to the cornea.

p. annula'ris, annular p.

p. of anterior cerebral artery, p. arteriae cerebri anterioris; an autonomic p. accompanying the anterior cerebral artery, derived from the internal carotid p.

anterior coronary p., the part of the cardiac p. that accompanies the coronary arteries on the anterior aspect of the heart.

aortic p., p. aorticus; a p. of lymph nodes and connecting vessels lying along the lower portion of the abdominal aorta.

p. aor'ticus, aortic p.

p. aor'ticus abdomina'lis [NA], abdominal aortic p.; an autonomic p. surrounding the abdominal aorta, directly continuous with the thoracic aortic p.

p. aor'ticus thora'cicus [NA], thoracic aortic p.; an autonomic p. surrounding the thoracic aorta and passing with it through the aortic opening in the diaphragm, to become continuous with the abdominal aortic p.

p. arte'riae cer'ebri anterio'ris, p. of anterior cerebral artery.

p. arte'riae cer'ebri me'diae, p. of middle cerebral artery.

p. arte'riae choroi'deae, p. of choroid artery.

ascending pharyngeal p., p. pharyngeus ascendens; an autonomic p. on the artery of the same name, formed of fibers from the superior cervical ganglion.

Auerbach's p., p. myentericus.

p. auricula'ris poste'rior, posterior auricular p.

autonomic p.'s, p. autonomici.

p. autono'mici [NA], autonomic p.'s; sympathetic p.'s; p.'s of nerves in relation to blood vessels and viscera, the component fibers of which are sympathetic, parasympathetic, and sensory.

p. axilla'ris, axillary p.

axillary p., p. axillaris; a lymphatic p. formed of the lymph nodes, with their afferent and efferent vessels, in the axilla.

basilar p., p. basilaris.

p. basila'ris [NA], basilar p.; basilar sinus; sinus basilaris; a venous p. on the clivus, connected with the cavernous and petrosal sinuses and the vertebral venous p.

Batson's p., p. venosi vertebrales.

brachial p., p. brachialis.

p. brachia'lis [NA], brachial p.; formed of the anterior rami of the fifth cervical to first thoracic nerves; the nerves converge in the posterior triangle of the neck between the scalenus anterior and medius and pass down on the lateral side of the subclavian artery behind the clavicle into the axilla.

cardiac p., p. cardiacus.

p. cardi'acus [NA], cardiac p.; a wide-meshed network of anastomosing cords from the sympathetic and vagus nerves, surrounding the arch of the aorta, the pulmonary artery, and continuing to the atria, ventricles, and coronary vessels.

p. cardi'acus profun'dus, deep cardiac p.

p. cardi'acus superficia'lis, superficial cardiac p.

p. carot'icus commu'nis [NA], common carotid p.; an autonomic p. accompanying the artery of the same name formed by fibers from the middle cervical ganglion.

p. carot'icus exter'nus [NA], external carotid p.; an autonomic p. formed by the external carotid nerves surrounding the artery of the same name, and giving origin to a number of secondary p.'s along the branches of this artery and to branches to the carotid body.

p. carot'icus inter'nus, internal carotid p.; **(1)** [NA], an autonomic p. surrounding the internal carotid artery in the carotid canal and cavernous sinus, and sending branches to the tympanic p., sphenopalatine ganglion, abducens and oculomotor nerves, the cerebral vessels, and the ciliary ganglion; **(2)** p. venosus caroticus internus.

p. caverno'si concha'rum [NA], cavernous p. of the conchae; corpus cavernosum conchae; erectile tissue in the mucous membrane covering the conchae of the nasal cavity.

p. caverno'sus, cavernous p.

cavernous p., p. cavernosus; Walther's p.; the portion of the internal carotid p. in the cavernous sinus.

cavernous p. of clitoris, *nervi* cavernosi clitoridis.

cavernous p. of conchae, p. cavernosi concharum.

cavernous p. of penis, *nervi* cavernosi penis.

celiac p., p. celiacus.

p. celi'acus, celiac p.; **(1)** [NA], solar p.; cerebrum abdominale; abdominal brain; Vieussens' ganglion; the largest of the autonomic p.'s lying in front of the aorta at the level of origin of the celiac artery, behind the stomach; it is formed by the splanchnic and the vagus nerves and cords from the celiac and superior mesenteric ganglia; through its connections with the other abdominal p.'s it sends branches to all the abdominal viscera; **(2)** a lymphatic p. formed of the superior mesenteric lymph nodes and the fifteen or twenty celiac nodes behind the stomach, duodenum, and pancreas, together with the connecting vessels.

cervical p., p. cervicalis.

p. cervica'lis [NA], cervical p.; formed by loops joining the anterior rami of the first four cervical nerves and receiving gray communicating rami from the superior cervical ganglion; it lies beneath the sternocleidomastoid muscle, and sends out numerous cutaneous, muscular, and communicating rami.

choroid p., p. choroideus.

p. of choroid artery, p. arteriae choroideae; an autonomic p. accompanying the artery of the same name, derived from the internal carotid p.

choroid p. of fourth ventricle, p. choroideus ventriculi quarti.

choroid p. of lateral ventricle, p. choroideus ventriculi lateralis.

choroid p. of third ventricle, p. choroideus ventriculi tertii.

p. choroi'deus [NA], choroid p.; tela vasculosa; a vascular proliferation or fringe of the tela choroidea in one of the cerebral ventricles; by secretion or absorption of cerebrospinal fluid the choroid p. serves to regulate the intraventricular pressure.

p. choroi'deus ventric'uli latera'lis [NA], choroid p. of lateral ventricle; the vascular fringe that projects from the choroidal fissure into each lateral ventricle.

p. choroi'deus ventric'uli quar'ti [NA], choroid p. of fourth ven-

tricle; one of two vascular fringes of pia mater projecting on either side from the lower part of the roof of the fourth cerebral ventricle.
p. choroi'deus ventric'uli ter'tii [NA], choroid p. of third ventricle; the double row of vascular projections from the undersurface of the tela choroidea where it roofs over the third ventricle.
ciliary ganglionic p., p. gangliosus ciliaris; an autonomic p. lying on the ciliary muscle, derived from the oculomotor, trigeminal, and sympathetic.
coccygeal p., p. coccygeus.
p. coccyg'eus [NA], coccygeal p.; a small p. formed by the fifth sacral and the coccygeal nerves; it gives origin to the anococcygeal nerves.
common carotid p., p. caroticus communis.
p. corona'rius cor'dis, coronary p.
coronary p., p. coronarius cordis; the continuation of the cardiac p. onto the coronary arteries.
Cruveilhier's p., a nerve p. formed by communications between the posterior rami of the first three cervical nerves; it lies deep to the semispinalis capitis muscle.
deep cardiac p., p. cardiacus profundus; the deeper part of the cardiac p.
deferential p., p. deferentialis.
p. deferentia'lis [NA], deferential p.; an autonomic p. on the seminal vesicle and ampulla of the ductus deferens on each side, derived from the inferior hypogastric p.
p. denta'lis infe'rior [NA], inferior dental p.; formed by branches of the inferior alveolar nerve interlacing before they supply the teeth; it gives off dental branches (rami dentales inferiores) and branches to the gums (rami gingivales inferiores).
p. denta'lis supe'rior [NA], superior dental p.; formed by branches of the infraorbital nerve; it gives off dental branches (rami dentales superiores) and branches to the gums (rami gingivales superiores).
enteric p., p. entericus.
p. enter'icus [NA], enteric p.; the autonomic p. in the wall of the intestine; it consists of three parts, p. submucosus, p. myentericus, and p. subserosus; ganglionic cells are scattered through the myenteric and submucous p.'s.
esophageal p., p. esophageus.
p. esopha'geus [NA], esophageal p.; p. gulae; one of two nervous p.'s, posterior and anterior on the walls of the esophagus; the first is formed by branches from the right vagus and left recurrent, the second by the anastomosing trunks of the vagus after leaving the pulmonary p.'s; branches supply the mucous and muscular coats of the esophagus.
Exner's p., a p. formed by tangential nerve fibers in the superficial plexiform or molecular layer of the cerebral cortex.
external carotid p., p. caroticus externus.
external iliac p., p. iliacus externus; a lymphatic p. formed by the lymph nodes along the external iliac artery on either side, and their afferent and efferent vessels.
external maxillary p., facial p.
facial p., external maxillary p.; p. maxillaris externus; an autonomic p. on the facial artery derived from the external carotid p.; it sends a branch to the submandibular ganglion.
femoral p., p. femoralis.
p. femora'lis [NA], femoral p.; an autonomic p. surrounding the femoral artery, derived from the iliac p.
p. ganglio'sus cilia'ris, ciliary ganglionic p.
gastric p.'s of autonomic system, p. gastrici systemati autonomici.
p. gas'trici systema'ti autono'mici [NA], gastric p.'s of autonomic system; the p.'s along the greater and lesser curvatures of the stomach derived from the celiac p.; also known as inferior and superior p.
p. gu'lae, p. esophageus.
Haller's p., a nervous p. of sympathetic filaments and branches of the external laryngeal nerve on the surface of the inferior constrictor muscle of the pharynx.
Heller's p., p. of small arteries in the wall of the intestine.
hemorrhoidal p., p. venosus rectalis. See also p. rectales inferiores, medii, and superior.
hepatic p., p. hepaticus.
p. hepat'icus [NA], hepatic p.; an unpaired autonomic p. lying on the hepatc artery and its branches in the liver.
p. hypogas'tricus infe'rior [NA], p. pelvinus; inferior hypogastric p.; pelvic p.; the autonomic p. in the pelvis that is distributed to the pelvic viscera; it receives the hypogastric nerves and the pelvic splanchnic nerves.
p. hypogas'tricus supe'rior [NA], nervus presacralis; superior hypogastric p.; presacral nerve; Latarjet's nerve; the continuation of the aortic p. downward across the fifth lumbar vertebra into the pelvis where it divides into two hypogastric nerves at the sides of the rectum; these join the inferior hypogastric p.'s to supply pelvic viscera.
iliac p., p. iliaci.
p. ili'aci [NA], iliac p.; the autonomic p. lying on the iliac arteries, derived from the aortic p.
p. ili'acus exter'nus, external iliac p.
inferior dental p., p. dentalis inferior.
inferior hemorrhoidal p.'s, p. rectales inferiores.
inferior hypogastric p., p. hypogastricus inferior.
inferior mesenteric p., p. mesentericus inferior.
inferior rectal p.'s, p. rectales inferiores.
inferior thyroid p., p. thyroideus inferior; an autonomic p. on the artery of this name, derived from the subclavian p.
inferior vesical p., p. vesicalis inferior; a venous p. in the female corresponding to the prostatic venous p. in the male.
inguinal p., p. inguinalis; a lymphatic p. formed of 10 to 15 lymph nodes with their connecting vessels lying superficially near the termination of the great saphenous vein and more deeply along the femoral artery and vein.
p. inguina'lis, inguinal p.
intermesenteric p., p. intermesentericus.
p. intermesenter'icus [NA], intermesenteric p.; the part of the aortic p. lying between the superior and inferior mesenteric p.'s.
internal carotid p., p. caroticus internus.
internal carotid venous p., p. venosus caroticus internus.
internal mammary p., internal thoracic p.
internal maxillary p., maxillary p.
internal thoracic p., internal mammary p.; p. mammarius internus; an autonomic p. on the internal thoracic artery derived from the subclavian p.
p. intraparoti'deus [NA], parotid p.; intraparotid p.; pes anserinus(1); the diverging branches of the facial nerve passing through the substance of the parotid gland, connected by numerous looped anastomoses.
ischiadic p., p. sacralis.
Jacobson's p., p. tympanicus.
Jacques' p., a nerve p. within the muscular coat of the uterine (fallopian) tube.
jugular p., p. jugularis; a lymphatic p. formed of many lymph nodes, with their afferent and efferent vessels, extending along the internal jugular vein.
p. jugula'ris, jugular p.
Leber's p., a small venous p. in the eye between the venous sinuses of the sclera (of Schlemm) and the spaces of the iridocorneal angle (of Fontana).
p. liena'lis [NA], splenic p.; the p. of autonomic nerves along the splenic artery.
lingual p., p. lingualis; an autonomic p. on the artery of this name, derived from the external carotid p.
p. lingua'lis, lingual p.
p. lumba'lis, lumbar p.; **(1)** [NA], a nervous p., formed by the ventral rami of the first four lumbar nerves; it lies in the substance of

the psoas muscle; **(2)** a lymphatic p. formed of about twenty lymph nodes and connecting vessels situated along the lower portion of the aorta and the common iliac vessels.
lumbar p., p. lumbalis.
lumbosacral p., p. lumbosacralis.
p. lumbosacra'lis [NA], lumbosacral p.; formed by the union of the anterior rami of the lumbar and sacral nerves; it is divided into lumbar and sacral p.'s.
lymphatic p., p. lymphaticus.
p. lymphat'icus [NA], lymphatic p. or network; a p. of lymphatic capillaries, usually without valves, that opens into one or more larger lymphatic vessels.
p. mamma'rius, mammary p.
p. mamma'rius inter'nus, internal thoracic p.
mammary p., p. mammarius; a lymphatic p., formed of small lymph nodes, with their vessels, situated along the course of the internal thoracic arteries.
p. maxilla'ris exter'nus, facial p.
p. maxilla'ris inter'nus, maxillary p.
maxillary p., internal maxillary p.; p. maxillaris internus; an autonomic p. on the maxillary artery derived from the external carotid p.
Meissner's p., p. submucosus.
meningeal p., p. meningeus.
p. menin'geus, meningeal p.; a nerve p. on the cerebral meninges, derived from the external carotid p.
p. mesenter'icus infe'rior [NA], inferior mesenteric p.; an autonomic p., derived from the aortic p., surrounding the inferior mesenteric artery and sending branches to the descending colon, sigmoid, and rectum.
p. mesenter'icus supe'rior [NA], superior mesenteric p.; an autonomic p., a continuation or part of the celiac p., sending nerves to the intestines and forming with the vagus the subserous, myenteric, and submucous p.'s.
p. of middle cerebral artery, p. arteriae cerebri mediae; an autonomic p. accompanying the middle cerebral artery, derived from the internal carotid p.
middle hemorrhoidal p.'s, p. rectales medii.
middle rectal p.'s, p. rectales medii.
middle sacral p., p. sacralis medius; a lymphatic p. formed of lymph nodes and connecting vessels situated chiefly in the mesorectum anterior and inferior to the sacral promontory.
myenteric p., p. myentericus.
p. myenter'icus [NA], myenteric p.; Auerbach's p.; a p. of unmyelinated fibers and postganglionic autonomic cell bodies lying in the muscular coat of the esophagus, stomach, and intestines; it communicates with the subserous and submucous p.'s, all subdivisions of the enteric p.
nerve p., p. nervosus; a p. formed by the interlacing of nerves by means of numerous communicating branches.
p. nervo'rum spina'lium [NA], p. of spinal nerves; an intermingling of fiber fascicles from adjacent spinal nerves to form a network; the major p.'s are the cervical, brachial, and lumbosacral.
p. nervo'sus, nerve p.
occipital p., p. occipitalis; an autonomic p. on the occipital artery derived from the external carotid p.
p. occipita'lis, occipital p.
ophthalmic p., p. ophthalmicus; an autonomic p., entering the orbit in company with the ophthalmic artery, derived from the internal carotid p.
p. ophthal'micus, ophthalmic p.
ovarian p., p. ovaricus.
p. ova'ricus [NA], ovarian p.; an autonomic p. derived from the aortic p. and accompanying the ovarian artery to the ovary, broad ligament, and uterine tube.
pampiniform p., p. pampiniformis.
p. pampinifor'mis [NA], pampiniform p.; a p. formed, in the male, by veins from the testicle and epididymis, consisting of eight or ten veins lying in front of the ductus deferens and forming part of the spermatic cord; in the female the ovarian veins form this p. between the layers of the broad ligament.
pancreatic p., p. pancreaticus.
p. pancreat'icus [NA], pancreatic p.; the autonomic p. that accompanies the pancretic arteries.
parotid p., p. parotideus.
pelvic p., p. hypogastricus inferior.
p. pelvi'nus [NA], official alternative name for p. hypogastricus inferior.
periarterial p., p. periarterialis.
p. periarteria'lis [NA], periarterial p.; an autonomic p. that accompanies an artery.
pharyngeal p., p. pharyngeus.
p. pharyn'geus [NA], pharyngeal p.; **(1)** the p. of nerves including branches of the glossopharyngeal, vagus, and accessory nerves, that lies along the posterior wall of the pharynx; **(2)** a venous p. on the posterolateral walls of the pharynx, emptying through the pharyngeal veins into the internal jugular.
p. pharyn'geus ascen'dens, ascending pharyngeal p.
phrenic p., p. phren'icus, an autonomic p. surrounding the inferior phrenic artery.
popliteal p., p. poplit'eus, p. popliteus; a nerve p. surrounding the popliteal artery, derived from the femoral p.
posterior auricular p., p. auricularis posterior; an autonomic p. on the artery of this name, derived from the external carotid p.
posterior coronary p., the portion of the cardiac p. that accompanies branches of the coronary arteries on the posteroinferior surface of the heart.
prostatic p., p. prostaticus.
prostatic venous p., p. venosus prostaticus.
p. prostaticovesica'lis, prostaticovesical p.
prostaticovesical p., p. prostaticovesicalis; a venous p. around the prostate gland and neck of the bladder; it communicates with the vesical and pudendal p.'s, and empties by one or more efferent vessels into the internal iliac (hypogastric) vein; it corresponds to the inferior vesical p. in the female.
p. prostat'icus [NA], prostatic p.; an autonomic p. of nerves on the prostate, derived from the inferior hypogastric p.
pterygoid p., p. pterygoideus.
p. pterygoi'deus [NA], pterygoid p.; a venous p. on the pterygoid muscles, receiving veins accompanying the branches of the maxillary artery, and terminating in the maxillary vein.
p. pudenda'lis, p. venosus prostaticus.
p. puden'dus nervo'sus, *nervus* pudendus.
p. pulmona'lis [NA], pulmonary p.; one of two autonomic p.'s, anterior and posterior, at the hilus of each lung, formed by branches of the sympathetic and bronchial rami of the vagus nerve; from them various branches accompany the bronchi and arteries into the lung.
pulmonary p., p. pulmonalis.
Quénu's hemorrhoidal p., lymphatic p.'s in the skin about the anus.
Ranvier's p., a subbasal stroma p. of the cornea. See stroma p.
rectal p.'s, see p. rectales inferiores, medii, and superior.
rectal venous p., p. venosus rectalis.
p. recta'les inferio'res [NA], inferior rectal p.'s; inferior hemorrhoidal p.'s; the autonomic p.'s along the anus derived from the inferior hypogastric p.
p. recta'les me'dii [NA], middle rectal p.'s; middle hemorrhoidal p.'s; the autonomic p.'s along the rectum derived from the inferior hypogastric p.
p. recta'lis supe'rior [NA], superior rectal p.; superior hemorrhoidal p.; the autonomic p. derived from the inferior mesenteric p. that accompanies the superior rectal artery.
Remak's p., p. submucosus.

renal p., p. renalis.
p. rena'lis [NA], renal p.; the autonomic p. surrounding the renal artery and extending with it into the substance of the kidney.
sacral p., p. sacralis.
sacral venous p., p. venosus sacralis.
p. sacra'lis [NA], sacral p.; sciatic p.; ischiadic p.; formed by the fourth and fifth lumbar and first, second, and third sacral nerves; it lies on the inner surface of the posterior wall of the pelvis; its nerves supply the lower limbs.
p. sacra'lis me'dius, middle sacral p.
Sappey's p., a network of lymphatics in the areola of the nipple.
sciatic p., p. sacralis.
solar p., p. celiacus (1).
spermatic p., p. testicularis.
p. of spinal nerves, p. nervorum spinalium.
splenic p., p. lienalis.
Stensen's p., the venous network surrounding the parotid (Stensen's) duct.
stroma p., a p. of nerves in the parenchyma of the cornea consisting of the primary or deep p., in the substance of the cornea, and the subbasal or superficial p. just beneath the anterior limiting membrane.
subclavian p., p. subclavius.
p. subcla'vius [NA], subclavian p.; the autonomic p. accompanying the artery of this name, formed by fibers from the cervicothoracic ganglion, and giving off secondary p.'s along the branches of the subclavian.
submucosal p., p. submucosus.
p. submuco'sus [NA], submucosal p.; Meissner's or Remak's p.; a gangliated p. of unmyelinated nerve fibers, derived chiefly from the superior mesenteric p., ramifying in the intestinal submucosa.
suboccipital venous p., p. venosus suboccipitalis.
p. subsero'sus [NA], subserous p.; the subserous part of the enteric plexus of autonomic nerves.
subserous p., p. subserosus.
superficial cardiac p., p. cardiacus superficialis; the superficial and smaller part of the cardiac p.
superficial temporal p., p. temporalis superficialis; an autonomic p. of nerves on the artery of this name, derived from the external carotid p.
superior dental p., p. dentalis superior.
superior hemorrhoidal p., p. rectalis superior.
superior hypogastric p., p. hypogastricus superior.
superior mesenteric p., p. mesentericus superior.
superior rectal p., p. rectalis superior.
superior thyroid p., p. thyroideus superior; an autonomic p. on the artery of the same name, derived from the external carotid p.
suprarenal p., p. suprarenalis.
p. suprarena'lis [NA], suprarenal p.; an autonomic p. formed mainly by branches from the celiac ganglion, lying at the hilus of the suprarenal gland.
sympathetic p.'s, p. autonomici.
p. tempora'lis superficia'lis, superficial temporal p.
testicular p., p. testicularis.
p. testicula'ris [NA], testicular p.; spermatic p.; the autonomic p. derived from the aortic p. and accompanying the testicular artery.
thoracic aortic p., p. aorticus thoracicus.
p. thyroi'deus im'par [NA], a venous p. in front of the lower portion of the trachea formed by anastomoses between the inferior thyroid veins; it terminates in the unpaired vena thyroidea ima.
p. thyroi'deus infe'rior, inferior thyroid p.
p. thyroi'deus supe'rior, superior thyroid p.
tympanic p., p. tympanicus.
p. tympan'icus [NA], tympanic p.; Jacobson's p.; a p. on the promontory of the labyrinthine wall of the tympanic cavity, formed by the tympanic nerve, an anastomotic branch of the facial, and sympathetic branches from the internal carotid p.; it supplies the mucosa of the middle ear, mastoid cells, and auditory (eustachian) tube, and gives off the lesser petrosal nerve to the otic ganglion.
ureteric p., p. uretericus.
p. ureter'icus [NA], ureteric p.; the autonomic p. derived from the celiac p. that accompanies the ureter.
uterine venous p., p. venosus uterinus.
uterovaginal p., p. uterovaginalis.
p. uterovagina'lis [NA], uterovaginal p.; Lee's or Frankenhäuser's ganglion; a gangliated autonomic p. on each side of the cervix uteri, derived from the inferior hypogastric p.
vaginal venous p., p. venosus vaginalis.
vascular p., p. vasculosus.
p. vasculo'sus [NA], vascular p.; a vascular network formed by frequent anastomoses between the blood vessels (arteries or veins) of a part.
p. veno'sus [NA], venous p.; a vascular network formed by numerous anastomoses between veins.
p. veno'sus areola'ris [NA], circulus venosus halleri; venous circle of the mammary gland; vascular circle (2); Haller's circle (2); a venous p. in the areola surrounding the nipple, formed by the mammary veins, and sending its blood to the lateral thoracic vein.
p. veno'sus cana'lis hypoglos'si [NA], venous p. of hypoglossal canal; circellus venosus hypoglossi; rete canalis hypoglossi; a small venous network around the hypoglossal nerve, connecting with the occipital sinus, inferior petrosal sinus, and internal jugular vein.
p. veno'sus carot'icus inter'nus [NA], internal carotid venous p.; p. caroticus internus (2); a venous network around the internal carotid artery in the carotid canal of the temporal bone, connecting with the cavernous sinus and internal jugular vein.
p. veno'sus foram'inis ova'lis [NA], venous p. of the foramen ovale; rete foraminis ovalis; a venous network around the mandibular nerve connecting the cavernous sinus and the pterygoid p.
p. veno'sus prostat'icus [NA], prostatic venous p.; p. pudendalis; Santorini's labyrinth; a venous p., arising chiefly from the dorsal vein of the penis, situated at the base of the bladder and sides of the prostate.
p. veno'sus recta'lis [NA], rectal venous p.; hemorrhoidal p.; a venous p. resting upon the posterior and lateral walls of the rectum; it drains into the superior rectal vein to the portal, the middle rectal to the internal iliac and the inferior rectal to the internal pudendal.
p. veno'sus sacra'lis [NA], sacral venous p.; a venous p. on the pelvic surface of the sacrum, formed by tributaries to the lateral sacral veins.
p. veno'sus suboccipita'lis [NA], suboccipital venous p.; the extensive p. of veins in the suboccipital region.
p. veno'sus uteri'nus [NA], uterine venous p.; the plexiform veins that lie along the sides of the uterus in the broad ligament.
p. veno'sus vagina'lis [NA], vaginal venous p.; the p. of veins that surrounds the vagina.
p. veno'sus vertebra'lis [NA], Batson's p.; vertebral venous p. or system; any of four interconnected venous networks surrounding the vertebral column; **p. v. v. exter'nus ante'rior,** the small p. around the vertebral bodies; **p. v. v. exter'nus poste'rior,** the extensive p. around the vertebral processes; **p. v. v. inter'nus ante'rior,** the p. running the length of the vertebral canal anterior to the dura; **p. v. v. inter'nus poste'rior,** the p. running the length of the vertebral canal posterior to the dura.
p. veno'sus vesica'lis [NA], venous p. of bladder; a p. of veins around the fundus and sides of the bladder.
venous p., p. venosus.
venous p. of bladder, p. venosus vesicalis.
venous p. of foramen ovale, p. venosus foraminis ovalis.
venous p. of hypoglossal canal, p. venosus canalis hypoglossi.
vertebral p., p. vertebralis.
p. vertebra'lis [NA], vertebral p.; a p. of autonomic nerves on the

vertebral artery derives from the subclavian p.
vertebral venous p., p. venosi vertebrales.
vesical p., p. vesicalis.
p. vesica'lis [NA], vesical p.; an autonomic p. on the bladder, derived from the inferior hypogastric p.
p. vesica'lis infe'rior, inferior vesical p.
Walther's p., cavernous p.

PLICA

plica, gen. and pl. **plicae** (plī'kă, plī'sē) [Mod. L. a plait or fold]. **1** [NA]. One of several anatomical structures in which there is a folding over of the parts. **2.** False *membrane.*
pli'cae adipo'sae, adipose folds of pleura; lobules of fat enveloped in the pleura, chiefly in the neighborhood of the costomediastinal sinus.
pli'cae ala'res [NA], alar folds; alar ligaments (2); winglike lateral fringes or expansions of the p. synovialis infrapatellaris.
p. ampulla'ris, one of the folds of mucous membrane at the fimbriated extremity of the uterine tube.
p. aryepiglot'tica [NA], aryepiglottic or arytenoepiglottidean fold; a prominent fold of mucous membrane stretching between the lateral margin of the epiglottis and the arytenoid cartilage on either side; it encloses the aryepiglottic muscle.
p. axilla'ris, axillary *fold.*
pli'cae ceca'les [NA], cecal folds; the two peritoneal folds that border the retrocecal fossa.
p. ceca'lis vascula'ris [NA], vascular fold of cecum; a peritoneal fold that arches over a branch of the ileocolic artery and bounds in front a narrow recess, the superior ileocecal (or ileocolic) recess.
p. chor'dae tym'pani [NA], fold of chorda tympani; the fold of mucosa that surrounds the chorda tympani nerve in its course through the tympanic cavity.
p. choroi'dea, in the embryo, an infolding of the chorion from which the choroid plexus develops.
pli'cae cilia'res [NA], ciliary folds; a number of low ridges in the furrows between the ciliary processes; together with the processes they constitute the corona ciliaris.
pli'cae circula'res [NA], circular folds; valvulae conniventes; Kerckring's folds or valves; the numerous folds of the mucous membrane of the small intestine, running transversely for about two-thirds of the circumference of the gut.
p. duodena'lis infe'rior [NA], p. duodenomesocolica; inferior duodenal fold; duodenomesocolic fold; a fold of peritoneum bounding the inferior duodenal recess.
p. duodena'lis supe'rior [NA], p. duodenojejunalis; superior duodenal fold; duodenojejunal fold; a fold of peritoneum bounding the superior duodenal recess.
p. duodenojejuna'lis [NA], p. duodenalis superior.
p. duodenomesocol'ica [NA], p. duodenalis inferior.
p. epigas'trica, p. umbilicalis lateralis.
p. epiglot'tica, one of the three folds of mucous membrane passing between the tongue and the epiglottis, p. glossoepiglottica lateralis on either side, and p. glossoepiglottica mediana.
p. fimbria'ta [NA], fimbriated fold; one of several folds running outward from the frenulum on the undersurface of the tongue.
pli'cae gas'tricae [NA], gastric folds; characteristic folds of the gastric mucosa.
pli'cae gastropancreat'icae [NA], gastropancreatic folds; the folds of peritoneum in the omental bursa that encase the hepatic and left gastric arteries as these vessels pass toward their destinations.
p. glossoepiglot'tica latera'lis [NA], lateral glossoepiglottic fold; pharyngoepiglottic fold; the fold of mucous membrane that extends from the margin of the epiglottis to the pharyngeal wall and base of the tongue on each side.
p. glossoepiglot'tica media'na [NA], middle glossoepiglottic fold; frenulum epiglottidis; a fold of mucous membrane in the midline that extends from the back of the tongue to the epiglottis.
p. guberna'trix, *ligamentum* genitoinguinale.
p. hypogas'trica, p. umbilicalis medialis.
p. ileoceca'lis [NA], ileocecal fold; Treves' fold; a fold of peritoneum bounding the ileocecal or ileoappendicular fossa.
p. in'cudis [NA], incudal fold; a variable fold of mucosa that passes from the roof of the tympanic cavity to the body and short limb of the incus.
p. inguina'lis, inguinal fold; an embryonic mesodermal thickening that joins the caudal end of the urogenital ridge to the anterior abdominal wall; the gubernaculum of the testis develops in it.
p. interdigita'lis, one of the folds of skin, or rudimentary web, between the fingers and toes.
p. interureter'ica [NA], interureteric fold; ureteric fold; p. ureterica; bar of bladder; Mercier's bar; a fold of mucous membrane extending from the orifice of the ureter of one side to that of the other side.
pli'cae ir'idis [NA], folds of iris; numerous very fine, almost microscopic, radial folds on the posterior surface of the iris that extend around the pupillary margin.
p. lacrima'lis [NA], lacrimal fold; Bianchi's, Huschke's, or Rosenmüller's valve; Hasner's valve or fold; a fold of mucous membrane guarding the lower opening of the nasolacrimal duct.
p. longitudina'lis duod'eni [NA], longitudinal fold of duodenum; a fold of mucosa on the medial wall of the descending part of the duodenum above the papilla duodeni major, probably caused by the relation to the ductus choledochus.
p. luna'ta, p. semilunaris conjunctivae.
p. mallea'ris [NA], mallear fold; Tröltsch's fold; p. membranae tympani; one of two ligamentous bands, anterior and posterior, making folds on the tympanic side of the tympanic membrane extending from each extremity of the tympanic notch to the malleolar prominence; they mark the boundary between the tense and the flaccid portions of the tympanic membrane.
p. membra'nae tym'pani, p. mallearis.
p. ner'vi laryn'gei [NA], fold of laryngeal nerve; the slight fold of mucosa in the piriform recess of the pharynx that encloses the superior laryngeal nerve.
p. palati'na transver'sa [NA], transverse palatine ridge; ruga palatina; a masticatory vestige on the hard palate; one of several irregular, sometimes branching, crests of soft tissue that radiate from the region of the incisive papillae at their most anterior parts and extend a slight distance backward, crossing the hard palate and reaching laterally for variable distances.
pli'cae palma'tae [NA], palmate folds; arbor vitae uteri; lyra uterina; the two longitudinal ridges, anterior and posterior, in the mucous membrane lining the cervix uteri, from which numerous secondary folds, or rugae, branch off.
p. palpebronasa'lis [NA], palpebronasal fold; mongolian fold; epicanthus; a fold of skin extending from the root of the nose to the medial termination of the eyebrow, overlapping the medial angle of the eye; its presence is normal in fetal life and in Orientals. See fig. on p. 1222.
p. paraduodena'lis [NA], paraduodenal fold; a sickle-shaped fold of peritoneum sometimes found to the left of the duodenojejunal flexure; its right free edge contains the inferior mesenteric vein and a branch of the left colic artery.
pli'cae rec'ti, plicae transversales recti.
p. rectouteri'na [NA], rectouterine fold; Douglas' fold; uterosacral ligament; Jajarvay's or Petit's ligament; a fold of peritoneum, containing the rectouterine muscle, passing from the rectum to the base of the broad ligament on either side, forming the lateral boundary of the rectouterine (Douglas') pouch.

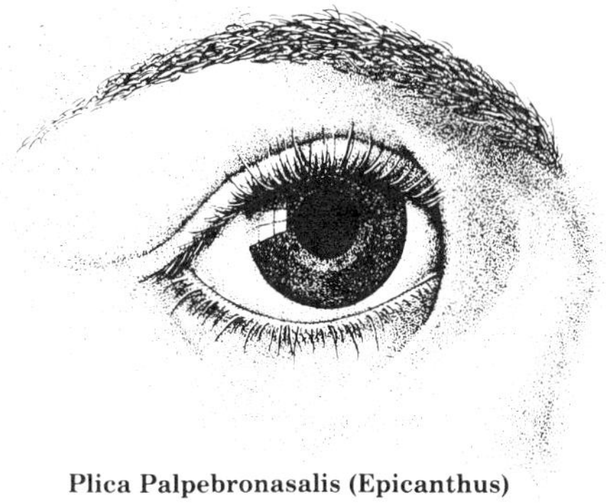

Plica Palpebronasalis (Epicanthus)

p. rectovagina'lis, rectovaginal fold; the lower part of the p. recto-uterina.
p. salpingopalatin'a [NA], salpingopalatine fold; p. tubopalatina; a ridge of mucous membrane passing from the anterior border of the opening of the auditory (eustachian) tube to the palate.
p. salpingopharyn'gea [NA], salpingopharyngeal fold; a ridge of mucous membrane extending from the lower end of the tubal elevation along the wall of the pharynx overlying the salpingopharyngeal muscle.
p. semiluna'ris [NA], semilunar fold; the curved fold connecting the arcus palatoglossus and arcus palatopharyngeus above the fossa supratonsillaris; it always contains lymphoid tissue.
p. semiluna'ris co'li [NA], semilunar fold of colon; p. sigmoidea; one of the folds of the wall of the colon between sacculations.
p. semiluna'ris conjuncti'vae, semilunar conjunctival fold; p. lunata; **(1)** [NA] the semilunar fold formed by the palpebral conjunctiva at the medial angle of the eye; **(2)** palpebra III or tertia; third eyelid; nictitating membrane; membrana nictitans; a fold of the conjunctival mucous membrane found in many animals; normally partially hidden in the medial canthus of the eye when at rest, it may be extended to cover part or all of the cornea in a winking-like action to clean the cornea, as in birds.
p. sigmoi'dea, p. semilunaris coli.
p. spira'lis duc'tus cys'tici [NA], spiral fold of cystic duct; valvula spiralis; Amussat's or Heister's valve; spiral valve; a series of crescentic folds of mucous membrane in the upper part of the cystic duct, arranged in a somewhat spiral manner.
p. stape'dis [NA], stapedial fold; a reflection of the delicate mucous membrane from the posterior wall of the tympanic cavity that covers the stapes.
p. sublingua'lis [NA], sublingual fold; an elevation in the floor of the mouth beneath the tongue, on either side, marking the site of the sublingual gland.
p. synovia'lis [NA], synovial fold; a projection from the synovial membrane of a joint extending toward or between the two articular surfaces.
p. synovia'lis infrapatella'ris [NA], infrapatellar synovial fold; p. synovialis patellaris; a fold of synovial membrane extending from below the level of the articular surface of the patella to the anterior part of the intercondylar fossa.
p. synovia'lis patella'ris, p. synovialis infrapatellaris.
pli'cae transversa'les rec'ti [NA], transverse folds of rectum; rectal folds; plicae recti; rectal valves; Houston's folds; Houston's or Kohlrausch's valves; the three or four crescentic folds placed horizontally in the rectal mucous membrane; one fold is situated near the beginning of the rectum on the left side; a second one projects from the right side about 8 cm above the anus; a third is on the left side about 5 cm above the anus.
p. triangula'ris [NA], triangular fold; a fold of mucous membrane anterior to the palatine tonsil arising from the palatoglossal arch.
pli'cae tuba'riae [NA], many longitudinal folds in the mucous membrane of the uterine (fallopian) tube.
p. tubopalati'na, p. salpingopalatina.
pli'cae tu'nicae muco'sae ves'icae fel'leae [NA], mucosal folds of gallbladder; the interlacing folds of the mucosa that produce a honeycomb appearance in the interior of the gallbladder.
p. umbilica'lis latera'lis [NA], lateral umbilical fold; epigastric fold; p. epigastrica; the ridge on the peritoneal surface of the anterior abdominal wall formed by the inferior epigastric vessels.
p. umbilica'lis me'dia, p. umbilicalis mediana.
p. umbilica'lis media'lis [NA], medial umbilical fold; p. hypogastrica; a fold of peritoneum on the lower part of the anterior abdominal wall that covers the obliterated umbilical artery on either side of the urachus.
p. umbilica'lis media'na [NA], middle umbilical fold; p. umbilicalis media; p. urachi; urachal fold; a fold of peritoneum on the anterior wall of the abdomen covering the urachus, or remains of the allantoic stalk.
p. ura'chi, p. umbilicalis mediana.
p. ureter'ica, p. interureterica.
p. uterovesica'lis, vesicouterine *ligament.*
p. ve'nae ca'vae sinis'trae [NA], fold of the left vena cava; Marshall's vestigial fold; vestigial fold; a pericardial fold lying between the left oblique vein of the atrium and the left superior pulmonary vein containing the obliterated remains of the left superior vena cava.
p. ventricula'ris, p. vestibularis.
p. vesica'lis transver'sa [NA], transverse vesical fold; a duplication of peritoneum passing over the empty bladder, but obliterated when the viscus is full.
p. vesicouteri'na, vesicouterine *ligament.*
p. vestibula'ris [NA], vestibular fold; p. ventricularis; ventricular fold; ventricular band of larynx; false vocal cord; one of the pair of folds of mucous membrane stretching across the laryngeal cavity from the angle of the thyroid cartilage to the arytenoid cartilage; they enclose a space called the rima vestibuli or false glottis.
p. vestib'uli, a fold of mucous membrane forming a ridge on the septum of the nose.
p. villo'sa [NA], one of the ridges of the mucous membrane of the stomach in the region of the pylorus.
p. voca'lis [NA], vocal fold, cord, or shelf; true vocal cord; chorda vocalis; labium vocale; one of Ferrein's cords; the sharp edge of a fold of mucous membrane stretching along either wall of the larynx from the angle between the laminae of the thyroid cartilage to the vocal process of the arytenoid cartilage; the vocal folds are the agents concerned in voice production.

---

plicate (plī'kāt). Folded; pleated; tucked.

plication (plī-kā'shŭn, pli-) [L. *plico,* pp. *-atus,* to fold]. A folding or putting together in pleats; specifically, an operation for reducing the size of a hollow viscus by taking folds or tucks in its walls.

plicotomy (plī-kot'ō-mē) [plica + G. *tomē,* incision]. Division of the plica mallearis.

Plimmer, Henry G., British protozoologist, 1857–1918. See P.'s *bodies.*

-ploid [G. *-plo-,* -fold, + *-ides,* in form; L. *-ploïdeus*]. Adjectival suffix denoting multiple in form; its combinations are used both adjectivally: and substantively of a (specified) multiple of chromosomes.

ploidy (ploy'dē) [see -ploid]. The state of a cell nucleus with respect to the number of genomes it contains. Gametes normally contain a single set of chromosomes or one genome and are haploid; autosomal cells normally contain two genomes and are diploid. See also polyploidy.

plombage (plom-bahzh') [Fr. lit. lead-work]. Formerly, the use of an inert material in collapse of the lung in the surgical treatment of pulmonary tuberculosis.

plosive (plō'siv). Speech sound made by impounding the air stream for a moment and then suddenly releasing it.

Plotz, Harry, U.S. physician, 1890–1947. See P. *bacillus.*

plug (plŭg). Any mass filling a hole or closing an orifice.
Dittrich's p.'s, Traube's p.'s; minute, dirty-grayish, ill-smelling masses of bacteria and fatty acid crystals in the sputum in pulmonary gangrene and fetid bronchitis.
epithelial p., a mass of epithelial cells temporarily occluding an embryonic opening; the term is most commonly used with reference to the external nares.
laminated epithelial p., *keratosis* obturans.
mucous p., a mass of mucus and cells filling the cervical canal between periods or during pregnancy.
Traube's p.'s, Dittrich's p.'s.
vaginal p., a p. formed by the coagulation of semen; found in the vagina after copulation in certain animals, such as the baboon, rat, and squirrel.

plug'ger. Packer (2); plugging instrument; a dental instrument used for condensing gold (foil), amalgam, or any plastic material in a cavity, and which is operated by hand or by mechanical means.
automatic p., automatic condenser; a mechanically or electrically activated device used to provide condensing pressure in the placement of amalgam or gold foil in a cavity preparation.
back-action p., an instrument for condensing gold foil or amalgam in areas that cannot be reached directly.
foot p., a p. the shape of which resembles a foot, used for condensing gold foil; the working surface may be flat or curved in the heel-toe direction.
root canal p., fine-tapered root canal instrument, blunt at the tip, used for pressing or forcing a gutta percha cone into a root canal.

plumbago (plŭm-bā'gō) [L. *plumbago,* black lead]. Graphite.

plumbic (plŭm'bik) [L. *plumbum,* lead]. **1.** Relating to or containing lead. **2.** Denoting the higher valence of the lead ion, Pb^{4+}.

plumbism (plŭm'bizm) [L. *plumbum,* lead]. Lead *poisoning.*

plumbum (plŭm'bŭm). [L.]. Lead.

Plummer, Henry S., U.S. physician, 1874–1937. See P.'s *bag, dilator, disease;* P.-Vinson *syndrome.*

plumose (plū'mōs). [L. *pluma,* feather]. Feathery.

pluri- [L. *plus, pluris,* more]. Combining form denoting several or more. See also multi-, poly-.

pluricausal (plūr-i-kaw'zăl). Having two or more causes; used in reference to the etiology of a disease; often indicates that a given disease develops only when two or more causative factors are operative simultaneously.

pluriglandular (plū-ri-glan'dū-lăr). Multiglandular; polyglandular; denoting several glands or their secretions.

plurilocular (plū-ri-lok'yū-lăr). Multilocular.

plurinuclear (plū-ri-nū'klē-ăr). Multinuclear.

pluripotent, pluripotential (plū-rip'ō-tent, plū'rē-pō-ten'shăl). **1.** Having the capacity to affect more than one organ or tissue. **2.** Not fixed as to potential development. See also pluripotent *cell.*

pluriresistant (plū'ri-rē-sis'tănt). Having multiple aspects of resistance.

plutomania (plū-tō-mā'nē-ă) [G. *ploutos,* wealth, + *mania,* frenzy]. A delusion that one has great wealth.

plutonism (plū'ton-izm). Effects produced, as demonstrated in experimental animals, by means of exposure to the radioactive element plutonium present in atomic piles; they consist of hepatic damage, bone changes, and graying of the hair.

plutonium (plū-tō'nē-ŭm) [planet, *Pluto*]. A transuranium artificial radioactive element, symbol Pu, atomic no. 94. The best-known α-emitting isotope is ^{239}Pu (half-life 24,000 years) which, like ^{235}U, is fissionable and can be used in atomic bombs and nuclear power plants; ^{238}Pu (half-life 86 years) is used as an energy source in pacemakers. Pu ions are bone-seekers; incorporation into body fluids is a radiation hazard in the same way as radium is.

Pm Symbol for promethium.

pm Symbol for picometer.

P-mitrale (mī-trā'lē). An electrocardiographic syndrome consisting of broad, notched P waves in many leads and with a prominent late negative component to the P wave in leads V_1 and V_2, presumed to be characteristic of mitral valvular disease. (Although this term is extensively used in electrocardiographic literature, it is actually a misnomer and would be more appropriately called P-sinistrocardiale, as it results from overload of the left atrium regardless of the cause and may occur independently of disease of the mitral valve.)

PMS Premenstrual *syndrome.*

PMSG Abbreviation for pregnant mare's serum *gonadotropin.*

-pnea [G. *pheō,* to breathe]. Suffix denoting breath or respiration.

pneo- [G. *pneō,* to breathe]. Combining form denoting breath or respiration. See also pneum-, pneumo-.

pneodynamics (nē'ō-dī-nam'iks). Pneumodynamics.

pneometer (nē-om'ĕter) [pneo- + G. *metron,* measure]. Obsolete term for spirometer.

pneometry (nē-om'ĕ-trē). Obsolete term for spirometry.

pneoscope (nē'ō-skōp). Pneumatoscope (1).

pneum-, pneuma-, pneumat-, pneumato- [G. *pneuma, pneumatos,* air, breath]. Combining forms denoting presence of air or gas, the lungs, or breathing. See also pneo-, pneumo-.

pneuma (nū'mă) [G. *pneuma,* air, breath]. In ancient Greek philosophy and medicine: **1.** Air or an all-pervading fiery essence in the air (which today would be identified with oxygen) which was the creative and animating spirit of the universe; drawn into the body through the lungs it generated and sustained the innate heat in the left ventricle of the heart and was distributed by the arteries to the brain and all parts of the body. **2.** Intelligence; breath; soul or psyche.

pneumarthrogram (nū-marth'rō-gram). Film records of pneumarthrography.

pneumarthrography (nū-marth-rog'ră-fē). Pneumoarthrography; arthropneumography; radiographic examination of a joint following the introduction of air, with or without another contrast medium.

pneumarthro'sis (nū-mar-thrō'sis) [G. *pneuma,* air, + *arthron,* joint, + *-osis,* condition]. Presence of air in a joint.

pneumatic (nū-mat'ik) [G. *pneumatikos*]. **1.** Relating to air or gas, or to a structure filled with air. **2.** Relating to respiration.

pneumatics (nū-mat'iks) [G. *pneuma,* air or gas]. The science concerned with the physical properties of air or gases.

pneumatinuria (nū-mă-ti-nū'rē-ă). Pneumaturia.

pneumatism (nū'mă-tizm). The doctrine of the pneumatists.

pneumatists (nū'mă-tists). The followers of the school whose physiology centered around the pneuma and who conceived the causes of disease as disturbances of this vital principle.

pneumatization (nū'mă-ti-zā'shŭn) [G. *pneuma,* air]. The development of air cells such as those of the mastoid and ethmoidal bones.

pneumatized (nū'mă-tīzd). Containing air.

pneumato-. See pneum-.

pneumatocardia (nū'mă-tō-kar'dē-ă). Presence of air bubbles or gas in the blood of the heart; produced by air embolism.

pneumatocele (nū'mă-tō-sēl) [G. *pneuma,* air, + *kēlē,* tumor, hernia]. **1.** An emphysematous or gaseous swelling. **2.** Pneumonocele. **3.** A thin-walled cavity forming within the lung, characteristic of staphylococcus pneumonia.

extracranial p., extracranial pneumocele; subgaleal emphysema; collection of gas beneath the galea aponeurotica, usually due to fracture into the paranasal sinuses.

intracranial p., intracranial pneumocele; a collection of gas within the skull, in the brain, or in the meninges.

pneumatohemia (nū'mă-tō-hē'mē-ă). Pneumohemia.

pneumatology (nū-mă-tol'ō-jē) [G. *pneuma,* air, + *logos,* study]. Obsolete term for the former science concerned with air or gases, their physical and chemical properties, and their therapeutic application (anesthesia, resuscitation, oxygen therapy).

pneumatometer (nū-mă-tom'ĕ-ter). Obsolete term for spirometer.

pneumatorrhachis (nū-mă-tōr'ă-kis) [G. *pneuma,* air, + *rhachis,* spine]. Pneumorrhachis.

pneumatoscope (nū'mă-tō-skōp, nū-mat'ō-skōp) [G. *pneuma,* air, + *skopeō,* to examine]. **1.** Pneoscope; pneumoscope; an instrument for measuring the extent of the respiratory excursions of the chest. **2.** An instrument for use in auscultatory percussion, the percussion sounds of the chest being heard at the mouth.

pneumatosis (nū-mă-tō'sis) [G. a blowing out]. Abnormal accumulation of gas in any tissue or part of the body.

p. cystoi'des intestina'lis, intestinal emphysema; a condition of unknown cause characterized by the occurrence of gas cysts in the intestinal mucous membrane; may produce intestinal obstruction.

pneumatothorax (nū'mă-tō-thōr'aks). Pneumothorax.

pneumaturia (nū-mă-tū'rē-ă) [G. *pneuma,* air, + *ouron,* urine]. Pneumatinuria; the passage of gas or air from the urethra during or after urination, resulting from decomposition of bladder urine or, more commonly, from an intestinal fistula.

pneumatype (nū'mă-tīp) [G. *pneuma,* breath, + *typos,* type]. A device for determining the permeability of the nasal fossae by exhaling through the nose against a plate of cooled glass.

pneumectomy (nū-mek'tō-mē). Pneumonectomy.

pneumo-, pneumon-, pneumono- [G. *pneumōn, pneumonos,* lung]. Combining forms denoting the lungs, air or gas, respiration, or pneumonia. See also aer-, pneo-, pneum-.

pneumoangiography (nū'mō-an-jē-og'ră-fē) [pneumo- + G. *angeion,* vessel, + *graphō,* to write]. Contrast roentgenographic study of the pulmonary and bronchial blood vessels.

pneumoarthrography (nū'mō-ar-throg'ră-fē) [G. *pneuma,* air, + *arthron,* joint, + *graphō,* to write]. X-ray study of a joint after injection of air.

pneumobacillus (nū'mō-bă-sil'ŭs). *Klebsiella pneumoniae.*

pneumobulbar (nū-mō-bŭl'bar) [G. *penumōn,* lung, + L. *bulbus,* bulb]. Relating to the lungs and their connection with the medulla oblongata by way of the vagus nerve.

pneumocardial (nū'mō-kar'dē-ăl). Cardiopulmonary.

pneumocele (nū'mō-sēl). Pneumonocele.

extracranial p., extracranial *pneumatocele.*

intracranial p., intracranial *pneumatocele.*

pneumocentesis (nū'mō-sen-tē'sis). Pneumonocentesis.

pneumocephalus (nū-mō-sef'ă-lŭs) [G. *pneuma,* air, + *kephalē,* head]. Presence of air or gas within the cranial cavity.

pneumocholecystitis (nū'mō-kō'lē-sis-tī'tis). Cholecystitis with gas-forming organisms giving rise to gas in the gallbladder.

pneumococcal (nū-mō-kok'ăl). Pertaining to or containing the pneumococcus.

pneumococcemia (nū'mō-kok-sē'mē-ă) [pneumococcus + G. *haima,* blood]. The presence of pneumococci in the blood.

pneumococcidal (nū'mō-kok-sī'dăl) [pneumococcus + L. *caedo,* to kill]. Destructive to pneumococci.

pneumococcolysis (nū'mō-kok-ol'i-sis) [pneumococcus + G. *lysis,* dissolution]. Lysis or destruction of pneumococci.

pneumococcosis (nū'mō-kok-ō'sis). Rarely used term for infection with pneumococci.

pneumococcosuria (nū'mō-kok-o-sū'rē-ă) [pneumococcus + G. *ouron,* urine]. The presence of pneumococci or their specific capsular substance in the urine.

pneumococcus, pl. **pneumococci** (nū-mō-kok'ŭs, -kok'sī) [G. *pneumōn,* lung, + *kokkos,* berry (coccus)]. *Streptococcus pneumoniae.*

Fraenkel's p., *Streptococcus pneumoniae.*

Fraenkel-Weichselbaum p., *Streptococcus pneumoniae.*

pneumocolon (nū-mō-kō'lŏn) [G. *pneuma,* air, + *kolon,* colon]. Gas in the colon or interstitial gas in the wall of the colon.

pneumoconiosis, pl. **pneumoconioses** (nū'mō-kō-nē-ō'sis, -sēz) [G. *pneumōn,* lung, + *konis,* dust, + *-osis,* condition]. Pneumonoconiosis; anthracotic tuberculosis; inflammation commonly leading to fibrosis of the lungs caused by the inhalation of dust incident to various occupations; characterized by pain in the chest, cough with little or no expectoration, dyspnea, reduced thoracic excursion, sometimes cyanosis, and fatigue after slight exertion; degree of disability depends on the type of particles inhaled, as well as the level of exposure to them. For such diseases not listed below, see entries under disease, lung.

bauxite p., Shaver's disease; a condition due to the occupational inhalation of bauxite fumes emitted during the manufacture of alumina abrasives; characterized by cough, shortness of breath, a combined obstructive and restrictive breathing pattern, and impairment of diffusing capacity.

pneumocranium (nū-mō-krā'nē-ŭm) [G. *pneuma,* air, + *kranion,* skull]. Air present between the cranium and the dura mater; the term is commonly used to indicate extradural or subdural air.

pneumocystiasis (nū'mō-sis-tī'ă-sis). Pneumocystosis.

Pneumocystis carinii (nū-mō-sis'tis kă-rī'nē-ī) [G. *pneuma,* air, breathing, + *kystis,* bladder, pouch]. A minute lung-infecting protozoa characterized by cysts which develop eight intracystic organisms; proliferation is within cysts and in the free trophozoite stage. These organisms are of worldwide distribution, are part of the normal flora of rodents, and are the cause of human pneumocystosis.

pneumocystography (nū'mō-sis-tog'ră-fē) [G. *pneuma,* air, + *kystis,* bladder, + *graphō,* to write]. Roentgenography of the bladder following injection of air.

pneumocystosis (nū'mō-sis-tō'sis). Interstitial plasma cell pneumonia; pneumocystiasis; pneumonia resulting from infection with *Pneumocystis carinii,* frequently seen in immunologically compromised or steroid-treated individuals, the elderly, or premature or debilitated babies during their first three months. The alveoli are filled with a honeycomb-like or foamy network of acidophilic material, apparently not fibrin and not stainable with silver, within which the organisms, individually or in aggregates, are enmeshed; throughout the alveolar walls and pulmonary sputa there is a diffuse infiltration of mononuclear inflammatory cells, chiefly plasma cells and macrophages, as well as a few lymphocytes. Patients may be only slightly febrile (or even afebrile), but are likely to be extremely weak, dyspneic, and cyanotic.

pneumocyte (nū'mō-sīt) [pneumo- + G. *kytos,* cell]. Alveolar *cell.*

pneumoderma (nū-mō-der'mă) [G. *pneuma,* air, + *derma,* skin]. Subcutaneous *emphysema.*

pneumodynamics (nū'mō-dī-nam'iks) [G. *pneuma,* breath, + *dynamis,* force]. Pneodynamics; the mechanics of respiration.

pneumoempyema (nū'mō-em'pī-ē'mă). Pyopneumothorax.

pneumoencephalogram (nū'mō-en-sef'ă-lō-gram). The roentgenographic record obtained by pneumoencephalography.

pneumoencephalography (nū'mō-en-sef'ă-log'ră-fē) [G. *pneuma,* air, + *enkephalos,* brain, + *graphō,* to write]. Radiographic visualization of cerebral ventricles and subarachnoid spaces by use of gas such as air.

pneumogastric (nū-mō-gas'trik) [G. *pneumōn,* lung, + *gastēr,* stomach]. Gastropneumonic; gastropulmonary. **1.** Relating to the lungs and the stomach. **2.** Obsolete term denoting the nervus vagus.

pneumogastrography (nū'mō-gas-trog'ră-fē) [G. *pneuma,* air, + *gastēr,* stomach, + *graphō,* to write]. Rarely used roentgenographic study of stomach after injection of air.

pneumogram (nū'mō-gram) [G. *pneumōn,* lung, + *gramma,* a drawing]. **1.** The record or tracing made by a pneumograph. **2.** Roentgenographic record of pneumography.

pneumograph (nū'mō-graf) [G. *pneumōn,* lung, + *graphō,* to write]. Generic term for any device that records respiratory excursions from movements on the body surface; *e.g.,* an impedance p., which applies the principles of impedance plethysmography to the chest.

pneumography (nū-mog'ră-fē) [G. *pneumōn,* lung, + *graphō,* to write]. **1.** Examination with a pneumograph. **2.** Pneumoradiography; pneumoroentgenography; a general term indicating radiography after injection of air.

pneumohemia (nū-mō-hē'mē-ă) [G. *pneuma,* air, + *haima,* blood]. Pneumatohemia; presence of air in blood vessels. See also air *embolism.*

pneumohemopericardium (nū'mō-hē-mō-per-i-kar'dē-ŭm). Hemopneumopericardium.

pneumohemothorax (nū'mō-hē-mō-thōr'aks). Hemopneumothorax.

pneumohydrometra (nū'mō-hī-drō-mē'tră) [G. *pneuma,* air, + *hydōr* (*hydr-*), water, + *mētra,* uterus]. The presence of gas and serum in the uterine cavity.

pneumohydropericardium (nū'mō-hī'drō-păr-i-kar'dē-ŭm). Hydropneumopericardium.

pneumohydroperitoneum (nū'mō-hī-drō-per-i-tō-nē'ŭm). Hydropneumoperitoneum.

pneumohydrothorax (nū-mō-hī-drō-thōr'aks). Hydropneumothorax.

pneumohypoderma (nū'mō-hī-pō-der'mă) [G. *pneuma,* air, + *hypo,* beneath, + *derma,* skin]. Subcutaneous *emphysema.*

pneumolith (nū'mō-lith) [G. *pneumōn,* lung, + *lithos,* stone]. Pulmolith; a calculus in the lung.

pneumolithiasis (nū-mō-li-thī'ă-sis). Formation of calculi in the lungs.

pneumology (nū-mol'ō-jē) [G. *pneuma,* lung, + *logos,* study]. Study of diseases of the lung and air passages.

pneumolysis (nū-mol'i-sis) [G. *pneumōn,* lung, + *lysis,* a loosening]. Separation of the lung and costal pleura from the endothoracic fascia.

pneumomalacia (nū-mō-mă-lā'shē-ă) [G. *pneumōn,* lung, + *malakia,* softness]. Softening of the lung tissue.

pneumomassage (nū'mō-mă-sahzh') [G. *pneuma,* air, + massage]. Compression and rarefaction of the air in the external auditory meatus, causing movement of the ossicles of the tympanum.

pneumomediastinum (nū'mō-mē'dē-ă-stī'nŭm) [G. *pneuma,* air, + mediastinum]. Escape of air into mediastinal tissues, usually from interstitial emphysema or from a ruptured pulmonary bleb.

pneumomelanosis (nū'mō-mel-ă-nō'sis) [G. *pneumōn,* lung, + *melanosis,* a becoming black]. Pneumonomelanosis; blackening of the lung tissue from the inhalation of coal dust or other black particles.

pneumometer (nū-mom'ĕ-ter). Obsolete term for spirometer.

pneumometry (nū-mom'ĕ-trē). Obsolete term for spirometry.

pneumomycosis (nū'mō-mī-kō'sis) [G. *pneumōn,* lung, + *mykēs,* fungus]. Pneumonomycosis; obsolete term denoting any disease of the lungs caused by the presence of fungi.

pneumomyelography (nū'mō-mī'ĕ-log'ră-fē) [G. *pneuma,* air, + *myelos,* marrow, + *graphō,* to write]. Rarely used roentgenographic examination of spinal canal after injection of air or gas into it.

pneumon-. See pneumo-.

pneumonectomy (nū'mō-nek'tō-mē) [G. *pneumōn,* lung, + *ektomē,* excision]. Pneumectomy; pulmonectomy; removal of all pulmonary lobes from a lung in one operation.

pneumonia (nū-mō'nē-ă) [G. fr. *pneumōn,* lung, + *-ia,* condition]. Inflammation of the lung parenchyma characterized by consolidation of the affected part, the alveolar air spaces being filled with exudate, inflammatory cells, and fibrin. Most cases are due to infection by bacteria or viruses, a few to inhalation of chemicals or trauma to the chest wall, and a small minority to rickettsias, fungi, and yeasts. Distribution may be lobar, segmental, or lobular; when lobular, in association with bronchitis, it is termed bronchopneumonia. See also pneumonitis.

acute interstitial p., a severe and usually fatal form of p. occurring in infants.

anthrax p., pulmonary *anthrax.*

apex p., apical p., p. of the apex or apices.

aspiration p., deglutition p.; bronchopneumonia resulting from the entrance of foreign material, usually food particles or vomit, into the bronchi.

atypical p., primary atypical p.

bronchial p., bronchopneumonia.

caseous p., a form of severe pulmonary tuberculosis in which tubercles are not prominent, but with a diffuse extensive cellular infiltration which undergoes caseation affecting large areas of lung.

central p., core p.; a form of p. in which exudation is confined for a time to the central portion of a lobe or the hilar region.

chemical p., p. caused by inhalation of toxic gas, such as the war gases phosgene or chlorine; the lungs are edematous and hemorrhagic, with large amounts of fluid which fill the air passages and may drown the patient; if recovery occurs, permanent damage of the lungs remains, and recurrent pulmonary infections are common.

congenital p., p. in the newborn, infection being contracted prenatally.

contusion p., traumatic p.; inflammation of the lungs following a severe blow on or compression of the chest, or following a wound of the lung itself.

core p., central p.

deglutition p., aspiration p.

desquamative interstitial p. (D.I.P.), diffuse proliferation of alveolar epithelial cells, which desquamate into the air sacs and become filled with macrophages, accompanied by interstitial cellular infiltration and fibrosis; gradual onset of dyspnea and nonproductive cough occurs.

p. dis'secans, p. interlobularis purulenta.

double p., lobar p. involving both lungs.

Eaton agent p., primary atypical p.

embolic p., infarction following embolization of a pulmonary artery or arteries.

eosinophilic p., an immunologic disorder characterized by radiologic evidence of infiltrates accompanied by either peripheral blood eosinophilia or histopathologic evidence of eosinophilic infiltrates in lung tissue.

Friedländer's p., a form of p. caused by infection with *Klebsiella*

pneumoniae (Friedländer's bacillus), characteristically severe and lobar in distribution.
gangrenous p., gangrene of the lungs.
giant cell p., giant interstitial p.; Hecht's p.; a rare complication of measles, with the postmortem finding of multinucleated giant cells lining alveoli.
Hecht's p., giant cell p.
hypostatic p., p. resulting from infection developing in the dependent portions of the lungs due to decreased ventilation of those areas, with resulting failure to drain bronchial secretions; occurs primarily in the aged or those debilitated by disease who lie in the same position for long periods.
influenzal p., **(1)** p. complicating influenza; **(2)** p. due to *Haemophilus influenzae.*
p. interlobula'ris purulen'ta, p. dissecans; p. in which the lobules of the lung are separated by collections of purulent exudate.
interstitial giant cell p., giant cell p.
interstitial plasma cell p., pneumocystosis.
intrauterine p., fetal p. contracted *in utero* and manifesting itself in the early neonatal period.
lipid p., lipoid p., a pulmonary condition marked by inflammatory and fibrotic changes in the lungs due to the inhalation of various oily or fatty substances, particularly liquid petrolatum, or resulting from accumulation in the lungs of endogenous lipid material, either cholesterol from obstructive pneumonitis or following fracture of a bone; phagocytes containing lipid are usually present.
lobar p., p. affecting one or more lobes, or part of a lobe, of the lung in which the consolidation is virtually homogeneous; commonly due to infection by *Streptococcus pneumoniae;* sputum is scanty and usually of a rusty tint from altered blood.
metastatic p., a purulent inflammation in the lungs due to infected emboli.
migratory p., wandering p.; a form of p. in which successive areas of the lung are affected; may occur in bronchopulmonary aspergillosis.
moniliasis p., p. due to species of *Candida,* usually *C. albicans.*
mycoplasma p. of pigs, virus p. of pigs; a worldwide chronic p. usually involving only the anterior lobes; it seldom causes death but is responsible for much unthriftiness; it is caused by *Mycoplasma hyopneumoniae.*
mycoplasmal p., primary atypical p.
oil p., lipid p.
organized p., unresolved p. in which fibrous tissue forms in the alveoli.
Pittsburgh p., a variant of Legionnaires' disease caused by *Legionella midadei.*
plague p., pneumonic *plague.*
pneumococcal p., p. due to infection by *Streptococcus pneumoniae;* often of lobar distribution.
postoperative p., p. occurring after an operation; may be an aspiration p., or p. due to ether anesthesia or to atelectasis; pulmonary infarction causes a similar syndrome.
primary atypical p., atypical, Eaton agent, or mycoplasmal p.; an acute systemic disease with involvement of the lungs, caused by *Mycoplasma pneumoniae* and marked by high fever, cough, relatively few physical signs, and scattered densities on x-rays; usually associated with development of cold agglutinins and antibodies to the bacteria.
rheumatic p., p. rarely occurring in severe acute rheumatic fever, even when the disease was common; consolidation occurs, the lungs being of a rubbery consistency, with fibrin exudate and small hemorrhages, as well as edema from left ventrical failure.
septic p., suppurative p.
staphylococcal p., p., usually caused by *Staphylococcus aureus,* usually commencing as a bronchopneumonia, and frequently leading to suppuration and distruction of lung tissue.
streptococcal p., p. due to *Streptococcus pyogenes.*
suppurative p., septic p.; any p. associated with the formation of pus and destruction of pulmonary tissue; abscess formation may occur.
terminal p., p. occurring in the course of some other disease toward its fatal termination.
traumatic p., contusion p.
tularemic p., tularemia with pulmonary lesions.
typhoid p., p. complicating typhoid fever.
unresolved p., p. in which the alveolar exudate persists and eventually undergoes fibrosis.
uremic p., **(1)** uremic *lung;* **(2)** terminal infective p. occurring in a patient with uremia.
virus p. of pigs, mycoplasma p. of pigs.
wandering p., migratory p.
wool-sorters' p., pulmonary *anthrax.*

pneumonic (nū-mon'ik). **1.** Pulmonary. **2.** Relating to pneumonia.

pneumonitis (nū-mō-nī'tis) [G. *pneumōn,* lung, + *-itis,* inflammation]. Pulmonitis; inflammation of the lungs. See also pneumonia.
feline p., an infectious respiratory illness of domesticated cats caused by *Chlamydia psittaci.*
hypersensitivity p., extrinsic allergic *alveolitis.*
uremic p., uremic *lung.*

pneumono-. See pneumo-.

pneumonocele (nū-mōn'ō-sēl). Pneumatocele (2); pneumocele; pleurocele; protrusion of a portion of the lung through a defect in the chest wall.

pneumonocentesis (nū'mō-nō-sen-tē'sis) [G. *pneumōn,* lung, + *kentēsis,* puncture]. Pneumocentesis; paracentesis of the lung.

pneumonococcal (nū'mō-nō-kok'ăl). Relating to or associated with *Streptococcus pneumoniae.*

pneumonococcus (nū'mō-nō-kok'ŭs). *Streptococcus pneumoniae.*

pneumonoconiosis (nū'mō-nō-kō-nē-ō'sis). Pneumoconiosis.

pneumonocyte (nū'mō-nō-sīt) [G. *pneumōn,* lung, + *kytos,* cell]. Nonspecific term referring to cells lining alveoli in the respiratory part of the lung.
granular p.'s, great alveolar *cells.*
phagocytic p., an alveolar phagocyte containing hemosiderin, carbon, or other foreign particles.

pneumonomelanosis (nū'mō-nō-mel-ă-nō'sis). Pneumomelanosis.

pneumonomoniliasis (nū'mō-nō-mon-i-lī'ă-sis). Rarely used term for candidiasis of the lung.

pneumonomycosis (nū'mō-nō-mī-kō'sis). Pneumomycosis.

pneumonopexy (nū'mō-nō-pek-sē) [G. *pneumōn,* lung, + *pēxis,* fixation]. Pneumopexy; fixation of the lung by suturing the costal and pulmonary pleurae or otherwise causing adhesion of the two layers.

pneumonorrhaphy (nū-mō-nōr'ă-fē) [G. *pneumōn,* lung, + *rhaphē,* suture]. Suture of the lung.

pneumonotomy (nū-mō-not'ō-mē) [G. *pneumōn,* lung, + *tomē,* incision]. Pneumotomy; incision of the lung.

Pneumonyssus simicola (nū-mō-nis'ŭs si-mik'ō-lă) [pneum- + G. *onyx* (*onychos*), nail; *simos,* flat-nosed]. A small mite (family Halarachnidae) that causes pulmonary acariasis in monkeys.

pneumo-orbitography (nū'mō-ōr'bi-tog'ră-fē). Radiographic visualization of the orbital contents following injection of a gas, usually air.

pneumopericardium (nū'mō-per-i-kar'dē-ŭm) [G. *pneuma,* air, + pericardium]. Presence of gas in the pericardial sac.

pneumoperitoneum (nū'mō-per-i-tō-nē'ŭm) [G. *pneuma,* air, + peritoneum]. Presence of air or gas in the peritoneal cavity as a result of disease, or produced artificially for treatment of pulmonary or intestinal tuberculosis, bronchiectasis, tuberculous empyema, and certain other conditions.

pneumoperitonitis (nū'mō-per-i-tō-nī'tis) [G. *pneuma,* air, + peritonitis]. Inflammation of the peritoneum with an accumulation of gas in the peritoneal cavity.

pneumopexy (nū'mō-pek-sē). Pneumonopexy.

pneumophagia (nū-mō-fā'jē-ă). Aerophagia.

pneumopleuritis (nū'mō-plū-ī'tis) [G. *pneuma,* air, + pleur- + *-itis,* inflammation]. Pleurisy with air or gas in the pleural cavity.

pneumopyelography (nū'mō-pī-ĕ-log'ră-fē) [G. *pneuma,* air, + *pyelos,* pelvis, + *graphō,* to write]. X-ray examination of the kidney after air or gas has been injected into the kidney pelvis.

pneumopyothorax (nū'mō-pī-ō-thōr'aks). Pyopneumothorax.

pneumoradiography (nu'mo-ra-dĭ-og'ră-fĭ). Pneumography (2).

pneumoresection (nū'mō-rē-sek'shŭn) [G. *pneumōn,* lung, + resection]. Excision of part of a lung.

pneumoretroperitoneum (nū'mō-ret'rō-per-i-tō-nē'ŭm). Escape of air into the retroperitoneal tissues.

pneumoroentgenography (nū'mō-rent'gĕ-nog'ră-fē). Pneumography (2).

pneumorrhachis (nū-mō-rā'kis, nū-mōr'ă-kis) [G. *pneuma,* air, + *rachis,* spinal column]. Pneumatorrhachis; the presence of gas in the spinal canal.

pneumoscope (nū'mō-skōp). Pneumatoscope.

pneumoserothorax (nū'mō-sēr-ō-thōr'aks). Hydropneumothorax.

pneumosilicosis (nū'mō-sil'i-kō'sis). Silicosis.

pneumotachogram (nū-mō-tak'ō-gram) [G. *pneuma,* air, + *tachys,* swift, + *gramma,* something written]. A recording of respired gas flow as a function of time, produced by a pneumotachograph.

pneumotachograph (nū-mō-tak'ō-graf). Pneumotachometer; an instrument for measuring the instantaneous flow of respiratory gases.

Fleisch p., a p. that measures flow in terms of the proportional pressure drop across a resistance consisting of numerous capillary tubes in parallel.

Silverman-Lilly p., a p. that measures flow in terms of the proportional pressure drop across a resistance consisting of a very fine mesh screen.

pneumotachometer (nū'mō-tă-kom'ĕ-ter) [G. *pneuma,* air, + *tachys,* swift, + *metron,* measure]. Pneumotachograph.

pneumothermomassage (nū-mō-ther'mō-mă-sahzh') [G. *pneuma,* air, + *thermē,* heat, + Fr. *massage*]. Application to the body of hot air under varying degrees of pressure.

pneumothorax (nū-mō-thōr'aks) [G. *pneuma,* air, + thorax]. Pneumatothorax; the presence of air or gas in the pleural cavity.

artificial p., p. produced by the injection of air, or a more slowly absorbed gas such as nitrogen, into the pleural space to collapse the lung.

extrapleural p., the presence of a gas between the endothoracic fascia-pleural layer and the adjacent chest wall.

open p., a free communication between the atmosphere and the pleural space either via the lung or through the chest wall. Also called blowing, sucking, or traumatopneic wound.

p. sim'plex, p., without known cause, in an otherwise healthy person.

spontaneous p., p. occurring secondary to parenchymal lung disease, usually from an emphysematous bulla which ruptures or occasionally from a lung abscess.

tension p., valvular p.; a variety of spontaneous p. in which air enters the pleural cavity and is trapped during expiration; intrathoracic pressure builds to values higher than atmospheric pressure, compresses the lung, and may displace the mediastinum and its structures toward the opposite side, with consequent disadvantageous effects on blood flow.

therapeutic p., p. designed to create some pulmonary parenchymal collapse, diaphragmatic immobilization, or both.

valvular p., tension p.

pneumotomy (nū-mot'ō-mē). Pneumonotomy.

pneumoventricle (nū-mō-ven'tri-kl). Air in the ventricular system of the brain; occurs as a complication of a fracture of the skull which passes through the accessory nasal sinuses.

Pneumovirus (nū'mō-vī'rŭs). A genus of viruses (family Paramyxoviridae) including respiratory syncytial virus and pneumonia virus of mice. Nucleocapsids are 12 to 15 nm in diameter and thus intermediate in size between other Paramyxoviridae and the Orthomyxoviridae; cytoplasmic inclusions are considerably more dense than those of other viruses in the family.

pneusis (nū'sis) [G. *pneuesthai,* to breathe]. Breathing.

pnigophobia (nī-gō-fō'bē-ă) [G. *pnigos,* choking, + *phobos,* fear]. Morbid fear of choking.

PNP Abbreviation for psychogenic nocturnal *polydipsia.*

PNPB Abbreviation for positive-negative pressure *breathing.*

Po Symbol for polonium.

Po_2, pO_2 Symbol for the partial pressure (tension) of oxygen. See partial *pressure.*

pock (pok) [A.S. *poc,* a pustule]. The specific pustular cutaneous lesion of smallpox.

pocket (pok'et) [Fr. *pochette*] **1.** A cul-de-sac or pouchlike cavity. **2.** A diseased gingival attachment; a space between the inflamed gum and the surface of a tooth, limited apically by an epithelial attachment. **3.** To enclose within a confined space, as the stump of the pedicle of an ovarian or other abdominal tumor between the lips of the external wound. **4.** A collection of pus in a nearly closed sac. **5.** To approach the surface at a localized spot, as with the thinned out wall of an abscess which is about to rupture.

gingival p., a diseased gingival attachment in which the increased depth of the sulcus is due to an increase in the bulk of its gingival wall.

infrabony p., intrabony p., subcrestal p.

periodontal p., a pathologic deepening of the gingival sulcus resulting from detachment of the gingiva from the tooth.

Rathke's p., pituitary *diverticulum.*

Seessel's p., Seessel's pouch; preoral gut; the part of the embryonic foregut extending cephalic to the level of the oral plate.

subcrestal p., infrabony or intrabony p.; a p. extending apically below the level of the adjacent alveolar crest.

Tröltsch's p.'s, *recessus* membranae tympani, anterior and posterior.

pockmark (pok'mark). The small depressed scar left after the healing of the smallpox pustule.

poculum (pok'yū-lŭm) [L.]. Cup (1).

p. diog'enis, Diogenes *cup.*

pod-, podo- [G. *pous, podos,* foot]. Combining forms meaning foot or foot-shaped.

podagra (pō-dag'ră) [G. fr. *pous,* foot, + *agra,* a seizure]. Severe pain in the foot, especially that of typical gout in the great toe.

podagral, podagric, podagrous (pod'ă-grăl, pō-dag'rik, pod'ă-grŭs). Relating to or characterized by podogra.

podalgia (pō-dal'jē-ă) [pod- + G. *algos,* pain]. Tarsalgia; pododynia; pain in the foot.

podalic (pō-dal'ik) [G. *pous* (*pod-*), foot]. Relating to the foot.

podarthritis (pod-ar-thrī'tis) [pod- + arthritis]. Inflammation of any of the tarsal or metatarsal joints.

podedema (pod-e-dē'mă). Edema of the feet and ankles.

podiatric (pō-dī'ă-trik). Relating to podiatry.

podiatrist (pō-dī'ă-trist) [pod- + G. *iatros*, physician]. Chiropodist; podologist; a practitioner of podiatry.

podiatry (pō-dī'ă-trē) [pod- + G. *iatreia*, medical treatment]. Podiatric medicine; chiropody; podology; the specialty concerned with the diagnosis and/or medical, surgical, mechanical, physical, and adjunctive treatment of the diseases, injuries, and defects of the human foot.

podismus (pō-diz'mŭs). Podospasm.

poditis (pō-dī'tis) [pod- + G. *-itis*, inflammation]. An inflammatory disorder of the foot.

tourniquet p., postischemic acute inflammatory edema in the foot (or paw), as the result of complete obstruction of the circulation to that member by use of a tourniquet; produced experimentally in animals as a means of evaluating the anti-inflammatory efficacy of drugs.

podo-. See pod-.

podobromidrosis (pod'ō-brō-mi-drō'sis) [podo- + G. *brōmos*, a foul smell, + *hidrōs*, sweat]. Foul-smelling perspiration of the feet.

podocyte (pod'ō-sīt) [podo- + G. *kytos*, a hollow (cell)]. An epithelial cell of the visceral layer of Bowman's capsule in the renal corpuscle, attached to the outer surface of the glomerular capillary basement membrane by cytoplasmic foot processes (pedicels); believed to play a role in the ultrafiltration of blood.

pododerm (pod'ō-derm) [podo- + G. *derma*, skin]. Corium ungulae; the corium of the foot; that portion of the skin which lies under the hoof and secretes the horny structure. The regions of the p. are the periople (corium limbi), coronary band (corium coronae), wall (corium parietis), and sole (corium solae).

pododermatitis (pod'ō-der-mă-tī'tis). Inflammation of the pododerm. See also laminitis (2).

pododynamometer (pod'ō-dī'nă-mom'ĕ-ter) [podo- + G. *dynamis*, force, + *metron*, measure]. An instrument for measuring the strength of the muscles of the foot or leg.

pododynia (pod-ō-din'ē-ă) [podo- + G. *odynē*, pain]. Podalgia.

podogram (pod'ō-gram) [podo- + G. *gramma*, written]. An imprint of the sole of the foot, showing the contour and the condition of the arch, or an outline tracing.

podograph (pod'ō-graf) [podo- + G. *graphō*, to write]. A device for taking an outline at the foot and an imprint of the sole.

podolite (pod'ō-līt). Dahllite.

podologist (pō-dol'ō-jist). Podiatrist.

podology (pō-dol'ō-jē) [podo- + G. *logos*, study]. Podiatry.

podomechanotherapy (pod-ō-mek'ă-nō-thār'ă-pē). Treatment of foot conditions with mechanical devices; *e.g.*, arch supports, ortheses.

podometer (pō-dom'ĕ-ter) [podo- + G. *metron*, measure]. Pedometer.

podophyllin (pod-ō-fil'in). Podophyllum *resin*.

podophyllotoxin (pod'ō-fil-ō-tok'sin). A toxic polycyclic substance, $C_{22}H_{22}O_8$, with cathartic properties present in podophyllum; has antineoplastic action.

podophyllum (pod-ō-fil'ŭm). Vegetable calomel; the rhizome of *Podophyllum peltatum* (family Berberidaceae), used as a laxative. Also called May-apple, American mandrake, umbrella plant, or duck's-foot.

Indian p., the dried rhizome and roots of *P. emodi*, a Himalayan plant; a cholagogue and cathartic.

podospasm, podospasmus (pod'ō-spazm, -spaz-mŭs) [podo- + G. *spasmos*, spasm]. Podismus; spasm of the foot.

POEMS Abbreviation for *p*olyneuropathy, *o*rganomegaly, *e*ndocrinopathy, *m*onoclonal gammopathy, and *s*kin changes. See POEMS *syndrome*.

pogoniasis (pō-gō-nī'ă-sis) [G. *pōgōn*, beard, + *-iasis*, condition]. Growth of a beard on a woman, or excessive hairiness of the face in men. See also hirsutism.

pogonion (pō-gō'ni-on) [G. dim. of *pōgōn*, beard]. Mental point; in craniometry, the most anterior point on the mandible in the midline; the most anterior, prominent point on the chin.

Pogonomyrmex (pō-gō'nō-mir'meks, -mer'meks) [G. *pōgōn*, beard, + *myrmex*, ant]. Harvester ant; a genus of ants that attack man and small animals.

-poiesis [G. *poiēsis*, a making]. Combining form denoting production.

poikilo- [G. *poikilos*, many colored, varied]. Combining form denoting irregular or varied.

poikiloblast (poy'ki-lō-blast) [poikilo- + G. *blastos*, germ]. A nucleated red blood cell of irregular shape.

poikilocyte (poy'ki-lō-sīt) [poikilo- + G. *kytos*, cell]. A red blood cell of irregular shape.

poikilocythemia (poy'ki-lō-sī-thē'mē-ă) [poikilocyte + G. *haima*, blood]. Poikilocytosis.

poikilocytosis (poy'ki-lō-sī-tō'sis) [poikilocyte + G. *-osis*, condition]. Poikilocythemia; the presence of poikilocytes in the peripheral blood.

poikilodentosis (poy'ki-lō-den-tō'sis) [poikilo- + L. *dens*, tooth, + G. *-osis*, condition]. Hypoplastic defects or mottling of enamel due to excessive fluoride in the water supply.

poikiloderma (poy'ki-lō-der'mă) [poikilo- + G. *derma*, skin]. A variegated hyperpigmentation and telangiectasia of the skin, followed by atrophy.

p. atroph'icans and cataract, Rothmund's *syndrome*.

p. atroph'icans vascula're, parakeratosis variegata; parapsoriasis lichenoides; a rare condition that simulates radiodermatitis in appearance; may eventuate as mycosis fungoides.

p. of Civatte, Civatte's disease; reticulated pigmentation and telangiectasia of the sides of the cheeks and neck; common in middle-aged women.

p. congenita'le, Rothmund's *syndrome*.

poikilotherm (poy'ki-lō-therm). Allotherm; warm-blooded animal; a poikilothermic animal.

poikilothermic, poikilothermal, poikilothermous (poy'ki-lō-ther'mic, -măl, -mŭs) [poikilo- + G. *thermē*, heat]. Cold-blooded; hematocryal. **1.** Varying in temperature according to the temperature of the surrounding medium; denoting the so-called cold-blooded animals, such as the reptiles and amphibians, and the plants. **2.** Capable of existence and growth in mediums of varying temperatures. *Cf.* heterothermic; homeothermic.

poikilothermy, poikilothermism (poy'ki-lō-ther'mē, -therm'izm) [poikilo- + G. *thermē*, heat]. The condition of plants and cold-blooded animals, the temperature of which varies with the changes in the temperature of the surrounding medium.

poikilothrombocyte (poy'ki-lō-throm'bō-sīt) [poikilo- + G. *thrombos*, clot, + *kytos*, cell]. A blood platelet of abnormal shape.

poikilothymia (poy'ki-lō-thī'mē-ă) [poikilo- + G. *thymos*, mind]. A mental state marked by abnormal variations in mood.

POINT

point (poynt) [Fr.; L. *punctum*, fr. *pungo*, pp. *punctus*, to pierce]. **1.** Punctum. **2.** A sharp end or apex. **3.** A slight projection. **4.** A stage or condition reached, as the boiling p. **5.** To become ready to

open, said of an abscess or boil the wall of which is becoming thin and is about to break.
p. A, subspinale.
absorbent p.'s, cones of paper or paper products used for drying or maintaining medicaments in conjunction with root canal therapy.
alveolar p., prosthion.
anterior focal p., the p. where parallel rays from the retina are focused.
apophysary p., apophysial p., **(1)** subnasal p.; **(2)** Trousseau's p.
auricular p., auriculare.
axial p., nodal p.
p. B, supramentale.
boiling p. (b.p.), the temperature at which the vapor pressure of a liquid equals the ambient atmospheric pressure.
Bolton p., the highest p. in the profile roentgenogram at the notches on the end of the occipital condyles.
Capuron's p.'s, the iliopubic eminences and the sacroiliac joints, constituting four fixed p.'s in the pelvic inlet.
cardinal p.'s, **(1)** the four p.'s in the pelvic inlet toward one of which the occiput of the baby is usually directed in case of head presentation: two sacroiliac articulations and the two iliopectineal eminences corresponding to the acetabula; **(2)** six p.'s of a compound optical system; the anterior focal p., the posterior focal p., the two principal p.'s, and the two nodal p.'s.
central-bearing p., the contact p. of a central-bearing device.
Clado's p., a p. at the junction of the interspinous and right semilunar lines, at the lateral border of the rectus abdominis muscle, where marked tenderness on pressure is felt in some cases of appendicitis.
cold-rigor p., the degree of lowered temperature at which the activity of a cell ceases and the cell passes into the narcotic or hibernating state.
congruent p.'s, the p. in each retina referred to the same external stimulus.
conjugate p., a p. so related to another that an object at one is imaged at the other.
contact p., contact *area.*
p.'s of convergence, see under convergence.
craniometric p.'s, fixed p.'s on the skull used as landmarks in craniometry.

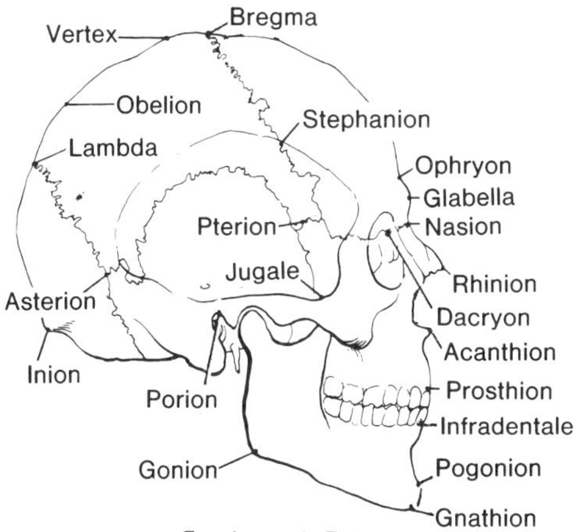

Craniometric Points

critical p., a p. at which two phases become identical; thus, at a given critical temperature and critical pressure, the liquid and gaseous state of a particular substance can no longer be differentiated.
dew p., the temperature at and below which moisture will condense for a specific humidity.
p. of elbow, olecranon.
end p., the completion of a reaction; usually evident by the first perceptible alteration of the color of an added indicator.
far p., punctum remotum; that p. in conjugate focus with the retina when the eye is not accommodating.
p. of fixation, p. of regard; the p. on the retina at which the rays coming from an object regarded directly are focused.
flash p., the lowest temperature at which vapors of a liquid may be ignited by a flame.
focal p., see anterior focal p.; posterior focal p.
freezing p., the temperature at which a liquid solidifies.
fusing p., see fusion *temperature.*
Guéneau de Mussy's p., a p., painful on pressure, at the junction of a line prolonging the left border of the sternum and a horizontal line at the level of end of the bony portion of the tenth rib; it is present in cases of diaphragmatic pleurisy.
gutta-percha p.'s, cones of a gutta percha compound used for filling root canals in conjunction with a cement, paste, or plastic.
Hallé's p., a p. at the intersection of a horizontal line touching the anterior superior spine of the ilium and a perpendicular line drawn from the spine of the pubis; here the ureter can be most readily palpated.
heat-rigor p., the degree of elevated temperature at which coagulation of protoplasm occurs with death of the cell.
incident p., the p. at which a light ray enters an optical system.
incisal p., the p. located between the incisal edges of the lower central incisors; the graphic projection of the excursions of the incisal p. in certain planes is generally used to illustrate the envelope of motion of mandibular movement.
isoelectric p., the pH at which an amphoteric substance, such as protein, is electrically neutral; below or above this pH, it acts as a base or acid, respectively.
isoionic p., the pH at which a zwitterion has an equal number of positive and negative charges; in water and in the absence of other solutes, this is the isoelectric p.
isosbestic p., in applied spectroscopy, a wavelength at which absorbance of two substances, one of which can be converted into the other, is the same.
J p., ST junction; the p. marking the end of the QRS complex and the beginning of the ST segment in the electrocardiogram.
jugal p., jugale.
lower alveolar p., infradentale.
malar p., apex of the tuberosity of the zygomatic (malar) bone.
p. of maximal impulse, the p. on the chest wall at which the maximal cardiac impulse is seen and/or felt.
maximum occipital p., the p. on the squama of the occipital bone farthest from the glabella.
Mayo-Robson's p., a p. just above and to the right of the umbilicus, where tenderness on pressure exists in disease of the pancreas.
McBurney's p., a p. between $1^1/_2$ and 2 inches superomedial to the anterior superior spine of the ilium, on a straight line joining that process and the umbilicus, where pressure elicits tenderness in acute appendicitis.
median mandibular p., a p. on the anteroposterior center of the mandibular ridge in the median sagittal plane.
melting p., the temperature at which a solid becomes a liquid.
mental p., pogonion.
metopic p., metopion.
motor p., a p. on the skin where the application of an electrode will cause the contraction of a particular muscle.
Munro's p., a p. at the right edge of the rectus abdominis muscle, between the umbilicus and the anterior superior spine of the ilium, where pressure elicits tenderness in appendicitis.
nasal p., nasion.
near p., punctum proximum; that p. in conjugate focus with the retina when the eye exerts maximal accommodation.
neutral p., the p. (pH 7) at which a solution is neither acid

nor alkaline.

nodal p., axial p.; one of two p.'s in a compound optical system so related that a ray directed toward the first p. will appear to have passed through the second p. parallel to its original direction.

occipital p., the most prominent posterior p. on the occipital bone above the inion.

p. of ossification, *punctum* ossificationis.

painful p., see Valleix's p.'s.

posterior focal p., the p. of a compound optical system where parallel rays entering the system are focused.

power p., in dentistry, the vertical dimension at which the greatest masticatory force may be registered.

preauricular p., a p. of the posterior root of the zygomatic arch lying immediately in front of the upper end of the tragus.

pressure p., a cutaneous locus having pressure-sensitive elements which when compressed, pressure is appreciated.

primary p. of ossification, *punctum* ossificationis primarium.

principal p., one of two p.'s on an optic axis so related that an object at one is exactly imaged at the other without magnification, minification, or inversion.

p. of proximal contact, contact *area.*

p. of regard, p. of fixation.

retention p., a provision made within a cavity preparation of a tooth to hold in place the first pieces of gold when placing a direct gold restoration.

secondary p. of ossification, *punctum* ossificationis secondarium.

silver p., a solid core cone of silver used in filling root canals in conjunction with a cement or paste.

spinal p., subnasal p.

subnasal p., apophysary or apophysial p. (1); spinal p.; the center of the root of the anterior nasal spine.

Sudeck's critical p., region in the colon between the supply of the sigmoid arteries and that of the superior rectal artery.

supra-auricular p., a craniometric p. on the posterior root of the zygomatic process of the temporal bone directly above the auricular p.

supranasal p., ophryon.

supraorbital p., ophryon.

sylvian p., the nearest p. on the skull to the lateral (sylvian) fissure, about 30 mm behind the zygomatic process of the frontal bone.

tender p.'s, Velleix's p.'s.

trigger p., trigger area; dolorogenic or trigger zone; a specific p. or area where, if stimulated by touch, pain, or pressure, a painful response will be induced.

Trousseau's p., apophysary or apophysial p. (2); a painful p., in neuralgia, at the spinous process of the vertebra below which arises the offending nerve.

Valleix's p.'s, tender p.'s; various p.'s in the course of a nerve, pressure upon which is painful in cases of neuralgia; these p.'s are: 1) where the nerve emerges from the bony canal; 2) where it pierces a muscle or aponeurosis to reach the skin; 3) where a superficial nerve rests upon a resisting surface where compression is easily made; 4) where the nerve gives off one or more branches; and 5) where the nerve terminates in the skin.

Weber's p., a p. situated 1 cm below the promontory of the sacrum; believed by Weber to represent the center of gravity of the body.

zygomaxillary p., zygomaxillare.

pointillage (pwan-tē-yazh') [Fr. dotting, stippling]. A massage manipulation with the tips of the fingers.

pointing (poynt'ing). Preparing to open spontaneously, said of an abscess or a boil.

point source. In photometry, a very small source of light which is regarded as a geometrical point from which light emanates in straight lines in all directions.

Poirier, Paul J., French surgeon, 1853–1907. See P.'s *gland, line.*

poise (poyz, pwahz) [J. *Poiseuille*]. In the CGS system, the unit of viscosity equal to 1 dyne-second per square centimeter.

Poiseuille, Jean Léonard Marie, Paris physiologist and physicist, 1797–1869. See poise; P.'s viscosity *coefficient, law, space.*

poison (poy'zŭn) [Fr., fr. L. *potio,* potion, draught]. Any substance, either taken internally or applied externally, that is injurious to health or dangerous to life.

acrid p., a p. which causes a destructive local irritation as well as systemic effects.

arrow p., curare.

fish p., **(1)** ichthyotoxicon; **(2)** fugu p.

fugu p. (fū'gū) [Jap. *fugu,* a poisonous fish], fish p. (2); a p. in the roe and other parts of various species of *Diodon, Triodon,* and *Tetradon,* fishes of eastern Asiatic waters.

poisoning (poy'zŏn-ing). Intoxication (1). **1.** The administering of poison. **2.** The state of being poisoned.

ackee p., Jamaican vomiting sickness; an acute and frequently fatal vomiting disease associated with central nervous system symptoms and marked hypoglycemia, caused by eating unripe ackee fruit of *Blighia spaida,* a tree common in Jamaica.

bacterial food p., a term commonly used to refer to conditions limited to enteritis or gastroenteritis (the enteric fevers and the dysenteries being excluded) caused by bacterial multiplication per se or by a soluble exotoxin.

blood p., see septicemia; pyemia.

bracken p., an acute fatal disease of cattle and horses caused by eating the bracken fern, *Pteridium aquilinum;* in horses, the disease is manifested by neurologic signs; in cattle, by pancytopenia.

carbon disulfide p., acute or chronic intoxication by CS_2, an industrial condition encountered among rubber workers and makers of artificial silk (rayon) by the viscose process; characterized by insomnia, listlessness, and irritability, followed by paralyses, impaired vision, peptic ulcer, and psychoses.

carbon monoxide p., a potentially fatal acute or chronic intoxication caused by inhalation of carbon monoxide gas which competes favorably with oxygen for binding with hemoglobin (carboxyhemoglobinemia) and thus interferes with the transportation of oxygen and carbon dioxide by the blood.

clay pigeon p., pitch p.

crotalaria p., crotalism; p. of man and animals with alkaloids of the plants *Senecio* (ragwort), *Crotalaria* (rattlebox), and *Heliotropum;* produces a veno-occlusive disease of the liver similar to Chiari's disease.

cyanide p., a fairly common disease of herbivorous animals, caused by eating cyanogenic plants containing glucosides which are hydrolyzed, yielding hydrocyanic acid; some farm chemicals, such as fungicides or insecticides, may be causes of cyanide p.; hydrogen cyanide and its salts are extremely poisonous to man, either by inhalation or by ingestion.

Datura p., p. resulting from ingestion of plants of the genus *Datura;* symptoms are parasympatholytic in nature and in severe p. include central nervous system depression, circulatory failure, and respiratory depression.

djenkol p., p. believed to result from eating excessive amounts of a bean, *Pitecolobium lobatum;* symptoms are pain in the renal region, dysuria, and later anuria; the djenkol bean has a high vitamin B content and is used for food despite its toxic qualities.

fescue p., fescue *foot.*

food p., poisoning in which the active agent is contained in ingested food.

lead p., plumbism; saturnism; acute or chronic intoxication by lead or any of its salts; symptoms of **acute l. p.** are usually those of acute gastroenteritis in adults or encephalopathy in children; **chronic l. p.** is manifested chiefly by anemia, constipation, colicky

abdominal pain, paralysis with wrist-drop involving the extensor muscles of the forearm, bluish lead line of the gums, and interstitial nephritis; saturnine gout, convulsions, and coma may occur.
lecheguilla p., swellhead (1); a plant toxemia of sheep and goats in western Texas, southeastern New Mexico, and northern Mexico caused by eating *Agave lecheguilla;* there is liver damage resulting in icterus, sometimes hemoglobinuria, and often death, and photosensitivity with edema, swelling, and crusting of the face and ears.
mercury p., mercurialism; hydrargyria; hydrargyrism; a disease usually caused by the ingestion of mercury or mercury compounds, which are toxic in relation to their ability to produce mercuric ions; **acute m. p.** is usually associated with ulcerations of the stomach and intestine, and toxic changes in the renal tubules; anuria and anemia may occur; **chronic m. p.** is usually a result of industrial p. and causes gastrointestinal or central nervous system manifestations including stomatitis, diarrhea, ataxia, tremor, hyperreflexia, sensorineural impairment, and emotional instability (Mad Hatter syndrome).
mushroom p., see subentries under mycetism.
oxygen p., oxygen *toxicity.*
pitch p., clay pigeon p.; a highly fatal disease of swine, usually caused by the ingestion of fragments of the clay pigeons used as targets by shooting clubs; some cases have been caused by consumption of other bituminous substances, such as road tar and tar paper.
salmon p., salmon disease; a disease of dogs and other canids in the northwest coastal region of the U.S., resulting from eating infected salmon and trout from streams flowing into the Pacific Ocean; these fish carry the encysted form or metacercaria of *Nanophyetus salmincola,* which infects the intestine and carries with it *Neorickettsia helmintheca,* the actual agent of the disease.
Salmonella food p., gastroenteritis caused by various strains of *Salmonella* that multiply freely in the gastrointestinal tract but do not produce septicemia; symptoms begin, usually, within 8 to 24 hours and include fever, headache, nausea, vomiting, diarrhea, and abdominal pain.
salt p., an often fatal disease of animals, especially pigs fed on garbage, resulting from the ingestion of excessive quantities of ordinary table salt, sodium chloride; this usually does not occur if the animals have access to sufficient quantities of fresh drinking water.
scombroid p., p. from ingestion of heat-stable toxins produced by bacterial action on inadequately preserved dark-meat fish of the order Scombroidea (tuna, bonito, mackerel, albacore, skipjack); characterized by epigastric pain, nausea and vomiting, headache, thirst, difficulty in swallowing, and urticaria.
selenium p., chronic p. of horses, cattle, and swine, caused by ingestion of grains and forage raised on soils high in selenium; it occurs only in arid regions, from eating certain plants which are selenium accumulators.
silver p., argyria.
Staphylococcus food p., outbreaks commonly caused by staphylococcal enterotoxin and characterized by an abrupt onset of gastroenteritis within several hours after ingestion of the food contaminated with the preformed exotoxin; vomiting is usually more severe and diarrhea less severe than in infectious forms of bacterial food p.
sweet clover p., a hemorrhagic disease of herbivores, especially cattle, occurring as a result of consuming damaged hay or silage containing sweet clover, but never as a result of eating freshly cut plants or pasturing on sweet clover. The causative agent is the anticoagulant, dicumarol, which is formed in the spoilage process from the harmless coumarin.
systemic p., toxicosis.
tetraethyl p., see tetraethyllead.
thallium p., a condition characterized by vomiting, diarrhea, leg pains, and severe sensorimotor polyneuropathy; about three weeks after p., temporary extensive loss of hair typically occurs; usually occurs after accidental ingestion of a rodenticide.
turpentine p., terebinthinism; p. from oil of turpentine; symptoms include hematuria, albuminuria, and coma; the urine may have an odor of violets.
wheat pasture p., grass *tetany.*

poison ivy, poison oak, poison sumac. **1.** See *Toxicodendron.* **2.** Common name for the cutaneous eruption (rhus dermatitis) caused by contact with these species of *Toxicodendron.*

poisonous (poy'zŭn-ŭs). Toxic (1); toxicant (1); toxiferous; venenous; characterized by, having the characteristics of, or containing a poison.

Poisson, Siméon Denis, French mathematician, 1781–1840. See P. *distribution;* P.-Pearson *formula.*

polar (pō'lăr) [Mod. L. *polaris,* fr. *polus,* pole]. **1.** Relating to a pole. **2.** Having poles, said of certain nerve cells having one or more processes.

polarimeter (pō'lăr-im'ĕ-ter) [Mod. L. *polaris,* polar, + G. *metron,* measure]. An instrument for measuring the angle of rotation in polarization or the amount of polarized light.

polarimetry (pō'lăr-im'ĕ-trē). Measurement by polarimeter.

polariscope (pō-lar'i-skōp) [Mod. L. *polaris,* polar, + G. *skopeō,* to examine]. An instrument for studying the phenomena of the polarization of light.

polariscopic (pō-lar-i-skop'ik). Relating to the polariscope or to polariscopy.

polariscopy (pō'lă-ris'kō-pē). Use of the polariscope in studying properties of polarized light.

polarity (pō-lar'i-tē) [Mod. L. *polaris,* polar]. **1.** The property of having two opposite poles, as that possessed by a magnet. **2.** The possession of opposite properties or characteristics. **3.** The direction or orientation of positivity relative to negativity. **4.** The direction along a polynucleotide chain.

polarization (pō'lăr-i-zā'shŭn). **1.** In electricity, coating of an electrode with a thick layer of hydrogen bubbles, with the result that the flow of current is weakened or arrested. **2.** A change effected in a ray of light passing through certain media, whereby the transverse vibrations occur in one plane only, instead of in all planes as in an ordinary light ray. **3.** Development of differences in potential between two points in living tissues, as between the inside and outside of a cell wall.

polarize (pō'lăr-īz). To put into a state of polarization.

polarizer (pō'lă-rīz'er). The first element of a polariscope that polarizes the light, as distinguished from the analyzer, the second polarizing element.

polarography (pō'lă-rog'ră-fē) [Mod. L. *polaris,* polar, + G. *graphō,* to write]. That branch of electrochemistry concerned with the variation in current flowing through a solution as the voltage is varied; this will vary with the ionic concentration of reducible substances so that p. can be used in chemical analysis. P. is commonly employed in the form of a reduction at a dropping mercury electrode.

poldine methylsulfate (pōl'dēn). 2-Benziloyloxymethyl-1,1-dimethylpyrrolidinium methylsulfate; an anticholinergic agent.

pole (pōl) [L. *polus,* the end of an axis, pole, fr. G. *polos*]. **1.** Polus. **2.** Either of the two points on a sphere at the greatest distance from the equator. **3.** One of the two points in a magnet or an electric battery or cell having extremes of opposite properties; the negative p. is a cathode, the positive p. an anode.
abapical p., in an ovum, the p. opposite the animal p.
animal p., germinal p.; the point in a telolecithal egg opposite the yolk, where most of the protoplasm is concentrated and where the nucleus is located; from this region, the polar bodies are extruded during maturation.

anterior p. of eyeball, *polus* anterior bulbi oculi.
anterior p. of lens, *polus* anterior lentis.
cephalic p., the head end of the fetus.
frontal p., *polus* frontalis cerebri.
germinal p., animal p.
inferior p., *extremitas* inferior.
lateral p., *extremitas* tubaria.
medial p., *extremitas* uterina.
occipital p., *polus* occipitalis cerebri.
pelvic p., the breech end of the fetus.
posterior p. of eyeball, *polus* posterior bulbi oculi.
posterior p. of lens, *polus* posterior lentis.
superior p., *extremitas* superior.
temporal p., *polus* temporalis cerebri.
vegetal p., vegetative p., the part of a telolecithal egg where the bulk of the yolk is situated.
vitelline p., the vegetative p. of an ovum.

Polenské number. See under number.

policeman (pō-lēs'man). An instrument, usually a rubber-tipped rod, for removing solid particles from a glass container.

polio- [G. *polios,* gray]. Combining form denoting gray or the gray matter (substantia grisea).

polio (pō'lē-ō). Abbreviated term for poliomyelitis.
French p., colloquialism for Guillain-Barré *syndrome.*

polioclastic (pō'lē-ō-klas'tik) [polio- + G. *klastos,* broken]. Destructive to gray matter of the nervous system.

poliodystrophia (pō'lē-ō-dis-trō'fē-ă). Poliodystrophy.
p. cer'ebri progressi'va infanta'lis, Christensen-Krabbe or Alpers disease; progressive cerebral poliodystrophy; familial progressive spastic paresis of extremities with progressive mental deterioration, with development of seizures, blindness and deafness, beginning during the first year of life, and with destruction and disorganization of nerve cells of the cerebral cortex.

poliodystrophy (pō'lē-ō-dis'trō-fē) [polio- + G. *dys-,* bad, + *trophē,* nourishment]. Poliodystrophia; wasting of the gray matter of the nervous system.
progressive cerebral p., *poliodystrophia* cerebri progressiva infantalis.

polioencephalitis (pō'lē-ō-en-sef'ă-lī'tis) [polio- + G. *enkephalos,* brain, + *-tis,* inflammation]. Inflammation of the gray matter of the brain, either of the cortex or of the central nuclei; an acute infectious disease marked at the onset by fever, headache, convulsions, or stupor, followed by ocular palsies, symptoms resembling those of bulbar paralysis, aphasia, or mental retardation.
p. infecti'va, von Economo's *disease.*
inferior p., p. with predominantly bulbar paralysis.
superior p., p. with ophthalmoplegia.
superior hemorrhagic p., Wernicke's *syndrome.*

polioencephalomeningomyelitis (pō'lē-ō-en-sef'ă-lō-mē-ning'gō-mī-ĕ-lī'tis) [polio- + G. *enkephalos,* brain, + *mēninx,* membrane, + *myelon,* marrow, + *-itis,* inflammation]. Inflammation of the gray matter of the brain and spinal cord and of the meningeal covering of the parts.

polioencephalomyelitis (pō'lē-ō-en-sef'ă-lō-mī'ĕ-lī'tis). Poliomyeloencephalitis.

polioencephalopathy (pō'lē-ō-en-sef'ă-lop'ă-thē) [polio- + G. *enkephalos,* brain, + *pathos,* suffering]. Any disease of the gray matter of the brain.

poliomyelencephalitis (pō'lē-ō-mī'el-en-sef'ă-lī'tis). Poliomyeloencephalitis.

poliomyelitis (pō'lē-ō-mī'ĕ-lī'tis) [polio- + G. *myelos,* marrow, + *-itis,* inflammation]. Inflammation of the gray matter of the spinal cord.
acute anterior p., acute atrophic or myogenic paralysis; inflammation of the anterior cornua of the spinal cord; an acute infectious disease caused by the poliomyelitis virus and marked by fever, pains, and gastroenteric disturbances, followed by a flaccid paralysis of one or more muscular groups, and later by atrophy.
acute bulbar p., poliomyelitis virus infection affecting nerve cells in the medulla oblongata and producing paralysis of the lower motor cranial nerves.
chronic anterior p., muscular atrophy of the upper extremities and neck, in which there are long intermissions of quiescence or improvement; not to be confused with poliomyelitis virus infections.
mouse p., mouse *encephalomyelitis.*

poliomyeloencephalitis (pō'lē-ō-mī'ĕ-lō-en-sef'ă-lī'tis) [polio- + G. *myelon,* marrow, + *enkephalos,* brain, + *-itis,* inflammation]. Polioencephalomyelitis; poliomyelencephalitis; acute anterior poliomyelitis with pronounced cerebral signs.

poliomyelopathy (pō'lē-ō-mī'ĕ-lop'ă-thē) [polio- + G. *myelon,* marrow, + *pathos,* suffering]. Any disease of the gray matter of the spinal cord.

poliosis (po-lē-ō'sis) [G., fr. *polios,* gray]. Trichopoliosis; an absence or lessening of melanin in groups of hair of the scalp, brows, or lashes, resulting from a hypomelanosis of the epidermis and appearing as patches or strands; it occurs in several hereditary syndromes or as an acquired abnormality following inflammation, irradiation, or infection such as herpes zoster.

poliovirus hominis (pō'lē-ō-vī'rŭs hom'i-nis). Poliomyelitis *virus.*

pol'ishing. In dentistry, the act or process of making a restoration smooth and glossy.

Politzer, Adam, Austrian otologist, 1835–1920. See P. *bag,* method; P.'s luminous *cone.*

politzerization (pol'it-zer-i-zā'shŭn). Inflation of the eustachian tube and middle ear by the Politzer method.
negative p., withdrawal of secretions from a cavity by suction, effected by attaching a compressed Politzer bag or rubber bulb to a tube inserted in the cavity.

polkissen of Zimmermann (pōl'kis-en) [Ger. *Polkissen,* pole + cushion]. Extraglomerular *mesangium.*

poll (pōl). The occipital region of an animal, especially the horse; high point of the head between the ears.

pollakidipsia (pol'ă-ki-dip'sē-ă) [G. *pollakis,* often, + *dipsa,* thirst]. Rarely used term for unduly frequent thirst.

pollakiuria (pol'ă-kē-yū'rē-ă) [G. *pollakis,* often, + *ouron,* urine]. Rarely used term for abnormally frequent micturition.

pollen (pol'en) [L. fine dust, fine flour]. Microspores of seed plants carried by wind or insects prior to fertilization; important in the etiology of hay fever.

pollenosis (pol-ĕ-nō'sis). Pollinosis.

pollex, gen. **pollicis,** pl. **pollices** (pol'eks, pol'i-sis, -sēz) [L.] [NA]. Digitus primus; thumb; the first digit of the hand.
p. pe'dis, hallux.

pollicization (pol'i-si-zā'shŭn) [L. *pollex,* thumb, + *-ize,* to make like, + *-ation,* state]. Construction of a substitute thumb.

pollinosis (pol-i-nō'sis) [L. *pollen,* pollen, + G. *-osis,* condition]. Pollenosis; hay fever excited by the pollen of various plants.

pollodic (pō-lō'dik) [G. *polloi,* many, + *hodos,* way]. Panodic.

pollutant (pō-lū'tănt). An undesired contaminant that results in pollution.

pollution (pō-lū'shŭn) [L. *pollutio,* fr. *pol-luo,* pp. *-lutus,* to defile]. Rendering unclean or unsuitable by contact or mixture with an undesired contaminant.
air p., contamination of air by smoke and harmful gases, mainly oxides of carbon, sulfur, and nitrogen, as from automobile exhausts, industrial emissions, burning rubbish, etc. See also smog.

noise p., annoying or physiologically damaging environmental noise levels, as from automobile engines, industrial machinery, amplified music, etc.

polocyte (pō'lō-sīt) [G. *polos,* pole, + *kytos,* cell]. Polar *body.*

polonium (pō-lō'nē-ŭm) [L. fr. Polonia, Poland, native country of Mme. Curie who with her husband discovered the substance]. A radioactive element, symbol Po, atomic no. 84, isolated from pitchblende; the longest-lived isotope is ^{209}Po (half-life 103 years; ^{210}Po is radium F (half-life 138 days), the only readily accessible isotope.

poloxalene (pŏl-ok'să-lēn). Poloxalkol; an oxyalkylene polymer, nonionic surface-active agent similar in actions and uses to dioctyl sodium sulfasuccinate; used in constipation due to hard dry stools.

poloxalkol (pŏl-ok'sal-kol). Poloxalene.

polster (pōl'ster) [G. cushion, bolster]. A bulge of smooth muscle cells, as in the penile arteries and veins, formerly thought to regulate blood flow.

polus, pl. **poli** (pō'lŭs, -lī) [L. pole] [NA]. Pole; one of the two points at the extremities of the axis of any organ or body.

p. ante'rior bul'bi oc'uli [NA], anterior pole of eyeball; the center of the corneal curvature of the eye.

p. ante'rior len'tis [NA], anterior pole of lens; the central point on the anterior surface of the lens of the eye.

p. fronta'lis cer'ebri [NA], frontal pole; the most anterior promontory of each cerebral hemisphere.

po'li liena'lis infe'rior et supe'rior, see *extremitas* anterior; *extremitas* posterior.

p. occipita'lis cer'ebri [NA], occipital pole; the most posterior promontory of each cerebral hemisphere; the apex of the occipital lobe.

p. poste'rior bul'bi oc'uli [NA], posterior pole of eyeball; the center of the posterior curvature of the eye.

p. poste'rior len'tis [NA], posterior pole of lens; the central point on the posterior surface of the lens.

poli rena'lis infe'rior et supe'rior, *extremitas* inferior; *extremitas* superior.

p. tempora'lis cer'ebri [NA], temporal pole; the most prominent part of the anterior extremity of the temporal lobe of each cerebral hemisphere, a short distance below the fissure of Sylvius.

poly- [G. *polys,* much, many]. **1.** Prefix denoting multiplicity; corresponds to the L. *multi-* See also pluri-. **2.** In chemistry, prefix meaning "polymer of," as in polypeptide, polysaccharide, polynucleotide; often used with symbols, as in poly(A) for poly(adenylic acid), poly(Lys) for poly(L- lysine).

poly (pol'ē). Abbreviated form and colloquialism for polymorphonuclear *leukocyte.*

Pólya, Jenö (Eugene), Hungarian surgeon, 1876–1944. See P. *gastrectomy;* P.'s *operation;* Reichel-P. stomach *resection.*

polyacid (pol-ē-as'id) [G. *polys,* much, many + acid]. An acid capable of liberating more than one hydrogen ion per molecule; *e.g.,* H_2SO_4, citric acid.

polyadenitis (pol'ē-ad-ĕ-nī'tis). Inflammation of many lymph nodes, especially with reference to the cervical group.

p. malig'na, bubonic *plague.*

polyadenopathy (pol'ē-ad-ĕ-nop'ă-thē). Polyadenosis; adenopathy affecting many lymph nodes.

polyadenosis (pol'ē-ad-ĕ-nō'sis). Polyadenopathy.

polyadenous (pol-ē-ad'ĕ-nŭs). Pertaining to or involving many glands.

polyalcohol (pol-ē-al'kō-hol) [G. *polys,* much, many + alcohol]. An aliphatic or alicyclic molecule characterized by the presence of two or more hydroxyl groups; *e.g.,* glycerol, inositol.

poly(alcohol) (pol-ē-al'kō-hol) [see poly- (2)]. A polymer of an alcohol.

polyallelism (pol'ē-ă-lēl'izm). The existence of multiple alleles at a genetic locus.

polyamine (pol-ē-am'ēn) [G. *polys,* much, many + amine]. Class name for substances of the general formula $H_2N(CH_2)_n$-NH_2, $H_2N(CH_2)_nNH(CH_2)_nNH_2$, $H_2N(CH_2)_nNH(CH_2)_nNH$-$(CH_2)_nNH_2$, where $n = 3$, 4, or 5. Many p.'s arise by bacterial action on protein; many are normally occurring body constituents of wide distribution, or are essential growth factors for microorganisms.

poly(amine) (pol-ē-ă-mēn, am'ēn) [see poly- (2)]. A polymer of an amine.

poly(amino acids) [see poly- (2)]. Polypeptides that are polymers of aminoacyl groups, *i.e.,* of –NH–CHR-CO–.

polyangiitis (pol'ē-an-jē-ī'tis). Inflammation of multiple blood vessels involving more than one type of vessel, *e.g.,* arteries and veins, or arterioles and capillaries.

polyanion (pol-ē-an'ī-on). Anionic sites on proteoglycans in the renal glomeruli that restrict filtration of anionic molecules and facilitate filtration of cationic proteins; loss of p. may cause albuminuria in lipoid nephrosis.

polyarteritis (pol'ē-ar-ter-ī'tis). Simultaneous inflammation of a number of arteries.

p. nodo'sa, Kussmaul's disease; arteritis or periarteritis nodosa; segmental inflammation, with infiltration by eosinophils, and necrosis of medium-sized or small arteries, most common in males, with varied symptoms related to involvement of arteries in the kidneys, muscles, gastrointestinal tract, and heart.

polyarthric (pol-ē-ar'thrik). Multiarticular.

polyarthritis (pol'ē-ar-thrī'tis) [poly- + G. *arthron,* joint, + *-itis,* inflammation]. Simultaneous inflammation of several joints.

p. chron'ica, obsolete term for rheumatoid *arthritis.*

p. chron'ica villo'sa, a chronic inflammation confined to the synovial membrane, involving a number of joints; it occurs in women at the menopause and in children.

epidemic p., epidemic exanthema; Murray Valley rash; Ross River fever; a mild febrile illness of humans in Australia characterized by polyarthralgia and rash, caused by the Ross River virus, and transmitted by mosquitoes.

p. rheumat'ica acu'ta, obsolete term for p. associated with rheumatic fever.

vertebral p., inflammation of a number of the intervertebral disks without involvement of the vertebral bodies.

polyarticular (pol-ē-ar-tik'yū-lăr) [poly- + L. *articulus,* joint]. Multiarticular.

polyavitaminosis (pol'ē-ā'vī-tă-mi-nō'sis). Avitaminosis with multiple deficiencies.

polybasic (pol-ē-bās'ik). Having more than one replaceable hydrogen atom, denoting an acid with a basicity greater than 1.

polyblast (pol'ē-blast) [poly- + G. *blastos,* germ]. One of a group of ameboid, mononucleated, wandering phagocytic cells found in inflammatory exudates.

polyblennia (pol-ē-blen'ē-ă) [poly- + G. *blennos,* mucus]. Excessive production of mucus.

polycarbophil (pol-ē-kar'bō-fil). A polyacrylic acid cross-linked with divinyl glycol; used as a gastrointestinal absorbent.

polycardia (pol-ē-kar'dē-ă). Tachycardia.

polycentric (pol-ē-sen'trik). Having several centers.

polycheiria, polychiria (pol-ē-kī'rē-ă) [poly- + G. *cheir,* hand]. Presence of supernumerary hands.

polychondritis (pol'ē-kon-drī'tis) [poly- + G. *chondros,* cartilage, + *-itis,* inflammation]. A widespread disease of cartilage.

chronic atrophic p., relapsing p.

relapsing p., a degenerative disease of cartilage producing a bizarre form of arthritis, with collapse of the ears, the cartilaginous portion of the nose, and the tracheobronchial tree; death may occur from chronic infection or suffocation because of loss of stability in the tracheobronchial tree. Also called chronic atrophic p.; relapsing perichondritis; generalized or systemic chondromalacia; (von) Meyenburg's disease; Meyenburg-Altherr-Uehlinger syndrome.

polychromasia (pol'ē-krō-mā'zē-ă). Polychromatophilia.

polychromatic (pol-ē-krō-mat'ik). Multicolored.

polychromatocyte (pol'ē-krō-mat'ō-sīt). Polychromatophil (2).

polychromatophil, polychromatophile (pol-ē-krō'mă-tō-fil, -fīl) [poly- + G. *chrōma*, color, + *phileō*, to love]. Polychromophil. **1.** Polychromatophilic; staining readily with acid, neutral, and basic dyes; denoting certain cells, especially certain red blood cells. **2.** Polychromatocyte; a young or degenerating erythrocyte that manifests acid and basic staining affinities.

polychromatophilia (pol-ē-krō'mă-tō-fil'ē-ă). Polychromasia; polychromatosis; polychromophilia. **1.** A tendency of certain cells, such as the red blood cells in pernicious anemia, to stain with basic and also acid dyes. **2.** Condition characterized by the presence of many red blood cells that have an affinity for acid, basic, or neutral stains.

polychromatophilic (pol-ē-krō'mă-tō-fil'ik). Polychromatophil (1).

polychromatosis (pol'ē-krō-mă-tō'sis). Polychromatophilia.

polychromemia (pol-ē-krō-mē'mē-ă). An increase in the total amount of hemoglobin in the blood.

polychromia (pol-ē-krō'mē-ă). Increased pigmentation in any part.

polychromophil (pol-ē-krō'mō-fil). Polychromatophil.

polychromophilia (pol-ē-krō-mō-fil'ē-ă). Polychromatophilia.

polychylia (pol-ē-kī'lē-ă) [poly- + G. *chylos*, chyle, + *-ia*, condition]. An increased production of chyle.

polycinematosomnography (pol'ē-sin'ē-mă-tō-som-nog'ră-fē). Somnocinematography.

polyclinic (pol-ē-klin'ik) [poly- + G. *klinē*, bed]. A dispensary for the treatment and study of diseases of all kinds.

polyclonal (pol-ē-klō'năl). In immunochemistry, pertaining to proteins from more than a single clone of cells, in contradistinction to monoclonal.

polyclonia (pol'ē-klō'nē-ă) [poly- + G. *klonos*, tumult]. *Myoclonus* multiplex.

polycoria (pol-ē-kō'rē-ă) [poly- + G. *korē*, pupil]. The presence of two or more pupils in one iris.

polycrotic (pol-ē-krot'ik). Relating to or marked by polycrotism.

polycrotism (pol-ik'rō-tizm) [poly- + G. *krotos*, a beat]. A condition in which the sphygmographic tracing shows several upward breaks in the descending wave.

polycyesis (pol'ē-sī-ē'sis) [poly- + G. *kyēsis*, pregnancy]. Multiple pregnancy.

polycystic (pol-ē-sis'tik). Composed of many cysts.

polycythemia (pol'ē-sī-thē'mē-ă) [poly- + G. *kytos*, cell, + *haima*, blood]. Erythrocythemia; hyperglobulia; hyperglobulism; an increase above the normal in the number of red cells in the blood.

compensatory p., a secondary p. resulting from anoxia, *e.g.*, in congenital heart disease, pulmonary emphysema, or prolonged residence at a high altitude.

p. hyperton'ica, Gaisböck's syndrome; p. associated with hypertension, but without splenomegaly.

relative p., a relative increase in the number of red blood cells as a result of loss of the fluid portion of the blood.

p. ru'bra, ru'bra ve'ra, or **ve'ra,** erythremia.

polydactylia (pol-ē-dak-til'ē-ă). Polydactyly.

polydactylism (pol-ē-dak'ti-lizm). Polydactyly.

polydactylous (pol-ē-dak'til-ŭs). Relating to polydactyly.

polydactyly (pol-ē-dak'ti-lē) [poly- + G. *daktylos*, finger]. Presence of more than five digits on either hand or foot. Also called hyperdactylia; hyperdactylism; hyperdactyly; polydactylia; polydactylism.

polydentia (pol-ē-den'shē-ă) [poly- + L. *dens*, tooth]. Polyodontia.

polydipsia (pol-ē-dip'sē-ă) [poly- + G. *dipsa*, thirst]. Excessive thirst that is relatively chronic.

hysterical p., psychogenic p.

psychogenic p., hysterical p.; excessive fluid consumption resulting from a disorder of the personality, without demonstrable organic lesion.

psychogenic nocturnal p. (PNP), see psychogenic nocturnal polydipsia *syndrome*.

polydispersoid (pol'ē-dis-per'soyd). A colloid system in which the dispersed phase is composed of particles having different degrees of dispersion.

polydysplasia (pol'ē-dis-plā'zē-ă) [poly- + G. *dys-*, bad, + *plasis*, a molding]. Tissue development abnormal in several respects.

polydystrophia (pol'ē-dis-trō'fē-ă). Polydystrophy.

polydystrophic (pol'ē-dis-trof'ik). Relating to polydystrophy.

polydystrophy (pol-ē-dis'trō-fē) [poly- + dystrophy]. Polydystrophia; a condition characterized by the presence of many congenital anomalies of the connective tissues.

polyembryony (pol-ē-em-brē'ō-nē) [poly- + G. *embryon*, embryo]. Condition of a zygote's giving rise to two or more embryos.

polyene (pol-ē-ēn'). A chemical compound having a series of conjugated (alternating) double bonds; *e.g.*, the carotenoids.

polyenic acids (pol-ē-ē'nik). Polyenoic acids.

polyenoic acids (pol-ē-en'ik). Polyenic acids; fatty acids with more than one double bonds in the carbon chain; *e.g.*, linoleic, linolenic, and arachidonic acids.

polyergic (pol-ē-er'jik) [poly- + G. *ergon*, work]. Capable of acting in several different ways.

polyesthesia (pol-ē-es-thē'zē-ă) [poly- + G. *aisthēsis*, sensation]. A disorder of sensation in which a single touch or other stimulus is felt as several.

polyestradiol phosphate (pol'ē-es-tră-dī'ol). An estradiol phosphate polymer, used as a long-acting estrogen for treatment of prostatic carcinoma.

polyestrous (pol-ē-es'trŭs). Having two or more estrous cycles in a mating season.

polyethylene glycols (pol-ē-eth'i-lēn). Poly(oxyethylene) glycols; condensation polymers of ethylene oxide and water, of the general formula $HO(CH_2CH_2O)_nH$, where *n* equals the average number of oxyethylene groups (300 - 6,000); they are waxlike solids, soluble in water, that are used as pharmaceutic aids.

polyfructose (pol-ē-fruk'tōs). Fructosan.

polygalactia (pol'ē-gă-lak'tē-ă, -shē-ă) [poly- + G. *gala*, milk]. Excessive secretion of breast milk, especially at the weaning period.

polygalacturonase (pol'ē-gă-lak'tū-ron-ās) [EC 3.2.1.15]. Pectinase; pectin depolymerase; a hydrolase cleaving 1,4-α-D-galacturonide links in pectate and other galacturonans.

polyganglionic (pol'ē-gang-glē-on'ik). Containing or involving many ganglia.

polygene (pol'ē-jēn). One of many genes that interact to produce a cumulative contribution to the value of a single measurable phenotype.

polygenic (pol-ē-jen'ik). Relating to a hereditary disease or normal characteristic controlled by interaction of genes at more than one locus.

polyglandular (pol-ē-glan′dū-lăr). Pluriglandular.

poly-β-glucosaminidase. Chitinase.

polyglutamate (pol-ē-glū′tă-māt). Poly(glutamic acid).

poly(glutamic acid) (pol′ē-glū-tam′ik) [see poly- (2)]. Polyglutamate; glutamic acid residues in the usual peptide linkage (α-carboxyl to α-amino). See also poly(γ-glutamic acid).

poly(γ-glutamic acid). A polypeptide formed of glutamic acid residues, the γ-carboxyl group of one glutamic acid being condensed to the amino group of its neighbor; occurs naturally in the anthrax bacillus capsule.

poly(glycolic acid) (pol′ē-glī-kol′ik) [see poly- (2)]. A polymer of glycolic acid, used in absorbable surgical sutures.

polygnathus (pol-ē-nath′ŭs, pŏ-lig′na-thŭs) [poly- + G. *gnathos*, jaw]. Unequal conjoined twins in which the parasite is attached to the jaw of the autosite.

polygraph (pol′ē-graf) [poly- + G. *graphō*, to write]. **1.** An instrument to obtain simultaneous tracings from several different pulsations; *e.g.*, radial and jugular pulse, apex beat of the heart. **2.** Lie detector; an instrument for recording changes in respiration, blood pressure, galvanic skin response, and other physiological changes while the person is questioned about some matter or asked to give associations to relevant and irrelevant words; the physiological changes are presumed to be indicators of emotional reactions, and thus whether the person is telling the truth.
Mackenzie's p., an instrument consisting of a system of tambours and a time-marker for recording simultaneously the jugular and arterial pulses and the apex beat; formerly used in the clinical investigation of cardiac arrhythmias.

polygyria (pol-ē-jī′rē-ă) [poly- + G. *gyros*, circle, gyre]. Condition in which the brain has an excessive number of convolutions.

polyhedral (pol-ē-hē′drăl) [G. *polyedros*, many-sided, fr. poly- + G. *hedra*, seat, facet]. Having many sides or facets.

polyhexoses (pol-ē-heks′ōs-ez). Hexosans.

polyhidrosis (pol′ē-hī-drō′sis). Hyperhidrosis.

polyhybrid (pol-ē-hī′brid). The offspring of parents differing from each other in more than three characters.

polyhydramnios (pol′ē-hī-dram′nē-os) [poly- + G. *hydōr*, water, + amnion]. Excess amount of amniotic fluid.

polyhydric (pol-ē-hī′drik). Containing more than one hydroxyl group, as in polyhydric alcohols (glycerol, $C_3H_5(OH)_3$) or polyhydric acids (*o*-phosphoric acid, $OP(OH)_3$).

polyhypermenorrhea (pol-ē-hī′per-men-ō-rē′ă) [poly- + G. *hyper*, above, + *mēn*, month, + *rhoia*, flow]. Frequent and excessive menstruation.

polyhypomenorrhea (pol-ē-hī′pō-men-ō-rē′ă) [poly- + G. *hypo*, below, + *mēn*, month, + *rhoia*, a flow]. Frequent but scanty menstruation.

polyidrosis (pol′ē-i-drō′sis). Hyperhidrosis.

polykaryocyte (pol-ē-kar′ē-ō-sīt) [poly- + G. *karyon*, kernel, + *kytos*, cell]. A cell containing many nuclei, such as the osteoclast.

polyleptic (pol-ē-lep′tik) [poly- + G. *lēpsis*, a seizing]. Denoting a disease occurring in many paroxysms, *e.g.*, malaria, epilepsy.

polylogia (pol-ē-lō′jē-ă) [poly- + G. *logos*, word]. Continuous and often incoherent speech.

polymastia (pol-ē-mas′tē-ă) [poly- + G. *mastos*, breast]. In humans, a condition in which more than two breasts are present. Also called polymazia; hypermastia (1); multimammae; pleomastia; pleomazia.

polymastigote (pol-ē-mas′ti-gōt) [poly- + G. *mastix*, a whip]. A mastigote having several grouped flagella.

polymazia (pol-ē-mā′zē-ă) [poly- + G. *mazos*, breast]. Polymastia.

polymelia (pol-ē-mē′lē-ă) [poly- + G. *melos*, limb]. Presence of supernumerary limbs or parts of limbs.

polymenorrhea (pol-ē-men-ō-rē′ă) [poly- + G. *mēn*, month, + *rhoia*, flow]. Occurrence of menstrual cycles of greater than usual frequency.

polymer (pol′i-mer) [see -mer (1)]. Polymerid; a substance of high molecular weight, made up of a chain of repeated units sometimes called "mers."
cross-linked p., cross-linked resin; a p. in which long chain molecules are attached to each other, forming a two- or three-dimensional network.

polymerase (po-lim′er-ās). General term for any enzyme catalyzing a polymerization, as of nucleotides to polynucleotides, thus belonging to EC class 2, the transferases.

polymeria (pol-ē-mĕr′ē-ă) [poly- + G. *meros*, part]. Condition characterized by an excessive number of parts, limbs, or organs of the body.

polymeric (pol-i-mer′ik). **1.** Having the properties of a polymer. **2.** Relating to or characterized by polymeria. **3.** Rarely used synonym for polygenic.

polymerid (po-lim′er-id). Polymer.

polymerization (po-lim′er-i-za′shŭn). A reaction in which a high-molecular-weight product is produced by successive additions to or condensations of a simpler compound; *e.g.*, polystyrene may be produced from styrene, or rubber from isoprene, or a polynucleotide from mononucleotides.

polymerize (pol′i-mer-īz, po-lim′er-īz). To bring about polymerization.

polymetacarpalia, polymetacarpalism (pol′ē-met-ă-kar-pā′lē-ă, -kar′pă-lizm). Congenital anomaly characterized by the presence of supernumerary metacarpal bones.

polymetatarsalia, polymetatarsalism (pol′ē-met-ă-tar-sā′lē-ă, -tar′să-lizm). Congenital anomaly characterized by the presence of supernumerary metatarsal bones.

polymicrolipomatosis (pol-ē-mī′krō-lip′ō-mă-tō′sis) [poly- + G. *mikros*, small, + lipoma + G. *-osis*, condition]. The occurrence of multiple, small, nodular, fairly discrete masses of lipid in the subcutaneous connective tissue.

polymitus (pŏ-lim′i-tŭs) [poly- + G. *mitos*, thread]. Exflagellation.

polymorph (pol′ē-mōrf). Colloquial term for polymorphonuclear *leukocyte*.

polymorphic (pol-ē-mōr′fik) [G. *polymorphos*, multiform]. Multiform; pleomorphic (1); pleomorphous; polymorphous; occurring in more than one morphologic form.

polymorphism (pol-ē-mōr′fizm). Pleomorphism; occurrence in more than one form; existence in the same species or other natural group of more than one morphologic type.
balanced p., a system of genes in which two alleles are maintained in stable equilibrium because the heterozygote is more fit than either of the homozygotes. See also overdominance.
DNA p., a condition in which one of two different but normal nucleotide sequences can exist at a particular site in DNA.
genetic p., the occurrence in the same population of two or more discontinuous variants or genotypes in such proportions that the rarest cannot be maintained by recurrent mutation alone.
lipoprotein p., heritable variations in low density β-lipoproteins; the variant lipoproteins exhibit different antigenic and chemical properties when compared with normal lipoproteins.
restriction (fragment) length p., the existence of allelic forms recognizable by the length of fragments that result when the nucleotide chain is treated by a specific (restriction) enzyme that cleaves wherever a particular sequence of nucleotides occurs. A mutation

in this sequence prevents cleaving and hence decreases the number of fragments; conversely, a new mutation can lead to a new cleavage (restriction) site.

restriction-site p., DNA p. in which the sequence of one form of the p. contains a recognition site for a particular endonuclease, but the sequence of the other form lacks such a site.

polymorphocellular (pol-ē-mōr′fō-sel′yū-lăr) [G. *polymorphos*, multiform, + L. *cellula*, cell]. Relating to or formed of cells of several different kinds.

polymorphonuclear (pol′ē-mōr-fō-nū′klē-ăr) [G. *polymorphos*, multiform, + L. *nucleus*, kernel]. Having nuclei of varied forms; denoting a variety of leukocyte.

polymorphous (pol-ē-mōr′fŭs). Polymorphic.

polymyalgia (pol′ē-mī-al′jē-ă) [poly- + G. *mys*, muscle, + *algos*, pain]. Pain in several muscle groups.

p. arterit′ica, p. rheumatica resulting from arteritis, especially disseminated giant cell arteritis.

p. rheumat′ica, a syndrome within the group of collagen diseases different from spondylarthritis or from humeral scapular periarthritis by the presence of an elevated sedimentation rate; much commoner in women than in men.

polymyoclonus (pol′ē-mī-ok′lō-nŭs). *Myoclonus* multiplex.

polymyositis (pol′ē-mī-ō-sī′tis) [poly- + G. *mys*, muscle, + *-itis*, inflammation]. Inflammation of a number of voluntary muscles simultaneously.

polymyxin (pol-ē-mik′sin). A mixture of antibiotic substances obtained from cultures of *Bacillus polymyxa* (*B. serosporus*), an organism found in water and soils, and obtainable as a crystalline hydrochloride; polypeptides containing various amino acids and a branched chain fatty acid, (+)-6-methyloctanoic acid. There are five different p.'s, designated A, B, C, D, and E, which are about equally effective against Gram-negative bacteria, but which differ in toxicity, p. E (colistin) and p. B being the least toxic. See also *colistin* sulfate; colistimethate sodium.

p. B sulfate, an antibacterial effective in tularemia, brucellosis, *Pseudomonas* infections, and urinary tract infections, but used systemically only for severe infections not responsive to less toxic agents; it is also used locally.

polynesic (pol-i-nē′sik) [poly- + G. *nēsos*, island]. Occurring in many separate foci; denoting certain forms of inflammation or infection.

polyneural (pol-ē-nū′răl) [poly- + G. *neuron*, nerve]. Relating to, supplied by, or affecting several nerves.

polyneuralgia (pol′ē-nū-ral′jē-ă). Neuralgia of several nerves simultaneously.

polyneuritis (pol′ē-nū-rī′tis). Multiple neuritis; simultaneous inflammation of a large number of the spinal nerves, marked by paralysis, pain, and wasting of muscles. See also nutritional *polyneuropathy*.

acute idiopathic p., Landry, Landry-Guillain-Barré, or Guillain-Barré syndrome; myeloradiculopolyneuronitis; polyradiculoneuropathy; polyradiculopathy; radiculoganglionitis; infectious p.; a neurological syndrome, probably an immune-mediated disorder, often a sequela of certain virus infections, marked by paresthesia of the limbs and muscular weakness or a flaccid paralysis; the characteristic laboratory finding is increased protein in the cerebrospinal fluid without increase in cell count.

chronic familial p., irritation of nerves related to infiltration by amyloid.

erythredema p., a chronic disease of childhood; vasomotor changes causing redness and edema of the extemities are constant.

infectious p., acute idiopathic p.

polyneuronitis (pol′ē-nū-rō-nī′tis). Inflammation of several groups of nerve cells.

polyneuropathy (pol′ē-nū-rop′ă-thē) [poly- + G. *neuron*, nerve, + *pathos*, disease]. A disease process involving a number of peripheral nerves.

buckthorn p., ascending p. resulting from ingestion of the fruit of *Karwinskia humboldtiana*.

nutritional p., a disorder of multiple peripheral nerves, noted in beriberi, chronic alcoholism, and other clinical states, resulting from thiamin deficiency.

uremic p., a distal sensory and motor p. without conspicuous inflammation and ascribed to the metabolic effects of chronic renal failure.

polynoxylin (pol-ē-nok′si-lin). Poly{methylenebis[*N,N*′-di(hydroxymethyl)urea]}a polymer of urea with formaldehyde, used as a topical antiseptic.

polynuclear, polynucleate (pol-ē-nū′klē-ăr, -klē-āt). Multinuclear.

polynucleosis (pol′ē-nū-klē-ō′sis). Multinucleosis; the presence of numbers of polynuclear, or multinuclear, cells in the peripheral blood.

polynucleotidases (pol′ē-nū′klē-ō-ti′dās-ez). **1.** Enzymes catalyzing the hydrolysis of polynucleotides to oligonucleotides or to mononucleotides; *e.g.*, phosphodiesterases, nucleases. **2.** Terms once applied to the two polynucleotide phosphatases, 2′ (3′)- and 5′-, which do not cleave internucleotide links.

polynucleotide (pol-ē-nū′klē-ō-tīd). A linear polymer containing an indefinite (usually large) number of nucleotides, linked from one ribose (or deoxyribose) to another via phosphoric residues. *Cf.* oligonucleotide.

p. phosphorylase, polyribonucleotide nucleotidyltransferase.

polyodontia (pol-ē-ō-don′shē-ă) [poly- + G. *odous*, tooth]. Polydentia; presence of supernumerary teeth.

polyol (pol′ē-ol). Polyhydroxy alcohol; a sugar that contains many -OH (-ol) groups, such as the sugar alcohols and inositols.

p. dehydrogenases, oxidizing enzymes that catalyze the dehydrogenation of sugar alcohols to monosaccharides (in EC class 1.1), specifically L-iditol dehydrogenase and aldose reductase.

Polyomavirus (pol-ē-ō′mă-vī′rŭs) [poly- + G. *-ōma*, tumor]. A genus of viruses (family Papovaviridae) containing DNA (MW 3×10^6), having virions about 45 nm in diameter, and including viruses oncogenic for animals; includes the polyoma virus of rodents, vacuolating viruses (SV40) of primates, and the BK and JC viruses of humans.

polyoncosis, polyonchosis (pol′ē-ong-kō′sis) [poly- + G. *onkos*, tumor, + *-osis*, condition]. Formation of multiple tumors.

cutaneomandibular p., basal cell nevus *syndrome*.

polyonychia (pol-ē-ō-nik′ē-ă) [poly- + G. *onyx*, nail]. Polyunguia; presence of supernumerary nails on fingers or toes.

polyopia, polyopsia (pol′ē-ō′pē-ă, -op′sē-ă) [poly- + G. *ōps*, eye]. Multiple vision; the perception of several images of the same object.

polyorchism, polyorchidism (pol-ē-ōr′kizm, -ōr′kid-izm) [poly- + G. *orchis*, testis]. Presence of one or more supernumerary testes.

polyostotic (pol′ē-os-tot′ik) [poly- + G. *osteon*, bone]. Involving more than one bone.

polyotia (pol-ē-ō′shē-ă) [poly- + G. *ous*, ear]. Presence of a supernumerary auricle on one or both sides of the head.

polyovular (pol-ē-ō′vyū-lăr). Containing more than one ovum.

polyovulatory (pol-ē-ō′vyū-lă-tōr-ē). Polyzygotic; discharging several ova in one ovulatory cycle.

polyoxyl 40 stearate (pol-ē-ok′sil). A mixture of the monostearate and distearate esters of a condensation polymer, $H(OCH_2CH_2)_n{\cdot}OCOC_{16}H_{32}CH_3$ (*n* is approximately 40); it is a nonionic surface-active agent used as an emulsifying agent in hydrophilic ointment and other emulsions.

polyp (pol′ip) [L. *polypus;* G. *polypous,* contr. fr. G. *polys,* many, + *pous,* foot]. Polypus; a general descriptive term used with reference to any mass of tissue that bulges or projects outward or upward from the normal surface level, thereby being macroscopically visible as a hemispheroidal, spheroidal, or irregular moundlike structure growing from a relatively broad base or a slender stalk; p.'s may be neoplasms, foci of inflammation, degenerative lesions, or malformations.
adenomatous p., polypoid adenoma; cellular p.; a p. that consists of benign neoplastic tissue derived from glandular epithelium.
bleeding p., vascular p.
bronchial p., a p. growing from the bronchial mucosa.
cardiac p., usually a rounded thrombus attached to the endocardium.
cellular p., adenomatous p.
choanal p., an antral-choanal p. that extends into the nasopharynx; generally originates in the antrum.
cystic p., hydatid p.; a pedunculated cyst.
dental p., hyperplastic *pulpitis.*
fibrinous p., a misnomer for a mass of fibrin retained within the uterine cavity after childbirth.
fibrous p., a p. consisting chiefly of cellular fibrous tissue, frequently with foci of fairly dense collagen or hyaline material (or both).
fleshy p., myomatous p.
gelatinous p., **(1)** a p. that consists of delicate, loose, edematous connective tissue; **(2)** a polypoid myxoma.
Hopmann's p., Hopmann's *papilloma.*
hydatid p., cystic p.
hyperplastic p., metaplastic p.; a benign small sessile p. of the large bowel showing lengthening and cystic dilation of mucosal glands; also applied to non-neoplastic gastric mucosal p.'s.
inflammatory p., pseudopolyp.
juvenile p., retention p.; a smoothly rounded mucosal hamartoma of the large bowel, which may be multiple and cause rectal bleeding, especially in the first decade of life; it is not precancerous.
laryngeal p., a p. projecting from the surface of one of the vocal cords.
lipomatous p., **(1)** a p. consisting chiefly of adipose tissue; **(2)** lipoma that bulges from the surface or is attached by means of a stalk.
lymphoid p., benign *lymphoma* of the rectum.
metaplastic p., hyperplastic p.
mucous p., **(1)** an adenomatous p. in which conspicuous amounts of mucin are formed; **(2)** a polypoid cyst that contains mucus.
myomatous p., fleshy p.; a p. that consists of benign neoplastic tissue derived from nonstriated (smooth) muscle.
nasal p., an inflammatory or allergic p., arising from one of the paranasal sinuses, which projects into the nasal cavity.
osseous p., a p. consisting in part of bony tissue.
pedunculated p., any form of p. that is attached to the base tissue by means of a slender stalk.

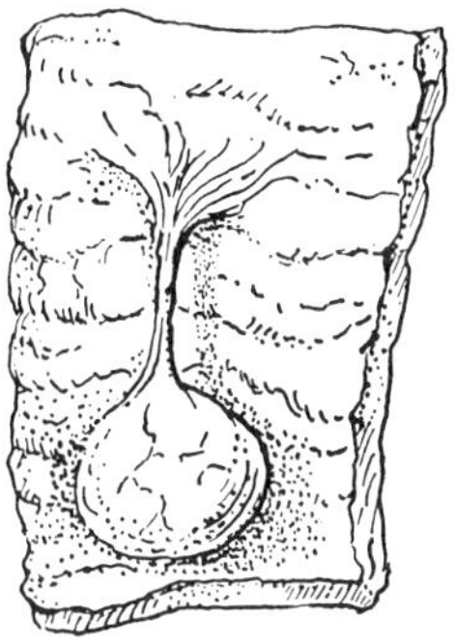

Pedunculated Polyp of Rectal Mucosa

placental p., a p. developed from a piece of retained placenta.
pulp p., hyperplastic *pulpitis.*
regenerative p., a hyperplastic p. of the gastric mucosa.
retention p., juvenile p.
sessile p., any form of p. that has a relatively broad base.
tooth p., hyperplastic *pulpitis.*
vascular p., bleeding p.; a bulging or protruding angioma of the nasal mucous membrane.

polypapilloma (pol′ē-pap-i-lō′mă). **1.** Multiple papillomas. **2.** Yaws.

polypathia (pol-ē-path′ē-ă) [poly- + G. *pathos,* disease]. A multiplicity of diseases or disorders.

polypectomy (pol-i-pek′tō-mē) [polyp + G. *ektomē,* excision]. Excision of a polyp.

polypeptide (pol-ē-pep′tīd). A peptide formed by the union of an indefinite (usually large) number of amino acids by peptide links (–NH–CO–).
gastric inhibitory p. (GIP), a peptide hormone, secreted by the stomach, that stimulates insulin release as part of the digestive process.
vasoactive intestinal p. (VIP), a p. hormone secreted most commonly by non-beta islet cell tumors of the pancreas, producing copious watery diarrhea and fecal electrolyte loss, particularly hypokalemia.

polyphagia (pol-ē-fā′jē-ă) [poly- + G. *phagein,* to eat]. Excessive eating; gluttony.

polyphalangism (pol′ē-fă-lan′jizm). Hyperphalangism.

polyphallic (pol-ē-fal′ik). Pertaining to the fantasy of possessing multiple penises.

polypharmacy (pol-ē-far′mă-sē). The mixing of many drugs in one prescription. See also shotgun *prescription.*

polyphenic (pol-ē-phēn′ik) [poly- + G. *phainō,* to display]. Pleiotropic.

polyphenol oxidase (pol-ē-fē′nol). Laccase.

polyphobia (pol-ē-fō′bē-ă) [poly- + G. *phobos,* fear]. Morbid fear of many things; a condition marked by the presence of many phobias.

polyphosphorylase (pol′ē-fos-fōr′i-lās). Phosphorylase.

polyphrasia (pol-ē-frā′zē-ă) [poly- + G. *phrasis,* speech]. Extreme talkativeness.

polyphyletic (pol′ē-fī-let′ik). **1.** Derived from more than one source, or having several lines of descent, in contrast to monophyletic. **2.** In hematology, relating to polyphyletism.

polyphyletism (pol-ē-fī′lĕ-tizm) [poly- + G. *phylē,* tribe]. Polyphyletic theory; in hematology, the theory that blood cells are derived from several different stem cells, depending on the particular blood cell type.

polyphyodont (pol-ē-fī′ō-dont) [poly- + G. *phyō,* to produce, + *odous* (*odont-*), tooth]. Having several sets of teeth formed in succession throughout life.

polypi (pol′i-pī). Plural of polypus.

polypiform (po-lip′i-fōrm). Polypoid.

polyplasmia (pol-ē-plaz′mē-ă). Hydremia.

polyplast (pol′ē-plast) [poly- + G. *plastos,* formed]. That which is polyplastic.

polyplastic (pol-ē-plas′tik) [poly- + G. *plastikos,* plastic]. **1.** Formed of several different structures. **2.** Capable of assuming several forms.

Polyplax (pol′ē-plaks) [poly- + G. *plax,* plate, plaque]. A sucking louse (order Anoplura) of rats and mice. The species *P. serratus* (the mouse louse) has been shown experimentally to be capable of transmitting tularemia and may also be a vector for murine typhus and *Trypanosoma lewisi.*

polyplegia (pol-ē-plē'jē-ă) [poly- + G. *plēgē,* a stroke]. Paralysis of several muscles.

polyploid (pol'ē-ployd). Characterized by or pertaining to polyploidy.

polyploidy (pol'ē-ploy'dē) [poly- + G. *polides,* in form]. The state of a cell nucleus containing three or a higher multiple of the haploid number of chromosomes. Cells containing three, four, five, or six multiples are referred to, respectively, as triploid, tetraploid, pentaploid, or hexaploid; higher multiples may be expressed by using the appropriate Greek number.

polypnea (pol-ip-nē'ă) [poly- + G. *pnoia,* breath]. Tachypnea.

polypodia (pol-i-pō'dē-ă). Presence of supernumerary feet.

polypoid (pol'i-poyd) [polyp + G. *eidos,* resemblance]. Polypiform; resembling a polyp in gross features.

polyporous (pol-ip'ōr-ŭs) [poly- + G. *poros,* pore]. Cribriform.

Polyporus (po-lip'ŏ-rŭs) [poly- + G. *poros,* pore]. A genus of mushrooms. See agaric.

polyposia (pol-ē-pō'zē-ă) [poly- + G. *posis,* drinking]. Rarely used term for sustained, excessive consumption of liquids.

polyposis (pol'i-pō'sis) [polyp + G. *-osis,* condition]. Presence of several polyps.

p. co'li, multiple intestinal p. (1).

familial intestinal p., multiple intestinal p.

multiple intestinal p., familial intestinal p.; **(1)** p. coli; p. of the colon characterized by polyps only of the mucosa, with no associated lesions, which begin to form usually in late childhood, increase in numbers, and may carpet the mucosal surface; there are symptoms of chronic colitis, and carcinoma of the colon almost invariably develops in untreated cases; autosomal dominant inheritance; **(2)** p. of the small or large intestine as a feature of Gardner's, Peutz-Jeghers, Turcot, and Zollinger-Ellison syndromes.

polypotome (po-lip'ō-tōm) [polyp + G. *tomos,* cutting]. An instrument used for cutting away a polyp.

polypotrite (pol-ip'ō-trīt) [polyp + L. *tero,* pp. *tritus,* to rub]. An instrument for crushing polyps.

polypous (pol'i-pŭs). Pertaining to, manifesting the gross features of, or characterized by the presence of a polyp or polyps.

polypragmasy (pol-ē-prag'mă-sē) [poly- + G. *pragma,* a thing]. Administration of many different remedies at the same time.

polyptychial (pol-ē-tik'ē-ăl) [G. *polyptychos,* having many folds or layers, fr. poly- + *ptychē,* fold or layer]. Folded or arranged so as to form more than one layer.

polypus, pl. **polypi** (pol'i-pŭs, -pī) [L.]. Polyp.

polyradiculitis (pol'ē-ra-dik'yū-lī'tis). Inflammation of nerve roots.

polyradiculomyopathy (pol'ē-ra-dik'yū-lō-mī-op'ă-thē). A combination of polyradiculitis (Guillain-Barré syndrome) with myositis.

polyradiculoneuropathy (pol-ē-ra-dik'yū-lō-nū-rop'ă-thē). Acute idiopathic *polyneuritis.*

polyradiculopathy (pol-ē-ra-dik'yū-lop'ă-thē). Acute idiopathic *polyneuritis.*

polyribonucleotide nucleotidyltransferase (pol'ē-rī-bō-nū'klē-ō-tīd) [EC 2.7.7.8]. Polynucleotide phosphorylase; an enzyme catalyzing phosphorolysis of polyribonucleotides or of RNA, yielding nucleoside diphosphates (or the reverse, the first artificial polynucleotide formation discovered).

polyribosomes (pol-ē-rī'bō-sōmz). Polysomes; conceptually, two or more ribosomes connected by a molecule of messenger RNA; structures satisfying this concept can be seen in electron micrographs and can be sedimented at rates consistent with aggregates of ribosomes (whence it is often, sometimes incorrectly, assumed that aggregates containing ribosomes are true p.); p. are active in protein synthesis.

polyrrhea (pol-i-rē'ă) [poly- + G. *rhoia,* a flow]. Profuse discharge of serous or other fluid.

polysaccharide (pol-ē-sak'ă-rīd). Glycan; a carbohydrate containing a large number of saccharide groups; *e.g.,* starch. *Cf.* oligosaccharide.

pneumococcal p., specific capsular *substance.*

specific soluble p., specific capsular *substance.*

polyscelia (pol-ē-sē'lē-ă) [poly- + G. *skelos,* leg]. A form of polymelia involving the presence of more than two legs.

polyscope (pol'ē-skōp). Diaphanoscope.

polyserositis (pol'ē-sēr-ō-sī'tis) [poly- + L. *serum,* serum, + G. *-itis,* inflammation]. Concato's disease; Bamberger's disease (2); multiple serositis; chronic inflammation with effusions in several serous cavities resulting in fibrous thickening of the serosa and constrictive pericarditis.

familial paroxysmal p., familial recurrent p., transient recurring attacks of abdominal pain, fever, pleurisy, arthritis, and rash; the condition is asymptomatic between attacks. Also called benign paroxysmal peritonitis; familial Mediterranean fever; Mediterranean fever (2); periodic p. or peritonitis.

periodic p., familial paroxysmal p.

polysinusitis (pol'ē-sī-nŭ-sī'tis). Simultaneous inflammation of two or more sinuses.

polysomes (pol'ē-sōmz). Polyribosomes.

polysomia (pol-ē-sō'mē-ă) [poly- + G. *sōma,* body]. Fetal malformation involving two or more imperfect and partially fused bodies.

polysomic (pol-ē-sō'mik). Pertaining to or characterized by polysomy.

polysomnogram (pol-ē-som'nō-gram) [poly- + L. *somnus,* sleep, + G. *gramma,* diagram]. The recorded physiologic function(s) obtained in polysomnography.

polysomnography (pol'ē-som-nog'ră-fē) [poly- + L. *somnus,* sleep, + G. *graphō,* to write]. Simultaneous and continuous monitoring of relevant normal and abnormal physiological activity during sleep.

polysomy (pol-ē-sō'mē) [poly- + G. *sōma,* body (chromosome)]. State of a cell nucleus in which a specific chromosome is represented more than twice. Cells containing three, four, or five homologous chromosomes are referred to, respectively, as trisomic, tetrasomic, or pentasomic.

polysorbate 80 (pol-ē-sōr'bāt). Polyoxethylene (20) sorbitan monooleate; a mixture of polyoxethylene ethers of mixed partial oleic esters of sorbitol anhydrides; used as an emulsifier, as in the preparation of pharmacologic products.

polyspermia, polyspermism (pol-ē-sper'mē-ă, -sper'mizm). **1.** Polyspermy. **2.** An abnormally profuse spermatic secretion.

polyspermy (pol'ē-sper-mē). Polyspermia (1); the entrance of more than one spermatozoon into the ovum.

polysplenia (pol-ē-sple'nē-ă) [poly- + G. *splēn,* spleen]. A condition in which splenic tissue is divided into two or more nearly equal masses. See also bilateral left-*sidedness.*

polysteraxic (pol'ē-ster-ak'sik). Denoting behavior characterized by its socially provocative quality.

polystichia (pol-ē-stik'ē-ă) [poly- + G. *stichos,* row]. Arrangement of the eyelashes in two or more rows.

polysulfide rubber (pol-ē-sŭl'fīd). Synthetic rubber used as a dental impression material.

polysuspensoid (pol-ē-sŭs-pen'soyd). A colloid system of solid phases having different degrees of dispersion.

polysymbrachydactyly (pol'ē-sim-brak-ē-dak'ti-lē) [poly- + symbrachydactyly]. Congenital malformation of the hand or foot in which the shortened digits are syndactylous and polydactylous.

polysynaptic (pol'ē-si-nap'tik). Multisynaptic; referring to neural pathways formed by a chain of a large number of synaptically connected nerve cells, as distinguished from oligosynaptic conduction systems.

polysyndactyly (pol'ē-sin-dak'ti-lē). Syndactyly of several fingers or toes.

polytendinitis (pol'ē-ten-di-nī'tis). Inflammation of several tendons.

polytene (pol'i-tēn). Consisting of many filaments of chromatin as the result of repeated division of chromonema without separation of filaments.

polythelia (pol-ē-thē'lē-ă) [poly- + G. *thēlē*, nipple]. Hyperthelia; presence of supernumerary nipples, either on the breast or elsewhere on the body.

polythiazide (pol-ē-thī'ă-zīd). 6-Chloro-3,4-dihydro-2-methyl-3-[(2,2,2-trifluoroethylthio)methyl] -2*H*- 1,2,4,-benzothiazine-7-sulfonamide 1,1-dioxide; a diuretic and antihypertensive of the benzothiadiazine group.

polytocous (pō-lit'ō-kŭs) [poly- + G. *tokos*, birth]. Producing multiple young at a birth.

polytomography (pol-i-tō-mog'ră-fē). Body section roentgenography using a machine specifically designed to effect complex motion.

polytrichia (pol-ē-trik'ē-ă) [poly- + G. *thrix* (*trich-*), hair]. Polytrichosis; excessive hairiness.

polytrichosis (pol'ē-tri-kō'sis). Polytrichia.

polyunguia (pol-ē-ŭng'gwē-ă) [poly- + L. *unguis*, nail]. Polyonychia.

polyuria (pol-ē-yū'rē-ă) [poly- + G. *ouron*, urine]. Hydruria; excessive excretion of urine resulting in profuse micturition.

polyvalent (pol-ē-vā'lent). **1.** Multivalent. **2.** Pertaining to a polyvalent antiserum.

polyvidone (pol-ē-vī'dōn). Povidone.

polyvinyl (pol-ē-vī'năl). Referring to a compound containing a number of vinyl groups in polymerized form.

polyvinyl alcohol. A compound, $CH_2(CHOH)_n$, that is soluble in water; an adhesive and emulsifier.

polyvinyl chloride (PVC). Chlorethene homopolymer; a substance used as a rubber substitute in many industrial applications, and suspected of being carcinogenic in man.

polyvinylpyrrolidone (PVP) (pol-ē-vī'nil-pi-rol'i-dōn). Povidone.

polyvinylpyrrolidone-iodine complex. Povidone-iodine.

polyzoic (pol-ē-zō'ik). Segmented body form, as in the higher tapeworms, subclass Cestoda. See also strobila; monozoic.

polyzygotic (pol-ē-zī-got'ik) [poly- + G. *zygōtos*, yoked]. Polyovulatory.

pomade (pō-mād', pō-mahd') [Fr. *pomade*, fr. L. *pomum*, apple]. Pomatum; an ointment or cream containing medicaments; usually used on the hair.

pomatum (pō-mā'tŭm) [Mod. L.]. Pomade.

pomegranate (pom'gran-at) [L. *pomum*, apple, + *granatus*, many seeded, fr. *granum*, grain or seed]. Granatum; fruit of *Punica granatum* (family Punicaceae), a reddish yellow fruit the size of an orange, containing many seeds enclosed in a reddish acidic pulp; used in diarrhea for its astringent properties; the bark of the tree and of the root contains pelletierine and other alkaloids, and has been used as a teniacide.

Pomeroy, Ralph H., U.S. obstetrician-gynecologist, 1867–1925. See P.'s *operation.*

POMP Abbreviation for Purinethol (6-mercaptopurine), Oncovin (vincristine sulfate), methotrexate, and prednisone, a cancer chemotherapy regimen.

Pompe, J.C., 20th century Dutch physician. See P.'s *disease.*

pompholyx (pom'fō-liks) [G. a bubble, fr. *pomphos*, a blister]. Dyshidrosis.

pomphus (pom'fŭs) [G. *pomphos*, blister]. A wheal or blister.

Ponceau de xylidine (pon-sō' dĕ zī'li-dēn) [C.I.-16151]. A monoazo acid dye originally employed as a red histological counterstain in Masson's trichrome stain.

Ponfick, Emil, German pathologist, 1844–1913. See P.'s *shadow.*

pono- [G. *ponos*, toil, fatigue, pain]. Combining form meaning bodily exertion, fatigue, overwork, pain.

ponograph (pō'nō-graf) [pono- + G. *graphō*, to write]. An instrument for recording graphically the progressive fatigue of a contracting muscle.

ponopalmosis (pō'nō-pal-mō'sis) [pono- + G. *palmos*, palpitation]. Rarely used term for a condition of irritable heart in which palpitation is excited by slight exertion.

ponophobia (pō-nō-fō'bē-ă) [pono- + G. *phobos*, fear]. Morbid fear of overwork or of becoming fatigued.

ponos (pō'nos) [G. toil, fatigue, pain]. A disease occurring in young children in certain of the islands of Greece, characterized by enlargement of the spleen, hemorrhages, fever, and cachexia; possibly the infantile form of visceral leishmaniasis.

pons, pl. **pontes** (ponz, pon'tēz) [L. bridge] **1** [NA]. In neuroanatomy, the pons varolii or pons cerebelli; that part of the brainstem between the medulla oblongata caudally and the mesencephalon rostrally, composed of the pars basilaris pontis and the tegmentum pontis. On the ventral surface of the brain the pars basilaris, the white pontine protuberance, is demarcated from both the medulla oblongata and the mesencephalon by distinct transverse grooves. **2.** Any bridgelike formation connecting two more or less disjoined parts of the same structure or organ.

p. cerebel'li, p. (1).

p. hep'atis, ponticulus hepatis; a bridge of liver tissue that sometimes overlaps the fossa venae cavae, converting it into a canal.

p. varo'lii, p. (1).

pontes (pon'tēz) [L.]. Plural of pons.

pontic (pon'tik). Dummy; an artificial tooth on a fixed partial denture; it replaces the lost natural tooth, restores its functions, and usually occupies the space previously occupied by the natural crown.

ponticulus (pon-tik'yū-lŭs) [L. dim. of *pons*, bridge]. A vertical ridge on the eminentia conchae giving insertion to the auricularis posterior muscle.

p. hep'atis, *pons* hepatis.

p. na'si, bridge of the nose.

p. promonto'rii, *subiculum* promontorii.

pontile, pontine (pon'tīl, -tēn, -tīn). Relating to a pons.

Pool, Eugene H., U.S. surgeon, 1874–1949. See P.'s *phenomenon;* P.-Schlesinger *sign.*

pool (pūl) [A.S. *pōl*] **1.** A collection of blood in any region of the body, due to a dilation and retardation of the circulation in the capillaries and veins of the part. **2.** A combination of resources.

abdominal p., the volume of blood within the abdomen.

gene p., the actual composition of the genes that are available for inheritance in a mating population.

metabolic p., the quantity of a given chemical compound or group of related compounds participating in metabolic reactions; may constitute only a portion of the total bodily content of such compounds.

vaginal p., the mucoid secretions and cellular material that accumulate in the posterior fornix of the vagina; used as a cellular specimen, principally for hormonal evaluation and cancer detection.

poplar (pop'lăr). *Populus.*

poples (pop'lēz) [L. the ham of the knee] [NA]. Ham (1); popliteus (2); popliteal region; the posterior region of the knee. See also *fossa* poplitea.

popliteal (pop-lit'ē-ăl, pop-li-tē'ăl). Relating to the poples.

popliteus (pop-li-tē'ŭs) [L.]. **1.** Popliteal. **2.** Poples. **3.** *Musculus* popliteus.

POPOP Abbreviation for 1,4-bis(5-phenyloxazol-2-yl)benzene.

poppy (pop'ē). *Papaver.*

p. oil, a fixed (drying) oil expressed from the seed of *Papaver somniferum;* sometimes used in the preparation of liniments and as a solvent of iodine in iodized oil.

population (pop-yū-lā'shŭn) [L. *populus,* a people, nation]. Statistical term denoting all the objects, events, or subjects in a particular class.

POR Abbreviation for problem-oriented *record.*

por-. See poro-.

porcelain (pōr'sĕ-lin). A powder composed of a clay, silica, and a flux which, when mixed with water, forms a paste that is molded to form artificial teeth, inlays, jacket crowns, and dentures. When heated, the materials fuse to form a ceramic.

porcine (pōr'sīn, -sin) [L. *porcinus,* fr. *porcus,* a hog]. Relating to pigs.

pore (pōr) [G. *poros,* passageway]. **1.** A hole, perforation, or foramen. See also porus. **2.** One of the minute openings of the sweat glands of the skin.

dilated p., acquired trichoepithelioma; an enlarged follicular opening of the skin, with a keratinous plug and occasional lanugo or mature hair.

external acoustic p., external auditory p., *porus* acusticus externus.

gustatory p., *porus* gustatorius.

interalveolar p.'s, Kohn's p.'s; openings in the interalveolar septa of the lung.

internal acoustic p., auditory p., *porus* acusticus internus.

Kohn's p.'s, interalveolar p.'s.

nuclear p., an octagonal opening, about 700 Å across, where the inner and outer membranes of the nuclear envelope are continuous.

slit p.'s, filtration slits; the intercellular clefts between the interdigitating pedicels of podocytes; they are part of the filtration barrier of renal corpuscles.

sweat p., *porus* sudoriferus.

taste p., *porus* gustatorius.

porencephalia (pōr'en-se-fā'lē-ă). Porencephaly.

porencephalic (pōr'en-se-fal'ik). Porencephalous; relating to or characterized by porencephaly.

porencephalitis (pōr'en-sef-ă-lī'tis) [G. *poros,* pore, + *enkephalos,* brain, + *-itis,* inflammation]. Chronic inflammation of the brain with the formation of cavities in the organ's substance.

porencephalous (pōr-en-sef'ă-lŭs). Porencephalic.

porencephaly (pōr-en-sef'ă-lē) [G. *poros,* pore, + *enkephalos,* brain]. Porencephalia; spelencephaly; the occurrence of cavities in the brain substance, communicating usually with the lateral ventricles.

Porges, O., Austrian bacteriologist, *1879. See P. *method;* P.-Meier *test.*

pori (pō'rī). Plural of porus.

poria (pōr'ē-ă). Plural of porion.

Porifera (pō-rif'er-ă) [L. *porus,* pore, + *fero,* to bear]. The sponges; a phylum of the Metazoa, comprising a group of sessile, aquatic animals possessing an endoskeleton and many branching canals, lined by flagellated collar cells; communication of the canals with the surface is made through many pores or through larger openings and oscula. See also Parazoa.

poriomania (pōr'ē-ō-mā'nē-ă) [G. *poreia,* a journey, + *mania,* frenzy]. A morbid impulse to wander or journey away from home.

porion, pl. poria (pōr'ē-on, -ē-ă) [G. *poros,* a passage]. The central point on the upper margin of the external auditory meatus; as a cephalometric landmark, it is located in the middle of the metal rods of the cephalometer.

pornolagnia (pōr-nō-lag'nē-ă) [G. *pornē,* prostitute, + *lagneia,* lust]. Sexual attraction toward prostitutes.

poro-, por-. **1** [G. *poros* (L. *porus*), passageway]. Combining form denoting a pore, duct, or opening. **2.** [G. *poreia,* a journey, passage]. Combining form denoting a going or passing through. **3** [G. *poros,* a kind of marble, a stone]. Combining form denoting a callus or induration.

porocele (pōr'ō-sēl) [G. *pōros,* callus, + *kēlē,* hernia]. A hernia with indurated coverings.

porocephaliasis (pō'rō-sef-ă-lī'ă-sis). Porocephalosis; infection with a species of *Porocephalus.*

Porocephalidae (pō'rō-se-fal'i-dē) [G. *poros,* pore, + *kephalē,* head]. A family of parasitic tongue worms (order Porocephalida, phylum Pentastomida) characterized by four hooks arranged in a curved line on either side of the mouth. Adults are found in the lungs of reptiles, and larvae or nymphs are found in the tissues of a great variety of vertebrates, including man. See also Linguatulidae; *Armillifer; Linguatula.*

porocephalosis (pō'rō-sef-ă-lō'sis). Porocephaliasis.

Porocephalus (pō-rō-sef'ă-lŭs) [G. *poros,* pore, + *kephalē,* head]. A genus of the family Porocephalidae, of which the adult worms or larvae cause porocephaliasis in a number of animal species including man.

P. armilla'tus, *Armillifer armillatus.*

poroconidium (pōr'ō-kō-nid'ē-ŭm). Porospore; in fungi, a spore produced through the microscopic pore of the condidiophore.

porokeratosis (pō'rō-ker-ă-tō'sis) [G. *poros,* pore, + keratosis]. A rare dermatosis in which there is a thickening of the stratum corneum with an annular keratotic rim or cornoid lamella and progressive centrifugal atrophy; cutaneous carcinoma has been reported to arise in the lesions. Also called Mibelli's disease; keratoderma eccentrica; hyperkeratosis eccentrica; hyperkeratosis figurata centrifuga atrophica; keratoatrophoderma.

actinic p., a lesion which occurs on exposed areas of extremities primarily; bears a resemblance to actinic keratosis but the histologic features are those of p.

poroma (pōrō'mă) [G. *pōrōma,* callus, fr. *pōros,* stone]. **1.** Callosity. **2.** Exostosis. **3.** Induration following a phlegmon. **4.** A tumor of cells lining the skin openings of sweat glands.

eccrine p., a p. or acrospiroma of the eccrine sweat glands, usually occurring on the sole of the foot.

porosis pl. **poroses** (pō-rō'sis, -sēz) [L. *porosus,* porous]. Porosity (1); a porous condition.

cerebral p., a porous condition of the brain caused by postmortem growth of *Clostridium perfringens* or other gas-forming organisms in the tissue.

porosity (pō-ros'i-tē) [G. *poros,* pore]. **1.** Porosis. **2.** A perforation.

porospore (pōr'ō-spōr). Poroconidium.

porotic (pō-rot'ik). Porous, as in osteoporotic.

porotomy (pō-rot'ō-mē) [G. *poros,* passage, + *tomē,* incision]. Meatotomy.

porous (pō'rŭs). Having openings that pass directly or indirectly through the substance.

porphin, porphine (pōr'fin). Porphyrin; the unsubstituted tetrapyrrole nucleus that is the basis of the porphyrins. *Cf.* phorbin; corrin. See also porphyrins.

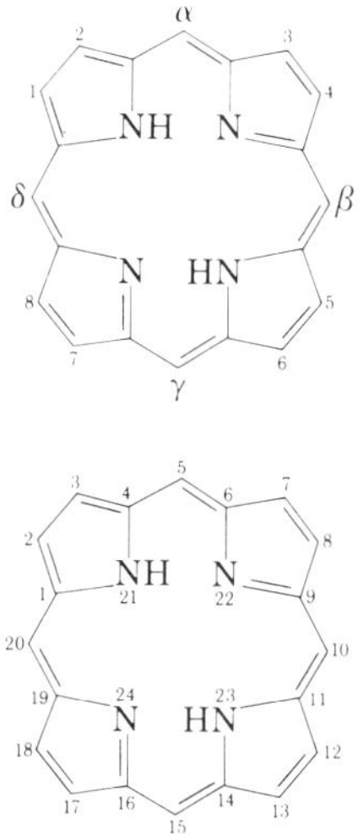

Porphin
Top, original Fischer numbering system
Bottom, modern (1–24) numbering system

porphobilin (pōr'fō-bī'lin). General term denoting intermediates between the monopyrrole, porphobilinogen, and the cyclic tetrapyrrole of heme (a porphin derivative). See also bilin.

porphobilinogen (PBG) (pōr'fō-bī-lin'ō-jen). 5-Aminomethyl-4-carboxymethylpyrrole-3-propionic acid; a porphyrin precursor of porphyrinogens, porphyrins, and heme; found in the urine in large quantities in cases of acute or congenital porphyria.
p. synthase [EC 4.2.1.24], δ-aminolevulinate dehydratase; a liver enzyme catalyzing the formation of porphobilinogen from 2 molecules of δ-aminolevulinate, an important reaction in porphyrin biosynthesis.

porphyria (pōr-fir'ē-ă). A group of disorders involving heme biosynthesis, characterized by excessive excretion of porphyrins or their precursors; may be inherited or may be acquired, as from the effects of certain chemical agents (*e.g.,* hexachlorobenzene).
acute intermittent p., acute p., intermittent acute p.
bovine p., p. as a mendelian recessive trait in certain breeds of cattle.
congenital erythropoietic p. (CEP), enhanced porphyrin formation by erythroid cells in bone marrow, leading to severe porphyrinuria, often in conjunction with hemolytic anemia and persistent cutaneous photosensitivity; caused by a deficiency of uroporphyrinogen III cosynthetase; autosomal recessive inheritance.
p. cuta'nea tar'da (PCT), symptomatic p.; p. characterized by liver dysfunction and photosensitive cutaneous lesions, with hyperpigmentation and scleroderma-like changes in the skin, and increased excretion of uroporphyrin; caused by a deficiency of uroporphyrinogen decarboxylase; autosomal dominant inheritance.
erythrohepatic p., see congenital erythrohepatic p.
erythropoietic p., a classification of p. that includes congenital erythropoietic p. and erythropoietic protoporphyria.
hepatic p., a category of p. that includes p. cutanea tarda, variegate p., and coproporphyria.
intermittent acute p. (IAP), acute p.; acute intermittent p.; p. caused by hepatic overproduction of δ-aminolevulinic acid, with greatly increased urinary excretion of it and of porphobilinogen, and some increase of uroporphyrin, due to a deficiency of porphobilingoen deaminase; characterized by intermittent acute attacks of hypertension, abdominal colic, psychosis, and neuropathy, but with no photosensitivity; autosomal dominant inheritance.
ovulocyclic p., acute episodic exacerbations of p. occurring in the premenstrual period.
South African type p., variegate p.
squirrel p., p. as an apparently normal metabolic state seen in the Florida fox squirrel (*Sciurus niger*).
swine p., p. as a dominant trait seen in swine.
symptomatic p., p. cutanea tarda.
variegate p. (VP), protocoproporphyria hereditaria; South African type p.; p. characterized by abdominal pain and neuropsychiatric abnormalities, by dermal sensitivity to light and mechanical trauma, by increased fecal excretion of proto- and coproporphyrin, and by increased urinary excretion of δ-aminolevulinic acid, porphobilinogen, and porphyrins; due to a deficiency of protoporphyrinogen oxidase; autosomal dominant inheritance.

porphyrin (pōr'fi-rin). Porphin.

porphyrinogens (pōr-fi-rin'ō-jenz). Intermediates in the biosynthesis of heme, as follows: four porphobilinogens condense to form uroporphyrinogens I and III (giving rise to side-products uroporphyrins I and III) which are decarboxylated to form coproporphyrinogens I and III (giving rise to side-products coproporphyrins I and III); coproporphyrinogen III is oxidized to protoporphyrin III (IX) which adds ferrous iron to yield heme.

porphyrins (pōr'fi-rinz). Pigments widely distributed throughout nature (*e.g.,* heme, bile pigments, cytochromes) consisting of four pyrroles joined in a ring (porphin) structure. They are substitution products of porphin (porphyrin) and comprise several varieties, differing for the most part in the sidechains (methyl, ethyl, vinyl, formyl, carboxyethyl, carboxymethyl, etc.) present at the eight available positions on the pyrrole rings. Depending on the nature of the side chains, the prefixes dentero-, etio-, meso-, proto-, etc., are attached to p.; distribution within each class is given by type I, II, III, and IV. P.'s combine with various metals (iron, copper, magnesium, etc.) to form metalloporphyrins, and with nitrogenous substances.

porphyrinuria (pōr'fir-i-nū'rē-ă). Porphyruria; purpurinuria; excretion of porphyrins and related compounds in the urine.

porphyrization (pōr'fi-ri-zā'shŭn). Grinding in a mortar (formerly on a slab of porphyry).

porphyruria (pōr-fi-rū'rē-ă). Porphyrinuria.

porrigo (pō-rī'gō) [L. scurf, dandruff]. Obsolete term for any disease of the scalp; *e.g.,* ringworm, favus, eczema.
p. decal'vans [L. *decalvo,* to make bald], *alopecia* areata.
p. favo'sa, favus.
p. fur'furans, *tinea* tonsurans.
p. larva'lis, eczema of the scalp.
p. lupino'sa, favus.
p. scutula'ta, favus.

Porro, Edoardo, Italian obstetrician, 1842–1902. See P. *hysterectomy, operation.*

porropsia (pō-rop'sē-ă) [G. *porrō,* at a distance, + *opsis,* vision]. A condition in which objects appear farther away than they are.

porta, pl. **portae** (pōr'tă, -tē) [L. gate]. **1.** Hilum (1). **2.** *Foramen* interventriculare.
p. hep'atis [NA], portal fissure; caudal transverse fissure; a transverse fissure on the visceral surface of the liver between the caudate and quadrate lobes, lodging the portal vein, hepatic artery, hepatic nerve plexus, hepatic ducts, and lymphatic vessels.
p. lie'nis, *hilum* splenicum.
p. pulmo'nis, *hilum* pulmonis.
p. re'nis, *hilum* renalis.

portacaval (pōr'tă-kā'văl). Concerning the portal vein and the inferior vena cava.

portal (pōr'tăl) [L. *portalis,* pertaining to a porta (gate)]. **1.** Relating to any porta or hilus, specifically to the porta hepatis and the p. vein. **2.** The point of entry into the body of a pathogenic microorganism.

intestinal p.'s, in young embryos, the communications from the midgut to the foregut (**anterior i. p.**; see *fovea* cardiaca), or to the hindgut (**posterior i. p.**).

Porter, Curt C., U.S. biochemist, *1914. See P.-Silber *chromogens, reaction,* chromogens *test.*

Porter, Thomas C., British scientist, 1860–1933. See Ferry-P. *law.*

Porter, William H., Irish surgeon, 1790–1861. See P.'s *fascia.*

portio, pl. **portiones** (pōr'shē-ō, -ō'nēz) [L. portion] [NA]. A part.

p. interme'dia, *nervus* intermedius.

p. ma'jor ner'vi trigem'ini, *radix* sensoria nervi trigemini.

p. mi'nor ner'vi trigem'ini, *radix* motoria nervi trigemini.

p. supravagina'lis [NA], the part of the cervix uteri lying above the attachment of the vagina.

p. vagina'lis [NA], the part of the cervix uteri contained within the vagina.

portiplexus (pōr-ti-plek'sŭs). The union of the choroid plexus of the lateral ventricle with that of the third ventricle at the interventricular foramen (of Monro).

porto- [L. *porta,* gate]. Combining form meaning portal.

portobilioarterial (pōr'tō-bil'ē-ō-ar-tēr'ē-ăl). Relating to the portal vein, biliary ducts, and hepatic artery, which have similar distributions. See also hepatic *triad.*

portoenterostomy (pōr'tō-en-ter-os'tō-mē). Kasai operation; an o. for biliary atresia in which a Roux-en-Y loop of jejunum is anastomosed to the hepatic end of the divided extravascular portal structures, including rudimentary bile ducts.

portogram (pōr'tō-gram) [porto- G. *gramma,* a writing]. Radiographic record of portography.

portography (pōr-tog'ră-fē) [porto- + G. *graphō,* to write]. Portovenography; delineation of the portal circulation by roentgenograms, using radiopaque material, usually introduced into the spleen or into the portal vein at operation.

portosystemic (pōr'tō-sis-tem'ik). Relating to connections between the portal and systemic venous systems.

portovenography (pōr'tō-vē-nog'ră-fē). Portography.

porus, pl. **pori** (pō'rŭs, -rī) [L. fr. G. *poros,* passageway] [NA]. A pore, meatus, or foramen.

p. acus'ticus exter'nus [NA], external acoustic or auditory pore or foramen; the orifice of the external acoustic meatus in the tympanic portion of the temporal bone.

p. acus'ticus inter'nus [NA], internal acoustic or auditory pore or foramen; the inner opening of the internal acoustic meatus on the posterior surface of the petrous part of the temporal bone.

p. crotaphy'tico-buccinato'rius, Hyrtl's foramen; an occasional foramen in the sphenoid bone through which passes the motor portion of the trigeminal nerve; it is formed by ossification of a ligament below and lateral to the foramen ovale.

p. gustato'rius [NA], gustatory or taste pore; the minute opening of a taste bud on the surface of the oral mucosa through which the gustatory hairs of the specialized neuroepithelial gustatory cells project.

p. op'ticus, *discus* nervi optici.

p. sudorif'erus [NA], sweat pore; the surface opening of the duct of a sweat gland.

Posadas, Alejandro, Argentine parasitologist, 1870–1902. See P.'s *disease.*

POSITION

position (pō-zish'ŭn) [L. *positio,* a placing, position, fr. *pono,* to place]. **1.** An attitude, posture, or place occupied. **2.** Posture or attitude assumed by a patient for comfort and to facilitate the performance of diagnostic, surgical, or therapeutic procedures. **3.** In obstetrics, the relation of an arbitrarily chosen portion of the fetus to the right or left side of the mother; with each presentation there may be a right or left p.; the fetal occiput, chin, and sacrum are the determining points of p. in vertex, face, and breech presentations, respectively. *Cf.* presentation.

anatomical p., the erect p. of the body with the face directed forward, the arms at the side and the palms of the hands directed forward; the terms posterior, anterior, lateral, medial, etc., are applied to the parts as they stand related to each other and to the axis of the body when in this p.

Bozeman's p., knee-elbow p., the patient being strapped to supports.

Casselberry p., a prone p. assumed when drinking, after intubation, in order to prevent the entrance of fluid into the tube.

centric p., the p. of the mandible in its most retruded relation to the maxillae. See also centric jaw *relation.*

condylar hinge p., **(1)** the p. of the condyles in the temporomandibular joints at which a hinge movement is possible; **(2)** the maxillomandibular relation from which a consciously stimulated true hinge movement can be executed.

dorsal p., supine p.

dorsosacral p., lithotomy p.

eccentric p., eccentric *relation.*

electrical heart p., heart p.; a description of the heart's electrical axis in the frontal plane, often based upon the form of the QRS complexes in leads aVL and aVF.

Elliot's p., a supine p. upon a double inclined plane or on a single inclined plane, with a cushion under the back at the level of the liver; used to facilitate abdominal section.

English p., Sims' p.

flank p., a lateral recumbent p., but with the lower leg flexed, the upper leg extended, and convex extension of the upper side of the body; used for nephrectomy.

Fowler's p., an inclined p. obtained by raising the head of the bed about 60 to 90 cm to promote better dependent drainage after an abdominal operation.

frontoanterior p., a cephalic presentation of the fetus with its forehead directed toward the right (**right frontoanterior, RFA**) or to the left (**left frontoanterior, LFA**) of the acetabulum of the mother.

frontoposterior p., a cephalic presentation of the fetus with its forehead directed toward the right (**right frontoposterior, RFP**) or to the left (**left frontoposterior, LFP**) sacroiliac articulation of the mother.

frontotransverse p., a cephalic presentation of the fetus with its forehead directed toward the right (**right frontotransverse, RFT**) or to the left (**left frontotransverse, LFT**) iliac fossa of the mother.

genucubital p., knee-elbow p.

genupectoral p., knee-chest p.

heart p., electrical heart p.

hinge p., in dentistry, the orientation of parts in a manner permitting hinge movement between them.

intercuspal p., the p. of the mandible when the cusps and sulci of the maxillary and mandibular teeth are in their greatest contact and the mandible is in its most closed position.

knee-chest p., genupectoral p.; a prone posture resting on the knees and upper part of the chest, assumed for gynecologic or rectal examination.

knee-elbow p., genucubital p.; a prone p. resting on the knees and elbows, assumed for gynecologic or rectal examination or operation.

lateral recumbent p., Sims' p.

leapfrog p., a stooping p., such as that taken by children in play-

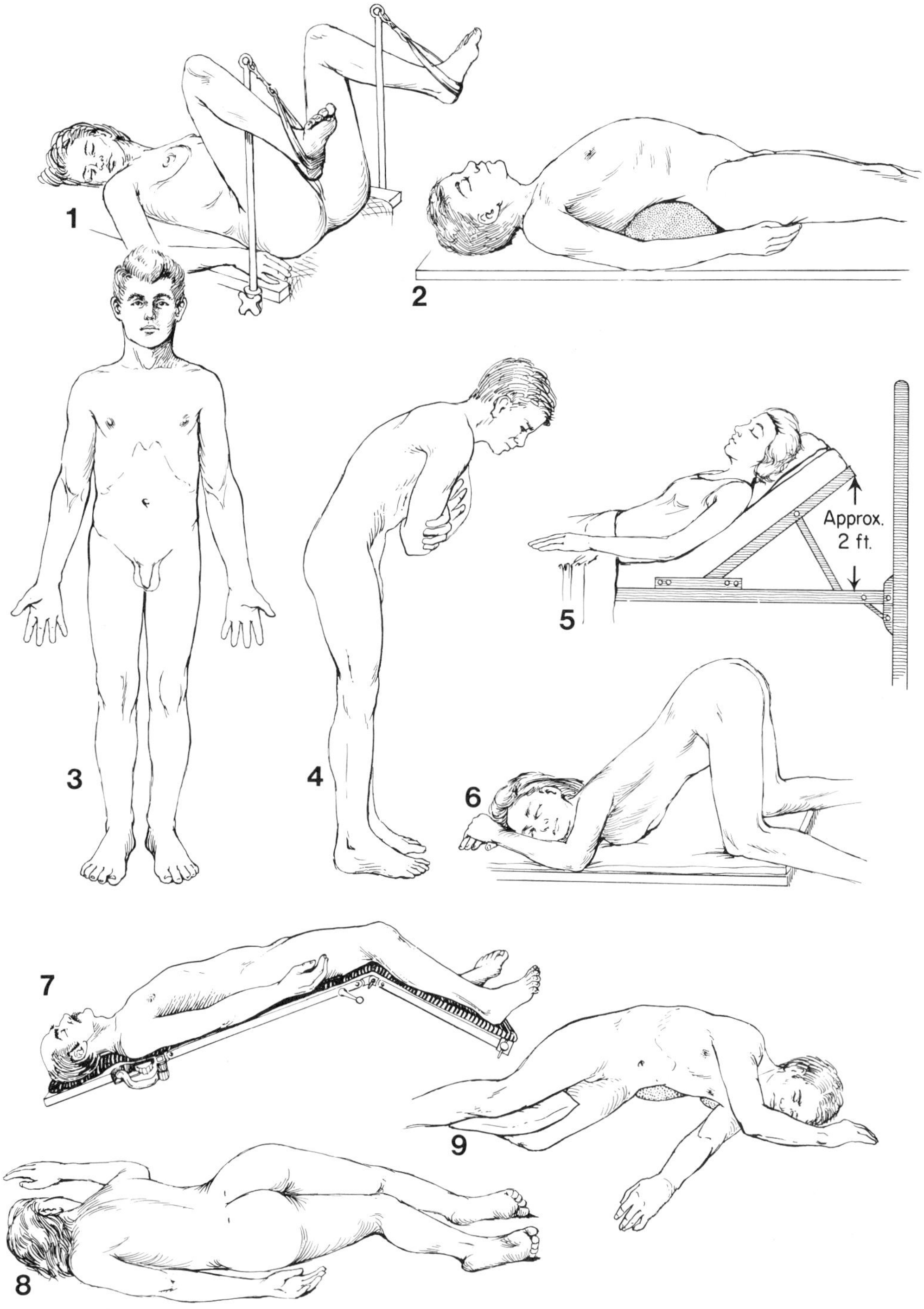

Positions

1, Lithotomy (dorsosacral); *2,* Elliot's; *3,* anatomical; *4,* Noble's; *5,* Fowler's; *6,* knee-chest (genupectoral); *7,* Trendelenburg's; *8,* Sim's (semiprone); *9,* lateral.

ing leapfrog, assumed for rectal examination.
lithotomy p., dorsosacral p.; a supine p. with buttocks at the end of the operating table, the hips and knees being fully flexed with feet strapped in p.
mandibular hinge p., any p. of the mandible which exists when the condyles are so situated in the temporomandibular joints that opening or closing movements can be made on the hinge axis.
Mayo-Robson's p., a supine p. with a thick pad under the loins, causing a marked lordosis in this region; used in operations on the gallbladder.
mentoanterior p., a cephalic presentation of the fetus with its chin pointing to the right (**right mentoanterior, RMA**) or to the left (**left mentoanterior, LMA**) acetabulum of the mother.
mentoposterior p., a cephalic presentation of the fetus with its chin pointing to the right (**right mentoposterior, RMP**) or to the left (**left mentoposterior, LMP**) sacroiliac articulation of the mother.
mentotransverse p., a cephalic presentation of the fetus with its chin pointing to the right (**right mentotransverse, RMT**) or to the left (**left mentotransverse, LMT**) iliac fossa of the mother.
Noble's p., patient standing and bent slightly forward; useful for inspection of a swelling of the loin that may occur with pyelonephritis.
obstetric p., the p. assumed by the parturient woman, either dorsal recumbent or lateral recumbent.
occipitoanterior p., a cephalic presentation of the fetus with its occiput turned toward the right (**right occipitoanterior, ROA**) or to the left (**left occipitoanterior, LOA**) acetabulum of the mother.
occipitoposterior p., a cephalic presentation of the fetus with its occiput turned toward the right (**right occipitoposterior, ROP**) or to the left (**left occipitoposterior, LOP**) sacroiliac joint of the mother.
occipitotransverse p., a cephalic presentation of the fetus with its occiput turned toward the right (**right occipitotransverse, ROT**) or to the left (**left occipitotransverse, LOT**) iliac fossa of the mother.
occlusal p., the relationship of the mandible and maxillae when the jaws are closed and the teeth are in contact; it may or may not coincide with centric occlusion.
physiologic rest p., postural, postural resting, or rest p.; the usual p. of the mandible when the patient is resting comfortably in the upright p. and the condyles are in a neutral unstrained p. in the glenoid fossae. See also rest *relation.*
postural p., postural resting p., physiologic rest p.
prone p., lying face down.
protrusive p., a forward p. of the mandible produced by muscular effort.
rest p., physiologic rest p.
Rose's p., the patient lies on his back with the head falling down over the end of the table; used in operations within the mouth, or the fauces, and on the fauciopharyngeal boundary.
sacroanterior p., a breech presentation of the fetus with the sacrum pointing to the right (**right sacroanterior, RSA**) or to the left (**left sacroanterior, LSA**) acetabulum of the mother.
sacroposterior p., a breech presentation of the fetus with the sacrum pointing to the right (**right sacroposterior, RSP**) or to the left (**left sacroposterior, LSP**) sacroiliac articulation of the mother.
sacrotransverse p., a breech presentation of the fetus with its sacrum pointing to the right (**right sacrotransverse, RST**) or to the left (**left sacrotransverse, LST**) sacroiliac articulation of the mother.
Scultetus' p., a supine p. on an inclined plane with head low, recommended by Scultetus for herniotomy and castration.
semiprone p., Sims' p. See also semiprone.
Simon's p., a p. for vaginal examination; a supine p. with hips elevated, thighs and legs flexed, and thighs widely separated.
Sims' p., English, lateral recumbent, or semiprone p.; a p. to facilitate a vaginal examination, the patient lying on the side with the under arm behind the back, the thighs flexed, the upper one more than the lower.
supine p., dorsal p.; lying upon the back.
terminal hinge p., the mandibular hinge p. from which further opening of the mandible would produce translatory rather than hinge movement.
Trendelenburg's p., a supine p. on the operating table, which is inclined at varying angles so that the pelvis is higher than the head with the knees flexed and legs hanging over the end of the table; used during and after operations in the pelvis or for shock.
Valentine's p., a supine p. on a table with double inclined plane so as to cause flexion at the hips; used to facilitate urethral irrigation.
Walcher p., a supine p. of the parturient woman with the lower extremities falling over the edge of the table.

---

positioner (pō-zish'ŭn-er). A resilient elastoplastic or rubber removable appliance fitting over the occlusal surface of the teeth, to obtain limited tooth movement and/or stabilization, usually used at the end of orthodontic treatment.

positive (+) (poz'i-tiv) [L. *positivus,* settled by arbitrary agreement, fr. *pono,* pp. *positus,* to set, place]. **1.** Affirmative; definite; not negative. **2.** Denoting a response, the occurrence of a reaction, or the existence of the entity or condition in question.
false p., a p. test result in a subject which does not possess the attribute for which the test is being conducted.

positive G. Gravity or acceleration in the usual head-to-foot direction in flying or in standing upright; the reverse of negative G.

positron (poz'i-tron). Positive electron; a subatomic particle of mass and charge equal to the electron but of opposite (*i.e.,* positive) charge.

posologic (pō-sō-loj'ik). Relating to posology.

posology (pō-sol'ō-jē) [G. *posos,* how much, + *logos,* study]. The branch of pharmacology and therapeutics concerned with a determination of the doses of remedies; the science of dosage.

post- [L. *post,* after]. Prefix, to words derived from L. roots, denoting after, behind, or posterior; corresponds to G. *meta-.*

post (pōst). In dentistry, a dowel or pin inserted into the root canal of a natural tooth as an attachment for an artificial crown.

postacetabular (pōst'as-ĕ-tab'yū-lăr). Posterior to the acetabular cavity.

postadolescence (pōst-ad-ō-les'ens). The period after adolescence or puberty.

postanal (pōst-ā'năl). Posterior to the anus.

postanesthetic (pōst'an-es-thet'ik). Occurring after anesthesia.

postapoplectic (pōst'ap-ō-plek'tik). Occurring after an attack of apoplexy.

postaxial (pōst-ak'sē-ăl). **1.** Posterior to the axis of the body or any limb, the latter being in the anatomical position. **2.** Denoting the portion of a limb bud which lies caudal to the axis of the limb.

postbrachial (pōst'brā'kē-ăl). On or in the posterior part of the upper arm.

postcardinal (pōst'kar'di-năl). Relating to the posterior cardinal veins.

postcava (pōst'kā'vă). *Vena* cava inferior.

postcaval (pōst'kā'văl). Relating to the inferior vena cava.

postcentral (pōst-sen'trăl). Referring to the cerebral convolution forming the posterior bank of the central sulcus: the postcentral gyrus.

postchroming (pōst'krōm'ing). Afterchroming.

postcibal (pōst-sī'bă) [L. *cibum,* food]. After a meal or the taking of food.

postclavicular (pōst'kla-vik'yū-lăr). Posterior to the clavicle.

postcoital (pōst-kō'i-tăl). After coitus.

postcoitus (pōst-kō'i-tŭs). The time immediately after coitus.

postcordial (pōst'kōr'jăl) [L. *cor* (*cord-*), heart]. Posterior to the heart.

postcostal (pōst-kos'tăl). Behind the ribs.

post'crown. A crown, replacing the natural crown, which is retained on the stump of the root of a tooth from which the pulp has been removed, by a post or pin integral with the crown and sealed in the treated root canal with a cement.

postcubital (pōst'kyū'bi-tăl). On or in the posterior or dorsal part of the forearm.

post'dam. Posterior palatal *seal.*

postdiastolic (pōst'dī-ă-stol'ik). Following the diastole of the heart.

postdicrotic (pōst-dī-krot'ik). Following the dicrotic wave in a sphygmogram; denoting an additional interruption in the descending line of the pulse tracing.

postdiphtheritic (pōst'dif-the-rit'ik). Following or occurring as a sequel of diphtheria.

postdormital (pōst-dōr'mi-tăl). Relating to the postdormitum.

postdormitum (pōst-dōr'mi-tŭm) [L. *dormire,* to sleep]. The period of increasing consciousness between sound sleep and waking.

postductal (pōst-dŭk'tăl). Relating to that part of tha aorta distal to the aortic opening of the ductus arteriosus.

postencephalitic (pōst-en-sef'ă-lit'ik). Following encephalitis.

postepileptic (pōst'ep-i-lep'tik). Following an epileptic seizure.

posterior (pos-tēr'ē-ōr) [L. comparative of *posterus,* following]. **1.** After, in relation to time or space. **2** [NA]. Dorsal (2); dorsalis; posticus; in human anatomy, denoting the back surface of the body. Often used to indicate the position of one structure relative to another, *i.e.,* nearer the back of the body. **3.** Near the tail or caudal end of certain embryos. **4.** An undesirable and confusing substitute for caudal in quadrupeds; in veterinary anatomy, p. is used only to denote some structures of the head.

posterius (pos-tēr'ē-ŭs) [L.]. Neuter of posterior.

postero- [L. *posterior*]. Combining form denoting posterior.

posteroanterior (pos'ter-ō-an-tēr'ē-ōr). A term denoting the direction of view or progression, from posterior to anterior, through a part.

posteroclusion (pos'ter-ō-klū'shŭn). Posterior *occlusion.*

posteroexternal (pos'ter-ō-ek-ster'năl). Posterolateral.

posterointernal (pos'ter-ō-in-ter'năl). Posteromedial.

posterolateral (pos'ter-ō-lat'ĕ-răl). Posteroexternal; behind and to one side, specifically to the outer side.

posteromedial (pos'ter-ō-mē'dē-ăl). Posterointernal; behind and to the inner side.

posteromedian (pos'ter-ō-mē'dē-an). Occupying a central position posteriorly.

posteroparietal (pos'ter-ō-pa-rī'ĕ-tăl). Relating to the posterior portion of the parietal lobe of the cerebrum.

posterosuperior (pos'ter-ō-sū-pē'rē-ōr). Situated behind and at the upper part.

posterotemporal (pos'ter-ō-tem'po-răl). Relating to or lying in the posterior portion of the temporal lobe of the cerebrum.

postesophageal (pōst'ē-sof'ă-jē'ăl, ē-sō-faj'ē-ăl). Behind the esophagus.

postestrus, postestrum (pōst-es'trŭs, -trŭm). The period in the estrus cycle following estrus; characterized by the growth of the corpus luteum and physiologic changes related to the production of progesterone. Sometimes called metestrus.

postfebrile (pōst-fē'brĭl). Metapyretic; occurring after a fever.

postganglionic (pōst'gang-glē-on'ik). Distal to or beyond a ganglion; referring to the unmyelinated nerve fibers originating from cells in an autonomic ganglion.

posthemiplegic (pōst'hem-i-plē'jik). Following hemiplegia.

posthemorrhagic (pōst-hem-ŏ-raj'ik). Following a hemorrhage.

posthepatic (pōst-he-pat'ik). Behind the liver.

posthetomy (pos-thet'ō-mē) [G. *posthē,* prepuce, + *tomē,* incision]. Circumcision (1).

posthioplasty (pos'thē-ō-plas-tē) [G. *posthion,* dim. form of *posthē,* prepuce, + *plastos,* formed]. Reparative or plastic surgery of the prepuce.

posthitis (pos-thī'tis) [G. *posthē,* prepuce, + *-itis,* inflammation]. Acroposthitis; inflammation of the prepuce.

postholith (pos'thō-lith) [G. *posthē,* prepuce, + *lithos,* stone]. Preputial *calculus.*

posthyoid (pōst-hī'oyd). Behind the hyoid bone.

posthypnotic (pōst-hip-not'ik). Following hypnotism; denoting an act suggested during hypnosis that is to be carried out at some time after the hypnotized subject is awakened.

postictal (pōst-ik'tăl). Following a seizure, *e.g.,* epileptic.

posticus (pos-tī'kŭs) [L. fr. *post,* after]. Posterior (2).

postinfluenzal (post'in-flū-en'zăl). Occurring as a sequel of influenza.

postischial (pōst-is'kē-ăl). Posterior to the ischium.

postmalarial (pōst-mă-lār'ē-ăl). Occurring as a sequel of malaria.

postmastoid (pōst'mas'toyd). Posterior to the mastoid process.

postmature (pōst-mă-tūr', mă-tyūr'). Remaining in the uterus longer than the normal gestational period; *i.e.,* longer than 42 weeks (288 days) in humans.

postmedian (pōst'mē'dē-an). Posterior to the median plane.

postmediastinal (pōst'mē'dē-as'ti-năl, -mē'dē-ă-stī'năl). **1.** Posterior to the mediastinum. **2.** Relating to the posterior mediastinum.

postmediastinum (pōst'mē'dē-ă-stī'nŭm). Posterior *mediastinum.*

postmenopausal (pōst-men-ō-paw'săl). Relating to the period following the menopause.

postminimus (pōst-min'i-mŭs). A small accessory appendage attached to the side of the fifth finger or toe; it may resemble a normal digit or be merely a fleshy mass.

postmortem (pōst-mōr'tem) [post- + L. acc. case of *mors* (*mort-*), death]. **1.** Pertaining to or occurring during the period after death. **2.** Colloquialism for autopsy (1).

postnarial (pōst'nā'rē-ăl). Relating to the posterior nares or choanae.

postnaris (pōst'nā'ris). Choana.

postnasal (pōst'nā'săl). **1.** Posterior to the nasal cavity. **2.** Relating to the posterior portion of the nasal cavity.

postnatal (pōst-nā'tăl) [L. *natus,* birth]. Occurring after birth.

postnecrotic (post-ne-krot'ik). Subsequent to the death of a tissue or part of the body.

postneuritic (pōst-nū-rit'ik). Following neuritis.

postocular (pōst'ok'yū-lăr) [L. *oculus,* eye]. Posterior to the eyeball.

postoperative (pōst-op'er-ă-tiv). Following an operation.

postoral (pos-tō'răl) [L. *os* (*or-*), mouth]. In the posterior part of, or posterior to, the mouth.

postorbital (pōst'ōr'bi-tăl). Posterior to the orbit.

postpalatine (pōst'pal'ă-tīn). Posterior to the palatine bones. Usually used to refer to the soft palate.

postparalytic (pōst'par-ă-lit'ik). Following or consequent upon paralysis.

postpartum (pōst-par'tŭm) [L. *partus,* birth (noun), fr. *pario,* pp. *partus,* to bring forth]. After childbirth. *Cf.* antepartem; intrapartem.

postpharyngeal (pōst'fă-rin'jē-ăl). Posterior to the pharynx.

postpneumonic (pōst-nū-mon'ik). Following or occurring as a sequel of pneumonia.

postprandial (pōst-pran'dē-ăl) [L. *prandium,* breakfast]. Following a meal.

postpuberal, postpubertal (pōst-pū'ber-ăl, -ber-tăl). Postpubescent.

postpuberty (pōst-pū'ber-tē). The period after puberty.

postpubescent (pōst-pū-bes'ent). Postpuberal; postpubertal; subsequent to the period of puberty.

postpyknotic (pōst-pik-not'ik). Following the stage of pyknosis in a red cell, denoting the disappearance of the nucleus (chromatolysis).

postrolandic (pos'trō-lan'dik). Behind the fissure of Rolando, or central sulcus. See postcentral.

postsacral (pōst'sā'krăl). Posterior or inferior to the sacrum; referring to the coccyx.

postscapular (pōst-skap'yū-lăr). Posterior to the scapula.

postscarlatinal (pōst'skar-lă-tē'năl). Occurring as a sequel of scarlatina.

postsphygmic (pōst-sfig'mik). [G. *sphygmos,* pulse]. Occurring after the pulse wave.

postsplenic (pōst'splen'ik). Posterior to the spleen.

postsynaptic (pōst-si-nap'tik). Pertaining to the area on the distal side of a synaptic cleft.

posttarsal (pōst'tar'săl). Relating to the posterior portion of the tarsus.

posttecta (pōst'tek'tă). Aboral to the hidden part of the duodenum.

posttibial (pōst'tib'ē-ăl). Posterior to the tibia; situated in the posterior portion of the leg.

posttransverse (pōst-tranz'vers). Behind a transverse process.

posttraumatic (pōst-traw-mat'ik). Temporally, and implied causally, related to a trauma.

posttrematic (pōst-trē-mat'ik) [post- + G. *trēma,* perforation]. Relating to the caudal surface of a branchial cleft.

posttussis (pōst-tŭs'is) [L. *tussis,* cough]. After coughing; referring usually to certain auscultatory sounds.

posttyphoid (pōst-tī'foyd). Occurring as a sequel of typhoid fever.

postulate (pos'tyū-lăt) [L. *postulo,* pp. *-atus,* to demand]. A proposition that is taken as self-evident or assumed without proof as a basis for reasoning. See also hypothesis; theory.
Ampère's p., Avogadro's *law.*
Avogadro's p., Avogadro's *law.*
Ehrlich's p., side-chain *theory.*
Koch's p.'s, Koch's law; to establish the specificity of a pathogenic microorganism, it must be present in all cases of the disease, inoculations of its pure cultures must produce disease in animals (when it is transmitted to such), and from these it must be again obtained and be propagated in pure cultures.

postural (pos'tyū-răl, pos'cher-ăl). Relating to or effected by posture.

posture (pos'chūr, pos'cher) [L. *positura,* fr. *pono,* pp. *positus,* to place]. Attitude; the position of the limbs or the carriage of the body as a whole.
Stern's p., a supine position with the head extended and lowered over the end of the table, by which the murmur is developed or made more distinct in cases of tricuspid insufficiency.

postuterine (pōst-yū'ter-in). Posterior to the uterus.

postvaccinal (pōst-vak'si-năl). After vaccination.

postvalvar, postvalvular (pōst-val'văr, -val'vyū-lăr). Relating to a position distal to the pulmonary or aortic valves.

potable (pō'tă-bl) [L. *potabilis,* fr. *poto,* to drink]. Drinkable; fit to drink.

Potain, Pierre C.E., French physician, 1825–1901. See P.'s *sign.*

potamophobia (pot'ă-mō-fō'bē-ă) [G. *potamos,* river, + *phobos,* fear]. Morbid fears aroused by the sight, and sometimes thought, of a river or any flow of water.

pot'ash [E. pot-ashes]. Pearl-ash; impure potassium carbonate.
caustic p., *potassium* hydroxide.
sulfurated p., liver of sulfur; a mixture composed chiefly of potassium polysulfides and potassium thiosulfate; used externally in scabies, acne, and psoriasis.

potassic (pō-tas'ik). Relating to or containing potassium.

potassiocupric (pō-tas'ē-ō-kyū'prik). Relating to or containing both potassium and copper.

potassiomercuric (pō-tas'ē-ō-mer-kyū'rik). Relating to or containing both potassium and mercury.

potassium (pō-tas'ē-ŭm) [Mod. L., fr. Eng. potash (fr. pot + ashes) + *-ium*]. Kalium; an alkaline metallic element, symbol K, atomic no. 19, atomic weight 39.100, occurring abundantly in nature but always in combination; its salts are used medicinally. For organic p. salts not listed below, see the name of the anion.
p. acetate, sal diureticum; $KC_2H_3O_2$; a diuretic, diaphoretic, and systemic and urinary alkalizer.
p. acid tartrate, p. bitartrate.
p. alum, *aluminum* potassium sulfate.
p. aminosalicylate, see *p*-aminosalicylic acid.
p. antimonyltartrate, *antimony* potassium tartrate.
p. atractylate, the p. salt of atractylic acid, the natural source of the latter.
p. bicarbonate, $KHCO_3$; used as a diuretic to decrease the acidity of the urine, and as an electrolyte replenisher.
p. bitartrate, p. acid tartrate; cream of tartar; $KHC_4H_4O_6$; a diuretic and laxative.
p. bromide, KBr; a sedative and hypnotic (sodium bromide is usually preferred).
p. chlorate, chlorate of potash, $KClO_3$, used as a mouthwash and gargle in stomatitis and follicular pharyngitis; it is incompatible in the dry state with all easily oxidizable substances.
p. chloride, used to correct p. deficiency.
p. citrate, Rivière's salt; $K_3C_6H_5O_7$; a deliquescent powder, soluble in water; used as a diuretic, diaphoretic, expectorant, and systemic and urinary alkalizer.
p. cyanide, KCN; a commercial fumigant.
dibasic p. phosphate, p. phosphate.
p. dichromate, p. bichromate, $K_2Cr_2O_7$; used externally as an astringent, antiseptic, and caustic.
effervescent p. citrate, a mixture of p. citrate, citric acid, sodium bicarbonate, and tartaric acid; used as a gastric antacid and urinary alkalizer.
p. ferrocyanide, yellow prussiate of potash; $K_4Fe(CN)_6 3H_2O$; used in the preparation of various cyanides and in medicine as an antidote to copper sulfate.
p. gluconate, gluconic acid p. salt; used in hypokalemia as a replenisher.
p. guai'acolsulfonate, $C_6H_3OHOCH_3SO_3K$; used as an expectorant.
p. hydroxide, caustic potash; KOH; a strong, penetrating caustic.
p. hypophosphite, KH_2PO_2; formerly believed to have a tonic effect upon the nervous system; may be explosive if triurated or heated with oxidizing agents.
p. iodate, KIO_3; an oxidizing agent and disinfectant.

p. iodide, KI; used as an alterative and expectorant, and in certain mycoses.
p. metaphosphate, $(KPO_3)_n$; a pharmaceutical aid (buffer).
monobasic p. phosphate, KH_2PO_4; used as a urinary acidifier and buffer.
p. nitrate, niter; saltpeter; KNO_3; sometimes used as a diuretic and diaphoretic; formerly it was included in asthmatic powders containing stramonium leaves.
penicillin G p., see under penicillin.
p. perchlorate, $KClO_4$; occasionally used, as an alternative to a thiouracil derivative, in the control of hyperthyroidism.
p. permanganate, $KMnO_4$; a strong oxidizing agent, used in solution as an antiseptic and deodorizing application for foul lesions, and as a gastric lavage in poisoning from morphine, strychnine, aconite, and picrotoxin; in electron microscopy, it stains cytomembranes well and gives results similar to head hydroxide staining; also used as a fixative (Luft's).
p. phosphate, dipotassium phosphate; dibasic p. phosphate; K_2HPO_4; a mild saline cathartic and diuretic.
p. rhodanate, p. thiocyanate.
p. sodium tartrate, sodium p. tartrate; Rochelle or Seignette's salt; $KNaC_4H_4O_6$; a mild saline cathartic, used as an ingredient in compound effervescent powders.
p. sorbate, 2,4-hexadienoic acid potassium salt; a mold and yeast inhibitor, used as a preservative.
p. succinate, a deliquescent powder used as a hemostatic.
p. sulfate, K_2SO_4; a laxative.
p. sulfocyanate, p. thiocyanate.
p. tartrate, soluble tartar; $K_2C_4H_4O_6 \cdot {}^1/_2H_2O$; a mild purgative and diuretic.
p. thiocyanate, p. sulfocyanate; p. rhodanate; used in the treatment of essential hypertension and as a reagent in the detection of copper, iron, and silver.

potassium-40 (^{40}K). A naturally occurring (0.0119 per cent) radioactive potassium isotope; beta emitter with half-life of 1.3 billion years; chief source of natural radioactivity of living tissue.

potassium-42 (^{42}K). An artificial potassium isotope; beta emitter with half-life of 12.47 hr, used as a tracer in studies of potassium distribution in body fluid compartments.

potassium-43 (^{43}K). An artificial potassium isotope; a beta emitter with a half-life of 22 hr, used as a tracer in myocardial perfusion studies.

potency (pō'ten-sē) [L. *potentia,* power]. **1.** Power, force, or strength; the condition or quality of being potent. **2.** Specifically, sexual p. **3.** In therapeutics, the pharmacological activity of a compound.
sexual p., the ability to carry out and consummate sexual intercourse, usually referring to the male.

potent (pō'tent). **1.** Possessing force, power, strength. **2.** Indicating the ability of a primitive cell to differentiate. See also totipotent; pluripotent. **3.** In psychiatry, possessing sexual potency.

potential (pō-ten'shăl) [L. *potentia,* power, potency]. **1.** Capable of doing or being, although not yet doing or being; possible, but not actual. **2.** A state of tension in an electric source enabling it to do work under suitable conditions; in relation to electricity, p. is analogous to the temperature in relation to heat.
action p., the change in membrane p. occurring in nerve, muscle, or other excitable tissue when excitation occurs.
after-p., see afterpotential.
bioelectric p., electrical p.'s occurring in living organisms.
biotic p., a theoretical measurement of the capacity of a species to survive or to compete successfully.
brain p., the electrical charge of the brain as compared to a point on the body; the p. may be steady (DC p.) or may fluctuate at specific frequencies when recorded against time, giving rise to the electroencephalogram.
demarcation p., injury p.; the difference in p. recorded when one electrode is placed on intact nerve fibers or muscle fibers and the other electrode is placed on the injured ends of the same fibers; the intact portion is positive with reference to the injured portion.
early receptor p. (ERP), a voltage arising across the eye from a charge displacement within photoreceptor pigment, in response to an intense flash of light.
evoked p., evoked *response.*
excitatory postsynaptic p. (EPSP), the change in p. which is produced in the membrane of the next neuron when an impulse which has an excitatory influence arrives at the synapse; it is a local change in the direction of depolarization; summation of these p.'s can lead to discharge of an impulse by the neuron.
extreme somatosensory evoked p. (ESEP), high voltage p. evoked by tapping the soles of the feet of young children, who, after a time, develop spontaneous motor adversive fits, less frequently generalized tonic-clonic seizures with focal or multifocal spikes in the the EEG. The seizures persist for about a year and disappear before 9 years of age; the EEG spiking also ceases 1-3 years after the seizures stop.
generator p., local depolarization of the membrane p. at the end of a sensory neurone in graded response to the strength of a stimulus applied to the associated receptor organ, *e.g.,* a pacinian corpuscle; if the generator p. becomes large enough (because the stimulus is at least of threshold strength), it causes excitation at the nearest node of Ranvier and a propagated action p.
inhibitory postsynaptic p. (IPSP), the change in p. produced in the membrane of the next neuron when an impulse which has an inhibitory influence arrives at the synapse; it is a local change in the direction of hyperpolarization; the frequency of discharge of a given neuron is determined by the extent to which impulses that lead to excitatory postsynaptic p.'s predominate over those that cause inhibitory postsynaptic p.'s.
injury p., demarcation p.
membrane p., transmembrane p.; the p. inside a cell membrane, measured relative to the fluid just outside; it is negative under resting conditions and becomes positive during an action p.
myogenic p., action p. of muscle.
oscillatory p., the variable voltage in the positive deflection of the electroretinogram (B-wave) of the dark-adapted eye arising from amacrine cells.
Ottoson p., electro-olfactogram.
oxidation-reduction p. (E_h), redox p.; the p. in volts of an inert metallic electrode measured in a system of an arbitrarily chosen ratio of [oxidant] to [reductant] and referred to the normal hydrogen electrode at absolute temperature; it is calculated from the following equation:

$$E_h = E_0 + \frac{RT}{nF} \ln \frac{[\text{oxidant}]}{[\text{reductant}]},$$

where R is the gas constant expressed in electrical units, T the absolute temperature (Kelvin), n the number of electrons transferred, F the faraday and E_0 the normal symbol for the p. of the system at pH 0.
S p., prolonged, slow, depolarizing or hyperpolarizing responses to illumination; initiated between the photoreceptor and ganglion cell layers of the retina.
redox p., oxidation-reduction p.
spike p., the main wave in the action p. of a nerve; it is followed by negative and positive afterpotentials.
thermodynamic p., see free *energy.*
transmembrane p., membrane p.
visual evoked p., voltage fluctuations that may be recorded from the occipital area of the scalp as the result of retinal stimulation by a light flashing at ${}^1/_4$-second intervals; commonly summated and

averaged by computer.
zeta p., the degree of negative charge on the surface of a red blood cell; *i.e.,* the p. difference between the negative charges on the red cell and the cation in the fluid portion of the blood.
zoonotic p., the p. for infections of subhuman animals to be transmissible to man.

potentiation (pō-ten′shē-ā′shŭn). Interaction between two or more drugs or agents resulting in a pharmacologic response greater than the sum of individual responses to each drug or agent.

potentiator (pō-ten′shē-ā-ter, -tōr). In chemotherapy, a drug used in combination with other drugs to produce deliberate potentiation.

potentiometer (pō-ten-shē-om′ĕ-ter) [L. *potentia,* power, + G. *metron,* measure]. **1.** An instrument used for measuring small differences in electrical potential. **2.** An electrical resistor of fixed total resistance between two terminals, but with a third terminal attached to a slider that can make contact at any desired point along the resistance.

potion (pō′shŭn) [L. *potio, potus,* fr. *poto,* to drink]. A draft or large dose of liquid medicine.

Pott, Sir Percivall, British surgeon, 1713–1788. See P.'s *abscess, aneurysm, curvature, disease, fracture, gangrene, paralysis, paraplegia,* puffy *tumor.*

Potter, Edith L., U.S. perinatal pathologist, *1901. See Potter's *disease, facies, syndrome.*

Potter, Irving White, U.S. obstetrician, 1868–1956. See P.'s *version.*

Potts, Willis J., U.S. pediatric surgeon, 1895–1968. See P.'s *anastomosis, clamp, operation.*

pouch (powch). A pocket or cul-de-sac.
antral p., a p. made in the antrum of the stomach of experimental animals.
branchial p.'s, pharyngeal p.'s.
Broca's p., pudendal *sac.*
celomic p.'s, lateral mesoderm-lined diverticula lying at either side of the notochord in the developing *Amphioxus.*
Denis Browne's p., superficial inguinal p.; a pocket formed in the tissues of the groin; a common lodging site for ectopic testes (as in cryptorchism).
Douglas' p., *excavatio* rectouterina.
endodermal p.'s, pharyngeal p.'s.
guttural p., a structure in the horse which is a diverticulum of the auditory (eustachian) tube; subject to chronic infections and inflammation and frequently necessitating surgery for relief.
Hartmann's p., pelvis of gallbladder; fossa provesicalis; a spheroid or conical p. at the junction of the neck of the gallbladder and the cystic duct.

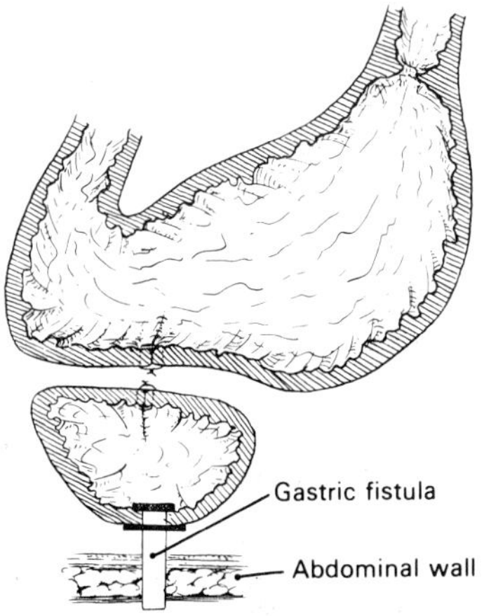

Cross Section of Heidenhain Pouch

Heidenhain p., a small sac or p. of the stomach, vagally denervated and closed off from the main cavity but with an opening through the abdominal wall, fashioned for the purpose of obtaining gastric juice and for studying gastric secretion in physiologic experiments.
hepatorenal p., *recessus* hepatorenalis.
hypophyseal p., pituitary *diverticulum.*
Kock p., a continent ileostomy with a reservoir and valved opening fashioned from doubled loops of ileum.
laryngeal p., *sacculus* laryngis.
Morison's p., *recessus* hepatorenalis.
paracystic p., the lateral portion of the uterovesical p.
pararectal p., the lateral portion of the rectouterine p.
paravesical p., the lateral portion of the uterovesical p.
Pavlov p., Pavlov or miniature stomach; a section of the stomach of a dog, retaining its vagal innervation but shut off from all communication with the main part of the organ and connected with the outside by a fistula; used in studies of gastric secretions.

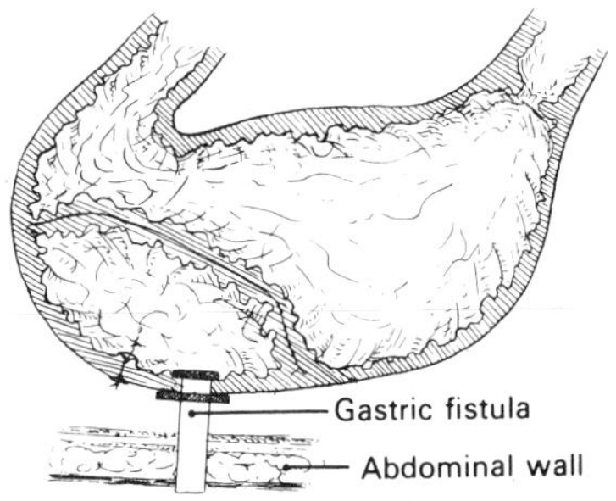

Cross Section of Pavlov Pouch

pharyngeal p.'s, branchial or endodermal p.'s; paired evaginations of embryonic pharyngeal endoderm, between the branchial arches, extending toward the corresponding ectodermally lined branchial grooves; during development they evolve into epithelial tissues and organs, such as thymus and thyroid glands.
Physick's p.'s, proctitis with mucous discharge and burning pain, involving especially the sacculations between the rectal valves.
Prussak's p., *recessus* membranae tympani superior.
Rathke's p., pituitary *diverticulum.*
rectouterine p., *excavatio* rectouterina.
rectovaginouterine p., *excavatio* rectouterina.
rectovesical p., *excavatio* rectovesicalis.
Seessel's p., Seessel's *pocket.*
superficial inguinal p., Denis Browne's p.
ultimobranchial p., a transient fifth pharyngeal p.; it is now considered to be incorporated into the caudal pharyngeal complex, the cells of which become the parafollicular cells of the thyroid.
uterovesical p., *excavatio* vesicouterina.
vesicouterine p., *excavatio* vesicouterina.
Willis' p., *omentum* minus.

poudrage (pū-drahzh′) [F.]. **1.** Powdering. **2.** Talc *operation.*
pericardial p., talc *operation.*
pleural p., covering the opposing pleural surfaces with a slightly irritating powder in order to secure adhesion.

poultice (pōl′tis) [L. *puls* (*pult-*), a thick pap; G. *poltos*]. Cataplasm; a soft magma or mush prepared by wetting various powders or other absorbent substances with oily or watery fluids, sometimes medicated, and usually applied hot to the surface; it exerts an emollient, relaxing, or stimulant, counterirritant effect upon the skin and underlying tissues.

pound (pownd) [A.S. *pund;* L. *pondus,* weight]. A unit of weight, containing 12 ounces, apothecaries' weight, or 16 ounces, avoirdupois.

poundal (pownd'ăl). The force required to give a mass of 1 lb. an acceleration of 1 ft./sec^2; equal to 1.13825 newtons.

Poupart, François, French anatomist, 1616– 1708. See P.'s *ligament, line.*

povidone (pō'vi-dōn). Polyvidone; polyvinylpyrrolidone; poly[1-(2-oxo-1-pyrrolidinyl)ethylene]; a synthetic polymer consisting mainly of linear 1-vinyl-2-pyrrolidone groups, with mean molecular weights ranging from 10,000 to 70,000; used as a dispersing and suspending agent; p. with molecular weight between 20,000 and 40,000 has been used as a plasma extender. It is not metabolized, but is excreted unchanged by the kidney.

po'vidone-i'odine. Polyvinylpyrrolidone-iodine complex; a topical anti-infective agent for the skin and mucous membranes; used for the prevention and control of infections susceptible to iodine.

pow'der [Fr. *poudre;* L. *pulvis*]. **1.** A dry mass of minute separate particles of any substance. **2.** In pharmaceutics, a homogenous dispersion of finely divided, relatively dry, particulate matter consisting of one or more substances; the degree of fineness of a p. is related to passage of the material through standard sieves. **3.** A single dose of a powdered drug, enclosed in an envelope of folded paper. **4.** To reduce a solid substance to a state of very fine division.
bleaching p., chlorinated *lime.*

pow'er. **1.** In optics, the refractive vergence of a lens. **2.** In physics and engineering, the rate at which work is done.
back vertex p., the effective p. of a lens as measured from a surface toward the eye; a standard for measurement of ophthalmic lenses.
equivalent p., the p. equal to an infinitely thin lens as measured on an optical bench.
resolving p., definition of a lens; in a microscope objective lens it is calculated by dividing the wavelength of the light used by twice the numerical aperture of the objective. See also definition.

pox (poks) [var. of pl. *pocks*]. **1.** An eruptive disease, usually qualified by a descriptive prefix; *e.g.,* smallpox, cowpox, chickenpox. See the specific term. **2.** An eruption, first papular then pustular, occurring in chronic antimony poisoning. **3.** Archaic or colloquial term for syphilis.
Kaffir p., alastrim.

Poxviridae (poks-vir'i-dē). A family of large complex viruses, with a marked affinity for skin tissue, that are pathogenic for man and other animals. Virions are 230 by 300 nm and enveloped (double membranes); some (avipoxviruses, orthopoxviruses) are ether-resistant, others ether-sensitive. Replication occurs entirely in the cytoplasm of infected cells. Capsids are of complex symmetry and contain double-stranded DNA (MW 160 $\times$ 10^6), the nucleoprotein antigen being common to all members of the family. Six genera are recognized: *Orthopoxvirus, Avipoxvirus, Capripoxvirus, Leporipoxvirus, Parapoxvirus,* and *Entomopoxvirus.*

poxvirus (poks'vī-rŭs). Any virus of the family Poxviridae.
p. officina'lis, vaccinia *virus.*

Pozzi, Samuel J., French gynecologist and anatomist, 1846–1918. See P.'s *muscle.*

PP Abbreviation for pyrophosphate.

PP$_i$ Abbreviation for inorganic pyrophosphate.

P.p. Abbreviation for *punctum proximum.*

PPCA Abbreviation for proserum prothrombin conversion *accelerator.*

PPCF Abbreviation for plasmin prothrombin conversion *factor.*

PPD Abbreviation for purified protein derivative of *tuberculin.*

PPLO Abbreviation for pleuropneumonia-like *organisms.*

ppm Abbreviation for parts per million.

PPO Abbreviation for 2,5-diphenyloxazole.

PPPPPP [*p*ain, *p*allor, *p*araesthesia, *p*ulselessness, *p*aralysis, *p*rostration]. A mnemonic of 6 P's designating the symptom complex of acute arterial occlusion.

PPRibp, PPRP Abbreviations for 5-phospho-α-D-ribosyl pyrophosphate.

P-pulmonale (pul-mō-nā'lē). An electrocardiographic syndrome of tall, narrow, peaked P waves in leads II, III, and aVF, and a prominent initial positive P wave component in V_1 and V_2, presumed to be characteristic of cor pulmonale. (Although this term is extensively used in the electrocardiographic literature, it is actually a misnomer and would be more appropriately called P-dextrocardiale, since it results from overload of the right atrium regardless of the cause, as in tricuspid stenosis, and may occur independently of cor pulmonale.)

PQ-9 Abbreviation for plastoquinone-9.

Pr **1.** Abbreviation for presbyopia. **2.** Symbol for praseodymium.

P.r. Abbreviation for *punctum remotum.*

PRA Abbreviation for plasma renin *activity.*

practice (prak'tis) [Mediev. L. *practica,* business, G. *praktikos,* pertaining to action]. The exercise of the profession of medicine or one of the allied health professions.
extramural p., delivery of health care services by university faculties or full-time hospital staff to persons beyond the confines of their respective medical centers.
group p., the p. of medicine by a group of physicians, each of whom as a rule specializes in some particular field; such a group often shares a common suite of consulting rooms, laboratories, staff, equipment, etc.
intramural p., delivery of health care services by university faculties or full-time hospital staff conducted within the confines of their respective medical centers.

practitioner (prak-tish'ŭn-er). A person who practices medicine or one of the allied health care professions.

practolol (prak'tō-lol). 4'-[2-Hydroxy-3- (isopropylamino)propoxy]acetanilide; a β-receptor blocking drug for treatment of cardiac arrhythmias.

Prader, A. See P.-Willi *syndrome.*

prae-. For words beginning thus, see pre-.

pragmatagnosia (prag'mat-ag-nō'sē-ă) [G. *pragma* (*pragmat-*), thing done, a deed, fr. *prassō,* to do, + *agnōsia,* ignorance]. Rarely used term for loss of the power of recognizing objects.

pragmatamnesia (prag'mat-am-nē'zē-ă) [G. *pragma,* a thing done, + *amnēsia,* forgetfulness]. Rarely used term for loss of the memory of the appearance of objects.

pragmatics (prag-mat'iks) [G. *pragmatikos,* fr. *pragma,* thing done]. A branch of semiotics; the theory that deals with the relation between signs and their users, both senders and receivers.

pragmatism (prag'mă-tizm) [G. *pragma* (*pragmat-*), thing done]. A philosophy emphasizing practical applications and consequences of beliefs and theories, that the meaning of anything derives from its usefulness.

pralidoxime chloride (pral-i-dok'sēm, prā-li-). 2-Formyl-1-methylpyridinium chloride oxime; used to restore the depressed cholinesterase activity resulting from organophosphate poisoning; has some limited value as an antagonist of the carbamate type of cholinesterase inhibitors that are used in the treatment of myasthenia gravis. Dizziness, blurred vision, drowsiness, nausea, tachycardia, and muscular weakness may occur.

pramoxine hydrochloride (pră-mok'sēn, -sin). 4-[3-(*p*-Butoxyphenoxy)propyl]morpholine hydrochloride; a surface anesthetic agent for dermal and rectal use.

prandial (pran'dē-ăl) [L. *prandium,* breakfast]. Relating to a meal.

praseodymium (prā-sē-ō-dim'ē-ŭm) [G. *prasios,* leekgreen, fr. *pra-*

son, a leek, + *didymos,* twin]. An element of the lanthanide or "rare earth" group; symbol Pr, atomic no. 59, atomic weight 140.91.

Pratt, Joseph H., U.S. physician, 1872–1956. See P.'s *method, symptom.*

Prausnitz, Otto Carl, German hygienist, 1876–1963. See P.-Küstner *antibody, reaction;* reversed P.-Küstner *reaction.*

praxiology (prak-sē-ol'ō-jē) [G. *praxis,* action, + *logos,* study]. The science or study of conduct.

praxis (prak'sis) [G. *praxis,* action]. The performance of an action.

prazepam (prā'zē-pam). 7-Chloro-1-(cyclopropylmethyl)-1,3-dihydro-5-phenyl-2*H*-1,4-benzodiazepin-2-one; an antianxiety agent.

praziquantel (prā-zi-kwahn'tel). $C_{19}H_{24}N_2O_2$; a pyrazinoisoquinoline derivative; a synthetic heterocyclic broad spectrum anthelmintic agent effective against all schistosome species of man as well as most other trematodes and adult cestodes.

prazosin hydrochloride (prā'zō-sin). 1-(4-Amino-6,7-dimethoxy-2-quinazolinyl)-4-(2-furoyl)piperazine monohydrochloride; an antihypertensive agent.

pre- [L. *prae,* before]. Prefix, to words formed from L. roots, denoting anterior or before in space or time. See also ante-, pro-(1).

preagonal (prē-ag'ō-năl) [pre- + G. *agōn,* struggle (agony)]. Immediately preceding death.

prealbumin (prē-al-byū'min). A protein component of plasma having a molecular weight of about 55,000 and containing 1.3% carbohydrate; estimated plasma concentration is 0.3 g/100 ml.

thyroxine-binding p., thyroxine-binding protein (2); a protein located in the "prealbumin" zone upon electrophoretic analysis of plasma proteins; its affinity for binding thyroxine is less than that of thyroxine-binding globulin but greater than that of albumin.

preanal (prē-ā'năl). Anterior to the anus.

preanesthetic (prē-an-es-thet'ik). Before anesthesia.

preantiseptic (prē'an-ti-sep'tik). Denoting the period, especially in relation to surgery, before the adoption of the principles of antisepsis.

preaortic (prē'ā-ōr'tik). Anterior to the aorta; denoting certain lymph nodes so situated.

preaseptic (prē-ā-sep'tik). Denoting the period, especially the early antiseptic period in relation to surgery, before the principles of asepsis were known or adopted.

preataxic (prē-ă-tak'sik). Denoting the early stages of tabes dorsalis prior to the appearance of ataxia.

preauricular (prē-aw-rik'yū-lăr). Anterior to the auricle of the ear; denoting lymphatic nodes so situated.

preaxial (prē-ak'sē-ăl). **1.** Anterior to the axis of the body or a limb, the latter being in the anatomical position. **2.** Denoting the portion of a limb bud which lies cranial to the axis of the limb.

precancer (prē-kan'ser). A lesion from which a malignant neoplasm is believed to develop in a significant number of instances, and which may or may not be recognizable clinically or by microscopic changes in the affected tissue.

precancerous (prē-kan'ser-ŭs). Premalignant; pertaining to any lesion that is interpreted as precancer.

precapillary (prē-kap'i-lār-ē). Preceding a capillary; an arteriole or venule.

precardiac (prē-kar'dē-ak). Anterior to the heart.

precardinal (prē-kar'di-năl). Relating to the anterior cardinal veins.

precartilage (prē-kar'ti-lij). A closely packed aggregation of mesenchymal cells just prior to their differentiation into embryonic cartilage.

precava (prē-kā'vă). *Vena* cava superior.

precentral (prē-sen'trăl). Referring to the cerebral convolution immediately anterior to the central sulcus: precentral gyrus.

prechordal (prē-kōr'dăl). Prochordal.

prechroming (prē-krōm'ing). Treatment of a tissue or fabric first with a metal mordant, followed by a dye.

precipitable (prē-sip'i-tă-bl). Capable of being precipitated.

precipitant (prē-sip'i-tant). Anything causing a precipitation from a solution.

precipitate (prē-sip'i-tāt) [L. *praecipito,* pp. *-atus,* to cast headlong]. **1.** To cause a substance in solution to separate as a solid. **2.** A solid separated out from a solution or suspension; a floc or clump, such as that resulting from the mixture of a specific antigen and its antibody. **3.** Accumulation of inflammatory cells on the corneal endothelium in uveitis (keratic precipitates).

keratic p.'s, punctate keratitis; keratitis punctata; inflammatory cells on the corneal endothelium.

mutton-fat keratic p.'s, coalescent p.'s forming small plaques that gradually become more translucent.

pigmented keratic p.'s, p.'s that occur in eyes with brown irides or after prolonged inflammation.

red p., mercuric oxide, red.

sweet p., calomel.

white mercuric p., ammoniated *mercury.*

yellow p., mercuric oxide, yellow.

precipitation (prē-sip-i-tā'shŭn) [see precipitate]. **1.** The process of formation of a solid previously held in solution or suspension in a liquid. **2.** The phenomenon of clumping of proteins in serum produced by the addition of a specific precipitin.

double antibody p., double antibody method or immunoassay; a method of separating antibody-bound antigen (*e.g.,* insulin) from free antigen by precipitating the former with antibody specific for immunoglobulin.

immune p., immunoprecipitation.

precipitin (prē-sip'i-tin). Precipitating antibody; an antibody that under suitable conditions combines with and causes its specific and soluble antigen to precipitate from solution.

precipitinogen (prē-sip-i-tin'ō-jen) [precipitin + G. *-gen,* producing]. Precipitogen. **1.** An antigen that stimulates the formation of specific precipitin when injected into an animal body. **2.** A precipitable soluble antigen.

precipitinogenoid (prē-sip-i-tin'ō-jĕ-noyd). A precipitinogen that is altered by means of heating, thereby resulting in a substance that combines with the specific precipitin, but does not lead to the formation of a precipitate.

precipitogen (prē-sip'i-tō-jen). Precipitinogen.

precipitoid (prē-sip'i-toyd) [precipitin + G. *eidos,* resemblance]. A heat-treated precipitin that when mixed with specific precipitinogen does not cause a precipitate and also interferes with the precipitating effect of additional nonheated precipitin.

precipitophore (prē-sip'i-tō-fōr) [precipitin + G. *phoros,* bearing]. In Ehrlich's side chain theory, the portion of a precipitin molecule that is required in the formation of a precipitate, as distinguished from the haptophore group.

preclinical (prē-klin'i-kăl). **1.** Before the onset of disease. **2.** A period in medical education before the student becomes involved with patients and clinical work.

precocious (prē-kō'shŭs) [L. *praecox,* premature]. Developing unusually early or rapidly.

precocity (prē-kos'i-tē) [see precocious]. Unusually early or rapid development of mental or physical traits.

precognition (prē-kog-nish'ŭn) [L. *praecogito,* to ponder before]. Advance knowledge, by means other than the normal senses, of a future event; a form of extrasensory perception.

preconscious (prē-kon'shŭs). In psychoanalysis, one of the three divisions of the psyche according to Freud's topographical psychology, the other two being the conscious and unconscious; includes all ideas, thoughts, past experiences, and other memory impressions that with effort can be consciously recalled. *Cf.* foreconscious.

preconvulsive (prē-kon-vŭl'siv). Denoting the stage in an epileptic paroxysm preceding convulsions.

precordia (prē-kōr'dē-ă) [L. *praecordia* (ntr. pl. only), the diaphragm, the entrails, fr. *prae,* before, + *cor* (*cord-*), heart]. Antecardium; the epigastrium and anterior surface of the lower part of the thorax.

precordial (prē-kōr'dē-ăl). Relating to the precordia.

precordialgia (prē'kōr-dē-al'jē-ă) [precordia + G. *algos,* pain]. Pain in the precordial region.

precordium (prē-kōr'dē-ŭm). Singular of precordia.

precostal (prē-kos'tăl) [pre- + L. *costa,* rib]. Anterior to the ribs.

precritical (prē-krit'i-kăl). Relating to the phase before a crisis.

precuneal (prē-kū'nē-ăl). Anterior to the cuneus.

precuneate (prē-kū'nē-āt). Relating to the precuneus.

precuneus (prē-kū'nē-ŭs) [pre- + L. *cuneus,* a wedge]]NA]. Quadrate lobe (3); quadrate lobule (2); lobulus quadratus (2); quader; a division of the medial surface of each cerebral hemisphere between the cuneus and the paracentral lobule; it lies above the subparietal sulcus and is bounded anteriorly by the pars marginalis of the sulcus cinguli and posteriorly by the parietooccipital sulcus.

precursor (prē-ker'ser) [L. *praecursor,* fr. *prae-,* pre- + *curro,* to run]. That which precedes another or from which another is derived, applied especially to a physiologically inactive substance that is converted to an active enzyme, vitamin, hormone, etc., or to a chemical substance that is built into a larger structure in the course of synthesizing the latter.

predecidual (prē-dē-sid'yū-ăl). Relating to the premenstrual or secretory phase of the menstrual cycle.

predentin (prē-den'tin). The organic fibrillar matrix of the dentin before its calcification.

prediabetes (prē'dī-ă-bē'tēz). A state of potential diabetes mellitus, with normal glucose tolerance but with an increased risk of developing diabetes.

prediastole (prē-dī-as'tō-lē). Late systole; the interval in the cardiac rhythm immediately preceding the diastole.

prediastolic (prē-dī-ă-stol'ik). Late systolic; relating to the interval preceding the cardiac diastole.

predicrotic (prē-dī-krot'ik). Preceding the dicrotic notch.

predigestion (prē-dī-jes'chŭn). The artificial initiation of digestion of proteins (proteolysis) and starches (amylolysis) before they are eaten.

predispose (prē'dis-pōz). To render susceptible.

predisposition (prē'dis-pō-zish'ŭn). A condition of special susceptibility to a disease.

prednisolone (pred-nis'ō-lōn). Metacortandrolone; Δ^1-dehydrocortisol; Δ^1-hydrocortisone; hydroretrocortine; 11β,17,21-trihydroxy-1,4-pregnadiene-3,20-dione; a dehydrogenated analogue of cortisol with the same actions and uses as cortisol.
p. acetate, prednisolone 21-acetate; same uses as p.; suitable for intramuscular administration.
p. butylacetate, p. tebutate.
p. sodium phosphate, prednisolone 21-(disodium phosphate); more soluble than p. and the other p. esters and useful when a rapid onset or a short duration of action is desired; suitable for intrasynovial, parenteral, and topical administration.
p. succinate, p. compound suitable for intramuscular, intravenous, or rectal administration.
p. tebutate, p. butylacetate; same actions and uses as p. but with longer duration of action and suitable for intrasynovial and soft tissue injection.

prednisone (pred'ni-sōn). Metacortandracin; deltacortisone; Δ^1-cortisone; retrocortine; 17α,21-dihydroxy-1,4-pregnadiene-3,11,20-trione; a dehydrogenated analogue of cortisone with the same actions and uses.

prednylidene (prĕd-nil'i-dēn). 16-Methyleneprednisolone; 11β,17,21-trihydroxy-16-methylenepregna-1,4-diene-3,20-dione; a glucocorticoid.

predormital (prē-dōr'mi-tăl). Pertaining to the predormitum.

predormitum (prē-dōr'mi-tŭm). [pre- + L. *dormire,* to sleep]. The stage of semi-unconsciousness preceding actual sleep.

preductal (prē-dŭk'tăl). Relating to that part of the aorta proximal to the aortic opening of the ductus arteriosus.

preeclampsia (prē-ē-klamp'sē-ă) [pre- + G. *eklampsis,* a shining forth (eclampsia)]. Development of hypertension with proteinuria or edema, or both, due to pregnancy or the influence of a recent pregnancy; it occurs after the 20th week of gestation, but may develop before this time in the presence of trophoblastic disease; it is predominantly a disorder of primigravidas.
superimposed p., superimposed eclampsia; the development of p. or eclampsia in a patient with chronic hypertensive vascular or renal disease; when the hypertension antedates the pregnancy as established by previous blood pressure recordings, a rise in the systolic pressure of 30 mm Hg or a rise in the diastolic pressure of 15 mm Hg and the development of proteinuria or edema, or both, are required during pregnancy to establish the diagnosis.

preepiglottic (prē'ep-i-glot'ik). Anterior to the epiglottis.

preeruptive (prē-e-rŭp'tiv). Denoting the stage of an exanthematous disease preceding the eruption.

preexcitation (prē'ek-sī-tā'shŭn). Premature activation of part of the ventricular myocardium by an impulse that travels by an anomalous path and so avoids physiological delay in the atrioventricular junction; an intrinsic part of the Wolff-Parkinson-White syndrome.

preformation (prē-fōr-mā'shŭn). See preformation *theory.*

prefrontal (prē-fron'tăl). **1.** Denoting the anterior portion of the frontal lobe of the cerebrum. **2.** Denoting the granular frontal cortex rostral to the premotor area.

preganglionic (prē'gang-glē-on'ik). Situated proximal to or preceding a ganglion; referring specifically to the preganglionic motor neurons of the autonomic nervous system (located in the spinal cord and brainstem) and the preganglionic, myelinated nerve fibers by which they are connected to the autonomic ganglia.

pregnancy (preg'nan-sē) [L. *praegnans* (*praegnant-*), pregnant, fr. *prae,* before, + *gnascor,* pp. *natus,* to be born]. Gestation; fetation; cyesis, graviditas; gravidism; the condition of a female after conception until the birth of the baby.
abdominal p., intraperitoneal p.; abdominocyesis (1); the implantation and development of the ovum in the peritoneal cavity, usually secondary to an early rupture of a tubal p.; very rarely, primary implantation may occur in the peritoneal cavity.
aborted ectopic p., tubal *abortion.*
ampullar p., tubal p. situated near the midportion of the oviduct.
bigeminal p., twin p.
cervical p., the implantation and development of the impregnated ovum in the cervical canal.
combined p., coexisting uterine and ectopic p.
compound p., development of a uterine p. in addition to a previously existing ectopic pregnancy (usually a lithopedion).
cornual p., the implantation and development of the impregnated ovum in one of the cornua of the uterus.

ectopic p., extrauterine p.; eccyesis; metacyesis; paracyesis; the development of an impregnated ovum outside the cavity of the uterus.

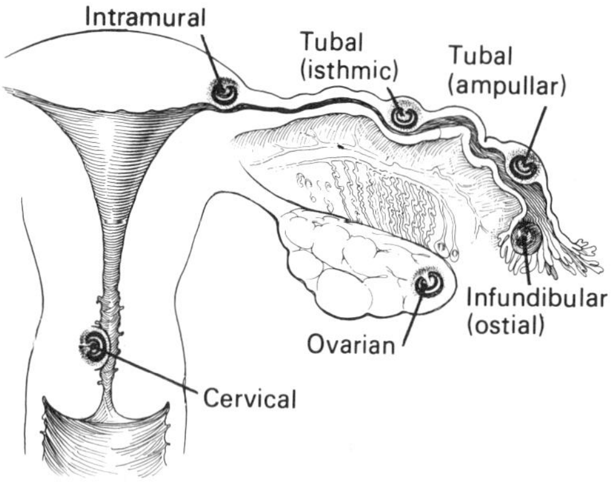

Sites of Ectopic Pregnancy

extraamniotic p., graviditas examnialis; a p. in which the chorion is intact, but the amnion has ruptured and shrunk.
extrachorial p., graviditas exochorialis; p. in which the membranes rupture and shrink, causing the fetus to develop outside the chorionic sac but within the uterus.
extramembranous p., a p. in which during the course of gestation the fetus has broken through its envelopes, coming directly in contact with the uterine walls.
extrauterine p., ectopic p.
fallopian p., tubal p.
false p., pseudocyesis; pseudopregnancy; phantom or spurious p.; a condition in which some signs and symptoms suggest pregnancy, although the woman is not pregnant.
heterotopic p., a p. not in the uterine cavity.
hydatid p., the presence of a hydiform mole in the pregnant uterus.
interstitial p., intramural p.
intraligamentary p., p. within the broad ligament.
intramural p., interstitial or tubouterine p.; development of the fertilized ovum in the uterine portion of the fallopian tube.
intraperitoneal p., abdominal p.
mesometric p., ectopic p. beginning as a tubal p., the amnotic sac being eventually formed by the mesometrium.
molar p., p. marked by a neoplasm within the uterus, whereby part or all of the chorionic villi are converted into a mass of clear vesicles.
multiple p., plural p.; condition of bearing two or more fetuses simultaneously.
mural p., p. in uterine muscular wall.
ovarian p., ovariocyesis; oocyesis; development of an impregnated ovum in an ovarian follicle. See also Spiegelberg's *criteria.*
ovarioabdominal p., ovarian p. which, as the result of the embryo's growth, becomes abdominal.
phantom p., false *pregnancy.*
plural p., multiple p.
secondary abdominal p., abdominocyesis (2); a condition in which the embryo or fetus continues to grow in the abdominal cavity after its expulsion from the fallopian tube or other seat of its primary development.
spurious p., false *pregnancy.*
tubal p., fallopian p.; salpingocyesis; development of an impregnated ovum in the fallopian tube.
tuboabdominal p., development of an ectopic p. partly in the fallopian tube and partly in the abdominal cavity.
tubo-ovarian p., development of the ovum at the fimbriated extremity of the fallopian and involving the ovary.
tubouterine p., intramural p.
twin p., bigeminal p.; a p. that may result from the fertilization of two separate ova or of a single ovum. See also twin.
uterine p., development of fetus within the uterus.
uteroabdominal p., development of the ovum primarily in the uterus and later, in consequence of the rupture of the uterus, in the abdominal cavity.

pregnane (preg'nān). Parent hydrocarbon of two series of steroids stemming from 5α-pregnane (originally allopregnane) and 5β-pregnane (17β-ethyletiocholane). 5β-Pregnane is the parent of the progesterones, pregnane alcohols, ketones, and several adrenocortical hormones, and is found largely in urine as a metabolic product of 5β-pregnane compounds. For structure, see steroids.

pregnanediol (preg-nān-dī'ol). 5β-Pregnane-3α,20α-diol; a steroid metabolite of progesterone that is biologically inactive and occurs as p. glucuronate in the urine.

pregnanedione (preg-nān-dī'ōn). 5β-Pregnane-3,20-dione; a metabolite of progesterone, formed in relatively small quantities, that occurs in 5α and 5β isomeric forms.

pregnanetriol (preg-nān-trī'ol). 5β-Pregnane-3α,17α,20α-triol; a urinary metabolite of 17-hydroxyprogesterone and a precursor in the biosynthesis of cortisol; its excretion is enhanced in certain diseases of the adrenal cortex and following administration of corticotropin.

preg'nant [see pregnancy]. Gravid; denoting a gestating female.

pregnene (preg'nēn). An unsaturated steroid of primarily terminological importance; utilized in systematic nomenclature of appropriate 21-carbon steroids.

pregneninolone (preg-nēn-in'ō-lōn, preg-nēn'in-). Ethisterone.

pregnenolone (preg-nēn'ō-lōn). 3β-Hydroxy-5-pregnen-20-one; a steroid that serves as an intermediate in the biosynthesis of numerous hormones.
p. succinate, a corticosteroid used for the treatment of rheumatoid arthritis.

prehallux (prē-hal'ŭks) [pre- + Mod. L. *hallux,* great toe]. A supernumerary digit, usually only partial, attached to the medial border of the great toe.

prehelicine (prē-hel'i-sēn). In front of the helix of the pinna.

prehemataminic acid (prē'hēm-ă-tin'ik). Neuraminic acid.

prehemiplegic (prē'hem-i-plē'jik). Preceding the occurrence of hemiplegia.

prehensile (prē-hen'sil) [L. *prehendo,* pp. *-hensus,* to lay hold of, seize]. Adapted for taking hold of or grasping.

prehension (prē-hen'shŭn). The act of grasping, or taking hold of.

prehormone (prē-hōr'mōn). A glandular secretory product, having little or no inherent biological potency, that is converted peripherally to an active hormone. *Cf.* prohormone (1).

prehyoid (prē-hī'oyd). Anterior or superior to the hyoid bone; denoting certain accessory thyroid glands lying superior to the mylohyoid muscle.

preictal (prē-ik'tăl) [pre- + L. *ictus,* a stroke]. Occurring before a convulsion or stroke.

preinduction (prē-in-dŭk'shŭn) [L. *prae,* before, + *inductio,* a bringing in, fr. *induco,* to lead in]. A modification in the third generation resulting from the action of environment on the germ cells of one or both individuals of the grandparental generation.

Preisz, Hugo von, Hungarian bacteriologist, 1860–1940. See P.-Nocard *bacillus.*

prelacrimal (prē-lak'ri-măl). Anterior to the lacrimal sac.

prelaryngeal (prē-lă-rin'jē-ăl). Anterior to the larynx; denoting especially one or two small lymphatic nodes.

preleptotene (prē-lep′tō-tēn) [pre- + leptotene, fr. G. *leptos,* slender, + *tainia,* band]. The earliest stage of prophase in meiosis, characterized by physiochemical changes in cytoplasm and karyoplasm and beginning contraction of chromosomes.

prelimbic (prē-lim′bik). Anterior to the limbus of the fossa ovalis.

preload (prē′lōd). The load to which a muscle is subjected before shortening.

ventricular p., formerly, the end-diastolic pressure stretching the ventricular walls, which determines the end-diastolic fiber length at the onset of ventricular contraction, or some other measure of this load on the muscle fibers before contraction; now, more rigorously expressed in terms of the wall stress at this moment, *i.e.,* the passive tension per unit cross-sectional area in the ventricular muscle fibers (calculated by Laplaces law from internal radius and wall thickness) that balances this transmural pressure at the moment before contraction begins.

premalignant (prē-mă-lig′nănt). Precancerous.

premaniacal (prē-mă-nī′ă-kăl). Preceding a manic attack.

premature (prē-mă-tūr′, -chūr) [L. *praematurus,* too early, fr. *prae-,* pre- + *maturus,* ripe (mature)]. **1.** Occurring before the usual or expected time. **2.** Denoting an infant born after less than 37 weeks of gestation; birth weight is no longer considered a critical criterion for use of this designation.

prematurity (prē-mă-tūr′i-tē, -chūr′i-tē). **1.** The state of being premature. **2.** In dentistry, deflective occlusal *contact.*

premaxilla (prē-mak-sil′ă) [pre- + L. *maxilla,* jawbone]. **1.** *Os* incisivum. **2.** The central isolated bony part in a complete bilateral cleft of the lip.

premaxillary (pre-mak′si-lār-ē). **1.** Anterior to the maxilla. **2.** Denoting the premaxilla.

premedication (prē′med-i-kā′shŭn). **1.** Administration of drugs prior to anesthesia to allay apprehension, produce sedation, and facilitate the administration of anesthesia. **2.** Drugs used for such purposes.

premelanosome (prē-mel′ă-nō-sōm). A nonpigmented membrane-bound vessicle in a melanocyte which contains tyrosine and matures into the melanin-filled melanosome; prominent in melanocytes of albinos.

premenstrual (prē-men′strū-ăl). Relating to the period preceding menstruation.

premenstruum (prē-men′strū-ŭm) [pre- + L. *menstruum,* ntr. of *menstruus,* monthly, pertaining to menstruation]. The period preceding menstruation.

premolar (prē-mō′lăr). **1.** Anterior to a molar tooth. **2.** A bicuspid tooth.

premonocyte (prē-mon′ō-sīt). Promonocyte; an immature monocyte not normally seen in the circulating blood.

premorbid (prē-mōr′bid) [pre- + L. *morbidus,* ill, fr. *morbus,* disease]. Preceding the occurrence of disease.

premunition (pre-mū-nish′ŭn) [Fr. fr. L. *praemunio,* pp. *-munitus,* to fortify beforehand]. Infection *immunity.*

premunitive (prē-mū′ni-tiv). Relating to premunition.

premyeloblast (prē-mī′ĕ-lō-blast). The earliest recognizable precursor of the myeloblast.

premyelocyte (prē-mī′ĕ-lō-sīt). Myeloblast.

prenaris, pl. **prenares** (prē-nā′ris, nā′rēz). Naris.

prenatal (prē-nā′tăl) [pre- + L. *natus,* born]. Antenatal; preceding birth.

preneoplastic (prē′nē-ō-plas′tik) [pre- + G. *neos,* new, + *plastikos,* formative]. Preceding the formation of any neoplasm, benign or malignant; a p. condition is not always precancerous, although the term is frequently used erroneously in that sense.

Prentice, Charles F., U.S. optician, 1854–1946. See P.'s *rule.*

prenyl (pren′il). 3-Methyl-2-buten-1-yl; $(CH_3)_2C{=}CH{-}CH_2{-}$; poly- or multiprenyl residues or derivatives thereof, apparently formed by end-to-end polymerization of isoprene molecules; found in the isoprenoids in nature.

prenylamine (pre-nil′ă-mēn). *N*-(3,3-Diphenylpropyl)-α-methylphenethylamine; an antianginal agent.

preoperative (prē-op′er-ă-tiv). Preceding an operation.

preoptic (prē-op′tik). Referring to the preoptic *region.*

preoral (prē-ō′răl) [pre- + L. *os* (*or-*), mouth]. In front of the mouth.

preosteoblast (prē-os′tē-ō-blast). Osteoprogenitor *cell.*

preoxygenation (prē′ok-sĕ-jĕ-nā′shŭn). Denitrogenation with 100% oxygen prior to induction of general anesthesia.

prepalatal (prē-pal′ă-tăl). Relating to the anterior part of the palate, or anterior to the palate bone.

preparalytic (prē-par-ă-lit′ik). Before the appearance of paralysis.

preparation (prep-ă-rā′shŭn) [L. *praeparatio,* fr. *prae,* before, + *paro,* pp. *-atus,* to get ready]. **1.** A getting ready. **2.** Something made ready, as a medicinal or other mixture, or a histologic specimen.

cavity p., **(1)** removal of dental caries and surgical p. of the remaining tooth structure to receive a dental restoration; **(2)** the final form of an excavation in a tooth resulting from such p.

corrosion p., a p. in which the hollow parts such as ducts, vessels, or alveoli of the lung are filled with a substance that hardens and persists after dissolving the tissues by digestion.

cytologic filter p., a cytologic specimen made by depositing a watery sample (obtained by a variety of methods from many body sites) upon a filter having pores of uniform size smaller than the cellular material to be concentrated; this is followed by fixation and staining, usually with 95% ethyl alcohol and Papanicolaou stain.

heart-lung p., an animal p. in which blood (rendered incoagulable) circulates through the heart and lungs and through an artificial system of vessels representing the systemic circulation; the latter is connected with the divided aorta on the one hand and with the superior vena cava on the other; used in physiologic studies of the heart and circulation.

prepatellar (prē-pă-tel′ăr). Anterior to the patella.

preperitoneal (prē′per-i-tō-nē′ăl). Denoting a fatty layer between the peritoneum and the transversalis fascia in the lower anterior abdominal wall.

prephenic acid (prē-fē′nik, -fen′ik). 1-Carboxy-4-hydroxy-2,5-cyclohexadiene-1-pyruvic acid; an intermediate in the microbial conversion of shikimic acid to phenylalanine and tyrosine.

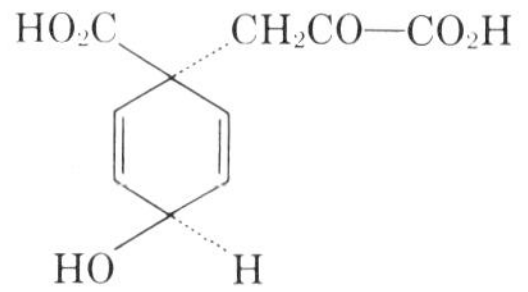

Prephenic acid

preplacental (prē-pla-sen′tăl). Before formation of a placenta.

prepotential (prē-pō-ten′shăl). A gradual rise in potential between action potentials as a phasic swing in electric activity of the cell membrane, which establishes its rate of automatic activity, as in the ureter or cardiac pacemaker.

prepsychotic (prē-sī-kot′ik). **1.** Relating to the period antedating the onset of psychosis. **2.** Denoting a potential for a psychotic episode, one that appears imminent under continued stress.

prepuberal, prepubertal (prē-pyū'ber-ăl, -ber-tăl). Before puberty.

prepubescent (prē-pyū-bes'ent). Immediately prior to the commencement of puberty.

prepuce (prē'pūs) [L. *praeputium,* foreskin]. Preputium.

preputial (pre-pyū'shē-ăl). Relating to the prepuce.

preputiotomy (prē-pyū'shē-ot'ō-mē) [preputium + G. *tomē,* incision]. Incision of prepuce.

preputium, pl. **preputia** (prē-pyū'shē-ŭm, shē-ă) [L. *praeputium*] [NA]. Prepuce; foreskin; the free fold of skin that covers more or less completely the glans penis.

p. clitor'idis [NA], the external fold of the labia minora, forming a cap over the clitoris.

prepyloric (prē-pī-lōr'ik). Anterior to or preceding the pylorus; denoting a temporary constriction of the wall of the stomach separating the fundus from the antrum during digestion.

prerectal (prē-rek'tăl). Anterior to or preceding the rectum.

prereduced (prē-rē-dūsd'). Pertaining to bacteriologic media that are boiled, tubed under oxygen-free gas with chemical reducing agents and colorimetric redox indicator in stoppered tubes or bottles, and then sterilized.

prerenal (prē-rē'năl) [L. *ren,* kidney]. Anterior to a kidney.

prereproductive (prē'rē-prō-dŭk'tiv). Obsolete term denoting the period of life before puberty.

preretinal (prē-ret'i-nal). Anterior to the retina.

presacral (prē-sā'krăl). Anterior to or preceding the sacrum.

presby-, presbyo- [G. *presbys,* old man]. Combining forms denoting old age. See also gero-.

presbyacousia (prez-bē-ă-kū'sē-ă). Presbyacusis.

presbyacusis, presbyacusia (prez'bē-ă-kū'sis) [presby- + G. *akousis,* hearing]. Presbyacousia; presbycusis; loss of ability to perceive or discriminate sounds as a part of the aging process; the pattern and age of onset may vary.

presbyatrics (prez-bē-at'riks) [presby- + G. *iatreia,* medical treatment]. Rarely used terms for geriatrics.

presbycusis (prez-bē-kū'sis). Presbyacusis.

presbyopia (Pr) (prez-bē-ō'pē-ă) [presby- + G. *ōps,* eye]. The physiologic loss of accommodation in the eyes in advancing age, said to begin when the near point has receded beyond 22 cm (9 inches).

presbyopic (prez'bē-op'ik, -ō'pik). Relating to or suffering from presbyopia.

prescribe (prē-skrīb) [L. *prae-scribo,* pp. *-scriptus,* to write before]. To give directions, either orally or in writing, for the preparation and administration of a remedy to be used in the treatment of any disease.

prescription (prē-skrip'shŭn) [L. *praescriptio;* see prescribe]. **1.** A written formula for the preparation and administration of any remedy. **2.** A medicinal preparation compounded according to formulated directions, said to consist of four parts: 1) *superscription,* consisting of the word *recipe,* take, or its sign, ℞; 2) *inscription,* the main part of the p., containing the names and amounts of the drugs ordered; 3) *subscription,* directions for mixing the ingredients and designation of the form (pill, powder, solution, etc.) in which the drug is to be made, usually beginning with the word, *misce,* mix, or its abbreviation, M.; 4) *signature,* directions to the patient regarding the dose and times of taking the remedy, preceded by the word *signa,* designate, or its abbreviation, S. or Sig.

shotgun p., a p. containing many ingredients, of which some may be inert, in an attempt to cover all possible types of therapy that may be needed.

presenile (prē-sē'nīl). Prior to the usual onset of senility, as in p. *dementia.*

presenility (prē-sĕ-nil'i-tē) [pre- + L. *senilis,* old]. Premature old age; the condition of an individual, not old in years, who displays the physical and mental characteristics of old age.

presenium (prē-sē'nē-ŭm). The period preceding old age.

present (prē-zent') [L. *praesens (-sent-),* pres. p. of *prae-sum,* to be before, be at hand]. **1.** To precede or appear first at the os uteri, said of the part of the fetus first felt during examination. **2.** To appear for examination, treatment, etc., said of a patient.

presentation (prē'zen-tā'shŭn, prez') [see present]. That part of the fetus presenting at the superior strait of the maternal pelvis; occiput, chin, and sacrum are, respectively, the determining points in vertex, face, and breech p. See also position (3), and subentries.

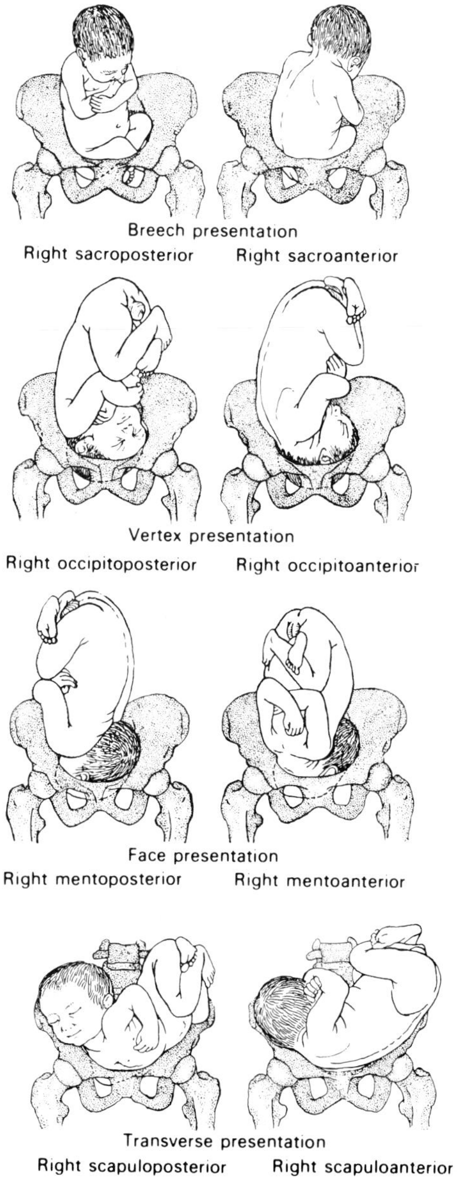

Presentations

acromion p., shoulder p.

breech p., pelvic p.; p. of any part of the pelvic extremity of the fetus, the nates, knees, or feet; more properly only of the nates;

frank b. p. occurs when the fetus presents by the pelvic extremity; the thighs may be flexed and the legs extended over the anterior surfaces of the body; in **full b. p.**, the thighs may be flexed on the abdomen and the legs upon the thighs, in **footling p., foot p.**, the feet may be the lowest part; in **incomplete foot p., knee p.**, one leg may retain the position which is typical of one of the above-mentioned presentations, while the other foot or knee may present.
brow p., see cephalic p.
cephalic p., head p.; p. of any part of the fetal head, usually the upper and back part as a result of flexion such that the chin is in contact with the thorax in vertex p.; there may be degrees of flexion so that the presenting part is the large fontanel in sincipital p., the brow in brow p., or the face in face p.
face p., see cephalic p.
footling p., foot p., see breech p.
frank breech p., see breech p.
full breech p., see breech p.
head p., cephalic p.
incomplete foot p., see breech p.
knee p., see breech p.
pelvic p., breech p.
placental p., *placenta* previa.
polar p., the p. of either pole of the fetal oval; may be either a cephalic or breech p., or a longitudinal lie.
shoulder p., acromion p.; transverse p. with the shoulder as the presenting part.
sincipital p., see cephalic p.
transverse p., an abnormal p., neither head nor breech, in which the fetus lies transversely in the uterus across the axis of the parturient canal.
vertex p., see cephalic p.

preservative (prē-zer′vă-tiv). A substance added to food products or to an organic solution to prevent chemical change or bacterial action.

presomite (prē-sō′mīt). Relating to the embryonic stage before the appearance of somites.

presphenoid (prē-sfē′noyd). In front of the sphenoid bone or cartilage.

presphygmic (prē-sfig′mik) [pre- + G. *sphygmos*, pulse]. Preceding the pulse beat; denoting a brief interval following the filling of the ventricles with blood before their contraction forces open the semilunar valves.

prespinal (prē-spī′năl). Anterior to the spine.

prespondylolisthesis (prē-spon-di-lō-lis′thē-sis). A condition predisposing to spondylolisthesis, consisting of a defect in the laminae of a lumbar vertebra but before development of any displacement of the vertebral body.

pressor (pres′er, -ōr) [L. *premo*, pp. *pressus*, to press]. Hypertensor; exciting to vasomotor activity; producing increased blood pressure; denoting afferent nerve fibers which, when stimulated, excite vasoconstrictors which increase peripheral resistance.

pressoreceptive (prcs′ō-rē-sep′tiv). Pressosensitive; capable of receiving as stimuli changes in pressure, especially changes of blood pressure.

pressoreceptor (pres′ō-rē-sep′ter, -tōr). Baroreceptor.

pressosensitive (pres-ō-sen′si-tiv). Pressoreceptive.

pressosensitivity (pres′ō-sen-si-tiv′i-tē). The state of being able to perceive changes in pressure. See also pressoreceptive.
reflexogenic p., p. also capable of initiating the regulation of heart rate, vascular tone, and blood pressure.

pressure (presh′ŭr) [L. *pressura*, fr. *premo*, pp. *pressus*, to press]. **1.** A stress or force acting in any direction against resistance. **2** (P, frequently followed by a subscript indicating location). In physics and physiology, the force per unit area exerted by a gas or liquid against the walls of its container or that would be exerted on a wall immersed at that spot in the middle of a body of fluid. The p. can be considered either relative to some reference p., such as that of the ambient atmosphere (imagined to be on the other side of the wall), or in absolute terms (relative to a perfect vacuum).
abdominal p., p. surrounding the bladder; estimated from rectal, gastric, or intraperitoneal p.
atmospheric p., barometric p.
back p., p. exerted upstream in the circulation as a result of obstruction to forward flow, as when congestion in the pulmonary circulation results from stenosis of the mitral valve or failure of the left ventricle.
barometric p., (P_B), atmospheric p.; the absolute p. of the ambient atmosphere, varying with weather, altitude, etc.; expressed in millibars (meteorology) or mm Hg or torr (respiratory physiology); at sea level, one atmosphere (atm) averages about 14.7 lb./sq. in., 1013.3 millibars, 1013×10^6 dynes/cm^2, 760 mm Hg or torr; in SI units, 101,325 pascals (Pa).
biting p., occlusal p.
blood p. (BP), arteriotony; piesis; the p. or tension of the blood within the arteries, maintained by the contraction of the left ventricle, the resistance of the arterioles and capillaries, the elasticity of the arterial walls, as well as the viscosity and volume of the blood; expressed as relative to the ambient atmospheric p.
central venous p. (CVP), the p. of the blood within the venous system in the superior and inferior vena cava, normally measured between 4 and 10 cm of water; it is depressed in circulatory shock and deficiencies of circulating blood volume, and increased with cardiac failure and congestion of the circulation.
cerebrospinal p., the p. of the cerebrospinal fluid, normally 100 to 150 mm of water, relative to the ambient atmospheric p.
continuous positive airway p. (CPAP), a technique of respiratory therapy, in either spontaneously breathing or mechanically ventilated patients, in which airway p. is maintained above atmospheric p. throughout the respiratory cycle by pressurization of the ventilatory circuit.
critical p., the minimum p. required to liquefy a gas at the critical temperature.
detrusor p., that component of intravesical pressure created by the tension (active and passive) exerted by the bladder wall; the transmural p. across the bladder wall estimated by subtracting abdominal p. from intravesical p.
diastolic p., the p. during or resulting from diastolic relaxation of a cardiac chamber; more specifically, the lowest arterial blood p. reached during any given ventricular cycle.
differential blood p., the arterial blood p. at corresponding points on the two sides of the body.
Donders' p., an increase of about 6 mm Hg shown by a manometer connected with the trachea when the thorax of the dead body is opened; it is caused by the collapse of the lungs when air is admitted to the thorax.
effective osmotic p., that part of the total osmotic p. of a solution that governs the tendency of its solvent to pass across a boundary, usually a semipermeable membrane; it is commonly represented by the product of the total osmotic p. of the solution and the ratio (corrected for activities) of the number of dissolved particles that do not permeate the bounding membrane to the total number of particles in the solution; equivalent in meaning to tonicity; commonly expressed in equivalent units of osmolality rather than p. per se.
gauge p., p. measured relative to ambient atmospheric p.; at sea level, it is 1 atm less than the p. in the atmosphere.
hydrostatic p., the p. exerted by a liquid as a result of its potential energy, ignoring its kinetic energy; frequently used to distinguish a true p. from an osmotic p. or to emphasize the variation in p. in a column of fluid due to the effect of gravity.
intracranial p. (ICP), p. within the cranial cavity.

intraocular p., the p. (usually measured in millimeters of mercury) of the intraocular fluid within the eye, measured by means of a manometer.
negative p., p. less than that of the ambient atmosphere.
negative end-expiratory p. (NEEP), a subatmospheric p. at the airway at the end of expiration.
occlusal p., biting p.; any force exerted upon the occlusal surfaces of teeth.
oncotic p., osmotic p. exerted by colloids in solution.
osmotic p., the p. that must be applied to a solution to prevent the passage into it of solvent when solution and pure solvent are separated by a membrane permeable only to the solvent. (Sometimes less correctly viewed as the force with which the solution attracts solvent through the semipermeable membrane.)
partial p., the p. exerted by a single component of a mixture of gases, commonly expressed in mm Hg or torr; for a gas dissolved in a liquid, the partial p. is that of a gas that would be in equilibrium with the dissolved gas. Formerly, symbolized by p, followed by the chemical symbol in capital letters (*e.g.,* pCO_2, pO_2); now, in respiratory physiology, P, followed by subscripts denoting location and/or chemical species (*e.g.,* P_{CO_2}, P_{O_2}, $P_{A_{CO_2}}$).
pleural p., the p. in the pleural space between the visceral and parietal pleurae.
positive end-expiratory p. (PEEP), a technique used in respiratory therapy in which airway p. greater than atmospheric p. is achieved at the end of exhalation by introduction of a mechanical impedance to exhalation.
pulmonary p., the blood p. in the pulmonary artery.
pulmonary capillary wedge p., an indirect indication of left atrial p. obtained by wedging a catheter into a small pulmonary artery sufficiently tightly to block flow from behind and thus to sample the p. beyond; normally it does not exceed 12 mm Hg; as the p. rises, signs of pulmonary congestion can be expected to appear, ordinarily when the hydrostatic p. exceeds the osmotic p. of the plasma.
pulp p., the p. in the dental pulp cavity associated with extracellular fluid p., but showing pulsatile variations during the cardiac cycle because of the encasement of the pulp within the tooth.
pulse p., the variation in blood p. occurring in an artery during the cardiac cycle; it is the difference between the systolic or maximum and diastolic or minimum p.'s.
selection p., reduction of effective reproduction due to environmental impact on the phenotype.
solution p., the force driving atoms or molecules to leave a solid particle and enter into solution (*i.e.,* to dissolve).
standard p., the absolute p. to which gases are referred under standard conditions (STPD), *i.e.,* 760 mm Hg, 760 torr, or 101,325 newtons/m^2.
systolic p., the p. during or resulting from systolic contraction of a cardiac chamber; more specifically, the highest arterial blood pressure reached during any given ventricular cycle.
transmural p., the p. inside a vessel or hollow viscus, measured relative to the p. just outside its wall; thus, the p. difference across the wall.
transpulmonary p., the difference between the p. of the respired gas at the mouth and the pleural p. around the lungs, measured when the airway is open; thus, it includes not only the transmural p. of the lung but also any drop in p. along the tracheobronchial tree during flow.
transthoracic p., the p. in the pleural space measured relative to the p. of the ambient atmosphere outside the chest; the transmural p. across the chest wall.
vapor p., the partial p. exerted by the vapor phase of a liquid.
ventricular filling p., the p. in the ventricle as it fills with blood, ordinarily equivalent to the atrial p. when there is no A-V valvular gradient; as the p. increases, congestion develops in the vascular bed behind the ventricle (the concept of "backward heart failure"); rising p. in the left ventricle leads to pulmonary congestion, while rising p. in the right ventricle leads to systemic congestion.
wedge p., the intravascular pressure reading obtained when a fine catheter is advanced until it completely occludes a small blood vessel or is sealed in place by inflation of a small cuff; commonly measured in the lung to estimate left atrial pressure.
zero end-expiratory p. (ZEEP), airway p. which, at the end of expiration, equals atmospheric p.

presternum (prē'ster'nŭm). *Manubrium* sterni.

presuppurative (prē-sŭp'yū-rā-tiv). Denoting an early stage in an inflammation prior to the formation of pus.

presynaptic (prē'si-nap'tik). Pertaining to the area on the proximal side of a synaptic cleft.

presystole (prē-sis'tō-lē). Perisystole; late diastole; that part of diastole immediately preceding systole.

presystolic (prē-sis-tol'ik). Perisystolic; late diastolic; relating to the interval immediately preceding systole.

pretarsal (prē-tar'săl). Denoting the anterior, or inferior, portion of the tarsus.

pretecta (prē-tek'tă). Orad to the hidden part of the duodenum.

pretectum (prē-tek'tŭm). Pretectal *area.*

prethyroid, prethyroideal, prethyroidean (prē-thī'royd, -thī-roy'dē-ăl, -thī-roy'dē-an). Anterior to or preceding the thyroid gland or cartilage.

pretibial (prē-tib'ē-ăl). Relating to the anterior portion of the leg; denoting especially certain muscles.

pretrematic (prē-trē-mat'ik) [pre- + G. *trēma,* perforation]. Relating to the cranial surface of a branchial cleft.

pretympanic (prē-tim-pan'ik). Anterior to the drum of the ear.

prevalence (prev'ă-lens). The number of cases of a disease existing in a given population at a specific period of time (*period p.*) or at a particular moment in time (*point p.*).

preventive (prē-ven'tiv) [L. *prae-venio,* pp. *-ventus,* to come before, prevent]. Prophylactic (1).

prevertebral (prē-ver'tē-brăl). Anterior to the body of a vertebra or of the vertebral column.

prevesical (prē-ves'i-kăl) [pre- + L. *vesica,* bladder]. Anterior to the bladder.

previus (prē'vē-ŭs) [L. *prae,* before, + *via,* way]. Obstructing; denoting anything blocking the passages in childbirth.

prezone (prē'zōn). Prozone.

PRF Abbreviation for prolactin releasing *factor.*

priapism (prī'ă-pizm) [see priapus]. Persistent erection of the penis, accompanied by pain and tenderness, resulting from a pathologic condition rather than sexual desire.

priapitis (prī-ă-pī'tis) [L. *priapus,* penis, + G. *-itis,* inflammation]. Penitis.

priapus (prī'ă-pŭs) [L. fr. L. *Priapus* (G. *Priapos*), god of procreation]. Penis.

Price, E.A. See Carr-P. *reaction.*

Price-Jones, Cecil, British hematologist, 1863–1943. See P.-J. *curve.*

Priestley, John Gillies, British physiologist, 1880–1941. See Haldane-P. *sample.*

prilocaine hydrochloride (pril'ō-kān). Propitocaine hydrochloride; 2-(propylamino)-*o*-propionotoluidide hydrochloride; a local anesthetic of the amide type, related chemically and pharmacologically to lidocaine hydrochloride; used for peridural, caudal, and nerve blocks, and for regional and infiltration anesthesia.

primaclone (prī'mă-klōn). Primidone.

primacy (prī'mă-sē) [see primary]. The state of being primary, or foremost in rank or importance.

genital p., in psychoanalysis, the primary characteristic of the genital phase of psychosexual development, *i.e.,* the libido becomes preponderantly concentrated in the penis.

oral p., in psychoanalysis, the primary characteristic of the oral phase of psychosexual development, *i.e.,* the libido is concentrated mainly in the oral zone.

primal (prī'măl). **1.** First or primary. **2.** Primordial (2).

primal scene. In psychoanalysis, the actual or fantasied observation by a child of sexual intercourse, particularly between the parents.

primaquine phosphate (prī'mă-kwin). 8-[(4-Amino-1-methylbutyl)amino]-6-methoxyquinoline phosphate (1:2); an antimalarial agent especially effective against *Plasmodium vivax,* terminating relapsing vivax malaria; usually administered with chloroquine.

primary (prī'mār-ē) [L. *primarius,* fr. *primus,* first]. **1.** The first or foremost, as a disease or symptoms to which others may be secondary or occur as complications. **2.** Relating to the first stage of growth or development. See primordial.

primate (prī'māt) [L. *primus,* first]. An individual of the order Primates.

Primates (prī-ma'tēz) [L. *primus,* first]. The highest order of mammals, including man, monkeys, and lemurs.

primerite (prī'mĕ-rīt) [L. *primus,* first, + G. *meris,* part]. Protomerite.

primidone (prī'mi-dōn). Primaclone; 5-ethyldihydro-5-phenyl-4,6-(1*H*,5*H*)-pyrimidenedione; an anticonvulsant drug used in the management of grand mal and psychomotor epilepsy.

primigravida (prī-mi-grav'i-dă) [L. fr. *primus,* first, + *gravida,* a pregnant woman]. See gravida.

primipara (prī-mip'ă-ră) [L. fr. *primus,* first, + *pario,* to bring forth]. See para.

primiparity (prī-mi-par'i-tē). Condition of being a primipara.

primiparous (prī-mip'ă-rŭs). Denoting a primipara.

primite (prī'mīt). The anterior member of a pair of gregarine gamonts in syzygy.

primitive (prim'i-tiv) [L. *primitivus,* fr. *primus,* first]. Primordial (2).

primordia (prī-mōr'dē-ă). Plural of primordium.

primordial (prī-mōr'dē-ăl). **1.** Relating to a primordium. **2.** Primitive; primal (2); relating to a structure in its first or earliest stage of development.

primordium, primordia (prī-mōr'-dē-ŭm, -dē-ă) [L. origin, fr. *primus,* first, + *ordior,* to begin]. Anlage (1); an aggregation of cells in the embryo indicating the first trace of an organ or structure.

primula (prim'yū-lă) [Mediev. L. primrose, fem. of L. *primulus,* first]. The rhizome and roots of a number of species of *Primula* (family Primulaceae), primrose or cowslip; has been used as expectorant, diuretic, and anthelmintic. In some sensitive persons contact with the plant causes a rash.

primulin (prī'myū-lin) [C.I. 49000]. An acid yellow thiazole dye, $C_{21}H_{14}N_3O_3Na$, used as a fluorescent vital stain.

primus (prī'mŭs) [L.]. First; denoting the first of a series of similar structures.

princeps, pl. **principes** (prin'seps, -si-pēz) [L. chief, fr. *primus,* first, + *capio,* to take, choose]. Principal; in anatomy, term used to distinguish several arteries.

p. cervi'cis, *ramus* descendens (2).

p. pol'licis, *arteria* princeps pollicis.

Princeteau, L.R., French physician, *1884. See P.'s *tubercle.*

principle (prin'si-pl) [L. *principium,* a beginning, fr. *princeps,* chief]. **1.** A general or fundamental doctrine or tenet. See also law; rule; theorem. **2.** The essential ingredient in a substance, especially one that gives it its distinctive quality or effect.

active p., a constituent of a drug, usually an alkaloid or glycoside, upon the presence of which the characteristic therapeutic action of the substance largely depends.

antianemic p., the material in liver (and certain other tissues) that stimulates hemopoiesis in pernicious anemia; for practical purposes, the antianemic effect of extracts from such tissues is approximately equivalent to the content of vitamin B_{12}.

azygos vein p., low flow p.; a p. based on the observation that animals can survive prolonged vena caval occlusion without sequelae: if blood from the azygos vein alone is permitted to enter the heart, patients are perfused during cardiac and pulmonary bypass at flows much less than the normal resting cardiac output.

Bernoulli's p., Bernoulli's *law.*

closure p., in psychology, the p. that when one views fragmentary stimuli forming a nearly complete figure (*e.g.,* an incomplete rectangle) one tends to ignore the missing parts and perceive the figure as whole.

consistency p., in psychology, the desire of the human being to be consistent, especially in his attitudes and beliefs; theories of attitude formation and change based on the consistency p. include balance theory, which suggests that the individual seeks to avoid incongruity in his various attitudes. See also cognitive dissonance *theory.*

Fick p., the basis of some indirect methods of measuring the output of the heart and of blood flow to some of the organs, *e.g.,* the kidneys; can be used when arterial and venous concentrations of a substance can be measured and the amount of uptake or removal of the substance can be determined. Oxygen consumption is equal to the product of the pulmonary blood flow and the increase in oxygen content of the blood passing through the lungs; usually rearranged so that flow equals O_2 consumption divided by the arteriovenous difference in blood O_2 concentration.

follicle-stimulating p., follitropin.

founder p., the conditional probability of the frequencies of a set of genes at any future date depends on the initial composition of the founders of the population and have in general no tendency to revert to the composition of the population from which the founders were themselves elected.

hematinic p., the p. previously thought to be produced by the action of Castle's intrinsic factor upon an extrinsic factor in food, now recognized as vitamin B_{12}.

p. of inertia, repetition-compulsion p.

Le Chatelier's p., Le Chatelier's *law.*

low flow p., azygos vein p.

luteinizing p., lutropin.

melanophore-expanding p., melanotropin.

nirvana p., in psychoanalysis, the p. that expresses the tendency toward the death instinct.

organic p., proximate p.

pain p., an unconscious striving for pain and death.

pain-pleasure p., pleasure p.; a psychoanalytic concept that, in man's psychic functioning, he tends to seek pleasure and avoid pain.

Pauli's p., the theory limiting the number of electrons in the orbit or shell of an atom; that it is not possible for any two electrons to have all four quantum numbers identical.

pleasure p., pain-pleasure p.

proximate p., organic p.; in chemistry, an organic compound that may exist already formed as a part of some other more complex substance (*e.g.,* various sugars, starches, and albumins).

reality p., the concept that the pleasure p. in personality development is modified by the demands of external reality; the p. or force that compels the growing child to adapt to the demands of external reality.

repetition-compulsion p., p. of inertia; in psychoanalysis, the impulse to redramatize or reenact earlier emotional experiences or situations.
ultimate p., one of the chemical elements.

Pringle, John J., British dermatologist, 1855–1922. See P.'s *disease;* Bourneville-P. *disease.*

Prinzmetal, Myron, U.S. cardiologist, *1908. See P.'s *angina.*

prion (prī'on) [proteinaceous infectious particle]. A small biological entity, with at least one protein but no demonstrable nucleic acid, which is resistant to inactivation by most procedures that modify nucleic acids, is resistant to inactivation by heat, and shows heterogeneity with respect to size (smallest forms possibly having MW 50,000 or less); these properties indicate that p.'s are novel infectious entities that differ from viruses, viroids, and plasmids; the agent causing scrapie in sheep and goats is considered to be a p.

prism (prizm) [G. *prisma*]. A transparent solid, with sides that converge at an angle, that deflects a ray of light toward the thickest portion (the base) and splits white light into its component colors; in spectacles, a p. corrects ocular muscle imbalance.

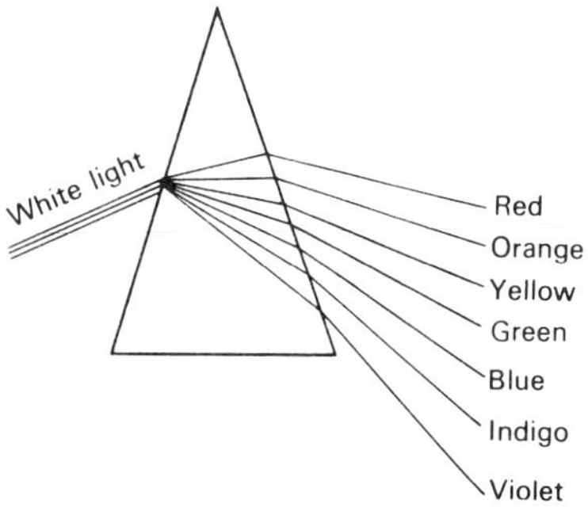

Splitting of White Light by a Prism

enamel p.'s, *prismata* adamantina.
Fresnel p., a p. composed of concentric annular rings.
Nicol p., a p. that transmits only polarized light.
Risley's rotary p., a p. with a circular base that is rotated in a metal frame marked with a scale; used in examination of ocular muscle imbalance.

prisma, pl. **prismata** (priz'mă, priz'mah-tă) [G. something sawed, a prism]. A structure resembling a prism.
pris'mate adaman'tina, enamel prisms, rods, or fibers; the calcified, microscopic rods radiating from the surface of the dentin, forming the substance of the enamel of a tooth.

prismatic (priz-mat'ik). Relating to or resembling a prism.

prism bar. A graduated series of p.'s mounted on a frame and used in ocular diagnosis.

privacy (prī'vă-sē). **1.** Being apart from others; confidentiality; seclusion; secrecy. **2.** Especially in psychiatry and clinical psychology, respect for the confidential nature of the therapist-patient relationship.

PRL Abbreviation for prolactin.

p.r.n. Abbreviation for L. *pro re nata,* as the occasion arises.

Pro Symbol for proline or its radicals.

pro- [L. and G. *pro,* before]. **1.** Prefix denoting before or forward. See also ante-; pre-. **2.** In chemistry, prefix indicating precursor of. See also -gen (2).

proaccelerin (prō-ak-sel'er-in). *Factor* V.

proacrosomal (prō-ak-rō-sō'măl). Relating to an early stage in the development of the acrosome.

proactinium (prō-ak-tin'ē-ŭm). Protactinium.

proactivator (prō-ak'ti-vā-ter). A substance that, when chemically split, yields a fragment (activator) capable of rendering another substance enzymically active.
C3 p., properdin *factor* B.
C3 p. convertase, properdin *factor* D.

proal (prō'ăl). Relating to a forward movement.

proamnion (prō-am'nē-on). An area of the extraembryonic membranes beneath, and in front of, the developing head of a young embryo which remains without mesoderm for some time.

proatlas (prō-at'las). A vertebral element intercalated between the atlas and occipital bone in crocodiles and alligators, traces of which are sometimes seen as an anomaly on the undersurface of the occipital bone in man.

probacteriophage (prō-bak-tēr'ē-ō-fāj). Prophage; the stage of a temperate bacteriophage in which the genome is incorporated in the genetic apparatus of the bacterial host.
defective p., see defective *bacteriophage.*

proband (prō'band) [L. *probo,* to test, prove]. Propositus (1); index case; in human genetics, the patient or member of the family that brings a family under study.

probang (prō'bang). A slender, flexible rod, tipped with a globular piece of sponge or some other material, used chiefly for making applications or removing obstructions in the larynx or esophagus.

probe (prōb) [L. *probo,* to test]. **1.** A slender rod of flexible material, with blunt bulbous tip, used for exploring sinuses, fistulas, other cavities, or wounds. **2.** A device or agent used to detect or explore a substance. **3.** To enter and explore, as with a p.
Anel's p., a p. for the punctum lacrimale and canaliculae.
Bowman's p., a double-ended p. for the lacrimal duct.
nucleic acid p., a nucleic acid fragment, labeled by a radioisotope, biotin, etc., that is complementary to a sequence in another nucleic acid (fragment) and that will, by hydrogen binding to the latter, locate or identify it and be detected; a diagnostic technique based on the fact that every species of microbe possesses some unique nucleic acid sequences which differentiate it from all others, and thus can be used as identifying markers or "fingerprints."
periodontal p., a calibrated instrument used to measure the depth and topography of periodontal pockets.
radioactive p., see nucleic acid p.
vertebrated p., a p. made up of a series of short sections hinged together for flexibility in penetrating convoluted tracts.
viral p., see nucleic acid p.

probenecid (prō-ben'ĕ-sid). *p*-Carboxy-*N,N*- diisopropylsulfonamide; a competitive inhibitor of the secretion of penicillin or *p*-aminohippurate by kidney tubules; a uricosuric agent used in chronic gouty arthritis.

probilifuscins (prō-bil'i-fŭs'in). See bilirubinoids.

probiosis (prō-bī-ō'sis) [pro- + G. *biōsis,* life]. An association of two organisms that enhances the life processes of both. *Cf.* antibiosis (1); symbiosis; mutualism.

probiotic (prō-bī-ot'ik). Relating to probiosis.

prob'lem. In the mental health professions, a term often used to denote life problems (the difficulties or challenges of life); sometimes used in preference to the terms mental illness or mental disorder.

proboscis, pl. **proboscides, proboscises** (prō-bos'is, prō-bos'i-dēz, -sēz) [G. *proboskis,* a means of providing food, fr. pro- + *boskein,* to feed]. **1.** A long flexible snout, such as that of a tapir or an elephant. **2.** In teratology, a cylindrical protuberance of the face which, in cyclopia or ethmocephaly, represents the nose.

Probstymayria vivipara (prob-sti-mā'rē-ă vi-vip'ă-ră). A nematode (family Atractidae) closely related to the true pinworms (family Oxyuridae) and still commonly considered the horse pinworm; it is distributed worldwide and is found often in tremendous numbers, because of internal autoreinfection, in the colon of horses and other equids.

probucol (prō'byū-kōl). Acetone bis(3,5-di-*tert*-butyl-4-hydroxyphenyl)mercaptole; an antihyperlipoproteinemic agent.

procainamide hydrochloride (pro-kān'ă-mīd, pro'kān-am'īd, -id). *p*-Amino-*N*-[2-(diethylamino)ethyl]benzamide hydrochloride; differs chemically from procaine by containing the amide group (CONH) instead of the ester group (COO). It depresses the irritability of the cardiac muscle, having a quinidine-like action upon the heart, and is used in ventricular arrhythmias.

procaine hydrochloride (prō'kān). 2-Diethylaminoethyl *p*-aminobenzoate monohydrochloride; a local anesthetic used for infiltration and spinal anesthesia.

procapsid (prō-kap'sid). A protein shell lacking a virus genome.

procarbazine hydrochloride (prō-kar'bă-zēn). Ibenzmethyzin hydrochloride; *N*-isopropyl-α-(2-methylhydrazino)-*p*-toluamide monohydrochloride; an antineoplastic agent.

procarboxypeptidase (prō'kar-bok-sē-pep'ti-dās). Inactive precursor of a carboxypeptidase.

Procaryotae (pro-kar-ē-ō'tē) [pro- + G. *karyon,* kernel, nut]. Prokaryotae.

procaryote (pro-kar'ē-ōt) [pro- + G. *karyon,* kernel, nut]. Prokaryote.

procaryotic (prō'kar-ē-ot'ik). Prokaryotic.

procatarctic (prō-kă-tark'tik) [G. *prokatarktikos,* beginning beforehand]. Denoting the exciting cause of a disease.

procatarxis (prō-kă-tark'sis) [G. a beginning beforehand, fr. *prokatararchō,* to begin first, fr. *pro,* before, + *kata,* upon, + *archō,* to begin]. **1.** Exciting *cause.* **2.** The beginning of a disease under the influence of the exciting cause, a predisposing cause already existing.

procedure (prō-sē'jūr). Act or conduct of diagnosis, treatment, or operation. See also entries under method, operation, technique.

Adson's p., Adson's *test.*

commando p., commando operation; an operation for malignant tumors of the floor of the oral cavity, involving resection of portions of the mandible in continuity with the oral lesion and radical neck dissection.

Eloesser p., transposition of a tonguelike pedicled skin flap from the chest wall into the depths of an incision that communicates with an empyema or peripheral lung abscess; used to prevent scar closure of the tract to insure long-term mandatory dependent drainage.

endorectal pull-through p., removal of diseased rectal mucosa along with resection of the lower bowel, followed by anastomosis of the proximal stump to the anus, in order to spare rectal muscle function.

Ewart's p., elevation of the larynx between the thumb and forefinger to elicit tracheal tugging.

Fontan p., Fontan operation; placement of a conduit (usually valved) from the right atrium to the main pulmonary artery as a bypass to an hypoplastic right ventricle, as in tricuspid atresia.

Girdlestone p., complete resection or excision of the head and neck of the femur.

Mustard p., Mustard *operation.*

Noble-Collip p., obsolete p. in which shock in rats is induced by rotating them in a drum.

Puestow p., longitudinal pancreaticojejunostomy for treatment of chronic pancreatitis.

push-back p., a surgical maneuver designed to reposition the soft palate posteriorly and reestablish velopharyngeal competence.

Putti-Platt p., Putti-Platt *operation.*

Rastelli p., placement of a valved conduit between the right ventricle and the main pulmonary artery to bypass an atretic pulmonary outflow tract.

shelf p., insertion of a graft from the ilium into the roof of the acetabulum for congenital dislocation of the hip.

Stanley Way p., a radical vulvectomy.

Sugiura p., esophageal transection with paraesophageal devascularization, for esophageal varices.

Thal p., correction of a benign stricturing of the lower esophagus in which the narrowed area is opened to full-thickness longitudinally and the adjacent external gastric wall is patch sutured over this defect to restore luminal circumference and continuity.

Vineberg p., implantation of the internal mammary artery into the myocardium to improve blood flow to the heart.

V-Y p., V-Y-plasty.

W p., W-plasty.

Z p., Z-plasty.

procelia (prō-sē'lē-ă) [pro- + G. *koilia,* a hollow]. A lateral ventricle of the brain; the hollow of the prosencephalon.

procelous (prō-sē'lŭs) [pro- + G. *koilos,* hollow]. Concave anteriorly.

procentriole (prō-sen'trē-ōl). The early phase in development *de novo* of centrioles or basal bodies from the centrosphere; p.'s form in relation to deuterosomes (p. organizers).

procephalic (prō-se-fal'ik) [pro- + G. *kephalē,* head]. Relating to the anterior part of the head.

procercoid (prō-ser'koyd) [pro- + G. *kerkos,* tail, + *eidos,* resemblance]. The first stage in the aquatic life cycle of certain tapeworms, such as the pseudophyllideans (family Diphyllobothriidae), following ingestion of the newly hatched larva (coracidium) by a copepod (water flea). The p. develops into a tailed larva in the body cavity of the crustacean first intermediate host; when the p. and its host are ingested by a fish, the p. enters the new host's tissues and becomes a plerocercoid. See also *Diphyllobothrium latum;* Pseudophyllidea.

procerus (prō-sē'rŭs) [L. long, stretched out]. *Musculus* procerus.

PROCESS

process (pros'es, prō'ses) [L. *processus,* an advance, progress, process, fr. *pro-cedo,* pp. *-cessus,* to go forward]. **1.** A method or mode of action used in the attainment of a certain result. **2.** An advance, progress, or method as of a disease. **3.** A projection or outgrowth. See processus. **4.** In dentistry, a series of operations which convert a wax pattern, such as that of a denture base, into a solid denture base of another material. See also dental *curing.*

A.B.C. p., purification of water or deodorization of sewage by a mixture of *alum, blood,* and *charcoal.*

accessory p., *processus* accessorius.

acromial p., acromion.

agene p., bleaching of flour with nitrogen trichloride (prohibited in the United States).

alar p., *ala* cristae galli.

alveolar p., *processus* alveolaris.

anterior p. of malleus, *processus* anterior mallei.

apical p., apical dendrite; the dendritic p. extending from the apex of a pyramidal cell of the cerebral cortex toward the surface.

articular p., *processus* articularis.

ascending p., *processus* ascendens.

auditory p., the roughened edge of the tympanic plate giving attachment to the cartilaginous portion of the external acoustic meatus.

axonal p., obsolete term for axon.

basilar p., *pars* basilaris ossis occipitalis.

Budde p., a method of milk sterilization; to the fresh milk, hydrogen peroxide is added in the proportion of 15 ml of a 3% solution to 1 liter of milk, and the mixture is heated to 51° or 52°C (124°F) for 3 hours, by which time the peroxide is decomposed and the nascent oxygen acts as an efficient germicide; the milk is then rapidly cooled and put into sealed bottles.
Burns' falciform p., *cornu* superius hiatus saphenus.
calcaneal p. of cuboid bone, *processus* calcaneus ossis cuboidei.
caudate p., *processus* caudatus.
ciliary p., *processus* ciliaris.
Civinini's p., *processus* pterygospinosus.
clinoid p., *processus* clinoideus.
cochleariform p., *processus* cochleariformis.
complex learning p.'s, those p.'s which require the use of symbolic manipulations, as in reasoning.
condylar p., *processus* condylaris.
condyloid p., *processus* condylaris.
conoid p., see *tuberculum* conoideum; *linea* trapezoidea.
coracoid p., *processus* coracoideus.
coronoid p., *processus* coronoideus.
costal p., *processus* costalis.
Deiters' p., obsolete term for axon.
dendritic p., dendrite (1).
dental p., *processus* alveolaris.
ensiform p., *processus* xiphoideus.
ethmoidal p., *processus* ethmoidalis.
falciform p., *processus* falciformis.
Folli's p., follian p., *processus* anterior mallei.
foot p., pedicel.
frontal p., *processus* frontalis.
frontonasal p., frontonasal *elevation.*
frontosphenoidal p., *processus* frontalis ossis zygomatici.
funicular p., the tunica vaginalis surrounding the spermatic cord.
globular p., obsolete term for intermaxillary *segment.*
hamular p. of lacrimal bone, hamulus lacrimalis.
hamular p. of sphenoid bone, *hamulus* pterygoideus.
head p., the primordium for the notochord.
intrajugular p., *processus* intrajugularis.
jugular p., *processus* jugularis.
lacrimal p., *processus* lacrimalis.
lateral p. of calcaneal tuberosity, *processus* lateralis tuberis calcanei.
lateral p. of malleus, *processus* lateralis mallei.
lateral nasal p., lateral nasal *elevation.*
lateral p. of talus, *processus* lateralis tali.
Lenhossék's p.'s, short p.'s ("aborted axons") possessed by some ganglion cells.
lenticular p. of incus, *processus* lenticularis incudis.
long p. of malleus, *processus* anterior mallei.
malar p., *processus* zygomaticus maxillae.
mamillary p., *processus* mamillaris.
mandibular p., mandibular *arch.*
mastoid p., *processus* mastoideus.
maxillary p., *processus* maxillaris.
maxillary p. (of embryo), the part of the first pharyngeal arch that lies cranial to the stomodeum and then develops into the upper jaw.
medial p. of calcaneal tuberosity, *processus* medialis tuberis calcanei.
medial nasal p., media nasal *elevation.*
mental p., *protuberantia* mentalis.
muscular p. of arytenoid cartilage, *processus* muscularis cartilaginis arytenoidei.
nasal p., *processus* frontalis maxillae.
notochordal p., in the embryo, a midline column of cells migrating forward from Hensen's node to form the notochord.
odontoblastic p., the extension of the odontoblast which lies within the dentinal tubule; application of painful stimuli to dentin may cause aspiration of odontoblast contents into the p.
odontoid p., dens (2).
odontoid p. of epistropheus, dens (2).
olecranon p., olecranon.
orbicular p., *processus* lenticularis incudis.
orbital p., *processus* orbitalis.
packing p., the method of placing denture base material in a flask for processing.
palatal p.'s, in the embryo, medially directed shelves from the oral surface of the maxillae; they develop into the palate after midline fusion.
palatine p., *processus* palatinus.
papillary p., *processus* papillaris.
paramastoid p., *processus* paramastoideus.
paroccipital p., *processus* paramastoideus.
posterior p. of septal cartilage, *processus* posterior cartilaginis septi nasi.
primary p., in psychoanalysis, the mental p. directly related to the functions of the id and characteristic of unconscious mental activity; marked by unorganized, illogical thinking and by the tendency to seek immediate discharge and gratification of instinctual demands. *Cf.* secondary p.
progressive p.'s, p.'s that continue after they no longer serve the needs of the organism, and after cessation of the stimulus that evoked the p.
pterygoid p., *processus* pterygoideus.
pterygospinous p., *processus* pterygospinosus.
pyramidal p., *processus* pyramidalis.
Rau's p., *processus* anterior mallei.
Ravius' p., *processus* anterior mallei.
secondary p., in psychoanalysis, the mental p. directly related to the functions of the ego and characteristic of conscious and preconscious mental activities; marked by logical thinking and by the tendency to delay gratification by regulation of the discharge of instinctual demands. *Cf.* primary p.
sheath p. of sphenoid bone, *processus* vaginalis ossis sphenoidalis.
short p. of malleus, *processus* lateralis mallei.
slender p. of malleus, *processus* anterior mallei.
sphenoid p., *processus* sphenoidalis.
sphenoid p. of septal cartilage, *processus* posterior cartilaginis septi nasi.
spinous p., (1) *spina* ossis sphenoidalis; **(2)** *processus* spinosus.
spinous p. of tibia, *eminentia* intercondylaris.
Stieda's p., *processus* posterior tali.
styloid p. of fibula, *apex* capitis fibulae.
styloid p. of radius, *processus* styloideus radii.
styloid p. of temporal bone, *processus* styloideus ossis temporalis.
styloid p. of third metacarpal bone, *processus* styloideus ossis metacarpalis III.
styloid p. of ulna, *processus* styloideus ulnae.
superior articular p. of sacrum, *processus* articularis superior ossis sacri.
supracondylar p., *processus* supracondylaris humeri.
supraepicondylar p., *processus* supraepicondylaris.
temporal p., *processus* temporalis.
Tomes' p.'s, p.'s of the enamel cells.
transverse p., *processus* transversus.
trochlear p., *trochlea* peronealis.
uncinate p. of ethmoid bone, *processus* uncinatus ossis ethmoidalis.
uncinate p. of pancreas, *processus* uncinatus pancreatis.
vaginal p., *vagina* processus styloidei.
vaginal p. of peritoneum, *processus* vaginalis peritonei.
vaginal p. of testis, *processus* vaginalis peritonei.
vermiform p., *appendix* vermiformis.
vocal p., *processus* vocalis cartilaginis artenoidei.

xiphoid p., *processus* xiphoideus.
zygomatic p., *processus* zygomaticus.

PROCESSUS

processus, pl. **processus** (prō-ses'ŭs) [L. see process] [NA]. A process; in anatomy, a projection or outgrowth.

p. accesso'rius [NA], accessory process; accessory tubercle; a small apophysis at the posterior part of the base of the transverse process of each of the lumbar vertebrae.

p. alveola'ris [NA], alveolar process, ridge, or body; alveolar bone (1); alveolar border (2); dental process; basal ridge (1); the projecting ridge on the inferior surface of the body of the maxilla containing the tooth sockets; the term is also applied to the superior aspect of the body of the mandible, containing the tooth sockets of the lower jaw. See also alveolar *bone* (2).

p. ante'rior mal'lei [NA], anterior or long process of the malleus; p. gracilis; slender p. of malleus; Folli's, Rau's, or Ravius' process; follian process; p. ravii; a slender spur running anteriorward from the neck of the malleus toward the petrotympanic fissure.

p. articula'ris [NA], articular process; zygapophysis; one of the small flat projections on the surfaces of the arches of the vertebrae on either side, at the point where the pedicles and laminae join, forming the zygapophysial joint surfaces; **p. a. supe'rior,** diapophysis; one of the p. a. on the superior surface of the vertebral arch; **p. a. infe'rior,** one of the p. a. on the inferior surface of the vertebral arch.

p. articula'ris supe'rior os'sis sa'cri [NA], superior articular process of the sacrum; the large process on each side of the sacrum posteriorly that articulates with the corresponding inferior articular process of the fifth lumbar vertebra.

p. ascen'dens, ascending process; an upward extension of the embryonic pterygoquadrate cartilage; it develops into the greater wing of the sphenoid bone.

p. bre'vis, p. lateralis mallei.

p. calca'neus os'sis cuboi'dei [NA], calcaneal process of the cuboid bone; the process projecting posteriorly from the plantar surface of the cuboid; it supports the anterior end of the calcaneus.

p. cauda'tus [NA], caudate process; a narrow band of hepatic tissue connecting the caudate and right lobes of the liver posterior to the porta hepatis.

p. cilia'ris [NA], ciliary process; one of the radiating pigmented ridges, usually seventy in number, on the inner surface of the ciliary body, increasing in thickness as they advance from the orbiculus ciliaris to the external border of the iris; these, together with the folds (plicae) in the furrows between them, constitute the corona ciliaris.

p. clinoi'deus [NA], clinoid process; clinoid (2); one of three pairs of bony projections from the sphenoid bone: **p. c. ante'rior,** the recurved posterior angle of the lesser wing; **p. c. me'dius,** a little spur of bone on the body of the sphenoid, posterolateral to the tuberculum sellae; **p. c. poste'rior,** a spur of bone at each superior angle of the dorsum sellae.

p. cochlearifor'mis [NA], cochleariform process; a bony angular process (the termination of the septum canalis musculotubarii) above the anterior end of the vestibular window, forming a pulley over which the tendon of the tensor tympani muscle plays.

p. condyla'ris [NA], condylar or condyloid process; mandibular condyle; the articular process of the ramus of the mandible; it contains the caput mandibulae, collum mandibulae, and fovea pterygoidea.

p. coracoi'deus [NA], coracoid process; a long curved projection from the neck of the scapula overhanging the glenoid cavity; it gives attachment to the short head of the biceps, the coracobrachialis, and the pectoralis minor muscles, and the conoid and coracoacromial ligaments.

p. coronoi'deus [NA], coronoid process; a sharp triangular projection from a bone; **p. c. mandib'ulae,** the triangular anterior process of the mandibular ramus, giving attachment to the temporal muscle; **p. c. ul'nae,** a bracket-like projection from the anterior portion of the proximal extremity of the ulna; its anterior surface gives attachment to the brachialis, its proximal surface enters into the formation of the trochlear notch.

p. costa'lis [NA], costal process; an apophysis extending laterally from the transverse process of a lumbar vertebra; it is the homologue of the rib.

p. ethmoida'lis [NA], ethmoidal process; a projection of the inferior concha, situated behind the lacrimal process and articulating with the uncinate process of the ethmoid.

p. falcifor'mis [NA], falciform process; falciform ligament; ligamentum falciforme; a continuation of the inner border of the sacrotuberous ligament upward and forward on the inner aspect of the ramus of the ischium.

p. ferrei'ni, *pars* radiata lobuli corticalis renis.

p. fronta'lis [NA], frontal process; **p. f. maxil'lae,** nasal process; the upward extension from the body of the maxilla, which articulates with the frontal bone; **p. f. os'sis zygomat'ici,** frontosphenoidal process; the process of the zygomatic bone which extends upward to form the lateral margin of the orbit and articulates with the frontal bone and greater wing of the sphenoid bone.

p. grac'ilis, p. anterior mallei.

p. intrajugula'ris [NA], intrajugular process; a small pointed process of bone extending from the middle of the jugular notch in both the occipital and the temporal bones, the two being joined by a ligament and dividing the jugular foramen into two portions.

p. jugula'ris [NA], jugular process; a short process jutting out from the posterior part of the condyle of the occipital bone, its anterior border forming the posterior boundary of the jugular foramen.

p. lacrima'lis [NA], lacrimal process; a projection from the anterior edge of the inferior concha which articulates with the lower border of the lacrimal bone.

p. latera'lis mal'lei [NA], lateral process of malleus; short process of malleus; p. brevis; tuberculum mallei; a short projection from the base of the manubrium of the malleus, attached firmly to the drum membrane.

p. latera'lis ta'li [NA], lateral process of the talus; a projection on the lateral side of the talus below the malleolar articular surface.

p. latera'lis tu'beris calca'nei [NA], lateral process of calcaneal tuberosity; the lateral projection from the posterior part of the calcaneus.

p. lenticula'ris incu'dis [NA], lenticular process, apophysis, or bone; orbicular bone or process; os orbiculare; os sylvii; a knob at the tip of the long limb of the incus which articulates with the stapes.

p. mamilla'ris [NA], mamillary process or tubercle; metapophysis; a small apophysis or tubercle on the dorsal margin of the superior articular process of each of the lumbar vertebrae and usually of the twelfth thoracic vertebra.

p. mastoi'deus [NA], mastoid process; mastoid bone; temporal apophysis; the nipple-like projection of the petrous part of the temporal bone.

p. maxilla'ris [NA], maxillary process; a thin plate of irregular form projecting from the middle of the upper border of the inferior concha, articulating with the maxilla bone and partly closing the orifice of the maxillary sinus.

p. media'lis tu'beris calca'nei [NA], medial process of calcaneal tuberosity; the medial projection from the posterior part of the calcaneus.

p. muscula'ris cartila'ginis arytenoi'dei [NA], muscular process of arytenoid cartilage; the blunt lateral projection of the arytenoid cartilage giving attachment to several intrinsic muscles of the larynx.

p. orbita'lis [NA], orbital process; the anterior and larger of the two processes at the upper extremity of the vertical plate of the palatine bone, articulating with the maxilla, ethmoid, and sphenoid bones.

p. palati'nus [NA], palatine process; the horizontal plate of the maxilla, forming with its fellow the anterior portion of the roof of the mouth.

p. papilla'ris [NA], papillary process; the left lower angle of the caudate lobe of the liver, opposite the caudate process.

p. paramastoi'deus [NA], paramastoid process; paroccipital process; an occasional process of bone extending downward from the jugular process of the occipital bone in man.

p. poste'rior cartila'ginis sep'ti na'si [NA], posterior or sphenoid process of the septal cartilage; p. sphenoidalis cartilaginis septi nasi; the tapering extension of the septal cartilage that lies between the perpendicular plate of the ethmoid and the vomer.

p. poste'rior ta'li [NA], Stieda's process; a projection of the talus bearing medial and lateral tubercles; it is posterior and inferior to the trochlea.

p. pterygoi'deus [NA], pterygoid process; os pterygoideum; a long process extending downward from the junction of the body and great wing of the sphenoid bone on either side; it is formed of two plates (lamina lateralis and lamina medialis), united anteriorly but separated below to form the pterygoid notch; the pterygoid fossa is formed by the divergence of these two plates posteriorly.

p. pterygospino'sus [NA], pterygospinous process; Civinini's process; a sharp projection from the posterior edge of the lateral pterygoid plate of the sphenoid bone.

p. pyramida'lis [NA], pyramidal process; the portion of the palatine bone passing lateral and posterior from the angle formed by the vertical and horizontal plates.

p. ra'vii, p. anterior mallei.

p. retromandibula'ris, that portion of the parotid salivary gland that is located behind the mandible and occupies the space between the ramus of the mandible and the mastoid process extending as far medially as the pharyngeal wall; also known as the p. retromandibularis glandulae parotidis.

p. sphenoida'lis [NA], spenoid process; the posterior and smaller of the two processes at the extremity of the vertical plate of the palatine bone; **p. s. cartila'ginis sep'ti na'si,** p. posterior cartilaginis septi nasi.

p. spino'sus [NA], spinous process (2); the dorsal projection from the center of a vertebral arch.

p. styloi'deus os'sis metacarpa'lis III [NA], styloid process of third metacarpal bone; a pointed projection from the dorsolateral angle of the base of the third metacarpal bone; it sometimes exists as a separate ossicle.

p. styloi'deus os'sis tempora'lis [NA], styloid process of temporal bone; a slender pointed projection running downward and slightly forward from the base of the inferior surface of the petrous portion of the temporal bone where it joins the tympanic portion; it gives attachment to the styloglossus, stylohyoid, and stylopharyngeus muscles and the stylohyoid and stylomandibular ligaments.

p. styloi'deus ra'dii [NA], styloid process of the radius; a thick, pointed projection on the lateral side of the distal extremity of the radius.

p. styloi'deus ul'nae [NA], styloid process of the ulna; a cylindrical, pointed projection from the medial and posterior aspect of the head of the ulna, to the tip of which is attached the ulnar collateral ligament of the wrist.

p. supraepicondyla'ris hu'meri [NA], supraepicondylar process; supracondylar process; an occasional spine projecting from the anteromedial surface of the humerus about 5 cm above the medial epicondyle to which it is joined by a fibrous band. The supracondylar foramen thus formed transmits the brachial artery and median nerve.

p. tempora'lis [NA], temporal process; the posterior projection of the zygomatic bone articulating with the zygomatic process of the temporal bone to form the zygomatic arch.

p. transver'sus [NA], transverse process; projecting on either side of the arch of a vertebra.

p. trochlea'ris, *trochlea* peronealis.

p. uncina'tus os'sis ethmoida'lis [NA], uncinate process of ethmoid bone; a sickle-shaped process of bone on the medial wall of the ethmoidal labyrinth below the middle concha; it articulates with the ethmoidal process of the inferior concha and partly closes the orifice of the maxillary sinus.

p. uncina'tus pancrea'tis [NA], uncinate process of pancreas; lesser, small, uncinate, or unciform pancreas; Willis' or Winslow's pancreas; pancreas minor; a portion of the head of the pancreas that hooks around posterior to the superior mesenteric vessels.

p. vagina'lis os'sis sphenoida'lis [NA], sheath process of sphenoid bone; a thin lamina of bone that extends medially under the body of the sphenoid bone from the medial lamina of the pterygoid process; it articulates with the vomer and the palatine bone.

p. vagina'lis peritone'i, vaginal process of peritoneum; vaginal process of testis; Nuck's diverticulum; a peritoneal diverticulum in the embryonic lower anterior abdominal wall that traverses the inguinal canal; in the male it forms the tunica vaginalis testis and normally loses its connection with the peritoneal cavity; a persistent p. vaginalis in the female is known as the canal of Nuck.

p. vermifor'mis, *appendix* vermiformis.

p. voca'lis cartila'ginis arytenoi'dei [NA], vocal process; the lower end of the anterior margin of the arytenoid cartilage to which the vocal cord is attached.

p. xiphoi'deus [NA], xiphoid or ensiform process or cartilage; ensisternum cartilage; mucro sterni; ensisternum; metasternum; xiphisternum; the cartilage at the lower end of the sternum.

p. zygomat'icus [NA], zygomatic process; **p. z. maxil'lae,** malar process; the rough projection from the maxilla that articulates with the zygomatic bone; **p. z. os'sis fronta'lis,** the massive projection of the frontal bone that joins the zygomatic bone to form the lateral margin of the orbit; **p. z. os'sis tempora'lis,** the anterior process of the temporal bone that articulates with the temporal process of the zygomatic bone to form the zygomatic arch.

---

procheilia, prochilia (prō-kī'lē-ă) [pro- + G. *cheilos,* lip]. Protruding lips.

procheilon, prochilon (prō-kī'lon). *Tuberculum* labii superioris.

prochlorperazine (prō-klōr-per'ă-zēn). 2-Chloro-10-[3-(1-methyl-4-piperazinyl)propyl]phenothiazine; a phenothiazine compound similar in structure, actions, and uses to chlorpromazine; used as a tranquilizer and antiemetic; available as the edisylate for oral and intramuscular administration and as the maleate for oral administration.

prochondral (prō-kon'drăl) [pro- + G. *chondros,* cartilage]. Denoting a developmental stage prior to the formation of cartilage.

prochordal (prō-kōr'dăl). Prechordal; located cephalic to the notochord.

prochymosin (prō-kī'mō-sin). The precursor of chymosin. Also called chymosinogen; pexinogen; prorennin; renninogen; rennogen.

procidentia (pros-i-den'shē-ă, prō'si-) [L. a falling forward, fr. *procido,* to fall forward]. A sinking down or prolapse of any organ or part.

p. u'teri, see *prolapse* of the uterus.

procollagen (prō-kol'ă-jen). Soluble precursor of collagen formed by fibroblasts and other cells in the process of collagen synthesis.

proconvertin (prō-kon-ver′tin). *Factor* VII.

procreate (prō′krē-āt) [L. *pro-creo,* pp. *-creatus,* to beget]. To beget; to produce by the sexual act; said usually of the male parent.

procreation (prō-krē-ā′shŭn). Reproduction (2).

procreative (prō′krē-ā-tiv). Having the power to beget or procreate.

proct-. See procto-.

proctagra (prok-tag′ră) [proct- + G. *agra,* a seizure]. Proctalgia.

proctalgia (prok-tal′jē-ă) [proct- + G. *algos,* pain]. Proctagra; proctodynia; rectalgia; pain at the anus, or in the rectum.

p. fu′gax, anorectal spasm; painful spasm of the muscle about the anus without known cause; probably a neurosis.

proctatresia (prok-tă-trē′zē-ă) [proct- + G. *a-* priv. + *trēsis,* a boring]. Anal *atresia.*

proctectasia (prok′tek-tā′zē-ă) [proct- + G. *ektasis,* extension]. Dilation of the anus or rectum.

proctectomy (prok-tek′tō-mē) [proct- + G. *ektomē,* excision]. Rectectomy; surgical resection of the rectum.

proctencleisis, proctenclisis (prok-ten-klī′sis) [proct- + G. *enkleisis,* enclosure]. Proctostenosis.

procteurynter (prok-tū-rin′ter) [proct- + G. *eurynō,* to dilate, fr. *eurys,* wide]. An inflatable bag for dilating the rectum.

proctitis (prok-tī′tis) [proct- + G. *-itis,* inflammation]. Rectitis; inflammation of the mucous membrane of the rectum.

chronic ulcerative p., idiopathic p.

epidemic gangrenous p., bicho; caribi; Indian sickness; a generally fatal disease affecting chiefly children in the tropics, characterized by gangrenous ulceration of the rectum and anus, accompanied by frequent watery stools and tenesmus.

idiopathic p., chronic ulcerative p.; probably a variant of ulcerative colitis involving the rectum; some cases progress to involve the remainder colon as well.

procto-, proct- [G. *prōktos,* anus]. Combining forms signifying anus or, more frequently, rectum. See also recto-.

proctocele (prok′tō-sēl) [procto- + G. *kēlē,* tumor]. Rectocele; prolapse or herniation of the rectum.

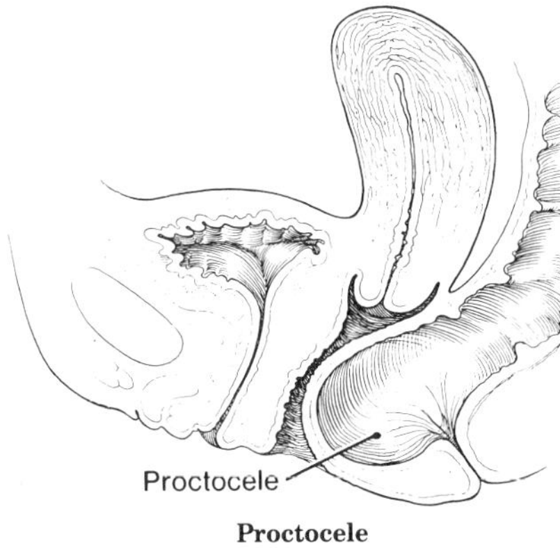

Proctocele

proctoclysis (prok-tok′li-sis) [procto- + G. *klysis,* a washing out]. Rectoclysis; Murphy drip; slow continuous administration of saline solution by instillation into the rectum and sigmoid colon.

proctococcypexy (prok-tō-kok′si-pek-sē) [procto- + G. *kokkyx,* coccyx, + *pēxis,* fixation]. Rectococcypexy; suture of a prolapsing rectum to the tissues anterior to the coccyx.

proctocolectomy (prok′tō-kō-lek′tō-mē) [procto- + G. *kolon,* colon, + *ektomē,* excision]. Surgical removal of the rectum together with part or all of the colon.

proctocolitis (prok′tō-kō-lī′tis). Coloproctitis.

proctocolonoscopy (prok′tō-kō′lō-nos′kŏ-pē) [procto- + G. *kolon,* colon, + *skopeō,* to view]. Inspection of interior of rectum and colon.

proctocolpoplasty (prok′tō-kol′pō-plas-tē) [procto- + G. *kolpos,* bosom (vagina), + *plastos,* formed]. Proctoelytroplasty; surgical closure of a rectovaginal fistula.

proctocystocele (prok′tō-sis′tō-sēl) [procto- + G. *kystis,* bladder, + *kēlē,* hernia]. Herniation of the bladder into the rectum.

proctocystoplasty (prok′tō-sis′tō-plas-tē) [procto- + G. *kystis,* bladder, + *plastos,* formed]. Surgical closure of a rectovesical fistula.

proctocystotomy (prok′tō-sis-tot′ō-mē) [procto- + G. *kystis,* bladder, + *tomē,* incision]. Incision into the bladder from the rectum.

proctodeal (prok′tō-dē-ăl). Relating to the proctodeum.

proctodeum, pl. **proctodea** (prok-tō-dē′ŭm, -dē′ă) [L. fr. G. *prōktos,* anus + *hodaios,* on the way, fr. *hodos,* a way]. **1.** Anal pit; an ectodermally lined depression under the root of the tail, adjacent to the terminal part of the embryonic hindgut; at its bottom, proctodeal ectoderm and cloacal endoderm form the cloacal plate. When this epithelial plate ruptures, the anal and urogenital external orifices are established. **2.** Terminal portion of the insect alimentary canal, extending from the pylorus (area of malpighian tubule attachment) to the anal opening; in certain diptera (flies) and other insects, the p. is divided into a tubular anterior intestine and an enlarged posterior intestine, or rectum, ending at the anus.

proctodynia (prok′tō-din′ē-ă) [procto- + G. *odynē,* pain]. Proctalgia.

proctoelytroplasty (prok-tō-el′i-trō-plas-tē) [procto- + G. *elytron,* sheath (vagina), + *plastos,* formed]. Proctocolpoplasty.

proctologic (prok-tō-loj′ik). Relating to proctology.

proctologist (prok-tol′ō-jist). A specialist in proctology.

proctology (prok-tol′ō-jē) [procto- + G. *logos,* study]. Surgical specialty concerned with the anus and rectum and their diseases.

proctoparalysis (prok′tō-pa-ral′i-sis). Paralysis of the anus, leading to incontinence of feces.

proctoperineoplasty (prok′tō-per-i-nē′ō-plas-tē) [procto- + perineum, + G. *plastos,* formed]. Proctoperineorrhaphy; rectoperineorrhaphy; plastic surgery of the anus and perineum.

proctoperineorrhaphy (prok′tō-per-i-nē-ōr′a-fē) [procto- + perineum, + G. *rhaphē,* suture]. Proctoperineoplasty.

proctopexy (prok′tō-pek-sē) [procto- + G. *pēxis,* fixation]. Rectopexy; surgical fixation of a prolapsing rectum.

proctophobia (prok-tō-fō′bē-ă) [procto- + G. *phobos,* fear]. Rectophobia; a morbid fear of rectal disease.

proctoplasty (prok′tō-plas-tē) [procto- + G. *plastos,* formed]. Rectoplasty; plastic surgery of the anus or rectum.

proctoplegia (prok′tō-plē′jē-ă) [procto- + G. *plēge,* stroke]. Paralysis of the anus and rectum occurring with paraplegia.

proctopolypus (prok-tō-pol′i-pŭs). Polypus of the rectum.

proctoptosia, proctoptosis (prok-top-tō′sē-ă, -tō′sis) [procto- + G. *ptōsis,* a falling]. Prolapse of the rectum and anus.

proctorrhagia (proc-tō-rā′jē-ă) [procto- + G. *rhēgnymi,* to burst forth]. State characterized by having a bloody discharge from the anus.

proctorrhaphy (prok-tōr′ă-fē) [procto- + G. *rhaphē,* suture]. Rectorrhaphy; repair by suture of a lacerated rectum or anus.

proctorrhea (prok-tō-rē′ă) [procto- + G. *rhoia,* a flow]. A mucoserous discharge from the rectum.

proctoscope (prok′tō-skōp) [procto- + G. *skopeō,* to view]. Rectoscope; a rectal speculum.

Tuttle's p., a tubular rectal speculum illuminated at its distal extremity; after introduction, the obturator is withdrawn and a glass window is inserted in the proximal end; then, by means of a rubber bulb and tube connected with the p., the rectal ampulla may be inflated.

proctoscopy (prok-tos'kō-pē). Rectoscopy; visual examination of the rectum and anus, as with a proctoscope.

proctosigmoidectomy (prok'tō-sig-moy-dek'tō-mē) [procto- + sigmoid, + G. *ektomē*, excision]. Excision of the rectum and sigmoid colon.

proctosigmoiditis (prok'tō-sig-moy-dī'tis) [procto- + sigmoid + G. *-itis*, inflammation]. Inflammation of the sigmoid colon and rectum.

proctosigmoidoscopy (prok'tō-sig-moy-dos'kō-pē) [procto- + sigmoid + G. *skopeō*, to view]. Direct inspection through a sigmoidoscope of the rectum and sigmoid colon.

proctospasm (prok'tō-spazm) [procto- + G. *spasmos*, spasm]. **1.** Spasmodic stricture of the anus. **2.** Spasmodic contraction of the rectum.

proctostasis (prok-tos'tă-sis) [procto- + G. *stasis*, a standing]. Constipation with stasis in the rectum.

proctostat (prok'tō-stat) [procto- + G. *statos*, standing]. A tube containing radium for insertion through the anus in the treatment of rectal cancer.

proctostenosis (prok'tō-stĕ-nō'sis) [procto- + G. *stenōsis*, a narrowing]. Proctenclisis; proctencleisis; rectostenosis; stricture of the rectum or anus.

proctostomy (prok-tos'tō-mē) [procto- + G. *stoma*, mouth]. Rectostomy; the formation of an artificial opening into the rectum.

proctotome (prok'tō-tōm). Rectotome; an instrument for use in proctotomy.

proctotomy (prok-tot'ō-mē) [procto- + G. *tomē*, incision]. Rectotomy; an incision into the rectum.

proctotresia (prok-tō-trē'zē-ă) [procto- + G. *trēsis*, a boring]. Operation for correction of an imperforate anus.

proctovalvotomy (prok'tō-val-vot'ō-mē). Incision of rectal valves.

procumbent (prō-kŭm'bent) [L. *procumbens*, falling or leaning forward]. In a prone position; lying face down.

procurvation (prō-ker-vā'shŭn) [L. *pro-curvo*, to bend forward]. A bending forward.

procyclidine hydrochloride (prō-sī'kli-dēn). 1-Cyclohexyl-1-phenyl-3-pyrrolidino-1-propanol hydrochloride; an anticholinergic agent used in the treatment of paralysis agitans and drug-induced parkinsonism.

procyclidine methochloride. Tricyclamol chloride; 1-(3-cyclohexyl-3-hydroxy-3-phenylpropyl)-1-methylpyrrolidinium chloride; an anticholinergic drug used in the treatment of functional gastrointestinal spasm.

α-prodine hydrochloride. See alphaprodine.

prodromal (prō-drō'măl, prod'rō'măl). Prodromic; prodromous; proemial; relating to a prodrome.

prodrome (prō'drōm) [G. *prodromos*, a running before, fr. pro- + *dromos*, a running, a course]. Prodromus; an early or premonitory symptom of a disease.

prodromic, prodromous (prō-drō'-mik, -mŭs; prod'rō). Prodromal.

prodromus, pl. **prodromi** (prod'rō-mŭs, -mī). Prodrome.

prodrug (prō'drŭg). A class of drugs the pharmacologic action of which results from conversion by metabolic processes within the body (biotransformation).

product (prod'ŭkt) [L. *productus*, fr. *pro-duco*, pp. *-ductus*, to lead forth]. **1.** Anything produced or made, either naturally or artificially. **2.** In mathematics, the result of multiplication.

cleavage p., a substance resulting from the splitting of a molecule into two or more simpler molecules.

double p., the p. of systolic blood pressure multiplied by the heart frequency; a measure of heart work load. See Robinson *index*.

fibrin/fibrinogen degradation p.'s (FDP), several poorly characterized small peptides, designated X, Y, D, and E, that result following the action of plasmin on fibrinogen and fibrin in the fibrinolytic process.

fission p., an atomic species produced in the course of the fission of a larger atom such as U^{235}.

orphan p.'s, drugs, biologicals, and medical devices (including diagnostic *in vitro* tests) that may be useful in common or rare diseases but which are not considered commercially viable.

spallation p., an atomic species produced in the course of the spallation of any atom.

substitution p., a p. obtained by replacing one atom or group in a molecule with another atom or group.

productive (prō-dŭk'tiv) [see product]. Producing or capable of producing; denoting especially an inflammation leading to the production of new tissue with or without an exudate.

proemial (prō-ē'mē-ăl) [L. *prooemium*, fr. G. *prooimion*, prelude]. Prodromal.

proencephalon (prō-en-sef'ă-lon). Prosencephalon.

proenzyme (prō-en'zīm). Zymogen; the precursor of an enzyme, requiring some change (usually the hydrolysis of an inhibiting fragment that masks an active grouping) to render it active; *e.g.*, pepsinogen, trypsinogen, profibrolysin.

proerythroblast (prō-ĕ-rith'rō-blast). Pronormoblast.

proerythrocyte (prō-ĕ-rith'rō-sīt). The precursor of an erythrocyte; an immature red blood cell with a nucleus.

proestrogen (prō-es'trō-jen). A substance that acts as an estrogen only after it has been metabolized in the body to an active compound.

proestrum (prō-es'trŭm). Proestrus.

proestrus (prō-es'trŭs). Proestrum; the period in the estrus cycle preceding estrus, characterized by the growth of the graafian follicles and physiologic changes related to estrogen production.

profenamine hydrochloride (pro-fen'ă-mēn). Ethopropazine hydrochloride.

proferment (prō-fer'ment). Obsolete term for proenzyme.

Profeta, Giuseppe, Italian dermatologist, 1840–1910. See P.'s *law*.

profibrinolysin (prō'fī-bri-nol'i-sin). Plasminogen. See plasmin.

Profichet, Georges C., French physician, *1873. See P.'s *disease*.

profile (prō'fīl) [It. *profilo*, fr. L. *pro*, forward, + *filum*, thread, line (contour)]. **1.** An outline or contour, especially one representing a side view of the human head. **2.** A summary, brief account, or record.

biochemical p., a combination of biochemical tests usually performed with automated instrumentation upon admission of a patient to a hospital or clinic.

facial p., **(1)** the outline form of the face from a lateral view; **(2)** the sagittal outline form of the face.

personality p., **(1)** a method by which the results of psychological testing are presented in graphic form; **(2)** a vignette or brief personality description.

test p., a combination of laboratory tests usually performed by automated methods and designed to evaluate organ systems of patients upon admission to a hospital or clinic.

urethral pressure p., the continual recording of pressure through a hole in the side of a small catheter as it is pulled (at a constant rate while either water or a gas is infused through the hole) from a point within the bladder, through the vesical neck, and down the entire urethra; a form of resistance measurement which gives a tracing indicative of the functional length of the urethra and the points of maximal urethral resistance.

profilometer (prō'fi-lom'ĕ-ter). An instrument for measuring the roughness of a surface, *e.g.,* of teeth.

proflavine (hemi)sulfate (prō-flā'vin, -vēn). The neutral sulfate of 3,6-diaminoacridine; a compound closely allied to acriflavine, having similar antiseptic properties.

profondometer (prō'fon-dom'ĕ-ter) [Fr. *profondeur,* depth, + G. *metron,* measure]. A rarely used device for fluoroscopically locating a foreign body by securing three lines of sight each of which passes through the foreign body.

proformiphen (prō-fōr'mi-fen). Phenprobamate.

profunda (prō-fŭn'dă) [L. fem. of *profundus,* deep]. A term applied to certain veins and arteries which lie deep in the tissues. See under arteria.

profundus (prō-fŭn'dŭs) [L.] [NA]. Deep; situated at a deeper level in relation to a specific reference point. *Cf.* superficialis.

progastrin (prō-gas'trin). Precursor of gastric secretion in the mucous membrane of the stomach.

progenia (prō-jē'nē-ă) [pro- + L. *gena,* cheek]. Prognathism.

progenitalis (prō-jen-i-tā'lis) [L.]. On any of the exposed surfaces of the genitalia.

progenitor (prō-jen'i-ter, -tōr) [L.]. A precursor, ancestor; one who begets.

progeny (proj'ĕ-nē) [L. *progenies,* fr. *progigno,* to beget]. Offspring; descendants.

progeria (prō-jēr'ē-ă) [pro- + G. *gēras,* old age]. Hutchinson-Gilford disease or syndrome; premature senility syndrome; a condition in which normal development in the first year is followed by gross retardation of growth, with a senile appearance characterized by dry wrinkled skin, total alopecia, and bird-like facies.

p. with cataract, p. with microphthalmia, *dyscephalia* mandibulo-oculofacialis.

progeroid (prō-jer'oyd) [pro + G. *geras,* old age + G. *eidos,* resemblance]. Resembling old age.

progestational (prō'jes-tā'shŭn-ăl). **1.** Favoring pregnancy; conducive to gestation; capable of stimulating the uterine changes essential for implantation and growth of a fertilized ovum. **2.** Referring to progesterone, or to a drug with progesterone-like properties.

progesterone (prō-jes'ter-ōn). Progestational or corpus luteum hormone; luteohormone; 4-pregnene-3,20-dione; an antiestrogenic steroid, believed to be the active principle of the corpus luteum, isolated from the corpus luteum and placenta or synthetically prepared; used to correct abnormalities of the menstrual cycle.

progestin (prō-jes'tin). **1.** A hormone of the corpus luteum. **2.** Generic term for any substance, natural or synthetic, that effects some or all of the biological changes produced by progesterone.

progestogen (prō-jes'tō-jen). **1.** Any agent capable of producing biological effects similar to those of progesterone; most p.'s are steroids like the natural hormones. **2.** A synthetic derivative from testosterone or progesterone that has some of the physiologic activity and pharmacologic effects of progesterone; progesterone is antiestrogenic, whereas some p.'s have estrogenic or androgenic properties in addition to progestational activity.

proglossis (prō-glos'is) [pro- + G. *glōssa,* tongue]. The anterior portion, or tip, of the tongue.

proglottid (prō-glot'id) [pro- + G. *glōssa,* tongue]. Proglottis; one of the segments of a tapeworm, containing the reproductive organs.

proglottis, pl. **proglottides** (prō-glot'is, -i-dēz). Proglottid.

prognathic (prog-nath'ik, -nā'thik) [pro- + G. *gnathos,* jaw]. Prognathous. **1.** Having a projecting jaw; having a gnathic index above 103. **2.** Denoting a forward projection of either or both of the jaws relative to the craniofacial skeleton.

prognathism (prog'nă-thizm). Progenia; the condition of being prognathic; abnormal forward projection of one or of both jaws beyond the established normal relationship with the cranial base; the mandibular condyles are in their normal rest relationship to the temporomandibular joints.

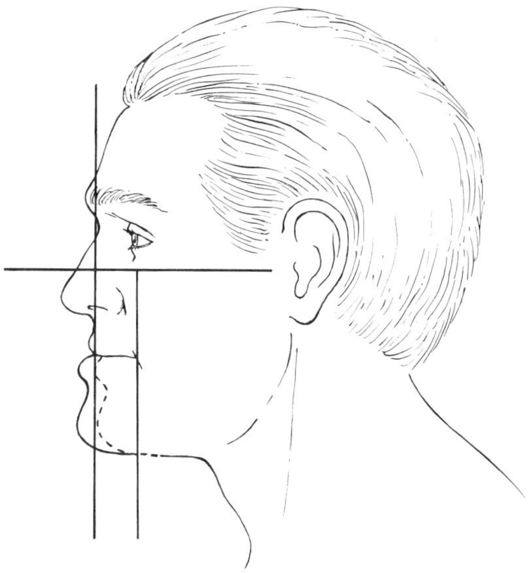

Prognathism

basilar p., the concave facial profile, or forward position of the chin, resembling mandibular p., created by the prominence of the bone of the mandible at the chin or menton.

prognathous (prog'nă-thŭs). Prognathic.

prognose (prog-nōs', -nōz'). Prognosticate.

prognosis (prog-nō'sis) [G. *prognōsis,* fr. *pro,* before, + *gignōskō,* to know]. A forecast of the probable course and/or outcome of a disease.

denture p., an opinion or judgment, given in advance of treatment, of the prospects for success in the construction and usefulness of a denture or restoration.

prognostic (prog-nos'tik) [G. *prognōstikos*]. **1.** Relating to prognosis. **2.** A symptom upon which a prognosis is based, or one indicative of the likely outcome.

prognosticate (prog-nos'ti-kāt). Prognose; to give a prognosis.

prognostician (prog-nos-tish'ŭn). One skilled in prognosis.

progonoma (prō-gon-ō'mă) [pro- + G. *gonōs,* offspring, + *-oma,* tumor]. A nodule or mass resulting from displacement of tissue when atavism occurs in embryonic development; represents a reversion to structures not normally occurring in the individuals of a species, but observed in ancestral forms of that species.

p. of jaw, melanotic neuroectodermal *tumor.*

melanotic p., a pigmented hairy nevus.

progranulocyte (prō-gran'yū-lō-sīt). Promyelocyte.

progress [L. *pro-gredior,* pp. *-gressus,* to go forth, fr. *gradior,* to step, go, fr. *gradus,* a step]. **1** (prog'res). An advance; the course of a disease. **2** (prō-gres'). To advance; to go forward; said of a disease, especially, when unqualified, of one taking an unfavorable course.

progressive (prō-gres'iv). Going forward; advancing; denoting the course of a disease, especially, when unqualified, an unfavorable course.

proguanil hydrochloride (prō-gwah'nil). Chloroguanide hydrochloride.

prohormone (prō-hōr'mōn). **1.** An intraglandular precursor of a hormone; *e.g.,* proinsulin. *Cf.* prehormone. **2.** Obsolete term formerly used to designate a substance developed in serum that antagonizes a specific antihormone, and thus enhances the action of the corresponding hormone.

proinsulin (prō-in'sŭ-lin). A single-chain precursor of insulin.

proiosystole (pro-ē-ō-sis'tō-lē) [G. *prōios,* early, + *systolē,* a contracting]. A heart beat occurring ahead of schedule. See also hysterosystole.

proiosystolia (prō-ē-ō-sis-tōl'ē-ă). Condition in which proiosystoles occur.

projection (prō-jek'shŭn) [L. *projectio;* fr. *pro- jicio,* pp. *-jectus,* to throw before]. **1.** A pushing out. **2.** The referring of a sensation to the object producing it. **3.** A defense mechanism by which a repressed complex in the individual is referred to another person, as when faults which the person tends to commit are perceived in or attributed to others. **4.** The conception by the consciousness of a mental occurrence belonging to the self as of external origin. **5.** Localization of visual impressions in space. **6.** In neuroanatomy, the system or systems of nerve fibers by which a group of nerve cells discharges its nerve impulses ("projects") to one or more other cell groups. **7.** The image of a three dimensional object on a plane; as in a radiograph.

axial p., axial view; base p.; base view; verticulosubmental view; radiographic p. devised to obtain direct visualization of the base of the skull.

base p., axial p.

Caldwell p., Caldwell view; radiographic p. devised to permit visualization of orbital structures unobstructed by the petrous ridges.

enamel p., extension of enamel into furcation.

erroneous p., false p.

false p., erroneous p.; the faulty visual sensation arising secondarily to underaction of an ocular muscle.

Stenvers p., Stenvers view; radiographic p. devised to provide an unobstructed view of the petrous bone, bony labyrinth, internal auditory canal, and meatus.

Towne p., Towne view; radiographic p. devised to permit demonstration of the entire occipital bone, foramen magnum, and dorsum sellae, as well as a view of the petrous ridges.

visual p., a perceptual synthesis involving visual mechanisms.

Prokaryotae (pro-kar-ē-ō'tē). Procaryotae; a superkingdom of organisms that includes the kingdom Monera (bacteria and blue-green algae) and, in some systems, a kingdom for viruses; characterized by the prokaryotic condition, minute size (10-300 nm for viruses, 0.2-10 μm for bacteria) and absence of the nuclear organization, mitotic capacities, and complex organelles that typify the superkingdom Eukaryotae.

prokaryote (prō-kar'ē-ōt). Procaryote; a member of the superkingdom Prokaryotae; an organismic unit consisting of a single and presumably primitive moneran cell, or a precellular organism, which lacks a nuclear membrane, paired organized chromosomes, a mitotic mechanism for cell division, microtubules, and mitochondria; viruses are often considered to be subcellular or even nonliving infectious units that require a host cell for replication and may have been derived from an ancestral cell. See also Prokaryotae; Monera; eukaryote.

prokaryotic (prō'kar-ē-ot'ik). Procaryotic; pertaining to or characteristic of a prokaryote.

prolabial (prō-lā'bē-ăl). Denoting the isolated central soft-tissue segment of the upper lip in the embryonic state and in an unrepaired bilateral cleft palate.

prolabium (prō-lā'bē-ŭm) [pro- + L. *labium,* lip]. **1.** The exposed carmine margin of the lip. **2.** The isolated central soft-tissue segment of the upper lip in the embryonic state and in an unrepaired bilateral cleft palate.

prolactin (PRL) (prō-lak'tin). A protein hormone of the anterior lobe of the hypophysis that stimulates the secretion of milk and possibly, during pregnancy, breast growth. Also called lactogenic, mammotropic, or galactopoietic factor or hormone; lactotropin.

prolactinoma (prō-lak-ti-nō'mă). Prolactin-producing *adenoma.*

prolactoliberin (prō-lak-tō-lib'er-in). Prolactin releasing factor or hormone; a substance of hypothalamic origin that stimulates the release of prolactin.

prolactostatin (prō-lak-tō-stat'in). Prolactin inhibiting factor or hormone; a substance of hypothalamic origin capable of inhibiting the synthesis and release of prolactin.

prolamines (prō-lam'ēnz, prō'lă-mēnz, -minz). Proteins insoluble in water or neutral salt solutions, soluble in dilute acids or alkalies, and in 70 to 90% alcohol; *e.g.,* gliadin, zein.

prolapse (prō-laps') [L. *prolapsus,* a falling]. **1.** To sink down, said of an organ or other part. **2.** A sinking of an organ or other part, especially its appearance at a natural or artificial orifice. See also procidentia; ptosis.

p. of the corpus luteum, ectropion of the corpus luteum, due to eversion of the granulosa membrane through the opening in the ruptured follicle; this occurs normally in certain animals.

mitral valve p., excessive retrograde movement of the mitral valve into the left atrium during left ventricular systole, often allowing mitral regurgitation; responsible for the click-murmur of Barlow syndrome, and may be due to rheumatic carditis or a connective tissue disorder such as Marfan's syndrome.

Morgagni's p., chronic inflammation of Morgagni's ventricle.

p. of umbilical cord, presentation of part of the umbilical cord ahead of the fetus; it may cause fetal death due to compression of the cord between the presenting part of the fetus and the maternal pelvis.

p. of the uterus, descensus uteri; falling of the womb; downward movement of the uterus due to laxity and atony of the muscular and fascial structures of the pelvic floor, usually resulting from injuries of childbirth or advanced age; p. occurs in three forms; **first degree p.,** the cervix of the prolapsed uterus is well within the vaginal orifice; **second degree p.,** the cervix is at or near the introitus; **third degree p.** (procidentia uteri), the cervix protrudes well beyond the vaginal orifice.

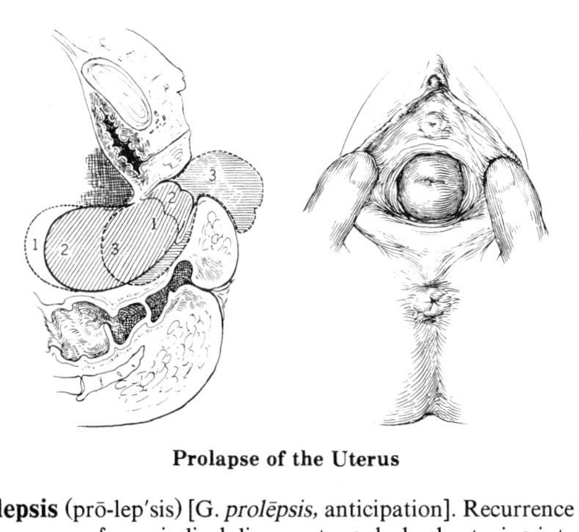

Prolapse of the Uterus

prolepsis (prō-lep'sis) [G. *prolēpsis,* anticipation]. Recurrence of the paroxysm of a periodical disease at regularly shortening intervals.

proleptic (prō-lep'tik). Subintrant; relating to prolepsis.

proleukocyte (prō-lū'kō-sīt). Leukoblast.

prolidase (prō'li-dās). *Proline* dipeptidase.

proliferate (prō-lif'ĕ-rāt) [L. *proles,* offspring, + *fero,* to bear]. To grow and increase in number by means of reproduction of similar forms.

proliferation (prō-lif-ĕ-rā'shŭn). Growth and reproduction of similar cells.
diffuse mesangial p., mesangial proliferative *glomerulonephritis.*
gingival p., gingival *hyperplasia.*

proliferative, proliferous (prō-lif'er-ă-tiv, -er-ŭs). Increasing the numbers of similar forms.

prolific (prō-lif'ik) [L. *proles,* offspring, + *facio,* to make]. Fruitful; bearing many children.

proligerous (prō-lij'er-ŭs) [L. *proles,* offspring, + *gero,* to bear]. Germinating; producing offspring.

prolinase (prō'li-nās). *Prolyl* dipeptidase.

proline (Pro) (prō'lēn). 2-Pyrrolidinecarboxylic acid; an amino acid that is a protein, especially collagens.

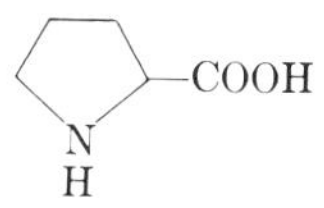

Proline

p. aminopeptidase, p. iminopeptidase.
p. dehydrogenase, pyrroline 2- or 5-carboxylate reductase.
p. dipeptidase [EC 3.4.13.9], prolidase; imidodipeptidase; an enzyme cleaving aminoacyl-proline bonds.
p. iminopeptidase [EC 3.4.11.5], p. aminopeptidase; a hydrolase cleaving L-proline residues from the N-terminal position in peptides.
p. oxidase, pyrroline 2- or 5-carboxylate reductase.
p. racemase [EC 5.1.1.4], an enzyme that converts D-proline to L-proline.

D-proline reductase [EC 1.4.1.6]. An oxidoreductase cleaving D-proline (not the natural form) to 5-aminovalerate, with dihydrolipoate as hydrogen donor.

prolyl (prō'lil). The acyl radical of proline.
p. dipeptidase [EC 3.4.13.8], iminodipeptidase; prolinase; prolylglycine dipeptidase; an enzyme cleaving L-prolyl-aminoacid bonds.

prolylglycine dipeptidase (prō'lil-glī'sēn). *Prolyl* dipeptidase.

promastigote (prō-mas'ti-gōt) [pro- + G. *mastix,* whip]. Term now generally used instead of "leptomonad" or "leptomonad stage," to avoid confusion with the flagellate genus *Leptomonas.* It denotes the flagellate stage of a trypanosomatid protozoan in which the flagellum arises from a kinetoplast in front of the nucleus and emerges from the anterior end of the organism; usually an extracellular phase, as in the insect intermediate host (or in culture) of *Leishmania* parasites.

promazine hydrochloride (prō'mă-zēn). 10-(3-Dimethylaminopropyl)phenothiazine hydrochloride; a phenothiazine tranquilizing agent with actions and uses similar to those of chlorpromazine.

promegaloblast (prō-meg'ă-lō-blast). The earliest of four maturation stages of the megaloblast. See discussion under erythroblast.

prometaphase (prō-met'ă-fāz). The stage of mitosis or meiosis in which the nuclear membrane disintegrates, the centrioles reach the poles of the cell, and the chromosomes continue to contract.

promethazine hydrochloride (prō-meth'ă-zēn). 10-(2-Dimethylaminopropyl)phenothiazine hydrochloride; an antihistaminic.

promethazine theoclate (prō-meth'ă-zēn). Promethiazine salt of 8-chlorotheophylline; an antihistaminic drug used for motion sickness.

promethestrol dipropionate (prō-meth'es-trol dī-prō'pē-ō-nāt). Dimethylhexestrol dipropionate; 4,4'-(1,2-diethylethylene)di-*o*-cresol dipropionate; a synthetic estrogen derived from stilbene.

promethium (prō-mē'thē-ŭm) [*Prometheus,* a Titan of G. myth.]. A radioactive element of the rare earth series, symbol Pm, atomic no. 61; isolated in 1948 among the fission products of uranium-235.

prominence (prom'i-nens) [L. *prominentia*]. Prominentia.
Ammon's p., an external p. in the posterior pole of the eyeball during early embryogenesis.
canine p., canine *eminence.*
cardiac p., the conspicuous external bulge appearing on the ventral aspect of the human embryo as early as at the fourth week, indicative of the precocious development of the heart.
p. of facial canal, *prominentia* canalis facialis.
forebrain p., frontonasal *elevation.*
hepatic p., the conspicuous external bulge appearing dorsocaudal to the cardiac p. on the body of the human embryo at about the fourth week, indicating the precocious development of the liver.
hypothenar p., hypothenar (1).
laryngeal p., *prominentia* laryngea.
p. of lateral semicircular canal, *prominentia* semicircularis lateralis.
mallear p., *prominentia* mallearis.
spiral p., *prominentia* spiralis.
styloid p., *prominentia* styloidea.
thenar p., thenar (1).

prominens (prom'i-nens) [L.]. Prominent; in anatomy, denoting a prominence.

prominentia, pl. **prominentiae** (prom-i-nen'shē-ă, -shē-ē) [L. fr. *promineo,* to jut out, be prominent] [NA]. Prominence; in anatomy, tissues or parts that project beyond a surface.
p. cana'lis facia'lis [NA], prominence of facial canal; the prominence on the medial wall of the tympanic cavity above the vestibular (oval) window produced by the presence of the facial canal.
p. cana'lis semicircula'ris latera'lis [NA], prominence of lateral semicircular canal; the slight bulge in the medial wall of the epitympanic recess caused by the proximity of the lateral semicircular canal.
p. laryn'gea [NA], laryngeal prominence; Adam's apple; thyroid eminence; protuberantia laryngea; the projection on the anterior portion of the neck formed by the thyroid cartilage of the larynx.
p. mallea'ris [NA], mallear prominence; a small prominence at the upper end of the stria mallearis produced by the lateral process of the malleus.
p. spira'lis [NA], spiral prominence; a projecting portion of the ligamentum spirale cochleae, bounding the lower edge of the stria vascularis and containing within it a blood vessel, the vas prominens.
p. styloi'dea [NA], styloid prominence; a rounded eminence on the posterior wall (paries mastoidea) of the tympanic cavity corresponding to the base of the styloid process.

promonocyte (prō-mon'ō-sīt). Premonocyte.

promontorium, pl. **promontoria** (prom'on-tō'rē-ŭm, -rē-ă) [L. a mountain ridge, a headland, fr. *promineo,* to jut out] [NA]. A projection of a part.
p. ca'vi tym'pani, tympanic promontory; tuber cochleae; a rounded eminence on the labyrinthine wall of the middle ear, caused by the first coil of the cochlea.
p. os'sis sa'cri, pelvic promontory; promontory of sacrum; the most prominent anterior projection of the base of the sacrum.

promontory (prom'on-tō-rē) [L. *promontorium*]. An eminence or projection. See promontorium.
pelvic p., *promontorium* ossis sacri.
p. of the sacrum, *promontorium* ossis sacri.

tympanic p., *promontorium* cavi tympani.

promoter (prō-mō'ter). **1.** In chemistry, a substance that increases the activity of a catalyst. **2.** In molecular biology, a DNA sequence at which RNA polymerase binds and initiates transcription.

promotion (prō-mō'shŭn). Stimulation of tumor induction, following initiation, by a promoting agent which may of itself be noncarcinogenic.

promyelocyte (prō-mī'ĕ-lō-sīt) [pro- + G. *myelos*, marrow, + *kytos*, cell]. Granular leukoblast; progranulocyte. **1.** The developmental stage of a granular leukocyte between the myeloblast and myelocyte, when a few specific granules appear in addition to azurophilic ones. **2.** A large uninuclear cell occurring in the circulating blood of persons with myelocytic leukemia.

pronasion (prō-nā'zē-on) [pro- + L. *nasus*, nose]. The point of the angle between the septum of the nose and the surface of the upper lip, found at the point where a tangent applied to the nasal septum meets the upper lip.

pronate (prō'nāt) [L. *pronatus*, fr. *prono*, pp. *-atus*, to bend forward, fr. *pronus*, bent forward]. **1.** To assume, or to be placed in, a prone position. **2.** To perform pronation of the forearm or foot.

pronation (prō-nā'shŭn). The condition of being prone; the act of assuming or of being placed in a prone position.
p. of foot, eversion and abduction of the foot, causing a lowering of the medial edge.
p. of forearm, rotation of the forearm in such a way that the palm of the hand faces backward when the arm is in the anatomical position, or downward when the arm is extended at a right angle to the body.

pronatis (prō-nā'tis) [L. *pro*, before, + *nasce*, born]. A baby born prematurely.

pronator (prō-nā'ter, tōr) [L.]. A muscle which turns a part into the prone position. See entries under musculus.

prone (prōn) [L. *pronus*, bending down or forward]. Denoting: **1.** The body when lying face downward. **2.** Pronation of the forearm or of the foot.

pronephros, pl. **pronephroi** (prō-nef'ros, -roy) [pro- + G. *nephros*, kidney]. Forekidney; primordial kidney. **1.** Head kidney; the definitive excretory organ of primitive fishes. **2.** In the embryos of higher vertebrates, a vestigial structure consisting of a series of tortuous tubules emptying into the cloaca by way of the primary nephric duct; in the human embryo, the p. is a very rudimentary and temporary structure, followed by the mesonephros and still later by the metanephros.

pronethalol hydrochloride (prō-neth'ă-lol). The hydrochloride of 2-isopropylamino-1-(2-naphthyl)ethanol; an adrenergic β-receptor blocking agent used as an antagonist of the cardiac action of epinephrine.

pronograde (prō'nō-grād) [L. *pronus*, inclined forward, + *gradior*, to walk]. Walking or resting with the body horizontal, denoting the posture of quadrupeds; opposed to orthograde.

pronometer (prō-nom'ĕ-ter). Goniometer (3).

pronormoblast (prō-nōr'mō-blast). Proerythroblast; rubriblast; the earliest of four stages in development of the normoblast. See also erythroblast.

pronucleus, pronuclei (prō-nū'klē-ŭs, -klē-ī). **1.** One of two nuclei undergoing fusion in karyogamy. **2.** In embryology, the nuclear material of the head of the spermatozoon (**male p.**) or of the ovum (**female p.**), after the ovum has been penetrated by the spermatozoon; each p. carries the haploid number of chromosomes, so that the merging of the pronuclei in fertilization reestablishes the diploid number of chromosomes characteristic of the species.

prootic (prō-ō'tik) [pro- + G. *ous*, ear]. In front of the ear.

propadiene (prō-pă-dī'ēn). Allene.

propagate (prop'ă-gāt) [L. *propago*, pp. *-atus*, to generate, reproduce]. **1.** To reproduce; to generate. **2.** To move along a fiber, *e.g.*, propagation of the nerve impulse.

propagation (prop-ă-gā'shŭn). The act of propagating.

propagative (prop-ă-gā'tiv). Relating to or concerned in propagation; denoting the sexual part of an animal or plant as distinguished from the soma.

propalinal (prō-pal'i-năl) [pro- + G. *palin*, backward]. Back and forth; denoting a forward and backward movement.

propamidine (prō-pam'i-dēn). 4,4'-Diamidino-1,3-diphenoxypropane; active against *Trypanosoma gambiensi* infections; also markedly bacteriostatic; used as a local anti-infective agent in 0.1% aqueous solution, and against systemic fungal infections such as blastomycosis.

propane (prō'pān). $CH_3CH_2CH_3$; one of the alkane series of hydrocarbons.

propanedioic acid (prō-pān-dī'ō-ik). Malonic acid.

1,2,3-**propanetriol** (prō-pān-trī'ol). Glycerol.

propanidid (prō-pan'i-did). Propyl{4- [(diethylcarbamoyl)-methoxy]-3-methoxyphenyl}acetate; a short-acting eugenol used intravenously for induction of general anesthesia.

propanoic acid (prō-pă-nō'ik). Propionic acid.

propanol (prō'pă-nol). *Propyl* alcohol.

propanolol (prō-pan'ō-lol). Propanolol hydrochloride.

propanoyl (prō'pă-nō-īl). Propionyl.

propantheline bromide (pro-pan'thĕ-lēn). β-Diisopropylmethylaminoethyl-9-xanthine carboxylate bromide; the isopropyl analogue of methantheline bromide; an anticholinergic agent.

proparacaine hydrochloride (prō-par'ă-kān). Proxymetacainehydrochloride; 2-diethylaminoethyl-3-amino-4-propoxybenzoate hydrochloride; a surface anesthetic agent used in ophthalmology.

propatyl nitrate (prō'pă-til). 2-Ethyl-2-(hydroxymethyl)-1,3-propanediol trinitrate; a coronary vasodilator.

propene (prō'pēn). Propylene.

propentdyopents (prō-pent-dī'ō-pentz). See bilirubinoids.

propenyl (prō'pē-nil). The radical, $-CH{=}CH-CH_3$.

propepsin (prō-pep'sin). Pepsinogen.

propeptone (prō-pep'tōn). A nondescript mixture of intermediate products in the conversion of native protein into peptone.

properdin (prō-per'din). A normal serum γ_2-globulin (MW 185,000) that participates, in conjunction with other factors, in an alternate pathway to the activation of the terminal components of complement. See also p. *system; component* of complement.

properitoneal (prō'per-i-tō-nē'ăl). In front of the peritoneum.

prophage (prō'fāj). Probacteriophage.
defective p., see defective *bacteriophage*.

prophase (prō'fāz) [G. *prophasis*, from *prophainō*, to foreshadow]. The first stage of mitosis or meiosis, consisting of linear contraction and increase in thickness of the chromosomes (each composed of two chromatids) accompanied by migration of the two daughter centrioles and their asters toward the poles of the cell. In meiosis, p. is complex and can be subdivided into stages: preleptotene, leptotene, zygotene, pachytene, diplotene, and diakinesis.

prophenpyridamine maleate (prō'fen-pi-rid'ă-mēn). Pheniramine maleate.

prophlogistic (prō-flō-jis'tik) [pro- + G. *phlogōsis*, inflammation]. Causing or producing tissue inflammation.

prophylactic (prō-fi-lak'tik) [G. *prophylaktikos;* see prophylaxis]. **1.** Preventive; preventing disease; relating to prophylaxis. **2.** An agent that acts to prevent a disease.

prophylaxis, pl. **prophylaxes** (prō-fi-lak'sis, -sēz) [Mod. L. fr. G. *pro-phylassō,* to guard before, take precaution]. Prevention of disease or of a process which can lead to disease.
active p., use of an antigenic (immunogenic) agent to actively stimulate the immunological mechanism.
chemical p., the administration of chemicals or drugs to members of a community to reduce the number of carriers of a disease and to prevent others contracting the disease.
dental p., a series of procedures whereby calculus, stain, and other accretions are removed from the clinical crowns of the teeth, and the enamel surfaces are polished.
passive p., use of an antiserum from another person or animal to provide temporary (a week to 10 days) protection against a specific infectious or toxic agent.

propicillin (prō-pi-sil'in). α-Phenoxypropylpenicillin potassium; a semisynthetic acid-stable penicillin that may be more effective than penicillin G.

propiolactone (prō'pē-ō-lak'tōn). β-Propiolactone; hydracrylic acid β-lactone; used to sterilize plasma, vaccines, and tissue grafts.

propiomazine (prō-pē-ō'mā-zēn). 1-[10-[2-(Dimethylamino)propyl]phenothiazin-2-yl]-1-propanone; used intramuscularly or intravenously as a preanesthetic sedative.

propionate (prō'pē-ō-nāt). A salt or ester of propionic acid.

Propionibacterium (prō-pē-on-i-bak-tēr'ē-ŭm). A genus of nonmotile, nonsporeforming, anaerobic to aerotolerant bacteria (family Propionibacteriaceae) containing Gram-positive rods which are usually pleomorphic, diphtheroid, or club-shaped with one end rounded, the other tapered or pointed. Some cells may be coccoid, elongate, bifid, or even branched. The cells usually occur singly, in pairs, in V and Y configurations, short chains, or clumps in "Chinese character" arrangement. The metabolism of these organisms is fermentative, and the products of fermentation include combinations of propionic and acetic acids. These organisms occur in dairy products, on the skin of man, and in the intestinal tract of man and other animals. They may be pathogenic. The type species is *P. freudenreichii.*
P. ac'nes, *Corynebacterium acnes;* acne bacillus; a species of bacteria commonly found in acne pustules, although it occurs in other types of lesions in humans and even as a saprophyte in the intestine, skin, hair follicles, and in sewage.
P. freudenrei'chii, a species found in raw milk, Swiss cheese, and other dairy products; it is the type species of the genus *P.*
P. jensen'ii, a species found in dairy products, silage, and occasionally in infections.

propionic acid (prō-pē-on'ik). Propanoic acid; methylacetic acid; ethylformic acid; CH_3CH_2COOH; found in sweat.

propionicacidemia (prō-pē-on'ik-as-i-dē'mē-ā). Presence of excess propionic acid in the blood, caused by a deficiency of propionyl-CoA carboxylase; characterized by vomiting, lethargy, ketoacidosis, and leukopenia.

propionyl (prō'pē-ō-nil). Propanoyl; CH_3CH_2CO–; the acyl radical of propionic acid.

propitocaine hydrochloride (prō-pit'ō-kān). Prilocaine hydrochloride.

proplasia (prō-plā'zē-ā) [pro- + G. *plassō,* to form]. That state of cell or tissue in which activity is increased above that of euplasia, *i.e.,* characterized by stimulation, repair, or regeneration.

proplasmacyte (prō-plaz'mā-sīt). A cell in the process of differentiating from a plasmablast to a mature plasma cell.

proplexus (prō-plek'sŭs). The choroid plexus in the lateral ventricle of the brain.

propositus, pl. **propos'iti** (prō'poz'i-tŭs, -tī) [L. fr. *propono,* pp. *-positus,* to lay out, propound]. **1.** Proband. **2.** A premise; an argument.

propoxycaine hydrochloride (prō-pok'sē-kān). 2'-Diethylaminoethyl-2-propoxy-4-aminobenzoate hydrochloride; a local anesthetic.

propoxyphene hydrochloride (prō-pok'si-fēn). Dextropropoxyphene hydrochloride; (+)-α-4-(dimethylamino)-3-methyl-1,2-diphenyl-2-butanol propionate hydrochloride; a nonantipyretic, orally effective analgesic structurally related to methadone and used for the relief of mild to moderate pain; it is less effective than codeine but with less liability for abuse.

propoxyphene napsylate (prō-pok'si-fēn). Dextropropoxyphene napsylate; mono-2-naphthalenesulfonate monohydrate salt of propoxyphene; an analgesic.

propranolol hydrochloride (prō-pran'ō-lōl). Propanolol; 1-(isopropylamino)-3-(1-naphthyloxy)-2-propanol hydrochloride; an adrenergic β-receptor blocking agent.

proprietary name (prō-prī'ĕ-tār-ē) [L. *proprietarius*]. The protected brand name or trademark, registered with the U.S. Patent Office, under which a manufacturer markets his product. It is written with a capital initial letter and is often further distinguished by a superscript R in a circle (®). *Cf.* generic name; nonproprietary name.

proprioceptive (prō'prē-ō-sep'tiv) [L. *proprius,* one's own, + *capio,* to take]. Capable of receiving stimuli originating in muscles, tendons, and other internal tissues.

proprioceptor (prō'prē-ō-sep'ter). One of a variety of sensory end organs (such as the muscle spindle and Golgi's tendon organ) in muscles, tendons, and joint capsules.

propriospinal (prō'prē-ō-spī'năl). Relating especially or wholly to the spinal cord; specifically, denoting those nerve cells and their fibers that connect the different segments of the spinal cord with each other (*e.g.,* spino-spinalis).

proptometer (prop-tom'ĕ-ter) [pro- + G. *ptōsis,* a falling, + *metron,* measure]. Exophthalmometer.

proptosis (prop-tō'sis) [G. *proptōsis,* a falling forward]. A forward displacement of any organ; specifically, exophthalmos or protrusion of the eyeball.

proptotic (prop-tot'ik). Referring to proptosis.

propulsion (prō-pŭl'shŭn) [G. *pro-pello,* pp. *-pulsus,* to drive forth]. The tendency to fall forward that causes the festination in paralysis agitans.

propyl (prō'pil). The alkyl radical of propane, $CH_3CH_2CH_2$–.
p. alcohol, propanol; ethylcarbinol; $CH_3CH_2CH_2OH$; a solvent for resins and cellulose esters.
p. gallate, propyl 3,4,5-trihydroxybenzoate; an antioxidant for emulsions.
p. hydroxybenzoate, propylparaben.

propylcarbinol (prō-pil-kar'bi-nol). Primary butyl alcohol. See butyl alcohol.

propylene (prō'pi-lēn). Propene; methylethylene; $CH_2{=}CHCH_3$; a gaseous olefinic hydrocarbon.
p. glycol, 1,2-propanediol; 1,2-dihydroxypropane; CH_3CHOH-CH_2OH; an ingredient of hydrophilic ointment; also used as a diluent, its toxicity being about the same as glycerin.

propylhexedrine (prō-pil-hek'se-drēn). *N*,α-Dimethylcyclohexaneethylamine; 1-cyclohexyl-2-methylaminopropane; a sympathomimetic and local vasoconstrictor.

propyliodone (prō-pil-ī'ō-dōn). Propyl-3,5-diiodo-4-oxo-1(4*H*)pyridineacetate; a radiopaque medium used for bronchography.

propylparaben (prō-pil-par'ă-ben). Propyl hydroxybenzoate; *p*-hydroxybenzoic acid propyl ester; an antifungal agent and pharmaceutical preservative.

propylthiouracil (PTU) (prō'pil-thī-ō-yū'ră-sil). 6-Propyl-2-thiouracil; an antithyroid agent that inhibits the synthesis of thyroid hormones; used in the treatment of hyperthyroidism.

propyromazine (prō-pi-rō'mă-zēn). 1-Methyl-1-[1-(phenothiazin-10-ylcarbonyl)ethyl]pyrrolidinium bromide; an intestinal antispasmodic with anticholinergic properties.

pro rat. aet. Abbreviation for L. *pro ratione aetatis,* according to (patient's) age.

pro re nata (p.r.n.) (prō rē nā'tă) [L.]. As the occasion arises.

prorennin (prō-ren'in). Prochymosin.

prorsad (prōr'sad) [L. *prorsum,* forward, + *ad,* to]. In a forward direction.

prorubricyte (prō-rū'bri-sīt) [pro- + rubricyte]. Basophilic normoblast. See discussion under erythroblast.

pernicious anemia type p., basophilic megaloblast. See discussion under erythroblast.

proscillaridin (prō-si-lar'i-din). Desglucotransvaaline; scillarenin 3β-rhamnoside; 14-hydroxy-3β-(rhamnosyloxy)bufa-4,20,22-trienolide; prepared from *Urginea maritima;* a cardiotonic agent, used for the treatment of congestive heart failure.

proscolex (prō-skō'leks) [pro- + G. *skōlēx,* a worm]. The embryonic form of a tapeworm.

prosecretin (prō-sē-krē'tin). Unactivated secretin.

prosect (prō-sekt') [L. *pro-seco,* pp. *-sectus,* to cut]. To dissect a cadaver or any part, that it may serve for a demonstration of anatomy before a class.

prosector (prō'sek'ter). One who prosects, or prepares the material for a demonstration of anatomy before a class.

prosectorium (prō'sek-tō'rē-ŭm) [L.]. A dissecting room; a place in which anatomical preparations are made for demonstration or for preservation in a museum.

prosencephalon (pros-en-sef'ă-lon) [G. *prosō,* forward, + *enkephalos,* brain] [NA]. Forebrain; proencephalon; forebrain vesicle; the anterior primitive cerebral vesicle and the most rostral of the three primary brain vesicles of the embryonic neural tube which divides in further development into diencephalon and telencephalon.

Proskauer, Bernhard, German bacteriologist, 1851–1915. See Voges-P. *reaction.*

prosodemic (pros-ō-dem'ik) [G. *prosō,* forward, + *dēmos,* people]. Denoting a disease that is transmitted directly from person to person.

prosop-. See prosopo-.

prosopagnosia (pros'ō-pag-nō'sē-ă) [prosop- + G. *a-* priv. + *gnōsis,* recognition]. Difficulty in recognizing familiar faces.

prosopagus (pro-sop'ă-gŭs). Prosopopagus.

prosopalgia (pros-ō-pal'jē-ă) [prosop- + G. *algos,* pain]. Trigeminal *neuralgia.*

prosopalgic (pros-ō-pal'jik). Relating to or suffering from trigeminal neuralgia.

prosopectasia (pros'ō-pek-tā'zē-ă) [prosop- + G. *ektasis,* extension]. Enlargement of the face, as in acromegaly.

prosoplasia (pros-ō-plā'zē-ă) [G. *prosō,* forward, + *plasis,* a molding]. Progressive transformation, such as the change of cells of the salivary ducts into secreting cells.

prosopo-, prosop- [G. *prosōpon,* face, countenance]. Combining forms denoting the face. See also facio-.

prosopoanoschisis (pros'ō-pō-ă-nos'ki-sis) [prosopo- + G. *anō,* upward, + *schisis,* fissure]. Facial *cleft.*

prosopodiplegia (pros'ō-pō-dī-plē'jē-ă) [prosopo- + diplegia]. Paralysis affecting both sides of the face.

prosoponeuralgia (pros'ō-pō-nū-ral'jē-ă). Trigeminal *neuralgia.*

prosopopagus (pros-ō-pop'ă-gŭs) [prosopo- + G. *pagos,* something fastened]. Prosopagus; unequal conjoined twins in which the parasite, in the form of a tumor-like mass, is attached to the orbit or cheek of the autosite.

prosopoplegia (pros'ō-pō-plē'jē-ă) [prosopo- + G. *plēgē,* stroke]. Facial *palsy.*

prosopoplegic (pros'ō-pō-plē'jik). Relating to, or suffering from, facial paralysis.

prosoposchisis (pros-ō-pos'ki-sis) [prosopo- + G. *schisis,* fissure]. Oblique facial cleft; congenital facial cleft from mouth to orbit.

prosopospasm (pros'ō-pō-spazm) [prosopo- + G. *spasmos,* spasm]. Facial *tic.*

prosopothoracopagus (pros'ō-pō-thōr-ă-kop'ă-gŭs) [prosopo- + G. *thōrax,* chest, + *pagos,* something fastened]. Conjoined twins attached by the face and chest; a variety of cephalothoracopagus.

prospermia (prō-sper'mē-ă) [pro- + G. *sperma,* seed]. Premature *ejaculation.*

prostacyclin (pros-tă-sī'klin). Prostaglandin I_2; a potent natural inhibitor of platelet aggregation and a powerful vasodilator.

prostaglandin (pros-tă-glan'din) [fr. genital fluids and accessory glands where discovered]. Any of a class of physiologically active substances present in many tissues, with effects such as vasodilation, vasoconstriction, stimulation of intestinal or bronchial smooth muscle, uterine stimulation, and antagonism to hormones influencing lipid metabolism. P.'s are prostanoic acids with ortho side-chains of varying degrees of unsaturation and varying degrees of oxidation. Often abbreviated PGA, PGB, PGC, PGD, etc. with numerical subscripts, according to structure.

p. E_1, alprostadil.

p. E_2, dinoprostone.

p. $F_{2\alpha}$, dinoprost.

p. $F_{2\alpha}$ tromethamine, *dinoprost* tromethamine.

prostanoic acid (pros'tă-nō-ik). 7-[2-(1-Octanyl)cyclopentyl]heptanoic acid; the 20-carbon acid that is the skeleton of the prostaglandins, with various hydroxyl and keto substitutions at positions 9, 11, and 15, and dehydrogenations (double bonds) in the long aliphatic chains.

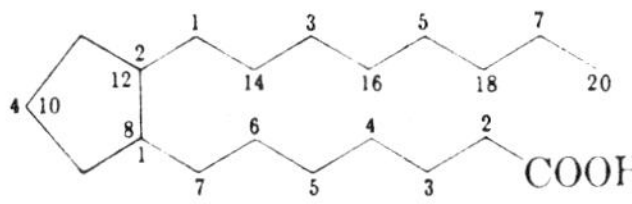

Prostanoic acid

Inner numbering, prostanoic acid; *outer numbering,* systematic.

prostat-. See prostato-.

prostata (pros'tah-tă) [Mod. L. from G. *prostatēs,* one standing before] [NA]. Prostate; prostate gland; glandula prostatica; a chestnut-shaped body, surrounding the beginning of the urethra in the male, that consists of two lateral lobes connected anteriorly by an isthmus and posteriorly by a middle lobe lying above and between the ejaculatory ducts. In structure, the prostate consists of 30 to 50 compound tubuloalveolar glands between which is abundant stroma consisting of collagen and elastic fibers and many smooth muscle bundles. The secretion of the glands is a milky fluid that is discharged by excretory ducts into the prostatic urethra at the time of the emission of semen.

prostatalgia (pros-tă-tal'jē-ă) [prostat- + G. *algos,* pain]. Prostatodynia; pain in the area of the prostate gland.

prostate (pros'tāt). Prostata.

female p., term sometimes applied to the periurethral glands in the upper part of the urethra in the female.

prostatectomy (pros-tă-tek'tō-mē) [prostat- + G. *ektomē,* excision]. Removal of a part or all of the prostate.

prostatic (pros-tat'ik). Relating to the prostate.

prostaticovesical (pros-tat'i-kō-ves'i-kăl). Relating to the prostate and the bladder.

prostatism (pros'tă-tizm). A clinical syndrome, occurring mostly in older men, usually caused by enlargement of the prostate gland and manifested by irritative (nocturia, frequency, decreased voided volume, sensory urgency, and urgency incontinence) and obstructive (hesitancy, decreased stream, terminal dribbling, double voiding, and urinary retention) symptoms.

prostatitic (pros-tă-tit'ik). Relating to prostatitis.

prostatitis (pros-tă-tī'tis) [prostat- + G. *-itis,* inflammation]. Inflammation of the prostate.

prostato-, prostat- [Med. L. *prostata* fr. G. *prostatēs,* one who stands before, protects]. Combining forms denoting the prostate gland.

prostatocystitis (pros'tă-tō-sis-tī'tis) [prostato- + G. *kystis,* bladder, + *-itis,* inflammation]. Inflammation of the prostate and the bladder; cystitis by extension of inflammation from the prostatic urethra.

prostatocystotomy (pros'tă-tō-sis-tot'ō-mē) [prostato- + G. *kystis,* bladder, + *tomē,* incision]. Incision through the prostate and bladder wall with drainage through the perineum.

prostatodynia (pros'tă-tō-din'ē-ă) [prostato- + G. *odynē,* pain]. Prostatalgia.

prostatolith (pros-tat'ō-lith) [prostato- + G. *lithos,* stone]. Prostatic *calculus.*

prostatolithotomy (pros'tă-tō-li-thot'ō-mē, pros-tat'ō-) [prostato- + G. *lithos,* stone, + *tomē,* incision]. Incision of the prostate for removal of a calculus.

prostatomegaly (pros'tă-tō-meg'ă-lē) [prostato- + G. *megas,* large]. Enlargement of the prostate gland.

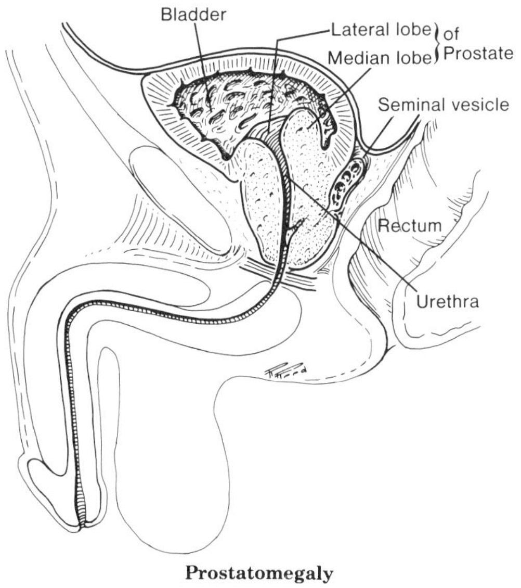

Prostatomegaly

prostatomy (pros-tat'ō-mē). Prostatotomy.

prostatorrhea (pros'tă-tō-rē'ă) [prostato- + G. *rhoia,* a flow]. An abnormal discharge of prostatic fluid.

prostatoseminalvesiculectomy (pros'tă-tō-sem'i-năl-ve-sik-yū-lek'tō-mē). Prostatovesiculectomy.

prostatotomy (pros'tă-tot'ō-mē) [prostato- + G. *tomē,* incision]. Prostatomy; an incision into the prostate.

prostatovesiculectomy (pros'tă-tō-ve-sik'yū-lek'tō-mē). Prostatoseminalvesiculectomy; surgical removal of the prostate gland and seminal vesicles.

prostatovesiculitis (pros'tă-tō-ve-sik'yū-lī'tis). Inflammation of the prostate gland and seminal vesicles.

prosternation (pros-ter-nā'shŭn). Camptocormia.

prostheon (pros'thē-on). Prosthion.

prosthesis, pl. **prostheses** (pros'thē-sis, pros-thē'sis, -sēz) [G. an addition]. Fabricated substitute for a diseased or missing part of the body.
cardiac valve p., see subentries under valve.
cochlear p., cochlear *implant.*
definitive p., a dental p. to be used over a prescribed period of time.
dental p., an artificial replacement of one or more teeth and/or associated structures. See also denture and subentries thereunder.
hybrid p., overlay *denture.*
mandibular guide p., a p. with an extension designed to direct a resected mandible into a functional relation with the maxilla.
ocular p., an artificial eye or implant.
provisional p., an interim dental p. worn for varying periods of time.
surgical p., an appliance prepared as an aid or as a part of a surgical proceeding, such as a heart valve or cranial plate.

prosthetic (pros-thet'ik). **1.** Relating to a prosthesis or to an artificial part. **2.** See prosthetic *group.*

prosthetics (pros-thet'iks). The art and science of making and adjusting artificial parts of the human body.
dental p., prosthodontics.
maxillofacial p., that branch of dentistry which provides prostheses or devices to treat or restore tissues of the stomatognathic system and associated facial structures that have been affected by disease, injury, surgery, or congenital defect, to provide all possible function and esthetics.

prosthetist (pros'the-tist). One skilled in constructing and fitting prostheses.

prosthetophacos (pros'thĕ-tō-fak'ōs) [G. *prosthesis,* an addition, + *phakos,* lens]. Lenticulus.

prosthion (pros'thē-on). [G. ntr. of *prosthios,* foremost]. Prostheon; alveolar point; the most anterior point on the maxillary alveolar process in the midline.

prosthodontia (pros-thō-don'shē-ă) [L.]. Prosthodontics.

prosthodontics (pros-thō-don'tiks) [L. *prosthodontia,* fr. G. *prosthesis* + *odous* (*odont-*), tooth]. Dental prosthetics; prosthetic dentistry; prosthodontia; the science of and art of providing suitable substitutes for the coronal portions of teeth, or for one or more lost or missing teeth and their associated parts, in order that impaired function, appearance, comfort, and health of the patient may be restored.

prosthodontist (pros-thō-don'tist). A dentist engaged in the practice of prosthodontics.

Prosthogonimus macrorchis (pros'thō-gon'i-mŭs mak-rōr'kis) [G. *prosō,* forward, + *thōs,* jackal, + *gonos,* progeny, seed; macro- + *orchis,* testicle]. A digenetic trematode (family Prosthogonimidae) located in the oviduct and bursa fabricii of poultry in North America, particularly common in states bordering the Great Lakes.

prosthokeratoplasty (pros'thō-ker'ă-tō-plas-tē). The surgical technique involved in utilizing a keratoprosthesis.

prostration (pros-trā'shŭn) [L. *pro-sterno,* pp. *-stratus,* to strew before, overthrow]. A marked loss of strength, as in exhaustion.
heat p., see heat *exhaustion.*

prot-. See proteo-; proto-.

protactinium (prō-tak-tin'ē-ŭm). Proactinium; protoactinium; a radioactive element, symbol Pa, atomic no. 91, atomic weight 231, formed in the decay of uranium and thorium; its most long-lived isotope, Pa-231, has a half-life of 32,400 years.

protalbumose (prō-tal'byū-mōs). Protoalbumose; intermediate products of protein digestion, derived from hemialbumose; soluble in water and not coagulable by heat, but precipitated by ammonium sulfate, cupric sulfate, and sodium chloride.

protaminase (prō-tam'i-nās). Carboxypeptidase B.

protamine (prō'tă-mēn, -min). Any of a class of proteins, highly basic because rich in arginine and simpler in constitution than the albumins and globulins, etc., found in fish spermatozoa in combination with nucleic acid; neutralizes anticoagulent action of heparin.

p. sulfate, p. sulphate injection; a purified mixture of simple protein principles from the sperm or testes of suitable species of fish; it is a heparin antagonist used in certain hemorrhagic states associated with increased amounts of heparin-like substances in the circulation and for the treatment of heparin overdosage.

protanomaly (prō'tă-nom'ă-lē) [G. *prōtos,* first, + *anōmalia,* anomaly]. A deficiency of color perception in which the red-sensitive pigment in cones is decreased.

protanopia (prō'tă-nō'pē-ă) [G. *prōtos,* first, + *a-* priv. + *ōps* (*ōp-*) eye]. A form of dichromatism characterized by absence of the red-sensitive pigment in cones, decreased luminosity for long wavelengths of light, and confusion in recognition of red and green.

protean (prō'tē-an) [G. *Prōteus,* a god having the power to change his form]. Changeable in form; having the power to change body form, like the ameba.

protease (prō'tē-ās). Descriptive term for proteolytic enzymes, both endopeptidases and exopeptidases.

protection (prō-tek'shŭn) [see protective]. Protective *block.*

proteid (prō'tē-id). Protein.

protein (prō'tēn, prō'tē-in) [G. *protein,* fr. *proteios,* primary]. Proteid; protide; macromolecules consisting of long sequences of α-amino acids [H_2N–CHR–COOH] in peptide (amide) linkage (elimination of H_2O between the α-NH_2 and α-COOH of successive residues). P. is three-fourths of the dry weight of most cell matter and is involved in structures, hormones, enzymes (all are p.'s), muscle contraction, immunological response, and essential life functions. The amino acids involved are generally the 20 "common" α-amino acids (glycine, alanine, etc.). Cross-links yielding globular forms of p. are often effected through the –SH groups of the two sulfur-containing amino acids, as well as by noncovalent forces (hydrogen bonds, lipophilic attractions, etc.).

acyl carrier p. (ACP), one of the p.'s of the complex in cytoplasm that contains all of the enzymes required to convert acetyl-CoA and malonyl-CoA to palmitic acid. This complex is tightly bound together in mammalian tissues and in yeast, but that from *Escherichia coli* is readily dissociated. The ACP thus isolated is a heat-stable p. with a molecular weight of about 10,000. It contains a free –SH that binds the acyl intermediates in the synthesis of fatty acids as thioesters. This –SH group is part of a 4'-phosphopantetheine, added to the apoprotein by ACP phosphodiesterase, which thus plays the same role that it does in coenzyme A. ACP is involved in every step of the fatty acid synthetic process.

antiviral p. (AVP), a human or animal factor, induced by interferon in virus-infected cells, which mediates interferon inhibition of virus replication.

autologous p., any p. found normally in the fluids or tissues of the body.

Bence Jones p., p. with unusual thermosolubility (see Bence Jones *reaction*) found in the urine of patients with multiple myeloma and occasional persons with other diseases of the reticuloendothelial system; similar in size and physical properties to the light chains of the myeloma p. synthesized by a given patient. See also immunoglobulin.

p. C, a vitamin K-dependent plasma p. which inhibits coagulation by enzymatic cleavage of the activated forms of factors V and VIII, and thus interferes with the regulation of intravascular clot formation.

cAMP receptor p. (CRP), catabolite (gene) activator p.

catabolite (gene) **activator p. (CAP),** cAMP receptor protein; catabolite gene activator; a p. that can be activated by cAMP, whereupon it affects the action of RNA polymerase by binding it with it or near it on the DNA to be transcribed.

compound p., conjugated p.

conjugated p., compound p.; p. attached to some other molecule or molecules (not amino acid in nature) otherwise than as a salt; *e.g.,* flavoproteins; chromoproteins, hemoglobins. *Cf.* simple p. See also prosthetic *group.*

corticosteroid-binding p., transcortin.

C-reactive p., a β-globulin found in the serum of various persons with certain inflammatory, degenerative, and neoplastic diseases; although the p. is not a specific antibody, it precipitates *in vitro* the C polysaccharide present in all types of pneumococci.

denatured p., a p. whose characteristics or properties have been altered in some way, as by heat, enzyme action, or chemicals.

derived p., a derivative of p. effected by chemical change, *e.g.,* hydrolysis.

fibrous p., any insoluble p., including the collagens, elastins, and keratins, involved in structural or fibrous tissues.

foreign p., heterologous p.; a p. that differs from any p. normally found in the organism in question.

globular p., any p. soluble in water, usually with added acid, alkali, salt, or ethanol, and roughly so classified (albumins, globulins, histones, protamines), in contrast to fibrous p.

heterologous p., foreign p.

immune p., antibody.

M p., **(1)** Streptococcus M *antigen.* See also β-hemolytic *streptococci; Streptococcus pneumoniae;* **(2)** monoclonal *immunoglobulin.*

monoclonal p., monoclonal *immunoglobulin.*

myeloblastic p., see human leukemia-associated *antigens.*

native p., the concept of a p. in its natural state, in the cell, unaltered by heat, chemicals, enzyme action, or the exigencies of extraction.

nonspecific p., a p. substance that elicits a response not mediated by specific antigen-antibody reaction.

phenylthiocarbamoyl p., PhNCS or PTC p.; formed by the reaction of phenylisothiocyanate with a terminal α-amino group of a peptide or p. See also phenylisothiocyanate; phenylthiohydantoin.

PhNCS p., phenylthiocarbamoyl p.

placenta p., human placental *lactogen.*

plasma p.'s, dissolved p.'s of blood plasma, mainly albumins and globulins (normally 6 to 8 g/100 ml); they hold fluid in blood vessels by osmosis and include antibodies and blood-clotting p.'s.

protective p., antibody.

PTC p., phenylthiocarbamoyl p.

purified placental p., human placental *lactogen.*

receptor p., an intracellular p. (or p. fraction) that has a high specific affinity for binding a known stimulus to cellular activity, such as a steroid hormone or adenosine 3',5' -cyclic phosphate.

S p., the major fragment produced from pancreatic ribonuclease by the limited action of subtilisin, which cleaves the ribonuclease between residues 20 and 21; the smaller fragment (residues 1-20) is S peptide.

p. S, a vitamin K-dependent antithrombotic p. that functions as a cofactor with activated p. C.

simple p., p. that yields only α-amino acids or their derivatives by hydrolysis; *e.g.*, albumins, globulins, glutelins, prolamines, albuminoids, histones, protamines. *Cf.* conjugated p.

strong silver p., see under silver.

Tamm-Horsfall p., see Tamm-Horsfall *mucoprotein.*

thyroxine-binding p. (TBP), (1) thyroxine-binding *globulin;* **(2)** thyroxine-binding *prealbumin.*

whey p., the soluble p. contained in the whey of milk clotted by rennin.

proteinaceous (prō'tē-nā'shŭs, prō'tē-i-nā'shŭs). Resembling a protein; possessing, to some degree, the physicochemical properties characteristic of proteins.

proteinases (prō'tē-in-ās-ez). Enzymes (EC sub-subclasses 3.4.21 – 3.4.24, 3.4.99) hydrolyzing native protein, or polypeptides, making internal cleavages (hence endopeptidases); *e.g.*, pepsin, chymosin, trypsin, papain.

protein hydrolysate. A sterile solution of amino acids and soft chain peptides prepared from a suitable protein by acid or enzymatic hydrolysis; used intravenously for the maintenance of positive nitrogen balance in severe illness, and after surgery involving the alimentary tract; or used orally in the diets of infants allergic to milk or as a supplement when high protein intake from ordinary foods cannot be accomplished.

proteinosis (pro-tē-nō'sis, prō'tē-i-nō'sis) [protein + G. *-osis,* condition]. A state characterized by disordered protein formation and distribution, particularly as manifested by the deposition of abnormal proteins in tissues.

lipid p., Urbach-Wiethe disease; lipoidosis cutis et mucosae; a disturbance of lipid metabolism in which there are deposits of a protein-lipid complex on the labial mucosa and sublingual and faucial areas, and characteristic papillomatous eyelid lesions; autosomal recessive inheritance.

pulmonary alveolar p., a chronic progressive lung disease of adults, characterized by alveolar accumulation of granular proteinaceous material that is PAS-positive and lipid rich, with little inflammatory cellular exudate; the cause is unknown.

proteinuria (prō-tē-nū'rē-ă, prō'tē-i-nū'rē-ă) [protein + G. *ouron,* urine]. **1.** Presence of urinary protein in concentrations greater than 0.3 g in a 24-hour urine collection or in concentrations greater than 1 g/l (1+ to 2+ by standard turbidometric methods) in a random urine collection on two or more occasions at least 6 hours apart; specimens must be clean, voided midstream, or obtained by catheterization. **2.** Albuminuria.

Bence Jones p., presence of Bence Jones proteins in the urine, usually indicative of a neoplastic process such as multiple myeloma, amyloidosis, or Waldenström's macroglobulinemia.

gestational p., the presence of p. during or under the influence of pregnancy in the absence of hypertension, edema, renal infection, or known intrinsic renovascular disease.

isolated p., p. in a patient who is asymptomatic, has normal renal function and urinary sediment, and has no manifestation of systemic disease upon initial examination.

nonisolated p., p. associated with other abnormalities.

orthostatic p., postural p., orthostatic *albuminuria.*

protensity (prō-ten'si-tē) [L. *protendo (-tensum),* to extend]. The time attribute of a mental process.

proteo-, prot-. Combining forms indicating protein.

proteoclastic (prō'tē-ō-klas'tik) [proteo- + G. *klastos,* broken]. Proteolytic.

proteoglycans (prō'tē-ō-glī'kanz). Glycoaminoglycans (mucopolysaccharides) bound to protein chains in covalent complexes; occur in the extracellular matrix of connective tissue.

proteohormone (prō'tē-ō-hōr'mōn). Obsolete term for a hormone possessing a protein structure.

proteolipids (prō'tē-ō-lip'idz). A class of lipid-soluble proteins found in brain tissue, insoluble in water but soluble in chloroform-methanol-water mixtures.

proteolysis (prō-tē-ol'i-sis) [proteo- + G. *lysis,* dissolution]. Albuminolysis; the decomposition of protein.

proteolytic (prō'tē-ō-lit'ik). Proteoclastic; relating to or effecting proteolysis.

proteometabolic (prō'tē-ō-met'ă-bol'ik). Relating to the metabolism of proteins.

proteometabolism (prō'tē-ō-mĕ-tab'ō-lizm). Protein *metabolism.*

Proteomyxidia (prō'tē-ō-mik-sid'ē-ă) [*Proteus* + G. *myxa,* mucus]. Former name for Eumycetozoea.

proteopectic, proteopexic (prō'tē-ō-pek'tik, -pek'sik). Relating to proteopexis.

proteopepsis (prō'tē-ō-pep'sis) [proteo- + G. *pepsis,* digestion]. The digestion of protein.

proteopexis (prō'tē-ō-pek'sis) [proteo- + G. *pēxis,* fixation]. The fixation of protein in the tissues.

proteose (prō'tē-ōs). A nondescript mixture of intermediate products of proteolysis between protein and peptone.

primary p., the first result of hydrolysis of metaprotein; two stages, protoproteose and heteroproteose, have been distinguished.

secondary p., p. derived from primary p. by further hydrolysis.

Proteus (prō'tē-ŭs) [G. *Prōteus,* a sea-god, who had the power to change his form]. **1.** A former genus of the Sarcodina, now termed *Amoeba.* **2.** A genus of motile, peritrichous, nonsporeforming, aerobic to facultatively anaerobic bacteria (family Enterobacteriaceae) containing Gram-negative rods; coccoid forms, large irregular involution forms, filaments, and spheroplasts occur under certain conditions. The metabolism is fermentative, producing acid or acid and visible gas from glucose; lactose is not fermented, and they rapidly decompose urea and deaminate phenylalanine. *P.* occurs primarily in fecal matter and in putrefying materials. The type species is *P. vulgaris.*

P. incon'stans, a species found in urinary tract infections and in sporadic cases of diarrhea in man; some strains cause gastroenteritis.

P. mirab'ilis, a species found in putrid meat, infusions, and abscesses; also reported to be a cause of gastroenteritis.

P. morgan'ii, Morgan's bacillus; a species found in the intestinal canal and in normal and diarrheal stools.

P. rettge'ri, a species found in chicken cholera and human gastroenteritis.

P. vulgar'is, the type species of the genus *P.*, found in putrefying materials and in abscesses; it is pathogenic for fish, dogs, guinea pigs, and mice; certain strains, the X strains of Weil and Felix, are agglutinated by typhus serum and are therefore of great importance in the diagnosis of typhus; strain X-19 is strongly agglutinated. See also Weil-Felix *reaction.*

prothipendyl (prō-thī'pen-dil). 10-(3-Dimethylaminopropyl)-10*H*-pyrido-[3,2-*b*][1,4]benzothiazine; an antipsychotic.

prothrombase (prō-throm'bās). Factor Xa. See *factor* X.

prothrombin (prō-throm'bin). Factor II (blood clotting); plasmozyme; serozyme; thrombinogen; thrombogen; a glycoprotein, molecular weight approximately 69,000, formed and stored in the parenchymal cells of the liver and present in blood in a concentration of approximately 20 mg/100 ml. In the presence of thromboplastin and calcium ion, p. is converted to thrombin, which in turn converts fibrinogen to fibrin, this process resulting in coagulation of blood.

prothrombinase (prō-throm'bi-nās). *Factor* X.

prothrombinogen (prō-throm'bi-nō-jen). *Factor* VII.

prothrombinopenia (prō-throm'bi-nō-pē'nē-ă). Hypoprothrombinemia.

prothrombokinase (prō'throm-bō-kī'nās). *Factors* V and VIII.

prothymia (prō-thī'mē-ă) [G. eagerness, fr. *pro,* before, + *thymos,* mind]. Mental alertness.

protide (prō'tīd). Protein.

protiodide (prō-tī'ō-dīd, -did). Protoiodide; obsolete term for the first of a series of compounds of iodine with a base, the compound that contains the fewest iodine atoms.

protirelin (prō-tī'rē-lin). 5-Oxo-L-propyl-L-histidyl-L-prolinamide; a synthetic form of thyroliberin.

protist (prō'tist). A member of the kingdom Protista.

Protista (prō-tis'tă) [G. ntr. pl. of *protistos,* the first of all]. Haeckel's term for a proposed third kingdom of living things to include the lowest orders of the animal and vegetable kingdoms, the Protozoa and the Protophyta. It has been proposed that the P. be divided into two groups according to complexity of structure: 1) the higher protists, the eukaryotes, including protozoa, fungi, and algae, which resemble plants and animals in cell structure (*i.e.,* the cells are eukaryotic; the nuclei include multiple chromosomes, are enclosed in a nuclear membrane, and undergo mitosis during replication; the cytoplasm contains mitochondria and vacuoles); higher protists differ from plants and animals in being unicellular, or, if multicellular, in having cells that are all similar with little or none of the tissue differentiation characteristic of plants and animals; 2) the lower protists, the prokaryotes (kingdom Monera, superkingdom Prokaryotae), which include the bacteria and blue-green bacteria; these have a genome consisting of a single long molecule of DNA not surrounded by a nuclear membrane, which does not undergo mitosis during replication, and which does not possess mitochondria; viruses, although they have similar genomes, are as a rule considered to form a separate kingdom of prokaryotic organisms in the superkingdom Prokaryotae, or are excluded as noncellular or nonliving.

protistologist (prō-tis-tol'ō-jist). Microbiologist.

protistology (prō-tis-tol'ō-jē) [G. *protistos,* first, + *logos,* study]. Microbiology.

protium (prō'tē-ŭm). Hydrogen-1.

proto-, prot- [G. *prōtos,* first]. Prefix, to words derived from Greek roots, denoting the first in a series or the highest in rank.

protoactinium (prō'tō-ak-tin'ē-um). Protactinium.

protoalbumose (prō-tō-al'byū-mōs). Protalbumose.

protobe (prō'tōb) [proto- + G. *bios,* life]. F. d'Herelle's term for bacteriophage.

protobiology (prō'tō-bī-ol'ō-jē). Bacteriophagology.

protocatechuic acid (prō'tō-kat'ē-chū'ik, -kū'ik). 3,4-Dihydroxybenzoic acid; 4-carboxycatechol; oxidation product of epinephrine.

protochloride (prō-tō-klōr'īd, -klōr'id). Obsolete term for the first of a series of chlorine compounds, the one containing the fewest chlorine atoms.

protocol (prō'tō-kol). A precise and detailed plan for the study of a biomedical problem or for a regimen of therapy.

protocone (prō'tō-kōn) [proto- + G. *kōnos,* cone]. The mesiolingual cusp of an upper molar tooth in a mammal.

protoconid (prō-tō-kon'id). The mesiolingual cusp of a lower molar tooth in a mammal.

protocoproporphyria (prō'tō-kop'rō-pōr-fir'ē-ă). Enhanced fecal excretion of proto- and coproporphyrins.

p. heredita'ria, variegate *porphyria.*

Protoctista (prō-tok-tis'tă) [G. *protos,* the first, + *ktistos,* to establish]. A kingdom of eukaryotes incorporating the algae and the protozoans that comprise the presumed ancestral stocks of the fungi, plant, and animal kingdoms; they lack the developmental pattern stemming from a blastula, typical of animals, the pattern of embryo development typical of plants, and development from spores as in the fungi. Included in P. are the nucleated algae and seaweeds, the flagellated water molds, slime molds and slime nets, and the protozoa; unicellular, colonial, and multicellular organisms are included, but the complex development of tissues and organs of plants and animals is absent. The term P. replaces the term Protista, which connotes single-celled or acellular organisms, whereas the basal pre-plant (Protophyta) and pre-animal (Protozoa) assemblages incorporated in P. include many multicellular forms, since multicellarity appears to have evolved independently a number of times within these primitive groups.

protoderm (prō'tō-derm) [proto- + G. *derma,* skin]. The undifferentiated cells of very young embryos from which the primary germ layers will evolve.

protodiastolic (prō'tō-dī-ă-stol'ik). Early diastolic; relating to the beginning of cardiac diastole.

protoduodenum (prō'tō-dū-ō-dē'nŭm, -dū-od'ē-nŭm). The first part of the duodenum extending from the gastroduodenal pylorus as far as the papilla duodeni major; it has no plicae circulares and is the seat of the duodenal glands.

protoerythrocyte (prō'tō-ē-rith'rō-sīt). A primitive erythroblast.

protofilament (prō-tō-fil'ă-ment) [proto- + L. *filum,* a thread]. Basic element of a contractile flagellar microtubule, approximately 5 nm thick.

protogen, protogen A (prō'tō-jen). Lipoic acid.

protoglobulose (prō-tō-glob'yū-lōs). Obsolete term for a product of the hydrolysis or digestion of a globulin.

protogonoplasm (prō-tō-gon'ō-plazm) [proto- + G. *gonos,* seed, + *plasma,* a thing formed]. A differentiated mass of cytoplasm in a protozoan, which forms the substance of later developing reproductive bodies.

protoheme (prō'tō-hēm). Heme.

protoiodide (prō-tō-ī'ō-dīd, -did). Protiodide.

protokylol hydrochloride (prō-tō-kī'lōl). α-[(α-Methyl-3,4-methylenedioxyphenethylamino)methyl]protocatechuyl alcohol hydrochloride; a derivative of isoproterenol with the selective β-receptor-stimulating activity of the parent compound; it is effective orally and is more stable in the body than isoproterenol; used as a bronchodilator in the treatment of bronchial asthma and status asthmaticus.

protoleukocyte (prō-tō-lū'kō-sīt). A primitive leukocyte; a leukocyte of the bone marrow.

protolysate (prō-tol'i-sāt). Obsolete term for a protein hydrolysate.

protomerite (prō-tom'ē-rīt, prō'tō-mēr'īt) [proto- + G. *meros,* part]. Primerite; the second segment (lacking a nucleus) of a septate gregarine, between the epimerite and the deutomerite; it becomes the anterior end of the gamont after it has broken free of its host cell, leaving the epimerite embedded (usually in the gut wall of an infected invertebrate).

protometrocyte (prō-tō-mē'trō-sīt) [proto- + G. *mētēr,* mother, + *kytos,* cell]. The ancestor cell of the protoleukocyte and protoerythrocyte, or of the cells of the leukocytic and erythrocytic series.

proton (prō'ton) [G. ntr. of *prōtos,* first]. The positively charged unit of the nuclear mass; p.'s form part (or in hydrogen-1 the whole) of the nucleus of the atom around which the negative electrons revolve.

protoneuron (prō-tō-nūr'on) [proto- + G. *neuron,* nerve]. Hypothetical primitive neuron lacking polarization.

proto-oncogene (prō-tō-on'kō-jēn). A preexisting gene, present in the normal human genome, that appears to have a role in normal cellular physiology and is often involved in regulation of normal cell growth or proliferation; involvement of these g.'s in a neoplastic process is a consequence of somatic mutations that convert them into oncogenic alleles.

protopathic (prō-tō-path'ik) [proto- + G. *pathos,* suffering]. Denoting a supposedly primitive set or system of peripheral sensory nerve fibers conducting a low order of pain and temperature sensibility which is poorly localized. *Cf.* epicritic.

protopectin (prō-tō-pek'tin). See pectin.

protopianoma (prō'tō-pē-an-ō'mă). Mother *yaw.*

protoplasm (prō'tō-plazm) [proto- + G. *plasma,* thing formed]. Living matter, the substance of which animal and vegetable cells are formed. See also cytoplasm; nucleoplasm.

totipotential p., living matter with the least recognizable differentiation of structure but with the greatest potential, all cell organs being formable by it.

protoplasmatic, protoplasmic (prō'tō-plaz-mat'ik, -plaz'mik). Relating to protoplasm.

protoplasmolysis (prō'tō-plaz-mol'i-sis). Plasmolysis.

protoplast (prō'tō-plast) [proto- + G. *plastos,* formed]. **1.** Archaic term meaning the first individual of a type or race. **2.** A bacterial cell from which the rigid cell wall has been completely removed; the bacterium loses its characteristic shape and becomes round.

protoporphyria (prō'tō-pōr-fir'ē-ă). Enhanced fecal excretion of protoporphyrin.

erythropoietic p., a benign disorder of porphyrin metabolism due to a deficiency of ferrochelatase and characterized by enhanced fecal excretion of protoporphyrin and elevated quantities of protoporphyrin IX in red blood cells, plasma, and feces; acute solar urticaria or more chronic solar eczema develops quickly upon exposure to sunlight; autosomal dominant inheritance with variable penetrance.

protoporphyrin type III (IX) (prō-tō-pōr'fi-rin). 2,7,12,18-Tetramethyl-3,8-divinylporphin-13, 17-dipropionic acid; the principal protoporphyrin found in nature (one of 15 possible isomers), characterized by the presence of 4 methyl groups, 2 vinyl groups, and 2 propionic acid side chains; a porphyrin derivative that, with iron, forms the heme of hemoglobin and the prosthetic groups of myoglobin, catalase, cytochromes, etc.

protoproteose (prō-tō-prō'tē-ōs). See primary *proteose.*

protosalt (prō'tō-sawlt). Acid *salt.*

protospasm (prō'tō-spazm) [proto- + G. *spasmos,* spasm]. A spasm beginning in one limb or one muscle and gradually becoming more general.

protospore (prō'tō-spōr) [proto- + G. *sporos,* seed]. The initial product of progressive cleavage, in which a multinucleate spore is produced.

Protostrongylus rufescens (prō-tō-stron'ji-lŭs rū-fes'ens) [proto- + G. *strongylos,* round]. The small lungworm of sheep, goats, and deer that occurs in the smaller bronchioles, where it causes plugging of the air passages by its presence and the formation of multiple areas of bronchopneumonia; symptoms produced generally are milder than those induced by the large lungworm, *Dictyocaulus filaria.*

protosulfate (prō-tō-sŭl'fāt). A compound of sulfuric acid with a protoxide of the metal.

protosyphilis (prō-tō-sif'i-lis). Obsolete term for primary *syphilis.*

prototaxic (prō-tō-tak'sik) [proto- + G. *taxis,* order, arrangement]. In interpersonal psychiatry, a term referring to primitive illogical thought.

Prototheca (prō-tō-thē'kă). A genus of microbes transitional between the fungi and achlorophyllous mutants of the green alga, *Chlorella.* Two species, *P. zopfii* and *P. wickerhamii,* cause protothecosis.

protothecosis (prō'tō-thē-kō'sis). A verrucous cutaneous or disseminated disease caused by *Prototheca zopfii* and *wickerhamii.*

prototoxin (prō'tō-tok-sin) [proto- + G. *toxikon,* poison (toxin)]. The obsolete concept of a hypothetical form of toxin in bacterial cultures possessing lethal properties and a very strong affinity for antitoxin.

prototoxoid (prō'tō-tok-soyd) [proto- + toxoid]. The obsolete concept of a hypothetical substance in a bacterial culture, nonpoisonous, but with a stronger affinity than toxin for antitoxin.

prototroph (prō'tō-trof, -trōf) [proto- + G. *trophē,* nourishment]. A bacterial strain that has the same nutritional requirements as the wild-type strain from which it was derived. See also wild-type *strain.*

prototrophic (prō-tō-trof'ik). **1.** Pertaining to a prototroph. **2.** Denoting the ability to undertake anabolism or to obtain nourishment from a single source, as with iron, sulfur, or nitrifying bacteria or photosynthesizing plants.

prototype (prō'tō-tīp) [proto- + G. *typos,* type]. The primitive form; the first form to which subsequent individuals of the class or species conform.

protoveratrine A and B (prō-tō-ver'ă-trēn). A mixture of two alkaloids isolated from *Veratrum album;* they exert their main effect upon the cardiovascular system through the carotid sinus receptors and vagal sensory endings in the heart; they cause vasodilation and are thought to bring about a redistribution to all vascular beds and thus to induce a fall in blood pressure; used in certain forms of hypertension; the maleates have the same actions.

protovertebra (prō'tō-ver'tē-bră). Provertebra. **1.** In the older literature, a mesodermic somite. **2.** More recently applied to the sclerotomal concentration which is the primordium of the centrum of a vertebra.

protovertebral (prō-tō-ver'tē-brăl). Relating to a protovertebra.

protoxide (prō-tok'sīd). Suboxide.

Protozoa (prō-tō-zō'ă) [proto- + G. *zōon,* animal]. Formerly considered a phylum, now regarded as a subkingdom of the animal kingdom, including all of the so-called acellular or unicellular forms. They consist of a single functional cell unit or aggregation of nondifferentiated cells, loosely held together and not forming tissues, as distinguishes the Animalia or Metazoa, which include all other animals. P. were formerly divided into four classes: Sarcodina, Mastigophora, Sporozoa, and Ciliata; new classifications employ higher taxa (phyla, subphyla, and superclasses) and a number of major subdivisions.

protozoal (prō-tō-zō'ăl). Protozoan (2).

protozoan (prō-tō-zō'an). **1.** Protozoon; a member of the phylum Protozoa. **2.** Protozoal; relating to protozoa.

protozoiasis (prō'tō-zō-ī'ă-sis). Infection with protozoans.

protozoicide (prō-tō-zō'i-sīd) [protozoa + L. *caedo,* to kill]. An agent used to kill protozoa.

protozoologist (prō'tō-zō-ol'ō-jist). A biologist who specializes in protozoology.

protozoology (prō'tō-zō-ol'ō-jē) [protozoa + G. *logos,* study]. The science concerned with all aspects of the biology and human interest in protozoa.

protozoon, pl. **protozoa** (prō-tō-zō'on, -zō'ă). Protozoan (1).

protozoophage (prō-tō-zō'ō-fāj) [protozoa + G. *phagein,* to eat]. A phagocyte that ingests protozoa.

protraction (prō-trak'shŭn) [see protractor]. In dentistry, the extension of teeth or other maxillary or mandibular structures into a position anterior to normal.

mandibular p., a type of facial anomaly in which the gnathion lies anterior to the orbital plane.

maxillary p., a type of facial anomaly in which the subnasion lies anterior to the orbital plane.

protractor (prō-trak'ter, -tōr) [L. *pro-traho,* pp. *-tractus,* to draw forth]. A muscle drawing a part forward, as antagonistic to a retractor.

protriptyline hydrochloride (prō-trip'ti-lēn). *N*-Methyl-5*H*-dibenzo[*a,d*]cycloheptene-5-propylamine hydrochloride; an antidepressant.

protrude (prō-trūd'). To thrust forward or project.

protrusio acetabuli (prō-trū'sē-ō as-ĕ-tab'yū-lī). Otto's *disease.*

protrusion (prō-trū'zhŭn) [L. *protrusio*]. **1.** The state of being thrust forward or projected. **2.** In dentistry, a position of the mandible forward from centric relation.

bimaxillary p., double p.; the excessive forward projection of both the maxilla and the mandible in relation to the cranial base.

bimaxillary dentoalveolar p., the positioning of the entire dentition forward with respect to the facial profile.

double p., bimaxillary p.

protrypsin (prō-trip'sin). Trypsinogen.

protuberance (prō-tū'ber-ans) [Mod. L. *protuberantia*]. A swelling or knoblike outgrowth. See also entries under protuberantia.

Bichat's p., *corpus* adiposum buccae.

external occipital p., *protuberantia* occipitalis externa.

internal occipital p., *protuberantia* occipitalis interna.

mental p., *protuberantia* mentalis.

protuberantia (prō-tū-ber-an'shē-ă) [Mod. L. fr. *protubero,* to swell out, fr. *tuber,* a swelling] [NA]. A bulging, swelling, or protruding part. See also entries under protuberance; prominence; eminence.

p. laryn'gea, *prominentia* laryngea.

p. menta'lis [NA], mental protuberance; mental process; the prominence of the chin at the anterior part of the mandible.

p. occipita'lis exter'na [NA], external occipital protuberance; a prominence about the center of the outer surface of the squamous portion of the occipital bone, giving attachment to the ligamentum nuchae.

p. occipita'lis inter'na [NA], internal occipital protuberance; a projection from about the center of the cruciform eminence on the inner surface of the occipital bone.

Proust, Louis J., French chemist, 1755–1826. See P.'s *law.*

Proust, P.T., 19th century French physician. See P.'s *space.*

proventriculus (prō-ven-trik'yū-lŭs) [L. *pro,* before, + *ventriculus,* dim. of *venter* (*ventr-*) belly]. **1.** In birds, the thin-walled glandular stomach preceding the muscular gizzard. **2.** In insects, the portion of the stomodeum that lies in front of the ventriculus or stomach; it is modified into a small proventricular valve in many diptera (flies).

provertebra (prō-ver'tĕ-bră). Protovertebra.

Providencia (prov'i-den'sē-ă). A genus of motile, peritrichous, nonsporeforming, aerobic or facultatively anaerobic bacteria (family Enterobacteriaceae) containing Gram-negative rods. These organisms do not hydrolyze urea or produce hydrogen sulfide; they produce indole and grow on Simmons' citrate medium. They do not decarboxylate lysine, arginine, or ornithine. These organisms occur in specimens from extraintestinal sources, particularly urinary tract infections; they have also been isolated from small outbreaks and sporadic cases of diarrheal disease. The type species is *P. alcalifaciens.*

P. alcalifa'ciens, a species found in extraintestinal sources, particularly in urinary tract infections; it has also been isolated from small outbreaks and sporadic cases of diarrheal disease; it is the type species of the genus *P.*

P. stuar'tii, a species isolated from urinary tract infections and from small outbreaks and sporadic cases of diarrheal disease.

provirus (prō-vī'rŭs). The precursor of an animal virus; theoretically analogous to the prophage in bacteria, the p. being integrated in the nucleus of infected cells.

provitamin (prō-vī'tă-min). A substance that can be converted into a vitamin.

p. A, trivial name for carotenoids exhibiting qualitatively the biological activity of β-carotene, *i.e.,* vitamin A precursors (α-, β-, and γ-carotene and cryptoxanthin); contained in fish liver oils, spinach, carrots, egg yolk, milk products, and other green leaf or yellow vegetables and fruits.

p. D_2, any substance that can give rise to ergocalciferol (vitamin D_2); *e.g.,* ergosterol.

p. D_3, 7-dehydrocholesterol.

Prowazek, Stanislas J.M. von, German protozoologist, 1876–1915. See *Prowazekia;* P.'s *bodies;* P.-Greeff *bodies;* Halberstaedter-P. *bodies.*

Prowazekia (prō-vă-zē'kē-ă) [S. *Prowazek*]. A genus of coprozoic flagellate protozoans, formerly part of the genus *Bodo;* the organisms may be parasitic but are not, so far as is known, pathogenic.

Prower. Surname of the patient in whom the Stuart-P. *factor* was first discovered.

prox-, proxi-. See proximo-.

proxemics (prok-sem'iks) [L. *proximus,* nearest, next]. The scientific discipline concerned with the various aspects of urban overcrowding.

proximad (prok'si-mad) [L. *proximus,* nearest, next, + *ad,* to]. In a direction toward a proximal part, or toward the center; not distad.

proximal (prok'si-măl) [Mod. L. *proximalis,* fr. L. *proximus,* nearest, next]. **1.** Proximalis; nearest the trunk or the point of origin, said of part of a limb, of an artery or a nerve, etc., so situated. **2.** Mesial. **3.** In dental anatomy, denoting the surface of a tooth in relation with its neighbor, whether mesial or distal, *i.e.,* nearer to or farther from the anteroposterior median plane.

proximalis (prok-si-mā'lis) [Mod. L.] [NA]. Proximal (1).

proximate (prok'si-māt). Immediate; next; proximal.

proximo-, prox-, proxi- [L. *proximus,* nearest, next (to)]. Combining forms denoting proximal.

proximoataxia (prok'si-mō-ă-tak'sē-ă) [proximo- + ataxia]. Ataxia or lack of muscular coordination in the proximal portions of the extremities, *i.e.,* arms and forearms, thighs and legs. *Cf.* acroataxia.

proximobuccal (prok'si-mō-bŭk'ăl). Relating to the proximal and buccal surfaces of a tooth; denoting the angle formed by their junction.

proximolabial (prok'si-mō-lā'bē-ăl). Relating to the proximal and labial surfaces of a tooth; denoting the angle formed by their junction.

proximolingual (prok'si-mō-ling'gwăl). Relating to the proximal and lingual surfaces of a tooth; denoting the angle formed by their junction.

proxymetacaine hydrochloride (prok-si-met'ă-kān). Proparacaine hydrochloride.

prozapine (prō'ză-pēn). Hexadiphane; 1-(3,3-diphenylpropyl)hexamethyleneimine; an intestinal antispasmodic with choleretic properties.

prozone (prō'zōn). Prezone; in the case of agglutination and of precipitation, the phenomenon in which visible reaction does not occur in mixtures of specific antigen and antibody because of either antibody excess or antigen excess.

prozygosis (prō-zī-gō'sis) [G. *pro,* before, + *zygōsis,* a yoking]. Syncephaly.

PRPP Abbreviation for 5-phospho-α-D-ribosyl pyrophosphate.

prune (prūn). The dried ripe fruit of *Prunus domestica* (family Rosaceae), a tree cultivated in warm temperate regions; a food with laxative properties.

Prunus (prū'nŭs) [L. a plum-tree]. A genus of trees (family Rosaceae) including the cherry, plum, peach, and apricot trees.

P. sero'tina, the wild black cherry; a botanical source of wild cherry. See *P. virginiana.*

P. virginia'na, (1) wild black cherry bark; the bark of *P. serotina,* used as a tonic and in cough mixtures as a bronchial sedative; **(2)** the choke cherry; the chief substitute and adulterant of *P. serotina.*

pruriginous (prū-rij'i-nŭs) [L. *pruriginosus,* having the itch]. Relating to or suffering from prurigo.

prurigo (prū-rī'gō) [L. itch, fr. *prurio,* to itch]. A chronic disease of the skin marked by a persistent eruption of papules that itch intensely.

p. aestiva'lis, summer p.; a form recurring each summer, becoming very severe as long as the hot weather continues.

p. a'gria, Hebra's p.

Besnier's p., an atopic form which may be associated with asthma, hay fever, or other allergic conditions.

p. fe'rox [L. wild, cruel], Hebra's p.

p. gestatio'nis, a papular skin disease occurring in pregnant women.

Hebra's p., p. ferox; p. agria; a severe form of chronic dermatitis in which there are constantly recurring, intensely itchy papules and nodules.

p. infanti'lis, *lichen* urticatus.

p. mi'tis, a mild form of a chronic dermatitis characterized by recurring, intensely itching papules and nodules, probably atopic.

p. nodula'ris, Hyde's disease; an eruption of hard nodules in the skin, accompanied by intense itching.

p. sim'plex, a mild form of p. having a pronounced tendency to relapse.

summer p., p. aestivalis.

pruritic (prū-rit'ik). Relating to pruritus.

pruritus (prū-rī'tŭs) [L. an itching, fr. *prurio,* to itch]. **1.** Itching. **2.** Itch. (3).

p. aestiva'lis, summer itch; p. occurring during hot weather; may be associated with prickly heat.

p. a'ni, itching of varying intensity at the anus; may be paroxysmal or constant, associated with seborrheic dermatitis or moniliasis, with irritated and enlarged hemorrhoidal veins, or may occur independently of any cutaneous lesions in association with systemic disease.

aquagenic p., intense itching produced by brief contact with water at any temperature without visible changes in the skin; associated with local release of acetylcholine, mast-cell degranulation, and raised histamine concentrations.

p. bal'nea, bath p.

bath p., bath itch; p. balnea; itching produced by inadequate rinsing off of soap or by overdrying of skin from excessive bathing.

essential p., itching that occurs independently of skin lesions.

p. hiema'lis, *dermatitis* hiemalis.

p. seni'lis, senile p., itching associated with degenerative changes in the skin of the aged.

symptomatic p., itching occurring as a symptom of some systemic disease.

p. vul'vae, itching of the external female genitalia, caused by a variety of factors, *e.g.,* seborrheic dermatitis, allergy to local contactants, senile atrophy of the vulva, and occasionally systemic disease.

Prussak, Alexander, Russian otologist, 1839–1897. See P.'s *fibers, pouch, space.*

Prussian blue [C.I. 77510]. Berlin blue.

prussiate (prŭsh'ē-āt, prŭs'ē-āt). **1.** A cyanide; a salt of hydrocyanic acid. **2.** A ferricyanide or ferrocyanide.

prussic acid (prŭs'ik). Hydrocyanic acid.

psalterial (sawl-ter'ē-ăl). Relating to the psalterium.

psalterium, pl. **psalteria** (sawl-ter'ē-ŭm, sawl-ter'ē-ă) [G. *psaltērion,* harp]. **1.** *Commissura* fornicis. **2.** Omasum.

psammo- [G. *psammos,* sand]. Combining form denoting sand.

psammocarcinoma (sam'ō-kar-si-nō'mă). A carcinoma that contains calcified foci resembling psammoma bodies.

psammoma (sa-mō'mă) [psammo- + G. *-oma,* tumor]. Angiolithic sarcoma; psammomatous meningioma; sand tumor; Virchow's p.; a firm cellular neoplasm derived from fibrous tissue of the meninges, choroid plexus, and certain other structures associated with the brain, characterized by the formation of multiple, discrete, concentrically laminated, calcareous bodies (psammoma bodies); most of these neoplasms are histologically benign, but may lead to severe symptoms as a result of compressing the brain.

Virchow's p., psammoma.

psammomatous (sa-mō'mă-tŭs). Possessing or characterized by the presence of psammoma bodies; refers usually to certain types of meningioma or to meningeal hyperplasia with psammoma bodies.

psammous (sam'ŭs) [G. *psammos,* sand]. Sandy.

Psaume, J., French physician. See Papillon-Léage and P. *syndrome.*

pselaphesis, pselaphesia (se-laf'ĕ-sis, sel-ă-fē'sis, sel-ă-fē'zē-ă) [G. *psēlaphēsis,* a touching]. The higher tactile sense, including the muscle sense.

psellism (sel'izm) [G. *psellismos,* a stammering]. Stammering.

pseud-. See pseudo-.

pseudacromegaly (sū-dak-rō-meg'ă-lē). Enlargement of the extremities and face, not caused by acromegaly.

pseudagraphia (sū-dă-graf'ē-ă) [pseud- + G. *a-* priv. + *graphō,* to write]. Pseudoagraphia; partial agraphia in which one can do no original writing, but can copy correctly.

pseudalbuminuria (sū'dal-byū-mi-nū'rē-ă). Cyclic *albuminuria.*

Pseudallescheria boydii (sūd'al-es-kĕ'rē-ă boy'dē-ī). A species of fungus that causes eumycotic mycetoma and pseuallescheriasis; its conidial (asexual) state is *Monosporium apiospermum.*

pseudallescheriasis (sūd'al-es-kĕ'ri-ă-sis). A variety of clinical diseases resulting from infection with *Pseudallescheria boydii; e.g.,* pulmonary colonization, fungoma, and invasive pneumonitis, as well as mycotic keratitis, endophthalmitis, endocarditis, meningitis, sinusitis, brain abscesses, cutaneous and subcutaneous infections, and disseminated systemic infections.

Pseudamphistomum (sū-dam-fis'tō-mŭm) [pseud- + G. *amphi,* two-sided, + *stoma,* mouth]. A genus of digenetic flukes of the family Opisthorchiidae; *P. truncatum* is a species that infects the bile ducts of the dog and cat (rarely of man) in Europe and India.

pseudangina (sū'dan-jī'nă, sū-dan'ji-nă). *Angina* pectoris vasomotoria.

pseudankylosis (sū-dang'ki-lō'sis). Fibrous *ankylosis.*

pseudaphia (sū-daf'ē-ă) [G. *haphē,* a touch]. Paraphia.

pseudarthrosis (sū-dar-thrō'sis) [pseud- + G. *arthrōsis,* a jointing]. Pseudoarthrosis; false joint; a new, false joint arising at the site of an ununited fracture.

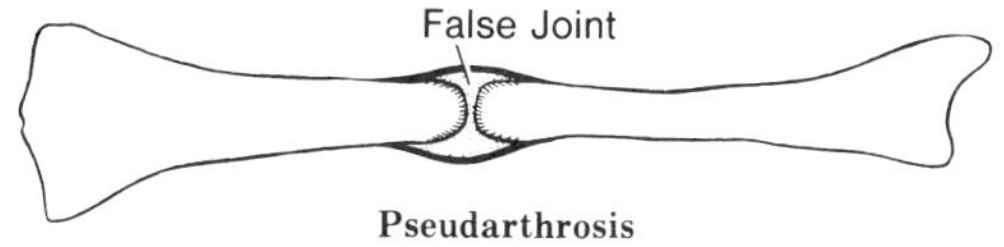

Pseudarthrosis

pseudelminth (sū-del'minth) [pseud- + G. *helmins,* worm]. Anything having the appearance of an intestinal worm.

pseudesthesia (sū-des-thē'zē-ă) [pseud- + G. *aisthēsis,* sensation]. Pseudoesthesia. **1.** Paraphia. **2.** A subjective sensation not arising from an external stimulus. **3.** Phantom *limb.*

pseudinoma (sū-di-nō'mă) [pseud- + G. *is* (*in*), fiber, + *-oma,* tumor]. An indurated swelling that grossly resembles a fibroma.

pseudo-, pseud- [G. *pseudēs,* false]. Prefix denoting a resemblance, often deceptive.

pseudoacanthosis nigricans (sū′dō-ak-an-thō′sis nī′gri-kanz). Acanthosis nigricans secondary to maceration of the skin from excessive sweating, or occurring in obese and dark-complexioned adults, or in association with endocrine disorders; not associated with visceral cancer.

pseudoacephalus (sū′dō-ă-sef′ă-lŭs) [pseudo- + G. *a-* priv. + *kephalē,* head]. An apparently headless placental parasitic twin which, however, has rudimentary cephalic structures that can be demonstrated by dissection.

pseudoachondroplasia (sū′dō-ă-kon-drō-plā′sē-ă). Dwarfism with short limbs and a relatively long trunk as in achondroplasia, but not evident at birth.

pseudoagglutination (sū′dō-ă-glū-ti-nā′shŭn). False agglutination. **1.** Agglomeration of particles in solution which does not involve antigen-antibody combination. **2.** Rouleaux *formation.*

pseudoagrammatism (sū′dō-ă-gram′ă-tizm) [pseudo- + G. *a-* priv. + *gramma,* writing, + *-ismos,* condition]. Paraphasia.

pseudoagraphia (sū′dō-ă-graf′ē-ă). Pseudagraphia.

pseudo-ainhum (sū′dō-in′yūm). Nonspontaneous amputation of a digit, caused by a variety of disorders such as neural leprosy, syringomyelia, and palmoplantar keratoderma.

pseudoalbuminuria (sū′dō-al-byū′mi-nū′rē-ă). Cyclic *albuminuria.*

pseudoallele (sū′dō-ă-lēl′). A gene exhibiting pseudoallelism.

pseudoallelic (sū′dō-ă-le′lik). Relating to pseudoallelism.

pseudoallelism (sū-dō-ă-lē′lizm). State of two or more genes that appear to occupy the same locus under certain conditions (*e.g.,* trans arrangement), but can be shown to occupy closely linked loci under other conditions (*e.g.,* cis arrangement).

pseudo-alopecia areata (sū′dō-al-ō-pē′shē-ă ar-ē-ā′tă). Alopecia in which mild inflammatory changes develop at the orifices of the affected hair follicles.

pseudoanaphylactic (sū′dō-an-ă-fī-lak′tik). Anaphylactoid.

pseudoanaphylaxis (sū′dō-an-ă-fī-lak′sis). A condition resembling anaphylaxis, but not due to specific antigen-antibody reaction.

pseudoanemia (sū′dō-ă-nē′mē-ă). False anemia; pallor of the skin and mucous membranes without the blood changes of anemia.

pseudoaneurysm (sū-dō-an′yū-rizm). False aneurysm (2); a dilation of an artery with actual disruption of one or more layers of its walls, as at the site of puncture as a complication of percutaneous arterial catheterization, rather than with expansion of all layers of the wall.

pseudoangina (sū′dō-an′ji-nă, -an-jī′nă). *Angina* pectoris vasomotoria.

pseudoangiosarcoma (sū′dō-an′jē-ō-sar-kō′mă). A benign vascular lesion that microscopically may be mistaken for an angiosarcoma.
Masson's p., intravascular papillary endothelial hyperplasia; a benign florid papillary endothelial proliferation within the veins of the skin or subcutis, less often in visceral blood vessels.

pseudoanodontia (sū′dō-an-ō-don′shē-ă) [pseudo- + G. *an-* priv. + *odous,* tooth]. Clinical absence of teeth due to a failure in eruption.

pseudoapoplexy (sū-dō-ap′ō-plek-sē). Parapoplexy; pseudoplegia; a condition simulating apoplexy, not due to cerebral hemorrhage or thrombosis.

pseudoappendicitis (sū′dō-ă-pen-di-sī′tis). A symptom-complex simulating appendicitis without inflammation of the appendix.

pseudoapraxia (sū′dō-ă-prak′sē-ă). A condition of exaggerated awkwardness in which the person makes wrong use of objects.

pseudoarthrosis (sū′dō-ar-thrō′sis). Pseudarthrosis.

pseudoataxia (sū′dō-ă-tak′sē-ă). Pseudotabes.

pseudoauthenticity (sū′dō-aw-then-ti′si-tē) [pseudo- + G. *authentikos,* original]. False or copied expression of thoughts and feelings.

pseudobacillus (sū′dō-bă-sil′ŭs). Any microscopic object, such as a poikilocyte, resembling a bacillus.

pseudobacterium (sū′dō-bak-tēr′ē-ŭm). Any microscopic object resembling a small bacillary organism or other bacterial form.

pseudoblepsia, pseudoblepsis (su-dō-blep′sē-ă, -blep′sis) [pseudo- + G. *blepsis,* vision]. Pseudopsia.

pseudobulbar (sū-dō-bŭl′bar). Denoting a supranuclear paralysis of the bulbar nerves.

pseudocartilage (sū-dō-kar′ti-lij). Chondroid *tissue* (1).

pseudocartilaginous (sū′dō-kar-ti-laj′i-nŭs). Composed of a substance resembling cartilage in texture.

pseudocast (sū′dō-kast). False *cast.*

pseudocele (sū′dō-sēl) [pseudo- + G. *koilia,* cavity]. *Cavum* septi pellucidi.

pseudocelom (sū-dō-sē′lom) [pseudo- + G. *koilōma,* hollow]. A partial or false celom, typical of Nematoda (roundworms) and related phyla, in which the body cavity is lined by mesoderm along only one surface (hypodermis, under the cuticular body wall). *Cf.* celom; acelom.

pseudocephalocele (sū-dō-sef′ă-lō-sēl) [pseudo- + G. *kephalē,* head, + *kēlē,* tumor]. Acquired herniation of intracranial tissues caused by injury or disease.

pseudochancre (sū-dō-shang′ker). A nonspecific indurated sore, usually located on the penis, resembling a chancre.

pseudocholinesterase (sū′dō-kol-in-es′ter-ās). Cholinesterase.
atypical p., a genetic variant of cholinesterase that fails to catalyze the hydrolysis of succinylcholine. See also dibucaine number; fluoride number.
typical p., a cholinesterase formed in the liver and present in plasma; it catalyzes the hydrolysis of succinylcholine, first into succinylmonocholine and choline, and then into choline and succinic acid.

pseudochorea (sū-dō-kōr-ē′ă). A spasmodic affection or extensive tic resembling chorea.

pseudochromesthesia (sū′dō-krō-mes-thē′zē-ă) [pseudo- + G. *chrōma,* color, + *aisthēsis,* sensation]. **1.** An anomaly in which each vowel in the printed word is seen as colored. See also photism. **2.** Color *hearing.*

pseudochromidrosis, pseudochromhidrosis (sū′dō-krō-mi-drō′sis, -hi-drō′sis) [pseudo- + G. *chrōma,* color, + *hidrōs,* sweat]. The presence of pigment on the skin in association with sweating, but due to the local action of pigment-forming bacteria and not to the excretion of colored sweat.

pseudochylous (sū-dō-kī′lŭs). Resembling chyle.

pseudocirrhosis (sū′dō-si-rō′sis). Cardiac *cirrhosis.*

pseudoclonus (sū-dō-klō′nŭs). Clonic response of short duration despite continued force to elicit it.

pseudocoarctation (sū′dō-kō-ark-tā′shŭn). Buckled or kinked aorta; distortion, often with slight narrowing, of the aortic arch at the level of insertion of the ligamentum arteriosum.

pseudocolloid (sū-dō-kol′oyd). A colloid-like or mucoid substance found in ovarian cysts, in the lips, and elsewhere.
p. of lips, Fordyce's *spots.*

pseudocollusion (sū′dō-co-lū′zhŭn) [pseudo- + Fr. *collusion,* fr. L. *colludere,* to play together]. A merely apparent sense of closeness emanating from a transference.

pseudocoma (sū-dō-kō'mă). Locked-in *syndrome.*

pseudocowpox (sū-dō-kow'poks). Paravaccinia; milkers' nodules or nodes; an infection of cows' udders by pseudocowpox virus that is transmitted to the fingers and hands of milkers, producing nodules and lymphangitis, and occasionally widespread papular or papulovesicular eruptions; human infection is transferable to uninfected cows.

pseudocoxalgia (sū'dō-kok-sal'jē-ă) [pseudo- + L. *coxa,* hip, + G. *algos,* pain]. Legg-Calvé-Perthes *disease.*

pseudocrisis (sū-dō-krī'sis). A temporary fall of the temperature in a disease usually ending by crisis; not a true crisis.

pseudocroup (sū-dō-krūp'). *Laryngismus* stridulus.

pseudocryptorchism (sū-dō-krip'tōr-kizm) [pseudo- + G. *kryptos,* hidden, + *orchis,* testis]. A condition in which the testes descend to the scrotum but continue to move up and down, rising high in the inguinal canal at one time and descending to the scrotum at another.

pseudocumene (sū-dō-kū'mēn). Pseudocumol; trimethyl benzene; a colorless liquid obtained from coal tar; used in the sterilization of catgut.

pseudocumol (sū-dō-kū'mol). Pseudocumene.

pseudocyesis (sū'dō-sī-ē'sis) [pseudo- + G. *kyēsis,* pregnancy]. False *pregnancy.*

pseudocylindroid (sū-dō-sil'in-droyd). A shred of mucus or other substance in the urine resembling a renal cast.

pseudocyst (sū'dō-sist) [pseudo- + G. *kystis,* bladder]. **1.** Adventitious or false cyst; an accumulation of fluid in a cystlike loculus, but without an epithelial or other membranous lining. **2.** A cyst whose wall is formed by a host cell and not by a parasite. **3.** A mass of 50 or more *Toxoplasma* bradyzoites, found within a host cell, frequently in the brain; formerly called a p., but now considered a true cyst enclosed in its own membrane within the host cell that may rupture to release particles that form new cysts, and apparently is infective to another vertebrate host. See also bradyzoite.

pseudodeciduosis (sū'dō-de-sid-yū-ō'sis) [pseudo- + L. *deciduus,* falling off]. A decidual response of endometrium in the absence of pregnancy.

pseudodementia (sū'dō-dē-men'shē-ă). A condition resembling dementia but usually due to a depressive disorder rather than brain dysfunction.

pseudodiabetes (sū'dō-dī-ă-bē'tēz). A condition in which a false positive test for sugar in the urine occurs.

pseudodiastolic (sū'dō-dī-as-tol'ik). Seemingly associated with the cardiac diastole.

pseudodigitoxin (sū'dō-dij-i-tok'sin). Gitoxin.

pseudodiphtheria (sū'dō-dif-thēr'ē-ă). Diphtheroid (1).

pseudodipsia (sū-dō-dip'sē-ă) [pseudo- + G. *dipsa,* thirst]. False *thirst.*

pseudodiverticulum (sū'dō-dī-ver-tik'yū-lūm). An outpouching from the lumen into an area of central necrosis within a large smooth muscle tumor, along any part of the intestinal wall.

pseudodysentery (sū-dō-dis'en-tār-ē). Occurrence of symptoms indistinguishable from those of bacillary dysentery, due to causes other than the presence of the specific microorganisms of bacillary dysentery.

pseudoedema (sū'dō-e-dē'mă) [pseudo- + G. *oidēma,* a swelling (edema)]. A puffiness of the skin not due to a fluid accumulation.

pseudoephedrine hydrochloride (sū'dō-e-fed'rin). *d*-Pseudoephedrine hydrochloride; the naturally occurring isomer of ephedrine; a sympathomimetic amine with actions and uses similar to those of ephedrine.

pseudoerysipelas (sū'dō-er-i-sip'ĕ-lăs). Erysipeloid.

pseudoesthesia (sū-dō-es-thē'zē-ă). Pseudesthesia.

pseudoexfoliation (sū'dō-eks-fō-lē-ā'shŭn). A condition simulating exfoliation in some respects, but in which the surface layer is not actually detached.

p. of lens capsule, a condition in which deposits on the lens resemble exfoliation of the lens capsule; frequently complicated by glaucoma.

pseudofluctuation (sū'dō-flŭk-chū-ā'shŭn). A wavelike sensation, resembling fluctuation, obtained by tapping muscular tissue.

pseudofolliculitis (sū'dō-fo-lik-yū-lī'tis). Follicular papules or pustules resulting from close shaving, or plucking, of very curly hair; growing tips of hairs consequently penetrate the follicle wall or reenter the skin adjacent to the follicle; p. of the beard area is very common in blacks.

pseudofracture (sū-dō-frak'chūr). A condition in which an x-ray shows formation of new bone with thickening of periosteum at site of an injury to bone.

pseudofructose (sū-dō-fruk'tōs). D-Psicose.

pseudoganglion (sū-dō-gang'glē-on). A localized thickening of a nerve trunk having the appearance of a ganglion.

pseudogene (sū'dō-jēn). A sequence of nucleotides that is not transcribed and therefore has no phenotypic effect.

pseudogeusesthesia (sū'dō-gyū-ses-thē'zē-ă) [pseudo- + G. *geusis,* taste, + *aisthēsis,* sensation]. Color *taste.*

pseudogeusia (sū-dō-gyū'sē-ă) [pseudo- + G. *geusis,* taste]. A subjective taste sensation not produced by an external stimulus.

pseudoglanders (sū-dō-glan'derz). Melioidosis.

pseudoglaucoma (sū'dō-glaw-kō'mă). Obsolete term for glaucoma with physiologically normal intraocular pressure.

pseudoglioma (sū'dō-glī-ō'mă). Any intraocular opacity liable to be mistaken for retinoblastoma.

pseudoglomerulus (sū'dō-glō-mer'yū-lūs). A structure within a neoplasm microscopically resembling a renal glomerulus but not representing renal glomerular differentiation.

pseudoglucosazone (sū'dō-glū-kō'să-zōn). A substance sometimes present in normal urine which gives a reaction in the phenylhydrazine test.

pseudogout (sū'dō-gowt). Calcium gout; acute episodes of synovitis caused by deposits of calcium pyrophosphate crystals rather than urate crytals as in true gout; associated with articular chondrocalcinosis.

pseudogynecomastia (sū'dō-gī-nĕ-kō-mas'tē-ă, -jin-ĕ-kō-) [pseudo- + G. *gynē,* woman, + *mastos,* breast]. Enlargement of the male breast by an excess of adipose tissue without any increase in breast tissue.

pseudohematuria (sū'dō-hem-ă-tū'rē-ă, -he-mă-). False hematuria; a red pigmentation of urine caused by certain foods or drugs, and thus not actually hematuria.

pseudohemoptysis (sū'dō-hē-mop'ti-sis) [pseudo- + G. haima, blood, + *ptysis,* a spitting]. Spitting of blood that does not come from the lungs or bronchial tubes.

pseudohermaphrodite (sū'dō-her-maf'rō-dīt). An individual exhibiting pseudohermaphroditism.

pseudohermaphroditism (sū'dō-her-maf'rō-dī-tizm). False hermaphroditism; a state in which the individual is of an unambiguous gonadal sex (*i.e.,* possessing either testes or ovaries) but has ambiguous external genitalia.

female p., androgynism; androgyny (1); p. in which the gonads are female in an individual with an XX karyotype.

male p., p. in which the gonads are male in an individual with a Y chromosome.

pseudohernia (sū-dō-her'nē-ă). Inflammation of the scrotal tissues or of an inguinal gland, simulating a strangulated hernia.

pseudoheterotopia (su'dō-het-er-ō-tō'pē-ă). A seeming displacement of certain tissues observed postmortem; actually an artifact, rather than a true heterotopia.

pseudohydrocephaly (sū'dō-hī-drō-sef'ă-lē). Condition characterized by an enlargement of the head without concomitant enlargement of the ventricular system.

pseudohydronephrosis (sū'dō-hī-drō-ne-frō'sis). Presence of a cyst near the kidney, simulating hydronephrosis.

pseudohyperparathyroidism (sū'dō-hī'per-par-ă-thī'roy-dizm). Hypercalcemia in a patient with a malignant neoplasm in the absence of skeletal metastases or primary hyperparathyroidism; believed to be due to formation of parathyroid hormone by nonparathyroid tumor tissue.

pseudohypertelorism (sū'dō-hī-per-tel'ōr-izm). An appearance of excessive distance between the eyes (ocular telorism) due to lateral displacement of the inner canthi.

pseudohypertrophic (sū'dō-hī-per-trof'ik). Relating to or marked by pseudohypertrophy.

pseudohypertrophy (sū'dō-hī-per'trō-fē). False hypertrophy; increase in size of an organ or a part, due not to increase in size or number of the specific functional elements but to that of some other tissue, fatty or fibrous.

pseudohypha (sū-dō-hī'fă) [pseudo- + G. *hyphē*, a web (hypha)]. A chain of easily disrupted fungal cells that is intermediate between a chain of budding cells and a true hypha, marked by constrictions rather than septa at the junctions.

pseudohyponatremia (sū'dō-hī-pō-nă-trē'mē-ă). A low serum sodium concentration due to volume displacement by massive hyperlipidemia or hyperproteinemia; also used to describe the low serum sodium concentration which may occur with high blood glucose.

pseudohypoparathyroidism (sū'dō-hī'pō-par-ă-thī'royd-izm). Sebright bantam syndrome; a disorder resembling hypoparathyroidism, but with signs and symptoms that are unresponsive to treatment with parathyroid hormone; characterized by short stature, round face, calcification of basal ganglia, true ectopic bone in fascial planes and skin, mental deficiency, hypocalcemia, hyperphosphatemia, and parathyroid tissue that is hyperplastic; not infrequently associated with moniliasis and manifestations of diabetes mellitis; assumed to represent refractoriness of target tissues to parathyroid hormone; most commonly inherited as a sex-linked dominant trait.

pseudoicterus (sū-dō-ik'ter-ŭs). Pseudojaundice; yellowish discoloration of the skin not due to bile pigments, as in Addison's disease.

pseudoileus (sū-dō-il'ē-ŭs). Absolute obstipation, stimulating ileus, due to paralysis of the intestinal wall.

pseudoinfluenza (sū'dō-in-flū-en'ză). An epidemic catarrh simulating influenza, but less severe.

pseudointraligamentous (sū'dō-in'tră-lig-ă-men'tŭs). Falsely giving the impression of lying within the broad ligament; *e.g.*, a p. tumor.

pseudoisochromatic (sū'dō-ī-sō-krō-mat'ik). Apparently of the same color; denoting certain charts containing colored spots mixed with figures printed in confusion colors; used in testing for color vision deficiency.

pseudojaundice (sū-dō-jawn'dis). Pseudoicterus.

pseudokeratin (sū-dō-kār'ă-tin). A protein extracted from epidermis and nervous tissue (glial fibrils), probably involved in keratinization.

pseudolipoma (sū'dō-li-pō'mă). Any circumscribed, soft, smooth, usually movable swelling or tumefaction that grossly resembles a lipoma.

pseudolithiasis (sū'dō-li-thī'ă-sis) [pseudo- + G. *lithos*, stone]. A disorder resembling one of the syndromes associated with a stone in a hollow viscus or elsewhere.

pseudologia (sū-dō-lō'jē-ă) [pseudo- + G. *logos*, word]. Pathological lying in speech or writing.

p. phantas'tica, an elaborate and often fantastic account of a patient's exploits, which are completely false but which the patient himself appears to believe.

pseudolymphocyte (sū-dō-lim'fō-sīt). A small neutrophilic leukocyte.

pseudolymphoma (sū'dō-lim-fō'mă). A benign infiltration of lymphoid cells or histiocytes which microscopically resembles a malignant lymphoma.

Spiegler-Fendt p., benign *lymphocytoma* cutis.

pseudolysogenic (sū'dō-lī-sō-jen'ik). Pertaining to pseudolysogeny.

pseudolysogeny (sū'dō-lī-soj'ĕ-nē). The condition in which a bacteriophage is maintained (carried) in a culture of a bacterial strain by infecting susceptible variants of the strain, in contradistinction to true lysogeny in which the bacteriophage genome multiplies as an integral part of the bacterial genome.

pseudomalignancy (sū'dō-mă-lig'nan-sē). A benign tumor that appears, clinically or histologically, to be a malignant neoplasm. See also pseudotumor.

pseudomamma (sū-dō-mam'ă). A glandular structure resembling the mammary gland, occurring in dermoid cysts.

pseudomania (sū-dō-mā'nē-ă). **1.** A factitious mental disorder. **2.** A mental disorder in which the patient alleges to have committed a crime, but of which he is innocent. **3.** Generally, the morbid impulse to falsify or lie, as in pseudologica.

pseudomasturbation (sū'dō-mas-ter-bā'shŭn). Peotillomania.

pseudomelanosis (sū'dō-mel-ă-nō'sis) [pseudo- + G. *melas*, black]. A dark greenish or blackish postmortem discoloration of the surface of the abdominal viscera, resulting from the action of sulfureted hydrogen upon the iron of disintegrated hemoglobin.

pseudomembrane (sū-dō-mem'brān). False *membrane*.

pseudomembranous (sū-dō-mem'bră-nŭs). Relating to or marked by the presence of a false membrane.

pseudomeningitis (sū'dō-men-in-jī'tis). Meningism.

pseudomenstruation (sū'dō-men-strū-ā'shŭn). Uterine bleeding without the typical premenstrual endometrial changes.

pseudometaplasia (sū'dō-met-ă-plā'zē-ă). Histologic *accommodation*.

pseudomnesia (sū-dom-nē'zē-ă) [pseudo- + G. *mnēsis*, memory]. A subjective impression of memory of events that have not occurred.

pseudomonad (sū-dō-mō'nad). A vernacular term used to refer to any member of the genus *Pseudomonas*.

Pseudomonas (sū-dō-mō'nas) [pseudo- + G. *monas*, unit, monad]. A genus of motile, polar flagellate, nonsporeforming, strictly aerobic bacteria (family Pseudomonadaceae) containing straight or curved, but not helical, Gram-negative rods which occur singly. The metabolism is respiratory, never fermentative. They occur commonly in soil and in fresh water and marine environments. Some species are plant pathogens. One species is a specialized mammalian parasite while others are occasionally pathogenic to animals. The type species is *P. aeruginosa*.

P. acidovo'rans, a species found in soil and occasionally in clinical specimens.

P. aerugino'sa, *P. pyocyanea;* blue pus bacillus; a species found in soil, water, and commonly in clinical specimens (wound infections, infected burn lesions, urinary tract infections); the causative agent of blue pus; occasionally pathogenic for plants; it is the type species of the genus *P.*

P. cepa'cia, a species found in rotted onions and in clinical specimens.
P. diminu'ta, a species found primarily in clinical specimens, rarely in water.
P. fluores'cens, a species found in soil and water; it is frequently found in clinical specimens and is commonly associated with food spoilage (eggs, cured meats, fish, and milk).
P. mal'lei, *Actinobacillus mallei;* glanders bacillus; a species infectious to horses and donkeys, causing glanders and farcy.
P. maltophil'ia, a species found primarily in clinical specimens but also in water, milk, and frozen food.
P. pseudoalcalig'enes, a species found in a sinus discharge.
P. pseudomal'lei, Whitmore's bacillus; a species found in cases of melioidosis in humans and other animals and in soil and water in tropical regions.
P. putrefa'ciens, a marine species implicated as a cause of fish spoilage but rarely as a human pathogen.
P. pyocyan'ea, *P. aeruginosa.*
P. stut'zeri, a species found in soil and water, frequently in clinical specimens.
P. vesicula're, a species found in the medicinal leech (*Hirudo medicinalis*) and in water from a stream.

pseudomorph (sū'dō-mōrf) [pseudo- + G. *morphē,* form]. A mineral found crystallized in a form that is not proper to it but to some other mineral.

pseudomycelium (sū'dō-mī-se'lē-ŭm). A mycelium-like mass of pseudohyphae.

pseudomyopia (sū'dō-mī-ō'pē-ă). A condition simulating myopia and due to spasm of the ciliary muscle.

pseudomyxoma (sū'dō-mik-sō'mă). A gelatinous mass resembling a myxoma but composed of epithelial mucus.
p. peritone'i, gelatinous ascites; the accumulation of large quantities of mucoid or mucinous material in the peritoneal cavity, either as a result of rupture of a mucocele of the appendix, or rupture of benign or malignant cystic neoplasms of the ovary; it will frequently persist because of the growth of mucus-secreting cells scattered on serosal surfaces, leading to intestinal adhesions and obstruction.

pseudonarcotic (sū'dō-nar-kot'ik). Inducing sleep by reason of a sedative effect, but not directly narcotic.

pseudoneoplasm (sū-dō-nē'ō-plazm). Pseudotumor.

pseudoneuritis (sū'dō-nū-rī'tis). Congenital blurring of margins of the optic disk simulating appearance of inflammation.

pseudoneuroma (sū'dō-nū-rō'mă). Traumatic *neuroma.*

pseudonit (sū'dō-nit). Hair *cast.*

pseudonystagmus (sū'dō-nis-tag'mŭs). Accentuation of the normal oscillatory eye movements occurring on shifting fixation.

pseudo-osteomalacia (sū'dō-os'tē-ō-mă-lā'shē-ă). Rachitic softening of bone.

pseudo-osteomalacic (sū'dō-os'tē-ō-mă-lā'sik). Marked by pseudo-osteomalacia.

pseudopapilledema (sū'dō-pap-il-e-dē'mă). Anomalous elevation of the optic disk; seen in severe hyperopia and optic nerve drusen.

pseudoparalysis (sū'dō-pă-ral'i-sis). Pseudoparesis (1); apparent paralysis due to voluntary inhibition of motion because of pain, to incoordination, or other cause, but without actual paralysis.
arthritic general p., Klippel's disease; a disease, occurring in arthritic subjects, having symptoms resembling those of general paresis, the lesions of which consist of diffuse changes of a degenerative and noninflammatory character due to intracranial atheroma.
congenital atonic p., *amyotonia* congenita.

pseudoparaplegia (sū'dō-par-ă-plē'jē-ă). Apparent paralysis in the lower extremities, in which the tendon and skin reflexes and the electrical reactions are normal; the condition is sometimes observed in rickets.
Basedow's p., weakness in the thigh muscles in thyrotoxicosis which may occur suddenly and cause the patient to fall; a specific form of myopathy is fairly common in thyrotoxicosis.

pseudoparasite (sū-dō-par'ă-sīt). A false parasite; may be either a commensal or a temporary parasite (the latter being an organism accidentally ingested and surviving briefly in the intestine).

pseudoparenchyma (sū'dō-pă-reng'ki-mă). In fungi, a tissue-like mass of modified hyphae.

pseudoparesis (sū'dō-pa-rē'sis, -par'ĕ-sis). **1.** Pseudoparalysis. **2.** A condition marked by the pupillary changes, tremors, and speech disturbances suggestive of early paresis, in which, however, the serologic tests are negative.

pseudopelade (sū'dō-pĕ-lahd') [pseudo- + Fr. *pelade,* disease that causes sporadic falling of hair]. Alopecia parviculata; a scarring type of alopecia; usually occurs in small areas preceded by folliculitis; assumed by many to be synonymous with folliculitis decalvans.

pseudopericarditis (sū'dō-per-i-kar-dī'tis). An artifact of auscultation resembling a friction rub, but due to movement of the tissue in the intercostal space when the diaphragm of the stethoscope is placed over the apex beat.

pseudoperitonitis (sū'dō-per'i-tō-nī'tis). Peritonism (2).

pseudophacos (sū'dō-fak'ōs) [pseudo- + G. *phakos,* lens]. Lenticulus.

pseudophakia (sū-dō-fak'ē-ă) [pseudo- + *phakos,* lentil (lens)]. An eye in which the natural lens is replaced with an intraocular lens.

pseudophakodonesis (sū-dō-fā'kō-dō-nē'sis). Excessive mobility of an intraocular lens implant.

pseudophlegmon (sū-dō-fleg'mon) [pseudo- + G. *phlegmonē,* inflammation]. A noninflammatory circumscribed redness of the skin.
Hamilton's p., a trophic affection of the subcutaneous connective tissue, marked by a circumscribed swelling which may become indurated and red, but never suppurates.

pseudophotesthesia (sū'dō-fō-tes-thē'zē-ă) [pseudo- + G. *phōs,* light, + *aisthēsis,* sensation]. Photism.

pseudophyllid (sū-dō-fī'lid). Common name for members of the order Pseudophyllidea.

Pseudophyllidea (sū'dō-fi-lid'ē-ă) [pseudo- + G. *phyllon,* leaf]. An order of tapeworms with an aquatic life cycle, passing through coracidium, procercoid, and plerocercoid stages before developing into adults in fish, marine mammals, or fish-eating mammals; includes the broad fish tapeworm of man, *Diphyllobothrium latum.*

pseudoplatelet (sū-dō-plāt'let). Any of the fragments of neutrophils which may be mistaken for platelets, especially in peripheral blood smears of leukemic patients.

pseudoplegia (sū-dō-plē'jē-ă) [pseudo- + G. *plēgē,* a stroke]. Pseudoapoplexy.

pseudopocket (sū'dō-pok'et). A pocket, adjacent to a tooth, resulting from gingival hyperplasia and edema but without apical migration of the epithelial attachment.

pseudopod (sū'dō-pod). Pseudopodium.

pseudopodium, pl. **pseudopodia** (sū-dō-pō'dē-ŭm, -pō'-dē-ă) [pseudo- + G. *pous,* foot]. Pseudopod; a temporary protoplasmic process, put forth by an ameboid stage or amebic protozoan for locomotion or for prehension of food.

pseudopolydystrophy (sū'dō-pol-ē-dis'trō-fē). Mucolipidosis III.

pseudopolyp (sū-dō-pol'ip). Inflammatory p.; a projecting mass of granulation tissue, large numbers of which may develop in ulcerative colitis; may become covered by regenerating epithelium.

pseudoporphyria (sū'dō-pōr-fir'ē-ă). A condition clinically and ultrastructurally identical to porphyria but with no abnormality in porphyrin excretion, consequent to drug ingestion or hemodialysis.

pseudopregnancy (sū-dō-preg'nan-sē). **1.** False pregnancy. **2.** A condition in which symptoms resembling those of pregnancy are present, but which is not pregnancy; occurs after sterile copulation in mammalian species in which copulation induces ovulation, and also in dogs, in which the estrus cycle includes a marked luteal phase.

pseudoprognathism (sū-dō-prog'nă-thizm). An acquired projection of the mandible due to occlusal disharmonies which force the mandible forward; the mandibular condyles are forward of their expected functional position.

pseudo-pseudohypoparathyroidism (sū'dō-sū-dō-hī'-pō-par-ă-thī'royd-ism). A heritable disorder that simulates pseudohypoparathyroidism; manifestations of hypoparathyroidism are mild or absent, hypocalcemia is not present, but changes in physical stature are present.

pseudopsia (sū-dop'sē-ă) [pseudo- + G. *opsis,* vision]. Pseudoblepsia; pseudoblepsis; visual hallucinations, illusions, or false perceptions.

pseudopterygium (sū'dō-tĕ-rij'ē-ŭm). Adhesion of the conjunctiva to the cornea, occurring after injury.

pseudoptosis (sū-dō-tō'sis, sū-dop'tō-sis) [pseudo- + G. *ptōsis,* a falling]. False blepharoptosis; a condition resembling an inability to elevate the eyelid, due to blepharophimosis, blepharochalasis, or some other affection.

pseudopuberty (sū-dō-pyū'ber-tē). Condition characterized by the development of a varying number of the somatic and functional changes typical of puberty; commonly caused by the hormonal secretions of a tumor and typically arises before the chronological age of puberty.

precocious p., the development of p. in very young children; commonly characterized by secretion of gonadal hormones, without stimulation of gametogenesis.

pseudorabies (sū-dō-rā'bēz) [pseudo- + rabies]. Aujeszky's disease; infectious bulbar paralysis; mad itch; a disease affecting cattle, horses, dogs, swine, and other mammalian species, caused by *Herpesvirus suis,* which has its reservoir in swine and is transmitted to wounds of other species by the nasal secretions. In species other than swine, it is highly fatal; in very young swine, it causes fatalities but in adult animals the disease is often inapparent.

pseudoreaction (sū'dō-rē-ak'shŭn). A false reaction; one not due to specific causes in a given test.

pseudoreplica (sū-dō-rep'li-kă). A specimen for electron microscopic examination obtained by depositing particles from a virus-containing suspension on an agarose surface, covering the surface with a plastic-containing solution, and, after evaporation of the solvent, removing the film along with enmeshed particles by floating it onto the surface of a uranyl acetate solution.

pseudoretinitis pigmentosa (sū'dō-ret-i-nī'tis pig-men-tō'să). A widespread pigmentary mottling of the retina that may follow severe eye trauma, especially from a penetrating injury.

pseudorheumatism (sū-dō-rū'mă-tizm). Joint or muscle symptoms without objective findings and with no apparent underlying causes.

pseudorickets (sū-dō-rik'ets). Renal *rickets.*

pseudorosette (sū'dō-rō-zet'). Perivascular radial arrangement of neoplastic cells around a small blood vessel. See rosette (2).

pseudorubella (sū'dō-rū-bel'ă). *Exanthema* subitum.

pseudosarcoma (sū-dō-sar-kō'mă). A bulky polyploid malignant tumor of the esophagus, composed of spindle cells with a focus of squamous cell carcinoma; spindle cells may be epithelial or metaplastic malignant fibroblasts.

pseudoscarlatina (sū'dō-skar-lă-tē'nă). Erythema with fever, due to causes other than *Streptococcus pyogenes.*

pseudosclerosis (sū'dō-sklĕr-ō'sis) [pseudo- + G. *sklērosis,* hardening]. **1.** Inflammatory induration or fatty or other infiltration simulating fibrous thickening. **2.** Westphal's p. or disease; Strümpell-Westphal disease; Westphal-Strümpell p.; the cerebral changes of hepatolenticular degeneration.

Westphal's p., Westphal-Strümpell p., pseudosclerosis (2).

pseudosmallpox (sū-dō-smawl'poks). Alastrim.

pseudosmia (sū-doz'me-ă) [pseudo- + G. *osmē,* smell]. Subjective sensation of an odor that is not present.

Pseudostertagia bullosa (sū'dō-ster-tā'jē-ă bŭl-ō'să). One of the medium stomach worms located in the abomasum of sheep, goats, and pronghorn; it is found chiefly in the western U.S.

pseudostoma (sū-dos'tō-mă) [pseudo- + G. *stoma,* mouth]. An apparent opening in a cell, membrane, or other tissue, due to a defect in staining or other cause.

pseudostrabismus (sū'dō-stra-biz'mŭs) [pseudo- + G. *strabismos,* a squinting]. The appearance of strabismus caused by epicanthus, abnormality in interorbital distance, or corneal light reflex not corresponding to the center of the pupil.

pseudotabes (sū-dō-tā'bēz). Pseudoataxia; Leyden's ataxia; peripheral tabes; a syndrome having the characteristics of tabes dorsalis but not due to syphilis.

pupillotonic p., Holmes-Adie *syndrome.*

pseudotrichinosis, pseudotrichiniasis (sū'dō-trik-i-nō'sis, -trik-i-nī'ă-sis). Multiple *myositis.*

pseudotruncus arteriosus (sū-dō-trŭng'kŭs ar-tēr-ē-ō'sŭs). Congenital cardiovascular deformity with atresia of the pulmonic valve and absence of the main pulmonary artery; the lungs are supplied with blood either through a patent ductus or via bronchial arteries arising from the aorta.

pseudotubercle (sū-dō-tū'ber-kl). A nodule histologically similar to a tuberculous granuloma, but due to infection by some microorganism other than *Mycobacterium tuberculosis.*

pseudotuberculosis (sū'dō-tū-ber'kyū-lō'sis). Pseudotubercular yersinosis; a disease of a wide variety of animal species caused by *Yersinia pseudotuberculosis.* Epizootics of p. are commonly seen in birds and rodents, often with high case fatality rates. In man, seven clinical entities are recognized: primary focalized infections (pseudoappendicitis, acute mesenteric lymphadenitis, or acute terminal ileitis), primary generalized infections (septicemia or scarlatiniform fever), and secondary immunological complexities (erythema nodosum or arthralgia).

pseudotumor (sū'dō-tū-mer). Pseudoneoplasm. **1.** An enlargement of nonneoplastic character which clinically resembles a true neoplasm so closely as to often be mistaken for such. **2.** A condition, commonly associated with obesity in young females, of cerebral edema with narrowed small ventricles but with increased intracranial pressure and frequently papilledema.

p. cer'ebri, a condition of the brain simulating the presence of an intracranial tumor, probably due either to vascular congestion or to swelling of the brain.

inflammatory p., a tumor-like mass in the lungs or other sites, composed of fibrous or granulation tissue infiltrated by inflammatory cells.

pseudouridine (**ψ, ψrd**) (sū-dō-yū'ri-dēn, -din). 5-Ribosyluracil; a naturally occurring isomer of uridine found in transfer ribonucleic acids; unique in that the ribosyl is attached to carbon rather than to nitrogen.

pseudovacuole (sū-dō-vak'yū-ōl). An apparent vacuole in a cell, either an artifact or an intracellular parasite.

pseudovariola (sū′dō-vă-rī′ō-lă) [pseudo- + L. *variola*, smallpox]. Alastrim.

pseudoventricle (sū-dō-ven′tri-kl). *Cavum* septi pellucidi.

pseudovitamin (sū-dō-vī′tă-min). A substance having a chemical structure very similar to that of a given vitamin, but lacking the usual physiologic action.

p. B_{12}, vitamin B_{12f}; ψ vitamin B_{12}; cobamide cyanide phosphate, 3′-ester with 7-α-D-ribofuranosyladenine, inner salt; vitamin B_{12} with adenine replacing dimethylbenzimidazole; one of several substances produced during anaerobic fermentation by certain organisms in bovine rumen contents; it is chemically closely similar to vitamin B_{12} (cyanocobalamin) but without, in man, the physiologic action of the vitamin.

pseudovomiting (sū-dō-vom′i-ting). Regurgitation of matter from the esophagus or stomach without expulsive effort.

pseudoxanthoma elasticum (sū′dō-zan-thō′mă e-las′ti-kŭm). Elastoma; an inherited disorder of connective tissue characterized by slightly elevated yellowish plaques on the neck, axillae, abdomen, and thighs, associated with angioid streaks of the retina and similar elastic tissue degeneration in other organs; two autosomal dominant and two autosomal recessive types have been described.

psi (sī). The 23rd letter (ψ) of the Greek alphabet. **1.** Symbol for pseudouridine. **2.** Symbol for pseudo-.

D-psicose (sī′kōs). D-Allulose; pseudofructose; D-ribo-2-hexulose; a ketohexose, isomeric with fructose.

psilocin (sī′lō-sin). 3-[2-(Dimethylamino)ethyl]indol-4-ol; a hallucinogenic agent related to psilocybin.

Psilocybe (sī-lō-sī′bē). A genus of mushrooms (family Agaricaceae) containing many species with psychotropic or hallucinogenic properties, including *P. mexicana*, of which the fruiting bodies are a source of the hallucinogen, psilocybin.

psilocybin (sī-lō-sī′bin, -sib′in). Indocybin; 3-(2-dimethylamino)-ethylindol-4-ol dihydrogen phosphate; the *N′,N′*-dimethyl derivative of 4-hydroxytryptamine; obtained from the fruiting bodies of the fungus *Psilocybe mexicana* and other species of *Psilocybe* and *Stropharia*. P. is a congener of 5-hydroxytryptamine, with striking central nervous system effects, and is readily hydrolyzed to 4-hydroxybufotenine; used as a hallucinogenic agent (and by Mexican aborigines to induce trances).

psilosis (sī-lō′sis) [G. *psilōsis*, a stripping, fr. *psilos*, bare]. **1.** Obsolete term for sprue (1). **2.** Falling out of the hair.

psilothin (sil′ō-thin) [see psilosis]. A depilatory plaster applied when warm to a hairy surface, and ripped off when cool, causing removal of the hairs.

psilotic (sī-lot′ik). **1.** Relating to psilosis. **2.** Epilatory (1).

P-sinistrocardiale (sin-is-trō-kar-dē-ā′lē). An electrocardiographic syndrome characteristic of overloading of the left atrium; often erroneously called P-mitrale, as the syndrome can result from any overloading of the left atrium from any cause.

psittacine (sit′ă-sēn). Referring to birds of the parrot family (parrots, parakeets, and budgerigars).

psittacosis (sit-ă-kō′sis) [G. *psittakos*, a parrot, + *-osis*, condition]. Parrot disease or fever; an infectious disease in psittacine birds and man caused by *Chlamydia psittaci*. Avian infections are mainly inapparent or latent, although acute or peracute disease do occur; human infections may result in mild disease with a flu-like syndrome or in severe disease, especially in older persons, with symptoms of bronchopneumonia.

psoas (sō′as) [G. *psoa*, the muscles of the loins]. See entries under musculus.

psomophagia, psomophagy (sō-mō-fā′jē-ă, sō-mof′ă-jē) [G. *psōmos*, morsel, bit, + *phagein*, to eat]. The practice of swallowing the food without thorough mastication.

psora (sō′ră) [G. *psōra*, itch]. Psoriasis.

psoralen (sōr′ă-len). Furo[3,2-*g*]coumarin; a phototoxic drug used by topical or oral administration for the treatment of vitiligo.

psorelcosis (sō-rel-kō′sis) [G. *psōra*, itch, + *helkōsis*, ulceration]. Ulceration resulting from scabies of the skin.

psorenteritis (sōr′en-ter-ī′tis) [G. *psōra*, itch (scabies), + *enteron*, intestine, + *-itis*, inflammation]. Inflammatory swelling of the solitary lymphatic follicles of the intestine.

Psorergates (psō-rer′gă-tēz) [G. *psōra*, itch]. A genus of itch mites (family Cheyletidae) parasitic on cattle, sheep, and goats. *P. bos* is the itch mite of cattle, described in New Mexico; *P. ovis* is the small itch mite of sheep in the U.S., Australia, New Zealand, and South Africa.

psoriasic (sō-rī′ă-sik). Psoriatic.

psoriasiform (sō-rī′ă-si-fōrm). Resembling psoriasis.

psoriasis (sō-rī′ă-sis) [G. *psōriasis*, fr. *psōra*, the itch]. Alphos; psora; a condition characterized by the eruption of circumscribed, discrete and confluent, reddish, silvery-scaled maculopapules; the lesions occur predominantly on the elbows, knees, scalp, and trunk, and microscopically show characteristic parakeratosis and elongation of rete ridges.

p. annula′ris, p. annula′ta, p. circinata.

p. arthrop′ica, p. associated with severe arthritis resembling rheumatoid arthritis, although serum rheumatoid factor is absent.

p. circina′ta, p. annularis, annulata, or orbicularis; p. in which healing is taking place at the center of the lesion while the process continues at the periphery, producing a ring-shaped or annular lesion.

p. diffu′sa, diffused p., a form of p. with extensive coalescence of the lesions.

p. discoi′dea, p. nummularis; p. in which the lesions are discrete and disklike.

generalized pustular p. of Zambusch, pustular p. (1).

p. geograph′ica, p. gyrata in which the lesions suggest the coast outline on a map.

p. gutta′ta, p. occurring in round patches of small size, giving the appearance of a rain-bespattered surface.

p. gyra′ta, p. circinata in which there is a coalescence of the rings giving rise to figures of various outlines.

p. invetera′ta, p. in which the lesions are confluent, the affected skin being thickened, indurated, and scaly.

p. nummula′ris, p. discoidea.

p. orbicula′ris, p. circinata.

p. ostrea′cea, p. rupioides; p. with concentric tiers of scales which give the appearance of the layering of an oyster shell.

p. puncta′ta, p. in which the individual lesions are papules, each red in color, and tipped with a single white scale.

pustular p., **(1)** generalized pustular p. of Zambusch; an extensive exacerbation of p., with pustule formation in the normal and psoriatic skin, fever, and granulocytosis; sometimes precipitated by oral steroids; **(2)** a local pustular eruption of the palms and soles, occurring most commonly in a patient with p.; difficult to distinguish from acrodermatitis continua.

p. rupioi′des, p. ostreacea.

p. spondylit′ica, p. associated with an ankylosing spondylitis.

p. universa′lis, a generalized p.

psoriatic (sō-rē-at′ik). Psoriasic; relating to psoriasis.

psoric (sō′rik). Psorous; relating to scabies.

psoroid (sō′royd) [G. *psōra*, itch (scabies), + *eidos*, resemblance]. Resembling scabies.

psorophthalmia (sō-rof-thal′mē-ă) [G. *psōra*, itch (scabies), + ophthalmia]. *Blepharitis* marginalis.

Psoroptes (sō-rop′tēz) [G. *psōra*, itch]. A genus of itch or mange mites (family Cheyletidae), including the species *P. cuniculi* (the scab mite of rabbits), *P. equi* (the mange or body mite of horses), and *P. ovis* (the common scab mite of sheep and cattle).

psorous (sō'rŭs). Psoric.

PSP Abbreviation for phenolsulfonphthalein.

psych-, psyche-. See psycho-.

psychagogy (sī'kă-go-jē) [psych- + G. *agōgia,* a tutor's office]. Psychotherapeutic reeducation stressing social adjustment of the individual.

psychalgalia (sī-kal-gā'lē-ă). Psychalgia (1).

psychalgia (sī-kal'jē-ă) [psych- + G. *algos,* pain]. **1.** Mind or soul pain; algopsychalia; phrenalgia (1); psychalgalia; distress attending a mental effort, noted especially in melancholia. **2.** Psychogenic *pain.*

psychalia (sī-kā'lē-ă). An emotional condition characterized by auditory and visual hallucinations.

psychanopsia (sī'kă-nop'sē-ă) [psych- + G. *an-* priv, + *opsis,* vision]. Mind *blindness.*

psychataxia (sī-kă-tak'sē-ă) [psych- + G. *ataxia,* confusion]. Mental confusion; inability to fix one's attention or to make any continued mental effort.

psyche (sī'kē) [G. mind, soul]. Obsolete term for the subjective aspects of the mind and of the individual.

psychedelic (sī-kē-del'ik) [psyche- + G. *dēloun,* to manifest]. **1.** Pertaining to a rather imprecise category of drugs with mainly central nervous system action, and with effects said to be the expansion or heightening of consciousness, *e.g.,* LSD, hashish, mescaline. **2.** A hallucinogenic substance, visual display, music, or other sensory stimulus having such action.

psychentonia (sī-ken-tō'nē-ă) [psych- + G. *en,* in, + *tonos,* tension]. Mental tension.

psychiatric (sī-kē-at'rik). Relating to psychiatry.

psychiatrics (sī-kē-at'riks). Psychiatry.

psychiatric trend. Benign or morbid emotional interests and urges as revealed by postures, gestures, actions, or speech.

psychiatrist (sī-kī'ă-trist). A physician who specializes in psychiatry.

psychiatry (sī-kī'ă-trē) [psych- + G. *iatreia,* medical treatment]. Psychiatrics. **1.** The medical specialty concerned with the diagnosis and treatment of mental illnesses. **2.** The diagnosis and treatment of mental illnesses. For some types of p. not listed below, see also subentries under therapy, psychotherapy, psychoanalysis.

analytic p., psychoanalytic p.

community p., p. focusing on the detection, prevention, early treatment, and rehabilitation of emotional disorders and social deviance as they develop in the community rather than as encountered one-on-one, in private practice, or at larger centralized psychiatric facilities; particular emphasis is placed on the social-interpersonal-environmental factors that contribute to mental illness.

contractual p., psychiatric intervention voluntarily assumed by the patient, who is prompted by his personal difficulties or suffering and who retains control over his participation with the psychiatrist.

dynamic p., psychoanalytic p.

existential p., existential *psychotherapy.*

forensic p., legal p., the application of p. in courts of law, *e.g.,* in determinations for commitment, fitness to stand trial, responsibility for crime.

psychoanalytic p., analytic or dynamic p.; psychiatric theory and practice emphasizing the principles of psychoanalysis.

social p., an approach to psychiatric theory and practice emphasizing the cultural and sociological aspects of mental disorder and treatment; the application of p. to social problems. See also community p.

psychic (sī'kik) [G. *psychikos*]. **1.** Psychical; relating to the phenomena of consciousness, mind, or soul. **2.** A person supposedly endowed with the power of communicating with spirits; a spiritualistic medium.

psychical (sī'ki-kăl). Psychic (1).

psychism (sī'kizm) [G. *psychē,* soul]. The theory that a principle of life pervades all nature.

psycho-, psych-, psyche- [G. *psychā,* soul, mind]. Combining forms denoting the mind.

psychoacoustics (sī'ko-ă-kūs'tiks) [psycho- + G. *akoustikos,* relating to hearing]. The science pertaining to the psychologic factors that influence one's awareness of sound.

psychoactive (sī-kō-ak'tiv). Possessing the ability to alter mood, anxiety, behavior, cognitive processes, or mental tension; usually applied to pharmacologic agents.

psychoallergy (sī-kō-al'er-jē). A sensitization to emotionally charged symbols.

psychoanalysis (sī'kō-ă-nal'i-sis) [psycho- + analysis]. **1.** Psychoanalytic therapy; a method of psychotherapy, originated by Freud, designed to bring preconscious and unconscious material to consciousness primarily through the analysis of transference and resistance. See also freudian p. **2.** A method of investigating the human mind and psychological functioning, especially through free association and dream analysis in the psychoanalytic situation. **3.** An integrated body of observations and theories on personality development, motivation, and behavior. **4.** An institutionalized school of psychotherapy, as in jungian or freudian p.

active p., p. in which the analyst intervenes directly and actively in the patient's life, *e.g.,* by making prohibitions, assigning tasks.

adlerian p., individual *psychology.*

freudian p., the theory and practice of p. and psychotherapy as developed by Freud, based on: 1) his theory of personality, which postulates that psychic life is made up of instinctual forces, or the id, the ego, and a superego, each of which must constantly accommodate to the other; 2) his discovery that the free association technique of verbalizing for the analyst all thoughts without censoring any of them is the therapeutic tactic which reveals the areas of conflict within a patient's personality; 3) that the vehicle for gaining this insight and next, on this basis, readjusting one's personality is the learning a patient does as he first develops a stormy emotional bond with the analyst (transference relationship) and next successfully learns to break his bond.

jungian p., analytical psychology; the theory of psychopathology and the practice of psychotherapy, according to the principles of Jung, which utilizes a system of psychology and psychotherapy emphasizing man's symbolic nature, and differs from freudian p. especially in placing less significance upon instinctual (sexual) urges.

psychoanalyst (sī-kō-an'ă-list). A psychotherapist, usually a psychiatrist or clinical psychologist, trained in psychoanalysis and employing its methods in the treatment of emotional disorders.

psychoanalytic (sī'kō-an-ă-lit'ik). Pertaining to psychoanalysis.

psychoauditory (sī-kō-aw'di-tōr-ē) [psycho- + L. *auditorius,* relating to hearing]. Relating to the mental perception and interpretation of sounds.

psychobiology (sī'kō-bī-ol'ō-jē). **1.** The study of the biology of the mind, including cognition and memory. **2.** Adolf Meyer's term for psychiatry.

psychocatharsis (sī'kō-kă-thar'sis). Catharsis (2).

psychochemistry (sī'kō-kem'is-trē). The alteration of affect or emotion by chemical means.

psychochrome (sī'kō-krōm) [psycho- + G. *chrōma,* color]. A certain color mentally conceived in response to a sense impression. See also psychochromesthesia.

psychochromesthesia (sī'kō-krō-mes-thē'zē-ă) [psycho- + G. *chrōma,* color, + *aisthēsis,* sensation]. A form of synesthesia in which a certain stimulus to one of the special organs of sense produces the mental image of a color. See also photism.

psychodiagnosis (sī'kō-dī-ag-nō'sis). **1.** Any method used to discover the factors which underlie behavior, especially malajusted or abnormal behavior. **2.** A subspecialty within clinical psychology that emphasizes the use of psychological tests and techniques for assessing psychopathology.

Psychodidae (sī-kod'i-dē) [G. *Psychē,* a Greek nymph, sometimes represented as a butterfly]. A family of small flies or gnats characterized by hairy mothlike body and the presence of 7 to 11 long parallel wing veins lacking cross-veins; includes the sandflies, *Phlebotomus* and *Lutzomyia,* vectors of all known forms of leishmaniasis.

psychodometry (sī-kō-dom'ĕ-trē) [psycho- + G. *hodos,* way, + *metron,* measure]. The measurement of the rapidity of mental action.

psychodrama (sī'kō-drah-mă). A method of psychotherapy in which patients act out their personal problems by taking diagnostically specific roles in spontaneous dramatic performances.

psychodynamics (sī'kō-dī-nam'iks) [psycho- + G. *dynamis,* force]. The systematized study and theory of human behavior, emphasizing unconscious motivation and the functional significance of emotion.

psychoendocrinology (sī'kō-en'dō-krĭ-nol'ō-jē). Study of the interrelationships between endocrine function and mental states.

psychoexploration (sī'kō-eks-plōr-ā'shŭn). Study of the attitudes and emotional life of a person.

psychogalvanic (sī'kō-gal-van'ik). Relating to changes in electric properties of the skin; *e.g.,* a change in skin resistance induced by psychologic stimulus.

psychogalvanometer (sī'kō-gal-vă-nom'ĕ-ter). A galvanometer that records changes in skin resistance related to emotional stress.

psychogender (sī-kō-jen'der). The attitudes adopted by an individual related to his personal identification as either a male or a female. See also gender *role.*

psychogenesis (sī-kō-jen'ĕ-sis) [psycho- + G. *genesis,* origin]. Psychogeny; the origin and development of the psychic processes including mental, behavioral, personality, and related psychological processes.

psychogenic, psychogenetic (sī'kō-jen'ik, -jĕ-net'ik). **1.** Of mental origin or causation. **2.** Relating to emotional development or to psychogenesis.

psychogeny (sī-koj'ĕ-nē). Psychogenesis.

psychogeusic (sī-kō-gū'sik) [psycho- + G. *geusis,* taste]. Pertaining to the mental perception and interpretation of taste.

psychogogic (sī-kō-goj'ik) [psycho- + G. *agōgos,* a leading away]. Acting as a stimulant to the emotions.

psychographic (sī-kō-graf'ik). Relating to psychography.

psychography (sī-kog'ră-fē) [psycho- + G. *graphē,* a writing]. The literary characterization of an individual, real or fictional, that uses psychoanalytical and psychological categories and theories; a psychological biography or character description.

psychohistory (sī-kō-his'tōr-ē). The combined use of psychology (especially psychoanalysis) and history in the writing especially of biography, as in the work of Erik Erikson. See also psychography.

psychokinesis, psychokinesia (sī'kō-ki-nē'sis, -nē'zē-ă) [psycho- + G. *kinēsis,* movement]. **1.** Impulsive behavior. **2.** The influence of mind upon matter, as the use of mental "power" to move or distort an object.

psychokym (sī'kō-kīm) [psycho- + G. *kyma,* wave]. Rarely used term for the physiologic substrate of psychic processes.

psycholagny (sī-kō-lag'nē) [psycho- + G. *lagneia,* lust]. Rarely used term for sexual excitement and satisfaction from mental imagery.

psycholepsy (sī'kō-lep-sē) [psycho- + G. *lepsis,* seizure]. Rarely used term for sudden mood changes accompanied by feelings of hopelessness and inertia.

psycholinguistics (sī'kō-ling-gwi'stiks) [psycho- + L. *lingua,* tongue]. Study of mental and intellectual factors that affect communication and understanding of language.

psychologic, psychological (sī-kō-loj'ik, -loj'i-kăl). **1.** Relating to psychology. **2.** Relating to the mind and its processes.

psychologist (sī-kol'ō-jist). A specialist in psychology licensed to practice professional psychology (*e.g.,* clinical p.), or qualified to teach psychology as a scholarly discipline (academic p.), or whose scientific specialty is a subfield of psychology (research p.).

psychology (sī-kol'ō-jē) [psycho- + G. *logos,* study]. The profession (*e.g.,* clinical p.), scholarly discipline (academic p.), and science (research p.) concerned with the behavior of man and animals, and related mental and physiological processes.

adlerian p., individual p.

analytical p., jungian *psychoanalysis.*

atomistic p., any psychologic system based on the doctrine that mental processes are built up through the combination of simple elements; *e.g.,* psychoanalysis, behaviorism.

behavioral p., behaviorism.

clinical p., a branch of p. that specializes in both discovering new knowledge and in applying the art and science of p. to persons with emotional or behavioral disorders; subspecialties include clinical child p. and pediatric p.

cognitive p., a branch of p. that attempts to integrate into a whole the disparate knowledge from the subfields of perception, learning, memory, intelligence, and thinking.

community p., the application of p. to community programs, *e.g.,* in the schools, correctional and welfare systems, and community mental health centers.

comparative p., a branch of p. concerned with the study and comparison of the behavior of organisms at different levels of phylogenic development to discover developmental trends.

constitutional p., the p. of the individual as related to body habitus.

criminal p., the study of the mind and its workings in relation to crime.

counseling p., p. with emphasis on facilitating the normal development and growth of the individual in coping with important problems of everyday living, as contrasted with clinical p.

depth p., the p. of the unconscious, especially in contrast with older (19th century) academic p. dealing only with conscious mentation; sometimes used synonymously with psychoanalysis.

developmental p., the study of the psychologic changes in an organism that occur with aging.

dynamic p., a psychologic approach that concerns itself with the causes of behavior.

educational p., the application of p. to education, especially to problems of teaching and learning.

environmental p., the study and application by behavioral scientists and architects of how changes in physical space and related physical stimuli impact upon the behavior of individuals. See also personal *space.*

existential p., a theory of p., based on the philosophies of phenomenology and existentialism, which holds that the proper study of p. is man's experience of the sequence, spatiality, and organization of his existence in the world.

experimental p., **(1)** a subdiscipline within the science of p. that is concerned with the study of conditioning, learning, perception, motivation, emotion, language, and thinking; **(2)** also used in relation to subject-matter areas in which experimental, in contrast to correlational or socio-experiential, methods are emphasized.
forensic p., the application of p. to legal matters in a court of law.
genetic p., a science dealing with the evolution of behavior and the relation to each other of the different types of mental activity.
gestalt p., see gestaltism.
holistic p., any psychologic system which postulates that the human mind or any mental process must be studied as a unit; *e.g.*, gestaltism, existential p.
humanistic p., an existential approach to psychology which emphasizes man's uniqueness, his subjectivity, and his capacity for psychological growth.
individual p., adlerian p. or psychoanalysis; a theory of human behavior emphasizing man's social nature, his strivings for mastery, and his drive to overcome, by compensation, feelings of inferiority.
industrial p., the application of the principles of p. to problems in business and industry.
medical p., the branch of p. concerned with the application of psychologic principles to the practice of medicine.
objective p., p. as studied by observation of the behavior and mental functions in others.
subjective p., the study of one's own mind and its various modes of action as a basis for psychologic deductions.

psychometrics (sī-kō-met'riks). Psychometry.

psychometry (sī-kom'ĕ-trē) [psycho- + G. *metron,* measure]. Psychometrics; the discipline pertaining to psychological and mental testing, and to any quantitative analysis of an individual's psychological traits or attitudes or mental processes.

psychomotor (sī-kō-mō'ter). **1.** Relating to the mental origin of muscular movement, and to the production of voluntary movements. **2.** Relating to the combination of psychic and motor events, including disturbances.

psychoneurosis (sī'kō-nū-rō'sis) [psycho- + G. *neuron,* nerve, + *-osis,* condition]. **1.** A mental or behavioral disorder of mild or moderate severity. **2.** Formerly a classification of neurosis including hysteria, psychasthenia, and neurasthenia.
p. mai'dica, pellagra.

psychoneurotic (sī'kō-nū-rot'ik). Pertaining to or suffering from psychoneurosis.

psychonomic (sī-kō-nom'ik). Relating to psychonomy.

psychonomy (sī-kon'ō-mē) [psycho- + G. *nomos,* law]. The branch of psychology concerned with the laws of behavior.

psychonosology (sī'kō-nō-sol'ō-jē) [psycho- + G. *nosos,* disease, + *logos,* study]. Psychiatric nosology; the classification of mental illnesses.

psychonoxious (sī-kō-nok'shŭs) [psycho- + L. *noxius,* harmful]. Rarely used term for: **1.** Having an unfavorable effect on the emotional life and reactions mediated by higher levels of the central nervous system; may be endogenous or exogenous. **2.** Denoting persons or situations that elicit fear, pain, or anxiety in an individual.

psychopath (sī'kō-path). Former designation for an individual with an antisocial type of personality disorder. See also antisocial *personality.*

psychopathic (sī-kō-path'ik). Relating to or characteristic of psychopathy.

psychopathist (sī-kop'ă-thist). Obsolete term for psychiatrist.

psychopathologist (sī'kō-pă-thol'ō-jist). One who specializes in psychopathology.

psychopathology (sī'kō-pă-thol'ō-jē) [psycho- + G. *pathos,* disease, + *logos,* study]. **1.** The science concerned with the pathology of the mind. **2.** The science of mental and behavioral disorders, including psychiatry and abnormal psychology.

psychopathy (sī-kop'ă-thē) [psycho- + G. *pathos,* disease]. Obsolete and inexact term referring to a pattern of antisocial or manipulative behavior engaged in by a psychopath. See also personality *disorder.*

psychopharmaceuticals (sī'kō-far-mă-sū'ti-kălz). Drugs used in the treatment of emotional disorders.

psychopharmacology (sī'kō-far'mă-kol'ō-jē) [psycho- + G. *pharmakon,* drug, + *logos,* study]. Neuropsychopharmacology. **1.** The use of drugs to treat mental disorders. **2.** The science of drug-behavior relationships.

psychophysical (sī-kō-fiz'i-kăl). **1.** Relating to the mental perception of physical stimuli. **2.** Psychosomatic.

psychophysics (sī-kō-fiz'iks). The science of the relation between the physical attributes of a stimulus and the measured, quantitative attributes of the mental perception of that stimulus.

psychophysiologic (sī'kō-fiz-ē-ō-loj'ik). **1.** Pertaining to psychophysiology. **2.** Denoting a so-called psychosomatic illness. **3.** Denoting a somatic disorder with significant emotional or psychological etiology.

psychophysiology (sī'kō-fiz-ē-ol'ō-jē). The science of the relation between psychological and physiological processes; *e.g.*, conscious elements of autonomic nervous system activity involved in emotion.

psychoprophylaxis (sī'kō-prō-fi-lak'sis) [psycho- + prophylaxis]. Psychotherapy directed toward the prevention of emotional disorders and the maintenance of mental health.

psychorelaxation (sī'kō-rē-lak-sā'shŭn). A method of treating anxiety and tension by practicing general bodily relaxation, as in systematic desensitization.

psychormic (sī-kōr'mik) [psycho- + G. *horman,* to set in motion]. Psychostimulant.

psychorrhea (sī-kō-rē'ă) [psycho- + G. *rhoia,* flow]. Rarely used term for a psychiatric syndrome characterized by incoherent and strange philosophical theories; a manifestation of schizophrenia.

psychorrhythmia, psychorhythmia (sī-kō-rith'mē-ă) [psycho- + G. *rhythmos,* rhythm]. Rarely used term for an involuntary repetition of formerly voluntary acts.

psychosensory, psychosensorial (sī'kō-sen'sōr-ē, -sen-sōr'ē-ăl). **1.** Denoting the mental perception and interpretation of sensory stimuli. **2.** Denoting a hallucination which by effort the mind is able to distinguish from reality.

psychosexual (sī-kō-sek'shū-ăl). Pertaining to the relationships among the emotional, mental, and physiologic components of sex or sexual development.

psychosine (sī'kō-sēn). Galactosylsphingosine, a constituent of cerebrosides, formed from UDPgalactose and sphingosine by UDP-galactose-sphingosine β-D-galactosyltransferase.

psychosis, pl. psychoses (sī-kō'sis, -sēz) [G. an animating]. **1.** A mental disorder causing gross distortion or disorganization of a person's mental capacity, affective response, and capacity to recognize reality, communicate, and relate to others to the degree of interfering with his capacity to cope with the ordinary demands of everyday life. The psychoses are divided into two major classifications according to their origins: 1) those associated with organic brain syndromes (*e.g.*, Korsakoff's syndrome); 2) those less strictly organic and having some functional component(s) (*e.g.*, the schizophrenias, bipolar disorder). **2.** Generic term for any of the so-called insanities, the most common forms being the schizophrenias. **3.** A severe emotional illness.
affective p., p. with predominant affective features.

alcoholic psychoses, mental disorders that result from alcholism and that involve organic brain damage, as in delirium tremens and Korsakoff's syndrome.
amnestic p., Korsakoff's *syndrome.*
arteriosclerotic p., psychotic disturbance in elderly persons suffering from cerebral arteriosclerosis.
Cheyne-Stokes p., a mental state characterized by anxiety and restlessness, accompanying Cheyne-Stokes respiration.
climacteric p., involutional p. associated with the climacteric.
drug p., p. following or precipitated by ingestion of a drug, *e.g.,* LSD.
dysmnesic p., Korsakoff's *syndrome.*
exhaustion p., a confusional emotional state following an exhausting event.
febrile p., infection-exhaustion p.
gestational p., psychotic reaction associated with pregnancy.
hysterical p., **(1)** a psychotic disturbance with predominantly hysterical symptoms; **(2)** a mental disorder resembling conversion hysteria but of psychotic severity; **(3)** a brief reactive p.
ICU p., psycotic episode(s), classically occurring in coronary care patients, occurring within 24 hours after entering the ICU in individuals with no previous history of p.; related to sleep deprivation, overstimulation in the ICU, and time spent on life support systems, and should be distinguished from exacerbation of a pre-existing p. or an organic p. such as delirium.
infection-exhaustion p., febrile p.; a p. following an acute infection, shock, or chronic intoxication; begins as delirium followed by pronounced mental confusion with hallucinations and unsystematized delusions, and sometimes stupor.
involutional p., mental disturbance occurring during the menopause or later life.
Korsakoff's p., Korsakoff's *syndrome.*
manic-depressive p., bipolar *disorder.*
polyneuritic p., Korsakoff's *syndrome.*
posthypnotic p., p. following or precipitated by hypnosis.
postinfectious p., psychotic disturbance following acute febrile disease such as pneumonia or typhoid fever.
postpartum p., puerperal p.; an acute mental disorder or p. in the mother following childbirth.
posttraumatic p., p. following trauma, especially to the head. *Cf.* traumatic p.
puerperal p., postpartum p.
schizo-affective p., psychotic disturbance in which there is a mixture of schizophrenic and manic-depressive symptoms.
senile p., mental disturbance occurring in old age and related to degenerative cerebral processes.
situational p., a transitory but severe emotional disorder caused in a predisposed person by a seemingly unbearable situation.
toxic p., a p. caused by some toxic substance, whether endogenous or exogenous.
traumatic p., a p. resulting from physical injury or emotional shock. *Cf.* posttraumatic p.
Windigo (Wittigo) p., severe anxiety neurosis with special reference to food, manifested in melancholia, violence, and obsessive cannibalism, occurring among Canadian Indians.

psychosocial (sī-kō-sō'shăl). Involving both psychological and social aspects.

psychosomatic (sī'kō-sō-mat'ik) [psycho- + G. *soma,* body]. Psychophysical (2); pertaining to the influence of the mind or higher functions of the brain (emotions, fears, desires, etc.) upon the functions of the body, especially in relation to bodily disorders or disease.

psychosomimetic (sī-kō'sō-mi-met'ik). Psychotomimetic.

psychostimulant (sī-kō-stim'yū-lant). Psychormic; an agent with antidepressant or mood-elevating properties.

psychosurgery (sī-kō-ser'jer-ē). The treatment of mental disorders by operation upon the brain, *e.g.,* lobotomy.

psychosynthesis (sī-kō-sin'thĕ-sis) [psycho- + synthesis]. A lay movement, the opposite of psychoanalysis, stressing therapy aimed at restoring useful inhibitions.

psychotechnics (sī-kō-tek'niks) [psycho- + G. *technē,* art, skill]. Practical application of psychologic methods in the study of economics, sociology, and other subjects.

psychotherapeutic (sī'kō-thār-ă-pyū'tik). Relating to psychotherapy.

psychotherapeutics (sī'kō-thār-ă-pyū'tiks). Psychotherapy.

psychotherapist (sī-kō-thār'ă-pist). A person, usually a psychiatrist or clinical psychologist, professionally trained and engaged in psychotherapy.

psychotherapy (sī-kō-thār'ă-pē) [psycho- + G. *therapeia,* treatment]. Psychotherapeutics; treatment of emotional, behavioral, personality, and psychiatric disorders based primarily upon verbal or nonverbal communication with the patient, in contrast to treatments utilizing chemical and physical measures. For some types of p. not listed here, see also subentries under psychoanalysis, psychiatry, psychology, therapy.
anaclitic p., a psychotherapeutic method characterized by encouragement and utilization of the patient's tendency to depend and lean upon the therapist as an authority figure; often contrasted with psychoanalytic therapy, which seeks to dissolve, rather than exploit, this phenomenon.
autonomous p., a type of psychoanalytic p. placing special emphasis on the value of the patient's self-determination in both the therapeutic situation and in real life.
contractual p., p. based on a firm agreement, or "contract," between therapist and patient as to the role of each in the therapeutic situation.
directive p., p. utilizing the authority of the therapist to direct the course of the patient's therapy, as contrasted with nondirective p.
dyadic p., individual therapy; a psychotherapeutic session involving only two persons, the therapist and the patient.
dynamic p., psychoanalytic p.
existential p., existential psychiatry; a type of therapy, based on existential philosophy, emphasizing confrontation, primarily spontaneous interaction, and feeling experiences rather than rational thinking, with less attention given to patient resistances; the therapist is involved on the same level and to the same degree as the patient.
group p., a type of psychological treatment involving two or more patients participating together in the presence of one or more psychotherapists who facilitate both emotional and rational congnitive interaction to effect changes in the maladaptive behavior of the individual patients in their everyday interpersonal exchanges. See also subentries under group.
heteronomous p., term embracing all forms of p. that foster the patient's dependence on others, especially dependence on the psychotherapist, in contrast to autonomous p.
hypnotic p., p. based on hypnosis.
intensive p., p. involving thorough exploration of the patient's life history and conflicts; often contrasted with supportive p.
marathon group p., a type of group p. characterized by prolonged sessions for periods of hours or days, with minimal interruptions for food and rest.
nondirective p., p. in which the therapist follows the lead of the patient during the interview rather than introducing his own theories and directing the course of the interview. See also client-centered *therapy.*
psychoanalytic p., dynamic p.; p. utilizing freudian principles. See also psychoanalysis.
reconstructive p., a form of therapy, such as psychoanalysis, that seeks not only to alleviate symptoms but also to produce alter-

ations in maladaptive character structure and to expedite new adaptive potentials; this aim is achieved by bringing into consciousness an awareness of and insight into conflicts, fears, inhibitions, and their manifestations.

suggestive p., p. utilizing the influence and authority of the therapist. See also directive p.

supportive p., p. aiming at bolstering the patient's psychological defenses and providing him reassurance, as in crisis intervention, rather than probing provocatively into his conflicts.

transactional p., p. with central emphasis on the actual relations (transactions) between the patient and other people in his life.

psychotic (sī-kot'ik). Relating to or affected by psychosis.

psychotogen (sī-kot'ō-jen) [psychotic + G. *-gen,* producing]. A drug that produces psychotic manifestations.

psychotogenic (sī-kot-ō-jen'ik). Inducing psychosis; particularly referring to drugs of the LSD series and similar substances.

psychotomimetic (sī-kot'ō-mi-met'ik). Psychosomimetic. **1.** A drug or substance that produces psychological and behavioral changes resembling those of psychosis; *e.g.,* LSD. **2.** Denoting such a drug or substance.

psychotropic (sī-kō-trop'ik) [psycho- + G. *tropē,* a turning]. Affecting the mind, denoting drugs used in the treatment of mental illnesses.

psychro- [G. *psychros,* cold]. Combining form relating to cold. See also cryo-, crymo-.

psychroalgia (sī-krō-al'jē-ă) [psychro- + G. *algos,* pain]. A painful sensation of cold.

psychroesthesia (sī'krō-es-thē'zē-ă) [psychro- + G. *aisthēsis,* sensation]. **1.** The form of sensation that perceives cold. **2.** A sensation of cold although the body is warm; a chill.

psychrometer (sī-krom'ĕ-ter) [psychro- + G. *metron,* measure]. Wet and dry bulb thermometer; a device for measuring the humidity of the atmosphere by the difference in temperature between two thermometers, the bulb of one kept moist, the other dry. Evaporation from the moist bulb lowers the reading of that thermometer; the greater the difference in readings, the drier the air; no difference indicates 100% relative humidity.

sling p., wet and dry bulb thermometers mounted on a hand sling, for use when a small portable psychrometer is required.

psychrometry (sī-krom'ĕ-trē) [psychro- + G. *metron,* measure]. Hygrometry; the calculation of relative humidity and water vapor pressures from wet and dry bulb temperatures and barometric pressure; whereas relative humidity is the value ordinarily employed, the vapor pressure is the measurement of physiological significance.

psychrophile, psychrophil (sī'krō-fīl) [psychro- + G. *phileō,* to love]. An organism which grows best at a low temperature (0 to 32°C; 32 to 86°F), with optimum growth occurring at 15 to 20°C (59 to 68°F).

psychrophilic (sī-krō-fil'ik). [psychro- + G. *phileō,* to love]. Pertaining to a psychrophile.

psychrophobia (sī-krō-fō'bē-ă) [psychro- + G. *phobos,* fear]. **1.** Extreme sensitiveness to cold. **2.** A morbid dread of cold.

psychrophore (sī'krō-fōr) [psychro- + G. *phoros,* bearing]. A double catheter through which cold water is circulated to apply cold to the urethra or another canal or cavity.

psyllium hydrophilic mucilloid (sil'ē-ŭm). See *plantago* seed.

PT Abbreviation for physical therapist or therapy.

Pt Symbol for platinum.

PTA Abbreviation for plasma thromboplastin *antecedent;* phosphotungstic acid.

PTAH Abbreviation for phosphotungstic acid *hematoxylin.*

ptarmic (tar'mik) [G. *ptarmikos,* causing to sneeze, fr. *ptarmos,* a sneezing]. Sternutatory.

ptarmus (tar'mŭs) [G. *ptarmos,* a sneezing]. Sneezing.

PTC Abbreviation for plasma thromboplastin *component;* phenylthiocarbamoyl.

Ptd Abbreviation for phosphatidyl.

PtdCho Abbreviation for phosphatidylcholine.

PtdEth Abbreviation for phosphatidylethanolamine.

PtdIns Abbreviation for phosphatidylinositol.

PtdSer Abbreviation for phosphatidylserine.

pter-, ptero- [G. *pteron,* wing, feather]. Combining forms meaning wing or feather.

pteridine (ter'i-dēn, -din). Azinepurine; benzotetrazine; pyrazino[2,3-*d*]pyrimidine; a two-ring heterocyclic compound found as a component of pteroic acid and the pteroylglutamic acids (folic acids, pteropterin, etc.); simple p. derivatives (*e.g.,* xanthopterin, leucopterin) occur as pigments in butterfly wings, whence the name.

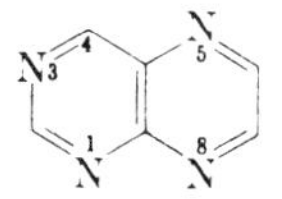

Pteridine

pterin (ter'in). Term loosely used for any of the compounds containing pteridine; specifically, 2-amino-4-hydroxypteridine. Some pteridines (*e.g.,* xanthopterin, leucopterin) still retain the pterin root.

p. deaminase [EC 3.5.4.11], an aminohydrolase catalyzing hydrolytic deamination of 2-amino-4-hydroxypteridine.

pterion (tē'rē-on) [G. *pteron,* wing]. A craniometric point in the region of the sphenoid fontanelle, at the junction of the greater wing of the sphenoid, the squamous temporal, the frontal, and the parietal bones.

pteroic acid (tĕ-rō'ik). A constituent of folic acid, containing *p*-aminobenzoic acid and pteridine linked by a $-CH_2-$group between the NH_2 of the former and C-6 of the latter.

pteropterin (ter-op'ter-in). Pteroyltriglutamic acid; pteroyl-γ-glutamyl-γ-glutamylglutamic acid; fermentation *Lactobacillus casei* factor; a folic acid conjugate, a principle chemically similar to folic acid except that it contains three molecules of glutamic acid instead of one, in γ linkage.

pteroylmonoglutamic acid (ter'ō-il-mon-ō'glū-tam'ik). Folic acid (2).

pteroyltriglutamic acid (ter'ō-il-trī'glū-tam'ik). Pteropterin.

pterygium (tĕ-rij'ē-ŭm) [G. *pterygion,* anything like a wing, a disease of the eye, dim. of *pteryx,* wing]. **1.** Web eye; a triangular patch of hypertrophied bulbar subconjunctival tissue, extending from the medial canthus to the border of the cornea or beyond, with apex pointing toward the pupil. **2.** A forward growth of the eponychium with adherence to the proximal portion of the nail. **3.** An abnormal skin web.

p. col'li, cervical patagium; a congenital, usually bilateral, web or tight band of skin of the neck extending from the acromion to the mastoid.

p. un'guis, overgrowth of cuticle onto the nail, with distortion and destruction of the nail.

pterygo- [G. *pteryx, pterygos,* wing]. Combining form denoting wing-shaped, usually the pterygoid process.

pterygoid (ter'i-goyd) [G. *pteryx* (*pteryg-*), wing, + *eidos,* resemblance]. Wing-shaped; resembling a wing; a term applied to various anatomical parts in the neighborhood of the sphenoid bone.

pterygomandibular (ter′i-gō-man-dib′yū-lăr). Relating to the pterygoid process and the mandible.

pterygomaxillare (ter′i-gō-mak-si-lār′ē). The point where the pterygoid process of the sphenoid bone and the pterygoid process of the maxilla begin to form the pterygomaxillary fissure; the lowest point of the opening is used in cephalometrics.

pterygomaxillary (ter′i-gō-mak′si-lār-ē). Relating to the pterygoid process and the maxilla.

pterygopalatine (ter′i-gō-pal′ă-tīn). Relating to the pterygoid process and the palatine bone.

pterygoquadrate (ter′i-gō-kwah′drāt). Relating to the pterygoid and quadrate bones in the upper jaw of lower vertebrates.

PTF Abbreviation for plasma thromboplastin *factor.*

PTH Abbreviation for parathyroid *hormone;* phenylthiohydantoin.

pthiriasis (thī-rī′a-sis) [G. *phtheiriasis,* fr. *phtheir,* a louse]. Pediculosis pubis; infestation with the pubic or crab louse, *Pthirus pubis.*

p. cap′itis, *pediculosis* capitis.

p. cor′poris, *pediculosis* corporis.

p. pu′bis, presence of crab lice in the pubis and other hairy areas of the trunk, and in the eyelashes of infants and young children.

Pthirus (thī′rŭs) [L. *phthir;* G. *phtheir,* a louse]. A genus of lice (family Pediculidae) formerly grouped in the genus *Pediculus.* The main species is *P. pubis* (*Pediculus pubis*), the crab or pubic louse, a parasite that infests the pubis and neighboring hairy parts of the body. Often incorrectly spelled *Phthirus* or *Phthirius.*

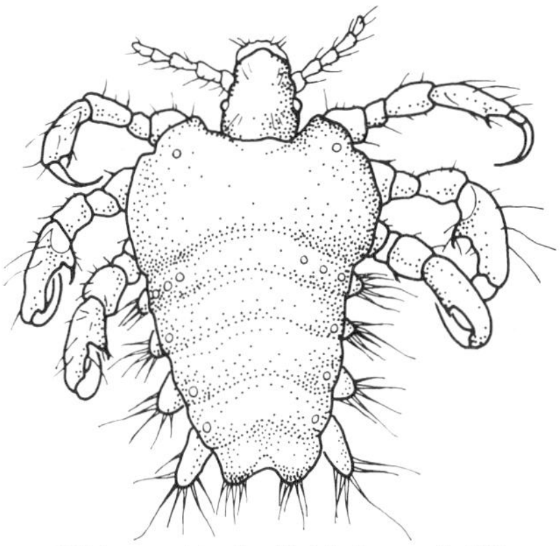

***Pthirus pubis,* the Pubic Louse (×25)**

ptilosis (ti-lō′sis) [G. *ptilōsis,* plumage, inflamed eyelids with falling lashes, fr. *ptilon,* soft feathers, down]. Loss of the eyelashes.

ptomaine (tō′mān) [G. *ptōma,* a corpse]. Ptomatine; an indefinite term applied to poisonous substances, *e.g.,* toxic amines, formed in the decomposition of protein by the decarboxylation of amino acids by bacterial action.

ptomainemia (tō-mā-nē′mē-ă) [ptomaine + G. *haima,* blood]. A condition resulting from the presence of a ptomaine in the circulating blood.

ptomatine (tō′mă-tēn). Ptomaine.

ptomatropine (tō-mat′rō-pēn). A ptomaine characterized by poisonous properties similar to those of atropine; formed by the action of bacteria in the decarboxylation of amino acids.

ptosed (tōzd). Ptotic.

-ptosis [G. *ptōsis,* a falling]. Suffix denoting a falling or downward displacement of an organ.

ptosis, pl. ptoses (tō′sis, tō′sēz) [G. *ptōsis,* a falling]. **1.** A sinking down or prolapse of an organ. **2.** Blepharoptosis.

p. adipo′sa, blepharochalasis.

p. sympathet′ica, Horner's *syndrome.*

ptotic (tot′ik). Ptosed; relating to or marked by ptosis.

PTU Abbreviation for propylthiouracil.

ptyal-, ptyalo- [G. *ptyalon,* saliva]. Combining forms denoting saliva, or the salivary glands. See also sialo-.

ptyalagogue (tī-al′ă-gog). Sialagogue.

ptyalectasis (tī′ă-lek′tă-sis) [ptyal- + G. *ektasis,* a stretching out]. Sialectasis.

ptyalin (tī′ă-lin). α-Amylase.

ptyalism (tī′al-izm) [G. *ptyalismos,* spitting]. Sialism.

ptyalocele (tī′ă-lō-sēl). Ranula (2).

ptyalography (tī-ă-log′ră-fē). Sialography.

ptyalolith (tī′ă-lō-lith). Sialolith.

ptyalolithiasis (tī′ă-lō-li-thī′ă-sis). Sialolithiasis.

ptyalolithotomy (tī′ă-lō-li-thot′ō-mē). Sialolithotomy.

ptychotis oil (tī-kō′tis). Ajowan oil.

ptyocrinous (tī-ok′ri-nŭs) [G. *ptyo,* to spit out, + *krinō,* to separate]. Secreting by discharge of the contents of the cell, as in mucous cells.

Pu Symbol for plutonium.

pubarche (pyū-bar′kē). Onset of puberty, particularly as manifested by the appearance of pubic hair.

puberal, pubertal (pyū′ber-ăl, -ber-tăl). Relating to puberty.

pubertas precox (pyū′ber-tahs prē′koks) [L.]. Puberty.

puberty (pyū′ber-tē) [L. *pubertas,* fr. *puber,* grown up]. Sequence of events by which a child becomes a young adult, characterized by the beginning of gametogenesis, secretion of gonadal hormones, development of secondary sexual characters, and reproductive functions; sexual dimorphism is accentuated. In girls, the first signs of p. may be evident at age 8 with the process largely completed by age 16; in boys, p. commonly begins at ages 10 to 12 and is largely completed by age 18. Ethnic and geographical factors may influence the time at which various events typical of p. occur. In law, the ages of presumptive puberty are 12 years in girls and 14 years in boys.

precocious p., pubertas precox; condition in which pubertal changes begin at an unexpectedly early age; often the result of a pathological process involving a gland capable of secreting estrogens or androgens, *e.g.,* the ovary or the adrenal cortex.

pubes (pyū′bēz) [L.]. Plural of pubis.

pubescence (pyū-bes′ens). **1** [L. *pubesco,* to attain puberty]. The approach of the age of puberty or sexual maturity. **2** [L. *pubes,* pubic hair]. Presence of downy or fine, short hair.

pubescent (pyū-bes′ent). Pertaining to pubescence.

pubic (pyū′bik). Relating to the os pubis.

pubiotomy (pyū-bē-ot′ō-mē) [L. *pubis,* pubic bone, + G. *tomē,* incision]. Gigli's operation; pelviotomy (2); severance of the pubic bone a few centimeters lateral to the symphysis, in order to increase the capacity of a contracted pelvis sufficiently to permit the passage of a living child.

pubis, pl. pubes (pyū′bis, pyū′bēz) [L. *pubes,* the hair on the genitals; the genitals]. **1.** *Os* pubis. **2** [NA]. One of the pubic hairs; the hair of the pubic region just above the external genitals. **3** [NA]. *Mons* pubis.

Public Health Service (PHS). See United States Public Health Service.

pubo- [L. *pubis*]. Combining form denoting pubis or pubic.

pubocapsular (pyū′bō-kap′sū-lăr). Relating to the pubis and the capsule of the hip joint.

pubococcygeal (pyū-bō-kok-sij'ē-ăl). Relating to the pubis and the coccyx.

pubofemoral (pyū'bō-fem'ō-răl). Relating to the os pubis and the femur.

pubomadesis (pyū'bō-mă-dē'sis) [L. *pubes,* pubic hair, + G. *madesis,* baldness]. Pubic baldness; loss of pubic hair.

puboprostatic (pyū'bō-pros-tat'ik). Relating to the pubic bone and the prostate.

puborectal (pyū'bō-rek'tăl). Relating to the pubis and the rectum.

pubovesical (pyū'bō-ves'i-kăl). Relating to the pubic bone and the bladder.

Puchtler-Sweat stains. See under stain.

pudenda (pyū-den'dă) [L.]. Plural of pudendum.

pudendal (pyū-den'dăl). Pudic; relating to the external genitals.

pudendum, pl. **pudenda** (pyū-den'dŭm, -dă) [L. ntr. of *pudendus,* particip. adj. of *pudeo,* to feel ashamed]. The external genitals, especially the female genitals (vulva). Used also in the plural.
p. femini'num [NA], vulva.
p. muli'ebre, vulva.

Pudenz, Robert H., U.S. neurosurgeon, *1911. See Heyer-P. *valve.*

pudic (pyū'dik) [L. *pudicus,* modest]. Pudendal.

puerpera, pl. **puerperae** (pyū-er'per-ă, -per-ē) [L., fr. *puer,* child, + *pario,* to bring forth]. Puerperant (2); a woman who has just given birth.

puerperal (pyū-er'per-ăl). Puerperant (1); relating to the puerperium, or period after childbirth.

puerperant (pyū-er'per-ant). **1.** Puerperal. **2.** A puerpera.

puerperium, pl. **puerperia** (pyū-er-pēr'ē-ŭm, -ē-ă) [L. childbirth, fr. *puer,* child, + *pario,* to bring forth]. Period from the termination of labor to complete involution of the uterus, usually defined as 42 days.

Puestow, Charles B., American surgeon, 1902–1973. See P.'s *procedure.*

puff (pŭf). A short blowing sound heard on auscultation, usually over the heart.
veiled p., a faint pulmonary murmur, simulating the muffled flapping of a cloth in the wind.

puffball (pŭf'bal). *Lycoperdon.*

Pulex (pyū'leks) [L. flea]. A genus of fleas (family Pulicidae, order Siphonaptera).
P. che'opis, former name for *Xenopsylla cheopis.*
P. fascia'tus, former name for *Nosopsyllus fasciatus.*
P. ir'ritans, the human flea, a common flea that infests man, many domestic animals (especially swine), and wild mammals and birds; a poor vector of plague.

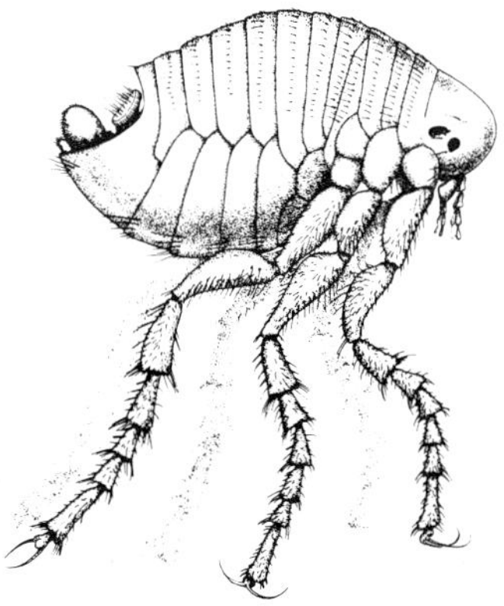

Pulex irritans, The Human Flea (×21)

P. pen'etrans, incorrect name for *Tunga penetrans.*
P. serra'ticeps, former name for *Ctenocephalides canis.*

pulicicide, pulicide (pyū-lis'i-sīd, pyū'li-sīd) [L. *pulex* (*pulic-*), flea, + *caedo,* to kill]. A chemical agent destructive to fleas.

pulley (pŭl'ē). See trochlea.
p. of humerus, *trochlea* humeri.
muscular p., *trochlea* muscularis.
peroneal p., *trochlea* peronealis.
p. of talus, *trochlea* tali.

pullulanase (pul'yū-lă-nās). α-Dextrin endo-1,6-α-glucoridase.

pullulate (pŭl'yū-lāt). To undergo pullulation.

pullulation (pŭl-yū-lā'shŭn) [L. *pullulo,* pp. *-atus,* to sprout forth]. The act of sprouting, or of budding as seen in yeast.

pulmo, gen. **pulmonis,** pl. **pulmones** (pŭl'mō, pŭl-mō'nis, -mō'nēz) [L.] [NA]. Lung.
p. dex'ter [NA], right lung.
p. sinis'ter [NA], left lung.

pulmo-, pulmon-, pulmono- [L. *pulmo,* lung]. Combining forms denoting the lungs. See also pneum-, pneumo-.

pulmoaortic (pŭl'mō-ā-ōr'tik). Relating to the pulmonary artery and the aorta.

pulmolith (pŭl'mō-lith) [L. *pulmo,* long, + G. *lithos,* stone]. Pneumolith.

pulmometer (pŭl-mom'ĕ-ter) [L. *pulmo,* lung, + G. *metron,* measure]. Obsolete term for spirometer.

pulmometry (pŭl-mom'ĕ-trē). Obsolete term for spirometry.

pulmonary (pŭl'mō-nār-ē) [L. *pulmonarius,* fr. *pulmo,* lung]. Pneumonic (1); pulmonic (1); relating to the lungs, to the pulmonary artery, or to the aperture leading from the right ventricle into the pulmonary artery.

pulmonectomy (pŭl-mō-nek'tō-mē) [L. *pulmo* (*pulmon-*), lung, + G. *ektomē,* excision]. Pneumonectomy.

pulmonic (pŭl-mon'ik). **1.** Pulmonary. **2.** Obsolete term for a remedy for diseases of the lungs.

pulmonitis (pŭl-mō-nī'tis). Pneumonitis.

pulmotor (pŭl'mō-ter) [L. *pulmo,* lung, + motor]. A medically obsolete term still used occasionally by lay personnel to refer to volume-limited or, more rarely, pressure-limited devices for the rhythmical inflation of lungs during resuscitation outside of hospitals.

pulp (pŭlp) [L. *pulpa,* flesh]. **1.** Pulpa; a soft, moist, coherent solid. **2.** *Pulpa* dentis. **3.** Chyme.
coronal p., *pulpa* coronale.
dead p., necrotic p.
dental p., dentinal p., *pulpa* dentis.
digital p., p. of finger.
enamel p., a layer of stellate cells in the enamel organ.
exposed p., p. that has been exposed or laid bare by a pathologic process, trauma, or a dental instrument.
p. of finger, digital p.; the fleshy mass at the extremity of the finger.
mummified p., a misnomer for a p. treated with a formaldehyde derivative.
necrotic p., nonvital or dead p.; necrosis of the dental p. which clinically does not respond to thermal stimulation; the tooth may be asymptomatic or sensitive to percussion and palpation.
nonvital p., necrotic p.
putrescent p., a decomposed p., often infected.
radicular p., *pulpa* radicularis.
red p., splenic p. seen grossly as a reddish brown substance, due to its abundance of red blood cells, consisting of splenic sinuses

and the tissue intervening between them (splenic cords).
splenic p., *pulpa* splenica.
tooth p., *pulpa* dentis.
vertebral p., *nucleus* pulposus.
vital p., a p. composed of viable tissue, either normal or diseased, that responds to the electric p. test and to heat and cold tests.
white p., that part of the spleen that consists of nodules and other lymphatic concentrations.

pulpa (pŭl'pă) [L. pulp] [NA]. Pulp (1).
p. corona'le [NA], coronal pulp; that portion of the p. dentis contained within the pulp chamber or crown cavity of the tooth.
p. den'tis [NA], dental, dentinal, or tooth pulp; pulp (2); the soft tissue within the pulp cavity, consisting of connective tissue containing blood vessels, nerves and lymphatics, and at the periphery a layer of odontoblasts capable of internal repair of the dentin.
p. lie'nis, p. splenica.
p. radicula'ris [NA], radicular pulp; that part of the p. dentis contained within the apical or root portion of the tooth.
p. splen'ica [NA], splenic pulp; p. lienis; the soft cellular substance of the spleen. See also red *pulp* and white *pulp.*

pulpal (pŭl'păl). Relating to the pulp.

pulpalgia (pŭl-pal'jē-ă) [L. *pulpa,* pulp, + G. *algos,* pain]. Pain arising from the dental pulp.

pulpation (pŭl-pā'shŭn). Pulpifaction.

pulpectomy (pŭl-pek'tō-mē) [L. *pulpa,* pulp, + G. *ektomē,* excision]. Removal of the entire pulp structure of a tooth, including the pulp tissue in the roots.

pulpifaction (pŭl-pi-fak'shŭn) [L. *pulpa,* pulp, + *facio,* pp. *factus,* to make]. Pulpation; reduction to a pulpy condition.

pulpiform (pŭl'pi-fōrm). Resembling pulp; pulpy.

pulpify (pŭl'pi-fī). To reduce to a pulpy state.

pulpitis (pŭl-pī'tis) [L. *pulpa,* pulp, + G. *-itis,* inflammation]. Odontitis; inflammation of the pulp of a tooth.
hyperplastic p., a dental, pulp, or tooth polyp; hyperplastic granulation tissue growing out of the exposed pulp chamber of a grossly decayed tooth.
hypertrophic p., a misnomer for hyperplastic p.
irreversible p., inflammation of the dental pulp from which the pulp is unable to recover; clinically, may be asymptomatic or characterized by pain which persists after thermal stimulation; microscopically, characterized by marked acute or chronic inflammation, sometimes with partial pulpal necrosis.
reversible p., minor inflammation from which the pulp is able to recover; characterized clinically by pain which disappears rapidly upon removal of thermal stimulation; characterized microscopically by vasodilation, hyperemia, and edema with minimal diapedesis of leukocytes.
suppurative p., obsolete term for a purulent irreversible p.

pulp'less. 1. Without a pulp. **2.** Denoting a tooth in which the pulp has died or from which the pulp has been removed. **3.** Denoting a tooth that gives no response to an electric pulp test or thermal test.

pulpodontia (pŭl-pō-don'shē-ă) [L. *pulpa,* pulp, + G. *odous,* tooth]. The science of root canal therapy. See also endodontics.

pulposus (pŭl-pō'sŭs) [L.]. Pulpy.

pulpotomy (pŭl-pot'ō-mē) [L. *pulpa,* pulp, + G. *tomē,* incision]. Pulp amputation; removal of a portion of the pulp structure of a tooth, usually the coronal portion.

pulpy (pŭl'pē). In the condition of a soft, moist solid.

pulsate (pŭl'sāt) [L. *pulso,* pp. *-atus,* to beat]. To throb or beat rhythmically; said of the heart or an artery.

pulsatile (pŭl'să-til). Throbbing or beating.

pulsation (pŭl-sā'shŭn) [L. *pulsatio,* a beating]. A throbbing or rhythmical beating, as of the pulse or the heart.

pulsator (pŭl-sā'ter, -tōr). A machine or device that operates in a throbbing, vibrating, or rhythmic manner.

pulse (pŭls) [L. *pulsus*]. Rhythmical dilation of an artery, produced by the increased volume of blood thrown into the vessel by the contraction of the heart. A p. may also at times occur in a vein or a vascular organ, such as the liver.
abdominal p., pulsus abdominalis; the soft, compressible aortic p. occurring in certain abdominal disorders.
alternating p., *pulsus* alternans.
anacrotic p., anadicrotic p., a small slow rising p. with a perceptible notch on the ascending limb, characteristic of aortic stenosis. See also plateau p.
bigeminal p., pulsus bigeminus; bigemina; coupled beats or p.; a p. in which the beats occur in pairs.
bisferious p., *pulsus* bisferiens.
bulbar p., a jugular p. supposed to indicate tricuspid insufficiency.
cannonball p., water-hammer p.
capillary p., the alternate rhythmical blanching and reddening of a capillary area, as seen under the nails or in the lip, upon gentle compression; a sign of arteriolar dilation, well seen in aortic insufficiency.
catacrotic p., pulsus catacrotus; a p. in which there is an upward notch interrupting the descending limb of the sphygmogram.
catadicrotic p., pulsus catadicrotus; a catacrotic p. in which there are two interrupting upward notches.
collapsing p., water-hammer p.
cordy p., tense p.
Corrigan's p., the water-hammer-type p. in aortic regurgitation or peripheral arterial dilation, characterized by an abrupt rise and rapid fall away.
coupled p., bigeminal p.
dicrotic p., pulsus duplex; a p. which is marked by a double beat, the second, due to a palpable dicrotic wave, being weaker than the first.
entoptic p., an intermittent phose synchronous with the p.
filiform p., a thready p.
gaseous p., a soft, full, but feeble p.
guttural p., a pulsation felt in the throat.
hard p., pulsus durus; a p. that strikes forcibly against the tip of the finger and is with difficulty compressed, indicating hypertension.
intermittent p., pulsus intercidens; irregularity of the heart due to extrasystoles which are too weak to open the semilunar valves; owing to the long pause following the premature beat, extra long pauses equal to two regular cycles occur from time to time between p. beats.
jugular p., the p. in the right internal jugular vein at the root of the neck, due to waves transmitted in the bloodstream from the right side of the heart.
Kussmaul's paradoxical p., see paradoxical p.
long p., a p. in which the impact is felt longer than usual.
monocrotic p., pulsus monocrotus; a p. without any perceptible dicrotism.
mousetail p., *pulsus* myurus.
movable p., the lateral movement of a strongly pulsating tortuous artery.
nail p., a capillary p. seen through the nail.
paradoxical p., p. paradoxus; p. respiratione intermittens; an exaggeration of the normal variation in the p. volume with respiration, becoming weaker with inspiration and stronger with expiration; characteristic of constrictive pericarditis or pericardial effusion, and so called because these changes are independent of changes in p. rate.
piston p., water-hammer p.
plateau p., the slow, sustained p. of aortic stenosis, producing a prolonged flat-topped curve in the sphygmogram.

pulmonary p., variation in intensity of the pulmonary second sound according to the tension in the pulmonary artery.
quadrigeminal p., pulsus quadrigeminus; a p. in which the beats are grouped in fours, a pause following every fourth beat.
Quincke's p., Quincke's sign; capillary pulsation, as shown by alternate reddening and blanching of the nailbed with each heart beat; a sign of arteriolar dilation and especially well seen in severe aortic insufficiency.
respiratory p., waxing and waning of venous pulsation produced by respiration.
reversed paradoxical p., a p. in which the amplitude increases with inspiration and decreases with expiration, as observed in some cases of tricuspid insufficiency.
Riegel's p., a p. that diminishes in volume during expiration.
soft p., a p. that is readily extinguished by pressure with the finger.
tense p., cordy p.; a hard, full p. but without very wide excursions, resembling the vibration of a thick cord.
thready p., filiform p.; pulsus filiformis; a small fine p., feeling like a small cord or thread under the finger.
trigeminal p., pulsus trigeminus; a p. in which the beats occur in trios, a pause following every third beat.
triphammer p., water-hammer p.
undulating p., pulsus fluens; a toneless p. in which there is a succession of waves without character or force.
vagus p., a slow p. due to the inhibitory action of the vagus nerve on the heart.
venous p., pulsus venosus; a pulsation occurring in the veins, especially the internal jugular vein.
vermicular p., a small rapid p., giving a wormlike sensation to the finger.
water-hammer p., cannonball p.; collapsing p.; piston p.; triphammer p.; pulsus celerimus; a p. with forcible impulse but immediate collapse, characteristic of aortic incompetency. See also Corrigan's p.
wiry p., a small, fine, incompressible p.

pulsellum (pŭl-sel'ŭm) [Mod. L. dim. of L. *pulsus,* a stroking]. A posterior flagellum constituting the organ of locomotion in certain protozoa.

pulsimeter, pulsometer (pŭl-sim'ĕ-ter, -som'ĕ-ter) [L. *pulsus,* pulse, + *metron,* measure]. An instrument for measuring the force and rapidity of the pulse.

pulsion (pŭl'shŭn) [L. *pulsio*]. A pushing outward or swelling.

pulsus (pŭl'sŭs) [L. a stroke, pulse]. Pulse.
p. abdomina'lis, abdominal *pulse.*
p. alter'nans, alternating pulse; mechanical alternation, a pulse regular in time but with alternate beats stronger and weaker, often detectable only with the sphygmomanometer and usually indicating serious myocardial disease.
p. anadic'rotus, anacrotic *pulse.*
p. bigem'inus, bigeminal *pulse.*
p. bisfer'iens, bisferious pulse; an arterial pulse with two palpable peaks, the second stronger than the first, as may be found in aortic insufficiency combined with aortic stenosis.
p. cap'risans, a bounding leaping pulse, irregular in both force and rhythm.
p. catac'rotus, catacrotic *pulse.*
p. catadic'rotus, catadicrotic *pulse.*
p. cel'er, a pulse beat swift to rise and fall.
p. celer'imus, water-hammer *pulse.*
p. cor'dis, the apex beat of the heart.
p. deb'ilis, a weak pulse.
p. dif'ferens, p. incongruens; a condition in which the pulses in the two radial arteries differ in strength.
p. du'plex, dicrotic *pulse.*
p. du'rus, hard *pulse.*
p. filifor'mis, thready *pulse.*
p. flu'ens, undulating *pulse.*
p. for'micans, a very small, nearly imperceptible pulse, the impression it gives to the finger being compared to formication.
p. for'tis, a full strong pulse.
p. fre'quens, a rapid pulse.
p. heterochron'icus, an arrhythmic pulse.
p. inaequa'lis, a pulse irregular in rhythm and force.
p. incon'gruens, p. differens.
p. infre'quens, a slow pulse.
p. inter'cidens, intermittent *pulse.*
p. intercur'rens, an occasional strong dicrotic pulse wave giving the impression of an intercurrent ventricular contraction.
p. irregula'ris perpet'uus, permanently irregular pulse often caused by, or characteristic of, atrial fibrillation; it may also be produced by a wide variety of other chaotic rhythms.
p. mag'nus, a large full pulse.
p. mol'lis, a soft, easily compressible pulse.
p. monoc'rotus, monocrotic *pulse.*
p. myu'rus, mousetail pulse; a pulse marked by a wave, the apex of which is reached suddenly and which then subsides very gradually.
p. paradox'us, paradoxical *pulse.*
p. par'vus, a small pulse.
p. quadrigem'inus, quadrigeminal *pulse.*
p. ra'rus, p. tardus.
p. respiratio'ne intermit'tens, paradoxical *pulse.*
p. tar'dus, p. rarus; a pulse beat slow to rise and fall. See also plateau *pulse.*
p. trem'ulus, a feeble fluttering pulse.
p. trigem'inus, trigeminal *pulse.*
p. vac'uus, a very weak pulse hardly distending the arterial wall.
p. veno'sus, venous *pulse.*

pultaceous (pŭl-tā'shŭs) [G. *poltos,* porridge]. Macerated; pulpy.

pulverization (pŭl'ver-i-zā'shŭn). Reduction to powder.

pulverize (pŭl'ver-īz) [L. *pulverizo,* fr. *pulvis, pulveris,* dust]. To reduce to a powder.

pulverulent (pŭl-ver'yū-lent). In a state of powder; powdery.

pulvinar (pŭl-vī'năr) [L. a couch made from cushions, fr. *pulvinus,* cushion] [NA]. The expanded posterior extremity of the thalamus which forms a cushion-like prominence overlying the geniculate bodies.

pulvinate (pŭl'vi-nāt) [L. *pulvinus,* cushion]. Raised or convex, denoting a form of surface elevation of a bacterial culture.

pumice (pŭm'is) [L. *pumex* (*pumic-*), a pumice stone]. Volcanic cinders ground to particles of varying sizes; used in dentistry for polishing restorations or teeth.

pump (pŭmp) **1.** An apparatus for forcing a gas or liquid from or to any part. **2.** Any mechanism for using metabolic energy to accomplish active transport of a substance.
breast p., a suction instrument for withdrawing milk from the breast.
Carrel-Lindbergh p., a perfusion device designed for use in culture of whole organs.
constant infusion p., an electrically driven device for delivery from a reservoir of a constant, often very small, volume of solution over a prolonged period of time.
dental p., saliva *ejector.*
intra-aortic balloon p., a pump connected to a balloon device which is inserted into the descending aorta as a counterpulsation device to provide temporary cardiac assistance in the management of left ventricular failure.
jet ejector p., a suction p. in which fluid under high pressure is forced through a nozzle into an abruptly larger tube where a high velocity jet, at a low pressure in accordance with Bernoulli's law, entrains gas or liquid from a side tube opening just beyond the end

of the nozzle to create suction; *e.g.*, the p. by which steam is used to evacuate an autoclave, a water aspirator.

saliva p., saliva *ejector.*

sodium p., a biologic mechanism that uses metabolic energy from ATP to achieve active transport of sodium across a membrane; sodium p.'s expel sodium from most cells of the body, sometimes coupled with the transport of other substances, and also serve to move sodium across multicellular membranes such as renal tubule walls.

sodium-potassium p., the biochemical mechanism that uses sodium-potassium ATPase to achieve (in most cells) transport of potassium opposite to that of the sodium p.

stomach p., an apparatus for removing the contents of the stomach by means of suction.

pump-oxygenator (pŭmp-ok'si-je-nā'ter). A mechanical device that can substitute for both the heart (pump) and the lungs (oxygenator) during open heart surgery.

puna (pū'nă) [Sp., fr. Quechua *puna,* a high, dry Andean plateau]. Altitude *sickness* (1).

punch (pŭnch) [L. *pungo,* pp. *punctus,* to stick, to punch]. An instrument for making a hole or indentation in some solid material or for driving out a foreign body in such material.

punchdrunk (pŭnch'drŭnk). See punchdrunk *syndrome.*

puncta (pŭngk'tă) [L.]. Plural of punctum.

punctate (pŭngk'tāt) [L. *punctum,* a point]. Marked with points or dots differentiated from the surrounding surface by color, elevation, or texture.

punctiform (pŭngk'ti-fōrm) [L. *punctum,* a point, + *forma,* shape]. Very small but not microscopic, having a diameter of less than 1 mm.

punctum, gen. **puncti,** pl. **puncta** (pŭngk'tŭm, -tī, -tă) [L. a prick, point, pp. ntr. of *pungo,* to prick, used as noun] [NA]. Point (1). **1.** The tip of a sharp process. **2.** A minute round spot differing in color or otherwise in appearance from the surrounding tissues. **3.** A point on the optic axis of an optical system. See also point.

p. ce'cum, the blind spot in the visual field corresponding to the location of the optic disk.

p. coxa'le, the highest point of the crest of the ilium.

p. doloro'sum, painful point; see Valleix's *points.*

lacrimal p., p. lacrimale.

p. lacrima'le [NA], lacrimal p. or opening; the minute circular opening of the lacrimal canaliculus, on the margin of each eyelid near the medial commissure.

p. lu'teum, *macula* retinae.

p. ossificatio'nis [NA], point or center of ossification; the site of earliest bone formation via accumulation of osteoblasts within connective tissue (membranous ossification) or of earliest destruction of cartilage prior to onset of ossification (endochondral ossification). **p. o. prima'rium** [NA], primary point or center of ossification, is the first site where bone begins to form in the shaft of a long bone, or in the body of an irregular bone; **p. o. seconda'rium** [NA], secondary point or center of ossification, is a center of bone formation appearing later than the p. o. primarium, usually in an epiphysis.

p. prox'imum (P.p.), near *point.*

p. remo'tum (P.r.), far *point.*

p. vasculo'sum, one of the minute dots seen on section of the brain, due to small drops of blood at the cut extremities of the arteries.

puncture (pŭnk'chūr) [L. *punctura,* fr. *pungo,* pp. *punctus,* to prick]. **1.** To make a hole with a small pointed object, such as a needle. **2.** A prick or small hole made with a pointed instrument.

Bernard's p., diabetic p.

cisternal p., passage of a hollow needle through the posterior atlantooccipital membrane into the cisterna cerebellomedullaris.

diabetic p., Bernard's p.; a p. at a point in the floor of the fourth ventricle of the brain which causes glycosuria.

lumbar p., a p. into the subarachnoid space of the lumbar region to obtain spinal fluid for diagnostic or therapeutic purposes. Also called Quincke's p.; spinal tap or p.; rachicentesis; rachiocentesis.

Quincke's p., lumbar p.

spinal p., lumbar p.

sternal p., removal of bone marrow from the manubrium by needle.

pungent (pŭn'jent) [L. *pungo,* pres. p. *-ens* (*-ent-*), to pierce]. Sharp; acrid; said of the taste or odor of a substance.

PUO Abbreviation for pyrexia of unknown (or uncertain) origin, a term applied to febrile illness before diagnosis has been established; also referred to as FUO (fever of unknown origin).

pupa, pl. **pupae** (pyū'pă, -pē) [L. *pupa,* doll]. The stage of insect metamorphosis following the larva and preceding the imago. See also complete *metamorphosis;* Holometabola.

pupil (p.) (pyū'pĭl) [L. *pupilla*]. Pupilla.

Adie's p., Holmes-Adie *syndrome.*

amaurotic p., p. in an eye that is blind because of ocular or optic nerve disease; this p. will not contract to light except when the normal fellow eye is stimulated with light.

Argyll Robertson p., Robertson or rigid p.; a form of reflex iridoplegia characterized by loss of the direct and consensual pupillary reflex to light, with normal pupillary constriction to convergence, with miosis, and with an irregular pupil; often present in tabes dorsalis.

artificial p., an opening made by excision of a portion of the iris in order to improve the vision in cases of central opacity of the cornea or lens.

bounding p., a rapid dilation and constriction of the pupil.

Bumke's p., dilation of the p. in response to psychic stimuli.

catatonic p., transient pupillary dilation with absence of pupillary reaction to light and convergence.

cat's-eye p., a distorted p. elongated in the vertical axis.

cogwheel p., pupillary constriction and dilation in a series of steps.

fixed p., a stationary pupil unresponsive to all stimuli.

Gunn p., Marcus Gunn p.

Holmes-Adie p., Holmes-Adie *syndrome.*

Horner's p., constricted p. due to impairment of sympathetic nerve innervation of the dilator muscle of the pupil.

Hutchinson's p., dilation of the p. on the side of the lesion with constriction of the fellow p., occurring in ipsilateral meningeal hemorrhage that compresses the oculomotor nerve in the brainstem.

keyhole p., a p. with a coloboma.

Marcus Gunn p., Gunn p.; afferent pupillary defect.

neurotonic p., contraction of the p. in response to light, not followed by equivalent redilation.

paradoxical p., see paradoxical pupillary *reflex.*

pinhole p., an extremely constricted p.

rigid p., Argyll Robertson p.

Robertson p., Argyll Robertson p.

Saenger p., delayed pupillary reaction to convergence.

tonic p., mydriatic rigidity; a p., usually large, which constricts very slowly, if at all, to light and convergence. See also Holmes-Adie *syndrome.*

pupilla, pl. **pupillae** (pyū-pil'ă, pyū-pil'ē) [L. dim. of *pupa,* a girl or doll] [NA]. Pupil; the circular orifice in the center of the iris, through which the light rays enter the eye.

pupillary (pyū'pi-lār-ē). Relating to the pupil.

pupillo- [L. *pupilla,* pupil]. Combining form relating to the pupils.

pupillography (pyū'pi-log'ră-fē) [pupillo- + G. *graphō,* to write]. The recording of pupillary reactions.

pupillometer (pyū'pi-lom'ĕ-ter) [pupillo- + G. *metron,* measure]. An instrument for measuring the diameter of the pupil.

pupillometry (pyū'pi-lom'ĕ-trē). Measurement of the pupil.

pupillomotor (pyū'pĭ-lō-mō'ter) [pupillo- + L. *motor,* mover]. Relating to the autonomic nerve fibers that supply the smooth muscle of the iris.

pupilloplegia (pyū'pĭ-lō-plē'jē-ă) [pupillo- + G. *plēgē,* stroke]. A condition in which the pupil reacts slowly to light stimuli, as in Holmes-Adie syndrome.

pupilloscopy (pyū'pi-los'kō-pē) [pupillo- + G. *skopeō,* to view]. Retinoscopy.

pupillostatometer (pyū'pi-lō-stă-tom'ĕ-ter) [pupillo- + G. *statos,* placed, + *metron,* measure]. An instrument for measuring the distance between the centers of the pupils.

pupiparous (pyū-pip'ă-rŭs). Pupae-bearing; denoting those insects that give birth to late-stage larvae that have already passed their larval development within the body of the female, as in flies of the family Hippoboscidae and in the Glossinidae (tsetse flies).

PUPPP Acronym for *p*ruritic *u*rticarial *p*apules and *p*laques of *p*regnancy, an intensely pruritic, occasionally vesicular, eruption of the trunk and arms appearing in the third trimester of pregnancy; spontaneous involution occurs within 10 days of term.

pure (pyūr) [L. *purus*]. Unadulterated; free from admixture or contamination with any extraneous matter.

purebred (pyūr'bred). An animal whose ancestors on both sides have been members of a recognized breed, and usually officially registered as such.

purgation (per-gā'shŭn) [L. *purgatio*]. Catharsis (1); evacuation of the bowels with the aid of a purgative or cathartic.

purgative (per'gă-tiv) [L. *purgativus,* purging]. An agent used for purging the bowels. See also cathartic (2).
saline p., Epsom salt, Rochelle salt, or any salt having p. properties.

purge (perj) [L. *purgo,* to cleanse, fr. *purus,* pure, + *ago,* to do]. **1.** To cause a copious evacuation of the bowels. **2.** A cathartic remedy.

purging cassia (perj'ing kash'yă). Cassia fistula.

puriform (pyū'ri-fōrm) [L. *pus (pur-),* pus, + *forma,* form]. Resembling pus.

purine (pyūr'ēn, -rin). The parent substance of adenine, guanine, and other naturally occurring purine "bases;" not known to exist as such in the body.

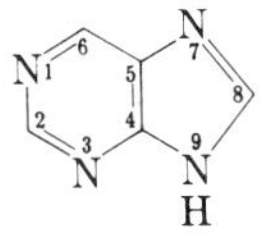

Purine

p.-nucleoside phosphorylase [EC 2.4.2.1], a ribosyltransferase that catalyzes the phosphorolysis of a purine nucleoside to a purine and ribose 1-phosphate.
p. ribonucleoside, nebularine.

purinemia (pyū-ri-nē'mē-ă) [purine + G. *haima,* blood]. The presence of purine or xanthine bases in the circulating blood.

purity (pyūr'i-tē). The state of being pure, free from contaminants or pollutants.
radiochemical p., the proportion of the total activity of a specific radionuclide in a specific chemical or biological form.
radioisotopic p., a loose term commonly used to denote radionuclidic p.
radionuclidic p., the proportion of the total radioactivity that is present as a specific radionuclide.
radiopharmaceutical p., the sterility and apyrogenicity of a radioactive tracer for human use.

Purkinje, Johannes E. von, Bohemian anatomist and physiologist, 1787–1869. See P. *conduction images, shift, system;* P.'s *cells, corpuscles, fibers, figures, layer, network, phenomenon;* P.-Sanson *images.*

Purmann, Matthaeus G., German surgeon, 1648–1721. See P.'s *method.*

puromucous (pyū-rō-myū'kŭs) [L. *pus (pur-),* pus, + *mucus,* mucus]. Mucopurulent.

puromycin (pyū-rō-mī'sin). 6-Dimethylamino-9-(3'-*p*-methoxy-L-phenylalanylamino-*β*-D-ribofuranosyl) purine; an antibiotic produced by the growth of *Streptomyces alboniger;* formerly used in the treatment of amebiasis and trypanosomiasis.

purple (per'pl) [L. *purpura*]. A color formed by a mixture of blue and red. For individual purple dyes see specific name.
visual p., rhodopsin.

purpura (pŭr'pū-ră) [L. fr. G. *porphyra,* purple]. Peliosis; a condition characterized by hemorrhage into the skin. Appearance of the lesions varies with the type of p., the duration of the lesions, and the acuteness of the onset. The color is first red, gradually darkens to purple, fades to a brownish yellow, and usually disappears in 2 or 3 weeks; color of residual permanent pigmentation depends largely on the type of unabsorbed pigment of the extravasated blood; extravasations may occur also into the mucous membranes and internal organs.
acute vascular p., Henoch-Schönlein p.
allergic p., anaphylactoid p. (1); nonthrombocytopenic p. due to foods, drugs, and insect bites.
anaphylactoid p., **(1)** allergic p.; **(2)** Henoch-Schönlein p.
p. angioneurot'ica, an eruption marked by angioneurotic edema, petechiae, and hyperesthesia of the skin and gastric mucous membrane.
p. annula'ris telangiecto'des, Majocchi's disease; annular lesions, principally of the lower extremities, in which the peripheral portion is composed of purpura or petechiae with brawny staining of hemosiderin deposits and minute telangiectasia.
factitious p., self-induced, often painful, ecchymoses.
fibrinolytic p., p. in which the bleeding is associated with rapid fibrinolysis of the clot.
p. ful'minans, a severe and rapidly fatal form of p. hemorrhagica, occurring especially in children, with hypotension, fever, and disseminated intravascular coagulation, usually following an infectious illness.
p. hemorrhag'ica, (1) idiopathic thrombocytopenic p.; **(2)** petechial fever; a noncontagious malady of horses, which occurs following suppurative infections, characterized by multiple hemorrhages and edema of the subcutaneous and submucous tissues.
Henoch's p., Henoch-Schönlein p.
Henoch-Schönlein p., Henoch's p., an eruption of nonthrombocytopenic purpuric lesions associated with joint pain and swelling, colic, and passage of bloody stools, and occurring characteristically in young children; glomerulonephritis may occur during an initial episode or develop later. Also called Schönlein's disease or p.; Henoch-Schönlein or Schönlein-Henoch syndrome; anaphylactoid p. (2); p. rheumatica or nervosa; acute vascular p.; hemorrhagic exudative erythema.
hyperglobulinemic p., Waldenström's *macroglobulinemia.*
idiopathic thrombocytopenic p. (ITP), Werlhof's disease; land scurvy; p. hemorrhagica (1); immune thrombocytopenic p.; a systemic illness characterized by extensive ecchymoses and hemorrhages from mucous membranes, and very low platelet counts; resulting from platelet destruction by macrophages due an antiplatelet factor; childhood cases are usually brief and rarely

with intracranial hemorrhages, but adult cases are often recurrent and have a higher incidence of grave bleeding, especially intracranial.

immune thrombocytopenic p., idiopathic thrombocytopenic p.

p. iod'ica, iodic p., an eruption of discrete miliary petechiae, usually confined to the lower extremities, appearing in rare instances on administration of any of the iodides.

p. nervo'sa, Henoch-Schönlein p.

nonthrombocytopenic p., p. simplex.

psychogenic p., autoerythrocyte sensitization *syndrome.*

p. pu'licans, p. pulico'sa, petechiae caused by the bites of insects and animal parasites.

p. rheumat'ica, Henoch-Schönlein p.

Schönlein's p., Henoch-Schönlein p.

p. seni'lis, the occurrence of petechiae and ecchymoses on the legs in aged and debilitated subjects.

p. sim'plex, nonthrombocytopenic p.; the eruption of petechiae or larger ecchymoses, usually unaccompanied by constitutional symptoms and not associated with systemic illness.

p. symptomat'ica, a petechial eruption in scarlet fever and other exanthemas.

thrombocytopenic p., see idiopathic thrombocytopenic p.

thrombotic thrombocytopenic p., Moschowitz' disease; a rapidly fatal or occasionally protracted disease with varied symptoms in addition to p., including signs of central nervous system involvement, due to formation of fibrin or platelet thrombi in arterioles and capillaries in many organs.

p. urti'cans, p. simplex accompanied by an urticarial eruption.

Waldenström's p., Waldenström's *macroglobulinemia.*

purpurea glycosides A and **B** (per'pū-rē'ă glī'kō-sīdz). The cardioactive precursor glycosides of *Digitalis* purpurea; they are structurally identical with desacetyl-lanatosides A and B, respectively. See also lanatoside.

purpuric (pŭr-pū'rik). Relating to or affected with purpura.

purpuriferous (per-pū-rif'er-ŭs) [L. *purpura,* purple, + *fero,* to bear]. Purpurigenous; purpuriparous. **1.** Forming a purple pigment. **2.** Obsolete term for forming visual purple (rhodopsin).

purpurigenous (per-pyū-rij'ĕ-nŭs) [L. *purpura,* purple, + G. *-gen,* producing]. Purpuriferous.

purpurin (per'pyū-rin). **1.** Uroerythrin. **2.** [C.I. 58205, 75410]. Alizarin purpurin; a violet stain related to alizarin by addition of a 4-OH group to alizarin.

purpurinuria (per'pyū-ri-nū'rē-ă). Porphyrinuria.

purpuriparous (per-pyū-rip'ă-rŭs) [L. *purpura,* purple, + *pario,* to bring forth]. Purpuriferous.

purr (per). A low vibratory murmur.

Purtscher, Otmar, German ophthalmologist, 1852–1927. See P.'s *disease.*

purulence, purulency (pyūr'ŭ-lens, pyūr'yū-lens, -len-sē) [L. *purulentia,* a festering, fr. *pus (pur-),* pus]. The condition of containing or forming pus.

purulent (pyūr'ŭ-lent, pyūr'yū-). Containing, consisting of, or forming pus.

puruloid (pyū'rŭ-loyd). Resembling pus.

pus (pŭs) [L.]. A fluid product of inflammation, consisting of a liquid containing leukocytes and the debris of dead cells and tissue elements liquefied by the proteolytic and histolytic enzymes (*e.g.,* leukoprotease) that are elaborated by polymorphonuclear leukocytes.

blue p., p. tinged with pyocyanin, a product of *Pseudomonas aeruginosa.*

cheesy p., a very thick almost solid p. resulting from the absorption of the liquor puris.

curdy p., p. containing flakes of caseous matter.

green p., blue p. when, as sometimes happens, it has more of a green hue.

ichorous p., thin p. containing shreds of sloughing tissue, and sometimes of a fetid odor.

laudable p., an obsolete term used when suppuration was considered a desirable stage in wound healing.

sanious p., ichorous p. stained with blood.

pustulant (pŭs'chū-lant). **1.** Causing a pustular eruption. **2.** An agent producing pustules.

pustular (pŭs'chū-lăr). Relating to or marked by pustules.

pustulation (pŭs'chū-lā'shŭn). The formation or the presence of pustules.

pustule (pŭs'chūl) [L. *pustula*]. A small circumscribed elevation of the skin, containing purulent material.

malignant p., cutaneous *anthrax.*

postmortem p., an ulcer, usually on the knuckle, resulting from infection during a dissection or the performance of an autopsy.

spongiform p. of Kogoj, an epidermal p. formed by infiltration of neutrophils into necrotic epidermis in which the cell walls persist as a spongelike network; seen in pustular psoriasis.

pustuliform (pŭs'chū-li-fōrm). Having the appearance of a pustule.

pustulocrustaceous (pŭs'chū-lō-krŭs-tā'shŭs). Marked by pustules crusted with dry pus.

pustulosis (pŭs-chū-lō'sis) [L. *pustula,* pustule, + G. *-osis,* condition]. **1.** An eruption of pustules. **2.** Term occasionally used to designate acropustulosis.

p. palmar'is et plantar'is, acrodermatitis continua or perstans; dermatitis repens; Hallopeau's disease (1); a sterile pustular eruption of the fingers and toes, variously attributed to dyshidrosis, pustular psoriasis, and unidentified bacterial infection.

p. vaccin'iformis acu'ta, *eczema* herpeticum.

putamen (pyū-tā'men) [L. that which falls off in pruning, fr. *puto,* to prune] [NA]. The outer, larger, and darker gray of the three portions into which the nucleus lentiformis is divided by laminae of white fibers; it is connected with the caudate nucleus by bridging bands of gray substance that penetrate the internal capsule. Its histological structure is similar to that of the caudate nucleus together with which it composes the striatum. See also *corpus* striatum; *nucleus* lentiformis.

Putnam, James J., U.S. neurologist, 1846–1918. See P.-Dana *syndrome.*

putrefaction (pyū-tri-fak'shŭn) [L. *putre-facio,* pp. *-factus,* to make rotten]. Decay (2); decomposition or rotting, the breakdown of organic matter usually by bacterial action, resulting in the formation of other substances of less complex constitution with the evolution of ammonia or its derivatives and hydrogen sulfide; characterized usually by the presence of toxic or malodorous products.

putrefactive (pyū-tri-fak'tiv). Relating to or causing putrefaction.

putrefy (pyū'tri-fī). To cause to become, or to become, putrid.

putrescence (pyū-tres'ens). The state of putrefaction.

putrescent (pyū-tres'ent) [L. *putresco,* to grow rotten, fr. *puter,* rotten]. Denoting, or in the process of, putrefaction.

putrescine (pyū-tres'ēn). 1,4-Diaminobutane; $NH_2(CH_2)_4NH_2$; a poisonous polyamine formed from the amino acid, arginine, during putrefaction.

putrid (pyū'trid) [L. *putridus*]. **1.** In a state of putrefaction. **2.** Denoting putrefaction.

Putti, Vittorio, Italian surgeon, 1880–1940. See P.-Platt *operation, procedure.*

PUVA Abbreviation for oral administration of *p*soralen and subsequent exposure to long wavelength ultraviolet light (*uv-a*); used to treat psoriasis.

PVC Abbreviation for polyvinyl chloride.

PVP Abbreviation for polyvinylpyrrolidone.

PWM Abbreviation for pokeweed *mitogen.*

pyarthrosis (pī-ar-thrō′sis) [G. *pyon,* pus, + *arthrōsis,* a jointing]. Suppurative *arthritis.*

pycno-. See pykno-.

pyel-. See pyelo-.

pyelectasis, pyelectasia (pī-ĕ-lek′tă-sis, pī-ĕ-lek-tā′zē-ă) [pyel- + G. *ektasis,* extension]. Dilation of the pelvis of the kidney.

pyelitic (pī-ĕ-lit′ik). Relating to pyelitis.

pyelitis (pī-ĕ-lī′tis) [pyel- + G. *-itis,* inflammation]. **1.** Inflammation of the renal pelvis. **2.** Obsolescent term for pyelonephritis.

pyelo-, pyel- [G. *pyelos,* trough, tub, vat (pelvis)]. Combining forms denoting pelvis, usually the renal pelvis.

pyelocaliceal (pī′ĕ-lō-kal′i-sē′ăl). Pyelocalyceal; relating to the renal pelvis and calices.

pyelocaliectasis (pī′ĕ-lō-kal′ē-ek′tă-sis). Caliectasis.

pyelocalyceal (pī′ĕ-lō-kal′i-sē′ăl). Pyelocaliceal.

pyelocystitis (pī-ĕ-lō-sis-tī′tis) [pyelo- + G. *kystis,* bladder, + *-itis,* inflammation]. Inflammation of the renal pelvis and the bladder.

pyelofluoroscopy (pī′ĕ-lō-flūr-os′kŏ-pē) [pyelo- + L. *fluo,* to flow, + G. *skopeō,* to view]. Fluoroscopic examination of the renal pelves and ureters, usually with a contrast medium.

pyelogram (pī′el-ō-gram). A roentgenogram of the renal pelvis and ureter, usually following injection of a contrast material.

pyelography (pī′ĕ-log′ră-fē) [pyelo- + G. *graphō,* to write]. Pelviureterography; pyeloureterography; ureteropyelography; radiologic study of the kidney and renal collecting system, usually performed with the aid of a contrast agent injected intravenously, or directly, through a ureteral catheter or percutaneously.
antegrade p., antegrade urography in which the contrast medium is injected into the renal calices or pelvis.

pyelolithotomy (pī′ĕ-lō-li-thot′ō-mē) [pyelo- + G. *lithos,* stone, + *tomē,* incision]. Pelvilithotomy; pelviolithotomy; operative removal of a calculus from the kidney through an incision in the renal pelvis.

pyelolymphatic (pī′ĕ-lō-lim-fat′ik). Pertaining to the lymphatics of the renal pelvis.

pyelonephritis (pī′ĕ-lō-ne-frī′tis) [pyelo- + G. *nephros,* kidney, + *-itis,* inflammation]. Nephropyelitis; inflammation of the renal parenchyma, calyces, and pelvis, particularly due to local bacterial infection.
acute p., acute inflammation of the renal parenchyma and pelvis characterized by small cortical abscesses and yellowish streaks in the medulla due to pus in the collecting tubules and interstitial tissue.
ascending p., p. due to bacterial infection from the lower urinary tract, particularly by reflux of infected urine.
contagious bovine p., a specific necrotizing inflammation of the renal pelvis and ureters of cattle, caused by infection with *Corynebacterium renale.*
chronic p., chronic inflammation of the renal parenchyma and pelvis resulting from bacterial infection, characterized by calyceal deformities and overlying large flat renal scars with patchy distribution.
xanthogranulomatous p., a chronic inflammatory condition diffusely involving the entire kidney and usually resulting in a grossly enlarged and functionless kidney which can grossly resemble a neoplasm or tuberculosis; histologically, it is characterized by an inflammatory reaction with numerous lipid-laden, foamy histiocytes mixed with lymphocytes and plasma cells to form multiple granulomas.

pyelonephrosis (pī′ĕ-lō-ne-frō′sis) [pyelo- + G. *nephros,* kidney, + *-osis,* condition]. Any disease of the pelvis of the kidney.

pyeloplasty (pī′e-lō-plas-tē) [pyelo- + G. *plastos,* formed]. Pelvioplasty (2); plastic surgery of the kidney pelvis to correct an obstruction.
Anderson-Hynes p., disjoined or dismembered p.
capsular flap p., a reconstructive procedure for correction of uteropelvic obstruction, whereby a flap of renal capsule is swung down from the renal hilus to enlarge an obstructed intrarenal pelvis and upper ureter; used to correct situations involving loss of renal pelvic tissue which preclude the use of renal pelvis for the reconstruction.
Culp p., a reconstructive technique for correction of uteropelvic obstruction, whereby a spiral flap of renal pelvis is brought down and interposed into a vertical incision in the ureter. See also Scardino vertical flap p.
disjoined p., dismembered p., Anderson-Hynes p.; a reconstructive procedure for correction of ureteropelvic obstruction, whereby the obstructed segment is resected and the upper ureter reanastomosed into the lower renal pelvis, usually utilizing a modified elliptical anastomotic technique.
Foley Y-plasty p., Foley operation; a reconstructive procedure for correction of ureteropelvic obstruction, whereby a Y-shaped flap of renal pelvis is advanced downward into a vertical incision in the upper ureter, thereby widening the ureteropelvic junction.
Scardino vertical flap p., a reconstructive technique for correction of uteropelvic obstruction, whereby a vertical flap of renal pelvis is brought down and interposed into a vertical incision in the ureter. *Cf.* Culp p.

pyeloplication (pī′ĕ-lō-pli-kā′shŭn) [pyelo- + L. *plico,* to fold]. An obsolete procedure of taking tucks in the wall of the renal pelvis when unduly dilated by a hydronephrosis.

pyeloscopy (pī-ĕ-los′kŏ-pē) [pyelo- + G. *skopeō,* to view]. Fluoroscopic observation of the pelvis and calices of the kidney, and the ureter, after the injection through the ureter of an opaque solution.

pyelostomy (pī-ĕ-los′tō-mē) [pyelo- + G. *stoma,* mouth]. Formation of an opening into the kidney pelvis to establish urinary drainage.

pyelotomy (pī-ĕ-lot′ō-mē) [pyelo- + G. *tomē,* incision]. Pelviotomy (3); incision into the pelvis of the kidney.
extended p., Gil-Vernet operation; extension of a standard p. into the lower pole infundibulum through the avascular plane between the posterior and basilar segmental renal arteries.

pyeloureterectasis (pī′ĕ-lō-yū-rē′ter-ek′tă-sis) [pyelo- + ureter + G. *ektasis,* a stretching]. Dilation of kidney pelvis and ureter, seen in hydronephrosis due to obstruction in the lower urinary tract.

pyeloureterography (pī′ĕ-lō-yū-rē′ter-og′ră-fē). Pyelography.

pyelovenous (pī′ĕ-lō-vē′nŭs) [pyelo- + venous]. Denoting the phenomenon of drainage from the renal pelvis into the renal veins from increased intrapelvic pressure.

pyemesis (pī-em′ĕ-sis) [G. *pyon,* pus, + *emesis,* vomiting]. The vomiting of pus.

pyemia (pī-ē′mē-ă) [G. *pyon,* pus, + *haima,* blood]. Pyogenic fever; pyohemia; septicemia due to pyogenic organisms causing multiple abscesses.
cryptogenic p., p. whose source is not evident.
portal p., suppurative pylephlebitis.

pyemic (pī-ē′mik), Relating to or suffering from pyemia.

Pyemotes tritici (pī-ĕ-mō′tēz tri-tī′kī). *Pediculoides ventricosus;* the straw or grain itch mite, a common parasite of insects in stored grain and a frequent cause of straw or grain itch from their bites; not to be confused with *P. ventricosus,* often called the straw itch mite, which is associated with the furniture beetle *Anobium punctatum* and is harmless to man.

pyencephalus (pī-en-sef′ă-lŭs) [G. *pyon,* pus, + *enkephalos,* brain]. Pyocephalus.

pyesis (pī-ē'sis) [G. *pyon,* pus, + *-esis,* condition or process]. Suppuration.

pyg-. See pygo-.

pygal (pī'găl) [G. *pygē,* buttocks]. Relating to the buttocks.

pygalgia (pī-gal'jē-ă) [pyg- + G. *algos,* pain]. Rarely used term meaning pain in the buttocks.

pygmalionism (pig-māl'yon-izm) [Pygmalion, G. myth. char.]. The state of being in love with an object of one's own creation.

pygmy (pig'mē) [G. *pygmaios,* dwarfish, fr. *pygmē,* fist, also a measure of length from elbow to knuckles]. Pigmy; a physiologic dwarf; especially one of a race of similar people, such as the p.'s of central Africa.

pygo-, pyg- [G. pygē, buttocks]. Combining forms denoting the buttocks.

pygoamorphus (pī'gō-ă-mōr'fŭs) [pygo- + G. *a-* priv. + *morphē,* form]. Conjoined twins in which the parasite, attached to the buttocks of the autosite, is reduced to a formless mass or embryoma.

pygodidymus (pī-gō-did'i-mŭs) [pygo- + G. *didymos,* twin]. Conjoined twins fused in the cephalothoracic region but with the buttocks and parts below doubled. See also *duplicitas* posterior.

pygomelus (pī-gom'ĕ-lŭs) [pygo- + G. *melos,* part]. Unequal conjoined twins in which the parasite is represented by a fleshy mass, or by a more fully developed limb, attached to the sacral or coccygeal region of the autosite.

pygopagus (pī-gop'ă-gŭs) [pygo- + G. *pagos,* something fixed]. Conjoined twins in which the two individuals are joined at the buttocks, most often back to back.

pyk-. See pykno-.

pyknic (pik'nik) [G. *pyknos,* thick]. Denoting a constitutional body type characterized by well rounded external contours and ample body cavities; virtually synonymous with endomorphic.

pykno-, pyk- [G. *pyknos,* thick, dense]. Combining forms meaning thick, dense, compact.

pyknodysostosis (pik'nō-dis-os-tō'sis) [pykno- + G. *dys-,* difficult, + *osteon,* bone, + *-osis,* condition]. Osteopetrosis acro-osteolytica; a condition characterized by short stature, delayed closure of the fontanelles, and hypoplasia of the terminal phalanges.

pyknoepilepsy, pyknolepsy (pik'nō-ep-i-lep-sē, pik'nō-lep-sē) [pykno- + G. *lepsis,* seizure]. Obsolete terms for absence.

pyknomorphous (pik'nō-mōr'fŭs) [pykno- + G. *morphē,* form, shape]. Denoting a cell or tissue that stains deeply because the stainable material is closely packed.

pyknophrasia (pik'nō-frā'zē-ă) [pykno- + G. *phrasis,* speech]. Thickness of utterance.

pyknosis (pik-nō'sis) [pykno- + G. *-osis,* condition]. A thickening or condensation; specifically, a condensation and reduction in size of the cell or its nucleus, usually associated with hyperchromatosis; nuclear p. is a stage of necrosis.

pyknotic (pik-not'ik). Relating to or characterized by pyknosis.

pyla (pī'lă) [G. *pylē,* gate]. The orifice of communication between the third ventricle and cerebral aqueduct (of Sylvius).

pylar (pī'lăr). Relating to the pyla.

pylemphraxis (pī-lem-frak'sis) [G. *pylē,* gate, + *emphraxis,* a stoppage]. Obstruction of the portal vein.

pylephlebectasis, pylephlebectasia (pī'lē-fle-bek'tă-sis, -bek-tā'sē-ă) [G. *pylē,* gate, + *phleps (phleb-),* vein, + *ektasis,* extension]. Dilation of the portal vein.

pylephlebitis (pī'lē-fle-bī'tis) [G. *pylē,* a gate, + *phleps,* vein, + *-itis,* inflammation]. Inflammation of the portal vein or any of its branches.

pylethrombophlebitis (pī-lē-throm'bō-phle-bī'tis) [G. *phylē,* gate, + *thrombos,* a clot, + *phleps,* vein, + *-itis,* inflammation]. Inflammation of the portal vein with the formation of a thrombus.

pylethrombosis (pī'lē-throm-bō'sis) [G. *pylē,* gate, + *thrombos,* a clot, + *-osis,* condition]. Thrombosis of the portal vein or its branches.

pylic (pī'lik). Relating to the portal vein.

pylon (pī'lon) [G. gateway]. A simple prosthesis, usually without joints, for a lower limb amputation.

pylor-. See pyloro-.

pyloralgia (pī-lō-ral'jē-ă) [pylor- + G. *algos,* pain]. Rarely used term for pain in the pyloric region of the stomach.

pylorectomy (pī'lōr-ek'tō-mē) [pylor- + G. *ektomē,* excision]. Excision of the pylorus. Also called gastropylorectomy; pylorogastrectomy.

pylori (pī-lōr'ī) [L.]. Plural of pylorus.

pyloric (pī-lōr'ik). Relating to the pylorus.

pyloristenosis (pī-lōr'i-ste-nō'sis) [pylor- + G. *stenōsis,* a narrowing]. Pylorostenosis; stricture or narrowing of the orifice of the pylorus.

pyloritis (pī-lō-rī'tis) [pylor- + G. *-itis,* inflammation]. Inflammation of the pyloric end of the stomach.

pyloro-, pylor- [G. *pyloros,* gatekeeper]. Combining forms denoting the pylorus.

pylorodiosis (pī-lōr'ō-dī-ō'sis) [pyloro- + G. *diōsis,* pushing apart]. Operative dilation of the pylorus.

pyloroduodenitis (pī-lōr'ō-dū'od-ĕ-nī'tis) [pyloro- + duodenitis]. Inflammation involving the pyloric outlet of the stomach and the duodenum.

pylorogastrectomy (pī-lōr'ō-gas-trek'tō-mē). Pylorectomy.

pyloromyotomy (pī-lōr'ō-mī-ot'ō-mē) [pyloro- + G. *mys,* muscle, + *tomē,* incision]. Ramstedt or Fredet-Ramstedt operation; longitudinal incision through the anterior wall of the pyloric canal to the level of the submucosa, to treat hypertrophic pyloric stenosis.

pyloroplasty (pī-lōr'ō-plas-tē) [pyloro- + G. *plastos,* formed]. Widening of the pyloric canal and any adjacent duodenal stricture by means of a longitudinal incision closed transversely.

Finney p., extension of a long full-thickness incision into the duodenum and proximally into the gastric antrum, with a C-shaped closure to provide a wider opening between stomach and duodenum.

Heineke-Mikulicz p., p. in which a short longitudinal incision is made over the pylorus and closed transversely.

Jaboulay p., a side-to-side gastroduodenostomy, useful when the pylorus and proximal duodenum are extensively scarred or indurated by peptic ulcer disease.

pyloroptosis, pyloroptosia (pī-lōr-ō-tō'sis, -tō'sē-ă) [pyloro- + G. *ptōsis,* a falling]. Downward displacement of the pyloric end of the stomach.

pylorospasm (pī-lōr'ō-spazm). Spasmodic contraction of the pylorus.

pylorostenosis (pī-lōr'ō-stĕ-nō'sis). Pyloristenosis.

pylorostomy (pī-lō-ros'tō-mē) [pyloro- + G. *stoma,* mouth]. Establishment of a fistula from the abdominal surface into the stomach near the pylorus.

pylorotomy (pī-lō-rot'ō-mē) [pyloro- + G. *tomē,* incision]. Incision of the pylorus.

pylorus, pl. **pylori** (pī-lōr'ŭs, pī-lōr'ī) [L. fr. G. *pylōros,* a gatekeeper, the pylorus, fr. *pylē,* gate, + *ouros,* a warder] [NA]. **1.** A muscular or myovascular device to open (musculus dilator) and to close (musculus sphincter) an orifice or the lumen of an organ. **2.** The muscular tissue surrounding and controlling the aboral outlet of the stomach.

Pym, Sir William, British physician, 1772–1861. See P.'s *fever.*

pyo- [G. *pyon,* pus]. Combining form denoting suppuration or an accumulation of pus.

pyocele (pī'ō-sēl) [pyo- + G. *kēlē,* tumor, hernia]. An accumulation of pus in the scrotum.

pyocelia (pī'ō-sē'lē-ă) [pyo- + G. *koilia,* a cavity]. Pyoperitoneum.

pyocephalus (pī'ō-sef'ă-lŭs) [pyo- + G. *kephalē,* head]. Pyencephalus; a purulent effusion within the cranium.
circumscribed p., abscess of the brain.
external p., meningeal suppuration.
internal p., intraventricular suppuration.

pyochezia (pī-ō-kē'zē-ă) [pyo- + G. *chezō,* to defecate]. A discharge of pus from the bowel.

pyocin (pī'ō-sin). Bacteriocin produced by strains of *Pseudomonas pyocyaneus.*

pyococcus (pī'ō-kok'ŭs) [pyo- + G. *kokkos,* berry (coccus)]. One of the cocci causing suppuration, especially *Streptococcus pyogenes.*

pyocolpocele (pī-ō-kol'pō-sēl) [pyo- + G. *kolpos,* bosom (vagina), + *kēlē,* tumor, hernia]. A vaginal tumor or cyst containing pus.

pyocolpos (pī-ō-kol'pos) [pyo- + G. *kolpos,* bosom (vagina)]. Accumulation of pus in the vagina.

pyocyanic (pī'ō-sī-an'ik) [pyo- + G. *kyanos,* blue]. Relating to blue pus or the organism that causes blue pus, *Pseudomonas aeruginosa.*

pyocyanogenic (pī'ō-sī'ă-nō-jen'ik) [pyo- + G. *kyanos,* blue, + *-gen,* producing]. Causing blue pus.

pyocyanolysin (pī'ō-sī-ă-nol'i-sin). A hemolysin formed by *Pseudomonas aeruginosa.*

pyocyst (pī'ō-sist) [pyo- + G. *kystis,* bladder]. A cyst with purulent contents.

pyocystis (pī-ō-sis'tis) [pyo- + G. *kystis,* bladder]. Chronic development and retention of excessive amounts of purulent matter in a urinary bladder that has been defunctionalized by prior supravesical diversion.

pyocyte (pī'ō-sīt) [pyo- + G. *kytos,* cell]. Pus *corpuscle.*

pyoderma (pī-ō-der'mă) [pyo- + G. *derma,* skin]. Pyodermatitis; pyodermatosis; any pyogenic infection of the skin; may be primary, as impetigo, or secondary to a previously existing condition.
chancriform p., a persistent, necrotizing, ulcerated, single pyogenic lesion, usually on the face or genitalia.
p. gangreno'sum, a chronic non-infective eruption of spreading, undermined ulcers showing central healing, with diffuse dermal neutrophil infiltration; often associated with ulcerative colitis.
primary p., a p., such as impetigo, in which pus formation is an essential part of the disease.
secondary p., a p. in which an existing skin lesion (eczema, herpes, seborrheic dermatitis, etc.) becomes secondarily infected.
p. veg'etans, *dermatitis* vegetans.

pyodermatitis (pī'ō-der-mă-tī'tis) [pyo- + G. *derma,* skin, + *-itis,* inflammation]. Pyoderma.

pyodermatosis (pī'ō-der-mă-tō'sis) [pyo- + G. *derma,* skin, + *-osis,* condition]. Pyoderma.

pyogen (pī'ō-jen) [pyo- + G. *-gen,* producing]. An agent that causes pus formation.

pyogenesis (pī'ō-jen'ĕ-sis) [pyo- + G. *genesis,* production]. Suppuration.

pyogenic, pyogenetic (pī-ō-jen'ik, -jĕ-net'ik). Pyogenous; pus-forming; relating to pus formation.

pyogenous (pī-oj'ĕ-nŭs). Pyogenic.

pyohemia (pī-ō-hē'mē-ă). Pyemia.

pyohemothorax (pī'ō-hē-mō-thōr'aks) [pyo- + G. *haima,* blood, + thorax]. Presence of pus and blood in the pleural cavity.

pyoid (pī'oyd) [G. *pyōdēs,* fr. *pyon,* pus, + *eidos,* resemblance]. Resembling pus.

pyolabyrinthitis (pī'ō-lab-i-rin-thī'tis) [pyo- + G. *labyrinthos,* labyrinth, + *-itis,* inflammation]. Suppurative inflammation of the labyrinth of the ear.

pyometra (pī-ō-mē'tră) [pyo- + G. *mētra,* uterus]. Accumulation of pus in the uterine cavity.

pyometritis (pī'ō-mē-trī'tis) [pyo- + G. *mētra,* womb, + *-itis,* inflammation]. Inflammation of uterine musculature associated with pus in the uterine cavity.

pyomyositis (pī'ō-mī-ō-sī'tis) [pyo- + G. *mys,* muscle, + *-itis,* inflammation]. Abscesses, carbuncles, or infected sinuses lying deep in muscles.
tropical p., *myositis* purulenta tropica.

pyonephritis (pī-ō-ne-frī'tis) [pyo- + G. *nephros,* kidney, + *-itis,* inflammation]. Suppurative inflammation of the kidney.

pyonephrolithiasis (pī'ō-nef'rō-li-thī'ă-sis) [pyo- + G. *nephros,* kidney, + *lithos,* stone, + *-iasis,* condition]. Presence in the kidney of pus and calculi.

pyonephrosis (pī'ō-ne-frō'sis) [pyo- + G. *nephros,* kidney, + *-osis,* condition]. Distention of the pelvis and calices of the kidney with pus, usually associated with obstruction.

pyo-ovarium (pī'ō-ō-var'ē-ŭm). Presence of pus in the ovary; an ovarian abscess.

pyopericarditis (pī'ō-per-i-kar-dī'tis). Suppurative inflammation of the pericardium.

pyopericardium (pī'ō-per-i-kar'dē-ŭm). Empyema of the pericardium; an accumulation of pus in the pericardial sac.

pyoperitoneum (pī'ō-per-i-tō-nē'ŭm). [G. *pyon,* pus]. Pyocelia; an accumulation of pus in the peritoneal cavity.

pyoperitonitis (pī'ō-per-i-tō-nī'tis) [pyo- + peritonitis]. Suppurative inflammation of the peritoneum.

pyophthalmia, pyophthalmitis (pī'of-thal'mē-ă, pī'of-thal-mī'tis) [pyo- + G. *ophthalmos,* eye, + *-ia,* condition, or *-itis,* inflammation]. Suppurative inflammation of the eye.

pyophysometra (pī'ō-fī-sō-mē'tră) [pyo- + G. *physa,* air, + *mētra,* uterus]. Presence of pus and gas in the uterine cavity.

pyopneumocholecystitis (pī'ō-nū'mō-kō'lē-sis-tī'tis) [pyo- + G. *pneuma,* air, + cholecystitis]. Combination of pus and gas in an inflamed gallbladder caused by gas-producing organisms or by the entry of air from the duodenum through the biliary tree.

pyopneumohepatitis (pī'ō-nū'mō-hep-ă-tī'tis) [pyo- + G. *pneuma,* air, + hepatitis]. Combination of pus and air in the liver, usually in association with an abscess.

pyopneumopericardium (pī'ō-nū'mō-per-i-kar'dē-ŭm) [pyo- + G. *pneuma,* air, + pericardium]. Presence of pus and gas in the pericardial sac.

pyopneumoperitoneum (pī'ō-nū'mō-per-i-tō-nē'ŭm) [pyo- + G. *pneuma,* air, + peritoneum]. Presence of pus and gas in the peritoneal cavity.

pyopneumoperitonitis (pī'ō-nū'mō-per-i-tō-nī'tis) [pyo- + G. *pneuma,* air, + peritonitis]. Peritonitis with gas-forming organisms or with gas introduced from a ruptured bowel.

pyopneumothorax (pī'ō-nū-mō-thōr'aks) [pyo- + G. *pneuma,* air, + thorax]. Pneumopyothorax; pneumoempyema; the presence of gas together with a purulent effusion in the pleural cavity.
subdiaphragmatic p., subphrenic p., subphrenic abscess associated with perforation of one of the hollow viscera, with gas in the chest, and abdomen.

pyopoiesis (pī'ō-poy-ē'sis) [pyo- + G. *poiēsis,* a making]. Suppuration.

pyopoietic (pī'ō-poy-et'ik). Pus-producing.

pyoptysis (pī-op'ti-sis) [pyo- + G. *ptysis,* a spitting]. A purulent expectoration.

pyopyelectasis (pī'ō-pī-ĕ-lek'tă-sis) [pyo- + G. *pyelos,* pelvis, + *ektasis,* a stretching]. Dilation of the renal pelvis with pus-producing inflammation.

pyorrhea (pī-ō-rē'ă) [pyo- + G. *rhoia,* a flow]. A purulent discharge.

pyosalpingitis (pi'o-sal-pin-ji'tis) [pyo- + salpingitis]. Suppurative inflammation of the fallopian tube.

pyosalpingo-oophoritis (pī-ō-sal'ping-gō-ō-of'ō-rī'tis) [pyo- + G. *salpinx,* trumpet (tube), + oophoritis]. Pyosalpingo-oothecitis; suppurative inflammation of the fallopian tube and the ovary.

pyosalpingo-oothecitis (pī-ō-sal'ping-gō-ō'ō-thē-sī'tis) [pyo- + G. *salpinx,* trumpet (tube), + Mod. L. *ootheca,* ovary, + G. *-itis,* inflammation]. Pyosalpingo-oophoritis.

pyosalpinx (pī-ō-sal'pingks) [pyo- + G. *salpinx,* trumpet (tube)]. Pus tube; distention of a fallopian tube with pus.

pyosemia (pī-ō-sē'mē-ă) [pyo- + L. *semen,* seed (of man)]. Pyospermia; presence of pus in seminal fluid, often associated with chronic prostatitis or other inflammatory conditions of the male genital tract.

pyosepticemia (pī'ō-sep-ti-sē'mē-ă) [pyo- + G. *sēptikos,* putrefying, + *haima,* blood]. Infection of the blood with several forms of bacteria, so-called pyogenic and also nonpyogenic organisms.

pyosis (pī-ō'sis) [G.]. Suppuration.
Manson's p., *pemphigus* contagiosus.
p. palma'ris, an affection observed in children in the East Indies, characterized by the presence of numerous discrete pustules on the palms.
p. trop'ica, Kurunegala ulcers; an affection seen in Sri Lanka, marked by the presence of dirty yellowish or blackish lesions, covered with a crust, the removal of which leaves a shallow granulating ulcer.

pyospermia (pī-ō-sper'mē-ă) [pyo- + G. *sperma,* seed, + *ia,* condition]. Pyosemia.

pyostatic (pī-ō-stat'ik) [pyo- + G. *statikos,* causing to stand]. **1.** Arresting the formation of pus. **2.** An agent that arrests the formation of pus.

pyostomatitis (pī'ō-stō-mă-tī'tis) [pyo- + G. *stoma,* mouth, + *-itis,* inflammation]. A suppurating inflammatory eruption of the mouth.
p. veg'etans, confluent pustular lesions of the mouth, with proliferative and verrucose eruptions of the buccal mucous membrane; associated with ulcerative colitis and other wasting diseases.

pyothorax (pī-ō-thōr'aks). Empyema in a pleural cavity.

pyourachus (pī-ō-yū'ră-kŭs). A purulent accumulation in the urachus.

pyoureter (pī-ō-yū-rē'ter). Distention of a ureter with pus.

pyoxanthin (pī'ō-zan'thin). A reddish yellow pigment obtained from blue pus by oxidation.

pyoxanthose (pī'ō-zan'thōs). A yellowish pigment obtained from blue pus by oxidation.

pyr- [G. *pyr,* fire]. Combining form denoting fire or heat. See also pyreto-, pyro- (1).

pyracin (pir'ă-sin). Pyridoxolactone, the lactone of 4-pyridoxic acid.

pyramid (pir'ă-mid) [G. *pyramis* (*pyramid-*), a pyramid]. **1.** Pyramis; a term applied to a number of anatomical structures having a more or less pyramidal shape. **2.** An obsolete term denoting the petrous portion of the temporal bone.
anterior p., *pyramis* medullae oblongatae.
cerebellar p., *pyramis* vermis.
Ferrein's p., *pars* radiata lobuli corticalis renis.
Lallouette's p., *lobus* pyramidalis glandulae thyroideae.
p. of light, cone of light; light reflex (3); Politzer's luminous cone; Wilde's triangle; a triangular area at the anterior inferior part of the tympanic membrane, running from the umbo to the periphery, where there is seen a bright reflection of light.
Malacarne's p., a lobule on the undersurface of the cerebellum, the posterior portion of the vermis.
malpighian p., *pyramis* renalis.
p. of medulla oblongata, *pyramis* medullae oblongatae.
medullary p., *pyramis* renalis.
olfactory p., a small area of gray matter situated between the roots of the olfactory tracts; it is continuous caudally with the anterior perforated substance.
petrous p., *pars* petrosa ossis temporalis.
posterior p. of the medulla, *fasciculus* gracilis.
renal p., *pyramis* renalis.
p. of thyroid, *lobus* pyramidalis glandulae thyroideae.
p. of tympanum, *eminentia* pyramidalis.
p. of vestibule, *pyramis* vestibuli.

pyramidal (pi-ram'i-dal). **1.** Of the shape of a pyramid. **2.** Relating to any anatomical structure called pyramid.

pyramidale (pi-ram'i-dā'lē) [Mod. L.]. *Os* triquetrum.

pyramidalis (pi-ram'i-dā'lis). See entries under musculus.

pyramidotomy (pi-ram'i-dot'ō-mē) [G. *pyramis,* pyramid, + *tomē,* incision]. Section of pyramidal tracts, in the spinal cord, for the relief of involuntary movements.
medullary p., see pyramidal *tractotomy.*
spinal p., see pyramidal *tractotomy.*

pyramin, pyramine (pir'ă-min). Toxopyrimidine.

pyramis, pl. **pyramides** (pir'ă-mis, pi-ram'i-dēz) [Mod. L. fr. G. pyramid] [NA]. Pyramid.
p. medul'lae oblonga'tae [NA], pyramid of medulla oblongata; anterior column of medulla oblongata; anterior pyramid; an elongated, white prominence on the ventral surface of the medulla oblongata on either side along the anterior median fissure, corresponding to the pyramidal tract.
p. rena'lis, pl. **pyram'ides rena'les** [NA], renal pyramid; malpighian or medullary pyramid; one of a number of pyramidal masses seen on longitudinal section of the kidney; they contain part of the secreting tubules and the collecting tubules.
p. tym'pani, *eminentia* pyramidalis.
p. ver'mis [NA], cerebellar pyramid; a subdivision of the inferior vermis of the cerebellum between the tuber and the uvula.
p. vestib'uli [NA], pyramid of vestibule; the upper triangular extremity of the crista vestibuli.

pyran (pī'ran). A cyclic compound that may be considered the formal parent of sugars with an oxygen bridge from carbon atoms 1 to 5 (the pyranoses).

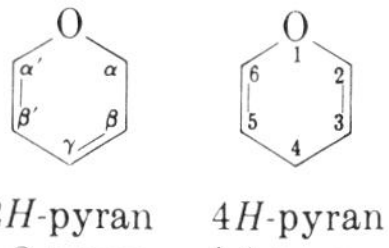

2*H*-pyran 4*H*-pyran
1,2-pyran 1,4-pyran
α-pyran γ-pyran

Pyran

pyranone (pir'ă-nōn, pī'-). Pyrone.

pyranose (pir'ă-nōs, pī'-). A cyclic form of a sugar in which the oxygen bridge forms a pyran.

pyrantel pamoate (pi-ran'tel). (*E*)-1,4,5,6-Tetrahydro-1-methyl-2-[2-(2-thienyl)vinyl]pyrimidine pamoate; an anthelmintic, especially useful drug for single or mixed intestinal nematode infections such as *Ascaris,* hookworm, pinworm, and *Trichostrongylus* species.

pyrathiazine hydrochloride (pir-ă-thī'ă-zēn). 10-[2-(1-Pyrrolidyl)ethyl]phenolthiazine hydrochloride; an antihistaminic.

pyrazinamide (pir-ă-zin'ă-mīd). Pyrazinoic acid amide; pyrazinecarboxamide; an antituberculous agent; the rapid development of resistance is delayed when given in combination with isoniazid; p. may produce hepatic damage.

pyrazolone (pir-ă-zō'lōn). A class of nonsteroidal anti-inflammatory agents used in the treatment of arthritic conditions; *e.g.,* phenylbutazone.

pyrectic (pī-rek'tik). Febrile.

pyrenemia (pī-rē-nē'mē-ă) [G. *pyrēn,* the pit of a fruit, + *haima,* blood]. A condition characterized by the presence of nucleated red blood cells.

Pyrenochaeta romeroi (pī'rĕ-nō-kē'tă rō'mĕ-roy). One of the numerous species of true fungi capable of causing mycetoma in man.

pyrenoid (pī'rē-noyd) [G. *pyrēn,* pit of a fruit, + *eidos,* resemblance]. One of the minute luminous bodies sometimes visualized in the chromatophores of some protozoa, such as *Euglena viridis.*

pyrethrins (pī-reth'rinz). Insecticidal constituents of pyrethrum flowers.

pyrethrolone (pī-reth'rō-lōn). 2-Methyl-4-oxo-3-(2,4-pentanedienyl)-2-cyclopentenol, a constituent of the pyrethrins.

pyrethrum (pī-rē'thrŭm) [G. *pyrethron,* feverfew, fr. *pyr,* fire, from the hot-tasting root]. Spanish chamomile; the root of *Anacyclus pyrethrum* (family Compositae), a shrub native to Morocco; has been used as a sialogogue; its flowers are a source of pyrethrins.

pyretic (pī-ret'ik) [G. *pyretikos*]. Febrile.

pyreto- [G. *pyretos,* fever, fr. *pyr,* fire]. Combining form denoting fever. See also pyr-, pyro- (1).

pyretogen (pī-ret'ō-jen) [pyreto- + G. *-gen,* producing]. Rarely used term for pyrogen.

pyretogenesis (pī'rĕ-tō-jen'ĕ-sis, pir'ĕ-tō-) [pyreto- + G. *genesis,* origin]. Rarely used term for the origin and mode of production of fever.

pyretogenetic, pyretogenic (pī'rĕ-tō-jĕ-net'ik, -jen'ik). Pyrogenic.

pyretogenous (pī-rĕ-toj'ĕ-nŭs). **1.** Caused by fever. **2.** Pyrogenic.

pyretotherapy (pī'rĕ-tō-thār'ă-pē) [pyreto- + G. *therapeia,* treatment]. **1.** Obsolete synonym for pyrotherapy. **2.** Treatment of fever.

pyrexia (pī-rek'sē-ă) [G. *pyrexis,* feverishness]. Fever.

pyrexial (pī-rek'sē-ăl). Relating to fever.

pyrexiophobia (pī-rek'sē-ō-fō'bē-ă) [G. *pyrexis,* feverishness, + *phobos,* fear]. Morbid fear of fever.

pyribenzyl methyl sulfate (pir-i-ben'zil). Bevonium methyl sulfate.

pyridine (pir'i-dēn, -din). C_5H_5N; a colorless volatile liquid of empyreumatic odor and burning taste, resulting from the dry distillation of organic matter containing nitrogen; used as an industrial solvent, in analytical chemistry, and for denaturing alcohol.

pyridofylline (pir-i-dof'i-lin). 7-(2-Hydroxyethyl)theophylline hydrogen sulfate compound with pyridoxol; a coronary vasodilator.

pyridostigmine bromide (pir'i-dō-stig'mēn). 3-Hydroxy-1-methylpyridinium bromide dimethylcarbamate; a cholinesterase inhibitor useful in the treatment of myasthenia gravis.

pyridoxal (pir'i-dok'săl). 4-Formyl-3-hydroxy-5-hydroxymethyl-2-methylpyridine; the 4-aldehyde of pyridoxine, having a similar physiologic action.

p. kinase [EC 2.7.1.35], an enzyme that catalyzes the phosphorylation by ATP of p. to pyridoxal 5′-phosphate, thus converting the food factor to the active coenzyme.

pyridoxal 5′-phosphate. Codecarboxylase; a coenzyme essential to many reactions in tissue, notably transaminations and amino acid decarboxylations.

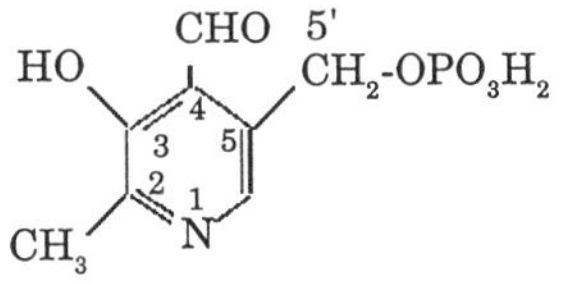

Pyridoxal phosphate

pyridoxamine (pir-i-dok'să-mēn). The amine of pyridoxine ($-CH_2NH_2$ replacing $-CH_2OH$ at position 4), having a similar physiologic action.

pyridoxamine-phosphate oxidase [EC 1.4.3.5]. An oxidoreductase catalyzing oxidative deamination of pyridoxamine 5′-phosphate (with O_2) to pyridoxal 5′-phosphate, H_2O_2, and NH_3.

4-pyridoxic acid (pir-i-dok'sik). The principal product of the metabolism of pyridoxal (–COOH replaces –CHO at position 4), appearing in the urine.

pyridoxine (pir-i-dok'sēn, -sin). 3-Hydroxy-4,5-bis(hydroxymethyl)-2-methylpyridine (with CH_2OH replacing CHO); the original vitamin B_6, which term now includes pyridoxal and pyridoxamine, associated with the utilization of unsaturated fatty acids. In rats, deficiency produces a nutritional dermatitis and acrodynia; in humans, deficiency may result in increased irritability, convulsions, and peripheral neuritis. The hydrochloride is used in pharmaceutical preparations.

pyridoxine 4-dehydrogenase [EC 1.1.1.65]. An oxidoreductase catalyzing oxidation of pyridoxine to pyridoxal by $NADP^+$.

pyridoxol (pir-i-dok'sol). Obsolete term for pyridoxine.

pyridoxonium (chloride) (pir'i-dok-sōn'ē-ŭm). Obsolete term for pyridoxine.

pyriform (pir'i-fōrm) [L. *pyrum* (prop. *pirum*), pear, + *forma,* form]. Piriform.

pyrilamine maleate (pī-ril'ă-mēn, pir'i-lă-). Mepyramine maleate; 2-[(2-dimethylaminoethyl) (*p*- methoxybenzyl)amino]pyridine maleate; an antihistaminic.

pyrimethamine (pir-i-meth'ă-mēn). 2,4-Diamino-5-*p*- chlorophenyl-6-ethylpyrimidine; a potent folic acid antagonist used as an antimalarial agent effective against *Plasmodium falciparum;* a valuable suppressant, active against the asexual erythrocytic and tissue forms; also used in the treatment of toxoplasmosis.

pyrimidine (pī-rim'i-dēn). A heterocyclic substance, the formal parent of several "bases" present in nucleic acids (uracil, thymine, cytosine) as well as of the barbiturates.

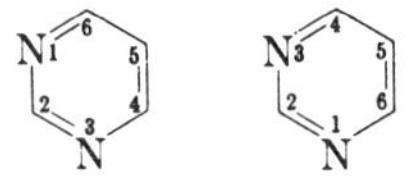

Pyrimidine

Left, original Fischer numbering system (*cf.* purine), now abandoned; *right,* current official numbering system.

p. transferase, *thiamin* pyridinylase.

pyrithiamin (pir'i-thī'ă-min). Neopyrithiamin; a thiamin antimetabolite, differing from thiamin in that the thiazole ring of the thiamin molecule is replaced by a pyridine ring.

pyro- [G. *pyr,* fire]. **1.** Combining form denoting fire, heat, or fever. See also pyr-, pyreto-. **2.** In chemistry, combining form denoting derivatives formed by removal of water (usually by heat) to form anhydrides. See also anhydro-.

pyroboric acid (pī-rō-bōr'ik). Tetraboric acid.

pyrocalciferol (pī'ro-kal-sif'er-ol). 10α-Ergosta-5,7,22-trien-3β-ol; 9-α-lumisterol; a thermal decomposition product of calciferol.

pyrocatechase (pī-rō-kat'ĕ-kās). Catechol 1,2-dioxygenase.

pyrocatechin (pī-rō-kat'ĕ-kin). Pyrocatechol.

pyrocatechol (pī-rō-kat'ĕ-kol). Catechol (1); pyrocatechin; 1,2-benzenediol; a constituent of the catecholamines, epinephrine and norepinephrine, and dopa; used externally as an antiseptic.

pyrogallic acid (pī-rō-gal'ik). Pyrogallol.

pyrogallol (pī-rō-gal'ol). Pyrogallic acid; $C_6H_3(OH)_3$; 1,2,3-trihydroxybenzene; used externally in the treatment of psoriasis, ringworm, and other skin affections.

pyrogallolphthalein (pī'rō-gal-ō-thal'ē-in, -thāl'ē-in). Gallein.

pyrogen (pī'rō-jen) [pyro- + G. *-gen,* producing]. An agent that causes a rise in temperature; p.'s are produced by bacteria, molds, viruses, and yeasts, and commonly occur in distilled water.

pyrogenic (pī-rō-jen'ik). Pyretogenic; pyretogenetic; pyretogenous (2); causing fever. See also febrifacient.

pyroglobulins (pī-rō-glob'yū-linz). Serum proteins (immunoglobulins), usually associated with multiple myeloma or macroglobulinemia, which precipitate irreversibly when heated to 56°C.

pyrolagnia (pī-rō-lag'nē-ă) [pyro- + G. *lagneia,* lust]. Sexual gratification from setting fires.

pyroligneous (pī-rō-lig'nē-ŭs) [pyro- + L. *lignum,* wood]. Relating to or produced by the dry distillation of wood.

pyrolysis (pī-rol'i-sis) [pyro- + G. *lysis,* dissolution]. Decomposition of a substance by heat.

pyromania (pī-rō-mā'nē-ă) [pyro- + G. *mania,* frenzy]. Incendiarism; a morbid impulse to set fires.

pyromaniac (pī-rō-mā'nē-ak). One affected with pyromania.

pyromen (pī'rō-men). Piromen.

pyrometer (pī-rom'ĕ-ter) [pyro- + G. *metron,* measure]. An instrument for measuring very high degrees of heat, beyond the capacity of a mercury or gas thermometer.

resistance p., resistance *thermometer.*

pyrone (pī'rōn). Pyranone; a keto derivative of pyran.

pyronin (pī'rō-nin). A fluorescent red basic xanthene dye, the chloride of tetramethyldiaminoxanthene, **p. Y** or **G** (C.I. 45005), or of tetraethyldiaminoxanthene, **p. B** (C.I. 45010). These dyes, especially p. Y, are used in combination with methyl green for differential staining of RNA (red) and DNA (green); difference in staining result is probably due to the higher degree of polymerization of DNA; p. Y is also used as a tracking dye for RNA in electrophoresis.

pyroninophilia (pī'rō-nin-ō-fil'ē-ă) [pyronin + G. *philos,* fond]. An affinity for the basic pyronin dyes; a useful indicator of intense protein synthesis accompanying RNA synthesis, as in the cytoplasm of an active plasma cell.

pyrophobia (pī-rō-fō'bē-ă) [pyro- + G. *phobos,* fear]. Morbid dread of fire.

pyrophosphatase (pī-rō-fos'fă-tās). Any enzyme cleaving a pyrophosphate between two phosphoric groups, leaving one on each of the two fragments; *e.g.,* inorganic p., NAD^+ p. (cleaves NAD, etc., to mononucleotides), ATP p. (cleaves inorganic pyrophosphate from ATP, leaving AMP)

inorganic p. [EC 3.6.1.1], a phosphohydrolase catalyzing hydrolysis of inorganic pyrophosphate to orthophosphate.

pyrophosphate (PP) (pī-rō-fos'fāt). A salt of pyrophosphoric acid.

pyrophosphokinases (pī'rō-fōs-fō-kī'nās-ez). Pyrophosphotransferases; enzymes (sub-subclass EC 2.7.6) transferring a pyrophosphoric group (*e.g.,* ribose-phosphate pyrophosphokinase, EC 2.7.6.1).

pyrophosphoric acid (pī'rō-fos-fōr'ik). $H_4P_2O_7$; an anhydride of phosphoric acid obtained by heating phosphoric acid to 213°C; it forms pyrophosphates with bases, and its esters are important in energy metabolism and in biosynthesis.

pyrophosphorylases (pī'rō-fos-fōr'il-ās-ez). Trivial name applied to the nucleotidyltransferases that catalyze the transfer of the AMP of ATP to another residue with the release of inorganic pyrophosphate, or the attachment of a nulceoside pyrophosphate to a polynucleotide with release of inorganic orthophosphate.

pyrophosphotransferases (pī'rō-fos-fō-trans'fer-ās-ez). Pyrophosphokinases.

pyroptothymia (pī-rop-tō-thī'mē-ă) [pyro- + G. *ptoein,* to frighten, + *thymos,* mind]. Rarely used term for a delusion in which one imagines being surrounded by flames.

pyroscope (pī'rō-skōp) [pyro- + G. *skopeō,* to view]. An instrument for measuring temperature by comparing the light of a heated object with a light standard.

pyrosis (pī-rō'sis) [G. a burning]. Heartburn; substernal pain or burning sensation, usually associated with regurgitation of acid-peptic gastric juice into the esophagus.

pyrotherapy (pī'rō-thār'ă-pē). Treatment of disease by inducing an artificial fever in the patient.

pyrotic (pī-rot'ik). **1.** Relating to pyrosis. **2.** Caustic.

pyrotoxin (pī'rō-tok'sin). A supposed toxic substance produced in the tissues during the progress of a fever.

pyrovalerone hydrochloride (pir-ō-val'er-ōn). 4'-Methyl-2-(1-pyrrolidinyl)valerophenone hydrochloride; an analeptic.

pyroxylin (pī-rok'si-lin) [pyro- + G. *xylon,* wood]. Colloxylin; soluble gun cotton; nitrocellulose; dinitrocellulose; xyloidin; consists chiefly of cellulose tetranitrate, obtained by the action of nitric and sulfuric acids on cotton; used in the preparation of collodion.

pyrrobutamine phosphate (pir-ō-byū'tă-mēn). 1-[4-(*p*-Chlorophenyl)-3-phenyl-2-butenyl]-pyrrolidine diphosphate; an antihistamine.

pyrrolase (pir'ō-lās). Tryptophan 2,3-dioxygenase.

pyrrol blue (pir'ol) [C.I. 42700]. Isamine blue; $C_4OH_3ON_3O_6Na$; an acid triarylmethane dye employed as a vital dye and as an elastin stain.

pyrrole (pir'ōl). Azole; imidole; divinylenimine; a heterocyclic compound found in many biologically important substances.

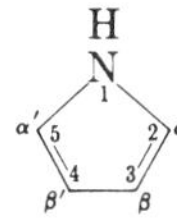

Pyrrole

pyrrolidine (pi-rol'i-dēn). Tetrahydropyrrole; pyrrole to which four H atoms have been added; the basis of proline and hydroxyproline.

pyrrolidone (pi-rol'i-dōn). 2-Pyrrolidinone; 2-ketopyrrolidine; 2-oxopyrrolidine; an industrial solvent, plasticizer, and coalescing agent.

pyrroline (pir'ō-lēn). 2,5-Dihydropyrrole; pyrrole to which two H atoms have been added.

pyrroline-2-carboxylate reductase [EC 1.5.1.1]. Proline dehydrogenase or oxidase; an oxidoreductase reducing 1-pyrroline-2-carboxylate to L-proline with NAD(P)H.

pyrroline-5-carboxylate reductase [EC 1.5.1.2]. Proline dehydrogenase or oxidase; an oxidoreductase reducing 1-pyrroline-5-carboxylate to L-proline with NAD(P)H.

pyrrolnitrin (pir-ol-nī'trin). 3-Chloro-4-(3-chloro-2-nitrophenyl)pyrrole; an antifungal agent.

pyruvaldoxine (pī'rū-văl-dok'sēn). Isonitrosoacetone.

pyruvate (pī'rū-vāt). A salt or ester of pyruvic acid.

p. carboxylase [EC 6.4.1.1], a ligase catalyzing reaction of ATP, p., and CO_2, to form ADP, inorganic phosphate, and oxaloacetate; biotin and acetyl-CoA are involved.

p. decarboxylase [EC 4.1.1.1], α-carboxylase; α-ketoacid carboxylase; a carboxy-lyase of yeast catalyzing decarboxylation of a 2-oxoacid (*e.g.,* p.) to an aldehyde (*e.g.,* acetaldehyde) without oxidoreduction and without lipoamide, in contrast to p. dehydrogenase (lipoamide).

p. dehydrogenase (cytochrome) [EC 1.2.2.2], an oxidoreductase catalyzing reaction between ferricytochrome b_1 and p. to yield acetate and CO_2.

p. dehydrogenase (lipoamide) [EC 1.2.4.1], an oxidoreductase catalyzing conversion of p. and (oxidized) lipoamide to CO_2 and S^6-acetyldihydrolipoamide in two successive reactions: the first between p. and thiamin pyrophosphate to yield CO_2 and α-hydroxyethylthiamin pyrophosphate; the second between the last named and lipoamide to regain the thiamin pyrophosphate and yield S^6-acetylhydrolipoamide.

p. kinase (PK) [EC 2.7.1.40], phospho*enol*pyruvate kinase; a phosphotransferase catalyzing transfer of phosphate from phospho*enol*pyruvate to ADP, forming ATP and p.; other nucleoside phosphates can participate in the reaction.

p. oxidase [EC 1.2.3.3], an oxidoreductase catalyzing the reaction of p., phosphate, and O_2 to yield acetyl phosphate, CO_2, and H_2O_2.

pyruvic acid (pī-rū'vik). 2-Oxopropanoic acid; α-ketopropionic acid; acetylformic acid; pyroacemic acid; CH_3–CO–COOH; an intermediate compound in the metabolism of carbohydrate; in thiamin deficiency, its oxidation is retarded and it accumulates in the tissues, especially in nervous structures. The enol form, *enol* pyruvic acid, $CH_2{=}C(OH)$–COOH, plays an important metabolic role. See phospho*enol* pyruvic acid.

pyruvic aldehyde. Methylglyoxal.

pyruvic-malic carboxylase. Malate dehydrogenase.

pyrvinium pamoate (pir-vin'i-ŭm). Viprynium embonate; 6-(dimethylamino)-2-[2-(2,5-dimethyl-1-phenylpyrrol-3-yl)-vinyl]-1-methylquinolinium 4,4′-methylenebis[3-hydroxy-2-naphthoate] (2:1); a highly effective drug used in the eradication of human pinworms.

Pythium insidiosum (pith'ē-ŭm in-sid'ē-um). *Hyphomyces destruens;* a species of fungi found in water or wet soil, and a cause of hyphomycosis.

pythogenesis (pī-thō-jen'ĕ-sis) [G. *pythō,* to decay, + *genesis,* origin]. **1.** Origination from decaying matter. **2.** The causation of decay.

pythogenic, pythogenous (pī-thō-jen'ik, pī-thoj'ĕ-nŭs). Originating from filth or putrescence.

pyuria (pī-yū'rē-ă) [G. *pyon,* pus, + *ouron,* urine]. Presence of pus in the urine when voided.

Q

Q Symbol for coulomb; quantity.

$\dot{Q}$ [quantity + an overdot denoting the time derivative] Symbol for blood flow. See flow (3).

Q_{10} Symbol for the increase in rate of a process produced by raising the temperature 10°C.

q In cytogenetics, symbol for long arm of a chromosome (in contrast to p for the short arm).

Q-banding. See Q-banding *stain.*

Q_{CO_2} Symbol for the microliters STPD of CO_2 given off per milligram of tissue per hour.

Q_O, Q_{O_2} Symbols for oxygen *consumption* (1).

q.d. Abbreviation for L. *quaque die,* every day.

$Q\text{-}H_2$ Symbol for ubiquinol.

q.h. Abbreviation for L. *quaque hora,* every hour.

q.i.d. Abbreviation for L. *quater in die,* four times a day.

q.l. Abbreviation for L. *quantum libet,* as much as desired.

q.s. Abbreviation for L. *quantum sufficiat* or *satis,* as much as desired.

quack (kwak). Charlatan.

quackery (kwak'er-ē). Charlatanism.

quader (kwah'der) [Ger. square]. The precuneus.

quadrangular (kwah-drang'yū-lăr) [L. *quadrangularis,* fr. *quadrangulum,* quadrangle]. Having four angles.

quadrant (kwah'drant) [L. *quadrans,* a quarter]. One quarter of a circle. In anatomy, roughly circular areas are divided for descriptive purposes into q.'s. The abdomen is divided into right upper and lower, and left upper and lower q.'s by a horizontal and a vertical line intersecting at the umbilicus. Q.'s of the fundus oculi (superior and inferior nasal, superior and inferior temporal) are demarcated by a horizontal and a vertical line intersecting at the optic disk. The tympanic membrane is divided into anterosuperior, anteroinferior, posterosuperior, and posteroinferior q.'s by a line drawn across the diameter of the drum in the axis of the handle of the malleus and another intersecting the first at right angles at the umbo.

quadrantanopsia (kwah'drant-an-op'sē-ă). Quadrantic *hemianopsia.*

quadrate (kwah'drāt) [L. *quadratus,* square]. Having four equal sides; square.

quadri- [L. *quattuor,* four]. Combining form denoting four.

quadribasic (kwah-dri-bā'sik). Denoting an acid having four hydrogen atoms that are replaceable by atoms or radicals of a basic character.

quadriceps (kwah'dri-seps) [L. fr. quadri- + *caput,* head]. Having four heads; denoting a muscle of the thigh, musculus q. femoris, and one of the calf, musculus q. surae or the combined gastrocnemius (with two heads), soleus, and plantaris, more commonly called musculus triceps surae, the plantaris being counted as a separate muscle.

quadricepsplasty (kwah-dri-seps'plas-tē). A corrective surgical procedure on the quadriceps femoris.

quadricuspid (kwah-dri-kŭs'pid). Tetracuspid.

quadridigitate (kwah'dri-dij'i-tāt) [quadri- + L. *digitus,* digit]. Tetradactyl.

quadrigeminal (kwah'dri-jem'i-năl) [quadri- + L. *geminus,* twin]. Four-fold.

quadrigeminum (kwah'dri-jem'i-nŭm). One of the corpora quadrigemina.

quadrigeminus (kwah-dri-jem'i-nŭs) [L.]. Quadruplet.

quadrigeminy (kwah'dri-jem'i-nē). Quadrigeminal *rhythm.*

quadriparesis (kwah'dri-pă-rē'sis). Tetraparesis.

quadriplegia (kwah'dri-plē'jē-ă) [quadri- + G. *plēgē,* stroke]. Tetraplegia; paralysis of all four limbs.

quadriplegic (kwah'dri-plē'jik). Tetraplegic; pertaining to or afflicted with quadriplegia.

quadripolar (kwah'dri-pō'lăr). Having four poles.

quadrisect (kwah'dri-sekt) [quadri- + L. *seco,* pp. *sectus,* to cut]. Quartisect; to divide into four parts.

quadrisection (kwah'dri-sek'shŭn). Division into four parts.

quadritubercular (kwah'dri-tū-ber'kyū-lăr) [quadri- + L. *tuberculum,* tubercle]. Having four tubercles or cusps, as a molar tooth.

quadrivalent (kwah-dri-vā'lent). Tetravalent; having the combining power (valency) of four.

quadruped (kwah'drū-ped) [L. *quattuor,* four, + *pes* (*ped-*), foot]. A four-footed animal.

quadruplet (kwah'drŭp-let, kwă-drū'plet) [L. *quadruplus,* four fold]. Quadrigeminus; one of four children born at one birth.

qualimeter (kwah-lim'ĕ-ter) [L. *qualis,* of what kind, + G. *metron,* measure]. An obsolete device for estimating the degree of hardness of x-rays.

Quant's sign. See under sign.

quanta (kwahn'tă) [L.]. Plural of quantum.

quantimeter (kwahn-tim'ĕ-ter) [L. *quantus,* how much, + G. *metron,* measure]. An obsolete device for determining the quantity of x-rays generated by a Crookes or Coolidge tube.

quantum, pl. **quanta** (kwahn'tŭm, -tă) [L. how much]. **1.** A unit of radiant energy (ϵ) varying according to the frequency (ν) of the radiation. **2.** A certain definite amount.

quarantine (kwar'an-tēn) [It. *quarantina* fr. L. *quadraginta,* forty]. **1.** A period (originally 40 days) of detention of vessels and their passengers coming from an area where an infectious disease prevails. **2.** To detain such vessels and their passengers until the incubation period of an infectious disease has passed. **3.** A place where such vessels and their passengers are detained. **4.** The isolation of a person with a known or possible contagious disease.

quart (kwōrt) [L. *quartus,* fourth]. **1.** A measure of fluid capacity; the fourth part of a gallon; the equivalent of 0.9468 liter. An imperial q. contains about 20% more than the ordinary q., or 1.1359 liters. **2.** A dry measure holding a little more than the fluid measure.

quartan (kwōr'tan) [L. *quartanus,* relating to a fourth (thing)]. Recurring every fourth day, including the first day of an episode in the computation.

double q., denoting malaria infection with two independent groups of q. parasites, so that paroxysms occur on two successive days followed by one day without fever.

triple q., denoting malaria infection with three independent groups of q. parasites, so that a paroxysm occurs every day, resembling a double tertian or a quotidian fever.

quarter-crack (kwōr'ter-krak). See sand-crack.

quartisect (kwōr'ti-sekt) [L. *quartus,* fourth, + *seco,* pp. *sectus,* to cut]. Quadrisect.

quartz (kwōrts). A crystalline form of silicon dioxide used in chemical apparatus and in optical and electric instruments.

quasidominance (kwā-si-dom'i-nans). False dominance; simulation by a recessive trait of the pattern of dominant inheritance (*i.e.*, recurrence in several generations) by repeated, and often occult, consanguineous matings.

quasidominant (kwā-si-dom'i-nănt). Denoting a trait in an inbred pedigree that simulates dominant inheritance.

quassation (kwah-sā'shŭn) [L. *quassatio*, fr. *quasso*, pp. *-atus*, to shake violently, fr. *quatio*, to shake]. The breaking up of crude drug materials, such as bark and woody stems, into small pieces to facilitate extraction and other treatment.

quassia (kwah'shē-ă) [*Quassi*, a resident of Surinam who used it as a tonic]. Bitterwood; the heartwood of *Picrasma excelsa* (*Picraena excelsa*), known as Jamaica q., or of *Quassia amara* (family Simarubaceae), known as Surinam q.; a bitter tonic; the infusion has been administered by enema in the treatment of threadworms.

quaternary (kwah'ter-nār-ē, kwah-ter'nĕ-rē) [L. *quaternarius*, containing four, fr. *quattuor*, four]. **1.** Denoting a chemical compound containing four elements; *e.g.*, $NaHSO_4$. **2.** Fourth in a series. **3.** Relating to organic compounds in which some central atom is attached to four functional groups; applied to the usually trivalent nitrogen in its "onium" state, R_4N^+, "quaternary nitrogen."

Quatrefages de Breau, Jean L.A. de, French naturalist, 1810–1892. See Q. de B.'s *angle.*

quazepam (kwā'zē-pam). 7-Chloro-5-(*o*-fluorophenyl)-1,3-dihydro-1-(2,2,2-trifluoroethyl)-2*H*-1,4-benzodiazepine-2-thione; a benzodiazepine derivative used as a sedative and hypnotic.

quebrachine (kē-brah'chēn). An alkaloid, $C_{21}H_{26}N_2O_3$, from quebracho and identical with yohimbine; formerly used in cardiac dyspnea.

quebracho (kē-brah'chō) [Port. *quebrahacho*, fr. *quebrar*, to break, + *hacha*, axe, referring to the hardness of the wood]. The dried bark of a genus of trees, *Aspidosperma quebrachoblanco* (family Apocynaceae); has been used as a respiratory stimulant in emphysema, dyspnea, and chronic bronchitis; the two chief alkaloids are aspidospermine and quebrachine.

Queckenstedt, Hans, German physician, 1876–1918. See Q.-Stookey *test.*

queen (kwēn). A female cat of breeding age.

quenching (kwench'ing). **1.** The process of extinguishing, removing, or diminishing a physical property such as heat or light; *e.g.*, the cooling of a hot metal rapidly by plunging it into water or oil. **2.** In beta liquid scintillation counting, the shifting of the energy spectrum from a true to a lower energy; it is caused by a variety of interfering materials in the counting solution, including foreign chemicals and coloring agents.

fluorescence q., a technique used in investigations dealing with binding of antigens (haptens) by purified antibodies, applicable in cases in which the bound antigen (hapten) absorbs (quenches) light emitted during fluorescence of protein (antibody) excited by ultraviolet light.

Quénu, Eduard A.V.A., French surgeon and anatomist, 1852–1933. See Q.'s hemorrhoidal *plexus;* Q.-Muret *sign.*

quercetin (kwer'sē-tin). Meletin; sophoretin; 3,3',4',5,7-pentahydroxyflavone; an aglycon of quercitrin, rutin, and other glycosides; occurs usually as the 3-rhamnoside; used in the treatment of abnormal capillary fragility.

quercus (kwer'kŭs) [L. oak]. The bark of *Quercus alba*, white oak or stone oak; formerly used as an astringent.

querulent (kwer'ū-lent) [L. *querulus*, complaining, fr. *queror*, to complain]. Denoting one who is ever suspicious, always opposing any suggestion, complaining of ill treatment and of being slighted or misunderstood, easily enraged, and dissatisfied; characteristic of paranoid personalities.

Quervain, Fritz de. See de Quervain.

questionnaire (kwes-chŭn-ār'). A list of questions submitted to obtain statistically useful data or personal information.

Holmes-Rahe q., a survey to measure in life change units the stressfulness of various life events.

Queyrat, Auguste, French dermatologist, *1872. See *erythroplasia* of Q.

Quick, Armand J., U.S. physician, *1894. See Q.'s *method, test.*

quick (kwik) [A.S. *cwic*, living]. **1.** Pregnant with a child whose fetal movements are recognizable. **2.** A sensitive part, painful to touch.

quickening (kwik'ĕn-ing) [A.S. *cwic*, living]. Signs of life felt by the mother as a result of the fetal movements, usually noted first in the fourth or fifth month of pregnancy.

quicklime (kwik'līm). Unslaked lime. See lime (2).

quicksilver (kwik'sil'ver). Mercury.

quiescent (kwi-es'ent). At rest or inactive.

quin-, quino-. Root of quinoline and quinone, hence used in many names of substances containing these structures (*e.g.*, quinine, quinol).

quina (kē'nă, kwē'nă) [Sp., fr. Peruv. *quina* or *kina*, cinchona]. Cinchona.

quinacrine hydrochloride (kwin'ă-krēn, -krin). Mepacrine hydrochloride; an acridine derivative, $C_{23}H_{30}ClN_3O{\cdot}2HCl{\cdot}2H_2O$, used as an antimalarial that destroys the trophozoites of *Plasmodium vivax* and *P. falciparum*, but does not affect the gametocytes, sporozoites, or exoerythrocytic stage of parasites; also used as an anthelmintic. As a dihydrochloride, it is used as a stain in cytogenetics to demonstrate Y chromatin by fluorescent microscopy.

quinaldic acid (kwin-al'dik). Quinaldinic acid; quinoline-2-carboxylic acid; a product of tryptophan catabolism, via kynurenic acid, found in human urine.

quinaldine red (kwin'al-dēn). A styrene-quinolinium iodide; used as a pH indicator (turns red at pH 3.2).

quinaldinic acid (kwin-al-din'ik). Quinaldic acid.

quinaquina (kē'nă-kē'nă, kwin'ă-kwin'ă) [a reduplication of Sp. *quina*, cinchona]. Cinchona.

quinate (kwī'nāt, kwin'āt). A salt or ester of quinic acid.

q. dehydrogenase [EC 1.1.1.24], an oxidoreductase catalyzing reaction of quinate and NAD to form 3-dehydroquinate.

quince (kwints). The edible fruit of *Cydonia oblongata* (family Rosaceae); the seeds have demulcent properties.

Quincke, Heinrich I., German physician, 1842–1922. See Q.'s *disease, edema, pulse, puncture, sign.*

quinestradiol, quinestradol (kwin'es-tră-dī'ol, kwin-es'tră-dol). 3-(Cyclopentyloxy)estra-1,3,5(10)-triene-16α,17β-diol; an estrogen.

quinethazone (kwin-eth'ă-zōn). 7-Chloro-2-ethyl-1,2,3,4-tetrahydro-4-oxo-6-quinazolinesulfonamide; a diuretic and antihypertensive agent.

quingestanol acetate (kwin-jes'tă-nol). 3-(Cyclopentyloxy)-19-nor-17α-pregna-3,5-dien-20-yn-17-ol acetate; a progestational agent.

quinhydrone (kwin-hī'drōn). A mixture of equimolecular quantities of quinone and hydroquinone; used in pH determinations (q. electrode).

quinic acid (kwin'ik). Chinic or kinic acid; L-quinic acid; 1,3,4,5-tetrahydroxycyclohexanecarboxylic acid; an acid found in cinchona bark and elsewhere in plants; 5-dehydroquinic acid is an intermediate in the biosynthesis of phenylalanine, tyrosine, and tryptophan from carbohydrate precursors.

quinidine (kwin'i-dēn, -din). Conquinine; β-quinine; one of the alkaloids of cinchona, a stereoisomer of quinine; used as an antimalarial; also used in the treatment of atrial fibrillation and flutter, and paroxysmal ventricular tachycardia.

quinine (kwī'nīn, -nēn; kwin'-īn, -ēn). $C_{20}H_{24}N_2O_23H_2O$; the most important of the alkaloids derived from cinchona; an antimalarial effective against the asexual and erythrocytic forms of the parasite, but having no effect on the exoerythrocytic (tissue) forms. It does not produce a radical cure of malaria produced by *Plasmodium vivax, P. malariae,* or *P. ovale,* but is used in the treatment of cerebral malaria and other severe attacks of malignant tertian malaria, and in malaria produced by chloroquine-resistant strains of *P. falciparum;* it is also used as an antipyretic, analgesic, sclerosing agent, stomachic, and oxytocic (occasionally), and in the treatment of atrial fibrillation, myotonia congenita, and other myopathies.

q. bisulfate, the acid sulfate of q., very soluble in water.

q. carbacrylic resin, see under resin.

q. ethylcarbonate, an almost tasteless form of q. that is poorly absorbed from the intestinal tract.

q. sulfate, the most frequently prescribed salt of q.

q. and urea hydrochloride, sclerosing agent for treatment of internal hemorrhoids, hydrocele, and varicose veins, containing not less than 58% and not more than 65% of anhydrous q.

q. urethan, a mixture of urethan and q. hydrochloride; a sclerosing agent for the treatment of varicose veins.

quininism (kwī'ni-nizm, kwin'i-). Cinchonism.

Quinlan's test. See under test.

quino-. See quin-.

quinocide hydrochloride (kwin'ō-sīd). 8-(4-Aminopentylamino)-6-methoxyquinoline hydrochloride; an antimalarial comparable to primaquine in effectiveness and scope.

quinol (kwin'ol). Hydroquinone.

quinoline (kwin'ō-lēn, -lin). Chinoleine; leucoline; benzo[*b*]pyridine; 1-benzazine; a volatile nitrogenous base obtained by the distillation of coal tar, bones, alkaloids, etc.; a basic structure of many dyes and drugs; also used as an antimalarial.

quinolinic acid (kwin-ō-lin'ik). 2,3-Pyridinedicarboxylic acid; a catabolite of tryptophan and a precursor of nicotinic acid.

quinology (kwin-ol'ō-jē) [Sp. *quina,* cinchona, + G. *logos,* study]. The botany, chemistry, pharmacology, and therapeutics of cinchona and its alkaloids.

quinolones (kwin'ō-lōnz). A class of synthetic broad spectrum antibacterial agents that exhibit bactericidal action.

quinone (kwin'ōn, kwī'nōn). **1.** General name for aromatic compounds bearing two oxygens in place of two hydrogens, usually in the *para* position; the oxidation product of a hydroquinone. **2.** Specific name for 1,4-benzoquinone.

q. reductase, NAD(P)H dehydrogenase (quinone).

quinovose (kwin'ō-vōs). D-Epirhamnose.

Quinquaud, Charles E., French physician, 1841–1894. See Q.'s *disease.*

quinquedigitate (kwin'kwē-dij'i-tāt) [L. *quinque,* five, + *digitus,* digit]. Pentadactyl.

quinquetubercular (kwin'kwē-tū-ber'kyū-lăr) [L. *quinque,* five, + *tuberculum,* tubercle, dim. of *tuber,* a swelling]. Having five tubercles or cusps, as certain molar teeth.

quinquevalent (kwin-kwē-vā'lent) [L. *quinque,* five, + *valentia,* strength]. Pentavalent.

quinquina (kwin-kwi'nă). Cinchona.

quinsy (kwin'zē) [M.E. *quinsie (quinesie),* a corruption of L. *cynanche,* sore throat]. Peritonsillar *abscess.*

lingual q., phlegmonous inflammation of the lingual tonsil and neighboring structures.

quintan (kwin'tan) [L. *quintus,* fifth]. Recurring every fifth day, including the first day of an episode in the computation, *i.e.,* after a free interval of three days.

quintuplet (kwin-tŭp'let) [L. *quintuplex,* fivefold]. One of five children born at one birth.

quittor (kwit'ŏr) [ME. *quetaur,* a boiling]. A fistulous tract leading from the coronet to the lateral cartilage of the horse, due to an injury, followed by bacterial infection and later by massive necrosis of cartilage and other tissues; the necrotic process may involve the joint capsule.

quotidian (kwō-tid'ē-ăn) [L. *quotidianus,* daily, fr. *quot,* as many as, + *dies,* day]. Daily; occurring every day.

quotient (kwo'shĕnt) [L. *quoties,* how often]. The number of times one amount is contained in another. See also index (2); ratio.

achievement q., a ratio, percentile rating, or related q. of the amount a child has learned in relation to his age, level of education, or peers.

Ayala's q., Ayala's *index.*

blood q., color *index.*

cognitive laterality q. (CIQ), test for difference in cognitive performance of left and right sides of the brain.

growth q., the fractional part or percentage of the entire food energy which is utilized for growth in the young animal.

intelligence q. (IQ), the psychologist's index of measured intelligence as one part of a two-part determination of intelligence, the other part being an index of adaptive behavior and including such criteria as school grades or work performance. IQ is a score, or similar quantitative index, used to denote a person's standing relative to his age peers on a test of general ability, ordinarily expressed as a ratio between the person's score on a given test and the score which the average individual his age attained on the same test, the ratio being computed by the psychologist or determined from a table of age norms, such as the various Wechsler intelligence scales.

respiratory q. (R.Q.), respiratory coefficient; the steady state ratio of carbon dioxide produced by tissue metabolism to oxygen consumed in the same metabolism; for the whole body, normally about 0.82 under basal conditions; in the steady state, the respiratory q. is equal to the respiratory exchange ratio.

spinal q., Ayala's *index.*

R

R Abbreviation or symbol for gas *constant;* electrical resistance; radical (usually an alkyl or aryl group, *e.g.,* ROH is an alcohol, RNH_2 an amine); Réaumur; respiration; respiratory exchange *ratio; roentgen;* the remainder of a chemical formula; the unit of resistance in the cardiovascular system.

R_f Symbol denoting movement of a substance in paper chromatography *r*elative to the solvent *f*ront.

℞ Symbol for recipe in a prescription.

r Abbreviation for racemic, occasionally used in naming compounds in place of the more common *dl,* as "r-alanine" (more often as the prefix rac.); roentgen.

Ra Symbol for radium.

rabbeting (rab'et-ing). [Fr. *raboter,* to plane]. Making congruous stepwise cuts on apposing bone surfaces for stability after impaction.

rabbitpox (rab'it-poks). Rabbit plague; a virulent epidemic disease among laboratory rabbits caused by the rabbitpox virus; it does not apparently occur among wild rabbits.

rab'id [L. *rabidus,* raving, mad]. Relating to or suffering from rabies.

rabies (rā'bēz) [L. rage, fury, fr. *rabio,* to rave, to be mad]. Highly fatal infectious disease that may affect all species of warm-blooded animals, including man, is transmitted almost exclusively by the bite of carnivorous animals, and is caused by a neurotropic lyssavirus in the central nervous system and the salivary glands. The symptoms are characteristic of a profound disturbance of the nervous system, *e.g.,* excitement, aggressiveness, and madness, followed by paralysis and death. Characteristic cytoplasmic inclusion bodies (Negri bodies) found in many of the neurons are an aid to rapid laboratory diagnosis.

dumb r., paralytic r.

furious r., the form or stage of r. in which the animal is markedly hyperactive, characterized by periods of agitation, thrashing, running, snapping, or biting.

paralytic r., dumb r.; a form or stage of r. marked by paralytic symptoms.

rabiform (rā'bi-fōrm). Resembling rabies.

rac-. Prefix for racemic.

race (rās). A group of animals or individuals within a species which has common somatic inherited characteristics.

racefemine (rā-sĕ-fem'ēn). *dl-threo-α*-Methyl-*N*-(1-methyl-2-phenoxyethyl)phenethylamine; used as a uterine relaxant for relief of postpartum pain.

racemase (rā'sē-mās). An enzyme capable of catalyzing racemization, *i.e.,* inversions of asymmetric groups; when more than one center of asymmetry is present, "epimerase" is used (*e.g.,* hydroxyproline, ribulose phosphate).

racemate (rā'sē-māt). A racemic compound, or the salt or ester of such a compound. See also racemic.

raceme (rā-sēm'). An optically inactive chemical compound. See also racemic.

racemic (r) (rā-sē'mik, -sem'ik). Denoting a mixture that is optically inactive, being composed of an equal number of dextro- and levorotatory substances, which are separable. Those compounds internally compensated, and therefore not separable into D and L (or *d* and *l*) forms, are termed "meso."

racemization (rā'sē-mi-zā'shŭn, ras-mi-). Partial conversion of one enantiomorph into another (as an L-amino acid to the corresponding D-amino acid) so that the specific optical rotation is decreased, or even reduced to zero, in the resulting racemate.

racemose (ras'ē-mōs) [L. *racemosus,* full of clusters]. Branching, with nodular terminations, resembling a bunch of grapes.

racephedrine hydrochloride (rās-ĕ-fed'rin). *dl*-Ephedrine hydrochloride; a sympathomimetic drug with peripheral effects similar to those of epinephrine, and with the same actions and uses as ephedrine.

rachi-, rachio- [G. *rhachis,* spine, backbone]. Combining form denoting the spine.

rachial (rā'kē-ăl). Spinal.

rachicentesis (rā-kē-sen-tē'sis) [rachi- + G. *kentēsis,* puncture]. Lumbar *puncture.*

rachidial (rā-kid'ē-ăl). Spinal.

rachidian (rā-kid'ē-an). Spinal.

rachigraph (rā'kē-graf) [rachi- + G. *graphō,* to write]. A graph for recording the curves of the vertebrae.

rachilysis (rā-kil'i-sis) [rachi- + G. *lysis,* a loosening]. Forcible correction of lateral curvature of the spine by lateral pressure against the convexity of the curve.

rachio-. See rachi-.

rachiocampsis (rā-kē-ō-kamp'sis) [rachio- + G. *kampsis,* a bending]. Curvature of the spine. See kyphosis; lordosis; scoliosis.

rachiocentesis (rā-kē-ō-sen-tē'sis) [rachio- + G. *kentēsis,* puncture]. Lumbar *puncture.*

rachiochysis (rā-kē-ok'i-sis) [rachio- + G. *chysis,* a pouring out]. A subarachnoid effusion of fluid in the spinal canal.

rachiometer (rā-kē-om'ĕ-ter) [rachio- + G. *metron,* measure]. An instrument for measuring the curvature of the spine, natural or pathologic, of the spinal column.

rachiopagus (rā-kē-op'ă-gŭs) [rachio- + G. *pagos,* something fixed]. Rachipagus; conjoined twins united back to back as a result of fusion of their spinal column.

rachiopathy (rā-kē-op'ă-thē) [rachio- + G. *pathos,* suffering]. Spondylopathy.

rachioplegia (rā'kē-ō-plē'jē-ă) [rachio- + G. *plēgē,* stroke]. Spinal *paralysis.*

rachioscoliosis (rā-kē-ō-skō-lē-ō'sis). Scoliosis.

rachiotome (rā'kē-ō-tōm) [rachio- + G. *tomē,* incision]. Rachitome; a specially devised instrument for dividing the laminae of the vertebrae.

rachiotomy (rā-kē-ot'ō-mē) [rachio- + G. *tomē,* incision]. Laminectomy.

rachipagus (rā-kip'ă-gŭs). Rachiopagus.

rachis, pl. rachides, rachises (rā'kis, rā'ki-dēz, rak-) [G. spine, backbone]. *Columna* vertebralis.

rachischisis (rā-kis'ki-sis) [G. *rhachis,* spine, + *schisis,* division]. Spondyloschisis.

r. partia'lis, merorachischisis.

posterior r., r. poste'rior, spondyloschisis of the entire vertebral column.

r. tota'lis, holorachischisis.

rachitic (ră-kit'ic). Rickety; relating to or suffering from rickets (rachitis).

rachitis (ră-kī'tis) [G. *rhachitis*]. Rickets.

r. feta'lis, r. intrauterina or uterina; congenital rickets.

r. feta'lis annula'ris, congenital enlargement of the epiphyses of the long bones.

r. feta'lis micromel'ica, a congenital condition in which develop-

ment of the long bones is deficient.
r. intrauteri'na, r. uteri'na, r. fetalis.
r. tar'da, adult *rickets*.

rachitism (rak'i-tizm). A rachitic state or tendency.

rachitogenic (ră-kit-ō-jen'ik) [rachitis + G. *genesis*, production]. Producing or causing rickets.

rachitome (rak'i-tōm). Rachiotome.

rachitomy (ră-kit'ŏ-mē). Laminectomy.

racoma (rā-kō'mă) [G. *rhakōma; rhakoō*, to tear in strips, fr. *rhakos*, a rag]. An excoriation.

rad 1. The unit for the dose absorbed from ionizing radiation, equivalent to 100 ergs per gram of tissue; 100 rad = 1 Gy. **2.** Symbol for radian.

radarkymography (rā'dar-kī-mog'ră-fē). Video tracking of heart motion by means of image intensification and closed circuit television during fluoroscopy; enables cardiac motion to be measured by reproducible linear graphic tracing.

radectomy (rā-dek'tō-mē) [L. *radix*, root, + G. *ektomē*, excision]. Root *amputation*.

Radford, Edward P., Jr., U.S. physiologist, *1922. See R. *nomogram*.

radiability (rā'dē-ă-bil'i-tē). The property of being radiable.

radiable (rā'dē-ă-bl). Capable of being penetrated or examined by rays, especially by x-rays.

radiad (rā'dē-ad). In a direction toward the radial side.

radial (rā'dē-ăl) [L. *radialis*, fr. *radius*, ray, lateral bone of the forearm]. **1.** Radialis; relating to the radius (bone of the forearm), to any structures named from it, or to the radial or lateral aspect of the upper limb as compared to the ulnar or medial aspect. **2.** Relating to any radius. **3.** Radiating; diverging in all directions from any given center.

radialis (rā-dē-ā'lis) [Mod. L.] [NA]. Radial(1).

radian (rad) (rā'dē-ăn) [L. *radius*, ray]. A supplementary SI unit of plane angle.

radiant (rā'dē-ant). **1.** Giving out rays. **2.** A point from which light radiates to the eye.

radiate (rā'dē-āt) [L. *radio*, pp. *-atus*, to shine]. **1.** To spread out in all directions from a center. **2.** To emit radiation.

radiatio, pl. **radiationes** (rā-dē-ā'shē-ō, -shē-ō'nēz) [L.]. Radiation (3); in neuroanatomy, a term applied to any one of the thalamocortical fiber systems that together compose the corona radiata of the cerebral hemisphere's white matter (*e.g.*, radiatio optica, acustica, etc.).
r. acus'tica [NA], acoustic radiation; the fibers that pass from the medial geniculate body to the transverse temporal gyri of the cerebral cortex by way of the sublentiform part of the internal capsule.
r. cor'poris callo'si [NA], radiation of the corpus callosum; the spreading out of the fibers of the corpus callosum in the centrum semiovale of each cerebral hemisphere.
r. op'tica [NA], optic or occipitothalamic radiation; geniculocalcarine radiation or tract; Gratiolet's radiation or fibers; Wernicke's radiation; the massive, fanlike fiber system passing from the lateral geniculate body of the thalamus to the visual cortex (striate or calcarine cortex, area 17 of Brodmann); the fibers follow the retrolenticular and sublenticular limbs of the internal capsule into the corona radiata but they curve back along the lateral wall of the temporal and occipital horns of the lateral ventricle to the striate cortex on the medial surface and pole of the occipital lobe.
r. pyramida'lis, pyramidal radiation; corticospinal fibers passing from the cortex into the pyramid.

radiation (rā'dē-ā'shŭn) [L. *radiatio*, fr. *radius*, ray, beam]. **1.** The act or condition of diverging in all directions from a center. **2.** The sending forth of light, short radio waves, ultraviolet or x-rays, or any other rays for treatment or diagnosis or for other purpose. *Cf.* irradiation (2). **3.** Radiatio. **4.** A ray. **5.** Radiant energy or a radiant beam.

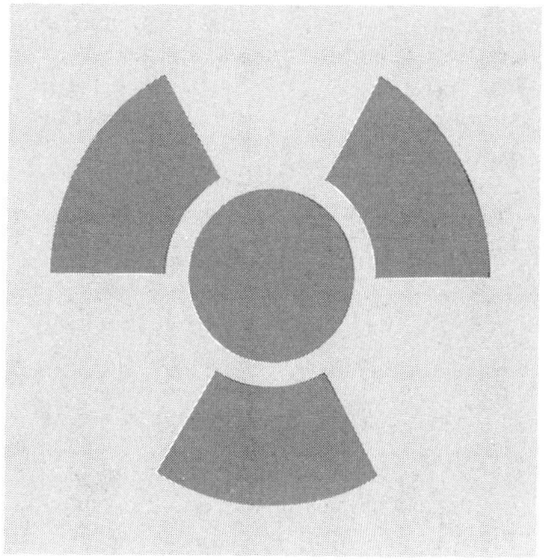

Symbol for Radiation
Purple figure on yellow background.

acoustic r., *radiatio* acustica.
annihilation r., when a positron from beta positive decay encounters an electron, they may annihilate each other and convert their energy, principally rest mass ($2M_eC^2$), into two antiparallel 0.51-MeV gamma rays.
background r., irradiation from environmental sources such as building materials, cosmic rays, etc.
beta r., radiant energy from a source of beta rays.
Cerenkov r., light given off by a high energy particle speeding through a transparent medium at a velocity greater than that of light in that medium.
r. of corpus callosum, *radiatio* corporis callosi.
corpuscular r., r. consisting of streams of subatomic particles such as protons, electrons, neutrons, etc.
electromagnetic r., r. originating in a varying electromagnetic field; *e.g.*, long and short radio waves; light, visible and invisible; x-radiation and gamma rays; cosmic rays.
geniculocalcarine r., *radiatio* optica.
Gratiolet's r., *radiatio* optica.
heterogeneous r., r. consisting of different frequencies, various energies, or a variety of particles.
homogeneous r., r. consisting of a narrow band of frequencies, the same energy, or a single type of particle.
ionizing r., corpuscular (*e.g.*, neutrons, electrons) or electromagnetic (*e.g.*, gamma) r. of sufficient energy to ionize the irradiated material.
K-r., usually a very penetrating form of x-r. excited by cathode rays (high speed electrons) impinging upon a metal anode such as tungsten; the energy of the r. is a function of the binding energy of the K-shell electrons of the metal anode.
L-r., an x-r. of slight penetrating power excited by cathode rays (high speed electrons) impinging on a metal anode; the energy of the r. is a function of the binding energy of the L-shell electrons of the metal anode.
occipitothalamic r., *radiatio* optica.
optic r., *radiatio* optica.
pyramidal r., *radiatio* pyramidalis.
scattered r., r. that during its passage through a substance has been deviated in direction, sometimes with an energy loss.
Wernicke's r., *radiatio* optica.

radical (rad'i-kăl) [L. *radix* (*radic-*), root]. **1.** In chemistry, a group of elements or atoms usually passing intact from one compound to another, but usually incapable of prolonged existence in a free state (*e.g.*, methyl, CH_3); in chemical formulas, a r. is often distinguished by being enclosed in parentheses or brackets. **2.** Thorough or extensive; relating or directed to the extirpation of the root or cause of a morbid process; *e.g.*, a r. operation. **3.** Denoting treatment by extreme, drastic, or innovative measures, as opposed to conservative.

acid r., a r. formed from an acid by loss of one or more hydrogen ions; *e.g.*, SO_4^-, NO_3^-.

color r., chromophore.

free r., a radical in its (usually transient) uncombined state; an atom or atom group carrying an unpaired elec- tron and no charge; *e.g.*, hydroxyl (·Ö:H) and methyl

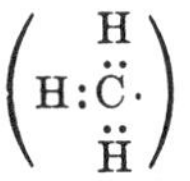

Free r.'s may be involved as short-lived, highly active intermediates in various reactions in living tissue, notably in photosynthesis.

radices (rā-dī'sēz). Plural of radix.

radicle (rad'i-kl) [L. *radicula,* dim. of *radix,* root]. A rootlet or structure resembling one, as the *r.* of a *vein,* a minute veinlet joining with others to form a vein, or the *r.* of a *nerve,* a nerve fiber which joins others to form a nerve.

radicotomy (rad-i-kot'ō-mē) [L. *radix* (*radic-*), root, + G. *tomē,* incision]. Rhizotomy.

radicul-. See radiculo-.

radicula (ră-dik'yū-lă) [L. dim of *radix,* root]. A spinal nerve root.

radiculalgia (ra-dik'yū-lal'jē-ă) [radicul- + G. *algos,* pain]. Neuralgia due to irritation of the sensory root of a spinal nerve.

radicular (ra-dik'yū-lăr). **1.** Relating to a radicle. **2.** Pertaining to the root of a tooth.

radiculectomy (ra-dik'yū-lek'tō-mē) [radicul- + G. *ektomē,* excision]. Rhizotomy.

radiculitis (ra-dik-yū-lī'tis) [radicul- + G. *-itis,* inflammation]. Inflammation of the intradural portion of a spinal nerve root prior to its entrance into the intervertebral foramen or of the portion between that foramen and the nerve plexus.

acute brachial r., brachial plexus *neuropathy.*

radiculo-, radicul- [L. *radicula,* radicle, dim. of *radix,* root]. Combining forms denoting radicle, radicular.

radiculoganglionitis (ra-dik'yū-lō-gang'glē-ō-nī'tis). Acute idiopathic *polyneuritis.*

radiculomeningomyelitis (ra-dik'yū-lō-mĕ-ning'gō-mī-ĕ-lī'tis). Rhizomeningomyelitis.

radiculomyelopathy (ra-dik'yū-lō-mī'ĕ-lop'ă-thē). Myeloradiculopathy.

radiculoneuropathy (ra-dik'yū-lō-nū-rop'ă-thē). Disease of the spinal nerve roots and nerves.

radiculopathy (ra-dik'yū-lop'ă-thē) [radiculo- + G. *pathos,* suffering]. Disease of the spinal nerve roots.

radiectomy (rā-dē-ek'tō-mē) [L. *radix,* root, + G. *ektomē,* excision]. Root *amputation.*

radiferous (rā-dif'er-ŭs). Containing radium.

radii (rā'dē-ī) [L.]. Plural of radius.

radio- [L. *radius,* ray]. Combining form denoting: **1.** Radiation, chiefly (in medicine) x-ray. **2.** The radioactive isotope of the element to which it is prefixed. **3.** Radius.

radioactive (rā'dē-ō-ak'tiv). Possessing radioactivity.

radioactive cow. Colloquialism for radionuclide *generator.* See also cow.

radioactivity (rā'dē-ō-ak-tiv'i-tē). The property of some atomic nuclei of spontaneously emitting gamma rays or subatomic particles (alpha and beta rays).

artificial r., induced r.; the r. of isotopes that exist only because man-made through the bombardment of naturally occurring isotopes by subatomic particles, or high levels of x- or gamma radiation.

induced r., artificial r.

radioanaphylaxis (rā'dē-ō-an'ă-fī-lak'sis). Sensitivity to radiant energy.

radioautogram (rā'dē-ō-aw'tō-gram). Obsolete term for autoradiograph.

radioautography (rā'dē-ō-aw-tog'ră-fē). Autoradiography.

radiobicipital (rā'dē-ō-bī-sip'i-tăl). Relating to the radius and the biceps muscle.

radiobiology (rā'dē-ō-bī-ol'ō-jē). The biologic study of the effects of ionizing radiation upon living tissue. Cf. radiopathology.

radiocalcium (rā'dē-ō-kal'sē-ŭm). A radioisotope of calcium, particularly calcium-45.

radiocarbon (rā'dē-ō-kar'bŏn). A radioactive isotope of carbon; *e.g.*, ^{14}C.

radiocardiogram (rā'dē-ō-kar'dē-ō-gram). A graphic record of the concentration of injected radioisotope within the cardiac chambers.

radiocardiography (rā'dē-ō-kar-dē-og'ră-fē). The technique of recording or interpreting radiocardiograms.

radiocarpal (rā'dē-ō-kar'păl). Cubitocarpal. **1.** Relating to the radius and the bones of the carpus. **2.** On the radial or lateral side of the carpus.

radiochemistry (rā'dē-ō-kem'is-trē). The science that uses radionuclides and their properties to study chemical applications and problems.

radiochlorine (rā'dē-ō-klōr'ēn). A radioactive isotope of chlorine, *e.g.*, ^{36}Cl.

radiocinematography (rā'dē-ō-sĭ-nē-mă-tog'ră-fē) [radio- + G. *kinēma,* motion, + *graphō,* to write]. Taking a motion picture of the movements of organs or other structures as revealed by an x-ray examination.

radiocobalt (rā'dē-ō-kō'balt). A radioactive isotope of cobalt; *e.g.*, ^{60}Co.

radiocurable (rā'dē-ō-kyūr'ă-bl). Curable by irradiation therapy.

radiode (rā'dē-ōd) [radium + G. *hodos,* way]. A metal container for radium.

radiodense (rā'dē-ō-dens). Radiopaque.

radiodensity (rā'dē-ō-den'si-tē). Radiopacity.

radiodermatitis (rā'dē-ō-der-mă-tī'tis). Dermatitis due to exposure to x-rays or gamma rays (ionizing radiation).

radiodiagnosis (rā'dē-ō-dī-ag-nō'sis). Diagnosis by means of x-rays.

radiodigital (rā'dē-ō-dij'i-tăl). Relating to the fingers on the radial or lateral side of the hand.

radioelectrophysiologram (ra'dē-ō-e-lek'trō-fiz-ē-ol'ō-gram). The record obtained by means of the radioelectrophysiolograph.

radioelectrophysiolograph (rā'dē-ō-ē-lek'trō-fiz-ē-ol'ō-graf). Formerly, an apparatus carried by a mobile individual by means of which changes in electrical potential from the brain or heart can be picked up and radio-transmitted to an electroencephalograph or an electrocardiograph. See telemeter.

radioelectrophysiolography (rā'dē-ō-ē-lek'trō-fiz'ē-ō-log'ră-fē). Formerly, recording the changes in the electrical potential of the brain or heart by means of the radioelectrophysiolograph. See telemetry.

radioelement (rā'dē-ō-el'ĕ-ment). Any element possessing radioactivity.

radioepidermitis (rā'dē-ō-ep'i-der-mī'tis). Destructive changes in the epidermis produced by ionizing radiation.

radioepithelitis (rā'dē-ō-ep'i-thē-lī'tis). Destructive changes in epithelium produced by ionizing radiation.

radiofrequency (rā'dē-o-frē'kwen-sē). Radiant energy of a certain frequency range; *e.g.*, radio and television employ radiant energy having a frequency between 10^5 10^{11} Hz, while diagnostic x-rays have a frequency in the range of 3×10^{18} Hz.

radiogallium (rā'dē-ō-gal'ē-ŭm). Gallium that is radioactive. See gallium-67; gallium-68.

radiogenesis (rā'dē-ō-jen'ĕ-sis) [radio- + G. *genesis,* production]. The formation or production of radioactivity resulting from radioactive transformation or disintegration of radioactive substances.

radiogenic (rā'dē-ō-jen'ik). **1.** Producing rays of any sort, especially dynamic rays. **2.** Caused by x- or gamma rays.

radiogenics (rā'dē-ō-jen'iks). The science of radiation.

radiogold colloid (rā'dē-ō-gōld kol'oyd). ^{198}Au colloid; colloidal radioactive gold; a radioactive isotope of gold emitting negative beta particles and gamma radiation, with a half-life of 2.7 days; used for irradiation of closed serous cavities in the palliative treatment of ascites and pleural effusion due to metastatic malignancies, and for liver scans.

radiogram (rā'dē-ō-gram) [radio- + G. *gramma,* something written]. Obsolete term for roentgenogram.

radiograph (rā'dē-ō-graf) [radio- + G. *graphō,* to write]. Roentgenogram.

bitewing r., intraoral dental film adapted to show the coronal portion and cervical third of the root of the teeth in near occlusion; especially useful in detecting interproximal caries and determining alveolar septal height.

occlusal r., intraoral section film positioned on the occlusal plane and used in visualizing entire sections of the jaw; especially useful in exploring calcifications of the sublingual salivary glands.

periapical r., a r. demonstrating tooth apices and surrounding structures in a particular intraoral area.

radiography (rā'dē-og'ră-fē). Roentgenography; examination of any part of the body for diagnostic purposes by means of x-rays with the record of the findings usually impressed upon a photographic film.

electron r., a radiographic imaging process in which the incident x-radiation is converted to a latent charge image subsequently developed by a special printing process; it improves detail enhancement by the virtual absence of background fog and image noise.

magnification r., r. using microfocus devices and high-speed intensifying screen/film combinations to enlarge the image without loss of sharpness and resolution or an undesirable increase in radiation exposure caused by increasing the distance between the subject and the film.

radiohumeral (rā'dē-ō-hyū'mer-ăl). Relating to the radius and the humerus; denoting the articulation between them.

radioimmunity (rā'dē-ō-i-myū'ni-tē). Lessened sensitivity to radiation.

radioimmunoassay (rā'dē-ō-im'u-nō-as'sā). An immunological (immunochemical) procedure in which radioisotope-labeled antigen (hormone or other substance) is reacted with specific antiserum and an aliquant part of the same antiserum previously treated with test fluid; any specific hormone or other substance in the test fluid sample would have reacted with antibody and, accordingly, a greater quantity of free labeled antigen (hormone) in the test fluid, with reference to the specific antiserum, would be a measure of hormone in the test fluid sample.

radioimmunodiffusion (rā'dē-ō-im'yū-nō-di-fyū'zhŭn). A method for the study of antigen-antibody reactions by gel diffusion using radioisotope-labeled antigen or antibody.

radioimmunoelectrophoresis (rā'dē-ō-im'yū-nō-ē-lek'trō-fō-rē'sis). Immunoelectrophoresis in which the antigen or antibody is labeled with a radioisotope; *e.g.,* in testing for insulin-binding antibodies by treating the test serum with radioactive iodine-labeled insulin, subjecting the mixture (antigen) to electrophoresis, precipitating the separated immunoglobulins with immunoglobulin-specific antiserum, and, then, with radiosensitive film, testing for bound insulin in the precipitates.

radioimmunoprecipitation (rā'dē-ō-im'yū-nō-prē-sip-i-tā'shŭn). Immunoprecipitation utilizing a radioisotope-labeled antibody or antigen.

radioiodinated (rā'dē-ō-ī'ō-din-ā-ted). Treated or combined with radioiodine.

radioiodine (rā'dē-ō-i'ō-dīn). A radioactive isotope of iodine; *e.g.,* ^{123}I.

radioiron (rā'dē-ō-ī'ern). A radioactive isotope of iron; *e.g.,* ^{59}Fe.

radioisotope (rā'dē-ō-ī'sō-tōp). An isotope that changes to a more stable state by emitting radiation.

radiolabeled (rā'dē-ō-lā'bld). See tag.

radiolead (rā'dē-ō-led'). Radioactive lead.

radiolesion (rā'dē-ō-lē'zhŭn). A lesion produced by ionizing radiation.

radioligand (rā'dē-ō-lig'and). A molecule with a radionuclide tracer attached; usually used for radioimmunoassay procedures.

radiologic, radiological (rā-dē-ō-log'ik, -loj'i-kăl). Pertaining to radiology.

radiologist (rā-dē-ol'ō-jist). A person skilled in the diagnostic and/or therapeutic use of x-rays and other forms of radiant energy.

radiology (rā-dē-ol'ō-jē) [radio- + G. *logos,* study]. The science of high energy radiation and of the sources and the chemical, physical, and biologic effects of such radiation; the term usually refers to the diagnosis and treatment of disease.

radiolucency (rā-dē-ō-lū'sen-sē). The state of being radiolucent.

radiolucent (rā-dē-ō-lū'sent) [radio- + L. *lucens,* shining]. Relatively penetrable by x-rays or other forms of radiation. *Cf.* radiopaque.

radiolus (rā-dē'ō-lŭs) [L. dim. of *radius,* spoke]. A probe or sound.

radiometer (rā-dē-om'ĕ-ter) [radio- + G. *metron,* measure]. Roentgenometer; a device for determining the penetrative power of x-rays.

pastil r., see Sabouraud's pastiles under *pastil.*

radiomicrometer (rā'dē-ō-mī-krom'ĕ-ter). A sensitive thermopile designed for the measurement of minute changes in radiant energy.

radiomimetic (rā'dē-ō-mi-met'ik) [radio- + G. *mimētikos,* imitative]. Imitating the action of radiation, as in the case of chemicals such as nitrogen mustards.

radiomuscular (rā'dē-ō-mŭs'kyū-lăr). Relating to the radius and the neighboring muscles; denoting certain nerves and muscular branches of the radial artery.

radionecrosis (rā'dē-ō-ne-krō'sis). Necrosis due to radiation; *e.g.,* after excessive exposure to x- or gamma rays. See radiation *burn.*

radioneuritis (rā'dē-ō-nū-rī'tis). Neuritis caused by prolonged or repeated exposure to x-rays or radium.

radionitrogen (rā'dē-ō-nī'trō-jen). A radioactive isotope of nitrogen; *e.g.,* ^{13}N.

radionuclide (rā'dē-ō-nū'klīd). A nuclide of artificial or natural origin that exhibits radioactivity.

radiopacity (rā'dē-ō-pas'i-tē). Radiodensity; state of being radiopaque.

radiopalmar (rā'dē-ō-pal'măr). Relating to the radial or lateral side of the palm.

radiopaque (rā-dē-ō-pāk') [radio- + Fr. opaque fr. L. *opacus*, shady]. Radiodense; exhibiting relative opacity to, or impenetrability by, x-rays or any other form of radiation. *Cf.* radiolucent.

radiopathology (rā'dē-ō-path-ol'ō-jē). A branch of radiology or pathology concerned with the effects of radioactive substances on cells and tissues. *Cf.* radiobiology.

radiopelvimetry (rā'dē-ō-pel-vim'ĕ-trē). Measurement of the pelvis by means of roentgen rays.

radiopharmaceuticals (rā'dē-ō-far-mă-sū'ti-kalz). Radioactive chemical or pharmaceutical preparations, used as diagnostic or therapeutic agents.

radiophobia (rā'dē-ō-fō'bē-ă) [radio- + G. *phobos*, fear]. Morbid fear of radiation, as from x-rays or nuclear energy.

radiophosphorus (rā'dē-ō-fos'fōr-ŭs). A radioactive isotope of phosphorus; *e.g.*, ^{32}P.

radiophylaxis (rā'dē-ō-fī-lak'sis) [radio- + G. *phylaxis*, protection]. The lessened effect of radiation after a previous small dose of radiation.

radiopill (rā'dē-ō-pil). Radiotelemetering *capsule*.

radiopotassium (rā'dē-ō-pō-tas'ē-ŭm). A radioactive isotope of potassium; *e.g.*, ^{40}K.

radiopraxis (rā'dē-ō-prak'sis) [radio- + G. *praxis*, a doing]. The use of light rays, x-rays, or radium in diagnosis or treatment.

radioreaction (rā'dē-ō-rē-ak'shŭn). A reaction of the body to radiation.

radioreceptor (rā'dē-ō-rē-sep'ter). A receptor that normally responds to radiant energy such as light or heat.

radioresistant (rā'dē-ō-rē-zis'tant). Indicating cells or tissues that are not destroyed by exposure to irradiation in the usual dosage range.

radioscopy (ra'dē-os'kō-pē) [radio- + G. *skopeō*, to view]. Archaic term for fluoroscopy.

radiosensitive (rā'dē-ō-sen'si-tiv). Readily affected by radiation.

radiosensitivity (rā'dē-ō-sen-si-tiv'i-tē). The condition of being readily acted upon by radiant energy.

radiosodium (rā'dē-ō-sō'dē-ŭm). A radioactive isotope of sodium; *e.g.*, ^{24}Na.

radiostereoscopy (rā'dē-ō-ster-ē-os'kŏ-pē) [radio- + G. *stereos*, solid, + *skopeō*, to view]. Inspection of two roentgenograms, taken at slightly different angles, with a device such that one roentgenogram is seen by the left eye, the other by the right eye, thus allowing a three-dimensional steroscopic x-ray visualization of the examination object to determine its position relative to (in front of or behind) another object.

radiostrontium (rā'dē-ō-stron'tē-ŭm). A radioactive isotope of strontium; *e.g.*, ^{90}Sr.

radiosulfur (rā'dē-ō-sŭl'fŭr). A radioactive isotope of sulfur; *e.g.*, ^{35}S.

radiotelemetry (rā'dē-ō-tē-lem'ĕ-trē). See telemetry; biotelemetry.

radiotherapeutic (rā'dē-ō-thār-ă-pyū'tik). Relating to radiotherapy or to radiotherapeutics.

radiotherapeutics (rā'dē-ō-thār-ă-pyū'tiks). The study and use of radiotherapeutic agents.

radiotherapist (rā'dē-ō-thār'ă-pist). One who practices radiotherapy or is versed in radiotherapeutics.

radiotherapy (rā'dē-ō-thār'ă-pē). The medical specialty concerned with the use of electromagnetic or particulate radiations in the treatment of disease.
mantle r., r. with protection of uninvolved radiosensitive structures or organs.

radiothermy (rā'dē-ō-ther'mē) [radio- + G. *thermē*, heat]. Diathermy effected by heat from radiant sources.

radiothyroidectomy (rā'dē-ō-thī'roy-dek-tō-mē). The destruction of thyroid tissue by administration of radioactive iodine.

radiothyroxin (rā'dē-ō-thī-rok'sin). Radioactive *thyroxin*.

radiotoxemia (rā'dē-ō-tok-sē'mē-ă) [radio- + G. *toxikon*, poison, + *haima*, blood]. Radiation sickness caused by the products of disintegration produced by the action of x-rays or other forms of radioactivity and by the depletion of certain cells and enzyme systems from the organism.

radiotransparent (rā'dē-ō-trans-par'ent). Allowing relatively free transmission of radiant energy.

radiotropic (rā'dē-ō-trop'ik) [radio- + G. *tropē*, a turning]. Affected by radiation.

radioulnar (rā'dē-ō-ŭl'năr). Relating to both radius and ulna.

radisectomy (rā-dē-sek'tō-mē) [L. *radix*, root, + G. *ektomē*, excision]. Root *amputation*.

radium (rā'dē-ŭm) [L. *radius*, ray]. A metallic element, symbol Ra, atomic no. 88, atomic weight 226.05, extracted in very minute quantities from pitchblende; **radium-226**, its longest lived isotope, is produced as an intermediate in the uranium series, being formed by the emission of an alpha particle by thorium-230 (ionium); radium emits alpha particles itself, breaking down to radon-222 with a half-life of 1,620 years; chemically, it is an alkaline earth metal with properties similar to those of barium. Its therapeutic action is similar to that of x-rays and is applied in the form of one of its salts, (*e.g.*, bromide, carbonate, chloride, or sulfate); improper use may lead to unwanted tissue destruction or malignant neoplasm.

radius, gen. and pl. **radii** (rā'dē-ŭs, rā'dē-ī) [L. spoke of a wheel, rod, ray]. **1.** A straight line passing from the center to the periphery of a circle. **2** [NA]. The lateral and shorter of the two bones of the forearm.
r. fix'us, a line passing from the hormion to the inion.
ra'dii len'tis [NA], lens sutures; lens stars (1); 9 to 12 faint lines on the anterior and posterior surfaces of the lens that radiate from the poles toward the equator; they mark the lines along which the ends of lens fibers abut.

radix, gen. **radicis**, pl. **radices** (rā'diks, rā-di'sis, rā'di-sēz or rā-dī'sēz) [L.] [NA]. Root (1); the primary or beginning portion of any part, as of a nerve at its origin from the brainstem or spinal cord.
r. ante'rior [NA], r. ventralis.
r. ar'cus ver'tebrae, *pediculus* arcus vertebrae.
r. bre'vis gan'glii cilia'ris, r. oculomotoria ganglii ciliaris.
r. clin'ica [NA], clinical root; that portion of a tooth embedded in the investing structures; the portion of a tooth not visible in the oral cavity.
r. cochlea'ris [NA], cochlear or inferior root of vestibulocochlear nerve; r. inferior nervi vestibulocochlearis; one of the components of nervus vestibulocochlearis; it is made up of the central processes of the bipolar neurons which compose the ganglion cochleare (Corti's ganglion) in the canalis spiralis modioli of the bony cochlea; the r. cochlearis enters the cranial cavity by passing in fascicles through the tractus spiralis foraminosus at the bottom of the internal auditory meatus; it enters the brainstem through the pontomedullary groove, closely adhering to the caudoventral aspect of the r. vestibularis, and distributes its fibers to the ventral and dorsal cochlear nuclei in the floor of the lateral recess of the fourth ventricle. See also *nervus* cochlearis.
ra'dices crania'les [NA], cranial roots; pars vagalis; vagal part of accessory nerve; the roots of the accessory nerve which arise from

the medulla.
r. den'tis [NA], root of a tooth; root (2); that part of a tooth below the neck, covered by cementum rather than enamel, and attached by the periodontal ligament to the alveolar bone.
r. dorsa'lis [NA], dorsal root; r. posterior; posterior root; r. sensoria; the sensory root of a spinal nerve.
r. facia'lis [NA], *nervus* canalis pterygoidei.
r. infe'rior [NA], inferior root; **r. i. an'sae cervica'lis** [NA], inferior root of cervical loop; descendens cervicalis; fibers from the second and third cervical nerves that pass forward and downward along the internal jugular vein; they contribute to the ansa cervicalis and innervate the infrahyoid muscles; **r. i. ner'vi vestibulocochlea'ris** [NA], r. cochlearis.
r. latera'lis ner'vi media'ni [NA], lateral root of the median nerve; the part of the median nerve arising from the lateral cord of the brachial plexus.
r. latera'lis trac'tus op'tici [NA], lateral root of the optic tract; the larger division of the posterior end of the optic tract that terminates in the lateral geniculate body.
r. lin'guae [NA], root or base of tongue; the posterior attached portion of the tongue.
r. lon'ga gan'glii cilia'ris, r. nasociliaris.
r. media'lis ner'vi media'ni [NA], medial root of median nerve; the part of the median nerve coming from the medial cord of the brachial plexus.
r. media'lis trac'tus op'tici [NA], the smaller division of the posterior end of the optic tract that disappears under the medial geniculate body.
r. mesenter'ii [NA], root of mesentery; the origin of the mesentery of the small intestine (jejunum and ileum) from the posterior parietal peritoneum.
r. moto'ria [NA], r. ventralis.
r. moto'ria ner'vi trigem'ini [NA], motor root of trigeminal nerve; portio minor nervi trigemini; masticator nerve; the smaller root of the trigeminal nerve, composed of fibers originating from the trigeminal motor nucleus and emerging from the pons medial to the much larger sensory root, to join the mandibular nerve; it carries motor and proprioceptive fibers to the muscles of mastication.
r. na'si [NA], root of nose; the upper portion of the external nose situated between the two orbits.
r. nasocilia'ris [NA], nasociliary root; sensory or long root of ciliary ganglion; r. longa ganglii ciliaris; ramus communicans cum ganglio ciliari; sensory fibers passing from the eyeball through the ciliary ganglion to their cell bodies in the trigeminal ganglion.
r. ner'vi facia'lis, root of the facial nerve; fibers running from the facial motor nucleus upward to the colliculus facialis where they curve around the abducens nucleus and then pass peripherally between the superior olive and sensory nucleus of the trigeminal, to emerge as the facial nerve from the pontomedullary groove.
ra'dices ner'vi trigem'ini, roots of trigeminal nerve; collective term for the r. sensoria nervi trigemini and r. motoria nervi trigemini.
r. oculomoto'ria gan'glii cilia'ris [NA], motor root of ciliary ganglion; r. brevis ganglii ciliaris; r. parasympathica ganglii ciliaris; short or parasympathetic root of ciliary ganglion; a branch of the oculomotor nerve supplying parasympathetic preganglionic nerve fibers to the ciliary ganglion.
r. parasympath'ica gan'glii cilia'ris [NA], r. oculomotoria ganglii ciliaris.
r. pe'nis [NA], root of penis; the proximal attached part of the penis, including the two crura and the bulb.
r. pi'li, hair root; the part of a hair which is embedded in the hair follicle, its lower succulent extremity capping the dermal papilla in the deep bulbous portion of the follicle.
r. poste'rior [NA], r. dorsalis.
r. pulmo'nis [NA], root of lung; all the structures entering or leaving the lung at the hilum, forming a pedicle invested with the pleura.
r. senso'ria [NA], r. dorsalis.
r. senso'ria ner'vi trigem'ini [NA], sensory root of trigeminal nerve; portio major nervi trigemini; the large sensory root of the trigeminal (or fifth cranial) nerve, extending from the semilunar ganglion of Gasser into the pons through the middle cerebellar peduncle or brachium pontis, immediately lateral to the small r. motoria or portio minor.
ra'dices spina'les [NA], spinal roots; the roots of the accessory nerve which arise from the ventrolateral part of the first five segments of the spinal cord.
r. supe'rior [NA], superior root; **r. s. an'sae cervica'lis** [NA], superior root of cervical loop; descendens hypoglossi; the fibers that arise from the first and second cervical nerves, accompany the hypoglossal nerve, then branch off to meet the inferior root in the ansa cervicalis; they innervate the infrahyoid muscles; **r. s. ner'vi vestibulocochlea'ris** [NA], r. vestibularis.
r. sympath'ica gan'glii cilia'ris [NA], sympathetic root of ciliary ganglion; postganglionic fibers from the carotid plexus passing through the ciliary ganglion without synapse to the eyeball.
r. un'guis [NA], root of nail; the proximal end of the nail, concealed under a fold of skin.
r. ventra'lis [NA], ventral root; r. anterior; anterior root; r. motoria; the motor root of a spinal nerve.
r. vestibula'ris [NA], vestibular or superior root of the vestibulocochlear nerve; r. superior nervi vestibulocochlearis; one of the components of nervus vestibulocochlearis; it is made up of the centrally directed axonal processes of the bipolar sensory neurons which compose the ganglion vestibulare (Scarpa's ganglion), located in the vestibule of the bony labyrinth; the r. vestibularis gains access to the cranial cavity by passing in fascicles through the vestibular areas and the foramen singulare at the bottom of the bony internal auditory meatus; continuing medially it enters the brainstem in the lateral extreme of the pontomedullary groove (cerebellopontine angle); root fibers passing dorsomedially between the pedunculus cerebellaris caudalis (inferior) and the tractus spinalis nervi trigemini are distributed to the nuclei vestibulares and to the flocculus, nodulus, and parts of the uvula of the cerebellum. See also *nervus* vestibularis.

radon (rā'don). A radioactive element, symbol Rn, atomic no. 86, atomic weight 222, resulting from the breakdown of radium; of the isotopes with mass numbers between 209 and 222, only the last is medically significant as an alpha-emitter with a half-life of 3.825 days.

Raeder, Georg Johan, Norwegian ophthalmologist, 1889–1956. See R.'s paratrigeminal *syndrome*.

raffinose (raf'i-nōs). Melitose; melitriose; gossypose; a dextrorotatory trisaccharide, occurring in cotton seed and in the molasses of beet root, composed of D-galactose, D-glucose, and D-fructose and formed by transfer of galactose from UDP-galactose to sucrose.

rage (rāj). Violent anger; a total discharge of the sympathetic portion of the autonomic nervous system.
sham r., a quasi-emotional state, characterized by manifestations of fear and anger upon trifling provocation; produced in animals by the removal of the cerebral cortex (decortication).

Rahn, Hermann, U.S. respiratory physiologist, *1912. See R.-Otis *sample*.

Raillietina (rī-li-ĕ-tē'nă). A genus of tapeworms (family Davaineidae, order Cyclophyllidea), three species of which, *R. madagascariensis* or *R. demerariensis, R. asiatica,* and *R. formsana,* have been found in man. However, the identification of many of these worms found in man has been questioned.

raillietiniasis (rī'li-ĕ-ti-nī'ă-sis). Infection of rodents and monkeys, and occasionally man, with tapeworms of the genus *Raillietina*.

Rainey, George, British anatomist, 1801–1884. See R.'s *corpuscles*.

rale (rahl) [Fr. rattle]. Ambiguous term for an added sound heard on auscultation of breath sounds; used by some to denote rhonchus and by others for crepitation.

amphoric r., sound heard through the stethoscope associated with the movement of fluid in a lung cavity communicating with a bronchus.

atelectatic r., transitory light crackling sound that disappears after deep breathing or coughing.

bubbling r., moist sound heard through the stethoscope as a result of air entering portions of lung tissue containing exudate and thus creating bubbles; sometimes associated with resolving pneumonia or small lung cavities.

cavernous r., cavernous rhoncus; a resonating bubbling sound caused by air entering a cavity partly filled with fluid.

clicking r., short sticking sound usually associated with opening of small bronchi on deep breathing, sometimes heard in early pulmonary tuberculosis.

consonating r., a resonant r. produced in a bronchial tube and heard through consolidated lung tissue.

crepitant r., vesicular r.; a fine bubbling or crackling sound produced by air mixing with very thin secretions in the smaller bronchial tubes.

dry r., a harsh or musical breath sound produced by a constriction in a bronchial tube or the presence of a viscid secretion narrowing the lumen.

gurgling r., coarse sound heard over large cavities or over trachea nearly filled with secretions.

guttural r., sound heard over the lung but resulting from upper airway obstruction.

metallic r., a r. of metallic quality caused by resonance in a large cavity.

moist r., a bubbling r. caused by air mixing with a fluid exudate in the bronchial tubes or a cavity.

mucous r., a bubbling r. heard on auscultation over bronchial tubes containing mucus.

palpable r., a vibration which can be felt accompanying a low-pitched, hard, musical, or sonorous r.

sibilant r., whistling r.; a whistling sound caused by air moving through a viscid secretion narrowing the lumen of a bronchus.

Skoda's r., a r. in a bronchus heard through an area of consolidated tissue in pneumonia.

sonorous r., a cooing or snoring sound often produced by the vibration of a projecting mass of viscid secretion in a large bronchus.

subcrepitant r., a very fine crepitant r.

vesicular r., crepitant r.

whistling r., sibilant r.

ram [A.S.]. A male sheep of breeding age.

ramal (rā'măl). Relating to a ramus.

Raman, Sir C.V., Indian physicist and Nobel laureate, *1888. See R. *effect, spectrum.*

Rambourg's stains. See under stain.

ramex (rā'meks) [L. hernia; pl. blood vessels of the lungs, fr. *ramus,* a branch]. Hernia, varicocele, or any scrotal tumor.

rami (rā'mī) [L.]. Plural of ramus.

Ramibacterium (rā'mī-bak-tēr'ē-ŭm) [L. *ramus,* branch, + bacterium]. An obsolete genus of bacteria, the type species of which, *R. ramosum,* is presently placed in the genus *Clostridium.*

R. ramo'sum, *Clostridium ramosum.*

ramicotomy (ram-i-kot'ō-mē) [L. *ramus,* branch, + G. *tomē,* incision]. Ramisection.

ramification (ram'i-fi-kā'shŭn). The process of dividing into a branchlike pattern.

ramify (ram'i-fī) [L. *ramus,* branch, + *facio,* to make]. To split into a branchlike pattern.

ramisection (ram-i-sek'shŭn) [L. *ramus,* branch, + L. *sectio,* section]. Ramicotomy; section of the rami communicantes of the sympathetic nervous system.

ramitis (ram-ī'tis) [L. *ramus,* branch, + G. *-itis,* inflammation]. Inflammation of a ramus.

Ramón y Cajal. See Cajal.

ramose, ramous (rā'mōs, rā'mŭs) [L. *ramosus,* fr. *ramus,* a branch]. Branching.

ramp. In electrical recording, a uniformly rising voltage or current. If reset to zero at regular intervals, it forms a sawtooth pattern used to provide the time sweep of a cathode ray oscilloscope beam; if reset to zero by a periodic event (*e.g.,* heart beats), the recorded height of the r.'s represents time between events.

Ramsay Hunt. See Hunt, James Ramsay.

Ramsden, Jesse, British optician, 1735–1800. See R.'s *ocular.*

Ramstedt, Conrad, German surgeon, 1867–1963. See R. *operation;* Fredet-R. *operation.*

ramulus, pl. ramuli (ram'yū-lŭs, -lī) [L. dim. of *ramus,* a branch]. A small branch or twig; one of the terminal divisions of a ramus.

RAMUS

ramus, pl. rami (rā'mŭs, rā'mī) [L.] [NA]. **1.** A branch. **2.** One of the primary divisions of a nerve or blood vessel. Arterial and nerve branches are also given under the major nerve or artery. See arteria and nervus. **3.** A part of an irregularly shaped bone (less slender than a "process") which forms an angle with the main body (*e.g.,* ramus of mandible). **4.** One of the primary divisions of a cerebral sulcus.

r. acetabula'ris [NA], acetabular branch; arteria acetabuli; acetabular artery; an arterial branch that supplies the acetabulum; two arteries, the obturator and the medial femoral circumflex, have such branches.

r. acromia'lis arte'riae thoracoacromia'lis [NA], acromial artery; acromial branch; a branch of the thoracoacromial artery that runs over the coracoid process and under the deltoid muscle.

ra'mi ad pon'tem [NA], branches to the pons; official alternate term for *arteriae* pontis.

ra'mi alveola'res superio'res anterio'res [NA], anterior superior alveolar branches; branches of the superior alveolar nerve that supply the incisors, canines, premolars, and first molar by their contributions to the superior dental plexus.

ra'mi alveola'res superio'res posterio'res [NA], posterior superior alveolar branches; branches of the superior alveolar nerves that supply the maxillary sinus and the molar tooth.

r. alveola'ris supe'rior me'dius [NA], middle superior alveolar branch; a branch of the superior alveolar nerve that contributes to the superior dental plexus.

r. anastomot'icus, anastomotic branch; a blood vessel that interconnects two neighboring vessels. It should not be used for the nervous system, because there is no analogy between a vascular anastomosing branch and a connection between nerves or their subdivisions. See also rami communicantes.

r. anastomot'icus cum lacrima'li [NA], r. orbitalis.

r. ante'rior [NA], anterior branch; each of the following structures has a branch so named: 1) great auricular nerve; 2) lateral cerebral sulcus; 3) left and right superior pulmonary veins; 4) medial cutaneous nerve of the forearm; 5) obturator artery; 6) obturator nerve; 7) renal artery; 8) right branch of portal vein; 9) right hepatic duct; 10) superior thyroid artery; 11) ulnar recurrent artery.

r. ante'rior ascen'dens [NA], ascending anterior branch; each of the following has a branch so named: 1) left pulmonary artery; 2) right pulmonary artery.
r. ante'rior descen'dens [NA], descending anterior branch; each of the following structures has a branch so named: 1) right pulmonary artery; 2) left pulmonary artery.
r. ante'rior latera'lis, lateral anterior branch; the former name for the ascending anterior branch of the left pulmonary artery.
r. apica'lis [NA], apical branch; each of the following has a branch so named; 1) r. superior (2); left and right inferior pulmonary veins; 2) left and right pulmonary arteries; 3) left superior pulmonary vein.
r. apica'lis lo'bi inferio'ris [NA], r. superior lobi inferioris.
r. apicoposte'rior [NA], apicoposterior branch of left superior pulmonary vein.
ra'mi articula'res [NA], articular branches of descending genicular artery.
r. ascen'dens [NA], ascending branch; each of the following has a branch so named: 1) deep circumflex iliac artery; 2) lateral cerebral sulcus; 3) lateral circumflex femoral artery.
ra'mi atria'les [NA], atrial branches; branches of the right coronary artery and the circumflex branch of the left coronary artery distributed to the right and left atrium, respectively.
ra'mi atrioventricula'res [NA], atrioventricular branches; nodal branches; the small arteries supplying the atrioventricular node; they usually arise from the right coronary artery where it turns to run in the posterior interventricular sulcus.
ra'mi auricula'res anterio'res [NA], anterior auricular branches of superficial temporal artery.
r. auricula'ris arte'riae occipita'lis [NA], auricular branch of occipital artery.
r. auricula'ris va'gi [NA], auricular r. of the vagus; Arnold's nerve; a branch of the superior ganglion of the vagus, supplying the back of the pinna and the external acoustic meatus.
r. basa'lis ante'rior [NA], anterior basal branch; each of the following has a branch so named: 1) left and right pulmonary arteries; 2) left and right inferior pulmonary veins.
r. basa'lis latera'lis [NA], lateral basal branch of the following: 1) basal part of right pulmonary artery; 2) basal part of left pulmonary artery.
r. basa'lis media'lis [NA], medial basal branch of r. cardiacus; a branch of the following: 1) basal part of left pulmonary artery; 2) basal part of right pulmonary artery.
r. basa'lis poste'rior [NA], posterior basal branch of the following: 1) basal part of left pulmonary artery; 2) basal part of right pulmonary artery.
ra'mi bronchia'les [NA], bronchial branches or arteries; vessels or nerves distributed to the bronchi; the following have branches so named: 1) thoracic aorta; 2) internal thoracic artery; 3) vagus nerves.
ra'mi bronchia'les segmento'rum [NA], branches of segmental bronchi.
ra'mi bucca'les [NA], buccal branches of facial nerves.
ra'mi calca'nei [NA], calcaneal branches or arteries; branches to the structures in the calcaneal region from 1) the posterior tibial artery and 2) the peroneal artery.
ra'mi calca'nei latera'les [NA], lateral calcaneal branches of sural nerve.
ra'mi calca'nei media'les [NA], medial calcaneal branches of tibial nerve.
r. calcari'nus [NA], calcarine branch; arteria calcarina; calcarine artery; a branch of the medial occipital artery that runs along the calcarine fissure.
ra'mi cap'sulae inter'nae [NA], internal capsular branches; branches of the anterior choroid artery to the internal capsule.
ra'mi capsula'res [NA], capsular branches of renal artery.
ra'mi cardi'aci cervica'les inferio'res [NA], inferior cervical cardiac branches of vagus nerve.
ra'mi cardi'aci cervica'les superio'res [NA], superior cervical cardiac branches of vagus nerve.
ra'mi cardi'aci thora'cici [NA], thoracic cardiac branches of vagus nerve.
r. cardi'acus, r. basalis medialis.
ra'mi caroticotympan'ici, *arteriae* caroticotympanici.
r. carpa'lis dorsa'lis arte'riae radia'lis [NA], r. carpeus dorsalis arteriae radialis.
r. carpa'lis dorsa'lis arte'riae ulna'ris [NA], r. carpeus dorsalis arteriae ulnaris.
r. carpa'lis palma'ris arte'riae radia'lis [NA], r. carpeus palmaris arteriae radialis.
r. carpa'lis palma'ris arte'riae ulna'ris [NA], r. carpeus palmaris arteriae ulnaris.
r. car'peus dorsa'lis arte'riae radia'lis [NA], dorsal carpal branch of radial artery; r. carpalis dorsalis arteriae radialis; a branch that passes to the back of the carpus to join the dorsal carpal rete.
r. car'peus dorsa'lis arte'riae ulna'ris [NA], dorsal carpal branch of the ulnar artery; r. carpalis dorsalis arteriae ulnaris; a branch that passes to the dorsal side of the carpus to enter the dorsal carpal rete.
r. car'peus palma'ris arte'riae radia'lis [NA], palmar carpal branch of radial artery; r. carpalis palmaris arteriae radialis; a small artery that passes medially across the wrist to supply the carpal joints; it anastomoses with the anterior carpal branch of the ulnar artery.
r. car'peus palma'ris arte'riae ulna'ris [NA], palmar carpal branch of ulnar artery; r. carpalis palmaris arteriae ulnaris; a branch that supplies the carpal joints and communicates with the anterior carpal branch of the radial artery.
ra'mi cau'dae nu'clei cauda'ti [NA], branches to the tail of the caudate nucleus; **(1)** branches from either the anterior choroid or the posterior communicating artery, or both, to supply the tail of the caudate nucleus; **(2)** a branch from the middle cerebral artery to the tail of the caudate nucleus.
ra'mi cauda'ti [NA], caudate branches of transverse part of left branch of portal vein.
ra'mi celi'aci [NA], celiac branches of vagus nerve.
ra'mi centra'les anteromedia'les [NA], anteromedial central branches; branches of the anterior communicating artery which supply part of the hypothalamus.
r. chiasmat'icus [NA], chiasmatic branch; a branch of the middle cerebral artery to the optic chiasm.
ra'mi choroi'dei [NA], choroid branches; **r. c. posterio'res latera'les** [NA], lateral posterior choroid branches of posterior cerebral artery distributed to the choroid plexus of the lateral ventricle; **r. c. posterio'res media'les** [NA], medial posterior choroid branches of posterior cerebral artery distributed to the choroid plexus of the third ventricle; **r. c. ventric'uli latera'lis** [NA], lateral ventricle choroid branch of anterior choroid artery distributed to the plexus of the lateral ventricle; **r. c. ventric'uli ter'tii** [NA], third ventricle choroid branch of anterior choroid artery to the third ventricle; **r. c. ventric'uli quar'ti** [NA], fourth ventricle choroid branch of posterior inferior cerebellar artery.
r. cingula'ris [NA], cingular branch; a branch of the callosomarginal artery supplying the gyrus cinguli.
r. circumflex'us [NA], circumflex branch of left coronary artery.
r. circumflex'us fib'ulae [NA], circumflex fibular branch or artery; a branch of the posterior tibial artery which winds around the neck of the fibula and joins the anastomoses around the knee joint.
r. clavicula'ris [NA], clavicular branch of thoracoacromial artery.
r. cli'vi [NA], branch to the clivus; a branch of the cerebral part of the internal carotid artery supplying the clivus.
r. cochlea'ris [NA], cochlear branch of labyrinthine artery.
r. collatera'lis [NA], collateral branch of posterior intercostal

arteries.

r. col'li, [NA], cervical branch of facial nerve.

r. commu'nicans, pl. **ra'mi communican'tes** [NA], communicating branch; a bundle of nerve fibers passing from one nerve to join another (*e.g.,* white r. communicans from mixed spinal nerve to sympathetic paravertebral ganglion and gray r. communicans from paravertebral ganglion to peripheral nerve). The term "ramus communicans" is used to replace the inadequate "ramus anastomoticus" in the nervous system.

r. commu'nicans arte'riae perone'ae [NA], r. communicans arteriae fibularis; communicating branch of the peroneal (fibular) artery.

r. commu'nicans cum chor'da tym'pani [NA], communicating branch with tympanic chord; **(1)** a small branch of the lingual nerve which joins the chorda tympani; **(2)** a small branch from the otic ganglion to the chorda tympani.

r. commu'nicans cum gan'glio cilia'ri [NA], *radix* nasociliaris.

r. commu'nicans cum ner'vo auriculotempora'li [NA], communicating branch of otic ganglion with auriculotemporal nerve.

ra'mi communican'tes cum ner'vo facia'li [NA], communicating branches of mandibular nerve with facial nerve.

r. commu'nicans cum ner'vo glossopharyn'geo [NA], communicating branch with glossopharyngeal nerve; **(1)** Haller's ansa; a small branch from the digastric branch of the facial nerve to the glossopharyngeal nerve; **(2)** a small branch from the auricular branch of the vagus to the glossopharyngeal nerve.

ra'mi communican'tes cum ner'vo hypoglos'so [NA], communicating branches between mandibular nerve and hypoglossal nerve.

r. commu'nicans cum ner'vo laryn'geo inferio're [NA], communicating branch of internal branch of superior laryngeal nerve with inferior laryngeal nerve.

ra'mi communican'tes cum ner'vo lingua'li [NA], communicating branches between submandibular ganglion and lingual nerve.

r. commu'nicans cum ner'vo pterygoi'dei media'lis [NA], communicating branch between the medial pterygoid nerve and the otic ganglion.

r. commu'nicans cum ner'vo ulna'ri [NA], communicating branch of median nerve with ulnar nerve in the hand.

r. commu'nicans cum ner'vo zygomat'ico [NA], communicating branch of lacrimal nerve with zygomatic nerve.

r. commu'nicans cum plex'u tympan'ico [NA], communicating branch of facial nerve with tympanic plexus.

r. commu'nicans cum ra'mo auricula'ri ner'vi vaga'lis [NA], communicating branch of glossopharyngeal nerve with auricular branch of the vagus nerve.

r. commu'nicans cum ra'mo laryn'geo inter'no [NA], communicating branch of inferior laryngeal nerve with internal laryngeal branch of superior laryngeal nerve.

r. commu'nicans cum ra'mo menin'geo [NA], communicating branch of otic ganglion with meningeal branch of mandibular nerve.

r. commu'nicans fibula'ris, r. communicans peroneus.

ra'mi communican'tes nervo'rum spina'lium [NA], communicating branches of spinal nerves; small bundles of nerve fibers connecting spinal nerves with sympathetic ganglia; the fibers passing from the ganglion to the spinal nerve are nonmyelinated and are called gray rami communicantes, those passing in the reverse direction are myelinated and are called white rami communicantes; see also sympathetic nervous *system.*

r. commu'nicans perone'us [NA], r. communicans fibularis; peroneal anastomotic r.; peroneal communicating nerve; nervus communicans peroneus (fibularis); the peroneal (fibular) communicating branch of the common peroneal (fibular) nerve; it arises from the common peroneal nerve in the popliteal space and passes over the lateral head of the gastrocnemius to the middle third of the leg, where it unites with the nervus cutaneus surae medialis to form the sural nerve.

r. commu'nicans ulna'ris [NA], ulnar communicating branch of superficial branch of radial nerve, joining the dorsal branch of the ulnar nerve in the hand.

ra'mi cor'poris amygdaloi'dei [NA], branches to the amygdaloid body; branches of the anterior choroid artery to the amygdaloid body.

r. cor'poris callo'si dorsa'lis [NA], dorsal corpus callosal branches; branches of the medial occipital artery to the dorsum of the corpus callosum.

ra'mi cor'poris genicula'ti latera'lis [NA], lateral geniculate body branches; branches of the anterior choroid artery to the lateral geniculate body.

r. costa'lis latera'lis [NA], lateral costal branch; a variable branch of internal thoracic artery that parallels the internal thoracic artery.

r. cricothyroi'deus [NA], cricothyroid branch or artery; a small branch of the superior thyroid artery that supplies the cricothyroid muscle.

ra'mi cuta'nei anterio'res ner'vi femora'lis [NA], anterior cutaneous branches of femoral nerve.

r. cuta'neus ante'rior ner'vi iliohypogas'trica [NA], anterior cutaneous branch of iliohypogastric nerve.

r. cuta'neus ante'rior (pectora'lis et abdomina'lis) nervo'rum thoracico'rum [NA], anterior cutaneous branch (pectoral and abdominal) of thoracic nerves.

ra'mi cuta'nei cru'ris media'les ner'vi saphe'ni [NA], medial crural cutaneous branches of saphenous nerve.

r. cuta'neus latera'lis [NA], lateral cutaneous branch of the following: 1) iliohypogastric nerve; 2) dorsal branch of thoracic nerves; 3) dorsal branch of posterior intercostal arteries.

r. cuta'neus media'lis [NA], medial cutaneous branch of the following: 1) dorsal branch of thoracic nerves; 2) dorsal branch of posterior intercostal arteries.

r. cuta'neus ra'mi anterio'ris ner'vi obturato'rii [NA], cutaneous branch of anterior branch of obturator nerve.

r. deltoi'deus [NA], deltoid branch of the following: 1) thoracoacromial artery; 2) deep brachial artery.

ra'mi denta'les [NA], dental branches of the following: 1) anterior superior alveolar arteries; 2) inferior alveolar artery; 3) posterior superior alveolar artery.

ra'mi denta'les inferio'res [NA], inferior dental branches of inferior dental plexus.

ra'mi denta'les superio'res [NA], superior dental branches of superior dental plexus.

r. descen'dens [NA], descending branch; **(1)** quadriceps artery of femur; descending branch of the lateral femoral circumflex artery; **(2)** princeps cervicis; princeps cervicis artery; descending branch of the occipital artery.

r. dex'ter [NA], right branch of the following: 1) portal vein; 2) proper hepatic artery.

r. digas'tricus [NA], digastric branch of the facial nerve.

ra'mi dorsa'les [NA], dorsal branches of the following: 1) cervical nerves; 2) lumbar nerves; 3) posterior intercostal arteries I and II; 4) sacral nerves; 5) thoracic nerves.

ra'mi dorsa'les lin'guae [NA], dorsal lingual branches of the lingual artery.

r. dorsa'lis [NA], dorsal branch of the following: 1) lumbar artery; 2) posterior intercostal arteries; 3) posterior intercostal veins; 4) spinal nerves; 5) subcostal artery; 6) ulnar nerve.

r. dorsa'lis nervo'rum spina'lium [NA], dorsal r. of spinal nerves; posterior primary division; the smaller division of each spinal nerve that innervates posterior axial musculature and part of the skin of the back.

ra'mi duodena'les [NA], duodenal branches of superior pancreaticoduodenal arteries.

ra'mi epiplo'ici, rami omentali.

ra'mi esophagea'les [NA], esophageal arteries; esophageal

branches of the following: 1) inferior thyroid artery; 2) left gastric artery; 3) thoracic aorta.
ra'mi esophage'i [NA], esophageal branches of recurrent laryngeal nerve.
r. exter'nus [NA], external branch of the following: 1) accessory nerve; 2) superior laryngeal nerve.
ra'mi faucia'les [NA], rami isthmi faucium.
r. femora'lis [NA], femoral branch of genitofemoral nerve.
r. fronta'lis [NA], frontal branch of superficial temporal artery.
r. fronta'lis anteromedia'lis [NA], anteromedial frontal branch of the callosomarginal artery.
r. fronta'lis interomedia'lis [NA], interomedial frontal branch of the callosomarginal artery.
r. fronta'lis posteromedia'lis [NA], posteromedial frontal branch of the callosomarginal artery.
ra'mi gangliona'res [NA], ganglionic branches; pterygopalatine nerves; nervi pterygopalatini; nervi sphenopalatini; two short sensory branches of the maxillary nerve in the pterygopalatine fossa, which pass through the pterygopalatine ganglion without synapse.
r. ganglio'nis trigem'ini [NA], branch to the trigeminal ganglion; a small branch of the cavernous part of the internal carotid artery to the trigeminal ganglion.
ra'mi gas'trici anterio'res ner'vi va'gi [NA], anterior gastric branches of the vagus; branches of the anterior vagal trunk to the anterior surface of the stomach.
ra'mi gas'trici posterio'res ner'vi va'gi [NA], posterior gastric branches; branches of the posterior vagal trunk to the posterior surface of the stomach.
r. genita'lis [NA], nervus spermaticus externus; genital branch of genitofemoral nerve.
ra'mi gingiva'les inferio'res [NA], inferior gingival branches of inferior dental plexus.
ra'mi gingiva'les superio'res [NA], superior gingival branches of superior dental plexus.
ra'mi glandula'res [NA], glandular branches; branches of various vessels, nerves, and ganglia distributed to glands.
ra'mi glo'bi pal'lidi [NA], branches to the globus pallidus; branches of the anterior choroid artery to the globus pallidus.
ra'mi hepat'ici [NA], hepatic branches of vagus nerve.
r. hypothalam'icus [NA], hypothalamic branch; a branch of the middle cerebral artery to the hypothalamus.
r. ili'acus [NA], iliac branch of iliolumbar artery.
r. infe'rior [NA], inferior branch of the following: 1) oculomotor nerve; 2) pubic bone; 3) superior gluteal artery.
ra'mi inferio'res ner'vi transver'si col'li [NA], inferior branches of the transverse nerve of the neck.
r. infrahyoi'deus [NA], infrahyoid branch of superior thyroid artery.
r. infrapatella'ris [NA], infrapatellar branch of saphenous nerve.
ra'mi inguina'les [NA], inguinal branches of external pudendal arteries.
ra'mi intercosta'les anterio'res [NA], anterior intercostal branches; two branches of the internal thoracic artery in each of the upper six intercostal spaces.
ra'mi intergangliona'res [NA], interganglionic branches; the nerve strands interconnecting the ganglia of the sympathetic trunk; they consist of pre- or postganglionic fibers passing to higher or lower levels of the trunk.
r. inter'nus [NA], internal branch of the following: 1) accessory nerve; 2) superior laryngeal nerve.
ra'mi interventricula'res septa'les, interventricular septal branches; septal branches; rami septales; branches of the anterior and posterior interventricular arteries distributed to the muscle of the interventricular septum.
r. interventricula'ris ante'rior [NA], anterior descending or interventricular artery; anterior interventricular branch of left coronary artery.
r. interventricula'ris poste'rior [NA], posterior descending or interventricular artery; posterior interventricular branch of right coronary artery.
ischiopubic r., the inferior r. of the os pubis and the r. of the ischium continuous with it.
ra'mi isth'mi fau'cium [NA], rami fauciales; faucial branches; branches to the isthmus of the fauces from the lingual nerve.
ra'mi labia'les anterio'res [NA], anterior labial branches; anterior labial arteries; arteriae labiales anteriores; branches of the external pudendal artery to the labium majus.
ra'mi labia'les inferio'res [NA], inferior labial branches; branches of mental nerve to lower lip.
ra'mi labia'les posterio'res [NA], posterior labial branches; posterior labial arteries; branches of the perineal artery to the labium majus.
ra'mi labia'les superio'res [NA], superior labial branches; branches of infraorbital nerve to upper lip.
ra'mi laryngopharyn'gei [NA], laryngopharyngeal branches; postganglionic fibers from the superior cervical ganglion to the pharyngeal plexus.
ra'mi latera'les [NA], lateral branches of the following: 1) the anterolateral central arteries; 2) the left branch of the portal vein.
r. latera'lis [NA], lateral branch of the following: 1) middle lobe branch of right pulmonary artery; 2) dorsal branches of cervical and lumbar nerves; 3) left hepatic duct; 4) supraorbital nerve.
ra'mi liena'les [NA], lienal or splenic branches of lienal, or splenic, artery.
ra'mi lingua'les [NA], lingual branches of 1) hypoglossal nerve; 2) lingual nerve.
r. lingua'lis [NA], lingual branch (inconstant) of the facial nerve.
r. lingula'ris [NA], lingular branch of 1) left pulmonary artery; 2) left pulmonary vein.
r. lingula'ris infe'rior [NA], inferior lingular branch of lingular branch of left pulmonary artery.
r. lingula'ris supe'rior [NA], superior lingular branch of lingular branch of left pulmonary artery.
r. lo'bi me'dii [NA], middle lobe branch of 1) the right pulmonary artery; 2) the right superior pulmonary vein.
r. lumba'lis [NA], lumbar branch of iliolumbar artery.
ra'mi malleola'res latera'les [NA], arteriae malleolares posteriores laterales; posterior peroneal arteries; lateral malleolar branches of peroneal artery.
ra'mi malleola'res media'les [NA], arteriae malleolares posteriores mediales; medial malleolar branches of posterior tibial artery.
ra'mi mamma'rii [NA], mammary branches of 1) lateral cutaneous branch of posterior intercostal arteries; 2) perforating branches of internal thoracic artery.
ra'mi mamma'rii latera'les [NA], lateral mammary branches of 1) lateral thoracic artery; 2) lateral cutaneous branches of intercostal nerve.
ra'mi mamma'rii media'les [NA], medial mammary branches of anterior cutaneous branches of intercostal nerve.
r. mandib'ulae [NA], r. of the mandible; the upturned perpendicular extremity of the mandible on either side; it gives attachment on its lateral surface to the masseter muscle.
r. margina'lis mandib'ulae [NA], mandibular marginal branch of facial nerve.
ra'mi mastoi'dei [NA], mastoid branches of posterior auricular artery.
r. mastoi'deus [NA], mastoid artery; mastoid branch of occipital artery.
r. mea'tus acu'stici inter'ni [NA], internal acoustic meatal branch. See *arteria* labyrinthi.
ra'mi media'les [NA], medial branches of 1) the anterolateral central arteries; 2) the left portal vein.
r. media'lis [NA], medial branch of 1) middle lobe branch of right pulmonary artery; 2) dorsal branches of cervical and lumbar

nerves; 3) left hepatic duct; 4) supraorbital nerve.
ra'mi mediastina'les [NA], medial branches; 1) arteriae mediastinales anteriores; medial branches of internal thoracic artery; 2) medial branches of thoracic aorta.
ra'mi medulla'res latera'les [NA], lateral medullary branches; branches of the posterior inferior cerebellar artery to the lateral part of the medulla oblongata.
ra'mi medulla'res media'les [NA], medial medullary branches; branches of the posterior inferior cerebellar artery to the medial part of the medulla oblongata.
r. membra'nae tym'pani [NA], nerve of tympanic membrane; a branch of the auriculotemporal nerve supplying the tympanic membrane.
r. meninge'us [NA], meningeal branch; **r. m. accesso'rius** [NA], accessory meningeal branch of middle meningeal artery; **r. m. ante'rior arte'riae vertebra'lis** [NA], anterior meningeal branch of the vertebral artery; **r. m. poste'rior** [NA], posterior meningeal branch of the vertebral artery; **r. m. arte'riae carot'is inter'nae** [NA], a branch from the cavernous part of the internal carotid artery to the meninges of the anterior cranial fossa; **r. m. arte'riae occipita'lis** [NA], meningeal branch of the occipital artery; **r. m. me'dius ner'vi maxilla'ris** [NA], middle or recurrent meningeal nerve; a recurrent branch of the maxillary nerve to the meninges of the middle cranial fossa; **r. m. ner'vi mandibula'ris** [NA], meningeal branch of the mandibular nerve; a branch from the mandibular nerve that enters the foramen spinosum to supply the meninges; **r. m. ner'vi va'gi** [NA], meningeal branch of the vagus; a branch from the superior ganglion of the vagus supplying the meninges of the posterior cranial fossa; **r. m. nervo'rum spina'lium** [NA], meningeal branch of the spinal nerves; sinuvertebral nerve; a branch from the proximal part of each spinal nerve passing back through the intervertebral foramen to supply the spinal meninges.
ra'mi menta'les [NA], mental branches of mental nerve.
ra'mi muscula'res [NA], branches of nerves or vessels that supply the muscles.
r. mus'culi stylopharyn'gei [NA], branch of the glossopharyngeal nerve to the stylopharyngeal muscle.
r. mylohyoi'deus [NA], branch of maxillary artery to the mylohyoid muscle.
ra'mi nasa'les [NA], nasal branches of anterior ethmoidal nerve.
ra'mi nasa'les exter'ni [NA], external nasal branches of 1) infraorbital nerve; 2) nasociliary nerve.
ra'mi nasa'les inter'ni [NA], internal nasal branches of 1) infraorbital nerve; 2) nasociliary nerve.
ra'mi nasa'les latera'les [NA], lateral nasal branches of nasociliary nerve.
ra'mi nasa'les media'les [NA], medial nasal branches of nasociliary nerve.
ra'mi nasa'les posterio'res inferio'res [NA], inferior posterior nasal branches of greater palatine nerve.
ra'mi nasa'les posterio'res superio'res latera'les [NA], lateral superior posterior nasal branches of pterygopalatine ganglion.
ra'mi nasa'les posterio'res superio'res media'les [NA], medial superior posterior nasal branches of pterygopalatine ganglion.
r. ner'vi oculomoto'rii [NA], branch to the oculomotor nerve; a branch of the middle cerebral artery to the oculomotor nerve.
r. no'di sinuatria'lis [NA], branch to the sinuatrial node; a small branch, usually the first, of the right coronary artery distributed to the sinuatrial node and adjacent portions of the right atrium.
ra'mi nucleo'rum hypothalamico'rum [NA], branches to hypothalamic nuclei; branches of the anterior choroid artery to the nuclei of the hypothalamus.
r. obturato'rius [NA], obturator branch of pubic branch of inferior epigastric artery; sometimes enlarged and named accessory obturator artery.
ra'mi occipita'les [NA], occipital branches of occipital artery.
r. occipita'lis [NA], occipital branch of 1) posterior auricular artery; 2) posterior auricular nerve.
r. occipitotempora'lis [NA], occipitotemporal branch; a branch of the medial occipital artery to the occipital and temporal regions of the cerebral cortex.
ra'mi omenta'li [NA], omental branches; epiploic branches; rami epiploici; branches of right and left gastro-omental arteries that supply the greater omentum.
ra'mi orbita'les [NA], orbital branches of pterygopalatine ganglion.
r. orbita'lis [NA], r. anastomoticus cum lacrimali; orbital branch of middle meningeal artery.
r. orbitofronta'lis latera'lis [NA], *arteria* frontobasalis lateralis.
r. orbitofronta'lis media'lis [NA], *arteria* frontobasalis medialis.
r. os'sis is'chii [NA], branch of the ischial bone; formerly called inferior branch of the ischium; the portion of the bone that passes forward from the ischial tuberosity to join the inferior r. of the pubic bone.
r. ova'ricus [NA], ovarian branch of uterine artery.
r. palma'ris ner'vi media'ni [NA], palmar branch of median nerve.
r. palma'ris ner'vi ulna'ris [NA], palmar branch of ulnar nerve.
r. palma'ris profun'dus arte'riae ulna'ris [NA], deep palmar branch of the ulnar artery; it supplies the hypothenar muscles then passes deep into the palm to the flexor tendons and anastomoses with the deep palmar arch from the radial artery.
r. palma'ris superficia'lis arte'riae radia'lis [NA], superficial palmar branch of radial artery; superficialis volae; superficial palmar or volar artery; it supplies the thenar muscles then enters the palm to communicate with the superficial palmar arch from the ulnar artery.
ra'mi palpebra'les [NA], palpebral branches of infratrochlear nerve.
ra'mi pancreat'ici [NA], pancreatic branches of 1) lienal artery; 2) superior pancreaticoduodenal arteries.
ra'mi parieta'les [NA], parietal branches of middle meningeal artery.
r. parieta'lis [NA], parietal branch of 1) superficial temporal artery; 2) medial occipital artery.
r. parieto-occipita'lis [NA], parieto-occipital branch of medial occipital artery.
ra'mi parotide'i [NA], parotid branches of 1) auriculotemporal nerve; 2) facial vein; 3) superficial temporal artery.
ra'mi pectora'les [NA], pectoral branches of thoracoacromial artery.
ra'mi peduncula'res [NA], peduncular branches; branches of the posterior cerebral artery to the cerebral peduncles.
r. per'forans [NA], anterior peroneal artery; perforating artery of peroneal; the branch of the peroneal artery that perforates the interosseous membrane just above the anterior tibiofibular ligament.
ra'mi perforan'tes [NA], perforating branches; **r. p. arte'riae metacarpa'lium palma'res,** perforating branches of palmar metacarpal arteries; perforating arteries of hand; three small arteries that pass dorsally through the second, third, and fourth interosseous spaces of the hand from the palmar metacarpal arteries; **r. p. arte'riae metatarsea'rum planta'res,** perforating branches of plantar metatarsal arteries; perforating arteries of foot; three small arteries that pass dorsally through the second, third, and fourth interosseous spaces of the foot from the plantar metatarsal arteries; **r. p. arte'riae thorac'icae inter'nae,** perforating branches of internal thoracic artery; perforating arteries of internal mammary; small branches of internal thoracic artery running between the costal cartilages to supply overlying skin and subcutaneous tissues.
ra'mi pericardi'aci aor'tae thora'cicae [NA], pericardiac branches of thoracic aorta.
r. pericardi'acus ner'vi phren'ici [NA], pericardiac branch of phrenic nerve.
ra'mi perinea'les [NA], perineal branches of posterior femoral

cutaneous nerve.

r. petro'sus [NA], petrous branch of middle meningeal artery.

ra'mi pharyngea'les [NA], pharyngeal branches of 1) ascending pharyngeal artery; 2) glossopharyngeal nerve; 3) inferior thyroid artery; 4) vagus nerve.

r. pharyn'geus [NA], Bock's nerve; nervus pharyngeus; pharyngeal branch of pterygopalatine ganglion.

ra'mi phrenicoabdomina'les [NA], phrenicoabdominal branches of phrenic nerve.

r. planta'ris profun'dus [NA], deep plantar branch of arcuate artery.

r. poste'rior [NA], posterior branch; each of the following has a branch so named; 1) great auricular nerve; 2) lateral cerebral sulcus; 3) left pulmonary artery; 4) obturator artery and nerve; 5) recurrent ulnar artery; 6) right branch of portal vein; 7) right hepatic duct; 8) right superior pulmonary vein; 9) superior thyroid artery; 10) renal artery.

r. poste'rior ascen'dens [NA], ascending posterior branch of right pulmonary artery.

r. poste'rior descen'dens [NA], descending posterior branch of right pulmonary artery.

r. profun'dus [NA], deep branch of 1) lateral plantar nerve; 2) medial femoral circumflex artery; 3) medial plantar artery; 4) radial nerve; 5) superior gluteal artery; 6) ulnar nerve.

r. profun'dus arte'ria scapula'ris descen'dens, *arteria* dorsalis scapulae.

r. profun'dus arte'riae transver'sae col'li, *arteria* dorsalis scapulae.

ra'mi pterygoi'dei [NA], pterygoid branches of middle meningeal artery.

pubic rami, see *os* pubis.

r. pu'bicus arte'riae epigas'tricae inferio'ris [NA], pubic branch of inferior epigastric artery,

r. pu'bicus arte'riae obturato'riae [NA], pubic branch of obturator artery.

ra'mi pulmona'les [NA], pulmonary branches of autonomic system.

ra'mi radicula'res [NA], rami spinales (1).

ra'mi rena'les ner'vi va'gi [NA], renal branches of vagus nerve.

r. rena'lis [NA], renal branch of lesser splanchnic nerve.

r. saphe'nus [NA], saphenous branch of descending genicular artery.

ra'mi scrota'les anterio'res [NA], anterior scrotal branches of external pudendal arteries.

ra'mi scrota'les posterio'res [NA], posterior scrotal branches of perineal artery.

ra'mi septa'les, rami interventricularis septales.

r. sinis'ter [NA], left branch of 1) portal vein; 2) proper hepatic artery.

r. si'nus carot'ici [NA], carotid sinus nerve; sinus nerve of Hering; Hering's sinus nerve; a branch of the glossopharyngeal nerve that innervates the baroreceptors in the wall of the carotid sinus and the chemoreceptors in the carotid body.

r. si'nus caverno'si [NA], cavernous sinus branch; a branch of the cavernous part of the internal carotid artery supplying the walls of the cavernous sinus.

ra'mi spina'les [NA], spinal branches; **(1)** radicular arteries; rami radiculares; branches of the following arteries which supply the meninges and spinal cord: 1) vertebral, 2) ascending cervical, 3) dorsal branch of posterior intercostal I to XI (also called arteries of Adamkiewicz), 4) dorsal branch of subcostal, 5) dorsal branch of lumbar arteries, 6) lumbar branch of iliolumbar, 7) lateral sacral; **(2)** veins draining the meninges and spinal cord, tributaries of the intervertebral veins.

r. stape'dius [NA], stapedial branch of posterior tympanic artery.

ra'mi sterna'les [NA], sternal arteries; sternal branches of internal thoracic artery.

ra'mi ster'noclei'domastoi'dei [NA], sternocleidomastoid branches of occipital artery.

r. ster'noclei'domastoi'deus [NA], sternocleidomastoid branch of superior thyroid artery.

r. stylohyoi'deus [NA], stylohyoid branch of facial nerve.

r. subapica'lis [NA], r. subsuperior; subapical or subsuperior branch of 1) basal part of left pulmonary artery; 2) basal part of right pulmonary artery.

ra'mi subscapula'res [NA], subscapular branches of axillary artery.

ra'mi substan'tiae ni'grae [NA], branches to the substantia nigra; branches of the anterior choroid artery to the substantia nigra.

r. subsupe'rior [NA], r. subapicalis.

r. superficia'lis [NA], superficial branch of 1) lateral plantar nerve; 2) medial plantar artery; 3) radial nerve; 4) superior gluteal artery; 5) ulnar nerve.

r. superficia'lis arte'riae transver'sae col'li [NA], arteria cervicalis superficialis; superficial branch of transverse artery of the neck.

r. supe'rior [NA], **(1)** superior branch of the deep branch of superior gluteal artery; the oculomotor nerve; the pubic bone; **(2)** r. apicalis (1).

r. supe'rior lo'bi inferio'ris [NA], r. apicalis lobi inferioris; superior branch of the inferior lobe of right and left pulmonary arteries.

ra'mi superio'res ner'vi transver'si col'li [NA], superior branches of transverse nerve of neck.

r. suprahyoi'deus [NA], suprahyoid branch of lingual artery.

r. sympath'icus ad gang'lion submandibula're [NA], sympathetic branch to the submandibular ganglion.

ra'mi tempora'les [NA], temporal branches of facial nerve.

ra'mi tempora'les anterio'res [NA], anterior temporal branches of lateral occipital artery, giving arterial supply to the cortex of the anterior part of the temporal lobe of the brain.

ra'mi tempora'les interme'dii media'les [NA], medial intermediate temporal branches of lateral occipital artery, giving arterial supply to the cortex of the intermediate and medial part of the temporal lobe of the brain.

ra'mi tempora'les posterio'res [NA], posterior temporal branches of lateral occipital artery giving arterial supply to the cortex of the posterior part of the temporal lobe of the brain.

ra'mi tempora'les superficia'les ner'vi auriculotempora'lis [NA], superficial temporal branches of auriculotemporal nerve.

r. tentor'ii [NA], tentorial branch; nervus tentorii; tentorial nerve; a branch of the ophthalmic nerve supplying the tentorium.

r. tento'rii basa'lis [NA], basal tentorial branch; a small branch from the cavernous part of the internal carotid artery to the base of the tentorium.

r. tento'rii margina'lis [NA], marginal tentorial branch; a small branch from the cavernous part of the internal carotid artery to the free margin of the tentorium.

ra'mi thalam'ici [NA], branches of the posterior cerebral artery to the thalamus.

r. thalam'icus [NA], a branch of the middle cerebral artery to the thalamus.

ra'mi thy'mici [NA], arteriae thymicae; thymic branches of internal thoracic artery.

r. thyrohyoi'deus [NA], thyrohyoid branch; a branch of the cervical ansa containing fibers of the first and second cervical nerves that accompany the hypoglossal nerve, then branch from it to reach the thyrohyoid muscle.

r. tonsil'lae cerebel'lae [NA], branch to the cerebellar tonsil; a branch from the posterior inferior cerebellar artery supplying the tonsil of the cerebellum.

ra'mi tonsilla'res [NA], tonsillar branches of glossopharyngeal nerve.

r. tonsilla'ris [NA], tonsillar branch of facial artery.

ra'mi trachea'les [NA], tracheal branches of 1) inferior thyroid artery; 2) recurrent laryngeal nerve.

ra'mi trac'tus op'tici [NA], optic tract branches; branches of the anterior choroid artery to the optic tract.
r. transver'sus [NA], transverse branch of 1) lateral femoral circumflex artery; 2) medial femoral circumflex artery.
r. tuba'rius [NA], tubal branch of 1) tympanic nerve; 2) uterine artery.
ra'mi tu'beris cine'rei [NA], branches to the tuber cinereum; branches of the anterior choroid artery to the tuber cinereum.
r. ulna'ris [NA], ulnar branch of medial cutaneous nerve of forearm.
ra'mi ureter'ici [NA], ureteral or ureteric branches of 1) artery of ductus deferens; 2) ovarian artery; 3) renal artery; 4) testicular artery.
ra'mi ventra'les nervo'rum cervica'lium [NA], ventral branches of cervical nerves.
ra'mi ventra'les nervo'rum lumba'lium [NA], ventral branches of lumbar nerves.
ra'mi ventra'les nervo'rum sacra'lium [NA], ventral branches of sacral nerves.
r. ventra'lis ner'vi spina'lis [NA], ventral r. of a spinal nerve; anterior primary division; the major division of each spinal nerve that contributes to the innervation of the limbs and the anterolateral parts of the body wall; the major plexuses (cervical, brachial and lumbosacral) are formed by the ventral rami.
ra'mi vestibula'res [NA], vestibular branches of labyrinthine artery.
ra'mi zygomat'ici [NA], zygomatic branches of facial nerve.
r. zygomaticofacia'lis [NA], zygomaticofacial branch of zygomatic nerve.
r. zygomaticotempora'lis [NA], zygomaticotemporal branch of zygomatic nerve.

ramycin (ră-mī'sin). Fusidic acid.

rancid (ran'sid) [L. *rancidus*, stinking, rank]. Having a disagreeable odor and taste, usually characterizing fat undergoing oxidation or bacterial decomposition to more volatile odiferous substances.

rancidify (ran-sid'i-fī). To make or become rancid.

rancidity (ran-sid'i-tē). The state of being rancid.

Rand, Gertrude, U.S. visual psychologist, 1886–1970. See Hardy-R.-Ritter *test*.

Rand, M.J. See Burn and R. *theory*.

Randall, Alexander, U.S. urologist, *1885. See R. stone *forceps*.

Raney Nickel. Raney catalyst; proprietary name for a finely powdered nickel catalyst made from Raney alloy by dissolving out the aluminum with alkali; used in the hydrogenation of organic substances.

range (rānj). A statistical measure of the dispersion or variation of values determined by the endpoint values; *e.g.*, in a group of children aged 6, 8, 9, 10, 13, and 16, the r. would be 10 (16 minus 6).

ranine (rā'nīn) [L. *rana*, a frog]. **1.** Relating to the frog. **2.** Relating to the undersurface of the tongue.

ranitidine (ră-nī'ti-dēn). *N*-[2-[[5-[(Dimethylamino) methyl]furfuryl]thio]ethyl]-*N*'-methyl-2-nitro-1,1-ethenediamine; a histamine H_2 antagonist used in the treatment of duodenal ulcers.

Ranke, Johannes, German anthropologist and physician, 1836–1916. See R.'s *angle*.

Ranke, Karl E. von, German chemist, 1870–1926. See R.'s *formula*.

Rankin, Fred Wharton, U.S. surgeon, 1886–1954. See R.'s *clamp*.

Rankine, William J. McQ., Scottish physicist, 1820–1870. See R. *scale*.

Ransohoff, Joseph, U.S. surgeon, 1853–1921. See R.'s *sign*.

ranula (ran'yū-lă) [L. tadpole, dim. of *rana*, frog]. **1.** Hypoclottis. **2.** Sublingual cyst; sialocele; ptyocele; ranine tumor; any cystic tumor of the undersurface of the tongue or floor of the mouth, especially one of the floor of the mouth due to obstruction of the duct of the sublingual glands.
r. pancreat'ica, a cystic tumor caused by obstruction of the pancreatic duct.

ranular (ran'yū-lăr). Relating to a ranula.

Ranvier, Louis A., French pathologist, 1835–1922. See R.'s *crosses, disks, node, plexus, segment*.

Raoult, François, M., French physicist, 1830–1899. See R.'s *law*.

rape (rāp) [L. *rapio*, to seize, to drag away]. **1.** Sexual intercourse by force, duress, intimidation, or deceit, or without legal consent (as with a minor). **2.** The performance of such an act.

rapeseed oil (rāp'sēd) [L. *rapa*, turnip]. The compressed oil from the seeds of *Brassica campestris* (family Cruciferae); used in the manufacture of soaps, margarine, and lubricants.

raphania (ră-fā'nē-ă). Rhaphania; a spasmodic disease supposed to be due to poisoning by the seeds of *Rhaphanus rhaphanistrum*, the wild radish.

raphe (rā'fē) [G. *rhaphē*, suture, seam] [NA]. Rhaphe; the line of union of two contiguous, bilaterally symmetrical structures.
amniotic r., the line of fusion of the amniotic folds over the embryo in reptiles, birds, and certain mammals.
r. anococcyg'ea, *ligamentum* anococcygeum.
anogenital r., in the male embryo the line of closure of the genital folds and swellings extending from the anus to the tip of the penis; it is differentiated in the adult into three regions: perineal r., scrotal r., and penile r.
r. cor'poris callo'si, a slight anteroposterior furrow on the median line of the upper surface of the corpus callosum.
lateral palpebral r., r. palpebralis lateralis.
r. lin'guae, *sulcus* medianus linguae.
median longitudinal r. of tongue, *sulcus* medianus linguae.
r. medul'lae oblonga'tae [NA], the seamlike median zone of the medulla oblongata, marked by intercrossing fiber bundles among which lie scattered neuronal cell bodies.
r. nuclei, see *nuclei* raphes.
r. pala'ti [NA], palatine r.; palatine ridge; a rather narrow, low elevation in the center of the hard palate that extends from the incisive papilla posteriorly over the entire length of the mucosa of the hard palate.
palatine r., r. palati.
palpebral r., r. palpebralis lateralis.
r. palpebra'lis latera'lis [NA], lateral palpebral r.; palpebral r.; a narrow fibrous band in the lateral part of the orbicularis oculi muscle formed by the interlacing of fibers passing through the upper and lower eyelids.
penile r., r. penis.
r. pe'nis [NA], penile r., the continuation of the r. of the scrotum onto the underside of the penis.
perineal r., r. perinei.
r. perine'i [NA], perineal r., the central anteroposterior line of the perineum, most marked in the male, being continuous with the r. of the scrotum.
r. pharyn'gis [NA], the central line of the pharynx posteriorly where the muscular fibers meet and partly interlace.
r. pon'tis [NA], the continuation of the r. medullae oblongatae into the pars dorsalis (or tegmentum) pontis.
pterygomandibular r., r. pterygomandibularis.
r. pterygomandibula'ris [NA], pterygomandibular r. or ligament; a tendinous thickening of the buccopharyngeal fascia, separating the buccinator muscle from the superior constrictor of the pharynx.
r. ret'inae, the horizontal line separating the superior and inferior portions of the temporal retina over which the retinal nerve fibers

do not course.

scrotal r., r. scroti.

r. scro'ti [NA], scrotal r.; Vesling line; a central line, like a cord, running over the scrotum from the anus to the root of the penis; it marks the position of the septum scroti.

Stilling's r., the transverse interdigitations of fiber bundles across the anterior median fissure of the medulla oblongata at the decussation of the pyramidal tracts.

Rapoport, Abraham, Canadian urologist, *1926. See R. *test.*

Rapoport, Samuel Mitja, Russian biochemist, *1912. See R.-Luebering *shunt.*

Rappaport classification. See under classification.

rapport (rap-ōr') [Fr.]. A feeling of relationship, especially when characterized by emotional affinity.

rapture of the deep (rap'chūr). See nitrogen *narcosis* (2).

rarefaction (rār-ĕ-fak'shŭn) [L. *rarus,* thin, + *facio,* to make]. The process of becoming light or less dense; the condition of being light; opposed to condensation.

rarefy (rār'ĕ-fī). To become light or less dense.

RAS Abbreviation for reticular activating *system.*

rasceta (ră-sē'tă) [Mod. L. *raseta,* fr. Ar. *rāhah,* palm of hand]. The transverse wrinkling on the anterior surface of the wrist.

rash [O. Fr. *rasche,* skin eruption, fr. L. *rado,* pp. *rasus,* to scratch, scrape]. Lay term for a cutaneous eruption.

ammonia r., diaper *dermatitis.*

antitoxin r., a cutaneous manifestation of serum sickness.

astacoid r., a massive exfoliation, sometimes occurring in malignant smallpox, the color of which resembles that of a boiled lobster.

black currant r., the cutaneous eruption seen in xeroderma pigmentosum.

butterfly r., butterfly (2).

caterpillar r., caterpillar *dermatitis.*

crystal r., *miliaria* crystallina.

diaper r., diaper *dermatitis.*

drug r., drug *eruption.*

heat r., *miliaria* rubra.

hydatid r., a toxic eruption occasionally following the rupture of a hydatid cyst.

Murray Valley r., epidemic *polyarthritis.*

napkin r., diaper *dermatitis.*

nettle r., urticaria.

serum r., a cutaneous manifestation of serum sickness.

summer r., *miliaria* rubra.

wildfire r., *miliaria* rubra.

rasion (rā'zhŭn) [L. *rasio,* a scraping, fr. *rado,* pp. *rasus,* to scrape, shave]. The subdivision of a crude drug by a rasp to prepare it for extraction.

Rasmussen, Fritz W., Danish physician, 1834–1881. See R.'s *aneurysm.*

raspatory (ras'pă-tōr-ē) [L. *raspatorium*]. A surgical instrument used to smooth the edges of a divided bone.

RAST Abbreviation for radioallergosorbent *test.*

Rastelli, Gian C., Italian cardiovascular surgeon, 1933–1970. See R. *procedure.*

rat. A rodent of the genus *Rattus* (family Muridae), involved in the spread of some diseases, including bubonic plague.

albino r.'s, r.'s with white fur and pink eyes; used extensively in laboratory experiments.

Wistar r.'s [*Wistar* Institute], an inbred strain of rats, homozygous at most loci, produced by strict brother-sister inbreeding over many generations to develop animals for research with the same general genetic composition.

rate (rāt) [L. *ratum,* a reckoning (see ratio)]. A record of the measurement of an event or process in terms of its relation to some fixed standard; measurement is expressed as the ratio of one quantity to another (*e.g.,* velocity, distance per unit time).

abortion r., the number of abortions per 1000 terminated pregnancies during a given period of time.

attack r., a cumulative incidence rate used for particular groups observed for limited periods under special circumstances, such as during an epidemic.

basal metabolic r. (BMR), basal *metabolism.*

baseline fetal heart r., the average heart r. for a particular fetus during the diastolic phase of uterine contractions.

birth r., the precise number of births for a year related to an exact population and place.

case fatality r., the proportion of individuals contracting a disease which die of that disease.

concordance r., the r. of occurrence of a trait, behavior action, etc. in members of a specified group, particularly in pairs of twins in genetic studies.

critical r., a heart r. at which aberration or incomplete block will occur; a result of shortening of cycle length so that it barely includes the refractory period.

death r., mortality r.

erythrocyte sedimentation r. (ESR), the rate of settling of red blood cells in anticoagulated blood utilizing the Westergren method; increased r.'s are often associated with anemia or inflammatory states.

fatality r., mortality r.

fetal death r., stillbirth r.; the number of fetal deaths divided by the sum of live births and fetal deaths occurring in the same population during the same time period.

fetal heart r., in the fetus, the number of heart beats per minute, normally 120 to 160.

glomerular filtration r. (GFR), the volume of water filtered out of the plasma through glomerular capillary walls into Bowman's capsules per unit time; it is considered to be equivalent to inulin clearance.

growth r., absolute or relative growth increase, expressed per unit of time.

heart r., r. of the heart's beat, recorded as the number of beats per minute.

infant mortality r., the number of deaths in the first year of life divided by the number of live births occurring in the same population during the same period of time.

lethality r., mortality r.

maternal death r., the number of maternal deaths that occur as the direct result of the reproductive process per 100,000 live births. See also maternal *death.*

mitotic r., the proportion of cells in a tissue that are undergoing mitosis, expressed as a mitotic index or, roughly, as the number of cells in mitosis in each microscopic high-power field in tissue sections.

morbidity r., the proportion of patients with a particular disease during a given year per given unit of population.

mortality r., mortality (2); death, fatality, or lethality r.; the ratio of the total number of deaths to the total population of a given community, usually expressed as deaths per 1000, 10,000, or 100,000 population per unit of time (*e.g.,* a year).

mutation r., the probability (or proportion) of progeny genes with a particular component of the genome not present in either biological parent; usually expressed as the number of mutants per generation occurring at one gene or locus.

neonatal mortality r., the number of deaths in the first 28 days of life divided by the number of live births occurring in the same population during the same period of time.

perinatal mortality r., the number of stillborn infants of 28 completed weeks or more plus the number of deaths occurring under 7 days of life divided by the number of stillborn infants of 28 weeks or more gestation plus all liveborn infants in the same population, regardless of the period of gestation.

pulse r., r. of the pulse as observed in an artery; recorded as beats per minute.

repetition r., the number of pulses per minute.

respiration r., frequency of breathing, recorded as the number of breaths per minute.

sedimentation r., the sinking velocity of blood cells, *i.e.,* the degree of rapidity with which the red cells sink in a mass of drawn blood.

shear r., the change in velocity of parallel planes in a flowing fluid separated by unit distance; units: $seconds^{-1}$.

slew r., in electronic pacemaker function, the maximum rate of change of an amplifier output voltage; important variable affecting heart function as controlled by an electronic pacemaker. Sensing circuits in the pacemaker often respond to the slew r. rather than to the absolute amplitude of the voltage pulse.

steroid metabolic clearance r. (MCR), a measure of the r. of metabolism of a given steroid within the body, usually expressed as liters of body fluid that contain the amount of steroid metabolized per day.

steroid production r., the total quantity of a given steroid formed in the body, usually expressed as milligrams per day; represents the sum of the glandular secretion of the steroid and extraglandular formation of it from various steroid precursors.

steroid secretory r., the r. of glandular secretion of a given steroid, usually expressed as milligrams per day; does not include any amount of the steroid that might be formed extraglandularly.

stillbirth r., fetal death r.

voiding flow r., urinary flow as a function of time during micturition, as graphically recorded by a flow meter.

rat-fish. Chimera (5).

Rathke, Martin H., German anatomist, physiologist, and pathologist, 1793–1860. See R.'s *bundles,* cleft *cyst, diverticulum, pocket, pouch,* pouch *tumor.*

ratio (ra'shē-ō) [L. *ratio (ration-)* a reckoning, reason, fr. *reor,* pp. *ratus,* to reckon, compute]. An expression of the relation of one quantity to another (*e.g.,* of a proportion or rate). See also index (2); quotient.

absolute terminal innervation r., the number of motor endplates divided by the number of terminal axons related to them.

accommodative convergence-accommodation r. (AC/A), the amount of convergence (measured in prism diopters of convergence) divided by the amount of accommodation (measured in diopters) required to direct both eyes upon an object.

A/G r., abbreviation for albumin-globulin r.

albumin-globulin r. (A/G r.), the r. of albumin to globulin in the serum or in the urine in kidney disease; the normal r. in the serum is approximately 1.55.

ALT:AST r., the r. of serum alanine aminotransferase to serum aspartate aminotransferase; elevated serum levels of both enzymes characterize hepatic disease; when both levels are abnormally elevated and the ALT:AST r. is greater than 1.0, severe hepatic necrosis or alcoholic hepatic disease is likely; when the r. is less than 1.0, an acute non-alcoholic hepatic condition is favored.

amylase-creatinine clearance r., a test for the diagnosis of acute pancreatitis; in apparently healthy individuals the renal clearance of amylase is less than 5% that of creatinine; it is determined by measuring amylase and creatinine in serum and urine; in acute pancreatitis the r. is said to be greater than 0.05 or 5% and to be specific for acute pancreatitis.

body-weight r., body weight (in grams) divided by stature (in centimeters).

cardiothoracic r., cardiothoracic index; the transverse diameter of the heart compared with that of the thoracic cage, as shown by x-ray examination.

r. of decayed and filled surfaces (RDFS), an index of decayed and filled permanent surfaces per person, per full complement of 122 tooth surfaces.

r. of decayed and filled teeth (RDFT), an index of decayed and filled permanent teeth per person, per full complement of 28 teeth.

extraction r. (E), the fraction of a substance removed from the blood flowing through the kidney; it is calculated from the formula $(A - V)/A$, where A and V, respectively, are the concentrations of the substance in arterial and renal venous plasma.

flux r., the r. of the two unidirectional fluxes through a particular boundary layer or membrane.

functional terminal innervation r., the number of muscle fibers divided by the number of axons that innervate them.

hand r., the r. of the length of the hand (measured on the dorsum from the styloid process of the ulna to the tip of the third finger) to the width across the knuckles.

IRI/G r., the r. of immunoreactive insulin to serum or plasma glucose; in hypoglycemic states a r. of less than 0.3 is usual with the exception of the hypoglycemia due to insulinoma, where the r. is often higher than 0.3.

K:A r., abbreviation for ketogenic-antiketogenic r.

ketogenic-antiketogenic (K:A) r., the proportion between substances that form ketones in the body and those that form glucose.

lecithin/sphingomyelin r. (L/S r.), a r. used to determine fetal pulmonary maturity, found by testing the amniotic fluid; when the lungs are mature, lecithin exceeds sphingomyelin by 2 to 1.

L/S r., abbreviation for lecithin/sphingomyelin r.

M:E r., the r. of myeloid to erythroid precursors in bone marrow; normally it varies from 2:1 to 4:1; an increased r. is found in infectious chronic myelogenous leukemia or erythroid hypoplasia; a decreased r. may mean a depression of leukopoiesis or normoblastic hyperplasia depending on the overall cellularity of the bone marrow.

mendelian r., the r. of contrasting phenotypes or genotypes expected in accordance with genetic principles among the offspring of matings specified as to genotype.

molecular weight r. (M_r), molecular *weight.*

nuclear-cytoplasmic r., r. of volume of nucleus to volume of cytoplasm, fairly constant for a particular cell type and usually increased in malignant neoplasms.

nutritive r., the ratio or proportion of digestible protein to digestible non-nitrogenous nutrients in a ration for livestock.

P/O r., a measure of oxidative phosphorylation; the r. of phosphate radicals esterified (forming adenosine triphosphate from adenosine diphosphate) to atoms of oxygen consumed by mitochondria; normally, the r. is 3.

respiratory exchange r. (R), the r. of the net output of carbon dioxide to the simultaneous net uptake of oxygen at a given site, both expressed as moles or STPD volumes per unit time; in the steady state, respiratory exchange r. is equal to the respiratory quotient of metabolic processes.

segregation r., in genetics, the proportion of progeny of a particular genotype or phenotype that may be expected.

sex r., **(1)** the r. of male to female progeny at some specified stage of the life cycle, notably at conception (primary), at birth (secondary), or at any stage between birth and death (tertiary); **(2)** the r. of the numbers of males to females affected by a particular disease or trait.

therapeutic r., the r. of the maximally tolerated dose of a drug to the minimal curative or effective dose; LD_{50} divided by ED_{50}.

ventilation/perfusion r. ($\dot{V}a/\dot{Q}$), the r. of alveolar ventilation to simultaneous alveolar capillary blood flow in any part of the lung; because both ventilation and perfusion are expressed per unit volume of tissue and per unit time, which cancel, the units become liters of gas per liter of blood.

zeta sedimentation r. (ZSR), the r. of the zetacrit to the hematocrit, normally 0.41 to 0.54 (41 to 54%); it is a sensitive indicator of the erythrocyte sedimentation rate (ESR) and, unlike the latter, is unaffected by anemia, which tends to elevate the ESR.

rational (rash'ŭn-ăl) [L. *rationalis,* fr. *ratio,* reason]. **1.** Pertaining to reasoning or to the higher thought processes; based on objective or scientific knowledge, in contrast to empirical (1). **2.** Influenced by reasoning rather than by emotion. **3.** Having the reasoning faculties; not delirious or comatose.

rationalization (ra-shŭn-ăl-i-zā'shŭn) [L. *ratio,* reason]. In psychoanalysis, a postulated defense mechanism through which irrational behavior, motives, or feelings are made to appear reasonable.

Ratner. See Kurzrok-R. *test.*

ratsbane (rats'bān). Arsenic.

rattlesnake (rat'l-snāk). A member of the crotalid genera *Crotalus* and *Sistrurus,* characterized by possession of cuticular warning rattles at the tip of the tail.

Rattus (rat'ŭs). The rats, a genus of rodents, family Muridae. *R. rattus,* the black r., is the species most commonly responsible for transmitting plague to man by means of its flea, *Xenopsylla cheopis;* it is smaller and darker in color than the Norwegian, sewer, or brown rat (*Rattus norvegicus*) and has longer ears and tail. See rat.

Rau (Ravius, Raw), Johann J., Dutch anatomist, 1668–1719. See R.'s *process, processus* ravii.

Rauber, August A., German anatomist, 1841–1917. See R.'s *layer.*

Rauscher, F.J., 20th century U.S. oncologist. See R.'s *virus.*

Rauwolfia (row-wool'fē-ă, raw-, rah-) [L. *Rauwolf,* German botanist, 16th century]. A genus of tropical trees and shrubs (family Apocynaceae). The powdered whole root of *R. serpentina* contains alkaloids that produce a sedative-antihypertensive-bradycrotic action; approximately 50% of the total activity is due to reserpine.

RAV Abbreviation for Rous-associated *virus.*

Ravius, Raw. See Rau.

ray (rā) [L. *radius*] **1.** A beam of light, heat, or other form of radiation. The r.'s from radium and other radioactive substances are produced by a spontaneous disintegration of the atom; they are electrically charged particles or electromagnetic waves of extremely short wavelength. **2.** A part or branch that extends radially from a structure.

actinic r., chemical r.; a light r. toward and beyond the violet end of the spectrum that acts upon a photograph plate and produces other chemical effects.

alpha r., alpha *particle.*

anode r.'s, positive r.'s; those originating in a gas discharge tube and moving in a direction opposite to that of cathode r.'s; made up of positively charged ions.

Becquerel r.'s, radiations given off by uranium and other radioactive substances; these include alpha, beta, and gamma r.'s.

beta r., beta *particle.*

borderline r.'s, obsolete term for grenz r.'s.

Bucky's r.'s, obsolete term for grenz r.'s.

cathode r.'s, a stream of electrons emitted from the negative electrode (cathode) in a Crookes tube; their bombardment of the anode or the glass wall of the tube gives rise to x-r.'s.

chemical r., actinic r.

cosmic r.'s, high velocity particles of enormous energies, bombarding earth from outer space; the "primary radiation" consists of protons and more complex atomic nuclei that, on striking the atmosphere, give rise to neutrons, mesons, and other less energetic "secondary radiation."

direct r.'s, primary r.'s (2).

Dorno r.'s, the ultraviolet r.'s with wavelengths below 289 nm; those biologically active.

dynamic r.'s, physically or therapeutically active r.'s.

gamma r.'s, electromagnetic radiation emitted from radioactive substances; they are high energy x-r's, but originate from the nucleus rather than the orbital shell, and are not deflected by a magnet.

glass r.'s, those formed by cathode r.'s striking the wall of an x-ray tube.

grenz r. (grents) [Ger. *Grenze,* borderline, boundary], very soft x-r.'s, closely allied to the ultraviolet r.'s in their wavelength (i.e., long) and in their biologic action upon tissues; they are produced by a specially built vacuum tube with a hot cathode operating from a transformer delivering not more than 8 kw.

H r.'s, a stream of hydrogen nuclei; *i.e.,* protons.

hard r.'s, r.'s of short wavelength and great penetrability.

incident r., the r. that strikes the surface before reflection.

indirect r.'s, x-r.'s generated at a surface other than the anode target.

infrared r., see infrared.

intermediate r.'s, W r.'s; those between ultraviolet and x-r.'s.

marginal r.'s, in geometric optics, those r.'s originating from the periphery.

medullary r., *pars* radiata lobuli corticalis renis.

monochromatic r.'s, light r.'s of a very narrow band of wavelengths (ideally, of a single wavelength).

Niewenglowski r.'s, radiation emitted from a phosphorescent body after exposure to sunlight.

parallel r.'s, r.'s parallel to the axis of an optical system.

paraxial r.'s, in geometric optics, those r.'s focused at the principal point.

positive r.'s, anode r.'s.

primary r.'s, **(1)** cosmic r.'s in the form in which they first strike the atmosphere; **(2)** direct r.'s; x-r.'s generated at the focal point of the tube.

reflected r., a r. of light or other form of radiant energy which is thrown back from a nonpermeable or nonabsorbing surface; the r. which strikes the surface before reflection is the incident r.

roentgen r., x-ray.

secondary r.'s, r.'s generated when primary r.'s impinge upon matter.

soft r.'s, r.'s of relatively long wavelength and slight penetrability.

supersonic r.'s, r.'s with a wavelength higher than that perceptible to the human ear, above 20,000 Hz.

transition r.'s, obsolete term for grenz r.'s.

ultrasonic r.'s, see ultrasonic.

ultraviolet r.'s, see ultraviolet.

W r.'s, intermediate r.'s.

x-r., see x-ray.

rayage (rā'ej). The dosage in radiotherapeutics.

Rayer, Pierre F., French physician, 1793–1867. See R.'s *disease.*

Rayleigh, Lord John W.S., British physicist, 1842–1919. See R. *equation, test.*

Raymond, Fulgence, French neurologist, 1844–1910. See R. type of *apoplexy.*

Raynaud, Maurice, French physician, 1834–1881. See R.'s *syndrome, disease, phenomenon.*

Rb Symbol for rubidium.

R-banding. See R-banding *stain.*

rbc, RBC Abbreviation for red blood *cell;* red *blood count.*

RBF Abbreviation for renal blood flow. See effective renal blood *flow.*

R.C.P. Abbreviation for Royal College of Physicians (of England).

R.C.P.(E) or **(Edin)** Abbreviation for Royal College of Physicians (Edinburgh).

R.C.P.(I) Abbreviation for Royal College of Physicians (Ireland).

R.C.S. Abbreviation for Royal College of Surgeons (England).

R.C.S.(E) or **(Edin)** Abbreviation for Royal College of Surgeons (Edinburgh).

R.C.S.(I) Abbreviation for Royal College of Surgeons (Ireland).

R.D. Abbreviation for *reaction* of degeneration; registered dietician.

RDFS Abbreviation for *ratio* of decayed and filled surfaces.

RDFT Abbreviation for *ratio* of decayed and filled teeth.

R.D.H. Abbreviation for Registered Dental Hygienist.

Re Symbol for rhenium.

R.E. Abbreviation for right eye.

re-. Prefix fr. Latin meaning again or backward.

react (rē-akt′) [Mod. L. *reactus*]. To take part in or to undergo a chemical reaction.

reactance (X) (rē-ak′tans). Inductive resistance; the weakening of an alternating electric current by passage through a coil of wire or a condenser.

reactant (rē-ak′tant). A substance taking part in a chemical reaction.
acute phase r.'s, alpha and beta serum proteins whose concentrations increase or decrease in response to acute inflammation.

REACTION

reaction (rē-ak′shŭn) [L. *re-*, again, backward, + *actio,* action]. **1.** The response of a muscle or other living tissue or organism to a stimulus. **2.** The color change effected in litmus and certain other organic pigments by contact with substances such as acids or alkalies; also the property that such substances possess of producing this change. **3.** In chemistry, the intermolecular action of two or more substances upon each other, whereby these substances are caused to disappear, new ones being formed in their place (chemical r.). **4.** In immunology, *in vivo* or *in vitro* action of antibody on specific antigen, with or without involvement of complement or other components of the immunological system.

accelerated r., vaccinoid r.; the cutaneous manifestations occurring during the period between the second and tenth day following smallpox vaccination; because it is intermediate between a primary r. and an immediate r., it is regarded as evidence of some degree of resistance, possible poor vaccination technique, or poor quality of vaccine.

acid r., **(1)** the change of blue litmus paper to red, indicating that the substance with which the litmus is brought into contact is acid; **(2)** an excess of hydrogen ions over hydroxide ions in aqueous solution indicated by a pH value less than 7.

acute situational r., stress r.

adverse r., a result of drug therapy which is neither intended nor expected in normal therapeutic use and which causes significant, sometimes life-threatening morbidity.

alarm r., the various phenomena, *e.g.*, stimulated endocrine activity, which the body exhibits as an adaptive response to injury or stress; first phase of the general adaptation syndrome.

aldehyde r., Ehrlich r.; the r. of the indole derivatives with aromatic aldehydes; *e.g.,* tryptophan and *p*-dimethylaminobenzaldehyde in H_2SO_4 give a red-violet color useful in assaying proteins for tryptophan content.

alkaline r., **(1)** the change of red litmus paper to blue, indicating that the substance with which the litmus is brought in contact is alkaline; **(2)** an excess of hydroxide ions over hydrogen ions in aqueous solution as indicated by a pH value greater than 7.

allergic r., hypersensitivity r.; a local or general r. of an organism following contact with a specific allergen to which it has been previously exposed and to which it has become sensitized; immunologic interaction of endogenous or exogenous antigen with antibody or sensitized lymphocytes gives rise to inflammation or tissue damage. Allergic r.'s are classified into four major types: type I, anaphylactic and IgE dependent; type II, cytotoxic; type III, immune-complex mediated; type IV, cell-mediated (delayed).

amphoteric r., a dôuble r. possessed by certain fluids, such as freshly drawn milk, which turns blue litmus paper red and red litmus paper blue.

anamnestic r., augmented production of an antibody due to previous response of the subject to stimulus by the same antigen.

antigen-antibody r., the phenomenon, occurring *in vitro* or *in vivo,* of antibody combining with antigen of the type that stimulated the formation of the antibody, thereby resulting in agglutination, precipitation, complement fixation, greater susceptibility to ingestion and destruction by phagocytes, or neutralization of exotoxin. See also skin *test.*

anxiety r., a psychological r. or experience involving the apprehension of danger accompanied by a feeling of dread and such physical symptoms as restlessness and tachycardia, in the absence of a clearly identifiable fear stimulus; when chronic, it is called generalized anxiety *disorder.* See also panic *attack.*

Arias-Stella r., Arias-Stella *phenomenon.*

arousal r., change in pattern of the brain waves when the subject is suddenly awakened and becomes alert.

Arthus r., **(1)** Arthus *phenomenon;* **(2)** Arthus-type r.'s, r.'s in man and other species that result from the same basic immunologic (allergic) mechanism which evokes, in the rabbit, the typical Arthus phenomenon. See also immune complex *disease.*

Ascoli r., a method for confirming the diagnosis of anthrax by means of a precipitin r. which indicates the presence of heat-stable *Bacillus anthracis* antigen in the extracted tissue.

associative r., a secondary or side r.

Bence Jones r., the classic means of identifying Bence Jones protein, which precipitates when urine (from patients with this type of proteinuria) is gradually warmed to 45 to 70°C and redissolves as the urine is heated to near boiling; as the specimen cools, the Bence Jones protein precipitates in the indicated range of temperature, and redissolves as the temperature of the specimen becomes less than 30 to 35°C.

Berthelot r., the r. of ammonia with phenol-hypochlorite to give indophenol; the principle is used to analyze ammonia concentration in body fluids.

bi-bi r., a r. catalyzed by a single enzyme in which two substrates and two products are involved; the ping-pong mechanism may be involved in such a r.

Bittorf's r., in cases of renal colic, pain on squeezing the testicle or pressing the ovary radiates to the kidney.

biuret r., the formation of biuret ($NH_2CONHCONH_2$), which gives a violet color due to the r. of a polypeptide of more than three amino acids with $CuSO_4$ in strongly alkaline solution; dipeptides and amino acids (except histidine, serine, and threonine) do not so react; used for the detection and quantitation of polypeptides, or proteins, in biological fluids.

Bloch's r., dopa r.

Brunn r., the increased absorption of water through the skin of the frog when the animal is injected with pituitrin and immersed in water; one of the physiological reactions used to study and classify posterior pituitary polypeptides and their analogues.

Burchard-Liebermann r., a blue-green color produced by acetic anhydride with cholesterol dissolved in chloroform, when a few drops of concentrated sulfuric acid are added. See Liebermann-Burchard *test.*

Cannizzaro's r., formation of an acid and an alcohol by the simultaneous oxidation of one aldehyde molecule and reduction of another; a dismutation: $2\ RCHO \rightarrow RCOOH + RCH_2OH$.

Carr-Price r., the r. of antimony trichloride with vitamin A to yield a brilliant blue color; this r. forms the basis of several quantitative techniques for the determination of vitamin A.

catalatic r., decomposition of H_2O_2 to O_2 and H_2O, as in the action of catalase; analogous to peroxidase r.
catastrophic r., the disorganized behavior that is the response to a severe shock or threatening situation with which the person cannot cope.
cell-mediated r., immunological r. of the delayed type, involving chiefly T lymphocytes. See also skin *test.*
chain r., a self-perpetuating r. in which a product of one step in the r. itself serves to bring about the next step in the r., and so on. *Cf.* autocatalysis.
Chantemesse r., a conjunctival r., especially as applied to typhoid.
cholera-red r., a test for cholera vibrio whereby the addition of 3 or 4 drops of sulfuric acid (concentrated, chemically pure) to an 18-hour-old bouillon or peptone culture of the organism produces a color from rose-pink to claret.
chromaffin r., production of a yellow-brown to brown coloration in normal and abnormal cells containing epinephrine and norepinephrine, when fresh tissue slices are placed in a dichromate-chromate mixture overnight; useful for detection of pheochromocytoma (adrenal medulla) and other tumors which produce catecholamines.
circular r., in sensorimotor theory, the tendency of an organism to repeat novel experiences.
cocarde r., cockade r., see Römer's *test.*
complement-fixation r., see complement *fixation.*
consensual r., indirect pupillary r.; consensual light reflex; contraction of the pupil of the fellow eye when light is directed into the other eye.
constitutional r., a generalized r. in contrast to a focal or local r.; in allergy the immediate or delayed response, following the introduction of an allergen, occurring at sites remote from that of injection.
conversion r., conversion *hysteria.*
cross r., a specific r. between an antiserum and an antigen complex other than the antigen complex that evoked the various specific antibodies of the antiserum, due to the two complexes including among their respective antigenic determinants at least one that is included also among the determinants of the other complex.
cutaneous r., cutireaction.
cytotoxic r., an immunologic (allergic) r. in which noncytotropic IgG or IgM antibody combines with specific antigen on cell surfaces; the resulting complex initiates the activation of complement which causes cell lysis or other damage, or which, in the absence of complement, may lead to phagocytosis or may enhance T lymphocyte involvement.
Dale r., see Schultz-Dale r.
dark r., in photosynthesis, the fixation of CO_2 into carbohydrate, which is independent in place and time of the absorption of light.
decidual r., the cellular and vascular changes occurring in the endometrium at the time of implantation.
r. of degeneration (DR or RD), the electrical r. in a degenerated nerve and the muscles supplied by it; characterized by absence of response to both galvanic and faradic stimulus in the nerve and to faradic stimulus in the muscles; the muscles may still respond to galvanic stimulation, but the cathodal closing contraction is greater than the anodal closing contraction, the reverse of normal.
delayed r., late r.; a local or generalized response that begins 24 to 48 hours after exposure to an antigen (allergen, immunogen) to which the individual has been sensitized (immunized); T lymphocytes, upon contact with the specific antigen, release lymphokines which in turn mobilize phagocytic cells and lymphocytes at the site of the r.
depot r., reddening of the skin at the point where the needle entered, in the subcutaneous tuberculin test.
dermotuberculin r., Pirquet's *test.*
diazo r., Ehrlich's diazo r.; the r. of diazotized sulfanilic acid with bilirubin to form azobilirubin, which forms the basis of quantitating the amount of bilirubin in biological fluids. See van den Bergh's *test.*
digitonin r., the r. of naturally occurring steroids with 3β-hydroxyl groups with digitonin, a steroid glycoside, resulting in the formation of an insoluble precipitate; useful in determining the presence of cholesterol and ergosterol.
Dische r., the assay of DNA by means of the blue color formed with diphenylamine in acid.
dissociative r., r. characterized by such dissociative behavior as amnesia, fugues, sleepwalking, and dream states.
dopa r., Bloch's r.; a dark staining observed in fresh tissue sections to which a solution of dopa has been applied, presumably due to the presence of dopa oxidase in the protoplasm of certain cells.
dystonic r., a state of abnormal tension or muscle tone, similar to dystonia, produced as a side effect of certain antipsychotic medication; a severe form, where the eyes appear to roll up into the head, is called oculogyric crisis.
early r., immediate r.
Ebbecke's r., dermatographism.
echo r., echolalia.
Ehrlich r., aldehyde r.
Ehrlich's benzaldehyde r., a test for urobilinogen in the urine, by dissolving 2 g of dimethyl-*p*-aminobenzaldehyde in 100 ml of 5% hydrochloric acid and adding this reagent to urine; a red color in the cold indicates the presence of an excessive amount of urobilinogen.
Ehrlich's diazo r., diazo r.
eosinopenic r., reduction in the numbers of circulating eosinophils by ACTH or by adrenal corticoids.
erythrophore r., fish test; a reddish coloration (nuptial coloration) caused in certain male fishes (bitterling) by the injection of the gonad hormone.
false-negative r., an erroneous or mistakenly negative response.
false-positive r., an erroneous or mistakenly positive response.
Fernandez r., a delayed hypersensitivity lepromin r., similar to a tuberculin r., at the site of intradermal injection of Dharmendra antigen in a lepromin test.
ferric chloride r. of epinephrine, an intense emerald green color in a neutral or slightly acid solution of epinephrine when ferric chloride is added to it; a r. typical of catechols.
Feulgen r., see Feulgen *stain.*
first-order r., a r. the rate of which is proportional to the concentration of the single substance undergoing change; radioactive decay is a first-order process, defined by the equation $-(dN/dt)=kN$, where N is the number of atoms subject to decay (reaction), t is time, and k is the first-order decay (reaction) constant, *i.e.,* the fraction of all atoms decaying per unit of time. See also decay *constant.*
fixation r., see complement *fixation.*
flocculation r., a form of precipitin r. in which precipitation occurs over a narrow range of antigen-antibody ratio, due chiefly to peculiarities of the antibody (precipitin).
focal r., local r.; a r. which occurs at the point of entrance of an infecting organism or of an injection, as in the Arthus phenomenon.
Folin's r., the r. of amino acids in alkaline solution with 1,2-naphthoquinone-4-sulfonate to yield a red color; useful for quantitative assay.
Forssman r., Forssman antigen-antibody r.
Forssman antigen-antibody r., Forssman r.; the combination of Forssman antibody with heterogenetic antigen of the Forssman type, as in the agglutination of sheep erythrocytes (which contain Forssman antigen) by serum from a person with infectious mononucleosis which contains Forssman antibody.
Frei-Hoffman r., Frei *test.*
fright r., after section and degeneration of the facial nerve of an

animal, the denervated facial muscles contract if the animal is frightened or becomes angry; due to the release of acetylcholine into the circulation.
fuchsinophil r., the property possessed by certain elements, when stained with acid fuchsin, of retaining the stain when treated with picric acid alcohol.
furfurol r., production of a red color on addition of furfurol to a solution of aniline.
galvanic skin r., galvanic skin *response*.
gel diffusion r.'s, gel diffusion precipitin *tests*.
Gell and Coombs r.'s, see allergic r.'s.
gemistocytic r., a r. to injury resulting in the proliferation of reactive, protoplastic, or gemistocytic astrocytes.
general adaptation r., see general adaptation *syndrome*.
Gerhardt's r., Gerhardt's *test* for acetoacetic acid.
graft versus host r., graft versus host *disease*.
group r., a r. with an agglutinin or other antibody that is common (though usually in varying concentrations) to an entire group of related bacteria, *e.g.,* the coli group.
Gruber's r., Gruber-Widal r., Widal's r.
Günning's r., the formation of iodoform from acetone by iodine and ammonia in alcohol.
harlequin r., sudden blanching of the lower half of the body of an infant lying on its side, leaving the remaining half of the body the normal pink color.
heel-tap r., see heel *tap*.
hemoclastic r., hemolysis as observed in the laking of the blood.
Henle's r., dark brown staining of the medullary cells of the adrenal bodies when treated with the salts of chromium, the cortical cells remaining unstained.
Herxheimer's r., Jarisch-Herxheimer r.; an inflammatory r. in syphilitic tissues (skin, mucous membrane, nervous system, or viscera) induced in certain cases by specific treatment with Salvarsan, mercury, or antibiotics; believed to be due to a rapid release of treponemal antigen with an associated allergic reaction in the patient.
Hill r., that portion of the photosynthesis r. that involves the photolysis of water and the liberation of oxygen and does not include carbon dioxide fixation. It involves the addition of oxidants (quinones or ferricyanide) to chloroplasts; upon illumination, O_2 is evolved and the added oxidant is reduced.
hunting r., hunting phenomenon; an unusual r. of digital blood vessels exposed to cold; vasoconstriction is alternated with vasodilation in irregular repeated sequences, in an apparent hunting of equilibrium of skin temperature.
hypersensitivity r., allergic r.
id r., an allergic manifestation of the dermatophytoses and of candidiasis, characterized by itching, vesicular lesions that appear in response to circulating antigens at sites that are often far distant from the primary fungal lesion itself. See also dermatophytid; -id (1).
r. of identity, see gel diffusion precipitin *tests* in two dimensions.
immediate r., early r.; local or generalized response that begins within a few minutes to about an hour after exposure to an antigen (allergen, immunogen) to which the individual has been sensitized (immunized). See also skin *test;* wheal-and-flare r.
immune r., antigen-antibody r. indicating a certain degree of resistance, usually in reference to the 36- to 48-hour reaction in vaccination against smallpox; because the degree of resistance indicated by the r. is not true immunity and may disappear relatively rapidly there is a tendency to refer to the immune r. as an allergic r.
incompatible blood transfusion r., a syndrome due to intravascular hemolysis of transfused blood by serum antibodies of the recipient, which react with an antigen of the donor red cells; characterized by chills, fever (often with urticaria), backache or muscle cramps, hemoglobinemia, hemoglobinuria, and oliguria which may result in acute renal failure.
indirect pupillary r., consensual r.
intracutaneous r., intradermal r., a r. following the injection of antigen into the skin of a sensitive subject, such as in the case of the tuberculin test.
iodate r. of epinephrine, a r. dependent upon the oxidation of epinephrine by iodine liberated from iodate, which is decomposed by the hormone; a faint pink color results.
iodine r. of epinephrine, a r. resulting from the oxidation of the hormone, a faint pink color appearing upon the addition of iodine.
irreversible r., a r. or response by the tissues to a pathogenic agent characterized by a permanent pathologic change.
Jaffe r., a bright orange-red complex resulting from the treatment of creatinine with alkaline picrate solution; the basis of most routine creatinine tests.
Jarisch-Herxheimer r., Herxheimer's r.
Jolly's r., myasthenic r.; rapid loss of response to faradic stimulation of a muscle with the galvanic response and the power of voluntary contraction retained.
late r., delayed r.
lengthening r., in the decerebrate animal, the rather sudden relaxation with lengthening of the extensor muscles when a limb is passively flexed; associated with clasp-knife spasticity.
lepromin r., a delayed hypersensitivity r. at the site of an intradermal injection of a lepromin, such as the Dharmendra antigen or Mitsuda antigen, in a lepromin test; the r.'s, such as the Fernandez or Mitsuda r., are variable, occurring in 48 hours or three to five weeks, but are uniformly negative in lepromatous leprosy, borderline leprosy, and mid-borderline leprosy.
leukemoid r., see *leukemoid reaction.*
lid closure r., constriction of the pupil on the side of forcible closure of the eyelid.
local r., focal r.
local anesthetic r., a toxic r. due to absorption of local anesthetic drug in regional anesthesia, ranging from drowsiness to convulsions and cardiovascular collapse.
Loewenthal's r., the agglutinative r. in relapsing fever.
magnet r., a r. seen in an animal deprived of its cerebellum; when the animal is placed upon its back and the head strongly flexed, the four limbs become flexed in all their joints. Due to stimulation of receptors in the deep layers of the skin, light pressure made upon a toe-pad with the finger causes reflex contraction of the limb extensors. The limb is thus pressed gently against the finger, and when the finger is withdrawn slightly, the experimenter has the sensation that his finger is raising the limb or drawing it out as by a magnet.
Marchi's r., failure of the myelin sheath of a nerve to blacken when submitted to the action of osmic acid.
Mazzotti r., Mazzotti *test.*
Millon r., the r. of phenolic compounds (*e.g.,* tyrosine in protein) with $Hg(NO_3)_2$ in HNO_3 (and a trace of HNO_2) to give a red color.
miostagmin r., a physiochemical immunity test, designed by Ascoli, consisting in determination of the surface tension of an immune serum to which its specific antigen has been added, before and after incubation at 37°C for 2 hours; in a positive r. the surface tension, as measured by the stalagmometer, is lowered.
Mitsuda r., a delayed hypersensitivity lepromin r., in the form of erythematous papular nodules, at the site of intradermal injection of Mitsuda antigen in a lepromin test.
mixed agglutination r., mixed agglutination; immune agglutination in which the aggregates contain cells of two different kinds but with common antigenic determinants; when used to identify isoantigens, the test cells are exposed to appropriate isoantibody, washed, and then mixed with indicator erythrocytes that combine with free sites on the test cell-attached isoantibody.
mixed lymphocyte culture r., see mixed lymphocyte culture *test.*
monomolecular r., unimolecular r.; a r. involving a single molecule (*e.g.,* decomposition, intramolecular rearrangement, intramolecular oxidation or reduction), even if a catalytic agent, such as

acid or alkali, is present in large excess, on a molecular basis, or is not rate determining; such r.'s are usually first order r.'s.
myasthenic r., Jolly's r.
Nadi r., peroxidase r.
near r., the pupillary constriction associated with ocular convergence.
Neufeld r., Neufeld capsular *swelling.*
neurotonic r., muscular contraction continuing well after cessation of stimulation.
neutral r., pH of 7.00; H and OH ion concentrations equal at 10^{-7} M.
ninhydrin r., triketohydrindene r.; a test for proteins, peptones, peptides, and amino acids possessing free carboxyl and α-amino groups that is based upon the r. with triketohydrinene hydrate; a blue color r. is used to quantitate free amino acids (*e.g.,* after hydrolysis and separation of the amino acids of a protein).
nitritoid r., a severe r. resembling that following the administration of nitrites, sometimes following intravenous administration of arsphenamine or other drugs; consists of flushing of the face, edema of the tongue and lips, vomiting, profuse sweating, a fall in blood pressure, and sometimes death.
r. of nonidentity, see gel diffusion precipitin *tests* in two dimensions.
nuclear r., the interaction of two atomic nuclei or of one such with a subatomic particle, or of the subatomic particles within an atomic nucleus, resulting in a change in the nature of the nuclei concerned or in the energy content of the nuclei or both, usually manifested by transmutation (accompanied by emission of α-, β-, or γ-rays) or by fission or fusion of the nuclei.
oxidase r., **(1)** the formation of indol blue when a blood smear containing myeloid leukocytes is treated with a mixture of α-naphthol and *p*-dimethylaniline sulfate; the myeloid leukocytes contain an oxidase that catalyzes this r., the lymphoid leukocytes do not; **(2)** in bacteriology, a r. that depends on the presence of certain oxidases in some bacteria that catalyze the transport of electrons between electron donors in the bacteria and an oxidation reduction dye, such as tetramethyl-*p*-phenylenediamine; the dye is reduced to a blue or black color.
oxidation-reduction r., see oxidation-reduction.
pain r., dilation of the pupil or any other involuntary act occurring in response to a stimulus causing sharp pain anywhere.
Pandy's r., Pandy's test; a test to determine the presence of proteins (chiefly globulins) in the spinal fluid, by adding one drop of spinal fluid to 1 ml of solution (*e.g.,* carbolic acid crystals in distilled water, cresol, or pyrogallic acid); the r. varies from a faint turbidity to a dense "milky" precipitate according to the degree of protein content.
r. of partial identity, see gel diffusion precipitin *tests* in two dimensions.
passive cutaneous anaphylactic r., see passive cutaneous *anaphylaxis.*
Paul's r., Paul's test; pus is rubbed into a scarification on a rabbit's eye; if the pus is from a variolous or vaccinal pustule a condition of epitheliosis develops in from 36 to 48 hours; the sputum of a smallpox patient is said to cause the same r.
performic acid r., oxidative destruction of the ethylene double bond (–HC=CH–) which is converted to a Schiff-reactive double aldehyde; used to indicate the presence of unsaturated lipids, such as phospholipids and cerebrosides, as well as cystine-rich substances, such as keratin, in tissue sections.
peroxidase r., Nadi r.; formation of indophenol blue by the action of an oxidizing enzyme present in certain cells and tissues when they are treated with a solution of α-naphthol and dimethylparaphenylenediamine; by this method, cells of the myelocyte series, which give a positive r., may be distinguished from those of the lymphocyte series, which give a negative r.; endothelial leukocytes give a variable r., probably positive when they have phagocytized the debris of myeloid cells.
phosphoroclastic r., cleavage of C–C bonds that involves phosphate transfer but not, as in phosphorolysis, directly to one of the products; *e.g.,* the decomposition of pyruvate to acetate + CO_2, in which P_i is added to ADP to form ATP.
Pirquet's r., Pirquet's *test.*
plasmal r., a histochemical technique that uses mercuric chloride to unmask the aldehyde group of acetalphosphatides and permit Schiff staining.
Porter-Silber r., the basis of the 17-hydroxycorticosteroid test; C-21 adrenocorticosteroids, which contain a dihydroxyacetone group at carbons 19, 20, and 21, react with phenylhydrazine.
Prausnitz-Küstner r., a test based on passive transfer of allergic sensitivity; blood serum from an allergic individual is injected into the skin of a normal person; 48 hours later the injected site shows an urticarial r. when injected with antigens to which the donor is allergic; other parts of the recipient's skin show no response.
precipitin r., see precipitin; precipitin *test.*
primary r., vaccinia.
prozone r., see prozone.
psychogalvanic r., psychogalvanic skin r., galvanic skin *response.*
quellung r. [Ger. *Quellung,* swelling], Neufeld capsular *swelling.*
reversed Prausnitz-Küstner r., the appearance of an urticarial r. at the site of injection when serum containing reaginic antibody is injected into the skin of a person in whom the allergen is already present.
reversible r., a chemical r. that takes place either from left to right or from right to left; ionization is such a r., as are, by definition, r.'s in which an enzyme (a catalyst) is involved.
Sakaguchi r., guanidines in alkaline solution develop an intense red color when treated with α-naphthol and sodium hypochlorite; a qualitative test for arginine, free or in a protein.
Schardinger r., the reduction of methylene blue to methylene white by formaldehyde is rapidly catalyzed by fresh milk but not by boiled milk, the catalyzing agent being xanthine oxidase; an example of oxidation in the absence of O_2 with an organic hydrogen acceptor (the dye).
Schultz r., see Schultz *stain.*
Schultz-Charlton r., Schultz-Charlton phenomenon; the specific blanching of a scarlatinal rash at the site of intracutaneous injection of scarlatina antiserum.
Schultz-Dale r., the contraction of an excised intestinal loop (Schultz) or of an excised strip of virginal uterus (Dale) from a sensitized animal (guinea pig) which occurs when the tissue is exposed to the specific antigen.
serum r., serum *sickness.*
shortening r., the adaptive shortening of the extensor muscles of the limb of a decerebrate animal when the limb is extended after it has been flexed. *Cf.* lengthening r.
Shwartzman r., Shwartzman *phenomenon.*
skin r., skin *test.*
specific r., the phenomena produced by an agent that is identical with or immunologically related to the one that has already caused an alteration in capacity of the tissue to react.
startle r., startle *reflex* (1).
Straus r., a diagnostic test for glanders. Male guinea pigs are inoculated intraperitoneally with suspected material; if the glanders organism is present, it will usually set up a necrotizing inflammation in the scrotal sac within a few days and the specific organism can be confirmed bacteriologically.
stress r., acute situational r.; an acute emotional r. related to extreme environmental stress.
supporting r.'s, supporting reflexes; described by Magnus, who distinguished two types: **positive supporting r.'s,** consisting of those reflex muscular contractions whereby the body is supported against gravity; seen in an exaggerated form in the decerebrate animal; **negative supporting r.'s,** consisting of inhibition of the exten-

sor muscles and unfixing of the joints which thus enable the limb to be flexed and moved into a new position.

symptomatic r., an allergic response similar to the original one, but occurring after the use of a test or therapeutic dose of an allergen or atopen.

thermoprecipitin r., the throwing down of a precipitate on the application of heat, as in the case of proteinaceous urine.

Treponema pallidum immobilization r., *Treponema pallidum* immobilization *test.*

triketohydrindene r., ninhydrin r.

unimolecular r., monomolecular r.

vaccinoid r., accelerated r.

Voges-Proskauer r., a chemical r. used in testing for the production of acetyl methyl carbinol by various bacteria; potassium hydroxide is added to a 24-hour culture in a suitable medium and thoroughly mixed; the treated culture is exposed to air and is observed at intervals of 2, 12, and 24 hours; a positive r. consists of the development of an eosin-like pink color, due to the production of acetylmethylcarbinol, which in the presence of alkali and oxygen is oxidized to diacetyl.

Wassermann r. (WR), Wassermann *test.*

Weidel's r., a r. showing the presence of xanthine; a solution of the suspected substance in chlorine water with a little nitric acid is evaporated in a water bath, and then exposed to the vapor of ammonia; the presence of xanthine is indicated when a red or purple color develops.

Weil-Felix r., Weil-Felix *test.*

Weinberg's r., a complement fixation test of the presence of hydatid disease.

Wernicke's r., hemiopic or hemiopic pupillary r.; Wernicke's sign; in hemianopsia, a r. due to damage of the optic tract, consisting in loss of pupillary constriction when the light is directed to the blind side of the retina; pupillary constriction is maintained when light stimulates the normal side.

wheal-and-erythema r., wheal-and-flare r., the characteristic immediate r. observed in the skin test; within 10 to 15 minutes after injection of antigen (allergen), an irregular, blanched, elevated wheal appears, surrounded by an area of erythema (flare).

Widal's r., Gruber's or Gruber-Widal r.; agglutination r. as applied to the diagnosis of typhoid.

Yorke's autolytic r., a test for paroxysmal hemoglobinuria; serum is placed in an ice chest and kept at 0°C for 5 to 7 minutes, then in an incubator at 37°C with erythrocytes for 1 hour, at which time, if the r. is positive, hemolysis occurs; if the serum is kept at 1°C for an hour and then placed in the incubator with erythrocytes there is little hemolysis.

zero-order r., a r. that proceeds at a particular rate independently of the concentration of the reactant or reactants.

Zimmermann r., Zimmermann test; a chemical r. between metadinitrobenzene and an active methylene group (carbon-16) of 17-ketosteroids; it is the basis of the 17-ketosteroid assay t.

---

reactivate (rē-ak'ti-vāt). To render active again; said of an inactivated immune serum to which normal serum (complement) is added.

reactivation (rē'ak-ti-vā'shŭn). Restoration of the lytic activity of an inactivated serum by means of the addition of complement.

reactivity (rē-ak-tiv'i-tē). **1.** The property of reacting, chemically or in any other sense. **2.** The process of reacting.

readthrough (rēd'thrū). In molecular biology, transcription of a nucleic acid sequence beyond its normal termination sequence.

reagent (rē-ā'jent) [Mod. L. *reagens*]. Any substance added to a solution of another substance to participate in a chemical reaction.

Benedict-Hopkins-Cole r., magnesium glyoxalate, made from a mixture of oxalic acid and magnesium, used for testing proteins for the presence of tryptophan.

biuret r., an alkaline solution of copper sulfate.

Cleland's r., dithioerythritol or dithiothreitol; HS–$CH_2(CHOH)_2CH_2SH$; used to reduce disulfide bonds in proteins.

diazo r., Ehrlich's diazo r.; two solutions, one of sodium nitrite, the other of acidified sulfanilic acid, used in bringing about diazotization.

Edlefsen's r., an alkaline permanganate solution used in the determination of sugar in the urine.

Edman's r., phenylisothiocyanate.

Ehrlich's diazo r., diazo r.

Erdmann's r., a mixture of sulfuric and nitric acids, used in testing alkaloids.

Esbach's r., picric acid, citric acid, and water (in the proportions 1, 2, and 97) used for the detection of albumin in the urine.

Exton r., 50 g sulfosalicylic acid and 200 g $Na_2SO_4 \cdot 10H_2O$ in a liter of water, used as a test for albumin.

Fehling's r., Fehling's *solution.*

Fouchet's r., a 25% solution of trichloroacetic acid, containing 0.9% ferric chloride; a drop of the r. added at the surface line of barium chloride-impregnated filter paper which has been dipped in urine for 10 sec will give a green color if bilirubin is present. See also Fouchet's *stain.*

Froehde's r., sodium molybdate 1, in strong sulfuric acid 1000; gives various color reactions with alkaloids.

Frohn's r., bismuth subnitrate (1.5) and water (20.0) heated to boiling, to which hydrochloric acid (10.0) and potassium iodide (7.0) are added; used to test for alkaloids and for sugar.

Girard's r., the hydrazine of betaine chloride, used to extract ketonic steroids by forming water-soluble hydrazones with them.

Günzberg's r., phloroglucin and vanillin used as a r. in Günzberg's test.

Hahn's oxine r., an alcoholic solution of 8-hydroxyquinoline used in the determination of zinc, aluminum, magnesium, etc.

Hammarsten's r., a mixture of 1 part of a 25% solution of nitric acid and 19 parts of a 25% solution of hydrochloric acid; the addition of a few drops to a mixture of 1 part of this r. and 4 parts of alcohol will give a green color if bile is present.

Ilosvay r., sulfanilic acid 0.5, dissolved in dilute acetic acid 150, mixed with naphthylamine 1, and dissolved in boiling water 20; the blue sediment which forms is dissolved in dilute acetic acid 150; a few drops of this r. added to water, saliva, or other fluid to be tested will produce a red color if nitrites are present.

Kasten's fluorescent Schiff r.'s, fluorescent analogues of Schiff's r. which are fluorescent basic dyes lacking acidic side groups and containing one or more primary amine groups; used in cytochemical detection of DNA in Kasten's fluorescent Feulgen stain, polysaccharides in Kasten's fluorescent PAS stain, and proteins in the ninhydrin-Schiff stain; such analogues include acriflavine, auramine O, and flavophosphine N.

Lloyd's r., precipitated aluminum silicate, used in the determination of alkaloids.

Mandelin's r., a solution of ammonium vanadate in sulfuric acid, used in color tests for alkaloids.

Marme's r., a solution of potassium iodide and cadmium iodide used in testing for alkaloids.

Marquis' r., a solution of formaldehyde in sulfuric acid used in color tests for formaldehyde.

Mecke's r., a solution of selenous acid in sulfuric acid, used for color tests of alkaloids.

Meyer's r., a solution of phenolphthalein 0.032, in decinormal sodium hydroxide 21, with water (distilled from glass) sufficient to make 100; in the presence of minute traces of blood, the solution becomes purple or blue-red.

Millon's r., mercuric nitrate and nitric acid as used in the Millon reaction.

Nessler's r., a solution of potassium hydroxide, mercuric iodide, and potassium iodide; it yields a yellow color with ammonia (a brown precipitate with larger amounts) that can be used for quantitive assay.

Rosenthaler-Turk r., a solution of potassium arsenate in sulfuric acid used in obtaining color tests for various opium alkaloids.

Sanger's r., fluoro-2,4-dinitrobenzene.

Schaer's r., an alcoholic or aqueous solution of chloral hydrate used as an extraction medium in investigations of alkaloids.

Scheibler's r., a solution of sodium tungstate in phosphoric acid used in tests for alkaloids.

Schiff's r., an aqueous solution of basic fuchsin or pararosaniline which is decolorized by sulfur dioxide, commonly prepared by addition of hydrochloric acid to a dye solution containing a metabisulphite or bisulphite salt; used for aldehydes and in histochemistry to detect polysaccharides, DNA, and proteins. See Feulgen *stain,* periodic acid-Schiff *stain;* ninhydrin-Schiff *stain* for proteins.

Scott-Wilson r., an alkaline solution of mercuric cyanide and silver nitrate used in the detection of acetone.

Sulkowitch's r., a r. for the detection of calcium in the urine, consisting of oxalic acid 2.5 g, ammonium oxalate 2.5 g, glacial acetic acid 5 cc, and distilled water to make 150 cc; a milky precipitate of calcium oxalate is formed when the r. is added to urine that contains calcium.

Uffelmann's r., to a 2% solution of phenol in water is added aqueous ferric chloride until the solution becomes violet in color; this turns lemon yellow in the presence of lactic acid, assumes an opaline tint in butyric acid, and is decolorized by hydrochloric acid.

Wurster's r., filter paper impregnated with tetramethyl-*p*-phenylenediamine, which turns blue in the presence of ozone or hydrogen peroxide.

reagin (rē-ā′jin). **1.** Wolff-Eisner's term for antibody. **2.** Old term for the "Wassermann" antibody; not to be confused with the Prausnitz-Küstner antibody.

atopic r., Prausnitz-Küstner *antibody.*

reaginic (rē-ā-jin′ik). Pertaining to a reagin.

reality (rē-al′i-tē) [L. *res,* thing, fact]. That which exists objectively and in fact, and can be consensually validated.

reality awareness. The ability to distinguish external objects as being different from oneself.

reality testing. In psychiatry and psychology, the ego function by which the objective or real world and one's relationship to it are evaluated and appreciated.

reamer (rē′mer) [A.S. *ryman,* to widen]. A rotating finishing or drilling tool used to shape or enlarge a hole.

engine r., an engine-mounted spirally-bladed instrument, used for enlarging the root canals of teeth.

intramedullary r., a rasp used for shaping the intramedullary portion of the metaphysis prior to the insertion of an appliance or a prosthesis.

reattachment (rē-ă-tach′ment). New epithelial or connective tissue attachment to the surface of a tooth that was surgically detached and not exposed to oral environment.

Réaumur, René A.F. de, French physicist, 1683–1757. See R. *scale.*

rebase (rē′bās). In dentistry, to refit a denture by replacing the denture base material without changing the occlusal relationship of the teeth. See also reline.

rebreathing (rē-brēdh′ing). Inhalation of part or all of gases previously exhaled.

Rebuck skin window technique. See under technique.

recalcification (rē-kal′si-fi-kā′shŭn). Restoration to the tissues of lost calcium salts.

recall (rē′kawl). The process of remembering thoughts, words, and actions of a past event in an attempt to recapture actual happenings.

Récamier, Joseph C.A., French gynecologist, 1774–1852. See R.'s *operation.*

recanalization (rē-kan′ăl-i-zā′shŭn). **1.** Restoration of a lumen in a blood vessel following thrombotic occlusion, by organization of the thrombus with formation of new channels. **2.** Spontaneous restoration of the continuity of the lumen of any occluded duct or tube, as with post-vasectomy r.

recapitulation (rē′kă-pit′yū-lā′shŭn). See recapitulation *theory.*

receiver (rē-sē′ver) [L. *receptor, fr. recipio,* to receive]. In chemistry, a vessel attached to a condenser to receive the product of distillation.

receptaculum, pl. **receptacula** (rē′sep-tak′yū-lŭm, -lă) [L. fr. *recipio,* pp. *-ceptus,* to receive, fr. *capio,* to take]. Reservoir; a receptacle.

r. chy′li, *cisterna* chyli.

r. gan′glii petro′si, *fossula* petrosa.

r. pecquet′i, *cisterna* chyli.

receptoma (rē-sep-tō′mă). Chemodectoma.

receptor (rē-sep′tŏr, tōr) [L. receiver, fr. *recipio,* to receive]. **1.** A structural protein molecule on the cell surface or within the cytoplasm that binds to a specific factor, such as a hormone, antigen, or neurotransmitter. **2.** Ceptor; C. Sherrington's term for any one of the various sensory nerve endings in the skin, deep tissues, viscera, and special sense organs.

adrenergic r.'s, adrenoreceptors; postulated reactive components of effector tissues, most of which are innervated by adrenergic postganglionic fibers of the sympathetic nervous system. Such r.'s can be activated by norepinephrine and/or epinephrine and by various adrenergic drugs; r. activation results in a change in effector tissue function, such as contraction of arteriolar muscles or relaxation of bronchial muscles; adrenergic r.'s are divided into α-r.'s and β-r.'s, on the basis of their response to various adrenergic activating and blocking agents.

α-adrenergic r.'s, postulated adrenergic r.'s in effector tissues capable of selective activation and blockade by drugs; conceptually derived from the ability of certain agents, such as phenoxybenzamine, to block only some adrenergic r.'s and of other agents, such as methoxamine, to activate only the same adrenergic r.'s. Such r.'s are designated as α-receptors. Their activation results in physiological responses such as increased peripheral vascular resistance, mydriasis, and contraction of pilomotor muscles.

β-adrenergic r.'s, postulated adrenergic r.'s in effector tissues capable of selective activation and blockade by drugs; conceptually derived from the ability of certain agents, such as propranolol, to block only some adrenergic r.'s and of other agents, such as isoproterenol, to activate only the same adrenergic r.'s. Such r.'s are designated as β-receptors. Their activation results in physiological responses such as increases in cardiac rate and force of contraction (β_1), and relaxation of bronchial and vascular smooth muscle (β_2).

cholinergic r.'s, chemical sites in effector cells or at synapses through which acetylcholine exerts its action.

Fc r., the site on B lymphocytes that is seemingly specific in the attachment of the Fc portion of immunoglobulin molecules.

opiate r.'s, regions of the brain which have the capacity to bind morphine; some, along the aqueduct of Sylvius and in the center median, are in areas related to pain, but others, as in the striatum, are not related.

sensory r.'s, peripheral endings of afferent neurons.

stretch r.'s, r.'s that are sensitive to elongation, especially those in Golgi tendon organs and muscle spindles, but also those found in visceral organs such as the stomach, small intestine, and urinary bladder; these r.'s have the function of detecting elongation, and this distinguishes them from baroreceptors, which actually are activated by stretching of the wall of the blood vessel but whose function is to elicit central reflex mechanism reducing the arterial blood pressure.

recess (rē'ses) [L. *recessus*]. Recessus.
anterior r. of tympanic membrane, *recessus* membranae tympani anterior.
cecal r., *recessus* retrocecalis.
cerebellopontine r., pontocerebellar r.; the angle formed at the junction of cerebellum, pons, and medulla.
cochlear r., *recessus* cochlearis.
costodiaphragmatic r., *recessus* costodiaphragmaticus.
costomediastinal r., *recessus* costomediastinalis.
duodenojejunal r., *recessus* duodenalis superior.
elliptical r., *recessus* ellipticus.
epitympanic r., *recessus* epitympanicus.
hepatoenteric r., a peritoneal r. at the caudal end of the embryonic pneumatoenteric r.; it separates the developing liver and stomach.
hepatorenal r., *recessus* hepatorenalis.
Hyrtl's epitympanic r., *recessus* epitympanicus.
inferior duodenal r., *recessus* duodenalis inferior.
inferior ileocecal r., *recessus* ileocecalis inferior.
inferior omental r., *recessus* inferior omentalis.
infundibular r., *recessus* infundibuli.
intersigmoid r., *recessus* intersigmoideus.
Jacquemet's r., a pouch of peritoneum between the gallbladder and the liver.
lateral r. of fourth ventricle, *recessus* lateralis ventriculi quarti.
mesentericoparietal r., parajejunal *fossa.*
optic r., *recessus* opticus.
pancreaticoenteric r., a r. of the embryonic peritoneal cavity that develops into the adult omental bursa.
paracolic r.'s, *sulci* paracolici.
paraduodenal r., *recessus* paraduodenalis.
parotid r., recessus parotideus; a deep hollow on the side of the head below and in front of the mastoid; it lodges the parotid gland.
pharyngeal r., *recessus* pharyngeus.
phrenicomediastinal r., *recessus* phrenicomediastinalis.
pineal r., *recessus* pinealis.
piriform r., *recessus* piriformis.
pleural r.'s, *recessus* pleurales.
pneumatoenteric r., pneumoenteric r., a r. of the embryonic celom between the right lung bud and the gut; it is normally largely obliterated before birth, leaving only the superior r. of the vestibule of the lesser peritoneal sac as a vestige.
pontocerebellar r., cerebellopontine r.
posterior r. of tympanic membrane, *recessus* membranae tympani posterior.
Reichert's cochlear r., *recessus* cochlearis.
retrocecal r., *recessus* retrocecalis.
retroduodenal r., *recessus* retroduodenalis.
Rosenmüller's r., *recessus* pharyngeus.
sacciform r., *recessus* sacciformis.
sphenoethmoidal r., *recessus* sphenoethmoidalis.
spherical r., *recessus* sphericus.
splenic r., *recessus* lienalis.
subhepatic r., *recessus* subhepatici.
subphrenic r.'s, *recessus* subphrenici.
subpopliteal r., *recessus* subpopliteus.
superior duodenal r., *recessus* duodenalis superior.
superior ileocecal r., *recessus* ileocecalis superior.
superior r. of lesser peritoneal sac, see pneumatoenteric r.
superior omental r., *recessus* superior omentalis.
superior r. of tympanic membrane, *recessus* membranae tympani superior.
suprapineal r., *recessus* suprapinealis.
supratonsillar r., *fossa* supratonsillaris.
triangular r., recessus triangularis; an occasional evagination of the anterior wall of the third ventricle of the brain between the anterior commissure and the diverging pillars of the fornix.
Tröltsch's r.'s, *recessus* membranae tympani, anterior and posterior.
tubotympanic r., the dorsal portion of the embryonic first endodermal pharyngeal pouch; it develops into the middle ear cavity.

recession (rē-sesh'ŭn) [L. *recessio* (see recessus)]. A withdrawal or retreating. See also retraction.
gingival r., gingival atrophy or resorption; apical migration of the gingiva along the tooth surface, with exposure of the tooth surface.
tendon r., curb tenotomy; surgical displacement of the tendon of an eye muscle posterior to its anatomic insertion.

recessitivity (rē'ses-i-tiv'i-tē). The state of being recessive (2).

recessive (rē-ses'iv). **1.** Drawing away; receding. **2.** In genetics, denoting a trait due to a particular allele that does not manifest itself in the presence of other alleles which generate traits dominant to it.

recessus, pl. **recessus** (rē-ses'sŭs) [L. a withdrawing, a receding] [NA]. Recess; a small hollow or indentation.
r. ante'rior, a circumscript deepening of the interpeduncular fossa in the direction of the mamillary bodies.
r. cochlea'ris [NA], cochlear recess; Reichert's cochlear recess; a small depression on the inner wall of the vestibule of the labyrinth at the portion of the pyramis vestibuli, between the two limbs into which the vestibular crest divides posteriorly; it is perforated by foramina giving passage to fibers which the cochlear branch of the vestibulocochlear nerve sends to the posterior extremity of the cochlear duct.
r. costodiaphragmat'icus [NA], costodiaphragmatic recess; phrenicocostal sinus; the cleftlike extension of the pleural cavity between the diaphragm and the rib cage.
r. costomediastina'lis [NA], costomediastinal recess or sinus; the recess of the pleural cavity between the costal cartilages and the mediastinum.
r. duodena'lis infe'rior [NA], inferior duodenal recess or fossa; Gruber-Landzert fossa; the variable peritoneal recess which lies behind the inferior duodenal fold and along the ascending part of the duodenum.

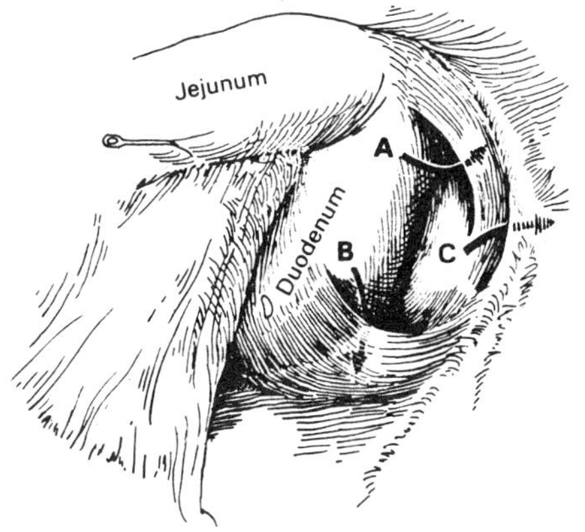

Duodenal Recess
A, superior duodenal recess; *B*, inferior duodenal recess; *C*, paraduodenal recess.

r. duodena'lis supe'rior [NA], superior duodenal fossa or recess; Jonnesco's fossa; duodenojejunal recess or fossa; a peritoneal recess extending upward behind the superior duodenal fold.
r. ellip'ticus [NA], elliptical recess; fovea hemielliptica; fovea elliptica; an oval depression in the roof and inner wall of the vestibule of the labyrinth, lodging the utriculus.
r. epitympan'icus [NA], epitympanic recess or space; epitympanum; Hyrtl's epitympanic recess; attic; tympanic attic; the upper portion of the tympanic cavity above the tympanic membrane; it

contains the head of the malleus and the body of the incus.

r. hepatorena'lis [NA], hepatorenal recess; hepatorenal pouch; Morison's pouch; the deep recess of the peritoneal cavity on the right side extending upward between the liver in front and the kidney and suprarenal behind.

r. ileoceca'lis infe'rior [NA], inferior ileocecal recess; a deep fossa sometimes found between the ileocecal fold, the mesoappendix, and the cecum.

r. ileoceca'lis supe'rior [NA], superior ileocecal recess; a shallow pouch occasionally existing between the terminal ileum, the cecum, and the ileocolic artery when the latter is present.

r. infe'rior omenta'lis [NA], inferior omental recess; a recess of the omental bursa extending into the great omentum.

r. infundib'uli [NA], infundibular recess; a funnel-shaped diverticulum leading from the anterior portion of the third ventricle down into the infundibulum of the hypophysis.

r. infundibulifor'mis, r. pharyngeus.

r. intersigmoi'deus [NA], intersigmoid recess; a peritoneal recess behind and below the sigmoid colon created by the attachment of the sigmoid mesocolon ascending across the left psoas then turning sharply to descend into the pelvis; the left ureter (pars tecta ureterica) passes posterior to this recess.

r. latera'lis ventric'uli quar'ti [NA], lateral recess of the fourth ventricle; the narrow recess of the ventricle that extends laterally over, and down along the side of, the inferior cerebellar peduncle and the overlying cochlear nuclei; at its tip it opens by way of Luschka's foramen into the cisterna basalis of the subarachnoid space. By way of this recess, part of the choroid plexus of the fourth ventricle protrudes into the subarachnoid space.

r. liena'lis [NA], splenic recess; the extension of the omental bursa toward the hilum of the spleen.

r. membra'nae tym'pani ante'rior [NA], anterior recess of tympanic membrane; Tröltsch's pocket or recess; a slitlike space on the tympanic wall between the anterior malleolar fold and the tympanic membrane.

r. membra'nae tym'pani poste'rior [NA], posterior recess of tympanic membrane; Tröltsch's pocket or recess; a narrow pocket in the tympanic wall between the posterior malleolar fold and the tympanic membrane.

r. membra'nae tym'pani supe'rior [NA], superior recess of tympanic membrane; Prussak's pouch or space; a space in the mucous membrane on the inner surface of the tympanic membrane between the flaccid part of the membrane and the neck of the malleus.

r. op'ticus [NA], optic recess; a diverticulum extending forward from the anterior part of the third ventricle above the optic chiasm.

r. paraduodena'lis [NA], paraduodenal recess; paraduodenal fossa; fossa venosa; an occasional recess in the peritoneum to the left of the terminal portion of the duodenum located behind a fold containing the inferior mesenteric vein.

r. parotide'us, parotid *recess.*

r. pharyn'geus [NA], pharyngeal recess; r. infundibuliformis; Rosenmüller's recess or fossa; a slitlike depression in the pharyngeal wall behind the opening of the auditory (eustachian) tube.

r. phrenicomediastina'lis [NA], phrenicomediastinal recess; the recess of the pleural cavity between the diaphragm and the mediastinum.

r. pinea'lis [NA], pineal recess; a diverticulum from the posterior part of the third ventricle extending back between the posterior commissure and the habenular commissure.

r. pirifor'mis [NA], piriform recess; piriform fossa or sinus; a recess in the pharynx on each side of the opening of the larynx.

r. pleura'les [NA], pleural recesses or sinuses; three recesses of the pleural cavity, one behind the sternum and costal cartilages (r. costomediastinalis), one between the diaphragm and chest wall (r. costodiaphragmaticus), and one between the diaphragm and mediastinum (r. phrenicomediastinalis).

r. poste'rior, a deepening of the interpeduncular fossa toward the pons.

r. retroceca'lis [NA], retrocecal or cecal recess; one of several small pockets sometimes found extending alongside the right margin of the ascending colon near the cecum.

r. retroduodena'lis [NA], retroduodenal recess or fossa; infraduodenal fossa; a peritoneal recess occasionally found behind the third part of the duodenum, between it and the aorta.

r. saccifor'mis, sacciform recess; **(1)** [NA], an extension of the cavity of the distal radioulnar articulation proximad between the two bones; **(2)** an extension of the capsule of the elbow joint at the neck of the radius.

r. sphenoethmoida'lis [NA], sphenoethmoidal recess; a small cleftlike pocket in the superior meatus of the nasal cavity above the superior concha.

r. spher'icus [NA], spherical recess; fovea hemispherica; fovea spherica; a rounded depression on the inner wall of the vestibule of the labyrinth, lodging the sacculus.

r. subhepat'ici [NA], subhepatic recess; the part of the peritoneal cavity between the visceral surface of the liver and the transverse colon.

r. subphren'ici [NA], subphrenic recesses; suprahepatic spaces; the recesses in the peritoneal cavity between the anterior part of the liver and the diaphragm, separated into right and left by the falciform ligament.

r. subpoplite'us [NA], subpopliteal recess; bursa of popliteus; the extension of the cavity of the knee joint between the tendon of the popliteus and lateral condyle of the femur.

r. supe'rior omenta'lis [NA], superior omental recess; a portion of the vestibule of the bursa omentalis that extends upward between the inferior vena cava and the esophagus.

r. suprapinea'lis [NA], suprapineal recess; a variable diverticulum from the posterior portion of the third ventricle of the brain, running backward some distance above and beyond the pineal r.

r. triangula'ris, triangular *recess.*

recidivation (rē-sid-i-vā'shŭn) [L. *recidivus,* falling back, recurring, fr. *re- cido,* to fall back]. Relapse of a disease, a symptom, or a behavioral pattern such as an illegal activity for which one was previously imprisoned.

recidivism (rē-sid'i-vizm) [L. *recidivus,* recurring]. The tendency of an individual toward recidivation.

recidivist (rē-sid'i-vist). A person who tends toward recidivation.

recipe (res'i-pē) [L. imperative *recipio,* to receive]. **1.** Take; the superscription of a prescription, usually indicated by the sign ℞ **2.** A prescription or formula.

recipiomotor (rē-sip'ē-ō-mō'ter) [L. *recipio,* to receive, + *motor,* mover]. Relating to the reception of motor stimuli.

reciprocation (rē-sip-rō-kā'shŭn) [L. *reciprocare,* pp. *reciprocatus,* to move back and forth]. In prosthodontics, the means by which one part of an appliance is made to counter the effect created by another part.

Recklinghausen, Friedrich D. von, German histologist and pathologist, 1833–1910. See R.'s *disease, disease* of bone, *tumor.*

reclination (rek-li-nā'shŭn) [L. *reclino,* pp. *-atus,* to bend back]. Turning the cataractous lens over into the vitreous to displace it from the line of vision; distinguished from couching, in which the lens is simply depressed into the vitreous.

recollection (rē-kō-lek'shŭn) [re- + L. *collectus,* pp. of *colligo,* to collect]. In renal physiology, a technique in which a known fluid is infused into a renal tubule lumen at one point and collected for analysis by a second micropipette further downstream.

recombinant (rē-kom'bi-nant). **1.** A microbe, or strain, that has received chromosomal parts from different parental strains. **2.** Pertaining to or denoting such organisms.

recombinant DNA. DNA resulting from the insertion into the chain, by chemical or biological means, of a sequence (a whole or partial chain of DNA) not originally (biologically) present in that chain.

recombination (rē-kom-bi-nā'shŭn). The process of reuniting of parts that had become separated.
genetic r., in microbial genetics, the inclusion of a chromosomal part or extrachromosomal element of one microbial strain in the chromosome of another; the interchange of chromosomal parts between different microbial strains.

recon (rē'kon). Rarely used term for the smallest unit (corresponding to a single DNA nucleotide) of recombination or crossing-over between two homologous chromosomes.

reconstitution (rē'kon-sti-tū'shŭn). **1.** The restitution or return to an original state of a substance, or combination of parts to make a whole. **2.** In the case of a lower organism, the restoration of a part of the body by regeneration.

record (rek'erd). **1.** In medicine, a chronologic written account that includes a patient's initial complaint(s) and medical history, the physician's physical findings, the results of diagnostic tests and procedures, and any therapeutic medications and/or procedures. **2.** In dentistry, a registration of desired jaw relations in a plastic material or on a device in order that such relations may be transferred to an articulator.
anesthesia r., a written account of drugs administered, procedures undertaken, and cardiovascular responses during the course of surgical or obstetrical anesthesia.
face-bow r., a registration by means of a face-bow of the position of the hinge axis and/or the condyles; the face-bow r. is used to orient the maxillary cast to the opening and closing axis of the articulator.
functional chew-in r., a r. of the natural chewing movements of the mandible made on an occlusion rim by teeth or scribing studs.
hospital r., the medical r. generated during a period of hospitalization, usually including written accounts of consultants' opinions as well as nurses' observations and treatments.
interocclusal r., checkbite; a r. of the positional relationship of the teeth or jaws to each other, recorded by placing a plastic material which hardens (such as plaster of Paris, wax, etc.) between the occlusal surfaces of the rims or teeth; the hardened material serves as the r.; it may be registered in centric or eccentric positions, as **centric i. r.,** a r. of centric jaw relation; **eccentric i. r.,** a r. of jaw position in other than centric relation; **lateral i. r.,** a r. of a lateral eccentric jaw position; and **protrusive i. r.,** a r. of a protruded eccentric jaw position.
maxillomandibular r., biscuit bite; maxillomandibular registration; **(1)** a r. of the relation of the mandible to the maxillae; **(2)** the act of recording the relation of the mandible to the maxillae.
medical r., see record (1).
occluding centric relation r., a registration of centric relation made at the established occlusal vertical dimension.
preextraction r., preoperative r.
preoperative r., pre-extraction r.; in dentistry, any r. made for the purpose of study or treatment planning. See also diagnostic *cast.*
problem-oriented r. (POR), a system of record keeping in which a list of the patient's problems is created and all history, physical findings, laboratory data, etc. pertinent to each problem are placed under that heading; especially useful for out-patient records of patients with multiple problems who are followed for long periods.
profile r., a registration or r. of the profile of a patient.
protrusive r., a registration of a forward position of the mandible with reference to the maxillae.
terminal jaw relation r., a r. of the relationship of the mandible to the maxillae made at the vertical relation of occlusion and at the centric position.
three-dimensional r., a maxillomandibular r. made at the occluding relation.

recording (rē-kōrd'ing). Preserving the results of a study.
clinical r., charting.
depth r., study of subcortical cerebral electrical activity after placing electrodes in these areas.

recovery (rē-kŏv'er-ē). **1.** A getting back or regaining; recuperation. **2.** Emergence from general anesthesia.
creep r., the time-dependent portion of the decrease in strain in a material or object following removal of the stress that has deformed it.
spontaneous r., the return of the conditioned response, after apparent extinction, in the presence of the conditioned stimulus without the unconditioned stimulus also being present.
ultrasonic egg r., obtaining an egg for *in vitro* fertilization by means of an ultrasonically guided needle biopsy of the ovary; may be performed transvesically or via the cul-de-sac.

recovery room. A hospital facility with special equipment and personnel for the immediate postoperative care of patients as they recover from anesthesia and surgery.

recrudescence (rē-krū-des'ens) [L. *re-crudesco,* to become raw again, break out afresh, fr. *crudus,* raw, harsh]. Resumption of a morbid process or its symptoms after a period of remission.

recrudescent (rē-krū-des'ent). Becoming active again, relating to a recrudescence.

recruitment (rē-krūt'ment) [Fr. *recrutement,* fr. L. *re-cresco,* pp. *-cretus,* to grow again]. **1.** A term used in the testing of hearing: the unequal reaction of the ear to equal steps of increasing intensity, measured in decibels, when such inequality of response results in a greater than normal increment of loudness. **2.** Recruiting response; the bringing into activity of additional motor neurons and thus causing greater activity in response to increased duration of the stimulus applied to a given receptor or afferent nerve. See also irradiation (4). **3.** The adding of parallel channels of flow in any system.

rect-. See recto-.

rectal (rek'tăl). Relating to the rectum.

rectalgia (rek-tal'jē-ă). Proctalgia.

rectectomy (rek-tek'tō-mē). Proctectomy.

rectify (rek'ti-fī) [L. *rectus,* right, straight]. **1.** To correct. **2.** To purify or refine by distillation; usually implies repeated distillations.

rectitis (rek-tī'tis). Proctitis.

recto-, rect- [L. *rectum,* fr. *rectus,* straight]. Combining forms denoting the rectum. See also procto-.

rectoabdominal (rek'tō-ab-dom'i-năl). Relating to the rectum and the abdomen; denoting a bimanual method of examination with one hand on the abdominal wall and a finger of the other hand in the rectum.

rectocele (rek'tō-sēl) [recto- + G. *kēlē,* tumor, hernia]. Proctocele.

rectoclysis (rek-tok'li-sis). Proctoclysis.

rectococcygeal (rek-tō-kok-sij'ē-ăl). Relating to the rectum and the coccyx.

rectococcypexy (rek-tō-kok'si-pek-sē). Proctococcypexy.

rectocolitis (rek'tō-kō-lī'tis). Coloproctitis.

rectoperineal (rek'tō-per-i-nē'ăl). Relating to the rectum and perineum.

rectoperineorrhaphy (rek'tō-per-i-nē-ōr'a-fē). Proctoperineoplasty.

rectopexy (rek'tō-pek-sē). Proctopexy.

rectophobia (rek-tō-fō'bē-ă) [recto- + G. *phobos,* fear]. Proctophobia.

rectoplasty (rek'tō-plas-tē). Proctoplasty.

rectorrhaphy (rek-tōr'ă-fē). Proctorrhaphy.

rectoscope (rek'tō-skōp). Proctoscope.

rectoscopy (rek-tos'kŏ-pē). Proctoscopy.

rectosigmoid (rek'tō-sig'moyd). The rectum and sigmoid colon considered as a unit; the term is also applied to the junction of the sigmoid colon and rectum.

rectostenosis (rek'tō-stĕ-nō'sis). Proctostenosis.

rectostomy (rek-tos'tō-mē). Proctostomy.

rectotome (rek'tō-tōm). Proctotome.

rectotomy (rek-tot'ō-mē). Proctotomy.

rectourethral (rek-tō-yū-rē'thrăl). Relating to the rectum and the urethra.

rectouterine (rek-tō-yū'ter-in). Relating to the rectum and the uterus.

rectovaginal (rek-tō-vaj'i-năl). Relating to the rectum and the vagina.

rectovesical (rek-tō-ves'i-kăl). Relating to the rectum and the bladder.

rectovestibular (rek'tō-ves-tib'yū-lăr). Relating to the rectum and the vestibule of the vagina.

rectum, pl. **rectums** or **recta** (rek'tŭm, rek'tă) [L. *rectus,* straight, pp. of *rego,* to make straight] [NA]. The terminal portion of the digestive tube, extending from the sigmoid colon to the anal canal.

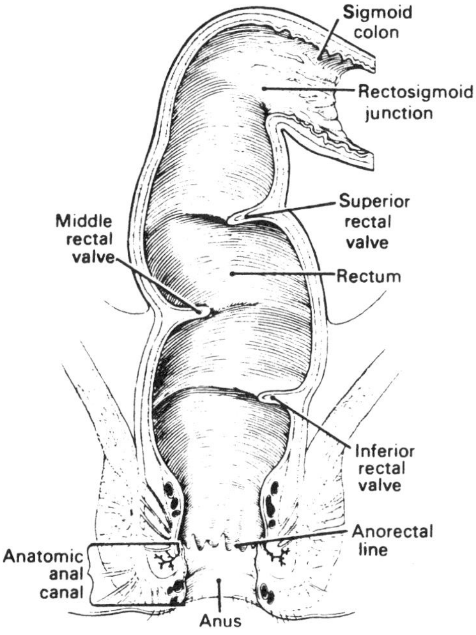

Rectum

recumbent (rē-kŭm'bent) [L. *recumbo,* to lie back, recline, fr. *re-,* back, + *cubo,* to lie]. Leaning; reclining; lying down.

recuperate (rē-kū'per-āt) [L. *recupero* (or *recip-*), pp. *-atus,* to take again, recover]. To undergo recuperation.

recuperation (rē-kū-per-ā'shŭn) [L. *recuperatio* (see recuperate)]. Recovery of or restoration to the normal state of health and function.

recurrence (rē-kŭr'ens) [L. *re-curro,* to run back, recur]. **1.** A return of the symptoms, occurring as a phenomenon in the natural history of the disease, as seen in recurrent fever. **2.** Relapse. **3.** Appearance of a genetic trait in a genetic relative of a proband.

recurrent (rē-kŭr'ent). **1.** In anatomy, turning back on itself. **2.** Denoting symptoms or lesions reappearing after an intermission or remission.

recurvation (rē-ker-vā'shŭn) [L. *re-curvus,* bent back]. A backward bending or flexure.

red [A.S. *reád*]. One of the primary colors, occupying the lower extremity of the spectrum at the other end from violet. For individual red dyes, see specific name.

Red Cross. A red Geneva cross on a white background, an international sign to identify medical and other personnel caring for the sick and wounded and facilities devoted to their care in times of war, also the emblem of the American Red Cross.

redia, pl. **rediae** (rē'dē-ă, -dē-ē) [F. *Redi*]. Intramolluscan development stage of a digenetic trematode, following the primary sporocyst stage, which forms after penetration of the snail tissues by the miracidium. Rediae are produced from cells within the sporocyst, are liberated from the latter, and develop in the tissues of the host snail as elongated, saclike, muscular organisms with a mouth and gut. The rediae may produce one or a number of additional generations in the snail, but they ultimately produce the final development stage, the cercaria. See also sporocyst (1); miracidium.

redifferentiation (rē-dif'er-en'shē-ā'shŭn). The return to a fully specialized condition for the performance of a particular function after a period of nonspecific activity.

redintegration (rē'din-tē-grā'shŭn) [L. *red-integro,* pp. *-atus,* to make whole again, renew, fr. *integer,* untouched, entire]. **1.** The restoration of lost or injured parts. **2.** Restoration to health. **3.** The recalling of a whole experience on the basis of a stimulus representing some item or portion of the original circumstances of the experience.

Redlich, Emil, Austrian neurologist, 1866–1930. See Obersteiner-R. *line, zone.*

redox (red'oks). Contraction of oxidation-reduction. See oxidation-reduction *potential.*

redressement forcé (rē-dres-mon' fōr-sā') [Fr.]. Straightening by force of a deformed part, as of knock-knee.

redressment (rē-dres'ment). **1.** Correction of a deformity; putting a part straight. **2.** A renewed dressing of a wound.

reduce (rē-dūs') [L. *re-duco,* to lead back, restore, reduce]. **1.** To perform reduction (1). **2.** In chemistry, to initiate reduction (2).

reducible (rē-dūs'i-bl). Capable of being reduced.

reductant (rē-dŭk'tant). The substance that is oxidized in the course of reduction.

reductase (rē-dŭk'tās). Reducing enzyme; an enzyme that catalyzes a reduction; since all enzymes catalyze reactions in either direction, any r. can, under the proper conditions, behave as an oxidase and vice versa, hence the term oxidoreductase. For individual r.'s, see the specific names.

reductic acid (rē-dŭk'tik). 2,3-Dihydroxy-2-cyclo-penten-1-one; a strong reducing product (antioxidant) formed in hot alkaline sugar solutions.

reduction (rē-dŭk'shŭn) [L. *reductio,* fr. *re-duco,* pp. *ductus,* to lead back]. **1.** Repositioning; the restoration, by surgical or manipulative procedures, of a part to its normal anatomical relation. **2.** In chemistry, a reaction involving a gain of one or more electrons by a substance, as when iron passes from the ferric (3+) to the ferrous (2+) state, or when hydrogen is added to the double bond of an organic compound, or when an aldehyde is converted to an alcohol.

r. of chromosomes, the process occurring during the meiotic cell division in gametogenesis whereby one member of each homologous pair of chromosomes is distributed to each sperm or ovum; the somatic number of chromosomes (46 in humans) is thus reduced to the haploid number (23 in humans) in each gamete; union of the sperm and ovum then restores the diploid or somatic number in the one-cell zygote.

closed r. of fractures, r. by manipulation of bone, without incision in the skin.

r. en masse, r. of hernial sac and contents, so that intestinal obstruction is still present.

open r. of fractures, r. by manipulation of bone, after incision in skin and muscle over the site of the fracture.

tuberosity r., the surgical excision of excessive fibrous or bony tissue in the area of the maxillary tuberosity prior to the construction of prosthetic appliances.

reduplication (rē'dū'pli-kā'shŭn) [L. *reduplicatio,* fr. *re-,* again, + *duplico,* to double, fr. *duplex,* two-fold]. **1.** A redoubling. **2.** A duplication or doubling, as of the sounds of the heart in certain morbid states or the presence of two instead of a normally, single part. **3.** A fold or duplicature.

reduviid (rē-dū'vĭ-id). A member of the family Reduviidae.

Reduviidae (rē-dū-vī'i-dē). A family (order Hemiptera) of predatory insects, the assassin bugs, which attack animals and humans. It includes the subfamily Triatominae, the kissing or conenosed bugs, whose type genus *Triatoma* includes species that are vectors of *Trypanosoma cruzi.*

Reed, Dorothy M., U.S. pathologist, 1874–1964. See R. *cells;* R.-Sternberg *cells.*

reefing (rēf'ing). Surgically reducing the extent of a tissue by folding it and securing with sutures, as in plication.

stomach r., gastroplication.

reenactment (rē-en-akt'ment). In psychodrama, the acting out of a past experience.

Reenstierna, John, Swedish dermatologist, *1882. See Ito-R. *test.*

reentry (rē-en'trē). Return of the same impulse into an area of heart muscle that it has recently activated but which is now no longer refractory, as seen in reciprocal rhythms.

Rees, H.M. See R.-Ecker *fluid.*

Reese, Algernon B., U.S. ophthalmologist, 1896–1981. See Cogan-R. *syndrome.*

refection (rē-fek'shŭn) [L. *refectio,* fr. *reficere,* to restore, fr. *re-* + *facio,* to do]. A restoring to the normal state.

Refetoff, S. See R. *syndrome.*

refine (rē-fīn'). To free from impurities.

reflect (rē-flekt') [L. *re- flecto,* pp. *-flexus,* to bend back]. **1.** To bend back. **2.** To throw back, as of radiant energy from a surface. **3.** To meditate; to think over a matter. **4.** To send back a motor impulse in response to a sensory stimulus. **5.** In psychotherapy, to repeat the patient's last phrase as a stimulus to him to continue his discourse.

reflection (rē-flek'shŭn) [L. *reflexio,* a bending back]. **1.** the act of reflecting. **2.** That which is reflected.

reflector (rē-flek'ter). Any surface that reflects light, heat, or sound.

REFLEX

reflex (rē'fleks) [L. *reflexus,* pp. of *re-flecto,* to bend back]. **1.** An involuntary reaction in response to a stimulus applied to the periphery and transmitted to the nervous centers in the brain or spinal cord. Most of the deep r.'s listed as subentries are stretch or myotatic r.'s, elicited by striking a tendon or bone, causing stretching, even slight, of the muscle which then contracts as a result of the stimulus applied to its proprioceptors. See also phenomenon. **2.** A reflection. **3.** Consensual.

abdominal r.'s, supraumbilical r. (2); contraction of the muscles of the abdominal wall upon stimulation of the skin (superficial a. r.'s) or tapping neighboring bony structures (deep a. r.'s).

abdominocardiac r., mechanical stimulation of the abdominal viscera causing changes (usually a slowing) in the heart rate or the occurrence of extrasystoles.

Abrams' heart r., a contraction of the myocardium when the skin of the precordial region is irritated.

accommodation r., increased convexity of the lens, due to contraction of the ciliary muscle and relaxation of the suspensory ligament, to maintain a distinct retinal image.

Achilles r., Achilles tendon r., ankle jerk or r.; tendo Achillis r.; triceps surae r.; a contraction of the calf muscles when the tendo calcaneus is sharply struck.

acousticopalpebral r., cochleopalpebral r.

acquired r., conditioned r.

acromial r., contraction of the biceps muscle caused by a tap on the acromion or the coracoid process.

adductor r., contraction of the adductors of the thigh caused by tapping the tendon of the adductor magnus muscle while the thigh is abducted.

allied r.'s, r.'s which, acting toward a common purpose, can traverse the final common path together.

anal r., contraction of the internal sphincter gripping the finger passed into the rectum.

ankle r., Achilles r.

antagonistic r.'s, r.'s which do not act toward a common purpose, and cannot together traverse the final common path.

aortic r., cardiac depressor r.

aponeurotic r., plantar flexion of the foot and toes elicited by tapping the sole near its outer edge; has the same significance as the Rossolimo toe flexion r. Also called Guillain-Barré, Weingrow's, or sole tap r.

Aschner's r., oculocardiac r.

Aschner-Dagnini r., oculocardiac r.

attitudinal r.'s, statotonic r.'s.

auditory r., any r. occurring in response to a sound, *e.g.,* cochleopalpebral r.

auditory oculogyric r., rotation of the eyes toward the source of a sudden sound.

auricular r., a movement of the ears in animals in response to a sound; part of the investigatory r.

auriculopalpebral r., Kisch's r.

auriculopressor r., Pavlov's r.; peripheral vasoconstriction and a rise in blood pressure in response to a fall in pressure in the great veins.

auropalpebral r., cochleopalpebral r.

axon r., an effect brought about by the passage of the nerve impulses from a sensory ending to the effector organ along divisions of a nerve fiber without traversing a nerve cell, *e.g.,* as in the vasodilation resulting from stimulation of the skin or the irritation of the conjunctiva; the reaction occurs even when the nerve fiber has been sectioned and thus isolated from the nervous centers.

Babinski r., Babinski's *sign* (1).

back (dorsum) of foot r., Mendel's instep r.

Bainbridge r., an increase in heart rate caused by a rise in pressure of the blood in the great veins at the entrance to the right atrium.

Barkman's r., contraction of the ipsilateral rectus muscle in response to a stimulus applied to the skin below a nipple.

basal joint r., finger-thumb or Mayer's r.; opposition and adduction of the thumb with flexion at its metacarpophalangeal joint and extension at its interphalangeal joint, when firm passive flexion of the third, fourth, or fifth finger is made; the r. is present normally but is absent in pyramidal lesions.

Bechterew-Mendel r., Mendel-Bechterew r.; dorsum pedis r.; percussion of the dorsum of the foot causes flexion of the toes; present

in a pyramidal lesion.
behavior r., conditioned r.
Benedek's r., plantar flexion of the foot by tapping the anterior margin of the lower part of the fibula, while the foot is slightly dorsiflexed.
Bezold-Jarisch r., a r. with afferent and efferent pathways in the vagus, originating in unidentified chemoreceptors in the heart and resulting in sinus bradycardia, hypotension, and probable peripheral vasodilation.
biceps r., contraction of the biceps muscle when its tendon is struck.
biceps femoris r., contraction of the biceps femoris upon tapping its lower part, just above its attachment to the head of the fibula, while the limb is partly flexed at hip and knee.
Bing's r., when the foot is passively dorsiflexed, plantar flexion occurs if any point on the ankle between the two malleoli is tapped.
bladder r., micturition r.
body righting r.'s, r. effects upon the neck muscles which bring the head into the correct position in space caused by stimulation of pressoreceptors in the body wall by contact with the ground.
bone r., a r. excited by a stimulus applied to a bone.
brachioradial r., with the arm supinated to 45° a tap near the lower end of the radius causes contraction of the brachioradial (supinator longus) muscle. Also called supinator jerk or r.; supination, styloradial, supinator longus, or radioperiosteal r.
Brain's r., quadripedal extensor r.
bregmocardiac r., in infants, pressure upon the anterior fontanelle causing cardiac slowing.
Brissaud's r., tickling the sole causes a contraction of the tensor fasciae latae muscle, even when there is no responsive movement of the toes.
bulbocavernosus r., a sharp contraction of the bulbocavernosus and ischiocavernosus muscles when the glans penis is suddenly compressed or tapped.
bulbomimic r., facial r.; Mondonesi's r.; in a case of coma from severe apoplexy, pressure on the eyeballs causes contraction of the facial muscles of expression on the side opposite to the lesion; in coma due to diabetes, uremia, or other toxic cause the r. is present on both sides.
Capps' r., Obsolete eponym for vasomotor collapse at the time of crisis in pneumonia.
cardiac depressor r., aortic or depressor r.; a fall in blood pressure due to peripheral vasodilation and cardiac inhibition by stimulations of terminations of a cardiac depressor nerve in the aortic arch and base of the heart.
carotid sinus r., carotid sinus *syndrome.*
celiac plexus r., arterial hypotension coincident with surgical manipulations in the upper abdomen during general anesthesia.
cephalic r.'s, r.'s associated with the cranial nerves.
cephalopalpebral r., contraction of the orbicularis muscle elicited by tapping the vertex of the skull.
cerebropupillary r., Haab's r.
Chaddock r., Chaddock *sign.*
chain r., a series of r.s, each serving as a stimulus for the next.
chin r., jaw r.
Chodzko's r., contractions of several muscles of the shoulder girdle and arm when the manubrium sterni is percussed.
ciliospinal r., pupillary-skin r.
clasping r., the strong flexion of the forelimbs of amphibia and certain other animals during the mating season when the chest or abdomen is stimulated; it is dependent upon the male sex hormone.
cochleo-orbicular r., cochleopalpebral r.
cochleopalpebral r., acousticopalpebral, auropalpebral, or cochleo-orbicular r.; startle r. (2); a form of the wink r. in which there is a contraction, sometimes very slight, of the orbicularis palpebrarum muscle when a sudden noise is made close to the ear; it is absent in labyrinthine disease with total deafness.
cochleopupillary r., constriction of the pupil in response to a sudden loud sound.
cochleostapedial r., contraction of the stapedius muscle in response to a loud sound; this is a protective r. which with the r. contraction of the tensor tympani reduces the amplitude of the vibrations of the tympanic membrane and ossicles.
conditioned r. (CR), acquired, behavior, or trained r.; a r. that is gradually developed by training and association through the frequent repetition of a definite stimulus.
conjunctival r., closure of the eyes in response to irritation of the conjunctiva.
consensual light r., consensual *reaction.*
contralateral r., Brudzinski's *sign* (1).
convulsive r., an incoordinated r. in which muscles, even those opposing one another as in strychnine poisoning, contract.
coordinated r., a r. in which several muscles take part in the performance of a purposeful act.
corneal r., **(1)** lid r.; a contraction of the eyelids when the cornea is lightly touched with a camel's hair pencil; **(2)** reflection of light from the surface of the cornea.
corticopupillary r., Haab's r.
costal arch r., contraction of the rectus abdominus muscle by tapping the costal margin inside the mammary line.
costopectoral r., pectoral r.
cough r., laryngeal r.; the r. which mediates coughing in response to irritation of the larynx or tracheobronchial tree.
craniocardiac r., stimulation of nerve endings of certain cranial nerves (*e.g.,* olfactory, ophthalmic branch of trigeminal), with resultant cardiac depressor r., manifested by bradycardia and hypotension, through the cardiac branch of the vagus.
cremasteric r., a drawing up of the scrotum and testicle of the same side when the skin over Scarpa's triangle or on the inner side of the thigh is scratched.
crossed r., crossed jerk; a r. movement on one side of the body in response to a stimulus applied to the opposite side.
crossed adductor r., crossed adductor jerk; contraction of the adductors of the thigh and inward rotation of the limb elicited by tapping the sole.
crossed extension r., extension of the contralateral hind limb when the paw of an animal is painfully stimulated or the central cut end of an afferent nerve, *e.g.,* the peroneal, is stimulated; sometimes occurs in man upon tapping the skin.
crossed knee r., crossed knee jerk; contraction of the contralateral quadriceps when a patellar r. is elicited.
crossed r. of pelvis, crossed spino-adductor r.; contraction of the contralateral adductors of the thigh upon tapping the anterior superior iliac spine.
crossed spino-adductor r., crossed r. of pelvis.
cry r., a sudden unconscious cry, during sleep, in a child with hip disease, long bone fractures, or other painful conditions of the extremities, elicited by movement of muscles that have relaxed after prolonged muscle spasms.
cuboidodigital r., metatarsal r.; flexion of the toes on tapping over the cuboid bone; almost identical with Guillain-Barré r., and fundamentally similar to Rossolimo's r.
cutaneous r., wrinkling of the skin, caused by a cutaneous stimulus, due to contraction of arrectores pilorum muscles.
cutaneous pupil r., cutaneous-pupillary r., pupillary-skin r.
darwinian r., the tendency of young infants to grasp a bar and hang suspended. *Cf.* grasping r.
deep r., jerk (2); an involuntary muscular contraction following percussion of a tendon or bone.
deep abdominal r.'s, contraction of abdominal muscles elicited by stimulation, such as tapping a deep structure; *e.g.,* the costal margin. See also Galant's r. (lower abdominal periosteal r.); upper abdominal periosteal r.
defense r., **(1)** flexor r.; **(2)** automatic reactions of an animal, *e.g.,*

raising of hair or feathers, dilation of the pupils, or baring of claws, when alarmed.
deglutition r., swallowing r.
Dejerine's r., Déjérine's hand *phenomenon.*
delayed r., a r. in which a little time elapses between stimulus and response. See also trace conditioned r.
depressor r., cardiac depressor r.
diffused r., one of several r.'s occurring in association with the main r.
digital r., Hoffmann's *sign* (2).
diving r., a r. by which immersing the face or body in water, especially cold water, tends to cause bradycardia and peripheral vasoconstriction; mean aortic pressure is little affected because the reduction in cardiac output tends to balance the increased peripheral resistance that reduces peripheral blood flow. Although relatively minor in most humans, the changes can be profound in some diving species of animal, *e.g.,* ducks and seals.
dorsal r., contraction of the muscles of the back elicited by cutaneous stimulation over the erector spinal muscle.
dorsum pedis r., Bechterew-Mendel r.
elbow r., triceps r.
enterogastric r., peristaltic contraction of the small intestine induced by the entrance of food into the stomach. See also gastrocolic r.
epigastric r., supraumbilical r. (1); a contraction of the upper portion of the rectus abdominis muscle when the skin of the epigastrium above is scratched.
erector-spinal r., a contraction of part of the erector spinae muscle following scratching of the skin on its outer border.
esophagosalivary r., Roger's r.; salivation caused by irritation of the lower end of the esophagus, as by carcinoma.
external oblique r., contraction of the external oblique and rectus abdominus muscles upon tapping the anterior and outer part of the lower thoracic wall.
eye r., light r. (2).
eye-closure r., wink r.
facial r., bulbomimic r.
faucial r., gag r.
femoral r., scratching the skin of the upper part of the front of the thigh causes extension of the knee and flexion of the foot.
femoroabdominal r., hypogastric r.; contraction of the abdominal muscles upon stroking the inner aspect of the thigh; in association with the cremasteric r.
finger-thumb r., basal joint r.
flexor r., withdrawal r.; nociceptive r.; defense r. (1); flexion of ankle, knee, and hip when the foot is painfully stimulated; the crossed extension r. occurs in association with it.
forced grasping r., grasping r.
front-tap r., periosteal r. (1); contraction of the gastrocnemius muscle when the shin is struck.
fundus r., light r. (2).
gag r., faucial r.; contact of a foreign body with the mucous membrane of the fauces causes retching or gagging.
Galant's r., lower abdominal periosteal r.; a deep abdominal r. in which there is a contraction of the abdominal muscles on tapping the anterior superior iliac spine.
galvanic skin r., galvanic skin *response.*
gastrocolic r., a mass movement of the contents of the colon, frequently preceded by a similar movement in the small intestine, that sometimes occurs immediately following the entrance of food into the stomach.
gastroileac r., opening of the ileocolic valve induced by entrance of food into the stomach.
Geigel's r., in the female, a contraction of the muscular fibers at the upper edge of Poupart's ligament on gently stroking the inner side of the thigh; analogue of the cremasteric r. in males.
Gifford's r., constriction of the pupils when an attempt is made to close the eyes while the lids are held open.
gluteal r., contraction of the gluteal muscles following irritation of the skin of the buttocks.
Gordon r., paradoxical flexor r.; dorsal flexion of the great toe produced by firm lateral pressure on the calf muscles.
grasp r., grasping r.
grasping r., grasp r.; forced grasping r.; an involuntary flexion of the fingers to tactile or tendon stimulation on the palm of the hand, producing an uncontrollable grasp; usually associated with frontal lobe lesions. *Cf.* darwinian r.
great-toe r., Babinski's *sign* (1).
Guillain-Barré r., aponeurotic r.
gustatory-sudorific r., sweating, especially over the face, when chewing food. See also auriculotemporal *syndrome.*
H r., a monosynaptic r. obtained by stimulating the tibial nerve; it short-circuits the neuromuscular spindle.
Haab's r., cerebropupillary or corticopupillary r.; constriction of the pupils when a dark-adapted subject looks at a bright object.
heart r., reduction of the cardiac area when the skin of the precordial region is irritated.
hepatojugular r., see hepatojugular *reflux.*
Hering-Breuer r., the effects of afferent impulses from the pulmonary vagi in the control of respiration, *e.g.,* inflation of the lungs arrests inspiration with expiration then ensuing, while deflation of the lungs brings on inspiration.
Hoffmann's r., Hoffmann's *sign* (2).
hypochondrial r., a quick inspiration induced by sharp pressure beneath the costal margin.
hypogastric r., femoroabdominal r.
innate r., unconditioned r.
interscapular r., scapular r.
intrinsic r., a r. muscular contraction elicited by the application of a stimulus, usually stretching, to the muscle itself as opposed to a muscular contraction caused by an extrinsic stimulus, *e.g.,* skin, as in the abdominal skin r.'s.
inverted r., paradoxical r.
inverted radial r., flexion of the fingers without flexion of the forearm, on tapping the lower end of the radius; regarded as indicating a lesion of the fifth cervical segment of the spinal cord.
investigatory r., orienting r.
ipsilateral r., a r. in which the response occurs on the side of the body that is stimulated.
Jacobson's r., flexion of the fingers elicited by tapping the flexor tendons over the wrist joint or the lower end of the radius.
jaw r., chin or jaw jerk; chin, mandibular, or masseter r.; a spasmodic contraction of the temporal muscles following a downward tap on the loosely hanging mandible.
jaw-working r., jaw-winking *syndrome.*
Joffroy's r., hip phenomenon; twitching of the glutei muscles when firm pressure is made on the nates, in cases of spastic paralysis.
Kisch's r., auriculopalpebral r.; closure of the eye in response to stimulation of the skin at the depth of the external auditory meatus.
knee r., patellar r.
knee-jerk r., patellar r.
labyrinthine r.'s, r.'s initiated through stimulation of receptors in the utricle or semicircular canals. See also statotonic, statokinetic, and righting r.'s.
labyrinthine righting r.'s, stimulation of the proprioceptors of the labyrinth causes changes in tone of the neck muscles which bring the head into its natural position in space.
lacrimal r., discharge of tears when the conjunctiva is irritated.
lacrimo-gustatory r., chewing of food causing secretion of tears. See also crocodile tears *syndrome.*
laryngeal r., cough r.
laryngospastic r., laryngospasm.

latent r., a r. which must be considered normal but which usually appears only under some pathologic circumstance that lowers its threshold.
laughter r., uncontrollable laughter excited by tickling.
lid r., corneal r. (1).
Liddell-Sherrington r., myotatic r.
light r., **(1)** pupillary r.; **(2)** fundus, light, or red r.; a red glow reflected from the fundus of the eye when a light is cast upon the retina, as in retinoscopy; **(3)** *pyramid* of light.
lip r., a pouting movement of the lips provoked in young infants by tapping near the angle of the mouth.
lordosis r., adoption of a copulatory posture when touched on the back; exhibited by female animals of certain species but only during the time of estrus.
Lovén r., a reaction in which a local dilation of vessels accompanies a general vasoconstriction; *e.g.,* when the central end of an afferent nerve to an organ is suitably stimulated, its efferent vasomotor fibers remaining intact, a general rise in blood pressure occurs together with a dilation of the vessels of the organ.
lower abdominal periosteal r., Galant's r.
magnet r., see magnet *reaction.*
mandibular r., jaw r.
mass r., in cases of gross injury to the spinal cord, as the stage of r. activity follows the primary flaccidity of the shock, a condition arises in which a strong stimulus to any part of one of the paralyzed limbs will be followed by contraction of the hip, knee, and ankle of the same side and often, when the stimulus is applied to the middle line of the body, of both sides, as well as of the abdominal wall, and even evacuation of the bladder and sweating over an area corresponding to the level of the lesion.
masseter r., jaw r.
Mayer's r., basal joint r.
McCarthy's r.'s, **(1)** spino-adductor r.; **(2)** supraorbital r.
mediopubic r., contraction of the adductors of the thigh upon tapping the pubic bone near the symphysis.
Mendel-Bechterew r., Bechterew-Mendel r.
Mendel's instep r., back (dorsum) of foot r.; the foot being firmly supported on its inner side, a sharp tap on the dorsal tendons causes extension of the second to the fifth toes.
metacarpohypothenar r., flexion of the little finger on tapping the dorsum of the hand; seen in pyramidal tract lesions and is similar to Starling's r.
metacarpothenar r., thumb r.
metatarsal r., cuboidodigital r.
micturition r., bladder, urinary, or vesical r.; contraction of the walls of the bladder and relaxation of the trigone and urethral sphincter in response to a rise in pressure within the bladder; the r. can be voluntarily inhibited and the inhibition readily abolished to control micturition.
milk-ejection r., release of milk from the breast following tactile stimulation of the nipple; the afferent path is postulated to exist from the nipple to the hypothalamus; the efferent limb is represented by the neurohypophysial release of oxytocin into the systemic circulation; contraction of myoepithelial elements within the breast, caused by oxytocin, moves milk into the collecting ducts and toward the nipple.
Mondonesi's r., bulbomimic r.
Moro r., startle r. (1).
muscular r., myotatic r.
myenteric r., law of intestine; contraction above and relaxation below a stimulated point in the intestine.
myotatic r., muscular, stretch, or Liddell-Sherrington r.; tonic contraction of the muscles in response to a stretching force, due to stimulation of muscle proprioceptors.
nasal r., sneezing caused by irritation of the nasal mucous membrane.
nasomental r., contraction of the mentalis muscle following a tap on the side of the nose.
near r., pupillary constriction with ocular convergence; an associated reaction, not a true r.
neck r.'s, changes in position of the head cause alterations in tone of the neck muscles through stimulation of proprioceptors in the labyrinth which bring the head into its correct position in space; stimulation of proprioceptors in the neck muscles causes in turn r. movements of the limbs which bring the animal into the normal position in relation to the head.
nociceptive r., flexor r.
nocifensor r., vascular dilation in a part surrounding an injury or in its neighborhood.
nose-bridge-lid r., orbicularis oculi r.
nose-eye r., orbicularis oculi r.
oculocardiac r., Aschner's r.; Aschner's phenomenon; Aschner-Dagnini r.; Ashley's phenomenon; a decrease in pulse rate associated with traction on extraocular muscles or compression of the eyeball.
oculocephalic r., oculocephalogyric r.
oculocephalogyric r., oculocephalic r.; turning of the eyes and head toward the source of an auditory, visual, or other form of stimulation.
olecranon r., paradoxical triceps r.; flexion of the forearm caused by tapping the olecranon.
Oppenheim's r., extension of the toes induced by scratching of the inner side of the leg or by following sudden flexion of the thigh on the abdomen and the leg on the thigh; a sign of cerebral irritation.
optical righting r.'s, visual stimuli that enable an animal to maintain the correct position of the head in space, by bringing about movements of the muscles of the neck and limbs.
opticofacial r., wink r.
orbicularis oculi r., nose-bridge-lid r.; nose-eye r.; contraction of the orbicularis oculi muscles upon tapping the margin of the orbit, or the bridge or tip of the nose.
orbicularis pupillary r., Galassi's pupillary phenomenon; constriction followed by dilation of the pupil upon forcible closure of the eyelids or on the attempt to close them while they are held apart.
orienting r., investigatory r.; orienting response; an aspect of attending in which an organism's initial response to a change or to a novel stimulus is such that the organism becomes more sensitive to the stimulation; *e.g.,* dilation of the pupil of the eye in response to dim light.
palatal r., palatine r., swallowing r. induced by stimulation of the palate.
palmar r., flexion of the fingers following tickling of the palm.
palm-chin r., palmomental r.
palmomental r., palm-chin r.; unilateral (sometimes bilateral) contraction of the mentalis and orbicularis oris muscles caused by a brisk scratch made on the palm of the ipsilateral hand.
parachute r., startle r.
paradoxical r., inverted r.; any r. in which the usual response is reversed or does not conform to the pattern characteristic of the particular r.
paradoxical extensor r., Babinski's *sign* (1).
paradoxical flexor r., Gordon r.
paradoxical patellar r., **(1)** a tap on the patellar tendon causes contraction of the adductor; **(2)** sudden passive extension of the leg causes a contraction of the extensor muscles of the leg.
paradoxical pupillary r., paradoxical pupillary phenomenon; a pupillary response to light, the reverse of that expected; *e.g.,* dilation of the pupil in response to photic stimulation.
paradoxical triceps r., olecranon r.
patellar r., a sudden contraction of the anterior muscles of the thigh, caused by a smart tap on the patellar tendon while the leg hangs loosely at a right angle with the thigh. Also called knee jerk; knee phenomenon; knee, knee-jerk, patellar tendon, or quadriceps r.

patellar tendon r., patellar r.
patello-adductor r., crossed adduction of the leg on tapping the quadriceps tendon.
Pavlov's r., auriculopressor r.
pectoral r., costopectoral r.; contraction of the pectoralis major muscle elicited by tapping the seventh rib between the anterior and the medial axillary lines while the arm is abducted; contraction of the deltoid and biceps may also occur.
Perez r., running a finger down the spine of an infant held supported in a prone position will normally cause the whole body to become extended.
pericardial r., a vagal r. seen during operations involving pericardial manipulation; characterized by signs of vagal stimulation (bradycardia and arterial hypotension).
periosteal r., **(1)** front-tap r.; **(2)** a muscular contraction in the arm following a tap on the radius or ulna.
pharyngeal r., **(1)** swallowing r.; **(2)** vomiting r.
phasic r., a coordinated complex response such as the scratch r. in the spinal animal.
Phillipson's r., a contraction of the extensors of the knee when the extensors of the opposite knee are inhibited.
pilomotor r., contraction of the smooth muscle of the skin resulting in "gooseflesh" caused by mild application of a tactile stimulus or by local cooling.
plantar r., sole r.; the response to tactile stimulation of the ball of the foot, normally plantar flexion of the toes; the pathologic response is Babinski's *sign* (1).

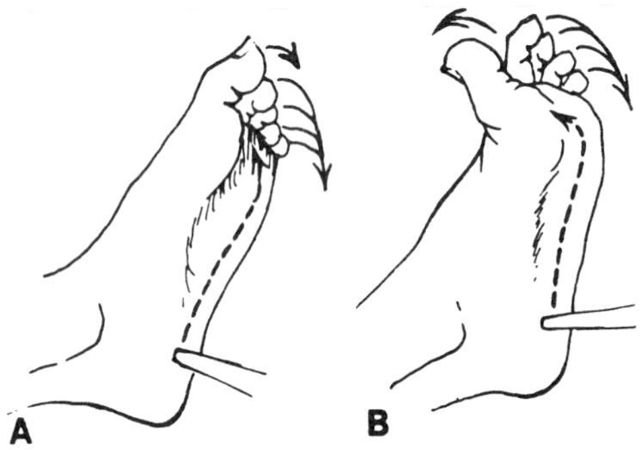

Plantar Reflex
A, normal; *B*, Babinski's sign.

plantar muscle r., Rossolimo's r. (1).
pneocardiac r., a modification in the blood pressure or heart rhythm caused by the inhalation of an irritating vapor.
pneopneic r., a modification of the respiratory rhythm caused by the inhalation of an irritating vapor.
postural r., static r. (1); responses that control the position of the trunk and extremities. See also righting r.
pressoreceptor r., carotid sinus *syndrome.*
pronator r., ulnar r.
proprioceptive r.'s, any r. brought about by stimulation of proprioceptors. See also proprioceptor.
proprioceptive-oculocephalic r., doll's eye *sign.*
protective laryngeal r., closure of the glottis to prevent entry of foreign substances into the respiratory tract.
psychocardiac r., a change in the circulatory rate and the consciousness of heart thumping resulting from a memory of, or a subconscious dream state recollection of, an emotional impression or experience.
psychogalvanic r., psychogalvanic skin r., galvanic skin *response.*
pulmonocoronary r., r. constriction of the coronary arteries as a result of vagal stimuli arising in the lungs, as in pulmonary embolism.
pupillary r., light r. (1); change in diameter of the pupil as a reflex response to any type of stimulus; *e.g.,* constriction caused by light.
pupillary-skin r., ciliospinal, cutaneous pupil, cutaneous-pupillary, or skin-pupillary r.; dilation of the pupil following scratching of the skin of the neck.
quadriceps r., patellar r.
quadripedal extensor r., Brain's r.; extension of the arm of a hemiplegic patient when turned prone as if on all fours.
radial r., on tapping the lower end of the radius, flexion of the forearm occurs, and sometimes, on strong percussion, flexion of the fingers. See also inverted radial r.
radiobicipital r., contraction of the biceps muscle which sometimes occurs in the elicitation of the brachioradial r.
radioperiosteal r., brachioradial r.
rectal r., the entrance of fecal matter into the rectum from the sigmoid colon causes an impulse to defecate.
rectocardiac r., a parasympathetic r. producing bradycardia and hypotension upon stimulation of the pelvic nerve, the afferent limb being the sacral outflow of the parasympathetic division of the autonomic nervous system, and the efferent limb, the cardiac vagus.
rectolaryngeal r., laryngeal spasm precipitated by stretching the anal sphincter.
red r., *pyramid* of light.
Remak's r., plantar flexion of the first three toes and, sometimes, the foot with extension of the knee induced by stroking of the upper anterior surface of the thigh; it occurs when the conducting paths in the cord are interrupted.
renal r., anuria caused by injury to a remote part of the body or by disease or injury to one kidney or ureter.
righting r.'s, static r. (2); r.'s which through various receptors, in labyrinth, eyes, muscles, or skin, tend to bring an animal's body into its normal position in space and which resist any force acting to put it into a false position, *e.g.,* on its back. See also neck r.'s; labyrinthine, optical, and body righting r.'s.
Roger's r., esophagosalivary r.
rooting r., in infants, rubbing or scratching about the mouth causes a puckering of the lips.
Rossolimo's r., Rossolimo's sign; **(1)** plantar muscle r.; flicking the tops of the toes from the plantar surface causes flexion of the toes; a stretch r. of the flexors of the toes seen in lesions of the pyramidal tracts; **(2)** Starling's reflex.
scapular r., interscapular r.; contraction of the upper muscles of the back by stimulation between the scapulae.
scapulohumeral r., scapuloperiosteal r.; contraction of muscles of the shoulder girdle and arm caused by tapping the lower part of the unilateral border of the scapula; the muscles which respond vary according to their degree of stretching at the time.
scapuloperiosteal r., scapulohumeral r.
Schäffer's r., in cases of injury to the corticospinal tract, the great toe is dorsiflexed when the skin over the Achilles tendon is pinched.
scratch r. in dogs, stimulus applied to the skin of a saddle-shaped area of the back, sides, and flanks produces a scratching movement of the hind leg of the side stimulated.
semimembranosus r., semitendinosus r., contraction of these muscles by tapping in the region of the tuberosity of the tibia.
shot-silk r., shot-silk *retina.*
sinus r., see carotid sinus *syndrome.*
skin r.'s, skin-muscle r.'s.
skin-muscle r.'s, skin r.'s; superficial or cutaneous r.'s, such as the superficial abdominal r.'s.
skin-pupillary r., pupillary-skin r.
snapping r., Hoffmann's *sign* (2).
snout r., pouting or pursing of the lips induced by light tapping of closed lips near the midline; seen in defective pyramidal innervation of facial musculature.

sole r., plantar r.
sole tap r., aponeurotic r.
spinal r., a r. arc involving the spinal cord. See reflex *arc.*
spino-adductor r., McCarthy's r. (1); contraction of the adductors of the thigh upon tapping the spinal column.
Starling's r., tapping the volar surfaces of the fingers causes flexion of the fingers; analogous to Rossolimo's r. (1), for the toes.
startle r., **(1)** Moro r.; parachute r.; startle reaction; the r. response of an infant (contraction of the limb and neck muscles) when allowed to drop a short distance through the air or startled by a sudden noise or jolt; **(2)** cochleopalpebral r.
static r., **(1)** postural r.; **(2)** righting r.
statokinetic r., a r. which, through stimulation of the receptors in the neck muscles and semicircular canals, brings about movements of the limbs and eyes appropriate to a given movement of the head in space.
statotonic r.'s, attitudinal r.'s; r.'s in which utricular receptors in the vestibular apparatus sense changes in the head's position in space in terms of linear acceleration and the earth's gravitational field while receptors in the neck muscles sense changes in the position of the head relative to the trunk; input from these receptors reflexly controls the tone of the limb muscles to maintain or regain the desired posture.
stepping r., if the plantar surface of a hind foot of a dog is pressed gently, a movement of extension of the limb will follow, accompanied sometimes by flexion of the opposite hind limb.
sternobrachial r., contraction of the adductors of the arm when the sternum is tapped.
stretch r., myotatic r.
Strümpell's r., stroking the abdomen or thigh causes flexion of the leg and adduction of the foot.
styloradial r., brachioradial r.
suckling r., the r. liberation of prolactin from the anterior lobe of the hypophysis evoked by stimulation of nerves in the nipple during the act of suckling by the newborn animal.
superficial r., any r., *e.g.,* the abdominal or cremasteric r., which is elicited by stimulation of the skin.
supination r., brachioradial r.
supinator r., supinator longus r., brachioradial r.
supporting r.'s, supporting *reactions.*
supraorbital r., McCarthy's r. (2); trigeminofacial r.; contraction of the orbicularis oculi muscle induced by tapping the supraorbital nerve.
suprapatellar r., the patella rises when a tap is given on the quadriceps tendon above the patella.
supraumbilical r., **(1)** epigastric r.; **(2)** abdominal r.'s.
swallowing r., deglutition r.; pharyngeal r. (1); the act of swallowing (second stage) induced by stimulation of the palate, fauces, or posterior pharyngeal wall.
synchronous r., subsidiary r. actions occurring in association with the main or leading r.
tapetal light r., the red glow from the eyes of some animals in the dark when a light illuminates the retina; due to the reflection of the light from the tapetum, an iridescent layer (containing guanidine crystals) in the choroid.
tarsophalangeal r., extension of all the toes except the first, when the outer part of the tarsus is tapped; in certain cerebral diseases the reverse takes place, the toes being flexed.
tendo Achillis r., Achilles r.
tendon r., a myotatic or deep r. in which the muscle stretch receptors are stimulated by percussing the tendon of a muscle.
thumb r., metacarpothenar r.; flexion of the thumb upon tapping the dorsum of the hand.
toe r., **(1)** strong passive flexion of the great toe excites contraction of the flexor muscles in the leg; **(2)** toe *clonus;* **(3)** Babinski's *sign* (1).
tonic r., Gordon's symptom; the occurrence of an appreciable interval after the production of a r. before relaxation, *e.g.,* the leg remains up for a time after a knee jerk.
trace conditioned r., a conditioned r. established by applying the stimulus a short time before reinforcement; in the conditioned r. of the animal so prepared, the response occurs at the same interval of time after the application of the stimulus as during the period of training.
trained r., conditioned r.
triceps r., elbow jerk or r.; a sudden contraction of the triceps muscle caused by a smart tap on its tendon when the forearm hangs loosely at a right angle with the arm.
triceps surae r., Achilles r.
trigeminofacial r., supraorbital r.
trochanter r., contraction of the adductor muscles of the thigh elicited by a tap on the trochanter.
Trömner's r., a modified Rossolimo r. in which, with the fingers of the patient partially flexed, the tapping of the volar aspect of the tip of the middle or index finger causes flexion of all four fingers and thumb; seen in pyramidal tract lesions with moderate spasticity.
ulnar r., pronator r.; pronation and adduction of the hand caused by tapping the styloid process of the ulna.
unconditioned r., innate r.; an instinctive r. not dependent on previous learning or experience.
upper abdominal periosteal r., percussing the lower margin of the costal cartilages in the nipple line causes a contraction of the ipsilateral abdominal muscles (inconstant).
urinary r., micturition r.
utricular r.'s, see statotonic r.'s.
vagovagal r., bradycardia with arterial hypotension, often with supraventricular arrhythmias; ascribed to stimulation, especially mechanical, of afferent vagal pathways in the abdomen, thorax, or airway, the efferent arc being vagal cardioinhibitory fibers.
vasopressor r., vasoconstriction caused by stimulation of certain afferent fibers, *e.g.,* in vagus nerve.
venorespiratory r., stimulation of respiration and increased pulmonary ventilation in response to an increase in venous pressure at the right auricle.
vertebra prominens r., pressure upon the last cervical vertebra of an animal, especially of one whose labyrinths have been destroyed and the vestibular nuclei isolated, causes relaxation or reduced tone of all four limbs.
vesical r., micturition r.
vestibulospinal r., the influence of vestibular stimulation on body posture.
visceral traction r., laryngeal spasm precipitated during an operation by traction on the stomach, gallbladder, or appendiceal mesentery.
viscerogenic r., any of a number of r.'s, such as headache, cough, disturbed pulse, etc., caused by disordered conditions of any of the viscera.
visceromotor r., contraction of the muscles of the thorax or abdomen in response to a stimulus from one of the viscera therein.
visceropannicular r., contraction of the panniculus carnosus muscle in the cat and certain other animals, in response to a stimulus applied to an abdominal viscus; the center for the r. is in the spinal cord, the afferent pathway is the splanchnic nerves.
viscerosensory r., an area of pain or sensitiveness to pressure in the external body wall due to disease of one of the viscera. See also Head's *lines.*
viscerotrophic r., a degenerative change in the skeletal soft tissues consequent upon a chronic inflammatory condition of any of the thoracic or abdominal viscera.
visual orbicularis r., contraction of the orbicularis oculi muscle caused by a sudden visual stimulus. See also wink r.
vomiting r., pharyngeal r. (2); vomiting (contraction of the abdominal muscles with relaxation of the cardiac sphincter of the

stomach and of the muscles of the throat) elicited by a variety of stimuli, especially one applied to the region of the fauces.
Weingrow's r., aponeurotic r.
Westphal's pupillary r., Westphal-Piltz *phenomenon.*
white pupillary r., leukocoria.
wink r., eye-closure or opticofacial r.; general term for r. closure of eyelids caused by any stimulus.
withdrawal r., flexor r.
wrist clonus r., sudden extension of the wrist induces a sustained clonic movement.

reflexogenic (rē-flek-sō-jen′ik). Reflexogenous; causing a reflex.

reflexogenous (rē-flek-soj′ĕ-nŭs). Reflexogenic.

reflexograph (rē-flek′sō-graf) [reflex + G. *graphō,* to write]. An instrument for graphically recording a reflex.

reflexology (rē-flek-sol′ō-jē) [reflex + G. *logos,* study]. The study of reflexes.

reflexometer (rē-flek-som′ĕ-ter) [reflex + G. *metron,* measure]. An instrument for measuring the force necessary to excite a reflex.

reflexophil, reflexophile (rē-flek′sō-fil, -fīl) [reflex + G. *phileō,* to love]. Having exaggerated reflexes.

reflexotherapy (rē-flek′sō-thār′ă-pē). Reflex *therapy.*

reflux (rē′flŭks) [L. *re-,* back, + *fluxus,* a flow]. **1.** A backward flow. See also regurgitation. **2.** In chemistry, to boil without loss of vapor because of the presence of a condenser that returns vapor as liquid.
abdominojugular r., hepatojugular r.
esophageal r., gastroesophageal r., regurgitation of the contents of the stomach into the esophagus, possibly into the pharynx where they can be aspirated between the vocal cords and down into the trachea; pulmonary complications are dependent upon the amount, content, and acidity of the aspirate.
hepatojugular r., abdominojugular r.; an elevation of venous pressure visible in the jugular veins and measurable in the veins of the arm, produced in active or impending congestive heart failure by firm pressure with the flat hand over the abdomen. Sometimes mistakenly called hepatojugular reflex.
ureterorenal r., backward flow of urine from ureter into renal pelvis.
vesicoureteral r., backward flow of urine from bladder into ureter.

refract (rē-frakt′) [L. *refringo,* pp. *-fractus,* to break up]. **1.** To change the direction of a ray of light. **2.** To detect an error of refraction and to correct it by means of lenses.

refraction (rē-frak′shŭn) [L. *refractio* (see refract)]. Refringence. **1.** The deflection of a ray of light when it passes from one medium into another of different optical density; in passing from a denser into a rarer medium it is deflected away from a line perpendicular to the surface of the refracting medium; in passing from a rarer to a denser medium it is bent toward this perpendicular line. **2.** The act of determining the nature and degree of the refractive errors in the eye and correction of the same by lenses.
double r., birefringence; the property of having more than one refractive index according to the direction of the transmitted light.
dynamic r., r. of the eye during accommodation.
static r., r. without accommodation.

refractionist (rē-frak′shŭn-ist). A person trained to measure the refraction of the eye and to determine the proper corrective lenses.

refractionometer (rē-frak-shŭn-om′ĕ-ter). Refractometer.

refractive (rē-frak′tiv). Refringent; pertaining to refraction.

refractivity (rē-frak-tiv′i-tē). Ability of a substance by which it refracts rays of light.

refractometer (rē-frak-tom′ĕ-ter) [refraction + G. *metron,* measure]. Objective optometer; refractionometer; an instrument for measuring the degree of refraction in translucent substances, especially the ocular media. See refractive *index.*

refractometry (rē-frak-tom′ĕ-trē). **1.** Measurement of the refractive index. **2.** Use of a refractometer to determine the refractive error of the eye.

refractory (rē-frak′tōr-ē) [L. *refractarius,* fr. *refringo,* pp. *-fractus,* to break in pieces]. **1.** Intractable (1); obstinate (2); resistant to treatment, as of a disease. **2.** Obstinate (1).

refracture (rē-frak′chūr) [re- + fracture]. Breaking a bone that has united after a previous fracture.

refrangible (rē-fran′ji-bl) [L. *refringo,* to break in pieces]. Capable of being refracted.

refresh (rē-fresh′) [O. Fr. *re-frescher*] **1.** To renew; to cause to recuperate. **2.** To perform revivification (2).

refrigerant (rē-frij′er-ănt) [L. *re-frigero,* pp. *-atus,* pr. p. *-ans,* to make cold, fr. *frigus (frigor-),* cold]. **1.** Cooling; reducing slight fever. **2.** An agent that gives a sensation of coolness or relieves feverishness.

refrigeration (rē-frij-er-ā′shŭn) [L. *refrigeratio* (see refrigerant)]. The act of cooling or reducing fever.

refringence (rē-frin′jens). Refraction.

refringent (rē-frin′jent). Refractive.

Refsum, Sigvald, Norwegian neurologist, *1907. See R.'s *disease, syndrome.*

refusion (rē-fū′zhŭn) [L. *re-fundo,* pp. *-fusus,* to pour back]. Return of the circulation of blood which has been temporarily cut off by ligature of a limb.

regainer (rē-gān′er). An appliance used in an attempt to regain space in the dental arches.

Regaud, Claude, French radiologist, 1870–1940. See R.'s *fixative;* residual *body* of R.

regenerate (rē-jen′er-āt) [L. *re- genero,* pp. *-atus,* to reproduce, fr. *genus (gener-),* birth, race]. To renew; to reproduce.

regeneration (rē′jen-er-ā′shŭn) [L. *regeneratio* (see regenerate)]. **1.** Neogenesis; reproduction or reconstitution of a lost or injured part. **2.** A form of asexual reproduction; *e.g.,* when a worm is divided into two or more parts, each segment is regenerated into a new individual.
aberrant r., misdirection phenomenon; misdirected regrowth of nerve fibers, commonly seen after oculomotor nerve injury and characterized by elevation of the eyelid with adduction of the eyeball, retraction and elevation of the lid on downward gaze, limita-

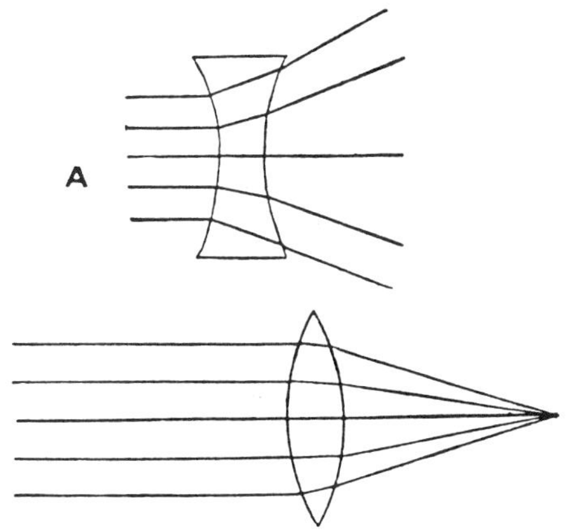

Refraction of Parallel Rays
A, by a concave lens; *B,* by a convex lens

tion of upward and downward gaze accompanied by adduction of the involved eyeball, and a dilated pupil nonresponsive to light but constricting on adduction.

regimen (rej'i-men) [L. direction, rule]. A program, including drugs, which regulates aspects of one's life-style for a hygienic or therapeutic purpose; sometimes mistakenly called regime.

REGIO

regio, gen. **regionis,** pl. **regiones** (rē'jē-ō, -ō'nis, -ō'nēz) [L.] [NA]. Region (1); an often arbitrarily limited portion of the surface of the body. See also region; area; space; spatium; zona; zone.

regio'nes abdo'minis [NA], abdominal regions or zones; the topographical subdivisions of the abdomen, including the right and left hypochondriac, right and left lateral, right and left inguinal, and the unpaired epigastric, umbilical and pubic regions.

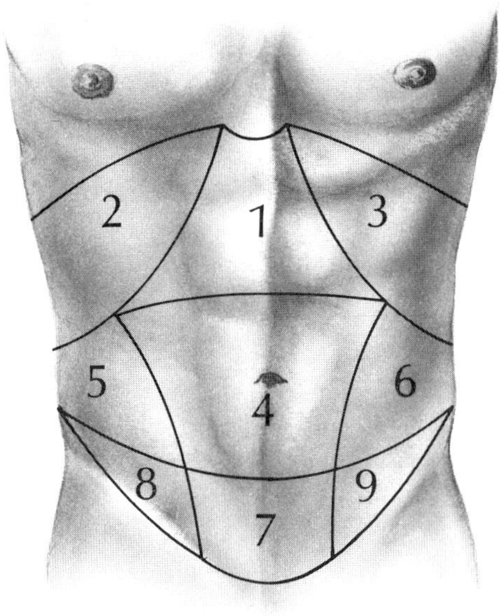

Regions of the Abdomen
1, Epigastric; *2* and *3*, hypochondriac (subcostal); *4*, umbilical; *5* and *6*, lateral; *7*, pubic; *8* and *9*, inguinal.

r. ana'lis [NA], anal region or triangle; the posterior portion of the perineal region through which the anal canal opens.

r. antebrachia'lis ante'rior [NA], anterior region of forearm; facies antebrachiales anterior; the area between the radial and ulnar borders of the forearm anteriorly.

r. antebrachia'lis poste'rior [NA], posterior region of forearm; facies antebrachiales posterior; the area between the radial and ulnar borders of the forearm posteriorly.

r. axilla'ris [NA], axillary region; the region of the axilla, including the axillary fossa.

r. brachia'lis ante'rior [NA], facies brachialis anterior; the anterior region of the arm.

r. brachia'lis poste'rior [NA], facies brachialis posterior; the posterior region of the arm.

r. bucca'lis [NA], buccal region; the region of the cheek, corresponding approximately to the outlines of the underlying buccinator muscle.

r. calca'nea [NA], calcaneal region; the region of the heel.

regio'nes cap'itis [NA], regions of head; the topographical division of the cranium in relation to the bones of the cranial vault; the regions include frontal, parietal, occipital, and temporal.

r. carpa'lis ante'rior [NA], anterior carpal region; the anterior part of the wrist.

r. carpa'lis poste'rior [NA], posterior carpal region; the posterior part of the wrist.

regio'nes cervica'les [NA], regions of neck; the topographical subdivisions of the neck; **r. c. ante'rior** [NA], anterior region of the neck; trigonum cervicale anterius; anterior triangle; the area of the neck bounded by the mandible, the anterior border of the sternocleidomastoid muscle, and the anterior midline of the neck; it is subdivided into carotid, muscular, submandibular, and submental triangles; **r. c. latera'lis** [NA], lateral region of the neck; trigonum cervicale posterius; posterior triangle of the neck; the region of the neck bounded by the sternocleidomastoid muscle, the trapezius muscle, and the upper border of the clavicle, including the omoclavicular triangle; **r. c. poste'rior** [NA], posterior region of the neck; nuchal region; r. nuchalis; the back of the neck.

regio'nes cor'poris [NA], regions of body; the topographical divisions of the body.

r. crura'lis ante'rior [NA], facies cruralis anterior; the anterior region of the leg.

r. crura'lis poste'rior [NA], facies cruralis posterior; the posterior region of the leg.

r. cubita'lis ante'rior [NA], anterior cubital region; facies cubitalis anterior; the area in front of the elbow, including the cubital fossa.

r. cubita'lis poste'rior [NA], posterior cubital region; facies cubitalis posterior; the posterior part of the elbow.

r. deltoi'dea [NA], deltoid region; the lateral aspect of the shoulder demarcated by the outlines of the deltoid muscle.

regio'nes dorsa'les [NA], regions of back; the topographical regions of the back of the trunk, including the r. vertebralis, r. sacralis, r. scapularis, r. infrascapularis, and r. lumbalis.

r. epigas'trica [NA], epigastrium; epigastric region; the region of the abdomen located between the costal margins and the subcostal plane.

regio'nes facia'les [NA], regions of face; the topographical subdivisions of the face, including nasal, oral, mental, orbital. infraorbital, buccal, and zygomatic.

r. femora'lis [NA], femoral region; **r. f. ante'rior** [NA], facies femoralis anterior; the anterior region of the thigh, including the femoral triangle; **r. f. poste'rior** [NA], facies femoralis posterior; the posterior region of the thigh.

r. fronta'lis cap'itis [NA], frontal region of head; the surface region of the head corresponding to the outlines of the frontal bone.

r. ge'nus ante'rior [NA], the anterior region of the knee.

r. ge'nus poste'rior [NA], the posterior region of the knee, including the popliteal fossa.

r. glutea'lis [NA], gluteal region; the region of the buttocks.

r. hypochondri'aca [NA], hypochondriac region; hypochondrium; the region on each side of the abdomen covered by the costal cartilages; it is lateral to the epigastric region.

r. infraclavicula'ris, *fossa* infraclavicularis.

r. inframamma'ria [NA], inframammary region; the region of the chest inferior to the mammary gland.

r. infraorbita'lis [NA], infraorbital region; the region of the face below the orbit and alongside the nose on each side.

r. infrascapula'ris [NA], infrascapular region; the region of the back lateral to the vertebral region and below the scapula.

r. inguina'lis [NA], inguinal region; groin; inguen; iliac region; the topographical area of the abdomen related to the inguinal canal, lateral to the pubic region.

r. latera'lis [NA], lateral region; the area of the abdomen on each side of the umbilical region.

r. lumba'lis [NA], lumbar region; the region of the back lateral to the vertebral region and between the rib cage and the pelvis.
r. mamma'ria [NA], mammary region; the region of the breast.
regio'nes mem'bri inferio'ris [NA], regions of inferior limb; the topographic divisions of the lower limb: buttock (r. glutealis), thigh (femur or r. femoralis), knee (genu), leg (crus or r. cruralis), ankle (r. talocruralis), and foot (pes).
regio'nes mem'bri superio'ris [NA], regions of superior limb; the topographic divisions of the upper limb: deltoid (r. deltoidea), arm (brachium), elbow (cubitus), forearm (antebrachium), and hand (manus).
r. menta'lis [NA], mental region; the region of the chin.
r. nasa'lis [NA], nasal region; the region of the nose.
r. nucha'lis [NA], r. cervicalis posterior.
r. occipita'lis cap'itis [NA], occipital region of head; the surface region of the head corresponding to the outlines of the occipital bone.
r. olfacto'ria tu'nicae muco'sae na'si [NA], olfactory region of tunica mucosa of the nose; Schultze's membrane; olfactory mucosa; the specialized olfactory receptive area that includes the upper one-third of the nasal septum and the lateral wall above the superior concha; it is lined with olfactory epithelium containing nerve cells whose axons form the filaments of the olfactory nerve; the lamina propria contains numerous olfactory glands (Bowman) that open to the surface.
r. ora'lis [NA], oral region; the region of the face including the lips and mouth.
r. orbita'lis [NA], orbital region; the region about the orbit.
r. parieta'lis cap'itis [NA], parietal region; the surface region of the head corresponding to the outlines of the underlying parietal bone.
regio'nes pectora'les [NA], regions of chest; pectoral regions; the topographic divisions of the chest: presternal (r. presternalis), mammary (r. mammaria), inframammary (r. inframammaria), and axillary (r. axillaris).
r. pectora'lis [NA], pectoral region; the region of the chest demarcated by the outline of the pectoralis major muscle.
r. perinea'lis [NA], perineal region; the r. at the lower end of the trunk, anterior to the sacral region between the thighs; it is divided into the anal region posteriorly and the urogenital region or perineum anteriorly.
r. presterna'lis [NA], presternal region; the part of the chest over the sternum.
r. pu'bica [NA], pubic region; hypogastrium; the lower central region of the abdomen below the umbilical region.
r. respirato'ria tu'nicae muco'sae na'si [NA], respiratory region of tunica mucosa of the nose; respiratory mucosa; an area consisting of pseudostratified ciliated columnar epithelium with goblet cells and a lamina propria containing, in addition to connective tissue, numerous seromucous glands and in some regions many thin-walled veins.
r. sacra'lis [NA], sacral region; the area of the back overlying the sacrum.
r. scapula'ris [NA], scapular region; the area of the back corresponding to the outlines of the scapula.
r. sternocleidomastoi'dea [NA], sternocleidomastoid region; the region overlying the sternocleidomastoid muscle, including the lesser supraclavicular fossa.
r. sura'lis [NA], sura.
r. talocrura'lis [NA], ankle region; the region of the lower limb between the leg (crus) and the foot (pes).
r. tempora'lis cap'itis [NA], temporal region; the surface region of the head corresponding approximately to the outlines of the temporal bone.
r. umbilica'lis [NA], umbilical region; the central region of the abdomen about the umbilicus.
r. urogenita'lis [NA], urogenital region or triangle; the anterior portion of the perineal region containing the openings of the urethra and vagina in the female and the urethra and root structures of the penis in the male.
r. vertebra'lis [NA], vertebral region; the central region of the back, corresponding to the underlying vertebral column.
r. zygomat'ica [NA], zygomatic region; the region of the face outlined by the zygomatic bone; the prominence above the cheek.

---

region (rē'jŭn) [L. *regio*]. **1.** Regio. **2.** A portion of the body having a special nervous or vascular supply, or a part of an organ having a special function. See also area; space; spatium; zona; zone.
abdominal r.'s, *regiones* abdominis.
anal r., *regio* analis.
ankle r., *regio* talocruralis.
anterior carpal r., *regio* carpalis anterior.
anterior cubital r., *regio* cubitalis anterior.
anterior r. of forearm, *regio* antebrachialis anterior.
anterior r. of neck, *regio* cervicalis anterior.
axillary r., *regio* axillaris.
r.'s of back, *regiones* dorsales.
r.'s of body, *regiones* corporis.
buccal r., *regio* buccalis.
calcaneal r., *regio* calcanea.
r.'s of chest, r. of chest, see *regiones* pectorales; *regio* pectoralis.
chromosomal r., that part of a chromosome defined either by anatomical details, notably banding, or by its linkages (linkage group).
constant r., see immunoglobulin.
deltoid r., *regio* deltoidea.
epigastric r., *regio* epigastrica.
r.'s of face, *regiones* faciales.
femoral r., *regio* femoralis.
frontal r. of head, *regio* frontalis capitis.
gluteal r., *regio* glutealis.
r.'s of head, *regiones* capitis.
hinge r., **(1)** that part of a tRNA structure that is deformed, bending a "cloverleaf" (two-dimensional) model to form an "L" model (crystal form, as seen by electron microscopy); **(2)** in an immunoglobulin, a short sequence of amino acids that lies between two longer sequences and allows the latter to bend about the former.
hypochondriac r., *regio* hypochondriaca.
iliac r., *regio* inguinalis.
r.'s of inferior limb, *regiones* membri inferioris.
inframammary r., *regio* inframammaria.
infraorbital r., *regio* infraorbitalis.
infrascapular r., *regio* infrascapularis.
inguinal r., *regio* inguinalis.
K r., carbons 9 and 10 of the phenanthrene ring system; thought by some to be the reactive spot in the various hydrocarbon carcinogens.
lateral r., *regio* lateralis.
lateral r. of neck, *regio* cervicalis lateralis.
lumbar r., *regio* lumbalis.
mammary r., *regio* mammaria.
mental r., *regio* mentalis.
nasal r., *regio* nasalis.
r.'s of neck, *regiones* cervicales.
occipital r. of head, *regio* occipitalis capitis.
olfactory r. of tunica mucosa of nose, *regio* olfactoria tunicae mucosae nasi.
oral r., *regio* oralis.
orbital r., *regio* orbitalis.
parietal r., *regio* parietalis capitis.
pectoral r., pectoral r.'s, see *regio* pectoralis; *regiones* pectorales.
perineal r., *regio* perinealis.
popliteal r., poples.
posterior carpal r., *regio* carpalis posterior.

posterior cubital r., *regio* cubitalis posterior.
posterior r. of forearm, *regio* antebrachialis posterior.
posterior r. of neck, *regio* cervicalis posterior.
preoptic r., preoptic area; the most anterior part of the hypothalamus surrounding the anterior or preoptic part of the third ventricle and including the lamina terminalis; containing the lateral and medial preoptic nucleus continuous caudally with, respectively, the lateral and anterior hypothalamic nucleus; rostrally the preoptic r. is continuous with the precommissural septum, laterally with the substantia innominata.
presternal r., *regio* presternalis.
presumptive r., in experimental embryology, the r. from which a specific structure or organ may be expected to develop.
pretectal r., prectectal *area.*
pubic r., *regio* pubica.
respiratory r. of tunica mucosa of nose, *regio* respiratoria tunicae mucosae nasi.
sacral r., *regio* sacralis.
scapular r., *regio* scapularis.
sternocleidomastoid r., *regio* sternocleidomastoidea.
r.'s of superior limb, *regiones* membri superioris.
sural r., sura.
temporal r. of head, *regio* temporalis capitis.
umbilical r., *regio* umbilicalis.
urogenital r., *regio* urogenitalis.
variable r., see immunoglobulin.
vertebral r., *regio* vertebralis.
Wernicke's r., Wernicke's *center.*
zygomatic r., *regio* zygomatica.

regional (rē'jŭn-ăl). Relating to a region.

regiones (rē'jē-ō'nēz) [L.]. Plural of regio.

registration (rej-is-trā'shŭn). In dentistry, a record.
maxillomandibular r., maxillomandibular *record.*
tissue r., in dentistry, **(1)** the accurate r. of the shape of tissues under any condition by means of a suitable material; **(2)** an impression.

regnancy (reg'nan-sē) [L. *regnant-, regnans,* pres. p. of *regno,* to rule]. The briefest unit of experience.

regression (rē-gresh'ŭn) [L. *re-gredio,* pp. *-gressus,* to go back]. **1.** A subsidence of symptoms. **2.** A relapse; a return of symptoms. **3.** Any retrograde movement or action. **4.** A return to a more primitive mode of behavior due to an inability to function adequately at a more adult level. **5.** An unconscious defense mechanism by which there occurs a return to earlier patterns of adaptation.
phonemic r., a decrease in intelligibility of speech associated with an increase in loudness.

regressive (rē-gres'iv). Relating to or characterized by regression.

regulation (reg'yū-lā'shŭn) [L. *regula,* a rule]. **1.** Control of the rate or manner in which a process progresses or a product is formed. **2.** In experimental embryology, the power of a very young embryo to continue approximately normal development after a part or parts have been manipulated or destroyed.

regurgitant (rē-ger'ji-tant). Regurgitating; flowing backward.

regurgitate (rē-ger'ji-tāt) [L. *re-,* back, + *gurgito,* pp. *-atus,* to flood, fr. *gurges (gurgit-),* a whirlpool]. **1.** To flow backward. **2.** To expel the contents of the stomach in small amounts, short of vomiting.

regurgitation (rē-ger'ji-tā'shŭn) [L. *regurgitatio* (see regurgitate)]. **1.** A backward flow, as of blood through an incompetent valve of the heart. **2.** The return of gas or small amounts of food from the stomach.
aortic r., Corrigan's disease; reflux of blood through an incompetent aortic valve into the left ventricle during ventricular diastole.
mitral r., reflux of blood through an incompetent mitral valve.

rehabilitation (rē'hă-bil-i-tā'shŭn) [L. *rehabilitare,* pp. *-tatus,* to make fit, fr. *re-* + *habilitas,* ability]. Restoration, following disease, illness, or injury, of the ability to function in a normal or near normal manner.
mouth r., restoration of the form and function of the masticatory apparatus to as nearly a normal condition as possible.

rehearsal (rē-her'săl). A process associated with short-term and long-term memory wherein newly presented information, such as a name or a list of words, is repeated to oneself one or more times in order not to forget it.

Rehfuss, Martin E., U.S. physician, 1887–1964. See R. *method,* stomach *tube.*

rehydration (rē-hī-drā'shŭn). The return of water to a system after its loss.

Reichel, Friedrich P., German gynecologist and surgeon, 1858–1934. See R.-Pólya stomach *resection.*

Reichert, Karl B., German anatomist, 1811–1884. See R.'s *cartilage,* cochlear *recess;* R.-Meissl *number.*

Reichstein, Tadeus, Polish biochemist in Switzerland and Nobel laureate *1897. See R.'s *substances.*

Reid, Robert W., Scottish anatomist, 1851–1939. See R.'s base *line.*

Reifenstein, Edward C. Jr., U.S. endocrinologist, *1908. See R.'s *syndrome.*

Reil, Johann C., German physician, neurologist, and histologist, 1759–1813. See R.'s *ansa, band, ribbon, triangle;* limiting or circular *sulcus* of R; *island* of R.

reimplantation (rē'im-plan-tā'shŭn). Replantation.

reinfection (rē-in-fek'shŭn). A second infection by the same microorganism, after recovery from or during the course of a primary infection.

reinforcement (rē-in-fōrs'ment). **1.** An increase of force or strength; denoting specifically the increased sharpness of the patellar reflex when the patient at the same time closes the fist tightly or pulls against the flexed fingers or contracts some other set of muscles. See also Jendrassik's *maneuver.* **2.** In dentistry, a structural addition or inclusion used to give additional strength in function; *e.g.,* bars in plastic denture base, or wire in silicate or amalgam. **3.** In conditioning, the totality of the process in which the conditioned stimulus is followed by presentation of the unconditioned stimulus which, itself, elicits the response to be conditioned. See also reinforcer; *schedules* of reinforcement.
primary r., satisfaction of physiological needs or drives, such as that supplied by food or sleep.
secondary r., r. through something which, while it does not satisfy the need directly, has been associated with direct satisfaction of the need.

reinforcer (rē-in-fōrs'er). Reward; in conditioning, a pleasant or satisfaction-yielding (**positive r.**) or painful or unsatisfying (**negative r.**), stimulus, object, or stimulus event that is obtained upon the performance of a desired or predetermined operant. See also reinforcement (3).

Reinke, Friedrich B., German anatomist, 1862–1919. See R.'s *crystalloids.*

reinnervation (rē-in-ner-vā'shŭn). Restoration of nerve control of a paralyzed muscle or organ by means of regrowth of nerve fibers either spontaneously or after anastomosis.

reinoculation (rē'i-nok-yū-lā'shŭn). Reinfection by means of inoculation.

Reinsch, Adolf, German physician, 1862–1916. See R.'s *test.*

reintegration (rē'in-tē-grā'shŭn). In psychiatry, the return to well adjusted functioning following disturbances due to mental illness.

reinversion (re-in-ver'shŭn). The correction, spontaneous or operative, of an inversion, as of the uterus.

Reisseisen, Franz D., German anatomist, 1773–1828. See R.'s *muscles.*

Reissner, Ernst, German anatomist, 1824–1878. See R.'s *fiber, membrane.*

Reitan, Ralph M., U.S. psychologist, *1922. See Halstead-R. *battery.*

Reiter, Hans, German bacteriologist, 1881–1969. See R. *test;* R.'s *disease, syndrome;* Fiessinger-LeRoy-R. *syndrome.*

rejection (rē-jek'shŭn) [L. *rejectio,* a throwing back]. **1.** The immunological response to incompatibility in a transplanted organ. **2.** A refusal to accept, recognize, or grant; a denial. **3.** Elimination of small ultrasonic echoes from display.

accelerated r., a transplant r. manifested in less than three days.

acute cellular r., a type of immunologically mediated injury to a transplant, typically a kidney graft, manifested by proliferation in the renal parenchyma of cells of the lymphoblastic series initially entering via peritubular capillaries in the vascular system, with eventual extension throughout the interstitium.

chronic r., a transplant r. occurring after a few or many months, mainly from persisting serum antibody action.

chronic allograft r., immunologically mediated damage to the allograft, typically a kidney allograft, manifested by diffuse interstitial fibrosis glomerular changes, typically membranous and sclerotic in nature, as well as intimal fibrosis of the blood vessels with tubular atrophy and loss of tubular structures.

hyperacute r., **(1)** a r. that usually develops in less than one hour from the implantation of a vascular graft; **(2)** a form of antibody-mediated, usually irreversible damage to a transplanted organ, particularly the kidney, manifested predominantly by diffuse thrombotic lesions, usually confined to the organ itself and only rarely disseminated; **(3)** for skin allograft rejection of this type, see white *graft.*

parental r., parental withholding or unacceptance of affection or attention from a child.

primary r., a r. occurring more than seven days after transplantation, mainly from a cellular immune response.

rejuvenescence (rē-jū-vĕ-nes'ens) [L. *re-,* again, + *juvenesco,* to grow young, fr. *juvenis,* a youth]. A renewal of youth; return of a cell or tissue to a state in which it was in an earlier stage of existence.

Rekoss, 19th century Prussian instrument maker. See R. *disk.*

relapse (rē'laps) [L. *re-labor,* pp. *-lapsus,* to slide back]. Recurrence (2); return of the manifestations of a disease after an interval of improvement.

relapsing (rē-lap'sing). Recurring; said of a disease or its manifestations that returns in a new attack after an interval of improvement.

relation (rē-lā'shŭn) [L. *relatio,* a bringing back]. **1.** An association or connection between or among people or objects. See also relationship and subentries. **2.** In dentistry, the mode of contact of teeth or the positional relationship of oral structures.

acquired centric r., see centric jaw r.

acquired eccentric r., an eccentric r. that is assumed by habit in order to bring the teeth into occlusion.

buccolingual r., the position of a space or tooth in r. to the tongue and the cheek.

centric jaw r., centric r., median or median retruded r.; **(1)** the most retruded physiologic r. of the mandible to the maxillae to and from which the individual can make lateral movements; it is a condition which can exist at various degrees of jaw separation, and it occurs around the terminal hinge axis; **(2)** the most posterior r. of the mandible to the maxillae at the established vertical r. See also eccentric r.

dynamic r.'s, relative movements between two objects, *e.g.,* the relationship of the mandible to the maxillae.

eccentric r., eccentric position; any r. of the mandible to the maxillae other than centric r.

intermaxillary r., maxillomandibular r.

maxillomandibular r., intermaxillary r.; any one of the many r.'s of the mandible to the maxillae, *e.g.,* centric jaw r., eccentric r.

median retruded r., median r., centric jaw r.

occluding r., the jaw r. at which the opposing teeth occlude.

protrusive r., the r. of the mandible to the maxillae when the lower jaw is thrust forward.

protrusive jaw r., a jaw r. resulting from a protrusion of the mandible.

rest r., rest jaw or unstrained jaw r.; the postural r. of the mandible to the maxillae when the patient is resting comfortably in the upright position and the condyles are in a neutral unstrained position in the glenoid fossa.

rest jaw r., rest r.

ridge r., the positional r. of the mandibular ridge to the maxillary ridge.

static r.'s, relationship between two parts that are not in motion.

unstrained jaw r., rest r.

relationship (rē-lā'shŭn-ship). The state of being related, associated, or connected.

blood r., consanguinity.

hypnotic r., r. between hypnotizer or hypnotist and the hypnotized or hypnotee.

object r., in the behavioral sciences, the emotional bond between an individual and another person, (or between two groups), as opposed to the individual's (or group's) interest in himself (itself).

sadomasochistic r., a r. characterized by the complementary enjoyment of inflicting and suffering cruelty.

relax (rē-laks') [L. *re-laxo,* to loosen]. **1.** To loosen; to slacken. **2.** To cause a movement of the bowels.

relaxant (rē-lak'sănt). **1.** Relaxing; causing relaxation; reducing tension, especially muscular tension. **2.** An agent that reduces muscular tension, usually referred to as a muscle r.

depolarizing r., an agent, *e.g.,* succinylcholine, that induces loss of polarity of the motor endplate and so paralyzes skeletal muscle by a phase I block.

muscular r., an agent that relaxes striated muscle; includes drugs acting at the spinal cord level or directly on muscle to decrease tone, as well as the neuromuscular r.'s.

neuromuscular r., an agent, *e.g.,* curare or succinylcholine, that produces relaxation of striated muscle by interruption of transmission of nervous impulses at the myoneural junction.

nondepolarizing r., an agent, *e.g.,* tubocurarine, that paralyzes skeletal muscle without altering polarity of the motor endplate, as in phase II block.

smooth muscle r., an agent, such as an antispasmodic, bronchodilator, or vasodilator, that reduces the tension or tone of a smooth (involuntary) muscle.

relaxation (rē-lak-sā'shŭn) [L. *relaxatio* (see relax)]. Loosening, lengthening, or lessening of tension in a muscle.

cardioesophageal r., r. of the lower esophageal sphincter which can allow reflux of acidic gastric contents into the lower esophagus, producing esophagitis.

isometric r., decrease in tension of a muscle while the length remains constant due to fixation of the ends.

isovolumetric r., isovolumic r.

isovolumic r., isovolumetric r.; that part of the cardiac cycle between the time of aortic valve closure and mitral opening, during which the ventricular muscle decreases its tension without lengthening so that ventricular volume remains unaltered.

relaxin (rē-lak'sin). A polypeptide hormone secreted from the corpus luteum of the ovary.

relearning (rē-lern'ing). The process of regaining a skill or ability that has been partially or entirely lost; savings involved in r., as compared with original learning, gives an index of the degree of retention.

reliability (rē-lī-ă-bil′i-tē). In psychology and statistics; the consistency of measurement or degree of dependability of a measuring instrument.

equivalent form r., in psychology, the consistency of measurement based on the correlation between scores on two similar forms of the same test taken by the same individual. See also reliability *coefficient.*

interjudge r., in psychology, the consistency of measurement obtained when different judges or examiners independently administer the same test to the same individual.

test-retest r., in psychology, the consistency of measurement based on the correlation between test and retest scores for the same individual. See also reliability *coefficient.*

relief (rē-lēf′) [see relieve]. **1.** Removal of pain or distress, physical or mental. **2.** In dentistry, reduction or elimination of pressure from a specific area under a denture base. See also r. *area;* r. *chamber.*

relieve (rē-lēv′) [thru O. Fr. fr. L. *re-levo,* to lift up, lighten]. To free wholly or partly from pain or discomfort, either physical or mental.

reline (rē′līn′). In dentistry, to resurface the tissue side of a denture with new base material to make it fit more accurately. See also rebase.

REM Acronym for rapid eye *movement;* reticular erythematous *mucinosis.*

rem Abbreviation for roentgen-equivalent-man. See under roentgen.

Remak, Ernst J., German neurologist, 1848–1911. See R.'s *paralysis, reflex, sign.*

Remak, Robert, German anatomist and histologist, 1815–1865. See R.'s nuclear *division, fibers, ganglia, plexus.*

remediable (rē-mē′dē-ă-bl) [L. *remediabilis,* fr. *remedio,* to cure]. Curable.

remedial (rē-mē′dē-ăl). Curative or acting as a remedy.

remedy (rem′ĕ-dē) [L. *remedium,* fr. *re-,* again, + *medeor,* cure]. An agent that cures disease or alleviates its symptoms.

remineralization (rē′min′er-ăl-i-zā′shŭn). **1.** The return to the body of necessary mineral constituents lost through disease or dietary deficiencies; commonly used in referring to the content of calcium salts in bone. **2.** In dentistry, a process enhanced by the presence of fluoride whereby partially decalcified enamel, dentin, and cementum become recalcified by mineral replacement.

reminiscence (rem-i-nis′sens). In the psychology of learning, an improvement in recall, over that shown on the last trial, of incompletely learned material after an interval without practice.

remission (rē-mish′ŭn) [L. *remissio,* fr. *re-mitto,* pp. *-missus,* to send back, slacken, relax]. **1.** Abatement or lessening in severity of the symptoms of a disease. **2.** The period during which such abatement occurs.

spontaneous r., in psychiatry and clinical psychology, disappearance of symptoms without formal treatment; causes of their disappearance are assumed to exist but are not known.

remit (rē-mit′) [see remission]. To become less severe for a time without absolutely ceasing.

remittence (rē-mit′ens). A temporary amelioration, without actual cessation, of symptoms.

remittent (rē-mit′ent). Characterized by temporary periods of abatement of the symptoms.

remodeling (rē-mod′el-ing). A cyclical process by which bone maintains a dynamic steady state through sequential resorption and formation of a small amount of bone at the same site.

ren, gen. **renis,** pl. **renes** (ren, rē′nis, rē′nēz) [L.] [NA]. Kidney.

renal (rē′năl). Nephric.

renculus (ren′kū-lŭs). Reniculus.

Rendu, Henri J.L.M., French physician, 1844–1902. See R.-Osler-Weber *disease, syndrome.*

reni-. See reno-.

renicapsule (ren′i-kap′sūl) [reni- + L. *capsula,* capsule]. The capsule of the kidney.

renicardiac (ren′i-kar′dē-ak) [reni- + G. *kardia,* heart]. Cardiorenal.

reniculus, pl. **reniculi** (rĕ-nik′yū-lŭs, -lī) [L. dim. of *ren,* kidney]. Renculus; renunculus. **1.** *Lobulus* corticalis renalis. **2.** A lobe of the human fetal kidney and that of some lower animals in which fibrous septa subdivide the organ.

renifleur (ren-i-fler′) [Fr.]. A sniffer; one who is sexually excited by odors.

reniform (ren′i-fōrm). Nephroid.

renin (rē′nin). Angiotensinogenase; a term originally used for a pressor substance obtained from rabbits' kidneys, now an enzyme (EC 3.4.99.19) that converts angiotensinogen to angiotensin.

reniportal (ren′i-pōr′tăl) [reni- + L. *porta,* gate]. **1.** Relating to the hilum of the kidney. **2.** Relating to the portal, or venous capillary circulation in the kidney.

rennase (ren′ās). Chymosin.

rennet (ren′et). Chymosin.

rennin (ren′in). Chymosin.

renninogen, rennogen (rĕ-nin′ō-jen, ren′ō-jen) [rennin + G. *-gen,* producing]. Prochymosin.

reno-, reni- [L. *ren,* kidney]. Combining forms denoting the kidney. See also nephro-.

renocutaneous (rē′nō-kyū-tā′nē-ŭs) [reno- + L. *cutis,* skin]. Relating to the kidneys and the skin.

renogastric (rē′nō-gas′trik) [reno- + G. *gastēr,* stomach]. Relating to the kidneys and the stomach.

renogenic (rē-nō-jen′ik). Originating in or from the kidney.

renogram (rē′nō-gram). The assessment of renal function by external radiation detectors after the administration of a radiopharmaceutical with renotropic characteristics.

renography (rē-nog′ră-fē). Radiography of the kidney.

renointestinal (rē′nō-in-tes′ti-năl). Relating to the kidneys and the intestine.

renomegaly (rē′nō-meg′ă-lē). Enlargement of the kidney.

renopathy (rē-nop′ă-thē). Nephropathy.

renoprival (rē-nō-prī′văl) [reno- + L. *privus,* deprived of]. Relating to, characterized by, or resulting from total loss of kidney function or from removal of all functioning renal tissue.

renopulmonary (rē′nō-pŭl′mo-nār-ē). Relating to the kidneys and the lungs.

renotrophic (rē-nō-trof′ik) [reno- + G. *trophē,* nourishment]. Renotropic; nephrotrophic; nephrotropic; relating to any agent influencing the growth or nutrition of the kidney or to the action of such an agent.

renotrophin (rē-nō-trō′fin). Renotropin; an agent affecting the growth or nutrition of the kidney.

renotropic (rē-nō-trop′ik) [reno- + G. *tropē,* a turning]. Renotrophic.

renotropin (rē-nō-trō′pin). Renotrophin.

renovascular (rē-nō-vas′kyū-ler). Pertaining to the blood vessels of the kidney, denoting especially disease of these vessels.

Renpenning, H., 20th century Canadian physician. See R.'s *syndrome.*

Renshaw, B., 20th century U.S. neurophysiologist. See R. *cells.*

renunculus (rē-nŭng'kyū-lŭs). [L. dim. of *ren*]. Reniculus.

Reoviridae (rē-ō-vir'i-dē) [*R*espiratory *E*nteric *O*rphan + viridae]. A family of double-stranded RNA viruses, some of which (*Reovirus*) previously were included with ECHO viruses, and others (*Orbivirus*), with arboviruses. Virions are 60 to 80 nm in diameter, usually naked, and ether-resistant; genomes contain double-stranded, segmented RNA (MW 10 to 16 $\times$ 10^6); capsids are of icosohedral symmetry with two layers of capsomeres. The family comprises six genera: *Reovirus, Orbivirus,* rotaviruses, cytoplasmic polyhedrosis virus group, and two plant reovirus groups.

Reovirus (rē'ōvī'rŭs). A genus of viruses (family Reoviridae) that are 75 to 80 nm in diameter, with distinct double layers of capsomeres, and have vertebrates as hosts but do not multiply therein. They have been recovered from children with mild fever and sometimes diarrhea, and from children with no apparent infection; from chimpanzees with coryza; monkeys and mice; and cattle feces. There are three antigenically distinct human types related by a common complement-fixing antigen.

rep Abbreviation for roentgen-equivalent-physical. See under roentgen.

repair (rē-pār'). Restoration of diseased or damaged tissues naturally by healing processes or artificially, as by surgical means.
chemical r., conversion of a free radical to a stable molecule.

repand (rē-pand') [L. *repandus,* bent or turned back, fr. *re-,* back, + *pandus,* curved]. Denoting a bacterial colony with edges marked by a series of slightly concave segments with angular projections at their points of union.

repellent (rē-pel'ent) [L. *re-pello,* pp. *-pulsus,* to drive back]. **1.** Capable of driving off or repelling; repulsive. **2.** An agent that drives away or prevents annoyance or irritation by insect pests. **3.** An astringent or other agent that reduces swelling.

repetition-compulsion (rep-e-tish'ŭn-kŏm-pŭl'shŭn). In psychoanalysis, the tendency to repeat earlier experiences or actions, in an unconscious effort to achieve belated mastery over them.

replant (rē'plant). **1.** To perform replantation. **2.** A part or organ so replaced or about to be so replaced.

replantation (rē-plan-tā'shŭn) [G. *re-,* again, + *planto,* pp. *-atus,* to plant, fr. *planta,* a sprout, slip]. Reimplantation; replacement of an organ or part back in its original site and reestablishing its circulation.
intentional r., elective extraction of a tooth, obturation of the root canal(s), and replacement of the tooth into the alveolus.

repletion (rē-plē'shŭn) [L. *repletio,* fr. *re-pleo,* pp. *-pletus,* to fill up]. Plethora.

replica (rep'li-kă). A specimen for electron microscopic examination obtained by coating a crystalline array or other virus material with carbon; the mold (the r.) obtained after the viral material has been dissolved provides details of structure and arrangement.

replicase (rep'li-kās). Descriptive term for RNA-directed RNA polymerase (EC 2.7.7.48) associated with replication of RNA viruses.

replicate (rep'li-kāt). **1.** One of several identical processes or observations. **2.** To repeat; to produce an exact copy.

replication (rep-li-kā'shŭn) [L. *replicatio,* a reply, fr. *replico,* pp. *-atus,* to fold back]. **1.** Repeating a process or observation; a word commonly used in describing experimental work. **2.** Autoreproduction.

replicator (rep'li-kā-ter). The specific site of a bacterial genome (chromosome) at which replication begins.

replicon (rep'li-kon). A segment of a chromosome (or of the DNA of a chromosome or similar entity) that can replicate, with its own initiation and termination codons, independently of the chromosome in which it may be located, and that has a unique function.

replisome (rep'li-sōm) [L. *replico,* to repeat + G. *sōma,* body]. Any of the sites on the matrix of a cell nucleus that contain series of enzyme complexes where DNA replication is thought to occur.

repolarization (rē'pō-lăr-i-zā'shŭn). The process whereby the membrane, cell, or fiber, after depolarization, is polarized again, with positive charges on the outer and negative charges on the inner surface.

repositioning (rē'pō-zish'ŭn-ing). Reduction (1).
gingival r., surgical relocation of the attached gingiva to eliminate pathosis or to establish more acceptable form and function.
jaw r., the changing of any relative position of the mandible to the maxillae, by altering the occlusion of the natural or artificial teeth or by surgical means.
muscle r., the surgical replacement of a muscle attachment into a more functional position.

repositor (rē-poz'i-ter, -tōr). An instrument used to reposition a displaced organ.

repressed (rē-prest'). Subjected to repression.

repression (rē-presh'ŭn) [L. *re-primo,* pp. *-pressus,* to press back, repress]. In psychotherapy, the defense mechanism by which ideas, impulses, and affects once available to conscious thought are removed from consciousness.
primal r., r. of material never in conscious thought.

repressor (rē-pres'er). The product of a regulator or repressor gene.
active r., a r. that combines directly with an operator gene to repress activity of the operator and its structural genes, thus repressing protein synthesis; active r. may be inactivated by an inducer, with resulting activation of protein synthesis; a homeostatic mechanism for regulation of inducible enzyme systems.
inactive r., aporepressor; a r. that is unable to combine with an operator gene until it has been activated by combination with a corepressor (usually a product of a protein pathway); after activation, the r. stops production of the proteins controlled by the operator gene; a homeostatic mechanism for regulation of repressible enzyme systems.

reproduction (rē-prō-dŭk'shŭn) [L. *re-,* again, + *pro-duco,* pp. *-ductus,* to lead forth, produce]. **1.** The recall and presentation in the mind of the steps of a former impression. **2.** Procreation; generation (1); the total process by which organisms produce offspring.
asexual r., agamogenesis; agamogony; r. other than by union of male and female sex cells.
cytogenic r., r. by means of unicellular germ cells; includes both sexual r. and asexual r. by means of spores.
sexual r., syngenesis; r. by union of male and female gametes to form a zygote.
somatic r., asexual r. by fission or budding of somatic cells.

reproductive (rē'prō-dŭk'tiv). Relating to reproduction.

Reptilia (rep-til'ē-ă) [L. *reptilis,* ntr. *-e,* creeping; ntr. as n., reptile]. A class of vertebrates comprising the alligators, crocodiles, lizards, turtles, tortoises, and snakes.

repullulation (rē-pul-yū-lā'shŭn) [L. *re-,* again, + *pullulo,* pp. *-atus,* to sprout]. Renewed germination; return of a morbid process or growth.

repulsion (rē-pŭl'shŭn) [L. *re-pello,* pp. *-pulsus,* to drive back]. **1.** The act of repelling or driving apart, in contrast to attraction. **2.** Strong dislike; aversion; repugnance. **3.** See coupling *phase.*

RES Abbreviation for reticuloendothelial *system.*

resazurin (rē-saz'yū-rin). A blue compound, 7-hydroxy-3*H*-phenoxazin-3-one 10-oxide, used as a redox indicator in the reductase test of milk and also as a pH indicator (orange at 3.8, violet at 6.5).

rescinnamine (rē-sin'ă-mēn, -min). 3,4,5-Trimethoxycinnamic acid ester of methyl reserpate; a purified ester alkaloid of the alseroxylon fraction of species of *Rauwolfia;* chemically and pharmacologically related to reserpine, with similar uses.

resect (rē-sekt') [L. *re-seco,* pp. *sectus,* to cut off]. **1.** To cut off, especially to cut off the articular ends of one or both bones forming a joint. **2.** To excise a segment of a part.

resectable (rē-sek'tă-bl). Amenable to resection.

resection (rē-sek'shŭn). **1.** Removal of articular ends of one or both bones forming a joint. **2.** Excision (1).
gum r., gingivectomy.
Miles r., Miles *operation.*
muscle r., shortening of the tendon of the ocular muscle in strabismus.
Reichel-Pólya stomach r., retrocolic anastomosis of the full circumference of the open stomach to the jejunum.
root r., apicoectomy.
scleral r., shortening of the outer coat of the eye in retinal separation.
transurethral r., endoscopic removal of the prostate gland or bladder lesions, usually for relief of prostatic obstruction or treatment of bladder malignancies.
wedge r., removal of a wedge-shaped portion of the ovary; used in the treatment of virilizing disorders of ovarian origin, such as the Stein-Leventhal syndrome.

resectoscope (rē-sek'tō-skōp). A special endoscopic instrument for the transurethral electrosurgical removal of lesions involving the bladder, prostate gland, or urethra.

reserpine (rē-ser'pēn, -pin). An ester alkaloid isolated from the root of certain species of *Rauwolfia;* it decreases the 5-hydroxytryptamine and catecholamine concentrations in the central nervous system and in peripheral tissues; used in conjunction with other hypotensive agents in the management of essential hypertension and is useful as a tranquilizer in psychotic states.

reserve (rē-zerv') [L. *re-servo,* to keep back, reserve]. Something available but held back for later use, as strength or carbohydrates.
alkali r., the sum total of the basic ions (mainly bicarbonates) of the blood and other body fluids which, acting as buffers, maintain the normal pH of the blood.
breathing r., the difference between the pulmonary ventilation (*i.e.,* the volume of air breathed under ordinary resting conditions) and the maximum breathing capacity.
cardiac r., the work which the heart is able to perform beyond that required under the ordinary circumstances of daily life, depending upon the state of the myocardium and the degree to which, within physiologic limits, the cardiac muscle fibers can be stretched by the volume of blood reaching the heart during diastole.

reservoir (rez'ĕv-wor) [Fr.]. Receptaculum.
r. of infection, living or nonliving material in or on which an infectious agent multiplies and/or develops and is dependent for its survival in nature.
Ommaya r., a plastic container placed in the subgaleal space which is connected to the lateral ventricle by tubing; it is used to instill medication into, or remove fluid from, the ventricle.
Pecquet's r., *cisterna* chyli.
r. of spermatozoa, the site where spermatozoa are stored; the distal portion of the tail of the epididymis and the beginning of the ductus deferens.
vitelline r., vitellarium.

reset nodus sinuatrialis (rē'set nō'dŭs sī'nū-ā-trē-ā'lis). Reset of the sinoatrial node produced by an atrial premature depolarization when the sum of the duration of the premature cycle and the return cycle is less than twice the spontaneous cycle length. *Cf.* nonreset nodus sinuatrialis.

resident (rez'i-dent) [L. *resideo,* to reside]. A house officer attached to a hospital for clinical training; formerly, one who actually resided in the hospital.

residua (rē-zid'yū-ă). Plural of residuum.

residual (rē-zid'yū-ăl). Relating to or of the nature of a residue.

residue (rez'i-dū) [L. *residuum*]. Residuum; that which remains after removal of one or more substances.
day r., psychoanalytic term for a dream related to an experience of the previous day.

residuum, pl. **residua** (rē-zid'yū-ŭm, -yū-ă) [L. ntr. of *residuus,* left behind, remaining, fr. *re- sideo,* to sit back, remain behind]. Residue.

resilience (rē-zil'yens) [L. *resilio,* to spring back, rebound]. **1.** Energy (per unit of volume) released upon unloading. **2.** Springiness or elasticity.

resin (rez'in) [L. *resina*]. **1.** An amorphous brittle substance consisting of the hardened secretion of a number of plants, probably derived from a volatile oil and similar to a stearoptene. **2.** Rosin. **3.** A precipitate formed by the addition of water to certain tinctures. **4.** A broad term used to indicate organic substances insoluble in water; these monomers are named according to their chemical composition, physical structure, and means for activation or curing, *e.g.,* acrylic r., autopolymer r.
acrylic r., a general term applied to a resinous material of the various esters of acrylic acid; used as a denture base material, for other dental restorations, and for trays.
activated r., autopolymer r.
anion-exchange r., see anion exchange; anion exchanger.
autopolymer r., autopolymerizing r., activated, cold cure, cold-curing, quick cure, or self-curing r.; any r. that can be polymerized by chemical catalysis rather than by the application of heat; used in dentistry for dental restoration, denture repair, and impression trays.
carbacrylamine r.'s, a mixture of the cation-exchange r.'s, carbacrylic r. and potassium carbacrylic r. (87.5%) and of the anion-exchange r., polyamine-methylene r. (12.5%), used to increase the fecal excretion of sodium in edema associated with excessive sodium retention by the kidneys, *e.g.,* in congestive heart failure, cirrhosis of the liver, and nephrosis.
cation-exchange r., see cation exchange; cation exchanger.
cholestyramine r., a strongly basic anion-exchange r. in the chloride form, consisting of a copolymer of styrene and divinylbenzene with quaternary ammonium functional groups; it lowers the blood cholesterol by binding the bile acids in the intestine, thus promoting their excretion in the feces instead of reabsorption from the bowel; used in the treatment of hypercholesterolemia, xanthomatous biliary cirrhosis, and other forms of xanthomatosis.
cold cure r., cold-curing r., autopolymer r.
composite r., composite dental *cement.*
copolymer r., synthetic r. produced by joint polymerization of two or more different monomers or polymers.
cross-linked r., cross-linked *polymer.*
direct filling r., an autopolymerizing r. especially designed as a dental restorative material.
epoxy r., any thermosetting r. based on the reactivity of epoxy; used as adhesives, protective coatings, and embedding media for electron microscopy.
gum r., the dry exudate from a number of plants, consisting of a mixture of a gum and a r., the former soluble in water but not alcohol, the latter soluble in alcohol but not water.
heat-curing r., r. that requires heat to initiate polymerization.
Indian podophyllum r., r. obtained from *Podophyllum emodi;* a cathartic and cholagogue.
ion-exchange r., see ion exchange; ion exchanger.
ipomea r., r. obtained from the dried root of *Ipomoea orizabensis;* a cathartic. See also scammony.

jalap r., r. extracted from the dried tuberous root of *Exogonium purga;* a purgative.
melamine r., melamine formaldehyde; a plastic material used mixed with plaster of Paris for casts. Such a cast is lighter and stronger than one made with plaster of Paris alone.
methacrylate r., polymerized methacrylic acid; a translucent plastic material, used for the manufacture of various medical appliances, surgical instruments, and seating components used in total joint replacement; it possesses the optical properties of fused quartz, and is readily molded when heated; formerly used in electron microscopy for embedding tissues, now superseded by epoxy r.'s.
podophyllum r., podophyllin; a mixture of r.'s obtained from the dried rhizomes and roots of *Podophyllum peltatum* or *P. hexandrum;* used as a laxative.
polyamine-methylene r., synthetic acid-binding r.; used as a gastric antacid.
polyester r., r. in which the polymers are insoluble in most organic solvents and are polymerized by light, heat, or oxygen; used in electron microscopy as a tissue embedding medium.
quick cure r., autopolymer r.
quinine carbacrylic r., azuresin.
self-curing r., autopolymer r.

resin acids. A class of organic compounds derived from various natural plant resins; diterpenes containing a phenanthrene ring system; *e.g.*, abietic acid, pimaric acid, ester gums.

resinoid (rez'i-noyd). **1.** A substance containing a resin or resembling one. **2.** An extract obtained by evaporating a tincture. **3.** Resembling rosin.

resinous (rez'i-nŭs). Relating to or derived from a resin.

resistance (rē-zis'tans) [L. *re-sisto,* to stand back, withstand]. **1.** A passive force exerted in opposition to another and active force. **2 (R).** The opposition in a conductor to the passage of a current of electricity, whereby there is a loss of energy and a production of heat; specifically, the potential difference in volts across the conductor per ampere of current flow; unit: ohm. *Cf.* impedance (1). **3.** The opposition to flow of a fluid through one or more passageways (*e.g.*, blood flow, respiratory gases in the tracheobronchial tree), analogous to (2); units are usually those of pressure difference per unit flow. *Cf.* impedance (2). **4.** In psychoanalysis, an individual's unconscious defense against bringing repressed thoughts to consciousness. **5.** The ability of red blood cells to resist hemolysis and to preserve their shape under varying degrees of osmotic pressure in the blood plasma. **6.** The natural or acquired ability of an organism to maintain its immunity to or to resist the effects of an antagonistic agent, *e.g.*, pathogenic microorganism, toxin, drug.
airway r., in physiology, the r. to flow of gases during ventilation due to obstruction or turbulent flow in the upper and lower airways; to be differentiated during inhalation from r. to inflation due to decreases in pulmonary or thoracic compliance.
bacteriophage r., r. of a bacterial mutant to infection by a bacteriophage to which the parent (wild type) strain is susceptible; due to bacterial surface changes that prevent adsorption by the phage, in contrast to bacteriophage immunity, which depends on lysogeny.
expiratory r., r. to flow of gas out of the lungs or the total r. to flow of gas during the expiratory phase of the respiratory cycle.
impact r., the ability of a lens for eyewear to withstand shattering or breakage upon impact, *i.e.*, of a $^3/_8$-inch steel ball dropped 50 feet; criteria for determination of impact r. are specified by U.S. regulations.
inductive r., reactance.
insulin r., diminished effectiveness of insulin in lowering blood sugar levels; arbitrarily defined as requiring 200 units or more of insulin per day to prevent hyperglycemia or ketosis; usually due to insulin binding by antibodies, but abnormalities in insulin receptors on cell surfaces also occur; associated with obesity, ketoacidosis, infection, and certain rare conditions.
mutual r., antagonism.
peripheral r., total peripheral r.
synaptic r., the ease or difficulty with which a nerve impulse can cross a synapse.
systemic vascular r., an index of arteriolar constriction throughout the body; equal to the blood pressure divided by the cardiac output.
total peripheral r. (TPR), peripheral r.; the total r. to flow of blood in the systemic circuit; the quotient produced by dividing the mean arterial pressure by the cardiac minute-volume.

resistor (rē-zis'ter, -tōr). An element included in an electrical circuit to provide resistance to the flow of current.

resolution (rez-ō-lū'shŭn) [L. *resolutio,* a slackening, fr. *re-solvo,* pp. *-solutus,* to loosen, relax]. **1.** The arrest of an inflammatory process without suppuration; the absorption or breaking down and removal of the products of inflammation or of a new growth. **2.** The optical ability to distinguish detail such as the separation of closely adjacent objects.

resolve (rē-zolv') [L. *resolvo,* to loosen]. To return or cause to return to the normal, particularly without suppuration, said of a phlegmon or other form of inflammation.

resolvent (rē-zol'vent). **1.** Causing resolution. **2.** An agent that arrests an inflammatory process or causes the absorption of a neoplasm.

resonance (rez'ō-nans) [L. *resonantia,* echo, fr. *re-sono,* to resound, to echo]. **1.** Sympathetic or forced vibration of air in the cavities above, below, in front of, or behind a source of sound; in speech, modification of the quality (*e.g.*, tone) of a sound by the passage of air through the chambers of the nose, pharynx, and head, without increasing the intensity of the sound. **2.** The sound obtained on percussing a part that can vibrate freely. **3.** The intensification and hollow character of the voice sound obtained on auscultating over a cavity. **4.** In chemistry, the manner in which electrons or electric charge are distributed among the atoms in compounds that are planar and symmetrical, particularly those with conjugated (alternating) double bonds; the existence of r. in the latter case lowers the energy content and increases the stability of a compound. **5.** The natural or inherent frequency of any oscillating system.
amphoric r., cavernous r.; a percussion sound, like that produced by blowing across the neck of an empty bottle, obtained by percussing over a pulmonary cavity with the patient's mouth open.
bandbox r., vesiculotympanitic r.
bellmetal r., coin test; anvil or bell sound; in cases of a large pulmonary cavity or of pneumothorax, a clear metallic sound obtained by striking a coin, held against the chest, by another coin, or by flicking the chest wall with one's fingernail, and is heard on auscultating the chest wall on the same side anteroposteriorly.
cavernous r., amphoric r.
cracked-pot r., cracked-pot sound; a peculiar sound, resembling that heard on striking a cracked pot, elicited on percussing over a pulmonary cavity that commmunicates with a bronchial tube, the patient having the mouth open.
electron spin r. (ESR), a spectrometric method, based on measurement of electron spins and magnetic moments, for detecting and estimating free radicals in organic reactions.
hydatid r., a peculiar vibratile r. heard on auscultatory percussion over a hydatid cyst.
nuclear magnetic r. (NMR), the phenomenon in which certain nuclei possessing a magnetic moment will gyrate around the axis of a strong external magnetic field, the frequency of gyration being specific for each specific nucleus at a particular strength of the magnetic field; gyrating nuclei induce their own oscillating magnetic fields and thereby emit electromagnetic radiation which under certain conditions can produce a detectable signal. NMR is

used as a method of defining the character of covalent bonds and is applied clinically as the technology underlying magnetic resonance *imaging* (*q.v.*).
skodaic r., Skoda's sign or tympany; a peculiar, high-pitched sound, less musical than that obtained over a cavity, elicited by percussion just above the level of a pleuritic effusion.
tympanitic r., tympany.
vesicular r., the sound obtained on percussing over the normal lungs.
vesiculotympanitic r., bandbox or wooden r.; a peculiar, partly tympanitic, partly vesicular sound, obtained on percussion in cases of pulmonary emphysema.
vocal r. (VR), the voice sounds as heard on auscultation of the chest.
wooden r., vesiculotympanitic r.

resonator (rez'ō-nā-ter). A device for employing inductance to create an electrical current of very high potential and small volume.

resorb (rē-sōrb') [L. *re-sorbeo,* to suck back]. To reabsorb; to absorb what has been excreted, as an exudate or pus.

resorcin (rē-zōr'sin). Resorcinol.

resorcinol (rē-zōr'si-nol). Resorcin; *m*-dihydroxybenzene; 1,3-benzenediol; used internally for the relief of nausea, asthma, whooping cough, and diarrhea, but chiefly as an external antiseptic in psoriasis, eczema, seborrhea, and ringworm; pyrocatechol and hydroquinone are isomers of r.
r. monoacetate, used externally in the treatment of acne, sycosis, seborrhea, and alopecia.
r. phthalic anhydride, fluorescein.

resorcinolphthalein (rē-zōr'si-nol-thal'ē-in). Fluorescein.
r. sodium, *fluorescein* sodium.

resorption (rē-sōrp'shŭn). **1.** The act of resorbing. **2.** A loss of substance by lysis, or by physiologic or pathologic means.
bone r., the removal of osseous tissue.
gingival r., gingival *recession.*
horizontal r., horizontal *atrophy.*
internal r., a loss of tooth structure originating within the pulp cavity.
ridge r., a loss in the volume and size of the alveolar portion of the mandible or maxilla.
root r., dissolution of the root of a tooth; either external, with loss or blunting of the apical portion, or internal, with loss of dentin from the inside (pulpal) part of the root area.

respirable (re-spīr'ă-bl, res'pĭ-ră-bl). Capable of being breathed.

respiration (R) (res-pi-rā'shŭn) [L. *respiratio,* fr. *re-spiro,* pp. *-atus,* to exhale, breathe]. **1.** A fundamental process of life characteristic of both plants and animals, in which oxygen is used to oxidize organic fuel molecules, providing a source of energy as well as carbon dioxide and water. In green plants, photosynthesis is not considered r. **2.** Ventilation (2).
abdominal r., breathing effected mainly by the action of the diaphragm.
aerobic r., a form of r. in which molecular oxygen is consumed and carbon dioxide and water are produced.
amphoric r., a sound like that made by blowing across the mouth of a bottle, heard on auscultation in some cases in which a large pulmonary cavity exists, or occasionally in pneumothorax.
anaerobic r., a form of r. in which molecular oxygen is not consumed; *e.g.* nitrate r., sulfate r.
artificial r., artificial *ventilation.*
assisted r., assisted *ventilation.*
Biot's r., Biot's breathing; abrupt, irregular alternating periods of apnea with constant rate and depth of breathing, as that resulting from lesions due to increased intracranial pressure.
bronchial r., a tubular blowing sound caused by the passage of air through a bronchus in an area of consolidated lung tissue.
bronchovesicular r., combined bronchial and vesicular r.
cavernous r., a hollow reverberating sound heard on auscultation over a cavity in the lung.
Cheyne-Stokes r., the pattern of breathing with gradual increase in depth and sometimes in rate to a maximum, followed by a decrease resulting in apnea; the cycles ordinarily are 30 seconds to 2 minutes in duration, with 5 to 30 seconds of apnea; characteristically seen in coma from affection of the nervous centers of respiration.

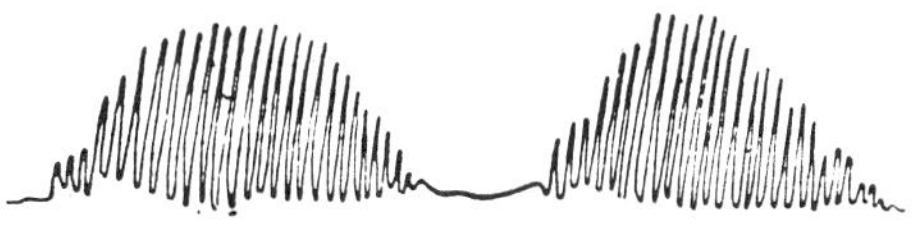

Cheyne-Stokes Respiration

cogwheel r., jerky or interrupted r.; the inspiratory sound being broken into two or three by silent intervals.
controlled r., controlled *ventilation.*
costal r., thoracic r.
diffusion r., apneic oxygenation; maintenance of oxygenation during apnea by intratracheal insufflation of oxygen at high flow rates.
electrophrenic r., the rhythmical electrical stimulation of the phrenic nerve by an electrode applied to the skin at the motor points of the phrenic nerve; it is used in paralysis of the respiratory center resulting from acute bulbar poliomyelitis.
external r., the exchange of respiratory gases in the lungs as distinguished from internal or tissue r.
forced r., voluntary hyperventilation.
internal r., tissue r.
interrupted r., jerky r., cogwheel r.
Kussmaul r., Kussmaul-Kien r., deep, rapid r. characteristic of diabetic or other causes of acidosis.
mouth-to-mouth r., a method of artificial ventilation involving an overlap of the patient's mouth (and nose in small children) with the operator's mouth to inflate the patient's lungs by blowing, followed by an unassisted expiratory phase brought about by elastic recoil of the patient's chest and lungs; repeated 12 to 16 times a minute; where the nose is not covered by the operator's mouth, the nostrils must be closed by pinching.
nitrate r., the process of r. used by some anaerobic organisms, in which nitrate rather than molecular oxygen is used to oxidize organic molecules to obtain energy.
paradoxical r., deflation of the lung during inspiration and inflation of the lung during the phase of expiration; seen in the lung on the side of an open pneumothorax.
puerile r., an exaggeration of the normal respiratory sounds, heard in children and in adults after exertion.
sulfate r., the process of r. used by some anaerobic organisms, in which sulfate rather than molecular oxygen is used to oxidize organic molecules to obtain energy.
thoracic r., costal r.; r. effected chiefly by the action of the intercostal and other muscles that raise the ribs, causing expansion of the chest.
tissue r., internal r.; the interchange of gases between the blood and the tissues.
tubular r., high-pitched bronchial r.
vesicular r., respiratory or vesicular murmur; the respiratory murmur heard on auscultating over the normal lung.
vesiculocavernous r., cavernous r., due to the presence of a cavity, mingled with the vesicular murmur of the surrounding normal lung tissue.

respirator (res'pi-rā-ter, -tōr). **1.** Inhaler (1); an appliance fitting over the mouth and nose, used for the purpose of excluding dust, smoke, or other irritants, or of otherwise altering the air before it enters the respiratory passages. **2.** An apparatus for administering artificial respiration, especially for a prolonged period, in cases of paralysis or inadequate spontaneous ventilation.

cuirass r., one of several types of r.'s producing alternating negative pressure about the thoracic cage; now rarely used.

Drinker r., iron lung; tank r.; a mechanical r. in which the body except the head is encased within a metal tank, which is sealed at the neck with an airtight gasket; artificial respiration is induced by making the air pressure inside negative.

pressure-controlled r., a r. that provides a predetermined pressure to gases during inhalation, the volume of gas moved being variable, depending upon resistance.

tank r., Drinker r.

volume-controlled r., a r. that provides a predetermined volume of gases during inhalation, with the pressure required to move that volume remaining variable, depending upon resistance.

respiratory (res'pi-rā-tōr-ē, rĕ-spīr'ă-tōr-ē). Relating to respiration.

respire (rĕ-spīr') [L. *respiro,* to breathe]. **1.** To breathe. **2.** To consume oxygen and produce carbon dioxide by metabolism.

respirometer (res-pĭ-rom'ĕ-ter) [L. *respiro,* to breathe, + G. *metron,* measure]. **1.** An instrument for measuring the extent of the respiratory movements. **2.** An instrument for measuring oxygen consumption or carbon dioxide production, usually of an isolated tissue.

Dräger r., an inferential meter to measure tidal and minute volume from the number of revolutions of a vane rotated by the gas stream as the latter passes through two light-weight lozenge-shaped meshing rotors.

Wright r., an inferential meter to measure tidal and minute volume from the number of revolutions of a vane rotated by the gas stream as the latter passes through 10 tangential slots in a cylindrical stator ring to turn a flat two-bladed rotor.

response (rē-spons') [L. *responsus,* an answer]. **1.** The reaction of a muscle, nerve, gland, or other excitable tissue to a stimulus. **2.** Operant behavior; any act or behavior, or its constituents, that an animal or human is capable of emitting. Reflexes are usually excluded because they are typically elicited by a specifiable (unconditioned or natural) stimulus rather than emitted under circumstances in which the stimulus was not specifiable.

biphasic r., immediate reaction to an antigenic challenge followed by a recurrence of symptoms after an interval of quiescence.

conditioned r., a r. already in an individual's repertoire but which, through repeated pairings with its natural stimulus, has been acquired or conditioned anew to a previously neutral or conditioned stimulus. *Cf.* unconditioned r.

curve r., computation of the spectral variation of red, green, and blue color pigments, believed to duplicate the photosensitivity of visual pigments.

Cushing r., Cushing *phenomenon.*

depletion r., subnormal metabolic r. to trauma in a person whose physiologic processes are already depressed by disease.

early-phase r., prompt onset of symptoms following an antigenic stimulus.

evoked r., evoked potential; an alteration in the electrical activity of a region of the nervous system through which an incoming sensory stimulus is passing; may be somatosensory (SER), auditory (BAER), or visual (VER).

flight or fight r., see emergency *theory.*

galvanic skin r. (GSR), a measure of changes in emotional arousal recorded by attaching electrodes to any part of the skin and recording changes in moment-to-moment perspiration and related autonomic nervous system activity. Also called psychogalvanic or psychogalvanic skin r.; galvanic skin, psychogalvanic, or psychogalvanic skin reaction or reflex.

Henry-Gauer r., inhibition of antidiuretic hormone secretion due to a rise in atrial pressure which stimulates atrial stretch receptors.

immune r., **(1)** the r. of previously sensitized tissue to an antigen; in the case of antigens produced by microbes and other parasitic organisms, the immune r. tends to resist infection; **(2)** the r. of the immunological mechanism to an antigen (immunogen) that leads to the condition of induced sensitivity, especially from the viewpoint of antibody (immunoglobulin) production; the immune r. to the initial antigenic exposure (**primary i. r.**) is serologically detectable, as a rule, only after a lag period of from several days to two weeks or more and is initiated by transient production of 19 S (IgM) immunoglobulins, followed by production of 7 S (mostly IgG) antibodies; the immune r. to a subsequent stimulus (**secondary i. r.**) by the same antigen (even in relatively small amounts) is more rapid than in the case of the primary immune r., and the antibodies produced reach higher titers, persist for a much longer period of time, and have a greater affinity for the antigen.

isomorphic r., Köbner's *phenomenon.*

late-phase r., recurrence of symptoms after an appreciable interval following challenge with an antigen; preceded by an initial early-phase r.

oculomotor r., widespread myogenic potential evoked by visual stimuli.

orienting r., orienting *reflex.*

psychogalvanic r. (PGR), psychogalvanic skin r., galvanic skin r.

recruiting r., recruitment (2).

relaxation r., an integrated hypothalamic reaction resulting in decreased sympathetic nervous system activity which, physiologically and psychologically, is almost a mirror image of the body's r.'s to Cannon's emergency theory (flight or fight r.); can be self-induced through the use of techniques associated with transcendental meditation, yoga, and biofeedback. See also emergency *theory.*

sonomotor r., widespread myogenic potential evoked by click stimulation.

target r., operant.

triple r., the triphasic r. to the firm stroking of the skin: Phase 1 is the sharply demarcated erythema that follows a momentary blanching of the skin, and is the result of release of histamine from the mast cells. Phase 2 is the intense red flare extending beyond the margins of the line of pressure but in the same configuration, and is the result of arteriolar dilation; also called axon flare because it is mediated by axon reflex. Phase 3 is the appearance of a line wheal in the configuration of the original stroking.

unconditioned r., a r., such as salivation, which is a part of the animal or human repertoire. *Cf.* conditioned r.

rest. 1 [A.S. *raest*]. Quiet; repose. **2** [A.S. *raestan*]. To repose; to cease from work. **3** [L. *restare,* to remain]. A group of cells or a portion of fetal tissue that has become displaced and lies embedded in tissue of another character. **4.** In dentistry, an extension from a prosthesis that affords vertical support for a restoration.

adrenal r., accessory *adrenal.*

cingulum r., the rigid part of a removable partial denture supported by a prepared r. area on the cingulum of an anterior tooth or crown.

incisal r., the portion of a removable partial denture supported by an incisal edge.

lingual r., a metallic extension onto the lingual surface of a tooth to provide support or indirect retention for a removable partial denture.

Malassez' epithelial r.'s, epithelial remains of Hertwig's root sheath in the periodontal ligament.

Marchand's r., Marchand's *adrenals.*

mesonephric r., wolffian r.

occlusal r., a rigid extension of a removable partial denture onto the occlusal surface of a posterior tooth for support of the prosthesis.

precision r., a r. consisting of closely interlocking parts.

Walthard's cell r., a nest of epithelial cells occurring in the peritoneum of the uterine tubes or ovary; when neoplastic, possibly comprising one of the components of the Brenner tumor.

wolffian r., mesonephric r.; remnants of the wolffian duct in the female genital tract that give rise to cysts; *e.g.,* Gartner's cyst.

restenosis (rē'sten-ō-sis) [re-, + G. *stenōsis,* a narrowing]. Recurrence of stenosis after corrective surgery on the heart valve.

restiform (res'ti-fōrm) [L. *restis,* rope, + *forma,* form]. Ropelike; rope-shaped; referring to the restiform body (pedunculus cerebellaris inferior).

restitution (res-ti-tū'shŭn) [L. *restitutio,* act of restoring]. In obstetrics, the return of the rotated head of the fetus to its natural relation with the shoulders after its emergence from the vulva.

restoration (res-tō-rā'shŭn) [L. *restauro,* pp. *-atus,* to restore, to repair]. In dentistry: **1.** A prosthetic r. or appliance; a broad term applied to any inlay, crown, bridge, partial denture, or complete denture which restores or replaces lost tooth structure, teeth, or oral tissues. **2.** A plug or stopping; any substance such as gold, amalgam, etc., used for restoring the portion missing from a tooth as a result of removing decay in the tooth.

acid-etched r., the r. of tooth structure with an autopolymerizing resin after the surface of the tooth has been treated with an acid solution that increases the retention of the r. by etching the surface.

combination r., a tooth r. of two or more materials applied in layers.

compound r., a r. of more than one surface of a tooth.

direct acrylic r., a direct resin r. of autopolymerizing acrylic.

direct composite resin r., a direct resin r. composed of an autopolymerizing epoxy resin and methacrylic acid matrix with as much as 78% of reinforcing fillers such as glass beads, rods, quartz, or lithium aluminum silicate.

direct resin r., a r. made by inserting a plastic mix of autopolymerizing resin(s) in a cavity prepared in a tooth, as opposed to curing a nonautopolymerizing resin in a matrix and cementing the completed r. in the cavity.

overhanging r., a r. with excessive material at the junction of the r. margin and the tooth.

permanent r., a r. designed to endure for as long a period as possible, in contradistinction to a temporary or provisional r.

root canal r., a gutta-percha, silver, or plastic cone that has been carried into a root canal, either alone or in conjunction with a cement, paste, or solvent, for the purpose of eliminating the canal space.

silicate r.'s, r.'s of lost tooth structure made with silicate cement.

temporary r., a r. to be used for a limited period of time, in contradistinction to a permanent r.

restorative (re-stōr'ă-tiv). **1.** Renewing health and strength. **2.** An agent that promotes a renewal of health or strength.

restraint (rē-strānt') [O. Fr. *restrainte*]. In psychiatry, intervention to prevent an excited or violent patient from doing harm to himself or others.

resuscitate (rē-sŭs'i-tāt) [L. *re-suscito,* to raise up again, revive]. To perform resuscitation.

resuscitation (rē-sŭs'i-tā'shŭn) [L. *resuscitatio*]. Revival from potential or apparent death.

cardiopulmonary r. (CPR), restoration of cardiac output and pulmonary ventilation following cardiac arrest and apnea, using artificial respiration and closed chest massage.

mouth-to-mouth r., mouth-to-mouth respiration employed as part of emergency cardiopulmonary r.

resuscitator (rē-sŭs'i-tā-ter, -tōr). An apparatus that forces gas (usually O_2) into lungs to produce artificial ventilation.

retainer (rē-tān'er). Any type of clasp, attachment, or device used for the fixation or stabilization of a prosthesis; an appliance used to prevent the shifting of teeth following orthodontic treatment.

continuous bar r., continuous clasp; a metal bar, usually resting on lingual surfaces of teeth, to aid in their stabilization and to act as indirect r.'s.

direct r., a clasp or attachment applied to an abutment tooth for the purpose of maintaining a removable appliance in position.

extracoronal r., a r. that depends upon contact with the outer circumference of the crown of a tooth for its retentive qualities.

Hawley r., Hawley appliance; a removable wire and acrylic palatal appliance used to retain or stabilize the teeth in their new position following orthodontic tooth movement; with modifications it can be used to move teeth as an active orthodontic appliance.

indirect r., a part of a removable partial denture which assists the direct r.'s in preventing occlusal displacement of the distal extension bases by functioning through lever action on the opposite side of the fulcrum line.

intracoronal r., a r. that depends upon components placed within the crown portion of a tooth for its retentive qualities.

matrix r., a mechanical device designed to hold a matrix around a tooth during restorative procedures, usually by engaging the ends of the matrix band and drawing the band tight.

space r., space *maintainer.*

retardate (rē-tahr'dāt) [L. *retardo,* to delay, hinder]. A person who has mental retardation.

retardation (rē-tahr-dā'shŭn). Slowness or limitation of development.

mental r., amentia (1); mental deficiency; subaverage general intellectual functioning that originates during the developmental period and is associated with impairment in adaptive behavior. The American Association on Mental Deficiency lists eight medical classifications and five psychological classifications; the latter five replace the three former classifications of moron, imbecile, and idiot. Mental r. classification requires assignment of an index for performance relative to a person's peers on two interrelated criteria: measured intelligence (IQ) and overall socio-adaptive behavior (a judgmental rating of the individual's relative level of performance in school, at work, at home, and in the community).

Psychological classifications of mental retardation

Classification	Stanford-Binet IQ	Wechsler IQ
Borderline	68–83	70–84
Mild	52–67	55–69
Moderate	36–51	40–54
Severe	20–35	25–39
Profound	below 20	below 25

psychomotor r., slowed psychic activity or motor activity, or both.

retarder (rē-tar'der). An agent used to slow the chemical hardening of gypsum, resins, or impression materials used in dentistry.

retch [A.S. *hraecan,* to hawk]. To make an involuntary effort to vomit.

retch'ing. Vomiturition; dry vomiting; gastric and esophageal movements of vomiting without expulsion of vomitus.

rete, pl. **retia** (rē'tē; rē'shē-ă, -tē-ă) [L. a net] [NA]. **1.** A network of nerve fibers or small vessels. **2.** A structure composed of a fibrous network or mesh.

r. acromia'le [NA], acromial network; a vascular network between the acromion and the skin of the shoulder, formed by anastomoses of the acromial branch of the suprascapular artery with the acromial branch of the thoracoacromial artery.

r. arterio'sum [NA], arterial network; a vascular network formed by anastomoses between minute arteries just before they become capillaries.

r. articula're cu'biti [NA], articular network of elbow; vascular networks in the region of the elbow, composed of anastomoses between branches of the radial and middle collateral, superior and inferior ulnar collateral, radial recurrent, interosseous recurrent, and recurrent ulnar arteries.

r. articula're ge'nus [NA], articular network of knee; an arterial network over the front and sides of the knee, formed by branches of the descending genicular artery, of the five genicular arteries from the popliteal, of the anterior tibial recurrent, and of the fibular circumflex branch of the posterior tibial.

r. calca'neum [NA], network of heel; a superficial network over the calcaneus, formed by branches of the peroneal and posterior tibial arteries and twigs from the malleolar retia.

r. cana'lis hypoglos'si, *plexus* venosus canalis hypoglossi.

r. car'pi dorsa'le [NA], dorsal carpal network; r. carpi posterius; a vascular network over the dorsal surface of the carpal joints, formed by anastomoses of branches of the anterior and posterior interosseous, and dorsal carpal branches of the radial and ulnar arteries.

r. car'pi poste'rius, r. carpi dorsale.

r. cuta'neum co'rii, the network of vessels parallel to the surface between the corium and the tela subcutanea.

r. foram'inis ova'lis, *plexus* venosus foraminis ovalis.

Haller's r., r. hal'leri, r. testis.

r. malleola're latera'le [NA], lateral malleolar network; a network over the lateral malleolus formed by branches of the posterior lateral malleolar, anterior lateral malleolar, peroneal, and lateral tarsal arteries.

r. malleola're media'le [NA], medial malleolar network; a network over the medial malleolus formed by branches from the anterior and posterior medial malleolar and medial tarsal arteries.

malpighian r., malpighian *stratum.*

r. mirab'ile [NA], a vascular network interrupting the continuity of an artery or vein, such as occurs in the glomeruli of the kidney (arterial) or in the liver (venous).

r. ova'rii, a transient network of cells in the developing ovary; homologous to the r. testis.

r. patel'lae [NA], patellar network; the superficial portion of the r. articulare genus.

r. subpapilla're, the network of vessels between the papillary and reticular strata of the corium.

r. tes'tis [NA], Haller's r.; r. halleri; the network of canals at the termination of the straight tubules in the mediastinum testis.

r. vasculosum articula're [NA], articular vascular network; a vascular r. in the neighborhood of a joint, where such arrangements are common.

r. veno'sum [NA], venous network.

r. veno'sum dorsa'le ma'nus [NA], dorsal venous network of hand; a superficial network of veins on the dorsum of the hand emptying into the cephalic and the basilic veins.

r. veno'sum dorsa'le pe'dis [NA], dorsal venous network of foot; a superficial network of fine veins on the dorsum of the foot.

r. veno'sum planta're [NA], plantar venous network; a fine superficial venous network in the sole of the foot.

retention (rē-ten'shŭn) [L. *retentio,* a holding back]. **1.** The keeping in the body of what normally belongs there, especially the retaining of food and drink in the stomach. **2.** The keeping in the body of what normally should be discharged, as urine or feces. **3.** Retaining that which has been learned so that it can be utilized later as in recall, recognition, or, if r. is partial, relearning. See also memory. **4.** Resistance to dislodgement. **5.** In dentistry, a passive period following treatment when a patient is wearing an appliance or appliances to maintain or stabilize the teeth in the new position into which they have been moved.

denture r., the means by which dentures are held in position in the mouth.

direct r., r. obtained in a removable partial denture by the use of attachments or clasps which resist their removal from the abutment teeth.

indirect r., r. obtained in a removable partial denture through the use of indirect retainers.

partial denture r., the fixation of a removable partial denture by the use of clasps, indirect retainers, or precision attachments.

retia (rē'shē-ă, -tē-ă) [L.]. Plural of rete.

retial (rē'shē-ăl). Relating to a rete.

reticul-. See reticulo-.

reticula (re-tik'yū-lă) [L.]. Plural of recticulum.

reticular, reticulated (re-tik'yū-lăr, -lāt-ed). Relating to a reticulum.

reticulation (re-tik-yū-lā'shŭn). The presence or formation of a reticulum or network, such as that observed in the red blood cells during active regeneration of blood.

reticulin (re-tik'yū-lin). Name given to the chemical substance of reticular fibers, which once were thought to be distinct from collagen by reason of their distinctive structure and staining properties but are now regarded as type III collagen (with its associated proteoglygans and structural glycoproteins).

reticulitis (re-tik'yū-lī'tis) [reticul- + G. *-itis,* inflammation]. Inflammation of the reticulum of ruminant animals.

reticulo-, reticul- [L. *reticulum,* a small net, dim. of *rete,* a net]. Combining forms denoting reticulum or reticular.

reticulocyte (re-tik'yū-lō-sīt) [reticulo- + G. *kytos,* cell]. Skein cell; reticulated corpuscle; a young red blood cell with a network of precipitated basophilic substance representing residual polyribosomes, and occurring during the process of active blood regeneration. See also erythroblast.

reticulocytopenia (re-tik'yū-lō-sī-tō-pē'nē-ă) [reticulocyte + G. *penia,* poverty]. Reticulopenia; paucity of reticulocytes in the blood.

reticulocytosis (re-tik'yū-lō-sī-tō'sis) [reticulocyte + G. *osis,* condition]. An increase in the number of circulating reticulocytes above the normal, which is less than 1% of the total number of red blood cells; it occurs during active blood regeneration (stimulation of red bone marrow) and in certain anemias, especially congenital hemolytic anemia.

reticuloendothelial (re-tik'yū-lō-en-dō-thē'lē-ăl). Denoting or referring to reticuloendothelium.

reticuloendothelioma (re-tik'yū-lō-en'dō-thē-lē-ō'mă) [reticuloendothelium + G. *-oma,* tumor]. A localized reticulosis, or neoplasm derived from reticuloendothelial tissue.

reticuloendotheliosis (re-tik'yū-lō-en'dō-thē-lē-ō'sis) [reticuloendothelium + G. *-osis,* condition]. Proliferation of the reticuloendothelium in any of the organs or tissues. See also reticulosis.

avian r., a leukosis-like disease of fowl caused by viruses of the avian type C oncovirus.

leukemic r., hairy cell *leukemia.*

reticuloendothelium (re-tik'yū-lō-en-dō-thē'lē-ŭm) [reticulo- + endothelium]. The cells making up the reticuloendothelial system.

reticulohistiocytoma (re-tik'yū-lō-his'tē-ō-sī-tō'mă) [reticulo- + histiocytoma]. Reticulohistiocytic granuloma; a solitary skin nodule composed of glycolipid-containing multinucleated large histiocytes; multiple lesions sometimes occur in association with arthritis.

reticulohistiocytosis (re-tik'yū-lō-his'tē-ō-sī-tō'sis). See reticulosis.

multicentric h., lipoid dermatoarthritis; a rare disease in which cutaneous papules composed of histiocytes containing glycolipids are associated with polyarthritis, often leading to shortening of the fingers.

reticuloid (re-tik'yū-loyd). **1.** Resembling a reticulosis. **2.** A condition resembling reticulosis.

actinic r., idiopathic photosensitivity occurring in elderly males, with erythroderma and marked thickening and ridging of exposed skin simulating lymphoma; there is infiltration by atypical mononuclear cells, and transformation to lymphoma may occur after several years.

reticulopenia (re-tik'yū-lō-pē'nē-ă). Reticulocytopenia.

reticulosis (re-tik-yū-lō'sis) [reticulo- + G. *-osis,* condition]. **1.** An increase in histiocytes, monocytes, or other reticuloendothelial elements. **2.** Lymphoma.

benign inoculation r., cat-scratch *disease.*

histiocytic medullary r., a malignant *histiocytosis.*

leukemic r., monocytic *leukemia.*

lipomelanic r., dermatopathic *lymphadenopathy.*

myeloid r., r. involving the bone marrow in which giant cells with a reticulated nucleus are found; they are thought to be derived from reticular cells of the reticuloendothelial system.

pagetoid r., Woringer-Kolopp *disease.*

polymorphic r., lymphomatoid *granulomatosis.*

reticulospinal (re-tik-yū-lō-spī'năl). Pertaining to the *tractus* reticulospinales.

reticulotomy (rē-tik-yū-lot'ō-mē) [reticulo- + G. *tomē,* incision]. Production of lesions in the reticular formation.

reticulum, pl. **reticula** (re-tik'yū-lŭm, -lă) [L. dim of *rete,* a net]. **1.** A fine network formed by cells, or formed of certain structures within cells or of connective tissue fibers between cells. **2.** Neuroglia. **3.** The second compartment of the stomach of a ruminant, a comparatively small chamber communicating with the rumen; sometimes called the honeycomb because of the characteristic structure of its wall.

agranular endoplasmic r., smooth-surfaced endoplasmic r.; endoplasmic r. that is lacking in ribosomal granules; involved in synthesis of complex lipids and fatty acids, detoxification of drugs, carbohydrate synthesis, and sequestering of Ca^{++}.

Ebner's r., a network of nucleated cells in the seminiferous tubules.

endoplasmic r., (ER), the network of tubules or flattened sacs (cisternae) with or without ribosomes on the surface of their membranes.

Golgi internal r., Golgi *apparatus.*

granular endoplasmic r., rough-surfaced endoplasmic r.; ergastoplasm; chromidial substance; endoplasmic r. in which ribosomal granules are applied to the cytoplasmic surface of the cisternae; involved in the synthesis and secretion of protein via membrane-bound vesicles to the extracellular space.

Kölliker's r., neuroglia.

rough-surfaced endoplasmic r., granular endoplasmic r.

sarcoplasmic r., the endoplasmic r. of skeletal and cardiac muscle; the complex of vesicles, tubules, and cisternae forming a continuous structure around striated myofibrils, with a repetition of structure within each sarcomere.

smooth-surfaced endoplasmic r., agranular endoplasmic r.

stellate r., a network of epithelial cells disposed in a fluid-filled compartment in the center of the enamel organ between the outer and inner enamel epithelium.

trabecular r., r. trabeculare.

r. trabecula're [NA], the network of fibers at the iridocorneal angle between the anterior chamber of the eye and the venous sinus of the sclera; it contains spaces between the fibers which are involved in drainage of the aqueous humor, and is composed of two portions; the pars corneoscleralis and the pars uvealis. Also called trabecular meshwork, network, reticulum; or zone; ligamentum anulare bulbi; ligamentum pectinatum; ligamentum pectinatum anguli iridocornealis; ligamentum pectinatum iridis; pectinate ligament; Hueck's ligament; pectinate ligament of iridocorneal angle or of iris; pillar of iris; Gerlach's valvula.

retiform (ret'i-fōrm) [L. *rete,* network]. Resembling a net or network.

retin-. See retino-.

retina (ret'i-nă) [Mediev, L. prob. fr. L. *rete,* a net] [NA]. Tunica interna bulbi; optomeninx; nervous tunic of eyeball; grossly, the r. consists of three parts: pars optica retinae, pars ciliaris retinae, and pars iridica retinae. The optic part, the physiologic portion that receives the visual light rays, is further divided into two parts, pars pigmentosa and pars nervosa, which are arranged in the following layers: 1) pigment layer; 2) layer of rods and cones; 3) external limiting membrane, actually a row of junctional complexes; 4) outer nuclear layer; 5) outer plexiform layer; 6) inner nuclear layer; 7) inner plexiform layer; 8) layer of ganglion cells; 9) layer of nerve fibers; 10) internal limiting membrane. Layers 2 through 10 comprise the pars nervosa. At the posterior pole of the visual axis is the macula, in the center of which is the fovea, the area of acute vision. Here layers 6, 7, 8, and 9 and blood vessels are absent, and only elongated cones are present. About 3 mm medial to the fovea is the optic disk, where axons of the ganglionic cells converge to form the optic nerve. The ciliary and iridial parts of the r. are forward prolongations of the pigmented layer and a layer of supporting columnar or epithelial cells over the ciliary body and the posterior surface of the iris, respectively.

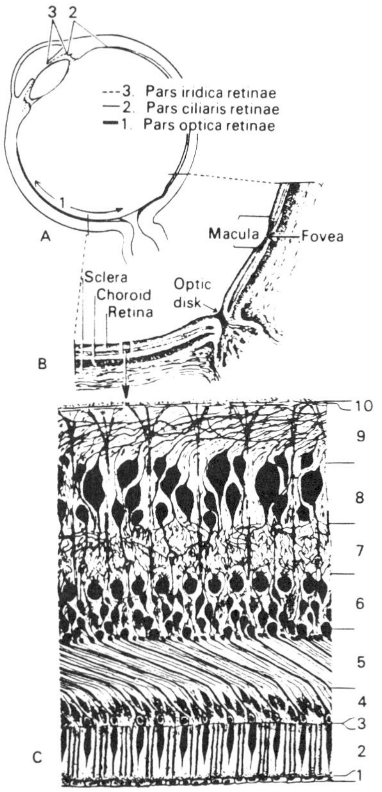

Retina

A, horizontal, meridional section of the eye, showing subdivisions of the retina; *B,* a posterior sector of the eye which includes the macula and optic disk; *C,* the layers of the pars optica retinae (after Polyak). For identification of layers, see definition of retina.

coarctate r., a ringlike effusion of fluid between the choroid and r., giving the latter a funnel shape.

detached r., retinal *detachment.*

fleck r. (of Kandori), an autosomal-recessive disorder of the retinal pigment epithelium occurring in Japanese people.

flecked r., an r. exhibiting fundus flavimaculatus, hereditary drusen, or fundus albipunctatus.
leopard r., tesselated *fundus.*
shot-silk r., shot-silk phenomenon or reflex; the appearance of numerous wavelike, glistening reflexes, like the shimmer of silk, observed sometimes in the r. of a young person.
tigroid r., tessellated *fundus.*

retinaculum, gen. **retinaculi,** pl. **retinacula** (ret-i-nak'yū-lŭm, -lī, -lă) [L. a band, a halter, fr. *retineo,* to hold back] [NA]. A frenum, or a retaining band or ligament.
r. cap'sulae articula'ris cox'ae, Weitbrecht's fibers; one of several longitudinal folds of the articular capsule of the hip joint reflected onto the femoral neck.
caudal r., r. caudale.
r. cauda'le [NA], caudal r. or ligament; ligamentum caudale; fibrous bands, remnants of the notochord, that extend from the skin to the coccyx, forming the coccygeal foveola.
r. cu'tis [NA], r. of skin; one of the numerous small fibrous strands that attaches the dermis to the underlying tela subcutanea; these are particularly well developed over the breast where they are known as ligamenta suspensoria mammae or suspensory ligaments of Cooper.
extensor r., r. extensorum.
retinacula of extensor muscles, r. musculorum extensorum inferius and superius.
r. extenso'rum [NA], extensor r.; dorsal carpal ligament; ligamentum carpi dorsale; a strong fibrous band stretching obliquely across the back of the wrist and binding down the extensor tendons of the fingers and thumb.
flexor r., r. flexorum.
r. of flexor muscles, r. musculorum flexorum.
r. flexo'rum [NA], flexor r.; ligamentum carpi volare; volar carpal ligament; ligamentum carpi transversum; transverse carpal ligament; a strong fibrous band crossing the front of the carpus and binding down the flexor tendons of the digits and the flexor carpi radialis tendon.
inferior r. of extensor muscles, r. musculorum extensorum inferius.
lateral r. of patella, r. patellae laterale.
medial r. of patella, r. patellae mediale.
Morgagni's r., *frenulum* valvae ileocecalis.
r. musculo'rum extenso'rum infe'rius [NA], inferior r. of extensor muscles; cruciate ligament of leg; ligamentum cruciatum cruris; a V-shaped ligament restraining the extensor tendons of the foot distal to the ankle joint.
r. musculo'rum extenso'rum supe'rius [NA], superior r. of extensor muscles; transverse crural ligament; ligamentum transversum cruris; transverse ligament of leg; the ligament that binds down the extensor tendons proximal to the ankle joint; it is continuous above with the deep fascia of the leg.
retinac'ula musculo'rum fibula'rium [NA], official alternate term for retinacula musculorum peroneorum.
r. musculo'rum flexo'rum [NA], r. of flexor muscles; ligamentum laciniatum; laciniate ligament; a wide band passing from the medial malleolus to the medial and upper border of the calcaneus and to the plantar surface as far as the navicular bone; it holds in place the tendons of the tibialis posterior, flexor digitorum longus, and flexor hallucis longus.
retinac'ula musculo'rum peroneo'rum [NA], retinacula of the peroneal or fibular muscles; retinacula musculorum fibularium; superior and inferior fibrous bands retaining the tendons of the peroneus longus and brevis in position as they cross the lateral side of the ankle.
retinacula of nail, retinacula unguis.
r. patel'lae latera'le [NA], lateral r. of patella; part of the aponeurosis of the vastus lateralis muscle passing lateral to the patella to attach to the tibial tuberosity.
r. patel'lae media'le, medial r. of patella; part of the aponeurosis of the vastus medialis muscle passing medial to the patella to attach to the medial condyle of the tibia.
retinacula of peroneal muscles, retinacula musculorum peroneorum.
r. of skin, r. cutis.
superior r. of extensor muscles, r. musculorum extensorum superius.
r. ten'dinum, the annular ligament of the ankle or wrist.
retinac'ula un' guis [NA], retinacula of nail; fibrous attachments of the nail-bed to the underlying phalanx.

retinal 1 (ret'i-năl). Relating to the retina. **2** (ret'i-nal). Retinaldehyde.
r. dehydrogenase [EC 1.2.1.36], retinaldehyde dehydrogenase; an oxidoreductase catalyzing the interconversion of retinaldehyde and retinoic acid.
r. isomerase [EC 5.2.1.3], retinaldehyde isomerase; an isomerase that catalyzes the *cis-trans* conversion of all-*trans*-retinal(dehyde) to 11-*cis*-retinal(dehyde).
r. reductase, alcohol dehydrogenase ($NAD(P)^+$).

11-*cis*-retinal. The isomer of retinaldehyde that can combine with opsin to form rhodopsin; it is formed from all-*trans*-retinal by retinal isomerase.

***trans*-retinal.** All-*trans*-retinal.

retinaldehyde (ret-i-nal'dĕ-hīd). Retinal; retinene; retinene-1; vitamin A_1 aldehyde; retinol oxidized to a terminal aldehyde; a carotene released (as all-*trans*-retinal(dehyde)) in the bleaching of rhodopsin by light and the dissociation of opsin.
r. dehydrogenase, *retinal* dehydrogenase.
r. isomerase, *retinal* isomerase.
r. reductase, alcohol dehydrogenase ($NAD(P)^+$).

retinene (ret'i-nēn). Retinaldehyde.

retinene-1. Retinaldehyde.

retinene-2. Dehydroretinaldehyde.

retinitis (ret-i-nī'tis) [retina + G. *-itis,* inflammation]. Inflammation of the retina.
albuminuric r., see hypertensive *retinopathy.*
apoplectic r., r. after occlusion of the central retinal vein.
azotemic r., see hypertensive *retinopathy.*
central angiospastic r., central serous *choroidopathy.*
circinate r., see circinate *retinopathy.*
diabetic r., see diabetic *retinopathy.*
exudative r., r. exudati'va, Coats' disease; a chronic abnormality characterized by deposition of cholesterol and cholesterol esters in outer retinal layers and subretinal space. In adults, often preceded by uveitis; in children, often preceded by retinal vascular abnormalities.
gravidic r., see toxemic *retinopathy* of pregnancy.
leukemic r., see leukemic *retinopathy.*
metastatic r., purulent or septic r. resulting from the arrest of septic emboli in the retinal vessels.
r. pigmento'sa, pigmentary or tapetoretinal retinopathy; a progressive abiotrophy of the neuroepithelium, with atrophy and pigmentary infiltration of the inner layers of the retina.
r. prolif'erans, proliferative *retinopathy.*
punctate r., see punctata albescens *retinopathy.*
purulent r., metastatic r.
recurrent central r., see central serous *retinopathy.*
r. sclopeta'ria, a severe contusion lesion of the retina.
secondary r., r. that follows uveal inflammation.
septic r., metastatic r.
serous r., simple r.; edema of the retina; an inflammation of the inner layers of the retina.
simple r., serous r.
r. syphilit'ica, syphilitic r., r. often associated with syphilitic cho-

roiditis, especially in congenital syphilis.

retino-, retin- [Med. L. *retina*]. Combining forms denoting the retina.

retinoblastoma (ret'i-nō-blas-tō'mă) [retino- + G. *blastos,* germ, + *-oma,* tumor]. Malignant ocular neoplasm of childhood usually occurring before the third year of life, composed of primitive retinal cells characterized by small round cells with deeply staining nuclei and by elongate cells forming rosettes. In familial forms, the disease is commonly bilateral and multiple within an eye; in sporadic cases, rarely so. The genetics are uncertain, but r. has been plausibly identified as a "two-hit" process in which the first stage or "hit" is inherited in familial cases, with the multiplicity of r. in such cases due to the large number of retinoblasts at risk of a second "hit."

retinochoroid (ret'i-nō-kō'royd). Chorioretinal.

retinochoroiditis (ret'i-nō-kō-roy-dī'tis) [retinochoroid + G. *-itis,* inflammation]. Chorioretinitis; choroidoretinitis; inflammation of the retina extending to the choroid.

bird shot r., bilateral diffuse retinal vasculitis with depigmentation of multiple areas of the choroid and retinal pigment epithelium posterior to the ocular equator, often with an associated papillitis or optic atrophy; vitiligo occurs occasionally.

r. juxtapapilla'ris, Jensen's disease; r. close to the optic disk.

retinodialysis (ret'i-nō-dī-al'i-sis) [retino- + G. *dialysis,* separation]. *Dialysis* retinae.

retinoic acid (ret-i-nō'ik). Vitamin A_1 acid; retinaldehyde in which the terminal –CHO has been oxidized to a –COOH; used topically in the treatment of acne.

retinoid (ret'i-noyd). **1** [G. *rētinē,* resin, + *eidos,* resemblance]. Resembling a resin; resinous. **2** [Mediev. L. *retina*]. Resembling the retina.

retinoids (ret'i-noydz). A class of keratolytic drugs derived from retinoic acid and used for treatment of severe acne and psoriasis.

retinol (ret'i-nol). Vitamin A (2); vitamin A_1; vitamin A_1 alcohol; 2,6,6-trimethyl-1-(9'-hydroxy-3',7'-dimethylnona-1',3',5',7'-tetraenyl)cyclohex-1-ene; a half-carotene bearing the β (or β-ionone) form of the cyclic end group and a CH_2OH at the C-15 position (numbering as in carotenoids) or 9' position (numbering as a nonyl side chain on a cyclohexene ring). See also dehydroretinol.

r. dehydrogenase [EC 1.1.1.105], an oxidoreductase catalyzing interconversion of retinal and retinol.

11-*cis*-retinol. Neoretinene B; retinol with *cis*-configuration at 11-position (carotenoid numbering) or 5'-position (retinol numbering) of side chain.

retinopapillitis (ret'i-nō-pap-i-lī'tis). Inflammation of the retina extending to the optic disk.

r. of premature infants, *retinopathy* of prematurity.

retinopathy (ret-i-nop'ă-thē) [retino- + G. *pathos,* suffering]. Noninflammatory degenerative disease of the retina.

angiopathic r., traumatic r.

arteriosclerotic r., r. distinguished by attenuated retinal arterioles with increased tortuosity, copper- or silver-wire appearance, perivascular sheathing, irregularity of lumen and scattered small hemorrhages, and small, sharp-edged deposits without surrounding edema.

central angiospastic r., central serous *choroidopathy.*

central serous r., central serous *choroidopathy.*

circinate r., a retinal degeneration marked by a girdle of sharply defined white exudates around an edematous macula; usually bilateral and typically affects the aged.

compression r., see traumatic r.

diabetic r., retinal changes occurring in diabetes of long duration, marked by hemorrhages, microaneurysms, and sharply defined waxy deposits, or by proliferative retinopathy.

dysoric r., r. associated with cotton-wool patches.

dysproteinemic r., retinal venous congestion due to increased blood viscosity in dysproteinemia.

eclamptic r., toxemic r. of pregnancy.

electric r., photoretinopathy.

external exudative r., see exudative *retinitis.*

gravidic r., toxemic r. of pregnancy.

hypertensive r., a retinal condition occurring in accelerated vascular hypertension, marked by arteriolar constriction, flame-shaped hemorrhages, cotton-wool patches, star-figure edema at the macula, and papilledema.

hypotensive r., see venous-stasis r.

Leber's idiopathic stellate r., a condition of unknown origin, showing unilaterally macular star with papilledema and spontaneous regression in 1 to 3 months.

leukemic r., appearance of the retina in all types of leukemia, characterized by engorgement and tortuosity of veins, scattered hemorrhages, and edema of the retina and disk.

lipemic r., the appearance of retinal vessels with a marked increase in serum triglycerides.

macular r., maculopathy.

photo r., see photoretinopathy.

pigmentary r., *retinitis* pigmentosa.

r. of prematurity, retrolental fibroplasia; retinopapillitis of premature infants; Terry's syndrome; abnormal replacement of the sensory retina by fibrous tissue and blood vessels, occurring mainly in premature infants having a birth weight of less than 1500 g who are placed in a high-oxygen environment.

proliferative r., retinitis proliferans; neovascularization of the retina extending into the vitreous humor.

puncta'ta al'bescens r., a familial disease in which both fundi show numerous white dots through the retina; causes night blindness.

renal r., hypertensive r. associated with chronic glomerulonephritis or nephrosclerosis.

rubella r., peripheral pigmentary retinal changes in congenital rubella, not affecting visual function.

sickle cell r., a condition marked by dilation and tortuosity of retinal veins, and by microaneurysms and retinal hemorrhages; advanced stages may show neovascularization, vitreous hemorrhage, or retinal detachment.

solar r., photoretinopathy.

stellate r., a r. that resembles hypertensive r., occurring as the result of trauma or obstruction of a retinal vessel.

tapetoretinal r., *retinitis* pigmentosa.

toxemic r. of pregnancy, gravidic or eclamptic r.; sudden angiospasm of retinal arterioles, later followed by retinal vascular signs of advanced hypertensive r; vascular changes disappear rapidly after termination of the pregnancy.

toxic r., retinal changes due to prolonged administration of various drugs.

traumatic r., angiopathic r.; islands of grayish white retinal opacities following extensive crushing or fracture injuries to the body.

venous-stasis r., a uniocular retinopathy associated with partial occlusion of the carotid or the ophthalmic artery.

retinopexy (ret'i-nō-pek'sē) [retino- + G. *pexis,* fixation]. Formation of chorioretinal adhesions surrounding a retinal tear for correction of retinal detachment.

retinopiesis (ret'i-nō-pī-ē'sis) [retino- + G. *piesis,* pressure]. Repositioning a detached retina by pressing it into position by gas or fluid.

retinoschisis (ret-i-nos'ki-sis) [retino- + G. *schisis,* division]. Degenerative splitting of the retina, with cyst formation between the two layers.

juvenile r., r. occurring before 10 years of age and within the nerve-fiber layer, with frequent macular involvement; at first, the inner wall is a translucent veil-like membrane, but it becomes more dense and may render the retina white; X-linked recessive inheritance.

senile r., r. occurring most often in the elderly and affecting the outer plexiform layer; it begins in the extreme inferotemporal periphery and is not significantly progressive; vision usually is good.

retinoscope (ret'i-nō-skōp) [retino- + G. *skopeō,* to view]. An optical device used to illuminate a subject's retina in retinoscopy.

luminous r., a portable optical device providing either a circular or linear (streak) beam of light.

reflecting r., a plane or concave mirror with a central perforation that allows the observer to see rays emerge from the subject's eye.

retinoscopy (ret'i-nos'kō-pē) [retino- + G. *skopeō,* to view]. Pupilloscopy; scotoscopy; skiascopy; shadow test; a method of determining errors of refraction by illuminating the retina and observing the rays of light emerging from the eye.

cylinder r., determination of spherical, astigmatic, and refractive error using cylindrical lenses.

fogging r., the method of reducing vision with convex lenses until accommodation is suspended; a static, noncycloplegic technique.

retoperithelium (rē'to-per-i-thē'lē-ŭm) [L. *rete,* net, + G. *peri,* around, + Mod. L. *thelium,* fr. G. *thēlē,* nipple]. The reticular cells related to the reticular fiber network, as in the stroma of lymphatic tissue.

retort (rē-tōrt') [Mediev. L. *retorta,* fem. pp. of *re- torqueo,* pp. *-tortus,* to twist or bend back]. **1.** A flasklike vessel with a long neck passing outward, once used in distilling. **2.** A small furnace.

Retortamonas (rē-tōr-tam'ō-nas) [L. *re-torqueo,* to twist back, + G. *monas,* single, a unit]. A genus of protozoan flagellates, one species of which, *R. intestinalis,* is found occasionally in the human intestine, although it is nonpathogenic and infrequently reported.

retothelioma (ret'ō-thē-lē-ō'mă). A neoplasm derived from reticular cells of the reticuloendothelial system.

retract (rē-trakt') [L. *re-traho,* pp. *-tractus,* a drawing back]. To shrink, draw back, or pull apart.

retractile (rē-trak'til). Retractable; capable of being drawn back.

retraction (rē-trak'shŭn) [L. *retractio,* a drawing back]. **1.** A shrinking, drawing back, or pulling apart. **2.** Posterior movement of teeth, usually with the aid of an orthodontic appliance.

gingival r., **(1)** lateral movement of the gingival margin away from the tooth surface; may be indicative of underlying inflammation or pocket formation; **(2)** displacement of the marginal gingivae away from the tooth by mechanical, chemical, or surgical means.

mandibular r., a type of facial anomaly in which the gnathion lies posterior to the orbital plane.

retractor (rē-trak'ter, -tōr). **1.** An instrument for drawing aside the edges of a wound or for holding back structures adjacent to the operative field. **2.** A muscle that draws a part backward.

retrad (rē'trad) [L. *retro,* backward, + *ad,* to]. Backward; toward the back part; directed posteriorly.

retrahens aurem, retrahens auriculam (rēt'ră-henz aw'rem, aw-rik'yū-lam) [L. drawing back the ear, or auricle]. See *musculus* auricularis posterior.

retreat from reality. Substitution of imaginary satisfactions or fantasy for relations with the real world.

retrenchment (rē-trench'-ment) [F. *re-,* back, + *trancher,* to cut]. The cutting away of superfluous tissue.

retrieval (rē-trē'văl). The third stage in the memory process, after encoding and storage, involving mental processes associated with bringing stored information back into consciousness.

retro- [L. back, backward]. Prefix, to words formed from L. roots, denoting backward or behind.

retroauricular (re'trō-aw-rik'yū-lăr). Behind the auricle.

retrobuccal (re'trō-bŭk'ăl). Relating to the back part of, or behind, the cheek.

retrobulbar (re'trō-bŭl'bar). Retro-ocular; behind the eyeball.

retrocalcaneobursitis (re'trō-kal-kā'nē-ō-ber-sī'tis) [retro- + L. *calcaneum* heel, + bursitis]. Achillobursitis.

retrocecal (re'trō-sē'kăl). Posterior to the cecum.

retrocervical (re'trō-ser'vi-kăl). Posterior to the cervix uteri.

retrocession (re-trō-sesh'ŭn) [L. *retro-cedo,* pp. *-cessus,* to go back, retire]. **1.** A going back; a relapse. **2.** Cessation of the external symptoms of a disease followed by signs of involvement of some internal organ or part. **3.** Denoting a position of the uterus or other organ further back than is normal.

retroclusion (re-trō-klū'zhŭn) [retro- + L. *claudo* (*cludo*) to close]. A form of acupressure for the arrest of bleeding; the needle is passed through the tissues above the cut end of the artery, is turned around, and then is passed backward beneath the vessel to come out near the point of entrance.

retrocolic (re'trō-kol'ik) [retro- + G. *kolon,* colon]. Posterior to the colon.

retrocollic (re'trō-kol'ik) [retro- + L. *collum,* neck]. Relating to the back of the neck; drawing back the head.

retrocollis (re-trō-kol'is). Retrocollic *spasm.*

retroconduction (re-trō-kon-dŭk'shŭn). Retrograde *conduction.*

retrocursive (re'trō-ker'siv) [retro- + L. *cursus,* a running]. Running backward.

retrodeviation (re'trō-dē-vē-ā'shŭn). A backward bending or inclining.

retrodisplacement (re'trō-dis-plās'ment). Any backward displacement, such as retroversion or retroflexion of the uterus.

retroesophageal (re'trō-ē-sof'ă-jē'ăl). Posterior to the esophagus.

retrofilling (re-trō-fil'ing). Placement of a sealing material into the apical foramen of a dental root from the apical end.

retroflected (re'trō-flek-ted). Retroflexed.

retroflection (re-trō-flek'shŭn). Retroflexion.

retroflexed (re'trō-flekst) [retro- + L. *flecto,* pp. *flexus,* to bend]. Retroflected; bent backward or posteriorly.

retroflexion (re-trō-flek'shŭn). Retroflection; backward bending, as of the uterus when the corpus is bent back, forming an angle with the cervix.

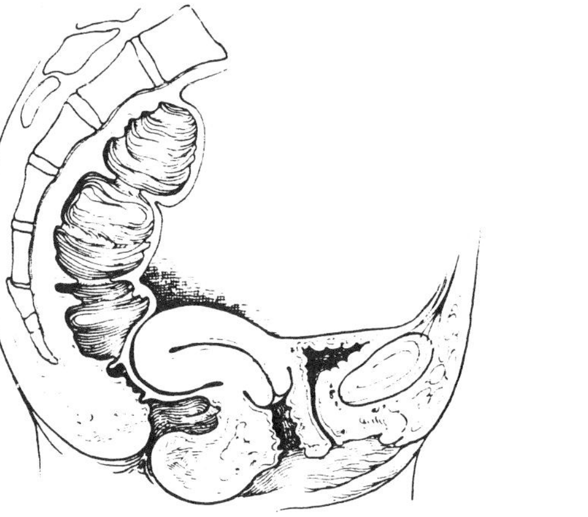

Retroflexion of the Uterus

r. of iris, abnormal position of the iris on the ciliary body after severe concussion.

retrognathic (re-trō-nath'ik). Denoting a state in which the mandible is located posterior to its normal position in relation to the maxillae.

retrognathism (re-trō-nath'izm) [retro- + G. *gnathos,* jaw]. A condition of facial disharmony in which one or both jaws are posterior to normal in their craniofacial relationships; usually used in reference to the mandible.

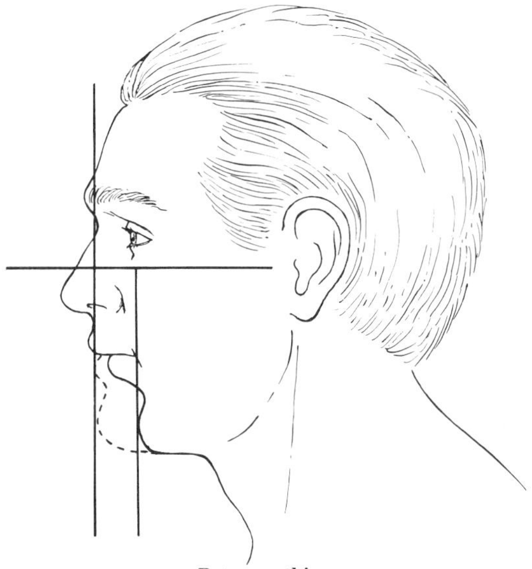

Retrognathism

retrograde (ret'rō-grād) [L. *retrogradus,* fr. retro- + *gradior,* to go]. **1.** Moving backward. **2.** Degenerating; reversing the normal order of growth and development.

retrography (re-trog'ră-fē) [retro- + G. *graphō,* to write]. Mirror-writing.

retrogression (re-trō-gresh'ŭn) [L. *retrogressus* fr. *retrogradior,* to go backwards]. Cataplasia.

retroiridian (re'trō-i-rid'ē-an). Posterior to the iris.

retrojection (re-trō-jek'shŭn) [L. *retro,* backward, + *jacio,* to throw]. The washing out of a cavity by the backward flow of an injected fluid.

retrojector (re'trō-jek-ter, -tōr). A form of syringe with long tubular attachment to the nozzle, used in retrojection.

retrolental (re'trō-len'tăl). Retrolenticular (1); posterior to the lens of the eye.

retrolenticular (re'trō-len-tik'yū-lăr). **1.** Retrolental. **2.** Behind the lentiform nucleus of the brain.

retrolingual (re'trō-ling'gwăl) [retro- + L. *lingua,* tongue]. Relating to the back part of the tongue; posterior to the tongue.

retromammary (re'trō-mam'ă-rē). Posterior to the mamma.

retromandibular (re'trō-man-dib'yū-lăr) [retro- + L. *mandibula,* lower jaw]. Posterior to the lower jaw.

retromastoid (re'trō-mas'toyd). Posterior to the mastoid process; relating to the posterior mastoid cells.

retromolar (re-trō-mō'lăr). Distal (or posterior) to the last erupted (or present) molar tooth.

retromorphosis (re-trō-mōr'fō-sis, -mōr-fō'sis) [retro- + G. *morphōsis,* process of forming]. Cataplasia.

retronasal (re'trō-nā'zăl). Posterior nasal; relating to the posterior nares.

retro-ocular (re'trō-ok'yū-lăr). Retrobulbar.

retroperitoneal (re'trō-per'i-tō-nē'ăl). External or posterior to the peritoneum.

retroperitoneum (re'trō-per'i-tō-nē'ŭm) [retro- + peritoneum]. *Spatium* retroperitoneale.

retroperitonitis (ret'rō-per-i-tō-nī'tis). Inflammation of the cellular tissue behind the peritoneum.
idiopathic fibrous r., idiopathic retroperitoneal *fibrosis.*

retropharyngeal (re'trō-fă-rin'jē-ăl). Posterior to the pharynx.

retropharynx (re'trō-făr'ingks). The posterior part of the pharynx.

retroplacental (re'trō-pla-sen'tăl). Behind the placenta.

retroplasia (ret-rō-plā'zē-ă) [retro- + G. *plasis,* a molding]. That state of cell or tissue in which activity is decreased below that considered normal; associated with retrogressive changes (*e.g.,* injury, degeneration, death, necrosis).

retroposed (re'trō-pōzd) [retro- + L. *pono,* pp. *positus,* to place]. Denoting retroposition.

retroposition (re'trō-pō-zish'ŭn) [retro- + L. *positio,* a placing]. Simple backward displacement of a structure or organ, as the uterus, without inclination, bending, retroversion, or retroflexion.

retroposon (re-trō-pōs'on). Term proposed for a transposition of sequences in a DNA that does not take place in the DNA by itself, but rather in an mRNA that is transcribed back into the genomic DNA, as in "retro" synthesis (RNA prescribing DNA).

retropubic (re-trō-pyū'bik). Posterior to the pubic bone.

retropulsion (re-trō-pŭl'shŭn) [retro- + L. *pulsio,* a pushing, fr. *pello,* pp. *pulsus,* beat, drive]. **1.** An involuntary backward walking or running, occurring in patients with the parkinsonian syndrome. **2.** A pushing back of any part.

retrospection (re-trō-spek'shŭn) [retro- + L. *specto,* pp. *-spectatus,* to look at]. The act or process of surveying the past.

retrospective (re-trō-spek'tiv). Relating to retrospection.

retrospondylolisthesis (re'trō-spon'di-lō-lis-thē'sis) [retro- + G. *spondylos,* vertebra, + *olisthēsis,* a slipping]. Slipping posteriorly of the body of a vertebra, bringing it out of line with the adjacent vertebrae.

retrosternal (re'trō-ster'năl). Posterior to the sternum.

retrosteroid (re-trō-stēr'oyd, -ster'oyd). A term sometimes used to designate a steroid in which the orientations of the substituents at carbons 9 and 10 are the opposite of those of the reference or "parent" compound.

retrotarsal (re'trō-tar'săl). Posterior to the tarsus, or edge of the eyelid.

retrouterine (re'trō-yū'ter-in). Posterior to the uterus.

retroversioflexion (re-trō-ver'sē-ō-flek'shŭn, -ver'zhō-). Combined retroversion and retroflexion of the uterus.

retroversion (re-trō-ver'zhŭn) [retro- + L. *verto,* pp. *versus,* to turn]. **1.** A turning backward, as of the uterus. **2.** Condition in which the teeth are located in a more posterior position than is normal. See fig. on p. 1356.

retroverted (re'trō-ver-ted). Denoting retroversion.

Retroviridae (re-trō-vir'i-dē). A family of viruses resembling the orthomyxoviruses in size and shape, but structurally more complex; they possess RNA-dependent DNA polymerases (reverse transcriptases) and are grouped in three subfamilies: Oncovirinae (RNA tumor viruses), Spumavirinae (foamy viruses), and Lentivirinae (visna and related agents). Virions are about 100 nm in diameter, enveloped, and ether-resistant, and contain segmented, single-stranded RNA of high molecular weight (5 to 10 $\times$ 10^6).

retrovirus (re'trō-vī'rŭs). Any virus of the family Retroviridae.

retrusion (rē-trū'zhŭn) [L. *re-trudo,* pp. *-trusus,* to push back]. **1.** Retraction of the mandible from any given point. **2.** The backward movement of the mandible.

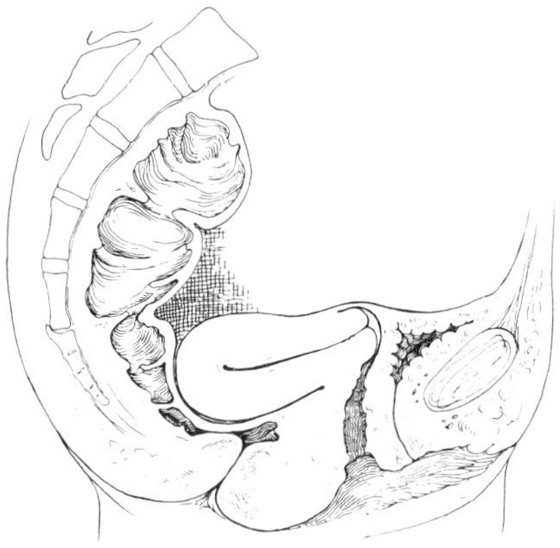

Retroversion of the Uterus

Rett, Andreas, 20th century Austrian pediatrician. See Rett's *syndrome.*

Retzius, Anders A., Swedish anatomist and anthropologist, 1796–1860. See R.'s *cavity, fibers, gyrus, ligament, space, veins.*

Retzius, Magnus G., Swedish anatomist and anthropologist, 1842–1919. See R.'s *striae; lines, foramen,* calcification *lines* of R.; Key-R. *corpuscles, foramen; sheath* of Key and R.

reunient (rē-yū'nē-ent) [L. *re-,* again, + *unio,* pp. *unitus,* to unite]. Connecting; denoting the ductus reuniens.

Reuss, August R. von, Austrian ophthalmologist, 1841–1924. See R.'s *formula,* color *tables, test.*

revaccination (rē'vak-si-nā'shŭn). Vaccination of an individual previously successfully vaccinated.

revascularization (rē-vas'kyū-lăr-i-zā'shŭn). Reestablishment of blood supply to a part.

Reverdin, Jacques L., Swiss surgeon, 1842–1929. See R. *graft;* R.'s *method.*

reversal (rē-ver'săl) [L. *re-verto,* pp. *-versus,* to turn back or about]. **1.** A turning or changing to the opposite direction, as of a process, disease, symptom, or state. **2.** The changing of a dark line or a bright one of the spectrum into its opposite. **3.** Denoting the difficulty of some persons in distinguishing the lower case printed or written letter *p* from *q* or *g, b* from *d,* or *s* from *z.* **4.** In psychoanalysis, the change of an instinct of affect into its opposite, as from love into hate.

adrenaline r., epinephrine r.

epinephrine r., adrenaline r.; the fall in blood pressure produced by epinephrine when given following blockage of α-adrenergic receptors by an appropriate drug such as phenoxybenzamine; the vasodilation reflects the ability of epinephrine to activate β-adrenergic receptors which, in vascular smooth muscle, are inhibitory; in the absence of α-receptor blockade, the β-receptor activation by epinephrine is masked by its predominant action on vascular α-receptors, which causes vasoconstriction.

narcotic r., the use of narcotic antagonists, such as naloxone, to terminate the action of narcotics.

pressure r., cessation of anesthesia by hyperbaric pressure; of major importance in understanding the mode of action of anesthetics.

relaxant r., use of acetylcholinesterase inhibitors to terminate the action of nondepolarizing neuromuscular relaxants.

sex r., a process whereby the sexual identity of an individual is changed from one sex to the other (*e.g.,* by a combination of surgical, pharmacologic, and psychiatric procedures); it may also occur in the life history of pseudohermaphroditic individuals whose sex at birth was uncertain; initially reared as members of one sex, such individuals may, upon subsequent medical examination and advice, be reared thereafter as members of the opposite sex.

reversible (rē-ver'si-bl). Capable of reversal; said of diseases or chemical reactions.

reversion (rē-ver'zhŭn) [L. *reversio* (see reversal)]. **1.** The manifestation in an individual of certain characteristics, peculiar to a remote ancestor, which have been suppressed during one or more of the intermediate generations. **2.** The return to the original phenotype, either by reinstatement of the original genotype (true r.) or by a mutation at a site different from that of the first mutation and which cancels the effect of the first mutation (suppressor mutation).

revertant (rē-ver'tant). In microbial genetics, a mutant that has reverted to its former genotype (true reversion) or to the original phenotype by means of a suppressor mutation.

Revilliod, Léon, Swiss physician, 1835–1919. See R.'s *sign.*

revivescence (re-vi-ves'ens) [L. *re-vivesco,* to come to life again, fr. *vivo,* to live]. Revivification (1).

revivification (rē-viv'i-fi-kā'shŭn) [L. *re-,* again, + *vivo,* to live, + *facio,* to make]. **1.** Revivescence; renewal of life and strength. **2.** Vivification; refreshening the edges of a wound by paring or scraping to promote healing.

revulsion (rē-vŭl'shŭn) [L. *revulsio,* art of pulling away, fr. *re-vello,* pp. *-vulsus,* to pluck or pull away]. **1.** Counterirritation. **2.** Derivation (1).

reward (rē-ward'). Reinforcer.

rewarming (rē-warm'ing). Application of heat to correct hypothermia.

Rexed lamina. See under lamina.

Reye, Ralph Douglas Kenneth, 20th century Australian pathologist. See R.'s *syndrome.*

Reymond. See Du Bois-Reymond.

RF Abbreviation for releasing *factor;* rheumatoid *factors;* replicative *form.*

RFA Abbreviation for right frontoanterior *position.*

RFP Abbreviation for right frontoposterior *position.*

RFT Abbreviation for right frontotransverse *position.*

RH Abbreviation for releasing *hormone.*

Rh **1.** Symbol for rhodium. **2.** See Rh blood group, Blood Groups appendix.

rhabarberone (ra-bar'ber-ōn). Aloe-emodin.

rhabd-. See rhabdo-.

Rhabditis (rab-dī'tis) [G. *rhabdos,* a rod]. A genus of small nematodes (family Rhabditidae, order Rhabditida), some of which are free-living, others parasitic on plants and animals; by dwelling on decaying organic matter, including putrefying flesh, some species have been viewed as parasitic or incipient parasites. *R. strongyloides* may invade the skin of dogs, cattle, and rodents, causing dermatitis.

rhabdo-, rhabd- [G. *rhabdos,* rod]. Combining forms denoting rod, rod-shaped (rhabdoid).

rhabdocyte (rab'dō-sīt) [rhabdo- + G. *kytos,* cell]. Rarely used term for band cell or metamyelocyte.

rhabdoid (rab'doyd) [rhabdo- + G. *eidos,* resemblance]. Rod-shaped.

rhabdomyoblast (rab-dō-mī'ō-blast) [rhabdo- + G. *mys,* muscle, + *blastos,* germ]. Large round, spindle-shaped, or strap-shaped cells with deeply eosinophilic fibrillar cytoplasm which may show cross striations; found in some rhabdomyosarcomas.

rhabdomyolysis (rab'dō-mī-ol'i-sis) [rhabdo- + G. *mys,* muscle, +

lysis, loosening]. An acute, fulminating, potentially fatal disease of skeletal muscle which entails destruction of skeletal muscle as evidenced by myoglobinemia and myoglobinuria.

acute recurrent r., familial paroxysmal r.; repeated paroxysmal attacks of muscle pain and weakness followed by passage of dark red-brown urine, diagnosed by demonstration of myoglobin in the urine; attributed to abnormal phosphorylase activity in skeletal muscle, but there may be more than one biological type; familial occurrence, but more common in males than females.

exertional r., r. produced in susceptible individuals by muscular exercise.

familial paroxysmal r., acute recurrent r.

idiopathic paroxysmal r., myoglobinuria.

rhabdomyoma (rab'dō-mī-ō'mă) [rhabdo- + G. *mys,* muscle, + *-oma,* tumor]. A benign neoplasm derived from striated muscle, occurring in the heart in children, probably as a harmatomatous process.

rhabdomyosarcoma (rab'dō-mī-ō-sar-kō'mă) [rhabdo- + G. *mys,* muscle, + *sarkōma,* sarcoma]. Rhabdosarcoma; a malignant neoplasm derived from skeletal (striated) muscle, occurring in children or, less commonly, in adults; classified as embryonal (*q.v.*). alveolar (composed of loose aggregates of small round cells), or pleomorphic (containing rhabdomyoblasts).

embryonal r.'s, malignant neoplasms occurring in children, consisting of loose, spindle-celled tissue with rare cross-striations, and arising in many parts of the body in addition to skeletal muscles.

rhabdophobia (rab-dō-fō'bē-ă) [rhabdo- + G. *phobos,* fear]. Morbid fear of a rod (or switch) as an instrument of punishment.

rhabdosarcoma (rab'dō-sar-kō'mă). Rhabdomyosarcoma.

rhabdosphincter (rab'dō-sfingk'ter) [rhabdo- + G. *sphinktēr,* sphincter]. Striated muscular sphincter; a sphincter made up of striated musculature.

Rhabdoviridae (rab'dō-vir'i-dē). A family of rod- or bullet-shaped viruses of vertebrates, insects, and plants, including rabies virus and vesicular stomatitis virus (of cattle). Virions (60 to 400 by 60 to 85 nm), formed by budding from surface membranes of cells, are enveloped and ether-sensitive, with surface spikes 10-nm long; nucleocapsids contain single-stranded RNA (MW 3 to 5 $\times$ 10^6) and are of helical symmetry. Two genera have been assigned names, *Vesiculovirus* and *Lyssavirus,* and there are possibly four others.

rhabdovirus (rab'dō-vī'rŭs). Any virus of the family Rhabdoviridae.

rhachi-. For words so beginning, see rachi-.

rhagades (rag'ă-dēz) [G. *rhagas,* pl. *rhagades,* a crack]. Chaps, cracks, or fissures occurring at mucocutaneous junctions; seen in vitamin deficiency diseases and in congenital syphilis.

rhagadiform (ră-gad'i-fōrm) [G. *rhagas* (*rhagad-*), crack, + L. *forma,* shape]. Resembling or characterized by rhagades.

-rhagia. See -rrhagia.

L-rhamnose (ram'nōs). Isodulcit; a methylpentose present in a number of plant glycosides, free in poison sumac, in lipopolysaccharides of *Enterobacteriaceae,* and in rutinose (a disaccharide).

rhamnoside (ram'nō-sīd). A glycoside of rhamnose.

rhamnoxanthin (ram-nō-zan'thin). Frangulin.

Rhamnus (ram'nŭs) [G. *rhamnos*]. Buckthorn; a genus of shrubs and trees (family Rhamnaceae). The bark and berries of *R. cathartica* are cathartic; *R. frangula* is the source of frangula; *R. purshiana* is the source of cascara sagrada.

rhaphania (ră-fā'nē-ă). Raphania.

rhaphe (rā'fē). Raphe.

-rhaphy. See -rrhaphy.

rhathymia (ră-thī'mē-ă) [G. *rhathymein,* to take a holiday, be relaxed]. Outgoing, carefree behavior.

rhe (rē) [G. *rheos,* a stream]. The absolute unit of fluidity, the reciprocal of the unit of viscosity.

-rhea. See -rrhea.

rhegma (reg'mă) [G. breakage]. A rent or fissure.

rhegmatogenous (reg-mă-toj'ĕ-nŭs) [G. *rhegma,* breakage, + *-gen,* producing]. Arising from a bursting or fractionating of an organ. See r. retinal *detachment.*

rheic (rē'ik). Relating to rheum (rhubarb).

Rheinberg microscope. See under microscope.

rhenium (rē'nē-ŭm) [Mod. L., fr. L. *Rhenus,* Rhine river]. A metallic element of the platinum group; symbol Re, atomic weight 186.21, atomic no. 75.

rheo- [G. *rheos,* stream, current, flow]. Combining form usually denoting blood flow or electrical current.

rheobase (rē'ō-bās) [rheo- + G. *basis,* a base]. Galvanic threshold; the minimal strength of an electrical stimulus of indefinite duration that is able to cause excitation of a tissue, *e.g.,* muscle or nerve. See also chronaxie.

rheobasic (rē-ō-bā'sik). Pertaining to or having the characteristics of a rheobase.

rheocardiography (rē'ō-kar-dē-og'ră-phē) [rheo- + cardiography]. Impedance plethysmography applied to the heart.

rheochrysidin (rē-ō-kris'i-din). The 3-methyl ether of emodin.

rheoencephalogram (rē'ō-en-sef'ă-lō-gram). Graphic registration of the changes in conductivity of tissue of the head caused by vascular factors.

rheoencephalography (rē'ō-en-sef-ă-log'ră-fē) [rheo- + encephalography]. The technique of measuring blood flow of the brain; commonly used to denote impedance r. which uses changes in electrical impedance and resistance as a measure of flow.

rheogram (rē'ō-gram) [rheo- + G. *gramma,* something written]. A plot of the shear stress versus the shear rate for a fluid.

rheologist (rē-ol'ō-jist). A specialist in rheology.

rheology (rē-ol'ō-jē) [rheo- + G. *logos,* study]. The study of the deformation and flow of materials.

rheometer (rē-om'ĕ-ter) [rheo- + G. *metron,* measure]. **1.** An instrument for measurement of the rheologic properties of materials, *e.g.,* of blood. **2.** A galvanometer.

rheometry (rē-om'ĕ-trē). Measurement of electrical current or blood flow.

rheopexy (rē'ō-pek-sē) [rheo- + G. *pexis,* fixation]. A property of certain materials in which an increased rate of shear favors an increase in viscosity.

rheostat (rē'ō-stat) [rheo- + G. *statos,* stationary]. A variable resistor used to adjust the current in an electrical circuit.

rheostosis (rē-os-tō'sis) [rheo- + G. *osteon,* bone, + *-osis,* condition]. Streak or flowing hyperostosis; a hypertrophying and condensing osteitis which tends to run in longitudinal streaks or columns, like wax drippings on a candle, and which involves a number of the long bones.

rheotaxis (rē-ō-tak'sis) [rheo- + G. *taxis,* orderly arrangement]. A form of positive barotaxis, in which a microorganism in a fluid is impelled to move against the current flow of its medium.

rheotropism (rē-ot'rō-pizm) [rheo- + G. *tropos,* a turning]. A movement contrary to the motion of a current, involving part of an organism, rather than the organism as a whole, as in rheotaxis.

rhestocythemia (res'tō-sī-thē'mē-ă) [G. *rhaiō,* to destroy, + *kytos,* a hollow (a cell), + *haima,* blood]. The presence of broken down red blood cells in the peripheral circulation.

rhesus (rē'sŭs) [Mod. L., fr. L. *Rhesus,* G. *Rhesos,* a mythical king of Thrace]. Generic name for *Macaca mulatta.*

rheum (rūm) [G. *rheuma,* a flux]. A mucous or watery discharge.

rheumatalgia (rū-mă-tal'jē-ă) [G. *rheuma,* flux, + *algos,* pain]. Obsolete term for rheumatic pain.

rheumatic (rū-mat'ik) [G. *rheumatikos,* subject to flux, fr. *rheuma,* flux]. Rheumatismal; relating to or characterized by rheumatism.

rheumatid (rū'mă-tid) [G. *rheum,* flux, + -id (1)]. Rheumatic nodules or other eruptions which may accompany rheumatism.

rheumatism (rū'mă-tizm) [G. *rheumatismos,* rheuma, a flux]. **1.** Obsolete term for rheumatic *fever.* **2.** Indefinite term applied to various conditions with pain or other symptoms which are of articular origin or related to other elements of the musculoskeletal system.

articular r., arthritis.

chronic r., a nonspecific disorder of the joints, slow in progress, producing a painful thickening and contraction of the fibrous structures, interfering with motion, and causing deformity.

gonorrheal r., an arthritis, often a polyarthritis, caused by systemic infection with the gonococcus.

inflammatory r., rheumatoid arthritis or other cause of joint inflammation.

lumbar r., lumbago.

Macleod's r., rheumatoid arthritis with abundant serous effusion in the affected joints.

muscular r., fibrositis (2).

nodose r., **(1)** rheumatoid *arthritis;* **(2)** an acute or subacute articular r., accompanied by the formation of nodules on the tendons, ligaments, and periosteum in the neighborhood of the affected joints.

subacute r., a mild, but usually protracted form of acute rheumatic fever, often resistant to treatment.

tuberculous r., an inflammatory condition of the joints or fibrous tissues during the course of tuberculosis.

rheumatismal (rū-mă-tiz'măl). Rheumatic.

rheumatocelis (rū'mă-tō-sē'lis) [G. *rheuma,* flux, + *kēlis,* spot]. Henoch-Schönlein *purpura.*

rheumatoid (rū'mă-toyd) [G. *rheuma,* flux, + *eidos,* resemblance]. Resembling r. arthritis in one or more features.

rheumatologist (rū-mă-tol'ō-jist). A specialist in rheumatology.

rheumatology (rū-mă-tol'ō-jē) [G. *rheum,* flux, + *logos,* study]. The medical specialty concerned with the study, diagnosis, and treatment of rheumatic conditions.

rhexis (rek'sis) [G. *rhēxis,* rupture]. Bursting or rupture of an organ or vessel.

rhigosis (ri-gō'sis) [G. *rhigoun,* to be cold, + *-osis,* condition]. The perception of cold.

rhigotic (ri-got'ik). Pertaining to rhigosis.

rhin-, rhino- [G. *rhis,* nose]. Combining forms denoting the nose.

rhinal (rī'năl). Nasal.

rhinalgia (rī-nal'jē-ă) [rhin- + G. *algos,* pain]. Rhinodynia; pain in the nose.

rhinarium, pl. **rhinaria** (rī-nā'rē-ŭm, -rē-ă). The area of hairless skin surrounding the nostrils in some mammals.

rhinedema (rī'ne-dē'mă) [rhin- + G. *oidema,* swelling]. Swelling of the nasal mucous membrane.

rhinencephalic (rī'nen-se-fal'ik). Relating to the rhinencephalon.

rhinencephalon (rī'nen-sef'ă-lon) [rhin- + G. *enkephalos,* brain]. Collective term denoting the parts of the cerebral hemisphere directly related to the sense of smell: the olfactory bulb, olfactory peduncle (together still listed as the first cranial nerve or olfactory nerve despite the fact that they form part of the central nervous system), olfactory tubercle, and olfactory or piriform cortex including the cortical nucleus of the amygdala. The term originally also encompassed the hippocampus, the entire amygdala, and the gyrus fornicatus, which are no longer believed to be specifically related to the sense of smell. See also limbic *system.*

rhinenchysis (rī-nen'kī-sis) [rhin- + G. *enchysis,* a pouring in]. A nasal douche; washing out the nasal cavities.

rhineurynter (rī-nū-rin'ter) [rhin- + G. *eurynō,* to dilate, fr. *eurys,* wide]. A dilatable bag used to make pressure within the nostril to arrest a profuse epistaxis.

rhinion (rin'ē-on) [G. *rhinion,* nostril, dim. of *rhis* (*rhin-*), nose]. A craniometric point: the lower end of the internal suture.

rhinism (rī'nizm). Rhinolalia.

rhinitis (rī-nī'tis) [rhin- + G. *-itis,* inflammation]. Nasal catarrh; inflammation of the nasal mucous membrane.

acute r., coryza; cold in the head; an acute catarrhal inflammation of the mucous membrane of the nose, marked by sneezing, lacrimation, and a profuse secretion of watery mucus; usually associated with infection by one of the common cold viruses.

allergic r., r. associated with hay fever.

atrophic r., chronic r. with thinning of the mucous membrane; often associated with crusts and foul-smelling discharge.

atrophic r. of swine, a disease manifested by atrophy, shrinkage, and often almost complete disappearance of the turbinate bones, accompanied by distortion of the facial bones, sneezing, and stunting of the growth of young animals; caused principally by *Bordetella bronchiseptica.*

r. caseo'sa, caseous r., a form of chronic r. in which the nasal cavities are more or less completely filled with an ill-smelling cheesy material.

chronic r., a protracted sluggish inflammation of the nasal mucous membrane; in the later stages the mucous membrane with its glands may be thickened (hypertrophic r.) or thinned (atrophic r.).

croupous r., membranous r.

eosinophilic nonallergic r., hyperplastic thickening of the nasal mucosa with abnormal numbers of eosinophilic leukocytes, not attributable to a specific allergen.

fibrinous r., membranous r.

gangrenous r., see cancrum nasi.

hypertrophic r., chronic r. with permanent thickening of the mucous membrane.

r. medicamento'sa, inflammation of the nasal mucosa secondary to excessive or improper topical medication.

membranous r., croupous, fibrinous, or pseudomembranous r.; a chronic inflammation of the nasal mucous membrane attended with a fibrinous or pseudomembranous exudate.

necrotic r. of pigs, bullnose; an infection of the subcutaneous structures of the snout of swine which causes malformation of the face; it is frequently due to infection of wounds made for the insertion of metal rings to discourage or prevent the animal from rooting in the soil; *Fusobacterium necrophorum* plays an important role in this disease.

r. nervo'sa, hay *fever.*

pseudomembranous r., membranous r.

r. purulen'ta, purulent r., a chronic r. in which pus formation is excessive.

scrofulous r., tuberculous infection of the nasal mucous membrane.

r. sic'ca, a form of chronic r. with little or no secretion.

vasomotor r., congestion of nasal mucosa without infection or allergy.

rhino-. See rhin-.

rhinoanemometer (rī'nō-an-ĕ-mom'ĕ-ter) [rhino- + G. *anemos,* wind, + *metron,* measure]. A variation of the pneumotachometer, used for measuring nasal air flow and nasal resistance to air flow.

rhinoantritis (rī'nō-an-trī'tis) [rhino- + g. *antron,* cave (antrum) + *-itis,* inflammation]. Inflammation of the nasal cavities and one or both maxillary antrums.

rhinobyon (rī-nō'bē-on, rī'nō-bī'on) [rhino- + G. *byō,* to stuff, plug]. A nasal plug or tampon.

rhinocanthectomy (rī'nō-kan-thek'tō-mē) [rhino- + G. *kanthos,* canthus, + *ektomē,* excision]. Excision of the inner canthus of the eye.

rhinocele (rī'nō-sēl) [rhino- + G. *koilia,* a hollow]. Cavity or ventricle of the rhinencephalon or primitive olfactory part of the telencephalon.

rhinocephaly, rhinocephalia (rī'nō-sef'ă-lē, -se-fā'lē-ă) [rhino- + G. *kephalē,* head]. Rhinencephaly; a form of cyclopia in which the nose is represented by a fleshy proboscis-like protuberance arising above the slitlike orbits, and the rhinencephalic lobes of the telencephalon are poorly developed with some tendency to become fused together.

rhinocheiloplasty, rhinochiloplasty (rī-nō-kī'lō-plas-tē) [rhino- + G. *cheilos,* lip, + *plastos,* formed]. Plastic surgery of the nose and upper lip.

Rhinocladiella (rī'nō-klad-ē-el'ă). A genus of dematiaceous (dark colored) fungi, characterized by acrotheca, that cause chromomycosis. See also *Phialophora.*

rhinocleisis (rī-nō-klī'sis) [rhino- + G. *kleisis,* a closure]. Rhinostenosis.

rhinodacryolith (rī-nō-dak'rē-ō-lith) [rhino- + G. *dakryon,* tear (duct), + *lithos,* stone]. A calculus in the nasolacrimal duct.

rhinodymia (rī-nō-dim'ē-ă) [rhino- + G. *-dymos,* fold]. Duplication of the nose on an otherwise normal face.

rhinodynia (rī-nō-din'ē-ă) [rhino- + G. *odynē,* pain]. Rhinalgia.

rhinoestrosis (rī'nō-es-trō'sis). Infection of horses and donkeys, rarely humans, with larvae of the fly *Rhinoestrus purpureus;* human infection is usually benign and of short duration, limited to the first stage of the larva and resulting in a mild ophthalmomyiasis.

Rhinoestrus purpureus (rī-nō-es'trŭs pŭr-pū'rē-ŭs). A species of fly of the family Oestridae, the nasal botflies, that causes rhinoestorsis.

rhinogenous (rī-noj'ĕ-nŭs) [rhino- + G. *-gen,* producing]. Originating in the nose.

rhinokyphectomy (rī'nō-kī-fek'tō-mē) [rhino- + G. *kyphōsis,* humped condition, + *ektomē,* excision]. Plastic surgery for rhinokyphosis.

rhinokyphosis (rī'nō-kī-fō'sis) [rhino- + G. *kyphōsis,* humped condition]. A humpback deformity of the nose.

rhinolalia (rī'nō-lā'lē-ă) [rhino- + G. *lalia,* talking]. Rhinism; rhinophonia; nasalized speech.
r. aper'ta, abnormal phonation attributable to inadequate velopharyngeal closure.
r. clau'sa, abnormal phonation attributable to nasal obstruction.

rhinolaryngitis (rī'nō-lar-in-jī'tis) [rhino- + G. *larynx,* larynx, + *-itis,* inflammation]. Inflammation of the nasal and laryngeal mucous membranes.

rhinolaryngology (rī'nō-lar-ing-gol'ō-jē). The medical study concerned with the relationship of the nose and larynx and their diseases.

rhinolite (rī'nō-līt). Rhinolith.

rhinolith (rī'nō-lith) [rhino- + G. *lithos,* stone]. Nasal calculus; rhinolite; a calcareous concretion in the nasal cavity.

rhinolithiasis (rī'nō-li-thī'ă-sis) [rhinolith + G. *-iasis,* condition]. The presence of a nasal calculus.

rhinologic (rī-nō-loj'ik). Relating to rhinology.

rhinologist (rī-nol'ō-jist). A specialist in diseases of the nose.

rhinology (rī-nol'ō-jē) [rhino- + G. *logos,* study]. The branch of medical science concerned with the nose and its diseases.

rhinomanometer (rī'nō-mă-nom'ĕ-ter) [rhino- + manometer]. A manometer used to determine the presence and amount of nasal obstruction, and the nasal air pressure and flow relationships.

rhinomanometry (rī'nō-mă-nom'ĕ-trē). **1.** The use of a rhinomanometer. **2.** The study and measurement of nasal air flow and pressures.

rhinomucormycosis (rī'nō-myū'kōr-mī-kō'sis) [rhino- + mucormycosis]. Entomophthoramycosis.

rhinomycosis (rī'nō-mī-kō'sis) [rhino- + mycosis]. Fungus infection of the nasal mucous membranes.

rhinonecrosis (rī'nō-ne-krō'sis) [rhino- + necrosis]. Necrosis of the bones of the nose.

rhinopathy (rī-nop'ă-thē) [rhino- + G. *pathos,* suffering]. Disease of the nose.

rhinopharyngeal (rī'nō-fă-rin'jē-ăl). **1.** Nasopharyngeal. **2.** Relating to the rhinopharynx.

rhinopharyngitis (rī'nō-far'in-jī'tis) [rhino- + pharynx, + G. *-itis,* inflammation]. Nasopharyngitis; inflammation of the mucous membrane of the upper part of the pharynx and posterior nares.
r. mu'tilans, gangosa.

rhinopharyngolith (rī'nō-fă-ring'gō-lith) [rhinopharynx + G. *lithos,* stone]. A concretion in the rhinopharynx.

rhinopharynx (rī'nō-far'ingks) [rhino- + pharynx]. *Pars* nasalis pharyngis.

rhinophonia (rī'nō-fō'nē-ă) [rhino- + G. *phōnē,* voice]. Rhinolalia.

rhinophycomycosis (rī'nō-fī'cō-mī-kō'sis). Entomophthoramycosis.

rhinophyma (rī'nō-fī'mă) [rhino- + G. *phyma,* tumor, growth]. Hypertrophy of the nose with follicular dilation, resulting from hyperplasia of sebaceous glands with fibrosis and increased vascularity. Also called hypertrophic rosacea; copper, rum, brandy, hammer, potato, or toper's nose; rum blossom.

rhinoplasty (rī'nō-plas-tē) [rhino- + G. *plastos,* formed]. **1.** Repair of a defect of the nose with tissue taken from elsewhere. **2.** Plastic surgery to change the shape or size of the nose.
English r., r. utilizing a flap from the cheek.
Indian r., Carpue's method; Indian method or operation; r. utilizing a flap from the forehead.
Italian r., Italian or tagliacotian operation; Italian method r. utilizing a flap from the arm.
Joseph r., obsolete term for reduction and reshaping of the nose.

rhinopneumonitis (rī'nō-nū-mō-nī'tis) [rhino- + G. *pneumōn,* lung, + *-itis,* inflammation]. Inflammation of the mucous membranes of the nose and lung in animals.
equine r., a mild respiratory disease of horses, caused by equine rhinopneumonitis virus, with fever, serous rhinitis, and leukopenia, sometimes resulting in abortion in mares.

rhinorrhagia (rī-nō-rā'jē-ă) [rhino- + G. *rhēgnymi,* to burst forth]. Epistaxis or nosebleed, especially if profuse.

rhinorrhea (rī-nō-rē'ă) [rhino- + G. *rhoia,* flow]. A discharge from the nasal mucous membrane.
cerebrospinal fluid r., a discharge of cerebrospinal fluid from the nose.
gustatory r., watery nasal discharge associated with stimulation of the sense of taste.

rhinosalpingitis (rī'nō-sal-pin-jī'tis) [rhino- + G. *salpinx,* tube, + *-itis,* inflammation]. Inflammation of the mucous membrane of the nose and eustachian tube.

rhinoscleroma (rī'nō-sklē-rō'mă) [rhino- + G. *sklērōma,* an induration]. A chronic granulomatous process involving the nose, upper lip, mouth, and upper air passages; starts usually as a growth of hard smooth nodules in the anterior nares which spreads backward into the pharynx, larynx, trachea, and even into the bronchi;

it may involve the external auditory meatus and is believed to be due to a specific bacterium, possibly a strain of *Klebsiella.*

rhinoscope (rī'nō-skōp). Nasoscope; a small mirror attached at a suitable angle to a rodlike handle, used in posterior rhinoscopy.

rhinoscopic (rī'nō-skop'ik). Relating to the rhinoscope or to rhinoscopy.

rhinoscopy (rī-nos'kŏ-pē) [rhino- + G. *skopeō,* to view]. Inspection of the nasal cavity.

anterior r., inspection of the anterior portion of the nasal cavity with or without the aid of a nasal speculum.

median r., inspection of the roof of the nasal cavity and openings of the posterior ethmoid cells and sphenoidal sinus by means of a long-bladed nasal speculum or nasopharyngoscope.

posterior r., inspection of the nasopharynx and posterior portion of the nasal cavity by means of the rhinoscope, or with a nasopharyngoscope. See also nasopharyngoscopy.

rhinosporidiosis (rī'nō-spō-rid-ē-ō'sis). Invasion of the nasal cavity by *Rhinosporidium seeberi,* resulting in a chronic granulomatous disease producing polyps or other forms of hyperplasia on mucous membranes; it is found in natives of North and South America, Pakistan, India, and Sri Lanka.

Rhinosporidium seeberi (rī'nōspō-rid'ē-ŭm sē-bē'rī) [rhino- + G. *sporidion,* dim. of *sporos,* seed]. A yeastlike organism, of worldwide distribution and uncertain taxonomic position, found in certain vascular raspberry-like tumors of the septum nasi (rhinosporidiosis).

rhinostenosis (rī'nō-ste-nō'sis) [rhino- + G. *stenōsis,* a narrowing]. Rhinocleisis; nasal obstruction.

rhinotomy (rī-not'ō-mē) [rhino- + G. *tomē,* incision, cutting]. **1.** Any cutting operation on the nose. **2.** Operative procedure in which the nose is incised along one side so that it may be turned away to provide full vision of the nasal passages for radical sinus operations.

rhinotracheitis (rī'nō-trā-kē-ī'tis) [rhino- + trachea + *-itis,* inflammation]. Inflammation of the nasal cavities and trachea.

feline viral r., an acute upper respiratory tract infection of cats caused by the feline rhinotracheitis virus; it is frequently fatal in kittens but mild in adults, who sometimes become convalescent carriers of the virus.

infectious bovine r. (IBR), an infectious disease of cattle characterized by tracheitis, rhinitis, and fever, and caused by bovine herpesvirus 1; other clinical manifestations include pustular vulvovaginitis or balanoposthitis, abortion, conjunctivitis and, rarely, encephalitis.

Rhinovirus (rī'nō-vī'rŭs). A proposed genus of acid-labile viruses (family Picornaviridae) of worldwide distribution, associated with the common cold in man and foot-and-mouth disease in cattle. There are more than 100 antigenic types, usually classified as M strains (culturable in rhesus monkey kidney cells) and H strains (growing only in cultures of human cells).

rhinovirus. Any virus of the genus *Rhinovirus.*

bovine r.'s, r.'s that cause widespread subclinical and occasionally mild clinical respiratory diseases of calves in the United States and Europe.

equine r.'s, r.'s that cause inapparent as well as mild to relatively severe upper respiratory tract disease in the United States and Europe; most prevalent in breeding stables, and associated with high morbidity but negligible mortality; all equine isolates are related serologically to the original isolate.

Rhipicephalus (rī-pi-sef'ă-lŭs) [G. *rhipis,* fan, + *kephalē,* head]. A genus of inornate hard ticks (family Ixodidae) consisting of about 50 species, all of which are Old World except *R. sanguineus.* Eyes and festoons are present in both sexes; short palpi and ventral plates are present only in the male. The genus includes important vectors of diseases in man and domestic animals.

R. appendicula'tus, the brown ear tick, a species that transmits *Theileria parva parva* the cause of East Coast fever, and *Theileria parva lawrencei,* the cause of Corridor disease, and *Theileria parva bovis,* the cause of Rhodesian malignant theileriosis.

R. evert'si, the red-legged or African red t., a vector of East Coast fever and of *Borrelia theileri.*

R. pulchel'lus, the yellow-backed or zebra tick; a vector of *Theileria taurotragi,* the cause of benign bovine theileriosis in Africa.

R. sanguin'eus, the brown dog tick, probably the most common and cosmopolitan species found on dogs in the U.S.; it may attack other animals but rarely attacks man; it is a vector of Rocky Mountain spotted fever in Mexico, the major vector of canine babesiosis, transmits canine ehrlichiosis, and is a vector of the rickettsia of boutonneuse fever.

rhizo- [G. *rhiza,* root]. Combining form denoting root.

rhizoid (rī'zoyd) [rhizo- + G. *eidos,* resemblance]. **1.** Rootlike. **2.** Irregularly branching, like a root; denoting a form of bacterial growth. **3.** In fungi, the rootlike hyphae which arise at the nodes of the hyphae of *Rhizopus* species.

rhizome (rī'zōm) [G. *rhizōma,* mass of roots, fr. *rhiza,* root, + *-oma,* mass]. The creeping underground stem of plants such as iris, calamus, and sanguinaria.

rhizomelia (rī-zō-mē'lē-ă) [rhizo- + G. *melos,* limb]. Disproportion in the length of the most proximal segment of the limbs (upper arms and thighs).

rhizomeningomyelitis (rī'zō-mĕ-ning'gō-mī-ĕ-lī'tis) [rhizo- + G. *mēninx,* membrane, + *myelon,* marrow, + *-itis,* inflammation]. Radiculomeningomyelitis; inflammation of the nerve roots, the meninges, and the spinal cord.

rhizoplast (rī'zō-plast) [rhizo- + G. *plastos,* formed]. A fine connection between the flagellum or blepharoplast and the nucleus of a protozoan.

Rhizopoda (rī-zō-pō'dă) [rhizo + G. *pous (pod-),* foot]. Rhizopodea; Rhizopodasida; a superclass in the subphylum Sarcodina that includes the amebae of humans, having pseudopodia of various forms but without axial filaments.

Rhizopodasida (rī'zō-pō-das'i-dă). Rhizopoda.

Rhizopodea (rī-zō-pō'dē-ă) [rhizo- + G. *pous (pod-),* foot]. Rhizopoda.

rhizopterin (rī-zop'ter-in). SLR factor; 10-formylpteroic acid; a folic acid factor for certain bacteria.

Rhizopus (rī-zō'pŭs). A genus of fungi (class Phycomycetes, family Mucoraceae); some species cause mucormycosis in man.

rhizotomy (rī-zot'ō-mē) [G. *rhiza,* root, + *tomē,* section]. Radiculectomy; radicotomy; section of the spinal nerve roots for the relief of pain or spastic paralysis.

anterior r., section of anterior spinal root.

facet r., a percutaneous radio frequency lysis of the innervation of a facet.

posterior r., Dana's operation; section of posterior spinal root.

trigeminal r., retrogasserian neurectomy or neurotomy; division or section of a sensory root of the fifth cranial nerve, accomplished through a subtemporal (Frazier-Spiller operation), suboccipital (Dandy operation), or transtentorial approach.

rhod-. See rhodo-.

rhodamine B (rō'dă-mēn, -min) [C.I. 45170]. A fluorescent red basic xanthene dye, tetraethylrhodamine chloride, used in histology as a contrasting stain to methylene blue and methyl green, and as a vital fluorochrome.

rhodanate (rō'dă-nāt). Thiocyanate.

rhodanese (rō'dă-nēz). *Thiosulfate* sulfurtransferase.

rhodanic acid (rō-dan'ik). Thiocyanic acid.

rhodanile blue (rō'dă-nīl). A dye mixture, considered by some to be a salt of rhodamine B and Nile blue, used to stain keratinized epithelium (red) and fibroblasts (blue), as well as spermatozoa and normal and pathologic acidophilic, basophilic, and certain neutrophilic elements of cells and tissues; used as a substitute for hematoxylin and eosin.

rhodeose (rō'dē-ōs). Fucose.

rhodin (rō'din). A dihydroporphyrin derivative (the two additional hydrogens being at positions 17 and 18) of the type found in chlorophyll *b* and with a formyl group on position 7 rather than a methyl group.

rhodium (rō'dē-ŭm) [Mod. L. fr. G. *rhodon,* a rose]. A metallic element, symbol Rh, atomic no. 45, atomic weight 102.91.

rhodo-, rhod- [G. *rhodon,* rose]. Combining forms denoting rose or red color.

rhodogenesis (rō'dō-jen'ĕ-sis) [rhodopsin + G. *genesis,* production]. The production of rhodopsin by the combination of 11-*cis*-retinal and opsin in the dark.

rhodophylactic (rō'dō-fī-lak'tik). Relating to rhodophylaxis.

rhodophylaxis (rō'dō-fī-lak'sis) [rhodopsin + G. *phylaxis,* a guarding]. The action of the pigment cells of the choroid in preserving or facilitating the reproduction of rhodopsin.

rhodopsin (rō-dop'sin). Visual purple; a red thermolabile protein, MW *ca.* 35,000, found in the external segments of the rods of the retina; it is bleached by the action of light, which converts it to opsin and all-*trans*- retinal, and is restored in the dark by rhodogenesis.

*meta***-rhodopsin I, II, III.** Precursors of opsin and all-*trans* -retinal, formed from lumirhodopsin in the visual cycle.

Rhodotorula (rō-dō-tōr'yū-lă). A genus of yeasts, usually pink to red and of questionable pathogenicity, which are generally introduced iatrogenically into severely compromised patients via intravenous catheters.

rhombencephalon (rom-ben-sef'ă-lon) [rhombo- + G. *enkephalos,* brain] [NA]. Hindbrain, hindbrain vesicle; that part of the brain developed from the most caudal of the three primary vesicles of the embryonic neural tube; secondarily divided into metencephalon and myelencephalon; the r. includes the pons, cerebellum, and medulla oblongata.

rhombic (rom'bik). **1.** Rhomboid. **2.** Relating to the rhombencephalon.

rhombo- [G. *rhombos,* a rhomb or rhombus]. Combining form denoting rhombic or rhomboid.

rhomboatloideus (rom'bō-at-lō-id'ē-ŭs). See under musculus.

rhombocele (rom'bō-sēl) [rhombo- + G. *koilia,* a hollow]. Rhomboidal *sinus.*

rhomboid, rhomboidal (rom'boyd, rom-boy'dăl) [rhombo- + G. *eidos,* appearance]. Rhombic (1); resembling a rhomb; *i.e.,* an oblique parallelogram, but having unequal sides; in anatomy, denoting especially a ligament and two muscles.

rhomboideus (rom-bō-id'ē-ŭs). See entries under musculus.

rhombomere (rom'bō-mēr) [rhombo- + G. *meros,* part]. Neuromere.

rhonchal, rhonchial (rong'kăl, rong'kē-ăl). Relating to or characteristic of a rhonchus.

rhonchus, pl. **rhonchi** (rong'kŭs, -kī) [L. fr. G. *rhenchos,* a snoring]. An added sound with a musical pitch occurring during inspiration or expiration, heard on auscultation of the chest, and caused by air passing through bronchi that are narrowed by inflammation, spasm of smooth muscle, or presence of mucus in the lumen; if low-pitched, it is called **sonorous r.;** if high-pitched, with a whistling or squeaky quality, **sibilant r.**

cavernous r., cavernous *rale.*

rhopheocytosis (rō'fē-ō-sī-tō'sis) [G. *rhophein,* to gulp down, or aspirate, + *kytos,* cell, + *-osis,* condition]. Formation of vacuoles at a cell surface without prior formation of cytoplasmic projections, by which the cell appears to aspirate surrounding material. See also pinocytosis.

rhoptry, pl. **rhoptries** (rŏp'trē, -trēs) [G. *rhopalon,* club]. Toxoneme; paired organelles; electron-dense club-shaped, tubular or saccular organelles extending back from the anterior end of sporozoites and other stages of certain sporozoans in the subphylum Apicomplexa.

rhotacism (rō'tă-sizm) [G. *rhō,* the letter r]. Mispronunciation of the "r" sound.

rhubarb (rū'barb). Any plant of the genus *Rheum* (family Polygonaceae), especially *R. rhaponticum,* garden rhubarb, and *R. officinale* or *R. palmatum;* the last two species or their hybrids, deprived of periderm tissues, dried, and powdered, are used for their astringent, tonic and laxative effects.

Rhus (rūs, rŭs) [L., fr. G. *rhous,* sumac]. A genus of vines and shrubs (family Anacardiaceae) containing various species that are used for their ornamental foliage; formerly used in tanning. Certain poisonous species are classified as *Toxicodendron.*

rhyparia (rī-pā'rē-ă) [G. filth, fr. *rhypos,* filth]. Sordes.

rhypophagy (rī-pof'ă-jē) [G. *rhypos,* filth, + *phagein,* to eat]. Scatophagy.

rhypophobia (rī-pō-fō'bē-ă) [G. *rhypos,* filth, + *phobos,* fear]. An abnormal aversion to or morbid fear of dirt or filth.

rhythm (ridh'ŭm) [G. *rhythmos*] **1.** Measured time or motion; the regular alternation of two different or opposite states. **2.** Rhythm *method.* **3.** Regular occurrence of an electrical event in the electroencephalogram. See also subentries under wave. **4.** Sequential beating of the heart generated by a single beat or sequence of beats in a different chamber than that controlling the resulting rhythm.

agonal r., an idioventricular r., characterized by unusually wide and bizarre ventricular complexes, often seen in moribund patients.

alpha r., Berger r.; alpha wave; a wave pattern in the encephalogram in the frequency band of 8 to 13 Hz.

atrioventricular (A-V) nodal r., nodal bradycardia; nodal r.; the cardiac r. when the heart is controlled by the A-V node; arising in the A-V node, the impulse ascends to the atria and descends to the ventricles simultaneously. In **upper nodal r.,** the P' wave precedes the QRS complex; in **lower nodal r.,** it follows the QRS complex; in **midnodal r.,** it is lost within the QRS complex.

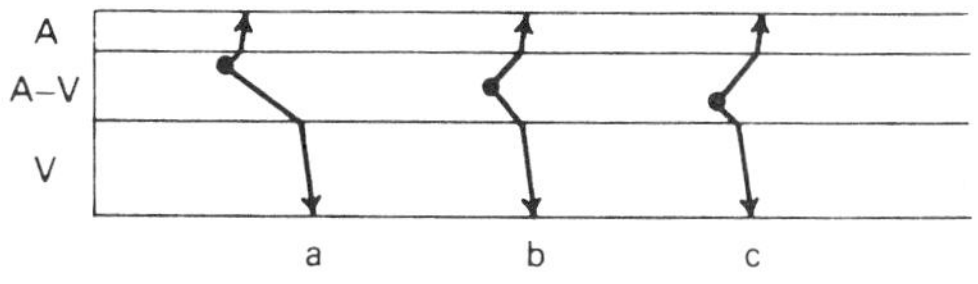

A-V Nodal Rhythms

a, Upper nodal rhythm; *b,* midnodal rhythm; *c,* lower nodal rhythm.

Berger r., alpha r.

beta r., beta wave; a wave pattern in the electroencephalogram in the frequency band of 18 to 30 Hz.

bigeminal r., coupling; coupled r.; that cardiac r. when each sinus beat is followed by a premature beat, with the result that the heartbeats occur in pairs (bigeminy).

cantering r., gallop.

circadian r., see circadian.

circus r., circus *movement.*

coronary nodal r., applied by some authorities to the electrocardiographic pattern of normal upright P waves in leads I and II with a short P-R interval.

coronary sinus r., an ectopic atrial r. supposedly originating from a pacemaker at the mouth of the coronary sinus; recognized in the electrocardiogram by a P-wave pattern similar to that of A-V nodal r. but with a normal or prolonged P-R interval.

coupled r., bigeminal r.

delta r., delta wave (2); a wave pattern in the electroencephalogram that lies in the frequency band of 1.5 to 4.0 Hz.

diurnal r., see diurnal.

ectopic r., any cardiac r. arising from a center other than the normal pacemaker, the sinus node.

escape r., three or more consecutive impulses at a rate not exceeding the upper limit of the inherent pacemaker; rate of impulse formation at the sinoatrial node is 60 to 100 impulses per minute, that of the atrioventricular node is 40 to 60 impulses per minute, and that of the ventricular myocardium is 20 to 40 impulses per minute.

fast r., a wave pattern in the electroencephalogram in the frequency bands above 13 Hz.

gallop r., gallop.

idionodal r., an independent ventricular r., the ventricles being under control of the A-V node.

idioventricular r., ventricular r.; a slow independent ventricular r. under control of an ectopic ventricular center.

nodal r., atrioventricular nodal r.

pendulum r., embryocardia.

quadrigeminal r., quadrigeminy; a cardiac dysrhythmia in which the heartbeats are grouped in fours, each usually composed of one sinus beat followed by three extrasystoles.

quadruple r., trainwheel r.; a quadruple cadence to the heart sounds due to the easy audibility of both third and fourth heart sounds, indicative of serious myocardial disease.

reciprocal r., a cardiac dysrhythmia in which the impulse arising in the A-V junction descends to and activates the ventricles and simultaneously ascends toward the atria; before reaching the atria, however, the impulse is reflected downward and again activates the ventricles, producing the echo or reciprocal beat; recognized in the electrocardiogram by the presence of an inverted P wave sandwiched between two normal ventricular complexes.

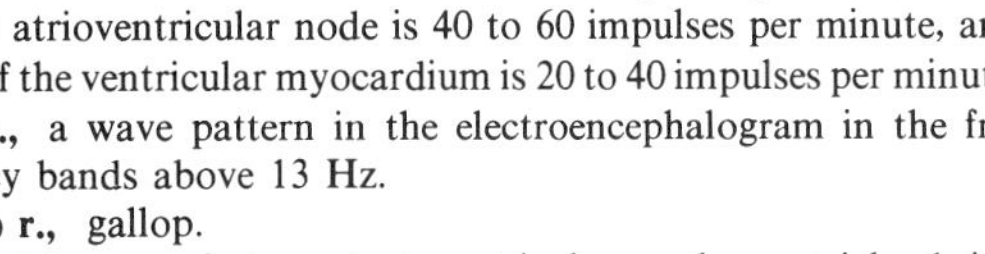

Reciprocal and Reciprocating Rhythms
Left, reciprocal; *center*, reversed reciprocal; *right*, reciprocating.

reciprocating r., a cardiac dysrhythmia initiated by an A-V nodal beat followed in turn by a reciprocal beat; the descending impulse of the reciprocal beat, before reaching the ventricles, is also reflected backward to the atria, but before reaching the atria is reflected downward again to the ventricles.

reversed reciprocal r., a cardiac dysrhythmia in which normal sinus impulse, before reaching the ventricles, is reflected backward to the atria; thus in the electrocardiogram a ventricular complex is sandwiched between a normal sinus P wave and a retrograde P wave; if the dysrhythmia continues, subsequent cycles are similar to those of reciprocating r.

sinus r., normal cardiac r. proceeding from the sinoatrial node.

theta r., theta wave; a wave pattern in the electroencephalogram in the frequency band of 4 to 7 Hz.

tic-tac r., embryocardia.

trainwheel r., quadruple r.

trigeminal r., trigeminy; a cardiac dysrhythmia in which the heartbeats are grouped in trios, usually composed of a sinus beat followed by two extrasystoles.

triple r., a triple cadence to the heart sounds at any rate, due to the easy audibility of a third or fourth heart sound.

ultradian r., see ultradian.

ventricular r., idioventricular r.

rhythmeur (rēt-mer'or ridh'mūr) [Fr.]. An apparatus for securing rhythmic interruptions of the electric current in an x-ray machine.

rhytidectomy (rit-i-dek'tō-mē) [G. *rhytis* (*rhytid-*), a wrinkle]. Rhytidoplasty; elimination of wrinkles from, or reshaping of, the face by excising any excess skin and tightening the remainder; the so-called face-lift.

rhytidoplasty (rit'i-dō-plas-tē) [G. *rhytis*, a wrinkle, + *plastos*, formed]. Rhytidectomy.

rhytidosis (rit-i-dō'sis) [G. a wrinkling, fr. *rhytis*, a wrinkle, + *-osis*, condition]. Rutidosis. **1.** Wrinkling of the face to a degree disproportionate to age. **2.** Laxity and wrinkling of the cornea, an indication of approaching death.

Rib Symbol for ribose.

rib- See ribo-.

rib [A.S. *ribb*] Costa (1).

bicipital r., fusion of first thoracic r. with cervical vertebra.

bifid r., one in which the body bifurcates.

cervical r., *costa* cervicalis.

false r.'s, *costae* spuriae.

floating r.'s, *costae* fluitantes.

lumbar r., an occasional r. articulating with the transverse process of the first lumbar vertebra.

slipping r., subluxation of a r. cartilage, with costochondral separation.

true r.'s, *costae* verae.

vertebral r.'s, *costae* fluitantes.

vertebrochondral r.'s, *costae* spuriae.

vertebrosternal r.'s, *costae* verae.

ribavirin (rī'bă-vī-rin). 1-β-D-Ribofuranosyl-1,2,4-triazole-3-carboxamide; a synthetic nucleoside antiviral agent which, by its inhibitory effect on the synthesis of guanosine 5'-phosphate, inhibits both DNA and RNA synthesis.

α-ribazole (rī'bă-zōl). 1-α-D-ribofuranosyl-5,6-dimethylbenzimidazole; the benzimidazole nucleoside in vitamin B_{12}.

Ribbert, Moritz W.H., German pathologist, 1855–1920. See R.'s *theory*.

ribbon (rib'ŏn) [M. E. *riban*]. A ribbon-shaped structure.

Reil's r., *lemniscus* medialis.

Ribes, François, French physician, 1765–1845. See R.'s *ganglion*.

ribitol (rī'bi-tol). Adonitol; $HOCH_2(CHOH)_3CH_2OH$; reduction product of ribose (–CHO at position 1 reduced to $-CH_2OH$).

ribityl (rī'bi-til). The radical of ribitol; a constituent of riboflavin.

ribo- **1.** The root of ribose, and thus part of its derivatives; *e.g.*, ribofuranose, ribopyranose. **2.** As an italicized prefix to the systematic name of a monosaccharide, *ribo-* indicates that the configuration of a set of three consecutive, but not necessarily contiguous, CHOH (or asymmetric) groups is that of ribose; *e.g.*, D-ribose, a trivial name, is D-*ribo*-pentose in systematic nomenclature.

riboflavin(e) (rī'bō-flā-vin). Flavin (1); lactoflavin (2); 7,8-dimethyl-10-ribitylisoalloxazine; a heat-stable factor of the vitamin B complex whose isoalloxazine nucleotides are coenzymes of the flavodehydrogenases. The daily human requirement is 1 to 2 mg, with higher daily requirement during pregnancy and lactation; dietary sources include green vegetables, liver, kidneys, wheat germ, milk, eggs, and cheese.

r. kinase [EC 2.7.1.26], flavokinase; an enzyme catalyzing the formation of flavin mononucleotide (r. phosphate) from r., utilizing ATP as phosphorylating agent.

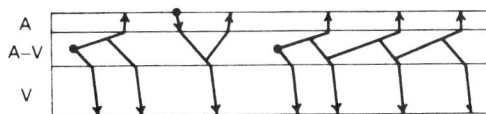

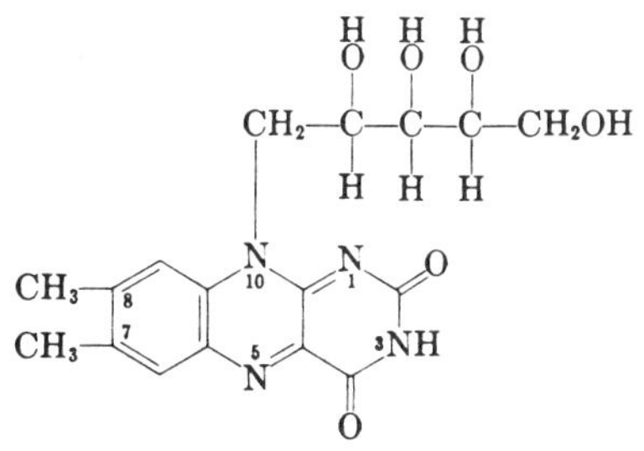

Riboflavin

methylol r., a mixture of methylol derivatives of r. formed by the action of formaldehyde on r. in weakly alkaline solution; it has the same action as r., but is preferred for parenteral administration.

riboflavin 5′-phosphate. *Flavin* mononucleotide.

ribofuranose (rī-bō-fūr′ă-nōs). The 1,4 cyclic furan form of ribose.

9-β-D-ribofuranosyladenine (rī′bō-fūr-an′o-sil-ad′ē-nēn). Adenosine.

1-β-D-ribofuranosylcytosine (rī′bō-fūr-an′o-sil-sī′tō-sēn). Cytidine.

9-β-D-ribofuranosylguanine (rī′bō-fūr-an′ō-sil-gwah′nēn). Guanosine.

ribofuranosylthymine (rī′bō-fūr-an′ō-sil-thī′mēn). Ribothymidine.

1-β-D-ribofuranosyluracil (rī′bō-fūr-an′ō-sil-yūr′ă-sil). Uridine.

ribonuclease (RNase) (rī-bō-nū′klē-ās). Ribonucleinase; a transferase or phosphodiesterase that catalyzes the hydrolysis of ribonucleic acid.

RNase I, ribonuclease (pancreatic).

RNase II [EC 3.1.13.1], an enzyme cleaving RNA exonucleolytically in the 3′ to 5′ direction, yielding 5′-phosphomononucleotides. See also microbial RNase II.

RNase III [EC 3.1.26.3], an enzyme hydrolyzing double-stranded RNA to 5′-nucleotides.

RNase A, ribonuclease (pancreatic).

alkaline RNase, ribonuclease (pancreatic).

RNase alpha [EC 3.1.26.2], an enzyme hydrolyzing *O*- methylated RNA to 5′-nucleotides.

Escherichia coli RNase I, RNase T_2.

microbial RNase II, RNase T_2.

RNase N_1, RNase T_1.

RNase N_2, RNase T_2.

RNase P [EC 3.1.26.5], an enzyme hydrolyzing tRNA precursors to 5′-nucleotides.

pancreatic RNase, see ribonuclease (pancreatic).

plant RNase, RNase T_2.

RNase T_1 [EC 3.1.27.3], guanyloribonuclease; RNase N_1; a nuclease cleaving ribonucleic acids at the 3′-5′ link of a guanosine 3′-phosphate residue, producing oligonucleotides terminating in this nucleotide; a transferase (endonuclease) in the first (cyclizing) step, a phosphodiesterase on the second (hydrolyzing) step.

RNase T_2 [EC 3.1.27.1], *Escherichia coli* RNase I; microbial RNase II; plant RNase; RNase N_2; an enzyme cleaving RNA to 3′-nucleotides with 2′,3′-cyclic nucleotides as intermediates.

RNase U_2 [EC 3.1.27.4], an enzyme cleaving RNA to 3′-phospho-mono- and oligonucleotides ending in adenylate or guanylate residues with 2′,3′-cyclic phosphate intermediates.

RNase U_4, yeast RNase.

yeast RNase [EC 3.1.14.1], RNase U_4; an enzyme hydrolyzing RNA to 3′-nucleotides.

ribonuclease (Bacillus subtilis) [EC 3.1.27.2]. Ribonuclease (*Azotobacter agilis*); ribonuclease (*Proteus mirabilis*); an enzyme hydrolyzing RNA to 2′3′-cyclic nucleotides endonucleolytically.

ribonuclease (pancreatic) [EC 3.1.27.5]. Alkaline r.; RNase A; an enzyme that transfers the 3′-phosphate of a pyrimidine ribonucleotide residue in a polynucleotide from the 5′-position of the adjoining nucleotide to the 2′-position of the pyrimidine nucleotide itself (a transferase, endonuclease action), thus breaking the chain and forming a pyrimidine 2′,3′-cyclic phosphate, then (or independently) hydrolyzing this phosphodiester to leave a pyrimidine nucleoside 3′-phosphate residue (phosphodiesterase action); used in cytochemistry to selectively degrade and remove RNA as a control for staining of RNA.

ribonucleic acid (RNA) (rī′bō-nū-klē′ik). A macromolecule consisting of ribonucleoside residues connected by phosphate from the 3′ hydroxyl of one to the 5′ hydroxyl of the next nucleoside. RNA is found in all cells, in both nuclei and cytoplasm and in particulate and nonparticulate form, and also in many viruses; polynucleotides made *in vitro* are generally called such. Various RNA fractions are identified by location, form, or function.

heterogeneous RNA, an ill-defined form of RNA, of high molecular weight, that never leaves the nucleus and is thought to be the precursor of messenger RNA.

informational RNA, messenger RNA.

messenger RNA (mRNA), informational or template RNA; the RNA reflecting the exact nucleoside sequence of the genetically active DNA and carrying the "message" of the latter, coded in its sequence, to the cytoplasmic areas where protein is made in amino-acid sequences specified by the mRNA, and hence primarily by the DNA; viral RNA's are considered to be natural messenger RNA's.

nuclear RNA (nRNA), RNA found in nuclei, or associated with DNA, or with nuclear structures (nucleoli).

RNA polymerase, see nucleotidyltransferases.

ribosomal RNA (rRNA), the RNA of ribosomes and polyribosomes.

soluble RNA (sRNA) [soluble in molar salt], transfer RNA.

template RNA, messenger RNA.

transfer RNA (tRNA), soluble RNA; short-chain RNA molecules present in cells in at least 20 varieties, each variety capable of combining with a specific amino acid (see aminoacyl-tRNA). By joining (through their anticodons) with particular spots (codons) along the messenger RNA molecule and carrying their amino acids along, they lead to the formation of protein molecules with a specific amino-acid arrangement—the one ultimately dictated by a segment of DNA in the chromosomes. Each tRNA has about 80 nucleotides (MW about 25,000); most of the 20 varieties occur in multiple "isoacceptor" forms, separable by chromatography. Further subvarieties exist in different strains of an organism, in subcellular organelles, in different metabolic states, etc.

ribonucleinase (rī-bō-nū′klē-i-nās). Ribonuclease.

ribonucleoprotein (RNP) (rī′bō-nū′klē-ō-prō′tēn). A combination of ribonucleic acid and protein.

ribonucleoside (rī-bō-nū′klē-ō-sīd). A nucleoside in which the sugar component is ribose; the common r.'s of RNA are adenosine, cytidine, guanosine, and uridine.

ribonucleotide (rī-bō-nū′klē-ō-tīd). A nucleotide (nucleoside phosphate) in which the sugar component is ribose; the major r.'s of RNA are adenylic acid, cytidylic acid, guanylic acid, and uridylic acid.

ribopyranose (rī-bō-pir′ă-nōs). The 1,5 cyclic form of ribose.

ribose (Rib) (rī′bōs). The pentose present in ribonucleic acid.

ribose-5-phosphate isomerase [EC 5.3.1.6]. Phosphopentose isomerase; phosphoriboisomerase; an enzyme catalyzing interconversion of ribose 5-phosphate and ribulose 5-phosphate; of importance in ribose metabolism.

riboside (rī′bō-sīd). The product formed by replacement of the H of the C-1 OH of ribose by an alcohol residue (which may be another sugar); differs from ribosyl compounds and does not occur in ribonucleic acids, where the radical is a ribosyl (1-OH missing entirely). See structure for methyl β-D-ribofuranoside below.

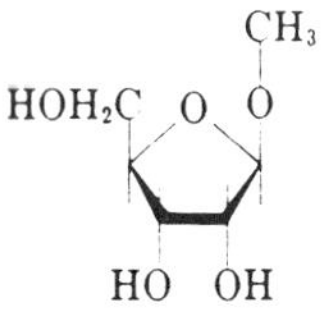

Methyl β-D-ribofuranoside

ribosome (rī'bō-sōm). Palade granule; a granule of ribonucleoprotein, 120 to 150 Å in diameter, that is the site of protein synthesis from aminoacyl-tRNAs as directed by mRNAs.

ribosuria (rī-bō-sū'rē-ă) [ribose + G. *ouron*, urine]. The enhanced urinary excretion of D-ribose; commonly one manifestation of muscular dystrophy.

ribosyl (rī'bō-sil). The radical formed by loss of the hemiacetal OH group from either of the two cyclic forms of ribose (yielding ribofuranosyl and ribopyranosyl compounds), by combination with an H of an –NH–or a –CH–group; the natural nucleosides are ribosyl compounds, not ribosides, as the bond between ribose and aglycon is C–N or C–C, not –C–O–X–.

1-ribosylorotate (rī'bō-sil-ōr'ō-tāt). Orotidine.

ribosylpurine (rī'bō-sil-pyūr'ēn). Nebularine.

ribothymidine (T, Thd, TTP) (rī-bō-thī'mi-dēn). Ribofuranosylthymine; 5-methyluridine; the ribosyl analogue of thymidine (deoxyribosylthymine); a nucleoside found in small amounts in ribonucleic acids.

ribothymidylic acid (TMP, rTMP) (rī'bō-thī-mi-dil'ik). Ribothymidine 5'-phosphate; the ribose analog of thymidylic acid; a rare component of transfer RNAs.

ribotide (rī'bō-tīd). A corruption of riboside, by analogy with nucleoside-nucleotide, to mean ribonucleotide.

ribovirus (rī'bō-vī'rŭs). RNA *virus.*

ribulose (rī'byū-lōs). D-*erythro*-Pentulose; D-adonose; D-*erythro*-2-ketopentose; the 2-keto isomer of ribose. As the 5-phosphate, it participates in the Dickens shunt; as the 1,5-bisphosphate, it combines with CO_2 at the start of the photosynthetic process in green plants ("carbon dioxide trap").

ribulose-bisphosphate carboxylase [EC 4.1.1.39]. Carboxydismutase; a dimerizing carboxy-lyase; an enzyme that catalyzes the addition of carbon dioxide to ribulose 1,5-bisphosphate and the hydrolysis of the addition product to two molecules of 3-phosphoglyceric acid, a key reaction in the fixation of CO_2 in photosynthesis.

ribulose-phosphate 3-epimerase [EC 5.1.3.1]. Phosphoribulose epimerase; an enzyme catalyzing the interconversion of xylulose 5-phosphate and its isomer, ribulose 5-phosphate.

Riccò, Annibale, Italian astrophysicist, 1844–1919. See R.'s law.

rice (rīs) [G. *oryza*]. The grain of *Oryza sativa* (family Gramineae), the rice plant; a food; also used, finely pulverized, as a dusting powder.

Rich, Arnold R., U.S. pathologist, *1893. See Hamman-R. *syndrome.*

Richard, Felix Adolphe, Paris surgeon, 1822–1872. See R.'s *fringes.*

Richards-Rundel syndrome. See under syndrome.

Richardson, J. Clifford, Canadian neurologist. See Steele-R.-Olszewski *disease; syndrome.*

Richter, August G., German surgeon, 1742–1812. See R.'s *hernia;* R.-Monro *line;* Monro-R. *line.*

Richter, Maurice N., U.S. pathologist, *1897. See R.'s *syndrome.*

ricin (rī'sin, ris'in). A highly toxic lectin and hemagglutin occurring in the seeds (castor beans) of the castor oil plant, *Ricinus communis;* if eaten, acts as a violent irritant and may be fatal.

ricinism (ris'i-nizm). Poisoning by ingestion of toxic principles from seeds (castor beans) or leaves of the castor oil plant, *Ricinus communis.*

ricinoleate (ris-i-nō'lē-āt). A salt of ricinoleic acid.

ricinoleic acid (ris-i-nō-lē'ik, rī-si-). $C_{18}H_{34}O_3$; an unsaturated hydroxy acid present in castor oil.

Ricinus (ris'i-nŭs) [L.]. Castor bean; a genus of plants (family Euphorbiaceae) with one species, *R. communis,* the castor oil plant, the source of castor oil; the leaves are said to be a galactagogue.

rickets (rik'ets) [E. *wrick,* to twist]. Rachitis; infantile or juvenile osteomalacia; a disease due to vitamin-D deficiency and characterized by overproduction and deficient calcification of osteoid tissue, with associated skeletal deformities, disturbances in growth, hypocalcemia, and sometimes tetany; usually accompanied by irritability, listlessness, and generalized muscular weakness; fractures are frequent.

acute r., hemorrhagic r.

adult r., osteomalacia.

celiac r., arrested growth, and osseous deformities associated with defective absorption of fat and calcium in celiac disease.

hemorrhagic r., acute r.; bone changes seen in infantile scurvy, consisting of subperiosteal hemorrhage and deficient osteoid tissue formation; often used to indicate simultaneous occurrence of r. and scurvy.

late r., adult r.

renal r., renal fibrocystic osteosis; renal osteitis fibrosa; renal infantilism; pseudorickets; a form of r. occurring in children in association with and apparently caused by renal disease with hyperphosphatemia.

scurvy r., infantile *scurvy.*

vitamin D-resistant r., X-linked hypophosphatemic osteomalacia; a heritable form of r., characterized by hypophosphatemia due to defective renal tubular reabsorption of phosphate and subnormal absorption of dietary calcium; not responsive to standard therapeutic doses of vitamin D, but may respond to very large doses of phosphate and of vitamin D.; X-linked recessive inheritance.

Rickettsia (ri-ket'sē-ă) [Howard T. *Ricketts,* U.S. pathologist, 1871–1910]. A genus of bacteria (order Rickettsiales) containing small (nonfilterable), often pleomorphic, coccoid to rod-shaped, Gram-negative organisms that usually occur intracytoplasmically in lice, fleas, ticks, and mites but do not grow in cell-free media; pathogenic species are parasitic in man and other animals, causing epidemic typhus, murine or endemic typhus, Rocky Mountain spotted fever, tsutsugamushi disease, rickettsialpox, and other diseases; type species is *R. prowazekii.*

R. ak'ari, a species causing human rickettsialpox; transmitted by the house mouse mite, *Liponyssoides sanguineus;* a mild febrile disease of 7 to 10 days is produced with an urban distribution in the northeastern U.S. and in wild or commensal rodents in the USSR and Africa.

R. austral'is, a species causing a spotted fever, North Queensland tick typhus, clinically and serologically similar to the disease caused by the agent of rickettsialpox; *Ixodes holocyclus* and *I. tasmani* are probable vectors. Small marsupials are suspected reservoirs of this agent, which is found over much of coastal Queensland, especially in secondary scrub and savannah.

R. burnet'ii, *Coxiella burnetii.*

R. conor'ii, R. conor'i, a widespread African species probably causing boutonneuse fever in man, transmitted by various ticks, such as the dog tick *Rhipicephalis sanguineus,* as well as ticks of several other genera; rodents as well as ticks serve as the reservoir

of human infection.
R. prowazek'ii, a species causing epidemic typhus, transmitted by body lice; type species of the genus *R.*
R. psitta'ci, *Chlamydia psittaci.*
R. ricketts'ii, the agent of Rocky Mountain spotted fever, South African tick-bite fever, São Paulo exanthematic typhus of Brazil, Tobia fever of Colombia, and spotted fevers of Minas Gerais and Mexico; transmitted by infected ixodid ticks, especially *Dermacentor andersoni* and *D. variabilis.*
R. ruminantium, *Cowdria ruminantium.*
R. sibir'ica, the agent of Siberian or North Asian tick typhus, transmitted by various ixodid ticks which also serve as reservoirs, possibly aided by rodents and hares; the disease resembles Rocky Mountain spotted fever.
R. tsutsugam'ushi, a species causing tsutsugamushi disease and scrub typhus; transmitted by trombiculid mites.
R. ty'phi, a species causing murine or endemic typhus fever, transmitted by the rat flea.

rickettsial (ri-ket'sē-ăl). Pertaining to or caused by rickettsiae.

rickettsialpox (ri-ket'sē-ăl-poks'). Kew Gardens fever; vesicular rickettsiosis; an acute disease caused by *Rickettsia akari* and transmitted by the mite *Liponnysoides sanguineus,* normally parasitic on the house mouse, with transmission to man by accidental biting by infected mites. A papule in the skin of a covered part of the body first appears, which develops into a deep-seated vesicle and then shrinks to form a black eschar; symptoms develop about a week after the appearance of the papule and consist of fever, chills, headache, backache, sweating, and local adenitis.

rickettsiosis (ri-ket-sē-ō'sis). Infection with rickettsiae.
vesicular r., rickettsialpox.

rickettsiostatic (ri-ket'sē-ō-stat'ik) [*Rickettsia* + G. *statikos,* bringing to a standstill]. An agent inhibitory to the growth of *Rickettsia.*

rickety (rik'ĕ-tē). Rachitic.

Rickles, Norman H., U.S. oral pathologist, *1920. See R. *test.*

RID Abbreviation for radial *immunodiffusion.*

Rideal, Samuel, British chemist and bacteriologist, 1863–1929. See R.-Walker *coefficient, method.*

Ridell's operation. See under operation.

ridge (rij) [A. S. *hyrcg,* back, spine]. **1.** A (usually rough) linear elevation. See also crest, crista. **2.** In dentistry, any linear elevation on the surface of a tooth. **3.** The remainder of the alveolar process and its soft tissue covering after the teeth are removed.
alveolar r., *processus* alveolaris.
apical ectodermal r., the layer of surface ectodermal cells at the apex of the embryonic limb bud; considered to exert an inductive influence on the condensation of underlying mesenchyme.
basal r., **(1)** *processus* alveolaris; **(2)** *cingulum* dentis.
bicipital r.'s, *crista* tuberculi majoris and minoris.
buccocervical r., a convexity within the cervical third of the buccal surface of molars.
buccogingival r., a distinct r. on the buccal surface of a deciduous molar tooth, approximately 1.5 mm from the crown-root junction.
bulbar r., one of two spiral subendocardial thickenings in the embryonic bulbus cordis; when they fuse, they divide the bulbus into the aorta and pulmonary artery.
bulboventricular r., an elevation on the inner surface of the embryonic heart at four to five weeks; it indicates the division between the developing ventricles and the bulbus cordis.
dental r., the prominent border of a cusp or margin of a tooth.
epidermal r.'s, *cristae* cutis.
epipericardial r., an elevation separating the developing pharyngeal region from the embryonic pericardium.
external oblique r., a horizontal bony crest on the external surface of the mandibular corpus, inferior to the alveolar bone, marking the site of attachment of the buccinator muscle.
ganglion r., neural *crest.*
genital r., gonadal r.
gluteal r., *tuberositas* glutea.
gonadal r., genital r.; an elevation of thickened mesothelium and underlying mesenchyme on the ventromedial border of the embryonic mesonephros; the primordial germ cells become embedded in it, establishing it as the primordium of the testis or ovary.
interpapillary r.'s, rete r.'s.
key r., zygomaxillare.
lateral epicondylar r., *crista* supracondylaris lateralis.
lateral supracondylar r., *crista* supracondylaris lateralis.
linguocervical r., linguogingival r.
linguogingival r., linguocervical r.; a r. occurring on the lingual surface, near the cervix, of the incisor and cuspid teeth.
Mall's r.'s, rarely used eponym for pulmonary r.'s.
mammary r., mammary fold; milk r.; bandlike thickening of ectoderm in the embryo extending on either side from just below the axilla to the inguinal region; in human embryos, the mammary glands arise from primordia in the thoracic part of the r., the balance of the r. disappearing; in some lower mammals which give birth to a litter of young, several milk glands develop along these lines.
marginal r., *crista* marginalis.
medial epicondylar r., *crista* supracondylaris medialis.
medial supracondylar r., *crista* supracondylaris medialis.
mesonephric r., a r. which, in early human embryos, comprises the entire urogenital r.; however, later in development a more medial genital r., the potential gonad, is demarcated from it. See also urogenital r.
milk r., mammary r.
mylohyoid r., *linea* mylohyoidea.
nasal r., *agger* nasi.
oblique r., a r. on the masticatory surface of an upper molar tooth from the mesiolingual to the distobuccal cusp.
oblique r. of trapezium, *tuberculum* ossis trapezii.
palatine r., *raphe* palati.
Passavant's r., Passavant's *cushion.*
pectoral r., *crista* tuberculi majoris.
primitive r., one of the paired r.'s on either side of the primitive groove.
pronator r., an oblique r. on the anterior surface of the ulna, giving attachment to the pronator quadratus muscle.
pterygoid r. of sphenoid bone, *crista* infratemporalis.
pulmonary r.'s, a pair of r.'s overlying the common cardinal veins and bulging from the lateral body wall into the embryonic celom; so called because they give early indication of where the pleuroperitoneal folds will develop.
residual r., that portion of the processus alveolaris remaining in the edentulous mouth following resorption of the section containing the alveoli.
rete r.'s, rete pegs; interpapillary r.'s; downward widening or thickening of the epidermis between the dermal papillae; peg is a misnomer because the dermal papillae are cylindrical but the epidermal thickening between papillae is not.
skin r.'s, *cristae* cutis.
superciliary r., *arcus* superciliaris.
supplemental r., a r. on the surface of a tooth that is not normally present.
supraorbital r., *margo* supraorbitalis.
taste r., one of the r.'s surrounding the vallate papillae of the tongue.
temporal r., *linea* temporalis inferior and superior.
transverse r., *crista* transversalis.
transverse palatine r., *plica* palatina transversa.
trapezoid r., *linea* trapezoidea.
triangular r., *crista* triangularis.

urogenital r., genital or mesonephric fold; wolffian r.; one of the paired longitudinal r.'s developing in the dorsal body-wall of the embryo on either side of the dorsal mesentery; the r. is formed at first by the growing mesonephros and later by the mesonephros and the gonad.
wolffian r., urogenital r.

Ridley, Humphrey, British anatomist, 1653–1708. See R.'s *circle, sinus;* R.'s *circulus* venosus ridleyi.

Riedel, Bernhard M.C.L., German surgeon, 1846–1916. See R.'s *disease, lobe, struma, thyroiditis.*

Rieder, Hermann, German pathologist, 1858–1932. See R. *cells; R.'s lymphocyte.*

Riegel, Franz, German physician, 1843–1904. See R.'s *pulse.*

Rieger, Herwigh, German ophthalmologist. See R.'s *anomaly, syndrome.*

Riehl, Gustav, Austrian dermatologist, 1855–1943. See R.'s *melanosis.*

rifampicin (rif'am-pi-sin). Rifampin.

rifampin (rif'am-pin). Rifaldazine; rifampicin; 3-[(4-methylpiperazinyl)iminomethyl] rifamycin SV; an antibacterial agent used in the treatment of tuberculosis.

rifamycin, rifomycin (rif-ă-mī'sin, rif-ō-). A complex antibiotic, isolated from *Nocardia mediterranei,* that is active against *Mycobacterium tuberculosis* and *Staphylococcus aureus;* it is poorly absorbed from the gastrointestinal tract and often causes irritation and severe pain at the sites of injection.

Riga, Antonio, Italian physician, 1832–1919. See R.-Fede *disease.*

right-eyed (rīt-īd). Dextrocular.

right-footed (rīt'fŭt-ed). Dextropedal.

right-handed (rīt'hand-ed). Dextral; dextromanual; denoting the habitual or more skillful use of the right hand for writing and most manual operations.

rigidity (ri-jid'i-tē) [L. *rigidus,* rigid, inflexible]. **1.** Rigor (1); stiffness or inflexibility. **2.** In psychiatry and clinical psychology, an aspect of personality characterized by an individual's resistance to change.
anatomic r., r. of the cervix uteri in labor, not due to any pathologic infiltration.
cadaveric r., *rigor* mortis.
catatonic r., r. associated with catatonic psychotic states in which all muscles exhibit flexibilitas cerea.
cerebellar r., increased tone of the extensor muscles, related to injury of the vermis of the cerebellum.
clasp-knife r., clasp-knife *spasticity.*
cogwheel r., a type of r. seen in parkinsonism in which the muscles respond with cogwheel-like jerks to the use of force in bending the limb.
decerebrate r., rigid contraction of the extensor and other muscles which maintain an animal in the standing position (antigravity muscles) following transection of the brain anywhere below the anterior corpora quadrigemina but above the vestibular nuclei.
lead-pipe r., the plastic type of r. resembling that of a pipe of lead seen in certain forms of parkinsonism.
mydriatic r., tonic *pupil.*
ocular r., the resistance offered by the eyeball to a change in intraocular volume; manifested as a change in intraocular pressure.
pathologic r., r. of the cervix uteri in labor, due to fibrosis, scarring, cancer, or other condition.
postmortem r., *rigor* mortis.
scleral r., the resistance of the eye to changes in shape with changes in intraocular pressure.

rigor (rig'er) [L. stiffness]. **1.** Rigidity (1). **2.** Chill (2).
acid r., coagulation of muscle protein induced by acids.
calcium r., arrest of the heart in the fully contracted state as a result of poisoning with calcium.
heat r., coagulation of muscle protein induced by heat.
r. mor'tis, cadaveric or postmortem rigidity; stiffening of the body, from 1 to 7 hours after death, from hardening of the muscular tissues in consequence of the coagulation of the myosinogen and paramyosinogen; it disappears after from 1 to 5 or 6 days, or when decomposition begins.
myocardial r. mortis, ischemic *contracture* of the left ventricle.

Riley, Conrad M., U.S. pediatrician, *1913. See R.-Day *syndrome.*

Riley, W.R. See Smith-Riley *syndrome.*

rim. A margin, border, or edge, usually circular in form.
bite r., occlusion r.
occlusal r., occlusion r.
occlusion r., bite, occlusal, or record r.; occluding surfaces built on temporary or permanent denture bases for the purpose of making maxillomandibular relation records and for arranging teeth.
record r., occlusion r.

rima, gen. and pl. **rimae** (rī'mă, rī'mē) [L. a slit] [NA]. A slit or fissure, or narrow elongated opening between two symmetrical parts.
r. glot'tidis [NA], glottis vera; true glottis; r. vocalis; the interval between the true vocal cords.
r. o'ris [NA], oral fissure; the mouth slit; the aperture of the mouth.
r. palpebra'rum [NA], palpebral fissure; the lid slit, or fissure between the eye lids.
r. puden'di [NA], r. vulvae; pudendal or vulvar slit; urogenital cleft; pudendal cleavage; fissura pudendi; the cleft between the labia majora.
r. respirato'ria, r. vestibuli.
r. vestib'uli [NA], glottis spuria; false glottis; r. respiratoria; the interval between the false vocal cords or vestibular folds.
r. voca'lis, r. glottidis.
r. vul'vae, r. pudendi.

Rimini's test. See under test.

rimose (rī'mōs) [L. *rimosus,* fr. *rima,* a fissure]. Fissured; marked by cracks in all directions, like the crackle of porcelain.

rimula (rim'yū-lă) [L. dim. of *rima*]. A minute slit or fissure.

rinderpest (rin'der-pest) [Ger. *rinder,* cattle]. Cattle plague; an acute, highly contagious, disease caused by rinderpest virus of the genus *Morbillivirus* and characterized by severe necrotizing inflammation of the alimentary canal and severe diarrhea; all ruminants and pigs are susceptible but natural infection occurs commonly only in cattle and buffaloes, sometimes in epizootic proportions.

Rindfleisch, Georg E., German physician, 1836–1908. See R.'s *cells, folds.*

ring [A.S. *hring*]. **1.** A circular band surrounding a wide central opening. **2.** In anatomy, annulus; sometimes anulus when used as an official alternate Nomina Anatomica term. **3.** The closed (*i.e.,* endless) chain of atoms in a cyclic compound; commonly used for "cyclic" or "cycle." **4.** A marginal growth on the upper surface of a broth culture of bacteria, adhering to the sides of the test tube in the form of a circle.
abdominal r., *annulus* inguinalis profundus.
amnion r., the r. formed by the attachment of the amnion to the umbilical cord at its point of emergence from the umbilicus.
anterior limiting r., Schwalbe's r.; the periphery of the cornea marking the termination of Descemet's membrane and the anterior border of the trabecular meshwork; an important landmark in gonioscopy.
Bandl's r., pathologic retraction r.
benzene r., the closed-chain arrangement of the carbon and hydrogen atoms in the benzene molecule. See also cyclic *compound.*

Bickel's r., lymphoid r.
Cannon's r., a tonically contracted muscular band in the transverse colon close to the hepatic flexure.
cardiac lymphatic r., *annulus* lymphaticus cardiae.
casting r., refractory *flask.*
choroidal r., a lightly pigmented crescent or r. adjacent to the optic disk.
ciliary r., *orbiculus* ciliaris.
common tendinous r., *annulus* tendineus communis.
conjunctival r., *annulus* conjunctivae.
constriction r., **(1)** true spastic stricture of the uterine cavity resulting when a zone of muscle goes into local tetanic contraction and forms a tight constriction about some part of the fetus; **(2)** amniotic *bands.*
crural r., *annulus* femoralis.
deep inguinal r., *annulus* inguinalis profundus.
Donders' r.'s, the iridescent r.'s observed by a patient with glaucoma.
external inguinal r., *annulus* inguinalis superficialis.
femoral r., *annulus* femoralis.
fibrocartilaginous r., *annulus* fibrocartilagineus.
fibrous r., *annulus* fibrosus.
Fleischer's r., an incomplete ring often present at the base of the keratoconus cone; it may be yellow or greenish from deposition of hemosiderin.
Flieringa's r., a stainless steel r. sutured to the sclera to prevent collapse of the globe in difficult intraocular operations.
glaucomatous r., glaucomatous *halo* (1).
Graefenberg r., a silver or silkworm gut r. designed for insertion into the uterine cavity as a means of contraception.
Imlach's r., that part of the inguinal canal which lodges the round ligament of the uterus.
internal inguinal r., *annulus* inguinalis profundus.
r. of iris, *annulus* iridis.
Kayser-Fleischer r., a greenish yellow pigmented r. encircling the cornea just within the corneoscleral margin, seen in hepatolenticular degeneration.
Liesegang r.'s, colored r.'s of precipitated silver chromate formed when a drop of concentrated silver nitrate is added to the surface of a gel (such as gelatin, agar, or silica gel) containing potassium dichromate.
Löwe's r., Maxwell's *spot.*
Lower's r., *annulus* fibrosus (1).
lymphatic r. of cardia, *annulus* lymphaticus cardiae.
lymphoid r., tonsillar r.; Waldeyer's throat r.; Bickel's r.; the broken r. of lymphoid tissue, formed of the lingual, faucial, and pharyngeal tonsils.
Maxwell's r., Maxwell's *spot.*
neonatal r., neonatal *line.*
pathologic retraction r., Baudelocque's uterine circle; Scanzoni's second os; Bandl's r.; a constriction located at the junction of the thinned lower uterine segment with the thick retracted upper uterine segment, resulting from obstructed labor; this is one of the classic signs of threatened rupture of the uterus.
physiologic retraction r., a ridge on the inner uterine surface at the boundary line between the upper and lower uterine segment that occurs in the course of normal labor.
polar r., a thickened, electron-dense ring at the anterior end of certain stages of the Apicomplexa; part of the apical complex characteristic of these sporozoans.
preputial r., annulus preputialis; the circular line of junction between the outer and the inner leaf of the prepuce at its distal extremity.
Schatzki's r., a contraction r. or incomplete diaphragm in the lower third of the esophagus which is occasionally symptomatic.
Schwalbe's r., anterior limiting r.
scleral r., the appearance of the sclera adjacent to the optic disk when the retinal pigment epithelium does not extend to the optic nerve.
signet r., the early stage of trophozoite development of the malaria parasite in the red blood cell; the parasite cytoplasm stains blue around its circular margin, and the nucleus stains red in Romanowsky stains, while the central vacuole is clear, giving the ringlike appearance.
r. of Soemmering, a mass of lenticular fibers enclosed between the anterior and posterior portion of the lenticular capsule, leaving the pupillary area relatively free.
subcutaneous r., *annulus* inguinalis superficialis.
superficial inguinal r., *annulus* inguinalis superficialis.
tonsillar r., lymphoid r.
tracheal r., *cartilagines* tracheales.
tympanic r., *annulus* tympanicus.
umbilical r., *annulus* umbilicalis.
vascular r., anomalous arteries congenitally encircling the trachea and esophagus, at times producing pressure symptoms.
Vieussens' r., *limbus* fossae ovalis.
Vossius' lenticular r., a ring-shaped opacity found on the anterior lens capsule after contusion of the eye, due to pigment and blood.
Waldeyer's throat r., lymphoid r.
Zinn's r., *annulus* tendineus communis.

ringbone (ring'bōn). Exostoses involving either the first or second phalanx of the horse, sometimes differentiated into high and low r., usually found in the foreleg; lameness may or may not result.
false r., an exostosis on the middle or upper part of the long pastern bone in the horse.

Ringer, Sydney, British physiologist, 1835–1910. See R.'s *injection, solution;* lactated R.'s *injection, solutions;* Krebs-R. *solution;* Locke-R. *solution.*

ring-knife (ring-nīf). Spoke-shave; a circular or oval ring with internal cutting edge, on the model of the carpenter's spoke-shave, for shaving off tumors in the nasal and other cavities.

ringworm (ring'werm). Tinea.
r. of beard, *tinea* barbae.
black-dot r., tinea capitis due most commonly to *Trichophyton tonsurans* or *T. violaceum.*
r. of body, *tinea* corporis.
crusted r., favus.
r. of foot, *tinea* pedis.
r. of genitocrural region, *tinea* cruris.
honeycomb r., favus.
hypertrophic r., *granuloma* trichophyticum.
r. of nails, onychomycosis.
Oriental r., *tinea* imbricata.
r. of scalp, *tinea* capitis.
scaly r., *tinea* imbricata.
Tokelau r., [*Tokelau* Islands in S. Pacific Ocean], *tinea* imbricata.

Riniker, Paul. See Glanzmann-R. *syndrome.*

Rinne, Friedrich Heinrich A., German otologist, 1819–1868. See R.'s *test.*

Riolan, Jean, French anatomist and botanist, 1577–1657. See R.'s *anastomosis, arcade, bones, bouquet, muscle.*

riparian (ri-pār'ē-an, rī-). Relating to a ripa; marginal.

Ripault, Louis H.A., French physician, 1807–1856. See R.'s *sign.*

ripening (rī'pen-ing). Denoting progressive oxidation of dye solutions, as in the r. of hematoxylin solutions to hematein or methylene blue to azure dyes.

RISA Abbreviation for radioiodinated serum *albumin.*

risk. The probability of some event seen in some sense as harmful or deleterious, expressed in various terms; *e.g.,* per person, per unit of time as an incidence, per event.
empiric r., r. that is based on empirical evidence alone, without

any appeal to formal theory or surmise.

recurrence r., r. that a disease will occur elsewhere in a pedigree, given that at least one member of the pedigree (the proband) exhibits the disease.

Risley, Samuel D., U.S. ophthalmologist, 1845–1920. See R.'s rotary *prism.*

risorius (ri-sōr'ē-ŭs) [L. *risor,* a laughter, fr. *rideo,* pp. *risus,* to laugh]. See under musculus.

ristocetin (ris-tō-sē'tin). An antibiotic produced by the fermentation of *Nocardia lurida,* comprising two substances; r. A and r. B; it is useful against staphylococcic and enterococcic infections refractory to other antibiotics.

risus caninus, risus sardonicus (rī'sŭs kā-nī'nŭs, sar-don'i-kŭs) [L. *risus,* laugh + *caninus,* doglike; G. *sardanios,* bitter laughter]. The semblance of a grin caused by facial spasm especially in tetanus. Also called canine or cynic spasm; sardonic grin; spasmus caninus; trismus sardonicus.

Ritgen, Ferdinand August Marie Franz von, German obstetrician, 1787–1867. See R.'s *maneuver.*

ritodrine (rī'tō-drēn). *erythro-p*-Hydroxy-α-{1-[(p-hydroxyphenethyl)amino]ethyl} benzyl alcohol; a sympathomimetic agent with β-adrenergic actions, used as a uterine relaxant.

Ritter, Gottfried Ritter von Rittershain, German physician, 1820–1883. See R.'s *disease.*

Ritter, Johann W., German physicist, 1776–1810. See R.'s *law,* opening *tetanus;* R.-Rollett *phenomenon.*

ritual (rich'ū-ăl) [L. *ritualis,* fr. *ritus,* rite]. In psychiatry and psychology, any psychomotor activity sustained by an individual to relieve anxiety or forestall its development; typically seen in obsessive-compulsive neurosis.

rivalry (rī'văl-rē) [L. *rivalis,* competitor, rival]. Competition between two or more individuals for the same object or goal.

binocular r., alteration in perception of portions of the visual field when the two eyes are simultaneously and rapidly exposed to targets containing dissimilar colors or borders.

r. of retina, simultaneous excitation of corresponding retinal areas of each eye by stimuli that differ in size, color, shape, or luminance, making fusion impossible.

sibling r., jealous competition among children, especially for the attention, affection, and esteem of their parents; by extension, a factor in both normal and abnormal competitiveness throughout life.

Rivea corymbosa (riv'ē-ă kō-rim-bō'să). Morning glory (2); Mexican bindweed, a plant of the family Convulvulaceae, the seeds of which were used in ceremonies by Aztec Indians in Mexico and contain lysergic acid amide, isolysergic acid, lysergic acid monoethylamide, chanoclavine, and other indole alkaloids; several hundred seeds must be ingested to produce hallucinatory and euphoric effects.

Riverius. See Rivière.

Rivero-Carvallo, J.M., 20th century Mexican cardiologist. See R. *effect.*

Rivers, William H., British physician, 1864–1922. See R.'s *cocktail.*

Rivière (Riverius), Lazare (Lazarus), French physician, 1589–1655. See R.'s *salt.*

Rivinus (Latin form of Bachmann), August Q., German anatomist, 1652–1723. See R.'s *canals, ducts, glands, incisure, membrane, notch.*

rivus lacrimalis (rī'vŭs lak-ri-mā'lis) [L. *rivus,* stream, + Mediev. L. *lacrimalis,* fr. L. *lacrima,* a tear] [NA]. Ferrein's canal; a space between the closed lids and the eyeball through which the tears flow to the punctum lacrimale.

riziform (riz'i-fōrm) [Fr. *riz,* rice]. Resembling rice grains.

RLL Abbreviation for right lower lobe (of lung).

RLQ Abbreviation for right lower quadrant (of abdomen).

RMA Abbreviation for right mentoanterior *position.*

RML Abbreviation for right middle lobe (of lung).

RMP Abbreviation for right mentoposterior *position.*

RMT Abbreviation for right mentotransverse *position.*

R.N. Abbreviation for registered *nurse.*

Rn Symbol for radon.

RNA Abbreviation for ribonucleic acid. For terms bearing this abbreviation, see subentries under ribonucleic acid.

RNase Abbreviation for ribonuclease. For terms bearing this abbreviation, see subentries under ribonuclease.

RNA splicing. Splicing (2).

RNP Abbreviation for ribonucleoprotein.

ROA Abbreviation for right occipitoanterior *position.*

Roach, F. Ewing, U.S. prosthodontist, 1868–1960. See R. *clasp.*

Roaf's syndrome. See under syndrome.

roaring (rōr'ing). A loud, rough, whistling or roaring sound emitted upon inspiration during active exercise by a horse that is suffering from laryngeal hemiplegia; caused by unilateral or bilateral paralysis of certain laryngeal muscles due to injury of the recurrent laryngeal nerve.

Robert, Heinrich, L.F., German gynecologist, 1814–1878. See R.'s *pelvis.*

Roberts, J.B., 20th century U.S. physician. See R. *syndrome.*

Robertshaw, Frank L., 20th century British anesthesiologist. See R. *tube.*

Robertson, Douglas Argyll, Scottish ophthalmologist, 1837–1909. See Argyll-R. *pupil;* R. *pupil.*

Robin, Charles P., French physician, 1821–1885. See Virchow-R. *space.*

Robin, Pierre, French pediatrician, 1867–1950. See Pierre Robin *syndrome.*

Robinson, Andrew R., U.S. dermatologist, 1845–1924. See R.'s *disease.*

Robinson, Brian F., 20th century British cardiologist. See R. *index.*

Robinson, Robert A., U.S. orthopedic surgeon, *1914. See Smith-R. *operation.*

Robinson catheter. See under catheter.

Robison, Robert, British chemist, 1884–1941. See R. *ester;* R. ester *dehydrogenase;* R.-Embden *ester.*

Robles, Rudolfo (Valverde R.), Guatemalan dermatologist, 1878–1939. See R.'s *disease.*

robotic (rō-bot'ik). Pertaining to or characteristic of a robot, an automatic mechanical device designed to duplicate a human function without direct human operation.

Robson. See Mayo-Robson.

roccellin (rok'sel-in) [C.I. 15620]. Archil.

Rochalimaea (rō-chă-lī'mā-ă). A genus of bacteria (family Rickettsiaceae) closely resembling *Rickettsia* in staining properties, morphology, and mode of transmission between hosts. They usually reside in the extracellular environment in the arthropod host and can be cultivated in cell-free media. The type species is *R. quintana,* which causes trench fever in humans.

Rocher, Henri Gaston Louis, French surgeon, *1876. See R.'s *sign.*

rock oil (rok oyl). Petroleum.

rod [A.S. *rōd*]. **1.** A straight slender cylindrical structure or device. For surgical r.'s, see also under nail, pin. **2.** R. cell of retina; the photosensitive, outward-directed process of a rhodopsin-containing r. cell in the external granular layer of the retina; many millions of such r.'s, together with the cones, form the photoreceptive layer of r.'s and cones.

analyzing r., a device used with a surveyor to determine the relative positions of parallel surfaces and undercuts when designing removable partial dentures.

Auer r.'s, Auer *bodies.*

basal r., costa (2).

Corti's r.'s, pillar *cells.*

enamel r.'s, *prismata* adamantina.

germinal r., sporozoite.

Maddox's r., a glass r., or a series of parallel glass r.'s, that converts the image of a light source into a streak of light perpendicular to the axis of the rod. The position of this streak in relation to the image of the light source seen by the fellow eye indicates the presence and amount of heterophoria.

Rodentia (rō-den'shē-ă) [Mod. L., fr. L. *rodo,* pres. p. *rodens,* to gnaw]. The rodents; the largest order of placental mammals (class Eutheria), all possessing one pair of chisel-like upper incisors for gnawing and flat-crowned premolars and molars for grinding; it includes the mice, rats, guinea pigs, squirrels, beavers, and many more.

rodenticide (rō-den'ti-sīd) [rodent + L. *caedo,* to kill]. An agent lethal to rodents.

rodonalgia (rō-don-al'jē-ă) [G. *rhodon,* rose, + *algos,* pain]. Erythromelalgia.

Roenne, Henning K.T., Danish ophthalmologist, 1878–1947. See R.'s nasal *step.*

Roentgen, Wilhelm K., German physicist, 1845–1923. See roentgen; R. *ray.*

roentgen (r, R) (rent'gen, rent'chen) [W. K. *Roentgen*]. The international unit of x- or gamma-radiation; the quantity of x- or gamma-radiation such that the associated corpuscular emission per 0.001293 g of air produces, in air, ions carrying 1 electrostatic unit (e.s.u.) of quantity of electricity of either sign or 86.9×10^{-4} J/kg in air.

r.-equivalent-man (rem), a unit of dose equal to that quantity of ionizing radiation of any type that produces in man the same biologic effect as one r. of x-rays or gamma rays; equal to the absorbed dose, measured in rads, multiplied by the relative biologic effectiveness of the radiation in question.

r.-equivalent-physical (rep), obsolete unit of measurement; that quantity of ionizing radiation of any kind which, upon absorption by living tissue, produces an energy gain per gram of tissue equivalent to that produced by 1 r. of x-rays or gamma-rays. See rad.

roentgenism (rent'gĕ-nizm). Obsolete. **1.** The use of roentgen rays in the diagnosis and treatment of disease. **2.** Any untoward effects of roentgen rays on the tissues.

roentgenization (rent'gen-ĭ-zā'shŭn). Obsolete term for roentgenism (1).

roentgenkymogram (rent'gen-kī'mō-gram). A record of the heart's movements taken with the roentgenkymograph.

roentgenkymograph (rent'gen-kī'mō-graf). An x-ray apparatus for recording the movements of the heart and great vessels on a single film. It consists essentially of a large, movable, lead sheet, called the grid, in which narrow horizontal slits, 0.4 mm wide, are cut at 12-mm intervals.

roentgenkymography (rent'gen-kī-mog'ră-fē). Recording the movements of the heart by means of the roentgenkymograph.

roentgenogram (rent'gen-ō-gram). Radiograph; roentogenograph; a representation made on a sensitized film by means of x-rays or by a radioactive substance.

cephalometric r., cephalogram; a radiographic view of the jaws and skull permitting measurement.

lateral oblique r., oblique lateral jaw r.; a radiographic view of the mandible, unilaterally revealing the mandible from symphysis to condyle.

lateral ramus r., a radiographic view of the mandibular ramus and condyle.

lateral skull r., a radiographic view of the sinuses and lateral aspects of the skeletal structures of the cranium.

maxillary sinus r., Waters' view r.; a radiographic view of the maxillary sinuses and the zygomas; permits direct comparison of the sides.

oblique lateral jaw r., lateral oblique r.

panoramic r., a radiographic view of the maxillae and mandible extending from the left to the right glenoid fossae.

periapical r., a radiographic view of one or several teeth and adjacent bony structures.

scout r., a preliminary r., frequently taken prior to injection of contrast material.

submental vertex r., a radiographic view used to visualize lateral movements of the condyle, lateral displacement of the condyle or coronoid process, or both, and the contour of the zygomatic arches.

Towne projection r., a radiographic view of the mandibular condyles and the midfacial skeleton.

transcranial r., a radiographic view of the temporomandibular articulation.

Waters' view r., maxillary sinus r.

roentgenograph (rent'gen-ō-graf). Roentgenogram.

roentgenography (rent'ge-nog'ră-fē). Radiography.

mucosal relief r., x-ray showing fine detail in gastrointestinal mucosa after introduction of a barium suspension, followed by air.

sectional r., tomography.

serial r., several x-ray exposures, over a period of time, of a region under study.

spot-film r., an x-ray of a localized region, usually under study by fluoroscopy.

roentgenologist (rent'gen-ol'ō-jist). A person skilled in the diagnostic or therapeutic application of roentgen rays.

roentgenology (rent'gen-ol'ō-jē). The study of roentgen rays in all their applications.

roentgenometer (rent'ge-nom'ĕ-ter). Radiometer.

roentgenometry (rent-ge-nom'ĕ-trē). X-ray dosimetry; measurement of the therapeutic dosage and the penetrating power of x-rays.

roentgenoscope (rent'gen-ō-scōp). Fluoroscope.

roentgenoscopy (rent-gen-os'kō-pē). Fluoroscopy.

roentgenotherapy (rent'gen-ō-thār'ă-pē). Treatment of disease by means of roentgen rays.

roetheln (ruht'eln). See röteln.

Roger, Georges Henri, French physiologist, 1860–1946. See R.'s *reflex.*

Roger, Henri L., French physician, 1809–1891. See R.'s *disease, murmur; bruit* de R., *maladie* de R.

Roger-Anderson pin fixation appliance. See under appliance.

Rogers, Oscar H., U.S. physician, *1857. See R.'s *sphygmomanometer.*

Rohr, Karl, Swiss embryologist and gynecologist, *1863. See R.'s *stria.*

Röhrer's index. See under index.

Rokitansky, Karl Freiherr von, Austrian pathologist, 1804–1878. See R.'s *disease, hernia;* R.-Aschoff *sinuses;* Mayer-R.-Küster-Hauser *syndrome.*

rolandic (rō-lan'dik). Relating to or described by Luigi Rolando.

Rolando, Luigi, Italian anatomist, 1773–1831. See R.'s *angle, area,* *cells, column, epilepsy,* gelatinous *substance, tubercle; fissure* of R.

role (rōl) [Fr.]. The pattern of behavior that a person exhibits in relationship to significant persons in his life; it has its roots in childhood and is influenced by significant people with whom the person had primary relationships.

complementary r., a r. in which the behavior pattern conforms with the expectations and demands of other people.

gender r., the sex of a child assigned by a parent; when opposite to the child's anatomical sex (*e.g.,* due to genital ambiguity at birth or to the parents' strong wish for a child of the opposite sex), the basis is set for postpubertal dysfunctions.

noncomplementary r., a r. that does not conform with the expectations and demands of other people.

sex r., the degree to which an individual acts out a stereotypical masculine or feminine r. in everyday behavior.

sick r., in medical sociology, the familially or culturally accepted behavior pattern or r. which one is permitted to exhibit during illness or disability, including sanctioned absence from school or work and a submissive, dependent relationship to family, health care personnel, and significant others.

role-playing. A psychotherapeutic method used in psychodrama to understand and treat emotional conflicts through the enactment or re-enactment of stressful interpersonal events.

rolitetracycline (rō'li-tet-ră-sī'klēn). *N*-(Pyrrolidinomethyl) tetracycline; a more soluble and less irritating derivative of tetracycline; uses and effectiveness are similar to those of tetracycline, and it may be administered intravenously or intramuscularly, which makes it useful when oral administration of a tetracycline is impossible or impracticable.

roll (rōl). A mass or structure in the shape of a roll.

iliac r., a sausage-shaped, often painful, nonfluctuating mass, with convexity to the right, palpable in the left iliac fossa, due to induration of the walls of the sigmoid flexure.

scleral r., scleral *spur.*

Roller, Christian F.W., German neurologist and psychiatrist, *1844. See R.'s *nucleus.*

roller (rō'ler). See roller *bandage.*

Rolleston, Sir Humphry D., British physician, 1862–1944. See R.'s *rule.*

Rollet, Alexander, Austrian physiologist, 1834–1903. See R.'s *stroma;* Ritter-R. *phenomenon.*

Romaña, C., Brazilian physician. See R.'s *sign.*

Romano, C., 20th century Italian physician. See R.-Ward *syndrome.*

Romanowsky, Dimitri L., Russian physician, 1861–1921. See R.'s blood *stain.*

Romberg, Moritz H., German physician, 1795–1873. See R. *test;* R.'s *disease, sign, symptom, syndrome, trophoneurosis;* R.-Howship *symptom.*

rombergism (rom'berg-izm). Romberg's *sign.*

Römer, Paul H., German bacteriologist, 1876–1916. See R.'s *experiment, test.*

rongeur (rawn-zhĕr') [Fr. *ronger,* to gnaw]. A strong biting forceps for nipping away bone.

roof (rūf) [A.S. *hrōf*]. A covering or rooflike structure; *e.g.,* a tectorium, tectum, tegmen, tegmentum, integument.

r. of fourth ventricle, *tegmen* ventriculi quarti.

r. of mouth, palatum.

r. of orbit, *paries* superior orbitae.

r. of skull, calvaria.

r. of tympanum, *tegmen* tympani.

roofplate (rūf'plāt). See roof *plate.*

root (rūt) [A.S. rot]. **1.** Radix. **2.** *Radix* dentis. **3.** The descending underground portion of a plant; it absorbs water and nutrients, provides support, and stores nutrients. For r.'s of pharmacological significance not listed below, see specific names.

anatomical r., that portion of a tooth extending from the cervical line to its apical extremity.

anterior r., *radix* ventralis.

clinical r., *radix* clinica.

cochlear r. of vestibulocochlear nerve, *radix* cochlearis.

cranial r.'s, *radices* craniales.

dorsal r., *radix* dorsalis.

facial r., *nervus* canalis pterygoidei.

r. of facial nerve, *radix* nervi facialis.

r. of foot, tarsus.

hair r., *radix* pili.

inferior r., *radix* inferior.

inferior r. of cervical loop, *radix* inferior ansae cervicalis.

inferior r. of vestibulocochlear nerve, *radix* cochlearis.

lateral r. of median nerve, *radix* lateralis nervi mediani.

lateral r. of optic tract, *radix* lateralis tractus optici.

long r. of ciliary ganglion, *radix* nasociliaris.

r. of lung, *radix* pulmonis.

medial r. of median nerve, *radix* medialis nervi mediani.

medial r. of optic tract, *brachium* colliculi superioris.

r. of mesentry, *radix* mesenterii.

motor r. of ciliary ganglion, *radix* oculomotoria ganglii ciliaris.

motor r. of trigeminal nerve, *radix* motoria nervi trigemini.

r. of nail, *radix* unguis.

nasociliary r., *radix* nasociliaris.

nerve r., one of the two bundles of nerve fibers (dorsal and ventral r.'s) emerging from the spinal cord which join to form a single segmental spinal nerve; some of the cranial nerves are similarly formed by the union of two r.'s, in particular the fifth or nervus trigeminus; in the case of the eighth cranial (vestibulocochlear) nerve, each of its two components (radix vestibularis and radix cochlearis) is referred to as a root even though they do not join each other and their central connections are distinctive; **conjoined n. r.,** two adjacent n. r.'s with the same common origin from the dura mater.

r. of nose, *radix* nasi.

olfactory r.'s, *striae* olfactoriae.

r.'s of olfactory tract, lateral and medial, the two fiber bands that form the caudal continuation of the olfactory tract which upon diverging, enclose the olfactory tubercle.

parasympathetic r. of ciliary ganglion, *radix* oculomotoria ganglii ciliaris.

r. of penis, *radix* penis.

posterior r., *radix* dorsalis.

sensory r. of ciliary ganglion, *radix* nasociliaris.

sensory r. of trigeminal nerve, *radix* sensoria nervi trigemini.

short r. of ciliary ganglion, *radix* oculomotoria ganglii ciliaris.

spinal r.'s, *radices* spinales.

superior r., *radix* superior.

superior r. of cervical loop, *radix* superior ansae cervicalis.

superior r. of vestibulocochlear nerve, *radix* vestibularis.

sympathetic r. of ciliary ganglion, *radix* sympathica ganglii ciliaris.

r. of tongue, *radix* linguae.

r. of tooth, *radix* dentis.

r.'s of trigeminal nerve, *radices* nervi trigemini.

tuberous r., a r. that is swollen for food storage; tuberous primary r.'s occur in aconite, beet, and carrot; tuberous secondary r.'s occur in plants of the Umbelliferae; and tuberous adventitious roots occur in jalap and sweet potato.

ventral r., *radix* ventralis.

vestibular r. of vestibulocochlear nerve, *radix* vestibularis.

rootlets (rūt'lets). In neuroanatomy, nerve rootlets (fila radicularis. See under filum).

root planing (plān'ing). In dentistry, abrading of rough root surfaces to achieve a smooth surface.

ROP Abbreviation for right occipitoposterior *position.*

ropalocytosis (rō-pal′ō-sī-tō′sis) [G. *ropalon,* club, + *kytos,* cell, + *-osis,* condition]. Formation of numerous processes of erythroid cells, which in ultrathin sections appear club-shaped, associated with cytoplasmic vesicles and found in some diseases of the blood.

Ropes test. See under test.

Rorschach, Hermann, Swiss psychiatrist, 1884–1922. See R. *test.*

Rosa (rō′ză) [L. rose]. A genus of plants including the roses (family Rosaceae); several varieties are the sources of rose oil: *R. alba,* cottage rose; *R. centifolia,* the pale rose or cabbage rose (source of official rose oil); *R. damascena,* damask rose; and *R. gallica,* red rose or French rose.

rosacea (rō-zā′shē-ă) [L. *rosaceus,* rosy]. Acne rosacea or erythematosa; vascular and follicular dilation involving the nose and contiguous portions of the cheeks; may vary from very mild but persistent erythema to extensive hyperplasia of the sebaceous glands with deep-seated papules and pustules; accompanied by telangiectasia at the affected erythematous sites.
hypertrophic r., rhinophyma.

rosanilin (rō-zan′i-lin) [C.I. 42510]. A tris(aminophenyl)methyl compound; together with pararosanilin it is a component of basic fuchsin; also used as an antifungal agent.

rosary (rō′zer-ē). A beadlike arrangement or structure.
rachitic r., beading of the ribs; a row of beading at the junction of the ribs with their cartilages, often seen in rachitic children.

Roscoe, Sir Henry E., British chemist, 1833–1915. See Bunsen-R. *law.*

Rose, Edmund, German physician, 1836–1914. See R.'s *position,* cephalic *tetanus.*

Rose, H.M., U.S. microbiologist, *1906. See R.-Waaler *test.*

rose (rōz) [L. *rosa*]. **1.** Erysipelas. **2.** Red r.; the petals of *Rosa gallica,* collected before expanding; used for its agreeable odor.
r. oil, attar of rose; a volatile oil from *Rosa centifolia;* used in perfumery and in ointments.

rose bengal (rōz′ ben′gal) [C.I. 45440]. The sodium salt of tetra-iodotetra-chlorfluorescein, $C_{20}H_2O_5I_4Cl_4Na_2$, used as a stain for bacteria, as a stain in the diagnosis of keratitis sicca, and in liver function tests.

Rose-Bradford kidney. See under kidney.

rosemary oil (rōz′mār-ē). The volatile oil distilled with steam from the fresh flowering tops of *Rosmarinus officinalis* (family Labiatae); used as a flavoring and in perfumery.

Rosenbach, Ottomar, German physician, 1851–1907. See R.'s *disease, law, sign, test;* R.-Gmelin *test.*

Rosenmüller, Johann C., German anatomist, 1771–1820. See R.'s *fossa, gland, node, recess, valve; organ* of R.

Rosenthal, Curt, 20th century German psychiatrist. See Melkersson-R. *syndrome.*

Rosenthal, Friedrich C., German anatomist, 1780–1829. See R.'s *canal, vein;* basal *vein* of R.

Rosenthal fiber. See under fiber.

Rosenthaler-Turk reagent. See under reagent.

roseola (rō-zē′ō-lă) [Mod. L. dim. of L. *roseus,* rosy]. Macular erythema; a symmetrical eruption of small closely aggregated patches of rose-red color.
epidemic r., rubella.
idiopathic r., r. not occurring as a symptom of a recognized general disease.
r. infan′tilis, r. infan′tum, *exanthema* subitum.
syphilitic r., macular or erythematous syphilid; usually the first eruption of syphilis, occurring 6 to 12 weeks after the initial lesion.

roseolous (rō-zē′ō-lŭs). Relating to or resembling roseola.

Roser, Wilhelm, German surgeon, 1817–1888. See R.-Nélaton *line.*

rosette (rō-zet′) [Fr. a little rose]. **1.** The quartan malarial parasite of *Plasmodium malariae* in its segmented or mature phase. **2.** A grouping of cells characteristic of neoplasms of neuroblastic or neuroectodermal origin; a number of nuclei form a ring from which neurofibrils, which can be demonstrated by silver impregnation, extend to interlace in the center. **3.** Roselike coiling of the uterus among certain pseudophyllidean tapeworms, such as *Diphyllobothrium latum.*
Wintersteiner r.'s, r.'s found only in retinal embryonic tumors, formed by a group of columnar cells with a peripheral basement membrane arranged in a radial manner around a central cavity, the spokes corresponding to the photoreceptors.

rosin (roz′in). Resin (2); colophony; the solid resin obtained from *Pinus palustris* and from other species of *Pinus* (family Pinaceae); used in plasters to render them adhesive, and also in ointments to render them locally stimulating.

***p*-rosolic acid** (rō-sol′ik). Aurin.

Ross, Sir George W., Canadian physician, 1841–1931. See R.-Jones *test.*

Rossolimo, Grigoriy I., Russian neurologist, 1860–1928. See R.'s *reflex, sign.*

rostellum (ros-tel′ŭm) [L. dim. of *rostrum,* a beak]. The anterior fixed or invertible portion of the scolex of a tapeworm, frequently provided with a row (or several rows) of hooks.
armed r., r. with one or more rows of hooks.
unarmed r., r. lacking hooks.

rostrad (ros′trăd) [L. *rostrum,* beak, + *-ad,* toward]. **1.** In a direction toward any rostrum. **2.** Situated nearer a rostrum or the snout end of an organism in relation to a specific reference point; opposite of caudad (2).

rostral (ros′trăl) [L. *rostralis,* fr. *rostrum,* beak]. Rostralis; relating to any rostrum or anatomical structure resembling a beak.

rostralis (ros′trā′lis) [L. fr. *rostrum,* beak] [NA]. Rostral.

rostrate (ros′trāt) [L. *rostratus*]. Having a beak or hook.

rostriform (ros′tri-fōrm) [L. *rostrum,* beak]. Beak-shaped.

rostrum, pl. rostra, rostrums (ros′trŭm, -tră) [L. a beak] [NA]. Any beak-shaped structure.
r. cor′poris callo′si [NA], beak of the corpus callosum; the recurved portion of the corpus callosum passing backward from the genu to the anterior commissure.
r. sphenoida′le [NA], the anterior projecting part of the body of the sphenoid bone which articulates with the vomer.

ROT Abbreviation for right occipitotransverse *position.*

rot [A.S. *rotian*]. To decay or putrify.
Barcoo r. [*Barcoo,* a river in S. Australia], desert *sore.*
foot r., **(1)** in sheep and goats, a highly contagious disease caused by the interaction of *Bacteroides nodusus* and *Fusobacterium necrophorum,* and characterized by lameness and bidigital separation of the hoof corneum from the basal epithelium and derma; **(2)** in cattle, a complex of diseases characterized by lameness and associated with a foul-smelling necrotic process of the feet from which *F. necrophorum* can invariably be isolated.

rotameter (rō-tam′ĕ-ter) [L. *rota,* wheel, + G. *metron,* measure]. A device for measuring the flow of gas or liquid; the fluid flowing up through a slightly tapered tube elevates a ball or other weight that partially obstructs the flow, until the wider cross-section allows that flow to pass around the floating obstruction.

rotation (rō-tā′shŭn) [L. *rotatio,* fr. *roto,* pp. *rotatus,* to revolve, rotate]. **1.** Turning or movement of a body round its axis. **2.** A recurrence in regular order of certain events, such as the symptoms of a periodic disease.

intestinal r., see malrotation.
molecular r., one hundredth of the product of the specific r. of an optically active compound and its molecular weight.
optical r., the change in the plane of polarization of polarized light upon passing through optically active substances; measured in terms of specific rotation by polarimetry, an important tool in organic chemical structural work, especially on carbohydrates.
specific r. ([α]), the arc through which the plane of polarized light is rotated by 1 gram of a substance per milliliter of water when the length of the light path through the solution is 1 decimeter.

rotator (rō-tā'ter, -tōr) [L. See rotation]. A muscle by which a part can be turned circularly. See *musculi* rotatores.
medial r., intortor.

rotavirus (rō'tă-vī'rŭs) [L. *rota,* wheel, + virus]. Duovirus; infantile gastroenteritis virus; gastroenteritis virus type B; reovirus-like agent; a group of RNA viruses (family Reoviridae) that are wheel-like in appearance and form a genus, *Rotavirus* which includes the human gastroenteritis viruses, Nebraska calf scours virus, epizootic diarrhea virus of infant mice, and others. They are fastidious, and *in vitro* culture is difficult.

Rotch, Thomas M., U.S. physician, 1848–1914. See R.'s *sign.*

röteln, roetheln (ruht'eln) [Ger. dim. of *rōte,* redness]. Rubella.

rotenone (rō'te-nōn). The principal insecticidal component of derris root, *Derris elliptica, D. malaccensis,* and other species of *D.,* and from *Lonchocarpus nicou* (family Leguminosae); used externally for the treatment of scabies and infestation with chiggers, and in veterinary medicine for follicular mange and infestation with lice, fleas, and ticks.

Roth. See Benedict-Roth *apparatus.*

Roth, Moritz, Swiss physician and pathologist, 1839–1914. See R.'s *spots, vas* aberrans.

Roth, Vladimir K., Russian neurologist, 1848–1916. See R.'s *disease,* R.-Bernhardt *disease,* Bernhardt-R. *syndrome.*

Rothera, Arthur C.H., British biochemist, 1880–1915. See R.'s nitroprusside *test.*

Rothia (roth'ē-ă) [G. D. *Roth*]. A genus of nonmotile, nonsporeforming, non-acid fast, aerobic to facultatively anaerobic bacteria (family Actinomycetaceae) containing Gram-positive, coccoid, diphtheroid, or filamentous cells; metabolism is fermentative, and glucose fermentation yields primarily lactic acid but no propionic acid. These organisms are normal inhabitants of the human oral cavity and are opportunistic pathogens. The type species is *R. dentocariosa.*

Rothmund, August von, German physician, 1830–1906. See R.'s *syndrome;* R.-Thomson *syndrome.*

Rotor, Arturo B., 20th century Philippine internist. See R.'s *syndrome.*

rotoscoliosis (rō'tō-skō-lē-ō'sis) [L. *roto,* to rotate, + G. *skoliōsis,* crookedness]. Curvature of the vertebral column by turning on its axis.

rototome (rō'tō-tōm). A rotating cutting instrument used in arthroscopic surgery.

rotoxamine (rō-tok'să-mēn). (—)-2-[*p*-Chloro-α-(2-dimethylaminoethoxy)benzyl]pyridine; active isomer of carbinoxamine; an antihistaminic.

Rouget, Antoine D., 19th century French physiologist. See R.'s *bulb.*

Rouget, Charles M.B., French physiologist, 1824–1904. See R. *cell; R.'s muscle;* R.-Neumann *sheath.*

rough (rŭf). Not smooth; denoting the irregular, coarsely granular surface of a certain bacterial colony type.

roughage (rŭf'ij). **1.** Anything in the diet, *e.g.,* bran, serving as a bulk stimulant of intestinal peristalsis. **2.** Hay or other coarse feed fed to cattle and other herbivores.

Roughton, Francis J.W., British scientist, 1899–1972. See R.-Scholander *apparatus, syringe.*

Rougnon de Magny, Nicholas F., French physician, 1727–1799. See R.-Heberden *disease.*

roundworm (rownd'werm). A nematode member of the phylum Nematoda, commonly confined to the parasitic forms.

Rous, F. Peyton, U.S. pathologist and Nobel laureate, 1879–1970. See R. *sarcoma,* sarcoma *virus, tumor;* R.-associated *virus.*

Roussy, Gustave, French pathologist, 1874–1948. See R.-Lévy *disease, syndrome;* Dejerine-R. *syndrome.*

Rouviere, Henri, French anatomist and embryologist, *1875. See *node* of R.

Roux, César, Swiss surgeon, 1857–1934. See R.-en-Y *anastomosis, operation.*

Roux, Philibert J., French surgeon, 1780–1854. See R.'s *method.*

Roux, Pierre P.E., French bacteriologist, 1853–1933. See R. *spatula; R.'s stain.*

Rovsing, Niels T., Danish surgeon, 1862–1927. See R.'s *sign.*

Rowntree, Leonard G., U.S. physician, *1883. See R. and Geraghty *test.*

RPF Abbreviation for renal plasma flow. See effective renal plasma *flow.*

R.Ph. Abbreviation for Registered Pharmacist.

rpm Abbreviation for revolutions per minute.

R.Q. Abbreviation for respiratory *quotient.*

-rrhagia [G. *rhēgnymi,* to burst forth]. Suffix denoting excessive or unusual discharge.

-rrhaphy [G. *rhaphā,* suture]. Suffix denoting surgical suturing.

-rrhea [G. *rhoia,* a flow]. Combining form (suffix) denoting a flowing or flux.

-rrhoea. See -rrhea.

rRNA Abbreviation for ribosomal *ribonucleic acid.*

RSA Abbreviation for right sacroanterior *position.*

RSP Abbreviation for right sacroposterior *position.*

RST Abbreviation for right sacrotransverse *position.*

RSV Abbreviation for Rous sarcoma *virus.*

RT_3 Symbol for reverse triiodothyronine.

rTMP Abbreviation for ribothymidylic acid.

Ru Symbol for ruthenium.

rub (rŭb). Friction encountered in moving one body over another.
friction r., friction *sound.*
pericardial r., pericardial friction r., pericardial friction *sound.*
pleuritic r., a friction sound produced by the rubbing together of the roughened surfaces of the costal and visceral pleurae.

Rubarth, Sven, 20th century Swedish veterinarian. See R.'s *disease;* R.'s disease *virus.*

rubber (rŭb'er). Caoutchouc; India r.; poly(*cis*-1,4-isoprene); the prepared inspissated milky juice of *Hevea brasiliensis* and other species of *Hevea* (family Euphorbiaceae), known in commerce as pure Para r.; used in the manufacture of various plasters, tissues, bandages, etc.

rubber policeman. See policeman.

rubeanic acid (rū'bē-an-ik). Dithiooxamide, which forms complete dark greenish-black complexes with copper in alkaline ethanolic solution; used histochemically for demonstrating pathologic copper deposits, as in Wilson's disease; also reacts with cobalt and nickel.

rubedo (rū-bē'dō) [L. redness, fr. *ruber,* red]. A temporary redness of the skin.

rubefacient (rū-bē-fā′shent) [L. *rubi-facio,* fr. *ruber,* red, + *facio,* to make]. **1.** Causing a reddening of the skin. **2.** A counterirritant that produces erythema when applied to the skin surface.

rubefaction (rū-bē-fak′shŭn) [see rubefacient]. Erythema of the skin caused by local application of a counterirritant.

rubella (rū-bel′ă) [L. *rubellus,* fem. *-a,* reddish, dim. of *ruber,* red]. German or three-day measles; röteln; roetheln; epidemic roseola; third disease; an acute exanthematous disease caused by rubella virus (*Rubivirus*), with enlargement of lymph nodes, but usually with little fever or constitutional reaction; a high incidence of abnormalities of children results from maternal infection during the first several months of fetal life.

rubellin (rū-bel′in). A cardiac glycoside with a digitalis-like action, obtained from *Urginia rubella* (family Liliaceae).

rubeola (rū-be′ō-lă, -bē-ō′lă) [Mod. L. dim. of *ruber,* red, reddish]. A term that been used as a synonym for two different virus diseases of man, measles and rubella; still used as a synonym for measles, but such usage should be avoided because of possible confusion.

rubeosis (rū-bē-ō′sis) [L. *ruber,* red, + G. *-osis,* condition]. Reddish discoloration, as of the skin.

r. i′ridis diabet′ica, neovascularization of the anterior surface of the iris in diabetes mellitus.

rubescent (rū-bes′ent) [L. *rubesco,* pr. p. *rubescens,* to become red]. Reddening.

rubidium (rū-bid′ē-ŭm) [L. *rubidus,* reddish, dark red, fr. *rubeo,* to be red]. An alkali element, symbol Rb, atomic no. 37, atomic weight 85.48; its salts have been used in medicine for the same purposes as the corresponding sodium or potassium salts.

Rubin, Isidor C., U.S. gynecologist, 1883–1958. See R. *test.*

rubin S, rubine (rū′bin, bēn) [C.I. 42685]. Acid *fuchsin.*

Rubinstein, Jack H., U.S. pediatrician, *1925. See R.-Taybi *syndrome.*

Rubivirus (rū′bi-vī′rŭs). A genus of viruses (family Togaviridae) that includes the rubella virus.

Rubner, Max, German hygienist and biochemist, 1854–1932. See R.'s *laws* of growth, *test.*

rubor (rū′bōr) [L.]. Redness, as one of the four signs of inflammation (r., calor, dolor, tumor) enunciated by Celsus.

rubratoxin (rū-bră-tok′sin). A mycotoxin produced by *Penicillium rubrum* and *P. purpurogenum,* which form readily on cereal grains; responsible for outbreaks of toxicosis in the U.S.

rubredoxins (rū-brē-dok′sinz). Ferredoxins without acid-labile sulfur and with the iron in a typical mercaptide coordination.

rubriblast (rū′bri-blast) [L. *ruber,* red, + G. *blastos,* germ]. Pronormoblast.

pernicious anemia type r., promegaloblast. See erythroblast.

rubricyte (rū′bri-sīt) [L. *ruber,* red, + *kytos,* cell]. Polychromatic normoblast. See discussion under erythroblast.

rubrospinal (rū′brō-spī′năl). Relating to the nerve fibers passing from the red nucleus to the spinal cord: the *tractus* rubrospinalis.

ructus (rŭk′tŭs) [L. fr. *ructo,* pp. *-atus,* to belch]. Eructation.

Rud, Einar, Danish physician, *1892. See R.'s *syndrome.*

rudiment (rū′di-ment) [L. *rudimentum, a beginning, fr. rudis,* unformed]. Rudimentum. **1.** An organ or structure that is incompletely developed. **2.** The first indication of a structure in the course of ontogeny.

rudimentary (rū-di-men′tăr-ē). Abortive (2); relating to a rudiment.

rudimentum, pl. **rudimenta** (rū′di-men′tŭm, -tă) [L.] [NA]. Rudiment.

r. hippocam′pi, tenia tecta; see *indusium* griseum.

Ruffini, Angelo, Italian histologist, 1864–1929. See R.'s *corpuscles;* flower-spray *organ* of R.

rufous (rū′fŭs) [L. *rufus,* reddish]. Erythristic.

ruga, pl. **rugae** (rū′gă, rū′gē) [L. a wrinkle] [NA]. A fold, ridge, or crease; a wrinkle.

r. gas′trica, one of the folds of the mucous membrane of the stomach when the organ is contracted.

r. palati′na, *plica* palatina transversa.

ru′gae vagina′les [NA], a number of transverse ridges in the mucous membrane of the vagina.

rugine (rū-zhēn′) [Fr.]. **1.** Periosteum *elevator.* **2.** A raspatory.

rugitus (rū′ji-tŭs) [L. a roaring, fr. *rugio,* to roar]. A rumbling sound in the intestines. See also borborygmus.

rugose (rū′gōs) [L. *rugosus*]. Rugous; marked by rugae; wrinkled.

rugosity (rū-gos′i-tē). **1.** The state of being thrown into folds or wrinkles. **2.** A ruga.

rugous (rū′gŭs). Rugose.

Ruiter. See Gougerot-R. *disease.*

RUL Abbreviation for right upper lobe (of lung).

rule (rūl) [O. Fr. *reule,* fr. L. *regula,* a guide, pattern]. A criterion, standard, or guide governing a procedure, arrangement, action, etc. See also law; principle; theorem.

Abegg's r., the tendency of the sum of the maximum positive and maximum negative valence of a particular element to equal 8; e.g., C may have a valence of +4 and −4, O of +6 and −2. Sometimes loosely stated as all atoms have the same number of valences, a consequence of the tendency of valence electron shells to be filled to 8.

American Law Institute r., a test of criminal responsibility (1962): "a person is not responsible for criminal conduct if at the time of such conduct as a result of mental disease or defect he lacks substantial capacity either to appreciate the wrongfulness of his conduct or to conform his conduct to the requirements of law."

r. of bigeminy, r. that a ventricular premature beat will follow the beat terminating a long cycle. Sudden prolongation of the ventricular cycle, by changing the refractoriness in the conduction system, causes a peripheral region of bidirectional block to become transiently unidirectional and thus opens the potential path for a reentry sweep.

Clark's weight r., an obsolete r. for an approximate child's dose, obtained by dividing the child's weight in pounds by 150 and multiplying the result by the adult dose.

Cowling's r., an obsolete r. for a child's dose: that fraction of the adult dose obtained by dividing the age of the child at the nearest birthday by 24.

Durham r., an American test of criminal responsibility (1954): "an accused is not criminally responsible if his unlawful act was the product of mental disease or mental defect."

Goriaew's r., a r. of a blood counting field by which it is marked off in a series of squares, some of which are again subdivided into sixteen smaller ones.

Haase's r., the length of the fetus in centimeters, divided by 5, is the duration of pregnancy in months, *i.e.,* the age of the fetus.

His' r., the duration of pregnancy is to be reckoned from the first day of the first omitted menstrual period.

isoprene r., the classical, outmoded statment that naturally occurring terpenes are built up by condensation of isoprene units by either a 1-4 linkage ("head to tail") or a 4-4 linkage ("tail to tail").

Jackson's r., after an epileptic attack, simple and quasiautomatic functions are less affected and more rapidly recovered than the more complex ones.

Le Bel-van't Hoff r., the number of stereoisomers of an organic compound is 2^n where *n* represents the number of asymmetric carbon atoms. A corollary of their simultaneously announced conclusions, in 1874, that the most probable orientation of the bonds of a carbon atom linked to four groups or atoms is toward the apexes of a tetrahedron, and that this accounted for all then-known phenomena of molecular asymmetry (which involved a carbon atom bearing four different atoms or groups). See also stereoisomerism.

Liebermeister's r., in adult febrile tachycardia, about eight pulse beats correspond to an increase of 1°C.

M'Naghten r., the classic English test of criminal responsibility (1843): "to establish a defense on the ground of insanity, it must be clearly proved that, at the time of committing the act, the party accused was laboring under such a defect of reasoning, from disease of the mind, as not to know the nature and quality of the act he was doing, or if he did know it, that he did not know he was doing what was wrong."

Nägele's r., means of estimating date of delivery by counting back three months from the first day of the last menstrual period and adding seven days.

New Hampshire r., pioneering American test of criminal responsibility (1871): "if the [criminal] act was the offspring of insanity, a criminal intent did not produce it."

Ogino-Knaus r., the time in the menstrual period when conception is most likely to occur is at about midway between two menstrual periods; fertilization of the ovum is least likely just before or just after menstruation; the basis for the rhythm method of contraception.

r. of outlet, an obstetric r. for determining whether the pelvic outlet will permit the passage of a fetus; the sum of the posterior sagittal diameter and the transverse diameter of the outlet must equal at least 15 cm if a normal-sized baby is to pass.

phase r., an expression of the relationships existing between systems in equilibrium: $P + V = C + 2$, where P is the number of phases, V the variance or degrees of freedom, and C the number of components; it also follows that the variance is, $V = C + 2 - P$. For H_2O at its triple point, $V = 1 + 2 - 3 = 0$, *i.e.*, both temperature and pressure are fixed.

Prentice's r., each centimeter of decentration of a lens results in 1 prism diopter of deviation of light for each diopter of lens power.

Rolleston's r., the ideal adult systolic blood pressure is 100 plus half the age, whereas the maximal physiologic pressure is 100 plus the age.

Schütz r., Schütz law; the rate of an enzyme reaction is proportional to the square root of the enzyme concentration; applied specifically to pepsin within a limited range.

Young's r., an obsolete r. to determine a child's dose: 12 is added to the child's age and the sum is divided by the age; the adult dose divided by the figure so obtained gives the proper dose.

ruler (rū'ler). A calibrated strip for measuring plane surfaces.

isometric r., a calibrated scale for eliminating distortion in the measurement of plane surfaces.

rum (rŭm). A spirit distilled from the fermented juice of the sugar cane.

rum-blossom (rŭm-blos'ŭm). Rhinophyma.

rumen, pl. **rumina** (rū'men, rū'mi-nă) [L. gullet, throat]. Paunch; the largest compartment of the stomach of a cow or other ruminant.

rumenitis (rū-mĕ-nī'tis) [rumen + G. *-itis,* inflammation]. Inflammation of the rumen of ruminant animals.

rumenotomy (rū-mĕ-not'ō-mē) [rumen + G. *tomē,* incision]. Incision into the rumen.

ruminant (rū'mi-nănt). An animal that chews the cud, material regurgitated from the rumen for rechewing; *e.g.,* the sheep, cow, deer, or antelope.

rumination (rū-mi-nā'shŭn) [L. *ruminatio,* fr. *rumino,* to chew the cud, think over, fr. *rumen,* throat]. **1.** The physiologic process in ruminant animals in which coarse, hastily eaten food is regurgitated from the rumen, thoroughly rechewed, reduced to finer particles, mixed with saliva, and reswallowed. **2.** A disorder of infancy characterized by repeated regurgitation of food, with weight loss or failure to thrive, developing after a period of normal functioning. **3.** Periodic reconsideration of the same subject.

ruminative (rū'min-ă-tiv). Characterized by a preoccupation with certain thoughts and ideas.

ruminoreticulum (rū'mi-nō-re-tik'yū-lŭm). The rumen and reticulum of the ruminant stomach taken together, since they freely communicate via the ruminoreticular orifice.

Rumpel, Theodor, German physician, 1862–1923. See R.-Leede *sign, test.*

runaround, runround (rŭn'ă-rownd, rŭn'rownd). Colloquialism for paronychia.

Rundel. See Richards-R. *syndrome.*

Runeberg, Johan W., Finnish physician, 1843–1918. See R.'s *formula.*

runt (rŭnt) [A.S.]. A stunted animal, occurring most frequently in species which give birth to large litters.

rupia (rū'pē-ă) [G. *rhypos,* filth]. **1.** Ulcers of late secondary syphilis, covered with yellowish or brown crusts which have been compared in their appearance to oyster shells. **2.** Yaws. **3.** Term occasionally used to designate a very scaly, heaped-up, and secondarily infected psoriatic lesion.

r. escharot'ica, *dermatitis* gangrenosa infantum.

rupial (rū'pē-ăl). Relating to rupia.

rupioid (rū'pē-oyd) [G. *rhypos,* filth (rupia), + *eidos,* resemblance]. Resembling rupia.

rupture (rŭp'chūr) [L. *ruptura,* a fracture (of limb or vein), fr. *rumpo,* pp. *ruptus,* to break]. **1.** Hernia. **2.** A solution of continuity or a tear; a break of any organ or other of the soft parts.

RUQ Abbreviation for right upper quadrant (of abdomen).

Russell, Alexander, 20th century British pediatrician. See R.'s *syndrome;* Silver-R. *dwarfism, syndrome.*

Russell, G.F.M., contemporary British physician. See B.'s *sign.*

Russell, James S. Risien, British physician, 1863–1939. See hooked *bundle* of R., uncinate *bundle* of R.

Russell, Patrick, Irish physician in India, 1727–1805. See R.'s viper *venom, viper.*

Russell, R. Hamilton, 20th century Australian surgeon. See R. *traction.*

Russell, William, Scottish physician, 1852–1940. See R. *bodies.*

Russell, William James, British chemist, 1830–1909. See R. *effect.*

Russell's Periodontal Index. An index that estimates the degree of periodontal disease present in the mouth by measuring both bone loss around the teeth and gingival inflammation; used frequently in the epidemiological investigation of periodontal disease.

Rust, Johann N., German surgeon, 1775–1840. See R.'s *disease, phenomenon.*

rusts (rŭsts). Species of *Puccinia* and other microbes comprising important pathogens of plants, especially cereal grains; they are important allergens for man when inhaled in large numbers, as in harvesting processes.

rut (rŭt) [O. F. *ruit,* roaring of deer in the breeding season]. A period of sexual excitement in the males of certain mammals, such as deer, camels, and elephants, which occurs seasonally. It is only during this season that spermatogenesis occurs and the males will mate; in most mammalian males spermatogenesis is continuous and breeding occurs whenever the females will accept the males. *Cf.* estrus.

ruthenium (rū-thē'nē-ŭm) [Mediev. L. *Ruthenia,* Russia, where first obtained]. A metallic element of the platinum group; symbol Ru, atomic no. 44, atomic weight 101.1.

ruthenium red. Ammoniated r. oxychloride, $Ru_3(NH_3)_{14}O_2Cl_6$, used in histology and electron microscopy as a stain for certain complex polysaccharides.

rutherford (rŭth'er-ferd) [Ernest *Rutherford,* British physicist, 1871–1937]. A unit of radioactivity, representing that quantity of radioactive material in which a million disintegrations are taking place per second; 37 r. equal 1 mCi.

rutidosis (rū-ti-dō'sis). Rhytidosis.

rutin (rū'tin). Rutoside; quercetin-3-rutinoside; quercetin-3-rhamnoglucoside; a flavonoid obtained from buckwheat, that causes decreased capillary fragility.

rutinose (rū'ti-nōs). 6-*O*-α-L-Rhamnosyl-D-glucose; a disaccharide of glucose and rhamnose, and a component of rutin.

rutoside (rū'tō-sīd). Rutin.

Ruysch, Frederik, Dutch anatomist, 1638–1731. See R.'s *membrane, muscle, tube, veins.*

RV Abbreviation for residual *volume.*

rye smut (rī' smŭt'). Ergot.

Ryle, John A., British physician, 1889–1950. See R.'s *tube.*

S

σ **1.** The 18th letter of the Greek alphabet, sigma. **2.** Symbol for reflection *coefficient;* standard *deviation.*

S **1.** Abbreviation for sacral vertebra (S1 to S5); spherical or spherical *lens;* Svedberg *unit.* **2.** Symbol for siemens; sulfur; entropy in thermodynamics; substrate in the Michaelis-Menton hypothesis; percentage saturation of hemoglobin (when followed by subscript O_2 or CO). **3.** Designation of a rare human antigen (hemagglutinogen) related genetically to the MNSs blood group. See Blood Groups appendix.

S_f Symbol for flotation *constant.*

s Abbreviation of L. *sinister,* left; L. *semis,* half; as a subscript, denotes steady *state.*

$\bar{s}$ Abbreviation for L. *sine,* without.

s Symbol for selection *coefficient.*

S-A Abbreviation for sinoatrial.

sabadilla (sab-ă-dil'ă) [Sp. *cevadilla,* ult. fr. L. *cibus,* food]. Cevadilla; the seed of *Schoenocaulon officinale* (family Liliaceae), a plant of the shores of the Gulf of Mexico and Caribbean Sea; it yields cevadine, veratridine, and several other alkaloids; has been used externally as a parasiticide.

Sabin, Albert B., U.S. virologist, *1906. See S. *vaccine.*

Sabin-Feldman dye test. See under test.

Sabouraud, Raymond J.A., French dermatologist, 1864–1938. See S.'s *agar, pastilles;* S.-Noiré *instrument.*

sabulous (sab'yū-lŭs) [L. *sabulosus,* fr. *sabulum,* coarse sand]. Sandy; gritty.

saburra (să-bŭr'ă) [L. sand]. **1.** Foulness of the stomach or mouth resulting from decomposed food. **2.** Sordes.

saburral (să-bŭr'ăl) Relating to saburra (1).

sac (sak) [L. *saccus,* a bag]. **1.** A pouch or bursa. See saccus; sacculus. **2.** An encysted abscess at the root of a tooth. **3.** The capsule of a tumor, or envelope of a cyst.

abdominal s., the part of the embryonic celom that becomes the abdominal cavity.

air s., *sacculus* alveolaris.

allantoic s., the dilated distal portion of the allantois.

alveolar s., *sacculus* alveolaris.

amniotic s., amnion.

anal s., a vesicular cutaneous invagination opening by a duct on each side of the anal canal in carnivores (best developed in skunks, but absent in some bears, the raccoon, kinkajou, coati, and sea otter), each lying between the external and internal anal sphincter muscles, which aid in emptying the contents. The s. stores odoriferous scent markers produced by glands that line its wall or duct; frequently the s. becomes impacted in the dog or cat, requiring manual emptying.

aneurysmal s., the dilated wall of an artery in a saccular aneurysm.

aortic s., in mammalian embryos, the endothelially lined dilation just distal to the truncus arteriosus; it is the primordial vascular channel from which the aortic arches arise and which becomes reshaped to form the ventral aortic roots.

chorionic s., chorion.

conjunctival s., *saccus* conjunctivae.

cupular blind s., *cecum* cupulare.

dental s., the outer connective tissue envelope surrounding a developing tooth; also applied to the mesenchymal concentration that is the primordium of the s. See also dental *follicle.*

endolymphatic s., *saccus* endolymphaticus.

heart s., pericardium.

hernial s., the peritoneal envelope of a hernia.

Hilton's s., *sacculus* laryngis.

lacrimal s., *saccus* lacrimalis.

lesser peritoneal s., *bursa* omentalis.

lymph s.'s, the earliest lymphatic vessels formed in the embryo.

nasal s.'s, deepened nasal pits that develop into definitive nasal cavities.

omental s., *bursa* omentalis.

preputial s., the space between the prepuce and the glans penis.

pudendal s., Broca's pouch; a pear-shaped encapsulated collection of connective tissue and fat in each labium majus.

tear s., *saccus* lacrimalis.

tooth s., a capsule that encloses the developing tooth.

vestibular blind s., *cecum* vestibulare.

vitelline s., yolk s.

yolk s., vitelline s.; umbilical vesicle; vesicula umbilicalis; the highly vascular layer of splanchnopleure surrounding the yolk of an embryo.

sacbrood (sak'brūd). A viral disease affecting the larvae of bees.

saccadic (să-kad'ik) [Fr. *saccade,* sudden check of a horse]. Jerky. See saccadic *movement.*

saccate (sak'āt) [L. *saccus,* sac]. Relating to a sac.

sacchar-. See saccharo-.

saccharase (sak'ă-rās). β-Fructofuranosidase.

saccharate (sak'ă-rāt). A salt or ester of saccharic acid.

saccharephidrosis (sak-ar-ef-i-drō'sis) [sacchar- + G. *ephidrōsis,* a slight perspiration]. The presence of sugar in the sweat.

sacchari-. See saccharo-.

saccharic (să-kar'ik). Relating to sugar.

saccharic acid (sak'ă-rik). Term used to denote the class of dicarboxy sugar acids.

saccharides (sak'ă-rīdz). Carbohydrates. S. are classified as mono-, di-, tri-, and polysaccharides according to the number of monosaccharide groups composing them.

sacchariferous (sak'ă-rif'er-ŭs). Producing sugar.

saccharification (să-kar'i-fi-kā'shŭn). The process of saccharifying.

saccharify (să-kar'i-fī) [sacchari- + L. *facio,* to make]. To convert starch into sugar.

saccharimeter (sak-ă-rim'ĕ-ter) (sacchari- + G. *metron,* measure]. Saccharometer; an instrument for determining the amount of sugar in a solution; it may be a polarimeter, a hygrometer, or a container in which the solution is fermented and the amount estimated by the volume of CO_2 produced.

saccharin (sak'ă-rin). Benzosulfimide; *o*-sulfobenzimide; 2,3-dihydro-3-oxobenzisosulfonazole; in dilute aqueous solution it is 300 to 500 times sweeter than sucrose; used as a sweetening agent (sugar substitute); s. sodium and s. calcium have the same use.

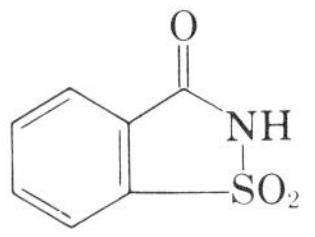

Saccharin

saccharine (sak'ă-rēn, -rin, -rīn). Relating to sugar; sweet.

saccharo-, sacchar-, sacchari- [G. *sakcharon,* sugar]. Combining forms denoting sugar (saccharide).

saccharogen amylase (sak'ă-rō-jen). β-Amylase.

saccharolytic (sak'ă-rō-lit'ik) [saccharo- + G. *lysis,* loosening]. Capable of hydrolyzing or otherwise breaking down a sugar molecule.

saccharometabolic (sak'ă-rō-met'ă-bol'ik). Relating to saccharometabolism.

saccharometabolism (sak-ă-rō-mĕ-tab'ō-lizm). Metabolism of sugar; the process of utilization of sugar in cells.

saccharometer (sak-ă-rom'ĕ-ter). Saccharimeter.

Saccharomyces (sak'ă-rō-mī'sēz) [saccharo- + G. *mykēs,* fungus]. A genus of budding yeasts (family Saccharomycetaceae); an ascomycete. *S. cerevisiae* is used to produce brewer's yeast.

Saccharomycetaceae (sak'ă-rō-mī-sē-tā'sē-ē). The family of yeasts; that group of fungi comprising the ascomycetes which possess a predominantly unicellular thallus, reproduce asexually by budding, transverse division, or both, and produce ascospores in an ascus, originating from a zygote or pathogenetically from a single somatic cell. The term yeastlike fungus is often applied to fungi that are not known to form ascospores, but otherwise possess the characteristics of yeasts; such forms are properly placed with the Fungi Imperfecti unless methods of sexual reproduction are known; *e.g., Cryptococcus neoformans.*

Saccharomycetales (sak'ă-rō-mī'sē-tā'lēz). Endomycetales.

saccharorrhea (sak'ă-rō-rē'ă) [saccharo- + G. *rhoia,* a flow]. Obsolete term for glycosuria.

saccharose (sak'ă-rōs). Sucrose.

saccharosuria (sak'ă-rō-sū'rē-ă) [saccharose + G. *ouron,* urine]. Obsolete term denoting the excretion of saccharose in the urine.

saccharum (sak'ă-rŭm) [Mod. L. fr. G. *sakcharon*] Sucrose.
s. canaden'se, maple sugar.
s. lac'tis, lactose.

sacciform (sak'si-fōrm) [L. *saccus,* sack, + *forma,* form]. Saccular; sacculated; pouched; sac-shaped.

saccular (sak'yū-lăr). Sacciform.

sacculated (sak'yū-lā'ted). Sacciform.

sacculation (sak'yū-lā'shŭn). **1.** A structure formed by a group of sacs. **2.** The formation of a sac or pouch.

saccule (sak'yūl) [L. *sacculus*]. Sacculus.
s. of larynx, *sacculus* laryngis.

sacculocochlear (sak'yū-lō-kok'lē-ăr). Relating to the sacculus and the membranous cochlea.

sacculus, pl. **sacculi** (sak'yū-lŭs, -lī) [L. dim. of *saccus,* sac] [NA]. Saccule; s. proprius or vestibuli; the smaller of the two membranous sacs in the vestibule of the labyrinth, lying in the spherical recess; it is connected with the cochlear duct by a very short tube, the ductus reuniens, and with the utriculus by the beginning of the ductus endolymphaticus and the ductus utriculosaccularis which joins it.
s. alveola'ris, pl. **sacculi alveola'res** **(1)** [NA], alveolar sac; air sac; terminal dilation of the ductuli aveolares which give rise to alveoli in the lung; a small air chamber in the pulmonary tissue from which the pulmonary alveoli project like bays and into which an alveolar duct opens; **(2)** in birds, air-containing extensions of bronchi which connect with bone cavities.
s. commu'nis, utriculus.
s. endolymphat'icus, *saccus* endolymphaticus.
s. lacrima'lis, *saccus* lacrimalis.
s. laryn'gis [NA], saccule of the larynx; appendix ventriculi laryngis; laryngeal pouch; Hilton's sac; a small diverticulum extending upward from the ventricle of the larynx between the vestibular fold and the lamina of the thyroid cartilage.
s. pro'prius, sacculus.
s. vestib'uli, sacculus.

saccus, pl. **sacci** (sak'ŭs, sak'sī) [L. a bag, sack] [NA]. A sac.
s. conjuncti'vae [NA], conjunctival sac; the space bound by the conjunctival membrane between the palpebral and bulbar conjunctiva; it opens anteriorly between the eyelids.
s. endolymphat'icus [NA], endolymphatic sac; Böttcher's or Cotunnius' space; sacculus endolymphaticus; the dilated blind extremity of the ductus endolymphaticus.
s. lacrima'lis [NA], lacrimal or tear sac; dacryocyst; sacculus lacrimalis; the upper portion of the nasolacrimal duct into which empty the two lacrimal canaliculi. See fig. under *apparatus* lacrimalis.
s. reu'niens, *sinus* venosus.
s. vagina'lis, an embryonic peritoneal fossa indicating the site where the processus vaginalis peritonei extends through the anterior abdominal wall during descent of the testis.

Sachs, Bernard, U.S. neurologist, 1858–1944. See Tay-S. *disease.*

Sachs, Hans, German bacteriologist, 1877–1945. See S.-Georgi *test.*

Sachs, M. See S.'s *bacillus,* Ghon-S. *bacillus.*

Sachs, Maurice D., U.S. radiologist, *1909. See S.-Hill *lesion.*

Sacks, Benjamin, U.S. physician, *1896. See Libman-S. *endocarditis, syndrome.*

sacr-. See sacro-.

sacrad (sā'krad) [sacr- + L. *ad,* to]. In the direction of the sacrum.

sacral (sā'krăl). Relating to or in the neighborhood of the sacrum.

sacralgia (sā-kral'jē-ă) [sacr- + G. *algos,* pain]. Sacrodynia; pain in the sacral region.

sacralization (sā'kral-i-zā'shŭn). Lumbar development of the first sacral vertebra.

sacrectomy (sā-krek'tō-mē) [sacr- + G. *ektomē,* excision]. Sacrotomy; resection of a portion of the sacrum to facilitate an operation.

sacro-, sacr- [L. *sacrum*]. Combining forms denoting the sacrum.

sacrococcygeal (sā-krō-kok-sij'ē-ăl). Relating to both sacrum and coccyx.

sacrococcygeus (sā'krō-kok-si-jē'ŭs). See entries under musculus.

sacrodynia (sā'krō-din'ē-ă) [sacro- + G. *odyne,* pain]. Sacralgia.

sacroiliac (sā-krō-il'ē-ak). Relating to the sacrum and the ilium.

sacroiliitis (sā'krō-il-ē-ī'tis). Inflammation of the sacroiliac joint.

sacrolisthesis (sā'krō-lis'thē-sis) [sacro- + G. *olisthēsis,* a slipping and falling]. Spondylolisthesis.

sacrolumbalis (sā'krō-lŭm-bā'lis). The musculus iliocostalis lumborum.

sacrolumbar (sā'krō-lŭm'băr). Lumbosacral.

sacrosciatic (sā'krō-sī-at'ik). Relating to both sacrum and ischium.

sacrospinal (sā'krō-spī'năl). Relating to the sacrum and the vertebral column above.

sacrotomy (sā-krot'ō-mē) [sacro- + G. *tomē,* incision]. Sacrectomy.

sacrovertebral (sā'krō-ver'tē-brăl). Relating to the sacrum and the vertebrae above.

sacrum, pl. **sacra** (sā'krŭm, sā'kră) [L. (lit. sacred bone), neuter of *sacer (sacr-),* sacred]. *Os* sacrum.
assimilation s., one which is composed of six segments, the last lumbar vertebra assuming the appearance of a sacral segment; or one which is composed of but four segments, the first sacral being free and having the characteristics of a lumbar vertebra.

SACT Abbreviation for sinoatrial conduction *time.*

saddle (sad'l). **1.** Sella; a structure shaped like, or suggestive of, a seat or s. used in riding horseback. **2.** Denture *base.*
Turkish s., *sella* turcica.

sadism (sā'dizm, sad'izm) [Marquis de *Sade,* 1740–1814, confessedly addicted to the practice]. Active algolagnia; a form of perversion, often sexual in nature, in which a person finds pleasure in inflicting abuse and maltreatment. *Cf.* masochism.

sadist (sā'dist, sad'ist). One who practices sadism.

sadistic (să-dis'tik). Pertaining to or characterized by sadism.

sadomasochism (sā-dō-mas'ō-kizm, sad-o-) [sadism + masochism]. A form of perversion marked by enjoyment of cruelty in its active and/or passive form.

Saemisch, Edwin T., German ophthalmologist, 1833-1909. See S.'s *operation, section, ulcer.*

Saenger, Alfred, German neurologist, 1860–1921. See S. *pupil;* S.'s *sign.*

Saenger, M., Prague obstetrician, 1853–1903. See S.'s *macula, operation.*

safflower (saf'low-er) [Ar. *safrā,* yellow]. Carthamus.

safflower oil. An oil extracted from the seeds of *Carthamus tinctorius,* containing 74.5% linoleic acid and 6.6% saturated fatty acids; used in hypercholesteremia, myocardial infarction, and coronary insufficiency.

saffron (saf'ron) [Ar. *zafarān,* fr. *safrā,* yellow]. Crocus.

meadow s., colchicum.

safranin O (saf'ră-nin) [C.I. 50240]. A mixture of dimethyl- and trimethylphenosafranin chloride, a basic red dye that exhibits orange metachromasia; used in histology as a nuclear stain, in microbiology as a counterstain in the Gram method, and to demonstrate enterochromaffin.

safranophil, safranophile (saf'ră-nō-fil, -fīl). Staining readily with safranin; denoting certain cells and tissues.

safrole (saf'rōl). The methylene ether of allyl pyrocatechol; $C_{10}H_{10}O_2$; contained in oil of sassafras, oil of camphor, and various other volatile oils; it is obtained chiefly from oil of camphor by fractional distillation; used as a tonic and carminative; prolonged administration causes fatty degeneration.

sage (sāj) [L. *salvia,* the sage plant, fr. *salvus,* safe]. Salvia.

sagitta (saj'i-tă). Statoconia.

sagittal (saj'i-tăl) [L. *sagitta,* an arrow]. Sagittalis; resembling an arrow; in the line of an arrow shot from a bow, *i.e.,* in an anteroposterior direction.

sagittalis (saj-i-tā'lis) [L.] [NA]. Sagittal; referring to a sagittal plane or direction.

Saint, Charles F.M., S. African roentgenologist, *1886. See S.'s *triad.*

Sainton, Paul, French physician, 1868–1958. See S.'s *sign.*

Sakaguchi reaction. See under reaction.

sal, pl. **sales** (sal, sal'ēz) [L.]. Salt.

s. alem'broth [an alchemist's term of unknown origin], salt of wisdom; the product obtained by crystallization from a solution of equal parts of ammonium chloride and mercuric chloride.

s. ammo'niac, *ammonium* chloride.

s. diuret'icum, *potassium* acetate.

s. soda, *sodium* carbonate.

s. vol'atile, smelling *salts.*

Salah, M., 20th century Egyptian surgeon. See S.'s sternal puncture *needle.*

salbutamol (sal-byū'tă-mol). Albuterol.

salicin (sal'i-sin). Saligenin-β-D-glucopyranoside; a glucoside of *o*-hydroxybenzylalcohol, obtained from the bark of several species of *Salix* (willow) and *Populus* (poplar); s. is hydrolyzed to glucose and saligenin (salicyl alcohol); formerly used in rheumatoid arthritis.

salicyl (sal'i-sil). The acyl radical of salicylic acid.

s. alcohol, saligenin; saligenol; *o*-hydroxybenzyl alcohol; obtained by the hydrolysis of salicin; a local anesthetic.

s. aldehyde, salicylic aldehyde; *o*-hydroxybenzaldehyde; obtained from *Spirea ulmaria* (meadow sweet), and made synthetically; used as a diuretic and antiseptic, and in perfumery.

salicylamide (sal-i-sil'ă-mīd). The amide of salicylic acid, *o*-hydroxybenzamide; an analgesic, antipyretic and antiarthritic, similar in action to aspirin.

salicylanilide (sal'i-sil-an'i-līd) *N*-Phenylsalicylamide; an antifungal agent especially useful in the treatment of tinea capitis caused by *Microsporum audouinii.*

salicylate (să-lis'i-lāt). **1.** A salt or ester of salicylic acid. **2.** Salicylize; to treat foodstuffs with salicylic acid as a preservative.

salicylated (să-lis'i-lāt-ĕd). Treated by the addition of salicylic acid as a preservative.

salicylazosulfapyridine (sal'i-sil-az'ō-sŭl-fă-pir'i-dēn). Sulfasalazine.

salicylic acid (sal-i-sil'ik). *o*-Hydroxybenzoic acid; a component of aspirin, derived from salicin and made synthetically; used externally as a keratolytic agent, antiseptic, and fungicide.

salicylic aldehyde (sal-i-sil'ik). *Salicyl* aldehyde.

salicylism (sal'i-sil-izm). Poisoning by salicylic acid or any of its compounds.

salicylize (sal'i-sil-īz). Salicylate (2).

salicylsalicylic acid (sal'i-sil-sal-i-sil'ik). The salicylic ester of salicylic acid; an antipyretic, analgesic, and antirheumatic.

salicylsulfonic acid (sal'i-sil-sŭl-fon'ik). Sulfosalicylic acid.

salicyluric acid (sal'i-sil-yūr'ik). The conjugation product of glycine with salicylic acid; excreted in urine after the administration of salicylic acid or some of its compounds.

salient (sā'lē-ent, sāl'yent) [L. *salio,* to leap or spring up]. Prominence; projection.

pulmonary s., pulmonary arc; the middle of the three convexities forming the left cardiovascular border in a roentgenogram or on fluoroscopy; it is composed of the main pulmonary artery and its left main branch.

salifiable (sal-i-fī'ă-bl). Capable of being made into salts; said of a base that combines with acids to make salts.

salify (sal'i-fī). To convert into a salt.

saligenin, saligenol (sal-i-jen'in, sal'i-jen-ol). *Salicyl* alcohol.

salimeter (să-lim'ĕ-ter). A hydrometer used to determine the specific gravity, or the concentration, of a saline solution.

saline (sā'lēn, -līn). **1.** Relating to, of the nature of, or containing salt; salty. **2.** A salt solution, usually sodium chloride.

physiological s., an isotonic aqueous solution of salts, containing 0.9% sodium chloride.

salinometer (sal-i-nom'ĕ-ter). A hydrometer so calibrated as to give a direct reading of the percentage of a particular salt present in solution.

saliva (să-lī'vă) [L. akin to G. *sialon*]. Spittle; a clear, tasteless, odorless, slightly acid (pH 6.8) viscid fluid, consisting of the secretion from the parotid, sublingual, and submaxillary salivary glands and the mucous glands of the oral cavity; its function is to keep the mucous membrane of the mouth moist, to lubricate the food during mastication, and, in a measure, to convert starch into maltose, the latter action being effected by a diastatic enzyme, ptyalin.

chorda s., the secretion of the submaxillary gland obtained by stimulation of the chorda tympani nerve.

ganglionic s., submaxillary s. obtained by direct irritation of the gland.

resting s., the s. found in the mouth in the intervals of food taking and mastication.

sympathetic s., submaxillary s. obtained by stimulation of the sympathetic fibers innervating the gland.

salivant (sal'i-vant). **1.** Causing a flow of saliva. **2.** Salivator; an agent that increases the flow of saliva.

salivary (sal'i-vār-ē) [L. *salivarius*]. Sialic; sialine; relating to saliva.

salivate (sal'i-vāt). To cause an excessive flow of saliva.

salivation (sal'i-vā'shŭn). Sialism.

salivator (sal'i-vā-ter). Salivant (2).

salivolithiasis (sa-lī'vō-li-thī'ă-sis). Sialolithiasis.

Salk, Jonas, U.S. immunologist, *1914. See S. *vaccine.*

Salmonella (sal'mō-nel'ă) [Daniel E. *Salmon,* U.S. pathologist, 1850–1914]. A genus of aerobic to facultatively anaerobic bacteria (family Enterobacteriaceae) containing Gram-negative rods that are either motile or nonmotile; motile cells are peritrichous. These organisms do not liquefy gelatin or produce indole and vary in their production of hydrogen sulfide; they utilize citrate as a sole source of carbon; their metabolism is fermentative, producing acid and usually gas from glucose, but they do not attack lactose; most are aerogenic, but *S. typhi* never produces gas; they are pathogenic for humans and other animals. The type species is *S. cholerae-suis.*
S. aborti'voequi'na, a species causing abortion in mares; also infects guinea pigs, rabbits, goats, and cows, producing abortion.
S. abor'tus-o'vis, a species causing abortion in sheep.
S. chol'erae-su'is, a species which occurs in pigs, where it is an important secondary invader in the virus disease hog cholera, but does not occur as a natural pathogen in other animals; occasionally causes acute gastroenteritis and enteric fever in humans; it is the type species of the genus *S.*
S. enterit'idis, Gärtner's bacillus; a widely distributed species that occurs in humans and in domestic and wild animals, especially rodents.
S. gallina'rum, a species causing fowl typhoid; it causes white diarrhea in young chicks and occasionally causes food poisoning or gastroenteritis in man.
S. hirschfeld'ii, a species causing enteric fever in man.
S. paraty'phi, a species causing enteric fever in man; not known to be pathogenic for other animals.
S. schottmül'leri, Schottmüller's bacillus; a species causing enteric fever in man; found rarely in cattle, sheep, swine, chickens, and lower primates.
S. ty'phi, *s. typhosa;* Eberth's bacillus; typhoid bacillus; a species found in human cases of typhoid fever and in contaminated water and food.
S. typhimu'rium, a species causing food poisoning in humans; it is a natural pathogen of all warm-blooded animals and is also found in snakes.
S. typho'sa, *S. typhi.*

salmonellosis (sal'mō-nel-ō'sis) [*Salmonella* + G. *-osis,* condition]. Infection with bacteria of the genus *Salmonella.*

salol (sal'ol). Phenyl salicylate.

salping-. See salpingo-.

salpingectomy (sal-pin-jek'tō-mē) [salping- + G. *ektomē,* excision]. Tubectomy; removal of the fallopian tube.
abdominal s., celiosalpingectomy; laparosalpingectomy; removal of one or both fallopian tubes through an abdominal incision.

salpingemphraxis (sal'pin-jem-frak'sis) [salping- + G. *emphraxis,* a stopping]. Obstruction of the eustachian or the fallopian tube.

salpinges (sal-pin'jēz). Plural of salpinx.

salpingian (sal-pin'jē-ăn). Relating to the fallopian tube or to the auditory tube.

salpingioma (sal-pin-jē-ō'mă) [salping- + G. *-oma,* tumor]. Any tumor arising in the tissues of a fallopian tube.

salpingitic (sal-pin-jit'ik). Relating to salpingitis.

salpingitis (sal-pin-jī'tis). [salping- + G. *-itis,* inflammation]. Inflammation of the fallopian or the eustachian tube.
chronic interstitial s., pachysalpingitis; s. in which fibrosis or mononuclear cell infiltration involves all layers of the fallopian or eustachian tube.
foreign body s., s. in which giant cells form in the tissue, as a result of introduction of foreign material into the fallopian tube.
gonorrheal s., inflammation of the fallopian tube following acute gonorrheal infection.
s. isth'mica nodo'sa, adenosalpingitis; a condition of the fallopian tube characterized by nodular thickening of the tunica muscularis of the isthmic portion of the tube enclosing gland-like or cystic duplications of the lumen.
pyogenic s., a form of acute s. usually occurring with puerperal infection.

salpingo-, salping- [G. *salpinx,* trumpet (tube)]. Combining forms denoting a tube, usually the fallopian or eustachian tubes. See also tubo-.

salpingocele (sal-ping'gō-sēl) [salpingo- + G. *kēle,* hernia]. Hernia of a fallopian tube.

salpingocyesis (sal-ping'gō-sī-ē'sis) [salpingo- + G. *kyēsis,* pregnancy]. Tubal *pregnancy.*

salpingography (sal-ping-gog'ră-fē) [salpingo- + G. *graphō,* to write]. Radiographic image of the fallopian tubes after the injection of a solution of a radiopaque substance.

salpingolysis (sal-ping-gol'i-sis) [salpingo- + G. *lysis,* loosening]. Freeing the fallopian tube from adhesions.

salpingo-oophor-, salpingo-oophoro- [salpingo- + Mod. L. *oophoron,* ovary, fr. G. *ōophoros,* egg-bearing]. Combining forms denoting the fallopian tube and ovary.

salpingo-oophorectomy (sal-ping'gō-ō-of-ō-rek'tō-mē). Salpingo-ovariectomy; tubo-ovariectomy; removal of the ovary and its fallopian tube.
abdominal s., laparosalpingo-oophorectomy.

salpingo-oophoritis (sal-ping'gō-ō-of-ō-rī'tis). Tubo-ovaritis; inflammation of both fallopian tube and ovary.

salpingo-oophorocele (sal-ping'gō-ō-of'ō-rō-sēl). Hernia of both ovary and fallopian tube.

salpingo-ovariectomy (sal-ping'gō-ō-var-ē-ek'tō-mē). Salpingo-oophorectomy.

salpingoperitonitis (sal-ping'gō-per-i-tō-nī'tis) [salpingo- + peritonitis]. Inflammation of the fallopian tube, perisalpinx, and peritoneum.

salpingopexy (sal-ping'gō-pek-sē) [salpingo- + G. *pēxis,* fixation]. Operative fixation of an oviduct.

salpingopharyngeal (sal-ping'gō-fă-rin'jē-ăl). Relating to the auditory tube and pharynx.

salpingopharyngeus (sal-ping'gō-far-in-jē'ŭs) [L.]. See under musculus.

salpingoplasty (sal-ping'gō-plas-tē) [salpingo- + G. *plastos,* formed]. Tuboplasty; plastic surgery of the fallopian tubes.

salpingorrhagia (sal-ping-gō-rā'jē-ă) [salpingo- + G. *rhēgnymi,* to burst forth]. Hemorrhage from a fallopian tube.

salpingorrhaphy (sal-ping-gōr'ă-fē) [salpingo- + G. *rhaphē,* stitching]. Suture of the fallopian tube.

salpingoscopy (sal-ping-gos'kō-pē) [salpingo- + G. *skopeō,* to view]. Visualization of fallopian tubes, usually by x-ray or by means of a culdoscope.

salpingostomatomy (sal-ping'gō-stō-mat'ō-mē) [salpingo- + G. *stoma,* mouth, + *tomē,* incision]. Salpingostomy.

salpingostomy (sal-ping-gos'tō-mē) [salpingo- + G. *stoma,* mouth]. Salpingostomatomy; establishment of an artificial opening in a fallopian tube in which the fimbriated extremity has been closed by inflammation.

salpingotomy (sal-ping-got'ō-mē) [salpingo- + G. *tomē,* incision]. Incision into a fallopian tube.
abdominal s., celiosalpingotomy; laparosalpingotomy; incision into the fallopian tube through an opening in the abdominal wall.

salpinx, pl. salpinges (sal'pingks, sal-pin'jēz) [G. a trumpet (tube)]. **1** [NA]. Official alternate term for *tuba* uterina. **2.** *Tuba* auditiva.
s. uteri'na [NA], *tuba* uterina.

salt [L. *sal*]. **1.** A compound formed by the interaction of an acid and a base, the ionizable hydrogen atoms of the acid being replaced by the positive ion of the base. **2.** Sodium chloride, the prototypical s. **3.** A saline cathartic, especially magnesium sulfate, sodium sulfate, or Rochelle s.; often denoted by the plural, salts.
acid s., bisalt; protosalt; a s. in which not all of the ionizable hydrogen of the acid is replaced by the electropositive element; *e.g.,* $NaHSO_4$, KH_2PO_4.
artificial Carlsbad s., a mixture of potassium sulfate, sodium chloride, sodium bicarbonate, and dried sodium sulfate; a laxative.
artificial Kissingen s., a mixture of potassium chloride, sodium chloride, anhydrous magnesium sulfate, and sodium bicarbonate; an antacid and laxative.
artificial Vichy s., a mixture of sodium bicarbonate, anhydrous magnesium sulfate, potassium carbonate, and sodium chloride; an antacid.
basic s., a s. in which there are one or more hydroxyl ions not replaced by the electronegative element of an acid; *e.g.,* $Fe(OH)_2Cl$.
bile s.'s, the s. forms of bile acids; *e.g.,* taurocholate, glycocholate.
bone s., see bone-salt.
common s., *sodium* chloride.
diazonium s.'s, s.'s of a theoretical base $R-\overset{+}{N}\equiv N$ or $R-N=NOH$ useful in histochemistry to demonstrate tissue phenols and aryl amines or with enzymatically released naphthols and naphthylamines to form the chromophore azo group $-N=N-$; diazonium s.'s contain only one $R-\overset{+}{N}\equiv N$ group, tetrazonium s.'s contain two, and hexazonium s.'s contain three; examples include fast garnet GBC base and naphthol AS.
double s., a s. in which two different positive ions are bonded to the same negative ion, or vice versa; *e.g.,* $NaKSO_4$.
effervescent s.'s, preparations made by adding sodium bicarbonate and tartaric and citric acids to the active s.; when thrown into water the acids break up the sodium bicarbonate, setting free the carbonic acid gas.
Epsom s.'s, *magnesium* sulfate.
Glauber's s., *sodium* sulfate.
hexazonium s.'s, diazonium s.'s that contain three azo groups.
Rivière's s., *potassium* citrate.
Rochelle s., Seignette's s., *potassium* sodium tartrate.
smelling s.'s, sal volatile; ammonium carbonate, scented with aromatic oils (lavender, nutmeg, etc.); sniffed as a general stimulant.
table s., *sodium* chloride.
tetrazonium s.'s, diazonium s.'s that contain three azo groups.
s. of wisdom, *sal* alembroth.

saltation (sal-tā'shŭn) [L. *saltatio,* fr. *salto,* pp. *-atus,* to dance, fr. *salio,* to leap]. A dancing or leaping, as in a disease (*e.g.,* chorea) or physiologic function (*e.g.,* saltatory conduction).

saltatory (sal'tă-tōr-ē). Pertaining to, or characterized by, saltation.

Salter, Robert, 20th century Canadian orthopedist. See S.-Harris *classification* of epiphysial fractures.

Salter, Sir Samuel J.A., British dentist, 1825–1897. See S.'s incremental *lines.*

salting out. The precipitation of a protein from its solution by saturation or partial saturation with such neutral salts as sodium chloride, magnesium sulfate, or ammonium sulfate.

saltpeter (salt'pē-ter). *Potassium* nitrate.
Chilean s., *sodium* nitrate.

salt substitute. A low-sodium food additive that tastes like salt, such as potassium chloride; useful as a dietary alternative to salt.

salubrious (să-lū'brē-ŭs) [L. *salubris,* healthy, fr. *salus,* health]. Healthful, usually in reference to climate.

saluresis (sal-yū-rē'sis) [L. *sal,* salt, + G. *ourēsis,* uresis (urination)]. Excretion of sodium in the urine.

saluretic (sal-yū-ret'ik). Facilitating the renal excretion of sodium.

salutarium (sal-yū-tār'ē-ŭm) [L. *salutaris,* healthful, fr. *salus* (*salut*), health]. Sanitarium.

salutary (sal'yū-tār-ē) [L. salutaris]. Healthful; wholesome.

Salvarsan (sal'var-san) [L. *salvare,* to preserve, + *sanitas,* health]. Historic proprietary name for arsphenamine.

salve (sav) [A.S. *sealf*]. Ointment.

salvia (sal'vē-ă) [L.]. Sage; the dried leaves of *Salvia officinalis* (family Labiatae), garden or meadow sage; it inhibits secretory activity, especially of the sweat glands, and is also used in bronchitis and inflammation of the throat.

Salzmann, Maximilian, Austrian ophthalmologist, 1862–1954. See S.'s nodular corneal *dystrophy.*

samarium (să-mār'ē-ŭm) [bands indicating its presence first found in the spectrum of *samarskite,* a mineral named after Col. Samarski]. A metallic element of the lanthanide group, symbol Sm, atomic no. 62, atomic weight 150.35.

sambucus (sam-byū'kŭs) [L. an elder-tree]. Elder flowers; the dried flowers of *Sambucus canadensis* or *S. nigra* (family Caprifoliaceae), the common elder or black elder; slightly laxative.

sam'ple. In statistics, a portion of a population selected, often randomly, for research.
end-tidal s., a s. of the last gas expired in a normal expiration, ideally consisting only of alveolar gas.
Haldane-Priestley s., an approximation of alveolar gas obtained from the end of a sudden maximal expiration into a Haldane tube.
Rahn-Otis s., an approximation of alveolar gas continuously provided by a simple device that admits just the latter part of each expiration.
random s., a selection on the basis of chance of individuals or items in a population for research; selection is made in such a way that all members presumably have the same chance of being selected.

SAN Abbreviation for sinoatrial *node.*

Sanarelli, Giuseppe, Italian bacteriologist, 1864–1940. See S. *phenomenon,* S.-Shwartzman *phenomenon.*

sanative (san'ă-tiv) [L. *sano,* to cure, heal]. Having a tendency to heal.

sanatorium (san'ă-tōr'ē-ŭm) [Mod. L. neuter of *sanatorius,* curative, fr. *sano,* to cure, heal]. An institution for the treatment of chronic disorders and a place for recuperation under medical supervision. *Cf.* sanitarium.

sanatory (san'ă-tōr-ē) [Mod. L. *sanatorius*]. Health-giving; conducive to health.

Sanchez Salorio, Manuel, Spanish ophthalmologist, *1930. See S. S. *syndrome.*

sand [A.S.]. The fine granular particles of quartz and other crystalline rocks, or a gritty material resembling s.
brain s., *corpora* arenacea.
hydatid s., the scoleces of *Echinococcus* tapeworms in the fluid within a primary or daughter hydatid cyst.
intestinal s., minute calculi or gritty material occurring in feces, composed of soaps, bile pigment, cholesterol, magnesium salts, succinic acid, etc.
urinary s., multiple small calculous particles passed in the urine of patients with nephrolithiasis; each particle is usually too small to cause significant symptoms or to be identified as a true calculus.

sandalwood oil (san'dăl-wŭd). Santal oil.

sand-crack (sand'krak). A crack or fissure in the hoof of the horse, occurring usually on the inside of the forefoot (quarter-crack) or in the forepart of the hindfoot (toe-crack); when the crack is deep enough to expose the sensitive laminae, or when it extends to the coronary band, lameness results.

sandfly (sand'flī). A small, biting, dipterous midge of the genus *Phlebotomus* or *Lutzomyia;* a vector of leishmaniasis.

Sandhoff, K., contemporary German biochemist. See S.'s *disease.*

Sandison, J. Calvin, U.S. surgeon, *1899. See S.-Clark *chamber.*

Sandström, I., Swedish anatomist, 1852–1889. See S.'s *bodies.*

sandworm (sand'werm). Any of the various dog and cat hookworms whose larvae cause cutaneous larva migrans.

sane (sān) [L. *sanus*] Denoting sanity.

Sanfilippo, Sylvester J., 20th century U.S. pediatrician. See S.'s *syndrome.*

Sanger's reagent. See under reagent.

sangui-, sanguin-, sanguino- [G. *sanguis,* blood]. Combining forms meaning blood, bloody.

sanguifacient (sang-gwi-fā'shent) [sangui- + L. *facio,* to make]. Hemopoietic.

sanguiferous (sang-gwif'er-ŭs) [sangui- + L. *fero,* to carry]. Circulatory (2); conveying blood.

sanguification (sang'gwi-fi-kā'shŭn) [sangui- + L. *facio,* to make]. Hemopoiesis.

sanguinarine (sang-gwi-nā'rēn). An alkaloid obtained from the bloodroot plant, *Sanguinaria canadensis,* used to treat and remove dental plaque.

sanguine (sang'gwin) [L. *sanguineus*]. **1.** Plethoric. **2.** Sanguineous (3); formerly, denoting a temperament characterized by a light, fair complexion, full pulse, good digestion, optimistic outlook, and a quick but not lasting temper.

sanguineous (sang-gwin'ē-ŭs) [L. *sanguineus*]. **1.** Relating to blood; bloody. **2.** Plethoric. **3.** Sanguine (2).

sanguinolent (sang-gwin'ō-lent) [L. *sanguinolentus*]. Bloody; tinged with blood.

sanguinopurulent (sang'gwi-nō-pū'rū-lent) [sanguino- + L. *purulentus,* festering (suppurative), fr. *pus,* pus]. Denoting exudate or matter containing blood and pus.

sanguis (sang'gwis) [L.]. Blood.

Sanguisuga (sang-gwi-sū'gă) [L. a leech, fr. *sanguis,* blood, + *sugo,* pp. *suctus,* to suck]. Former name for *Hirudo.*

sanguivorous (sang-gwiv'er-ŭs) [sangui- + L. *voro,* to devour]. Bloodsucking, as applied to certain bats, leeches, insects, etc.

sanies (sā'nē-ēz) [L.]. A thin, blood-stained, purulent discharge.

saniopurulent (sā'nē-ō-pū'rū-lent) [L. *sanies,* thin, bloody matter, + *purulentus,* festering (suppurative), fr. *pus,* pus]. Characterized by bloody pus.

sanioserous (sā'nē-ō-sēr'ŭs). Characterized by blood-tinged serum.

sanious (sā'nē-ŭs). Relating to sanies; ichorous and blood-stained.

sanitarian (san-i-tăr'ē-ăn) [L. *sanitas,* health, fr. *sanus,* sound]. One who is skilled in sanitation and public health.

sanitarium (san-i-tăr'ē-ŭm) [L. *sanitas,* health]. Salutarium; a health resort. *Cf.* sanatorium.

sanitary (san'i-tăr-ē) [L. *sanitus,* health]. Healthful; conducive to health; usually in reference to a clean environment.

sanitation (san-i-tā'shŭn) [L. *sanitas,* health]. Use of measures designed to promote health and prevent disease; development and establishment of conditions in the environment favorable to health.

sanitization (san'i-ti-zā'shŭn). The process of making something sanitary.

sanity (san'i-tē) [L. *sanitas,* health]. Soundness of mind, emotions, and behavior; mental health.

San Jose. See Maldonado-S.J. *stain.*

Sansom, Arthur E., British physician, 1838–1907. See S.'s *sign.*

Sanson, Louis J., French physician, 1790–1841. See S.'s *images;* Purkinje-S. *images.*

santal oil (san'tăl). Sandalwood oil; a volatile oil distilled from the wood of *Santalum album* (family Santalaceae), a tree of India; used in subacute bronchitis and in gonorrhea.

Santini's booming sound. See under sound.

santonin (san'tō-nin) [G. *santonikon,* wormwood]. The inner anhydride or lactone of santoninic acid, obtained from santonica, the unexpanded flower heads of *Artemisia cina* and other species of *Artemisia* (family Compositae); has been used to effect expulsion of roundworms (*Ascaris lumbricoides*); and in the treatment of urinary incontinence.

Santorini, Giandomenico (Giovanni Domenico), Italian anatomist, 1681–1737. See S.'s *canal, cartilage,* major and minor *caruncle, concha, duct, fissures, incisure, labyrinth, muscle, tubercle, vein.*

sap. The juice or tissue fluid of a living organism.
nuclear s., karyolymph.

saphena (să-fē'nă) [Med. L. attributed by some as derived fr. Ar. *safin,* standing; by others, fr. G. *saphēnēs,* manifest, clearly visible]. See entries under vena.

saphenectomy (saf-ĕ-nek'tō-mē) [saphena + G. *ektomē,* excision]. Excision of a saphenous vein.

saphenous (să-fē'nŭs) [see saphena]. Relating to or associated with a saphenous vein; denoting a number of structures in the leg.

sapo-, sapon- [L. *sapo,* soap]. Combining forms relating to soap.

sapogenin (să-poj'ĕ-nin). The aglycon of a saponin; one of a family of steroids of the spirostan type (a 16,22:22,26-diepoxycholestane).

saponaceous (sap-ō-nā'shŭs). Soapy; relating to or resembling soap.

saponatus (sap-ō-nā'tŭs) [L.]. Mixed with soap.

saponification (să-pon'i-fi-kā'shŭn) [sapo- (*sapon-*) + L. *facio,* to make]. Conversion into soap, denoting the hydrolytic action of an alkali upon fat; in histochemistry, s. is used to demethylate or reverse blockage of carboxylic acid groups, thus permitting basophilia to occur.

saponify (să-pon'i-fī). To perform or undergo saponification.

saponins (sap'ō-ninz). Glycosides of plant origin characterized by properties of foaming in water and of lysing cells (as in hemolysis of erythrocytes when s. are injected into the bloodstream).

Sappey, Marie P.C., French anatomist, 1810–1896. See S.'s *fibers, plexus, veins.*

sapphism (saf'izm) [*Sapphō,* homosexual Greek poetess, queen of the island of Lesbos]. Lesbianism.

sapr-. See sapro-.

sapremia (să-prē'mē-ă) [sapr- + G. *haima,* blood]. Septicemia.

sapro-, sapr- [G. *sapros,* rotten]. Combining forms denoting rotten, putrid, decayed.

saprobe (sap'rōb) [sapro- + G. *bios,* life]. An organism that lives upon dead organic material. This term is preferable to saprophyte, since bacteria and fungi are no longer regarded as plants.

saprobic (sap-rō'bik). Pertaining to a saprobe.

saprodontia (sap-rō-don'shē-ă) [sapro- + G. *odous,* tooth]. Dental *caries.*

saprogen (sap'rō-jen) [sapro- + G. *-gen,* producing]. An organism living on dead organic matter and causing the decay thereof.

saprogenic, saprogenous (sap-rō-jen'ik, să-proj'ĕ-nŭs). Causing or resulting from decay.

saprophilous (să-prof′i-lŭs) [sapro- + G. *philos*, fond]. Thriving on decaying organic matter.

saprophyte (sap′rō-fīt) [sapro- + G. *phyton*, plant]. Necroparasite; an organism that grows on dead organic matter, plant or animal. See saprobe.

facultative s., an organism, usually parasitic, that occasionally may live and grow as a s.

saprophytic (sap-rō-fit′ik). Relating to a saprophyte.

saprozoic (sap-rō-zō′ik) [sapro- + G. *zōikos*, relating to animals]. Living in decaying organic matter; especially denoting certain protozoa.

saprozoonosis (sap′rō-zō-ō-nō′sis) [sapro- + G. *zōon*, animal, + *nosos*, disease]. A zoonosis the agent of which requires both a vertebrate host and a nonanimal (food, soil, plant) reservoir or developmental site for completion of its cycle. Combination terms may be used, such as saprometazoonoses for fluke infections, when metacercariae encyst on plants, or saprocyclozoonoses for tick infestations, whose agents complete part of their life cycles in soil.

saralasin acetate (sar-al′ă-sin). An angiotensin II derivative used in the treatment of essential hypertension.

Sarcina (sar′si-nă) [L. *sarcina*, a pack, bundle, fr. *sarcio*, to mend, patch]. A genus of nonmotile, strictly anaerobic bacteria (family Micrococcaceae) containing Gram-positive cocci, 1.8 to 3.0 μm in diameter, which divide in three perpendicular planes, producing regular packets of eight or more cells. The metabolism of these chemoorganotrophic organisms is fermentative. Saprophytic and facultatively parasitic species occur. The type species is *S. ventriculi.*

S. max′ima, a species from the hull or outer coat of cereal grains such as wheat, oat, rice, and rye, and from horse manure and soil.

S. ventric′uli, a species found in soil, mud, the contents of a diseased human stomach, rabbit and guinea pig stomach contents, and on the surfaces of cereal seeds; it is the type species of the genus *S.*

sarcine (sar′sēn). **1.** Hypoxanthine. **2.** A packet of cocci of the genus *Sarcina.*

sarco- [G. *sarx* (*sark*-), flesh]. Combining form denoting muscular substance or a resemblance to flesh.

sarcoblast (sar′kō-blast) [sarco- + G. *blastos*, germ]. Myoblast.

sarcocele (sar′kō-sēl) [sarco- + G *kēlē*, tumor]. A fleshy tumor or sarcoma of the testis.

Sarcocystis (sar-kō-sis′tis) [sarco- + G. *kystis*, bladder]. A genus of protozoan parasites, related to the sporozoan genera *Eimeria, Isospora,* and *Toxoplasma,* and placed in a distinct family, Sarcocystidae, but with the above genera in the same suborder, Eimeriina, within the subclass Coccidia, class Sporozoea, and phylum Apicomplexa. Tissue stages of *S.* are usually seen as thick-walled cylindrical or fusiform cysts (Miescher's tubes) in reptile, bird, or mammal striated muscles. Cysts are smooth in the house mouse form or with radial spines (cytophaneres) in sheep or rabbit cysts; contents may be compartmentalized by septa. Variably-shaped spores (Rainey's corpuscles) probably are peripheral rounded cells (sporoblasts, cytomeres) that divide to form mature "spores" (bradyzoites), motile bodies when released from the cyst; sexual stages have been described in tissue cultures. These parasites are abundant but rarely of pathogenic significance.

S. fusifor′mis, a species found in the striated and heart muscle of cattle and water buffalo.

S. hom′inis, a species now recognized as a two-host infection, with beef serving as the intermediate host source of infective tissue cysts to humans who serve as the final host. Gamogony and sporogony occur in mucosal cells of the human small intestine; cattle become infected from human feces contaminated with *S. hominis* sporocysts.

S. lindeman′ni, a species described on rare occasions from the striated and heart muscles of humans, probably as an infection due to various species, possibly from domestic dogs or other final hosts from which infective oocysts or sporocysts were passed to man via water or direct exposure; in these instances man serves as an intermediate rather than a final host.

S. miescheria′na, a common species of worldwide distribution that is found in the striated and heart muscle of pigs; it is the type species of the genus *S.*

S. suihom′inis, a recently described form of *S.* in which man serves as the final host, with the pig serving as intermediate host, the source of infected tissues to humans. The life cycle and moderate disease induced follow the pattern of *S. hominis,* though the disease appears to be somewhat more pathogenic. Human infection is widespread, having been reported in Europe, the Mediterranean area, northern and western Africa, Indonesia, and South America.

S. tenel′la, an extremely common species of worldwide distribution that is found in the striated and heart muscle of sheep and goats.

sarcocystosis (sar′kō-sis-tō′sis). Infection with *Sarcocystis.*

sarcode (sar′kōd) [sarco- + G. *eidos*, resemblance]. A term of historical interest (1835), applied to the protoplasm of protozoa before the term protoplasm was coined.

Sarcodina (sar′kō-dī′nă, -dē′nă) [Mod. L. fr. G. *sarx*, flesh]. The amebae; a subphylum of protozoa in the phylum Sarcomastigophora, possessing pseudopodia or locomotive protoplasmic flow for movement. Includes forms that possess flagella during development and forms with an internal or external test or skeleton and others lacking such a structure; asexual reproduction occurs by fission, and sexual reproduction, if present, by flagellate or ameboid gametes; most species are free-living.

sarcoglia (sar-kog′lē-ă) [sarco- + G. *glia*, glue]. The accumulation of neurolemma cells at the motor endplate.

sarcoid (sar′koyd) [sarco- + G. *eidos*, resemblance]. **1.** Sarcoidosis. **2.** Obsolete term for a tumor resembling a sarcoma.

Boeck's s., sarcoidosis.

Spiegler-Fendt s., benign *lymphocytoma* cutis.

sarcoidosis (sar-koy-dō′sis) [sarcoid + G. *-osis*, condition]. Sarcoid (1); Boeck's disease or sarcoid; Besnier-Boeck-Schaumann syndrome or disease; Schaumann's syndrome; a systemic granulomatous disease of unknown cause, especially involving the lungs with resulting fibrosis, but also involving lymph nodes, skin, liver, spleen, eyes, phalangeal bones, and parotid glands; granulomas are composed of epithelioid and multinucleated giant cells with little or no necrosis.

hypercalcemic s., s. with hypercalcemia of unknown cause, not necessarily associated with detectable bone involvement by s.

sarcolemma (sar′kō-lem′ă) [sarco- + G. *lemma*, husk]. Myolemma; the plasma membrane of a muscle fiber; formerly, the delicate connective tissue of the endomysium was included under this term by some.

sarcolemmal, sarcolemmic, sarcolemmous (sar′kō-lem′ăl, -lem′ik, -lem′ŭs). Relating to the sarcolemma.

sarcology (sar-kol′ō-jē) [sarco- + G. *logos*, study]. **1.** Myology. **2.** The anatomy of the soft parts, as distinguished from osteology.

sarcolysine (sar-kō-lī′sēn). Merphalan.

sarcoma (sar-kō′mă) [G. *sarkōma*, a fleshy excrescence, fr. *sarx*, flesh, + *-oma*, tumor]. A connective tissue neoplasm, usually highly malignant, formed by proliferation of mesodermal cells.

alveolar soft part s., a malignant tumor formed of a reticular stroma of connective tissue enclosing aggregates of large round or polygonal cells; occurs in subcutaneous and fibromuscular tissues.

ameloblastic s., ameloblastic *fibrosarcoma.*

angiolithic s., psammoma.

avian s., Rous s.
botryoid s., a polypoid form of embryonal rhabdomyosarcoma which occurs in children, most frequently in the urogenital tract, characterized by the formation of grossly apparent grapelike clusters of neoplastic tissue that consist of rhabdomyoblasts, spindle, and stellate cells in a myxomatous stroma; neoplasms of this type grow relatively rapidly and are highly malignant.
endometrial stromal s., stromatosis; a term sometimes used for a relatively rare s. believed to be a form of endometriosis in which the lesions form multiple foci in the myometrium and in vascular spaces in other sites, and which consist of histologic and cytologic elements that resemble those of the endometrial stroma.
Ewing's s., Ewing's *tumor.*
fascicular s., spindle cell s.
giant cell s., a malignant giant cell tumor of bone.
granulocytic s., myeloid s.; a malignant tumor of immature myeloid cells, frequently subperiosteal, associated with or preceding granulocytic leukemia.
immunoblastic s., immunoblastic *lymphoma.*
Jensen's s., a mouse tumor transmissible by inoculation.
juxtacortical osteogenic s., periosteal s.; a form of osteogenic s. of relatively low malignancy, probably arising from the periosteum and initially involving cortical bone and adjacent connective tissue, which occurs in middle-aged as well as young adults and most commonly affects the lower part of the femoral shaft.
Kaposi's s., multiple idiopathic hemorrhagic s.; a multifocal malignant neoplasm of primitive vasoformative tissue, occurring in the skin and sometimes in lymph nodes or viscera, consisting of spindle cells and irregular small vascular spaces frequently infiltrated by hemosiderin-pigmented macrophages and extravasated red cells; clinically manifested by cutaneous lesions consisting of reddish-purple to dark blue macules, plaques, or nodules; seen most commonly in men over 60 years of age and as an opportunistic disease in AIDS patients.
leukocytic s., leukemia.
lymphatic s., lymphosarcoma.
medullary s., a soft, extremely vascular s.
multiple idiopathic hemorrhagic s., Kaposi's s.
myelogenic s., s. originating in the bone marrow.
myeloid s., granulocytic s.
osteogenic s., osteosarcoma; the most common and malignant of bone s.'s, which arises from bone-forming cells and affects chiefly the ends of long bones; its greatest incidence is in the age group between 10 and 25 years.
periosteal s., juxtacortical osteogenic s.
reticulum cell s., histiocytic *lymphoma.*
round cell s., an undifferentiated malignant neoplasm, believed to be of mesenchymal origin, composed chiefly of closely packed round cells.
Rous s., Rous tumor; avian s.; a fibrosarcoma, originally observed in a Plymouth Rock hen, now thought to be an expression of infection by the avian leukosis-sarcoma complex.
spindle cell s., fascicular s.; a malignant neoplasm, believed to be of mesenchymal origin, composed of elongated, spindle-shaped cells.
synovial s., malignant synovioma; a rare malignant tumor of synovial origin, most commonly involving the knee joint and composed of spindle cells usually enclosing slits or pseudoglandular spaces that may be lined by radially disposed epithelial-like cells.
telangiectatic osteogenic s., a lytic cystic variant of osteogenic s. composed of aneurysmal blood-filled spaces lined by sarcoma cells producing osteoid.

Sarcomastigophora (sar'kō-mas-ti-gof'ō-ră) [sarco- + G. *mastix* (*mastig-*), whip, + *phoros,* to bear]. A phylum of the subkingdom Protozoa characterized by flagellae, pseudopodia, or both types of locomotory organelles; includes both the flagellates (subphylum Mastigophora) and the amebae (subphylum Sarcodina) in a single large assemblage.

sarcomatoid (sar-kō'mă-toyd) [sarcoma + G. *eidos,* resemblance]. Resembling a sarcoma.

sarcomatosis (sar'kō-mă-tō'sis) [sarcoma + G. *-osis,* condition]. Occurrence of several sarcomatous growths on different parts of the body.

sarcomatous (sar-kō'mă-tŭs). Relating to or of the nature of sarcoma.

sarcomere (sar'kō-mēr) [sarco- + G. *meros,* part]. The segment of a myofibril between two adjacent Z lines, representing the functional unit of striated muscle.

sarconeme (sar'kō-nēm) [sarco- + G. *nema,* thread]. Microneme.

sarcoplasm (sar'kō-plazm) [sarco- + G. *plasma,* a thing formed]. The nonfibrillar cytoplasm of a muscle fiber.

sarcoplasmic (sar-kō-plaz'mik). Relating to sarcoplasm.

sarcoplast (sar'kō-plast) [sarco- + G. *plastos,* formed]. Satellite *cell* of skeletal muscle.

sarcopoietic (sar'kō-poy-et'ik) [sarco- + G. *poiēsis,* a making]. Forming muscle.

Sarcopsylla penetrans (sar-kō-sil'ă pen'ĕ-tranz). *Tunga penetrans.*

Sarcopsyllidae (sar-kop-sil'li-dē) [sarco- + G. *psylla,* flea]. Older name for Tungidae.

Sarcoptes scabiei (sar-kop'tēz skā'bē-ī) [sarco- + G. *koptō,* to cut; L. *scabies,* scurf]. *Acarus scabiei;* the itch mite, varieties of which are distributed worldwide and affect man, horses, cattle, swine, sheep, dogs, cats, and many wild animals; serious and fatal infections are not uncommon in untreated animals. Although considered to belong to a single species, they do not readily pass from one host to another of a different animal species; transitory infections of this type do occur, however, especially from various animals to man, and are spread by direct contact. The mite burrows into the skin and lays eggs within the burrow; intense itching and rash develop near the burrow in about a month. See scabies; mange.

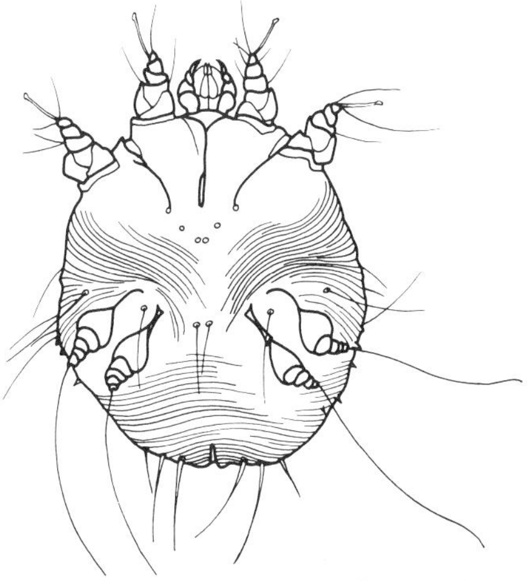

Sarcoptes scabiei, **Scabies or Itch Mite** (×100)

sarcoptic (sar-kop'tik). Of, relating to, or caused by mites of the genus *Sarcoptes* or other members of the family Sarcoptidae.

sarcoptid (sar-kop'tid). Common name for members of the Sarcoptidae, a family of mites that includes the genera *Sarcoptes, Knemidokoptes,* and *Notoedres.*

sarcosine (sar'kō-sēn). *N*-Methylglycine; an intermediate in the metabolism of choline; it can donate a methyl group to tetrahydrofolate, yielding 5,10-methylenetetrahydrofolate; demethylation by s.

dehydrogenase yields formaldehyde, glycine, and a reduced acceptor.

s. dehydrogenase [EC 1.5.99.1], an enzyme that cleaves s. to glycine, formaldehyde, and a reduced acceptor molecule.

sarcosinemia (sar'kō-si-nē'mē-ă). Hypersarcosinemia; a disorder of amino acid metabolism due to deficiency of sarcosine dehydrogenase, causing sarcosine to be elevated in blood plasma and excreted in urine; affected infants fail to thrive, are irritable, may have muscle tremors, and have retarded motor and mental development; autosomal recessive inheritance.

sarcosis (sar-kō'sis) [G. *sarkōsis,* the growth of flesh, fr. *sarx,* flesh]. **1.** An abnormal increase of flesh. **2.** A multiple growth of fleshy tumors. **3.** A diffuse sarcoma involving the whole of an organ.

sarcosome (sar'kō-sōm) [sarco- + G. *soma,* body]. **1.** Formerly, any granule in a muscle fiber. **2.** Now, sometimes used synonymously with myomitochondrion.

sarcostosis (sar-kos-tō'sis) [sarco- + G. *osteon,* bone, + *-osis,* condition]. Ossification of muscular tissue.

sarcotic (sar-kot'ik). **1.** Relating to sarcosis. **2.** Causing an increase of flesh.

sarcotripsy (sar'kō-trip-sē) [sarco- + G. *tripsis,* a rubbing]. Use of a crushing forceps to stop hemorrhage.

sarcotubules (sar-kō-tū'būlz). The continuous system of membranous tubules in striated muscle which corresponds to the smooth endoplasmic reticulum of other cells.

sarcous (sar'kŭs) [G. *sarx,* flesh]. Relating to muscular tissue; muscular; fleshy.

sardonic grin (sar-don'ik). *Risus* sardonicus or caninus.

sarin (zah-rēn') [Ger.]. Isopropyl methylphosphonofluoridate; a nerve poison similar to diisopropyl fluorophosphate and tetraethyl pyrophosphate; a very potent irreversible cholinesterase inhibitor and a more toxic nerve gas than tabun or soman.

sarmassation (sar-mă-sā'shŭn) [G. *sarx,* flesh, + *massein,* to knead]. Erotic squeezing, kneading, or caressing of female tissues and organs.

sarsaparilla (sar'să-per-il'ă, sas-per-il'ă) [Sp. *zarza,* a bramble]. The dried root of *Smilax aristolochioefolia* (Mexican s.), *S. regelii* (Honduras s.), *S. febrifuga* (Ecuadorian s.), or of undetermined species of *Smilax* (family Liliaceae), a thorny vine widely distributed throughout the tropical and semitropical world; it has been used in psoriasis, gout, rheumatism, and syphilis, and popularly as a "blood purifier."

SART Abbreviation for sinoatrial recovery *time.*

sartorius (sar-tōr'ē-ŭs) [L. *sartor,* a tailor, the muscle being used in crossing the legs in the tailor's position, fr. *sarcio,* pp. *sartus,* to patch, mend]. See under musculus.

sassafras (sas'ă-fras). The dried bark of the root of *Sassafras albidum* (family Lauraceae), a tree of the eastern U.S.; a flavoring agent, diuretic, and diaporetic; s. oil, a volatile oil obtained by distillation from the bark of *S. albidum* and *S. variifolium,* is used as a carminative, topical antiseptic, pediculicide, and flavoring agent.

sat Abbreviation for saturated.

satellite (sat'ĕ-līt) [L. *satelles (sattelit-),* attendant]. **1.** A minor structure accompanying a more important or larger one; *e.g.,* a vein accompanying an artery, or a small or secondary lesion adjacent to a larger one. **2.** The posterior member of a pair of gregarine gamonts in syzygy, several of which may be found in some species. See also primite.

chromosome s., a small chromosomal segment separated from the main body of the chromosome by a secondary constriction; in man it is usually associated with the short arm of an acrocentric chromosome.

nucleolar s., term originally given by Murray Barr to a small dot of chromatin found adjacent to the nucleolus in nerve cells of females but not in those of males. See sex *chromatin.*

perineuronal s., an oligodendroglia cell surrounding the neuron.

satellitosis (sat'ĕ-lī-tō'sis) [L. *satelles (satellit-),* an attendant, + G. *-ōsis,* condition]. A condition marked by an accumulation of neuroglia cells around the neurons of the central nervous system; often as a prelude to neuronophagia.

satiation (sā-shē-ā'shŭn) [L. *satio,* pp. *-atus,* to fill, satisfy]. The state produced by fulfillment of a specific need, such as hunger or thirst.

sat. sol., sat. soln. Abbreviation for saturated *solution.*

Sattler, Hubert, Austrian ophthalmologist, 1844–1928. See S.'s elastic *layer,* S.'s *veil.*

saturate (satch'ŭ-rāt) [L. *saturo,* pp. *-atus,* to fill, fr. *satur,* sated]. **1.** To impregnate to the greatest possible extent. **2.** To neutralize; to satisfy all the chemical affinities of a substance (as by converting all double bonds to single bonds). **3.** To dissolve a substance up to that concentration beyond which the addition of more results in two phases.

saturation (satch-ŭ-rā'shŭn). **1.** Impregnation of one substance by another to the greatest possible extent. **2.** Neutralization, as of an acid by an alkali. **3.** That concentration of a dissolved substance that cannot be exceeded. **4.** In optics, see saturated *color.* **5.** Filling of all the available sites on an enzyme molecule by its substrate, or on a hemoglobin molecule by oxygen (symbol So_2) or carbon monoxide (symbol Sco).

secondary s., a technique of nitrous oxide anesthesia consisting of an abrupt curtailment of the oxygen in the inhaled mixture to produce a deep plane of anesthesia, following which oxygen is administered to correct hypoxia.

saturnine (sat'er-nīn) [Mediev. L. *saturninus,* fr. *saturnus,* lead, fr. L. *saturnis,* the god and planet Saturn]. **1.** Relating to lead. **2.** Due to or symptomatic of lead poisoning.

saturnism (sat'er-nizm) [Mediev. L. *saturnus,* alchemical term for lead]. Lead *poisoning.*

satyriasis (sat-i-rī'ă-sis) [G. *satyros,* a satyr]. Satyrism; satyromania; excessive sexual excitement and behavior in the male; the counterpart of nymphomania in the female.

satyrism (sat'i-rizm). Satyriasis.

saucerization (saw'ser-i-zā'shŭn). Craterization; excavation of tissue to form a shallow depression, performed in wound treatment to facilitate drainage from infected areas.

Sauerbruch, Ernst Ferdinand, German surgeon, 1875–1951. See S.'s *cabinet.*

Saundby, Robert, British physician, 1849–1918. See S.'s *test.*

sauriasis (saw-rī'ă-sis) [G. *sauros,* lizard, + *-iasis,* condition]. Ichthyosis.

sauriderma (saw-ri-der'mă) [G. *sauros,* lizard, + *derma,* skin]. Ichthyosis.

sauriosis (saw-ri-ō'sis) [G. *sauros,* lizard, + *-osis,* condition]. Ichthyosis.

sauroderma (saw'rō-der'mă) [G. *sauros,* lizard, + *derma,* skin]. Ichthyosis.

Savage, Henry, British anatomist and gynecologist, 1810–1900. See S.'s perineal *body.*

saw [A.S. *saga*] A metal operating instrument having an edge of sharp, toothlike projections, for dividing bone, cartilage, or plaster; edges may be attached to a rigid band, a flexible wire or chain, or a motorized oscillator.

Gigli's s., a chain s. for use in craniotomy or pubiotomy.

Stryker s., a rapidly oscillating s. used for cutting bone or plaster casts; it cuts hard matter, but soft tissues give and thus are not injured.

saxitoxin (sak-si-tok'sin). A potent neurotoxin found in shellfish, such as the mussel or the clam, produced by the dinoflagellate *Gonyaulax catenella,* which is ingested by the shellfish.

Sayre, George P., U.S. ophthalmologist, *1911. See Kearns-S. *syndrome.*

Sayre, Lewis A., U.S. surgeon, 1820–1900. See S.'s suspension *traction, apparatus, jacket.*

Sb Symbol for antimony.

SBE Abbreviation for subacute bacterial *endocarditis.*

Sc Symbol for scandium.

s.c. Abbreviation for subcutaneous; subcutaneously.

scab (skab) [A.S. *scaeb*] A crust formed by coagulation of blood, pus, serum, or a combination of these, on the surface of an ulcer, erosion, or other type of wound.

scabicidal (skā-bi-sī'dăl). Destructive to itch mites.

scabicide (skā'bi-sīd). Scabieticide; an agent lethal to itch mites.

scabies (skā'bēz) [L. *scabo,* to scratch]. **1.** An eruption due to *Sarcoptes scabiei* var. *hominis;* the female of the species burrows into the skin, producing a vesicular eruption with intense pruritus between the fingers, on the male genitalia, buttocks, and elsewhere on the trunk and extremities. **2.** In animals, s. or scab is usually applied to cutaneous acariasis in sheep, which may be caused by *Sarcoptes, Psoroptes,* or *Chorioptes.* Mite infections causing dermatitis in wild and domestic animals, including sheep, are more commonly called mange, and may be caused by species and varieties of the genera listed above and of others such as *Demodex, Notoedres,* and *Otodectes.* See also mange.

Norwegian s., Norway itch; a severe form of s. caused by *Sarcoptes scabiei* var. *crustosae.*

scabieticide (skā-bē-et'i-sīd). Scabicide.

scabious (skā'bē-ŭs). Relating to or suffering from scabies.

scabrities (skā-brish'i-ēz) [L., fr. *scaber,* scurfy]. Roughness of the skin.

s. un'guium, thickening and distortion of the nails.

scabwort (skab'wōrt). Elecampane.

scala, pl. scalae (skā'lă, -lē) [L. a stairway] [NA]. One of the cavities of the cochlea winding spirally around the modiolus.

Löwenberg's s., *ductus* cochlearis.

s. me'dia, *ductus* cochlearis.

s. tym'pani [NA], the division of the spiral canal of the cochlea lying below the lamina spiralis.

s. vestib'uli [NA], vestibular canal; the division of the spiral canal of the cochlea lying above the lamina spiralis and vestibular membrane.

scald (skawld) [L. *excaldo,* to wash in hot water]. **1.** To burn by contact with a hot liquid or steam. **2.** The lesion resulting from such contact. **3.** Scall.

scalding (skawl'ding). A burning pain in urinating.

scale (skāl). [L. *scala,* a stairway] **1.** A strip of metal, glass, or other substance, marked off in lines, for measuring. **2.** A standardized test for measuring psychological, personality, or behavioral characteristics. See also subentries under test. [O.E. *scealu,* fr. O.Fr. *escale,* shell, husk] **3.** Squama. **4.** A small thin plate of horny epithelium, resembling a fish s., cast off from the skin. **5.** To desquamate. **6.** To remove tartar from the teeth.

absolute s., obsolete term for Kelvin s.

adaptive behavior s.'s, a behavioral assessment device to quantify the levels of skills of mentally retarded and developmentally delayed individuals in interacting with the environment; consists of three developmentally related factors: 1) personal self-sufficiency, *e.g.,* eating, dressing; 2) community self-sufficiency, *e.g.,* shopping, communicating; 3) personal and social responsibility, *e.g.,* use of leisure time, job performance.

Ångström s., a table of wavelengths of a large number of light rays corresponding to as many Fraunhofer's lines in the spectrum.

Baumé s., a hydrometer s. for determining the specific gravity of liquids heavier and lighter than water,respectively:for liquids lighter than water divide 140 by 130 plus the Baumé degree; for liquids heavier than water divide 145 by 145 minus the Baumé degree.

Bayley S.'s of Infant Development, a device used to measure the developmental progress of infants over the first two and one-half years of life; consists of three scales: mental, motor, and behavior record.

Benois s., an obsolete s. for measuring penetrability of x-rays.

Binet s., a measure of intelligence designed for both children and adults.

Binet-Simon s., forerunner of individual intelligence tests, particularly the Stanford-Binet intelligence s.

Celsius s., centigrade s.; a thermometer s. in which there are 100 degrees between the freezing point (0°C) and boiling point (100°C) of water at sea level.

centigrade s., Celsius s.

Charrière s., French s.

Columbia Mental Maturity S. [*Columbia University,* NY], an individually administered intelligence test that provides an estimate of the intellectual ability of children; provides mental ages ranging from three to 12 years, and requires no verbal response and minimal or no motor response.

coma s., a clinical s. to assess impaired consciousness; assessment may include motor responsiveness, verbal performance, and eye opening, as in the Glasgow (Scotland) c.s., or the same three items and dysfunction of cranial nerves, as in the Maryland (U.S.) c.s.

Fahrenheit s., a thermometer s. in which the freezing point of water is 32°F and the boiling point of water 212°F; 0°F indicates the lowest temperature Fahrenheit could obtain by a mixture of ice and salt.

French s. (Fr), Charrière s.; a s. for grading sizes of sounds, tubules, and catheters as based on a measurement of $^1/_3$ mm and equaling 1 fr on the scale (*e.g.,* 3 fr = 1 mm); grading to scale is carried out using a metal plate with holes ranging from $^1/_3$ mm to 1 cm in diameter.

Gaffky s., Gaffky *table.*

gray s., see gray-scale *ultrasonography.*

hardness s., Mohs s.; a qualitative s. in which minerals are classified in order of their increasing hardness, based on the fact that the harder of two materials will scratch the softer and will not be scratched by it. The s. lists 15 substances: 1, talc; 2, gypsum; 3, calcite; 4, fluorite; 5, apatite; 6, orthoclase, periclase; 7, vitreous pure silica; 8, quartz, stellite; 9, topaz; 10, garnet; 11, tantalum carbide, fused zirconia; 12, fused alumina; 13, silicon carbide; 14, boron carbide; 15, diamond.

homigrade s., a special thermometer s. in which 100° indicates the normal temperature of man (98.6°F, 37°C), 0° the freezing point, and 270° the boiling point (212°F., 100°C).

interval s., like a temperature s. in centigrade or Fahrenheit units, a s. on which the intervals are equal but which has an arbitrary zero point; *e.g.,* intelligence quotient values are values along an interval s.

Karnofsky s., a performance s. for rating a person's usual activities; used to evaluate a patient's progress after a therapeutic procedure.

Kelvin s., temperature measured in degrees Celsius from absolute zero (−273.16°C).

Leiter International Performance S., a nonverbal (performance) test for measuring intelligence which contains norms for each age between 2 and 18; originally developed as a method of assessing the comparative intellectual abilities of Caucasian, Chinese, and Japanese children, but now occasionally used for assessing slow learners and those who are blind, deaf, or verbally handicapped.

masculinity-femininity s., any s. on a psychological test that assesses the relative masculinity or femininity of an individual; s.'s vary and may focus, for example, on basic identification with either sex or preference for a particular sex role.

Mohs s., hardness s.

pH s., Sorensen s.

Rankine s., a thermometer s. in which each degree Rankine (°Rank.) is equal to the Fahrenheit but applied to the absolute temperature s. with its zero point at absolute zero.

ratio s., a s. that involves physical units and demonstrates their relations.

Réaumur s., a thermometer s. in which each degree Réaumur (°R) is $^{1}/_{80}$ of the temperature difference between the freezing point and boiling point of pure water at 1 atmosphere pressure, with 0°R set at the freezing point and 80°R set at the boiling point of water.

Shipley-Hartford s. [*Hartford* Retreat, CT, where Shipley employed]. a test of conceptual aptitude and flexibility.

Sörensen s., pH s.; the negative logarithm of the hydrogen ion concentration, used as a s. for expressing acidity and alkalinity. See also pH.

Stanford-Binet intelligence s., Binet or Binet-Simon test; a standardized test for the measurement of intelligence consisting of a series of questions, graded according to the intelligence of normal children at different ages, the answers to which indicate the mental age of the person tested; primarily with children, but also contains norms for adults standardized against adult age levels rather than those of children, as formerly was the case.

Wechsler-Bellevue s., a measure of general intelligence superseded by the Wechsler adult intelligence s. See also Wechsler intelligence s.'s.

Wechsler intelligence s.'s, standardized s.'s for the measurement of general intelligence in preschool children (Wechsler preschool and primary s. of intelligence), in children (Wechsler intelligence s. for children), and in adults (Wechsler adult intelligence s., the successor to the Wechsler-Bellevue s.).

scalene (skā'lēn) [G. *skalēnos,* uneven]. Scalenus. **1.** Having sides of unequal length, said of a triangle so formed. **2.** One of several muscles so named. See scalenus entries under musculus.

scalenectomy (skā'lĕ-nek'tō-mē) [scalene + G. *ektomē,* excision]. Resection of the scalene muscles.

scalenotomy (skā'lĕ-not'ō-mē) [scalene + G. *tomē,* incision]. Division or section of the anterior scalene muscle.

scalenus (skā-lē'nŭs) [L.]. Scalene.

scaler (skā'ler). **1.** An instrument for removing tartar from the teeth. **2.** A device for counting electrical impulses, as in the assay of radioactive materials.

hoe s., a hoe-shaped s. with a very short blade.

sonic s., a s. utilizing sonic speed vibration to remove calculus from teeth.

scaling (skā'ling). In dentistry, removal of accretions from the crowns and roots of teeth by use of special instruments.

scall (skawl) [Ice. *skalli,* bald-head]. Scald (3); any crusted or pustular scaly eruption or lesion of the skin or scalp, *e.g.,* favus.

honeycomb s., archaic term for an eruption of minute contiguous ulcers separated by raised edges.

milk s., *crusta* lactea.

scalloping (skal'ō-ping). A series of indentations or erosions on a normally smooth margin of a structure.

scalp (skalp) [M. E. fr. Scand. *skalpr,* sheath]. The skin covering the cranium.

scalpel (skal'pl) [L. *scalpellum;* dim. of *scalprum,* a knife]. A knife used in surgical dissection.

plasma s., a s. that uses a fine high-temperature gas jet, instead of a blade, for cutting.

scalpriform (skal'pri-fōrm) [L. *scalprum,* chisel, + *forma,* shape]. Chisel-shaped.

scalprum (skal'prŭm) [L. chisel, penknife, fr. *scalpo,* pp. *scalptus,* to carve]. **1.** A large strong scalpel. **2.** A raspatory.

scaly (skā'lē). Squamous.

scammony (skam'ō-nē) [G. *skammōnia*]. The plant, *Convolvulus scammonia* (family Convolvulaceae), the dried root of which contains a cathartic resin. See also ipomea.

scan (skan). **1.** Abbreviated form of scintiscan, usually preceded by the organ or structure examined; *e.g.,* brain s., bone s., etc. **2.** To survey by traversing with an active or passive sensing device. **3.** The image, record, or data obtained by scanning, usually preceded by the technology or device employed; *e.g.,* CT (CAT) s., radionuclide s., etc.

Meckel s., use of technetium-99m pertechnetate in a s. of the gastric mucosa to detect ectopic gastric mucosa in Meckel's diverticulum; the pertechnetate anion is secreted by epithelial cells in the gastric mucosa.

ventilation-perfusion s., a diagnostic test for pulmonary embolism employing an inhaled radionuclide followed by an intravenous radionuclide; their respective distribution and perfusion in the lung are recorded radiographically.

scandium (skan'dē-ŭm) [L. *Scandia,* Scandinavia, where discovered]. A metallic element, symbol Sc, atomic no. 21, atomic weight 44.96.

scanner (skan'er). A device or instrument that scans.

scanning (skan'ing). The act of surveying by traversing with an active or passive sensing device, often preceded by the technology or device employed.

scansorius (skan-sōr'ē-ŭs) [L. relating to climbing, fr. *scando,* to climb]. See under musculus.

Scanzoni, Friedrich W., German obstetrician, 1821–1891. See S.'s *maneuver,* second *os.*

scapha (skaf'ă, skā'fă) [L. fr. G. *skaphē,* skiff] [NA]. **1.** A boat-shaped structure. **2.** Fossa of the helix; scaphoid fossa (2); fossa navicularis auris; the longitudinal furrow between the helix and the antihelix of the auricle.

scapho- [G. *skaphē,* skiff, boat]. Combining form denoting scapha or scaphoid.

scaphocephalic (skaf-ō-se-fal'ik). Scaphocephalous; tectocephalic; denoting or relating to scaphocephaly.

scaphocephalism (skaf-ō-sef'ă-lizm). Scaphocephaly.

scaphocephalous (skaf-ō-sef'ă-lŭs). Scaphocephalic.

scaphocephaly (skaf-ō-sef'ă-lē) [scapho- + G. *kephalē,* head]. Scaphocephalism; tectocephaly; a form of craniosynostosis presenting a long, narrow head in which the parietal eminences are absent and frontal and occipital protrusions are conspicuous; a crest may exist indicating the site of a prenatally closed sagittal suture; sometimes accompanied by mental retardation.

scaphohydrocephalus, scaphohydrocephaly (skaf'ō-hī'drō-sef'ă-lŭs, -lē). Occurrence of hydrocephalus in a scaphocephalic individual.

scaphoid (skaf'oyd) [scapho- + G. *eidos,* resemblance]. Navicular; boat-shaped; hollowed.

scapula, gen. and pl. **scapulae** (skap'yū-lă, -lē) [L. *scapulae,* the shoulder blades] [NA]. Shoulder blade; blade bone; a large triangular flattened bone lying over the ribs, posteriorly on either side, articulating laterally with the clavicle and the humerus.

s. ala'ta, winged s.

s. eleva'ta, Sprengel's *deformity.*

scaphoid s., a s. in which the vertebral border below the level of the spine presents concavity instead of the normal convexity; the **scaphoid type of s.** (Graves) is a s. in which the vertebral border between the spine and the teres major process is either straight or tends toward concavity.

winged s., s. alata; condition wherein the medial border of the scapula protrudes away from the thorax; the protrusion is posterior and lateral, as the scapula rotates out; caused by paralysis of the serratus anterior muscle.

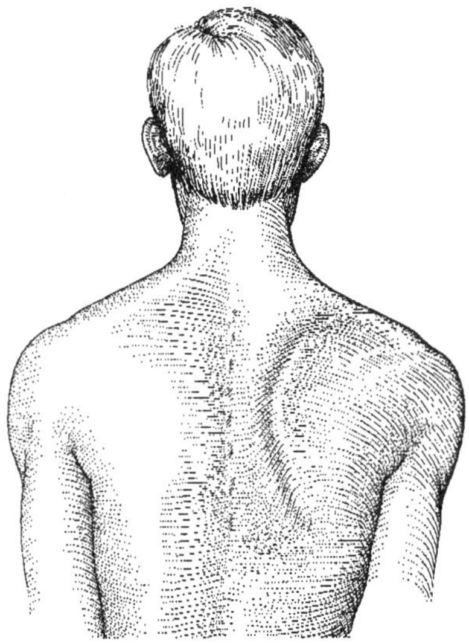

Winged Scapula

scapulalgia (skap′yū-lal′jē-ă) [scapula + G. *algos,* pain]. Scapulodynia; rarely used term meaning pain in the shoulder blades.

scapular (skap′yū-lăr). Relating to the scapula.

scapulary (skap′yū-lăr-ē). A form of brace or suspender for keeping a belt or body bandage in place.

scapulectomy (skap′yū-lek′tō-mē) [scapula + G. *ektomē,* excision]. Excision of the scapula.

scapulo- [L. *scapulae,* shoulder blades]. Combining form denoting scapula or scapular.

scapuloclavicular (skap′yū-lō-klă-vik′yū-lăr). **1.** Acromioclavicular. **2.** Coracoclavicular.

scapulodynia (skap′yū-lō-din′ē-ă) [scapulo- + G. *odynē,* pain]. Scapulalgia.

scapulohumeral (skap′yū-lō-hyū′mer-ăl). Relating to both scapula and humerus.

scapulopexy (skap′yū-lō-pek-sē) [scapulo- + G. *pēxis,* fixation]. Operative fixation of the scapula to the chest wall or to the spinous process of the vertebrae.

scapus, pl. **scapi** (skā′pŭs, -pī) [L. shaft, stalk]. A shaft or stem.

s. pe′nis, *corpus* penis.

s. pi′li, a hair shaft.

scar (skar) [G. *eschara,* scab]. Cicatrix; the fibrous tissue replacing normal tissues destroyed by injury or disease.

cigarette-paper s.'s, papyraceous s.'s; atrophic s.'s in the skin over the knees, shins, and elbows of persons with Ehlers-Danlos syndrome.

hypertrophic s., an elevated s. resembling a keloid but which does not spread into surrounding tissues, is rarely painful, and regresses spontaneously; collagen bundles run parallel to the skin surface.

papyraceous s.'s, cigarette-paper s.'s.

radial s., radial sclerosing *lesion.*

shilling s.'s, round, well healed s.'s that follow involution of rupial syphilids.

Scardino, Peter L., U.S. urologist, *1915. See S. vertical flap *pyeloplasty.*

Scarff, John E., U.S. neurosurgeon, *1898. See Stookey-S. *operation.*

scarification (skar-i-fi-kā′shŭn) [L. *scarifico,* to scratch, fr. G. *skariphos,* a style for sketching]. The making of a number of superficial incisions in the skin.

scarificator (skar′i-fi-kā-tōr). An instrument for scarification, consisting of a number of concealed spring-projected cutting blades, set near together, that make superficial incisions in the skin.

scarify (skar′i-fī). To produce scarification.

scarlatina (skar′lă-tē′nă) [through It. fr. Mediev. L. *scarlatum,* scarlet, a scarlet cloth]. Scarlet fever; an acute exanthematous disease, caused by infection with streptococcal organisms producing erythrogenic toxin, marked by fever and other constitutional disturbances, and a generalized eruption of closely aggregated points or small macules of a bright red color followed by desquamation in large scales, shreds, or sheets; mucous membrane of the mouth and fauces is usually also involved.

anginose s., s. angino′sa, Fothergill's disease (2); a form of s. in which the throat affection is unusually severe.

s. hemorrhag′ica, a form of s. in which blood extravasates into the skin and mucous membranes, giving to the eruption a dusky hue; frequently bleeding from the nose and into the intestine also occurs.

s. la′tens, latent s., a form of s. in which the rash is absent, the action of the specific toxin being manifested in acute nephritis.

s. malig′na, a severe scarlet fever in which the patient is early overcome with the intensity of the systemic intoxication.

s. rheumat′ica, dengue.

s. sim′plex, a mild form of the disease.

scarlatinal (skar-lă-tē′năl). Relating to scarlatina.

scarlatinella (skar-lă-ti-nel′ă) [dim. of *scarlatina*]. Fourth *disease.*

scarlatiniform (skar-lă-tē′ni-fōrm, -tin′i-fōrm). Scarlatinoid (1); resembling scarlatina, denoting a rash.

scarlatinoid (skar-lă-tē′noyd, skar-lat′i-noyd) [scarlatina + G. *eidos,* resemblance]. **1.** Scarlatiniform. **2.** Fourth *disease.*

scarlet (skar′let) [Mediev. L. *scarlatum,* scarlet cloth]. Denoting a bright red color tending toward orange.

scarlet red [C.I. 26905]. Medicinal scarlet red; scharlach red; Sudan IV; Biebrich scarlet red; *o*-tolylazo-*o*-tolylazo-β-naphthol. An azo dye; a dark, brownish red powder, soluble in oils, fats, and chloroform, but insoluble in water; used in medicine as a vulnerary, in histology to stain fat in tissue sections and basic proteins at high pH, and in immunoelectrophoresis.

scarlet red sulfonate. An azo dye that has been used to stimulate healing of chronic superficial wounds and ulcers.

Scarpa, Antonio, Italian anatomist, orthopedist, and ophthalmologist, 1747–1832. See S.'s *fascia, fluid, foramina, fossa* (scarpae major), *ganglion, habenula, hiatus, liquor, membrane, method, sheath, staphyloma, triangle.*

scatemia (skă-tē′mē-ă) [scato- + G. *haima,* blood]. Intestinal autointoxication.

scato- [G. *skōr* (*skat-*), feces, excrement]. Combining form denoting feces. See also copro-, sterco-.

scatologic (skat-ō-loj′ik). Pertaining to scatology.

scatology (skă-tol′o-jē) [scato- + G. *logos,* study]. **1.** Coprology; the scientific study and analysis of feces, for physiologic and diagnostic purposes. **2.** The study relating to the psychiatric aspects of excrement or excremental (anal) function.

scatoma (ska-tō′mă) [scato- + G. *-oma,* tumor]. Coproma.

scatophagy (skă-tof′ă-jē) [scato- + G. *phagein,* to eat]. Coprophagy; rhypophagy; the eating of excrement.

scatoscopy (skă-tos'kō-pē) [scato- + G. *skopeō,* to view]. Examination of the feces for purposes of diagnosis.

scatter (skat'er). A change in direction of a photon or subatomic particle, as the result of a collision or interaction.

scatula (skat'yū-lă) [Mediev. L. a rectangular figure whose width is one-tenth of its length]. A square pillbox.

Scedosporium apiospermum (sked-os-pōr'ē-ŭm ā-pē-os'per-mŭm). *Monosporium apiospermum;* the imperfect state of the fungus *Pseudallescheria boydii,* one of the 16 species of true fungi that may cause mycetoma in man.

scelalgia (se-lal'jē-ă) [G. *skelos,* leg, + *algos,* pain]. Pain in the leg.

scelotyrbe (sel-ō-ter'bē) [G. *skelos,* leg, + *tyrbē,* disorder]. Spastic paralysis of the legs.

scent (sent). Odor.

Schacher, Polycarp G., German physician, 1674–1737. See S.'s *ganglion.*

Schaer's reagent. See under reagent.

Schäfer, Sir Edward A. Sharpey-, British physiologist and histologist, 1850–1935. See S.'s *method.*

Schäffer, Max, German neurologist, 1852–1923. See S.'s *reflex.*

Schaffer's test. See under test.

Schamberg, Jay F., U.S. dermatologist, 1870–1934. See S.'s *dermatitis, disease.*

Schanz, Alfred, German orthopedic surgeon, 1868–1931. See S.'s *syndrome.*

Schapiro, Heinrich, Russian physician, 1852–1901. See S.'s *sign.*

Schardinger, Franz, 19th century Austrian scientist. See S. *enzyme, reaction.*

scharlach red (shar'lak). Scarlet red.

Schatzki, Richard, U.S. radiologist, *1901. See S.'s *ring.*

Schaudinn, Fritz R., German bacteriologist, 1871–1906. See S.'s *fixative.*

Schaumann, Jörgen, Swedish physician, 1879–1953. See S.'s *bodies, lymphogranuloma, syndrome;* Besnier-Boeck-S. *disease, syndrome.*

Schaumberg, H.H., U.S. neuropathologist, *1912. See S.'s *disease.*

Schauta, Friedrich, Austrian gynecologist, 1849–1919. See S. vaginal *operation.*

Schede, Max, German surgeon, 1844–1902. See S.'s *clot, method.*

schedule (sked'jūl) [L. *scheda,* fr. *scida,* a strip of papyrus, leaf of paper]. A procedural plan for a proposed objective, especially the sequence and time allotted for each item or operation required for its completion.
s.'s of reinforcement, in the psychology of conditioning, established procedures or sequences for reinforcing operant behavior; *e.g.,* in a lever pressing situation, every displacement of the lever will bring a reinforcer (**continuous reinforcement s.**), or the reinforcer will come at every 5 seconds, regardless of how many displacements occur earlier (**fixed-interval reinforcement s.**), at every 10th displacement (**fixed-ratio reinforcement s.**), or on an average of every 5 seconds (**variable-interval reinforcement s.**), or the reinforcer will come in a noncontinuous fashion in which less than 100% of the displacements bring a reinforcer (**intermittent reinforcement s.**).

Scheele, Karl W., Swedish chemist, 1742–1786. See S.'s *green.*

Scheibe's deafness. See under deafness.

Scheibler's reagent. See under reagent.

Scheie, Harold G., U.S. ophthalmologist, *1909. See S.'s *syndrome.*

Scheiner, Christoph, German physicist, 1575–1650. See S.'s *experiment.*

Schellong, Fritz, German physician, *1891. See S. *test;* S.-Strisower *phenomenon.*

schema, pl. schemata (skē'mă, skē-mah'tă) [G. *schēma,* shape, form]. **1.** Scheme; a plan, outline, or arrangement. **2.** In sensorimotor theory, the organized unit of cognitive experience.
body s., body *image.*

schematic (skē-mat'ik) [G. *schēmatikos,* in outward show, fr. *schēma,* shape, form]. Made after a definite type of formula; representing in general, but not with absolute exactness; denoting an anatomical drawing or model.

schematograph (skē-mat'ō-graf) [G. *schēma,* form, + *graphō,* to write]. An instrument for making a tracing in reduced size of the outline of the body.

scheme (skēm). Schema (1).
occlusal s., occlusal *system.*

Schenck, Benjamin R., U.S. surgeon, 1873–1920. See S.'s *disease.*

Scheuermann, Holger W., Danish surgeon, 1877–1960. See S.'s *disease.*

Schick, Bela, Austrian pediatrician in U.S., 1877–1967. See S. *method, test,* test *toxin.*

Schiff, Hugo, German chemist in Florence, 1834–1915. See S. *base; S.'s reagent;* periodic acid-S. *stain;* ninhydrin-S. *stain* for proteins.

Schiff, Moritz, German physiologist, 1823–1896. See S.-Sherrington *phenomenon.*

Schilder, Paul, German-American psychiatrist, 1886–1940. See S.'s *disease;* Flatau-S. *disease.*

Schiller, Walter, Austrian pathologist in U.S., 1887–1960. See S.'s *test.*

Schilling, Victor, German hematologist, 1883–1960. See S.'s *blood count,* band *cell, index, test;* S. type of monocytic *leukemia.*

schindylesis (skin-dī-lē'sis) [G. *schindylēsis,* splintering] [NA]. Schindyletic joint; wedge-and-groove joint or suture; a form of fibrous joint in which the sharp edge of one bone is received in a cleft in the edge of the other, as in the articulation of the vomer with the rostrum of the sphenoid.

Schiötz, Hjalmar, Norwegian physician, 1850–1927. See S. *tonometer.*

Schirmer, Otto W.A., German ophthalmologist, 1864–1917. See S. *test.*

Schirmer, Rudolph, German ophthalmologist, 1831–1896. See S.'s *syndrome.*

schisto- [G. *schistos,* split]. Combining form denoting split or cleft. See also schizo-.

schistocelia (skis-tō-sē'lē-ă) [schisto- + G. *koilia,* a hollow]. Congenital fissure of the abdominal wall.

schistocormia (skis-tō-kōr'mē-ă) [schisto- + G. *kormos,* trunk of a tree]. Schistosomia; congenital cleft of the trunk, the lower extremities of the fetus usually being imperfectly developed.

schistocystis (skis-tō-sis'tis) [schisto- + G. *kystis,* bladder]. Fissure of the bladder.

schistocyte (skis'tō-sīt) [schisto- + G. *kytos,* cell]. Schizocyte; a variety of poikilocyte that owes its abnormal shape to fragmentation occurring as the cell flows through damaged small vessels.

schistocytosis (skis'tō-sī-tō'sis). Schizocytosis; the occurrence of many schistocytes in the blood.

schistoglossia (skis-tō-glos'ē-ă) [schisto- + G. *glōssa,* tongue]. Congenital fissure or cleft of the tongue.

schistorrhachis (skis-tōr'ă-kis) [schisto- + G. *rhachis,* spine]. *Spina* bifida.

Schistosoma (skis-tō-sō'mă) [schisto- + G. *sōma,* body]. A genus of digenetic trematodes, including the important blood flukes of man and domestic animals, that cause schistosomiasis; characterized by elongate shape, by separate sexes with marked sexual dimorphism, by their unusual location in the smaller blood vessels of their host, and by utilization of water snails as intermediate hosts.

S. bo'vis, a species infecting cattle, buffalo, sheep, goats, and wild ruminants in Africa, the Middle East, southern Europe, and Asia; characterized by long spindle-shaped eggs with a terminal spine.

S. haemato'bium, the vesical blood fluke, a species with terminally spined eggs that occurs as a parasite in the portal system and mesenteric veins of the bladder (causing human schistosomiasis haematobium) and rectum; common in the Nile delta but is found along waterways, irrigation ditches, or streams throughout Africa and in parts of the Middle East; the intermediate host is *Bulinus truncatus* in Egypt; elsewhere, other snails of the subfamily Bulininae (*Bulinus, Physopsis, Pyrgophysa*) are involved.

S. in'dicum, a species that occurs in the portal and mesenteric veins of cattle, sheep, goats, horses, and camels in Indo-Pakistan.

S. intercala'tum, a blood fluke species related to *S. haematobium* and found in natives of Zaire causing mild dysentery and abdominal pains, with enlargement of the spleen and liver; a planorbid snail, *Bulinus (Physopis) africanus,* serves as the intermediate host.

S. japon'icum, the Oriental or Japanese blood fluke, a species having eggs with small lateral spines, usually only a small knob; causes schistosomiasis japonica, with extensive pathology from encapsulation of the eggs, particularly in the liver, and is the most pathogenic of the three common schistosome species afflicting man, possibly owing to greater egg production per female worm; it is also the most intractable to treatment and the most difficult to control, as the intermediate hosts are amphibious snails (species of *Oncomelania,* family Hydrobiidae) that can leave the water to avoid molluscicides, and also because many other animals, such as pigs, oxen, cattle, and dogs, serve as reservoir hosts.

S. manso'ni, a common species characterized by large eggs with a strong lateral spine and transmitted by planorbid snails of the genus *Biomphalaria;* causes schistosomiasis mansoni in man in Africa, parts of the Middle East, and West Indies, South America, and certain Caribbean islands.

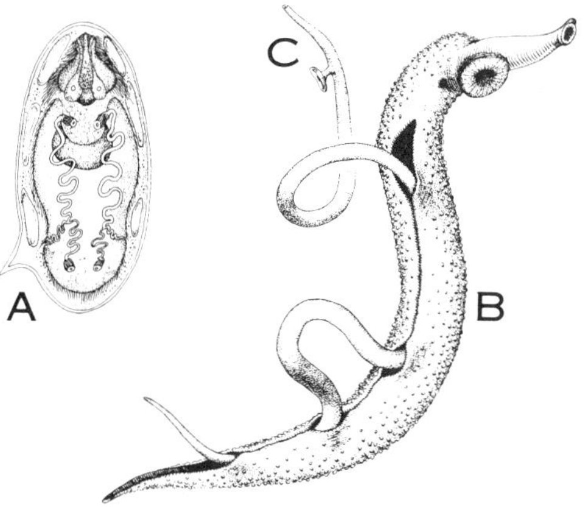

Schistosoma mansoni

A, egg containing miracidium (×200); *B,* adult male (×8); *C,* adult female (×8).

S. mat'theei, a species found in the portal and mesenteric veins of ruminants, primates (including man), zebra, and rodents in Africa.

S. mekon'gi, the Mekong schistosome, a species recently described from the Mekong delta near Khong Island in southern Laos and northern Cambodia. Infection rates are highest for ages 7 to 15; dogs appear to be the chief reservoir host; the intermediate host snail is the 3 mm-long operculid snail, *Tricula aperta.* Pathology is similar to that of *S. japonicum.*

S. spinda'le, a species parasitic in the portal and mesenteric veins of ruminants, and occasionally horses and dogs, in Africa, Indo-Pakistan, and Southeast Asia.

schistosome (skis'tō-sōm). Common name for a member of the genus *Schistosoma.*

schistosomia (skis-tō-sō'mē-ă) [schisto- + G. *sōma,* body]. Schistocormia.

schistosomiasis (skis'tō-sō-mī'ă-sis). Bilharziasis; bilharziosis; hemic distomiasis; snail fever; infection with a species of *Schistosoma;* manifestations of this often chronic and debilatory disease vary with the infecting species but depend in large measure upon tissue reaction (granulation and fibrosis) to the eggs deposited in venules and in the hepatic portals, the latter resulting in portal hypertension and esophageal varices, as well as liver damage leading to cirrhosis. See also schistosome *dermatitis;* Symmers' clay pipestem *fibrosis.*

Asiatic s., s. japonica.

bladder s., s. haematobium.

ectopic s., a clinical form of s. that occurs outside of the normal site of parasitism (mesenteric vein or hepatic portals); may result from accidental blood-borne transport of schistosome eggs or, rarely, adult worms, to various unusual sites such as the skin, brain, or spinal cord.

s. haemato'bium, urinary or bladder s.; endemic or Egyptian hematuria; infection with *Schistosoma haematobium,* the eggs of which invade the urinary tract, causing cystitis and hematuria, and possibly an increased likelihood of bladder cancer.

intestinal s., s. mansoni.

s. japon'ica, Japanese s., Oriental s.; infection with *Schistosoma japonicum,* characterized by dysenteric symptoms, painful enlargement of the liver and spleen, dropsy, urticaria, and progressive anemia. Also called Asiatic or Oriental s.; Katayama disease or syndrome; Kinkiang, Yangtze Valley, or urticarial fever; kabure; kabure itch.

s. manso'ni, Manson's s., Manson's disease; intestinal s.; infection with *Schistosoma mansoni,* the eggs of which invade the wall of the large intestine and the liver, causing irritation, inflammation, and ultimately fibrosis.

s. mekon'gi, infection with *Schistosoma mekongi* which chiefly afflicts children in the Mekong delta, where it was discovered; the disease is similar to s. japonica.

Oriental s., s. japonica.

urinary s., s. haematobium.

schistosomulum, pl. **schistosomula** (skis-tō-sō'myū-lŭm, -lă). The stage in the life cycle of a blood fluke of the genus *Schistosoma* immediately after penetration of the skin as a cercaria; marked by loss of the tail and gaining of physiological modifications allowing it to survive in a mammalian bloodstream.

schistosternia (skis-tō-ster'nē-ă) [schisto- + G. *sternon,* sternum]. Congenital cleft of the sternum.

schistothorax (skis-tō-thōr'aks) [schisto- + G. *thōrax,* thorax]. Congenital cleft of the chest wall.

schiz-. See schizo-.

schizamnion (skiz-am'nē-on) [schiz- + amnion]. An amnion developing, as in the human embryo, by the formation of a cavity within the inner cell mass.

schizaxon (skiz-ak'son) [schiz- + G. *axōn,* axis]. An axon divided into two branches.

schizencephaly (skiz-en-sef'ă-lē) [schiz- + G. *enkephalos,* brain]. Abnormal divisions or clefts of the brain substance.

schizo-, schiz- [G. *schizō,* to split or cleave]. Combining forms denoting split, cleft, division. See also schisto-.

schizo-affective (skiz'ō-ă-fek'tiv). Having an admixture of symptoms suggestive of both schizophrenia and affective disorder.

schizocyte (skiz'ō-sīt) [schizo- + G. *kytos,* cell]. Schistocyte.

schizocytosis (skiz'ō-sī-tō'sis). Schistocytosis.

schizogenesis (skiz-ō-jen'ĕ-sis) [schizo- + G. *genesis,* origin]. Fissiparity; scissiparity; origin by fission.

schizogony (ski-zog'ō-nē) [schizo- + G. *gonē,* generation]. Agamocytogeny; multiple fission in which the nucleus first divides and then the cell divides into as many parts as there are nuclei; called merogony if daughter cells are merozoites, sporogony if daughter cells are sporozoites, or gametogony if daughter cells are gametes.

schizogyria (skiz-ō-jī'rē-ă, -jir'ē-ă) [schizo- + G. *gyros,* circle (convolution)]. Deformity of the cerebral convolutions marked by occasional interruptions of their continuity.

schizoid (skiz'oyd) [schizo(phrenia), + G. *eidos,* resemblance]. Socially isolated, withdrawn, having few (if any) friends or social relationships; resembling the personality features characteristic of schizophrenia, but in a milder form. See also s. *personality.*

schizoidism (skiz'oy-dizm). A schizoid state; the manifestation of schizoid tendencies.

schizomycete (skiz'ō-mī-sēt). A member of the class Schizomycetes; a bacterium.

Schizomycetes (skiz'ō-mī-sē'tēz) [schizo- + G. *mykēs,* fungus]. Fission fungi; Naegeli's term for a class comprised of all the bacteria; a misnomer, since bacteria are generally not considered to be fungi. The bacteria are now classified in the kingdom Prokaryotae.

schizomycetic (skiz-ō-mī-sē'tik). Relating to or caused by fission fungi (bacteria).

schizomycosis (skiz-ō-mī-kō'sis). Any schizomycetic or bacterial disease.

schizont (skiz'ont) [schizo- + G. *ōn (ont-),* a being]. Agamont, segmenting body; a sporozoan trophozoite (vegetative form) that reproduces by schizogony, producing a varied number of daughter trophozoites or merozoites. See also meront; segmenter.

schizonticide (ski-zon'ti-sīd) [schizont + L. *caedo,* to kill]. An agent that kills schizonts.

schizonychia (skiz-ō-nik'ē-ă) [schizo- + G. *onyx,* nail]. Splitting of the nails.

schizophasia (skiz-ō-fā'zē-ă) [schizo- + G. *phasis,* speech]. The disordered speech (word salad) of the schizophrenic individual.

schizophrenia (skiz-ō-frē'nē-ă, skit'sō-) [schizo- + G. *phrēn,* mind]. A term, coined by Bleuler, synonymous with and replacing dementia precox; a common type of psychosis, characterized by a disorder in the thinking processes, such as delusions and hallucinations, and extensive withdrawal of the individual's interest from other people and the outside world, and the investment of it in his own; now considered a group of mental disorders rather than as a single entity, with distinction sometimes made between process s. and reactive s.

ambulatory s., a milder form of s. in which the patient is capable of maintaining himself in society and need not be hospitalized.

catatonic s., s. characterized by marked disturbances in activity, with either generalized inhibition or excessive activity.

disorganized s., hebephrenic s.; a severe form of s. characterized by the predominance of incoherence, blunted, inappropriate or silly affect, and the absence of systematized delusions.

hebephrenic s., disorganized s.

latent s., a preexisting susceptibility for developing overt s. under strong emotional stress.

paranoid s., s. characterized predominantly by delusions of persecution and megalomania.

process s., those forms of severe schizophrenic disorders in which chronic and progressive organic brain changes are considered to be the primary cause and in which prognosis is poor, as contrasted with reactive s.

pseudoneurotic s., s. in which the underlying psychotic process is masked by complaints ordinarily regarded as neurotic.

reactive s., those forms of severe schizophrenic disorders which are distinguished from process s. by their more acute onset, greater relation to environmental stress, and better prognosis.

residual s., blunted or inappropriate affect, social withdrawal, eccentric behavior, or loose associations, but without prominent psychotic symptoms, as the remains of former psychotic symptoms of s.

simple s., s. characterized by withdrawal, apathy, indifference, and impoverishment of human relationships.

schizophrenic (skiz-ō-fren'ik, -frē'nik; skit-sō-). Relating to, characteristic of, or suffering from one of the schizophrenias.

schizothemia (skiz-ō-thē'mē-ă) [schizo- + G. *thema,* theme]. Repeated interruptions in a conversation by the speaker introducing other topics.

schizotonia (skiz-ō-tō'nē-ă) [schizo- + G. *tonos,* tension, tone]. Division of the distribution of tone in the muscles.

schizotrichia (skiz-ō-trik'ē-ă) [schizo- + G. *thrix,* hair]. Scissura pilorum; a splitting of the hairs at their ends.

Schizotrypanum cruzi (skiz-ō-trī'pan-ŭm krū'zī) [schizo- + G. *trypanon,* a borer, an auger]. A distinct generic designation used for *Trypanosoma cruzi,* used frequently by workers in the endemic area of South American trypanosomiasis; also used as a subgeneric designation, *i.e., Trypanosoma (Schizotrypanum) cruzi.*

schizozoite (skiz-ō-zō'īt) [schizo- + G. *zōn,* animal]. A merozoite prior to schizogony, as in the exoerythrocytic phase of the development of the *Plasmodium* agent after sporozoite invasion of the hepatocyte and before multiple division.

Schlatter, Carl, Swiss surgeon, 1864–1934. See Osgood-S. *disease.*

Schlemm, Friedrich S., German anatomist, 1795–1858. See S.'s *canal.*

Schlesinger, Hermann, Austrian physician, 1868–1934. See S.'s *sign;* Pool-S. *sign.*

Schmid, Rudi, Swiss-American internist and biochemist, *1922. See McArdle-S.-Pearson *disease.*

Schmid, W. See S.-Fraccaro *syndrome.*

Schmidel, Kasimir C., German anatomist, 1718–1792. See S.'s *anastomoses.*

Schmidt, Gerhard, U.S. biochemist, *1900. See S.-Thannhauser *method.*

Schmidt, Henry D., U.S. anatomist and pathologist, 1823–1888. See S.-Lanterman *clefts, incisures.*

Schmidt, Johann F.M., German laryngologist, 1838–1907. See S.'s *syndrome.*

Schmidt, Martin Benno, German physician, 1863–1949. See S.'s *syndrome.*

Schmorl, Christian G., German pathologist, 1861–1932. See S.'s *bacillus, furrow, nodule, stains.*

Schneider, Franz C., German chemist, 1813–1897. See S.'s *carmine.*

Schneidersitz (shnī'der-zitz) [Ger.]. A typical sitting position with legs crossed in front, exhibited by severely defective patients with phenylketonuria and resembling the position which was commonly attributed to tailors.

Scholander, Per F., Norwegian physiologist. See S. *apparatus;* Roughton-S. *apparatus, syringe.*

Scholz, Willibald, German neurologist, *1889. See S. *disease.*

Schönbein, Christian F., German chemist, 1799–1868. See S.'s *test.*

Schönlein, Johann L., German physician, 1793–1864. See S.'s *disease, purpura;* Henoch-S. *purpura.*

school (skūl) [O. E. *scōl*]. A set of beliefs, teachings, methods, etc.

biometrical s., a group of British geneticists, followers of Galton and Karl Pearson, whose approach to genetics was quantitative rather than enumerative.
dogmatic s., ancient Greek s. or tradition in medicine whose members were the successors to or followers of Hippocrates; they based their conceptions of disease upon the humoral theory and their practice upon experience and sound reasoning, and were comparatively free from fads, speculative theories, and dogma, which the term dogmatic falsely implies.
dynamic s., a group of theorists founded by Stahl, who professed the belief that all vital action is the result of an internal force independent of anything external to the body.
hippocratic s., the followers of the teachings of Hippocrates. See also dogmatic s.
iatromathematical s., mechanistic s.; a group of academicians, of whom Descartes was one of the foremost proponents, who maintained that all physiologic processes were the result of physical laws.
mechanistic s., iatromathematical s.

Schott, Theodor, 1850–1921, German physician in Bad Nauheim. See S. *treatment.*

Schottmüller, Hugo A.G., German physician, 1867–1936. See *Salmonella shottmülleri;* S.'s *bacillus, disease.*

Schreger, Christian H.T., German anatomist and chemist, 1768–1833. See S.'s *lines;* Hunter-S. *bands, lines.*

Schridde, Hermann, German pathologist, *1875. See S.'s cancer *hairs.*

Schroeder, Karl L.E., German gynecologist, 1838–1887. See S.'s *operation.*

Schuchardt, Karl A., German surgeon, 1856–1901. See S.'s *operation.*

Schüffner, Wilhelm, German pathologist in Sumatra, 1867–1949. See S.'s *granules, dots.*

Schüller, Artur, Austrian neurologist, *1874. See S.'s *disease, phenomenon, syndrome;* Hand-S.-Christian *disease.*

Schüller, Karl H.L.A. Max, German surgeon, 1843–1907. See S.'s *ducts.*

Schultes, Johann. See Scultetus.

Schultz, Arthur R.H., German physician, *1890. See S. *reaction, stain.*

Schultz, Werner, German internist, 1878–1947. See S.-Charlton *phenomenon, reaction;* S.-Dale *reaction.*

Schultze, Bernhard S., German obstetrician, 1827–1919. See S.'s *fold, mechanism, phantom, placenta.*

Schultze, Max J., German histologist and zoologist, 1825–1874. See S.'s *cells, membrane, sign;* comma *bundle* of S.; comma *tract* of S.

Schütz, Erich, German biochemist, *1902. See S. *law, rule.*

Schütz, Hugo, 19th century German anatomist. See S.'s *bundle.*

Schwabach, Dagobert, German otologist, 1846–1920. See S. *test.*

Schwachman syndrome. See under syndrome.

Schwalbe, Gustav A., German anatomist, 1844–1916. See S.'s *corpuscle, nucleus, rings, spaces.*

Schwann, Theodor, German histologist and physiologist, 1810–1882. See S. *cells;* S.'s white *substance; sheath* of S.

schwannoma (shwah-nō'mă) [Theodor *Schwann* + -oma]. **1.** Neurofibroma. **2.** Neurilemoma.
acoustic s., acoustic *neurinoma.*

schwannosis (shwah-nō'sis). A non-neoplastic proliferation of Schwann cells in the perivascular spaces of the spinal cord; seen particularly in older patients, especially those with diabetes mellitus.

Schwartz, Henry, U.S. neurosurgeon, *1909. See S. *tractotomy.*

Schwartz, Oscar, U.S. pediatrician, *1919. See S. *syndrome.*

Schwarz, Karl L.H., German chemist, 1824–1890. See S.'s *test.*

Schweigger-Seidel, Franz, German physiologist, 1834–1871. See *sheath* of S.-S.

Schweninger, Ernst, German dermatologist, 1850–1924. See S.-Buzzi *anetoderma.*

sciage (sē-ahzh') [Fr. *scie,* saw]. A to-and-fro, sawlike movement of the hand in massage.

sciatic (sī-at'ik) [Mediev. L. *sciaticus,* a corruption of G. *ischiadikos,* fr. *ischion,* the hip joint]. **1.** Ischiadic; ischial; ischiatic; relating to or situated in the neighborhood of the ischium or hip. **2.** Relating to sciatica.

sciatica (sī-at'i-kă) [see sciatic]. Cotunnius disease; ischialgia (2); sciatic neuralgia; pain in the lower back and hip radiating down the back of the thigh into the leg, usually due to herniated lumbar disk.

scilla (sil'ă) [G.]. Squill.

scillaren (sil'lă-ren). A mixture of glycosides, possessing digitalis-like actions, present in squill.
s. A., a crystalline steroidal glycoside, present in squill, that can be hydrolyzed to glucose and proscillaridin A; the latter can be hydrolyzed to rhamnose and the steroid aglycone scillaridin A; same actions and uses as digitalis glycosides.
s. B, an amorphous glycosidal fraction obtained from squill, consisting of at least seven cardioactive glycosides: glucoscillaren A, scillipheoside, glucoscillipheoside, scillicryptoside, scilliglaucoside, scillicyanoside, and scillazuroside.

scinticisternography (sin'ti-sis-tern-og'ră-fē). Cisternography performed with a radiopharmaceutical and recorded with a stationary imaging device.

scintigram (sin'ti-gram) [L. *scintilla,* spark, + G. *gramma,* something written]. Scintiscan.

scintigraphic (sin'ti-graf'ik). Relating to or obtained by scintigraphy.

scintigraphy (sin-tig'ră-fē). A diagnostic procedure employing intravenous injection of a radionuclide, with an affinity for the organ or tissue of interest, followed by determination of the distribution of the radioactivity by an external scintillation detector.

scintillascope (sin-til'ă-skōp) [L. *scintilla,* spark, + G. *skopeō,* to observe]. Scintillation *counter.*

scintillation (sin-ti-lā'shŭn) [L. *scintilla,* a spark]. **1.** A flashing or sparkling; a subjective sensation as of sparks or flashes of light. **2.** In radiation measurement, the light produced by an ionizing event in a phosphor, as in a crystal or liquid scintillator. See also scintillation *counter.*

scintillator (sin'ti-lā-ter, -tōr). A substance that emits visible light when hit by a subatomic particle or x- or gamma ray. See also scintillation *counter.*

scintillometer (sin-ti-lom'ĕ-ter) [L. *scintilla,* spark, + G. *metron,* measure]. Scintillation *counter.*

scintiphotograph (sin-ti-fō'tō-graf). The photographic display obtained by scintiphotography. See also scintiscan.

scintiphotography (sin'ti-fō-tog'ră-fē). The process of obtaining a photographic recording of the distribution of an internally administered radiopharmaceutical with the use of a stationary scintillation detector device, a gamma camera.

scintiscan (sin'ti-skan). Gammagram; scintigram; the record obtained by scintigraphy. See also scan.

scintiscanner (sin'ti-skan'er). The apparatus used to make a scintiscan.

scion (sī'on) [O. Fr. *sion,* shoot, sprig, fr. L. *seco,* to cut]. In experimental embryology, an embryonic tissue or part grafted to another embryo of the same or of another species. See also chimera.

sciosophy (sī-os'ō-fē) [G. *skia,* shadow, + *sophia,* wisdom]. A system of beliefs that are claimed to be facts but are not supported by scientific data.

scirrhencanthis (skir-en-kan'this, sir-en-) [G. *skirrhos,* hard, a hard tumor, + *en,* in, + *kanthos,* canthus]. An indurated tumor of the lacrimal gland.

scirrhosity (skir-os'i-tē, sir-). A scirrhous state or hardness of a tumor.

scirrhous (skir'us, sir'). Hard; relating to a scirrhus.

scirrhus (skir'ŭs, sir') [G. *skirrhos,* hard, a hard tumor]. Obsolete term for any fibrous indurated area, especially an indurated carcinoma.

scission (sizh'ŭn) [L. *scissio,* fr. *scindo,* pp. *scissus,* to cleave]. **1.** A separation, division, or splitting, as in fission. **2.** Cleavage (2).

scissiparity (sis-i-par'i-tē) [L. *scissio,* cleavage, + *pario,* to bring forth]. Schizogenesis.

scissors (siz'erz) [L. *scindo,* pp. *scissus,* to cut]. Shears; an instrument with two blades, moving on a pivot, that cut against each other.
de Wecker's s., a small s. with sharp points for intraocular cutting of the iris and lens capsule.
Smellie's s., lance-pointed shears, with external cutting edges, used for fetal craniotomy.

scissors-shadow. A distorted image seen in mixed astigmatism by retinoscopy.

scissura, pl. **scissurae** (si-sū'ră, -rē) [L.]. Scissure. **1.** Cleft or fissure. **2.** A splitting.
s. pilo'rum, schizotrichia.

scissure (sish'ūr). Scissura.

scler-. See sclero-.

sclera, pl. **scleras, sclerae** (sklēr'ă, -ăz, -ē) [Mod. L. fr. G. *sklēros,* hard] [NA]. Sclerotica; sclerotic coat; tunica albuginea oculi; tunica sclerotica; white of eye; a fibrous tunic forming the outer envelope of the eye, except for its anterior sixth which is occupied by the cornea.
blue s., see van der Hoeve's *syndrome.*

scleradenitis (sklēr'ad-ĕ-nī'tis) [scler- + G. *adēn,* gland, + *-itis,* inflammation]. Inflammatory induration of a gland.

scleral (sklēr'ăl). Sclerotic (2); relating to the sclera.

scleratogenous (sklēr-ă-toj'ĕ-nŭs). Sclerogenous.

sclerectasia (sklēr-ek-tā'zē-ă) [scler- + G. *ektasis,* an extension]. Scleral ectasia; localized bulging of the sclera lined with uveal tissue.
partial s., partial protrusion of a portion of the sclera, typically seen in severe myopia.
total s., uniform stretching of the entire sclera, typically seen in buphthalmos.

sclerectoiridectomy (sklĕ-rek'tō-ir-i-dek'tō-mē). A combined sclerectomy and iridectomy used in glaucoma to form a filtering cicatrix.

sclerectoiridodialysis (sklĕ-rek'tō-ir'i-dō-dī-al'i-sis). A combined operation of sclerectomy and iridodialysis for the relief of glaucoma.

sclerectomy (sklĕ-rek'tō-mē) [scler- + G. *ektomē,* excision]. **1.** Excision of a portion of the sclera. **2.** Removal of the fibrous adhesions formed in chronic otitis media.

scleredema (sklēr-e-dē'mă) [scler- + G. *oidēma,* a swelling (edema)]. Hard nonpitting edema of the skin, giving a waxy appearance and no sharp demarcation.
s. adulto'rum, Buschke's disease (1); a benign spreading induration of the skin and subcutaneous tissue, possibly streptoccocal in origin, that may follow a febrile illness, appearing first on the head and neck and extending over the trunk; a misnomer, because the disease is not restricted to adults.

sclerema (sklĕ-rē'mă) [scler- + edema]. Induration of subcutaneous fat.
s. adipo'sum, s. neonatorum.
s. neonato'rum, s. adiposum; subcutaneous fat necrosis of newborn; Underwood's disease; s. appearing at birth or in early infancy, usually in premature and debilitated infants, as sharply demarcated and yellowish white indurated plaques that usually involve the cheeks, buttocks, shoulders, and calves; subcutaneous fat has a high proportion of saturated fatty acids; microscopically, there is thickening of interlobular fibrous tissue and formation of triglyceride crystals and foreign body giant cells; prognosis is poor for widespread lesions, but localized lesions may resolve slowly over a period of many months.

sclerencephaly, sclerencephalia (sklēr-en-sef'ă-lē, -en-sĕ-fā'lē-ă) [scler- + G. *enkephalos,* brain]. Sclerosis and shrinkage of the brain substance.

scleriasis (sklĕ-rī'ă-sis) [scler- + G. *-iasis,* condition]. A diffuse, symmetrical scleroderma.

scleriritomy (sklēr-i-rit'ō-mē), An incision into the iris and sclera.

scleritis (sklĕ-rī'tis). Leucitis; inflammation of the sclera.
annular s., an often protracted inflammation of the anterior portion of the sclera, forming a ring around the corneoscleral limbus.
anterior s., inflammation of the sclera adjacent to the cornea.
brawny s., gelatinous s.; a gelatinous-appearing swelling surrounding the cornea with a tendency to involve the periphery of the cornea.
deep s., severe inflammation of the sclera, with involvement of the underlying uvea.
gelatinous s., brawny s.
malignant s., progressive inflammation of the anterior sclera and adjacent choroid with associated uveitis.
necrotizing s., fibrinoid degeneration and necrosis of the sclera.
nodular s., firm, immobile, single or multiple areas of localized s.
posterior s., inflammation, often monocular, of the sclera adjacent to the optic nerve, with frequent extension to the retina and choroid.

sclero-, scler- [G. *sklēros,* hard]. Combining forms denoting hardness (induration), sclerosis, relationship to the sclera.

scleroatrophy (sklēr-ō-at'rō-fē). Sclerotylosis.

scleroblastema (sklēr-ō-blas-tē'mă) [sclero- + G. *blastēma,* sprout]. The embryonic tissue entering into the formation of bone.

sclerochoroidal (sklēr-ō-kō-roy'dăl). Relating to both the sclera and the choroid.

sclerochoroiditis (sklēr'ō-kō-roy-dī'tis). Scleroticochoroiditis; inflammation of the sclera and choroid.
s. ante'rior, a secondary inflammation of the sclera by an extension of a process from the uvea.
s. poste'rior, posterior *staphyloma.*

scleroconjunctival (sklēr'ō-kon-jŭngk-tī'văl). Relating to the sclera and the conjunctiva.

sclerocornea (sklēr-ō-kōr'nē-ă). **1.** The cornea and sclera regarded as forming together the hard outer coat of the eye, the tunica fibrosa bulbi. **2.** A congenital anomaly in which the whole or part of the cornea is opaque and resembles the sclera; other ocular abnormalities are frequently present.

sclerodactyly, sclerodactylia (sklēr-ō-dak'ti-lē, -dak-til'ē-ă) [sclero- + G. *daktylos,* finger or toe]. Acrosclerosis.

scleroderma (sklēr-ō-der'mă) [sclero- + G. *derma,* skin]. Dermatosclerosis; sclerosis cutanea or corii; hidebound or skinbound disease; thickening of the skin caused by swelling and thickening of fibrous tissue, with atrophy of pilosebaceous follicles; a manifestation of progressive systemic sclerosis and used synonymously for that disease.

localized s., morphea.

sclerodermatitis (sklĕr′ō-der-mă-tī′tis) [sklero- + G. *derma,* skin + *-itis,* inflammation]. Inflammation and thickening of the skin.

sclerodermatous (sklĕr-ō-der′mă-tŭs). Marked by, or resembling, scleroderma.

sclerogenous, sclerogenic (skle-roj′ĕ-nŭs, sklĕr-ō-jen′ik) [sclero- + G. *-gen,* producing]. Scleratogenous; producing hard or sclerotic tissue; causing sclerosis.

scleroid (sklĕr′oyd) [sclero- + G. *eidos,* resemblance]. Sclerous; sclerosal; indurated or sclerotic, of unusually firm texture, leathery, or scar-like texture.

scleroiritis (sklĕr′ō-ī-rī′tis). Inflammation of both sclera and iris.

sclerokeratitis (sklĕr′ō-ker-ă-tī′tis) [sclero- + G. *keras,* horn]. Inflammation of the sclera and cornea.

sclerokeratoiritis (sklĕr-ō-ker′ă-tō-ī-rī′tis). Inflammation of sclera, cornea, and iris.

scleroma (skle-rō′mă) [G. *sklērōma,* an induration]. A circumscribed indurated focus of granulation tissue in the skin or mucous membrane.

respiratory s., rhinoscleroma in which the lesion involves the mucous membrane of the greater part or all of the upper respiratory tract.

scleromalacia (sklĕr′ō-mă-lā′shē-ă) [sclero- + G. *malakia,* a softening]. Degenerative thinning of the sclera, occurring in persons with rheumatoid arthritis and other collagen disorders.

scleromere (sklĕr′ō-mēr) [sclero- + G. *meros,* part]. Any metamere of the skeleton, such as a vertebral segment.

sclerometer (sklē-rom′ĕ-ter) [sclero- + G. *metron,* measure]. A device for determining the density or hardness of any substance.

scleromyxedema (sklĕr′ō-mik-se-dē′mă). Arndt-Gottron syndrome; lichen myxedematosus with diffuse thickening of the skin underlying the papules.

scleronychia (sklĕr-ō-nik′ē-ă) [sclero- + G. *onyx,* nail, + *-ia,* condition]. Induration and thickening of the nails.

sclero-oophoritis (sklĕr′ō-ō-of′ō-rī′tis) [sclero- + Mod. L. *oophoron,* ovary + G. *-itis,* inflammation]. Inflammatory induration of the ovary.

sclerophthalmia (sklĕr-of-thal′mē-ă) [sclero- + G. *opthalmos,* eye]. A congenital abnormality in which the normally transparent cornea resembles the opaque sclera.

scleroplasty (sklĕr′ō-plas-tē) [sclero- + G. *plastos,* formed]. Plastic surgery of the sclera.

scleroprotein (sklĕr-ō-prō′tēn). Albuminoid (3). See also fibrous *protein.*

sclerosal (sklĕ-rō′săl). Scleroid.

sclerosant (sklĕr′ō-sant). An injectable irritant used to treat varices by producing thrombi in them.

sclerose (sklĕ-rōz′). To harden; to undergo sclerosis.

sclerosis, pl. **scleroses** (sklĕ-rō′sis, -sēz) [G. *sklērōsis,* hardness]. **1.** Induration (2). **2.** In neuropathy, induration of nervous and other structures by a hyperplasia of the interstitial fibrous or glial connective tissue.

Alzheimer's s., hyaline degeneration of the medium and smaller blood vessels of the brain.

amyotrophic lateral s. (ALS), Charcot's disease; a disease of the motor tracts of the lateral columns and anterior horns of the spinal cord, causing progressive muscular atrophy, increased reflexes, fibrillary twitching, and spastic irritability of muscles.

arterial s., arteriosclerosis.

arteriocapillary s., arteriosclerosis, especially of the finer vessels.

arteriolar s., arteriolosclerosis.

bone s., eburnation.

Canavan's s., spongy *degeneration.*

central areolar choroidal s., areolar *choroidopathy.*

combined s., a form of s. of the spinal cord involving both posterior and lateral columns, often associated with severe anemia, particularly pernicious anemia.

s. co′rii, scleroderma.

s. cuta′nea, scleroderma.

diffuse infantile familial s., globoid cell *leukodystrophy.*

disseminated s., multiple s.

endocardial s., endocardial *fibroelastosis* (1).

focal s., multiple s.

glomerular s., glomerulosclerosis.

hippocampal s., a loss of cortical neurons and a reactive astrocytosis in the hippocampal regions of some persons with epilepsy.

idiopathic hypercalcemic s. of infants, see idiopathic *hypercalcemia* of infants.

insular s., multiple s.

laminar cortical s., a degeneration of nerve fibers in the corona radiata in a laminar pattern.

lateral spinal s., a degenerative state of the lateral tracts of the spinal cord causing spastic paraplegia; a clinical variant of amyotrophic lateral s.

lobar s., s. of the brain involving the greater part or all of a lobe; typically caused by perinatal hypoxia.

mantle s., a common cerebral lesion in the palsied states of early life characterized by nodular cortical atrophy.

menstrual s., physiologic s.

Mönckeberg's s., Mönckeberg's *arteriosclerosis.*

multiple s. (MS), disseminated, focal, or insular s.; the occurrence of patches of s. (plaques) in the brain and spinal cord, causing some degree of paralysis, tremor, nystagmus, and disturbances of speech, the various symptoms depending upon the seat of the lesions; it occurs chiefly in early adult life, with characteristic exacerbations and remissions.

nodular s., atherosclerosis.

nuclear s., increased refractivity of the central portion of the lens of the eye. See nuclear *cataract.*

ovulational s., physiologic s.

physiologic s., menstrual or ovulational s.; a slowly progressive s. in the walls of the ovarian arteries which commences after puberty.

posterior s., *tabes* dorsalis.

posterior spinal s., *tabes* dorsalis.

progressive systemic s., a systemic disease characterized by formation of hyalinized and thickened collagenous fibrous tissue, with thickening of the skin and adhesion to underlying tissues (especially of the hands and face), dysphagia due to loss of peristalsis and submucosal fibrosis of the esophagus, dyspnea due to pulmonary fibrosis, myocardial fibrosis, and renal vascular changes resembling those of malignant hypertension; Raynaud's phenomenon, atrophy of the soft tissues, and osteoporosis of the distal phalanges (acrosclerosis), sometimes with gangrene at the ends of the digits, are common findings. Also called scleroderma.

tuberous s., epiloia; Bourneville's disease; multisystem hamartomas producing the typical triad of seizures, mental retardation, and skin nodules of the face, originally considered to be sebaceous adenomas but since shown to be angiofibromas; the cerebral and retinal lesions are glial nodules; other skin lesions are white macules, shagreen patches, and periungual fibromas; autosomal dominant inheritance with variable penetrance and expression.

unicellular s., a growth of fibrous tissue between and isolating the individual cells of a part.

vascular s., arteriosclerosis.

s. of white matter, leukodystrophy.

sclerostenosis (sklĕr-ō-ste-nō′sis) [sclero- + G. *stenōsis,* a narrowing]. Induration and contraction of the tissues.

Sclerostoma (sklĕ-ros'tō-mă) [sclero- + G. *stoma,* mouth]. A former generic name for strongyle (hookworm) nematodes and for trichostrongyle worms of horses; now replaced by other genera but still used as a collective term for this group. Species include *S. duodenale* (*Ancylostoma duodenale*) and *S. syngamus* (*Syngamus trachea*).

sclerostomy (sklĕ-ros'tō-mē) [sclero- + G. *stoma,* mouth]. Surgical perforation of the sclera, as for the relief of glaucoma.

sclerotherapy (sklĕr-ō-thār'ă-pē). Sclerosing therapy; treatment involving the injection of a sclerosing solution into vessels or tissues.

sclerothrix (sklĕr'ō-thriks) [sclero- + G. *thrix,* hair]. Sclerotrichia; induration and brittleness of the hair.

sclerotic (sklĕ-rot'ik). **1.** Relating to or characterized by sclerosis. **2.** Scleral.

sclerotica (sklĕ-rot'i-kă) [Mod. L. *scleroticus,* hard]. Sclera.

scleroticochoroiditis (sklĕ-rot'i-kō-kō-roy-dī'tis). Sclerochoroiditis.

sclerotium, pl. **sclerotia** (sklĕ-rō'shē-ŭm, -shē-ă). **1.** In fungi, a variably sized resting body composed of a hardened mass of hyphae with or without host tissue, usually with a darkened rind, from which fruit bodies, stromata, conidiophores, or mycelia may develop. **2.** The hardened resting condition of the plasmodium of Myxomycetes.

sclerotome (sklĕr'ō-tōm) [sclero- + G. *tomos,* a cutting]. **1.** A knife used in sclerotomy. **2.** The group of mesenchymal cells emerging from the ventromesial part of a mesodermic somite and migrating toward the notochord. Sclerotomal cells from adjacent somites become merged in intersomitically located masses that are the primordia of the centra of the vertebrae.

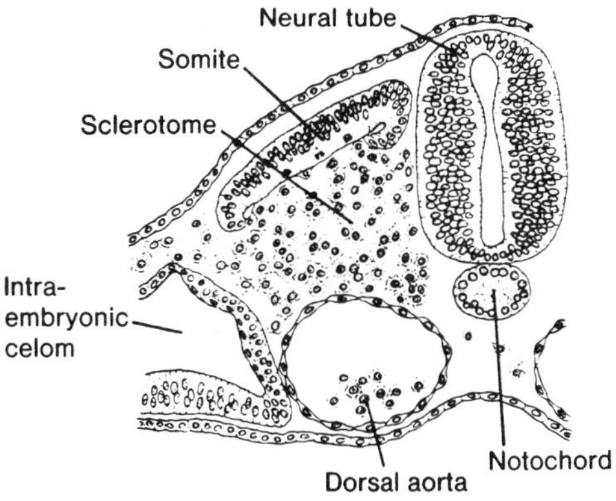

Sclerotome

sclerotomy (sklĕ-rot'ō-mē) [sclero- + G. *tomē,* incision]. An incision through the sclera.
anterior s., incision into the anterior chamber of the eye.
posterior s., incision through the sclera into the vitreous humor.

sclerotrichia (sklĕr-ō-trik'ē-ă). Sclerothrix.

sclerotylosis (sklĕr'ō-tī-lō'sis) [sclero- + G. *tylosis,* a becoming callous]. Scleroatrophy; atrophic fibrosis of the skin, hypoplasia of the nails, and palmoplantar keratoderma; associated with gastrointestinal cancer; autosomal dominant inheritance.

sclerous (sklĕr'ŭs) [G. *sklēros,* hard]. Scleroid.

scoleces (skō'le-sez). Plural of scolex.

scoleciasis (skō-lē-sī'ă-sis) [G. *skōlēx,* worm, + *-iasis,* condition]. Infection of the intestine by larvae of lepidopterans (moths and butterflies).

scoleciform (skō-lē'si-fōrm). Scolecoid.

scolecoid (skō'lē-koyd) [G. *skōlēkoeidēs,* fr. *skōlēx,* worm, + *eidos,* appearance]. Scoleciform. **1.** Resembling a tapeworm scolex. **2.** Wormlike. See also lumbricoid (1), vermiform.

scolecology (skō-lē-kol'ō-jē) [G. *skōlēx,* worm, + *logos,* study]. Helminthology.

scolex, pl. **scoleces** or **scolices** (skō'leks, skō'le-sēz, skō'li-sēz) [G. *skōlēx,* a worm]. The head or anterior end of a tapeworm attached by suckers, and frequently by rostellar hooks, to the wall of the intestine; it is formed within the hydatid cyst in *Echinococcus,* within a cysticercus in *Taenia,* a cysticercoid in *Hymenolepis,* or by a plerocercoid, as in *Diphyllobothrium latum.* The form of the s. varies greatly, the most familiar being rounded or club-shaped with four circular muscular suckers and an armed or unarmed rostellum, or a spatulate flattened s. with a pair of slitlike suckers (bothria) and no rostellum, as in *Diphyllobothrium* and its allies. Other forms have complex leaflike, cup-shaped, or fimbriated shapes, or retractile, multiply spined proboscides. These varied forms characterize the orders of cestodes, which are particularly well developed as parasites of sharks and skates or rays.

scoliokyphosis (skō'lē-ō-kī-fō'sis) [G. *scolios,* curved, + *kyphōsis,* kyphosis]. Lateral and posterior curvature of the spine.

scoliometer (skō-lē-om'ĕ-ter) [G. *skolios,* curved, + *metron,* measure]. An instrument for measuring curves, especially those in lateral curvature of the spine.

scoliosis (skō-lē-ō'sis) [G. *skoliōsis,* a crookedness]. Rachioscoliosis; lateral curvature of the spine; depending on the etiology, there may be one curve, or primary and secondary compensatory curves; s. may be "fixed" as a result of muscle and/or bone deformity or "mobile" as a result of unequal muscle contraction.

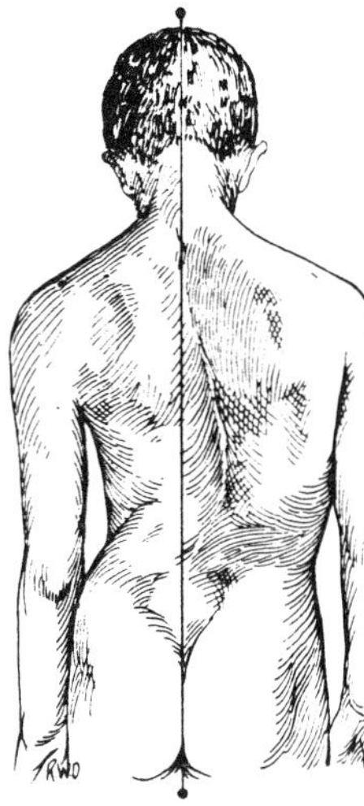
Scoliosis

coxitic s., s. in the lumbar spine resulting from tilting of the pelvis in a case of hip disease.
empyemic s., s. due to retraction of one side of the chest following an empyema.
habit s., s. supposedly due to habitual standing or sitting in an improper position.
myopathic s., lateral curvature due to weakness of the spinal muscles, as in poliomyelitis.
ocular s., ophthalmic s., s. supposed to be due to head tilting, caused by ophthalmological dysfunction.
osteopathic s., lateral curvature of the spine due to vertebral disease.

paralytic s., lateral curvature of the spine due to paralysis of spinal muscles.
rachitic s., s. occurring as a result of rickets.
sciatic s., s. caused by asymmetric spasm of spinal muscles usually associated with sciatica, usually presenting as a list toward one side.
static s., lateral curvature of the spine due to inequality in length of the legs.

scoliotic (skō'lē-ot'ik). Relating to or suffering from scoliosis.

scoliotone (skō'lē-ō-tōn) [G. *skolios,* crooked, + *tonos,* tension]. An apparatus for stretching the spine and reducing the curve in scoliosis.

Scolopendra (skō-lō-pen'dră) [Mod. L., fr. G. *skōlopendra,* multipede]. A genus of centipedes characterized by 21 to 23 pairs of legs. Common U.S. species are *S. heros* (the western house centipede) and *S. morsitans.*

scoop (skūp) [A.S. *skopa*] A narrow, spoonlike instrument for extracting the contents of cavities or cysts.

-scope [G. *skopeō,* to view]. Suffix usually denoting an instrument for viewing but extended to include other methods of examination.

scopine (skō'pēn). Scopolamine less the tropic acid side chain, *i.e.,* 6,7-epoxytropine, or 6,7-epoxy-3-hydroxytropane.

scopolamine (skō-pol'ă-mēn, -min). Hyoscine; scopine tropate; an alkaloid found in the leaves and seeds of *Hyoscyamus niger, Duboisia myoproides, Scopolia japonica, Scopolia carniolica, Atropa belladonna,* and other solanaceous plants; the 6,7-epoxide of atropine, *i.e.,* 6,7-epoxytropine tropate. For structure, see tropine.
s. hydrobromide, hyoscine hydrobromide; anticholinergic action is similar to that of atropine.
s. methylbromide, a quaternary ammonium derivative of s.; used when spasmolytic or antisecretory effects are desired.

scopolia (skō-pō'lē-ă) [G.A. *Scopoli,* Italian naturalist, 1723–1788]. The dried rhizome and roots of *Scopolia carniolica* (family Solanaceae), a herb of Austria and neighboring countries of Europe; it resembles belladonna in pharmacologic action.
s. japon'ica, Japanese belladonna, the leaves, root, and seeds of which contain scopolamine.

scopoline (skō'pō-lēn). 3β,7β-Epoxy-1β*H*,5β*H*-tropan-6α-ol; a decomposition product of scopolamine, and an isomer of scopine, in that the expoxy and hydroxyl groups are in different locations.

scopometer (skō-pom'ĕ-ter) [G. *skopeō,* to view, + *metron,* measure]. A device for determining the density of a precipitate by the degree of translucency of a fluid containing it. See also nephelometer.

scopomorphinism (skō-pō-mōr'fi-nizm). Associated chronic addiction to scopolamine and morphine.

scopophilia (skō-pō-fil'ē-ă) [G. *skopeō,* to view, + *philos,* fond]. Voyeurism.

scopophobia (skō-pō-fō'bē-ă) [G. *skopeō,* to view, + *phobos,* fear]. Morbid dread of being stared at.

Scopulariopsis (skō'pyū-lar-ē-op'sis) [Mod. L. *scopula,* a small broom, + G. *opsis,* appearance]. A genus of filamentous fungi of doubtful pathogenicity for man, although several species have been implicated in onychomycosis, ulcerating granuloma, and other "mycotic" entities. *Penicillium*-like, it is common in nature and generally a contaminant in laboratory cultures of human tissues.

-scopy [G. *skopeō,* to view]. Suffix denoting an action or activity involving the use of an instrument for viewing.

scorbutic (skōr-byū'tik). Relating to, suffering from, or resembling scurvy (scorbutus).

scorbutigenic (skōr-byū-ti-jen'ik). Scurvy-producing.

scorbutus (skōr-byū'tŭs) [Mediev. L. form of Teutonic *schorbuyck,* scurvy]. Scurvy.

scordinema (skōr'di-nē'mă) [G. *skordinēma,* yawning]. Heaviness of the head with yawning and stretching, occurring as a prodrome of an infectious disease.

score (skōr) [M. E. *scor,* notch, tally]. An evaluation, usually expressed numerically, of status, achievement, or condition in a given set of circumstances.
Apgar s., evaluation of a newborn infant's physical status by assigning numerical values (0 to 2) to each of 5 criteria: 1) heart rate, 2) respiratory effort, 3) muscle tone, 4) response stimulation, and 5) skin color; a score of 10 indicates the best possible condition.
Dubowitz s., a method of clinical assessment of gestational age in the newborn that includes neurological criteria for the infant's maturity and other physical criteria to determine the gestational age of the infant; useful from birth to 5 days of life.
Gleason's s., see Gleason's tumor *grade.*
raw s., the actual s., measurement, or value obtained before any statistics are applied to it. *Cf.* standard s.
recovery s., a number expressing the condition of an infant at various stipulated intervals greater than 1 minute after birth and based on the same features assessed by the Apgar s. at 60 seconds after birth.
standard s., a derived s. representing the deviation of a raw s. from its mean in standard deviation units.

scorpion (skōr'pē-on) [G. *skorpios*]. A member of the order Scorpionida; includes the devil s., *Vejovis,* and the hairy s., *Hadrurus.*

Scorpionida (skōr-pē-on'i-dă) [Mod. L.]. The scorpions; an order of venomous, predaceous, arachnid arthropods characterized by a distinctly segmented bony abdomen terminating in a sharply recurved stinging spine equipped with a poison gland; causes a severely painful but rarely fatal sting. North American genera include *Centruroides, Hadrurus,* and *Vejovis.*

scoto- [G. *skotos,* darkness]. Combining form denoting darkness.

scotochromogens (skō'tō-krō'mō-jenz) [scoto- + G. *chrōma,* color, + *-gen,* producing]. Group II *mycobacteria.*

scotograph (skō'tō-graf) [scoto- + G. *graphō,* to write]. **1.** An appliance for aiding one to write in straight lines in the dark or for aiding the blind to write. **2.** An impression made on a photographic film by a radioactive substance without the intervention of any opaque object other than the screen of the film.

scotoma, pl. **scotomata** (skō-tō'mă, skō-tō'mă-tă) [G. *skotōma,* vertigo, fr. *skotos,* darkness]. **1.** An isolated area of varying size and shape, within the visual field, in which vision is absent or depressed. **2.** A blind spot in psychological awareness.
absolute s., a s. in which there is no perception of light.
annular s., a circular s. surrounding the center of the field of vision.
arcuate s., a s. extending from the blind spot and arching into the nasal field following the lines of retinal nerve fibers.
Bjerrum's s., sickle s.; Bjerrum's sign; a comet-shaped s., occurring in glaucoma, attached at the temporal end to the blind spot or separated from it by a narrow gap; the defect widens as it extends above and nasally curves around the fixation spot, and then extends downward to end exactly at the nasal horizontal meridian.
cecocentral s., a s. involving the optic disk area (blind spot) and the papillomacular fibers; there are three forms: 1) the cecocentral defect which extends from the blind spot toward or into the fixation area; 2) angioscotoma; 3) glaucomatous nerve-fiber bundle s., due to involvement of nerve-fiber bundles at the edge of the optic disk. See also Bjerrum's s.; Roenne's nasal *step.*
central s., a s. involving the fixation point.
color s., an area of depressed color vision in the visual field.
flittering s., scintillating s.
glaucomatous nerve-fiber bundle s., see cecocentral s.
hemianopic s., a s. involving half of the central field.

insular s., a small area of blindness surrounded by an area of normal vision.
mental s., blind spot (2); absence of insight into, or inability to comprehend, items relative to a subject whose content is highly emotional to the individual.
negative s., a s. that is not ordinarily perceived, but is detected only on examination of the visual field.
paracentral s., a s. adjacent to the fixation point.
pericentral s., a s. that surrounds the fixation point more or less symmetrically.
peripheral s., a s. outside of the central 30 degrees of the visual field.
physiologic s., blind spot (1); the negative s. in the visual field, corresponding to the optic disk.
positive s., a s. that is perceived as a black spot within the field of vision.
quadrantic s., a s. involving a quarter segment of the central visual field.
relative s., a s. in which there is visual depression but not complete loss of light perception.
ring s., an annular area of blindness in the visual field surrounding the fixation point in pigmentary degeneration of the retina and in glaucoma.
scintillating s., flittering s.; a localized area of blindness that may follow the appearance of brilliantly colored shimmering lights (teichopsia); usually a prodromal symptom of migraine. See also fortification *spectrum.*
Seidel's s., a form of Bjerrum's s. See also Seidel's *sign.*
sickle s., Bjerrum's s.
zonular s., a curved s. not corresponding to the path of retinal nerve fibers.

scotomata (skō-tō'mă-tă). Plural of scotoma.

scotomatous (skō-tō'mă-tŭs). Relating to scotoma.

scotometer (skō-tom'ĕ-ter). An instrument for determining the size, shape, and intensity of a scotoma.

scotometry (skō-tom'ĕ-trē) [scoto- + G. *metron,* measure]. The plotting and measuring of a scotoma.

scotophilia (skō-tō-fil'ē-ă) [scoto- + G. *philos,* fond]. Nyctophilia.

scotophobia (skō-tō-fō'bē-ă) [scoto- + G. *phobos,* fear]. Nyctophobia.

scotopia (skō-tō'pē-ă) [scoto- + G. *opsis,* vision]. Scotopic *vision.*

scotopic (skō-tō'pik, -top'ik). Referring to low illumination to which the eye is dark-adapted. See scotopic *vision.*

scotopsin (skō-top'sin). The protein moiety of the pigment in the rods of the retina.

scotoscopy (skō-tos'kŏ-pē) [scoto- + G. *skopeō,* to view]. Retinoscopy.

Scott, Charles I., Jr., U.S. pediatrician, *1934. See Aarskog-S. *syndrome.*

Scott, H. William, U.S. surgeon, *1916. See S. *operation.*

Scott-Wilson, H., British scientist. See S.-W. *reagent.*

scrape (skrāp). A specimen scraped from a lesion or specific site, for cytological examination. See also smear and subentries.

scrapie (skrap'ē, skrā'pē). A communicable degenerative disorder of the central nervous system of sheep and goats caused by a virus-like agent (classified as a prion) and characterized by a very long incubation period followed by pruritus, abnormalities of gait, and frequently death; it resembles Kuru in man.

scratches (skratch'ez). Grease *heel* (2).

screen (skrēn) [Fr. *écran*]. **1.** A sheet of any substance used to shield an object from any influence, such as heat, light, x-rays, etc. **2.** A sheet upon which an image is projected. **3.** Formerly, to make a fluoroscopic examination. **4.** In psychoanalysis, concealment, as one image or memory concealing another. See also screen *memory.* **5.** To examine, evaluate; to process a group to select or separate certain individuals from it. **6.** A thin layer of crystals which converts x-rays to light photons to expose film; used in a cassette to produce radiographic images on film.
Bjerrum s., tangent s.
fluorescent s., a s. coated with fluorescent crystals such as the calcium tungstate used in the fluoroscope.
Hess s., a s. used in the measurement of ocular deviation.
tangent s., Bjerrum s.; a flat, usually black surface used to measure the central 30 degrees of the field of vision.
vestibular s., a s. made of acrylic resin that covers the labial or buccal surfaces of one or both dental arches; used to treat oral habits and to stimulate tooth movement by using perioral muscle force.

screening (skrēn'ing). **1.** To screen (5). **2.** Examination of a group of usually asymptomatic individuals to detect those with a high probability of having a given disease, typically by means of an inexpensive diagnostic test. **3.** In psychiatry, initial patient evaluation that includes medical and psychiatric history, mental status evaluation, and diagnostic formulation to determine the patient's suitability or a particular treatment modality.
carrier s., indiscriminate examination of members of a population to detect heterozygotes for serious disorders and discourage marriage with other carriers, and by antenatal diagnosis where a married couple are both carriers; often sacrifices precision to simplicity and is most effectively applied to populations which are known to be at high risk.
cytologic s., a s. for the detection of early disease, usually cancer, through microscopic examination of a cellular specimen by inspecting each cell and structure present, usually at ×100 magnification with a mechanical stage, so that all areas are screened; the findings are evaluated and significant abnormalities are flagged (*e.g.,* by dotting the cover slip) for further evaluation by a cytopathologist. This s. is usually performed by a cytotechnologist, but at times is done by automated machine prescreening.
familial s., s. directed at close relatives of patients who have diseases that may lie latent, as in age-dependent dominant traits, or that may involve risk to progeny, as X-linked traits.
multiphasic s., the routine use of multiple tests, usually biochemical, for the purpose of detecting disease at a preventable or curable stage.
neonatal s., testing of newborns for the detection of preventable or curable disease.
prenatal s., s. for the detection of fetal disease, usually by testing amniotic fluid obtained by amniocentesis.

screw (skrū). A helically grooved cylinder for fastening two objects together or for adjusting the position of an object resting on one end of the s.
afterloading s., a device for setting the length at which a contracting muscle encounters an afterload.

screw-worm (skrū'werm). The larva of the botfly, *Cochliomyia hominivorax,* and other similar forms that causes human and animal myiasis.
primary s., an obligatory s. that can penetrate normal tissues and feed as a primary invader. The important myiasis flies of man that serve as p. s.'s are *Cochliomyia hominivorax, Chrysomya bezziana,* and *Wohlfahrtia magnifica.*
secondary s., an accidental or facultative s. that enters a prior wound or suppurated condition and feeds on infected rather than intact tissues. Many blowflies are included, such as *Calliphora vicina, Phaenicia sericata, Phormia regina, Cochliomyia macellaria, Chrysomya* species, and other fleshflies.

scribe (skrīb) [L. *scribo,* pp. *scripto,* to write]. **1.** To write, trace, or mark by making a line with a marker or pointed instrument, as in surveying a dental cast for a removable prosthesis. **2.** To form, by instrumentation, negative areas within a master cast to provide a positive beading in the framework of a removable partial denture, or the posterior palatal seal area for a complete denture.

Scribner, Belding H., U.S. nephrologist, *1921. See S. *shunt.*

scrobiculate (skrō-bik'yū-lāt) [L. *scrobiculus;* dim. of *scrobis,* a trench]. Pitted; marked with minute depressions.

scrobiculus cordis (skrō-bik'yū-lŭs kōr'dis) [L. pit or fossa of the heart]. Epigastric *fossa.*

scrofula (skrof'yū-lă) [L. *scrofulae* (pl. only), a glandular swelling, scrofula, fr. *scrofa,* a breeding sow]. Obsolete term for cervical tuberculous lymphadenitis.

scrofuloderma (skrof'yū-lō-der'mă) [scrofula + G. *derma,* skin]. Cutaneous *tuberculosis.*
s. gummo'sa, a deep cutaneous tuberculous lesion.
papular s., papular *tuberculid.*
tuberculous s., scrofulotuberculosis; ulcerative s.; a granulating ulcer surrounding the orifice of a sinus extending from a tuberculous gland or focus of bone tuberculosis.
ulcerative s., tuberculous s.
verrucous s., *tuberculosis* cutis verrucosa.

scrofulotuberculosis (skrof'yū-lō-tū-ber-kyū-lō'sis). Tuberculous *scrofuloderma.*

scrofulous (skrof'yū-lŭs). Relating to or suffering from scrofula.

scrotal (skrō'tăl). Oscheal; relating to the scrotum.

scrotectomy (skrō-tek'tō-mē) [scrotum, + G. *ektomē,* excision]. Removal of all or part of scrotum.

scrotiform (skrō'ti-fōrm). Having the shape or form of a scrotum.

scrotitis (skrō-tī'tis). Inflammation of the scrotum.

scrotocele (skrō'tō-sēl) [scrotum + G. *kēlē,* hernia]. Obsolete term for scrotal *hernia.*

scrotoplasty (skrō'tō-plas-tē) [scrotum + G. *plastos,* formed]. Oscheoplasty; reparative or plastic surgery of the scrotum.

scrotum, pl. **scrota, scrotums** (skrō'tŭm, -tă, -tŭmz) [L.] [NA]. Bursula testium; marsupium (1); a musculocutaneous sac containing the testes; it is formed of skin, containing a network of nonstriated muscular fibers (the dartos), cremasteric fascia, cremaster muscle, and the serous coverings of the testes and epididymides.

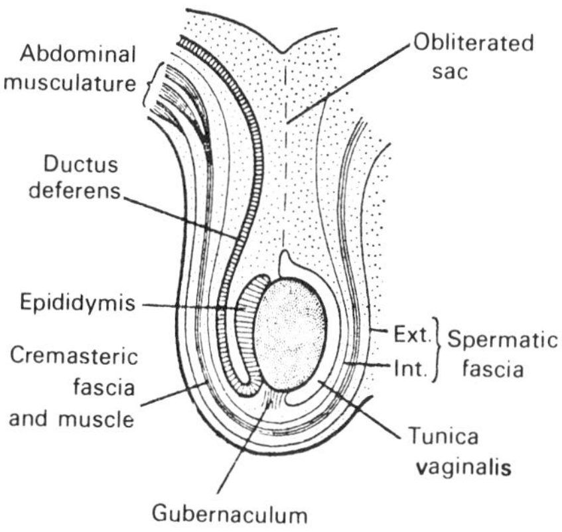

Scrotum
Diagrammatic drawing of the testis, epididymis, ductus deferens, and the various layers of the abdominal wall that surround the testis in the scrotum.

lymph s., *elephantiasis* scroti.
watering-can s., urinary sinuses in scrotum and perineum, resulting from disease of the perineal urethra.

scruple (skrū'pl) [L. *scrupulus,* a small sharp stone, a weight, the 24th part of an ounce, a scruple, dim. of *scrupus,* a sharp stone]. An apothecaries' weight of 20 grains or one-third of a dram.

SCUBA Acronym for *s*elf-*c*ontained *u*nderwater *b*reathing *a*pparatus.

Scultetus (Scultet), originally Schultes, Johann, German surgeon, 1595–1645. See S.'s *bandage, position.*

scum (skŭm) [M.E.]. A film of insoluble material that rises to the surface of a liquid, as in epistasis.

scurf (skerf) [A.S.]. Dandruff.

scurvy (sker'vē) [fr. A. S. scurf]. Scorbutus; sea s.; a disease marked by inanition, debility, anemia, edema of the dependent parts, a spongy condition, sometimes with ulceration, of the gums, and hemorrhages into the skin and from the mucous membranes; due to a monotonous diet especially lacking in sources of vitamin C.
Alpine s., pellagra.
infantile s., Barlow's or Cheadle's disease; scurvy rickets; osteopathia hemorrhagia infantum; a cachectic condition in infants, resulting from malnutrition and marked by pallor, fetid breath, coated tongue, diarrhea, and subperiosteal hemorrhages; probably a combination of s. and rickets due to combined deficiency of vitamins C and D.
land s., idiopathic thrombocytopenic *purpura.*
sea s., s.

scutate (skū'tāt). Scutiform.

scute (skūt) [L. *scutum,* shield]. Scutum (1); a thin lamina or plate.
tympanic s., the thin bony plate separating the epitympanic recess from the mastoid cells.

scutiform (skū'ti-fōrm) [L. *scutum,* shield, + *forma,* form]. Scutate; shield-shaped.

Scutigera (skū-tij'er-ă) [L. *scutum,* an oblong shield]. A genus of centipedes commonly found in the eastern U.S.; the eastern house centipede is a member of the species *S. cleopatra.*

scutular (skū'tyū-lăr). Relating to a scutulum.

scutulum, pl. **scutula** (skū'tyū-lŭm, skū'chū-lŭm, -lă) [L. dim. of *scutum,* shield]. A yellow saucer-shaped crust, the characteristic lesion of favus, consisting of a mass of hyphae and spores.

scutum, pl. **scuta** (skū'tŭm, -tă) [L. shield]. **1.** Scute. **2.** In ixodid (hard) ticks, a plate that largely or entirely covers the dorsum of the male and forms an anterior shield behind the capitulum of the female or immature ticks.

scybala (sib'ă-lă). Plural of scybalum.

scybalous (sib'ă-lŭs). Relating to scybala.

scybalum, pl. **scybala** (sib'ă-lŭm, -lă) [G. *skybalon,* excrement]. A hard round mass of inspissated feces.

scyphiform (sī'fi-fōrm) [G. *skyphos,* goblet, cup, + L. *forma,* form]. Scyphoid.

scyphoid (sī'foyd) [G. *skyphos,* cup, + *eidos,* resemblance]. Scyphiform; cup-shaped.

SD Abbreviation for streptodornase; standard *deviation.*

SDA Abbreviation for specific dynamic *action.*

Se Symbol for selenium.

seal (sēl). **1.** An airtight closure. **2.** To effect an airtight closure.
border s., peripheral s.; the contact of the denture border with the underlying or adjacent tissues to prevent the passage of air or other substances.
palatal s., posterior palatal s.
peripheral s., border s.
posterior palatal s., postdam; palatal s.; postpalatal s.; the s. at the posterior border of a denture. See also posterior palatal s. *area.*
postpalatal s., posterior palatal s.
velopharyngeal s., closure between the oral and nasopharyngeal cavities.

sealant (sē'lănt). A material used to effect an airtight closure.
fissure s., a dental material usually made from interaction between bisphenol A and glycidyl methacrylate; such s.'s are used to seal nonfused, noncarious pits and fissures on surfaces of teeth.

searcher (ser'cher). A form of sound used to determine the presence of a calculus in the bladder.

Seashore, Carl E., U.S. psychologist, 1866–1949. See S. *test.*

seasickness (sē'sik-nes). Naupathia; mal de mer; vomitus marinus; a form of motion sickness caused by the motion of a floating platform, such as a ship, boat, or raft.

season (sē'zŏn). A particular phase of some slow cyclic phenomenon, especially the annual weather cycle.
mating s., the period during which an animal will mate, *i.e.,* the period during which estrus occurs.

seat (sēt). A surface against which an object may rest to gain support.
basal s., denture *foundation.*
rest s., rest *area.*

seatworm (sēt'werm). Pinworm.

seb-, sebi-. See sebo-.

sebaceous (sē-bā'shŭs) [L. *sebaceus*]. Relating to sebum; oily; fatty.

sebaceus (sē-bā'shŭs) [L.]. Sebaceous.

sebiagogic (seb'ē-ă-goj'ik) [sebi- + G. *agōgos,* leading]. Sebiferous.

sebiferous (sē-bif'er-ŭs) [sebi- + L. *fero,* to bear]. Sebiagogic; sebiparous; producing sebaceous matter.

Sebileau, Pierre, French anatomist, 1860–1953. See S.'s *hollow, muscle.*

sebiparous (sē-bip'ă-rŭs) [sebi- + L. *pario,* to produce]. Sebiferous.

sebo-, seb-, sebi- [L. *sebum,* suet, tallow]. Combining forms denoting sebum, sebaceous.

sebolith (seb'ō-lith) [sebo- + G. *lithos,* stone]. A concretion in a sebaceous follicle.

seborrhea (seb-ō-rē'ă) [sebo- + G. *rhoia,* a flow]. Overactivity of the sebaceous glands, resulting in an excessive amount of sebum.
s. adipo'sa, s. oleosa.
s. cap'itis, branny tetter (2); s. of the scalp.
s. ce'rea, waxy secretion of sebum.
concrete s., thick, oily crusts on scalp and eyebrows.
s. cor'poris, seborrheic *dermatitis.*
eczematoid s., seborrheic eczema in which lesions have lost definition and have become confluent, usually as a result of trauma and overzealous use of soap and medication.
s. fa'ciei, s. of face, s. oleosa affecting especially the nose and forehead.
s. furfura'cea, s. sicca (1).
s. ni'gra, a form of s. characterized by a pigmented secretion.
s. oleo'sa, a greasy condition of the skin due to excessive secretion of the sebaceous glands. Also called s. adiposa; cutis unctuosa; acne sebacea; hyperhidrosis oleosa.
s. sic'ca, **(1)** s. furfuracea; an accumulation on the skin, especially the scalp, of dry scales; **(2)** dandruff.
s. squamo'sa neonato'rum, seborrheic dermatitis in infants.

seborrheic (seb-ō-rē'ik). Relating to seborrhea.

sebum (sē'bŭm) [L. tallow]. The secretion of the sebaceous glands.
s. cuta'neum, cutaneous fatty secretion.
s. palpebra'le, lema.
s. preputia'le, *smegma* preputii.

Secernentasida (se-ser-nen-tas'i-dă) [L. *secerno,* to separate, hide]. Secernentia; Phasmidia; a class of nematodes possessing lateral canals opening into the excretory system and phasmids; it includes most of the familiar nematode parasites of man and domestic animals, including the soil-borne nematodes, strongyles, and filiariae. See also Adenophorasida.

Secernentia (se-ser-nen'shē-ă). Secernentasida.

Seckel, Helmut P.G., German physician, *1900. See S. *dwarfism, syndrome.*

seclusion of pupil (se-klū'zhŭn). *Exclusion* of pupil.

secobarbital (sē-kō-bar'bi-tahl). 5-Allyl-5-(1-methylbutyl)barbituric acid; a sedative and short-acting hypnotic.

secondaries (sek'ŏn-dăr-ēz). The lesions of secondary syphilis.

secreta (se-krē'tă) [L. neuter pl. of *secretus,* pp. of *se-cerno,* to separate]. Secretions.

secretagogue (se-krē'tă-gog) [secreta + G. *agōgos,* drawing forth]. Secretogogue; an agent that promotes secretion.

Secrétan, H., Swiss surgeon, 1856–1916. See S.'s *syndrome.*

secrete (se-krēt') [L. *se-cerno,* pp. *-cretus,* to separate]. To elaborate or produce some physiologically useful substance (*e.g.,* enzyme, hormone, metabolite) by a cell and to deliver it into blood, body cavity, or sap, either by direct diffusion or by means of a duct.

secretin (se-krē'tin). Oxykrinin; a hormone, formed by the epithelial cells of the duodenum under the stimulus of acid contents from the stomach, that incites secretion of pancreatic juice; used as a diagnostic aid in the diagnosis of pancreatic exocrine disease and as an adjunct in obtaining desquamated pancreatic cells for cytological examination.

secretion (se-krē'shŭn) [L. *se-cerno,* pp. *-cretus,* to separate]. **1.** Production by a cell or aggregation of cells (a gland) of a physiologically useful substance and its introduction into the body by direct diffusion or by a duct. **2.** The product, solid, liquid, or gaseous, of cellular or glandular activity that is stored up in or utilized by the organism in which it is produced. *Cf.* excretion.
cytocrine s., the transfer of secretory material from one cell to another, such as the transfer of melanin granules from melanocytes to epidermal cells.
neurohumoral s., transmission of a nerve impulse across a synapse or to an end-organ by s. of a minute amount of a chemical transmitter such as acetylcholine.

secretogogue (se-krē'tō-gog). Secretagogue.

secretomotor, secretomotory (se-krē'tō-mō'ter, -mō'ter-ē). Stimulating secretion.

secretor (se-krē'ter, tōr). An individual whose saliva and other body fluids contain a water-soluble form of the antigens of the ABO blood group found in his erythrocytes.

secretory (se-krēt'ĕ-rē, sē'krĕ-tōr-ē). Relating to secretion or the secretions.

sectile (sek'til, tīl) [L. *sectilis,* fr. *seco,* to cut]. **1.** Capable of being cut or divided. **2.** Having the appearance of being divided.

sectio, pl. **sectiones** (sek'shēō, sek-shē-ō'nēz) [L.] [NA]. Section; in anatomy, a subdivision or segment.

section (sek'shŭn) [L. *sectio,* a cutting, fr. *seco,* to cut]. **1.** The act of cutting. **2.** A cut or division. **3.** A segment or part of any organ or structure delimited from the remainder. **4.** A cut surface. **5.** A thin slice of tissue, cells, microorganisms, or any material for examination under the microscope.
abdominal s., celiotomy.
attached cranial s., attached *craniotomy.*
cesarean s., cesarean operation; incision through the abdominal wall and the uterus (abdominal hysterotomy) for extraction of the fetus.
classical cesarean s., a cesarean s. in which the uterus is entered through a vertical fundal incision.
coronal s., a vertical s. of the skull at right angles to the sagittal s.
detached cranial s., detached *craniotomy.*
frozen s., a thin slice of tissue cut from a frozen specimen, often used for rapid microscopic diagnosis.
Latzko's cesarean s., a cesarean s. in which the uterus is entered

by paravesical blunt dissection without entering the peritoneal cavity.
low cervical cesarean s., a cesarean s. in which the uterus is entered in its lower segment by a transperitoneal approach with extraperitoneal closure.
microscopic s., s. (5).
perineal s., any s. through the perineum, either lateral or median lithotomy or external urethrotomy.
pituitary stalk s., transection of the neurovascular connection between the hypothalamus and the pituitary gland.
Saemisch's s., procedure of transfixing the cornea beneath an ulcer and then cutting from within outward through the base.
sagittal s., a vertical s. of the skull or part of the body in an anteroposterior direction, dividing it into two lateral halves.
serial s., one of a number of consecutive microscopic s.'s.
thin s., ultrathin s., a s. of tissue for electron microscopic examination; the specimen is fixed, typically in gluteraldehyde and/or in osmium tetroxide, embedded in a plastic resin, and sectioned at less than 0.1μm in thickness with a glass or diamond knife in an ultramicrotome.

sectiones (sek-shē-ō'nēz). Plural of sectio.

sectoranopia (sek'tŏr-an-ō'pē-ă) [sector + G. *an-* priv. + *opsis,* vision]. Loss of vision in a sector of the visual field.

sectorial (sek-tōr'ē-ăl) [L. *sector,* cutter]. **1.** Relating to a sector. **2.** Cutting or adapted for cutting; denoting the carnassial or shearing molar and premolar teeth of carnivores.

secundigravida (sek'ŭn-di-grav'i-dă). See gravida.

secundina, pl. **secundinae** (sek-ŭn-dī'nă, -nē) [L. *secundinae,* the afterbirth, fr. *secundus,* second]. Afterbirth.

secundines (sek'ŭn-dēnz) [L. *secundinae,* the afterbirth]. Afterbirth.

secundipara (sek'ŭn-dip'ă-ră). See para.

sedate (sĕ-dāt') [L. *sedatus;* see sedation]. To bring under the influence of a sedative.

sedation (sĕ-dā'shŭn) [L. *sedatio,* to calm, allay]. **1.** The act of calming, especially by the administration of a sedative. **2.** The state of being calm.

sedative (sed'ă-tiv) [L. *sedatious;* see sedation]. **1.** Calming; quieting. **2.** A drug that quiets nervous excitement; designated according to the organ or system upon which specific action is exerted; *e.g.,* cardiac, cerebral, nervous, respiratory, spinal.

sedigitate (se-dij'i-tāt) [L. *sex,* six, + *digitus,* digit]. Sexdigitate.

sediment (sed'i-ment) [L. *sedimentum,* a settling, fr. *sideo,* to sit, settle down]. **1.** Sedimentum; insoluble material that tends to sink to the bottom of a liquid, as in hypostasis. **2.** Sedimentate; to cause or effect the formation of a sediment or deposit, as in the case of centrifugation or ultracentrifugation.

sedimentate (sed'i-men-tāt). Sediment (2).

sedimentation (sed'i-men-tā'shŭn). Formation of a sediment.
s. rate, sinking velocity of the blood cells, *i.e.,* the degree of rapidity with which the red cells sink in a mass of drawn blood.

sedimentator (sed'i-men-tā'ter, tōr). A centrifuge.

sedimentometer (sed'ĭ-men-tom'ĕ-ter) [sediment + G. *metron,* measure]. A photographic apparatus for the automatic recording of the blood sedimentation rate.

sedimentum (sed-i-men'tŭm). [L.]. Sediment (1).
s. laterit'ium, brickdust *deposit.*

sedoheptulose (sē-dō-hep'tyū-lōs). D-*altro*-2-Heptulose; a 2-ketoheptulose formed metabolically as the 7-phosphate by condensation of xylulose 5-phosphate and ribose 5-phosphate, splitting out glyceraldehyde 3-phosphate.

seed (sēd) [A.S. *soed*]. **1.** Semen (2); the reproductive body of a flowering plant; the mature ovule. **2.** In bacteriology, to inoculate a culture medium with microorganisms.

Seeligmüller, Otto L.G.A., German neurologist, 1837–1912. See S.'s *sign.*

Seessel, Albert, U.S. embryologist, 1850–1910. See S.'s *pocket, pouch.*

seg'ment [L. *segmentum,* fr. *seco,* to cut]. **1.** Segmentum. See also metamere. **2.** To divide and redivide into minute equal parts.
anterior s., *segmentum* anterius.
anterior basal s., *segmentum* basale anterius.
anterior inferior s., *segmentum* anterius inferius.
anterior ocular s., that portion of the eye comprising the cornea, iris, lens, and their associated chambers and adnexa.
anterior superior s., *segmentum* anterius superius.
apical s., *segmentum* apicale.
apicoposterior s., *segmentum* apicoposterius.
arterial s.'s of kidney, *segmenta* renalia.
bronchopulmonary s., *segmentum* bronchopulmonalis.
cardiac s., *segmentum* cardiacum.
hepatic s.'s, segmenta hepatis; segments of liver; territories of the liver with independent portobilioarterial distribution or independent venous drainage. The naming of segments in the NA is based upon the portobilioarterial distribution. See *segmentum* anterius (1), *segmentum* laterale (1), *segmentum* mediale (1), *segmentum* posterius (1).
hepatic venous s.'s, venous s.'s of liver.
inferior s., *segmentum* inferius.
inferior lingular s., *segmentum* lingulare inferius.
interannular s., internodal s.
intermaxillary s., the primordial mass of tissue formed by the merging of the medial nasal elevations of the embryo; it contributes to the intermaxillary portion of the upper jaw, the prolabial portion of the upper lip and the primary palate.
internodal s., segmentum internodale; interannular s.; Ranvier's s.; internode; the portion of a myelinated nerve fiber between two successive nodes.
Lanterman's s.'s, the divisions of the nerve fiber between the Schmidt-Lanterman incisures.
lateral s., *segmentum* laterale.
lateral basal s., *segmentum* basale laterale.
s.'s of liver, hepatic s.'s.
lower uterine s., the inferior portion or isthmus of the uterus, the lower extremity of which joins with the cervical canal and, during pregnancy, expands to become the lower part of the uterine cavity.
medial s., *segmentum* mediale.
medial basal s., *segmentum* basale mediale.
mesoblastic s., somite.
neural s., neuromere.
P-R s., that part of the electrocardiographic curve between the end of the P wave and the beginning of the QRS complex.
posterior s., *segmentum* posterius.
posterior basal s., *segmentum* basale posterius.
Ranvier's s., internodal s.
renal s.'s, *segmenta* renalia.
RST s., the part of the electrocardiogram between the QRS complex and T wave.
s.'s of spinal cord, *segmenta* medullae spinalis.
s.'s of spleen, segmenta lienis; splenic territories receiving independent arterial supply or drained by independent roots of the splenic vein.
ST s., that part of the electrocardiographic tracing immediately following the QRS complex and merging into the T wave.
subapical s., *segmentum* subapicale; segmentum subsuperius; subsuperior segment; an inconstant segment of the inferior lobe of the right and left lungs.
subsuperior s., subapical s.
superior s., *segmentum* superius.

superior lingular s., *segmentum* lingulare superius.
sympathetic s., a divison of the sympathetic trunks based on the origins of the gray rami communicantes.
upper uterine s., the main portion of the body of the gravid uterus, the contraction of which furnishes the chief force of expulsion in labor.
venous s.'s of the kidney, anatomical s.'s of the kidney drained by tributaries of the renal vein; not a true segmental distribution, since cross communication exists between the various tributaries within the kidney.
venous s.'s of liver, hepatic venous s.'s; each of the four territories of the liver separately drained by the hepatic veins.

segmenta (seg-men'tă). Plural of segmentum.

segmental (seg-men'tăl). Relating to a segment.

segmentation (seg'men-tā'shŭn). **1.** The act of dividing into segments; the state of being divided into segments. **2.** Cleavage (1).

segmentectomy (seg-men-tek'tō-mē). Excision of a segment of any organ or gland.

segmenter (seg'men-ter). A schizont; usually applied to the malaria parasite developing in a red blood cell after having undergone nuclear and cytoplasmic division, just before cell rupture and release of the merozoites.

Segmentina (seg-men-tī'nă) [L. *segmentum,* fr. *seco,* to cut]. A genus of freshwater pulmonate snails (family Planorbidae, subfamily Segmentininae); includes the species *S. hemisphaerula,* an important intermediate host of *Fasciolopsis buski.*

segmentum, pl. **segmenta** (seg-men'tŭm, -tă) [L. segment] [NA]. Segment (1). **1.** A section; a part of an organ or other structure delimited naturally, artificially, or by invagination from the remainder. **2.** A territory of an organ having independent function, supply, or drainage.
s. ante'rius [NA], anterior segment; **(1)** anterior segment of the right lobe of the liver; **(2)** anterior segment of the superior lobe of right and left lungs.
s. ante'rius infe'rius [NA], inferior anterior segment of kidney.
s. ante'rius supe'rius [NA], superior anterior segment of kidney.
s. apica'le [NA], apical segment; **(1)** apical segment of the superior lobe of the right lung; **(2)** s. superius (2); apical segment of the inferior lobe of the right and left lungs.
s. apicoposte'rius [NA], apicoposterior segment of superior lobe of left lung.
s. basa'le ante'rius [NA], anterior basal segment of inferior lobe of right and left lung.
s. basa'le latera'le [NA], lateral basal segment of inferior lobe of right and left lung.
s. basa'le media'le [NA], s. cardiacum; medial basal segment of inferior lobe of right and left lung.
s. basa'le poste'rius [NA], posterior basal segment of inferior lobe of right and left lungs.
s. bronchopulmona'lis [NA], bronchopulmonary segment; the largest subdivision of a lobe of the lung; it is supplied by a direct branch of a lobar bronchus and is separated from adjacent segments by connective tissue septa.
s. cardi'acum [NA], cardiac segment; official alternative term for s. basale mediale.
segmen'ta hep'atis, hepatic *segments.*
s. infe'rius [NA], inferior segment of kidney.
s. internoda'le, internodal *segment.*
s. latera'le [NA], lateral segment; **(1)** of the left lobe of the liver; **(2)** of the middle lobe of the right lung.
segmen'ta lien'is, *segments* of spleen.
s. lingula're infe'rius [NA], inferior lingular segment of superior lobe of left lung.
s. lingula're supe'rius [NA], superior lingular segment of the superior lobe of the left lung.
s. media'le [NA], medial segment; **(1)** medial segment of the left lobe of the liver; **(2)** medial segment of the middle lobe of the right lung.
segmen'ta medul'lae spina'lis [NA], segments of spinal cord; portions of the spinal cord corresponding to the line of attachment of the roots of the individual spinal nerves; **s. m. s. cervica'lia** [NA], *pars* cervicalis medullae spinalis; **s. m. s. coccyg'ea** [NA], *pars* coccygea medullae spinalis; **s. m. s. lumba'lis** [NA], *pars* lumbalis medullae spinalis; **s. m. s. sacra'lis** [NA], *pars* sacralis medullae spinalis; **s. m. s. thora'cica** [NA], *pars* thoracica medullae spinalis.
s. poste'rius [NA], posterior segment; **(1)** posterior segment of the right lobe of the liver; **(2)** posterior segment of the superior lobe of the right lung; **(3)** posterior segment of the kidney.
segmen'ta rena'lia [NA], renal segments; arterial segments of the kidney; regions of the kidney supplied by end arteries branching from the renal arteries; they are named s. anterius inferius, s. anterius superius, s. inferius, s. posterius, and s. superius.

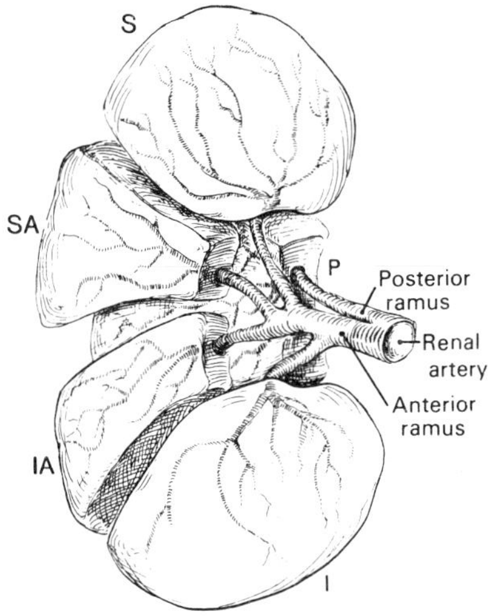

Renal Segments (Segmenta Renalia)
Shown with segmental arteries that supply them. *S,* superior; *SA,* superior anterior; *IA,* inferior anterior; *I,* inferior; *P,* posterior.

s. subapica'le, subapical *segment.*
s. subsupe'rius, subapical *segment.*
s. supe'rius [NA], **(1)** superior segment of the kidney; **(2)** official alternative term for s. apicale (2).

segregation (seg-rĕ-gā'shŭn) [L. *segrego,* pp. *-atus,* to set apart from the flock, separate]. **1.** Separation; removal of certain parts from a mass. **2.** Separation of contrasting characters in the offspring of heterozygotes. **3.** Separation of the paired state of genes which occurs at the reduction division of meiosis; only one member of each somatic gene pair is included in each sperm or ovum; *e.g.,* an individual heterozygous for a gene pair, *Aa,* will form gametes half containing gene *A* and half containing gene *a.*

segregator (seg're-gā-ter, tōr). Separator (2).

Seidel, Erich, German ophthalmologist, 1882–1946. See S.'s *scotoma, sign.*

Seignette, Pierre, French apothecary, 1660–1719. See S.'s *salt.*

Seiler, Carl, Swiss laryngologist and anatomist in U.S., 1849–1905. See S.'s *cartilage.*

Seip, Martin, 20th century Scandinavian physician. See Lawrence-S. *syndrome.*

seismotherapy (sīz-mō-thār'ă-pē) [G. *seismos,* a shaking, vibration]. Vibratory *massage.*

Seitelberger, Franz, 20th century Austrian neuropathologist. See S.'s *disease.*

seizure (sē′zher) [O. Fr. *seisir,* Med. L. *sacire,* to grasp, take possession of]. **1.** An attack; the sudden onset of a disease or of certain symptoms. **2.** Convulsion; an epileptic attack.

absence s., *absence.*

anosognosic s., anosognosic epilepsy.

complex partial s., psychomotor *epilepsy.*

generalized tonic-clonic s., generalized tonic-clonic *epilepsy.*

partial s., focal *epilepsy.*

psychic s., an attack of morbid sensations, such as fullness in the head, vertigo, palpitation, etc., with temporary disturbance of consciousness, not amounting to unconsciousness.

psychomotor s., psychomotor *epilepsy.*

sejunction (sē-jŭngk′shŭn) [L. *se-jungo,* pp. *-junctus,* to disjoin]. A separation; a breaking of continuity in the mental processes.

selaphobia (sē-lă-fō′bē-ă) [G. *selas,* light, + *phobos,* fear]. Rarely used term for a morbid fear of a flash of light.

Seldinger, S.I., Swedish radiologist, *1921. See S. *technique.*

selection (sĕ-lek′shŭn) [L. *se-ligo,* to separate, select, fr. *se,* apart + *lego,* to pick out]. The combined effect of the causes and consequences of genetic factors that determine the average number of progeny of a species that attain sexual maturity; phenotypes that are lethal early in life (*e.g.,* Tay-Sachs disease), that cause sterility (*e.g.,* Turner's syndrome), or that produce sterile progeny are selected against. When s. is used of individual pedigrees, other factors, notably variance of the number of progeny and number that survive to maturity, are significant; in large populations, these factors even out and the mean only is of importance.

artificial s., interference by man with natural s. by purposeful breeding of animals or plants of specific genotype or phenotype to produce a strain with desired characteristics; *e.g.,* breeding of dairy cattle for high milk production.

medical s., preservation, by medical care and treatment, of individuals of pathologic genotypes who would not otherwise reproduce, thus tending to increase the frequency of pathologic genes in the population; conversely, reduction of the frequency of pathologic genes by preventing reproduction of individuals of specified genotype by surgical sterilization or other means.

natural s., "survival of the fittest," the principle that in nature those individuals best able to adapt to their environment will survive and reproduce, while those less able will die without progeny, and the genes carried by the survivors will increase in frequency.

sexual s., a form of natural s. in which, according to Darwin's theory, the male or female is attracted by certain characteristics, form, color, behavior, etc., in the opposite sex; thus modifications of a special nature are brought about in the species.

selene unguium (sē-lē′nē ŭng′gwi-ŭm) [G. *selēnē,* moon; gen. pl. of L. *unguis,* nail]. Lunula (1).

selenium (sĕ-lē′nē-ŭm) [G. *selēnē,* moon]. A metallic element chemically similar to sulfur, symbol Se, atomic no. 34, atomic weight 78.96; an essential trace element toxic in large quantities.

s. sulfide, a mixture of crystalline s. monosulfide and solid solutions of s. and sulfur in an amorphous form, containing 52 to 55.5% Se; used in the treatment of seborrhea of the scalp or dandruff; it is applied to the scalp as a suspension.

selenocysteine (sĕ-lē-nō-sis′tēn). Cysteine containing selenium in place of one sulfur atom, found in nature and, at least in part, responsible for certain curative effects of cysteine.

selenodont (sĕ-lē′nō-dont) [G. *selēnē,* moon, + *odous* (*odont-*), tooth]. Denoting an animal, or man, having teeth, as the human molars, with longitudinal crescent-shaped ridges.

selenomethionine (sĕ-lē′nō-me-thī′ō-nēn). Methionine containing selenium in place of sulfur.

Selenomonas (sĕ-lē′nō-mō′nas) [G. *selēnē,* moon, + *monas,* single (unit)]. A genus of bacteria of uncertain taxonomic affiliation, containing curved to crescentic or helical, Gram-negative, strictly anaerobic rods that are motile with an active tumbling motion. Several flagella are present in a tuft, often near the center of the concave side. The type species, *S. sputigena,* is found in the human buccal cavity.

self. **1.** A sum of the attitudes and behavioral predispositions that make up the personality. **2.** The individual as represented in his own awareness and in his environment. **3.** In immunology, an individual's autologous cell components as contrasted with non-s., or foreign, constituents; the basic mechanism underlying recognition of s. from non-s. is unknown, but serves to protect the host from an immunologic attack on his own antigenic constituents, as opposed to immune system destruction or elimination of foreign antigens.

subliminal s., subconscious mind; the sum of the mental processes which take place without the conscious knowledge of the individual.

self-accusation. A common psychiatric symptom, encountered most characteristically in agitated depression.

self-analysis. Autoanalysis.

self-awareness. Realization of one's ongoing emotional experience; a major goal of all psychotherapy.

self-centeredness. Autosynnoia.

self-commitment. Voluntary mental hospitalization.

self-control. **1.** Self-regulation of one's behavior in accordance with personal beliefs, goals, and attitudes. **2.** Use by an individual of active coping strategies to deal with problem situations, in contrast to passive conditioning strategies which do things to the individual and require no action by the person.

self-differentiation. Differentiation resulting from the action of intrinsic causes.

self-discovery. In psychoanalysis, the freeing of the repressed ego in a person raised to be submissive to those around him.

self-fertilization. Fecundation of the ovules by the pollen of the same flower, or of the ova by the spermatozoa of the same animal in hermaphrodite forms; denoting an extreme type of inbreeding seen in certain plants and animal forms which produce both male and female gametes.

self-infection. Autoinfection.

self-knowledge. Autognosis.

self-limited. Denoting a disease that tends to cease after a definite period; *e.g.,* pneumonia.

self-love. Narcissism.

self-poisoning. Autointoxication.

self-stimulation. A technique for electrical stimulation of peripheral nerves, spinal cord, or brain by the patient himself to relieve pain.

Selivanoff, Feodor, Russian chemist, *1859. See S.'s *test.*

sella (sel′ă) [L. saddle]. Saddle (1).

empty s., a sella turcica, often enlarged, that contains no discernible pituitary gland; may be primarily due to an incompetent sellar diaphragm with compression of the pituitary gland by herniating arachnoid or secondarily due to surgery or radiotherapy.

s. tur′cica [NA], Turkish saddle; pars sellaris; a saddle-like prominence on the upper surface of the sphenoid bone, situated in the middle cranial fossa and dividing it into two halves.

sellar (sel′ăr). Relating to the sella turcica.

Sellick, Brian A., 20th century British anesthetist. See S.'s *maneuver.*

Selter, Paul, German pediatrician, 1866–1941. See S.'s *disease.*

Selye, Hans, Austrian endocrinologist in Canada, 1907–1982. See adaptation *syndrome* of Selye.

semantics (se-man'tiks) [G. *sēmainein,* to show]. A branch of semiotics: **1.** The study of the significance and development of the meaning of words. **2.** The study concerned with the relations between signs and their referents; the relations between the signs of a system; and human behavioral reaction to signs, including unconscious attitudes, influences of social institutions, and epistemological and linguistic assumptions.

semelincident (sem-el-in'si-dent) [L. *semel,* once, + *incido,* to happen, fr. *cado,* to fall]. Happening once only; said of an infectious disease, one attack of which confers permanent immunity.

semen, pl. **semina, semens** (sē'men, sē-mi'nă, sē'menz) [L. *semen (semin-),* seed (of plants, men, animals)]. **1** [NA]. Seminal fluid; sperm (2); the penile ejaculate; a thick, yellowish white, viscid fluid containing spermatozoa; a mixture produced by secretions of the testes, seminal vesicles, prostate, and bulbourethral glands. **2.** Seed (1).

semenuria (sē-mĕ-nū'rē-ă). Seminuria; spermaturia; the excretion of urine containing semen.

semi- [L. *semis,* half]. Prefix denoting one-half or partly, used with words derived from L. roots; corresponds to G. *hemi-.*

semialdehyde (sem-ē-al'dĕ-hīd). The monoaldehyde of a dicarboxylic acid, so called because half the COOH groups of the original acid are reduced to the aldehyde while the other half are unchanged; *e.g.,* glutamic acid s., $CHO–CH_2CH_2CH(NH_2)–COOH$. Many s.'s are intermediates in the biosynthesis and metabolic degradation of amino acids (*e.g.,* lysine, aspartate, glutamate, valine).

semicanal (sem'ē-kă-nal'). Semicanalis.

semicanalis, pl. **semicanales** (sem'ē-kă-nal'is, -ēz) [L.]. Semicanal; a half canal; a deep groove on the edge of a bone which, uniting with a similar groove or part of an adjoining bone, forms a complete canal.

s. mus'culi tensor'is tym'pani [NA], semicanal of the tensor muscle of the tympanum; the superior division of the canalis musculotubarius containing the tensor tympani muscle.

s. tu'bae auditi'vae [NA], semicanal of the auditory tube; the inferior division of the canalis musculotubarius which forms the bony part of the auditory (eustachian) tube.

semicartilaginous (sem'ē-kar-ti-laj'i-nŭs). Composed partly of cartilage.

semicircular (sem'ē-sir'kyū-lăr). Semiorbicular; forming a half circle or an incomplete circle.

semicoma (sem-ē-kō'mă). A mild degree of coma from which it is possible to arouse the patient. See also consciousness.

semicomatose (sem-ē-kō'mă-tōs). In a condition of unconsciousness from which one can be aroused.

semiconductor (sem'ē-kon-dŭk'ter). A metalloid, in one form or another, that conducts electricity more easily than a true nonmetal but less easily than a metal; *e.g.,* silicon, germanium.

semiconscious (sem-ē-kon'shŭs). Partly conscious.

semicrista (sem'ē-kris'tă) [semi- + L. *crista,* crest, tuft]. A small or imperfect ridge or crest.

s. incisi'va, *crista* nasalis.

semidecussation (sem'ē-dē-kŭs-sā'shŭn). Incomplete decussation such as occurs in the human optic chiasm.

semiflexion (sem-ē-flek'shŭn). The position of a joint or segment of a limb midway between extension and flexion.

semilunar (sem-ē-lū'năr) [semi- + L. *luna,* moon]. Lunar (2).

semilunare (sem-ē-lū-nā'rē). *Os* lunatum.

semiluxation (sem-ē-lŭk-sā'shŭn). Subluxation.

semimembranosus (sem'ē-mem-bră-nō'sŭs). See under musculus.

semimembranous (sem'ē-mem'brā-nŭs). Consisting partly of membrane; denoting the musculus semimembranosus.

seminal (sem'i-năl). **1.** Relating to the semen. **2.** Original or influential of future developments.

semination (sem-i-nā'shŭn). Insemination.

seminiferous (sem'i-nif'er-ŭs) [L. *semen,* seed (semen) + *fero,* to carry]. Carrying or conducting the semen; denoting the tubules of the testis.

seminoma (sem-i-nō'mă) [L. *semen,* seed (semen) + G. *-oma,* tumor]. A radiosensitive malignant testicular neoplasm arising from germ cells in young male adults which metastasizes to the paraortic lymph nodes; a counterpart of dysgerminoma of the ovary.

spermacytic s., a relatively slow-growing, locally invasive type of testicular s. that does not metastasize and has no ovarian counterpart.

seminomatous (sem-i-nō'mă-tŭs). Relating to a seminoma.

seminormal (N/2) (sem-ē-nōr'măl). Denoting a solution one-half the strength of a normal solution (0.5 N).

seminose (sem'i-nōs) [L. *semen,* seed + -ose (1)]. Mannose.

seminuria (sē-mi-nū'rē-ă). Semenuria.

semiography, semeiography (sē-mē-og'ră-fē) [G. *sēmeion,* sign, + *graphē,* a description]. Obsolete term for a treatise on symptomatology or a description of the symptoms of a disease.

semiologic, semeiologic (sē'mē-ō-loj'ik). Obsolete term for symptomatic.

semiology, semeiology (sē-mē-ol'ō-jē) [G. *sēmeion,* sign, + *logos,* study]. Obsolete term for symptomatology.

semiopathic, semeiopathic (sē'mē-ō-path'ik) [G. *sēmeion,* sign, + *pathos,* disease]. Denoting the disordered use of symbols.

semiorbicular (sē-mē-ōr-bik'yū-lăr). Semicircular.

semiosis, semeiosis (sē-mē-ō'sis) [G. *sēmeiōsis,* fr. *sēmeion,* sign]. The mental or symbolic process in which something (*e.g.,* word, symbol, nonverbal cue) functions as a sign for the organism.

semiotic, semeiotic (sē-mē-ot'ik, sem-ē-) [G. *sēmeiōtikos,* fr. *sēmeion,* sign]. **1.** Relating to semiotics. **2.** Relating to signs, linguistic or bodily.

semiotics, semeiotics (sē-mē-ot'iks, sem-e-) [see semiotic]. **1.** Obsolete term for symptomatology. **2.** The general philosophical theory of signs and symbols, having three branches: syntactics, semantics, and pragmatics.

semipenniform (sem'ē-pen'i-fōrm). Penniform on one side. See *musculus* unipennatus.

semipermeable (sem-ē-per'mē-ă-bl). Freely permeable to water (or other solvent) but relatively impermeable to solutes. Depending on the context, it has been used to imply impermeability to all solutes except very small uncharged molecules (*e.g.,* a cell membrane), or merely impermeability to very large molecules such as proteins (*e.g.,* a capillary membrane).

semiplacenta (sem'ē-pla-sen'tă). The type of placenta in ruminants, horse and pig, in which the maternal and fetal placentas do not grow together but can be easily separated without tearing; an apposed or contact placenta.

semipronation (sem'ē-prō-nā'shŭn) The attitude or assumption of a partly prone position, as in Sims' position.

semiprone (sem-ē-prōn'). Denoting semipronation.

semiquinone (sem-ē-kwin'ōn). A free radical resulting from the removal of one hydrogen atom with its electron during the process of dehydrogenation of a hydroquinone to quinone or similar compound (*e.g.,* flavin mononucleotide).

semispinal (sem-ē-spī'năl). Half spinal; denoting muscles attached in part to the spinous processes of the vertebrae.

Semisulcospina (sem′ē-sŭl-kō-spī′nă) [semi- + L. *sulcus,* a furrow + *spina,* thorn, spine]. A genus of operculate snails (family Pleuroceriidae, subclass Prosobranchiata). An oriental form, *S. libertina,* is the first intermediate host of a number of trematodes, including *Paragonimus westermani.*

semisulcus (sem′ē-sŭl′kŭs). A slight groove on the edge of a bone or other structure, which, uniting with a similar groove on the corresponding adjoining structure, forms a complete sulcus.

semisupination (sem′ē-sū-pi-nā′shŭn). The attitude or assumption of a partly supine position.

semisupine (sem-ē-sū-pīn′). Denoting semisupination.

semisynthetic (sem′ē-sin-thet′ik). Describing the process of synthesizing a particular chemical utilizing a naturally occurring chemical as a starting material, thus obviating part of a total synthesis; *e.g.,* the conversion of cholesterol (obtained from a natural source) into a corticosteroid.

semisystematic name (sem′ē-sis-tĕ-mat′ik). Semitrivial name; a name of a chemical of which at least one part is systematic and at least one part is not (*i.e.,* is trivial). For example, calciferol includes the -ol suffix denoting an -OH radical, while calcifer-, which has no systematic meaning, is used only in this word. Cortisone contains the -one suffix, indicating a ketone group, but the rest of the term derives from cortex (adrenal). Hippuric acid (trivial) may be defined as *N*-benzoylglycine (semitrivial name); benzoyl is systematic for the C_6H_5–CO– radical, whereas glycine is the trivial name for α-aminoacetic (or 2-aminoethanoic, to be completely systematic) acid, and the *N* signifies that the benzoyl is attached to the N in the glycine; from this, the structure C_6H_5–CO–NH–CH_2–COOH is uniquely defined. Many generic or nonproprietary names of drugs, including USAN names, hormones, etc., are semitrivial in this chemical sense, although often termed trivial names; distinction between trivial and semitrivial is not often made.

semitendinosus (sem′ē-ten-di-nō′sŭs) [L.]. Semitendinous.

semitendinous (sem′ē-ten′di-nŭs) [L. *semitendinosus*]. Composed in part of tendon; denoting the musculus semitendinosus.

semitertian (sem-ē-ter′shē-ăn, -ter′shŭn). Partly tertian, partly quotidian; denoting a malarial fever in which two paroxysms occur on one day and one on the succeeding day.

semitrivial name (sem-ē-triv′ē-ăl). Semisystematic name.

semivalent (sem-ē-vā′lent). Denoting the ability to form a one-electron bond.

Semon, Sir Felix, German laryngologist in Britain, 1849–1921. See S.'s *law;* Gerhardt-S. *law.*

Semon, Richard W., German biologist, 1859–1908. See S.-Hering *theory.*

Semple, Sir David, British physician, 1856–1937. See S. *vaccine.*

Senear, Francis E., U.S. dermatologist, 1889–1958. See S.-Usher *disease, syndrome.*

Senecio (sĕ-nē′sē-ō, -shē-ō) [L. a plant, groundsel, fr. *senecio,* an old man]. **1.** A large genus of plants (family Compositae), many species of which contain alkaloids that produce hepatic necrosis. **2.** *Senecio aureus;* life-root; sqaw-weed; ragwort; a common weed of the eastern U.S., formerly used in the treatment of amenorrhea and other menstrual irregularities.

senecioic acid (sĕ-nē′si-ō-ik). 3-Methyl-2-butenoic acid; 3,3-dimethylacrylic acid; methylcrotonic acid; $(CH_3)_2C{=}CH{-}COOH$; a polymer precursor and a precursor of isoprenoid and terpene compounds; the acid component of binapacryl in which it is esterfied with 4,6-dinitro-2-(1-methylpropyl)phenol; an intermediate in leucine degradation; used as a fungicide and miticide.

seneciosis (sĕ-nē-sē-ō′sis). Liver degeneration and necrosis caused by ingestion of plants of the genus *Senecio,* such as ragwort and groundsel; similar hepatotoxic properties have been observed after ingestion of some kinds of *Crotalaria* and *Heliotropium.*

senega (sen′ē-gă) [*Seneca,* an Indian tribe]. Seneca snakeroot; the dried root of *Polygala senega* (family Polygalaceae), a herb of eastern and central North America; an expectorant.

senescence (se-nes′ens) [L. *senesco,* to grow old, fr. *senex,* old]. The state of being old.

dental s., that condition of the teeth and associated structures in which there is deterioration due to normal or premature aging processes.

senescent (sē-nes′ent). Growing old.

Sengstaken, Robert W., U.S. neurosurgeon, *1923. See S.-Blakemore *tube.*

senile (sē′nīl, sen′īl) [L. *senilis*] Relating to or characteristic of old age.

senility (se-nil′i-tē) [see senile]. Old age; the cognitive and physiologic expressions of the sum of the physical and mental changes occurring in advanced life.

senium (sē′nē-ŭm) [L. the feebleness of age, fr. *seneo,* to be old, feeble]. Rarely used term for old age; especially the debility of advanced age.

senna (sen′ă) [Ar. *senā*]. The dried leaflets or legumes of *Cassia acutifolia* (Alexandrine s.) and *C. angustifolia* (Tinnevelly or Indian s.); a laxative.

s. pod, s. fruit.

sennosides A and B (sen′ō-sīdz). Two anthraquinone glucosides that are the laxative principles of senna.

sensate (sen′sāt). Able to perceive touch and other sensations; used in reference to patients who have had partial nerve or spinal cord injuries.

sensation (sen-sā′shŭn) [L. *sensatio,* perception, feeling, fr. *sentio,* to perceive, feel]. A feeling; the translation into consciousness of the effects of a stimulus exciting any of the organs of sense.

cincture s., zonesthesia.

delayed s., a s. that is not perceived until the lapse of an appreciable interval following the application of the stimulus.

general s., a s. referred to the body as a whole rather than to any particular part.

girdle s., zonesthesia.

objective s., a s. caused by a verifiable stimulus.

primary s., a s. that is the direct result of a stimulus.

referred s., reflex or transferred s.; a s. felt in one place in response to a stimulus applied in another.

reflex s., referred s.

special s., a s. referred to a stimulus produced by an external body and acting on any of the sense organs.

subjective s., a s. not readily referrable to a verifiable stimulus.

transferred s., referred s.

sense (sens) [L. *sentio,* pp. *sensus,* to feel, to perceive]. Feeling; sensation; consciousness; the faculty of perceiving any stimulus.

color s., the ability to perceive variations in hue, luminosity, and saturation of light

s. of equilibrium, static s.; the s. that makes possible a normal physiologic posture.

joint s., articular *sensibility.*

kinesthetic s., myesthesia.

light s., the ability to perceive variations in the degree of light or brightness.

muscular s., myesthesia.

obstacle s., the ability, often found in the blind, to avoid objects without visual warning.

posture s., position s.; the ability to recognize the position in which a limb is passively placed, with the eyes closed.

pressure s., baresthesia; piesesthesia; the faculty of discriminating various degrees of pressure on the surface.

seventh s., visceral s.
sixth s., cenesthesia.
space s., the faculty of perceiving the relative positions of objects in the external world.
special s., one of the five senses related respectively to the organs of sight, hearing, smell, taste, and touch.
static s., s. of equilibrium.
tactile s., touch (1).
temperature s., thermoesthesia.
thermal s., thermic s., thermoesthesia.
time s., the faculty by which the passage of time is appreciated.
visceral s., seventh s.; splanchnesthesia; splanchnesthetic sensibility; the perception of the existence of the internal organs.

sensibility (sen-si-bil'i-tē) [L. *sensibilitas*]. The consciousness of sensation; the capability of perceiving sensible stimuli.
articular s., arthresthesia; joint sense; appreciation of sensation in joint surfaces.
bone s., pallesthesia.
cortical s., the integration of sensory stimuli by the cerebral cortex.
deep s., myesthesia.
dissociation s., the loss of the pain and the thermal senses with preservation of tactile sensibility.
electromuscular s., s. of muscular tissue to stimulation by electricity.
epicritic s., see epicritic.
mesoblastic s., myesthesia.
pallesthetic s., pallesthesia.
proprioceptive s., see proprioceptive.
protopathic s., see protopathic.
splanchnesthetic s., visceral *sense.*
vibratory s., pallesthesia.

sensible (sen'si-bl) [L. *sensibilis,* fr. *sentio,* to feel, perceive]. **1.** Perceptible to the senses. **2.** Capable of sensation. **3.** Sensitive. **4.** Having reason or judgment; intelligent.

sensiferous (sen-sif'er-ŭs) [L. *sensus,* sense, + *fero,* to carry]. Conducting a sensation.

sensigenous (sen-sij'e-nŭs) [L. *sensus,* sense, + G. *-gen,* to produce]. Giving rise to sensation.

sensimeter (sen-sim'ĕ-ter) [L. *sensus,* sense, + G. *metron,* measure]. An instrument that measures degrees of cutaneous sensation.

sensitive (sen'si-tiv). **1.** Capable of perceiving sensations. **2.** Responding to a stimulus. **3.** Acutely perceptive of interpersonal situations. **4.** One who is readily hypnotizable. **5.** Readily undergoing a chemical change, with but slight change in environmental conditions, as a s. reagent. **6.** In immunology, denoting: 1) a sensitized *antigen;* 2) a person (or animal) rendered susceptible to immunological reactions (especially those reactions not associated directly with resistance to infection) by previous exposure of the immunological system to the antigen concerned.

sensitivity (sen-si-tiv'i-tē) [L. *sentio,* pp. *sensus,* to feel]. **1.** The ability to appreciate by one or more of the senses. **2.** Esthesia (2); state of being sensitive. **3.** In clinical pathology and medical screening, the proportion of individuals with a positive test result for the disease that the test is intended to reveal, *i.e.,* true positive results as a proportion of the total of true positive and false negative results. *Cf.* specificity (2).
acquired s., allergy (1).
antibiotic s., microbial susceptibility to antibiotics. See also antibiotic sensitivity *test,* minimum inhibitory *concentration.*
contrast s., in optics, the ability to discern the difference in brightness of adjacent areas.
diagnostic s., the probability (P) that, given the presence of disease (D), an abnormal test result (T) indicates the presence of disease; *i.e.,* P(T/D).
idiosyncratic s., a type I allergic reaction (atopic).
induced s., allergy (1)
pacemaker s., the minimum cardiac activity required to consistently trigger a pulse generator.
photoallergic s., see photosensitization.
phototoxic s., see photosensitization.
primaquine s., nonimmunological inborn s. to primaquine, causing hemolysis on exposure to the drug, due to deficiency of glucose 6-phosphate dehydrogenase in red cells.
relative s., the s. of a medical screening test as determined by comparison with the same type of test; *e.g.,* s. of a new serological test relative to s. of an established serological test.
salt s., the tendency of certain bacterial suspensions to agglutinate spontaneously in physiological saline solution.
spectral s., the reciprocal of the amount of monochromatic radiation that produces a fixed response.

sensitization (sen'si-ti-zā'shŭn). Immunization, especially with reference to antigens (immunogens) not associated with infection; the induction of acquired sensitivity or of allergy.
autoerythrocyte s., see autoerythrocyte sensitization *syndrome.*
covert s., aversive conditioning or training during which the patient is taught to imagine unpleasant and related aversive consequences while engaging in an unwanted habit.
photodynamic s., photosensitization (2); the action by which certain substances, notably fluorescing dyes (acridine, eosin, methylene blue, rose bengal) absorb visible light and emit the energy at wavelengths that are deleterious to microbes or other organisms in the dye-containing suspension.

sensitize (sen'si-tīz). To render sensitive (7); to induce acquired sensitivity, to immunize. See also sensitized *antigen.*

sensitizer (sen'si-tīz-er). **1.** Antibody. **2.** A substance that causes dermatitis only after alteration (sensitization) of the skin by previous exposure to that substance.

sensomobile (sen-sō-mō'bēl). Capable of movement in response to a stimulus.

sensomobility (sen-sō-mō-bil'i-tē). The state of being sensomobile.

sensomotor (sen-sō-mō'ter). Sensorimotor.

sensor (sen'sŏr) [see sense]. A device designed to respond to physical stimuli such as temperature, light, magnetism, or movement, and transmit resulting impulses for interpretation, recording, movement, or operating control.

sensori- [L. *sensorius,* sensory]. Combining form denoting sensory.

sensorial (sen-sōr'ē-ăl). Relating to the sensorium.

sensoriglandular (sen'sōr-i-glan'dyū-lăr). Relating to glandular secretion excited by stimulation of the sensory nerves.

sensorimotor (sen'sōr-i-mō'ter). Sensomotor; both sensory and motor; denoting a mixed nerve with afferent and efferent fibers.

sensorimuscular (sen'sōr-i-mŭs'kyū-lăr). Denoting muscular contraction in response to a sensory stimulus.

sensorium, pl. **sensoria, sensoriums** (sen-sōr'ē-ŭm, -ă, -ŭmz) [Late L.]. **1.** An organ of sensation. **2.** Perceptorium; the hypothetical "seat of sensation." **3.** In human biology and psychology, consciousness; sometimes used as a generic term for the intellectual functions.

sensorivascular (sen'sōr-i-vas'kyū-lăr). Sensorivasomotor.

sensorivasomotor sen'sōr-i-vas-ō-mō'ter). Sensorivascular; denoting contraction or dilation of the blood vessels occurring as a sensory reflex.

sensory (sen'sō-rē) [L. *sensorius,* fr. *sensus,* sense]. Relating to sensation.

sensual (sen'shū-ăl) [L. *sensualis,* endowed with feeling]. **1.** Relating to the body and the senses, as distinguished from the intellect or spirit. **2.** Denoting bodily or sensory pleasure, not necessarily sexual.

sensualism (sen'shū-ăl-izm) [L. *sensualis,* endowed with feeling, fr. *sentio,* to feel]. **1.** Domination by the emotions. **2.** Indulgence in sensory pleasures.

sensuality (sen-shŭ-al'i-tē). The state or quality of being sensual.

sentient (sen'shent, sen'shē-ent) [L. *sentiens,* pres. p. of *sentio,* to feel, perceive]. Capable of, or characterized by, sensation.

sentiment (sen'ti-ment) [L. *sentio,* to feel]. **1.** Feeling or emotion in relation to one idea. **2.** A complex disposition or organization of a person with reference to a given object (a person, thing, or abstract idea) that makes the object what it is for him.

sentisection (sen-ti-sek'shŭn). Vivisection of an animal that is not anesthetized.

separation (sep-ă-rā'shŭn). **1.** The act of keeping apart or dividing, or the state of being held apart. **2.** In dentistry, the process of gaining slight spaces between the teeth preparatory to adapting and cementing bands.
jaw s., the amount of space between the jaws at any degree of opening.
s, of retina, see retinal *detachment.*
s. of teeth, **(1)** loss of proximal contact of teeth; **(2)** in orthodontics, the creation of interproximal spaces for the fitting of an appliance.

separator (sep'er-ā-ter) [L. *se-paro,* pp. *-atus,* to separate, fr. *se,* apart, + *paro,* to prepare]. **1.** That which divides or keeps apart two or more substances or prevents them from mingling. **2.** In dentistry, an instrument for forcing two teeth apart, so as to gain access to adjacent proximal walls.

sepsis, pl. **sepses** (sep'sis, -sēz) [G. *sēpsis,* putrefaction]. The presence of various pus-forming and other pathogenic organisms, or their toxins, in the blood or tissues; septicemia is a common type of s.
intestinal s., s. associated with autointoxication of intestinal origin.
s. len'ta, a slowly developing and more or less localized infection.
puerperal s., puerperal *fever.*

sept-. See septi-; septico-; septo-.

septa (sep'tă) [L.]. Plural of septum.

septal (sep'tăl). Relating to a septum.

septan (sep'tăn) [L. *septem,* seven]. Denoting a malarial fever the paroxysms of which recur every seventh day, counting the day of the occurrence as the first day.

septate (sep'tāt) [L. *saeptum,* septum]. Having a septum; divided into compartments.

septectomy (sep-tek'tō-mē) [L. *saeptum,* septum, + G. *ektomē,* excision]. Operative removal of the whole or a part of a septum, specifically of the nasal septum.

septemia (sep-tē'mē-ă). Septicemia.

septi-, sept- [L. *septem,* seven]. Combining forms meaning seven.

septic (sep'tik). Relating to or caused by sepsis.

septicemia (sep-ti-sē'mē-ă) [G. *sēpsis,* putrefaction, + *haima,* blood]. Septemia; sapremia; septic fever; hematosepsis; septic intoxication; systemic disease caused by the spread of microorganisms and their toxins via the circulating blood. See also pyemia.
acute fulminating meningococcal s., Waterhouse-Friderichsen *syndrome.*
anthrax s., anthracemia.
cryptogenic s., a form of s. in which no primary focus of infection can be found.
hemorrhagic s., s. pluriformis; a disease in animals caused by members of the genus *Pasteurella;* occurs in cattle, sheep, swine, rabbits, and fowls.
s. pluriform'is, hemorrhagic s.
puerperal s., a severe bloodstream infection resulting from an obstetric delivery or procedure.
typhoid s., typhosepsis; typhoid during the phase when the organism can be cultured from the blood.

septicemic (sep-ti-sē'mik). Relating to, suffering from, or resulting from septicemia.

septico-, septic- [G. *sēptikos,* putrifying, fr. *sēpsis,* putrefaction]. Combining forms meaning sepsis, septic.

septicopyemia (sep'ti-kō-pī-ē'mē-ă). Pyemia and septicemia occurring together.

septicopyemic (sep'ti-kō-pī-ē'mik). Relating to septicopyemia.

septimetritis (sep'ti-mē-trī'tis) [G. *sēptikōs,* septic, + *mētra,* uterus, + *-itis,* inflammation]. Septic inflammation of the uterus.

septivalent (sep-ti-vā'lent, sep-tiv'ă-lent). Having a combining power (valency) of seven.

septo-, sept- [L. *saeptum,* septum]. Combining forms meaning septum.

septodermoplasty (sep-tō-der'mō-plas-tē) [septo- + dermo- + G. *plastos,* formed]. Operation to graft squamous epithelium to replace the mucosa of the nasal septum, especially in cases of hereditary hemorrhagic telangiectasia.

septomarginal (sep'tō-mar'ji-năl). Relating to the margin of a septum, or to both a septum and a margin.

septonasal (sep'tō-nā'săl). Relating to the nasal septum.

septoplasty (sep'tō-plas-tē) [septo- + G. *plastos,* formed]. Operation to correct defects or deformities of the nasal septum, often by alteration or partial removal of supporting structures.

septorhinoplasty (sep-tō-rī'nō-plas-tē) [septo- + G. *rhis,* nose, + *plastos,* formed]. Combined operation to repair defects or deformities of the nasal septum and of the external nasal pyramid.

septostomy (sep-tos'tō-mē) [septo- + G. *stoma,* mouth]. Surgical creation of a septal defect.

septotomy (sep-tot'ō-mē) [septo- + G. *tomē,* incision]. Incision of a septum, as of the nasal septum.

septulum, pl. **septula** (sep'tyū-lŭm, -lă) [Mod. L. dim. of *septum*]. A minute septum.
s. tes'tis [NA], trabecula testis; one of the trabeculae of the testis; imperfect septa and fibrous cords radiating toward the surface of the gland from the mediastinum testis.

SEPTUM

septum, gen. **septi,** pl. **septa** (sep'tŭm, -tī, -tă) [L. *saeptum,* a partition]. **1** [NA]. A thin wall dividing two cavities or masses of softer tissue. **2.** For terms in neuroanatomy, see septal *area; septum* pellucidum. **3.** In fungi, a wall; usually a cross-wall in a hypha.
s. accesso'rium, an additional ridge forming the lower border of the limbus fossae ovalis.
alveolar s., s. interalveolare.
aortopulmonary s., the spiral s. which, during development, separates the truncus arteriosus into a ventral pulmonary trunk and dorsal aorta.
atrioventricular s., s. atrioventriculare.
s. atrioventricula're [NA], atrioventricular s.; pars membranacea septi atriorum; the small part of the membranous s. of the heart just above the septal cusp of the tricuspid valve that separates the right atrium from the left ventricle.
s. of auditory tube, s. canalis musculotubarii.
Bigelow's s., *calcar* femorale.

bony nasal s., s. nasi osseum.
bulbar s., old term for spiral s.
s. bul'bi ure'thrae, a fibrous s. in the interior of the bulb of the penis which divides it into two hemispheres.
s. cana'lis musculotuba'rii [NA], s. of musculotubal canal; s. tubae; s. of auditory tube; a very thin horizontal plate of bone forming two semicanals, the upper, smaller, for the tensor tympani muscle, the lower, larger for the auditory tube; its termination in the middle ear is the processus cochleariformis.
cartilaginous s., *cartilago* septi nasi.
s. cervica'le interme'dium [NA], a thin s. composed of glia fiber and leptomeningeal connective tissue in the cervical spinal cord marking the border between the fasciculi gracilis and cuneatus of the dorsal funiculus.
s. clitor'idis, s. corporum cavernosorum.
Cloquet's s., s. femorale.
comblike s., pectiniform s.
s. corpo'rum cavernoso'rum [NA], s. clitoridis; an incomplete fibrous s. between the corpora cavernosa of the clitoris.
crural s., s. femorale.
endovenous s., s. endoveno'sum, a remnant of the primitive separation between veins which fused to form the definitive trunk, such as the trunk leading to the left common iliac and the left renal veins.
femoral s., s. femorale.
s. femora'le [NA], femoral s.; crural s.; Cloquet's s.; the delicate fibrous membrane that closes the femoral ring at the base of the femoral canal.
s. of frontal sinuses, s. sinuum frontalium.
gingival s., interdental *papilla.*
s. glan'dis [NA], s. of glans; a fibrous partition extending through the glans penis from the lower surface of the tunica albuginea to the urethra.
s. of glans, s. glandis.
hanging s., the deformity caused by an abnormal width of the septal portion of the alar cartilages.
interalveolar s., **(1)** the tissue intervening between two adjacent pulmonary alveoli; it consists of a close-meshed capillary network covered on both surfaces by very thin alveolar epithelial cells; **(2)** s. interalveolare.
s. interalveola're, pl. **sep'ta interalveola'ria** [NA], interalveolar s. (2); alveolar s.; septal bone (1); one of the bony partitions between the tooth sockets.
interatrial s., s. interatriale.
s. interatria'le [NA], interatrial s.; the wall between the atria of the heart. See also s. primum and s. secundum.
interdental s., the bony portion separating two adjacent teeth in a dental arch.
s. interme'dium, old term for the s. of the atrioventricular canal of the embryonic heart formed by the fusion of the dorsal and ventral atrioventricular canal cushions.
intermuscular s., s. intermusculare.
s. intermuscula're [NA], intermuscular s.; a term applied to aponeurotic sheets separating various muscles of the limbs; these are anterior and posterior crural, lateral and medial femoral, lateral and medial humeral.
interpulmonary s., mediastinum (2).
interradicular septa, septa interradicularia.
sep'ta interradicula'ria [NA], interradicular septa; septal bone (2); the bony partitions that project into the alveoli between the roots of the molar teeth.
interventricular s., s. interventriculare.
s. interventricula're [NA], interventricular s.; ventricular s.; the wall between the ventricles of the heart.
s. lin'guae [NA], lingual s.; s. of tongue; nucleus fibrosus linguae; the median vertical fibrous partition of the tongue merging posteriorly into the aponeurosis of the tongue.
s. lu'cidum, s. pellucidum.
s. mediastina'le, mediastinum (2).
s. membrana'ceum ventriculo'rum, *pars* membranacea septi interventricularis.
membranous s., **(1)** *pars* membranacea septi nasi; **(2)** *pars* membranacea septi interventricularis.
s. mo'bile na'si, *pars* mobilis septi nasi.
s. muscula're ventriculo'rum, *pars* muscularis septi interventricularis.
s. of musculotubal canal, s. canalis musculotubarii.
nasal s., s. nasi.
s. na'si [NA], nasal s.; the wall dividing the nasal cavity into halves; it is composed of a central supporting skeleton covered on each side by a mucous membrane.
s. na'si oss'eum [NA], bony nasal s.; the bones supporting the pars ossea septi nasi; these are the perpendicular plate of the ethmoid, the vomer, the sphenoidal rostrum, the crest of the nasal bones, the frontal spine, and the median crest formed by the apposition of the maxillary and palatine bones.
s. orbita'le [NA], a fibrous membrane attached to the margin of the orbit and extending into the lids, constituting in great part the posterior fascia of the musculus orbicularis oculi.
pectiniform s., s. pectinifor'me, comblike s.; the anterior portion of the s. penis which is broken by a number of slitlike perforations.
s. pellu'cidum [NA], transparent s.; s. lucidum; a thin plate of brain tissue, containing nerve cells and numerous nerve fibers, that is stretched like a flat, vertical sheet between the columna and corpus fornicis below, the corpus callosum above and anteriorly; it is usually fused in the median plane with its partner on the opposite side so as to form a thin, median partition between the left and right frontal horn of the lateral ventricles; in less than 10% of humans there is a blind, slitlike, fluid-filled space between the two septa pellucidi, the cavum septi pellucidi. The s. pellucidum is continuous ventralward through the interval between the corpus callosum and the anterior commissure with the precommissural septum, gyrus subcallosus, or corpus paraterminale. See also *cavum* septi pellucidi; septal *area.*
s. pe'nis [NA], the portion of the tunica albuginea separating the two corpora cavernosa of the penis.
placental septa, incomplete partitions between placental cotyledons; they are covered with trophoblast and contain a core of maternal tissue.
precommissural s., see septal *area.*
s. pri'mum, a crescentic s. in the embryonic heart that develops on the dorsocephalic wall of the originally single atrium and initiates its partitioning into right and left chambers; the tips of the s. grow toward and fuse with the atrioventricular canal cushions.
proximal spiral s., see spiral s.
rectovaginal s., s. rectovaginale.
s. rectovagina'le [NA], rectovaginal s.; the fascial layer between the vagina and the lower part of the rectum.
rectovesical s., s. rectovesicale.
s. rectovesica'le [NA], rectovesical s.; rectovesical fascia; Denonvilliers' aponeurosis; Tyrrell's fascia; a fascial layer that extends from the central tendon of the perineum to the peritoneum between the prostate and rectum.
scrotal s., s. scroti.
s. scro'ti [NA], scrotal s.; an incomplete wall of connective tissue and nonstriated muscle dividing the scrotum into two sacs, each containing a testis.
s. secun'dum, the second of two major septal structures involved in the partitioning of the atrium, developing later than s. primum and located to the right of it; like s. primum, it is crescentic, but its tips are directed toward the sinus venosus, and it is more heavily muscular; it remains an incomplete partition until after birth, with its unclosed area constituting the foramen ovale.
sinus s., a small fold forming the medial end of the valve of the

inferior vena cava; it is developed from the dorsal wall of the embryonic sinus venosus.

s. sin'uum fronta'lium [NA], s. of frontal sinuses; the bony partition between the two frontal sinuses; it is often deflected to one side of the middle line.

s. sin'uum sphenoida'lium [NA], s. of sphenoidal sinuses; the bony partition between the two sphenoidal sinuses, often deflected to one side of the middle line.

s. of sphenoidal sinuses, s. sinuum sphenoidalium.

spiral s., a s. dividing the embryonic bulbus cordis into pulmonary and aortic outflow tracts from the developing heart; the **distal s.s.** is derived from the right and left endocardial cushions and so separates the pulmonary and aortic orifices; the **proximal s.s.** is the portion of the s. that is incorporated into the membranous part of the interventricular s.

spiral bulbar s., see spiral s.

s. spu'rium, a s. in the right atrium of the embryonic heart formed by the right venous valve and its continuation onto the dorsocephalic wall of the atrium; in human embryos, it reaches its fullest development during the third month and then undergoes regression, taking no part in atrial partitioning (hence its designation as false); reduced portions persist as the valve of the inferior vena cava and the valve of the coronary sinus.

s. of tongue, s. linguae.

transparent s., s. pellucidum.

transverse s., (1) *crista* ampullaris; **(2)** the mesodermal mass separating pericardial and peritoneal cavities; it is covered with mesothelium except where intimately associated with the liver, which originally developed within it; the s. is definitively incorporated into the diaphragm as the central tendon.

s. tu'bae, s. canalis musculotubarii.

urogenital s., the coronally placed ridge formed by the caudal portion of the urogenital ridges fusing in the midline of the embryo; it lies between the hindgut dorsally and the bladder ventrally.

urorectal s., urorectal fold; in embryos, a partition dividing the cloaca into a dorsal, rectal portion and a ventral portion called the urogenital sinus; reaching the cloacal membrane at about the time of its disintegration, the urorectal s. divides the cloacal exit into an anal and a urogenital orifice.

ventricular s., s. interventriculare.

sequela, pl. sequelae (sē-kwel'ă, sē-kwel'ē) [L. *sequela,* a sequel, fr. *sequor,* to follow]. A condition following as a consequence of a disease.

sequence (sē'kwens) [L. *sequor,* to follow]. The succession, or following, of one thing or event after another.

coding s., the portion of DNA that codes for transcription of messenger RNA. See exon.

insertion s., discrete DNA s.'s of approximately 1000 nucleotides which are repeated at various sites on a bacterial chromosome, certain plasmids, and bacteriophages, and which can move from one site to another on the chromosome, to another plasmid in the same bacterium, or to a bacteriophage.

intervening s., intron.

palindromic s., see palindrome.

regulatory s., any DNA s. that is responsible for the regulation of gene expression, such as promoters and operators.

termination s., termination *codon.*

sequence ladder. The array of bands, made conspicuous by labeling, when DNA fragmented by endonucleases is subject to gel electrophoresis; corresponds to the nucleotide sequence.

sequential (sē-kwen'shăl). Occurring in sequence.

sequester (sē-kwes'ter). To separate off from the main mass of tissue.

sequestra (sē-kwes'tră). Plural of sequestrum.

sequestral (sē-kwes'trăl). Relating to a sequestrum.

sequestration (sē-kwes-trā'shŭn) [L. *sequestratio,* fr. *sequestro,* pp. *-atus,* to lay aside]. **1.** Formation of a sequestrum. **2.** Loss of blood or of its fluid content into spaces within the body so that it is withdrawn from the circulating volume, resulting in hemodynamic impairment, hypovolemia, hypotension, and reduced venous return to the heart.

bronchopulmonary s., a congenital anomaly in which a mass of lung tissue becomes isolated, during development, from the rest of the lung; the bronchi in the mass are usually dilated or cystic and are not connected with the bronchial tree; it is supplied by a branch of the aorta.

sequestrectomy (sē-kwes-trek'tō-mē) [sequestrum + G. *ektomē,* excision]. Sequestrotomy: operative removal of a sequestrum.

sequestrotomy (sē-kwes-trot'ō-mē) [sequestrum + G. *tomē, incision*]. Sequestrectomy.

sequestrum, pl. sequestra (sē-kwes'trŭm, -tră) [Mod. L. use of Mediev. L. *sequestrum,* something laid aside, fr. L. *sequestro,* to lay aside, separate]. A piece of necrotic tissue, usually bone, that has become separated from the surrounding healthy tissue.

primary s., a completely detached s.

sequoiosis (sē-kwoy-ō'sis). Extrinsic allergic alveolitis caused by inhalation of redwood sawdust containing spores of *Graphium, Pullularia, Aureobasidium,* and other fungi.

SER Abbreviation for somatosensory evoked response. See under evoked *response.*

Ser Symbol for serine and its radical.

sera (sēr'ă). Plural of serum.

seralbumin (sēr-al-byū'min). Serum *albumin.*

serendipity (ser-en-dip'i-tē) [coined by Horace Walpole and relates to *The Three Princes of Serendip,* fr. alternate spelling of *Serendib,* ancient name for Ceylon]. Accidental discovery; finding one thing while looking for something else, as in Fleming's discovery of penicillin.

Sergent, Emile, French physician, 1867–1943. See S.'s white *line;* Bernard-S. *syndrome.*

series, pl. series (sēr'ēz) [L. fr. *sero,* to join together]. **1.** A succession of similar objects following one another in space or time. **2.** In chemistry, a group of substances, either elements or compounds, having similar properties or differing from each other in composition by a constant ratio.

aromatic s., all the compounds derived from benzene, or similar cyclic compounds, distinguished from those compounds that are acyclic or that contain rings that lack the conjugated double bond structure characteristic of benzene.

erythrocytic s., the cells in the various stages of development in the red bone marrow leading to the formation of the erythrocyte, *e.g.,* erythroblasts, normoblasts, erythrocytes.

fatty s., the alkanes; all the acyclic compounds in the methane, ethane, propane, etc., group, distinguished from the aromatic s.

granulocytic s., the cells in the several stages of development in the bone marrow leading to the mature granulocyte of the circulation, *e.g.,* myeloblasts, different stages of the myelocyte, granulocytes.

Hofmeister s., lyotropic s.; the series of cations Mg^{2+}, Ca^{2+}, Sr^{2+}, Ba^{2+}, Li^{+}, Na^{+}, K^{+}, Rb^{+}, Cs^{+}, and of anions citrate^{3-}, tartrate^{2-}, $SO_4{}^{2-}$, acetate^{-}, $NO_3{}^{-}$, $ClO_3{}^{-}$, I^{-}, CNS^{-} (among others), each series arranged in order of decreasing ability to: 1) precipitate the dispersed substance of lyophilic sols; 2) "salt out" organic substances (*e.g.,* aniline, ethyl acetate) from aqueous solutions; or 3) inhibit the swelling of gels. These effects, among other related ones, are ascribable to the abstraction and binding of water by these ions (*i.e.,* hydration), which also decreases in the orders given, so that (in the monovalent cation series) Li^{+}, with the smallest crystal radius, has the largest hydrated radius, and vice versa for Cs^+.

homologous s., a s. of organic compounds, the succeeding members of which differ from each other by the radical CH_2 (as in the fatty series).

lymphocytic s., lymphoid s., the cells at various states in the development in lymphoid tissue of the mature lymphocytes, *e.g.,* lymphoblasts, young lymphocytes, mature lymphocytes.

lyotropic s., Hofmeister s.

myeloid s., the granulocytic and the erythrocytic s.

thrombocytic s., the cells of successive stages in thrombocytic (platelet) development in the bone marrow, *e.g.,* thromboblasts, thrombocytes.

serine (Ser) (ser'ēn). 2-Amino-3-hydroxypropanoic acid; one of the amino acids occurring in proteins.

s. deaminase, *threonine* dehydratase.

s. dehydrase, L-serine dehydratase.

s. diazoacetate, azaserine.

s. sulfhydrase, cystathionine β-synthase.

L-serine dehydratase [EC 4.2.1.13]. L-Hydroxyamino acid dehydratase; serine dehydrase; a deaminating hydro-lyase converting L-serine to pyruvate and NH_3. See also *threonine* dehydratase.

seriograph (sēr'ē-ō-graf) [series + G. *graphō,* to write]. An instrument for taking a series of radiographs; used in cerebral angiography.

seriography (sēr-ē-og'ră-fē). The taking of a series of radiographs by means of the seriograph.

serioscopy (sēr-ē-os'kō-pē) [series + G. *skopeō,* to view]. Formerly, a series of x-rays of a region taken from different directional points and later matched to a target area.

seriscission (ser-i-sish'ŭn) [L. *sericum,* silk, + *scissio,* a cleaving]. Division of the pedicle of a tumor or other tissue by a silk ligature.

sero- [L. *serum,* whey]. Combining form denoting serum, serous.

serocolitis (sēr'ō-kō-lī'tis) [Mod. L. *serosa,* serous membrane, + colitis]. Pericolitis.

seroconversion (sēr'ō-kon-ver'zhŭn). Development of detectable specific antibodies in the serum as a result of infection or immunization.

serocystic (sēr-ō-sis'tik). Relating to one or more serous cysts.

serodiagnosis (sēr'ō-dī-ag-nō'sis). Diagnosis by means of a reaction in the blood serum or other serous fluids in the body.

seroenteritis (sēr'ō-en-ter-ī'tis) [Mod. L. *serosa,* serous membrane, + enteritis]. Perienteritis.

seroepidemiology (sēr'ō-ep-i-dē-mē-ol'ō-jē). Epidemiological study based on the detection of infection by serological testing.

serofast (sēr'ō-fast). Serum-fast.

serofibrinous (sēr-ō-fī'bri-nŭs). Denoting an exudate composed of serum and fibrin.

serofibrous (sēr-ō-fī'brŭs). Relating to a serous membrane and a fibrous tissue.

serologic (sēr-ō-loj'ik). Relating to serology.

serology (sĕ-rol'ō-jē) [sero- + G. *logos,* study]. The branch of science concerned with serum, especially with specific immune or lytic serums.

seroma (sē-rō'mă) [sero- + G. *-oma,* tumor]. A mass or tumefaction caused by the localized accumulation of serum within a tissue or organ.

seromembranous (sēr'ō-mem'bră-nŭs). Relating to a serous membrane.

seromucoid (sēr-ō-myū'koyd). General term for a mucoprotein (glycoprotein) from serum.

acid s., orosomucoid.

seromucous (sēr-ō-myū'kŭs). Pertaining to a mixture of watery and mucinous material, such as that of certain glands.

seronegative (sēr-ō-neg'ă-tiv). Lacking an antibody of a specific type in serum; used to mean absence of prior infection with a specific agent (*e.g.,* rubella virus), disappearance of antibodies after treatment of a disease (*e.g.,* syphilis), or absence of antibody usually found in a given syndrome (*e.g.,* rheumatoid arthritis without rheumatoid factor).

seropositive (sēr-ō-poz'i-tiv). Containing antibody of a specific type in serum; used to indicate presence of immunological evidence of a specific infection (*e.g.,* Lyme disease, syphilis) or presence of a diagnostically useful antibody (*e.g.,* rheumatoid arthritis with rheumatoid factor).

seropurulent (sēr'ō-pū'rū-lent). Composed of or containing both serum and pus; denoting a discharge of thin watery pus (seropus).

seropus (sēr'ō-pŭs). Purulent serum, *i.e.,* pus largely diluted with serum.

serosa, pl. serosae (se-rō'să, -sē) [fem. of Mod. L. *serosus,* serous]. **1.** *Tunica* serosa. **2.** Membrana serosa (2); the outermost of the extraembryonic membranes that encloses the embryo and all its other membranes; it consists of somatopleure, *i.e.,* ectoderm reinforced by somatic mesoderm; the serosa of mammalian embryos is frequently called the trophoderm.

serosamucin (se-rō-să-myū'sin). Mucoid material found in serous fluids, *e.g.,* in ascitic or synovial fluid.

serosanguineous (sēr'ō-sang-gwin'ē-ŭs). Denoting an exudate or a discharge composed of or containing serum and also blood.

seroserous (sēr-ō-sēr'ŭs). **1.** Relating to two serous surfaces. **2.** Denoting a suture, as of the intestine, in which the edges of the wound are infolded so as to bring the two serous surfaces in apposition.

serositis (sēr-ō-sī'tis). Inflammation of a serous membrane.

multiple s., polyserositis.

serosity (se-ros'i-tē). **1.** A serous fluid or a serum. **2.** The condition of being serous. **3.** The serous quality of a liquid.

serosynovial (sēr'ō-si-nō'vē-ăl). Relating to serum and also synovia.

serosynovitis (sēr'ō-sin-ō-vī'tis). Synovitis attended with a copious serous effusion.

serotaxis (sēr-ō-tak'sis) [sero- + G. *taxis,* an arranging]. Edema of the skin induced by the application of a strong cutaneous irritant.

serotherapy (sēr-ō-thār'ă-pē). Serum therapy; treatment of an infectious disease by injection of an antitoxin or specific serum.

serothorax (sēr-ō-thōr'aks). Hydrothorax.

serotina (sēr'ō-tī'nă) [L. fem. of *serotinus,* late]. See under decidua.

serotonergic (sēr-ō-tō-ner'jik, sēr-). Related to the action of serotonin or its precursor tryptophan.

serotonin (sēr-ō-tō'nin). 5-Hydroxytryptamine; enteramine; thrombocytin; thrombotonin; 3-(2-aminoethyl)-5-indolol; a vasoconstrictor, liberated by the blood platelets, that inhibits gastric secretion and stimulates smooth muscle; present in relatively high concentrations in some areas of the central nervous system (hypothalamus, basal ganglia), and occurs in many peripheral tissues and cells and in carcinoid tumors.

serotype (sēr'ō-tīp). Serovar.

serous (sēr'ŭs). Relating to, containing, or producing serum or a substance having a watery consistency.

serovaccination (sēr'ō-vak-si-nā'shŭn). A process for producing mixed immunity by the injection of a serum, to secure passive immunity, and by vaccination with a modified or killed culture to acquire active immunity later.

serovar (sēr'ō-var). Serotype; a subdivision of a species or subspecies distinguishable from other strains therein on the basis of antigenic character.

serozyme (sēr'ō-zīm). Prothrombin.

serpentaria (ser-pen-tā'rē-ă, -tar'ē-ă) [L. snakeweed]. Snakeroot; the dried rhizome and roots of *Aristolochia serpentaria,* Virginia snakeroot, or of *A. reticulata,* Texas snakeroot (family Aristolochiaceae); a stomachic.

serpiginous (ser-pij'i-nŭs) [Mediev. L. *serpigo- (-gin),* ringworm, fr. L. *serpo,* to creep]. Creeping; denoting an ulcer or other cutaneous lesion that extends with an arciform border; the margin has a wavy or serpent-like border.

serpigo (ser-pī'gō) [Mediev. L. *serpigo* (*-gin*), ringworm, fr. L. *serpo,* to creep]. **1.** Tinea. **2.** Herpes. **3.** Any creeping or serpiginous eruption.

serrate, serrated (ser'āt, -ā'ted) [L. *serratus,* fr. *serra,* a saw]. Notched; dentate; toothed.

Serratia (se-rā'shē-ă) [Serafino *Serrati,* 18th century Italian physicist]. A genus of motile, peritrichous, aerobic to facultatively anaerobic bacteria (family Enterobacteriaceae) which contain small, Gram-negative rods. Some strains are encapsulated. Many strains produce a pink, red, or magenta pigment; their metabolism is fermentative and they are saprophytic on decaying plant and animal materials. The type species is *S. marcescens.*
S. marces'cens, a species found in water, soil, milk, foods, and silkworms and other insects; hospital-acquired infection has been reported in patients with impaired immunity; it is the type species of the genus *S.*

serration (se-rā'shŭn) [L. *serra,* saw]. **1.** The state of being serrated or notched. **2.** Any one of the processes in a serrate or dentate formation.

serrefine (ser-e-fēn') [Fr.]. A small spring forceps used for approximating the edges of a wound or for temporarily closing an artery during an operation.

serrenoeud (ser-e-no-ūd') [Fr. *serrer,* to press, + *noeud,* knot]. An instrument for tightening a ligature.

Serres, Antoine E.R.A., French anatomist, 1786–1868. See S.'s *angle, glands.*

serrulate, serrulated (ser'yū-lāt, -lā'ted) [L. *serrula,* a small saw, dim. of *serra*]. Finely serrate.

Sertoli, Enrico, Italian histologist, 1842–1910. See S.'s *cells, columns;* S. cell *tumor.*

serum, pl. **serums, sera** (sēr'ŭm, -ŭmz, -ă) [L. whey]. **1.** A clear watery fluid, especially that moistening the surface of serous membranes, or exuded in inflammation of any of those membranes. **2.** The fluid portion of the blood obtained after removal of the fibrin clot and blood cells, distinguished from the plasma in circulating blood. Sometimes used as a synonym for antiserum or antitoxin.
anticomplementary s., s. that destroys or inactivates complement.
antiepithelial s., an antiserum (cytotoxin) for epithelial cells.
antilymphocyte s. (ALS), antiserum against lymphoid tissue, used to suppress rejection of grafts or organ transplants; when used in man, the globulin fraction of the heterologous s. (prepared in horse or other animals) is usually used in conjunction with other immunosuppressive agents (drugs or chemicals) and for a limited period of time.
antirabies s., a sterile solution containing antiviral substances obtained from the blood s. or plasma of a healthy animal, usually the horse, that has been immunized against rabies by means of vaccine; administered immediately after severe or multiple bites by domestic animals suspected to be rabid and in all wild animal bites, to be followed by a regimen of rabies vaccine.
antireticular cytotoxic s., an antiserum specific for cells of the reticuloendothelial system.
antitoxic s., an antitoxin.
bacteriolytic s., an antiserum (bacteriolysin) that sensitizes a bacterium to the lytic action of complement.
blood s., see s. (2).
convalescent s., s. from patients recently recovered from a disease; useful in preventing or modifying by passive immunization the same disease in exposed susceptible individuals.
Coombs' s., antihuman *globulin.*
dried human s., s. prepared by drying liquid human s. by freeze-drying or by any other method that will avoid denaturation of the proteins and will yield a product readily soluble in a quantity of water equal to the volume of liquid human s. from which it was prepared.
foreign s., a s. derived from an animal and injected into an animal of another species or into man.
human s., see dried human s.; liquid human s.; normal human s.
human measles immune s., measles convalescent s.; obtained from the blood of a healthy person who has survived an attack of measles.
human pertussis immune s., the sterile s. prepared from the pooled blood of healthy adult human beings who have received repeated courses of phase I pertussis vaccine; administered intravenously or intramuscularly for the prophylaxis or treatment of whooping cough.
human scarlet fever immune s., scarlet fever convalescent s.; obtained from healthy persons who have survived an attack of scarlet fever.
immune s., antiserum.
s. lactis, whey.
liquid human s., the pool of fluids separated from blood withdrawn from human subjects and allowed to clot in the absence of any anticoagulant; not more than 10 separate donations are pooled; the contributions from donors of A, O, and either B or AB groups are represented in approximately the ratio 9:9:2.
measles convalescent s., human measles immune s.
muscle s., the fluid remaining after the coagulation of muscle plasma and the separation of myosin.
nonimmune s., a s. from a subject that is not immune; a s. that is free of antibodies to a given antigen.
normal s., a nonimmune s., usually with reference to a s. obtained prior to immunization.
normal horse s., the sterile and filtered s. of a healthy, unvaccinated horse.
normal human s., sterile s. obtained by pooling approximately equal amounts of the liquid portion of coagulated whole blood from eight or more persons who are free from any disease transmissible by transfusion.
polyvalent s., an antiserum obtained by inoculating an animal with several species or strains of the bacterium in question.
pooled s., pooled blood s., the mixed s. from a number of individuals.
salted s., salted *plasma.*
specific s., a monovalent antiserum, *i.e.,* one obtained by inoculating an animal with only one species or strain of the bacterium in question.
thyrotoxic s., an antiserum obtained by injecting into animals the nucleoproteins of the thyroid gland.
truth s., colloquialism for a drug, such as amobarbital sodium or thiopental sodium, intravenously injected for the purpose of eliciting information from the subject under its influence; a misnomer because the subject's revelations may or may not be factually true, and its legal status and use is questionable.

serumal (sēr'ŭm-ăl). Relating to or derived from serum.

serum-fast (sēr'ŭm-fast). Serofast; pertaining to a serum in which there is little or no change in the titer of antibody, even under conditions of treatment or immunologic stimulation.

serum glutamic-oxaloacetic transaminase (SGOT). *Aspartate* aminotransferase.

serum glutamic-pyruvic transaminase (SGPT). Alanine aminotransferase.

servation (ser-vā'shŭn). The use or function of an organ.

Servetus (Servet, Servide), Miguel, Spanish anatomist and theologian, 1511–1553. See S.'s *circulation.*

servomechanism (ser'vō-mek'ă-nizm) [L. *servus,* servant, + G. *mēchanē,* contrivance]. **1.** A control system using negative feedback to operate another system. **2.** A process that behaves as a self-regulatory device; *e.g.,* the reaction of the pupil to light.

seryl (Ser) (ser'il). A radical of serine.

sesame (ses'ă-mē) [G. *sēsamē,* sesame, an eastern leguminous plant]. Benne plant; an herb, *Sesamum indicum* (family Pedaliaceae), the seeds of which are used as a food, and which are the source of sesame oil.

s. oil, benne, gingili, or teel oil; the refined fixed oil obtained from the seed of one or more cultivated varieties of *Sesamum indicum;* a solvent for intramuscular injections.

sesamoid (ses'ă-moyd) [G. *sēsamoeidēs,* like sesame]. **1.** Resembling in size or shape a grain of sesame. **2.** Denoting the sesamoid bone (*os* sesamoideum).

sesamoiditis (ses-ă-moy-dī'tis). Inflammation of the proximal sesamoid bones in the horse.

sesqui- [L.]. Prefix denoting $1^1/_2$; at one time used in chemistry to indicate a ratio of 3 to 2 between the two parts of a compound (*e.g.,* sesquisulfide, sesquibasic), but presently used only for sesquihydrates.

sesquihydrates (ses-kwi-hī'drāts). Compounds crystallizing with (nominally) 1.5 molecules of water.

sessile (ses'il) [L. *sessilis,* low-growing, fr. *sedeo,* pp. *sessus,* to sit]. Having a broad base of attachment; not pedunculated.

set. 1. A readiness to perceive or to respond in some way; an attitude which facilitates or predetermines an outcome; *e.g.,* prejudice or bigotry as a s. to respond independently of the merits of the stimulus. **2.** To reduce a fracture; *i.e.,* to bring the bones back into a normal position or alignment.

learning s., a readiness or predisposition to learn developed from previous learning experiences, as when an organism learns to solve each successive problem (of equal or increasing difficulty) in fewer trials.

postural s., an overall motor readiness to respond, as in a runner instructed to get set and on the mark.

seta, pl. **setae** (sē'tă, -tē) [L. *saeta* or *seta,* a stiff hair or bristle]. Chaeta; a bristle or a slender, stiff, bristle-like structure.

setaceous (sē-tā'shŭs) [L. *seta,* a bristle]. **1.** Having bristles. **2.** Resembling a bristle.

Setaria (sē-tā'rē-ă, -tar'ē-ă) [L. *seta,* a bristle]. A nematode genus of the family Stephanofilariidae (superfamily Filarioidea). Adults are long and thin, typically occur in the peritoneal cavity, and produce sheathed microfilariae in the blood that are transmitted to other hosts after cyclical development in appropriate mosquito hosts. They are parasitic in cattle or equines (wild or domestic) and generally are nonpathogenic, although occasionally young worms may wander into the anterior chamber of the eye.

S. cer'vi, a species that occurs in the abdominal cavity of cattle, buffalo, bison, yak, and various deer, but rarely in sheep.

S. equi'na, a species that is a common parasite of horses and other equids in all parts of the world; they are slender whitish filaments, several inches in length, usually found free in the peritoneal cavity, but occasionally reported in the pleural cavity, lungs, scrotum, eye, and intestine.

setariasis (sē'tā-rē-ā'-sis). An infection with filarial parasites of the genus *Setaria,* usually of little pathogenic significance; aberrant migration in horses, sheep, and goats can lead to paralysis and blindness.

setback (set'bak). A surgical operation for treatment of a bilateral cleft of the palate in which the premaxilla is moved posteriorly; the procedure is often accompanied by bone grafting.

setiferous (sē-tif'er-ŭs) [L. *seta,* bristle, + *fero,* to carry]. Setigerous; bristly or having bristles.

setigerous (sē-tij'er-ŭs) [L. *seta,* bristle, + *gero,* to bear]. Setiferous.

seton (sē'tŏn) [L. *seta,* bristle]. A wisp of threads, a strip of gauze, a length of wire, or other foreign material passed through the subcutaneous tissues or a cyst to form a sinus or fistula.

set'ting. Hardening, as of amalgam.

set-up. 1. The arrangement of teeth on a trial denture base. **2.** A procedure in dental case analysis involving cutting off and repositioning of teeth in the desired positions on a plaster cast.

Severinghaus, John W., U.S. physiologist and anesthesiologist, *1922. See S. *electrode.*

sevoflurane (sev-ō-flūr'ān). Fluoromethyl 2,2,2-trifluoro-1-(trifluoromethyl)ethyl ether; a halogenated ether for inhalation anesthesia.

sevum (sē'vŭm) [L.]. Suet or tallow.

sex (seks) [L. *sexus*]. **1.** The biological character or quality that distinguishes male and female from one another as expressed by analysis of the individual's gonadal, morphological (internal and external), chromosomal, and hormonal characteristics. *Cf.* gender. **2.** The physiological and psychological processes within an individual which prompt behavior related to procreation and/or erotic pleasure.

sexdigitate (seks-dij'i-tāt) [L. *sex,* six, + *digitus,* finger or toe]. Sedigitate; having six digits on one or both hands or feet.

sexduction (seks'dŭk-shŭn). F *duction.*

sex-influenced. Denoting a class of genetic disorders in which the same genotype has differing manifestations in the two sexes; the variation may be rational (*e.g.,* breast cancer occurs less frequently in males) or have only empirical support (*e.g.,* pattern baldness behaves as a dominant trait in the male and as a recessive trait in the female). See also sex-influenced *inheritance.*

sexivalent (sek-sĭ-vā'lent, sek-siv'ă-lent) [L. *sex,* six, + *valencia,* strength]. Having a valence of six.

sex-limited. Occurring in one sex only. See sex-limited *inheritance.*

sex-linked. See sex *linkage;* sex-linked *gene.*

sexology (sek-sol'ō-jē) [L. *sexus,* sex, + G. *logos,* study]. The study of all aspects of sex and, in particular, sexual behavior.

sextan (seks'tăn) [L. *sextus,* sixth]. Denoting a malarial fever the paroxysms of which recur every sixth day, counting the day of the episode as the first.

sexual (sek'shū-ăl) [L. *sexualis,* fr. *sexus,* sex]. **1.** Relating to sex; erotic; genital. **2.** A person considered in his or her s. relations or tendencies.

contrary s., a homosexual.

sexuality (sek-shū-al'i-tē). **1.** The sum of a person's sexual behaviors and tendencies, and the strength of such tendencies. **2.** One's degree of sexual attractiveness. **3.** The quality of having sexual functions or implications.

infantile s., in psychoanalytic personality theory, the concept concerning psychosexual development in infants and children; encompasses the overlapping oral, anal, and phallic phases during the first five years of life.

sexualization (sek'shū-ăl-i-zā'shŭn). **1.** The state characterized by the presence of sexual energy or drive. **2.** The act of acquiring sexual energy or drive.

sexual preference. The biologic sex preferred in one's sexual partners.

Sézary, A., French dermatologist, 1880–1956. See S. *cell, erythroderma, syndrome.*

S.G.O. Abbreviation for Surgeon General's Office.

SGOT Abbreviation for serum glutamic-oxaloacetic transaminase.

SGPT Abbreviation for serum glutamic-pyruvic transaminase.

SH Abbreviation for serum *hepatitis.*

shadow (shad'ō). **1.** A surface area defined by the interception of light rays by a body. See also density (3). **2.** In jungian psychology, the archetype consisting of collective animal instincts. **3.** Achromocyte.
Gumprecht's s.'s, smudge *cells.*
Ponfick's s., achromocyte.

shadow-casting. Deposition of a film of carbon or certain metals such as palladium, platinum, or chromium on a contoured microscopic object in order to allow the object to be seen in relief with the electron microscope or sometimes with the light microscope.

Shaffer, A., U.S. biochemist, 1881–1960. See S.-Hartman *method.*

shaft [A.S. *sceaft*] An elongated rodlike structure, as the part of a long bone between the epiphysial extremities.
s. of femur, *corpus* ossis femoris.
hair s., *scapus* pili.
s. of humerus, *corpus* humeri.
s. of radius, *corpus* radii.
s. of tibia, *corpus* tibiae.

shank [A.S. *sceanca*] **1.** The tibia; the shin; the leg. **2.** The portion of an instrument that connects the cutting or functional portion to a handle; with rotary tools, such as burrs and drills, the end that fits into the chuck.

shaping (shāp'ing). In operant conditioning, when the operant is not in the organism's repertoire, a procedure in which the experimenter breaks down the operant into those parts which appear most frequently, begins reinforcing them, and then slowly and successively withholds the reinforcer until more and more of the operant is emitted.

shark liver oil. Oil extracted from the livers of sharks, mainly of the species *Hypoprion brevirostris;* a rich source of vitamins A and D.

Sharpey, William, Scottish physiologist and histologist, 1802–1880. See S.'s *fibers.*

Sharpey-Schäfer. See Schäfer.

Shaver, Cecil Gordon, Canadian physician, *1901. See S.'s *disease.*

shear (shēr) [A.S.]. The distortion of a body by two oppositely directed parallel forces. The distortion consists of a sliding over one another of imaginary planes (within the body) parallel to the planes of the forces.

shears (shērz). Scissors.
Liston's s., strong s. for cutting plaster of Paris bandages.

sheath (shēth) [A.S. *scaeth*] **1.** Any enveloping structure, such as the membranous covering of a muscle, nerve, or blood vessel. **2.** Vagina (1). **3.** The prepuce of male animals, especially of the horse. **4.** A specially designed tubular instrument through which special obturators or cutting instruments can be passed, or through which blood clots, tissue fragments, calculi, etc. can be evacuated. **5.** A tube used as an orthodontic appliance, usually on molars.
carotid s., *vagina* carotica.
caudal s., a group of microtubules arranged cylindrically around the caudal pole of the nucleus in a developing spermatozoon.
common flexor s., *vagina* communis musculorum flexorum.
crural s., femoral s.
dentinal s., Neumann's s.; a layer of tissue relatively resistant to the action of acids, which forms the walls of the dentinal tubules.
dural s., an extension of the dura mater which ensheathes the roots of spinal nerves or, more particularly, the vagina externa nervi optici.
enamel rod s., organic covering of the individual enamel rod.
s. of eyeball, *vagina* bulbi.
femoral s., crural or infundibuliform s.; the fascia enclosing the femoral vessels, formed by the fascia transversalis anteriorly and the fascia iliaca posteriorly; two septa divide the s. into three compartments, the lateral of which contains the femoral artery and the femoral branch of the genitofemoral nerve, the middle the femoral vein, and the medial is the femoral canal.
fenestrated s., a s. with a window cut in the tip or lateral convexity, through which special cutting instruments can be passed.
fibrous s.'s, see entries under *vagina* fibrosa.
Henle's s., endoneurium.
Hertwig's s., the merged outer and inner epithelial layers of the enamel organ which extends beyond the region of the anatomical crown and initiates formation of dentin in the root of a developing tooth; it atrophies as the root is formed, and any of the cells that persist are called Malassez' epithelial rests.
Huxley's s., Huxley's *layer.*
infundibuliform s., femoral s.
intertubercular s., *vagina* intertubercularis.
s. of Key and Retzius, endoneurium.
Mauthner's s., axolemma.
medullary s., myelin s.
microfilarial s., the membrane surrounding the embryos of certain blood-borne microfilariae, such as *Wuchereria, Brugia,* and *Loa* of man; thought to be derived from the vitelline membrane.
mitochondrial s., the spirally arranged mitochondria in the middle piece of a spermatozoon.
mucous s. of tendon, *vagina* synovialis tendinis.
myelin s., medullary s.; the lipoproteinaceous envelope in vertebrates surrounding most axons of more than 0.5-μm diameter; it consists of a double plasma membrane wound tightly around the axon in a variable number of turns, and supplied by oligodendroglia cells (in the brain and spinal cord) or Schwann cells (in peripheral nerves); unwound, the double membrane would appear as a sheetlike cell expansion that is empty of cytoplasm but for a few narrow cytoplasmic strands corresponding to apparent interruptions of the regular myelin structure, the incisures of Schmidt-Lanterman; the myelin s. of each axon is composed of a fairly regular longitudinal sequence of segments, each corresponding to the length of s. supplied by a single oligodendroglia or Schwann cell; in the short interval between each two neighboring segments, the nodes of Ranvier, the axon is unmyelinated even though enclosed by complex finger-like plasmatic expansions of the neighboring oligodendroglia or Schwann cells.
Neumann's s., dentinal s.
notochordal s., the fibrous outer covering of the notochord.
resectoscope s., an operative s. through which transurethral electroresection of bladder tumors or prostate gland can be performed.

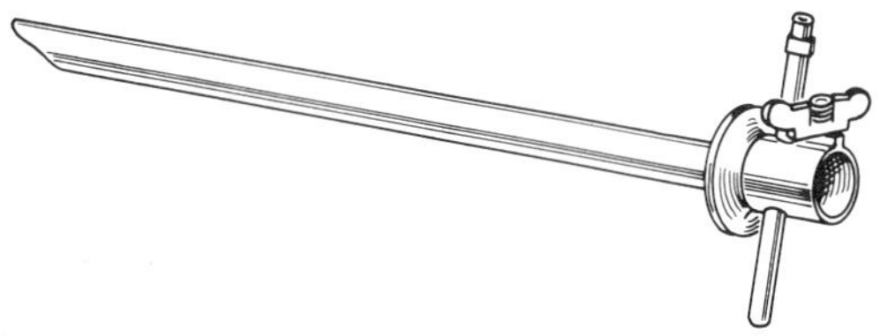

Resectoscope Sheath With Terminal Fenestra

root s., one of the epidermic layers of the hair follicle: external **r. s.** is continuous with the stratum basale and stratum spinosum of the epidermis; internal **r. s.** comprises the cuticle of the internal roots, Huxley's layer, and Henle's layer.
Rouget-Neumann s., the amorphous ground substance between an osteocyte and the lacunar or canalicular wall.

Scarpa's s., *fascia* cremasterica.
s. of Schwann, neurilemma.
s. of Schweigger-Seidel, ellipsoid.
s. of styloid process, *vagina* processus styloidei.
s. of superior oblique muscle, *vagina* musculorum obliqui superioris.
synovial s., see entries under *vagina* synovialis.
synovial s.'s of digits of foot, *vaginae* synoviales digitorum pedis.
synovial s.'s of digits of hand, *vaginae* synoviales digitorum manus.
tail s., the protoplasmic envelope in the tail of a spermatozoon.
s.'s of vessels, *vaginae* vasorum.
Waldeyer's s., Waldeyer's space; the tubular space between the bladder wall and the intramural portion of the ureter as it courses obliquely through this structure; actually a space and not a true s.

Sheehan, H.L., 20th century British pathologist. See S.'s *syndrome.*

sheep-pox (shēp'poks). Ovinia; a highly contagious disease of sheep, chiefly in parts of Asia, Africa, the Middle East, and southern Europe, caused by the sheep-pox virus.

Sheldon, J.H. See Freeman-S. *syndrome.*

shelf. In anatomy, a structure resembling a shelf.
Blumer's s., rectal s.
dental s., dental *ledge.*
palatal s., a medially directed outgrowth of the embryonic maxilla; when fused with its opposite number it forms the secondary palate.
rectal s., Blumer's s.; a s. palpable by rectal examination, due to metastatic tumor cells gravitating from an abdominal cancer and growing in the rectovesical or rectouterine pouch.
vocal s., *plica* vocalis.

shell. An outer covering.
cytotrophoblastic s., the external layer of fetally derived trophoblastic cells on the maternal surface of the placenta.
diffusion s., a small vessel made of a semipermeable membrane through which peptone, but not serum albumin, can pass; used in performing the Abderhalden test.

shellac (shĕ-lak'). Lacca; a resinous excretion of an insect, *Laccifer (Tachardia) lacca* (family Coccidae). The insects suck the juice of various resiniferous Asiatic (chiefly Indian) trees and excrete and deposit "stick-lac." S. softens at a low temperature. It has many nonmedicinal uses and is also used to coat confections and tablets and in dental materials, *e.g.,* impression compound and denture base plates.

Shenton, Edward W.H., British radiologist, 1872–1955. See S.'s *line.*

Shepherd, Francis J., Canadian surgeon, 1851–1929. See S.'s *fracture.*

Sherman, Henry C., U.S. biochemist, 1875–1955. See S. *unit;* S.-Bourquin *unit* of vitamin B_2; S.-Munsell *unit.*

Sherrington, Charles, British physiologist and Nobel laureate, 1857–1952. See S. *phenomenon;* S.'s *law;* Schiff-S. *phenomenon;* Liddell-S. *reflex.*

shield (shēld) [A.S. *scild*]. A protecting screen; lead sheet for protecting the operator from x-rays.
embryonic s., a thickened area of the embryonic blastoderm within which the primitive streak appears.
nipple s., a cap or dome placed over the nipple to protect it during nursing.
oral s.'s, removable appliances used in orthodontic treatment, usually placed between the labial and buccal mucosa and the teeth.

shift. Transfer; change. See also deviation.
antigenic s., sudden and major changes (mutation) in the antigenic structure of a virus, occurring at longer intervals than with antigenic drift and associated with pandemics.
axis s., axis *deviation.*
chloride s., Hamburger's phenomenon; when CO_2 enters the blood from the tissues, it passes into the red blood cell and is converted by carbonate dehydratase to carbonic acid (H_2CO_3); HCO_3^- ion passes out into the plasma while Cl^- migrates into the red blood cell. Reverse changes occur in the lungs when CO_2 is eliminated from the blood.
Doppler s., the magnitude of the frequency change in hertz when sound and observer are in relative motion away from or toward each other. See also Doppler *effect.*
s. to the left, **(1)** deviation to the left; a marked increase in the percentage of immature cells in the circulating blood, based on the premise in hematology that the bone marrow with its immature myeloid cells is on the left, while the circulating blood with its mature neutrophils is on the right; **(2)** see maturation *index.*
luteoplacental s., the change in site of production of the estrogen and progesterone essential for human pregnancy from the corpus luteum to the placenta; ovariectomy always terminates pregnancy in most mammals because their placentas never produce enough estrogen and progesterone, but, after the sixth week of pregnancy, a human placenta can produce enough of these hormones to prevent abortion despite ovariectomy.
Purkinje s., Purkinje's *phenomenon.*
s. to the right, **(1)** deviation to the right; in a differential count of white blood cells in the peripheral blood, the absence of young and immature forms; **(2)** see maturation *index.*
threshold s., measurement of the degree of hearing loss or impairment in terms of a decibel s. from an individual's previous audiogram.

Shiga, Kiyoshi, Japanese bacteriologist, 1870–1957. See *Shigella;* S. *bacillus;* S.-Kruse *bacillus.*

Shigella (shē-gel'lă) [K. *Shiga*] A genus of nonmotile, aerobic to facultatively anaerobic bacteria (family Enterobacteriaceae) containing Gram-negative nonencapsulated rods. These organisms cannot use citrate as a sole source of carbon; their growth is inhibited by potassium cyanide and their metabolism is fermentative; they ferment glucose and other carbohydrates with the production of acid but not gas; lactose is ordinarily not fermented, although it is sometimes slowly attacked; the normal habitat is the intestinal tract of humans and of higher monkeys; all of the species produce dysentery. The type species is *S. dysenteriae.*
S. boy'dii, a species found only in feces of symptomatic individuals; occurs in a low proportion of cases of bacillary dysentery.
S. dysenter'iae, Shiga or Shiga-Kruse bacillus; a species causing dysentery in humans and in monkeys, found only in feces of symptomatic individuals; the type species of the genus *S.*
S. flexne'ri, Flexner's bacillus; paradysentery bacillus; *S. paradysenteriae;* a species found in the feces of symptomatic individuals and of convalescents or carriers; the most common cause of dysentery epidemics and sometimes of infantile gastroenteritis.
S. paradysenter'iae, *S. flexneri.*
S. son'nei, Sonne bacillus; a species causing mild dysentery and also summer diarrhea in children.

shigellosis (shig-ĕ-lō'sis). Bacillary dysentery caused by bacteria of the genus *Shigella,* often occurring in epidemic patterns.

shikimate dehydrogenase (shi-kim'āt) [EC 1.1.1.25]. An oxidoreductase reducing 3-dehydroshikimic acid to shikimic acid, by transfer of hydrogens from NADPH, in phenylalanine and tyrosine biosynthesis.

shikimic acid (shi-kim'ik). $3\alpha,4\alpha,5\beta$-Trihydroxy-1-cyclohexene-1-carboxylic acid, a cyclic trihydroxy acid that acts as an intermediate in the bacterial synthesis of phenylalanine and tyrosine.

shin [A.S. *scina*] Cnemis; the anterior portion of the leg.
saber s., the sharp-edged anteriorly convex tibia in congenital syphilis.

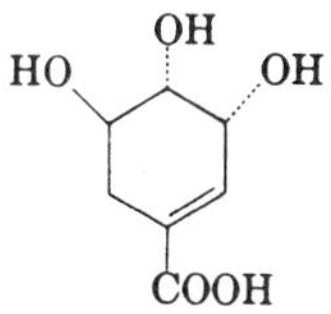

Shikimic acid

sore s.'s, a condition seen most frequently in young thoroughbred horses during early training, and characterized by periostitis of the dorsal surface of the third metacarpal or metatarsal bone.
toasted s.'s, *erythema* caloricum.

shingles (shing'glz) [L. *cingulum,* girdle]. *Herpes* zoster.

shin-splints. Tenderness and pain with induration and swelling of pretibial muscles, following athletic overexertion by the untrained; it may be a mild form of anterior tibial compartment syndrome.

ship. A structure resembling the hull of a ship.
Fabricius' s., the outlines of the sphenoid, occipital, and frontal bones, from their fancied resemblance to the hull of a s.

Shipley, Walter C., U.S. psychiatrist, *1903. See S.-Hartford *scale.*

Shirodkar, N.V., Indian obstetrician and gynecologist, 1900–1971. See S. *operation.*

shiv'er. **1.** To shake or tremble, especially from cold. **2.** A tremor; a slight chill.

shiv'ering. **1.** Trembling from cold or fear. **2.** A spasmodic affection, resembling chorea, affecting the thigh muscles of the horse.

shoat (shōt). Shote; a young hog.

shock (shok). **1.** A sudden physical or mental disturbance. **2.** A state of profound mental and physical depression consequent upon severe physical injury or an emotional disturbance. **3.** The abnormally palpable impact, appreciated by a hand on the chest wall, of an accentuated heart sound. See diastolic and systolic s.
anaphylactic s., a severe, often fatal form of s. characterized by smooth muscle contraction and capillary dilation initiated by cytotropic (IgE class) antibodies; typically an antibody-associated phenomenon that does not occur in sensitivities of the delayed kind (type IV allergic reaction). See also anaphylaxis; serum *sickness.*
anaphylactoid s., anaphylactoid crisis; pseudoanaphylactic s.; a reaction that is similar to anaphylactic s., but which does not require the incubation period characteristic of induced sensitivity (anaphylaxis); it may result from intravenous injection of serum that is pretreated with kaolin or starch, trypsin, organic colloids, peptone, or other materials; it is unrelated to antigen-antibody reactions.
anesthetic s., s. produced by the administration of anesthetic drug(s), usually in relative overdosage.
break s., the s. produced by breaking a constant current passing through the body.
cardiogenic s., s. resulting from decline in cardiac output secondary to serious heart disease, usually myocardial infarction.
chronic s., the state of peripheral circulatory insufficiency developing in elderly patients with a debilitating disease, *e.g.,* carcinoma; a subnormal blood volume makes the patient susceptible to hemorrhagic s. as a result of even a moderate blood loss such as may occur during an operation.
counter-s., see countershock.
cultural s., a form of stress associated with the beginning of an individual's assimilation into a new culture vastly different from that in which he was raised.
declamping s., declamping *phenomenon.*
deferred s., delayed s., a state of s. coming on at a considerable interval after the receipt of the injury.
delirious s., erethistic s.
diastolic s., the abnormally palpable impact, appreciated by a hand on the chest wall, of an accentuated second heart sound.
electric s., a sudden violent impression caused by the passage of a current of electricity through any portion of the body.
endotoxin s., s. produced by bacterial endotoxins, especially of *Escherichia coli.*
erethistic s., delirious s.; traumatic or toxic delirium following s.
hemorrhagic s., hypovolemic s. resulting from acute hemorrhage, characterized by hypotension, tachycardia, pale, cold, and clammy skin, and oliguria.
histamine s., the s. state produced in animals by the injection of histamine; characterized by bronchiolar spasm in the guinea pig and constriction of hepatic veins in the dog.
hypovolemic s., s. caused by a reduction in volume of blood, as from hemorrhage or dehydration.
insulin s., wet s.; severe hypoglycemia produced by administration of insulin, manifested by sweating, tremor, anxiety, vertigo, and diplopia, followed by delirium, convulsions, and collapse.
irreversible s., s. that has progressed beyond the stage when it will respond to transfusion or other form of treatment, and recovery is impossible.
nitroid s., a syndrome resembling that produced by the administration of a large dose of a nitrite, sometimes caused by a too rapid intravenous injection of arsphenamine or some other drug.
oligemic s., s. associated with pronounced fall in blood volume, sometimes resulting from increased permeability of blood vessels.
osmotic s., a sudden change in the osmotic pressure to which a cell (or virus particle) is subjected, usually in order to cause it to lyse and lose its contents.
primary s., s. mainly nervous in nature, from pain, anxiety, etc., which ensues almost immediately upon the receipt of a severe injury.
protein s., the systemic reaction following the parenteral administration of a protein.
reversible s., s. that will respond to treatment and from which recovery is possible.
septic s., **(1)** s. associated with sepsis, usually associated with abdominal and pelvic infection complicating trauma or operations; **(2)** s. associated with septicemia caused by Gram-negative bacteria.
serum s., anaphylactic or anaphylactoid s. caused by the injection of antitoxic or other foreign serum.
shell s., battle *fatigue.*
spinal s., transient depression or abolition of reflex activity below the level of an acute spinal cord injury or transection.
systolic s., the abnormally palpable impact, appreciated by a hand on the chest wall, of an accentuated first heart sound.
toxic s., see toxic shock *syndrome.*
vasogenic s., s. resulting from depressed activity of the higher vasomotor centers in the brain stem and the medulla, producing vasodilation without loss of fluid so that the container is disproportionately large. In oligemic s., blood volume is reduced; in both, return of venous blood is inadequate.
wet s., insulin s.

Shone, John D. See S.'s *anomaly.*

shook jong (shuk-yong'). Koro.

Shope, Richard E., U.S. pathologist, *1902. See S. *fibroma,* fibroma *virus.*

shortsightedness (shōrt'sīt-ed-nes). Myopia.

shote (shōt). Shoat.

shot-feel (shot'fēl). A peculiar sensation as of a nervous discharge or electric shock passing rapidly from the top of the head to the feet, sometimes described as a sensation of rolling of shot down the body, occurring in acromegaly.

shoulder (shōl'der) [A.S. *sculder*]. **1.** The lateral portion of the scapular region, where the scapula joins with the clavicle and humerus

and is covered by the rounded mass of the deltoid muscle. **2.** In dentistry, the ledge formed by the junction of the gingival and axial walls in extracoronal restorative preparations.
frozen s., adhesive *capsulitis.*

shoulder blade (shōl'der blād). Scapula.

show (shō) [A.S. *sceáwe*]. An appearance. **1.** First appearance of blood in beginning menstruation. **2.** Sign of impending labor, characterized by the discharge from the vagina of a small amount of blood-tinged mucus representing the extrusion of the mucous plug which has filled the cervical canal during pregnancy.

Shrapnell, Henry J., British anatomist, 1761–1841. See S.'s *membrane.*

shudder (shŭd'er). A convulsive or involuntary tremor.
carotid s., vibrations at the height of the carotid pulse tracing, seen in aortic stenosis.

Shulman, Lawrence E., U.S. rheumatologist, *1919. See S.'s *syndrome.*

shunt (shŭnt). Bypass. **1.** To bypass or divert. **2.** A bypass or diversion of accumulations of fluid to an absorbing or excreting system by fistulation or a mechanical device. The nomenclature commonly includes origin and terminus, *e.g.,* atriovenous, splenorenal, ventriculocisternal. See also bypass.
arteriovenous s., the passage of blood directly from arteries to veins, without going through the capillary network.
Denver s., LeVeen-type s. with an implanted, valved, manually compressible chamber used to determine and maintain patency.
dialysis s., arteriovenous s. connecting the arterial and venous cannulas in arm or leg.
Dickens s., pentose phosphate *pathway.*
distal splenorenal s., Warren s.
H s., H graft; a side-to-side s. between adjacent vessels which utilizes a connecting conduit.
hexose monophosphate s., pentose phosphate *pathway.*
jejunoileal s., jejunoileal *bypass.*
left-to-right s., a diversion of blood from the left side of the heart to right (as through a septal defect), or from the systemic circulation to the pulmonary (as through a patent ductus arteriosus).
LeVeen s., a plastic tube used to transport ascitic fluid from the abdomen, via a jugular vein, to the superior vena cava.
mesocaval s., **(1)** anastomosis of the side of the superior mesenteric vein to the proximal end of the divided inferior vena cava, for control of portal hypertension; **(2)** H-shunt anastomosis of the inferior vena cava to the superior mesenteric vein, using a synthetic conduit or autologous vein.
peritoneovenous s., a s., usually by a catheter, between the peritoneal cavity and the venous system.
portacaval s., **(1)** surgical anastomosis between portal and systemic veins; **(2)** surgical anastomosis between the portal vein and the vena cava, as in an Eck fistula.
portasystemic s., a s. between any parts of the portal and systemic venous systems, including portacaval, mesocaval, splenorenal s.'s or spontaneously occurring s.'s.
Rapoport-Luebering s., part of the glycolytic pathway characteristic of human erythrocytes in which 2,3-diphosphoglycerate (2,3-P_2Gri) is formed as an intermediate between 1,3-P_2Gri and 3-phosphoglycerate; 2,3-P_2Gri is an important regulator of the affinity of hemoglobin for oxygen.
renal-splenic venous s., splenorenal s.
reversed s., right-to-left s.
right-to-left s., reversed s.; the passage of blood from the right side of the heart into the left (as through a septal defect), or from the pulmonary artery into the aorta (as through a patent ductus arteriosus); such a shunt can occur only when the pressure on the right side exceeds that in the left, as in advanced pulmonic stenosis, or when the pulmonary artery pressure exceeds aortic pressure, as in one form of Eisenmenger's syndrome or in tricuspid atresia.
Scribner s., connection of an artery, customarily the radial, to the cephalic vein via a short extracorporeal catheter.
splenorenal s., renal-splenic venous s.; anastomosis of the splenic vein to the left renal vein, usually end-to-side, for control of portal hypertension.
Torkildsen s., a ventriculocisternal s.; see s. (2).
Warburg-Lipmann-Dickens s., pentose-phosphate *pathway.*
Warren s., distal splenorenal s.; anastomosis of the splenic end of the divided splenic vein to the left renal vein.
Waterston s., creation of a narrow (about 3 mm) opening between the ascending aorta and the subjacent right pulmonary artery to increase pulmonary circulation in cyanotic heart disease with decreased pulmonary flow.

Shwartzman, Gregory, Russian bacteriologist in U.S., 1896–1965. See S. *phenomenon, reaction;* generalized S. *phenomenon;* Sanarelli-S. *phenomenon.*

Shy, G. Milton, U.S. neurologist, 1919–1967. See S.-Drager *syndrome.*

SI Abbreviation for International System of Units (Système International d'Unités).

Si Symbol for silicon.

SIADH Abbreviation for *syndrome* of inappropriate secretion of antidiuretic hormone.

siagonantritis (sī'ă-gon-an-trī'tis) [G. *siagōn,* jaw, + *antron,* cave, + *-itis,* inflammation]. Inflammation of the maxillary sinus.

sial-. See sialo-.

sialaden (sī-al'ă-den) [sial- + G. *adēn,* gland]. A salivary gland.

sialadenitis (sī'al-ad-ĕ-nī'tis) [sial- + G. *adēn,* gland, + *-itis,* inflammation]. Sialoadenitis; inflammation of a salivary gland.

sialadenoncus (si'al-ad-ĕ-nong'kŭs) [sial- + G. *adēn,* gland, + *onkos,* bulk (tumor)]. A neoplasm of salivary tissue.

sialadenosis (sī'al-ad-ĕ-nō'sis) [sial- + G. *aden,* gland, + *-osis,* condition]. Enlargement of the salivary glands, usually the parotids; seen in alcoholism, malnutrition, and other conditions.

sialadenotropic (sī'al-ad'ĕ-nō-trop'ik) [sial- + G. *adēn,* gland, + *tropē,* a turning]. Having an influence on the salivary glands.

sialagogue (sī-al'ă-gog) [sial- + G. *agōgos,* drawing forth]. Sialogogue; ptyalagogue. **1.** Promoting the flow of saliva. **2.** An agent having this action.

sialaporia (sī'al-ă-pō'rē-ă) [sial- + G. *aporia,* difficulty of passage]. A deficient secretion of saliva.

sialectasis (sī'ă-lek'tă-sis) [sial- + G. *ektasis,* a stretching]. Ptyalectasis; dilation of a salivary duct.

sialemesis, sialemesia (sī'al-em'ĕ-sis, -ĕ-mē'zē-ă) [sial- + G. *emesis,* vomiting]. Vomiting of saliva, or vomiting caused by or accompanying an excessive secretion of saliva.

sialic (sī-al'ik). Salivary.

sialic acids (sī-al'ik). Esters and other *N-* and *O-*acyl derivatives of neuraminic acid; radicals of s. a. are sialoyl, if the OH of the COOH is removed, and sialosyl, if the OH comes from the anomeric carbon (C-2) of the cyclic structure.

sialidase (sī-al'i-dās) [EC 3.2.1.18]. Neuraminidase; an enzyme that cleaves terminal acylneuraminic residues from oligosaccharides, glycoproteins, or glycolipids; present as a surface antigen in myxoviruses; used in histochemistry to selectively remove sialomucins, as from bronchial mucous glands and the small intestine.

sialidosis (sī-al-i-dō'sis). Cherry-red spot myoclonus *syndrome.*

sialine (sī'ă-lēn). Salivary.

sialism, sialismus (sī'ă-lizm, sī'ă-liz'mŭs) [G. *sialismos*]. Ptyalism; hygrostomia; salivation; sialorrhea; sialosis; an excess secretion of saliva.

sialo-, sial- [G. *sialon,* saliva]. Combining forms denoting saliva, salivary glands. See also ptyal-.

sialoadenectomy (sī'ă-lō-ad-ĕ-nek'tō-mē) [sialo- + G. *adēn,* gland, + *ektomē,* excision]. Excision of a salivary gland.

sialoadenitis (sī'ă-lō-ad-ĕ-nī'tis). Sialadenitis.

sialoadenotomy (sī'ă-lō-ad-ĕ-not'ō-mē) [sialo- + G. *adēn,* gland, + *tomē,* incision]. Incision of a salivary gland.

sialoaerophagy (sī'ă-lō-ār-of'ă-jē) [sialo- + G. *aēr,* air, + *phagein,* to eat]. Aerosialophagy; a habit of frequent swallowing whereby quantities of saliva and air are taken into the stomach.

sialoangiectasis (sī'ă-lō-an-jē-ek'tă-sis) [sialo- + G. *angeion,* vessel, + *ektasis,* a stretching]. Dilation of salivary ducts.

sialoangiitis (sī'ă-lō-an-jē-ī'tis) [sialo- + G. *angeion,* vessel, + *-itis,* inflammation]. Inflammation of a salivary duct.

sialocele (sī'ă-lō-sēl) [sialo- + G. *kēlē,* tumor]. Ranula (2).

sialodochitis (sī'ă-lō-dō-kī'tis) [sialo- + G. *dochē,* receptacle, + *-itis,* inflammation]. Inflammation of the duct of a salivary gland.

sialodochoplasty (sī'ă-lō-dō'kō-plas'tē) [sialo- + G. *dochē,* receptacle, + *plassō,* to fashion]. Repair of a salivary duct.

sialogenous (sī'ă-loj'ĕ-nŭs) [sialo- + G. *-gen,* producing]. Producing saliva. See also sialagogue.

sialogogue (sī-al'ă-gog). Sialagogue.

sialogram (sī-al'ō-gram) [sialo- + G. *gramma,* a writing]. The recorded display following sialography.

sialography (sī-ă-log'ră-fē) [sialo- + G. *graphō,* to write]. Ptyalography; x-ray examination of the salivary glands and ducts after the introduction of a radiopaque material into the ducts.

sialolith (sī'ă-lō-lith) [sialo- + G. *lithos,* stone]. Ptyalolith; a salivary calculus.

sialolithiasis (sī'ă-lō-li-thī'ă-sis) [sialolith + G. *-iasis,* condition]. Ptyalolithiasis; salivolithiasis; the formation or presence of a salivary calculus.

sialolithotomy (sī'ă-lō-li-thot'ō-mē) [sialolith + G. *tomē,* incision]. Ptyalolithotomy; incision of a salivary duct or gland to remove a calculus.

sialometaplasia (sī'ă-lō-met-ă-plā'zē-ă). Squamous cell metaplasia in the salivary ducts.
necrotizing s., squamous metaplasia of the salivary gland ducts and lobules, with ischemic necrosis of the salivary gland lobules; seen most frequently in the hard palate.

sialometry (sī-ă-lom'ĕ-trē) [sialo- + G. *metron,* measure]. A measurement of salivary secretion function, generally for a comparison of a denervated or diseased gland with its healthy counterpart.

sialorrhea (sī'ă-lō-rē'ă) [sialo- + G. *rhoia,* a flow]. Sialism.

sialoschesis (sī'ă-los'kĕ-sis) [sialo- + G. *schesis,* retention]. Suppression of the secretion of saliva.

sialosemiology, sialosemeiology (sī-ă-lō-sē-mē-ol'ō-jē) [sialo- + G. *sēmeion,* sign, + *logos,* study]. The study and analysis of saliva as an aid to diagnosis.

sialosis (sī'ă-lō'sis). Sialism.

sialostenosis (sī'ă-lō-ste-nō'sis) [sialo- + G. *stenōsis,* a narrowing]. Stricture of a salivary duct.

sialosyrinx (sī'ă-lō-sir'ingks) [sialo- + G. *syrinx,* a pipe, fistula]. A salivary fistula; a pathologic communication between the outside via the skin or the oral tissues and the salivary gland or duct.

sib. A member of a sibship.

sibilant (sib'i-lănt) [L. *sibilans (-ant-),* pres. p. of *sibilo,* to hiss]. Hissing or whistling in character; denoting a form of rale.

sibilus (sib'i-lŭs) [L. a hissing]. A sibilant rale.

sib'ling [A. S. *sib,* relation, + *-ling,* diminutive]. One of two or more children of the same parents.

sib'ship [A.S. *sib,* relationship]. **1.** The reciprocal state between individuals who have the same pair of parents. **2.** All progeny of one pair of parents.

Sibson, Francis, British anatomist, 1814–1876. See S.'s *aponeurosis, fascia, groove, muscle,* and aortic *vestibule.*

siccant (sik'ant) [L. *siccans (-ant-),* pres. p. of *sicco,* pp. *-atus,* to dry]. Siccative. **1.** Drying; removing moisture from surrounding substances. **2.** A substance with such properties.

siccative (sik'ă-tiv). Siccant.

sicchasia (sĭ-kā'zē-ă) [G. *sikchasia,* loathing, fr. *sicchos,* squeamish]. **1.** Nausea. **2.** Loathing for food.

siccolabile (sik-ō-lā'bil, -bīl) [L. *siccus,* dry, + *labilis,* perishable]. Subject to alteration or destruction on drying.

siccostabile, siccostable (sik-ō-stā'bil, -bīl; -bl) [L. *siccus,* dry, + *stabilis,* stable]. Not subject to alteration or destruction on drying.

sick (sik) [A.S. *seóc*] **1.** Ill; unwell; suffering from disease. **2.** Nauseated.

sicklemia (sik-lē'mē-ă). Presence of sickle- or crescent-shaped erythrocytes in peripheral blood; seen in sickle cell anemia and sickle cell trait.

sickling (sik'ling). Production of sickle-shaped erythrocytes in the circulation, as in sickle cell anemia.

sickness (sik'nes). Disease (1).
acute African sleeping s., Rhodesian *trypanosomiasis.*
African horse s., a disease of horses and other equids in Africa, caused by an orbivirus which is transmitted by biting gnats of several *Culicoides* species; the disease may be mild, subacute, or acute; in severe cases, death results from pulmonary edema.
African sleeping s., see Gambian *trypanosomiasis;* Rhodesian *trypanosomiasis.*
air s., a form of motion s. caused by flying in an airplane.
altitude s., **(1)** Acosta's disease; mountain s.; puna; soroche; a syndrome caused by low inspired oxygen pressure (as at high altitude) and characterized by nausea, headache, dyspnea, malaise, and insomnia; in severe instances, pulmonary edema and adult respiratory distress syndrome can occur; formerly attributed to toxic emanations of ores in mountains; **(2)** a similar disease in cattle, characterized by subcutaneous edema and congestive heart failure.
black s., visceral *leishmaniasis.*
bush s., anemia of sheep and cattle due to deficiency of cobalt.
car s., a form of motion s. caused by riding on a train or in an automobile or bus.
chronic African sleeping s., Gambian *trypanosomiasis.*
chronic mountain s., altitude erythremia; chronic soroche; Monge's disease; loss of high altitude tolerance after prolonged exposure (*e.g.,* by residence), characterized by extreme polycythemia, exaggerated hypoxemia, and reduced mental and physical capacity; relieved by descent.
decompression s., bends; caisson or decompression disease; a symptom complex caused by the escape from solution in the body fluids of nitrogen bubbles absorbed originally at high atmospheric pressure, as a result of abrupt reduction in atmospheric pressure (either rapid ascent to high altitude or return from a compressed-air environment); it is characterized by headache, pain in the arms, legs, joints, and epigastrium, itching of the skin, vertigo, dyspnea, coughing, choking, vomiting, weakness and sometimes paralysis, and severe peripheral circulatory collapse.
East African sleeping s., Rhodesian *trypanosomiasis.*
falling s., epilepsy.
green s., chlorosis.
Indian s., epidemic gangrenous *proctitis.*
Jamaican vomiting s., ackee *poisoning.*
lambing s., pregnancy *disease* of sheep.
laughing s., see pseudobulbar *paralysis.*
milk s., lactimorbus; a disease of humans caused by ingesting con-

taminated milk from cows suffering from trembles; clinical manifestations include severe vomiting, labored breathing, delirium, convulsions, coma, and death; recovery from nonlethal illness is slow.

Monday morning s., *azoturia* of horses.

morning s., nausea gravidarum; the nausea and vomiting of early pregnancy.

motion s., kinesia; the syndrome of pallor, nausea, weakness, and malaise which may progress to vomiting and incapacitation, caused by stimulation of the semicircular canals during travel or motion as on a boat, plane, train, car, swing, or rotating amusement ride.

mountain s., altitude s. (1).

radiation s., the condition that follows therapeutic x-radiation. In mild forms there are anorexia, nausea, vomiting, malaise, and leukopenia; in more severe forms there are reduction or disappearance of platelets with bleeding, reduction or disappearance of leukocytes with risk of infection, and reduction of new red cells leading to anemia. The severity of the effect is dose dependent, although it varies among individuals.

serum s., serum disease or reaction; an immune complex disease appearing some days after injection of a foreign protein, with local and systemic reactions such as urticaria, fever, general lymphadenopathy, edema, joint pains, and occasionally albuminuria.

sleeping s., see Gambian *trypanosomiasis;* Rhodesian *trypanosomiasis.*

spotted s., pinta.

sweating s., an acute febrile disease of cattle in Africa; it is induced by the tick, *Hyalomma truncatum,* but the precise causative agent has not been identified.

West African sleeping s., Gambian *trypanosomiasis.*

side (sīd) [A.S. *sīde*]. One of the two lateral margins or surfaces of a body, midway between the front and back.

balancing s., in dentistry, the nonfunctioning s. from which the mandible moves during the working bite.

working s., in dentistry, the lateral segment of a dentition toward which the mandible is moved during occlusal function.

sidebones (sīd'bōnz). Ossification of the lateral cartilages of the horse's foot, seen most often in the forefeet of the heavier working breeds; exostoses often appear, and may be seen and palpated above the hoof line.

side effect. A result of drug or other therapy in addition to or in extension of the desired therapeutic effect; usually but not necessarily, connoting an undesirable effect. Although technically the therapeutic effect carried beyond the desired limit (*e.g.,* a hemorrhage from an anticoagulant) is a s.e., the term more often refers to pharmacologic results of therapy unrelated to the usual objective (*e.g.,* a development of signs of Cushing's syndrome with steroid therapy).

sideration (sid-er-ā'shŭn) [L. *sideror,* pp. *sideratus,* to be blasted or palsied by a constellation, fr. *sidus* (*sider-*), a constellation, the heavens]. Any sudden attack, as of apoplexy.

sidero- [G. *sidērŏs,* iron]. Combining form denoting iron.

sideroblast (sid'er-ō-blast) [sidero- + G. *blastos,* germ]. An erythroblast containing granules of ferritin stained by the Prussian blue reaction.

siderocyte (sid'er-ō-sīt) [sidero- + G. *kytos,* cell]. An erythrocyte containing granules of free iron, as detected by the Prussian blue reaction, in the blood of normal fetuses, where they constitute from 0.10 to 4.5% of the erythrocytes.

sideroderma (sid'er-ō-der'mă) [sidero- + G. *derma,* skin]. Brownish discoloration of the skin on the legs due to hemosiderin deposits.

siderofibrosis (sid'er-ō-fī-brō'sis). Fibrosis associated with small foci in which iron is deposited.

siderogenous (sid-er-oj'ĕ-nŭs) [sidero- + G. *-gen,* producing]. Iron-forming.

sideropenia (sid'er-ō-pē'nē-ă) [sidero- + G. *penia,* poverty]. An abnormally low level of serum iron.

sideropenic (sid'er-ō-pē'nik). Characterized by sideropenia.

siderophage (sid'er-ō-fāj) [sidero- + G. *phagein,* to eat]. Siderophore.

siderophil, siderophile (sid'er-ō-fil, -fīl) [sidero- + G. *philos,* fond]. **1.** Siderophilous; absorbing iron. **2.** A cell or tissue that contains iron.

siderophilin (sid-er-ō-fil'in, -of'ĭ-lin). Transferrin (1).

siderophilous (sid-er-of'i-lŭs). Siderophil (1).

siderophone (sid'er-ō-fōn, sĭ-der'ō-fōn) [sidero- + G. *phōnē,* sound]. Obsolete term for an electrical device for detecting a bit of iron in the eyeball, its presence causing the instrument to sound.

siderophore (sid'er-ō-fōr) [sidero- + G. *phoros,* bearing]. Siderophage; heart failure cell; a large extravasated mononuclear phagocyte containing granules of hemosiderin, found in the sputum or in the lungs of individuals with longstanding pulmonary congestion from left ventricular failure.

sideroscope (sid'er-ō-skōp) [sidero- + G. *skopeō,* to view]. Obsolete term for a very delicately poised magnetic needle for the detection of the presence and location of a particle of iron or steel imbedded in the eyeball.

siderosilicosis (sid'er-ō-sil'i-kō'sis) [sidero- + silicosis]. Silicosiderosis; silicosis due to inhalation of dust containing iron and silica.

siderosis (sid-er-ō'sis) [sidero- + G. *-osis,* condition]. **1.** A form of pneumoconiosis due to the presence of iron dust. **2.** Discoloration of any part by disposition of an iron pigment; usually called hemosiderosis. **3.** An excess of iron in the circulating blood. **4.** Degeneration of the retina, lens, and uvea as a result of the deposition of intraocular iron.

siderotic (sid-er-ot'ik). Related to siderosis; pigmented by iron or containing an excess of iron.

SIDS Abbreviation for sudden infant death *syndrome.*

Siegert, Ferdinand, German pediatrician, 1865–1946. See S.'s *sign.*

Siegle, Emil, German otologist, 1833–1900. See S.'s *otoscope.*

Siemens, Hermann Werner, German dermatologist, *1891. See Christ-S. *syndrome.*

siemens (S) (sē'menz) [Sir William *Siemens,* Ger. born British engineer, 1823–1883]. Mho; the SI unit of electrical conductance; the conductance of a body with an electrical resistance of 1 ohm, allowing 1 ampere of current to flow per volt applied.

Siemerling, Ernst, 20th century German physician, 1857–1931. See S.-Creutzfeldt *disease.*

sieve (siv) [O.E. *sive*]. A meshed or perforated device for separating fine particles from coarser ones.

molecular s., a gel-like material with pore sizes of such ranges as to exclude molecules above certain sizes; used in fractionating or purifying macromolecules.

sievert (Sv) (sē'vert). The SI derived unit of ionizing radiation absorbed dose equivalent, producing the same biologic effect on a tissue as one gray; 1 Sv = 100 rem.

Sig. Abbreviation for L. *signa,* label, write, or *signetur,* let it be labeled.

Siggaard-Andersen, Ole, Danish clinical biochemist, *1932. See S.-A. *nomogram.*

sigh (sī) [A.S. *sīcan*] **1.** An audible inspiration and expiration under the influence of some emotion. **2.** To perform such an act.

sight (sīt) [A.S. *gesihth*] The ability or faculty of seeing. See also vision.

day s., nyctalopia.
far s., hyperopia.
long s., hyperopia.
near s., myopia.
night s., hemeralopia.
second s., senile lenticular myopia; improved near vision in the aged as a result of increased refractivity of the nucleus of the lens causing myopia.
short s., myopia.

sigma (sig′mă). The 18th letter of the Greek alphabet, σ (*q.v.*).

sigmatism (sig′mă-tizm) [G. *sigma,* the letter S]. Lisping.

sigmoid (sig′moyd) [G. *sigma,* the letter S, + *eidos,* resemblance]. Resembling in outline the letter S or one of the forms of the Greek sigma.

sigmoid-. See sigmoido-.

sigmoidectomy (sig-moy-dek′tō-mē) [sigmoid- + G. *ektomē,* excision]. Excision of the sigmoid colon.

sigmoiditis (sig-moy-dī′tis) [sigmoid- + G. *-itis,* inflammation]. Inflammation of the sigmoid colon.

sigmoido-, sigmoid- [G. *sigma,* the letter S, + *eidos,* resemblance]. Combining forms denoting sigmoid, usually the sigmoid colon.

sigmoidopexy (sig-moy′dō-pek-sē) [sigmoido- + G. *pēxis,* fixation]. Operative attachment of the sigmoid colon to a firm structure to correct rectal prolapse.

sigmoidoproctostomy (sig-moy′dō-prok-tos′tō-mē) [sigmoido- + G. *prōktos,* anus, + *stoma,* mouth]. Sigmoidorectostomy; anastomosis between the sigmoid colon and the rectum.

sigmoidorectostomy (sig-moy′dō-rek-tos′tō-mē). Sigmoidoproctostomy.

sigmoidoscope (sig-moy′dō-skōp) [sigmoido- + G. *skopeō,* to view]. Sigmoscope; an endoscope for viewing the cavity of the sigmoid colon.

sigmoidoscopy (sig′moy-dos′kŏ-pē). Inspection, through an endoscope, of the interior of the sigmoid colon.

sigmoidostomy (sig′moy-dos′tō-mē) [sigmoido- + G. *stoma,* mouth]. Establishment of an artificial anus by opening into the sigmoid colon.

sigmoidotomy (sig′moy-dot′ō-mē) [sigmoido- + G. *tomē,* incision]. Surgical opening of the sigmoid.

sigmoscope (sig′mō-skōp). Sigmoidoscope.

SIGN

sign (sīn) [L. *signum,* mark]. **1.** Any abnormality indicative of disease, discoverable on examination of the patient; an objective symptom of disease, a symptom being a subjective s. of disease. **2.** An abbreviation or symbol. **3.** In psychology, any object or artifact (stimulus) that represents a specific thing or conveys a specific idea to the person who perceives it.

Aaron's s., in acute appendicitis, a referred pain or feeling of distress in the epigastrium or precordial region, on continuous firm pressure over McBurney's point.

Abadie's s. of exophthalmic goiter, spasm of the musculus levator palpebrae superioris in Graves' disease.

Abadie's s. of tabes dorsalis, insensibility to pressure over the tendo achillis.

Abrahams' s., an obsolete s.: **(1)** rales and other adventitious sounds, changes in the respiratory murmurs, and increase in the whispered sounds which can be heard on auscultation over the acromial end of the clavicle some time before they become audible at the apex; heard primarily in pulmonary tuberculosis; **(2)** a dull-flat note, *i.e.,* one between the normal dullness at the right apex and absolute flatness, heard on percussion in that region, indicating progress from incipient to advanced tuberculosis.

accessory s., assident s.; a finding frequently but not consistently present in a disease.

Allis' s., in fracture of the neck of the femur, the trochanter rides up, relaxing the fascia lata, so that the finger can be sunk deeply between the great trochanter and the iliac crest.

Amoss' s., in painful flexion of the spine, it is necessary to support a sitting position by extending the arms behind the torso with the weight placed on the hands.

Anghelescu's s., in vertebral tuberculosis, painful or impossible flexion of the spine when the patient attempts to rest weight on the heels and occiput.

antecedent s., prodromic s.

Arroyo's s., asthenocoria.

assident s., accessory s.

Auenbrugger's s., an epigastric prominence seen in cases of marked pericardial effusion.

Aufrecht's s., an obsolete s.: diminished breath sounds in the trachea just above the jugular notch, in cases of stenosis.

Babinski's s., **(1)** extension of the great toe and abduction of the other toes instead of the normal flexion reflex to plantar stimulation, considered indicative of pyramidal tract involvement ("positive" Babinski). Also called Babinski's reflex or phenomenon; paradoxical extensor reflex; great toe reflex; toe reflex (3); toe phenomenon; **(2)** in hemiplegia, weakness of the platysma muscle on the affected side, as is evident in such actions as blowing or opening the mouth; **(3)** when the patient is lying upon his back, with arms crossed on the front of his chest, and attempts to assume the sitting posture, the thigh on the side of an *organic* paralysis is flexed and the heel raised, whereas the limb on the sound side remains flat; **(4)** in hemiplegia, the forearm on the affected side turns to a pronated position when placed in a position of supination.

Baccelli's s., aphonic pectoriloquy; an obsolete s.: good conduction of the whisper in nonpurulent pleural effusions.

Ballance's s., the presence of a dull percussion note in both flanks, constant on the left side but shifting with change of position on the right, said to indicate ruptured spleen; the dullness is due to the presence of blood, fluid on the right side but coagulated on the left.

Ballet's s., partial or complete external ophthalmoplegia in Graves' disease.

Bamberger's s., **(1)** jugular pulse in tricuspid insufficiency; **(2)** allesthesia; **(3)** dullness on percussion at the angle of the scapula, clearing up as the patient leans forward, indicating pericarditis with effusion.

bandage s., Rumpel-Leede *test.*

Bárány's s., in cases of ear disease, in which the vestibule is healthy, injection into the external auditory canal of water below the body temperature (18°C or lower) will cause rotary nystagmus toward the opposite side; when the injected fluid is above the body temperature (41°C or higher) the nystagmus will be toward the injected side; if the labyrinth is diseased or nonfunctional there may be diminished or absent nystagmus.

Bard's s., in organic nystagmus, increased rapidity of the oscillations in an attempt to fixate a moving target.

Barré's s., if the hemiplegic is placed in the prone position with the limbs flexed at the knees, he is unable to maintain the flexed position on the side of the lesion but extends the leg.

Bassler's s., in chronic appendicitis, pinching the appendix between the thumb and the iliacus muscle causes sharp pain.

Bastedo's s., an obsolete s.: in chronic appendicitis, pain and tenderness in the right iliac fossa on inflation of the colon with air.

Battle's s., postauricular ecchymosis in cases of fracture of the base of the skull.
Bechterew's s., paralysis of automatic facial movements, the power of voluntary movement being retained.
Beevor's s., with paralysis of the lower portions of the recti abdominis muscles the umbilicus moves upward.
Bezold's s., Bezold's *symptom.*
Biederman's s., a dusky redness of the lower portion of the anterior pillars of the fauces in certain cases of syphilis.
Bielschowsky's s., in paralysis of a superior oblique muscle, tilting the head to the side of the involved eye causes that eye to rotate upward.
Biermer's s., Gerhardt's s.
Biernacki's s., analgesia of the ulnar nerve (the "funny-bone" sensation being absent) in tabes dorsalis and dementia paralytica.
Bird's s., the presence of a zone of dullness on percussion with absence of respiratory s.'s in hydatid cyst of the lung.
Bjerrum's s., Bjerrum's *scotoma.*
Blumberg's s., pain felt upon sudden release of steadily applied pressure on a suspected area of the abdomen, indicative of peritonitis.
Bonhoeffer's s., loss of normal muscle tone in chorea.
Boston's s., jerky downward movement of the upper eyelid on downward rotation of the eye, characteristic of Graves' disease.
Bozzolo's s., pulsating vessels in the nasal mucous membrane, noted occasionally in thoracic aneurysm.
Branham's s., bradycardia following compression or excision of an arteriovenous fistula.
Braxton Hicks s., irregular uterine contractions occurring after the third month of pregnancy.
Broadbent's s., a retraction of the thoracic wall, synchronous with cardiac systole, visible in the left posterior axillary line; a s. of adherent pericardium.
Brockenbrough s., absolute decrease in pulse pressure of the beat immediately following a premature beat; a s. of idiopathic hypertrophic subaortic stenosis.
Brudzinski's s., **(1)** contralateral reflex or s.; in meningitis, on passive flexion of the leg on one side, a similar movement occurs in the opposite leg; **(2)** neck s.; in meningitis, if the neck is passively flexed, flexion of the legs occurs.
Bryant's s., in dislocation of the shoulder, an abnormal position of axillary folds occurs.
burning drops s., in certain cases of perforated gastric ulcer, a sensation as of drops of hot liquid falling into the abdominal cavity or as of a stream of intensely hot liquid being poured into the cavity.
Calkins' s., the change of shape of the uterus from discoid to ovoid, indicating placental separation from the uterine wall.
Cantelli's s., see doll's eye s.
Carnett's s., disappearance of abdominal tenderness to palpation when the anterior abdominal muscles are contracted, indicating pain of intra-abdominal origin; its persistence suggests a source in the abdominal wall, which is also indicated when tenderness is caused by gently pinching a fold of skin and fat between the thumb and forefinger.
Carvallo's s., in right ventricular disease, an increase in the intensity of the pansystolic murmur of tricuspid regurgitation during or at the end of inspiration distinguishes tricuspid from mitral involvement.
Castellani-Low s., a fine tremor of the tongue observed in sleeping sickness.
Chaddock s., Chaddock reflex; external malleolar s.; when the external malleolar skin area is irritated, extension of the great toe occurs in cases of organic disease of the corticospinal reflex paths.
Chadwick's s., a bluish discoloration of the cervix and vagina which characterizes pregnancy.
Chaussier's s., severe pain in the epigastrium, a prodrome of eclampsia; may be of central origin or caused by distention of the capsule of liver by hemorrhage.
Chvostek's s., Weiss s.; facial irritability in tetany, unilateral spasm of the orbicularis oculi or oris muscle being excited by a slight tap over the facial nerve just anterior to the external auditory meatus.
Claybrook's s., in rupture of abdominal viscus, transmission of breath and heart sounds through abdominal wall.
Cleemann's s., in fracture of the femur with overriding of the fragments, wrinkling of the skin occurs directly above the patella.
clenched fist s., in angina pectoris, pressing of the clenched fist against the chest to indicate the constricting, pressing quality of the pain.
Codman's s., in the absence of rotator cuff function, hunching of the shoulder occurs when the deltoid muscle contracts.
Comby's s., an early s. of measles, consisting in thin whitish patches on the gums and buccal mucous membrane, formed of desquaminating epithelial cells.
commemorative s., a phenomenon pointing to the previous existence of some disease other than the one present at the time.
Comolli's s., in cases of fracture of the scapula, a typical triangular cushion-like swelling appears, corresponding to the outline of the scapula.
contralateral s., Brudzinski's s. (1).
conventional s.'s, s.'s that acquire their function through social (linguistic) custom; *e.g.,* words, mathematical symbols. See also symbol (4).
Coopernail's s., in fracture of the pelvis, occurrence of ecchymosis of the perineum and scrotum, or labia.
Courvoisier's s., Courvoisier's *law.*
Crichton-Browne's s., a slight tremor at the angles of the mouth and at the outer canthus of each eye in general paresis.
Cruveilhier-Baumgarten s., a murmer over the umbilicus in the presence of caput medusae, resulting from hepatic cirrhosis with portal hypertension; recanalization of the umbilical vein with reverse blood flow from the liver into the abdominal wall veins creates the murmur.
Cullen's s., periumbilical darkening of the skin from blood, a s. of intraperitoneal hemorrhage, especially in ruptured ectopic pregnancy.
Dalrymple's s., retraction of the upper eyelid in Graves' disease, causing abnormal wideness of the palpebral fissure.
Dance's s., a slight retraction in the neighborhood of the right iliac fossa in some cases of intussusception.
Danforth's s., shoulder pain on inspiration, due to hemoperitoneum in ruptured ectopic pregnancy.
Darier's s., urtication on stroking of cutaneous lesions of urticaria pigmentosa (mastocytosis).
Dawbarn's s., pain of subacromial bursitis disappears when the arm is abducted.
Dejerine's s., aggravation of symptoms of radiculitis by the acts of coughing, sneezing, or straining to defecate.
Delbet's s., in a case of aneurysm of a main artery, efficient collateral circulation if the nutrition of the part below is well maintained, despite the fact that the pulse has disappeared.
D'Espine's s., an obsolete s.: **(1)** bronchophony over the spinous processes heard, at a lower level than in health, in pulmonary tuberculosis; **(2)** an echoed whisper following a spoken word, heard in the stethoscope placed over the seventh cervical or first or second dorsal spine, in cases of tuberculosis of the mediastinal glands.
dimple s., in dermatofibroma, dimpling elicited when the lesion is squeezed.
doll's eye s., proprioceptive-oculocephalic reflex; reflex movement of the eyes in the opposite direction to that which the head is moved, *e.g.,* the eyes being lowered as the head is raised, and the reverse (Cantelli); an indication of functional integrity of the brainstem tegmental pathways and cranial nerves involved in eye movement.

Dorendorf's s., fullness of one supraclavicular groove in aneurysm of the aortic arch.
drawer s., Rocher's s.; drawer test; in a knee examination, the forward or backward sliding of the tibia indicating laxity or tear of the anterior (forward slide) or posterior (backward slide) cruciate ligaments of the knee.
Drummond's s., in certain cases of aortic aneurysm, a puffing sound, synchronous with the cardiac systole, heard from the nostrils, when the mouth is closed.
Duchenne's s., falling in of the epigastrium during inspiration in paralysis of the diaphragm.
Dupuytren's s., **(1)** in congenital dislocation, free up and down movement of the head of the femur occurs upon intermittent traction; **(2)** a crackling sensation on pressure over the bone in certain cases of sarcoma.
ear s., in cases of subcutaneous inflammation, the ears are not involved because of the close adhesion of the skin and cartilage; in erysipelas and certain other skin inflammations the ears may be involved.
Ebstein's s., in pericardial effusion, obtuseness of the cardiohepatic angle on percussion.
s. of edema of lower eyelid, swelling of the lower lid found in congestive failure, myxedema, or nephrosis.
Enroth's s., in Graves' disease, edema of the eyelids, especially of the upper eyelid near the supraorbital margin.
Erb's s., **(1)** increased electric excitability of the muscles to the galvanic current, and frequently to the faradic, in tetany; **(2)** Erb-Westphal s.
Erb-Westphal s., Erb's s. (2); abolition of the patellar tendon reflex, in tabes and certain other diseases of the spinal cord, and occasionally also in brain disease.
Erichsen's s., in sacroiliac disease, pain is felt when sudden pressure approximates the iliac bones; this s. is not present in hip disease.
Escherich's s., in hypoparathyroidism (latent tetany) tapping the skin at the angle of the mouth causes protrusion of the lips.
Ewart's s., Pins s.; in large pericardial effusions, an area of dullness with bronchial breathing and bronchophony below the angle of the left scapula.
Ewing's s., **(1)** dullness on percussion to the inner side of the angle of the left scapula, denoting an accumulation of fluid in the pericardium behind the heart; **(2)** tenderness at the upper inner angle of the orbit at the point of attachment of the pulley of the superior oblique muscle, denoting closure of the outlet of the frontal sinus.
external malleolar s., Chaddock s.
eyelash s., in a case of apparent unconsciousness due to functional disease, such as conversion hysteria, stroking the eyelashes will occasion movement of the lids, but no such reflex will occur in case of severe organic brain lesion such as apoplexy, fracture of the skull, or other traumatism.
Faget's s., a slow pulse with an elevated temperature, often seen in yellow fever.
fan s., the spreading apart of the toes in the complete Babinski's sign.
Fischer's s., an obsolete s.: in tuberculosis of the bronchial glands, after bending the patient's head as far back as possible, auscultation over the manubrium sterni will sometimes reveal a continuous loud murmur caused by the pressure of the enlarged glands on the large mediastinal vessels.
flag s., bands of discoloration of hair (reddish, blonde, or gray, depending on original color) resulting from fluctuations in nutrition characteristic of kwashiorkor and in diseases of protein depletion such as ulcerative colitis.
Forchheimer's s., the presence, in German measles, of a reddish maculopapular eruption on the soft palate.
Fothergill's s., in rectus sheath hematoma, the hematoma produces a mass that does not cross the midline and remains palpable when the rectus muscle is tense.
Friedreich's s., in adherent pericardium, sudden collapse of the previously distended veins of the neck at each diastole of the heart.
Froment's s., flexion of the distal phalanx of the thumb when a sheet of paper is held between the thumb and index finger in ulnar nerve palsy.
Gaenslen's s., pain on hyperextension of the hip with pelvis fixed by flexion of opposite hip; causes a torsion stress at the sacroiliac and lumbosacral joints.
Gauss' s., marked mobility of the uterus in the early weeks of pregnancy.
Gerhardt's s., Biermer's s.; complete bilateral paralysis of the adductor muscles of the larynx with severe inspiratory dyspnea.
Gifford's s., difficulty in everting the upper eyelid in Graves' disease.
Glasgow's s., a systolic murmur heard over the brachial artery in aneurysm of the aorta.
Goggia's s., the fibrillation of the biceps muscle, when pinched and tapped, is confined to a limited area in cases of debilitating disease, whereas in health it is general.
Goldstein's toe s., increased space between the great toe and its neighbor, seen in mongolism and occasionally in cretinism.
Goldthwait's s., in sprain of sacroiliac ligaments, flexion of hip with extended knee elicits pain in sacroiliac region; not now considered specific.
Goodell's s., softening of the cervix and vagina as being usually indicative of pregnancy.
Goppert's s., pupillary dilation elicited by mild stimulation of the skin.
Gordon's s., finger *phenomenon.*
Gorlin's s., unusual ease in touching the tip of the nose with the tongue; seen in Ehlers-Danlos syndrome.
Graefe's s., von Graefe's s.; in Graves disease, lag of the upper eyelid as it follows the rotation of the eyeball downward.
Grasset's s., normal contraction of the sternocleidomastoid muscle on the paralyzed side in cases of hemiplegia.
Grey Turner's s., local areas of discoloration about the umbilicus and in the region of the loins, in acute hemorrhagic pancreatitis and other causes of retroperitoneal hemorrhage.
Griffith's s., lagging of the lower eyelid on upward gaze in Graves' disease.
Grisolle's s., in smallpox, the continued presence and palpability of papules when the skin is stretched.
Grocco's s., **(1)** acute dilation of the heart following a muscular effort, noted in Graves disease; **(2)** extension of the liver dullness several centimeters to the left of the midspinal line in cases of enlargement of that organ; **(3)** Grocco's *triangle.*
groove s., large, hard, fixed, and extremely tender lymph nodes in the groin above and below the inguinal ligament, with a groove along the ligament; characteristic of lymphogranuloma venereum.
Gunn's s., Marcus Gunn's s.; **(1)** compression of the underlying vein at arteriovenous crossings seen ophthalmoscopically in arteriolar sclerosis; **(2)** on alternate stimulation with light, the pupil of an eye with optic nerve transmission defect dilates when stimulated (afferent pupillary defect).
Guyon's s., **(1)** ballottement of the kidney in cases of nephroptosis, especially when there is also a renal tumor; **(2)** the hypoglossal nerve lies directly upon the external carotid artery, whereby this vessel may be distinguished from the internal carotid when ligation is necessary.
halo s., elevation of the subcutaneous fat layer over the fetal skull in a dead or dying fetus; said to be the most common radiologic sign of fetal death.
halo s. of hydrops, a discredited roentgenographic s. of fetal hydrops caused by scalp edema so that a definite corona surrounds the skull.
Hamman's s., an obsolete s.: a crunching, rasping sound, syn-

chronous with heart beat, heard over the precordium and sometimes at a distance from the chest in interstitial emphysema of the lungs.

Hegar's s., softening and compressibility of the lower segment of the uterus in early pregnancy (about the seventh week) which, on bimanual examination, is felt by the finger in the vagina as though the neck and body of the uterus were separated, or connected by only a thin band of tissue.

Heim-Kreysig s., Kreysig's s.; in adherent pericardium, an indrawing of the intercostal spaces, synchronous with the cardiac systole.

Helbings' s., a malalignment of the Achilles tendon associated with a valgus deformity of the os calcis.

Higoumenakia s., sternoclavicular swelling in late congenital syphilis.

Hill's s., Hill's phenomenon; in aortic insufficiency, greater systolic blood pressure in the legs than in the arms; normal arterial systolic pressure in the leg is 10 to 20 mm of Hg above that in the arm, whereas in aortic insufficiency the difference may be 60 to 100 mm of Hg.

Hoffmann's s., (1) in latent tetany mild mechanical stimulation of the trigeminal nerve causes severe pain; **(2)** Hoffmann's, digital, or snapping reflex; flexion of the terminal phalanx of the thumb and of the second and third phalanges of one or more of the fingers when the volar surface of the terminal phalanx of the fingers is flicked.

Hoglund's s., eyelid edema in infectious mononucleosis.

Homans' s., slight pain at the back of the knee or calf when the ankle is slowly and gently dorsiflexed (with the knee bent), indicative of incipient or established thrombosis in the veins of the leg.

Hoover's s.'s, (1) a person lying supine on a couch, when asked to raise one leg, involuntarily makes counterpressure with the heel of the other leg; if this leg is paralyzed, whatever muscular power is preserved in it will be exerted in this way; or if the patient attempts to lift a paralyzed leg, counterpressure will be made with the other heel, whether any movement occurs in the paralyzed limb or not; not present in hysteria or malingering; **(2)** a modification in the movement of the costal margins during respiration, caused by a flattening of the diaphragm; suggestive of empyema or other intrathoracic condition causing a change in the contour of the diaphragm.

Hueter's s., in a case of fracture, the vibration expected on tapping the bone is not transmitted when tissue intervenes between the fractured parts of bone.

iconic s.'s, s.'s that acquire their function through similarity to what they signify; *e.g.,* a photograph as a s. of the person in the picture.

indexical s.'s, s.'s that acquire their function through a causal connection with what they signify; *e.g.,* smoke as a s. of fire.

Jackson's s. [J. H. Jackson], during quiet respiration the movement of the paralyzed side of the chest may be greater than that of the opposite side, while in forced respiration the paralyzed side moves less than the other.

Jellinek's s., in Graves' disease, a brownish pigmentation of the eyelids, especially the upper one.

Joffroy's s., (1) immobility of the facial muscles when the eyeballs are rolled upward, in exophthalmic goiter; **(2)** disorder of the arithmetical faculty (the person being unable to do simple sums in addition or multiplication) in the early stages of organic brain disease.

Keen's s., increased width at the malleoli in Pott's fracture.

Kehr's s., violent pain in the left shoulder in a case of rupture of the spleen.

Kernig's s., when the subject lies upon the back and the thigh is flexed to a right angle with the axis of the trunk, complete extension of the leg on the thigh is impossible; present in various forms of meningitis.

Kestenbaum's s., a decrease in the number of arterioles crossing optic disk margins as a s. of optic neuritis.

Knies' s., inequality of pupillary dilation in Graves' disease.

Kocher's s., in Graves' disease, on upward gaze, the globe lags behind the movement of the upper eyelid.

Kreysig's s., Heim-Kreysig s.

Kussmaul's s., in cardiac tamponade, a paradoxical increase in venous distention and pressure during inspiration.

Lancisi's s., a large systolic jugular venous wave caused by tricuspid regurgitation replacing the normal negative systolic trough ("x" descent).

Landolfi's s., in aortic insufficiency, systolic contraction and diastolic dilation of the pupil.

Lasègue's s., when patient is supine with hip flexed, dorsiflexion of the ankle causing pain or muscle spasm in the posterior thigh indicates lumbar root or sciatic nerve irritation.

Laugier's s., in fracture of the lower portion of the radius, the styloid processes of the radius and of the ulna are on the same level.

Legendre's s., in facial hemiplegia of central origin, when the examiner raises the lids of the actively closed eyes the resistance is less on the affected side.

Leichtenstern's s., Leichtenstern's phenomenon; tapping gently one of the bones of the extremities causes the patient to draw back violently, sometimes with a loud cry; noted in cases of cerebrospinal meningitis.

Leri's s., voluntary flexion of the elbow is impossible in a case of hemiplegia when the wrist on that side is passively flexed.

Leser-Trélat s., the sudden appearance and rapid increase in the number and size of seborrheic keratoses with pruritus; associated with internal malignancy.

Lhermitte's s., sudden electric-like shocks extending down the spine on flexing the head.

Lichtheim's s., Déjérine-L. phenomenon; in subcortical aphasia, the patient can indicate by use of the fingers the number of syllables of a word he has in mind but cannot speak.

local s., the characteristic of a sensation that permits distinguishing it from another sensation by locating its position in space.

Loewi's s., ready dilation of the pupil with epinephrine in Graves' disease.

Lorenz' s., an obsolete s.: stiffness of the thoracic spine in early pulmonary tuberculosis.

Lovibond's profile s., Lovibond's *angle.*

Ludloff's s., in traumatic separation of the epiphysis of the small trochanter: **(1)** swelling and ecchymosis appears at the base of Scarpa's triangle; **(2)** inability to raise the thigh in the sitting posture.

Macewen's s., Macewen's symptom; percussion of the skull gives a cracked-pot sound in cases of hydrocephalus.

Magendie-Hertwig s., Magendie-Hertwig syndrome; skew deviation of the eyes in acute cerebellar lesions.

Magnan's s., paresthesia in the psychosis of cocaine addicts, who imagine they have a foreign body, in the shape of a powder or fine sand, under the skin, and that it is constantly changing its position.

Magnus' s., an obsolete s.: after death, constriction of a limb or one of its segments is not followed by venous congestion of the distal part.

Mannkopf's s., acceleration of the pulse when a painful point is pressed upon.

Marañón's s., in Graves' disease, a vasomotor reaction following stimulation of the skin over the throat.

Marcus Gunn's s., Gunn's s.

Masini's s., a marked degree of dorsal extension of the fingers on the metacarpals and of the toes on the metatarsals, noted in children with mental instability.

Means' s., globe lag in Graves' disease, with the upper eyelid moving prior to and faster than the globe in upward gaze.

Metenier's s., easy eversion of the upper eyelid in Ehlers-Danlos syndrome.

Mirchamp's s., a premonitory symptom of mumps; if a strongly flavored substance is placed on the tongue a painful reflex secretion of saliva occurs in the gland which is the seat of the incipient affection.
Möbius' s., impairment of ocular convergence in Graves' disease.
Müller's s., in aortic insufficiency, rhythmical pulsatory movements of the uvula, synchronous with the heart's action; accompanied by swelling and redness of the velum palati and tonsils.
Munson's s., in keratoconus, the angulation of the lower eyelid caused by the cornea as the eye rotates downward.
Musset's s., in incompetence of the aortic valve, rhythmical nodding of the head, synchronous with the heart beat.
neck s., Brudzinski's s. (2).
Néri's s., in hemiplegia, the knee bends spontaneously when the leg is passively extended.
Nikolsky's s., a peculiar vulnerability of the skin in pemphigus vulgaris; the apparently normal epidermis may be separated at the basal layer and rubbed off when pressed with a sliding motion.
objective s., a s. that is evident to the examiner.
s. of the orbicularis, Revilliod's s.; in hemiplegia, inability to voluntarily close the eye on the paralyzed side except in conjunction with closure of the other eye.
Osler's s., in acute bacterial endocarditis, circumscribed painful erythematous swellings, ranging in size from that of a pinhead to that of a pea, in the skin and subcutaneous tissues of the hands and feet.
Pastia's s., Thomson's s.; the presence of pink or red transverse lines at the bend of the elbow in the preeruptive stage of scarlatina; they persist through the eruptive stage and remain as pigmented lines after desquamation.
Payr's s., pain on pressure over the sole of the foot; a s. of thrombophlebitis.
Perez' s., rales audible over the upper part of the chest when the arms are alternately raised and lowered; common in cases of fibrous mediastinitis and also of aneurysm of the aortic arch.
Pfuhl's s., the pressure of pus within a subphrenic abscess rises during inspiration and falls during expiration, the reverse of what happens in the case of a purulent collection above the diaphragm; when the diaphragm is paralyzed this distinction is lost.
physical s., a s. that is elicited by auscultation, percussion, or palpation.
Piltz s., Westphal-Piltz pupillary *phenomenon.*
Pins' s., Ewart's s.
Pitres' s., **(1)** haphalgesia; **(2)** diminished sensation in the testes and scrotum in tabes dorsalis.
placental s., slight endometrial oozing of blood which occurs in certain animals and sometimes in women at the time of implantation of the fertilized ovum; in women, if the blood appears externally it may be mistaken for a scanty menstrual period.
Pool-Schlesinger s., Pool's *phenomenon* (1).
Potain's s., in dilation of the aorta, dullness on percussion extending from the manubrium sterni toward the second intercostal space and the third costal cartilage on the right, the upper limit extending from the base of the sternum in the segment of a circle to the right.
prodromic s., antecedent s.; a s. that appears during the prodrome of a disease.
pseudo-Graefe s., a phenomenon similar to Graefe's s., due to aberrant regeneration of fibers of the oculomotor nerve following its paresis or paralysis.
puddle s., a s. of free abdominal fluid: the patient assumes a position on all fours; one flank is percussed by repeated light flicking of constant intensity while a Bowles type stethoscope is placed over the most dependent portion of the abdomen and gradually moved towards the flank opposite the percussion; a sharp increase in the intensity of the sound picked up by the stethescope indicates the level of fluid.
pyramid s., any of the symptoms indicating a morbid condition of the pyramidal tracts, such as the Babinski or Gordon s., spastic spinal paralysis, foot clonus, etc.
Quant's s., a T-shaped depression in the occipital bone occurring in many cases of rickets.
Quénu-Muret s., in aneurysm, well-maintained collateral circulation indicated by issue of blood when the main artery of the limb is compressed and a puncture is made at the periphery.
Quincke's s., Quincke's *pulse.*
Ransohoff's s., yellow pigmentation in the umbilical region in rupture of the common bile duct.
Remak's s., dissociation of the sensations of touch and of pain in tabes dorsalis and polyneuritis.
Revilliod's s., s. of the orbicularis.
Ripault's s., a s. of death, consisting in a permanent change in the shape of the pupil produced by unilateral pressure on the eyeball.
Rocher's s., drawer s.
Romaña's s., marked edema of one or both eyelids, usually a unilateral palpebral edema, thought to be a sensitization response to the bite of a triatomine bug infected with *Trypanosoma cruzi,* and a strong suggestion of acute Chagas' disease.
Romberg's s., rombergism; Romberg's symptom (1); Romberg or station test; if closing the eyes increases the unsteadiness of a standing patient, a loss of proprioceptive control is indicated.
Rosenbach's s., **(1)** in Graves' disease, fine tremor of the upper eyelids, when the eyes are gently closed; **(2)** loss of the abdominal reflex in cases of acute inflammation of the viscera.
Rossolimo's s., Rossolimo's *reflex.*
Rotch's s., in pericardial effusion, percussion dullness in the fifth intercostal space on the right.
Rovsing's s., pain at McBurney's point induced in cases of appendicitis, by pressure exerted over the descending colon.
Rumpel-Leede s., Rumpel-Leede *test.*
Russell's s., abrasions and scars on the back of the hands of individuals with bulimia, usually due to manual attempts at self-induced vomiting.
Saenger's s., a lost light reflex of the pupil returns after a short time in the dark, noted in cerebral syphilis but absent in tabes dorsalis.
Sainton's s., contraction of the musculus frontalis after cessation of action of the musculus levator palpebrae superioris on upward gaze in Graves' disease.
Sansom's s., in mitral stenosis, reduplication of the second heart sound.
Schapiro's s., in myocardial weakness, no slowing of the pulse occurs when the patient lies down.
Schlesinger's s., Pool's *phenomenon* (1).
Schultze's s., tongue phenomenon; in latent tetany, tapping the tongue causes its depression with a concave dorsum.
scimitar s., a curvilinear structure seen roentgenographically in the lung and associated with anomalous pulmonary venous drainage, suggesting the sickle shape, of a Turkish saber.
Seeligmüller's s., contraction of the pupil on the affected side in facial neuralgia.
Seidel's s., a sickle-shaped scotoma appearing as an upward or downward extension of the blind spot.
Siegert's s., shortness and inward curvature of the terminal phalanges of the fifth fingers in Down's syndrome.
Signorelli's s., tenderness on pressure in the glenoid fossa in front of the mastoid process in meningitis.
Simon's s., in incipient meningitis in children, the movements of the diaphragm are dissociated from those of the thorax.
Skoda's s., skodaic *resonance.*
spinal s., in pleurisy, the spinal muscles are in a state of tonic contraction on the affected side.
spine s., resistance to flexion of the spine in cases of meningitis.
Steinberg thumb s., in Marfan's syndrome, when the thumb is held across the palm of the same hand, it projects well beyond the

ulnar surface of the hand.
Stellwag's s., infrequent and incomplete blinking in Graves' disease.
Stewart-Holmes s., rebound phenomenon (1); in cerebellar disease, the inability to check a movement when passive resistance is suddenly released.
Stierlin's s., constant emptying of the cecum, seen on x-ray, with barium remaining in the terminal part of the ileum and in the transverse colon; due to irritation of the cecum, frequently caused by tuberculous cecitis.
Straus' s., in facial paralysis, if an injection of pilocarpine is followed by sweating on the affected side later than on the other, the lesion is peripheral.
subjective s., a s. that is perceived only by the patient.
Sumner's s., a slight increase in tonus of the abdominal muscles, an early indication of inflammation of the appendix, stone in the kidney or ureter, or a twisted pedicle of an ovarian cyst; it is detected by exceedingly gentle palpation of the right or left iliac fossa.
ten Horn's s., pain caused by gentle traction on the right spermatic cord, indicative of appendicitis.
Thomson's s., Pastia's s.
Tinel's s., a sensation of tingling, or of "pins and needles," felt in the distal extremity of a limb when percussion is made over the site of an injured nerve; it indicates a partial lesion or early regeneration in the nerve. Sometimes called distal tingling on percussion.
Toma's s., to distinguish between inflammatory and noninflammatory ascites: in inflammatory conditions of the peritoneum, the mesentery contracts, drawing the intestines over to the right side; consequently, when the patient lies on his back, tympany is elicited on the right side, dullness on the left.
Topolanski's s., congestion of the pericorneal region of the eye in Graves' disease.
Tournay s., dilation of the pupil in the abducting eye on extreme lateral fixation.
Trélat's s., an obsolete s.; the presence of disseminated yellowish spots in the neighborhood of tuberculous ulcers of the mouth; they are minute tubercles or miliary abscesses.
Trendelenburg's s., in congenital dislocation of the hip or in hip abductor weakness, the pelvis will sag on the side opposite to the dislocation when the hip and knee of the normal side is flexed; without dislocation or weakness, the pelvis will rise on the side of the flexed hip and knee.
Tresilian's s., a reddish prominence at the orifice of Stenson's duct, noted in mumps.
Trousseau's s., in latent tetany, the occurrence carpopedal spasm accompanied by paresthesia elicited when the upper arm is compressed, as by a tourniquet or a blood pressure cuff.
Uhthoff s., in multiple sclerosis, vasodilation from exposure to heat or from exertion may cause transient visual impairment or weakness.
Vierra's s., yellowing and canalization of the nail in fogo selvagem.
Vipond's s., a generalized adenopathy occurring during the period of incubation of various of the exanthemas of childhood, affording an early diagnostic s. in a case of known exposure.
vital s.'s, manifestation of breathing, heart beat, and sustained blood pressure.
von Graefe's s., Graefe's s.
Weber's s., Weber's *syndrome.*
Weiss' s., Chvostek's s.
Wernicke's s., Wernicke's *reaction.*
Westphal's s., Westphal-Erb s., Westphal's phenomenon; abolition of the patellar reflex.
Wilder's s., a slight twitch of the eyeball when changing its movement from abduction to adduction or the reverse, noted in Graves' disease.
Winterbottom's s., swelling of the posterior cervical lymph nodes, characteristic of early stages of African trypanosomiasis; useful for surveys or control of migrations from endemic areas of persons with preclinical infections.
wrist s., in Marfan's syndrome, when the wrist is gripped with the opposite hand, the thumb and fifth finger overlap appreciably.

---

signature (sig'nă-chūr, -tūr) [Mediev. L. *signatura,* fr. L. *signum,* a sign, mark]. The part of a prescription containing the directions to the patient.

significant (sig-nif'i-kant) [L. *significo,* to make known, signify, fr. *signum,* sign, + *facio,* to make]. In statistics, denoting the reliability of a finding or, conversely, the probability of the finding being the result of chance (generally less than 5%).

Signorelli, Angelo, Italian physician, 1876–1952. See S.'s *sign.*

silane (sī'lān). Silicon tetrahydride; SiH_4; the first member of a series of s.'s that are analogous in structure to the alkanes.

Silber, Robert H., U.S. biochemist, *1915. See Porter-S. *chromogens, reaction,* chromogens *test.*

silent (sī'lent). Producing no detectable signs or symptoms, said of certain diseases or morbid processes.

silica (sil'ī-kă) [Mod. L. fr. L. *silex* (*silic-*), flint]. Silicon dioxide; silicic anhydride; SiO_2; the chief constituent of sand, hence of glass.
s. gel, a precipitated form of silicic acid, used for adsorption of various gases.

silicate (sil'i-kāt). **1.** A salt of silicic acid. **2.** The term sometimes applied to dental restorations of synthetic porcelain.

silicatosis (sil'i-kă-tō'sis). Silicosis.

siliceous (si-lish'ŭs). Silicious; containing silica.

silicic (si-lis'ik). Relating to silica or silicon.

silicic acid. $Si(OH)_4$; obtained in water as a colloid by treating silicates; precipitated s. a. is silica gel.

silicic anhydride. Silica.

silicious (si-lish'ŭs). Siliceous.

silicofluoride (sil'i-kō-flūr'īd). A compound of silicon and fluorine with another element.

silicon (sil'i-kon). A very abundant nonmetallic element, symbol Si, atomic no. 14, atomic weight 28.086, occurring in nature as silica and silicates; in pure form, used as a semiconductor and in solar batteries.

silicon dioxide. Silica.
colloidal s. d., a submicroscopic fumed silica prepared by the vapor-phase hydrolysis of a silicon compound; used as a tablet diluent and as a suspending and thickening agent.

silicone (sil'i-kōn). A polymer of organic silicon oxides, which may be a liquid, gel, or solid, depending on the extent of polymerization; widely used in surgical implants, in intracorporeal tubes to conduct fluids, as dental impression material as a grease or sealing substance, as a coating on the inside of glass vessels for blood collection, and in various ophthalmological procedures.

silicoproteinosis (sil'i-kō-prō'tē-i-nō'sis). An acute pulmonary disorder, radiographically and histologically similar to pulmonary alveolar proteinosis, resulting from relatively short exposure to high concentrations of silica dust; pulmonary symptoms are of rapid onset and the condition is invariably fatal.

silicosiderosis (sil'i-kō-sid'er-ō'sis). Siderosilicosis.

silicosis (sil-i-kō'sis) [L. *silex,* flint, + *-osis,* condition]. Silicatosis; a form of pneumoconiosis resulting from occupational exposure to and inhalation of silica dust over a period of years; characterized by a slowly progressive fibrosis of the lungs, which may result in impairment of lung function; s. predisposes to pulmonary tuberculosis.

silicotuberculosis (sil'i-kō-tū-ber-kyū-lō'sis). Silicosis associated with tuberculous pulmonary lesions.

siliqua olivae (sil'i-kwă ō-lī'vē) [L. the husk of the olive]. The arcuate fibers, which appear to encircle the inferior olive in the medulla oblongata.

siliquose (sil'i-kwōs). Resembling a silique, or long slender pod; denoting a form of cataract resulting in shriveling of the lens with calcareous deposit in the capsule.

silk. The fibers or filaments obtained from the cocoon of the silkworm.

floss s., dental *floss.*

surgical s., thread prepared from the cocoon filaments of glutinous gum which are spun by the mulberry silkworm *Bombyx mori;* used as suture material in 14 sizes from 0.025 mm to 1.016 mm in diameter and numbered accordingly from 7-0 to 7.

virgin s., an extremely fine ophthalmic suture material consisting of two to seven natural s. filaments bonded together by sericin, a natural adhesive.

Silver, Henry K., U.S. pediatrician, *1918. See S.-Russell *dwarfism, syndrome.*

sil'ver [A.S. *seolfor*] Argentum; a metallic element, symbol Ag, atomic no. 47, atomic weight 107.873.

s. chloride, used in the preparation of antiseptic silver preparations.

colloidal s. iodide, an antiseptic used for treatment of inflammation of the mucous membranes.

s. fluoride, $AgF_2 \cdot H_2O$; an antiseptic.

fused s. nitrate, toughened s. nitrate.

s. iodate, a reagent for the determination of chloride.

s. lactate, has been used as an astringent and antiseptic.

mild s. protein, rendered colloidal by the presence of or combination with protein; it contains not less than 19 and not more than 23% of s.; used externally as an antiseptic devoid of irritating properties.

s. nitrate, an antiseptic and astringent; used externally, in solution, in the prevention of ophthalmia neonatorum; also used in the special staining of the nervous system, spirochetes, reticular fibers, Golgi apparatus, nucleolar organizer region, and calcium.

s. oxide, has been used in epilepsy and chorea; it is explosive when mixed with readily combustible substances.

s. picrate, an ionizable salt of s., used in the treatment of trichomoniasis and moniliasis of the vagina.

strong s. protein, a compound of s. and protein containing not less than 7.5 and not more than 8.5% of s.; used externally as an antiseptic, devoid of astringent and nearly so of irritant properties.

s. sulfadiazine, the s. derivative of sulfadiazine, used externally as a topical antibacterial agent in preventing and treating infections in burns.

toughened s. nitrate, fused s. nitrate; an escharotic and germicide for local application.

silver impregnation. Silver complexes employed to demonstrate reticulin in normal and diseased tissues, as well as neuroglia, neurofibrillae, argentaffin cells, and Golgi apparatus.

Silverman, Leslie, U.S. engineer, 1914–1966. See S.-Lilly *pneumotachograph.*

Silverman, William A., 20th century U.S. pediatrician. See Caffey-S. *syndrome.*

Silverskiöld, Nils G., Swedish orthopedist, 1888–1957. See S.'s *syndrome.*

simethicone (si-meth'i-kōn). A mixture of dimethyl polysiloxanes and silica gel; an antiflatulent.

similia similibus curantur (si-mil'ē-ă si-mil'i-bŭs ker-an'ter) [L. likes are cured by likes]. The homeopathic formula expressing the law of similars, the doctrine that any drug which is capable of producing morbid symptoms in the healthy will remove similar symptoms occurring as an expression of disease. Another reading of the formula, employed by Hahnemann, the founder of homeopathy, is *similia similibus curentur,* let likes be cured by likes.

similimum, simillimum (si-mil'i-mŭm) [L. *simillimus,* most like, superl. of *similis,* like]. In homeopathy, the remedy indicated in a certain case because the same drug, when given to a healthy person, will produce the symptom complex most nearly approaching that of the disease in question.

Simmonds, Morris, German physician, 1855–1925. See S.'s *disease.*

Simmons, J.S., U.S. bacteriologist, 1890–1954. See S.'s citrate *medium.*

Simon, Charles E., U.S. physician, 1866–1927. See S.'s *sign.*

Simon, Gustav, German surgeon, 1824–1876. See S.'s *position.*

Simon, Théodore, French physician, 1873–1961. See Binet-S. *scale, test.*

Simonart, Pierre J.C., Belgian obstetrician, 1817–1847. See S.'s *bands, ligaments, threads.*

Simonea folliculorum (si-mō'nē-ă fō-lik-yū-lōr'ŭm). *Demodex folliculorum.*

Simons, Arthur, German physician, *1877. See S.'s *disease.*

simple (sim'pl) [L. *simplex*]. **1.** Not complex or compound. **2.** In anatomy, composed of a minimum number of parts. **3.** A medicinal herb.

Simplified Oral Hygiene Index (OHI-S). An index that measures the current oral hygiene status based upon the amount of debris and calculus occurring on six representative tooth surfaces in the mouth; often used in field surveys of periodontal disease.

Simpson, Sir James Y., Scottish obstetrician, 1811–1870. See S. uterine *sound;* S.'s *forceps.*

Simpson, William S., British civil engineer, †1917. See S. *light.*

Sims, J. Marion, U.S. gynecologist, 1813–1883. See S. *position,* uterine *sound.*

simulation (sim-yū-lā'shŭn) [L. *simulatio,* fr. *simulo,* pp. *-atus,* to imitate, fr. *similis,* like]. Imitation; said of a disease or symptom that resembles another, or of the feigning of illness as in factitious illness or malingering.

computer s., computer *model.*

simulator (sim'yū-lā-ter, tōr). An apparatus designed to produce effects simulating those of specific environmental conditions; used in experimentation and training.

Simulium (si-myū'lē-ŭm) [L. *simulo,* to simulate]. Eusimulium; a genus of biting gnats or midges, the black flies, humpbacked flies, or buffalo gnats in the dipteran family Simuliidae. The aquatic larvae require swift-flowing streams or highly oxygenated waters for their development, a critical epidemiological factor in the role of these flies as disease vectors. In Central and South America, Mexico, and across central Africa, various species transmit *Onchocerca volvulus,* agent of human onchocerciasis; in North America, *Onchocerca gutturosa* and other onchocercid infections of cattle, horses, and various wild ruminants are transmitted by other black flies.

S. damno'sum, species that is an important vector of onchocerciasis in central Africa.

S. neav'ei, species that is an important vector of onchocerciasis in eastern Africa where its larvae and pupae are attached to the shells of crabs of the genus *Potamonantes.*

S. ochra'ceum, species that is a vector of human onchocerciasis in Central America.

S. orna'tum, species that is a vector of bovine onchocerciasis in Australia.

S. ruggle'si, species that is a vector of *Leucocytozoon simondi* in Canada and the northern U.S.

simultanagnosia (sī-mŭl-tan-ag-nō'sē-ă). Inability to recognize multiple elements in a simultaneously displayed visual presentation, *i.e.,* the ability to appreciate elements of a scene but not the display as a whole.

SIMV Abbreviation for spontaneous or synchronized intermittent mandatory *ventilation.*

sincalide (sin'kă-līd). The C-terminal octapeptide of cholecystokinin; it causes smooth muscle contraction of the gallbladder and small intestine, relaxation of the choledoduodenal junction, and stimulates pancreatic and gastric secretions; also used as a diagnostic aid to retrieve bile for analysis.

sincipital (sin-sip'i-tăl). Relating to the sinciput.

sinciput, pl. **sincipita, sinciputs** (sin'si-put, sin-sip'i-tă) [L. half of the head]. The anterior part of the head just above and including the forehead.

sinew (sin'ū) [A.S. *sinu*]. Tendon.

singultation (sing'gŭl-tā'shŭn) [L. *singulto,* pp. *-atus,* to hiccup]. Hiccupping.

singultous (sing-gŭl'tŭs). Relating to hiccups.

singultus (sing-gŭl'tŭs) [L.]. A hiccup.

sinigrase, sinigrinase (sin'i-grās, -gri-nās). Thioglucosidase.

sinister (si-nis'ter) [L.] [NA]. Left.

sinistrad (sin'is-trad, si-nis'trad) [L. *sinister,* left, + *ad,* to]. Toward the left side.

sinistral (sin'is-trăl, sĭ-nis'trăl). **1.** Sinistrous; relating to the left side. **2.** Denoting a left-handed person.

sinistrality (sin-is-tral'i-tē). The condition of being left-handed.

sinistro- [L. *sinister,* left]. Combining form denoting left, toward the left.

sinistrocardia (sin'is-trō-kar'dē-ă) [sinistro- + G. *kardia,* heart]. Displacement of the heart beyond the normal position on the left side.

sinistrocerebral (sin'is-trō-ser'ĕ-brăl) [sinistro- + L. *cerebrum,* brain]. Relating to the left cerebral hemisphere.

sinistrocular (sin-is-trok'yū-lăr) [sinistro- + L. *oculus,* eye]. Left-eyed; denoting one who prefers the left eye in monocular work, such as in the use of a microscope. *Cf.* dominant *eye.*

sinistrogyration (sin'is-trō-jī-rā'shŭn) [sinistro- + L. *gyratio,* a turning around (gyration)]. Sinistrotorsion.

sinistromanual (sin'is-trō-man'yū-ăl) [sinistro- + L. *manus,* hand]. Left-handed.

sinistropedal (sin-is-trop'ĕ-dăl) [sinistro- + L. *pes (ped-),* foot]. Left-footed; denoting one who uses the left leg by preference.

sinistrorotation (sin'is-trō-rō-tā'shŭn). Sinistrotorsion.

sinistrorse (sin'is-trors) [L. *sinistrorsus,* on the left side, fr. *sinister,* left, + *verto,* pp. *versus,* to turn]. Turned or twisted to the left.

sinistrotorsion (sin'is-trō-tōr'shŭn) [sinistro- + L. *torsio,* a twisting (torsion)]. Sinistrogyration; sinistrorotation; levorotation (2); levotorsion (1); a turning or twisting to the left.

sinistrous (sin'is-trŭs, si-nis'trŭs). Sinistral (1).

sinoatrial (S-A) (sī'nō-ā'trē-ăl). Sinuatrial; relating to the sinus venosus and the right atrium of the heart.

sinography (sī-nog'ră-fē) [sinus + G. *graphō,* to write]. Radiographic use of a contrasting medium to visualize a sinus tract.

sinopulmonary (sī'nō-pŭl'mō-nār-ē). Relating to the paranasal sinuses and the pulmonary airway.

sinovaginal (sī-nō-vaj'i-năl). Relating to that part of the vagina derived from the urogenital sinus.

sin'ter [Ger. dross, slag]. To heat a powdered substance without thoroughly melting it, causing it to fuse into a solid but porous mass.

sinuatrial (sin'yū-ā'trē-ăl, sī'nū-). Sinoatrial.

SINUS

sinus, pl. **sinus, sinuses** (sī'nŭs, -ĕz) [L. *sinus,* cavity, channel, hollow]. **1** [NA]. A channel for the passage of blood or lymph, without the coats of an ordinary vessel; *e.g.,* blood passages in the gravid uterus or those in the cerebral meninges. **2.** A hollow in bone or other tissue. **3.** A fistula or tract leading to a suppurating cavity.

s. a'lae par'vae, s. sphenoparietalis.

anal s.'s, s. anales.

s. ana'les, anal s.'s; **(1)** [NA] rectal s.'s; Morgagni's crypts; Morgagni's s. (1); the grooves between the anal columns; **(2)** pockets or crypts in the columnar zone of the anal canal between the anocutaneous line and the anorectal line; the s.'s give the mucosa a scalloped appearance.

anterior s.'s, s. anteriores.

s. anterio'res [NA], anterior s.'s; anterior cells; cellulae anteriores; the anterior group of air cells of the ethmoidal s.'s; each s. communicates with the middle meatus of the nasal cavity.

s. aor'tae [NA], aortic s.; Valsalva's or Petit's s.; the space between each semilunar valve and the wall of the aorta.

aortic s., s. aortae.

Arlt's s., an inconstant depression on the internal surface of the lacrimal sac.

barber's pilonidal s., pilonidal s. occurring in barbers, usually in the web between the fingers, due to the burying of hairs by the alternate loosening and tightening of tissues of the hand by the manipulation of scissors.

basilar s., *plexus* basilaris.

Breschet's s., s. sphenoparietalis.

s. carot'icus [NA], carotid s.; carotid bulb; a slight dilation of the common carotid artery at its bifurcation into external and internal carotids; it contains baroreceptors which, when stimulated, cause slowing of the heart, vasodilation, and a fall in blood pressure.

carotid s., s. caroticus.

s. caverno'sus [NA], cavernous s.; a paired dural s. on either side of the sella turcica, the two being connected by anastomoses, the anterior and posterior intercavernous s., in front of and behind the hypophysis, respectively, making thus the circular s.

cavernous s., s. cavernosus.

cerebral s.'s, s. durae matris.

cervical s., precervical s.; in young mammalian embryos a depression in the nuchal region caudal to the hyoid arch, with the third and fourth branchial arches and grooves in its floor; normally it is obliterated after the second month, but occasionally cervical fistulae persist as vestiges of it.

circular s., s. circularis.

s. circula'ris, circular s.; **(1)** s. intercernosi; **(2)** a venous s. at the periphery of the placenta; **(3)** s. venosus sclerae.

coccygeal s., a fistula opening in the region of the coccyx, being the result of incomplete closure of the caudal end of the neural tube. See also pilonidal s.

s. corona'rius [NA], coronary s.; a short trunk receiving most of the veins of the heart, running in the posterior part of the coronary sulcus and emptying into the right atrium between the inferior vena cava and the atrioventricular orifice.

coronary s., s. coronarius.

costomediastinal s., *recessus* costomediastinalis.

cranial s.'s, s. durae matris.

dermal s., a s. lined with epidermis and skin appendages extending from the skin to some deeper-lying structure, most frequently

the spinal cord.
s.'s of dura mater, s. durae matris.
s. du'rae ma'tris [NA], s.'s of dura mater; cerebral, cranial, dural, or venous s.'s; endothelium-lined venous channels in the dura mater.
dural s.'s, s. durae matris.
Englisch's s., s. petrosus inferior.
s. epididym'idis [NA], a narrow space between the body of the epididymis and the testis.
ethmoidal s.'s, s. ethmoidales.
s. ethmoida'les [NA], ethmoidal s.'s; antra ethmoidale; evaginations of the mucous membrane of the middle and superior meatuses of the nasal cavity; they are subdivided into s. anteriores, s. mediae, and s. posteriores.
frontal s., s. frontalis.
s. fronta'lis [NA], frontal s.; a hollow formed on either side in the lower part of the squama of the frontal bone; it communicates by the ethmoidal infundibulum with the middle meatus of the nasal cavity of the same side.
Guérin's s., a cul-de-sac or diverticulum behind the valvula fossae navicularis.
Huguier's s., *fossula* fenestrae vestibuli.
inferior longitudinal s., s. sagittalis inferior.
inferior petrosal s., s. petrosus inferior.
inferior sagittal s., s. sagittalis inferior.
s. intercaverno'si [NA], intercavernous s.'s; s. circularis (1); circulus venosus ridleyi; Ridley's s.'s or circle; the anterior and posterior anastomoses between the cavernous s.'s.
intercavernous s.'s, s. intercavernosi.
jugular s., s. jugula'ris, one of three enlargements of the jugular veins; the external jugular s. is between the two sets of valves; the internal jugular s.'s are at the origin (superior bulb) and near the termination (inferior bulb).
s. lactif'eri [NA], lactiferous s.; ampulla of milk duct; ampulla lactiferi; a circumscribed spindle-shaped dilation of the lactiferous duct just before it enters the nipple.
lactiferous s., s. lactiferi.
laryngeal s., *ventriculus* laryngis.
s. laryn'geus, *ventriculus* laryngis.
lateral s., s. transversus.
s. lie'nis [NA], splenic sinus; an elongated venous channel, 12 to 40 μm wide, lined by rod-shaped cells.
longitudinal s., see s. sagittalis inferior and superior.
Luschka's s., venous s. in the petrosquamous suture.
lymph s., lymphatic s.
lymphatic s., lymph s.; the channels in a lymph node crossed by a reticulum of cells and fibers and bounded by littoral cells; there are subcapsular, trabecular, and medullary s.'s.
Maier's s., an infundibuliform depression on the internal surface of the lacrimal sac which receives the lacrimal canaliculi.
marginal s. of placenta, discontinuous venous lakes at the margin of the placenta.
mastoid s.'s, *cellulae* mastoideae.
s. maxilla'ris [NA], maxillary s.; antrum of Highmore; maxillary antrum; genyantrum; an air cavity in the body of the maxilla, communicating with the middle meatus of the nose.
maxillary s., s. maxillaris.
s. me'diae [NA], middle s.'s; middle cells; cellulae mediae; the middle group of air cells of the ethmoidal s.'s; each s. communicates with the middle meatus of the nasal cavity.
Meyer's s., a small concavity in the floor of the external auditory canal near the membrana tympani.
middle s.'s, s. mediae.
Morgagni's s., (1) s. anales (1); **(2)** *utriculus* prostaticus; **(3)** *ventriculus* laryngis.
s. of nail, s. unguis.
oblique s. of pericardium, s. obliquus pericardii.
s. obli'quus pericar'dii [NA], oblique s. of pericardium; the recess in the pericardial cavity behind the heart bounded by the pericardial reflections on the pulmonary veins and inferior vena cava.
occipital s., s. occipitalis.
s. occipita'lis [NA], occipital s.; an unpaired dural s. commencing at the confluens sinuum and passing downward in the base of the falx cerebelli to the foramen magnum.
Palfyn's s., a space within the crista galli of the ethmoid described as communicating with the ethmoidal and frontal s.'s.
paranasal s.'s, s. paranasales.
s. paranasa'les [NA], paranasal s.'s; the paired cavities in the bones of the face lined by mucous membrane continuous with that of the nasal cavity; these s.'s are the frontal, sphenoidal, maxillary, and ethmoidal.
parasinoidal s.'s, *lacunae* laterales.
Petit's s., s. aortae.
petrosal s., see s. petrosus inferior and superior.
s. petro'sus infe'rior [NA], inferior petrosal s.; Englisch's s.; a paired s. of the dura mater running in the groove on the petrooccipital fissure connecting the cavernous s. with the superior bulb of the internal jugular vein.
s. petro'sus supe'rior [NA], superior petrosal s.; a paired s. of the dura mater in the groove on the superior margin of the petrous part of the temporal bone, connecting the cavernous s. with the transverse s.
phrenicocostal s., *recessus* costodiaphragmaticus.
pilonidal s., pilonidal fistula; a fistula or pit in the sacral region, communicating with the exterior, containing hair which may act as a foreign body producing chronic inflammation.
piriform s., *recessus* piriformis.
pleural s.'s, *recessus* pleurales.
s. pocula'ris, *utriculus* prostaticus.
s. poste'rior [NA], a deep groove above the pyramidal eminence in the posterior wall of the tympanic cavity.
s. posterio'res [NA], posterior s.'s; posterior cells; cellulae posteriores; the posterior group of air cells of the ethmoidal s.'s; each s. communicates with the superior meatus of the nasal cavity.
precervical s., cervical s.
prostatic s., s. prostaticus.
s. prostat'icus [NA], prostatic s.; the groove on either side of the urethral crest in the prostatic part of the urethra.
rectal s.'s, s. anales.
s. rec'tus [NA], straight s.; tentorial s.; an unpaired s. of the dura mater in the posterior part of the falx cerebri where it is attached to the tentorium cerebelli; it passes horizontally to the confluens sinuum.
renal s., s. renalis.
s. rena'lis [NA], renal s.; the cavity of the kidney, containing the calyces and pelvis.
s. reu'niens, obsolete term for s. venosus.
rhomboidal s., s. rhomboidalis, rhombocele; a dilation of the central canal of the spinal cord in the lumbar region.
Ridley's s., s. intercavernosi.
Rokitansky-Aschoff s.'s, small outpocketings of the mucosa of the gallbladder which extend through the muscular layer; they may be congenital.
s. sagitta'lis infe'rior [NA], inferior sagittal s.; inferior longitudinal s.; an unpaired dural s. in the lower margin of the falx cerebri, running parallel to the superior saggital s. and emptying into the straight s.
s. sagitta'lis supe'rior [NA], superior sagittal s.; superior longitudinal s.; an unpaired dural s. in the sagittal groove, beginning at the foramen caecum and terminating at the confluens sinuum.
sigmoid s., s. sigmoideus.
s. sigmoi'deus [NA], sigmoid s.; the S-shaped dural s. lying on the mastoid process of the temporal bone and the jugular process of the occipital bone; it is continuous with the transverse s. and emp-

ties into the internal jugular vein.
sphenoidal s., s. sphenoidalis.
s. sphenoida'lis [NA], sphenoidal s.; one of a pair of cavities in the body of the sphenoid bone communicating with the nasal cavity.
sphenoparietal s., s. sphenoparietalis.
s. sphenoparieta'lis [NA], sphenoparietal s.; s. alae parvae; Breschet's s.; a paired s. of the dura mater beginning on the parietal bone, running along the posterior margin of the lesser wing of the sphenoid, and emptying into the cavernous s.
splenic s., s. lienis.
straight s., s. rectus.
superior longitudinal s., s. sagittalis superior.
superior petrosal s., s. petrosus superior.
superior sagittal s., s. sagittalis superior.
tarsal s., s. tarsi.
s. tar'si [NA], tarsal s. or canal; a hollow or canal formed by the groove of the talus and the groove of the calcaneus.
tentorial s., s. rectus.
terminal s., s. termina'lis, the vein bounding the area vasculosa in the blastoderm.
s. tonsilla'ris, *fossa* tonsillaris.
Tourtual's s., *fossa* supratonsillaris.
transverse s., s. transversus.
transverse s. of pericardium, s. transversus pericardii.
s. transver'sus [NA], transverse s.; lateral s.; a paired dural s. that begins at the confluens sinuum and terminates in the sigmoid s.
s. transver'sus pericar'dii [NA], transverse s. of pericardium; Theile's canal; a passage in the pericardium between the origins of the great vessels and the atria.
s. trun'ci pulmona'lis [NA], the space at the origin of the pulmonary trunk between the wall of the vessel and each cusp of the semilunar valve.
s. tym'pani [NA], tympanic s.; a depression in the tympanic cavity posterior to the tympanic promontory.
tympanic s., s. tympani.
s. un'guis, s. of the nail; the deep cleft housing the root of the nail.
urogenital s., s. urogenitalis (1).
s. urogenita'lis, **(1)** urogenital s.; the ventral part of the cloaca after its separation from the rectum by the growth of the urorectal septum; from it develops the lower part of the bladder in both sexes, the prostatic portion of the male urethra, and the urethra and vestibule in the female; **(2)** persistent *cloaca.*
uterine s., uterine sinusoid; a small irregular vascular channel in the endometrium.
uteroplacental s., irregular vascular spaces in the zone of the chorionic attachment to the decidua basalis.
Valsalva's s., s. aortae.
s. vena'rum cava'rum [NA], the portion of the cavity of the right atrium of the heart that receives the blood from the venae cavae; it is separated from the rest of the atrium by the crista terminalis.
s. veno'sus [NA], a cavity at the caudal end of the embryonic cardiac tube in which the veins from the intra- and extraembryonic circulatory arcs unite; in the course of development it forms the portion of the right atrium known in adult anatomy as the sinus venarum cavarum.
s. veno'sus scle'rae [NA], venous s. of sclera; Schlemm's, Fontana's or Lauth's canal; s. circularis (3); the vascular structure encircling the anterior chamber of the eye and through which anterior aqueous humor leaves the eye.
venous s.'s, s. durae matris.
venous s. of sclera, s. venosus sclerae.
s. vertebra'les longitudina'les, portions of the internal vertebral venous plexus lying on the posterior surfaces of the vertebral bodies on either side of the posterior longitudinal ligament.

sinusitis (sī-nŭ-sī'tis) [sinus + G. *-itis,* inflammation]. Inflammation of the lining membrane of any sinus, especially of one of the paranasal sinuses.
s. abscen'dens, s. complicated with caries or necrosis of the bony wall directly beneath the affected portion of the mucous lining of the sinus.
frontal s., infection in one or both frontal sinuses.
infectious s. of turkeys, see chronic respiratory *disease.*

sinusoid (si'nŭ-soyd) [sinus + G. *eidos,* resemblance]. **1.** Resembling a sinus. **2.** A thin-walled terminal blood vessel having an irregular and larger caliber than an ordinary capillary; its endothelial cells have large gaps and the basal lamina is either discontinuous or absent.
uterine s., uterine *sinus.*

sinusoidal (sī-nŭ-soy'dăl). Relating to a sinusoid.

sinusotomy (sin-ŭ-sot'ō-mē) [sinus + G. *tomē,* incision]. Incision into a sinus.

si op. sit Abbreviation for L. *si opus sit,* if needed.

siphon (sī'fōn) [G. *siphōn,* tube]. A tube bent into two unequal lengths, used to remove fluid from a cavity or vessel by atmospheric pressure.

siphonage (sī'fōn-ij). Emptying of the stomach or other cavity by means of a siphon.

Siphona irritans (sī-fō'nă ir'i-tanz) [G. *siphōn,* tube]. The horn fly, a bloodsucking muscoid fly that causes great irritation and annoyance to cattle, and transmits *Stephanofilaria stilesi.*

Siphonaptera (sī-fō-nap'tĕ-ră) [G. *siphōn,* tube, + G. *a-* priv. + *pteron,* wing]. The fleas, an order of wingless insect ectoparasites highly adapted for survival in mammalian fur; they are flattened laterally, spined, and equipped with well-developed metathoracic legs for jumping.

Sipple, J.H., U.S. physician, *1930. See S.'s *syndrome.*

Sippy, Bertram W., U.S. physician, 1866–1924. See S. *diet.*

sireniform (sī-ren'i-fōrm). Denoting a malformation with the appearance of sirenomelia.

sirenomelia (sī'rĕ-nō-mē'lē-ă) [L. *siren,* G. *seirēn,* a siren]. Mermaid deformity; symmelia; union of the legs with partial or complete fusion of the feet. See also sympus.

siriasis (si-rī'ă-sis) [G. *seiriasis,* from *seiriaō,* to be hot]. Sunstroke.

Siris, Evelyn, U.S. radiologist, *1914. See Coffin-S. *syndrome.*

sirup (sir'ŭp). Syrup.

sismotherapy (sis-mō-thār'ă-pē) [G. *seismos,* a shaking, fr. *seiō,* fut. *seisō,* to shake]. Vibratory *massage.*

sisomicin sulfate (sis-ō-mī'sin). $(C_{19}H_{37}N_5O_7)_2 \cdot 5H_2SO_4$; an antibiotic produced by *Micromonospora inyoensis* that has a spectrum of activity and application similar to that of gentamicin.

sis'ter. In Great Britain: **(1)** the title of a head nurse in a public hospital or in a ward or the operating room of a hospital; **(2)** any registered nurse in private practice.

Sister Joseph, superintendent at Saint Mary's hospital, Mayo Clinic, and surgical assistant to Dr. William Mayo, c. 1928. See S. J.'s *nodule.*

Sistrunk, Walter Ellis, U.S. surgeon, 1880–1933. See S. *operation.*

site (sīt) [L. *situs*]. Place; seat; situation; location. See also situs.
active s., that portion of an enzyme molecule at which the actual reaction proceeds; considered to consist of one or more residues or atoms in a spatial arrangement that permits interaction with the substrate to effect the reaction of the latter.
allosteric s., postulated as the place on an enzyme where a nonsubstrate, which may be the product of the biosynthetic pathway involving the enzyme, may bind and influence the activity of the enzyme by changing the enzyme's shape; the influence of CTP on aspartate carbamoyltransferase activity exemplifies the concept of

an allosteric site on an allosteric protein.
cleavage s., restriction s.
fragile s., a non-staining gap at a specific point on a chromosome, usually involving both chromatids, always at the same point on chromosomes of different cells from an individual or kindred; it results in *in vitro* production of acentric fragments, deleted chromosomes, or other chromosome anomalies; inherited as a dominant chromosome marker.
privileged s., an anatomic area lacking lymphatic drainage, such as the brain, cornea, and hamster cheek pouch, in which heterologous tumors may grow because the host does not become sensitized.
receptor s., point of attachment of viruses, hormones, or other activators to cell membranes.
restriction s., cleavage s.; a s. in nucleic acid in which the bordering bases are of such a type as to leave them vulnerable to the cleaving action of an endonuclease.
switching s., the break point in a DNA sequence at which a gene segment unites with another gene segment, as in the production of the immunoglobulins.

sito- [G. *sitos, sition,* food, grain]. Combining form relating to food or grain.

sitostane (sī'tō-stān). Stigmastane.

β-sitosterol (sī-tō-stēr'ol). Cinchol; stigmast-5-en-3β-ol; (24*R*)-24-ethyl-5-cholesten-3β-ol; an anticholesteremic.

sitotaxis (sī-tō-tak'sis) [sito- + G. *taxis,* orderly arrangement]. Sitotropism.

sitotoxin (sī-tō-tok'sin) [sito- + G. *toxikon,* poison]. Any food poison, especially one developing in grain.

sitotoxism (sī-tō-tok'sizm) [sito- + G. *toxikon,* poison]. **1.** Poisoning by spoiled or fungous grain. **2.** Food poisoning in general.

sitotropism (sī-tot'rō-pizm) [sito- + G. *tropē,* a turning]. Sitotaxis; turning of living cells to or away from food.

situation (sich-yū-ā'shŭn). The aggregate of biological, psychological, and sociological factors that affect an individual's behavioral pattern.
psychoanalytic s., the relationship, characteristically restricted to the therapist's office, between patient and therapist.

situs (sī'tŭs) [L.]. Site.
s. inver'sus, s. transversus; reversal of position or location; **s. i. viscerum,** visceral inversion; a transposition of the viscera, *e.g.,* the liver developing on the left side or the heart on the right.
s. perver'sus, malposition of any viscus.
s. sol'itus, the normal visceral arrangement.
s. transver'sus, s. inversus.

Siwe, Sture A., Swedish pediatrician, 1897–1966. See Letterer-S. *disease.*

sizer (sī'zer) A cylinder of variable diameter, with rounded ends, used to measure the internal diameter of the bowel in preparation for stapling.

Sjögren, Henrik S.C., Swedish ophthalmologist, *1899. See S.'s *disease, syndrome;* Gougerot-S. *disease.*

Sjögren, Torsten, Swedish physician, 1859–1939. See S.-Larsson *syndrome,* Torsten S.'s *syndrome,* Marinesco-S. *syndrome.*

Sjöqvist, O., Swedish neurosurgeon, 1901–1954. See S. *tractotomy.*

SK Abbreviation for streptokinase.

skato-. Obsolescent spelling of scato-.

skatole (skat'ōl). 3-Methyl-1*H*-indole, formed in the intestine by the bacterial decomposition of tryptophan and found in fecal matter, to which it imparts its characteristic odor.

skatoxyl (skă-tok'sil). 3-Hydroxymethylindole, formed in the intestine by the oxidation of skatole; some undergoes conjugation in the body with sulfuric or gluronic acids and is excreted in the urine in conjugated form.

skein (skān) [Gael. *sgeinnidh,* hempen thread]. The coiled threads of chromatin seen in the prophase of mitosis.
choroid s., *glomus* choroideum.
test s.'s, s.'s of wool of various colors used in testing for color vision deficiency.

skeletal (skel'ĕ-tăl). Relating to the skeleton.

skeletology (skel-ĕ-tol'ō-jē). The branch of anatomy and of mechanics dealing with the skeleton.

skeleton (skel'ĕ-tŏn) [G. *skeletos,* dried, ntr. *skeleton,* a mummy, a skeleton]. **1.** The bony framework of the body in vertebrates (endoskeleton) or the hard outer envelope of insects (exoskeleton or dermoskeleton). **2.** All the dry parts remaining after the destruction and removal of the soft parts; this includes ligaments and cartilages as well as bones. **3.** All the bones of the body taken collectively.
appendicular s., s. appendiculare.
s. appendicula're [NA], appendicular s.; the bones of the limbs including the pectoral and pelvic girdles.
articulated s., mounted s., one with the various parts connected in such a way as to allow of motion as in the living body.
axial s., s. axiale.
s. axia'le [NA], axial s.; the bones of the head and trunk excluding the pectoral and pelvic girdles.
cardiac s., the dense supporting connective tissue of the heart; it consists of the four anuli fibrosi from which some of the myocardial fibers take origin, the right and left trigona fibrosa, and the membranous part of the interventricular septum.
s. of free inferior limb, the bones of the lower limb except the hip bones.
s. of free superior limb, the bones of the upper limb except the scapula and clavicle.
gill arch s., cartilages associated with the visceral portion of the embryonic mammalian chondrocranium, representing the gill arch (branchial) skeletons as seen in shark-type fishes; they are the primordia of Meckel's cartilage, styloid, hyoid, cricoid, thyroid, and arytenoid cartilages and the auditory ossicles. See also branchial *arch.*
jaw s., viscerocranium.
visceral s., visceroskeleton (2).

Skene, Alexander J.C., U.S. gynecologist, 1838–1900. See S.'s *glands, tubules; ducts* of S.'s glands.

skeneitis, skenitis (skē-nī'tis). Inflammation of Skene's glands.

skeneoscope (skēn'ō-skōp). A form of endoscope for inspecting Skene's glands.

skew (skyū). In statistics, departure from symmetry of a frequency distribution.

skia- [G. *skia,* shadow]. Combining form denoting shadow; in radiology, superseded by radio-.

skiascopy (skī-as'kŏ-pē). Retinoscopy.

skiascotometry (skī'ă-skō-tom'ĕ-trē) [G. *skia,* shadow, + scotometry]. A method of plotting scotomas in the visual field by using an adaptation of the Goldmann perimeter.

Skillern's fracture. Penn Gaskell, U.S. surgeon, *1882. See S.'s *fracture.*

skin [A.S. *scinn*] Cutis.
alligator s., ichthyosis.
bronzed s., the dark s. in Addison's disease.
deciduous s., keratolysis (2).
diamond s., the appearance of the affected site in erysipeloid.
elastic s., see Ehlers-Danlos *syndrome.*
farmer's s., sailor's s.; dry, wrinkled s. with presence of dry premalignant keratoses; observed most commonly in fair-skinned,

blue-eyed persons who are exposed to sunshine for prolonged periods and over many years.
fish s., ichthyosis.
glabrous s., s. that is normally devoid of hair.
glossy s., atrophoderma neuriticum; shiny atrophy of the s., usually of the hands, following nerve injury.
loose s., *cutis* laxa.
nail s., eponychium (2).
parchment s., parchment-like appearance of the s. caused by loss of underlying connective and elastic tissue, or by the relatively rapid and persistent loss of water from the horny layer.
piebald s., vitiligo.
pig s., soft s. in which follicles are widely dilated; seen in pretibial myxedema.
porcupine s., epidermolytic *hyperkeratosis.*
sailor's s., farmer's s.
sex s., the s. of the genital regions of the *Macaca mulatta* and other primates which becomes hyperemic during estrus; at the same time the dermis becomes gelatinous and the epidermis thickened.
shagreen s., shagreen patch; an oval-shaped nevoid plaque, skin-colored or occasionally pigmented, smooth or crinkled, appearing on the trunk or lower back in early childhood; sometimes seen with other signs of tuberous sclerosis.
s. of teeth, *cuticula* dentis.
toad s., phrynoderma.
yellow s., xanthoderma.

Skinner, Burrhus F., U.S. psychologist, *1904. See skinnerian *conditioning;* S. *box.*

skin writing. Dermatographism.

Sklowsky, E.L., 20th century German physician. See S. *symptom.*

Skoda, Joseph, Bohemian clinician in Vienna, 1805–1881. See skodaic *resonance;* S.'s *rale, sign, tympany.*

skodaic (skō-dā'ik). Relating to Skoda.

skull (skŭl) [Early Eng. *skulle,* a bowl]. Cranium.
cloverleaf s., see cloverleaf skull *syndrome.*
maplike s., various defects in the s., especially in the temporal bone, the anterior fossa, and orbits, forming irregular outlines resembling the national boundaries on an atlas.
steeple s., tower s., oxycephaly.

skullcap (skŭl'kap). Calvaria.

sky blue (skī' blū'). A pigment mixture of cobaltous stannate and calcium sulfate; used biologically as an injection mass.

sl Symbol for slyke.

slab-off. A process by which prism base-up is produced in the reading field of a spectacle lens through bicentric grinding.

SLE Abbreviation for systemic *lupus* erythematosus.

sleep (slēp) [A.S. *slaep*]. A physiologic state of relative unconsciousness and inaction of the voluntary muscles, the need for which recurs periodically. The stages of sleep have been variously defined in terms of depth (light, deep, dreaming), EEG characteristics (delta waves, synchronization), physiological characteristics (REM, NREM, orthodox), and presumed anatomical level (pontine, mesencephalic, rhombencephalic, Rolandic, etc.).
crescendo s., normal s., marked by a gradual increase in movements of the sleeper during the course of the night.
electric s., a condition of unconsciousness induced by the passage of an electric current through the brain.
electrotherapeutic s., see electrotherapeutic s. *therapy.*
hypnotic s., hypnosis.
light s., dysnystaxis.
paradoxical s., a deep s., with a brain wave pattern more like that of waking states than of other states of s., which occurs during rapid eye movement s.
paroxysmal s., narcolepsy.
rapid eye movement (REM) s., that state of deep s. in which rapid eye movements, alert EEG pattern, and dreaming occur; several central and autonomic functions are distinctive during this state.
twilight s., formerly a method of producing s. for delivery by a combination of morphine and scopolamine.
winter s., hibernation.

sleepiness (slēp'i-nes). Somnolence (1).

sleeplessness (slēp'les-nes). Insomnia.

sleep'talking. **1.** Somniloquence (1). **2.** Somniloquy.

sleep'walker. Somnambulist.

sleep'walking. Somnambulism (1).

slide (slīd). A rectangular glass plate on which is placed an object to be examined under the microscope.

sling. A supporting bandage or suspensory device; especially a loop suspended from the neck and supporting the flexed forearm.

slit. A long, narrow opening, incision, or aperture.

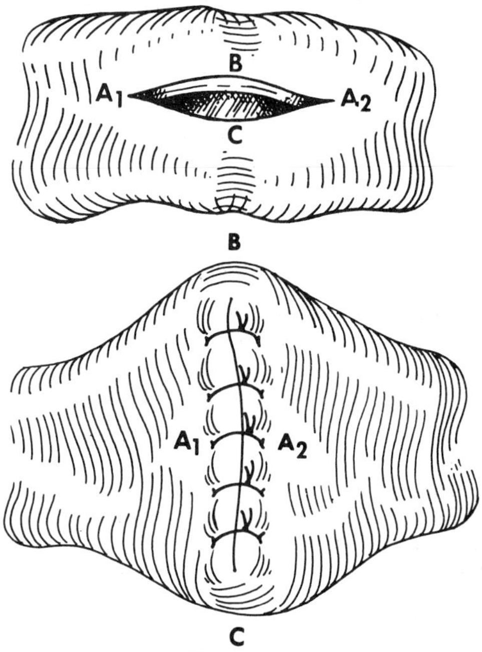

Cheatle Slit

Cheatle s., a longitudinal incision into the antimesenteric border of the small intestine, which when closed transversely creates a larger lumen than would be possible by simple end-to-end anastomosis; currently modified to include longitudinal incisions into the cut ends of the transected small intestine or other tubular structures, allowing a wide caliber elliptical anastomosis to be performed.
filtration s.'s, slit *pores.*
pudendal s., *rima* pudendi.
vulvar s., *rima* pudendi.

slit'lamp. Biomicroscope.

slope (slōp). An inclination or slant.
lower ridge s., the s. of the mandibular residual ridge in the second and third molar as seen from the buccal side.

slough (slŭf). **1.** Necrosed tissue separated from the living structure. **2.** To separate from the living tissue, said of a dead or necrosed part.

Sluder's neuralgia. See under neuralgia.

sludge (slŭdj). A muddy sediment. See also sludged *blood.*
activated s., see activated sludge *method.*

sluice (slūs). Waterfall.

sluiceway (slūs'wā). Spillway.

slurry (sler'ē). A thin semifluid suspension of a solid in a liquid.

slyke (sl) (slīk) [D.D. Van *Slyke,* U.S. physician and chemist, 1883–1971]. A unit of buffer value, the slope of the acid-base titration curve of a solution; the millimoles of strong acid that must be added per unit of change in pH.

Sm Symbol for samarium.

SMA Abbreviation for sequential multichannel *autoanalyzer.*

smallpox (smawl'poks) [E. *small pocks,* or pustules]. Variola; variola major; an acute eruptive contagious disease caused by a poxvirus (*Orthopoxvirus*) and marked at the onset by chills, high fever, backache, and headache; in from 2 to 5 days the constitutional symptoms subside and the eruption appears as papules which become umbilicated vesicles, develop into pustules, dry, and form scabs which on falling off leave a permanent marking of the skin (pock marks); average incubation period is 8 to 14 days.
confluent s., a severe form in which the lesions run into each other, forming large suppurating areas.
discrete s., the usual form in which the lesions are separate and distinct from each other.
fulminating s., a rare form of s. with moderate initial fever, fatigue, early appearance of purpura characteristically predominant in the axillae and lower trunk, and terminal hemorrhages in the mucosal surfaces.
hemorrhagic s., variola hemorrhagica; a severe form of s. accompanied by extravasation of blood into the skin in the early stage, or into the pustules at a later stage, accompanied often by nosebleed and hemorrhage from other orifices of the body.
malignant s., a type of s. occurring in one of two forms: confluent, with moderate initial fever, soft, hot, and tender hemorrhagic lesions of the face and arms, no pustules, and 70% mortality, or semiconfluent, with similar onset but with eruption confined to the face and 25% mortality.
modified s., varicelloid s., varioloid (2).
West Indian s., alastrim.

smear (smēr). A thin specimen for examination; it is usually prepared by spreading material uniformly onto a glass slide, fixing it, and staining it before examination.
alimentary tract s., a group of cytologic specimens containing material from the mouth (oral s.), esophagus and stomach (gastric s.), duodenum (paraduodenal s.), and colon, obtained by specialized lavage techniques; used principally for the diagnosis of cancer of those areas.
bronchoscopic s., lower respiratory tract s.
buccal s., a cytologic s. containing material obtained by scraping the lateral buccal mucosa above the dentate line, smearing, and fixing immediately; used principally for determining somatic sex as indicated by the presence of the sex chromocenter (Barr body).
cervical s., a generic name for different types of FGT s.'s of the cervix uteri, *e.g.,* ectocervical, endocervical, pancervical; used principally for cervical screening.
colonic s., see alimentary tract s.
cul-de-sac s., an FGT cytologic specimen of material obtained by aspirating the pouch of Douglas from the posterior vaginal fornix and prepared by smearing, centrifuging, or filtering; used principally for ovarian cancer.
cytologic s., cytosmear; a type of cytologic specimen made by smearing a sample (obtained by a variety of methods from a number of sites), then fixing it and staining it, usually with 95% ethyl alcohol and Papanicolaou stain.
duodenal s., see alimentary tract s.
ectocervical s., a cytologic s. of material obtained from the ectocervix, usually by scraping; used principally for the diagnosis of late cervical cancers involving the ectocervix.
endocervical s., a cytologic s. of material obtained from the endocervical canal by swab, aspiration, or scraping; used principally for the detection of early cervical cancer.
endometrial s., a group of FGT cytologic s.'s containing material obtained directly from the endometrium by aspiration, lavage, or brushing of the uterine cavity.
esophageal s., see alimentary tract s.
fast s., an FGT cytologic smear containing material from the vaginal pool and pancervical scrapings, mixed and prepared on one microscopic slide, smeared, and fixed immediately; used principally for routine FGT screening of ovaries, endometrium, cervix, vagina, and hormonal states.
FGT (female genital tract) cytologic s., any cytologic s. obtained from the female genital tract.
gastric s., see alimentary tract s.
lateral vaginal wall s., a cytologic s. containing material obtained by scraping the lateral wall of the vagina near the junction of its upper and middle third; used for cytohormonal evaluation.
lower respiratory tract s., bronchoscopic or sputum s.; a group of cytologic specimens containing material from the lower respiratory tract and consisting mainly of sputum (spontaneous, induced) and material obtained at bronchoscopy (aspirated, lavaged, brushed); used for cytologic study of cancer and other diseases of the lungs.
oral s., see alimentary tract s.
pancervical s., a cytologic s. of material obtained from the endocervical canal, external os, and ectocervix by scraping these areas with a properly designed cervical spatula; used principally for early cervical cancer detection.
Pap s., Papanicolaou s., a s. of vaginal or cervical cells obtained for cytological study.
sputum s., lower respiratory tract s.
urinary s., a group of cytologic specimens containing processed urine obtained from bladder, ureters, or renal pelvis; used for cytologic study of cancer and other diseases of the urinary tract.
vaginal s., a s. of debris from the vaginal lumen of mammals, used to determine the stage of their reproductive cycle. It is most useful in subprimate mammals having short estrous cycles; nucleated epithelial cells and leukocytes prevail in the s. during diestrus and proestrus, and cornified cells during estrus.
VCE s., a cytologic s. of material obtained from the vagina, ectocervix, and endocervix, smeared separately (in that order) on one slide, and fixed immediately; used principally for the detection of cervical cancer and identification of the sites of diseases of those areas, and for hormonal evaluation.

smegma (smeg'mă) [G. unguent]. A foul-smelling pasty accumulation of desquamated epidermal cells and sebum that has collected in moist areas of the genitalia.
s. clitor'idis, the secretion of the apocrine glands of the clitoris, in combination with desquamating epithelial cells.
s. prepu'tii, sebum preputiale; whitish secretion that collects under the prepuce of the foreskin of the penis or of the clitoris; it is comprised chiefly of desquamating epithelial cells.

smegmalith (smeg'mă-lith) [smegma + G. *lithos,* stone]. A calcareous concretion in the smegma.

smell. **1.** To scent; to perceive by means of the olfactory apparatus. **2.** Olfaction (1). **3.** Odor.

smell-brain (smel'brān). Rhinencephalon.

Smellie, William, British obstetrician, 1697–1763. See S.'s *scissors.*

Smith, David W., U.S. pediatrician, *1926. See S.-Lemli-Opitz *syndrome.*

Smith, G.W., U.S. neurosurgeon, 1917–1964. See S.-Robinson *operation.*

Smith, H.D. See S.-Riley *syndrome.*

Smith, Henry, British military surgeon in India, 1862–1948. See S.'s *operation;* S.-Indian *operation.*

Smith, Robert W., Irish surgeon, 1807–1873. See S.'s *fracture.*

Smith, Theobald, U.S. pathologist, 1859–1934. See Theobald S.'s *phenomenon.*

Smith-Petersen, Marius N., U.S. surgeon, 1886–1953. See S.-P. *nail.*

smog [smoke + fog]. Air pollution characterized by a hazy and often highly irritating atmosphere resulting from a mixture of fog with smoke and other air pollutants.

smut (smŭt). A fungus disease of cereal grains caused by species of Ustilago and characterized by dark brown or black masses of spores on the plants; *e.g.,* corn s. (*U. maydis*); loose s. of wheat (*U. nuda*).

Sn Symbol for tin.

***sn*-.** Prefix meaning stereospecifically numbered; a system of numbering the glycerol carbon atoms in lipids, so that the locant numbers remain constant regardless of chemical substitutions, as opposed to systematic numbering.

snail (snāl) [M.E. *snaile*]. Common name for members of the class Gastropoda (phylum Mollusca). The freshwater pulmonate (nonoperculated, air-breathing) s.'s (subclass Pulmonata, order Basommatophora) include the majority of intermediate hosts of trematodes parasitic in humans and domestic birds and mammals, chiefly in the families Lymnaeidae and Planorbidae. The subclass Prosobranchiata, the operculate snails, includes the order Neogastropoda, which includes the venomous stinging cone snails (genus *Conus*), and the order Mesagastropida, of which the family Hydrobiidae includes most of the medically important host snails.

snake (snāk). An elongated, limbless, scaly reptile of the suborder Ophidia.

snakeroot (snāk'rūt). Serpentaria.
Canada s., *Asarum canadense.*
European s., *Asarum europaeum.*
Seneca s., senega.
Texas s., *Aristolochia reticulata;* botanical source of serpentaria.
Virginia s., *Aristolochia serpentaria;* botanical source of serpentaria.

snap. A short sharp sound; a click; said especially of cardiac sounds.
closing s., the accentuated first heart sound of mitral stenosis, related to closure of the abnormal valve.
opening s., a sharp, high-pitched click in early diastole, usually best heard between the cardiac apex and the lower left sternal border, related to opening of the abnormal valve in cases of mitral stenosis.

snare (snār) [A.S. *snear,* a cord]. An instrument for removing polyps and other projections from a surface, especially within a cavity; it consists of a wire loop passed around the base of the tumor and gradually tightened.
cold s., an unheated s.
galvanocaustic s., hot s., a s. the wire of which is heated to a high temperature by an electric current.

Sneddon, I.B., 20th century British dermatologist. See S.'s *syndrome;* S.-Wilkinson *disease.*

sneeze (snēz) [A.S. *fneōsan*]. **1.** To expel air from the nose and mouth by an involuntary spasmodic contraction of the muscles of expiration. **2.** An act of sneezing; a reflex excited by an irritation of the mucous membrane of the nose or, sometimes, by a bright light striking the eye.

Snell, Simeon, British ophthalmologist, 1851–1909. See S.'s *law.*

Snellen, Hermann, Dutch ophthalmologist, 1834–1908. See S.'s *test types.*

snore (snōr) [A.S. *snora*]. **1.** A rough, rattling, inspiratory noise produced by vibration of the pendulous palate, or sometimes of the vocal cords, during sleep or coma. See also stertor; rhonchus. **2.** To breathe noisily, or with a s.

snout (snowt) [M.E.]. In veterinary anatomy, the rostral extremity of the face and rhinarium, frequently elongate and related to specialized feeding habits as in the gar, soft-shelled turtle, pig, etc.

snow (snō). See *carbon* dioxide snow.

snuff (snŭf). **1.** To inhale forcibly through the nose. **2.** Finely powdered tobacco used by inhalation through the nose or applied to the gums. **3.** Any medicated powder applied by insufflation to the nasal mucous membrane.

snuff-box (snŭf'boks). See *anatomical* snuff-box.

snuffles (snŭf'lz). Obstructed nasal respiration, especially in the newborn infant, sometimes due to congenital syphilis.
rabbit s., acute inflammation of the upper nasal passages, usually associated with *Pasteurella* organisms; in outbreaks of s. in rabbitries there usually are some deaths from pneumonia.

Snyder, Marshall L., U.S. microbiologist, *1907. See S.'s *test.*

SOAP Acronym for *s*ubjective, *o*bjective, *a*ssessment, and *p*lan; used in problem-oriented records for organizing follow-up data, evaluation, and planning.

soap (sōp) [A.S. *sape,* L. *sapo,* G. *sapōn*]. The sodium or potassium salts of long chain fatty acids (*e.g.,* sodium stearate); used for cleansing purposes and as an excipient in the making of pills and suppositories.
animal s., tallow, curd, or domestic s.; s. made with sodium hydroxide and a purified animal fat consisting chiefly of stearin; used in pharmacy in the preparation of certain liniments.
Castile s., hard s.
curd s., domestic s., animal s.
green s., medicinal soft s.
hard s., Castile s.; a s. made with olive oil, or some other suitable oil or fat, and sodium hydroxide; used as a detergent, as an antidote in poisoning by mineral acids, and in the form of a suppository or soapsuds enema for constipation; used also as an excipient in pills.
insoluble s., s. made with a fatty acid and an earthy or metallic base.
marine s., salt water s.; a s. made of palm or coconut oil for use with sea water in which it is soluble.
medicinal soft s., soft or green s.; a s. made with vegetable oils, potassium hydroxide, oleic acid, glycerin, and purified water; used as a stimulant in chronic skin diseases.
salt water s., marine s.
soft s., medicinal soft s.
soluble s., any s. made with potassium, sodium, or ammonium hydroxide: ordinary animal s., Castile s., green s., etc.
superfatted s., a s. containing an excess (3 to 5%) of fat above that necessary to completely neutralize all the alkali; used in the manufacture of medicated s., and in the treatment of skin diseases.
tallow s., animal s.

soapstone (sōp'stōn). Talc.

Soave, F., 20th century Italian pediatric surgeon. See S. *operation.*

socaloin (sō-kal'ō-in). $C_{15}H_{16}O_7$; an aloin obtained from aloes of the island of Socotra.

socialization (sō'shăl-i-zā'shŭn) [L. *socia,* partner, companion]. **1.** The process of learning interpersonal and interactional skills which are in conformity with the values of one's society. **2.** In a group therapy setting, a way of learning to effectively participate in the group.

socia parotidis (sō'shē-ă pa-rot'i-dis) [L. companion of the parotid]. *Glandula* parotidea accessoria.

socio- [L. *socius,* companion]. Combining form denoting social, society.

sociocentric (sō'sē-ō-sen'trik) [socio- + L. *centrum,* center]. Outgoing; reactive to the social or cultural milieu.

sociocentrism (sō'sē-ō-sen'trizm). Taking one's own social group as the standard by which others are measured.

sociocosm (sō'sē-ō-kozm) [socio- + G. *kosmos,* universe]. The totality that includes human society, human thought, and the relationship of man to nature.

sociogenesis (sō'sē-ō-jen'ĕ-sis) [socio- + G. *genesis,* origin]. The origin of social behavior from past interpersonal experiences.

sociogram (sō'sē-ō-gram) [socio- + G. *gramma,* something written]. A diagrammatic representation of the interpersonal interactions of members of a group.

sociomedical (sō'sē-ō-med'i-kăl). Pertaining to the relation of the practice of medicine to society.

sociometry (sō-sē-om'ĕ-trē) [socio- + G. *metron,* measure]. The study of interpersonal relationships in a group.

sociopath (sō'sē-ō-path). Former designation for a person with an antisocial personality type of disorder. See also antisocial *personality.*

sociopathy (sō-sē-op'ă-thē) [socio- + G. *pathos,* suffering]. Obsolete term for the behavioral pattern exhibited by persons with an antisocial personality type of disorder. See also personality disorder.

socket (sok'et) [thr. O. Fr. fr. L. *soccus,* a shoe, a sock]. **1.** The hollow part of a joint; the excavation in one bone of a joint which receives the articular end of the other bone. **2.** Any hollow or concavity into which another part fits, as the eye s.

dry s., alveoalgia.

eye s., orbita.

tooth s., *alveolus* dentalis.

soda (sō'dă) [It., possibly fr. Mediev. L. barilla plant]. *Sodium* carbonate.

baking s., *sodium* bicarbonate.

caustic s., *sodium* hydroxide.

s. lime, a mixture of calcium and sodium hydroxides used to absorb carbon dioxide in situations in which rebreathing occurs; *e.g.,* in basal determinations or in certain types of anesthesia circuits.

washing s., *sodium* carbonate.

sodic (sō'dik). Relating to or containing soda or sodium.

sodio-. Prefix denoting a compound containing sodium; as sodiocitrate, sodiotartrate, a citrate or tartrate of some element containing sodium in addition.

SODIUM

sodium (sō'dē-ŭm) [Mod. L. fr. *soda*]. Natrium; a metallic element, symbol Na, atomic no. 11, atomic weight 22.99; an alkali metal oxidizing readily in air or water; its salts are extensively used in medicine and industry. For organic s. salts not listed below, see under the name of the organic acid portion.

s. acetate, $CH_3COONa{\cdot}3H_2O$; a systemic and urinary alkalizer, expectorant, and diuretic.

s. acid carbonate, s. bicarbonate.

s. acid citrate, s. citrate.

s. acid phosphate, s. biphosphate.

s. alginate, algin.

s. *p*-aminohippurate, used intravenously in renal function tests, to determine the renal plasma flow and the tubular excretion.

s. *p*-aminophenylarsonate, s. arsanilate; $H_2N{-}C_6H_4{-}AsO(OH)(ONa){\cdot}3H_2O$: a compound that was one of the first modern pentavalent arsenicals.

s. aminosalicylate, $C_6H_3(p\text{-}NH_2)(o\text{-}OH){-}COONa{\cdot}2H_2O$; used for the same purposes as aminosalicylic acid.

s. antimonylgluconate, stibogluconate sodium (2).

s. antimonyl tartrate, *antimony* sodium tartrate.

s. arsanilate, s. *p*-aminophenylarsonate.

s. ascorbate, same actions and uses as ascorbic acid; it is preferred for intramuscular administration.

s. aurothiomalate, *gold* sodium thiomalate.

s. aurothiosulfate, *gold* sodium thiosulfate.

s. benzoate, C_6H_5COONa; used in chronic and acute rheumatism and as a liver function test.

s. bicarbonate, baking soda; s. acid carbonate; s. hydrogen carbonate; $NaHCO_3$; used as a gastric and systemic antacid, to alkalize urine, and for washes of body cavities.

s. biphosphate, s. acid phosphate; s. dihydrogen phosphate; primary s. phosphate; $NaH_2PO_4{\cdot}H_2O$; used to increase urinary acidity.

s. bisulfite, s. pyrosulfite; s. hydrogen sulfite; $NaHSO_3$; acid s. sulfite, used in gastric and intestinal fermentation, externally in the treatment of parasitic diseases, and as an antioxidant in certain injections (s. metabisulfite).

s. borate, borax; s. pyroborate; s. tetraborate; $Na_2B_4O_7{\cdot}10H_2O$; used in lotions, gargles, mouthwashes, and as a detergent.

s. bromide, NaBr; a hypnotic and sedative; used in epilepsy and other functional disorders of the nervous system.

s. cacodylate, s. dimethylarsenate; $(CH_3)_2AsOONa{\cdot}3H_2O$; used in anemia, leukemia, and malaria.

s. calcium edetate, *edetate* calcium disodium.

s. carbonate, soda; sal soda; washing soda; $Na_2CO_3{\cdot}10H_2O$; used in the treatment of scaly skin diseases; otherwise rarely used in medicine because of its irritant action.

s. carboxymethyl cellulose, the s. salt of a polycarboxymethyl ether of cellulose; used as a gastric antacid and laxative.

s. chloride, common or table salt; NaCl; the chief component of blood and other body fluids, and urine; used to make isotonic and physiological saline solutions, as an emetic, in the treatment of salt depletion, and topically for inflammatory lesions.

s. chromate Cr 51, anionic hexavalent radioactive chromium in the form of s. chromate ($Na_2{}^{51}CrO$) with a half-life of 27.8 days; used for the determination of circulating red cell volume and red cell survival time.

s. citrate, s. acid citrate; trisodium citrate; $Na_3C_6H_5O_7{\cdot}2H_2O$; used as diuretic, antilithic, systemic and urinary alkalizer, expectorant, and anticoagulant (*in vitro*).

s. citrate, acid, disodium hydrogen citrate; $C_6H_6O_7Na{\cdot}1^1/_2H_2O$; same actions and uses as s. citrate; in addition, it may be used in solutions of glucose without producing caramelization of the latter during autoclaving.

s. cromoglycate, cromolyn sodium.

s. dehydrocholate, a cholagogue; also used to determine circulation time.

s. diatrizoate, s. 3,5-diacetamido-2,4,6-triiodobenzoate; a water-soluble organic iodine compound used for intravenous excretory urography and angiography.

dibasic s. phosphate, s. phosphate.

s. dihydrogen phosphate, s. biphosphate.

s. dimethylarsenate, s. cacodylate.

s. dodecyl sulfate, a widely used detergent, identical with s. lauryl sulfate.

effervescent s. phosphate, exsiccated s. phosphate 200, s. bicarbonate 477, tartaric acid 252, and citric acid 162, mixed and passed through a sieve to make a granular salt.

s. ethylsulfate, s. sulfovinate; $Na(C_2H_5SO_4){\cdot}H_2O$; a laxative.

exsiccated s. sulfite, anhydrous s. sulfite, used as a preservative in

pharmaceutical preparations.
s. fluoride, used as a dental prophylactic in drinking water, and topically as a 2% solution applied on the teeth.
s. fluosilicate, s. hexafluorosilicate.
s. folate, s. pteroylglutamate; the s. salt of folic acid; action and uses are the same as those of folic acid, but it is preferred for parenteral administration.
s. fusidate, fusidate sodium.
s. glycerophosphate, $C_3H_5(OH)_2PO_4Na$; has been used as a tonic.
s. hexafluorosilicate, s. fluosilicate; s. silicofluoride; Na_2SiF_6; used (in dilute solutions) as an antiseptic and deodorant, and for fluoridation of drinking water.
s. hydrogen carbonate, s. bicarbonate.
s. hydrogen sulfite, s. bisulfite.
s. hydroxide, caustic soda; NaOH; used externally as a caustic.
s. hypophosphite, $NaPH_2O_2{\cdot}H_2O$; formerly used as a nerve tonic.
s. hyposulfite, s. thiosulfate.
s. ichthyolsulfonate, an alterative and antiseptic.
s. indigotindisulfonate, *indigo* carmine.
s. iodide, NaI; used as a source of iodine.
s. iodide I 131, prepared from radioactive iodine (^{131}I); practically carrier-free, with a half-life of 8.0 days; used as a diagnostic agent in suspected thyroid disease and in the treatment of selected thyroid diseases.
s. lactate, $C_3H_5NaO_3$; a systemic and urinary alkalizer.
s. lauryl sulfate, $CH_3(CH_2)_{10}CH_2OSO_3Na$; a surface-active agent of the anionic type.
s. levothyroxine, 3,3′,5,5′-tetraiodothyronine pentahydrate; it is twice as effective as the racemic form; used in the treatment of thyroid deficiency syndromes.
s. liothyronine, s. L-triiodothyronine, the physiologically active isomer of triiodothyronine, twice as active as the racemic form; used in the treatment of thyroid deficiency syndromes.
s. metabisulfite, $Na_2S_2O_5$; used as an antioxidant in injectable solutions.
s. methicillin, *methicillin* sodium.
s. methylarsonate, disodium monomethyl arsonate; $Ch_3H_5O(ONa)_2{\cdot}5H_2O$; formerly used in tuberculosis, chorea, and other affections in which the cacodylates were used.
s. nitrate, cubic niter; Chilean saltpeter; $NaNO_3$; formerly used for dysentery and as a diuretic.
s. nitrite, $NaNO_2$; used to lower systemic blood pressure, to relieve local vasomotor spasms, especially in angina pectoris and Raynaud's disease, to relax bronchial and intestinal spasms, and as an antidote for cyanide poisoning.
s. nitroprusside, s. nitroferricyanide, $(Na_2FeCCN)_5NO{\cdot}5H_2O$; used as a reagent for detection of organic compounds in the urine; also a potent hypotensive agent used by dilute intravenous infusion in induced hypotension.
s. nucleate, s. nucleinate, s. salts of yeast acids, used in the treatment of anemias, rheumatism, and gout.
s. orthophosphate, s. phosphate.
s. perborate, $NaBO_2H_2O_2{\cdot}3H_2O$; used in the extemporaneous preparation of hydrogen peroxide; a 2% solution is equivalent in germicidal action to 0.4% of hydrogen peroxide.
s. peroxide, Na_2O_2; used externally as a paste or soap in the treatment of comedones and acne.
s. pertechnetate, Na-99m TeO_4; a radiopharmaceutical used for brain, thyroid, and salivary gland scanning.
s. phenolsulfonate, s. sulfocarbolate; has been used in tonsillitis and as an intestinal antiseptic; has no antiseptic properties.
s. phosphate, s. orthophosphate; dibasic s. phosphate; $Na_2HPO_4{\cdot}H_2O$; a laxative.
s. phosphate P 32, anionic radioactive phosphorus in the form of a solution of s. acid phosphate and s. basic phosphate; a beta emitter with a half-life of 14.3 days; pH between 5.0 and 6.0; after administration, highest concentrations are found in rapidly proliferating tissues with high phosphorus content; it is used in the treatment of polycythemia vera and chronic myelogenous leukemia, and in colloid form to control malignant pleural or peritoneal effusions.
s. polyanhydromannuronic acid sulfate, an anticoagulant drug prepared from alginic acid and having an action similar to that of heparin.
s. polystyrene sulfonate, a cationic exchange resin used in hyperpotassemia.
s. potassium tartrate, *potassium* sodium tartrate.
primary s. phosphate, s. biphosphate.
s. propionate, the s. salt of propionic acid; used for fungus infections of the skin, usually in combination with calcium propionate.
s. psylliate, the s. salt of the liquid fatty acids of psyllium oil, prepared by dissolving the fatty acid in dilute s. hydroxide solution; used like morrhuate s. as a sclerosing agent in the treatment of varicose veins.
s. pteroylglutamate, s. folate.
s. pyroborate, s. borate.
s. pyrosulfite, s. *bisulfite.*
s. rhodanate, s. thiocyanate.
s. ricinoleate, s. ricinate, the s. salt of ricinoleic acid; a sclerosing agent similar in action to morrhuate s.
s. salicylate, an analgesic, antipyretic, and antirheumatic.
s. silicofluoride, s. hexafluorosilicate.
s. stearate, stearic acid sodium salt, used as a pharmaceutical adjuvant in ointments, creams, and suppositories.
s. succinate, disodium succinate; used as an analeptic in barbiturate poisoning, and as a hepatic stimulant, urinary alkalizer, and diuretic; also used to measure circulation time.
s. sulfate, Glauber's salt; $Na_2SO_4{\cdot}10H_2O$; an ingredient of many of the natural laxative waters, and also used as a hydragogue cathartic.
s. sulfite, $Na_2SO_3{\cdot}7H_2O$; has been used for the relief of intestinal fermentation, and externally for aphthous stomatitis.
s. sulfocarbolate, s. phenolsulfonate.
s. sulfocyanate, s. thiocyanate.
s. sulforicinate, s. sulforicinoleate, made by combining castor oil, sulfuric acid, and s. hydroxide and chloride; used as a solvent for iodine, iodoform, resorcinol, pyrogallol, and a number of other substances for external use.
s. sulfovinate, s. ethylsulfate.
s. tartrate, $Na_2C_4H_4O_6{\cdot}2H_2O$; a laxative.
s. taurocholate, the s. salt of taurocholic acid, extracted from the bile of carnivora; a cholagogue.
s. tetraborate, s. borate.
s. tetradecyl sulfate, an anionic surface-active agent used for its wetting properties to enhance the surface action of certain antiseptic solutions; also used as a sclerosing agent similar to morrhuate s. in the treatment of varicose veins.
s. thiocyanate, s. rhodanate or sulfocyanate; NaSCN; used in the management of essential hypertension.
s. thiosulfate, s. hyposulfite; $Na_2S_2O_3{\cdot}5H_2O$; an antidote in cyanide poisoning in conjunction with s. nitrite; used as a prophylactic agent against ringworm infections in swimming pools and baths, and to measure the extracellular fluid volume of the body.
s. tungstoborate, used in electron microscopy as a negative stain.

---

sodium-24 (^{24}Na). The isotope of sodium with an atomic weight of 24, and a half-life of 14.8 hr; it emits beta and gamma rays, and is more easily prepared than the longer-lived, positron-emitting ^{22}Na (half-life, 2.6 yr). It is used to measure the extracellular fluid.

sodium group. The alkali metals: cesium, lithium, potassium, rubidium, and sodium.

sodoku (sō-dō′kū) [Jap. rat poison]. Rat-bite *fever.*

sodomist, sodomite (sod'ō-mist, -mīt) [G. *sodomitēs,* an inhabitant of the biblical city of Sodom, which was destroyed by fire because of the wickedness of its people]. One who practices sodomy.

sodomy (sod'ŏm-ē) [see sodomist]. Buggery; a term denoting a variety of sexual practices considered abnormal, especially bestiality, fellatio, and anal intercourse.

Soemmering, Samuel T. von, German anatomist, 1755–1830. See S.'s *ganglion, ligament, muscle, spot; ring* of S.

Soffer, Louis J., U.S. internist, *1904. See Sohval-S. *syndrome.*

Sohval, Arthur R., U.S. internist, *1904. See S.-Soffer *syndrome.*

soja (sō'yah). Soybean.

sokosho (sō-kō'shō) [Jap. *so,* rat, + *ko,* bite, + *sho,* malady]. Rat-bite *fever.*

sol. 1. A colloidal dispersion of a solid in a liquid. *Cf.* gel. **2.** Abbreviation for solution.

Solanaceae (sō-lă-nā'sē-ē). A family of plants that includes the genus *Solanum* (nightshade) and some 84 other genera comprising 1,800 species, including the tomato and potato plants.

solanaceous (sō-lă-nā'shŭs, sol'ă-). Pertaining to plants of the family Solanaceae, or to drugs derived from them.

solanochromene (sol'ă-nō-krō'mēn). Plastochromenol-8.

solapsone (sō-lap'sōn). Solasulfone.

solasulfone (sol-ă-sŭlf'ōn). Solapsone; tetrasodium 1,1'-[sulfonylbis(*p*-phenyleneimino)] bis [3-phenyl-1,3-propanedisulfonate]; a leprostatic agent.

solation (sol-ā'shŭn). In colloidal chemistry, the transformation of a gel into a sol, as by melting gelatin.

solder (sod'er) [L. *solidare,* to make solid, through Fr., various forms]. **1.** A fusible alloy used to unite edges or surfaces of two pieces of metal of higher melting point; hard s.'s, usually containing gold or silver as their main constituent, are usually used in dentistry to connect noble metal alloys. **2.** To join two pieces of metal with such an alloy.

sole (sōl) [A.S.]. Planta pedis.

Solenoglypha (sō-lē-nog'li-fă) [L., fr. G. *sōlēn,* pipe channel, + *glyphein,* to carve]. A major category of snakes that includes the viper and rattlesnake families.

solenoid (sol'ĕ-noyd). A helical coil of wire energized electrically to produce a magnetic field, which induces a current in any conductor placed within or near the coil.

Solenopotes capillatus (sō-lĕ-nō-pō'tēz kap-i-lā'tŭs) [G. *solen,* pipe, + *potos,* a drinking]. A sucking louse of cattle, called the little blue cattle louse in the U.S. and the tubercle-bearing louse in Australia.

solenopsin A (sō-lĕ-nop'sin). *trans*-2-Methyl-6-*n*-undecylpiperidine; one of several, probably five, alkaloidal constituents present in the venom of the imported fire ant, *Solenopis saevissima;* the venom has necrotoxic, hemolytic, insecticidal, and antibiotic properties.

soleus (sō-lē'ŭs) [Mod. L. fr. L. *solea,* a sandal, sole of the foot (of animals), fr. *solum,* bottom, floor, ground]. See under musculus.

sol'id [L. *solidus*] **1.** Firm; compact; not fluid; without interstices or cavities; not cancellous. **2.** A body that retains its form when not confined; one that is not fluid, neither liquid nor gaseous.

solidism (sol'i-dizm). Methodism; the theory propounded by Asclepiades and his followers that disease was due to an imbalance between solid particles (atoms) of the body and the spaces (pores) between them, a doctrine which opposed the humoral conception of Hippocrates.

solidist (sol'i-dist). An adherent of the doctrine of solidism.

solidistic (sol-i-dis'tik). Relating to solidism.

solidus (sol'i-dŭs). That line on a constitution diagram indicating the temperature below which all metal is solid.

soliped (sol'i-ped) [L. solus, alone, + pes, foot]. A solid-hoofed animal such as the horse.

solipsism (sō'lip-sizm, sol'ip-) [L. *solus,* alone, + *ipse,* self]. A philosophical concept that only one's own experience is real.

soln. Abbreviation for solution.

solubility (sol-yū-bil'i-tē). The property of being soluble.

soluble (sol'yū-bl) [L. *solubilis,* fr. *solvo,* to dissolve]. Capable of being dissolved.

solum (sō'lŭm) [L.]. Bottom; floor; the lowest part.

solute (sol'yūt, sō'lūt) [L. *solutus,* dissolved, pp. of *solvo,* to dissolve]. The dissolved substance in a solution.

solutio (sō-lū'shē-ō) [L.]. Solution.

solution (sol., soln.) (sō-lū'shŭn) [L. *solutio*]. **1.** The incorporation of a solid, a liquid, or a gas in a liquid or noncrystalline solid resulting in a homogeneous single phase. See dispersion; suspension. **2.** Generally, an aqueous s. of a nonvolatile substance. **3.** In the language of the Pharmacopeia, an aqueous s. of a nonvolatile substance is called a solution or liquor; an aqueous s. of a volatile substance is a water (aqua); an alcoholic s. of a nonvolatile substance is a tincture (tinctura); an alcoholic s. of a volatile substance is a spirit (spiritus); a s. in vinegar is a vinegar (acetum); a s. in glycerin is a glycerol (glyceritum); a s. in wine is a wine (vinum); a s. of sugar in water is a syrup (syrupus); a s. of a mucilaginous substance is a mucilage (mucilago); a s. of an alkaloid or metallic oxide in oleic acid is an oleate (oleatum). **4.** The termination of a disease by crisis. **5.** A break, cut, or laceration of the solid tissues. See s. of contiguity; s. of continuity.

acetic s., a vinegar.

Benedict's s., an aqueous solution of sodium citrate, sodium carbonate, and copper sulfate which changes from its normal blue color to orange, red, or yellow in the presence of a reducing sugar such as glucose. See also Benedict's *test.*

Burow's s., a preparation of albumin subacetate and glacial acetic acid, used for its antiseptic and astringent action on the skin.

chemical s., see solution (1).

colloidal s., colloidal dispersion; a dispersoid, emulsoid, or suspensoid.

s. of contiguity, the breaking of contiguity; a dislocation or displacement of two normally contiguous parts.

s. of continuity, dieresis; division of bones or soft parts that are normally continuous, as by a fracture, a laceration, or an incision.

Dakin's s., Dakin's fluid; buffered sodium hypochlorite s.; a bactericidal wound irrigant.

disclosing s., a s. that selectively stains all soft debris, pellicle, and bacterial plaque on teeth; used as an aid in identifying bacterial plaque after rinsing with water.

Earle's s., a tissue culture medium containing $CaCl_2$, $MgSO_4$, KCl, $NaHCO_3$, NaCl, $NaH_2PO_4{\cdot}H_2O$, and glucose.

ethereal s., a s. of any substance in ether.

Fehling's s., Fehling's reagent; an alkaline copper tartrate s. formerly used for detection of reducing sugars.

Fonio's s., a diluent with magnesium sulfate, used for stained smears of blood platelets.

Gallego's differentiating s., a dilute s. of formaldehyde and acetic acid used in a modified Gram stain to differentiate and enhance the basic fuchsin binding to Gram-negative microorganisms.

Gey's s., a salt s. usually used in combination with naturally occurring body substances (*e.g.,* blood serum, tissue extracts) and/or more complex chemically defined nutritive s.'s for culturing animal cells.

Hanks' s., a salt s. usually used in combination with naturally occurring body substances (*e.g.,* blood serum, tissue extracts) and/or more complex chemically defined nutritive s.'s for culturing animal cells; two variations contain $CaCl_2$, $MgSO_4 \cdot 7H_2O$, KCl, KH_2PO_4, $NaHCO_3$, NaCl, $Na_2HPO_4 \cdot 2H_2O$, and glucose.

Hartman's s., a s. used to desensitize dentin in dental operations; contains thymol, ethyl alcohol, and sulfuric ether.

Hartmann's s., lactated Ringer's s.

Hayem's s., a blood diluent used prior to counting red blood cells.

Krebs-Ringer s., a modification of Ringer's s., prepared by mixing NaCl, KCl, $Cacl_2$, $MgSO_4$, and phosphate buffer, pH 7.4.

lactated Ringer's s., Hartmann's s.; a s. containing NaCl, sodium lactate, $CaCl_2$ (dihydrate), and KCl in distilled water; used for the same purposes as Ringer's s.

Lange's s., a colloidal gold s. used to demonstrate protein abnormalities in spinal fluid. See Lange's *test.*

Locke's s.'s, s.'s containing, in varying amounts, NaCl, $CaCl_2$, KCl, $NaHCO_3$, and glucose; used for irrigating mammalian heart and other tissues, in laboratory experiments; also used in combination with naturally occurring body substances (*e.g.,* blood serum, tissue extracts) and/or more complex chemically defined nutritive s.'s for culturing animal cells.

Locke-Ringer s., a s. containing NaCl, $CaCl_2$, KCl, $MgCl_2$, $NaHCO_3$, glucose, and water; used in the laboratory for physiological and pharmacological experiments.

Lugol's iodine s., an iodine-potassium iodide s. used as an oxidizing agent, for removal of mercurial fixation artifacts, and also in histochemistry and to stain amebas.

molecular dispersed s., dispersoid.

normal s., see normal (3).

ophthalmic s.'s, sterile s.'s, free from foreign particles and suitably compounded and dispensed for instillation into the eye.

Ringer's s., **(1)** a s. resembling the blood serum in its salt constituents; it contains 8.6 g of NaCl, 0.3 g of KCl, and 0.33 g of $CaCl_2$ in each 1000 ml of distilled water; used topically for burns and wounds; **(2)** a salt s. usually used in combination with naturally occurring body substances (*e.g.,* blood serum, tissue extracts) and/or more complex chemically defined nutritive s.'s for culturing animal cells; **(3)** see Ringer's *injections.*

saline s., **(1)** salt s.; a s. of any salt; **(2)** specifically, an isotonic sodium chloride s.

salt s., saline s. (1).

saturated s. (sat. sol., sat. soln.), a s. that contains all of a substance capable of dissolving; a solution of a substance in equilibrium with an excess undissolved substance.

standard s., standardized s., a s. of known concentration, used as a standard of comparison or analysis.

supersaturated s., a s. containing more of the solid than the liquid would ordinarily dissolve; it is made by heating the solvent when the substance is added, and on cooling the latter is retained without precipitation; addition of a crystal or solid of any kind usually results in precipitation of the excess solute, leaving a saturated s.

test s., a s. of some reagent, in definite strength, used in chemical analysis or testing.

Tyrode's s., a modified Locke's s.; it contains 8 g of NaCl, 0.2 g of KCl, 0.2 g of $CaCl_2$, 0.1 g of $MgCl_2$, 0.05 g of NaH_2PO_4, 1 g of $NaHCO_3$, 1 g of glucose, and water to make 1000 ml; used to irrigate the peritoneal cavity, and in laboratory work.

volumetric s. (VS), a s. made by mixing measured volumes of the components.

Weigert's iodine s., an iodine-potassium iodide mixture used as a reagent to alter crystal and methyl violet so that they are retained by certain bacteria and fungi.

solvate (sol'vāt). A nonaqueous solution or dispersoid in which there is a noncovalent or easily reversible combination between solvent and solute, or dispersion means and disperse phase; when water is the solvent or dispersion medium, it is called a hydrate.

solvation (sol-vā'shŭn). Noncovalent or easily reversible combination of a solvent with solute, or of a dispersion means with the disperse phase; if the solvent is water, s. is called hydration. S. affects the size of ions in solution, thus Na^+ is much larger in H_2O than in solid NaCl.

sol'vent [L. *solvens,* pres. p. of *solvo,* to dissolve]. A liquid that holds another substance in solution, *i.e.,* dissolves it.

amphiprotic s., a s. capable of acting as an acid or a base; *e.g.,* H_2O. See solvolysis.

fat s.'s, nonpolar s.'s; organic liquids notable for their ability to dissolve lipids; usually, but not always, immiscible in water; *e.g.,* diethyl ether, carbon tetrachloride.

nonpolar s.'s, fat s.'s.

polar s.'s, s.'s that exhibit polar forces on solutes, due to high dipole moment, wide separation of charges, or tight association; *e.g.,* water, alcohols, acids.

universal s., a substance sought by the alchemists, and claimed by some to have been found, supposedly capable of dissolving all substances; sometimes, in a physiological sense, applied to water.

solvolysis (sol-vol'i-sis). The reaction of a dissolved salt with the solvent to form an acid and a base; the (partial) reverse of neutralization. If the solvent is water, an amphiprotic solvent, s. is called hydrolysis.

soma (sō'mă) [G. *sōma,* body]. **1.** The axial part of the body, *i.e.,* head, neck, trunk, and tail. **2.** All of an organism with the exception of the germ cells. See also body; corpus.

soman (sō'man). Methylphosphonofluoridic acid 1,2,2-trimethylpropyl ester; an extremely potent cholinesterase inhibitor. See also sarin; tabun.

somasthenia (sō-mas-thē'nē-ă). Somatasthenia.

somat-, somatico-. See somato-.

somatagnosia (sō'mă-tag-nō'sē-ă) [somat- + G. *a-* priv. + *gnōsis,* recognition]. Somatotopagnosis.

somatalgia (sō-mă-tal'jē-ă) [somat- + G. *algos,* pain]. **1.** Pain in the body. **2.** Pain due to organic causes, as opposed to psychogenic pain.

somatasthenia (sō'mă-tas-thē'nē-ă) [somat- + G. *asthenia,* weakness]. Somasthenia; a condition of chronic physical weakness and fatigability.

somatesthesia (sō'mă-tes-thē'zē-ă) [somat- + G. *aisthēsis,* sensation]. Somesthesia; bodily sensation, the conscious awareness of the body.

somatesthetic (sō'mat-es-thet'ik). Relating to somatesthesia.

somatic (sō-mat'ik) [G. *sōmatikos,* bodily]. **1.** Relating to the soma or trunk, the wall of the body cavity, or the body in general. **2.** Relating to the vegetative, as distinguished from the generative, functions.

somaticosplanchnic (sō-mat-i-kō-splangk'nik) [G. *sōmatikos,* relating to the body, + *splanchnikos,* relating to the viscera]. Somaticovisceral; relating to the body and the viscera.

somaticovisceral (sō-mat-i-kō-vis'er-ăl). Somaticosplanchnic.

somatist (sō'mă-tist). One who considers that neuroses and psychoses are manifestations of organic disease.

somatization (sō'mat-i-zā'shŭn). Conversion of anxiety into physical symptoms.

somato-, somat-, somatico- [G. *sōma,* body]. Combining forms denoting the body, bodily.

somatochrome (sō'mă-tō-krōm) [somato- + G. *chrōma,* color]. Denoting the group of neurons or nerve cells in which there is an abundance of cytoplasm completely surrounding the nucleus.

somatogenic (sō'mă-tō-jen'ik) [somato- + G. *genesis,* origin]. **1.** Originating in the soma or body under the influence of external forces. **2.** Having origin in body cells.

somatoliberin (sō′mă-tō-lib′er-in). Somatotropin-releasing factor; growth hormone-releasing factor or hormone; a decapeptide released by the hypothalamus which induces the release of human growth hormone (somatotropin).

somatology (sō-mă-tol′ō-jē) [somato- + G. *logos,* study]. The science concerned with the study of the body; includes both anatomy and physiology.

somatomammotropin (sō′mă-tō-mam′ō-trō-pin). A peptide hormone, closely related to somatotropin in its biological properties, produced by the normal placenta and by certain neoplasms. **human chorionic s. (HCS),** human placental *lactogen.*

somatomedin (sō′mă-tō-mē′din). Insulin-like growth factor; sulfation factor; a peptide (MW of about 4,000), synthesized in the liver and probably in the kidney, that is capable of stimulating certain anabolic processes in bone and cartilage, such as synthesis of DNA, RNA, and protein (including chondromucoprotein), and the sulfation of mucopolysaccharides; secretion and/or biological activity of s. is known to be dependent on somatotropin.

somatomegaly (sō′mă-tō-meg′ă-lē) [somato- + G. *megas* (*megal-*), great]. Gigantism.

somatometry (sō-mă-tom′ĕ-trē) [somato- + G. *metron,* measure]. Classification of persons according to body form, and relation of the types to physiologic and psychologic characteristics.

somatopagus (sō-mă-top′ă-gŭs) [somato- + G. *pagos,* something fixed]. Conjoined twins united in their body regions.

somatopathic (sō′mă-tō-path′ik) [somato- + G. *pathos,* suffering]. Relating to bodily or organic illness, as distinguished from nervous (neurologic) or mental (psychologic) disorder.

somatopathy (sō-mă-top′ă-thē) [somato- + G. *pathos,* suffering]. Obsolete term for any disease of the body.

somatophrenia (sō′mă-tō-frē′nē-ă) [somato- + G. *phrēn,* mind]. A tendency to imagine or exaggerate body ills.

somatoplasm (sō′mă-tō-plazm, sō-mat′ō-) [somato- + G. *plasma,* something formed]. Aggregate of all the forms of specialized protoplasm entering into the composition of the body, other than germ plasm.

somatopleural (sō′mă-tō-plūr′ăl). Relating to the somatopleure.

somatopleure (sō′mă-tō-plūr) [somato- + G. *pleura,* side]. Embryonic layer formed by association of the parietal layer of the lateral mesoderm with the ectoderm.

somatoprosthetics (sō′ma-tō-pros-thet′iks) [somato- + G. *prosthesis,* an addition]. The art and science of prosthetically replacing external parts of the body that are missing or deformed.

somatopsychic (sō′mă-tō-sī′kik) [somato- + G. *psychē,* soul]. Relating to the body-mind relationship; the study of the effects of the body upon the mind, as opposed to psychosomatic.

somatopsychosis (sō′mă-tō-sī-kō′sis) [somato- + G. *psychōsis,* an animating]. An emotional disorder associated with an organic disease.

somatoscopy (sō-mă-tos′kŏ-pē) [somato- + G. *skopeō,* to view]. Examination of the body.

somatosensory (sō-mă-tō-sen′sō-rē). Sensation relating to the body's superficial and deep parts as contrasted to specialized senses such as sight.

somatosexual (sō′mă-tō-sek′shū-ăl). Denoting the somatic aspects of sexuality as distinguished from its psychosexual aspects.

somatostatin (sō′mă-tō-stat′in). Somatotropin release-inhibiting factor; a tetradecapeptide capable of inhibiting the release of somatotropin by the anterior lobe of the pituitary gland.

somatostatinoma (sō′mă-tō-stat-i-nō′mă). A somatostatin-secreting tumor of the pancreatic islets.

somatotherapy (sō′mă-tō-thār′ă-pē). **1.** Therapy directed at physical disorders. **2.** In psychiatry, a variety of therapeutic interventions employing chemical or physical, as opposed to psychological, methods.

somatotopagnosis (sō′mă-tō-top′ag-nō′sis) [somato- + top- + G. *a-* priv. + G. *gnosis,* knowledge]. Somatagnosia; the inability to identify any part of the body, either one's own or another's body. *Cf.* autotopagnosia.

somatotopic (sō-mă-tō-top′ik). Relating to somatotopy.

somatotopy (sō-mă-tot′ō-pē) [somato- + G. *topos,* place]. The topographic association of positional relationships of receptors in the body via respective nerve fibers to their terminal distribution in specific functional areas of the cerebral cortex; the continuation of these positional relationships in all stages of the ascent of nerve fibers through the central nervous system enables the brain and spinal cord to function on a basis of spatially designated units.

somatotroph (sō′mă-tō-trof). A cell of the adenohypophysis that produces somatotropin.

somatotrophic (sō′mă-tō-trof′ik) [somato- + G. *trophē,* nourishment]. Somatotropic.

somatotropic (sō′mă-tō-trop′ik) [somato- + G. *tropē,* a turning]. Somatotrophic; having a stimulating effect on body growth.

somatotropin (sō′mă-tō-trō′pin). Growth or pituitary growth hormone; somatotropic hormone; a protein hormone of the anterior lobe of the pituitary, produced by the acidophil cells, that promotes body growth, fat mobilization, and inhibition of glucose utilization; diabetogenic when present in excess.

somatotype (sō′mă-tō-tīp). **1.** The constitutional or body type of an individual. **2.** The particular constitutional or body type associated with a particular personality type.

somatotypology (sō′mă-tō-tī-pol′ō-jē) [somato- + G. *typos,* form, + *logos,* study]. The study of somatotypes.

somatrem (sō′mă-trem). *N*-L-Methionyl growth hormone (human); a purified polypeptide hormone, made by recombinant DNA techniques, that contains the identical sequence of 191 amino acids constituting naturally occurring somatotropin, plus an additional amino acid, methionine; used in long-term treatment of children deficient in somatotropin.

somesthesia (sō-mes-thē′zē-ă). Somatesthesia.

somite (sō′mīt) [G. *sōma,* body, + *-ite*]. Mesoblastic segment; one of the paired, metamerically arranged cell masses formed in the early embryonic paraxial mesoderm; commencing in the third or early fourth week in the region of the hindbrain, they develop in a caudal direction until 42 pairs are formed; their presence is considered evidence that metameric segmentation is a vertebrate characteristic. **occipital s.,** one of the four most rostral s.'s which become incorporated into the occipital region of the embryonic skull.

somnambulance (som-nam′byū-lans). Somnambulism (1).

somnambulism (som-nam′byū-lizm) [L. *somnus,* sleep, + *ambulo,* to walk]. **1.** Sleepwalking; somnambulance; oneirodynia activa; noctambulation; noctambulism; a disorder of sleep involving complex motor acts which occurs primarily during the first third of the night but not during rapid eye movement sleep. **2.** A form of hysteria in which purposeful behavior is forgotten.

somnambulist (som-nam′byū-list). Sleepwalker; one who is subject to somnambulism (1).

somnifacient (som-ni-fā′shent) [L. *somnus,* sleep, + *facio,* to make]. Soporific (1).

somniferous (som-nif′er-ŭs) [L. *somnus,* sleep, + *fero,* to bring]. Soporific (1).

somnific (som-nif′ik). Soporific (1).

somnifugous (som-nif′yū-gŭs) [L. *somnus,* sleep, + *fugo,* to put to flight]. Dispelling sleep.

somniloquence, somniloquism (som-nil'ō-kwens, -kwizm) [L. *somnus,* sleep, + *loquor,* to talk]. **1.** Sleeptalking (1); talking or muttering in one's sleep. **2.** Somniloquy.

somniloquist (som-nil'ō-kwist). A habitual sleep-talker.

somniloquy (som-nil'ō-kwē) [L. *somnus,* sleep, + *loquor,* to speak]. Sleeptalking (2); somniloquence (2); talking under the influence of hypnotic suggestion.

somnipathist (som-nip'ă-thist). One affected by or under the influence of somnipathy.

somnipathy (som-nip'ă-thē) [L. *somnus,* sleep, + G. *pathos,* suffering]. **1.** Any disorder of sleep. **2.** Hypnotism (1).

somnocinematograph (som'nō-sin-ĕ-mat'ō-graf) [L. *somnos,* sleep, + G. *kinēma,* motion, + G. *graphō,* to write]. Hypnocinematograph; a device for recording the movements made by sleepers.

somnocinematography (som'nō-sin-ĕ-mă-tog'ră-fē). Polycinematosomnography; the process or technique of recording movements during sleep.

somnolence, somnolency (som'nō-lens, -len-sē) [L. *somnolentia*]. Somnolentia (1). **1.** Drowsiness; sleepiness; an inclination to sleep. **2.** A condition of semiconsciousness approaching coma.

somnolent (som'nō-lent) [L. *somnus,* sleep]. **1.** Drowsy; sleepy; having an inclination to sleep. **2.** In a condition of incomplete sleep; semicomatose.

somnolentia (som-nō-len'shē-ă) [L.]. **1.** Somnolence. **2.** Sleep *drunkenness.*

somnolescent (som-nō-les'ent). Inclined to sleep; drowsy.

somnolism (som'nō-lizm). Hypnotism (1).

Somogyi, Michael, U.S. biochemist, 1883–1971. See S. *effect, method, unit.*

soncogene (son'kō-jēn). One of a number of genes on specific chromosomes that can suppress the action of oncogenes.

Sondermann, R., 20th century German ophthalmologist. See S.'s *canal.*

sone (sōn) [L. *sonus,* sound]. A unit of loudness; a pure tone of 1000 Hz at 40 dB above the normal threshold of audibility has a loudness of 1 s.

sonic (son'ik) [L. *sonus,* sound]. Of, pertaining to, or determined by sound; *e.g.,* s. vibration.

sonicate (son'i-kāt). To expose a suspension of cells or microbes to the disruptive effect of the energy of high frequency sound waves.

sonication (son-i-kā'shŭn). The process of disrupting biologic materials by use of sound wave energy.

sonification (son'i-fi-kā'shŭn). The production of sound, or of sound waves.

sonifier (son'i-fī-er). An instrument which produces sound waves, especially those of the frequencies used in sonification procedures.

sonify (son'i-fī). To produce sound.

Sonne, Carl, Danish bacteriologist, 1882–1948. See S. *bacillus, dysentery.*

sonochemistry (son-ō-kem'is-trē). The branch of chemistry concerned with chemical changes caused by, or involving, sound, particularly ultrasound.

sonogram (son'ō-gram) [L. *sonus,* sound, + G. *gramma,* a drawing]. Ultrasonogram.

sonograph (son'ō-graf) [L. *sonus,* sound, + G. *graphō,* to write]. Ultrasonograph.

sonographer (sŏ-nog'ră-fer). Ultrasonographer.

sonography (sŏ-nog'ră-fī) [L. *sonus,* sound. + G. *graphō,* to write]. Ultrasonography.

sonolucent (son-o-lu'sent). Anechoic; echo-free; not containing internal interfaces that reflect high frequency sound waves.

sonomotor (son-ō-mō'ter). Related to movements caused by sound. See sonomotor *response.*

sophisticate (sō-fis'ti-kāt) [Mod. L. *sophisticare,* pp. *sophisticatus,* to alter deceptively, fr. G. *sophistikos,* deceitful]. To adulterate.

sophoretin (sof-ŏ-rē'tin). Quercetin.

sopor (sō'pōr) [L.]. An unnaturally deep sleep.

soporiferous (sō-pōr-if'er-ŭs, sop'ōr-) [L. *soporifer,* fr. *sopor,* deep sleep, + *fero,* to bring]. Soporific (1).

soporific (sō-pōr-if'ik, sop'ōr-) [L. *sopor,* deep sleep, + *facio,* to make]. **1.** Causing sleep. Also called somnifacient; somniferous; somnific; soporiferous. **2.** An agent that produces sleep.

soporose, soporous (sō'pŏ-rōs, -rŭs) [L. *sopor,* deep sleep]. Relating to or causing sopor.

sorbefacient (sōr-bĕ-fā'shent) [L. *sorbeo,* to suck up, + *facio,* to make]. **1.** Causing absorption. **2.** An agent that causes or facilitates absorption.

sorbic acid (sōr'bik). 2,4-Hexadienoic acid; obtained from berries of the mountain ash, *Sorbus aucuparia* (family Rosaceae), or prepared synthetically; it inhibits growth of yeast and mold and is nearly nontoxic to humans; used as a preservative.

sorbin, sorbinose (sōr'bin, -bin-ōs). L-Sorbose.

sorbitan (sōr'bi-tan). Sorbitol or sorbose and related compounds in ester combination with fatty acids, and with short oligo (ethylene oxide) side chains and an oleate terminus, to form detergents such as polysorbate 80.

sorbite (sōr'bīt). Sorbitol.

sorbitol (sōr'bi-tol). D-Sorbitol; D-glucitol; L-gulitol; sorbite; a reduction product of glucose and sorbose found in the berries of the mountain ash, *Sorbus aucuparia* (family Rosaceae), and in many fruits and seaweeds. It has many industrial and pharmaceutical uses; medicinally, it is used as a diuretic and as a sweetening agent, and is almost completely metabolized (to CO_2).

D-sorbitol-6-phosphate dehydrogenase [EC 1.1.1.140]. Ketose reductase; an oxidoreductase that interconverts the 6-phosphates of D-sorbitol and D-fructose, with NAD as hydrogen acceptor or donor.

sorbitose (sōr'bi-tōs). L-Sorbose.

L-sorbose (sōr'bōs). Sorbitose; sorbin; sorbinose; a very sweet reducing, but not fermentable, 2-ketohexose obtained from the berries of the mountain ash, *Sorbus aucuparia* (family Rosaceae), and from sorbitol by fermentation with *Acetobacter suboxydans;* it is isomeric with fructose and is used in manufacture of vitamin C.

sordes (sōr'dēz) [L. fifth, fr. *sordeo,* to be foul]. Rhyparia; saburra (2); a dark brown or blackish crustlike collection on the lips, teeth, and gums of a person with dehydration associated with a chronic debilitating disease.

sore (sōr) [A.S. *sār*] **1.** A wound, ulcer, or any open skin lesion. **2.** Painful; aching; tender.
bay s., chiclero's ulcer.
bed s., see bedsore.
canker s.'s, aphthae (2).
cold s., colloquialism for *herpes* simplex.
desert s., Barcoo rot; veldt s.; any of a variety of chronic nonspecific cutaneous ulcers, most commonly on the shins, knees, hands, and forearms, and probably a variant of ecthyma, that occur in tropical and desert areas.
fungating s., a granulating chancroid.
hard s., chancre.
Oriental s., the lesion occurring in cutaneous leishmaniasis.
pressure s., decubitus *ulcer.*
soft s., chancroid.
summer s.'s, cutaneous *habronemiasis.*
tropical s., the lesion occurring in cutaneous leishmaniasis.

veldt s., desert s.
venereal s., chancroid.
water s., cutaneous *ancylostomiasis.*

sorehead (sōr'hed). Filarial *dermatosis.*

soremouth (sōr'mowth). Contagious *ecthyma.*

soremuzzle (sōr'mŭz-l). Bluetongue.

Sörensen, Sören P.L., Danish chemist, 1868–1939. See S. *scale.*

Soret, C., French radiologist, †1931. See S. *band;* S.'s *phenomenon.*

soroche (sō-rō'chē) [Sp. (orig. ore, formerly attributed to toxic emanations of ores in mountains)]. Altitude *sickness* (1).
chronic s., chronic mountain *sickness.*

sorption (sōrp'shŭn). Adsorption or absorption.

Sorsby, Arnold, British ophthalmologist, *1900. See S.'s macular *degeneration, syndrome.*

s.o.s. Abbreviation for L. *si opus sit,* if needed.

sotalol hydrochloride (sō'tă-lol). 4'-[1-Hydroxy-2-(isopropylamino)ethyl]methanesulfonanilide monohydrochloride; a β-receptor blocking agent with uses similar to those of propanolol.

Sotos, J.F., U.S. pediatrician, *1927. See S. *syndrome.*

Sottas, Jules, French neurologist, 1866–1943. See Dejerine-S. *disease.*

souffle (sū'fl) [Fr. *souffler,* to blow]. A soft blowing sound heard on auscultation.
cardiac s., a soft puffing heart murmur.
fetal s., funic, funicular, or umbilical s.; a blowing murmur, synchronous with the fetal heart beat, sometimes only systolic and sometimes continuous, heard on auscultation over the pregnant uterus.
funic s., funicular s., fetal s.
mammary s., a blowing murmur heard late in pregnancy and during lactation at the medial border of the breast, sometimes only systolic and sometimes continuous.
placental s., uterine s.
umbilical s., fetal s.
uterine s., placental s.; a blowing sound, synchronous with the cardiac systole of the mother, heard on auscultation of the pregnant uterus.

Soulier, J.P. See Bernard-S. *syndrome.*

sound (sownd). **1.** The vibrations produced by a sounding body, transmitted by the air or other medium, and perceived by the internal ear. **2.** An elongated cylindrical, usually curved, instrument of metal, used for exploring the bladder or other cavities of the body, for dilating strictures of the urethra, esophagus, or other canal, for calibrating the lumen of a body cavity, or for detecting the presence of a foreign body in a body cavity. **3.** To explore or calibrate a cavity with a s. **4.** Whole; healthy; not diseased or injured.
after-s., see aftersound.
amphoric voice s., see amphoric *voice.*
anvil s., bellmetal *resonance.*
atrial s., fourth heart s.; see heart s.
auscultatory s., a rale, murmur, bruit, fremitus, or other s. heard on auscultation of the chest or abdomen.
bell s., bellmetal *resonance.*
Béniqué's s., a s. of lead or block of tin of wide curve, used to dilate strictures in the male urethra.
bowel s.'s, relatively high pitched abdominal s.'s caused by propulsion of intestinal contents through the lower alimentary tract.
Campbell s., a miniature s. with a short round-tipped beak, especially curved for the deep urethra of the young male.
cannon s., *bruit* de canon.
cardiac s., heart s.
cavernous voice s., see cavernous *voice.*
coconut s., a s. like that produced when a cracked coconut is tapped; it is elicited by percussing the skull of a patient with osteitis deformans.
cracked-pot s., cracked-pot *resonance.*
Davis interlocking s., a s. comprised of two instruments with curved male and female tips, used to introduce a catheter into the bladder in the treatment of ruptured urethra; the male s. is introduced into the distal urethra via the meatus and the female s. is passed downward through the bladder neck into the proximal urethra via an open cystotomy; the ends of the two instruments are engaged, with the female s. guiding the male s. upward into the bladder; a catheter is then sutured to the tip of the male s. and withdrawn through the urethra to restore continuity of its lumen.
double-shock s., *bruit* de rappel.
eddy s.'s, s.'s that punctuate the continuous murmur of patent ductus arteriosus, imparting to it a characteristically "uneven" quality.
ejection s., a sharp s. heard in early systole over the aortic or pulmonic area when the aorta or pulmonary artery is dilated.
friction s., friction rub; the s., heard on auscultation, made by the rubbing of two opposed serous surfaces roughened by an inflammatory exudate.
gallop s., the abnormal third or fourth heart s. which, when added to the first and second s.'s, produces the triple cadence of gallop rhythm. See also gallop.
heart s., cardiac sound; any of the s.'s heard on auscultation over the region of the heart: the **first h. s.** occurs with ventricular systole and is mainly produced by closure of the atrioventricular valves; the **second h. s.** signifies the beginning of diastole and is due to closure of the semilunar valves; the **third h. s.** occurs in early diastole and corresponds with the first phase of rapid ventricular filling; the **fourth h. s.** occurs in late diastole, corresponds with atrial contraction, and is rarely audible in normal hearts.
hippocratic succussion s., a splashing s. elicited by shaking a patient with hydro- or pyopneumothorax, the physician's ear being applied to the chest.
Jewett s., a short straight s. for dilating the anterior urethra.
Korotkoff s.'s, s.'s heard over an artery when pressure over it is

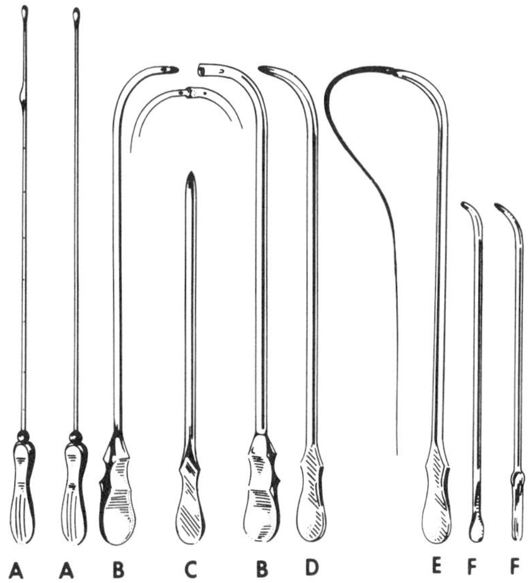

Sounds
A, uterine (Simpson, Sims); *B*, Davis interlocking; *C*, Jewett; *D*, Van Buren; *E*, Le Fort, with threaded filiform bougie; *F*, miniature infant (Campbell, McCrea).

reduced, as when blood pressure is determined by the auscultatory method.
Le Fort s., a curved s. threaded for a filiform bougie, used for dilation of urethral strictures in the male when small caliber or presence of false passages prevents safe passage of a standard s. or catheter.
McCrea s., a gently curved s. used to dilate the urethra in infants or children.
Mercier's s., a catheter the beak of which is short and bent almost at a right angle.
muscle s., a fine murmur heard on auscultation over the belly of a contracting muscle.
percussion s., any s. elicited on percussing over one of the cavities of the body.
pericardial friction s., pericardial rub; pericardial friction rub; a to-and-fro creaking s. heard over the heart in some cases of pericarditis, due to rubbing of the inflamed pericardial surfaces as the heart contracts and relaxes.
pistol-shot femoral s., a shotlike systolic s. heard over the femoral artery in high output states, especially aortic insufficiency; presumably due to sudden stretching of the elastic wall of the artery.
posttussis suction s., a s. produced by the falling back of a drop of mucus or pus into a pulmonary cavity after the latter has been emptied by coughing.
respiratory s., a murmur, bruit, fremitus, rhoncus, or rale heard on auscultation over the lungs or any part of the respiratory tract.
sail s., a s., likened to the snapping of a sail, heard in early systole in some patients with Ebstein's anomaly.
Santini's booming s., a sonorous booming s. heard on auscultatory percussion of a hydatid cyst.
Simpson uterine s., a slender flexible metal rod used to calibrate or dilate the cervical canal, or to hold the uterus in various positions during gynecologic surgery.
Sims uterine s., a slender flexible s. with a small projection about 7 cm from its tip, used to estimate the size and caliber of the uterine cavity.
tambour s., a heart s., usually the aortic or pulmonic valve closure s. when it has a booming and ringing quality like that of a tambour or drum; the aortic s. commonly has a tambour quality in systemic hypertension, the pulmonic s. in pulmonary hypertension.
tic-tac s.'s, embryocardia.
Van Buren s., a standard s., available in several calibers, with a gently curved tip designed to follow the contour of the deep bulbous urethra in the male; used for urethral calibration or dilation.
water-whistle s., a bubbling whistle heard on auscultation over a bronchial or pulmonary fistula.
Winternitz' s., a double-current catheter in which water at any desired temperature circulates.
xiphisternal crunching s., see Hamman's *sign.*

Southern, M.E., 20th century British biologist. See S. blot *analysis.*

Southey, Reginald S., British physician, 1835–1899. See S.'s *tubes.*

sow [M.E.]. A female hog of breeding age.

soya (soy'ă) [Hind. *soyā,* fennel]. Soybean.

soybean (soy'bēn) [Hind. *soyā,* fennel]. Soya; soja; the bean of the climbing herb *Glycine soja* or *G. hispida* (family Leguminosae); a bean rich in protein and containing little starch; it is the source of s. oil; s. flour is used in preparing a bread for diabetics, in feeding formulas for infants who are unable to tolerate cow's milk, and for adults allergic to cow's milk.
s. oil, obtained from s.'s by expression or solvent extraction; contains triglycerides of linoleic acid, oleic acid, linolenic acid, and saturated fatty acids; used as a food and in the manufacture of margarine and other food products.

sp. Abbreviation for subspecies; L. *spiritus,* spirit.

spa (spah) [*Spa,* a mineral spring health resort in Belgium]. A health resort, especially one where there are one or more mineral springs whose waters possess therapeutic properties.

SPACE

space (spās) [L. *spatium,* room, space]. Any demarcated portion of the body, either an area of the surface, a segment of the tissues, or a cavity. See also area; regio; region; zona; zone.
alveolar dead s., the difference between physiologic dead s. and anatomical dead s.; it represents that part of the physiologic dead s. resulting from ventilation of relatively underperfused or nonperfused alveoli; it differs specifically in being placed so as to fill and empty in parallel with functional alveoli, rather than being interposed in the conducting tubes between functional alveoli and the external environment.
anatomical dead s., the volume of the conducting airways from the external environment (at the nose and mouth) down to the level at which inspired gas exchanges oxygen and carbon dioxide with pulmonary capillary blood; formerly presumed to extend down to the beginning of alveolar epithelium in the respiratory bronchioles, but more recent evidence indicates that effective gas exchange extends some distance up the thicker-walled conducting airways because of rapid longitudinal mixing. *Cf.* alveolar dead s.; physiologic dead s.
antecubital s., *fossa* cubitalis.
apical s., the s. between the alveolar wall and the apex of the root of a tooth where an alveolar abscess usually has its origin.
axillary s., *fossa* axillaris.
Berger's s., the s. between the patellar fossa of the vitreous and the lens.
Bogros' s., retroinguinal s.
Böttcher's s., *saccus* endolymphaticus.
Bowman's s., capsular s.
Burns' s., suprasternal s.
capsular s., Bowman's s.; filtration s.; the slitlike s. between the visceral and parietal layers of the capsule of the renal corpuscle; it opens into the proximal tubule of the nephron at the neck of the tubule.
cartilage s., cartilage *lacuna.*
Chassaignac's s., s. between the pectoralis major and the mammary gland.
Cloquet's s., a s. between the zonula ciliaris and the vitreous body.
Colles' s., *spatium* perinei superficiale.
corneal s., lacuna (4); one of the stellate s.'s between the lamellae of the cornea, each of which contains a cell or corneal corpuscle.
Cotunnius' s., *saccus* endolymphaticus.
dead s., **(1)** a cavity, potential or real, remaining after the closure of a wound which is not obliterated by the operative technique; **(2)** see anatomical dead s.; physiologic dead s.
deep perineal s., *spatium* perinei profundum.
denture s., **(1)** that portion of the oral cavity which is, or may be, occupied by maxillary and/or mandibular denture(s); **(2)** the s. between the residual ridges which is available for dentures. See also interarch *distance.*
Disse's s., perisinusoidal s.
s. of Donders, the space between the dorsum of the tongue and the hard palate when the mandible is in rest position following the expiratory cycle of respiration.
epidural s., *cavum* epidurale.
episcleral s., *spatium* episclerale.
epitympanic s., *recessus* epitympanicus.
filtration s., capsular s.

Fontana's s.'s, *spatia* anguli iridocornealis.
freeway s., interocclusal distance (2); interocclusal clearance or gap; the s. between the occluding surfaces of the maxillary and mandibular teeth when the mandible is in physiologic resting position.
gingival s., *sulcus* gingivalis.
haversian s.'s, s.'s in bone formed by the enlargement of haversian canals.
Henke's s., a s., filled with connective tissue, between the vertebral column and the pharynx and esophagus.
His' perivascular s., Virchow-Robin s.
infraglottic s., *cavitas* infraglotticum.
interalveolar s., interarch *distance.*
intercostal s., *spatium* intercostale.
interfascial s., *spatium* episclerale.
interglobular s., *spatium* interglobulare.
interglobular s. of Owen, *spatium* interglobulare.
interocclusal rest s., interocclusal *distance.*
interpleural s., mediastinum (2).
interproximal s., the s. between adjacent teeth in a dental arch; it is divided into the embrasure occlusal to the contact area, and the septal s. gingival to the contact area.
interradicular s., the s. between the roots of multirooted teeth.
interseptovalvular s., the interval in the developing embryonic heart between the septum primum and the left valve of the sinus venosus.
intersheath s.'s of optic nerve, *spatia* intervaginalia nervi optici.
intervillous s.'s, the s.'s containing maternal blood, located between placental villi.
intraretinal s., the potential cleft between the pigmented and neural layers of the retina; it represents the cavity of the embryonic optic vesicle.
s.'s of iridocorneal angle, *spatia* anguli iridocornealis.
Kiernan's s., interlobular s. in the liver.
Kretschmann's s., a slight depression in the epitympanic recess below the recessus membranae tympani superior.
Kuhnt's s.'s, shallow diverticula or recesses between the ciliary body and ciliary zonule which open into the posterior chamber of the eye.
lateral pharyngeal s., *spatium* lateropharyngeum.
leeway s., the difference between the combined mesiodistal widths of the deciduous cuspids and molars and their successors.
lymph s., a s., in tissue or a vessel, filled with lymph.
Magendie's s.'s, s.'s between the pia and arachnoid at the level of the fissures of the brain.
Malacarne's s., *substantia* perforata posterior.
Meckel's s., *cavum* trigeminale.
mediastinal s., mediastinum (2).
medullary s., the central cavity and the cellular intervals between the trabeculae of bone, filled with marrow.
Mohrenheim's s., *fossa* infraclavicularis.
Nuel's s., an interval in the spiral organ (of Corti) between the outer pillar cells on one side and the phalangeal cells and hair cells on the other.
palmar s., one of two fascial s.'s in the palm; one, toward the ulnar side, is called the middle palmar s., the other, toward the radial side, is called the thenar s.
parapharyngeal s., pharyngomaxillary s.
Parona's s., a s. between the superficial and deep muscles of the forearm.
perforated s., see *substantia* perforata anterior and posterior.
perichoroid s., *spatium* perichoroideale.
perilymphatic s., *spatium* perilymphaticum.
perineal s.'s, see *spatium* perinei profundum; *spatium* perinei superficiale.
perinuclear s., *cisterna* caryothecae.
peripharyngeal s., *spatium* peripharyngeum.
periportal s. of Mall, a tissue s. between the limiting lamina and the portal canal in the liver.
perisinusoidal s., Disse's s.; the potential extravascular s. between the liver sinusoids and liver parenchymal cells.
perivitelline s., the s. between the vitelline membrane and the zona pellucida, appearing in an ovum immediately following fertilization.
personal s., a term used in psychology and psychiatry to denote the physical area immediately surrounding an individual who is in proximity to one or more others, whether known or unknown, and which serves as a body buffer zone in such interpersonal transactions.
pharyngeal s., the area occupied by the pharynx (naso-, oro-, and laryngopharnynx). Not to be confused with the retropharyngeal s.
pharyngomaxillary s., parapharyngeal s.; the s. limited by the lateral wall of the pharynx, the cervical vertebrae, and the medial pterygoid muscle.
physiologic dead s. (V_D), the sum of anatomic and alveolar dead s.; the dead s. calculated when the carbon dioxide pressure in systemic arterial blood is used instead of that of alveolar gas in Bohr's equation; it is a virtual or apparent volume that takes into account the impairment of gas exchange because of uneven distributions of lung ventilation and perfusion.
plantar s., one of four areas between fascial layers in the foot, where pus may be confined when the foot is infected.
pleural s., *cavitas* pleuralis.
pneumatic s., any one of the paranasal sinuses.
Poiseuille's s., still *layer.*
popliteal s., *fossa* poplitea.
postpharyngeal s., *spatium* retropharyngeum.
Proust's s., *excavatio* rectovesicalis.
Prussak's s., *recessus* membranae tympani superior.
pterygomandibular s., the area between the mandibular ramus and the pterygoid process of the sphenoid bone.
respiratory dead s., that part of the respiratory tract or of a single breath which fails to exchange oxygen and carbon dioxide with pulmonary capillary blood; a nonspecific term which fails to distinguish between anatomical dead s. and physiologic dead s.
retroinguinal s., spatium retroinguinale; Bogros' s.; a triangular s. between the peritoneum and the transversalis fascia, at the lower angle of which is the inguinal ligament; it contains the lower portion of the external iliac artery.
retromylohyoid s., the sulcus at the posterior end of the mylohyoid line.
retroperitoneal s., *spatium* retroperitoneale.
retropharyngeal s., *spatium* retropharyngeum.
retropubic s., *spatium* retropubicum.
Retzius' s., *spatium* retropubicum.
Schwalbe's s.'s, *spatia* intervaginalia nervi optici.
subarachnoid s., *cavum* subarachnoidale.
subchorial s., subchorial lake; the part of the placenta adjacently beneath the chorion.
subdural s., *spatium* subdurale.
subgingival s., *sulcus* gingivalis.
suprahepatic s.'s, *recessus* subphrenici.
suprasternal s., Burns' s.; a narrow interval between the deep and superficial layers of the cervical fascia above the manubrium sterni through which pass the anterior jugular veins.
Tarin's s., *cisterna* interpeduncularis.
Tenon's s., *spatium* episclerale.
thenar s., see palmar s.
Traube's s., a semilunar s. about 12 cm wide, bounded medially by the left border of the sternum, above by an oblique line from the sixth costal cartilage to the lower border of the eighth or ninth rib, and below by the costal margin; the percussion tone here is normally tympanitic, because of the underlying stomach, but is modified by pulmonary emphysema, a pleural effusion, or an enlarged spleen.

Trautmann's triangular s., the area of the temporal bone bounded by the sinus sigmoideus, the sinus petrosus superior, and a tangent to the posterior semicircular canal.
Virchow-Robin s., His' perivascular s.; a tunnel-like extension of the subarachnoid s. surrounding blood vessels that pass into the brain or spinal cord from the subarachnoid s.; the lining of the channel is composed of pia and glial feet of astrocytes; a continuation of the s. around capillaries and nerve cells probably does not occur.
Waldeyer's s., Waldeyer's *sheath.*
Westberg's s., the s. surrounding the origin of the aorta which is invested with the pericardium.
zonular s.'s, *spatia* zonularia.

---

spagyric (spă-jir'ik) [G. *spaō,* to tear open, + *ageiro,* to collect]. Relating to the paracelsian or alchemical system of medicine, which stressed the treatment of disease by various types of chemical substances.

spagyrist (spaj'ĭ-rist). A physician of the 16th century, a follower of the teachings of Paracelsus who believed in the essential importance of chemical or alchemical knowledge in the understanding and treatment of disease.

spall (spawl). **1.** A fragment. **2.** To break up into fragments.

Spallanzani, Lazaro, Italian priest and scientist, 1729–1799. See S.'s *law.*

spallation (spaw-lā'shŭn) [M.E. *spalle,* fragment]. **1.** Fragmentation. **2.** Nuclear reaction in which nuclei, on being bombarded by high energy particles, liberate a number of protons and alpha particles.

span. The amount, distance, or length between two points; the full extent or reach of anything.
memory s., the maximum number of items recalled after a single presentation (auditory or visual).

spannungs-P (spahn'nŭngz) [Ger. *Spannung,* tightening; stretching or straining, + P wave]. Prominent prolonged and high voltage P waves recorded in electrocardiograms of patients with hypertrophy of both atria, particularly in those with congenital heart disease. See also P-congenitale.

sparganoma (spar-gă-nō'mă). A localized mass resulting from sparganosis.

sparganosis (spar-gă-nō'sis). Infection with the plerocercoid or sparganum of a pseudophyllidean tapeworm, usually in a dermal sore resulting from application of infected flesh as a poultice; infection may also occur from ingestion of uncooked frog, snake, mammal, or bird intermediate or transport host bearing the spargana, but not from fish with *Diphyllobothrium* larvae, since s. is an infection with nonhuman pseudophyllidean tapeworms, usually species of *Spirometra.* S. may also develop from ingestion of water containing procercoid-infected *Cyclops.*
ocular s., infestation of the orbits with the sparganum of *Spirometra mansoni;* characterized by redness and edema of the eyelids, lacrimation, and blepharoptosis; acquired by application of infected raw frog flesh against the eye as a poultice.

sparganum (spar'gă-nŭm) [G. *sparganon,* a swathing band, fr. *spargo,* to swathe]. Originally described as a genus, but now restricted to the plerocercoid stage of certain tapeworms.

sparteine (spar'tē-ēn, -tē-in). *l*-Sparteine; lupinidine; an alkaloid obtained from scoparius, *Cytisus scoparius* and *Lupinus luteus;* s. sulfate is used as an oxytocic drug.

spasm (spazm) [G. *spasmos*]. Spasmus. **1.** An involuntary muscular contraction; if painful, usually referred to as a cramp; if violent, a convulsion. **2.** Muscle s.; increased muscular tension and shortness that cannot be released voluntarily and that prevent lengthening of the muscles involved; s. is due to pain stimuli to the lower motor neuron.
s. of accommodation, excessive contraction of the ciliary muscle.
affect s.'s, spasmodic attacks of laughing, weeping, and screaming, accompanied by marked tachypnea.
anorectal s., *proctalgia* fugax.
Bell's s., facial *tic.*
cadaveric s., rigor mortis occurring irregularly in the different muscles, causing movements of the limbs.
canine s., *risus* caninus.
carpopedal s., carpopedal contraction; s. of the feet and hands observed in hyperventilation, calcium deprivation, and tetany: flexion of the hands at the wrists and of the fingers at the metacarpophalangeal joints and extension of the fingers at the phalangeal joints; the feet are dorsiflexed at the ankles and the toes plantar flexed.
clonic s., alternate involuntary contraction and relaxation of a muscle.
cynic s., *risus* caninus.
dancing s., saltatory s.
epidemic transient diaphragmatic s., epidemic *pleurodynia.*
facial s., facial *tic.*
functional s., occupational *neurosis.*
habit s., tic.
histrionic s., facial *tic.*
infantile s., brief (1 to 3 seconds) muscular s.'s in infants with West's syndrome, which often appear as nodding or salaam s.'s.
intention s., a spasmodic contraction of the muscles occurring when a voluntary movement is attempted.
masticatory s., involuntary convulsive muscular contraction affecting the muscles of mastication.
mimic s., facial *tic.*
mobile s., a tonic s. occurring in spastic infantile hemiplegia on attempted movement.
muscle s., spasm (2).
nictitating s., winking s.; spasmus nictitans; involuntary spasmodic winking.
nodding s., salaam s., attack, or convulsions; spasmus nutans (1); **(1)** in infants, a drop of the head on the chest due to loss of tone in the neck muscles as in epilepsia nutans, or to tonic spasm of anterior neck muscles as in West's syndrome; **(2)** in adults, a psychogenic nodding of the head from clonic s.'s of the sternomastoid muscles.
occupational s., professional s., occupational *neurosis.*
phonic s., *dysphonia* spastica.
progressive torsion s., *dystonia* musculorum deformans.
retrocollic s., retrocollis; torticollis in which the s. affects the posterior neck muscles.
rotatory s., spasmodic *torticollis.*
salaam s., nodding s.
saltatory s., Gower's disease (1); Bamberger's disease (1); static convulsion; dancing spasm; a spasmodic affection of the muscles of the lower extremities.
sewing s., seamstress's *cramp.*
synclonic s., clonic s. of two or more muscles.
tailor's s., tailor's *cramp.*
tonic s., entasia; entasis; a continuous involuntary muscular contraction.
tonoclonic s., convulsive contraction of muscles.
tooth s.'s, infantile convulsions associated with teething.
torsion s., a spasmodic twisting of the body and pelvis.
vasomotor s., spasmodic contraction of the smaller arteries.
winking s., nictitating s.

spasmo- [G. *spasmos,* spasm]. Combining form denoting spasm.

spasmodic (spaz-mod'ik) [G. *spasmōdes,* convulsive, fr. *spasmos,* + *eidos,* form]. Relating to or marked by spasm.

spasmogen (spaz'mō-jen). A substance causing contraction of smooth muscle; *e.g.,* histamine.

spasmogenic (spaz-mō-jen'ik) [spasmo- + G. *-gen,* producing]. Causing spasms.

spasmology (spaz-mol'ō-jē) [spasmo- + G. *logos,* study]. Study of the nature, causation, and means of relief of spasms.

spasmolygmus (spaz-mō-lig'mŭs) [spasmo- + G. *lygmos,* a sobbing, hiccup, fr. *lyzō,* to hiccup, sob]. **1.** Spasmodic sobbing. **2.** Spasmodic hiccup.

spasmolysis (spaz-mol'i-sis) [spasmo- + G. *lysis,* dissolution]. The arrest of a spasm or convulsion.

spasmolytic (spaz'mō-lit'ik). **1.** Relating to spasmolysis. **2.** Antispasmodic; denoting a chemical agent that relieves smooth muscle spasms.

spasmophilia (spaz-mō-fil'ē-ă) [spasmo- + G. *phileō,* to love]. Spasmophilic *diathesis.*

spasmophilic (spaz-mō-fil'ik). Relating to spasmophilic *diathesis.*

spasmus (spaz'mŭs) [L. fr. G. *spasmos,* spasm]. Spasm.

s. ag'itans, parkinsonism (1).

s. cani'nus, *risus* sardonicus.

s. coordina'tus, compulsive movements, such as imitative or mimic tics, festination, etc.

s. glot'tidis, *laryngismus* stridulus.

s. nic'titans, nictitating *spasm.*

s. nu'tans, **(1)** nodding *spasm;* **(2)** nystagmus associated with head-nodding movements.

spastic (spas'tik) [L. *spasticus,* fr. G. *spastikos,* drawing in]. **1.** Hypertonic (1). **2.** Relating to spasm or to spasticity.

spasticity (spas-tis'i-tē). A state of increased muscular tone with exaggeration of the tendon reflexes.

clasp-knife s., clasp-knife effect or rigidity; rigidity of the extensor muscles of a joint which thus offer resistance to passive flexion up to a point, when they give way rather suddenly allowing the joint then to be easily flexed; the rigidity is due to an exaggeration of the stretch reflex. See also lengthening reaction.

s. of conjugate gaze, an oblique or horizontal deviation of the eyes evoked during forcible lid closure or while fixating on an object 30 or 40 cm in front, the eyelids being opened and closed at 4 to 5 second intervals; usually associated with a temporal lobe lesion opposite to the direction of deviation.

spatia (spā'shē-ă) [L.]. Plural of spatium.

spatial (spā'shăl). Relating to space or a space.

spatium, pl. **spatia** (spā'shē-ŭm, -shē-ă) [L.] [NA]. Space.

spa'tia an'guli iridocornea'lis [NA], spaces of iridocorneal angle; Fontana's spaces; ciliary canals; irregularly shaped endothelium-lined spaces within the trabecular meshwork.

s. episclera'le [NA], episcleral space; s. intervaginale bulbi oculi; Tenon's space; interfascial space; s. interfasciale; the space between the vagina bulbi and the sclera.

s. intercosta'le [NA], intercostal space; an interval between the ribs.

s. interfascia'le, s. episclerale.

s. interglobula're, pl. **spa'tia interglobula'ria** [NA], interglobular s.; interglobular s. of Owen; one of a number of irregularly branched spaces near the periphery of the dentin of the crown of a tooth, through which pass the ramifications of the tubules; they are caused by failure of calcification of the dentin.

spa'tia interos'sea metacar'pi [NA], the spaces between the metacarpal bones in the hand.

spa'tia interos'sea metatar'si [NA], the spaces between the metatarsal bones in the foot.

s. intervagina'le bulb'i oc'uli, s. episclerale.

spa'tia intervagina'lia ner'vi op'tici [NA], intersheath spaces of optic nerve; Schwalbe's spaces; the spaces between the internal and external sheaths of the optic nerve, filled with cerebrospinal fluid and continuous with the subarachnoid space.

s. lateropharynge'um [NA], lateral pharyngeal space; that part of the s. peripharyngeum located at the sides of the pharynx. See also s. retropharyngeum.

s. perichoroidea'le [NA], perichoroid space; the interval between the choroid and the sclera filled by the loose meshes of the lamina fusca and the lamina suprachoroidea.

s. perilymphat'icum [NA], perilymphatic space; cisterna perilymphatica; space between the bony and membranous portions of the labyrinth.

s. perine'i profun'dum [NA], deep perineal space or pouch; the region between the perineal membrane and the endopelvic fascia of the floor of the pelvis occupied by the membranous part of the urethra, the bulbourethral gland (in the male), the deep transverse perineal and sphincter urethrae muscles, and the dorsal nerve and artery of the penis or clitoris.

s. perine'i superficia'le [NA], Colles' space; the superficial compartment of the perineum; the space bounded above by the perineal membrane (inferior fascia of the urogenital diaphragm) and below by the superficial perineal fascia (Colles' fascia); it contains the root structure of the penis or clitoris.

s. peripharynge'um [NA], peripharyngeal space; the space, filled with loose areolar tissue, around the pharynx; it is divided into two portions, s. lateropharyngeum and s. retropharyngeum.

s. retroinguina'le, retroinguinal *space.*

s. retroperitonea'le [NA], retroperitoneal space; retroperitoneum; the space between the parietal peritoneum and the muscles and bones of the posterior abdominal wall.

s. retropharynge'um [NA], retropharyngeal space; postpharyngeal space; that part of the s. peripharyngeum located posterior to the pharynx. See also s. lateropharyngeum.

s. retropu'bicum [NA], retropubic space; cavum retzii; Retzius' cavity or space; the area of loose connective tissue between the bladder with its related fascia and the pubis and anterior abdominal wall.

s. subdura'le [NA], subdural space or cavity; cavum subdurale; the very narrow interval between the dura and arachnoid; it contains only sufficient fluid to moisten the opposing surfaces of the two membranes.

spa'tia zonula'ria [NA], zonular spaces; Petit's canals; the spaces between the fibers of the zonula ciliaris at the equator of the lens of the eye.

spatula (spach'ŭ-lă) [L. dim. of *spatha,* a broad, flat wooden instrument, fr. G. *spathē*] A flat blade, like a knife blade but without a sharp edge, used in pharmacy for spreading plasters and ointments.

Roux s., a very small nickeled steel s. used to transfer bits of infected material, such as diphtheritic membrane, to culture tubes.

spatulate (spach'ŭ-lāt). **1.** Spatulated; shaped like a spatula. **2.** To manipulate or mix with a spatula. **3.** To incise the cut end of a tubular structure longitudinally and splay it open, to allow creation of an elliptical anastomosis of greater circumference than would be possible with conventional transverse or oblique (bevelled) end-to-end anastomoses. See fig. on p. 1442.

spatulated (spach'ŭ-lāt-ed). Spatulate.

spatulation (spach'ŭ-lā'shŭn). Manipulation of material with a spatula.

Spatz, Hugo, German neurologist and psychiatrist, 1888–1969. See Hallervorden-S. *disease.*

spav'in [M.E. *spavayne,* swelling fr. O. Fr. *esparvain*]. A disease of the tarsal joints of the horse.

blood s., a distention of the veins in the vicinity of the tarsus in a horse, due to pressure from the swelling of bog s. impeding the return flow of blood.

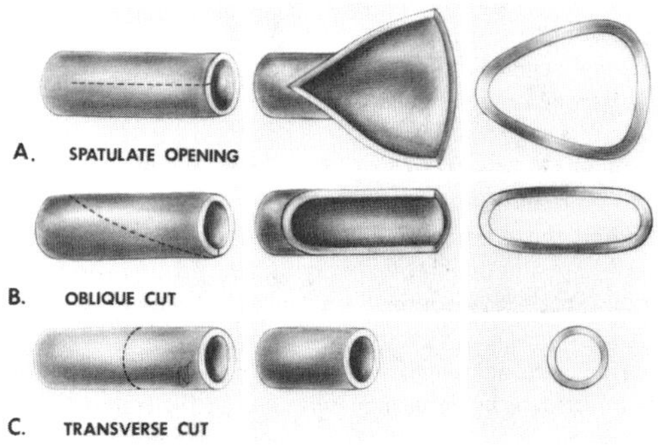

Spatulate
Spatulated opening (*A*) in ureter compared with oblique (*B*) and transverse (*C*) sections.

bog s., a chronic synovitis of the tibiotarsal joint in the horse resulting in distention of the joint capsule with fluid; it usually causes little or no lameness.
bone s., a rarefying osteitis involving the bones of the tarsus of the horse, usually those on the medial surface, resulting in exostoses and ankylosis.

spavined (spav'ind). Affected with spavin.

spay (spā) [Gael. *spoth,* castrate, or G. *spadōn,* eunuch]. To remove the ovaries of an animal.

SPCA Abbreviation for serum prothrombin conversion *accelerator.*

spearmint (spĕr'mint). The leaves and flowering tops of *Mentha viridis* (green garden or lamb mint) or *M. cardiaca* (family Labiatae); a carminative and flavoring agent.
s. oil, the volatile oil, distilled with steam from the fresh overground parts of the flowering plant of *Mentha viridis* or *M. cardiaca,* a flavoring agent.

specialist (spesh'ă-list). One who devotes professional attention to a particular specialty or subject area.

specialization (spesh'ă-li-zā'shŭn). **1.** Professional attention limited to a particular specialty or subject area for study, research, and/or treatment. **2.** Differentiation (1).

specialize (spesh'ă-līz). To engage in specialization (1).

specialty (spesh'al-tē) [L. *specialitas* fr. *specialis,* special]. The particular subject area or branch of medical science to which one devotes professional attention.

speciation (spē-shē-ā'shŭn). The evolutionary process by which new species of animals or plants are formed from preexisting species.

species, pl. **species** (spē'shēz) [L. appearance, form, kind, fr. *specio,* to look at]. **1.** A biological division between the genus and a variety or the individual; a group of organisms which generally bear a close resemblance to one another in the more essential features of their organization, and with sexual forms which produce fertile progeny. **2.** A class of pharmaceutical preparations consisting of a mixture of dried plants, not pulverized, but in sufficiently fine division to be conveniently used in the making of extemporaneous decoctions or infusions, as a tea.
type s., the name of the single s. or of one of the s. of a genus or subgenus when the name of the genus or subgenus was originally validly published.

species-specific. Indicating a serum that is produced by the injection of cells, protein, or other material into an animal, and that acts only upon the cells, protein, etc., of a member of the same species as that from which the original antigen was obtained.

specific (spĕ-sif'ik) [L. *specificus* fr. *species* + *facio,* to make]. **1.** Relating to a species. See also s. *epithet,* **2.** Relating to an individual infectious disease, one caused by a special microorganism. **3.** A remedy having a definite therapeutic action in relation to a particular disease or symptom, as quinine in relation to malaria.

specificity (spes-i-fis'i-tē). **1.** The condition or state of being specific, of having a fixed relation to a single cause or to a definite result; manifested in the relation of a disease to its pathogenic microorganism, of a reaction to a certain chemical union, or of an antibody to its antigen or the reverse. **2.** In clinical pathology and medical screening, the proportion of individuals with negative test results for the disease that the test is intended to reveal, *i.e.,* true negative results as a proportion of the total of true negative and false-positive results. *Cf.* sensitivity (2).
diagnostic s., the probability (P) that, given the absence of disease (D), a normal test result (T) excludes disease; *i.e.,* P(T/D).
relative s., the s. of a medical screening test as determined by comparison with the same type of test (*e.g.,* s. of a new serological test relative to s. of an established serological test).

specillum, pl. **specilla** (spe-sil'ŭm, -lă) [L. a probe, fr. *specio,* to look at]. A probe or small sound.

specimen (spes'ĭ-men) [L. fr. *specio,* to look at]. A small part, or sample, of any substance or material obtained for testing.
cytologic s., a s. obtainable by a variety of methods from many areas of the body, including the female genital tract, respiratory tract, urinary tract, alimentary tract, and body cavities; used for cytologic examination and diagnosis (*e.g.,* cytologic smears, filter preparations, centrifuged buttons).

SPECT Abbreviation for single photon emission *tomography.*

spectacles (spek'tĭ-klz) [L. *specto,* pp. *-atus,* to watch, observe]. Eyeglasses; glasses (1); lenses set in a frame that holds them in front of the eyes, used to correct errors of refraction or to protect the eyes. The parts of the s. are the *lenses;* the *bridge* between the lenses, resting on the nose; the *rims* or *frames,* encircling the lenses; the *sides* or *temples* that pass on either side of the head to the ears; the *bows,* the curved extremities of the temples; the *shoulders,* short bars attached to the rims or the lenses and jointed with the sides.
Bartels' s., markedly convex or concave s. used to study nystagmus.
bifocal s., s. with bifocal lenses. See under lens.
clerical s., half-glass s.
divers' s., strongly convex lenses for clear vision underwater.
divided s., Franklin s.
Franklin s., divided s.; an early form of bifocal s. in which the lower half of the lens is for near vision, the upper half for distant vision.
half-glass s., clerical, pantoscopic, or pulpit s.; s., used for reading, in which the upper portion of the lenses are removed.
hemianopic s., s. with a prism to allow the individual with homonymous hemianopsia to see objects in his blind half field.
Masselon's s., s. with little offsets of metal with smooth edges, which engage below the upper eyelid and keep it raised above the pupil in cases of paralytic blepharoptosis.
orthoscopic s., convex lenses with base-in prisms for close work.
pantoscopic s., half-glass s.
photochromic s., s. with lenses that darken on exposure to ultraviolet light.
protective s., safety s.; s. which protect against ultraviolet or infrared rays or against mechanical injuries.
pulpit s., half-glass s.
safety s., protective s.
stenopeic s., stenopaic s., **(1)** opaque disks with narrow slits in the center allowing only a minimum amount of light to enter; used as a protection against snow blindness; **(2)** s. having opaque disks with multiple perforations used to aid vision in incipient cataract and in discrete opacities of the cornea; occasionally used as a substitute for corrective lenses or sunglasses.

telescopic s., magnifying s. obtained by using a convex objective lens and a concave eyepiece separated by the difference in their focal lengths.

spectinomycin hydrochloride (spek'ti-nō-mī'sin). Actinospectacin; espectinomicina; decahydro-4a,7,9-trihydroxy-2-methyl-6,8-bis(methylamino)-4*H*-pyrano [2,3-*b*] [1,4]benzodioxin-4-one dihydrochloride; an antibacterial agent.

spectra (spek'tră) [L.]. Plural of spectrum.

spectral (spek'trăl). Relating to a spectrum.

spectrin (spek'trin). A filamentous contractile protein that together with actin and other cytoskeleton proteins forms a network that gives the red blood cell membrane its shape and flexibility.

spectro- [L. *spectrum,* an image]. Combining form denoting a spectrum.

spectrochemistry (spek'trō-kem'is-trē). The study of chemical substances and their identification by means of spectroscopy, *i.e.,* by light emitted or absorbed.

spectrocolorimeter (spek'trō-kŏl-er-im'ĕ-ter). A colorimeter using a source of light from a selected portion of the spectrum, *i.e.,* of a selected wavelength.

spectrofluorometer (spek-trō-flūr-om'ĕ-ter). An instrument for measuring the intensity and quality of fluorescence.

spectrogram (spek'trō-gram) [spectro- + G. *gramma,* something written]. A graphic representation of a spectrum.

spectrograph (spek'trō-graf). An instrument used in spectography.
mass s., an instrument that subjects charged and accelerated ions (atomic or molecular) to a magnetic field that imparts a curved path that differs for each mass-to-charge ratio, thus separating individual species; used in detecting and assaying isotopic ratios and in molecular structure determinations.

spectrography (spek-trog'ră-fē) [spectro- + G. *graphō,* to write]. The procedure of photographing or tracing a spectrum.

spectrometer (spek-trom'ĕ-ter) [spectro- + G. *metron,* measure]. An instrument for determining the wavelength or energy of light or other electromagnetic emission.

spectrometry (spek-trom'ĕ-trē). The procedure of observing and measuring the wavelengths of light or other electromagnetic emissions.
clinical s., biospectrometry.

spectrophobia (spek-trō-fō'bē-ă) [spectro- + G. *phobos,* fear]. Morbid fear of mirrors or of one's mirrored image.

spectrophotofluorimetry (spek'trō-fō'tō-flūr-im'ĕ-trē). Measurement of the intensity and quality of fluorescence by means of a spectrophotometer.

spectrophotometer (spek'trō-fō-tom'ĕ-ter) [spectro- + photometer]. An instrument for measuring the intensity of light of a definite wavelength transmitted by a substance or a solution, giving a quantitative measure of the amount of material in the solution absorbing the light; a colorimeter with a choice of wavelength and photometric measurement.

spectrophotometry (spek'trō-fō-tom'ĕ-trē). Analysis by means of a spectrophotometer.
atomic absorption s., determination of concentration by the ability of atoms to absorb radiant energy of specific wavelengths.
flame emission s., determination of the concentration of an element by measurement of light emitted when the element is excited by energy in the form of heat.

spectropolarimeter (spek'trō-pō-lar-im'ĕ-ter) [spectro- + polarimeter]. An instrument for measuring the rotation of light of specific wavelength upon passage through a solution or translucent solid.

spectroscope (spek'trō-skōp) [spectro- + G. *skopeō,* to view]. An instrument for resolving light from any luminous body into its spectrum, and for the analysis of the spectrum so formed. It consists of a prism that refracts the light or a grating for diffraction of the light, an arrangement for rendering the rays parallel, and a telescope that magnifies the spectrum.
direct vision s., a s. consisting of a single tube containing a series of prisms; one end of the tube is placed in as close contact as possible with the substance to be examined while the observer places his eye at the opposite end; it can be used to make a spectroscopic examination of the blood *in vivo,* as in the ear lobe or web of the thumb.

spectroscopic (spek-trō-skop'ik). Relating to or performed by means of a spectroscope.

spectroscopy (spek-tros'kŏ-pē). Observation and study of spectra of absorbed or emitted light by means of a spectroscope.
clinical s., biospectroscopy.
infrared s., the study of the specific absorption in the infrared region of the electromagnetic spectrum; used in the study of the chemical bonds within molecules.

spectrum, pl. **spectra, spectrums** (spek'trŭm, -ă, -ŭmz) [L. an image, fr. *specio,* to look at]. **1.** The range of colors presented when white light is resolved into its constituent colors by being passed through a prism or through a diffraction grating: red, orange, yellow, green, blue, indigo, and violet, arranged according to the increasing frequency of vibration or decreasing wavelength. **2.** Figuratively, the pathogenic microorganisms against which an antibiotic or other antibacterial agent is active. **3.** The plot of intensity vs. wavelength of light emitted or absorbed by a substance, usually characteristic of the substance and used in qualitative and quantitative analysis.
absorption s., the s. observed after light has passed through, and been partially absorbed by a solution or translucent substance; many molecular groupings have characterisitic light absorption patterns, which can be used for detection and quantitative assay.
antimicrobial s., see s. (2).
broad s., a term indicating a broad range of activity of an antibiotic against a wide variety of microorganisms.
chromatic s., color s.; the continuum of colors that white light forms on passing through a prism or diffraction grating.
color s., chromatic s.
continuous s., a s. in which there are no absorption bands or lines.
excitation s., fluorescence produced over a range of wavelengths of the exciting light.
fluorescence s., fluorescence evoked over a range of wavelengths when the excitation wavelength is at a maximum.
fortification s., fortification figures; the zigzag banding of light that marks the margin of the scintillating scotoma (teichopsia).
infrared s., thermal s.
invisible s., the radiation lying to either side of the chromatic s.; *e.g.,* the infrared and ultraviolet radiation.
Raman s., the characteristic array of light produced by the Raman effect.
thermal s., infrared s.; the invisible part of the s. outside of the red rays.
toxin s., a figure in the form of a s. used by Ehrlich to represent the neutralizing power of antitoxin in the presence of toxin, prototoxoid, toxone, etc.
visible s., that part of electromagnetic radiation that is visible to the human eye; it extends from extreme red, 7606 Å (760.6 nm), to extreme violet, 3934 Å (393.4 nm).
wide s., see s. (3).

speculum, pl. **specula** (spek'yū-lŭm, -lă) [L. a mirror, fr. *specio,* to look at]. An instrument for enlarging the opening of any canal or cavity in order to facilitate inspection of its interior.
bivalve s., a s. with two adjustable blades.
Cooke's s., a three-pronged s. for rectal examinations and operations.

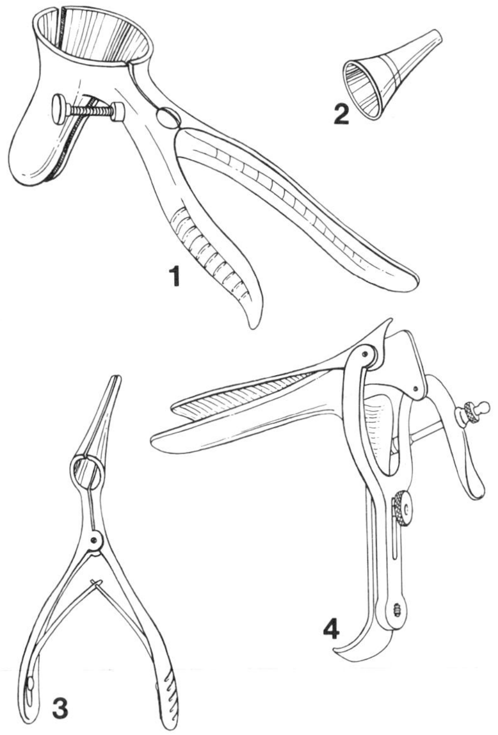

Speculum
1, rectal; *2,* ear; *3,* nasal; *4,* vaginal duckbill.

duckbill s., a bivalve s., the blades of which are broad and flattened, resembling a duck's bill, used in inspection of the vagina and cervix.
eye s., blepharostat; an instrument for keeping the eyelids apart during inspection of or operation on the eye.
Kelly's rectal s., a tubular s. with obturator for rectal examination.
Pedersen's s., a narrow flat s. used in vaginas with a small introitus.
stop-s., a dilating s., as a s. of the eyelids, which is provided with a catch to prevent its being opened too wide.

Spee, Ferdinand Graf von, German embryologist, 1855–1937. See *curve* of S.

speech [A.S. *spaec*]. Speaking; talk; the use of the voice in conveying ideas.
cerebellar s., an explosive type of utterance, with slurring of words.
clipped s., scamping s.
echo s., echolalia.
esophageal s., a technique for speaking following total laryngectomy; consists of swallowing air and regurgitating it, producing a vibration in the hypopharynx.
explosive s., logospasm (2); loud, sudden s. related to injury of the nervous system.
helium s., the peculiar high-pitched, often unintelligible speech sounds produced when one breathes a mixture of up to 80 per cent helium and 20 per cent oxygen.
mirror s., a reversal of the order of syllables in a word, analogous to mirror writing.
scamping s., clipped s.; a form of lalling in which consonants or syllables that are difficult to pronounce are omitted.
scanning s., measured or metered, often slow s.
slurring s., slovenly articulation of the more difficult letter sounds.
spastic s., labored s. related to increased tone of muscles.
staccato s., syllabic s.; an abrupt utterance, each syllable being enunciated separately; noted especially in multiple sclerosis.
subvocal s., slight movements of the muscles of s. related to thinking but producing no sound.
syllabic s., staccato s.

spelencephaly (spē-len-sef'ă-lē) [*spēlaion,* cave, + *enkephalos,* brain]. Porencephaly.

speleostomy (spē'lē-os'tō-mē) [G. *spēlaion,* cave, + *stoma,* mouth]. Cavernostomy.

Spens, Thomas, Scottish physician, 1764–1842. See S.'s *syndrome.*

sperm [G. *sperma,* seed] [NA]. **1.** Spermatozoon. **2.** Semen.

sperma-, spermato-, spermo- [G. *sperma,* seed]. Combining forms denoting semen or spermatozoa.

spermaceti (sper-mă-set'ē) [sperma- + G. *ketos, whale*]. Cetaceum; a peculiar fatty, waxy substance, chiefly cetin (cetyl palmitate), obtained from the head of the sperm whale, *Physeter macrocephalus;* used to impart firmness to ointment bases.

spermagglutination (sperm'ă-glū-ti-nā'shŭn). Agglutination of spermatozoa.

sperm-aster (sperm'as-ter) [sperm + G. *astēr,* a star (aster)]. Cytocentrum with astral rays in the cytoplasm of an inseminated ovum; it is brought in by the penetrating spermatozoon and evolves into the mitotic spindle of the first cleavage division.

spermatic (sper-mat'ik). Relating to the sperm or semen.

spermatid (sper'mă-tid) [spermat- + *-id* (2)]. A cell in a late stage of the development of the spermatozoon; it is a haploid cell derived from the secondary spermatocyte and evolves by spermiogenesis into a spermatozoon.

spermatin (sper'mă-tin). Name proposed for an albuminoid in the seminal fluid.

spermato-. See sperma-.

spermatoblast (sper'mă-tō-blast) [spermato- + G. *blastos,* germ]. Spermatogonium.

spermatocele (sper'mă-tō-sēl) [spermato- + G. *kēlē,* tumor]. Cyst of the epididymis containing spermatozoa.

spermatocidal (sper'mă-tō-sī'dăl). Spermicidal; destructive to spermatozoa.

spermatocide (sper'mă-tō-sīd) [spermato- + L. *caedo,* to kill]. Spermicide; an agent destructive to spermatozoa.

spermatocyst (sper'mă-tō-sist) [spermato- + G. *kystis,* bladder]. Obsolete term for *vesicula* seminalis; spermatocele.

spermatocytal (sper-mă-tō-sī'tăl). Relating to spermatocytes.

spermatocyte (sper'mă-tō-sīt) [spermato- + G. *kytos,* cell]. Parent cell of a spermatid, derived by mitotic division from a spermatogonium.
primary s., the s. derived by a growth phase from a spermatogonium, and which undergoes the first division of meiosis.
secondary s., the s. derived from a primary s. by the first meiotic division; each secondary s. produces two spermatids by the second meiotic division.

spermatocytogenesis (sper'mă-tō-sī'tō-jen'ĕ-sis). Spermatogenesis.

spermatogenesis (sper'mă-tō-jen'ĕ-sis) [spermato- + G. *genesis,* origin]. Spermatocytogenesis; spermatogeny; the entire process by which spermatogonial stem cells divide and differentiate into spermatozoa. See also spermiogenesis.

spermatogenetic (sper'mă-tō-jĕ-net'ik). Spermatogenic.

spermatogenic (sper'mă-tō-jen'ik). Spermatogenetic; spermatogenous; spermatopoietic (1); relating to spermatogenesis; sperm-producing.

spermatogenous (sper-mă-toj'ĕ-nŭs). Spermatogenic.

spermatogeny (sper-mă-toj'ĕ-nē). Spermatogenesis.

spermatogone (sper'mă-tō-gōn). Spermatogonium.

spermatogonium (sper'mă-tō-gō'nē-ŭm) [spermato- + G. *gonē,* generation]. Spermatoblast; spermatogone; the primitive sperm cell derived by mitotic division from the germ cell; increasing several times in size, it becomes a primary spermatocyte.

spermatoid (sper'mă-toyd) [spermato- + G. *eidos,* resemblance]. Resembling a sperm or sperm tail.

spermatology (sper-mă-tol'ō-jē) [spermato- + G. *logos,* study]. The branch of histology, physiology, and embryology concerned with sperm and/or seminal secretion.

spermatolysin (sper-mă-tol'i-sin). A specific lysin (antibody) formed in response to the repeated injection of spermatozoa.

spermatolysis (sper-mă-tol'i-sis) [spermato- + G. *lysis,* dissolution]. Spermolysis; destruction, with dissolution, of the spermatozoa.

spermatolytic (sper'mă-tō-lit'ik). Relating to spermatolysis.

spermatophobia (sper'mă-tō-fō'bē-ă) [spermato- + G. *phobos,* fear]. Morbid fear of spermatorrhea or loss of semen.

spermatophore (sper'mă-tō-fōr) [spermato- + G. *phoros,* bearing]. A capsule containing spermatozoa; found in a number of invertebrates.

spermatopoietic (sper'mă-tō-poy-et'ik) [spermato- + G. *poieō,* to make]. **1.** Spermatogenic. **2.** Secreting semen.

spermatorrhea (sper'mă-tō-rē'ă) [spermato- + G. *rhoia,* a flow]. An involuntary discharge of semen, without orgasm.

spermatoxin (sper-mă-tok'sin). Spermotoxin; a cytotoxic antibody specific for spermatozoa.

spermatozoa (sper'mă-tō-zō'ă). Plural of spermatozoon.

spermatozoal, spermatozoan (sper'ma-tō-zō'ăl, -zō'ăn). Relating to spermatozoa.

spermatozoon, pl. **spermatozoa** (sper'mă-tō-zō'on, -zō'ă) [G. *sperma,* seed, + *zoōn,* animal]. Sperm (1); sperm cell; the male gamete or sex cell that contains the genetic information to be transmitted by the male, exhibits autokinesia, and is able to effect zygosis with an ovum. The human s. is composed of a head and a tail, the tail being divisible into a neck, a middle piece, a principal piece, and an end piece; the head, 4 to 6 μm in length, is a broadly oval, flattened body containing the nucleus; the tail is about 55 μm in length.

spermaturia (sper-mă-tū'rē-ă). Semenuria.

spermia (sper'mē-ă). Plural of spermium.

spermicidal (sper-mi-sī'dăl). Spermatocidal.

spermicide (sper'mi-sīd). Spermatocide.

spermidine (sper'mi-dēn). *N*-(3-Aminopropyl)butanediamine; $NH_2(CH_2)_4NH(CH_2)_3NH_2$; a polyamine found with spermine in a wide variety of organisms and tissues.

spermiduct (sper'mi-dŭkt). **1.** *Ductus* deferens. **2.** *Ductus* ejaculatorius.

spermine (sper'mēn). Gerontine; neuridine; musculamine; *N,N'*-bis(3-aminopropyl)-1,4-butanediamine; $NH_2(CH_2)_3NH(CH_2)_4NH(CH_2)_3NH_2$; an essential growth factor in some bacteria; associated with nucleic acids in some viruses.

spermiogenesis (sper'mē-ō-jen'ĕ-sis) [sperm- + G. *genesis,* origin]. That segment of spermatogenesis during which immature spermatids become spermatozoa.

spermism (sper'mizm). The belief by preformationists that the male sex cell (sperm) contains a miniature preformed body called the homunculus.

sper'mist. A preformationist who believed in the concept of spermism.

spermium, pl. **spermia** (sper'mē-ŭm, -ă). H.W.G. Waldeyer's term for the mature male germ cell or spermatozoon.

spermo-. See sperma-.

spermolith (sper'mō-lith) [spermo- + G. *lithos,* stone]. A concretion in the ductus deferens.

spermolysis (sper-mol'i-sis). Spermatolysis.

spermatoxin (sper-mō-tok'sin). Spermatoxin.

SPF Abbreviation for sun protection *factor.*

sp. gr. Abbreviation for specific *gravity.*

sph. Abbreviation for spherical, or spherical *lens.*

sphacelate (sfas'ĕ-lāt) [G. *sphakelos,* gangrene]. To become gangrenous or necrotic.

sphacelation (sfas-ĕ-lā'shŭn) [G. *sphakelos,* gangrene]. **1.** The process of becoming gangrenous or necrotic. **2.** Gangrene or necrosis.

sphacelism (sfas'ĕ-lizm). The condition manifested by a sphacelus.

sphaceloderma (sfas'ĕ-lō-der'mă) [G. *sphakelos,* gangrene, + *derma,* skin]. Gangrene of the skin.

sphacelous (sfas'ĕ-lŭs). Sloughing, gangrenous, or necrotic.

sphacelus (sfas'ĕ-lŭs) [G. *sphakelos,* gangrene]. A mass of sloughing, gangrenous, or necrotic matter.

Sphaerophorus (sfē-rof'er-ŭs) [L. fr. G. *sphaira,* sphere, + *phoros,*

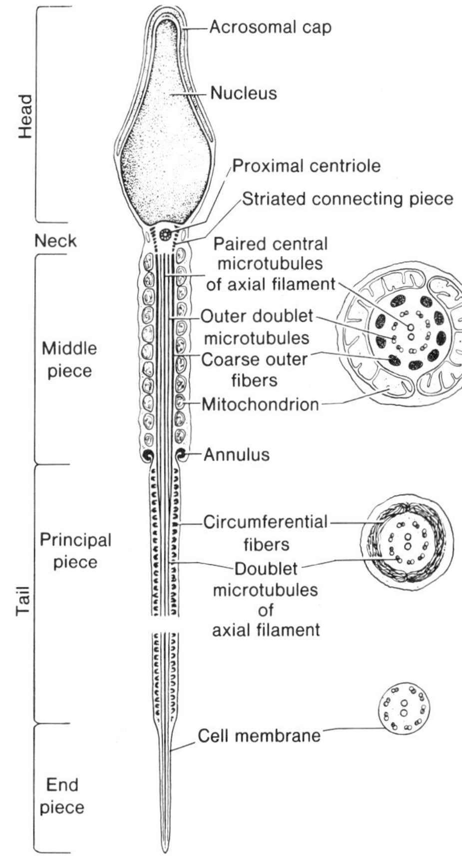

Mature Human Spermatozoon
Left, longitudinal section; *right,* transverse sections of the middle, principal, and end pieces of the tail.

bearing]. *Spherophorus;* an illegitimate bacterial generic name; organisms previously placed in this genus have been transferred to *Fusobacterium* or *Bacteroides.* The type species, *S. necrophorus,* has been transferred to *Fusobacterium.*

sphenethmoid (sfē-neth'moyd). Sphenoethmoid.

sphenion (sfē'nē-on) [Mod. L. fr. G. *sphēn,* wedge, + dim. *-iōn*]. The tip of the sphenoidal angle of the parietal bone; a craniometric point.

spheno- [G. *sphēn,* wedge]. Combining form denoting wedge, wedge-shaped, the sphenoid bone.

sphenobasilar (sfē'nō-bas'i-lăr). Sphenoccipital; spheno-occipital; relating to the sphenoid bone and the basilar process of the occipital bone.

sphenoccipital (sfē'nok-sip'i-tăl). Sphenobasilar.

sphenocephaly (sfē'nō-sef'ă-lē) [spheno- + G. *kephalē,* head]. Condition characterized by a deformation of the skull giving it a wedge-shaped appearance.

sphenoethmoid (sfē-nō-eth'moyd). Sphenethmoid; relating to the sphenoid and ethmoid bones.

sphenofrontal (sfē'nō-fron'tăl). Relating to the sphenoid and frontal bones.

sphenoid (sfē'noyd) [G. *sphēnoeidēs,* fr. *sphēn,* wedge, + *eidos,* resemblance]. Sphenoidal.

sphenoidal (sfē-noy'dăl). Sphenoid. **1.** Relating to the sphenoid bone. **2.** Wedge-shaped.

sphenoidale (sfē-noy-dā'lē). The point of greatest convexity between the anterior contour of the sella turcica and the planum sphenoidale.

sphenoiditis (sfē-noy-dī'tis) [sphenoid + G. *-itis,* inflammation]. **1.** Inflammation of the sphenoid sinus. **2.** Necrosis of the sphenoid bone.

sphenoidostomy (sfe-noy-dos'tō-mē) [sphenoid + G. *stoma,* mouth]. An operative opening made in the anterior wall of the sphenoid sinus.

sphenoidotomy (sfē'noy-dot'ō-mē) [sphenoid + G. *tomē,* a cutting]. Any operation on the sphenoid bone or sinus.

sphenomalar (sfē'nō-mā'lăr). Sphenozygomatic.

sphenomaxillary (sfē'nō-mak'si-lār-ē). Relating to the sphenoid bone and the maxilla.

spheno-occipital (sfē'nō-ok-sip'i-tăl). Sphenobasilar.

sphenopalatine (sfē-nō-pal'ă-tīn). Relating to the sphenoid and the palatine bones.

sphenoparietal (sfē'nō-pă-rī'ă-tăl). Relating to the sphenoid and the parietal bones.

sphenopetrosal (sfē'nō-pe-trō'săl). Relating to the sphenoid bone and the petrous portion of the temporal bone.

sphenorbital (sfē-nōr'bi-tăl). Denoting the portions of the sphenoid bone contributing to the orbits.

sphenosalpingostaphylinus (sfē'nō-sal-ping'gō-staf-i-lī'nŭs) [L.]. See under musculus.

sphenosquamosal (sfē'nō-skwā-mō'săl). Squamosphenoid.

sphenotemporal (sfē'nō-tem'pō-răl). Relating to the sphenoid and the temporal bones.

sphenotic (sfē-nō'tik) [spheno- + G. *ous,* ear]. Relating to the sphenoid bone and the bony case of the ear.

sphenoturbinal (sfē'nō-ter'bi-năl). Denoting the concha sphenoidalis.

sphenovomerine (sfē'nō-vō'mer-ēn, -īn). Relating to the sphenoid bone and the vomer.

sphenozygomatic (sfē'nō-zī-gō-mat'ik). Sphenomalar; relating to the sphenoid and the zygomatic bones.

sphere (sfēr) [G. *sphaira*] A ball or globular body.
attraction s., astrosphere.
Morgagni's s.'s, Morgagni's *globules.*

spheresthesia (sfēr-es-thē'zē-ă) [G. *sphaira,* sphere, + *aisthēsis,* sensation]. *Globus* hystericus.

spherical (sfēr'i-kăl). Pertaining to, or shaped like, a sphere.

sphero- [G. *sphaira,* globe, sphere]. Combining form denoting spherical, a sphere.

spherocylinder (sfēr'ō-sil'in-der). Spherocylindrical *lens.*

spherocyte (sfēr'ō-sīt) [sphero- + G. *kytos,* cell]. A small, spherical red blood cell.

spherocytosis (sfēr'ō-sī-tō'sis) [spherocyte + G. *-osis,* condition]. Presence of sphere-shaped red blood cells in the blood, a feature of familial hemolytic anemia.
hereditary s., a congenital defect of the erythrocyte cell membrane, which is abnormally permeable to sodium, resulting in thickened and almost spherical erythrocytes that are fragile and susceptible to spontaneous hemolysis, with decreased survival in the circulation; results in chronic anemia with reticulocytosis, episodes of mild jaundice due to hemolysis, and acute crises with fever and abdominal pain; symptomatology is highly variable; autosomal dominant inheritance. Also called congenital hemolytic jaundice or icterus; chronic familial jaundice or icterus; spherocytic or icterohemolytic anemia, globe cell anemia; chronic acholuric jaundice.

spheroid, spheroidal (sfēr'oyd, sfē-royd'ăl, sfir-) [L. *spheroideus*]. Shaped like a sphere.

spherometer (sfēr-om'ĕ-ter) [sphero- + G. *metron,* measure]. An instrument to determine the curvature of a sphere or a spherical lens.

spherophakia (sfēr-ō-fā'kē-ă) [sphero- + G. *phakos,* lens]. A congenital bilateral aberration in which the lenses are small, spherical, and subject to subluxation; may occur as an independent anomaly or may be associated with the Weill-Marchesani syndrome.

Spherophorus (sfē-rof'ō-rŭs). *Sphaerophorus.*

spheroplast (sfēr'ō-plast) [sphero- + G. *plastos,* formed]. A bacterial cell from which the rigid cell wall has been incompletely removed. The bacterium loses its characteristic shape and becomes round.

spheroprism (sfēr'ō-prizm). A spherical lens decentered to produce a prismatic effect, or a combined spherical lens and prism.

spherospermia (sfēr'ō-sper'mē-ă) [sphero- + G. *sperma,* seed]. Spheroid spermatozoa lacking an elongated tail, in contrast to the threadlike, tailed sperm of man and other mammals (nematospermia).

spherule (sfer'ūl) [LL. *sphaerula,* dim. of L. *sphaera,* sphere, ball]. **1.** A small spherical structure. **2.** A sporangial-like structure filled with endospores at maturity, produced within tissue and *in vitro* by *Coccidioides immitis.*

sphincter (sfingk'ter) [G. *sphinktēr,* a band or lace]. *Musculus* sphincter.
anatomical s., an accumulation of muscular circular fibers or specially arranged oblique fibers the function of which is to reduce partially or totally the lumen of a tube, the orifice of an organ, or the cavity of a viscus; the closing component of a pylorus.
s. angula'ris, angular s., thickening of the circular muscular layer forming the so-called s. intermedius at the level of the incisura angularis of the stomach.
s. a'ni, anal s., see *musculus* sphincter ani externus, *musculus* sphincter ani internus.
s. a'ni ter'tius, the third s. of the anus, a physiological s. at the sigmoidorectal junction.
annular s., a short thickening of circular muscular fibers, similar

to a ring; a ring-shaped s. as opposed to a segmental s.
antral s., s. antri.
s. an'tri, s. of antrum; antral s.; s. of gastric antrum; s. intermedius; a portion of the circular muscular layer of the stomach acting as a s. between the corpus and the antrum.
s. of antrum, s. antri.
artificial s., a s. produced by surgical procedures to reduce speed of flow in the digestive system or to maintain continence of the intestine.
basal s., sphincteroid tract of ileum; the thickening of the circular muscular coat at the base of the ileal papilla at the terminal ileum.
bicanalicular s., a s. encircling two canals, such as the terminal portions of the common bile duct and the main pancreatic duct.
Boyden's s., *musculus* sphincter ductus choledochi.
canalicular s., a s. located somewhere along the course of an organ, a tube, or a duct, as opposed to ostial s.
choledochal s., *musculus* sphincter ductus choledochi.
colic s., one of the s.'s of the colon.
s. of common bile duct, *musculus* sphincter ductus choledochi.
s. constric'tor car'diae, a s. supposedly present at the esophagogastric junction.
duodenal s., one of the physiological s.'s described in the duodenum.
duodenojejunal s., the s. supposedly present at the duodenojejunal flexure.
extrinsic s., a s. provided by circular muscular fibers extraneous to the organ.
first duodenal s., the s. supposedly located at the level of the aboral extremity of the duodenal bulb.
functional s., physiological s.
s. of gastric antrum, s. antri.
Glisson's s., *musculus* sphincter ampullae hepatopancreaticae.
s. of hepatic flexure of colon, s. at the level of the flexura coli dextra.
Hyrtl's s., a band, generally incomplete, of circular muscular fibers in the rectum about 10 cm above the anus.
ileal s., ileocecocolic s.; marginal s.; a thickening of circular musculature at the free margin of the ileal papilla.
ileocecocolic s., ileal s.
iliopelvic s., midsigmoid s.
s. intermedius, s. antri.
intrinsic s., a thickening of the circular fibers of the tunica muscularis of an organ.
macroscopic s., a s. visible to the naked eye.
marginal s., ileal s.
mediocolic s., a physiological s. located midway in the ascending colon.
microscopic s., a s. visible only under the microscope.
midgastric transverse s., a s. described at the level of the junction between the body of the stomach and the antrum.
midsigmoid s., iliopelvic s.; the s. midway in the sigmoid colon.
myovascular s., a s. having a muscular and a vascular (usually venous) component.
myovenous s., a s. having a muscular and a venous component, *e.g.,* at the pharyngoesophageal junction and anal canal.
Nélaton's s., Nélaton's fibers; an inconstant band of circular muscular fibers in the wall of the rectum 8 to 10 cm above the anus.
O'Beirne's s., pelvirectal or rectosigmoid s.; a circular band of muscular fibers in the upper part of the rectum.
s. oc'uli, *musculus* orbicularis oculi.
Oddi's s., *musculus* sphincter ampullae hepatopancreaticae.
s. o'ris, *musculus* orbicularis oris.
ostial s., a thickening of circular muscular fibers at the level of an orifice.
pancreatic s., a s. at the level of the termination of the main and of the accessory pancreatic duct.
pathologic s., a thickening of circular musculature caused by disease.
pelvirectal s., O'Beirne's s.
physiological s., functional s.; radiological s.; a section of a tubular structure that acts as if it has a specialized band of circular muscle to constrict it, although no such specialized structure can be found on morphological examination.
postpyloric s., the duodenal portion of the s. or closing mechanism of the gastroduodenal pylorus.
prepapillary s., a s. of duodenum described in the location oral to the major duodenal papilla.
prepyloric s., a band of circular muscular fibers in the wall of the stomach near the gastroduodenal pylorus.
s. pupil'lae, *musculus* sphincter pupillae.
pyloric s., *musculus* sphincter pylori.
radiological s., physiological s.
rectosigmoid s., O'Beirne's s.
segmental s., a s. of a segment of an organ, a tube, or a canal, and longer than an annular s.
smooth muscular s., lissosphincter.
striated muscular s., rhabdosphincter.
s. of third portion of duodenum, a physiological s. supposedly located at the horizontal (inferior) portion of the duodenum.
unicanalicular s., a s. limited to one visceral canal or tube.
s. ure'thrae, *musculus* sphincter urethrae.
s. vagi'nae, *musculus* bulbospongiosus.
Varolius' s., operculum ilei; the sphincter muscle at the terminal ileum.
s. vesi'cae, *musculus* sphincter vesicae.
s. vesi'cae fel'leae, the s. of the gallbladder, at the transition between the neck of the gallbladder and the cystic duct.

sphincteral (sfingk'ter-ăl). Sphincterial; sphincteric; relating to a sphincter.

sphincteralgia (sfingk-ter-al'jē-ă) [sphincter + G. *algos,* pain]. Pain in the sphincter ani muscles.

sphincterectomy (sfingk-ter-ek'tō-mē) [sphincter + G. *ektomē,* excision]. **1.** Excision of a portion of the pupillary border of the iris. **2.** Dissecting away any sphincter muscle.

sphincterial, sphincteric (sfingk-tēr'ē-ăl, -ter-ik). Sphincteral.

sphincterismus (sfingk-ter-iz'mŭs). Spasmodic contraction of the sphincter ani muscles.

sphincteritis (sfingk'ter-ī'tis). Inflammation of any sphincter.

sphincteroid (sfingk'ter-oyd) [sphincter + G. *eidos,* resemblance]. Denoting similarity to a musculus sphincter.

sphincterolysis (sfingk-ter-ol'i-sis) [sphincter, + G. *lysis,* loosening]. An operation for freeing the iris from the cornea in anterior synechia involving only the pupillary border.

sphincteroplasty (sfingk'ter-ō-plas-tē) [sphincter + G. *plastos,* formed]. Plastic surgery of any sphincter muscle.

sphincteroscope (sfingk'ter-ō-skōp) [sphincter + G. *skopeō,* to view]. A speculum to facilitate inspection of the internal sphincter ani muscle.

sphincteroscopy (sfingk'ter-os'kŏ-pē). Visual examination of a sphincter.

sphincterotome (sfingk'ter-ō-tōm). An instrument for incising a sphincter.

sphincterotomy (sfingk-tĕ-rot'ō-mē) [sphincter + G. *tomē,* incision]. Incision or division of a sphincter muscle.
transduodenal s., division of Oddi's sphincter; an operation to open the lower end of the common duct to remove impacted stones or to relieve spasm or stricture of the terminal bile and pancreatic ducts.
urethral s., incision of the urethral closure musculature, usually performed transurethrally with a special resectoscope and electrode.

sphinganine (sfing'gă-nēn). Dihydrosphingosine; 2*D*- or D-*erythro*-2- or (2*S*,3*R*)-2-amino-1,3-octadecanediol; a constituent of the sphingolipids.

(4*E*)-**sphingenine** (sfing'gen-ēn). Sphingosine.

sphingol (sfing'gol). Sphingosine.

sphingolipid (sfing'gō-lip-id). Any lipid containing a long chain base like that of sphingosine (*e.g.*, ceramides, cerebrosides, gangliosides, sphingomyelins); a constituent of nerve tissue.

sphingolipidosis (sfing'gō-lip-i-dō'sis). Sphingolipodystrophy; collective designation for a variety of diseases characterized by abnormal sphingolipid metabolism, *e.g.*, gangliosidosis, Gaucher's disease, Niemann-Pick disease.

cerebral s., cerebral lipidosis; any one of a group of inherited diseases characterized by failure to thrive, hypertonicity, progressive spastic paralysis, loss of vision and occurrence of blindness, usually with macular degeneration and optic atrophy, convulsions, and mental deterioration; associated with abnormal storage of sphingomyelin and related lipids in the brain. Four types are recognized as clinically and enzymatically distinct: 1) **infantile type** (Tay-Sachs disease, G_{M2} gangliosidosis); 2) **early juvenile type** (Jansky-Bielschowsky or Bielschowsky's disease); 3) **late juvenile type** (Spielmeyer-Vogt disease; Spielmeyer-Sjögren disease; Batten-Mayou disease; ceroid lipofuscinosis); and 4) **adult type** (Kufs disease).

sphingolipodystrophy (sfing'gō-lip-ō-dis'trō-fē). Sphingolipidosis.

sphingomyelinase (sfing'gō-mi'ĕ-li-nās). Sphingomyelin phosphodiesterase.

sphingomyelin phosphodiesterase (sfing'gō-mī'ĕ-lin) [EC 3.1.4.12]. Sphingomyelinase; an enzyme catalyzing hydrolysis of sphingomyelin to *N*-acylsphingosine (a ceramide) and phosphocholine.

sphingomyelins (sfing'gō-mī'ĕ-linz). Phosphosphingosides; a group of phospholipids, found in brain, spinal cord, kidney, and egg yolk, containing 1-phosphocholine (choline *O*-phosphate) combined with a ceramide (an *N*-acyl long-chain base, such as sphingosine).

sphingosine (sfing'gō-sēn). (4*E*)-Sphingenine; sphingol; (2*S*,3*R*,4*E*)-2-amino-4-octadecene-1,3-diol; $CH_3(CH_2)_{12}CH{=}CHCH(OH)$-$CH(NH_2)CH_2OH$; the principal long-chain base found in sphingolipids.

sphygm-. See sphygmo-.

sphygmic (sfig'mik). Relating to the pulse.

sphygmo-, sphygm- [G. *sphygmos*, pulse]. Combining forms denoting pulse.

sphygmocardiograph (sfig'mō-kar'dē-ō-graf) [sphygmo- + G. *kardia*, heart, + *graphō*, to write]. Sphygmocardioscope; a polygraph recording both the heartbeat and the radial pulse.

sphygmocardioscope (sfig'mō-kar'dē-ō-skōp) [sphygmo- + G. *skopeō*, to view]. Sphygmocardiograph.

sphygmochronograph (sfig'mō-kron'ō-graf) [sphygmo- + G. *chronos*, time, + *graphō*, to write]. A modified sphygmograph that represents graphically the time relations between the beat of the heart and the pulse; one recording the character of the pulse as well as its rapidity.

sphygmogram (sfig'mō-gram) [sphygmo- + G. *gramma*, something written]. Pulse curve; the graphic curve made by a sphygmograph.

sphygmograph (sfig'mō-graf) [sphygmo- + G. *graphō*, to write]. An instrument consisting of a lever, the short end of which rests on the radial artery at the wrist, its long end being provided with a stylet which records on a moving ribbon of smoked paper the excursions of the pulse.

sphygmographic (sfig-mō-graf'ik). Relating to or made by a sphygmograph; denoting the s. tracing, or sphygmogram.

sphygmography (sfig-mog'ră-fē). Use of the sphygmograph in recording the character of the pulse.

sphygmoid (sfig'moyd) [sphygmo- + G. *eidos*, resemblance]. Pulselike; resembling the pulse.

sphygmomanometer (sfig'mō-mă-nom'ĕ-ter) [sphygmo- + G. *manos*, thin, scanty, + *metron*, measure]. Sphygmometer; an instrument for measuring arterial blood pressure consisting of an inflatable cuff, inflating bulb, and a guage showing the blood pressure.

Mosso's s., an apparatus for measuring the blood pressure in the digital arteries.

Rogers' s., an s. with an aneroid barometer guage.

sphygmomanometry (sfig'mō-mă-nom'ĕ-trē). Determination of the blood pressure by means of a sphygmomanometer.

sphygmometer (sfig-mom'ĕ-ter). Sphygmomanometer.

sphygmometroscope (sfig-mō-met'rō-skōp) [sphygmo- + G. *metron*, measure, + *skopeō*, to view]. An instrument for auscultating the pulse, used especially in the auscultatory method of reading the blood pressure, particularly the diastolic pressure.

sphygmo-oscillometer (sfig'mō-os'i-lom'ĕ-ter) [sphygmo- + L. *oscillo*, to swing, + G. *metron*, measure]. An instrument resembling an aneroid sphygmomanometer used in the measurement of the systolic and diastolic blood pressure.

sphygmopalpation (sfig'mō-pal-pa'shŭn) [sphygmo- + L. *palpatio*, palpation]. Feeling the pulse.

sphygmophone (sfig'mō-fōn) [sphygmo- + G. *phōnē*, sound]. An instrument by which a sound is produced with each beat of the pulse.

sphygmoscope (sfig'mō-skōp) [sphygmo- + G. *skopeō*, to view]. An instrument by which the pulse beats are made visible by causing fluid to rise in a glass tube, by means of a mirror projecting a beam of light, or simply by a moving lever as in the sphygmograph.

Bishop's s., an instrument for measuring the blood pressure, with special reference to diastolic pressure; the tube is filled with a solution of cadmium borotungstate, and the scale is the reverse of that of a mercurial manometer, the pressure being made directly by the weight of the liquid and not by compressed air.

sphygmoscopy (sfig-mos'kō-pē) [sphygmo- + G. *skopeō*, to view]. Examination of the pulse.

sphygmosystole (sfig-mō-sis'tō-lē) [sphygmo- + G. *systolē*, a contracting]. That segment of the pulse wave corresponding to the cardiac systole.

sphygmotonograph (sfig-mō-tō'nō-graf) [sphygmo- + G. *tonos*, tension, + *graphō*, to write]. An instrument for recording graphically both the pulse and the blood pressure.

sphygmotonometer (sfig-mō-tō-nom'ĕ-ter) [sphygmo- + G. *tonos*, tension, + *metron*, measure]. An instrument, like the sphygmotonograph, for determining the degree of blood pressure.

sphygmoviscosimetry (sfig-mō-vis-kō-sim'ĕ-trē). Measurement of the pressure and the viscosity of the blood.

sphyrectomy (sfī'rek'tō-mē) [G. *sphyra*, malleus, + *ektomē*, excision]. Seldom used term for exsection of the malleus.

sphyrotomy (sfī-rot'ō-mē) [G. *sphyra*, malleus, + *tomē*, incision]. Seldom used term for malleotomy.

spica, pl. **spicae** (spī'kă, spī'kē) [L. a point, an ear of grain]. See under bandage.

spicula (spik'yū-lă) [L.]. Plural of spiculum.

spicular (spik'yū-lăr). Relating to or having spicules.

spicule (spik'yūl) [L. *spiculum*, dim. of *spica*, or *spicum*, a point]. A small needle-shaped body.

spiculum, pl. **spicula** (spik'yū-lŭm, -lă) [L.]. A spicule or small spike.

spider (spī'der) [O. E. *spinnan*, to spin]. **1.** An arthropod of the order Araneida (subclass Arachnida) characterized by four pairs of legs, a cephalothorax, a globose smooth abdomen, and a complex of web-spinning spinnerets. Among the venomous s.'s found in the New World are the black widow s., *Latrodectus mactans;* red-legged widow s., *Latrodectus bishopi;* pruning s., or Peruvian tarantula, *Glyptocranium gasteracanthoides;* Chilean brown s., *Loxosceles laeta;* Peruvian brown s., *Loxosceles rufiper;* brown recluse s. of North America, *Loxosceles reclusus.* **2.** Arterial s. **3.** An obstructive growth in the teat of a cow.

arterial s., vascular s., a telangiectatic arteriole in the skin with radiating capillary branches simulating the legs of a s.; characteristic, but not pathognomonic of, parenchymatous liver disease; also seen in pregnancy, often disappearing after delivery, and at times in normal persons. Also called nevus arachnoideus or araneus; spider angioma, nevus, mole, or telangiectasia.

spider-burst (spī'der-berst). Radiating dull red capillary lines on the skin of the leg, usually without any visible or palpable varicose veins, but nevertheless due to deep-seated venous dilation; sometimes referred to as skyrocket capillary ectasis.

Spiegelberg, Otto, German gynecologist, 1830–1881. See S.'s *criteria.*

Spieghel, Adrian van der. See Spigelius.

Spiegler, Eduard, Austrian dermatologist, 1860–1908. See S.'s *reagent;* S.-Fendt *pseudolymphoma, sarcoid.*

Spielmeyer, Walter, Munich neurologist, 1879–1935. See S.'s acute *swelling;* S.-Stock *disease,* S.-Vogt *disease.*

spigelian (spī-jē'lē-an). Relating to or described by Spigelius.

Spigelius, Adrian (van der Spieghel), Flemish anatomist in Padua, 1578–1625. See spigelian *hernia;* S.'s *line, lobe.*

spike (spīk). A brief electrical event of 3 to 25 msec that gives the appearance in the electroencephalogram of a rising and falling vertical line.

spill. An overflow; a scattering of fluid or finely divided matter.

cellular s., a dissemination of cells through the lymph or blood, thereby resulting in metastases or implantation of foreign tissue in any part or organ.

Spiller, William G., U. S. neurologist, 1864–1940. See Frazier-S. *operation.*

spill'way. Sluiceway; a groove or channel through which food may pass from the occlusal surfaces of teeth during the masticatory process.

spiloma (spī-lō'mă) [G. *spilos,* spot, + *-oma,* tumor]. Nevus.

spiloplaxia (spī-lō-plak'sē-ă) [G. *spilos,* spot, + *plax,* a plaque, plate]. A red spot observed in leprosy or pellagra.

spilus (spī'lŭs) [Mod. L. fr. G. *spilos,* a spot]. Nevus.

spin-. See spino-.

spina, gen. and pl. **spinae** (spī'nă, -nē) [L. a thorn, the backbone, spine]. **1** [NA]. Any spine or sharp thornlike process. **2.** *Columna* vertebralis.

s. angula'ris, s. ossis sphenoidalis.

s. bif'ida, bi'fida, hydrocele spinalis; schistorrhachis; a limited defect in the spinal column, characterized by absence of the vertebral arches, through which the spinal membranes, with or without spinal cord tissue, may protrude.

s. bif'ida aper'ta, s. bifida manifesta.

s. bif'ida cys'tica, s. bifida associated with a meningeal cyst (meningocele) or a cyst containing both meninges and spinal cord (meningomyelocele) or only spinal cord (myelocele).

s. bif'ida manifes'ta, s. bifida aperta; s. bifida in which the vertebral defect is apparent and may be associated with a meningeal or myelic anomaly.

s. bif'ida occul'ta, s. bifida in which there is a spinal defect, but no protrusion of the cord or its membrane, although often some abnormality in their development.

s. dorsa'lis, *columna* vertebralis.

s. fronta'lis, s, nasalis ossis frontalis.

s. hel'icis [NA], spine of helix; apophysis helicis; an anteriorly directed spine at the extremity of the crus of the helix of the auricle.

s. ili'aca ante'rior infe'rior [NA], anterior inferior iliac spine; spine on the anterior border of the ilium between the s. iliaca anterior superior and the acetabulum.

s. ili'aca ante'rior supe'rior [NA], anterior superior iliac spine; the anterior extremity of the iliac crest.

s. ili'aca poste'rior infe'rior [NA], posterior inferior iliac spine; spine on the posterior border of the ilium between the s. iliaca posterior superior and the greater sciatic notch.

s. ili'aca poste'rior supe'rior [NA], posterior superior iliac spine; the posterior extremity of the iliac crest.

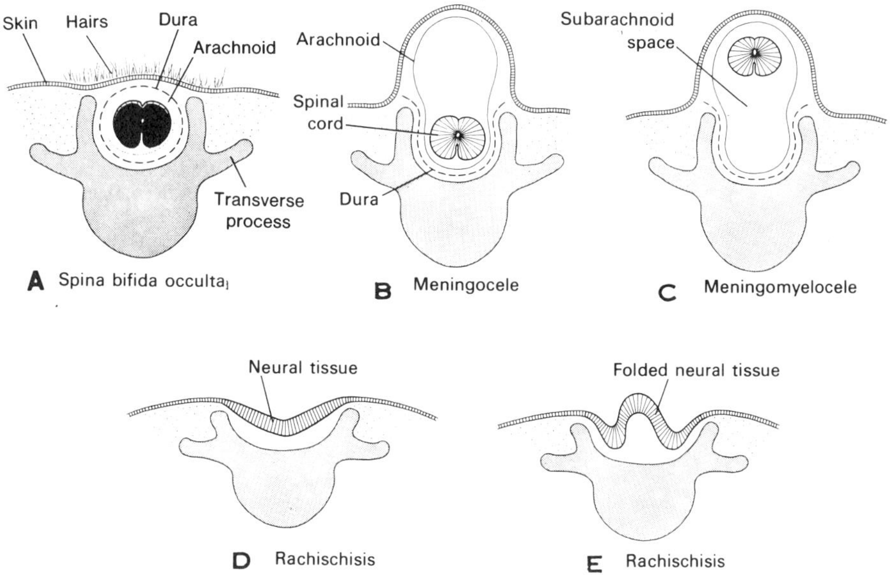

Spina Bifida

s. ischiad'ica [NA], ischiadic or sciatic spine; a pointed process from the posterior border of the ischium on a level with the lower border of the acetabulum.
s. mea'tus, s. suprameatica.
s. menta'lis [NA], mental spine; genial tubercle; a slight projection, sometimes two, in the middle line of the posterior surface of the body of the mandible, giving attachment to the geniohyoid muscle (below) and the genioglossus (above).
s. nasa'lis ante'rior [NA], anterior nasal spine; a pointed projection at the anterior extremity of the intermaxillary suture; the tip, as seen on a lateral cephalometric radiograph, is used as a cephalometric landmark.
s. nasa'lis os'sis fronta'lis [NA], nasal spine of frontal bone; s. frontalis; a projection from the center of the nasal part of the frontal bone, which lies between and articulates with the nasal bones and the perpendicular plate of the ethmoid.
s. nasa'lis poste'rior [NA], posterior nasal spine; posterior palatine spine; the sharp posterior extremity of the nasal crest.
s. os'sis sphenoida'lis [NA], sphenoidal spine; alar or angular spine; spina angularis; spinous process (1); a posterior and downward projection from the greater wing of the sphenoid bone on either side.
spi'nae palati'nae [NA], palatine spines; the longitudinal ridges along the palatine grooves on the inferior surface of the palatine process of the maxilla.
s. pe'dis, a hard or soft corn.
s. peronea'lis, *trochlea* peronealis.
s. pu'bis, *tuberculum* pubicum.
s. scap'ulae [NA], spine of scapula; the prominent triangular ridge on the dorsal aspect of the scapula.
s. supramea'tica [NA], suprameatal or meatal spine; Henle's spine; spina meatus; spina suprameatum; small bony prominence anterior to the supramastoid pit at the posterosuperior margin of the bony external acoustic meatus.
s. suprамea'tum, s. suprameatica.
s. trochlea'ris [NA], trochlear spine; a spicule of bone arising from the edge of the fovea trochlearis, giving attachment to the pulley of the superior oblique muscle of the eyeball.
s. tympan'ica ma'jor [NA], greater tympanic spine; the anterior edge of the tympanic notch (of Rivinus).
s. tympan'ica mi'nor [NA], lesser tympanic spine; the posterior edge of the tympanic notch (of Rivinus).
s. vento'sa, a condition occasionally seen in tuberculosis or tuberculous dactylitis, in which there is absorption of bone bordering the medulla, with a new deposit under the periosteum, resulting in a change that is suggestive of bone being inflated with gas.

spinacene (spin'ă-sēn). Squalene.

spinal (spī'năl) [L. *spinalis*]. Rachial; rachidial; rachidian. **1.** Relating to any spine or spinous process. **2.** Relating to the vertebral column.

spinalis (spī-nā'lis) [L.]. Spinal.

spinant (spī'nant). An agent increasing the reflex irritability of the spinal cord.

spinate (spī'nāt). Spined; having spines.

spindle (spin'dl) [A.S.]. In anatomy and pathology, any fusiform cell or structure.
aortic s., His s.; a fusiform dilation of the aorta immediately beyond the isthmus.
central s., a central group of microtubules (continuous fibers) that course uninterrupted, between the asters, in contrast to the microtubules attached to the individual chromosomes (s. fibers).
cleavage s., the s. formed during the cleavage of a zygote or its blastomeres.
His' s., aortic s.
Krukenberg's s., a vertical fusiform area of melanin pigmentation on the posterior surface of the central cornea.
Kühne's s., neuromuscular s.
mitotic s., nuclear s.; the fusiform figure characteristic of a dividing cell; it consists of microtubules (s. fibers), some of which become attached to each chromosome at its centromere and provide the mechanism for chromosomal movement; other microtubules (continuous fibers) pass from pole to pole.
muscle s., neuromuscular s.
neuromuscular s., muscle s.; Kühne's s.; a fusiform end organ in skeletal muscle in which afferent and a few efferent nerve fibers terminate; it contains from 3 to 10 striated muscle fibers (intrafusal fibers) which are much smaller than the ordinary muscle fibers, are separated from them by a capsule that encloses the organ, and are innervated by the thin axon of a gamma motoneuron (gamma motor fiber); the sensory endings that occur on the intrafusal fibers are either annulospiral or flower spray endings (see under ending); this sensory end organ is particularly sensitive to passive stretch of the muscle in which it is enclosed.

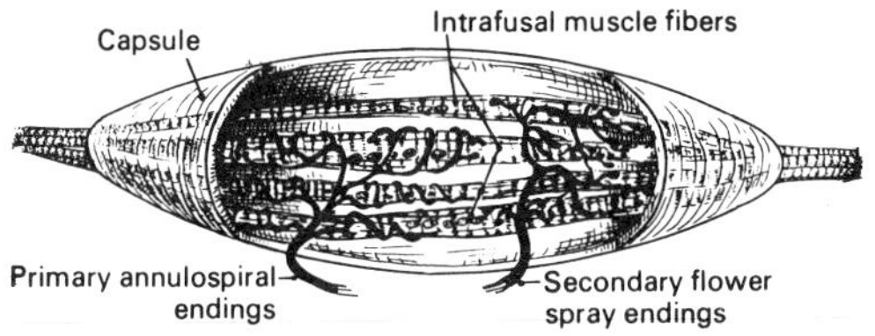

Neuromuscular Spindle, with Capsule Cut Open

neurotendinous s., Golgi tendon *organ.*
nuclear s., mitotic s.
sleep s., the electroencephalographic record of 14-per-second bursts of wave frequency occurring during sleep.

spine (spīn) [L. *spina*] **1.** A short sharp process of bone; a spinous process. **2.** *Columna* vertebralis. **3.** The bar or stay in a horse's hoof.
alar s., *spina* ossis sphenoidalis.
angular s., *spina* ossis sphenoidalis.
anterior inferior iliac s., *spina* iliaca anterior inferior.
anterior nasal s. (ANS), *spina* nasalia anterior.
anterior superior iliac s., *spina* iliaca anterior superior.
cleft s., spondyloschisis.
dendritic s.'s, gemmules (2); dendritic thorns; variably long excrescences of nerve cell dendrites, varying in shape from small knobs to thornlike or filamentous processes, usually more numerous on distal dendrite arborizations than on the proximal part of dendritic trunks; they are a preferential site of synaptic axodendritic contact; sparse or absent in some types of nerve cells (motor neurons; the large cells of the globus pallidus; stellate cells of the cerebral cortex), they are exceedingly numerous in others such as the pyramidal cells of the cerebral cortex and the Purkinje cells of the cerebellar cortex.
dorsal s., *columna* vertebralis.
greater tympanic s., *spina* tympanica major.
s. of helix, *spina* helicis.
hemal s., the middle point of the hemal arch of the typical vertebra; considered by some to be represented by the sternum in man.
Henle's s., *spina* suprameatica.
iliac s., see *spina* iliaca anterior inferior, anterior superior, posterior inferior, and posterior superior.
ischiadic s., *spina* ischiadica.
lesser tympanic s., *spina* tympanica minor.
meatal s., *spina* suprameatica.
mental s., *spina* mentalis.
nasal s. of frontal bone, *spina* nasalis ossis frontalis.
neural s., the middle point of the neural arch of the typical verte-

bra, represented by the spinous process.

palatine s.'s, *spinae* palatinae.

penis s.'s, penis thorns; epithelial excrescences on the glans of the p. of the guinea pig and cat; they are under the influence of the male hormone.

poker s., stiff s. resulting from widespread joint immobility or overwhelming muscle spasm as might be evoked by an osteomyelitis of a vertebra.

posterior inferior iliac s., *spina* iliaca posterior inferior.

posterior nasal s., *spina* nasalis posterior.

posterior palatine s., *spina* nasalis posterior.

posterior superior iliac s., *spina* iliaca posterior superior.

pubic s., *tuberculum* pubicum.

s. of scapula, *spina* scapulae.

sciatic s., *spina* ischiadica.

sphenoidal s., *spina* ossis sphenoidalis.

Spix's s., *lingula* mandibulae.

suprameatal s., *spina* suprameatica.

thoracic s., the thoracic region of the columna vertebralis; the vertebrae thoracicae as a whole; that part of the vertebral column which enters into the formation of the thorax.

trochlear s., *spina* trochlearis.

Spinelli, Pier G., Italian gynecologist, 1862–1929. See S. *operation.*

spinifugal (spī-nif'yū-găl) [spine + L. *fugio,* to flee]. Conducting in a direction away from the spinal cord; denoting the efferent fibers of the spinal nerves.

spinipetal (spī-nip'ĕ-tăl) [spine + L. *peto,* to seek]. Conducting in a direction toward the spinal cord; denoting the afferent fibers of the spinal nerves.

spinnbarkeit (spin'bahr-kīt) [Ger. *Spinnbarkeit,* capable of forming a thread (spinning), viscosity]. The stringy, elastic character of cervical mucus during the ovulatory period; in contrast to other times in the menstrual cycle, cervical secretions at midcycle are clear, abundant, and of low viscosity.

spino-, spin- [L. *spina*]. Combining forms denoting: **1.** The spine. **2.** Spinous.

spinobulbar (spī'nō-bŭl'bar) Bulbospinal.

spinocerebellum (spī'nō-sār-ĕ-bel'ŭm). Paleocerebellum.

spinocollicular (spī'nō-col-ik'yū-lar) Spinotectal.

spinocostalis (spī'nō-kos-tā'lis) [L.]. The superior and inferior serratus posterior muscles regarded as one.

spinogalvanization (spī'nō-gal-van-i-zā'shŭn). Application of the constant electrical current to the spinal cord.

spinoglenoid (spī'nō-glē'noyd). Relating to the spine and the glenoid cavity of the scapula.

spinomuscular (spī'nō-mŭs'kyū-lăr). Relating to the spinal cord and the muscles supplied by the spinal nerves.

spinoneural (spī-nō-nū'răl). Relating to the spinal cord and the nerves given off from it.

spinose (spī'nōs). Spinous.

spinotectal (spī-nō-tek'tăl). Spinocollicular; passing upward from the spinal cord to the tectum.

spinotransversarius (spī'nō-trans-ver-sār'ē-ŭs). The splenius and obliquus capitis major muscles regarded as one.

spinous (spī'nŭs). Relating to, shaped like, or having a spine or spines.

spintharicon (spin-thăr'i-kon) [G. *spinthēr,* spark]. A spark chamber device used to record the distribution of low energy emissions from radiopharmaceuticals administered internally, especially for thyroid scans using iodine-125.

spinthariscope (spin-thăr'i-skōp) [G. *spinthēr,* spark, + *skopeō,* to view]. Scintillation *counter.*

spiperone (spip'ĕ-rōn). 8-[3-(*p*-Fluorobenzoyl)propyl]-1-phenyl-1,3,8-triazaspiro[4.5]decan-4-one; an antipsychotic.

spir-. See spiro-.

spiracle (spī'ră-kl, spir-) [L. *spiraculum,* fr. *spiro,* to breathe]. An aperture for breathing in arthropods and in sharks and related fishes.

spiradenitis (spī'rad-ĕ-nī'tis) [L. *spiro,* to breathe or perspire, + G. *adēn,* gland, + *-itis,* inflammation]. *Hidradenitis* suppurativa.

spiradenoma (spī-rad-ĕ-nō'mă) [G. *speira,* coil, + adenoma]. A benign tumor of sweat glands.

eccrine s., a painful skin tumor composed of two cell types derived from the secretory part of sweat glands.

spiral (spī'răl) [Mediev. L. *spiralis,* fr. G. *speira,* a coil]. **1.** Coiled; winding around a center like a watch spring; winding and ascending like a wire spring. **2.** A structure in the shape of a coil.

Curschmann's s.'s, spirally twisted masses of mucus occurring in the sputum in bronchial asthma.

s. of Tillaux, an imaginary line connecting the insertions of the recti muscles of the eye.

spiramycin (spir-ă-mī'sin). An antibiotic substance (almost identical to leucomycin) produced by *Streptomyces ambofaciens;* an antimicrobial agent.

spirem, spireme (spī'rem, spī'rēm) [G. *speirēma,* a coil 1]. Term formerly applied to the first stage of mitosis (prophase) when extended chromosome filaments have the appearance of a loose ball of yarn, under the incorrect hypothesis that the filaments were continuous and later broke apart to form individual chromosomes.

spirilla (spī-ril'ă). Plural of spirillum.

Spirillaceae (spī-ri-lā'sē-ē) [see *Spirillum*]. A family of usually motile, aerobic to facultatively anaerobic bacteria (order Pseudomonadales) containing Gram-negative, rod-shaped cells which are curved or spirally twisted. Motile cells contain a single polar flagellum or a tuft of polar flagella. These organisms are primarily water forms, although some are parasitic or pathogenic on humans and other higher animals. The type genus is *Spirillum.*

spirillar (spī-ril'ăr). S-shaped; referring to a bacterial cell with an S shape.

spirillicidal (spī-ril-i-sī'dăl) [spirilla + L. *caedo,* to kill]. Destructive to spirilla or spirochetes.

spirillosis (spī'ri-lō'sis). Any disease caused by the presence of spirilla in the blood or tissues.

Spirillum (spī-ril'ŭm) [Mod. L. dim. of L. *spira,* coil, fr. G. *speira*]. A genus of large (1.4 to 1.7 μm in diameter), rigid, helical, Gram-negative bacteria (family Spirillaceae) which are motile by means of bipolar fascicles of flagella. These freshwater organisms are obligately microaerophilic and chemoorganotrophic, possessing a strictly respiratory metabolism; they neither oxidize nor ferment carbohydrates. This genus contains only a single species, *S. volutans,* the type species.

S. mi'nus, a species of uncertain taxonomic classification that causes a form of rat-bite fever.

S. vol'utans, a species found in fresh water; it is the type species of *S.*

spirillum, pl. **spirilla** (spī-ril'ŭm, -ă). A member of the genus *Spirillum.*

Obermeier's s., *Borrelia recurrentis.*

Vincent's s., the s. or spirochete found in association with Vincent's bacillus.

spirit (spir'it) [L. *spiritus,* a breathing, life soul, fr. *spiro,* to breathe]. **1.** An alcoholic liquor stronger than wine, obtained by distillation. **2.** Any distilled liquid. **3.** An alcoholic or hydroalcoholic solution of volatile substances; some s.'s are used as flavoring agents, others have medicinal value.

ardent s.'s, brandy, whiskey, and other forms of distilled alcoholic liquors.
industrial methylated s., methylated s., denatured *alcohol.*
proof s., dilute alcohol, specific gravity 0.920, containing 49.5% by weight (57.27% by volume) of C_2H_5OH at 15.56°C. Originally in Great Britain it was the weakest alcohol that would permit ignition of gunpowder moistened with it. British proof s. has a specific gravity of 0.9198 and contains 49.2% C_2H_5OH by weight, or 57.1% by volume at the temperature of 10.56°C.
pyroligneous s., pyroxylic s., *methyl* alcohol.
rectified s., alcohol (2).
vital s.'s, in the galenical teachings, a vital essence or principle supposed to be generated from the air or pneuma in the left ventricle of the heart; carried in the blood to the brain, it was converted to animal s.'s which then flowed along the nerves to all parts of the body.
wine s., alcohol (2).
wood s., *methyl* alcohol.

spirituous (spir'i-chū-ŭs). Containing alcohol in large amount, denoting liquors.

spiritus, gen. and pl. **spiritus (sp.)** (spir'i-tŭs) [L.]. Spirit.

spiro-, spir-. **1** [G. *speira,* a coil]. Combining forms denoting a coil, coil-shaped. **2** [L. *spiro,* to breathe]. Combining forms denoting breathing.

Spirocerca lupi (spi-rō-ser'kă lū'pī) [L., fr. G. *speira,* coil, + G. *kerkos,* tail; L. *lupus,* wolf]. The esophageal worm of dogs and other carnivores, a red spiruroid nematode that occurs in nodules in the wall of the esophagus, stomach, and aorta of dogs, foxes, and wolves; intermediate hosts are various coprophagic beetles. Clinical symptoms occur only in very heavy infections, which are associated with esophageal carcinomata in dogs and with hypertrophic pulmonary osteoarthropathy.

Spirochaeta (spī'rō-kē'tă) [Mod. L. fr. G. *speira,* a coil, + *chaitē,* hair]. A genus of motile bacteria (order Spirochaetales) containing presumably Gram-negative, flexible, undulating, spiral-shaped rods which may or may not possess flagelliform, tapering ends. The protoplast is spirally wound around an axial filament. No obvious periplast membrane or cross-striations occur. These organisms are motile by means of a creeping motion over the surfaces of supporting objects. They are not parasitic but are found free-living in fresh or sea water slime; they are commonly found in sewage and foul waters. At present the genus contains five species. The type species is *S. plicatilis.*
S. obermei'eri, *Borrelia recurrentis.*
S. plicat'ilis, a very large species (sometimes as long as 200 μm) of bacteria; it is nonparasitic, so far as known; it is the type species of the genus *S.*

Spirochaetaceae (spī-rō-kē-tā'sē-ē) [see *Spirochaeta*]. A family of bacteria (order Spirochaetales) consisting of coarse, spiral cells, 30 to 50 μm in length and possessing definite protoplasmic structures. These organisms occur in stagnant, fresh, or salt water and in the intestinal tracts of bivalve molluscs. The type genus is *Spirochaeta.*

Spirochaetales (spī-rō-kē-tā'lēz). An order of bacteria containing slender, flexuous cells, 6 to 500 μm in length, in the form of spirals with at least one complete turn. Some species may have an axial filament, a lateral crista, or ridge, or transverse striations. All of these organisms are motile, whirling or spinning about the long axis, thus driving the organism forward or backward. Free-living, saprophytic, and parasitic forms occur. The type family is Spirochaetaceae.

spirochetal (spī-rō-kē'tăl). Relating to spirochetes, especially to infection with such organisms.

spirochete (spī'rō-kēt) A vernacular term used to refer to any member of the genus *Spirochaeta.*

spirochetemia (spī'rō-kē-tē'mē-ă) [spirochete + G. *haima,* blood]. Presence of spirochetes in the blood.

spirocheticide (spiī-rō-kē'tĭ-sīd) [spirochete + L. *caedo,* to kill]. An agent destructive to spirochetes.

spirochetolysis (spī'rō-kē-tol'i-sis) [spirochete + G. *lysis,* a loosening]. Destruction of spirochetes, as by chemotherapy or by specific antibodies.

spirochetosis (spī'rō-kē-tō'sis). Any disease caused by a spirochete.
avian s., a highly fatal disease of chickens, turkeys, pheasants, and other birds caused by *Borrelia anserina* and transmitted chiefly by the fowl tick, *Argas persicus.*
bronchopulmonary s., hemorrhagic *bronchitis.*

spirochetotic (spī'rō-kē-tot'ik). Relating to or marked by spirochetosis.

spirogram (spī'rō-gram). The tracing made by the spirograph.

spirograph (spī'rō-graf) [L. *spiro,* to breathe, + G. *graphō,* to write]. A device for representing graphically the depth and rapidity of respiratory movements.

spiro-index (spī'rō-in-deks). Vital capacity divided by the height of the individual.

spirometer (spī-rom'ĕ-ter) [L. *spiro,* to breathe, + G. *metron,* measure]. A gasometer used for measuring respiratory gases; usually understood to consist of a counterbalanced cylindrical bell sealed by dipping into a circular trough of water. In physiology, a gasometer is more commonly used for vessels of large capacity (*e.g.,* 100 liters), while a s. is more commonly used for small vessels (*e.g.,* 10 liters).
chain-compensated s., a Tissot s. in which compensation for change in bell buoyancy is accomplished automatically by a suspending chain of correct mass per unit length.
Krogh s., a water-sealed s. in which the bell is a large, shallow, rectangular box rotating slightly around a horizontal axis extending along one edge, with an arm extending beyond that axis to a counterbalancing weight; comparable to a wedge s.
Tissot s., a very large water-sealed s. designed for accumulating expired gas over a long period of time; the counterbalancing of the bell (almost frictionless) is compensated for the bell's change in buoyancy as it emerges from the water, keeping the contained gas precisely at ambient atmospheric pressure.
wedge s., a waterless s. constructed of two large rectangular plates with edges connected by accordion-pleated rubber so that large changes in volume are accommodated by small changes in the acute angle of the wedge-shaped interior, sensed by an electrical transducer; designed for rapid response by reducing the acceleration of the moving parts.

Spirometra (spī-rō-mē'tră) [G. *speira,* coil, + *metra,* womb (uterus)]. A genus of pseudophyllid tapeworms.
S. manso'ni, *Diphyllobothrium linguloides; D. mansoni;* a species of pseudophyllid tapeworms of wild and feral cats, the larval form of which (sparganum) may survive in human tissues; it has been commonly found in man in the Orient, but is also reported from widely scattered areas elsewhere; infection of man with the sparganum occurs from active migration of the larva from freshly split infected frogs used as a poultice for wounds, sore eyes (see ocular *sparganosis*), bruises, or ulcerations; it is also likely that man may be infected with sparganum larvae from eating any vertebrate harboring these plerocercoids.
S. mansonoi'des, *Diphyllobothrium mansonoides;* a species of pseudophyllid tapeworms from North America, whose larva (sparganum) may be a cause of sparganosis of man in Florida and the Gulf States.

spirometry (spī-rom'ĕ-trē). Making pulmonary measurements with a spirometer.

spironolactone (spī'rō-nō-lak'tōn). 3-(3-Oco-7α-acetylthio-17β-hydroxy-4-androsten-17α-yl)propionic acid-α-lactone; a diuretic agent that blocks the renal tubular actions of aldosterone. It increases the urinary excretion of sodium and chloride, decreases the excretion of potassium and ammonium, and reduces the titratable acidity of the urine; most effectively used to potentiate the natriuretic action and reduce the potassium excretion produced by other diuretics.

spiroscope (spī'rō-skōp) [L. *spiro,* to breathe, + G. *skopeō,* to view]. A device for measuring the air capacity of the lungs.

spirostan (spī'rō-stan). A 16,22;22,26-diepoxycholestane.

spiruroid (spī'rū-royd). Common name for a member of the superfamily Spiruroidea.

Spiruroidea (Spī-rū-roy'dē-ă) [G. *speiroeidēs,* spiral]. A superfamily of arthropod-borne nematode parasites of the alimentary tract, respiratory system, or orbital, nasal, or oral cavities of vertebrates. They are common and frequently pathogenic parasites of domestic mammals and birds, producing ulcerations from penetration of the anterior end of these spiny worms through the alimentary lining; includes the families Acuariidae, Gnathostomatidae, Rictulariidae, Seuratidae, Physalopteridae, Spiruridae, and Thelaziidae.

spissitude (spis'i-tūd) [L. *spissitudo,* fr. *spissus,* thick]. The state of being inspissated; the condition of a fluid thickened almost to a solid by evaporation or inspissation.

spit'ting. Expectoration (2).

spittle (spit'l) [A.S. *spātl*]. Saliva.

Spitz, S., 20th century U.S. pathologist. See S. *nevus.*

Spitzer, Alexander, Austrian anatomist, 1868–1943. See S.'s *theory.*

Spitzka, Edward C., U.S. neurologist, 1852–1914. See S.'s *nucleus,* marginal *tract,* marginal *zone.*

Spix, Johann B., German anatomist, 1781–1826. See S.'s *spine.*

SPL Abbreviation for sound pressure *level.*

splanchn-, splanchni-. See splanchno-.

splanchnapophysial, -physeal (splangk'nă-pō-fiz'ē-ăl). Relating to a splanchnapophysis.

splanchnapophysis (splangk'nă-pof'i-sis) [splanchn- + G. *apophysis,* offshoot]. An apophysis of the typical vertebra, on the side opposite to the neural apophysis, and enclosing any viscera.

splanchnectopia (splangk-nek-tō'pē-ă) [splanchn- + G. *ektopos,* out of place]. Splanchnodiastasis; displacement of any of the viscera.

splanchnemphraxis (splangk-nem-frak'sis) [splanchn- + G. *emphraxis,* a stoppage]. Intestinal obstruction.

splanchnesthesia (splangk-nes-thē'zē-ă) [splanch- + G. *aisthēsis,* sensation]. Visceral *sense.*

splanchnic (splangk'nik). Visceral.

splanchnicectomy (splangk-ni-sek'tō-mē) [splanchni- + G. *ektomē,* excision]. Resection of the splanchnic nerves and usually of the celiac ganglion as well.

splanchnicotomy (splangk-ni-kot'ō-mē) [splanchni- + G. *tomē,* incision]. Section of a splanchnic nerve or nerves, a surgical procedure used in the treatment of hypertension.

splanchno-, splanchn-, splanchni- [G. *splanchnon,* viscus]. Combining forms denoting the viscera. See also viscero-.

splanchnocele (splangk'nō-sēl). **1** [G. *koilos,* hollow]. The primitive body cavity or celom in the embryo. **2** [G. *kēlē,* hernia]. Hernia of any of the abdominal viscera.

splanchnocranium (splangk-nō-krā'nē-ŭm). Viscerocranium.

splanchnodiastasis (splangk'nō-dī-as'tă-sis) [splanchno- + G. *diastasis,* separation]. Splanchnectopia.

splanchnography (splangk-nog'ră-fē) [splanchno- + G. *graphō,* to write]. A treatise on or description of the viscera.

splanchnolith (splangk'nō-lith) [splanchno- + G. *lithos,* stone]. An intestinal calculus.

splanchnologia (splangk'nō-lō'jē-ă) [NA]. Splanchnology.

splanchnology (splangk-nol'ō-jē) [splanchno- + G. *logos,* study]. Splanchnologia; the branch of medical science dealing with the viscera.

splanchnomegaly (splangk-nō-meg'ă-lē) [splanchno- + G. *megas,* large]. Visceromegaly.

splanchnomicria (splangk-nō-mik'rē-ă) [splanchno- + G. *mikros,* small]. Condition in which the splanchnic organs are of smaller than normal size.

splanchnopathy (splangk-nop'ă-thē) [splanchno- + G. *pathos,* disease]. Any disease of the abdominal viscera.

splanchnopleural (splangk-nō-plūr'ăl). Splanchnopleuric.

splanchnopleure (splangk'nō-plūr) [splanchno- + G. *pleura,* side]. The embryonic layer formed by association of the visceral layer of the lateral mesoderm with the endoderm.

splanchnopleuric (splangk-nō-plūr'ik). Splanchnopleural; relating to the splanchnopleure.

splanchnoptosis, splanchnoptosia (splangk'nō-tō'sis, -tō'sē-ă) [splanchno- + G. *ptosis,* a falling]. Visceroptosis.

splanchnosclerosis (splangk'nō-skle-rō'sis) [splanchno- + G. *sklērōsis,* hardening]. Hardening, through connective tissue overgrowth, of any of the viscera.

splanchnoskeletal (splangk-nō-skel'ĕ-tăl). Visceroskeletal.

splanchnoskeleton (splangk-nō-skel'ĕ-tŏn). Visceroskeleton (2).

splanchnosomatic (splangk'nō-sō-mat'ik) [splanchno- + G. *sōma,* body]. Viscerosomatic.

splanchnotomy (splangk-not'ō-mē) [splanchno- + G. *tomē,* incision]. Dissection of the viscera by incision.

splanchnotribe (splangk'nō-trīb) [splanchno- + G. *tribō,* to rub, bruise]. An instrument resembling a large angiotribe used for occluding the intestine temporarily, prior to resection.

splay (splā). **1.** To lay open the end of a tubular structure by making a longitudinal incision to increase its potential diameter. See also spatulate. **2.** The rounding of the corner on the graph relating rate of renal tubular secretion or reabsorption of a substance to its arterial plasma concentration, due primarily to the fact that some nephrons reach their tubular maximum before others do.

splayfoot (splā'fŭt). *Talipes* planus.

spleen (splēn) [G. *splēn*]. Splen.

accessory s., *splen* accessorius.

diffuse waxy s., a condition of amyloid degeneration of the s., affecting chiefly the extrasinusoidal tissue spaces of the pulp.

floating s., movable s.; lien mobilis; a s. that is palpable because of excessive mobility from a relaxed or lengthened pedicle rather than because of enlargement.

lardaceous s., waxy s.

movable s., floating s.

sago s., amyloidosis in the s. affecting chiefly the malpighian bodies.

sugar-coated s., hyaloserositis involving the s.

waxy s., lardaceous s.; amyloidosis of the s.

splen-. See spleno-.

splen [G. *splen,* spleen] [NA]. Spleen; lien; a large vascular lymphatic organ lying in the upper part of the abdominal cavity on the left side, between the stomach and diaphragm, composed of white and red pulp; the white consists of lymphatic nodules and diffuse lymphatic tissue; the red consists of venous sinusoids between which are splenic cords; the stroma of both red and white pulp is reticular fibers and cells. A framework of fibroelastic trabeculae extending from the capsule subdivides the structure into poorly defined lobules. It is a blood-forming organ in early life and a storage organ for red corpuscles; because of the large number of macrophages, it also acts as a blood filter.

s. accessorius [NA], accessory spleen; lien succenturiatus; lien accessorius; splenule; spleneolus; spleniculus; splenunculus; splenulus; lienculus; lienunculus; one of the small globular masses of splenic tissue occasionally found in the region of the spleen, in one of the peritoneal folds or elsewhere.

splenalgia (splē-nal'jē-ă) [splen- + G. *algos,* pain]. Splenodynia; a painful condition of the spleen.

splenauxe (splē-nawk'sē) [splen- + G. *auxē,* increase]. Splenomegaly.

Splendore, A., 20th century Italian physician. See S.-Hoeppli *phenomenon,* Lutz-S.-Almeida *disease.*

splenectomy (splē-nek'tō-mē) [splen- + G. *ektomē,* excision]. Removal of the spleen.

splenectopia, splenectopy (splen'ek-tō'pē-ă, splē-nek'tō-pē) [splen- + G. *ektopos,* out of place]. **1.** Displacement of the spleen, as in a floating spleen. **2.** The presence of rests of splenic tissue, usually in the region of the spleen.

splenelcosis (splen-el-kō'sis) [splen- + G. *helkōsis,* ulceration]. Abscess of the spleen.

splenemphraxis (splen-em-frak'sis) [splen- + G. *emphraxis,* stoppage]. Congestion of the spleen.

spleneolus (splē-nē'ō-lŭs) [Mod. L. dim. of G. *splēn*]. *Splen* accessorius.

splenetic (splē-net'ik). **1.** Splenic. **2.** Fretfully surly.

splenial (splē'nē-ăl) [G. *splēnion,* bandage]. **1.** Relating to the splenium. **2.** Relating to a splenius muscle.

splenic (splen'ik). Lienal; splenetic (1); relating to the spleen.

spleniculus (splen-ik'yū-lŭs) [Mod. L.]. *Splen* accessorius.

spleniform (splen'i-fōrm, splē'ni-). Splenoid.

spleniserrate (splen'i-ser'at). Relating to the splenius and serratus muscles.

splenitis (splē-nī'tis) [splen- + G. *-itis,* inflammation]. Inflammation of the spleen.

splenium, pl. **splenia** (splē'nē-ŭm, -ă) [Mod. L. fr. G. *splēnion,* bandage]. **1.** A compress or bandage. **2** [NA]. A structure resembling a bandaged part.

s. cor'poris callo'si [NA], tuber corporis callosi; the thickened posterior extremity of the corpus callosum.

splenius (splē'nē-ŭs) [Mod. L. fr. G. *splēnion,* a bandage]. See entries under musculus.

spleno-, splen- [G. *splēn,* spleen]. Combining forms denoting the spleen.

splenocele (splē'nō-sēl) [spleno- + G. *kēlē,* tumor, hernia]. **1.** Splenoma. **2.** A splenic hernia.

splenocleisis (splē-nō-klī'sis) [spleno- + G. *kleisis,* closure]. Inducing the formation of new fibrous tissue on the surface of the spleen by friction or wrapping with gauze.

splenocolic (splē'nō-kol'ik). Relating to the spleen and the colon; denoting a ligament or fold of peritoneum passing between the two viscera.

splenodynia (splē'nō-din'ē-ă) [spleno- + G. *odynē,* pain]. Splenalgia.

splenography (splē-nog'ră-fē) [spleno- + G. *graphō,* to write]. Splenic *venography.*

splenohepatomegaly, splenohepatomegalia (splē'nō-hep'ă-tō-meg'ă-lē, -mĕ-gā'ē-ă) [spleno- + G. *hēpar,* liver, + *megas,* large]. Enlargement of both spleen and liver.

splenoid (splē'noyd) [spleno- + G. *eidos,* resemblance]. Spleniform; resembling the spleen.

splenolymphatic (splē'nō-lim-fat'ik). Relating to the spleen and the lymph nodes.

splenoma (splē-nō'mă) [spleno- + G. *-oma,* tumor]. Splenocele (1); splenoncus; general nonspecific term for an enlarged spleen.

splenomalacia (splē'nō-mă-lā'shē-ă) [spleno- + G. *malakia,* softness]. Softening of the spleen.

splenomedullary (splē-nō-med'ū-lār-ē) [spleno- + L. *medulla,* marrow]. Splenomyelogenous.

splenomegaly, splenomegalia (splē-nō-meg'ă-lē, -mĕ-gā'lē-ă) [spleno- + G. *megas (megal-),* large]. Megalosplenia; splenauxe; enlargement of the spleen.

congestive s., enlargement of the spleen due to passive congestion; sometimes used as a synonym for Banti's syndrome.

Egyptian s., term sometimes used as a synonym for schistosomiasis mansoni, although hepatomegaly and fibrosis are more consistently found than is an enlarged spleen.

hemolytic s., s. associated with congenital hemolytic jaundice.

hyperreactive malarious s., tropical s. syndrome; a syndrome characterized by persistent splenomegaly, exceptionally high serum IgM and malaria antibody levels, and hepatic sinusoidal lymphocytosis; believed to be a disturbance in the T-lymphocyte control of the humoral response to recurrent malaria.

tropical s., visceral *leishmaniasis.*

splenomyelogenous (splē'nō-mī-ĕ-loj'ĕ-nŭs) [spleno- + G. *myelos,* marrow, + *-gen,* producing]. Splenomedullary; lienomedullary; lienomyelogenous; originating in the spleen and bone marrow, denoting a form of leukemia.

splenomyelomalacia (splē'nō-mī'ĕ-lō-mă-lā'shē-ă) [spleno- + G. *myelos,* marrow, + *malakia,* softness]. Pathologic softening of the spleen and bone marrow.

splenoncus (splē-nong'kŭs) [spleno- + G. *onkos,* mass]. Splenoma.

splenonephric (splē'nō-nef'rik) [spleno- + G. *nephros,* kidney]. Lienorenal.

splenopancreatic (splē'nō-pan-krē-at'ik). Lienopancreatic; relating to the spleen and the pancreas.

splenopathy (splē-nop'ă-thē) [spleno- + G. *pathos,* suffering]. Any disease of the spleen.

splenopexy, splenopexia (splē'nō-pek-sē, splē-nō-pek'sē-ă) [spleno- + G. *pēxis,* fixation]. Splenorrhaphy (2); suturing in place an ectopic or floating spleen.

splenophrenic (splē'nō-fren'ik) [spleno- + G. *phrēn,* diaphragm]. Relating to the spleen and the diaphragm; denoting a ligament or fold of peritoneum extending between the two structures.

splenoportogram (splē-nō-pōr'tō-gram). X-ray demonstration of the outline of the portal vascular bed obtained by injection of radiopaque material into the spleen.

splenoportography (splē'nō-pōr-tog'ră-fē) [spleno- + portography]. Introduction of radiopaque material into the spleen to obtain an x-ray visualization of the portal vessel of the portal circulation.

splenoptosis, splenoptosia (splē-nop-tō'sis, -tō'sē-ă) [spleno- + G. *ptōsis,* falling]. Downward displacement of the spleen, as in a floating spleen.

splenorenal (splē'nō-rē'năl). Lienorenal.

splenorrhagia (splē'nō-rā'jē-ă) [spleno- + G. *rhēgnymi,* to burst forth]. Hemorrhage from a ruptured spleen.

splenorrhaphy (splē-nōr'ă-fē) [spleno- + G. *rhaphē,* suture]. **1.** Suturing a ruptured spleen. **2.** Splenopexy.

splenotomy (splē-not'ō-mē) [spleno- + G. *tomē,* incision]. **1.** Anatomy or dissection of the spleen. **2.** Surgical incision of the spleen.

splenotoxin (splē-nō-tok'sin) [spleno- + G. *toxikon,* poison]. A cytotoxin specific for cells of the spleen.

splenule (splen'yūl) [Mod. L. *splenulus*]. *Splen* accessorius.

splenulus, pl. **splenuli** (splen'yū-lŭs, -lī) [Mod. L. dim. of L. *splen,* spleen]. *Splen* accessorius.

splenunculus, pl. **splenunculi** (splē-nŭng'kyū-lŭs, -lī) [Mod. L. dim. of L. *splen,* spleen]. *Splen* accessorius.

splicing (splīs'ing). **1.** Gene s.; attachment of one DNA molecule to another. **2.** RNA s.; removal of introns from mRNA precursors.

splint [Middle Dutch *splinte*]. **1.** An appliance for preventing movement of a joint or for the fixation of displaced or movable parts. **2.** The s. bone, or fibula.

acid etch cemented s., a s. of heavy wire which is cemented to the labial surfaces of teeth with any of the acid etch cement techniques; used to stabilize traumatically displaced or periodontally diseased teeth.

active s., dynamic s.

air s., inflatable s.; a plastic s. inflated by air used to immobilize part or all of an extremity.

airplane s., a complicated s. that holds the arm in abduction at about shoulder level with the forearm midway in flexion, generally with an axillary strut for support.

anchor s., a s. used for fracture of the jaw, with wires around teeth and a rod to hold it in place.

Anderson s., a skeletal traction s. with pins inserted into proximal and distal ends of a fracture; reduction is obtained by an external plate attached to the pins.

backboard s., a board s. with slots for fixation by straps; shorter ones are used for neck injuries, longer ones for back injuries.

Balkan s.'s, Balkan *frame.*

cap s., a plastic or metallic fracture appliance designed to cover the crowns of the teeth and usually cemented to them.

coaptation s., a short s. designed to prevent overriding of the ends of a fractured bone, usually supplemented by a longer s. to fix the entire limb.

contact s., a slotted plate, held by screws, used in the treatment of fracture of long bones.

Cramer wire s., ladder s.

Denis Browne s., a light aluminum s. applied to the lateral aspect of the leg and foot; used for clubfoot.

dynamic s., active s.; functional s. (1); a s. utilizing springs or elastic bands that aids in movements initiated by the patient by controlling the plane and range of motion.

Essig s., a stainless steel wire passed labially and lingually around a segment of the dental arch and held in position by individual ligature wires around the contact areas of the teeth; used to stabilize fractured or repositioned teeth and the involved alveolar bone.

Frejka pillow s., a pillow s. used for abduction and flexion of the femurs in treatment of congenital hip dysplasia or dislocation in infants.

functional s., **(1)** dynamic s.; **(2)** the joining of two or more teeth into a rigid unit by means of fixed restorations that cover all or part of the abutment teeth.

Gunning s., a prosthesis fabricated from models of endentulous maxillary and mandibular arches in order to aid in reduction and fixation of a fracture.

Hodgen s., a suspension leg s. for fractures of the middle or lower end of the femur; it provides support for traction.

inflatable s., air s.

interdental s., a s. for a fractured jaw, consisting of two metal or acrylic resin bands wired to the teeth of the upper and lower jaws, respectively, and then fastened together to keep the jaws immovable.

Kingsley s., reverse Kingsley s.; a winged maxillary s. used to apply traction to reduce maxillary fractures as well as immobilize

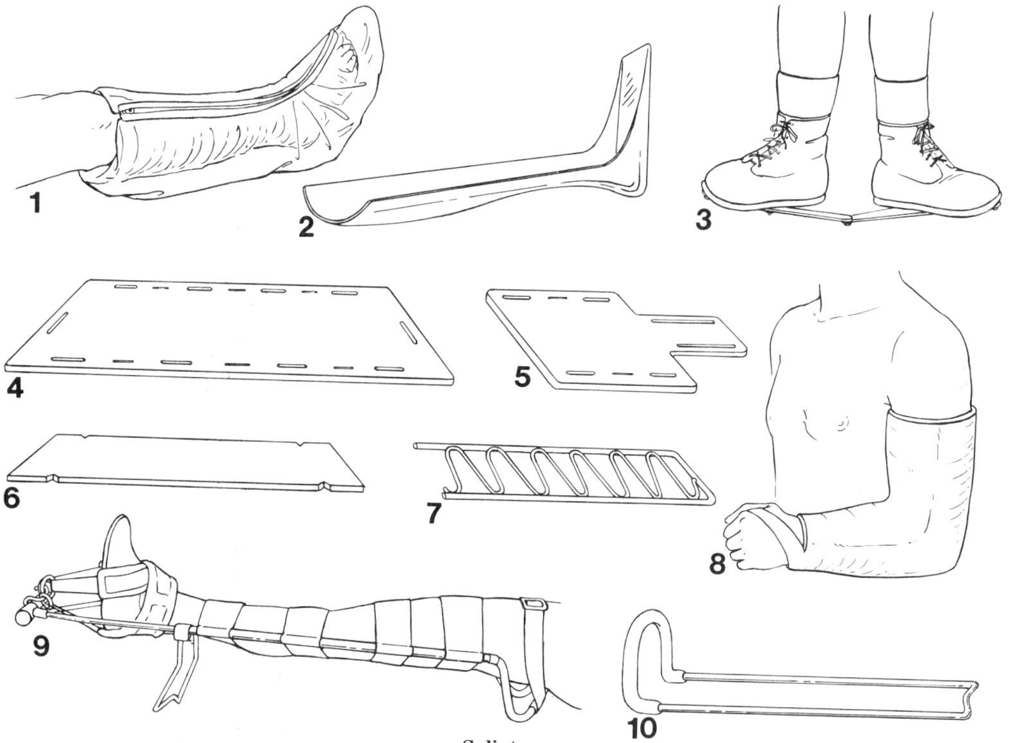

Splints
1, air; *2,* aluminium; *3,* Denis Browne; *4* and *5,* backboard; *6,* board; *7,* ladder; *8,* plaster of Paris; *9,* traction; *10,* Thomas.

them by having the wings attached to a head appliance by elastics.
labial s., an appliance of plastic, metal, or in combination, made to conform to the outer aspect of the dental arch and used in the management of jaw and facial injuries.
ladder s., Cramer wire s.; a flexible s. consisting of two stout parallel wires with finer cross wires.
lingual s., one similar to the labial s., but conforming to the inner aspect of the dental arch.
Liston's s., a long s. extending from the axilla to the sole of the foot.
plaster s., a s. constructed of bandages impregnated with plaster of Paris.
reverse Kingsley s., Kingsley s.
shin s.'s, see shin-splints.
Stader s., a s. used primarily in veterinary medicine; with metal pins through the proximal and distal segments of a long bone fracture, the fixation of the pins is maintained by the apparatus which is external to the limb.
surgical s., general term for a device used to maintain tissues in a new position following surgery.
Taylor's s., Taylor's back *brace.*
Thomas s., a long leg s. extending from a ring at the hip to beyond the foot, allowing traction to a fractured leg, for emergencies and transportation.
Tobruk s., [port of *Tobruk,* Libya]. a Thomas s., applied and held in plaster with plaster of Paris dressings; a s. first used during World War II to immobolize the limb during hazardous conditions such as transport from small to large boats.
wire s., a device to stabilize teeth loosened by accident or by a periodontal condition in the maxilla or mandible; a device to reduce and stabilize maxillary or mandibular fractures by applying it to both jaws and connecting it by intermaxillary wires or rubber bands.

splint'ing. **1.** Application of a splint or treatment using a splint. **2.** In dentistry, the joining of two or more teeth into a rigid unit by means of fixed or removable restorations or applicances. **3.** Stiffening of a body part to avoid pain caused by movement of the part, as from a fracture.

splints [see splint]. Exostoses occurring along the course of the small metacarpal and metatarsal bones of the horse.

split'ting. In chemistry, the cleavage of a covalent bond, fragmenting the molecule involved.

spm Abbreviation for a gene that leads to *su*ppression and *m*utation of mutants that are unstable.

spodogenous (spŏ-doj'ĕ-nŭs) [G. *spodos,* ashes, + *-gen,* producing]. Caused by waste material.

spodogram (spō'dō-gram) [G. *spodos,* ashes, + *gramma,* a drawing]. The pattern of ash residue formed by microincineration of a minute tissue specimen, usually a thin section.

spodography (spŏ-dog'-ră-fē) [G. *spodos,* ashes, + *graphō,* to write]. Microincineration.

spodophorous (spŏ-dof'ō-rŭs) [G. *spodos,* ashes, + *phoros,* bearing]. Removing or carrying off waste materials from the body.

spoke-shave (spōk' shāv). Ring-knife.

spondaic (spon-dā'ik). Relating to spondee.

spondee (spon'dē) [Fr.]. A bisyllabic word with generally equivalent stress on each of the two syllables; used in the testing of speech hearing.

spondyl-. See spondylo-.

spondylalgia (spon-di-lal'jē-ă) [spondyl- + G. *algos,* pain]. Pain in the spine.

spondylarthritis (spon'dil-ar-thrī'tis) [spondyl- + G. *arthron,* joint, + *-itis,* inflammation]. Inflammation of the intervertebral articulations.

spondylarthrocace (spon-dil-ar-throk'ă-sē) [spondyl- + G. *arthron,* joint, + *kakē,* badness]. Spondylocace. **1.** Tuberculous *spondylitis.* **2.** Rust's *disease.*

spondylitic (spon-di-lit'ik). Relating to spondylitis.

spondylitis (spon-di-lī'tis) [spondyl- + G. *-itis,* inflammation]. Inflammation of one or more of the vertebrae.
ankylosing s., arthritis of the spine, resembling rheumatoid arthritis, that may progress to bony ankylosis with lipping of vertebral margins; the disease is more common in the male often with the rheumatoid factor absent and the HLA antigen present. Also called Strümpell-Marie or Marie-Strümpell disease; rheumatoid s.
s. defor'mans, poker back; Bechterew's disease; Strümpell's disease (1); arthritis and osteitis deformans involving the spinal column; marked by nodular deposits at the edges of the intervertebral disks with ossification of the ligaments and bony ankylosis of the intervertebral articulations, it results in a rounded kyphosis with rigidity.
Kümmell's s., late posttraumatic collapse of vertebral body.
rheumatoid s., ankylosing s.
tuberculous s., tuberculous infection of the spine associated with a sharp angulation of the spine at the point of disease. Also called Pott's disease; trachelocyrtosis; trachelokyphosis; spondylarthrocace (1).

spondylo-, spondyl- [G. *spondylos,* vertebra]. Combining forms denoting the vertebrae.

spondylocace (spon-di-lok'ă-sē) [spondylo- + G. *kakē,* badness]. Spondylarthrocace.

spondylolisthesis (spon'di-lō-lis-thē'sis) [spondylo- + G. *olisthēsis,* a slipping and falling]. Sacrolisthesis; spondyloptosis; forward movement of the body of one of the lower lumbar vertebrae on the vertebra below it, or upon the sacrum.

spondylolisthetic (spon'di-lō-lis-thet'ik). Relating to or marked by spondylolisthesis.

spondylolysis (spon-di-lol'i-sis) [spondylo- + G. *lysis,* loosening]. Degeneration of the articulating part of a vertebra.

spondylomalacia (spon'di-lō-mă-lā'shē-ă) [spondylo- + G. *malakia,* softness]. Softening of vertebrae with multiple collapsed vertebral bodies.

spondylopathy (spon-di-lop'ă-thē) [spondylo- + G. *pathos,* suffering]. Rachiopathy; any disease of the vertebrae or spinal column.

spondyloptosis (spon'di-lō-tō'sis) [spondylo- + G. *ptōsis,* a falling]. Spondylolisthesis.

spondylopyosis (spon'di-lō-pī-ō'sis) [spondylo- + G. *pyōsis,* suppuration]. Suppurative inflammation of one or more of the vertebral bodies.

spondyloschisis (spon-di-los'ki-sis) [spondylo- + G. *schisis,* fissure]. Rachischisis; cleft spine; congenital fissure of one or more of the vertebral arches.

spondylosis (spon-di-lō'sis) [G. *spondylos,* vertebra]. Ankylosis of the vertebra; often applied nonspecifically to any lesion of the spine of a degenerative nature.
cervical s., general term indicating reactive changes in the vertebral bodies about the interspace, usually associated with chronic discopathy.
hyperostotic s., diffuse idiopathic skeletal *hyperostosis.*

spondylosyndesis (spon'di-lō-sin-dē'sis) [spondylo- + G. *syndesis,* binding together]. Spinal *fusion.*

spondylothoracic (spon'di-lō-thō-ras'ik). Relating to the vertebra and the thorax.

spondylotomy (spon-di-lot'ō-mē) [spondylo- + G. *tomē,* incision]. Laminectomy.

spondylous (spon'di-lŭs). Relating to a vertebra.

sponge (spŭnj) [G. *spongia*]. **1.** Absorbent material, such as gauze or prepared cotton, used to absorb fluids. **2.** A member of the phylum Porifera, the cellular endoskeleton of which is a source of commercial s.'s.

absorbable gelatin s., a sterile, absorbable, water-insoluble gelatin base s., used to control capillary bleeding in surgical operations; it is left *in situ* and is absorbed in from 4 to 6 weeks.

Bernays' s., a compressed disk of aseptic cotton that swells when moistened; used in packing cavities.

bronchoscopic s., a small fold of gauze used on a long applicator to apply medication or remove secretions through a bronchoscope.

compressed s., s. tent; a s. is impregnated with thin mucilage of acacia, wrapped with twine to the desired shape, and then dried; used to dilate sinuses, the os uteri, etc. by absorbing moisture after insertion.

contraceptive s., a resilient, hydrophilic s. of polyurethane foam impregnated with a spermicide; contraception is achieved by action of the spermicide, absorption of sperm into the s., and blockage of the cervix.

spongia (spŭn'jē-ă) [G.]. Sponge.

spongiform (spŭn'ji-fōrm). Spongy.

spongio- [G. *spongia,* sponge]. Combining form denoting sponge, spongelike, spongy.

spongioblast (spŭn'jē-ō-blast) [spongio- + G. *blastos,* germ]. A neuroepithelial, filiform ependyma cell extending across the entire thickness of the wall of the brain or spinal cord, *i.e.,* from the internal to the external limiting membrane.

spongioblastoma (spŭn'jē-ō-blas-tō'mă) [spongioblast + G. *-oma* tumor]. A glioma consisting of cells (elongated, spindle-shaped, and sometimes pleomorphic, with one or two fibrillary processes) that resemble the embryonic spongioblasts, occurring normally around the neural canal of the human embryo; it grows relatively slowly, usually originating in the brainstem, optic chiasm, or infundibulum, and infiltrates adjacent structures or causes compression of the third and fourth ventricle. S.'s were formerly subclassified as s. polare and s. unipolare. See also glioblastoma; astrocytoma grade IV.

spongiocyte (spŭn'jē-ō-sīt) [spongio- + G. *kytos,* cell]. **1.** A neuroglial cell. **2.** A cell in the zona fasciculata of the adrenal containing many droplets of lipid material which, after staining with hematoxylin and eosin, show pronounced vacuolization.

spongioid (spŭn'jē-oyd) [spongio- + G. *eidos,* resemblance]. Spongy.

spongiose (spŭn'jē-ōs) [L. *spongiosus*]. Resembling or characteristic of a sponge.

spongiosis (spŭn-jē-ō'sis). Intercellular edema of the epidermis.

spongiositis (spŭn-jē-ō-sī'tis). Inflammation of the corpus spongiosum, or corpus cavernosum urethrae.

spongy (spŭn'jē). Spongiform; spongioid; of spongelike texture or appearance.

spontaneous (spon-tā'nē-ŭs) [L. *spontaneus,* voluntary, capricious]. Without apparent cause; said of disease processes or remissions.

spoon (spūn) [A.S. *spōn,* chip]. An instrument with a handle and a small bowl- or cup-shaped extremity.

cataract s., a small concave instrument for removing a cataractous lens.

Daviel's s., a small oval-shaped instrument for removing the remains of a cataract after discission.

sharp s., an instrument with a small cup-shaped extremity having sharpened edges, used for scraping skin lesions.

Volkmann's s., a sharp s. for scraping away carious bone or other diseased tissue.

spor-, spori-. See sporo-.

sporadic (spō-rad'ik) [G. *sporadikos,* scattered]. Occurring singly, not grouped; neither epidemic nor endemic.

sporadin (spōr'ă-din). Gamont stage of a gregarine parasite after it has lost its epimerite or mucron.

sporangiophore (spō-ran'jē-ō-fōr) [sporangium + G. *phoros,* bearing]. In fungi, a specialized hypha that bears a sporangium at its tip.

sporangium, pl. **sporangia** (spō-ran'jē-ŭm, -ă) [L. fr. G. *sporos,* seed, + *angeion,* vessel]. A cell within a fungus, in which asexual spores are borne by progressive cleavage.

spore (spōr) [G. *sporos,* seed]. **1.** The asexual or sexual reproductive body of fungi or sporozoan protozoa. **2.** A cell of a plant lower in organization than the seed-bearing spermatophytic plants. **3.** A resistant form of certain species of bacteria. **4.** The highly modified reproductive body of certain protozoa, as in the phyla Microspora and Myxozoa.

black s., a degenerating malarial or other blood parasite in the body of the mosquito.

sporicidal (spōr-i-sī'dăl) [spori- + L. *caedo,* to kill]. Lethal to spores.

sporicide (spōr'i-sīd). An agent that kills spores.

sporidium, pl. **sporidia** (spō-rid'ē-ŭm, -ă) [Mod. L. dim., fr. G. *sporos,* seed]. A protozoan spore; an embryonic protozoan organism.

sporo-, spori-, spor- [G. *sporos,* seed]. Combining forms denoting seed, spore.

sporoagglutination (spōr'ō-ă-glū-ti-nā'shŭn). A diagnostic method in relation to the mycoses, based upon the fact that the blood of patients with diseases caused by fungi contains specific agglutinins that cause clumping of the spores of these organisms.

sporoblast (spōr'ō-blast) [sporo- + G. *blastos,* germ]. Zygotomere; an early stage in the development of a sporocyst prior to differentiation of the sporozoites. See also oocyst; sporocyst (2); pansporoblast.

sporocyst (spōr'ō-sist) [sporo- + G. *kystis,* bladder]. **1.** A larval form of digenetic trematode (fluke) that develops in the body of its molluscan intermediate host, usually a snail; the s. forms a simple saclike structure with germinal cells that bud off internally and develop into other larval types that continue this process of larval multiplication (considered to be a form of polyembryony). See also miracidium; redia; cercaria. **2.** A secondary cyst that develops within the oocyst of Coccidia, a group of sporozoans that includes many of the most important disease agents of domestic animals and fowl; the s. develops from a sporoblast and produces within itself one or several sporozoites, the infective agents for infection and multiplication in the next host.

Sporocystinea (spōr'ō-sis-tin'ē-ă). [sporo + G. *kystis,* bladder]. In older classification schemes, a suborder of Coccidia in which the sporoblasts develop sporocysts.

sporodochium (spō-rō-dō'kē-ŭm). In fungi, a cushion-shaped stroma covered with conidiophores.

sporogenesis (spōr-ō-jen'ĕ-sis) [sporo- + G. *genesis,* production]. Sporogony.

sporogenous (spō-roj'ĕ-nŭs). Relating to or involved in sporogony.

sporogeny (spō-roj'ĕ-nē). Sporogony.

sporogony (spō-rog'ō-nē) [sporo- + G. *goneia,* generation]. Sporogenesis; sporogeny; the formation of sporozoites in sporozoan protozoa, a process of asexual division within the sporoblast, which becomes the sporocyst within an oocyst; follows fusion of gametes (gametogony) and zygote (sporont) formation.

sporont (spōr'ont) [sporo- + G. *ōn* (*ont-*), being]. The zygote stage within the oocyst wall in the life cycle of coccidia; gives rise to sporoblasts, which form sporocysts, within which the infective sporozoites are produced.

sporophore (spōr'ō-fōr) [sporo- + G. *phoros,* bearing]. Any specialized hyphae in fungi that give rise to spores.

sporoplasm (spōr'ō-plazm) [sporo- + G. *plasma,* thing formed]. The protoplasm of a spore.

sporotheca (spōr'o-the'ka) [sporo- + G. *thēkē,* case]. The envelope enclosing the minute needle-like spores of certain Sporozoa.

Sporothrix (spōr'ō-thriks) [Mod. L., fr. G. *sporos,* seed, + *thrix,* hair]. A genus of dimorphic imperfect fungi, including the species *S. schenckii,* an organism of worldwide distribution and the causative agent of sporotrichosis in man and animals, which grows in soil or vegetation, especially in thorny bushes, and is acquired by man when infected thorns are introduced into subcutaneous tissues; at 37°C it grows as a yeast and parasitizes tissues as a yeast.

sporotrichosis (spōr'ō-tri-kō'sis). Schenck's disease; a chronic subcutaneous mycosis spread by way of the lymphatics and caused by *Sporothrix schenckii.* The disease may remain localized or may become generalized, involving bones, joints, lungs, and the central nervous system; lesions may be granulomatous or suppurative, ulcerative, or draining.

Sporotrichum (spō-rot'ri-kŭm) [Mod. L. fr. G. *sporos,* seed, + *thrix,* hair]. A genus of imperfect fungi (Hyphomycetes) that are usually common contaminants.

sporozoan (spōr-ō-zō'an). **1.** Sporozoon; an individual organism of the class Sporozoea. **2.** Relating to the Sporozoea.

Sporozoasida (spōr'ō-zō-as'i-dă). Sporozoea.

Sporozoea (spōr-ō-zō'ē-ă) [Mod. L., fr. G. *sporos,* seed, + *zōon,* animal]. Sporozoasida; Telosporea; Telosporidia; a large class of protozoans (phylum Apicomplexa, subkingdom Protozoa) consisting of obligatory parasites with simple spores lacking polar filaments; cilia and flagella are absent (except for microgametes, found in some groups), and locomotion is by undulation, gliding, or body flexion; sexuality, when present, is by syngamy, forming oocysts with infective sporozoites from sporogony. The class includes the gregarines and coccidia, the latter including many agents of human and animal disease, such as the plasmodia of malaria.

sporozoite (spōr-ō-zō'īt) [sporo- + G. *zōon,* animal]. Oxyspore; germinal rod; zoite; zygotoblast; one of the minute elongated bodies resulting from the repeated division of the oocyst during sporogony. In the case of the malarial parasite, it is the form that is concentrated in the salivary glands and introduced into the blood by the bite of a mosquito; it enters the liver cells (exoerythrocytic cycle), whose progeny, the merozoites, infect the red blood cells to initiate clinical malaria.

sporozooid (spōr-ō-zō'oyd) [sporo- + G. *zōon,* animal, + *eidos,* resemblance]. Obsolete term for a falciform figure seen in certain cancerous tumors, formerly regarded by some as a sporozoan spore or sporozoite.

sporozoon (spōr-ō-zō'on) Sporozoan (1).

sport (spōrt). An organism varying in whole or in part, without apparent reason, from others of its type; this variation may be transmitted to the descendants or the latter may revert to the original type.

sporular (spōr'yū-lăr). Relating to a spore or sporule.

sporulation (spōr'ū-lā'shŭn). Multiple *fission.*

sporule (spōr'ūl) [Mod. L. *sporula;* dim. of G. *sporos,* seed]. A spore; a small spore.

spot. 1. Macula. **2.** To lose a slight amount of blood through the vagina.

acoustic s.'s, see *macula* utriculi and *macula* sacculi.

Bitot's s.'s, small, circumscribed, lusterless, grayish white, foamy, greasy, triangular deposits on the bulbar conjunctiva adjacent to the cornea in the area of the palpebral fissure of both eyes; occurs in vitamin A deficiency.

blind s., **(1)** physiologic *scotoma;* **(2)** mental *scotoma;* **(3)** *discus* nervi optici.

blood s.'s, hemorrhagic graafian follicles seen in ovaries of mice, caused by injection of urine of pregnant women; a positive result in the now obsolete Aschheim-Zondek test for pregnancy.

blue s., **(1)** *macula* cerulea; **(2)** mongolian s.

Brushfield's s.'s, mottled, marbled, or speckled s.'s on the iris in mongolism.

café au lait s.'s, uniformly light brown, sharply defined, and usually oval-shaped patches of the skin that are characteristic of neurofibromatosis, but also found in normal individuals.

cherry-red s., Tay's cherry-red s; the ophthalmoscopic appearance of the normal choroid beneath the fovea centralis, appearing as a red s. surrounded by white retinal edema in central artery closure or lipid infiltration in sphingolipidosis.

corneal s., *macula* corneae.

cotton-wool s.'s, cotton-wool *patches.*

De Morgan's s.'s, senile *hemangioma.*

Elschnig's s.'s, isolated choroidal bright yellow or red s.'s with black pigment flecks at their borders, seen ophthalmoscopically in advanced hypertensive retinopathy.

Filatov's s.'s, Koplik's s.'s.

flame s.'s, hemorrhagic areas occurring in the nerve fiber layer of the retina.

Fordyce's s.'s, Fordyce's disease or granules; pseudocolloid of lips; a condition marked by the presence of numerous small, yellowish white bodies or granules on the inner surface and vermilion border of the lips; histologically the lesions are ectopic sebaceous glands.

Fuchs' black s., an area of pigment proliferation in the macular region in degenerative myopia.

Gaule's s.'s, sharply circumscribed areas of central corneal degeneration in neuroparalytic keratitis.

germinal s., archaic term for the nucleolus in the nucleus of an ovum.

Graefe's s.'s, small areas over the vertebrae or near the supraorbital foramen, pressure upon which causes relaxation of blepharofacial spasm.

hot s., a region in a gene in which there is a putatively high rate of mutation; its existence involves a consideration of the size of the region concerned, the readiness with which the mutation could be detected, and the possibility that selection against mutants at that point is less than against mutants elsewhere.

hypnogenic s., a pressure-sensitive point on the body of certain susceptible persons, which, when pressed, causes the induction of sleep.

Koplik's s.'s, Filatov's s.'s; small red s.'s on the buccal mucous membrane, in the center of each of which may be seen, in a strong light, a minute bluish white speck; they occur early in measles (morbilli), before the skin eruption, and are regarded as a pathognomonic sign of the disease.

liver s., senile *lentigo.*

Mariotte's blind s., *discus* nervi optici.

Maxwell's s., Maxwell's or Löwe's ring; entoptic projection of the macula and fovea, elicited by a dichromic purple filter and an alternating neutral filter while the patient is gazing at transilluminated opal glass.

milk s.'s, **(1)** soldier's patches; white plaques of hyalinized fibrous tissue situated in the epicardium overlying the right ventricle of the heart where it is not covered by lung; **(2)** white macroscopic areas in the omentum, due to accumulation of macrophages and lymphocytes.

mongolian s., mongolian macula; blue s. (2); any of a number of dark bluish or mulberry-colored rounded or oval s.'s on the sacral region due to the ectopic presence of melanocytes in the dermis. These congenital lesions are frequent in black, Amerindian, and

Oriental children from 2 to 12 years, after which time they gradually recede; they do not disappear on pressure and are sometimes mistaken for bruises from child abuse.
mulberry s.'s, the abdominal eruption in typhus fever.
rose s.'s, characteristic exanthema of typhoid fever.
Roth's s.'s, a round white retina s. surrounded by hemorrhage in bacterial endocarditis.
ruby s.'s, senile *hemangioma.*
saccular s., *macula* sacculi.
Soemmering's s., *macula* retinae.
spongy s., vascular *zone.*
Tardieu's s.'s, Tardieu's *ecchymoses.*
Tay's cherry-red s., cherry-red s.
temperature s., one of a number of definitely arranged s.'s on the skin sensitive to heat and cold, but not to ordinary pressure or pain stimuli.
tendinous s., *macula* albida.
Trousseau's s., meningitic *streak.*
utricular s., *macula* utriculi.
white s., *macula* albida.
yellow s., *macula* retinae.

spp. Plural of sp., abbreviation for subspecies.

sprain (sprān). **1.** Stremma; an injury to a ligament when the joint is carried through a range of motion greater than normal, but without dislocation or fracture. **2.** To cause a s. of a joint.

spray (sprā). A jet of liquid in fine drops, coarser than a vapor; it is produced by forcing the liquid from the minute opening of an atomizer, mixed with air.

spreader (spred'er). **1.** An instrument used to distribute a substance over a surface or area. **2.** A device for spacing or parting structures.
gutta-percha s., an instrument used in dentistry for condensing gutta-percha laterally in a root canal.
rib s., an instrument for widening the space between ribs in intrathoracic operations.
root canal s., a tapered instrument utilized for condensing root filling materials laterally.

Sprengel, Otto G.K., German surgeon, 1852–1915. See S.'s *deformity.*

Sprinz, Helmuth, 20th century German physician in the U.S., *1911. See S.-Nelson *syndrome.*

Sprinz-Nelson syndrome. See under syndrome.

sprout (sprowt). A structure resembling the s. of a plant.
syncytial s., syncytial *knot.*

sprue (sprū) [D. *spruw*]. **1.** Cachexia aphthosa; primary intestinal malabsorption with steatorrhea. **2.** In dentistry, wax or metal used to form the aperture(s) for molten metal to flow into a mold to make a casting; also, the metal that later fills the s. hole(s).
nontropical s., s. occurring in persons away from the tropics; usually called celiac disease.
tropical s., Cochin China or tropical diarrhea; s. occurring in the tropics, often associated with enteric infection and nutritional deficiency, and frequently complicated by folate deficiency with macrocytic anemia.

sprue-former (sprū fōr'mer). The base to which the sprue (2) is attached while the wax pattern is being invested in a refractory investment in a casting flask; it is sometimes referred to as a crucible-former.

spud (spŭd). A triangular knife used for removing foreign bodies from the cornea.

Spumavirinae (spū'mă-vir'i-nē) [L. *spuma,* foam]. A subfamily of viruses (family Retroviridae) that includes the foamy viruses (agents) of primates and other mammals; in common with other retroviruses, they possess RNA-dependent DNA polymerases (reverse transcriptase).

Spumavirus (spū'mă-vī'rŭs). A genus of viruses of the subfamily Spumavirinae.

spur (sper) [A.S. *spora*] Calcar.
Fuchs' s., epithelial outgrowth of the dilator muscle of the pupil about midway in the breadth of the sphincter.
Grunert's s., epithelial outgrowth of the dilator muscle of the pupil at the junction of the iris and the ciliary body.
Michel's s., epithelial outgrowth of the dilator muscle of the pupil at the peripheral border of the sphincter.
Morand's s., *calcar* avis.
scleral s., scleral roll; a ridge of the sclera at the internal scleral sulcus from which ciliary muscle fibers take origin.
vascular s., partial septum between vessels (arteries and veins) at the level of fusion or branching at acute angle.

spurious (spū'rē-ŭs) [L. *spurius*]. False; not genuine.

sputum, pl. **sputa** (spū'tŭm, -tă) [L. *sputum,* fr. *spuo,* pp. *sputus,* to spit]. **1.** Expectorated matter, especially mucus or mucopurulent matter expectorated in diseases of the air passages. See also expectoration (1). **2.** An individual mass of such matter.
s. aerogeno'sum, green s.; a green expectoration seen occasionally in jaundice, due to staining of the s. by bile pigments.
globular s., nummular s.
green s., s. aeruginosum.
nummular s., globular s.; a thick, coherent mass expectorated in globular shape which does not run at the bottom of the cup but forms a discoid mass resembling a coin.
prune-juice s., prune-juice expectoration; a thin reddish expectoration, characteristic of gangrene or cancer of the lung and certain cases of pneumonia; due to hemorrhage caused by destruction of the lung parenchyma.
rusty s., a reddish brown, blood-stained expectoration characteristic of lobar pneumonococcal pneumonia.

SQ Abbreviation for subcutaneous.

squalene (skwā'lēn). Spinacene; a hexaisoprenoid (triterpenoid) hydrocarbon found in shark oil and in some plants; intermediate in the biosynthesis of cholesterol.

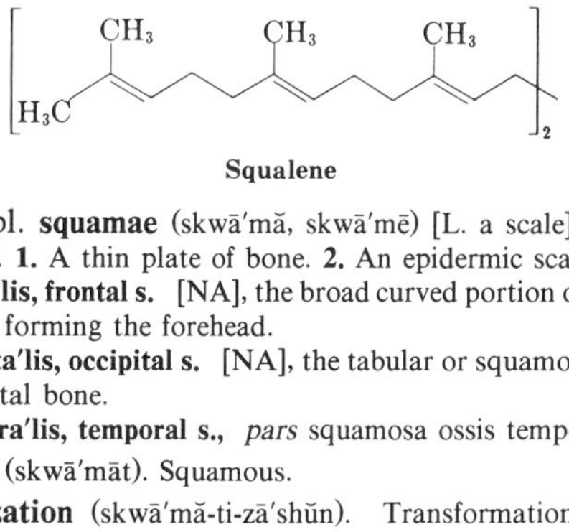

Squalene

squama, pl. **squamae** (skwā'mă, skwā'mē) [L. a scale]. Squame; scale (3). **1.** A thin plate of bone. **2.** An epidermic scale.
s. fronta'lis, frontal s. [NA], the broad curved portion of the frontal bone forming the forehead.
s. occipita'lis, occipital s. [NA], the tabular or squamous portion of occipital bone.
s. tempora'lis, temporal s., *pars* squamosa ossis temporalis.

squamate (skwā'māt). Squamous.

squamatization (skwā'mă-ti-zā'shŭn). Transformation of other types of cells into squamous cells.

squame (skwām). Squama.

squamo- [L. *squama,* a scale]. Combining form denoting squama, squamous.

squamocellular (skwā-mō-sel'yū-lăr). Relating to or having squamous epithelium.

squamocolumnar (skwā-mō-kol'ŭm-nar). Pertaining to the junction between a stratified squamous epithelial surface and one lined by columnar epithelium; *e.g.,* the cardia of the stomach or anus.

squamofrontal (skwā'mō-frŏn'tăl). Relating to the squama frontalis.

squamomastoid (skwā'mō-mas'toyd). Relating to the squamous and petrous portions of the temporal bone.

squamo-occipital (skwā'mō-ok-sip'i-tăl). Relating to the squamous portion of the occipital bone, developing partly in membrane and partly in cartilage.

squamoparietal (skwā'mō-pă-rī'ĕ-tăl). Relating to the parietal bone and the squamous portion of the temporal bone.

squamopetrosal (skwā'mō-pē-trō'săl). Petrosquamosal.

squamosa, pl. squamosae (skwā-mō'să, -sē) [L. *squamosus,* scaly, fr. *squama,* scale]. The squama of the frontal, occipital, or temporal bone, especially the latter.

squamosal (skwā-mō'săl). Relating especially to the squama of the temporal bone.

squamosphenoid (skwā'mō-sfē'noyd). Sphenosquamosal; relating to the sphenoid bone and the squama of the temporal bone.

squamotemporal (skwā'mō-tem'pō-răl). Relating to the pars squamosa ossis temporalis.

squamous (skwā'mŭs) [L. *squamosus*]. Squamate; squarrose; squarrous; scaly; relating to or covered with scales.

squamozygomatic (skwā'mō-zī-gō-mat'ik). Relating to the squama and the zygomatic process of the temporal bone.

squarrose, squarrous (skwar'ōs, skwar'ŭs) [L. *squarrosus*]. Squamous.

squill (skwil) [L. *squilla* or *scilla*]. Scilla; the cut and dried fleshy inner scales of the bulb of the white variety of *Urginea maritima* (Mediterranean s.), or of *U. indica* (Indian s.) (family Liliaceae); the central portion of the bulb is excluded during its processing; s. contains cardiac glycosides (scillaren-A and scillaren-B).

squint (skwint). **1.** Strabismus. **2.** To suffer from strabismus.
convergent s., esotropia.
divergent s., exotropia.
external s., exotropia.
internal s., esotropia.

Sr Symbol for strontium.

SRF Abbreviation for somatotropin-releasing *factor.*

SRF-A Abbreviation for slow-reacting *factor* of anaphylaxis.

SRIF Abbreviation for somatotropin release-inhibiting *factor.*

sRNA Abbreviation for soluble *ribonucleic acid.*

S roma'num (rō-mā'nŭm). *Colon* sigmoideum.

SRS, SRS-A Abbreviation for slow-reacting *substance* or slow-reacting *substance* of anaphylaxis.

SSS Abbreviation for soluble specific *substance.*

stab [Gael. *stob*]. To pierce with a pointed instrument, as a knife or dagger.

stabilate (stā'bi-lāt). A sample of organisms preserved alive on a single occasion.

stabile (stā'bīl, -bil) [L. *stabilis*]. Stable; steady; fixed; denoting: 1) certain constituents of serum unaffected by ordinary degrees of heat; 2) an electrode held steadily on a part during the passage of an electric current.

stabilimeter (stā-bi-lim'ĕ-ter) [L. *stabilitas,* firmness, + G. *metron,* measure]. An instrument to measure the sway of the body when standing with feet together and usually with eyes closed.

stability (stă-bil'i-tē). The condition of being stable or resistant to change.
denture s., stabilization (2); the quality of a denture to be firm, steady, constant, and resist change of position when functional forces are applied.
dimensional s., the property of a material to retain its size and form.
endemic s., enzootic s.; a situation in which all factors influencing disease occurrence are relatively stable, resulting in little fluctuation in disease incidence over time; changes in one or more of these factors (*e.g.,* reduction in proportion of individuals exposed to infectious agent) can lead to an unstable situation in which major disease outbreaks occur.
enzootic s., endemic s.
suspension s., a very slow sedimentation rate.

stabilization (stā'bĭ-li-zā'shŭn). **1.** The accomplishment of a stable state. **2.** Denture *stability.*

stabilizer (stā'bĭ-lī-zer). **1.** That which renders something else more stable. **2.** An agent that retards the effect of an accelerator, thus preserving a chemical equilibrium. **3.** A part possessing the quality of rigidity or creating rigidity when added to another part.
endodontic s., a pin implant passing through the apex of a tooth from its root canal and extending well into the underlying bone to provide immobilization of periodontally involved teeth.

stable (stā'bl). Steady; not varying; resistant to change. See also stabile.

stachybotryotoxicosis (stak-ē-bot'rē-ō-tok-si-kō'sis). A type of mycotoxicosis seen in horses and cattle following ingestion of hay and fodder overgrown by the fungus *Stachybotrys atra;* may also occur in persons exposed to hay either by inhalation or by absorbing the toxin through the skin, and is manifested by skin rash, pharyngitis, and mild leukopenia.

stachydrine (stak'i-drēn). *N*- methylproline methylbetaine; the betaine of proline found in alfalfa, chrysanthemum, and citrus plants.

stachyose (stak'ē-ōs). A raffinosegalactopyranoside; a tetrasaccharide that yields glucose, fructose, and 2 moles of galactose upon hydrolysis; present in certain tubers and other plant tissues.

stactometer (stak-tom'ĕ-ter) [G. *staktos,* dropping, fr. *stazō,* to let fall by drops, + *metron,* measure]. Stalagmometer.

Stader, Otto, U.S. veterinary surgeon. See S. *splint.*

Staderini, Rutilio, 19th century Italian neuroanatomist. See S.'s *nucleus.*

stadiometer (stā-dē-om'ĕ-ter) [L. *stadium,* fr. G. *stadion,* a fixed length, + G. *metron,* measure]. An instrument for measuring standing or sitting height.

stadium, pl. stadia (stā'dē-ŭm, -dē-ă) [L. fr. G. *stadion,* a fixed standard length]. Obsolete term for a stage in the course of a disease, especially of an acute pyretic disease.

staff [A.S. *staef*] **1.** A specific group of workers. **2.** Director (1).
attending s., physicians and surgeons who are members of a hospital s. and regularly attend their patients at the hospital; may also supervise and teach house s., fellows, and medical students.
consulting s., specialists affiliated with a hospital who serve in an advisory capacity to the attending s.
house s., physicians and surgeons in specialty training at a hospital who care for the patients under the direction and responsibility of the attending s.

staff of Aesculapius [L. *Aesculapius,* G. *Asklēpios,* god of medicine]. A rod with only one serpent encircling it and without wings; correct symbol of medicine and emblem of the American Medical Association, Royal Army Medical Corps (Britain), and Royal Canadian Medical Corps. See also caduceus.

Stafne, Edward C., U.S. oral pathologist, *1894. See S. bone *cyst.*

stage (stāj) [M.E. thr. O. Fr. *estage,* standing-place, fr. L. *sto,* pp. *status,* to stand]. **1.** A period in the course of a disease; a description of the extent of involvement of a disease process or the status of a patient with a specific disease, as of the distribution and extent of dissemination of a malignant neoplastic disease. See also period. **2.** The part of a microscope on which the microslide bears the object to be examined. **3.** A particular step, phase, or position in a developmental process. For psychosexual s.'s, see subentries under phase.

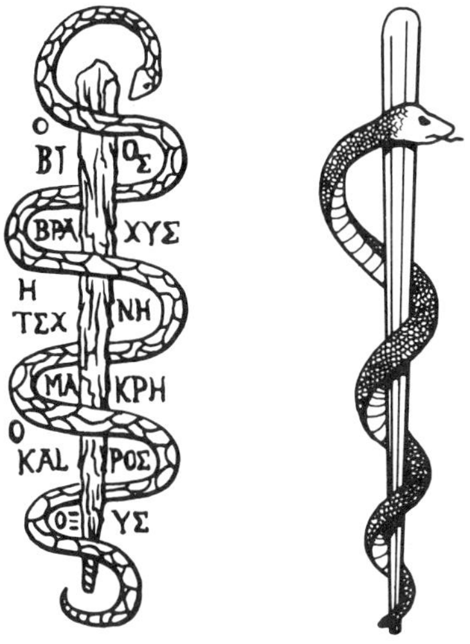

Staff of Aesculapius

algid s., the s. of collapse in cholera.

Arneth s.'s, a differential grouping of polymorphonuclear neutrophils in accordance with the number of lobes in their nuclei, *i.e.*, cells with 1, 2, 3, 4, or 5 (or more) lobes are designated, respectively, as class I, II, and so on. See also Arneth formula.

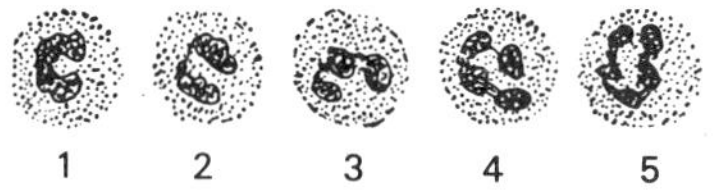

Arneth Stages

cap s., the second s. in the proliferative phase of tooth development.

cold s., the s. of chill in a malarial paroxysm.

defervescent s., see defervesence.

end s., the late, fully developed phase of a disease; *e.g.*, in end-stage renal disease, shrunken and scarred kidney that may result from a variety of chronic diseases which have become indistinguishable in their effect on the kidney.

exoerythrocytic s., developmental s. of the malaria parasite (*Plasmodium*) in liver parenchyma cells of the vertebrate host before erythrocytes are invaded. The initial generation produces cryptozoites, the next generation metacryptozoites; reinfection of liver cells from blood cells apparently does not occur. Delayed development of the sporozoite (hypnozoite) of *Plasmodium vivax* and *P. ovale* appears to be responsible for malarial relapse that may occur with these disease agents.

imperfect s., a mycological term used to describe the asexual life cycle phase of a fungus.

incubative s., incubation period (2); s. of invasion; latent or prodromal s.; the primary s. of certain infectious diseases during which the prodromal symptoms are appearing, and usually synchronous with the induction of sensitivity.

intuitive s., in psychology, a s. of development, usually occurring between 4 and 7 years of age, in which a child's thought processes are determined by the most prominent aspects of the stimuli to which he is exposed, rather than by some form of logical thought.

s. of invasion, incubative s.

s.'s of labor, see labor.

latent s., incubative s.

perfect s., a mycological term used to describe the sexual life cycle phase of a fungus in which spores are formed after nuclear fusion.

preconceptual s., in psychology, the s. of development in an infant's life, prior to actual conceptual thinking, in which sensorimotor activity predominates.

prodromal s., incubative s.

resting s., vegetative s.; the quiescent s. of a cell or its nucleus in which no karyokinetic changes are taking place.

Tanner s., a s. of puberty in the Tanner growth chart, based on pubic hair growth, development of genitalia in boys, and breast development in girls.

trypanosome s., see trypomastigote.

tumor s., the extent of the spread of a malignant neoplasm from its site of origin. See also TMN *staging*.

vegetative s., resting s.

stagger (stag'er) To walk unsteadily; to reel.

staggers (stag'erz). **1.** A form of decompression sickness in which vertigo, mental confusion, and muscular weakness are the chief symptoms. **2.** Gid; a disease in sheep, marked by swaying and uncertain gait, caused by the presence of the larva of *Multiceps multiceps* in the brain, or by other cerebral lesions.

blind s., subacute selenium poisoning in animals.

bracken s., a condition occurring in horses as a result of eating bracken; characterized by locomotor incoordination; due to thiamin deficiency (bracken contains thiaminase).

staging (stāj'ing). The determination or classification of distinct phases or periods in the course of a disease or pathological process.

Jewett and Strong s., s. of bladder carcinoma: O, noninvasive; A, with submucosal invasion; B, with muscle invasion; C, with invasion of merivascular fat; D, with lymph node metastasis.

TNMs., a system of clinicopathologic evaluation of tumors based on the extent of tumor involvement at the primary site (T, followed by a number indicating size and depth of invasion), and lymph node involvement (N) and metastasis (M) each followed by a number starting at 0 for no evident metastasis; numbers used depend on the organ involved and influence the prognosis and choice of treatment.

stagnation (stag-nā'shŭn) [L. *stagnum,* a pool]. Retardation or cessation of flow of blood in the vessels, as in passive congestion; accumulation in any part of a normally circulating fluid.

Stahl, Friedrich K., German physician, 1811–1873. See S.'s *ear.*

Stahl, George E., German physician and chemist, 1660–1734. He promulgated the phlogiston theory. See phlogiston.

Stähli, Jean, Swiss ophthalmologist, *1890. See S.'s *line,* Hudson-S. *line.*

STAIN

stain (stān) [M.E. *steinen*]. **1.** To discolor. **2.** To color; to dye. **3.** A discoloration. **4.** A dye used in histologic and bacteriologic technique. **5.** A procedure in which a dye or combination of dyes and reagents is used to color the constituents of cells and tissues. For individual dyes or staining substances, see the specific names.

Abbott's s. for spores, spores are stained blue with alkaline methylene blue; bodies of the bacilli become pink with eosin counterstain.

aceto-orcein s., a s. used for chromosomes in air-dried or squashed cytologic material.

acid s., a dye in which the anion is the colored component of the dye molecule, *e.g.*, sodium eosinate (eosin).

Ag-AS s., silver-ammoniacal silver s.

Albert's s., a s. for diphtheria bacilli and their metachromatic

granules; contains toluidine blue, methyl green, glacial acetic acid, alcohol, and distilled water.
Altmann's anilin-acid fuchsin s., a mixture of picric acid, anilin, and acid fuchsin which stains mitochondria crimson against a yellow background.
auramine O fluorescent s., a rapid and accurate technique for *Mycobacterium tuberculosis,* using auramine O-phenol and a methylene blue counterstain.
basic s., a dye in which the cation is the colored component of the dye molecule that binds to anionic groups of nucleic acids ($PO_4\equiv$) or acidic mucopolysaccharides (*e.g.,* chondroitin sulfate).
basic fuchsin-methylene blue s., a s. for intact epoxy sections; semi-thick sections of plastic-embedded tissues have nuclei stained purple; collagen, elastic lamina, and connective tissue are stained blue; mitochondria, myelin, and lipid droplets are stained red; cytoplasm, smooth muscle cells, axoplasm, and chrondroblasts are stained pink.
Bauer's chromic acid leucofuchsin s., a s. for glycogen and fungi utilizing chromic acid as an oxidizing agent of polysaccharides, followed by Schiff's reagent; glycogen and fungi cell walls appear deep red.
Becker's s. for spirochetes, a s. applied to thin films fixed in formaldehyde-acetic acid; preparations are treated successively with tannin, carbolic acid, and carbol fuchsin.
Bennhold's Congo red s., an amyloid s. useful for amyloid detection in pathologic tissue; gives red staining of amyloid; also induces green birefringence to amyloid under polarized light.
Berg's s., a method for staining spermatozoa, utilizing a carbolfuchsin solution followed by dilute acetic acid and methylene blue; spermatozoa are stained a brilliant red and most other structures appear blue to purple.
Best's carmine s., a method for the demonstration of glycogen in tissues.
Bielschowsky's s., a method of treating tissues with silver nitrate to demonstrate reticular fibers, neurofibrils, axons, and dendrites.
Biondi-Heidenhain s., an obsolete s. for spirochetes, using acid fuchsin and orange G.
Birch-Hirschfeld s., an obsolete s. for demonstrating amyloid, using Bismarck brown and crystal violet; amyloid is usually stained a bright ruby red, whereas the cytoplasm of cells is not stained and nuclei are brown.
Bodian's copper-PROTARGOL s., a s. employing a silver proteinate complex (PROTARGOL) to demonstrate axis cylinders and neurofibrils.
Borrel's blue s., a s. for demonstrating spirochetes, treponemes, and Borrelia organisms, using silver oxide (prepared by means of mixing solutions of silver nitrate and sodium bicarbonate) and methylene blue.
Bowie's s., a s. for juxtaglomerular granules in which the kidney sections are stained in a mixture of Biebrich scarlet red and ethyl violet; juxtaglomerular granules and elastic fibers are stained a deep purple, erythrocytes are amber, and background tissue appears in shades of red.
Brown-Brenn s., a method for differential staining of Gram-positive and Gram-negative bacteria in tissue sections; it utilizes a modified Gram s. of crystal violet, Gram's iodine, and basic fuchsin.
Cajal's astrocyte s., a method for demonstrating astrocytes by impregnation in a solution containing gold chloride and mercuric chloride.
carbol-thionin s., a s. useful for demonstrating typhoid bacilli in films and sections, and for Nissl substance.
C-banding s., centromere banding s.; a selective chromosome banding s. used in human cytogenetics, employing Giemsa s. after most of the DNA is denatured or extracted by treatment with alkali, acid, salt, or heat; only heterochromatic regions close to the centromeres and rich in satellite DNA stain, with the exception of the Y chromosome whose long arm usually stains throughout.
centromere banding s., C-banding s.
chromate s. for lead, a method in which tissues preserved in chromate-containing fixatives, such as Regaud's or Orth's fixatives, precipitate lead as yellow lead chromate crystals; formalin-fixed sections are treated with potassium chromate acidified with acetic acid.
chrome alum hematoxylin-phloxine s., a s. used to demonstrate pancreatic islet cells; alpha cells appear red, beta cells blue or unstained.
Ciaccio's s., a method for demonstrating complex insoluble intracellular lipids using fixation in a formalin-dichromate solution, embedding in paraffin, staining with Sudan III or IV, and examination in aqueous mountant.
contrast s., differential s.; a dye used to color one portion of a tissue or cell which remained unaffected when the other part was stained by a dye of different color.
Da Fano's s., a silver s. that produces a blackening of Golgi elements after tissues are fixed in a mixture of nitrate and formalin.
Dane's s., a s. for prekeratin, keratin, and mucin which employs hemalum, phloxine, Alcian blue, and orange G; nuclei appear orange to brown, acid mucopolysaccharides pale blue, and keratins orange to red-orange.
DAPI s., a sensitive fluorescent probe for DNA, 4′6-diamidino-2-phenylindole·2HCl, used in fluorescence microscopy to detect DNA in yeast mitochondria, chloroplasts, viruses, mycoplasma, and chromosomes; DNA is visualized in vitally stained living cells and after cells are fixed in formaldehyde.
diazo s. for argentaffin granules, in enterochromaffin cells, a variety of diazonium salts are used to blacken the cells.
Dieterle's s., s. used to demonstrate spirochetes and Leishman-Donovan bodies; employs silver nitrate and uranium nitrate.
differential s., contrast s.
double s., a mixture of two dyes, each of which stains different portions of a tissue or cell.
Ehrlich's acid hematoxylin s., an alum type of hematoxylin s. used as a regressive staining method for nuclei, followed by differentiation to required staining intensity; the solution may be allowed to ripen naturally in sunlight or partially oxidized with sodium iodate.
Ehrlich's aniline crystal violet s., a s. for Gram-positive bacteria.
Ehrlich's triacid s., a differential leukocytic s. comprised of saturated solutions of orange G, acid fuchsin, and methyl green.
Ehrlich's triple s., a mixture of indulin, eosin Y, and aurantia.
Einarson's gallocyanin-chrome alum s., a method for staining both RNA and DNA a deep blue; with proper controls, nucleic acid content of stained cells and nuclei may be estimated by cytophotometry; also useful for Nissl substance.
Eranko's fluorescence s., exposure of frozen sections to formaldehyde which produces a strong yellow-green fluorescence from cells containing norepinephrine.
Feulgen s., a selective cytochemical reaction for DNA in which sections or cells are first hydrolyzed with hydrochloric acid to produce apurinic acid and then are stained with Schiff's reagent to produce magenta-stained nuclei; generally the concentration of DNA in nucleoli and mitochondria is too low to permit detection by this s. See also Kasten's fluorescent Feulgen s.
Field's rapid s., a s. to permit rapid positive diagnosis of malaria in endemic areas by using thick films; it employs methylene blue and azure B in a phosphate buffer, with the preparation counterstained by eosin in a phosphate buffer.
Fink-Heimer s., a method used for histologic demonstration of degenerating nerve fibers and terminals of the central nervous system (black on a yellow background).
Flemming's triple s., a s. comprised of safranin, methyl violet, and orange G.
fluorescence plus Giemsa s., a s. used to demonstrate sister chromatid exchange; cells are grown in 5-bromodeoxyuridine, followed

by chromosome preparation, staining in Hoechst 33258, exposure to light, and staining in Giemsa; chromosomes exhibit a "harlequin" appearance.

fluorescent s., a s. or staining procedure using a fluorescent dye or substance that will combine selectively with certain tissue components and that will then fluoresce upon irradiation with ultraviolet or violet-blue light.

Fontana's s., a traditional method for silver-impregnation of treponemes and other spirochetal forms.

Fontana-Masson silver s., Masson-Fontana ammoniacal silver s.

Foot's reticulin impregnation s., a silver s. in which reticulin stains black and collagen stains golden brown; sections are floated on the surface of solutions to avoid contamination with silver debris.

Fouchet's s., Fouchet's reagent employed to demonstrate bile pigments; paraffin sections are used for conjugated bile pigments, frozen sections for unconjugated ones.

Fraser-Lendrum s. for fibrin, a multistaining procedure after Zenker's fixation in which fibrin, keratin, and some cytoplasmic granules appear red, erythrocytes appear orange, and collagen appears green.

Friedländer's s. for capsules, an obsolete s. employing gentian violet.

G-banding s., Giemsa chromosome banding s.; a unique chromosome staining technique, used in human cytogenetics to identify individual chromosomes, which produces characteristic bands; it utilizes acetic acid fixation, air drying, denaturing chromosomes mildly with proteolytic enzymes, salts, heat, detergents, or urea, and finally Giemsa s.; chromosome bands appear similar to those fluorochromed by Q-banding s.

Giemsa s., compound of methylene blue-eosin and methylene blue used for demonstrating Negri bodies, *Tunga* species, spirochetes and protozoans, and differential staining of blood smears; also used for chromosomes, sometimes after hydrolyzing the cytologic preparation in hot hydrochloric acid, and for showing chromosome G bands; often used in glycerol-methanol buffer solution.

Giemsa chromosome banding s., G-banding s.

Glenner-Lillie s. for pituitary, a modification of Mann's methyl blue-eosin s. which changes the dye proportions, buffering the dye mixture, and staining at 60°C; basophils are stained blue to black, acidophils are dark red, chromophobe granules are gray to pink, and erythrocytes are orange; with modification, the method is also useful for enterochromaffin cells, goblet cells, Paneth cells, and pancreatic islet cells.

Golgi's s., any of several methods for staining nerve cells, nerve fibers, and neuroglia using fixation and hardening in formalin-osmic-dichromate combinations for various times, followed by impregnation in silver nitrate.

Gomori's aldehyde fuchsin s., a s. used to demonstrate beta cells of the pancreas, storage form of thyrotrophic hormone in beta cells of the anterior pituitary, hypophyseal neurosecretory substance, mast cells, granules, elastic fibers, sulfated mucins, and gastric chief cells.

Gomori's chrome alum hematoxylin-phloxine s., a technique used to demonstrate cytoplasmic granules, after Bouin's or formalin-Zenker fixations, using oxidized hematoxylin plus phloxine; in the pancreas, beta cells are blue, alpha and delta cells are red, and zymogen granules are red to unstained; in the pituitary, alpha cells are pink, beta cells and chromophobes are gray-blue, and nuclei are purple to blue.

Gomori's methenamine-silver (GMS) s.'s, techniques for 1) *argentaffin cells:* a method using a methenamine-silver solution in combination with gold chloride, sodium thiosulphate, and safranin O; argentaffin granules appear brown-black against a green background; 2) *urates:* warm sections are treated directly with a hot methenamine-silver solution to produce a blackening of urates; 3) *fungi:* see Grocott-Gomori methenamine-silver s.; 4) *melanin,* which reduces silver nitrate.

Gomori's nonspecific acid phosphatase s., a method in which formalin-fixed frozen sections are incubated in a substrate containing sodium β-glycerophosphate and lead nitrate at pH 5.0; the insoluble lead phosphate produced is treated with ammonium sulfide to give a black lead sulfide.

Gomori's nonspecific alkaline phosphatase s., a calcium-cobalt sulfide method using frozen sections or cold acetone- or formalin-fixed paraffin sections, plus sodium β-glycerophosphate as a substrate at pH 9.0 to 9.5 with Mg^{++} as activator; calcium ions precipitate the liberated phosphate, cobalt salt replaces the calcium phosphate, and ammonium sulfide converts the product to a black cobalt sulfide.

Gomori's one-step trichrome s., a connective tissue s. that uses hematoxylin and a dye mixture containing chromotrope 2R and light green or aniline blue; muscle fibers appear red, collagen is green (or blue if aniline blue is used), and nuclei are blue to black.

Gomori's silver impregnation s., a reliable method for reticulin, as an aid in the diagnosis of neoplasm and early cirrhosis of the liver; the staining solution employs silver nitrate, potassium hydroxide, and ammonia water carefully prepared to avoid having silver precipitate.

Gomori-Jones periodic acid-methenamine-silver s., a staining method using methenamine silver, periodic acid, gold chloride, hematoxylin, and eosin to delineate basement membrane, reticulin, collagen, and nuclei; used in renal histopathology. See also Rambourg's periodic acid-methenamine-silver s.

Goodpasture's s., a s. for Gram-negative bacteria, using aniline fuchsin.

Gordon and Sweet s., a s. for reticulin, using acidified potassium permanganate, oxalic acid, iron alum, silver nitrate, formaldehyde, gold chloride, and sodium thiosulfate.

Gram's s., a method for differential staining of bacteria; smears are fixed by flaming, stained in a solution of crystal violet, treated with iodine solution, rinsed, decolorized, and then counterstained with safranin O; Gram-positive organisms stain purple black and Gram-negative organisms stain pink; useful in bacterial taxonomy and identification, and also in indicating fundamental differences in cell wall structure.

green s., a deposit, produced by chromogenic bacteria, found on the cervicolabial portions of the teeth, usually in children. See also acquired *pellicle.*

Gridley's., a silver staining method for reticulum.

Gridley's s. for fungi, a method for fixed tissue sections based on Bauer's chromic acid leucofuchsin s. with the addition of Gomori's aldehyde fuchsin s. and metanil yellow as counterstains; against a yellow background, hyphae, conidia, yeast capsules, elastin, and mucin appear in different shades of blue to purple.

Grocott-Gomori methenamine-silver s., a modification of Gomori's methenamine-silver s. for fungi in which sections are pretreated with chromic acid before addition of the methenamine-silver solution and then counterstained with light green to demonstrate black-brown fungi against a pale green background.

Hale's colloidal iron s., a s. used to distinguish acid mucopolysaccharides such as hyaluronic acid; may be combined with PAS to also visualize carbohydrate-containing proteins and glycoproteins.

Heidenhain's azan s. [*azo*carmine +*an*iline blue], a technique using azocarmine B or G followed by aniline blue to stain nuclei and erythrocytes red, muscle orange, glia fibrils reddish, mucin blue, and collagen and reticulum dark blue.

Heidenhain's iron hematoxylin s., an iron alum hematoxylin s. used for staining muscle striations and mitotic structures blue-black.

hematoxylin and eosin s., probably the most generally useful of all staining methods for tissues; nuclei are stained a deep blue-black with hematoxylin, and cytoplasm is stained pink after counterstaining with eosin, usually in water.

hematoxylin-malachite green-basic fuchsin s., a s. for epoxy resin-extracted sections; semi-thick sections have their plastic dissolved out and the residual tissue is stained sequentially with the various dyes; nuclei and astrocytes are purplish-pink and myelin, lipid droplets, nucleoli, and oligodendrocytes are bright blue-green.

hematoxylin-phloxine B s., a s. for intact epoxy sections; semi-thick sections of plastic-embedded tissues have the following structures stained blue to black; chromatin, nucleoli, basophilic cytoplasm, mitochondria, plasma and nuclear membranes, anisotropic myofibrils, mast cell granules, and elastic membranes of blood vessels; appearing pink to red are collagen fibrils, reticulum, goblet cell mucins, hyalin cartilage matrix, stereocilia, cytoplasm, and erythrocytes; fat droplets and perichondrocyte matrix are green.

Hirsch-Peiffer s., a s. used for cytologic demonstration staining of metachromatic leukodystrophy; excess sulfatides stain metachromatically (golden brown) with cresyl violet in acetic acid.

Hiss' s., a s. for demonstrating the capsules of microorganisms, using gentian violet or basic fuchsin followed by a copper sulphate wash.

Holmes' s., a silver nitrate staining method for nerve fibers.

Hortega's neuroglia s., one of several silver carbonate methods to demonstrate astrocytes, oligodendroglia, and microglia.

Hucker-Conn s., a crystal violet-ammonium oxalate mixture used in Gram's stain.

immunofluorescent s., s. resulting from combination of fluorescent antibody with antigen specific for the antibody portion of the fluorochrome conjugate.

India ink capsule s., a negative s. for crystal bacteria in which cells appear purple (Gram's crystal violet) and the capsules appear clear against a dark background.

iodine s., a s. to detect amyloid, cellulose, chitin, starch, carotenes, and glycogen, and to stain amebas by virtue of their glycogen; feces and other wet preparations are stained directly with Lugol's iodine solution; smears are treated with Schaudinn's fixative and then stained with alcoholic iodine, followed by Heidenhain's iron hematoxylin.

intravital s., a s. which is taken up by living cells after parenteral administration, *e.g.,* intravenously or subcutaneously.

Jenner's s., a methylene blue eosinate similar to Wright's s. but differing in not using polychromed methylene blue; used for staining of blood smears.

Kasten's fluorescent Feulgen s., a fluorescent modification of the Feulgen s., utilizing any one of a variety of fluorescent basic dyes to which SO_2 is added; the brilliant fluorescence makes this method unusually sensitive and adaptable to cytofluorometric quantification of DNA.

Kasten's fluorescent PAS s., a fluorescent modification of the periodic acid Schiff s. for polysaccharides which uses one of Kasten's fluorescent Schiff reagents.

Kinyoun s., a method for demonstrating acid-fast microorganisms, using carbol fuchsin, acid alcohol, and methylene blue; acid-fast microorganisms appear red against a blue background.

Kittrich's s., a cytodiagnostic method for detecting amniotic discharge by staining a fresh vaginal smear with 0.05% Nile blue sulfate; any fetal epidermal cells present will be stained orange to red and all other cells will be stained blue.

Kleihauer's s., a combination of aniline blue and Biebrich scarlet red used for detection of fetal cells in the maternal blood.

Klinger-Ludwig acid-thionin s. for sex chromatin, a method using a preliminary acid treatment on buccal smears, prior to staining with buffered thionin, to differentiate Barr body.

Klüver-Barrera Luxol fast blue s., in combination with cresyl violet, a s. useful for demonstrating myelin and Nissl substance.

Kossa s., von Kossa s.

Kronecker's s., a 5% sodium chloride s. rendered faintly alkaline with sodium carbonate, used in the examination of fresh tissues under the microscope.

Laquer's s. for alcoholic hyalin, a combination of Altmann's aniline-acid fuchsin s. with a Masson trichrome s. which, on a gray-brown background, stains alcoholic hyalin red, collagen green, and nuclei brown.

Lawless' s., an acid fuchsin-light green s. for *Entamoeba histolytica* from fecal or cultured material.

lead hydroxide s., a s. for electron microscopy; after aldehyde fixation, alkaline lead hydroxide preferentially stains RNA, but after OsO_4 fixation, it reacts largely with osmium in tissues to give a general s.; in addition to binding to cytomembranes, it also stains carbohydrates (*e.g.,* glycogen).

Leishman's s., a polychromed eosin-methylene blue s. used in the examination of blood films.

Lendrum's phloxine-tartrazine s., a s. for demonstrating acidophilic inclusion bodies, which appear red on a yellow background; nuclei stain blue, but Negri bodies do not stain.

Lepehne-Pickworth s., a staining technique for hemoglobin and other heme-containing substances in cryostat or frozen sections, which utilizes the presence of tissue peroxidase to oxidize benzidine to a blue quinhydrone.

Levaditi s., a silver nitrate s. for blackening spirochetes in tissue sections.

Lillie's allochrome connective tissue s., a procedure using PAS, hematoxylin, picric acid, and methyl blue; used for distinction between basement membrane and reticulin, and for demonstration of arteriosclerotic lesions.

Lillie's azure-eosin s., a s. in which an azure eosinate solution is used to s. bacteria and rickettsiae in tissues.

Lillie's ferrous iron s., a method using potassium ferrocyanide in acetic acid which demonstrates melanins as a deep green color; lipofuscins and heme pigments are unreactive.

Lillie's sulfuric acid Nile blue s., a technique for showing fatty acids when present in high concentrations.

Lison-Dunn s., a technique using leuco patent blue V and hydrogen peroxidase to demonstrate hemoglobin peroxidase on time sections and smears.

Loeffler's s., a s. for flagella; the specimen is treated with a mixture of ferrous sulfate, tannic acid, and alcoholic fuchsin, then stained with aniline-water fuchsin or gentian violet made alkaline with sodium hydroxide solution.

Loeffler's caustic s., a s. for flagella, utilizing an aqueous solution of tannin and ferrous sulfate with the addition of an alcoholic fuchsin s.

Luna-Ishak s., a staining method using celestine blue and acid fuchsin in which bile canaliculi s. pink to red.

Macchiavello's s., a basic fuchsin-citric acid-methylene blue sequence in smears which produces red staining of rickettsiae and inclusion bodies, with nuclei staining blue.

MacNeal's tetrachrome blood s., a s. for blood smears comprised of a mixture of methylene blue, azure A, methylene violet, and eosin Y.

malarial pigment s., a s. using phloxine-toluidine blue O sequence; malarial pigment and nuclei are bluish, erythrocytes and cytoplasm are red to orange; found in phagocytic cells of the reticuloendothelial system.

Maldonado-San Jose s., a staining method for staining pancreatic islet cells, using a phloxine-azure B-hematoxylin sequence; alpha cells are purple, beta cells are violet-blue, delta cells are light blue, and exocrine cells are grayish blue with red secretion granules.

Mallory's s. for actinomyces, a s. using alum hematoxylin, followed by eosin; immersion in Ehrlich's aniline crystal violet s., and Weigert's iodine solution; mycelia stain blue and clubs stain red.

Mallory's aniline blue s., Mallory's trichrome s.

Mallory's collagen s., one of a number of staining methods using phosphomolybdic or phosphotungstic acid with an acid stain, such as aniline blue, or with hematoxylin for connective tissue staining.

Mallory's s. for hemofuchsin, sections are stained sequentially in alum hematoxylin and basic fuchsin; the lipofuchsin-like pigment and ceroid stain bright red, nuclei stain blue, while melanin and hemosiderin appear unstained in their natural browns.
Mallory's iodine s., amyloid appears red-brown after Gram's iodine, then violet and blue after flooding with dilute sulfuric acid.
Mallory's phloxine s., a technique based on retention of phloxine by hyaline after overstaining and then decolorizing with lithium carbonate, used in combination with alum hematoxylin to give nuclear staining; hyaline appears red, older hyaline is pink to colorless, amyloid is pale pink, and nuclei are blue-black.
Mallory's phosphotungstic acid hematoxylin s., phosphotungstic acid *hematoxylin.*
Mallory's trichrome s., Mallory's aniline blue s.; Mallory's triple s.; a method especially suitable for studying connective tissue; sections are stained in acid fuchsin, aniline blue-orange G solution, and phosphotungstic acid; fibrils of collagen are blue, fibroglia, neuroglia, and muscle fibers are red, and fibrils of elastin are pink or yellow.
Mallory's triple s., Mallory's trichrome s.
Mann's methyl blue-eosin s., a s. useful for anterior pituitary and viral inclusion bodies; a mixture of the two dyes stains alpha cell granules red, beta cell granules dark blue, chromophobes gray to pink, colloid red, erythrocytes orange-red, and collagen fibers blue; this method is also useful for enterochromaffin, goblet, Paneth, and pancreatic islet cells; Negri bodies appear red while their nuclei and central granules are blue.
Marchi's s., a staining method in which the specimen is hardened for 8 to 10 days in a modified Müller's fixative, followed by immersion for 1 to 3 weeks in the same with the addition of osmic acid; fat and degenerating nerve fibers stain black.
Masson's argentaffin s., a s. used to stain enterochromaffin granules brown-black.
Masson-Fontana ammoniacal silver s., Fontana-Masson silver s.; a s. used to demonstrate melanin and argentaffin granules.
Masson's trichrome s., original composition for multicolored tissue preparations included Ponceau de xylidine, acid fuchsin, iron alum hematoxylin, and either aniline blue or fast green FCF; chromatin stains black, cytoplasm is in shades of red, granules of eosinophils and mast cells are deep red, erythrocytes are black, elastic fibers are red, and collagen fibers and mucus are dark blue (aniline blue) or green (fast green FCF); modifications substitute other dyes, such as Biebrich scarlet red and wool green S.
Maximow's s. for bone marrow, an alum-hematoxylin and azure II-eosin s. used to distinguish granulated leukocytes, mast cells, and cartilage.
May-Grünwald s., a German equivalent of Jenner's s., used for blood staining and in cytology; often used in combination with Giemsa s.; valuable in demonstrating parasitic flagellates.
Mayer's hemalum s., a progressive nuclear s. also used as a counterstain.
Mayer's mucicarmine s., see mucicarmine.
Mayer's mucihematein s., see mucihematein.
metachromatic s., a s., such as methylene blue, thionin, or azure A, that has the ability to produce different colors with various histological or cytological structures.
methyl green-pyronin s., a staining method useful for identification of plasma cells which are intensely pyroninophilic; a mixture of a green and a red dye that has the property of staining highly polymerized nucleic acid (DNA) green and low molecular weight nucleic acids (RNA) red. See Unna-Pappenheim s.
Mowry's colloidal iron s., a s. used for demonstrating acid mucopolysaccharides.
MSB trichrome s., a s. for fibrin using martius yellow, brilliant crystal scarlet 6R, and soluble blue; fibrin is selectively stained red and connective tissue appears blue.
multiple s., a mixture of several dyes each having an independent selective action on one or more portions of the tissue.
Nakanishi's s., a method for vital staining of bacterial in which a slide is treated with hot methylene blue solution until it acquires a sky-blue color, after which a drop of an emulsion of the bacteria is put on the cover glass and the latter laid on the slide; the bacteria are stained differentially, some parts more intensely than others.
Nauta's s., a s. for degenerating axons in which they stain with silver and appear as fragmented and swollen fibers.
negative s., s. forming an opaque or colored background against which the object to be demonstrated appears as a translucent or colorless area; in electron microscopy, an electron opaque material, such as phosphotungstic acid or sodium phosphotungstate, is used to give detail as to surface structure.
Neisser's s., a s. for the polar nuclei of the diphtheria bacillus which uses a mixture of methylene blue and crystal violet.
neutral s., salt dye; a compound of an acid s. and a basic s., such as the eosinate of methylene blue, in which the anion and cation each contains a chromophore group.
Nicolle's s. for capsules, s. in a mixture of a saturated solution of gentian violet in alcohol-phenol.
ninhydrin-Schiff s. for proteins, proteins are revealed by using ninhydrin or alloxan to produce aldehydes from primary aliphatic amines by oxidative deamination; the aldehydes are shown by reaction with Schiff's reagent.
Nissl's s., **(1)** a method for staining nerve cells with basic fuchsin; **(2)** a method for staining aggregates of rough endoplasmic reticulum and ribosomes in neuronal cell bodies and dendrites with basic dyes such as cresyl violet (or cresyl echt violet), thionine, toluidin blue O, or methylene blue.
Noble's s., a basic fuchsin-orange G staining technique for detection of viral inclusion bodies in fixed tissues.
nuclear s., a s. for cell nuclei, usually based on the binding of a basic dye to DNA or nucleohistone.
Orth's s., a lithium carmine s. for nerve cells and their processes.
oxytalan fiber s., an orcein staining method in which tissue sections are first oxidized in potassium peroxymonosulphate.
Padykula-Herman s. for myosin ATPase, a technique similar to that of Gomori's nonspecific alkaline phosphatase s., except that incubation is carried out with ATP as the substrate at pH 9.4 in the absence of Mg^{++}; enzyme activity is demonstrated as blackened deposits in the A band of striated muscle sarcomeres; control tissue sections lacking substrate and containing sulfhydryl inhibitors are necessary.
Paget-Eccleston s., an aldehyde-thionin-PAS-orange G staining technique modified to identify seven different cell types in the anterior pituitary gland.
panoptic s., a s. in which a Romanowsky-type s. is combined with another s.; such a combination improves the staining of cytoplasmic granules and other bodies.
Papanicolaou s., a multichromatic s. used principally on exfoliated cytologic specimens and based on aqueous hematoxylin with multiple counterstaining dyes in 95% ethyl alcohol, giving great transparency and delicacy of detail; important in cancer screening, especially of gynecologic smears.
Pappenheim's s., a method for differentiating tubercle and smegma bacilli; the preparation is stained with hot carbol-fuchsin solution, then treated with an alcoholic solution of rosolic acid and methylene blue to which glycerin is added; tubercle bacilli are stained bright red, but smegma bacilli are decolorized.
paracarmine s., a staining fluid consisting of a solution of calcium chloride and carminic acid in 75% alcohol.
PAS s., periodic acid-Schiff s.
periodic acid-Schiff s., PAS s.; a tissue-staining procedure in which 1,2-glycol groupings are first oxidized with periodic acid to aldehydes, which then react with the sulfite leucofuchsin reagent of Schiff, and become colored red-violet; strong staining occurs with polysaccharides, such as glycogen, and mucopolysaccharides of

epithelial mucins, basement membranes, and connective tissue.
Perls' Prussian blue s., a s. for ferric iron as in hemosiderins, using potassium ferrocyanide in acetic acid or dilute hydrochloric acid followed by a red counterstain such as safranin O or neutral red; various hemosiderins and most mineral irons give a blue-green reaction, while nuclei stain red.
peroxidase s., a method for demonstrating peroxidase granules in some neutrophils and in eosinophils; the enzyme promotes the oxidation of benzidine by hydrogen peroxide; tissues treated with horseradish peroxidase can also have the enzyme detected in the electron microscope.
phosphotungstic acid s., PTA s.; the first general s. used for electron microscopy; a selective s. for extracellular components such as elastin, collagen, and basement membrane mucopolysaccharides; it can be followed by uranyl acetate or lead.
picrocarmine s., a red crystalline powder derived from a solution of carmine, ammonia, and picric acid which is evaporated, leaving the powder (soluble in water); it produces excellent staining of keratohyaline granules.
picro-Mallory trichrome s., a modification of Mallory's trichrome s. that involves the addition of picric acid.
picronigrosin s., a solution of nigrosin in picric acid, used for staining connective tissue.
plasma s., plasmatic s., plasmic s., a s. whose principal affinity is for the cytoplasm of cells.
plastic section s., (1) for electron microscopy, a s. (*e.g.,* osmic acid, PTA, potassium permanganate) used on thin sections of plastic-embedded tissues, utilizing differential attachment of heavy atoms to various cellular and tissue structures so that electrons will be absorbed and scattered by these structures to produce an image; to achieve differential staining, the s. must penetrate nonwettable plastic embedments; **(2)** for light microscopy, a s. (*e.g.,* alkaline toluidine blue, silver methenamine) used on plastic-embedded tissues to attain higher resolution and more detail than normally possible; semi-thick (0.5-1.5 μm) sections are particularly useful in renal pathology, especially in combination with the phase microscope.
port-wine s., *nevus* flammeus.
positive s., direct binding of a dye with a tissue component to produce contrast; in electron microscopy, heavy metals like uranyl and lead salts are used to bind to selective cell constituents to produce increased density to the electron beam, *i.e.,* contrast.
Prussian blue s., a s. employing acid potassium ferrocyanide to demonstrate iron, as in siderocytes.
PTA s., phosphotungstic acid s.
Puchtler-Sweat s. for basement membranes, a staining method using resorcin-fuchsin and nuclear fast red solutions after Carnoy's fixation; basement membranes are gray to black and nuclei pink to red.
Puchtler-Sweat s. for hemoglobin and hemosiderin, a complex staining method in which, on a yellow background, hemoglobin is stained red, hemosiderin blue to green and elastic fibers are pink.
Q-banding s., quinacrine chromosome banding s.; a fluorescent s. for chromosomes which produces specific banding patterns for each pair of homologous chromosomes; the acridine dye derivative, quinacrine hydrochloride, or other derivatives like quinacrine mustard dihydrochloride produces a green-yellow fluorescence at pH 4.5 in chromosome segments rich in constitutive heterochromatin with deoxyadenylate-deoxythymidilate (A-T) bases of DNA; centromeric regions of human chromosomes 3, 4, and 13 are specifically stained, as are satellites of some acrocentric chromosomes and the end of the long arm of the Y chromosome; banding patterns are similar to those obtained with G-banding stain; similar fluorescent s. results are seen with the antibiotics adriamycin and daunomycin, as well as the tertiary dyes butyl proflavine and DAPI, and the bisbenzimidazole dye HOECHST 33258.
quinacrine chromosome banding s., Q-banding s.
Rambourg's chromic acid-phosphotungstic acid s., a s. for glycoproteins, used with an electron microscope, with which ultrathin tissue sections reveal complex carbohydrates in the same locations as shown by Rambourg's periodic acid-chromic methenamine-silver s.
Rambourg's periodic acid-chromic methenamine-silver s., a s. for glycoproteins, used with an electron microscope, adapted from the Gomori-Jones periodic acid-methenamine-silver s.; it produces silver deposits in mature saccules of the Golgi apparatus, lysosomal vesicles, cell coat, and basement membranes.
R-banding s., a reverse Giemsa chromosome banding method that produces bands complementary to G-bands; induced by treatment with high temperature, low pH, or acridine orange staining; often used together with G-banding on human karyotype to determine whether there are deletions.
Romanowsky's blood s., prototype of the eosin-methylene blue s.'s for blood smears, using agueous solutions made of a mixture of methylene blue (saturated) and eosin. Romanowsky-type s.'s depend for their action on compounds formed by interaction of methylene blue and eosin; most are of no value if water is present in the alcohol because neutral dyes become precipitated.
Roux's s., a double s. for diphtheria bacilli which employs crystal violet or dahlia and methyl green.
Schaeffer-Fulton s., a s. for bacterial spores using malachite green and safranin so that bacterial bodies are red to pink and spores are green.
Schmorl's ferric-ferricyanide reduction s., a s. to test for reducing substances in tissues, including melanin, argentaffin granules, thyroid colloid, keratin, keratohyalin, and lipofucsin pigments; ferricyanide is converted into ferrocyanide which is converted to insoluble Prussian blue in the presence of ferric ions.
Schmorl's picrothionin s., a s. for compact bone which employs thionin and picric acid solutions to produce blue to blue-black staining of bone canaliculi and cells; bone matrix is yellowish and cartilage ground substance is purple.
Schultz s., a s. for cholesterol; a relatively specific but insensitive histochemical test for cholesterol and cholesterol esters in which frozen sections of formalin-fixed tissues are oxidized in iron alum, hydrogen peroxide, or sodium iodate, then treated with sulfuric acid to give a blue-green to red color in a positive reaction; the presence of glycerol inhibits the reaction.
selective s., a s. that colors one portion of a tissue or cell exclusively or more deeply than the remaining portions.
silver s., any of a variety of s.'s (*e.g.,* Bielschowsky's, Gomori's silver, impregnation s.'s) which employ alkaline silver nitrate solutions to stain connective tissue fibers (reticulin, collagen), calcium salt deposits, spirochaetes, neurological tissue, and nucleolar organizer regions.
silver-ammoniacal silver s., Ag-As s.; a s. for the acid protein component of nucleolar regions which are active or which were transcriptionally active in the preceding interphase; uses silver nitrate, ammoniacal silver, and formalin.
silver protein s., a silver proteinate complex used in staining nerve fibers, nerve endings, and flagellate protozoa; also used to demonstrate phagocytosis in living animals by the cells of the reticuloendothelial system.
Stirling's modification of Gram's s., a stable aniline-crystal violet s.
supravital s., a procedure in which living tissue is removed from the body and cells are placed in a nontoxic dye solution so that their vital processes may be studied.
Taenzer's s., Unna-Taenzer s.; an orcein solution used for staining elastic tissue.
Takayama's s., a s. containing pyridine, sodium hydrate, and dextrose; used for identification of blood stains; a drop added to a suspected blood stain results in the formation of hemochromogen crystals.

telomeric R-banding s., a modified R-banding s. in which the telomeres become strongly stained and faint R-banding still occurs over the rest of the chromosomes; uses air-dried slides, aging for several days, and staining in hot phosphate-buffered Giemsa s.
thioflavine T s., a s. employed to detect amyloid, which induces specific yellow fluorescence; tissue sections are first put in alum-hematoxylin to quench nuclear fluorescence and then stained in thioflavine T.
Tizzoni's s., a s. used as a test for iron in tissue; the tissue is treated with a solution of potassium ferrocyanide and then with dilute hydrochloric acid; a blue coloration indicates the presence of iron.
Toison's s., a blood diluent and leukocyte stain containing methyl violet, sodium chloride, sodium sulfate, and glycerin; also used for erythrocyte counts.
trichrome s., staining combinations which usually contain three dyes of contrasting colors selected to stain connective tissue, muscle, cytoplasm, and nuclei in bright colors; generally, tissue sections are first dyed in iron hematoxylin before being treated with the other dyes.
trypsin G-banding s., see G-banding s.
Unna's s., **(1)** an alkaline methylene blue s. for plasma cells; **(2)** a polychrome methylene blue s. with which mast cells are stained red (metachromatic).
Unna-Pappenheim s., a contrast s. consisting of a methyl green-pyronin solution; originally used for gonococci, but later used to detect RNA and DNA in tissue sections; RNA is stained red and DNA appears green; used to demonstrate plasma cells during chronic inflammation. See methyl green-pyronin s.
Unna-Taenzer s., Taenzer's s.
uranyl acetate s., a s. used in electron microscopy; uranyl acetate binds specifically to nucleic acids but selectively tends to be abolished by osmium fixation; proteins are well stained, but cytomembranes are poorly stained.
urate crystals s., a s. using silver methenamine to detect crystals, which polarize light in contrast with calcium crystals; useful in diagnosing gout and kidney infarcts resulting from uric acid build-up.
van Ermengen's s., a method for staining flagella which utilizes glacial acetic acid, osmic acid, tannic acid, silver nitrate, gallic acid, and potassium acetate.
van Gieson's s., a mixture of acid fuchsin in saturated picric acid solution, used in collagen staining.
Verhoeff's elastic tissue s., a s. for tissue sections in which a mixture of hematoxylin, ferric chloride, and Lugol's iodine solution is used; tissue may be counterstained, if desired, with eosin or van Gieson's s.; elastic fibers and nuclei appear blue-black to black while collagen and other components are shades of pink to red.
vital s., a s. applied to cells or parts of cells while they are still living.
von Kossa s., Kossa s.; a s. for calcium in mineralized tissue, utilizing a silver nitrate solution followed by sodium thiosulfate; calcified bone but not osteoid is stained brown to black.
Wachstein-Meissel s. for calcium-magnesium-ATPase, a method similar to that of Gomori's nonspecific acid phosphatase s., except that incubation is carried out with ATP as substrate at neutral pH; enzyme activity is generally demonstrated at cell membranes.
Warthin-Starry silver s., a s. for spirochetes in which preparations are incubated in 1% silver nitrate solution followed by a developer.
Weigert's s. for actinomyces, a staining method using immersion in a dark red orsellin solution in alcohol, then staining in crystal-violet solution. See also Weigert's iron *hematoxylin.*
Weigert's s. for elastin, a staining solution of fuchsin, resorcin, and ferric chloride; elastic fibers stain blue-black.
Weigert's s. for fibrin, a staining method using solutions of aniline-crystal violet and iodine-potassium iodide, then decolorizing in aniline oil and xylol; the fibrin is stained dark blue.
Weigert's iron hematoxylin s., a nuclear staining solution containing hematoxylin, ferric chloride, and hydrochloric acid; useful in combination with von Gieson's s., especially for demonstrating connective tissue elements or *Entamoeba histolytica* in sections.
Weigert's s. for myelin, a staining method using ferric chloride and hematoxylin; myelin stains deep blue, degenerated portions a light yellowish color.
Weigert's s. for neuroglia, a complicated process in which the final treatment is like that for staining fibrin; neuroglia and nuclei stain blue.
Weigert-Gram s., a s. for bacteria in tissues in which sections are stained in alum-hematoxylin, then in eosin, aniline methyl violet, and Lugol's solution.
Wilder's s. for reticulum, a silver impregnation technique in which reticulum appears as black, well-defined fibers without beading and with a relatively clear background.
Williams' s., a s. for Negri bodies which utilizes picric acid, fuchsin, and methylene blue; Negri bodies are magenta, granules and nerve cells blue, and erythrocytes yellowish.
Wright's s., a staining mixture of eosinates of polychromed methylene blue used in staining of blood smears.
Ziehl's s., a carbol-fuchsin solution of phenol and basic fuchsin used as a s. to demonstrate bacteria and cell nuclei.
Ziehl-Neelsen s., a method for staining acid-fast bacteria using Ziehl's s., decolorizing in acid alcohol, and counterstaining with methylene blue; acid-fast organisms appear red, other tissue elements light blue; a modification of this s. is also used for *Actinomycetes* and *Brucella.*

staining (stān'ing). **1.** The act of applying a stain. See also entries under stain. **2.** In dentistry, modification of the color of the tooth or denture base.
progressive s., a procedure in which s. is continued until the desired intensity of coloring of tissue elements is attained.
regressive s., a type of s. in which tissues are overstained and the excess dye is then removed selectively until the desired intensity is obtained.

stains-all (stainz'awl). 4,5,4′,5′-Dibenzo-3,3′-diethyl-9-methylthiocarbocyanine bromide; a dye that stains phosphoproteins blue, proteins red, nucleic acids purple, and mucoproteins and mucopolysaccharides various colors on acrylamide gels; also used on tissue sections.

staircase (stār'kās). A series of reactions that follow one another in progressively increasing or decreasing intensity, so that a chart shows a continuous rise or fall. See treppe.

stalagmometer (stal-ă-gom'ĕ-ter) [G. *stalagma,* a drop, + *metron,* measure]. Stactometer; an instrument for determining exactly the number of drops in a given quantity of liquid; used as a measure of the surface tension of a fluid (the lower the tension, the smaller the drops and, consequently, the more numerous in a given quantity of the fluid).

stalk (stawk). A narrowed connection with a structure or organ.
allantoic s., the narrow connection between the intraembryonic portion of the allantois and the extraembryonic allantoic vesicle.
body s., the extraembryonic precursor of the connecting s. or umbilical cord by which the embryo is attached to its trophoblastic chorion.
connecting s., body s.
infundibular s., infundibular *stem.*
optic s., the constricted proximal portion of the optic vesicle in the embryo; it develops into the optic nerve.
pineal s., the attachment of the pineal body to the roof of the third ventricle; it contains the pineal recess of the third ventricle.
pituitary s., a process comprising the pars tuberalis investing the

infundibular stem which attaches the hypophysis to the tuber cinereum at the base of the brain.
yolk s., the narrowed connection between the intraembryonic gut and the yolk sac; its walls are splanchnopleure.

staltic (stawl'tik) [G. *staltikos,* contractile]. Styptic.

Stamey, Thomas A., U.S. urologist, *1928. See S. *test.*

stammer (stam'er) [A.S. *stamur*]. **1.** To hesitate in speech, halt, repeat, and mispronounce, by reason of embarrassment, agitation, or unfamiliarity with the subject. *Cf.* stutter. **2.** To mispronounce or transpose certain consonants in speech.

stammering (stam'er-ing). **1.** Psellism; paralalia literalis; a speech disorder characterized by hesitation and repetition of words, or by mispronunciation or transposition of certain consonants, especially *l, r,* and *s.* **2.** Sounds other than speech, that are similar to stammering.
s. of the bladder, urinary *stuttering.*

Stamnosoma (stam-nō-sō'mă) [G. *stamnos,* a jar, + *sōma,* body]. A genus of flukes of the family Heterophyidae, identical with *Centrocestus.* Two species, *S. armatum* and *S. formosanum,* have been described as sometimes infecting man.

standardization (stan'dard-i-zā'shŭn). **1.** The making of a solution of definite strength so that it may be used for comparison and in tests. **2.** Making any drug or other preparation conform to the type or standard.
s. of a test, in psychology, the following of definite procedures for administering, scoring, evaluating, and reporting the results of a new test which is under development.

stand'still. Arrest; cessation of activity.
atrial s., auricular s.; cessation of atrial contractions, marked by absence of atrial waves in the electrocardiogram.
auricular s., atrial s.
cardiac s., asystole.
sinus s., cessation of sinus node activity, marked by absence of normal P waves in the electrocardiogram.
ventricular s., cessation of ventricular contractions, marked by absence of ventricular complexes in the electrocardiogram.

Stanley, Edward, English surgeon, 1793–1862. See S.'s cervical *ligaments.*

Stanley Way. See Way, Stanley.

stannic (stan'ik) [L. *stannum,* tin]. Relating to tin, especially when in combination in its higher valency.

stannic chloride. $SnCl_4$; a fuming liquid (fuming spirit of Libavius), specific gravity 2.23, boiling point 115°C, that forms several hydrates; the pentahydrate (butter of tin) is used for mordanting and "loading" or "weighting" silk.

stannic oxide. Tin oxide; SnO_2; used in industry; it is a cause of pneumoconiosis.

Stannius, Herman F., German biologist, 1808–1883. See S.'s *ligature.*

stannous (stan'ŭs) [L. *stannum,* tin]. Relating to tin, especially when in combination in its lower valency.

stannous fluoride. A preparation containing not less than 71.2% of stannous tin and not less than 22.3% and not more than 25.5% of fluoride; used as a prophylactic in dentistry.

stannum (stan'ŭm) [L.]. Tin.

stanolone (stan'ō-lōn). Dihydrotestosterone; 17β-hydroxy-5α-androstane-3-one; an androgen with the same actions and uses as testosterone; used for its anabolic and tumor-suppressing effects, specifically, in carcinoma of the breast.

stanozolol (stan-ō'zō-lol, -lōl). Androstanozole; stanozol, 17α-methyl-5α-androstan-17β-ol carrying a pyrazole ring (=CH–NH–N=) attached to C-2 and C-3 (see steroids for androstane structure). A semisynthetic, orally effective anabolic agent.

stapedectomy (stā-pĕ-dek'tō-mē) [stapes + G. *ektomē,* excision]. Operation to remove the stapes footplate in whole or part with replacement of the stapes superstructure (crura) by metal or plastic prosthesis; used for otosclerosis with stapes fixation.

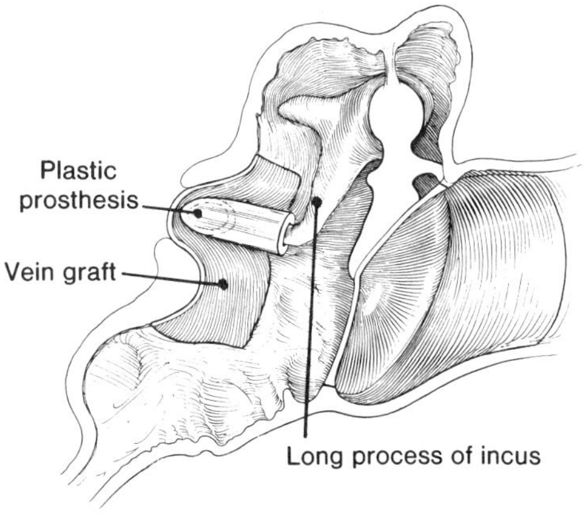

Stapedectomy
Stapes and oval window membrane have been replaced with a vein graft; plastic prosthesis connects graft with incus.

stapedial (stā-pē'dē-ăl). Relating to the stapes.

stapediotenotomy (stā-pē'dē-ō-tĕ-not'ō-mē) [stapedius + G. *tenōn,* tendon, + *tomē,* incision]. Division of the tendon of the stapedius muscle.

stapediovestibular (stā-pē'dē-ō-ves-tib'yū-lăr). Relating to the stapes and the vestibule of the ear.

stapedius, pl. stapedii (stā-pē'dē-ŭs, stā-pē'dē-ī) [Mod. L.]. *Musculus* stapedius.

stapes, pl. **stapes, stapedes** (stā'pēz, stā'pē-dēz) [Mod. L. stirrup] [NA]. Stirrup; the smallest of the three auditory ossicles; its base, or footpiece, fits into the vestibular (oval) window, while its head is articulated with the lenticular process of the long limb of the incus.

staphyl-. See staphylo-.

staphylagra (staf'i-lag'ră) [staphyl- + G. *agra,* seizure]. A forceps for holding the uvula.

staphylectomy (staf-i-lek'tō-mē) [staphyl- + G. *ektomē,* excision]. Uvulectomy.

staphyledema (staf'il-e-dē'mă) [staphyl- + G. *oidēma,* swelling (edema)]. Edema of the uvula.

staphyline (staf'i-līn, -lēn). Botryoid.

staphylion (stă-fil'ē-on) [G. dim. of *staphylē,* a bunch of grapes]. The midpoint of the posterior edge of the hard palate; a craniometric point.

staphylo-, staphyl- [G. *staphylē,* a bunch of grapes]. Combining forms denoting resemblance to a grape or a bunch of grapes, hence relating usually to staphylococci or, in obsolescent image, to the uvula palatina. See also uvulo-.

staphylococcal (staf'i-lō-kok'ăl). Relating to or caused by any organism of the genus *Staphylococcus.*

staphylococcemia (staf'i-lō-kok-sē'mē-ă) [staphylo- + G. *haima,* blood]. Staphylohemia; the presence of staphylococci in the circulating blood.

staphylococci (staf'i-lō-kok'sī). Plural of staphylococcus.

staphylococcia (staf'i-lō-kok'sē-ă). Any staphylococcic infection.

staphylococcic (staf'i-lō-kok'sik). Relating to or caused by any species of *Staphylococcus.*

staphylococcolysin (staf'i-lō-kō-kol'i-sin). Staphylolysin.

staphylococcolysis (staf′i-lō-kŏ-kol′i-sis) [staphylo- + G. *lysis,* dissolution]. Lysis or destruction of staphylococci.

staphylococcosis, pl. **staphylococcoses** (staf′i-lō-kok-ō′sis, -sēz). Infection by species of *Staphylococcus.*

Staphylococcus (staf′i-lō-kok′ŭs) [staphylo- + G. *kokkos,* a berry]. A genus of nonmotile, nonsporeforming, aerobic to facultatively anaerobic bacteria (family Micrococcaceae) containing Gram-positive, spherical cells, 0.5 to 1.5 μm in diameter, which divide in more than one plane to form irregular clusters. These organisms are chemoorganotrophic, and their metabolism is respiratory and fermentative. Under anaerobic conditions, lactic acid is produced from glucose; under aerobic conditions, acetic acid and small amounts of CO_2 are produced. Coagulase-positive strains produce a variety of toxins and are therefore potentially pathogenic and may cause food poisoning. These organisms are usually susceptible to antibiotics such as the β-lactam and macrolide antibiotics, tetracyclines, novobiocin, and chloramphenicol but are resistant to polymyxin and polyenes. They are susceptible to antibacterials such as phenols and their derivatives, surface-active compounds, salicylanilides, carbanilides, and halogens (chlorine and iodine) and their derivatives, such as chloramines and iodophors. They are found on the skin, in skin glands, on the nasal and other mucous membranes of warm-blooded animals, and in a variety of food products. The type species is *S. aureus.*
S. au′reus, *S. pyogenes aureus;* a common species found especially on nasal mucous membrane and skin (hair follicles); causes furunculosis, cellulitis, pyemia, pneumonia, osteomyelitis, endocarditis, suppuration of wounds, other infections, and food poisoning; the type species of the genus *S.*
S. epider′midis, a species, originally found in small stitch abscesses and other skin wounds, which occurs on parasitic skin and mucous membranes of man and other animals; it is parasitic rather than pathogenic.
S. hyi′cus, a species whose porcine subspecies are opportunistic pathogens associated with epidermites such as greasy pig disease.
S. pyog′enes al′bus, *S. aureus;* a name formerly applied to the organisms which are now regarded as the mutants of *S. aureus* which form white colonies.
S. pyog′enes au′reus, *S. aureus.*

staphylococcus pl. **staphylococci** (staf′i-lō-kok′ŭs, kok′sī). A vernacular term used to refer to any member of the genus *Staphylococcus.*

staphyloderma (staf′i-lō-der′mă) [staphylo- + G. *derma,* skin]. Pyoderma due to staphylococci.

staphylodermatitis (staf′i-lō-der-mă-tī′tis). Inflammation of the skin due to the action of staphylococci.

staphylodialysis (staf′i-lō-dī-al′i-sis) [staphylo- + G. *dialysis,* a separation]. Uvuloptosis.

staphylohemia (staf′i-lō-hē′mē-ă). Staphylococcemia.

staphylohemolysin (staf′i-lō-hē-mol′i-sin). A mixture of hemolysins (alpha, beta, gamma, and delta), included in staphylococcal exotoxin; the α hemolysin has a marked effect on vascular muscle.

staphylokinase (staf′i-lō-kī′nās) [EC 3.4.24.4]. A microbial metalloenzyme from *Staphylococcus aureus,* with action similar to that of urokinase and streptokinase, that can convert plasminogen to plasmin but requires Ca^{2+}.

staphylolysin (staf-i-lol′i-sin). Staphylococcolysin. **1.** A hemolysin elaborated by a staphylococcus. **2.** An antibody causing lysis of staphylococci.

staphyloma (staf-i-lō′mă) [staphylo- + G. *-ōma,* tumor]. A bulging of the cornea or sclera containing uveal tissue.
annular s., a s. extending around the periphery of the cornea.
anterior s., corneal s.; a bulging near the anterior pole of the eyeball.
ciliary s., scleral s. occurring in the region of the ciliary body.
corneal s., anterior s.
equatorial s., scleral s.; a s. occurring in the area of exit of the vortex veins.
intercalary s., a scleral s. occurring between the insertion of the ciliary body and the root of the iris.
posterior s., Scarpa's s.; sclerochoroiditis posterior; a bulging near the posterior pole of the eyeball due to degenerative changes in severe myopia.
Scarpa's s., posterior s.
scleral s., equatorial s.
uveal s., protrusion of the iris through a rupture of the sclera.

staphylomatous (staf-i-lō′mă-tŭs). Relating to or marked by staphyloma.

staphyloncus (staf-i-long′kŭs) [staphy- + G. *onkos,* bulk, mass]. A tumor or swelling of the uvula.

staphylopharyngorrhaphy (staf′i-lō-far-in-gōr′ă-fē) [staphylo- + pharynx + G. *rhaphē,* suture]. Palatopharyngorrhaphy; surgical repair of defects in the uvula or soft palate and the pharynx.

staphyloplasty (staf′i-lō-plas-tē) [staphylo- + G. *plassō,* to form]. Palatoplasty.

staphyloplegia (staf′i-lō-plē′jē-ă). Palatoplegia.

staphyloptosis (staf′i-lop-tō′sis) [staphylo- + G. *ptōsis,* a falling]. Uvuloptosis.

staphylorrhaphy (staf-i-lōr′ă-fē) [staphylo- + G. *rhaphē,* suture]. Palatorrhaphy.

staphyloschisis (staf-i-los′ki-sis) [staphylo- + G. *schisis,* fissure]. Bifid uvula with or without cleft of soft palate.

staphylotome (staf′i-lō-tōm). Uvulotome.

staphylotomy (staf-i-lot′ō-mē) [staphylo- + G. *tomē,* incision]. **1.** Uvulotomy. **2.** Excision of a staphyloma.

staphylotoxin (staf′i-lō-tok′sin) [staphylo- + G. *toxikon,* poison]. The toxin elaborated by any species of *Staphylococcus.* See also staphylohemolysin.

stapling (stāp′ling). Use of a stapling device that unites two tissues, such as the two ends of bowel, by applying a row or circle of staples.
gastric s., partitioning of the stomach by rows of staples; used to treat morbid obesity.

star [A.S. *steorra*] Any star-shaped structure. See also aster, astrosphere, stella, stellula.
daughter s., polar s.; one of the figures forming the diaster.
lens s.'s, **(1)** *radii* lentis; **(2)** congenital cataracts with opacities along the suture lines of the lens; may be anterior or posterior, or both.
mother s., monaster.
polar s., daughter s.
venous s., a small, red nodule formed by a dilated vein in the skin; caused by increased venous pressure.
Verheyen's s.'s, *venulae* stellatae.
Winslow's s.'s, *stellulae* winslowii.

starch [A.S. *stearc,* strong]. Amylum; a polysaccharide built up of glucose residues in α-1,4 linkage, differing from cellulose in the presence of α- rather than β-glucoside linkages, that exists in most plant tissues; converted into dextrin when subjected to the action of dry heat, and into dextrin and glucose by amylases and glucoamylases in saliva and pancreatic juice; used as a dusting powder, an emollient, and an ingredient in medicinal tablets, and is an important raw material for the manufacture of alcohol, acetone, *n*-butanol, lactic acid, citric acid, glycerine, and gluconic acid by fermentation.
animal s., glycogen.
liver s., glycogen.
moss s., lichenin.

soluble s., a high-molecular-weight, water-soluble dextrin produced by the partial acid hydrolysis of s.; useful in iodimetry, as it gives an easily visible purple-black end point in the presence of free iodine.

starch-eating. Amylophagia.

stare (stār) [A.S. *starian*]. **1.** To look intently or fixedly. **2.** An intent gaze.

postbasic s., gaze in children with posterior basic meningitis, due to retraction of the upper eyelid and downward rotation of the eye.

Stargardt, Karl, German ophthalmologist, 1875–1927. See S.'s *disease.*

Starling, Ernest H., British physiologist, 1866–1927. See S.'s *curve, hypothesis, law, reflex;* Frank-S. *curve.*

Starry. See Warthin-S. silver *stain.*

starvation (star-vā'shŭn). Lengthy and continuous deprivation of food.

starve [A.S. *steorfan,* to die]. **1.** To suffer from lack of food. **2.** To deprive of food so as to cause suffering or death. **3.** Formerly, to die of cold.

Stas, Jean-Servais, Belgian chemist, 1813–1891. See S.-Otto *method.*

stasimorphia (stas-i-mōr'fē-ă) [G. *stasis,* a standing still, + *morphē,* shape]. Deformity due to arrested development.

stasis, pl. stases (stā'sis, stas'is; -ēz) [G. a standing still]. Stagnation of the blood or other fluids.

papillary s., papilledema.

pressure s., traumatic *asphyxia.*

stat-. Prefix applied to electrical units in the cgs-electrostatic system to distinguish them from units in the cgs-electromagnetic system (prefix ab-) and those in the metric system or SI system (no prefix).

-stat [G. *statēs,* stationary]. Suffix indicating an agent intended to keep something from changing or moving.

stat. Abbreviation for L. *statim,* at once, immediately.

statampere (stat-am'pēr) [G. *statos,* standing (stationary), + ampere]. The electrostatic unit of current; the flow of 1 electrostatic unit of charge (1 statcoulomb) per second; equal to 3.3 $\times 10^{-10}$ ampere.

statcoulomb (stat-kū'lom) [G. *statos,* standing (stationary), + coulomb]. The electrostatic unit of charge, such that two objects, each carrying such a charge and separated (center to center) by 1 cm in a vacuum, will repel each other with a force of 1 dyne (or 10^{-5} newton); equal to 3.3 $\times$ 10^{10} coulomb.

state (stāt) [L. *status,* condition, state]. Condition; situation; status.

absent s., dreamy s.

apallic s., apallic syndrome; a s. of unresponsiveness due to diffuse cortical or brain stem damage as in persistent vegetative s.

activated s., excited s.

anxiety s., generalized anxiety *disorder.*

carrier s., the s. of being a carrier of pathogenic organisms; *i.e.,* one who is infected but free of disease.

central excitatory s., the building up of excitatory influences produced by individual impulses finally causes firing of the next neuron.

convulsive s., epilepsy.

dreamy s., absent s.; the semiconscious s. associated with an epileptic attack.

eunuchoid s., an imprecisely delineated condition of a male manifesting signs of inadequate androgen secretion, regardless of the cause; usually referring to long legs, short trunk, and boyish beardless faces.

excited s., activated s.; the condition of an atom or molecule after absorbing energy, which may be the result of exposure to light, electricity, elevated temperature, or a chemical reaction; such activation may be a necessary prelude to a chemical reaction or to the emission of light.

ground s., the normal, inactivated s. of an atom from which, on activation, the singlet, triplet, and other excited s.'s are derived.

hypnotic s., hypnosis.

hypometabolic s., a rare s. of reduced metabolism with symptoms resembling hypothyroidism but with some tests for thyroid gland function normal; also used to describe the reduced metabolic activity seen in true hypothyroidism.

imperfect s., in fungi, the s. or stage at which only asexual spores such as conidia are formed; most such species are classified as Deuteromycetes (Fungi Imperfecti).

local excitatory s., increased irritability of a nerve fiber or muscle fiber which is produced by an ineffective electrical stimulus; summation of the stimuli may occur, resulting in a propagated impulse if two or more subliminal stimuli are applied in rapid succession.

multiple ego s.'s, various psychological organizational s.'s reflecting different life experiences.

perfect s., in fungi, that portion of the life cycle in which spores are formed after nuclear fusion.

refractory s., subnormal excitability immediately following a response to previous excitation; the s. is divided into absolute and relative phases.

singlet s., a transient, excited s. of a molecule (*e.g.,* of chlorophyll, upon absorbing light) that can release energy as heat or light (fluorescence) and thus return to the initial (ground) s.; it may alternatively assume a slightly more stable, but still excited s. (triplet s.), with an electron still dislocated as before but with reversed spin.

steady s. (subscript s), a s. obtained in moderate muscular exercise, when the removal of lactic acid by oxidation keeps pace with its production, the oxygen supply being adequate, and the muscles do not go into debt for oxygen; more generally, any condition in which the formation or introduction of substances just keeps pace with their destruction or removal so that all volumes, concentrations, pressures, and flows remain constant.

triplet s., a second excited s. of a molecule (*e.g.,* chlorophyll) produced by absorption of light to produce the singlet s., then loss of some energy (fluorescence) to arrive at the longer-lived triplet s. The molecule may remain sufficiently long in the triplet s. for a second activating light quantum to be effective in producing a "second triplet" s., obviously at still a higher level of excitation, hence reactivity. Alternatively, it may lose the triplet s. energy directly and return to the ground s.

twilight s., a condition of disordered consciousness during which actions may be performed without the conscious volition of the individual and with no memory of such actions. *Cf.* somnabulic *epilepsy.*

statfarad (stat-fa'rad). The electrostatic unit of capacitance, equal to 1.1 $\times$ 10^{-12} farad.

stathenry (stat-hen'rē). Electrostatic unit of inductance, equal to 9 $\times$ 10^{11} henries.

stathmokinesis (stath'mō-ki-nē'sis) [G. *stathmos,* standing place, + *kinēsis,* motion]. Condition of arrested mitosis after treatment with an agent, such as colchicine, which effectively alters the mitotic spindle to prevent typical rearrangement of the chromosomes preceding cell division.

statim (stat.) (stā'tim) [L.]. At once; immediately.

statistics (stă-tis'tiks). A collection of facts numerically grouped into definite classes and subject to analysis, particularly analysis of the probability of findings being due to chance.

descriptive s., numerical values which describe the chief features of a group of scores, without regard to a larger population; *e.g.,* mean, median, mode.

inferential s., s. from which an inference is made about the nature of a population; the purpose is to generalize about the population, based upon data from the sample selected from the population.

vital s., the branch of s. concerned with data relating to human birth, health, disease, and death.

statoacoustic (stat'ō-ă-kū'stik) [G. *statos,* standing, + *akoustikos,* acoustic]. Vestibulocochlear (2); relating to equilibrium and hearing.

statoconia, sing. **statoconium** (stat'ō-kō'nē-ă, -nē-ŭm) [L. fr. G. *statos,* standing, *konis,* dust] [NA]. Statoliths; otoconia; otoliths (1); otolites (1); sagitta; ear crystals; crystalline particles of calcium carbonate and a protein adhering to the gelatinous membrane of the maculae of the utricle and saccule.

statokinetic (stat'ō-ki-net'ik). Pertaining to statokinetics.

statokinetics (stat'ō-ki-net'iks) [G. *statos,* standing, + *kinēsis,* movement]. The adjustment made by the body in motion to maintain stable equilibrium.

statoliths (stat'ō-liths) [G. *statos,* standing, + *lithos,* stone]. Statoconia.

statometer (stă-tom'ĕ-ter) [G. *statos,* standing, + *metron,* measure]. Exophthalmometer.

statosphere (stat'ō-sfēr). Centrosphere.

stature (statch'er) [L. *statura,* fr. *statuo,* pp. *statutus,* to cause to stand]. The height of a person.

status (stā'tŭs, stat'ŭs) [L. a way of standing]. State; condition.

s. angino'sus, prolonged angina pectoris refractory to treatment.

s. arthrit'icus, obsolete term for gouty diathesis or predisposition.

s. asthmat'icus, a condition of severe, prolonged asthma.

s. cholera'icus, the cold stage of shock and depression in cholera, due to fluid and electrolyte loss and resulting hypovolemia; characterized by weak pulse, cold clammy skin, confusion, and depression.

s. chore'icus, a very severe form of chorea in which the persistence of the movements prevents sleep and the patient may die of exhaustion.

s. convul'sivus, epilepsy.

s. cribro'sus, a condition marked by dilations of the perivascular spaces in the brain.

s. crit'icus, a very severe and persistent form of crisis in tabes dorsalis.

s. dysmyelinisa'tus, a condition marked by disease of myelinated fibers in the globus pallidus and substantia nigra with accumulation of iron pigment in the cells; affected children show motor disturbances (dyskinesias) and often mental deficiency.

s. dysra'phicus, a condition in which there is failure of fusion of midline structures; related to syringomyelia and perhaps to Marfan's syndrome or arachnodactyly.

s. epilep'ticus, a repeated seizure or a seizure prolonged for at least 30 minutes; may be convulsive (tonic-clonic), nonconvulsive (absence) or partial (epilepsia partialis continuans).

s. hemicra'nicus, a condition in which attacks of migraine succeed each other with such short intervals as to be almost continuous.

s. hypnot'icus, hypnosis.

s. lacuna'ris, a condition, occurring in cerebral arteriosclerosis, in which there are numerous small areas of degeneration in the brain.

s. lymphat'icus, s. thymicolymphaticus.

s. marmora'tus, a congenital condition due to maldevelopment of the corpus striatum associated with choreoathetosis, in which the striate nuclei have a marblelike appearance caused by altered myelination.

s. nervo'sus, s. typhosus.

s. prae'sens, obsolete term for the part of the history of a case describing the condition of the patient at the time when he comes under observation.

s. rap'tus, ecstasy.

s. spongio'sus, multiple fluid-filled spaces of microscopic size in the cerebral white matter; seen in certain hypoxic, toxic, and metabolic diseases.

s. ster'nuens, a state of continual sneezing.

s. thymicolymphat'icus, s. lymphaticus or thymicus; a syndrome of supposed enlargement of the thymus and lymph nodes in infants and young children, formerly believed to be associated with unexplained sudden death; it was also erroneously believed that pressure of the thymus on the trachea might cause death during anesthesia. Prominence of these structures is now considered normal in young children, including those who have died suddenly without preceding illnesses that might lead to atrophy of lymphoid tissue. See also sudden infant death *syndrome.*

s. thy'micus, s. thymicolymphaticus.

s. typho'sus, s. nervosus; an erethistic or typhoidal state.

s. vertigino'sus, chronic vertigo; a condition in which attacks of vertigo occur in rapid succession.

statuvolence (stat-yū-vō'lens, stă-tū'vō-lens) [status (hypnoticus) + L. *volens,* pres. p. of *volo,* to wish]. Autohypnosis.

statuvolent (stat-yū-vō'lent). Relating to or capable of statuvolence.

statvolt (stat'vōlt) [G. *statos,* standing (stationary), + volt]. The electrostatic unit of potential or electromotive force, equal to 300 volts.

Staub, Hans, Swiss internist, *1890. See S.-Traugott *effect.*

staurion (staw'rē-on) [G. dim. of *stauros,* cross]. A craniometric point at the intersection of the median and transverse palatine sutures.

stauroplegia (staw-rō-plē'jē-ă) [G. *stauros,* cross, + *plēgē,* stroke]. Alternate *hemiplegia.*

STD Abbreviation for sexually transmitted *disease.*

steal (stēl). Diversion of blood via alternate routes or reversed flow, from a vascularized tissue to one deprived by proximal arterial obstruction.

iliac s., the decrease in flow in one common iliac artery when an occlusion of the other common iliac artery is released.

renal-splanchnic s., diversion of blood from the right renal artery via the inferior adrenal branch into splanchnic collaterals distal to a stenosis of the celiac axis.

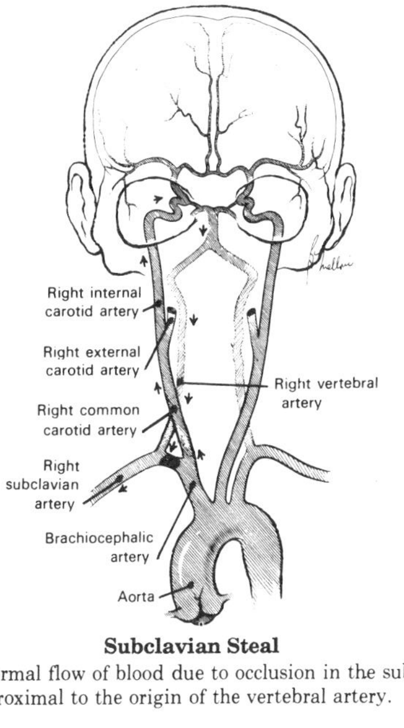

Subclavian Steal

Abnormal flow of blood due to occlusion in the subclavian artery proximal to the origin of the vertebral artery.

subclavian s., obstruction of the subclavian artery proximal to the origin of the vertebral artery; blood flow through the vertebral artery is reversed and the subclavian artery thus "steals" cerebral blood, causing symptoms of cerebrovascular insufficiency (subclavian steal syndrome). See fig. on p. 1471.

steapsin (stē-ap′sin). Triacylglycerol lipase.

stear-. See stearo-.

stearal (stē′ă-răl). Stearaldehyde; octadecanal(dehyde); the aldehyde of stearic acid.

stearaldehyde (stē-ă-ral′dĕ-hīd). Stearal.

stearate (stē′ă-rāt). A salt of stearic acid.

stearic acid (stē′ă-rik). Octadecanoic acid; one of the most abundant fatty acids found in animal lipids; used in pharmaceutical preparations, ointments, soaps, and suppositories.

stearin (stē′ă-rin). Tristearin; tristearoylglycerol; the "triglyceride" of stearic acid present in solid animal fats and in some vegetable fats; source of stearic acid.

Stearns, A. Warren, U.S. physician, 1885–1959. See S.'s alcoholic *amentia.*

stearo-, stear- [G. *stear,* tallow]. Combining forms denoting fat. See also steato-.

stearrhea (stē-ă-rē′ă). Steatorrhea.

stearyl alcohol (ste′ă-ril). Octadecyl alcohol; octadecanol; an ingredient of hydrophilic ointment and hydrophilic petrolatum; also used in the preparation of creams.

steatite (stē′ă-tīt). Talc in the form of a mass.

steatitis (stē-ă-tī′tis) [G. *stear* (*steat-*), tallow, + *-itis,* inflammation]. **1.** Inflammation of adipose tissue. **2.** A disease of young mink characterized by a brownish yellow discoloration of the adipose tissues; believed to be caused by feeding diets containing too much unsaturated fatty acid and too little vitamin E.

steato- [G. *stear* (*steat-*), tallow]. Combining form denoting fat. See also stearo-.

steatocystoma (stē′ă-tō-sis-tō′mă). **1.** A cyst with sebaceous gland cells in its wall. **2.** Pilar *cyst.*

s. mul′tiplex, widespread, multiple, thin-walled cysts of the skin that are lined by squamous epithelium, including lobules of sebaceous cells.

steatogenesis (stē′ă-tō-jen′ĕ-sis) [steato- + G. *genesis,* production]. Biosynthesis of lipids. The term is used specifically to designate lipid accumulation in the testes of nonmammalian vertebrates on completion of spermatogenesis in the breeding period.

steatolysis (stē-ă-tol′i-sis) [steato- + G. *lysis,* dissolution]. The hydrolysis or emulsion of fat in the process of digestion.

steatolytic (stē-ă-tō-lit′ik). Relating to steatolysis.

steatonecrosis (stē′ă-tō-ne-krō′sis) [steato- + G. *nekrōsis,* death]. Fat *necrosis.*

steatopyga, steatopygia (stē′ă-tō-pī′gă, -pij′ē-ă) [steato- + G. *pygē,* buttocks]. Excessive accumulation of fat on the buttocks.

steatopygous (stē-ă-top′ă-gŭs). Having excessively fat buttocks.

steatorrhea (stē′ă-tō-rē′ă) [steato- + G. *rhoia,* a flow]. Stearrhea; fat indigestion; passage of fat in large amounts in the feces, as noted in pancreatic disease and the malabsorption syndromes.

biliary s., s. due to the absence of bile from the intestine; usually accompanied by jaundice.

intestinal s., s. due to malabsorption resulting from intestinal disease. See also sprue; celiac *disease.*

pancreatic s., s. due to the absence of pancreatic juice from the intestine.

steatosis (stē-ă-tō′sis) [steato- + G. *-osis,* condition]. **1.** Adiposis. **2.** Fatty *degeneration.*

s. cor′dis, fatty degeneration of the heart.

hepatic s., fatty *liver.*

steatozoon (stē′ă-tō-zō′on) [steato- + G. *zōon,* animal]. Common name for *Demodex folliculorum.*

Steele, John C., Canadian neurologist. See S.-Richardson-Olszewski *disease, syndrome.*

Steell. See Graham Steell.

Steenbock, Harry, U.S. physiologist and chemist, 1886–1967. See S. *unit.*

stege (stē′gē) [G. *stegos,* roof, a house]. The internal pillar of Corti's organ.

stegnosis (steg-nō′sis) [G. stoppage]. **1.** A stoppage of any of the secretions or excretions. **2.** A constriction or stenosis.

stegnotic (steg-not′ik). **1.** Astringent or constipating. **2.** An astringent or constipating agent.

Steidele, Raphael, 18th century Austrian obstetrician. See S.'s *complex.*

Stein, Irving F., U.S. gynecologist, *1887. See S.-Leventhal *syndrome.*

Stein, Stanislav A.F. von, Russian otologist, *1855. See S.'s *test.*

Steinberg, I. See S. thumb *sign.*

Steinbrinck, W. See Chédiak-S.-Higashi *anomaly, syndrome.*

Steinert, Hans, 19th century German physician. See S.'s *disease.*

Steinmann, Fritz, Swiss surgeon, 1872–1932. See S. *pin.*

STEL Abbreviation for short-term exposure *limit.*

stella, pl. stellae (stel′ă, -ē) [Mod. L.]. A star or star-shaped figure.

s. len′tis hyaloi′dea, the posterior pole of the lens. See *radii* lentis.

s. len′tis irid′ica, the anterior pole of the lens. See *radii* lentis.

stellate (stel′āt) [L. *stella,* a star]. Star-shaped.

stellectomy (stel-ek′tō-mē). Stellate ganglionectomy.

stellula, pl. stellulae (stel′yū-lă, -lē) [L. dim. of *stella,* star]. A small star or star-shaped figure.

stel′lulae vasculo′sae, stellulae winslowii.

stel′lulae verheyen′ii, *venulae* stellatae.

stel′lulae winslo′wii, Winslow's stars; stellulae vasculosae; capillary whorls in the lamina choroidocapillaris from which arise the venae vorticosae.

Stellwag, Carl von C., Austrian ophthalmologist, 1823–1904. See S.'s *sign.*

stem. A supporting structure similar to the stalk of a plant.

brain s., see under B.

infundibular s., infundibular stalk; the neural component of the pituitary stalk which contains nerve tracts passing from the hypothalamus to the pars nervosa.

sten. A statistical term which uses the standard deviation in a method of converting data into standardized scores which define 10 steps along a normal distribution, with five steps on either side of the mean.

Stender, Wilhelm P., 19th century Leipzig manufacturer of scientific apparatus. See S. *dish.*

Stenger test. See under test.

stenion (sten′ē-on) [G. *stenos,* narrow, + dim. *-iōn*]. The termination in either temporal fossa of the shortest transverse diameter of the skull; a craniometric point.

Steno. See Stensen.

steno- [G. *stenos,* narrow]. Combining form denoting narrowness or constriction.

stenobregmatic (sten′ō-breg-mat′ik) [steno- + G. *bregma*]. Denoting a skull narrow anteriorly, at the part where the bregma is.

stenocardia (sten-ō-kar′dē-ă) [steno- + G. *kardia,* heart]. *Angina* pectoris.

stenocephalia (sten-ō-se-fā′lē-ă). Stenocephaly.

stenocephalous, stenocephalic (sten-ō-sef'ă-lŭs, -se-fal'ik). Pertaining to, or characterized by, stenocephaly.

stenocephaly (sten-ō-sef'ă-lē) [steno- + G. *kephalē*, head]. Stenocephalia; marked narrowness of the head.

stenochoria (sten-ō-kō'rē-ă) [G. *stenochōria*, narrowness, fr. steno- + *chōra*, place, room]. Abnormal contraction of any canal or orifice, especially of the lacrimal ducts.

stenocompressor (sten'ō-kom-pres'er, ōr). An instrument for compressing the ducts of the parotid glands (Stensen's duct) in order to keep back the saliva during dental operations.

stenocrotaphy, stenocrotaphia (sten'ō-krot'ă-fē, -krō-tā'fē-ă) [steno- + G. *krotaphos*, temple]. Narrowness of the skull in the temporal region; the condition of a stenobregmate skull.

Stenon [*Stenonius*, Latin form of Stensen]. See Stensen.

stenopeic, stenopaic (sten-ō-pē'ik, sten-ō-pā'ik) [steno- + G. *opē*, opening]. Provided with a narrow opening or slit, as in s. spectacles.

stenosal (ste-nō'săl). Stenotic.

stenosed (sten'ōzd). Narrowed; contracted: strictured.

stenosis, pl. stenoses (ste-nō'sis, -sēz) [G. *stenōsis*, a narrowing]. A stricture of any canal; especially, a narrowing of one of the cardiac valves.
- **aortic s.,** pathologic narrowing of the aortic valve orifice.
- **buttonhole s.,** extreme narrowing, usually of the mitral valve.
- **calcific nodular aortic s.,** most common type of aortic s., occurring usually in elderly men, in which the cusps contain calcified fibrous nodules on both surfaces; the causes include rheumatic fever and atherosclerosis.
- **congenital pyloric s.,** hypertrophic pyloric s.
- **coronary ostial s.,** narrowing of the mouths of the coronary arteries, usually as a result of syphilitic aortitis.
- **Dittrich's s.,** infundibular s.
- **double aortic s.,** subaortic s. associated with s. of the valve itself, both lesions being congenital.
- **fish-mouth mitral s.,** extreme mitral s.
- **hypertrophic pyloric s.,** congenital pyloric s.; muscular hypertrophy of the pyloric sphincter, associated with projectile vomiting appearing in the second or third week of life, usually in males.
- **idiopathic hypertrophic subaortic s.,** muscular subaortic s.; left ventricular outflow obstruction due to hypertrophy of the ventricular septum.
- **infundibular s.,** Dittrich's s.; narrowing of the outflow tract of the right ventricle below the pulmonic valve; may be due to a localized fibrous diaphragm just below the valve or, more commonly, to a long narrow fibromuscular channel.
- **laryngeal s.,** narrowing or stricture of any or all areas of the larynx; may be congenital or acquired.
- **mitral s.,** pathologic narrowing of the orifice of the mitral valve.
- **muscular subaortic s.,** idiopathic hypertrophic subaortic s.
- **pulmonary s.,** narrowing of the opening into the pulmonary artery from the right ventricle.
- **pyloric s.,** narrowing of the gastric pylorus, especially by congenital muscular hypertrophy or scarring resulting from a peptic ulcer. See also hypertrophic pyloric s.
- **subaortic s.,** subvalvar s.; congenital narrowing of the outflow tract of the left ventricle by a ring of fibrous tissue or by hypertrophy of the muscular septum shortly below the aortic valve.
- **subvalvar s.,** subaortic s.
- **supravalvar s.,** narrowing of the aorta above the aortic valve by a constricting ring or shelf, or by coarctation or hypoplasia of the ascending aorta.
- **tricuspid s.,** pathologic narrowing of the orifice of the tricuspid valve.

stenostenosis (sten'ō-stĕ-nō'sis). Stricture of the parotid duct (Steno's or Stensen's duct).

stenostomia (sten-ō-stō'mē-ă) [steno- + G. *stoma*, mouth]. Narrowness of the oral cavity.

stenothermal (sten-ō-ther'măl) [steno- + G. *thermē*, heat]. Thermostable through a small range; able to withstand only slight changes in temperature.

stenothorax (sten'ō-thōr'aks) [steno- + thorax]. A narrow contracted chest.

stenotic (ste-not'ik). Stenosal; narrowed; affected with stenosis.

stenoxenous (sten-ok'sĕ-nŭs) [steno- + G. *xenos*, a stranger, foreigner]. Denoting a parasite with a narrow host range; *e.g.*, *Eimeria* (among the Coccidia), hookworm, biting and sucking lice.

Stensen (Steno, Stenon, Stenonius), Niels (Nicholaus), Danish anatomist, 1638–1686. See S.'s *duct, experiment, foramen, plexus, veins.*

Stent, C., 19th century British dentist, See stent; S. *graft.*

stent [C. *Stent*]. **1.** Device used to maintain a bodily orifice or cavity during skin grafting, or to immobilize a skin graft after placement. **2.** Slender thread, rod, or catheter, lying within the lumen of tubular structures, used to provide support during or after their anastomosis, or to assure patency of an intact but contracted lumen.

Stenvers projection, Stenvers view. See under projection, view.

step. 1. In dentistry, a dove-tailed or similarly shaped projection of a cavity prepared in a tooth into a surface perpendicular to the main part of the cavity for the purpose of preventing displacement of the restoration (filling) by the force of mastication. **2.** A change in direction resembling a stair-step in a line, a surface, or the construction of a solid body.
- **Krönig's s.'s,** extension of the lower part of the right border of absolute cardiac dullness in hypertrophy of the right heart.
- **Roenne's nasal s.,** a nasal visual field defect with one margin corresponding to the retinal horizontal medium; seen in glaucoma.

stephanial (ste-fā'nē-ăl). Pertaining to the stephanion.

stephanion (ste-fā'nē-on) [G. dim. of *stephanos*, crown]. A craniometric point where the coronal suture intersects the inferior temporal line.

Stephanofilaria stilesi (stef'ă-nō-fi-lar'ē-ă stī-le'sī) [G. *stephanos*, crown, + filaria]. A skin-infecting species of filaria parasitic in cattle and transmitted by the horn fly, *Siphona irritans;* the only species known to occur in the U.S.; characterized by a row of spines behind the mouth of the adult worm, which is 6 to 8 mm in the female, 2 to 3 mm in the male. Both adults and larvae are found in granulomatous skin lesions in cattle, usually on the underside of the abdomen.

Stephanurus dentatus (stef-ă-nū'rŭs den-tā'tŭs) [G. *stephanos*, crown, + *oura*, tail]. The kidney worm or lard worm of swine, a strongyle nematode parasite species that also occurs, though rarely, in the liver of cattle. Adult worms in swine live in the perirenal fat, the kidney pelvis, or as erratic forms in many other locations. Eggs are passed through the urine and infection is direct, by ingestion of infective larvae or by skin infection, or indirect, by ingestion of earthworms in which the larvae can survive.

steppage (step'aj) [Fr.]. The peculiar, high steppage gait of sufferers from neuritis of the peroneal nerve and from tabes dorsalis; because the ankle cannot be dorsiflexed when walking, the foot is raised very high in order that the drooping toes clear the ground.

steradian (stē-rā'dē-ăn) [G. *stereos*, solid, + *radion*, radius]. The unit of solid angle; the solid angle that encloses an area on the surface of a sphere equivalent to the square of the radius of the sphere.

sterane (ster'ān, stēr'ān). The hypothetical parent molecule for any steroid hormone; a saturated hydrocarbon compound that contains no oxygen. The name was originally conceived to achieve forms of systematic nomenclature, but is now supplanted by the fundamental variants: gonane, estrane, androstane, norandrostane (etiane), cholane, cholestane, ergostane, and stigmastane. See also steroids.

sterco- [L. *stercus*, feces, excrement]. Combining form denoting feces. See also copro-, scato-.

stercobilin (ster'kō-bī'lin, -bil'in). A brown degradation product of hemoglobin, present in the feces. See also bilirubinoids.

l-**stercobilinogen** (ster'kō-bī-lin'ō-jen). Reduction product of *l*-urobilinogen, precursor of *l*-stercobilin in the final stages of bilirubin metabolism; excreted in feces, wherein it is oxidized to stercobilin. See also bilirubinoids.

stercolith (ster'kō-lith) [sterco- + G. *lithos*, stone]. Coprolith.

stercoraceous (ster-kō-rā'shŭs). Stercoral; stercorous; relating to or containing feces.

stercoral (ster'kō-răl). Stercoraceous.

stercorin (ster'kō-rin). Coprosterol.

stercoroma (ster-kō-rō'mă) [stereo- + G. *-oma*, tumor]. Coproma.

stercorous (ster'kō-rŭs). Stercoraceous.

stercus (ster'kŭs) [L. feces, excrement]. Feces.

stere (stēr, stār) [Fr. fr. G. *stereos*, solid]. A measure of capacity; equivalent to a cubic meter or a kiloliter.

stereo- [G. *stereos*, solid]. **1.** Combining form denoting a solid, or a solid condition or state. **2.** Prefix denoting spatial qualities, three-dimensionality.

stereoagnosis (ster'ē-ō-ag-nō'sis). Astereognosis.

stereoanesthesia (ster'ē-ō-an-es-thē'zē-ă) [stereo- + G. *an*- priv. + *aisthēsis*, sensation]. Astereognosis.

stereoarthrolysis (ster'ē-ō-ar-throl'i-sis) [stereo- + G. *arthron*, joint, + *lysis*, loosening]. Production of a new joint with mobility in cases of bony ankylosis.

stereocampimeter (ster'ē-ō-kam-pim'ĕ-ter) [stereo- + L. *campus*, field, + G. *metron*, measure]. An apparatus for studying the central visual fields.

stereochemical (ster'ē-ō-kem'i-kăl). Relating to stereochemistry.

stereochemistry (ster-ē-ō-kem'is-trē). The branch of chemistry concerned with the spatial three-dimensional relations of atoms in molecules, *i.e.*, the positions the atoms in a compound bear in relation to one another in space.

stereocilium, pl. **stereocilia** (ster'ē-ō-sil'ē-ŭm, -ă) [stereo- + L. *cilium*, eyelid]. A nonmotile cilium or long microvillus.

stereocinefluorography (ster'ē-ō-sin'ĕ-flūr-og'ră-fē). Motion picture recording of x-ray images obtained by stereoscopic fluoroscopy; three-dimensional views are obtained.

stereocolpogram (ster'ē-ō-kol'pō-gram). Picture taken with the stereocolposcope.

stereocolposcope (ster'ē-ō-kol'pō-skōp) [stereo- + G. *kolpos*, a hollow (vagina), *skopeō*, to view]. Instrument that provides the observer with a magnified three-dimensional gross inspection of the vagina and cervix.

stereoelectroencephalography (ster-ē-ō-ē-lek'trō-en-sef-ă-log'ră-fē). Recording of electrical activity in three planes of the brain, *i.e.*, with surface and depth electrodes.

stereoencephalometry (ster'ē-ō-en-sef'ă-lom'ĕ-trē). The localization of brain structures by use of three-dimensional coordinates.

stereoencephalotomy (ster'ē-ō-en-sef'ă-lot'ō-mē) [stereo- + G. *encephalos*, brain, + *tomē*, a cutting]. Stereotaxy.

stereognosis (ster'ē-og'nō'sis) [stereo- + G. *gnōsis*, knowledge]. The appreciation of the form of an object by means of touch.

stereognostic (ster'ē-og-nos'tik). Relating to stereognosis.

stereogram (ster'ē-ō-gram). A stereoscopic x-ray image.

stereograph (ster'ē-ō-graf). A stereoscopic x-ray apparatus.

stereoisomer (ster'ē-ō-ī'sō-mer) [stereo- + G. *isos*, equal, + *meros*, part]. A molecule containing the same number and kind of atom groupings as another but in a different arrangement in space, by virtue of which it exhibits different properties; *e.g.*, as between D and L amino acids, 5α and 5β steroids.

stereoisomeric (ster'ē-ō-ī-sō-mer'ik). Relating to stereoisomerism.

stereoisomerism (ster'ē-ō-ī-som'er-izm). Stereochemical isomerism; molecular asymmetry; isomerism involving different spatial arrangements of the same groups (*e.g.*, androsterone and isoandrosterone, differing only in that one has a 3α OH, the other a 3β OH). See also stereoisomer; LeBel-van't Hoff *rule*.

stereology (ster'ē-ol'ō-jē) [stereo- + G. *logos*, study]. A study of the three-dimensional aspects of a cell or microscopic structure.

stereometer (ster-ē-om'ĕ-ter) [stereo- + G. *metron*, measure]. An instrument used in stereometry.

stereometry (ster-ē-om'ĕ-trē). **1.** Measurement of a solid object or the cubic capacity of a vessel. **2.** Determination of the specific gravity of a liquid.

stereo-orthopter (ster'ē-ō-ōr-thop'ter) [stereo- + G. *orthos*, straight, + *optikos*, optical]. A type of stereoscope used in visual training.

stereopathy (ster-ē-op'ă-thē). Persistent stereotyped thinking.

stereophantoscope (ster'ē-ō-fan'tō-skōp) [stereo- + G. *phantos*, visible, + *skopeō*, to view]. A stereophoroscope with rotating disks of different colors instead of pictures.

stereophorometer (ster'ē-ō-fō-rom'ĕ-ter). A phorometer with a stereoscopic attachment.

stereophoroscope (ster'ē-ō-fōr'ō-skōp) [stereo- + G. *phoros*, bearing, *skopeō*, to view]. Obsolete term for a stereoscope producing images having apparent motion.

stereophotomicrograph (ster'ē-ō-fō'tō-mī'krō-graf). A stereoscopic photomicrograph which, when viewed with a stereoscope, appears three-dimensional.

stereopsis (ster-ē-op'sis) [stereo- + G. *opsis*, vision]. Stereoscopic *vision*.

stereoradiography (ster'ē-ō-rā-dē-og'ră-fē). Stereoroentgenography.

stereoroentgenography (ster'ē-ō-rent'gen-og'ră-fē). Stereoradiography; the utilization of x-ray images made from two slightly different positions to obtain a three-dimensional effect.

stereoscope (ster'ē-ō-skōp) [stereo- + G. *skopeō*, to view]. An instrument producing two horizontally separated images of the same object, providing a single image with an appearance of depth.

stereoscopic (ster'ē-ō-skop'ik). Relating to a stereoscope, or giving the appearance of three dimensions.

stereoscopy (ster-ē-os'kō-pē). An optical technique by which two images of the same object are blended into one, giving a three-dimensional appearance to the single image.

stereoselective (ster'ē-ō-sĕ-lek'tiv). As applied to a reaction, denoting a process in which of two or more possible stereoisomeric products only one predominates; a s. process is not necessarily stereospecific.

stereospecific (ster'ē-ō-spĕ-sif'ik). As applied to a reaction, denoting a process in which stereoisomerically different starting materials give rise to stereoisomerically different products; a s. process is thus necessarily stereoselective, but not all stereoselective processes are s.

stereotactic, stereotaxic (ster'ē-ō-tak'tik, -tak'sik). Relating to stereotaxis or stereotaxy.

stereotaxis (ster'ē-ō-tak'sis) [stereo- + G. *taxis*, orderly arrangement]. **1.** Three-dimensional arrangement. **2.** Stereotropism, but applied more exactly where the organism as a whole, rather than a part only, reacts. **3.** Stereotaxy.

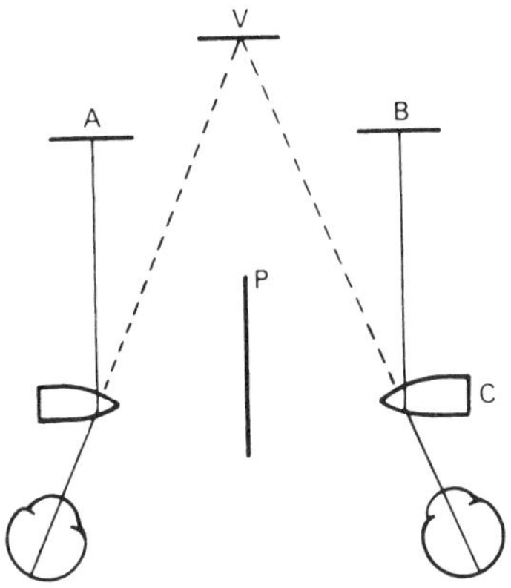

Diagram Illustrating the Principle of the Stereoscope
A and *B* represent photographs of two views taken from slightly different angles; *C*, prisms; *P*, partition to prevent one eye seeing the picture opposite the other eye; *V*, the image formed when the two views are fused by the instrument appears to be at *V*.

stereotaxy (ster'ē-ō-tak'sē). Stereotaxis (3); stereoencephalotomy; stereotactic surgery; a precise method of destroying deep-seated brain structures located by use of three-dimensional coordinates.

stereotropic (ster'ē-ō-trop'ik). Relating to or exhibiting stereotropism.

stereotropism (ster'ē-ot'rō-pizm) [stereo- + G. *tropos,* a turning]. Growth or movement of a plant or animal toward (**positive s.**) or away from (**negative s.**) a solid body, usually applied where a part of the organism rather than the whole reacts.

stereotypy (ster'ē-ō-tī-pē) [stereo- + G. *typos,* impression, type]. **1.** Maintenance of one attitude for a long period. **2.** Constant repetition of certain meaningless gestures or movements, as in certain forms of schizophrenia.
oral s., verbigeration.

steric (ster'ik, stēr-). Pertaining to stereochemistry.

steric hindrance. Interference with or inhibition of a seemingly feasible reaction (usually synthetic) because the size of one or another reactant prevents approach to the required interatomic distance.

sterid (ster'id, stēr-). Steroid (2).

sterigma, pl. **sterigmata** (ste-rig'mă, -mă-tă) [G. *stērigma,* a support]. A slender, pointed structure arising from a basidium upon which a basidiospore will develop.

sterile (ster'il) [L. *sterilis,* barren]. Relating to or characterized by sterility.

sterility (stĕ-ril'i-tē) [L. *sterilitas*]. **1.** In general, the incapabiity of fertilization or reproduction. See female s.; male s. **2.** Condition of being aseptic, or free from all living microorganisms and their spores.
absolute s., female s.
adolescent s., a period following the menarche, and lasting up to approximately 18 months, during which menstrual cycles may be markedly irregular and are often anovulatory.
aspermatogenic s., s. due to a failure to produce living spermatozoa.
dysspermatogenic s., male s. due to some abnormality in production of spermatozoa.
female s., absolute s.; infecundity; the inability of the female to conceive, due to inadequacy in structure or function of the genital organs.
male s., the inability of the male to fertilize the ovum; it may or may not be associated with impotence.
normospermatogenic s., male s. due to some cause other than failure to produce live, normal spermatozoa, *e.g.*, blockage of the seminiferous passages.
one-child s., s. occurring in a woman who has borne one child.
relative s., infertility.

sterilization (ster'ĭ-li-zā'shŭn). **1.** The act or process by which an individual is rendered incapable of fertilization or reproduction, as by vasectomy, salpingectomy, or castration. **2.** The destruction of all microorganisms in or about an object, as by steam (flowing or pressurized), chemical agents (alcohol, phenol, heavy metals, ethylene oxide gas) high-velocity electron bombardment, ultraviolet light radiation.
discontinuous s., fractional s.
fractional s., tyndallization; discontinuous or intermittent s.; exposure to a temperature of 100°C (flowing steam) for a definite period, usually an hour, on each of several days; at each heating the developed bacteria are destroyed; spores, which are unaffected, germinate during the intervening periods and are subsequently destroyed.
intermittent s., fractional s.

sterilize (ster'ĭ-līz). To produce sterility.

sterilizer (ster'i-lī-zer). An apparatus for rendering objects aseptic.
glass bead s., a s. for root canal equipment; the heat is transmitted to the instruments, absorbent points, or cotton pellets by means of glass beads.
hot salt s., a s. for endodontic equipment in which table salt is heated in a container at 218 to 246°C; the dry heat is transmitted to root canal instruments, absorbent points, or cotton pellets for their rapid (5 to 10 seconds) sterilization.

Stern, Heinrich, U.S. physician, 1868–1918. See S.'s *posture.*

stern-. See sterno-.

sterna (ster'nă). Plural of sternum.

sternad (ster'nad). In a direction toward the sternum.

sternal (ster'năl). Relating to the sternum.

sternalgia (ster-nal'jē-ă) [stern- + G. *algos,* pain]. Sternodynia; pain in the sternum or the sternal region.

sternalis (ster-nā'lis). See under musculus.

Sternberg, George M., U.S. bacteriologist, 1838– 1915. See S. *cells;* S.-Reed *cells,* Reed-S. *cells.*

sternebra, pl. **sternebrae** (ster'nē-bră, -brē) [Mod. L. fr. stern(um) + (vert)ebra]. One of the four segments of the primordial sternum of the embryo by the fusion of which the body of the adult sternum is formed.

ster'nen [stern- + G. *en,* in]. Relating to the sternum independent of any other structures.

sterno-, stern- [G. *sternon,* chest (sternum)]. Combining forms denoting the sternum.

sternochondroscapularis (ster'nō-kon'drō-skap-yū-lā'ris) [Mod. L.]. See under musculus.

sternoclavicular (ster'nō-kla-vik'yū-lăr). Relating to the sternum and the clavicle.

sternoclavicularis (ster'nō-kla-vik'yū-lā'ris). See under musculus.

sternocleidal (ster'nō-klī'dăl) [sterno- + G. *kleis,* key (clavicle)]. Relating to the sternum and the clavicle.

sternocleidomastoid (ster'nō-klī'dō-mas'toyd). Relating to sternum, clavicle, and mastoid process.

sternocleidomastoideus (ster'nō-klī'dō-mas-tō-id'-ē-ŭs) [Mod. L.]. See under musculus.

sternocostal (ster'nō-kos'tăl). [L. *costa,* rib]. Relating to the sternum and the ribs.

sternodynia (ster-nō-din'ē-ă) [sterno- + G. *odynē,* pain]. Sternalgia.

sternofascialis (ster'nō-fash-ē-ā'lis). See under musculus.

sternoglossal (ster-nō-glos'ăl). Denoting muscular fibers which occasionally pass from the sternohyoid muscle to join the hyoglossal muscle.

sternohyoideus (ster'nō-hī-oyd'ē-ŭs) [Mod. L.]. See under musculus.

sternoid (ster'noyd) [sterno- + G. *eidos,* resemblance]. Resembling the sternum.

sternomastoid (ster'nō-mas'toyd). Relating to the sternum and the mastoid process of the temporal bone; applied to the musculus sternocleidomastoideus.

sternopagia (ster-nō-pā'jē-ă) [sterno- + G. *pagos,* something fixed]. Condition shown by conjoined twins united at the sterna or more extensively at the ventral walls of the chest.

sternopericardial (ster'nō-per'i-kar'dē-ăl). Relating to the sternum and the pericardium.

sternoschisis (ster-nos'ki-sis) [sterno- + G. *schisis,* a cleaving]. Congenital cleft of the sternum.

sternothyroideus (ster'nō-thī-royd'ē-ŭs) [Mod. L.]. See under musculus.

sternotomy (ster-not'ō-mē) [sterno- + G. *tomē,* incision]. Incision into or through the sternum.

sternotracheal (ster'nō-trā'kē-ăl). Relating to the sternum and the trachea.

sternotrypesis (ster'nō-trī-pē'sis) [sterno- + G. *trypēsis,* a boring]. Trephining of the sternum.

sternovertebral (ster'nō-ver'tĕ-brăl). Vertebrosternal; relating to the sternum and the vertebrae; denoting the true ribs, or the seven upper ribs on either side, which articulate with the vertebrae and with the sternum.

sternum, gen. **sterni,** pl. **sterna** (ster'nŭm, -nī, -nă) [Mod. L. fr. G. *sternon,* the chest] [NA]. Breast bone; a long flat bone, articulating with the cartilages of the first seven ribs and with the clavicle, forming the middle part of the anterior wall of the thorax; it consists of three portions: the corpus or body, the manubrium, and the xiphoid process.

sternutation (ster'nū-tā'shŭn) [L. *sternutatio,* fr. *sternuo (sternuto),* pp. *sternutatus,* to sneeze]. The act of sneezing.

sternutator (ster'nū-tā-ter, -tōr). Sneezing gas; a substance, such as a gas, that induces sneezing.

sternutatory (ster-nū'tă-tōr-ē). Ptarmic. **1.** Causing sneezing. **2.** An agent that provokes sneezing.

steroid (stēr'oyd, ster'oyd). **1.** Steroidal; pertaining to the steroids. **2.** Sterid; one of the steroids. **3.** Generic designation for compounds closely related in structure to the steroids, such as sterols, bile acids, cardiac glycosides, and precursors of the vitamins D. **4.** Jargon for a compound having biological actions similar to a steroid hormone, of semisynthetic or synthetic origin, and whose structure may or may not resemble that of a steroid.

s. hydroxylases, s. monooxygenases.

s. monooxygenases, s. hydroxylases; enzymes catalyzing addition of hydroxyl groups to the s. rings utilizing O_2; differentiated into s. 11β-monooxygenase (EC 1.14.15.4), s. 17α-monoxygenase (EC 1.14.99.9), and s. 21-monooxygenase (EC 1.14.99.10), in accordance with the position of the catalytically introduced hydroxyl group.

steroidal (stēr'oy-dăl, ster'). Steroid (1).

steroidogenesis (stēr'oy-dō-jen'ĕ-sis, ster'). [steroid + G. *genesis,* production]. The formation of steroids; commonly referring to the biological synthesis of steroid hormones, but not to the production of such compounds in a chemical laboratory.

steroids (stēr'oydz, ster-). A large family of chemical substances, comprising many hormones, vitamin D, body constituents, and drugs, each containing the tetracyclic cyclopenta[α]phenanthrene skeleton. Formula I of the accompanying page of structures shows the numbering and lettering of the rings, which are retained even if, in a given compound, any of the atoms shown are absent or involved in ring closures, or if rings are expanded ("homo," see below) or contracted ("nor," see below). Stereoisomerism among steroids is not only common but of critical biological significance, and the isomeric groups are usually represented as shown in II. The conventions are that the nucleus is presented as if projected onto the plane of the paper, with groups then lying above that plane being denoted by thickened bonds and called β, those then lying below that plane by broken bonds and called α; the letter ξ indicates unknown or unspecified orientation. Depending on the situation at C-5, the molecule is sometimes represented in perspective as in III and IV; 5α, 5β, or 5ξ should be included in the name. Unless otherwise stated, it is assumed that atoms or groups attached to the other ring-junctions (8, 9, 10, 13, 14) are as in II, *i.e.,* 8β, 9α, 10β, 13β, 14α.

The principal classes of steroids, with names for the unsubstituted, saturated hydrocarbon forms that are clearly related to physiological functions or sources, are shown in V, VI, VII, and VIII. The digitaloid lactone derivatives known as cardanolides have the basic structure IX. The squill-toad poison group of lactones are called bufanolides (X). Spirostans and furostans (the basic structures of many "genins," including the sapogenins) are derived from XI and XII, respectively.

The natural and synthetic derivatives are named by adding conventional chemical prefixes and suffixes for substituents; *e.g.,* -ol for a hydroxyl group, -on(e) for a keto group, -al for an aldehyde group. "Nor" indicates loss of a $-CH_2$-group; "homo," the addition of a $-CH_2$-group; each is preceded by the letter indicating which ring is contracted or expanded, respectively, or, in the case where the $-CH_2$-is lost from a methyl group, the number of the carbon atom lost. "Seco" indicates fission of a ring with addition of hydrogen atoms at the positions indicated by numerals preceding the term. Unsaturation is denoted, as usual, by substituting appropriate terms, *e.g.,* -en(e), -yn(e), -adien(e), for the -ane or -an parts of the hydrocarbon or parent class names, with numerals indicating locations of the unsaturated bonds. The locations of double bonds are specified by the lower of the two (consecutive) numbers of the carbon atoms involved. When a double bond is formed between two nonconsecutive carbon atoms, the second is indicated in parentheses after the first; *e.g.,* estriol and the estradiols possess three double bonds, between C1 and C2, between C3 and C4, and between C5 and C10, respectively.

Steroid alkaloids may be named from the steroid parent, as above, or from trivial family names usually ending in -anine if the steroid is saturated or in -enine, -adienine, etc., if it is not saturated (*e.g.,* conanine, tomatanine).

sterol (stēr'ol). A steroid of 27 or more carbon atoms with one OH (alcohol) group; the systematic names contain either the prefix hydroxy- or the suffix -ol, *e.g.,* cholesterol, ergosterol.

stertor (ster'tōr) [L. *sterto,* to snore]. A noisy inspiration occurring in coma or deep sleep, sometimes due to obstruction of the larynx or upper airways.

hen-cluck s., a breath sound like the clucking of a hen, sometimes heard in cases of postpharyngeal abscess.

stertorous (ster'tōr-ŭs). Relating to or characterized by stertor or snoring.

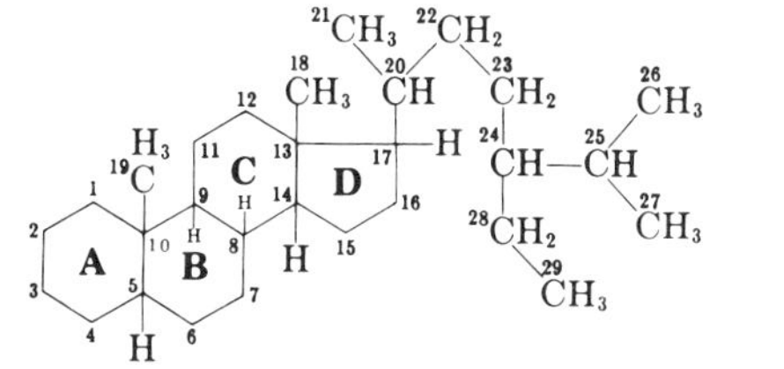

I. Numbering of atoms and rings of steroids and conventional orientation.

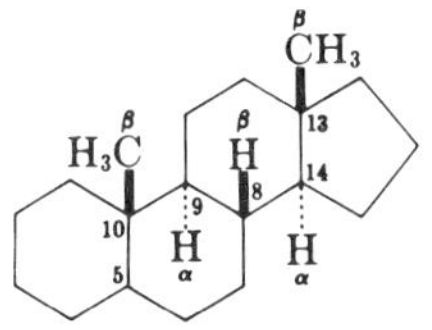

II. Depiction of α and β exocyclic atoms of steroids. These orientations are assumed to prevail in a steroid unless specifically otherwise indicated in the name.

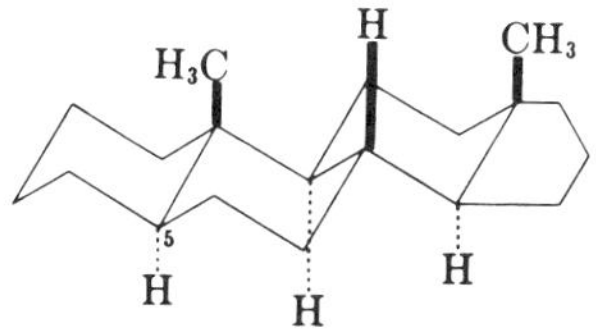

III. Perspective view of a 5α-steroid

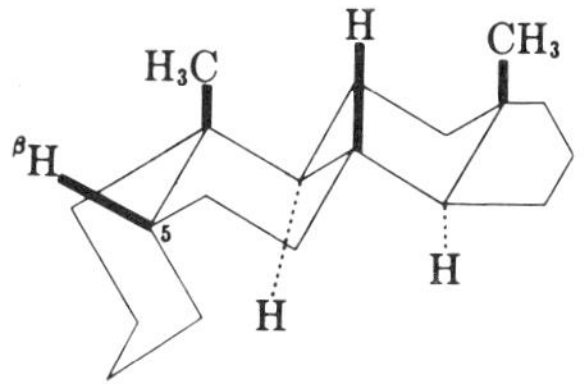

IV. Perspective view of a 5β-steroid

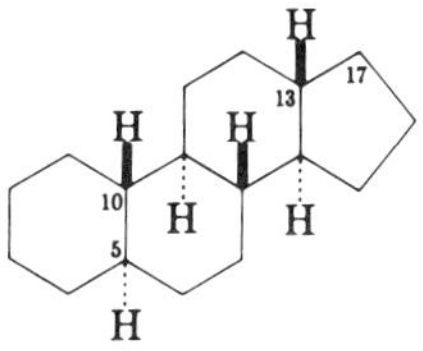

V. 5α-gonane

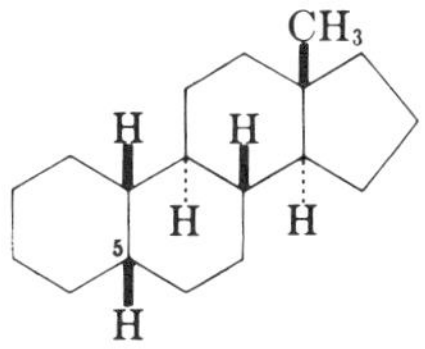

VI. 5β-estrane

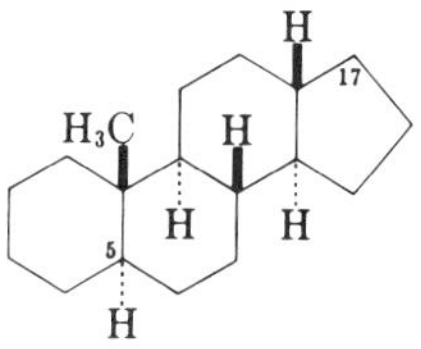

VII. 5α-18-norandrostane (= 10-methyl-5α-gonane)

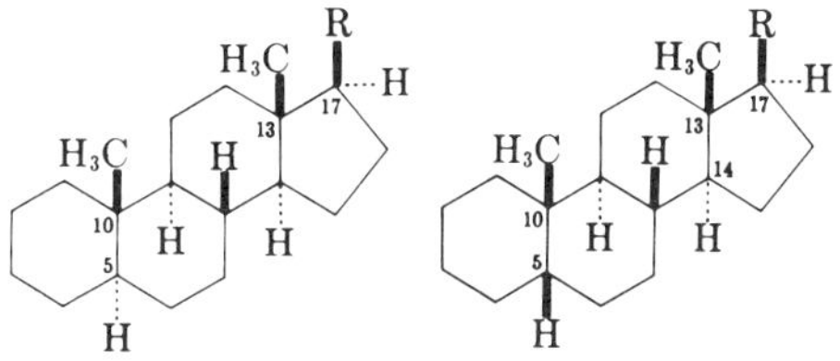

VIII. Steroids with methyl groups at both C-10 and C-13. *Left*, 5α series; *right*, 5β series. The names listed below are used for these steroids.

R (at position 17)	5α Series	5β Series
H	5α-Androstane (*not* etioallocholane)	5β-Androstane (*not* testane or etiocholane or etiane)
C_2H_5	5α-Pregnane (*not* allopregnane)	5β-Pregnane
$CH(CH_3)CH_2CH_2CH_3$	5α-Cholane (*not* allocholane)	5β-Cholane
$CH(CH_3)CH_2CH_2CH_2CH(CH_3)_2$	5α-Cholestane	5β-Cholestane (*not* coprostane)
$CH(CH_3)CH_2CH_2CH(CH_3)CH(CH_3)_2$	5α-Ergostane	5β-Ergostane
$CH(CH_3)CH_2CH_2CH(C_2H_5)CH(CH_3)_2$	5α-Stigmastane	5β-Stigmastane

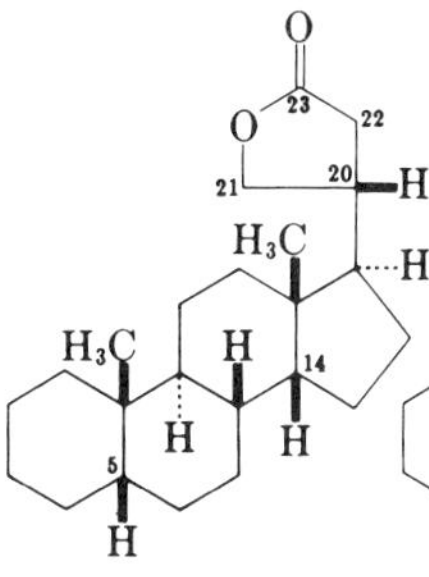

IX. 5β, 14β-cardanolide

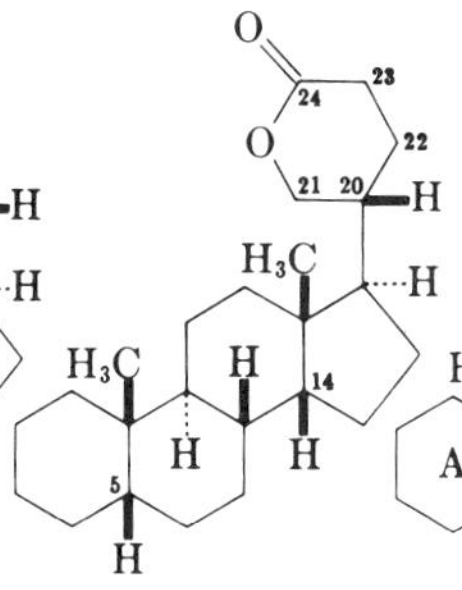

X. 5β, 14β-bufanolide

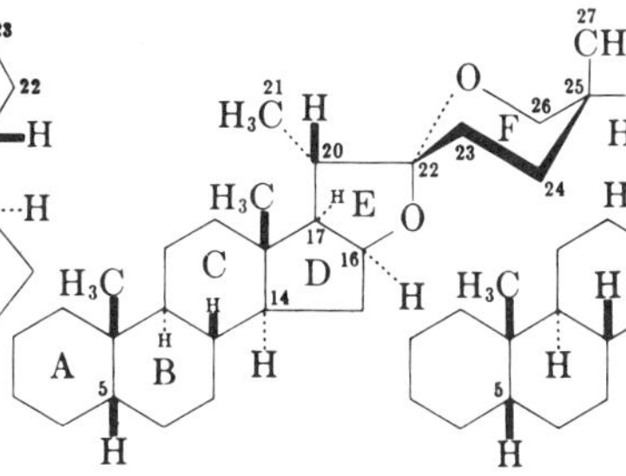

XI. 5β-spirostan

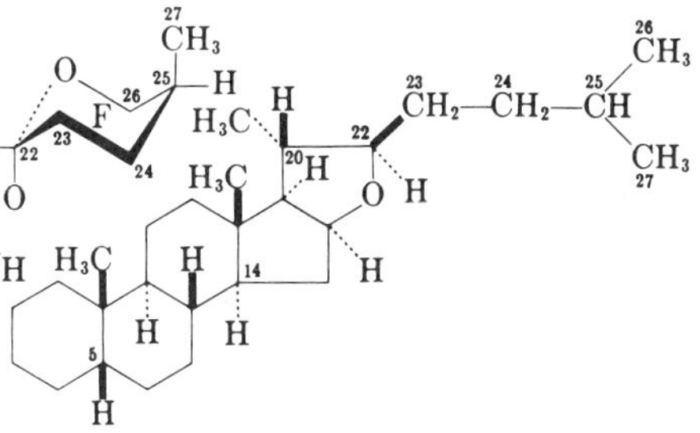

XII. 5β-furostan

Steroids

steth-. See stetho-.

stethalgia (ste-thal'jē-ă) [steth- + G. *algos,* pain]. Pain in the chest.

stetharteritis (steth'ar-ter-ī'tis) [steth- + L. *arteria,* artery, + G. *-itis,* inflammation]. Inflammation of the aorta or other arteries in the chest.

stethendoscope (steth-en'do-skōp) [steth- + endoscope]. An obsolete fluoroscope for examination of the chest.

stetho-, steth- [G. *stēthos,* chest]. Combining forms denoting the chest.

stethocyrtograph (steth'ō-ser'tō-graf) [stetho- + G. *kyrtos,* bent, + *graphō,* to write]. Stethokyrtograph; an apparatus for measuring and recording the curvatures of the thorax.

stethocyrtometer (steth'ō-ser-tom'ĕ-ter) [stetho- + G. *kyrtos,* bent, + *metron,* measure]. An instrument for measuring curvature or deformity of the vertebral column in kyphosis.

stethogoniometer (steth'ō-gō-nē-om'ĕ-ter) [stetho- + G. *gōnia,* angle, + *metron,* measure]. An apparatus for measuring the curvatures of the thorax.

stethograph (steth'ō-graf) [stetho- + G. *graphō,* to write]. An apparatus for recording the respiratory movements of the chest.

stethokyrtograph (steth'ō-ker'tō-graf). Stethocyrtograph.

stethomyitis, stethomyositis (steth'ō-mī-ī'tis, steth'ō-mī-ō-sī'tis) [stetho- + G. *mys,* muscle, + *-itis,* inflammation]. Inflammation of the muscles of the chest wall.

stethoparalysis (steth'ō-pă-ral'i-sis). Paralysis of the respiratory muscles.

stethoscope (steth'ō-skōp) [stetho- + G. *skopeō,* to view]. An instrument originally devised by Laennec for aid in hearing the respiratory and cardiac sounds in the chest, but now modified in various ways and used in auscultation of any of vascular or other sounds anywhere in the body.

binaural s., a s. in which the two ear pieces connect with a single bell.

Bowles type s., a s. in which the chest piece is a shallow metal cup about 4.5 cm. in diameter, the mouth of which is covered by a hard rubber or celluloid diaphragm.

differential s., a s. having two chest pieces so that two sounds in different parts of the chest may be heard simultaneously and compared.

stethoscopic (steth-ō-skop'ik). **1.** Relating to or effected by means of a stethoscope. **2.** Relating to an examination of the chest.

stethoscopy (stĕ-thos'kō-pē). **1.** Examination of the chest by means of auscultation, either mediate or immediate, and percussion. **2.** Mediate auscultation with the stethoscope.

stethospasm (steth'ō-spazm). Spasm of the chest.

Stevens, Albert M., U.S. pediatrician, 1884–1945. See S.-Johnson *syndrome.*

Stewart, Fred D. See S.-Treves *syndrome.*

Stewart, George N., Canadian-American scientist, 1860–1930. See S.'s *test.*

Stewart, R.M., 20th century British neurologist. See S.-Morel *syndrome.*

Stewart, Thomas Grainger, 20th century British neurologist, 1877–1957. See S.-Holmes *sign.*

STH Abbreviation for somatotropic *hormone.*

sthenia (sthē'nē-ă) [G. *sthenos,* strength, + *-ia,* condition]. A condition of activity and apparent force, as in an acute sthenic fever.

sthenic (sthen'ik). Strong; active; marked by sthenia; said of a fever with strong bounding pulse, high temperature, and active delirium.

stheno- [G. *sthenos,* strength]. Combining form denoting strength, force, power.

sthenometer (sthĕ-nom'ĕ-ter) [stheno- + G. *metron,* measure]. An instrument for measuring muscular strength.

sthenometry (sthĕ-nom'ĕ-trē) [stheno- + G. *metrin,* to measure]. The measurement of muscular strength.

stibamine glucoside (stib'ă-mēn). A pentavalent antimony compound; a nitrogen glycoside of sodium *p*-aminobenzenestibonate; has been used in leishmaniasis (kala azar) and certain other tropical diseases, but is no longer marketed.

stibenyl (stib'ĕ-nil). Sodium 4-acetamidobenzenestibonate; the first pentavalent antimonial used in the treatment of leishmaniasis (kala azar).

stibialism (stib'ē-ă-lizm) [L. *stibium,* antimony]. Chronic antimonial poisoning.

stibiated (stib'ē-ā-ted). Impregnated with or containing antimony.

stibiation (stib-ē-ā'shŭn). Impregnation with antimony.

stibium (stib'ē-ŭm) [L. fr. G. *stibi*]. Antimony.

stibocaptate (stib-ō-kap'tāt). *Antimony* dimercaptosuccinate.

stibogluconate sodium (stib-ō-glū'kō-nāt). **1.** Antimony sodium gluconate; pentavalent sodium stibogluconate; used in the treatment of all types of leishmaniasis; toxic effects are frequent. **2.** Trivalent antimony sodium gluconate; trivalent sodium stibogluconate; sodium antimonylgluconate; used in the treatment of schistosomiasis; toxic effects are frequent.

stibonium (sti-bō'nē-ŭm). The hypothetical radical, SbH_4^+, analogous to ammonium.

stibophen (stib'ō-fen). Pentasodium bis[4,5-dihydroxybenz-1,3-disulfonate]antimonate; an organic trivalent antimony compound, used in the treatment of schistosomiasis, filariasis, leishmaniasis, and lymphogranuloma inguinale.

stichochrome (stik'ō-krōm) [G. *stichos,* a row, + *chrōma,* color]. Denoting a nerve cell in which the chromophil substance, or stainable material, is arranged in roughly parallel rows or lines.

Sticker, Georg, German physician, 1860–1960. See S.'s *disease.*

Stickler, G.B. See S. *syndrome.*

Stieda, Alfred, German surgeon, 1869–1945. See Pellegrini-S. *disease.*

Stieda, Ludwig, German anatomist, 1837–1918. See S.'s *process.*

Stierlin, Eduard, German surgeon, 1878–1919. See S.'s *sign.*

stifle (stī'fl). Stifle *joint.*

stigma, pl. **stigmas, stigmata** (stig'mă, -mă-tă) [G. a mark. fr. *stizō,* to prick]. **1.** Visible evidence of a disease. **2.** Follicular s. **3.** Any spot or blemish on the skin. **4.** A bleeding spot on the skin which is considered a manifestation of conversion hysteria. **5.** The orange pigmented eyespot of certain chlorophyll-bearing protozoa, such as *Euglena viridis;* which serves as a light filter by absorbing certain wavelengths. **6.** A mark of shame or discredit.

follicular s., stigma (2); macula pellucida; the point where the graafian follicle is about to rupture on the surface of the ovary.

malpighian s.'s, the points of entrance of the smaller veins into the larger veins of the spleen.

s. ventric'uli, one of a number of miliary ecchymoses of the gastric mucosa.

stigmastane (stig-mas'tān). Sitostane; the parent substance of sitosterol.

stigmata (stig'mă-tă). Alternate plural of stigma.

stigmata maydis (stig'mă-tă mā'dis). Zea.

stigmatic (stig-mat'ik). Relating to or marked by a stigma.

stigmatism (stig'mă-tizm). Stigmatization (1); the condition of having a stigma.

stigmatization (stig'mă-ti-zā'shŭn). **1.** Stigmatism. **2.** Production of stigmas, especially of a hysterical nature. **3.** Debasement of a person by attributing a stigma to him.

stigmatometer (stig-mă-tom'ĕ-ter). Astigmatometer.

stilbamidine (stil-bam'i-dēn). Stilbene-4,4'-dicarbonamidine; a compound used in the treatment of leishmaniasis (kala azar), in infections due to *Blastomyces dermatitidis,* and in actinomycosis; also used in multiple myeloma for the relief of bone pain.

stilbazium iodide (stil-baz'ē-ŭm). 1-Ethyl-2,6-bis[(*p*-pyrrolidinylstyryl)] pyridinium iodide; an anthelmintic.

stilbene (stil'bēn). α,β-Diphenylethylene; $C_6H_5CH{=}CHC_6H_5$; an unsaturated hydrocarbon, the nucleus of stilbestrol and other synthetic estrogenic compounds.

stilbestrol (stil-bes'trol). Diethylstilbestrol.

Stiles, Walter S., British physicist, *1901. See S.-Crawford *effect.*

stilet, stilette (stī'let, stī-let'). See stylet.

Still, Sir George F., British physician, 1868–1941. See S.'s *disease, murmur;* S.-Chauffard *syndrome.*

stillbirth (stil'berth). The birth of an infant who shows no evidence of life after birth.

stillborn (stil'bōrn). Born dead; denoting an infant dead at birth.

Stilling, Benedict, German anatomist, 1810–1879. See S.'s *canal, column, nucleus, raphe,* gelatinous *substance.*

Stilling, Jakob, German ophthalmologist, 1842–1915. See S. color *tables.*

stilus (stī'lŭs). Stylus.

stimulant (stim'yū-lănt) [L. *stimulans,* pres. p. of *stimulo,* pp. *-atus,* to goad, incite, fr. *stimulus,* a goad]. Excitant. **1.** Stimulating; exciting to action. **2.** Excitor; stimulator; an agent that arouses organic activity, strengthens the action of the heart, increases vitality, and promotes a sense of well-being; classified according to the parts upon which they chiefly act: cardiac, respiratory, gastric, hepatic, cerebral, spinal, vascular, genital, etc. See also stimulus.

diffusible s., a s. that produces a rapid but temporary effect.

general s., a s. that affects the entire body.

local s., a s. whose action is confined to the part to which it is applied.

stimulation (stim-yū-lā'shŭn) [see stimulant]. **1.** Arousal of the body or any of its parts or organs to increased functional activity. **2.** The condition of being stimulated. **3.** In neurophysiology, the application of a stimulus to a responsive structure, such as a nerve or muscle, regardless of whether the strength of the stimulus is sufficient to produce excitation.

dorsal column s., electrical s., either percutaneously or by direct application of electrodes to the dorsal columns of the spinal cord.

Ganzfeld s. [Ger. *Ganzfeld,* whole field], illumination of the entire retina in the electroretinogram.

percutaneous s., electrical s. of the peripheral nerves or spinal cord by the application of electrodes to the skin.

photic s., the use of a flickering light to influence the pattern of the electroencephalogram and also to bring out latent abnormalities.

stimulator (stim'yū-lā-ter, -tōr). Stimulant (2).

long-acting thyroid s. (LATS), a substance, found in the blood of some hyperthyroid patients, that exerts a prolonged stimulatory effect on the thyroid gland; associated in plasma with the IgG (7S γ-globulin) fraction and seems to be an antibody or, perhaps, an immune complex.

stimulus, pl. **stimuli** (stim'yū-lŭs, -lī) [L. a goad]. **1.** A stimulant. **2.** That which can elicit or evoke action (response) in a muscle, nerve, gland or other excitable tissue, or cause an augmenting action upon any function or metabolic process.

adequate s., a s. to which a particular receptor responds effectively and that gives rise to a characteristic sensation; *e.g.,* light and sound waves that stimulate, respectively, visual and auditory receptors.

conditioned s., **(1)** a s. applied to one of the sense organs (*e.g.,* receptors of vision, hearing, touch) which are an essential and integral part of the neural mechanism underlying a conditioned reflex; **(2)** a neutral s., when paired with the unconditioned s. in simultaneous presentation to an organism, capable of eliciting a given response.

discriminant s., a s. which can be differentiated from all other s. in the environment because it has been, and continues to serve as, an indicator of a potential reinforcer.

heterologous s., a s. that acts upon any part of the sensory apparatus or nerve tract.

homologous s., a s. that acts only on the nerve terminations in a special sense organ.

inadequate s., subthreshold or subliminal s.; a s. too weak to evoke a response.

liminal s., threshold s.

maximal s., a s. strong enough to evoke a maximal response.

square wave stimuli, electrical stimulation in which the intensity of the current is brought suddenly to a given level and maintained at that level until it suddenly is cut off; this type of s. is particularly useful in obtaining a strength-duration curve.

subliminal s., inadequate s.

subthreshold s., inadequate s.

supramaximal s., a s. having strength significantly above the minimum required to activate all of the nerve or muscle fibers in contact with the electrode; used when response of all the fibers is desired despite a general decrease in their irritability.

threshold s., liminal s.; a s. of threshold strength, *i.e.,* one just strong enough to excite. See also adequate s.

train-of-four s., a method for measuring magnitude and type of neuromuscular blockade, based upon the ratio of the amplitude of the fourth evoked mechanical response to the first one, when four supramaximal 2-Hz electrical currents are applied for 2 seconds to a peripheral motor nerve.

unconditioned s., a s. that elicits an unconditioned response; *e.g.,* food is an unconditioned s. for salivation, which in turn is an unconditioned response in a hungry animal.

stimulus word. The word used in association tests to evoke a response.

sting. **1.** Sharp momentary pain, most commonly produced by the puncture of the skin by many species of arthropods, including hexapods, myriapods, and arachnids; can also be produced by jellyfish, sea urchins, sponges, mollusks, and several species of venomous fish, such as the stingray, toadfish, rabbitfish, and catfish. See also bites. **2.** The venom apparatus of a stinging animal, consisting of a chitinous spicule or bony spine and a venom gland or sac. **3.** To introduce (or the process of introducing) a venom by stinging.

stink weed. *Datura stramonium.*

stippling (stip'ling). **1.** Punctate basophilia; a speckling of a blood cell or other structure with fine dots when exposed to the action of a basic stain, due to the presence of free basophil granules in the cell protoplasm. **2.** An orange peel appearance of the attached gingiva. **3.** A roughening of the surfaces of a denture base to stimulate natural gingival s.

geographic s. of nails, regularly arranged longitudinal s. found

commonly in psoriasis and occasionally in alopecia areata.
Ziemann's s., Ziemann's *dots.*

Stirling, William, British histologist and physiologist, 1851–1932. See S.'s modification of Gram's *stain.*

stirrup (ster'ŭp, stir'ŭp) [A.S. *stīrāp*]. Stapes.

stitch [A.S. *stice,* a pricking]. **1.** A sharp sticking pain of momentary duration. **2.** A single suture. **3.** Suture (2).

STM Abbreviation for short-term *memory.*

Stock, Wolfgang, German ophthalmologist, 1874–1956. See Spielmeyer-S. *disease.*

stock (stok) [A.S. *stoc*] All the populations of organisms derived from an isolate without any implication of homogeneity or characterization.

Stocker, Frederick William, U.S. ophthalmologist, 1893–1974. See S.'s *line.*

stocking (stok'ing). Edema of the leg in the horse.

Stoerk, Karl, Austrian laryngologist, 1832–1899. See S.'s *blennorrhea.*

Stoffel, Adolf, German orthopedic surgeon, 1880–1937. See S.'s *operation.*

stoichiology (stoy-kē-ol'-ō-jē) [G. *stoicheion,* element (lit. one of a row), fr. *stoichos,* a row, + *logos,* study]. The science concerned with the elements or principles in any branch of knowledge, especially in chemistry, cytology, or histology.

stoichiometric (stoy'kē-ō-met'rik). Pertaining to stoichiometry.

stoichiometry (stoy-kē-om'ĕ-trē) [G. *stoicheion,* element, + *metron,* measure]. Determination of the relative quantities of the substances concerned in any chemical reaction; *e.g.,* with the laws of definite proportions in chemistry, as in the molar proportions in a reaction.

stoke (stōk) [Sir George Gabriel *Stokes,* British mathematician and physicist, 1819–1903]. A unit of kinematic viscosity, that of a fluid with a viscosity of 1 poise and a density of 1 g/ml.

Stokes, Sir William, Irish surgeon, 1839–1900. See S.'s or Gritti-S. *amputation.*

Stokes, William, Irish physician, 1804–1878. See S.'s *law;* Cheyne-S. *psychosis, respiration;* S.-Adams, Adams-S. *disease;* Morgagni-Adams-S. *syndrome.*

stolon (stō'lon) [L. *stolō,* branch, shoot, twig]. A runner or connective aerial hypha that forms a cluster of rhizoids when it touches the substrate, and then sends out other runners to produce the aerial mycelium and sporangiosphores typical of *Rhizopus.*

stom-. See stomato-.

stoma, pl. **stomas, stomata** (stō'mă, stō'maz, stō'mă-tă) [G. a mouth]. **1.** A minute opening or pore. **2.** Mouth. **3.** An artificial opening between two cavities or canals, or between such and the surface of the body.
Fuchs' s.'s, small depression on the surface of the iris near the margin of the pupil.
loop s., a specialized s. of intestine or ureter by which a loop of the hollow viscus is brought through an opening in the abdominal wall, with an opening created in the apex of the viscus to allow egress of its contents.

stomach (stŭm'ŭk) [G. *stomachos,* L. *stomachus*]. Ventriculus (1); gaster; a large irregularly piriform sac between the esophagus and the small intestine, lying just beneath the diaphragm; when distended it is 25 to 28 cm in length and 10 to 10.5 cm in its greatest diameter, and has a capacity of about 1 liter. Its wall has four coats or tunics: mucous, submucous, muscular, and peritoneal; the muscular coat is composed of three layers, the fibers running longitudinally in the outer, circularly in the middle, and obliquely in the inner layer.

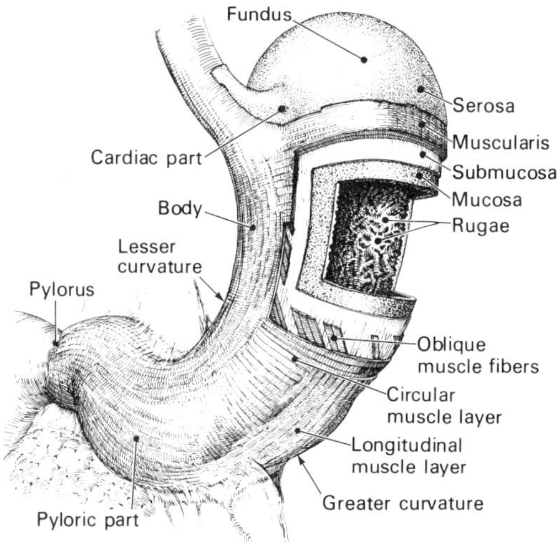

Parts of Human Stomach

bilocular s., hourglass s.
cascade s., a radiographic diagnosis in which the gastric cardia serves as a reservoir until sufficient volume is present to spill (cascade) into the antrum; previously said to cause symptoms of postprandial distention and inability to belch, but probably normal.
drain-trap s., water-trap s.
hourglass s., bilocular s.; ectasia ventriculi paradoxa; a condition in which there is a central constriction of the wall of the s. dividing it into two cavities, cardiac and pyloric.

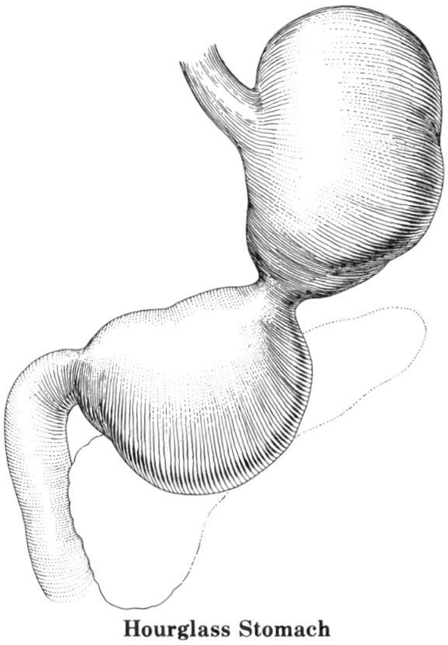

Hourglass Stomach

leather-bottle s., sclerotic s.; marked thickening and rigidity of the s. wall, with reduced capacity of the lumen although often without obstruction; nearly always due to scirrhous carcinoma, as in linitis plastica.
miniature s., Pavlov *pouch.*
Pavlov s., Pavlov *pouch.*
powdered s., the dried and powdered defatted wall of the s. of the hog, *Sus scrofa;* it contains thermolabile factors including native vitamin B_{12} and intrinsic factor; has been used in the treatment of pernicious anemia.

sclerotic s., leather-bottle s.
thoracic s., a condition in which part or all of the s. is contained within the thorax; a variant of hiatal hernia.
trifid s., a condition in which the s. is divided by two constrictions into three pouches.
wallet s., a form of dilated s. in which there is a general baglike distention, the antrum and fundus being indistinguishable.
water-trap s., drain-trap s.; a ptotic and dilated s., having a relatively high (though normally placed) pyloric outlet which is held up by the gastrohepatic ligament.

stomachal (stŭm'ă-kăl). Stomachic (1); relating to the stomach.

stomachalgia (stŭm-ă-kal'jē-ă) [stomach + G. *algos,* pain]. Obsolete term for stomach *ache.*

stomachic (sto'mak'ik). **1.** Stomachal. **2.** An agent that improves appetite and digestion.

stomachodynia (stŭm'ă-kō-din'ē-ă) [stomach + G. *odynē,* pain]. Obsolete term for stomach *ache.*

stomal (stō'măl). Relating to a stoma.

stomat-. See stomato-.

stomata (stō'mă-tă). Alternate plural of stoma.

stomatal (stō'mă-tăl). Relating to a stoma.

stomatalgia (stō-mă-tal'jē-ă) [stomat- + G. *algos,* pain]. Stomatodynia; pain in the mouth.

stomatic (stō-mat'ik). Relating to the mouth; oral.

stomatitis (stō-mă-tī'tis) [stomat- + G. *-itis,* inflammation]. Inflammation of the mucous membrane of the mouth.
angular s., angulus infectiosus; an inflammation at the corners of the mouth usually associated with a wrinkled or fissured epithelium, stopping at the mucocutaneous junction and not involving the mucosa; variously caused by riboflavin deficiency, monilial infection, and maceration from overhang of the upper lips, common in denture wearers.
aphthobullous s., the type of s. occurring in foot-and-mouth disease, characterized by vesication and ulceration.
aphthous s., aphthae (2).
bovine papular s., s. papulosa; a *Parapoxvirus* infection of cattle causing oral lesions.
gangrenous s., s. characterized by necrosis of oral tissue. See noma.
gonococcal s., inflammatory and ulcerative oral lesions resulting from infection with *Neisseria gonorrhoeae;* usually primary as a result of oral-genital contact, but occasionally is the result of gonococcemia.
lead s., oral manifestation of lead poisoning consisting of a bluish-black line following the contours of the marginal gingiva where lead sulfide has precipitated due to the inflamed environment.
s. medicamento'sa, inflammatory alterations of the oral mucosa associated with a systemic drug allergy; lesions may consist of erythema, vesicles, bullae, ulcerations, or angioneurotic edema.
mercurial s., alterations of the oral mucosa arising from chronic mercury poisoning; may consist of mucosal erythema and edema, ulceration, and deposition of mercurial sulfide in inflamed tissues, resulting in oral pigmentation resembling that of lead s.
s. papulo'sa, bovine papular s.
primary herpetic s., first infection of oral tissues with herpes simplex virus; characterized by gingival inflammation, vesicles, and ulcers.
recurrent aphthous s., aphthae (2).
recurrent herpetic s., reactivation of herpes simplex virus inflection, characterized by vesticles and ulceration limited to the hard palate and attached gingiva.
recurrent ulcerative s., aphthae (2).
ulcerative s., aphthae (2).
s. venena'ta, localized allergic alterations of the oral mucous membranes (*e.g.,* erythema, edema, vesiculation, and ulceration) caused by direct contact with the offending agent, (*e.g.,* drugs, dentifrices).
vesicular s., a vesicular disease of horses, cattle, swine, and occasionally man caused by a vesiculovirus (vesicular stomatitis virus); in horses and cattle the disease usually causes mouth vesicles which, in cattle, cannot be differentiated clinically from those of foot-and-mouth disease.

stomato-, stom-, stomat- [G. *stoma,* mouth]. Combining forms denoting mouth.

stomatocatharsis (stō'mă-tō-kă-thar'sis) [stomato- + G. *katharsis,* purgation, cleansing]. Disinfection of the oral cavity.

stomatocyte (stō'mă-tō-sīt). A red blood cell that exhibits a slit or mouth-shaped pallor rather than a central one on air-dried smears; *e.g.,* Rh null cells.

stomatocytosis (stō'mă-tō-sī-tō'sis). A hereditary deformation of red blood cells, which are swollen and cup-shaped, causing congenital hemolytic anemia. See also Rh null *syndrome.*

stomatodeum (stō'mă-tō-dē'ŭm). Stomodeum (1).

stomatodynia (stō'mă-tō-din'ē-ă) [stomato- + G. *odynē,* pain]. Stomatalgia.

stomatodysodia (stō'mă-tō-di-sō'dē-ă) [stomato- + G. *dysōdia,* bad odor]. Halitosis.

stomatognathic (stō'mă-tog-nath'ik) [stomato- + G. *gnathos,* jaw]. Pertaining to the physiology of the mouth.

stomatologic (stō'mă-tō-loj'ik). Relating to stomatology.

stomatologist (stō-mă-tol'ō-jist). A specialist in diseases of oral cavity, membranes, and tissues.

stomatology (stō-mă-tol'ō-jē) [stomato- + G. *logos,* study]. The study of the structures, functions, and diseases of the mouth.

stomatomalacia (stō'mă-tō-mă-lā'shē-ă) [stomato- + G. *malakia,* softness]. Pathologic softening of any of the structures of the mouth.

stomatomy (stō-mat'ō-mē). Stomatotomy.

stomatomycosis (stō'mă-tō-mī-kō'sis) [stomato- + G. *mykēs,* fungus, + *-osis,* condition]. Disease of the mouth due to the presence of a microscopic fungus.

stomatonecrosis (stō'mă-tō-nĕ-krō'sis) [stomato- + G. *nekrōsis,* death]. Noma.

stomatonoma (stō'mă-tō-nō'mă) [stomato- + G. *nomē,* a spreading (sore)]. Noma.

stomatopathy (stō-mă-top'ă-thē) [stomato- + G. *pathos,* suffering]. Stomatosis; any disease of the oral cavity.

stomatoplastic (stō'mă-tō-plas'tik). Relating to stomatoplasty.

stomatoplasty (stō'mă-tō-plas-tē) [stomato- + G. *plastos,* formed]. Plastic surgery of the mouth.

stomatorrhagia (stō'mă-tō-rā'jē-ă) [stomato- + G. *rhēgnymi,* to burst forth]. Bleeding from the gums or other part of the oral cavity.

stomatoscope (stō'mă-tō-skōp) [stomato- + G. *skopeō,* to view]. An apparatus for illuminating the interior of the mouth to facilitate examination.

stomatosis (stō-mă-tō'sis) [stomato- + G. *-osis,* condition]. Stomatopathy.

stomatotomy (stō-mă-tot'ō-mē) [stomato- + G. *tomē,* incision]. Stomatomy; surgical incision of the cervix uteri to facilitate labor.

stomion (stō'mē-on). The median point of the oral slit when the lips are closed.

stomocephalus (stō'mō-sef'ă-lŭs) [G. *stoma,* mouth, + *kephalē,* head]. Malformed individual with undeveloped jaw and a snoutlike mouth; likely to be combined with an ethmocephalic type of cyclopia.

stomodeal (stō'mō-dē'ăl). Relating to a stomodeum.

stomodeum (stō-mō-dē'ŭm) [Mod. L. fr. G. *stoma,* mouth, + *hodaios,* on the way, fr. *hodos,* a way]. **1.** Stomatodeum; a midline ectodermal depression ventral to the embryonic brain and surrounded by the mandibular arch; when the buccopharyngeal membrane disappears it becomes continuous with the foregut and forms the mouth. **2.** The anterior portion of the insect alimentary canal, consisting of mouth, buccal cavity, pharynx, esophagus, crop (frequently a diverticulum), and the proventriculus.

Stomoxys calcitrans (stō-mok'sis kal'si-tranz) [Mod. L., fr. C. *stoma,* mouth, + *oxys,* sharp; L. pres. p. of *calcitro,* to kick, fr. *calx,* the heel]. The stable fly, a species of biting fly, resembling in size and general appearance the common housefly, which is an annoying pest of man and domestic animals worldwide and is implicated in the mechanical transmission of diseases such as trypanosomiasis, anthrax, and equine infectious anemia. It is especially important in the spread of surra by transmitting *Trypanosoma evansi,* and also serves as intermediate host for *Habronema,* and for the deer filaria, *Setaria cervi.*

-stomy [G. *stoma,* mouth]. Combining form denoting artificial or surgical opening.

stone (stōn) [A.S. *stān*] **1.** Calculus. **2.** An English unit of weight of the human body, equal to 14 pounds.
artificial s., a specially calcined gypsum derivative similar to plaster of Paris, but stronger, because the grains are nonporous.
philosopher's s., a s. sought by the alchemists of the Middle Ages which was supposedly able to transmute base metals into gold, to make precious s.'s, and to cure all ills, and thus confer longevity; it was also believed to be a universal solvent.
pulp s., endolith.
skin s.'s, *calcinosis* cutis.
tear s., dacryolith.
vein s., phlebolith.

Stookey, Byron, U.S. neurosurgeon, 1887–1966. See S.-Scarff *operation,* Queckenstedt-S. *test.*

stool (stūl) [A.S. *stōl,* seat]. Movement (2); motion (3). **1.** A discharging of the bowels. **2.** Evacuation (2); the matter discharged at one movement of the bowels.
butter s.'s, fatty s.'s, occurring especially in steatorrhea.
rice-water s., a watery fluid containing whitish flocculi, discharged from the bowel in cholera and occasionally in other cases of serous diarrhea.
spinach s.'s, dark greenish porridge-like s.'s, resembling chopped spinach.
Trélat's s.'s, glairy s.'s streaked with blood, occurring in proctitis.

stops. Bends in, or wires soldered to, an archwire to limit passage through a bracket or tube.

storage (stōr'ij). The second stage in the memory process, following encoding and preceding retrieval, involving mental processes associated with retention of stimuli that have been registered and modified by encoding.

storax (stōr'aks) [G. *styrax,* a sweet-smelling gum]. Styrax; a liquid balsam obtained from the wood and inner bark of *Liquidamber orientalis,* a tree of Asia Minor, or *L. styraciflua* (family Hamamelidaceae); has been used in the treatment of chronic inflammation of the mucous membranes, and externally for scabies.

storiform (stōr'i-fōrm) [L. *storea,* woven mat, + *-formis,* form]. Having a cartwheel pattern, as of spindle cells with elongated nuclei radiating from a center.

storm (stōrm). An exacerbation of symptoms or a crisis in the course of a disease.
thyroid s., thyrotoxic *crisis.*

Stout's wiring. See under wiring.

STPD Symbol indicating that a gas volume has been expressed as if it were at standard temperature (0°C), standard pressure (760 mm Hg absolute), dry; under these conditions a mole of gas occupies 22.4 liters.

strabismal, strabismic (stra-biz'măl, -mik). Relating to or affected with strabismus.

strabismometer (stra-biz-mom'ĕ-ter) [G. *strabismos,* a squinting, + *metron,* measure]. Strabometer; an obsolete instrument having a plate with the upper margin curved, to conform with the lower lid, and marked in millimeters or fractions of an inch, used to measure the lateral deviation in strabismus.

strabismus (stra-biz'mŭs) [Mod. L., fr. G. *strabismos,* a squinting]. Crossed eyes; heterotropia; squint (1); a manifest lack of parallelism of the visual axes of the eyes.
A-s., **(1)** s. in which esotropia is more marked in looking upward than downward; **(2)** s. in which exotropia is more marked on looking downward than upward.
accommodative s., s. in which the severity of deviation varies with accomodation.
alternate day s., cyclic *esotropia.*
alternating s., a form of s. in which either eye fixes.
concomitant s., a condition in which the degree of s. is the same in all directions of gaze.
convergent s., esotropia.

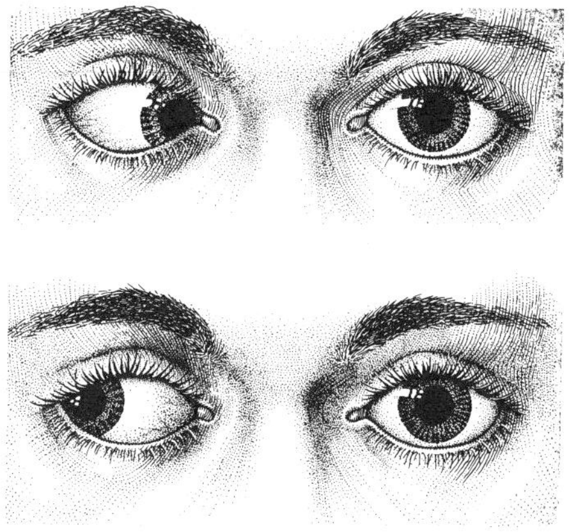

Strabismus
Upper, esotropia; *lower,* exotropia.

cyclic s., a s. that appears and disappears in rhythym, most frequently at 48-hour intervals.
s. deor'sum ver'gens, hypotropia; vertical s. in which the visual axis of one eye deviates downward.
divergent s., exotropia.
external s., exotropia.
incomitant s., paralytic s.
internal s., esotropia.
kinetic s., s. due to spasm of an extraocular muscle.
manifest s., evident deviation of one eye or the other; may be alternating or monocular.
mechanical s., s. due to restriction of action of the ocular muscle within the orbit.
monocular s., s. in which one eye habitually deviates.
paralytic s., incomitant s.; s. due to weakness or adhesion of ocular muscles.
s. sur'sum ver'gens, hypertropia; vertical s. in which the visual axis of one eye deviates upward.
vertical s., a form of s. in which the visual axis of one eye deviates upward (s. sursum vergens) or downward (s. deorsum vergens).

X-s., s. in which exotropia is more marked when looking upward or downward than when looking straight ahead.

strabometer (stră-bom'ĕ-ter). Strabismometer.

strabotome (strab'ō-tōm). An obsolete knife for use in performing strabotomy.

strabotomy (stra-bot'ō-mē) [G. *strabismos,* strabismus, + *tomē,* a cutting]. Obsolete term for division of one or more of the ocular muscles or their tendons for the correction of squint.

strain (strān) [A.S. *stryand; streōnan,* to beget]. **1.** A population of homogeneous organisms possessing a set of defined characters; in bacteriology, the set of descendants that originates from a common ancestor and retains the characteristics of the ancestor; members of a s. that subsequently differ from the original isolate are regarded as belonging either to a substrain of the original s., or to a new s. **2.** A hereditary tendency. **3.** [L. *stringere,* to bind]. To make an effort to the limit of one's strength. **4.** To injure by overuse or improper use. **5.** An act of straining. **6.** Injury resulting from s. or overuse. **7.** The change in shape that a body undergoes when acted upon by an external force. **8.** To filter; to percolate.

auxotrophic s.'s, s.'s which are derived from the prototrophic s. but which require extra growth factors.

carrier s., pseudolysogenic s.; a bacterial s. that is contaminated with a bacteriophage of low infectivity.

cell s., in tissue culture, cells derived from a single cell (clone) and possessing a specific feature such as a marker chromosome, antigen, or resistance to a virus.

congenic s., an inbred s. of animals produced by continued crossing of a gene of one line onto another inbred (isogenic) line.

HFR s., Hfr s. [*h* igh *f* reguency of *r* ecombination], a s., or clone, in which a conjugative plasmid (such as an F'), integrated in the bacterial genome, is instrumental in the transfer (along with plasmid DNA) of integrated bacterial DNA in a sequential manner to a suitable recipient.

hypothetical mean s. (HMS), a hypothetical s. that possesses the characteristics of a calculated mean organism.

isogenic s., pure line; a s. of animals inbred for many generations and homozygous for certain specified genes.

lysogenic s., a s. of bacterium that is infected with a temporate bacteriophage. See lysogeny.

neotype s., neotype culture; a s. accepted by international agreement to replace a type s. which is no longer in existence or to serve as the type s. if a type s. was not designated and if no s. exists which can be designated as the type.

prototrophic s.'s, s.'s that have the same nutritional requirements as the wild-type s.

pseudolysogenic s., carrier s.

recombinant s., see recombinant (1).

stock s., a bacterial or other microbial s. that has been maintained under laboratory conditions as representative of its type.

type s., the nomenclatural type of a species or subspecies.

wild-type s., a s. found in nature or a standard s. See also auxotrophic s.'s and protrophic s.'s.

strait (strāt) [M.E. *streit* thr. O. Fr. fr. L. *strictus,* drawn together, tight]. A narrow passageway. **Inferior s.,** *apertura* pelvis superior; **superior s.,** *apertura* pelvis superior.

straitjacket (strāt'jak-et). Camisole; a garment-like device with long sleeves that can be secured to restrain a violently disturbed person.

stramonium (stra-mō'nē-ŭm) [Mod. L.]. The dried leaves and flowering or fruiting tops with branches of *Datura stramonium* or *D. tatula* (family Solanaceae), a herb abounding in temperate and subtropical countries; it contains an alkaloid, daturine, identical with hyoscyamine. It is an antispasmodic and has been used in the treatment of asthma and parkinsonism; when abused or taken inadvertently, it may cause an atropine-like toxic psychosis.

strand. In microbiology, a filamentous or threadlike structure.

complementary s., minus s., see replicative *form.*

viral s., plus s., see replicative *form.*

Strandberg, J.V., 20th century Swedish dermatologist. See Grönblad-S. *syndrome.*

strangalesthesia (strang'gal-es-thē'zē-ă) [G. *strangalē,* halter, + *aisthēsis,* sensation]. Zonesthesia.

strangle (strang'gl) [G. *strangaloō,* to choke, fr. *strangalē,* a halter]. To suffocate; to choke; to compress the trachea so as to prevent sufficient passage of air.

strangles (strang'glz). An acute infectious disease in the horse, marked by mucopurulent nasal catarrh and edematous and hemorrhagic nasal and pharyngeal respiratory passages with enlargement and suppuration of associated lymph nodes; it is caused by *Streptococcus equi* and affects chiefly horses under the age of five years.

strangulated (strang'gyū-lā-ted) [L. *strangulo,* pp. *-atus,* to choke, fr. G. *strangaloō,* to choke (strangle)]. Constricted so as to prevent sufficient passage of air, as through the trachea, or to cut off venous return, as in the case of a hernia.

strangulation (strang'gyū-lā'shŭn). The act of strangulating or the condition of being strangulated, in any sense.

strangury (strang'gyū-rē) [G. *stranx* (*strang-*), something squeezed out, a drop, + *ouron,* urine]. Difficulty in micturition, the urine being passed drop by drop with pain and tenesmus.

strap [A.S. *stropp*] **1.** A strip of adhesive plaster. **2.** To apply overlapping strips of adhesive plaster.

Strassburg, Gustav A., German physiologist, *1848. See S.'s *test.*

Strassman, Paul F., German gynecologist, 1866–1938. See S.'s *phenomenon.*

strata (strā'tă, strat'ă). Plural of stratum.

stratification (strat'i-fi-kā'shŭn) [L. *stratum,* layer, + *facio,* to make]. An arrangement in the form of layers or strata.

stratified (strat'i-fīd). Arranged in the form of layers or strata.

stratigraphy (stra-tig'ră-fē) [L. *stratum,* layer, + G. *graphē,* a writing]. Tomography.

STRATUM

stratum, gen. **strati,** pl. **strata** (strat'ŭm, strā'tŭm, tī, tă) [L. *sterno,* pp. *stratus,* to spread out, strew, ntr. of pp. as noun, *stratum,* a bed cover, layer]. One of the layers of differentiated tissue, the aggregate of which forms any given structure, such as the retina or the skin. See also lamina, layer.

s. aculea'tum, obsolete term for s. spinosum.

s. al'bum profun'dum, a layer of myelinated fibers, the deepest layer of the colliculus superior, delimiting the latter from the central gray substance surrounding the cerebral aqueduct.

s. basa'le, basal layer; **(1)** the outermost layer of the endometrium which undergoes only minimal changes during the menstrual cycle; **(2)** s. basale epidermidis.

s. basa'le epider'midis, s. cylindricum or germinitivum; s. basale (2); palisade, columnar, or basal cell layer; the deepest layer of the epidermis, composed of dividing stem cells and anchoring cells.

s. cerebra'le ret'inae, pars optica retinae; cerebral or neural layer of the retina; optic part of the retina; the internal layer of the retina containing the neural elements, as distinguished from the outer leaf of the retina, or stratum pigmenti.

s. cine'reum collic'uli superio'ris, s. griseum colliculi superioris.

s. circula're membra'nae tym'pani, circular layer of tympanic membrane; circular fibers deep to the radiate layer of the mem-

brane which are more abundant near the periphery; not present in the pars flaccida.
s. circula're tu'nicae muscula'ris co'li [NA], circular layer of the muscular tunic of the colon.
s. circula're tu'nicae muscula'ris intesti'ni ten'uis [NA], circular layer of the muscular tunic of the small intestine.
s. circula're tu'nicae muscula'ris rec'ti [NA], circular layer of the muscular tunic of the rectum.
s. circula're tu'nicae muscula'ris ventric'uli [NA], circular layer of the muscular tunic of the stomach.
s. compac'tum, compacta; the superficial layer of decidual tissue in the pregnant uterus, in which the interglandular tissue preponderates.
s. cor'neum epider'midis, corneal or horny layer of epidermis; the outer layer of the epidermis, consisting of several layers of flat keratinized non-nucleated cells.
s. cor'neum un'guis, cornified or horny layer of the nail; the outer, horny layer of the nail.
s. cuta'neum membra'nae tym'pani, cutaneous layer of the tympanic membrane; the thin layer of skin on the external surface of the tympanic membrane.
s. cylin'dricum, s. basale epidermidis.
s. disjunc'tum, the layer of partly detached cells on the free surface of the s. corneum, as seen in sections under the microscope; an artifact of fixation.
s. fibro'sum [NA], *membrana* fibrosa.
s. functiona'le, the endometrium except for the s. basale; formerly believed to be lost during menstruation but now considered to be only partially disrupted.
s. gangliona're ner'vi op'tici, ganglionic layer of the optic nerve; the inner layer of multipolar neurons in the retina consisting of the relatively large neurons that give rise to the fibers of the optic nerve.
s. gangliona're ret'inae, ganglionic layer of the retina; s. nucleare internum retinae; the intermediate layer of neurons in the retina composed largely of bipolar cells.
s. ganglio'sum cerebel'li, s. gangliosum cerebelli.
s. germinati'vum, s. basale epidermidis.
s. germinati'vum un'guis, germinative layer of nail; the deeper layer of the nail that is continuous with the s. germinativum of the surrounding skin and from which the nail plate is continuously formed.
s. granulo'sum cerebel'li [NA], granular layer of the cerebellar cortex; the deepest of the three layers of the cortex; it contains large numbers of granule cells, the dendrites of which synapse with incoming mossy fibers in cerebellar glomeruli. Thin, unmyelinated axons of granule cells ascend perpendicularly into the s. moleculare in which they bifurcate into fibers coursing parallel to the long axis of the cerebellar folia. Parallel fibers form numerous synapses with the dendrites of Purkinje cells, basket cells, and stellate cells.
s. granulo'sum epider'midis [NA], granular layer of epidermis; a layer of somewhat flattened cells containing granules of keratohyalin and lying just above the s. spinosum and deeply to the s. corneum.
s. granulo'sum follic'uli ova'rici vesiculo'si, granular layer of a vesicular ovarian follicle; s. granulosum ovarii; granulosa; membrana granulosa; the layer of small cells that forms the wall of an ovarian follicle.
s. granulo'sum ova'rii, s. granulosum folliculi ovarici vesiculosi.
s. gris'eum collic'uli superio'ris [NA], gray layer(s) of the superior colliculus; s. cinereum colliculi superioris; term applied to any one of the three major layers of gray matter of the superior colliculus that alternate with layers composed chiefly of nerve fibers: 1) the s. griseum superficiale, superficial gray layer, above the largely white layer of the incoming fibers of the optic tract (s. opticum); 2) s. griseum medium, placed between the s. opticum and a more deeply located layer of fibers, the s. lemnisci; 3) s. griseum profundum, between the s. lemnisci and the central gray substance surrounding the cerebral aqueduct, and containing the large nerve cells from which most of the colliculus descending connections (tractus tectobulbaris, tectopontinus, and tectospinalis) originate.
s. gris'eum me'dium, see s. griseum colliculi superioris.
s. gris'eum profun'dum, see s. griseum colliculi superioris.
s. gris'eum superficia'le, see s. griseum colliculi superioris.
s. interoliva're lemnis'ci, the medial region of the medulla oblongata between the left and right olivary nucleus, traversed longitudinally by the left and right medial lemniscus, and transversally by the decussating olivocerebellar fibers.
s. lemnis'ci, fillet layer; a largely fibrous (hence whitish) layer of the superior colliculus separating the s. griseum medium from the s. griseum profundum and containing, among others, fibers from the spinal and trigeminal lemnisci.
s. longitudina'le tu'nicae muscula'ris co'li [NA], longitudinal layer of the muscular tunic of the colon.
s. longitudina'le tu'nicae muscula'ris intesti'ni ten'uis [NA], longitudinal layer of the muscular tunic of the small intestine.
s. longitudina'le tu'nicae muscula'ris rec'ti [NA], longitudinal layer of the muscular tunic of the rectum.
s. longitudina'le tu'nicae muscula'ris ventric'uli [NA], longitudinal layer of the muscular tunic of the stomach.
s. lu'cidum, clear layer of epidermis; a layer of lightly staining corneocytes in the deepest level of the s. corneum; found only in the thick epidermis of the palmar and plantar skin.
malpighian s., malpighian layer or rete; the living layer of the epidermis comprising the s. basale, s. spinosum, and s. granulosum.
s. molecula're, molecular or plexiform layer; term applied to any layer of brain tissue that contains few nerve-cell bodies and is composed largely of terminal arborizations of dendrites and axons; notable examples are the superficial layer (first layer) of the cerebral cortex (see *cortex* cerebri) and the s. moleculare cerebelli.
s. molecula're cerebel'li [NA], molecular layer of the cerebellar cortex; the outer lamina of the cortex, containing the cell bodies and dendrites of Purkinje cells, the axons of the granule cells, and the cell bodies, dendrites, and axons of basket cells.
s. molecula're ret'inae, name applied to each of the plexiform layers of the retina.
s. neuroepithelia'le ret'inae, neuroepithelial layer of the retina; s. nucleare externum retinae; the outermost layer of the pars optica retinae, composed of the primary receptor cells of the retina; the s. consists of two sublayers: 1) an external layer made up of the rods and cones, the photosensitive processes of the receptor cells, and 2) the external nuclear layer containing the cell bodies of these cells; the external limiting membrane forms a perforated supporting plate between the two sublayers; the name refers to the fact that the retinal receptor cells are a specialized form of (epithelial) ependyma cell and thus, in a sense, are comparable to the neuroepithelial cells (*e.g.,* hair cells) of other sense organs.
s. neurono'rum pirifor'mium [NA], layer of piriform neurons; s. gangliosum cerebelli; ganglionic layer of the cerebellar cortex; Purkinje's layer; the layer of Purkinje cells between the molecular and granular layers of the cerebellar cortex. See also Purkinje *cell.*
s. nuclea're exter'num et inter'num ret'inae, nuclear *layers* of the retina.
s. nuclea're exter'num ret'inae, s. neuroepitheliale retinae.
s. nuclea're inter'num ret'inae, s. ganglionare retinae.
s. op'ticum, optic layer; **(1)** a layer of white matter interspersed with nerve-cell bodies, immediately below the s. griseum superficialis of the superior colliculus, composed of myelinated fibers originating in the retina and striate cortex; **(2)** the inner layer of the retina, consisting of the fibers originating from the cells of the s. ganglionare nervi optici; in their further course these fibers combine to form the optic nerve or optic tract.
s. papilla're cor'ii, papillary layer; corpus papillare; the more superficial layer of the corium whose papillae interdigitate with the

epidermis.
s. pigmen'ti bul'bi, s. pigmenti retinae.
s. pigmen'ti cor'poris cilia'ris, pigmented layer of the ciliary body; the continuation of the pigment layer of the retina onto the posterior aspect of the ciliary body.
s. pigmen'ti i'ridis, pigmented layer of the iris; the double layer of pigmented epithelium on the posterior surface of the iris.
s. pigmen'ti ret'inae, pigmented layer of the retina; s. pigmenti bulbi; tapetum nigrum; tapetum oculi; ectoretina; the outer layer of the retina, consisting of pigmented epithelium.
s. plexifor'me exter'num et inter'num ret'inae, plexiform *layers* of the retina.
s. radia'tum membra'nae tym'pani, radiate layer of tympanic membrane; the connective tissue layer of the tympanic membrane beneath the stratum cutaneum, the fibers of which radiate from the manubrium of the malleus to the peripheral fibrocartilaginous ring of the membrane; absent from the pars flaccida.
s. reticula're co'rii, s. reticulare cutis; reticular layer of corium; tunica propria corii; the thicker deep layer of the corium consisting of dense irregularly arranged connective tissue.
s. reticula're cu'tis, s. reticulare corii.
s. spino'sum epider'midis, spinous or prickle cell layer; the layer of polyhedral cells in the epidermis; shrinkage artifacts and adhesion of these cells at their desmosomal junctions gives a spiny or prickly appearance.
s. spongio'sum, the middle layer of the endometrium formed chiefly of dilated glandular structures; it is flanked by the compacta on the luminal side and the basalis on the myometrial side.
s. subcuta'neum, *tela* subcutanea.
s. synovia'le [NA], *membrana* synovialis.
s. zona'le [NA], zonular layer; **(1)** a thin layer of white substance covering the upper surface of the thalamus and forming part of the floor of the body of the lateral ventricle; **(2)** a layer of white substance on the surface of the superior colliculus.

Straus, Isidore, French physician, 1845–1896. See S. *reaction;* S.'s *sign.*

Strauss, Lotte, U.S. pathologist, *1913. See Churg-S. *syndrome.*

Straüssler. See Gerstman-S. *syndrome.*

streak (strēk) [A.S. *strica*]. A line, stria, or stripe, especially one that is indistinct or evanescent.
angioid s.'s, Knapp's s.'s or striae; breaks in the lamina vitrea of the eye occurring in a variety of systemic disorders affecting elastic tissue.
gonadal s., streaked gonad; a form of aplasia in which the ovary is replaced by a functionless tissue, as found in Turner's syndrome.
Knapp's s.'s, angioid s.'s.
meningitic s., Trousseau's spot; tache méningéale or cérébrale; a line of redness resulting from drawing a point across the skin, especially notable in cases of meningitis.
Moore's lightning s.'s, photopsia manifested by vertical flashes of light, seen usually on the temporal side of the affected eye, caused by the involutional shrinkage of vitreous humor.
primitive s., an ectodermal ridge in the midline at the caudal end of the embryonic disk from which arises the intraembryonic mesoderm; achieved by inward and then lateral migration of cells; in human embryos, it appears on day 15 and gives a cephalocaudal axis to the developing embryo.

stream (strēm). Flumen.
hair s.'s, *flumina* pilorum.

streaming (strēm'ing). See streaming *movement.*

streblodactyly (streb-lō-dak'ti-lē) [G. *streblos,* twisted, + *daktylos,* finger]. Campylodactyly.

Streeter, George L., U.S. embryologist, 1873–1948. See S.'s *bands, horizon(s).*

Streeter's horizon(s) [G.L. Streeter]. A term borrowed from geology and archeology by Streeter to define 23 developmental stages in young human embryos, from fertilization through the first 2 months; each horizon spanned 2 to 3 days and emphasized specific anatomic characteristics, to avoid discrepancies in the determination of age and body dimensions.

Streiff, E.B., Swiss ophthalmologist. See Hallermann-S. *syndrome.*

stremma (strem'ă) [G. a twist, fr. *strephō,* to twist]. Sprain.

strength. 1. The quality of being strong or powerful. **2.** The degree of intensity. **3.** The property of materials by which they endure the application of force without yielding or breaking.
associative s., in psychology, the s. of a stimulus response linkage as measured by the frequency with which a stimulus elicits a particular response.
biting s., *force* of mastication.
compressive s., tensile s., except that the stress is in compression.
fatigue s., the stress level below which a particular component will survive an indefinite number of load cycles (typically about 50% of the ultimate s. of the component).
ionic s., symbolized as $\Gamma/2$ and set equal to $\Sigma {}^1/_2\, c_i z_i^2$, where c_i equals the concentration and z_i the charge of each ion present in solution; a number of biochemically important events (*e.g.,* protein solubility and rate of enzyme action) vary with the ionic s. of a solution.
tensile s., the maximum tensile stress or load that a material is capable of sustaining; usually expressed in pounds per square inch.
ultimate s., the maximum stress achieved prior to failure of a component on a single application of the load.
yield s., the amount of stress at which a permanent (plastic) deformation in a component becomes measurable (usually taken as 0.2% permanent strain).

strephosymbolia (stref'ō-sim-bō'lē-ă) [G. *strephō,* to turn, + *symbolon,* a mark or sign]. **1.** Generally, the perception of objects reversed as if in a mirror. **2.** Specifically, difficulty in distinguishing written or printed letters that extend in opposite directions but are otherwise similar, such as *p* and *d,* or related kinds of mirror reversal.

strepitus (strep'i-tŭs) [L.]. Rarely used term for a noise, usually an auscultatory sound.

strepticemia (strep-ti-sē'mē-ă). Streptococcemia.

strepto- [G. *streptos,* twisted, fr. *strephō,* to twist]. Combining form denoting curved or twisted, usually relating to organisms thus described.

Streptobacillus (strep-tō-ba-sil'ŭs) [strepto- + bacillus]. A genus of nonmotile, nonsporeforming, aerobic to facultatively anaerobic bacteria (family Bacteroidaceae) containing Gram-negative, pleomorphic cells which vary from short rods to long, interwoven filaments which have a tendency to fragment into chains of bacillary and coccobacillary elements. These organisms are parasitic to pathogenic for rats, mice, and other mammals. The type species is *S. moniliformis.*
S. monilifor'mis, a species commonly found as an inhabitant of the nasopharynx of rats; it occurs as the etiologic agent of an epizootic septic polyarthritis in mice and of one type of rat-bite fever; it is the type species of the genus *S.*

streptobiosamine (strep'tō-bī-ō'să-mēn). A methylamino disaccharide (streptose + *N*-methyl-L-glucosamine), with the oxygen link between C-2 of streptose and C-1 of the glucosamine; with streptidine, it forms streptomycin.

streptobiose (strep-tō-bī'ōs). Old term for streptose.

streptocerciasis (strep'tō-ser-kī'ă-sis). Infection of man and higher primates with the nematode *Dipetalonema streptocerca.*

streptococcal (strep'tō-kok'ăl). Relating to or caused by any organism of the genus *Streptococcus.*

streptococcemia (strep'tō-kok-sē'-mē-ă) [streptococcus + G. *haima,* blood]. Strepticemia; streptosepticemia; the presence of streptococci in the blood.

streptococci (strep'tō-kok'sī). Plural of streptococcus.

streptococcic (strep'tō-kok'sik). Relating to or caused by any organism of the genus *Streptococcus.*

streptococcosis (strep'tō-kŏ-kō'sis). Any streptococcal infection.

Streptococcus (strep-tō-kok'ŭs) [strepto- + G. *kokkus,* berry (coccus)]. *Diplococcus;* a genus of nonmotile (with few exceptions), nonsporeforming, aerobic to facultatively anaerobic bacteria (family Lactobacillaceae) containing Gram-positive, spherical or ovoid cells which occur in pairs or short or long chains. Dextrorotatory lactic acid is the main product of carbohydrate fermentation. These organisms occur regularly in the mouth and intestines of humans and other animals, in dairy and other food products, and in fermenting plant juices. Some species are pathogenic. The type species is *S. pyogenes.*
S. acidomin'imus, a species found in the bovine vagina and on the skin of calves.
S. agalac'tiae, a species found in the milk and tissues from udders of cows with mastitis; also reported to be associated with a variety of human infections, especially those of the urogenital tract.
S. angino'sus, a species found in the human throat, sinuses, abscesses, vagina, skin, and feces; this organism has been associated with glomerular nephritis and various types of mild respiratory diseases.
S. bo'vis, a species found in the bovine alimentary tract; this organism may also be found in blood and heart lesions in cases of subacute endocarditis.
S. dur'ans, a species found in dried milk powder and in the intestines of humans and other animals.
S. dysgalac'tiae, a species causing acute mastitis in cattle.
S. e'qui, a species causing strangles in horses.
S. equi'nus, a species which is the predominant organism in the intestines of horses.
S. equisim'ilis, a species found in the normal human nose and throat, vagina, and skin; sometimes found in the respiratory tract of domestic animals; occasionally associated with erysipelas and puerperal fever.
S. faeca'lis, a species found in human feces and in the intestines of many warm-blooded animals; occasionally found in urinary infections and in blood and heart lesions in cases of subacute endocarditis; associated with European foul brood of bees and with mild outbreaks of food poisoning.
S. lac'tis, a species found commonly as a contaminant in milk and dairy products; a common cause of the souring and coagulation of milk; some strains produce nisin, a powerful antibiotic that inhibits the growth of many other Gram-positive organisms.
S. mi'tis, a species found in the human mouth, throat, and nasopharynx; ordinarily, it is not considered to be pathogenic, but this organism may be recovered from ulcerated teeth and sinuses and from blood and heart lesions in cases of subacute endocarditis.
S. mu'tans, a species associated with the production of dental caries in humans and in some other animals.
S. pneumo'niae, pneumococcus; Fraenkel's or Fraenkel-Weichselbaum pneumococcus; pneumonococcus; a species of Gram-positive, lancet-shaped diplococci frequently occurring in chains; cells are readily lysed by bile salts. Virulent forms are enclosed in type-specific polysaccharide capsules; there is also a specific somatic antigen (M protein) for each of the approximately 85 types, and a somatic C carbohydrate common to all types. Normal inhabitants of the respiratory tract, and perhaps the most common cause of lobar pneumonia, they are relatively common causative agents of meningitis, sinusitis, and other infections. It is the type species of the genus *Diplococcus.*
S. pyog'enes, a species found in the human mouth, throat, and respiratory tract and in inflammatory exudates, bloodstream, and lesions in human diseases; it is sometimes found in the udders of cows and in dust from sickrooms, hospital wards, schools, theaters, and other public places; it causes the formation of pus or even fatal septicemias. It is the type species of the genus *S.*
S. saliva'rius, a species found in the human mouth, throat, and nasopharynx.
S. san'guis, a species originally found in the so-called vegetation on heart valves from cases of subacute bacterial endocarditis; occasionally found in infected sinuses and teeth and in house dust.
S. u'beris, a species causing mastitis in cattle.
S. vir'idans, a name applied not to a distinct species but rather to the group of α-hemolytic streptococci as a whole; viridans streptococci have been isolated from the mouth and intestines of humans, the intestines of horses, the milk and feces of cows, milk and milk products, and the sputum and lungs in cases of primary atypical pneumonia.
S. zooepidem'icus, a species causing mastitis in cattle.

streptococcus, pl. **streptococci** (strep'tō-kok'ŭs, -kok'sī). A term used to refer to any member of the genus *Streptococcus.*
α-streptococci, streptococci that form a green variety of reduced hemoglobin in the area of the colony on a blood agar medium.
β-hemolytic streptococci, hemolytic streptococci; those that produce active hemolysins (O and S) which cause a zone of clear hemolysis on the blood agar medium in the area of the colony; β-hemolytic streptococci are divided into groups (A to O) on the basis of cell wall C carbohydrate (see Lancefield *classification*); Group A (strains pathogenic for man) comprises more than 50 types (designated by Arabic numerals) determined by cell wall M protein, which seems to be associated closely with virulence and is produced chiefly by strains with matt or mucoid colonies, in contrast to nonvirulent, glossy colony-producing strains; other surface protein antigens such as R and T (T substance), and the nucleoprotein fraction (P substance) seem to be of less importance. The more than 20 extracellular substances elaborated by strains of β-hemolytic streptococci include erythrogenic toxin (elaborated only by lysogenic strains), deoxyribonuclease (streptodornase), hemolysins (streptolysins O and S), hyaluronidase, and streptokinase.
hemolytic streptococci, β-hemolytic streptococci.

streptoderma (strep-tō-der'mă). Pyoderma due to streptococci.

streptodermatitis (strep'tō-der-mă-tī'tis). Inflammation of the skin caused by the action of streptococci.

streptodornase (SD) (strep-tō-dōr'nās). A "dornase" (deoxyribonuclease) obtained from streptococci; used with streptokinase to facilitate drainage in septic surgical conditions.

streptofuranose (strep-tō-fūr'ă-nōs). Streptose.

streptokinase (SK) (strep-tō-kī'nās) [EC 3.4.24.4]. Streptococcal fibrinolysin; plasminokinase; an extracellular metalloenzyme from hemolytic streptococci that cleaves plasminogen, producing plasmin, which causes the liquefaction of fibrin (same activity as staphylokinase and urokinase); usually used in conjunction with streptodornase.

streptokinase-streptodornase. A purified mixture containing streptokinase, streptodornase, and other proteolytic enzymes; used by topical application or by injection into body cavities to remove clotted blood and fibrinous and purulent accumulations of exudate.

streptolysin (strep-tol'i-sin). A hemolysin produced by streptococci.
s. O, a hemolysin that is produced by β-hemolytic streptococci and is hemolytically active only in the reduced state; anti-s. O produced during infection is of diagnostic significance.

Streptomyces (strep-tō-mī'sēz) [strepto- + G. *mykēs,* fungus]. A genus of nonmotile, aerobic, Gram-positive bacteria (family Streptomycetaceae) that grow in the form of a much-branched mycelium; conidia are produced in chains on aerial hyphae. These organisms (several hundred species in the genus) are predominantly saprophytic soil forms; some are parasitic on plants or animals; many produce antibiotics. The type species is *S. albus.*

S. al'bus, a species found in dust, soil, grains, and straw; some strains produce actinomycetin; others produce thiolutin or endomycin; it is the type species of the genus *S.*

S. gibso'nii, *Nocardia gibsonii;* a species found in human infections.

S. somalien'sis, a species that causes Bouffardi's white mycetoma.

Streptomycetaceae (strep'tō-mī-sĕ-tā'sē-ē). A family of aerobic Gram-positive bacteria (order Actinomycetales) that produce a vegetative mycelium which does not fragment into bacillary or coccoid forms; they produce conidia which are borne on sporophores. These organisms occur primarily in the soil; some are thermophiles found in rotting manure, a few are parasitic, and many produce antibiotics. The type genus is *Streptomyces.*

streptomycete (strep'tō-mī'sēt). A term used to refer to a member of the genus *Streptomyces;* it is sometimes improperly used to refer to any member of the family Streptomycetaceae.

streptomycin, streptomycin A (strep-tō-mī'sin). An antibiotic agent obtained from *Streptomyces griseus* that is active against the tubercle bacillus and a large number of Gram-positive and Gram-negative bacteria; also used in the form of dihydrostreptomycin (aldehyde of s. reduced to CH_2OH). It is a glucoside and contains streptidine and streptobiosamine linked by an oxygen bridge between C-4 of the inositol residue and C-1 of the streptose residue; s. B has a mannose residue attached to the glucosamine and is a natural product, with less activity than s. A.

streptomycosis (strep'tō-mī-kō'sis) [strepto- + G. *mykēs,* fungus, + *-osis,* condition]. Old term for streptococcemia.

streptonivicin (strep'tō-ni-vī'sin). Novobiocin.

streptose (strep'tōs). Streptofuranose; 5-deoxy-3-*C*-formyl-L-lyxose; an unusual pentose that is a component of streptobiosamine, hence of streptomycin.

streptosepticemia (strep'tō-sep-ti-sē'mē-ă). Streptococcemia.

streptothrichosis (strep'tō-thri-kō'sis). Streptotrichosis; streptotrichiasis; an infectious disease originally attributed to any of a variety of species of the now obsolete genus *Streptothrix* (*q.v.*); frequently characterized by a chronic suppurative inflamation with pus containing granules composed chiefly of colonies of the causal microorganism.

Streptothrix (strep'tō-thriks). An obsolete generic name of bacteria; the type species, *S. foersteri,* is not recognizable by modern standards. A number of the pathogenic species that were placed in this genus have subsequently been transferred to other genera (*e.g., Actinomyces israelii, Dermatophilus congolensis,* Nocardia madurae, *Streptobacillus moniliformis*).

streptotrichiasis (strep'tō-tri-kī'ă-sis). Streptothrichosis.

streptotrichosis (strep'tō-tri-kō'sis). Streptothrichosis.

streptozocin (strep-tō-zō'sin). 2-Deoxy-2-(3-methyl-3-nitrosoureido)-D-glucopyranose; an antineoplastic agent used in the treatment of mestatic islet-cell carcinoma of the pancreas.

stress (stres) [L. *strictus,* tight, fr. *stringo,* to draw together]. **1.** Reactions of the body to forces of a deleterious nature, infections, and various abnormal states that tend to disturb its normal physiologic equilibrium (homeostasis). **2.** The resisting force set up in a body as a result of an externally applied force. **3.** In dentistry, the forces set up in teeth, their supporting structures, and structures restoring or replacing teeth as a result of the force of mastication. **4.** The force or pressure applied or exerted between portions of a body or bodies, generally expressed in pounds per square inch. **5.** In rheology, the force in a material transmitted per unit area to adjacent layers. **6.** In psychology, a physical or psychological stimulus which, when impinging upon an individual, produces strain or disequilibrium.

life s., events or experiences that produce severe strain, *e.g.,* failure on the job, marital separation, loss of a love object.

shear s., the force acting in shear flow expressed in force per unit area; units in the CGS system: dynes/cm^2.

tensile s., a s. acting on a body per unit cross-sectional area so as to elongate the body.

yield s., the critical s. that must be applied to a material before it begins to flow, as in a Bingham plastic.

stress breaker. A device that relieves the abutment teeth, to which a fixed or removable partial denture is attached, of all or part of the forces generated by occlusal function.

stress riser. A mechanical defect, such as a hole, in bone or other materials that concentrates stress in the area.

stress shielding. Osteopenia occurring in bone as the result of removal of normal stress from the bone by an implant.

stretch'er [A.S. *streccan,* to stretch]. A litter, usually a sheet of canvas stretched to a frame with four handles, used for transporting the sick or injured.

stria, gen. and pl. **striae** (strī'ă, strī'ē) [L. channel, furrow]. Vergeture. **1.** Striation (1); a stripe, band, streak, or line, distinguished by color, texture, depression, or elevation from the tissue in which it is found. **2.** *Striae* cutis distensae.

acoustic striae, striae medullares ventriculi quarti.

stri'ae atroph'icae, striae cutis distensae.

auditory striae, striae medullares ventriculi quarti.

brown striae, Retzius' striae.

stri'ae cilia'res, shallow radial grooves on the surface of the orbiculus ciliaris extending from the teeth of the ora serrata and leading into the valleys between the ciliary processes.

stri'ae cu'tis disten'sae, bands of thin wrinkled skin, initially red but becoming purple and white, which occur commonly on the abdomen, buttocks, and thighs at puberty and/or during and following pregnancy, and result from atrophy of the dermis and overextension of the skin; also associated with ascites and Cushing's syndrome. Also called lineae albicantes or atrophicae; linear or traction atrophy; striae (2); striae atrophicae or gravidarum; vergeture.

s. for'nicis, s. medullaris thalami.

Gennari's s., *line* of Gennari.

stri'ae gravida'rum, striae cutis distensae.

Knapp's striae, angioid *streaks.*

stri'ae lanci'si, the s. longitudinalis lateralis and the s. longitudinalis medialis.

Langhans' s., fibrinoid that accumulates on the chorionic plate between the bases of placental villi during the first half of pregnancy.

lateral longitudinal s., s. longitudinalis lateralis.

s. longitudina'lis latera'lis [NA], lateral longitudinal s.; s. tecta; a thin longitudinal band of nerve fibers accompanied by gray matter, near each outer edge of the upper surface of the corpus callosum under cover of the gyrus cinguli.

s. longitudina'lis media'lis [NA], medial longitudinal s.; a thin longitudinal band of nerve fibers accompanied by gray matter, running along the surface of the corpus callosum on either side of the median line. Together with the s. longitudinalis lateralis it forms part of a thin layer of gray matter on the dorsal surface of the corpus callosum, the indusium griseum, a rudimentary component of the hippocampus.

s. mallea'ris [NA], mallear stripe; a bright line seen through the membrana tympani, produced by the attachment of the manubrium of the malleus.

medial longitudinal s., s. longitudinalis medialis.

s. medulla'ris thal'ami [NA], medullary s. of the thalamus; s. fornicis; s. ventriculi tertii; a narrow, compact fiber bundle that extends along the line of attachment of the roof of the third ventricle to the thalamus on each side and terminates posteriorly in the habenular nucleus. It is composed of fibers originating in the septal area, the substantia perforata anterior, the lateral preoptic nucleus, and the medial segment of the globus pallidus.

stri'ae medulla'res ventric'uli quar'ti [NA], medullary striae of the fourth ventricle; acoustic or auditory striae; teniae acusticae; medullary teniae; Bergmann's cords; slender fascicles of fibers extending transversally below the ependymal floor of the ventricle from the median sulcus to enter the inferior cerebellar peduncle. They arise from the arcuate nuclei on the ventral surface of the medullary pyramid.

medullary striae of the fourth ventricle, striae medullares ventriculi quarti.

medullary s. of the thalamus, s. medullaris thalami.

s. na'si transver'sa, transverse nasal groove; a single deep horizontal groove at the level of the alae, with no associated defects; autosomal dominant inheritance.

Nitabuch's s., Nitabuch's *membrane.*

stri'ae olfacto'riae [NA], olfactory striae or roots; three distinct fiber bands (s. medialis, s. intermedia, s. lateralis) that caudally extend the olfactory tract beyond its attachment to the olfactory trigone. The medial s. curves dorsally into the tenia tecta; the intermediate, often barely visible, extends straight back and terminates in the olfactory tubercle; the lateral olfactory s., the largest of the three, passes along the lateral side of the olfactory tubercle, curving laterally as far as the limen insulae, then sharply medially to reach the uncus of the parahippocampal gyrus where it terminates in the plexiform layer of the olfactory cortex. See also s. longitudinalis medialis.

olfactory striae, striae olfactoriae.

stri'ae paral'lelae, Retzius' striae.

striae ret'inae, concentric lines on the surface of an abnormal retina.

Retzius' striae, striae parallelae; brown striae; dark concentric lines crossing the enamel prisms of the teeth, seen in axial cross sections of the enamel.

Rohr's s., layer of fibrinoid in the intervillous spaces of the placenta.

s. spino'sa, Lucas' groove; sulcus spinosus; a faint groove occasionally caused by the chorda tympani nerve on the spine of the sphenoid.

s. tec'ta, s. longitudinalis lateralis.

terminal s., s. terminalis.

s. termina'lis [NA], terminal s.; tenia semicircularis; Foville's fasciculus; Tarin's tenia; a slender, compact fiber bundle that connects the amygdala (corpus amygdaloideum) with the hypothalamus and other basal forebrain regions. Originating from the amygdala, the bundle passes first caudalward in the roof of the temporal horn of the lateral ventricle; it follows the medial side of the caudate nucleus forward in the floor of the ventricle's pars centralis (or body) until it reaches the interventricular foramen, in the posterior wall of which it curves steeply down to enter the hypothalamus, with fibers passing both rostral and caudal to the anterior commissure. Coursing caudalward in the medial part of the hypothalamus, the bundle terminates in the anterior and ventromedial hypothalamic nuclei.

s. vascula'ris duc'tus cochlea'ris [NA], vascular stripe; psalterial cord; the stratified epithelium lining the upper part of the ligamentum spirale cochleae; it is penetrated by capillaries and is believed to be the site of production of endolymph.

s. ventric'uli ter'tii, s. medullaris thalami.

Wickham's striae, fine whitish lines, having a network arrangement, on the surface of lichen planus papules.

striae of Zahn, *lines* of Zahn.

striatal (strī'ā-tăl). Relating to the corpus striatum.

striate, striated (strī'āt, -ā-ted) [L. *striatus,* furrowed]. Striped; marked by striae.

striation (strī-ā'shŭn). **1.** Stria (1). **2.** A striate appearance. **3.** The act of streaking or making striae.

basal s.'s, the vertical infranuclear s.'s due to the infolded plasma membrane and mitochondria; they are seen in kidney tubules and certain intralobular salivary ducts.

tigroid s., tabby cat s., linear whitish or yellowish markings on the fatty degenerated heart muscle.

striatonigral (strī-ā-tō-nī'grăl). Referring to the efferent connection of the striatum with the *substantia* nigra (*q.v.*).

striatum (strī-ā'tŭm) [L. neut. of *striatus,* furrowed]. Collective name for the caudate nucleus and putamen which together with the globus pallidus or pallidum form the corpus striatum.

stricture (strik'chūr) [L. *strictura,* fr. *stringo,* pp. *strictus,* to draw tight, bind]. A circumscribed narrowing or stenosis of a hollow structure, usually consisting of cicatricial contracture or deposition of abnormal tissue.

anastomotic s., narrowing, usually by scarring, of an anastomotic suture line.

annular s., a ringlike constriction encircling the wall of a canal.

bridle s., narrowing of a canal by a band of tissue stretching across part of its lumen.

contractile s., recurrent s.

functional s., spasmodic s.

Hunner's s., bladder s. produced by interstitial cystitis (Hunner's ulcer).

organic s., permanent s.; a s. due to the presence of cicatricial or other new tissue, not spasmodic.

permanent s., organic s.

recurrent s., contractile s.; a s. due to the presence of contractile tissue which may be dilated but soon returns.

spasmodic s., functional or temporary s.; a s. due to localized spasm of muscular fibers in the wall of the canal.

temporary s., spasmodic s.

urethral s., a stenosing lesion of the urethra, due usually to inflammation or to iatrogenic instrumentation and resulting in reduction of urethral caliber which may be focal or may involve virtually the entire length of the urethra.

stricturotome (strik'chūr-ō-tōm). A stricture knife; an instrument for use in dividing a stricture.

stricturotomy (strik-chūr-ot'ō-mē) [stricture + G. *tomē,* incision]. Surgical opening or division of a stricture.

strident (strī'dent) [L. *stridens,* pres. p. of *strideo,* to creak]. Creaking; grating; harsh-sounding; denoting an auscultatory sound or rale.

stridor (strī'dōr) [L. a harsh, creaking sound]. A high-pitched, noisy respiration, like the blowing of the wind; a sign of respiratory obstruction, especially in the trachea or larynx.

congenital s., laryngeal s.; crowing inspiration occurring at birth or within the first few months of life; sometimes without apparent cause and sometimes due to abnormal flaccidity of epiglottis or arytenoids.

s. den'tium, grinding of the teeth.

expiratory s., a singing sound due to the semi-approximated vocal cords offering resistance to the escape of air; arises in response to somatic sensory stimulation or pathology involving the larynx.

inspiratory s., a crowing sound during the inspiratory phase of respiration due to pathology involving the epiglottis or larynx.

laryngeal s., congenital s.

s. serrat'icus, a rough grating like the sound of a saw.

stridulous (strid'yū-lŭs) [L. *stridulus,* fr. *strideo,* to creak, to hiss]. Having a shrill or creaking sound.

string. A slender cord or cordlike structure.

auditory s.'s, bundles of parallel filaments in the zona pectinata of the lamina basilaris of the cochlea; the length of the s.'s varies from 64 μm in the basal coil to 480 μm in the apex.

strip [A.S. *strypan,* to rob]. **1.** Milk (4); to express the contents from a collapsible tube or canal, such as the urethra, by running the finger along it. **2.** Subcutaneous excision of a vein in its longitudinal axis, performed with a stripper. **3.** Any narrow piece, relatively long and of uniform width.

abrasive s., a ribbon-like piece of linen on one side of which is bonded abrasive particles; used in dentistry for contouring and polishing proximal surfaces of restorations.

amalgam s., a linen s. without abrasive used to smooth proximal contours of newly placed amalgam restorations.

celluloid s., a clear plastic s. used as a matrix when inserting a silicate cement or acrylic resin cement in proximal cavity preparations of anterior teeth.

lightning s., a s. of metal with abrasive on one side, used to open rough or improper contacts of proximal restorations.

stripe (strīp) In anatomy, a streak, line, band, or stria.

s. of Gennari, *line* of Gennari.

Hensen's s., a band on the undersurface of the membrana tectoria of the cochlear duct.

mallear s., *stria* mallearis.

Mees' s.'s, Mees' *lines.*

vascular s., *stria* vascularis ductus cochlearis.

strip'per. An instrument used to strip a vein.

Strisower. See Schellong-S. *phenomenon.*

strobila, pl. **strobilae** (strō'bi-lă, -lē) [G. *stobilē,* a twist of lint]. A chain of segments, less the scolex and unsegmented neck portion, of a tapeworm; in the monozoic tapeworms (subclass Cestodaria and some members of the subclass Cestoda), it may consist of a single proglottid.

strobilocercus (strō'bi-lō-ser'kŭs) [G. *strobilē,* a twist of lint, + *kerkos,* tail]. A taenioid tapeworm larva of the cysticercus type, but with a conspicuous segmented neck, small terminal bladder, and everted scolex; the larval form of *Taenia taeniaeformis,* called *Cysticercus fasciolaris.*

strobiloid (strō'bi-loyd) [G. *strobilē,* strobile, + *eidos,* resemblance]. Resembling a chain of segments of a tapeworm.

stroboscope (strō'bō-skōp). An electronic instrument that produces intermittent light flashes of controlled frequency; used to influence electrical activity of the cerebral cortex.

stroboscopic (strō-bō-skop'ik) [G. *strobos,* a twisting around, fr. *strephō,* to twist, + *skopeō,* to view]. Pertaining to the illusion of motion, retarded or accelerated, produced by visual images observed intermittently in rapid succession.

Stroganoff, Vasili V., Russian obstetrician, 1857–1938. See S.'s *method.*

stroke (strōk) [A.S. *strāc*]. **1.** Lay term denoting a sudden neurological affliction usually related to the impaired cerebral blood supply as in paralytic, aphasic, or amnesic s. More appropriate terms indicate the nature of the disturbance; *e.g.,* thrombosis, hemorrhage, or embolism. **2.** A pulsation. **3.** To pass the hand or any instrument gently over a surface. See also stroking. **4.** A gliding movement over a surface.

heart s., **(1)** impact of the apex of the heart against the wall of the chest; **(2)** *angina* pectoris.

heat s., see heatstroke.

spinal s., acute hemorrhage, embolism, thrombosis, or ischemia of the spinal cord causing necrosis and loss of function, producing a paralysis of one or more extremities with or without sensory changes.

sun s., see sunstroke.

stroking (strōk'ing). The nonverbal fondling and nurturance accorded infants or the nonverbal and verbal forms of acceptance, reassurance, and positive reinforcement accorded to children and adults either by an individual to himself or to another person in order to satisfy a basic biopsychological need of all developing humans; various psychopathological conditions are believed to result when such s. is absent or faulty.

stroma, pl. **stromata** (strō'mă, strō'mă-tă) [G. *strōma,* bed] [NA]. The framework, usually of connective tissue, of an organ, gland, or other structure, as distinguished from the parenchyma or specific substance of the part.

s. glan'dulae thyroi'deae [NA], s. of thyroid gland; the connective tissue that supports the lobules and follicles of the thyroid gland.

s. i'ridis [NA], s. of iris; the delicate vascular connective tissue that lies between the anterior surface of the iris and the pars iridica retinae.

s. of iris, s. iridis.

lymphatic s., the network of reticular fibers and associated reticular cells of lymphatic tissue.

s. ova'rii [NA], s. of ovary; the fibrous tissue of the medulla of the ovary.

s. of ovary, s. ovarii.

Rollet's s., the colorless s. of the red blood cells.

s. of thyroid gland, s. glandulae thyroideae.

s. of vitreous, s. vitreum.

s. vit'reum [NA], s. of vitreous; the delicate framework of the vitreous body.

stromal, stromic (strō'măl, strō-mat'ik). Stromatic; relating to the stroma of an organ or other structure.

stromatin (strō'mă-tin). An insoluble protein in the stroma of erythrocytes.

stromatolysis (strō-mă-tol'i-sis) [stroma + G. *lysis,* dissolution]. Destruction of the enveloping membrane of a bacterial or other cell, the cell body not being affected.

stromatosis (strō-mă-tō'sis). Endometrial stromal *sarcoma.*

stromuhr (strōm'ūr) [Ger. *Strom,* stream, + *Uhr,* clock]. An instrument for measuring the quantity of blood that flows per unit of time through a blood vessel.

Ludwig's s., one of the first devices for measuring flow in blood vessels.

thermo-s., see thermostromuhr.

Strong, Edward K., Jr., U.S. psychologist, *1884. See S. vocational interest *test.*

strongyle (stron'jil) [G. *strongylos,* round]. Common name for members of the family Strongylidae.

Strongylidae (stron-jil'i-dē) [see *Strongyloides*]. A family of parasitic nematode worms (order Strongyloidea) including the genera *Strongylus* and *Oesophagostomum.*

Strongyloidea (stron-ji-loy'dē-ă) [see *Strongyloides*]. A superfamily of strongyle nematode parasites including the genera *Ancylostoma, Necator, Ostertagia, Haemonchus,* and *Strongylus,* as well as the gapeworms of fowl, the lungworms of carnivores, and some of the most important helminth pathogens of man and domestic animals.

Strongyloides (stron-ji-loy'dēz) [G. *strongylos,* round, + *eidos,* resemblance]. The threadworm, a genus of small nematode parasites (superfamily Rhabditoidea), commonly found in the small intestine of mammals (particularly ruminants), that are characterized by an unusual life cycle that involves one or several generations of free-living adult worms. Species include *S. fulleborni,* occurring in primates; *S. papillosus,* in cattle, sheep, and goats; *S. ransomi,* in swine; *S. stercoralis,* in dogs, primates, and humans; and *S. westeri,* in horses.

strongyloidiasis, strongyloidosis (stron'ji-loy-dī'ă-sis, -dō'sis). Infection with nematodes of the genus *Strongyloides,* considered to be a parthenogenetic female. Larvae passed to the soil form free-living adults or develop directly into infective third stage strongyliform or filariform larvae, which penetrate the skin or buccal mucosa via drinking water. Infection can occur by larvae of a new generation developed in the soil (indirect cycle), by infective larvae developed without an intervening adult stage (direct cycle), or by larvae that develop directly in the feces within the intestine of the host, penetrate the mucosa, and pass by blood-lung migration back to the intestine (autoreinfection); most serious human infections and nearly all fatalities result from autoreinfection, which commonly follow immunosuppression by steroids, ACTH, or other immunosuppressive agents. Autoreinfection also may develop in patients with AIDS.

strongylosis (stron-ji-lō'sis). Disease caused by infection with a species of *Strongylus;* effects may be extreme from worm-caused lesions, nodules, and aneurysms.

Strongylus (stron'ji-lŭs) [G. *strongylos,* round]. The palisade worm, a genus of large strongyle nematodes (subfamily Strongylinae, family Strongylidae) parasitic in horses and other equids, and the cause of strongylosis.
S. asi'ni, a species that occurs in the large intestine of the ass and other wild equids.
S. edenta'tus, a bloodsucking species occurring in the cecum and colon of the horse, ass, mule, and zebra.
S. equi'nus, a cosmopolitan bloodsucking species found in the cecum and (rarely) colon of horses and other equids.
S. radia'tus, *Cooperia oncophora.*
S. ventrico'sus, *Cooperia oncophora.*
S. vulga'ris, a bloodsucking species found chiefly in the cecum of horses and other equids; in the course of their migration, larvae commonly lodge in the wall of the posterior aorta, causing wall damage and the development of verminous aneurysms in this vessel, especially in the anterior mesenteric arteries.

strontium (stron'shē-ŭm) [*Strontian,* a town in Scotland]. A metallic element, symbol Sr, atomic no. 38, atomic weight 87.62; one of the alkaline earth series and similar to calcium in chemical and biological properties. Various salts of s. are used therapeutically for their anions; *e.g.,* s. bromide, iodide, lactate.

strontium-89 (^{89}Sr). A radioactive strontium isotope; a beta emitter with half-life of 51 days; used as a tracer in studies of strontium absorption by the body, strontium incorporation in bone, etc.

strontium-90 (^{90}Sr). A radioactive strontium isotope; a beta emitter with half-life of 29 years; a major component (about 5%) of the uranium fission products; it is incorporated into bone tissue where turnover is slow.

strophanthin (strō-fan'thin). K-strophanthin; a glycoside or mixture of glycosides from *Strophanthus kombé;* a cardiac tonic, like ouabain (G-s.); extremely toxic.

Strophanthus (strō-fan'thŭs) [G. *strophos,* a twisted cord, + *anthos,* flower]. A genus of vines of east Africa (family Apocynaceae); the dried ripe seeds of *S. kombé* or *S. hispidus* contain the cardiac glycoside strophanthin, and were used as an arrow poison; the seeds of *S. gratus* are the botanical source of ouabain.

strophocephaly (strof-ō-sef'ă-lē) [G. *strophē,* a twist, + *kephalē,* head]. Condition characterized by a congenitally distorted head and face, in which there is a tendency toward cyclopia and malformation of the oral region.

strophosomia (strof-ō-sō'mē-ă) [G. *strophē,* a twist, + *sōma,* body]. Severe form of a congenital ventral fissure, extremely rare in humans.

strophulus (strof'yū-lŭs) [Mod. L. dim. of G. *strophus,* colic]. *Miliaria* rubra.
s. can'didus, a form of s. in which the papules are colorless and shining.
s. intertinc'tus, s. prurigino'sus, a form of s. marked by an eruption of itching papules.

Stroud, Bert B., 19th century U.S. physiologist, anatomist, and zoologist. See S.'s pectinated *area.*

struck (strŭk). A disease of adult sheep in Britain caused by *Clostridium perfringens* type C.

structural (strŭk'chūr-ăl). Relating to the structure of a part; having a structure.

structuralism (strŭk'chūr-ăl-ism. A branch of psychology interested in the basic structure of the mind, including intellect and feeling, and behavior of man. *Cf.* functionalism.

structure (strŭk'chūr) [L. *structura,* fr. *struo,* pp. *structus,* to build]. **1.** The arrangement of the details of a part; the manner of formation of a part. **2.** A tissue or formation made up of different but related parts. **3.** In chemistry, the specific connections of the atoms in a given molecule.
brush heap s., haphazard interlocking of fibrils in a gel or hydrocolloid impression material.
crystal s., the arrangement in space and the interatomic distances and angles of the atoms in crystals, usually determined by x-ray diffraction measurements.
denture-supporting s.'s, the tissues, teeth, and/or residual ridges, which serve as the foundation for removable partial or complete dentures.
fine s., ultrastructure.
gel s., brush heap s. of fibrils giving firmness to hydrocolloids.
mental s., mental *apparatus.*
tuboreticular s., tubules 20–30 nm in length that lie within cisterns of smooth endoplasmic reticulum; observed in connective tissue diseases such as SLE, and in various cancers and virus infections.

struma, pl. **strumae** (strū'mă, -mē) [L. a scrofulous tumor, fr. *struo,* to pile up, build]. **1.** Goiter. **2.** Formerly, any enlargement of a tissue.
s. aberra'ta, aberrant *goiter.*
s. colloi'des, colloid goiter.
Hashimoto's s., Hashimoto's *thyroiditis.*
ligneous s., Riedel's *thyroiditis.*
s. lymphomato'sa, Hashimoto's *thyroiditis.*
s. malig'na, cancer of the thyroid gland.
s. medicamento'sa, goiter due to the use of some therapeutic agent.
s. ova'rii, a rare ovarian tumor, regarded as teratomatous, in which thyroid tissue has surpassed the other elements; occasionally associated with hyperthyroidism.
Riedel's s., Riedel's *thyroiditis.*

strumectomy (strū-mek'tō-mē) [struma + G. *ektomē,* excision]. Surgical removal of all or a portion of a goitrous tumor.
median s., removal of a median goiter or an enlarged isthmus of the thyroid gland.

strumiform (strū'mi-fōrm) [struma + L. *forma,* form]. Resembling a goiter.

strumitis (strū-mī'tis) [struma + G. *-itis,* inflammation]. Inflammation, with swelling, of the thyroid gland. See also thyroiditis.

strumous (strū'mŭs). Denoting or characteristic of a struma.

Strümpell, Ernst Adolf von, German physician, 1853–1925. See S.'s *disease, phenomenon, reflex;* S.-Marie, Marie-S., S.-Westphal *disease;* Westphal-S. *pseudosclerosis.*

strychnine (strik'nin, -nēn, -nīn). An alkaloid from *Strychnos nux-vomica;* $C_{21}H_{22}N_2O_2$; colorless crystals of intensely bitter taste, nearly insoluble in water. It stimulates all parts of the central nervous system, and is used as a stomachic, an antidote for depressant poisons, and in the treatment of myocarditis; however, its therapeutic popularity is unwarranted. The commonly used salts of s. are s. hydrochloride, s. phosphate, and s. sulfate. It is a potent chemical capable of producing acute or chronic poisoning of man or animals.

strychninism (strik′nin-izm). Chronic strychnine poisoning, the symptoms being those that arise from central nervous system stimulation; the first signs are tremors and twitching, progressing to severe convulsions and respiratory arrest.

Strychnos (strik′nos) [G. nightshade]. A genus of tropical shrubs or trees (family Loganiaceae); most South American species contain chiefly quaternary neuromuscular blocking alkaloids, *e.g.,* curare; the African, Asiatic, and Australian species contain tertiary strychnine-like alkaloids.

Stryker, Garold V., U.S. pathologist, *1896. See S.-Halbeisen *syndrome.*

Stryker, Homer H., U.S. orthopedic surgeon. See S. *frame, saw.*

Stuart. Surname of the patient in whom the S. or S.-Prower *factor* was first discovered.

Student. Pseudonym for William Sealy Gosset, British statistician, and chemist, 1876–1937. See S.'s *t test.*

study (stŭd′ē) [L. *studium,* study, inquiry]. Research, detailed examination, and/or analysis of an organism, object, or phenomena.
blind s., a s. in which the experimenter is unaware of which group is subject to which maneuver.
case-control s., a s. using epidemiological methods in which a group of people or animals with a disease is compared retrospectively with a similar group without the disease for possession by each group of some particular attribute (*e.g.,* age, sex, exposure to some environmental factor). *Cf.* cohort s.
cohort s., a s. using epidemiological methods, such as a clinical trial, in which a cohort with a particular attribute (*e.g.,* smokers, recipients of a drug) is followed prospectively and compared for some outcome (*e.g.,* disease, cure) with another cohort not possessing the attribute.
cross-sectional s., synchronic s.
diachronic s., longitudinal s.; a s. of the natural course of a life or disorder in which a cohort of subjects is serially observed over a period of time and no assumptions need be made about the stability of the system.
double blind s., a s. in which neither the experimenter nor any other assessor of the results, including patients, know which group is subject to which procedure.
longitudinal s., diachronic s.
multivariate s.'s, simultaneous investigations of the influence of several variables.
synchronic s., cross-sectional s.; a s. of the structure of a population at one instant in time. If the natural history remains constant, and the entry of new cases and the loss of old cases (by death or attrition) are equal and unvarying, the results so obtained will correspond exactly to those of a diachronic s.

stump (stŭmp). **1.** The extremity of a limb left after amputation. **2.** The pedicle remaining after removal of the tumor attached to it.

stun (stŭn) [A.S. *stunian,* to make a loud noise]. To stupefy; to render unconscious by cerebral trauma.

stupe (stūp) [L. stupa, oakum, tow]. A compress or cloth wrung out of hot water, usually impregnated with turpentine or other irritant, applied to the surface to produce counterirritation.

stupefacient, stupefactive (stū-pĕ-fā′shent, -fak′tiv). [L. *stupefacio*]. Causing stupor.

stupor (stū′per) [L. fr. *stupeo,* to be stunned]. A state of impaired consciousness in which the individual shows a marked diminution in his reactivity to environmental stimuli.
benign s., depressive s.; a stuporous syndrome from which recovery is the rule, as opposed to malignant s.
catatonic s., s. associated with catatonia.
depressive s., benign s.
malignant s., a stuporous condition from which recovery is infrequent, as opposed to benign s.

stuporous (stū′per-ŭs). Carotic (2); relating to or marked by stupor.

Sturge, William A., British physician, 1850–1919. See S.'s *disease;* S.-Weber *syndrome.*

Sturm, Johann C., 1635–1703. See S.'s *conoid, interval.*

Sturmdorf, A., U.S. gynecologist, 1861–1934. See S.'s *operation.*

stutter (stŭt′er) [frequentative of *stut,* from Goth. *stautan,* to strike]. To enunciate certain words with difficulty and with frequent halting and repetition of the initial consonant of a word or syllable.

stuttering (stŭt′er-ing). Logospasm (1); a phonatory or articulatory disorder, characteristically beginning in childhood, with intense anxiety about the efficiency of oral communications, and characterized by hesitations, repetitions, and prolongations of sounds and syllables, interjections, broken words, circumlocutions, and words produced with excess tension.
urinary s., stammering of the bladder; frequent involuntary interruption occurring during the act of urination.

sty, stye, pl. sties, styes (stī, stīz). *Hordeolum* externum.
meibomian s., *hordeolum* internum.
zeisian s., inflammation of one of Zeis' glands.

style (stīl). Stylet.

stylet, stylette (stī′let, stī-let′) [It. *stilletto,* a dagger; dim. of L. *stilus* or *stylus,* a stake, a pen]. Stylus (3); style. **1.** A flexible metallic rod inserted in the lumen of a flexible catheter to stiffen it and give it form during its passage. **2.** A slender probe.
endotracheal s., a rod of malleable metal used to maintain the desired curve of an endotracheal tube for its insertion into the trachea.

styliform (stī′li-fōrm) [L. *stilus* (*stylus*), a stake, + *forma,* form]. Styloid.

stylo- [G. *stylos,* pillar, post]. Prefix denoting styloid; specifically, the styloid process of the temporal bone.

styloauricularis (stī′lō-aw-rik-yū-lā′ris). See under musculus.

styloglossus (stī′lō-glos′ŭs). Relating to the styloid process and the tongue. See under musculus.

stylohyal (stī-lō-hī′ăl). Stylohyoid (1); relating to the styloid process of the temporal bone and to the hyoid bone.

stylohyoid (stī-lō-hī′oyd). **1.** Stylohyal. **2.** Relating to the musculus stylohyoideus.

styloid (stī′loyd) [stylo- + G. *eidos,* resemblance]. Styliform; peg-shaped; denoting one of several slender bony processes. See entries for *processus* styloideus.

styloiditis (stī-loy-dī′tis). Inflammation of a styloid process.

stylolaryngeus (stī′lō-lar-in-jē′ŭs) See under musculus.

stylomandibular (stī′lō-man-dib′yū-lăr). Stylomaxillary; relating to the styloid process of the temporal bone and the mandible; denoting the ligamentum stylomandibulare.

stylomastoid (stī′lō-mas′toyd). Relating to the styloid and the mastoid processes of the temporal bone; denoting especially a small artery and a foramen.

stylomaxillary (stī′lō-mak′si-lăr-ē). Stylomandibular.

stylopharyngeus (stī′lō-far-in-jē′ŭs). See under musculus.

stylopodium (stī-lō-pō′dē-ŭm) [stylo- + G. *podion,* small foot]. The proximal intermediate segment of the limb skeleton, the humerus and the femur, in the embryo.

stylostaphyline (stī-lō-staf′i-līn). Relating to the styloid process of the temporal bone and the uvula.

stylosteophyte (stī-los′tē-ō-fīt) [G. *stylos,* post, + *osteon,* bone, + *phyton,* growth]. A peg-shaped bony outgrowth.

Styloviridae (stī-lō-vir′i-dē) [G. *stylos,* pillar, column]. Provisional name for a family of bacterial viruses with long, noncontractile tails and isometric or elongated heads, containing double-stranded DNA (MW 25 to 79 × 10^6); includes the λ temperate phage group and probably other genera.

stylus (stī'lŭs) [L. *stilus* or *stylus,* a stake or pen]. Stilus. **1.** Any pencil-shaped structure. **2.** A pencil-shaped medicinal preparation for external application; *e.g.,* a medicated bougie, or a pencil or stick of silver nitrate or other caustic. **3.** Stylet.

stype (stīp) [G. *stypē,* tow]. A tampon.

styptic (stip'tik) [G. *styptikos,* astringent]. Staltic. **1.** Having an astringent or hemostatic effect. **2.** Hemostyptic; an astringent hemostatic agent used topically to stop bleeding.

styramate (stī'ră-māt). Carbamic acid β-hydroxyphenethyl ester; an orally effective skeletal muscle relaxant with a relatively long duration of action.

styrax (stī'raks). Storax.

styrene (stī'rēn). Styrol; cinnamene; ethenylbenzene; vinylbenzene; phenylethylene; $C_6H_5CH{=}CH_2$; the monomer from which polystyrenes, plastics, and synthetic rubber are made; together with divinylbenzene (for cross-linking), it is the basis of many synthetic ion exchangers.

styrol (stī'rol). Styrene.

styrone (stī'rōn). Cinnamic alcohol; $C_9H_{10}O$; obtained from storax by distillation with potassium hydroxide; used as a deodorant in 12% glycerin solution, and as a decolorizing agent in histology.

sub- [L. *sub,* under]. Prefix, to words formed from L. roots, denoting beneath, less than the normal or typical, inferior; corresponds to G. *hypo-.*

subabdominal (sŭb-ab-dom'i-năl). Below the abdomen.

subabdominoperitoneal (sŭb-ab-dom'i-nō-per-i-tō-nē'-ăl). Subperitoneoabdominal; beneath the abdominal, as distinguished from the pelvic, peritoneum.

subacetate (sŭb-as'ĕ-tāt). A mixture or complex of a base and its acetate.

subacromial (sŭb-ă-krō'mē-ăl). Beneath the acromion process.

subacute (sŭb-ă-kyūt'). Between acute and chronic; denoting the course of a disease of moderate duration or severity.

subalimentation (sŭb'al-i-men-tā'shŭn). Hypoalimentation; a condition of insufficient nourishment.

subanal (sŭb-ā'năl). Below the anus.

subaortic (sŭb'ā-ōr'tik). Below the aorta.

subapical (sŭb-ap'i-kăl). Below the apex of any part.

subaponeurotic (sŭb-ap-ō-nū-rot'ik). Beneath an aponeurosis.

subarachnoid (sŭb-ă-rak'noyd). Underneath the arachnoid membrane.

subarcuate (sŭb-ar'kyū-āt). Slightly arcuate or bowed.

subareolar (sŭb-ă-rē'ō-lăr). Beneath an areola; especially the areola of the mamma.

subastragalar (sŭb-as-trag'ă-lăr). Beneath the calcaneus (astragalus).

subatomic (sŭb-ă-tom'ik). Pertaining to particles making up the intra-atomic structure; *e.g.,* protons, electrons, neutrons.

subaural (sŭb-aw'răl). Below the ear.

subauricular (sŭb-aw-rik'yū-lăr). Below an auricle; especially the concha or pinna of the ear.

subaxial (sŭb-ak'sē-ăl). Below the axis of the body or any part.

subaxillary (sŭb-ak'si-lār-ē). Infra-axillary; below the axillary fossa.

subbasal (sŭb-bā'săl). Beneath any base or basal membrane.

subbrachycephalic (sŭb-brak-ē-se-fal'ik). Slightly brachycephalic; having a cephalic index of 80.01 to 83.33.

subcalcarine (sŭb-kal'kă-rīn). Below the calcarine fissure; denoting the gyrus lingualis.

subcallosal (sŭb-ka-lō'săl). Below the corpus callosum; denoting either the gyrus or the fasciculus subcallosus.

subcapsular (sŭb-kap'sū-lăr). Beneath any capsule.

subcarbonate (sŭb-kar'bon-āt). A mixture or complex of a base and its carbonate.

subcardinal (sŭb-kar'di-năl). Lying ventral to the anterior or posterior cardinal veins in the embryo.

subcartilaginous (sŭb'kar-ti-laj'i-nŭs). **1.** Partly cartilaginous. **2.** Beneath a cartilage.

subcecal (sŭb-sē'kăl). Below the cecum; denoting a fossa.

subcellular (sŭb-sel'yū-lăr). Noncellular (1).

subception (sŭb-sep'shŭn) [sub- + L. *-ceptum,* perceived]. The reaction to a stimulus not fully perceived.

subchloride (sŭb-klōr'īd). The chloride of a series that contains proportionally the greatest amount of the other element in the compound; *e.g.,* s. of mercury is Hg_2Cl_2, whereas chloride or perchloride of mercury is $HgCl_2$.

subchondral (sŭb-kon'drăl). Beneath or below the cartilages of the ribs.

subchorionic (sŭb'kō-rē-on'ik). Beneath the chorion.

subchoroidal (sŭb-kō-roy'dăl). Beneath the choroid coat of the eye.

subclass (sŭb'klas). In biologic classification, a division between class and order.

subclavian (sŭb-klā'vē-an). **1.** Infraclavicular; beneath the clavicle. **2.** Pertaining to the s. artery or vein.

subclavicular (sŭb-kla-vik'yū-lăr). Pertaining to the region beneath the clavicle.

subclavius (sŭb-klā'vē-ŭs). See under musculus.

subclinical (sŭb-klin'i-kăl). Denoting the presence of a disease without manifest symptoms; may be an early stage in the evolution of a disease.

subcollateral (sŭb-kō-lat'er-ăl). Below the collateral fissure; denoting a cerebral convolution, or gyrus.

subconjunctival (sŭb'kon-jŭnk-tī'văl). Beneath the conjunctiva.

subconjunctivitis (sŭb'kon-jŭnk-ti-vī'tis). *Episcleritis* periodica fugax.

subconscious (sŭb-kon'shŭs). **1.** Not wholly conscious. **2.** Denoting an idea or impression which is present in the mind, but of which there is at the time no conscious knowledge or realization.

subconsciousness (sŭb-kon'shŭs-nes). **1.** Partial unconsciousness. **2.** The state in which mental processes take place without the conscious perception of the individual.

subcoracoid (sŭb-kōr'ă-koyd). Beneath the coracoid process.

subcortex (sŭb-kōr'teks). Any part of the brain lying below the cerebral cortex, and not itself organized as cortex.

subcortical (sŭb-kōr'ti-kăl). Relating to the subcortex; beneath the cerebral cortex.

subcostal (sŭb-kos'tăl). **1.** Infracostal; beneath a rib or the ribs. **2.** Denoting certain arteries, veins, and nerves.

subcostalgia (sŭb-kos-tal'jē-ă) [subcostal + G. *algos,* pain]. Pain in the subcostal region.

subcostosternal (sŭb-kos'tō-ster'năl). Below or beneath the ribs and sternum.

subcranial (sŭb-krā'nē-ăl). Beneath or below the cranium.

subcrepitant (sub-krep'i-tănt). Nearly, but not frankly, crepitant; denoting a rale.

subcrepitation (sŭb'krep-i-tā'shŭn). **1.** The presence of subcrepitant rales. **2.** A sound approaching crepitation in character.

subcrureus, subcruralis (sŭb-krū-rē-ŭs, -krū-rā'lis) [sub- + L.

crus, leg]. *Musculus* articularis genu.

subculture (sŭb-kŭl′chūr). **1.** A culture made by transferring to a fresh medium microorganisms from a previous culture; a method used to prolong the life of a particular strain where there is a tendency to degeneration in older cultures. **2.** To make a fresh culture with material obtained from a previous one.

subcurative (sŭb-kyūr′ă-tiv). Denoting a dose less than that necessary for a curative effect.

subcutaneous (s.c., SQ) (sŭb-kyū-tā′nē-ŭs) [sub- + L. *cutis,* skin]. Beneath the skin. Also called hypodermatic; hypodermic (1); subdermic; subintegumental; subtegumental.

subcuticular (sŭb-kyū-tik′yū-lăr). Subepidermal; subepidermic; beneath the cuticle or epidermis.

subcutis (sŭb-kyū′tis). *Tela* subcutanea.

subdelirium (sŭb-dē-lir′ē-ŭm). Slight or not continuous delirium.

subdeltoid (sŭb-del′toyd). Beneath the deltoid muscle; denoting a bursa.

subdental (sŭb-den′tăl). Beneath the roots of the teeth.

subdermic (sŭb-der′mik). Subcutaneous.

subdiaphragmatic (sŭb′dī-ă-frag-mat′ik). Infradiaphragmatic; subphrenic; beneath the diaphragm.

subdorsal (sŭb-dōr′săl). Below the dorsal region.

subduce, subduct (sŭb-dūs′, sŭb-dŭkt′) [L. *sub-duco,* pp. *-ductus,* to lead away]. To pull or draw downward.

subdural (sŭb-dū′răl). Beneath the dura mater or between it and the arachnoid.

subendocardial (sŭb-en-dō-kar′dē-ăl). Beneath the endocardium.

subendothelial (sŭb′en-dō-thē′lē-ăl). Beneath the endothelium.

subendothelium (sŭb′en-dō-thē′lē-ŭm). The connective tissue between the endothelium and inner elastic membrane in the intima of arteries.

subendymal, subependymal (sŭb-en′di-măl, sŭb-ep-en′di-mal). Beneath the endyma, or ependyma.

subependymoma (sŭb-ep-en-di-mō′mă). Discrete lobulated ependymal nodules in the walls of the anterior third or posterior fourth ventricles commonly found at autopsy.

subepidermal, subepidermic (sŭb′ep-i-der′măl, -der′mik). Subcuticular.

subepithelial (sŭb′ep-i-thē′lē-ăl). Beneath the epithelium.

subepithelium (sŭb′ep-i-thē′lē-ŭm). Any structure beneath the epithelium.

suberosis (sū-ber-ō′sis) [L. *suber,* cork, + G. *-osis,* condition]. Extrinsic allergic alveolitis caused by inhalation of mold spores from contaminated cork.

subfamily (sŭb-fam′i-lē). In biologic classification, a division between family and tribe or between family and genus.

subfascial (sŭb-fash′ē-ăl). Beneath a fascia.

subfertility (sŭb-fer-til′i-tē). Less than normal capacity for reproduction.

subfissure (sŭb-fish′er). A cerebral fissure beneath the surface, concealed by overlapping convolutions.

subfolium (sŭb-fō′lē-ŭm). A secondary division of a cerebellar folium.

subgallate (sŭb-gal′āt). Partially neutralized gallic acid; a basic gallate, such as bismuth s.

subgemmal (sŭb-jem′ăl). Below a gemma or bud (*e.g.,* a taste bud).

subgenus (sŭb-jē′nŭs). In biologic classification, a division between genus and species.

subgingival (sŭb-jin′ji-văl). Below the gingival margin.

subglenoid (sŭb-glē′noyd). Infraglenoid.

subglossal (sŭb-glos′ăl). Sublingual; hypoglossal; below or beneath the tongue.

subglossitis (sŭb-glo-sī′tis). Inflammation of the tissues beneath the tongue.

subglottic (sŭb-glot′ik). Infraglottic.

subgranular (sŭb-gran′yū-lăr). Slightly granular.

subgrundation (sŭb-grŭn-dā′shŭn) [sub- + A.S. *grund,* bottom, foundation]. The depression of one fragment of a broken cranial bone below the other.

subhepatic (sŭb-he-pat′ik). Infrahepatic; below the liver.

subhyaloid (sŭb-hī′ă-loyd). Beneath, on the vitreous side of, the hyaloid (vitreous) membrane.

subhyoid, subyoidean (sŭb-hī′oyd, sŭb-hī-oyd′ē-an). Infrahyoid.

subicteric (sŭb-ik′ter-ik) [sub- + G. *ikterikos,* jaundiced]. Slightly jaundiced.

subicular (sū-bik′yū-lăr, sū-bik′). Relating to the subiculum.

subiculum, pl. **subicula** (sū-bik′yū-lŭm, -lă, sū-bik′) [L. dim. of *subex,* support]. **1.** A support or prop. **2.** The zone of transition between the parahippocampal gyrus and Ammon's horn of the hippocampus.

s. promonto′rii [NA], support of the promontory; ponticulus promontorii; a bony ridge bounding the fossula fenestrae cochleae posteriorly.

subiliac (sŭb-il′ē-ak). **1.** Below the ilium. **2.** Relating to the subilium.

subilium (sŭb-il′ē-ŭm). The portion of the ilium contributing to the acetabulum.

subinfection (sŭb-in-fek′shŭn). A secondary infection occurring in one exposed to and successfully resisting an epidemic of another infectious disease.

subinflammatory (sŭb-in-flam′ă-tō-rē). Denoting a slightly inflammatory irritation of the tissues.

subintegumental (sŭb′in-teg-yū-men′tăl). Subcutaneous.

subintimal (sŭb-in′ti-măl). Beneath the intima.

subintrant (sŭb-in′trant) [L. *sub-intro,* pres. p. *-ans,* to enter by stealth]. Proleptic.

subinvolution (sŭb-in-vō-lū′shŭn). Arrest of the normal involution of the uterus following childbirth with the organ remaining abnormally large.

subiodide (sŭb-ī′ō-dīd). That one of a series of iodine compounds with a given cation containing the least iodine; analogous to subchloride.

subjacent (sŭb-jā′sent) [L. *sub-jaceo,* to lie under]. Below or beneath another part.

subject (sŭb′jekt) [L. *subjectus,* lying beneath]. An organism that is the object of research, treatment, experimentation, or dissection.

subjective (sŭb-jek′tiv) [L. *subjectivus,* fr. *subjicio,* to throw under]. **1.** Perceived by the individual only and not evident to the examiner; said of certain symptoms, such as pain. **2.** Colored by one's personal beliefs and attitudes. *Cf.* objective (2).

subjugal (sŭb-jū′găl). Below the zygomatic (jugal) bone.

subkingdom (sŭb-king′dom). In biologic classification, a division between kingdom and phylum.

sublation (sŭb-lā′shŭn) [L. *sublatio,* a lifting up]. Detachment, elevation, or removal of a part.

sublethal (sŭb-lē′thăl). Not quite lethal.

subleukemia (sŭb-lū-kē′mē-ă). Subleukemic *leukemia.*

sublimate (sŭb′lim-āt) [L. *sublimo,* pp. *-atus,* to raise on high, fr. *sublimis,* high]. **1.** To perform or accomplish sublimation. **2.** Any substance that has been submitted to sublimation.

corrosive s., mercuric chloride.

sublimation (sŭb-lim-ā'shŭn). **1.** The process of converting a solid into a gas without passing through a liquid state; analogous to distillation. **2.** In psychoanalysis, an unconscious defense mechanism in which unacceptable instinctual drives and wishes are modified into more personally and socially acceptable channels.

sublime (sŭb-līm'). **1.** To sublimate. **2.** To undergo a process of sublimation.

subliminal (sŭb-lim'i-năl) [sub- + L. *limen* (*limin-*), threshold]. Below the threshold of perception or excitation; below the limit or threshold of consciousness.

sublimis (sŭb-lī'mis) [L.]. **1.** At the top. **2.** Superficialis.

sublingual (sŭb-ling'gwăl). Subglossal.

sublinguitis (sŭb-ling-gwī'tis). Inflammation of the sublingual salivary gland.

sublobular (sŭb-lob'yū-lăr). Beneath a lobule, as of the liver.

sublumbar (sŭb-lŭm'băr). Below the lumbar region.

subluminal (sŭb-lū'mi-năl). Below or beneath the structure facing the lumen of an organ.

subluxation (sŭb-lŭk-sā'shŭn) [sub- + L. *locatio,* luxation (dislocation)]. Semiluxation; an incomplete luxation or dislocation; though a relationship is altered, contact between joint surfaces remains.

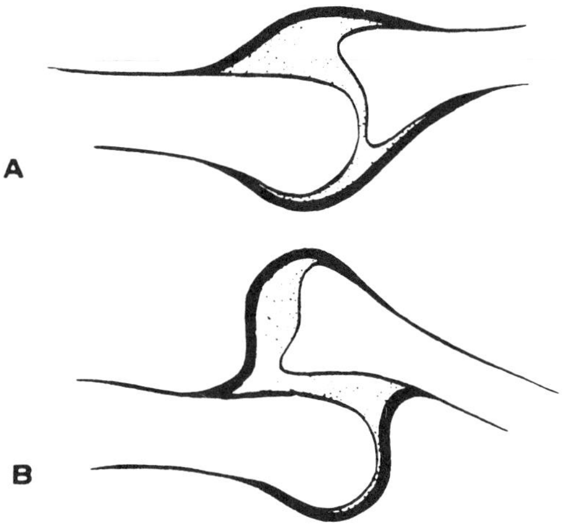

Subluxation
Diagram of subluxation (*A*) shows partial contact of apposing articular surfaces; in dislocation (*B*) there is complete loss of contact.

sublymphemia (sŭb-lim-fē'mē-ă) [sub- + L. *lympha,* lymph, + G. *haima,* blood]. A blood state in which there is a great increase in the proportion of lymphocytes although the total number of white cells is normal.

submammary (sŭb-mam'ă-rē). **1.** Deep to the mammary gland. **2.** Inframammary.

submandibular (sŭb-man-dib'yū-lăr). Inframandibular; submaxillary (2); beneath the mandible or lower jaw.

submarginal (sŭb-mar'ji-năl). Near the margin of any part.

submaxilla (sŭb-mak-sil'ă). Mandibula.

submaxillaritis (sŭb-mak'sil-ă-rī'tis) [sub- + maxilla + G. *-itis,* inflammation]. Submaxillitis; inflammation, which may be due to mumps virus, affecting the submandibular salivary gland.

submaxillary (sŭb-mak'si-lăr-ē). **1.** Mandibular. **2.** Submandibular.

submaxillitis (sŭb-mak'si-lī'tis). Submaxillaritis.

submedial, submedian (sŭb-mē'dē-ăl, sŭb-mē'dē-an). Almost, but not exactly in the middle.

submembranous (sŭb-mem'bră-nŭs). Partly or nearly membranous.

submental (sŭb-men'tăl). Beneath the chin.

submerged (sŭb-merjd'). In dentistry, describing a field of operation covered by saliva.

submetacentric (sŭb'met-ă-sen'trik). See submetacentric *chromosome.*

submicronic (sŭb-mī-kron'ik). Smaller than 1 micron in size.

submicroscopic (sŭb'mī-krō-skop'ik). Amicroscopic; ultramicroscopic; too minute to be visible with a light microscope.

submorphous (sŭb-mōr'fŭs). Neither definitely amorphous nor definitely crystalline, denoting the structure of certain calculi.

submucosa (sŭb-mū-kō'să). A layer of tissue beneath a mucous membrane.

submucous (sŭb-myū'kŭs). Beneath a mucous membrane.

subnarcotic (sŭb-nar-kot'ik). Slightly narcotic.

subnasal (sŭb-nā'săl). Under the nose.

subnasion (sŭb-nā'zē-on). The point of the angle between the septum of the nose and the surface of the upper lip.

subneural (sŭb-nū'răl). Below the neural axis.

subnitrate (sŭb-nī'trāt). A basic nitrate; a salt of nitric acid having one or more atoms of the base still capable of combining with the acid.

subnormal (sub-nōr'măl). Below the normal standard of some quality.

subnormality (sŭb-nōr-mal'i-tē). A subnormal state or condition.

subnucleus (sŭb-nū'klē-ŭs). A secondary nucleus.

suboccipital (sŭb-ok-sip'i-tăl). Below the occiput or the occipital bone.

suboptimal (sŭb-op'ti-măl). Below or less than the optimum.

suborbital (sŭb-ōr'bi-tăl). Infraorbital.

suborder (sŭb-ōr'der). In biologic classification, a division between order and family.

suboxidation (sŭb'oks-i-dā'shŭn). Deficient oxidation.

suboxide (sŭb-ok'sīd). Protoxide; that one of a series of oxides containing the least oxygen.

subpapular (sŭb-pap'yū-lăr). Denoting the eruption of few and scattered papules, in which the lesions are very slightly elevated, being scarcely more than macules.

subparietal (sŭb-pa-rī'ĕ-tăl). Below or beneath any structure called parietal: bone, lobe, layer of a serous membrane, etc.

subpatellar (sŭb-pa-tel'ăr). **1.** Deep to the patella. **2.** Infrapatellar.

subpectoral (sŭb-pek'tō-răl). Beneath the pectoralis muscle.

subpelviperitoneal (sŭb-pel'vi-per-i-tō-nē'ăl). Subperitoneopelvic; beneath the pelvic, as distinguished from the abdominal, peritoneum.

subpericardial (sŭb-per-i-kar'dē-ăl). Beneath the pericardium.

subperiosteal (sŭb-per-ē-os'tē-ăl). Beneath the periosteum.

subperitoneal (sŭb-per-i-tō-nē'ăl). Beneath the peritoneum.

subperitoneoabdominal (sŭb-per-i-tō-nē'ō-ab-dom'i-năl). Subabdominoperitoneal.

subperitoneopelvic (sŭb-per-i-tō-nē'ō-pel'vik). Subpelviperitoneal.

subpetrosal (sŭb-pe-trō'săl). **1.** Denoting the inferior petrosal. **2.** Denoting a dural venous sinus.

subpharyngeal (sŭb-fă-rin'jē-ăl). Below the pharynx.

subphrenic (sŭb-fren'ik). Subdiaphragmatic.

subphylum (sŭb-fī'lŭm). In biologic classification, a division between phylum and class.

subpial (sŭb-pī'ăl). Beneath the pia mater.

subplacental (sŭb-pla-sen'tăl). Beneath the placenta; denoting the decidua basalis.

subpleural (sŭb-plu'răl). Beneath the pleura.

subplexal (sŭb-plek'săl). Below or beneath any plexus.

subpreputial (sŭb-prē-pyū'shē-ăl). Beneath the prepuce.

subpubic (sŭb-pyū'bik). Beneath the pubic arch; denoting a ligament, ligamentum arcuatum pubis, connecting the two pubic bones below the arch.

subpulmonary (sŭb-pŭl'mō-nār-ē). Below the lungs.

subpyramidal (sūb-pi-ram'i-dăl). **1.** Below any pyramid; denoting especially the sinus tympani. **2.** Nearly pyramidal in shape.

subretinal (sŭb-ret'i-năl). **1.** Between the sensory retina and the retinal pigment epithelium. **2.** Between the retinal pigment epithelium and the choroid.

subsalt (sŭb'salt). A basic salt; a salt in which the base has not been completely neutralized by the acid.

subsartorial (sŭb-sar-tō'rē-ăl). Beneath the sartorius muscle; denoting a nerve plexus.

subscapular (sŭb-skap'yū-lăr). **1.** Deep to the scapula. **2.** Infrascapular.

subscapularis (sŭb-skap-yū-lā'ris). See under musculus.

subscleral (sŭb-sklē'răl). Subsclerotic (1); beneath the sclera of the eye, *i.e.,* on the choroidal side of this layer.

subsclerotic (sŭb-skle-rot'ik). **1.** Subscleral. **2.** Partly or slightly sclerotic or sclerosed.

subscription (sŭb-skrip'shŭn) [L. *subscriptio,* fr. *subscribo,* pp. *-scriptus,* to write under, subscribe].The part of a prescription preceding the signature, in which are the directions for compounding.

subserous, subserosal (sŭb-sē'rŭs, sŭb-se-rō'săl). Beneath a serous membrane.

subsibilant (sŭb-sib'i-lănt). Rarely used term denoting a rale with a quality between blowing and whistling.

subsidence (sŭb-sī'dens). Sinking or settling in bone, as of a prosthetic component of a total joint implant.

subspinale (sŭb-spi-nā'lē). Point A; in cephalometrics, the most posterior midline point on the premaxilla between the anterior nasal spine and the prosthion.

subspinous (sŭb-spī'nŭs). **1.** Infraspinous. **2.** Tendency to spininess.

substage (sŭb'stāj). An attachment to a microscope, below the stage, supporting the condenser or other accessory.

substance (sŭb'stans) [L. *substantia,* essence, material, fr. *sub- sto,* to stand under, be present]. Matter; stuff; material. See also subentries under substantia.

alpha s., reticular s. (1).

anterior perforated s., *substantia* perforata anterior.

bacteriotropic s., opsonin or other s. that alters bacterial cells in such a manner that they are more susceptible to phagocytic action.

basophil s., Nissl s.

beta s., Heinz *bodies.*

blood group s., blood group *antigen.*

blood group-specific s.'s A and B, solution of complexes of polysaccharides and amino acids that reduces the titer of anti-A and anti-B isoagglutinins in serum from group O persons; used to render group O blood reasonably safe for transfusion into persons of group A, B, or AB, but does not affect any incompatibility that results from various other factors, such as Rh.

central gray s., *substantia* grisea centralis.

chromidial s., granular endoplasmic *reticulum.*

chromophil s., Nissl s.

compact s., *substantia* compacta.

controlled s., a s. subject to the Controlled Substances Act (1970), which regulates the prescribing and dispensing, as well as the manufacturing, storage, sale, or distribution of s.'s assigned to five schedules according to their 1) potential for or evidence of abuse, 2) potential for psychic or physiologic dependence, 3) contributing a public health risk, 4) harmful pharmacologic effect, or 5) role as a precursor of other controlled s.'s.

cortical s., *substantia* corticalis.

exophthalmos-producing s. (EPS), a compound postulated to be a pituitary hormone responsible for exophthalmos in hyperthyroidism.

filar s., reticular s. (1).

gelatinous s., *substantia* gelatinosa.

glandular s. of prostate, *substantia* glandularis prostatae.

gray s., *substantia* grisea.

ground s., substantia fundamentalis; the amorphous material in which structural elements occur; in connective tissue, it is composed of proteoglycans, plasma constituents, metabolites, water, and ions present between cells and fibers.

H s., released s.; designation given by Sir Thomas Lewis to a diffusible s. in skin, indistinguishable in action from histamine, that is liberated by injury and causes the triple response.

innominate s., *substantia* innominata.

interspongioplastic s., obsolete term for cytochylema.

s. of lens of eye, *substantia* lentis.

medullary s., substantia medullaris (2); **(1)** Schwann's white s.; the lipid material present in the myelin sheath of nerve fibers; **(2)** medulla of bones and other organs.

muscular s. of prostate, *substantia* muscularis prostatae.

neurosecretory s., the secretion of nerve cell bodies located in the hypothalamus; the s. is transported by way of hypothalamo-hypophysial tract fibers into the neurohypophysis where the terminals of the nerve fibers contain the secretion. As seen in the fibers and terminals with a light microscope, the s. appears as Herring bodies or hyaline bodies of the pituitary (see under body).

Nissl s., the material consisting of granular endoplasmic reticulum and ribosomes which occurs in nerve cell bodies and dendrites. Also called Nissl bodies or granules; chromophil or basophil s.; tigroid bodies or s.; substantia basophilia.

s. P, a peptide neurotransmitter composed of eleven amino acids, present in minute quantities in the brain and intestines of man and various animals, that is primarily involved in pain transmission and is one of the most potent compounds affecting smooth muscle (dilation of blood vessels and contraction of intestine).

posterior perforated s., *substantia* perforata posterior.

pressor s., pressor *base.*

proper s., see *substantia* propria corneae, propria membranae tympani, and propria sclerae.

released s., H s.

reticular s., **(1)** substantia reticularis (1); substantia reticulofilamentosa; filar s. or mass; alpha s.; a filamentous plasmatic material, beaded with granules, demonstrable by means of vital staining in the immature red blood cells; **(2)** *formatio* reticularis.

Rolando's gelatinous s., Rolando's s., *substantia* gelatinosa.

Schwann's white s., medullary s. (1).

sensitizing s., complement-fixing *antibody.*

slow-reacting s. (of anaphylaxis) (SRS, SRS-A), slow-reacting factor of anaphylaxis; a leukotriene of low molecular weight which is released in anaphylactic shock and produces slower and more prolonged contraction of muscle than does histamine; it is active in the presence of antihistamines (but not epinephrine) and seems not to occur preformed in mast cells, but as a result of an antigen-antibody reaction on the granules.

soluble specific s. (SSS), specific capsular s.

specific capsular s., soluble specific s.; pneumococcal polysaccharide; specific soluble polysaccharide or sugar; a soluble type-specific polysaccharide produced during active growth of virulent pneumococci composing a large part of the capsule.

spongy s., *substantia* spongiosa.
Stilling's gelatinous s., *substantia* intermedia centralis et lateralis.
threshold s., threshold body; any material (*e.g.,* glucose) that is excreted in the urine only when its plasma concentration exceeds a certain value, termed its threshold.
tigroid s., Nissl s.
white s., *substantia* alba.
zymoplastic s., thromboplastin.

substantia, pl. **substantiae** (sŭb-stan'shē-ă, -shē-ē) [L.] [NA]. Substance.
s. adamanti'na, enamelum.
s. al'ba [NA], alba; white substance; white matter; those regions of the brain and spinal cord which are largely or entirely composed of nerve fibers and contain few or no neuronal cell bodies or dendrites.
s. basophi'lia, Nissl *substance.*
s. cine'rea, s. grisea.
s. compac'ta [NA], compact substance or bone; s. compacta ossium; the compact, noncancellous portion of bone that consists largely of concentric lamellar osteons and interstitial lamellae.
s. compac'ta os'sium, s. compacta.
s. cortica'lis [NA], cortical bone or substance; the superficial thin layer of compact bone.
s. ebur'nea, dentinum.
s. ferrugin'ea [NA], *locus* ceruleus.
s. fundamenta'lis, ground *substance.*
s. gelatino'sa [NA], gelatinous substance; Rolando's gelatinous substance; Rolando's substance; the apical part of the posterior horn (dorsal horn; posterior gray column) of the spinal cord's gray matter, composed largely of very small nerve cells; its gelatinous appearance is due to its very low content of myelinated nerve fibers.
s. gelatino'sa centra'lis, s. intermedia centralis et lateralis.
s. glandula'ris prosta'tae, glandular substance of prostate; numerous compound tubuloalveolar glands interspersed through the fibromuscular tissue of the gland and draining into the urethra through 20 or more ductules.
s. gris'ea [NA], s. cinerea; gray substance; gray matter; those regions of the brain and spinal cord which are made up primarily of the cell bodies and dendrites of nerve cells rather than myelinated axons.
s. gris'ea centra'lis [NA], central gray substance; **(1)** in general: the predominantly small-celled gray matter adjoining or surrounding the central canal of the spinal cord and the third and fourth ventricles of the brainstem; **(2)** in particular: the thick sleeve of gray matter surrounding the cerebral sylvian aqueduct in the midbrain, rostrally continuous with the posterior nucleus of the hypothalamus; in sections stained for myelin it stands out from the adjoining tectum and tegmentum by the poverty of its myelinated fibers.
s. innomina'ta, innominate substance; the region of the forebrain that lies ventral to the anterior half or so of the lentiform nucleus, extending in the frontal plane from the lateral preopticohypothalamic zone laterally over the optic tract to the amygdala (corpus amygdaloideum); rostrally it tapers off over the dorsal border of the olfactory tubercle, caudally it ends where the internal capsule reaches the surface to form the cerebral peduncle or pes pedunculi. Notable among its polymorphic cell population is the large-celled nucleus basalis of Meynert. These magnocellular elements within the s. i. are present in the medial septum and the diagonal band of Broca, but occur in largest numbers ventral to the globus pallidus. Histochemical evidence indicates that magnocellular elements distribute cholinergic fibers widely in the cerebral cortex and that these cells undergo selective degeneration in Alzheimer's disease.
s. interme'dia centra'lis et latera'lis [NA], Stilling's gelatinous substance; s. gelatinosa centralis; commissura anterior and posterior grisea; the central gray matter of the spinal cord surrounding the central canal.
s. len'tis [NA], substance of lens of eye.
s. medulla'ris, **(1)** medulla; **(2)** medullary *substance.*
s. metachromaticogranula'ris, Heinz *bodies.*
s. muscula'ris prosta'tae [NA], muscular substance of prostate; musculus prostaticus; the smooth muscle in the stroma of the prostate.
s. ni'gra [NA], nucleus or locus niger; nigra; Soemmering's ganglion; a large cell mass, crescentic on transverse section, extending forward over the dorsal surface of the crus cerebri from the rostral border of the pons into the subthalamic region; it is composed of a dorsal stratum of closely spaced pigmented (*i.e.,* melanin-containing) cells, the pars compacta, and a larger ventral region of widely scattered cells, the pars reticulata; the pars compacta in particular includes numerous cells that project forward to the striatum (caudate nucleus and putamen) and contain dopamine, which acts as the transmitter substance at their synaptic endings; other, apparently non-dopaminergic cells of the s. nigra project to a rostral part of the nucleus ventralis thalami, the middle layers of the superior colliculus and to restricted parts of the reticular formation of the midbrain; the nigrostriatal projection is reciprocated by a massive striatonigral fiber system with multiple neurotransmitters, chief among which is γ-aminobutyric acid (GABA); s. n. receives smaller afferent projections from the subthalamic nucleus, the lateral segment of the globus pallidus, the dorsal nucleus of the raphe and the pedunculopontine nucleus of the midbrain. The pars reticulata forms part of the output system for the corpus striatum. The s. n. is involved in the metabolic disturbances associated with Parkinson's disease and Huntington's disease.
s. os'sea den'tis, cementum.
s. perfora'ta ante'rior [NA], anterior perforated substance; olfactory area; area olfactoria; locus perforatus anticus; a region at the base of the brain through which numerous small branches of the anterior and middle cerebral arteries (lenticulostriate arteries) enter the depth of the cerebral hemisphere; it is bordered medially by the optic chasm and anterior half of the optic tract, rostrally and laterally by the lateral olfactory stria; its anteromedial part corresponds to the olfactory tubercle.
s. perfora'ta poste'rior [NA], posterior perforated substance; locus perforatus posticus; Malacarne's space; the bottom of the interpeduncular fossa at the base of the midbrain, extending from the anterior border of the pons forward to the mamillary bodies, and containing numerous openings for the passage of perforating branches of the posterior cerebral arteries.
s. pro'pria cor'neae [NA], proper substance of cornea; modified transparent connective tissue, between the layers of which are open spaces or lacunae nearly filled with the corneal cells or corpuscles.
s. pro'pria membra'nae tym'pani, proper substance of tympanic membrane; the layer of radial and circular collagenous fibers of the tympanic membrane.
s. pro'pria scle'rae [NA], proper substance of the sclera; the dense white fibrous tissue arranged in interlacing bundles that forms the main mass of the sclera, continuous anteriorly with the substantia propria corneae.
s. reticula'ris, **(1)** reticular *substance* (1); **(2)** *formatio* reticularis.
s. reticulofilamento'sa, reticular *substance* (1).
s. spongio'sa [NA], spongy bone (1); spongy substance; cancellous or trabecular bone; s. trabecularis; bone in which the spicules or trabeculae form a three-dimensional latticework (cancellus) with the interstices filled with embryonal connective tissue or bone marrow.
s. trabecula'ris [NA], s. spongiosa.
s. vit'rea, enamelum.

substernal (sŭb-ster'năl). **1.** Deep to the sternum. **2.** Infrasternal.

substernomastoid (sŭb-ster'nō-mas'toyd). Beneath the sternomastoid muscle; denoting a group of deep cervical lymph nodes.

substitute (sŭb'sti-tūt). **1.** Anything that takes the place of another.

2. In psychology, a surrogate.
blood s., any material (*e.g.,* human plasma, serum albumin, or a solution of such substances as dextran) used for transfusion in hemorrhage and shock.
plasma s., plasma expander; a solution of a substance (*e.g.,* dextran) used for transfusion in hemorrhage or shock as a s. for plasma.
volume s., infusion of cell-free or volume-expanding fluids such as dextran for replacement of fluid lost from the circulation as part of the prevention or treatment of circulatory shock.

substitution (sŭb-sti-tū'shŭn) [L. *substitutio,* to put in place of another]. **1.** In chemistry, the replacement of an atom or group in a compound by another atom or group (*e.g.,* s. of H by Cl in CH_4 to give CH_3Cl). **2.** In psychoanalysis, an unconscious defense mechanism by which an unacceptable or unattainable goal, object, or emotion is replaced by one that is more acceptable or attainable; the process is more acute and direct, and less subtle, than sublimation.
stimulus s., classical *conditioning.*
symptom s., symptom formation; an unconscious psychological process by which a repressed impulse is indirectly manifested through a particular symptom, *e.g.,* anxiety, compulsion, depression, hallucination, obsession.

substrate (sŭb'strāt) [L. *sub-sterno,* pp. *-stratus,* to spread under]. The substance acted upon and changed by an enzyme; the reactant considered to be attacked in a chemical reaction.

substratum (sŭb-strā'tŭm) [L. see substrate]. Any layer or stratum lying beneath another.

substructure (sŭb-strŭk'chŭr). A tissue or structure wholly or partly beneath the surface.
implant denture s., the metal framework which is placed beneath the soft tissues in contact with, or embedded into, bone for the purpose of supporting an implant denture superstructure.

subsulfate (sŭb-sŭl'fāt). A basic sulfate; a sulfate that contains some base unneutralized and still capable of combining with the acid.

subsultus (sŭb-sŭl'tŭs) [L. *subsilio,* pp. *-sultus,* to leap up, fr. *salio,* to leap]. A twitching or jerking.
s. clo'nus, s. tendinum.
s. ten'dinum, s. clonus; tremor tendinum; a twitching of the tendons, especially noticeable at the wrist, occurring in low fevers.

subtarsal (sŭb-tar'săl). Below the tarsus.

subtegumental (sŭb'teg-yū-men'tăl). Subcutaneous.

subtentorial (sŭb-ten-tō'rē-ăl). Beneath the tentorium cerebelli.

subterminal (sŭb-ter'mi-năl). Situated near the end or extremity of an oval or rod-shaped body.

subtetanic (sŭb-te-tan'ik). Denoting tonic muscular spasms or convulsions that are not entirely sustained but have brief remissions.

subthalamic (sŭb-thă-lam'ik). Related to the subthalamus region or to the subthalamic nucleus.

subthalamus (sŭb-thal'ă-mŭs). That part of the diencephalon that lies wedged between the thalamus on the dorsal side and the cerebral peduncle ventrally, lateral to the dorsal half of the hypothalamus from which it cannot be sharply delineated. It is composed of the nucleus subthalamicus (corpus luysi), the zona incerta, and the fields of Forel; laterally it expands in a winglike fashion into the nucleus reticularis thalami; caudally it is continuous with the midbrain tegmentum.

subthyroideus (sŭb-thī-royd'ē-ŭs). A muscular bundle formed of fibers derived from the thyroarytenoideus and the vocalis muscles.

subtilisin (sŭb-ti-lī'sin) [EC 3.4.21.14]. Subtilopeptidase; a proteinase formed by *Bacillus subtilis,* similar to the serine proteinases of other molds and bacteria; it catalyzes the hydrolysis of a few specific peptide bonds in certain proteins, converting chymotrypsinogen to chymotrypsin and ovalbumin to plakalbumin in this manner, and cleaves pancreatic ribonuclease into S-peptide and S-protein.

subtilopeptidase (sŭb'ti-lō-pep'ti-dās). Subtilisin.

subtraction (sŭb-trak'shŭn). A technique used to improve detectability of abnormalities on radiographic or scintigraphic images; a negative mask of one image is photographically or electronically separated and removed from a second image. See also digital subtraction *angiography.*

subtrapezial (sŭb-tra-pē'zē-ăl). Beneath the trapezius muscle; denoting a nerve plexus.

subtribe (sŭb-trīb). In biologic classification, a division between tribe and genus.

subtrochanteric (sŭb-trō-kan-ter'ik). Below any trochanter.

subtrochlear (sŭb-trok'lē-ar). Below any trochlea.

subtuberal (sŭb-tū'ber-ăl). Lying below any tuber.

subtympanic (sŭb-tim-pan'ik). Below the tympanic cavity.

subumbilical (sŭb-ŭm-bil'i-kăl). Infraumbilical.

subungual, subunguial (sŭb-ŭng'gwăl, sŭb-ŭng'gwi-ăl) [L. *unguis,* nail]. Hyponychial (1); beneath the finger or toe nail.

suburethral (sŭb-yū-rē'thrăl). Beneath the male or female urethra.

subvaginal (sŭb-vaj'i-năl). **1.** Below the vagina. **2.** On the inner side of any tubular membrane serving as a sheath.

subvalvar, subvalvular (sŭb-val'văr, sŭb-val'vyū-lăr). Below any valve.

subvertebral (sŭb-ver'tē-brăl). Beneath, or on the ventral side, of a vertebra or the vertebral column.

subvirile (sŭb-vir'il). Deficient in virility.

subvitrinal sŭb-vit'ri-năl). Beneath the vitreous body.

subvolution (sŭb-vō-lū'shŭn) [L. *sub,* under, + *volvo,* pp. *volutus,* to turn]. Turning over a flap of mucous membrane, as in the operation for pterygium, to prevent adhesion.

subwaking (sŭb-wāk'ing). Denoting the mental state between sleeping and waking.

subzonal (sŭb-zō'năl). Below or beneath any zona or zone, such as the zona radiata or zona pellucida.

subzygomatic (sŭb-zī-gō-mat'ik). Below or beneath the zygomatic bone or arch.

succagogue (sŭk'ă-gog) [L. *succus,* juice, + G. *agōgos,* leading]. **1.** Stimulating the flow of juice. **2.** An agent having such an effect.

succedaneous (sŭk-sē-dā'nē-ŭs) [see succedaneum]. **1.** Relating to a succedaneum. **2.** Relating to the permanent or second teeth that replace the deciduous or primary teeth.

succedaneum (sŭk-sē-dā'nē-ŭm) [L. *succedaneus,* following after, substituting, fr. *suc-cedo,* to follow, to take the place of, fr. *sub,* under, + *cedo,* to go]. A substitute; a drug or any therapeutic agent that has the properties of and can be used in place of another.

succenturiate (sŭk-sen-tyū'rē-āt) [L. *suc-centurio,* pp. *-atus,* to substitute]. In anatomy, substituting for, or accessory to, some organ.

succinate (sŭk'si-nāt). A salt of succinic acid.
s. dehydrogenase [EC 1.3.99.1], fumarate reductase; fumaric hydrogenase; a flavoenzyme that catalyzes the removal of hydrogen from succinic acid and converts it into fumaric acid.

succinate-CoA ligase. Succinyl-CoA synthetase; succinic thiokinase. **1** [EC 6.2.1.5]. A ligase combining succinate and CoA with the splitting of ATP to ADP and inorganic phosphate. **2** [EC 6.2.1.4]. A similar ligase, but one able to use itaconate as well as succinate and GTP (or ITP) in place of ATP.

succinic acid (sŭk-sin'ik). 1,4-Butanedioic acid; ethylenedicarboxylic acid; $HOOC(CH_2)_2COOH$; an intermediate in the tricarboxylic acid cycle; several of its salts have been variously used in medicine.

succinic thiokinase. Succinate-CoA ligase.

succinylcholine (sŭk'si-nil-kō'lēn). Diacetylcholine; succinyldicholine; a neuromuscular relaxant with short duration of action which characteristically first depolarizes the motor endplate (phase I block) but which is often later associated with a curare-like, nondepolarizing neuromuscular block (phase II block); used to produce relaxation during surgical anesthesia.

succinyl-CoA (sŭk'sin-il). Succinylcoenzyme A.

succinyl-CoA synthetase. Succinate-CoA ligase.

succinylcoenzyme (sŭk'si-nil-kō-en'zīm). Succinyl-CoA; "active succinate," the condensation product of succinic acid and CoA; one of the intermediates of the tricarboxylic acid cycle.

succinyldicholine (sŭk'si-nil-dī-kō'lēn). Succinylcholine chloride.

***O*- succinylhomoserine (thiol)-lyase** (sŭk'si-nil-hō'mō-ser'ēn) [EC 4.2.99.9]. Cystathionine γ-synthase; an enzyme catalyzing the reaction between cystathionine and succinate to form cysteine and *O*- succinylhomoserine.

succinylsulfathiazole (sŭk'si-nil-sŭl'fă-thī'ă-zōl). 4'-(2-Thiazolylsulfamoyl)succinanilic acid; the most effective of the poorly absorbed bacteriostatic sulfonamides used for sterilization of the intestinal tract.

succisulfone iminodiethanol (sŭk-si-sŭl'fōn im'i-nō-dī-eth'ă-nol). 4'-Sulfanilylsuccinanilic acid 2,2'-iminodiethanol salt; an antimicrobial agent.

succorrhea (sŭk-ō-rē'ă) [L. *succus,* juice, + G. *rhoia,* a flow]. An abnormal increase in the secretion of a digestive fluid.

succubus (sŭk'yū-bŭs) [L. *succubo,* to lie under]. A demon, in female form, believed to have sexual intercourse with a man during sleep. *Cf.* incubus.

succus, gen. and pl. succi (sŭk'ŭs, sŭk'sī) [L.]. **1.** Obsolete term for the fluid constituents of the body tissues. **2.** Obsolete term for a fluid secretion, especially the digestive fluid. **3.** Formerly, a pharmacopeial preparation obtained by expressing the juice of a plant and adding to it sufficient alcohol (1 part to 3 of juice) to preserve it. See also juice.

succuss (sŭ-kŭs'). To make succussion.

succussion (sŭ-kŭsh'ŭn) [L. *suceussio,* fr. *suc-cutio* (*subc-*), pp. *-cussus,* to shake up, fr. *quatio,* to shake]. A diagnostic procedure that consists in shaking the body so as to elicit a splashing sound in a cavity containing both gas and fluid.

hippocratic s., a splashing noise produced by shaking the body when there is gas or air and fluid in the stomach or intestine, or free in the peritoneum, thorax, and rarely the pericardium.

suck (sŭk) [A.S. *sūcan*] **1.** To draw a fluid through a tube by exhausting the air in front. **2.** To draw a fluid into the mouth; specifically, to draw milk from the breast.

suckle (sŭk'l). **1.** To nurse; to feed by milk from the breast. **2.** To suck; to draw sustenance from the breast.

Sucquet, J.P., French anatomist, 1840–1870. See S.'s *anastomoses, canals;* S.-Hoyer *anastomoses, canals.*

sucralfate (sū-kral'fāt). Sucrose octakis (hydrogen sulfate) aluminum complex; a polysaccharide with antipeptic activity, used to treat duodenal ulcers.

sucrase (sū'krās). Sucrose α-D-gluchohydrolase.

sucrate (sū'krāt). A compound of sucrose.

sucrose (sū'krōs). Saccharum; beet or cane sugar; saccharose; a nonreducing disaccharide made up of glucose and fructose obtained from sugar cane, *Saccharum officinarum* (family Gramineae), from several species of sorghum, and from the sugar beet, *Beta vulgaris* (family Chenopodiaceae); the common sweetener, used in pharmacy in the manufacture of syrup, confections, etc.

s. octaacetate, an alcohol denaturant.

sucrose α-D-glucohydrolase [EC 3.2.1.48]. Sucrase; an enzyme hydrolyzing sucrose and maltose.

sucrosemia (sū-krō-sē'mē-ă) [sucrose + G. *haima,* blood]. The presence of sucrose in the blood.

sucrosuria (sū-krō-sū'rē-ă) [sucrose + G. *ouron,* urine]. The excretion of sucrose in the urine.

suction (sŭk'shŭn) [L. *sugo,* pp. *suctus,* to suck]. The act or process of sucking. See also aspiration (1, 2).

posttussive s., a s. sound heard on auscultation over a pulmonary cavity at the end of a cough.

Wangensteen s., Wangensteen tube; a modified siphon that maintains constant negative pressure, used with a duodenal tube for the relief of gastric and intestinal distention.

suctorial (sŭk-tō'rē-ăl). Relating to suction, or the act of sucking; adapted for sucking.

sudamen, pl. **sudamina** (sū-dā'men, -dam'i-nă) [Mod. L., fr. L. *sudo,* to sweat]. A minute vesicle due to retention of fluid in a sweat follicle, or in the epidermis.

sudamina (sū-dam'i-nă). **1.** Plural of sudamen. **2.** *Miliaria* crystallina.

sudaminal (sū-dam'i-năl). Relating to sudamina.

Sudan III, Sudan red III [C.I. 26100]. A red stain, $(C_6H_5)N{=}N(C_6H_4)N{=}N(C_{10}H_6)OH$, used for neutral fat in histologic technique; it also stains the fatty envelope of the tubercle bacillus.

Sudan IV [C.I. 26105]. Scarlet red.

Sudan black B [C.I. 26150]. A diazo dye, $C_{29}H_{24}N_6$, used as a stain for fats.

Sudan brown [C.I. 12020]. A brown stain, $(C_{10}H_7)N{=}N(C_{10}H_6)OH$, derived from α-naphthylamine and used as a stain for fats.

sudanophilia (sū-dan-ō-fil'ēă). **1.** Affinity for an oil-soluble or Sudan dye. **2.** A condition in which leukocytes contain minute fat droplets which take a brilliant red stain when treated with 0.2% Sudan III and 0.1% cresyl blue in absolute alcohol.

sudanophilic (sū-dan-ō-fil'ik). Staining easily with Sudan dyes, usually referring to lipids in tissues.

sudanophobic (sū-dan-ō-fō'bik). Denoting tissue that fails to stain with a Sudan or fat-soluble dye.

Sudan yellow. Metadioxyazobenzene; a yellow stain for fats.

sudation (sū-dā'shŭn) [L. *sudatio,* fr. *sudo,* pp. *-atus,* to sweat]. Perspiration (1).

Sudeck, Paul H.M., German surgeon, 1866–1938. See S.'s *atrophy,* critical *point, syndrome.*

sudomotor (sū-dō-mō'ter) [L. *sudor,* sweat, + *motor,* mover]. Denoting the nerves that stimulate the sweat glands to activity.

sudor- [L. *sudor,* sweat]. Combining form denoting sweat, perspiration.

sudor (sū'dōr) [L.]. Perspiration (3).

s. sanguin'eus, hematidrosis.

s. urino'sus, uridrosis.

sudoral (sū'dōr'ăl). Relating to perspiration.

sudoresis (sū-dō-rē'sis) [sudor- + G. *-ēsis,* condition]. Profuse sweating.

sudoriferous (sū-dō-rif'er-ŭs) [sudor- + L. *fero,* to bear]. Carrying or producing sweat.

sudorific (sū-dō-rif'ik) [sudor- + L. *facio,* to make]. Causing sweat.

sudorikeratosis (sū'dōr-i-ker-ă-tō'sis). Keratosis of the sudoriferous ducts.

sudoriparous (sū-dō-rip'ă-rŭs) [sudor- + L. *pario,* to produce]. Secreting sweat.

sudorometer (sū-dō-rom′ĕ-ter) [sudor- + G. *metron,* measure]. An instrument for measuring the amount of perspiration.

sudorrhea (sū-dō-rē′ă) [sudor- + G. *rhoia,* a flow]. Hyperhidrosis.

suet (sū′et). The hard fat around the kidneys of cattle and sheep; when rendered it yields tallow.

prepared s., prepared mutton tallow; the internal fat of the abdomen of the sheep, *Ovis aries,* purified by melting and straining; used in pharmacy in making ointments.

sufentanil citrate (sū-fen′tă-nil). *N*-[4-(Methoxymethyl)-1-[2-(2-thienyl)ethyl]-4-piperidyl]proprionanilide; an injectable general anesthetic with narcotic action, used to induce and maintain anesthesia.

suffocate (sŭf′ō-kāt) [L. *suffoco (subf-),* pp. *-atus,* to choke, strangle]. **1.** To impede respiration; to asphyxiate. **2.** To be unable to breathe; to suffer from asphyxiation.

suffocation (sŭf-ō-kā′shŭn). The act or condition of suffocating or of asphyxiation.

suffusion (sŭ-fyū′zhŭn) [L. *suffusio,* fr. *suffundo* (*subf-*), to pour out]. **1.** The act of pouring a fluid over the body. **2.** A reddening of the surface. **3.** The condition of being wet with a fluid. **4.** Extravasate (2).

sugar (shu-ger) [G. *sakcharon;* L. *saccharum*] One of the sugars, *q.v.* Pharmaceutical forms are compressible s. and confectioner's s.

amino s.'s, s.'s that contain an amino group; *e.g.,* glucosamine.

beechwood s., xylose.

beet s., sucrose.

blood s., glucose.

brain s., galactose.

cane s., sucrose.

corn s., glucose.

deoxy s., a s. containing fewer oxygen atoms than carbon atoms and in which, consequently, one or more carbons in the molecule lack an attached hydroxyl group.

fruit s., fructose.

gelatin s., glycine.

grape s., glucose.

invert s., a mixture of equal parts of glucose and fructose produced by hydrolysis of sucrose (inversion).

s. of lead, *lead* acetate.

malt s., maltose.

manna s., mannitol.

maple s., saccharum canadense; sucrose extracted from the sap of the sugar maple, *Acer saccharinum.*

milk s., lactose.

oil s., oleosaccharum.

pectin s., arabinose.

reducing s., a s., such as glucose in the urine, that has the property of reducing various inorganic ions, notably cupric ion to cuprous ion.

specific soluble s., specific capsular *substance.*

starch s., glucose.

wood s., xylose.

sugar acids. Acids, such as gluconic, glycuronic, and saccharic acid, produced by the oxidation of glucose.

sugar alcohol. The polyalcohol resulting from the reduction of the carbonyl group in a monosaccharide to a hydroxyl group.

sugars (shug′erz) Those carbohydrates (saccharides) having the general composition $(CH_2O)_n$ and simple derivatives thereof. Although the simple monomeric s. (glycoses) are often written as polyhydroxy aldehydes or ketones, *e.g.,* $CH_2OH–(CHOH)_4–CHO$ for aldohexoses (*e.g.,* glucose) or $CH_2OH–(CHOH)_3–CO–CH_2OH$ for 2-ketoses (*e.g.,* fructose), cyclization can give rise to varied structures as described below. S. are generally identifiable by the ending -ose or, if in combination with a nonsugar (aglycon), -oside or -osyl. S. especially glucose, are the chief source of energy, by oxidation, in nature, and they and their derivatives (*e.g.,* glucosamine, glucuronic acid), in polymeric form, are major constituents of mucoproteins, bacterial cell walls, and plant structural material (*e.g.,* cellulose). S. are often found in combination with steroids (steroid glycosides) and other aglycons.

Fischer projection formulas of s., representations, by projection, of cyclic s., or derivatives thereof, in which the carbon chain is depicted vertically. The lowest-numbered asymmetric carbon atom (C-1 in aldoses; C-2 in 2-ketoses, *e.g.,* fructose) is drawn at the top, and the rest of the carbon atoms of the chain are drawn in sequence below the top carbon atom. For each carbon atom, depicted in projection as lying in the plane of the paper, the carbon-to-carbon bond(s), which actually point away from the viewer, are drawn as vertical lines. The left-hand and right-hand bonds of each carbon atom, which actually point toward the viewer, are, in projection, depicted as horizontal lines.

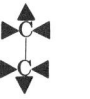

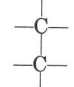

Actual Fischer projection

The conventions for the Fischer formulas of cyclic s. are as follows: 1) Asymmetric carbon atoms having O to the right are D carbon atoms (*i.e.,* are related in configuration to D-glyceraldehyde, the prototype). 2) If the highest-numbered asymmetric carbon atom has its OH (or its replacement) lying to the right, as is the 2-OH of D-glyceraldehyde, the sugar has the D configuration; if the OH is to the left, the sugar has the L configuration. 3) On the anomeric carbon atom (C-1 in the aldoses; C-2 in the 2-ketoses, *e.g.,* fructose), an OH or substituted OH that lies to the right, with the OH of the highest-numbered asymmetric carbon atom also to the right (*i.e.,* D s.) is α; if it is to the left, with the OH of the highest-numbered carbon atom still to the right, it is β; the reverse applies if the latter OH is to the left (L s.). 4) The orientation of a terminal CH_2OH group in the aldoses carries no configurational significance, as it contains no asymmetric carbon atom. See fig. on p. 1500.

Haworth conformational formulas of cyclic s., for the pyranoses, these depict those shapes (conformations) on which none, one, or two ring-atoms lie outside the plane of the ring. If there are two such atoms *para* to each other, they can lie 1) on opposite sides of the plane (*trans*), giving chair forms, or 2) on the same side of the plane (*cis*), giving boat forms. For β-D-ribopyranose, the two chair forms ($^4C_1$ and $^1C_4$) are depicted.

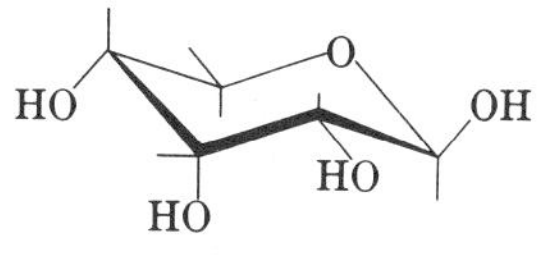

$^4C_1$

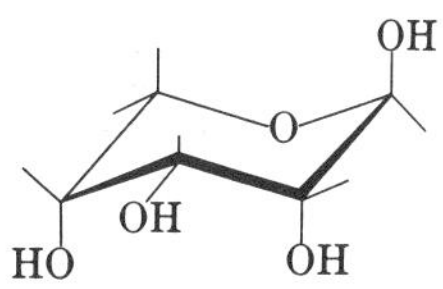

$^1C_4$

Similarly, there are six boat conformations. If the two (*trans*) exoplanar atoms are *meta* to each other, the conformation is a skew form; if the two atoms are *ortho* to each other, the conformation is a half-chair form.

For the furanoses, the envelope conformations have one ring-atom exoplanar. If there are three adjacent, coplanar ring-atoms (the two exoplanar ring-atoms on opposite sides of the plane), the conformations are twist forms.

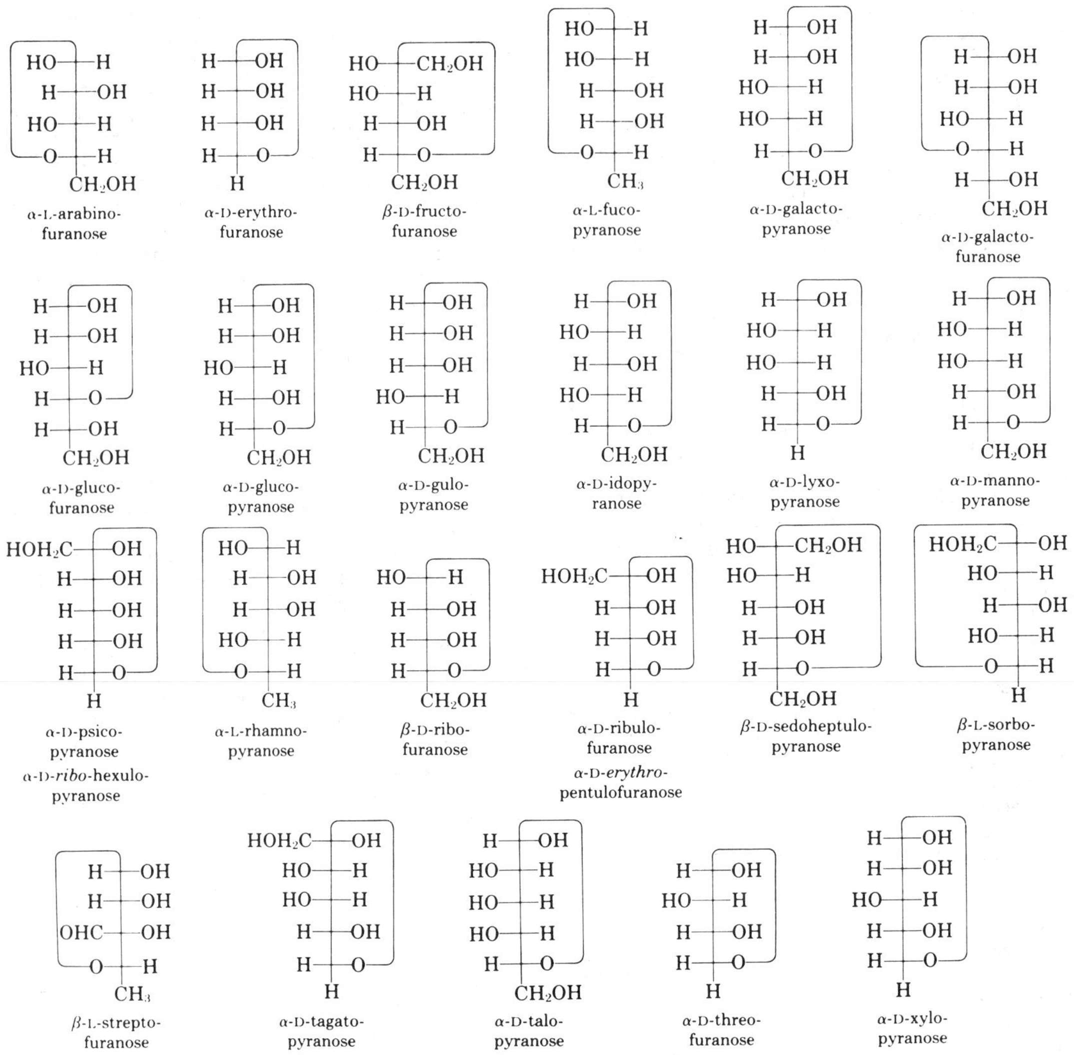

Fischer projection formulas for some cyclic sugars

Haworth perspective formulas of cyclic s., perspective representations of furanose or pyranose structures as pentagons or hexagons, respectively, with the connecting bonds so shaded as to make them appear as though the plane of the ring is at an angle of 30° to the plane of the paper, and the bonds to H and OH are at right angles to the plane of the ring. These formulas depict the planar conformation, a situation not usually met. Other conformational formulas *e.g.,* Haworth conformational formulas of cyclic s. attempt to depict the many deviations from planarity. See also Fischer projection formulas of s.

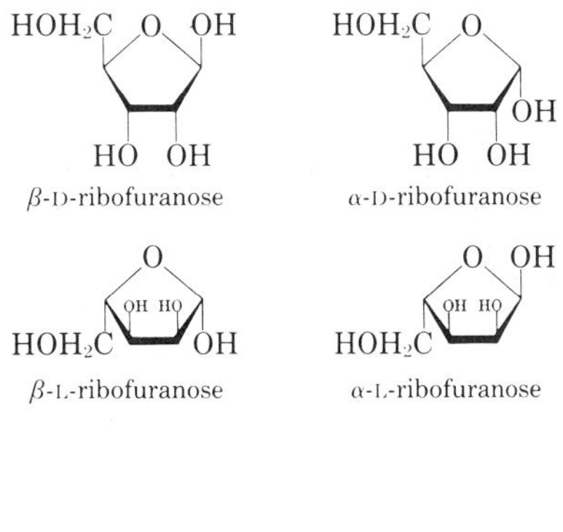

The basic conventions in Haworth formulas of cyclic s. (cyclic glycoses) are as follows: 1) The lowest-numbered asymmetric ring-carbon atom is depicted at the right. 2) Ring-carbon atoms having the exocyclic O atom below the plane of the ring are D carbons (*i.e.,* are configurationally identical to D-glyceraldehyde, the prototype), whereas those having this O atom above the plane are L. 3) If the highest-numbered asymmetric carbon atom is D, the sugar is D; the formula of an L-glycose may be derived from that of its D isomer by reversing the up or down direction of all groups attached to the ring-carbon atoms. 4) If the hydroxyl group attached to the anomeric carbon (C-1 in aldoses; C-2 in 2-ketoses, *e.g.,* fructose) is below the plane of the ring of a D-glycose, it is α; if above, it is β; the reverse applies if the sugar is L.

suggestibility (sŭg-jes′tĭ-bil′i-tē). Sympathism; responsiveness or susceptibility to a psychological process whereby an idea is induced into, or adopted by, an individual without argument, command, or coercion.

suggestible (sŭg-jes′tĭ-bl). Susceptible to suggestion.

suggestion (sŭg-jes′chŭn) [L. *sug-gero* (*subg-*), pp. *-gestus,* to bring under, supply]. The implanting of an idea in the mind of another by some word or act on one's part, the subject's conduct or physical

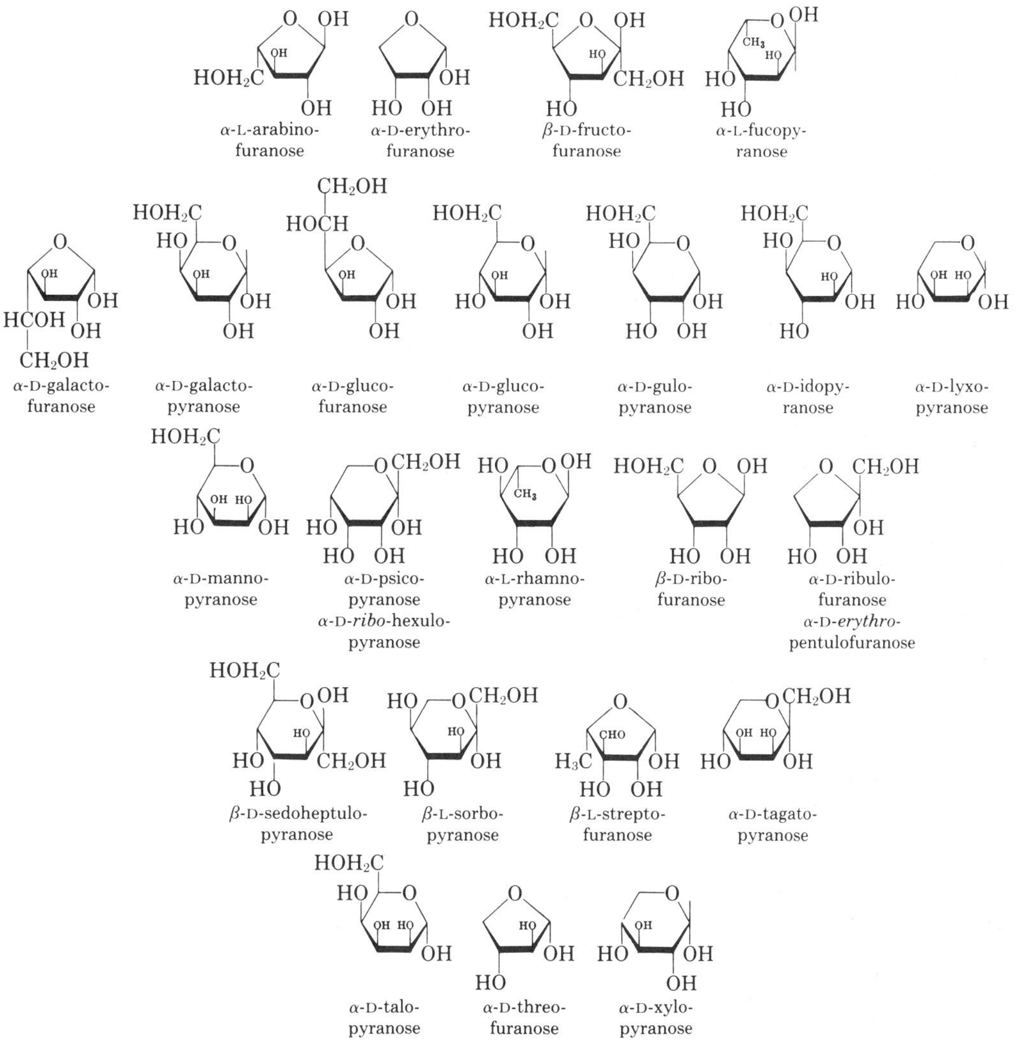

Haworth perspective formulas for some cyclic sugars

condition being influenced to some degree by the implanted idea. See also autosuggestion.

posthypnotic s., s. given to a subject who is under hypnosis for certain actions to be performed by him after he is "awakened" from the hypnotic trance.

suggestive (sŭg-jes'tiv). Relating to suggestion.

suggillation (sŭg-ji-lā'shŭn, sŭj-i-) [L. *sugillo,* pp. *-atus,* to beat black and blue]. A bruise or livedo. See also contusion.

postmortem s., postmortem *livedo.*

Sugiura, M., 20th century Japanese surgeon. See S. *procedure.*

suicide (sū'i-sīd) [L. *sui,* self, + *caedō,* to kill]. **1.** The act of taking one's own life. **2.** A person who commits such an act.

suicidology (sū'i-sī-dol'ō-jē) [suicide + G. *logos,* study]. A branch of the behavioral sciences devoted to the study of the nature, causes, socioeconomic correlates, and prevention of suicide.

suint (swint) [Fr. wool-grease]. The natural grease in sheep's wool, from which the official wool fat is extracted.

suit (sūt). An outer garment designed for protection against specific environmental conditions.

anti-G s., a garment with bladders that expand to apply external pressure to the abdomen and lower extremities during positive G maneuvers in flight or on a human centrifuge; the anti-G s. is worn to prevent the pooling of blood and serves to increase the wearer's ability to withstand exposure to higher G forces.

sulbentine (sŭl-ben'tēn). Dibenzthione.

sulcal (sŭl'kăl). Relating to a sulcus.

sulcate, sulcated (sŭl'kāt, -kā-ted). Grooved; furrowed; marked by a sulcus or sulci.

sulciform (sŭl'si-fōm). Having the form of a groove or sulcus.

sulculus, pl. **sulculi** (sŭl'kŭ-lŭs, -lī) [Mod. L. dim. of L. *sulcus,* furrow]. A small sulcus.

SULCUS

sulcus, gen. and pl. **sulci** (sŭl'kŭs, sŭl'sī) [L. a furrow or ditch]. **1** [NA]. One of the grooves or furrows on the surface of the brain, bounding the several convolutions or gyri; a fissure. See also fissura. **2** [NA]. Any long narrow groove, furrow, or slight depression. **3.** A groove or depression in the oral cavity or on the surface of a tooth.

alveolobuccal s., alveolobuccal *groove.*

alveololabial s., alveololabial *groove.*

alveololingual s., alveololingual *groove.*

s. ampulla'ris [NA], ampullary s.; the groove on the external surface of the ampulla of each semicircular duct where the nerve enters the crista ampullaris.

ampullary s., s. ampullaris.

s. angula'ris, *incisura* angularis.

anterior parolfactory s., s. parolfactorius anterior.

anterolateral s., s. lateralis anterior.

s. anthel'icis transver'sus [NA], a deep groove on the cranial surface of the auricle separating the eminences of the triangular fossa and of the concha.

aortic s., s. aor'ticus, a broad deep groove on the medial aspect of the left lung above and behind the hilum receiving the arch of the aorta and the thoracic aorta.

s. arte'riae occipita'lis [NA], s. of occipital artery; occipital groove; a narrow groove medial to the mastoid notch of the temporal bone that lodges the occipital artery.

s. arte'riae subcla'viae [NA], groove for subclavian artery; a groove immediately posterior to the scalene tubercle on the upper surface of the first rib across which the subclavian artery passes.

s. arte'riae tempora'lis me'diae [NA], s. for middle temporal artery; a vertical groove located above the external acoustic meatus on the external surface of the squamous part of the temporal bone.

s. arte'riae vertebra'lis [NA], s. for vertebral artery; the s. on the superior aspect of the posterior arch of the atlas that transmits the vertebral artery medially toward the foramen magnum.

sul'ci arterio'si [NA], arterial grooves; branching grooves on the interior surface of the cranial vault in which the meningeal arteries course, the most prominent of which are related to branches of the middle meningeal artery.

atrioventricular s., s. coronarius.

s. auric'ulae ante'rior, *incisura* anterior auris.

s. auric'ulae poste'rior [NA], posterior auricular groove; the s. between the antitragus and cauda helicis overlying the antitragicohelicine fissure.

basilar s., s. basilaris pontis.

s. basila'ris pon'tis [NA], basilar s.; a median groove on the ventral surface of the pons varolii in which lies the basilar artery.

s. bicipita'lis latera'lis [NA], lateral bicipital groove; at the cubital fossa, the groove separating the biceps brachii and brachialis muscles on the lateral side.

s. bicipita'lis media'lis [NA], medial bicipital groove; at the cubital fossa, the groove separating the biceps brachii and brachialis muscles on the medial side.

calcaneal s., s. calcanei.

s. calca'nei [NA], calcaneal s.; interosseous groove (1); the groove on the upper part of the calcaneus, which with a corresponding groove on the talus forms the sinus tarsi.

calcarine s., s. calcarinus.

s. calcari'nus [NA], calcarine s.; calcarine or posthippocampal fissure; fissura calcarina; a deep fissure on the medial aspect of the cerebral cortex, extending on an arched line from the isthmus of the fornicate gyrus back to the occipital pole, marking the border between the lingual gyrus below and the cuneus above it. The cortex in the depth of the sulcus corresponds to the horizontal meridian of the contralateral half of the visual field.

callosal s., s. corporis callosi.

s. callosomargina'lis, s. cinguli.

s. carot'icus [NA], carotid s. or groove; cavernous groove; the groove on the body of the sphenoid bone in which the internal carotid artery lies in its course through the cavernous sinus.

carotid s., s. caroticus.

s. car'pi [NA], carpal groove; carpal canal (2); the concavity on the anterior surface of the arch formed by the carpal bones.

central s., s. centralis.

s. centra'lis [NA], central s.; fissure of Rolando; a double-S-shaped fissure extending obliquely upward and backward on the lateral surface of each cerebral hemisphere at the boundary between frontal and parietal lobes.

cerebellar sulci, grooves between the folia cerebelli.

cerebral sulci, sulci cerebri.

sul'ci cer'ebri [NA], cerebral sulci; the grooves between the cerebral gyri or convolutions.

chiasmatic s., s. prechiasmatis.

s. cin'guli [NA], s. of the cingulum; s. callosomarginalis; callosomarginal fissure; a fissure on the mesial surface of the cerebral hemisphere, bounding the upper surface of the gyrus cinguli (callosal convolution); the anterior portion is called the pars subfrontalis; the posterior portion which curves up to the superomedial margin of the hemisphere and borders the paracentral lobule posteriorly, the pars marginalis.

s. of cingulum, s. cinguli.

circular s. of Reil, s. circularis insulae.

s. circula'ris in'sulae [NA], circular or limiting s. of Reil; a semicircular fissure demarcating the insula from the opercula above, below, and behind.

collateral s., s. collateralis.

s. collatera'lis [NA], s. occipitotemporalis; collateral or occipitotemporal s.; collateral fissure; fissura collateralis; a long, deep sagittal fissure on the undersurface of the temporal lobe, marking the border between the fusiform gyrus laterally and the hippocampal and lingual gyri medially; the great depth of the s. collateralis results in a bulging of the floor of the occipital and temporal horn of the lateral ventricle, the eminentia collateralis.

s. corona'rius [NA], coronary s.; atrioventricular s. or groove; auriculoventricular groove; a groove on the outer surface of the heart marking the division between the atria and the ventricles.

coronary s., s. coronarius.

s. cor'poris callo'si [NA], s. of the corpus callosum; callosal s.; the fissure between the corpus callosum and the gyrus cinguli.

s. of corpus collasum, s. corporis callosi.

s. cos'tae [NA], costal or subcostal groove; a groove in the lower inner border of the rib, lodging the intercostal vessels and nerve.

s. cru'ris heli'cis [NA], groove of crus of helix; a transverse fissure on the cranial surface of the auricle corresponding to the crus of the helix.

sul'ci cu'tis [NA], skin grooves; the numerous grooves of variable depth on the surface of the epidermis.

s. ethmoida'lis [NA], ethmoidal groove; a groove on the inner surface of each nasal bone, lodging the external nasal branch of the anterior ethmoid nerve.

external spiral s., s. spiralis externus.

fimbriodentate s., s. fimbriodenta'tus, a shallow groove between the fimbria and the dentate fascia of the hippocampus.

s. fronta'lis infe'rior [NA], inferior frontal s.; a sagittal fissure on the lateral convex surface of each frontal lobe of the cerebrum demarcating the middle from the inferior frontal gyrus.

s. fronta'lis me'dius, middle or median frontal s.; a relatively shallow sagittal fissure dividing the middle frontal convolution into an upper and lower part; this s. is found only in man and the anthropoid apes; at its anterior extremity it bifurcates, the two branches spreading out laterally and constituting the frontomarginal s.

s. fronta'lis supe'rior [NA], superior frontal s.; a sagittal fissure on the superior surface of each frontal lobe of the cerebrum starting from the precentral s.; it forms the lateral boundary of the superior frontal convolution.

s. frontomargina'lis, see s. frontalis medius.

gingival s., s. gingivalis.

s. gingiva'lis [NA], gingival s., crevice, or space; subgingival space; the space between the surface of the tooth and the free gingiva.

gingivobuccal s., alveolobuccal *groove.*

gingivolabial s., alveololabial *groove.*

gingivolingual s., alveololingual *groove.*

s. glute'us [NA], gluteal furrow; the furrow between the buttock and thigh.

s. for greater palatine nerve, s. palatinus major.

s. ham'uli pterygoi'dei [NA], s. of pterygoid hamulus; a groove at the base of the hamular process which forms a pulley for the tendon of the tensor veli palatini.

s. hippocam'pi [NA], hippocampal fissure; fissura hippocampi; dentate fissure; fissura dentata; a shallow groove between the gyrus dentatus (dentate gyrus or fascia dentata) and the parahippocampal gyrus; the remains of a fissure extending deep into the hippocampus between Ammon's horn and the dentate gyrus which becomes obliterated during fetal development.

hypothalamic s., s. hypothalamicus.

s. hypothalam'icus [NA], hypothalamic s.; Monro's s.; a groove in the lateral wall of the third ventricle on either side leading from the interventricular foramen to the aditus ad aqueductum cerebri; the s.-demarcated boundary between dorsal thalamus and hypothalamus.

inferior frontal s., s. frontalis inferior.

inferior petrosal s., s. sinus petrosi inferioris.

inferior temporal s., s. temporalis inferior.

s. infraorbita'lis [NA], infraorbital groove; a gradually deepening groove on the orbital surface of the maxilla, which leads to the infraorbital canal.

s. infrapalpebra'lis, the hollow or furrow below the lower eyelid.

s. interme'dius ante'rior, anterior intermediate groove; a furrow occasionally seen in the adult between the anterior median fissure and the anterior lateral s. of the spinal cord but usually present only in the fetus. It indicates the lateral border of the anterior corticospinal fasciculus.

s. interme'dius poste'rior [NA], posterior intermediate groove; a longitudinal furrow between the posterior median and the posterolateral sulci of the spinal cord in the cervical region, marking the funiculus gracilis from the funiculus cuneatus.

internal spiral s., s. spiralis internus.

interparietal s., s. intraparietalis.

intertubercular s., s. intertubercularis.

s. intertubercula'ris [NA], intertubercular s.; intertubercular groove; bicipital groove; a furrow running down the shaft of the humerus between the two tubercles, lodging the tendon of the long head of the biceps, and giving attachment in its floor to the latissimus dorsi muscle.

s. interventricula'ris ante'rior [NA], anterior interventricular groove; crena cordis (1); a groove on the anterosuperior surface of the heart, marking the location of the septum between the two ventricles.

s. interventricula'ris cor'dis, see s. interventricularis anterior and s. interventricularis posterior.

s. interventricula'ris poste'rior [NA], posterior interventricular groove; crena cordis (2); a groove on the diaphragmatic surface of the heart, marking the location of the septum between the two ventricles.

s. intragra'cilis, a fissure between the gracilis minor and gracilis posterior lobuli of the cerebellum.

intraparietal s., s. intraparietalis.

intraparietal s. of Turner, s. intraparietalis.

s. intraparieta'lis [NA], intraparietal or interparietal s.; Turner's s.; intraparietal s. of Turner; a horizontal s. extending back from the postcentral s. over some distance, then dividing perpendicularly into two branches so as to form, with the postcentral s., a figure H. It divides the parietal lobe into superior and inferior parietal lobules.

labial s., lip s.; primary labial groove; a furrow between the developing lip and gum.

s. lacrima'lis [NA], lacrimal groove; (2) the groove in the nasal surface of the maxilla which, together with the lacrimal bone, forms the fossa for the lacrimal sac.

lateral cerebral s., s. lateralis cerebri.

lateral occipital s., s. occipitalis lateralis; one of several variable sulci on the lateral aspect of the occipital lobe of each cerebral hemisphere, bounding the lateral occipital convolutions.

s. latera'lis ante'rior [NA], anterolateral groove or s.; an indistinct furrow on the ventral surface of the spinal cord and medulla oblongata, on either side marking the line of exit of the anterior nerve roots.

s. latera'lis cer'ebri [NA], lateral cerebral s. or fissure; fissura cerebri lateralis; fissure of sylvius; sylvian fissure; the deepest and most prominent of the cortical fissures, extending from the anterior perforated substance first laterally at the deep incisure between the frontal and temporal lobes, then back and slightly upward over the lateral aspect of the cerebral hemisphere, with the superior temporal gyrus as its lower bank, the insula forming its greatly expanded floor. Two short side branches, the ramus anterior and ramus ascendens, divide the inferior frontal gyrus into a pars orbitalis, pars triangularis, and pars opercularis.

s. latera'lis poste'rior [NA], posterolateral groove or s.; a longitudinal furrow on either side of the posterior median s. of the spinal cord marking the line of entrance of the posterior nerve roots.

s. lim'itans [NA], the medial longitudinal groove on the inner surface of the neural tube separating the alar and basal plates.

s. lim'itans fos'sae rhomboi'deae [NA], limiting s. of rhomboid fossa; a lateral groove running the whole length of the floor of the rhomboid fossa on either side of the midline, the remains of the s. demarcating the alar (dorsal) from the basal (ventral) plate of the embryonic rhombencephalon.

limiting s. of Reil, s. circularis insulae.

limiting s. of rhomboid fossa, s. limitans fossae rhomboideae.

lip s., labial s.

longitudinal s. of heart, see s. interventricularis anterior and s. interventricularis posterior.

lunate s., s. lunatus cerebri.

s. luna'tus cer'ebri [NA], ape, lunate, or simian fissure; lunate s.; a small, inconstant semilunar groove on the cortical convexity near the occipital pole, marking the anterior border of the striate cortex (area 17) and considered homologous with the major s. of the same name that is a more constant feature of the cerebral cortex in monkeys and apes.

malleolar s., s. malleolaris.

s. malleola'ris [NA], malleolar s.; a broad groove on the posterior surface of the medial malleolus, through which the tendon of the tibialis posterior muscle runs.

s. ma'tricis un'guis, groove of the nail matrix; vallecula unguis;

the cutaneous furrow in which the lateral border of the nail is situated.
s. media'lis cru'ris cer'ebri [NA], s. nervi oculomotorii; a groove in the lateral wall of the interpeduncular fossa of the midbrain from which the rootlets of the oculomotor nerve emerge.
median s. of fourth ventricle, s. medianus ventriculi quarti.
median frontal s., s. frontalis medius.
s. media'nus lin'guae [NA], median groove or median longitudinal raphe of tongue; raphe linguae; a slight longitudinal depression running forward on the dorsal surface of the tongue from the foramen cecum.
s. media'nus poste'rior medul'lae oblonga'tae [NA], posterior median s. or fissure of the medulla oblongata; the longitudinal groove marking the posterior midline of the medulla oblongata; continuous below with the posterior median s. of the spinal cord.
s. media'nus poste'rior medul'lae spina'lis [NA], posterior median s. or fissure of the spinal cord; a shallow furrow in the median line of the posterior surface of the spinal cord.
s. media'nus ventric'uli quar'ti [NA], median s. of the fourth ventricle; the shallow midline groove in the floor of the ventricle.
s. mentolabia'lis, mentolabial furrow; the indistinct line separating the lower lip from the chin.
middle frontal s., s. frontalis medius.
middle temporal s., s. temporalis medius.
s. for middle temporal artery, s. arteriae temporalis mediae.
Monro's s., s. hypothalamicus.
s. mus'culi subcla'vii [NA], subclavian s. or groove; s. subclavianus; a groove on the inferior surface of the body of the clavicle to which is attached the subclavius muscle.
s. mylohyoi'deus [NA], mylohyoid groove or fossa; a groove on the medial surface of the ramus of the mandible beginning at the lingula; it lodges the mylohyoid artery and nerve.
s. nasolabia'lis, nasolabial groove; a furrow between the ala nasi and the lip.
s. ner'vi oculomoto'rii, s. medialis cruris cerebri.
s. ner'vi petro'si majo'ris [NA], groove of greater petrosal nerve; the groove on the anterior surface of the petrous part of the temporal bone that lodges the greater petrosal nerve.
s. ner'vi petro'si mino'ris [NA], groove of lesser petrosal nerve; the groove on the anterior surface of the petrous part of the temporal bone that accommodates the lesser petrosal nerve in its course to the otic ganglion.
s. ner'vi radia'lis [NA], groove for radial nerve; musculospiral or spiral groove; the shallow groove that passes around the shaft of the humerus; it lodges the radial nerve and deep brachial artery.
s. ner'vi spina'lis [NA], groove for spinal nerve; the laterally directed groove on the superior surface of the transverse processes of typical cervical vertebrae between the anterior and posterior tubercles along which the emerging spinal nerve passes.
s. ner'vi ulna'ris [NA], groove for ulnar nerve; a furrow on the posterior surface of the medial epicondyle of the humerus, lodging the ulnar nerve.
nymphocaruncular s., s. nymphocaruncula'ris, nymphohymenal s.; a groove between the labium minus and the border of the remains of the hymen, in which is the opening of the duct of the glandula vestibularis major (Bartholin's gland) on either side.
nymphohymenal s., nymphocaruncular s.
s. obturato'rius [NA], obturator groove; a deep groove on the inner surface of the superior ramus of the pubis.
s. of occipital artery, s. arteriae occipitalis.
s. occipita'lis latera'lis, lateral occipital s.
s. occipita'lis supe'rior, superior occipital s.
s. occipita'lis transver'sus [NA], transverse occipital s.; the posterior, vertical limb of the intraparietal s.
occipitotemporal s., s. collateralis.
s. occipitotempora'lis [NA], s. collateralis.
s. olfacto'rius [NA], olfactory s. or groove; the sagittal s. on the inferior or orbital surface of each frontal lobe of the cerebrum, demarcating the gyrus rectus from the orbital gyri, and covered on the orbital surface by the bulbus and tractus olfactorii.
s. olfacto'rius na'si [NA], olfactory s. of nose; the narrow groove in the nasal cavity above the agger nasi that leads from the atrium to the olfactory area.
olfactory s., s. olfactorius.
olfactory s. of nose, s. olfactorius nasi.
orbital sulci, sulci orbitales.
sul'ci orbita'les [NA], orbital sulci; a number of irregularly disposed, variable sulci dividing the inferior or orbital surface of each frontal lobe of the cerebrum into the orbital gyri.
s. palati'nus, pl. **sul'ci palati'ni** [NA], palatine groove; one of a number of grooves on the lower surface of the palatine process of the maxilla in which the palatine vessels and nerves lie.
s. palati'nus ma'jor [NA], greater palatine groove; s. for greater palatine nerve; pterygopalatine groove; s. pterygopalatinus; a groove on both the body of the maxilla and the perpendicular plate of the palatine bone; when the bones are articulated the grooves form the greater palatine canal.
s. palatovagina'lis [NA], palatovaginal groove; a furrow on the inferior aspect of the vaginal process of the sphenoid bone that is bridged below by the sphenoidal process of the palatine bone to form the palatovaginal canal.
sul'ci paraco'lici [NA], paracolic recesses; the grooves between the lateral aspect of the ascending or descending colon and the abdominal wall.
paraglenoid s., preauricular *groove.*
s. paraglenoida'lis, preauricular *groove.*
parieto-occipital s., s. parieto-occipitalis.
s. parieto-occipita'lis [NA], parieto-occipital fissure or s.; fissura parieto-occipitalis; a very deep, almost vertically oriented fissure on the medial surface of the cerebral cortex, marking the border between the parietal lobe and the cuneus of the occipital lobe; its lower part curves forward and fuses with the anterior extent of the calcarine fissure (sulcus calcarinus); the great depth of this combined fissure causes a bulge in the medial wall of the occipital horn of the lateral ventricle, the calcar avis.
s. parolfacto'rius ante'rior, anterior parolfactory s.; a fissure marking the anterior border of the parolfactory area.
s. parolfacto'rius poste'rior, posterior parolfactory s.; a shallow groove on the medial surface of the hemisphere demarcating the subcallosal gyrus or precommissural septum from the parolfactory area.
periconchal s., *fossa* anthelicis.
s. poplite'us, popliteal *groove.*
postcentral s., s. postcentralis.
s. postcentra'lis [NA], postcentral s.; the s. that demarcates the postcentral gyrus from the superior and inferior parietal lobules.
posterior median s. of medulla oblongata, s. medianus posterior medullae oblongatae.
posterior median s. of spinal cord, s. medianus posterior medullae spinalis.
posterior parolfactory s., s. parolfactorius posterior.
posterolateral s., s. lateralis posterior.
preauricular s., preauricular *groove.*
precentral s., s. precentralis.
s. precentra'lis [NA], precentral s.; s. verticalis; an interrupted fissure anterior to and in general parallel with the s. centralis, marking the anterior border of the precentral gyrus.
prechiasmatic s., s. prechiasmatis.
s. prechias'matis [NA], chiasmatic s.; prechiasmatic s.; optic groove; a groove on the upper surface of the sphenoid bone between the optic canals in which the optic chiasm lies.
s. promonto'rii [NA], a narrow branched groove running vertically over the surface of the promontory in the middle ear, lodging the tympanic plexus.

s. of pterygoid hamulus, s. hamuli pterygoidei.
s. pterygopalati'nus, s. palatinus major.
s. pulmona'lis [NA], pulmonary s.; the deep recess on either side of the vertebral column formed by the posterior sweep of the curvature of the ribs.
pulmonary s., s. pulmonalis.
rhinal s., s. rhinalis.
s. rhina'lis [NA], rhinal s. or fissure; the shallow rostral continuation of the collateral s. that delimits the rostral part of the parahippocampal gyrus from the fusiform or lateral occipitotemporal gyrus. One of the oldest sulci of the pallium, it marks the border between the neocortex and the allocortical (olfactory).
sagittal s., s. sinus sagittalis superioris.
s. of sclera, s. sclerae.
s. scle'rae [NA], s. of sclera; a slight groove on the external surface of the eyeball indicating the line of union of the sclera and cornea.
sigmoid s., s. sinus sigmoidei.
s. si'nus petro'si inferio'ris [NA], inferior petrosal s. or groove; a groove lodging the inferior petrosal sinus, formed by union of similarly named grooves in the petrous part of the temporal bone and the basilar part of the occipital bone.
s. si'nus petro'si superio'ris [NA], superior petrosal s.; a groove on the superior border of the petrous portion of the temporal bone in which rests the superior petrosal sinus.
s. si'nus sagitta'lis superio'ris [NA], sagittal s. or groove; groove for superior sagittal sinus; superior longitudinal s.; the groove in the midline of the inner table of the calvaria lodging the superior sagittal sinus.
s. si'nus sigmoi'dei [NA], sigmoid s.; sigmoid fossa or groove; a broad groove in the posterior cranial fossa, first situated on the lateral portion of the occipital bone, then curving around the jugular process on to the mastoid portion of the temporal bone, and finally turning sharply on the posterior inferior angle of the parietal bone and becoming continuous with the transverse groove; it lodges the transverse sinus.
s. si'nus transver'si [NA], s. for the transverse sinus; the groove on the inner surface of the occipital bone marking the course of the transverse sinus; the tentorium is attached to its margins.
s. spino'sus, *stria* spinosa.
s. spira'lis exter'nus [NA], external spiral s.; a concavity in the outer wall of the cochlear duct between the prominentia spiralis and the spiral organ.
s. spira'lis inter'nus [NA], internal spiral s.; a concavity in the floor of the cochlear duct formed by the overhanging labium vestibulare.
subclavian s., s. musculi subclavii.
s. subclavia'nus, s. musculi subclavii.
s. subcla'vius, a groove on the surface of the lung just below the apex, corresponding to the course of the subclavian artery.
subparietal s., s. subparietalis.
s. subparieta'lis [NA], subparietal s.; a s. continuing the direction of the s. cinguli from where the pars marginalis of that fissure bends upward; it forms the upper boundary of the posterior portion of the gyrus cinguli.
superior frontal s., s. frontalis superior.
superior longitudinal s., s. sinus sagittalis superioris.
superior occipital s., s. occipitalis superior; one of several small and variable sulci bordering the superior occipital gyri on the upper aspect of the occipital lobe of the cerebrum.
superior petrosal s., s. sinus petrosi superioris.
superior temporal s., s. temporalis superior.
supra-acetabular s., s. supra-acetabularis.
s. supra-acetabula'ris [NA], supra-acetabular s. or groove; a groove, posterosuperior to the acetabulum, that is the attachment for the reflected head of the rectus femoris muscle.
talar s., s. tali.
s. ta'li [NA], talar s.; interosseous groove (2); the groove on the inferior surface of the talus which with a corresponding groove on the calcaneus forms the sinus tarsi.
s. tempora'lis infe'rior [NA], inferior temporal s.; Clevenger's fissure; the s. on the basal aspect of the temporal lobe that separates the fusiform gyrus from the inferior temporal gyrus on its lateral side.
s. tempora'lis me'dius, middle temporal s.; the s. between the gyrus temporalis medius and gyrus temporalis inferior.
s. tempora'lis supe'rior [NA], superior temporal s.; superior temporal fissure; the longitudinal s. that separates the superior and middle temporal gyri.
sul'ci tempora'les transver'si [NA], transverse temporal sulci; the shallow sulci that demarcate the transverse temporal gyri on the opercular surface of the superior temporal gyrus.
s. ten'dinis mus'culi fibula'ris lon'gi [NA], official alternate term for s. tendinis musculi peronei longi.
s. ten'dinis mus'culi flexo'ris hal'lucis lon'gi [NA], groove for tendon of the flexor hallucis longus; a vertical s. on the posterior process of the talus continuous with a similar groove on the underside of the sustentaculum tali of the calcaneus.
s. ten'dinis mus'culi perone'i lon'gi [NA], s. tendinis musculi fibularis longi; groove for tendon of long peroneal muscle; **(1)** the groove below the peroneal trochlea of the calcaneus; **(2)** the groove distal to the tuberosity of the cuboid bone.
terminal s., s. terminalis.
s. termina'lis [NA], terminal s.; **(1)** a V-shaped groove, with apex pointing backward, on the surface of the tongue, marking the separation between the oral, or horizontal, and the pharyngeal, or vertical, parts; **(2)** a groove on the surface of the right atrium of the heart, marking the junction of the primitive sinus venosus with the atrium.
tonsillolingual s., the space between the palatine tonsil and the tongue.
transverse occipital s., s. occipitalis transversus.
s. for transverse sinus, s. sinus transversi.
transverse temporal sulci, sulci temporales transversi.
s. tu'bae auditi'vae [NA], groove for auditory tube; pharyngotympanic groove; a furrow on the inner surface of the posterior border of the greater wing of the sphenoid bone, for the cartilaginous auditory tube.
Turner's s., s. intraparietalis.
s. tympan'icus [NA], tympanic groove; the s. on the inner aspect of the tympanic part of the temporal bone in which the tympanic membrane is fixed.
s. for vena cava, s. venae cavae.
s. ve'nae ca'vae [NA], s. for vena cava; fossa venae cavae; a groove on the posterior surface of the liver between the caudate lobe and the right lobe which gives passage to the inferior vena cava.
s. ve'nae ca'vae crania'lis, a groove on the surface of the right lung, above the hilum, in which runs the superior vena cava.
s. ve'nae subcla'viae [NA], groove for subclavian vein; a groove just anterior to the scalene tubercle of the first rib marking the course of the subclavian vein across the rib.
s. ve'nae umbilica'lis [NA], the s. on the fetal liver occupied by the umbilical vein.
sul'ci veno'si [NA], venous grooves; grooves occasionally found on the internal surface of the parietal bone, in which veins lie.
s. ventra'lis, *fissura* mediana anterior medullae spinalis.
s. for vertebral artery, s. arteriae vertebralis.
s. vertica'lis, s. precentralis.
vomeral s., s. vomeris.
s. vomera'lis [NA], s. vomeris.
s. vo'meris [NA], vomeral s. or groove; s. vomeralis; the groove on the anterior border of the vomer that receives the septal cartilage.
s. vomerovagina'lis [NA], vomerovaginal groove; a s. on the infe-

rior aspect of the vaginal process of the sphenoid bone that, together with ala of the vomer forms the vomerovaginal canal.

sulf-, sulfo- **1.** Prefix denoting that the compound to the name of which it is attached contains a sulfur atom. This spelling (rather than sulph-, sulpho-) is preferred by the American Chemical Society and has been adopted by the USP and NF, but not by the BP. **2.** Prefix form of sulfonic acid or sulfonate.

sulfa (sŭl′fă). Denoting the sulfa drugs, or sulfonamides.

sulfabenzamide (sŭl-fă-ben′ză-mīd). *N*-sulfanilylbenzamide; an antimicrobial of the sulfonamide group.

sulfacetamide (sŭl-fă-set′ă-mīd). *N*-Sulfanilylacetamide; N^1-acetylsulfanilamide; an antibacterial agent of the sulfonamide group, primarily used topically; s. sodium has the same uses as s. and also is used locally for eye infections and for prevention of gonorrheal ophthalmia in newborn infants.

sulfacid (sŭlf-as′id). Thioacid.

sulfactam (sŭl-fak′tam). A β-lactamase inhibitor with weak antibacterial action; when used in conjunction with penicillins (*e.g.,* ampicillin) with little β-lactamase inhibiting action, it greatly increases their effectiveness against organisms which would ordinarily not be susceptible.

sulfacytine (sŭl-fă-sī′tēn). A sulfonamide used as an oral antibiotic in the treatment of urinary tract infections.

sulfadiazine (sŭl-fă-dī′ă-zēn). N^1-2-Pyrimidinylsulfanilamide; one of a group of diazine derivatives of sulfanilamide, the pyrimidine analogue of sulfapyridine and sulfathiazole; one of the components of the triple sulfonamide mixture. It is highly effective against pneumococcal, staphylococcal, and streptococcal infections, against infections with *Escherichia coli* and *Klebsiella pneumoniae,* and in acute gonococcal arthritis; s. sodium has the same uses.

sulfadimethoxine (sŭl′fă-dī-mĕ-thok′sēn). 2,4-Dimethoxy-6-sulfanilamide-1,3-diazine; a long-acting sulfonamide that is rapidly absorbed after oral administration and is slowly excreted by the kidney; it accumulates in the tissue and requires lower doses to attain effective tissue concentrations than do the other sulfonamides.

sulfadimidine (sŭl-fă-dim′i-dēn). Sulfamethazine.

sulfadoxine (sŭl-fă-dok′sēn). Sulformethoxine; N^1-(5,6-dimethoxy-4-pyrimidyl)sulfanilamide; a long-acting sulfonamide, used with quinine and pyrimethamine to reduce the relapse rate of malaria.

sulfaethidole (sŭl-fă-eth′i-dōl). N^1-(5-Ethyl-1,3,4-thiadiazole-2-yl)sulfanilamide; a sulfonamide used in the treatment of systemic and urinary tract infections.

sulfafurazole (sŭl-fă-fyūr′ă-zōl). Sulfisoxazole.

sulfaguanidine (sŭl-fă-gwahn′i-dēn). Sulfanilylganidine; N^1-amidinosulfanilamide; the guanidine derivative of sulfanilamide. It is poorly absorbed from the gastroenteric tract; useful for bacterial infections of the lower intestinal tract and for preoperative sterilization of the intestinal tract.

sulfalene (sŭl′fă-lēn). N^1-(3-Methoxy-2-pyrimidyl)sulfanilamide; a very long-acting sulfonamide that enhances, as do other sulfonamides and sulfones, the effectiveness of antimalarial agents such as pyrimethamine, chloroguanide, or cycloguanil.

sulfamerazine (sŭl-fă-mer′ă-zēn). N^1-(4-Methyl-2-pyrimidinyl)sulfanilamide; an antibacterial agent; one of the components of the triple sulfonamide mixtures.

sulfameter (sŭlf′ă-mē-ter). Sulfamethoxydiazine; 2-(4-aminobenzenesulfon-amido)-5-methoxypyrimidine; a slowly excreted sulfonamide used in the treatment of acute and chronic urinary tract infections.

sulfamethazine (sŭl-fă-meth′ă-zēn). Sulfadimidine; N^1-(4,6-dimethyl-2-pyrimidinyl)sulfanilamide; an antibacterial agent; one of the components of the triple sulfonamide mixture.

sulfamethizole (sŭl-fă-meth′i-zōl). N^1-(5-Methyl-1,3,4-thiadiazol-2-yl)sulfanilamide; a sulfonamide useful for the treatment of urinary tract infection, because of its high solubility.

sulfamethoxazole (sŭl′fă-meth-ok′să-zōl). N^1-(5-Methyl-3-isoxazoyl)sulfanilamide; a sulfonamide related chemically to sulfisoxazole, with a similar antibacterial spectrum, but a slower rate of absorption from the gastrointestinal tract and urinary excretion.

sulfamethoxydiazine (sŭl′fă-me-thok′si-dī′ă-zēn). Sulfameter.

sulfamethoxypyridazine (sŭl′fă-me-thok′si-pi-rid′ă-zēn). A long-acting sulfonamide that requires a single daily dose for maintaining effective tissue concentrations. S. acetyl is a preparation well suited for pediatric use because it is tasteless; it is also used to enhance the actions of quinine and other suppressants in the chemoprophylaxis of malaria.

sulfamoxole (sŭl-fă-mok′sōl). Sulfadimethyloxazole; N^1-(4,5-dimethyl-2-oxazolyl)sulfanilamide; an antimicrobial agent of the sulfonamide group.

***p*-sulfamylacetanilide** (sŭl′fă-mil-as-e-tan′il-īd). N^4-Acetylsulfanilamide.

sulfanilamide (sŭl-fă-nil′ă-mīd). *p*-Aminobenzenesulfonamide; the first sulfonamide used for its chemotherapeutic effect in infections caused by some β-hemolytic streptococci, meningococci, gonococci, *Clostridium welchii,* and in certain infections of the urinary tract, especially those due to *Escherichia coli* and *Proteus vulgaris;* less effective than sulfapyridine in the treatment of pneumococcic, staphylococcic, and *Klebsiella pneumoniae* infections. Toxic manifestations include acidosis, cyanosis, hemolytic anemia, and agranulocytosis.

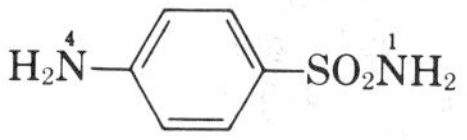

Sulfanilamide

***N*-sulfan′ilylacet′amide** (sŭl-fan′i-lil-ă-set′ă-mīd). Sulfacetamide.

***N*-sulfan′ilylben′zamide** (sŭl-fan′i-lil-ben′ză-mīd). Sulfabenzamide.

sulfanilylguanidine (sŭl-fan′i-lil-gwahn′i-dēn). Sulfaguanidine.

sulfanitran (sŭl-fă-nī′tran). 4′-[(*p*-Nitrophenyl) sulfamoyl]acetanilide; an antimicrobial agent of the sulfonamide group.

sulfaperin (sŭl′fă-per-in). Isosulfamerazine; N'-(5-methyl-2-pyrimidinyl)sulfanilamide; an antimicrobial agent of the sulfonamide group.

sulfaphenazole (sŭl-fă-fen′ă-zōl). A long-acting sulfonamide that is rapidly absorbed after oral administration; one dose is sufficient to maintain effective tissue concentration for 24 hours.

sulfapyrazine (sŭl-fă-pir′ă-zēn). N^1-2-Pyrazinylsulfanilamide; an antibacterial agent of the sulfonamide group.

sulfapyridine (sŭl-fă-pir′i-dēn). An antibacterial agent of the sulfonamide group.

sulfasalazine (sŭl-fă-sal′ă-zēn). Salicylazosulfapyridine; 5-[*p*-(2-pyridylsulfamyl)phenylazo]salicylic acid; a sulfonamide (acid-azo-sulfa compound) with a marked affinity for connective tissues, especially for those rich in elastin, used in chronic ulcerative colitis; it is broken down in the body to amino salicylic acid and sulfapyridine.

sulfatase (sŭl′fă-tās). **1.** Trivial name for enzymes in EC group 3.1.6, the sulfuric ester hydrolases, which catalyze the hydrolysis of sulfuric esters (sulfates) to the corresponding alcohols plus inorganic sulfate; includes aryl-, sterol, glycol-, chondroitin, choline-, cellulose, cerebroside, and chondro- sulfatases. **2.** Arylsulfatase.

sulfate (sŭl′fāt). A salt or ester of sulfuric acid.
acid s., bisulfate.
active s., adenosine 3′-phosphate 5′-phosphosulfate.

sulfathiazole (sŭl-fă-thī′ă-zōl). 2-Sulfanilylaminothiazole; 2-(*p*-aminobenzenesulfonamido)thiazole; an antibacterial agent of the sulfonamide group.

sulfatidates (sŭl′fă-ti-dāts). Cerebroside sulfuric esters containing sulfate groups in the sugar portion of the molecule.

sulfatides (sŭl′fă-tīdz). Obsolete term for sulfatidates.

sulfatidosis (sŭl′fă-ti-dō′sis). Metachromatic *leukodystrophy.*

sulfation (sŭl-fā′shŭn). Addition of sulfate groups as esters to pre-existing molecules.

sulfhemoglobin (sŭlf-hē′mō-glō-bin). Sulfmethemoglobin.

sulfhemoglobinemia (sulf-hē′mō-glō-bi-nē′mē-ă). A morbid condition due to the presence of sulfhemoglobin in the blood; it is marked by a persistent cyanosis, but the blood count does not reveal any special abnormality in that fluid; it is thought to be caused by the action of hydrogen sulfide absorbed from the intestine.

sulfhydrate (sŭlf-hī′drāt). Sulfohydrate; a compound (hydrosulfide) containing the ion HS^-.

sulfhydryl (sŭlf-hī′dril). The radical –SH; contained in glutathione, cysteine, coenzyme A, lipoamide (all in the reduced state), and in mercaptans (R–SH).

sulfide (sŭl′fīd). Sulfuret; a compound of sulfur in which the sulfur has a valence of −2; *e.g.,* Na_2S, HgS.

sulfindigotic acid (sŭl′fin-dī-got′ik). $C_8H_5NOSO_3$; formed by the action of sulfuric acid on indigo, a reaction that also yields indigo carmine.

sulfinpyrazone (sŭl-fin-pir′ă-zōn). 1,2-Diphenyl-4-(2-phenylsulfinylethyl)pyrazolidine-3,5-dione; an analgesic and uricosuric agent that promotes the excretion of uric acid, probably by interfering with the tubular reabsorption of uric acid.

β-sulfinylpyruvic acid (sŭl′fi-nil-pī-rū′vik). $HO_2S–CH_2–CO–COOH$, an intermediate product of cysteine catabolism in mammalian tissue.

sulfisomidine (sŭl-fi-sō′mi-dēn). N^1-(2,6-Dimethyl-4-pyrimidinyl)-sulfanilamide; the structural isomer of sulfamethazine, used in the treatment of systemic and urinary tract infections.

sulfisoxazole (sŭl-fi-sok′să-zōl). Sulfafurazole; N^1-(3,4-dimethyl-5-isoxazolyl)sulfanilamide; a sulfonamide used chiefly in bacterial infections of the urinary tract.
s. diolamine, the 2,2′-iminodiethanol salt of s.; used for intravenous, subcutaneous, or intramuscular administration.

sulfite (sŭl′fīt). A salt of sulfurous acid.
s. dehydrogenase [EC 1.8.2.1], an oxidoreductase catalyzing oxidation of sulfite to sulfate with the reduction of ferricytochrome *c.*
s. oxidase [EC 1.8.3.1], a liver oxidoreductase (hemoprotein) catalyzing the oxidation of inorganic sulfite ion to sulfate ion with O_2, producing H_2O_2.
s. reductase [EC 1.8.99.1], oxidoreductase catalyzing reduction of sulfite to H_2S.

sulfmethemoglobin (sŭlf-met-hē′mō-glō-bin). Sulfhemoglobin; the complex formed by H_2S (or sulfides) and ferric ion in methemoglobin.

sulfo-. See sulf-.

sulfoacid (sŭl′fō-as-id). **1.** Thioacid. **2.** Sulfonic acid.

3-sulfoalanine (sŭl-fō-al′ă-nēn). Cysteic acid.

sulfobromophthalein sodium (sŭl′fō-brō-mō-thal′ē-in). Bromosulfophthalein; bromsulfophthalein; a triphenylmethane derivative excreted by the liver, used in testing hepatic function, particularly of the reticuloendothelial cells.

sulfocyanate (sŭl-fō-sī′ă-nāt). Thiocyanate.

sulfocyanic acid (sŭl-fō-sī-an′ik). Thiocyanic acid.

sulfogel (sŭl′fō-jel). A hydrogel with sulfuric acid instead of water as the dispersion means.

sulfohydrate (sŭl-fō-hī′drāt). Sulfhydrate.

sulfolysis (sul-fol′i-sis). Lysis brought on or accelerated by sulfuric acid.

sulfomucin (sŭl-fō-myū′sin). A mucin containing sulfuric esters in its mucopolysaccharides or glycoproteins.

sulfomyxin sodium (sŭl-fō-mik′sin). A mixture of sulfomethylated polymyxin B and sodium bisulfite; an antibacterial agent.

sulfonamides (sŭl-fon′ă-mīdz). The sulfa drugs, a group of bacteriostatic drugs containing the sulfanilamide group (sulfanilamide, sulfapyridine, sulfathiazole, sulfadiazine, and other sulfanilamide derivatives).

sulfonate (sŭl′fō-nāt). A salt or ester of sulfonic acid.

sulfone (sŭl-fōn). A compound of the general structure $R'–SO_2–R''$.

sulfonic acid (sŭl-fon′ik). Sulfoacid (2); any of the compounds in which a hydrogen atom of a CH group is replaced by the s. a. group, $–SO_3H$; general formula: $R–SO_3H$.

sulfonylureas (sŭl′fō-nil-yū-rē′ăz). Derivatives of isopropylthiodiazylsulfanilamide, chemically related to the sulfonamides, which possess hypoglycemic action. Belonging to this series are acetohexamide, azepinamide, chlorpropamide, fluphenmepramide, glymidine, hydroxyhexamide, heptolamide, indylamide, thiohexamide, tolazamide, and tolbutamide.

sulfoprotein (sŭl-fō-prō′tēn). A protein molecule containing sulfate groups.

6-sulfoquinovosyl diacylglycerol (sŭl′fō-kwī′nō-vō-sil, -kwin′ō). Quinovose containing an SO_3H on C-6 and a doubly substituted glycerol on C-1; the sulfolipid occurring in all photosynthetic tissues.

sulforhodamine B (sŭl-fō-rō′dă-mēn) [C.I. 45100]. Lissamine rhodamine B 200; $C_{27}H_{29}N_2O_7S_2Na$; a xanthene dye derivative, a fluorochrome used for tagging proteins by a sulfamido condensation; employed in immuno-fluorescence alone or in combination with fluorescein isothiocyanate for the simultaneous microscopic detection of two antigens in contrasting red and green colors.

sulformethoxine (sŭl′fōr-me-thok′sēn). Sulfadoxine.

sulfosalicylic acid (sŭl′fō-sal-i-sil′ik). Salicylsulfonic acid; 3-carboxy-4-hydroxybenzenesulfonic acid; $HOC_6H_3(CO_2H)SO_3H$; used as a test for albumin and ferric ion.

sulfosol (sŭl′fō-sol). A hydrosol with sulfuric acid instead of water as the dispersion means.

sulfotransferase (sŭl-fō-trans′fer-ās). Generic term for enzymes in EC sub-subclass 2.8.2 catalyzing the transfer of a sulfate group from 3′-phosphoadenylyl sulfate (active sulfate) to the hydroxyl group of an acceptor.

sulfoxide (sŭl-fok′sīd). The sulfur analogue of a ketone, $R'–SO–R''$.

sulfoxone sodium (sŭl-fok′sōn). Disodium sulfonyl-*bis*(*p*-phenyleneimino)dimethanesulfinate; an antileprotic.

sulfur (sŭl′fer) [L. *sulfur,* brimstone, sulfur]. Brimstone; an element, symbol S, atomic no. 16, atomic weight 32.066, that combines with oxygen to form s. dioxide (SO_2) and s. trioxide (SO_3), and these with water to make strong acids, and with many metals and nonmetallic elements to form sulfides; mildly laxative; has been used to treat rheumatism, gout, and bronchitis, and externally in the treatment of skin diseases.
s. dioxide, sulfurous oxide; SO_2; a colorless, nonflammable gas with a strong, suffocating odor; a powerful reducing agent used to prevent oxidative deterioration of food and medicinal products. See also sulfurous acid.
s. iodide, has been used in the treatment of certain skin diseases.

liver of s., sulfurated *potash.*
precipitated s., milk of s.; lac sulfuris; sublimed s. boiled with lime water, the lime being removed from the precipitate by washing with diluted hydrochloric acid; used in preparing s. ointment and in the treatment of various skin disorders.
roll s., sublimed s. melted and cast in cylindrical molds; sometimes called brimstone.
soft s., an allotropic form obtained by dropping very hot melted s. into water; it is then temporarily of a viscid or waxy consistency.
sublimed s., flowers of s.; used in preparing s. ointment and in the treatment of various skin disorders.
s. trioxide, sulfuric oxide; SO_3; forms sulfuric acid, H_2SO_4, by its reaction with water.
vegetable s., lycopodium.
washed s., sublimed s. macerated in diluted ammonia water to remove the free acid; same therapeutic uses as sublimed s.
wettable s., s. prepared from calcium polysulfide solution containing a protective colloid such as casein; it is easily dispersed and suspended in water.

sulfur-35 (^{35}S). A radioactive sulfur isotope; a beta emitter with half-life of 87.1 days; used as a tracer in study of metabolism of cysteine, cystine, methionine, etc.

sulfuret (sŭl'fer-et). Sulfide.

sulfur group The elements sulfur, selenium, and tellurium; they form dibasic acids with hydrogen, and their oxyacids are also dibasic.

sulfuric acid (sŭl-fyūr'ik). Oil of vitriol; H_2SO_4; a colorless, nearly odorless, heavy, oily, corrosive liquid containing 96% of the absolute acid; used occasionally as a caustic.
fuming s. a., Nordhausen s. a.
Nordhausen s. a. [named for *Nordhausen,* a town in Saxony where it was first prepared], fuming s. a.; s. a. containing sulfurous acid gas in solution.

sulfuric ether (sul-fyūr'ik). Diethyl ether.

sulfuric oxide. *Sulfur* trioxide.

sulfurous (sŭl'fŭr-ŭs). Designating a sulfur compound in which sulfur has a valence of +4 as contrasted to sulfuric compounds in which sulfur has a valence of +6, or sulfides (−2).

sulfurous acid. H_2SO_3; a solution of about 6% sulfur dioxide in water; used chiefly as a disinfectant and bleaching agent, and occasionally as a spray in tonsillitis; it has been used externally for its parasiticidal effect in various skin diseases.

sulfurous oxide. *Sulfur* dioxide.

sulfuryl (sŭl'fŭr-il). The bivalent radical, $-SO_2-$.

sulfydrate (sŭl-fī'drāt). Sulfohydrate; a compound of SH^-.

sulindac (sŭl-in'dak). *cis*-5-Fluoro-2-methyl-1-[(*p*-methylsulfinyl]benzylidene)]indene-3-acetic acid; a nonsteroidal anti-inflammatory agent with analgesic and antipyretic actions.

sulisobenzone (sū-lī'sō-ben'zōn). 5-Benzoyl-4-hydroxy-2-methoxybenzene sulfonic acid; a sunscreen agent.

Sulkowitch, Hirsh W., U.S. physician, *1906. See S.'s *reagent.*

sulph-, sulpho-. See sulf-.

sulpiride (sŭl'pir-īd). *N*-[(1-Ethyl-2-pyrrolidinyl)methyl]-5-sulfamoyl-*o*-anisamide; an antidepressant.

sulthiame (sŭl-thi'ām). *p*-Tetrahydro-2*H*-1,2-thiazin-2-yl)-benzenenesulfonamide, *S,S*-dioxide; an anticonvulsant used in the treatment of temporal lobe epilepsy and grand mal with psychomotor seizures; may cause ataxia, paresthesias, and psychotic episodes.

Sulzberger, Marion B., U.S. dermatologist, 1895–1983. See Bloch-S *disease, syndrome;* S.-Garbe *disease, syndrome.*

summation (sŭm-ā'shŭn) [Mediev. L. *summatio,* fr. *summo,* pp. *-atus,* to sum up, fr.L. *summa,* sum].The aggregation of a number of similar neural impulses or stimuli.
s. of stimuli, muscular or neural effects produced by the frequent repetition of slight stimuli, one of which alone might be without evident response.

Sumner, F.W., 20th century British surgeon. See S.'s *sign.*

sunburn (sŭn'bern). Erythema solare; erythema caused by exposure to critical amounts of ultraviolet light, usually within the range of 2600 to 3200 Å.

sunflower seed oil (sŭn'flow-er). Oil from the seeds of *Helianthus annuus* (family Compositae); the glycerides consist mainly of the mixed triglycerides, each containing one or two linoleic acid radicals; used as a food, and in dietary supplements.

sunscreen (sŭn'skrēn). A topical product that protects the skin from ultraviolet-induced erythema and resists washing off; its use may also reduce ultraviolet-B-induced skin cancer and wrinkling.

sunstroke (sŭn'strōk). Insolation (2); solar fever (2); heliosis; ictus solis; siriasis; thermoplegia; a form of heatstroke resulting from undue exposure to the sun's rays, probably caused by the action of actinic rays combined with high temperature; symptoms are those of heatstroke, but often without fever.

super- [L. *super,* above, beyond]. Prefix, to words of L. derivation, denoting in excess, above, superior, or in the upper part of; often the same usage as L. *supra-;* corresponds to G. *hyper-.*

superabduction (sū-per-ab-dŭk'shŭn). Abduction of a limb beyond the normal limit.

superacidity (sū'per-a-sid'i-tē). An excess of acid; excessive acidity.

superacromial (sū-per-ă-krō'mē-ăl). Supra-acromial; above the acromion process.

superactivity (sū-per-ak-tiv'i-tē). Hyperactivity (1); abnormally great activity.

superacute (sū'per-ă-kyūt'). Extremely acute; marked by extreme severity of symptoms and rapid progress, as of the course of a disease.

superalimentation (sū'per-al'i-men-tā'shŭn). Hyperalimentation.

superanal (sū-per-ā'năl). Supra-anal.

superciliary (sū-per-sil'ē-ār-ē). Supraciliary; relating to or in the region of the eyebrow.

supercilium, pl. supercilia (sū'per-sil'ē-ŭm, -ă) [L. fr. *super,* above, + *cilium,* eyelid] [NA]. **1.** Eyebrow; the crescentic line of hairs at the superior edge of the orbit. **2.** An individual hair of the eyebrow.

superdicrotic (sū-per-dī-krot'ik). Hyperdicrotic.

superdistention (sū'per-dis-ten'shŭn). Hyperdistention.

superduct (sūper-dŭkt) [L. *super-duco,* pp. *-ductus,* to lead over]. To elevate or draw upward.

superego (sū-per-ē'gō). In psychoanalysis, one of the three components of the psychic apparatus in the freudian structural framework, the other two being the ego and the id. It is an outgrowth of the ego that has identified itself unconsciously with important persons, such as parents, from early life, and which results from incorporating the values and wishes of these persons as part of one's own standards to form the "conscience."

superexcitation (sū'per-ek-sī-tā'shŭn). **1.** The act of exciting or stimulating unduly. **2.** A condition of extreme excitement or stimulation.

superextension (sū-per-eks-ten'shŭn). Hyperextension.

superfatted (sū'per-fat'ed). With additional fat added, as in the case of soap.

superfetation (sū'per-fe-tā'shŭn). Hypercyesis; multifetation; superimpregnation; the presence of two fetuses of different ages, not twins, in the uterus, due to the impregnation of two ova liberated at successive periods of ovulation; an obsolete concept.

superficial (sū-per-fish'ăl) [L. *superficialis,* fr. *superficies,* surface]. **1.** Cursory; not thorough. **2.** Pertaining to or situated near the surface. **3.** Superficialis.

superficialis (sū'per-fish-ē-ā'lis) [L.] [NA]. Superficial (3); sublimis (2); situated nearer the surface of the body in relation to a specific reference point. *Cf.* profundus.

s. vo'lae, *ramus* palmaris superficialis arteriae radialis.

superficies (su-per-fish'ĭ-ēz) [L. the top surface, fr. *super,* above, + *facies,* figure, form]. Outer surface; facies.

superflexion (sū-per-flek'shŭn). Hyperflexion.

superfuse (sū-per-fyūs'). To flush a fluid over the top of a tissue. *Cf.* perfuse; perifuse.

superfusion (sū-per-fyū'zhŭn). The act of superfusing.

supergenual (sū-per-jen'yū-ăl). Above the knee or any genu.

superimpregnation (sū'per-im-preg-nā'shŭn). Superfetation.

superinduce (sū'per-in-dūs). To induce or bring on in addition to something already existing.

superinfection (sū'per-in-fek'shŭn). A fresh infection added to one of the same nature already present.

superinvolution (sū'per-in-vō-lū'shŭn). Hyperinvolution; an extreme reduction in size of the uterus, after childbirth, below the normal size of the nongravid organ.

superior (sū-pēr'ē-ōr) [L. comparative of *superus,* above]. **1.** Situated above or directed upward. **2** [NA]. Cranial (2); in human anatomy, situated nearer the vertex of the head in relation to a specific reference point; opposite of inferior.

superlactation (sū'per-lak-tā'shŭn). Hyperlactation; the continuance of lactation beyond the normal period.

superligamen (sū-per-lig'ă-men) [L. *ligamen,* bandage]. A retentive dressing; a bandage retaining a surgical dressing in place.

supermedial (sū-per-mē'dē-ăl). Above the middle of any part.

supermotility (sū'per-mō-til'i-tē). Hyperkinesis.

supernatant (sū-per-nā'tănt) [super- + L. *natare,* to swim]. See supernatant *fluid.*

supernumerary (sū-per-nū'mer-ār-ē) [super- + L. *numerus,* number]. Epactal; exceeding the normal number.

supernutrition (sū'per-nū-trish'ŭn). Hypernutrition; overeating leading to obesity.

superolateral (sū-per-ō-lat'er-ăl). At the side and above.

superovulation (sū'per-ō-vyū-lā'shŭn). Ovulation of a greater than normal number of ova; usually the result of the administration of exogenous gonadotropins.

superoxide (sū-per-oks'īd). Hyperoxide; the molecule HO_2, a strong acid, hence often written as $H^+ + O_2^-$, the latter being the s. radical.

s. dismutase [EC 1.15.1.1], a copper-containing protein ensyme decomposing the superoxide radical to $O_2 + H_2O_2$ (with consumption of hydrogen ion).

superparasite (sū-per-par'ă-sīt). A member of a large population of parasites living on a host, usually a parasitic hymenopteran larva in its insect host. See also parasitoid.

superparasitism (sū-per-par'ă-si-tizm). **1.** Association between parasitic Hymenoptera and their insect hosts. **2.** An excess of parasites of the same species in a host, overtaxing the defense mechanism to the degree that disease or death results, in contrast to multiple parasitism.

superpetrosal (sū-per-pe-trō'săl). Above or at the upper part of the petrous portion of the temporal bone.

superpigmentation (sū'per-pig-men-tā'shŭn). Hyperpigmentation.

supersaturate (sū-per-sach'ŭ-rāt). To make a solution hold more of a salt or other substance in solution than it will dissolve when in equilibrium with that salt in the solid phase; such solutions are usually unstable with respect to precipitating the excess salt or substance and becoming saturated.

superscription (sū'per-skrip'shŭn) [L. *super-scribo,* pp. *-scriptus,* to write upon or over]. The beginning of a prescription, consisting of the injunction, *recipe,* take, usually denoted by the sign ℞.

supersonic (sū'per-son'ik) [super- + L. *sonus,* sound]. **1.** Pertaining to or characterized by a speed greater than the speed of sound. See also hypersonic. **2.** Pertaining to sound vibrations of high frequency, above the level of human audibility. See also ultrasonic.

superstructure (sū-per-strŭk'chūr). A structure above the surface.

implant denture s., the denture which is retained and stabilized by the implant denture substructure.

supertension (sū-per-ten'shŭn). Extreme tension; incorrectly used as a synonym of high blood pressure, or hyperpiesis.

supervoltage (sū'per-vol'tij). In radiation therapy, a vague term for voltage between one thousand and one million volts.

supinate (sū'pi-nāt) [L. *supino,* pp. *-atus,* to bend backwards, place on back, fr. *supinus,* supine]. **1.** To assume, or to be placed in, a supine (face upward) position. **2.** To perform supination of the forearm or of the foot.

supination (sū'pi-nā'shŭn). The condition of being supine; the act of assuming or of being placed in a supine position.

s. of the foot, inversion and abduction of the foot, causing an elevation of the medial edge.

s. of the forearm, rotation of the forearm in such a way that the palm of the hand faces foreward when the arm is in the anatomical position, or upward when the arm is extended at a right angle to the body.

supinator (sū'pi-nā-ter, -tōr). A muscle that produces supination of the forearm. See under musculus.

supine (sū-pīn') [L. *supinus*]. **1.** Denoting the body when lying face upward. **2.** Supination of the forearm or of the foot.

suppedanium, pl. **suppedania** (sŭp-ĕ-dā'nē-ŭm, -ă) [Late L., a footstool, fr. L. *sub,* beneath, + *pes,* foot]. An application to the sole of the foot.

support (sŭ-pōrt') [L. *supporto,* to carry]. **1.** Supporter. **2.** In dentistry, a term used to denote resistance to vertical components of masticatory force.

supporter (sŭ-pōrt'er) [see support]. Support (1); an apparatus intended to hold in place a dependent or pendulous part, prolapsed organ, or joint.

suppository (sŭ-poz'i-tōr-ē) [L. *suppositorium,* fr. *suppositorius,* placed underneath]. A small solid body shaped for ready introduction into one of the orifices of the body other than the oral cavity (*e.g.,* rectum, urethra, vagina), made of a substance, usually medicated, which is solid at ordinary temperatures but melts at body temperature. S. bases usually used are theobroma oil, glycerinated gelatin, hydrogenated vegetable oils, mixtures of polyethylene glycols of various molecular weights, and fatty acid esters of polyethylene glycol.

suppression (sŭ-presh'ŭn) [L. *sub-primo* (*subp-*), pp. *-pressus,* to press down]. **1.** Deliberately excluding from conscious thought. *Cf.* repression. **2.** Arrest of the secretion of a fluid, such as urine or bile. *Cf.* retention (2). **3.** Checking of an abnormal flow or discharge, as in s. of a hemorrhage. **4.** The effect of a second mutation which cancels a phenotypic change caused by a previous mutation at a different point on the chromosome. See epistasis. **5.** Inhibition of vision in one eye when dissimilar images fall on corresponding retinal points.

suppurant (sŭp'yūr-ant) [L. *suppurans,* causing suppuration]. **1.** Causing or inducing suppuration. **2.** An agent with this action.

suppurate (sŭp'yūr-āt) [L. *sup-puro* (*subp-*), pp. *-atus,* to form *pus* (*pur*), pus]. To form pus.

suppuration (sŭp'yŭ-rā'shŭn) [L. *suppuratio* (see suppurate)]. Pyesis; pyosis; pyopoiesis; pyogenesis; the formation of pus.

suppurative (sŭp'yŭr-ă-tiv). Forming pus.

supra- [L. *supra,* on the upper side]. Prefix denoting a position above the part indicated by the word to which it is joined; in this sense, the same as super-.

supra-acromial (sū-pră-ă-krō'mē-ăl). Superacromial.

supra-anal (sū-pră-ā'năl). Superanal; above the anus.

supra-auricular (sū-pră-aw-rik'yū-lăr). Above the auricle or pinna of the ear.

supra-axillary (sū'pră-ak'si-lār'ē). Above the axilla.

suprabuccal (sū-pră-bŭk'ăl). Above the cheek.

suprabulge (sū'pră-bŭlj). The portion of the crown of a tooth that converges toward the occlusal surface of the tooth.

supracardinal (sū-pră-kar'di-năl). Lying dorsal to the anterior or posterior cardinal veins in the embryo.

supracerebellar (sū-pră-ser-ĕ-bel'ar). On or above the surface of the cerebellum.

supracerebral (sū-pră-ser'ĕ-brăl, -sĕ-rē'brăl). On or above the surface of the cerebrum.

suprachoroid (sū-pră-kō'royd). On the outer side of the choroid of the eye.

suprachoroidea (sū'pră-kō-roy'dē-ă). *Lamina* suprachoroidea.

supraciliary (sū-pră-sil'ē-ār-ē). Superciliary.

supraclavicular (sū-pră-kla-vik'yū-lăr). Above the clavicle.

supraclavicularis (sū'pră-kla-vik'yū-lār'is). See under musculus.

supracondylar, supracondyloid (sū-pră-kon'di-lăr, -kon'di-loyd). Above a condyle.

supracostal (sū-pră-kos'tăl). Above the ribs.

supracotyloid (sū-pră-kot'i-loyd). Above the cotyloid cavity, or acetabulum.

supracristal (sū-pră-kris'tăl). Above a crest.

supradiaphragmatic (sū-pră-dī-ă-frag-mat'ik). Above the diaphragm.

supraduction (sū-pră-dŭk'shŭn). Sursumduction; the upward rotation of one eye.

supraepicondylar (sū-pră-ep'i-kon'di-lăr). Above an epicondyle.

supraglenoid (sū-pră-glē'noyd). Above the glenoid cavity or fossa.

supraglottic (sū-pră-glot'ik). Above the glottis.

suprahepatic (sū-pră-he-pat'ik). Above the liver.

suprahyoid (sū-pră-hī'oyd). Above the hyoid bone.

suprainguinal (sū-pră-ing'gwin-ăl). Above the inguinal region, or groin.

supraintestinal (sū-pră-in-tes'ti-năl). Above the intestine.

supraliminal (sū-pră-lim'i-năl) [supra- + L. *limen,* threshold]. More than just perceptible; above the threshhold for conscious awareness.

supralumbar (sū-pră-lŭm'bar). Above the lumbar region.

supramalleolar (sū-pră-mal-ē-ō-lăr). Above a malleolus.

supramammary (sū-pră-mam'ă-rē). Above the mammary gland.

supramandibular (sū-pră-man-dib'yū-lăr). Above the mandible.

supramarginal (sū-pră-mar'jin-ăl). Above any margin; denoting especially the s. gyrus.

supramastoid (sū-pră-mas'toyd). Above the mastoid process of the temporal bone.

supramaxilla (sū'pră-mak-sil'ă). Obsolete term for maxilla.

supramaxillary (sū-pră-mak'si-lār-ē). Above the maxilla.

supramental (sū-pră-men'tăl). Above the chin.

supramentale (sū'pră-men-tā'lē) [supra- + L. *mentum,* chin]. Point B; in cephalometrics, the most posterior midline point, above the chin, on the mandibula between the infradentate and the pogonion.

supranasal (sū-pră-nā'săl). Above the nose.

supraneural (sū-pră-nū'răl). Above the neural axis.

supranuclear (sū-pră-nū'klē-er) Above (cranial to) the level of the motor neurons of the spinal or cranial nerves; as used in clinical neurology, s. indicates disorders of movement caused by destruction or functional impairment of brain structures other than the motor neurons, such as the motor cortex, pyramidal tract, or corpus striatum; *e.g.,* supranuclear palsy, as distinguished from the nuclear (or flaccid, or "lower motor neuron") paralysis that results from destruction or functional impairment of the motor neurons or their axons in a peripheral nerve.

supraocclusion (sū'pră-ō-klū'zhŭn). An occlusal relationship in which a tooth extends beyond the occlusal plane.

supraorbital (sū-pră-ōr'bi-tăl). Above the orbit, either on the face or within the cranium; denoting numerous structures. See canalis, foramen, incisura, nerve, etc.

suprapatellar (sū-pră-pă-tel'ăr). Above the patella.

suprapelvic (sū-pră-pel'vik). Above the pelvis.

supraphysiologic, supraphysiological (sū'pră-fiz-ē-ō-loj'ik, -loj'i-kăl). Denoting any dose (of a chemical agent that either is or mimics a hormone, neurotransmitter, or other naturally-occurring agent) that is larger or more potent than would occur naturally, or the effects of such a dose. *Cf.* homeopathic (2), pharmacologic (2), physiologic (4).

suprapubic (sū-pră-pyū'bik). Above the pubic bone.

suprarenal (sū'pră-rē'năl) [supra- + L. *ren,* kidney]. **1.** Surrenal; above the kidney. **2.** Pertaining to the glandula suprarenalis.

suprarenalectomy (sū'pră-rē-năl-ek'tō-mē). Adrenalectomy.

suprascapular (sū-pră-skap'yū-lăr). Above the scapula.

suprascleral (sū-pră-sklēr'ăl). On the outer side of the sclera, denoting the s. or perisclerotic space between the sclera and the fascia bulbi.

suprasellar (sū-pră-sel'ăr). Above or over the sella turcica.

supraspinal (sū-pră-spī'năl). Above the vertebral column or any spine.

supraspinalis (sū-pră-spi-nā'lis). See under musculus.

supraspinatus (sū-pră-spī-nā'tŭs). See under musculus.

supraspinous (sū-pră-spī'nŭs). Above any spine; especially above one or more of the vertebral spines or the spine of the scapula.

suprastapedial (sū-pră-sta-pēd'ē-ăl). Above the stapes.

suprasternal (sū-pră-ster'năl). Above the sternum.

suprasylvian (sūp-ră-sil'vē-an). Above the fissure of Sylvius or lateral cerebral sulcus.

suprasymphysary (sū-pră-sim-phiz'ă-rē). Above the symphysis pubis.

supratemporal (sū-pră-tem'pŏ-răl). Above the temporal region.

supratentorial (sū'pră-ten-tōr'ē-ăl). Denoting cranial contents located above the tentorium cerebelli.

suprathoracic (sū-pră-thō-ras'ik). Above or in the upper part of the thorax.

supratonsillar (sū-pră-ton'si-lăr). Above the tonsil; denoting a recess above and slightly back of the tonsil.

supratrochlear (sū-pră-trok'lē-ăr). Above a trochlea.

supraturbinal (sū-pră-ter'bi-năl). *Concha* nasalis suprema.

supratympanic (sū-pră-tim-pan'ik). Above the tympanic cavity.

supravaginal (sū-pră-vaj'i-năl). Above the vagina, or above any sheath.

supravalvar, supravalvular (sū-pră-val'văr, -val'vyū-lăr). Above the valves, either pulmonary or aortic.

supraventricular (sū-pră-ven-trik'yū-lăr). Above the ventricles; especially applied to rhythms originating from centers proximal to the ventricles, namely in the atrium or A-V node, in contrast to rhythms arising in the ventricles themselves.

supravergence (sū-pră-ver'jens) [supra- + L. *vergo,* to incline or turn]. Sursumvergence; upward rotation of an eye.

supraversion (sū-pră-ver'zhŭn) [supra- + L. *verto,* pp. *versus,* to turn]. **1.** A turning (version) upward. **2.** In dentistry, the position of a tooth when it is out of the line of occlusion in an occlusal direction; a deep overbite. **3.** In ophthalmology, binocular conjugate rotation upward.

suprofen (sū-prō'fen). *p*-2-Thenoylhydratropic acid; a nonsteroidal anti-inflammatory agent with antipyretic and analgesic properties.

sura (sū'ră) [L.] [NA]. Calf (1); regio suralis; sural region; the muscular swelling of the back of the leg below the knee, formed chiefly by the bellies of the gastrocnemius and soleus muscles.

sural (sū'răl). Relating to the calf of the leg.

suralimentation (ser-al'i-men-tā'shŭn) [Fr. *sur,* fr. L. *super,* above]. Hyperalimentation.

suramin sodium (sū'ră-min). A complex derivative of urea; $C_{51}H_{34}N_6O_{23}S_6Na_6$; used in the treatment of trypanosomiasis, onchocerciasis, and pemphigus.

surface (ser'făs) [F. fr. L. *superficius,* see superficial]. Facies (2); the outer part of any solid.

acromial articular s. of clavicle, *facies* articularis acromialis claviculae.
anterior s., *facies* anterior.
anterior articular s. of dens, *facies* articularis anterior dentis.
anterior calcaneal articular s., *facies* articularis calcanea anterior.
anterior s. of eyelids, *facies* anterior palpebrarum.
anterior s. of leg, *facies* anterior cruris.
anterior s. of maxilla, *facies* anterior corporis maxillae.
anterior s. of petrous part, *facies* anterior partis petrosae.
anterolateral s. of humerus, *facies* anterior lateralis humeri.
anteromedial s. of humerus, *facies* anterior medialis humeri.
articular s. of acromion, *facies* articularis acromii.
articular s. of arytenoid cartilage, *facies* articularis cartilaginis arytenoideae.
articular s. of head of fibula, *facies* articularis capitis fibulae.
articular s. of head of rib, *facies* articularis capitis costae.
articular s. of patella, *facies* articularis patellae.
articular s. of temporal bone, *facies* articularis ossis temporalis.
articular s. of tubercle of rib, *facies* articularis tuberculi costae.
arytenoidal articular s. of cricoid, *facies* articularis arytenoidea cricoideae.
auricular s. of ilium, *facies* auricularis ossis ilii.
auricular s. of sacrum, *facies* auricularis ossis sacri.
axial s., the s. of a tooth parallel with its long axis; the axial s.'s are the vestibular (labial or buccal), lingual, and contact (mesial or distal).
balancing occlusal s., balancing *contact.*
basal s., the s. of the denture of which the detail is determined by the impression and which rests upon the basal seat.
buccal s., **(1)** *facies* vestibularis dentis; **(2)** the mucosa of the cheek; **(3)** in prosthodontics, the side of a denture adjacent to the cheek.
calcaneal articular s. of talus, *facies* articularis calcanea tali.
carpal articular s. of radius, *facies* articularis carpi radii.
cerebral s., *facies* cerebralis.
colic s. of spleen, *facies* colica lienis.
contact s. of tooth, *facies* contactus dentis.
costal s., *facies* costalis.
costal s. of lung, *facies* costalis pulmonis.
costal s. of scapula, *facies* costalis scapulae.
cuboidal articular s. of calcaneus, *facies* articularis cuboidea calcanei.
denture basal s., denture foundation s.
denture foundation s., denture basal s.; that portion of the s. of a denture which has its contour determined by the impression and bears the greater part of the occlusal load.
denture impression s., that portion of the s. of a denture which has its contour determined by the impression; it includes the borders of the denture and extends to the polished s.
denture occlusal s., occlusal s. (2); that portion of the s. of a denture that makes contact or near contact with the corresponding s. of an opposing denture or tooth.
denture polished s., that portion of the denture which extends in an occlusal direction from the border of the denture and includes the palatal s.; it is the part of the denture base which is usually polished and includes the buccal and lingual s.'s of the teeth.
diaphragmatic s., *facies* diaphragmatica.
distal s. of tooth, *facies* distalis dentis.
dorsal s. of digit, *facies* digitalis dorsalis.
dorsal s. of sacrum, *facies* dorsalis ossis sacri.
dorsal s. of scapula, *facies* dorsalis scapulae.
external s. of frontal bone, *facies* externa ossis frontalis.
external s. of parietal bone, *facies* externa ossis parietalis.
facial s. of tooth, *facies* vestibularis dentis.
fibular articular s. of tibia, *facies* articularis fibularis tibiae.
gastric s. of spleen, *facies* gastrica splenis.
glenoid s., *cavitas* glenoidalis.
gluteal s. of ilium, *facies* glutea ossis ilii.
grinding s., *facies* occlusalis dentis.
incisal s., *margo* incisalis.
inferior articular s. of tibia, *facies* articularis inferior tibiae.
inferior s. of cerebellar hemisphere, *facies* inferior hemispherii cerebelli.
inferior s. of pancreas, *facies* inferior pancreatis.
inferior s. of petrous part of temporal bone, *facies* inferior partis petrosae.
inferior s. of tongue, *facies* inferior linguae.
inferolateral s. of prostate, *facies* inferolateralis prostatae.
infratemporal s. of maxilla, *facies* infratemporalis maxillae.
interlobar s.'s of lung, *facies* interlobares pulmonis.
internal s., *facies* interna.
internal s. of frontal bone, *facies* interna ossis frontalis.
internal s. of parietal bone, *facies* interna ossis parietalis.
intestinal s. of uterus, *facies* intestinalis uteri.
labial s., **(1)** *facies* vestibularis dentis; **(2)** the inner s. of the lip.
lateral s., *facies* lateralis.
lateral s. of leg, *facies* lateralis cruris.
lateral malleolar s. of talus, *facies* malleolaris lateralis tali.
lateral s. of ovary, *facies* lateralis ovarii.
lingual s., *facies* lingualis.
lunate s. of acetabulum, *facies* lunata acetabuli.
malleolar articular s. of fibula, *facies* articularis malleoli fibulae.
malleolar articular s. of tibia, *facies* articularis malleoli tibiae.
masticating s., *facies* occlusalis dentis.
masticatory s., *facies* occlusalis dentis.
maxillary s., *facies* maxillaris.
medial s., *facies* medialis.
medial s. of arytenoid cartilage, *facies* medialis cartilaginis arytenoideae.
medial s. of cerebral hemisphere, *facies* medialis cerebri.
medial s. of fibula, *facies* medialis fibulae.
medial s. of lung, *facies* medialis pulmonis.
medial malleolar s. of talus, *facies* malleolaris medialis tali.
medial s. of ovary, *facies* medialis ovarii.
medial s. of tcstis, *facies* medialis testis.

medial surface of tibia, *facies* medialis tibiae.
medial s. of ulna, *facies* medialis ulnae.
mesial s. of tooth, *facies* mesialis dentis.
middle calcaneal articular s., *facies* articularis calcanea media.
nasal s. of maxilla, *facies* nasalis maxillae.
nasal s. of palatine bone, *facies* nasalis ossis palatini.
navicular articular s. of talus, *facies* articularis navicularis tali.
occlusal s., **(1)** *facies* occlusalis dentis; **(2)** denture occlusal s.
orbital s., *facies* orbitalis.
palatine s., *facies* palatina.
patellar s. of femur, *facies* patellaris femoris.
pelvic s. of sacrum, *facies* pelvina ossis sacri.
popliteal s. of femur, *facies* poplitea femoris.
posterior s., *facies* posterior.
posterior articular s. of dens, *facies* articularis posterior dentis.
posterior calcaneal articular s., *facies* articularis calcanea posterior.
posterior s. of eyelids, *facies* posterior palpebrarum.
posterior s. of petrous part, *facies* posterior partis petrosae.
pulmonary s. of heart, *facies* pulmonalis cordis.
renal s., *facies* renalis.
sacropelvic s. of ilium, *facies* sacropelvina ossis ilii.
sternal articular s. of clavicle, *facies* articularis sternalis claviculae.
sternocostal s. of heart, *facies* sternocostalis cordis.
subocclusal s., a portion of the occlusal s. of a tooth which is below the level of the occluding portion of the tooth.
superior s. of talus, *facies* superior tali.
superior articular s. of tibia, *facies* articularis superior tibiae.
superior s. of cerebellar hemisphere, *facies* superior hemispherii cerebelli.
superolateral s. of cerebrum, *facies* superolateralis cerebri.
symphysial s. of pubis, *facies* symphysialis.
talar articular s. of calcaneus, *facies* articularis talaris calcanei.
temporal s., *facies* temporalis.
thyroidal articular s. of cricoid, *facies* articularis thyroidea cricoideae.
urethral s. of penis, *facies* urethralis penis.
ventral s. of digit, *facies* digitalis ventralis.
vesical s. of uterus, *facies* vesicalis uteri.
vestibular s. of tooth, *facies* vestibularis dentis.
visceral s. of liver, *facies* visceralis hepatis.
visceral s. of the spleen, *facies* visceralis lienis.
working occlusal s.'s, the s.'s of teeth upon which mastication can occur.

surface-active (ser'fās-ak'tiv). Indicating the property of certain agents of altering the physicochemical nature of surfaces and interfaces, bringing about lowering of interfacial tension; they usually possess both lipophilic and hydrophilic groups. See also surfactant.

surfactant (ser-fak'tănt). **1.** A surface-active agent, including substances commonly referred to as wetting agents, surface tension depressants, detergents, dispersing agents, emulsifiers, quaternary ammonium antiseptics, etc. **2.** Those surface-active agents forming a monomolecular layer over pulmonary alveolar surfaces; lipoproteins that include lecithins and sphygmomyelins that stabilize alveolar volume by reducing surface tension and altering the relationship between surface tension and surface area.

surgeon (ser'jŭn) [G. *cheirougos;* L. *chirurgus*]. **1.** A physician who treats disease, injury, and deformity by operation or manipulation. **2.** In England, formerly a practitioner without a degree of M.D. but with the license of the Royal College of Surgeons.
attending s., a surgical member of the attending staff of a hospital.
dental s., a general practitioner of dentistry; a dentist with the D.D.S. or D.M.D. degree.
house s., the senior member of the surgical house staff responsible for the execution of the orders of the attending s., and who also substitutes when the latter is absent.
oral s., a dentist who specializes in oral surgery.

surgeon-general (ser'jŭn-jen'ĕ-răl). The chief medical officer in the U.S. Army, Navy, Air Force, or Public Health Service. In some foreign military services any member of the medical corps who has the rank of general, not necessarily the chief medical officer.

surgery (ser'jer-ē) [L. *chirurgia;* G. *cheir,* hand, + *ergon,* work]. **1.** The branch of medicine concerned with the treatment of disease, injury, and deformity by operation or manipulation. **2.** The performance or procedures of an operation.
ambulatory s., operative procedures performed on patients who are admitted to and discharged from a hospital on the same day.
aseptic s., the performance of an operation with sterilized hands, instruments, etc., and utilizing precautions against the introduction of infectious microorganisms from without.
closed s., s. without incision into skin, *e.g.*, reduction of a fracture or dislocation.
cosmetic s., esthetic s.; s. in which the principal purpose is to improve the appearance, usually with the connotation that the improvement sought is beyond the normal appearance, and its acceptable variations, for the age and the ethnic origin of the patient.
craniofacial s., simultaneous s. on the cranium and facial bones.
esthetic s., cosmetic s.
featural s., rarely used term for plastic s. of the face, for correction or improvement of appearance.
major s., see major *operation.*
minor s., see minor *operation.*
open heart s., operative procedure(s) performed on or within the exposed heart.
oral s., the branch of dentistry concerned with the diagnosis and surgical and adjunctive treatment of diseases, injuries, and deformities of the oral and maxillofacial region.
orthognathic s., surgical *orthodontics.*
orthopaedic s., orthopedic s., the branch of s. that embraces the treatment of deformities and of chronic joint diseases. See also orthopaedics.
plastic s., the surgical specialty or procedure concerned with the restoration, construction, reconstruction, or improvement in the shape and appearance of body structures that are missing, defective, damaged, or misshapen.
reconstructive s., see plastic s.
stereotactic s., stereotaxic s., stereotaxy.
transsexual s., procedures designed to alter a patient's external sexual characteristics so that they resemble those of the other sex.

surgical (ser'ji-kăl). Relating to surgery.

surra (ser'ă) [East Indian name]. A disease of camels, horses, mules, dogs, cattle, and other mammals in Africa, Asia, and Central and South America, caused by *Trypanosoma evansi;* infection is generally by mechanical transmission by a bloodsucking species of *Stomoxys* or *Tabanus,* or both; signs depend upon the virulence of the strain of pathogen and the susceptibility of the host. See also murrina.

surrenal (ser-rē'năl). Suprarenal (1).

surrogate (ser'ō-gāt) [L. *surrogare,* to put in another's place]. **1.** A person who functions in another's life as a substitute for some third person. **2.** A person who reminds one of another person so that one uses the first as an emotional substitute for the second.
mother s., one who substitutes for or takes the place of the mother.

sursanure (ser-sā'nūr) [Fr., fr. L. *super,* over, + *sanus,* healthy]. A superficially healed ulcer, with pus beneath the surface.

sursumduction (ser-sŭm-dŭk'shŭn) [L. *sursum,* upward, + *duco,* pp. *-ductus,* to draw]. Supraduction.

sursumvergence (ser-sŭm-ver'jens) [L. *sursum,* upward, + *vergo,* to bend]. Supravergence.

sursumversion (ser-sŭm-ver'zhŭn) [L. *sursum,* upward, + *verto,* pp. *versus,* to turn]. The act of rotating the eyes upward.

surveillance (ser-vā'lans) [Fr. *surveiller,* to watch over, fr. L. *super-* + *vigilo,* to watch]. The collection, collation, analysis, and dissemination of data; a type of observational study that involves continuous monitoring of disease occurrence within a population.

immunological s., immune s., the concept that the immunologic mechanism "recognizes" (because of antigenic change) and removes malignant cells as they arise.

surveying (ser-vā'ing). In dentistry, the procedure of locating and delineating the contour and position of the abutment teeth and associated structures before designing a removable partial denture.

surveyor (ser-vā'er, ōr). In dentistry, the instrument used in surveying.

survival (ser-vī'văl). Continued existence; persistence of life.

suspension (sŭs-pen'shŭn) [L. *suspensio,* fr. *sus-pendo,* pp. *-pensus,* to hang up, suspend]. **1.** A temporary interruption of any function. **2.** A hanging from a support, as used in the treatment of spinal curvatures or during the application of a plaster jacket. **3.** Fixation of an organ, such as the uterus, to other tissue for support. **4.** Coarse dispersion; the dispersion through a liquid of a solid in finely divided particles of a size large enough to be detected by purely optical means; if the particles are too small to be seen by microscope but still large enough to scatter light (Tyndall phenomenon), they will remain dispersed indefinitely and are then called a colloidal s. **5.** A class of pharmacopeial preparations of finely divided, undissolved drugs (*e.g.,* powders for s.) dispersed in liquid vehicles for oral or parenteral use.

amorphous insulin zinc s., prompt insulin zinc s.

Coffey s., an operative technique following partial excision of the cornu as in salpingectomy whereby the broad and the round ligament are sutured over the cornual wound to restore continuity of the peritoneum and to suspend the uterus on the operated side.

crystalline insulin zinc s., extended insulin zinc s.

extended insulin zinc s., crystalline insulin zinc s.; ultralente i.; a long-acting insulin s., obtained from beef, with an approximate time of onset of 7 hours and a duration of action of 36 hours.

insulin zinc s., lente i.; a sterile buffered s. with zinc chloride, containing 40 or 80 units per ml; the solid phase of the s. consists of a mixture of 7 parts of crystalline insulin and 3 parts of amorphous insulin.

magnesia and alumina oral s., a mixture of magnesium hydroxide and variable amounts of aluminum oxide; used as an antacid.

prompt insulin zinc s., amorphous insulin zinc s.; semilente i.; a sterile s. of insulin in buffered water for injection, modified by the addition of zinc chloride such that the solid phase of the s. is amorphous; it contains 40 or 80 units per ml; the duration of action is equivalent to that of insulin injection.

suspensoid (sŭs-pen'soyd) [suspension + G. *eidos,* resemblance]. Hydrophobic, lyophobic, or suspension colloid; a colloidal solution in which the disperse particles are solid and lyophobe or hydrophobe, and are therefore sharply demarcated from the fluid in which they are suspended.

suspensory (sŭs-pen'sō-rē). **1.** Suspending; supporting; denoting a ligament, a muscle, or other structure that keeps an organ or other part in place. **2.** A supporter applied to uplift a dependent part, such as the scrotum or a pendulous breast.

sustentacular (sŭs-ten-tak'yū-lăr). Relating to a sustentaculum; supporting.

sustentaculum, pl. **sustentacula** (sŭs'ten-tak'yū-lŭm, -lă) [L. a prop, fr. *sustento,* to hold upright] [NA]. A structure that serves as a stay or support to another.

s. li'enis, *ligamentum* phrenicocolicum.

s. ta'li [NA], support of the talus; a bracket-like lateral projection from the medial surface of the calcaneus, the upper surface of which presents a facet for articulation with the talus.

susurrus (sŭ-ser'ŭs) [L.]. Murmur (1).

s. au'rium, murmur in the ear.

Sutter blood group. See Blood Groups appendix.

Sutton, Richard L., U. S. dermatologist, 1878–1952. See S.'s *disease* (1), *nevus.*

Sutton, Richard L., Jr., U.S. dermatologist, *1908. See S.'s *disease* (2), *ulcer.*

SUTURA

sutura, pl. **suturae** (sū'tū'ră, -rē) [L. a sewing, a suture, fr. *suo,* pp. *sutus,* to sew] [NA]. Suture joint; suture (1); a form of fibrous joint in which two bones formed in membrane are united by a fibrous membrane continuous with the periosteum.

s. corona'lis [NA], coronal suture; the line of junction of the frontal with the two parietal bones of the skull.

sutu'rae cra'nii [NA], cranial sutures; the sutures between the bones of the skull.

s. ethmoidolacrima'lis [NA], ethmoidolacrimal suture; the line of union of the orbital plate of the ethmoid and the posterior margin of the lacrimal bone.

s. ethmoidomaxilla'ris [NA], ethmoidomaxillary suture; line of apposition of the orbital surface of the body of the maxilla with the orbital plate of the ethmoid bone.

s. fronta'lis [NA], frontal suture; the suture between the two halves of the frontal bone, usually obliterated by about the sixth year; if persistent it is called s. metopica.

s. frontoethmoida'lis [NA], frontoethmoidal suture; line of union between the cribriform plate of the ethmoid and the orbital plate and posterior margin of the nasal process of the frontal bone.

s. frontolacrima'lis [NA], frontolacrimal suture; line of union between the upper margin of the lacrimal and the orbital plate of the frontal bone.

s. frontomaxilla'ris [NA], frontomaxillary suture; articulation of the frontal process of the maxilla with the frontal bone.

s. frontonasa'lis [NA], frontonasal suture; s. nasofrontalis; line of union of the frontal and of the two nasal bones.

s. frontozygomat'ica [NA], frontozygomatic suture; s. zygomaticofrontalis; line of union between the zygomatic process of the frontal and the frontal process of the zygomatic bone.

s. inci'siva [NA], incisive suture; premaxillary suture; line of union of the two portions of the maxilla (pre- and postmaxilla); it is present at birth but may persist into old age.

s. infraorbita'lis, infraorbital suture; an inconstant suture running from the infraorbital foramen to the infraorbital groove.

s. intermaxilla'ris [NA], intermaxillary suture; the line of union of the two maxillae.

s. internasa'lis [NA], internasal suture; line of union between the two nasal bones.

s. interparieta'lis, s. sagittalis.

s. lacrimoconcha'lis [NA], lacrimoconchal suture; line of union of the lacrimal bone with the inferior nasal concha.

s. lacrimomaxilla'ris [NA], lacrimomaxillary suture; linc of union, on the medial wall of the orbit, between the anterior and inferior margin of the lacrimal bone and the maxilla.

s. lambdoi'dea [NA], lambdoid suture; line of union between the occipital and the parietal bones.

s. meto'pica [NA], metopic suture; a persistent frontal suture, sometimes discernible a short distance above s. frontonasalis.

s. nasofronta'lis, s. frontonasalis.

s. nasomaxilla'ris [NA], nasomaxillary suture; line of union of the lateral margin of the nasal bone with the frontal process of the maxilla.

s. no'tha (nō'tă) [G. fem. of *nothos,* spurious], false *suture.*

s. occipitomastoi'dea [NA], occipitomastoid suture; continuation of the lambdoid suture between the posterior border of the petrous portion of the temporal bone and the occipital.

s. palati'na media'na [NA], median palatine suture; line of union between the horizontal plates of the palatine bones, continuing the intermaxillary suture posteriorly.

s. palati'na transver'sa [NA], transverse palatine suture; line of union of the palatine processes of the maxillae with the horizontal plates of the palatine bones.

s. palatoethmoida'lis [NA], palatoethmoidal suture; line of junction of the orbital process of the palatine bone and the orbital plate of the ethmoid.

s. palatomaxilla'ris [NA], palatomaxillary suture; line of union, in the floor of the orbit, between the orbital process of the palatine bone and the orbital surface of the maxilla.

s. parietomastoi'dea [NA], parietomastoid suture; articulation of the posterior inferior angle of the parietal with the mastoid process of the temporal bone.

s. pla'na [NA], plane suture; harmonic suture; harmonia; a simple firm apposition of two smooth surfaces of bones, without overlap, as seen in the lacrimomaxillary suture.

s. sagitta'lis [NA], sagittal suture; s. interparietalis; interparietal suture; line of union between the two parietal bones.

s. serra'ta [NA], serrate suture; dentate suture; one whose opposing margins present deep sawlike indentations, as most of the sagittal suture.

s. sphenoethmoida'lis [NA], sphenoethmoidal suture; line of union between the crest of the sphenoid bone and the perpendicular and cribriform plates of the ethmoid.

s. sphenofronta'lis [NA], sphenofrontal suture; line of union between the orbital plate of the frontal and the lesser wings of the sphenoid on either side.

s. sphenomaxilla'ris [NA], sphenomaxillary suture; an inconstant suture between the pterygoid process of the sphenoid bone and the body of the maxilla.

s. spheno-orbita'lis, spheno-orbital *suture.*

s. sphenoparieta'lis [NA], sphenoparietal suture; line of union of the lower border of the parietal with the upper edge of the greater wing of the sphenoid.

s. sphenosquamo'sa [NA], sphenosquamous suture; articulation of the greater wing of the sphenoid with the squamous portion of the temporal bone.

s. sphenovomeria'na [NA], sphenovomerine suture; the line of union of the vaginal process of the sphenoid with the wing of the vomer.

s. sphenozygoma'tica [NA], sphenozygomatic suture; junction of the zygomatic bone and greater wing of the sphenoid.

s. squamo'sa [NA], squamous suture; **(1)** a scalelike suture, one whose opposing margins are scalelike and overlapping; **(2)** squamoparietal suture; the articulation of the parietal with the squamous portion of the temporal bone.

s. squamosomastoi'dea [NA], squamomastoid suture; line of union of the squamous and petrous portions of the temporal bone during development; it sometimes persists in the region of the mastoid process.

s. temporozygomat'ica [NA], temporozygomatic suture; s. zygomaticotemporalis; line of junction of the zygomatic process of the temporal and the temporal process of the zygomatic bone.

s. zygomaticofronta'lis, s. frontozygomatica.

s. zygomaticomaxilla'ris [NA], zygomaticomaxillary suture; articulation of the zygomatic bone with the zygomatic process of the maxilla.

s. zygomaticotempora'lis, s. temporozygomatica.

sutural (sū'chūr-ăl). Relating to a suture in any sense.

SUTURE

suture (sū'chūr) [L. *sutura,* a seam]. **1.** Sutura. **2.** Stitch (3); to unite two surfaces by sewing. **3.** The material (silk thread, wire, catgut, etc.) with which two surfaces are kept in apposition. **4.** The seam so formed, a surgical s.

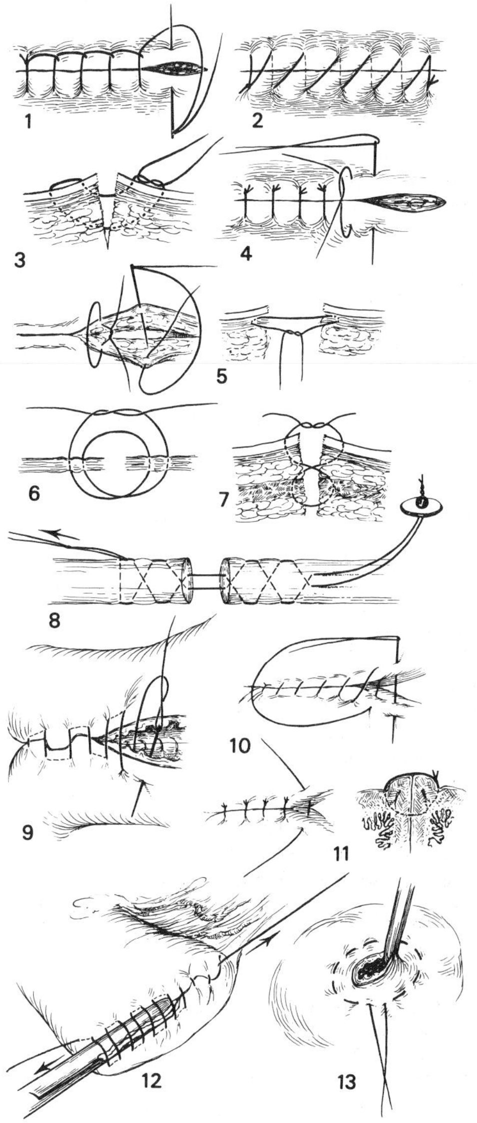

Sutures

Skin sutures: 1, lock-stitch; 2, continuous; 3, vertical mattress; 4, interrupted; 5, Halsted subcuticular. *Fascial sutures:* 6, far-and-near; 7, figure-of-8. *Tendon suture:* 8, Bunnell wire pull-out. *Intestinal sutures:* 9, Connell; 10, Lembert, continuous; 11, Lembert, interrupted; 12, Parker-Kerr; 13, pursestring.

absorbable surgical s. a surgical s. material prepared from a substance that can be digested by body tissues and is therefore not permanent; it is available in various diameters and tensile strengths, and can be treated to modify its resistance to absorption and be impregnated with antimicrobial agents.
Albert's s., a modified Czerny s., the first row of stitches passing through the entire thickness of the wall of the gut.
apposition s., coaptation s.; a s. of the skin only.
approximation s., a s. that pulls together the deep tissues.
atraumatic s., a s. swaged onto the end of an eyeless needle.
blanket s., a continuous lock-stitch used to approximate the skin of a wound.
bridle s., a s. passed through the superior rectus muscle to rotate the globe downward in eye surgery.
Bunnell's s., a method of tenorrhaphy using a pull-out wire affixed to buttons.
buried s., any s. placed entirely below the surface of the skin.
button s., a s. in which the threads are passed through the holes of a button and then tied; used to reduce the danger of the threads cutting through the flesh.
catgut s., see catgut.
coaptation a., apposition s.
cobbler's s., doubly-armed s.
Connell's s., a continuous s. used for inverting the gastric or intestinal walls in performing an anastomosis.
continuous s., spiral s.; an uninterrupted series of stitches using one s.; the stitching is fastened at each end by a knot.
coronal s., *sutura* coronalis.
cranial s.'s, *suturae* cranii.
Cushing's s., a running horizontal mattress s. used to approximate two adjacent surfaces.
Czerny's s., the first row of the Czerny-Lembert intestinal s.; the needle enters the serosa and passes out through the submucosa or muscularis, and then enters the submucosa or muscularis of the opposite side and emerges from the serosa.
Czerny-Lembert s., an intestinal s. in two rows combining the Czerny s. (first) and the Lembert s. (second).
delayed s., a suturing of a wound after an interval of days.
dentate s., *sutura* serrata.
doubly armed s., cobbler's s.; a s. with a needle attached at both ends.
Dupuytren's s., a continuous Lembert s.
end-on mattress s., a vertical mattress s. used for exact skin approximation.
ethmoidolacrimal s., *sutura* ethmoidolacrimalis.
ethmoidomaxillary s., *sutura* ethmoidomaxillaris.
Faden s. [Ger. *Faden,* thread, twine], an s. placed between an ocular rectus muscle and the posterior sclera to limit excessive action of the eyeball.
false s., sutura notha; one whose opposing margins are smooth or present only a few ill-defined projections.
far-and-near s., a s. utilizing alternate near and far stitches, used to approximate fascial edges.
figure-of-8 s., a s. utilizing criss-cross stitches, used to approximate fascial edges or the musculofascial and outer layers of an abdominal wound.
frontal s., *sutura* frontalis.
frontoethmoidal s., *sutura* frontoethmoidalis.
frontolacrimal s., *sutura* frontolacrimalis.
frontomaxillary s., *sutura* frontomaxillaris.
frontonasal s., *sutura* frontonasalis.
frontozygomatic s., *sutura* frontozygomatica.
Frost s., intermarginal s. between the eyelids to protect the cornea.
Gély's s., a cobbler's s. used in closing intestinal wounds.
glover's s., a continuous s. in which each stitch is passed through the loop of the preceding one.
Gould's s., an intestinal mattress s. in which each loop is invaginated in such a way that the tissue at the loop is bulged out, becoming convex instead of concave.
Gussenbauer's s., a figure-of-8 s. for the intestine, resembling the Czerny-Lembert s. but not including the mucous membrane.
Halsted's s., a s. placed through the subcuticular fascia; used for exact skin approximation.
harmonic s., *sutura* plana.
implanted s., passage of a pin through each lip of the wound parallel to the line of incision, the pins then being looped together with s.'s.
incisive s., *sutura* incisiva.
infraorbital s., *sutura* infraorbitalis.
intermaxillary s., *sutura* intermaxillaris.
internasal s., *sutura* internasalis.
interparietal s., *sutura* sagittalis.
interrupted s., a single stitch fixed by tying ends together.
Jobert de Lamballe's s., an interrupted intestinal s., used for invaginating the margins of the intestines in circular enterorrhaphy.
lacrimoconchal s., *sutura* lacrimoconchalis.
lacrimomaxillary s., *sutura* lacrimomaxillaris.
lambdoid s., *sutura* lambdoidea.
Lembert s., the second row of the Czerny-Lembert intestinal s.; an inverting s. for intestinal surgery, used either as a continuous s. or interrupted s., producing serosal apposition and including the collagenous submucosal layer but not entering the lumen of the intestine.
lens s.'s, *radii* lentis.
mattress s., quilted s.; a s. utilizing a double stitch that forms a loop about the tissue on both sides of a wound, producing eversion of the edges when tied.
median palatine s., *sutura* palatina mediana.
metopic s., *sutura* metopica.
nasomaxillary s., *sutura* nasomaxillaris.
nerve s., neurorrhaphy.
neurocentral s., neurocentral *synchondrosis.*
nonabsorbable surgical s., surgical s. material that is relatively unaffected by the biological activities of the body tissues and is therefore permanent unless removed; *e.g.,* stainless steel, silk, cotton, nylon, and other synthetic materials.
occipitomastoid s., *sutura* occipitomastoidea.
palatoethmoidal s., *sutura* palatoethmoidalis.
palatomaxillary s., *sutura* palatomaxillaris.
Pancoast's s., in plastic surgery, union of two edges by a tongue-and-groove arrangement.
Paré's s., the approximation of the edges of a wound by pasting strips of cloth to the surface and stitching them instead of the skin.
parietomastoid s., *sutura* parietomastoidea.
Parker-Kerr s., a continuous inverting s. used to close an open end of intestine.
petrosquamous s., see *fissura* petrosquamosa.
plane s., *sutura* plana.
premaxillary s., *sutura* incisiva.
purse-string s., a continuous s. placed in a circular manner either for inversion (as for an appendiceal stump) or closure (as for a hernia).
quilted s., mattress s.
relaxation s., a s. so arranged that it may be loosened if the tension of the wound becomes excessive.
retention s., tension s.; a heavy reinforcing s. placed deep within the muscles and fasciae of the abdominal wall to relieve tension on the primary s. line and thus obviate postoperative wound disruption.
sagittal s., *sutura* sagittalis.

secondary s., delayed closure of a wound.
serrate s., *sutura* serrata.
shotted s., a s. in which the ends are fastened by passing through a split shot (a partially divided lead pellet) which is then compressed.
sphenoethmoidal s., *sutura* sphenoethmoidalis.
sphenofrontal s., *sutura* sphenofrontalis.
sphenomaxillary s., *sutura* sphenomaxillaris.
spheno-occipital s., *synchondrosis* sphenooccipitalis.
spheno-orbital s., sutura spheno-orbitalis; articulation between the orbital process of the palatine bone and the outer surface of the body of the sphenoid.
sphenoparietal s., *sutura* sphenoparietalis.
sphenosquamous s., *sutura* sphenosquamosa.
sphenovomerine s., *sutura* sphenovomeriana.
sphenozygomatic s., *sutura* sphenozygomatica.
spiral s., continuous s.
squamomastoid s., *sutura* squamosomastoidea.
squamoparietal s., *sutura* squamosa (2).
squamous s., *sutura* squamosa.
subcuticular s., see Halsted s.
temporozygomatic s., *sutura* temporozygomatica.
tendon s., tenorrhaphy.
tension s., retention s.
transfixion s., **(1)** a criss-cross stitch so placed as to control bleeding from a tissue surface or small vessel when tied; **(2)** a s. used to fix the columella to the nasal septum.
transverse palatine s., *sutura* palatina transversa.
tympanomastoid s., *fissura* tympanomastoidea.
uninterrupted s., continuous s.
wedge-and-groove s., schindylesis.
zygomaticomaxillary s., *sutura* zygomaticomaxillaris.

suturectomy (sū-chūr-ek′tō-mē). Removal of cranial suture.

Suzanne, Jean G., French physician, *1859. See S.'s *gland.*

SV Abbreviation for simian *virus, numbered serially; e.g.,* SV1.

Sv Abbreviation for sievert.

Svedberg, Theodor, Swedish chemist, 1884–1971. See *Svedberg* of flotation, S. *unit.*

Svedberg of flotation. Flotation *constant.*

swab (swob). A wad of cotton, gauze, or other absorbent material attached to the end of a stick or clamp, used for applying or removing a substance from a surface.

swage (swāj) [Old F. *souage*]. **1.** To fuse suture thread to suture needles. **2.**To shape metal by hammering or adapting it onto a die, often by using a counterdie.

swallow (swawl′ō) [A.S. *swelgan*]. To pass anything through the fauces, pharynx, and esophagus into the stomach; to perform deglutition.
somatic s., a swallowing pattern with muscular contractions which appear to be under control of the person at a subconscious level; distinguished from visceral s.
visceral s., the immature swallowing pattern of an infant or a person with tongue thrust, resembling peristaltic wavelike muscular contractions observed in the gut; adult or mature swallowing is more volitional and therefore somatic.

Swan, Harold James C., U.S. cardiologist, *1922. See S.-Ganz *catheter.*

swarming (swōrm′ing) [A.S. *swearm*]. A progressive spreading by motile bacteria over the surface of a solid medium.

sway-back (swā′bak). Enzootic *ataxia.*

Sweat. See Puchtler-S. *stains.*

sweat (swet) [*A.S. swāt*] **1.** Perspiration (3); especially sensible perspiration. **2.** To perspire.
colliquative s., profuse clammy s.
night s.'s, profuse sweating at night, occurring in pulmonary tuberculosis and other chronic debilitating affections with low-grade fever.
red s., reddening of s., especially in the axilla, due to pigment produced by *Rhodococcus roseofulvis.* See also chromidrosis.

sweating (swet′ing). Perspiration (1).

Swediauer, Francois X., Austrian physician, 1748–1824. See S.'s *disease.*

sweep (swēp). The travel of the beam of a cathode ray oscilloscope from left to right, representing the time axis, produced by an artificially generated sawtooth voltage.

Sweet, R.D., 20th century British dermatologist. See S.'s *disease.*

Sweet. See Gordon and S. *stain.*

swellhead (swel′hed). **1.** Lecheguilla *poisoning.* **2.** In turkeys, distention of the sinuses due to accumulation of exudate in infectious sinusitis.

swelling (swel′ing). **1.** An enlargement, *e.g.,* a protuberance or tumor. **2.** In embryology, a primordial elevation that develops into a fold, ridge, or process.
albuminous s., cloudy s.
arytenoid s., paired primordial elevations, on either side of the embryonic larynx, within which the arytenoid cartilages are formed.
brain s., a pathologic entity, localized or generalized, characterized by an increase in bulk of brain tissue, due to expansion of the intravascular (congestion) or extravascular (edema) compartments that may coexist or may occur separately and be clinically indistinguishable; clinical manifestations depend on disturbed neuronal function due to local s., shifting of intracranial structures, and the effects of intracranial hypertension or circulatory disturbance.
Calabar s., loiasis.
cloudy s., albuminous s.; granular hydropic, or parenchymatous degeneration; s. of cells due to injury to the membranes affecting ionic transfer; causes an accumulation of intracellular water.
fugitive s., loiasis.
genital s.'s, labioscrotal s.'s; paired primordial elevations flanking the genital tubercle and the urogenital orifice of the embryo; they develop into the labioscrotal folds which become the labia majora in the female, and unite to form the scrotal pouch of the male.
hunger s., starvation edema caused by many factors, primarily reduced serum albumin.
labial s., the female embryonic genital s. which elongates to become the definitive labium majus. See also genital s.'s.
labioscrotal s.'s, genital s.'s.
lateral lingual s.'s, in the embryo, paired oval elevations that appear in the floor of the mouth at mandibular arch level; the primordial elevations, composed of mesenchyme covered by ectoderm of stomodeal origin, merge to form the greater part of the body of the tongue.
levator s., *torus* levatorius.
Neufeld capsular s., Neufeld reaction; quellung reaction, phenomenon, or test; increase in opacity and visibility of the capsule of capsulated organisms exposed to specific agglutinating anticapsular antibodies.
scrotal s., the embryonic genital s. after it has become spherical and has migrated caudally to the base of the penis; just before birth the testis comes to lie within it.
Spielmeyer's acute s., a form of degeneration of nerve cells in which the cell body and its processes swell and stain palely and diffusely.

Swift, H., 20th century Australian physician. See S.'s *disease.*

swinepox (swīn′poks). A usually mild disease occurring in swine, caused by swinepox virus (family Poxviridae) and characterized by papulopustular lesions; usually transmitted by lice.

Swyer, Paul R., U.S. pediatrician, *1921. See S.-James *syndrome.*

sycoma (sī-kō'mă) [G. *sykōma,* fr. *sykon,* fig, + *-oma,* tumor]. **1.** A pendulous figlike growth. **2.** A large soft wart.

sycosiform (sī-kō'si-fōrm). Resembling sycosis.

sycosis (sī-kō'sis) [G. *sykōsis,* fr. *sykōn,* fig, + *-osis,* condition]. Mentagra; ficosis; a pustular folliculitis, particularly of the bearded area.

s. frambesifor'mis, acne *keloid.*

lupoid s., ulerythema sycosiforme; a papular or pustular inflammation of the hair follicles of the beard, followed by punctuate scarring and loss of the hair.

s. nu'chae necroti'sans, acne keloid on the back of the neck at the hairline.

Sydenham, Thomas, English physician, 1624–1689. See S.'s *chorea, disease.*

Sydney crease, Sydney line. See under crease, line.

syllable-stumbling (sil'ă-bl stŭm'bling) [L. *syllabē,* several letters or sounds taken together]. Dyssyllabia; a form of stuttering in which the patient halts before certain syllables that he finds difficult to enunciate.

sylvatic (sil-vat'ik) [L. *silva,* woods]. Occurring in or affecting wild animals.

Sylvest, Ejnar, Norwegian physician, 1880–1931. See S.'s *disease.*

sylvian (sil'vē-an). Relating to Franciscus or Jacobus Sylvius or to any of the structures described by either of them.

Sylvius (Dubois, de le Boë), Franciscus (François), Dutch physician, anatomist, and physiologist, 1614–1672. See sylvian *angle, aqueduct, fissure, line, point, valve, ventricle; fossa* of S.; *vallecula* sylvii.

Sylvius (Dubois), Jacobus (Jacques), French anatomist, 1478–1555. See *caro* quadrata sylvii, *os* sylvii.

sym-. See syn-.

symballophone (sim-bal'ō-fōn) [G. *symballō,* to throw together, + *phōnē,* sound]. A stethoscope having two chest pieces, designed to lateralize sound and produce a stereophonic effect.

symbion, symbiont (sim'bē-on, -ont) [G. *symbiōn,* neut. of *symbiōs,* living together]. Mutualist; symbiote; an organism associated with another in symbiosis.

symbiosis (sim-bē-ō'sis) [G. *symbiōsis,* state of living together, fr. sym- *bios,* life, + *-osis,* condition]. **1.** Any intimate association between two species; sometimes used as a synonym of mutualism which, like commensalism and parasitism, is a symbiotic state. **2.** The mutual cooperation or interdependence of two persons, as mother and infant, or husband and wife; sometimes used to denote excessive or pathological interdependence of two persons.

dyadic s., s. between a child and one parent.

triadic s., s. between a child and both parents.

symbiote (sim'bē-ōt). Symbion.

symbiotic (sim-bē-ot'ik). Relating to symbiosis.

symblepharon (sim-blef'ă-ron) [sym- + G. *blepharon,* eyelid]. Atretoblepharia; adhesion of one or both eyelids to the eyeball, partial or complete, resulting from burns or other trauma but rarely congenital.

anterior s., union between the lid and eyeball by a fibrous band not involving the fornix.

posterior s., adhesion between the eyeball and eyelid involving the fornix.

symblepharopterygium (sim-blef'ă-rō-tĕ-rij'ē-ŭm) [symblepharon + pterygium]. Adhesion of the eyelid to the eyeball.

symbol (sim'bŏl) [G. *symbolon,* a mark or sign, fr. *sym-ballō,* to throw together]. **1.** A conventional sign serving as an abbreviation. **2.** In chemistry, an abbreviation of the name of an element, radical, or compound, expressing in chemical formulas one atom or molecule of that element (*e.g.,* H and O in H_2O); in biochemistry, an abbreviation of trivial names of molecules used primarily in combination with other similar s.'s to construct larger assemblies (*e.g.,* Gly for glycine, Ado for adenosine, Glc for glucose). **3.** In psychoanalysis, an object or action that is interpreted to represent some repressed or unconscious desire, often sexual. **4.** A philosophical-linguistic sign. See also conventional *sign.*

symbolia (sim-bō'lē-ă) [G. *symbolon,* a mark or sign]. The capability of recognizing the form and nature of an object by touch.

symbolism (sim'bō-lizm). **1.** In psychoanalysis, the process involved in the disguised representation in consciousness of unconscious or repressed contents or events. **2.** A mental state in which everything that happens is regarded by the individual as symbolic of his own thoughts. **3.** The description of the emotional life and experiences in abstract terms.

symbolization (sim'bō-li-zā'shŭn). An unconscious mental mechanism whereby one object or idea is represented by another.

symbrachydactyly (sim-brak'i-dak'ti-lē) [sym- + G. *brachys,* short, + *daktylos,* finger]. Condition in which abnormally short fingers are joined or webbed in their proximal portions.

Syme, James, Scottish surgeon, 1799–1870. See S.'s *amputation, operation.*

Symington, Johnson, Scottish anatomist, 1851–1924. See S.'s anococcygeal *body.*

symmelia (si-mē'lē-ă) [sym- + G. *melos,* limb]. Sirenomelia.

Symmers, Douglas, U.S. pathologist, 1879–1952. See Brill-S. *disease.*

Symmers, W. St. C., British pathologist, 1863–1937. See S.'s clay pipestem *fibrosis.*

symmetry (sim'ĕ-trē) [G. *symmetria,* fr. sym- + *metron,* measure]. Equality or correspondence in form of parts distributed around a center or an axis, at the extremities or poles, or on the opposite sides of any body.

inverse s., correspondence of the right or left side of an asymmetrical individual to the left or right side of another.

sympath-, sympatheto-, sympathico-, sympatho- [see sympathetic]. Combining forms relating to the sympathetic part of the autonomic nervous system.

sympathectomy, sympathetectomy (sim-pă-thek'tō-mē, sim-pă-thĕ-tek'tō-mē) [sympath- + G. *ektomē,* excision]. Sympathicectomy; excision of a segment of a sympathetic nerve or of one or more sympathetic ganglia.

chemical s., destruction of the periareterial sympathetic nerves, as in Doppler's operation, by a corrosive such as phenol.

periarterial s., histonectomy; Leriche's operation; sympathetic denervation by arterial decortication.

presacral s., presacral *neurectomy.*

sympathetic (sim-pă-thet'ik) [G. *sympathētikos,* fr. *sympatheō,* to feel with, sympathize, fr. *syn,* with, + *pathos,* suffering]. Sympathic. **1.** Relating to or exhibiting sympathy. **2.** Denoting the sympathetic part of the autonomic nervous system.

sympathetoblast (sim-pă-thet'ō-blast). Sympathoblast.

sympathetoblastoma (sim-pă-thet'ō-blas-tō'mă). Sympathoblastoma.

sympathic (sim-path'ik). Sympathetic.

sympathicectomy (sim-path'i-sek'tō-mē). Sympathectomy.

sympathico-. See sympath-.

sympathicoblast (sim-path'i-kō-blast). Sympathoblast.

sympathicoblastoma (sim-path'i-kō-blas-tō'mă). Sympathoblastoma.

sympathicogonioma (sim-path'i-kō-gō-nē-ō'mă). Sympathoblastoma.

sympathicolytic (sim-path'i-kō-lit'ik). Sympatholytic.

sympathicomimetic (sim-path'i-kō-mi-met'ik). Sympathomimetic.

sympathiconeuritis (sim-path'i-kō-nū-rī'tis). Inflammation of the autonomic nerves.

sympathicopathy (sim-path-i-kop'ă-thē) [sympathico- + G. *pathos,* suffering]. A disease resulting from disordered action of the autonomic nervous system.

sympathicotonia (sim-path'i-kō-tō'nē-ă) [sympathico- + G. *tonos,* tone, tension]. A condition in which there is increased tonus of the sympathetic system and a marked tendency to vascular spasm and high blood pressure; opposed to vagotonia.

sympathicotonic (sim-path'i-kō-ton'ik). Relating to or characterized by sympathicotonia.

sympathicotripsy (sim-path'i-kō-trip'sē) [sympathico- + G. *tripsis,* a rubbing]. Operation of crushing the sympathetic ganglion.

sympathicotropic (sim-path'i-kō-trop'ik) [sympathico- + G. *tropikos,* inclined, fr. *tropē,* a turning]. Having a special affinity for the sympathetic nervous system.

sympathin (sim'pă-thin). Sympathetic hormone; the substance diffusing into circulation from sympathetic nerve terminals when they are active. The term was introduced by W. B. Cannon, who thought that this substance differed from the mediator produced by the nerve ending (now known to be incorrect); the mediator itself (norepinephrine) diffuses into circulation.

sympathism (sim'pă-thizm) [G. *sympatheia,* sympathy]. Suggestibility.

sympathist (sim'pă-thist). One susceptible to suggestibility.

sympathizer (sim'pă-thī-zer). **1.** An eye affected with sympathetic ophthalmia. **2.** One who exhibits sympathy.

sympatho-. See sympath-.

sympathoadrenal (sim'pă-thō-ă-drē'năl). Relating to the sympathetic part of the autonomic nervous system and the medulla of the adrenal gland, as the postganglionic neurons.

sympathoblast (sim'pă-thō-blast) [sympatho- + G. *blastos,* germ]. Sympathetoblast; sympathicoblast; a primitive cell derived from the neural crest glia; with the pheochromoblasts, s.'s enter into the formation of the adrenal medulla.

sympathoblastoma (sim'pă-thō-blas-tō'mă) [sympathoblast + G. *-oma,* tumor]. Sympathicoblastoma; sympathetoblastoma; sympathicogonioma; sympathogonioma; a completely undifferentiated malignant tumor, composed of sympathoblasts, which originates from embryonal cells of the sympathetic nervous system.

sympathogonia (sim'pă-thō-gō'nē-ă) [sympatho- + G. *gonē,* seed]. The completely undifferentiated cells of the sympathetic nervous system.

sympathogonioma (sim'pă-thō-gō-nē-ō'mă) [sympathogonia + G. *-ōma,* tumor]. Sympathoblastoma.

sympatholytic (sim'pă-thō-lit'ik) [sympatho- + G. *lysis,* a loosening]. Sympathoparalytic; sympathicolytic; denoting antagonism to or inhibition of adrenergic nerve activity. See also adrenergic blocking *agent.*

sympathomimetic (sim'pă-thō-mi-met'ik) [sympatho- + G. *mimikos,* imitating]. Sympathicomimetic; denoting mimicking of action of the sympathetic system. See also adrenomimetic.

sympathoparalytic (sim'pă-thō-par-ă-lit'ik). Sympatholytic.

sympathy (sim'pă-thē) [G. *sympatheia,* fr. sym- + *pathos,* suffering]. **1.** The mutual relation, physiologic or pathologic, between two organs, systems, or parts of the body. **2.** Mental contagion, as seen in mass hysteria or in the yawning induced by seeing another person yawn. **3.** An expressed sensitive appreciation or emotional concern for and sharing of the mental and emotional state of another person. *Cf.* empathy (1).

symperitoneal (sim'per-i-tō-nē'ăl). Relating to the surgical induction of adhesion between two portions of the peritoneum.

sympexis (sim-pek'sis) [G. concretion]. A term proposed by R.P. Heidenhain to denote the deposition of red blood cells according to the laws of surface tension.

symphalangism, symphalangy (sim-fal'an-jizm, sim-fal'an-jē) [sym- + phalanx]. **1.** Syndactyly. **2.** Ankylosis of the finger or toe joints.

symphyogenetic (sim'fē-ō-jĕ-net'ik) [G. *symphyēs,* grown together, + *genesis,* origin]. Relating to the combined effects of hereditary and environmental factors in determining the structure and function of the organism.

symphysial, symphyseal (sim-fiz'ē-ăl). Symphysic; relating to a symphysis; grown together; fused.

symphysic (sim-fiz'ik). Symphysial.

symphysion (sim-fiz'ē-on). A craniometric point, the most anterior point of the alveolar process of the mandible.

symphysiotome, symphyseotome (sim-fiz'ē-ō-tōm). Instrument for use in symphysiotomy.

symphysiotomy, symphyseotomy (sim-fiz-ē-ot'ō-mē) [symphysis + G. *tomē,* incision]. Pelviotomy (1); synchondrotomy; division of the pubic joint to increase the capacity of a contracted pelvis sufficiently to permit passage of a living child.

symphysis, gen. **symphyses** (sim'fi-sis, -sēz) [G. a growing together]. **1** [NA]. Amphiarthrosis; form of cartilaginous joint in which union between two bones is effected by means of fibrocartilage. **2.** A union, meeting point, or commissure of any two structures. **3.** A pathologic adhesion or growing together.

cardiac s., adhesion between the parietal and visceral layers of the pericardium.

intervertebral s., s. intervertebralis.

s. intervertebra'lis [NA], intervertebral s.; the union between adjacent vertebral bodies composed of the nucleus pulposus, annular ligament, and the anterior and posterior longitudinal ligaments.

s. mandib'ulae, s. mentalis.

manubriosternal s., s. manubriosternalis.

s. manubriosterna'lis [NA], manubriosternal s.; the later union, by fibrocartilage, of the manubrium and the body of the sternum; it begins as a synchondrosis and becomes a symphysis, occasionally fusing to become a synostosis.

mental s., s. mentalis.

s. menta'lis, mental s.; s. menti; s. mandibulae; the fibrocartilaginous union of the two halves of the mandible in the fetus; it becomes an osseous union during the first year.

s. men'ti, s. mentalis.

pubic s., s. pubica.

s. pu'bica, s. pu'bis [NA], pubic s.; the firm fibrocartilaginous joint between the two pubic bones.

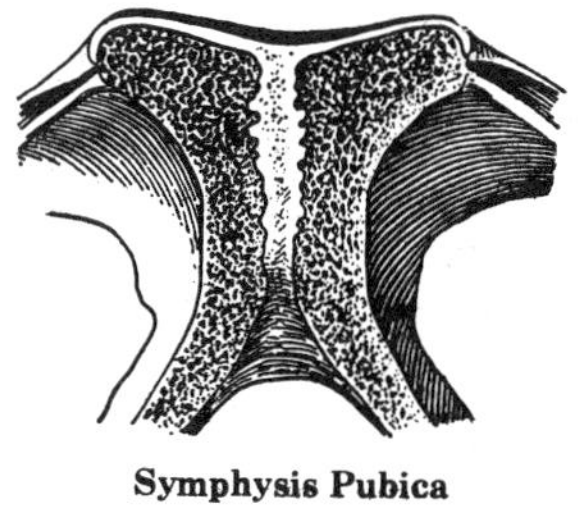

Symphysis Pubica

s. sacrococcyg'ea, *articulatio* sacrococcygea.

symplasmatic (sim-plaz-mat'ik) [G. *sym- plassō,* to mold together]. Relating to the union of protoplasm as in giant cell formation.

symplast (sim'plast) [sym- + G. *plastos,* formed]. A multinucleated cell which has formed by fusion of separate cells.

sympodia (sim-pō'dē-ă) [sym- + G. *pous,* foot]. Condition characterized by union of the feet. See also sirenomelia and sympus.

symport (sim'pōrt) [sym- + L. *porto,* to carry]. Coupled transport of two different molecules or ions through a membrane in the same direction by a common carrier mechanism (symporter). *Cf.* antiport; uniport.

symporter (sim-pōrt'er). The common carrier mechanism of symport.

symptom (simp'tŏm) [G. *symptōma*]. Any morbid phenomenon or departure from the normal in structure, function, or sensation, experienced by the patient and indicative of disease. See also phenomenon; reflex; sign; syndrome.

abstinence s.'s, withdrawal s.'s.

accessory s., assident or concomitant s.; a s. that usually but not always accompanies a certain disease, as distinguished from a pathognomonic s.

accidental s., any morbid phenomenon coincidentally occurring in the course of a disease, but having no relation with it.

assident s., accessory s.

Baumès s., pain behind the sternum in angina pectoris.

Bezold's s., Bezold's sign; inflammatory edema at the tip of the mastoid process in mastoiditis.

Bolognini's s., a feeling of crepitation on gradually increasing pressure on the abdomen in cases of measles.

cardinal s., the primary or major s. of diagnostic importance.

concomitant s., accessory s.

constitutional s., a s. indicating a systemic effect of a disease; *e.g.,* weight loss.

deficiency s., manifestation of a lack, in varying degrees, of some substance (*e.g.,* hormone, enzyme, vitamin) necessary for normal structure and/or function of an organism.

Demarquay's s., absence of elevation of the larynx during deglutition, said to indicate syphilitic induration of the trachea.

Duroziez' s., Duroziez' murmur; a double murmur (systolic and diastolic) heard over the femoral artery, when compressed by the stethoscope, in cases of aortic insufficiency.

Epstein's s., a neurologic eyelid s., resembling Graefe's sign, occurring in infants and giving them a frightened expression, characterized by Epstein as a "wild glance."

equivocal s., a s. that points definitely to no special disease, being associated with any one of a number of morbid states, or whose presence is uncertain or indefinite.

first rank s.'s (FRS), Schneider's (schneiderian) first rank s.'s.

Fischer's s., a presystolic nonvalvular murmur audible in cases of pericardial adhesions.

Frenkel's s., lowered muscular tonus in tabes dorsalis.

Gordon's s., tonic *reflex.*

Griesinger's s., edema of the superficial tissues at the tip of the mastoid process in cases of thrombosis of the sigmoid sinus.

Haenel's s., absence of sensation on pressure of the eyeball in tabes.

incarceration s., Dietl's *crisis.*

induced s., a s. excited by a drug, exercise, or other means, often intentionally for diagnostic purposes.

Kerandel's s., deep-seated hyperesthesia observed in cases of sleeping sickness.

Kussmaul's s., filling of the veins of the neck during inspiration in cases of pericardial effusion or constrictive pericarditis.

local s., a s. of limited extent, caused by disease of a particular organ or part.

localizing s., a s. indicating clearly the seat of the morbid process.

Macewen's s., Macewen's *sign.*

objective s., a s. that is evident to the observer.

Oehler's s., a sudden pallor and coldness in the arm with slight disability, occurring on lifting of a heavy weight.

pathognomonic s., a s. that, when present, points unmistakably to the presence of a certain definite disease.

Pratt's s., rigidity in the muscles of an injured limb, which precedes the occurrence of gangrene.

rainbow s., glaucomatous *halo* (2).

reflex s., sympathetic s.; a disturbance of sensation or function in an organ or part more or less remote from the morbid condition giving rise to it; *e.g.,* muscle spasm due to joint inflammation.

Romberg's s., (1) Romberg's *sign;* **(2)** Romberg-Howship s.

Romberg-Howship s., Romberg's s. (2); in cases of incarcerated obturator hernia; lancinating pains along the inner side of the thigh to the knee, or down the leg to the foot; caused by compression of the obturator nerve.

Schneider's (schneiderian) first rank s.'s, first rank s.'s; those s.'s that, when present, are specific for the diagnosis of schizophrenia, provided that organic or toxic etiology is ruled out: delusion of control, thought broadcasting, thought withdrawal, thought insertion, hearing one's thoughts spoken aloud, auditory hallucinations that comment on one's behavior, and auditory hallucinations in which two voices carry on a conversation.

Sklowsky s., the rupture of a varicella vesicle on very slight pressure with the finger, greater pressure being necessary to break the vesicles of smallpox, herpes, or other affections.

subjective s., a s. apparent only to the patient.

sympathetic s., reflex s.

Trendelenburg's s., a waddling gait in paresis of the gluteal muscles, as in progressive muscular dystrophy.

Trunecek's s., palpable impulse of the subclavian artery near the point of origin of the sternomastoid muscle in cases of aortic sclerosis.

Wartenberg's s., (1) intense pruritus of the tip of the nose and nostrils in cases of cerebral tumor; **(2)** flexion of the thumb when the patient attempts to flex the four fingers against resistance, a "pyramid sign."

withdrawal s.'s, abstinence s.'s; a group of morbid s.'s, predominantly erethistic, occurring in an addict who is deprived of his accustomed dose of the addicting agent.

symptomatic (simp-tō-mat'ik). Indicative; relating to or constituting the aggregate of symptoms of a disease.

symptomatology (simp'tō-mă-tol'ō-jē) [symptom + G. *logos,* study]. **1.** The science of the symptoms of disease, their production, and the indications they furnish. **2.** The aggregate of symptoms of a disease.

symptomatolytic, symptomolytic (simp'tō-mat-ō-lit'ik, -tō-mō-lit'ik) [symptom + G. *lytikos,* dissolving]. Removing symptoms.

symptosis (sim-tō'sis) [G. a falling together, collapse, fr. *syn,* together, + *ptōsis,* a falling]. A localized or general wasting of the body.

sympus (sim'pŭs) [G. *sympous,* fr. sym- + *pous,* foot]. A sirenomelus in which the fusion of the legs has extended to involve the feet.

s. a'pus, a sirenomelus without feet.

s. di'pus, a sirenomelus with both feet more or less distinct.

s. mo'nopus, a sirenomelus with but one foot externally visible.

Syms, Parker, U.S. surgeon, 1860–1933. See S.'s *tractor.*

syn- [G. *syn,* with, together]. Prefix, to words of G. derivation, indicating together, with, joined; appears as sym- before b, p, ph, or m; corresponds to L. *con-*.

synadelphus (sin-ă-del'fŭs) [syn- + G. *adelphos,* brother]. Cephalothoracoiliopagus; conjoined twins with single head, partially united trunk, and four upper and four lower limbs.

synalgia (si-nal'jē-ă) [syn- + G. *algos,* pain]. Referred *pain.*

synalgic (sin-al'jik). Relating to or marked by referred pain.

synanastomosis (sin'an-as-tō-mō'sis). An anastomosis between several blood vessels.

synanche (si-nang'kē). Sore *throat.*

synandrogenic (sin'an-drō-jen'ik). Relating to any agent or condition that enhances the effects of androgens.

synanthem, synanthema (si-nan'them, sin'an-thē'mă) [G. *syn- antheō,* to blossom together]. An exanthem consisting of several different forms of eruption.

synaphoceptors (si-naf-ō-sep'terz) [G. *synaphe,* contact, + L. *recipio,* to receive]. Receptors stimulated by direct contact.

synapse, pl. **synapses** (sin'aps, sĭ-naps'; sĭ-nap'sēz) [syn- + G. *haptein,* to clasp]. The functional membrane-to-membrane contact of the nerve cell with another nerve cell, an effector (muscle, gland) cell, or a sensory receptor cell. The s. subserves the transmission of nerve impulses, commonly from a variably large (1 to 12 μm), generally knob-shaped or club-shaped axon terminal (the presynaptic element) to the circumscript patch of the receiving cell's plasma membrane (the postsynaptic element) on which the s. occurs. In most cases the impulse is transmitted by means of a chemical transmitter substance (such as acetylcholine, γ-aminobutyric acid, dopamine, norepinephrine, etc.) released into a synaptic cleft (15 to 50 nm wide) which separates the presynaptic from the postsynaptic membrane; the transmitter is stored in quantal form in synaptic vesicles: round or ellipsoid, membrane-bound vacuoles (10 to 50 nm in diameter) in the presynaptic element. In other s.'s transmission takes place by direct propagation of the bioelectrical potential from the presynaptic to the postsynaptic membrane; in such electrotonic s.'s ("gap junctions"), the synaptic cleft is no more than about 2 nm wide. In most cases, synaptic transmission takes place in only one direction ("dynamic polarity" of the s.), but in some s.'s synaptic vesicles occur on both sides of the synaptic cleft, suggesting the possibility of reciprocal chemical transmission.
axoaxonic s., the synaptic junction between an axon terminal of one neuron and either the initial axon segment or an axon terminal of another nerve cell.
axodendritic s., the synaptic contact between an axon terminal of one nerve cell and a dendrite of another nerve cell.
axosomatic s., pericorpuscular s.; the synaptic junction of an axon terminal of one nerve cell to the cell body of another nerve cell.
electrotonic s., gap *junction.* See also synapse.
pericorpuscular s., axosomatic s.

synapsis (si-nap'sis) [G. a connection, junction]. Synaptic phase; the point-for-point pairing of homologous chromosomes during the prophase of meiosis.

synaptic (si-nap'tik). **1.** Relating to a synapse. **2.** Relating to synapsis.

synaptology (sin'ap-tol'ō-jē). Study of the synapse.

synaptosome (si-nap'tō-sōm). Membrane-bound sac containing synaptic vesicles which breaks away from axon terminals when brain tissue is homogenized under controlled conditions; such particles can be separated from other subcellular particles by differential and density gradient centrifugation.

synarthrodia (sin'ar-thrō'dē-ă). *Articulatio* fibrosa.

synarthrodial (sin-ar-thrō'dē-ăl). Relating to synarthrosis; denoting an articulation without a joint cavity.

synarthrophysis (sin-ar-thrō-fī'sis) [syn- + G. *arthron,* joint, + *physis,* growth]. The process of ankylosis.

synarthrosis, pl. **synarthroses** (sin'ar-thrō'sis, -sēz) [G. fr. *syn,* together, + *arthrōsis,* articulation]. In the BNA, this class of joints has included those that in the NA are classified as articulatio fibrosa and articulatio cartilaginis. See under articulatio.

syncanthus (sin-kan'thŭs) [syn- + L. *canthus,* wheel]. Adhesion of the eyeball to orbital structures.

syncaryon (sin-kar'ē-on). Synkaryon.

syncephalus (sin-sef'ă-lŭs) [syn- + G. *kephalē,* head]. Monocephalus; monocranius; conjoined twins having a single head with two bodies. *Cf.* craniopagus, janiceps.
s. asymmet'ros, *janiceps* asymmetrus.

syncephaly (sin-sef'ă-lē). Prozygosis; the condition exhibited by a syncephalus.

syncheilia, synchilia (sin-kī'lē-ă) [syn- + G. *cheilos,* lip]. A more or less complete adhesion of the lips; atresia of the mouth.

syncheiria, synchiria (sin-kī'rē-ă) [syn- + G. *cheir,* hand]. A form of dyscheiria in which the subject refers a stimulus applied to one side of the body to both sides.

synchondroseotomy (sin-kon'drō-sē-ot'ō-mē) [synchondrosis + G. *tomē,* cutting]. Operation of cutting through a synchondrosis; specifically, cutting through the sacroiliac ligaments and forcibly closing the arch of the pubes; used in the treatment of exstrophy of the bladder.

synchondrosis, pl. **synchondroses** (sin'kon-drō'sis, -sēz) [Mod. L. fr. G. *syn,* together, + *chondros,* cartilage, + *-osis,* condition] [NA]. Synchondrodial joint; a union between two bones formed either by hyaline cartilage or fibrocartilage.
s. arycornicula'ta, the junction of the corniculate cartilage (of Santorini) with the arytenoid.
cranial synchondroses, synchondroses cranii.
synchondro'ses cra'nii [NA], cranial synchondroses; the cartilaginous joints of the skull; these include s. sphenoethmoidalis, s. spheno-occipitalis, s. sphenopetrosa, s. petro-occipitalis, s. intraoccipitalis anterior, and s. intraoccipitalis posterior.
s. epiphy'seos, *linea* epiphysialis.
synchrondoses intersternebra'les, intersternebral joints; persisting cartilages uniting the bony elements of the sternum, as in some domestic animals such as the dog.
s. intraoccipita'lis ante'rior [NA], anterior intraoccipital joint; cartilaginous union in the newborn between the lateral and the basilar portions of the occipital bone.
s. intraoccipita'lis poste'rior [NA], posterior intraoccipital joint; Budin's obstetrical joint; cartilaginous union between the squamous and lateral parts of the occipital bone in the newborn.
s. manubriosterna'lis [NA], manubriosternal joint; the early union, by hyaline cartilage, of the manubrium and the body of the sternum, which later becomes a symphysial type of joint.
neurocentral s., neurocentral joint; neurocentral suture; the cartilaginous union on either side between the body and arch of a vertebra in the young child.
s. petro-occipita'lis [NA], petro-occipital joint; fibrocartilage filling the petro-occipital fissure.
sphenoethmoidal s., s. sphenoethmoidalis.
s. sphenoethmoida'lis [NA], sphenoethmoidal s.; cartilaginous union between the body of the sphenoid and the posterior part of the ethmoidal labyrinth.
s. spheno-occipita'lis [NA], spheno-occipital joint or suture; cartilaginous union between the body of the sphenoid and the basilar portion of the occipital; it fuses by the twentieth year; incorrectly called spheno-occipital suture.
s. sphenopetro'sa [NA], sphenopetrous or sphenopetrosal s.; fi-

brocartilage filling the sphenopetrosal fissure.
sphenopetrosal s., sphenopetrous s., s. sphenopetrosa.
sternal synchondroses, synchondroses sternales.
synchondro'ses sterna'les [NA], sternal synchondroses; sternal joints; the cartilaginous junctions between the body of the sternum and the manubrium, and the xiphoid process; in domestic animals, there may be several, *e.g.,* s. manubriosternalis, s. intersternebralis, and s. xiphosternalis.
s. xiphosterna'lis [NA], xiphisternal joint; the cartilaginous union between the xiphoid process and the body of the sternum.

synchondrotomy (sin-kon-drot'ō-mē). Symphysiotomy.

synchorial (sin-kōr'ē-ăl) [syn- + chorion]. Relating to fused chorions.

synchronia (sin-krō'nē-ă) [syn- + G. *chronos,* time]. **1.** Synchronism. **2.** Origin, development, involution, or functioning of tissues or organs at the usual time for such an event. *Cf.* heterochronia.

synchronism (sin'krō-nizm) [syn- + G. *chronos,* time]. Sychronia (1); occurrence of two or more events at the same time; the condition of being simultaneous.

synchronous (sin'krō-nŭs) [G. *synchronos*]. Homochronous (1); occurring simultaneously.

synchrony (sin'krō-nē) [syn- + G. *chronos,* time]. The simultaneous appearance of two separate events.
bilateral s., simultaneous normal or abnormal electroencephalographic activity derived from electrodes situated at homologous points on the two sides of the head.

synchrotron (sin'krō-tron). A machine for generating high speed electrons or protons, as for nuclear studies.

synchysis (sin'kĭ-sis) [G. a mixing together, fr. syn- + *chysis,* a pouring]. Collapse of the collagenous framework of the vitreous humor, with liquefaction of the vitreous body.
s. scintil'lans, an appearance of glistening spots in the eye, due to cholesterol crystals floating in a fluid vitreous.

syncinesis (sin-si-nē'sis). Synkinesis.

synclinal (sin'klĭ-năl) [G. *syn- klinō,* to incline together]. Denoting two structures inclined one toward the other.

synclitic (sin-klit'ik). Relating to or marked by synclitism.

synclitism (sin'kli-tizm) [G. *syn-klinō,* to incline together]. Condition of parallelism between the planes of the fetal head and of the pelvis, respectively.

synclonus (sin'klō-nŭs) [syn- + G. *klonos,* tumult]. Clonic spasm or tremor of several muscles.

syncopal (sin'kō-păl). Syncopic; relating to syncope.

syncope (sin'kō-pē) [G. *synkopē,* a cutting short, a swoon]. A fainting or swooning; a sudden fall of blood pressure or failure of the cardiac systole, resulting in cerebral anemia and subsequent loss of consciousness.
carotid sinus s., s. resulting from overactivity of the carotid sinus; attacks may be spontaneous or produced by pressure on a sensitive carotid sinus.
hysterical s., fainting due to, or to avoid, emotional stress.
laryngeal s., laryngeal or Charcot's vertigo; a paroxysmal neurosis characterized by attacks of coughing, with unusual sensations, as of tickling, in the throat, followed by a brief period of unconsciousness.
local s., limited numbness in a part, especially of the fingers; one of the symptoms, usually associated with local asphyxia, of Raynaud's disease.
micturition s., fainting or s. occurring in association with the act of emptying the bladder; also called psychomotor epilepsy associated with micturition.
postural s., s. upon assuming an upright position caused by inadequate blood flow to the brain resulting from failure of normal vasoconstrictive mechanisms.
vasovagal s., vagal *attack.*

syncopic (sin-kop'ik). Syncopal.

syncretio (sin-krē'shē-ō) [L. a growing together]. Development of adhesion between inflamed opposing surfaces.

syncyanin (sin-sī'ă-nin). A blue pigment produced by *Pseudomonas syncyanea.*

syncytial (sin-sish'ăl, -sish'ē-ăl, -sit'ē-ăl). Relating to a syncytium.

syncytiotrophoblast (sin-sish'ē-ō-trō'fō-blast) [syncytium + trophoblast]. Syntrophoblast; plasmodiotrophoblast; plasmodial or syncytial trophoblast; placental plasmodium; the syncytial outer layer of the trophoblast. See also trophoblast.

syncytium, pl. **syncytia** (sin-sish'ē-ŭm, -sit'ē-ŭm, -ă) [Mod. L. fr. syn- + G. *kytos,* cell]. A multinucleated protoplasmic mass formed by the secondary union of originally separate cells.

syndactyl, syndactyle (sin-dak'til, -dak'tīl). Syndactylous.

syndactylia, syndactylism (sin-dak-til'ē-ă, -dak'ti-lizm). Syndactyly.

syndactylous (sin-dak'ti-lŭs). Syndactyl; syndactyle; having fused or webbed fingers or toes.

syndactyly (sin-dak'ti-lē) [syn- + G. *daktylos,* finger or toe]. Any degree of webbing or fusion of fingers or toes, involving soft parts only or including bone structure; usually autosomal dominant inheritance. Also called dactylia; dactylium; syndactylia; syndactylism; symphalangism (1); zygodactyly.

syndesis (sin-dē'sis) [syn- + G. *desis,* a binding]. Arthrodesis.

syndesm-. See syndesmo-.

syndesmectomy (sin-dez-mek'tō-mē) [syndesm- + G. *ektomē,* excision]. Cutting away a section of a ligament.

syndesmectopia (sin-dez-mek-tō'pē-ă) [syndesm- + G. *ektopos,* out of place]. Displacement of a ligament.

syndesmitis (sin-dez-mī'tis) [syndesm- + G. *-itis,* inflammation]. Inflammation of a ligament.
s. metatar'sea, inflammation of the metatarsal ligaments.

syndesmo-, syndesm- [G. *syndesmos,* a fastening, fr. *syndeo-,* to bind]. Combining forms denoting a ligament, ligamentous.

syndesmochorial (sin-dez-mō-kōr'ē-ăl) [syndesmo- + G. *chorion,* membrane]. Relating to the placenta in ruminant animals. See s. *placenta.*

syndesmodial (sin-des-mō'dē-ăl). Syndesmotic.

syndesmography (sin-dez-mog'ră-fē) [syndesmo- + G. *graphō,* to write]. A treatise on or description of the ligaments.

syndesmologia (sin-dez'mō-lō'jē-ă). Arthrology.

syndesmology (sin-dez-mol'ō-jē) [syndesmo- + G. *logos,* study]. Arthrology.

syndesmopexy (sin-dez'mō-pek-sē) [syndesmo- + G. *pēxis,* fixation]. The joining of two ligaments, or attachment of a ligament in a new place.

syndesmophyte (sin-dez'mō-fīt) [syndesmo- + G. *phyton,* plant]. An osseous excrescence attached to a ligament.

syndesmoplasty (sin-dez'mō-plas-tē) [syndesmo- + G. *plastos,* formed]. Rarely used term for plastic surgery of a ligament.

syndesmorrhaphy (sin-dez-mōr'ă-fē) [syndesmo- + G. *rhaphē,* suture]. Suture of ligaments.

syndesmosis, pl. **syndesmoses** (sin'dez-mō'sis, -sēz) [syndesmo- + G. *-osis,* condition] [NA]. Syndesmodial or syndesmotic joint; a form of fibrous joint in which opposing surfaces that are relatively far apart are united by ligaments; *e.g.,* the union of the styloid process of the temporal bone and the hyoid bone via the stylohyoid ligament, and the union between the distal ends of the tibia and fibula.

radioulnar s., s. radioulnaris.

s. radioulna'ris [NA], radioulnar s.; the fibrous union of the radius and ulna consisting of the oblique cord and the interosseous membrane.

tibiofibular s., s. tibiofibularis.

s. tibiofibula'ris [NA], tibiofibular s.; inferior tibiofibular joint; the fibrous union of the tibia and fibula consisting of the interosseous membrane and the anterior and posterior tibiofibular ligaments at the distal extremities of the bones.

s. tympanostape'dia [NA], tympanostapedial junction; the connection of the base or foot-plate of the stapes with the vestibular (oval) window.

syndesmotic (sin-des-mot'ik). Syndesmodial; relating to syndesmosis.

syndesmotomy (sin-dez-mot'ō-mē) [syndesmo- + G. *tomē,* incision]. Surgical division of a ligament.

SYNDROME

syndrome (sin'drōm) [G. *syndromē,* a running together, tumultuous concourse; (in med.) a concurrence of symptoms, fr. *syn,* together, + *dromos,* a running]. The aggregate of signs and symptoms associated with any morbid process, and constituting together the picture of the disease. See also disease.

Aarskog-Scott s., faciodigitogenital *dysplasia.*

abdominal muscle deficiency s., prune belly s.; triad s.; congenital absence (partial or complete) of abdominal muscles, in which the outline of the intestines is visible through the protruding abdominal wall; in males, genitourinary anomalies (urinary tract dilatation and cryptorchidism) are also found.

Achard s., arachnodactyly with small receding mandible, broad skull, and joint laxity limited to the hands and feet.

Achard-Thiers s., one form of a virilizing disorder of adrenocortical origin in women, characterized by masculinization and menstrual disorders in association with manifestations of diabetes mellitus, such as glucosuria.

Achenbach s., hematoma of the finger pad with accompanying edema; of unknown cause in the absence of disturbances in blood coagulation mechanisms.

acquired immunodeficiency s., AIDS.

acrofacial s., acrofacial *dysostosis.*

acroparesthesia s., abnormal sensation such as numbness and tingling in the extremities.

acute radiation s., a s. caused by exposure of the body to large amounts of radiation, (*e.g.,* from certain forms of therapy, accidents, and nuclear explosions; it is categorized into three major forms which are, in ascending order of severity, the hematogic, gastrointestinal, and central nervous system-cardiovascular forms; its clinical manifestations are divided into prodromal, latent, overt, and recovery stages.

Adams-Stokes s., Adams-Stokes disease; Stokes-Adams s. or disease; Morgagni's disease; Morgagni-Adams-Stokes s.; Spens s.; a s. characterized by slow or absent pulse, vertigo, syncope, convulsions, and sometimes Cheyne-Stokes respiration; usually as a result of heart block.

adaptation s. of Selye, general nonspecific adaptation of the organism in response to specific stimuli.

adherence s., restriction action of an ocular muscle owing to adhesions between the muscle and its fascial sheath.

Adie s., Holmes-Adie s.

adiposogenital s., *dystrophia* adiposogenitalis.

adrenal cortical s., an inexact (and obsolete) term that has been applied to Cushing's s., Addison's disease, or the adrenogenital s.

adrenal virilizing s., adrenal *virilism.*

adrenogenital s., generic designation for a group of disorders caused by adrenocortical hyperplasia or malignant tumors and characterized by masculinization of women, feminization of men, or precocious sexual development of children; representative of excessive or abnormal secretory patterns of adrenocortical steroids, especially those with androgenic or estrogenic effects.

adult respiratory distress s. (ARDS), acute lung injury from a variety of causes, characterized by interstitial and/or alveolar edema and hemorrhage as well as perivascular pulmonary edema associated with hyaline membrane, proliferation of collagen fibers, and swollen epithelium with increased pinocytosis.

afferent loop s., gastrojejunal loop obstruction s.; acute or chronic obstruction of the duodenum and jejunum proximal to the gastrojejunostomy performed in a Billroth II type gastrectomy; a distended afferent loop causes symptoms of pain and fullness.

aglossia-adactylia s., congenital absence or hypoplasia of the tongue, associated with absence of the digits.

Ahumada-Del Castillo s., Argonz-Del Castillo s.; unphysiological lactation and amenorrhea not following pregnancy characterized by hyperprolactinemia and a pituitary adenoma.

Aicardi's s., multiple genetic central nervous system anomalies and infantile spasms in female babies.

Albright's s., **(1)** McCune-Albright s.; **(2)** Albright's hereditary *osteodystrophy.*

alcohol amnestic s., an amnestic s. resulting from alcoholism and vitamin deficiency; usually, other neurological complications of alcohol and malnutrition may result, such as peripheral neuropathy and cerebellar ataxia. *Cf.* Korsakoff's s.

Aldrich s., Wiskott-Aldrich s.

Alezzandrini's s., a rare s. appearing in adolescents and young adults, characterized by unilateral degenerative retinitis, followed by ipsilateral poliosis and facial vitiligo, and occasionally bilateral perceptive deafness.

Alice in Wonderland s., the illusion of dreams, feelings of levitation, and alteration in the sense of the passage of time, sometimes associated with migraine, epilepsy, and various diseases of the parietal lobe of the brain.

Allen-Masters s., pelvic pain resulting from an old laceration of the broad ligament received during delivery.

Alport's s., progressive microscopic hematuria leading to chronic renal failure in males, accompanied by defects such as sensorineural hearing loss, lenticonus, and maculopathy; autosomal dominant inheritance.

Alström's s., retinal degeneration with nystagmus and loss of central vision, associated with obesity in childhood; sensorineural hearing loss and diabetes mellitus usually occur after age 10; autosomal recessive inheritance.

amenorrhea-galactorrhea s., unphysiologic lactation from endocrinological causes or from a pituitary tumor.

amnestic s., **(1)** Korsakoff's s.; **(2)** an organic brain s. with short term (but not immediate) memory disturbance, regardless of the etiology.

amniotic fluid s., pulmonary embolic phenomena due to infusion of a considerable volume of amniotic fluid containing epithelial squames into maternal blood vessels; shock ensues and sudden death may occur.

Amsterdam s. [*Amsterdam,* the Netherlands], de Lange s.

Angelucci's s., extreme excitability, vasomotor disturbances, and palpitation associated with vernal conjunctivitis.

angio-osteohypertrophy s., Klippel-Trenaunay-Weber s.

ankyloglossia superior s., a congenital condition in which the tongue adheres to the hard palate.

anorectal s., soreness, burning, itching, or other irritation of the rectum together with redness about the anus, and sometimes ac-

companied by diarrhea, occurring as a toxic effect of the oral administration of certain broad spectrum antibiotics.
anterior chamber cleavage s., Peters' anomaly; a congenital disorder originating from faulty separation of embryonic structures; it results in bilateral central corneal opacities, with an anterior ring attachment of the iridic pupillary border and anterior polar cataracts.
anterior tibial compartment s., ischemic necrosis of the muscles of the anterior tibial compartment of the leg, presumed due to compression of arteries by swollen muscles following unaccustomed exertion.
antibody deficiency s., antibody deficiency disease; any of a group of disorders associated with a defective antibody production due to defects in the B-type lymphocyte system or in T-type lymphocytes; chief manifestation is an increased susceptibility to infection by various microorganisms.
Anton's s., in cortical blindness, lack of awareness of being blind.
anxiety s., the constellation of signs and symptoms accompanying anxiety (1).
aortic arch s., Martorell's s.; thrombotic obliteration of the branches of the arch of the aorta leading to diminished or absent pulses in the neck and arms. See also pulseless *disease;* reversed *coarctation.*
apallic s., apallic *state.*
Apert's s., type I *acrocephalosyndactyly.*
Apert-Crouzon s., type II *acrocephalosyndactyly.*
s. of approximate relevant answers, Ganser's s.
Argonz-Del Castillo s., Ahumada-Del Castillo s.
Arndt-Gottron s., scleromyxedema.
Arnold-Chiari s., Arnold-Chiari *deformity.*
Ascher's s., a condition in which a congenital double lip is associated with blepharochalasis and nontoxic thyroid gland enlargement.
Asherman's s., synechiae within the endometrial cavity, often causing amenorrhea and infertility.
auriculotemporal nerve s., gustatory sweating s.; Frey's s.; localized flushing and sweating of the ear and cheek in response to eating.
autoerythrocyte sensitization s., psychogenic purpura; Gardner-Diamond s.; painful-bruising s.; a condition, usually occurring in women, in which the individual brusies easily (purpura simplex) and the ecchymoses tend to enlarge and involve adjacent tissues, resulting in pain in the affected parts; so-called because similar lesions are produced by inoculation of the individual's blood and it is assumed to be a form of autosensitization, although no specific antibodies have been demonstrable; in some individuals, there seems to be a psychogenic mechanism.
Avellis' s., jugular foramen s.; unilateral paralysis of the larynx and velum palati, with contralateral loss of pain and temperature sensibility in the parts below.
A-V strabismus s., strabismus in which the angle of deviation is more marked on looking upward or downward. See also A-*esotropia,* V-*esotropia,* A-*exotropia,* V-*exotropia.*
Axenfeld's s., a congenital ocular dysgenesis expressed as widened trabecular meshwork, large iridial bands, and glaucoma.
Ayerza's s., cardiopathia nigra; sclerosis of the pulmonary arteries in chronic cor pulmonale; associated with severe cyanosis, it is a condition resembling polycythemia vera but resulting from primary pulmonary arteriosclerosis or primary pulmonary hypertension and characterized by plexiform lesions of arterioles.
Balint's s., ocular motor *apraxia.*
Bamberger-Marie s., hypertrophic pulmonary *osteoarthropathy.*
Banti's s., Banti's disease; splenic anemia; chronic congestive splenomegaly that occurs primarily in children as a sequel to hypertension in the portal or splenic veins, usually as a result of thrombosis of the veins; anemia, splenomegaly, and irregular episodes of gastrointestinal bleeding are usually observed, with ascites, jaundice, leukopenia, and thrombocytopenia developing in various instances.
Bardet-Biedl s., mental retardation, pigmentary retinopathy, polydactyly, obesity, and hypogenitalism; recessive inheritance. See also Laurence-Moon s.
bare lymphocyte s., absence of HLA antigens on peripheral mononuclear cells, which may result in immunodeficiency.
Barlow s., late apical systolic murmur or (so-called "mid-late") systolic click, or both, due to massive protrusion of the posterior (mural) mitral valvular leaflet into the left atrial cavity (floppy valve s.); electrocardiographically, signs of posteroinferior myocardial ischemia, probably resulting from distortion of a circumflex coronary artery, and rhythm disturbances frequently coexist with this s.
Barrett s., Barrett esophagus; chronic peptic ulcer of the lower esophagus, which is lined by columnar epithelium, resembling the mucosa of the gastric cardia, acquired as a result of long-standing chronic esophagitis; esophageal stricture with reflux, and adenocarcinoma, have also been reported.
Bart's s., a form of epidermolysis bullosa with blistering of the extremities and intertriginous areas, erosions of the mouth, and deformed nails; probably autosomal dominant with occasional variable penetrance or spontaneous mutation; there is often spontaneous improvement with no residual scarring.
Bartter's s., primary juxtaglomerular cell hyperplasia with secondary hyperaldosteronism, reported in children with hypokalemic alkalosis and elevated renin or angiotensin levels; however, the blood pressure is low or normal, edema is absent, and growth is usually retarded; recessive inheritance.
basal cell nevus s., Gorlin's s.; cutaneomandibular polyoncosis; a s. of myriad basal cell nevi, odontogenic keratocysts, erythematous pitting of the palms and soles, calcification of the cerebral falx, and frequently skeletal anomalies, particularly ribs that are bifid or broadened anteriorly; autosomal dominant inheritance.
Basan's s., ectodermal dysplasia with hypotrichosis, hypohidrosis, defective teeth, and unusual dermatoglyphics.
Basex's s., paraneoplastic acrokeratosis; erythematous to plum-colored scaly acral skin lesions, paronychia, and nail dysplasia; associated with cancer of the upper respiratory or upper alimentary tract.
Bassen-Kornzweig s., abetalipoproteinemia.
battered child s., the clinical presentation of child abuse: various injuries to the skeleton, soft tissues, or organs of a child sustained as a result of repeated mistreatment or beating, usually by an individual responsible for its care.
Bauer's s., aortitis and aortic endocarditis as a little recognized manifestation of rheumatoid arthritis.
Beckwith-Wiedemann s., EMG s.
Behçet's s., triple symptom complex; Behçet's disease; recurrent hypopyon; iridocyclitis septica; cutaneomucouveal, oculobuccogenital, or uveo-encephalitic s.; a s. characterized by simultaneously or successively occurring recurrent attacks of genital and oral ulcerations (aphthae) and uveitis or iridocyclitis with hypopyon, often with arthritis; a phase of a generalized disorder, occurring more often in men than in women, with variable manifestations, including dermatitis, erythema nodosum, thrombophlebitis, and cerebral involvement.
Behr's s., Behr's disease; adult or presenile form of heredomacular degeneration.
Benedikt's s., hemiplegia with clonic spasm or tremor and oculomotor paralysis on the opposite side.
Beradinelli's s., accelerated growth, lipodystrophy with muscular hypertrophy, hepatomegaly, and lipemia.
Bernard-Horner s., Horner's s.
Bernard-Sergent s., acute adrenocortical *insufficiency.*
Bernard-Soulier s., a coagulation disorder characterized by thrombocytopenia, giant platelets, and a bleeding tendency.

Bernhardt-Roth s., *meralgia* paraesthetica.
Bernheim's s., right heart failure (enlarged liver, distended neck veins, and edema) without pulmonary congestion in subjects with left ventricular enlargement from any cause, *e.g.,* hypertension; reduction in the size of the right ventricular cavity is found postmortem and is due to encroachment by the hypertrophied septum.
Besnier-Boeck-Schaumann s., sarcoidosis.
Beuren s., supravalvular aortic stenosis with multiple areas of peripheral pulmonary arterial stenosis, mental retardation, and dental anomalies.
Biemond s., iris coloboma, mental retardation, obesity, hypogenitalism, and postaxial polydactyly; a recessive inheritance disorder resembling Laurence-Moon and Bardet-Biedel s.'s.
Bjornstad's s., pili torti associated with sensorineural hearing loss, the severity of distortion and brittleness of the hair correlated with the degree of deafness; autosomal dominant inheritance.
B-K mole s. [initials of patients' surnames], irregularly shaped, variously colored, distinctively melanocytic, 5- to 10-mm nevi occurring in large numbers (to over 100) primarily on the trunk and extremities, with a high incidence of conversion to malignant melanoma; reported in several members and three generations of a family.
Blatin's s., hydatid *thrill.*
blind loop s., stagnation of intestinal contents with bacterial overgrowth producing substances which interfere with absorption of fat, vitamins and other nutrients, usually occurring in the small intestine following operations that produce a blind loop or pouch.
Bloch-Sulzberger s., *incontinentia* pigmenti.
Bloom's s., congenital telangiectatic erythema, primarily in butterfly distribution, of the face and occasionally of the hands and forearms, with sensitivity of skin lesions and dwarfism with normal body proportions except for a narrow face and dolichocephalic skull; chromosomes are excessively fragile; autosomal recessive inheritance.
Boerhaave's s., spontaneous rupture of the lower esophagus, a variant of Mallory-Weiss s.
Bonnevie-Ullrich s., pseudo-Turner's s.
Bonnier's s., a s. due to a lesion of Deiters nucleus and its connection; the symptoms include ocular disturbances (*e.g.,* paralysis of accommodation, nystagmus, diplopia), as well as deafness, nausea, thirst, anorexia, and symptoms referable to the involvement of the vagus centers.
Böök s., PHC s.; premolar aplasia, hyperhidrosis, and premature canities associated as a dominantly inherited trait.
Börjeson-Forssman-Lehmann s., a condition characterized by mental deficiency, epilepsy, hypogonadism, hypometabolism, obesity, and narrow palpebral fissures; X-linked recessive inheritance.
bowel bypass s., fever, chills, malaise, and inflammatory cutaneous papules and pustules on the extremities and upper trunk, sometimes with polyarthralgia, with recurrent symptoms following bowel bypass surgery.
Briquet's s., a chronic but fluctuating mental disorder, usually of young women, characterized by frequent complaints of physical illness involving multiple organ systems simultaneously.
Brissaud-Marie s., unilateral spasm of the tongue and lips, of hysterical nature.
Brock's s., middle lobe s.
Brown's s., tendon sheath s.
Brown-Séquard's s., Brown-Séquard's paralysis; hemiparaplegia and hyperesthesia, but with loss of joint and muscle sense on the side of the lesion, and hemianesthesia of the opposite side, in case of a unilateral involvement of the spinal cord.
Brugsch's s., acropachyderma.
Budd's s., Budd-Chiari s., Chiari's s.
Bürger-Grütz s., type I familial *hyperlipoproteinemia.*
Burnett's s., milk-alkali s.
Buschke-Ollendorf s., osteodermatopoikilosis.
Caffey's s., infantile cortical *hyperostosis.*
Caffey-Silverman s., infantile cortical *hyperostosis.*
Capgras' s., illusion of doubles; Capgras' phenomenon; the delusional belief that a person (or persons) close to the schizophrenic patient has been substituted for by one or more imposters.
Caplan's s., Caplan's nodules; intrapulmonary nodules, histologically similar to subcutaneous rheumatoid nodules, associated with rheumatoid arthritis and pneumoconiosis in coal workers.
carcinoid s., malignant or metastatic carcinoid s.; a combination of symptoms and lesions usually produced by the release of serotonin from carcinoid tumors of the gastrointestinal tract which have metastasized to the liver; consists of irregular mottled blushing, angiomas of the skin, acquired tricuspid and pulmonary stenosis with some minor involvement of valves on the left side of the heart, diarrhea, bronchial spasm, mental aberration, and excretion of large quantities of 5-hydroxyindoleacetic acid.
carotid sinus s., Charcot-Weiss-Baker s.; pressoreceptor reflex; carotid sinus reflex; stimulation of a hyperactive carotid sinus, causing a marked fall in blood pressure due to vasodilation and cardiac slowing; syncope with or without convulsions or heart block may occur.
carpal tunnel s., pain and paresthesia (tingling, burning, and numbness) in the hand in the area of distribution of the median nerve, caused by compression of the median nerve by fibers of the flexor retinaculum.
Carpenter's s. [C. C. J. Carpenter], the association of primary hypothyroidism, primary adrenocortical insufficiency, and diabetes mellitus.
Carpenter's s. [G. Carpenter], acrocephalopolysyndactyly.
cataract-oligophrenia s., Marinesco-Sjögren s.
cat-cry s., cri-du-chat s.
cat's-eye s., Schmid-Fraccaro s.; a s. characterized by iris colobomas (resembling the vertical pupils of a cat) and anal atresia, associated with an additional acrocentric chromosome; other malformations and mental retardation may be present.
cauda equina s., dull pain in upper sacral region with anesthesia or analgesia in buttocks, genitalia, or thigh; accompanied by disturbed bowel and bladder function.
cavernous sinus s., a s. caused by thrombosis of the cavernous intracranial sinus characterized by edema of eyelids and conjunctivae, and paralysis of the third, fourth and sixth nerves.
Ceelen-Gellerstadt s., idiopathic pulmonary *hemosiderosis.*
cellular immunity deficiency s., a s. marked by increased susceptibility to infection, especially to viral infection, associated with defective functioning of the mechanism responsible for acquired immunity of the cell-mediated kind. See also immunodeficiency.
central cord s., paraplegia most severely involving the upper extremities, with or without sensory loss and bladder dysfunction, probably due to ischemia from osteophytic or traumatic compression of the central part of the cervical spinal cord and/or artery.
cerebellar s., the signs and symptoms of cerebellar deficiency: dysmetria, dysarthria, asynergia, nystagmus, ataxia, staggering gait, and adiadochokinesia.
cerebellomedullary malformation s., Arnold-Chiari *deformity.*
cerebellopontine angle s., a s. due most commonly to an acoustic tumor in the region between the cerebellum and pons, and marked by ataxia and hypotension of muscles on the side of the lesion together with nystagmus, tinnitus, deafness, disturbances of labyrinth function, and involvement of any of the cranial nerves, fifth, sixth, seventh, ninth, or tenth.
cerebrohepatorenal s., Zellweger s.; a neonatal s. characterized by muscular hypotonia, incomplete myelinization of nervous tissue, craniofacial malformations, hepatomegaly, and small glomerular cysts of the kidney; autosomal recessive inheritance.
cervical compression s., cervical disc s.
cervical disc s., cervical compression s.; pain, paresthesias, and muscular spasms in the area of the distribution of the cervical spi-

nal nerve roots, due to pressure of a protruded cervical intervertebral disc.
cervical fusion s., Klippel-Feil s.
cervical rib s., symptoms due to pressure upon nerves of the brachial plexus by a supernumerary rib which arises from the seventh cervical vertebra (costa cervicalis); the chief symptoms are pain and tingling along the forearm and hand over the distribution of the first thoracic nerve root and, later, anesthesia with cyanosis and coldness over the ulnar area of the hand; wasting of the intrinsic muscles of the hand may occur.
cervical tension s., posttraumatic neck s.
cervico-oculo-acoustic s., Wildervanck s.; a congenital short neck associated with paralysis of the external ocular muscles and with perceptive deafness; occurs in girls.
Cestan-Chenais s., contralateral hemiplegia, hemianesthesia, and loss of pain and temperature sensibility, with ipsilateral hemiasynergia and lateropulsion, paralysis of the larynx and soft palate, enophthalmia, miosis, and ptosis, due to lesions of the brain stem.
chancriform s., an ulcerative lesion at the site of primary infection by microorganisms, with regional lymph node enlargement; it occurs not only in chancroid infections but also in various bacterial and fungal infections.
Chandler s., iridocorneal s.; iris atrophy with corneal edema.
Charcot's s., intermittent *claudication.*
Charcot-Weiss-Baker s., carotid sinus s.
Charlin's s., neuritis of the nasal ciliary nerve with paroxysmal congestion of the eye, rhinorrhea, and neuralgic pain.
Chauffard's s., Still-Chauffard s.; the symptoms of Still's disease in one suffering from bovine or other nonhuman form of tuberculosis.
Chédiak-Steinbrinck-Higashi s., Chédiak-Steinbrinck-Higashi anomaly; Chédiak-Higashi disease; Béguez César disease; abnormalities of granulation and nuclear structure of all types of leukocytes with malformation of peroxidase-positive granules, cytoplasmic inclusions, and Döhle bodies, often with hepatosplenomegaly, lymphadenopathy, anemia, thrombocytopenia, roentgenologic changes of bones, lungs and heart, skin and psychomotor abnormalities, and susceptibility to infection, usually resulting in death in childhood; occurs in mink, cattle, and mice, as well as man; autosomal recessive inheritance.
Cheney s., acro-osteolysis with osteoporosis and changes in the skull and mandible.
cherry-red spot myoclonus s., sialidosis; a neuronal storage disorder in children characterized by a cherry red spot at the macula, progressive myoclonus, and easily controlled seizures; the result of sialidase deficiency. Type 1 is characterized by normal body habitus, cherry red macula, myoclonus, and normal β-galactosidase levels; type 2 by short stature, bony abnormalities, and deficient β-galactosidase.
Chiari's s., Chiari-Budd s., thrombosis of the hepatic vein with great enlargement of the liver and extensive development of collateral vessels, intractable ascites, and severe portal hypertension. Also called Chiari's disease; Rokitansky's disease (2); Budd's or Budd-Chiari s.
Chiari II s., elongation of medulla and cerebellar tonsils and vermis with displacement through the foramen magnum into the upper spinal canal; often associated with other cerebral anomalies.
Chiari-Frommel s., unphysiological lactation and amenorrhea following pregnancy, but not caused by infant's nursing; characterized by hyperprolactinemia and a pituitary adenoma.
chiasma s., a s. characterized by a bitemporal visual field defect and optic nerve atrophy due to a lesion in or about the chiasm.
Chilaiditi's s., interposition of the colon between the liver and the diaphragm.
CHILD s., *c*ongenital *h*emidysplasia with *i*chthyosiform erythroderma and *l*imb *d*efects.
"Chinese restaurant" s., development of chest pain, feelings of facial pressure, and sensation of burning over variable portions of the body surface after ingestion of food containing monosodium L-glutamate by persons sensitive to this food additive.
Chotzen s., type III *acrocephalosyndactyly.*
Christian's s., Hand-Schüller-Christian *disease.*
Christ-Siemens s., anhidrotic ectodermal *dysplasia.*
chromosomal s., general designation for s.'s due to chromosomal aberrations; typically associated with mental retardation and multiple congenital anomalies.
chromosomal instability s.'s, chromosomal breakage s.'s, a group of mendelian conditions associated with chromosomal instability and breakage *in vitro,* and often manifest an increased tendency to certain types of malignancies.
chronic hyperventilation s., reduced CO_2 content of the blood (hypocapnia) as a result of hyperventilation of prolonged duration; may occur in anxiety states and in some chronic organic, usually cardiovascular, disease; alkalemia, paresthesia, and tetany may occur.
Churg-Strauss s., allergic granulomatosis; allergic granulomatous angiitis; asthma, fever, eosinophilia, and varied symptoms and signs of vasculitis, primarily affecting small arteries, with vascular and extravascular granulomas.
Clarke-Hadfield s., cystic *fibrosis.*
Claude's s., midbrain s. with oculomotor palsy on the side of the lesion and incoordination on the opposite side.
climacteric s., menopausal s.
cloverleaf skull s., intrauterine bone dysplasia and synostosis of the coronal and lambdoid sutures producing a trilobar head shape, with various craniofacial and long-bone anomalies.
Cobb s., cutaneomeningospinal angiomatosis; cutaneous angiomas associated with vascular abnormality of the spinal cord and resulting neurologic symptoms.
Cockayne's s., Cockayne's disease; dwarfism, precociously senile appearance, pigmentary degeneration of the retina, optic atrophy, deafness, sensitivity to sunlight, and mental retardation; autosomal recessive inheritance.
Coffin-Siris s., Coffin-Lowry s., mental retardation with wide bulbous (pugilistic) nose, low nasal bridge, moderate hirsutism, and digital anomalies with nail hypoplasia (especially of the fifth fingers); the full s. occurs only in males, but female relatives may have abnormal fingers and mild mental retardation; X-linked inheritance, incompletely recessive.
Cogan's s., oculovestibulo-auditory s.
Cogan-Reese s., iridocorneal endothelial s.
Collet-Sicard s., unilateral lesions of the ninth, tenth, eleventh, and twelfth cranial nerves producing Vernet syndrome and paralysis of the tongue on the same side.
compartmental s., a condition in which increased pressure in a confined anatomical space adversely affects the circulation and threatens the function and viability of the tissues therein.
compression s., crush s. (1).
Conn's s., primary *aldosteronism.*
Cornelia de Lange s., de Lange s.
corpus luteum deficiency s., functional disturbances caused by insufficient ovarian luteinization; reflected by inadequate luteal phase endometrial response.
Costen's s., a symptom complex of loss of hearing, otalgia, tinnitis, dizziness, headache, and burning sensation of the throat, tongue, and side of the nose; originally attributed to temporomandibular joint dysfunction resulting from occlusal disharmony, but currently recognized as not being well founded on anatomic and physiologic principles.
costochondral s., pain in the chest with tenderness over one or more costochondral junctions.
costoclavicular s., a s. resulting from compression of the neurovascular bundle between the medial portions of the clavicle and the first rib.

Cotard's s., psychotic depression involving delusion of the existence of one's body, along with ideas of negation and suicidal impulses.
Crandall's s., pili torti and hearing defects associated with hypogonadism; a sex-linked trait in which there is a deficiency of luteinizing and of growth hormone.
CREST s., a variant of scleroderma characterized by *c*alcinosis, *R*aynaud's phenomenon, *e*sophageal motility disorders, *s*clerodactyly, and *t*elangiectasia.
cri-du-chat s., cat-cry s.; Lejune s.; a disorder due to deletion of the short arm of chromosome 5, characterized by microcephaly, antimongoloid palpebral fissures, epicanthal folds, micrognathia, strabismus, mental and physical retardation, and a characteristic high-pitched catlike whine.
Crigler-Najjar s., Crigler-Najjar disease; a rare defect in ability to form bilirubin glucuronide due to deficiency of bilirubin-glucuronside glucuronosyltransferase; characterized by familial nonhemolytic jaundice and, in its severe form, by irreversible brain damage that resembles kernicterus and may be fatal; autosomal recessive inheritance.
crocodile tears s., residual facial paralysis with profuse lacrimation during eating, caused by a lesion of the seventh nerve central to the geniculate ganglion; there is misdirection of regenerating autonomic fibers, which formerly innervated the salivary gland, to the lacrimal glands.
Cronkhite-Canada s., a sporadically occurring s. of gastrointestinal polyps with diffuse alopecia and nail dystrophy.
Crouzon's s., craniofacial *dysostosis.*
CRST s., a s. characterized by *c*alcinosis cutis, *R*aynaud's phenomenon, *s*clerodactyly, and *t*elangiectasia; usually due to scleroderma.
crush s., compression s.; the shocklike state that follows release of a limb or limbs or the trunk and pelvis after a prolonged period of compression, as by a heavy weight; characterized by suppression of urine, probably the result of damage to the renal tubules by myoglobin from the damaged muscles.
Cruveilhier-Baumgarten s., Cruveilhier-Baumgarten disease; cirrhosis of the liver with patent umbilical or paraumbilical veins and varicose periumbilical veins (caput medusae).
cryptophthalmus s., Fraser's s.
Cushing's s., Cushing's or pituitary basophilism; a disorder resulting from increased adrenocortical secretion of cortisol, caused by ACTH-dependent adrenocortical hyperplasia or tumor, ectopic ACTH-secreting tumor, or ACTH-independent adrenocortical tumor or nodular hyperplasia; characterized by trunkal obesity, moon face, acne, abdominal striae, hypertension, decreased carbohydrate tolerance, protein catabolism, psychiatric disturbances, and amenorrhea and hirsutism in females; when associated with an ACTH producing adenoma, sometimes called Cushing's disease.
Cushing's s. medicamentosus, a variable number of the signs and symptoms of Cushing's s.; produced by the chronic administration of large doses of any steroid that is a potent glucocorticoid.
cutaneomucouveal s., Behçet's s.
DaCosta's s., neurocirculatory *asthenia.*
Dandy-Walker s., hydrocephalus in infants associated with atresia of the foramina of Luschka and Magendie.
dead fetus s., s. characterized by lengthy intrauterine retention of a dead fetus and loss of incoagulable blood; persistent tachycardia is usually present before hemorrhage occurs; fibrinogen levels are usually chronically depressed.
de Clerambault s., erotomania accompanied by the delusional belief that a certain person is in love with you.
Degos s., malignant atrophic *papulosis.*
Dejerine-Roussy s., thalamic s.
de Lange s., Cornelia de Lange s.; a congenital anomaly characterized by impaired development, mental retardation, characteristic facies with eyebrows growing across base of nose and hairline well down on forehead, depressed bridge of nose with uptilted tip of nose, and small head with low-set ears, and flat spadelike hands with simian crease and short tapering fingers.
Del Castillo s., Sertoli-cell-only s.
de Morsier's s., septo-optic *dysplasia.*
dengue shock s., dengue fever of grade III or IV severity.
De Sanctis-Cacchione s., xeroderma pigmentosum with mental deficiency, dwarfism, and gonadal hypoplasia; recessive inheritance.
De Toni-Fanconi s., cystinosis.
s. of deviously relevant answers, Ganser's s.
dialysis disequilibrium s., nausea, vomiting, and hypertension, occasionally with convulsions, developing within several hours after starting hemodialysis for renal failure; apparently caused by too rapid removal of urea from the extracellular fluid compartment, with movement of water into cells, and cerebral edema.
dialysis encephalopathy s., dialysis dementia; a progressive, often fatal, diffuse encephalopathy occurring in a few patients on chronic hemodialysis; to be differentiated from the relatively acute, self-limited dialysis disequilibrium s.
Diamond-Blackfan s., congenital hypoplastic *anemia.*
diencephalic s. of infancy, profound emaciation after initial normal growth, locomotor hyperactivity and euphoria, usually with skin pallor, hypotension and hypoglycemia; usually due to neoplasm involving the anterior hypothalamus.
DiGeorge s., third and fourth pharyngeal pouch s.; congenital absence of the thymus and parathyroid glands, without agammaglobulinemia but with frequent infections and delayed development. See also *immunodeficiency* with hypoparathyroidism.
Di Guglielmo's s., eponym for the acute form of erythremic *myelosis.*
disconnection s., general term for various neurological disorders due to interruption of fiber pathways of the cerebrum.
disk s., low back pain, pain in the thigh, and sciatica sometimes with wasting and loss of achilles and patellar reflexes, as the result of a compressive radiculopathy from intervertebral disk pressure.
Doose s., a rare familial type of primary, generalized myoclonic astatic epilepsy characterized by 2 to 3 or 4 to 6 Hz spike and wave complexes in the EEG; the condition usually responds to medication.
Dorfman-Chanarin s., neutral lipid storage disease; congenital ichthyosis, leukocyte vacuoles, and variable involvement of other organ systems.
Down's s., mongolism; trisomy 21 s.; a syndrome of mental retardation associated with a variable constellation of abnormalities caused by representation of at least a critical portion of chromosome 21 three times instead of twice in some or all cells; no single physical sign is diagnostic and most stigmata are found in some normal persons; the abnormalities include retarded growth, flat hypoplastic face with short nose, prominent epicanthic skin folds, protruding lower lip, small rounded ears with prominent antihelix, fissured and thickened tongue, laxness of joint ligaments, pelvic dysplasia, broad hands and feet, stubby fingers usually with dysplasia of the middle phalanx of the fifth finger, transverse palmar crease, dermatoglyphic changes including distal displacement of the palmar axial triradius, dry rough skin in older patients and abundant slack neck skin in newborns, and muscle hypotonia and absence of Moro reflex in newborns; most patients are trisomic for chromosome 21 as a result of nondisjunction; some patients are mosaic, with both normal and trisomic cell lines; a few patients have 46 chromosomes but are effectively trisomic because of translocation of a major portion of chromosome 21 to another chromosome; in rare patients no chromosome abnormality can be detected.
Dressler's s., postmyocardial infarction s.
dry eye s., *keratoconjunctivitis* sicca.
Duane's s., retraction s.

Dubin-Johnson s., chronic idiopathic jaundice; Sprinz-Nelson s.; familial recurrence of mild jaundice, with unconjugated bilirubin as the major pigment, accumulation of pigment of undefined nature in hepatic cells, impaired excretion of sulfobromophthalein sodium, and nonvisualization of gallbladder.
Dubreuil-Chambardel s., simultaneous caries of the upper incisor teeth occurring in either sex between the ages of 14 and 17; after an interval of varying length the other teeth also become involved.
Duchenne's s., subacute or chronic anterior spinal paralysis combined with multiple neuritis.
dumping s., postgastrectomy s.; the s. that occurs after eating in patients with shunts of the upper alimentary canal; characterized by flushing, sweating, dizziness, weakness, and vasomotor collapse, occasionally with pain and headache; results from rapid passage of large amounts of food into the small intestine, with an osmotic effect removing fluid from plasma and causing hypovolemia.
Dyggve-Melchior-Clausen s., an osteochondrodysplasia that clinically resembles Morquio's s., but without excretion of mucopolysaccharides; characterized by mental retardation, short stature, progressive sternal bulging, flattening of vertebral bodies and iliac crests, shortening of metacarpals, and changes in long bones; autosomal recessive inheritance.
dysmnesic s., Korsakoff's s.
dysplastic nevus s., clinically atypical nevi (usually exceeding 5 mm in diameter and having variable pigmentation and ill defined borders) with an increased risk for development of non-familial cutaneous malignant melanoma; biopsies show melanocytic dysplasia; nevi are clinically and histologically identical to the precursor lesions for melanoma in the B-K mole s.
Eagle s., facial pain due to an elongated styloid process.
Eaton-Lambert s., Lambert-Eaton s.
ectopic ACTH s., the association of Cushing's s. with a non-pituitary neoplasm, usually a lung carcinoma that produces ACTH.
Edwards' s., trisomy 18 s.
effort s., neurocirculatory *asthenia.*
egg-white s., egg-white injury; dermatitis, loss of hair, and loss of muscle coordination, produced in rats by diets containing large amounts of raw egg white, the avidin of which combines with biotin producing a deficiency of the latter.
Ehlers-Danlos s., cutis hyperelastica; a group of inherited generalized connective tissue diseases characterized by overelasticity and friability of the skin, excessive extensibility of the joints, and fragility of the cutaneous blood vessels and sometimes large arteries, due to deficient quality or quantity of collagen; the most common is inherited as an autosomal dominant trait; some recessive cases have hydroxylysine-deficient collagen due to deficiency of collagen lysyl hydroxylase.
Eisenlohr's s., numbness and weakness in the extremities, paralysis of the lips, tongue, and palate, and dysarthria.
Eisenmenger s., pulmonary hypertension associated with a congenital communication between the two circulations (*e.g.,* atrial or ventricular septal defect, patent ductus arteriosus) so that a right-to-left shunt results.
Ekbom s., restless legs s.
Ellis-van Creveld s., chondroectodermal *dysplasia.*
EMG s., Beckwith-Wiedemann s.; exomphalos, macroglossia, and gigantism, often with neonatal hypoglycemia; autosomal recessive inheritance.
encephalotrigeminal vascular s., angiomatosis of the brain accompanied by nevi in the trigeminal area.
endocrine polyglandular s., familial endocrine *adenomatosis,* type 1.
erythrodysesthesia s., tingling sensation of the palms and soles, progressing to severe pain and tenderness with erythema and edema; caused by continuous infusion therapy.
Evans' s., acquired hemolytic anemia and thrombocytopenia.
extrapyramidal s., abnormalities of movement related to injury of motor pathways other than the pyramidal tract.
Faber's s., achlorhydric *anemia.*
Fanconi's s., **(1)** Fanconi's *anemia;* **(2)** a group of conditions with characteristic disorders of renal tubular function, which may be classified as: 1) cystinosis, a recessive hereditary disease of early childhood; 2) adult Fanconi s., a rare hereditary form, probably due to a recessive gene different from that found in cystinosis, characterized by the tubular malfunction seen in cystinosis and by osteomalacia, but without cystine deposit in tissues; 3) acquired Fanconi s., which may be associated with multiple myeloma or may result from chemical poisoning, injury, or persisting damage of proximal tubular epithelium due to various causes, leading to multiple defects of tubular function.
Farber's s., disseminated *lipogranulomatosis.*
Felty's s., rheumatoid arthritis with splenomegaly and leukopenia.
fetal alcohol s., a specific pattern of fetal malformation with growth deficiency, craniofacial anomalies, and limb defects, found among offspring of mothers who are chronic alcoholics; mental retardation is often demonstrated later.
fetal aspiration s., a s. resulting from uterine aspiration of amniotic fluid and meconium by the fetus, usually caused by hypoxia and often leading to aspiration pneumonia.
fetal face s., a s. of facies resembling an early fetus with short forearms, and genital hypoplasia at birth, but without evidence of achondroplasia; leads to dwarfism without mental retardation.
fetal hydantoin s., a fetal s. resulting from maternal ingestion of hydantoin analogues, characterized by growth deficiency, mental deficiency, dysmorphic facies, cleft palate or lip, cardiac defects, or abnormal genitalia.
fetal trimethadione s., a fetal s. resulting from maternal ingestion of trimethadione during the early weeks of pregnancy and characterized by developmental delay, v-shaped eyebrows, epicanthus, low-set ears with anteriorly folded helix, palatal anomaly, and irregular teeth.
fetal warfarin s., fetal bleeding, nasal hypoplasia, optic atrophy, and fetal death resulting from administration of warfarin to the pregnant patient.
fibrinogen-fibrin conversion s., a s. characterized by hypofibrinogenemia with incoagulable blood; it may be seen in abruptio placentae, prolonged retention of a dead fetus in an Rh-isosensitized mother, Sheehan's syndrome, hemolytic blood reactions, bilateral renal cortical necrosis, and cases of trauma.
Fiessinger-Leroy-Reiter s., Reiter's s.
Figueira's s., weakness of the neck muscles with slight spasticity of the muscles of the lower extremities and increased tendon reflexes; supposed to be an attenuated sporadic form of acute poliomyelitis.
first arch s., generic term including s.'s of malformations involving derivatives of the first branchial arch, with or without associated malformations; includes mandibulofacial dysostosis, micrognathia with peromelia, otomandibular dystosis, acrofacial dysostosis, and others.
Fisher's s., a s. characterized by ophthalmoplegia, ataxia, and areflexia; a form of polyneuroradiculitis.
Fitz-Hugh and Curtis s., gonococcal perihepatitis in women with a history of gonorrheal salpingitis.
flashing pain s., sudden, intermittent, and severe brief episodes of pain, without apparent cause, in the distribution of a spinal dermatome; resembles in character the pain of tic douloureux.
flecked retina s., hereditary retinal disorder with abnormal transmission of fluorescence through the retinal pigment epithelium on angiography.
floppy valve s., retrograde slippage of degenerating mitral valve leaflets into the valve's orifice beyond the point of closure during systole of the left ventricle; a feature of Barlow's s.
Flynn-Aird s., a familial s. characterized by muscle wasting,

ataxia, dementia, skin atrophy, and ocular anomalies.
focal dermal hypoplasia s., widely distributed linear areas of dermal hypoplasia resembling striae distensae, with soft yellow nodules of fat herniation.
Foix's s., total ophthalmoplegia, paresis of the sympathetic nerves, and neuroparalytic keratitis from compression within the lateral wall of the cavernous sinus.
folded-lung s., round atelectasis; collapse of part of the lung caught between shrinking fibrous pleura scars, sometimes resulting from pleural asbestosis.
Forbes-Albright s., pituitary tumor in a patient without acromegaly which secretes excessive amounts of prolactin (LTH) and produces persistent lactation.
Forney's s., familial mitral insufficiency, conductive hearing loss, short stature, and bony fusion of the cervical vertebrae and carpal and tarsal bones.
Foster Kennedy's s., Kennedy's s.
Foville's s., a form of alternating hemiplegia characterized by abducens paralysis on one side, paralysis of the extremities on the other.
fragile X s., see fragile X *chromosome.*
Fraley s., dilation of the upper pole renal calices due to stenosis of the upper infundibulum, usually caused by compression from vessels supplying the upper and middle segments of the kidney.
Franceschetti's s., mandibulofacial *dysostosis,* when complete or nearly complete.
Franceschetti-Jadassohn s., Naegeli s.
Fraser's s., cryptophthalmus s.; an association of cryptophthalmus with multiple anomalies, including middle and outer ear malformations, cleft palate, laryngeal deformity, displacement of umbilicus and nipples, digital malformations, separation of symphysis pubis, maldevelopment of kidneys, and masculinization of genitalia in females; autosomal recessive inheritance.
Freeman-Sheldon s., craniocarpotarsal *dystrophy.*
Frenkel's anterior ocular traumatic s., a s. with mydriasis, hyphema, small iris tears near the pupil, discrete punctate opacities of the lens, and occasionally iridodialysis.
Frey's s., auriculotemporal nerve s.
Friderichsen-Waterhouse s., Waterhouse-Friderichsen s.
Fröhlich's s., Launois-Cléret s.; dystrophia adiposogenitalis, originally involving an adenohypophysial tumor.
Froin's s., loculation s.; an alteration in the cerebrospinal fluid, which is yellowish in hue and coagulates spontaneously in a few seconds after withdrawal, owing to its greatly increased protein (albumin and globulin) content; noted in loculated portions of the subarachnoid space isolated from spinal fluid circulation by an inflammatory or neoplastic obstruction.
Fuchs' s., a s. characterized by heterochromia of the iris, iridocyclitis, keratic precipitates, and cataract.
functional prepubertal castration s., a s. characterized by the absence of testes from the scrotum but in their place mesonephric duct derivatives, pronounced gynecomastia and eunuchoid habitus, and increased urinary excretion of gonadotrophins.
G s. [first letter of surname of affected person reported], a s. of characteristic facies associated with hypospadias, ventral curvature of the penis, and dysphagia.
Gaisböck's s., *polycythemia* hypertonica.
Ganser's s., s. of approximate relevant answers; s. of deviously relevant answers; nonsense s.; a psychotic-like condition, without the symptoms and signs of a traditional psychosis, occurring typically in prisoners who feign insanity; *e.g.,* such a person, when asked to multiply 6 by 4, will give 23 as the answer, or he will call a key a lock.
Gardner's s., the development of multiple tumors, inherited as a dominant trait, including osteomas of the skull, epidermoid cysts, and fibromas before 10 years of age, and multiple polyposis predisposing to carcinoma of the colon.
Gardner-Diamond s., autoerythrocyte sensitization *syndrome.*
gastrocardiac s., disturbances of the heart's action due to faulty action of the digestive system, especially of the stomach.
gastrojejunal loop obstruction s., afferent loop s.
Gélineau's s., narcolepsy.
general-adaptation s., term given by H. Selye to the nonspecific reactions of organisms to organic and mental injury or stress; it comprises three stages: 1) alarm reaction; 2) stage of resistance, which includes all those nonspecific systemic adaptive reactions called forth by prolonged exposure to injurious stimuli; 3) state of exhaustion, in which the adaptation can no longer be maintained.
Gerstmann s., finger agnosia, agraphia, confusion of laterality of body, and acalculia; caused by lesions between the occipital area and the angular gyrus.
Gerstmann-Sträussler s., a more chronic cerebellar form of spongiform encephalopathy.
Gianotti-Crosti s., papular acrodermatitis of childhood; a cutaneous manifestation of hepatitis B infection occurring in young children; an exanthem comprised of dusky papules on the legs, buttocks, and extensors of the arms; it lasts 2 to 8 weeks and is associated with adenopathy and malaise.
Gilbert's s., familial nonhemolytic *jaundice.*
Gilles de la Tourette's s., Gilles de la Tourette's, Tourette's, or Guinon's disease; Tourette's s.; motor incoordination with echolalia and coprolalia; a form of tic.
Glanzmann-Riniker s., X-linked *hypogammaglobulinemia.*
glomangiomatous osseous malformation s., a congenital association of glomus tumors with osteoporosis of limb bones.
glucagonoma s., necrolytic migratory erythema, stomatitis, anemia, weight loss, and hyperglycemia resulting from glucagon-secreting pancreatic islet cell tumors.
Goldberg-Maxwell s., testicular feminization s.
Goldenhar's s., oculoauriculovertebral *dysplasia.*
Goltz s., focal dermal *hypoplasia.*
Goodpasture's s., glomerulonephritis of the anti-basement membrane type associated with or preceded by hemoptysis; the nephritis usually progresses rapidly to produce death from renal failure, and the lungs at autopsy show extensive hemosiderosis or recent hemorrhage.
Gopalan's s., severe discomfort of the feet associated with elevated skin temperature and excessive sweating.
Gorlin's s., basal cell nevus s.
Gorlin-Chaudhry-Moss s., a very rare congenital condition in which are associated craniofacial dysostosis, patent ductus arteriosus, hypertrichosis, hypoplasia of labia majora, and dental and ocular abnormalities.
Gorman's s., hemangiomatosis of the skeletal system with or without involvement of the overlying skin, resulting in osteolysis and fibrous replacement of bone.
Gougerot-Carteaud s., confluent and reticulate *papillomatosis.*
Gowers' s., vagal *attack.*
gracilis s., osteonecrosis of the pubic bone following trauma.
Gradenigo's s., petrositis with abducens paralysis and pain in the temporal region, due to localized meningitis involving the fifth and sixth nerves.
Graham Little s., *lichen* planopilaris.
gray s., gray baby s., gray appearance of an infant at birth and during the neonatal period which can be caused by transplacental toxic effects of the drug chloramphenicol taken by the mother during late pregnancy; the s. may be fatal.
Greig's s., ocular *hypertelorism.*
Grönblad-Strandberg s., angioid streaks of the retina together with pseudoxanthoma elasticum of the skin.
Gruber's s., dysencephalia splanchnocystica.
Gubler's s., Gubler's hemiplegia or paralysis; Millard-Gubler s.; a form of alternating hemiplegia characterized by contralateral hemiplegia and ipsilateral facial paralysis.

Guillain-Barré s., acute idiopathic *polyneuritis.*
Gunn's s., jaw-winking s.
gustatory sweating s., auriculotemporal nerve s.
Haber's s., a permanent flushing and telangiectasia of the cheeks, nose, forehead, and chin, with prominent follicular openings, small papules with scaling, and minute pitted areas; occasionally accompanied by scaly and keratotic lesions of the trunk; appears in childhood as an autosomal dominant inherited trait.
Hallermann-Streiff s., *dyscephalia* mandibulo-oculofacialis.
Hallervorden-Spatz s., Hallervorden s., a pathologic process in which the nerve fibers connecting the striatum and pallidum are completely demyelinated.
Hallgren's s., vestibulocerebellar ataxia, pigmentary retinal dystrophy, congenital deafness, and cataract.
Hamman's s., Hamman's disease; spontaneous mediastinal emphysema, resulting from rupture of alveoli.
Hamman-Rich s., acute or chronic interstitial fibrosis of the lung, giving rise to serious right ventricular failure and cor pulmonale.
hand-and-foot s., sickle cell dactylitis; recurrent painful swelling of the hands and feet occurring in infants and young children with sickle cell anemia.
Hanhart's s., *micrognathia* with peromelia.
happy puppet s., a s. of unknown cause characterized by mental retardation, ataxia, hypotonia, epileptic seizures, easily provoked and prolonged spasms of laughter, prognathism, and an open-mouthed expression.
Harada's s., Harada's disease; uveoencephalitis; uveomeningitis s.; bilateral retinal edema, uveitis, choroiditis, and retinal detachment, with temporary or permanent deafness, graying of the hair (poliosis), and alopecia; related to the Vogt-Koyanagi s. and sympathetic ophthalmia.
Hartnup s., Hartnup *disease.*
Hayem-Widal s., Widal's s.; icteroanemia; acquired hemolytic icterus; a s. in which icterus and anemia occur in association with a moderate degree of splenomegaly, increased fragility of red blood cells, and increased amounts of urobilin in the urine.
head-bobbing doll s., bobbing motion of the head usually due to cysts in or about the third ventricle.
heart-hand s., Holt-Oram s.
Hegglin's s., dissociation between hemodynamic systole and electrical (Q-T interval) systole so that the second heart tone is sounded before the end of the T wave; described by Hegglin as an energy-dynamic cardiac insufficiency during diabetic coma.
Helweg-Larssen s., familial anhidrosis present from birth with neurolabyrinthitis developing in the fourth or fifth decade.
hemangioma-thrombocytopenia s., Kasabach-Merritt s.
hemolytic uremic s., hemolytic anemia and thrombocytopenia occurring with acute renal failure. In children, characterized by sudden onset of gastrointestinal bleeding, hematuria, oliguria, and microangiopathic hemolytic anemia; in adults, associated with complications of pregnancy following normal delivery, or associated with oral contraceptive use or with infection.
Henoch-Schönlein s., Henoch-Schönlein *purpura.*
hepatorenal s., hepatonephoric s., the occurrence of acute renal failure in patients with disease of the liver or biliary tract, apparently due to decreased renal blood flow; conditions which damage both organs, such as carbon tetrachloride poisoning and leptospirosis.
Herlitz s., *epidermolysis* bullosa lethalis.
Herrmann's s., a nervous system disorder beginning in late childhood or early adolescence, characterized by photomyoclonus and hearing loss followed by diabetes mellitus, progressive dementia, pyelonephritis, and glomerulonephritis; progressive sensorineural hearing loss is of later onset; dominant inheritance.
Hinman s., pseudoneurogenic bladder; detrusor-sphincter incoordination of psychologic basis.
Hirschowitz s., acanthosis nigricans associated with hypovitaminosis; responds well to topical retinoic acid therapy.
holiday s., regression, development of diffuse anxiety, feelings of helplessness, irritability, and depression; said to occur in certain psychoanalytic patients before Thanksgiving and continuing into the Christmas holiday season, ending a few days after January first.
holiday heart s., dysrhythmias of the heart, sometimes apparent after a vacation or weekend away from work, and coupled with excessive alcohol consumption.
Holmes-Adie s., pupillotonic pseudotabes; Adie's pupil; Adie s.; Holmes-Adie pupil; tonic pupillary reactions with absent or diminished tendon reflexes. See also tonic *pupil.*
Holt-Oram s., atriodigital dysplasia; heart-hand s.; atrial septal defect in association with finger-like or absent thumb and other deformities of the forearm; autosomal dominant inheritance.
Horner's s., ptosis sympathetica; Bernard-Horner s.; ptosis, miosis, anidrosis, and enophthalmos due to a lesion of the cervical sympathetic chain or its central pathways.
Houssay s., the amelioration of diabetes mellitus by a destructive lesion in, or surgical removal of, the pituitary gland.
Hunt's s., Ramsay Hunt's s.; **(1)** progressive cerebellar tremor; dyssynergia cerebellaris progressiva; an intention tremor beginning in one extremity, gradually increasing in intensity, and subsequently involving other parts of the body; **(2)** facial paralysis, otalgia, and herpes zoster resulting from viral infection of the seventh cranial nerve and geniculate ganglion; **(3)** paleostriatal or pallidal s.; a form of juvenile paralysis agitans associated with primary atrophy of the pallidal system.
Hunter's s., type II mucopolysaccharidosis; an error of mucopolysaccharide metabolism characterized by deficiency of iduronate sulfatase, with excretion of dermatan sulfate and heparan sulfate in the urine; clinically similar to Hurler's s. but distinguished by less severe skeletal changes, no corneal clouding, and X-linked recessive inheritance.
Hurler's s., mucopolysaccharidosis in which there is a deficiency of α-L-iduronidase, an accumulation of an abnormal intracellular material, and excretion of dermatan sulfate and heparan sulfate in the urine; characterized by severe abnormality in development of skeletal cartilage and bone, with dwarfism, kyphosis, deformed limbs, limitation of joint motion, spadelike hand, corneal clouding, hepatosplenomegaly, mental retardation, and gargoyle-like facies; autosomal recessive inheritance. Also called dysostosis multiplex; Hurler's disease; lipochondrodystrophy; type I mucopolysaccharidosis; Pflaundler-Hurler s. See also mucolipidosis.
Hutchinson-Gilford s., progeria.
Hutchison s., adrenal neuroblastoma of infants with metastasis to the orbit; at one time erroneously believed to arise predominantly from the left adrenal gland. See also Pepper s.
hydralazine s., a s. simulating systemic lupus erythematosus, occurring during protracted therapy of hypertension with hydralazine.
17-hydroxylase deficiency s., congenital deficiency of adrenocortical, and possibly ovarian, steroid C-17α hydroxylase; the resulting excessive secretion of corticosterone and deoxycorticosterone produces hypertension and hypokalemic alkalosis; absence of aldosterone secretion in such patients may indicate a multiple enzymic deficiency.
hyperabduction s., pain running down the arm, numbness, paresthesias, and erythema, with weakness of the hands; due to abduction of the arm for a prolonged period (*e.g.*, during sleep or necessitated by occupation) which stretches the axillary vessels and the nerves of the brachial plexus.
hypereosinophilic s., persistent peripheral eosinophilia with later infiltration into bone marrow, heart, and other organ systems; accompanied by nocturnal sweating, coughing, anorexia and weight loss, itching and various skin lesions, and symptoms of Loffler's endocarditis.
hyperimmunoglobulin E s., Job's s.; an immunodeficiency disor-

der characterized by high levels of plasma IgE concentrations, a leukocyte chemotactic defect, and recurrent staphylococcal infections of the skin, upper respiratory tract, and other sites.
hyperkinetic s., a condition marked by pathologically excessive energy seen sometimes in young children with brain injury, mental illness, and attention deficit disorder, and in epileptics; hypermotility and emotional instability are the chief characteristics; distractibility, inattention, and lack of shyness and of fear are common accompaniments.
hypersensitive xiphoid s., abnormal tenderness of the xiphoid, often associated with spontaneous pains in the chest, upper abdomen, and shoulders.
hypertrophied frenula s., a condition marked by abnormal frenula, pseudoclefts in lip, tongue and palate, mental retardation, and syndactyly.
hyperventilation s., see chronic hyperventilation s.
hyperviscosity s., a s. resulting from increased viscosity of the blood; an increase in serum proteins may be associated with bleeding from mucous membranes, retinopathy, and neurological symptoms, and is sometimes seen in Waldenström's macroglobulinemia and in multiple myeloma; an increased viscosity secondary to polycythemia may be associated with organ congestion and decreased capillary perfusion.
hypometabolic s., a clinical situation suggesting hypothyroidism or myxedema, in which some tests of thyroid function may be normal and the gland is not obviously atrophic or diseased; indicative of a failure of peripheral tissues to react to thyroid hormone.
hypoparathyroidism s., a s. characterized by fatigue, muscular weakness, paresthesia and cramps of the extremities, tetany, and laryngeal stridor; due to hypocalcemia resulting from a lack of parathyroid hormone; may be idiopathic, postoperative, or caused by organic lesions of the parathyroids.
hypophysial s., *dystrophia* adipsogenitalis.
hypophysio-sphenoidal s., neoplastic invasion of the base of the skull in the region of the sphenoidal sinus, often with destruction of the dorsum sellae.
hypoplastic left heart s., association of underdevelopment of the left heart chambers with atresia or stenosis of the aortic and/or mitral valve and hypoplasia of the ascending aorta.
immotile cilia s., an inherited disorder characterized by recurrent sinopulmonary infections, reduced fertility in women, and sterility in men due to the inability of ciliated structures to beat effectively because of the absence of one or both dynein arms; when associated with situs inversus, it is known as Kartagener's s.
immunodeficiency s., immunological deficiency s., a s. associated with an immunological deficiency or disorder, of which the chief symptom is an increased susceptibility to infection, the pattern of susceptibility being dependent upon the kind of deficiency. See also immunodeficiency.
s. of inappropriate secretion of antidiuretic hormone (SIADH), continued secretion of antidiuretic hormone despite low serum osmolality and expanded extracellular volume.
indifference to pain s., congenital insensitivity to pain, possibly due to an absence of organized nerve endings in the skin.
internal capsule s., hemianopsia with contralateral hemianesthesia of the face.
inversed jaw-winking s., when there are supranuclear lesions of the trigeminal nerve, touching the cornea may produce a brisk movement of the mandible to the opposite side.
iridocorneal endothelial s., Cogan-Reese s.; iris-nevus s.; s. of glaucoma, iris atrophy, decreased corneal endothelium, anterior peripheral synechia, and multiple iris nodules.
iris-nevus s., iridocorneal endothelial s.
Irvine-Gass s., macular edema, aphakia, and vitreous humor adherent to incision for cataract extraction.
Ivemark's s., a possibly heritable disorder in which organs of the left side of the body are a mirror image of their counterpart on the right side (*e.g.,* normal asymmetry of the lungs is lost and the left lung has three lobes); splenic agenesis and cardiac malformations are associated.
Jacod's s., total ophthalmoplegia, blindness, and trigeminal neuralgia.
Jadassohn-Lewandowski s., *pachyonychia* congenita.
Jahnke's s., Sturge-Weber s. without glaucoma.
jaw-winking s., an increase in the width of the eye lids during chewing, sometimes with a rhythmic elevation of the upper lid when the mouth is open and ptosis when the mouth is closed. Also called jaw-winking phenomenon; Gunn's or Marcus Gunn phenomenon or syndrome; jaw-working reflex.
Jeghers-Peutz s., Peutz-Jeghers s.
Jervell and Lange-Nielsen s., surdocardiac s.
Jeune's s., asphyxiating thoracic *dysplasia.*
Job s. [*Job,* biblical char.], hyperimmunoglobulin E s.
Joubert's s., agenesis of the cerebellar vermis; characterized clinically by attacks of tachypnea or prolonged apnea, abnormal eye movements, ataxia, and mental retardation.
jugular foramen s., Avellis s.
Kallmann's s., *hypogonadism* with anosmia.
Kanner's s., infantile *autism.*
Kartagener's s., Kartagener's triad; complete situs inversus associated with bronchiectasis and chronic sinusitis associated with ciliary dysmotility and impaired ciliary mucous transport in the respiratory epithelium; autosomal recessive inheritance with variable penetrance. See also immotile cilia s.
Kasabach-Merritt s., hemangioma-thrombocytopenia s.; capillary hemangioma associated with thrombocytopenic purpura.
Katayama s., *schistosomiasis* japonica.
Kearns-Sayre s., pigmentary retinal dystrophy, myopathic ophthalmoplegia, cardiomyopathy, and varied cranial nerve impairment; typically occurring before 20 years of age.
Kennedy's s., Foster Kennedy's s; ipsilateral optic atrophy with central scotoma and contralateral choked disk or papilledema, caused by a meningioma of the ipsilateral optic nerve.
Kimmelstiel-Wilson s., Kimmelstiel-Wilson disease; nephrotic syndrome and hypertension in diabetics, associated with diabetic glomerulosclerosis.
Kleine-Levin s., a rare form of periodic hypersomnia associated with bulimia, occurring in males aged 10 to 25 years, characterized by periods of ravenous appetite alternating with prolonged sleep (as long as 18 hours), along with behavioral disturbances, impaired thought processes, and hallucinations; acute illness or fatigue may precede an episode which may occur as often as several times a year.
Klinefelter's s., XXY s.; a chromosomal anomaly with chromosome count 47, XXY sex chromosome constitution; buccal and other cells are usually sex chromatin-positive; patients are male in development, but with seminiferous tubule dysgenesis, elevated urinary gonadotropins, variable gynecomastia, and eunuchoid habitus; some patients are chromosomal mosaics, with two or more cell lines of different chromosome constitution; male tortoiseshell cat (calico cat) is an animal model.
Klippel-Feil s., cervical fusion s.; a congenital defect manifest as a short neck, extensive fusion of the cervical vertebrae, and abnormalities of the brain stem and cerebellum.
Klippel-Trenaunay-Weber s., an anomaly of the extremity in which there is a combination of angiomatosis and anomalous development of the underlying bone and muscle, sometimes associated with localized gigantism. Also called angio-osteohypertrophy s.; congenital dysplastic angiectasia; elephantiasis congenita angiomatosa; hemangiectatic hypertrophy.
Klumpke-Dejerine s., Klumpke's *paralysis.*
Klüver-Bucy s., a s. characterized by psychic blindness or hyperreactivity to visual stimuli, increased oral and sexual activity, and depressed drive and emotional reactions; reported in monkeys after

bilateral temporal lobe ablation, but rarely reported in man.
Kniest s., a type of metatropic dwarfism characterized by short limbs, round face with central depression, enlargement and stiffness of joints, contracture of fingers, and often cleft palate, scoliosis, retinal detachment and myopia, and deafness; autosomal dominant inheritance.
Koenig's s., alternating attacks of constipation and diarrhea, with colic, meteorism, and gurgling in the right iliac fossa, said to be symptomatic of cecal tuberculosis.
Koerber-Salus-Elschnig s., retraction *nystagmus.*
Korsakoff's s., Korsakoff's psychosis; amnestic, dysmnesic, or polyneuritic psychosis; amnestic s. (1); dysmnesic s.; an alcohol amnestic s. characterized by confusion and severe impairment of memory, especially for recent events, for which the patient compensates by confabulation; typically encountered in chronic alcoholics; delirium tremens may precede the s., and Wernicke's s. often coexists; the precise pathogenesis is uncertain, but direct toxic effects of alcohol are probably less important than severe nutritional deficiencies often associated with chronic alcoholism.
Krabbe's s., an incomplete form of Sturge-Weber s. consisting of angiomas of face and meninges only.
Krause's s., encephalo-ophthalmic *dysplasia.*
Kuskokwim s., congenital joint contractures resembling arthrogryposis, found in Eskimos of the Kuskokwim river delta in Alaska.
Laband's s., fibromatosis of the gingivae associated with hypoplasia of the distal phalanges, nail dysplasia, joint hypermotility, and sometimes hepatosplenomegaly; autosomal dominant inheritance.
Labbé's neurocirculatory s., an anxiety neurosis that may occur in Basedow's disease but may be associated with tachycardia and exophthalmos without increase of basal metabolic rate or other evidence of hyperthyroidism.
LAMB s., the concurrence of lentigines, atrial myxoma, mucocutaneous myxomas, and blue nevi. See also NAME *syndrome.*
Lambert-Eaton s., Eaton-Lambert s.; carcinomatous myopathy; progressive proximal muscle weakness in patients with carcinoma, in the absence of dermatomyositis or polymyositis; caused by antibodies directed against motor-nerve axon terminals.
Landau-Kleffner s., acquired epileptic aphasia; childhood generalized and psychomotor seizures associated with acquired aphasia; multifocal spikes and spike and wave discharges in the electroencephalogram.
Landry s., acute idiopathic *polyneuritis.*
Landry-Guillain-Barré s., acute idiopathic *polyneuritis.*
Larsen's s., a s. characterized by multiple congenital dislocations with osseous anomalies, including characteristic flattened facies and cleft soft palate.
Lasègue's s., in conversion hysteria, inability to move an anesthetic limb, except under control of the sight.
lateral medullary s., posterior inferior cerebellar artery s.
Launois-Bensaude s., multiple symmetric *lipomatosis.*
Launois-Cléret s., Fröhlich's s.
Laurence-Biedl s., Laurence-Moon-Bardet-Biedl s.
Laurence-Moon s., a s. of mental retardation, pigmentary retinopathy, hypogenitalism, and spastic paraplegia; recessive inheritance.
Laurence-Moon-Bardet-Biedl s., Laurence-Biedl s.; a suggested combination of the Laurence-Moon s. and Bardet-Biedl s.
Lawford's s., an incomplete form of Sturge-Weber s. consisting of angiomas of the face and choroid only, with late glaucoma.
Lawrence-Seip s., lipoatrophy.
Lejeune s., cri-du-chat s.
Lenègre's s., Lenègre's disease; isolated damage of the cardiac conduction system as a result of sclerodegenerative lesion; characterized ordinarily as idiopathic atrioventricular nodal, His bundle, or bundle branch block.
Lennox-Gastaut s., Lennox s., a generalized myoclonic astatic epilepsy in children, with mental retardation, resulting from various cerebral afflictions such as perinatal hypoxia, cerebral hemorrhage, encephalitides, maldevelopment or metabolic disorders of the brain; characterized by generalized tonic seizures or akinetic attacks and mental deterioration with diffuse, slow spike and wave patterns in the EEG.
Leri-Weill s., dyschondrosteosis.
Leriche's s., aortoiliac occlusive *disease.*
Lermoyez' s., labyrinthine angiospasm; increasing deafness, interrupted by a sudden attack of dizziness, after which the hearing improves.
Lesch-Nyhan s., a disorder, associated with failure to form hypoxanthine phosphoribosyltransferase, characterized by hyperuricemia and uric acid urolithiasis, choreoathetosis, mental retardation, spastic cerebral palsy, and self-mutilation of fingers and lips by biting; X-linked recessive inheritance.
Lev's s., bundle branch block in a patient with normal myocardium and normal coronary arteries resulting from fibrosis or calcification of the conducting system; involves the membranous septum, the apex of the muscular septum, and the mitral and aortic rings.
Libman-Sacks s., Libman-Sacks *endocarditis.*
Li-Fraumeni cancer s., familial breast cancer in young women, with soft-tissue sarcomas in children and other cancers in close relatives.
Lignac-Fanconi s., cystinosis.
Lobstein's s., a variation of osteogenesis imperfecta, with blue sclera.
locked-in s., pseudocoma; quadriplegia and paralysis of lower cranial nerves without loss of consciousness, communication being made with the eyes; due to a mesencephalic lesion.
loculation s., Froin's s.
Löffler's s., **(1)** simple pulmonary *eosinophilia;* **(2)** Löffler's *endocarditis.*
Lorain-Lévi s., pituitary *dwarfism.*
Louis-Bar s., *ataxia* telangiectasia.
Lowe's s., Lowe-Terrey-MacLachlan s., oculocerebrorenal s.
Lown-Ganong-Levine s., electrocardiographic s. of a short P-R interval with normal duration of the QRS complex; it lacks the slurred delta wave of the Wolff-Parkinson-White s., but resembles it in its frequent association with paroxysmal tachycardia.
low salt s., low sodium s., salt depletion s.; a s. resulting from salt restriction in treatment of congestive heart failure and hypertension, characterized by weakness, drowsiness, muscle cramps, and a reduction in glomerular filtration with consequent nitrogen retention, renal failure, and death; occurs also in cirrhosis of the liver with ascites and in adrenal insufficiency.
Lutembacher's s., a congenital cardiac abnormality consisting of a defect of the interatrial septum, mitral stenosis, and enlarged right atrium.
Lyell's s., toxic epidermal *necrolysis.*
Macleod's s., abnormally increased radiolucency of one lung; characterized by normal or reduced size, underventilation and underperfusion of the lung with blood, panacinar emphysema, and some obstruction of the bronchioles; cause is unknown, but bronchiolitis in childhood is a possibility.
Mad Hatter s. [fr. char. in *Alice in Wonderland],* gastrointestinal and central nervous system manifestations of chronic mercury poisoning, including stomatitis, diarrhea, ataxia, tremor, hyperreflexia, sensorineural impairment, and emotional instability.
Maffucci's s., dyschondroplasia with hemangiomas; enchondromatosis with multiple cavernous hemangiomas.
Magendie-Hertwig s., Magendie-Hertwig *sign.*
malabsorption s., a state characterized by diverse features such as diarrhea, weakness, edema, lassitude, weight loss, poor appetite, protuberant abdomen, pallor, bleeding tendencies, paresthesias,

muscle cramps, etc., caused by any of several conditions in which there is ineffective absorption of nutrients, *e.g.*, sprue, gastroileostomy, tuberculosis, and certain fistulas.
male Turner's s., Noonan's s.
malignant carcinoid s., carcinoid s.
Mallory-Weiss s., laceration of the lower end of the esophagus associated with bleeding, or penetration into the mediastinum, with subsequent mediastinitis; caused usually by severe retching and vomiting.
mandibulofacial dysotosis s., mandibulofacial *dysostosis.*
mandibulo-oculofacial s., *dyscephalia* mandibulo-oculofacialis.
Marañón's s., a s. characterized by ovarian insufficiency, scoliosis, and flat-feet.
Marchesani s., Weill-Marchesani s.
Marchiafava-Micheli s., paroxysmal nocturnal *hemoglobinuria.*
Marcus Gunn s., jaw-winking s.
Marfan's s., Marfan's disease; a s. of congenital changes in the mesodermal and ectodermal tissues, skeletal changes (arachnodactyly, excessive length of extremities, laxness of joints), bilateral ectopia lentis, and vascular defects (particularly aneurysm of the aorta, dissecting or diffuse); iris transillumination is marked due to a deficiency of posterior epithelium pigment; autosomal dominant inheritance.
Marie-Robinson s., insomnia and mild melancholia associated with alimentary levulosuria.
Marinesco-Garland s., Marinesco-Sjögren s.
Marinesco-Sjögren s., a rare neurologic disorder characterized by cerebellolental degeneration with mental retardation; autosomal recessive inheritance. Also called Marinesco-Garland, Torsten Sjögren's, or cataract-oligophrenia s.
Maroteaux-Lamy s., type VI mucopolysaccharidosis; polydystrophic dwarfism; an error of mucopolysaccharide metabolism characterized by excretion of dermatan sulfate in the urine, growth retardation, lumbar kyphosis, sternal protrusion, genu valgum, usually hepatosplenomegaly, and no mental retardation; onset occurs after two years of age; autosomal recessive inheritance.
Marshall s., s. of mid-face hypoplasia, cataract, sensorineural hearing loss, and hypohidrosis.
Martorell's s., aortic arch s.
massive bowel resection s., malabsorption following extensive resection of the bowel, particularly the small intestine, characterized by diarrhea, steatorrhea, hypoproteinemia, and malnutrition.
Mauriac's s., dwarfism with obesity and hepatosplenomegaly in children with poorly controlled diabetes mellitus.
Mayer-Rokintansky-Küster-Hauser s., Rokintansky-Küster-Hauser s.; primary amenorrhea, absence of vagina, or presence of a short vaginal pouch, and absence of the uterus with normal karyotype and ovaries.
May-White s., progressive myoclonus epilepsy with lipomas, deafness, and ataxia; probably a familial form of mitochondrial encephalomyopathy.
McCune-Albright s., Albright's s. (1); Albright's disease; polyostotic fibrous dysplasia with irregular brown patches of cutaneous pigmentation and endocrine dysfunction, especially precocious puberty in girls.
Meadows' s., cardiomyopathy developing during pregnancy or the puerperium.
Meckel s., Meckel-Gruber s., dysencephalia splanchnocystica.
meconium blockage s., low intestinal obstruction in newborn infants resulting from blockage of meconium.
megacystic s., a combination of a large smooth thin-walled bladder, vesicoureteral regurgitation, and dilated ureters.
Meigs' s., fibromyoma of the ovary associated with hydroperitoneum and hydrothorax.
Melkersson-Rosenthal s., cheilitis granulomatosum, fissured tongue, and facial nerve paralysis.
Melnick-Needles s., osteodysplasty.
Mendelson's s., pulmonary disorders resulting from aspiration of gastric contents into the lungs following vomiting or regurgitation in obstetrical patients.
Ménétrièr's., Ménétrièr's *disease.*
Ménière's s., Ménière's *disease.*
Menkes' s., kinky-hair *disease.*
menopausal s., climacteric s.; recurring symptoms experienced by some women during the climacteric period; they include hot flashes, chills, headache, irritability, and depression.
metastatic carcinoid s., carcinoid s.
Meyenburg-Altherr-Uehlinger s., relapsing *polychondritis.*
Meyer-Betz s., myoglobinuria.
Meyer-Schwickerath and Weyers s., oculodentodigital *dysplasia.*
middle lobe s., Brock's s.; atelectasis with chronic pneumonitis of the middle lobe of the (right) lung, due to compression of the middle lobe bronchus, usually by enlarged lymph nodes, which may be tuberculous; chief symptoms are chronic cough, wheezing, recurrent respiratory infections, hemoptysis, chest pain, malaise, easy fatigability, and loss of weight; sometimes confused with interlobar accumulation of fluid in the lateral x-ray view.
Mikulicz' s., the symptoms characteristic of Mikulicz' disease occurring as a complication of some other disease, such as lymphosarcoma, leukemia, or uveoparotid fever.
milk-alkali s., Burnett's s.; a chronic disorder of the kidneys, reversible in its early stages, induced by ingestion of large amounts of calcium and alkali in the therapy of peptic ulcer; can progress to renal failure.
Milkman's s., osteoporosis with multiple fractures, occurring most frequently in middle-aged women.
Millard-Gubler s., Gubler's s.
Milles' s., an incomplete form of Sturge-Weber s. consisting of angiomas of face and choroid, without glaucoma.
minimal-change nephrotic s., nephrotic s. with minimal glomerular changes, occurring most frequently in children, marked by edema, albuminuria, and an increase in cholesterol in the blood, but otherwise with fairly good renal function; tubular epithelium is vacuolated by cholesterol droplets, but the glomeruli show only that the foot processes of the glomerular epithelial cells are fused, probably secondary to the proteinuria; the cause of the increased glomerular permeability to plasma protein is unknown.
Mirizzi's s., benign obstruction of the hepatic ducts due to spasm and/or fibrous scarring of surrounding connective tissue; often associated with a stone in the cystic duct and chronic cholecystitis.
Möbius' s., congenital facial diplegia; a developmental bilateral facial paralysis usually associated with oculomotor or other neurological disorders.
Monakow's s., contralateral hemiplegia, hemianesthesia, and homonomous hemianopsia due to occlusion of the anterior choroidal artery.
Morgagni's s., Stewart-Morel s.; metabolic craniopathy; hyperostosis frontalis interna in elderly women, with obesity and neuropsychiatric disorders of uncertain cause.
Morgagni-Adams-Stokes s., Adams-Stokes s.
morning glory s., a funnel-shaped hypoplastic optic nerve with a dot of white tissue at its center; surrounded by an elevated anulus of chorioretinal pigment.
Morquio's s., type IV mucopolysaccharidosis; Morquio's, Morquio-Ullrich, or Brailsford-Morquio disease; an error of mucopolysaccharide metabolism with excretion of keratan sulfate in urine; characterized by severe skeletal defects with short stature, severe deformity of spine and thorax, long bones with irregular epiphyses but with shafts of normal length, enlarged joints, flaccid ligaments, and waddling gait; autosomal recessive inheritance.
Morris s., testicular feminization s.
Morton's s., congenital shortening of the first metatarsal causing metatarsalgia.

Mounier-Kuhn s., tracheobronchomegaly.
Mucha-Habermann s., *pityriasis* lichenoides et varioliformis acuta.
Muckle-Wells s., a s. characterized by familial amyloidosis, notably involving the kidneys, progressive hearing loss of neural origin and unknown cause, and periods of febrile urticaria associated with pain in joints and muscles of the extremities; autosomal dominant inheritance.
mucocutaneous lymph node s., Kawasaki disease; a polymorphous erythematous febrile disease of unknown etiology occurring in children, especially under two years of age; accompanied by conjunctivitis, pharyngitis, strawberry tongue, cervical lymphadenopathy, perivasculitis and vasculitis, and other systemic toxic involvement, with characteristic desquamation of fingers and toes, and a furrowing depression of the nails.
Muir-Torre s., Torre's s.
multiple hamartoma s., Cowden's *disease.*
multiple lentigines s., LEOPARD s.
multiple mucosal neuroma s., multiple submucosal neuromas or neurofibromas of the tongue, lips, and eyelids in young persons; sometimes associated with tumors of the thyroid or adrenal medulla, or with subcutaneous neurofibromatosis.
Munchausen (Münchhausen) s., repeated fabrication of clinically convincing simulations of disease for the purpose of gaining medical attention.
myeloproliferative s.'s, a group of conditions that result from a disorder in the rate of formation of cells of the bone marrow, including chronic granulocytic leukemia, erythremia, myelosclerosis, panmyelosis, and erythremic myelosis and erythroleukemia.
myofacial pain-dysfunction s., temporomandibular joint pain-dysfunction s.; dysfunction of the masticatory apparatus related to spasm of the muscles of mastication precipitated by occlusal dysharmony or alteration in vertical dimension of the jaws, and exacerbated by emotional stress; characterized by pain in the preauricular region, muscle tenderness, popping noise in the temporomandibular joint, and limitation of jaw motion.
myofascial s., irritation of the muscles and fascia of the back and neck causing acute and chronic pain not associated with any neurological or bony evidence of disease; presumed to arise primarily from poorly understood changes in the muscle and fascia themselves.
Naegeli s., Franceschetti-Jadassohn s.; reticular skin pigmentation, diminished sweating, hypodontia, and hyperkeratosis of the palms and soles; autosomal dominant inheritance.
Naffziger s., scalenus-anticus s.
nail-patella s., onycho-osteodysplasia; arthro-onychodysplasia; a congenital skeletal disorder characterized by hypoplasia of the patella, iliac horns, dysplasia of the fingernails and toenails, and thickening of the glomerular lamina densa; the lower ends of the femur have a shape very similar to Erlenmeyer flask deformity; autosomal dominant inheritance.
NAME s., the concurrence of nevi, atrial myxoma, myxoid neurofibromas, and ephilides.
Nelson s., postadrenalectomy s.; a s. of hyperpigmentation, third nerve damage, and enlarging sella turcica caused by pituitary adenomas presumably present before adrenalectomy for Cushing's s. but enlarging and symptomatic afterward.
nephritic s., the clinical symptoms of acute glomerulonephritis, particularly hematuria, hypertension, and renal failure.
nephrotic s., nephrosis (3); a clinical state characterized by edema, albuminuria, decreased plasma albumin, doubly refractile bodies in the urine, and usually increased blood cholesterol; lipid droplets may be present in the cells of the renal tubules, but the basic lesion is increased permeability of the glomerular capillary basement membranes, of unknown cause or resulting from glomerulonephritis, diabetic glomerulosclerosis, systemic lupus erythematosus, amyloidosis, renal vein thrombosis, or hypersensitivity to various toxic agents.
Netherton's s., congenital ichthyosiform erythroderma or ichthyosis linearis circumscripta associated with bamboo hair, and irregularly with atopy, urticaria, intermittent aminoaciduria, and mental retardation; probably an autosomal recessive trait.
neural crest s., s. consisting of loss of pain sensibility, autonomic dysfunction, pupillary abnormalities, neurogenic anhidrosis, vasomotor instability, aplasia of dental enamel, meningeal thickening, hyperflexion, and a degree of albinism; may reflect developmental abnormalities of the neural crest.
neurocutaneous s., the occurrence of nevi and sometimes various skeletal deformities with symptoms pointing to gliosis or abiotrophy of the central nervous system.
neuroleptic malignant s., hyperthermia with extrapyramidal and autonomic disturbances which may result in death, following the use of neuroleptic agents.
Nezelof s., cellular *immunodeficiency* with abnormal immunoglobulin synthesis.
Nieden's s., multiple telangiectasis of the face, forearms, and hands, with cataract and aortic stenosis.
nonsense s., Ganser's s.
Noonan's s., male Turner's s.; the male phenotype of Turner's s., characterized by congenital heart disease, especially pulmonary stenosis, pigeon breast, webbing of the neck, antimongoloid slanting of the palpebrae, and other less regular minor features; autosomal dominant inheritance.
Nothnagel's s., dizziness, staggering, and rolling gait, with irregular forms of oculomotor paralysis and often nystagmus, seen in cases of tumor of the midbrain.
nystagmus blockage s., strabismus with eyes and head in a position to minimize associated nystagmus.
OAV s., oculoauriculovertebral *dysplasia.*
ocular-mucous membrane s., Stevens-Johnson s. with associated ocular lesions (conjunctivitis, panophthalmitis, iritis), oral lesions (bullae, erosions, superficial ulcers), and genital lesions (urethritis, balanitis circinata, blebs).
oculobuccogenital s., Behçet's s.
oculocerebrorenal s., Lowe's or Lowe-Terrey-MacLachlan s.; a congenital s. with hydrophthalmia, cataracts, mental retardation, aminoaciduria, reduced ammonia production by the kidney, and vitamin D-resistant rickets; X-linked recessive inheritance.
oculocutaneous s., Vogt-Koyanagi s.
oculodentodigital s., oculodentodigital *dysplasia.*
oculopharyngeal s., a myopathic disorder with a slowly progressive blepharoptosis and dysphagia, beginning late in life; autosomal dominant inheritance.
oculovertebral s., oculovertebral *dysplasia.*
oculovestibulo-auditory s., Cogan's s.; a nonsyphilitic interstitial keratitis characterized by an abrupt onset with vertigo and tinnitus followed by deafness; about 50% of patients have an associated systemic disease, most commonly polyarteritis nodosa.
ODD s., oculodentodigital *dysplasia.*
OFD s., orodigitofacial *dysostosis.*
Omenn's s., a rapidly fatal familial immunodeficiency disease characterized by erythroderma, diarrhea, repeated infections, hepatosplenomegaly, and leukocytosis with eosinophilia.
OMM s., ophthalmomandibulomelic *dysplasia.*
Oppenheim's s., *amyotonia* congenita.
orbital s., neoplastic tissue formation involving the apex of the orbit, causing ophthalmoplegia and optic nerve atrophy.
organic brain s. (OBS), organic mental s. (OMS), a constellation of behavioral or psychological signs and symptoms caused by transient or permanent dysfunction of the brain.
orofaciodigital (OFD) s., orodigitofacial *dysostosis.*
osteomyelofibrotic s., myelofibrosis.
Othello s. [*Othello,* Shakespearian char.], a delusional belief in the infidelity of one's spouse.

otomandibular s., otomandibular *dysostosis.*
otopalatodigital s., conduction deafness and cleft palate with characteristic facies consisting of broad nasal root and frontal bossing, wide spacing of toes, broad thumbs and great toes, and often other signs of generalized bone dysplasia; X-linked recessive inheritance.
pachydermoperiostosis s., see pachydermoperiostosis.
Paget-von Schrötter s., *thrombose* par effort.
painful-bruising s., an intense inflammatory reaction to slight extravasation of blood, due to an allergic sensitivity to red blood cells; more commonly seen in adult women.
paleostriatal s., Hunt's s. (3).
pallidal s., Hunt's s. (3).
Pancoast s., pain and tingling of the arm over the area of distribution of the ulnar nerve, constriction of the pupil, and paralysis of the levator palpebrae superioris muscle, due to pressure on the brachial plexus by a malignant tumor (as shown by x-ray imaging) in the region of the superior pulmonary sulcus.
papillary muscle s., papillary muscle *dysfunction.*
Papillon-Léage and Psaume s., orodigitofacial *dysostosis.*
Papillon-Lefèvre s., a congenital hyperkeratosis of the palms and soles, with progessive destruction of alveolar bone about the deciduous and permanent teeth beginning as early as 2 years of age, and also with premature exfoliation of teeth.
paraneoplastic s., a s. directly resulting from a malignant neoplasm, but not resulting from the presence of tumor cells in the affected parts.
Parinaud's s., Parinaud's opthalmoplegia; paralysis of conjugate upward gaze with a lesion at the level of the superior colliculi; Bell's phenomenon is present.
Parinaud's oculoglandular s., unilateral conjunctival granuloma with preauricular adenopathy in tularemia, chancre, and tuberculosis.
Patau's s., trisomy 13 s.
Paterson-Kelly s., Plummer-Vinson s.
Pellizzi's s., *macrogenitosomia* precox.
Pendred's s., a type of familial goiter; congenital nerve deafness with goiter (usually small) due to defective organic binding of iodine in the thyroid; afflicted individuals are usually euthyroid; autosomal recessive inheritance.
Pepper s., obsolete eponym for neuroblastoma of the adrenal gland with metastases in the liver; formerly believed to occur more frequently when the primary tumor was in the right adrenal, whereas tumors of the left adrenal tended to metastasize to the skull (Hutchison's syndrome).
pericolic membrane s., a symptom complex simulating chronic appendicitis, caused by congenital constricting pericolic membranes.
petrosphenoidal s., neoplastic infiltration of the apex of the petrous bone and the anterior part of the foramen lacerum.
Peutz-Jeghers s., Peutz's s., Jeghers-Peutz s.; periorificial lentiginosis. Generalized hamartomatous multiple polyposis of the intestinal tract, consistently involving the jejunum, associated with melanin spots of the lips, buccal mucosa, and fingers; autosomal dominant inheritance.
Pfaundler-Hurler s., Hurler's s.
Pfeiffer s., type V *acrocephalosyndactyly.*
pharyngeal pouch s., *immunodeficiency* with hypoparathyroidism.
PHC s., Böök s.
Picchini's s., a form of polyserositis involving the three great serosae in contact with the diaphragm, sometimes also the meninges, tunica vaginalis testis, synovial sheaths, and bursae, caused by the presence of a trypanosome.
Pick's s., Pick's *disease* (1).
Pickwickian s. [after the "fat boy" in Dickens' *Pickwick Papers],* a combination of severe, grotesque obesity, somnolence, and general debility, theoretically resulting from hypoventilation induced by the obesity; pulmonary hypertension and cor pulmonale can result.
Pierre Robin s., Robin's s.; micrognathia and abnormal smallness of the tongue, often with cleft palate, severe myopia, congenital glaucoma, and retinal detachment.
Pins' s., dullness, diminution of vocal fremitus and of the vesicular murmur, and a slight distant blowing sound, heard in the posteroinferior region of the chest on the left side, in cases of pericardial effusion; there is sometimes also a fine rale in this region, but all the adventitious auscultatory signs disappear when the patient assumes the genupectoral position.
placental dysfunction s., fetal malnutrition and hypoxia resulting from impaired transfer of oxygen and various nutritive materials from mother to fetus.
Plummer-Vinson s., sideropenic dysphagia; Patterson-Kelly s.; iron deficiency anemia, dysphagia, esophageal web, and atrophic glossitis.
POEMS s., a condition characterized by *p*olyneuropathy, *o*rganomegaly, *e*ndocrinopathy, *m*onoclonal gammopathy, and *s*kin changes.
polycystic ovary s., Stein-Leventhal s.; sclerocystic disease of the ovary; a condition commonly characterized by hirsutism, obesity, menstrual abnormalities, infertility, and enlarged ovaries; thought to reflect excessive androgen secretion of ovarian, and possibly adrenocortical, origin.
polyendrocrine deficiency s., polyglandular deficiency s., associated pathologic dysfunction of several endocrine glands, as in Schmidt's s.
polysplenia s., bilateral *left-sidedness.*
popliteal entrapment s., a crush s. resulting from compression of the popliteal artery and impairment of its blood flow by structures of the popliteal space.
postadrenalectomy s., Nelson s.
postcardiotomy s., postpericardiotomy s.
postcholecystectomy s., the persistence of signs and symptoms that led to removal of the gallbladder, as a sequel to cholecystectomy.
postcommissurotomy s., a s. of uncertain cause appearing within a few weeks after a cardiac valvar operation, characterized by fever, chest pain, pericardial rub or effusion, and pleural rub or effusion.
postconcussion s., see posttraumatic s.
posterior inferior cerebellar artery s., Wallenberg's s.; lateral medullary s.; a s. due usually to thrombosis, characterized by dysarthria, dysphagia, staggering gait, and vertigo, and marked by hypotonia, incoordination of voluntary movement, nystagmus, Horner's s. on the ipsilateral side, and loss of pain and temperature senses on the side of the body opposite to the lesion.
postgastrectomy s., dumping s.
postmaturity s., gestation extending 43 weeks or longer; sometimes associated with fetal dysmaturity.
postmyocardial infarction s., Dressler's s.; a complication developing several days to several weeks after myocardial infarction; its clinical features are fever, leukocytosis, chest pain, evidence of pericarditis, pleurisy and pneumonitis, and a tendency to recurrence.
postpartum pituitary necrosis s., Sheehan's s.
postpericardiotomy s., postcardiotomy s.; the occurrence of the symptoms of pericarditis, with or without fever and often in repeated episodes, weeks to months after cardiac surgery.
postphlebitic s., a state characterized by edema, pain, stasis dermatitis, cellulitis, and varicose veins, and ending in ulceration of the lower leg, developing as a sequel to deep venous thrombosis of the lower extremity.
postrubella s., a group of congenital defects resulting from maternal rubella during the first trimester of pregnancy and including microphthalmos, cataracts, deafness, mental retardation, patent ductus arteriosus, and pulmonary arterial stenosis.

posttraumatic s., traumatic neurasthenia; a clinical complex, caused by injury to the head, characterized by headache, dizziness, neurasthenia, hypersensitivity to stimuli, and diminished concentration.
posttraumatic neck s., a clinical complex of pain, tenderness, tight neck musculature, vasomotor instability, and ill-defined symptoms such as dizziness and blurred vision as the result of trauma to the neck. Also variously termed occipital or suboccipital neuralgia or neuritis; cervical tension s.; cervical myospasm, myositis, or fibrositis.
posttraumatic stress s., a disorder appearing after a psychologically traumatic event, characterized by symptoms of re-experiencing the event, numbing of responsiveness to the environment, exaggerated startle response, guilt feelings, impairment of memory, and difficulties in concentration and sleep.
Potter's s., renal agenesis with hypoplastic lungs and associated neonatal respiratory distress, hemodynamic instability, acidosis, cyanosis, edema, and characteristic (Potter's) facies; death usually occurs from respiratory insufficiency which develops before uremia.
Prader-Willi s., a congenital s. of unknown etiology characterized by short stature, mental retardation, polyphagia with marked obesity, and sexual infantilism; initially severe muscular hypotonia and poor responsiveness to external stimuli decrease with age.
precordial catch s., a benign s. of uncertain origin, characterized by intense pain in the region of the cardiac apex on inspiration, yet usually relieved by forcing a deeper breath; tenderness is absent.
preexcitation s., Wolff-Parkinson-White s.,
preinfarction s., abrupt development of angina pectoris or worsening of existing angina by increases in its frequency or severity; often heralds myocardial infarction.
premature senility s., progeria.
premenstrual s., (PMS), premenstrual tension; premenstrual tension syndrome; menstrual molimina; in women of reproductive age, the regular monthly experience of physiological and emotional distress, usually during the several days preceding menses; characterized by nervousness, depression, fluid retention, and weight gain.
premenstrual salivary s., glandular abnormalities occurring prior to the onset of menses, including swelling of the breast tissues and enlargement of the salivary glands.
premenstrual tension s., premenstrual s.
premotor s., hemiplegia with spasticity, Rossolimo's reflex, but not the Babinski sign, together with forced grasping and vasomotor disturbances.
prune belly s., abdominal muscle deficiency s.
pseudothalidomide s., Roberts s.
pseudo-Turner's s., Bonnevie-Ullrich s.; a s. characterized by short stature and a webbed neck; unlike Turner's s., patients with this disorder may be of either sex, have normal chromosomes, have no renal abnormalities, often be mentally retarded, and have various forms of congenital heart disease.
psychogenic nocturnal polydipsia (PNP) s., emotionally induced excessive water drinking at night.
pterygium s., webbing of the neck, antecubital fossae, and popliteal fossae with flection deformities of the extremities and anomalies of the vertebrae; observed in pseudo-Turner's s. and Turner's s.
pulmonary dysmaturity s., Wilson-Mikity s.; a respiratory disorder occurring in small, premature infants who are incapable of normal pulmonary ventilation and who often die of hypoxia after an illness of 6 to 8 weeks; the lungs contain widespread focal emphysematous blebs and the parenchyma has thickened alveolar walls; diagnosed principally on the basis of the clinical history, chest radiographic findings, and the findings at autopsy, which must include the absence of pathological changes characteristic of other pulmonary disorders commonly encountered in this age group.
punchdrunk s., a condition seen in boxers and alcoholics, presumably caused by repeated cerebral concussions, characterized by weakness in the lower limbs, unsteadiness of gait, slowness of muscular movements, tremors of hands, hesitancy of speech, and slow cerebration.
Putnam-Dana s., subacute combined *degeneration* of the spinal cord.
radial aplasia-thrombocytopenia s., thrombocytopenia-absent radius s.
radicular s., a group of symptoms resulting from any interference with the intradural portion of one or more spinal nerve roots; the chief symptoms are pain, paresthesia, hypesthesia, or hyperesthesia, motor, trophic, and reflex disturbances.
Raeder's paratrigeminal s., an incomplete Horner's s. with cranial nerve disturbance caused by involvement of the carotid sympathetic plexus.
Ramsay Hunt's s., Hunt's s.
Raynaud's s., Raynaud's disease; symmetric asphyxia; idiopathic paroxysmal bilateral cyanosis of the digits due to arterial and arteriolar contraction; caused by cold or emotion. See also Raynaud's *phenomenon.*
Refetoff s., a condition characterized by goiter and elevated serum level of thyroid hormones without manifestations of thyrotoxicosis, due to target organ unresponsiveness to thyroid hormones.
Refsum's s., Refsum's *disease.*
Reifenstein's s., a familial form of male pseudohermaphroditism characterized by varying degrees of ambiguous genitalia or hypospadias, postpubertal development of gynecomastia, and infertility associated with semeniferous tubular sclerosis; cryptorchidism may be present, and Leydig cell hypofunction may lead to impotence in later years; chromosomal studies are usually normal; X-linked recessive or autosomal dominant male-linked trait.
Reiter's s., Reiter's disease; Fiessinger-Leroy-Reiter s.; the association of urethritis, iridocyclitis, and arthritis, sometimes with diarrhea; one or more of these conditions may recur at intervals of months or years, but the arthritis may be persistent.
REM s., reticular erythematous mucinosis; a reticular erythematous dermatitis of the upper trunk, more common in women, in which there is perivascular infiltrate of lymphocytes, few plasma cells, and deposits of mucopolysaccharide; worsens on exposure to ultraviolet light.
Rendu-Osler-Weber s., hereditary hemorrhagic *telangiectasia.*
Renpenning's s., familial X-linked mental retardation due to the presence of the fragile X chromosome and occurring more frequently in males, although some females may also be affected.
residual ovary s., the development of a pelvic mass, pelvic pain, and occasionally dyspareunia following hysterectomy without removal of both ovaries.
resistant ovary s., Savage s.
respiratory distress s. of the newborn, hyaline membrane *disease* of the newborn.
restless legs s., Ekbom s.; restless legs; a sense of indescribable uneasiness, twitching, or restlessness that occurs in the legs after going to bed, frequently leading to insomnia, which may be relieved temporarily by walking about; thought to be caused by inadequate circulation or as a side effect of antipsychotic medication. See also akathisia.
retraction s., Duane's s.; inability to abduct the affected eye with retraction of the globe and pseudoptosis on attempted adduction; due to abnormal narrowing of the palpebral fissure and innervation of the horizontal recti causing simultaneous contraction of both muscles on adduction and relaxation on abduction; more rarely, the vertical muscles are similarly affected, producing a vertical retraction.
Rett's s., cerebroatrophic hyperammonemia; a progressive s. of autism, dementia, ataxia, and purposeless hand movements; associated with hyperammonemia, principally in girls.

Reye's s., a disorder of young children following an acute febrile illness, usually influenza or varicella infection, characterized by recurrent vomiting beginning within a week after onset of the infection and from which the child either recovers within a day or two or lapses into a coma with intracranial hypertension; serum transaminases are elevated; death may result from edema of the brain and resulting cerebral herniation.
Rh null s., a lack of all Rh antigens, compensated hemolytic anemia, and stomatocytosis.
Richards-Rundel s., a nervous system disorder beginning in early childhood and characterized by congenital severe, progressive sensorineural hearing loss, ataxia, muscle wasting nystagmus, absent deep tendon reflexes, mental retardation, and failure to develop secondary sexual characteristics; autosomal recessive inheritance.
Richter's s., a high-grade lymphoma developing during the course of chronic lymphocytic leukemia; associated with cachexia, pyrexia, dysproteinemia, and lymphomas with multinucleated tumor cells.
Rieger's s., iridocorneal mesodermal dysgenesis combined with hypodontia or anodontia and maxillary hypoplasia.
right ovarian vein s., a condition characterized by intermittent abdominal pain due to ureteral compression by the right ovarian vein, occurring with overwhelming frequency on the right side, and thought to be due to aberrant crossing of the right ovarian vein over the ureter, generally at the level of the first sacral vertebra; dilation of the ovarian vein during pregnancy and unilateral ptosis of the kidney are thought to be contributing factors leading to intermittent ureteral obstruction and recurring bouts of pain and pyelonephritis.
Riley-Day s., familial *dysautonomia.*
Roaf's s., a nonhereditary craniofacial-skeletal disorder characterized by congenital or early retinal detachment, cataracts, myopia, shortened long bones, and mental retardation; sensorineural progressive hearing loss is of later onset.
Roberts s., pseudothalidomide s.; phocomelia or lesser degrees of hypomelia, microbrachycephaly, midfacial defect, prenatal growth deficiency, and cryptorchidism; autosomal recessive inheritance.
Robin's s., Pierre Robin s.
Rokintansky-Küster-Hauser s., Mayer-Rokintansky-Küster-Hauser s.
Romano-Ward s., a prolonged Q-T interval in the electrocardiogram, found in children subject to attacks of unconsciousness that result from Adams-Stokes syndrome and ventricular fibrillation; differs from the surdocardiac s. only in the absence of congenital deafness; autosomal dominant inheritance.
Romberg's s., facial *hemiatrophy.*
Rothmund's s., Rothmund-Thomson s., poikiloderma congenitale; poikiloderma atrophicans and cataract; atrophy, pigmentation, and telangiectasia of the skin, usually with juvenile cataract, saddle nose, congenital bone defects, disturbance of hair growth, hypogonadism; autosomal recessive inheritance.
Rotor's s., jaundice appearing in childhood due to impaired biliary excretion inherited as an autosomal recessive trait; most of the plasma bilirubin is conjugated, liver fraction tests are usually normal, and there is no hepatic pigmentation.
Roussy-Lévy s., Roussy-Lévy *disease.*
Rubinstein-Taybi s., a constellation of congenital defects including mental retardation, broad thumb and great toe, antimongoloid slant to the eyes, thin and beaked nose, prominent forehead, low set ears, high arched palate, and cardiac anomaly.
Rud's s., ichthyosiform erythroderma associated with acanthosis nigricans, dwarfism, hypogonadism, and epilepsy; probably a recessive trait.
Russell's s., failure of infants and young children to thrive due to suprasellar lesions, commonly astrocytomas of the anterior third ventricle; although the growth hormone may be elevated, the child is emaciated and has loss of body fat.
salt depletion s., low salt s.
Sanchez Salorio s., a s. characterized by retinal pigmentary dystrophy, cataract, hypotrichosis of the lashes, mental deficiencies, and retarded somatic development.
Sanfilippo's s., type III mucopolysaccharidosis; an error of mucopolysaccharide metabolism, with excretion of large amounts of heparan sulfate in the urine and severe mental retardation with hepatomegaly; skeleton may be normal or may present mild changes similar to those in Hurler's s.; several different types (A, B, C, and D) have been identified according to the enzyme deficiency; autosomal recessive inheritance.
Savage s. [after the surname of the first reported patient], resistant ovary s.; amenorrhea associated with hypergonadotrophism and normal ovarian follicles.
scalded skin s., see staphylococcal scalded skin s.
scale'nus anter'ior s., Naffziger s.; a disorder having symptoms identical with those of cervical rib, due, however, to compression of the brachial plexus and subclavian artery against the first thoracic rib by a hypertonic scalenus anticus muscle; pressure upon sympathetic nerves may cause vascular spasm resembling Raynaud's disease.
scapulocostal s., pain of insidious development in the upper or posterior part of the shoulder radiating into the neck and occiput, down the arm, or around the chest; there may be numbness or tingling in the fingers; attributed to an alteration from the normal relationship between the scapula and posterior wall of the thorax.
Schanz s., spinal muscle weakness, marked by quick fatigue, pain on pressure over the spinous processes, pain produced by the prone position, and a tendency to curvature of the spine.
Schaumann's s., sarcoidosis.
Scheie's s., type IS mucopolysaccharidosis; a variant of Hurler's s. characterized by α-L-iduronidase deficiency, corneal clouding, deformity of the hands, aortic valve involvement, and normal intelligence.
Schirmer's s., an incomplete form of Sturge-Weber s. consisting of angiomas of the face and choroid only, with early glaucoma (buphthalmia).
Schmid-Fraccaro s., cat's-eye s.
Schmidt's s. [J. F. M. Schmidt], unilateral paralysis of a vocal cord, the velum palati, trapezius, and sternocleidomastoid.
Schmidt's s. [M. B. Schmidt], the association of primary hypothyroidism, primary adrenocortical insufficiency, and insulin-dependent diabetes mellitus.
Schönlein-Henoch s., Henoch-Schönlein *purpura.*
Schüller's s., Hand-Schüller-Christian *disease.*
Schwachman s., an inherited disorder, probably autosomal recessive, characterized by sinusitis and bronchiectasis with pancreatic insufficiency, resulting in malnutrition; associated with neutropenia and defect in neutrophile chemotaxis, short stature, and bone abnormalities.
Schwartz s., a congenital disorder characterized by myotonic myopathy, dystrophy of epiphyseal cartilages resulting in dwarfism, joint contractures, blepharophimosis, and characteristic facies; autosomal recessive inheritance.
Sebright bantam s., pseudohypoparathyroidism.
Seckel s., Seckel dwarfism; an autosomal recessive disorder characterized by low birth weight, dwarfism, microcephaly, large eyes, beaked nose, receding mandible, and moderate mental retardation.
Secrétan's s., factitious, traumatic, recurrent edema or hemorrhage of the dorsum of the hand.
Senear-Usher s., *pemphigus* erythematosus.
Sertoli-cell-only s., Del Castillo s.; the absence from the seminiferous tubules of the testes of germinal epithelium, Sertoli cells alone being present; there is sterility due to azoospermia but no other sexual abnormality, Leydig cells are normal, and the output of gonadotrophins in the urine is increased; probably represents one form of seminiferous tubule dysgenesis.

Sézary s., Sézary erythroderma; exfoliative dermatitis with intense pruritus, resulting from cutaneous infiltration by atypical mononuclear cells (T lymphocytes with markedly convoluted or cerebriform nuclei) also found in the peripheral blood, and associated with alopecia, edema, and nail and pigmentary changes; a variant of mycosis fungoides.

Sheehan's s., postpartum pituitary necrosis s.; thyrohypophysial s.; hypopituitarism arising from a severe circulatory collapse postpartum, with resultant pituitary necrosis.

shoulder-girdle s., brachial plexus *neuropathy.*

shoulder-hand s., brachial plexus *neuropathy.*

Shulman's s., eosinophilic *fasciitis.*

Shy-Drager s., a progressive encephalomyelopathy involving the autonomic system, characterized by hypotension, external ophthalmoplegia, iris atrophy, incontinence, anhidrosis, impotence, tremor, and muscle wasting.

sicca s., Sjögren's s.

sick sinus s., chaotic atrial activity characterized by continual changes in P wave configuration, with bradycardia alternating with recurring ectopic beats and runs of supraventricular tachycardia.

Silver-Russell s., Silver-Russell dwarfism; a disorder characterized by low birth weight, late closure of the anterior fontanel, bilateral bodily asymmetry, clinodactyly of the fifth fingers, triangular facies, and carp mouth.

Silverskiöld's s., a type of osteochondrodystrophy with only slight vertebral changes but with shortened and curved long bones of the extremities.

Sipple's s., familial endocrine *adenomatosis,* type 2.

Sjögren's s. [H. S. C. Sjögren], Sjögren's or Gougerot-Sjögren disease; sicca s.; keratoconjunctivitis sicca, dryness of mucous membranes, telangiectasias or purpuric spots on the face, and bilateral parotid enlargement, seen in menopausal woman, and often associated with rheumatoid arthritis, Raynaud's phenomenon, and dental caries; there are changes in the lacrimal and salivary glands resembling those of Mikulicz' disease.

Sjögren-Larsson s., congenital ichthyosis in association with oligophrenia and spastic paraplegia autosomal recessive inheritance.

slit ventricle s., in shunt dependent patients, a state characterized by intermittent or chronic headaches, small ventricles, and slow reflux of the valve mechanism.

Smith-Lemli-Opitz s., mental retardation, small stature, anteverted nostrils, ptosis, male genital anomalies, and syndactyly of the second and third toes, often in breech-born babies with delayed fetal activity.

Smith-Riley s., multiple hemangiomas, macrocephaly, and blurred optic discs; angiomas appear at birth or later, and enlarge and multiply.

smoker's respiratory s., a triad of symptoms seen in smokers, consisting of chronic pharyngitis, wheezing and dyspnea, and a susceptibility to respiratory infections; small lymphoid nodules may appear in the pharynx; there is also often cough, pain in the chest, and hoarseness of the voice; edema of the vocal cords and later an edematous fibroma may be found.

Sneddon's s., a genetic cerebral arteriopathy of unknown etiology, characterized by non-inflammatory intimal hyperplasia of medium-sized vessels associated with diffuse cutaneous livedo reticularis.

Sohval-Soffer s., hypogonadism, gynecomastia, skeletal anomalies, and mental retardation without chromosomal abnormality.

Sorsby's s., congenital macular coloboma and apial dystrophy of the extremities.

Sotos s., cerebral gigantism and generalized large muscles in childhood, with mental retardation and defective coordination; of unknown etiology.

spastic s. in cattle, a disease of the nervous system manifested by spastic contractions of the muscles of one or both hind legs, most common in old bulls; the cramps usually become more frequent and severe, eventually resulting in decreasing the usefulness of the animal.

Spens' s., Adams-Stokes s.

spherophakia-brachymorphia s., Weill-Marchesani s.

splenic flexure s., symptoms of pain, gas, bloating, a sense of fullness experienced in the left upper abdominal quadrant, sometimes beneath the ribs, in some instances radiating upward, and in some instances producing anterior chest pain central or predominantly on the left. It may be induced experimentally by the introduction and trapping of air in the splenic flexure.

Sprinz-Nelson s., Dubin-Johnson *syndrome.*

staphylococcal scalded skin s., Lyell's disease; Ritter's disease (1); a disease affecting infants in which large areas of skin peel off, as in a second-degree burn, as a result of upper respiratory staphylococcal infection even though the skin lesions may be sterile; the level of skin separation is subcorneal, unlike the clinically similar toxic epidermal necrolysis which occurs in children and adults and which involves subepidermal cleavage.

Steele-Richardson-Olszewski s., Steele-Richardson-Olszewski disease; a progressive neurologic disorder in the sixth decade characterized by paralysis of downward gaze rendering ambulation impossible, retraction of eyelids, exophoria under cover, dysarthria, and dementia.

Stein-Leventhal s., polycystic ovary s.

steroid withdrawal s., a condition exhibited by persons who previously had been receiving large therapeutic doses of glucocorticoid hormones for long periods of time; pituitary-adrenocortical insufficiency is manifested, particularly during stress, for as long as a year or more thereafter and varying degrees of emotional disturbance may be exhibited.

Stevens-Johnson s., erythema multiforme bullosum or exudativum; ectodermosis erosiva pluriorificialis; a bullous form of erythema multiforme which may be extensive, involving the mucous membranes and large areas of the body; it may produce serious subjective symptoms and may have a fatal termination. See also ocular-mucous membrane s.

Stewart-Morel s., Morgagni's s.

Stewart-Treves s., angiosarcoma arising in arms affected by postmastectomy lymphedema.

Stickler s., hereditary progressive *arthro-ophthalmopathy.*

stiff-man s., a chronic, progressive, but variable, central nervous system disorder of unknown cause, associated with fluctuating painful muscle spasm and rigidity involving muscles of the limbs, trunk, and neck.

Still-Chauffard s., Chauffard s.

Stockholm s. [*Stockholm,* Sweden, where early case reported], a form of bonding between a captive and captor in which the captive begins to identify with, and may even sympathize with, the captor.

Stokes-Adams s., Adams-Stokes s.

straight back s., loss of the normal anterior concavity of the thoracic spine with resulting compression of the heart between spine and sternum and consequent prominent precordial pulsations, an ejection murmur, and radiologic evidence of a widened cardiac silhouette.

Stryker-Halbeisen s., reddish, scaling, macular eruption on the head and upper trunk due to vitamin B complex deficiency; associated with macrocytic anemia.

Sturge-Kalischer-Weber s., Sturge-Weber s.

Sturge-Weber s., in full, a triad: 1) congenital cutaneous angioma (flame nevus) in the distribution of the trigeminal nerve, usually unilateral; 2) homolateral meningeal angioma with intracranial calcification and neurologic signs; 3) angioma of choroid, often with secondary glaucoma. Incomplete forms of the s. may exhibit any two of the major features in variable degree, occasionally with angiomas elsewhere. Also called cephalotrigeminal or encephalotrigeminal angiomatosis; Sturge-Kalischer-Weber s.; Sturge's or

Sturge-Weber disease.
subclavian steal s., symptoms of cerebrovascular insufficiency resulting from subclavian steal.
sudden infant death s. (SIDS), crib death; abrupt and inexplicable death of an apparently healthy infant; various theories have been advanced to explain such deaths (*e.g.,* sleep-induced apnea, laryngospasm, overwhelming infectious disease) but none has been generally accepted or demonstrated at autopsy.
Sudeck's s., Sudeck's *atrophy.*
Sulzberger-Garbe s., Sulzberger-Garbe *disease.*
sump s., a complication of side-to-side choledochoduodenostomy in which the lower end of the common bile duct at times acts as a diverticulum, resulting in stasis, trapping of food particles, and infection.
superior cerebellar artery s., s. due to thrombosis of the superior cerebellar artery which supplies the spinothalamic tract and the superior cerebellar peduncle; there is incoordination in performing skilled movements, with loss of pain and temperature senses on the side of the face and body opposite to that of the lesion.
superior mesenteric artery s., Wilkie's disease; partial or complete block of the superior mesenteric artery, with pain, vomiting, blood in the stool and/or vomitus, and abdominal distention with characteristic radiologic appearance (thumbprinting); often culminates in bowel infarction.
superior vena caval s., obstruction of the superior vena cava or its main tributaries by bronchogenic carcinoma, mediastinal neoplasm or lymphoma, or, rarely, substernal goiter, causing edema and engorgement of the vessels of the face, neck, and arms, nonproductive cough, and dyspnea; bluish looking venous stars may be found in the early phases, overlying the large veins to which they are tributary, but they tend to diminish in size and disappear after collateral circulation has been reestablished.
supine hypotensive s., in the supine pregnant woman at or near term, maternal hypotension and fetal hypoxia; maternal hypotension is due to obstruction by the gravid uterus of the inferior vena cava with resulting decrease in venous return to the heart; fetal hypoxia is due to maternal hypotension and obstruction of the maternal aorta by the gravid uterus with resulting decrease in placental perfusion.
supraspinatus s., pain on abduction of the shoulder and tenderness upon deep pressure over the supraspinatus tendon; due to pressure of an injured tendon or inflamed subacromial bursa coming into contact or pressing upon the overlying acromial process when the arm is abducted within an arc of 60° to 120°.
supravalvar aortic stenosis s., supravalvar aortic stenosis sometimes associated with pulmonary valvular or peripheral arterial stenosis but with normal facies and mentality; autosomal dominant inheritance.
supravalvar aortic stenosis-infantile hypercalcemia s., supravalvar aortic stenosis associated with elfin facies, mental retardation, and hypercalcemia; usually nonfamilial.
surdocardiac s., Jervell and Lange-Nielsen s.; a prolonged Q-T interval recorded in the electrocardiogram of certain congenitally deaf children subject to attacks of unconsciousness resulting from Adams-Stokes seizures and ventricular fibrillation; autosomal recessive inheritance.
Swyer-James s., decrease in size of one lung due to obliterating bronchiolitis, a congenital abnormality, or some other disorder, resulting in compensatory overinflation of the normal lung; appears on a radiograph as a unilateral hyperlucency of the lung.
tachycardia-bradycardia s., alternating periods of slow and rapid heart beat; often associated with disturbances of both sinoatrial and atrioventricular conduction. See also sick sinus s.
Takayasu's s., pulseless *disease.*
Tapia's s., unilateral paralysis of the larynx, the velum palati, and the tongue, with atrophy of the latter.
tarsal tunnel s., s. produced by entrapment neuropathy of posterior tibial nerve at the ankle.
Taussig-Bing s., Taussig-Bing disease; complete transposition of the aorta, which arises from the right ventricle, with a left sided pulmonary artery overriding the left ventricle, and with high ventricular septal defect, right ventricular hypertrophy, anteriorly situated aorta, and posteriorly situated pulmonary artery.
tegmental s., a s. usually caused by a vascular lesion in the tegmentum; marked by contralateral hemiplegia and ipsilateral ocular paresis.
temporomandibular s., Costen's s.; those various symptoms of discomfort, pain, or pathosis stated to be caused by loss of vertical dimension, lack of posterior occlusion, or other malocclusion, trismus, muscle tremor, arthritis, or direct trauma to the temporomandibular joint.
temporomandibular joint pain-dysfunction s., myofacial pain-dysfunction s.
tendon sheath s., Brown's s.; limited elevation of the eye in adduction, appearing clinically as a paresis of the inferior oblique muscle, due to fascia contracting the superior oblique muscle on the same side.
Terry's s., *retinopathy* of prematurity.
testicular feminization s., Goldberg-Maxwell s.; Morris s.; a type of male pseudohermaphroditism characterized by female external genitalia (may be ambiguous if the s. is incomplete), incompletely developed vagina often with rudimentary uterus and fallopian tubes, female habitus at puberty but with scanty or absent axillary and pubic hair and amenorrhea, and testes present within the abdomen or in the inguinal canals or labia majora; epididymis and vas deferens are usually present; androgens and estrogens are formed, but target tissues are largely unresponsive to androgens; individuals are sex chromatin-negative and have a normal male karyotype; x-linked recessive inheritance.
tethered cord s., sacral retention of the spinal cord by the filum terminale producing incontinence, progressive motor and sensory impairment in the legs and associated with pain, or scoliosis, or both.
thalamic s., Dejerine-Roussy s.; a s. produced by infarction of the postero-inferior thalamus causing transient hemiparesis, severe loss of superficial and deep sensation with preservation of crude pain in the hypalgic limbs which frequently have vasomotor or trophic disturbances.
third and fourth pharyngeal pouch s., DiGeorge s.
thoracic outlet s., compression of brachial plexus and subclavian artery by attached muscles in the region of the first rib and clavicle.
Thorn's s., salt-losing *nephritis.*
thrombocytopenia-absent radius (TAR) s., radial aplasia-throbocytopenia s.; congenital absence of the radius associated with thrombocytopenia that is symptomatic in infancy but later improves; congenital heart disease and renal anomalies occur in some cases; autosomal recessive inheritance.
thrombopathic s., a nondescript term to describe any of a number of bleeding diseases in which clot formation is deficient rather than those in which there is an organic fault of the blood vessels.
thyrohypophysial s., Sheehan's s.
Tietze's s., peristernal perichondritis; inflammation and painful, tender nonsuppurative swelling of a costochondral junction.
Tolosa-Hunt s., Cavernous sinus s. produced by an idiopathic granuloma.
tooth-and-nail s., hypodontia associated with absent or very small nails at birth.
TORCH s., a group of congenital infections whose clinical manifestations are similar, although symptoms may vary in degree and time of appearance: *t*oxoplasmosis, *o*ther infections, *r*ubella, *c*ytomegalovirus infection, and *h*erpes simplex.
Tornwaldt's s., nasopharyngeal discharge, occipital headache, and stiffness of posterior cervical muscles, with halitosis due to chronic infection of the pharyngeal bursa.

Torre's s., Muir-Torre s.; multiple sebaceous gland neoplasms associated with multiple visceral malignancies.
Torsten Sjögren's s., Marinesco-Sjögren s.
Tourette's s., Gilles de la Tourette's s.
toxic shock s., infection with staphylococci producing an endotoxin, occurring most often in the vagina of menstruating women using superabsorbent tampons, and characterized by high fever, vomiting, diarrhea, a scarlatiniform rash followed by desquamation, and decreasing blood pressure and shock which can result in death; hyperemia of the conjunctival, oropharyngeal, and vaginal mucous membranes also occurs.
transplant lung s., a s. associated with fever and diffuse bilateral pulmonary infiltration mainly at the base or at the hilum of the lung; can accompany rejection of an organ (kidney) transplant or follow a reduction in dosage of an immunosuppressive drug.
Treacher Collins' s., mandibulofacial *dysostosis,* when limited to the orbit and malar region.
triad s., abdominal muscle deficiency s.
trichorhinophalangeal s., a condition characterized by sparse fine hair, broad nose with a long philtrum, swollen middle phalanges with cone-shaped epiphyses, and growth retardation.
triple X s., in principle, the phenotypic features characteristic of trisomy of the X chromosome. Original observations (made in mental institutions) were seriously biased and the phenotypic changes spurious; now, even the remaining claim, that there is mild mental retardation, is suspect. The outstanding feature of the s. is the occurance of twin Barr bodies in a typical cell.
trisomy C s., trisomy for any chromosome of group C, numbers 6 through 12, most often number 8.
trisomy D s., trisomy 13 s.
trisomy E s., trisomy 18 s.
trisomy 8 s., the most common of the trisomy C s.'s, involving chromosome number 8 and resulting in multiple malformations including craniofacial dysmorphia, short wide neck but narrow cylindrical trunk, and multiple joint and digital defects.
trisomy 13 s., Patau's s.; trisomy D s.; a variable s. of malformation in infants with 47 chromosomes, the extra chromosome being of group D, no. 13, which is usually fatal within two years; more than 30 signs have been described, including apparent mental retardation and malformed ears in all patients, and in most patients cleft lip or palate, microphthalmia or coloboma, small mandible, polydactyly, cardiac defects, convulsions, renal anomalies, umbilical hernia, malrotation of intestines, and dermatoglyphic anomalies.
trisomy 18 s., Edwards' s.; trisomy E s.; a variable s. of malformations in infants with 47 chromosomes, the extra chromosome being of group E, no. 18, which is usually fatal within two to three years; more than 30 signs have been described, including mental retardation, abnormal skull shape, lowset and malformed ears, small mandible, cardiac defects, short sternum, diaphragmatic or inguinal hernia, Meckel's diverticulum, abnormal flexion of fingers, and dermatoglyphic anomalies.
trisomy 20 s., profound mental retardation with coarse facies, macrostomia and macroglossia, minor anomalies of the ears, pigmentary dysplasia of the skin, dorsal kyphoscoliosis, and other skeletal defects.
trisomy 21 s., Down's s.
trochanteric s., tendonitis and bursitis around the trochanter major.
tropical splenomegaly s., hyperreactive malarious *splenomegaly.*
Trousseau's s., **(1)** gastric *vertigo;* **(2)** thrombophlebitis migrans associated with visceral cancer.
tumor lysis s., hyperphosphatemia, hypocalcemia, hyperkalemia, and hyperuricemia following induction chemotherapy of malignant neoplasms; believed to be due to the release of intracellular products by cell lysis.
Turcot s., a rare and perhaps distinct form of multiple intestinal polyposis in which brain tumors are present.
Turner's s., XO s.; a chromosomal anomaly with chromosome count 45, including only a single X chromosome (XO sex chromosome constitution); buccal and other cells are usually sex chromatin-negative; anomalies include dwarfism, webbed neck, valgus of elbows, pigeon chest, infantile sexual development, and amenorrhea; the ovary has no primordial follicles and may be represented only by a fibrous streak; some individuals are chromosomal mosaic, with two or more cell lines of different chromosome constitution; seen in many animal species, in the meadow vole it is the normal female state.
Uehlinger's s., acropachyderma.
Ulysses s. [L. *Ulysses,* fr. G. *Odysseus,* myth. char.], the ill effects of extensive diagnostic investigations conducted because of a false-positive result in the course of routine laboratory screening.
Usher's s., congenital nerve deafness and retinitis pigmentosa; autosomal recessive inheritance.
uveocutaneous s., Vogt-Koyanagi s.
uveo-encephalitic s., Behçet's s.
uveomeningitis s., Harada's s.
VACTERL s., abnormalities of *v*ertebrae, *a*nus, *c*ardivovascular tree, *t*rachea, *e*sophagus, *r*enal system, and *l*imb buds associated with administration of sex steroids during early pregnancy.
Van Buchem's s., generalized cortical hyperostosis; an inherited skeletal dysplasia, with mandibular enlargement and thickening of the diaphyses and calvaria, and increased serum alkaline phosphatase; autosomal recessive inheritance.
van der Hoeve's s., a variation of osteogenesis imperfecta with blue sclera and deafness due to osteosclerosis.
vanishing lung s., a radiologic sign, common to many diseases, of progressive decrease of radiologic density of the lung due to a variety of pathophysiologic conditions.
vasculocardiac s. of hyperserotonemia, rarely used term for carcinoid s.
vasovagal s., vagal *attack.*
Verner-Morrison s., WDHA s.; watery diarrhea, hypokalemia, and achlor-hydria associated with secretion of vasoactive intestinal polypeptide by a pancreatic islet-cell tumor in the absence of gastric hypersecretion.
Vernet's s., a s. characterized by paralysis of the motor components of the glossopharyngeal, vagus, and accessory cranial nerves as they lie in the posterior fossa; it is most commonly the result of head injury.
vertical retraction s., see retraction s.
vibration s., tingling, numbness, and blanching of the fingers with progressive peripheral neurologic effects resulting from hand-transmitted vibration tools; persisting without further exposure to vibration.
virus-associated hemophagocytic s., a s. closely resembling malignant histiocytosis but potentially reversible, following a herpes group virus infection such as by the Epstein-Barr virus.
vitreoretinal choroidopathy s., an ocular condition characterized by peripheral pigmentary retinopathy, retinal vascular abnormalities, vitreous opacities, choroidal atrophy, and presenile cataracts; autosomal dominant inheritance.
vitreoretinal traction s., traction on the internal limiting membrane of the retina by adherent vitreous fibrils in vitreous humor detachment.
Vogt s. [Cècile and Oscar Vogt], double athetosis; spastic diplegia with athetosis and pseudobulbar paralysis associated with a lesion of the caudate nucleus and putamen.
Vogt-Koyanagi s., oculocutaneous or uveocutaneous s.; bilateral uveitis with iritis and glaucoma, premature graying of the hair, and alopecia, vitiligo, and dysacusia; related to Harada's s. and sympathetic ophthalmia.
Vohwinkel s., mutilating *keratoderma.*
von Hippel-Lindau s., Lindau's *disease.*

von Willebrand's s., von Willebrand's *disease.*
vulnerable child s., a reaction characterized by disturbance in psychosocial development, often occurring in children whose parents expect them to die prematurely.
Waardenburg s., dystopia canthorum; lateral dystopia of medial canthi and lacrimal puncta, increased width of the root of the nose, heterochromia or hypochromia iridis, cochlear deafness, white forelock, and synophrys; autosomal dominant inheritance.
Wagner's s., hyaloretinal *degeneration.*
Waldenström's s., Waldenström's *macroglobulinemia.*
Wallenberg's s., posterior inferior cerebellar artery s.
Waterhouse-Friderichsen s., Friderichsen-Waterhouse s.; acute fulminating meningococcal septicemia; a condition occurring mainly in children under 10 years of age, characterized by vomiting, diarrhea, extensive purpura, cyanosis, toniclonic convulsions, and circulatory collapse, usually with meningitis and hemorrhage into the adrenal glands.
WDHA s. [*w*atery *d*iarrhea, *h*ypokalemia, *a*chlorhydria], Verner-Morrison *syndrome.*
Weber's s., Weber's sign; a form of alternating paralysis characterized by paralysis of the oculomotor nerve on the side of the lesion and paralysis of the extremities and of the face and tongue on the opposite side due to a lesion in the ventral and internal part of a cerebral peduncle.
Weber-Cockayne s., *epidermolysis* bullosa, of the hands and feet.
Weill-Marchesani s., spherophakia-brachymorphia or Marchesani s; ectopia lentis (lens abnormally round and small), short stature, and brachydactyly; recessive autosomal inheritance.
Wells' s., eosinophilic cellulitis; recurrent cellulitis followed by brawny edematous skin lesions, or a less acute presentation of papular, annular, or gyrate skin lesions which are sometimes urticarial; affected skin and subcutis are heavily infiltrated by eosinophils and histiocytes, with scattered small necrotic areas (flame figures).
Wermer's s., familial endocrine *adenomatosis,* type 1.
Werner's s., a disorder consisting of scleroderma-like skin changes, bilateral juvenile cataracts, progeria, hypogonadism, and diabetes mellitus; autosomal recessive inheritance.
Wernicke's s., Wernicke's disease or encephalopathy; superior hemorrhagic polioencephalitis; a condition frequently encountered in chronic alcoholics, largely due to thiamin deficiency and characterized by disturbances in ocular motility, pupillary alterations, nystagmus, and ataxia with tremors; an organic-toxic psychosis is often an associated finding, and Korsakoff's s. often coexists.
Wernicke-Korsakoff s., the coexistence of Wernicke's and Korsakoff's s.'s.
West's s., an encephalopathy in infancy characterized by infantile spasms, arrest of psychomotor development, and hypsarrhythmia.
Weyers-Thier s., oculovertebral *dysplasia.*
whistling face s., craniocarpotarsal *dystrophy.*
white-out s., a psychosis which occurs in Arctic explorers or others similarly exposed to the stimulus deprivation of a snow-clad environment. See also sensory *deprivation.*
Widal's s., Hayem-Widal s.
Wildervanck s., cervico-oculo-acoustic s.
Williams s., a congenital disorder characterized by mental deficiency, mild growth deficiency, elfin facies, supravalvular aortic stenosis, and, occasionally, elevated blood calcium; may be associated with hypersensitivity to vitamin D or excess ingestion of the vitamin during pregnancy.
Wilson's s., hepatolenticular *degeneration.*
Wilson-Mikity s., pulmonary dysmaturity s.
Wiskott-Aldrich s., Aldrich s.; an X-linked immunodeficiency disorder occurring in male children and characterized by thrombocytopenia, eczema, melena, and susceptibility to recurrent bacterial infections; death occurs from severe hemorrhage or overwhelming infection.
Wissler's s., high intermittent fever, irregularly recurring macular and maculo-papular eruption of the face, chest and limbs, leukocytosis, arthralgia, occasionally eosinophilia, and raised erythrocyte sedimentation rate; occurs in children and adolescents, with varying duration.
Wolff-Parkinson-White s., preexcitation s., an electrocardiographic pattern sometimes associated with paroxysmal tachycardia; it consists of short P-R interval (0.1 second or less) together with a prolonged QRS complex with a slurred initial component (delta wave).
Wyburn-Mason s., arteriovenous malformation on the cerebral cortex, retinal arteriovenous angioma and facial nevus, usually occurring in mentally retarded individuals.
XO s., Turner's s.
XXY s., Klinefelter's s.
XYY s., a chromosomal anomaly with chromosome count 47, with a supernumerary Y chromosome; controversial evidence associates tallness, aggressiveness, and acne with this condition.
Zellweger s., cerebrohepatorenal s.
Zieve's s., transient jaundice, hemolytic anemia, and hyperlipemia associated with acute alcoholism in patients with cirrhosis or a fatty liver.
Zollinger-Ellison s., peptic ulceration with gastric hypersecretion and non-beta cell tumor of the pancreatic islets, sometimes associated with familial polyendocrine adenomatosis.

syndromic (sin-drom'ik, -drō'mik). Relating to a syndrome.

synechia, pl. synechiae (si-nek'ē-ă, si-nē'kē-ă, -kē-ē) [G. *synecheia,* continuity, fr. *syn,* together, + *echō,* to have, hold]. Any adhesion; specifically, anterior or posterior s.
annular s., adhesion of the entire pupillary margin of the iris to the capsule of the lens.
anterior s., adhesion of the iris to the cornea.
s. pericar'dii, concretio cordis.
peripheral anterior s., goniosynechia.
posterior s., adhesion of the iris to the capsule of the lens.
total s., adhesion of the entire surface of the iris to the lens capsule.

synechiotomy (si-nek'ē-ot'ō-mē) [synechia + G. *tomē,* incision]. Division of the adhesions in synechia.

synechotome (si-nek'ō-tōm). A small knife for use in synechiotomy.

synectenterotomy (si-nek'ten-ter-ot'ō-mē) [G. *synektos,* held together (see synechia), + *enteron,* intestine, + *tomē,* incision]. Division of intestional adhesions.

synencephalocele (sin-en-sef'ă-lō-sēl) [syn- + G. *enkephalos,* brain, + *kēlē,* hernia]. Protrusion of brain substance through a defect in the skull, with adhesions preventing reduction.

syneresis (si-ner'ĕ-sis) [G. *synairesis,* a taking or drawing together]. **1.** The contraction of a gel, *e.g.,* a blood clot, by which part of the dispersion medium is squeezed out. **2.** Degeneration of the vitreous humor with loss of gel consistency to become partially or completely fluid.

synergetic (sin-er-jet'ik). Synergistic.

synergia (si-ner'jē-ă). Synergism.

synergic (si-ner'jik). Synergistic.

synergism (sin'er-jizm) [G. *synergia,* fr. *syn,* together, + *ergon,* work]. Synergia; synergy; coordinated or correlated action of two or more structures, agents, or physiologic processes so that the combined action is greater than that of each acting separately. *Cf.* antagonism.

synergist (sin'er-jist). A structure, agent, or physiologic process that aids the action of another. *Cf.* antagonist.

synergistic (sin-er-jis'tik). Synergic; synergetic. **1.** Pertaining to synergism. **2.** Denoting a synergist.

synergy (sin'er-jē). Synergism.

synesthesia (sin-es-thē'zē-ă) [syn- + G. *aisthēsis,* sensation]. A condition in which a stimulus, in addition to exciting the usual and normally located sensation, gives rise to a subjective sensation of different character or localization; *e.g.,* color hearing, color taste.
s. al'gica, synesthesialgia.
auditory s., phonism; a second sensation associated with a sound.

synesthesialgia (sin'es-thē-zē-al'jē-ă). Synesthesia algica; painful synesthesia.

Syngamidae (sin-gam'i-dē) [see *Syngamus*]. A family of nematodes (order Strongyloidea) parasitic in the respiratory system of birds and mammals.

Syngamus (sin'gă-mŭs) [syn- + G. *gamos,* marriage]. A genus of moderate-sized, bloodsucking, strongyle nematodes (family Syngamidae) that live in the bronchi and tracheae of birds, and are especially important parasites of gallinaceous birds. They are called gapeworms because the host often gapes with open mouth due to the presence of the worms in the throat, or forked worms because the male is permanently attached to the midregion of the female, where the bursa of the male is clasped over the female vulva.
S. tra'chea, a worldwide parasite of the trachea of domestic fowl and many wild birds, causing gapes.

syngamy (sin'gă-mē) [syn- + G. *gamos,* marriage]. Conjugation of the gametes in fertilization.

syngeneic (sin'jĕ-nē'ik) [G. *syngenēs,* congenital]. Syngenic; isogeneic; isogenic; isologous; isoplastic; relating to genetically identical individuals.

syngenesioplasty (sin-jĕ-nē'zē-ō-plas-tē) [syn- + G. *genesis,* origin, + *plastos,* formed]. Plastic surgery involving syngenesiotransplantation.

syngenesiotransplantation (sin-jĕ-nē'zē-ō-trans-plan-tā'shŭn) [syn- + G. *genesis,* origin, + transplantation]. Transplantation in which the donor and recipient of a graft are closely related, *e.g.,* parent and child or siblings.

syngenesis (sin-jen'ĕ-sis) [syn- + G. *genesis,* origin]. Sexual *reproduction.*

syngenetic (sin-jĕ-net'ik). Relating to syngenesis.

syngenic (sin-jen'ik). Syngeneic.

syngnathia (sin-nath'ē-ă) [syn- + G. *gnathos,* jaw]. Congenital adhesion of the jaws by fibrous bands.

syngraft (sin'graft). Syngeneic, isogeneic, isologous, or isoplastic graft; isograft; a tissue or organ transplanted between genetically identical individuals.

synidrosis (sin-i-drō'sis) [syn- + G. *hidrosis,* sweating]. A condition in which excessive sweating is part of the clinical manifestation.

synizesis (sin-i-zē'sis) [G. collapse]. **1.** Closure or obliteration of the pupil. **2.** The massing of chromatin at one side of the nucleus that occurs usually at the beginning of synapsis.

synkaryon (sin-kar'ē-on) [syn- + G. *karyon,* kernel (nucleus)]. Syncaryon; the nucleus formed by the fusion of the two pronuclei in karyogamy.

synkinesis (sin-ki-nē'sis) [syn- + G. *kinēsis,* movement]. Syncinesis; involuntary movement accompanying a voluntary one, as the movement of a closed eye following that of the uncovered one, or the movement occurring in a paralyzed muscle accompanying motion in another part.

synkinetic (sin-ki-net'ik). Relating to or marked by synkinesis.

synnematin B (sin-ĕ-mā'tin, si-nē'mă-tin). *Cephalosporin* N.

synonychia (sin-ō-nik'ē-ă) [sin- + G. *onyx* (*onych-*), nail]. Fusion of two or more nails of the digits, as in syndactyly.

synonym (sin'ō-nim). In biologic nomenclature, a term used to denote one of two or more names for the same species or taxonomic group (taxon).
objective s.'s, different names for the same organism, based on one and the same nomenclatural type, as when a species is transferred from one genus to another (*e.g.,* the transfer of *Diplococcus pneumoniae* to the genus *Streptococcus* as *Streptococcus pneumoniae*), in contrast to subjective s.'s.
senior s., the earliest published of two or more available names for the same organism, usually used as the correct name (law of priority).
subjective s.'s, different names, based on different nomenclatural types, for organisms that were originally regarded as different but were later regarded to be identical, or nearly so, as a matter of personal opinion, in contrast to objective s.'s

synophrys (sin-of'ris) [syn- + G. *ophrys,* eyebrow]. Hypertrophy and fusion of the eyebrows.

synophthalmia, synophthalmus (sin-of-thal'mē-ă, -mŭs) [syn- + G. *ophthalmos,* eye]. Cyclopia.

synoptophore (sin-op'tō-fōr) [syn- + G. *ōps,* eye, + *phoros,* bearing]. A modified form of Wheatstone stereoscope used in orthoptic training.

synorchidism, synorchism (sin-ōr'ki-dizm, sin-ōr'kizm) [syn- + G. *orchis,* testis]. Congenital fusion of the testes in the abdominal cavity.

synoscheos (sin-os'kē-os) [syn- + G. *oschē,* scrotum]. Partial or complete adhesion of the penis and scrotum, a malformation in hermaphroditism.

synosteology (sin-os'tē-ol'ō-jē) [syn- + G. *osteon,* bone, + *logos,* study]. Arthrology.

synosteosis (sin-os-tē-ō'sis). Synostosis.

synostosis (sin-os-tō'sis) [syn- + G. *osteon,* bone, + *-osis,* condition]. Synosteosis; bony or true ankylosis; osseous union between the bones forming a joint.
tribasilar s., fusion in early life of the three bones at the base of the skull, resulting in interference with the development of the brain.

synostotic (sin-os-tot'ik). Relating to synostosis.

synotia (si-nō'shē-ă) [syn- + G. *ous,* ear]. Fusion or abnormal approximation of the lobes of the ears in otocephaly.

synovectomy (sin-ō-vek'tō-mē) [synovia + G. *ektomē,* excision]. Villusectomy; exsection of a portion or all of the synovial membrane of a joint.

synovia (si-nō'vē-ă) [Mod. L., a word coined by Paracelsus, fr. G. *syn,* together, + *ōon* (L. *ovum*), egg] [NA]. Joint oil; synovial fluid; a clear thixotropic fluid, the function of which is to serve as a lubricant in a joint, tendon sheath, or bursa; consists mainly of mucin with some albumin, fat, epithelium, and leukocytes.

synovial (si-nō'vē-ăl). **1.** Relating to, containing, or consisting of synovia. **2.** Relating to the membrana synovialis.

synovioma (si-nō-vē-ō'mă) [sinovia + G. *-oma,* tumor]. A tumor of synovial origin involving joint or tendon sheath.
malignant s., synovial *sarcoma.*

synoviparous (sin'ō-vip'ă-rŭs) [synovia + L. *pario,* to produce]. Producing synovia.

synovitis (sin-ō-vī'tis) [synovia + G. *-itis,* inflammation]. Inflammation of a synovial membrane, especially that of a joint; in general, when unqualified, the same as arthritis.
bursal s., bursitis.
chronic hemorrhagic villous s., pigmented villonodular s.
dry s., s. sicca; s. with little serous or purulent effusion.
filarial s., synovial inflammation often followed by fibrotic ankylosis due to microfilariae in the joint.
pigmented villonodular s., chronic hemorrhagic villous s.; diffuse outgrowths of synovial membrane of a joint, usually the knee,

composed of synovial villi and fibrous nodules infiltrated by hemosiderin- and lipid-containing macrophages and multinucleated giant cells; the condition may be inflammatory, although recurrence is likely to follow incomplete removal.

purulent s., suppurative *arthritis.*

serous s., s. with a large effusion of nonpurulent fluid.

s. sic'ca, dry s.

suppurative s., suppurative *arthritis.*

tendinous s., tenosynovitis.

vaginal s., tenosynovitis.

synovium (si-nō'vē-ŭm). *Membrana* synovialis.

synpolydactyly (sin'pol-ē-dak'ti-lē). Associated syndactyly and polydactyly.

syntactics (sin-tak'tiks) [syn- + G. *taxis,* order]. A branch of semiotics concerned with the formal relations between signs, in abstraction from their meaning and their interpreters.

syntality (sin-tal'i-tē) [prob. telescoped from syn- + mentality]. The consistent and predictable behavior of a social group.

syntectic (sin-tek'tik). Pertaining to or marked by syntexis.

syntenic (sin-ten'ik). Pertaining to synteny.

synteny (sin'ten-ē) [syn- + G. *tainia,* ribbon]. The relationship between two genetic loci (not genes) represented on the same chromosomal pair or (for haploid chromosomes) on the same chromosome; an anatomic rather than a segregational relationship.

syntexis (sin-tek'sis) [G. *syn-tēxis,* a melting together]. Emaciation or wasting.

synthase (sin'thās). Trivial name used in Enzyme Commission Report for a lyase reaction going in the reverse direction. See also synthetase. For individual s.'s, see the specific names.

synthermal (sin-ther'măl) [syn- + G. *thermē,* heat]. Having the same temperature.

synthesis, pl. **syntheses** (sin'thĕ-sis, -sēz) [G. fr. *syn,* together, + *thesis,* a placing, arranging]. **1.** A building up, putting together, composition. **2.** In chemistry, the formation of compounds by the union of simpler compounds or elements. **3.** A period in the cell *cycle.*

s. of continuity, healing of the edges of a wound or fracture.

enzymatic s., s. by enzymes. See biosynthesis.

protein s., The process in which individual amino acids, whether of exogenous or endogenous origin, are connected to each other in peptide linkage in a specific order dictated by the sequence of nucleotides in DNA; this governing sequence is conveyed to the synthesizing apparatus in the ribosomes by mRNA, formed by base-pairing on the DNA template. See fig. on p. 1543.

synthesize (sin'thĕ-sīz). To make something by synthesis, *i.e.,* synthetically.

synthetase (sin'thĕ-tās). An enzyme catalyzing the synthesis of a specific substance. S. is limited, in the Enzyme Commission Report, to use as a trivial name for the ligases (EC class 6), which in turn are those synthesizing enzymes that require the cleavage of a pyrophosphate linkage in ATP or a similar compound. Reversal of lyase (EC class 4) reactions, producing a synthesis, is indicated (in trivial names) by synthase; such reactions do not involve pyrophosphate cleavage. For individual s.'s, see the specific names.

synthetic (sin-thet'ik). Relating to or made by synthesis.

synthorax (sin-thōr'aks). Thoracopagus.

syntonic (sin-ton'ik) [G. *syntonos,* in harmony, fr. *syn,* together, + *tonos,* tone]. Having even tone or temperament.

syntrophism (sin'trō-fizm) [syn- + G. *trophē,* nourishment]. State of mutual dependence, with reference to food supply, of organs or cells of a plant or an animal.

syntrophoblast (sin-trō'fō-blast, -trof'ō-). Syncytiotrophoblast.

syntropic (sin-trop'ik). Relating to syntropy.

syntropy (sin'trō-pē) [syn- + G. *tropē,* a turning]. **1.** The tendency sometimes seen in two diseases to coalesce into one. **2.** The state of wholesome association with others. **3.** In anatomy, a number of similar structures inclined in one general direction; *e.g.,* the spinous processes of a series of vertebrae, the ribs.

inverse s., a situation in which the presence of one disease tends to decrease the possibility of another.

Syphacia (si-fā'shē-ă) [fr. L. *siphon,* tube]. Genus of oxyurid nematode pinworms of rodents; *S. obvelata* is the common cecal pinworm of mice, and *S. muris,* of rats. See also *Aspiculuris tetraptera.*

syphil-, syphili-. See syphilo-.

syphilemia (sif-i-lē'mē-ă) [syphilis + G. *haima,* blood]. A state in which the specific organism, *Treponema pallidum,* is present in the bloodstream.

syphilid (sif'i-lid) [syphilis + *-id* (1)]. Syphiloderm; any of the several kinds of cutaneous and mucous membrane lesions of secondary and tertiary syphilis, but most commonly denoting the former.

acneform s., pustular s.

acuminate papular s., follicular s.

annular s., cutaneous lesions of secondary syphilis in which the papules form annular lesions with raised papular borders and clear central portions.

bullous s., pemphigoid s.; a rare manifestation of congenital syphilis.

corymbose s., a secondary syphilitic eruption consisting of a large central papule surrounded by a more or less complete ring of smaller papules.

ecthymatous s., pustular s.

erythematous s., syphilitic *roseola.*

flat papular s., lenticular s.

follicular s., lichen syphiliticus; acuminate papular s.; miliary papular s.; secondary eruption of small follicular papules, usually appearing as groups of lesions.

frambesiform s., rupial s.

gummatous s., gumma.

impetiginous s., pustular s.

lenticular s., flat papular s.; eruption of flattened, dull reddish papules, 5 mm to 1 cm in diameter, occurring in secondary syphilis.

macular s., syphilitic *roseola.*

miliary papular s., follicular s.

nodular s., gumma.

nummular s., flat, disk-shaped papules of secondary syphilis.

palmar s., dull red papules in the palms, occurring in secondary syphilis.

papular s., see follicular s.; lenticular s.

papulosquamous s., scaling papules of secondary syphilis.

pemphigoid s., bullous s.

pigmentary s., lesions of secondary syphilis consisting of rounded white macules on the trunk.

plantar s., dull red papules on the soles in secondary syphilis.

pustular s., acne syphilitica; acneform, impetiginous, varioliform, or ecthymatous s.; a type of pustular eruption occurring in secondary syphilis.

rupial s., frambesiform s.; lesions that appear granulomatous and crusted, resembling those of yaws.

secondary s., a syphilitic skin lesion characteristic of the second stage of the disease.

tertiary s., a syphilitic skin lesion characteristic of the third stage

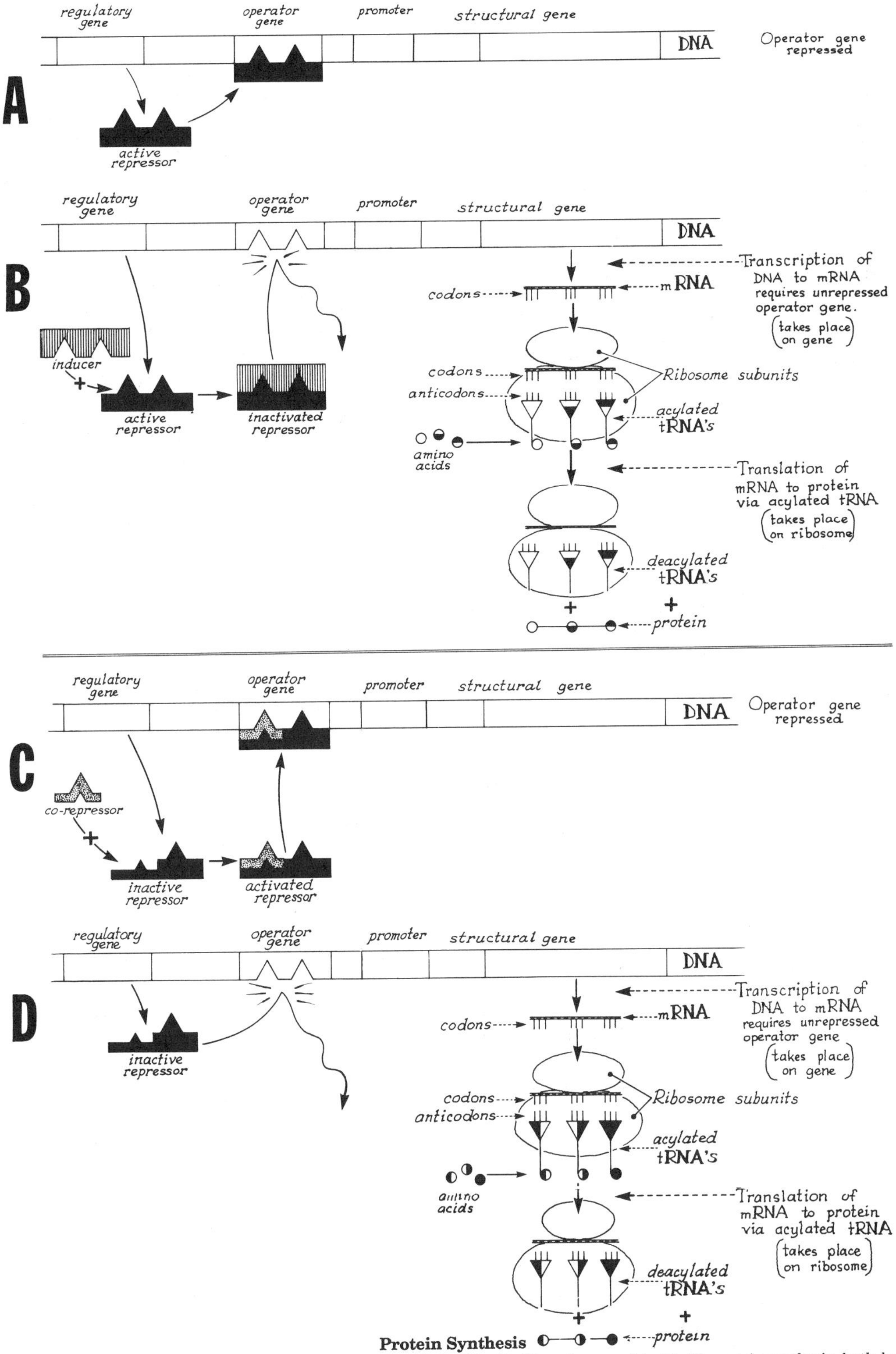

Protein Synthesis

The operon concept for the regulation, in bacteria, of inducible (A, B) and repressible (C, D) protein synthesis, both by "negative control". "Positive control" is the situation where the combination called "inactivated repressor" in B causes activation of the promoter gene by combining with a gene lying between the operator and promoter genes, or with the latter, thus bypassing the inactivated operator gene (shown in A).

of the disease.
varioliform s., pustular s.

syphilimetry (sif-i-lim'ĕ-trē) [syphilis + G. *metron,* measure]. A test designed to determine intensity of syphilitic infection, *e.g.,* titered serologic test.

syphilionthus (sif'i-li-on'thŭs) [syphilid + G. *ionthos,* acne of adolescence]. A copper-colored syphilid with branny scales.

syphilis (sif'i-lis) [Mod. L. *syphilis* (*syphilid-*), (?) fr. a poem, *Syphilis sive Morbus Gallicus,* by Fracastorius, *Syphilus* being a shepherd and principal char.]. Lues venerea; malum venereum; an acute and chronic infectious disease caused by *Treponema pallidum* and transmitted by direct contact, usually through sexual intercourse. After an incubation period of 12 to 30 days, the first symptom is a chancre, followed by slight fever and other constitutional symptoms (*primary s.*), followed by a skin eruption of various appearances with mucous patches (*secondary s.*), and subsequently by the formation of gummas, cellular infiltration, and functional abnormalities resulting from cardiovascular and central nervous system lesions (*tertiary s.*).
congenital s., s. hereditaria; hereditary s.; s. acquired by the fetus *in utero,* thus present at birth.
s. d'emblée (dom-blā') [Fr. right away], s. occurring without an initial sore.
equine s., dourine.
s. heredita'ria, hereditary s., congenital s.
s. heredita'ria tar'da, s., believed to be congenital, but not manifesting itself until several years after birth.
meningovascular s., a rare manifestation of secondary or tertiary s. characterized by mild, nonsuppurative, chronic inflammation of the leptomeninges and an intracranial or spinal angiitis.
primary s., the first stage of s. See under syphilis.
quaternary s., parasyphilis.
secondary s., mesosyphilis; the second stage of s. See under syphilis.
tertiary s., the final stage of s. See under syphilis.

syphilitic (sif-i-lit'ik). Luetic; relating to, caused by, or suffering from syphilis.

syphilo-, syphil-, syphili- [see syphilis]. Combining forms relating to syphilis.

syphiloderm, syphiloderma (sif'i-lō-derm, -der'mă) [syphilo- + G. *derma,* skin]. Syphilid.

syphiloid (sif'i-loyd) [syphilo- + G. *eidos,* resemblance]. Resembling syphilis.

syphilologist (sif-i-lol'o-jist). One who specializes in the study, diagnosis, and treatment of syphilis.

syphilology (sif-i-lol'ō-jē) [syphilo- + G. *logos,* study]. The branch of medical science concerned with the origin, prevention, and treatment of syphilis.

syphiloma (sif-i-lō'mă) [syphilo- + G. *-oma,* tumor]. Gumma.
s. of Fournier, Fournier's *disease.*

syphilomatous (sif-i-lō'mă-tŭs). Gummatous.

syr. Abbreviation of Mod. L. *syrupus,* syrup.

syrigmus (sĭ-rig'mŭs) [L. fr. G. *syrigmos,* a hissing]. *Tinnitus* aurium.

syring-. See syringo-.

syringadenoma (sir'ing-ad-ĕ-nō'mă) [syring- + G. *adēn* gland, + *-oma,* tumor]. Syringoadenoma; a benign sweat gland tumor showing glandular differentiation typical of secretory cells.

syringadenosus (sir'ing-ad-ĕ-nō'sŭs) [L. fr. syring- + G. *adēn,* gland]. Relating to the sweat glands.

syringe (sĭ-rinj', sir'inj) [G. *syrinx,* pipe or tube]. An instrument used for injecting or withdrawing fluids.
air s., chip s.

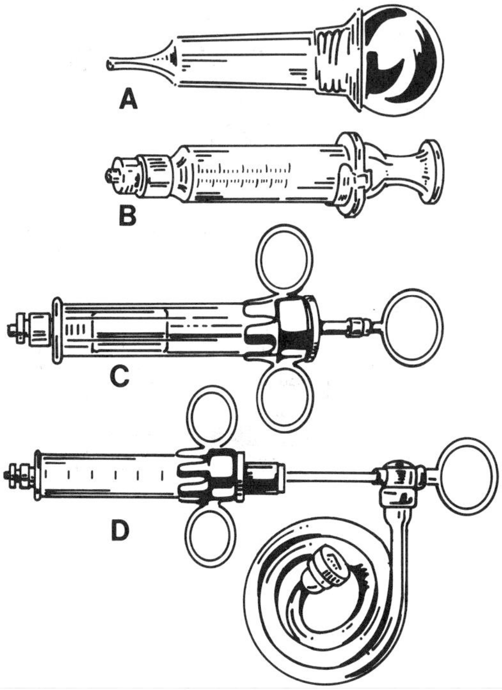

Syringes
A, Asepto; *B,* Luer; *C,* control; *D,* Pitkin.

chip s., air s.; a tapered metal tube through which air is forced from a rubber bulb or pressure tank to blow debris from, or to dry, a cavity in preparing teeth for restoration.
control s., ring s.; a type of Luer-Lok s. with thumb and finger rings attached to the proximal end of the barrel and to the tip of the plunger, allowing operation of the s. with one hand.
Davidson s., a rubber tube, armed with an appropriate nozzle, intersected with a compressible bulb, with valves so arranged that compression forces the fluid, into which one end of the tube is inserted, forward to the nozzle end.
dental s., a breech-loading metal cartridge s. into which fits a hermetically sealed glass cartridge containing the anesthetic solution.
fountain s., an apparatus consisting of a reservoir for holding fluid, to the bottom of which is attached a tube with a suitable nozzle; used for vaginal or rectal injections, irrigating wounds, etc., the force of the flow being regulated by the height of the reservoir above the point of discharge.
hypodermic s., hypodermic (3); a small s. with a barrel (which may be calibrated), perfectly matched plunger, and tip; used with a hollow needle for subcutaneous injections and for aspiration.
Luer s., Luer-Lok s., a glass s. with a metal tip and locking device to secure the needle; used for hypodermic and intravenous purposes.
Neisser's s., a urethral s. used in treatment of gonococcal urethritis.
Pitkin s., a self-filling s., with a rubber tube attached to the plunger that allows continuous injection of large amounts of solution; used to administer anesthesia.
probe s., a s. with an olive-shaped tip, used in treatment of diseases of the lacrimal passages.
ring s., control s.
Roughton-Scholander s., Roughton-Scholander *apparatus.*
rubber-bulb s., a s. with a hollow rubber bulb and cannula provided with a check valve, used to obtain a jet of air or water.

syringeal (sĭ-rin'jē-ăl). Relating to a syrinx.

syringectomy (si-rin-jek'tō-mē) [syring- + G. *ektomē*, excision]. Fistulectomy.

syringitis (si-rin-jī'tis) [syring- + G. *-itis*, inflammation]. Inflammation of the eustachian tube.

syringo-, syring- [G. *syrinx*, pipe or tube]. Combining forms relating to a syrinx.

syringoadenoma (sĭ-ring'gō-ad-ĕ-nō'mă). Syringadenoma.

syringobulbia (sĭ-ring'gō-bŭl'bē-ă) [syringo- + L. *bulbus*, bulb (medulla oblongata)]. A fluid-filled cavity of the brainstem, analogous to syringomyelia.

syringocarcinoma (sĭ-ring'gō-kar-si-nō'mă) [syringo- + carcinoma]. A malignant epithelial neoplasm which has undergone cystic change (cystic carcinoma).

syringocele (sĭ-ring'gō-sēl) [syringo- + G. *koilia*, a hollow]. **1.** *Canalis* centralis. **2.** A meningomyelocele in which there is a cavity in the ectopic spinal cord.

syringocystadenoma (sĭ-ring'gō-sis-tad-ĕ-nō'mă) [syringo- + cystadenoma]. A cystic benign sweat gland tumor.

s. papillif'erum, a s. characterized by numerous finger-like projections of proliferated neoplastic epithelial cells in two layers on a stromal core of fibrous connective tissue infiltrated by plasma cells.

syringocystoma (sĭ-ring'gō-sis-tō'mă) [syringo- + cystoma]. Hidrocystoma.

syringoencephalomyelia (sĭ-ring'gō-en-sef'ă-lō-mī-ē'lē-ă) [syringo- + G. *enkephalos*, brain, + *myelos*, marrow]. A tubular cavity involving both brain and spinal cord and etiologically unrelated to vascular insufficiency.

syringoid (sĭ-ring'goyd) [syringo- + G. *eidos*, resemblance]. Resembling a tube or fistula.

syringoma (si-ring-gō'mă) [syringo- + G. *-ōma*, tumor]. A benign, often multiple, neoplasm of the sweat glands composed of very small round cysts.

chondroid s., mixed tumor of skin; a benign tumor of sweat glands with a mucoid stroma showing cartilaginous metaplasia.

syringomeningocele (sĭ-ring'gō-mē-ning'gō-sēl) [syringo- + meningocele]. A form of spina bifida in which the dorsal sac consists chiefly of membranes, with very little cord substance, enclosing a cavity that communicates with a syringomyelic cavity.

syringomyelia (sĭ-ring'gō-mī-ē'lē-ă) [syringo- + G. *myelos*, marrow]. Hydrosyringomyelia; Morvan's disease; myelosyringosis; syringomyelus; the presence in the spinal cord of longitudinal cavities lined by dense, gliogenous tissue, which are not caused by vascular insufficiency. S. is marked clinically by pain and paresthesia, followed by muscular atrophy of the hands and analgesia with thermoanesthesia of the hands and arms, but with the tactile sense preserved; later marked by painless whitlows, spastic paralysis in the lower extremities, and scoliosis of the lumbar spine. Some cases are associated with low grade astrocytomas or vascular malformations of the spinal cord.

syringomyelocele (sĭ-ring'gō-mī'ĕ-lō-sēl) [syringo- + myelocele]. A form of spina bifida, consisting in a protrusion of the membranes and spinal cord through a dorsal defect in the vertebral column, the fluid of the syrinx of the cord being increased and expanding the cord tissue into a thin-walled sac which then expands through the vertebral defect.

syringomyelus (sĭ-ring'gō-mī'ĕ-lŭs) [syringo- + G. *myelos*, marrow]. Syringomyelia.

syringopontia (sĭ-ring'gō-pon'shē-ă) [syringo- + L. *pons*, bridge]. A condition of cavity formation in the pons, of the same nature as syringomyelia.

syringotome (sĭ-rin'gō-tōm). Fistulatome.

syringotomy (si-rin-got'ō-mē). Fistulotomy.

syrinx, pl. **syringes** (sir'ingks, sĭ-rin'jēz) [G. a tube, pipe]. **1.** A rarely used synonym for fistula. **2.** A pathologic tube-shaped cavity in the brain or spinal cord.

syrosingopine (sir-ō-sin'gō-pēn). Carbethoxysyringoyl methyl reserpate; prepared from reserpine by hydrolysis and reesterification; an antihypertensive agent with actions similar to those of reserpine.

syrup (ser'ŭp, sir'ŭp) [Mod. L. *syrupus*, fr. Ar. *sharāb*]. Sirup. **1.** Refined molasses; the uncrystallizable saccharine solution left after the refining of sugar. **2.** Any sweet fluid; a solution of sugar in water in any proportion. **3.** A liquid preparation of medicinal or flavoring substances in a concentrated aqueous solution of a sugar, usually sucrose; other polyols, such as glycerin or sorbitol, may be present to retard crystallization of sucrose or to increase the solubility of added ingredients. When the s. contains a medicinal substance, it is termed a medicated s.; a s. may contain antimicrobial agents to prevent bacterial and mold growth.

syrupus (syr.) (sir'ŭ-pŭs) [Mod. L.]. Syrup.

syrupy (ser'ŭ-pē, sir'). Relating to syrup; of the consistency of syrup.

syssarcosic (sis'ar-kō'sik). Syssarcotic.

syssarcosis (sis'ar-kō'sis) [G. *syssarkōsis*, a being overgrown with flesh, fr. *syn*, with, + *sarx*, flesh]. Union of bones by muscle; a muscular articulation; *e.g.*, in man, the muscular connections of the patella.

syssarcotic (sis'ar-kot'ik). Syssarcosic; relating to or characterized by syssarcosis.

systaltic (sis-tahl'tik, -tal'tik) [G. *systaltikos*, contractile]. Pulsating; alternately contracting and dilating; denoting the action of the heart.

SYSTEM

system (sis'tĕm) [G. *systēma*, an organized whole]. **1.** A consistent and complex whole made up of correlated and semi-independent parts. **2.** The entire organism seen as a complex organization of parts. **3.** Any complex of structures anatomically related (*e.g.* vascular s.) or functionally related (*e.g.*, digestive s.). **4.** A scheme of medical theory. See also apparatus; classification; systema.

absolute s. of units, a s. based on absolute units accepted as being fundamental (length, mass, time) and from which other units (force, energy or work, power) are derived; such s.'s in common use are the foot-pound-second, centimeter-gram-second, and meter-kilogram-second s.'s.

absorbent s., *systema* lymphaticum.

alimentary s., *apparatus* digestorius.

arch-loop-whorl (A.L.W.) s., see Galton's system of classification of *fingerprints*.

association s., groups or tracts of nerve fibers interconnecting different regions of one and the same major subdivision of the central nervous system, such as the various areas of the cerebral cortex or the various segments of the spinal cord.

autonomic nervous s., *pars* autonomica.

blood group s.'s, see Blood Groups appendix.

blood-vascular s., cardiovascular s.

bulbosacral s., *pars* parasympathica.

cardiovascular s., blood-vascular s.; the heart and blood vessels considered as a whole.

caudal neurosecretory s., urohypophysis.

centimeter-gram-second (CGS, cgs) s., the scientific s. of expressing the fundamental physical units of length, mass, and time, and those units derived from them, in centimeters, grams, and seconds; currently being replaced by the International System of Units

based on the meter, kilogram, and second.
central nervous s. (CNS), *pars* centralis.
cerebrospinal s., the combined central nervous s. and peripheral nervous s.
chromaffin s., the cells of the body which stain with chromium salts and occur in the medullary portion of the adrenal body, paraganglia, and in relation to certain sympathetic nerves.
circulatory s., vascular s.
colloid s., a combination of the two phases, internal and external, of a colloid solution; the various s.'s are: gas + liquid (foam); gas + solid (meerschaum); liquid + gas (fog); solid + gas (smoke); solid + liquid (sol); liquid + solid (gel); liquid + liquid (emulsion); solid + solid (colored glass).
conducting s. of heart, the s. of atypical cardiac muscle fibers comprising the sinoatrial node, internodal tracts, atrioventricular node and bundle, the bundle branches, and their terminal ramifications into the Purkinje network. Sometimes also called cardionector.
craniosacral s., *pars* parasympathica.
cytochrome s., respiratory *chain.*
dermal s., dermoid s., the skin and its appendages, the nails and hair.
digestive s., *apparatus* digestorius.
ecological s., ecosystem.
electron-transport s., respiratory *chain.*
endocrine s., collective designation for those tissues capable of secreting hormones.
esthesiodic s., a s. of neurons and fiber tracts in the spinal cord and brain subserving sensation.
exterofective s., name applied by Cannon to the somatic nervous s. as opposed to the interofective or autonomic s.
extrapyramidal motor s., literally: all of the brain structures affecting bodily (somatic) movement, excluding the motor neurons, the motor cortex, and the pyramidal (corticobulbar and corticospinal) tract. Despite its very wide literal connotation, the term is commonly used to denote in particular the corpus striatum (basal ganglia), its associated structures (substantia nigra; subthalamic nucleus), and its descending connections with the midbrain.
feedback s., **(1)** a complex of neuronal circuits whereby a part of the efferent path returns to the input to modulate its activity, thus acting as a governor on the s.; **(2)** see feedback.
foot-pound-second (FPS, fps) s., a s. of absolute units based on the foot, pound, and second.
Galton's s. of classification of fingerprints, see under fingerprint.
gamma motor s., gamma *loop.*
genital s., reproductive s.; the complex s. consisting of the male or female gonads, associated ducts, and external genitalia dedicated to the function of reproducing the species.
genitourinary s., *apparatus* urogenitalis.
glandular s., all the glands of the body collectively.
haversian s., osteon.
hematopoietic s., the blood-making organs; in the embryo at different ages these are the yolk sac, liver, thymus, spleen, lymph nodes, and bone marrow; after birth they are principally the bone marrow, spleen, thymus, and lymph nodes.
heterogeneous s., in chemistry, a s. that contains various distinct and mechanically separable parts or phases; *e.g.,* a suspension or an emulsion.
hexaxial reference s., the figure resulting if the lines of derivation of the unipolar limb leads of the electrocardiogram are added to the triaxial reference s.
His-Tawara s., the complex s. of interlacing Purkinje fibers within the ventricular myocardium. See also conducting s. of the heart.
homogeneous s., in chemistry, a s. whose parts cannot be mechanically separated, and is therefore uniform throughout and possesses in every part identically physical properties; *e.g.,* a solution of sodium chloride in water.
hypothalamohypophysial portal s., a s. of veins that originate from the capillary tufts of the median eminence, pass downward along the stalk and pars tuberalis of the hypophysis, and enter the anterior lobe of the hypophysis where they arborize into a secondary capillary bed; these portal vessels convey to the anterior lobe releasing factors, chemical transmitters synthesized by certain neurons of the hypothalamus. See also hypophysis; median *eminence.*
hypoxia warning s., a device designed to produce an audio or visual signal at a predetermined level of oxygen partial pressure; ideally, the system would warn of impending hypoxia in time for corrective action to be taken.
immune s., an intricate complex of interrelated cellular, molecular, and genetic components which provides a defense (immune response) against foreign organisms or substances and aberrant native cells.
indicator s., in *in vitro* immunological tests, a combination of reagents used to determine the degree to which immunological reagents have combined (*e.g.,* sensitized erythrocytes in complement-fixation tests; enzyme and substrate in enzyme-linked immunosorbent assays).
integumentary s., the skin and its associated derivatives; it is derived from ectoderm and subjacent mesoderm.
intermediary s, interstitial *lamella.*
International System of Units, see at International.
interofective s., term applied by W. Cannon to the autonomic nervous s. as opposed to the somatic nervous s. or exterofective s.
involuntary nervous s., *pars* autonomica.
kallikrein s., a blood serum s., the activity of which is initiated by factor XII (Hageman factor) leading to the production of prekallikrein activator and then to kallikrein which, after activation by plasmin, splits bradykinin from kininogen.
kinetic s., **(1)** a term proposed by G.W. Crile to denote the chain of organs through which latent energy is transformed into motion and heat: it includes the brain, the thyroid, the adrenals, the liver, the pancreas, and the muscles; **(2)** that part of the neuromuscular s. whereby active movements are effected; distinguished from the static s.
lateral line s., a series of sense organs that detect pressure or vibrations along the head and side of cyclostomes, fishes, and some amphibians.
limbic s., visceral brain; collective term denoting a heterogeneous array of brain structures at or near the edge (limbus) of the medial wall of the cerebral hemisphere, in particular the hippocampus, amygdala, and gyrus fornicatus; the term is often used so as to include also the interconnections of these structures, as well as their connections with the septal area, the hypothalamus, and a medial zone of mesencephalic tegmentum. By way of the latter connections, the limbic s. exerts an important influence upon the endocrine and autonomic motor s.'s; its functions also appear to affect motivational and mood states.
linnaean s. of nomenclature [Carl von *Linné,* Swedish botanist, 1707–1778], binary or binomial nomenclature; the s. of nomenclature in which the names of species are composed of two parts, a generic name and a specific epithet (species name, in botany).
lymphatic s., *systema* lymphaticum.
s. of macrophages, mononuclear phagocytic s.
masticatory s., masticatory apparatus (1); dental apparatus; the organs and structures primarily functioning in mastication: the jaws, teeth with their supporting structures, temporomandibular articulation, mandibular musculature, tongue, lips, cheeks, and oral mucosa.
metameric nervous s., paleencephalon; that part of the nervous s. which innervates body structures developed in ontogeny from the segmentally arranged somites or, in the head region, branchial arches. The term implies reference to the neural mechanisms intrinsic to the spinal cord and brainstem (represented by the sensory

nuclei, motoneuronal cell groups, and their associated interneurons in the reticular formation); by strict definition it should exclude the autonomic nervous system.

meter-kilogram-second (MKS, mks) s., an absolute s. based on the meter, kilogram, and second; the basis of the International System of Units.

metric s., a s. of weights and measures, universal for scientific use, based upon the meter, which was originally intended to be one ten-millionth of a quadrant of the earth's meridian, equivalent to 39.37 inches. Fractions of a meter (prefixes) are expressed in Latin: deci- (d, 10^{-1}), centi- (c, 10^{-2}), milli- (m, 10^{-3}), micro- (μ, 10^{-6}), nano- (n, 10^{-9}), pico- (p, 10^{-12}), femto- (f, 10^{-15}), atto- (a, 10^{-18}). Multiples (prefixes) are expressed in Greek: deca- (dk, 10), hecto- (h, 10^2), kilo- (k, 10^3), mega- (M, 10^6), giga- (G, 10^9), tera- (T, 10^{12}). The unit of weight is the gram, which is the weight of one cubic centimeter of distilled water, equivalent to 15.432+ grains. The unit of volume is the liter or one cubic decimeter, equal to 1.056 quarts; a cubic centimeter is about 15 minims.

mononuclear phagocyte s. (MPS), s. of macrophages; a widely distributed collection of both free and fixed macrophages derived from bone marrow precursor cells by way of monocytes; their substantial phagocytic activity is mediated by immunoglobulin and the serum complement system. In both connective and lymphoid tissue, they may occur as free and fixed macrophages; in the sinusoids of the liver, as Kupffer cells; in the lung, as alveolar macrophages; and in the nervous system, as microglia.

muscular s., all the muscles of the body collectively.

nervous s., *systema* nervosum.

neuromuscular s., the muscles of the body collectively and the nerves supplying them.

nonspecific s., reticular activating s.

occlusal s., occlusal scheme; the form or design and arrangement of the occlusal and incisal units of a dentition or the teeth on a denture.

oculomotor s., that part of the central nervous s. having to do with eye movements; it is composed of pathways connecting various regions of the cerebrum, brainstem, and ocular nuclei, utilizing multisynaptic articulations.

O-R s., abbreviation for oxidation-reduction s.

oxidation-reduction s. (O-R s.), redox s.; an enzyme s. in the tissues by which oxidation and reduction proceed simultaneously through the transference of hydrogen or of one or more electrons from one metabolite to another. See also oxidation-reduction.

parasympathetic nervous s., *pars* parasympathica. See also *pars* autonomica.

pedal s., efferent fibers connecting the forebrain with more caudal structures.

periodic s., the arrangement of the chemical elements in a definite order as indicated by their respective atomic numbers in such a way that groups of elements with similar chemical properties (similar valence shell electron number) are grouped together. See Mendeléeff's *law*.

peripheral nervous s., *pars* peripherica.

Pinel's s., the abolition of forcible restraint in the treatment of the mental hospital patient.

portal s., a s. of vessels in which blood, after passing through one capillary bed, is conveyed through a second capillary network, as in the hepatic portal system in which blood from the intestines passes through the liver sinusoids.

pressoreceptor s., the pressoreceptive areas which with their afferent fibers and connections with the autonomic system react to a rise in arterial blood pressure and serve to buffer it by inhibiting the heart rate and vascular tone. See also baroreceptor.

projection s., the s. of axons carrying stimuli from one portion of the nervous system to other portions.

properdin s., an immunological s. that is the alternative pathway for complement, composed of several distinct proteins that react in a serial manner and activate C3 (third component of complement), seemingly without utilizing components C1, C4, and C2; in addition to properdin, the s. includes properdin factors A (native C3), B (C3 proactivator), D (C3 proactivator convertase), and perhaps at least one other, E; the s. can be activated, in the absence of specific antibody, by bacterial endotoxins, by a variety of polysaccharides and lipopolysaccharides, and by a component of cobra venom.

Purkinje s., terminal ramifications in the ventricles of the specialized conducting s. of the heart.

redox s., oxidation-reduction s.

reproductive s., genital s.

renin-angiotensin s., a selective regulator of the aldosterone biosynthetic pathway that acts by increasing aldosterone production and sodium retention as a result of volume depletion, with resulting increased renin production in the kidney and conversion of angiotensin I in the plasma to angiotensin II.

respiratory s., *apparatus* respiratorius.

reticular activating s. (RAS), nonspecific s.; a physiological term denoting that part of the brainstem reticular formation that plays a central role in the organism's bodily and behavorial alertness; it extends as a diffusely organized neural apparatus through the central region of the brainstem into the subthalamus and the intralaminar nuclei of the thalamus; by its ascending connections it affects the function of the cerebral cortex in the sense of behavioral responsiveness; its descending (reticulospinal) connections transmit its activating influence upon bodily posture and reflex mechanisms (*e.g.,* muscle tonus), in part by way of the gamma motor neurons. See also *formatio* reticularis.

reticuloendothelial s. (RES), a collection of putative macrophages, first described by Aschoff, which included most of the true macrophages (now classified under the mononuclear phagocytic s.) as well as cells lining the sinusoids of the spleen, lymph nodes, and bone marrow, and the fibroblastic reticular cells of hematopoietic tissues; all of these latter cells are only weakly phagocytic and are not true macrophages. The term persists in the literature and is often erroneously equated with the mononuclear phagocytic s.

second signaling s., pavlovian term for speech in which words are considered to be the "second signals" capable of producing conditioned responses.

skeletal s., *systema* skeletale.

somesthetic s., sensory data derived from skin, muscles, and body organs in contrast to that derived from the five special senses.

static s., that part of the neuromuscular s. whereby the animal organism is maintained in posture and equilibrium, and counteracts the forces of gravity and atmospheric pressure; distinguished from the kinetic s. (2).

stomatognathic s., masticatory apparatus (2); all of the structures involved in speech and in the receiving, mastication, and deglutition of food. See also masticatory s.

sympathetic nervous s., **(1)** originally, the entire autonomic nervous s.; **(2)** *pars* sympathica. See also *pars* autonomica.

T s., the transverse tubules which are continuous with the sarcolemma in skeletal and cardiac muscle fibers.

thoracolumbar s., *pars* sympathica. See also *pars* autonomica.

triaxial reference s., the figure resulting from rearranging the lines of derivation of the three standard limb leads of the electrocardiogram (as represented in Einthoven's triangle) so that, instead of forming the sides of an equilateral triangle, they bisect one another. See fig. on p. 1548.

urinary s., *apparatus* urogenitalis.

urogenital s., *apparatus* urogenitalis.

uropoietic s., the kidneys, ureters, bladder, and urethra, considered as a s. for the secretion and excretion of urine.

vascular s., circulatory s.; the cardiovascular and lymphatic s.'s collectively.

vegetative nervous s., *pars* autonomica.

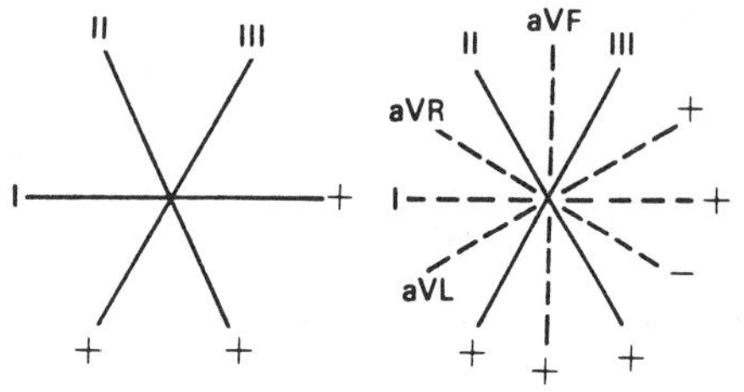

Triaxial (*left*) and Hexaxial (*right*) Reference Systems

vertebral-basilar s., the arterial complex comprising the two vertebral arteries joining to form the basilar artery, and their immediate branches.
vertebral venous s., *plexus* venosi vertebrales.
visceral nervous s., *pars* autonomica.

systema (sis'tē'mă) [L. fr. G. systēma]. [NA]. A complex of anatomical structures functionally related. See also system, apparatus.
s. digesto'rium [NA], official alternate term for *apparatus* digestorius.
s. lymphat'icum [NA], lymphatic system; absorbent system; it consists of lymphatic vessels, nodes, and lymphoid tissue; it empties into the veins at the level of the superior aperture of the thorax.
s. nervo'sum [NA], nervous system; the entire nerve apparatus, composed of a central part, the brain and spinal cord, and a peripheral part, the cranial and spinal nerves, autonomic ganglia, and plexuses.
s. nervo'sum autonom'icum [NA], official alternative term for *pars* autonomica.
s. nervo'sum centra'le [NA], official alternative term for *pars* centralis.
s. nervo'sum peripher'icum [NA], official alternative term for *pars* peripherica.
s. respirato'rium [NA], official alternate term for *apparatus* respiratorius.
s. skeleta'le [NA], skeletal system; the bones and cartilages of the body.
s. urogenita'le [NA], official alternate term for *apparatus* urogenitalis.

systematic (sis'tĕ-mat'ik). Relating to a system in any sense; arranged according to a system.

systematic name. As applied to chemical substances, a s. n. is composed of specially coined or selected words or syllables, each of which has a precisely defined chemical structural meaning, so that the structure may be derived from the name. Water (trivial name) is hydrogen oxide (systematic). The s. n. of histamine (a semisystematic name) is imidazolethylamine, which indicates that a radical of imidazole replaces one hydrogen atom of ethylamine, which in turn is an ethyl group attached to an amine group. Dimethyl sulfoxide states that two methyl radicals are attached to a sulfur atom that holds an oxygen atom. Carbolic acid (trivial name) or phenol (semisystematic name) are, systematically, benzeneol or phenyl hydroxide or hydroxycyclohexatriene (cyclohexa indicating that six carbon atoms, attached as in hexane, are in a ring; triene indicating that three double bonds occur between them, thus yielding CH=CH—CH=CH—CH=CH or benzene; hydroxy indicating OH in place of one H). See also semisystematic name.

systematization (sis-tĕ-mat'i-zā'shŭn, sis-tem'ă-ti-). The arrangement of ideas into orderly sequence.

Système International d'Unités. See International System of Units.

systemic (sis-tem'ik). Relating to a system; specifically somatic, relating to the entire organism as distinguished from any of its individual parts.

systemoid (sis'tĕ-moyd). Resembling a system; denoting a tumor of complex structure resembling an organ.

systole (sis'tō-lē) [G. *systolē,* a contracting]. Miocardia; contraction of the heart, especially of the ventricles, by which the blood is driven through the aorta and pulmonary artery to traverse the systemic and pulmonary circulations, respectively; its occurrence is indicated physically by the first sound of the heart heard on auscultation, by the palpable apex beat, and by the arterial pulse.
aborted s., a loss of the systolic beat in the radial pulse through weakness of the ventricular contraction.
s. alter'nans, hemisystole.
atrial s., auricular s.; contraction of the atria.
auricular s., atrial s.
electromechanical s., Q-S_2 interval; the period from the beginning of the QRS complex to the first vibration of the second heart sound.
extra-s., see extrasystole.
late s., prediastole.
premature s., extrasystole.
ventricular s., contraction of the ventricles.

systolic (sis-tol'ik). Relating to, or occurring during cardiac systole.

systolometer (sis'tō-lom'ĕ-ter) [systole + G. *metron,* measure]. **1.** An apparatus for determining the force of the cardiac contraction. **2.** An instrument for analyzing the sounds of the heart.

systremma (sis-trem'ă) [G. anything twisted]. A muscular cramp in the calf of the leg, the contracted muscles forming a hard ball.

syzygial (si-zij'ē-ăl). Relating to syzygy.

syzygiology (si-zij'ē-ol'ō-jē) [G. *syzygios,* yoked (see syzygy), + *logos,* study]. The study of interrelationships, or interdependencies, especially of the whole, as opposed to the study of separate parts or isolated functions.

syzygium (si-zij'ē-ŭm). Syzygy.

syzygy (siz'i-jē) [G. *syzygios,* yoked, bound together, fr. *syn,* together, + *zygon,* a yoke]. Syzygium. **1.** The association of gregarine protozoans end-to-end or in lateral pairing (without sexual fusion). **2.** Pairing of chromosomes in meiosis.

T

T 1. Symbol for ribothymidine; tension (T+, increased tension; T−, diminished tension); tera-; tesla; tritium. **2.** As a subscript, refers to tidal *volume.* **3.** Abbreviation for thoracic vertebra (T1 to T12); tocopherol.

T_3 Symbol for 3,5,3′-triiodothyronine.

T_4 Symbol for thyroxine.

2,4,5-T Abbreviation for (2,4,5-trichlorophenoxy)acetic acid.

T Symbol for absolute temperature (Kelvin).

T_m Symbol for *temperature* midpoint (Kelvin).

t Abbreviation for metric ton.

t Symbol for temperature (Celsius); tritium.

t_m Symbol for *temperature* midpoint (Celsius).

Ta Symbol for tantalum.

tabanid (tab′ă-nid) [L. *tabanus,* gadfly]. Common name for flies of the family Tabanidae.

Tabanidae (tă-ban′i-dē) [L. *tabanus,* gadfly]. A family of blood-sucking flies that includes the genera *Tabanus* (horsefly) and *Chrysops* (deerfly and mango fly), which are involved in transmission of several blood-borne parasites.

Tabanus (tă-bā′nŭs) [L. a gadfly]. The gadflies and horseflies; a genus of biting flies, some species of which transmit surra, infectious equine anemia, anthrax, and other diseases.

tabardillo (tah-bar-dē′yō). Mexican term for typhus.

tabatière anatomique (tab-ah-tē-ār′ an-ah-to-mēk′) [Fr. snuffbox]. Anatomical snuffbox.

tabella, pl. **tabellae** (tă-bel′lă, -lē) [L. dim. of *tabula,* tablet]. A medicated tablet or lozenge.

tabes (tā′bēz) [L. a wasting away]. Progressive wasting or emaciation.

t. diabet′ica, diabetic neuropathy, especially of the motor nerves of the lower extremities, marked by muscular atrophy and a steppage gait.

t. dorsa′lis, locomotor ataxia (2); posterior or posterior spinal sclerosis; t. spinalis; spinal atrophy; a chronic inflammation and progressive sclerosis of the posterior proximal spinal roots, the posterior columns of the spinal cord, and the peripheral nerves; the symptoms include ataxia, or muscular incoordination, anesthesia, neuralgia, lancinating pains, visceral crises, and muscular atrophy; atrophy of the optic nerve is not uncommon, trophic disorders of the joints (arthropathies) are frequent, and paralysis is a late symptom; the disease begins usually in middle life and is a tertiary form of syphilis.

t. ergot′ica, ataxia, amyotrophy, and neuralgic pain seen in ergot intoxication.

t. mesenter′ica, tuberculosis of the mesenteric and retroperitoneal lymph nodes.

peripheral t., pseudotabes.

t. spasmod′ica, spastic *diplegia.*

t. spina′lis, t. dorsalis.

tabescence (ta-bes′ens). The state of progressive wasting away.

tabescent (ta-bes′ent) [L. *tabesco,* to waste away, fr. *tabes,* a wasting away]. Characteristic of tabes.

tabetic (ta-bet′ik). Tabic; tabid; relating to or suffering from tabes, especially tabes dorsalis.

tabetiform (ta-bet′i-fōrm) [irreg. formed fr. L. *tabes,* a wasting, + *forma,* form]. Resembling tabes, especially tabes dorsalis.

tabic (tab′ik). Tabetic.

tab′id [L. *tabidus,* wasting away]. Tabetic.

tablature (tab-lă-chūr) [L. *tabula,* tablet]. The state of division of the cranial bones into two plates separated by the diploë.

table (tā′bl) [L. *tabula*]. **1.** One of the two plates or laminae, separated by the diploë, into which the cranial bones are divided. **2.** An arrangement of data in parallel columns, showing the essential facts in a readily appreciable form. **3.** A piece of furniture with a flat surface supported by legs.

Aub-DuBois t., t. of basal metabolic rates in calories per square meter of body surface per hour or day for different ages.

examining t., a t. on which the patient lies during a medical examination.

Gaffky t., Gaffky scale; a numerical rating for the classification of tuberculosis according to the number of tubercle bacilli in the sputum, ranging from 1 (one to four organisms in the whole preparation) to 9 (an average of 100 per field).

inner t. of skull, *lamina* interna cranii.

life t., a representation of the survivorship of a defined population of subjects; since survivorship is changed by new methods of prevention or treatment, a diachronic study is commonly used because the main interest lies in the composite structure of the current population.

occlusal t., the occlusal or grinding surfaces of the bicuspid and molar teeth.

operating t., a t. on which the patient lies during a surgical operation.

outer t. of skull, *lamina* externa cranii.

Reuss' color t.'s, Stilling color t.'s; charts in which colored letters are printed on colored backgrounds in such combination that some of them are invisible to a person with deficient color vision.

Stilling color t.'s, Reuss' color t.'s.

tilt t., a t. with a top capable of being rotated on its transverse axis so that a patient lying upon it can be brought into the erect position as desired; used in experimental investigation and in physical therapy.

vitreous t., the inner t. of one of the cranial bones; it is more compact and harder than the outer t.

tablespoon (tā′bl-spūn). A large spoon, used as a measure of the dose of a medicine, equivalent to about 4 fluidrams or $^1/_2$ fluidounce or 15 ml.

tab′let [Fr. *tablette,* L. *tabula*]. Tabule; a solid dosage form containing medicinal substances with or without suitable diluents; it may vary in shape, size, and weight, and may be classed according to the method of manufacture, as molded t. and compressed t.

buccal t., usually a small, flat t. intended to be inserted in the buccal pouch, where the active ingredient is absorbed directly through the oral mucosa; such a t. dissolves or erodes slowly.

compressed t., a t. prepared, usually as a large-scale production, by means of great pressure; most compressed t.'s consist of the active ingredient and a diluent, binder, disintegrator, and lubricant.

dispensing t., a t. prepared by molding or by compression; used by the dispensing pharmacist to obtain certain potent substances in a convenient form for accurate compounding.

enteric coated t., a t. with a coating that delays release of the medication until the t. has entered the intestine.

hypodermic t., a compressed or molded t. that dissolves completely in water (for injection) to form an injectable solution.

prolonged action t., repeat action t., sustained action t.

sublingual t., usually a small, flat t. intended to be inserted beneath the tongue, where the active ingredient is absorbed directly through the oral mucosa; such a t. dissolves very promptly.

sustained action t., sustained release t., prolonged or repeat action t.; a drug product formulation that provides the required dos-

age initially and then maintains or repeats it at desired intervals.
t. triturate, a small, usually cylindrical, molded or compressed disk of varying size, containing a diluent usually consisting of dextrose (glucose) or of a mixture of lactose and powdered sucrose and a moistening agent or excipient, such as dilute alcohol.

taboo, tabu (tă-bū') [Tongan, set apart]. Restricted, prohibited, or forbidden; set apart for religious or ceremonial purposes.

taboparesis (tā'bō-pă-rē'sis, -par'ē-sis). A condition in which the symptoms of tabes dorsalis and general paresis are associated.

tabular (tab'yū-lăr) [L. *tabularis*, fr. *tabula*, table]. **1.** Laminar; tablelike. **2.** Arranged in the form of a table (2).

tabule (tab'yūl) [L. *tabula*]. Tablet.

tabun (tä'bŭn). Dimethylphosphoramidocyanidic acid, ethyl ester; an extremely potent cholinesterase inhibitor; the lethal dose for man is believed to be as low as 0.01 mg per kg.

tache (tash) [Fr. spot]. A circumscribed discoloration of the skin or mucous membrane, such as a macule or freckle.
t. blanche, *macula* albida.
t. bleuâtre, *macula* cerulea.
t. cérébrale, meningitic *streak*.
t. laiteuse, **(1)** milk *spot;* **(2)** *macula* albida.
t. méningéale, meningitic *streak*.
t. noire, a necrotic area covered with black crust, characteristic of the tick bite lesion in certain tick-borne diseases.
t. spina'le, a trophic bulla forming on the skin in certain cases of disease of the spinal cord.

tachetic (tă-ket'ik) [Fr. *tache*, spot]. Marked by bluish or brownish spots.

tachistesthesia (tă-kis'tes-thē'zē-ă) [G. *tachistos*, very rapid, from *tachys*, rapid, + *aesthēsis*, perception]. Recognition of light flicker.

tachistoscope (tă-kis'tō-skōp) [G. *tachistos*, very rapid, fr. *tachys*, rapid, + *skopeō*, to view]. An instrument to determine the shortest time an object must be exposed in order to be perceived.

tachogram (tak'ō-gram) [G. *tachos*, speed, + *gramma*, mark]. Record made by a tachometer.

tachograph (tak'ō-graf) [G. *tachos*, speed, + *graphō*, to write]. A tachometer designed to provide a continuous record of speed or rate.

tachography (tă-kog'ră-fē) [G. *tachos*, speed, + *graphō*, to write]. The recording of speed or rate.

tachometer (tă-kom'ē-ter) [G. *tachos*, speed, + *metron*, measure]. An instrument for measuring speed or rate; *e.g.*, revolutions of a shaft, heart rate (cardiotachometer), arterial blood flow (hemotachometer), respiratory gas flow (pneumotachometer).

tachy- [G. *tachys*, quick, rapid]. Combining form denoting rapid.

tachyarrhythmia (tak'ē-ă-ridh'mē-ă) [tachy- + G. *a-* priv. + *rhythmos*, rhythm]. Any disturbance of the heart's rhythm, regular or irregular, resulting in a rate over 100 beats per minute.

tachyauxesis (tak'ē-awk-sē'sis) [tachy- + G. *auxō*, to increase]. Type of growth in which a part grows more rapidly than the whole.

tachycardia (tak'i-kar'dē-ă) [tachy- + G. *kardia*, heart]. Polycardia; tachyrhythmia; tachysystole; rapid beating of the heart, usually applied to rates over 100 per minute.
atrial t., auricular t.; paroxysmal t. originating in an ectopic focus in the atrium.
atrial chaotic t., multifocal origin of tachycardia within the atrium; often confused with atrial fibrillation.
atrioventricular (A-V) nodal t., nodal t.; t. originating in the A-V junction.
auricular t., atrial t.
bidirectional ventricular t., ventricular t. in which the QRS complexes in the electrocardiogram are alternately mainly positive and

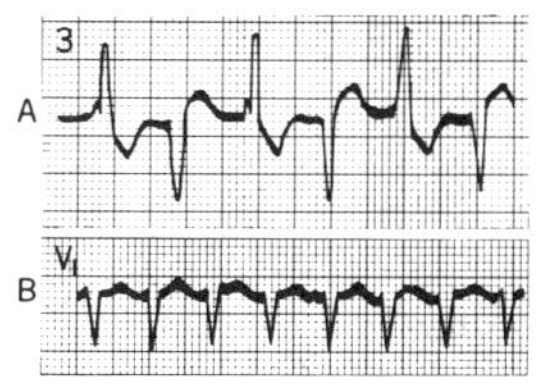

Tachycardia
A, bidirectional ventricular tachycardia; *B*, double tachycardia.

mainly negative; many such cases may represent A-V t. with alternating forms of aberrant ventricular conduction.
double t., the simultaneous t. of two ectopic t.'s, *e.g.*, atrial and A-V nodal t.
ectopic t., a t. originating in a focus other than the sinus node, *e.g.*, atrial, A-V nodal, or ventricular t.
t. en salves [Fr. *t. in salvos*], short runs of paroxysmal t. of the Gallavardin type. *Cf.* Gallavardin *phenomenon*.
essential t., persistent rapid action of the heart due to no discoverable organic lesion.
t. exophthal'mica, rapid heart action occurring as one of the symptoms of exophthalmic goiter.
fetal t., a fetal heart rate of 160 or more beats per minute.
nodal t., atrioventricular nodal t.
paroxysmal t., recurrent attacks of t., with abrupt onset and termination, originating from an ectopic focus which may be atrial, A-V nodal, or ventricular.
sinus t., t. originating in the sinus node.
ventricular t., paroxysmal t. originating in an ectopic focus in the ventricle. See also torsade de pointes.

tachycardiac (tak-i-kar'dē-ak). Relating to or suffering from excessively rapid action of the heart.

tachycrotic (tak'i-krot'ik) [tachy- + G. *krotos*, a striking]. Relating to, causing, or characterized by a rapid pulse.

tachykinin (tak-ē-kī'nin). Any member of a group of polypeptides, widely scattered in vertebrate and invertebrate tissues, that have in common four of the five terminal amino acids: Phe-Xaa-Gly-Leu-Met-NH_2; pharmacologically, they all cause hypotension in mammals, contraction of gut and bladder smooth muscle, and secretion of saliva.

tachylalia (tak-i-lā'lē-ă) [tachy- + G. *lalia*, talking]. Tachylogia.

tachylogia (tak-ĭ-lō'jē-ă) [tachy- + G. *logos*, word]. Rapid or voluble speech. Also called tachylalia, tachyphasia, tachyphemia, tachyphrasia.

tachypacing (tak'ĭ-pā'sing). Rapid pacing of the heart by an artificial electronic pacemaker operating faster than 100 beats per minute.

tachyphagia (tak-i-fā'jē-ă) [tachy- + G. *phagein*, to eat]. Rapid eating; bolting of food.

tachyphasia (tak-i-fā'zē-ă) [tachy- + G. *phasis*, speaking]. Tachylogia.

tachyphemia (tak-ĭ-fē'mē-ă) [tachy- + G. *phēme*, speech]. Tachylogia.

tachyphrasia (tak-ĭ-frā'zē-ă) [tachy- + G. *phrasis*, speaking]. Tachylogia.

tachyphylaxis (tak'i-fī-lak'sis) [tachy- + G. *phylaxis*, protection]. Rapid appearance of progressive decrease in response following repetitive administration of a pharmacologically or physiologically active substance.

tachypnea (tak-ip-nē'ă) [tachy- + G. *pnoē* (*pnoiē*), breathing]. Polypnea; rapid breathing.

tachyrhythmia (tak-i-ridh'mē-ă) [tachy- + G. *rhythmos,* rhythm]. Tachycardia.

tachysterol (tă-kis'ter-ōl). Sterol(s) formed by ultraviolet irradiation of any 5,7-diene-3β-sterol, which breaks the 9,10 bond, but usually from either or both of ergosterol and lumisterol to produce t.$_2$ (ertacalciol, (6*E*,22*E*)-9,10-secoergosta-5(10),6,8,22-tetraen-3β-ol) and from 7-dehydrocholesterol to produce t.$_3$ (tacalciol,(6*E*)-(3*S*)-9,10-secocholesta-5(10),6,8-trien-3β-ol). When reduced to the 5,7-diene (or 5,7,22-triene) form, dihydrotachysterol$_3$ (10,19-dihydrocalciol) or dihydrotachysterol$_2$ (10,19-dihydroercalciol), antirachitic action appears. This property has been of therapeutic interest, but t. is being replaced by the true vitamin D hormone (calcitriol) and its derivatives.

tachysystole (tak-i-sis'tō-lē) [tachy- + G. *systolē,* contracting]. Tachycardia.

tachyzoite (tak-ĭ-zō'īt) [tachy- + G. *zōon,* animal]. A rapidly multiplying stage in the development of the tissue phase of certain coccidial infections, as in *Toxoplasma gondii* development in acute infections of toxoplasmosis.

tacrine (tak'rēn). 9-Amino-1,2,3,4-tetrahydroacridine; an anticholinesterase agent with nonspecific central nervous system stimulatory effects.

tactile (tak'til) [L. *tactilis,* fr. *tango,* pp. *tactus,* to touch]. Relating to touch or to the sense of touch.

taction (tak'shŭn) [L. *tactio,* fr. *tango,* pp. *tactus,* to touch]. **1.** The sense of touch. **2.** The act of touching.

tactometer (tak-tom'ĕ-ter) [L. *tactus,* touch, + G. *metron,* measure]. Esthesiometer.

tactor (tak'tăr, -tōr) [L. one who or that which touches]. A tactile end organ.

tactual (tak'chūl). Relating to or caused by touch.

TAD Acronym for transient acantholytic *dermatosis.*

Taenia (tē'nē-ă) [see taenia]. A genus of cestodes that formerly included most of the tapeworms, but is now restricted to those species infecting carnivores with cysticercus found in tissues of various herbivores, rodents, and other animals of prey. See also tapeworm.
T. africa'na, a tapeworm found in native Africans, the cysticercus of which is unknown.
T. arma'ta, *T. solium.*
T. crassic'ollis, *T. taeniformis.*
T. demerarien'sis, former name for *Davainea madagascariensis.*
T. denta'ta, *T. solium.*
T. equi'na, *Anoplocephala perfoliata.*
T. hom'inis, unusual form of *T. saginata.*

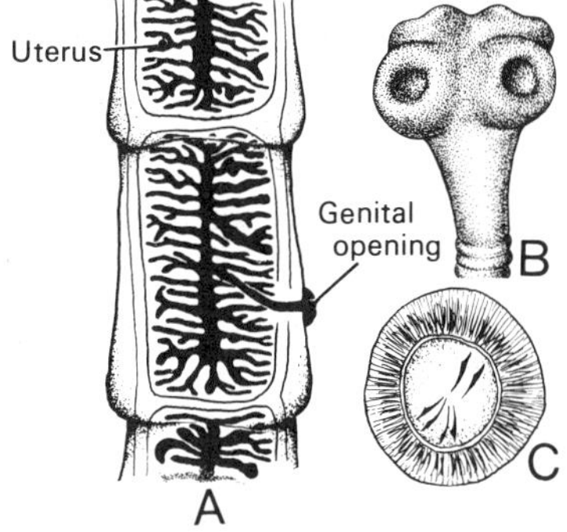

***Taenia saginata,* the beef tapeworm**
*A,*proglottid or body segment showing reproductive organs (X1.7); *B,*scolex (X12); *C,*egg (X550).

T. hydatig'ena, a tapeworm of dogs, cats, wolves, foxes, and other carnivores; the larva is known as *Cysticercus tenuicollis.*
T. madagascarien'sis, former name for *Davainea madagascariensis.*
T. min'ima, former name for *Hymenolepis nana.*
t. o'vis, a tapeworm of dogs and foxes whose larval form is found in the muscles of sheep; heavy larval infections in sheep can have severe economic consequences due to condemnation of carcasses at meat inspection.
T. philippi'na, atypical form of *T. saginata.*
T. pisifor'mis, a common tapeworm of dogs, foxes, and other carnivores; the larval form is *Cysticercus pisiformis.*
T. quadriloba'ta, *Anoplocephala perfoliata.*
T. sagina'ta, the beef, hookless, or unarmed tapeworm of man, acquired by eating insufficiently cooked flesh of cattle infected with *Cysticercus bovis.*
T. so'lium, *T. armata; T. dentata;* the pork, armed, or solitary tapeworm of man, acquired by eating insufficiently cooked pork infected with *Cysticercus cellulosae;* hatching of ova within the human intestine may result in establishment of cysticerci in human tissues, resulting in cysticercosis.

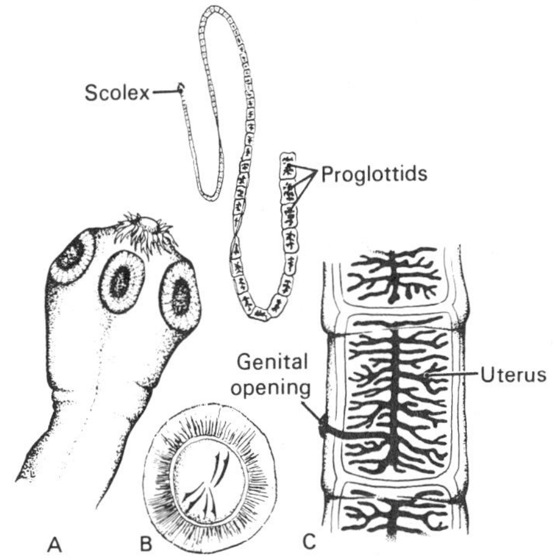

***Taenia solium,* the pork tapeworm**
A, enlarged scolex (X18); *B.,*egg (X375); *C,*enlarged proglottid (X1.5).

T. taeniaefor'mis, *Hydatigera taeniaeformis; T. crassicollis;* one of the common tapeworms of household cats; the larval form is called *Cysticercus fasciolaris.*

taenia (tē'nē-ă) [L., fr. G. *tainia,* band, tape, a tapeworm]. **1.** A coiled bandlike anatomical structure. See tenia (1). **2.** Tenia (2); common name for a tapeworm, especially of the genus *Taenia.*

Taeniarhynchus (tē'nē-ă-ring'kŭs) [G. *tainia,* band, + *rhynchos,* snout]. A genus established for the *Taenia* species having a rudimentary rostellum but lacking the rostellar hooklets typical of *Taenia.* The best known example is *Taeniarhynchus saginatus,* but the older name, *Taenia saginata,* is more commonly used.

taeniasis (tē-nē-ī'ă-sis). Infection with cestodes of the genus *Taenia.*

taeniid (tē-nē'id). Common name for a member of the family Taeniidae.

Taeniidae (tē-nē'i-dē). A family of parasitic cestodes (order Cyclophyllidea) that includes the genera *Taenia, Taeniarhynchus, Multiceps,* and *Echinococcus.*

taenioid (tē'nē-oyd). Denoting members of the genus *Taenia.*

Taeniorhynchus (tē-nē-ō-ring'kŭs) [G. *tainia,* band, + *rhynchos,* snout]. A genus and subgenus of mosquitoes now considered synonymous with *Mansonia.*

Taenzer, Paul R., German dermatologist, 1858–1919. See T.'s *stain,* Unna-T. *stain.*

TAF Abbreviation for tumor angiogenic *factor.*

tag. 1. Label; to incorporate into a compound a substance that is readily detected, such as a radioactive isotope, whereby its metabolic or chemical history can be followed. **2.** The substance so incorporated. See also tracer. **3.** A small outgrowth or polyp.

anal skin t., a fibrous polyp of the anus.

sentinel t., projecting edematous skin at the lower end of an anal fissure.

skin t., acrochordon; fibroma molle; soft wart; senile fibroma; fibroepithelial papilloma; a polypoid outgrowth of both epidermis and dermal fibrovascular tissue.

tagatose (tag'ă-tōs). A ketohexose isomeric with fructose. For structure, see sugars.

tagliacotian (tal-yah-cō'shē-an). Pertaining to or described by Tagliacozzi.

Tagliacozzi, Gasparo, Italian surgeon, 1546–1599. See tagliacotian *operation.*

tail (tāl) [A.S. *taegl*]. Cauda.

t. of caudate nucleus, *cauda* nuclei caudati.

t. of dentate gyrus, uncus *band* of Giacomini.

t. of epididymis, *cauda* epididymidis.

t. of helix, *cauda* helicis.

t. of pancreas, *cauda* pancreatis.

tailgut (tāl'gŭt). Postanal *gut.*

Tait, Robert L., British gynecologist, 1845–1899. See T.'s *law.*

Takahara, Shigeo, 20th century Japanese otolaryngologist. See T.'s *disease.*

Takayama, Masao, Japanese physician, *1871. See T.'s *stain.*

Takayasu (Takayashu), Michishige, Japanese ophthalmologist, *1872. See T.'s *disease, syndrome.*

take (tāk). A successful grafting operation or vaccination.

talalgia (tă-lal'jē-ă) [L. *talus,* heel, + G. *algos,* pain]. Pain in the heel.

talar (tā'lăr). Relating to the talus.

Talbot, William Henry Fox, British scientist, 1800–1877. See Plateau-T. *law.*

talbutal (tal'byū-tăl). 5-Allyl-5-*sec*-butylbarbituric acid; a short-acting hypnotic and sedative.

talc (tălk) [Ar. *talq*]. Talcum; soapstone; French chalk; native hydrous magnesium silicate, sometimes containing small proportions of aluminum silicate, purified by boiling powdered t. with hydrochloric acid in water; used in pharmacy as a filter aid, as a dusting powder, and in cosmetic preparations.

talcosis (tal-kō'sis). A pulmonary disorder related to silicosis, occurring in workers exposed to talc mixed with silicates; characterized by restrictive or obstructive disorders of breathing or the two in combination.

talcum (tal'kŭm) [L.]. Talc.

talion (tal'ē-on, tal'yŭn) [Welsh *tal,* compensation]. The principle of retribution in intrapsychic behavior.

talion dread. The symbolic anxieties that represent the unconscious dread of penalties for an act.

talipedic (tal-i-ped'ik). Clubfooted.

talipes (tal'i-pēz) [L. *talus,* heel, ankle, + *pes,* foot]. Pes (4); any deformity of the foot involving the talus.

t. arcua'tus, t. cavus.

t. calcaneoval'gus, t. calcaneus and t. valgus combined; the foot is dorsiflexed, everted, and abducted.

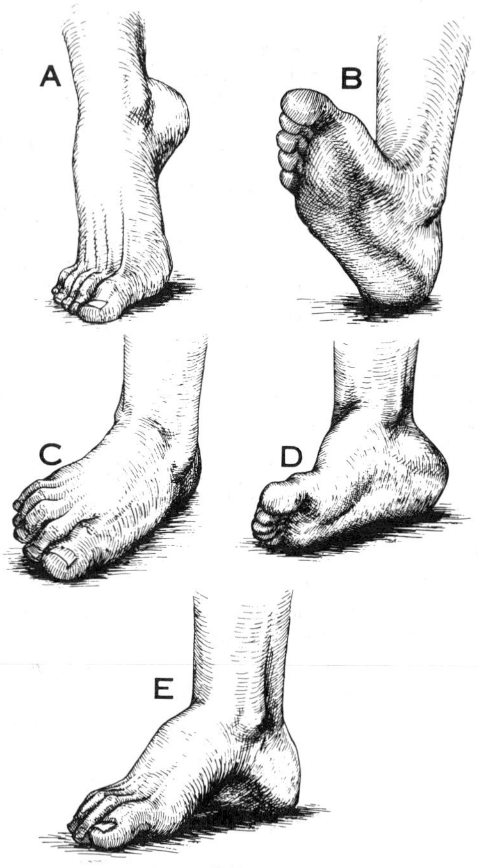

Talipes
A, equinus; *B,* calcaneus; *C,* valgus; *D,* varus; *E.* cavus.

t. calcaneova'rus, t. calcaneus and t. varus combined; the foot is dorsiflexed, inverted, and adducted.

t. calca'neus, calcaneus (2); a deformity due to weakness or absence of the calf muscles, in which the axis of the calcaneus becomes vertically oriented; commonly seen in poliomyelitis.

t. ca'vus, contracted foot (1); t. arcuatus or plantaris; pes cavus; an exaggeration of the normal arch of the foot.

t. equinoval'gus, equinovalgus; pes equinovalgus; t. equinus and t. valgus combined; the foot is plantarflexed, everted, and abducted.

t. equinova'rus, clubfoot; equinovarus; reel foot; pes equinovarus; t. equinus and t. varus combined; the foot is plantarflexed, inverted, and adducted.

t. equi'nus, permanent extension of the foot so that only the ball rests on the ground; it is commonly combined with t. varus.

t. planta'ris, t. cavus.

t. pla'nus, flatfoot; splayfoot; pes planus; a condition in which the arch of the foot is broken down, the entire sole touching the ground.

t. spasmod'icus, a temporary distortion of the foot, usually t. equinus, due to muscular spasm.

t. transversopla'nus, *metatarsus* latus.

t. val'gus, pes pronatus, valgus, or abductus; permanent eversion of the foot, the inner side alone of the sole resting on the ground; it is usually combined with a breaking down of the plantar arch.

t. va'rus, pes adductus or varus; inversion of the foot, the outer side of the sole only touching the ground; usually some degree of t. equinus is associated with it, and often t. cavus.

talipomanus (tal-ĭ-pom'ă-nŭs, -pō-mā'nŭs) [Mod. L. *talipes* + *manus,* hand]. Clubhand; a fixed deformity of the hand, either congenital or acquired. The spatial relationship of the hand to the forearm determines the names of the conditions. See subentries under manus.

Tallerman, Lewis A., 19th century British inventor. See T. *apparatus.*

tallow (tal'ō). The rendered fat from mutton suet.
prepared mutton t., prepared *suet.*

Talma, Sape, Dutch physician, 1847–1918. See T.'s *disease.*

talo- [L. *talus,* ankle, ankle bone]. Combining form denoting the talus.

talocalcaneal, talocalcanean (tā-lō-kal-kā'nē-ăl, tā-lō-kal-kā'nē-an). Relating to the talus and the calcaneus.

talocrural (tā'lō-krū'răl). Relating to the talus and the bones of the leg; denoting the ankle joint.

talofibular (tā'lō-fib'yū-lăr). Relating to the talus and the fibula.

tal'on [Mediev. L. *talo,* claw of a bird]. The caudally directed digit on the foot, particularly of a bird of prey.

talonavicular (tā'lō-nă-vik'yū-lăr). Taloscaphoid; astragaloscaphoid; relating to the talus and the navicular bone.

taloscaphoid (tā'lō-skaf'oyd). Talonavicular.

talose (tal'ōs). An aldohexose, isomeric with glucose.

talotibial (tā'lō-tib'ē-ăl). Relating to the talus and the tibia.

talus, gen. **tali** (tā'lŭs, -lī) [L. ankle bone, heel] [NA]. Ankle bone; ankle (3); astragalus; the bone of the foot that articulates with the tibia and fibula to form the ankle joint.

tamarind (tam'ă-rind) [Mediev. L. fr. Ar. *tamr*]. The pulp of the fruit of *Tamarindus indica* (family Leguminosae), a large tree of India; mildly laxative.

tambour (tahm-bur') [Fr. drum]. The recording part of a graphic apparatus, such as a sphygmograph, consisting of a membrane stretched across the open end of a cylinder and the recording stile attached to it.

Tamm, Igor, U.S. virologist, *1922. See T.-Horsfall *mucoprotein, protein.*

tamoxifen citrate (tă-mok'si-fen). (*Z*)-2-[*p*-(1,2-Diphenyl-1-butenyl)phenoxy]-*N,N*-dimethylethylamine citrate (1:1); an antiestrogen agent used in the palliative treatment of advanced breast cancer.

tam'pon [O. Fr.]. **1.** A cylinder or ball of cotton-wool, gauze, or other loose substance; used as a plug or pack in a canal or cavity to restrain hemorrhage, absorb secretions, or maintain a displaced organ in position. **2.** To insert such a plug or pack.
Corner's t., a plug of omentum stuffed into a wound of the stomach or intestine as a temporary t.

tamponade, tamponage (tam-pŏ-nād', tam'pŏ-nij). The insertion of a tampon.
cardiac t., compression of venous return to the heart due to increased volume of fluid in the pericardium.

tamponing, tamponment (tam'pon-ing, tam-pon'ment). The act of inserting a tampon.

tanacetol, tanacetone (ta-nās'tol, tan-ă-sē'tōn). Thujone.

tangentiality (tan-jen'shē-al'i-tē) [L. *tangeno,* to touch, take away]. A disturbance in the associative thought process in which one tends to digress readily from one topic under discussion to other topics which arise in the course of associations; observed in schizophrenia and certain types of organic brain disorders. *Cf.* circumstantiality.

tannase (tan'ās) [EC 3.1.1.20]. Tannin acyl-hydrolase; an enzyme produced in cultures of *Penicillium glaucum* and found in certain tannin-forming plants; it hydrolyzes digallate to gallate, and also acts on ester links in other tannins.

tannate (tan'āt). A salt of tannic acid.

Tanner growth chart, Tanner stage. See under chart; stage.

tannic (tan'ik). Relating to tan (tan-bark) or to tannin.

tannic acid. A tannin, $C_{76}H_{52}O_{46}$, that occurs in many plants, particularly in the bark of oaks and other members of the Fagaceae; used as a styptic and astringent, and in the treatment of diarrhea; available also as tannic acid glycerite. Sometimes used synonymously with tannin.

tannin (tan'in). Any one of a group of complex nonuniform plant constituents that can be classified into hydrolyzable t.'s (esters of a sugar, usually glucose, and one or several trihydroxybenzenecarboxylic acids) and condensed t.'s (derivatives of flavonols). T.'s are used in tanning, dyeing, photography, and as clarifying agents for beer and wine. Sometimes used synonymously with tannic acid.

tannylacetate (tan-il-as'ē-tāt). Acetyltannic acid.

tantalum (tan'tă-lŭm) [mythical king *Tantalus*]. A heavy metal of the vanadium group, symbol Ta, atomic no. 73, atomic weight 180.95; used in surgical prostheses because of its noncorrosive properties.

tantrum (tan'trŭm). A fit of bad temper, especially in children.

tanycyte (tan'i-sīt). A variety of ependymal cell found principally in the walls of the third ventricle of the brain; the t.'s may have branched or unbranched processes, some of which end on capillaries or neurons.

tanyphonia (tan-i-fō'nē-ă) [G. *tanyō,* to stretch, + *phonē,* sound]. A thin, weak voice resulting from tension of vocal muscles.

tap. 1. To withdraw fluid from a cavity by means of a trocar and cannula, hollow needle, or catheter. **2.** To strike lightly with the finger or a hammerlike instrument in percussion or to elicit a tendon reflex. **3.** A light blow. **4.** An East Indian fever of undetermined nature. **5.** An instrument to cut threads in a hole in bone prior to inserting a screw.
heel t., a reflex movement of the toes when the heel is tapped, present in multiple sclerosis and other diseases of the pyramidal tract.
mitral t., the palpable equivalent of the opening snap of the mitral valve.
spinal t., lumbar *puncture.*

tape (tāp). A thin flat strip of fascia or tendon, or of synthetic material, used as a tie or suture.
adhesive t., fabric or film evenly coated on one side with a pressure-sensitive adhesive mixture.

tapetochoroidal (tă-pē'tō-kō-roy'dăl). Relating to the tapetum and the choroid.

tapetoretinal (tă-pē'tō-ret'i-năl). Relating to the retinal pigment epithelium and the sensory retina.

tapetoretinopathy (tă-pē'tō-ret-in-op'ă-thē) [tapetum + retinopathy]. Hereditary degeneration of the sensory retina and pigmentary epithelium; seen in pigmentary retinopathy, choroideremia, gyrate atrophy, congenital nyctalopia, congenital amaurosis, and heredomacular degeneration.

tapetum, pl. **tapeta** (tă-pē'tŭm, -tă) [L. *tapēte,* a carpet]. **1.** In general, any membranous layer or covering. **2.** Membrana versicolor; Fielding's membrane; in neuroanatomy, a thin sheet of fibers in the lateral wall of the temporal and occipital horns of the lateral ventricle, continuous with the corpus callosum. **3.** A dense layer in the choroidea of the eye of many mammalian species, including the cat and dog but not man, that forms a discrete or diffuse area of reflective cells, rodlets, and fibers; its strong light-reflecting properties cause the metallic hue and light-glow of such eyes in the dark.
t. alve'oli, periodontal *ligament.*
t. ni'grum, *stratum* pigmenti retinae.

t. oc'uli, *stratum* pigmenti retinae.

tapeworm (tāp'werm). An intestinal parasitic worm, adults of which are found in the intestine of vertebrates; the term is commonly restricted to members of the class Cestoidea. T.'s consist of a scolex, variously equipped with spined or sucking structures by which the worm is attached to the intestinal wall of the host, and strobila having several to many proglottids that lack a digestive tract at any stage of development. The ovum, entering the intestine of an appropriate intermediate host, hatches and the hexacanth penetrates the gut wall and develops into a specific larval form (*e.g.,* cysticercoid, cysticercus, hydatid, strobilocercus), which develops into an adult when the intermediate host is ingested by the proper final host. A three-host cycle with a swimming coracidium, procercoid and plerocercoid (sparganum) larva, and adult intestinal worm is found in aquatic life cycles, as in *Diphyllobothrium latum* (broad fish t.) and other pseudophyllid cestodes. Other important species of t. are *Echinococcus granulosus* (hydatid t.), *Hymenolepis nana* or *H. nana* var. *fraterna* (dwarf or dwarf mouse t.), *Taenia saginata* (beef, hookless, or unarmed t.), *T. solium* (armed, pork, or solitary t.), and *Thysanosoma actinoides* (fringed t. of sheep).

taphophilia (taf-ō-fil'ē-ă) [G. *taphos,* grave, + *phileō,* to love]. Morbid attraction for graves.

taphophobia (taf-ō-fō'bē-ă) [G. *taphos,* the grave, + *phobos,* fear]. Morbid fear of being buried alive.

Tapia, Antonio, Spanish otolaryngologist, 1875–1950. See T.'s *syndrome.*

tapinocephalic (tap'i-nō-sĕ-fal'ik, tă-pī'nō-). Having a low flat head; relating to tapinocephaly.

tapinocephaly (tă-pi-nō-sef'ă-lē) [G. *tapeinos,* low, + *kephalē,* head]. A condition of flat head in which the skull has a vertical index below 72; similar to chamecephaly.

tapioca (tap'ē-ō'kă) [Braz. *tipioca*]. Cassava starch; a starch from the root of *Janipha manihot* and other species of *J.* (family Euphorbiaceae), plants of tropical America; an easily digested starch, free of irritant properties.

tapiroid (tā'pir-oyd) [tapir + G. *eidos,* resemblance]. Resembling a tapir's snout; sometimes applied to an elongated cervix uteri.

tapotement (tă-pot-mawn') [Fr. fr. *tapoter,* to tap]. Tapping (1); a massage movement consisting in striking with the side of the hand, usually with partly flexed fingers.

tapping (tap'ing). **1.** Tapotement. **2.** Paracentesis.

TAR Acronym for thrombocytopenia and absent radius. See thrombocytopenia-absent radius *syndrome.*

tar. A thick, semisolid, blackish brown mass, of complex hydrocarbon composition, obtained by the destructive distillation of carbonaceous materials. For individual t.'s, see specific names.

rectified t. oil, a volatile oil distilled from pine t.; used externally in the treatment of skin diseases such as eczema and psoriasis.

tarantism (tar'an-tizm). A form of mass hysteria which originated in Taranto, Italy, in the late Middle Ages as a dancing mania to cure the madness allegedly caused by the bite of a tarantula.

tarantula (tă-ran'chū-lă) [see tarantism]. A very large, hairy spider, considered highly venomous and often greatly feared; the bite, however, is usually no more harmful than a bee sting, and the creature is relatively inoffensive.

American t., *Eurypelma hentzii,* the Arkansas t.; although greatly feared, its bite is relatively uncommon and harmless to man.

black t., *Sericopelma communis,* a large black t. of Panama and the Canal Zone, whose bite is poisonous, although the effect is localized.

European t., *Lycosa tarentula,* the large European wolf spider or true t. Its bite was once believed to cause madness, which inspired frenzied contortions and dancing to rid the body of the venom, though the bite is, in fact, harmless, as is that of most of the large, hairy "tarantula spiders" of the tropics.

Peruvian t., Pruning spider; *Glyptocranium gasteracanthoides,* a poisonous Peruvian spider whose bite causes local gangrene, hematuria, and neurotoxic symptoms.

taraxacum (tă-rak'să-kŭm) [Mod. L. fr. Ar. *tarakshagūn,* wild chicory]. The dried rhizome and root of *Taraxacum officinale* (family compositae), the dandelion, a wild plant of wide distribution throughout the temperate regions of the northern hemisphere; a tonic and hepatic stimulant.

Tardieu, Auguste A., French physician, 1818–1879. See T.'s *ecchymoses, petechiae, spots.*

tardive (tar'div). Late; tardy.

target (tar'get) [It. *targhetta,* a small shield]. **1.** An object fixed as goal or point of examination. **2.** In the ophthalmometer, the mire. **3.** Target *organ.* **4.** Anode of an x-ray tube. See also x-ray.

Tarin (Tarini, Tarinus), Pierre, French anatomist, 1725–1761. See T.'s *space, tenia, valve; valvula* semilunaris tarini; *velum* tarini.

tariric acid (tă-rī'rik). An 18-carbon acid, $CH_3(CH_2)_{10}C{\equiv}C(CH_2)_4COOH$, notable for the presence of a triple bond.

Tarlov, Isadore Max, U. S. surgeon, *1905. See T.'s *cyst.*

Tarnier, Étienne Stephane, French obstetrician, 1828–1897. See T.'s *forceps.*

tarragon oil (tar'ă-gon). Estragon oil; a volatile oil distilled from the leaves of *Artemisia dranculus* (family Compositae); a flavoring.

tars-. See tarso-.

tarsadenitis (tar'sad-ĕ-nī'tis) [tarsus + G. *adēn,* gland, + *-itis,* inflammation]. Inflammation of the tarsal borders of the eyelids and meibomian glands.

tarsal (tar'săl). Relating to a tarsus in any sense.

tarsale, pl. **tarsalia** (tar-sā'lē, tar-sā'lē-ă) [Mod. L. fr. G. *tarsos,* sole of the foot]. Any tarsal bone.

tarsalgia (tar-sal'jē-ă) [tarsus + G. *algos,* pain]. Podalgia.

tarsalis (tar-sā'lis). See entries under musculus.

tarsectomy (tar-sek'tō-mē) [tarsus + G. *ektomē,* excision]. Excision of the tarsus of the foot or of a segment of the tarsus of an eyelid.

tarsectopia, tarsectopy (tar-sek-tō'pē-ă, -sek'tō-pē) [tarsus + G. *ektopos,* out of place]. Subluxation of one or more tarsal bones.

tar'sen [tarsus + G. *en,* in]. Within the tarsus; relating to the tarsus independent of other structures.

tarsitis (tar-sī'tis). **1.** Inflammation of the tarsus of the foot. **2.** Inflammation of the tarsal border of an eyelid.

tarso-, tars- [See tarsus]. Combining forms relating to a tarsus.

tarsochiloplasty (tar-sō-kī'lō-plas-tē) [tarso- + G. *cheilos,* lip, + *plassō,* to form]. Blepharoplasty of the tarsal margin of the eyelid.

tarsoclasia, tarsoclasis (tar-sō-klā'zē-ă, tar-sok'lă-sis) [tarso- + G. *klasis,* a breaking]. Instrumental fracture of the tarsus, for the correction of talipes equinovarus.

tarsomalacia (tar'sō-mă-lā'shē-ă) [tarso- + G. *malakia,* softness]. Softening of the tarsal cartilages of the eyelids.

tarsomegaly (tar-sō-meg'ă-lē) [tarso- + G. *megas,* large]. Dysplasia epiphysialis hemimelia; a congenital maldevelopment and overgrowth of a tarsal or carpal bone.

tarsometatarsal (tar-sō-met'ă-tar'săl). Relating to the tarsal and metatarsal bones; denoting the articulations between the two sets of bones, and the ligaments in relation thereto.

tarsometatarsus (tar'sō-met-ă-tar'sŭs). The lowermost long bone or shank in the leg of a bird; the distal tarsal elements fuse with the metatarsals, resulting in a compound bone unlike that in mammals.

tarso-orbital (tar'sō-ōr'bi-tăl). Relating to the eyelids and the orbit.

tarsophalangeal (tar-sō-fă-lan′jē-ăl). Relating to the tarsus and the phalanges.

tarsophyma (tar-sō-fī′mă) [tarso- + G. *phyma,* a tumor, boil]. A tarsal tumor.

tarsorrhaphy (tar-sōr′ă-fē) [tarso- + G. *rhaphē,* suture]. Blepharorrhaphy; the suturing together of the eyelid margins, partially or completely, to shorten the palpebral fissure or to protect the cornea in keratitis or in paralysis of the orbicularis oculi muscle.

tarsotarsal (tar′sō-tar′săl). Mediotarsal.

tarsotibial (tar′sō-tib′ē-al). Tibiotarsal; relating to the tarsal bones and the tibia.

tarsotomy (tar-sot′ō-mē) [tarso- + G. *tomē,* incision]. **1.** Incision of the tarsal cartilage of an eyelid. **2.** Any operation on the tarsus of the foot.

tarsus, gen. and pl. **tarsi** (tar′sŭs, -sī) [G. *tarsos,* a flat surface, sole of the foot, edge of eyelid] [NA]. **1.** Root of foot; as a division of the skeleton, the seven bones of the instep: talus, calcaneus, navicular, three cuneiform (wedge), and cuboid bones. **2.** The fibrous plates giving solidity and form to the edges of the eyelids; often erroneously called tarsal or ciliary cartilages.
t. infe′rior [NA], the fibrous plate in the lower eyelid.
t. supe′rior [NA], the fibrous plate in the upper eyelid.

tartar (tar′tăr). [Mediev. L. *tartarum,* ult. etym. unknown]. **1.** A crust on the interior of wine casks, consisting essentially of potassium bitartrate. **2.** Dental calculus; a white, brown, or yellow-brown deposit at or below the gingival margin of teeth, chiefly hydroxyapatite in an organic matrix.
cream of t., *postassium* bitartrate.
t. emetic, *antimony* potassium tartrate.
soluble t., *potassium* tartrate.

tartaric acid (tar-tar′ik). Dihydroxysuccinic acid; HOOC–CHOH–CHOH–COOH; made from crude tartar; a laxative and refrigerant; used in the manufacture of various effervescing powders, tablets, and granules.

tartrate (tar′trāt). A salt of tartaric acid.
acid t., a salt of tartaric acid which contains an acid group still capable of combining with a base; *e.g.,* bitartrate.
normal t., t. that contains no uncombined acid groups.

tartrated (tar′trāt-ed). Combined with or containing tartar or tartaric acid.

tartrazine (tar′tră-zēn) [C.I. 19140]. Hydrazine yellow; a yellow acid dye, $C_{16}H_9N_4O_9S_2Na_3$, used in place of orange G in a variant of Mallory's aniline blue stain for collagen and cellular inclusion bodies.

taste (tāst) [It. *tastare;* L. *tango,* to touch]. **1.** To perceive through the medium of the gustatory nerves. **2.** The sensation produced by a suitable stimulus applied to the gustatory nerve endings in the tongue.
after-t., see aftertaste.
color t., pseudogeusesthesia; a form of synesthesia in which the color sense and t. are associated, with stimulation of either sense inducing a subjective sensation in the associated sense.
franklinic t., voltaic t.; a metallic or sour t. produced by the application of static electricity to the tongue.
voltaic t., franklinic t.

TAT Abbreviation for thematic apperception *test.*

tattoo (tă-tū′) [Tahiti, *tatu*]. **1.** A tinctorial and pictorial effect of deliberate (and occasionally accidental) implanting or injecting of indelible pigments into the skin. **2.** To produce such an effect.
amalgam t., a bluish-black or gray macular lesion of the oral mucous membrane caused by accidental implantation of silver amalgam into the tissue during tooth restoration or extraction.

taurine (taw′rin, -rēn). A crystallizable substance, $NH_2CH_2CH_2SO_3H$, formed by the decomposition of taurocholic acid.

taurocholate (taw-rō-kō′lāt). A salt of taurocholic acid.

taurocholic acid (taw-rō-kō′lik). Cholaic acid; cholyltaurine; *N*-choloyltaurine; a compound of cholic acid and taurine, involving the –COOH group of the former and the NH_2– of the latter; a common bile salt in carnivores.

taurodontism (taw-rō-don′tizm) [L. *taurus,* bull, + G. *odous,* tooth]. A developmental anomaly involving molar teeth in which the bifurcation or trifurcation of the roots is very near the apex, resulting in an abnormally large and long pulp chamber with exceedingly short pulp canals.

Taussig, Helen B., U.S. pediatrician, *1898. See T.-Bing *disease, syndrome;* Blalock-T. *operation.*

tautomenial (taw-tō-mē′nē-ăl) [G. *tautos,* the same, + *mēn,* month]. Relating to the same menstrual period.

tautomeric (taw-tō-mer′ik) [G. *tautos,* the same, + *meros,* part]. **1.** Relating to the same part. **2.** Relating to or marked by tautomerism.

tautomerism (taw-tom′er-izm) [G. *tautos,* the same, + *meros,* part]. A phenomenon in which a chemical compound exists in two forms of different structure (isomers) in equilibrium, the two forms differing, usually, in the position of a hydrogen atom; *e.g.,* keto-enol t., $R{-}CH_2{-}C(O){-}R' \rightleftarrows R{-}CH{=}C(OH){-}R'$.

Tawara, K. Sunao, Japanese pathologist, 1873–1952. See T.'s *node;* His-T. *system; node* of Aschoff and T.

taxa (tak′să). Plural of taxon.

taxis (tak′sis) [G. orderly arrangement]. **1.** Reduction of a hernia or of a dislocation of any part by means of manipulation. **2.** Systematic classification or orderly arrangement. **3.** The reaction of protoplasm to a stimulus, by virtue of which animals and plants are led to move or act in certain definite ways in relation to their environment; the various kinds of t. are designated by a prefix denoting the stimulus governing them; *e.g.,* chemotaxis, electrotaxis, thermotaxis.
bipolar t., repositioning of a retroverted uterus by making traction on the cervix in the vagina, and pushing up the fundus by the finger in the rectum.
negative t., the repulsion of protoplasm away from a stimulus.
positive t., the attraction of protoplasm toward a stimulus.

taxon, pl. **taxa** (tak′son, tak′să). The name given to a particular level or grouping in a systematic classification of living things or organisms (taxonomy).

taxonomic (tak-sō-nom′ik). Relating to taxonomy.

taxonomy (tak-sawn′ō-mē) [G. *taxis,* orderly arrangement, + *nomos,* law]. The systematic classification of living things or organisms. Kingdoms of living organisms are divided into groups (taxa) to show degrees of similarity or presumed evolutionary relationships, with the higher categories being larger, more inclusive, and more broadly defined, the lower categories being more restricted, with fewer species more closely related. The divisions below kingdom are, in descending order: phylum, class, order, family, genus, species, and subspecies (variety). Infra- and supra- or sub- and super- categories can be used when needed; additional categories, such as tribe, section, level, group, etc., are also used.
numerical t., an approach to the classification of organisms that strives for objectivity, wherein characters of organisms are given equal weight (adansonian classification) and the relationships of the organisms are numerically determined, usually with the aid of a computer.

Tay, Warren, British physician, 1843–1927. See T.'s cherry red *spot;* T.-Sachs *disease.*

Taybi, Hooshang, U.S. pediatrician and radiologist, *1919. See Rubinstein-T. *syndrome.*

Taylor, Charles F., U.S. orthopedic surgeon, 1827–1899. See T.'s back *brace, apparatus, splint.*

Taylor, Robert W., U.S. dermatologist, 1842–1908. See T.'s *disease.*

TB Colloquial abbreviation for tuberculosis.

Tb Symbol for terbium.

TBG Abbreviation for thyroxine-binding *globulin.*

TBP Abbreviation for thyroxine-binding *protein.*

TBV Abbreviation for total blood volume.

Tc Symbol for technetium.

2,3,7,8-TCDD Abbreviation for 2,3,7,8-tetrachlorodibenzo[*b,e*]-[1,4]dioxin. See dioxin (3).

TCG Abbreviation for time compensation *gain.*

$TCID_{50}$, TCD_{50} Abbreviation for tissue culture infectious *dose.*

TDP Abbreviation for ribothymidine 5′-diphosphate. The thymidine analogue is dTDP.

Te **1.** In electrodiagnosis, abbreviation denoting tetanic contraction. **2.** Symbol for tellurium.

tea (tē) [Chinese (Amoy dial.) *t'e,* Mod. L. *thea*]. **1.** The dried leaves of various genera of the family Theaceae, including *Thea* (*T. senensis*), *Camellia,* and *Gordonia,* a shrub indigenous to China, southern and southeastern Asia, and Japan. Its chief constituent, upon which its stimulating action largely depends, is the alkaloid caffeine, which is present in the amount of 1% to 4%. **2.** The infusion made by pouring boiling water upon t. leaves. **3.** Any infusion or decoction made extemporaneously. See also species (2).
Hottentot t., buchu.
Jesuit t., Mexican t., chenopodium.
Paraguay t., maté.

TEAE-cellulose. Triethylaminoethyl-substituted cellulose, used in ion-exchange chromatography.

Teale, Thomas P., British surgeon, 1801–1868. See T.'s *amputation.*

tear (tēr) [A.S. *teár*]. The fluid secreted by the lacrimal glands by means of which the conjunctiva and cornea are kept moist.
artificial t.'s, mixtures of fluid compounds to substitute for naturally produced t's.
crocodile t.'s, see crocodile t.'s *syndrome.*

tear (tār). A discontinuity in substance of a structure. *Cf.* laceration.
bucket-handle t., a t. in the central part of a semilunar cartilage.
Mallory-Weiss t., Mallory-Weiss *lesion.*

tearing (tēr'ing). Epiphora.

tease (tēz) [A. S. *taesan*]. To separate the structural parts of a tissue by means of a needle, in order to prepare it for microscopic examination.

teaspoon (tē'spūn). A small spoon, holding about 1 dram (or about 5 ml) liquid; used as a measure in the dosage of fluid medicines.

teat (tēt) [A.S. *tit*]. **1.** *Papilla* mammae. **2.** Mamma. **3.** Papilla.

tebutate (teb'yū-tāt). USAN-approved contraction for tertiary butylacetate, $(CH_3)_3C–CH_2–CO_2^-$.

technetium (tek-nē'shē-um) [G. *technetos,* artificial]. An artificial radioactive element, symbol Tc, atomic no. 43, artificially produced in 1937 by bombardment of molybdenum by neutrons; also a product of the fission of uranium-235.

technetium-99 (^{99}Tc). A radioisotope of technetium which is the decay product of technetium-99m and has a weak beta emission and a physical half-life of 215,000 years.

technetium-99m (^{99m}Tc). A radioisotope of technetium which decays by isomeric transition, emitting an essentially monoenergetic gamma ray of 140 keV with a physical half-life of 6 hr. It is usually obtained from a radionuclide generator of molybdenum-99 and is used to prepare radiopharmaceuticals for scanning the brain, parotid, thyroid, lungs, blood pool, liver, spleen, kidney, lacrimal drainage apparatus, bone, and bone marrow.

technic (tek-nik'). Technique.

technical (tek'ni-kăl). **1.** Relating to technique. **2.** Pertaining to some particular art, science, or trade. **3.** In connection with a chemical substance, denoting that the substance contains appreciable quantities of impurities.

technician (tek-nish'ŭn) [G. *technē,* an art]. Technologist.

technique (tek-nēk') [Fr., fr. G. *technikos,* relating to *technē,* art, skill]. Technic; the manner of performance, or the details, of any surgical operation, experiment, or mechanical act. See also entries under method; operation; procedure.
airbrasive t., a method of grinding or cutting tooth structure, now little used, by means of a device utilizing a gas-impelled jet of fine Al_2O_3 particles which, after striking the tooth, are removed by a powerful aspirator.
atrial-well t., a closed surgical t. for repairing atrial septal defects.
Barcroft-Warburg t., see Warburg's *apparatus.*
Begg light wire differential force t., see light wire *appliance.*
direct t., direct *method* for making inlays.
Ficoll-Hypaque t., a density-gradient centrifugation t. for separating lymphocytes from other formed elements in the blood; the sample is layered onto a Ficoll-sodium metrizoate gradient of specific density; following centrifugation, lymphocytes are collected from the plasma-Ficoll interface.
flicker fusion frequency t., flicker *perimetry.*
fluorescent antibody t., a t. used to test for antigen with a fluorescent antibody, performed by one of two methods: *direct,* in which immunoglobulin (antibody) conjugated with a fluorescent dye is added to tissue and combines with specific antigen (microbe, or other), the resulting antigen-antibody complex being located by fluorescence microscopy, or *indirect,* in which unlabeled immunoglobulin (antibody) is added to tissue and combines with specific antigen, after which the antigen-antibody complex may be labeled with fluorescein-conjugated anti-immunoglobulin antibody, the resulting triple complex then being located by fluorescence microscopy.
flush t., a t. for determining the systolic blood pressure in infants; the elevated limb is "milked" of blood from the hand or foot proximally; the blood pressure cuff is then inflated above the likely systolic pressure and the limb lowered; the cuff pressure is then gradually released until the blanched limb flushes.
Hampton t., obsolete term for atraumatic, nonpalpation, fluoroscopic examination of the upper gastrointestinal tract in peptic ulcer disease with acute hemorrhage.
Hartel t., a method of reaching the gasserian ganglion by passing a needle from the mouth, inserting it about the level of the upper midmolar tooth, and passing it inward until the point reaches the bone in front and to the outer side of the foramen ovale, allowing an alcohol injection to be made for the relief of trigeminal neuralgia.
immunoperoxidase t., a method using horseradish peroxidase to label antigen-antibody complexes in tissues; a colored reaction product is deposited at the site of peroxidase activity; has high specificity, and can be used on paraffin-embedded tissue; important tool in pathology to demonstrate hormones, unique tissue-specific antigens, structural proteins, tissue enzymes, oncofetal antigens, and microorganisms and viruses; see PAP *technique.*
indirect t., indirect *method* for making inlays.
Judkins t., a method of selective coronary artery catheterization utilizing the standard Seldinger t. through a percutaneous femoral artery puncture.
long cone t., the use of a cone distance of 14 inches or more in making oral roentgenographs.
McGoon's t., plastic reconstruction of an incompetent mitral valve, when the incompetence is due to rupture of chordae to the

posterior leaflet, by plication of the redundant leaflet.
Merendino's t., plastic reconstruction of an incompetent mitral valve using heavy silk sutures to narrow the annulus in the region of the medial commissure.
Mohs' fresh tissue chemosurgery t., chemosurgery in which superficial cancers are excised after fixation *in vivo.*
PAP t., an unlabeled antibody peroxidase method which reacts both with the rabbit antihorseradish peroxidase antibody and free horseradish peroxidase to form a soluble complex of peroxidase antiperoxidase or PAP; a uniquely sensitive immunohistochemical method that is applicable to paraffin-embedded tissues.
rebreathing t., use of a breathing or anesthesia circuit in which exhaled air is subsequently inhaled either with or without absorption of CO_2 from the exhaled air.
Rebuck skin window t., an *in vivo* test of the inflammatory response in which the skin is abraded and a slide applied to the abraded area to permit visualization of leukocyte mobilization.
sealed jar t., a t. for producing suspended animation in small experimental animals, consisting of sealing the animal in a jar which is then refrigerated.
Seldinger t., a method of percutaneous insertion of a catheter into an artery or vein; a needle is used to puncture the vessel in question and to thread a small wire into it; when the needle is withdrawn, the catheter is threaded over the wire into the vessel; the wire is withdrawn, leaving the catheter in place.
sterile insect t., a t. used to control or eradicate insect pests or vectors, utilizing induction by irradiation of dominant lethality in the chromosomes of the released insects.
supersonic vibration t., an oscillatory method used for the fragmentation of bacteria and spermatozoa preparatory to study of their antigenic composition.
washed field t., the cutting of cavity preparations in teeth utilizing a constant irrigant which is immediately removed from the mouth by means of a vacuum device.

technocausis (tek-nō-kaw'sis) [G. *technē,* art, + *kausis,* a burning]. Actual *cautery.*

technologist (tek-nol'ō-jist). Technician; one trained in and using the techniques of a profession, art, or science.

technology (tek-nol'ō-jē) [G. *technē,* an art, + *logos,* study]. The knowledge and use of the techniques of a profession, art, or science.

teclothiazide (tek-lō-thī'ă-zīd). Tetrachlormethiazide.

tectal (tek'tăl). Relating to a tectum.

tectiform (tek'ti-fōrm). Roof-shaped.

tectocephalic (tek'tō-sĕ-fal'ik). [L. *tectum,* roof, + G. *kephalē,* head]. Scaphocephalic.

tectocephaly (tek'tō-sef'ă-lē). Scaphocephaly.

tectology (tek-tol'ō-jē) [G. *tektōn,* builder, + *-logia*]. Structural morphology.

tectonic (tek-ton'ik) [G. *tektonikos,* relating to building]. **1.** Relating to variations in structure in the eye, particularly the cornea. **2.** Obsolete term denoting plastic surgery or the restoration of lost parts by grafting.

tectorial (tek-tōr'ē-ăl). Relating to or characteristic of a tectorium.

tectorium (tek-tōr'ē-ŭm) [L. an overlaying surface (plaster, stucco), fr. *tego,* pp. *tectus,* to cover]. **1.** An overlaying structure. **2.** *Membrana* tectoria ductus cochlearis.

tectospinal (tek-tō-spī'năl). Denoting nerve fibers passing from the tectum mesencephali to the spinal cord.

tectum, pl. **tecta** (tek'tŭm, tek'tă) [L. roof, roofed structure, fr. *tego,* pp. *tectus,* to cover] [NA]. Any rooflike covering or structure.
t. mesenceph'ali [NA], *lamina* tecti mesencephali.

TEDD Abbreviation for total end-diastolic *diameter.*

teel oil (tēl). Sesame oil.

teeth (tēth). Plural of tooth.

teething (tē'thing). Odontiasis; eruption or "cutting" of the teeth, especially of the deciduous teeth.

teflurane (tef'lū-rān). 2-Bromo-1,1,1,2-tetrafluoroethane; a nonexplosive and nonflammable inhalation anesthetic of moderate potency.

tegmen, gen. **tegminis,** pl. **tegmina** (teg'men, -mi-nis, -mi-nă) [L. a covering, fr. *tego,* to cover] [NA]. A structure that covers or roofs over a part.
t. cru'ris, old term for *tegmentum* mesencephali.
t. mastoi'deum, the lamina of bone roofing over the mastoid cells.
t. tym'pani [NA], roof of tympanum; the roof of the middle ear, formed by the thinned anterior surface of the petrous portion of the temporal bone.
t. ventric'uli quar'ti [NA], roof of fourth ventricle, formed in its upper part by the superior medullary velum stretching between the two brachia conjunctiva (superior cerebellar peduncles), in its lower part by the inferior medullary velum composed of the choroid membrane and choroid plexus of the fourth ventricle.

tegmental (teg-men'tăl). Relating to, characteristic of, or placed or oriented toward a tegmentum or tegmen.

tegmentotomy (teg-men-tot'ō-mē) [tegmentum + G. *tomē,* incision]. Production of lesions in the reticular formation of the midbrain tegmentum.

tegmentum, pl. **tegmenta** (teg-men'tŭm, -tă) [L. covering structure, fr. *tego,* to cover] [NA]. **1.** A covering structure. **2.** T. mesencephali.
t. mesenceph'ali [NA], tegmentum (2); mesencephalic or midbrain t.; that major part of the substance of the mesencephalon or midbrain that extends from the substantia nigra to the level of the cerebral aqueduct.
mesencephalic t., t. mesencephali.
midbrain t., t. mesencephali.
t. of pons, *pars* dorsalis pontis.
t. rhombenceph'ali [NA], t. of rhombencephalon; the portion of the pons continuous with the t. mesencephali; it consists of reticular formation, tracts, and cranial nerve nuclei, and forms the dorsal part of the pons (pars dorsalis pontis).
t. of rhombencephalon, t. rhombencephali.

tegument (teg'yū-ment) [L. *tegumentum,* a collat. form of *tegmentum*]. Integument.

tegumental, tegumentary (teg-yū-men'tăl, teg-yū-ment-ă-rē). Relating to the integument.

Teichmann, Ludwig, German histologist, 1823–1895. See T.'s *crystals.*

teichoic acids (tī-kō'ik). One of two classes (the other being the muramic acids or mucopeptides) of polymers constituting the cell walls of Gram-positive bacteria, but also found intracellularly; linear polymers of a polyol (ribitol phosphate or glycerol phosphate) carrying D-alanine residues esterified to OH groups and glycosidically linked sugars.

teichopsia (tī-kop'sē-ă) [G. *teichos,* wall, + *opsis,* vision]. A transient visual sensation of bright shimmering colors, such as that which precedes scintillating scotoma in migraine.

tel-, tele-, telo- [G. *tēle,* distant, *telos,* end]. Combining forms denoting distance, end, or other end.

tela, gen. and pl. **telae** (tē'lă, tē'lē) [L. a web]. **1.** Any thin weblike structure. **2.** A tissue; especially one of delicate formation.
choroid t. of fourth ventricle, t. choroidea ventriculi quarti.
choroid t. of third ventricle, t. choroidea ventriculi tertii.
t. choroi'dea, that portion of the pia mater which covers the ependymal roof or, in the case of the lateral ventricle, medial wall of a cerebral ventricle.

t. choroi'dea inferior, t. choroidea ventriculi quarti.
t. choroi'dea superior, t. choroidea ventriculi tertii.
t. choroi'dea ventric'uli quar'ti [NA], choroid t. of fourth ventricle; t. choroidea inferior; the sheet of pia mater covering the lower part of the ependymal roof of the fourth ventricle.
t. choroi'dea ventric'uli ter'tii [NA], choroid t. of third ventricle; t. choroidea superior; velum interpositum or triangulare; diatela; triangular lamella; a double fold of pia mater, enclosing subarachnoid trabeculae, between the fornix above and the epithelial roof of the third ventricle and the thalami below; at each lateral margin is a vascular fringe projecting into the fissura choroidea of the lateral ventricle; on its undersurface are several small vascular projections filling the folds of the ependymal roof of the third ventricle.
t. conjuncti'va, connective *tissue.*
t. elas'tica, elastic *tissue.*
t. subcuta'nea [NA], superficial fascia; subcutis; stratum subcutaneum; hypoderm; hypodermis; a loose fibrous envelope beneath the skin, containing fat in its meshes (panniculus adiposus) or fasciculi of muscular tissue (panniculus carnosus); it contains the cutaneous vessels and nerves and is in relation by its undersurface with the deep fascia.
t. submuco'sa [NA], tunica submucosa; the layer of connective tissue beneath the tunica mucosa.
t. submuco'sa pharyn'gis, *fascia* pharyngobasilaris.
t. subsero'sa [NA], the layer of connective tissue beneath a serous membrane.
t. vasculo'sa, *plexus* choroideus.

Teladorsagia davtiani (tē'lă-dōr-sā'jē-ă dav-shē-ān'ī) [tele- + L. *dorsum,* back]. One of the medium stomach worm species (family Trichostrongylidae) of sheep, goats, and deer occurring in the abomasum; it is similar to *Ostertagia trifurcata.*

telalgia (tel-al'jē-ă) [G. *tēle,* distant, + *algos,* pain]. Referred *pain.*

telangiectasia (tel-an'jē-ek-tā'zē-ă) [G. *telos,* end, + *angeion,* vessel, + *ektasis,* a stretching out]. Dilation of the previously existing small or terminal vessels of a part.
cephalo-oculocutaneous t., an angioma involving the skin of the face, orbit, meninges, and brain. See also Sturge-Weber *syndrome.*
essential t., (1) localized capillary dilation of undetermined origin; **(2)** *angioma* serpiginosum.
hereditary hemorrhagic t., Osler's disease (2); Rendu-Osler-Weber disease or syndrome; a disease with onset usually after puberty, marked by multiple small telangiectases and dilated venules that develop slowly on the skin and mucous membranes; the face, lips, tongue, nasopharynx, and intestinal mucosa are frequent sites, and recurrent bleeding may occur; autosomal dominant inheritance.
t. lymphat'ica, lymphangiectasia.
t. macula'ris erupti'va per'stans, a disseminated eruption of telangiectases associated with erythematous and edematous macules.
spider t., arterial *spider.*
t. verruco'sa, angiokeratoma.

telangiectasis, pl. **telangiectases** (tel-an'jē-ek'tă-sis, -sēz). A lesion formed by a dilated capillary or terminal artery, most commonly on the skin. See telangiectasia.

telangiectatic (tel-an'jē-ek-tat'ik). Relating to or marked by telangiectasia.

telangiectodes (tel-an'jē-ek-tō'dēz) [telangiectasis + G. *-odes,* fr. *eidos,* resemblance]. A term used to qualify highly vascular tumors.

telangioma (tel-an'jē-ō'mă). Angioma due to dilation of the capillaries or terminal arterioles.

telangion (tel-an'jē-on) [G. *telos,* end, + *angeion,* vessel]. Trichangion; one of the terminal arterioles or a capillary vessel.

telangiosis (tel'an-jē-ō'sis). Any disease of the capillaries and terminal arterioles.

tele-. See tel-.

telecanthus (tel-ĕ-kan'thŭs) [G. *tēle,* distant, + *kanthos,* canthus]. Canthal hypertelorism; increased distance between the medial canthi of the eyelids.

telecardiogram (tel-ĕ-kar'dē-ō-gram). Telelectrocardiogram.

telecardiophone (tel-ĕ-kar'dē-ō-fōn) [G. *tēle,* distant, + *kardia,* heart, + *phōnē,* sound]. A specially constructed stethoscope by means of which heart sounds can be heard by listeners at a distance from the patient.

telecobalt (tel'ĕ-kō'bawlt). Radioactive cobalt for use at a long distance from the region being treated.

telediagnosis (tel'ĕ-dī-ag-nō'sis). Detection of a disease by evaluation of data transmitted to a receiving station, a process normally involving patient-monitoring instruments and a transfer link to a diagnostic center at some distance from the patient.

telediastolic (tel'ĕ-dī-ă-stol'ik) [G. *telos,* end, + *diastolē,* dilation]. Pertaining to or occurring toward the end of cardiac diastole.

telelectrocardiogram (tel'ē-lek-trō-kar'dē-ō-gram) [G. *tēle,* distant, + electrocardiogram]. Telecardiogram; an electrocardiogram recorded at a distance from the subject being tested; *e.g.,* the electrocardiogram obtained through telemetry, or, as with a galvanometer in the laboratory, being connected by a wire with the patient in another room.

telemeter (tĕ-lem'ĕ-ter) [G. *tēle,* distant, + *metron,* measure]. An electronic instrument that senses and measures a quantity, then transmits radio signals to a distant station for recording and interpretation.

telemetry (tĕ-lem'ĕ-trē). The science of measuring a quantity, transmitting the results by radio signals to a distant station, and there interpreting, indicating, and/or recording the results. See also biotelemetry.
cardiac t., transmission of electrocardiographic signals to a receiving location where the electrocardiogram is displayed for monitoring.

telencephalic (tel'en-se-fal'ik). Relating to the telencephalon or endbrain.

telencephalization (tel-en-sef'ăl-i-zā'shŭn). Corticalization.

telencephalon (tel-en-sef'ă-lon) [G. *telos,* end, + *enkephalos,* brain] [NA]. Endbrain; the anterior division of the prosencephalon which develops into the olfactory lobes, the cortex of the cerebral hemispheres and the subcortical telencephalic nuclei, the basal ganglia, particularly the striatum and the amygdala.

teleology (tel-ē-ol'ō-jē) [G. *telos,* end, + *logos,* study]. The philosophical doctrine according to which events, especially in biology, are explained in part by reference to final causes or end goals.

teleomitosis (tel'ē-ō-mī-tō'sis) [G. *teleos,* complete, + mitosis]. A completed mitosis.

teleonomic (tel'ē-ō-nom'ik). **1.** Pertaining to teleonomy. **2.** In psychology, pertaining to those patterns of behavior that are a function of an inferred purpose or motive; *e.g.,* a child's behavior pattern may be classified teleonomically by an observer as attention-getting.

teleonomy (tel-ē-on'ō-mē) [G. *telos,* end, + *nomos,* law]. The doctrine that life is characterized by endowment with a project or purpose; *i.e.,* the existence in an organism of a structure or function implies that it has had evolutionary survival value.

teleopsia (tel-ē-op'sē-ă) [G. *tēle,* distant, + *opsis,* vision]. An error in judging the distance of objects arising from lesions in the parietal temporal region.

teleorganic (tel'ē-ōr-gan'ik) [G. *teleos,* complete, + *organikos,* organic]. Vital; manifesting life.

teleost (tel'ē-ost) [G. *teleos,* complete, perfect, + *osteon,* bone]. One of the bony or true fishes.

telepathine (tel-ĕ-path'ēn). Harmine.

telepathy (tĕ-lep'ă-thē) [G. *tēle,* distant, + *pathos,* feeling]. Extrasensory thought transference; mind-reading; transmittal and reception of thoughts by means other than through the normal senses, as a form of extrasensory perception.

teleradiography (tel-ĕ-rā-dē-og'ră-fē) [G. *tēle,* distant, + radiography]. Teleroentgenography; roentgenography with the tube positioned about 2 m from the body, thereby securing practical parallelism of the rays and minimum distortion.

teleradium (tel'ĕ-rā'dē-ŭm). See teleradium *therapy.*

telereceptor (tel'ĕ-rē-sep'ter, -tōr). An organ, such as the eye, that can receive sense stimuli from a distance.

telergy (tel'er-jē) [G. *tēle,* far off, + *ergon,* work]. Automatism.

teleroentgenogram (tel-ĕ-rent'gen-ō-gram). The image obtained by teleroentgenography.

teleroentgenography (tel'ĕ-rent-gen-og'ră-fē). Teleradiography.

teleroentgentherapy (tel'ĕ-rent'gen-thār'ă-pē). Teletherapy.

telesis (tel-ē'sis) [G. *telos,* end, + *-osis,* condition]. A goal to be attained by planned conduct.

telesystolic (tel'ĕ-sis-tol'ik) [G. *telos,* end, + *systolē,* a contracting]. Relating to the end of cardiac systole.

teletactor (tel-ĕ-tak'ter) [G. *telos,* end, + L. *tactus,* touch]. An instrument to transmit sound waves to the skin.

teletherapy (tel-ĕ-thār'ă-pē) [G. *tēle,* distant, + *terapeia,* treatment]. Teleroentgentherapy; x-ray therapy administered at a distance from the body.

TeLinde, Richard W., U.S. gynecologist, *1894. See T. *operation.*

telluric (tĕ-lūr'ik) [L. *tellus (tellur-),* the earth]. **1.** Relating to or originating in the earth. **2.** Relating to the element tellurium, especially in its 6^+ valence state.

tellurism (tel'ū-rizm) [L. *tellus (tellur-),* the earth]. The alleged influence of soil emanations in producing disease.

tellurium (tel-ū'rē-ŭm) [L. *tellus (tellur-),* the earth]. A rare semimetallic element, symbol Te, atomic no. 52, atomic weight 127.60, belonging to the sulfur group.

telo-. See tel-.

telodendron (tel-ō-den'dron) [G. *telos,* end, + *dendron,* tree]. End-brush; an anomalous term which refers to the terminal arborization of an axon.

telogen (tel'ō-jen) [G. *telos,* end, + *-gen,* producing]. Resting phase of hair cycle.

teloglia (tĕ-log'lē-ă) [G. *telos,* end, + *glia,* glue]. Accumulation of neurolemmal cells at the myoneural junction.

telognosis (tel-og-nō'sis) [G. *tēle,* distant, + *gnosis,* a knowing]. Obsolete term denoting diagnosis by means of roentgenograms or other diagnostic tests transmitted by telephone or radio.

telokinesia (tel'ō-ki-nē'zē-ă) [G. *telos,* end, + *kinēsis,* movement]. Telophase.

telolecithal (tel-ō-les'i-thăl) [G. *telos,* end, + G. *lekithos,* yolk]. Denoting an ovum in which a large amount of deutoplasm accumulates at the vegetative pole, as in the eggs of birds and reptiles.

telomere (tel'ō-mēr) [G. *telos,* end, + *meros,* part]. The distal extremity of a chromosome arm.

telopeptide (tel-ō-pep'tīd). A peptide covalently bound in or on a protein, protruding therefrom and therefore subject to enzyme attack and maturation modification or cross-linking, and conferring immunogenic specificity.

telophase (tel'ō-fāz) [G. *telos,* end, + *phasis,* appearance]. Telokinesia; the final stage of mitosis or meiosis that begins when migration of chromosomes to the poles of the cell is completed; the chromosomes progressively lengthen while the nuclear membranes of the two daughter nuclei are reconstructed and the cytoplasm becomes divided at the equator by formation of cell membrane to complete the separation of the two daughter cells.

Telosporea (tel-ō-spō'rē-ă). Sporozoea.

Telosporidia (tel'ō-spō-rid'ē-ă) [G. *telos,* end, + *sporos,* seed]. A former order of Sporozoea.

telotism (tel'ō-tizm) [G. *telos,* end]. The perfect performance of a function, as that of sight or hearing.

TEM Abbreviation for triethylenemelamine.

temazepam (te-maz'ĕ-pam). A benzodiazepine sedative-hypnotic primarily used to relieve insomnia.

tem'per. 1. Mood; disposition; temperament (2); in general, any characteristic or particular state of mind. **2.** A display of irritation or anger. See tantrum. **3.** To treat metal by application of heat, as in annealing or quenching.

temperament (tem'per-ă-ment) [L. *temperamentum,* proper measure, moderation, disposition]. **1.** The psychophysical organization peculiar to the individual, including one's character or personality predispositions, which influence the manner of thought and action, and general views of life. **2.** Temper (1).

temperance (tem'per-ans) [L. *temperantia,* moderation]. Moderation in all things; especially, abstinence from the use of alcoholic beverages.

temperate (tem'per-ăt). Moderate; restrained in the indulgence of any appetite or activity.

temperature (tem'per-ă-chŭr) [L. *temperatura,* due measure, temperature, fr. *tempero,* to proportion duly]. The sensible intensity of heat of any substance; the measure of the average kinetic energy of the molecules making up a substance. See also entries under scale.

absolute t., (***T***), t. reckoned in Kelvins (degrees Celsius) from the absolute zero.

critical t., the t. of a gas above which it is no longer possible by use of any pressure, however great, to convert it into a liquid.

denaturation t. of DNA, melting t. of DNA; that t. at which, under a given set of conditions, double-stranded DNA is changed (50%) to single-stranded DNA; under standard conditions, the base composition of the DNA can be estimated from the denaturation t., since the greater the denaturation t., the greater the guanine-plus-cytosine content of the DNA.

effective t., a comfort index or scale which takes into account the t. of air, its moisture content, and movement.

equivalent t., the t. of a thermally uniform enclosure in which, under still air conditions, a "sizable" black body loses heat at the same rate as in the nonuniform environment.

eutectic t., the t. at which a eutectic mixture becomes fluid (melts).

fusion t. (wire method), the recorded t. at which a 20-gauge metal wire will collapse under a 3-ounce load; the recorded t. at which porcelain becomes glazed.

maximum t., in bacteriology, denoting a t. above which growth will not take place.

mean t., the average atmospheric t. in any locality for a designated period of time, as a month or a year.

melting t., t. midpoint.

melting t. of DNA, denaturation t. of DNA.

t. midpoint (**T_m**, Kelvin; **t_m**, Celsius), melting t.; the midpoint in the change in optical properties (absorbance, rotation) of a structured polymer (*e.g.,* DNA) with increasing t.

minimum t., in bacteriology, denoting a t. below which growth will not take place.

optimum t., the t. at which any operation, such as the culture of any special microorganism, is best carried on.

room t., the ordinary t. (65° to 80°F, 18.3° to 26.7° C) of the atmosphere in the laboratory; a culture kept at room t. is one kept in the laboratory, not in an incubator.

sensible t., the atmospheric t. as felt by the individual, supposed to be that recorded by the wet-bulb thermometer.

standard t., a t. of 0°C or 273° absolute (Kelvin).

template (tem'plăt). **1.** A pattern or guide that determines the shape of a substance. **2.** Metaphorically, the specifying nature of a nucleic acid or polynucleotide with respect to the primary structure of the nucleic acid or polynucleotide or protein made from it *in vivo* or *in vitro.* **3.** In dentistry, a curved or flat plate utilized as an aid in setting teeth. **4.** An outline used to trace teeth, bones, or soft tissue in order to standardize their form. **5.** A pattern or guide that determines the specificity of antibody globulins.

surgical t., **(1)** a thin, transparent, resin base shaped to duplicate the form of the impression surface of an immediate denture, used as a guide for surgically shaping the alveolar process to fit an immediate denture; **(2)** a guide for various osteotomy procedures; **(3)** a guide for duplicating size and shape for an autogenic (free) gingival graft.

temple (tem'pl) [L. *tempus (tempor-),* time, the temple]. **1.** The area of the temporal fossa on the side of the head above the zygomatic arch. **2.** The part of a spectacle frame passing from the rim backward over the ear.

tempolabile (tem-pō-lā'bil, -bīl) [L. *tempus,* time, + *labilis,* perishable]. Undergoing spontaneous change or destruction during the passage of time.

tempora (tem'pō-ră) [L. pl. of *tempus*]. The temples.

temporal (tem'pō-răl) [L. *temporalis,* fr. *tempus (tempor-),* time, temple]. **1.** Relating to time; limited in time; temporary. **2.** Relating to the temple.

temporalis (tem-pō-rā'lis) [L.]. See under musculus; regio.

temporo- [L. *temporalis,* temporal]. Combining form denoting temporal (2).

temporoauricular (tem'pō-rō-aw-rik'yū-lăr). Relating to the temporal region and the auricle.

temporohyoid (tem'pō-rō-hī'oyd). Relating to the temporal and the hyoid bones or regions.

temporomalar (tem'pō-rō-mā'lăr). Temporozygomatic.

temporomandibular (tem'pō-rō-man-dib'yū-lăr). Temporomaxillary (2); relating to the temporal bone and the mandible; denoting the articulation of the lower jaw.

temporomaxillary (tem'pō-rō-mak'si-lăr'ē). **1.** Relating to the regions of the temporal and maxillary bones. **2.** Temporomandibular.

temporo-occipital (tem'pō-rō-ok-sip'i-tăl). Relating to the temporal and the occipital bones or regions.

temporoparietal (tem'pō-rō-pă-rī'ĕ-tăl). Relating to the temporal and the parietal bones or regions.

temporopontine (tem-pō-rō-pon'tīn). Referring to the projection fibers from the temporal lobe of the cerebral cortex to the basilar part of the pons.

temporosphenoid (tem'pō-rō-sfē'noyd). Relating to the temporal and sphenoid bones.

temporozygomatic (tem'pō-rō-zī'gō-mat'ik). Temporomalar; relating to the temporal and zygomatic bones or regions.

tempostabile, tempostable (tem-pō-stā'bil, -stā'bl) [L. *tempus,* time + *stabilis,* stable]. Not subject to spontaneous alteration or destruction.

temps utile (temp' ū-tēl') [Fr. service or utilization time]. Utilization *time.*

tempus, gen. **temporis,** pl. **tempora** (tem'pŭs, -pō-ris, -pō-ră) [L. time]. **1.** The temple. **2.** Time.

TEN Abbreviation for toxic epidermal *necrolysis.*

tenacious (tĕ-nā'shŭs) [L. *tenax (tenac-),* fr. *teneo,* to hold]. Sticky; glutinous; viscid; denoting tenacity.

tenacity (tĕ-nas'i-tē) [L. *tenacitas,* fr. *teneo,* to hold]. Adhesiveness; the character or property of holding fast.

cellular t., the inherent property of all cells to persist in a given form or direction of activity.

tenaculum, pl. **tenacula** (tĕ-nak'yū-lŭm, -lă) [L. a holder, fr. *teneo,* to hold]. A surgical clamp designed to hold or grasp tissue during dissection.

tenac'ula ten'dinum, *vincula* tendinum.

tenalgia (te-nal'jē-ă) [G. *tenōn,* tendon, + *algos,* pain]. Tenontodynia; tenodynia; pain referred to a tendon.

t. crep'itans, *tenosynovitis* crepitans.

ten'der [L. *tener,* soft, delicate]. Sensitive or painful as a result of pressure or contact which is not sufficent to cause discomfort in normal tissues.

tenderness (ten'der-nes). The condition of being tender.

pencil t., strictly localized t., elicited by pressure with the rubber tip of a pencil, *e.g.,* in cases of incomplete or subperiosteal fracture.

rebound t., t. felt when pressure, particularly pressure on the abdomen, is suddenly released.

tendinitis (ten-di-nī'tis). Tendonitis.

tendinoplasty (ten'din-ō-plas-tē) [Mediev. L. *tendo (tendin-),* tendon, + G. *plastos,* formed]. Tenontoplasty.

tendinosuture (ten'di-nō-sū'chūr). Tenorrhaphy.

tendinous (ten'di-nŭs). Relating to, composed of, or resembling a tendon.

tendo- [L. *tendo,* tendon]. Combining form denoting a tendon. See also teno-.

tendo, gen. **tendinis,** pl. **tendines** (ten'dō, -di-nis, -di-nēz) [Mediev. L., fr. L. *tendo,* to stretch out, extend] [NA]. Tendon; a fibrous cord or band of variable length that connects a muscle with its bony attachment; it may unite with the muscle at its extremity or may run along the side or in the center of the muscle for a longer or shorter distance, receiving the muscular fibers along its lateral border. For histological description, see tendon.

t. Achil'lis [NA], official alternative term for t. calcaneus.

t. calca'neus [NA], calcanean tendon; Achilles tendon; heel tendon; t. Achillis; chorda magna; the tendon of insertion of the triceps surae (gastrocnemius and soleus) into the tuberosity of the calcaneus.

t. calca'neus commu'nis, see hamstring (2).

t. conjuncti'vus [NA], official alternate term for *falx* inguinalis.

t. cricoesophage'us [NA], cricoesophageal tendon; suspensory ligament of esophagus; Gillette's suspensory ligament; longitudinal fiber of the esophagus that attaches to the posterior aspect of the cricoid cartilage of the larynx.

t. oc'uli, *ligamentum* palpebrale mediale.

t. palpebra'rum, *ligamentum* palpebrale mediale.

tendolysis (ten-dol'i-sis) [tendo- + G. *lysis,* dissolution]. Tenolysis; release of a tendon from adhesions.

tendomucin, tendomucoid (ten-dō-myū'sin, -myū'koyd). A form of mucin found in tendons.

tendon (ten'dŏn) [L. *tendo*]. Tendo; a fibrous cord or band that connects a muscle to a bone or other structure; it consists of fascicles of very densely arranged, almost parallel collagenous fibers, rows of elongated tendon cells, and a minimum of ground substance. For gross anatomical description, see tendo.

Achilles t., *tendo* calcaneus.

bowed t., a condition caused by severe strain of the digital flexor tendons, the outer osseus (suspensory ligament), or the accessory ligament (distal cheek ligament) of the horse's limb and characterized by swelling, pain, and lameness; it occurs most frequently in race horses under stress of running.

calcanean t., *tendo* calcaneus.

central t. of diaphragm, *centrum* tendineum diaphragmae.
central t. of perineum, *centrum* tendineum perinei.
conjoined t., conjoint t., *falx* inguinalis.
contracted t., a condition of young horses in which the flexor t.'s of the leg are shortened.
coronary t., *annulus* fibrosus (1).
cricoesophageal t., *tendo* cricoesophageus.
Gerlach's annular t., *annulus* fibrocartilagineus.
hamstring t., see hamstring.
heel t., *tendo* calcaneus.
slipped t., see perosis.
Todaro's t., an inconstant tendinous structure that extends from the right fibrous trigone of the heart toward the valve of the inferior vena cava.
trefoil t., *centrum* tendineum diaphragmae.
Zinn's t., *annulus* tendineus communis.

tendonitis (ten-dō-nī'tis). Tendinitis; tenonitis (2); tenontitis; tenositis; inflammation of a tendon.

tendophony (ten-dof'ō-nē). Tenophony.

tendoplasty (ten'dō-plas-tē). Tenontoplasty.

tendosynovitis (ten'dō-si-nō-vī'tis). Tenosynovitis.

tendotomy (ten-dot'ō-mē). Tenotomy.

tendovaginal (ten-dō-vaj'i-năl) [tendo- + L. *vagina,* sheath]. Relating to a tendon and its sheath.

tendovaginitis (ten'dō-vaj-i-nī'tis) [tendo- + L. *vagina,* sheath, + G. *-itis,* inflammation]. Tenosynovitis.
radial styloid t., de Quervain's *disease.*

tenectomy (tĕ-nek'tō-mē) [G. *tenōn,* tendon, + *ektomē,* excision]. Tenonectomy; resection of part of a tendon.

tenesmic (tĕ-nez'mik). Relating to or marked by tenesmus.

tenesmus (te-nez'mŭs) [G. *teinesmos,* ineffectual effort to defecate, fr. *teinō,* to stretch]. A painful spasm of the anal sphincter with an urgent desire to evacuate the bowel or bladder, involuntary straining, and the passage of but little fecal matter or urine.

ten Horn, C., Dutch surgeon. See t. H.'s *sign.*

tenia, pl. **teniae** (tē'nē-ă, tē'nē-ē) [L. fr. G. *tainia,* band, tape, a tapeworm]. **1.** Any anatomical bandlike structure. **2.** Taenia (2).
te'niae acus'ticae, *striae* medullares ventriculi quarti.
t. choroi'dea [NA], tenia telae [NA]; the somewhat thickened line along which a choroid membrane or plexus is attached to the rim of a brain ventricle.
te'niae co'li [NA], bands of colon; colic teniae; teniae of Valsalva; the three bands in which the longitudinal muscular fibers of the large intestine, except the rectum, are collected; these are t. mesocolica, situated at the place corresponding to the mesenteric attachment; t. libera, free band, opposite the mesocolic band; and t. omentalis, at the place corresponding to the site of adhesion of the greater omentum to the transverse colon.
colic teniae, teniae coli.
t. fim'briae, t. fornicis.
t. for'nicis [NA], t. of the fornix; t. fimbriae; the line of attachment of the choroid plexus of the lateral ventricle to the fornix.
t. of the fornix, t. fornicis.
t. of fourth ventricle, t. ventriculi quarti.
t. hippocam'pi, *fimbria* hippocampi.
t. lib'era [NA], see teniae coli.
medullary teniae, *striae* medullares ventriculi quarti.
t. mesocol'ica, [NA], see teniae coli.
t. omenta'lis, [NA], see teniae coli.
t. semicircula'ris, *stria* terminalis.
Tarin's t., *stria* terminalis.
t. tec'ta, rudimentum hippocampi; see *indusium* griseum.
t. te'lae [NA], t. choroidea [NA].
t. termina'lis, *crista* terminalis.
t. thal'ami [NA], t. of the thalamus; thalamic t.; t. ventriculi tertii; the sharp edge or angle between the superior and medial surface of the thalamus on either side; to it is attached the epithelial lamina forming the roof of the third ventricle.
thalamic t., t. thalami.
teniae of Valsalva, teniae coli.
t. ventric'uli quar'ti [NA], t. of the fourth ventricle; the line of attachment of the choroid roof to the rim of the fourth ventricle.
t. ventric'uli ter'tii, t. thalami.

teniacide (tē'nē-ă-sīd) [L. *taenia,* tapeworm, + *caedo,* to kill]. Tenicide; an agent destructive to tapeworms.

teniafuge (tē'nē-ă-fūj) [L. *taenia,* tapeworm, + *fugo,* to put to flight]. Tenifuge; an agent that causes the expulsion of tapeworms.

tenial (ten'ē-ăl). **1.** Relating to a tapeworm. **2.** Relating to one of the structures called tenia.

teniasis (tē-nī'ă-sis). Presence of a tapeworm in the intestine.
somatic t., invasion of the body by the cysticercus of a tenioid worm.

tenicide (ten'i-sīd). Teniacide.

teniform (ten'i-fōrm). Tenioid.

tenifugal (te-nif'yū-găl). Having the power to expel tapeworms.

tenifuge (ten'i-fyūj). Teniafuge.

tenioid (tē'nē-oyd) [G. *tainia,* a tape, + *eidos,* resemblance]. Teniform. **1.** Band-shaped; ribbon-shaped. **2.** Resembling a tapeworm.

teniola (tē-nī'ō-lă) [L. dim. of *taenia,* ribbon]. A slender tenia or bandlike structure.
t. cor'poris callo'si, *lamina* rostralis.

teno-, tenon-, tenont-, tenonto- [G. *tenōn,* tendon]. Combining forms meaning tendon. See also tendo-.

tenodesis (tĕ-nod'ē-sis, ten'ō-dē'sis) [teno- + G. *desis,* a binding]. Stabilizing a joint by anchoring the tendons which move that joint.

tenodynia (ten-ō-din'ēă) [teno- + G. *odynē,* pain]. Tenalgia.

tenofibril (ten-ō-fī'bril) [teno- + Mod. L. *fibrilla,* a small fiber]. Tonofibril.

tenolysis (ten-ol'i-sis). Tendolysis.

tenomyoplasty (ten-ō-mī'ō-plas-tē). Tenontomyoplasty.

tenomyotomy (ten-ō-mī-ot'ō-mē). Myotenotomy.

Tenon, Jacques R., French pathologist and oculist, 1724–1816. See T.'s *capsule, space.*

tenon-, tenont-. See teno-.

tenonectomy (ten-ō-nek'tō-mē) [tenon- + G. *ektomē,* excision]. Tenectomy.

tenonitis (ten-ō-nī'tis). **1.** Inflammation of Tenon's capsule or the connective tissue within Tenon's space. **2.** Tendonitis.

tenonometer (ten-ō-nom'ĕ-ter). Tonometer (1).

tenontitis (ten'on-tī'tis) [tenont- + G. *-itis,* inflammation]. Tendonitis.

tenonto-. See teno-.

tenontodynia (te-non'tō-din'ē-ă). Tenalgia.

tenontography (ten'on-tog'ră-fē) [tenonto- + G. *graphē,* description]. A treatise on or description of the tendons.

tenontolemmitis (te-non'tō-lĕ-mī'tis) [tenonto- + G. *lemma,* husk, + *-itis*]. Tenosynovitis.

tenontology (ten'on-tol'ō-jē) [tenonto- + G. *logos,* study]. The branch of science that has to do with the tendons.

tenontomyoplasty (te-non'tō-mī'ō-plas-tē) [tenonto- + G. *mys,* muscle, + *plastos,* formed]. Tenomyoplasty; a combined tenontoplasty and myoplasty, used in the radical correction of a hernia.

tenontomyotomy (te-non'tō-mī-ot'ō-mē). Myotenotomy.

tenontoplastic (te-non'tō-plas-tik). Relating to tenontoplasty.

tenontoplasty (te-non'tō-plas-tē) [tenonto- + G. *plastos,* formed]. Tenoplasty; tendinoplasty; tendoplasty; reparative or plastic surgery of the tendons.

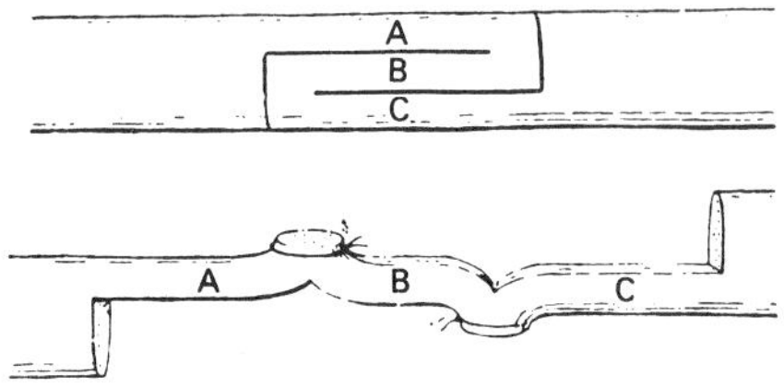

One Type of Tenontoplasty

tenontothecitis (te-non'tō-thē-sī'tis) [tenonto- + G. *thēkē,* case, box, + *-itis*]. Tenosynovitis.

tenophony (te-nof'ō-nē) [teno- + G. *phōnē,* sound]. Tendophony; a heart murmur assumed to be due to an abnormal condition of the chordae tendineae.

tenophyte (ten'ō-fīt) [teno- + G. *phyton,* plant]. Bony or cartilaginous growth in or on a tendon.

tenoplastic (ten-ō-plas'tik). Relating to tenoplasty.

tenoplasty (ten'ō-plas-tē). Tenontoplasty.

tenoreceptor (ten'ō-rē-sep'ter, -tōr). A receptor in a tendon, activated by increased tension.

tenorrhaphy (te-nōr'ă-fē) [teno- + G. *raphē,* suture]. Tendinosuture; tenosuture; tendon suture; suture of the divided ends of a tendon.

tenositis (ten-ō-sī'tis). Tendonitis.

tenostosis (ten-os-tō'sis) [teno- + G. *osteon,* bone, + *-osis,* condition]. Ossification of a tendon.

tenosuspension (ten'ō-sŭs-pen'shŭn). Using a tendon as a suspensory ligament, sometimes as a free graft or in continuity.

tenosuture (ten-ō-sū'chūr). Tenorrhaphy.

tenosynovectomy (ten'ō-sin-ō-vek'tō-mē) [teno- + synovia + G. *ektomē,* excision]. Excision of a tendon sheath.

tenosynovitis (ten'ō-sin-ō-vī'tis) [teno- + synovia + G. *-itis,* inflammation]. Inflammation of a tendon and its enveloping sheath. Also called tendosynovitis; tendovaginitis; tenontothecitis; tenontolemmitis; tenovaginitis; vaginal or tendinous synovitis.

t. crep'itans, tenalgia crepitans; inflammation of a tendon sheath in which movement of the tendon is accompanied by a cracking sound.

localized nodular t., giant cell *tumor* of tendon sheath.

villonodular pigmented t., villous t.

villous t., villonodular pigmented t.; a condition resembling pigmented villonodular synovitis but arising in periarticular soft tissue rather than in joint synovia; occurs most commonly in the hands.

tenotomy (te-not'ō-mē) [teno- + G. *tomē,* incision]. Tendotomy; the surgical division of a tendon for relief of a deformity caused by congenital or acquired shortening of a muscle, as in clubfoot or strabismus.

curb t., tendon *recession.*

graduated t., partial incisions of the tendon of an eye muscle for correction of strabismus.

subcutaneous t., division of a tendon by means of a small pointed knife introduced through skin and subcutaneous tissue without an open operation.

tenovaginitis (ten'ō-vaj-i-nī'tis) [teno- + L. *vagina,* sheath, + G. *-itis,* inflammation]. Tenosynovitis.

tense (tens) [L. *tensus,* pp. of *tendo,* to stretch]. Tight, rigid, or strained; characterized by anxiety.

tensiometer (ten-sē-om'ĕ-ter) [L. *tensio,* tension, + G. *metron,* measure]. A device for measuring tension.

tension (ten'shŭn) [L. *tensio,* fr. *tendo,* pp. *tensus,* to stretch]. **1.** The act of stretching. **2.** The condition of being stretched or tense, or a stretching or pulling force. **3.** The partial pressure of a gas, especially that of a gas dissolved in a liquid such as blood. **4.** Mental, emotional, or nervous strain; strained relations or barely controlled hostility between persons or groups.

arterial t., the blood pressure within an artery.

interfacial surface t., the t. or resistance to separation possessed by the film of liquid between two well-adapted surfaces, as of the thin film of saliva between the denture base and the tissues.

ocular t. (Tn), resistance of the tunics of the eye to deformation; it can be estimated digitally or measured by means of a tonometer.

premenstrual t., premenstrual *syndrome.*

surface t., the expression of intermolecular attraction at the surface of a liquid, in contact with air or another gas, a solid, or another immiscible liquid, tending to pull the molecules of the liquid inward from the surface; dimensional formula: mt^{-2}.

tissue t., a theoretical condition of equilibrium or balance between the tissues and cells whereby overaction of any part is restrained by the pull of the mass.

tensor, pl. **tensores** (ten'sōr, ten-sō'rēz). [Mod. L. fr. L. *tendo,* pp. *tensus,* to stretch]. A muscle the function of which is to render a part firm and tense.

tent [L. *tendo,* pp. *tensus,* to stretch]. **1.** Canopy used in various types of inhalation therapy to control humidity and concentration of oxygen in inspired air. **2.** Cylinder of some material, usually absorbent, introduced into a canal or sinus to maintain its patency or to dilate it. **3.** To elevate or pick up a segment of skin, fascia, or tissue at a given point, giving it the appearance of a t.

oxygen t., a transparent enclosure, suspended over the bed and enclosing the patient, used to supply a high concentration of oxygen.

sponge t., compressed *sponge.*

tentacle (ten'tă-kl) [Mod. L. *tentaculum,* a feeler, fr. *tento,* to feel]. A slender process for feeling, prehension, or locomotion in invertebrates.

tentorial (ten-tō'rē-ăl). Relating to a tentorium.

tentorium, pl. **tentoria** (ten-tō'rē-ŭm, -rē-ă) [L. tent, fr. *tendo,* to stretch] [NA]. A membranous cover or horizontal partition.

t. cerebel'li [NA], a strong fold of dura mater roofing over the posterior cranial fossa with an anterior median opening, the incisura tentorii, through which the midbrain passes; the t. cerebelli is attached along the midline to the falx cerebri and separates the cerebellum from the basal surface of the occipital and temporal lobes of the cerebral hemisphere.

t. of hypophysis, *diaphragma* sellae.

TEPA Abbreviation for triethylenephosphoramide.

tephromalacia (tef'rō-mă-lā'shē-ă) [G. *tephros,* ashen-gray, + *malakia,* softness]. Softening of the gray matter of the brain or spinal cord.

tephrylometer (tef-ri-lom'ĕ-ter) [G. *tephros,* ashen, + *hylē,* stuff, + *metron,* measure]. An instrument for measuring the thickness of the cerebral cortex; it consists of a graduated tube of thin glass which is inserted into the brain substance, so the depth of the gray matter can be read off on the scale.

TEPP Abbreviation for tetraethyl pyrophosphate.

teprotide (tē'prō-tīd). Bradykinin-potentiating peptide; 2-L-tryptophan-3-de-L-leucine-4-de-L-proline-8-L-glutamine-bradykinin-potentiator B; a nonapeptide in which glycine is replaced by tryptophan, leucine and the first proline are missing, and the lysine is replaced by glutamine; an angiotensin-converting enzyme inhibitor.

tera- [G. *teras,* monster]. **1.** (T) Prefix used in the SI and metric systems to signify one trillion. **2.** Combining form denoting a teras. See also terato-.

teras, pl. **terata** (ter'as, ter'ă-tă) [G.]. Fetus with deficient, redundant, misplaced, or grossly misshapen parts.

teratic (ter-at'ik). Relating to a teras.

teratism (ter'ă-tizm) [G. *teratisma,* fr. *teras*]. Teratosis.

terato- [G. *teras,* monster]. Combining form denoting a teras. See also tera- (2).

teratoblastoma (ter'ă-tō-blas-tō'mă) [terato- + G. *blastos,* germ, + *-oma,* tumor]. Teratoma.

teratocarcinoma (ter'ă-tō-kar-si-nō'mă). **1.** A malignant teratoma, occurring most commonly in the testis. **2.** A malignant epithelial tumor arising in a teratoma.

teratogen (ter'ă-tō-jen) [terato- + G. *-gen,* producing]. A drug or other agent that causes abnormal fetal development.

teratogenesis (ter'ă-tō-jen'ĕ-sis) [terato- + G. *genesis,* origin]. Teratogeny; the origin or mode of production of a malformed fetus; the disturbed growth processes involved in the production of a malformed fetus.

teratogenic, teratogenetic (ter'ă-tō-jen'ik, -jĕ-net'ik). **1.** Relating to teratogenesis. **2.** Causing abnormal fetal development.

teratogenicity (ter'ă-tō-jĕ-nis'i-tē) [terato- + G. *genesis,* generation]. The property or capability of producing fetal malformation.

teratogeny (ter-ă-toj'ĕ-nē). Teratogenesis.

teratoid (ter'ă-toyd) [G. *teratōdēs,* fr. *teras* (*terat-*), monster, + *eidos,* resemblance]. Resembling a teras.

teratologic (ter'ă-tō-loj'ik). Relating to teratology.

teratology (ter-ă-tol'ō-jē) [terato- + G. *logos,* study]. The branch of science concerned with the production, development, anatomy, and classification of malformed fetuses. See also dysmorphology.

teratoma (ter-ă-tō'mă) [terato- + G. *-oma,* tumor]. Teratoblastoma; teratoid tumor; a neoplasm composed of multiple tissues, including tissues not normally found in the organ in which it arises. T.'s occur most frequently in the ovary, where they are usually benign and form dermoid cysts; in the testis, where they are usually malignant; and, uncommonly, in other sites, especially the midline of the body.

t. or'bitae, orbitopagus.

triphyllomatous t., tridermoma; a t. composed of tissues derived from all three germ layers, *i.e.,* a teratoma.

teratomatous (ter'ă-tō'mă-tŭs). Relating to or of the nature of a teratoma.

teratophobia (ter'ă-tō-fō'bē-ă) [terato- + G. *phobos,* fear]. Morbid fear of carrying and giving birth to a malformed infant.

teratosis (ter'ă-tō'sis) [terato- + G. *-osis,* condition]. Teratism; an anomaly producing a teras.

atresic t., a t. in which any of the normal orifices, such as the nares, mouth, anus, or vagina, is imperforate.

ceasmic t., a t. in which there is a failure of the lateral halves of a part to unite, as in cleft palate.

ectogenic t., a t. in which there is a deficiency of parts.

ectopic t., a t. in which the organs or other parts are misplaced.

hypergenic t., a t. in which there is a redundancy of parts.

symphysic t., a t. in which there is a fusion of normally separated parts.

teratospermia (ter'ă-tō-sper'mē-ă) [terato- + G. *sperma,* seed]. Condition characterized by the presence of malformed spermatozoa in the semen.

terazosin hydrochloride (tĕ-rā'zō-sin). 1-(4-Amino-6,7-dimethoxy-2-quinazolinyl)-4-(tetrahydro-2-furoyl)piperazine monohydrochloride dihydrate; a peripherally acting antiadrenergic used to treat hypertension.

terbium (ter'bē-ŭm) [fr. *Ytterby,* a place in Sweden]. A metallic element of the lanthanide or rare earth series, symbol Tb, atomic no. 65, atomic weight 158.93.

terbutaline sulfate (ter-byū'tă-lēn). α-[(*tert*-Butylamino)methyl]-3,5-dihydroxybenzyl alcohol sulfate; a sympathomimetic drug, used principally as a bronchodilator.

terebene (ter'ĕ-bēn). A thin colorless liquid of an aromatic odor and taste, a mixture of terpene hydrocarbons, chiefly dipentene and terpinene, obtained from oil of turpentine; used as an expectorant and in cystitis and urethritis.

terebinthinate (ter-ĕ-bin'thĭ-nāt) [G. *terebinthos,* the terebinth or turpentine-tree]. Terebinthine. **1.** Containing or impregnated with turpentine. **2.** A preparation containing turpentine.

terebinthine (ter-ĕ-bin'thin). Terebinthinate.

terebinthinism (ter-ĕ-bin'thin-izm). Turpentine *poisoning.*

terebrant, terebrating (ter'ĕ-brant, -brā-ting) [L. *terebro,* pp. *-atus,* to bore, fr. *terebra,* an auger]. Boring; piercing; used figuratively, as in the term t. pain.

terebration (ter-ĕ-brā'shŭn) [L. *terebro,* to bore, fr. *terebra,* an auger]. **1.** The act of boring, or of trephining. **2.** A boring, piercing pain.

teres, gen. **teretis,** pl. **teretes** (ter'ēz, ter'ĕ-tis, ter'ĕ-tēz, -tēr-) [L. round, smooth, fr. *tero,* to rub]. Round and long; denoting certain muscles and ligaments.

terfenadine (ter-fen'ă-dēn). α-(*p*-*tert*-Butylphenyl)-4-(hydroxydiphenylmethyl)-1-piperidinebutanol; an antihistamine used to treat a variety of allergic conditions; has less sedative effects than other antihistamines.

tergal (ter'găl) [L. *tergum,* back]. Dorsal (1).

tergum (ter'gŭm) [L.]. Dorsum.

term [L. *terminus,* a limit, an end]. **1.** A definite or limited period. **2.** A name or descriptive word or phrase. See also terminus; term *infant.*

terminad (ter'mi-nad). Toward the terminus.

terminal (ter'mi-năl) [L. *terminus,* a boundary, limit]. **1.** Relating to the end; final. **2.** Relating to the extremity or end of any body. **3.** A termination, extremity, end, or ending.

axon t.'s, end-feet; terminal, synaptic, or axonal terminal boutons; boutons or pieds terminaux; synaptic endings or t.'s; neuropodia; the somewhat enlarged, often club-shaped endings by which axons make synaptic contacts with other nerve cells or with effector cells (muscle or gland cells). As isolated, by homogenizing brain or spinal cord, they contain acetylcholine and the related enzymes. T.'s contain neurotransmitters of various kinds, sometimes more than one. These can be demonstrated by chemical analysis and immunocytochemical methods. See also synapse.

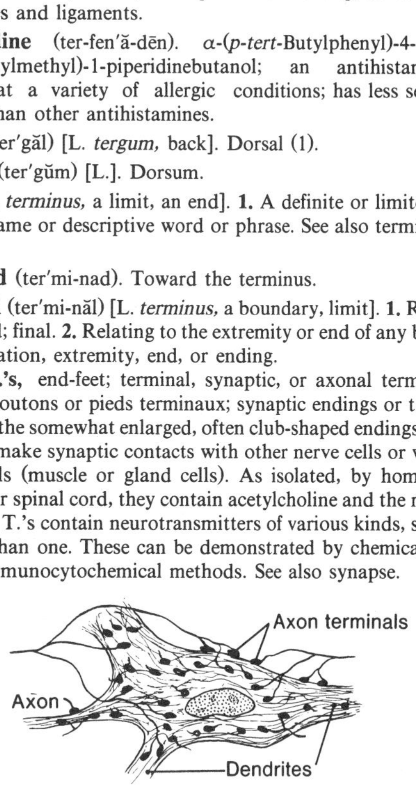

Axon Terminals

synaptic t.'s, axon t.'s.

terminal deoxynucleotidyltransferase. (dē-ok'sē-nū'klē-ō-tī-dil-trans'fer-ās). DNA nucleotidylexotransferase.

terminatio, pl. **terminationes** (ter'mi-nā'shē-ō, -ō'nēz) [L.] [NA].

A termination or ending, particularly a nerve ending. See also ending.
terminatio'nes nervo'rum li'berae [NA], free nerve endings; a form of peripheral ending of sensory nerve fibers in which the terminal filaments end freely in the tissue.

termination (ter'mi-nā'shŭn) [L. *terminatio*]. An end or ending. See terminatio; ending.

terminationes (ter-mi-nā-shē-ō'nēz) [L.]. Plural of terminatio.

terminus, pl. termini (ter'mi-nŭs, -nī) [L.]. A boundary or limit.
C-t., that end of a polypeptide chain that has a free carboxyl group.
ter'mini genera'les [NA], general terms; words that are of general use in descriptive anatomy.

termone (ter'mōn) [L. *ter,* thrice, threefold, + hormone]. A type of ectohormone, secreted by some invertebrate organisms, that stimulates gametogenesis.

ternary (ter'nār-ē) [L. *ternarius,* of three]. Denoting or comprised of three compounds, elements, molecules, etc.

teroxide (ter-ok'sīd). Trioxide.

terpene (ter'pēn). One of a class of and camphene. hydrocarbons with an empirical formula of $C_{10}H_{16}$, occurring in essential oils and resins. Acyclic t.'s may be regarded as isomers and polymers of diisoprene, $[(CH_3)_2C{=}CH{-}CH]_2$; cyclic forms include menthane, bornane, and camphene. T.'s containing 15, 20, 30, 40, etc., carbon atoms are called sesquiterpenes, diterpenes, triterpenes, tetraterpenes, etc.

***p*-terphenyl** (ter-fen'il). $C_6H_5{-}C_6H_4{-}C_6H_5$; useful as a scintillator in scintillation counting of radioactive decompositions.

ter'pin. Dipenteneglycol; *p*-menthane-1,8-diol; a cyclic terpene alcohol, $C_{10}H_{18}(OH)_2$, obtained by the action of nitric acid and dilute sulfuric acid on pine oil.
t. hydrate, terpinol; a monohydrate of terpin; an expectorant.

terpineol (ter-pin'ē-ol). *p*-Menth-1-en-8-ol; an unsaturated alcoholic terpene obtained by heating terpin hydrate with diluted phosphoric acid; an active antiseptic and a perfume.

terpinol (ter'pin-ol). *Terpin* hydrate.

terra japonica (ter'ră jă-pon'i-kă). See gambir.

terrace (ter'as) [thr. O. Fr. fr. L. *terra,* earth]. To suture in several rows, in closing a wound through a considerable thickness of tissue.

Terrey, Mary. See Lowe-T.-MacLachlan *syndrome.*

Terrien, Felix, French ophthalmologist, *1872. See T.'s marginal *degeneration.*

Terrier, Louis F., French surgeon, 1837–1908. See T.'s *valve.*

territoriality (ter'i-tōr-ē-al'i-tē). **1.** The tendency of individuals or groups to defend a particular domain or sphere of interest or influence. **2.** The tendency of an individual animal to define a finite space as his own habitat from which he will fight off trespassing animals of his own species.

Terry, Theodore L., U.S. ophthalmologist, 1899–1946. See T.'s *syndrome.*

Terry's nails. See under nail.

Terson, Albert, French ophthalmologist, 1867–1935. See T.'s *glands.*

tertian (ter'shăn) [L. *tertianus,* fr. *tertius,* third]. Recurring every third day, counting the day of an episode as the first; actually, occurring every 48 hours or every other day.
double t., denoting malarial infections with two different sets of organisms producing daily paroxysms. See also quotidian *malaria.*

tertiarism, tertiarismus (ter'shē-ă-rizm, -riz'mŭs). All the symptoms of the tertiary stage of syphilis taken collectively.

TESD Abbreviation for total end-systolic *diameter.*

Tesla, Nikola, Serbian-American electrical engineer, 1856–1943. See tesla; T. *current.*

tesla (T) (tes'lă) [N. *Tesla*]. In the SI system, the unit of magnetic field intensity expressed as $kg/sec^{-2}/A^{-1}$.

tessellated (tes'ĕ-lāt-ed) [L. *tessella,* a small square stone]. Made up of small squares; checkered.

TEST

test [L. *testum,* an earthen vessel]. **1.** To try a substance; to prove; to determine the chemical nature of a substance by means of reagents. **2.** A method of examination, as to determine the presence or absence of a definite disease or of some substance in any of the fluids, tissues, or excretions of the body. **3.** A reagent used in making a t. **4.** Testa. See also entries under assay; reaction; reagent; scale; stain.
ABLB t., alternate binaural loudness balance t.
abortus-Bang-ring t., milk-ring t.
acetone t., a t. for ketonuria; the suspected urine is shaken up with a few drops of sodium nitroprusside, and strong ammonia water is then gently poured over the mixture; if acetone is present, a magenta ring forms at the line of contact; tablets containing sodium nitroprusside and alkali are now more commonly used.
achievement t., a standardized t. used to measure acquired learning, *e.g.,* competence in a specific subject area, in contrast to an intelligence t. which is a useful index of potential learning.
acidified serum t., Ham's t.; lysis of the patient's red cells in acidified fresh serum, specific for paroxysmal nocturnal hemoglobinuria.
acid perfusion t., Bernstein t.
acid phosphatase t. for semen, a screening t. for semen by determining acid phosphatase content; because seminal fluid contains high concentrations of acid phosphatase, while other body fluids and extraneous foreign materials have very low concentrations, high values of acid phosphatase on vaginal aspirate or lavage, or on wash fluid from stains, render positive identification of semen, even if the male is aspermic.
acid reflux t., a t. to detect gastroesophageal reflux by monitoring esophageal pH by an electrode in the distal esophagus either basally or after acid is instilled into the stomach.
ACTH stimulation t., a t. for adrenal cortical function; ACTH administered by continuous intravenous infusion, or intramuscularly, evokes an increase in plasma cortisol in normal persons; in adrenal cortical insufficiency, the expected increase in plasma cortisol is limited or nonexistent.
active rosette t., a t. for rosette-forming cells (T-lymphocytes) in which these cells and sheep erythrocytes, suspended in serum, are incubated and centrifuged lightly, then examined under a microscope for rosette formation.
adhesion t., immune adhesion t.; red cell adherence t.; erythrocyte adherence t.; the diagnostic application of the immune adhesion phenomenon.
Adler's t., benzidine t.
adrenal ascorbic acid depletion t., a t. used to measure the quantity of corticotrophin in tissue, blood, or urine.
Adson's t., Adson's maneuver; a t. for thoracic outlet syndrome; the patient is seated, with head extended and turned to the side of the lesion; with deep inspiration there is a diminution or total loss of radial pulse on the affected side.
Albarran's t., polyuria t.; a t. for renal insufficiency wherein the drinking of large quantities of water will cause a proportionate increase in the volume of urine if the kidneys are sound, but not if the epithelium of the secreting tubules is damaged.

alkali denaturation t., a t. for hemoglobin F (Hb F), based on the fact that hemoglobins, with the exception of Hb F, are denatured by alkali to alkaline hematin; the t. is sensitive to 2% or more Hb F.
Allen's t. [A.H. Allen], **(1)** for phenol: upon the addition of 5 or 6 drops of hydrochloric acid and then 1 of nitric acid to the suspected fluid, a red color develops; **(2)** for strychnine: fluid is extracted with ether, which is then evaporated by means of "drop-by-drop" pipetting into a warmed porcelain dish or crucible; the residue is treated with a small bit of manganese dioxide and dilute sulfuric acid; a red-blue or violet color develops if strychnine is present.
Allen t. [E.V. Allen], a t. for radial or ulnar patency; either the radial or ulnar artery is digitally compressed by the examiner after blood has been forced out of the hand by clenching it into a fist; failure of the blood to diffuse into the hand when opened indicates that the artery not compressed is occluded.
Allen-Doisy t., a t. for estrogenic activity; the material to be investigated is injected repeatedly into immature or spayed rats or mice; the disappearance of leukocytes from the vaginal smear and the appearance of cornified cells constitutes a positive reaction.
Almén's t. for blood, Schönbein's, van Deen's, or guaiac t.; glacial acetic acid, gum guaiac solution, and hydrogen peroxide are added to an aqueous suspension of the suspected stain; if occult blood or blood pigment is present, a blue color develops.
alternate binaural loudness balance (ABLB) t., a t. for recruitment in one ear; the comparison of relative loudness of a series of intensities presented alternately to either ear.
alternate cover t., a t. to detect phoria or strabismus; attention is directed to a small fixation object, and one eye is covered for several seconds; then the fellow eye is immediately covered; if the eye moves when it is uncovered, a strabismus or phoria is present.
Ames t., Ames assay; a screening t. for possible carcinogens using strains of *Salmonella typhinium* that are unable to synthesize histidine; if the test substance produces mutations that regain the ability to synthesize histidine, the substance is carcinogenic.
Amsler t., projection of a visual field defect onto an Amsler chart.
Anderson-Collip t., a procedure for evaluating the thyrotropic activity of an extract of the anterior lobe of the pituitary gland, as indicated by an increased basal metabolic rate or histologic evidence of stimulation of the thyroid gland in a hypophysectomized rat injected with the t. extract.
anoxemia t., hypoxemia t.; a t. for coronary insufficiency; the patient breathes a mixture of 10% oxygen and 90% nitrogen; if anginal pain or electrocardiographic abnormalities are induced, the t. is positive.
antibiotic sensitivity t., the *in vitro* testing of bacterial cultures with antibiotics to determine susceptibility of bacteria to antibiotic therapy.
antiglobulin t., Coombs' t.
antihuman globulin t., see Coombs' t. t.
aptitude t., an occupation-oriented intelligence t. used to evaluate a person's abilities, talents, and skills; particularly valuable in vocational counseling.
Aschheim-Zondek t. (A.-Z. t.), Zondek-Ascheim t.; an obsolete t. for pregnancy; repeated injections of small quantities of urine voided during the first months of pregnancy produce in infantile mice, within 100 hours, minute intrafollicular ovarian hemorrhages, and the development of lutein cells.
ascorbate-cyanide t., a t. for glucose 6-phosphate-deficient red blood cells; blood is incubated with sodium cyanide and ascorbate; the hydrogen peroxide generated is free to oxidize hemoglobin to methemoglobin, since cyanide inhibits catalase; a brown color is produced more rapidly in glucose 6-phosphate-deficient cells.
association t., a word (stimulus word) is spoken to the subject, who is to reply immediately with another word (reaction word) suggested to him by the first; used as a diagnostic aid in psychiatry and psychology, clues being given by the length of time (association time) between the stimulus and reaction words, and also by the nature of the reaction words.
Astwood's t., metrotrophic t.
atropine t., Dehio's t.
augmented histamine t., histamine t.
aussage t. (ows'zah-gă) [Ger. *Aussage,* a declaration], a t. of ability to reproduce correctly something that has been seen for a brief interval.
autohemolysis t., when sterile defibrinated blood is incubated at 37°C, normal red blood cells hemolyze slowly; cells with membrane or metabolic defects do so to a greater extent.
A.-Z. t., Aschheim-Zondek t.
Bachman-Pettit t., a modification of Kober's t. for the detection of estradiol and similar estrogenic hormones in the urine.
Bagolini t., a t. for retinal correspondence with the subject observing a figure through two striated lenses.
BALB t., binaural alternate loudness balance t.
Bárány's caloric t., caloric or nystagmus t.; a t. for vestibular function, made by irrigating the external auditory meatus with either hot or cold water; this normally causes stimulation of the vestibular apparatus, resulting in nystagmus and past-pointing; in vestibular disease, the response may be reduced or absent.
BEI t., butanol-extractable iodine t.
belt t., an obsolete t.: firm upward pressure on the lower part of the abdomen will remove the feeling of discomfort in cases of enteroptosia.
Bender gestalt t., a psychological t. used by neurologists and clinical psychologists to measure a person's ability to visually copy a set of geometric designs; useful for measuring visuospatial and visuomotor coordination to detect brain damage.
Benedict's t. for glucose, a copper-reduction t. for glucose in the urine, which involves thiocyanate in addition to copper sulfate for qualitative or quantitative use.
bentiromide t., a t. of pancreatic exocrine function that does not require duodenal intubation: orally administered bentiramide is cleaved by chymotrypsin within the lumen of the small intestine, releasing *p*-aminobenzoic acid which is absorbed and excreted in the urine; diminished urinary excretion of *p*-aminobenzoic acid suggests pancreatic insufficiency.
bentonite flocculation t., a flocculation t. for rheumatoid arthritis in which sensitized bentonite particles are added to inactivated serum; the t. is positive if half of the particles are clumped while the other half remain in suspension.
benzidine t., Adler's t.; a t. for blood; the suspected fluid is treated with glacial acetic acid and ether, and the latter is then decanted and treated with hydrogen peroxide and a solution of benzidine in acetic acid; the presence of blood is indicated by a bluish color turning to purple.
Bernstein t., acid perfusion t.; a t. to establish that substernal pain is due to reflux esophagitis, performed by instillation of a weak hydrochloric acid solution directly into the lower esophagus; symptoms disappear when the acid solution is replaced by normal saline solution.
Berson t., a t. of thyroid clearance of ^{131}I from the plasma by the thyroid gland.
Betke-Kleihauer t., a slide t. for the presence of fetal red blood cells among those of the mother; hemoglobins other than Hb F are eluted from the red blood cells on an air-dried blood film by a buffer of pH 3.3.
Bettendorff's t., a t. for arsenic; after mixing the suspected fluid with hydrochloric acid a solution of stannous chloride is added; when a piece of tin foil is then added, a brown precipitate forms.
Bial's t., orcinol t.; a t. for pentoses with orcinol.
bile acid tolerance t., a sensitive t. of hepatic dysfunction; following oral administration of labeled or unlabeled bile acid, the measured fractional disappearance rate or 10-minute retention is measured.

binaural alternate loudness balance t., BALB t.; a t. for recruitment in one ear; the comparison of relative loudness of a series of intensities presented alternately to either ear.
Binet t., Stanford-Binet intelligence *scale.*
Binz' t., a qualitative t. for the presence of quinine in the urine; a precipitate is formed on the addition of an aqueous solution of iodine and potassium iodide if quinine is present.
biuret t., a t. for the determination of serum proteins, based on the reaction of an alkaline copper reagent with substances containing two or more peptide bonds to produce a violet-blue color.
blind t., a method of testing in which an independent observer records the results of any t., drug, placebo, or procedure without knowing the identity of the samples or what result might be expected.
block design t., a performance t. using colored blocks to match standard designs; one of the subtests of the Wechsler intelligence scales.
breath analysis t., a t. of hepatic and intestinal absorptive function; aminopyrine labeled with radioactive carbon is administered orally; expired $^{14}CO_2$ is a measure of aminopyrine absorption and its metabolism in the liver.
breath-holding t., a rough index of cardiopulmonary reserve measured by the length of time that a subject can voluntarily stop breathing; normal duration is 30 seconds or more; diminished cardiac or pulmonary reserve is indicated by a duration of 20 seconds or less.
bromphenol t., a colorimetric t. for measurement of protein, albumin, and globulin in the urine by use of reagent strips.
bromsulphalein t., BSP t., a t. for liver function (hepatic excretory capacity) in which a known amount of dye, usually 5 mg/kg of body weight, is injected intravenously; subsequently (usually after 45 minutes elapsed time), the amount of dye remaining in the serum is measured; a concentration of 0.4 mg or less of bromsulphalein per 100 ml of serum or less than 4% of the injected dye is considered normal; bromsulphalein retention may follow decreased hepatic blood flow or biliary obstruction as well as hepatic cell damage.
butanol-extractable iodine t., BEI t.; a t. for thyroid function, applicable in patients who have received large amounts of iodine or iodized products.
California psychological inventory t., a personality inventory, used with normal persons, in which emphasis is upon social interaction variables.
Calmette t., conjuctival reaction to tuberculin.
caloric t., Bárány's caloric t.
CAMP t. [*C*hristie, *A*tkins, and *M*unch-*P*etersen, discoverers of the t.], a t. to identify Group B β-streptococci based on their formation of a substance (CAMP factor) that enlarges the area of hemolysis formed by streptococcal β-hemolysin.
capillary fragility t., vitamin C or capillary resistance t.; a tourniquet t. used to determine presence of vitamin C deficiency or thrombocytopenia; a circle 2.5 cm in diameter, the upper edge of which is 4 cm below the crease of the elbow, is drawn on the inner aspect of the forearm, pressure midway between the systolic and diastolic blood pressure is applied above the elbow for 15 minutes, and a count of petechiae within the circle is made: 10, normal; 10 to 20, marginal zone; over 20, abnormal. See also Rumpel-Leede t.
capillary resistance t., capillary fragility t.
capon-comb-growth t., comb-growth t.
carbohydrate utilization t., a t. for the definitive identification of clinically important yeasts and yeastlike organisms.
Casoni intradermal t., Casoni skin t., a t. for hydatid disease in which hydatid fluid is injected intracutaneously; immediate or delayed wheal and flare reaction is positive.
catatorulin t., an assay method for thiamine based upon its effect in increasing the uptake of oxygen by incubated slices of brain tissue to which it has been added.
Chick-Martin t., a method of testing the *in vitro* efficiency of a bactericidal agent; a standard culture of *Salmonella typhi* which has been added to a fixed amount of sterilized feces or yeast is tested for a fixed period (30 minutes), against various concentrations of phenol solution and various concentrations of the disinfectant; the result is expressed as a ratio: the phenol coefficient, which is the highest dilution of the disinfectant under t. at which the bacteria are killed, divided by the highest dilution of phenol which sterilizes the solution in the same length of time.
chi square t., a statistical method of assessing the significance of a difference, as when the date from two or more samples is represented by a discrete number.
Clauberg t., a t. for progestational activity; immature rabbits are treated with 8 daily injections of estrogen and then given 5 daily injections of the t. substance; the amount required to produce definite progestational changes in the endometrium is taken as the unit; it is equivalent to 0.75 mg of progesterone.
clomiphene t., a t. of pituitary gonadotropin reserve using clomiphene.
coccidioidin t., an intracutaneous t. for determining the presence of infection with the fungus *Coccidioides immitis;* a reaction of delayed hypersensitivity indicates a positive t. and is interpreted as meaning past or present infection with the fungus.
coin t., bellmetal *resonance.*
cold bend t., a t. of the ability of a wire to be shaped; performed by counting the number of times a wire can be bent to a right angle and reversed at the same point before breaking; important in establishing specifications for orthodontic wires.
colorimetric caries susceptibility t., Snyder's t.
comb-growth t., capon-comb-growth t.; a t. for androgenic activity, based upon the stimulation of comb growth in capons (castrated cockerels) or immature roosters.
complement-fixation t., an immunological t. for determining the presence of a particular antigen or antibody when one of the two is known to be present, based on the fact that complement is "fixed" in the presence of antigen and its specific antibody. See also Bordet-Gengou *phenomenon.*
Coombs' t., antiglobulin t.; a t. for antibodies, the so-called antihuman globulin t. using either the direct or indirect Coombs' t.'s.
Corner-Allen t., a t. for progestational activity; adult female rabbits are mated during estrus and spayed 18 hours later; the t. substance is injected subcutaneously on 5 successive days; the minimal amount required to produce complete progestational proliferation of the endometrium is taken as a unit, equivalent to 1.25 mg of progesterone.
cover t., a t. used for objective demonstration of ocular deviation in strabismus; may be performed by two methods: the cover-uncover t. and the alternate cover t.
cover-uncover t., a t. to detect strabismus; attention is directed to a small fixation object, and one eye is covered; if the uncovered eye moves to see the picture, strabismus is present.
CO_2-withdrawal seizure t., hyperventilation t.; utilization of hyperventilation to demonstrate abnormalities in the brain waves or even to precipitate a convulsion.
Crampton t., a test for physical condition and resistance; a record is made of the pulse and the blood pressure in the recumbent and in the standing position, and the difference is graded from the theoretical perfection of 100 (seldom attained) downward (a reading of 75 is considered excellent, 65 poor); high values indicate a good physical resistance but low ones indicate weakness and a liability to shock after an operation.
t.'s of criminal responsibility, in forensic psychiatry, legal precedents upon which are based decisions concerning insanity in criminals. See also American Law Institute *rule,* Durham *rule,* M'Naghten *rule,* and New Hampshire *rule.*
cutaneous t., skin t.
cutaneous tuberculin t., see tuberculin t.

cutireaction t., skin t.
cyanide-nitroprusside t., a qualitative t. for diagnosis of cystinuria; the addition of fresh sodium cyanide formed by sodium nitroprusside to a sample of urine gives rise to a stable red-purple color in the presence of cystine.
cytotropic antibody t., a rosette t. for macrophage cytotropic antibody: monolayers of macrophages are exposed first to antibody cytotropic for macrophages, then to the antigen (for which the antibody is specific), and indicator sheep erythrocytes; if the antibody is specific for sheep erythrocytes, the latter will form a rosette around the macrophages directly, but if not, and the antigen is soluble, the antigen must be coupled to the sheep erythrocytes by an agent such as bis-diazotized benzidine.
DA pregnancy t., direct agglutination latex t. for pregnancy. See immunologic pregnancy t.
Day's t., a t. for blood by adding to the suspected fluid, or the washing of a suspected stain, tincture of guaiac and then hydrogen peroxide; the presence of blood results in a blue color.
Dehio's t., atropine t.; if an injection of atropine relieves bradycardia, the condition is due to action of the vagus; if it does not, the condition is due to an affection of the heart itself.
dehydrocholate t., a method of determining the speed of the blood circulation; a solution of sodium dehydrocholate is injected intravenously, and the time that elapses before a bitter taste is noted in the mouth is recorded; the average of this time is normally about 13 seconds.
dexamethasone suppression t., a t. for the detection and diagnosis of Cushing's syndrome; following administration of 1.0 mg of dexamethasone at 11 p.m., normal persons suppress plasma cortisol to low levels; patients with Cushing's syndrome do not. Higher dose regimens distinguish between Cushing's syndrome due to tumor and due to hyperplasia.
Dick t., Dick method; an intracutaneous t. of susceptibility to the erythrogenic toxin of *Streptococcus pyogenes* responsible for the rash and other manifestations of scarlet fever.
differential renal function t., differential ureteral catheterization t.
differential ureteral catheterization t., differential or split renal function t.; a study performed to determine various functional parameters of one kidney compared to the contralateral kidney; ureteral catheters are inserted at cystoscopy into the ureter or renal pelvis bilaterally, and simultaneous measurements are made of urine flow rate, insulin, or PAH (if infused), endogenous creatinine, or various urinary solutes.
dinitrophenylhydrazine t., a screening t. for maple syrup urine disease; the addition of 2,4-dinitrophenylhydrazine in HCl to urine gives a chalky white precipitate in the presence of ketoacids.
direct Coombs' t., a t. for detecting sensitized erythrocytes in erythroblastosis fetalis and in cases of acquired hemolytic anemia: the patient's erythrocytes are washed with saline to remove serum and unattached antibody protein, then incubated with Coombs' anti-human globulin (usually serum from a rabbit or goat previously immunized with human globulin); after incubation, the system is centrifuged and examined for agglutination, which indicates the presence of so-called incomplete or univalent antibodies on the surface of the erythrocytes.
direct fluorescent antibody t., see fluorescent antibody *technique*.
discontinuation t., a t. to determine whether a certain drug is responsible for a reaction by observation of a remission of symptoms following cessation of its use.
Doerfler-Stewart (D-S) t., examination of the patient's ability to respond to spondee words in the presence of a masking noise of the saw-tooth type; used especially in differentiating between functional and organic hearing loss.
double (gel) diffusion precipitin t. in one dimension, see gel diffusion precipitin t.'s in one dimension.
double (gel) diffusion precipitin t. in two dimensions, see gel diffusion precipitin t.'s in two dimensions.
Dragendorff's t., a qualitative t. for bile; a play of colors is produced by adding a drop of nitric acid to white filter paper or unglazed porcelain, moistened with a fluid containing bile pigments. The t. is essentially the same as Gmelin's t. for bile in urine.
drawer t., drawer *sign.*
D-S t., Doerfler-Stewart t.
Ducrey t., Ito-Reenstierna t.; an intradermal t., using inactivated *Haemophilus ducreyi,* for diagnosis of chancroid; a positive delayed reaction is indicative of present or past infection; false-positive results occur.
Dugas' t., in the case of an injured shoulder, if the elbow cannot be made to touch the chest while the hand rests on the opposite shoulder, the injury is a dislocation and not a fracture of the humerus.
dye exclusion t., a t. to determine cell viability in which a dilute solution of certain dyes (*e.g.,* trypan blue, eosin Y, nigrosin, Alcian blue) is mixed with a suspension of live cells; cells that exclude dye are considered to be alive while cells that stain are considered dead; it is not always an accurate t. because it indicates only the structural integrity of the cell membrane.
Ebbinghaus t., a psychological t. in which the patient is asked to complete certain sentences from which several words have been left out.
Ellsworth-Howard t., measurement of serum and urinary phosphorus after intravenous administration of parathyroid extract; used in the diagnosis of pseudohypoparathyroidism.
Emmens' S/L t., a t. for distinguishing estrogenic precursors from active estrogens; a number of mice are divided into two groups, one of which is treated subcutaneously with the estrogen; the other group receives the estrogen intravaginally. The systemic and local effective doses are expressed as a ratio (S/L); the ratio is unity for the precursors but much greater than unity for active estrogens.
E-rosette t., a t. to identify T lymphocytes by mixing purified blood lymphocytes with serum and sheep erythrocytes; rosettes of erythrocytes form around human T lymphocytes on incubation.
erythrocyte adherence t., adhesion t.
erythrocyte fragility t., fragility t.
ether t., a t. to determine arm-to-lung circulation time; diluted ether is injected intravenously and the end point taken when the subject coughs or tastes ether or the observer smells ether on the subject's breath.
exercise t., two-step exercise t.
Farnsworth-Munsell color t., a t. for color perception using 84 color disks arranged in order of increasing hue.
fern t., a t. for estrogenic activity; cervical mucus smears form a fern pattern at those times when estrogen secretion is elevated, as at the time of ovulation.
ferric chloride t., a qualitative t. for the detection of phenylketonuria; the addition of ferric chloride to urine gives rise to a blue-green color in the presence of phenylketonuria.
Fevold t., a t. for relaxin; based on the degree of relaxation of the pelvic ligaments of the guinea pig upon injection of extracts of the corpus luteum.
Finckh t., a psychological t. in which the patient is asked to explain certain proverbial expressions, such as "burn the candle at both ends," "the early bird catches the worm," etc.
finger-nose t., a t. of voluntary eye-motor coordination of the upper limb(s); the subject is asked to slowly touch the tip of his nose with his extended index finger.
finger-to-finger t., a t. for coordination and position sense of the upper limbs; the subject is asked to approximate the ends of his index fingers.
fish t., erythrophore *reaction.*
Fishberg concentration t., a t. of renal water conservation; after overnight fluid deprivation, morning urine samples are collected

and specific gravity is measured.
fistula t., compression or rarefaction of the air in the external auditory canal excites nystagmus when there is an erosion of the inner bony wall of the tympanum, so long as the labyrinth is still capable of functioning; when the tympanic wall is intact, no nystagmus occurs.
FIT t., fusion-inferred threshold t.
Fleitmann's t., a t. for arsenic; hydrogen is generated in a t. tube containing the suspected fluid; the fluid is heated and a piece of filter paper moistened with silver nitrate solution is held over the top; if arsenic is present, the moistened paper is blackened.
flocculation t., see flocculation *reaction.*
fluorescein instillation t., a t. for patency of the lacrimal system; fluorescein instilled in the conjunctival sac can be recovered from the inferior nasal meatus.
fluorescein string t., a string t. in which fluorescein is given intravenously to determine gastrointestinal hemorrhage; if the string fluoresces after removal, it has been contaminated by blood that has appeared since injection of the fluorescein.
fluorescent antinuclear antibody (FANA) t., a t. for antinuclear antibody components; used, in particular, for the diagnosis of collagen-vascular diseases.
fluorescent treponemal antibody-absorption t., FTA-ABS t.; a sensitive and specific serologic t. for syphilis using a suspension of the Nichols strain of *Treponema pallidum* as antigen; the presence or absence of antibody in the patient's serum is indicated by an indirect fluorescent antibody technique.
foam stability t., shake t.; a t. for fetal pulmonary maturity, determined by the ability of pulmonary surfactant in amniotic fluid to generate stable foam in the presence of ethanol after mechanical agitation.
Folin's t., **(1)** a quantitative t. for uric acid by means of the color produced with phosphotungstic acid and a base; **(2)** a quantitative t. for urea; the urea is decomposed by boiling with magnesium chloride, and the freed ammonia is measured.
Folin-Looney t., a t. for tyrosine that gives a blue color in alkaline solution with a reagent consisting of sodium tungstate, phosphomolybdic acid, and phosphoric acid.
Fosdick-Hansen-Epple t., a t. for determining dental caries activity based on a solution of powdered human enamel in a saliva-glucose-enamel mixture.
Foshay t., an intradermal t. for cat-scratch disease, using material prepared from suppurative lymph nodes of persons known to have had the disease.
fragility t., erythrocyte fragility t.; a t. that measures the resistance of erythrocytes to hemolysis in hypotonic saline solutions; erythrocytes to be tested are added to varying concentrations of saline (usually ranging from 0.85 to 0.10% sodium chloride with 0.05% increments), and beginning and complete hemolysis are measured; normal erythrocytes show initial hemolysis at concentrations of 0.45 to 0.39% and complete hemolysis at 0.33 to 0.30%; in hereditary spherocytosis the fragility of the erythrocytes is markedly increased, whereas in thalassemia, sickle cell anemia, and obstructive jaundice the fragility of the erythrocytes is usually reduced.
Frei t., Frei-Hoffman reaction; an intracutaneous diagnostic t. for lymphogranuloma Venereum: originally, the antigen was prepared from a softened, partially liquefied bubo, but the modern Frei antigen is usually a sterile preparation of inactivated chlamydiae from domestic fowl; a positive delayed type reaction is not diagnostically specific for lymphogranuloma venereum because of a group antigen also present in related chlamydiae.
Fridenberg's stigometric card t., a t. of vision and accommodation for illiterates, using a card containing a series of dots and squares of graduated size, to be counted at various distances.
FTA-ABS t., fluorescent treponemal antibody-absorption t.
fusion-inferred threshold (FIT) t., employment of the phenomenon of cerebral fusion of binaural sounds to substitute for conventional masking in hearing testing.
Gaddum and Schild t., a sensitive method for identification of epinephrine in tissue or other material, based on the fluorescence of epinephrine exposed to ultraviolet light in the presence of alkali and oxygen; sensitivity ranges from 1:50 to 1:100 million.
galactose tolerance t., a liver function t., based on the ability of the liver to convert galactose to glycogen, measured by the rate of excretion of galactose following ingestion or intravenous injection of a known amount; normally, less than 3 g appear in the urine within 5 hours after the ingestion of 40 g.
gel diffusion precipitin t.'s, gel diffusion reactions; precipitin t.'s in which the immune precipitate forms in a gel medium (usually agar) into which one or both reactants have diffused; generally classified in two types, in one dimension, and in two dimensions.
gel diffusion precipitin t.'s in one dimension, precipitin t.'s in which antigen solution and antibody incorporated in agar are layered in tubes, permitting effective diffusion in the vertical dimension; the antibody-containing agar may be overlaid directly with antigen solution (*single (gel) diffusion in one dimension*), or the antigen (fluid or in agar) layer and the antibody-containing agar layer may be separated by a layer of plain agar into which both antigen and antibody diffuse (*double (gel) diffusion in one dimension*).
gel diffusion precipitin t.'s in two dimensions, precipitin t.'s made in a uniform flat layer of agar that permits radial diffusion, in both of the horizontal dimensions, of one or both reactants. *Single (gel) diffusion in two dimensions* incorporates antibody in which agar and antigen solutions are placed in wells from which the agar has been removed. *Double (gel) diffusion in two dimensions* (Ouchterlony test, technique, or method) incorporates antigen and antibody solutions placed in separate wells in a sheet of plain agar, permitting radial diffusion of both reactants; this method is widely used to determine antigenic relationships; the bands of precipitate that form where the reactants meet in optimal concentration are of three patterns, referred to as reaction of identity, reaction of partial identity (cross-reaction), and reaction of nonidentity.
Gellé t., a vibrating tuning fork is applied over the mastoid process; if it is heard, the air in the external auditory canal is compressed, by means of a rubber tube inserted into the canal and a hand bulb, thereby fixing the stapes in the oval window, and the sound ceases to be heard, but is again perceived if the air pressure is removed; a t. of the mobility of the ossicles.
Geraghty's t., phenolsulfonphthalein t.
Gerhardt's t. for acetoacetic acid, Gerhardt's reaction; in fresh urine a red color develops upon addition of $FeCl_3$; no color develops if the urine has first been boiled; this t. has low specificity and sensitivity.
Gerhardt's t. for urobilin in the urine, the urobilin is extracted with chloroform and then treated with iodine and potassium hydrate, a fluorescent green color being produced.
germ tube t., a t. for the identification of *Candida albicans;* after a 3-hr incubation in serum, an inoculum of *Candida* develops tube-like appendages.
glucose oxidase paper strip t., a qualitative t. for glucose in the urine, in which glucose is oxidized to gluconic acid by glucose oxidase; a specific t., unless ascorbic acid is present.
glucose tolerance t., a t. for diabetes, based upon the ability of the normal liver to absorb and store excessive amounts of glucose as glycogen; following ingestion of 100 g of glucose, the fasting blood sugar promptly rises and then falls to normal within 2 hours, but in a diabetic patient the increase is greater and the return to normal unusually prolonged.
Gmelin's t., Rosenbach-Gmelin t.; a t. for bile in the urine or other body fluid; nitric acid, with a little nitrous acid, is cautiously added to a few milliliters of the material to be tested; if bile (bilirubin) is present, it is oxidized to varying degrees, thereby re-

sulting in disklike zones that are (from the interface outward) yellow, red, violet, blue, and green; development of green and violet layers is essential to the validity of the t.

Gofman t., a t. for various serum lipoproteins that contain cholesterol, as an index of the tendency to the development of atheromatous lesions and arteriosclerosis; the t. is based on the differential flotation of molecules of various sizes when the serum is treated in an ultracentrifuge.

Goldscheider's t., determination of the temperature sense by touching the skin with a sharp-pointed metallic rod, heated to varying degrees.

gold sol t., Lange's t.

Göthlin's t., a capillary fragility t. to determine the presence or absence of scurvy.

group t., in psychology, a t. designed to be administered to more than one individual at a time; *e.g.,* scholastic achievement t., medical college admissions t.

guaiac t., Almén's t. for blood.

Günzberg's t., a t. for hydrochloric acid utilizing phloroglucin vanillin (Gunzberg's reagent), with which a bright red color is produced in the presence of the acid.

Guthrie t., bacterial inhibition assay for direct measurement of serum phenylalanine; in widespread use for detection of phenylketonuria in the newborn.

Gutzeit's t., a t. for arsenic; a piece of zinc and a little sulfuric acid are added to the suspected liquid which is then boiled; a bit of filter paper with a silver nitrate solution is held in the vapor and will turn yellow if arsenic is present.

Habel t., a method of determining the antigenic efficacy of inactivated rabies vaccines.

Hallion's t., Tuffier's t.; a t. of collateral circulation; when the main artery and vein of a limb are compressed, in a case of aneurysm, swelling of the veins of the hand or foot will take place only when the collateral circulation is free.

Ham's t., acidified serum t.

Hardy-Rand-Ritter t., a t. for color vision deficiency similar to the Ishihara t.

Harrington-Flocks t., a rapid screening t. for visual field defects; patterns are viewed tachistoscopically, and the patterns are visible only when illuminated by a flash of ultraviolet light.

Harris t., Harris and Ray t.

Harris and Ray t., a t. for vitamin C in the urine; a microtitration t. of the urine against a known amount of 0.05% aqueous solution of the dye 2,6-dichloroindophenol in 10% acetic acid (usually 0.05 ml of dye is used, roughly equivalent to 0.025 mg of ascorbic acid).

head-dropping t., a t. used in the diagnosis of disease of the extrapyramidal or striatal system (*e.g.,* parkinsonism, Wilson's disease); with the patient supine, relaxed, and his attention diverted, the examiner briskly lifts the patient's head with the right hand and then allows it to drop upon the palm of his left hand; the head of a normal person drops suddenly like a dead weight, whereas, in striatal disease the head falls slowly, gently, and almost hesitantly.

heat coagulation t., a t. for measurement of protein in urine; albumin and globulin are coagulated by heat at an acid pH, and the amount of turbidity present provides a qualitative estimation of the degree of proteinuria.

heat instability t., a t. for the presence of unstable hemoglobins; fresh red blood cells lysed in distilled water develop a precipitate within one hour at 50°C if unstable hemoglobin is present.

heel-tap t., see heel *tap.*

Heinz body t., a t. for glucose 6-phosphate dehydrogenase-deficient red blood cells; an oxidant (acetylphenylhydrazine) is added to blood; after incubation at 37°C, glucose 6-phosphate dehydrogenase-deficient samples exhibit more than 30% Heinz bodies.

hemadsorption virus t., a procedure for titrating viral antibodies in a serum (using a known virus), or for identifying a virus (using a known antiserum); the t. is based on the fact that some viruses are adsorbed on the surface of red blood cells during an appropriate incubation period, and cells treated in this manner may be used in an agglutination t. with serum that contains antibody for the virus that is on the surface of the erythrocytes.

hemoccult t., a qualitative t. for occult blood in stool based upon detecting the peroxidase activity of hemoglobin; a t. kit can be used at home and the specimen mailed to a laboratory for evaluation.

Hering's t., a t. of binocular vision; the subject looks through an apparatus having at its farther end a thread about which a small sphere is dropped; with binocular vision the observer recognizes the location of the sphere in front of or behind the thread; with monocular vision this is not possible.

Hess' t., Rumpel-Leede t.

Hinton t., a formerly widely used precipitin (flocculation) t. for syphilis in which the "antigen" consisted of glycerol, cholesterol, and beef heart extract.

Histalog t., maximal Histalog t; a t. for measurement of maximal production of gastric acidity or anacidity; it is similar to the histamine t., but uses Histalog (betazole hydrochloride), an analogue of histamine.

histamine t., augmented histamine t.; a t. for maximal production of gastric acidity or anacidity; after preliminary administration of an antihistamine, histamine acid phosphate is injected subcutaneously in a dose of 0.04 mg/kg of body weight, followed by analysis of gastric contents. See also Histalog t.

histoplasmin-latex t., a passive agglutination t. for histoplasmosis; latex particles, sensitized with antigen extracted from *Histoplasma capsulatum,* are used in a flocculation reaction with the patient's serum.

Hollander t., insulin hypoglycemia t.

Holmgren's t., Holmgren method; a t. for color blindness in which the subject matches variously colored skeins of wool.

homovanillic acid t., HVA t.; a t. for homovanillic acid based upon the fact that dopamine is present in sympathetic nervous tissue as precursor of norepinephrine; since norepinephrine has a metabolic pathway which yields homovanillic acid, tumors such as neuroblastomas and ganglioneuromas may cause elevations of urinary dopamine and homovanillic acid.

Hooker-Forbes t., a t. for compounds with progestational activity; such compounds cause hypertrophy of the stromal nuclei of the endometrium in uteri obtained from spayed mice; a sensitive t. capable of detecting 0.0002 μg of progesterone.

Howard t., a differential ureteral catheterization t. performed by the insertion of bilateral ureteral catheters to measure simultaneous urinary volume and sodium concentration in patients with suspected renovascular hypertension; patients with unilateral obstruction of the main renal artery are found to have a decrease in urine volume of at least 50%, and of urinary sodium concentration by at least 15% from the ipsilateral kidney when compared to the normal side.

Huhner t., determination of sperm quantity and motility in specimens obtained from the cervical canal following coitus.

HVA t., homovanillic acid t.

17-hydroxycorticosteroid t., 17-OH-corticoids t.; Porter-Silber chromogens t.; a t., dependent on the Porter-Silber reaction, that is used as a measure of adrenocortical function and is performed on urine. Low values are seen in Addison's disease and hypopituitarism; high values are seen in Cushing's syndrome and extreme stress.

hyperemia t., Moszkowicz t.

hyperventilation t., CO_2-withdrawal seizure t.

hypoxemia t., anoxemia t.

^{131}I uptake t., radioactive iodide uptake t.; RAI t.; a t. of thyroid function in which ^{131}I-iodide is given orally; after 24 hours, the amount present in the thyroid gland is measured and compared with normal values.

immune adhesion t., adhesion t.

immunologic pregnancy t., a general term for t.'s for detection of increased human chorionic gonadotropin in plasma or urine by immunologic techniques including latex particle agglutination, radioimmunoassay, and radioreceptor assays.
indirect t., see Prausnitz-Küstner *reaction*.
indirect Coombs' t., a t. routinely performed in cross-matching blood or in the investigation of transfusion reaction: test or patient's serum is incubated with a suspension of donor erythrocytes; if specific antibodies are present, they become attached to the antigen in donor's cells; after a washing with saline, Coombs' antihuman globulin is added; agglutination at this point indicates that antibodies present in the original test serum had indeed become attached to donor erythrocytes.
indirect fluorescent antibody t., see fluorescent antibody *technique*.
indirect hemagglutination t., passive *hemagglutination*.
insulin hypoglycemia t., Hollander t.; a t. to determine the completeness of vagotomy for peptic ulcer; after the surgical procedure is performed, insulin is administered to cause hypoglycemia; if vagotomy is complete, the acid output from the stomach following administration of insulin is less than that before insulin administration; if the reverse if true, incomplete vagotomy is likely.
intelligence t., a t., using well researched items and involving a systematic method of administration and scoring, used to assess an individual's global aptitude or level of competence, in contrast to an achievement t.
Ishihara t., a t. for color vision deficiency that utilizes a series of pseudoisochromatic plates on which numbers or letters are printed in dots of primary colors surrounded by dots of other colors; the figures are discernable by individuals with normal color vision.
isopropanol precipitation t., a t. using the principle that the internal bonds of hemoglobin are weakened by nonpolar solvents; thus, unstable hemoglobins will precipitate more rapidly than other hemoglobins in isopropanol.
Ito-Reenstierna t., Ducrey t.
Jacquemin's t., a t. for phenol; to the suspected fluid an equal amount of aniline is added, and, after thorough admixture, a little solution of sodium hypochlorite; if phenol is present the fluid becomes blue in color.
Jaffe's t., a qualitative t. for the presence of indicanuria; after an equal amount of HCl is added to the urine, the further addition of chloroform and $CaCl_2$ gives rise to blue or purple chloroform droplets which sink to the bottom if indican is present.
Janet's t., a t. for functional or organic anesthesia; the patient (with eyes closed) is told to say "yes" or "no" when he feels or does not feel the touch of the examiner's finger; in the case of functional anesthesia he may say "no" when an anesthetic area is touched, but will say nothing, being unaware that he is touched, in cases of organic anesthesia.
Jolles' t., a t. for bile; a precipitate is obtained by agitation with chloroform, a solution of barium chloride, and hydrochloric acid; the precipitate is removed, and the addition of a drop or two or sulfuric acid will produce a play of color if bile pigments are present.
Katayama's t., a qualitative colorimetric t. for the presence of carboxyhemoglobin in the blood.
ketogenic corticoids t., 17-ketogenic steroid assay t.
17-ketogenic steroid assay t., ketogenic corticoids t.; a t., performed on the urine, that is valuable in diagnosis of adrenogenital syndrome and in some cases of Cushing's syndrome.
17-ketosteroid assay t., a colorimetric t., based on the Zimmermann reaction, that indicates metabolites or adrenal and testicular steroids excreted as 17-ketones in the urine; increased values are most striking in adrenocortical tumors, decreased values in Addison's disease or in panhypopituitarism.
Knoop hardness t., see Knoop hardness *number*.
Kober t., a t. for naturally occurring estrogens, based upon the production of a pink color (absorption maximum: 520 mμ) when an estrogen is heated in a mixture of phenol and sulfuric acid.
Kolmer t., a former standard quantitative method for the Wassermann t., with numerous modifications (especially as to antigen).
Korotkoff's t., a t. of collateral circulation; while the artery above an aneurysm is compressed, the blood pressure in the distal circulation is estimated; if it is fairly high, the collateral circulation is good.
Kurzrok-Ratner t., a t. for estrogens in the urine; the urine is extracted with ethyl acetate and, after purification, the extract is subjected to bioassay as in the Allen-Doisy t.
Kveim t., Kveim-Stilzbach t., Nickerson-Kveim t.; an intradermal t. for the detection of sarcoidosis, done by injecting Kveim antigen (obtained from spleens of persons with sarcoidosis) and examining skin biopsies after three and six weeks; a positive t. is indicated by typical nodules showing evidence of sarcoid tissue.
Landsteiner-Donath t., see Donath-Landsteiner *phenomenon*.
Lange's t., gold sol t.; Zsigmondy's t.; an obsolete, nonspecific t. for altered proteins in spinal fluid. As originally used by Lange in 1912, the t. was thought to be specific for neurosyphilis; however, this proved to be incorrect. Dilutions of spinal fluid are made in saline and to these a colloidal gold solution is added; if altered proteins are present, there is a color change or precipitate formed. At present, its chief use is to demonstrate cerebrospinal fluid protein abnormalities in multiple sclerosis.
latex agglutination t., latex fixation t., a passive agglutination t. in which antigen is adsorbed onto latex particles which then clump in the presence of antibody specific for the adsorbed antigen.
LE cell t., lupus erythematosus cell t.; *in vitro* incubation of blood or bone marrow of patients with systemic lupus erythematosis, or action of their serum on normal leukocytes, causes formation of characteristic LE cells.
Legal's t., a t. for acetone; the urine is rendered alkaline by a few drops of a solution of potassium hydroxide, and to this are added 2 or 3 drops of a freshly prepared 10% solution of sodium nitroprusside; it is colored red, then yellow; then a few drops of acetic acid are trickled down the side of the t. tube and at the line of junction of the two fluids is formed a carmine or purple ring.
lepromin t., a t. utilizing an intradermal injection of a lepromin, such as the Dharmendra antigen or Mitsuda antigen, to classify the stage of leprosy based on the lepromin reaction, such as the Fernandez reaction or Mitsuda reaction; it differentiates tuberculoid leprosy, in which there is a positive delayed reaction at the injection site, from lepromatous leprosy, in which there is no reaction (*i.e.*, a negative t. result) despite the active malignant *Mycobacterium leprae* infection; the t. is not diagnostic, since normal uninfected persons may react.
leukocyte adherence assay t., a t. to detect the ability of leukocytes to adhere to bacteria, performed *in vitro* using nylon fibers to measure adherence.
leukocyte bactericidal assay t., a t. of leukocytes to determine their ability to kill a culture of live bacteria.
Liebermann-Burchard t., a colorimetric t. for unsaturated sterols, notably cholesterol; a blue-green color develops when such substances are added to acetic anhydride and sulfuric acid in chloroform.
limulus lysate t., a t. for the rapid detection of Gram-negative bacterial meningitis; Gram-negative endotoxin induces gel formation of *Limulus polyphemus* (horseshoe crab) lysates.
line t., a t. for rickets, based on observation of the lines of calcification in the growing ends of rachitic long bones in rats given vitamin D preparations under standard t. conditions; used in biological assay of vitamin D by the USP.
Lombard voice-reflex t., the observation of fluctuations in the intensity of a patient's voice when a masking noise is increased or decreased; a t. useful in assessing functional hearing loss.
Lücke's t., a t. for hippuric acid; hot nitric acid is added to the urine and evaporated to dryness; the presence of hippuric acid is

indicated by an odor of nitrobenzol upon further heating.
lupus band t. (LBT), a direct immunofluorescent technique for demonstrating a band of immunoglobulins at the dermal-epidermal junction of the skin of patients with lupus erythematosus.
lupus erythematosus cell t., LE cell t.
Machado-Guerreiro t., a complement-fixation t. for infection with *Trypanosoma cruzi.*
macrophage migration inhibition t., migration inhibition t.
Mantoux t., see tuberculin t.
Master's t., Master's two-step exercise t., two-step exercise t.
Mauthner's t., an obsolete t. for color perception similar to Holmgren's, but made with vials filled with pigments instead of with skeins of wool.
maximal Histalog t., Histalog t.
Mazzotti t., Mazzotti reaction; a t. for onchocerciasis using an oral t. dose of diethylcarbamazine (50 or 100 mg), resulting in the appearance of an acute rash in 2 to 24 hours from death of microfilariae in the skin.
McMurray t., rotation of the tibia on the femur to determine injury to meniscal structures.
McPhail t., a t. for progesterone and like substances; immature female rabbits are treated with 150 IU of estrone over a period of 6 days; the t. material is then given in five daily subcutaneous doses; progestational proliferation of the endometrium is noted and the results estimated according to a scale from 0 to ++++; the amount required to produce an average (++) response is taken as a unit, equivalent to 0.25 mg of progesterone.
Meinicke t., the first successful application (1917–1918) of immune precipitation to diagnosis of syphilis, now obsolete.
Meltzer-Lyon t., a t. used in diagnosis of gallbladder conditions: 25 ml of a 25% solution of magnesium sulfate are delivered into the region of the sphincter of Oddi through a duodenal tube, causing contraction of the gallbladder, relaxation of the sphincter, and the expulsion of bile from the common duct and gallbladder; bile from the common duct is pale and is expelled first, that from the gallbladder follows; samples aspirated from the tube are examined for pus cells, pigment granules, epithelial cells, cholesterol, etc.
metabisulfite t., a t. for sickle cell hemoglobin (Hb S); deoxygenation of cells containing Hb S is enhanced by addition of sodium metabisulfite to the blood, causing sickling visible on a slide; certain other abnormal hemoglobins (Hb C_{Harlem} and Hb I) also sickle in this t.
3-methoxy-4-hydroxymandelic acid t., vanillylmandelic acid t.
metrotrophic t., Astwood's t.; a t. for the assay of estrogenic substances; immature female rats (25 to 49 g) are injected subcutaneously with the hormone and killed after 6 hours, when the increase in uterine weight (due largely to imbibation of water) is taken as the criterion of estrogenic activity.
MHA-TP t., microhemagglutination-*Treponema pallidum* t.
microhemagglutination-Treponema pallidum t., MHA-TP t.; a microtechnical version of the *Treponema pallidum* hemagglutination t.
microprecipitation t., a precipitation t. in which reduced quantities of t. reagents are used.
migration inhibition t., macrophage migration inhibition t.; an *in vitro* method of testing for cellular (delayed type) sensitivity; when specific antigen is present, peritoneal exudate cells (macrophages) from a sensitized animal do not migrate from the capillary tube in which they have been packed, or from a well in agar, in the manner characteristic of similar cells from a normal animal.
milk-ring t., abortus-Bang-ring t.; a special form of agglutination t. done on the pooled milk of many cows, usually entire herds, for the detection of herds containing individuals infected with bovine brucellosis.
Millon-Nasse t., a t. for protein, the tyrosine of which reacts with nitrite after a brief treatment with mercuric ion in acid to give a color.
Minnesota multiphasic personality inventory t., (MMPI), a questionnaire type of psychological test for ages 16 and over, with 550 true-false statements coded in 14 personality scales in both individual and group forms.
mixed agglutination t., see mixed agglutination *reaction.*
mixed lymphocyte culture t., MLC t.; a t. for histocompatibility of HL-A antigens in which donor and recipient lymphocytes are mixed in culture; the degree of incompatibility is indicated by the number of cells that have undergone transformation and mitosis, or by the uptake of radioactive isotope-labeled thymidine.
MLC t., mixed lymphocyte culture t.
Molisch's t., a color t. for sugar, which condenses with α-naphthol or thymol in the presence of strong sulfuric acid, which converts the sugar to furfural derivatives.
Moloney t., a t. to detect a high degree of sensitivity to diphtheria toxoid; more than a minimal local reaction to diluted ($^1/_{20}$) toxoid given intradermally indicates that prophylactic toxoid should be inoculated in fractional doses at suitable intervals.
Morner's t., **(1)** for cysteine, which gives a brilliant purple color with sodium nitroprusside; **(2)** for tyrosine, which gives a green color on boiling with sulfuric acid containing formaldehyde.
Moszkowicz' t., hyperemia t.; a t. for arteriosclerosis; a lower limb is made anemic with an Esmarch tourniquet bandage, which is removed at the end of 5 minutes; color normally reaches the tips of the toes in a few seconds, but in arteriosclerosis with sufficient obstruction the color returns slowly, requiring sometimes several minutes to suffuse the entire limb.
Motulsky dye reduction t., a t. for glucose 6-phosphate dehydrogenase deficiency in the blood, using a mixture of brilliant cresyl blue, glucose 6-phosphate, and NADP.
mucin clot t., Ropes t.; a t. that reflects the polymerization of synovial fluid hyaluronate; a few drops of synovial fluid added to acetic acid form a clot; poor clot formation occurs in a variety of inflammatory conditions including septic arthritis, gouty arthritis, and rheumatoid arthritis.
multiple puncture tuberculin t., a kind of tine t. See tuberculin t.
mumps sensitivity t., a skin t. for sensitivity to mumps, in which inactivated mumps virus is used as antigen.
Nagel's t., a t. for color vision in which the observer determines the relative amounts of red and green necessary to match spectral yellow.
NBT t., abbreviation for nitroblue tetrazolium t.
neutralization t., protection t.
niacin t., a t. of the ability of mycobacteria to elaborate niacin; used to distinguish different strains.
Nickerson-Kveim t., Kveim t.
Nicklès' t., a t. for cane sugar; heating with carbon tetrachloride to the boiling point produces a black color if the sugar is cane sugar (sucrose), but not if it is glucose.
nitroblue tetrazolium (NBT) t., a t. to detect the phagocytic ability of polymorphonuclear leukocytes by measuring the capacity of the oxygen-dependent leukocytic bactericidal system.
nitroprusside t., a qualitative t. for cystinuria; following the addition of sodium cyanide to the urine, the further addition of nitroprusside produces a red-purple color if the cyanide has reduced any cystine present to cysteine.
nystagmus t., Bárány's caloric t.
Obermayer's t., a t. for indican; solids in the urine are precipitated by means of a 20% solution of acetate of lead and then filtered, and to the filtrate is added fuming hydrochloric acid containing a small amount of ferric chloride solution; if indican is present, the addition of chloroform causes the formation of indigo, indicated by the blue color.
17-OH-corticoids t., 17-hydroxycorticosteroid t.
oral lactose tolerance t., a t. for lactose deficiency; the plasma glucose response to an oral lactose load is measured as in the (oral) glucose tolerance t.

orcinol t., Bial's t.
Ouchterlony t., double (gel) diffusion t. in two dimensions. See gel diffusion precipitin t.'s in two dimensions.
ovarian ascorbic acid depletion t., a t. used to measure the quantity of luteinizing hormone in tissue, blood, or urine.
P and P t., prothrombin and proconvertin t.
Pachon's t., in a case of aneurysm, determination of the collateral circulation by estimation of the blood pressure.
Palmer acid t. for peptic ulcer, in duodenal ulcer, the administration of acid by duodenal tube causes severe pain.
palmin t., palmitin t., a t. of pancreatic efficiency, based upon the fact that the presence of fat in the stomach causes the pylorus to open and admit the pancreatic juice; this splits the palmin so that an examination of the stomach contents, after a t. meal containing palmin, will reveal the presence of fatty acids.
pancreozymin-secretin t., see secretin t.
Pandy's t., Pandy's *reaction.*
Pap t., Papanicolaou smear t., microscopic examination of cells exfoliated or scraped from a mucosal surface after staining with Papanicolaou's stain; used especially for detection of cancer of the uterine cervix.
parallax t., measurement of the deviation in strabismus by the alternate cover t. combined with neutralization of the deviation using prisms.
patch t., a t. of skin sensitiveness: a small piece of blotting paper or cloth, wet with the t. fluid, is applied to the skin and after 48 hours the area previously covered is compared with the uncovered surface; an eczematous reaction occurs if the substance causes contact allergy. See also photo-patch t.
Patrick's t., a t. to determine the presence or absence of sacroiliac disease; with the patient supine, the thigh and knee are flexed and the external malleolus is placed above the patella of the opposite leg; this can ordinarily be done without pain, but, on depressing the knee, pain is promptly elicited in sacroiliac disease.
Paul's t., Paul's *reaction.*
PBI t., protein-bound iodine t.
pentagastrin t., an alternative to histamine for stimulation of acid secretion in gastric analysis.
performance t., a t., such as five of the eleven Wechsler adult intelligence scale subtests, requiring little or no verbal instruction from the examiner and virtually no verbal response by the examinee.
Perls' t., a t. for hemosiderin, utilizing Perls' Prussian blue *stain.*
personality t., any of the category of psychological t.'s designed to test the characteristics of the personality, emotional status, mental disorder, etc., in contrast to an intelligence t.
Perthes' t., a t. for patency of deep femoral vein; with the patient standing, a tourniquet is applied above the knee; after walking, if deep circulation is competent, the superficial varicosities remain unchanged and legs become painful.
phenolsulfonphthalein t., Geraghty's t.; phthalein, red, or Rowntree and Geraghty t.; a t. for renal function; after the patient has drunk a glass or two of water, 1 ml of a 0.6% solution of dye is injected hypodermically; the time between this injection and the appearance of a pink tinge in the urine as it falls into an alkaline solution is noted; the amount excreted in each of the next 2 hours is then estimated colorimetrically.
phentolamine t., a t. for pheochromocytoma; intravenous administration of phentolamine (5 mg) reduces hypertension due to a pheochromocytoma but not that due to other causes, *e.g.,* essential hypertension; the blood pressure is raised by the drug in the latter form of hypertension.
photo-patch t., a t. of contact photosensitization: after application of a patch with the suspected sensitizer for 48 hours, if there is no reaction the area is exposed to an erythema dose of ultraviolet light; if positive, a more severe reaction develops at the patch site than in surrounding skin.
photostress t., measurement of visual acuity before and after exposure of the eyes to intense light.
phrenic pressure t., pressure is made on the phrenic nerve on each side, above the clavicles where the nerve passes over the scalenus anticus muscle; if pain is felt and the patient inclines his head to the painful side, the problem is in the pleural space; if his head does not incline to one side, the problem is in the abdominal cavity.
phthalein t., phenolsulfonphthalein t.
Pirquet's t., Pirquet's reaction; dermotuberculin reaction; a cutaneous tuberculin t. See tuberculin t.
pivot shift t., a maneuver to detect a deficiency of the anterior cruciate ligament of the knee; when the knee is extended, a sudden subluxation of the lateral tibial condyle upon the distal femur is positive.
plasmacrit t., a serologic screening method used as an aid in the diagnosis of syphilis; after only a few drops of heparinized blood (obtained from a pricked finger) are collected in a special capillary tube, the capillary tube is centrifugated in order to collect plasma, which is then mixed with a 0.01-ml drop of antigen (cardiolipin previously treated with choline chloride as an anti-inhibitor, in order to avoid falsely negative results that may occur with nonheated plasma or serum). After mechanically agitating the antigen-plasma mixture for 4 min, the presence or absence of flocculation is observed. A positive result should not be regarded as conclusively diagnostic, but a negative result excludes the likelihood of syphilis.
platelet aggregation t., a t. of the ability of platelets to adhere to each other and hence form a hemostatic plug to prevent bleeding; failure to aggregate occurs in several conditions, *e.g.,* thrombasthenia, Von Willebrand's disease, and following administration of aspirin, phenylbutazone, and indomethacin; the t. is conducted by quantitating the decrease in turbidity that occurs in platelet-rich plasma following the *in vitro* addition of one or several platelet-aggregating agents (*e.g.,* ADP, epinephrine, or serotonin).
polyuria t., Albarran's t.
Porges-Meier t., an early flocculation t. for syphilis; of significance in having introduced as antigens acetone-insoluble, alcohol-soluble fractions of tissue, and lecithin.
Porter-Silber chromogens t., 17-hydroxycorticosteroid t.
precipitation t., precipitin t.
precipitin t., precipitation t.; an *in vitro* t. in which antigen is in soluble form and precipitates when it combines with added specific antibody in the presence of an electrolyte. See also gel diffusion precipitin t.'s; ring precipitin t.
prism vergence t., measurement of the amplitude of fusion by placing prisms of gradually increasing power in the direction tested until diplopia occurs.
projective t., a loosely structured psychological t. containing many ambiguous stimuli that require the subject to reveal his own feelings, personality, or psychopathology in response to them; *e.g.,* Rorschach t., thematic apperception t.
protection t., neutralization t.; a t. to determine the antimicrobial activity of a serum by inoculating a susceptible animal with a mixture of the serum and the virus or other microbe being tested.
protein-bound iodine t., PBI t.; a formerly used t. of thyroid function in which serum protein-bound iodine is measured to provide an estimate of hormone bound to protein in peripheral blood.
prothrombin t., Quick's t. or method; a quantitative t. for prothrombin in the blood based on the clotting time of oxalated blood plasma in the presence of thromboplastin and calcium chloride. See also prothrombin *time.*
prothrombin and proconvertin t., P and P t.; a t. used by some to control anticoagulant therapy with bishydroxycoumarin and indandione drugs.
provocative t., a t. for pheochromocytoma, *e.g.,* histamine t., which when positive provokes a paroxysm of hypertension.
provocative Wassermann t., an obsolete t. of historical interest only; the use of the Wassermann test from one or two days to one or two weeks after the administration of arsphenamine or neoars-

phenamine; the result may then be positive when before the giving of arsphenamine it was negative.
psychological t.'s, t.'s designed to measure a person's achievements, intelligence, skills, personality, or individual and occupational characteristics, or potentialities. See also subentries under scale.
psychomotor t.'s, psychological t.'s which, although based on other psychological processes (*e.g.,* sensory, perceptual), require a motor reaction such as copying designs, building blocks, or manipulating controls.
pulp t., vitality t.
Queckenstedt-Stookey t., compression of the jugular vein in a healthy person causes an increase in the pressure of the spinal fluid in the lumbar region within 10 to 12 seconds, and an equally rapid fall to normal on release of the pressure on the vein; when there is a block of subarachnoid channels, compression of the vein causes little or no increase of pressure in the cerebrospinal fluid.
quellung t., Neufeld capsular *swelling.*
Quick's t., prothrombin t.
quinine carbacrylic resin t., a t. for gastric anacidity. See quinine carbacrylic *resin.*
Quinlan's t., a t. for bile; when a thin layer of bile is examined through a spectroscope, absorption lines appear in the violet.
radioactive iodide uptake t., ^{131}I uptake t.
radioallergosorbent t. (RAST), a radioimmunoassay t. to detect IgE-bound allergens responsible for tissue hypersensitivity: the allergen is bound to insoluble material and the patient's serum is reacted with this conjugate; if the serum contains antibody to the allergen, it will be complexed to the allergen.
RAI t., ^{131}I uptake t.
rapid plasma reagin t., RPR t.; a group of serologic t.'s for syphilis in which unheated serum or plasma is reacted with a standard test antigen containing charcoal particles; positive t.'s yield a flocculation. A modification, called the RPR (circle) card t., is widely used as a screening t.
Rapoport t., a differential ureteral catheterization t. used in evaluation of suspected renovascular hypertension; urine specimens from each kidney are obtained by bilateral ureteral catheterization, and the tubular rejection fraction ratio is determined by measuring concentrations of sodium and creatinine in the urine from each kidney; urine from kidneys in which significant renal artery senosis is present will have a decrease in urine sodium concentration and an increase in creatinine concentration when compared to the normal contralateral kidney; a positive t. suggests a decrease in renal blood flow to the involved kidney and correlates well with reduction in blood pressure following corrective surgery.
Rayleigh t., Rayleigh *equation.*
red t., phenolsulfonphthalein t.
red cell adherence t., adhesion t.
Reinsch's t., a t. for arsenic in which a strip of copper is placed in the suspected fluid, which is then acidulated with hydrochloric acid and boiled; if arsenic is present a gray deposit occurs on the copper, and this deposit on heating is sublimated and deposited as a crystalline layer on a piece of glass held above the copper strip.
Reiter t., a complement-fixation t. for syphilis using as antigen material prepared from the Reiter strain of *Treponema pallidum;* the t. has been largely replaced in laboratory medicine by the fluorescent treponemal antibody-absorption (FTA-ABS) t.
resorcinol t., Selivanoff's t.; a t. for furctosuria; fresh urine treated with resorcinol in acid gives a red precipitate in the presence of fructose; the precipitate should form a red solution in ethanol.
Reuss' t., a t. for atropine; the addition of oxidizing agents and sulfuric acid to a liquid containing atropine produces an odor of orange-flowers and roses.
Rh blocking t., a t. for nonagglutinating Rh antibodies: an Rh agglutination t. is first carried out; if the t. for Rh agglutinins is negative, then 1 drop of anti-Rh_0 agglutinating serum of moderate titer is mixed with the patient's serum containing Rh-positive t. cells; if after incubating for from 1 to 2 hr at 37°C no agglutination occurs, Rh_0-blocking antibodies are assumed to be present in the patient's serum.
Rickles t., a colorimetric t. for predicting dental caries activity by incubating saliva in sucrose and determining pH changes.
Rimini's t., a t. for formaldehyde in urine, milk, and other fluids, by the use of dilute solution of phenylhydrazine hydrochloride, sodium nitroprusside, and sodium hydroxide.
ring t., ring precipitin t.
ring precipitin t., ring t.; a precipitin t. in which antigen solution is carefully layered over antibody solution in a tube; as diffusion proceeds, a disk of precipitate forms where the antibody ratio is optimal.
Rinne's t., **(1)** as a positive t.: a vibrating tuning fork is held in contact with the skull (usually the mastoid process) until the sound is lost, its prongs are then brought close to the auditory orifice when, if the hearing is normal, a faint sound will again be heard; **(2)** as a negative t.: a vibrating tuning fork is heard longer and louder when in contact with the skull than when held near the auditory orifice, indicating some disorder of the sound conducting apparatus.
Romberg t., Romberg's *sign.*
Römer's t., a t. of historical interest: tuberculin, either pure or diluted, is injected intracutaneously into a guinea pig; if the animal is tuberculous, a large papule with a necrotic hemorrhagic center appears in about 24 hours (cocarde of cockade reaction).
Ropes t., mucin clot t.
Rorschach t., a projective psychological t. in which the subject reveals his attitudes, emotions, and personality by reporting what he sees in each of 10 inkblot pictures.
rose bengal radioactive (^{131}I) t., a t. of liver function used as a means of measuring hepatic blood flow and for scintillation scanning of the liver to determine size and contour of the liver, or the presence of space-occupying masses in the liver.
Rosenbach's t., a t. for bile in the urine; the suspected urine is passed several times through the same filter paper, which is then dried and touched with a drop of slightly fuming nitric acid; the presence of bile is indicated by the resulting play of colors characteristic of the bile pigments (a yellow spot surrounded by rings of red, violet, blue, and green).
Rosenbach-Gmelin t., Gmelin's t.
Rose-Waaler t., a t. of historical interest: when sheep red cells are suspended in a concentration of antiserum to sheep red cells which is too low to cause agglutination, the addition of serum from a patient with rheumatoid arthritis will cause agglutination.
Ross-Jones t., a t. for an excess of globulin in the cerebrospinal fluid; 1 ml of cerebrospinal fluid is carefully floated over 2 ml of a concentrated ammonium sulfate solution; if globulin is present in excess, a fine white ring appears at the line of junction in about 3 min.
Rothera's nitroprusside t., a t. for ketone bodies; 5 ml of fresh urine are saturated with solid ammonium sulfate and mixed with 10 drops of freshly prepared 2% sodium nitroprusside solution, which is then mixed with 10 drops of concentrated ammonia water and allowed to stand for 15 min; the presence of acetoacetic acid, or of larger concentrations of acetone, is indicated by the development of a blue-purple color.
Rowntree and Geraghty t., phenolsulfonphthalein t.
RPR t., rapid plasma reagin t.
rubella HI t., a hemagglutination inhibition (HI) t. for rubella, often performed routinely as part of a prenatal workup of the pregnant woman; the presence of any detectable HI titer in the absence of disease indicates previous infection and immunity to reinfection; if HI antibody is undetected, the patient is considered potentially susceptible and is followed accordingly. See also hemagglutination *inhibition.*

Rubin t., tubal insufflation; a t. of patency of the fallopian tubes; a cannula is introduced into the cervix uteri, and carbon dioxide gas is passed through the cannula by means of a syringe with manometer attachment; if the tubes are patent, the escape of gas into the abdominal cavity is evidenced by a high-pitched bubbling sound heard on auscultation over the lower abdomen, or free gas under the diaphragm can be demonstrated by x-ray.
Rubner's t., a t. for lactose or glucose in the urine; lead acetate is added to the suspected urine which is then filtered; ammonia is added until a permanent precipitate is formed; if lactose is present, the precipitate will take on a pink to red color when the fluid is heated; if there is glucose, the color will be yellow to brown.
Rumpel-Leede t., bandage or Rumpel-Leede sign; Hess' t.; a tourniquet t. for capillary fragility, often positive in the presence of severe thrombocytopenia. See also capillary fragility t.
Sabin-Feldman dye t., a method for the detection of anti-toxoplasma antibody in serum, based on the fact that *Toxoplasma gondii* cells (from peritoneal exudate in mice) are fairly well stained with alkaline methylene blue, whereas organisms in a serum that contains specific antibody have no affinity for the dye; furthermore, normal toxoplasma cells become rounded, and the nucleus and cytoplasm deeply stained, when treated with the methylene blue; on the other hand, when dye is mixed with organisms and antibody, the cells retain their crescent shape and only the shrunken nuclear endosome is stained.
Sachs-Georgi t., the first precipitin t. for syphilis of diagnostic practicality, the significant innovation having been the addition of cholesterol to the lipoidal antigen (alcoholic tissue extract) used in the earlier Meinicke t.
Saundby's t., a t. for blood in the stools; on the addition of 30 drops of a 20-volume hydrogen peroxide solution to a mixture of 10 drops of a saturated benzidine solution and a small quantity of feces in a test tube, a persistent dark blue color denotes the presence of blood.
scarification t., a t., *e.g.,* Pirquet's t., in which a material is pricked or scratched into the skin.
Schaffer's t., a t. for nitrites in the urine; urine is decolorized with animal charcoal and then 4 ml of a 10% solution of acetic acid and 3 drops of a 5% solution of potassium ferrocyanide are added; if nitrites are present, an intense yellow color will be produced.
Schellong t., a test for circulatory function; the subject is required to stand for 10 to 20 minutes, during which time the blood pressure is measured continuously; a fall of systolic pressure of 20 mm Hg or more indicates poor circulatory function.
Schick t., Schick method; a t. for susceptibility to *Corynebacterium diphtheriae* toxin: 0.1 ml of Schick test toxin is injected into the skin of one forearm (test site) and the same quantity of the same, but heat-inactivated, material into the skin of the other forearm (control site); individuals with toxin-neutralizing antibodies either will have no reaction at either injection site (negative test) or may have a pseudoreaction due to antibodies for substances (antigens) in the test materials other than diphtheria toxin; individuals lacking toxin-neutralizing antibodies either may have a simple positive reaction or a positive reaction may occur along with a pseudoreaction (combined reaction).
Schiller's t., a test for nonglycogen-containing areas of the portio vaginalis of the cervix, which may be the site of early carcinoma; such areas fail to stain dark brown with iodine solution; loss of glycogen due to erosion and other benign conditions may also give a positive result.
Schilling t., a procedure for determining the amount of vitamin B_{12} excreted in the urine using cyanocobalamin tagged with a radioisotope of cobalt.
Schirmer t., a t. for tear production using a strip of filter paper; a measurement of basal and reflex lacrimal gland function.
Schönbein's t., Almén's t. for blood.
Schwabach t., a series of five tuning forks of different tones is used and the number of seconds is noted in which the patient can hear each by air and bone conduction.
Schwarz's t., a t. for sulfonmethane, heating of which with charcoal gives rise to the odor of mercaptan.
scratch t., a form of skin t. in which antigen is applied through a scratch in the skin.
screening t., any testing procedure designed to separate people or objects according to a fixed characteristic or property.
Seashore t., a t. in which the sense of pitch, intensity, rhythm, and other components of innate musical ability can be measured.
secretin t., pancreozymin-secretin t.; a t. of pancreatic exocrine function, variably performed and standardized, in which the bicarbonate, amylase, and volume of the duodenal aspirate are measured after intravenous administration of secretin.
Selivanoff's t., resorcinol t.
shadow t., retinoscopy.
shake t., foam stability t.
sickle cell t., in an anaerobic wet preparation containing equal amounts of blood and 2% sodium bisulfite, erythrocytes containing hemoglobin S undergo a change in shape to a sickle cell form; the number of sickled red cells per 1000 red blood cells is determined, and expressed as a percentage.
single (gel) diffusion precipitin t. in one dimension, see gel diffusion precipitin t.'s in one dimension.
single (gel) diffusion precipitin t. in two dimensions, see gel diffusion precipitin t.'s in two dimensions.
SISI (small increment sensitivity index) t., the sounding of a tone 20 dB above threshold, followed by a series of 200-msec tones 1 dB louder; perception of these is indicative of cochlear damage.
situational t., in psychology and psychiatry, a t. situation in which a subject is observed as he performs a daily task or an actual sample of the job or role he will fill.
skin t., skin reaction; cutireaction or cutaneous t.; a method for determining induced sensitivity (allergy) by applying an antigen (allergen) to, or inoculating it into, the skin; induced sensitivity (allergy) to the specific antigen is indicated by an inflammatory reaction of one of two general kinds: 1) immediate, appears in minutes to an hour or so and in general is dependent upon circulating immunoglobulins (antibodies); 2) delayed (microbial), appears in 12 to 72 hours and is not dependent upon these soluble substances but upon cellular response and infiltration.
skin-puncture t., t. for Behçet's syndrome; after pricking the skin with a sterile needle, pustulation follows within 24 hours owing to the dermal sensitivity in this disease.
Snyder's t., colorimetric caries susceptibility t.; a colorimetric t. for determining dental caries activity or susceptibility based on the rate of acid production by acidogenic oral microorganisms (*e.g.,* lactobacillus) in a glucose medium, using bromcresol green as the indicator, and producing a color change from green to yellow.
solubility t., a screening t. for sickle cell hemoglobin (Hb S), which is reduced by dithionite and is insoluble in concentrated inorganic buffer; addition of blood showing Hb S to buffer and dithionite causes opacity of the solution.
spironolactone t., administration of spironolactone (400 mg orally) for 4 consecutive days: an increase in serum potassium during the t., and a decrease afterward, strongly suggests primary aldosteronism.
split renal function t., differential ureteral catheterization t.
spot t. for infectious mononucleosis, a slide t. widely used for the diagnosis of infectious mononucleosis, based on the principle that the heterophil antibodies that occur in the serum of patients with infectious mononucleosis are absorbed by beef red cells but not by guinea pig kidney cells; thus, when horse red cells (which provoke heterophil antibodies) are mixed with patient serum and agglutination occurs in the presence of beef red cells, the presumptive diagnosis is infectious mononucleosis.
Stamey t., a modified Howard t.

standard serologic t.'s (STS) for syphilis, nontreponemal antigen t.'s giving presumptive but not conclusive evidence of syphilis, including the Wassermann and VDRL t.'s.
standing t., a t. for the effect of a hypotensive drug, carried out by the patient: after taking the drug, he stands perfectly still for one minute commencing from the time that the maximal action of the drug should be manifested; if the dose is adequate, the patient should experience a slight hypotensive reaction.
standing plasma t., if plasma is stored at 4°C upright in a t. tube, chylomicrons will float to the top and form a creamy layer.
starch-iodine t., a t. for sweating in which iodine in oil is painted on the skin, followed by dusting with a starch powder which turns blue-black in the presence of iodine and moisture.
station t., Romberg's *sign.*
Stein's t., in cases of labyrinthine disease the patient is unable to stand or to hop on one foot with his eyes shut.
Stenger t., a test for detecting simulation of unilateral deafness.
Stewart's t., estimation of the amount of collateral circulation, in case of an aneurysm of the main artery of a limb, by means of a calorimeter.
Strassburg's t., a t. for bile in the urine; albumin, if present, is precipitated, then cane sugar is added and filter paper is dipped in the fluid and dried; if bile pigments are present in the urine sulfuric acid will turn the filter paper a reddish violet color.
string t., **(1)** a t. to locate gastrointestinal hemorrhage; a string is repeatedly swallowed and removed, each time allowing the string to go further down the gut until blood is encountered. See also fluorescein string t. **(2)** a procedure to obtain a specimen of duodenal juices; a weighted string is swallowed, withdrawn after four hours, and the duodenal secretions extracted from the string for examination.
Strong vocational interest t., a t. that matches an individual's specific interests to those characteristic of persons working in each of a number of vocations.
Student's *t* t., *t* t.; a statistical method analogous to the calculation of the normal deviate; the formula is $t = (x - x)/s$, where the numerator is the deviation from the mean, and the denominator is the standard deviation for sample sizes of less than 30 cases.
sucrose hemolysis t., isotonic sucrose promotes binding of complement to red blood cells; in paroxysmal nocturnal hemoglobinuria a proportion of the cells is sensitive to complement-mediated lysis, and hemolysis ensues.
sulfosalicylic acid turbidity t., a t. for measurement of protein in the urine; sulfosalicylic acid precipitates protein in the urine with a turbidity that is approximately proportional to the concentration of protein in a solution.
sweat t., a test for cystic fibrosis of the pancreas in which electrolytes are measured in collected sweat; sodium chlorid concentration above 50 mEq/l (children) or 60 mEq/l (adults) is positive.
sweating t., a t. for locating the level of a lesion in the spinal cord; when the body is heated or the patient is given a diaphoretic, sweat secretion is absent below the level of the lesion.
swimming t., a t. for activity of adrenal cortical preparations; two days after adrenalectomy, rats are placed in water and the time during which they can swim is recorded; they are then injected with the material to be tested; the response is termed "positive" if the swimming time is doubled.
swordfish t., *Xiphophorus* t.; a rarely used t. for androgenic activity, based upon the fact that androgens cause the development of the sword, a male structure, in female swordfish (*Xiphophorus helleri*).
***t* t.,** Student's *t* t.
thematic apperception t. (TAT), a projective psychological t. in which the subject is asked to tell a story about standard ambiguous pictures depicting life-situations to reveal his own attitudes and feelings.
thermostable opsonin t., a t. for opsonic activity of antibody in the absence of effect of heat-labile complement.
Thompson's t., two-glass t.; the urine, in a case of gonorrhea, is passed into two glasses; if the gonococci and gonorrheal threads are found only in the first glass the probability is that the process is limited to the anterior urethra.
Thormählen's t., a t. for melanin; the suspected liquid is treated with sodium nitroprusside, caustic potash, and acetic acid; if melanin is present, the solution takes on a deep blue color.
Thorn t., a putative t. of adrenal cortical function; stimulation of a normally functioning adrenal cortex by the adrenocorticotrophic hormone is followed by a reduction in the number of circulating eosinophils and lymphocytes and an increase in the excretion of uric acid. The t. lacks sufficient specificity and is rarely used.
three-glass t., Valentine's t.; the bladder is emptied by passing urine into a series of 3-ounce test tubes, and the contents of the first and the last are examined; the first tube contains the washings from the anterior urethra, the second, material from the bladder, and the last, material from the posterior urethra, prostate, and seminal vesicles.
thyroid-stimulating hormone (TSH) stimulation t., a t. that measures the uptake of ^{131}I in the thyroid gland before and after administration of thyroid-stimulating hormone; useful in distinguishing primary hyperthyroidism (increased TSH serum concentration) from secondary or tertiary hyperthyroidism (low TSH serum concentrations).
thyroid suppression t., Werner's t.; a thyroid function t. used to diagnose difficult cases of hyperthyroidism, now largely replaced by the thyrotropin-releasing hormone stimulation t.; triiodothyronine is administered for a week to 10 days, and a reduction of its uptake by the thyroid gland to less than half of the initial uptake is a normal response.
thyrotropin-releasing hormone (TRH) stimulation t., a t. of pituitary response to injection of thyrotropin-releasing hormone, which normally stimulates pituitary secretion of thyroid-stimulating hormone (TSH, thyrotropin), used primarily to distinguish pituitary from hypothalamic causes of thyroid disorders; TSH does not rise in cases of pituitary dysfunction, but does rise in cases of hypothalamic disorders.
tine t., see tuberculin t.
titratable acidity t., the number of milliliters of 0.1 N NaOH required to neutralize a 24-hr specimen of urine.
tolbutamide t., a t. to detect insulin-producing tumors; after a 1-g intravenous dose of tolbutamide, plasma insulin and glucose are measured at intervals up to 3 hr; higher insulin responses and lower glucose values characterize patients with such tumors.
tone decay t., the sounding of a continuous tone at threshold for 1 min; if the intensity must be increased by more than 5 dB for continued perception, it may be a sign of retrocochlear damage.
Töpfer's t., an obsolete t. for free hydrochloric acid in the gastric contents; dimethylaminoazobenzene is used as the indicator.
total catecholamine t., a fluorometric determination of catecholamines in 24-hr urine specimens; elevated values are seen in patients with pheochromocytoma and neuroblastoma; spurious elevations may be seen due to excretion products of medication containing adrenaline, tetracyclines, quinidine, and some antihypertensive agents; false-positive elevations may be seen in persons with extensive burns, in vigorous exercise, or in progressive muscular dystrophy.
tourniquet t., see capillary fragility t.; Rumpel-Leede t.
TPHA t., *Treponema pallidum* hemagglutination t.
TPI t., *Treponema pallidum* immobilization t.
Trendelenburg's t., a t. of the valves of the leg veins; the leg is raised above the level of the heart until the veins are empty and is then rapidly lowered; in varicosity and incompetence of the valves the veins will at once become distended.
Treponema pallidum hemagglutination t., TPHA t.; a highly sensitive and specific t. for the serologic diagnosis of syphilis; tanned

sheep red blood cells are coated with the antigen of *Treponema pallidum* and, following absorption of nonspecific patient serum antibody, a positive reaction with tanned sheep red blood cells and patient serum indicates the presence of specific antibody for *Treponema pallidum* in patient serum.
Treponema pallidum immobilization (TPI) t., *Treponema pallidum* immobilization reaction; TPI t.; a t. for syphilis in which an antibody other than Wassermann antibody is present in the serum of a syphilitic patient, which in the presence of complement causes the immobilization of actively motile *Treponema pallidum* obtained from testes of a rabbit infected with syphilis.
triiodothyronine uptake t., T_3 uptake t.; a t. of thyroid function in which triiodothyronine (T_3) is added to a patient's serum *in vitro* to measure the relative affinities of serum proteins and of an added competitive substance for T3; higher T3 uptakes are associated with hyperthyroidism.
tuberculin t., application of the skin t. to the diagnosis of infection by *Mycobacterium tuberculosis* in which tuberculin or its "purified" protein derivative serves as an antigen (allergen); injection of graduated doses of tuberculin or of purified protein derivative into the skin, most often by means of a needle and syringe (Mantoux t.) or by means of tines (tine t.); t. material may also be applied by means of a "patch" in which it is absorbed but this method (patch t.) is viewed as being less reliable; the t. is read on the basis of induration and erythema, the former being considered the more diagnostic of infection with the tubercle bacillus (*M. tuberculosis*); the t. does not distinguish between infection in a resistant person without disease and an individual with clinical manifestations of disease.
Tuffier's t., Hallion's t.
T_3 uptake t., triiodothyronine uptake t.
two-glass t., Thompson's t.
two-step exercise t., Master's t.; Master's two-step exercise t.; exercise t.; a t. for coronary insufficiency; the subject makes two steps 9 in. high repeatedly for $1^1/_2$ min; the total number of steps to be made in the time is determined by the age, weight, and sex of the subject; significant depression of RS-T in the electrocardiogram is considered abnormal and suggests coronary insufficiency.
Tzanck t., in the fluid in the bullae of pemphigus vulgaris, the characteristic finding of Tzanck cells (altered epithelial cells, rounded and devoid of intercellular attachments); the periphery is basophilic and the nucleus is spherical and enlarged, with prominent nucleoli.
urea clearance t., a t. of renal function based on urea clearance.
urease t., a t. for the identification of cryptococci, common species of which elaborate urease.
urinary concentration t., a t. of renal tubular function whereby the patient is dehydrated for a measured period of time and the specific gravity of the urine is subsequently determined.
vaginal cornification t., a t. for estrogenic activity, in which the appearance of cornified epithelial cells in a vaginal smear of a test animal is an indication of the action of an estrogen.
vaginal mucification t., a t. for progestational activity; stimulation of mucus production by the vaginal epithelium in rats, guinea pigs, or mice by progestogens.
Valentine's t., three-glass t.
Valsalva t., the heart is observed fluoroscopically while the patient performs the Valsalva maneuver; the heart becomes smaller in normal persons but may dilate in the patient with impaired myocardial reserve.
van Deen's t., Almén's t. for blood.
van den Bergh's t., a t. for bile pigments (bilirubin) by reaction with diazotized sulfanilic acid (diazo reaction).
van der Velden's t., a t. for free hydrochloric acid, the presence of which turns an added solution of methylene blue from violet to green.
vanillylmandelic acid t., VMA t.; 3-methoxy-4-hydroxymandelic acid t.; a t. for catecholamine-secreting tumors (pheochromocytoma and neuroblastoma) performed on a 24-hr urine specimen; it is based on the fact that vanillylmandelic acid is the major urinary metabolite of norepinephrine and epinephrine.
VDRL t., a flocculation t. for syphilis, using cardiolipin-lecithin-cholesterol antigen as developed by the Venereal Disease Research Laboratory of the United States Public Health Service.
vitality t., pulp t.; a group of thermal and electrical t.'s used to aid in assessment of dental pulp health.
vitamin C t., capillary fragility t.
VMA t., vanillylmandelic acid t.
Volhard's t., a t. for renal function: the patient drinks 1500 ml of water on an empty stomach; if the patient was not dehydrated beforehand and the kidneys are normal, this fluid will be excreted by the end of 4 hr, with specific gravity of the urine being from 1.001 to 1.004.
Vollmer t., a tuberculin patch t.
Wada t., intracarotid injection of amobarbital to determine the laterality of speech; injection on the dominant side temporarily abolishes the power of speech.
Waldenström's t., a t. for porphyrin in the urine; 2 ml of urine are mixed with an equal amount of 2% dimethyl-*p*-aminobenzaldehyde in 50/100 HCl. A red color appears if urobilinogen (Ehrlich's benzaldehyde reaction) or porphobilinogen is present.
Wang's t., a quantitative t. for indican, which is transformed into indigo-sulfuric acid and then titrated by a solution of potassium permanganate.
washout t., a means of estimating renal obstruction by the rate of disappearance of excreted radioactive material from the kidney.
Wassén t., a nonspecific t. for the diagnosis of lymphogranuloma venereum; it consists of causing a fatal encephalitis in mice by the injection of chlamydia obtained from humans.
Wassermann t., Wassermann reaction; a complement-fixation t. used in the diagnosis of syphilis; originally the "antigen" was an extract of liver from a syphilitic fetus, but later the active substance, referred to as cardiolipin, was found to be present in normal tissues, including heart, and has been identified as a diphosphatidylglycerol.
Watson-Schwartz t., a qualitative screening t. for diagnosis of acute intermittent porphyria by the addition of Ehrlich's reagent and saturated sodium acetate to the urine; a pink or red color indicates the presence of porphobilinogen or urobilinogen; the former indicates porphyria, the latter does not; therefore, positive results require further differential extraction with butanol and chloroform to eliminate false-positive results due to urobilinogen.
Weber's t. for hearing, the application of a vibrating tuning fork to one of several points in the midline of the head or face, to ascertain in which ear the sound is heard best by bone conduction, that ear being the affected one if the sound-conducting apparatus (middle ear) is at fault (positive t.), but probably the normal one if the neurosensory apparatus is diseased (negative t.).
Webster's t., a t. for trinitrotoluene in the urine.
Weil-Felix t., Weil-Felix reaction; a t. for the presence and type of rickettsial disease based on the agglutination of X-strains of *Proteus vulagris* with suspected rickettsia in a patient's blood serum.
Werner's t., thyroid suppression t.
Wheeler-Johnson t., cystosine or uracil when treated with bromine yields dialuric acid which gives a green color with excess of barium hydroxide.
Wormley's t., a t. for alkaloids, by treating the solution with picric acid or a dilute iodine-potassium-iodide solution, the presence of alkaloids being shown by a color reaction.
Wurster's t., a t. for tyrosine; the substance is dissolved in boiling water and quinone is added; if tyrosine is present a ruby-colored reaction takes place, the solution changing to brown after a few hours.
Xiphophorus t., swordfish t.

xylose t., a laboratory aid in diagnosing alimentary or essential pentosuria, conditions in which xylose (a pentose) is excreted; the xylose may be identified by rapid reduction of Benedict's solution, by nonfermentation by yeasts, or by a positive Bial's t. for pentose.
Yvon's t., **(1)** for alkaloids; to the suspected solution is added a mixture of bismuth subnitrate, potassium iodide, and hydrochloric acid in water; a positive reaction is indicated by the appearance of a red color; **(2)** for acetanilid in the urine; the suspected fluid is extracted with chloroform and heated with yellow nitrate of mercury; if acetanilid is present, the fluid will be colored green.
Zimmermann t., Zimmermann *reaction.*
Zondek-Aschheim t., Aschheim-Zondek t.
Zsigmondy's t., Lange's t.

testa (tes'tă) [L. shell]. **1.** Eggshell. **2.** In protozoology, usually termed test; an envelope of certain forms of ameboid protozoa, consisting of various earthy materials cemented to a chitinous base (as in the testate rhizopods of the subclass Testacealobosia) or the calcareous, siliceous, organic, or strontium sulfate skeletons in the rhizopod subclass Foraminifera. **3.** In botany, the outer, sometimes the only, coat of a seed.

Testacealobosia (tes-tā'shē-ă-lō-bō'zē-ă) [L. *testa,* shell]. A subclass of the subphylum Sarcodina (amebae), in which the cells are provided with a firm chitinous envelope, often containing earthy material, with an opening through which the pseudopodia are protruded.

testalgia (tes-tal'jē-ă) [testis + G. *algos,* pain]. Orchialgia.

testane (tes'tān). Etiane.

testectomy (tes-tek'tō-mē) [testis + G. G. *ektomē,* excision]. Orchiectomy.

testes (tes'tēz) [L.]. Plural of testis.

testicle (tes'tĭ-kl) [L. *testiculus,* dim. of *testis*] Testis.

testicular (tes-tik'yū-lăr). Relating to the testes.

testiculus (tes-tik'yū-lŭs) [L.]. Testicle.

testis, pl. testes (tes'tis, -tēz) [L.] [NA]. Testicle; orchis; didymus; one of the two male reproductive glands, located in the cavity of the scrotum.

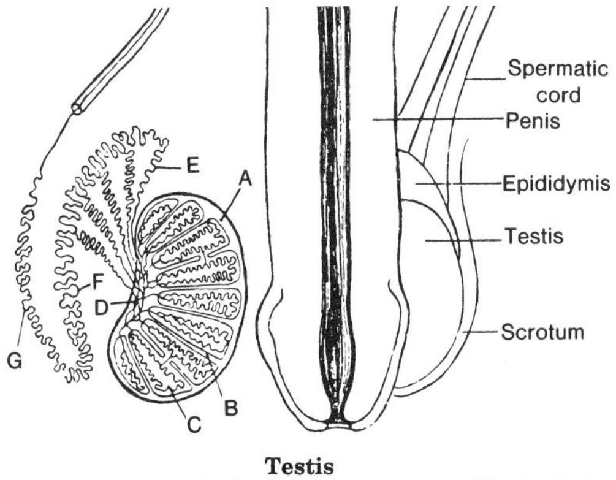

Testis
External male genitalia showing structures of the testis: *A*, tunica albuginea; *B*, septum; *C*, seminiferous tubule; *D*, mediastinum with rete testis; *E*, ductus efferens; *F*, ductus epididymidis; *G*, ductus deferens (After Dickinson).

cryptorchid t., undescended t.
ectopic t., *ectopia* testis.
inverted t., a t. that is rotated in the scrotum, with the epididymis being directed anteriorly instead of in its normal position.
irritable t., neuralgia of the t.
movable t., t. redux; a condition in which there is a tendency in the testis to ascend to the upper part of the scrotum or into the inguinal canal.
obstructed t., a t. whose descent has been prevented by fascial bands at the inguinal canal or upper scrotum.
t. re'dux, movable t.
retained t., undescended t.
retractile t., a t. that periodically disappears from the scrotum, as contrasted with an undescended t.
undescended t., cryptorchid or retained t.; a t. that has failed to descend into the scrotum, having been retained in the abdomen or inguinal canal; sperm formation does not occur in the adult.

testitis (tes-tī'tis). Orchitis.

test letter. See test types.

testoid (tes'toyd) [testis + G. *eidos,* resemblance]. **1.** Androgenic. **2.** Androgen.

testolactone (tes-tō-lak'tōn). D-Homo-17α-oxa-1,4-androstadiene-3,17-dione; an androgenic agent used as an antineoplastic agent for treatment of mammary carcinoma.

testopathy (tes-top'ă-thē) [testis + G. *pathos,* disease]. Orchiopathy.

testosterone (tes-tos'tĕ-rōn). 17βHydroxy-4-androstene-3-one; the most potent naturally occurring androgen, formed in greatest quantities by the interstitial cells of the testes, and possibly secreted also by the ovary and adrenal cortex; may be produced in nonglandular tissues from precursors such as androstenedione; used in the treatment of hypogonadism, cryptorchism, certain carcinomas, and menorrhagia.
t. cypionate, t. cyclopentylpropionate; a preparation with the same actions and uses as t. propionate, but with a prolonged duration of action.
t. enanthate, a preparation with the same actions and uses as t., but with a prolonged duration of action, being administered in oil.
t. phenylpropionate, an alternate preparation for the propionate.
t. propionate, a preparation that has an action similar to but more pronounced and prolonged than that of t.; used in the treatment of undescended testes and in menorrhagia.

test symbols. See test types.

test types. Letters of various sizes used to test visual acuity.
Jaeger's t. t., type of different sizes used for testing the acuity of near vision.
point system t. t., a near-vision test chart in which the various test types are multiples of a point ($^1/_{72}$ inch), lower-case letters being one-half the designated point size; reading 4-point at 16 inches is normal, and is designated N-4.
Snellen's t. t., square black symbols employed in testing the acuity of distant vision; the letters vary in size in such a way that each one subtends a visual angle of 5′ a particular distance. See fig. on p. 1578.

tetan-. See tetano-.

tetania (te-tā'nē-ă). Obsolete synonym for tetany.
t. epidem'ica, rheumatic *tetany.*
t. gas'trica, gastric *tetany.*
t. gravida'rum, tetany in pregnant women.
t. neonato'rium, neonatal *tetany.*
t. parathyreopri'va, parathyroid *tetany.*
t. rheumat'ica, rheumatic *tetany.*

tetanic (te-tan'ik) [G. *tetanikos*]. **1.** Relating to or marked by a sustained muscular contraction, as in tetanus. **2.** An agent, such as strychnine, that in poisonous doses produces tonic muscular spasm.

tetaniform (te-tan'i-fōrm). Tetanoid (1).

tetanigenous (tet-ă-nij'ĕ-nŭs) [tetanus + G. *-gen,* producing]. Causing tetanus or tetaniform spasms.

tetanilla (tet-ă-nil'ă) [Mod. L. dim. of L. *tetanus*] **1.** Fibrillary *myoclonia.* **2.** Tetany.

tetanism (tet'ă-nizm). Neonatal *tetany.*

tetanization (tet'ă-ni-zā'shŭn). **1.** The act of tetanizing the muscles. **2.** A condition of tetaniform spasm.

tetanize (tet'ă-nīz). To stimulate a muscle by a rapid series of stimuli so that the individual muscular responses (contractions) are fused into a sustained contraction; to cause tetanus (2) in a muscle.

tetano-, tetan- [G. *tetanos,* convulsive tension]. Combining forms denoting tetanus, tetany.

tetanode (tet'ă-nōd) [G. *tetanōdēs*]. Denoting the quiet interval between the recurrent tonic spasms in tetanus.

tetanoid (tet'ă-noyd) [tetano- + G. *eidos,* resemblance]. **1.** Tetaniform; resembling or of the nature of tetanus. **2.** Resembling tetany.

tetanolysin (tet-ă-nol'i-sin). A hemolytic principle, elaborated by *Clostridium tetani,* which seems to have no role in the etiology of tetanus.

tetanometer (tet-ă-nom'ĕ-ter) [tetano- + G. *metron,* measure]. An instrument for measuring the force of tonic muscular spasms.

tetanomotor (tet'ă-nō-mō'ter) [tetano- + L. *motor,* a mover]. An instrument by means of which tonic spasms are produced by the mechanical irritation of a hammer striking the motor nerve of the muscle affected.

tetanospasmin (tet'ă-nō-spaz'min). The neurotoxin of *Clostridium tetani,* which causes the characteristic signs and symptoms of tetanus; chief action is on the anterior horn cells, and the spasms seem to be due to action at inhibitory synapses.

tetanotoxin (tet'ă-nō-tok'sin) [tetano- + G. *toxikon,* poison]. Tetanus *toxin.*

tetanus (tet'ă-nŭs) [L. fr. G. *tetanos,* convulsive tension]. **1.** A disease marked by painful tonic muscular contractions, caused by the neurotropic toxin (tetanospasmin) of *Clostridium tetani* acting upon the central nervous system. **2.** A sustained muscular contraction caused by a series of stimuli repeated so rapidly that the individual muscular responses are fused; motor impulses reach intact muscles in the body at such a rate, usually, as to produce a tetanic contraction. See emprosthotonos; opisthotonos; pleurothotonos.

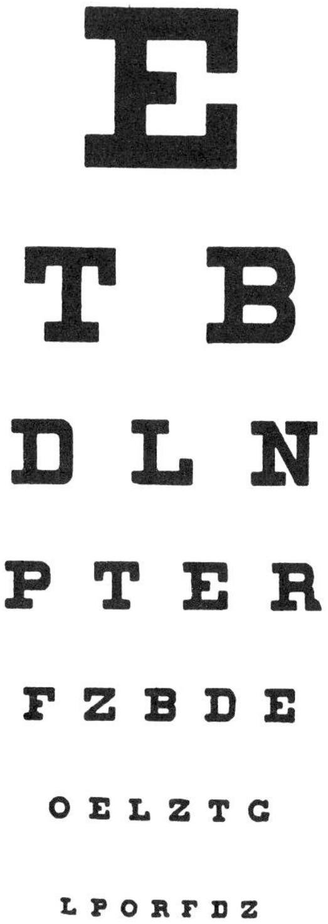

Snellen's Test Types

acoustic t., experimental t. induced by a faradic current, the speed of which is estimated by the pitch of the vibrations.

anodal closure t. (ACTe), obsolete term for a tetanic muscular contraction occurring during the time the circuit is closed, the current then running, while the positive pole is applied.

anodal duration t. (ADTe, AnDTe), obsolete term for the period of muscular contraction occurring at the anode when the electric circuit is closed.

anodal opening t., obsolete term for a tonic contraction in a muscle, to which the anode is applied, when the circuit is opened.

t. anti'cus, emprosthotonos.

apyretic t., tetany.

benign t., tetany.

cathodal closure t. (CCTe), obsolete term for a tetanic muscular contraction occurring during the time the circuit is closed, the current then running, while the negative pole is applied.

cathodal duration t. (CaDTe), obsolete term for a tetanic contraction occurring on application of the cathode or negative pole, while the circuit is closed.

cathodal opening t. (COTe), obsolete term for a tonic contraction in a muscle, to which the cathode is applied; when the circuit is opened, the contraction is suddenly interrupted.

cephalic t., cerebral t.; head, hydrophobic, or Rose's cephalic t.; tonic spasms in the face and throat due to a tetanus-infected wound of the head, usually injuring the facial nerve.

cerebral t., cephalic t.

complete t., t. (2) in which stimuli to a particular muscle are repeated so rapidly that decrease of tension between stimuli cannot be detected.

t. comple'tus, generalized t.; t. involving most of the muscles of the body.

t. dorsa'lis, opisthotonos.

drug t., toxic t.; tonic spasms caused by strychnine or other tetanic.

extensor t., t. affecting chiefly the extensor muscles.

flexor t., t. affecting chiefly the flexor muscles.

generalized t., t. completus.

head t., cephalic t.

hydrophobic t., cephalic t.

imitative t., conversion hysteria that resembles t.

incomplete t., t. (2) in which each stimulus causes a contraction to be initiated when the muscle has only partly relaxed from the previous contraction.

intermittent t., tetany.

local t., an early stage of t. affecting a group of muscles in close proximity to an infected wound, due to the action of the neurotoxin on the anterior horn cells at that level.

t. neonato'rum, a form of t. affecting newborn infants, usually due to infection through the open end of the severed umbilical cord.

t. posti'cus, opisthotonos.

postpartum t., puerperal t.

puerperal t., postpartum or uterine t.; t. occurring during the puerperium from infection of the obstetric wound.

Ritter's opening t., the tetanic contraction that occasionally occurs when a strong current, passing through a long stretch of nerve, is suddenly interrupted.

Rose's cephalic t., cephalic t.

toxic t., drug t.

traumatic t., t. following infection of a wound.

uterine t., puerperal t.

tetany (tet'ă-nē) [G. *tetanos,* tetanus]. Intermittent cramp or tetanus; tetanilla (2); apyretic or benign tetanus; a disorder marked by intermittent tonic muscular contractions, accompanied by fibrillary tremors, paresthesias, and muscular pains; the hands are usually first affected, followed by spasms in the face, the trunk, and sometimes in the laryngeal muscles, with increased irritability of the motor and sensory nerves to electrical and mechanical stimuli; results from decreased ionized calcium in the plasma and occurs with gastric and intestinal disorders, alkalosis, or a deficiency of vitamin D and parathyroid function.

t. of alkalosis, t. due to a loss of acid from the body or an increase in alkali, resulting in a reduction of ionized calcium in plasma and body fluids, *e.g.,* hyperventilation t. (loss of CO_2), gastric t. (loss of HCl by vomiting), or injection or ingestion of excessive amounts of sodium bicarbonate.

duration t. (DT), a tonic spasm occurring in degenerated muscles upon application of a strong galvanic current.

epidemic t., rheumatic t.

gastric t., tetania gastrica; t. associated with a gastric disorder, especially with loss of HCl by vomiting.

grass t., wheat pasture poisoning; a highly fatal disease of cows and sheep occurring generally during the first two weeks in the spring after the animals have been out on lush pastures; it is characterized by convulsions, hypomagnesemia, and usually hypocalcemia.

hyperventilation t., t. caused by forced overbreathing, due to a reduction in CO_2 in the blood.

hypoparathyroid t., parathyroid t.

infantile t., t. of infants occurring usually in rickets in the healing stage when the blood calcium is reduced.

latent t., t. that is made manifest only when certain procedures are used. See Trousseau's *sign;* Chvostek's *sign;* Erb's *sign.*

manifest t., t. from any cause in which the symptoms (as under main title) referable to neuromuscular hyperexcitability are clearly evident, as opposed to latent t.

neonatal t., tetania neonatorium; tetanism; myotonia neonatorum; a general muscular hypertonicity in neonates or young infants.

parathyroid t., tetania parathyreopriva; hypoparathyroid or parathyroprival t.; t. due to lack of parathyroid function, spontaneous or following excision of the parathyroid glands.

parathyroprival t., parathyroid t.

phosphate t., t. due to the ingestion of an excess of alkaline phosphates (Na_2HPO_4 or K_2HPO_4); most commonly produced experimentally in animals by the injection of alkaline phosphate which reduces the ionized calcium of the blood.

postoperative t., parathyroid t. caused by injury to or excision of the parathyroids during thyroid removal.

rheumatic t., tetania rheumatica or epidemica; epidemic t.; an acute epidemic form of t., of several weeks' duration, occurring chiefly in winter.

transport t., an acute disease seen in cattle and sheep during and shortly after shipping; it appears most often in females in advanced pregnancy and is believed to be precipitated by stress, lack of food and water, and perhaps heat.

tetartanopia (te-tar'tă-nō'pē-ă). Tetartanopsia.

tetartanopsia (te-tar'tă-nop'sē-ă) [G. *tetartos,* fourth, + *an-* priv. + *opsis,* vision]. Tetartanopia; a homonymous form of quadrantic hemianopsia.

tetra- [G. *tetra-,* four]. Prefix, to words formed from G. roots, meaning four.

tetra-amelia (tet'ră-ă-mē'lē-ă) [tetra- + G. *a-* priv. + *melos,* limb]. Absence of upper and lower limbs.

tetrabasic (tet-ră-bā'sik). Denoting an acid having four acid groups and thereby being able to neutralize four equivalents of base.

tetrabenazine (tet'ră-ben'ă-zen). 2-Oxo-3-isobutyl-9,10-dimethoxy-1,2,3,4,6,7-hexahydro-11b*H*-benzo[α]quinolizine; formerly used as a tranquilizer; now used in the management of chorea and other disorders of motion.

tetraboric acid (tet'ră-bōr'ik). Perboric or pyroboric acid.

tetrabrachius (tet'ră-brā'kē-ŭs) [tetra- + G. *brachiōn,* arm]. A malformed individual with four arms.

tetrabromophenolphthalein sodium (tet'ră-brō'mō-fē'nol-thal'ēn, -ē-in). The sodium salt of a dibasic dye; it has been used for x-ray examination of the gallbladder.

tetracaine hydrochloride (tet'ră-kān). 2-(Dimethylamino)ethyl *p*-(butylamino)benzoate monohydrochloride; a highly potent local anesthetic used for spinal, nerve block, and topical anesthesia.

tetrachirus (tet'ră-kī'rŭs) [tetra- + G. *cheir,* hand]. A malformed individual having four hands.

tetrachlorethylene (tet'ră-klōr-eth'i-lēn). Tetrachloroethylene; carbon dichloride; ethylene tetrachloride; an anthelmintic against hookworm and other nematodes.

tetrachloride (tet'ră-klōr'īd). A compound containing four atoms of chlorine to one atom of the other element or one radical equivalent; *e.g.,* carbon t., CCl_4.

tetrachlormethiazide (tet'ră-klōr-me-thī'ă-zīd). Teclothiazide; 6-chloro-3,4-dihydro-3-trichloromethyl-2*H*-1,2,4-benzothiadiazine-7-sulfonamide 1,1-dioxide; a diuretic.

tetrachloroethane (tet'ră-klōr-ō-eth'ān). Cellon; acetylene tetrachloride; $Cl_2HC—CHCl_2$; a nonflammable solvent for fats, oils, waxes, resins, etc.; used in the manufacture of paint and varnish removers, photographic films, lacquers, and insecticides. Its toxicity exceeds that of chloroform and carbon tetrachloride, and produces narcosis, liver damage, kidney damage, and gastroenteritis.

tetrachloroethylene (tet'ră-klōr-ō-eth'i-lēn). Tetrachlorethylene.

tetrachloromethane. (tet'tră-klōr-ō-meth'ān). *Carbon* tetrachloride.

tetracoccus, pl. **tetracocci** (tet'ră-kok'ŭs, -kok'sī) [tetra- + G. *kokkos,* berry]. A spherical bacterium that divides in two planes and characteristically forms groups of four cells.

tetracosactide, tetracosactin (tet'ră-kō-sak'tid, -tin). Cosyntropin.

tetracosanoic acid (tet'ră-kō-să-nō'ik). Lignoceric acid.

tetracrotic (tet'ră-krot'ik) [tetra- + G. *krotos,* a striking]. Denoting a pulse curve with four upstrokes in the cycle.

tetracuspid (tet-ră-kŭs'pid). Quadricuspid; having four cusps.

tetracycline (tet-ră-sī'klēn, -klin). A broad spectrum antibiotic (a naphthacene derivative), the parent of oxytetracycline, prepared from chlortetracycline and also obtained from the culture filtrate of several species of *Streptomyces;* also available as t. hydrochloride and t. phosphate complex. T. fluorescence has been used in studies of growing tumors and calcium deposition in developing bone and teeth.

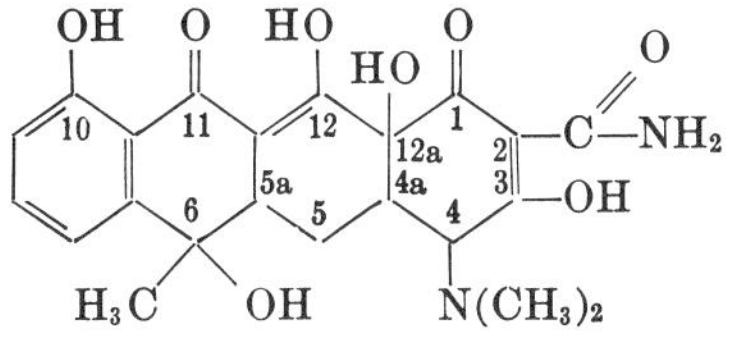

Tetracycline

tet'rad [G. *tetras (tetrad-),* the number four]. **1.** Tetralogy; a collection of four things having something in common. **2.** In chemistry, a quadrivalent element. **3.** In heredity, a bivalent chromosome that divides into four during meiosis.

Fallot's t., Fallot's *tetralogy.*
narcoleptic t., uncontrollable sleep, cataplexy, and hypnagogic hallucinations.

tetradactyl (tet-ră-dak'til) [tetra- + G. *daktylos,* finger or toe]. Quadridigitate; having only four fingers or toes on a hand or foot.

tetradecanoic acid (tet'ră-dek-ă-nō'ik). Myristic acid.

12-O-**tetradecanoylphorbol** 13-**acetate (TPA)** (tet'ră-dek'ă-nō-il-fōr'bol). A double ester of phorbol found in croton oil; a cocarcinogen or tumor promoter.

tetradic (te-trad'ik). Relating to a tetrad.

tetraethylammonium chloride (tet-ră-eth'il-ă-mō'nē-ŭm). $(C_2H_5)_4N^+Cl^-$; a quaternary ammonium compound that partially blocks transmission of impulses through parasympathetic and sympathetic ganglia; its clinical usefulness is limited.

tetraethyllead (tet'ră-eth'i-led). Lead tetraethyl; tetraethylplumbane; $Pb(C_2H_5)_4$; an anti-knock compound added to motor fuel; has a toxic action causing anorexia, nausea, vomiting, diarrhea, tremors, muscular weakness, insomnia, irritability, nervousness, and anxiety; death may occur.

tetraethylmonothionopyrophosphate (tet-ră-eth'il-mon-ō-thī'ō-nō-pī-rō-fos'fāt). An anticholinesterase agent used in the treatment of glaucoma.

tetraethyl pyrophosphate (TEPP) (tet'ră-eth'il). $Et_4P_2O_7$; $[(EtO)_2PO]_2O$; an organic phosphoric compound used as an insecticide; a potent irreversible cholinesterase inhibitor.

tetraethylthiuram disulfide (tet'ră-eth-il-thī'yū-ram). Disulfiram.

tetraglycine hydroperiodide (tet-ră-glī'sēn hī'drō-per-ī'ō-dīd). $(NH_2CH_2COOH)_4HI{\cdot}1^1/_4I_2$; dissolves in water to the extent of 380 g per liter; used for the emergency disinfection of drinking water in amounts to yield 8 p.p.m. of active iodine.

tetragon, tetragonum (tet'ră-gon, tet'ră-gō'nŭm) [tetra- + G. *gōnia,* angle]. A figure having four sides.
t. lumba'le, a quadrangular space bounded laterally by the obliquus externus abdominis muscle, medially by the erector spinae, above by the serratus posterior inferior, and below by the obliquus internus abdominis.

tetragonus (tet'ră-gō'nŭs). Platysma.

tetrahydric (tet-ră-hī'drik). Denoting a compound containing four ionizable hydrogen atoms (four acid groups).

tetrahydro-. Prefix denoting attachment of four hydrogen atoms; *e.g.,* tetrahydrofolate, H_4folate.

tetrahydrocannabinol (tet'ră-hī'drō-kă-nab'i-nol). $C_{21}H_{30}O_2$; the Δ^1-3,4-*trans* isomer and the Δ^6-3,4-*trans* isomer are believed to be the active isomers present in *Cannabis,* having been isolated from marihuana. See also *Cannabis.*

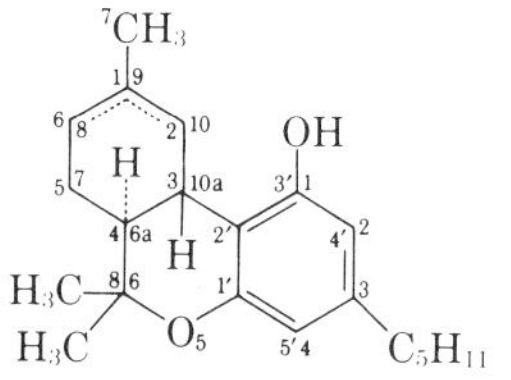

Tetrahydrocannabinol
(*Dotted lines* indicate Δ^1 and Δ^6 isomers, by left-hand numbers; alternate numbering shown by right hand numbers.)

tetrahydrofolate dehydrogenase (tet'ră-hī-drō-fō'lāt). Dihydrofolate reductase.

tetrahydrozoline hydrochloride (tet-ră-hī-droz'ō-lēn). A sympathomimetic agent related to ephedrine, used as a topical nasal and conjunctival decongestant; excessive amounts may convert an acute congestion into a chronic reactive hyperemia.

Tetrahymena pyriformis (tet-ră-hī'mē-nă pir-i-fōr'mis) [tetra- + G. *hymēn,* membrane]. A ciliate belonging to a large group characterized by three membranes on one side of the buccal cavity and one on the other; it somewhat resembles the paramecium and, like it, is readily cultured and used extensively for experimental studies.

tetraiodophenolphthalein sodium (tet'ră-ī-ō'dō-fē'nol-thal'ēn, -thal'ē-in). Iodophthalein.

tetralogy (tet-ral'ō-jē) [G. *tetralogia*]. Tetrad (1).
Eisenmenger's t., Eisenmenger's *complex.*
Fallot's t., Fallot's tetrad; the most common form of cyanotic congenital heart disease, the t. consisting of high pulmonic stenosis, ventricular septal defect, dextroposition of the aorta, and right ventricular hypertrophy.

tetramastia (tet'ră-mas'tē-ă) [tetra- + G. *mastos,* breast]. Presence of four breasts on an individual.

tetramastigote (tet-ră-mas'ti-gōt) [tetra- + G. *mastix,* whip]. A protozoan or other microorganism possessing four flagella.

tetramastous (tet'ră-mas'tŭs). Having four breasts.

tetramelus (tē-tram'ĕ-lŭs) [tetra- + G. *melos,* limb]. Conjoined twins possessing four arms (tetrabrachius), or four legs (tetrascelus).

Tetrameres (tet-ram'ĕ-rēz) [see tetrameric]. A genus of stomach-infecting parasitic nematodes (family Spiruridae) of birds. When filled with eggs, the female worm is enormously enlarged and has a globular, blood-red appearance. Species include *T. americana,* found in the proventriculus of chickens (sometimes severely pathogenic in young chicks), turkeys, grouse, and quail, and transmitted by infected cockroaches and grasshoppers, and *T. fissispina,* found in the proventriculum of ducks, geese, wild waterfowl, pigeons, and doves but rarely in gallinaceous birds.

tetrameric, tetramerous (tet'ră-mer'ik, tē-tram'ĕ-rŭs) [tetra- + G. *meros,* part]. Having four parts, or parts arranged in groups of four, or capable of existing in four forms.

tetramethylammonium iodide (tet-ră-meth'il-ă-mō'nē-ŭm). $(CH_3)_4NI_3$; dissolves in water to the extent of 0.25 gm per liter; used for the emergency disinfection of drinking water.

tetramethyldiarsine (tet'ră-meth'il-dī-ar'sēn). Cacodyl.

tetramethylputrescine (tet-ră-meth'il-pyū-tres'ēn). A derivative of putrescine, $C_8H_{20}N_2$, similar in its action to muscarine.

tetranitrol (tet-ră-nī'trol). Erythrityl tetranitrate.

tetranucleotide (tet'ră-nū'klē-ō-tīd). A compound of four nucleotides; once thought to represent the actual structure of nucleic acid (tetranucleotide theory).

tetraparesis (tet'ră-pă-rē'sis). Weakness of all four extremities.

tetrapeptide (tet'ră-pep'tīd). A compound of four amino acids in peptide linkage.

tetraperomelia (tet'ră-pē-rō-mē'lē-ă) [tetra- + G. *peros,* maimed, + *melos,* limb]. Peromelia involving all four extremities.

tetraphocomelia (tet'ră-fō-kō-mē'lē-ă). Phocomelia involving all four limbs.

tetraplegia (tet'ră-plē'jē-ă) [tetra- + G. *plēgē,* stroke]. Quadriplegia.

tetraplegic (tet'ră-plē'jik). Quadriplegic.

tetraploid (tet'ră-ployd) [G. *tetraploos,* fourfold, + *eidos,* form]. See polyploidy.

tetrapus (tet'ră-pŭs) [G. *tetrapous,* fr. tetra- + *pous,* foot]. A malformed individual with four feet.

tetrapyrrole (tet'ră-pir'ōl). A molecule containing four pyrrole nuclei; *e.g.,* porphyrin.

tetrasaccharide (tet'ră-sak'ă-rīd). A sugar containing four molecules of a monosaccharide; *e.g.,* stachyose.

tetrascelus (te-tras'ĕ-lŭs) [tetra- + G. *skelos,* leg]. A malformed individual with four legs.

tetrasomic (tet'ră-sō'mik) [tetra- + chromosome]. Relating to a cell nucleus in which one chromosome is represented four times while all others are present in the normal number.

tetraster (tet-ras'ter) [tetra- G. *astēr,* star]. A figure exceptionally and abnormally occurring in mitosis, in which there are four asters.

tetrastichiasis (tet'ră-sti-kī'ă-sis) [tetra- + G. *stichos,* row]. Duplication of the growth of the eyelashes (in four rows).

tetraterpenes (tet'ră-ter'pēnz). Hydrocarbons or their derivatives formed by the condensation of eight isoprene units (*i.e.,* four terpenes) and therefore containing 40 carbon atoms; *e.g.,* various carotenoids.

tetratomic (tet'ră-tom'ik) [tetra- + G. *atomos,* atom]. Denoting a quadrivalent element or radical.

Tetratrichomonas (tet'ră-tri-kom'ŏ-nas) [tetra- + *Trichomonas*]. A genus of parasitic protozoan flagellates, formerly part of the genus *Trichomonas* but now separated into a distinct genus by the presence of four anterior and one trailing flagella, a pelta, and a disc-shaped parabasal body. See *Trichomonas.*

T. o'vis, a species that occurs in the cecum or rumen of domestic sheep.

tetravalent (tet'ră-vā'lent) [tetra- + L. *valentia,* strength]. Quadrivalent.

tetrazole (tet'ră-zōl). The compound CN_4H_2 with the structure of tetrazolium.

tetrazolium (tet'ră-zō'lē-ŭm). Any of a group of organic salts having the general structure

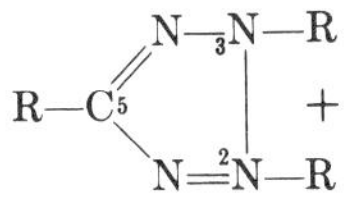

which on reduction (cleaving the 2,3 bond) yields a colored insoluble formazan; used as a reagent in oxidative enzyme histochemistry.

nitroblue t. (NBT), a pale yellow dye that is converted on reduction to colored formazans in the histochemical demonstration of dehydrogenases; used in hematology for staining of neutrophils to help indicate the presence of bacterial infections.

tetrodotoxin (tet'rō-dō-tok'sin). A potent neurotoxin found in the liver and ovaries of the Japanese pufferfish, *Sphoeroides rubripes,* other species of pufferfish, and certain newts; produces axonal blocks of the preganglionic cholinergic fibers and the somatic motor nerves.

tetrose (tet'rōs). A monosaccharide containing only four carbon atoms in the main chain; *e.g.,* erythrose, threose.

tetrotus (te-trō'tŭs) [tetra- + G. *ous* (*ōt-*), ear]. A malformed individual with four ears.

tetroxide (te-trok'sīd). An oxide containing four oxygen atoms; *e.g.,* OsO_4.

tetter (tet'er) [A.S. *teter*] A colloquial term, popularly applied to ringworm and eczema, and occasionally applied to other eruptions.

branny t., **(1)** dandruff; **(2)** seborrhea capitis.

crusted t., impetigo.

dry t., colloquialism for eczema.

honeycomb t., favus.

humid t., *eczema* madidans.

milk t., *crusta* lactea.

moist t., *eczema* madidans.

scaly t., colloquialism for eczema.

wet t., *eczema* madidans.

Teutleben, F.E.K. von, 19th century German anatomist. See T.'s *ligament.*

textiform (teks'tĭ-fōrm) [L. *textum,* something woven]. Weblike.

textural (teks'chŭr-ăl). Relating to the texture of the tissues.

texture (teks'chŭr) [L. *textura,* fr. *texo,* pp. *textus,* to weave]. The composition or structure of a tissue or organ.

textus (teks'ŭs) [L.]. A tissue.

TGC Abbreviation for time-varied gain *control.*

TGE Abbreviation for transmissible *gastroenteritis* of swine.

Th Symbol for thorium.

Thal, Alan P., U.S. surgeon, *1925. See T. *procedure.*

thalam-. See thalamo-.

thalamectomy (thal-ă-mek'tō-mē) [thalamus + G. *ektomē,* excision]. See chemothalamectomy.

thalamencephalic (thal'ă-men-se-fal'ik). Relating to the thalamencephalon.

thalamencephalon (thal'ă-men-sef'ă-lon) [thalamus + G. *enkephalos,* brain]. That part of the diencephalon comprising the thalamus and its associated structures.

thalamic (tha-lam'ik). Relating to the thalamus.

thalamo-, thalam- [G. *thalamos,* bedroom (thalamus)]. Combining forms relating to the thalamus.

thalamocortical (thal'ă-mō-kōr'ti-kăl). Relating to the efferent connections of the thalamus with the cerebral cortex.

thalamotomy (thal-ă-mot'ō-mē) [thalamus + G. *tomē,* incision]. Destruction of a selected portion of the thalamus by stereotaxy for the relief of pain, involuntary movements, epilepsy, and, rarely, emotional disturbances; produces few, if any, neurological deficits or undesirable personality changes.

thalamus, pl. **thalami** (thal'ă-mŭs, -mī) [G. *thalamos,* a bed, a bedroom] [NA]. The large, ovoid mass of gray matter that forms the larger dorsal subdivision of the diencephalon; it is placed medial to the internal capsule and the body and tail of the caudate nucleus. Its medial aspect forms the dorsal half of the lateral wall of the third ventricle; its dorsal surface can be subdivided into a lateral triangle forming the floor of the body (pars centralis) of the lateral ventricle, and a medial triangle covered by the velum interpositum; its taillike caudal part curves ventralward around the posterolateral aspect of the cerebral peduncle and ends in the lateral geniculate body. The t. is composed of a large number of anatomically and functionally distinct cell groups or nuclei, usually classified as 1) sensory relay nuclei (nucleus ventralis posterior, corpus geniculatum laterale and mediale) each receiving a modally specific sensory conduction system and in turn projecting each to the corresponding primary sensory area of the cortex; 2) "secondary" relay nuclei (nucleus ventralis lateralis and ventralis anterior) receiving fibers from the medial segment of the globus pallidus, the contralateral deep cerebellar nuclei (*i.e.,* cerebellothalamic fibers) and the pars reticulata of the substantia nigra which project to various regions of the motor cortex; 3) a nucleus associated with the limbic system: the composite nucleus anterior receiving the mamillothalamic tract and projecting to the gyrus fornicatus; 4) association nuclei (nucleus medialis dorsalis, nucleus lateralis including the large pulvinar) each projecting to a particular large expanse of association cortex; 5) the midline and intralaminar nuclei or "nonspecific" nuclei (nucleus centromedianus, centralis lateralis, paracentralis, reuniens).

thalassemia, thalassanemia (thal-ă-sē'mē-ă, thă-las-ă-nē'mē-ă) [G. *thalassa,* the sea, + *haima,* blood]. Any of a group of inherited disorders of hemoglobin metabolism in which there is a decrease in net synthesis of a particular globin chain without change in the structure of that chain; several genetic types exist, and the corresponding clinical picture may vary from barely detectable hematologic abnormality to severe and fatal anemia.

A_2 t., β t., heterozygous state.

α t., t. due to one of two or more genes that depress (severely or moderately) synthesis of α-globin chains by the chromosome with the abnormal gene. Heterozygous state: severe type, t. minor with 5 to 15% of Hb Barts at birth, only traces of Hb Barts in adult; mild type, 1 to 2% of Hb Barts at birth, not detectable in adult. Homozygous state: severe type, erythroblastosis fetalis and fetal death, only Hb Barts and Hb H present; mild type not clinically defined. See also *hemoglobin* H.

α t. interme'dia, hemoglobin H disease. See *hemoglobin* H.

β t., t. due to one of two or more genes that depress (partially or completely) synthesis of β-globin chains by the chromosome bearing the abnormal gene. Heterozygous state (A_2 t.): t. minor with Hb A_2 increased, Hb F normal or variably increased, Hb A normal or slightly reduced. Homozygous state: t. major with Hb A reduced to very low but variable levels, Hb F very high level.

β-δ t., F t.; t. due to a gene that depresses synthesis of both β- and δ-globin chains by the chromosome bearing the abnormal gene. Heterozygous state: t. minor with Hb F comprising 5 to 30% of total hemoglobin but distributed unevenly among cells, Hb A_2 reduced or normal. Homozygous state: moderate anemia with only Hb F present, no Hb A or Hb A_2.

F t., β-δ t.

Lepore t., t. syndrome due to production of abnormally structured Lepore hemoglobin. Heterozygous state: t. minor with about 10% of Hb Lepore, Hb F moderately increased, Hb A_2 normal. Homozygous state: t. major with only Hb F and Hb Lepore produced, no Hb A or Hb A_2.

t. ma'jor, Cooley's anemia; primary erythroblastic anemia; the syndrome of severe anemia resulting from the homozygous state of one of the t. genes or one of the hemoglobin Lepore genes with onset, in infancy or childhood, of pallor, icterus, weakness, splenomegaly, cardiac enlargement, thinning of inner and outer tables of skull, microcytic hypochromic anemia with poikilocytosis, anisocytosis, stippled cells, target cells, and nucleated erythrocytes; types of hemoglobin are variable and depend on the gene involved.

t. mi'nor, the heterozygous state of a t. gene or a hemoglobin Lepore gene; usually asymptomatic, and quite variable hematologically, with leptocytosis, mild hypochromic microcytosis, and often slightly reduced hemoglobin level with slightly increased erythrocyte count; types of hemoglobin are variable and depend on the gene involved.

thalassophobia (thal'ă-sō-fō'bē-ă, thă-las'ō-) [G. *thalassa,* the sea, + *phobos,* fear]. Morbid fear of the sea.

thalassoposia (thal'ă-sō-pō'zē-ă, thă-las'ō-) [G. *thalassa,* the sea, + *posis,* drinking]. Mariposia.

thalassotherapy (thal'ă-sō-thār'ă-pē) [G. *thalassa,* the sea]. Treatment of disease by exposure to sea air, by sea bathing, or by a sea voyage.

thalidomide (thă-lid'ō-mīd). α-Phthalimidoglutarimide; *N*-phthalylglutamimide; *N*-(2,6-dioxo-3-(piperidyl)phthalimide; a hypnotic drug which, if taken in early pregnancy, may cause the birth of infants with phocomelia and other defects.

thallic (thal'lik). Denoting conidia produced with no enlargement or growth after delimitation by septa in the hypha (thallus); the entire parent cell becomes an arthroconidium.

thallium (thal'ē-ŭm) [G. *thallos,* a green shoot (it gives a green line in the spectrum)]. A white metallic element, symbol Tl, atomic no. 81, atomic weight 204.37.

Thallophyta (thă-lof'i-tă) [G. *thallos,* a green shoot, + *phyton,* plant]. In older classification systems, a primary division of the plant kingdom whose members, with a few exceptions, were devoid of true roots, stems, and leaves; it included bacteria, fungi, and algae.

thallophyte (thal'ō-fīt). A member of the division Thallophyta.

thallospore (thal'ō-spōr) [G. *thallos,* a green twig, + *sporos,* seed]. Obsolete term for a reproductive asexual type of spore formed as an integral part of the thallus or mycelium, in contrast to a conidium formed on a specialized hypha.

thallotoxicosis (thal'ō-tok-si-kō'sis) [thallium + G. *toxikon,* poison, + *-osis,* condition]. Poisoning by thallium; marked by stomatitis, gastroenteritis, peripheral and retrobulbar neuritis, endocrine disorders, and alopecia.

thallus (thal'ŭs) [G. *thallos,* a young shoot]. A simple plant or fungus body which is devoid of roots, stems, and leaves.

thamuria (tha-myū'rē-ă) [G. *thama,* often, + *ouron,* urine]. Obsolete term for frequent micturition.

thanato- [G. *thanatos,* death]. Combining form denoting death.

thanatobiologic (than'ă-tō-bī-ō-loj'ik) [thanato- + G. *bios,* life, + *logos,* study]. Relating to the processes involved in life and death.

thanatognomonic (than'ă-tō-nō-mon'ik) [thanato- + G. *gnōmē,* a sign]. Of fatal prognosis, indicating the approach of death.

thanatography (than-ă-tog'ră-fē) [thanato- + G. *graphē,* a writing]. **1.** A description of one's symptoms and thoughts while dying. **2.** A treatise on death.

thanatoid (than'ă-toyd) [thanato- + G. *eidos,* resemblance]. **1.** Resembling death. **2.** Mortal; deadly.

thanatology (than-ă-tol'ō-jē) [thanato- + G. *logos,* study]. The branch of science concerned with the study of death and dying.

thanatomania (than'ă-tō-mā'nē-ă) [thanato- + G. *mania,* frenzy]. Illness or death resulting from belief in the efficacy of magic; a phenomenon observed among those primitive societies or illiterate and superstitious people who believe in the power of evil spirits, spells, curses, and individuals over one's bodily processes, with such belief and resulting fear manifesting itself as psychosomatic illness and even death.

thanatophidia (than'ă-tō-fid'ē-ă) [thanato- + G. *ophidion,* dim. of *ophis,* a serpent]. Venomous snakes.

thanatophobia (than'ă-tō-fō'bē-ă) [thanato- + G. *phobos,* fear]. Morbid fear of death.

thanatophoric (than'ă-tō-fōr'ik) [thanato- + G. *phoros,* bearing]. Lethal; leading to death.

thanatopsy (than'ă-top-sē) [thanato- + G. *opsis,* view]. Autopsy (1).

thanatos (than'ă-tos) [G. death]. In psychoanalysis, the death principle, representing all instinctual tendencies toward senescence and death. *Cf.* eros. See also subentries under instinct.

Thane, Sir George D., British anatomist, 1850–1930. See T.'s *method.*

thaumatropy (thaw-mat'rō-pē) [G. *thauma* (*thaumat-*), a wonder, + *tropē,* a turning]. The transformation of one form of tissue into another.

Thayer, J.D., See T.-Martin *medium.*

Thd Symbol for ribothymidine.

thea (thēă) [Mod. L.]. Tea.

theaism (thē'ă-izm). Theinism.

theater (thē'ă-ter) [G. *theatron,* a place for seeing, theater, fr. *theomai,* to look at]. **1.** A large room for lectures and demonstrations; sometimes applied to an operating room equipped for observation by persons other than the surgical team. **2.** Any operating room or suite of such rooms.

thebaic (thē-bā'ik) [L. *Thebaicus,* relating to Thebes, whence opium was formerly obtained]. Relating to or derived from opium.

thebaine (thē-bā'ēn, -in). Paramorphine; $C_{19}H_{21}NO_3$; an alkaloid obtained from opium (0.3 to 1.5%); it resembles strychnine in its action, causing tetanic convulsions.

Thebesius, Adam C., German physician, 1686–1732. See thebesian *foramina, valve, veins.*

theca, pl. **thecae** (thē'kă, thē'sē) [G. *thēkē,* a box]. A sheath or capsule.

t. cor'dis, pericardium.

t. exter'na, *tunica* externa thecae folliculi.

t. follic'uli, the wall of a vesicular ovarian follicle. See also *tunica* externa; *tunica* interna thecae folliculi.

t. inter'na, *tunica* interna thecae folliculi.

t. ten'dinis, *vagina* synovialis tendinis.

t. vertebra'lis, *dura mater* spinalis.

thecal (thē'kăl) [see theca]. Relating to a sheath, especially a tendon sheath.

thecitis (thē-sī'tis) [G. *thēkē,* box (sheath), + *-itis,* inflammation]. Inflammation of the sheath of a tendon.

thecodont (thē'kō-dont) [G. *thēkē,* box, + *odous (odont-),* tooth]. Having the teeth inserted in alveoli.

thecoma (thē-kō'mă) [G. *thēkē,* box (theca), + *-oma,* tumor]. Theca cell tumor; a neoplasm derived from ovarian mesenchyme, consisting chiefly of spindle-shaped cells that frequently contain small droplets of fat; gross features generally resemble those of a granulosa cell tumor, *i.e.,* firm, yellow, encapsulated mass, ordinarily about 10 cm or less in diameter, but it tends to be less malignant; it may form considerable quantities of estrogens, thereby resulting in precocious development of secondary sexual features in prepubertal girls, or hyperplasia of the endometrium in older patients.

thecomatosis (thē'kō-mă-tō'sis). A stromal hyperplasia or increase in the number of connective tissue elements of an ovary.

thecostegnosia, thecostegnosis (thē'kō-steg-nō'sē-ă, -nō'sis) [G. *thēkē,* box (sheath), + *stegnōsis,* a narrowing]. Constriction of a tendon sheath.

Theden, Johann C.A., German surgeon, 1714–1797. See T.'s *method.*

Theile, Friedrich W., German anatomist, 1801– 1879. See T.'s *canal, glands, muscle.*

Theiler, Max, South African microbiologist in the U.S. and Nobel laureate, 1899–1972. See T.'s *disease, virus.*

Theileria (thī-lēr'ē-ă) [A. *Theiler*]. Cytauxzoon; a genus of piroplasmid sporozoan protozoa (family Theileriidae, order Piroplasmida, class Sporozoea) that are tick-borne parasites and among the most important pathogens of domestic animals; they multiply asexually in lymphocytes or other cells and then invade the erythrocytes, where they remain without multiplying until ingested by a transmitting tick.

T. annula'ta, a species that causes Mediterranean or tropical theileriosis in cattle.

T. bo'vis, *T. parva bovis.*

T. fe'lis, a highly pathogenic species that causes theileriosis in domestic cats and bobcats.

T. hir'ci, a species that causes malignant theileriosis in sheep and goats.

T. lawren'cei, *T. parva lawrencei.*

T. mu'tans, a species that causes benign bovine theileriosis in Africa and the Carribbean; occasionally causes fatal disease in cattle.

T. orienta'lis, *T. sergenti;* a bovine species found worldwide which, in some regions, has been reported to cause clinical disease in cattle.

T. par'va, a species now divided into three subspecies: *T. p. bovis, T. p. lawrencei,* and *T. p. parva.*

T. par'va bo'vis, *T. bovis;* a parasite causing Rhodesian malignant theileriosis in cattle.

T. par'va lawren'cei, *T. lawrencei;* a parasite of the wild African buffalo (*Syncerus caffer*); it is highly pathogenic to cattle, causing Corridor disease.

T. par'va par'va, a highly pathogenic parasite causing East Coast fever in cattle.

T. sergen'ti, *T. orientalis.*

T. taurotra'gi, a species that causes benign bovine theileriosis, and is infective to sheep and goats; transmitted by *Rhipicephalus pulchellus* in Africa.

theileriasis (thī-le-rī'ă-sis). Theileriosis.

Theileriidae (thī-lē'rē-i-dē). A family of sporozoan protozoa which, combined with the family Babesiidae, comprises the order Piroplasmida; it consists of one recognized genus, *Theileria,* transmitted by ixodid ticks; some species are highly pathogenic to domestic and wild ruminants, causing theileriosis.

theileriosis (thī-lēr-ē-ō'sis). Theileriasis; disease of cattle, sheep, and goats caused by infection with *Theileria,* and transmitted by ixodid ticks.

benign bovine t., t. in cattle, caused either by *Theileria mutans* (transmitted by ticks of the genus *Amblyomma* in Africa and the *Caribbean*) or by *T. taurotragi* (transmitted by *Rhipicephalus appendiculatus* and *R. pulchellus* in Africa).

malignant ovine and caprine t., a highly pathogenic disease of sheep and goats in southeastern Europe, northern Africa, and the Near and Middle East; it is caused by *Theileria hirri* and transmitted by *Hyalomma anatolicum anatolicum.*

Mediterranean t., tropical t.

Rhodesian malignant t., a highly pathogenic disease of cattle in Zimbabwe caused by *Theileria parva bovis* and transmitted by *Rhipicephalus appendiculatus.*

tropical t., Mediterranean t; a highly pathogenic disease of cattle in northern Africa, southern Europe, the Near and Middle East, and central Asia; caused by *Theileria annulata* and transmitted by ticks of the genus *Hyalomma.*

thein (thē'in, tē'in). Caffeine.

theinism, theism (thē'i-nizm, thē'izm; tē'-) [Mod. L. *thea,* tea]. Theaism; chronic poisoning resulting from immoderate tea-drinking, marked by palpitation, insomnia, nervousness, headache, and dyspepsia.

thel-. See thelo-.

thelarche (thē-lar'kē) [thel- + G. *archē,* beginning]. The beginning of development of the breasts in the female.

Thelazia (thē-lā'zē-ă) [G. *thēlazō,* to suck]. The eye worms, a genus of spiruroid nematodes that inhabit the lacrimal ducts and surface of the eyes of various domestic and wild animals, but rarely man; a number of species have been reported from wild birds. Cyclic development occurs in muscoid flies; infective larvae emerge from the fly mouthparts while the fly is feeding on or near the eyes of the host.

T. californien'sis, a species occurring in the tear ducts, conjunctival sac, or under the nictitating membrane of dogs, coyotes, black bears, sheep, deer, jack rabbits, cats, and occasionally man in the western and southwestern U.S.; heavy infections cause photophobia, lacrimation, eyelid edema, conjunctivitis, and even blindness.

T. callip'aeda, a species reported from man in Southeast Asia and California; the worm, embedded in a subconjunctival tumor or swimming in the aqueous humor after penetrating the corneoscleral limbus, causes pain, photophobia, and tearing.

thelaziasis (thē-lă-zī'ă-sis, thel-ă-). Infection with *Thelazia.*

thele (thē'lē) [G.]. *Papilla* mammae.

theleplasty (thē'lē-plas-tē) [thel- + G. *plastos,* formed]. Mammillaplasty.

thelium, pl. **thelia** (thē'lē-ŭm, -lē-ă) [Mod. L., fr. G. *thēlē,* nipple]. **1.** A nipple-like structure. **2.** A cellular layer. **3.** *Papilla* mammae.

thelo-, thel- [G. *thēlē,* nipple]. Combining forms denoting the nipples.

theloncus (thē-long'kŭs) [thelo- + G. *onkos,* a mass]. A neoplasm involving the nipple.

thelorrhagia (thē-lō-rā'jē-ă) [thelo- + G. *rhēgnymi,* to burst forth]. Bleeding from the nipple.

thenad (thē'nad) [G. *thenar,* the palm of the hand, + L. *ad,* to]. Toward the thenar or lateral side of the palm of the hand.

thenal (thē'năl). Thenar (2).

thenaldine (thē-nal'dēn). Thenophenopiperidine; 1-methyl-4-*N*-2-thenylanilinopiperidine; an antihistaminic and antipruritic agent (as the tartrate).

thenar (thē'nar) [G. the palm of the hand]. **1** [NA]. Thenar eminence or prominence; the fleshy mass on the lateral side of the palm; the radial palm; the ball of the thumb. **2.** Thenal; applied to any structure in relation with this part.

thenen (thē'nen) [G. *thenar,* palm, + *en,* in]. Relating only to the palm, specifically to the radial side.

thenyl (then'il). The radical of 2-methylthiophene, $(SC_4H_3)CH_2$–. *Cf.* thienyl.

thenyldiamine hydrochloride (then-il-dī'ă-mēn). 2-[(2-Dimethylaminoethyl)-3-thenylamino]pyridine hydrochloride; $C_{14}H_{19}N_3S$ HCl; an antihistaminic.

theobroma (thē-ō-brō'mă) [G. *theos,* a god, + *brōma,* food]. Cacao.
t. oil, cacao oil or butter; cocoa butter; the fat obtained from the wasted seed of *Theobroma cacao* (family Sterculiaceae); it contains the glycerides of stearic, palmitic, oleic, arichidic, and linoleic acids; used as a base for suppositories and ointments and, in operative dentistry, as a lubricant and protective.

theobromine (thē-ō-brō'mēn). 3,7-Dimethyl-2,6-dihydroxypurine; 3,7-di-methylxanthine; an alkaloid resembling caffeine in its action, prepared from the dried ripe seed of *Theobroma cacao* or made synthetically; used as a diuretic, myocardial stimulant, dilator of coronary arteries, and smooth muscle relaxant. Compounds with calcium gluconate, calcium salicylate, sodium acetate, sodium lactate, and sodium salicylate have been listed.

theomania (thē-ō-mā'nē-ă) [G. *theos,* god, + *mania,* frenzy]. A delusion in which one believes that he is God.

theophobia (thē-ō-fō'bē-ă) [G. *theos,* god, + *phobos,* fear]. Morbid fear of God.

theophylline (thē-of'i-lēn, -lin). 1,3-Dimethylxanthine; an alkaloid found with caffeine in tea leaves (commercial t. is prepared synthetically); a smooth muscle relaxant, diuretic, cardiac stimulant, and vasodilator; used in angina pectoris, peripheral vascular disease, and bronchial asthma.
t. aminoisobutanol, ambuphylline.
t. calcium salicylate, a mixture of calcium t. and sodium salicylate in molecular proportion; has the same actions and uses as t.
t. ethanolamine, t. monoethanolamine, with the same actions and uses as t.
t. ethylenediamine, aminophylline.
t. isopropanolamine, has the same actions and uses as aminophylline, but a more rapid onset and a longer duration of action.
t. sodium acetate, a mixture of t. sodium and sodium acetate, with 60% of t.; has the same uses as t.
t. sodium glycinate, equilibrium mixture containing t. sodium and glycine in approximately molecular proportions, buffered with an additional mole of glycine; similar in action and uses to aminophylline but more stable in air, and less irritating to the gastric mucosa.

theorem (thē'ō-rem). A proposition that can be proved, and so is established as a law or principle. See also entries under law; principle; rule.
Bayes t., relates the probability of an item (*e.g.,* a patient) being a member of a particular group (*e.g.,* clinical class), given the presence of an attribute (*e.g.,* an abnormal test result), to the probability of known group members having the attribute and the probability of obtaining a group member when picking at random an item from the universe of items. See also diagnostic *sensitivity;* diagnostic *specificity;* predictive *value.*
Bernoulli's t., Bernoulli's *law.*
Gibbs' t., substances that lower the surface tension of the pure dispersion medium tend to collect in its surface, whereas substances that raise the surface tension tend to remain out of the surface film.

THEORY

theory (thē'ōr-ē) [G. *theōria,* a beholding, speculation, theory, fr. *theōros,* a beholder]. A reasoned explanation of known facts or phenomena that serves as a basis of investigation by which to reach the truth. See also hypothesis; postulate.
adsorption t. of narcosis, that a drug becomes concentrated at the surface of the cell as a result of adsorption, and thus alters permeability and metabolism.
Altmann's t., that protoplasm is composed of a number of granular elements (bioblasts) surrounded by an indifferent substance.
Arrhenius-Madsen t., that the reaction of an antigen with its antibody is a reversible reaction, the equilibrium being determined according to the law of mass action by the concentrations of the reacting substances.
atomic t., that chemical compounds are formed by the union of atoms in certain definite proportions; in its modern form, first advanced in 1803 by John Dalton.
Baeyer's t., that carbon bonds are set at fixed angles (109°) and that those carbon rings are most stable that least distort those angles; for this reason, planar rings composed of 5 or 6 carbon atoms (*e.g.,* cyclopentane, benzene) are more common than rings containing less than 5 or more than 6 carbon atoms.
balance t., in social psychology, a t. which assumes that steady and unsteady states can be specified for cognitive units, such as an individual and his attitudes or acts, and that such units tend to seek steady states (balance); *e.g.,* balance exists when both parts of a unit are evaluated the same, but disequilibrium arises when both parts are not evaluated the same, which causes either cognitive reevaluation of the parts or their segregation. See also cognitive dissonance t.; consistency *principle.*
balance t. of sex, a t. of sex determination that attributes female differentiation of the embryo to a 1:1 balance of X chromosomes to haploid autosome sets (*i.e.,* 2 X chromosomes + 2 sets of autosomes = female), male differentiation to a 1:2 balance (*i.e.,* 1 X chromosome + 2 autosome sets =male), and intersexual development to ratios other than 1:1 and 1:2.
beta-oxidation-condensation t., that the two carbon fragments split from the fatty acid molecule by beta-oxidation are converted to acetic acid and then condensed to acetoacetic acid.
Bohr's t., that spectrum lines are produced 1) by the emission of radiant energy when electrons drop from an orbit of a higher to one of a lower energy level, or 2) by absorption of radiation when an electron rises from a lower to a higher energy level.
Bordeau t., Bordeu t., see de Bordeau t.
Bowman's t., that the urine is formed by passive filtration through the glomeruli and secretion by the epithelium of the tubules, the water and salts being separated from the plasma in the former situation, the urea and other urinary constituents in the latter. Parts of this t. are now known to be wrong.
Brønsted t., that an acid is a substance, charged or uncharged,

liberating hydrogen ions in solution, and that a base is a substance that removes them from solution (*e.g.,* NH_4^+, CH_3COOH, and HSO_4^- are acids; NH_3, CH_3COO^-, and $SO_4^=$ are bases); useful in the concept of weak electrolytes and buffers.
Burn and Rand t., that stimulation of sympathetic fibers results first in the production of acetylcholine in the postganglionic nerve endings, which then release norepinephrine to act on the active site of the effector cell.
Cannon's t., emergency t.
Cannon-Bard t., the view that the feeling aspect of emotion and the pattern of emotional behavior are controlled by the hypothalamus.
celomic metaplasia t. of endometriosis, that endometrial tissue arises directly from the peritoneal mesothelium.
cloacal t., the belief sometimes held by neurotics or children that a child is born, as a stool is passed, from a common opening.
clonal selection t., that mutation of stem cells produces all possible templates for antibody production. Exposure to a specific antigen will then selectively stimulate proliferation of the cell with the appropriate template to form a clone or colony of specific antibody-forming cells.
cognitive dissonance t., a t. of attitude formation and behavior which indicates that persons try to achieve consistency (consonance) and avoid dissonance which, when it arises, may be coped with by changing one's attitudes, rationalizing, selective perception, and other means. See also balance t. and consistency *principle.*
Cohnheim's t., emigration t.; that neoplasms originate from various cell rests, *i.e.,* embryonal cells thought to persist in various sites after the development of the fetal organs and tissues.
colloid t. of narcosis, that coagulation or flocculation of protein causes dehydration and reduction of metabolism.
darwinian t., the t. of the origin of species and of the development of higher organisms from lower forms through natural selection (survival of the fittest in the struggle for existence), and of the evolution of man from an ancestor common to himself and the apes.
de Bordeau t., Bordeau or Bordeu t.; that each organ of the body manufactured a specific humor which it secreted into the bloodstream.
decay t., a t. of forgetting based on the premise that an engram deteriorates progressively with time during the interval when it is not activated.
De Vries' t., see mutation (2).
Dieulafoy's t., an obsolete t. that appendicitis is always the result of the transformation of the appendicular canal into a closed cavity.
dipole t., a t. in which the activation current of the heart is conceived as a moving dipole, the positive pole leading.
duplicity t. of vision, that the cones of the retina function in bright light and the rods function in dim light.
Ehrlich's t., Ehrlich's side-chain t., see side-chain t.
t. of electrolytic dissociation, see Arrhenius *doctrine.*
emergency t., Cannon's t.; a t. of the emotions, advanced by W.B. Cannon, that animal and human organisms respond to emergency situations by increased sympathetic nervous system activity including an increased catecholamine production with associated increases in blood pressure, heart and respiratory rates, and skeletal muscle blood flow. See also relaxation *response.*
emigration t., Cohnheim's t.
enzyme inhibition t. of narcosis, that narcotics inhibit respiratory enzymes by suppression of the formation of high energy phosphate bonds within the cell.
Flourens' t., that thought is a process depending upon the action of the entire cerebrum.
Frerich's t., that uremia represents a toxic condition caused by ammonium carbonate, which is formed as the result of the action of a plasma enzyme on the increased amounts of urea.
Freud's t., a comprehensive t. of how personality is formed and develops in normal and emotionally disturbed individuals; *e.g.,* that an attack of conversion hysteria is due to a psychic trauma which was not adequately reacted to at the time it was received, and persists as an affect memory. See also psychoanalysis.
gametoid t., that the malignancy of a tumor results from the neoplastic cells having developed sexual characteristics, by means of which they multiply and grow autonomously as parasites on the host's tissues.
gastrea t., Haeckel's gastrea t.
gate-control t., gate-control hypothesis; that afferent stimuli, particularly pain, entering the substantia gelatinosa are modulated by other afferent stimuli and descending spinal pathways so that their transmission to ascending spinal pathways is blocked (gated).
germ t., the t., now a doctrine, that infectious diseases are due to the presence and functional activity of microorganisms within the body.
germ layer t., the concept that young embryos differentiate three primary germ layers (ectoderm, mesoderm, and endoderm), each of which has the potentiality of forming different characteristic structures and organs in the developing body.
gestalt t., see gestaltism.
Haeckel's gastrea t., gastrea t.; that the two-layered gastrula is the ancestral form of all multicellular animals.
Helmholtz t. of accommodation, that the ciliary muscle relaxes for near vision and allows the anterior aspect of the lens to become more convex.
Helmholtz t. of color vision, Young-Helmholtz t. of color vision.
Helmholtz-Gibbs t., see Gibbs-Helmholtz *equation.*
Helmholtz t. of hearing, resonance t. of hearing.
hematogenous t. of endometriosis, that endometrial tissue is carried, like metastases of a malignant tumor, through the blood stream.
Hering's t. of color vision, that there are three opponent visual processes: blue-yellow, red-green, and white-black.
humoral t., see humoral *doctrine.*
hydrate microcrystal t. of anesthesia, Pauling's t.; a t. of narcosis pertaining to nonhydrogen-bonding agents; postulates the interaction of the molecules of the anesthetic drug with water molecules in the brain.
implantation t. of the production of endometriosis, that, at the time of menstruation, cells of the uterine mucosa pass through the uterine tubes and escape into the pelvic cavity where they implant themselves on the peritoneum.
information t., in the behavioral sciences, a system for studying the communication process through the detailed analysis, often mathematical, of all aspects of the process including the encoding, transmission, and decoding of signals; not concerned in any direct sense with the meaning of a message.
incasement t., preformation t.
James-Lange t., that bodily changes, such as tachycardia or sweating, precede rather than follow the conscious perception of an emotion and by themselves evoke the emotional feeling.
kern-plasma relation t. [Ger. *kern,* kernel, nucleus], a t. enunciated by Hertwig (1903) that a definite relation as to size normally exists in every cell between the mass of nuclear material and that of the protoplasm.
Knoop's t., that the catabolism of fatty acids occurs in stages in each of which there is a loss of two carbon atoms as a result of oxidation at the β-carbon atom, *e.g.,*

$$C_6H_5 - \overset{\beta}{CH_2} - \overset{\alpha}{CH_2} - COOH \rightarrow C_6H_5 - COOH.$$

Ladd-Franklin t., molecular dissociation t.
lamarckian t., that acquired characteristics may be transmitted to the descendants.
learning t., any of several prominent theories designed to explain

learning, especially those promulgated by Pavlov, Thorndike, Guthrie, Hull, Kohler, Spence, Miller, Skinner, and their modern followers. See also conditioning.

libido t., Freud's t. that man's psychic life results mainly from instinctual or libidinal needs and the attempts to satisfy them.

Liebig's t., that the hydrocarbons that oxidize readily and burn are aliments that produce the greatest quantity of animal heat.

lipoid t. of narcosis, Meyer-Overton t. of narcosis; that narcotic efficiency parallels the coefficient of partition between oil and water, and that lipoids in the cell and on the cell membrane absorb the drug because of this affinity.

lymphatic dissemination t. of endometriosis, that endometrial tissue is transmitted by the lymphatic channels.

mass action t., that large areas of brain tissue function as a whole in learned or intelligent action.

t. of medicine, the science, as distinguished from the art, or practice, of medicine.

membrane expansion t., that adsorption of anesthetics into membranes so alters membrane volume and/or configuration that membrane function is affected in such a way as to produce anesthesia.

Metchnikoff's t., the phagocytic t., that the body is protected against infection by the leukocytes and other cells that engulf and destroy the invading microorganisms.

Meyer-Overton t. of narcosis, lipoid t. of narcosis.

migration t., obsolete t. that sympathetic ophthalmia is caused by a migration of the pathogenic agent through the lymph channels of the optic nerve.

Miller's chemicoparasitic t., that dental caries is caused by microorganisms of the mouth fermenting dietary carbohydrates and producing acids that demineralize the teeth.

mnemic t., mnemic *hypothesis.*

molecular dissociation t., Ladd-Franklin t.; a t., pertaining to color vision, that gray is the earliest of color sensations, from which are derived, by molecular change, two paired substances that, respectively, detect yellow and blue, and that the yellow gives rise to paired substances for detection of red and green.

monophyletic t., monophyletism.

myoelastic t., a t. stating that sound of the human voice is produced by vibrations of the vocal cords resulting from folding upward due to air pressure below, and subsequent movement downward due to elastic tension of cords.

myogenic t., that cardiac movements are due mainly to stimuli originating in the heart muscle itself and that the heart does not act solely in response to nerve stimulation.

Nernst's t., that the passage of an electric current through the tissues causes a dissociation of the ions, with consequent concentration of salts in the solution bathing the cell membranes, the electric stimulus being thereby effected.

neurochronaxic t., t. stating that variations in pitch of the human voice are produced by active muscular contractions synchronized with cycles per second of pitch, no longer believed to be true.

neurogenic t., that cardiac movements are due solely to stimuli conveyed by the nerves. *Cf.* myogenic t.

Ollier's t., a t. of compensatory growth; after resection of the articular extremity of a bone, the articular cartilage of the other bone entering into the structure of the joint takes on an increased growth.

omega-oxidation t., that the oxidation of fatty acids commences at the CH_3 group, *i.e.,* the terminal or omega-group; beta-oxidation then proceeds at both ends of the fatty acid chain.

overproduction t., Weigert's *law.*

oxygen deprivation t. of narcosis, that narcotics inhibit oxidation, which causes the cell to be narcotized.

Pauling's t., hydrate microcrystal t. of anesthesia.

permeability t. of narcosis, that the permeability of the cell membrane is decreased by narcotic concentrations of aliphatic and other central nervous system depressants.

phlogiston t., see phlogiston.

pithecoid t., the t. of man's descent with the ape from a common ancestor. See also darwinian *theory.*

place t., a t. of pitch perception which states that the perception of the pitch of a sound depends upon the level or region of the basilar membrane of the cochlea which is set into vibration by the sound waves. See also resonance t.

Planck's t., quantum t.

polyphyletic t., polyphyletism.

preformation t., emboitment; incasement t.; archaic t. that the embryo was fully formed in miniature within a gamete at the time of conception. See also homunculus.

quantum t., Planck's t.; that energy can be emitted, transmitted, and absorbed only in discrete quantities (quanta), so that atoms and subatomic particles can exist only in certain energy states.

recapitulation t., the t. formulated by E.H. Haeckel that individuals in their embryonic development pass through stages similar in general structural plan to the stages their species passed through in its evolution; more technically phrased, the t. that ontogeny is an abbreviated recapitulation of phylogeny. Also called law of biogenesis or recapitulation; biogenetic or Haeckel's law.

reed instrument t., a no longer tenable t. stating that in human voice production the larynx functions in a manner similar to a reed musical instrument.

reentry t., that extrasystoles are due to reentry of the sinus impulse, to which the extrasystole is coupled, into the ectopic focus.

resonance t. of hearing, Helmholtz t. of hearing; that the basilar membrane of the cochlea acts as a resonating structure, recording low tones from its apical turns and high tones from its basal turns.

Ribbert's t., that a neoplasm may result when a reduction in tension (exerted by adjacent tissues) leads to conditions favorable to uncontrolled growth of cell rests.

Semon-Hering t., mnemic *hypothesis.*

sensorimotor t., in the developmental t. of Piaget, the postulation that during the first 18 months of life there occurs a transformation of action into thought; at first there is a gradual shift from inborn to acquired behavior, then from body-centered to object-centered activity, ultimately permitting intentional behavior and inventive thinking.

side-chain t., Ehrlich's postulate; the t. advanced by Ehrlich to explain the phenomena of infection, immunity, nutrition, etc.; it assumes that the protoplasmic molecule is analogous in constitution to the benzene molecule, or benzene nucleus, with its linked hydrogen atoms capable of being displaced by various groups to form side chains; linked to the protoplasmic molecule are numerous "side chains," or receptors, capable of seizing upon certain bodies (*e.g.,* foodstuffs, poisons) and incorporating them in the molecule. See also receptor.

somatic mutation t. of cancer, that cancer is caused by a mutation or mutations in the body cells (as opposed to germ cells), especially nonlethal mutations associated with increased proliferation of the mutant cells.

Spitzer's t., an interpretation of the partitioning of the heart of mammalian embryos primarily on the basis of recapitulations of the adult structural pattern of lower forms; most frequently cited in relation to the partitioning of the truncus arteriosus to form ascending aorta and pulmonary trunk.

stringed instrument t., a no longer tenable t. stating that in human voice production the vocal cords function in a manner similar to the strings in a stringed musical instrument.

surface tension t. of narcosis, that substances which lower the surface tension of water pass more readily into the cell and cause narcosis by decreasing metabolism.

telephone t., a t. of pitch perception which states that the cochlea possesses no faculty of sound analysis, but that the frequency of the impulses transmitted over the auditory nerve fibers corresponds to

the frequency of the sound vibrations, and is the sole basis for pitch discrimination.
thermodynamic t. of narcosis, that the interposition of narcotic molecules in nonaqueous cellular phase causes changes that interfere with facilitation of ionic exchange.
two-sympathin t., a t., now obsolete, advanced by Cannon and Rosenblueth that two different types of substances (sympathin E and I) diffuse into circulation when adrenergic nerves are stimulated, although the mediator itself is the same.
van't Hoff's t., that substances in dilute solution obey the gas laws.
Warburg's t., that the development of cancer is due to irreversible damage to the respiratory mechanism of cells, leading to the selective multiplication of cells with increased glycolytic metabolism, both aerobic and anaerobic.
Weismann's t., that the vehicle of inheritance is the germ plasm transmitted from one generation to another, and that modifications in the offspring can be effected only by the mingling of the germ plasm of the parents; acquired characters, which affect only the somatic cells, are never transmitted since the somatic cells are mortal and perish with the individual, only the germ cells passing down the succeeding generations and transmitting the inheritance.
Wollaston's t., semidecussation of the optic nerves, proved by the hemianopsia in brain lesions.
Young-Helmholtz t. of color vision, Helmholtz t. of color vision; a t. that there are three color-perceiving elements in the retina: red, green, and blue. Perception of other colors arises from the combined stimulation of these elements; deficiency or absence of any one of these elements results in inability to perceive that color and a misperception of any other color of which it forms a part.

theotherapy (thē-ō-thār'ă-pē) [G. *theos,* god, + *therapeia,* therapy]. Treatment of disease by prayer or religious exercises.

thèque (tek) [Fr. a small box]. A nest or aggregation of nevocytes or other cells in the epidermis.

therapeusis (thār-ă-pyū'sis). **1.** Therapeutics. **2.** Therapy.

therapeutic (thār-ă-pyū'tik) [G. *therapeutikos*] Relating to therapeutics or to the treatment of disease.

therapeutics (thār-ă-pyū'tiks) [G. *therapeutikē,* medical practice]. Therapeusis (1); therapia (2); the practical branch of medicine concerned with the treatment of disease.
ray t., radiotherapy.
suggestive t., treatment of disease by means of suggestion.

therapeutist (thār-ă-pyū'tist). One skilled in therapeutics.

therapia (thār-ă-pē'ă) [L. fr. G. *therapeia,* therapy]. **1.** Therapy. **2.** Therapeutics.
t. mag'na sterili'sans, Ehrlich's concept that an infectious disease, especially one of protozoal origin, can be cured by one large dose of a suitable remedy, large enough to sterilize all the tissues and to destroy the microorganism contained therein.
t. sterili'sans cover'gens, in chemotherapy, a rapid decrease in the number of the parasites, following the administration of the remedy.
t. sterili'sans diver'gens, in chemotherapy, a primary increase in the number of the parasites preceding their final disappearance. See also anamnestic *reaction.*
t. sterili'sans fractiona'ta, in chemotherapy, the use of small repeated doses of a microparasiticide when the organism does not become refractory to the drug so given.

therapist (thār'ă-pist). One professionally trained and/or skilled in the practice of a particular type of therapy.

THERAPY

therapy (ther'ă-pē) [G. *therapeia,* medical treatment]. Therapeusis (2); therapia (1). **1.** The treatment of disease by various methods. See also therapeutics. **2.** In psychiatry, and clinical psychology, a short term for psychotherapy. See also subentries under psychotherapy; psychiatry; psychology; psychoanalysis.
alkali t., see alkalitherapy.
analytic t., short term for psychoanalytic t.
anticoagulant t., the use of anticoagulant drugs in order to reduce or prevent any tendency toward intravascular or intracardiac clotting.
autoserum t., t. with serum obtained from the patient's own blood.
aversion t., a form of behavior t. that pairs an unpleasant stimulus with undesirable behavior(s) so that the patient learns to avoid the latter. See also aversive *training.*
behavior t., an offshoot of psychotherapy involving the use of procedures and techniques associated with research in the fields of conditioning and learning for the treatment of a variety of psychological conditions; distinguished from psychotherapy because specific symptoms (*e.g.,* phobia, enuresis, high blood pressure) are selected as the target for change, planned interventions or remedial steps to extinguish or modify these symptoms are then employed, and the progress of changes is continuously and quantitatively monitored.
client-centered t., a system of nondirective psychotherapy based on the assumption that the client (patient) both has the internal resources to improve and is in the best position to resolve his own personality dysfunction, provided that the therapist can establish a permissive, accepting, and genuine atmosphere in which the client feels free to discuss his problems and to obtain insight into them in order to achieve self-actualization.
cognitive t., any of a variety of techniques in psychotherapy that utilizes guided self-discovery, imaging, self-instruction, symbolic modeling, and related forms of explicitly elicited cognitions as the principal mode of treatment.
collapse t., the surgical treatment of pulmonary tuberculosis whereby the diseased lung is placed, totally or partially, temporarily or permanently, in a nonfunctional respiratory state of retraction and immobilization.
conjoint t., a type of marriage t. in which a therapist sees the partners together in joint sessions.
cytoreductive t., t. with the intention of reducing the number of cells in a lesion, usually a malignancy.
depot t., injection of a drug together with a substance that slows the release and prolongs the action of the drug.
diathermic t., treatment of various lesions by diathermy.
electroconvulsive t. (ECT), electroshock t.
electroshock t., electroconvulsive t.; a form of treatment of mental disorders in which convulsions are produced by the passage of an electric current through the brain.
electrotherapeutic sleep t., treatment by inducing sleep by means of nonconvulsive electric stimulation of the brain.
extended family t., a type of family t. that involves family members outside the nuclear family and who are closely associated with it and affect it.
family t., a type of group psychotherapy in which a family in conflict meets as a group with the therapist and explores its relationships and processes; focus is on the resolution of current interactions between members rather than on individual members.
fever t., see pyrotherapy.

foreign protein t., protein shock t.
functional orthodontic t., functional jaw *orthopedics.*
geriatric t., gerontotherapy.
gestalt t., a type of psychotherapy, used with individuals or groups, that emphasizes treatment of the person as a whole: his biological component parts and their organic functioning, his perceptual configuration, and his interrelationships with the external world; it focuses on the sensory awareness of the person's immediate experiences rather than on past recollections or future expectations, employing role playing and other techniques to promote the patient's growth process and to develop his full potential.
heterovaccine t., t. with a vaccine obtained from organisms not directly concerned with the disorder being treated.
hyperbaric oxygen t., treatment in which oxygen is provided in a sealed chamber at an ambient pressure greater than 1 atmosphere. See also hyperbaric *oxygenation.*
implosive t., a type of behavior t. using implosion.
individual t., dyadic *psychotherapy.*
inhalation t., therapeutic use of gases or aerosols by inhalation.
insulin coma t., see insulin coma *treatment.*
intralesional t., t. by injection directly into a lesion, as in corticosteroid injections into skin lesions.
maintenance drug t., in chemotherapy, systematic dosage at a level which maintains protection against exacerbation.
marriage t., a type of family t. that involves both husband and wife and focuses on the marital relationship as it affects the individual psychopathologies of the partners; the rationale for this method is the assumption that psychopathological processes within the family structure and in the social matrix of the marriage perpetuate individual pathological personality structures, which find expression in the disturbed marriage and are aggravated by the feedback between partners.
microwave t., microkymatotherapy.
milieu t., psychiatric treatment employing manipulation of the social environment for the benefit of the patient.
myofunctional t., t. of malocclusion and other dental and speech disorders utilizing muscular exercises of the tongue and lips; most often intended to alter a tongue thrust swallowing pattern.
nonspecific t., phlogotherapy; the injection of a foreign protein, typhoid vaccine, etc., to induce fever in the treatment of certain diseases, especially those of a parasyphilitic nature.
occupational t. (OT), therapeutic use of self-care, work, and recreational activities to increase independent function, enhance development, and prevent disability; may include adaptation of tasks or environment to achieve maximum independence and optimum quality of life.
orthodontic t., see orthodontics.
orthomolecular t., treatment designed to remedy deficiencies in any of the normal chemical constituents of the body.
oxygen t., treatment in which an increased concentration of oxygen is made available for breathing, through a nasal catheter, tent, chamber, or mask.
parenteral t., t. introduced usually by a needle through some other route than the alimentary canal.
photoradiation t., photoradiation.
physical t. (PT), **1.** Physiotherapy; treatment of pain, disease, or injury by physical means. **2.** The health profession concerned with promotion of health, with prevention of physical disabilities, with evaluation and rehabilitation of persons disabled by pain, disease, or injury, and with treatment by physical therapeutic measures as opposed to medical, surgical, or radiologic measures.
plasma t., treatment with plasma.
play t., a type of t. used with children in which they can express or reveal their problems and fantasies by playing with dolls or other toys, drawing, etc.
proliferation t., rehabilitation of an incompetent structure (ligament or tendon) by the induced proliferation of new cells; accomplished by injecting an irritating substance into the loose ligament or tendon, the resulting scar formation and contracture serving to tighten up the ligament or tendon as scar tissue proliferates.
protein shock t., foreign protein t.; the injection of a foreign protein to induce fever as a means of treating certain diseases.
psychedelic t., psychiatric t. utilizing psychedelic drugs.
psychoanalytic t., psychoanalysis (1).
pulse t., a short, intensive course of pharmacotherapy, usually given at intervals such as weekly or monthly; often used in chemotherapy of malignancy.
quadrangular t., marriage t. involving the husband and wife and their respective therapists.
radiation t., radiotherapy.
radium beam t., teleradium t.
rational t., therapeutic procedures introduced by Albert Ellis and based on the premise that lack of information or illogical thought patterns are basic causes of a patient's difficulties; it is assumed that the patient can be assisted in overcoming his problems by a direct, prescriptive, advice-giving approach by the therapist.
reflex t., reflexotherapy; treatment of some morbid condition by exciting a reflex action, as in the household treatment of nosebleed by a piece of ice applied to the cervical spine.
replacement t., t. designed to compensate for a lack or deficiency arising from inadequate nutrition, from certain dysfunctions (*e.g.,* glandular hyposecretion), or from losses (*e.g.,* hemorrhage); replacement may be physiological or may entail administration of a substitute (*e.g.,* a synthetic estrogen in place of estradiol).
root canal t., dental t. for damaged pulp by sterilization and filling of the root canal.
sclerosing t., sclerotherapy.
serum t., serotherapy.
shock t., see shock *treatment.*
social t., a psychiatric rehabilitative t. to improve a patient's social functioning.
social network t., a type of t. involving the assembling of all persons emotionally or functionally important to the patient.
substitution t., replacement t., particularly when replacement is not physiological but entails administration of a substitute.
substitutive t., allopathy.
teleradium t., radium beam t.; therapeutic use of radium rays, the source of which is a large quantity of radium situated at a distance from the patient.
thyroid t., the treatment of hypothyroidism.
total push t., the application of all available t.'s to the treatment of a psychiatric patient in a hospital setting.
ultrasonic t., t. for musculoskeletal disease using ultrasonic waves to produce heat.
x-ray t., t. administered by using x-rays.

therencephalous (thĕr-en-sef′ă-lŭs, -ther-) [G. *thēr,* wild beast, + *enkephalos,* brain]. Denoting a skull in which the angle at the hormion, formed by lines converging from the inion and nasion, measures from 116° to 129°.

theriaca (thē-rī′ă-kă) [L. antidote to snake bite, fr. G. *thēriakos,* pertaining to wild beasts]. A mixture containing a great number of ingredients, used in the Middle Ages and believed to possess antidotal and curative powers to an almost miraculous degree.

theriatrics (thĕr-ē-at′riks) [G. *thērion,* beast, + *iatrikē,* medical treatment]. The medical treatment of animals in a zoo or menagerie.

therio- [G. *thēr, thērion,* beast]. Combining form denoting animals.

theriogenologic, theriogenological (thē′rē-ō-jen-ō-loj′ik, -loj′i-kăl). Pertaining to theriogenology.

theriogenology (thĕr′ē-ō-jen-ol′ōjē) [therio- + G. *genos* birth, + *logos,* study]. The study of reproduction in animals, especially domestic animals; includes the study of obstetrics and genital diseases in male and female animals, as well as the physiology of animal reproduction.

theriomorphism (thēr′ē-ō-mōr′fizm) [therio- + *morphē*, form]. Ascription of animal characteristics to human beings. *Cf.* anthropomorphism.

therm [G. *thermē*, heat]. A unit of heat used indiscriminately for: 1) a small calorie, 2) a large calorie, 3) 1000 large calories, 4) 100,000 British thermal units.

therm-. See thermo-.

thermacogenesis (ther′mă-kō-jen′ĕ-sis) [G. *thermē*, heat, + *pharmakon*, drug, + *genesis*, production]. The elevation of body temperature by drug action.

thermal (ther′măl). Pertaining to heat.

thermalgesia (ther-mal-jē′zē-ă) [therm- + G. *algēsis*, sense of pain]. Thermoalgesia; high sensibility to heat; pain caused by a slight degree of heat.

thermalgia (ther-mal′jē-ă) [therm- + G. *algos*, pain]. Burning pain. See also causalgia.

thermanalgesia (therm′an-al-jē′zē-ă) [therm- + analgesia]. Thermoanesthesia.

thermanesthesia (therm′an-es-thē′zē-ă). Thermoanesthesia.

thermatology (ther-mă-tol′ō-jē) [therm- + G. *logos*, study]. The branch of therapeutics concerned with the application of heat. See also thermotherapy.

thermelometer (ther-mĕ-lom′ĕ-ter) [therm- + electric + G. *metron*, measure]. An electric thermometer, especially used for recording slight variations of temperature.

thermesthesia (therm-es-thē′zē-ă). Thermoesthesia.

thermesthesiometer (therm′es-thē-zē-om′ĕ-ter). Thermoesthesiometer.

thermistor (ther′mis-ter, -tōr) [G. *thermē*, heat]. A device for determining temperature; also may be used to monitor control of temperature.

thermo-, therm- [G. *therme*, heat; *thermos*, warm or hot]. Combining forms denoting heat.

thermoalgesia (ther′mō-al-jē′zē-ă). Thermalgesia.

thermoanalgesia (ther′mō-an′al-jē′zē-ă). Thermoanesthesia.

thermoanesthesia (ther′mō-an-es-thē′zē-ă) [thermo- + G. *an-* priv. + *aisthēsis*, sensation]. Ardanesthesia; thermanesthesia; thermoanalgesia; thermanalgesia; loss of the temperature sense or of the ability to distinguish between heat and cold; insensibility to heat or to temperature changes.

thermocauterectomy (ther′mō-kaw-ter-ek′tō-mē) [thermocautery + G. *ektomē*, excision]. Removal of tissue by thermocautery.

thermocautery (ther′mō-kaw′ter-ē) [thermo- + G. *kau- tērion*, branding iron (cautery)]. The use of an actual cautery, such as an electrocautery.

thermochemistry (ther-mō-kem′is-trē). The interrelation of chemical action and heat.

thermochroic (ther-mō-krō′ik). **1.** Relating to thermochrose. **2.** Exerting a selective action on heat rays.

thermochroism (ther-mok′rō-izm). Thermochrosis.

thermochrose (ther′mō-krōz) [thermo- + G. *chrōsis*, coloring]. Thermocrosy; the property possessed by heat rays of reflection, refraction, and absorption, similar to that of light rays.

thermochrosis (ther-mō-krō′sis) [thermo- + G. *chrōsis*, coloring]. Thermochroism; the selective action of certain substances on radiant heat, absorbing some of the rays, reflecting or transmitting others.

thermochrosy (ther-mok′rō-sē). Thermochrose.

thermocoagulation (ther′mō-kō-ag-yū-lā′shŭn). The process of converting tissue into a gel by heat.

thermocouple (ther-mō-kŭp′l). Thermojunction; a device for measuring slight changes in temperature, consisting of two wires of different metals, one wire being kept at a certain low temperature, the other in the tissue or other material whose temperature is to be measured; a thermoelectric current is set up which is measured by a potentiometer.

thermocurrent (ther-mō-ker′ent). A current of thermoelectricity.

thermodiffusion (ther′mō-di-fyū′zhŭn). Diffusion of fluids, either gaseous or liquid, as influenced by the temperature of the fluid.

thermodilution (ther′mō-di-lū′shŭn). Reduction in temperature in a liquid that occurs when it is introduced into a colder liquid; the volume of the latter liquid can be calculated from the amount of rise in its temperature.

thermoduric (ther-mō-dū′rik) [thermo- + L. *durus*, hard, enduring]. Resistant to the effects of exposure to high temperature; used especially with reference to microorganisms.

thermodynamics (ther′mō-dī-nam′iks) [thermo- + G. *dynamis*, force]. **1.** The branch of physicochemical science concerned with heat and energy and their conversions one into the other involving mechanical work. **2.** The study of the flow of heat.

thermoelectric (ther′mō-ē-lek′trik). Relating to thermoelectricity.

thermoelectricity (ther′mō-ē-lek-tris′i-tē). An electrical current generated in a thermopile.

thermoesthesia (ther′mō-es-thē′zē-ă) [thermo- + G. *aisthēsis*, sensation]. Thermesthesia; thermal or thermic sense; temperature sense; the ability to distinguish differences of temperature.

thermoesthesiometer (ther′mō-es-thē′zē-om′ĕ-ter) [thermo- + G. *aisthēsis*, sensation, + *metron*, measure]. Thermesthesiometer; an instrument for testing the temperature sense, consisting of a metal disk with thermometer attached, by which the exact temperature of the disk at the time of application may be known.

thermoexcitory (ther′mō-ek-sī′tō-rē). Stimulating the production of heat.

thermogenesis (ther′mō-jen′ĕ-sis) [thermo- + G. *genesis*, production]. The production of heat; specifically the physiologic process of heat production in the body.

thermogenetic, thermogenic (ther′mō-je-net′ik, -jen′ik). **1.** Thermogenous; relating to thermogenesis. **2.** Calorigenic (2).

thermogenics (ther-mō-jen′iks). The science of heat production.

thermogenous (ther-moj′ĕ-nŭs). Thermogenetic (1).

thermogram (ther′mō-gram) [thermo- + G. *gramma*, a writing]. **1.** A regional temperature map of a body part or organ obtained by infrared sensing devices; it measures radiant heat, and thus the blood flow, if the environment is constant. **2.** The record made by a thermograph.

thermograph (ther′mō-graf) [thermo- + G. *graphō*, to write]. The instrument or device used in producing a thermogram.

thermography (ther-mog′ră-fē). A process for measuring the regional temperature of a body part or organ.

infrared t., measurement of the regional skin temperature by collection of radiated heat with an infrared sensing device.

liquid crystal t., measurement of the regional skin temperature with a flexible plate containing liquid crystals that appear to change color with changes in temperature.

thermohyperalgesia (ther′mō-hī′per-al-jē′zē-ă) [thermo- + G. *hyper*, over, *algēsis*, sense of pain]. Excessive thermalgesia.

thermohyperesthesia (ther′mō-hī′per-es-thē′zē-ă) [thermo- + G. *hyper*, over, + *aisthēsis*, sensation]. Very acute thermoesthesia or temperature sense.

thermohypesthesia (ther-mō-hip′es-thē′zē-ă, -hī′pes-thē′zē-ă) [thermo- + G. *hypo*, under, + *aisthēsis*, sensation]. Thermohypoesthesia; diminished heat perception.

thermohypoesthesia (ther-mō-hī′pō-es-thē′zē-ă). Thermohypesthesia.

thermoinhibitory (ther′mō-in-hib′i-tōr-ē). Inhibiting or arresting thermogenesis.

thermointegrator (ther-mō-in′tĕ-grā-ter, -tōr). Any device for assessing the effective warmth or coldness of an environment as it might be experienced by a living organism, taking into account radiation and convection as well as conduction. Conceived of as a thermal model of an organism, the device usually consists of a standard object (*e.g.*, sphere, cylinder), the surface temperature of which is measured while it is being heated internally at a standard rate.

thermojunction (ther-mō-jŭngk′shŭn). Thermocouple.

thermokeratoplasty (ther-mō-ker′ă-tō-plas-tē) [thermo- + G. *keras*, horn, + *plassō*, to form]. A treatment of keratoconus, based on the hydrothermal shrinkage of collagen fibers; corneal flattening occurs after an instrument at 130°C. is applied to the cornea.

thermolabile (ther-mō-lā′bīl, -bil) [thermo- + L. *labilis*, perishable]. Subject to alteration or destruction by heat.

thermolamp (ther′mō-lamp). Heat lamp.

thermology (ther-mol′ō-jē) [thermo- + G. *logos*, study]. Thermotics; the science of heat.

thermolysis (ther-mol′i-sis) [thermo- + G. *lysis*, dissolution]. **1.** Loss of body heat by evaporation, radiation, etc. **2.** Chemical decomposition by heat.

thermolytic (ther-mō-lit′ik). **1.** Relating to thermolysis. **2.** An agent promoting heat dissipation.

thermomassage (ther′mō-mă-sahzh′). Combination of heat and massage in physical therapy.

thermometer (ther-mom′ĕ-ter) [thermo- + G. *metron*, measure]. An instrument for indicating the temperature of any substance; usually a sealed vacuum tube containing mercury, which expands with heat and contracts with cold, its level accordingly rising or falling in the tube, with the exact degree of variation of level being indicated by a scale. See also entries under scale.

air t., see gas t.

clinical t., a small, self-registering t., consisting of a simple scaled glass tube containing mercury, used for taking the temperature of the body.

differential t., thermoscope.

gas t., a t. filled with dry air or a gas, the expansion or increased pressure of which indicates the degree of heat; used to measure high temperatures.

resistance t., resistance pyrometer; a device measuring temperature by the change of the electrical resistance of a metal wire.

self-registering t., a t. in which the maximum or minimum temperature, during the period of observation, is registered by means of a special appliance; in the clinical t. only the highest temperature is registered, usually by a steel bar above the column of mercury or by a segment of the mercury separated from the main column by a bubble of air; after the maximum temperature is registered, the bar or segment of mercury remains in place as the column of mercury contracts.

spirit t., a t. filled with alcohol, used to measure extreme degrees of cold.

surface t., a t. in the form of a disk or strip which indicates the temperature of the portion of the skin to which it is applied.

wet and dry bulb t., psychrometer.

thermometric (ther-mō-met′rik). Relating to thermometry or to a thermometer reading.

thermometry (ther-mom′ĕ-trē) [thermo- + G. *metron*, measure]. The measurement of temperature.

thermoneurosis (ther′mō-nū-rō′sis). Elevation of the temperature of the body due to an emotional influence.

thermonuclear (ther-mō-nū′klē-er). Pertaining to nuclear reactions brought about by nuclear fission; *e.g.*, the fusion of hydrogen to helium at temperatures of over 100,000,000°C. (the reaction in the "hydrogen bomb").

thermopenetration (ther′mō-pen-ĕ-trā′shŭn). Medical *diathermy*.

thermophile, thermophil (ther′mō-fīl, -fil) [thermo- + G. *phileō*, to love]. An organism that thrives at a temperature of 50°C or higher.

thermophilic (ther-mō-fil′ik). Pertaining to a thermophile.

thermophobia (ther-mō-fō′bē-ă) [thermo- + G. *phobos*, fear]. Morbid fear of heat.

thermophore (ther′mō-fōr) [thermo- + G. *phoros*, bearing]. **1.** An arrangement for applying heat to a part; consists of a water heater, a tube conveying hot water to a coil, and another tube conducting the water back to the heater. **2.** A flat bag containing certain salts that produce heat when moistened; used as a substitute for the hot-water bag.

thermophylic (ther-mō-fī′lik) [thermo- + G. *phylaxis*, protection]. Resistant to heat, denoting certain microorganisms.

thermopile (ther′mō-pīl) [thermo- + pile]. Thermoelectric pile; a thermoelectric battery, consisting usually of a series of bars of antimony and bismuth joined together, that generates a thermoelectric current when the junctions are heated; used as a thermoscope.

thermoplacentography (ther′mō-plă-sen-tog′ră-fē) [thermo- + L. *placenta*, placenta, + G. *graphō*, to write]. Determination of placental position by detection of infrared rays from the large amounts of blood flowing through the placenta.

Thermoplasma (ther′mō-plaz′mă) [thermo- + G. *plasma*, something formed]. A genus of bacteria (order Mycoplasmatales) which possess the same characteristics as the organisms in the genus *Mycoplasma* except that the thermoplasmas do not require sterol for growth, have an optimal temperature of 55 to 59°C, have an optimal pH of 1.0 to 2.0, and reproduce by budding. The type species is *T. acidophilum*.

T. acidoph′ilum, a species found in a coal refuse pile which had undergone self-heating; it is also found in acid hot springs; it is the type species of the genus *T.*

thermoplasma, pl. **thermoplasmata** (ther′mō-plaz′mă, -plaz′mah-tă). A vernacular term used to refer to any member of the genus *Thermoplasma*.

thermoplastic (ther-mō-plas′tik). A classification for materials that can be made soft by the application of heat and harden upon cooling.

thermoplegia (ther-mō-plē′jē-ă) [thermo- + G. *plēgē*, stroke]. Sunstroke.

thermoreceptor (ther′mō-rē-sep′ter, -tōr). A receptor that is sensitive to heat.

thermoregulation (ther′mō-reg-yū-lā′shŭn). Temperature control, as by a thermostat.

thermoregulator (ther-mō-reg′yū-lā-ter, -tōr). Thermostat.

thermoscope (ther′mō-skōp) [thermo- + G. *skopeō*, to view]. Differential thermometer; an instrument for indicating slight differences of temperature, without registering or recording them.

thermoset (ther′mō-set). A classification for materials that become hardened or cured by the application of heat.

thermostabile, thermostable (ther-mō-stā′bil, -stā′bl) [thermo- + L. *stabilis*, stable]. Not subject to alteration or destruction by heat.

thermostat (ther′mō-stat) [thermo- + G. *statos*, standing]. Thermoregulator; an apparatus for the automatic regulation of heat, as in an incubator.

thermosteresis (ther'mō-stĕ-rē'sis) [thermo- + G. *sterēsis,* deprivation, loss]. The abstraction or deprivation of heat.

thermostromuhr (ther-mō-strom'ūr). A stromuhr that consists of a heating element between two thermocouples, which are applied to the outside of a vessel; blood flow is calculated from the difference in temperatures recorded by the proximal and distal thermocouples.

thermosystaltic (ther'mō-sis-tal'tik) [thermo- + G. *systaltikos,* contractile]. Relating to thermosystaltism.

thermosystaltism (ther-mō-sis'tal-tizm) [see thermosystaltic]. Contraction, as of the muscles, under the influence of heat.

thermotactic, thermotaxic (ther-mō-tak'tik, tak'sik). Relating to thermotaxis.

thermotaxis (ther-mō-tak'sis) [thermo- + G. *taxis,* orderly arrangement]. **1.** Reaction of living protoplasm to the stimulus of heat. *Cf.* thermotropism. **2.** Regulation of the temperature of the body.
negative t., repulsion of a plant or animal from heat.
positive t., attraction of a plant or animal to heat.

thermotherapy (ther'mō-thār'ă-pē) [thermo- + G. *therapeia,* treatment]. Treatment of disease by therapeutic application of heat.

thermotic (ther-mot'ik). Relating to thermotics.

thermotics (ther-mot'iks) [G. *thermotēs,* heat]. Thermology.

thermotonometer (ther'mō-tō-nom'ĕ-ter) [thermo- + G. *tonos,* tone, tension, + *metron,* measure]. An instrument for measuring the degree of thermosystaltism, or muscular contraction under the influence of heat.

thermotropism (ther-mot'rō-pizm) [thermo- + G. *tropē,* a turning]. The motion by a part of an organism (*e.g.,* leaves or stems) toward or away from a source of heat. *Cf.* thermotaxis.

theroid (thē'royd) [G. *thēr,* a wild beast, + *eidos,* resemblance]. Resembling an animal in instincts or propensities.

therology (thē-rol'ō-jē) [G. *thēr,* a wild beast, + *logos,* study]. The study of mammals.

thesaurismosis (thē-saw-riz-mō'sis) [G. *thēsauros,* store, storehouse, + G. *-osis,* condition]. Rarely used term for a metabolic disorder in which a substance accumulates or is stored in certain cells, usually in large amounts.

thesaurismotic (thē'saw-riz-mot'ik). Pertaining to thesaurismosis.

thesaurosis (thē-saw-rō'sis) [G. *thēsauros,* store, storehouse]. Abnormal or excessive storage in the body of normal or foreign substances.

thesis, pl. **theses** (thē'sis, -sēz) [G. a placing, a position, thesis]. **1.** An essay on a medical topic prepared by the graduating student. **2.** A proposition submitted by the candidate for a doctoral degree in some universities, which must be sustained by argument against any objections offered. **3.** Any theory or hypothesis advanced as a basis for discussion.

thetins (thē'tinz). Methyl sulfonium compounds, abundant in marine algae, in which the *S*-methyl group is "active," and that therefore act as methyl donors in some plants; *e.g.,* dimethylpropriothetin, $(CH_3)_2S^+–CH_2–CH_2–COO^-$.

thia-. Prefix indicating the replacement of carbon by sulfur in a ring or chain. *Cf.* thio-.

thiabendazole (thī-ă-ben'dă-zōl). 2-(4-Thiazolyl)benzimidazole; a broad spectrum anthelmintic especially useful against *Strongyloides stercoralis* and, with corticosteroids, against *Trichinella* infection (trichina worm).

thiabutazide (thī-ă-byū'tă-zīd). Buthiazide.

thiacetazone (thī-ă-set'ă-zōn, -ă-se'tă-zōn). Amithiozone.

thialbarbital (thī-al-bar'bi-tawl). 5-Allyl-5-(2-cyclohexen-1-yl)-2-thiobarbituric acid; an ultra-short acting thiobarbiturate for induction of general anesthesia by intravenous injection; used as the sodium salt.

thiambutosine (thī-am-byū'tō-sēn). 4-Butoxy-4'-(dimethylamino)thiocarbanilide; an antileprotic agent.

thiamin (thī'ă-min). Thiamine; vitamin B_1; aneurine; antineuritic vitamin or factor; antiberiberi vitamin or factor; a heat-labile vitamin contained in milk, yeast, synthesized; in the germ and husk of grains, also artifically synthesized; essential for growth.

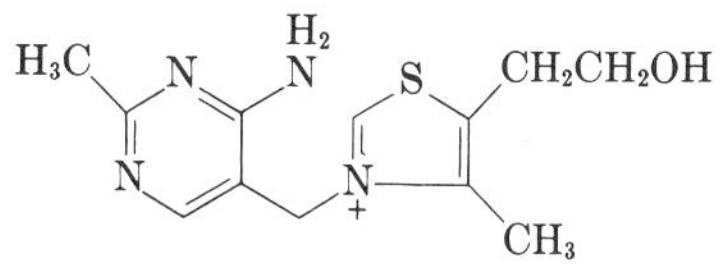

Thiamin

t. hydrochloride, aneurine hydrochloride; a coenzyme used in the prevention of beriberi and other conditions associated with a deficiency of t. in the diet.
t. mononitrate, same action as t. hydrochloride.
t. pyridinylase [EC 2.5.1.2], thiaminase I; pyrimidine transferase; an enzyme catalyzing transfer of a pyridine or other bases into the position of the pyrimidine in t.
t. pyrophosphate (TPP), diphosphothiamin; cocarboxylase; the diphosphoric ester of t., a coenzyme of several (de)carboxylases.

thiaminase (thī-am'i-nās). **1.** An enzyme present in raw fish that destroys thiamin and may produce thiamin deficiency in animals on a diet largely composed of raw fish. **2** [EC 3.5.99.2]. Thiaminase II; a hydrolase cleaving thiamin into a pyrimidine moiety and a thiazole moiety; the pyrimidine moiety may appear in the urine as pyramin.
t. I, *thiamin* pyridinylase.
t. II, thiaminase (2).

thiamine (thī'ă-min, -mēn). Thiamin.

thiamphenicol (thī-am-fen'i-kol). Thiophenicol; dextrosulphenidol; D-(+)- *threo-* 2,2-dichloro-*N-* [β-hydroxy-α- (hydroxymethyl)-*p*-(methylsulfonyl)phenethyl]acetamide; an antibiotic with uses and toxicity similar to those of chloramphenicol.

thiamylal sodium (thī-am'i-lawl). Sodium 5-allyl-5-(1-methylbutyl)-2-thiobarbiturate; a short-acting barbiturate, prepared as a mixture with sodium bicarbonate, used intravenously to produce anesthesia of short duration.

thiaphorases (thī-ă-fōr'ās-ez). CoA transferases. See under coenzyme A.

Thiara (thī-ah'ră). A widespread genus of operculate snails (family Thiaridae, subclass Prosobranchiata) found in fresh and brackish waters, chiefly in tropical and subtropical Africa and Asia. *T. tuberculata* is one of the initial intermediate hosts of the human lung fluke, *Paragonimus westermani,* and of several fish-borne heterophyid flukes of man and fish-eating mammals.

thiazides (thī'ă-zīdz). Abbreviated form of benzothiadiazides.

thiazin (thī'ă-zin). Iminothiodiphenylimine; $C_{12}H_{10}SN_2$; parent substance of a family of biological blue dyes; *e.g.,* methylene blue, thionin, toluidine blue.

thiazolsulfone (thī-ă-zol-sŭl'fōn). 2-Amino-5-sulfanylthiazole; it has the same uses as glucosulfone sodium, but is less toxic and also less effective in the treatment of leprosy.

thickness (thik'nes). **1.** The measure of the depth of something, as opposed to its length or width. **2.** A layer or stratum.
Breslow's t., maximal t. of a primary cutaneous melanoma measured in tissue sections from the top of the epidermal granular layer, or from the ulcer base (if the tumor is ulcerated), to the bottom of the tumor; metastatic rates correlate closely with tumor t.

thiemia (thī-ē'mē-ă) [G. *theion,* sulfur, + *haima,* blood]. The presence of sulfur in the circulating blood.

thienyl (thī'en-il). The radical of thiophene, SC_4H_3–. *Cf.* thenyl.

thienylalanine (thī'ĕ-nil-al'ă-nēn). 3-(3-Thienyl)alanine; a compound structurally similar to phenylalanine that inhibits the growth of *Escherichia coli,* presumably by competitive inhibition of enzymes for which phenylalanine is the substrate.

Thier, Carl Jorg. See Weyers-T. *syndrome.*

Thiers, Joseph, French physician, *1885. See Achard-T. *syndrome.*

Thiersch, Karl, German surgeon, 1822–1895. See T. *graft;* T.'s *canaliculi, method;* Ollier-T. *graft.*

thiethylperazine maleate (thī-eth'il-per'ă-zēn). 2-Ethyl-mercapto-10-3-(1-methyl-4-piperazinyl)propyl phenothiazine dimaleate; an antiemetic agent used to control nausea and vomiting associated with vertigo, the administration of general anesthetics, and with several other clinical conditions; it also has weak hypotensive, spasmolytic, antihistaminic, and hypothermic actions.

thigh (thī). Femur (1); the part of the inferior limb, between the hip and the knee.

driver's t., neuralgia or neuritis of the sciatic nerve, due to pressure on the nerve produced by the long-continued use of the accelerator pedal in driving a vehicle.

Heilbronner's t., in cases of organic paralysis, flattening and broadening of the t., when the patient lies supine on a hard mattress; absent in hysterical paralysis.

thigmesthesia (thig-mes-thē'zē-ă) [G. *thigma,* touch, + *aisthēsis,* sensation]. Sensibility to touch.

thigmotaxis (thig-mō-tak'sis) [G. *thigma,* touch, + *taxis,* orderly arrangement]. A form of barotaxis; denoting the reaction of plant or animal protoplasm to contact with a solid body. *Cf.* thigmotropism.

thigmotropism (thig-mot'rō-pizm) [G. *thigma,* touch, + *tropē,* a turning]. A movement toward or away from a touch stimulus on the part of a portion of an organism, such as leaves or tendrils. *Cf.* thigmotaxis.

thimerosal (thī-mer'ō-săl). Thiomersalate; thiomersal; [(*o*-carboxyphenyl)thio]ethylmercury sodium salt; an antiseptic.

think'ing. The act of reasoning.

abstract t., t. in terms of concepts and general principles (*e.g.,* a table and a chair as furniture), as contrasted with concrete t.

archaic-paralogical t., prelogical t.

concrete t., t. of objects as specific items rather than as an abstract representation of a more general concept, as contrasted with abstract t.

creative t., productive t., with novel rather than routine results.

magical t., the irrational equating of t. with doing.

prelogical t., archaic-paralogical t.; prelogical mind; a concrete type of t., characteristic of children and primitives, to which schizophrenic persons are sometimes said to regress.

thinking through. The psychological process of understanding, with insight, one's own behavior.

thinning (thin'ing). Causing a decrease in viscosity by chemical means, as by the addition of a solvent, or by mechanical means, as in shear t.

shear t., decreasing the viscosity of a polymer or macromolecule or gel by increasing the rate of shear; not ordinarily a function of time. See also thixotropy.

thio- [G. *theion,* sugar]. Prefix denoting the replacement of oxygen by sulfur in a compound. *Cf.* thia-.

thioacid (thī-ō-as'id). Sulfacid; sulfoacid (1); an organic acid in which one or more of the oxygen atoms have been replaced by sulfur atoms; *e.g.,* thiosulfuric acid.

thioalcohol (thī-ō-al'kō-hol). Mercaptan (1).

thioamide (thī-ō-am'īd). An amide in which S replaces O.

thioate (thī'ō-āt). A salt or ester of a -thioic acid.

thiobarbiturates (thī'ō-bar-bich'yūr-āts). Hypnotics of the barbiturate group, *e.g.,* thiopental, in which the oxygen atom at carbon-2 is replaced by sulfur.

thiocarbamide (thī-ō-kar'bă-mīd). Thiourea.

thiocarlide (thī-ō-kar'līd). 4,4'-Di(isoamyloxy)thiocarbanilide; a synthetic compound whose molecule contains the three antituberculous groups *p*-aminosalicylic acid, *p*-aminobenzaldehyde thiosemicarbazone, and the thiocarbamide group; an antitubercular agent.

thiochrome (thī'ō-krōm). A fluorescent compound, $C_{12}H_{14}N_4OS$, produced by the oxidation of thiamin; used in methods for detection and determination of thiamin.

thioctic acid (thī-ok'tik). Lipoic acid.

thiocyanate (thī-ō-sī'ă-nāt). Rhodanate; sulfocyanate; a salt of thiocyanic acid.

thiocyanic acid (thī-ō-sī-an'ik). Rhodanic or sulfocyanic acid; HS–CN; hydrogen thiocyanate.

thiodiphenylamine (thī'ō-dī-fen'il-am'ēn). Phenothiazine.

thioethanolamine acetyltransferase (thī'ō-eth-ă-nol'ă-mēn) [EC 2.3.1.11]. Thiotransacetylase B; an enzyme transferring acetyl from acetyl-CoA to the sulfur atom of thioethanolamine.

thioether (thī-ō-ē'ther). An organic sulfide; an ether in which the oxygen is replaced by sulfur.

thioflavine S (thī-ō-flā'vin) [C.I. 49010]. A methylated and sulfonated derivative of primulin; a yellowish dye used in fluorescence microscopy as a vital stain.

thioflavin T (thī-ō-flā'vin) [C.I. 49005]. A yellow thiazole dye, $C_{17}H_{19}N_2SCl$, used in histopathology as a fluorochrome for hyaline and amyloid.

thiofuran (thī'ō-fūr'an). Thiophene.

thioglucosidase (thī-ō-glū'kō-si-dās) [EC 3.2.3.1]. Myrosinase; sinigrinase; sinigrase; an enzyme in mustard seed that converts thioglycosides into thiols plus sugars.

thioglycerol (thī-ō-glis'er-ol). Monothioglycerol.

thioglycolate, thioglycollate (thī-ō-glī'kō-lāt). A salt or ester of thioglycolic acid; frequently used in bacterial media to reduce their oxygen content so as to create favorable conditions for the growth of anaerobes; the t. will also inactivate any mercurial that might be carried over with the inoculum.

thioglycolic acid (thī'ō-glī-kol'ik). Mercaptoacetic acid; $HSCH_2COOH$; used as a reagent for the detection of metals such as iron, molybdenum, silver, and tin; the ammonium and sodium salts are used in home permanents, the calcium salt as a depilatory.

thioguanine (thī-ō-gwah'nēn). 2-Aminopurine-6-thiol; an antineoplastic agent used for leukemias and nephrosis.

-thioic acid. Suffix denoting the radical, –C(S)OH or –C(O)SH, the sulfur analogue of a carboxylic acid, *i.e.,* a thiocarboxylic acid.

thiokinase (thī-ō-kī'nās). Group term for enzymes that form acyl-CoA compounds from the corresponding fatty acids and CoA; the bond is through the sulfur atom of the CoA.

thiol (thī'ol). **1.** The monovalent radical –SH when attached to carbon; a hydrosulfide. **2.** A mixture of sulfurated and sulfonated petroleum oils purified with ammonia; used in the treatment of skin diseases.

thiolase (thī'ō-lās). Acetyl-CoA acetyltransferase.

thiole (thī'ōl). Thiophene.

thiolhistidylbetaine (thī'ol-his'ti-dil-bē'tă-ēn). Ergothioneine.

thioltransacetylase A (thī'ol-trans-ă-set'i-lās). Dihydrolipoamide acetyltransferase.

thiolysis (thī-ol'i-sis). The cleavage of a chemical bond with the addition of coenzyme A to one part; analogous to hydrolysis and phosphorolysis.

thiomersal (thī-ō-mer′săl). Thimerosal.

thiomersalate (thī-ō-mer′să-lāt). Thimerosal.

thiomethyladenosine (thī′ō-meth′il-ă-den′ō-sēn). Methylthioadenosine.

β-thionase (thī′ō-nās). Cystathionine β-synthase.

-thione. Suffix denoting the radical >C=S, the sulfur analogue of a ketone, *i.e.,* a thiocarbonyl group.

thioneine (thī′ō-ne′in). Ergothioneine.

thionic (thī-on′ik). Relating to sulfur.

thionine (thī′ō-nin) [C.I. 52000]. Lauth's violet; amidophenthiazine; a dark green powder, giving a purple solution in water; useful as a basic stain in histology for chromatin and mucin because of its metachromatic properties.

thiono-. Prefix sometimes used for thioxo-.

thiopanic acid (thī-ō-pan′ik). Pantoyltaurine.

thiopental sodium (thī-ō-pen′tawl). Sodium 5-ethyl-5-(1-methylbutyl)-2-thiobarbiturate; an ultra-short-acting barbiturate administered intravenously or rectally for induction of anesthesia. .

thiophene (thī′ō-fēn). Thiofuran; thiole; the fundamental ring compound:

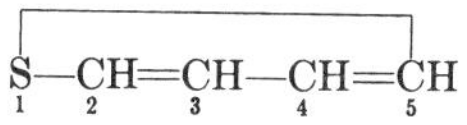

thiophenicol (thī-ō-fen′i-kol). Thiamphenicol.

thiophorases (thī-ō-fōr′ās-ez). CoA transferases. See under coenzyme A.

thiopropazate hydrochloride (thī-ō-prō′pă-zāt). 2-Chloro-10-{3-[4-(2-acetoxyethyl)piperazinyl]propyl}phenothiazine dihydrochloride; a phenothiazine derivative related chemically and pharmacologically to prochlorperazine and perphenazine; an antipsychotic.

thioproperazine (thī′ō-prō-per′ă-zēn). *N,N*-Dimethyl-10-[3-(4-methyl-1-piperazinyl)propyl]phenothiazine-2-sulfonamide; an antiemetic and antianxiety agent.

thioridazine hydrochloride (thī-ō-rid′ă-zēn). 10-[2-(1-Methyl-2-piperidylethyl]-2-(methylthio)phenothiazine monohydrochloride; an antipsychotic with action similar to that of chlorpromazine.

thiosemicarbazide (thī′ō-sem′ē-kar′bă-zīd). One of the group of thiosemicarbazones with a tuberculostatic action; used as a reagent in the detection of metals.

thiosemicarbazone (thī′ō-sem′ē-kar′bă-zōn). **1.** A compound containing the thiosemicarbazide radical, $=N—NH—C(S)—NH_2$. **2.** One of a group of tuberculostatic drugs that includes thiosemicarbazide, benzaldehyde thiosemicarbazone, and 4-aminoacetylbenzaldehyde thiosemicarbazone.

thiosulfate (thī-ō-sŭl′fāt). $S_2O_3{}^{=}$; the anion of thiosulfuric acid.

t. cyanide transsulfurase, t. sulfurtransferase.

t. sulfurtransferase [EC 2.8.1.1], rhodanese; t. thiotransferase; t. cyanide transsulfurase; a transferase that catalyzes the formation of thiocyanate and sulfite from cyanide and t.

t. thiotransferase, t. sulfurtransferase.

thiosulfuric acid (thī′ō-sŭl-fyūr′ik). $H_2S_2O_3$; sulfuric acid in which an atom of oxygen has been replaced by one of sulfur.

thiotepa (thī-ō-tep′ă). Triethylenethiophosphoramide.

thiothixene (thī-ō-thik′sēn). *N,N*- Dimethyl-9-[3-(4-methyl-1-piperazinyl)propylidene]thioxanthene-2-sulfonamide; an antipsychotic.

thiotransacetylase B (thī′ō-trans-ă-set′i-lās). Thioethanolamine acetyltransferase.

2-thiouracil (thī-ō-yūr′ă-sil). 2-Mercapto-4-pyrimidinone; a rare component of transfer RNA's; a thioamide derivative that inhibits the synthesis of thyroid hormones.

4-thiouracil. Uracil with S replacing O in position 4, isomeric with 2-thiouracil; a rare component of transfer RNA's.

thiourea (thī′ō-yū-rē′ă). Thiocarbamide; $SC(NH_2)_2$; an antithyroid compound of the thioamide group, with the same actions and uses as thiouracil. Several derivatives of t. are useful in the treatment of leprosy.

thioxanthene (thī-ō-zan′thēn). A class of tricyclic compounds resembling phenothiazine, but with the central ring nitrogen replaced by a carbon atom; current use emphasizes the antipsychotic and antiemetic properties of this class.

thioxo-. Prefix indicating =S in a thioketone.

thioxolone (thī-ok′sō-lōn). 6-Hydroxy-1,3-benzoxathiol-2-one; an antiseborrheic.

thiphenamil hydrochloride (thī-fen′ă-mil). Diphenylthioacetic acid *S*-(2-diethylaminoethyl) ester hydrochloride; an anticholinergic drug.

thirst [A.S. *thurst*] A desire to drink associated with uncomfortable sensations in the mouth and pharynx.

false t., pseudodipsia; t. that is not satisfied by drinking or taking water; t. associated with a dry mouth but not with a bodily need for water.

insensible t., hypodipsia.

morbid t., dipsesis.

subliminal t., hypodipsia.

true t., t. that can be satisfied by drinking water.

Thiry, Ludwig, Austrian physiologist, 1817–1897. See T.'s *fistula,* T.-Vella *fistula.*

thixolabile (thik-sō-lā′bil, -bīl). Susceptible to thixotropy.

thixotropic (thik-sō-trop′ik). Pertaining to, or characterized by, thixotropy.

thixotropy (thik-sot′rō-pē) [G. *thixis,* a touching, + *tropē,* turning]. Reclotting phenomenon; the property of certain gels of becoming less viscous when shaken or subjected to shearing forces and returning to the original viscosity upon standing (*e.g.,* synovial fluid, ferrous hydroxide gel); a characteristic of a system exhibiting a decrease in viscosity with an increase in the rate of shear, usually a function of time.

Thoma, Richard, German histologist, 1847–1923. See T.'s *ampulla,* counting *chamber, fixative, laws.*

Thomas, Hugh Owen, British surgeon, 1834–1891. See T. *splint.*

Thompson, Sir Henry, British surgeon, 1820–1904. See T.'s *test.*

Thomsen, Asmus J., Danish physician, 1815–1896. See T.'s *disease.*

Thomson, F.H., British physician, 1867–1938. See T.'s *sign.*

Thomson, Matthew Sidney, British dermatologist, *1894. See Rothmund-T. *syndrome.*

thonzonium bromide (thon-zō′nē-ŭm). Hexadecyl[2-[(*p*-methoxybenzyl)-2-pyrimidinylamino]ethyl]dimethylammonium bromide; a surface-active agent used in ear drops and aerosols.

thonzylamine hydrochloride (thon-zil′ă-mēn). 2-[(2-Dimethylaminoethyl)(*p*-methoxybenzyl)amino]pyrimidine hydrochloride; an antihistamine.

thorac-. See thoraco-.

thoracal (thor′ă-kăl). Thoracic.

thoracalgia (thōr-ă-kal′jē-ă) [thoraco- + G. *algos,* pain]. Thoracodynia; pain in the chest.

thoracectomy (thōr-ă-sek′tō-mē) [thoraco- + G. *ektomē,* excision]. Resection of a portion of a rib.

thoracentesis (thōr′ă-sen-tē′sis) [thoraco- + G. *kentēsis,* puncture].

Pleuracentesis; pleurocentesis; thoracocentesis; paracentesis of the pleural cavity.

thoracic (thō-ras'ik). Thoracal; relating to the thorax.

thoracico-. See thoraco-.

thoracicoabdominal (thō-ras'i-kō-ab-dom'i-năl). Thoracoabdominal; relating to the thorax and the abdomen.

thoracicoacromial (thō-ras'i-kō-ă-krō'mē-ăl). Acromiothoracic.

thoracicohumeral (thō-ras'i-kō-hyū'mer-ăl). Relating to the thorax and the humerus.

thoraco-, thorac-, thoracico- [G. *thōrax,* chest]. Combining forms denoting the chest (thorax).

thoracoabdominal (thōr'ă-kō-ab-dom'i-năl). Thoracicoabdominal.

thoracoacromial (thōr'ă-kō-ă-krō'mē-ăl). Acromiothoracic.

thoracoceloschisis (thōr'ă-kō-sē-los'ki-sis) [thoraco- + G. *koilia,* belly, + *schisis,* fissure]. Thoracogastroschisis; a congenital fissure of the trunk embracing both the thoracic and abdominal cavities.

thoracocentesis (thōr'ă-kō-sen-tē'sis). Thoracentesis.

thoracocyllosis (thōr'ă-kō-si-lō'sis) [thoraco- + G. *kyllōsis,* a crippling]. A deformity of the chest.

thoracocyrtosis (thōr'ă-kō-ser-tō'sis) [thoraco- + G. *kyrtōsis,* a being crooked]. Abnormally wide curvature of the chest wall.

thoracodelphus (thōr'ă-kō-del'fŭs). Thoradelphus.

thoracodynia (thōr'ă-kō-din'ē-ă) [thoraco- + G. *odynē,* pain]. Thoracalgia.

thoracogastroschisis (thōr'ă-kō-gas-tros'ki-sis) [thoraco- + G. *gastēr,* belly, + *schisis,* fissure]. Thoracoceloschisis.

thoracograph (thōr'ă-kō-graf) [thoraco- + G. *graphō,* to record]. An instrument for determining the horizontal contour of the chest.

thoracolaparotomy (thōr'ă-kō-lap-ă-rot'ō-mē) [thoraco- + laparotomy]. Exposure of diaphragmatic region by an incision that opens both thorax and abdomen.

thoracolumbar (thōr'ă-kō-lŭm'bar). **1.** Relating to the thoracic and lumbar portions of the vertebral column. **2.** Relating to the origins of the sympathetic division of the autonomic nervous system. See *systema* nervosum autonomicum.

thoracolysis (thōr-ă-kol'i-sis) [thoraco- + G. *lysis,* dissolution]. Breaking up of pleural adhesions.

thoracomelus (thōr-ă-kom'ĕ-lŭs) [thoraco- + G. *melos,* limb]. Unequal conjoined twins in which the parasite, often only a single arm or leg, is attached to the thorax of the autosite.

thoracometer (thōr-ă-kom'ĕ-ter) [thoraco- + G. *metron,* measure]. An instrument for measuring the circumference of the chest or its variations in respiration.

thoracomyodynia (thōr'ă-kō-mī-ō-din'ē-ă) [thoraco- + G. *mys,* muscle, + *odynē,* pain]. Pain in the muscles of the chest wall.

thoracopagus (thōr-ă-kop'ă-gŭs) [thoraco- + G. *pagos,* something fastened]. Synthorax; conjoined twins with fusion in the thoracic region.

thoracoparacephalus (thōr'ă-kō-par-ă-sef'ă-lŭs) [thoraco- + G. *para,* beside, + *kephalē,* head]. Unequal conjoined twins in which a rudimentary parasitic head is attached to the thorax of the autosite.

thoracopathy (thōr-ă-kop'ă-thē) [thoraco- + G. *pathos,* suffering]. Any disease of the thoracic organs or tissues.

thoracoplasty (thōr'ă-kō-plas-tē) [thoraco- + G. *plastos,* formed]. Plastic surgery of the thorax.
conventional t., resection of ribs to allow inward retraction of the chest wall to reduce size of the pleural space; may be used in the treatment of empyema.

thoracopneumoplasty (thōr'ă-kō-nū'mō-plas-tē) [thoraco- + G. *pneumōn,* lung, + *plastos,* formed]. Plastic surgery of the chest in which the lung is also involved.

thoracoschisis (thōr-ă-kos'ki-sis) [thoraco- + G. *schisis,* fissure]. Congenital fissure of the chest wall.

thoracoscope (thō-rak'ō-skōp) [thoraco- + G. *skopeō,* to view]. An endoscope used for examination of the pleural cavity.

thoracoscopy (thōr-ă-kos'kŏ-pē) [thoraco- + G. *skopeō,* to view]. Examination of the pleural cavity with an endoscope.

thoracostenosis (thōr'ă-kō-stĕ-nō'sis). [thoraco- + G. *stenōsis,* narrowing]. Narrowness of the chest.

thoracostomy (thōr-ă-kos'tō-mē) [thoraco- + G. *stoma,* mouth]. Establishment of an opening into the chest cavity, as for the drainage of an empyema.

thoracotomy (thōr-ă-kot'ō-mē) [thoraco- + G. *tomē,* incision]. Pleurotomy; incision into the chest wall.

thoradelphus (thōr-ă-del'fŭs) [thoraco- + G. *adelphos,* brother]. Thoracodelphus; duplicitas posterior in which, from the navel upward, the conjoined twins are fused into one.

thorax, gen. **thoracis,** pl. **thoraces** (thō'raks, thō'rā-sis, -rā'sēz) [L. fr. G. *thōrax,* breastplate, the chest, fr. *thōrēssō,* to arm] [NA]. Chest; the upper part of the trunk between the neck and the abdomen; it is formed by the 12 thoracic vertebrae, the 12 pairs of ribs, the sternum, and the muscles and fasciae attached to these; below it is separated from the abdomen by the diaphragm; it contains the chief organs of the circulatory and respiratory systems, as distinguished from the abdomen which encloses those of the digestive apparatus.

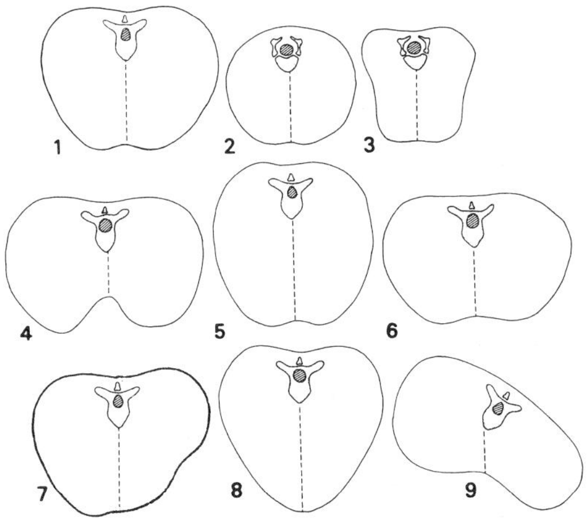

Thorax
Types of abnormal thorax compared with normals in cross section: *1,* normal adult; *2,* normal infant; *3,* rachitic; *4,* funnel chest; *5,* emphysematous; *6,* phthisical; *7,* unilaterally retracted; *8,* pigeon breast; *9,* in scoliosis.

Peyrot's t., an obliquely oval deformity of the chest in cases of a very large pleural effusion.

thorium (thōr'ē-ŭm) [*Thor,* Norse god of thunder]. A radioactive metallic element; symbol Th, atomic no. 90, atomic weight 232.05. Th-232, the only naturally occurring nuclide, with a half-life of 14 $\times 10^9$ years, is used in colloidal form in electron microscopy as a stain for acid mucopolysaccharides.

Thormählen, Johann, 19th century German physician. See T.'s *test.*

Thorn, George W., U.S. physician, *1906. See T. *test;* T.'s *syndrome.*

thorn (thōrn). In anatomy, a thornlike or spinous structure.
dendritic t.'s, dendritic *spines.*
penis t.'s, penis *spines.*

thorn apple. *Datura stramonium.*

Thornwaldt, Gustavus Ludwig. See Tornwaldt.

thoroughbred (ther'ō-bred). A breed of light horses used for racing purposes; often used erroneously for purebred.

thorough-pin (ther'ō-pin). Synovial distention of the sheath of the flexor perforans tendon of the horse, causing a swelling on each side of the hollow of the hock.

thought broadcasting (thot brod'kas'ting). The delusion of experiencing one's thoughts, as they occur, as being broadcast from one's head to the external world where other people can hear them.

thought insertion (thot in-ser'shŭn). The delusion that one's thoughts are not really one's own but are being placed into one's mind by an external force.

thought withdrawal (thot with-draw'ăl). The delusion that one's thoughts have been removed from one's head resulting in a diminished number of thoughts remaining.

Thr Symbol for threonine or its radical forms.

thread (thred). **1.** A fine strand of suture material. **2.** A filamentous structure.
Simonart's t.'s, amniotic *bands.*
terminal t., *filum* terminale.

threadworm (thred'werm). Common name for species of the genus *Strongyloides;* sometimes applied to any of the smaller parasitic nematodes.

threonic acid (thrē-on'ik). The acid derived by oxidation of the CHO group of threose to COOH; a product of the oxidation of ascorbic acid by hypoiodite.

threonine (Thr) (thrē'ō-nēn). $CH_3CH(OH)–CH(NH_2)$ COOH; 2-amino-3-hydroxybutyric acid; one of the naturally occurring amino acids, included in the structure of most proteins, and essential to the diet of man and other mammals.
t. deaminase, t. dehydratase.
t. dehydratase [EC 4.2.1.16], t. deaminase; serine deaminase; an enzyme catalyzing the anaerobic deamination of t. to 2-ketobutyric acid.

threose (thrē'ōs). An aldotetrose; one of the two aldoses (the other is erythrose) containing four carbon atoms. See structure under sugars.

threshold (thresh'ōld) [A.S. *therxold*] **1.** The point where a stimulus begins to produce a sensation, the lower limit of perception of a stimulus. **2.** The minimal stimulus that produces excitation of any structure; more specifically, the minimal stimulus eliciting a motor response. **3.** Limen.
absolute t., stimulus t.; the lowest limit of any perception whatever. *Cf.* differential t.
achromatic t., visual t.
auditory t., the intensity of any barely perceptible sound.
brightness difference t., light difference (2); the smallest difference that can be perceived as a difference in brightness.
t. of consciousness, the lowest point at which a stimulus sensation can be perceived.
convulsant t., the smallest amount of stimulation, electric current, or drug required to induce a convulsion.
differential t., t. differential; the lowest limit at which two stimuli can be differentiated.
displacement t., the least distinguishable break in the contour of a line.
double-point t., the least degree of separation of two points applied to the body surface that permits of their being felt as two.
erythema t., the point where erythema of the skin is produced by irradiation with ultraviolet or other kinds of rays.
fibrillation t., least intensity of an electrical stimulus that will initiate fibrillation.
galvanic t., rheobase.
light differential t., the smallest difference in light intensity that can be appreciated.
minimum light t., visual t.
t. of nose, *limen* nasi.
pain t., the smallest intensity of a stimulus at which the subject perceives pain.
relational t., the smallest degree of difference between two stimuli that permits them to be perceived as different.
renal t., concentration of plasma substance above which the substance appears in the urine.
stimulus t., absolute t.
swallowing t., **(1)** the moment that the act of swallowing begins after the mastication of food; **(2)** the critical moment of reflex action initiated by minimum stimulation, prior to the act of deglutition.
visual t., t. of visual sensation, achromatic or minimum light t.; the minimal light intensity evoking a visual sensation.

thrill. A vibration accompanying a cardiac or vascular murmur that can be felt on palpation. See also fremitus.
diastolic t., a t. felt over the precordium or over a blood vessel during ventricular diastole.
hydatid t., hydatid fremitus; Blatin's syndrome; the peculiar trembling or vibratory sensation felt on palpation of a hydatid cyst.
presystolic t., a t. immediately preceding the ventricular contraction, that is sometimes felt on palpation over the apex of the heart.
systolic t., a t. felt over the precordium or over a blood vessel during ventricular systole.

thrix (thriks) [G.]. Hair.
t. annula'ta, ringed *hair.*

throat (thrōt) [A.S. *throtu*]. **1.** Gullet; the fauces and pharynx. **2.** Jugulum; the anterior aspect of the neck. **3.** Any narrowed entrance into a hollow part.
putrid t., gangrenous *pharyngitis.*
septic sore t., a severe pseudomembranous inflammation of the fauces and tonsils, usually occurring in epidemic form, caused by the hemolytic streptococcus transmitted in an infected milk supply.
sore t., angina (1); cynanche; synanche; a condition characterized by pain or discomfort on swallowing; it may be due to any of a variety of inflammations of the tonsils, pharynx, or larynx.

throb. 1. To pulsate. **2.** A beating or pulsation.

thromb-. See thrombo-.

thrombase (throm'bās). Thrombin.

thrombasthenia (throm-bas-thē'nē-ă) [thromb- + G. *asthenia,* weakness]. Thromboasthenia; an abnormality of platelets characteristic of Glanzmann's t. See also Bernard-Soulier *syndrome.*
Glanzmann's t., Glanzmann's disease; constitutional thrombopathy (2); hereditary hemorrhagic t.; a hemorrhagic diathesis of autosomal recessive inheritance in almost all cases, characterized by normal or prolonged bleeding time, normal coagulation time, defective clot retraction, normal platelet count but morphologic or functional abnormality of platelets; several different kinds of platelet abnormalities have been described.
hereditary hemorrhagic t., Glanzmann's t.

thrombectomy (throm-bek'tō-mē) [thromb- + G. *ektomē,* excision]. The excision of a thrombus.

thrombi (throm'bī). Plural of thrombus.

throm'bin. Thrombosin; thrombase; fibrinogenase. **1** [EC 3.4.21.5]. An enzyme (proteinase), formed in shed blood, that converts fibrinogen into fibrin by hydrolyzing peptides (and amides and esters) of L-arginine; formed from prothrombin by the action of prothrombinase (factor Xa, another proteinase). **2.** A sterile protein substance prepared from prothrombin of bovine origin through interaction with thromboplastin in the presence of calcium; causes clotting of whole blood, plasma, or a fibrinogen solution; used as a topical hemostatic for capillary bleeding with or without fibrin foam in general and plastic surgical procedures.

human t., t. obtained from human plasma by precipitation with suitable salts and organic solvents; same uses as t.

thrombinogen (throm-bin'ō-jen). Prothrombin.

thrombinogenesis (throm'bi-nō-jen'ĕ-sis). Thrombin production.

thrombintimectomy (throm'bin-ti-mek'tō-mē) [thromb- + L. *intima (tunica)*, innermost tunic, + G. *ektomē*, excision]. Old term for thromboendarterectomy.

thrombo-, thromb- [G. *thrombos*, clot (thrombus)]. Combining forms denoting blood clot or relation thereto.

thromboangiitis (throm'bō-an-ji-ī'tis) [thrombo- + G. *angeion*, vessel, + *-itis*, inflammation]. Inflammation of the intima of a blood vessel, with thrombosis.

t. oblit'erans, Buerger's or Winiwarter-Buerger disease; inflammation of the entire wall and connective tissue surrounding medium-sized arteries and veins, especially of the legs of young and middle-aged men; associated with thrombotic occlusion and commonly resulting in gangrene.

thromboarteritis (throm'bō-ar-ter-ī'tis). Arterial inflammation with thrombus formation.

thromboasthenia (throm'bō-as-thē'nē-ă). Thrombasthenia.

thromboblast (throm'bō-blast) [thrombo- + G. *blastos*, germ]. Megakaryocyte.

thromboclasis (throm-bok'lă-sis) [thrombo- + G. *klasis*, a breaking]. Thrombolysis.

thromboclastic (throm-bō-klas'tik). Thrombolytic.

thrombocyst, thrombocystis (throm'bō-sist, -sis'tis) [thrombo- + G. *kystis*, a bladder]. A membranous sac enclosing a thrombus.

thrombocytasthenia (throm'bō-sī-tas-thē'nē-ă) [thrombocyte + G. *astheneia*, weakness]. A term for a group of hemorrhagic disorders in which the platelets may be only slightly reduced in number, or even within the normal range, but are morphologically abnormal, or are lacking in factors that are effective in the coagulation of blood.

thrombocyte (throm'bō-sīt) [thrombo- + G. *kytos*, cell]. Platelet.

thrombocythemia (throm'bō-sī-thē'mē-ă) [thrombocyte + G. *haima*, blood]. Thrombocytosis.

thrombocytin (throm-bō-sī'tin). Serotonin.

thrombocytopathy (throm'bō-sī-top'ă-thē) [thrombocyte + G. *pathos*, suffering]. General term for any disorder of the coagulating mechanism that results from dysfunction of the blood platelets.

thrombocytopenia (throm'bō-sī-tō-pē'nē-ă) [thrombocyte + G. *penia*, poverty]. Thrombopenia; a condition in which there is an abnormally small number of platelets in the circulating blood.

autoimmune t., immune t. in which antibodies produced by the mother against her own platelets cross the placenta to sensitize the fetal platelets.

essential t., a primary form of t., in contrast to secondary forms that are associated with metastatic neoplasms, tuberculosis, and leukemia involving the bone marrow, or with direct suppression of bone marrow by the use of chemical agents, or with other conditions.

immune t., t. associated with antiplatelet antibodies. See autoimmune t.; isoimmune t.

isoimmune t., immune t. resulting from maternal-fetal platelet incompatibility.

thrombocytopoiesis (throm'bō-sī-tō-poy-ē'sis) [thrombocyte + G. *poiēsis*, a making]. The process of formation of thrombocytes or platelets.

thrombocytosis (throm'bō-sī-tō'sis) [thrombocyte + G. *-osis*, condition]. Thrombocythemia; an increase in the number of platelets in the circulating blood.

thromboelastogram (throm'bō-ē-las'tō-gram). Registration of coagulation process by a thromboelastograph.

thromboelastograph (throm'bō-ē-las'tō-graf) [thromb- + G. *elastreō*, to push, + *graphō*, to write]. Apparatus for registering elastic variations of a thrombus during the process of coagulation.

thromboembolectomy (throm'bō-em-bō-lek'tō-mē) [thrombo- + G. *embolos*, embolus, + *ektomē*, excision]. Extraction of an embolic thrombus.

thromboembolism (throm'bō-em'bō-lizm) [thrombo- + G. *embolismos*, embolism]. Embolism from a thrombus.

thromboendarterectomy (throm'bō-end-ar-ter-ek'tō-mē) [thrombo- + endarterectomy]. An operation that involves opening an artery, removing an occluding thrombus along with the intima and atheromatous material, and leaving a clean, fresh plane internal to the adventitia.

thromboendocarditis (throm'bō-en'dō-kar-dī'tis). Nonbacterial thrombotic *endocarditis*.

thrombogen (throm'bō-jen) [thrombo- + G. *-gen*, producing]. Prothrombin.

thrombogene (throm'bō-jēn). *Factor* V.

thrombogenic (throm-bō-jen'ik). **1.** Relating to thrombogen. **2.** Causing thrombosis or coagulation of the blood.

thromboid (throm'boyd) [thrombo- + G. *eidos*, resemblance]. Resembling a thrombus.

thrombokatilysin (throm'bō-kat-i-lī'sin). *Factor* VIII.

thrombokinase (throm-bō-kī'nās). Thromboplastin.

thrombolic (throm-bol'ik). Relating to a thrombolus.

thrombolus (throm'bō-lŭs) [thrombo- + G. *embolos*, embolus]. An embolus composed of agglutinated platelets.

thrombolymphangitis (throm'bō-lim-fan-jī'tis). Inflammation of a lymphatic vessel with the formation of a lymph clot.

thrombolysis (throm-bol'i-sis) [thrombo- + G. *lysis*, a dissolving]. Thromboclasis; fluidifying or dissolving of a thrombus.

thrombolytic (throm-bō-lit'ik). Thromboclastic; breaking up or dissolving a thrombus.

throm'bon. An all-inclusive term for circulating thrombocytes (blood platelets) and the cellular forms from which they arise (thromboblasts or megakaryocytes). It is analogous to erythron and leukon of the red and white blood cells, respectively.

thrombonecrosis (throm'bō-ne-krō'sis). Necrosis of the walls of a blood vessel, with thrombosis in the lumen.

thrombopathy (throm-bop'ă-thē) [thrombo- + G. *pathos*, disease]. A nonspecific term applied to disorders of blood platelets resulting in defective thromboplastin, without obvious change in the appearance or number of platelets.

constitutional t., **(1)** von Willebrand's *disease;* **(2)** Glanzmann's *thrombasthenia.*

thrombopenia (throm-bō-pē'nē-ă). Thrombocytopenia.

thrombophilia (throm-bō-fil'ē-ă) [thrombo- + G. *philos*, fond]. A disorder of the hemopoietic system in which there is a tendency to the occurrence of thrombosis.

thrombophlebitis (throm'bō-flĕ-bī'tis) [thrombo- + G. *phleps*, vein, + *-itis*, inflammation]. Venous inflammation with thrombus formation.

t. mi'grans, creeping or slowly advancing t., appearing in first one vein and then another.

t. sal'tans, t. occurring in the same vein, but at a distance from the original lesion, or appearing suddenly in a distant vein.

thromboplastid (throm-bō-plas'tid) [thrombo- + G. plastos, formed]. **1.** Platelet. **2.** A nucleated spindle cell in submammalian blood.

thromboplastin (throm-bō-plas′tin). Thrombokinase; thrombozyme; platelet tissue factor; zymoplastic substance; a substance present in tissues, platelets, and leukocytes necessary for the coagulation of blood; in the presence of calcium ions t. is necessary for the conversion of prothrombin to thrombin, an important step in coagulation of blood. It is now generally believed that t. activity may be developed through blood (intrinsic) or tissue (extrinsic) systems. Tissue t. (factor III) interacts with factor VII and calcium to activate factor X; active factor X combines with factor V in the presence of calcium and phospholipid to produce t. activity (also commonly called t.).

thromboplastinogen (throm′bō-plas-tin′ō-jen). *Factor* VIII.

thromboplastinogenase (throm′bō-plas-tin′ō-jĕ-nās, -ti-noj′ĕ-nās). An enzyme in blood that catalyzes the conversion of inactive thromboplastinogen to thromboplastin.

thromboplastinogenemia (throm′bō-plas-tin′ō-jĕ-nē′mē-ă) [thromboplastinogen + G. *haima,* blood]. The presence of thromboplastinogen in the circulating blood.

thrombopoiesis (throm′bō-poy-ē′sis) [thrombo- + G. *poiēsis,* a making]. Precisely, the process of a clot forming in blood, but generally used with reference to the formation of blood platelets (thrombocytes).

thrombosed (throm′bōsd). **1.** Clotted. **2.** Denoting a blood vessel that is the seat of thrombosis.

thrombose par effort (throm-bōs′ par eh-fōr′) [Fr. thrombosis from stress]. Paget-von Schröttler syndrome; stress thrombosis or spontaneous thrombosis of the subclavian or axillary vein; a thoracic-outlet syndrome.

thromboses (throm-bō′sēz). Plural of thrombosis.

thrombosin (throm′bō-sin). Thrombin.

thrombosis, pl. thromboses (throm-bō′sis, -sēz) [G. *thrombōsis,* a clotting, fr. *thrombos,* clot]. Formation or presence of a thrombus; clotting within a blood vessel which may cause infarction of tissues supplied by the vessel.

atrophic t., marantic or marasmic t.; t. due to feebleness of the circulation, as in marasmus.

cerebral t., clotting of blood in a cerebral vessel.

compression t., t. due to arrest of the circulation in a vessel by compression, as from a tumor.

coronary t., coronary occlusion by thrombus formation, usually the result of atheromatous changes in the arterial wall and usually leading to myocardial infarction.

creeping t., a gradually increasing t. involving one section of a vein after another in continuity.

dilation t., t. due to slowed circulation consequent upon dilation of a vein.

effort t., see thrombose par effort.

jumping t., t. occurring in one vein and another in different regions.

marantic t., marasmic t., atrophic t.

mural t., the formation of a thrombus in contact with the endocardial lining of a cardiac chamber, or a large blood vessel, if not occlusive.

placental t., t. of the veins of the uterus at the placental site.

plate t., platelet t., t. due to an abnormal accumulation of platelets.

posttraumatic arterial t., posttraumatic venous t., intravascular clotting due to injury to a vessel wall.

thrombostasis (throm-bos′tă-sis) [thrombo- + G. *stasis,* a standing]. Local arrest of the circulation by thrombosis.

thrombosthenin (throm-bō-sthē′nin). Platelet *actomyosin.*

thrombotic (throm-bot′ik). Relating to, caused by, or characterized by thrombosis.

thrombotonin (throm-bō-tō′nin). Serotonin.

thromboxane (throm′bok-zān). Homo-11a-oxaprostane; (2*R*-*trans*)-3-heptyltetrahydro-2-octyl-2*H*-pyran; the formal parent of the thromboxanes; prostanoic acid in which the –COOH has been reduced to $-CH_3$ and an oxygen atom has been inserted between carbons 11 and 12.

thromboxanes (throm′bok-zānz). A group of compounds, included in the eicosanoids, formally based on thromboxane, but with the terminal COOH group present; biochemically related to the prostaglandins and formed from them through a series of steps involving the formation of an endoperoxide (an O–O bridge between carbons 9 and 11 in the prostaglandins) by a cyclooxygenase, followed by a rearrangement (catalyzed by thromboxane synthase) that inserts one of the two oxygen atoms between carbons 11 and 12, leaving the other still bridging carbons 9 and 11. T. are so named from their influence on platelet aggregation and the formation of the oxygen-containing six-membered ring (pyran or oxane). Like the prostaglandins, individual t. (abbreviated TX) are designated by letters (A, B, C, etc.) and subscripts indicating structural features.

thrombozyme (throm′bō-zīm). Thromboplastin.

thrombus, pl. thrombi (throm′bŭs, -bī) [L. fr. G. *thrombos,* a clot]. A clot in the cardiovascular systems formed during life from constituents of blood; it may be occlusive or attached to the vessel or heart wall without obstructing the lumen (mural t.).

agglutinative t., hyaline t.

agonal t., a heart clot formed during the act of dying after prolonged heart failure.

antemortem t., a clot formed in the circulation during life.

ball t., an antemortem t. found in the left atrium in certain cases of mitral stenosis.

ball-valve t., ball t. intermittently occluding the mitral orifice.

bile t., an intracanalicular deposit of bile, usually a result of obstruction to bile drainage.

fibrin t., a t. formed by repeated deposits of fibrin from the circulating blood; it usually does not completely occlude the vessel.

globular t., one of a number of thrombi of varying size, from a pea to a walnut, within the heart cavity, connected by a delicate fibrinous network.

hyaline t., agglutinative t.; a translucent colorless plug, partly or filling a capillary or small artery or vein, formed by agglutination of red blood corpuscles.

infective t., a t. formed in septic phlebitis.

laminated t., a t. formed gradually by clotting of the blood in successive layers.

marantic t., marasmic t., a t. formed in cases of marasmus or general debility.

mixed t., stratified t.; a laminated t., the layers of different ages being of different color or consistency.

mural t., a t. formed on and attached to a diseased patch of endocardium, not on a valve or on one side of a large blood vessel.

obstructive t., a t. due to obstruction in the vessel from compression or other cause.

pale t., white t.

parietal t., an arterial t. adhering to one side of the wall of the vessel.

postmortem t., a clot formed within the heart or in a blood vessel after death.

propagated t., see creeping *thrombosis.*

red t., a t. formed rapidly by the coagulation of stagnating blood.

secondary t., a t. formed about an embolus as a nucleus.

stratified t., mixed t.

valvular t., a parietal t. that projects into the lumen of the vessel.

white t., pale t.; a t. of opaque dull white color composed essentially of blood platelets.

throwback (thrō′bak). Atavus.

thrush (thrŭsh) [fr. the thrush fungus, *Candida albicans*]. **1.** Infection of the oral tissues with *Candida albicans.* **2.** A rare foul-smelling infective process of the horse's foot, involving the frog and sole; the affected parts degenerate and soften, and a black exudate is present; generally occurs when horses are made to stand in wet, unhygienic stalls.

thuja (thū'jă, -yă) [G. *thyia,* an African tree with sweet-smelling wood]. Thuya; the fresh tops of *Thuja occidentalis* (family Pinaceae), an ornamental evergreen tree of eastern North America, a source of cedar leaf oil; has been used internally as an expectorant, emmenagogue, and anthelmintic, and externally as a mild counterirritant.
t. oil, cedar leaf oil.

thujol (thū'jol). Thujone.

thujone (thū'jōn). Thujol; thuyol; thuyone; absinthol; tanacetol; tanacetone; $C_{10}H_{16}O$; the chief constituent of cedar leaf oil; a stimulant similar to camphor.

thulium (thū'lē-ŭm) [L. *Thule,* an island in extreme north of Europe]. A metallic element of the lanthanide series, symbol Tm, atomic no. 69, atomic weight 168.94.

thumb (thŭmb) [A.S. *thuma*]. Pollex; first finger; the first digit on the radial side of the hand.
gamekeeper's t., chronic subluxation of the metacarpophalangeal joint of the t.
hitchhiker t.'s, congenital elongation of the t.'s.
tennis t., tendinitis with calcification in the tendon of the long flexor of the t. (flexor pollicis longus) caused by friction and strain as in tennis playing, but also occurring in other exercises in which the t. is subject to repeated pressure or strain.

thumbprinting (thŭm'print-ing). A radiographic sign of intestinal abnormality frequently associated with hematoma formation in the bowel wall.

thumps (thŭmps). **1.** Spasmodic contractions of the diaphragm, or hiccups, occasionally seen in animals. **2.** In swine, a type of irregular jerky breathing seen in swine influenza, in severely anemic pigs, and in young pigs when ascarid larvae are migrating through the tissues.

thus (thŭs, thūs) [L. incense]. Olibanum.

thuya (thū'yă). Thuja.

thuyol, thuyone (thū'yol, thū'yōn). Thujone.

Thygeson, Phillips, U.S. ophthalmologist, *1903. See T.'s *disease.*

thylacitis (thī-lă-sī'tis) [G. *thylax,* bag, + *-itis,* inflammation]. Inflammation of the sebaceous glands of the skin.

thym-. See thymo-.

thyme (tīm) [G. *thymon,* thyme]. The dried leaves and flowering tops of *Thymus vulgaris* (family Labiatae), used as a condiment; it contains a volatile oil (t. oil) and is a source of thymol.
t. oil, oil of t., a volatile oil distilled from the flowering plants of *Thymus vulgaris* or *T. zygis;* a flavoring agent.

thymectomy (thī-mek'tō-mē) [thymus + G. *ektomē,* excision]. Removal of the thymus gland.

thymelcosis (thī-mel-kō'sis) [thymus + G. *helkōsis,* ulceration]. Obsolete term for suppuration of the thymus gland.

thymi-. See thymo-.

-thymia [G. *thymos,* the mind or heart as the seat of strong feelings or passion]. Suffix denoting relation to the mind, soul, emotions. See also thymo-(2).

thymic (thī'mik). Relating to the thymus gland.

thymic acid [see thyme]. Thymol.

thymicolymphatic (thī'mi-kō-lim-fat'ik). Relating to the thymus and the lymphatic system.

thymidine (dThd, dT) (thī'mi-dēn). Thymine deoxyribonucleoside; 1-(2-deoxyribosyl)thymine; one of the four major nucleosides in DNA (the others being deoxyadenosine, deoxycytidine, and deoxyguanosine).
t. phosphorylase [EC 2.4.2.4], phosphorylase that catalyzes the phosphorolysis of t.
tritiated t., t. containing the hydrogen radioisotope, tritium; used as a radioactive marker in cell and tissue studies for new formation of DNA, into which it is incorporated.

thymidine 5'-diphosphate (dTDP). Thymidine esterfied at its 5' position with diphosphoric acid.

thymidine 5'-phosphate. Thymidylic acid.

thymidine 5'-triphosphate (dTTP). Thymidine esterfied at its 5' position with triphosphoric acid; the immediate precursor of thymidylic acid in DNA.

thymidylate synthase (thī-mi-dil'āt) [EC 2.1.1.45]. An enzyme catalyzing conversion of deoxyuridine 5'-phosphate to thymidine 5'-phosphate, the methyl group coming from methylenetetrahydrofolate.

thymidylic acid (thī'mi-dil'ik). Thymidine 5'-phosphate; thymine nucleotide; a major constituent of DNA.

thymin (thī'min). Thymic lymphopoietic *factor.*

thymine (thī'mēn, -min). 5-Methyluracil; a constituent of thymidylic acid and DNA.

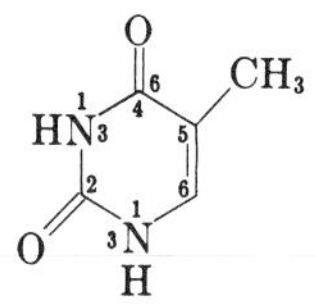

Thymine

Inner numbering, official international (IUPAC); *outer numbering,* original Fischer (abandoned).

t. deoxyribonucleoside, thymidine.
t. deoxyribonucleotide, deoxythymidylic acid.
t. nucleotide, thymidylic acid.

thymion (thī'mē-on) [G. dim. of *thymos,* a warty excrescence]. A wart.

thymiosis (thī-mē-ō'sis) [G. *thymion,* a wart]. Obsolete term for: **1.** A warty condition. **2.** Yaws.

thymitis (thī-mī'tis). Inflammation of the thymus gland.

thymo-, thym-, thymi-. **1** [G. *thymos,* thymus]. Combining forms denoting the thymus. **2** [G. *thymos,* the mind or heart as the seat of strong feelings or passions]. Combining forms denoting relation to the mind, soul, emotions.

thymocyte (thī'mō-sīt) [thymus + G. *kytos,* cell]. A cell that develops in the thymus, seemingly from a stem cell of bone marrow and of fetal liver, and is the precursor of the thymus-derived lymphocyte (T lymphocyte) that effects cell-mediated (delayed type) sensitivity.

thymogenic (thī-mō-jen'ik) [G. *thymos,* mind, + *genesis,* origin]. Of affective origin.

thymokinetic (thī'mō-ki-net'ik) [thymus + G. *kinēsis,* movement]. Activating the thymus gland.

thymol (thī'mol). Thymic acid; thyme camphor; 1-methyl-3-hydroxy-4-isopropylbenzene; $C_{10}H_{14}O$; a phenol present in the volatile oil of *Thymus vulgaris* (thyme), *Monarda punctata* (horsemint), and other volatile oils; used externally and internally as an antiseptic, as a deodorizer of offensive discharges, and as a specific for ancylostomiasis.
t. blue [C.I. 52025], a dye used as an acid-base indicator, with a pK value at 1.7 and another at 8.9; red at pH values below 1.2, yellow between 2.8 and 8.0, and blue above 9.6.
t. iodide, $C_{20}H_{24}I_2O_2$; has been used as a substitute for iodoform in skin diseases, wounds, ulcers, purulent rhinitis, otitis, etc.

thymoma (thī-mō′mă) [thymus + G. *-oma,* tumor]. A neoplasm in the anterior mediastinum, originating from thymic tissue, usually benign, and frequently encapsulated; occasionally invasive, but metastases are extremely rare; histologically, consists of any type of thymic epithelial cell as well as lymphocytes that are usually abundant and probably not neoplastic. Malignant lymphoma that involves the thymus, *e.g.,* lymphosarcoma, Hodgkin's disease (previously termed granulomatous t.), should not be regarded as t., and most neoplasms formerly classified as thymic carcinoma seem to be examples of mediastinal seminoma.

thymonuclease (thī-mō-nū′klē-ās). Deoxyribonuclease I.

thymopoietin (thī′mō-poy-ē′tin). Thymic lymphopoietic *factor.*

thymoprival, thymoprivic, thymoprivous (thī-mō-prī′văl, -priv′ik, -prī′vŭs) [thymus + L. *privus,* deprived of]. Relating to or marked by premature atrophy or removal of the thymus.

thymosin (thī′mō-sin). Thymic lymphopoietic *factor.*

thymoxamine (thī-mok′să-mēn). Moxisylyte.

thymus, pl. **thymi, thymuses** (thī′mŭs, thī′mī) [G. *thymos,* excrescence, sweetbread]. Thymus gland. **1** [NA]. A lymphoid organ, located in the superior mediastinum and lower part of the neck, that is necessary in early life for the normal development of immunological function. It reaches its greatest relative weight shortly after birth and its greatest absolute weight at puberty; it then begins to involute, and much of the lymphoid tissue is replaced by fat. The t. consists of two irregularly shaped parts united by a connective tissue capsule. Each part is partially subdivided by connective tissue septa into lobules, 0.5 to 2 mm in diameter, which consist of an inner medullary portion, continuous with the medullae of adjacent lobules, and an outer cortical portion. It is supplied by the inferior thyroid and internal thoracic arteries, and its nerves are derived from the vagus and sympathetic nerves. **2.** The t. of the calf or lamb.

thyr-. See thyro-.

thyreo-. Obsolete spelling for thyro-.

thyro-, thyr- [see thyroid]. Combining forms denoting the thyroid gland.

thyroacetic acid (thī′rō-ă-sē′tik). A degradation product of thyronine (alanine side chain reduced to acetic acid), itself a degradation product (or precursor) of thyroxine.

thyroadenitis (thī′rō-ad-ĕ-nī′tis) [thyro- + G. *adēn,* gland, + *-itis,* inflammation]. Thyroiditis.

thyroaplasia (thī′rō-ă-plā′zē-ă) [thyro- + G. *a-* priv. + *plasis,* a molding]. Anomalies observed in individuals with congenital defects of the thyroid gland and deficiency of its secretion.

thyroarytenoid (thī′rō-ar′i-tē′noyd). Relating to the thyroid and arytenoid cartilages.

thyrocalcitonin (thī′rō-kal-si-tō′nin). Calcitonin.

thyrocardiac (thī-rō-kar′dē-ak). Affecting the heart as a result of hyperthyroidism.

thyrocele (thī′rō-sēl) [thyro- + G. *kēlē,* tumor]. A tumor of the thyroid gland, such as a goiter.

thyrocervical (thī′rō-ser′vi-kăl). Relating to the thyroid gland and the neck.

thyrochondrotomy (thī′rō-kon-drot′ō-mē) [thyro- + G. *chondros,* cartilage, + *tomē,* incision]. Laryngofissure.

thyrocolloid (thī-rō-kol′oyd). A colloid substance in the thyroid gland.

thyrocricotomy (thī′rō-krī-kot′ō-mē). Division of the cricothyroid membrane.

thyroepiglottic (thī′rō-ep-i-glot′ik). Relating to the thyroid cartilage and the epiglottis.

thyroesophageus (thī′rō-e-sof-ă-jē′ŭs). A small, inconstant band of muscular fibers passing between the esophagus and the thyroid cartilage.

thyrofissure (thī′rō-fish′er). Laryngofissure.

thyrogenic, thyrogenous (thī-rō-jen′ik, -roj′ĕ-nŭs) [thyroid + G. *-gen,* producing]. Of thyroid gland origin.

thyroglobulin (thī-rō-glob′yū-lin). **1.** Iodoglobulin; thyroprotein (1); a thyroid hormone-containing protein, usually stored in the colloid within the thyroid follicles; biosynthesis of thyroid hormone entails iodination of the tyrosine moieties of this protein and the combination of two iodotyrosines to form thyroxine, the fully iodinated thyronine; secretion of thyroid hormone requires proteolytic degradation of t., with the attendant release of free hormone. **2.** A substance obtained by the fractionation of thyroid glands from the hog, *Sus scrofa,* containing not less than 0.7% of total iodine; used as a thyroid hormone in the treatment of hypothyroidism.

thyroglossal (thī-rō-glos′ăl). Thyrolingual; relating to the thyroid gland and the tongue.

thyrohyal (thī-rō-hī′ăl). The greater cornu of the hyoid bone.

thyrohyoid (thī-rō-hī′oyd). Hyothyroid; relating to the thyroid cartilage and the hyoid bone. See musculus thyrohyoideus.

thyroid (thī′royd) [G. *thyreoeidēs,* fr. *thyreos,* an oblong shield, + *eidos,* form]. **1.** Resembling a shield; scutiform; denoting a gland (glandula thyroidea) and a cartilage of the larynx (cartilago thyroidea) having such a shape. **2.** Dried t. gland; the cleaned, dried, and powdered t. gland obtained from one of the domesticated animals used for food and containing 0.17 to 0.23% of iodine; used in the treatment of cretinism and myxedema, in certain cases of obesity, and in skin disorders.

accessory t., *glandula* thyroidea accessoria.

thyroidea (thī-roy′dē-ă). *Glandula* thyroidea.

t. accesso′ria, t. i′ma, *glandula* thyroidea accessoria.

thyroidectomy (thī-roy-dek′tō-mē) [thyroid + G. *ektomē,* excision]. Removal of the thyroid gland.

"chemical" t., jargon for the reduction of thyroid function produced by the administration of antithyroid drugs. See also radiothyroidectomy.

thyroidism (thī′roy-dizm). Obsolete designation for: **1.** Hyperthyroidism. **2.** Poisoning by overdoses of a thyroid extract.

thyroiditis (thī-roy-dī′tis) [thyroid + G. *-itis,* inflammation]. Thyroadenitis; inflammation of the thyroid gland.

autoimmune t., Hashimoto's t.

chronic atrophic t., replacement of the thyroid gland by fibrous tissue, the commonest cause of myxedema in older persons.

de Quervain's t., subacute granulomatous t.

focal lymphocytic t., focal infiltration of the thyroid by lymphocytes and plasma cells. See also Hashimoto's t.

giant cell t., subacute granulomatous t.

Hashimoto's t., Hashimoto's disease, struma, or t.; autoimmune t.; lymphadenoid goiter; struma lymphomatosa; diffuse infiltration of the thyroid gland with lymphocytes, resulting in diffuse goiter and progressive destruction of the parenchyma and hypothyroidism.

ligneous t., Riedel's t.

parasitic t., chronic South American trypanosomiasis with involvement of the thyroid gland, causing myxedema.

Riedel's t., Riedel's disease or struma; ligneous struma or t.; a rare fibrous induration of the thyroid gland, with adhesion to adjacent structures, which may cause tracheal compression.

subacute granulomatous t., de Quervain's t.; giant cell t.; t. with round cell (usually lymphocytes) infiltration, destruction of thyroid cells, epithelial giant cell proliferation, and evidence of regeneration; thought by some to be a reflection of a systemic infection and not an example of true chronic t.

thyroidology (thī-roy-dol′ō-jē) [thyroid + G. *logos,* study]. The study of the thyroid gland, both normal and pathological.

thyroidotomy (thī′roy-dot′ō-mē) [thyroid + G. *tomē,* incision]. Laryngofissure.

thyrolaryngeal (thī′rō-lă-rin′jē-ăl). Relating to the thyroid gland or cartilage and the larynx.

thyroliberin (thī-rō-lib′er-in). Thyrotropin-releasing *hormone;* thyroid-stimulating hormone-releasing factor; a tripeptide hormone from the hypothalamus which stimulates the anterior lobe of the hypophysis to release thyrotropin.

thyrolingual (thī′rō-ling′gwăl) [thyro- + L. *lingua,* tongue]. Thyroglossal.

thyrolytic (thī-rō-lit′ik) [thyro- + G. *lytikos,* dissolving]. Causing destruction of thyroid gland cells.

thyromegaly (thī-rō-meg′ă-lē) [thyro- + G. *megas,* large]. Enlargement of the thyroid gland.

thyronine (thī′rō-nēn, -nin). $HOC_6H_4–O–C_6H_4–CH_2–CHNH_2–COOH$; an amino acid with a diphenyl ether group in the side chain; occurs in proteins only in the form of iodinated derivatives (iodothyronines), such as thyroxine.

thyropalatine (thī-rō-pal′ă-tīn). Denoting the musculus palatopharyngeus.

thyroparathyroidectomy (thī′rō-par-ă-thī′roy-dek′tō-mē). Excision of thyroid and parathyroid glands.

thyropathy (thī-rop′ă-thē) [thyro- + G. *pathos,* suffering]. A disorder of the thyroid gland.

thyropharyngeal (thī-rō-fă-rin′jē-ăl). Denoting the thyropharyngeal portion of the musculus constrictor pharyngis inferior.

thyroprival (thī-rō-prī′văl) [thyro- + L. *privus,* deprived of]. Thyroprivic; thyroprivous; relating to thyroprivia, denoting hypothyroidism produced by disease or thyroidectomy.

thyroprivia (thī-rō-priv′ē-ă). A state characterized by reduced activity of the thyroid.

thyroprivic, thyroprivous (thī-rō-priv′ik, -priv′ŭs). Thyroprival.

thyroprotein (thī-rō-prō′tēn). **1.** Thyroglobulin (1). **2.** An iodinated protein, usually casein, that has thyroxine activity.

thyroptosis (thī-rop-tō′sis) [thyro- + G. *ptōsis,* a falling]. Downward dislocation of the thyroid gland.

thyrotomy (thī′rot′ō-mē) [thyro- + G. *tomē,* a cutting]. **1.** Any cutting operation on the thyroid gland. **2.** Laryngofissure.

thyrotoxic (thī-rō-tok′sik). Denoting thyrotoxicosis.

thyrotoxicosis (thī′rō-tok-si-kō′sis) [thyro- + G. *toxikon,* poison, + *-osis,* condition]. The state produced by excessive quantities of endogenous or exogenous thyroid hormone.
apathetic t., chronic t., presenting as cardiac disease or as a wasting syndrome, with weakness of proximal muscles and depression but with few of the more typical clinical manifestations of t.
t. medicamento′sa, a hyperthyroid state resulting from excessive doses of thyroid hormone preparation.

thyrotoxin (thī-rō-tok′sin). **1.** A hypothetical substance formerly believed to be an abnormal product of diffusely hyperplastic thyroid glands in persons with Graves' disease, and presumed to be the cause of the distinctive signs and symptoms of that condition (in contrast to simple hyperthyroidism). **2.** A complement-fixing antigenic factor associated with certain diseases of the thyroid gland. See also thyrotoxic complement-fixation *factor.* **3.** Rarely used term referring to any material toxic to thyroidal tissue.

thyrotroph (thī′rō-trof). A cell in the anterior lobe of the pituitary that produces thyrotropin.

thyrotrophic (thī-rō-trof′ik) [thyro- + G. *trophē,* nourishment]. Thyrotropic.

thyrotrophin (thī-rot′rō-fin, thī-rō-trō′fin). Thyrotropin.

thyrotropic (thī-rō-trop′ik) [thyro- + G. *tropē,* a turning]. Thyrotrophic; stimulating or nurturing the thyroid gland.

thyrotropin (thī-rot′rō-pin, thī-rō-trō′pin). Thyrotrophin; thyrotropic hormone; thyroid-stimulating hormone; a glycoprotein hormone produced by the anterior lobe of the hypophysis which stimulates the growth and function of the thyroid gland; it also is used as a diagnostic test to differentiate primary and secondary hypothyroidism.

thyroxine, thyroxin (T_4) (thī-rok′sēn, -sin). 3,3′,5,5′-Tetraiodothyronine; β-[(3,5-diiodo-4-hydroxyphenoxy) -3,5-diiodophenyl]-alanine; the active iodine compound existing normally in the thyroid gland and extracted therefrom in crystalline form for therapeutic use; also prepared synthetically; used for the relief of hypothyroidism, cretinism, and myxedema.
radioactive t., radiothyroxin; t. in which a radioisotope of iodine (I-125 or I-131) is incorporated into its molecule; used in experiments tracing the metabolism of t.
t. sodium, a preparation obtained by the action of a limited amount of sodium carbonate upon t.; it contains between 61 and 65% of iodine. See *sodium* levothyoxine; *sodium* liothyronine.

Thysanosoma actinoides (this-ă-nō-sō′mă ak-ti-noyd′ēz). Fringed tapeworm of sheep, a relatively short, thick tapeworm (family Anocephalidae) in which the posterior borders of the proglottids are fringed. It inhabits the small intestine, but often invades the bile ducts and causes many livers to be condemned for human food. It is essentially nonpathogenic and is common in stock-raising countries, where it infects a wide variety of ruminants; oribatid mites are probably the vectors.

Ti Symbol for titanium.

TIA Abbreviation for transient ischemic *attack.*

tibia, gen. and pl. **tibiae** (tib′ē-ă, tib′ē-ē) [L. the large shinbone] [NA]. Shin bone; shank bone (2); the medial and larger of the two bones of the leg, articulating with the femur, fibula, and talus.
saber t., deformity of the t. occurring in tertiary syphilis or yaws, the bone having a marked forward convexity as a result of the formation of gummas and periostitis.
t. val′ga, *genu* valgum.
t. va′ra, *genu* varum.

tibiad (tib′ē-ad) [tibia + L. *ad,* to]. In a direction toward the tibia.

tibial (tib′ē-ăl) [L. *tibialis*]. Tibialis.

tibiale posticum (tib-ē-ā′lē pos-tī′kŭm). *Os* tibiale posterius.

tibialgia (tib′ē-al′jē-ă) [tibia + G. *algos,* pain]. Pain in the shin.

tibialis (tib-ē-ā′lis) [L.] [NA]. Tibial; relating to the tibia or to any structure named from it; also denoting the medial or tibial aspect of the lower limb.

tibio- [L. *tibia,* the large shinbone]. Combining form denoting the tibia.

tibiocalcanean (tib′ē-ō-kal-kā′nē-an). Relating to the tibia and the calcaneus.

tibiofascialis (tib-ē-ō-fas-ē-ā′lis). See under musculus.

tibiofemoral (tib-ē-ō-fem′ō-răl). Relating to the tibia and the femur.

tibiofibular (tib-ē-ō-fib′yū-lăr). Peroneotibial; tibioperoneal; relating to both tibia and fibula.

tibionavicular (tib-ē-ō-na-vik′yū-lăr). Tibioscaphoid; relating to the tibia and the navicular bone of the tarsus.

tibioperoneal (tib′ē-ō-per′ō-nē′ăl). Tibiofibular.

tibioscaphoid (tib′ē-ō-skaf′oyd). Tibionavicular.

tibiotarsal (tib-ē-ō-tar′săl). Tarsotibial.

tic (tik) [Fr.]. Habit chores or spasm; Brissaud's disease; a more or less involuntary repeated contraction of a certain group of associated muscles; a habitual spasmodic movement or contraction of

any part. See also spasm.
convulsive t., facial t.
t. douloureux (dū-lū-rĕ′) [Fr. painful], trigeminal *neuralgia.*
facial t., involuntary twitching of the facial muscles, sometimes unilateral. Also called convulsive or mimic t.; palmus (1); facial, histrionic, mimic, or Bell's spasm; prosopospasm; mimic convulsion.
glossopharyngeal t., glossopharyngeal *neuralgia.*
habit t., a habitual repetition of some grimace, shrug of the shoulder, twisting or jerking of the head, or the like.
local t., a t. of very limited extent, as the winking of an eye or a twitch of a finger.
mimic t., facial t.
t. de pensée (dĕ pahn-sā′) [Fr. of thought], the habit of involuntarily giving expression to any thought that comes to mind.
psychic t., a gesture or exclamation made under the influence of an irresistible morbid impulse.
rotatory t., spasmodic *torticollis.*
spasmodic t., Henoch's chorea; a disorder in which sudden spasmodic coordinated movements of certain muscles or groups of physiologically related muscles occur at irregular intervals.

ticarcillin disodium (tī-kar-sil′in). The disodium salt of 6-(α-carboxy-α-thien-3-ylacetamido)penicillanic acid; a bactericidal antibiotic useful in treating *Pseudomonas aeruginosa* infections and similar in effect to carbenicillin disodium.

tick (tik). An acarine of the families Ixodidae (hard t.'s) or Argasidae (soft t.'s), which contain many bloodsucking species that are important pests of man and domestic birds and mammals, and that probably exceed all other arthropods in the number and variety of disease agents that they transmit. T.'s are differentiated from the much smaller true mites by possession of an armed hypostome and a pair of tracheal spiracular openings located behind the basal segment of the third or fourth pair of walking legs; the larva (seed t.) has six legs, and after molting appears as an eight-limbed nymph. Some important t.'s are *Amblyomma americanum* (Lone Star t.) and *A. hebraeum* (South African bont t.); *Argas persicus* (adobe, fowl, or Persian t.) and *A. reflexus* (pigeon t.); *Boophilus* (cattle t.'s); *Dermacentor albopictus* (horse or winter t.), *D. andersoni* (Rocky Mountain, spotted-fever, or wood t.), *D. nitens* (tropical horse t.), *D. occidentalis* (Pacific or wood t.), and *D. variabilis* (American dog t.); *Haemaphysalis chordeilis* (bird t.) and *H. leporis-palustris* (rabbit t.); *Ixodes pacificus* (California black-legged t.), *I. pilosus* (paralysis t.), *I. ricinus* (castor bean t.), and *I. scapularis* (black-legged or shoulder t.); *Ornithodoros coriaceus* (pajaroello t.) and *O. moubata* (African relapsing fever or tampan t.); and *Rhipicephalus everti* (African red t.), *R. sanguineus* (brown dog t.), and *R. simus* (black-pitted t.).

tickling (tik′ling). Denoting a peculiar itching or tingling sensation caused by excitation of surface nerves, as of the skin by light stroking.

ticrynafen (tī-krin′ă-fen). [2,3-Dichloro-4-(2-thenoyl)phenoxy]acetic acid; an antihypertensive diuretic and uricosuric agent; its clinical use is associated with an unusually high incidence of hepatitis.

t.i.d. Abbreviation for L. *ter in die,* three times a day.

tidal (tī′dăl). Relating to or resembling the tides, alternately rising and falling.

tide (tīd) [A.S. *tīd,* time]. An alternate rise and fall, ebb and flow, or an increase or a decrease.
acid t., acid wave; a temporary increase in the acidity of the urine occurring during fasting.
alkaline t., alkaline wave; a period of urinary neutrality or even alkalinity after meals due to withdrawal of hydrogen ion for the purpose of secretion of the highly acid gastric juice.
fat t., an increase in the fat content of blood and lymph following a meal.

Tièche, Max, 20th century Swiss dermatologist. See Jadassohn-T. *nevus.*

Tiedemann, Friedrich, German anatomist, 1781–1861. See T.'s *gland, nerve.*

Tierfellnaevus (tēr′fel-nē-vŭs) [Ger. a nevus simulating the pelt of an animal]. Bathing trunk *nevus.*

Tietze, Alexander, German surgeon, 1864–1927. See T.'s *syndrome.*

tiglate (tig′lāt). A salt or ester of tiglic acid.

tiglian (tig′lē-ăn) [fr. *Croton tiglium* (Euphorbiaceae)]. Original trivial name for the saturated form of phorbol.

tiglic acid (tig′lik). (*E*)-2-Methyl-2-butenoic acid; *trans*-2,3-dimethyl-acrylic acid; $CH_3CH{=}C(CH_3)COOH$; an unsaturated fatty acid present in glycerides in croton oil.

tigretier (tē-grĕ-ty-ā′) [Fr.]. A form of saltatory chorea or dancing mania occurring in certain parts of Abyssinia.

tigroid (tī′groyd) [G. *tigroeidēs,* fr. *tigris,* tiger, + *eidos,* appearance]. See chromophil *substance.*

tigrolysis (tī-grol′i-sis) [tigroid + G. *lysis,* dissolution]. Chromatolysis.

Tillaux, Paul J., French surgeon, 1834–1904. See *spiral* of T.

timbre (tam′br, tim′br) [Fr.]. Tone color; the distinguishing quality of a sound, by which one may determine its source.

time (tīm) [A.S. *tima*]. **1.** That relation of events which is expressed by the terms past, present, and future, and measured by units such as minutes, hours, days, months, or years. **2.** A certain period during which something definite or determined is done.
activated partial thromboplastin t., the t. needed for plasma to form a fibrin clot following the addition of calcium and a phospholipid reagent; used to evaluate the intrinsic clotting system.
A-H conduction t., see under atrioventricular *conduction.*
association t., t. elasping between a stimulus and the verbalized mental association.
biologic t., the concept that our appreciation of t. varies with age and is governed by the neural organization of the individual; it obeys a logarithmic rather than an arithmetic law.
bleeding t., the t. interval between the appearance of the first drop of blood and the removal of the last drop following puncture of the ear lobe or the finger, usually 1 to 3 minutes; it is prolonged in cases of thrombocytopenia, diminished prothrombin, phosphorus poisoning, or chloroform poisoning, and in some liver diseases; it is normal in hemophilia. Since the earlier techniques were not well controlled, better controlled modifications such as that of Ivy are now employed to determine the bleeding.

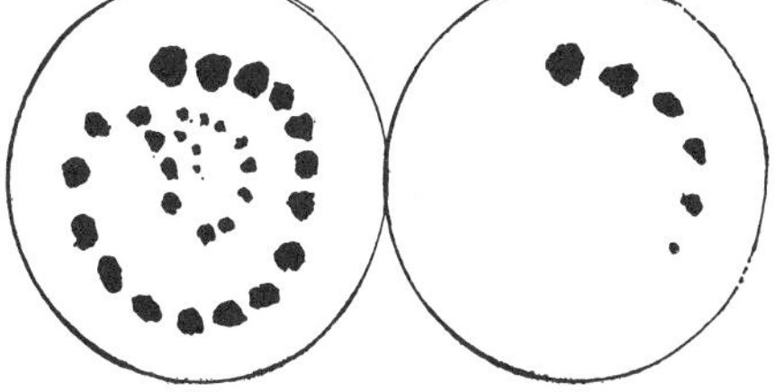

Bleeding Time
Right, normal; *left,* in thrombocytopenic purpura; blood samples at 20-second intervals. (After Quick.)

calcium t., the t. required for the coagulation of blood to which calcium chloride has been added; if this t. is less than the coagulation t. for the same blood without the added calcium, then the delay is probably the result of a deficiency of calcium in the patient.
circulation t., the t. taken for the blood to pass through a given

circuit of the vascular system, *e.g.,* the pulmonary or systemic circulation, from one arm to another, from arm to tongue, or from arm to lung; it is measured by the injection into an arm vein of a substance, such as sodium dehydrocholate, ether, fluorescein, histamine, or a radium salt, which can be detected when it arrives at another point in the vascular system.
clot retraction t., the t. required for a blood clot to separate from the tube wall and express serum, usually completed in 18 to 24 hours, but retarded or absent in persons with thrombocytopenic purpura.
clotting t., coagulation t.
coagulation t., clotting t.; the t. required for blood to coagulate; prolonged in hemophilia and in the presence of obstructive jaundice, some anemias and leukemias, and some of the infectious diseases.
euglobulin clot lysis t., a measure of the ability of plasminogen activators and plasmin to lyse a clot; normally, clot lysis is determined by the balance of factors which activate fibrinolysis (plasminogen activators and plasmin) and those which inhibit lysis; in certain conditions (*e.g.,* carcinoma or hepatic insufficiency) activating factors predominate and can be measured by noting the t. it takes the euglobulin fraction of plasma (excluding inhibitors of fibrinolysis) to clot.
fading t., the t. required for a constant stimulus applied to a fixed area of the peripheral visual field to stop.
forced expiratory t. (FET), the t. taken to expire a given volume or a given fraction of vital capacity during measurement of forced vital capacity; subscripts specify the exact parameters measured.
half-t., see half-time.
H-R conduction t., see under intraventricular *conduction.*
H-V conduction t., see under intraventricular *conduction.*
inertia t., the interval elapsing between the reception of the stimulus from a nerve and the contraction of the muscle.
intra-atrial conduction t., the total duration of electrical activity of the atrium in one cardiac cycle.
left ventricular ejection t. (LVET), the t. measured from onset to incisural notch of the carotid pulse.
P-A conduction t., see under atrioventricular *conduction.*
partial thromboplastin t., see activated partial thromboplastin t.
P-H conduction t., see under atrioventricular *conduction.*
prothrombin t., the t. required for clotting after thromboplastin and calcium are added in optimal amounts to blood of normal fibrinogen content; if prothrombin is diminished, the clotting t. increases. See also prothrombin *test.*
reaction t., the interval between the presentation of a stimulus and the responsive reaction to it.
recognition t., the interval between the application of a stimulus and the recognition of its nature.
rise t., the t. required for a pulse or echo to rise from 10% to 90% of its peak amplitude.
sensation t., the minimal t. a visual image must be exposed in order to be perceived.
sinoatrial conduction t. (SACT), the t. required for an impulse to travel from sinus node to atrium; estimated indirectly during reset nodus sinuatrialis period by halving the average interval from the premature beat to the following normal sinus beat of the atrium.
sinoatrial recovery t. (SART), interval from the last paced P wave to the first succeeding spontaneous P wave (after 2 to 5 minutes of right atrial pacing at 120 to 140 beats per minute, and when expressed as percentage of control cycle length, it normally ranges from 115 to 159%).
survival t., **(1)** the period elapsing between the completion or institution of any procedure and death; **(2)** the life-span of biologically or physically marked erythrocytes or other cells.
thrombin t., the t. needed for a fibrin clot to form after the addition of thrombin to citrated plasma; prolonged thrombin t. is seen in patients receiving heparin therapy.
tissue thromboplastin inhibition t., a test used to identify lupus anticoagulant; the thromboplastin source used in the prothrombin test is diluted to increase sensitivity to inhibitors.
utilization t., temps utile; the minimum duration of a stimulus of rheobasic strength that is just sufficient to produce excitation.

timolol maleate (tī'mō-lōl). (−)-1-(*tert*-Butylamino)-3-[(4-morpholino-1,2,5-thiadiazol-3-yl)oxy]-2-propanol maleate; a β-adrenergic blocking agent used in the treatment of hypertension and used in eyedrops in the treatment of chronic open-angle glaucoma.

tin. Stannum; a metallic element, symbol Sn, atomic no. 50, atomic weight 118.69.
t. oxide, stannic oxide.

tin-113 (^{113}Sn). A radioisotope of tin with a physical half-life of 115 days; used in the manufacture of radionuclide generators for the production of indium-113m.

tinct. Abbreviation of L. *tinctura,* tincture.

tinctable (tingk'tă-bl). Stainable.

tinction (tingk'shŭn) [L. *tingo,* pp. *tinctus,* to dye]. **1.** A stain; a preparation for staining. **2.** The act of staining.

tinctorial (tingk-tōr'ē-ăl) [L. *tinctorius,* fr. *tingo,* to dye]. Relating to coloring or staining.

tinctura, gen. and pl. **tincturae (tinct., tr.)** (tingk-tū'ră, -rē) [L. a dyeing, fr. *tingo,* pp. *tinctus,* to dye]. Tincture.

tincturation (tingk-chū-rā'shŭn). The making of a tincture from a crude drug.

tincture (tr.) (tingk'chūr) [see *tinctura*] An alcoholic or hydroalcoholic solution prepared from vegetable materials or from chemical substances; most t.'s are prepared by percolation or by maceration. The proportions of drug represented in the different t.'s are not uniform, but vary according to the established standards for each. T.'s of potent drugs essentially represent the activity of 10 g of the drug in each 100 ml of t., the potency being adjusted after assay; most other t.'s represent 20 g of drug in each 100 ml of t. Compound t.'s are made according to long-established formulas.
alcoholic t., a t. made with undiluted alcohol.
ammoniated t., a t. made with ammoniated alcohol.
ethereal t., a class of preparations consisting of 10% percolations of drugs in a menstruum of ether 1 and alcohol 2.
glycerinated t., a t. made with diluted alcohol to which glycerin is added to facilitate the extraction or to preserve the preparation.
hydroalcoholic t., a t. made with diluted alcohol in various proportions with water.

tine (tīn) [A.S. *tind,* a prong]. **1.** In dentistry, the slender, pointed end of an explorer. **2.** An instrument used to introduce antigen, such as tuberculin into the skin, and usually containing several individual t.'s.

tinea (tin'ē-ă) [L. worm, moth]. Ringworm; serpigo (1); a fungus infection (dermatophytosis) of the hair, skin, or nails. Genera of fungi causing such infection are *Microsporum, Trichophyton,* and *Epidermophyton.*
t. amianta'cea, pityriasis amiantacea; an inflammatory condition of the scalp in which heavy scales extend onto the hairs and bind the proximal portions together; it is not caused by a fungus.
t. axilla'ris, obsolete term for a fungus infection of the hair and skin of the axillary region.
t. bar'bae, t. of the beard, occurring as a follicular infection or as a granulomatous lesion; the primary lesions are papules and pustules. Also called ringworm of beard; barber's itch; folliculitis barbae; tinea sycosis; trichophytosis barbae.
t. cap'itis, ringworm of scalp; trichophytosis capitis; a common form of fungus infection of the scalp caused by various species of *Microsporum* and *Trichophyton,* occurring almost exclusively in children and characterized by irregularly placed and variously sized patches of apparent baldness because of hairs breaking off at

the surface of the scalp, scaling, black dots (see black-dot *ringworm*), and occasionally erythema and pyoderma.

t. cilio'rum, obsolete fungus infection of the eyelashes.

t. circina'ta, t. corporis.

t. cor'poris, t. circinata; trichophytosis corporis; ringworm of body; a well-defined, scaling, macular eruption that frequently forms annular lesions and may appear on any part of the body.

t. cru'ris, t. inguinalis; trichophytosis cruris; dhobie or jock itch; eczema marginatum; ringworm of genitocrural region; a form of t. imbricata occurring in the genitocrural region, including the inner side of the thighs, the perineal region, and the groin.

t. favo'sa, favus.

t. furfura'cea, obsolete term for t. versicolor.

t. glabro'sa, ringworm or fungus infection of the hairless skin.

t. imbrica'ta, an eruption consisting of a number of concentric rings of overlapping scales forming papulosquamous patches scattered over the body; it occurs in tropical climates and is caused by the fungus *Trichophyton concentricum.* Also called herpes desquamans; Oriental, scaly, or Tokelau ringworm; t. tropicalis, Malabar itch.

t. inguina'lis, t. cruris.

t. ke'rion, Celsus' kerion; an inflammatory fungus infection of the scalp and beard, marked by pustules and a boggy infiltration of the surrounding parts; most commonly caused by *Microsporum audouinii.*

t. ma'nus, ringworm of the hand, usually referring to infections of the palmar surface. See also t. corporis.

t. ni'gra, pityriasis nigra; a fungus infection due to *Exophiala werneckii,* marked by dark lesions giving a spattered appearance and occurring most commonly on the palms of the hands.

t. pe'dis, dermatomycosis pedis; athlete's foot; Hong Kong foot or toe; ringworm of foot; dermatophytosis of the feet, especially of the skin between the toes, and the nails, caused by one of the dermatophytes, usually a species of *Trichophyton* or *Epidermophyton;* the disease consists of small vesicles, fissures, scaling, maceration, and eroded areas between the toes and on the plantar surface of the foot; other skin areas may be involved.

t. syco'sis, t. barbae.

t. tar'si, obsolete term for fungus infection of eyelids.

t. ton'dens, obsolete term for t. tonsurans.

t. tonsu'rans, porrigo furfurans; t. capitis or t. corporis caused by *Trichophyton tonsurans;* characterized by small plaques and fewer broken off hairs than in t. capitis caused by other species.

t. tropica'lis, t. imbricata.

t. un'guium, onychomycosis.

t. ve'ra, obsolete term for favus.

t. versic'olor, pityriasis versicolor; an eruption of tan or brown branny patches on the skin of the trunk, often appearing white, in contrast with hyperpigmented skin after exposure to the summer sun; caused by *Malassezia furfur.*

Tinel, Jules, French neurologist, 1879–1952. See T.'s *sign.*

tinfoil (tin'foyl). **1.** Tin rolled into extremely thin sheets. **2.** A base metal foil used as a separating material, as between the cast and denture base material during flasking and curing procedures.

tingibility (tin'ji-bil'i-tē). The property of being tingible.

tingible (tin'ji-bl) [L. *tingo,* to dye]. Capable of being stained.

tingle (ting'gl). To feel a peculiar pricking sensation.

ting'ling. A peculiar pricking thrill, caused by cold, by an emotional shock, or striking a nerve, such as the ulnar at the elbow (the "funny bone").

tinidazole (ti-nid'ă-zōl). 1-[2-(Ethylsulfonyl)ethyl]-2-methyl-5-nitroimidazole; an antiprotozoal agent.

tinnitus (ti-nī'tŭs) [L. a jingling, fr. *tinnio,* pp. *tinnitus,* to jingle, clink]. Noises (ringing, whistling, booming, etc.) in the ears. Also called t. aurium.

t. au'rium, syrigmus; tympanophonia (1); sensation of sound in one or both ears usually associated with disease in the middle ear, the inner ear, or the central auditory apparatus.

t. cere'bri, subjective sensation of noise in head rather than ears.

clicking t., an objective clicking sound in the ear in cases of chronic catarrhal otitis media; it may be audible to the bystander as well as to the patient and is supposed to be due to an opening and closing of the mouth of the eustachian tube, or to a rhythmical spasm of the velum palati.

Leudet's t., a dry spasmodic click, audible also through the otoscope, heard in catarrhal inflammation of the eustachian tube; caused by reflex spasm of the tensor palati muscle.

tint [L. *tingo,* pp. *tinctus,* to dye]. A shade of color varying according to the amount of white admixed with the pigment.

tioconazole (tī-ō-kon'ă-zōl). 1-[2,4-Dichloro-β-[(2-chloro-3-thenyl)-oxy]phenethyl]imidazole; an antifungal agent.

tip. 1. A point; a more or less sharp extremity. **2.** A separate, but attached, piece of the same or another structure, forming the extremity of a part.

t. of auricle, *apex* auriculae.

t. of elbow, olecranon.

t. of nose, *apex* nasi.

t. of posterior horn, *apex* cornus posterioris.

root t., *apex* radicis dentis.

t. of tongue, *apex* linguae.

Woolner's t., the extremity of the helix of the auricle.

tip'ping. A tooth movement in which the angulation of the long axis of the tooth is altered.

tiprenolol hydrochloride (tip-ren'ō-lol). (+)-1-(Isopropylamino)-3-[*o*-(methylthio)phenoxy]-2-propanol hydrochloride; a β-receptor blocking agent.

tiring (tīr'ing). Cerclage.

Tiselius, Arne, Swedish biochemist, 1902–1971. See T. *apparatus,* electrophoresis *cell.*

Tissot, Jules, early 20th century French physiologist. See T. *spirometer.*

tissue (tish'ū) [Fr. *tissu,* woven, fr. L. *texo,* to weave]. A collection of similar cells and the intercellular substances surrounding them. There are four basic tissues in the body: 1) epithelium; 2) the connective tissues, including blood, bone, and cartilage; 3) muscle tissue; and 4) nerve tissue.

adenoid t., lymphatic t.

adipose t., fat (1); white fat (1); fatty t. (1); a connective t. consisting chiefly of fat cells surrounded by reticular fibers and arranged in lobular groups or along the course of one of the smaller blood vessels. See fig. on p. 1604.

areolar t., loose, irregularly arranged connective t. that consists of collagenous and elastic fibers, a protein polysaccharide ground substance, and connective t. cells (fibroblasts, macrophages, mast cells, and sometimes fat cells, plasma cells, leukocytes, and pigment cells).

bone t., osseous t.

cancellous t., latticelike or spongy osseous t.

cardiac muscle t., see cardiac *muscle.*

cartilaginous t., see cartilage.

cavernous t., erectile t.

chondroid t., (1) fibrohyaline t.; pseudocartilage; in an adult, t. resembling cartilage; **(2)** in an embryo, an early stage in cartilage formation.

chromaffin t., a cellular t., vascular and well supplied with nerves, made up chiefly of chromaffin cells; it is found in the medulla of the suprarenal glands and, in smaller collections, in the paraganglia.

connective t., interstitial t.; tela conjunctiva; the supporting or framework t. of the animal body, formed of fibrous and ground substance with more or less numerous cells of various kinds; it is

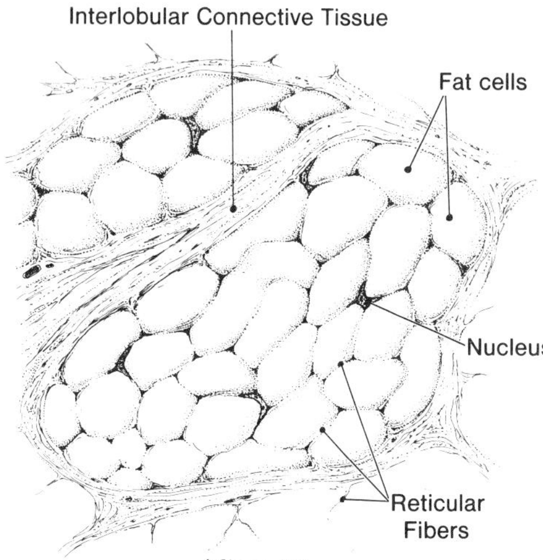

Adipose Tissue

derived from the mesenchyme, and this in turn from the mesoderm; the varieties of connective t. are: areolar or loose; adipose; dense, regular or irregular, white fibrous; elastic; mucous; and lymphoid t.; cartilage; and bone; the blood and lymph may be regarded as connective t.'s the ground substance of which is a liquid.
dartoic t., t. resembling tunica dartos.
elastic t., elastica (2); tela elastica; a form of connective t. in which the elastic fibers predominate; it constitutes the ligamenta flava of the vertebrae and the ligamentum nuchae, especially of quadrupeds; it occurs also in the walls of the arteries and of the bronchial tree, and connects the cartilages of the larynx.
epithelial t., see epithelium.
erectile t., cavernous t.; a t. with numerous vascular spaces which may become engorged with blood.
fatty t., **(1)** adipose t.; **(2)** in some animals, brown *fat.*
fibrohyaline t., chondroid t. (1).
fibrous t., a t. composed of bundles of collagenous white fibers between which are rows of connective t. cells; the tendons, ligaments, aponeuroses, and some of the membranes, such as the dura mater.
Gamgee t., a thick layer of absorbent cotton between two layers of absorbent gauze, used in surgical dressings.
gelatinous t., mucous connective t.
gingival t.'s, see gingiva.
granulation t., vascular connective t. forming granular projections on the surface of a healing wound, ulcer, or inflamed t. surface. See also granulation.
Haller's vascular t., *lamina* vasculosa choroideae.
hard t., **(1)** t. that has become mineralized; **(2)** t. having a firm intercellular substance, *e.g.,* cartilage and bone.
hemopoietic t., t. in which there is a development of blood cells or other formed elements.
indifferent t., undifferentiated, nonspecialized, embryonic t.
interstitial t., connective t.
investing t.'s, the t.'s covering or enclosing a structure.
islet t., *islets* of Langerhans.
lymphatic t., lymphoid t., adenoid t.; a three-dimensional network of reticular fibers and cells the meshes of which are occupied in varying degrees of density with lymphocytes; there is nodular, diffuse, and loose lymphatic t.
mesenchymal t., see mesenchyme.
mesonephric t., intermediate mesoderm situated in the thoracic and lumbar regions of the embryo or fetus; it evolves into the mesonephros and associated structures.
metanephrogenic t., t. derived from the intermediate mesoderm caudal to mesonephric levels, and concerned with the formation of the nephrons of the metanephros.
mucous connective t., gelatinous t.; a type of connective t. little differentiated beyond the mesenchymal stage; its ground substance of glycoproteins is abundant and contains fine collagenous fibers and fibroblasts; in its most characteristic form, it appears in the umbilical cord as Wharton's jelly.
multilocular adipose t., brown *fat.*
muscular t., flesh (2); a t. characterized by the ability to contract upon stimulation; its three varieties are skeletal, cardiac, and smooth. See under muscle.
myeloid t., bone marrow consisting of the developmental and adult stages of erythrocytes, granulocytes, and megakaryocytes in a stroma of reticular cells and fibers, with sinusoidal vascular channels.
nasion soft t., the outer point of intersection between the nasion-sella line and the soft tissue profile.
nephrogenic t., the t. from which the pronephros, mesonephros, and metanephros develop.
nervous t., a highly differentiated t. composed of nerve cells, nerve fibers, dendrites, and a supporting t. (neuroglia).
nodal t., see *nodus* atrioventricularis; *nodus* sinuatrialis.
osseous t., bone t.; a connective t., the matrix of which consists of collagen fibers and ground substance and in which are deposited calcium salts (phosphate, carbonate, and some fluoride) in the form of an apatite.
osteogenic t., a connective t. with the property of forming osseous t.
osteoid t., osseous t. prior to calcification.
periapical t., the structures adjacent to a root apex, particularly the periodontal ligament and bone.
reticular t., retiform t., a t. in which the argyrophilic collagenous fibers form a network and which usually has a network of reticular cells associated with the fibers.
rubber t., a thin sheet of rubber used as a cover in surgical dressings.
skeletal muscle t., see skeletal *muscle.*
smooth muscle t., see smooth *muscle.*
subcutaneous t., a layer of loose, irregular, connective t. immediately beneath the skin and closely attached to the corium by coarse fibrous bands, the retinacula cutis; it contains fat cells except in the auricles, eyelids, penis, and scrotum.

tissue-trimming. Border *molding.*

tissular (tish'yū-lăr). Relating or pertaining to a tissue.

titanium (tī-tā'nē-ŭm) [*Titan,* in G. myth., one of a race of giants]. A metallic element, symbol Ti, atomic no. 22, atomic weight 47.90.
t. dioxide, TiO_2; contains not less than 99.0% and not more than 100.5% of TiO_2, calculated on the dry basis; used in creams and powders as a protectant against external irritations and solar rays.

titer (tī'ter) [Fr. *titre,* standard]. The standard of strength of a volumetric test solution; the assay value of an unknown measure by volumetric means.

TITh Abbreviation for 3,5,3′-triiodothyronine.

titillation (tit-i-lā'shŭn) [L. *titillatio,* fr. *titillo,* pp. *-atus,* to tickle]. The act or sensation of tickling.

titrant (tī'trant). In chemistry, the solution that is added (titrated with) in a titration.

titrate (tī'trāt). To analyze volumetrically by a solution (the titrant) of known strength to an end point.

titration (tī-trā'shŭn) [Fr. *titre,* standard]. Volumetric analysis by means of the addition of definite amounts of a test solution to a solution of the substance being assayed.
colorimetric t., a t. in which the end point is marked by a color

change.
formol t., a method of titrating the amino groups of amino acids, by adding formaldehyde to the neutral solution; the formaldehyde reacts with the NH_3^+ group, liberating an equivalent quantity of H^+, which may then be estimated by t. with NaOH.
potentiometric t., a t. during which the pH is continually measured with some value of the pH serving as end point.

titubation (tit-yū-bā'shŭn) [L. *titubo,* pp. *-atus,* to stagger]. **1.** A staggering or stumbling in trying to walk. **2.** A tremor or shaking of the head, of cerebellar origin.

Tizzoni, Guido, Italian physician 1853–1932. See T.'s *stain.*

Tl Symbol for thallium.

TLC Abbreviation for thin-layer *chromatography;* total lung *capacity.*

TLE Abbreviation for thin-layer *electrophoresis.*

TLV Abbreviation for threshold limit *value.*

Tm Symbol for thulium; transport or tubular *maximum.*

TMJ Abbreviation for temporomandibular joint *dysfunction.*

TM-mode. M-mode.

TMP Abbreviation for ribothymidylic acid.

T-mycoplasma. *Ureaplasma.*

Tn Abbreviation for ocular *tension.*

TNM Abbreviation for tumor-node-metastasis. See TNM *staging.*

TNT Abbreviation for trinitrotoluene.

TO Abbreviation for Theiler's Original, Theiler's original strain of mouse encephalomyelitis virus.

tobacco (tō-bak'ō). A South American herb, *Nicotiana tabacum,* that has large ovate to lanceolate leaves and terminal clusters of tubular white or pink flowers. T. leaves contain 2 to 8% of nicotine and are the source of smoking and chewing t.
wild t., lobelia.

tobramycin (tō-bră-mī'sin). An antibiotic produced by *Streptomyces tenebrarius,* having bactericidal effects and used mainly in the treatment of *Pseudomonas* infections.

tocamphyl (tō-kam'fil). *p,α*-Dimethylbenzyl camphorate, diethanolamine salt; a choleretic.

tocainide hydrochloride (tō-kā-'nid). 2-Amino-2',6'-propionoxylidide hydrochloride; an oral antiarrhythmic agent, similar in action to lidocaine,used in the treatment of ventricular arryhthmias.

toco- [G. *tokos,* birth]. Combining form denoting childbirth.

tocochromanol-3 (tō'kō-krō'mă-nol). α-Tocotrienol.

tocodynagraph (tō-kō-dī'nă-graf, tok-ō-) [toco- + G. *dynamis,* force, + *graphē,* a writing]. Tocograph; a recording of the force of uterine contractions.

tocodynamometer (tō'kō-dī-nă-mom'ĕ-ter, tok'ō-) [toco- + G. *dynamis,* force, + *metron,* measure]. Tocometer; an instrument for measuring the force of uterine contractions.

tocograph (tō'kō-graf). Tocodynagraph.

tocography (tō-kog'ră-fē) [toco- + G. *graphō,* to write]. The process of recording uterine contractions.

tocol (tō'kol). Fundamental unit of the tocopherols; 6-phytylhydroquinone (see structure *A,* below) becomes, in the chromanol form, 2-methyl-2-(4,8,12-trimethyltridecyl)chroman-6-ol (structure *B*).

tocology (tō-kol'ō-jē) [toco- + G. *logos,* study]. Obstetrics.

tocolytic (tō-kō-lit'ik). Denoting any pharmacological agent used to arrest uterine contractions; often used in an attempt to arrest premature labor contractions.

tocometer (tō-kom'ĕ-ter). Tocodynamometer.

tocopherol (T) (tō-kof'er-ōl). **1.** Name given to vitamin E by its discoverer, but now a generic term for vitamin E and compounds chemically related to it, with or without biological activity; similar in chemical structure and properties to vitamins K and coenzyme Q. **2.** A methylated tocol or methylated tocotrienol.
mixed t.'s concentrate, a source of vitamin E, obtained by vacuum distillation of edible vegetable oils or their by-products.

α-tocopherol (α-T). Vitamin E (1);2,5,7,8-tetramethyl-2-(4',8',12'-trimethyltridecyl)-6-chromanol; 5,7,8-trimethyltocol; a light yellow, viscous, odorless, oily liquid that deteriorates on exposure to light, is obtained from wheat germ oil or by synthesis, biologically exhibits the most vitamin E activity of the t.'s, and is an antioxidant retarding rancidity by interfering with the autoxidation of fats. Prepared from natural phytol, it is called 2-*ambo*-α-tocopherol; from synthetic phytol, *all-rac*-α-tocopherol or *synt*-α-tocopherol; also available are *d*-α-tocopheryl acetate, *dl*-α-tocopheryl acetate, *d*-α-tocopheryl acid succinate, and *d*-α-tocopheryl acetate concentrate.

β-tocopherol (β-T). 5,8-Dimethyltocol; a lower homologue of α-tocopherol, that contains one less methyl group in the aromatic nucleus and is less active biologically; accompanies α-T and γ-T.

γ-tocopherol (γ-T). 7,8-Dimethyltocol; a form biologically less active than α-T.

tocopherolquinone (tō-kof'er-ol-kwī'nōn). Tocopherylquinone; an oxidized tocopherol, formed from the isomeric 2-methyl-2-phytyl-6-chromenol with methyl groups in one or more of positions 5,7, and 8, by migration of H atom from 6-OH to C-4, which yields a 1,4-benzoquinone. Abbreviated TQ and preceded by α-, β-, etc., as in the tocopherols, to indicate degree of methylation.

tocopherylquinone (tō-kof'er-il-kwī'nōn). Tocopherolquinone.

tocophobia (tō'kō-fō'bē-ă, tok'ō-) [toco- + G. *phobos,* fear]. Morbid dread of childbirth.

tocoquinone (tō-kō-kwī'nōn). Class name for the 2,3,5-trimethyl-6-multiprenyl-1,4-benzoquinones.

tocotrienol (tō-kō-trī'en-ol). A tocol with three double bonds in the side chain, *i.e.,* with three additional double bonds in the phytyl chain, thus a 6-(3',7',11',15'-tetramethyl-2',6',10',14'-hexadecatetraenyl)-1,4-hydroquinone or a 2-methyl-2-(4,8,12-trimethyltrideca-3,7,11-trienyl)chroman-6-ol. The natural products carry methyls at one or more of positions 5, 7, and 8 of the chromanol and are thus identical, except for the unsaturation in the phytyl-like side chain, to the tocopherols; also analogous is the cyclization to form a chromanol derivative and oxidation to form the tocotrienolquinones (or chromenols). Abbreviated T-*n* (hydroquinone form) or TQ-*n* (quinone form) and preceded by α-, β-, etc., as in the tocopherols, to indicate degree of methylation (the *n* indicates the number of intact isoprene or prenyl units remaining in the chromanol or chromenol form). T. terminology is used to indicate relationships to tocols and tocoenols (vitamin E-like), the chromanol terminology to indicate relationship to the isoprenoidal com-

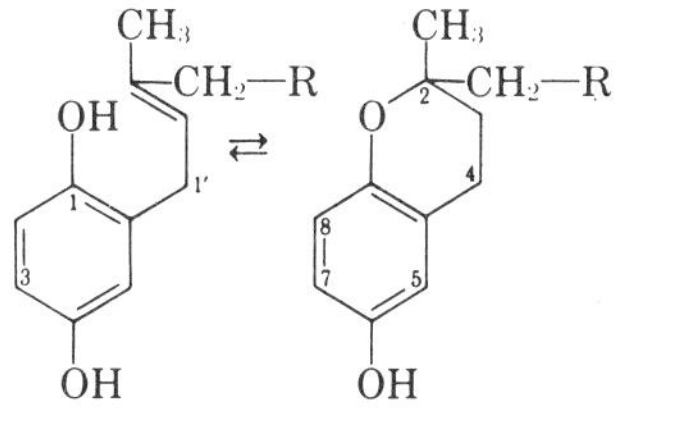

(A) (B)

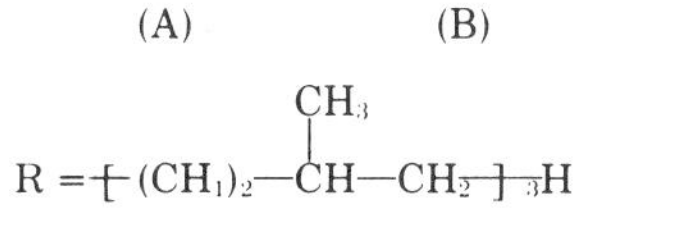

Tocol

pounds of the vitamin K and coenzyme Q series.

tocotrienolquinone (tō-kō-trī'en-ol-kwī'nōn). A tocotrienol in which the hydroquinone has been oxidized to a quinone (the chromanol has become a chromenol); the t.'s carry α, β, γ, and δ prefixes in accordance with the degree of methylation, as do the tocotrienols.

Tod, David, British surgeon, 1794–1856. See T.'s *muscle.*

Todaro, Francesco, Italian anatomist, 1839–1918. See T.'s *tendon.*

Todd, Robert B., English physician, 1809–1860. See T.'s *paralysis,* postepileptic *paralysis.*

toe (tō) [A.S. *ta*]. Digitus pedis; one of the digits of the feet.
great t., hallux.
hammer t., permanent flexion at the midphalangeal joint of one or more of the t.'s.
Hong Kong t., *tinea* pedis.
painful t., *hallux* dolorosus.
stiff t., *hallux* rigidus.
webbed t.'s, syndactyly involving the toes.

toe-crack (tō'krak'). See sand-crack.

toe-drop (tō'drop). A drooping of the anterior portion of the foot, due to paralysis of the muscles that dorsally flex the foot.

toenail (tō'nāl). See unguis.
ingrowing t., ingrown *nail.*

tofenacin hydrochloride (tō-fen'ă-sin). *N*-Methyl-2-[(*o*-methyl-α-phenylbenzyl)oxy]ethylamine hydrochloride; an anticholinergic drug.

Togaviridae (tō-gă-vir'i-dē). The family of viruses that includes the antigenic groups A and B arboviruses, which constitute the genera *Alphavirus* and *Flavivirus* respectively, the rubella virus (***Rubivirus***), hog cholera virus, and related cattle and pig viruses of the genus *Pestivirus.* Virions are 40 to 70 nm in diameter, enveloped, and ether-sensitive; the capsid is of icosahedral symmetry, containing probably 32 capsomeres; genomes contain single-stranded messenger RNA.

togavirus (tō'gă-vī'rŭs). Any virus of the family Togaviridae.

toilet (toy-let') [Fr. *toilette*]. **1.** Cleansing of the obstetrical patient after childbirth or of a wound after an operation preparatory to the application of the dressing. **2.** In dentistry, cavity debridement, the final step before placing a restoration in a tooth whereby the cavity is cleaned and all debris is removed.

Toison, J., French histologist, 1858–1950. See T.'s *stain.*

toko-. See toco-.

tolazamide (tō-laz'ă-mīd). 1-(Hexahydro-1*H*-azeprin-1-yl)-3-(*p*-tolylsulfonyl)urea; an oral hypoglycemic agent similar in use to tolbutamide.

tolazoline hydrochloride (tō-laz'ō-lēn). 2-Benzyl-2-imidazoline hydrochloride; an adrenergic α-receptor blocking agent used to augment blood flow in peripheral vascular disorders.

tolbutamide (tol-byū'tă-mīd). 1-Butyl-3-*p*- tolylsulfonylurea; an orally active hypoglycemic agent used in the management of adult-onset diabetes mellitus; it appears to stimulate the synthesis and release of endogenous insulin from functional islets; available as t. sodium for injection.

tolcyclamide (tol-sī'klă-mīd). Glycyclamide.

Toldt, Karl, Austrian anatomist, 1840–1920. See T.'s *fascia, membrane.*

tolerance (tol'er-ăns) [L. *tolero,* pp. *-atus,* to endure]. **1.** The ability to endure or be less responsive to a stimulus, especially over a period of continued exposure. **2.** The power of resisting the action of a poison, or of taking a drug continuously or in large doses without injurious effects.
acoustic t., the maximum sound pressure level that can be experienced without producing pain or permanent defect of hearing in a normal individual.
cross t., the resistance to one or several effects of a compound as a result of t. developed to a pharmacologically similar compound.
frustration t., the level of an individual's ability to withstand frustration without developing inadequate modes of response, such as "going to pieces" emotionally or becoming neurotic.
immunological t., immunotolerance; acquired, specific failure of the immunological mechanism to respond, induced by exposure to the given antigen.
individual t., t. to a drug that the person has never received before.
pain t., the greatest intensity of painful stimulation that an individual is able to tolerate.
species t., the insensitivity to a particular drug exhibited by a particular species.
split t., immune *deviation.*
vibration t., the maximum vibratory or oscillatory movements that an individual can experience and bear without pain; the limit of t. is a function of amplitude and frequency of the vibration and varies with the direction of application.

tolerant (tol'er-ănt). Having the property of tolerance.

tolerogenic (tol'er-ō-jen'ik). Producing immunologic tolerance.

tolhexamide (tol-hek'să-mīd). Glycyclamide.

tolmetin (tol'met-in). 1-Methyl-5-*p*-toluoylpyrrole-2-acetic acid; an anti-inflammatory drug used in the treatment of rheumatoid arthritis.

tolnaftate (tol-naf'tāt). *o*- 2-Naphthyl *m,N*-dimethylthiocarbanilate; a topical antifungal agent.

tolonium chloride (tō-lō'nē-ŭm). 3-Amino-7-dimethylamino-2-methylphenazothionium chloride; the medicinal grade of toluidine blue O, used as an antiheparin compound.

Tolosa, E., 20th century Spanish neurosurgeon. See T.-Hunt *syndrome.*

tolpropamine (tol-prō'pă-mēn). *N,N*-Dimethyl-3-phenyl-3-*p*-tolylpropylamine; a topical antipruritic agent.

toluene (tol'yū-ēn). Toluol; methylbenzene; a colorless liquid obtained by the dry distillation of tolu and other resinous bodies, and also derived from coal tar; its physical and chemical properties resemble those of benzene. Used in explosives and dyes, and in the extraction of various principles from plants.

toluic acid (tō-lū'ik). Methylbenzoic acid; $CH_3C_6H_4COOH$; an oxidation product of xylene.

toluidine (tō-lū'i-dēn, -din). Aminotoluene; one of three isomeric substances, $CH_3C_6H_4NH_2$, derived from toluene.
alkaline t. blue O, t. blue O in borax solution, used with heat on semithick sections of epoxy embedded tissues.
t. blue O [C.I. 52040], a blue basic dye, $C_{15}H_{16}N_3SCl$, used as an antibacterial agent, as a nuclear stain, and to stain metachromatically certain structures (*e.g.,* the granules in mast cells which are believed to contain heparin and cartilage matrix which is rich in chondroitin sulfate), and in electrophoresis to stain RNA, RNase, and mucopolysaccharides; it also antagonizes the anticoagulant action of heparin. See also tolonium chloride.

toluol (tol'ū-ol). Toluene.

toluoyl (tol-ū'ō-il). $CH_3C_6H_4CO$–; the radical of toluic acid.

toluylene red (tol-ū'i-lēn). Neutral red.

tolyl (tol'il). $CH_3C_6H_4$–; the univalent radical of toluene.

Toma's sign. See under sign.

-tome [G. *tomos,* cutting, sharp; a cutting (section or segment)]. Suffix denoting: **1.** A cutting instrument, the first element in the compound usually indicating the part that the instrument is designed to cut. **2.** Segment, part, section.

tomentum, tomentum cerebri (tō-men'tŭm, tō-men'tŭm ser'ĕ-brī) [L. a stuffing for cushions]. The numerous small blood vessels passing between the cerebral surface of the pia mater and the cortex of the brain.

Tomes, Sir Charles S., British dentist, 1846–1928. See T.'s *processes.*

Tomes, Sir John, British dentist and anatomist, 1815–1895. See T.'s *fibers,* granular *layer.*

Tommaselli, Salvatore, Italian physician, 1834–1906. See T.'s *disease.*

tomogram (tō'mō-gram) [G. *tomos,* a cutting (section) + *gramma,* a writing]. The roentgenogram obtained by tomography.

tomograph (tō'mō-graf) [G. *tomos,* a cutting (section), + *graphō,* to write]. The radiographic equipment used in tomography.

tomography (tō-mog'ră-fē). Sectional roentgenography; planigraphy; planography; stratigraphy; laminagraphy; the taking of sectional roentgenograms by having the x-ray tube in a curvilinear motion synchronous with reciprocal film motion while the patient remains motionless; the selected plane for imaging remains stationary on the moving film while the structures in all other planes have a relative displacement on the film and are therefore obliterated or blurred.

computed t. (CT), computerized axial t.; the gathering of anatomical information from a cross-sectional plane of the body, presented as an image generated by a computer synthesis of x-ray transmission data obtained in many different directions through the given plane.

computerized axial t. (CAT), computed t.

hypocycloidal t., body section radiography using a complex film and tube motion with a pattern resembling a three-leaf clover.

positron emission t. (PET), tomographic imaging of local metabolic and physiological functions in tissues, the image being formed by computer synthesis of data transmitted by positron-emitting radionuclides, often incorporated into natural biochemical substances and administered to the patient; a computer traces the path of photons (produced by the collision of positrons emitted by the radioactive biochemical with the negatively charged electrons normally present in the tissue cells) and produces a composite image, often in color, representing the metabolism level of the biochemicals in the tissue, as an indicator of the presence or absence of disease.

single photon emission computed t. (SPECT), tomographic imaging of local metabolic and physiological functions in tissues, the image being formed by computer synthesis of data transmitted by single gamma photons emitted by radionucleides administered in suitable form to the patient.

tomolevel (tō'mō-lev-el). The level at which tomography is performed.

tomomania (tō-mō-mā'nē-ă) [G. *tomos,* cutting, + *mania,* frenzy]. An irrational desire to use operative procedures by a doctor or a patient.

-tomy [G. *tomē,* incision]. Termination denoting a cutting operation. See also -ectomy.

tonaphasia (tōn-ă-fā'zē-ă) [G. *tonos,* tone, + *a-* priv. + *phasis,* speech]. Loss, through cerebral lesion, of the ability to remember tunes.

tone (tōn) [G. *tonos,* tone, or a tone]. **1.** A musical sound. **2.** The character of the voice expressing an emotion. **3.** The tension present in resting muscles. **4.** Firmness of the tissues; normal functioning of all the organs. **5.** To perform toning.

affective t., emotional t., feeling t.

feeling t., emotional or affective t.; affectivity; the mental state (pleasure, repugnance, etc.) that accompanies every act or thought.

fundamental t., the component of lowest frequency in a complex t.

Traube's double t., a double sound heard on auscultation over the femoral vessels in cases of aortic and tricuspid insufficiency.

toner (tō'ner). A solution used in toning.

tongue (tŭng) [A.S. *tunge*]. Lingua (1).

baked t., the dry blackish t. noted when patients with typhoid fever or other disorders are allowed to become dehydrated.

bald t., atrophic *glossitis.*

beet-t., sometimes used of the t. in pellagra, where intense erythema appears, first at the tip, then along the edges, and finally over the dorsum; there may be pain and increased elevation; the shiny appearance results from edema, not atrophy, except in chronic pellagra.

bifid t., cleft t.; a structural defect of the t. in which the extremity is divided longitudinally for a greater or lesser distance. See diglossia.

black t., nigrities linguae; melanoglossia; lingua nigra; black to yellowish brown discoloration of the dorsum of the t. due to staining by exogenous material such as the components of tobacco; usually superimposed on hairy t.

t. of cerebellum, *lingula* cerebelli.

cleft t., bifid t.

coated t., furred t.; a t. with a whitish layer on its upper surface, composed of epithelial debris, food particles, and bacteria; often an indication of indigestion or of fever.

dotted t., stippled t.; one in which each separate papilla is capped with a whitish deposit.

fissured t., lingua fissurata or plicata; furrowed, grooved, or scrotal t.; a painless condition of the t. characterized by numerous grooves or furrows on the dorsal surface.

furred t., coated t.

geographic t., asymptomatic erythematous circinate macules, often bounded peripherally by a white band, as a result of atrophy of the filiform papillae; with time the lesions resolve, coalesce, and change in distribution. Also called benign migratory glossitis; lingua geographica or dissecta; pityriasis linguae; glossitis areata exfoliativa; erythema migrans or migrans linguae.

grooved t., fissured t.

hairy t., glossotrichia; trichoglossia; a t. with abnormal elongation of the filiform papillae, resulting in a thickened furry appearance.

hobnail t., interstitial glossitis with hypertrophy and verrucous changes in papillae; seen in some cases of late acquired syphilis.

magenta t., purplish red coloration of the t., with edema and flattening of the filiform papillae, occurring in riboflavin deficiency. *Cf.* cyanosis.

mandibular t., *lingula* mandibulae.

raspberry t., strawberry t. that is a dark red color.

scrotal t., fissured t.

smoker's t., obsolete term for leukoplakia.

stippled t., dotted t.

strawberry t., a t. with a whitish coat through which the enlarged fungiform papillae project as red points, characteristic of scarlet fever and of mucocutaneous lymph node syndrome.

wooden t. of cattle, actinobacillosis.

tongue crib. An appliance used to control visceral (infantile) swallowing and tongue thrusting and to encourage the mature or somatic tongue posture and function.

tongue-swallowing. A slipping back of the tongue against the pharynx, causing choking.

tongue thrust. The infantile pattern of the suckle-swallow movement in which the tongue is placed between the incisor teeth or the alveolar ridges during the initial stage of swallowing, resulting sometimes in an anterior open bite.

tongue-tie. Ankyloglossia; abnormal shortness of the frenulum linguae.

tonic (ton'ik) [G. *tonikos,* fr. *tonos,* tone]. **1.** In a state of continuous unremitting action; denoting especially a muscular contraction. **2.** Invigorating; increasing physical or mental tone or strength. **3.** A remedy purported to restore enfeebled function and promote vigor and a sense of well being; qualified, according to the organ or system on which they are presumed to act, as cardiac, digestive, hematic, vascular, nervine, uterine, general, etc.

bitter t., a t. of bitter taste, such as quinine, gentian, quassia, etc., which acts chiefly by stimulating the appetite and improving digestion.

tonicity (tō-nis'i-tē) [G. *tonos,* tone]. **1.** Tonus; a state of normal tension of the tissues by virtue of which the parts are kept in shape, alert, and ready to function in response to a suitable stimulus. In the case of muscle, it refers to a state of continuous activity or tension beyond that related to the physical properties; *i.e.,* it is active resistance to stretch; in skeletal muscle it is dependent upon the efferent innervation. **2.** The osmotic pressure or tension of a solution, usually relative to that of blood. See also isotonicity.

tonicoclonic (ton-i-kō-klon'ik). Tonoclonic; both tonic and clonic, referring to muscular spasms.

tonin (tō'nin). An enzyme converting angiotensin I to angiotensin II, thus similar to or identical with angiotensin-converting enzyme.

toning (tōn'ing). The replacing of a silver deposit with one of gold in an impregnated histologic section, by treatment with a solution of gold chloride.

tonitrophobia (tō'ni-trō-fō'bē-ă) [L. *tonitrus,* thunder, + G. *phobos,* fear]. Brontophobia.

tono- [G. *tonos,* tone, tension]. Combining form relating to tone, tension, pressure.

tonoclonic (ton-ō-klon'ik). Tonicoclonic.

tonofibril (ton-ō-fī'bril). Epitheliofibril; tenofibril; one of a system of fibers found in the cytoplasm of epithelial cells. See cytoskeleton.

tonofilament (ton-ō-fil'ă-ment). A structural cytoplasmic protein, of a class known as intermediate filaments, bundles of which together form a tonofibril; a t. is made up of a variable number or related proteins, keratins, and is found in all epithelial cells, but is particularly well developed in the epidermis.

tonograph (ton'ō-graf, tō'nō-) [tono- + G. *graphō,* to write]. A recording tonometer.

tonography (tō-nog'ră-fē). Continuous measurement of intraocular pressure by means of a recording tonometer, in order to determine the facility of aqueous outflow.

tonometer (tō-nom'ĕ-ter) [tono- + G. *metron,* measure]. **1.** Tenonometer; an instrument for determining pressure or tension, especially an instrument for determining ocular tension. **2.** Aerotonometer (2); a vessel for equilibrating a liquid (*e.g.,* blood) with a gas, usually at a controlled temperature; originally so named because it was used with a very small gas/blood ratio to allow the gas to approach blood oxygen tension and thus serve as a measure of it; now commonly used with a very large gas/blood ratio to adjust the blood to the oxygen pressure of the gas.

applanation t., an instrument for determining ocular tension by application of a small flat disk to the cornea.

Gärtner's t., an apparatus for estimating the blood pressure by noting the force, expressed by the height of a column of mercury, needed to arrest pulsation in a finger encircled by a compressing ring.

Goldmann's applanation t., an applanation t. that flattens only 3 sq mm of cornea, used with a slitlamp.

Mackay-Marg t., a recording electronic applanation t.

Mueller electronic t., a Schiötz type t. that electronically indicates the extent of corneal indentation; may also have an attached recorder for continuous pressure readings (tonography).

pneumatic t., a recording applanation t. operated by compressed gas.

Schiötz t., an instrument that measures ocular tension by indicating the ease with which the cornea is indented.

tonometry (tō-nom'ĕ-trē). **1.** Measurement of the tension of a part, *e.g.,* intravascular tension or blood pressure. **2.** Measurement of ocular tension.

tonophant (tō'nō-fant, ton'ō-) [tono- + G. *phainō,* to appear]. An instrument for visualizing sound waves.

tonoplast (tō'nō-plast, ton'ō-) [tono- + G. *plastos,* formed]. An intracellular structure or vacuole.

tonoscillograph (tō-nos'i-lō-graf) [tono- + L. *oscillo,* to swing, + G. *graphō,* to write]. An instrument that produces graphic records of arterial and capillary pressures as well as of individual pulse characters.

tonotopic (tō-nō-top'ik). Denoting a spatial arrangement of structures such that certain tone frequencies are transmitted, as in the auditory pathway.

tonotropic (tō-nō-trop'ik) [G. *tonikos, tonos,* tone, + *tropos,* a turning]. Denoting the shortening of the resting length of a muscle.

tonsil (ton'sil) [L. *tonsilla,* a stake, in pl. the tonsils]. **1.** Tonsilla. **2.** *Tonsilla* palatina.

cerebellar t., *tonsilla* cerebelli.

eustachian t., *tonsilla* tubaria.

faucial t., *tonsilla* palatina.

Gerlach's t., *tonsilla* tubaria.

laryngeal t.'s, *folliculi* lymphatici laryngei.

lingual t., *tonsilla* lingualis.

Luschka's t., *tonsilla* pharyngea.

palatine t., *tonsilla* palatina.

pharyngeal t., *tonsilla* pharyngea.

submerged t., a faucial t. that is flat and lying below the level of the pillars of the fauces.

third t., *tonsilla* pharyngea.

tubal t., *tonsilla* tubaria.

tonsilla, pl. **tonsillae** (ton-sil'ă, -ē) [L. (see tonsil)] [NA]. Tonsil (1); amygdala (2); any collection of lymphoid tissue.

t. cerebel'li [NA], cerebellar tonsil; amygdala cerebelli; a rounded lobule on the undersurface of each cerebellar hemisphere, continuous medially with the uvula of the cerebellar vermis.

t. intestina'lis, see *folliculi* lymphatici aggregati.

t. lingua'lis [NA], lingual tonsil; a collection of lymphoid follicles on the posterior or pharyngeal portion of the dorsum of the tongue.

t. palati'na [NA], faucial or palatine tonsil; tonsil (2); a large oval mass of lymphoid tissue embedded in the lateral wall of the oral pharynx on either side between the pillars of the fauces.

t. pharyn'gea [NA], pharyngeal tonsil; third tonsil; Luschka's tonsil; Luschka's gland (1); a collection of more or less closely aggregated lymphoid nodules on the posterior wall of the nasopharynx, the hypertrophy of which constitutes the morbid condition called adenoids.

t. tuba'ria [NA], tubal tonsil; Gerlach's or eustachian tonsil; a collection of lymphoid nodules near the pharyngeal opening of the auditory tube.

tonsillar, tonsillary (ton'si-lăr, ton'si-lă-rē). Amygdaline (3); relating to a tonsil, especially the palatine tonsil.

tonsillectomy (ton'si-lek'tō-mē) [tonsil + G. *ektomē,* excision]. Removal of the entire tonsil.

tonsillith (ton'si-lith). Tonsillolith.

tonsillitis (ton'si-lī'tis) [tonsil + G. *-itis,* inflammation]. Inflammation of a tonsil, especially of the palatine tonsil.

lacunar t., inflammation of the mucous membrane lining the tonsillar crypts.

parenchymatous t., inflammation of the entire substance of the faucial tonsil, often passing into quinsy.

superficial t., inflammation simply of the mucous membrane covering the tonsil.

Vincent's t., angina limited chiefly to the tonsils, caused by Vincent's organisms (bacillus and spirillum).

tonsillo- [L. *tonsilla,* tonsil]. Combining form denoting tonsil.

tonsillolith (ton-sil'ō-lith) [tonsillo- + G. *lithos,* stone]. Tonsillar calculus; tonsillith; a calcareous concretion in a distended tonsillar crypt.

tonsillopathy (ton'si-lop'ă-thē) [tonsillo- + G. *pathos,* suffering]. Disease of the tonsil.

tonsillotome (ton-sil'ō-tōm) [tonsillo- + G. *tomos,* cutting]. An instrument, sometimes modelled after a guillotine, for use in cutting away a portion or all of a hypertrophied tonsil.

tonsillotomy (ton'si-lot'ō-mē) [tonsillo- + G. *tomē,* incision]. The cutting away of a portion or all of a hypertrophied faucial tonsil.

tonus (tō'nŭs) [L., fr. G. *tonos*]. Tonicity (1).

baseline t., uterine tension between contractions during labor.

Tooth, Howard H., British physician, 1856–1925. See Charcot-Marie-T. *disease.*

TOOTH

tooth, pl. **teeth** (tūth, tēth) [A.S. *tōth*]. Dens (1); one of the hard conical structures set in the alveoli of the upper and lower jaws, used in mastication and assisting in articulation. A t. is a dermal structure composed of dentin (dentinum) and encased in cement (cementum) on the covered portion and enamel (enamelum) on its exposed portion. It consists of a root (radix) buried in the alveolus, a neck (collum) covered by the gum, and a crown (corona), the exposed portion. In the center is the pulp cavity (cavum dentis) filled with a connective tissue reticulum containing a jelly-like substance (pulpa dentis) and blood vessels and nerves which enter through a canal at the apex of the root. The 20 deciduous teeth or primary teeth appear between the sixth or ninth and the 24th month of life; these exfoliate and are replaced by the 32 permanent teeth appearing from the fifth or seventh to the 17th or 23rd year. There are four kinds of teeth: incisor (dens incisivus), canine (dens caninus), premolar (dens premolaris), and molar (dens molaris). See also subentries under dens.

acrylic resin t., a t. made of acrylic resin.

anatomic teeth, artificial teeth that duplicate the anatomic forms of natural teeth.

ankylosed t., see dental *ankylosis.*

anterior teeth, oral teeth; the central incisor, lateral incisor, and cuspid teeth, which comprise the organs for incision and are located in the front portion of the jaws.

auditory teeth, *dentes* acustici.

baby t., *dens* deciduus.

back teeth, all teeth posterior to the canines.

bicuspid t., *dens* premolaris.

buck t., an anterior t. in labioversion.

canine t., *dens* caninus.

carnassial t., **(1)** a t. adapted to shear flesh; **(2)** the last upper premolar or first lower molar t. of certain carnivores.

cheek t., *dens* molaris.

Corti's auditory teeth, *dentes* acustici.

cross-bite teeth, posterior teeth designed to permit the modified cusps of the upper teeth to be positioned in the fossae of the lower teeth.

cuspid t., cuspidate t., *dens* caninus.

cuspless t., **(1)** a t. devoid of cusp formation; **(2)** severe abrasion of an occlusal surface; **(3)** a type of artificial denture t.

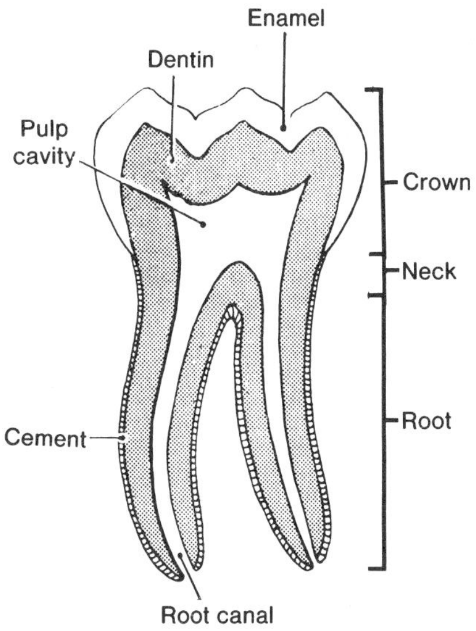

Tooth
Cross section of a human molar.

cutting teeth, the maxillary and mandibular anterior teeth.

dead t., a misnomer for pulpless t.

deciduous t., *dens* deciduus.

devitalized t., a misnomer for an extirpated pulpless t.

extruded teeth, See *extrusion* of a tooth.

eye t., *dens* caninus.

fluoridated teeth, teeth exposed to fluorine salts during odontogenesis.

fused teeth, teeth joined by dentin as a result of embryological fusion or juxtaposition of two adjacent tooth germs.

geminated teeth, a developmental anomaly arising from the attempted division of one t. bud, resulting in incomplete formation of two teeth and usually manifest as a bifid crown upon a single root.

ghost t., a t. with reduced radiodensity seen in regional odontodysplasia.

green t., green to brown discoloration of the primary teeth associated with erythroblastosis fetalis and caused by deposition of hemoglobin pigments into the developing teeth.

Horner's teeth, incisor teeth having a horizontal hypoplastic groove.

Huschke's auditory teeth, *dentes* acustici.

Hutchinson's teeth, notched, screwdriver, or syphilitic teeth; the teeth of congenital syphilis in which the incisal edge is notched and narrower than the cervical area. See also Hutchinson's crescentic *notch.*

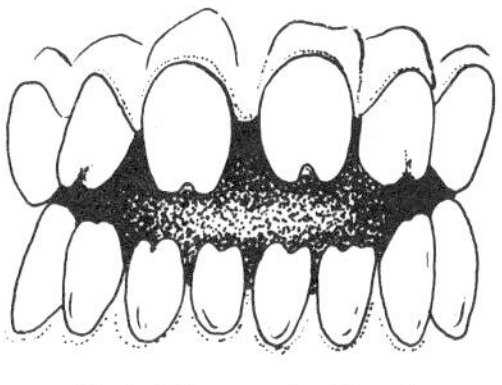

Hutchinsons's Teeth

impacted t., **(1)** a t. whose normal eruption is prevented by adjacent teeth or bone; **(2)** a t. that has been driven into the alveolar process or surrounding tissue as a result of trauma.

incisor t., *dens* incisivus.
metal insert teeth, prosthetic teeth containing metal cutting surfaces in the occlusal surfaces.
migrating teeth, teeth which are changing position under natural forces.
milk t., *dens* deciduus.
molar t., *dens* molaris.
mottled t., see mottled *enamel.*
multicuspid t., *dens* molaris.
natal t., a predeciduous supernumerary t. present at birth.
neonatal t., a t. erupting up to 30 days after birth.
nonanatomic teeth, **(1)** teeth with occlusal surfaces not based on anatomic forms; **(2)** artificial teeth so designed that the occlusal surfaces are not copied from natural forms, but rather are given forms which in the opinion of the designer seem more nearly to fulfill the requirements of mastication, tissue tolerance, etc.
nonvital t., a t. with a nonvital pulp.
normally posed t., a t. in correct spatial relationship with its antagonist.
notched teeth, Hutchinson's teeth.
oral teeth, anterior teeth.
pegged t., a conical t. whose sides converge from the cervical to the incisal region.
permanent t., *dens* permanens.
perpetually growing t., persistently growing t., a physiologic phenomenon whereby the t. continually or constantly grows, calcifies, and erupts; *e.g.,* the rat incisor t.
plastic teeth, artificial teeth constructed of synthetic resins.
posterior teeth, the bicuspid and molar teeth which comprise the organs of mastication and are located in the back part of the jaws.
premolar t., *dens* premolaris.
primary t., *dens* deciduus.
protruding teeth, teeth extending beyond the normal contour of the dental arches; usually in an anterior direction.
pulpless t., a t. with a nonvital or necrotic pulp, or one from which the pulp has been extirpated.
sclerotic teeth, teeth that are naturally hard and resistant to caries.
screwdriver teeth, Hutchinson's teeth.
second t., *dens* permanens.
spaced teeth, teeth which have separated and lost proximal contact with adjacent teeth.
stomach t., one of the lower canine teeth.
succedaneous t., *dens* permanens.
syphilitic teeth, Hutchinson's teeth.
temporary t., *dens* deciduus.
triangularity of the teeth, a well-marked indication of advancing age in the horse, shown by increasing depth from front to rear in the occlusal surfaces of the incisor teeth; at nine years, when the marks fail, this sign is of use in determining the age of the animal.
tricuspid t., a t. having a crown with three cusps.
tube teeth, artificial teeth constructed with a vertical, cylindric aperture extending from the center of the base up into the body of the t. into which a pin may be placed or cast for the attachment of the t. to a denture base.
Turner's t., enamel hypoplasia involving a solitary permanent t.; related to infection in the primary t. that preceded it or to trauma during odontogenesis.
unerupted t., **(1)** a t. prior to emergence; **(2)** a t. unable to break out or emerge from the dental alveolar tissues into the oral cavity.
vital t., a t. with a living pulp.
wisdom t., *dens* serotinus.
wolf t., a rudimentary first premolar t. of the horse, usually appearing in the upper jaw.
zero degree teeth, prosthetic teeth having no cusp angles in relation to the horizontal.

toothache (tūth'āk). Dentalgia; odontalgia; odontodynia; pain in a tooth due to the condition of the pulp or periodontal membrane resulting from caries, infection, or trauma.

tooth arrangement. Articulation (5). **1.** The placement of teeth on a denture base with definite objectives in mind. **2.** The setting of teeth on temporary bases.

tooth-borne. A term used to describe a prosthesis or part of a prosthesis which depends entirely upon the abutment teeth for support.

top-. See topo-.

topagnosis (top-ag-nō'sis) [top- + G. *a-* priv. + *gnosis,* recognition]. Topoanesthesia; inability to localize tactile sensations.

topalgia (tō-pal'jē-ă) [top- + G. *algos,* pain]. Pain localized in one spot; a symptom occurring in neuroses whereby localized pain, without evident organic basis, is experienced.

topectomy (tō-pek'tō-mē) [top- + G. *ektomē,* excision]. Corticectomy; frontal gyrectomy; removal of a specific portion of the cerebral cortex.

topesthesia (top'es-thē'zē-ă) [top- + G. *aisthēsis,* sensation]. The ability to localize a light touch applied to any part of the skin.

Töpfer, Alfred E., German physician, *1858. See T.'s *test.*

tophaceous (tō-fā'shŭs) [L. *tophaceus*]. Sandy; gritty; pertaining to or manifesting the features of a tophus.

tophi (tō'fī). Plural of tophus.

tophus, pl. tophi (tō'fŭs, tō'fī) [L. a calcareous deposit from springs, tufa]. **1.** See gouty t. **2.** A salivary calculus, or tartar.
gouty t., arthritic calculus; uratoma; a deposit of uric acid and urates in periarticular fibrous tissue, cartilage of the external ear, or kidney, in gout.

topica (top'i-kă) [neut. pl. of Mod. L. *topicus,* local]. Remedies for local external use.

topical (top'i-kăl) [G. *topikos,* fr. *topos,* place]. Relating to a definite place or locality; local.

Topinard, Paul, French anthropologist, 1830–1912. See T.'s facial *angle, line.*

topistic (tō-pis'tik) [G. *topos,* place]. Denoting an anatomically defined region in the nervous system.

topo-, top- [G. *topos,* place]. Combining forms denoting place, topical.

topoanesthesia (top'ō-an-es-thē'zē-ă, tō'pō-) [topo- + anesthesia]. Topagnosis.

topognosis, topognosia (top-og-nō'sis, -nō'zē-ă) [topo- + G. *gnōsis,* knowledge]. Recognition of the location of a sensation; in the case of touch, topesthesia.

topogometer (top-ō-gom'ĕ-ter) [topo- + G. *gonia,* angle, + *metron,* measure]. A movable fixation target attached to the front of a keratometer, used in fitting contact lenses to measure the curvatures of the cornea in its peripheral zones.

topography (tō-pog'ră-fē) [topo- + G. *graphē,* a writing]. In anatomy, the description of any part of the body, especially in relation to a definite and limited area of the surface.

Topolanski, Alfred, Austrian ophthalmologist, 1861–1960. See T.'s *sign.*

topology (tō-pol'ō-jē) [topo- + G. *logos,* study]. **1.** Regional *anatomy.* **2.** The study of the dimensions of personality.

toponarcosis (top'ō-nar-kō'sis) [topo- + narcosis]. A localized cutaneous anesthesia.

toponym (tō'pō-nim) [topo- + G. *onyma,* name]. A regional term; one designating a region as distinguished from the name of a structure, system, or organ.

toponymy (tō-pon'i-mē) [topo- + G. *onyma,* name]. Topical or regional nomenclature, as distinguished from organonymy.

topopathogenesis (tō'pō-path-ō-jen'ĕ-sis) [topo- + pathogenesis]. Topography of lesions related to their pathogenesis.

topophobia (tō-pō-fō'bē-ă) [topo- + G. *phobos,* fear]. A neurotic dread of or related to a particular place or locality.

topophylaxis (tō'pō-fi-lak'sis) [topo- + G. *phylaxis,* protection]. Prevention of arsphenamine shock by a tourniquet applied to the limb above the site of injection, and its slow release 5 or 6 minutes later.

toposcope (top'ō-skōp) [topo- + G. *skopeō,* to view]. An apparatus to project the electrical activity of the cerebral cortex as a spatial coordinate visual system.

topothermesthesiometer (top'ō-therm'es-thē-zē-om'ĕ-ter) [topo- + G. *thermē,* heat, + *aisthēsis,* sensation, + *metron,* measure]. A device for determining the temperature sense in different parts of the surface.

TORCH Acronym for *t*oxoplasmosis, *o*ther infections, *r*ubella, *c*ytomegalorvirus infection, and *h*erpes simplex. See TORCH *syndrome.*

torcular herophili (tōr'kyū-lăr hĕ-rof'i-lī) [L. wine-press of *Herophilus,* fr. *torqueo,* to twist]. *Confluens* sinuum.

Torek, Franz J.A., U.S. surgeon, 1861–1938. See T. *operation.*

toric (tō'rik). Relating to, or having the curvature of, a torus.

Torkildsen, Arne, 20th century Norwegian neurosurgeon. See T. *shunt.*

Tornwaldt, Gustavus Ludwig, German physician, 1843–1910. See T.'s *abscess, cyst, disease, syndrome.*

torose, torous (tō'rōs, -rŭs) [L. *torosus,* fleshy, fr. *torus,* a knot, bulge]. Bulging; tubercular; knobby.

torpent (tōr'pent) [L. *torpeo,* pres. p. *-ens,* to be sluggish]. **1.** Torpid. **2.** A benumbing agent.

torpid (tōr'pid) [L. *torpidus,* fr. *torpeo,* to be sluggish]. Torpent (1); inactive; sluggish.

torpidity (tōr-pid'i-tē). Torpor.

torpor (tōr'per, pōr) [L. sluggishness, numbness]. Inactivity, sluggishness.
t. ret'inae, a form of nyctalopia, the retina responding only to bright luminous stimuli.

torque (tōrk) [L. *torqueo,* to twist]. **1.** A rotatory force. **2.** In dentistry, a torsion force applied to a tooth to produce or maintain crown or root movement.

torr (tōr) [Evangelista *Torricelli,* Italian scientist, 1608–1647]. A unit of pressure sufficient to support a 1-mm column of mercury at 0°C against the standard acceleration of gravity at 45° north latitude (980.6 cm/sec^2); equivalent to 1333.22 $dynes/cm^2$, 1.333 millibars, 1.36 cm H_2O, 133.322 $newtons/m^2$; one standard atmosphere equals 760 t.

Torre, Douglas P., U.S. dermatologist, *1919. See T.'s *syndrome.*

torrefaction (tōr-ē-fak'shŭn) [L. *torre-facio,* pp. *-factus,* to make dry by heat, fr. *torreo,* to parch]. Parching or drying by heat; a pharmaceutical operation for rendering drugs friable.

torrefy (tōr'ē-fī). To parch.

torsade de pointes (tōr-sahd-dĕ-pwant') [Fr. *torsade,* fringe, twist, or coil, + *pointe,* point or tip (euphonious for "wave burst")]. Paroxysms of ventricular tachycardia in which the electrocardiogram shows a steady undulation in the QRS axis in runs of 5 to 20 beats with progressive changes in direction.

torsiometer (tōr-si-om'ĕ-ter). An instrument for measuring ocular torsion, cycloductions, and cyclophorias.

torsion (tōr'shŭn) [L. *torsio,* fr. *torqueo,* to twist]. **1.** A twisting or rotation of a part upon its long axis. **2.** Twisting of the cut end of an artery to arrest hemorrhage. **3.** Rotation of the eye around its anteroposterior axis. See also intorsion; extorsion; dextrotorsion; levotorsion.
t. of testis, rotation producing ischemia of testis.
t. of a tooth, rotation of a tooth in its socket.

torsionometer (tōr-shŭn-om'ĕ-ter). A device for measuring the degree of rotation of the spinal column.

torsiversion (tōr-si-ver'shŭn). Torsive occlusion; torsoclusion (2); a malposition of a tooth in which it is rotated on its long axis.

torso (tōr'sō) [It.]. The trunk; the body without relation to head or extremities.

torsoclusion (tōr'sō-klū-zhŭn) [L. *torqueo,* to twist, + *claudo* or *cludo,* to close]. **1.** Acupressure performed by entering the needle in the tissues parallel with the artery, then turning it so that it crosses the artery transversely, and passing it into the tissues on the opposite side of the vessel. **2.** Torsiversion.

torticollar (tōr-ti-kol'ăr). Relating to or marked by torticollis.

torticollis (tōr-ti-kol'is) [L. *tortus,* twisted, + *collum,* neck]. Collum distortum; accessory cramp; loxia; wryneck; stiff neck; a contraction, often spasmodic, of the muscles of the neck, chiefly those supplied by the spinal accessory nerve; the head is drawn to one side and usually rotated so that the chin points to the other side.

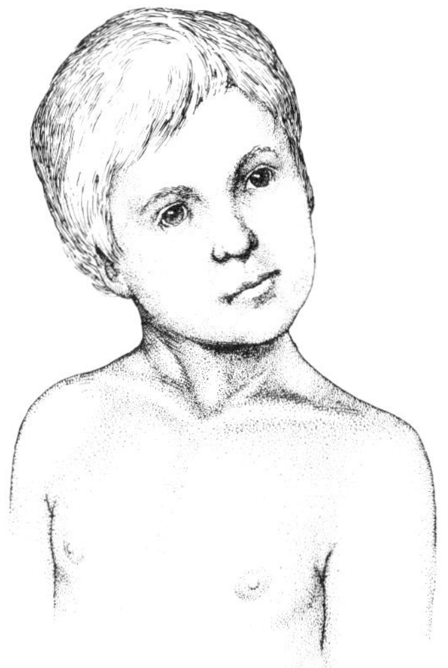

Torticollis

congenital t., fibromatosis colli; t. due to a unilateral fibrous tumor in the sternocleidomastoid muscle, present at birth as a swelling that may subside or may lead to t. by shortening of the muscle.
dermatogenic t., painful stiff neck with limitation of motion due to extensive skin lesion in the area.
dystonic t., spasmodic t.
fixed t., persistent contracture of cervical muscles on one side.
intermittent t., t. spastica.
labyrinthine t., t. due to vestibular disorder.
ocular t., t. incident to paralysis of an extraocular muscle, especially an oblique muscle.
psychogenic t., spasmodic contractions of the neck muscles, of psychosomatic origin. See also spasmodic t.
rheumatic t., symptomatic t.
spasmodic t., rotatory spasm or tic; dystonic t.; rotatory spasm of the head on the neck due to intermittent contraction of the neck muscles.
t. spas'tica, intermittent t.; stiff neck due to hypertonicity of the neck muscles.

spurious t., stiffness of the neck due to caries, malformation, or fracture of the cervical vertebrae.

symptomatic t., rheumatic t.; stiff neck due to cervical or neck myositis, chiefly of the sternocleidomastoid, occurring especially in children.

tortipelvis (tōr-ti-pel'vis). Twisted pelvis.

tortuous (tōr'chū-ŭs) [L. *tortuosus,* fr. *torqueo,* to twist]. Having many curves; full of turns and twists.

toruloma (tōr-yū-lō'mă) [fr. *Torula,* old name for *Cryptococcus,* + G. *-oma,* tumor]. Cryptococcoma.

Torulopsis (tōr-ū-lop'sis). A genus of yeasts morphologically similar to *Cryptococcus,* but with smaller blastospores (2 to 4 nm); the species *T. glabrata* is the causative agent of torulopsosis, usually in compromised hosts.

torulopsosis (tōr-ū-lop'sō-sis). A usually opportunistic infection caused by *Torulopsis glabrata* and seen in patients with severe underlying disease or in immunocompromised patients; the pattern of disease may be bronchopulmonary, genitourinary, or septicemic.

torulus, pl. **toruli** (tōr'yū-lŭs, -lī) [L. dim. of *torus,* a protuberance, swelling]. A minute elevation or papilla.

tor'uli tact'iles [NA], tactile elevations; small areas in the skin of the palms and soles especially rich in sensory nerve endings.

torus, pl. **tori** (tō'rŭs, tō'rī) [L. swelling, knot, bulge]. **1.** A geometrical figure formed by the revolution of a circle round the base of any of its arcs, such as the convex molding at the base of a pillar. **2** [NA]. A rounded swelling, such as that caused by a contracting muscle.

t. fronta'lis, a slight prominence on the frontal bone at the root of the nose.

t. levator'ius [NA], levator swelling; levator cushion; the bulge in the lateral wall of the nasopharynx, below the opening of the auditory tube, produced by the levator veli palatini muscle.

mandibular t., t. mandibula'ris, an exostosis protruding from the lingual aspect of the mandible, usually opposite the premolar teeth.

t. ma'nus, the carpal bones.

t. occipita'lis, an occasional ridge near the superior nuchal line of the occipital bone.

palatine t., t. palati'nus, an exostosis protruding from the midline of the hard palate.

t. tuba'rius [NA], eustachian cushion; a ridge in the pharyngeal wall posterior to the opening of the auditory (eustachian) tube, caused by the projection of the cartilaginous portion of this tube.

t. ureter'icus, a smooth ridge in the bladder wall stretching between the ureteral orifices.

t. uteri'nus, a transverse ridge on the back part of the cervix uteri, formed by the junction of the rectouterine folds.

tosyl (tō'sil). Toluenesulfonyl radical, widely used to block $-NH_2$ groups in the course of organic syntheses of drugs and other biologically active compounds.

tosylate (tō'si-lāt). USAN-approved contraction for *p*-toluenesulfonate.

totem (tō'tem) [Amer. Indian]. An object (usually an animal or plant) serving as the emblem of a family or clan and often as a reminder of its ancestry; something that serves as a revered symbol.

totemism (tō'tem-izm). Belief in a kinship with, or a mystical relationship between, a group or individual and a totem.

totemistic (tō-tem-is'tik). Relating to totemism.

totipotency, totipotence (tō-ti-pō'ten-sē, tō-tip'ō-tens) [L. *totus,* entire, + *potentia,* power]. The ability of a cell to differentiate into any type of cell and thus form a new organism or regenerate any part of an organism; *e.g.,* a fertilized ovum, or a small excised portion of a *Planaria,* which is capable of regenerating a complete new organism.

totipotent, totipotential (tō-tip'ō-tent, tō'ti-pō-ten'shăl). Relating to totipotency.

touch (tŭch) [Fr. *toucher*]. **1.** Tactile sense; the sense by which slight contact with the skin or mucous membrane is appreciated. **2.** Digital examination.

Tourette. See Gilles de la Tourette.

Tournay, Auguste, French ophthalmologist, 1878–1969. See T. *sign.*

tourniquet (tūr'ni-ket) [Fr. fr. *tourner,* to turn]. An instrument for temporarily arresting the flow of blood to or from a distal part by pressure applied with an encircling device.

Dupuytren's t., an instrument for compression on the abdominal aorta.

Esmarch t., a narrow hard rubber t. with a chain fastener.

Tourtual, Kaspar T., Prussian anatomist, 1802–1865. See T.'s *membrane, sinus.*

Touton, Karl, German dermatologist, *1858. See T. giant *cell.*

Tovell, Ralph M., U.S. anesthesiologist, 1901–1967. See T. *tube.*

Towne, E.B., U.S. otolaryngologist, 1883–1957. See T. *projection,* T. projection *roentgenogram, T. view.*

tox-. See toxico-.

toxanemia (tok-să-nē'mē-ă) [G. *toxikon,* poison, + anemia]. Anemia resulting from the effects of a hemolytic poison.

toxaphene (tok'să-fēn). A chlorinated hydrocarbon insecticide.

Toxascaris leonina (tok-sas'kă-ris lē-ō-nī'nă) [G. *toxon,* bow, + *Ascaris*]. An ascarid nematode of the dog that differs from *Toxocara* in that the larvae do not migrate through the lungs; the entire developmental cycle occurs in the gut. This parasite has been found in man in a few instances and is a cause of visceral larva migrans in children, though less frequently implicated than is *Toxocara canis.*

toxemia (tok-sē'mē-ă) [G. *toxikon,* poison, + *haima,* blood]. Toxicemia. **1.** Clinical manifestations observed during certain infectious diseases, assumed to be caused by toxins and other noxious substances elaborated by the infectious agent; in certain infections by Gram-negative bacteria, endotoxins probably play a role when the bacterial cell wall breaks down, releasing the complex lipopolysaccharide; however, the role of other bacterial substances is unclear, except in the case of the specific exotoxins such as those of diphtheria and tetanus. **2.** The clinical syndrome caused by toxic substances in the blood. **3.** An ill-defined term referring to metabolic disorders of pregnancy characterized by hypertension, edema, and albuminuria; *e.g.,* preeclampsia.

toxemic (tok-sē'mik). Pertaining to, affected with, or manifesting the features of toxemia.

toxi-. See toxico-.

toxic (tok'sik) [G. *toxikon,* an arrow-poison]. **1.** Poisonous. **2.** Pertaining to a toxin.

toxicant (tok'si-kant). **1.** Poisonous. **2.** Any poisonous agent, specifically an alcoholic or other poison, causing symptoms of what is popularly called intoxication.

toxicemia (tok-si-sē'mē-ă). Toxemia.

toxicity (tok-sis'i-tē). The state of being poisonous.

oxygen t., oxygen poisoning; a body disturbance resulting from breathing high partial pressures of oxygen; characterized by visual and hearing abnormalities, unusual fatigue while breathing, muscular twitching, anxiety, confusion, incoordination, and convulsions; although the mechanism for development of the condition is obscure, a disruption of enzymatic activity is likely, perhaps as a result of free radical formation.

toxico-, tox-, toxi-, toxo- [G. *toxikon,* bow, hence (arrow) poison]. Combining forms denoting poison, toxin.

Toxicodendron (tok'si-kō-den'dron) [toxico- + G. *dendron,* tree]. A genus of poisonous plants (family Anacardiaceae) comprising those members of the genus *Rhus* with smooth fruits and foliage that contain urushiol, which produces a contact dermatitis (rhus dermatitis); species include poison ivy (*T. radicans*), poison oak (*T. diversilobum*), and poison sumac (*T. vernix*).

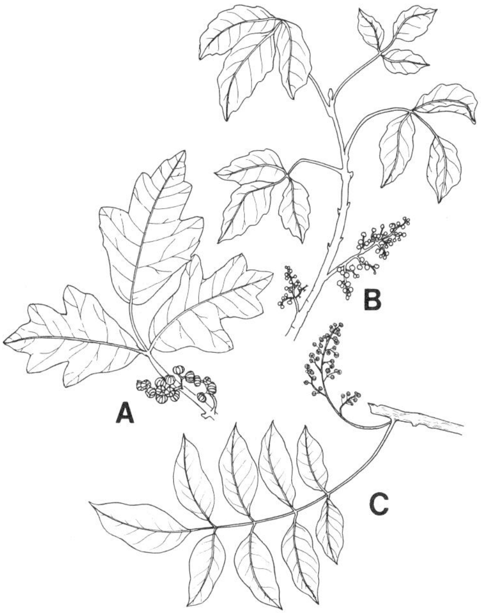

Toxicodendron
A, *T. diversilobum*, poison oak; B, *T. radicans*, poison ivy; C, *T. vernix*, poison sumac.

toxicoderma (tok′si-kō-der′mă) [toxico- + G. *derma*, skin]. Toxicodermatosis; any skin disease caused by a poison or by a toxin-producing microorganism.

toxicodermatitis (tok′si-kō-der′mă-tī′tis). Inflammation of the skin caused by the action of a poison.

toxicodermatosis (tok′si-kō-der′mă-tō′sis). Toxicoderma.

toxicogenic (tok′si-kō-jen′ik) [toxico- + G. *-gen*, producing]. **1.** Producing a poison. **2.** Caused by a poison.

toxicoid (tok′si-koyd) [toxico- + G. *eidos*, resemblance]. Having an action like that of a poison; temporarily poisonous.

toxicologic (tok′si-kō-loj′ik). Relating to toxicology.

toxicologist (tok-si-kol′ō-jist). A specialist or expert in toxicology.

toxicology (tok-si-kol′ō-jē) [toxico- + G. *logos*, study]. The science of poisons, including their source, chemical composition, action, tests, and antidotes.

toxicopathic (tok′si-kō-path′ik). Denoting any morbid state caused by the action of a poison.

toxicophobia (tok′si-kō-fō′bē-ă) [toxico- + G. *phobos*, fear]. Toxiphobia; morbid fear of being poisoned.

toxicosis (tok-si-kō′sis) [toxico- + G. *-osis*, condition]. Systemic poisoning; any disease of toxic origin.
endogenic t., autointoxication.
exogenic t., any disease caused by a poison introduced from without and not generated within the body.
thyroid t., triiodothyronine t.
triiodothyronine (T_3) t., thyroid t.; hyperthyroidism resulting from excessive circulating 3,5,3′-triiodothyronine.

toxiferines (tok-sif′er-ēnz). The most potent group of the curare alkaloids; the principle source is *Strychnos toxifera*.

toxiferous (tok-sif′er-ŭs) [toxi- + L. *fero*, to bear]. Poisonous.

toxigenic (tok-si-jen′ik). Toxinogenic.

toxigenicity (tok′si-jĕ-nis′i-tē). Toxinogenicity.

toxilic acid (tok-sil′ik). Maleic acid.

toxin (tok′sin) [G. *toxikon*, poison]. A noxious or poisonous substance that is formed or elaborated either as an integral part of the cell or tissue, as an extracellular product (exotoxin), or as a combination of the two, during the metabolism and growth of certain microorganisms and some higher plant and animal species.
animal t., zootoxin.
anthrax t., *Bacillus anthracis* t.; a culture filtrate of *Bacillus anthracis* containing at least three different substances: edema factor, lethal factor, and protective antigen.
Bacillus anthracis t., anthrax t.
bacterial t., any intracellular or extracellular t. formed in or elaborated by bacterial cells.
botulinus t., botuline; botulismotoxin; a potent neurotoxin from *Clostridium botulinum*.
cholera t., see *Vibrio cholerae*.
diagnostic diphtheria t., Schick test t.
Dick test t., streptococcus erythrogenic t.
dinoflagellate t., a potent neurotoxin that is thought to act similarly to botulinus t. by impairing the synthesis or the release of acetylcholine.
diphtheria t., see *Corynebacterium diphtheriae*.
erythrogenic t., streptococcus erythrogenic t.
extracellular t., exotoxin.
intracellular t., endotoxin.
normal t., a t. solution holding exactly 100 lethal doses in 1 ml.
plant t., phytotoxin.
scarlet fever erythrogenic t., streptococcus erythrogenic t.
Schick test t., diagnostic diphtheria t.; *Corynebacterium diphtheriae* t. diluted so that the inoculated dose (0.1 or 0.2 ml) will contain $^{1}/_{50}$th of guinea pig minimal lethal dose. See also Schick *test*.
streptococcus erythrogenic t., Dick test t.; erythrogenic t.; scarlet fever erythrogenic t.; a culture filtrate of lysogenized group A strains of β-hemolytic streptococci, erythrogenic when inoculated into the skin of susceptible persons, and neutralized by antibodies that appear during scarlet fever convalescence; three immunological types (A, B, and C) are recognized.
tetanus t., tetanotoxin; the neurotropic, heat-labile exotoxin of *Clostridium tetani* and the cause of tetanus; it has been isolated as a crystalline protein (molecular weight 67,000), is one of the most poisonous substances known, and seems to function by blocking inhibitory synaptic impulses.

toxinic (tok-sin′ik). Relating to a toxin.

toxinogenic (tok′si-nō-jen′ik) [toxin + G. *-gen*, producing]. Toxigenic; producing a toxin, said of an organism.

toxinogenicity (tok′si-nō-jĕ-nis′i-tē). Toxigenicity; the capacity to produce toxin.

toxinology (tok′si-nol′ō-jē) [toxin + G. *logos*, study]. The study of toxins, in a restricted sense, with reference to the relatively unstable proteinaceous substances of microbial, plant, or animal origins.

toxinosis (tok-si-nō′sis) [toxin + G. *-osis*, condition]. Toxonosis; any disease or lesion caused by the action of a toxin.

toxipathic (tok-si-path′ik). Relating to any diseased state caused by a poison, *e.g.*, neuritis or hepatitis caused by arsenic.

toxipathy (tok-sip′ă-thē) [toxi- + G. *pathos*, suffering]. Any disease due to poisoning, especially chronic poisoning.

toxiphobia (tok-si-fō′bē-ă). Toxicophobia.

toxisterol (tok-sis′ter-ol). A toxic substance formed by excessive irradiation of ergosterol or calciferol.

toxo-. See toxico-.

Toxocara (tok'sō-kar'ă) [G. *toxon,* bow, + *kara,* head]. A genus of ascarid nematodes, chiefly found in carnivores, that cause toxocariasis.

T. ca'nis, the common ascarid species in the small intestine of the dog, where prenatal infection is a common mode of infection of pups; it is also reported from cats, wolves, foxes, coyotes, and badgers; the second-stage larva is the most frequent cause of visceral larva migrans in the liver of children.

T. mys'tax, a common ascarid species of cats, but not reported from dogs; prenatal infection of kittens does not occur, infection being by infective eggs, which hatch in the intestine, releasing second-stage larvae, which then undergo migration through the heart, lung, trachea, mouth, and gut, as with *Ascaris lumbricoides* in man; mice and other vertebrates, and also some invertebrates (*e.g.,* earthworms, cockroaches) may serve as transport hosts, in which the migrating larvae encyst in the tissues.

toxocariasis (tok'sō-kă-rī'ă-sis). Infection with nematodes of the genus *Toxocara;* parenterally migrating larvae, chiefly of *Toxocara canis,* may cause visceral larva migrans; ocular involvement results in either a solitary granuloma in the retina, peripheral inflammatory masses, or chronic endophthalmitis.

toxoid (tok'soyd) [toxin + G. *eidos,* resemblance]. Anatoxin; a toxin that has been treated (commonly with formaldehyde) so as to destroy its toxic property but retain its antigenicity, *i.e.,* its capability of stimulating the production of antitoxin antibodies and thus of producing an active immunity. For specific t.'s, see under vaccine.

toxon, toxone (tok'sŏn, tok'sōn). A hypothetical bacterial product, of feeble toxicity and weak affinity for antitoxin.

toxoneme (tok'sō-nēm) [G. *toxon,* bow, + *nema,* thread]. Rhoptry.

toxonosis (tok-sō-nō'sis) [toxo- + G. *nosos,* disease]. Toxinosis.

toxophil, toxophile (tok'sō-fil, -fīl) [toxo- + G. *philos,* fond]. Susceptible to the action of a poison.

toxophore (tok'sō-fōr) [toxo- + G. *phoros,* bearing]. Denoting the atomic group of the toxin molecule which carries the poisonous principle.

toxophorous (tok-sof'ăr-ŭs). Relating to the toxophore group of the toxin molecule.

Toxoplasma gondii (tok-sō-plaz'mă gon'dē-ī) [G. *toxon,* bow or arc, + *plasma,* anything formed]. An abundant, widespread sporozoan species (family Eimeriidae) that is an intracellular, nonhost-specific parasite in a great variety of vertebrates. It develops its sexual cycle, leading to oocyst production, exclusively in cats and other felids; proliferative stages (tachyzoites) and tissue cysts (containing bradyzoites) develop in a wide variety of animal species that acquire the infection from ingestion of oocysts, tissue cysts from infected meat, or by transplacental migration, leading to infection in utero.

Toxoplasmatidae (tok'sō-plaz-mat'i-dē). A family of coccidian sporozoa including the genera *Toxoplasma* and *Frankelia,* characterized by endodyogeny and by the presence of cysts (sometimes termed pseudocysts) containing bradyzoites in parenteral cells of the host; schizonts and gamonts are produced in intestinal cells, and gamonts give rise to oocysts. Final hosts of *Toxoplasma* are cats and other felids; final hosts of *Frankelia* are unknown.

toxoplasmosis (tok'sō-plaz-mō'sis). Disease caused by the protozoan parasite *Toxoplasma gondii* which can produce abortion in sheep, encephalitis in mink, and a variety of syndromes in man. Prenatally acquired human infection can result in the presence of abnormalities such as microcephalus or hydrocephalus at birth, the development of jaundice with hepatosplenomegaly or meningoencephalitis in early childhood, or the delayed appearance of ocular lesions such as chorioretinitis in later childhood. Postnatally acquired human infections typically remain subclinical; if clinical disease does occur, symptoms include fever, lymphadenopathy, headache, myalgia, and fatigue, with eventual recovery, except in the immunocompromised patient where fatal encephalitis often develops.

acquired t. in adults, a form of t. that may result in fever, encephalomyelitis, chorioretinopathy, maculopapular rash, arthralgia, myalgia, myocarditis, and pneumonitis; a lymphadenopathic form seems to be more prevalent in adults, and such persons may manifest fever, lymphadenopathy, malaise, and headache, a form frequently found in patients with AIDS.

congenital t., t. apparently resulting from parasites in an infected mother being transmitted *in utero* to the fetus, observed as three syndromes: 1) acute, most of the organs contain foci of necrosis in association with fever, jaundice, hydrocephaly, encephelomyelitis, pneumonitis, cutaneous rash, ophthalmic lesions, hepatomegaly, and splenomegaly; 2) subacute, most of the lesions are partly healed or calcified, but those in the brain and eye seem to remain active, inasmuch as chorioretinitis is observed in more than 80% of diseased infants; 3) chronic, usually not recognized during the newborn period, but chorioretinitis and cerebral lesions may be detected weeks to years later.

toxopyrimidine (toks'ō-pi-rim'i-dēn). Pyramin; pyramine; 4-amino-5-hydroxymethyl-2-methylpyrimidine; one of the products resulting from the hydrolysis of thiamin by thiaminase and appearing in the urine.

Toynbee, Joseph, British otologist, 1815–1866. See T.'s *corpuscles, experiment, muscle, tube.*

TPA Abbreviation for 12-*O*-tetradecanoylphorbol 13-acetate; tissue plasminogen *activator.*

TPC Abbreviation for thromboplastic plasma *component.*

TPI Abbreviation for *Treponema pallidum* immobilization *test.*

TPN Abbreviation for total parenteral *nutrition.*

TPN, TPNH Abbreviation for triphosphopyridine nucleotide and its reduced form (the oxidized form is TPN^+).

TPP Abbreviation for *thiamin* pyrophosphate.

TPR Total peripheral *resistance.*

TQ Abbreviation for tocopherolquinone.

tr. Abbreviation for L. *tinctura,* or tincture.

trabecula, gen. and pl. **trabeculae** (tră-bek'yū-lă, -lē) [L. dim. of *trabs,* a beam]. **1.** One of the supporting bundles of fibers traversing the substance of a structure, usually derived from the capsule or one of the fibrous septa. **2.** A small piece of the spongy substance of bone usually interconnected with other similar pieces. **3.** In histopathology, a band of neoplastic tissue two or more cells wide.

anterior chamber t., tissue at the angle of the anterior chamber through which aqueous humor exits from the eye.

trabec'ulae car'neae [NA], Rathke's bundles; columnae carneae; muscular bundles on the lining walls of the ventricles of the heart.

trabec'ulae cor'poris spongio'si pe'nis [NA], the fibrous bands interlacing between the vascular spaces of the corpus spongiosum and glans penis.

trabec'ulae cor'porum cavernoso'rum [NA], fibromuscular bands and cords given off from the fibrous envelopes and septum of the corpora cavernosa penis and which separate the cavernous veins.

trabec'ulae cra'nii, a pair of chondrification centers in the base of the embryonic cartilaginous neurocranium, lying in front of the developing hypophysis.

trabec'ulae, li'enis, trabec'ulae sple'nicae [NA], small fibrous bands given off from the capsule of the spleen and constituting the framework of that organ.

septomarginal t., t. septomarginalis.

t. septomargina'lis [NA], septomarginal t.; moderator band; Reil's band (1); one of the trabeculae carneae in the right ventricle of the heart; it carries the right branch of the A-V bundle from the septum to the opposite wall of the ventricle.

t. tes'tis, *septulum* testis.

trabecular, trabeculate (tră-bek'yū-lăr, -yū-lāt). Relating to or containing trabeculae.

trabeculation (tră-bek'yū-lā'shŭn). **1.** The occurrence of trabeculae in the walls of an organ or part. **2.** The process of forming trabeculae, as in spongy bone.

trabeculectomy (tră-bek'yū-lek'tō-mē) [trabecula + G. *ektomē,* excision]. A filtering operation for glaucoma by creation of a fistula between the anterior chamber of the eye and the subconjunctival space, through a subscleral excision of a portion of the trabecular meshwork.

trabeculoplasty (tră-bek'yū-lō-plas-tē). Photocoagulation of the trabecular meshwork of the eye using the laser in the treatment of glaucoma.

laser t., an operation for glaucoma in which laser energy is applied to trabecular meshwork.

trabeculotomy (tră-bek-yū-lot'ō-mē) [trabekula + G. *tomē,* incision]. Surgical opening of the sinus venosus sclerae (canal of Schlemm) to treat glaucoma.

trace (trās). **1.** Evidence of the former existence, influence, or action of an object, phenomenon, or event. **2.** An extremely small amount or barely discernible indication of something.

memory t., see engram.

tracer (trā'ser). **1.** An element or compound containing atoms that can be distinguished from their normal counterparts by physical means (*e.g.,* radioactivity assay or mass spectrography or scintillation counter) and that can thus be used to follow (trace) the course of the normal substances in metabolism or similar chemical changes. A colored substance (*e.g.,* a dye) can be used as a t. to follow the flow of water. However, most t.'s are radioactive or "heavy" nuclides (^{32}P, ^{14}C, ^{2}H, etc.). **2.** An instrument used in dissecting out nerves and blood vessels. **3.** A mechanical device with a marking point attached to one jaw and a graph plate or tracing plate attached to the other jaw; used to record the direction and extent of movements of the mandible. See also tracing (2).

trache-. See tracheo-.

trachea, pl. **tracheae** (trā'kē-ă, -kē-ē) [G. *tracheia artēria,* rough artery] [NA]. Windpipe; the air tube extending from the larynx into the thorax (level of the fifth or sixth thoracic vertebra) where it bifurcates into the right and left main bronchi. The t. is composed of from 16 to 20 rings of hyaline cartilage connected by a membrane (annular ligament); posteriorly, the rings are deficient for one-fifth to one-third of their circumference, the interval forming the membranous wall being closed by a fibrous membrane containing smooth muscular fibers. Internally, the mucosa is composed of a pseudostratified ciliated columnar epithelium with mucous goblet cells; numerous small mixed mucous and serous glands occur, the ducts of which open to the surface of the epithelium.

scabbard t., a deformity of the t. caused by flattening and approximation of the lateral walls, producing more or less pronounced stenosis.

tracheal (trā'kē-ăl). Relating to the trachea.

trachealgia (trā-kē-al'jē-ă) [trachea + G. *algos,* pain]. Pain in the trachea.

trachealis (trā-kē-ā'lis). See under musculus.

tracheitis (trā-kē-ī'tis) [trachea + G. *-itis,* inflammation]. Trachitis; inflammation of the lining membrane of the trachea.

trachel-. See trachelo-.

trachelagra (trak-ē-lag'ră) [trachel- + G. *agra,* seizure]. A gouty or rheumatic affection of the muscles of the neck, producing torticollis.

trachelalis (trak-ĕ-lā'lis). *Musculus* longissimus capitis.

trachelectomy (trak-ĕ-lek'tō-mē) [trachel- + G. *ektomē,* excision]. Cervicectomy.

trachelematoma (trak'ĕ-lē-mă-tō'mă) [trachel- + hematoma]. A hematoma of the neck.

trachelian (tră-kē'lē-an) [G. *trachēlos,* neck]. Cervical.

trachelism, trachelismus (trak'ĕ-lizm, -liz'mŭs) [G. *trachēlismos,* a seizing by the throat]. A bending backward of the neck, such as sometimes ushers in an epileptic attack.

trachelitis (trak-ĕ-lī'tis). Cervicitis.

trachelo-, trachel- [G. *trachēlos,* neck]. Combining forms denoting neck.

trachelocele (trak'ĕ-lō-sēl) [trachelo- + G. *kēlē,* tumor, hernia]. Tracheocele.

trachelocyrtosis (trak'ĕ-lō-ser-tō'sis) [trachelo- + G. *kyrtos,* bent]. Tuberculous *spondylitis.*

trachelocystitis (trak'ĕ-lō-sis-tī'tis) [trachelo- + G. *kystis,* bladder, + *-itis,* inflammation]. Obsolete term for inflammation of the neck of the bladder.

trachelodynia (trak'ĕ-lō-din'ē-ă) [trachelo- + G. *odynē,* pain]. Cervicodynia.

trachelokyphosis (trak'ĕ-lō-kī-fō'sis) [trachelo- + G. *kyphōsis,* hump-back]. Tuberculous *spondylitis.*

trachelology (trak-ĕ-lol'ō-jē) [trachelo- + G. *logos,* study]. The study of the neck and its injuries and diseases.

trachelomastoid (trak'ĕ-lō-mas'toyd). *Musculus* longissimus capitis.

trachelomyitis (trak'ĕ-lō-mī-ī'tis) [trachelo- + G. *mys,* muscle, + *-itis,* inflammation].Obsolete term for inflammation of the muscles of the neck.

trachelo-occipitalis (trak'ĕ-lō-ok-sip'i-tā'lis). *Musculus* semispinalis capitis.

trachelopanus (trak'ĕ-lō-pā'nŭs) [trachelo- + L. *panus,* tumor, swelling]. **1.** Swelling of the lymphatic vessels of the neck. **2.** Lymphatic engorgement of the cervix uteri.

trachelopexia, trachelopexy (trak'ĕ-lō-pek'sē-ă, -pek-sē) [trachelo- + G. *pēxis,* fixation]. Surgical fixation of the cervix uteri.

trachelophyma (trak'ĕ-lō-fī'mă) [trachelo- + G. *phyma,* tumor]. A tumor or swelling of the neck.

tracheloplasty (trak'ĕ-lō-plas-tē) [trachelo- + G. *plastos,* formed]. Rarely used term for plastic surgery of the cervix uteri.

trachelorrhaphy (trak-ĕ-lōr'ă-fē) [trachelo- + G. *rhaphē,* suture]. Emmet's operation; repair by suture of a laceration of the cervix uteri.

trachelos (trak'ĕ-los) [G. *trachēlos*]. Collum.

tracheloschisis (trak-ĕ-los'ki-sis) [trachelo- + G. *schisis,* fissure]. Congenital fissure in the neck.

trachelotomy (trak-ĕ-lot'ō-mē) [trachelo- + G. *tomē,* incision]. Cervicotomy.

tracheo-, trache- [see trachea]. Combining forms denoting the trachea.

tracheoaerocele (trā'kē-ō-ār'ō-sēl) [tracheo- + G. *aēr,* air, + *kēlē,* hernia]. An air cyst in the neck caused by distention of a tracheocele.

tracheobiliary (trā'kē-ō-bil'ē-ār-ē). Relating to the trachea or bronchi and the biliary duct system.

tracheobronchial (trā'kē-ō-brong'kē-ăl). Relating to both trachea and bronchi.

tracheobronchitis (trā'kē-ō-brong-kī'tis). Inflammation of the mucous membrane of the trachea and bronchi.

tracheobronchomegaly (trā'kē-ō-brong'kō-meg'ă-lē) [tracheo- + bronchus + G. *megas,* large]. Mounier-Kuhn syndrome; gross widening of the trachea and main bronchi, usually congenital.

tracheobronchoscopy (trā'kē-ō-brong-kos'kŏ-pē) [tracheo- + bronchus, + G. *skopeō,* to view]. Inspection of the interior of the trachea and bronchi.

tracheocele (trā'kē-ō-sēl) [tracheo- + G. *kēlē,* hernia]. Trachelocele; a protrusion of the mucous membrane through a defect in the wall of the trachea.

tracheoesophageal (trā'kē-ō-ē-sof'ă-jē'ăl). Relating to the trachea and the esophagus.

tracheolaryngeal (trā'kē-ō-lă-rin'jē-ăl). Relating to the trachea and the larynx.

tracheomalacia (trā'kē-ō-mă-lā'shē-ă) [tracheo- + G. *malakia,* softness]. Degeneration of elastic and connective tissue of the trachea.

tracheomegaly (trā'kē-ō-meg'ă-lē) [tracheo- + G. *megas (megal-),* large]. An abnormally dilated trachea which may, like bronchiectasis, result from infection.

tracheopathia, tracheopathy (trā'kē-ō-path'ē-ă, -op'ă-thē) [tracheo- + G. *pathos,* disease]. Any disease of the trachea.

t. osteoplas'tica, a rare disease characterized by cartilaginous and bony growths in the trachea and bronchi which produce sessile polyps and plaques projecting into and partly obstructing the lumina.

tracheopharyngeal (trā'kē-ō-fă-rin'jē-ăl). Relating to both trachea and pharynx; denoting an occasional band of muscular fibers passing from the inferior constrictor of the pharynx to the trachea.

tracheophonesis (trā'kē-ō-fō-nē'sis) [tracheo- + G. *phōnēsis,* a sounding]. Auscultation of the heart sounds at the sternal notch.

tracheophony (trā-kē-of'ō-nē) [tracheo- + G. *phōnē,* voice]. The hollow voice sound heard in auscultating over the trachea. See also bronchophony.

tracheoplasty (trā'kē-ō-plas-tē) [tracheo- + G. *plastos,* formed]. Plastic surgery of the trachea.

tracheopyosis (trā-kē-ō-pī-ō'sis) [tracheo- + G. *pyōsis,* suppuration]. Suppurative inflammation of the trachea.

tracheorrhagia (trā-kē-ō-rā'jē-ă) [tracheo- + G. *rhēgnymi,* to burst forth]. Hemorrhage from the mucous membrane of the trachea.

tracheoschisis (trā-kē-os'ki-sis) [tracheo- + G. *schisis,* fissure]. A fissure into the trachea.

tracheoscope (trā'kē-ō-skōp). An instrument used in tracheoscopy.

tracheoscopic (trā-kē-ō-skop'ik). Relating to tracheoscopy.

tracheoscopy (trā-kē-os'kŏ-pē) [tracheo- + G. *skopeō,* to examine]. Inspection of the interior of the trachea.

tracheostenosis (trā'kē-ō-stĕ-nō'sis) [tracheo- + G. *stenōsis,* constriction]. Narrowing of the lumen of the trachea.

tracheostoma (trā'kē-os'tō-mă) [tracheo- + G. *stoma,* mouth]. Opening into the trachea through the neck; generally applied to such an opening after tracheotomy or laryngectomy.

tracheostomy (trā'kē-os'tō-mē) [tracheo- + G. *stoma,* mouth]. Formation of an opening into the trachea or that opening.

tracheotome (trā'kē-ō-tōm). A knife used in the operation of tracheotomy.

tracheotomy (trā-kē-ot'ō-mē) [tracheo- + G. *tomē,* incision]. The operation of opening into the trachea.

trachitis (trā-kī'tis). Tracheitis.

trachoma (tră-kō'mă) [G. *trachōma,* fr. *trachys,* rough, harsh]. Contagious granular conjunctivitis; granular lids; granular or Egyptian ophthalmia; chronic contagious microbial inflammation, with hypertrophy, of the conjunctiva, marked by the formation of minute grayish or yellowish translucent granules caused by *Chlamydia trachomatis.*

follicular t., granular t., the ordinary form of t. marked by the presence of granulations on the conjunctiva.

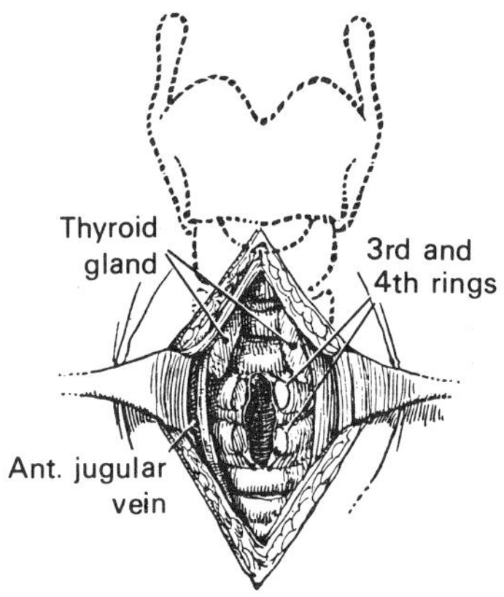

Tracheotomy

trachomatous (tră-kō'mă-tŭs). Relating to or suffering from trachoma.

trachychromatic (trak-i-krō-mat'ik) [G. *trachys,* rough, + *chrōmatikos,* chromatic]. Denoting a nucleus with very deeply staining chromatin.

trachyphonia (trak'ē-fō'nē-ă) [G. *trachys,* rough, + *phōnē,* voice]. Roughness of voice.

tracing (trās'ing). **1.** Any graphic display of electrical or mechanical cardiovascular events, *e.g.,* electrocardiogram, phlebogram. See also curve. **2.** In dentistry, a line or lines, scribed on a table or plate by a pointed instrument, representing a record of movements of the mandible; may be extraoral (made outside the oral cavity) or intraoral (made within the oral cavity).

arrow point t., needle point t.

cephalometric t., an overlay drawing or t. of the teeth, facial bones, and anthropometric landmarks made directly from a cephalometric radiograph and used as a basis for cephalometric analysis.

Gothic arch t., needle point t.

needle point t., Gothic arch; arrow point, Gothic arch, or stylus t.; a t. of mandibular movements made by means of a device attached to the opposing arches; its shape resembles that of an arrowhead or a Gothic arch, and when the instrument's marking point is at the apex of the arch, the jaws are considered to be in centric relation.

stylus t., needle point t.

TRACT

tract (trakt) [L. *tractus,* a drawing out]. Tractus; an elongated area, *e.g.,* path, track, way. See fasciculus.

alimentary t., digestive t.

anterior corticospinal t., *tractus* pyramidalis anterior.

anterior pyramidal t., *tractus* pyramidalis anterior.

anterior spinocerebellar t., *tractus* spinocerebellaris anterior.

anterior spinothalamic t., *tractus* spinothalamicus anterior.

Arnold's t., *tractus* temporopontinus.

association t., see association *system.*

auditory t., *lemniscus* lateralis.

Burdach's t., *fasciculus* cuneatus.

central tegmental t., *tractus* tegmentalis centralis.

cerebellorubral t., *tractus* cerebellorubralis.
cerebellothalamic t., *tractus* cerebellothalamicus.
Collier's t., *fasciculus* longitudinalis medialis.
comma t. of Schultze, *fasciculus* semilunaris.
corticobulbar t., *tractus* corticobulbaris.
corticopontine t., *tractus* corticopontini.
corticospinal t., *tractus* pyramidalis.
crossed pyramidal t., *tractus* pyramidalis lateralis.
cuneocerebellar t., the nerve fiber system originating from the nucleus cuneatus accessorius and entering the cerebellum as a component of the inferior caudal cerebellar peduncle.
dead t.'s, dentin areas characterized by degenerated odontoblastic processes; may result from injury caused by caries, attrition, erosion, or cavity preparation.
deiterospinal t., *tractus* vestibulospinalis.
dentatothalamic t., *tractus* cerebellothalamicus.
descending t. of trigeminal nerve, *tractus* spinalis nervi trigemini.
digestive t., alimentary t. or canal; digestive tube; tubus digestorius; the passage leading from the mouth to the anus through the pharynx, esophagus, stomach, and intestine.
direct pyramidal t., *tractus* pyramidalis anterior.
dorsal spinocerebellar t., *tractus* spinocerebellaris posterior.
dorsolateral t., *fasciculus* dorsolateralis.
fastigiobulbar t., *tractus* fastigiobulbaris.
Flechsig's t., *tractus* spinocerebellaris posterior.
frontopontine t., *tractus* frontopontinus.
frontotemporal t., *fasciculus* uncinatus.
gastrointestinal t., the stomach, small intestine, and large intestine; often used as a synonym of digestive t.
geniculocalcarine t., *radiatio* optica.
genital t., genital duct; the genital passages of the urogenital apparatus.
t. of Goll, *fasciculus* gracilis.
Gowers' t., *tractus* spinocerebellaris anterior.
habenulointerpeduncular t., *fasciculus* retroflexus.
Hoche's t., see *fasciculus* semilunaris.
hypothalamohypophysial t., a fiber t. that connects the paraventricular and supraoptic nuclei of the hypothalamus with the neurohypophysis; the oxytocin vasopressin synthetized by the paraventricular and the supraoptic nuclei pass down the axons of the hypothalamohypophysial t. and are stored in the terminals of these fibers in the neurohypophysis, from which they are released into the systemic circulation.
James t.'s, James *fibers.*
lateral corticospinal t., *tractus* pyramidalis lateralis.
lateral pyramidal t., *tractus* pyramidalis lateralis.
lateral spinothalamic t., *tractus* spinothalamicus lateralis.
Lissauer's t., *fasciculus* dorsolateralis.
Loewenthal's t., *tractus* tectospinalis.
mamillothalamic t., *fasciculus* mamillothalamicus.
Marchi's t., *tractus* tectospinalis.
mesencephalic t. of trigeminal nerve, *tractus* mesencephalicus nervi trigemini.
Monakow's t., *tractus* rubrospinalis.
t. of Münzer and Wiener, *tractus* tectopontinus.
nerve t., a bundle or group of nerve fibers in the brain or spinal cord.
occipitocollicular t., occipitotectal t.
occipitopontine t., *tractus* occipitopontinus.
occipitotectal t., the system of nerve fibers by which the occipital cortex projects to the superior colliculus.
olfactory t., *tractus* olfactorius.
olivocerebellar t., *tractus* olivocerebellaris.
olivospinal t., Helweg's bundle; a slender bundle of nerve fibers in the peripheral zone of the lateral funiculus of the spinal cord, composed of spino-olivary fibers more likely than olivospinal fibers.
optic t., *tractus* opticus.
parietopontine t., *tractus* parietopontinus.
posterior spinocerebellar t., *tractus* spinocerebellaris posterior.
prepyramidal t., *tractus* rubrospinalis.
pyramidal t., *tractus* pyramidalis.
respiratory t., the air passages from the nose to the pulmonary alveoli, through the pharynx, larynx, trachea, and bronchi.
reticulospinal t., *tractus* reticulospinalis.
rubrobulbar t., **(1)** that component of the rubrospinal t. which distributes its fibers to lateral parts of the rhombencephalic tegmentum rather than the spinal cord; **(2)** uncrossed rubro-olivary fibers.
rubroreticular t., fibers that pass from the red nucleus to the reticular formation of the pons and medulla.
rubrospinal t., *tractus* rubrospinalis.
t. of Schütz, *fasciculus* longitudinalis dorsalis.
sensory t., see lemniscus.
septomarginal t., see *fasciculus* semilunaris.
solitary t., *tractus* solitarius.
sphincteroid t. of ileum, basal *sphincter.*
spinal t., any one of a multitude of fiber bundles ascending or descending in the spinal cord.
spinal t. of trigeminal nerve, *tractus* spinalis nervi trigemini.
spinocerebellar t.'s, see *tractus* spinocerebellaris anterior and posterior.
spino-olivary t., multiple spinal tracts terminating in the accessory olivary nuclei. See olivospinal t.
spinotectal t., *tractus* spinotectalis.
spinothalamic t., *tractus* spinothalamicus.
spiral foraminous t., *tractus* spiralis foraminosus.
Spitzka's marginal t., *fasciculus* dorsolateralis.
sulcomarginal t., collective term for those fiber t.'s which descend in the anterior funiculus of the spinal cord along the wall of the anterior median fissure: tectospinal t., medial longitudinal fasciculus, and anterior pyramidal t.
supraopticohypophysial t., *tractus* supraopticohypophysialis.
tectobulbar t., *tractus* tectobulbaris.
tectopontine t., *tractus* tectopontinus.
tectospinal t., *tractus* tectospinalis.
temporofrontal t., *fasciculus* uncinatus.
temporopontine t., *tractus* temporopontinus.
tuberoinfundibular t., *tractus* tuberoinfundibularis.
Türck's t., *tractus* pyramidalis anterior.
urinary t., the passage from the pelvis of the kidney to the urinary meatus through the ureters, bladder, and urethra.
uveal t., *tunica* vasculosa bulbi.
ventral spinocerebellar t., *tractus* spinocerebellaris anterior.
ventral spinothalamic t., *tractus* spinothalamicus anterior.
vestibulospinal t., *tractus* vestibulospinalis.
Waldeyer's t., *fasciculus* dorsolateralis.

---

tractellum, pl. **tractella** (trak-tel'ŭm, -ă) [Mod. L. dim. of L. *tractus*]. An anterior locomotor flagellum of a protozoon.

traction (trak'shŭn) [L. *tractio,* fr. *traho,* pp. *tractus,* to draw]. **1.** The act of drawing or pulling, as by an elastic or spring force. **2.** A pulling or dragging force exerted on a limb in a distal direction.
axis t., rarely used procedure to apply t. upon the fetal head in the line of the birth canal by means of axis t. forceps.
Bryant's t., t. upon the lower limb placed vertically, employed especially in fractures of the femur in children.
Buck's t., Buck's *extension.*
external t., a pulling force created by using fixed anchorage (*e.g.,* a headcap or bed frame) outside the oral cavity; principally used in the management of midfacial fractures.
halo t., application of skeletal t. to the head by means of a halo device.

intermaxillary t., maxillomandibular t.
internal t., a pulling force created by using one of the cranial bones, above the point of fracture, for anchorage.
isometric t., t. in which the length of the limb does not change.
isotonic t., t. in which the amount of force does not change.
maxillomandibular t., intermaxillary t.; a pulling force developed by using elastic or wire ligatures and interdental wiring or splints, or both.
Russell t., an improvement of Buck's extension for fracture of femur.
Sayre's suspension t., Sayre's suspension apparatus; spinal t. obtained by vertical suspension of the patient by means of a head halter.
skeletal t., skeletal extension; t. pull on a bone structure mediated through pin or wire inserted into the bone to reduce a fracture of long bones.
skin t., t. on an extremity by means of adhesive tape or other types of strapping applied to the limb.

tractor (trak'ter, tōr) [Mod. L. a drawer, see traction]. An instrument for exerting traction upon, or pulling out, an organ or structure.
Lowsley t., a slender curved instrument with flexible blades at its tip, which can be opened or closed by rotation at the proximal end of the t.; it is passed per urethram into the bladder and used to retract the prostate gland downward into the operative field in the initial stages of perineal prostatectomy.
Syms t., a collapsible rubber bag attached to the extremity of a tube; the tube is introduced into the bladder through the perineal wound and the bag is inflated; traction produced draws the enlarged prostate into the wound where it is more accessible.
Young prostatic t., a short, straight tubular instrument with blades at its tip, which can be rotated open and closed; it is passed into the prostatic urethra, through a prostatotomy incision made during the later stages of open perineal prostatectomy, with its tip into the bladder; direct traction on the instrument brings the prostate gland down into the operative field where enucleation can be more easily performed.

tractotomy (trak-tot'ō-mē) [L. *tractus,* tract, + G. *tomē,* incision]. Interruption of a nerve tract in the brainstem or spinal cord by laminectomy, craniotomy, or stereotaxy.
anterolateral t., anterolateral *cordotomy.*
intramedullary t., trigeminal t.
pyramidal t., division of a pyramidal tract; may be mesencephalic (pedunculotomy or crusotomy), medullary (medullary pyramidotomy), or spinal (spinal pyramidotomy).
Schwartz t., (medullary) spinothalamic t.
Sjöqvist t., trigeminal t.
spinal t., anterolateral *cordotomy.*
spinothalamic t., division of a spinothalamic tract; may be spinal (cordotomy), medullary (Schwartz t.), or mesencephalic (Walker t.).
trigeminal t., intramedullary or Sjöqvist t.; division of the descending root of the trigeminal nerve.
Walker t., (mesencephalic) spinothalamic t.

TRACTUS

tractus, gen. and pl. **tractus** (trak'tŭs) [L. a drawing, drawing out, extent, tract, fr. *traho,* pp. *tractus,* to draw]. Tract.
t. centra'lis tegmen'ti, t. tegmentalis centralis.
t. cerebellorubra'lis [NA], cerebellorubral tract; that component of the superior cerebellar peduncle (brachium conjunctivum) which distributes fibers within the nucleus ruber of the opposite side.
t. cerebellothalam'icus [NA], cerebellothalamic tract; dentatothalamic tract; that component of the superior cerebellar peduncle (brachium conjunctivum) which originates in the cerebellar nuclei, crosses completely in the decussation of the brachia conjunctiva, bypasses the red nucleus, and terminates in parts of the ventralis anterior, ventralis lateralis, ventralis posterolateralis, and centralis lateralis nuclei of the thalamus.
t. corticobulba'ris, corticobulbar tract; collective term for those fibers (corticonuclear fibers) which separate from the corticospinal tract in the course of the latter's descent through the pons and medulla oblongata. Fibers of this tract innervate the motor nuclei of the trigeminal, facial, and hypoglossal nerves (perhaps also the nucleus ambiguus), directly and by way of interneurons in the lateral part of the rhombencephalic tegmentum. No direct supranuclear cortical innervation of the motor nuclei innervating the external eye muscles (oculomotor, trochlear, abducens) has been identified. Fibers of the corticobulbar tract also project into the formatio reticularis (*i.e.,* corticoreticular fibers) and terminate upon sensory relay nuclei (*e.g.,* nuclei gracilis and cuneatus, nucleus spinalis trigeminalis and nucleus solitarius).
t. corticoponti' ni [NA], corticopontine tract; collective term for the multitude of fibers which, originating in all of the major subdivisions of the cerebral cortex, descend in the internal capsule and crus cerebri to terminate in the nuclei pontis or pars ventralis pontis. Individual components of this massive fiber system are indicated, according to their origin in the cerebral cortex, as t. frontopontinus, t. parietopontinus, t. occipitopontinus, and t. temporopontinus.
t. corticospina'lis [NA], t. pyramidalis.
t. corticospina'lis ante'rior [NA], t. pyramidalis anterior.
t. corticospina'lis latera'lis [NA], t. pyramidalis lateralis.
t. descen'dens ner'vi trigem'ini, t. spinalis nervi trigemini.
t. dorsolatera'lis [NA], *fasciculus* dorsolateralis.
t. fastigiobulba'ris, fastigiobulbar tract; a fiber bundle originating in the nucleus fastigii (nucleus tecti) of both sides, passing out of the cerebellum in the inferior cerebellar peduncle (corpus restiforme), and distributing its fibers to the vestibular nuclei and other cell groups in the medulla oblongata. Prominent crossed fibers loop over the dorsal surface of the superior cerebellar peduncle before turning ventrally, forming the uncinate bundle of Russell.
t. frontoponti'nus [NA], frontopontine tract; Türck's tract or bundle; a large group of fibers arising from the frontal lobe of the cerebral hemisphere, especially the precentral gyrus, descending in the capsula interna, farther caudally composing the medial part of the crus cerebri in which they extend caudalward to end in the gray matter (pontine nuclei) of the pars ventralis pontis.
t. habenulopeduncula'ris, *fasciculus* retroflexus.
t. iliotibia'lis [NA], iliotibial band; Maissiat's band; a fibrous reinforcement of the fascia lata on the lateral surface of the thigh, extending from the crest of the ilium to the lateral condyle of the tibia.
t. mesencephal'icus ner'vi trigem'ini [NA], mesencephalic tract of the trigeminal nerve; located alongside the substantia grisea centralis and composed of primary sensory fibers, the cells of origin of which compose the mesencephalic nucleus of the trigeminus.
t. occipitoponti'nus [NA], occipitopontine tract; a group of fibers originating in the occipital lobe of the cerebral hemisphere and descending in the internal capsule and lateral part of the crus cerebri to the pontine nuclei or pars ventralis pontis.
t. olfacto'rius [NA], olfactory tract; olfactory peduncle; a nerve-like, white band composed primarily of nerve fibers originating from the mitral cells and tufted cells of the olfactory bulb but also containing the scattered cells of the anterior olfactory nucleus. The tract is closely applied to the ventral surface of the frontal lobe, and attaches itself to the base of the cerebral hemisphere at the olfac-

tory trigone, beyond which it extends in the form of the olfactory striae which distribute their fibers to the olfactory tubercle and, in largest number, to the olfactory cortex on and around the uncus of the parahippocampal gyrus. See also *nervi* olfactorii.

t. olivocerebella'ris [NA], olivocerebellar tract; a large group of loosely arranged fiber fascicles emerging from the hilus of the olivary nucleus, crossing to the opposite side of the medulla oblongata through the stratum interolivare lemnisci and the contralateral olive, and joining the contralateral inferior (caudal) cerebellar peduncle; its fibers terminate in all parts of the cerebellar cortex as climbing fibers.

t. op'ticus [NA], optic tract; the continuation of the optic nerve fibers beyond (behind) the latter's hemidecussation in the optic chiasm; each of the two symmetrical optic tracts is composed of fibers originating from the temporal half of the retina of the ipsilateral eye and a nearly equal number of fibers from the nasal half of the contralateral retina; it forms a compact, somewhat flattened fiber band passing caudolaterally alongside the base of the hypothalamus and over the basal surface of the crus cerebri; most of its fibers terminate in the lateral geniculate body; a smaller number of fibers enter the brachium of the superior colliculus, to terminate in the superior colliculus and the pretectal region.

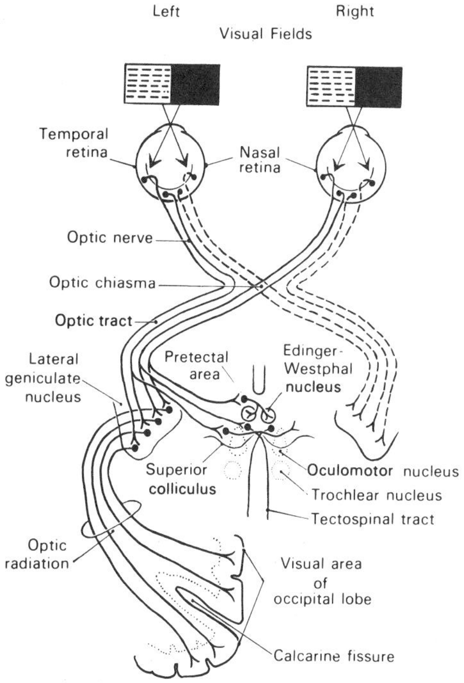

Tractus Opticus (Optic Tract)

t. parietoponti'nus [NA], parietopontine tract; a system of fibers originating in the parietal lobe of the cerebral hemisphere which descend in the internal capsule and lateral part of the crus cerebri to terminate in the nuclei pontis or pars ventralis pontis.

t. pyramida'lis [NA], t. corticospinalis; pyramidal or corticospinal tract; a massive bundle of fibers originating from pyramidal cells of various sizes in the fifth layer of the precentral motor (area 4), the premotor area (area 6), and to a lesser extent from the postcentral gyrus. Cells of origin in area 4 include the gigantopyramidal cells of Betz. Fibers from these cortical regions descend through the internal capsule, the middle third of the crus cerebri, and the pars ventralis pontis to emerge on the ventral surface of the medulla oblongata as the pyramis. Continuing caudally, most of the fibers cross to the opposite side in the pyramidal decussation and descend in the dorsal half of the lateral funiculus of the spinal cord as the t. pyramidalis lateralis, which distributes its fibers throughout the length of the spinal cord to interneurons of the zona intermedia of the spinal gray matter. In the (extremity-related) spinal cord enlargements, fibers also pass directly to motoneuronal groups that innervate distal extremity muscles subserving particular hand-and-finger or foot-and-toe movements. The uncrossed fibers form a small bundle, the t. pyramidalis anterior, which descends in the anterior funiculus of the spinal cord and terminates in synaptic contact with interneurons in the medial half of the anterior horn on both sides of the spinal cord. Interruption of the pyramidal tract at or below its cortical origin causes impairment of movement in the opposite body-half, especially severe in the arm and leg; characterized by muscular weakness, spasticity and hyperreflexia, and a loss of discrete finger and hand movements. Babinski's sign is associated with this condition of hemiplegia.

t. pyramida'lis ante'rior [NA], t. corticospinalis anterior; anterior or direct pyramidal tract; anterior corticospinal tract; Türck's bundle, tract, column; fasciculus corticospinalis anterior; fasciculus pyramidalis anterior. See t. pyramidalis.

t. pyramida'lis latera'lis [NA], t. corticospinalis lateralis; lateral or crossed pyramidal tract; lateral corticospinal tract; fasciculus corticospinalis lateralis; fasciculus pyramidalis lateralis. See t. pyramidalis.

t. reticulospina'lis [NA], reticulospinal tract; collective term denoting a variety of fiber tracts descending to the spinal cord from the reticular formation of the pons and medulla oblongata. Part of these fibers conduct impulses from the neural mechanisms regulating autonomic functions to the corresponding somatic and visceral motor neurons of the spinal cord; others form links in nonpyramidal motor mechanisms affecting muscle tonus, reflex activity, and somatic movement.

t. rubrospina'lis [NA], rubrospinal tract; prepyramidal tract; Monakow's tract or bundle; a somatotopically organized fiber bundle, relatively small in man, arising from the red nucleus, immediately crossing in the ventral tegmental decussation, descending near the lateral surface of the brainstem into the lateral funiculus of the spinal cord at the ventral border of the lateral pyramidal tract. It terminates in the zona intermedia of the spinal cord where its distribution coincides with that of the lateral pyramidal tract; in contrast to the latter it appears not to have direct connections with spinal motor neurons. Impulses conveyed by this tract indirectly increase flexor muscle tone.

t. solita'rius [NA], solitary tract or bundle; Gierke's or Krause's respiratory bundle; fasciculus rotundus or solitarius; funiculus solitarius; a slender, compact fiber bundle extending longitudinally through the dorsolateral region of the medullary tegmentum, surrounded by the nucleus of the solitary tract, below the obex decussating over the canalis centralis, and descending over some distance into the upper cervical segments of the spinal cord. It is composed of primary sensory fibers that enter with the vagus, glossopharyngeal, and facial nerves, and in part convey information from stretch receptors and chemoreceptors in the walls of the cardiovascular, respiratory, and intestinal tracts; in rostral parts of the tract impulses are generated by the receptor cells of the taste buds in the mucosa of the tongue. Its fibers are distributed to the nucleus of the solitary tract.

t. spina'lis ner'vi trigem'ini [NA], spinal tract of the trigeminal nerve; descending tract of the trigeminal nerve; t. descendens nervi trigemini; a compact fiber bundle, comma-shaped on transverse section, composed of primary sensory fibers of the portio major of the trigeminal nerve, descending from the level of the entrance of the trigeminus in the upper pons down through the dorsolateral region of the rhombencephalic tegmentum along the lateral side of the descending or spinal nucleus of the trigeminus, emerging on the

dorsolateral surface of the lower medulla oblongata as the tuberculum cinereum, and continuing as far as the second cervical segment of the spinal cord. Its fibers are distributed to the descending or spinal nucleus of the trigeminus.
t. spinocerebella′ris ante′rior [NA], anterior or ventral spinocerebellar tract; Gowers' tract or column; a bundle of fibers originating in the base of the posterior horn and zona intermedia throughout lumbosacral segments of the spinal cord, crossing to the opposite side and ascending in a peripheral position in the ventral half of the lateral funiculus. In its ascent through the rhombencephalon, the tract curves sharply dorsalward along the rostral border of the trigeminal motor nucleus, entering the cerebellum in a caudal direction over the dorsal surface of the superior cerebellar peduncle, and terminating as mossy fibers in the granular layer of the cortex of the cerebellar vermis. The bundle conveys proprioceptive and exteroceptive information largely from the opposite lower extremity.
t. spinocerebella′ris poste′rior [NA], posterior or dorsal spinocerebellar tract; Flechsig's tract; a compact bundle of heavily myelinated, thick fibers at the periphery of the dorsal half of the lateral funiculus of the spinal cord, originating in the ipsilateral nucleus thoracicus (column of Clarke) and ascending by way of the inferior cerebellar peduncle. Terminals end as mossy fibers in the granular layer of the cortex of the cerebellar vermis. The bundle conveys largely proprioceptive information originating from the annulospiral nerve endings surrounding muscle spindles and from Golgi tendon organs.
t. spinotecta′lis [NA], spinotectal tract; the relatively small component of the t. spinothalamicus that terminates in the intermediate and deep layers of the superior colliculus and in parts of the periaqueductal gray.
t. spinothalam′icus, spinothalamic tract; lemniscus spinalis; a large ascending fiber bundle in the ventral half of the lateral funiculus of the spinal cord, arising from cells in the posterior horn at all levels of the cord, which cross within their segments of origin in the commissura alba. In their contralateral ascent, the bundle is intermingled with numerous intersegmental fibers. The t. spinothalamicus continues from the spinal cord into the brainstem, occupying a ventrolateral position and issuing numerous fibers to the rhombencephalic and mesencephalic reticular formation, to the lateral part of the central gray substance of the mesencephalon, and to the deep and intermediate layers of the superior colliculus; the relatively few fibers (10 to 20%) that remain form the true spinothalamic tract which enters the diencephalon and ends in the nucleus ventralis posterior (pars caudalis) and intralaminar nuclei of the thalamus. In its ascent in the spinal cord the tract is composed of a dorsal part, the t. spinothalamicus lateralis, which conveys impulses associated with pain and temperature sensation, and a more ventral part, the t. spinothalamicus anterior, involved in tactile sensation.
t. spinothalam′icus ante′rior [NA], anterior or ventral spinothalamic tract; see t. spinothalamicus.
t. spinothalam′icus latera′lis [NA], lateral spinothalamic tract; see t. spinothalamicus.
t. spira′lis foramino′sus [NA], spiral foraminous tract; t. spiralis foraminulosis; openings in the cochlear area of the bottom of the internal acoustic meatus through which the fibers of the cochlear nerve leave the bony labyrinth to enter the cranial cavity.
t. spira′lis foraminulo′sus, t. spiralis foraminosus.
t. supraopticohypophysia′lis [NA], supraopticohypophysial tract; a bundle of unmyelinated fibers originating from all cells of the supraoptic nucleus and an estimated 20% of those of the paraventricular nucleus of the hypothalamus, which extend through the infundibulum and pituitary stalk to their endings in the posterior lobe of the hypophysis; the fibers convey neurosecretory substances, vasopressin and oxytocin which are stored in (and can be released into the circulating blood from) their terminals. See also hypophysis; neurosecretion.
t. tectobulba′ris, tectobulbar tract; fibers originating in the deep layers of the superior colliculus and accompanying the t. tectospinalis but, unlike the latter, terminating in medial regions of the pontine and medullary tegmentum.
t. tectoponti′nus, tectopontine tract; tract of Münzer and Wiener; a fiber bundle arising in the superior colliculus, passing caudoventrally on the same side along the medial side of the lateral lemniscus, issuing fibers terminating in the lateral zone of the mesencephalic tegmentum, and ending in the lateral part of the gray matter of the pars ventralis pontis.
t. tectospina′lis [NA], tectospinal tract; predorsal bundle; Held's bundle; Loewenthal's tract or bundle; Marchi's tract; a bundle of thick, heavily myelinated fibers originating in the deep layers of the superior colliculus, crossing to the opposite side in the dorsal tegmental decussation, descending along the median plane, between the medial longitudinal fasciculus dorsally, the medial lemniscus ventrally, into the anterior funiculus of the spinal cord. The tract ends in the medial region of the anterior horn of the cervical spinal cord, and appears to be involved in head movements during visual and auditory tracking. Throughout its course in the brainstem it is accompanied by fibers of the tectobulbar tract.
t. tegmenta′lis centra′lis [NA], t. centralis tegmenti; central tegmental tract or fasciculus; a large fiber bundle passing longitudinally through the central mesencephalic and pontine tegmentum, distinguished from adjacent longitudinal groups of fiber-fascicles of the reticular formation by a more compact composition. In transverse sections of the mesencephalon the bundle occupies a large triangular area lateral to the medial longitudinal fasciculus; farther caudally it expands ventralward and finally passes over the lateral side of the (inferior) olivary nucleus, becoming part of the latter's fiber capsule. The bundle contains fibers from the mesencephalic tegmentum and regions surrounding the central gray substance descending to the olivary nucleus; it also includes numerous fibers ascending from the medullary, pontine, and mesencephalic reticular formation to the thalamus and subthalamus region.
t. temporoponti′nus [NA], temporopontine tract; Arnold's tract or bundle; a fiber group originating in the cerebral cortex of the temporal lobe, particularly the superior and middle temporal gyri, following the sublenticular limb of the internal capsule into the lateral margin of the crus cerebri in which it descends to its termination in the pontine nuclei or pars ventralis pontis.
t. tuberoinfundibula′ris, tuberoinfundibular tract; a system of fine, unmyelinated fibers apparently originating from small-celled nuclei of the tuber cinereum, especially the nucleus arcuatus, and terminating in the median eminence of the infundibulum, in contact with modified ependymal cells and the capillary tufts from which the hypothalamohypophysial portal veins originate. See also hypophysis; neurosecretion.
t. vestibulospina′lis [NA], vestibulospinal tract; deiterospinal tract; a somatopically organized fiber bundle originating from the lateral vestibular nucleus (nucleus of Deiters) which descends uncrossed into the anterior funiculus of the spinal cord lateral to the anterior median fissure; the t. extends throughout the length of the cord, distributing fibers at all levels to the medial part of the anterior horn. Excitatory impulses conveyed by the t. v. increase extensor muscle tone.

tragacanth, tragacantha (trag′ă-kanth, -santh, -kan′thă) [G. *tragakantha,* a gum-producing shrub, fr. *tragos,* goat, + *akanthos,* thorn]. A gummy exudation from *Astragalus* species, including *A. gummifer,* shrubs of the eastern end of the Mediterranean; it occurs as bands or strings of a tough gummy substance, forming a jelly-like mucilage with 50 parts of water; used as a demulcent and excipient in emulsions and suspensions.

tragal (trā′găl). Relating to the tragus.

tragi (trā′jī). **1.** Plural of tragus. **2** [NA]. The hairs growing at the entrance to the external acoustic meatus.

tragicus (trā'ji-kŭs). See under musculus.

tragion (trā'jē-on). A cephalometric point in the notch just above the tragus of the ear; it lies 1 to 2 mm below the spina helicis, which can be palpated.

tragomaschalia (trag-ō-mas-kal'ē-ă) [G. *tragomaschalos,* with smelling armpits, fr. *tragos,* goat, + *maschalē,* the axilla]. Bromidrosis of the axillae.

tragophonia, tragophony (trag'ō-fō'nē-ă, tră-gof'ō-nē) [G. *tragos,* goat, + *phōnē,* voice]. Egophony.

tragus, pl. **tragi** (trā'gŭs, -jī) [G. *tragos,* goat, in allusion to the hairs growing on the part, like a goatee]. **1** [NA]. Antilobium; hircus (3); a tonguelike projection of the cartilage of the auricle in front of the opening of the external acoustic meatus and continuous with the cartilage of this canal. **2.** See tragi (2).

train (trān) [Fr. *trainer,* fr. L. *traho,* to draw]. To increase the virulence of bacteria by successive inoculations in animals.

training (trān'ing). An organized system of education, instruction, or discipline.

assertive t., assertive conditioning; a form of behavior modification or therapy in which a client is taught to feel free to make legitimate demands and refusals in situations which previously elicited diffident responses.

aversive t., aversive conditioning; a form of behavior t. or modification in which a noxious event is used to punish or extinguish undesirable behavior. See also aversion *therapy.*

toilet t., t. directed at teaching a child proper control of his bladder and bowel functions; in psychoanalytic personality theory, it is believed that the attitudes of both parent and child concerning this t. may have important psychological implications for the child's later development.

trait (trāt) [Fr. from L. *tractus,* a drawing out, extension]. A characteristic, especially one that distinguishes an individual from others.

Bombay t., See Bombay *phenomenon.*

categorical t., qualitative t.; in genetics, a feature that can conveniently and effectively be analyzed by sorting into classes either because there is no satisfactory way of measuring it (as with blood groups) or because it falls into natural classes so that the variation among classes far exceeds that within classes (*e.g.,* the phenotypic effects of many enzyme polymorphisms); existence of categories suggests the operation of a major, simple, underlying cause.

chromosomal t., a t. dependent on a chromosomal aberration.

codominant t., see codominant.

dominant t., **(1)** an outstanding mental or physical characteristic; **(2)** see *dominance* of genes.

intermediate t., a measurable t. in which there is some evidence of the operation of a simple major cause, but in which the variation within the putative categories is such as to cause overlap and hence ambiguity in classification of any particular reading.

liminal t., a t. that falls into natural groups that originate not in categorically distinct causes but in whether or not the outcome attains critical values; *e.g.,* gallstones may result from a categorical cause or from unusual levels of causal factors that themselves show no evidence of grouping.

marker t., a t. that may be of little importance in itself but which by association, linkage, or other means facilitates the detection, anticipation, or understanding of the disease or (for genetic diseases) the localization of the causative gene on the karyotype.

nonpenetrant t., a genetic t. that is not phenotypically manifest because of factors outside its own locus; does not include recessivity or lyonization.

qualitative t., categorical t.

recessive t., see *dominance* of genes.

sickle cell t., the heterozygous state of the gene for hemoglobin S in sickle cell anemia.

trajector (tră-jek'ter, -tōr) [L. fr. *tra-jicio,* pp. *-jectus,* to throw over or across]. An instrument for locating the course of a bullet in a wound.

tramazoline hydrochloride (tră-maz'ō-lēn). 2-[(5,6,7,8-Tetrahydro-1-naphthyl)amino]-2-imidazoline hydrochloride; an adrenergic and sympathomimetic agent used for nasal decongestion.

trance (trans) [L. *trans-eo,* to go across]. An altered state of consciousness as in hypnosis, catalepsy, or ecstacy.

death t., a condition of suspended animation, marked by unconsciousness and barely perceptible respiration and heart action.

induced t., the artificially induced state of hypnosis or of somnambulistic t.

somnambulistic t., a state of somnambulism, paralysis, anesthesia, or catalepsy induced by suggestion in major hypnosis.

tranexamic acid (tran-eks-am'ik). *trans*-4(Aminomethyl)cyclohexanecarboxylic acid; a competitive inhibitor of plasminogen activation and of plasmin; used in hemophilia to reduce or prevent hemorrhage.

tranquilizer (trang'kwi-lī-zer). A drug that promotes tranquility by calming, soothing, quieting, or pacifying without sedating or depressant effects.

major t., antipsychotic *agent.*

minor t., antianxiety *agent.*

trans- [L. *trans,* through, across]. **1.** Prefix meaning across, through, beyond; opposite of cis-. **2.** In genetics, denoting the location of two genes on opposite chromosomes of a homologous pair. **3.** In organic chemistry, a form of isomerism in which the atoms attached to two carbon atoms, joined by double bonds, are located on opposite sides of the molecule. **4.** In biochemistry, a prefix to group name in an enzyme name or a reaction denoting transfer of that group from one compound to another; *e.g.,* transformylase (transfers formyl group), transpeptidation.

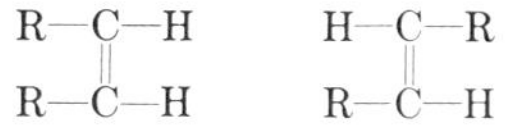

cis- *trans-*

transacetylase (trans-ă-set'i-lās). Acetyltransferase.

transacetylation (trans'ă-set-i-lā'shŭn). Transfer of an acetyl group (CH_3CO–), from one compound to another; such reactions, usually involving formation of acetyl-CoA, occur notably in the initiation of the tricarboxylic acid cycle by the transfer of an acetyl group to oxaloacetate to form citrate.

transaction (tranz-ak'shŭn). **1.** Interaction arising from the encounter of two or more persons. **2.** In transactional analysis, the unit of analysis involving a social stimulus and a response.

transacylases (trans-as'i-lā-sez). Acyltransferases.

transaldolase (trans-al'dō-lās) [EC 2.2.1.2]. Dihydroxyacetonetransferase; glycerone-transferase; transferase interconverting sedoheptulose 7-phosphate plus glyceraldehyde 3-phosphate and erythrose 4-phosphate plus fructose 6-phosphate. See also transketolase.

transaldolation (trans'al-dō-lā'shŭn). A reaction involving the transfer of an aldol group (CH_2OH–CO–CHOH–) from one compound to another; such reactions generally involve the sugar phosphates and occur in the phosphogluconate oxidation pathway of carbohydrate catabolism.

transamidinases (trans-am'i-di-nās-ez). Amidinotransferases.

transamidination (trans-am'i-di-nā'shŭn). A reaction involving the transfer of an amidine group ($NH_2C{=}NH$) from one compound to another; the amidine donor is generally arginine and the reaction is of significance in the biosynthesis of creatine.

transaminases (trans-am'i-nās-ez). Aminotransferases.

transamination (trans-am'i-nā'shŭn). The reaction between an α-amino acid and an α-keto acid through which the amino group is transferred from the former to the latter.

transanimation (trans-an'i-mā'shŭn) [trans- + L. *anima,* breath, life]. Resuscitation of a stillborn infant.

transaudient (trans-aw'dē-ent) [trans- + L. *audio,* pres. p. *audiens,* to hear]. Permeable to sound waves.

transcalent (trans-kā'lent) [trans- + L. *caleo,* to be warm]. Diathermanous.

transcapsidation (trans-kap-si-dā'shŭn). The phenomenon whereby the adenovirus capsid of the SV40 adenovirus "hybrid" is replaced by the capsid of another type of adenovirus; extended to include a similar phenomenon in other viruses.

transcarbamoylases (trans-kar-bam'ō-i-lā-sez). Carbamoyltransferases.

transcarboxylases (trans-kar-boks'i-lās-ez). Carboxyltransferases.

transcobalamins (trans-kō-bal'ă-minz). Substances included in "R binder," the name given a family of cobalamin-binding proteins; deficiencies have been associated with low serum cobalamin levels.

transcondylar (trans-kon'di-lăr). Across or through the condyles; denoting the line of bone incision in Carden's amputation.

transcortical (tranz-kōr'ti-kăl). **1.** Across or through the cortex of the brain, ovary, kidney, or other organ. **2.** From one part of the cerebral cortex to another; denoting the various association tracts.

transcortin (trans-kōr'tin). Corticosteroid-binding globulin or protein; an α_2-globulin in blood that binds cortisol and corticosterone.

transcriptase (tran-skrip'tās). A polymerase associated with the process of transcription; especially the DNA-dependent RNA polymerase.
reverse t., RNA-dependent DNA polymerase, present in virions of RNA tumor viruses.

transcription (tran-skrip'shŭn). Transfer of genetic code information from one kind of nucleic acid to another, especially with reference to the process by which a base sequence of messenger RNA is synthesized (by an RNA polymerase) on a template of complementary DNA.

transcutaneous (trans-kyū-tā'nē-ŭs). Percutaneous.

transcytosis (trans-sī-tō'sis). Cytopempsis; vesicular transport; a mechanism for transcellular transport in which a cell encloses extracellular material in an invagination of the cell membrane to form a vesicle (endocytosis), then moves the vesicle across the cell to eject the material through the opposite cell membrane by the reverse process (exocytosis).

transdermic (trans-der'mik). Percutaneous.

transduce (trans-dūs'). To effect transduction.

transducer (trans-dū'ser) [see transduction]. A device designed to convert energy from one form to another.

transducing (trans-dūs'ing). Pertaining to the mediation of transduction (*e.g.,* a transducing bacteriophage).

transductant (trans-dŭk'tănt). A cell that has acquired a new character by means of transduction; may be *complete,* with integration of the transferred genetic fragment in its genome, or *abortive,* in which case the genetic fragment is not integrated and passes to only one of the two daughter cells on division.

transduction (trans-dŭk'shŭn) [trans- + L. *duco,* pp. *ductus,* to lead across]. **1.** Transfer of genetic material (and its phenotypic expression) from one cell to another by viral infection. **2.** Conversion of energy from one form to another.
abortive t., t. in which the genetic fragment from the donor bacterium is not integrated in the genome of the recipient bacterium, and, when the latter divides, is transmitted to only one of the daughter cells.
complete t., t. in which the transferred genetic fragment is fully integrated in the genome of the recipient bacterium.
general t., t. in which the transducing bacteriophage is able to transfer any gene of the donor bacterium.
high frequency t., specialized t. in which the donor bacterium contains not only the transducing, defective probacteriophage but also nondefective prophage that serves as "helper" virus, enabling most of the defective prophage particles to develop sufficiently to function as transducing agents.
low frequency t., specialized t. in which only a small portion of the prophage particles, because of their defectiveness, are able to develop sufficiently to serve as effective transducing agents.
specialized t., specific t.; t. in which the bacteriophage strain is able to transfer only some, or only one, of the donor bacterium genes.
specific t., specialized t.

transection (tran-sek'shŭn) [trans- + L. *seco,* pp. *sectus,* to cut]. Transsection. **1.** A cross section. **2.** Cutting across.

transethmoidal (trans'eth-moy'dăl). Across or through the ethmoid bone.

transfection (trans-fek'shŭn). A method of gene transfer utilizing artificial infection of a cell nucleus with nucleic acid (as from a retrovirus) resulting in integration of the endogenous nucleic acid with the host nucleic acid, with subsequent replication in the transfected cell and cloning of the genetically engineered cell.

trans'fer [L. *trans-fero,* to bear across]. **1.** Process of removal or transferral. **2.** A condition in which learning in one situation influences learning in another situation; a carry-over of learning which may be positive in effect, as when learning one behavior facilitates the learning of something else, or may be negative, as when one habit interferes with the acquisition of a later one.
embryo t., after either in vitro or in vivo artificial insemination, the fertilized ovum is transferred at the blastocyst stage to the recipient's uterus.

transferases (trans'fer-ās-ez). Transferring enzymes; enzymes (EC class 2) transferring: one-carbon groups (2.1, including methyltransferases, 2.1.1; formyltransferases, 2.1.2; carboxyl- and carbamoyltransferases, 2.1.3, and amidinotransferases, 2.1.4); acyl residues (acyltransferases, 2.3); glycosyl residues (glycosyltransferases, 2.4, including hexosyltransferases, 2.4.1, and pentosyltransferases, 2.4.2); alkyl or aryl groups (2.5); nitrogenous groups (2.6); phosphorus-containing groups (2.7, phosphotransferases); and sulfur-containing groups (2.8, including sulfurtransferases, 2.8.1; sulfotransferases, 2.8.2; and CoA-transferases, 2.8.3).

transference (trans-fer'ens). **1.** Conveyance of an object from one place to another. **2.** Shifting of symptoms from one side of the body to the other, as seen in certain cases of conversion hysteria. **3.** Displacement of affect from one person or one idea to another; in psychoanalysis, generally applied to the projection of feelings, thoughts and wishes onto the analyst, who has come to represent some person from the patient's past.
extrasensory thought t., telepathy.
negative t., t. characterized by predominantly hostile feelings on the part of the patient toward the analyst.
passive t., the passage of an immunity or allergic susceptibility by the injection of serum of an animal or individual who has acquired an active immunity to the disease.
positive t., t. characterized by predominantly friendly, respectful, and positive feelings on the part of the patient toward the analyst.

transference love. Love expressed by the patient for the psychoanalyst as a manifestation of transference (3).

transferrin (trans-fer'in). **1.** Siderophilin; a non-heme β_1-globulin of the plasma, capable of associating reversibly with up to 1.25 μg of iron per g, and acting therefore as an iron-transporting protein. **2.** A glycoprotein, found in mammalian milk (lactoferrin) and egg white (conalbumin, ovotransferrin), that binds and transports iron (Fe^{3+}).

transfer-RNA. See under ribonucleic acid.

transfix (trans'fiks) [L. *trans-figo,* pp. *-fixus,* to pierce through, fr. *figo,* to fasten]. To pierce with a sharp instrument.

transfixion (trans-fik'shŭn) [L. *transfixio* (see transfix)]. A maneuver in amputation in which the knife is passed from side to side through the soft parts, close to the bone, and the muscles are then divided from within outward.

transformant (trans-fōr'mănt). A bacterium that has received genetic material (and its phenotypic expression) from another bacterium by means of transformation.

transformation (trans-fōr-mā'shŭn) [L. *trans-formo,* pp. *-atus,* to transform]. **1.** Metamorphosis. **2.** A change of one tissue into another, as cartilage into bone. **3.** In metals, a change in phase and physical properties in the solid state caused by heat treatment. **4.** In microbial genetics, transfer of genetic information between bacteria by means of "naked" intracellular DNA fragments derived from bacterial donor cells and incorporated into a competent recipient cell.

cell t., morphological and physiological changes resulting from infection of the cell by an oncogenic virus, and the subsequent cell-virus coexistence.

Haldane t., the multiplication of inspired oxygen concentration by the ratio of expired to inspired nitrogen concentrations in the calculation of oxygen consumption or respiratory quotient by the open circuit method.

Lobry de Bruyn-van Ekenstein t., the conversion of glucose to fructose and mannose in dilute alkali by enolization adjacent to the carbonyl group to form an enediol, a reaction analogous to certain biochemical transformations.

logit t., a method of linearizing dose-response curves for radioimmunoassay techniques; *i.e.,* Logit B (bound)/B_0(initial binding) = Log ($B/B_0/1\text{-}B/B_0$).

lymphocyte t., the t. into large, blastlike forms (immunoblasts) that occurs when lymphocytes are exposed to histoincompatible antigen either *in vitro* (mixed lymphocyte culture) or *in vivo* (organ transplant). See also mixed lymphocyte culture *test.*

nodular t. of the liver, nodular regenerative hyperplasia; a rare condition in which nodules of hyperplastic hepatocytes develop without fibrosis or general loss of lobular architecture.

transfuse (trans-fyūz'). To perform transfusion.

transfusion (trans-fyū'zhŭn) [L. *trans-fundo,* pp. *-fusus,* to pour from one vessel to another]. **1.** Transfer of blood or blood component of an individual (donor) to another individual (receptor). **2.** Intravascular injection of physiologic saline solution.

arterial t., direct t. from an artery of the donor into an artery of the receptor.

direct t., immediate t.; t. of blood from the donor to the receptor, either through a tube connecting their blood or by suturing the vessels together.

drip t., t. slow enough to measure by drops.

exchange t., exsanguination, substitution, or total t.; removal of most of a patient's blood followed by introduction of an equal amount from donors.

exsanguination t., exchange t.

immediate t., direct t.

indirect t., mediate t.; t. into a patient of blood previously obtained from a donor and stored in a suitable container.

mediate t., indirect t.

peritoneal t., the injection of saline solution or other fluid into the peritoneal cavity.

reciprocal t., an attempt to confer immunity by transfusing blood taken from a donor just recovered from an infectious disease into a receptor suffering from the same affection, the balance being maintained by transfusing an equal amount from the sick to the well person.

subcutaneous t., an infusion of absorbable solutions beneath the skin.

substitution t., total t., exchange t.

twin-twin t., direct vascular anastomosis, arterial or venous, between placental circulation of twins.

transglucosylase (trans-glū'kō-si-lās). Glucosyltransferase.

transglycosylase (trans-glī'kō-si-lās). Glycosyltransferase.

transhiatal (trans-hī-ā'tăl). By way of a hiatus; said of a surgical procedure.

transient (trans'shĕnt, -sē-ĕnt) [L. *transeo,* pres. p. *transiens,* to cross over]. **1.** Short-lived; passing; not permanent; said of a disease or an attack. **2.** A short-lived cardiac sound having little duration (less than 0.12 second) as distinct from a murmur; *e.g.,* first, second, third, and fourth heart sounds, clicks, and opening snaps.

transiliac (tran-sil'ē-ak). Extending from one ilium or iliac crest or spine to the other.

transilient (tran-sil'yent, -zil-) [L. *trans-silio,* to leap across, fr. *salio,* to leap]. Jumping across; passing over; pertaining to those cortical association fibers in the brain that pass from one convolution to another nonadjacent one.

transillumination (trans-i-lū'mi-nā'shŭn) [trans- + L. *illumino,* pp. *-atus,* to light up]. Method of examination by the passage of light through tissues or a body cavity.

transinsular (tranz-in'sū-lăr). Across the insula or island of Reil.

transischiac (trans-is'kē-ak). Extending from one ischium to the other.

transisthmian (trans-is'mē-an). Across any isthmus; specifically, across the isthmus of the gyrus fornicatus, denoting the gyrus transitivus.

transition (tran-sish'ŭn, -zish'ŭn) [L. *transitio,* fr. *transeo,* pp. *-itus,* to go across]. Change; passage from one condition or one part to another.

cervicothoracic t., the junction between the last cervical vertebra and first thoracic vertebra.

isomeric t., the t. of a nuclear isomer to a lower quantum state; *e.g.,* $^{131m}Xe \rightarrow {}^{131}Xe + \gamma$.

transitional (tran-sish'ŭn-ăl, -zish-). Relating to or marked by a transition; transitory.

transketolase (trans-kē'tō-lās) [EC 2.2.1.1]. Glycolaldehydetransferase; a transferase bringing about the interconversion of sedoheptulose 7-phosphate plus glyceraldehyde 3-phosphate and ribose 5-phosphate plus xylulose 5-phosphate, and also other similar reactions, such as hydroxypyruvate and an aldehyde into CO_2 and an extended hydroxypyruvate. See also transaldolase.

transketolation (trans'kē-tō-lā'shŭn). A reaction involving the transfer of a ketole group ($HOCH_2CO$–) from one compound to another.

translation (trans-lā'shŭn) [L. *translatio,* a transferring, fr. *transfero,* pp. *-latus,* to carry across]. **1.** A change or conversion into another form. **2.** The rather complex process by which messenger RNA, transfer RNA, and ribosomes effect the production of protein from amino acids, the specificity of synthesis being controlled by the base sequences of the messenger RNA. **3.** In dentistry, the movement of a tooth through alveolar bone without change in axial inclination.

translocation (trans-lō-kā'shŭn). Transposition of two segments between nonhomologous chromosomes as a result of abnormal breakage and refusion of reciprocal segments.

balanced t., t. of the long arm of an acrocentric chromosome to another chromosome, accompanied by loss of the small fragment containing the centromere; an individual with a balanced t. is clinically normal but has a chromosome count of 45 and is capable of having children with an unbalanced t.

reciprocal t., t. without demonstrable loss of genetic material.

robertsonian t. [W.R.B. *Robertson,* U.S. geneticist, *1881], centric fusion; t. in which the centromeres of two acrocentric chromosomes appear to have fused, forming an abnormal chromosome consisting of the long arms of two different chromosomes; if the t. is balanced, the individual is clinically normal but a carrier of the t.; if the t. is unbalanced, the individual is trisomic for the major part of a chromosome.

unbalanced t., condition resulting from fertilization of a gamete containing a t. chromosome by a normal gamete; if this abnormality is compatible with life, the individual would have 46 chromosomes but a segment of the t. chromosome would be represented three times in each cell and a partial or complete trisomic state would exist.

translucent (trans-lū'sent) [L. *translucens,* fr. trans- + *luceo,* to shine through]. Partially transparent; permitting light to pass through diffusely.

transmembrane (trans-mem'brān). Through or across a membrane.

transmethylase (trans-meth'i-lās). Methyltransferase.

transmethylation (trans'meth-i-lā'shŭn). Transfer of a methyl group from one compound to another; *e.g.,* homocysteine is converted to methionine by the transfer to the latter of a methyl group derived from choline.

transmigration (trans-mī-grā'shŭn) [L. *trans-migro,* pp. *-atus,* to remove from one place to another]. Movement from one site to another; may entail the crossing of some usually limiting barrier, as in the passage of blood cells through the walls of the vessels (diapedesis).

ovular t., the passage of an ovum from one ovary into the fallopian tube of the other side; **external o.t., direct o.t.** occurs when the ovum passes across the pelvic cavity; **internal o.t., indirect o.t.** when the ovum crosses the uterine cavity and so enters the tube of the opposite side.

transmissible (trans-mis'i-bl). Capable of being transmitted (carried across) from one person to another, as a t. disease, an infectious or contagious disease.

transmission (trans-mish'ŭn) [L. *transmissio,* a sending across]. **1.** Transfer. **2.** The conveyance of disease from one person to another. **3.** The passage of a nerve impulse across an anatomic cleft, as in autonomic or central nervous system synapses and at myoneural junctions, by activation of a specific chemical mediator which stimulates or inhibits the structure across the synapse. See neurohumeral t.; transmitter *substance.*

duplex t., the passage of impulses in both directions through a nerve trunk.

horizontal t., t. of infectious agents from an infected individual to a susceptible contemporary, in contradistinction to vertical t.

iatrogenic t., t. of infectious agents due to medical interference (*e.g.,* t. by contaminated needles).

neurohumoral t., neurotransmission; a process by which a presynaptic cell, upon excitation, releases a specific chemical agent (a neurotransmitter) to cross a synapse to stimulate or inhibit the postsynaptic cell.

transovarial t., passage of parasites or infective agents from the maternal body to eggs within the ovaries; commonly used to describe certain arthropods, to explain the ability of larvae of the next generation to transmit disease pathogens, as with the infection of larval mites or ticks with rickettsiae or viruses.

transstadial t., passage of a microbial parasite, such as a virus or rickettsia, from one developmental stage (stadium) of the host to its subsequent stage or stages, particularly as seen in mites. See also transovarial.

vertical t., **(1)** t. of a virus (*e.g.,* RNA tumor virus) by means of the genetic apparatus of a cell in which the viral genome is integrated; **(2)** for infectious agents in general, t. of an agent from an individual to its offspring. *i.e.,* from one generation to the next. *Cf.* horizontal *t.*

transmural (trans-myū'răl) [trans- + L. *murus,* wall]. Through any wall, as of the body or of a cyst or any hollow structure.

transmutation (trans-myū-tā'shŭn) [L. *trans-muto,* pp. *-atus,* to change, transmute]. A change; transformation.

transocular (trans-ok'yū-lăr). Across the eye.

transonance (trans'ō-nans) [trans- + L. *sonans,* sounding]. Transmission of a sound arising in one organ through another.

transparietal (trans-pă-rī'ĕ-tăl). Through or across a parietal region, area, or structure.

transpeptidase (trans-pep'ti-dās). An enzyme catalyzing a transpeptidation reaction; many proteolytic enzymes (*e.g.,* trypsin, papain) act as t.'s in the course of proteolysis, forming an acylated enzyme as an intermediate in the process.

transpeptidation (trans'pep-ti-dā'shŭn). A reaction involving the transfer of one or more amino acids from one peptide chain to another, as by transpeptidase action, or of a peptide chain itself, as in bacterial cell wall synthesis.

transperitoneal (trans'per-i-tō-nē'ăl). Through the peritoneum; *e.g.* denoting a nephrectomy performed by abdominal section.

transphosphatases (trans-fos'fă-tās-ez). Phosphotransferases.

transphosphorylases (trans-fos-fōr'i-lā-sez). See phosphotransferases; phosphorylases; kinase.

transphosphorylation (trans'fos-fōr-i-lā'shŭn). A reaction involving the transfer of a phosphoric group from one compound to another, often with the involvement of ATP. as by the action of a phosphotransferase or kinase.

transpirable (trans-pī'ră-bl). Capable of transpiring or being transpired.

transpiration (trans-pi-rā'shŭn) [trans- + L. *spiro,* pp. *-atus,* to breathe]. Passage of watery vapor through the skin or any membrane. See also insensible *perspiration.*

pulmonary t., the passage of water vapor from the blood into the air via the respiratory tract.

transpire (trans-pīr') [trans- + L. *spiro,* to breathe]. To exhale vapor from the skin or respiratory mucous membrane.

transplacental (tranz-pla-sen'tăl). Crossing the placenta.

transplant (tranz'plant) [trans- + L. *planto,* to plant]. **1.** To transfer from one part to another, as in grafting and transplantation. **2.** The tissue or organ in grafting and transplantation. See also graft and its subentries.

Gallie's t., narrow strips of the femoral fascia lata used for suture material.

transplantar (trans-plan'tar). Across the sole of the foot; denoting certain muscular fibers or ligamentous structures.

transplantation (tranz-plan-tā'shŭn) [L. *trans-planto,* pp. *-atus,* to transplant]. Implanting in one part a tissue or organ taken from another part or from another individual. See also subentries under graft.

bone marrow t., grafting of bone marrow tissue; of value in aplastic anemia, primary immunodeficiency, and acute leukemia (following total body irradiation).

corneal t., t. of cornea, keratoplasty.

heart t., replacement of a severely damaged heart by: 1) a healthy donated heart from a victim of trauma or other morbid process not incompatible with t.; 2) an artifical heart.

pancreaticoduodenal t., a technically feasible t. including both the duodenum and pancreas.

renal t., t. of a kidney from a compatible donor to restore kidney function in a recipient suffering from renal failure.

tendon t., **(1)** insertion of a slip from the tendon of a sound muscle into the tendon of a paralyzed muscle; **(2)** replacement of a length of tendon by a free graft.

tooth t., the transfer of a tooth from one alveolus to another.

transpleural (trans-plū′răl). Through the pleura or across the pleural cavity; on the other side of the pleura.

transport (trans′pōrt) [L. *transporto,* to carry over, fr. trans- + *porto,* to carry]. The movement or transference of biochemical substances in biologic systems.

active t., the passage of ions or molecules across a cell membrane, not by passive diffusion but by an energy-consuming process at the expense of catabolic processes proceeding within the cell; in active t., movement takes place against an electrochemical gradient.

axoplasmic t., transport by way of flow of axoplasm toward cell soma (retrograde) or toward axon terminal (anterograde).

hydrogen t., the transfer of hydrogen from one metabolite (hydrogen donor) to another (hydrogen acceptor) through the action of an enzyme system; the donor is thus oxidized and the acceptor reduced.

vesicular t., transcytosis.

transposase (tranz-pōz′ās). An enzyme that is required for transposition of DNA segments.

transpose (tranz-pōz) [L. *trans-pono,* pp. *-positus,* to place across, transfer]. To transfer one tissue or organ to the place of another and *vice versa.*

transposition (tranz-pō-zish′ŭn). **1.** Removal from one place to another; transference; metathesis. **2.** The condition of being transposed to the wrong side of the body, as in t. of the viscera, in which the viscera are located opposite their normal position; *e.g.,* the liver on the left, the apex of the heart on the right. **3.** Positioning of teeth out of their normal sequence in an arch.

t. of arterial stems, t. of the great vessels.

t. of the great vessels, t. of arterial stems; a cyanotic form of congenital cardiovascular malformation in which the aorta arises from the right ventricle while the pulmonary artery arises from the left ventricle; for life to exist there must be an associated septal defect or patent ductus arteriosus to permit some crossflow between the two circulations.

transposon (trans-pō′son). Transposable element; a segment of DNA (*e.g.,* an R-factor gene) which has a repeat of an insertion sequence element at each end that can migrate from one plasmid to another within the same bacterium, to a bacterial chromosome, or to a bacteriophage; the mechanism of transposition seems to be independent of the host's usual recombination mechanism.

transsection (trans-sek′shŭn). Transection.

transsegmental (trans-seg-men′tăl). Across or through a segment.

transseptal (trans-sep′tăl). Across or through a septum; on the other side of a septum.

transsexual (trans-sek′shū-ăl). **1.** A person with the external genitalia and secondary sexual characteristics of one sex, but whose personal identification and psychosocial configuration is that of the opposite sex; a study of morphologic, genetic, and gonadal structure may be genitally congruent or incongruent. **2.** Denoting or relating to such a person. **3.** Relating to medical and surgical procedures designed to alter a patient's external sexual characteristics so that they resemble those of the opposite sex.

transsexualism (tranz-sek′shū-ă-lizm). **1.** The state of being a transsexual. **2.** The desire to change one's anatomic sexual characteristics to conform physically with one's perception of self as a member of the opposite sex.

transsphenoidal (trans-sfē-noy′dăl). Through or across the sphenoid bone.

transsulfurase (trans-sŭl′fer-ās). Transulfurase; descriptive term applied to the enzymes catalyzing, among others, the following reactions involving sulfur-containing compounds: 1) cystathionine → cysteine + α-ketobutyrate + NH_3 (cystathionine γ-lyase); 2) cystathionine → homocysteine + pyruvate + NH_3 (cystathionine β-lyase); 3) cystine → thiocysteine + pyruvate + NH_3 (cystathionine γ-lyase); 4) cystathionine → serine + homocysteine (cystathionine synthase).

transsynaptic (trans-si-nap′tik). Indicating transmission of a nerve impulse across a synapse.

transtentorial (trans-ten-tōr′ē-ăl). Passing across or through either the tentorial notch or tentorium cerebelli.

transthalamic (trans-tha-lam′ik). Passing across the thalamus.

transthermia (trans-ther′mē-ă) [trans- + G. *thermē,* heat]. Diathermy.

transthoracic (trans-thōr-as′ik). Passing through the thoracic cavity.

transthoracotomy (trans-thōr′ă-kot′ō-mē) [trans- + thorax + G. *tomē,* incision]. A surgical procedure carried out through an incision into the chest wall.

transubstantiation (tran′sŭb-stan-shē-ā′shŭn) [trans- + L. *substantia,* substance]. Substitution of one tissue for another, as in the experimental patching of an artery with peritoneal membrane.

transudate (tran′sū-dāt) [trans- + L. *sudo,* pp. *-atus,* to sweat]. Transudation (2); any fluid (solvent and solute) that has passed through a presumably normal membrane, such as the capillary wall, as a result of imbalanced hydrostatic and osmotic forces; characteristically low in protein unless there has been secondary concentration. *Cf.* exudate.

transudation (tran-sū-dā′shŭn) [see transudate]. **1.** Passage of a fluid or solute through a membrane by a hydrostatic or osmotic pressure gradient. **2.** Transudate.

transude (tran-sūd′) [see transudate]. In general, to ooze or to pass gradually a liquid through a membrane, more specifically, through a normal membrane, as a result of imbalanced hydrostatic and osmotic forces.

transulfurase (tran-sŭl′fer-ās). Transsulfurase.

transureteroureterostomy (tranz-yū-rē′ter-ō-yū-rē-ter-os′tō-mē). Ureteroureterostomy; anastomosis of the transsected end of one ureter into the intact contralateral ureter, by direct or elliptical end-to-side technique.

transurethral (trans-yū-rē′thrăl). Through the urethra.

transvaginal (trans-vaj′i-năl). Across or through the vagina.

transvector (trans-vek′tōr, tōr). An animal that transmits a toxic substance that it does not produce, but that may be accumulated from animal (dinoflagellate) or plant (algae) sources; *e.g.,* filter-feeding mollusks.

transversalis (trans-ver-sā′lis) [L.] [NA]. Transverse.

transverse (trans-vers′) [L. *transversus*]. Transversalis; transversus; crosswise; lying across the long axis of the body or of a part.

transversectomy (trans-ver-sek′tō-mē) [transverse + G. *ektomē,* excision]. Exsection of the transverse process of a vertebra.

transversion (trans-ver′zhŭn). **1.** Substitution in DNA and RNA of a pyrimidine for a purine, or vice-versa, by mutation. **2.** In dentistry, the eruption of a tooth in a position normally occupied by another; transposition of a tooth.

transversocostal (trans-ver′sō-kos′tăl). Costotransverse.

transversourethralis (trans-ver-sō-yū-rē-thrā′lis). Denoting the transverse fibers of the sphincter urethrae muscle, arising from the arch of the pubes.

transversus (trans-ver′sŭs) [L. fr. *trans,* across, + *verto,* pp. *versus,* to turn] [NA]. Transverse.

transvestism (trans-ves′tizm) [trans- + L. *vestio,* to dress]. Transvestitism; the practice of dressing or masquerading in the clothes of the opposite sex; especially the adoption of feminine mannerisms and costume by a male.

transvestite (trans-ves'tīt). A person who practices transvestism.

transvestitism (trans-ves'ti-tizm). Transvestism.

Trantas, Alexios, Greek ophthalmologist, 1867–1960. See T.'s *dots;* Horner-T. *dots.*

tranylcypromine sulfate (tran-il-sip'rō-mēn). (+)-*trans*- 2-Phenylcyclopropylamine sulfate; a monoamine oxidase inhibitor; an antidepressant used in the treatment of severe mental depression.

trapezial (tra-pē'zē-ăl). Relating to any trapezium.

trapeziform (tra-pē'zi-form). Trapezoid (1).

trapeziometacarpal (tra-pē'zē-ō-met'ă-kar'păl). Relating to the trapezium and the metacarpus.

trapezium, pl. **trapezia, trapeziums** (tra-pē'zē-ŭm, -ă) [G. *trapezoin,* a table or counter, a trapezium, dim. of *trapeza,* a table, fr. *tra-* (=*tetra-*), four, + *pous* (*pod-*), foot]. **1.** A four-sided geometrical figure having no two sides parallel. **2.** *Os* trapezium.

trapezius (tra-pē'zē-ŭs). *Musculus* trapezius.

trapezoid (trap'ĕ-zoyd) [G. *trapezōdēs,* fr. *trapezoin,* trapezium, + *eidos,* resemblance]. **1.** Trapeziform; resembling a trapezium. **2.** A geometrical figure resembling a trapezium except that two of its opposite sides are parallel. **3.** *Os* trapezoideum. **4.** *Corpus* trapezoideum.

trapidil (trap'ĭ-dil). *N,N*-Diethyl-5-methyl-[1,2,4]triazolo-[1,5-a]pyrimidin-7-amine; an antagonist and selective synthesis inhibitor of thromboxane A_2; used to prevent cerebral vasospasm.

Trapp, Julius, Russian pharmacist, 1815–1908. See T.'s *formula;* T.-Häser *formula.*

Traube, Ludwig, German physician and pathologist, 1818–1876. See T.'s *bruit, corpuscle, dyspnea, plugs, space,* double *tone;* T.-Hering *curves, waves.*

Traugott, Carl, German internist, *1885. See Staub-T. *effect.*

traum-, traumat-. See traumato-.

trauma, pl. **traumata, traumas** (traw'mă, -mă-tă) [G. wound]. Traumatism; an injury, physical or mental.

birth t., **(1)** physical injury to an infant during its delivery; **(2)** the supposed emotional injury, inflicted by events incident to birth, upon an infant which allegedly appears in symbolic form in patients with mental illness.

occlusal t., abnormal occlusal stresses capable of producing or which have produced pathologic changes in the tooth and its surrounding structures.

t. from occlusion, a reversible lesion in the periodontium caused by excessive movement of teeth.

psychic t., an upsetting experience precipitating or aggravating an emotional or mental disorder.

traumasthenia (traw-mas-thē'nē-ă) [traum- + G. *astheneia,* weakness]. Nervous exhaustion following an injury.

traumata (traw'mă-tă). Plural of trauma.

traumatic (traw-mat'ik) [G. *traumatikos*]. Relating to or caused by trauma.

traumatism (traw'mă-tizm). Trauma (1).

traumatize (traw'mă-tīz) [G. *traumatizō,* to wound]. To cause or inflict trauma.

traumato-, traumat-, traum- [G. *trauma,* wound]. Combining forms denoting wound, injury.

traumatology (traw-mă-tol'ō-jē) [traumato- + G. *logos,* study]. The branch of surgery concerned with the injured.

traumatonesis (traw'mă-tō-nē'sis, -ton'ē-sis) [traumato- + G. *neois,* a spinning]. Surgical repair of an accidental wound.

traumatopathy (traw-mă-top'ă-thē) [traumato- + G. *pathos,* suffering]. Any pathologic condition resulting from violence or wounds.

traumatopnea (traw'mă-top-nē'ă) [traumato- + G. *pnoē,* breath]. Passage of air in and out through a wound of the chest wall.

traumatopyra (traw'mă-tō-pī'ră) [traumato- + G. *pyr,* fire, fever]. Obsolete synonym of traumatic *fever.*

traumatosepsis (traw'mă-tō-sep'sis) [traumato- + G. *sēpsis,* putrefaction]. Infection of a wound; septicemia following a wound.

traumatotherapy (traw'mă-tō-ther'ă-pē). Treatment of trauma or the result of injury.

Trautmann, Moritz F., German otologist, 1832–1902. See T.'s triangular *space.*

traverse (trav'ers). In computed tomography, one complete linear movement of the gantry across the object being scanned, as occurs in translate and rotate CT machines.

tray (trā). A flat receptacle with raised edges.

acrylic resin t., a plastic impression t. used in dentistry; usually fashioned for the individual patient from an autopolymerizing acrylic resin.

annealing t., an electrically heated, thermostatically controlled device used to drive off the protective NH_3 gas coating from the surface of cohesive gold foil.

impression t., a receptacle used to carry and confine plastic impression material when making an impression of oral structures.

trazodone hydrochloride (traz'ō-dōn). 2-[3-[4-(*m*-Chlorophenyl)-1-piperazinyl]propyl]-*s*-triazolo[4,3-*a*]pyridin-3(2*H*)one monohydrochloride; an antidepressant structurally unrelated to other antidepressants.

Treacher Collins. See Collins, Edward Treacher.

treacle (trē'kl) [M.E. *triacle,* antidote, fr. L. *theriaca,* antidote to snake bite, fr. G. *thēriakos,* pertaining to wild beasts]. **1.** Molasses, a viscid syrup that drains from sugar-refining molds. **2.** A saccharine fluid. **3.** Formerly, a remedy for poison, hence any effective remedy. See also theriaca.

treat (trēt) [Fr. *traiter,* fr. L. *tracto,* to drag, handle, perform]. To manage a disease by medicinal, surgical, or other measures; to care for a patient medically or surgically.

treatment (trēt'ment) [Fr. *traitment* (see treat)]. Medical or surgical management of a patient. See also therapy; therapeutics.

Carrel's t., Dakin-Carrel t., t. of wound surfaces by intermittent flushing with Dakin's solution.

Goeckerman t., a t. for psoriasis; the involved areas are painted with a solution of coal tar, or are covered with coal tar ointment and subsequently irradiated with ultraviolet.

heat t., in dentistry, a method of controlled temperature handling of metals so as to change the microscopic structure and thus the physical properties. See also temper; anneal.

insulin coma t., rarely used t. of major mental illness by means of hypoglycemic coma induced by insulin.

isoserum t., therapeutic use of serum taken from a person having or having had the same disease as the patient under treatment.

Kenny's t., a method for the t. of anterior poliomyelitis; the affected parts are wrapped in woolen cloth wrung out with hot water; after the acute stage of the disease has passed, the limbs are passively exercised to reeducate the paralyzed muscles.

light t., phototherapy.

medical t., conservative t. of disease by hygienic and pharmacologic remedies, as distinguished from invasive surgical procedures.

Mitchell's t., Weir Mitchell t.; t. of mental illness by rest, nourishing diet, and a change of environment.

moral t., a type of milieu therapy utilized in the 19th century, emphasizing religious doctrine and benevolent guidance in activities of daily living; as such it was a form of psychotherapy as opposed to somatic t.'s such as bloodletting and purging.

Nauheim t. [*Bad Nauheim,* W. Germany], Nauheim bath; Schott t; t. of certain cardiac affections by baths in water through which carbonic acid gas is bubbling, followed by resisting exercises.
palliative t., t. to alleviate symptoms without curing the disease.
preventive t., prophylactic t.
prophylactic t., preventive t.; the institution of measures designed to protect a person from an attack of a disease to which he has been, or is liable to be exposed.
root canal t., **(1)** the means by which painful or diseased teeth, in which the pulp is involved, are restored to a healthy state; **(2)** removal of a normal, diseased, or dead pulp by biochemical and mechanical means, enlargement and sterilization of the root canal, followed by filling the canal, to effect healing of diseased periapical tissues; **(3)** the diagnosis and t. of diseases of the pulp and their sequelae.
Schott t., Nauheim t.
shock t., see electroshock *therapy.*
Tweed edgewise t., see edgewise *appliance.*
Weir Mitchell t., Mitchell's t.

trehala (trē-hah'lă). A saccharine substance containing trehalose and resembling manna, excreted by a parasitic beetle, *Larinus maculatus.*

trehalose (trē'hă-lōs). Mycose; a nonreducing disaccharide, (α-D-glucosido)-α-D-glucoside, contained in trehala; also found in fungi, such as *Amanita muscaria.*

Treitz, Wenzel, Bohemian pathologist, 1819–1872. See T.'s *arch, fascia, fossa, hernia, ligament, muscle.*

Trélat, Ulysse, French surgeon, 1828–1890. See T.'s *stools;* Leser-T. *sign.*

trema (trē'mă) [G. *trēma,* a hole]. **1.** Foramen. **2.** Vulva.

Trematoda (trem'ă-tō'dă) [G. *trēmatōdēs,* full of holes, fr. *trēma,* a hole, + *eidos,* appearance]. A class in the phylum Platyhelminthes (the flatworms), consisting of flukes with a leaf-shaped body and two muscular suckers, and an acelomate parenchyma-filled body cavity. Circulatory system and sense organs are not present, but an incomplete alimentary canal is found (lacking an anus). Flukes of interest to human or veterinary medicine are members of the order Digenea, with complete life cycles involving embryonic multiplication in a mollusk first intermediate host. The other order, Monogenea, consists chiefly of parasites of fish that have a simpler pattern of direct development on a single host.

trematode, trematoid (trem'ă-tōd, trem'ă-toyd). **1.** Common name for a fluke of the class Trematoda. **2.** Relating to a fluke of the class Trematoda.

trembles (trem'blz) [L. *tremulus,* trembling, fr. *tremo,* to tremble]. An intoxication of cattle, caused by eating white snakeroot, *Eupatorium urticaefolium,* or the rayless goldenrod; the active agent is a higher alcohol, tremetol, which intoxicated cows eliminate in their milk, causing milk sickness when ingested by man.

tremb'ling. The shaking or quaking of a tremor.

tremelloid, tremellose (trem'ĕ-loyd, -lōs) [L. *tremulus,* trembling]. Jelly-like.

tremogram (trem'ō-gram). Tremorgram; the graphic representation of a tremor taken by means of the tremograph or kymograph.

tremograph (trem'ō-graf) [L. *tremor,* a shaking, + G. *graphō,* to write]. An apparatus for making a graphic record of a tremor.

tremolabile (trem-ō-lā'bil, -bīl) [L. *tremor,* a shaking, + *labilis,* perishable]. Inactivated or destroyed by shaking.

tremophobia (trem-ō-fō'bē-ă) [L. *tremor,* trembling, + G. *phobos,* fear]. Morbid fear of trembling.

tremor (trem'er, -ōr) [L. a shaking]. **1.** An involuntary trembling movement. **2.** Minute ocular movement occurring during fixation on an object.
action t., intention t.
alternating t., a form of hyperkinesia characterized by regular, symmetrical, to-and-fro movements (at about 4 per second) that are produced by patterned, alternating contraction of muscles and their antagonists.
arsenical t., a t. caused by chronic poisoning by arsenic.
t. ar'tuum, trembling of the extremities, especially of the hands.
benign essential t., heredofamilial t.
coarse t., a t. in which the amplitude is large and the oscillations are usually irregular and slow.
continuous t., persistent t.
epidemic t., avian infectious *encephalomyelitis.*
fibrillary t., isolated twitching of the fine strands or fasciculi of a muscle.
fine t., a t. in which there are 10 to 12 vibrations per second.
flapping t., asterixis.
head t.'s, head-nodding.
heredofamilial t., benign essential t.; a benign t. inherited as a dominant character; it may be a rapid oscillation resembling that seen in thyrotoxicosis, a coarse t. during rest and inhibited by a voluntary effort, or one which appears only upon movement.
intention t., action t.; volitional t. (2); a t. that occurs when a voluntary movement is made.
kinetic t., a t. occurring during active movement of the limb.
mercurial t., a t. caused by chronic mercury poisoning.
metallic t., a t. caused by poisoning with metal.
t. opiophago'rum, a t. occurring in opium addicts.
passive t., a t. that occurs when the subject is at rest, and diminishes or ceases during voluntary movement.
persistent t., continuous t.; a t. that is constant, whether the subject is at rest or moving.
postural t., static t.
t. potato'rum, a t. occurring in the subjects of chronic alcoholism.
progressive cerebellar t., Hunt's *syndrome* (1).
saturnine t., a t. caused by chronic lead poisoning.
senile t., a t., usually an intention t., but sometimes a persistent t., occurring in the aged.
static t., postural t.; a t. excited when the person makes an effort to hold a limb in a certain position.
t. ten'dinum, *subsultus* tendinum.
volitional t., **(1)** a t. that can be arrested by a strong effort of the will; **(2)** intention t.

tremorgram (trem'ōr-gram). Tremogram.

tremostable (trem-ō-stā'bl) [L. *tremor,* a shaking, + *stabilis,* stable]. Not subject to alteration or destruction by being shaken.

tremulor (trem'yū-ler, -lōr). An instrument for giving vibratory massage.

tremulous (trem'yū-lŭs). Characterized by tremor.

Trenaunay, Paul, French physician, *1875. See Klippel-T.-Weber *syndrome.*

Trendelenburg, Friedrich, German surgeon, 1844–1924. See T.'s *operation, position, sign, symptom, test.*

trend of thought. Thinking with a tendency toward or centering on a particular idea with a particular affect.

trepan (trē-pan') [G. *trypanon,* a borer]. Trephine.

trepanation (trep-ă-nā'shŭn). Trephination.
corneal t., t. of cornea, keratoplasty.

trephination (tref-i-nā'shŭn). Trepanation; removal of a circular piece ("button") of cranium by a trephine.

trephine (trē-fīn', -fēn') [contrived fr. L. *tres fines,* three ends]. Trepan. **1.** A cylindrical or crown saw used for the removal of a disc of bone, especially from the skull, or of other firm tissue as that of the cornea. **2.** To remove a disc of bone or other tissue by means of a t.

trephocyte (tref'ō-sīt) [G. *trephō,* to nourish, + *kytos,* cell]. Trophocyte.

trepidant (trep'i-dant) [L. *trepidans,* pres. p. of *trepido,* to tremble, to be agitated]. Trembling; marked by tremor.

trepidatio cordis (trep-i-dā'shē-ō kōr'dis). Palpitation.

trepidation (trep-i-dā'shŭn) [L. *trepidatio,* fr. *trepido,* to tremble, to be agitated]. **1.** Trembling; tremor. **2.** Anxious fear.

Treponema (trep-ō-nē'mă) [G. *trepō,* to turn, + *nēma,* thread]. A genus of anaerobic bacteria (order Spirochaetales) consisting of cells, 3 to 8 μm in length, with acute, regular, or irregular spirals and no obvious protoplasmic structure. A terminal filament may be present. They stain with difficulty except with Giemsa's stain or silver impregnation. Some species are pathogenic and parasitic for humans and other animals, generally producing local lesions in tissues. The type species is *T. pallidum.*

T. callig'yrum, a species found in lesions and membranes of the pudenda.
T. cara'teum, a species that causes pinta, or carate.
T. cunic'uli, a species which causes spirochetosis in rabbits.
T. genita'lis, a nonpathogenic species found on the genitalia of humans.
T. hyodysente'riae, an enteropathogenic species that causes swine dysentery.
T. microden'tium, a species found in the normal oral cavity.
T. muco'sum, a species found in pyorrhea alveolaris; it possesses pyogenic properties.
T. pal'lidum, a species which causes syphilis in man; this organism can be experimentally transmitted to anthrapoid apes and to rabbits; it is the type species of the genus *T.*
T. perten'ue, a species that causes yaws; patients with this disease give positive results in serologic screening tests for syphilis.

treponematosis (trep'ō-nē-mă-tō'sis). Treponemiasis.

treponeme (trep'ō-nēm). A vernacular term used to refer to any member of the genus *Treponema.*

treponemiasis (trep'ō-nē-mī'ă-sis). Treponematosis; infection caused by *Treponema.*

treponemicidal (trep'ō-nē'mi-sī'dăl) [*Treponema* + L. *caedo,* to kill]. Antitreponemal; destructive to any species of *Treponema,* but usually with reference to *T. pallidum.*

treppe (trep'eh) [Ger. *Treppe,* staircase]. Staircase phenomenon; a phenomenon in cardiac muscle first observed by H.P. Bowditch; if a number of stimuli of the same intensity are sent into the muscle after a quiescent period, the first few contractions of the series show a successive increase in amplitude.

Tresilian, Frederick J., British physician, 1862–1926. See T.'s *sign.*

tresis (trē'sis) [G. *trēsis,* a boring]. Perforation.

tretinoin (tret'i-nō-in). All-*trans*-retinoic acid; a keratolytic agent. See retinoic acid.

Treves, Sir Frederick, British surgeon, 1853–1923. See T.'s *fold.*

Treves, Norman, U.S. surgeon, *1894. See Stewart-T. *syndrome.*

TRF Abbreviation for thyrotropin-releasing *factor.*

TRH Abbreviation for thyrotropin-releasing *hormone.*

tri- [L. and G.] Prefix denoting three. *Cf.* tris-.

triacetic acid (trī-ă-sē'tik). 3,5-Dioxohexanoic acid; $CH_3COCH_2COCH_2COOH$; formed by condensation of acetyl and malonyl CoA's in the course of fatty acid synthesis.

triacetin (trī-as'ĕ-tin). Glyceryl triacetate; triacetylglycerol; used as a solvent of basic dyes, as a fixative in perfumery, and as a topical antifungal agent.

triacetylglycerol (trī-as'i-til-glis'er-ol). Triacetin.

triacetyloleandomycin (trī-as'ĕ-til-ō'lē-an-dō-mī'sin). Troleandomycin.

triacylglycerol (trī-as'il-glis'er-ol). Triglyceride; glycerol esterified at each of its three hydroxyl groups by a fatty (aliphatic) acid; *e.g.,* tristearoylglycerol.

t. lipase [EC 3.1.1.3], tributyrase; tributyrinase; steapsin; the fat-splitting enzyme in pancreatic juice.

triad (trī'ad) [G. *trias (triad-),* the number 3, fr. *tries,* three]. **1.** A collection of three things having something in common. **2.** The transverse tubule and the terminal cisternae on each side of it in skeletal muscle fibers. **3.** The branches of the portal vein, hepatic artery, and bile duct in a portal tract. **4.** The father, mother, and child relationship projectively experienced in group psychotherapy.

acute compression t., Beck's triad; the rising venous pressure, falling arterial pressure, and decreased heart sounds of pericardial tamponade.
Beck's t., acute compression t.
Bezold's t., diminished perception of the deeper tones, retarded bone conduction, and negative Rinne's test, pointing, in the absence of objective signs, to otosclerosis.
Charcot's t., in multiple (disseminated) sclerosis, the three symptoms: nystagmus, tremor, and scanning speech.
Fallot's t., *trilogy* of Fallot.
hepatic t., branches of the portal vein, hepatic artery, and the biliary ducts bound together in the perivascular fibrous capsule as they ramify within the substance of the liver.
Hull's t., the association of diastolic gallop, anasarca, and small pulse pressure.
Hutchinson's t., parenchymatous keratitis, labyrinthine disease, and Hutchinson's teeth, significant of congenital syphilis.
Kartagener's t., Kartagener's *syndrome.*
Saint's t., the concurrence of hiatal hernia, diverticulosis, and cholelithiasis.

triage (trē'ahzh) [Fr. sorting]. Medical screening of patients to determine their relative priority for treatment; the separation of a large number of casualties, in military or civilian disaster medical care, into three groups: 1) those who cannot be expected to survive even with treatment; 2) those who will recover without treatment; 3) the highest priority group of those who need treatment in order to survive.

trial and error. The apparently random, haphazard, hit-or-miss exploratory activity which often precedes the acquisition of new information or adjustments; it may be overt, as in a rat running in a maze, or covert (vicarious), as when one thinks of various ways of coping with a situation.

triamcinolone (trī-am-sin'ō-lōn). 9α-Fluoro-16α-hydroxyprednisolone; a glucocorticoid with actions and uses similar to those of prednisolone.

t. acetonide, a potent glucocorticoid for topical treatment of dermatoses.
t. diacetate, an anti-inflammatory and antiallergic agent for parenteral use.

tri-amelia (trī'ă-mē'lē-ă) [tri- + G. *a-* priv. + *melos,* limb]. Absence of three limbs.

triamterene (trī-am'ter-ēn). 2,4,7-Triamino-6-phenylpteridine; a diuretic agent.

TRIANGLE

triangle (trī'ang-gl) [L. *triangulum,* fr. *tri-,* three, + *angulus,* angle]. In anatomy and surgery, a three-sided area with arbitrary or natural boundaries. See also trigone; trigonum.

anal t., *regio* analis.
anterior t., *regio* cervicalis anterior.

Assézat's t., a t. formed by lines connecting the nasion with the alveolar and nasal point; used to indicate prognathism in comparative craniology.
auricular t., a t. formed by the base of the auricle and by lines drawn from the true tip of the auricle to the extremities of the base.
t. of auscultation, space bounded by the lower border of the trapezius, the latissimus dorsi, and the medial margin of the scapula.
axillary t., a triangular area embracing the medial aspect of the arm, the axilla, and the pectoral region which is one of the seats of predilection for the petechial initial rash of smallpox.
Béclard's t., area bounded by the posterior border of the hyoglossus muscle, the posterior belly of the digastric and the greater horn of the hyoid bone.
Bonwill t., an equilateral t. formed by lines from the contact points of the lower central incisors, or the medial line of the residual ridge of the mandible, to the condyle on either side and from one condyle to the other.
Bryant's t., iliofemoral t.; in fracture of the neck of the femur to determine upward displacement of the trochanter, lines are drawn on the body to form a t.: line *a* is drawn around the body at the level of the anterior superior iliac spines; line *b,* perpendicular to line *a,* is drawn to the great trochanter of the femur; line *c* is drawn from the trochanter to the iliac spine; upward displacement is measured along line *b.*
Burow's t., a triangle of skin and subcutaneous fat excised so that a pedicle flap can be advanced without buckling the adjacent tissue.
Calot's t., t. bounded by the cystic artery, cystic duct, and hepatic duct; its dissection early in cholecystectomy safeguards essential structures, should there be anatomic variations from the norm.
cardiohepatic t., cardiohepatic *angle.*
carotid t.'s, see *trigonum* musculare; *trigonum* caroticum.
cephalic t., a t. on the cranium formed by lines connecting the metopion, the pogonion, and the occipital point.
cervical t., *trigonum* cervicale.
Codman's t., in radiology, the interface between growing bone tumor and normal bone, presenting as an incomplete triangle formed by periosteum.
crural t., an area of predilection for the petechial initial rash of smallpox; it occupies the lower abdominal, inguinal, and genital regions and the inner aspects of the thighs, the base of the t. traversing the umbilicus.
deltoideopectoral t., *fossa* infraclavicularis.
digastric t., *trigonum* submandibulare.
Einthoven's t., an imaginary equilateral t. with the heart at its center, formed by lines representing the three standard limb leads of the electrocardiogram.

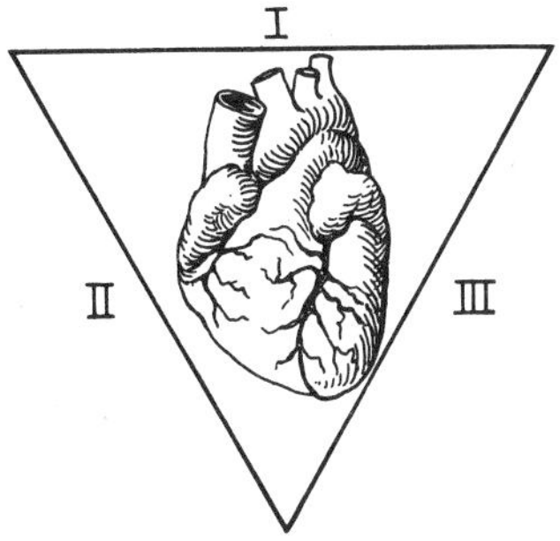

Einthoven's Triangle

Elaut's t., t. formed by the iliac arteries and the promontory of the sacrum.
t. of elbow, a space between the pronator teres and the brachioradialis muscles on the flexor side of the elbow.
facial t., a t. formed by lines connecting the basion, the prosthion, and the nasion.
Farabeuf's t., the t. formed by the internal jugular and facial veins and the hypoglossal nerve.
femoral t., *trigonum* femorale.
t. of fillet, *trigonum* lemnisci.
frontal t., a t. bounded above by the maximum frontal diameter and laterally by lines joining the extremities of this diameter with the glabella.
Garland's t., a triangular area of relative resonance in the lower back near the spine, found in the same side as a pleural effusion.
Gombault's t., see *fasciculus* semilunaris.
Grocco's t., Grocco's sign (3); paravertebral t.; a triangular patch of dullness at the base of the chest alongside the spinal column, on the side opposite a pleural effusion.
Grynfeltt's t., Lesshaft's t.; a triangular space bounded above by the end of the last rib and the serratus posterior inferior muscle, anteriorly by the obliquus internus, and posteriorly by the quadratus lumborum; lumbar hernia occurs in this space.
Hesselbach's t., *trigonum* inguinale.
iliofemoral t., Bryant's t.
inferior carotid t., *trigonum* musculare.
inferior occipital t., a t. with its apex at the external occipital protuberance; its base is formed by a line joining the two mastoid processes.
infraclavicular t., *fossa* infraclavicularis.
inguinal t., *trigonum* inguinale.
Koch's t., a triangular area of the wall of the right atrium of the heart, that marks the situation of the atrioventricular node.
Labbé's t., an area bounded below by a horizontal line touching the lower edge of the cartilage of the left ninth rib, laterally by the line of the false ribs, and to the right side by the liver; here the stomach is normally in contact with the abdominal wall.
Langenbeck's t., a t. formed by lines drawn from the anterior superior iliac spine to the surface of the great trochanter and to the surgical neck of the femur; a penetrating wound in this area probably involves the joint.
Lesser's t., the space between the bellies of the digastric muscle and the hypoglossal nerve.
Lesshaft's t., Grynfeltt's t.
Lieutaud's t., *trigonum* vesicae.
lumbar t., *trigonum* lumbale.
lumbocostoabdominal t., an irregular area bounded by the serratus posterior inferior, obliquus externus, obliquus internus, and erector spinae muscles.
Macewen's t., suprameatal t.
Malgaigne's t., *trigonum* caroticum.
Marcille's t., an area bounded by the medial border of the psoas major, the lateral margin of the vertebral column, and the iliolumbar ligament below; it is crossed by the obturator nerve.
muscular t., *trigonum* musculare.
occipital t., a t. of the neck bounded by the trapezius, the sternocleidomastoid, and the omohyoid muscles. See also inferior occipital t.
omoclavicular t., *trigonum* omoclaviculare.
omotracheal t., *trigonum* musculare.
palatal t., trigonum palati; a triangular area bounded by the greatest transverse diameter of the palate and by lines converging from its extremities to the alveolar point.
paravertebral t., Grocco's t.
Petit's lumbar t., *trigonum* lumbale.
Philippe's t., see *fasciculus* semilunaris.
Pirogoff's t., a t. formed by the intermediate tendon of the digastric muscle, the posterior border of the mylohyoid muscle, and the hypoglossal nerve.
posterior t. of neck, *regio* cervicalis lateralis.
pubourethral t., a t. in the perineum bounded by the transversus

perinei, the ischiocavernosus, and the bulbocavernosus muscles.
Reil's t., *trigonum* lemnisci.
sacral t., the surface area over the sacrum.
t. of safety, the area at the lower left sternal border where the pericardium is not covered by lung; preferred site for aspiration of pericardial fluid.
Scarpa's t., *trigonum* femorale.
sternocostal t., *trigonum* sternocostale.
subclavian t., *trigonum* omoclaviculare.
subinguinal t., *trigonum* femorale.
submandibular t., *trigonum* submandibulare.
submaxillary t., *trigonum* submandibulare.
submental t., *trigonum* submentale.
suboccipital t., a t. bounded by the obliquus inferior, the obliquus superior, and the rectus capitis posterior major muscles.
superior carotid t., *trigonum* caroticum.
suprameatal t., Macewen's t.; a t. formed by the root of the zygomatic arch, the posterior wall of the bony external acoustic meatus, and an imaginary line connecting the extremities of the first two lines; used as a guide in mastoid operations.
tracheal t., *trigonum* musculare.
Tweed t., a t. defined by facial and dental landmarks on a lateral cephalometric film, using the Frankfort horizontal plane as a base and intended for use as a guide in the evaluation and planning of orthodontic treatment.
umbilicomammillary t., a t. with its apex at the umbilicus and its base at the line joining the nipples.
urogenital t., *regio* urogenitalis.
vesical t., *trigonum* vesicae.
Ward's t., an area of diminished density in the trabecular pattern of the neck of the femur evident by x-ray as well as by direct inspection.
Weber's t., on the sole of the foot, an area indicated by the heads of the first and fifth metatarsal bone and the center of the plantar surface of the heel.
Wilde's t., *pyramid* of light.

triangularis (trī-ang'gū-lā'ris) [L.]. See entries under musculus.

triangulum (trī-ang'gū-lŭm) [L.]. Triangle; trigone.

Triatoma (trī-ă-tō'mă). A genus of insects (subfamily Triatominae, family Reduviidae) that includes important vectors of *Trypanosoma cruzi,* such as *T. dimidiata, T. infestans,* and *T. maculata.*

Triatominae (trī-ă-tō'mi-nē). A subfamily of insects (family Reduviidae, suborder Heteroptera) that are vertebrate bloodsuckers and include such important disease vector species as *Panstrongylus, Rhodnius,* and *Triatoma;* they are commonly called conenose or kissing bugs.

triazolam (trī-ā'zō-lam). 8-Chloro-6-(*o*-chlorophenyl)-1-methyl-4*H*-*s*-triazolo[4,3-*a*][1,4]benzodiazepine; a benzodiazepine derivative used as a sedative and hypnotic.

triazologuanine (trī'ă-zol-ō-gwah'nēn). 8-Azaguanine.

tribade (trib'ăd) [G. *tribō,* to rub]. A lesbian, especially one who obtains sexual pleasure by rubbing her external genitalia against those of another woman.

tribadism, tribady (trib'ăd-izm, -ă-dē) [G. *tribō,* to rub]. Lesbianism, particularly as practiced by a tribade.

tribasic (trī-bā'sik). Having three titratable hydrogen atoms; denoting an acid with a basicity of 3.

tribasilar (trī-bas'i-lăr). Having three bases.

tribe (trīb) [L. *tribus*]. In biological classification, an occasional division between the family and the genus; often the same as the subfamily.

tribology (tri-bol'ō-jē) [G. *tribō,* to rub, + *logos,* study]. The study of friction and its effects in biological systems, especially in regard to articulated surfaces of the skeleton.

triboluminescence (trib'ō-lū-mi-nes'ens) [G. *tribō,* to rub, + luminescence]. Luminosity produced by friction.

tribrachia (trī-brā'kē-ă) [tri- + G. *brachiōn,* arm]. Condition seen in conjoined twins when the fusion has merged the adjacent arms to form a single one, so that there are only three arms for the two bodies.

tribrachius (trī-brā'kē-ŭs). Conjoined twins exhibiting tribrachia.

tribromoethanol (trī-brō-mō-eth'ă-nol). $Br_3C—CH_2OH$; a basal anesthetic agent administered rectally.

tribromsalan (trī-brom'să-lan). 3,4',5-Tribromosalicylanilide; a disinfectant used in soaps.

tributyrase (trī-byū'ti-rās). *Triacylglycerol* lipase.

tributyrin (trī-byū'ti-rin). Tributyrylglycerol; glyceryl tributyrate; a synthetic substrate for lipase assays.

tributyrinase (trī-byū'ti-ri-nās). *Triacylglycerol* lipase.

tributyrylglycerol (trī-byū'ti-ril-glis'er-ol). Tributyrin.

TRIC Acronym for *tr*achoma and *i*nclusion *c*onjunctivitis. See TRIC *agents.*

tricalcium phosphate (trī-kal'sē-ŭm). Tribasic *calcium* phosphate.

tricephalus (trī-sef'ă-lŭs) [tri- + G. *kephalē,* head]. Fetus with three heads.

triceps (trī'seps) [L. fr. *tri-,* three, + *caput,* head]. Three-headed; denoting especially two muscles: t. brachii and t. surae. See entries under musculus.

trich-. See tricho-.

trichalgia (trik-al'jē-ă) [trich- + G. *algos,* pain]. Trichodynia; pain produced by touching the hair.

trichangion (trik-an'jē-on) [trich- + G. *angeion,* vessel]. Telangion.

trichatrophia (trik-ă-trō'fē-ă) [trich- + G. *atrophia,* atrophy]. Atrophy of the hair bulbs, with brittleness, splitting, and falling out of hair.

trichauxis (trik-awk'sis) [trich- + G. *auxis,* increase]. Excessive growth of hair in length and quantity.

trichi-. See tricho-.

-trichia [G. *thrix* (*trich-*), hair, + *-ia,* condition]. Combining form denoting condition or type of hair.

trichiasis (tri-kī'ă-sis) [trich- + G. *-iasis,* condition]. Trichoma; trichomatosis; a condition in which the hair adjacent to a natural orifice turns inward and causes irritation; *e.g.,* in inversion of an eyelid (entropion), eyelashes irritate the eye.

trichilemmoma (trik'i-le-mō'mă) [trichi- + G. *lemma,* husk, + *-ōma,* tumor]. Tricholemmoma; a benign tumor derived from outer root sheath epithelium of a hair follicle, consisting of cells with pale-staining cytoplasm containing glycogen; multiple t.'s are present on the face in Cowden's disease.

Trichina (tri-kī'nă). Old name for a genus of nematode worms, correctly called *Trichinella.*

trichina, pl. **trichinae** (tri-kī'nă, -nē) [Mod. L., fr. G. *thrix* (*trich-*), a hair]. A larval worm of the genus *Trichinella;* the infective form in pork.

Trichinella (trik'i-nel'ă) [Mod. L. fr. trichina + dim. suffix *ella*]. A nematode genus in the aphasmid group that causes trichinosis in man and carnivores.
T. spira'lis, the pork or trichina worm, a species of parasites that cause trichinosis, found in most regions of the world but more frequently in the Northern Hemisphere; transmission occurs as a result of ingesting raw or inadequately cooked meat (especially pork) that contains encysted larvae which develop into adults that survive in the jejunum and ileum for approximately six weeks; the female worm is viviparous, and bears approximately 1500 embryonic

larvae that are laid deep in the mucosa so that they are picked up in the submucosal capillaries and are transported via the liver to the heart, lungs, and systemic circulation; eventually the larvae break out of the body capillaries, penetrate a muscle fiber, coil, and encyst, thereby inducing the strong sensitization, pain, fever, edema, and eosinophilic reaction characteristic of trichinosis.

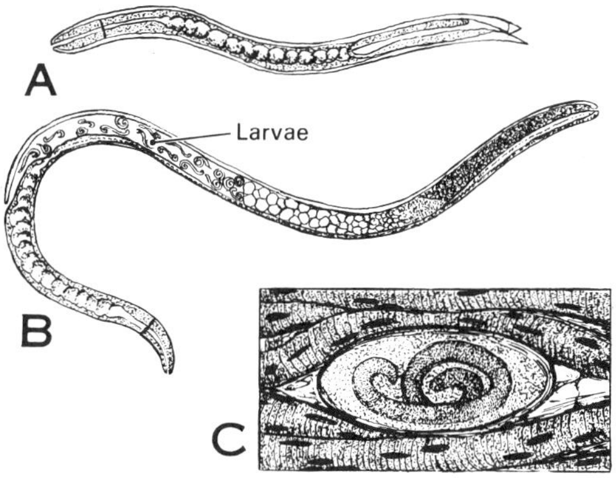

Trichinella spiralis
A, male (X30.5); *B*, female (X30.0); *C*, larvae encysted in muscle (X75).

trichinelliasis (trik'i-nel-ī'ă-sis). Trichinosis.

Trichinellicae (tri-ki-nel'i-kē). Trichinelloidea.

Trichinelloidea (trik'i-nel-oy'dē-ă). Trichinellicae; a superfamily of nematodes, including the following roundworms that are parasitic in man: *Trichinella spiralis*, the trichina worm (family Trichinellidae); *Trichuris trichiura*, the human whipworm; *Capillaria hepatica*, the capillary liver worm; and *C. philippinensis* (family Trichuridae).

trichinellosis (trik'i-nel-ō'sis). Trichinosis.

trichiniasis (trik-i-nī'ă-sis). Trichinosis.

trichiniferous (trik-i-nif'ĕ-rŭs). Containing trichina worms.

trichinization (trik'i-ni-zā'shŭn). Infection with trichina worms.

trichinoscope (trik'i-nō-skōp) [trichina + G. *skopeō*, to view]. A magnifying glass used in the examination of meat suspected of being trichinous.

trichinosis (trik-i-nō'sis) [*Trichinella* (trichina) + G. *-osis*, condition]. Trichinelliasis; trichiniasis; trichinellosis; the disease resulting from ingestion of raw or inadequately cooked pork (or bear or walrus meat in Alaska) that contains encysted larvae of the nematode parasite *Trichinella spiralis*. The initial symptoms of human disease are abdominal pain, cramping, and diarrhea, associated with the development of the parasites in the small intestine. Once the resultant larval parasites migrate and invade muscular tissue, a second set of symptoms is manifest, including facial and periorbital edema, myalgia, fever, pruritus, urticaria, conjunctivitis, and signs of myocarditis.

trichinous (trik'i-nŭs). Infected with trichina worms.

trichion (trik'ē-on) [G. *thrix*, hair]. A cephalometric point at the midpoint of the hairline at the top of the forehead.

trichite (trik'īt). Trichocyst.

trichitis (tri-kī'tis) [trich- + G. *-itis*, inflammation]. Inflammation of the hair bulbs.

trichloral (trī-klōr'ăl). *m*-Chloral.

trichlorfon (trī-klōr'fon). Metrifonate; $C_4H_8Cl_3O_4P$; an organophosphorus compound effective against immature and mature stages of *Schistosoma haematobium*, but ineffective against other species of *Schistosoma* in man.

trichloride (trī-klōr'īd). A chloride having three chlorine atoms in the molecule; *e.g.*, PCl_3.

trichlormethiazide (trī-klōr-me-thī'ă-zīd). 6-Chloro-3-(dichloromethyl)- 3,4-dihydro-2*H*- 1,2,4-benzothiadiazine-7-sulfonamide; an orally effective benzothiazide diuretic and antihypertensive agent.

trichlormethine (trī-klōr-meth'ēn). 2,2',2''-Trichlorotriethylamine hydrochloride; tris(2-chloroethyl)amine hydrochloride; a nitrogen mustard used in the treatment of leukemia.

trichloroacetic acid (trī-klōr'ō-ă-sē'tik). CCl_3COOH; used as an astringent antiseptic in 1 to 5% solution or as an escharotic for venereal and other warts; a widely used protein precipitant.

trichloroethane (trī-klōr-ō-eth'ān). 1,1,1-Trichloroethane; methylchloroform; CH_3CCl_3; an industrial solvent with pronounced inhalation anesthetic activity.

trichloroethanol (trī-klōr-ō-eth'ă-nol). 2,2,2-Trichloroethanol; trichloroethyl alcohol; CCl_3CH_2OH; a hypnotic and sedative; as a metabolite of chloral hydrate, it contributes to the depressant activity of chloral hydrate.

trichloroethene (trī-klōr-ō-eth'ēn). Trichloroethylene.

trichloroethyl alcohol (trī-klōr-ō-eth'il). Trichloroethanol.

trichloroethylene (trī-klōr-ō-eth'i-lēn). Trichloroethene; ethinyl trichloride; $ClCH{=}CCl_2$; an analgesic and inhalation anesthetic used in minor surgical operations and in obstetrical practice.

trichlorofluoromethane (trī-klōr'ō-flūr-ō-meth'ān). Trichloromonofluoromethane; CCl_3F; a propellant used for aerosol sprays; has anesthetic and arrhythmogenic activity if inhaled in high concentration.

trichloromethane (trī-klōr-ō-meth'ān). Chloroform.

trichloromonofluoromethane (trī-klōr-ō-mon'ō-flūr-ō-meth'ān). Trichlorofluoromethane.

trichlorophenol (trī-klōr-ō-fē'nol). 2,4,5-Trichlorophenol or 2,4,6-trichlorophenol; used as an antiseptic, disinfectant, and fungicide.

(2,4,5-**trichlorophenoxy) acetic acid (2,4,5-T)** (trī-klōr-ō-fe-nok'sē). An herbicide, synthesized by condensation of chloracetic acid and 2,4,5-trichlorophenol, used as the principal constituent of Agent Orange.

tricho-, trich-, trichi- [G. *thrix* (*trich-*), hair]. Combining forms denoting the hair or a hairlike structure.

trichobezoar (trik-ō-bē'zōr) [tricho- + bezoar]. Pilobezoar; hair ball; a hair cast in the stomach or intestinal tract, common in cats.

Trichocephalus (trik-ō-sef'ă-lŭs) [tricho- + G. *kephalē*, head]. Incorrect name for *Trichuris*.

trichoclasia, trichoclasis (trik-ō-klā'zē-ă, tri-kok'lă-sis) [tricho- + G. *klasis*, breaking off]. *Trichorrhexis* nodosa.

trichocryptosis (trik'ō-krip-tō'sis) [tricho- + G. *kryptos*, concealed]. Any disease of the hair follicles.

trichocyst (trik'ō-sist) [tricho- + G. *kystis*, bladder]. Trichite; one of a number of structures, in the form of minute elongated cysts, arranged radially around the periphery of a protozoan cell and containing fluid which when discharged serves for offense or defense; found in ciliates, such as *Paramecium* species.

Trichodectes (trik-ō-dek'tēz) [tricho- + G. *dektēs*, a beggar]. A genus of biting lice that includes the species *T. canis* (*T. latus*), the biting louse of dogs that commonly serves as an intermediate host for the dog tapeworm, *Dipylidium caninum*, as well as the species *T. climax* (*Bovicola caprae*), *T. parumpilosus* (*B. equi*), *T. scalaris* (*B. bovis*), and *T. sphaerocephalus* (*B. ovis*). See also *Bovicola; Damalinia*.

Trichoderma (trik-ō-der'mă) [tricho- + G. *derma*, skin]. A genus of fungi in soil that furnishes the antibiotic gliotoxin.

trichodiscoma (trik'ō-dis-kō'mă). Haarscheibe *tumor.*

trichodynia (trik-ō-din'ē-ă) [tricho- + G. *odynē,* pain]. Trichalgia.

trichoepithelioma (trik'ō-ep-i-thē-lē-ō'mă) [tricho- + epithelioma]. Multiple small benign nodules, occurring mostly on the skin of the face, derived from basal cells of hair follicles enclosing keratin pearls; autosomal dominant inheritance. Also called acanthoma or epithelioma adenoides cysticum; Brooke's tumor; hereditary multiple t.; t. papillosum multiplex.
acquired t., dilated *pore.*
desmoplastic t., a solitary, hard, annular, centrally depressed papule, occurring usually in women on the face, consisting of dermal strands of baseloid cells and small keratinous cysts within desmoplastic stroma.
hereditary multiple t., trichoepithelioma.
t. papillo'sum mul'tiplex, trichoepithelioma.

trichoesthesia (trik'ō-es-thē'zē-ă) [tricho- + G. *aisthēsis,* sensation]. **1.** The sensation felt when a hair is touched. **2.** A form of paresthesia in which there is a sensation as of a hair on the skin, on the mucous membrane of the mouth, or on the conjunctiva.

trichofolliculoma (trik'ō-fol-ik-yū-lō'mă) [tricho- + L. *folliculus,* fountain, spring, + G. *-oma,* tumor]. A usually solitary tumor or hamartoma in which multiple abortive hair follicles open into a central cyst or space opening on the skin surface.

trichogen (trik'o-jen) [tricho- + G. *-gen,* producing]. An agent that promotes the growth of hair.

trichogenous (tri-koj'ĕ-nŭs). Promoting the growth of the hair.

trichoglossia (trik-ō-glos'ē-ă) [tricho- + G. *glōssa,* tongue]. Hairy *tongue.*

trichohyalin (trik-ō-hī'ă-lin). A substance of the nature of keratohyalin found in the developing inner root sheath of the hair follicle.

trichoid (trik'oyd) [tricho- + G. *eidos,* resemblance]. Hairlike.

tricholemmoma (trik'ō-le-mō'mă). Trichilemmoma.

tricholith (trik'ō-lith) [tricho- + G. *lithos,* stone]. A concretion on the hair; the lesion of piedra.

trichologia (trik-ō-lō'jē-ă) [G. *trichologeo,* to pluck hairs, fr. tricho- + *lego,* to pick out, gather]. Trichology (2); a nervous habit of plucking at the hair.

trichology (tri-kol'ō-jē). **1** [tricho- + G. *logos,* study]. The study of the anatomy, growth, and diseases of the hair. **2** [G. *trichologeo,* fr. tricho- + *legō,* to pick out]. Trichologia.

trichoma (tri-kō'mă) [tricho- + G. *-oma,* tumor]. Trichiasis.

trichomatose (tri-kō'mă-tōs). Trichomatous.

trichomatosis (tri-kō'mă-tō'sis). Trichiasis.

trichomatous (tri-kō'mă-tŭs). Trichomatose; relating to or suffering from trichoma.

trichomegaly (trik'ō-meg'ă-lē) [tricho- + G. *megas,* large]. Congenital condition characterized by abnormally long eyelashes.

trichomonacide (trik-ō-mō'nă-sīd)., An agent that is destructive to *Trichomonas* organisms.

trichomonad (trik-ō-mō'nad). Common name for members of the family Trichomonadidae.

Trichomonadidae (trik'ō-mō-nad'i-dē). A family of protozoan flagellates that includes the genus *Trichomonas.*

Trichomonas (trik-ō-mō'nas) [tricho- + G. *monas,* single (unit)]. A genus of parasitic protozoan flagellates (subfamily Trichomonidinae, family Trichomonadidae) that have four anterior flagella and a posterior flagellum along the margin of an undulating membrane (which is not free posteriorly), a filamentous costa along the basal portion of the membrane, a typical pelta, a sausage-shaped parabasal body (Golgi body), a rodlike axostyle, and a large single anterior nucleus in a pyriform cell body with a pointed posterior end. Species cause trichomoniasis in man, other primates, and birds; specificity is more marked for precise microhabitat than for host species. This genus has been divided into several genera: *Trichomonas, Pentatrichomonas, Tetratrichomonas,* and *Tritrichomonas.*
T. bucca'lis, *T. tenax.*
T. foe'tus, former name for *Tritrichomonas foetus.*
T. gal'linae, the species that causes avian trichomoniasis; the pigeon is the natural host, but the organism also occurs in turkeys, chickens, doves, hawks, falcons, and other birds; infection is most serious in young domestic pigeons, who acquire it from pigeon milk produced in the pigeon crop; other birds are infected from contaminated water or by feeding on infected birds.
T. gallina'rum, former name for *Tetratrichomonas gallinarium.*
T. hom'inis, former name for *Pentatrichomonas hominis.*
T. o'vis, former name for *Tetratrichomonas ovis.*
T. su'is, former name for *Tritrichomonas suis.*
T. te'nax, *T. buccalis;* a species that lives as a commensal in the mouth of man and other primates, especially in the tartar around the teeth or in the defects of carious teeth; there is no evidence of direct pathogenesis, but it is frequently associated with pyogenic organisms in pus pockets or at the base of teeth.
T. vagina'lis, a species frequently found in the vagina and urethra of women and in the urethra and prostate gland of men (the only known natural hosts), in whom it causes trichomoniasis vaginitis; considerable differences in pathogenicity exists among various strains of this species.

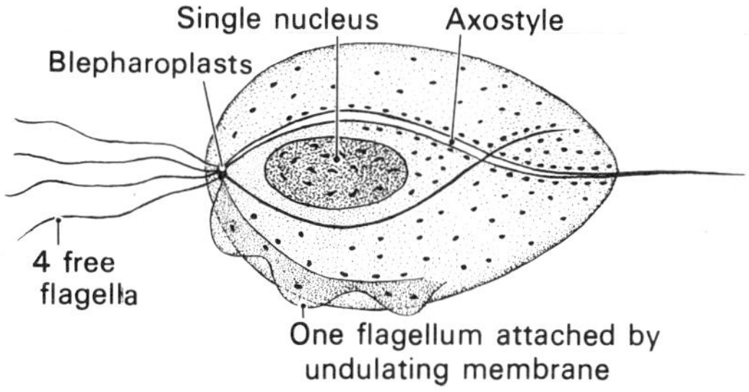

Trichomonas vaginalis (×1440)

trichomoniasis (trik'ō-mō-nī'ă-sis). Disease caused by infection with a species of *Trichomonas* or related genera; often used to designate t. vaginitis.
avian t., t. occurring in the upper digestive tract in a variety of birds and caused by *Trichomonas gallinae;* it causes necrotic ulceration in the mouth, esophagus, crop, and proventriculus, frequently with rapid weight loss and death.
bovine t., a venereal infection in cattle caused by *Tritrichomonas foetus;* in the bull, the infection is usually asymptomatic, the organisms being present in small or moderate numbers, chiefly in the preputial sheath; infection in the female may result in delayed conception, abortion early in pregnancy, or pyometra; transmission occurs during copulation or by artificial insemination from infected bulls.
t. vagini'tis, acute or subacute vaginitis or urethritis caused by infection with *Trichomonas vaginalis,* which does not invade the mucosa or the tissue but provokes an inflammatory reaction; infection is venereal or by other forms of contact; widespread infection in human populations is usually asymptomatic but may produce vaginitis, with vaginal and vulvar pruritis, leukorrhea with frothy watery discharge, and (rarely) purulent urethritis in males.

trichomycetosis (trik'ō-mī-sē-tō'sis). Trichomycosis.

trichomycosis (trik'ō-mī-kō'sis) [tricho- + G. *mykēs,* fungus, + G. *-osis,* condition]. Trichomycetosis; formerly used to mean any disease of the hair caused by a fungus; presently synonymous with trichonocardiosis or t. axillaris. In present usage, t. is a misnomer

because the causative agent of the disease is a nocardia (an entity intermediate between fungus and bacterium) and not a true fungus.
t. axilla'ris, Paxton's disease; lepothrix; t. chromatica, nodosa, nodularis, or palmellina; trichonodosis; trichonocardiasis axillaris; infection of axillary and pubic hairs with development of yellow (flava), black (nigra), or red (rubra) concretions around the hair shafts.
t. chromat'ica, t. axillaris.
t. nodo'sa, t. nodula'ris, t. axillaris.
t. palmelli'na, t. axillaris.
t. pustulo'sa, any parasitic disease of the hair marked by pustule formation at the orifices of the hair follicles.

trichonocardiosis (trik'ō-nō-kar'dē-ō'sis) [tricho- + *Nocardia* + G. *-osis,* condition]. An infection of hair shafts, especially of the axillary and pubic regions, with nocardiae. Yellow, red, or black concretions develop around the infected hair shafts and contain the causative agent and, frequently, micrococci; the micrococci probably account for the variety of the colors of the concretions and for the resultant varieties of t. which have been described. See also trichomycosis; *trichomycosis* axillaris.
t. axilla'ris, *trichomycosis* axillaris.

trichonodosis (trik'ō-nō-dō'sis) [tricho- + L. *nodus,* node (swelling), + G. *-osis,* condition]. *Trichomycosis* axillaris.

trichonosis (trik'ō-nō'sis). Trichopathy.

trichonosus (tri-kon'ō-sŭs) [tricho- + G. *nosos,* disease]. Trichopathy.
t. versic'olor, ringed *hair.*

trichopathic (trik-ō-path'ik). Relating to any disease of the hair.

trichopathophobia (trik'ō-path-ō-fō'bē-ă) [tricho- + G. *pathos,* suffering, + *phobos,* fear]. Excessive worry regarding disease of the hair, its color, or abnormalities of its growth.

trichopathy (tri-kop'ă-thē) [tricho- + G. *pathos,* suffering]. Trichonosus; trichonosis; trichosis; any disease of the hair.

trichophagy (tri-kof'ă-jē) [tricho- + G. *phagein,* to eat]. Habitual biting of the hair.

trichophobia (trik-ō-fō'bē-ă) [tricho- + G. *phobos,* fear]. Morbid disgust caused by the sight of loose hairs on clothing or elsewhere.

trichophytic (trik-ō-fit'ik). Relating to trichophytosis.

trichophytid (tri-kof'i-tid, trik-ō-fī'tid) [tricho- + G. *phyton,* plant, + *-id* (1)]. An eruption remote from the site of infection, which is the expression of allergic response to *Trichophyton* infection.

trichophytin (tri-kof'i-tin). An extract of cultures of several species of *Trichophyton,* the ringworm fungus, formerly used in the diagnosis and treatment of a number of varieties of ringworm infection; now used only as a measure of general immune response in a compromised person.

trichophytobezoar (trik'ō-fī'tō-bē'zōr) [tricho- + G. *phyton,* plant, + bezoar]. Phytotrichobezoar; a mixed hair and food ball, consisting of vegetable fibers, seeds and skins of fruits, and animal hair that are matted together to form a ball in the stomach of man or animals, especially ruminants.

Trichophyton (tri-kof'i-tŏn) [tricho- + G. *phyton,* plant]. A genus of pathogenic fungi causing dermatophytosis in man and animals; species may be anthropophilic, zoophilic, or geophilic, and attack the hair, skin, and nails, and are characterized by their growth in hair. Endothrix species grow from the skin into the hair follicle, penetrate the shaft, and grow into it, producing rows of arthroconidia as the hyphae septate; there is no growth on the external surface of the shaft. Ectothrix species are of two kinds, large spored and small spored. In both, the fungus grows into the hair follicle, surrounds the hair shaft, and penetrates it, but continues to grow both within and outside the hair shaft, producing arthroconidia externally.
T. concen'tricum, an anthropophilic species which is the causative agent of tinea imbricata; it closely resembles the branching mycelium of *T. schoenleinii.*
T. equi'num, a zoophilic species causing endothrix infections of hair in horses, from which man may also be infected; it requires nicotinic acid for growth.
T. megnin'ii, an anthropophilic ectothrix species of dermatophyte with spores in chains, causing infection in man; it requires histidine, which differentiates it from *Microsporum gallinae.*
T. mentagrophy'tes, a zoophilic small-spored ectothrix species that causes infection of the hair, skin, and nails; it is a cause of ringworm in dogs, horses, rabbits, mice, rats, chinchillas, foxes, and man.

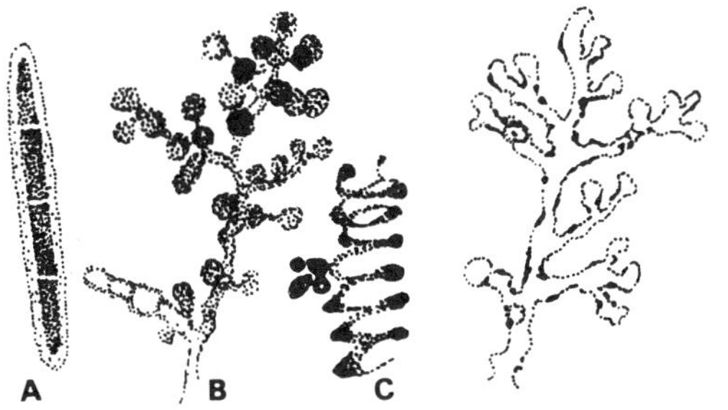

Trichophyton
A, clavate macroconidium; *B,* microconidium; *C,* coiled hypha.

T. ru'brum, a widely distributed anthropophilic species that causes persistent infections in the nails that are unusually resistant to therapy; it rarely invades the hair, where it is endoectothrix in nature; occasional subcutaneous and systemic infections have been reported.
T. schoenlei'nii, an anthropophilic endothrix species of dermatophyte causing favus in man; it is endemic throughout Eurasia and Africa and, because of travel, is seen more frequently in the Western Hemisphere; it produces tunnels within the hair shaft which are filled with air bubbles after the hyphae disintegrate.
T. sim'ii, a zoophilic species that causes infection in rhesus monkeys, dogs, and man; most infections have had their origin in India.
T. ton'surans, an anthropophilic endothrix species that causes epidemic dermatophytosis in Europe, South America, and the U.S.; it infects some animals and requires thiamin for growth.
T. verrucos'um, a zoophilic species that causes ringworm in cattle, from which man can become infected.
T. viola'ceum, an anthropophilic species that causes black-dot ringworm or favus infection of the scalp; hair infection is of the endothrix type; usually found in South America, Europe, Asia, and Africa.

trichophytosis (trik'ō-fī-tō'sis) [tricho- + G. *phyton,* plant, + *-osis,* condition]. Superficial fungus infection caused by species of *Trichophyton.*
t. bar'bae, *tinea* barbae.
t. cap'itis, *tinea* capitis.
t. cor'poris, *tinea* corporis.
t. cru'ris, *tinea* cruris.
t. un'guium, fungus infection of the nail plates. See also onychomycosis.

Trichopleuris (tri-kō-plū'ris) [tricho- + G. *pleura,* rib, side]. A genus of biting lice that infest ruminants, *e.g., T. lipeuroides* and *T. parallelus* in American deer; considered by some to be a subgenus of *Damalinia.*

trichopoliosis (trik′ō-pō-lē-ō′sis) [tricho- + G. *polios,* gray, + *-osis,* condition]. Poliosis.

Trichoptera (tri-kop′ter-ă) [tricho- + G. *pteron,* wing]. An order of insects in which the aquatic larvae (caddis flies) construct a protective case (caddis) of bits of submerged material in a highly specific form; commonly found attached under stones in freshwater streams. The adult caddis flies, having hairy wings, shed their hairs and epithelia, causing hay fever-like (allergic) symptoms in sensitive people.

trichoptilosis (trik′ō-ti-lō′sis, tri-kop-ti-lō′sis) [tricho- + G. *ptilōsis,* plumage, + *-osis,* condition]. A condition of splitting of the shaft of the hair, giving it a feathery appearance.

trichorrhexis (trik-ō-rek′sis) [tricho- + G. *rhēxis,* a breaking]. A condition in which the hairs tend to readily break or split.
t. invagina′ta, bamboo *hair.*
t. nodo′sa, trichoclasia; trichoclasis; clastothrix; nodositas crinium; a condition in which minute nodes are formed in the hair shafts; splitting and breaking, complete or incomplete, may occur at these points or nodes.

trichoschisis (tri-kos′ki-sis) [tricho- + G. *schisis,* a cleaving]. The presence of broken or split hairs. See also trichorrhexis.

trichoscopy (tri-kos′kō-pē) [tricho- + G. *skopeō,* to examine]. Examination of the hair.

trichosis (tri-kō′sis) [tricho- + G. *-osis,* condition]. Trichopathy.
t. carun′culae, a growth of hair on the lacrimal caruncle.
t. sensiti′va, hyperesthesia of the hairy parts.
t. seto′sa, coarseness of the hair.

trichosomatous (trik-ō-sō′mă-tŭs) [tricho- + G. *sōma,* body]. Having flagella with a small body; denoting certain protozoan organisms. See *Trichomonas.*

Trichosporon (tri-kos′pō-ron, trik-ō-spōr′on) [tricho- + G. *sporos,* seed (spore)]. A genus of imperfect fungi that possess branching septate hyphae with arthrospores and blastopores; these organisms are part of the normal flora of the intestinal tract of man. *T. beigelii* is the causative agent of white piedra or trichosporosis.

trichosporosis (trik′ō-spō-rō′sis) [*Trichosporon* + G. *-osis,* condition]. A superficial mycotic infection of the hair in which nodular masses of causative fungi become attached to the hair shafts; it may be a disseminated infection in debilitated individuals. This disease is commonly called white piedra, caused by *Trichosporon beigelii;* so called black piedra is caused by *Piedraia hortae.*

trichostasis spinulosa (tri-kos′tă-sis spī′nū-lō′să) [tricho- + G. *stasis,* a standing; L. *spinulosus,* thorny]. A condition in which hair follicles are blocked with a keratin plug containing lanugo hairs.

trichostrongyle (trik-ō-stron′jil). Common name for members of the family Trichostrongylidae.

Trichostrongylidae (trik′ō-stron-jil′i-dē) [see *Trichostrongylus*]. A family of nematodes (order Strongylida or, in older terminology, Strongylata); includes the important genera *Cooperia, Ostertagia, Haemonchus, Trichostrongylus, Nematodirus,* and *Hippostrongylus.*

trichostrongylosis (trik′ō-stron-ji-lō′sis). Infection with *Trichostrongylus.*

Trichostrongylus (trik-ō-stron′ji-lŭs) [tricho- + G. *strongylos,* round]. The hairworm, or bankrupt or black scour worm; an economically important genus (about 30 species) of small slender nematodes (family Trichostrongylidae) that inhabit the small intestine, in some cases the stomach, of a variety of herbivorous animals and gallinaceous birds. They burrow into the mucosa and suck blood; in large numbers they do serious damage, especially to young hosts.
T. ax′ei, the most common species in cattle, occurring also in the abomasum of sheep, horses, antelope, bison, llama, and deer, and in the stomach of pigs and horses.
T. capric′ola, a species that occurs in the small intestine and abomasum of sheep, goats, deer, and pronghorn.
T. colubrifor′mis, a species that occurs in anterior portions of the small intestine and sometimes in the abomasum of sheep, goats, cattle, camels, and some wild ruminants, and in the stomach of primates (including man), rabbits, and squirrels; it is distributed worldwide and is common in the U.S., especially in sheep.
T. longispicula′ris, a species found in the small intestine of cattle, sheep, and goats; it is distributed worldwide but uncommon in the U.S.
T. ten′uis, a species that is a widespread pathogenic parasite of the ceca and small intestines of fowl, including ducks, geese, turkeys, pheasants, and partridges.
T. vitri′nus, a species that is an important pathogen of lambs, found chiefly in the duodenum of sheep, camels, rabbits, and goats but also reported from man and pigs.

Trichothecium (tri-kō-thē′sē-ŭm). A genus of imperfect fungi generally considered a common saprophyte.

trichothiodystrophy (trik′ō-thī′ō-dis′trō-fē) [tricho- + thio- + G. *dys,* bad, + *trophē,* nourishment]. An abnormality of the hair shaft, probably inherited, characterized by fine brittle hairs with abnormally low sulfur content.

trichotillomania (trik′ō-til-ō-mā′nē-ă) [tricho- + G. *tillo,* pull out, + *mania,* insanity]. A compulsion to pull out one's own hair.

trichotomy (tri-kot′ō-mē) [G. *trichia,* threefold, + *tomē,* a cutting]. A division into three parts.

trichotoxin (trik′ō-tok′sin). A cytotoxin having an injurious effect specifically for ciliated epithelium.

trichotrophy (tri-kot′rō-fē) [tricho- + G. *trophē,* nourishment]. Nutrition of the hair.

trichroic (trī-krō′ik). Relating to or marked by trichroism.

trichroism (trī′krō-izm) [G. *trichroos,* three-colored, fr. tri- + *chroa,* color]. The property of some crystals of emitting different colors in three different directions.

trichromat (trī-krō′mat) [tri- + G. *chrōma,* color]. A person who sees three primary colors; hence, one with normal color vision.

trichromatic (trī-krō-mat′ik). Trichromic. **1.** Having, or relating to, the three primary colors, red, green, and blue. **2.** Capable of perceiving the three primary colors; having normal color vision.

trichromatism (trī-krō′mă-tizm) [tri- + G. *chrōma,* color]. The state of being trichromatic.
anomalous t., a defect in color perception in which there appears to be an abnormality or deficiency in one of the three primary pigments of the retinal cones. See protanomaly; deuteranomaly; tritanomaly.

trichromatopsia (trī-krō′mă-top′sē-ă) [tri- + G. *chrōma,* color, + *opsis,* vision]. Normal color vision; the ability to perceive the three primary colors.

trichromic (trī-krō′mik). Trichromatic.

trichterbrust (tricht′er-brŭst) [Ger. *Trichterbrust,* funnel chest]. *Pectus* excavatum.

trichuriasis (tri-kū-rī′ă-sis). Infection with a species of *Trichuris.* In man, intestinal parasitization by *T. trichiura* is usually asymptomatic and not associated with peripheral eosinophilia; in massive infections it frequently induces diarrhea or rectal prolapse.

Trichuris (tri-kū′ris) [tricho- + G. *oura,* tail]. A genus of aphasmid nematodes (sometimes improperly termed *Trichocephalus*) related to the trichina worm, *Trichinella spiralis,* and having a body with a slender, elongated, anterior portion threaded into the mucosa of the colon or large intestine of the host and a thick posterior portion bearing reproductive organs and their products. *T.* contains about 70 species, all in mammals.
T. trichiu′ra, the whipworm of man, a species that causes trichuri-

asis; the body is filiform and slender in the anterior three-fifths, and more robust posteriorly; females are 4 or 5 cm long, males are shorter (with coiled caudal extremity and a single eversible spicule); eggs are barrel-shaped, 50 to 56 by 20 to 22 μm, with double shell and translucent knobs at each of the two poles; humans are the only susceptible hosts and usually acquire infection by direct finger-to-mouth contact or by ingestion of soil, water, or food that contains larvated eggs (development in the soil takes 3 to 6 weeks under proper conditions of warmth and moisture, hence distribution is chiefly tropical); larvae escape from eggs in the ileum, mature in approximately a month, and then pass directly into the cecum without undergoing a parenteral migration as occurs with *Ascaris lumbricoides;* adults may persist for 2 to 7 years.

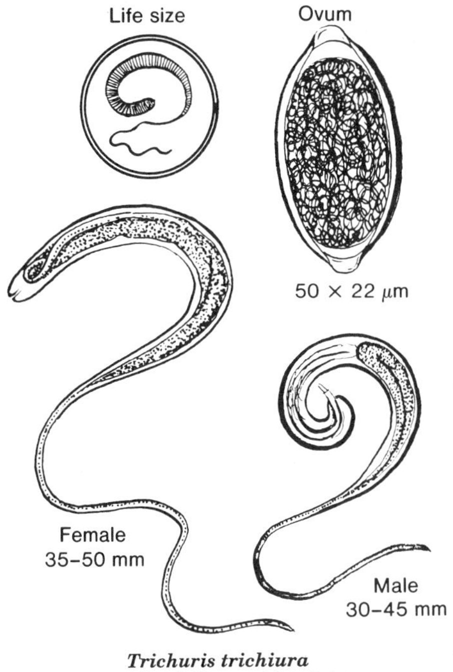

Trichuris trichiura
(After Jeffrey and Leach.)

tricipital (trī-sip'i-tăl). Having three heads; denoting a triceps muscle.

triclobisonium chloride (trī'klō-bi-sō'nē-ŭm). Hexamethylenebis[dimethyl[1-methyl- 3-(2,2,6-trimethylcyclohexyl)- propyl]ammonium chloride]; a bisquaternary ammonium compound used topically in the treatment of superficial infections of the skin and vagina; a cationic antiseptic effective against both Gram-negative and Gram-positive organisms. It is inactivated by soap and pH changes.

triclofenol piperazine (trī-klō'fen-ol). Bis(2,4,5-trichlorophenol) piperazine; an anthelmintic.

tricorn (trī'kōrn) [tri- + L. *cornu,* horn]. **1.** One of the lateral ventricles of the brain. **2.** Tricornute.

tricornute (trī-kōr'nūt) [tri- + L. *cornutus,* horned, fr. *cornu,* a horn]. Tricorn (2); having three cornua or horns.

tricresol (trī-krē'sol). Cresol.

tricrotic (trī-krot'ik) [tri- + G. *krotos,* a beat]. Tricrotous; thrice-beating; marked by three waves in the arterial pulse tracing.

tricrotism (trī'krō-tizm). The condition of being tricrotic.

tricrotous (trī'krō-tŭs). Tricrotic.

Tricula (trik'yū-lă). A genus of operculate freshwater snails related to *Oncomelania* (the *Schistosoma japonicum* intermediate hosts) of the family Hydrobiidae, subclass Prosobranchiata; it includes *T. aperta,* intermediate host of *Schistosoma mekongi.*

tricuspid, tricuspidal, tricuspidate (trī-kŭs'pid, -kŭs'pi-dăl, -kŭs'pi-dāt). **1.** Having three points, prongs, or cusps, as the tricuspid valve of the heart. **2.** Tritubercular; having three tubercles or cusps, as the second upper molar tooth (occasionally) and the upper third molar (usually).

tricyclamol chloride (trī-sī'klă-mol). Procyclidine methochloride.

tridactylous (trī-dak'ti-lŭs). Tridigitate.

trident (trī'dent). Tridentate.

tridentate (trī-den'tāt) [tri- + L. *dentatus,* toothed]. Trident; three-toothed; three-pronged.

tridermic (trī-der'mik) [tri- + G. *derma,* skin]. Relating to or derived from the three primary germ layers of the embryo: ectoderm, endoderm, and mesoderm.

tridermoma (trī-der-mō'mă) [tri- + G. *derma,* skin, + *-oma,* tumor]. Triphyllomatous *teratoma.*

tridigitate (trī-dij'i-tāt) [tri- + L. *digitus,* digit]. Tridactylous; having three fingers.

tridihexethyl chloride (trī'dī-heks-eth'il). 3-Diethylamino-1-phenyl-1-cyclohexyl 1-propanol ethylchloride; an anticholinergic drug.

tridymite (trid'i-mīt) [fr. G. *tridymos,* threefold]. A form of silica used in dental casting investment.

tridymus (trid'ĭ-mŭs) [L. fr. G. *tridymos,* threefold]. Triplet (1).

trielcon (trī-el'kon) [tri- + G. *helkō,* to draw]. A long, three-jawed forceps for the extraction of foreign bodies from wounds or canals.

trientine hydrochloride (trī'en-tēn). Triethylenetetramine dihydrochloride; $C_6H_{18}N_4 \cdot 2HCl$; a chelating agent used to remove excess copper from the body in Wilson's disease.

triethanolamine (trī'eth-ă-nol'ă-mēn). A mixture of mono-, di-, and triethanolamine, used as an emulsifying agent in the preparation of medicated ointments and lotions and as an aid in the absorption of such medicaments through the skin.

triethylene glycol (trī-eth'i-lēn). 2,2'-Ethylenedioxybis(ethanol); $C_6H_{14}O_4$; used in the vapor state as an air-sterilizing agent; toxic to bacteria, fungi, and viruses in very low concentrations in air; variations in the humidity of the air limit the germicidal effectiveness.

triethylenemelamine (TEM) (trī-eth'i-lēn-mel'ă-mēn). 2,4,6-Tris(ethyleneimino)-*s*-triazine; an antineoplastic agent chemically related to the nitrogen mustards; used in the treatment of leukemia.

triethylenephosphoramide (TEPA) (trī-eth'i-lēn-fos-fōr'ă-mīd). A drug with the same actions and uses as triethylenemelamine in the treatment of leukemias.

triethylenetetramine dihydrochloride (trī-eth'i-lēn-tet'ră-am'ēn). Trientine hydrochloride.

triethylenethiophosphoramide (trī-eth'i-lēn-thī'ō-fos-fōr'ă-mīd). Thiotepa; tris(1-aziridinyl)phosphine sulfide; an alkylating agent used for the palliative treatment of malignant diseases such as leukemia, lymphoma, and carcinoma.

trifacial (trī-fā'shăl) [tri- + L. *facies,* face]. Denoting the fifth pair of cranial nerves, nervus trigeminus.

trifid (trī'fid) [L. *trifidus,* three-cleft]. Split into three.

trifluoperazine hydrochloride (trī'flū-ō-per'ă-zēn). 10-[3-(4-Methyl-1-piperazinyl)propyl]-2-(trifluoromethyl)phenothiazine hydrochloride; an antipsychotic.

2,2,2-**trifluoroethyl vinyl** (trī-flūr-ō-eth'il). Fluroxene.

5-**trifluoromethyldeoxyuridine** (trī-flūr'ō-meth'il-dē-ok-si-yū'ri-dēn). A pyrimidine analogue used topically in the treatment of herpes simplex keratitis.

trifluperidol hydrochloride (trī-flū-per'i-dol). 4'-Fluoro-4-[4-hydroxy-4-(α,α,α-trifluoro-*m*-tolyl)piperidino]butyrophenone hydrochloride; a tranquilizer.

triflupromazine hydrochloride (trī-flū-prō'mă-zēn). 10-[3-(Dimethylamino)propyl]-2-trifluoromethylphenothiazine hydrochloride; an antipsychotic closely related chemically and pharmacologically to chlorpromazine.

trifluridine (trī-flūr'i-dēn). 2'-Deoxy-5-(trifluoromethyl)uridine; an antiviral agent used in eye drops to treat herpes simplex infections of the eye.

trifocal (trī'fō-kăl). Having three foci. See t. *lens.*

trifoliosis (trī-fō-lē-ō'sis) [L. *trifolium,* trefoil, clover]. Trefoil dermatitis; clover disease; a form of photosensitization that occurs in horses, cattle, sheep, and pigs from eating several types of clover and alfalfa.

trifurcation (trī-fŭr-kā'shŭn) [tri- + L. *furca,* fork]. **1.** A division into three branches. **2.** The area where the tooth roots divide into three or more distinct portions.

trigastric (trī-gas'trik) [tri- + G. *gastēr,* belly]. Having three bellies; denoting a muscle with two tendinous interruptions.

trigeminal (trī-jem'i-năl) [L. *trigeminus,* threefold]. Relating to the fifth cranial or trigeminus nerve.

trigeminus (trī-jem'i-nŭs) [L. threefold, fr. tri- + *geminus,* twin]. Trigeminal.

trigeminy (trī-jem'i-nē) [L. *trigeminus,* threefold]. Trigeminal *rhythm.*

trigenolline (trig-ĕ-nol'ēn). Trigonelline.

trigger (trig'er). Term describing a system in which a relatively small input turns on a relatively large output, the magnitude of which is unrelated to the magnitude of the input.

triglyceride (trī-glis'er-īd). Triacylglycerol.

trigona (trī-gō'nă) [L.]. Plural of trigonum.

trigonal (trig'ō-năl). Triangular; relating to a trigonum.

trigone (trī'gōn) [L. *trigonum,* fr. G. *trigōnon,* triangle]. **1.** Trigonum. **2.** The first three dominant cusps (protocone, paracone, and metacone), taken collectively, of an upper molar tooth.
t. of auditory nerve, trigonum acustici; acoustic tubercle; the slight prominence of the floor of the lateral recess of the fourth ventricle, corresponding to the underlying cochlear and vestibular nuclei.
t. of bladder, *trigonum* vesicae.
collateral t., *trigonum* collaterale.
deltoideopectoral t., *fossa* infraclavicularis.
fibrous t.'s of heart, see *trigonum* fibrosum dextrum; *trigonum* fibrosum sinistrum.
t. of fillet, *trigonum* lemnisci.
t. of habenula, *trigonum* habenulae.
t. of hypoglossal nerve, *trigonum* nervi hypoglossi.
inguinal t., *trigonum* inguinale.
t. of lateral ventricle, *trigonum* collaterale.
left fibrous t., *trigonum* fibrosum sinistrum.
Lieutaud's t., *trigonum* vesicae.
Müller's t., the floor of the supraoptic recess of the third ventricle.
olfactory t., *trigonum* olfactorium.
right fibrous t., *trigonum* fibrosum dextrum.
t. of vagus nerve, *trigonum* nervi vagi.
vertebrocostal t., trigonum lumbocostale; Bochdalek's gap; a triangular area in the diaphragm near the lateral arcuate ligament that is devoid of muscle fibers; it is covered by pleura superiorly and by peritoneum inferiorly.

trigonelline (trig-ō-nel'ēn). Caffearine; trigenolline; *N*-methylnicotinic acid; the methyl betaine of nicotinic acid; a product of the metabolism of nicotinic acid; excreted in the urine.

trigonid (trī-gon'id, -gō'nid) [see *trigonum*]. The first three dominant cusps, taken collectively, of a lower molar tooth. See also trigone.

trigonitis (trī'gō-nī'tis) [trigone + G. *-itis,* inflammation]. Inflammation of the urinary bladder, localized in the mucous membrane at the trigone.

trigonocephalic (trig'ō-nō-se-fal'ik). Pertaining to trigonocephaly.

trigonocephaly (trig'ō-nō-sef'ă-lē, trī'gō-nō-) [trigone + G. *kephalē,* head]. Malformation characterized by a triangular configuration of the skull, due in part to premature synostosis of the cranial bones with compression of the cerebral hemispheres.

trigonum, pl. **trigona** (trī-gō'nŭm, -nă) [L., fr. G. *trigōnon,* a triangle]. Trigone; any triangular area. See triangle (2).
t. acus'tici, *trigone* of the auditory nerve.
t. carot'icum [NA], superior carotid triangle; fossa carotica; Gerdy's hyoid fossa; Malgaigne's fossa or triangle; a space bounded by the superior belly of the omohyoid muscle, anterior border of the sternocleidomastoid, and posterior belly of the digastric; it contains the bifurcation of the common carotid artery.
t. cerebra'le, fornix (2).
t. cervica'le, cervical triangle; t. colli; any one of the triangles of the neck; **(1) t. c. ante'rius** [NA], *regio* cervicalis anterior; **(2) t. c. poste'rius** [NA], *regio* cervicalis lateralis.
t. collatera'le [NA], collateral trigone; t. ventriculi; trigone of the lateral ventricle; a triangular prominence of the floor of the lateral ventricle at the transition between occipital and temporal horn, continuous rostrally with the collateral eminence and, like the latter, caused by the deep penetration of the collateral sulcus from the ventral surface of the temporal lobe.
t. col'li, t. cervicale.
t. deltoideopectora'le, *fossa* infraclavicularis.
t. femora'le [NA], femoral or subinguinal triangle; Scarpa's triangle; fossa scarpae major; a triangular space at the upper part of the thigh, bounded by the sartorius and adductor longus muscles and the inguinal (Poupart's) ligament.
trigo'na fibro'sa cor'dis, see t. fibrosum dextrum; t. fibrosum sinistrum.
t. fibro'sum dex'trum [NA], right fibrous trigone; part of the fibrous skeleton of the heart located between the aortic fibrous ring and rings surrounding the right and left atrioventricular ostia.
t. fibro'sum sinis'trum [NA], left fibrous trigone; the part of the fibrous skeleton of the heart located in the interval between the left side of the left atrioventricular ring and the aortic ring.
t. haben'ulae [NA], trigone of the habenula; a small triangular area on the dorsomedial surface of the thalamus at the caudal end of the stria medullaris, corresponding to the underlying habenula.
t. hypoglos'si, t. nervi hypoglossi.
t. inguina'le [NA], inguinal triangle or trigone; Hesselbach's triangle; the triangular area in the lower abdominal wall bounded by the inguinal ligament below, the border of the rectus abdominis medially and the inferior epigastric vessels laterally. It is the site of direct inguinal hernia.
t. lemnis'ci, triangle of Reil; triangle or trigone of the fillet; a triangular area on the lateral surface of the caudal half of the mesencephalon, bordered caudally by the slight prominence of the lateral lemniscus, dorsally by the base of the inferior colliculus and brachium colliculi superioris, and ventrally by the crus cerebri.
t. lumba'le [NA], lumbar triangle; Petit's lumbar triangle; an area in the posterior abdominal wall bounded by the edges of the latissimus dorsi and external oblique muscles and the iliac crest; herniations occasionally occur here.
t. lumbocosta'le, vertebrocostal *trigone.*
t. muscula're [NA], muscular triangle; inferior carotid, omotracheal, or tracheal triangle; t. omotracheale; the triangle bounded by the sternocleidomastoid muscle, the superior belly of the omo-

hyoid muscle, and the anterior midline of the neck; the infrahyoid muscles occupy most of it.

t. ner'vi hypoglos'si [NA], trigone of the hypoglossal nerve; t. hypoglossi; tuberculum hypoglossi; hypoglossal eminence; eminentia hypoglossi; a slight elevation in the floor of the inferior recess of the fourth ventricle, beneath which is the nucleus of origin of the twelfth cranial nerve.

t. ner'vi va'gi [NA], trigone of the vagus nerve; ala cinerea; ashen or gray wing; a prominence in the floor of the fovea inferior of the fourth ventricle that overlies the dorsal motor nucleus of the vagus.

t. olfacto'rium [NA], olfactory trigone; a grayish triangular area corresponding to the attachment of the olfactory peduncle ("olfactory nerve" or tractus olfactorius) to the base of the brain, at the anterior border of the anterior perforated substance.

t. omoclavicula're [NA], omoclavicular triangle; subclavian triangle; greater supraclavicular fossa; fossa supraclavicularis major; the triangle bounded by the clavicle, the omohyoid muscle, and the sternocleidomastoid muscle; it contains the subclavian artery and vein.

t. omotrachea'le [NA], t. musculare.

t. pala'ti, palatal *triangle.*

t. sternocosta'le, sternocostal triangle; Larrey's cleft; a muscular defect in the diaphragm between the costal and the sternal portions.

t. submandibula're [NA], submandibular triangle; digastric or submaxillary triangle; the triangle of the neck bounded by the mandible and the two bellies of the digastric muscle; it contains the submandibular gland.

t. submenta'le [NA], submental triangle; a triangle bounded by the anterior belly of the digastric muscles, and the hyoid bone; the mylohyoid muscle forms its floor.

t. ventric'uli, t. collaterale.

t. vesi'cae [NA], vesical triangle; trigone of bladder; Lieutaud's trigone or body; a triangular smooth area at the base of the bladder between the openings of the two ureters and that of the urethra.

trihybrid (trī-hī'brid) [tri- + L. *hybrida,* hybrid]. The offspring of parents which differ in three mendelian characters.

trihydric (trī-hī'drik). Denoting a chemical compound containing three replaceable hydrogen atoms.

trihydroxyestrin (trī'hī-drok'sē-es'trin). Estriol.

triiniodymus (trī-in'i-od'i-mŭs) [tri- + G. *inion,* nape of the neck, + *didymos,* twin]. A grossly malformed fetus with three heads, joined at the occiput, and a single body.

triiodide (trī-ī'ō-did, -dīd). An iodide with three atoms of iodine in the molecule; *e.g.,* KI_3.

triiodomethane (trī-ī'ō-dō-meth'ān). Iodoform.

3,5,3'-**triiodothyronine (TITh, T_3)** (trī-ī'ō-dō-thī'rō-nēn). Liothyronine; a thyroid hormone normally synthesized in smaller quantities than thyroxine; present in blood and in thyroid gland and exerts the same biological effects as thyroxine but, on a molecular basis, is more potent and the onset of its effect is more rapid.

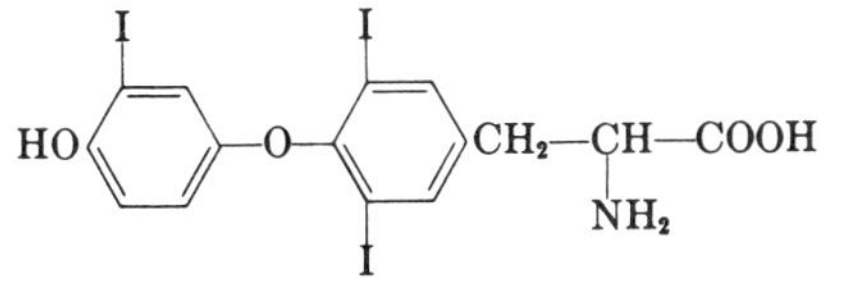

3,5,3'-Triiodothyronine

triketohydrindene hydrate (trī-kē-tō-hī'drin-dēn). Former name for ninhydrin.

triketopurine (trī-kē-tō-pyūr'ēn). Uric acid.

trilabe (trī'lāb) [tri- + G. *labē,* a handle, hold]. A three-pronged forceps for removal of foreign bodies from the bladder.

trilaminar (trī-lam'i-nar). Having three laminae.

trilateral (tri-lat'ĕ-răl). Having three sides.

trilobate, trilobed (trī-lō'bāt, trī'lobd). Having three lobes.

trilocular (trī-lok'yū-lăr). Having three cavities or cells.

trilogy (tril'ō-jē) [G. *trilogia,* fr. tri- + *logos,* study, discourse]. A triad of related entities.

t. of Fallot, Fallot's triad; atrial septal defect associated with pulmonic stenosis and right ventricular hypertrophy.

trilostane (trī'lō-stān). 4α,5-Epoxy-3,17β-dihydroxy-5α-androst-2-ene-2-carbonitrile; an adrenal steroid inhibitor used for amelioration of adrenal hyperfunction in Cushing's syndrome.

trimastigote (trī-mas'ti-gōt) [tri- + G. *mastix,* whip]. Having three flagella, as observed in certain protozoan organisms.

trimeprazine tartrate (trī-mep'ră-zēn). 10-[3-(Dimethylamino)-2-methylpropyl]phenothiazine tartrate; a phenothiazine compound related chemically and pharmacologically to promazine but with a more pronounced histamine-antagonizing action; used for the symptomatic relief of pruritus.

trimester (trī'mes-ter, trī-mes'ter) [L. *trimestris,* of three-month duration]. A period of 3 months; one-third of the length of a pregnancy.

trimetaphan camsylate (trī-met'ă-fan). Trimethaphan camsylate.

trimetazidine (trī-me-taz'i-dēn). 1-(2,3,4-Trimethoxybenzyl)piperazine; a coronary vasodilator.

trimethadione (trī'meth-ă-dī'ōn). Troxidone; 3,5,5-trimethyl-2,4-oxazolidinedione; an anticonvulsant used for the treatment of petit mal (absence seizures) and psychomotor epilepsy.

trimethaphan camsylate (trī-meth'ă-fan). Trimetaphan camsylate; *d-* 1,3-dibenzyldecahydro-2-oxoimidazo[*c*]thieno[1,2-α]thiolium camphorsulfonate; a ganglionic blocking agent that produces vasodilation of brief duration; used in surgery, particularly neurosurgery, to produce a relatively bloodless operative field (controlled hypotension).

trimethidium methosulfate (trī-me-thid'ē-ŭm meth-ō-sŭl'fāt). (+)-[*N*-Methyl-*N*-(γ-trimethylammoniumpropyl)]-1,8,8-trimethyl-3-azabicyclo[3.2.1]octane dimethosulfate; a quaternary ammonium compound that blocks ganglionic transmission at sympathetic and parasympathetic ganglia; used in the treatment of severe hypertension.

trimethobenzamide hydrochloride (trī'meth-ō-ben'ză-mīd). *N*-[(2-Dimethylaminoethoxy)benzyl]-3,4,5-trimethoxybenzamide hydrochloride; an antiemetic.

trimethoprim (trī-meth'ō-prim). 2,4-Diamino-5-(3,4,5-trimethoxybenzyl)pyrimidine; an antimicrobial agent that potentiates the effect of sulfonamides and sulfones.

trimethylamine (trī-meth'il-am'ēn). $N(CH_3)_3$; a degradation product, often by putrefaction, of nitrogenous plant and animal substances such as beet sugar residue or herring brine; in the body, it probably results from decomposition of choline.

trimethylaminuria (trī-meth'il-am-i-nūr'ē-ă). Increased excretion of trimethylamine in urine and sweat, with characteristic offensive, fishy body odor.

trimethylcarbinol (trī-meth'il-kar'bin-ol). Tertiary butyl alcohol. See *butyl* alcohol.

trimethylene (trī-meth'il-ēn). Cyclopropane.

trimethylethylene (trī-meth-il-eth'il-ēn). Amylene.

trimethylglycocoll anhydride (trī-meth'il-glī'kō-kol). Betaine.

trimethylomelamine (trī'meth-i-lō-mel'ă-mēn). (*s*-Triazine-2,4,6-triyltriimino)trimethanol; an antineoplastic agent.

trimetozine (trī-met'ō-zēn). 4-(3,4,5-Trimethoxybenzoyl)morpholine; an antianxiety agent.

trimetrexate (trī-me-treks'āt). 2,4-Diamino-5-methyl-6-[(3,4,5-trimethoxyanilino)methyl]quinazoline; an antineoplastic agent and antiprotozoal orphan drug used in the treatment of *Pneumocystis carinii* pneumonia in AIDS patients.

trimipramine (trī-mip'ră-mēn). 5-[3-(Dimethylamino)-2-methylpropyl]-10,11-dihydro-5*H*-dibenz[*b,f*]azepine; an antidepressant.

trimorphic (trī-mōr'fik). Trimorphous.

trimorphism (trī-mōr'fizm) [tri- + G. *morphē*, form]. Existence under three forms, as in holometabolous insects that pass through larval, pupal, and imago stages.

trimorphous (trī-mōr'fŭs). Trimorphic; existing under three forms; marked by trimorphism.

trinitrocellulose (trī'nī-trō-sel'yū-lōs). A constituent of soluble guncotton; used in the preparation of collodion and of pyroxylin.

trinitroglycerin (trī'nī-trō-glis'ĕ-rin). Nitroglycerin.

trinitrotoluene (TNT) (trī'nī-trō-tol'yū-ēn). Trinitrotoluol; $CH_3C_6H_2(NO_2)_3$; an explosive made by the nitrification of toluene; it causes gastric and intestinal disturbances and dermatitis in workers in munition factories.

trinitrotoluol (trī'nī-trō-tol'yū-ol). Trinitrotoluene.

trinucleotide (trī-nū'klē-ō-tīd). A combination of three adjacent nucleotides, free or in a polynucleotide or nucleic acid molecule; often used with specific reference to the unit (codon or anticodon) specifying a particular amino acid in expression of the genetic code.

triokinase (trī-ō-kī'nās) [EC 2.7.1.28]. Triosekinase; a phosphotransferase catalyzing the phosphorylation of glyceraldehyde to glyceraldehyde 3-phosphate by ATP.

triolein (trī-ō'lē-in). Olein.

triophthalmos (trī-of-thal'mos) [tri- + G. *ophthalmos*, eye]. Conjoined twins with fusion in the facial region such that the eyes on the joined sides have merged to form a single one; a variety of opodidymus.

triorchism (trī-ōr'kizm). Condition of having three testes.

triose (trī'ōs). A three-carbon monosaccharide; *e.g.*, glyceraldehyde.

triosekinase (trī'ōs-kī'nās). Triokinase.

triosephosphate isomerase (trī'ōs-fos'fāt) [EC 5.3.1.1]. Phosphotriose isomerase; an isomerizing enzyme that catalyzes the interconversion of glyceraldehyde 3-phosphate and dihydroxyacetone phosphate, a reaction of importance in glycolysis.

triotus (trī-ō'tŭs) [tri- + G. *ous*, ear]. Diprosopus in which three ears are present.

trioxide (trī-oks'īd). Teroxide; a molecule containing three atoms of oxygen.

trioxsalen (trī-ok'să-len). 4,5,8-Trimethylpsoralen; 2,5,9-trimethyl-7*H*-furo[3,2-g][1]benzopyrano-7-one; an orally effective pigmenting, photosensitizing agent; used as a tanning agent and in the treatment of vitiligo.

trioxymethylene (trī'ok-sē-meth'i-lēn). Paraformaldehyde.

tripalmitin (trī-pal'mi-tin). Palmitin.

triparanol (trī-par'ă-nol). 1-[*p*-(2-Diethylaminoethoxy)phenyl]-1-(*p*-tolyl)-2-(*p*-chlorophenyl)ethanol; formerly used as inhibitor of cholesterol biosynthesis but withdrawn from the market because it promoted the formation of cataracts.

tripelennamine hydrochloride (trī-pē-len'ă-mēn). 2-[Benzyl[2-(dimethylamino)ethyl]amino]pyridine monohydrochloride; an antihistamine. Also available, with the same actions, is t. citrate; it is less bitter than the hydrochloride salt, and is therefore used in elixir.

triphalangia (trī-fă-lan'jē-ă) [tri- + phalanx]. Malformation in which three phalanges are present in the thumb or great toe.

triphosphatase (trī-fos'fă-tās). Adenosinetriphosphatase.

triphosphopyridine nucleotide (TPN, TPNH) (trī-fos'fō-pir'i-dēn). Former name for nicotinamide adenine dinucleotide phosphate.

Tripier, Léon, French surgeon, 1842–1891. See T.'s *amputation*.

triplant (trī'plant). See triplant *implant*.

triplegia (trī-plē'jē-ă) [tri- + G. *plēgē*, stroke]. Paralysis of an upper and a lower extremity and of the face, or of both extremities on one side and of one on the other.

trip'let. 1. Tridymus; one of three children delivered at the same birth. **2.** A set of three similar objects, as a compound lens in a microscope, formed of three planoconvex lenses. **3.** Codon.

nonsense t., a trinucleotide (codon) in which a base change results in premature termination of the growing polypeptide chain and, consequently, incomplete protein molecules.

triploblastic (trip-lō-blas'tik) [G. *triploos*, threefold, + *blastos*, germ]. Formed of three primary germ layers (ectoderm, mesoderm, endoderm), or containing tissue derived from all three layers.

triploid (trip'loyd) [G. *triploos*, threefold, + *eidos*, form]. Pertaining to or characteristic of triploidy.

triploidy (trip'loy-de). The presence of three complete sets of chromosomes, instead of two, in all cells; results in fetal or neonatal death.

triplopia (trip-lō'pē-ă) [G. *triploos*, triple, + *opsis*, sight]. Triple vision; visual defect in which three images of the same object are seen.

tripod (trī'pod) [G. *tripous*, fr. tri- + *pous*, foot]. **1.** Three-legged. **2.** A stand having three legs or supports.

Haller's t., *truncus* celiacus.

vital t., the brain, the heart, and the lungs, regarded as the three organs essential to life.

tripodia (trī-pō'dē-ă) [tri- + G. *pous*, foot]. Condition seen in conjoined twins when fusion has merged the lower extremities on the joined sides to form a single foot, so that there are only three feet for the two bodies.

triprolidine hydrochloride (trī-prol'i-dēn). *trans*-2-[3-(1-Pyrrolidinyl)-1-(*p*-tolyl)propenyl]pyridine hydrochloride; an antihistaminic used in the management of allergic and pruritic conditions.

triprosopus (trī'prō-sō'pŭs) [tri- + G. *prosōpon*, face]. Fetus with three heads fused, leaving only parts of three faces.

tripsis (trip'sis) [G. a rubbing]. **1.** Trituration (1). **2.** Massage.

triquetrous (trī-kwē'trŭs, -kwet-) [L. *triquetrus*, three-cornered]. Triangular.

triquetrum (trī-kwē'trŭm, -kwet-) [L. *triquetrus*, three-cornered]. *Os* triquetrum.

triradial, triradiate (trī-rā'dē-ăl, trī-rā'dē-āt). Radiating in three directions.

triradius (trī-rā'dē-ŭs). Galton's delta (2); in dermatoglyphics, the figure at the base of each finger in the palm, produced by rows of papillae running in three directions so as to form a triangle.

Tris Abbreviation for tris(hydroxymethyl)aminomethane; used as a trivial name.

tris-. Chemical prefix indicating three of the substituents that follow, independently linked. *Cf.* tri-.

trisaccharide (trī-sak'ă-rīd). A carbohydrate containing three monosaccharide residues, *e.g.*, raffinose.

tris(hydroxymethyl)methylamine (Tris). Tromethamine.

triskaidekaphobia (tris'kī-dek-ă-fō'bē-ă) [G. *triskaideka*, thirteen, + *phobos*, fear]. Superstitious dread of the number thirteen.

trismic (triz'mik). Relating to or marked by trismus.

trismoid (triz'moyd) [trismus + G. *eidos*, resemblance].

1. Resembling trismus. 2. Trismus nascentium, formerly regarded as a distinct variety due to pressure on the occiput during birth.

trismus (triz'mŭs) [L. fr. G. *trismos,* a creaking, rasping]. Lockjaw; ankylostoma; a firm closing of the jaw due to tonic spasm of the muscles of mastication from disease of the motor branch of the trigeminus; usually associated with and due to general tetanus.

t. capistra'tus, congenital adhesion of the cheeks to the gums.

t. dolorif'icus, trigeminal *neuralgia.*

t. nascen'tium, t. neonato'rum, stiffness of the jaw muscles in neonates, usually as the beginning of tetanus neonatorum.

t. sardon'icus, risus sardonicus. See risus caninus.

trisomic (trī-sō'mik). Relating to trisomy.

trisomy (trī'sō-mē) [tri- + (chromo)some]. The state of an individual or cell with an extra chromosome instead of the normal pair of homologous chromosomes; in man, the state of a cell containing 47 normal chromosomes.

trisplanchnic (trī-splangk'nik) [tri- + G. *splanchnon,* viscus]. Relating to the three visceral cavities: skull, thorax, and abdomen.

tristearin (trī-stē'ă-rin). Stearin.

tristichia (trī-stik'i-ă) [G. *tristichos,* in three rows, fr. *tri-,* three, + *stichos,* row]. Presence of three rows of eyelashes.

trisulcate (trī-sŭl'kāt). Marked by three grooves.

trisymptome (trī-simp'tōm). Cutaneous *vasculitis.*

tritanomaly (trī'tă-nom'ă-lē) [G. *tritos,* third, + *anōmalia,* irregularity]. A type of partial color deficiency due to a deficiency or abnormality of blue-sensitive retinal cones.

tritanopia (trī'tă-nō'pē-ă) [G. *tritos,* third, + *an-* priv. + *ōps,* eye]. Deficient color perception in which there is an absence of blue-sensitive pigment in the retinal cones.

triterpenes (trī-ter'pēnz). Hydrocarbons or their derivatives formed by the condensation of six isoprene units (equivalent to three terpene units) and containing, therefore, 30 carbon atoms; *e.g.,* squalene.

tritiated (trit'ē-ā-ted). Containing atoms of tritium (hydrogen-3) in the molecule.

triticeoglossus (tri-tish'ē-ō-glos'ŭs) [L. *triticeum,* + G. *glōssa,* tongue]. See under musculus.

triticeous (tri-tish'ŭs) [L. *triticeus,* fr. *triticum,* a grain of wheat]. Resembling or shaped like a grain of wheat.

triticeum (tri-tish'ē-ŭm) [L. *triticeus,* triticeous, like a grain of wheat]. *Cartilago* triticea.

tritium (T, *t*) (trit'ē-ŭm, trish'-). Hydrogen-3.

tritocaline (trit-ō-kal'ēn). Tritoqualine.

tritoqualine (trit-ō-kwal'ēn). Tritocaline; 7-amino-4,5,6-triethoxy-3-(5,6,7,8- tetrahydro-4-methoxy-6-methyl- 1,3-dioxolo[4,5-*g*]isoquinolin-5-yl)phthalide; an antihistaminic.

Tritrichomonas (trī'trĭk-ō-mō'nas) [G. *tri-,* three, + *Trichomonas*]. A genus of parasitic protozoan flagellates, formerly part of the genus *Trichomonas* but now separated as a distinct genus by the absence of a pelta and the presence of three anterior flagella. Species include *T. foetus,* which causes bovine trichomoniasis, and *T. suis,* which occurs in the nasal passages, stomach, cecum, and colon of pigs. See also *Trichomonas.*

tritubercular (trī-tū-ber'kyū-lăr). Tricuspid (2).

triturable (trit'yū-ră-bl). Capable of being triturated.

triturate (trit'yū-rāt). 1. To accomplish trituration. 2. A triturated substance.

tablet t., a compressed tablet of a medicated powder rubbed up with milk sugar.

trituration (trit-yū-rā'shŭn) [L. *trituratio,* fr. *trituro,* to thresh, fr. *tero,* pp. *tritus,* to rub]. 1. Tripsis (1); the act of reducing a drug to a fine powder and incorporating it thoroughly with sugar of milk by rubbing the two together in a mortar. 2. Mixing of dental amalgam in a mortar and pestle or with a mechanical device.

trityl (trī'til). The triphenylmethyl radical, Ph_3C–.

trivalence, trivalency (trī-vā'lens, -len-sē). The property of being trivalent.

trivalent (trī-vā'lent). Having the combining power (valence) of 3.

trivalve (trī'valv). Provided with three valves, as a speculum with three diverging blades.

trivial name. A name of a chemical, no part of which is necessarily used in a systematic sense; *i.e.,* it gives little or no indication as to chemical structure. Such names are common for drugs, hormones, proteins and other biologicals, and are used by the general public. They may not be officially sanctioned, in contrast to nonproprietary names, but may be adopted as official nonproprietary names as a result of widespread usage. Examples are water, aspirin, chlorophyll, heme, methotrexate, folic acid, caffeine, thyroxine, epinephrine, barbital, etc.; also common abbreviations for chemically defined substances, such as ACTH, MSH, BAL, DDT, which are spoken as such and not in terms of the words they represent. The distinction between trivial and semitrivial names is seldom made; thus tetrahydrofolate, methylglycine, glucosamine, etc., are often termed trivial even though each contains a systematic part that is used in the correct systematic sense (tetrahydro for four hydrogen atoms, methyl for a $-CH_3$ group, amine for $-NH_2$ in the above). Trivial names are often assigned arbitrarily to chemical compounds, especially from natural sources, before the chemical structures, hence systematic names, can be assigned; also, they afford useful shortenings of long systematic names even when these can be stated (although most such shortenings turn out to be semisystematic, as they incorporate some portion of the systematic name).

trizonal (trī-zō'năl). Having, or arranged in, three zones or layers.

tRNA Abbreviation for transfer *ribonucleic acid.*

trocar (trō'kar) [Fr. *trocart,* fr. *trois,* three, + *carre,* side (of a sword blade)]. An instrument for withdrawing fluid from a cavity, or for use in paracentesis; it consists of a metal tube (cannula) into which fits an obturator with a sharp three-cornered tip, which is withdrawn after the instrument has been pushed into the cavity; the name t. is usually applied to the obturator alone, the entire instrument being designated t. and cannula.

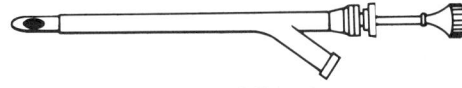

Trocar and Cannula

troch. Abbreviation for trochiscus.

trochanter (trō-kan'ter) [G. *trochantēr,* a runner, fr. *trechō,* to run]. One of the bony prominences developed from independent osseous centers near the upper extremity of the femur; there are two in man, three in the horse.

greater t., t. major.

lesser t., t. minor.

t. ma'jor [NA], greater t.; a strong process at the proximal and lateral part of the shaft of the femur, overhanging the root of the neck; it gives attachment to the gluteus medius and minimus, piriformis, obturator internus and externus, and gemelli muscles.

t. mi'nor [NA], lesser or small t.; trochantin; a pyramidal process projecting from the medial and proximal part of the shaft of the femur at the line of junction of the shaft and the neck; it receives the insertion of the psoas major and iliacus (iliopsoas) muscles.

small t., t. minor.

t. ter'tius [NA], third t.; gluteal tuberosity (2); an occasional process at the proximal end of the lateral lip of the linea aspera of the femur, about on a level with the lesser t., giving insertion to the greater part of the gluteus maximus muscle.

third t., t. tertius.

trochanterian, trochanteric (trō-kan-ter'ē-an, -ter'ik). Relating to a trochanter; especially the trochanter major.

trochanterplasty (trō-kan'ter-plas-tē). Plastic surgery of the trochanters and neck of the femur.

trochantin (trō-kan'tin). *Trochanter* minor.

trochantinian (trō-kan-tin'ē-an). Relating to the trochanter minor.

troche (trōk, trō'kē) [L. *trochiscus*]. Lozenge; pastil (2); trochiscus; morsulus; a small, disk-shaped or rhombic body composed of solidifying paste containing an astringent, antiseptic, or demulcent drug, used for local treatment of the mouth or throat, the t. being held in the mouth until dissolved. The vehicle or base of the t. is usually sugar, made adhesive by admixture with acacia or tragacanth, fruit paste, made from black or red currants, confection of rose, or balsam of tolu.

trochiscus, pl. **trochisci (troch.)** (trō-kis'kŭs) [L., fr. G. *trochiskos,* a small wheel, a lozenge, fr. *trochos,* a wheel]. Troche.

trochlea, pl. **trochleae** (trok'lē-ă, -lē-ē) [L. pulley, fr. G. *trochileia,* a pulley, fr. *trechō,* to run] [NA]. **1.** A structure serving as a pulley. **2.** A smooth articular surface of bone upon which another glides. **3.** A fibrous loop in the orbit, near the nasal process of the frontal bone, through which passes the tendon of the superior oblique muscle of the eye.

t. fem'oris, *facies* patellaris femoris.

t. fibula'ris calca'nei [NA], official alternative term for t. peronealis.

t. hu'meri [NA], t. or pulley of humerus; the grooved surface at the lower end of the humerus articulating with the trochlear notch of the ulna.

t. of humerus, t. humeri.

t. muscula'ris [NA], muscular pulley; a fibrous loop through which the tendon of a muscle passes; the intermediate tendon of the digastric and omohyoid muscles pass through such a t.

t. peronea'lis [NA], t. fibularis calcanei; peroneal pulley; trochlear process; processus trochlearis; spina peronealis; a projection from the lateral side of the calcaneus between the tendons of the peroneus longus and brevis.

t. phalan'gis, [NA], official alternative term for *caput* phalangis.

t. ta'li [NA], pulley of talus; the rounded articular surface of the talus articulating with the distal ends of the tibia and fibula.

trochlear (trok'lē-ar). **1.** Relating to a trochlea, especially the trochlea of the superior oblique muscle of the eye. **2.** Trochleiform.

trochleariform (trok-lē-ar'i-fōrm). Trochleiform.

trochlearis (trok-lē-ā'ris) [L.]. Trochlear.

trochleiform (trok'lē-i-fōrm). Trochleariform; trochlear (2); pulley-shaped.

trochocardia (trok-ō-kar'dē-ă) [G. *trochos,* wheel, + *kardia,* heart]. Rotary displacement of the heart around its axis.

trochoid (trō'koyd) [G. *trochōdēs,* fr. *trochos,* wheel, + *eidos,* resemblance]. Revolving; rotating; denoting a revolving or wheel-like articulation.

trochorizocardia (trō-kōr-ī'zō-kar'dē-ă). Combined trochocardia and horizocardia.

Troglotrema salmincola (trog-lō-trē'mă sal-mingk'ō-lă). *Nanophyetus salmincola.*

Troisier, Charles-Emile, French physician, 1844–1919. See T.'s *ganglion, node.*

trolamine (trō'lă-mēn). USAN-approved contraction for triethanolamine, $N(CH_2CH_2OH)_3$.

troland (trō'land) [L.T. *Troland,* U.S. physicist, 1889–1932]. Photon (1); a unit of visual stimulation at the retina equal to the illumination per square millimeter of pupil received from a surface of 1 lux brightness.

Trolard, Paulin, French anatomist, 1842–1910. See T.'s *vein.*

troleandomycin (trō'lē-an-dō-mī'sin). Triacetyloleandomycin; the triacetyl ester of oleandomycin, with a potency of not less than 760 μg per mg; an orally effective antibiotic for infections produced by Gram-positive, penicillin-resistant bacteria.

trolnitrate phosphate (trol-nī'trāt). Triethanolamine trinitrate diphosphate; an organic nitrate with mild but persistent vasodilator action on smooth muscle of the smaller vessels of postarteriolar vascular beds; used to prevent attacks of angina pectoris.

Tröltsch, Anton F. von, German otologist, 1829–1890. See T.'s *corpuscles, fold, pockets, recesses.*

Trombicula (trom-bik'yū-lă). The chigger mite, a genus of mites (family Trombiculidae) whose larvae (chiggers, red bugs) include pests of man and other animals, and vectors of rickettsial and probably viral diseases.

T. akamu'shi, *Leptotrombidium akamushi.*

T. alfredduge'si, a species common in second growth and grassy brush areas of the Americas; the larvae attack man (as well as reptiles, birds, and wild and domestic animals), causing an intensely itching dermatitis.

T. delien'sis, *Leptotrombidium deliensis.* See *Leptotrombidium akamushi.*

trombiculiasis (trom-bik-yū-lī'ă-sis). Infestation by *Trombicula.*

trombiculid (trom-bik'yū-lid). Common name for members of the family Trombiculidae.

Trombiculidae (trom-bik-ū-lī'dē). A family of mites whose larvae (redbugs, rougets, harvest mites, scrub mites, or chiggers) are parasitic on vertebrates and whose nymphs and adults are bright red and free-living, living on insect eggs or minute organisms in the soil. The six-legged larvae are barely visible red or orange parasites that attach to the skin for a few days to a month, producing an exceedingly irritating reaction. In the Orient, trombiculid chiggers of the genus *Leptotrombidium* transmit tsutsugamushi disease caused by *Rickettsia tsutsugamushi,* which is transovarially transmitted in these mites.

Trombidiidae (trom-bi-dī'i-dē). A family of mites that formerly included the subfamily Trombiculinae, now raised to the family Trombiculidae (including the vectors of tsutsugamushi disease). T. larvae are characteristically parasitic on insects, not on vertebrates as with the larvae of Trombiculidae.

tromethamine (trō-meth'ă-mēn). Tris(hydroxymethyl)methylamine; 2-amino-2-(hydroxymethyl)-1,3-propanediol; $H_2N{-}C(CH_2OH)_3$; a weakly basic compound used as an alkalizing agent and as a buffer in enzymic reactions.

Trömner, Ernest L.O., German neurologist, *1868. See T.'s *reflex.*

trona (trō'nă). A native sodium carbonate.

tropaic acid (trō-pā'ik). Tropic acid.

tropane (trō'pān). A bicyclic hydrocarbon, the fundamental structure of tropine, atropine, and other physiologically active substances.

tropate (trō'pāt). A salt or ester of tropic acid.

tropeic acid (trō-pē'ik). Tropic acid.

tropeine (trō'pē-in). An ester of tropine; either a naturally occurring alkaloid or prepared synthetically.

tropentane (trō-pen'tān). 1-Phenylcyclopentanecarboxylic acid 3α-tropanyl ester hydrochloride; an antispasmodic with anticholinergic properties.

tropeolins (trō-pē'ō-linz) [G. *tropaios,* pertaining to a turning or change, fr. *tropē,* a turn]. A group of azo dyes used as indicators; *e.g.,* methyl orange.

troph-. See tropho-.

trophectoderm (trof-ek'tō-derm) [troph- + ectoderm]. Outermost layer of cells in the mammalian blastodermic vesicle that will make contact with the endometrium and take part in establishing the embryo's means of receiving nutrition; the cell layer from which the trophoblast differentiates.

trophedema (trof-e-dē'mă). Hereditary *lymphedema.*

trophesic (trō-fē'sik). Pertaining to trophesy.

trophesy (trof'ĕ-sē). The results of any disorder of the trophic nerves.

trophic (trof'ik, trō'fik) [G. *trophē,* nourishment]. **1.** Relating to or dependent upon nutrition. **2.** Resulting from interruption of nerve supply.

-trophic [G. *trophē,* nourishment]. Suffixed combining form denoting nutrition. *Cf.* -tropic.

trophicity (trō-fis'i-tē). Trophism (1); a trophic influence or condition.

trophism (trof'izm) [G. *trophē,* nourishment]. **1.** Trophicity. **2.** Nutrition (1).

tropho-, troph- [G. *trophē,* nourishment]. Combining forms denoting food or nutrition.

trophoblast (trof'ō-blast, trō'fō-blast) [tropho- + G. *blastos,* germ]. The mesectodermal cell layer covering the blastocyst that erodes the uterine mucosa and through which the embryo receives nourishment from the mother; the cells do not enter into the formation of the embryo itself, but contribute to the formation of the placenta. The t. develops processes that later receive a core of vascular mesoderm and are then known as the chorionic villi; the t. soon becomes two-layered: the syncytiotrophoblast, an outer layer comprised of a multinucleated protoplasmic mass (syncytium), and the cytotrophoblast, the inner layer next to the mesoderm in which the cells retain their membranes.
plasmodial t., syncytiotrophoblast.
syncytial t., syncytiotrophoblast.

trophoblastic (trō-fō-blas'tik). Relating to the trophoblast.

trophoblastoma (trof'ō-blas-tō'mă). Choriocarcinoma.

trophochromatin (trof-ō-krō'mă-tin) [tropho- + G. *chrōma,* color]. Trophochromidia.

trophochromidia (trof'ō-krō-mid'ē-ă). Trophochromatin; nongerminal or vegetative extranuclear masses of chromatin, found in certain protozoan forms; *e.g.,* the macronucleus of certain ciliates, such as *Paramecium.*

trophocyte (trof'ō-sīt) [tropho- + G. *kytos,* cell]. Trephocyte; a cell that supplies nourishment; *e.g.,* Sertoli cells in the seminiferous tubules.

trophoderm (trof'ō-derm) [tropho- + G. *derma,* skin]. The trophectoderm, or trophoblast, together with the vascular mesodermal layer underlying it. See also serosa (2).

trophodermatoneurosis (trof'ō-der'mă-tō-nū-rō'sis). Cutaneous trophic changes due to neural involvement.

trophodynamics (trof'ō-dī-nam'iks) [tropho- + G. *dynamis,* power]. Nutritional energy; the dynamics of nutrition or metabolism.

trophoneurosis (trof'ō-nū-rō'sis) [tropho- + G. *neuron,* nerve, + *-osis,* condition]. A trophic disorder, such as atrophy, hypertrophy, or a skin eruption, occurring as a consequence of disease or injury of the nerves of the part.
facial t., facial *hemiatrophy.*
lingual t., progressive lingual *hemiatrophy.*
muscular t., progressive muscular *atrophy.*
Romberg's t., facial *hemiatrophy.*

trophoneurotic (trof-ō-nū-rot'ik). Relating to a trophoneurosis.

trophonucleus (trof-ō-nū'klē-ŭs). Macronucleus (2).

trophoplasm (trof'ō-plazm) [tropho- + G. *plasma,* a thing formed]. Obsolete term referring to the achromatin or supposed formative substance of a cell.

trophoplast (trof'ō-plast) [tropho- + G. *plastos,* formed]. Plastid (1).

trophospongia (trof'ō-spon'jē-ă) [tropho- + G. *spongia,* a sponge]. Canalicular structures described by A.F. Holmgren in the protoplasm of certain cells.

trophotaxis (trof-ō-tak'sis) [tropho- + G. *taxis,* arrangement]. Trophotropism.

trophotropic (trof-ō-trop'ik). Relating to trophotropism.

trophotropism (trō-fot'rō-pizm) [tropho- + G. *tropē,* a turning]. Trophotaxis; chemotaxis of living cells in relation to nutritive material; it may be positive (toward nutritive material) or negative (away from nutritive material).

trophozoite (trof-ō-zō'īt) [tropho- + G. *zōon,* animal]. The ameboid, vegetative, asexual form of certain Sporozoea, such as the schizont of the plasmodia of malaria and related parasites.

-trophy [G. *trophē,* nourishment]. Suffix meaning food, nutrition.

tropia (trō'pē-ă) [G. tropē, a turning]. Abnormal deviation of the eye. See strabismus.

-tropic [G. *tropē,* a turning]. Suffixed combining form denoting a turning toward, having an affinity for. *Cf.* -trophic.

tropic acid (trop'ik). Tropaic or tropeic acid; α-phenylhydracrylic acid; 2-phenyl-3-hydroxypropionic acid; $HOCH_2CH(C_6H_5)$-COOH; a constituent of atropine and of scopolamine, in which it is esterified through its COOH to the 3-CHOH of tropine.

tropicamide (trō-pik'ă-mīd). *N*-Ethyl-2-phenyl-*N*-4-pyridylmethyl)hydracrylamide; an anticholinergic agent used to effect a rapid and brief mydriasis for eye examinations.

tropine (trō'pēn). 3α-Tropanol; 3α-hydroxytropane; the major constituent of atropine and scopolamine, from which it is obtained on hydrolysis.

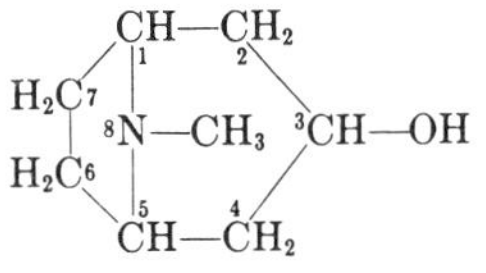

Tropine

t. mandelate, homatropine.
t. tropate, atropine.

tropism (trō'pizm) [G. *tropē,* a turning]. The phenomenon, observed in living organisms, of moving toward (**positive t.**) or away from (**negative t.**) a focus of light, heat, or other stimulus; usually applied to the movement of a portion of the organism as opposed to taxis, the movement of an entire organism.
viral t., the specificity of a virus for a particular host tissue, determined in part by the interaction of viral surface structures with host cell-surface receptors.

tropocollagen (trō-pō-kol'ă-jen, trop'ō-). The fundamental units of collagen fibrils, consisting of three helically arranged polypeptide chains.

tropometer (trō-pom'ĕ-ter) [G. *tropē,* a turning, + *metron,* measure]. Any instrument for measuring the degree of rotation or torsion, as of the eyeball or the shaft of a long bone.

tropomyosin (trō-pō-mī'ō-sin). A fibrous protein extractable from muscle; sometimes specified as t. B to distinguish it from t. A (paramyosin) prominent in mollusks.

troponin (trō'pō-nin). A globular protein of muscle that binds to tropomyosin and has considerable affinity for calcium ions.

trough (trawf). A long, narrow, shallow channel or depression.

gingival t., the formation of a crater as a result of destruction of interdental tissues so that, in effect, there exists a labial and lingual curtain of gingiva with no interproximal connection at all.
Langmuir t., a t. with a movable surface barrier for studying the compression of surface films.
synaptic t., the depression of the surface of the striated muscle fiber that accommodates the motor endplate.

Trousseau, Armand, French physician, 1801–1867. See T.'s *point, sign, spots, syndrome;* T.-Lallemand *bodies.*

troxerutin (troks'ē-rū-tin). 7,3′,4′-Tris[*O*-(2-hydroxyethyl)]rutin; used for treatment of venous disorders.

troxidone (trok'si-dōn). Trimethadione.

Trp Symbol for tryptophan and its radicals.

truncal (trŭng'kăl). Relating to the trunk of the body or to any arterial or nerve trunk, etc.

truncate (trŭng'kāt) [L. *trunco,* pp. *-atus,* to maim, cut off]. Truncated; cut across at right angles to the long axis, or appearing to be so cut.

truncus, gen. and pl. **trunci** (trŭng'kŭs, -kī) [L. stem, trunk].
1. The body (trunk or torso), excluding the head and extremities.
2. A primary nerve, vessel, or collection of tissue before its division.
3. A large collecting lymphatic vessel.
t. arterio'sus (commu'nis), the common arterial trunk opening out of both ventricles in early fetal life, later destined to be divided into aorta and pulmonary artery by development of the spiral septum.
t. atrioventricula'ris [NA], atrioventricular trunk, bundle, or band; bundle of His; Gaskell's bridge; His' band or bundle; Keith's or Kent-His bundle; Kent's bundle (1); fasciculus atrioventricularis; ventriculonector; the bundle of modified cardiac muscle fibers that begins at the atrioventricular node and passes through the right atrioventricular fibrous ring to the membranous part of the interventricular septum where it divides into two branches, crus dextrum truncus atrioventricularis and crus sinistrum truncus atrioventricularis; the two crura ramify in the subendocardium of their respective ventricles. See also conducting *system* of heart.
t. brachiocepha'licus [NA], brachiocephalic trunk; innominate artery; arteria anonyma; anonymous artery; *origin,* arch of aorta; *branches,* right subclavian and right common carotid; occasionally it gives off the thyroidea ima.
t. bronchiomediastina'lis [NA], bronchomediastinal trunk; a lymphatic vessel arising from the union of the efferent lymphatics from the bronchial and mediastinal nodes on either side.
t. celi'acus [NA], celiac trunk; arteria celiaca; celiac artery or axis; Haller's tripod; *origin,* abdominal aorta just below diaphragm; *branches,* left gastric, common hepatic, splenic.
t. cor'poris callo'si [NA], trunk of the corpus callosum; the main arched portion of the corpus callosum.
t. costocervica'lis [NA], costocervical trunk; costocervical artery; a short artery that arises from the subclavian artery on each side and divides into deep cervical and highest intercostal branches, the latter dividing usually to form the first and second posterior intercostal arteries.
t. infe'rior [NA], inferior trunk; the nerve bundle formed by the union of the ventral branches of the eighth cervical and first thoracic nerves; it provides fibers to the posterior and inferior cords (fasciculi) of the brachial plexus.
trun'ci intestina'les [NA], intestinal trunks; the vessels conveying lymph from the lower part of the liver, the stomach, spleen, pancreas, and small intestine; they discharge into the cisterna chyli and are sometimes duplicated.
t. jugula'ris [NA], jugular trunk or duct; lymphatic vessel on each side, conveying the lymph from the head and neck; that on the right side empties into the right lymphatic duct, that on the left into the thoracic duct.
t. linguofacia'lis [NA], the common trunk by which the lingual and facial arteries frequently arise from the external carotid artery.
trun'ci lumba'les [NA], lumbar trunks; two lymphatic ducts conveying lymph from the lower limbs, pelvic viscera and walls, large intestine, kidneys, and suprarenal glands; they discharge into the cisterna chyli.
t. lum'bosacra'lis [NA], lumbosacral trunk; a large nerve, formed by the union of the fifth lumbar and first sacral nerves, with a branch from the fourth lumbar nerve, which enters into the formation of the sacral plexus.
t. me'dius [NA], middle trunk; the continuation of the ventral branch of the seventh cervical nerve; it contributes fibers to the posterior and lateral cords (fasciculi) of the brachial plexus.
persistent t. arterio'sus, a congenital cardiovascular deformity resulting from failure of development of the spiral septum and consisting of a common arterial trunk opening out of both ventricles, the pulmonary arteries being given off from the ascending common trunk.
trun'ci plex'us brachia'lis [NA], trunks of the brachial plexus; the superior, middle, and inferior trunks; they divide distally to form the cords (fasciculi) of the plexus.
t. pulmona'lis [NA], pulmonary trunk; arteria pulmonalis; venous or pulmonary artery; *origin,* right ventricle of heart; *distribution,* it divides into the arteria pulmonalis dextra and the arteria pulmonalis sinistra, which enter the corresponding lungs and branch along with the segmental bronchi.
t. subcla'vius [NA], subclavian trunk or duct; it is formed by the union of the vessels draining the lymph nodes of either upper limb, emptying into the thoracic duct at the root of the neck on the left or into the right lymphatic duct.
t. supe'rior [NA], superior trunk; the nerve bundle formed by the union of the ventral branches of the fifth and sixth cervical nerves and some fibers from the fourth; it contributes fibers to the posterior and lateral cords (fasciculi) of the brachial plexus.
t. sympath'icus [NA], sympathetic trunk; gangliated cord; one of the two long ganglionated nerve strands alongside the vertebral column that extend from the base of the skull to the coccyx; they are connected to each spinal nerve by gray rami and receive fibers from the spinal cord through white rami connecting with the thoracic and upper lumbar spinal nerves.
t. thyrocervica'lis [NA], thyrocervical trunk; thyroid axis; a short arterial trunk arising from the subclavian artery and dividing generally into three branches: thyroidea inferior, transversa colli, and suprascapularis.
t. vaga'lis [NA], vagal trunk; one of the two nerve bundles, anterior and posterior, into which the esophageal plexus continues as it passes through the diaphragm.

Trunecek, Karel, Czechoslovakian physician, *1865. See T.'s *symptom.*

trunk (trŭnk) [L. *truncus*]. Truncus.
atrioventricular t., *truncus* atrioventricularis.
t.'s of brachial plexus, *trunci* plexus brachialis.
brachiocephalic t., *truncus* brachiocephalicus.
bronchomediastinal t., *truncus* bronchomediastinalis.
celiac t., *truncus* celiacus.
t. of corpus callosum, *truncus* corporis callosi.
costocervical t., *truncus* costocervicalis.
inferior t., *truncus* inferior.
intestinal t.'s, *trunci* intestinales.
jugular t., *truncus* jugularis.
lumbar t.'s, *trunci* lumbales.
lumbosacral t., *truncus* lumbosacralis.
middle t., *truncus* medius.
nerve t., a collection of funiculi or bundles of nerve fibers enclosed in a connective tissue sheath, the epineurium.
pulmonary t., *truncus* pulmonalis.

subclavian t., *truncus* subclavius.
superior t., *truncus* superior.
sympathetic t., *truncus* sympathicus.
thyrocervical t., *truncus* thyrocervicalis.
vagal t., *truncus* vagalis.

trusion (trū'zhŭn) [L. *trudo,* pp. *trusus,* to thrust]. Displacement of a body, *e.g.,* a tooth, from an initial position.

truss (trŭs) [Fr. *trousser,* to tie up, to pack]. An appliance designed to prevent the return of a reduced hernia or the increase in size of an irreducible hernia; it consists of a pad attached to a belt and kept in place by a spring or straps.

Try Former abbreviation for tryptophan.

try-in (trī'in). Preliminary insertion of a complete denture wax-up (trial denture), of a partial denture casting, or of a finished restoration to determine the fit, esthetics, maxillomandibular relation, etc.

trypan blue (trī'pan, trip') [C.I. 23850]. An acid azo dye, $C_{34}H_{34}N_6O_{14}S_4Na_4$, used for vital staining of the reticuloendothelial system, uriniferous tubules, and cells in tissue culture, and as an experimental teratogen; formerly used as a trypanocide.

trypanicidal (tri-pan-i-sī'dăl). Trypanocidal.

trypanicide (tri-pan'i-sīd). Trypanocide.

trypanid (trip'ă-nid). Trypanosomatid.

trypanocidal (tri-pan'ō-sī'dăl, trip'ă-nō-). Trypanicidal; destructive to trypanosomes.

trypanocide (tri-pan'ō-sīd, trip'ă-nō-) [trypanosome + L. *caedo,* to kill]. Trypanicide; trypanosomicide; an agent that kills trypanosomes.

Trypanoplasma (tri-pan-ō-plaz'mă, trip'ă-nō-) [G. *trypanon,* auger, + *plasma,* anything formed]. A genus of flagellate Protozoa (family Cryptobiidae), the members of which have a body of varying shape, an undulating membrane, and a flagellum projecting from either extremity; parasitic in the blood of fishes.

Trypanosoma (tri-pan'ō-sō'mă, trip'ă-nō-) [G. *trypanon,* an auger, + *sōma,* body]. A genus of asexual digenetic protozoan flagellates (family Trypanosomatidae) that have a spindle-shaped body with an undulating membrane on one side, a single anterior flagellum, and a kinetoplast; they are parasitic in the blood plasma of many vertebrates (only a few being pathogenic) and as a rule have an intermediate host, a bloodsucking invertebrate, such as a leech, tick, or insect; pathogenic species cause trypanosomiasis in man and a number of other diseases in domestic animals.

T. a'vium, a species that occurs in owls, crows, and other birds; various bloodsucking arthropods are the vectors, including mosquitoes, black flies, and hippoboscids; this species was reported under a large number of names now considered to be physiologic strains of the species.

T. bru'cei, a species now divided into three subspecies: *T. b. brucei, T. b. rhodesiense,* and *T. b. gambiense.*

T. bru'cei bru'cei, a subspecies causing nagana in Africa; it produces fatal disease in camels, acute disease in equines, dogs, and cats, and chronic disease in swine, cattle, sheep, and goats; it is transmitted primarily by tsetse flies of the genus *Glossina.*

T. bru'cei gambien'se, *T. gambiense; T. hominis; T. ugandense;* a subspecies causing Gambian trypanosomiasis; transmitted by tsetse flies, especially *Glossina palpalis.*

T. bru'cei rhodesien'se, *T. rhodesiense;* a subspecies causing Rhodesian trypanosomiasis; it is transmitted by tsetse flies, especially *Glossina morsitans;* various game animals can act as reservoir hosts.

T. congolen'se, a species transmitted primarily by tsetse flies of the genus *Glossina* and causing nagana in Africa, with anemia as a prominent feature; most domestic mammals (cattle, sheep, goats, equines, camels, dogs, and cats) are highly susceptible to infection, with the resultant disease taking an acute to chronic course with or without recovery; swine are more resistant, with clinical disease running a mild course.

T. cru'zi, *T. escomelis; T. triatomae;* a species that causes South American trypanosomiasis and is endemic in Mexico and various countries of Central and South America; transmission and infection are common only where the triatomine bug vector defecates while taking blood, as the bug feces contains the infective agents that are scratched into the skin or brought in contact with mucosal surfaces. Trypomastigotes are found in the blood, and amastigotes occur intracellularly in clusters or colonies in the tissues; heart muscle fibers and cells of many other organs are attacked, the organisms not being restricted to macrophages as in visceral leishmaniasis; man, dogs, cats, house rats, armadillos, bats, certain monkeys, and opossums are the usual vertebrate hosts; vectors are members of the family Triatominae. Also known as *Schizotrypanum cruzi,* a distinct generic designation widely used in the endemic regions.

T. dimor'phon, an African species found in horses, cattle, sheep, goats, pigs, and dogs, formerly thought to be the same as *T. congolense* but now recognized as a distinct and more pathogenic species in cattle, sheep, and dogs; it is spread by tsetse flies across central Africa.

T. equi'num, a species that causes mal de caderas of horses in Central and South America; except for being akinetoplastic, it is transmitted mechanically by bloodsucking flies.

T. equiper'dum, a species that causes dourine.

T. escome'lis, *T. cruzi.*

T. ev'ansi, *T. hippicum;* a parasite chiefly of cattle, camels, horses, and dogs, causing surra and murrina; it is transmitted mechanically by tabanid and other bloodsucking flies.

T. gambien'se, *T. brucei gambiense.*

T. hip'picum, *T. evansi.*

T. hom'inis, *T. gambiense.*

T. igno'tum, old name for *T. simiae.*

T. lew'isi, species that is a worldwide nonpathogenic parasite in the blood of rats widely used for laboratory study; it is transmitted by the rat flea, *Nosopsyllus fasciatus.*

T. melopha'gium, a nonpathogenic species (related to *T. theileri*) found in sheep throughout the world, and probably in goats as well; the vector is *Melophagus ovinus.*

T. range'li, a species that parasitizes a wide variety of mammals, including man, in South America and is transmitted by the triatomid bugs *Rhodnius prolixus* and *Tiratoma dimidiata,* and probably others; it is apparently nonpathogenic but may be pathogenic in the bug host.

T. rhodesien'se, *T. brucei rhodesiense.*

T. simi'ae, a species normally found in warthogs; it is highly pathogenic in pigs and camels, and is transmitted cyclically by tsetse flies and mechanically by bloodsucking flies.

T. su'is, a species pathogenic for swine in Africa; it is transmitted by tsetse flies.

T. thei'leri, a large, relatively nonpathogenic species found in African antelopes and in cattle in many parts of the world; the parasites are spread by bloodsucking tabanid horseflies.

T. triatom'ae, *T. cruzi.*

T. uganden'se, *T. gambiense.*

T. vi'vax, a species causing nagana in cattle, sheep, and goats in Africa, and trypanosomiasis in cattle and water buffalo in South America; it is transmitted cyclically by tsetse flies (*Glossina* spp.) in Africa and presumably mechanically by bloodsucking flies in South America.

trypanosomatid (trī-pan'ō-sō-mat'id). Common name for a member of the family Trypanosomatidae.

Trypanosomatidae (trī-pan'ō-sō-mat'i-dē). A protozoan family of hemoflagellates (order Kinetoplastida, class Zoomastigophorea, subphylum Mastigophora); asexual blood and/or tissue parasites of leeches, insects, and vertebrates and sap inhabitants of plants, characterized by a rounded or elongate form, a single nucleus, elongate mitochondrion (its position in relation to the nucleus is a characteristic of each genus), and an anteriorly directed single flagellum (in some genera, it borders an undulating membrane). T. includes the genera *Crithidia, Herpetomonas, Leptomonas,* and *Blastocrithidia,* all of which are monogenetic and found in insects, and *Phytomonas* (found in plants), *Endotrypanum, Leishmania,* and *Trypanosoma,* all of which are digenetic; *Leishmania* and *Trypanosoma* include important pathogens of man and animals. Many trypanosomes pass through developmental or life cycle stages similar to the body forms characteristic of the genera; these forms include amastigote, choanomastigote, opisthomastigote, promastigote, epimastigote, and trypomastigote.

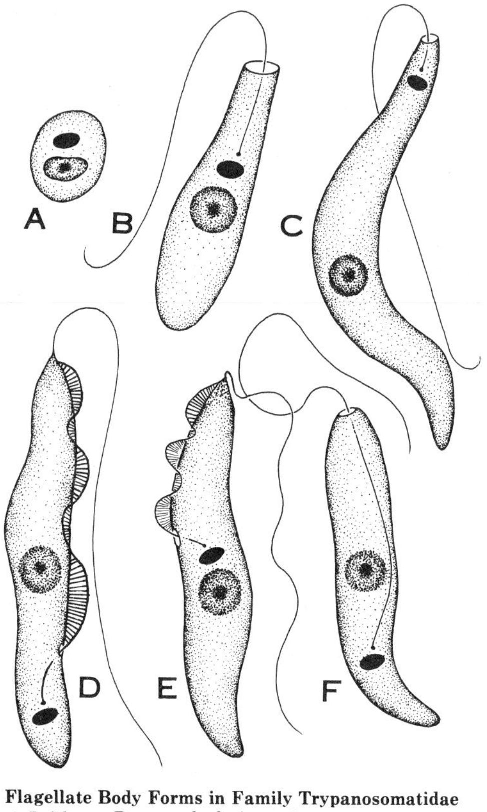

Flagellate Body Forms in Family Trypanosomatidae
A, Leishman-Donovan body (amastigote); *B*, choanomastigote; *C*, promastigote; *D*, trypomastigote; *E*, epimastigote; *F*, opisthomastigote.

trypanosome (tri-pan′ō-sōm, trip′ă-nō-) [G. *trypanon,* an auger, + *sōma,* body]. Common name for any member of the genus *Trypanosoma* or of the family Trypanosomatidae.

trypanosomiasis (tri-pan′ō-sō-mī′ă-sis, trip′ă-nō-). Any disease caused by a trypanosome.
acute t., Rhodesian t.
African t., African sleeping sickness; a serious endemic disease in tropical Africa, of two types: Gambian t. and Rhodesian t.
chronic t., Gambian t.
Cruz t., South American t.
East African t., Rhodesian t.
Gambian t., West African t. or sleeping sickness; chronic African t. or sleeping sickness; a chronic disease of man caused by *Trypanosoma brucei gambiense* in northern and sub-Saharan Africa from Senegal east to Sudan and Uganda; characterized by splenomegaly, drowsiness, an uncontrollable urge to sleep, and the development of psychotic changes; basal ganglia and cerebellar involvement commonly lead to chorea and athetosis; the terminal phase of the disease is characterized by wasting, anorexia, and emaciation that gradually leads to coma and death, usually from intercurrent infection.
Rhodesian t., East African t. or sleeping sickness; chronic African t. or sleeping sickness; a disease of man caused by *Trypanosoma brucei rhodesiense* in eastern Africa from Ethiopia and Uganda south to Zimbabwe; it is clinically similar to Gambian t. but of shorter duration and more acute in form; patients suffer repeated episodes of pyrexia, become anemic, and die commonly from cardiac failure.
South American t., Chagas' or Chagas-Cruz disease; Cruz t.; t. caused by *Trypanosoma* (or *Schizotrypanum*) *cruzi* and transmitted by certain species of reduviid (triatomine) bugs. In its acute form, it is seen most frequently in young children, with swelling of the skin at the site of entry, most often the face, and regional lymph node enlargement; in its chronic form it can assume several aspects, commonly cardiomyopathy, but megacolon and megaesophagus also occur; natural reservoirs include dogs, armadillos, rodents, and other domestic, domiciliated, and wild mammals.
West African t., Gambian t.

trypanosomic (tri-pan-ō-sō′mik, trip′ă-nō-). Relating to trypanosomes, especially denoting infection by such organisms.

trypanosomicide (tri-pan′ō-sō′mi-sīd). Trypanocide.

trypanosomid (tri-pan′ō-sō-mid) [trypanosome + G. *-id* (1)]. Trypanid; a skin lesion resulting from immunologic changes from trypanosome disease.

trypan red (trī′pan, trip′) [C.I. 22850]. An azo dye formerly used in the treatment of trypanosomiasis.

tryparsamide (trī-par′să-mīd). Sodium *N*-carbamylmethyl-*p*-aminobenzenearsonate; used in the treatment of trypanosomic and spirochetal infections, especially neurosyphilis, and the late stages of African sleeping sickness.

trypomastigote (trip-ō-mas′ti-gōt) [G. *trypanon,* auger, + *mastix,* whip]. Term to replace the older term, "trypanosome stage," which was often confused with the flagellate genus *Trypanosoma.* It denotes the stage (infective stage for South American trypanosomiasis and African trypanosomiasis, and the only stage found in man in the latter illness) in which the flagellum arises from a posteriorly located kinetoplast and emerges from the side of the body, with an undulating membrane running along the length of the body.

trypsin (trip′sin) [EC 3.4.21.4]. A proteolytic enzyme formed in the small intestine from trypsinogen by the action of enteropeptidase; a serine proteinase that hydrolyzes peptides, amides, esters, etc., at bonds of the carboxyl groups of L-arginine or L-lysine; it also produces the meromyosins.
crystallized t., a purified preparation of the pancreatic enzyme; used as an adjunct to surgery for débridement of necrotic wounds and ulcers.

trypsinogen, trypsogen (trip-sin′ō-jen, trip′sō-jen). Protrypsin; an inactive protein secreted by the pancreas that is converted into trypsin by the action of enteropepsidase.

tryptamine (trip′tă-mēn, -min). 3-(2-Aminoethyl)indole; a decarboxylation product of tryptophan that occurs in plants and certain foods (*e.g.,* cheese). It raises the blood pressure through vasoconstrictor action, by the release of norepinephrine at postganglionic sympathetic nerve endings, and is believed to be one of the agents responsible for hypertensive episodes following therapy with monoamine oxidase inhibitors (*e.g.,* pargyline hydrochloride).

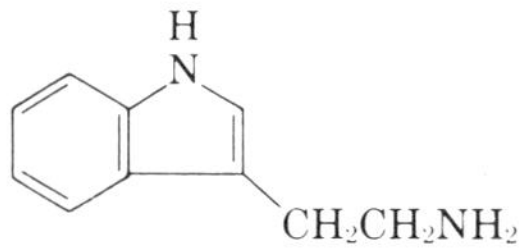

Tryptamine

tryptamine-strophanthidin (trip'ta-mēn-strō-fan'thi-din). A semisynthetic cardiac glycoside that is a condensation product of strophanthidin and tryptamine; given orally, it has a rapid onset and short duration of cardiac action.

tryptic (trip'tik). Relating to trypsin, as t. digestion.

tryptone (trip'tōn). A peptone produced by proteolytic digestion with trypsin.

tryptonemia (trip-tō-nē'mē-ă). The presence of tryptone in the circulating blood.

tryptophan (Trp) (trip'tō-fan). 2-Amino-3-(3-indolyl)propionic acid; a component of proteins.
t. decarboxylase, aromatic L-amino-acid decarboxylase.
t. desmolase, t. synthase.
t. oxygenase, tryptophan 2,3-dioxygenase.
t. pyrrolase, tryptophan 2,3-dioxygenase.
t. synthase [EC 4.2.1.20], t. desmolase or synthetase; a hydro-lyase condensing L-serine (or glyceraldehyde phosphate) and indole (or indole-3-glycerol phosphate) to L-tryptophan; pyridoxal phosphate is required.
t. synthetase, t. synthase.

tryptophanase (trip'to-fă-nās). **1.** Tryptophan 2,3-dioxygenase. **2.** [EC 4.1.99.1]. An enzyme found in bacteria that catalyzes the cleavage of tryptophan to indole, pyruvic acid, and ammonia; pyridoxal phosphate is a coenzyme.

tryptophan 2,3-dioxygenase [EC 1.13.11.11]. Tryptophan oxygenase or pyrrolase; tryptophanase (1); pyrrolase; an oxidoreductase catalyzing reductive closure of the side chain on the benzene ring in *N*-formylkynurenine to the pyrrole ring of tryptophan; an adaptive enzyme, the level (in the liver) being controlled by adrenal hormones.

tryptophanuria (trip'tō-fă-nū'rē-ă). Enhanced urinary excretion of tryptophan.
t. with dwarfism, a syndrome of dwarfism, mental defect, cutaneous photosensitivity, and gait disturbance associated with t.; autosomal recessive inheritance.

tsetse (tset'sē, tsē'tsē) [S. African native name]. See *Glossina.*

TSH Abbreviation for thyroid-stimulating *hormone.*

TSH-RF Abbreviation for thyroid-stimulating hormone-releasing *factor.*

TSS Abbreviation for toxic shock *syndrome.*

TSTA Abbreviation for tumor-specific transplantation *antigens.*

TTP Abbreviation for ribothymidine 5'-triphosphate.

T.U. Abbreviation for toxic or toxin *unit.*

tuaminoheptane (tū'am-i-nō-hep'tān). 2-Aminoheptane; a sympathomimetic volatile amine, used by inhalation as a nasal decongestant; available also as t. sulfate, with the same actions, and more potent as a vasoconstrictor than ephedrine.

tuba, gen. and pl. **tubae** (tū'bă, tū'bē) [L. a straight trumpet]. Tube; a hollow cylindrical structure or canal.
t. acus'tica, t. auditiva.
t. auditi'va [NA], t. auditoria; auditory, eustachian, otopharyngeal, or pharyngotympanic tube; t. eustachiana or eustachii; guttural duct; t. acustica; otosalpinx; salpinx (2); a tube leading from the tympanic cavity to the nasopharynx; it consists of an osseous (posterolateral) portion at the tympanic end, and a fibrocartilaginous (anteromedial) portion at the pharyngeal end; where the two portions join, in the region of the sphenopetrosal fissure, is the narrowest portion of the tube (isthmus).
t. audito'ria [NA], official alternative term for t. auditiva.
t. eustachia'na, t. eusta'chii, t. auditiva.
t. fallopia'na, t. fallo'pii, t. uterina.
t. uteri'na [NA], uterine tube; oviduct; fallopian tube; gonaduct (2); salpinx uterina; t. fallopiana; salpinx (1); one of the tubes leading on either side from the fundus of the uterus to the upper or outer extremity of the ovary; it consists of infundibulum, ampulla, isthmus, and uterine parts.

tubage (tū'baj). Introduction of a tube into a canal. See also intubation.

tubal (tū'băl). Relating to a tube, especially the uterine tube.

tubatorsion (tū-bă-tōr'shŭn). Tubotorsion.

tubba, tubbae (tŭb'ă, tŭb'bē). foot *yaws.*

Tubbs, Oswald S., British surgeon, *1908. See T. *dilator.*

TUBE

tube (tūb) [L. *tubus*]. **1.** Tuba. **2.** A hollow cylinder or pipe.
Abbott's t., Miller-Abbott t.
air t., the trachea, or a bronchus or any of its branches conveying air to the lungs.
auditory t., *tuba* auditiva.
Babcock t., a t. in which milk, after treatment with sulfuric acid, is centrifuged and its fat content then determined in a graduated neck.
Bouchut's t., a short cylindrical t. used in intubation of the larynx.
Bourdon t., a curved and partially flattened t. that tends to straighten out in proportion to internal pressure; used as a transducer to move the pointer of an aneroid manometer.
bronchial t.'s, bronchia.
Cantor t., a long, single-lumen intestinal t. with a sealed rubber bag tip; mercury is injected into the rubber bag with a needle and syringe.
cardiac t., the primitive tubular heart in the embryo, before its division into chambers.
Carlen's t., a double lumen flexible endobronchial t. used for bronchospirometry, for isolation of one lung to prevent contamination or secretions from the contralateral lung, or for ventilation of one lung.
cathode ray t. (CRT), an evacuated t. containing a beam of electrons which can be deflected to various parts of a fluorescent screen; used in the cathode ray oscilloscope.
Celestin t., a plastic tube introduced through a tumor in the esophagus; it permits maintenance of swallowing certain substances when the lesion is unresectable.
Coolidge t., an x-ray t., in which the cathode consists of a tungsten wire spiral surrounded by a molybdenum t.; the tungsten spiral is heated by an electric current; the quantity and quality of the x-ray so generated is regulated by varying the temperature of the cathode and the applied voltage.
digestive t., digestive *tract.*
drainage t., a t. introduced into a wound or cavity to facilitate removal of a fluid.
Durham's t., a jointed tracheotomy t.
empyema t., a rubber drainage t., piercing a sheet rubber shield, passed through the chest wall in order to drain an empyema.
endobronchial t., a single or double lumen t. with an inflatable cuff at the distal end that, after being passed through the larynx and trachea, is positioned so that ventilation is restricted to one lung; a single lumen t. is placed in the main stem bronchus of the

lung; a double lumen t. is positioned at the tracheal carina to permit ventilation of either or both lungs.
endotracheal t., intratracheal or tracheal t.; a flexible t. inserted nasally or orally into the trachea to provide an airway, as in tracheal intubation.
eustachian t., *tuba* auditiva.
fallopian t., *tuba* uterina.
feeding t., a flexible t. passed through the oral pharynx and into the esophagus and stomach, through which liquid food is fed.
Ferrein's t., *tubulus* renalis contortus.
Geiger-Müller t., see Geiger-Müller *counter.*
germ t., a young hypha growing out of a yeast cell or spore, the beginning of a mycelium; also used as a rapid test for differentiating *Candida albicans* from other *Candida* species.
Haldane t., a t. for securing human alveolar air samples; consisting of a narrow hosepipe with a mouthpiece from which a t. is attached for the withdrawal of expired air at the end of a sudden, maximal expiration.
intratracheal t., endotracheal t.
Levin t., a t. introduced through the nose into the upper alimentary canal, to facilitate intestinal decompression.
Martin's t., a drainage t. with a cross piece near the extremity to keep it from slipping out of a cavity.
medullary t., neural t.
Miescher's t.'s, elongate fusiform or cylindrical bodies forming the encapsulated cystic intramuscular stage of the protozoan *Sarcocystis.*
Miller-Abbott t., Abbott's t.; a t. with two lumens, one ending in a small collapsible balloon and the other in a metallic tip with numerous perforations; used for intestinal decompression.
Moss t., **(1)** a triple-lumen, nasogastric, feeding-decompression t., that utilizes a gastric balloon to occlude cardioesophageal junction, with simultaneous esophageal aspiration and intragastric feeding; **(2)** a double-lumen, gastric lavage t., that provides continuous delivery of saline via a small bore, with simultaneous aspiration of fluid and some particles via a large bore.
nasogastric t., a stomach tube passed through the nose.
nasotracheal t., an endotracheal t. inserted through the nasal passages.
neural t., medullary t.; the epithelial t. formed from the neuroectoderm of the early embryo by the closure of the neural groove; by complex processes of cell proliferation and organization the neural t. develops into the spinal cord and brain.
O'Dwyer's t., a metal t. formerly used for intubation of the larynx in diphtheria.
orotracheal t., an endotracheal t. inserted through the mouth.
otopharyngeal t., *tuba* auditiva.
pharyngotympanic t., *tuba* auditiva.
photomultiplier t., a detector which magnifies the signal (by as much as 10^6) received from the electromagnetic radiation by a system of electron acceleration from a photocathode through a series of dynodes.
Pitot t., a stationary L-shaped t. inserted in a fluid stream, with its opening upstream, and used for measuring the velocity of fluid movement at that point in terms of the pressure developed in the t. by the fluid impinging on it, compared to a second t. opening laterally or downstream.
pus t., pyosalpinx.
Rehfuss stomach t., a t. with a calibrated syringe, formerly used for aspiration of stomach contents in gastric analysis; replaced by plastic disposable stomach t.'s.
Robertshaw t., a variation of Carlen's t. that eliminates some mechanical disadvantages of the latter.
roll t., a modification of the plate culture; a seeded medium containing agar is placed in a test t. which is rolled or spun horizontally until the medium solidifies evenly on the interior of the t.
Ruysch's t., a minute tubular cavity opening in the lower and anterior portion of each surface of the nasal septum; best seen in the early fetal period when it is associated with the organum vomeronasale.
Ryle's t., a thin rubber t., with about the lumen of a no. 8 catheter, and an olive-tipped extremity, used in the giving of a test meal.
Sengstaken-Blakemore t., a t. with three lumens, one for drainage of the stomach and two for inflation of attached gastric and esophageal balloons; used for emergency treatment of bleeding esophageal varices.
Southey's t.'s, obsolete cannulas of small, almost capillary, caliber, thrust by a trocar into the subcutaneous tissues to drain the fluid of anasarca.
stomach t., a flexible t. passed into the stomach for lavage or feeding.
T t., a self-retaining t. with side extensions, shaped like a T.
test t., a t. of thin glass closed at one end, used in the examination of urine and other chemical operations, for bacterial cultures, etc.
Tovell t., an armored endotrachial t. with a wire spiral embedded in the wall to prevent both obstruction of the lumen when the t. is compressed and kinking when the t. is bent at a sharp angle.
Toynbee's t., a t. by which an otologist can listen to the sounds in a patient's ear during politzerization.
tracheal t., endotracheal t.
tracheotomy t., a curved t. used to keep the opening free after tracheotomy.
tympanostomy t., a small t. inserted through the tympanic membrane after myringotomy to aerate the middle ear; often used for serous otitis media.
uterine t., *tuba* uterina.
vacuum t., a glass t. from which the air has been nearly removed, containing two or more electrodes, used in the experimental passage of an electrical current or spark, in the production of x-rays, and to control circuits. Previously in wide use, the v.t. has been supplanted by transistors for some uses.
Venturi t., a t. with a specially streamlined constriction to minimize energy losses in the fluid flowing through it while maximizing the fall in pressure in the constriction in accordance with Bernoulli's law; the basis of the Venturi meter.
Wangensteen t., Wangensteen *suction.*
x-ray t., see x-ray.

---

tubectomy (tū-bek'tō-mē) [L. *tuba,* tube, + G. *ektomē,* excision]. Salpingectomy.

tuber, pl. **tubera** (tū'ber, tū'ber-ă) [L. protuberance, swelling]. **1.** A localized swelling; a knob. **2.** A short, fleshy, thick, underground stem of plants, such as the potato.
t. ante'rius, t. cinereum.
ashen t., t. cinereum.
calcaneal t., t. calcanei.
t. calca'nei [NA], calcaneal t. or tuberosity; t. calcis; the posterior extremity of the calcaneus, or os calcis, forming the projection of the heel.
t. cal'cis, t. calcanei.
t. cine'reum [NA], ashen or gray t.; t. anterius; a prominence of the base of the hypothalamus, bordered caudally by the mamillary bodies, rostrally by the optic chiasm, and laterally by the optic tract, extending ventrally into the infundibulum and hypophysial stalk.
t. coch'leae, *promontorium* cavi tympanum.
t. cor'poris callo'si, *splenium* corporis callosi.
t. dorsa'le, t. vermis.
eustachian t., a slight projection from the labyrinthine wall of the middle ear below the fenestra vestibuli (ovalis).
frontal t., t. frontale.
t. fronta'le [NA], eminentia frontalis; frontal t.; frontal eminence; the most prominent portion of the frontal bone on either side.

gray t., t. cinereum.
t. ischiad'icum [NA], t. of ischium; ischial tuberosity; the rough bony projection at the junction of the lower end of the body of the ischium and its ramus.
t. of ischium, t. ischiadicum.
t. maxil'lae [NA], maxillary tuberosity; eminentia maxillae; maxillary eminence; the bulging lower extremity of the posterior surface of the body of the maxilla, behind the root of the last molar tooth.
omental t., t. omentale.
t. omenta'le [NA], omental t.; **(1)** an eminence on the visceral surface of the left hepatic lobe to the left of the fossa for the ductus venosus; **(2)** a bulge on the anterior surface of the body of the pancreas to the left of the superior mesenteric vessels.
parietal t., t. parietale.
t. parieta'le [NA], parietal t.; parietal eminence; eminentia parietalis; a prominent portion of the parietal bone, a little above the center of its external surface, usually corresponding to the point of maximum width of the head.
t. ra'dii, *tuberositas* radii.
t. val'vulae, t. vermis.
t. ver'mis [NA], t. of the vermis; t. valvulae; t. dorsale; the posterior division of the inferior vermis of the cerebellum located between the folium and the pyramis.
t. zygomat'icum, a slight prominence near the origin of the zygomatic process of the temporal bone.

tubercle (tū'ber-kl) [L. *tuberculum,* dim. of *tuber,* a swelling]. **1.** Tuberculum. **2.** In dentistry, a small elevation arising on the surface of a tooth. **3.** A granulomatous lesion due to infection by *Mycobacterium tuberculosis.* Although somewhat variable in size (0.5 to 2 or 3 mm in diameter) and in the proportions of various histologic components, t.'s tend to be fairly well circumscribed, spheroidal, firm lesions that usually consist of three irregularly outlined but moderately distinct zones: 1) an inner focus of necrosis, coagulative at first, and then becoming caseous; 2) a middle zone that consists of a fairly dense accumulation of large mononuclear phagocytes (macrophages), frequently arranged somewhat radially (with reference to the necrotic material) resembling an epithelium, and hence termed epithelioid cells—multinucleated giant cells of Langhans type may also be present; 3) an outer zone of numerous lymphocytes, and a few monocytes and plasma cells. In instances where healing has begun, a fourth zone of fibrous tissue may form at the periphery. Morphologically indistinguishable lesions may occur in diseases caused by other agents; many observers use the term nonspecifically, *i.e.,* with reference to any such granuloma; others use "tubercle" only for tuberculous lesions, and then designate those of undetermined causes as epithelioid-cell granulomas.
accessory t., *processus* accessorius.
acoustic t., *trigone* of the auditory nerve.
adductor t., *tuberculum* adductorium.
amygdaloid t., a projection from the roof of the anterior end-portion of the temporal horn of the lateral ventricle, marking the location of the amygdaloid nucleus.
anatomical t., postmortem *wart.*
anterior t. of atlas, *tuberculum* anterius atlantis.
anterior t. of cervical vertebrae, tuberculum anterius vertebrarum cervicalium; the anterior projection from the transverse process.
t. of anterior scalene muscle, *tuberculum* musculi scaleni anterioris.
anterior t. of thalamus, *tuberculum* anterius thalami.
articular t., *tuberculum* articulare.
ashen t., *tuberculum* cinereum.
auricular t., *tuberculum* auriculae.
calcaneal t., *tuberculum* calcanei.
Carabelli t., a small t., resembling a supernumerary cusp, found

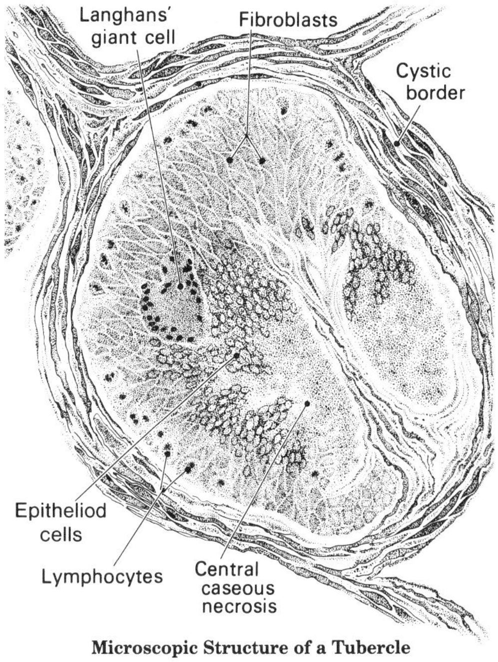

Microscopic Structure of a Tubercle

occasionally on the lingual surface of the mesiolingual cusp of a permanent maxillary first molar.
carotid t., *tuberculum* caroticum.
caseous t., soft t.
Chassaignac's t., *tuberculum* caroticum.
conoid t., *tuberculum* conoideum.
corniculate t., *tuberculum* corniculatum.
crown t., *tuberculum* dentis.
t. of cuneate nucleus, *tuberculum* nuclei cuneati.
cuneiform t., *tuberculum* cuneiforme.
darwinian t., *tuberculum* auriculae.
dental t., *tuberculum* dentis.
dissection t., postmortem *wart.*
dorsal t., *tuberculum* dorsale.
epiglottic t., *tuberculum* epiglotticum.
fibrous t., a t. in which fibroblasts proliferate about the periphery (and into the cellular zones), eventually resulting in a rim or wall of cellular fibrous tissue or collagenous material around the t.
genial t., *spina* mentalis.
genital t., phallic t.; the median elevation just cephalic to the urogenital orifice of an embryo; it is the primordium of the penis of the male or the clitoris of the female.
Gerdy's t., a t. on the lateral side of the upper end of the tibia giving attachment to the tractus iliotibialis and some fibers of the tibialis anterior muscle.
Ghon's t., Ghon's focus or primary lesion; the pulmonary lesion of primary tuberculosis.
gracile t., *tuberculum* nuclei gracilis.
gray t., *tuberculum* cinereum.
greater t. of humerus, *tuberculum* majus humeri.
hard t., a t. lacking necrosis.
hyaline t., a form of fibrous t. in which the cellular fibrous tissue and collagenous fibers become altered and merged into a fairly homogeneous, acellular, deeply acidophilic, firm mass.
iliac t., *tuberculum* iliacum.
t. of iliac crest, *tuberculum* iliacum.
inferior thyroid t., *tuberculum* thyroideum inferius.

infraglenoid t., *tuberculum* infraglenoidale.
intercondylar t., *tuberculum* intercondylare.
intervenous t., *tuberculum* intervenosum.
jugular t., *tuberculum* jugulare.
labial t., *tuberculum* labii superioris.
lateral t. of posterior process of talus, *tuberculum* laterale processus posterioris tali.
lesser t. of humerus, *tuberculum* minus humeri.
Lisfranc's t., *tuberculum* musculi scaleni anterioris.
Lister's t., *tuberculum* dorsale.
Lower's t., *tuberculum* intervenosum.
mamillary t., *processus* mamillaris.
mamillary t. of hypothalamus, *corpus* mamillare.
marginal t., *tuberculum* marginale ossis zygomatici.
medial t. of posterior process of talus, *tuberculum* mediale processus posterioris tali.
mental t., *tuberculum* mentale.
Montgomery's t.'s, elevated reddened areolar glands, usually associated with pregnancy.
Morgagni's t., *cartilago* cuneiformis.
Müller's t., sinus t.; a median protuberance projecting into the embryonic urogenital sinus from its dorsal wall; it is formed from the fused caudal ends of the paramesonephric ducts, and is the first evidence of the embryonic uterus and vagina.
nuchal t., *vertebra* prominens.
t. of nucleus gracilis, *tuberculum* nuclei gracilis.
obturator t., *tuberculum* obturatorium.
olfactory t., *tuberculum* olfactorium.
orbital t., orbital eminence; eminentia orbitalis; Whitnall's t.; a small elevation on the orbital surface of the zygomatic bone, just within the orbital margin, about 1 cm below the zygomaticofrontal suture; it gives attachment to the lateral check ligament, the lateral palpebral ligament, and the suspensory ligament of the eyeball.
phallic t., genital t.
pharyngeal t., *tuberculum* pharyngeum.
posterior t. of atlas, *tuberculum* posterius atlantis.
posterior t. of cervical vertebrae, tuberculum posterius vertebrarum cervicalium; a posterior projection from the transverse processes.
postmortem t., postmortem *wart.*
Princeteau's t., a slight prominence on the temporal bone near the apex of the petrous part where the superior petrosal sinus commences.
prosector's t., postmortem *wart.*
pterygoid t., a slight prominence on the posterior surface of the lamina medialis of the sphenoid bone, inferior and to the medial side of the pterygoid canal.
pubic t., *tuberculum* pubicum.
t. of rib, *tuberculum* costae.
Rolando's t., *tuberculum* cinereum.
t. of saddle, *tuberculum* sellae.
Santorini's t., *tuberculum* corniculatum.
scalene t. of Lisfranc, *tuberculum* musculi scaleni anterioris.
t. of scaphoid bone, *tuberculum* ossis scaphoidei.
sebaceous t., milium.
sinus t., Müller's t.
soft t., caseous t.; a t. showing caseous necrosis.
superior thyroid t., *tuberculum* thyroideum superius.
supraglenoid t., *tuberculum* supraglenoidale.
supratragic t., *tuberculum* supratragicum.
t. of tooth, *tuberculum* dentis.
t. of trapezium, *tuberculum* ossis trapezii.
t. of upper lip, *tuberculum* labii superioris.
wedge-shaped t., *tuberculum* nuclei cuneati.
Whitnall's t., orbital t.
Wrisberg's t., *tuberculum* cuneiforme.

tubercul-. See tuberculo-.

tubercula (tū-ber'kyū-lă). Plural of tuberculum.

tubercular, tuberculate, tuberculated (tū-ber'kyū-lăr, -lāt, -lāt-ed). Pertaining to or characterized by tubercles or small nodules. *Cf.* tuberculous.

tuberculation (tū-ber-kyū-lā'shŭn). **1.** Tuberculization; the formation of tubercles or nodules. **2.** The arrangement of tubercles or nodules in a part.

tuberculid (tū-ber'kyū-lid) [tubercul- + G. *-id* (1)]. A lesion of the skin or mucous membrane resulting from an immunologic response to a previous infection with tubercle bacilli at a remote site, resulting from specific sensitization to the organism.
nodular t., *erythema* induratum.
papular t., papular scrofuloderma; lichen scrofulosorum; an allergic manifestation of tuberculous infection in the body, consisting of small to medium-sized papules which have tuberculoid architecture but do not contain the bacteria.
papulonecrotic t., acne scrofulosorum; tuberculosis papulonecrotica; tuberculosis cutis follicularis disseminata; dusky-red papules followed by crusting and ulceration primarily on the extremities and predominantly in young adults with a deep focus of tuberculosis or with a history of preceding infection.
rosacea-like t., acne telangiectodes; a facial t. consisting of small papules or nodules which appear yellowish brown on diascopic pressure, with dermal tubercles not related to hair follicles.

tuberculin (tū-ber'kyū-lin). **1.** A glycerin-broth culture of *Mycobacterium tuberculosis* evaporated to $^{1}/_{10}$ volume at 100°C and filtered; introduced by Robert Koch for the treatment of tuberculosis but now used chiefly for diagnostic tests; originally known as Koch's old t. (OT) or Koch's original t. **2.** One or another of a relatively large number of extracts of *Mycobacterium tuberculosis* cultures, different from OT and now obsolete.
Koch's old t. (OT), Koch's original t., see t. (1).
purified protein derivative of t. (PPD), purified t. containing the active protein fraction; the t. from which it is prepared differs from t. (1) chiefly in that the bacteria are grown in a synthetic rather than in a broth medium.

tuberculitis (tū-ber-kyū-lī'tis) [tubercul- + G. *-itis,* inflammation]. Inflammation of any tubercle.

tuberculization (tū-ber'kyū-li-zā'shŭn). Tuberculation (1).

tuberculo-, tubercul- [L. *tuberculum,* tubercle]. Combining forms denoting a tubercle, tuberculosis.

tuberculocele (tū-ber'kyū-lō-sēl) [tuberculo- + G. *kēlē,* tumor, hernia]. Tuberculosis of the testes.

tuberculochemotherapeutic (tū-ber'kyū-lō-kē'mō-ther-ă-pyū'tik). Relating to the treatment of tuberculosis by tuberculostatic or tuberculocidal drugs.

tuberculocidal (tū-ber'kyū-lō-sī'dăl). Destructive to the tubercle bacillus.

tuberculoderma (tū-ber'kyū-lō-der'mă). **1.** Any tubercular process of the skin. **2.** The cutaneous manifestation of tuberculosis.

tuberculofibroid (tū-ber'kyū-lō-fī'broyd). A discrete, well circumscribed, usually spheroidal, moderately to extremely firm, encapsulated nodule that is formed during the process of healing in a focus of tuberculous granulomatous inflammation.

tuberculoid (tū-ber'kyū-loyd) [tuberculo- + G. *eidos,* resemblance]. Resembling tuberculosis, or a tubercle.

tuberculoma (tū-ber-kyū-lō'mă) [tuberculo- + G. *-oma,* tumor]. A rounded tumorlike but non-neoplastic mass, usually in the lungs or brain, due to localized tuberculous infection.

tuberculoprotein (tū-ber'kyū-lō-prō'tēn). Any one, or a mixture of any or all of the proteins present in the body of the tubercle bacillus, all of which have been found to possess certain properties of tuberculin.

tuberculosis (tū-ber-kyū-lō'sis) [tuberculo- + G. *-osis,* condition]. A specific disease caused by the presence of *Mycobacterium tuberculosis* which may affect almost any tissue or organ of the body, the most common seat of the disease being the lungs; the anatomical lesion is the tubercle, which can undergo caseation necrosis; local symptoms vary according to the part affected; general symptoms are those of sepsis: hectic fever, sweats, and emaciation.
acute t., acute miliary t., disseminated t.; a rapidly fatal disease due to the general dissemination of tubercle bacilli in the blood, resulting in the formation of miliary tubercles in various organs and tissues, and producing symptoms of profound toxemia.
adult t., secondary t.
anthracotic t., pneumoconiosis.
arrested t., healed t.
attenuated t., a mild chronic form marked by caseous tubercles of the skin and the occurrence of cold abscesses.
basal t., t. of the basilar portions of the lungs.
cerebral t., **(1)** tuberculous *meningitis;* **(2)** cerebral tuberculoma.
childhood type t., primary t.
cutaneous t., scrofuloderma; t. cutis; dermal t.; pathologic lesions of the skin caused by *Mycobacterium tuberculosis.*
t. cu'tis, cutaneous t.
t. cu'tis follicula'ris dissemina'ta, papulonecrotic *tuberculid.*
t. cu'tis lupo'sa, *lupus* vulgaris.
t. cu'tis orificia'lis, t. ulcerosa; any tuberculous lesion in or about the mouth or anus.
t. cu'tis verruco'sa, lupus verrucosus or papillomatosus; tuberculous wart; verrucous scrofuloderma; a tuberculous skin lesion having a warty surface with a chronic inflammatory base. See also postmortem *wart.*
dermal t., cutaneous t.
disseminated t., acute miliary t.
enteric t., a complication of cavitary pulmonary t. resulting from expectoration and swallowing of bacilli which then infect areas of the digestive tract where there is relative stasis or abundant lymphoid tissue. See also tuberculous *enteritis.*
general t., miliary t.
healed t., arrested or inactive t.; a scar or a calcified, fibrous, or caseous nodule in the lung pleura, lymph node, or other organ, resulting from previous t. that has regressed; reactivation is possible.
inactive t., healed t.
miliary t., general t.; a general dissemination of tubercle bacilli with the production of countless minute discrete tubercles in various organs and tissues; evident in the lung as numerous tiny densities on the radiograph.
open t., pulmonary t., tuberculous ulceration, or other form in which the tubercle bacilli are present in the excretions or secretions; in the lung, usually the result of cavity formation.
t. papulonecrot'ica, papulonecrotic *tuberculid.*
postprimary t., secondary t.
primary t., childhood type t.; first infection by *Mycobacterium tuberculosis,* typically seen in children but also occurs in adults, characterized in the lungs by the formation of a primary complex consisting of small peripheral pulmonary focus and hilar or paratracheal lymph node involvement; may cavitate or heal with scarring or may progress.
pulmonary t., t. of the lungs.
reinfection t., secondary t.
secondary t., adult, postprimary, or reinfection t.; t. found in adults and characterized by lesions near the apex of an upper lobe, which may cavitate or heal with scarring, without spreading to lymph nodes; theoretically, secondary t. may be due to exogenous reinfection or to reactivation of a dormant endogenous infection.
t. ulcero'sa, t. cutis orificialis.

tuberculostat (tū-ber'kyū-lō-stat). A tuberculostatic agent.

tuberculostatic (tū-ber'kyū-lō-stat'ik) [tuberculo- + G. *statikos,* causing to stand]. Relating to an agent that inhibits the growth of tubercle bacilli.

tuberculous (tū-ber'kyū-lŭs). Relating to or affected by tuberculosis. *Cf.* tubercular.

TUBERCULUM

tuberculum, pl. **tubercula** (tū-ber'kyū-lŭm, -lă) [L. dim. of *tuber,* a knob, swelling, tumor] [NA]. Tubercle (1). **1.** A nodule, especially in an anatomical, not pathologic, sense. **2.** A circumscribed, rounded, solid elevation on the skin, mucous membrane, or surface of an organ. **3.** A slight elevation from the surface of a bone giving attachment to a muscle or ligament.
t. adducto'rium [NA], adductor tubercle; the prominence above the medial epicondyle of the femur to which the tendon of the adductor magnus attaches.
t. ante'rius atlan'tis [NA], anterior tubercle of atlas; a conical protuberance on the anterior surface of the arch of the atlas.
t. ante'rius thal'ami [NA], anterior tubercle of the thalamus; a prominence at the anterior extremity of the thalamus which corresponds to the nuclei anteriores.
t. ante'rius vertebra'rum cervica'lium, anterior *tubercle* of cervical vertebrae.
t. arthrit'icum, **(1)** Heberden's *nodes;* **(2)** any gouty concretion in or around a joint.
t. articula're [NA], articular tubercle or eminence; eminentia articularis; articular eminence of the temporal bone which bounds the mandibular fossa anteriorly; it forms the anterior root of the zygomatic process.
t. auric'ulae [NA], auricular tubercle; darwinian tubercle; t. superius; a small projection from the upper end of the posterior portion of the incurved free margin of the helix.
t. calca'nei [NA], calcaneal tubercle; the projection, often double, on the inferior aspect of the calcaneus at the anterior end of the area for attachment of the long plantar ligament.
t. carot'icum [NA], carotid tubercle; Chassaignac's tubercle; the anterior tubercle of the transverse process of the sixth cervical vertebra, against which the carotid artery may be compressed by the finger.
t. cine'reum, ashen or gray tubercle; Rolando's tubercle; a longitudinal prominence on the dorsolateral surface of the medulla oblongata along the lateral border of the tuberculum cuneatum; it is the surface profile of the tractus spinalis nervi trigemini, continuous caudally with the fasciculus dorsolateralis (Lissauer's tract).
t. conoi'deum [NA], conoid tubercle; the prominence near the lateral end of the inferior surface of the clavicle that gives attachment to the conoid ligament.
t. cornicula'tum [NA], corniculate tubercle; Santorini's tubercle; a rounded eminence on the posterior part of the aryepiglottic fold, formed by the underlying corniculate cartilages.
t. coro'nae, t. dentis.
t. cos'tae [NA], tubercle of rib; the knob on a rib, near its head, which articulates with the transverse process of a vertebra.
t. cuneifor'me [NA], cuneiform tubercle; Wrisberg's tubercle; a rounded eminence on the posterior part of the aryepiglottic fold, formed by the underlying cuneiform cartilage.
t. den'tis [NA], tubercle of tooth; t. coronae; crown or dental tubercle; a small elevation on some portions of a crown produced by an extra formation of enamel.
tuber'cula doloro'sa, obsolete term for multiple cutaneous myomas or neuromas which are painful on pressure.
t. dorsa'le [NA], dorsal tubercle; Lister's tubercle; a small prominence on the dorsal aspect of the distal end of the radius lateral to

the groove for the extensor pollicis longus tendon.
t. epiglot'ticum [NA], epiglottic tubercle; cushion of epiglottis; a convexity at the lower part of the epiglottis over the upper part of the thyroepiglottic ligament.
t. hypoglos'si, *trigonum* nervi hypoglossi.
t. ili'acum [NA], iliac tubercle; tubercle of iliac crest; a prominence on the outer lip of the iliac crest about 5 cm behind the anterior superior iliac spine.
t. im'par, median tongue bud; a small median protuberance on the floor of the oral cavity of the embryo, which plays a minor role in the development of the tongue.
t. infraglenoida'le [NA], infraglenoid tubercle or tuberosity; a rough surface below the glenoid cavity of the scapula, giving attachment to the long tendon of the triceps.
t. intercondyla're [NA], intercondylar tubercle; one of two projections, medial and lateral, springing from the central lip of each articular surface of the tibia on either side of the intercondylar eminence.
t. interveno'sum [NA], intervenous tubercle; Lower's tubercle; the slight projection on the wall of the right atrium between the orifices of the venae cavae.
t. jugula're [NA], jugular tubercle; an oval elevation on the cerebral surface of the lateral part of the occipital bone, on either side of the foramen magnum above the hypoglossal canal.
t. la'bii superio'ris [NA], tubercle of upper lip; labial tubercle; procheilon; the slight projection on the free edge of the center of the upper lip at the lower extent of the philtrum.
t. latera'le proces'sus posterio'ris ta'li [NA], lateral tubercle of posterior process of talus; the prominence lateral to the groove for the flexor hallucis longus tendon.
t. ma'jus hu'meri [NA], greater tubercle or tuberosity of humerus; the larger of the two tubercles next to the head of the humerus; it gives attachment to the supraspinatus, infraspinatus, and teres minor muscles.
t. mal'lei, *processus* lateralis mallei.
t. margina'le os'sis zygomat'ici [NA], marginal tubercle; a prominence on the temporal border of the zygomatic bone to which the temporal fascia is attached.
t. media'le proces'sus posterio'ris ta'li [NA], medial tubercle of posterior process of talus; the eminence medial to the sulcus for the flexor hallucis longus tendon.
t. menta'le [NA], mental tubercle; eminentia symphysis; a paired eminence on the mental protuberance of the mandible.
t. mi'nus hu'meri [NA], lesser tubercle or tuberosity of humerus; the anterior of the two tubercles of the neck of the humerus on which the subscapularis is inserted.
t. mus'culi scale'ni anterio'ris [NA], tubercle of anterior scalene muscle; Lisfranc's tubercle; scalene tubercle of Lisfranc; a small spine on the inner edge of the first rib, giving attachment to the scalenus anterior muscle.
t. nu'clei cunea'ti [NA], tubercle of the cuneate nucleus; wedge-shaped tubercle; the bulbous rostral extremity of the fasciculus cuneatus corresponding to the position of the nucleus cuneatus, lying lateral to the clava and separated from the t. cinereum on its lateral side by the posterior lateral sulcus.
t. nu'clei gra'cilis [NA], tubercle of the nucleus gracilis; gracile tubercle; clava; the somewhat expanded upper end of the fasciculus gracilis, corresponding to the position of the nucleus gracilis.
t. obturato'rium [NA], obturator tubercle; one of two processes, anterior and posterior, on the margin of the pubic portion of the obturator foramen, bounding the termination of the obturator groove.
t. olfacto'rium, olfactory tubercle; a small, oval area at the base of the cerebral hemisphere, between the diverging medial and lateral olfactory striae, in the anteromedial part of the anterior perforated substance; it is formed by a small area of allocortex characterized by the presence of the islands of Calleja. Corresponding to a much more prominent structure in nonprimate mammals (especially rodents and insectivores), the olfactory tubercle receives fibers from the olfactory bulb by way of the stria olfactoria intermedia; it has efferent connections with the hypothalamus and the mediodorsal nucleus of the thalamus.
t. os'sis scaphoi'dei [NA], tubercle of scaphoid bone; a projection at the inferior lateral angle of the scaphoid (navicular) bone; it can be felt at the root of the thumb.
t. os'sis trape'zii [NA], tubercle of trapezium; oblique ridge of trapezium; a prominent ridge on the trapezium (os multangulum majus) forming the lateral border of the groove in which runs the tendon of the flexor carpi radialis.
t. pharyn'geum [NA], pharyngeal tubercle; a projection from the undersurface of the basilar portion of the occipital bone, giving attachment to the fibrous raphe of the pharynx.
t. poste'rius atlan'tis [NA], posterior tubercle of atlas; a protuberance of the posterior extremity of the arch of the atlas, a rudiment of the spinous process giving attachment to the musculus rectus capitis posterior minor.
t. poste'rius vertebra'rum cervica'lium, posterior *tubercle* of cervical vertebrae.
t. pu'bicum [NA], pubic tubercle; pubic spine; spina pubis; a small projection at the anterior extremity of the crest of the pubis about 2 cm from the symphysis.
t. seba'ceum, milium.
t. sel'lae [NA], tubercle of saddle; the slight elevation in front of the pituitary fossa on the body of the sphenoid bone.
t. sep'ti na'rium, a flat elevation on the septum in each naris opposite the anterior end of the middle concha; it is due to an aggregation of glands.
t. supe'rius, t. auriculae.
t. supraglenoida'le [NA], supraglenoid tubercle; a rough surface above the glenoid cavity of the scapula, giving attachment to the tendon of the long head of the biceps.
t. supratra'gicum [NA], supratragic tubercle; a small elevation often present on the edge of the upper tragus.
t. syphilit'icum, gumma of the skin.
t. thyroi'deum infe'rius [NA], inferior thyroid tubercle; a slight lateral projection from the lower margin of the lamina of the thyroid cartilage on either side, at the inferior end of the oblique line.
t. thyroi'deum supe'rius [NA], superior thyroid tubercle; a blunt projection on the lamina of the thyroid cartilage on either side at the superior end of the oblique line.

tuberiferous (tū-ber-if'er-ŭs) [tuber + L. *ferro,* to bear]. Tuberous.
tuberose (tū'ber-ōs). Tuberous.
tuberositas (tū'ber-os'i-tas) [LL., fr. L., *tuberosus,* full of lumps, fr. *tuber,* a knob]. Tuberosity; a large tubercle or rounded elevation, especially from the surface of a bone.
t. coracoi'dea, replaced by the NA terms *tuberculum* conoideum and *linea* trapezoidea.
t. costa'lis, *impressio* ligamenti costoclavicularis.
t. deltoi'dea [NA], deltoid tuberosity; deltoid eminence; deltoid crest or impression; a rough elevation about the middle of the lateral side of the shaft of the humerus, giving attachment to the deltoid muscle.
t. glu'tea [NA], gluteal tuberosity (1); crista glutea; gluteal crest or ridge; the point of insertion in the upper portion of the shaft of the femur of the greater part of the gluteus maximus muscle; when markedly developed this tuberosity is called the third trochanter.
t. ili'aca [NA], iliac tuberosity; a rough area above the auricular surface on the medial aspect of the ala of the ilium, giving attachment to the posterior sacroiliac ligament.
t. masseter'ica [NA], masseteric tuberosity; a roughened surface on the external aspect of the angle of the mandible, giving attachment to fibers of the masseter muscle.

t. mus'culi serra'ti anterio'ris [NA], a rough oval area, about the middle of the outer surface and lower border of the second rib, for the attachment of the serratus anterior muscle.
t. os'sis cuboi'dei [NA], tuberosity of cuboid bone; a slight eminence on the lateral surface of the cuboid bone, capped with an articular facet for a sesamoid bone in the tendon of the peroneus longus muscle.
t. os'sis metatarsa'lis pri'mi [NA], tuberosity of first metatarsal; a tubercle at the base of the bone to which is attached the tendon of the peroneus longus muscle.
t. os'sis metatarsa'lis quin'ti [NA], tuberosity of fifth metatarsal; a tubercle at the base of this bone to the posterior part of which is attached the tendon of the peroneus brevis muscle.
t. os'sis navicula'ris [NA], tuberosity of navicular bone; scaphoid tuberosity; a rounded eminence on the medial surface of the navicular bone, giving attachment to a part of the tendon of the tibialis posterior muscle.
t. phalan'gis dista'lis [NA], ungual tuberosity; t. unguicularis; a roughened raised surface of horseshoe shape on the palmar surface of the distal end of the terminal or ungual phalanx of each finger and toe, which serves to support the pulp of the digit.
t. pterygoi'dea [NA], pterygoid tuberosity; a roughened area on the internal aspect of the mandible, giving attachment to fibers of the medial pterygoid muscle.
t. ra'dii [NA], tuberosity of radius; bicipital tuberosity; tuber radii; an oval projection from the medial surface of the radius just distal to the neck, giving attachment on its posterior half to the tendon of the biceps.
t. sacra'lis [NA], sacral tuberosity; a rough prominence on the lateral surface of the sacrum posterior to the auricular surface for attachment of posterior sacroiliac ligaments.
t. tib'iae [NA], tibial tuberosity; an oval elevation on the anterior surface of the tibia about 3 cm distal to the articular surface, giving attachment at its distal part to the ligamentum patellae.
t. ul'nae [NA], tuberosity of ulna; a prominence at the lower border of the anterior surface of the coronoid process, giving attachment to the brachialis muscle.
t. unguicula'ris, t. phalangis distalis.

tuberosity (tū'ber-os'i-tē). Tuberositas.
bicipital t., *tuberositas* radii.
calcaneal t., *tuber* calcanei.
coracoid t., see *linea* trapezoidea; *tuberculum* conoideum.
costal t., *impressio* ligamenti costoclavicularis.
t. of cuboid bone, *tuberositas* ossis cuboidei.
deltoid t., *tuberositas* deltoidae.
t. of fifth metatarsal, *tuberositas* ossis metatarsalis quinti.
t. of first metatarsal, *tuberositas* ossis metatarsalis primi.
gluteal t., **(1)** *tuberositas* glutea; **(2)** *trochanter* tertius.
greater t. of humerus, *tuberculum* majus humeri.
iliac t., *tuberositas* iliaca.
infraglenoid t., *tuberculum* infraglenoidale.
ischial t., *tuber* ischiadicum.
lateral femoral t., *epicondylus* lateralis ossis femoris.
lesser t. of humerus, *tuberculum* minus humeri.
masseteric t., *tuberositas* masseterica.
maxillary t., *tuber* maxillae.
medial femoral t., *epicondylus* medialis ossis femoris.
t. of navicular bone, *tuberositas* ossis navicularis.
pterygoid t., *tuberositas* pterygoidea.
t. of radius, *tuberositas* radii.
sacral t., *tuberositas* sacralis.
scaphoid t., *tuberositas* ossis navicularis.
tibial t., *tuberositas* tibiae.
t. of ulna, *tuberositas* ulnae.
ungual t., *tuberositas* phalangis distalis.

tuberous (tū'ber-ŭs) [L. *tuberosus*]. Tuberiferous; tuberose; knobby, lumpy, or nodular; presenting many tubers or tuberosities.

tubo- [L. *tubus, tuba,* tube]. Combining form denoting tubular, a tube. See also salpingo-.

tuboabdominal (tū'bō-ab-dom'i-năl). Relating to a uterine (fallopian) tube and the abdomen.

tubocurarine chloride (tū'bō-kūr-ar'ēn). *d*-Tubocurarine chloride; $C_{38}H_{44}Cl_2N_2O_6 \cdot 5H_2O$; an alkaloid (obtained from the stems of *Chondodendron,* particularly *C. tomentosum*) that raises the threshold for acetylcholine at the myoneural junction by occupying the receptors competitively, and that also blocks ganglionic transmission and releases histamine; used to produce muscular relaxation during surgical operations.

tuboligamentous (tū'bō-lig-ă-men'tŭs). Relating to the uterine (fallopian) tube and the broad ligament of the uterus.

tubo-ovarian (tū'bō-ō-vā'rē-an). Relating to the uterine (fallopian) tube and the ovary.

tubo-ovariectomy (tū'bō-ō-var-ē-ek'to-mĭ). Salpingo-oophorectomy.

tubo-ovaritis (tū'bō-ō-va-rī'tis). Salpingo-oophoritis.

tuboperitoneal (tū'bō-per-i-tō-nē'ăl). Relating to the uterine (fallopian) tubes and the peritoneum.

tuboplasty (tū'bō-plas-tē). Salpingoplasty.

tubotorsion (tū'bō-tōr-shŭn) [tubo- + L. *torsio,* torsion]. Tubatorsion; twisting of a tubular structure, such as a uterine tube.

tubotympanic, tubotympanal (tū'bō-tim-pan'ik, -tim'pă-năl). Relating to the auditory (eustachian) tube and the tympanic cavity of the ear.

tubouterine (tū'bō-ū'ter-in). Relating to a uterine (fallopian) tube and the uterus.

tubovaginal (tū-bō-vaj'i-năl). Relating to a uterine (fallopian) tube and the vagina.

tubular (tū'byū-lăr). Tubuliform; relating to or of the form of a tube or tubule.

tubulature (tu'byū-lă-chūr). The short neck of a retort.

tubule (tū'byūl) [L. *tubulus,* dim. of *tubus,* tube]. Tubulus.
Albarran y Dominguez' t.'s, Albarran's *glands.*
collecting t., *tubulus* renalis rectus.
connecting t., a narrow arching t. of the kidney joining the distal convoluted t. and the collecting t.
convoluted t. of kidney, *tubulus* renalis contortus.
convoluted seminiferous t., *tubulus* seminiferus contortus.
dental t.'s, dentinal t.'s, *canaliculi* dentales.
discharging t., a urinary t. formed by the union of several collecting t.'s and terminating as a papillary duct.
Henle's t.'s, the straight portions of the uriniferous t.'s which form Henle's loop, distinguished as the descending and ascending t.'s of Henle.
Kobelt's t.'s, wolffian t.'s; remnants of the mesonephric t.'s in the female, contained within the epoophoron.
malpighian t.'s, in insects, slender tubular or hairlike excretory structures that emerge from the alimentary canal between the mesenteron (midgut) and proctodeum (hindgut) in a region frequently termed the pylorus; they vary in number from 1 to over 100, and may be assorted in equally sized bundles in some insects.
mesonephric t., an excretory t. of the mesonephros.
metanephric t., an excretory unit of the metanephros or permanent kidney.
paragenital t.'s, remnants of embryonic mesonephric t.'s, some of which form the paradidymis.
pronephric t., an excretory unit of the pronephros, present only in vestigial form in human embryos.
seminiferous t., see *tubulus* seminiferus contortus; *tubulus* seminiferus rectus.

Skene's t.'s, the embryonic urethral glands which are the female homologue of the prostate.
spiral t., the segment of urinary t. coming next after the proximal convoluted t.
straight t., **(1)** *tubulus* renalis rectus; **(2)** *tubulus* seminiferus rectus.
T t., the transverse t. that passes from the sarcolemma across a myofibril of striated muscle; it is the intermediate t. of the triad.
uriniferous t., the functional unit of the kidney, composed of a long convoluted portion (nephron) and an intrarenal collecting duct.
wolffian t.'s, Kobelt's t.'s.

tubuli (tū'byū-lī). Plural of tubulus.

tubuliform (tū'byū-li-fōrm). Tubular.

tubulin (tū'byū-lin). A protein subunit of microtubules which is a dimer composed of two globular polypeptides, α-tubulin and β-tubulin. See also dynein.

tubulization (tū'byū-li-zā'shŭn). Enclosing the joined ends of a divided nerve, after neurorrhaphy, in a cylinder of paraffin or of some slowly absorbable material to keep the surrounding tissues from pushing in and preventing union.

tubulocyst (tū'byū-lō-sist). Tubular cyst; a cyst formed by the dilation of any occluded canal or tube.

tubulodermoid (tū'byū-lō-der'moyd). A dermoid cyst arising from a persistent embryonal tubular structure.

tubuloracemose (tū'byū-lō-ras'ĕ-mōs). Denoting a gland of combined tubular and racemose structure.

tubulorrhexis (tū'byū-lō-rek'sis) [tubule + G. *rhēxis,* a breaking]. A pathologic process characterized by necrosis of the epithelial lining in localized segments of renal tubules, with focal rupture or loss of the basement membrane.

tubulose, tubulous (tū'byū-lōs, -lŭs). Having many tubules.

tubulus, pl. **tubuli** (tū'byū-lŭs, -lī) [L. dim. of *tubus,* a pipe]. Tubule; a small tube.
tu'buli bilif'eri, *ductuli* biliferi.
t. contor'tus, **(1)** t. renalis contortus; **(2)** t. seminiferus contortus.
tu'buli denta'les, *canaliculi* dentales.
tu'buli epooph'ori, *ductuli* transversi epoophori.
tu'buli galactoph'ori, *ductus* lactiferi.
tu'buli lactif'eri, *ductus* lactiferi.
tu'buli parooph'ori, *ductuli* paroophori.
t. rec'tus, **(1)** t. renalis rectus; **(2)** t. seminiferus rectus.
t. rena'lis contor'tus [NA], convoluted tubule of kidney; t. contortus (1); Ferrein's tube; the highly convoluted segments of the nephron in the renal labyrinth comprising the proximal convoluted tubule, which leads from Bowman's capsule to the descending limb of Henle's loop, and the distal convoluted tubule, which leads from the ascending limb of Henle's loop to the collecting tube.
t. rena'lis rec'tus [NA], collecting tubule; straight tubule (1); t. rectus (1); one of the straight tubules of the kidney, present in the medulla and pars radiata of the cortex.
t. seminif'erus contor'tus [NA], convoluted seminiferous tubule; t. contortus (2); one of two or three twisted curved tubules in each lobule of the testis, in which spermatogenesis occurs.
t. seminif'erus rec'tus [NA], straight seminiferous tubule; straight tubule (2); t. rectus (2); the t. seminiferus contortus which becomes straight just before entering the mediastinum to form the rete testis.

tubus, pl. **tubi** (tū'bŭs, -bī) [L.]. A tube or canal.
t. digesto'rius, digestive *tract.*
t. medulla'ris, *canalis* centralis.
t. vertebra'lis, *canalis* vertebralis.

Tucker, Ervin Alden, U.S. obstetrician, 1862–1902. See T.-McLean *forceps.*

Tuffier, Marin Théodore, French surgeon, 1857–1929. See T.'s *test.*

tuft (tŭft). A cluster, clump, or bunch, as of hairs.
enamel t., a group of structures representing defects in tooth mineralization that extend from the dentino-enamel junction into the enamel to about one-half its thickness.
malpighian t., glomerulus (2).
synovial t.'s, *villi* synoviales.

tug, tugging (tŭg, tŭg'ing). A pulling or dragging movement or sensation.
tracheal t., **(1)** a downward pull of the trachea, manifested by a downward movement of the thyroid cartilage, synchronous with the action of the heart and symptomatic of aneurysm of the aortic arch; the sign is elicited most easily by drawing the cricoid cartilage upward with the thumb and forefinger while the patient sits with head thrown back and mouth closed; **(2)** a jerky type of inspiration seen when the intercostal muscles and the sternocostal parts of the diaphragm are paralyzed by deep general anesthesia or muscle relaxants; due to the unopposed action of the crura pulling on the dome of the diaphragm and thence on the pericardium, lung roots, and tracheobronchial tree during each inspiration.

tularemia (tū-lă-rē'mē-ă) [*Tulare,* Lake and County, CA, + G. *haima,* blood]. Deer-fly disease or fever; rabbit fever; Pahvant Valley plague or fever; a disease caused by *Francisella tularensis* and transmitted to man from rodents through the bite of a deer fly, *Chrysops discalis,* and other bloodsucking insects; can also be acquired directly through the bite of an infected animal or through handling of an infected animal carcass; symptoms, similar to those of undulant fever and plague, consist of a prolonged intermittent or remittent fever and often swelling and suppuration of the lymph nodes draining the site of infection; rabbits are an important reservoir host.

tulle gras (tūl-gră') [Fr. oily net]. A dressing for wounds, used chiefly in France, comprised of wide-mesh curtain net cut into squares and impregnated with soft paraffin (98 parts), balsam of Peru (1 part), and olive oil (1 part).

Tulp (Tulpius), Nicholas (Nicolaus), Dutch anatomist, 1593–1674. See T.'s *valve.*

tumefacient (tū-mĕ-fā'shent) [L. *tume-facio,* to cause to swell, fr. *tumeo,* to swell]. Causing or tending to cause swelling.

tumefaction (tū-mĕ-fak'shŭn) [see tumefacient]. **1.** Tumentia; a swelling. **2.** Tumescence.

tumefy (tū'mĕ-fī). To swell or to cause to swell.

tumentia (tū-men'shē-ă) [L. fr. *tumeo,* to swell]. Tumefaction (1).

tumescence (tū-mes'ens) [L. *tumesco,* to begin to swell]. Tumefaction (2); turgescence; the condition of being or becoming tumid.

tumescent (tū-mes'ent). Turgescent; denoting tumescence.

tumid (tū'mid) [L. *tumidus*] Turgid; swollen, as by congestion, edema, hyperemia.

TUMOR

tumor (tū'mŏr) [L. *tumor,* a swelling]. **1.** Any swelling or tumefaction. **2.** Neoplasm. **3.** One of the four signs of inflammation (t., calor, dolor, rubor) enunciated by Celsus.
acinar cell t., a solid and cystic t. of the pancreas, occurring in young women; t. cells contain zymogen granules.
acute splenic t., acute splenitis, enlargement, and softening of the spleen, usually due to bacteremia or severe bacterial toxemia.
adenoid t., adenoma, or neoplasm with glandlike spaces.
adenomatoid t., adenofibromyoma; adenoleiomyofibroma; angi-

omatoid t.; Recklinghausen's t.; benign mesothelioma of genital tract; a small benign t. of the male epididymis and female genital tract, consisting of fibrous tissue or smooth muscle enclosing anastomosing glandlike spaces containing acid mucopolysaccharide lined by flattened cells that have ultra-structural characteristics of mesothelial cells.
adenomatoid odontogenic t., adenoameloblastoma; ameloblastic adenomatoid t.; a benign epithelial odontogenic t. appearing radiographically as a well-circumscribed radiolucent-radiopaque lesion usually surrounding the crown of an impacted tooth in an adolescent or young adult; characterized histologically by columnar cells organized in a duct-like configuration interspersed with spindle-shaped cells and calcification; inductive change in the connective tissue varies.
adipose t., lipoma.
ameloblastic adenomatoid t., adenomatoid odontogenic t.
amyloid t., nodular *amyloidosis.*
angiomatoid t., adenomatoid t.
aortic body t., chemodectoma.
Bednar t., pigmented *dermatofibrosarcoma protuberans.*
benign t., innocent t.; a t. that does not form metastases and does not invade and destroy adjacent normal tissue.
blood t., term sometimes used to denote an aneurysm, hemorrhagic cyst, or hematoma.
Brenner t., a relatively infrequent benign neoplasm of the ovary, consisting chiefly of fibrous tissue that contains nests of cells resembling transitional type epithelium, as well as glandlike structures that contain mucin; origin is controversial, but it may arise from Walthard's cell rest; ordinarily found incidentally in ovaries removed for other reasons, especially in postmenopausal women.
Brooke's t., trichoepithelioma.
brown t., a mass of fibrous tissue containing hemosiderin-pigmented macrophages and multinucleated giant cells, replacing and expanding part of a bone in primary hyperparathyroidism.
Buschke-Löwenstein t., giant *condyloma.*
calcifying epithelial odontogenic t., Pindborg t.; a benign epithelial odontogenic neoplasm derived from the stratum intermedium of the enamel organ; a painless, slowly growing, mixed radiolucent-radiopaque lesion characterized histologically by cords of polyhedral epithelial cells, deposits of amyloid, and spherical calcifications.
carcinoid t., argentaffinoma; a usually small, slow-growing neoplasm composed of islands of rounded, oxyphilic, or spindle-shaped cells of medium size, with moderately small vesicular nuclei, and covered by intact mucosa with a yellow cut surface; neoplastic cells are frequently palisaded at the periphery of the small groups, and the latter have a tendency to infiltrate surrounding tissue. Such neoplasms occur anywhere in the gastrointestinal tract (and in the lungs and other sites), with approximately 90% in the appendix and the remainder chiefly in the ileum, but also in the stomach, other parts of the small intestine, the colon, and the rectum; those of the appendix and small t.'s seldom metastasize, but reported incidences of metatases from other primary sites and from t.'s exceeding 2.0 cm in diameter vary from 25 to 75%; lymph nodes in the abdomen and the liver may be conspicuously involved, but metastases above the diaphragm are rare. See also carcinoid *syndrome.*
carotid body t., chemodectoma.
cellular t., a t. composed mainly of closely packed cells.
cerebellopontine angle t., acoustic *neurinoma.*
chemoreceptor t., chemodectoma.
chromaffin t., chromaffinoma.
Codman's t., chondroblastoma of the proximal humerus.
collision t., two originally separate t.'s, especially a carcinoma and a sarcoma, that appear to have developed by chance in close proximity, so that an area of mingling exists. See also carcinosarcoma.
connective t., any t. of the connective tissue group, such as osteoma, fibroma, sarcoma.
dermal duct t., a benign small eccrine tumor occurring often on the head and neck.
dermoid t., dermoid *cyst.*
desmoid t., desmoid (2).
eighth nerve t., acoustic *neurinoma.*
embryonal t., embryonic t., embryoma; a neoplasm, usually malignant, which arises during intrauterine or early postnatal development from an organ rudiment or immature tissue; it forms immature structures characteristic of the part from which it arises, and may form other tissues as well. The term includes neuroblastoma and Wilms' t., and is also used to include certain neoplasms presenting in later life, this usage being based on the belief that such tumors arise from embryonic rests. See also teratoma.
embryonal t. of ciliary body, embryonal *medulloepithelioma.*
endodermal sinus t., yolk sac t.; a malignant neoplasm occurring in the gonads, in sacrococcygeal teratomas, and in the mediastinum; produces α-fetoprotein and is thought to be derived from primitive endodermal cells.
endometrioid t., a t. of the ovary containing epithelial or stromal elements resembling t.'s of the endometrium.
Erdheim t., craniopharyngioma.
Ewing's t., Ewing's sarcoma; endothelial myeloma; a malignant neoplasm which occurs usually before the age of 20 years, about twice as frequently in males, and in about 75% of patients involves bones of the extremities, including the shoulder girdle, with a predilection for the metaphysis; histologically, there are conspicuous foci of necrosis in association with irregular masses of small, regular, rounded, or ovoid cells (2 to 3 times the diameter of erythrocytes), with very scanty cytoplasm.
fecal t., coproma.
fibroid t., old term for certain fibromas and leiomyomas.
giant cell t. of bone, giant cell myeloma; osteoclastoma; a soft, reddish brown, sometimes malignant, osteolytic t. composed of multinucleated giant cells and ovoid or spindle-shaped cells, occurring most frequently in an end of a long tubular bone of young adults.
giant cell t. of tendon sheath, localized nodular tenosynovitis; a nodule, possibly inflammatory in nature, arising commonly from the flexor sheath of the fingers and thumb; composed of fibrous tissue, lipid- and hemosiderin-containing macrophages, and multinucleated giant cells.
glomus t., angiomyoneuroma; angioneuromyoma; glomangioma; an unusual vascular neoplasm composed of specialized pericytes (sometimes termed glomus cells), usually in single encapsulated nodular masses which may be several millimeters in diameter and occur almost exclusively in the skin; it is exquisitely tender and may be so painful that patients voluntarily immobilize an extremity, sometimes leading to atrophy of muscles; multiple glomus t.'s occur, sometimes with autosomal dominant inheritance.
glomus jugulare t., chemodectoma.
Godwin t., benign lymphoepithelial *lesion.*
granular cell t., granular cell myoblastoma; a microscopically specific, benign t., often involving peripheral nerves in skin, mucosa, or connective tissue, derived from Schwann cells; the abundant cytoplasm contains lysosomal granules, the cells infiltrate between adjacent tissues although growth is slow, and adjacent surface epithelium may show hyperplasia.
granulosa cell t., folliculoma (1); a benign or malignant t. of the ovary arising from the membrana granulosa of the graafian follicle and frequently secreting estrogen; it is soft, solid, white or yellow, and consists of small round cells sometimes enclosing Call-Exner bodies; larger lipid-containing cells may be present.
Grawitz' t., old eponym for renal *adenocarcinoma.*
Gubler's t., a fusiform swelling on the wrist in lead palsy.
haarscheibe t. [Ger. *Haar,* hair, +*Scheibe,* disk], trichodiscoma;

hamartoma of the mesodermal portion of the hair disk.
heterologous t., a t. composed of a tissue unlike that from which it springs.
hilar cell t. of ovary, a small benign masculinizing ovarian t. derived from hilar cells, which resemble Leydig cells of the testis.
histoid t., a t. composed of a single type of differentiated tissue.
homologous t., a t. composed of tissue of the same sort as that from which it springs.
Hürthle cell t., a neoplasm of the thyroid gland composed of polyhedral acidophilic cells, thought by some to be oncocytes; it may be benign or malignant, the behavior of the latter depending on the general microscopic pattern, whether follicular, papillary, or undifferentiated.
hylic t., hyloma.
innocent t., benign t.
interstitial cell t. of testis, Leydig cell *adenoma.*
Koenen's t., periungual *fibroma.*
Krukenberg's t., a metastatic carcinoma of the ovary, usually bilateral and secondary to a mucous carcinoma of the stomach, which contains signet ring cells filled with mucus.
Landschutz t., a transplantable, possibly isoantigenic, highly virulent neoplasm which can be grown in any strain of mice; the host is killed in a few days by what is apparently an anaplastic carcinoma.
Lindau's t., hemangioblastoma.
malignant t., a t. that invades surrounding tissues, is usually capable of producing metastases, may recur after attempted removal, and is likely to cause death of the host unless adequately treated. See also cancer.
melanotic neuroectodermal t., melanoameloblastoma; retinal anlage t.; progonoma of the jaw; pigmented ameloblastoma or epulis; a benign neoplasm of neuroectodermal origin that most often involves the anterior maxilla of infants in the first year of life. It presents clinically as a rapidly growing bluish-black lesion producing a destructive radiolucency; histologically, it is characterized by small round undifferentiated t. cells interspersed with larger polyhedral melanin-producing cells arranged in an alveolar configuration.
Merkel cell t., trabecular carcinoma of the skin; a rare malignant cutaneous tumor composed of dermal nodules of small round cells with scanty cytoplasm in a trabecular pattern; the tumor cells usually contain cytoplasmic dense core granules resembling neurosecretory granules seen in Merkel cells.
mesonephroid t., mesonephroma.
mixed t., a t. composed of two or more varieties of tissue.
mixed mesodermal t., a sarcoma of the body of the uterus arising in older women, composed of more than one mesenchymal tissue, especially including striated muscle cells.
mixed t. of salivary gland, pleomorphic adenoma; a t. composed of salivary gland epithelium and fibrous tissue with mucoid or cartilaginous areas.
mixed t. of skin, chondroid *syringoma.*
mucoepidermoid t., mucoepidermoid *carcinoma.*
Nelson t., a pituitary t. causing the symptoms of Nelson *syndrome.*
oil t., lipogranuloma.
oncocytic hepatocellular t., fibrolamellar liver cell *carcinoma.*
organoid t., a t. of complex structure, glandular in origin, containing epithelium, connective tissue, etc.
Pancoast t., superior pulmonary sulcus t.; an adenocarcinoma of a lung apex causing Pancoast syndrome.
papillary t., papilloma.
paraffin t., paraffinoma.
pearl t., obsolete term for cholesteatoma.
phantom t., accumulation of fluid in the interlobar spaces of the lung, secondary to congestive heart failure, radiologically simulating a neoplasm.
phyllodes t., *cystosarcoma* phyllodes.
pilar t. of scalp, proliferating tricholemmal cyst; a solitary t. of the scalp in elderly women that may ulcerate; microscopically resembles squamous cell carcinoma composed of glycogen-rich clear cells, but is benign.
Pindborg t., calcifying epithelial odontogenic t.
pontine angle t., a t. growing in the proximal portion of the acoustic nerve, in the angle formed by the cerebellum and the lateral pons.
potato t. of neck, a firm nodular mass in the neck, usually a carotid body tumor (chemodectoma).
Pott's puffy t., a circumscribed swelling of the scalp indicating an underlying osteitis of the skull or an extradural abscess.
pregnancy t., *granuloma* gravidarum.
ranine t., ranula (2).
Rathke's pouch t., craniopharyngioma.
Recklinghausen's t., adenomatoid t.
retinal anlage t., melanotic neuroectodermal t.
Rous t., Rous *sarcoma.*
sand t., psammoma.
Sertoli cell t., androblastoma (1).
squamous odontogenic t., a benign epithelial odontogenic t. thought to arise from the epithelial cell rests of Malassez; appears clinically as a radiolucent lesion closely associated with the tooth root and histologically as islands of squamous epithelium enclosed by a peripheral layer of flattened cells.
sugar t., a benign clear cell t. of the lung containing abundant glycogen.
superior pulmonary sulcus t., Pancoast t.
teratoid t., teratoma.
theca cell t., thecoma.
transmissible venereal t., canine venereal *granuloma.*
triton t., a peripheral nerve t. with striated muscle differentiation, seen most often in neurofibromatosis; named after Masson's theory of transformation of motor nerve fibers into muscle in triton salamanders.
turban t., cylindroma of the scalp which, when overgrown, may resemble a turban.
villous t., villous *papilloma.*
Warthin's t., adenolymphoma.
Wilms' t., adenomyosarcoma; embryoma of the kidney; mesoblastic nephroma; nephroblastoma; renal carcinosarcoma; a malignant renal t. of young children, composed of small spindle cells and various other types of tissue, including tubules and, in some cases, structures resembling fetal glomeruli, and striated muscle and cartilage; it is radiosensitive, but may have already metastasized to the lungs or elsewhere when a renal mass or hematuria is noted.
Yaba t., a poxvirus-induced neoplasm of monkeys caused by the Yaba monkey virus; tumor-like growths occur chiefly on the head and limbs; the natural disease has been reported only in Africa in monkeys kept outdoors.
yolk sac t., endodermal sinus t.
Zollinger-Ellison t., a non-beta cell tumor of pancreatic islets causing the Zollinger-Ellison syndrome.

tumoraffin (tū'mōr-af'in) [tumor + L. *affinis,* related to]. Oncotropic.

tumor burden. The total mass of tumor tissue carried by a patient with cancer.

tumoricidal (tū'mōr-i-sī'dăl) [tumor + L. *caedo,* to kill]. Denoting an agent destructive to tumors.

tumorigenesis (tū'mōr-i-jen'ĕ-sis) [tumor + G. *genesis,* origin]. Production of a new growth or growths.
foreign body t., induction of malignant tumors in tissues by nonviable, nonabsorbable solid material not known to contain a chemical carcinogen.

tumorigenic (tū'mŏr-i-jen'ik). Causing or producing tumors.

tumorlets (tū'mŏr-lets). Minute foci of atypical bronchiolar epithelial hyperplasia that are found multifocally; although now considered benign, they were once believed to be precursors of carcinoma.

tumorous (tū'mŏr-ŭs). Swollen; tumor-like; protuberant.

tumultus cordis (tū-mŭl'tŭs kōr'dis). Palpitation and irregular action of the heart.

Tunga penetrans (tŭng'ă pen'ĕ-tranz). *Sarcopsylla penetrans;* a member of the flea family, Tungidae, commonly known as chigger flea, sand flea, chigoe, or jiggers; the minute female penetrates the skin, frequently under the toenails; as she becomes distended with eggs to about pea size, a painful ulcer with inflammation develops at the site.

tungiasis (tŭng-ī'ă-sis). Infestation with sand fleas (*Tunga penetrans*).

Tungidae (tŭng'i-dē). A family of fleas containing the jigger or chigoe flea species, *Tunga penetrans.*

tungsten (tŭng'sten) [Swed. *tung,* heavy, + *sten,* stone]. Wolfram; wolframium; a metallic element, symbol W, atomic no. 74, atomic weight 183.85.

t. carbide, one of the hardest known materials, used as an abrasive and in the manufacture of dental cutting instruments.

tunic (tū'nik) [L. *tunica*] Tunica.

Bichat's t., the tunica intima of the blood vessels.

Brücke's t., *tunica* nervea.

fibrous t. of corpus spongiosum, *tunica* albuginea corporis spongiosi.

fibrous t. of eye, *tunica* fibrosa bulbi.

mucosal t.'s, mucous t.'s, see entries under *tunica* mucosa.

muscular t.'s, see entries under *tunica* muscularis.

nervous t. of eyeball, retina.

serous t., *tunica* serosa.

TUNICA

tunica, pl. **tunicae** (tū'ni-kă, -kē) [L. a coat] [NA]. Tunic; coat or covering; one of the enveloping layers of a part, especially one of the coats of a blood vessel or other tubular structure.

t. abdomina'lis, the aponeurosis of the abdominal muscles of quadrupeds.

t. adventi'tia [NA], membrana adventitia (1); the outermost fibrous coat of a vessel or an organ that is derived from the surrounding connective tissue.

t. albugin'ea [NA], a dense, white, collagenous tunic surrounding a structure.

t. albugin'ea cor'poris spongio'si [NA], fibrous tunic of corpus spongiosum; the thick layer of fibrous tissue surrounding the corpus spongiosum penis; it is thinner than the corresponding layer around each corpus cavernosum.

t. albugin'ea cor'porum cavernoso'rum [NA], a strong, fibrous membrane enveloping each corpus cavernosum penis.

t. albugin'ea oc'uli, sclera.

t. albugin'ea tes'tis [NA], peridldymis; a thick white fibrous membrane forming the outer coat of the testis.

t. car'nea, t. dartos.

t. conjuncti'va [NA], conjunctiva; the mucous membrane investing the anterior surface of the eyeball and the posterior surface of the lids: **t. c. bul'bi** [NA], conjunctival layer of bulb; bulbar conjunctiva; the part of the conjunctiva covering the anterior surface of the sclera and the surface epithelium of the cornea; **t. c. palpebra'rum** [NA], palpebral conjunctiva; conjunctival layer of eyelids; the part of the conjunctiva lining the posterior surface of the eyelids and continuous with the bulbar conjunctiva at the conjunctival fornices.

t. dar'tos [NA], t. carnea; membrana carnosa; dartos muscle; a layer of smooth muscular tissue in the integument of the scrotum. See also *dartos* muliebris.

t. elas'tica, t. media of large arteries.

t. exter'na [NA], t. extima; **(1)** the outer of two or more enveloping layers of any structure; **(2)** specifically, the outer fibroelastic coat of a blood or lymph vessel.

t. exter'na oc'uli, t. fibrosa bulbi.

t. exter'na the'cae follic'uli, theca externa; the external fibrous layer of the theca of a well-developed vesicular ovarian follicle; the cells and fibers are arranged in a concentric fashion.

t. ex'tima, t. externa.

t. fibro'sa [NA], any fibrous envelope of a part.

t. fibro'sa bul'bi [NA], t. externa oculi; fibrous tunic of eye; the outer layer of the eyeball composed of the sclera and cornea.

t. fibro'sa hep'atis [NA], the fibrous layer that surrounds the liver.

t. fibro'sa lie'nis [NA], official alternate term for t. fibrosa splenis.

t. fibro'sa re'nis, *capsula* fibrosa renis.

t. fibro'sa sple'nis [NA], t. fibrosa lienis; t. propria lienis; capsula lienis; the fibrous capsule of the spleen, containing collagen, elastic fibers, and smooth muscle.

tu'nicae funic'uli spermat'ici [NA], coverings of the spermatic cord, including external and internal spermatic fasciae, and cremasteric muscle and fascia.

Haller's t. vasculosa, t. vasculosa bulbi.

t. inter'na bul'bi [NA], retina.

t. inter'na the'cae follic'uli, theca interna; the inner cellular and vascular layer of the vesicular ovarian follicle; there is evidence that the epithelioid cells produce estrogen and contribute to the formation of the corpus luteum after ovulation.

t. in'tima [NA], the innermost coat of a blood or lymphatic vessel; it consists of endothelium, usually a thin fibroelastic subendothelial layer, and an inner elastic membrane or longitudinal fibers.

t. me'dia [NA], media (1); the middle, usually muscular, coat of an artery or other tubular structure.

t. muco'sa [NA], mucous membrane; membrana mucosa; a mucous tissue lining various tubular structures, consisting of epithelium, lamina propria, and, in the digestive tract, a layer of smooth muscle.

t. muco'sa bronchio'rum [NA], the inner coat of the bronchi.

t. muco'sa cavita'tis tym'pani [NA], the mucous layer of the tympanic cavity and the structures in it.

t. muco'sa co'li [NA], the inner mucous coat of the colon.

t. muco'sa duc'tus deferen'tis [NA], the inner layer of the ductus deferens.

t. muco'sa esoph'agi [NA], the inner coat of the esophagus.

t. muco'sa intesti'ni ten'uis [NA], the mucous coat of the small intestine.

t. muco'sa laryn'gis [NA], the mucous coat of the larynx.

t. muco'sa lin'guae [NA], mucous membrane of the tongue; the mucosa of the dorsum of the tongue appears velvety due to the presence of vast numbers of papillae; that of the inferior surface is smooth and thinner.

t. muco'sa na'si [NA], pituitary membrane; schneiderian membrane; membrana pituitosa; the mucous membrane of the nose; it is continuous with the skin in the vestibule of the nose and with the mucosa of the nasopharynx, the paranasal sinuses, and the nasolacrimal duct, and contains goblet cells; it is subdivided into the *regio* olfactoria and *regio* respiratoria.

t. muco'sa o'ris [NA], the mucous membrane of the oral cavity, including the gingiva.

t. muco'sa pharyn'gis [NA], the mucous coat of the pharynx.

t. muco'sa tra'cheae [NA], the inner mucous layer of the trachea.

t. muco'sa tu'bae auditi'vae [NA], the lining coat of the auditory tube.
t. muco'sa tu'bae uteri'nae [NA], the mucous layer of the uterine tube.
t. muco'sa ure'teris [NA], the inner layer of the ureter.
t. muco'sa ure'thrae femini'nae [NA], the inner mucosal layer of the female urethra.
t. muco'sa u'teri [NA], endometrium.
t. muco'sa vagi'nae [NA], the mucous membrane of the vagina.
t. muco'sa ventric'uli [NA], the mucous layer of the stomach.
t. muco'sa ves'icae bilia'ris [NA], t. mucosa vesicae felleae; the inner coat of the gallbladder.
t. muco'sa ves'icae fel'leae [NA], official alternate term for t. mucosa vesicae biliaris.
t. muco'sa ves'icae urina'riae [NA], the inner coat of the urinary bladder.
t. muco'sa vesic'ulae semina'lis [NA], the mucous membrane of the seminal vesicle.
t. muscula'ris [NA], the muscular, usually middle, layer of a tubular structure.
t. muscula'ris bronchio'rum [NA], muscular tunic of the bronchi.
t. muscula'ris co'li [NA], muscular tunic of the colon.
t. muscula'ris duc'tus deferen'tis [NA], muscular tunic of the ductus deferens.
t. muscula'ris esoph'agi [NA], muscular tunic of the esophagus.
t. muscula'ris intesti'ni ten'uis [NA], muscular tunic of the small intestine.
t. muscula'ris pharyn'gis [NA], muscular tunic of the pharynx.
t. muscula'ris rec'ti [NA], muscular tunic of the rectum.
t. muscula'ris tra'cheae [NA], muscular tunic of the trachea.
t. muscula'ris tu'bae uteri'nae [NA], muscular tunic of the uterine tube.
t. muscula'ris ure'teris [NA], muscular tunic of the ureter.
t. muscula'ris ure'thrae femini'nae [NA], muscular tunic of the female urethra.
t. muscula'ris u'teri [NA], muscular tunic of the uterus.
t. muscula'ris vagi'nae [NA], muscular tunic of the vagina.
t. muscula'ris ventric'uli [NA], muscular tunic of the stomach; it consists of smooth muscles arranged in three fairly well defined layers: an outer stratum longitudinale, comprising the musculus dilator pylori gastroduodenalis, a middle stratum circulare, continuous with the musculus sphincter pylori, and an inner incomplete layer consisting of fibrae obliquae arching over the cardiac notch.
t. muscula'ris ves'icae bilia'ris [NA], t. muscularis vesicae felleae; muscular tunic of the gallbladder.
t. muscula'ris ves'icae fel'leae [NA], official alternate term for t. muscularis vesicae biliaris.
t. muscula'ris ves'icae urina'riae [NA], muscular tunic of the urinary bladder.
t. ner'vea, Brücke's tunic; an older term, formerly used to designate the retina exclusive of the layer of rods and cones.
t. pro'pria, the special envelope of a part as distinguished from the peritoneal or other investment common to several parts.
t. pro'pria co'rii, *stratum* reticulare corii.
t. pro'pria lie'nis, t. fibrosa splenis.
t. reflex'a, the reflected layer of the t. vasculosa testis that lines the scrotum.
t. sclerot'ica, sclera.
t. sero'sa [NA], serous tunic, coat, or membrane; membrana serosa (1); serosa (1); the outermost coat or serous layer of a visceral structure that lies in the body cavities of abdomen or thorax; it consists of a surface layer of mesothelium reinforced by irregular fibroelastic connective tissue.
t. sero'sa co'li [NA], serous tunic of the colon.
t. sero'sa hep'atis [NA], serous tunic of the liver.
t. sero'sa intesti'ni ten'uis [NA], serous tunic of the small intestine.
t. sero'sa peritone'i [NA], serous tunic of the peritoneum.
t. sero'sa tu'bae uteri'nae [NA], serous tunic of the uterine tube.
t. sero'sa u'teri [NA], official alternate term for perimetrium.
t. sero'sa ventric'uli [NA], serous tunic of the stomach.
t. sero'sa ves'icae bilia'ris [NA], t. serosa vesicae felleae; serous tunic of the gallbladder.
t. sero'sa ves'icae fel'leae [NA], official alternate term for t. serosa vesicae biliaris.
t. sero'sa ves'icae urina'riae [NA], serous tunic of the urinary bladder.
t. submuco'sa, *tela* submucosa.
t. vagina'lis commu'nis, *fascia* spermatica interna.
t. vagina'lis tes'tis [NA], the serous sheath of the testis and epididymis, derived from the peritoneum; it consists of an outer and inner serous layer, lamina parietalis and lamina visceralis, respectively.
t. vasculo'sa, any vascular layer.
t. vasculo'sa bul'bi [NA], uvea; uveal tract; t. vasculosa oculi; Haller's t. vasculosa; the vascular, pigmentary, or middle coat of the eye, comprising the choroid, ciliary body, and iris.
t. vasculo'sa len'tis, a nutrient vascular layer enveloping the lens of the eye in the fetus.
t. vasculo'sa oc'uli, t. vasculosa bulbi.
t. vasculo'sa tes'tis, the vascular layer enveloping the testis beneath the t. albuginea.
t. vit'rea, *membrana* vitrea.

---

tunnel (tŭn'ĕl). An elongated passageway, usually open at both ends.
carpal t., *canalis* carpi.
Corti's t., Corti's canal; the spiral canal in the organ of Corti, formed by the outer and inner pillar cells or rods of Corti; it is filled with fluid and occasionally crossed by nonmedullated nerve fibers.

Tuohy, Edward B., 20th century U.S. anesthesiologist. See T. *needle.*

turanose (tūr'ă-nōs). 3-*O*-α-D-Glucopyranosyl-D-fructose; a reducing disaccharide.

Turbatrix (ter-bā'triks) [L. *turbare,* to disturb]. A genus of free-living nematodes in the family Cephalobidae; it includes the species *T. aceti* (the vinegar eel), found in old vinegar or in rotting fruits and vegetables.

turbid (ter'bid) [L. *turbidus,* confused, disordered]. Cloudy, as by sediment or insoluble matter in a solution.

turbidimeter (ter-bi-dim'ĕ-ter). An instrument for measuring turbidity.

turbidimetric (ter'bid-i-met'rik). Pertaining to the measurement of turbidity.

turbidimetry (ter-bi-dim'ĕ-trē) [turbidity + G. *metron,* measure]. A method for determining the concentration of a substance in a solution by the degree of cloudiness or turbidity it causes or by the degree of clarification it induces in a turbid solution.

turbidity (ter-bid'i-tē) [L. *turbiditas,* fr. *turbidus,* turbid]. The quality of being turbid, of losing transparency because of sediment or insoluble matter.

turbinal (ter'bi-năl). Turbinated *body* (1).

turbinate (ter'bi-nāt). A bone shaped like a top, especially referring to turbinated bones. See entries under *concha* nasalis.

turbinated (ter'bi-nāt-ed) [L. *turbinatus,* shaped like a top]. Scroll-shaped.

turbinectomy (ter'bi-nek'tō-mē) [turbinate + G. *ektomē,* excision]. Surgical removal of a turbinated bone.

turbinotome (ter'bi-nō-tōm). An instrument for use in turbinotomy or turbinectomy.

turbinotomy (ter'bi-not'ō-mē) [turbinate + G. *tomē,* incision]. Incision into or excision of a turbinated body.

Türck, Ludwig, Austrian neurologist, 1810–1868. See T.'s *bundle, column, degeneration, tract.*

Turcot syndrome. See under syndrome.

turgescence (ter-jes'ens) [L. *turgesco,* to begin to swell, fr. *turgeo,* to swell]. Tumescence.

turgescent (ter-jes'ent). Tumescent.

turgid (ter'jid) [L. *turgidus,* swollen, fr. *turgeo,* to swell]. Tumid.

turgometer (ter-gom'ĕ-ter) [turgor + G. *metron,* measure]. A device for measuring turgor, or turgescence, particularly of the skin.

turgor (ter'gōr) [L., fr. *turgeo,* to swell]. Fullness.
t. vita'lis, the normal fullness of the capillaries.

turista (tū-rēs'tă). Mexican term for traveler's *diarrhea.*

Türk, Siegmund, 20th century Swiss ophthalmologist. See Ehrlich-T. *line.*

Türk, Wilhelm, Austrian hematologist, 1871–1916. See T. *cell;* T.'s *leukocyte.*

turkey red (ter'kē). Madder.

turmeric (ter'mer-ik). Curcuma.

turn (tern) [A.S. *tyrnan*] To revolve or cause to revolve; specifically, to change the position of the fetus within the uterus to convert a malpresentation into a presentation permitting normal delivery.

Turner, George Grey, British surgeon, 1877–1951. See Grey Turner's *sign.*

Turner, Henry H., U.S. endocrinologist, *1892. See T.'s *syndrome;* male T's *syndrome;* pseudo-T.'s *syndrome.*

Turner, Joseph G., British dentist, †1955. See T.'s *tooth.*

Turner, Sir William, British anatomist, 1832–1916. See T.'s *sulcus.*

turnover (tern'ō-ver). The quantity of a material metabolized or processed, usually within a given length of time.

turpentine (ter'pen-tīn) [G. *terebinthinos,* pertaining to *terebinthos,* the terebinth tree]. An oleoresin from *Pinus palustris* and other species of *Pinus;* source of t. oil and a constituent of stimulating ointments.
Canada t., Canada *balsam.*
Chian t., an exudation from *Pistacia terebinthus,* a small tree of Chios and regions eastward; on exposure to air it thickens and forms translucent yellow masses similar to mastic.
larch t., Venice t.; a transparent, yellowish, thick liquid, the oleoresin obtained from *Larix europaea* (family Pinaceae).
Venice t., larch t.
white t., t. from *Pinus palustris.*

turpentine oil. Turpentine spirit; a volatile oil, distilled from turpentine, that has been used as a diuretic, carminative, vermifuge, expectorant, rubefacient, and counterirritant.
rectified t. o., obtained by treating t. o. with sodium hydroxide, and redistilling; used externally as a counterirritant.

turpentine spirit. Turpentine oil.

turps (terps). Popular name for turpentine oil.

turricephaly (tūr-i-sef'ă-lē) [L. *turris,* tower, + G. *kephalē,* head]. Oxycephaly.

turunda, pl. **turundae** (tū-rŭn'dă, -dē) [L.]. A surgical tent, gauze drain, or tampon.

tush, tusk (tŭsh, tŭsk). A canine tooth in the horse, pig, or musk-deer; an incisor in the elephant and walrus.

tussal (tŭs'ăl). Tussive.

tussicular (tŭ-sik'yū-lăr) [L. *tussicularis,* fr. *tussicula,* a slight cough, dim. of *tussis,* cough]. Tussive.

tussiculation (tŭ-sik'yū-lā'shŭn). A hacking cough.

tussis (tŭs'is) [L.]. A cough.

tussive (tŭs'siv) [L. *tussis,* a cough]. Tussal; tussicular; relating to a cough.

tutamen, pl. **tutamina** (tū-tā'men, -tā'mi-nă) [L. protection]. Any defensive or protective structure.
tuta'mina cer'ebri, the scalp, cranium, and cerebral meninges.
tuta'mina oc'uli, the eyebrows, eyelids, and eyelashes.

Tuttle, James P., U.S. surgeon, 1857–1913. See T.'s *proctoscope.*

TVG Abbreviation for time-varied *gain.*

Tweed, Charles H., U.S. orthodontist, 1895–1970. See T. edgewise *treatment, triangle.*

tweezers (twē'zerz) [A.S. *twisel,* fork]. An instrument with pincers that are squeezed together to grasp or extract fine structures.

twig [A.S.]. One of the finer terminal branches of an artery; a small branch or small ramus.

twilight (twī'līt) [A.S. *twi-,* two]. **1.** Figuratively, a faint light. **2.** Pertaining to faint or indistinct mental perception, as in twilight *state.*

twin [A.S. *getwin,* double]. **1.** One of two children born at one birth. **2.** Double; growing in pairs.
allantoidoangiopagous t.'s, unequal monochorial t.'s with fusion of their allantoic vessels within the placenta; the lesser t. is essentially a parasite on the placental circulation of the larger t.
conjoined t.'s, monozygotic t.'s with varying extent of union and different degrees of residual duplication. The various types of union are named by the use of a prefix designating the region that is united and adding the suffix *-pagus,* meaning fused (*e.g.,* craniopagus, thoracopagus); the various types of residual duplication are named by designating the parts duplicated and adding the suffix *-didymus,* or *-dymus,* meaning twin (*e.g.,* cephalodidymus, or cephalodymus).
conjoined equal t.'s, conjoined symmetrical t.'s, conjoined t.'s in which both members are approximately of the same size, and nearly normal except for the areas of fusion.
conjoined unequal t.'s, conjoined asymmetrical t.'s, conjoined t.'s with one member nearly normal (host or autosite) and the other (parasite) small, incomplete, and dependent for its nutrition upon the more nearly normal member.
dichorial t.'s, dizygotic t.'s.
diovular t.'s, dizygotic t.'s.
dizygotic t.'s, t.'s derived from two separate zygotes. Also called dichorial, diovular, fraternal, or heterologous t.'s.
enzygotic t.'s, monozygotic t.'s.
fraternal t.'s, dizygotic t.'s.
heterologous t.'s, dizygotic t.'s.
identical t.'s, monozygotic t.'s.
incomplete conjoined t.'s, conjoined t.'s, the two components of which equal one another but are less than entire individuals.
monoamniotic t.'s, t.'s within a common amnion; such t.'s are monovular in origin and may be conjoined.
monochorial t.'s, monozygotic t.'s.
monovular t.'s, monozygotic t.'s.
monozygotic t.'s, t.'s resulting from a single fertilized ovum that at an early stage of development becomes separated into independently growing cell aggregations giving rise to two individuals of the same sex and identical genetic constitution. Also called enzygotic, identical, monochorial, uniovular, or monovular t.'s.
omphaloangiopagous t.'s, obsolete term for allantoidoangiopagous t.'s.
parasitic t., the smaller of unequal conjoined t.'s.
placental parasitic t., omphalosite.
polyzygotic t.'s, t.'s resulting from fertilization of more than two ova which have been discharged in a single ovulating cycle.
Siamese t.'s, originally, much publicized conjoined t.'s (xiphopagus) from Siam in the 19th century; this term has since come into general lay usage for any type of conjoined t.'s.

uniovular t.'s, monozygotic t.'s.

twinge (twinj). A sudden momentary sharp pain.

twin'ning. Production of equivalent structures by division; the tendency of divided parts to assume symmetrical relations.

twitch [A.S. *twiccian*]. **1.** To jerk spasmodically. **2.** A momentary spasmodic contraction of a muscle fiber.

Twort, Frederick W., British bacteriologist, 1877–1950. See T. *phenomenon;* T.-d'Herelle *phenomenon.*

TX Abbreviation for individual thromboxanes, designated by capital letters with subscripts indicating structural features.

tybamate (tī'bă-māt). 2-(Hydroxymethyl)-2-methylpentyl butylcarbamate carbamate; a tranquilizer related to meprobamate.

tyle (tī'lē) [G. *tylē,* a swelling, a callus]. Callosity.

tylectomy (tī-lek'tō-mē) [G. *tylē,* lump, + *ektomē,* excision]. Lumpectomy; surgical removal of a localized swelling or tumor. See also lumpectomy.

tylion, pl. **tylia** (til'ē-on, tī'lē-on, -lē-ă) [G. a small pin, dim. of *tylē,* a lump]. A craniometric point at the middle of the anterior edge of the sulcus chiasmatis.

tyloma (tī-lō'mă) [G. a callus]. Callosity.

t. conjuncti'vae, localized keratinization of the conjunctiva, occurring in xerosis of the conjunctiva.

tylosis, pl. **tyloses** (tī-lō'sis, -sēz) [G. a becoming callous]. Formation of a callosity (tyloma).

t. cilia'ris, pachyblepharon.

t. ling'uae, leukoplakia of the tongue.

t. palma'ris et planta'ris, palmoplantar *keratoderma.*

tylotic (tī-lot'ik). Relating to or marked by tylosis.

tyloxapol (tī-lok'să-pol). Oxyethylated *tert*-octylphenol formaldehyde polymer; a detergent and mucolytic agent used as an aerosol to liquify sputum.

tymazoline (tī-maz'ō-lēn). 2-[(Thymyloxy)methyl]-2-imidazoline; a nasal decongestant.

tympan-, tympani-. See tympano-.

tympanal (tim'pă-năl). Tympanic.

tympanectomy (tim'pă-nek'tō-mē) [tympan- + G. *ektomē,* excision]. Excision of the tympanic membrane.

tympania (tim-pan'ē-ă). Tympanites.

tympanic (tim-pan'ik). Tympanal. **1.** Relating to the tympanic cavity or membrane. **2.** Resonant. **3.** Tympanitic (2).

tympanichord (tim-pan'i-kōrd). *Chorda* tympani.

tympanichordal (tim-pan-i-kōr'dăl). Relating to the chorda tympani nerve.

tympanicity (tim'pă-nis'i-tē). The quality of being tympanic or drumlike in tone.

tympanism (tim'pă-nizm). Tympanites.

tympanites (tim-pă-nī'tēz) [L. fr. G. *tympanitēs,* a dropsy in which the belly is stretched like a drum, *tympanon*] Meteorism; tympania; tympanism; swelling of the abdomen from gas in the intestinal or peritoneal cavity.

uterine t., physometra.

tympanitic (tim-pă-nit'ik). **1.** Tympanous; referring to tympanites. **2.** Tympanic (3); denoting the quality of sound elicited by percussing over the inflated intestine or a large pulmonary cavity.

tympanitis (tim-pă-nī'tis). Myringitis.

tympano-, tympan-, tympani- [G. *tympanon,* drum]. Combining forms denoting tympanum, tympanites.

tympanocentesis (tim'pă-nō-sen-tē'sis) [tympano- + G. *kentēsis,* puncture]. Puncture of the tympanic membrane with a needle to aspirate middle ear fluid.

tympanoeustachian (tim'pă-nō-ū-stā'shŭn, -stā'kē-an). Relating to the tympanic cavity and the auditory (eustachian) tube.

tympanohyal (tim'pă-nō-hī'ăl). Relating to that part of the tympanic cavity developed from the hyoid arch.

tympanomalleal (tim'pă-nō-mal'ē-ăl). Relating to the tympanic membrane and the malleus.

tympanomandibular (tim'pă-nō-man-dib'yū-lăr). Relating to the tympanic cavity and the mandible.

tympanomastoid (tim'pă-nō-mas'toyd). Relating to the tympanic cavity and the mastoid cells.

tympanomastoiditis (tim'pă-nō-mas-toy-dī'tis). Inflammation of the middle ear and the mastoid cells.

tympanomeatomastoidectomy (tim'pă-nō-mē'ă-tō-mas-toy-dek'-tō-mē). Radical *mastoidectomy.*

tympanophonia, tympanophony (tim'pă-nō-fō'nē-ă, tim'pă-nof'ō-nē) [tympano- + G. *phōne,* sound]. **1.** *Tinnitus* aurium. **2.** Autophony.

tympanoplasty (tim'pă-nō-plas-tē) [tympano- + G. *plassō,* to form]. Operative correction of a damaged middle ear.

tympanosquamosal (tim'pă-nō-skwă-mō'săl). Relating to the tympanic and squamous parts of the temporal bone.

tympanostapedial (tim'pă-nō-stā-pē'dē-ăl). Relating to the tympanic cavity and the stapes.

tympanostomy (tim-pan-os'tō-mē) [tympano- + G. *ostium,* mouth]. Myringotomy.

tympanotemporal (tim'pă-nō-tem'pō-răl). Relating to the tympanic cavity and the temporal region or bone.

tympanotomy (tim'pă-not'-ō-mē) [tympano- + G. *tomē,* incision]. Myringotomy.

tympanous (tim'pă-nŭs). Tympanitic (1).

tympanum, pl. **tympana, tympanums** (tim'pă-nŭm, tim'pă-nă) [L., fr. G. *tympanon,* a drum]. *Cavitas* tympanica.

tympany (tim'pă-nē). Tympanitic resonance; a low-pitched, resonant, drumlike note obtained by percussing the surface of a large air-containing space, such as the distended abdomen or the thorax with or without pneumothorax.

Skoda's t., skodaic *resonance.*

Tyndall, John, British physicist, 1820–1893. See T. *phenomenon.*

tyndallization (tin'dăl-i-zā'shŭn) [John *Tyndall*]. Fractional *sterilization.*

type (tīp) [G. *typos,* a mark, a model]. **1.** The usual form, or a composite form, that all others of the class resemble more or less closely; a model, denoting especially a disease or a symptom complex giving the stamp or characteristic to a class. See also constitution; habitus; personality. **2.** In chemistry, a substance in which the arrangement of the atoms in a molecule may be taken as representative of other substances in that class.

basic personality t., **(1)** an individual's unique, covert, or underlying personality propensities, whether or not they are behaviorally manifest or overt; **(2)** personality characteristics of an individual which are also shared by a majority of the members of a social group.

blood t., see *blood type.*

nomenclatural t., the constituent element of a taxon to which the name of the taxon is permanently attached; the t. of a species is preferably a strain (in special cases it may be a description, a preserved specimen or preparation, or an illustration); the t. of a genus is a species; and the t. of an order, family, or tribe is the genus on whose name the name of the higher taxon is based.

test t., see *test types.*

wild t., a gene, phenotype, or genotype that is overwhelmingly common among those possible at a locus of interest, and therefore presumably not harmful.

typhinia (tī-fin′ē-ă) [G. *typhos,* smoke, stupor arising from fever]. Relapsing *fever.*

typhl-. See typhlo-.

typhlectasis (tif-lek′tă-sis) [G. *typhlon,* cecum, + *ektasis,* a stretching out]. Dilation of the cecum.

typhlectomy (tif-lek′tō-mē). Cecectomy.

typhlenteritis (tif′len-ter-ī′tis). Cecitis.

typhlitis (tif′lī′tis). Cecitis.

typhlo-, typhl-. **1** [G. cecum]. Combining form denoting the cecum. See also ceco-. **2** [G. *typhlos,* blind]. Combining form denoting blindness.

typhlodicliditis (tif-lō-dik-li-dī′tis) [G. *typhlon,* cecum, + *diklis (diklid-),* double-folding (of doors), + *-itis,* inflammation]. Inflammation of the ileocecal valve.

typhloempyema (tif′lō-em-pī-ē′mă) [G. *typhlon,* cecum, + *empyēma,* abscess]. Presence of an abscess following typhlitis.

typhloenteritis (tif′lō-en-ter-ī′tis). Cecitis.

typhlolithiasis (tif′lō-li-thī′ă-sis) [G. *typhlon,* cecum, + *lithos,* stone]. Presence of fecal concretions in the cecum.

typhlology (tif-lol′ō-jē) [G. *typhlos,* blind, + *logos,* study]. The branch of science concerned with the causes and prevention of blindness, and the rehabilitation of those afflicted.

typhlomegaly (tif′lō-meg′ă-lē) [G. *typhlon,* cecum, + *megas (megal-),* large]. Enlargement of the cecum.

typhlon (tif′lon) [G.]. Cecum.

typhlopexy, typhlopexia (tif′lō-pek-sē, tif-lō-pek′sē-ă). Cecopexy.

typhlorrhaphy (tif-lōr′ă-fē). Cecorrhaphy.

typhlosis (tif-lō′sis) [G. *typhlos,* blind]. Blindness.

typhlostomy (tif-los′tō-mē). Cecostomy.

typhlotomy (tif-lot′ō-mē). Cecotomy.

typhloureterostomy (tif′lō-yū-rē′ter-os′tō-mē) [G. *typhlon,* cecum, + ureter, + *stoma,* mouth]. Obsolete anastomosis of a ureter into the cecum.

typho- [G. *typhos*]. Combining form denoting typhus, typhoid.

typhoid (tī′foyd) [typhus + G. *eidos,* resemblance]. **1.** Typhus-like; stuporous from fever. **2.** Typhoid *fever.*
abdominal t., typhoid *fever.*
ambulatory t., walking t.
apyretic t., t. fever in which the temperature does not rise more than a degree or two.
bilious t. of Griesinger, relapsing *fever.*
fowl t., a septicemic disease of chickens and turkeys, caused by *Salmonella gallinarum;* some human infections with this organism have been reported.
latent t., walking t.
provocation t., an accelerated onset of t. fever, sometimes of unusual severity, resulting from typhoid-paratyphoid A and B (T.A.B.) vaccination late in the incubation period.
walking t., ambulatory or latent t.; t. fever without much prostration, the patient being up and around and sometimes working.

typhoidal (tī-foyd′ăl). Relating to or resembling typhoid fever.

typholysin (tī-fol′i-sin). A hemolysin formed by *Salmonella typhosa.*

typhomania (tī-fō-mā′nē-ă) [typho- + G. *mania,* frenzy]. A muttering delerium characteristic of that in typhoid fever and typhus.

typhosepsis (tī-fō-sep′sis). Typhoid *septicemia.*

typhous (tī′fŭs). Relating to typhus.

typhus (tī′fŭs) [G. *typhos,* smoke, stupor]. An acute infectious and contagious disease, caused by rickettsiae, and occurring in two principal forms: epidemic t. and endemic (murine) t. Also called jail, camp, ship fever.
endemic t., murine t.
epidemic t., louse-borne t.; t. caused by *Rickettsia prowazekii* and spread by body lice; marked by high fever, mental and physical depression, and a macular and papular eruption; lasts for about two weeks and occurs when large crowds are brought together and personal hygiene is at a low ebb; recrudescences occur.
flea-borne t., murine t.
louse-borne t., epidemic t.
mite t., tsutsugamushi *disease.*
t. mit′ior, a mild or abortive t.
murine t., a milder form of epidemic t. caused by *Rickettsia typhi* and transmitted to man by rat or mouse fleas. Also called endemic or flea-borne t.; red or congolian red fever; red fever of the congo.
North Queensland tick t., t. caused by *Rickettsia australis.*
recrudescent t., Brill-Zinsser *disease.*
scrub t., tsutsugamushi *disease.*
tick t., Marseilles or eruptive fever; collective term for the tick-borne rickettsial diseases involving many strains (or species) placed in the subgenus *Dermacentroxenus* and identified by their immunological reactions and, in some cases, by their pathogenicity; the tick-borne rickettsiae invade the nuclei as well as cytoplasm of host cells, whereas true t. rickettsiae are found in cytoplasm only.
tropical t., tsutsugamushi *disease.*

typing (tīp′ing) [see type]. Classification according to type.
bacteriophage t., a microbiological procedure, of epidemiological importance, for distinguishing types within a seemingly homogeneous bacterial species or strain by the use of type-specific bacteriophage.
blood t., *blood grouping.*

Tyr Symbol for tyrosine and its radicals.

tyraminase (tī′ră-mi-nās, tir′ă-). *Amine* oxidase (flavin-containing).

tyramine (tī′ră-mēn, tir′ă-). 4-Hydroxyphenylethylamine; decarboxylated tyrosine, a sympathomimetic amine having an action in some respects resembling that of epinephrine; present in ergot, mistletoe, ripe cheese, and putrefied animal matter.
t. oxidase, *amine* oxidase (flavin-containing).

tyrannism (tir′ă-nizm) [G. *tyrannos,* a tyrant]. A form of sadism characterized by a lust for domination and cruelty, with subsequent humiliation of the partner.

tyremesis (tī-rem′ĕ-sis) [G. *tyros,* cheese, + *emesis,* vomiting]. Tyrosis (1); vomiting of curdy material by infants.

tyrocidin, tyrocidine (tī-rō-sī′din). An antibacterial cyclopeptide obtained from *Bacillus brevis.* See also tyrothricin.

Tyrode, Maurice V., U.S. pharmacologist, 1878–1930. See T.'s *solution.*

tyrogenous (tī-roj′ĕ-nŭs) [G. *tyros,* cheese, + G. -gen, producing]. Produced by, or originating in, cheese.

Tyroglyphus longior (tī-rog′li-fŭs lon′gē-ōr, tī′rō-glif′ŭs) [G. *tyros,* cheese, + *glyphe,* carving]. *Tyrophagus putrescentiae.*

tyroid (tī′royd) [G. *tyrōdēs,* fr. *tyros,* cheese, + *eidos,* resemblance]. Cheesy; caseous.

tyroketonuria (tī′rō-kē-tō-nū′rē-ă). The urinary excretion of ketonic metabolites of tyrosine, such as *p*-hydroxyphenylpyruvic acid.

tyroma (tī-rō′mă) [G. *tyros,* cheese, + *-ōma,* tumor]. A caseous tumor.

tyropanoate sodium (tī′rō-pă-nō′āt). 3-Butyramido-α-ethyl-2,4,6-triiodohydrocinnamic acid, sodium salt; a radiographic medium for cholecystography.

Tyrophagus putrescentiae (tī-rof′ă-gŭs pyū′tre-sen′tē-ē) [G. *tyros,* cheese, + *phagein,* to eat]. *Tyroglyphus longior;* one of the grain mite species that cause various forms of dermatitis resulting from infestation by grain mites in food and produce, which sensitizes and causes dermatitis in storage and handling personnel.

tyrosinase (tī'rō-si-nās, tir'ō-). Monophenol monooxygenase.

β-tyrosinase. *Tyrosine* phenol-lyase.

tyrosine (Tyr) (tī'rō-sēn, -sin). 2-Amino-3-(4-hydroxyphenyl)propionic acid; 3-(4-hydroxyphenyl)alanine; an α-amino acid present in most proteins.

t. iodinase, a postulated enzyme in the thyroid catalyzing iodination of t., a reaction important in the eventual biosynthesis of thyroxine. See also peroxidases.

t. phenol-lyase [EC 4.1.99.2], β-tyrosinase; an enzyme cleaving L-tyrosine to phenol, pyruvate, and NH_3.

tyrosinemia (tī'rō-si-nē'mē-ă) [tyrosine + G. *haima,* blood]. Hypertyrosinemia; a disorder consisting of elevated blood concentrations of tyrosine, enhanced urinary excretion of tyrosine and tyrosyl compounds, hepatosplenomegaly, nodular cirrhosis of the liver, multiple renal tubular reabsorptive defects, and vitamin D-resistant rickets; autosomal recessive inheritance.

tyrosinosis (tī'rō-si-nō'sis) [tyrosine + G. *-osis,* condition]. A very rare, possibly heritable disorder of tyrosine metabolism that may be caused by defective formation of *p*-hydroxyphenylpyruvic acid oxidase or of tyrosine transaminase; characterized by enhanced urinary excretion of *p*-hydroxyphenylpyruvic acid and of other tyrosyl metabolites upon ingestion of tyrosine.

tyrosinuria (tī'rō-si-nū'rē-ă) [tyrosine + G. *ouron,* urine]. The excretion of tyrosine in the urine.

tyrosis (tī-rō'sis) [G. *tyros,* cheese]. **1.** Tyremesis. **2.** Caseation.

tyrosyluria (tī'rō-si-lū'rē-ă). Enhanced urinary excretion of certain metabolites of tyrosine, such as *p*-hydroxyphenylpyruvic acid; present in tyrosinosis, scurvy, pernicious anemia, and other diseases.

tyrothricin (tī-rō-thrī'sin). An antibacterial mixture obtained from peptone cultures of *Bacillus brevis;* bactericidal and bacteriostatic, and active against Gram-positive bacteria. It yields the crystalline antibacterial agents gramicidin and tyrocidin; the gramicidin component is a polypeptide containing L-tryptophan, D-leucine, D-valine, L-valine, L-alanine, glycine, and an aminoethanol; the tyrocidin component is a cyclopolypeptide containing tyrosine, ornithine, and several other amino acids.

tyrotoxism (tī-rō-tok'sizm) [G. *tyros,* cheese, + *toxikon,* poison]. Poisoning by cheese or any milk product.

Tyrrell, Frederick, British anatomist and surgeon, 1797–1843. See T.'s *fascia.*

Tyson, Edward, British anatomist, 1649–1708. See T.'s *glands.*

Tyzzeria (tī-zē'rē-ă). A genus of coccidia (family Eimeriidae) in which the oocyst contains eight naked sporozoites. Important species are *T. anseris,* a relatively nonpathogenic species found in the small intestine of domestic and wild geese, whistling swans, and certain wild ducks, and *T. perniciosa,* which occurs in the small intestine of the domestic duck in North America and Europe, and is pathogenic in ducklings.

Tzanck, Arnault, Russian dermatologist, 1886–1954. See T. *cells, test.*

U

U **1.** Abbreviation for unit. **2.** Symbol for kilurane; uranium; uridine in polymers; urinary *concentration,* followed by subscripts indicating location and chemical species.

ubihydroquinone (yū'bi-hī-drō-quī'nōn). Ubiquinol.

ubiquinol (Q-H_2, H_2Q) (yū'bi-kwī'nol, yū-bik'wi-nol). Ubihydroquinone; the reduction product of a ubiquinone.

ubiquinone (yū'bi-kwī'nōn, yū-bik'wi-nōn). A 2,3-dimethoxy-5-methyl-1,4-benzoquinone with a multiprenyl side chain.

ubiquinone-6 (-Q_6). Ubiquinone-30; coenzyme Q_6; 2,3-dimethoxy-5-methyl-6-hexaprenyl-1,4 benzoquinone.

ubiquinone-10 (-Q_{10}). Ubiquinone-50; coenzyme Q_{10}; 2,3-dimethoxy-5-methyl-6-decaprenyl-1,4-benzoquinone.

ubiquitin (yū-bik'kwi-tin). A small (76 amino acid residues) protein found in all cells of higher organisms and one whose structure has changed minimally during evolutionary history; involved in at least two processes; histone modification and intracellular protein breakdown.

udder (ŭd'er) [A.S., *ūder*]. The large complex of mammary glands of the cow and other ungulates.

UDP Abbreviation for *uridine* diphosphate.

UDPG Abbreviation for uridinediphosphoglucose.

UDPGal Abbreviation for uridinediphosphogalactose.

UDPgalactose. Uridinediphosphogalactase.

UDPgalactose 4-epimerase. UDPglucose 4-epimerase.

UDPGlc Abbreviation for uridinediphosphoglucose.

UDP-GlcUA Abbreviation for uridinediphosphoglucuronic acid.

UDPglucose. Uridinediphosphoglucose.

UDPglucose 4-epimerase [EC 5.1.3.2]. Galactowaldenase; UDPgalactose 4-epimerase; an enzyme that catalyzes the Walden inversion of UDPglucose to UDPgalactose.

UDPglucose–hexose-1-phosphate uridylyltransferase [EC 2.7.7.12]. Hexose-1-phosphate uridylyltransferase; uridyltransferase; phosphogalactoisomerase; an enzyme that catalyzes the interconversion of glucose 1-phosphate and galactose 1-phosphate with simultaneous interconversion of UDPglucose and UDPgalactose. See also UDPglucose 4-epimerase.

UDPglucuronate–bilirubin glucuronosyltransferase, UDP-glucuronate bilirubinglucuronoside glucuronosyltransferase. Hepatic transferases (EC 2.4.1.76 and .77 respectively) that catalyze the transfer of the glucuronic moiety of UDP-glucuronic acid to bilirubin or bilirubin glucuronide for biliary excretion.

Uehlinger, E. See U.'s *syndrome;* Meyenburg-Altherr-U. *syndrome.*

Uffelmann, Jules, German physician, 1837–1894. See U.'s *reagent.*

Uhl, Henry S.M., U.S. internist, *1921. See U. anomaly.

Uhthoff, Wilhelm, German ophthalmologist, 1853–1927. See U. *sign.*

ukambin (ū-kam'bin). An African arrow poison from plants of the family Apocynaceae; a heart poison resembling digitalis or strophanthus in its action.

ULCER

ulcer (ŭl'ser) [L. *ulcus* (*ulcer-*), a sore, ulcer]. A lesion on the surface of the skin or a mucous surface, caused by superficial loss of tissue, usually with inflammation. A wound with superficial loss of tissue from trauma is not primarily an u., but may become ulcerated if infection occurs.

acute decubitus u., a severe form of bedsore, of neutrophic origin, occurring in hemiplegia or paraplegia.

Aden u., the lesion occurring in cutaneous leishmaniasis.

amputating u., an u. encircling a limb.

anastomotic u., an u. of jejunum, after gastroenterostomy.

atonic u., an u. that shows little or no tendency to heal.

Buruli u. [*Buruli,* district in Uganda], an u. of the skin, with widespread necrosis of subcutaneous fat, due to infection with *Mycobacterium ulcerans;* occurs in Uganda in persons living on the Nile river banks.

chiclero's u., bay sore; a form of New World cutaneous leishmaniasis found among forest workers in parts of Mexico, Guatemala, and Belize; usually a mild zoonotic disease, commonly eroding the pinna of the ear over a long course of infection, which frequently is difficult to cure; the causative agent is *Leishmania mexicana,* which is transmitted to man from arboreal rodents and other forest mammals by the night-biting sandfly *Lutzomyia olmeca.*

chrome u., tanner's u.; an u. produced by exposure to chromium compounds.

chronic u., a longstanding u. with fibrous scar tissue in the floor of the u.

cockscomb u., an u. that may occur in association with condylomata acuminata.

cold u., a small gangrenous u. on the extremities; due to defective circulation.

constitutional u., symptomatic u.; an u. due to systemic disease, such as tuberculosis.

corrosive u., noma.

creeping u., serpiginous u.

Curling's u., stress u.; an u. of the duodenum in a patient with extensive superficial burns, intracranial lesions, or severe bodily injury.

decubitus u., a chronic u. that appears in pressure areas in debilitated patients confined to bed or otherwise immobilized, due to a circulatory defect in the area under pressure. Also called bedsore; pressure sore; decubital, nosocomial, pressure, or hospital gangrene; sloughing phagedena; ulcus hypostaticum.

dendritic corneal u., keratitis caused by herpes simplex virus.

dental u., an u. on the oral mucuous membrane caused by biting or by rubbing against the edge of a broken tooth.

diphtheritic u., an u. covered with a gray adherent membrane, caused by *Corynebacterium diphtheriae.*

distention u., an u. of the intestine in the dilated part above a stricture.

elusive u., Hunner's u.

fascicular u., a localized vascularization of the cornea to the site of a corneal u.

Fenwick-Hunner u., Hunner's u.

Gaboon u. [*Gaboon,* a region in Africa], a form of tropical u. affecting the residents of this region; it resembles a syphilitic u., especially in the appearance of its scar.

gastric u., an u. of the stomach.

gravitational u., a chronic u. of the leg with impaired healing because of the dependent position of the extremity and the incompetence of the valves of the varicosed veins; the venous return stagnates and creates hypoxemia. See also varicose u.

groin u., *granuloma* inguinale tropicum.

gummatous u., lesion of the skin occurring in late syphilis.

hard u., chancre.

healed u., an u. covered by epithelial regeneration, beneath which there may be scarring and absence of glands or appendages.
herpetic u., u. caused by herpes simplex virus.
Hunner's u., elusive u.; Fenwick-Hunner u.; a focal and often multiple lesion involving all layers of the bladder wall in chronic interstitial cystitis; the surface epithelium is destroyed by inflammation and the initially pale lesion cracks and bleeds with distention of the bladder.
hypopyon u., **(1)** an advancing central suppurative u. of the cornea. See also hypopyon; **(2)** a corneal u. with pus in the anterior chamber; **(3)** serpiginous *keratitis.*
indolent u., a chronic u., with hard elevated edges and few or no granulations, and showing no tendency to heal.
inflamed u., an u. with a purulent discharge and inflamed borders.
Kurunegala u.'s [*Kurunegala,* a district in Sri Lanka], *pyosis* tropica.
Lipschütz' u., a simple acute ulceration of the vulvae or lower vagina of nonvenereal origin.
lupoid u., an u. resembling that of cutaneous tuberculosis.
Mann-Williamson u., see Mann-Williamson *operation.*
marginal ring u. of cornea, a slowly advancing intermittent u. involving the circumference of the corneal margin.
Marjolin's u., warty u.; a malignant, verrucose, ulcerating growth occurring in cicatricial tissue or at the epithelial edge of a chronic benign u.
Meleney's u., Meleney's *gangrene.*
Mooren's u., chronic inflammation of the peripheral cornea that slowly progresses centrally with corneal thinning and sometimes perforation.
Oriental u., the lesion occurring in cutaneous leishmaniasis.
penetrating u., an u. extending into deeper tissues of an organ.
peptic u., an u. of the alimentary mucosa, usually in the stomach or duodenum, exposed to acid gastric secretion.

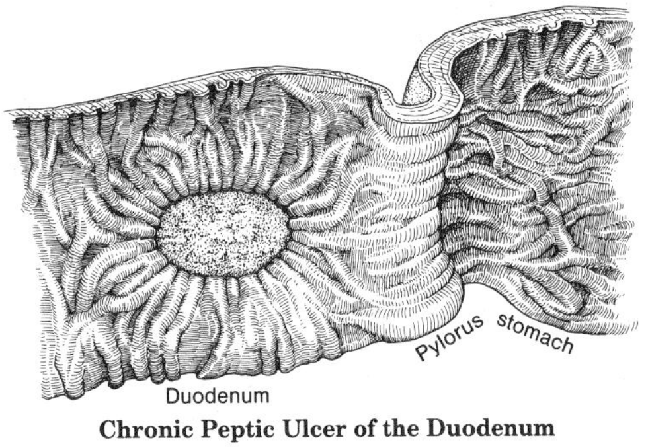

Chronic Peptic Ulcer of the Duodenum

perambulating u., phagedenic u.
perforated u., an u. extending through the wall of an organ.
perforating u. of foot, mal perforant; a round, deep, trophic u. of the sole of the foot, following disease or injury, in any part of its course from the center to the periphery of the nerve supplying the part.
phagedenic u., perambulating or sloughing u.; ulcus ambulans; a rapidly spreading u. attended by the formation of extensive sloughing.
phlegmonous u., a u. accompanied by inflammation of the neighboring tissues.
pneumococcus u., serpiginous *keratitis.*
pudendal u., *granuloma* inguinale.
recurrent aphthous u.'s, aphthae (2).
ring u. of cornea, inflammation of the greater part or the whole of the corneal periphery.
rodent u., a slowly enlarging ulcerated basal cell carcinoma, usually on the face.
Saemisch's u., a form of serpiginous keratitis, frequently accompanied by hypopyon.
serpent u. of cornea, serpiginous *keratitis.*
serpiginous u., creeping u.; an u. extending on one side while healing at the opposite edge, forming an undulating margin.
simple u., a local, not constitutional, u. not accompanied by marked pain or inflammation.
sloughing u., phagedenic u.
soft u., chancroid.
stasis u., varicose u.
stercoral u., an u. of the colon due to pressure and irritation of retained fecal masses.
steroid u., an u., usually on the leg or foot, developing from a wound in patients undergoing long-term steroid therapy; results from the wound-healing inhibitory effects characteristic of steroids.
stomal u., an intestinal u. occurring after gastrojejunostomy in the jejunal mucosa near the opening (stoma) between the stomach and the jejunum.
stress u.'s, Curling's u.
Sutton's u., a solitary, deep, painful u. of the buccal or genital mucous membrane.
symptomatic u., constitutional u.
syphilitic u., **(1)** chancre, **(2)** any ulceration caused by a syphilitic infection.
Syriac u., Syrian u., old names for diphtheria.
tanner's u., chrome u.
transparent u. of the cornea, obsolete term for an u. of the cornea, occurring usually in children, that heals without opacity.
trophic u., an u. due to impaired nutrition of the part.
tropical u., **(1)** the lesion occurring in cutaneous leishmaniasis; **(2)** tropical phagedenic ulceration caused by a variety of microorganisms, including mycobacteria; common in northern Nigeria.
undermining u., a chronic cutaneous u. with overhanging margins; due to hemolytic streptococci or other bacteria.
varicose u., stasis u.; the loss of skin surface in the drainage area of a varicose vein, usually in the leg, resulting from stasis and infection.
venereal u., chancroid.
warty u., Marjolin's u.
Zambesi u., an u., usually single, about 3 cm in diameter, on the foot or leg, occurring in laborers in the Zambesi Delta; it has a sloughing surface, but does not spread and produces no constitutional symptoms or glandular enlargement; it is associated with the presence of a spirillum and a large fusiform bacillus; one attack seems to confer a partial immunity.

---

ulcera (ŭl'ser-ă). Plural of ulcus.

ulcerate (ŭl'ser-āt). To form an ulcer.

ulcerated (ŭl'ser-āt-ed). Having undergone ulceration.

ulceration (ŭl-ser-ā'shŭn). **1.** The formation of an ulcer. **2.** An ulcer or aggregation of ulcers.
lip and leg u., ulcerative *dermatosis.*
tracheal u., erosion of the tracheal mucous membrane with, in some cases, exposure of the rings, at the site at which a cuffed tracheostomy tube has been present for some time.

ulcerative (ŭl'ser-ă-tiv). Relating to, causing, or marked by an ulcer or ulcers.

ulcerogenic (ŭl'ser-ō-jen'ik). Ulcer-producing.

ulceroglandular (ŭl'ser-ō-gland'yū-lăr). Denoting a local ulceration at a site of infection followed by regional or generalized lymphadenopathy.

ulceromembranous (ŭl'ser-ō-mem'bră-nŭs). Relating to or characterized by ulceration and the formation of a false membrane.

ulcerous (ŭl'ser-ŭs) [L. ulcerosus]. Relating to, affected with, or containing an ulcer.

ulcus, pl. **ulcera** (ŭl'kŭs, ŭl'ser-ă) [L.]. Ulcer.
u. am'bulans, phagedenic *ulcer.*
u. hypostat'icum, decubitus *ulcer.*
u. ser'pens cor'neae, serpiginous *keratitis.*
u. tere'brans, obsolete term for an invasive basal cell carcinoma, usually around the eye, nose, or ear, and extending to underlying bony tissue.
u. vene'reum, **(1)** chancre; **(2)** chancroid.
u. vul'vae acu'tum, Lipschütz *ulcer.*

ule-. See ulo-.

ulectomy (yū-lek'tō-mē) [G. *oulē,* scar, + *ektomē,* excision]. Obsolete synonym for cicatrectomy.

ulegyria (yū'lē-jī'rē-ă) [G. *oulē,* scar, + *gyros,* ring]. A defect of the cerebral cortex characterized by narrow and distorted gyri; may be congenital or the result of scars.

ulerythema (ū'ler-i-thē'mă) [G. *oulē,* scar, + *erythēma,* redness of the skin]. Scarring with erythema.
u. ophryog'enes, folliculitis of the eyebrows resulting in scarring and alopecia.
u. sycosifor'me, lupoid *sycosis.*

uletic (yū-let'ik) [G. *oulē,* a scar]. Obsolete synonym for cicatricial.

uletomy (yū-let'ō-mē) [G. *oulē,* scar, + *tomē,* incision]. Obsolete synonym for cicatricotomy.

Ullman, Emerich, Hungarian surgeon, 1861–1937. See U.'s *line.*

Ullrich, Otto, German physician, 1894–1957. See Morquio-U. *disease;* Bonnevie-U. *syndrome.*

ulna, gen. and pl. **ulnae** (ŭl'nă, ŭl'nē) [L. elbow, arm, fr. G. *ōlenē*] [NA]. Elbow bone; cubitus (2); the medial and larger of the two bones of the forearm.

ulnad (ŭl'nad) [ulna + L. *ad,* to]. In a direction toward the ulna.

ulnar (ŭl'năr). Ulnaris; relating to the ulna, or to any of the structures (artery, nerve, etc.) named from it.

ulnaris (ŭl-nā'ris) [Mod. L.] [NA]. Ulnar; relating to the ulna or to the ulnar or medial aspect of the upper limb.

ulnen (ŭl'nen) [ulna + G. *en,* in]. Relating to the ulna independent of other structures.

ulnocarpal (ŭl'nō-kar'păl). Relating to the ulna and the carpus, or to the ulnar side of the wrist.

ulnoradial (ŭl'nō-rā'dē-ăl). Relating to both ulna and radius; denoting the two articulations, ligaments, etc.

ulo-, ule-. **1** [G. *oulē,* scar]. Combining forms denoting scar or scarring. **2** [G. *oulon,* gums]. Obsolescent combining forms denoting the gums. See also gingivo-.

ulodermatitis (ū'lō-der-mă-tī'tis) [G. *oulē,* scar, + *derma,* skin, + *-itis,* inflammation]. Inflammation of the skin resulting in destruction of tissue and the formation of scars.

uloid (yū'loyd) [G. *oulē,* scar + *eidos,* resemblance]. **1.** Resembling a scar. **2.** A scarlike lesion due to a degenerative process in deeper layers of skin.

ulotomy (yū-lot'ō-mē) [G. *oulē,* scar, + *tomē,* incision]. Obsolete term for cicatricotomy.

ulotrichous (yū-lot'ri-kŭs) [G. *oulotrichos,* curly haired, fr. *oulos,* wooly, + *thrix* (*trich-*), hair]. Having curly hair. *Cf.* leiotrichous.

ultimobranchial (ŭl'ti-mō-brang'kē-ăl) [L. *ultimus,* last, + G. *branchia,* gills]. In embryology, relating to the caudal pharyngeal pouch.

ultimum moriens (ŭl'ti-mŭm mōr'ī-enz) [L. the last thing dying]. The right atrium of the heart, said to contract after the rest of the heart is still.

ultra- [L. beyond]. Prefix denoting excess, exaggeration, beyond.

ultrabrachycephalic (ŭl-tră-brak-ē-se-fal'ik). Denoting an extremely short skull, one with an index of at least 90.

ultracentrifuge (ŭl-tră-sen'-tri-fyūj). A high speed centrifuge (up to 100,000 rpm) by means of which large molecules, *e.g.,* of protein or nucleic acids, are caused to sediment at practicable rates; used for determinations of molecular weights, separation of large molecules, criteria of homogeneity of large molecules, etc.

ultracytostome (ŭl-tră-sī'tō-stōm) [ultra- + G. *kytos,* cell, + *stoma,* mouth]. Former name for micropore.

ultradian (ŭl-tră'dē-ăn) [ultra- + L. *dies,* day]. Relating to biologic variations or rhythms occurring in cycles more frequent than every 24 hours. *Cf.* circadian; infradian.

ultradolichocephalic (ŭl-tră-dol-i-kō-se-fal'ik). Denoting a very long skull, one with a cephalic index of less than 65.

ultrafilter (ŭl'tră-fil-ter). A semipermeable membrane (collodion, fish bladder, or filter paper impregnated with gels) used as a filter to separate colloids and large molecules from water and small molecules, which pass through.

ultrafiltration (ŭl'tră-fil-tră'shŭn). Filtration through a semipermeable membrane or any filter that separates colloid solutions from crystalloids or separates particles of different size in a colloid mixture.

ultraligation (ŭl-tră-lī-gā'shŭn). Ligation of a blood vessel beyond the point where a branch is given off.

ultramicroscope (ŭl-tră-mī'krō-skōp). A microscope that utilizes refracted light for visualizing objects too small for the ordinary microscope when direct light is used.

ultramicroscopic (ŭl'tră-mī-krō-skop'ik). Submicroscopic.

ultramicrotome (ŭl-tră-mī'krō-tōm). A microtome used in cutting sections 0.1 μm thick, or less, for electron microscopy.

ultramicrotomy (ŭl'tră-mī-krot'ō-mē). The cutting of ultrathin sections for electron microscopy by use of an ultramicrotome.

ultrasonic (ŭl-tră-son'ik) [ultra- + L. *sonus,* sound]. Relating to energy waves similar to those of sound but of higher frequencies (above 30,000 Hz).

ultrasonics (ŭl-tră-son'iks). The science and technology of ultrasound, its characteristics and phenomena.

ultrasonogram (ŭl-tră-son'ō-gram). Echogram; sonogram; the image obtained by ultrasonography. See also echogram.

ultrasonograph (ŭl'tră-son'ō-graf) [ultra- + L. *sonus,* sound, + G. *graphō,* to write]. Echograph; sonograph; instrument used to create an image using ultrasound in ultrasonography.

ultrasonographer (ŭl'tră-sō-nog'ră-fer). Echographer; sonographer; a person who performs and interprets ultrasonographic examinations.

ultrasonography (ŭl'tră-sō-nog'ră-fē) [ultra- + L. *sonus,* sound, + G. *graphō,* to write]. Echography; sonography; the location, measurement, or delineation of deep structures by measuring the reflection or transmission of high frequency or ultrasonic waves. See also subentries under ultrasound.
Doppler u., u. applying the Doppler effect, with frequency-shifted ultrasound reflections produced by moving targets (usually red blood cells) in the bloodstream along the ultrasound axis in direct proportion to the velocity of movement of the targets, to determine both direction and velocity of blood flow.
gray-scale u., the display of small differences in acoustical impedance as different shades of gray, thus improving the quality of the image obtained by u.
See fig. on p. 1664.

ultrasonosurgery (ŭl'tră-son-ō-ser'jer-ē). Use of ultrasound techniques to disrupt cells, tissues, or tracts, particularly in the central nervous system.

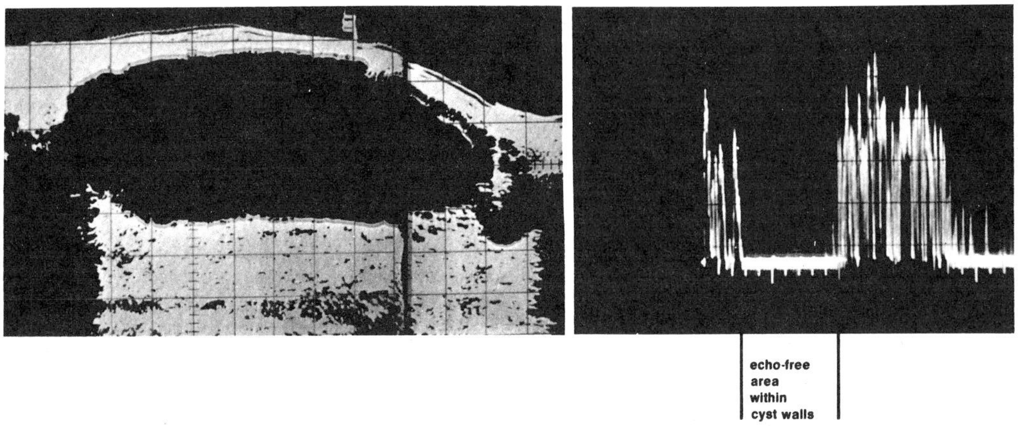

Ultrasonography

A, Image of large ovarian cyst filling most of abdominal cavity (white on black); *B*, A-mode representation of cyst.

ultrasound (ŭl'tră-sownd). Sound having a frequency greater than 30,000 Hz.
diagnostic u., the use of u. to obtain images for medical diagnostic purposes, employing frequencies ranging from 1.6 to about 10 MHz.
real-time u., the production of individual B-mode u. images rapidly, so that a moving video display results.

ultrastructure (ŭl-tră-strŭk'chŭr). Fine structure; structures or particles seen with the ultramicroscope or the electron microscope.

ultratherm (ŭl'tră-therm) [ultra- + G. *thermē*, heat]. A short-wave diathermy machine.

ultraviolet (ŭl-tră-vī'ō-let). Denoting electromagnetic rays beyond the violet end of the visible spectrum.
extravital u., having wavelengths of 2900 to 1850 Å.
intravital u., having wavelengths of 3900 to 3200 Å.
vital u., rays necessary or helpful to normal growth, promoting calcium metabolism, and antirachitic in action, having wavelengths between 3200 and 2900 Å.

ultravirus (ŭl'tră-vī'rŭs). Virus (2).

ultromotivity (ŭl'trō-mō-tiv'i-tē) [L. *ultro*, beyond, on one's own part + L. *motio*, movement]. Power of spontaneous movement.

ululation (ū-lū-lā'shŭn) [L. *ululo*, pp. *-atus*, to howl]. The inarticulate crying of emotionally disturbed persons.

umbilical (ŭm-bil'i-kăl). Omphalic; relating to the umbilicus.

umbilicate, umbilicated (ŭm-bil'i-kāt, -kāt-ed) [L. *umbilicatus*]. Of navel shape; pitlike; dimpled.

umbilication (ŭm-bil-i-kā'shŭn). **1.** A pit or navel-like depression. **2.** Formation of a depression at the apex of a papule, vesicle, or pustule.

umbilicus, pl. **umbilici** (ŭm-bil'i-kŭs, -i-sī; ŭm-bi-lī-kŭs, -lī'kī) [L. navel] [NA]. Navel; belly-button; the pit in the center of the abdominal wall marking the point where the umbilical cord entered in the fetus.

umbo, gen. **umbonis,** pl. **umbones** (ŭm'bō, -bō-nis, -bō-nēs) [L. boss of a shield, a knob] [NA]. A projecting point of a surface.
u. membra'nae tym'pani [NA], the projection on the inner surface of the tympanic membrane at the end of the manubrium of the malleus; this corresponds to the most depressed point of the membrane, viewed laterally, that is commonly called the umbo.

UMP Abbreviation for *uridine* phosphate.

un- [M.E.]. **1.** Prefix meaning not, akin to L. *in-* and G. *a-*, *an-*. **2.** Prefix denoting reversal, removal, release, deprivation. **3.** Prefix expressing an intensive action.

uncal (ŭng'kăl). Denoting or relating to the uncus.

unci (ŭn'sī). Plural of uncus.

uncia (ŭn'sē-ă) [L. a twelfth part, an ounce]. An ounce.

unciform (ŭn'si-fōrm) [L. *uncus*, hook, + *forma*, form]. Uncinate.

unciforme (ŭn-si-fōr'mē) [Mod. L. unciform]. *Os* hamatum.

Uncinaria (ŭn-si-nar'ē-ă) [LL. *uncinus*, a hook]. A genus of nematode hookworms that infect various mammals. Species include *U. stenocephala*, the European hookworm of dogs, cats, and various wild carnivores, also found in North America, where it is much less common than *Ancylostoma caninum*, though it has been implicated in human cutaneous larva migrans.

uncinariasis (ŭn'si-nă-rī'ă-sis). Ancylostomiasis.

uncinate (ŭn'si-nāt) [L. *uncinatus*]. **1.** Unciform; hooklike or hook-shaped. **2.** Relating to an uncus or, specifically, to the u. gyrus (2).

uncinatum (ŭn-si-nā'tŭm). *Os* hamatum.

uncipressure (ŭn'si-presh-ŭr) [L. *uncus*, hook]. Arrest of hemorrhage from a cut artery by pressure with a blunt hook.

uncomplemented (ŭn-kom'plĕ-men-ted) Not united with complement and therefore inactive.

unconscious (ŭn-kon'shŭs). **1.** Insensible (1); not conscious. **2.** In psychoanalysis, the psychic structure comprising the drives and feelings of which one is unaware.
collective u., in jungian psychology, the combined engrams or memory potentials inherited from an individual's phylogenetic past.

unconsciousness (ŭn-kon'shŭs-ness). A state of impaired consciousness in which the individual shows a total lack of responsiveness to environmental stimuli; such an individual may respond to deep pain with involuntary movements.

unco-ossified (ŭn-kō-os'i-fīd). Not co-ossified; not united into one bone.

uncouplers (ŭn-kŭp'lerz). Substances such as dinitrophenol that allow oxidation in mitochondria to proceed without the usual concomitant phosphorylation to produce ATP; these poisons thus "uncouple" oxidation and phosphorylation.

uncovertebral (ŭn-kō-ver'tĕ-brăl). Pertaining to or affecting the uncinate process of a vertebra.

unction (ŭngk'shŭn) [L. *unctio*, fr. *ungo*, pp. *unctus*, to anoint]. The action of anointing or rubbing with an ointment or oil.

unctuous (ŭngk'shū-ŭs, -chū-ŭs) [L. *unctuosus,* fr. *unctio,* unction]. Greasy or oily.

uncture (ŭnk'chūr). Ointment.

uncus, pl. **unci** (ŭn'kŭs, ŭn'sī) [L. a hook, fr. G. *onkos*]. [NA]. **1.** Any hook-shaped process or structure. **2.** Uncinate gyrus; u. gyri parahippocampalis; the anterior, hooked extremity of the parahippocampal gyrus on the basomedial surface of the temporal lobe; the anterior face of the u. corresponds to the olfactory cortex, its ventral surface to the entorhinal area; deep to the uncus lies the amygdala (corpus amygdaloideum).
u. gy'ri parahippocampa'lis, u. (2).

undecenoic acid (ŭn'des-ĕ-nō'ik). Undecylenic acid.

undecoylium chloride (ŭn-de-kō-il'ē-ŭm). Acylcolaminoformylmethylpyridinium chloride; a topical antiseptic.

undecoylium chloride-iodine. A complex of iodine with undecoylium chloride; a cationic detergent used topically as a germicidal agent.

undecylenate (ŭn-des'i-li-nāt). A salt of undecylenic acid.

undecylenic acid (ŭn-des-i-len'ik). Undecenoic acid; $CH_2CH(CH_2)_8COOH$; an acid present in small amounts in sweat; used with its zinc salt in ointments, or as a powder in the treatment of fungus diseases of the skin, psoriasis, and certain other cutaneous affections.

underachievement (ŭn'der-ă-chēv'ment). Failure to achieve as well as one's abilities would seem to allow.

underachiever (ŭn'der-ă-chēv'er). One who manifests underachievement.

underbite (ŭn'der-bīt). A nontechnical term applied to mandibular underdevelopment or to excessive maxillary development.

undercut (ŭn'der-kŭt). **1.** That portion of a tooth that lies between the survey line (height of contour) and the gingivae. **2.** The contour of a cross-section of a residual ridge or dental arch which would prevent the insertion of a denture. **3.** The contour of a flasking stone which interlocks in such a way as to prevent the separation of the parts.

underdrive pacing (ŭn'der-drīv pās'ing). Electrical stimulation of the heart at a rate lower than that of an existing tachycardia; designed to capture the heart between beats, *i.e.,* to interrupt a reentry pathway in order to terminate the tachycardia.

underhorn (ŭn'der-hōrn). *Cornu* inferius.

undernutrition (ŭn'der-nū-tri'shŭn). A form of malnutrition resulting from a reduced supply of food or from inability to digest, assimilate, and utilize the necessary nutrients.

undershoot (ŭn'der-shūt). A temporary decrease below the final steady-state value that may occur immediately following the removal of an influence that had been raising that value, *i.e.,* overshoot in a negative direction.

underventilation (ŭn'der-ven-ti-lā'shŭn). Hypoventilation.

Underwood, Michael, English pediatrician, 1737–1820. See U.'s *disease.*

undifferentiated (ŭn'dif-er-en'shē-ā-ted). Not differentiated; *e.g.,* primitive, embryonic, immature, or having no special structure or function.

undine (ŭn'dēn, -dīn) [Mod. L. *undina,* fr. L. *unda,* wave]. A small glass flask used in irrigation of the conjunctiva.

undinism (ŭn'di-nizm) [Mod. L. *undina,* fr. L. *unda,* wave]. A condition in which sexual thoughts are aroused by water, urine, and urination.

undiversion (ŭn-di-ver'shŭn). Surgical restoration of continuity in any organ system, the flow through which had previously been diverted; *e.g.,* between the upper urinary tract and bladder after supravesical urinary diversion.

undoing (ŭn-dū'ing). In psychology and psychiatry, an unconscious defense mechanism by which one symbolically acts out in reverse some earlier unacceptable behavior.

undulate (ŭn'dū-lāt) [Mod. L. *undula,* dim. of *unda,* wave]. Having an irregular, wavy border; denoting the shape of a bacterial colony.

undulipodium, pl. **undulipodia** (ŭn'dū-li-pō'dē-um, -ă) [L. *undul,* waving, + *podium,* foot]. A flexible whiplike intracellular extension of many eukaryotic cells, with a characteristic nine-fold symmetry, an arrangement of nine paired peripheral microtubules and one central pair, often termed 9 + 2 symmetry; it appears to grow out from a basal body (kinetosome) in the cell and is a fundamental component of the eukaryotic cell. Both the cilium and the eukaryotic flagellum (not the bacterial flagellum which lacks the 9 + 2 pattern) are considered u.

ung. Abbreviation of L. *unguentum,* ointment.

ungual (ŭng'gwăl) [L. *unguis,* nail]. Unguinal; relating to a nail or the nails.

unguent (ŭng'gwent) [L. *unguentum*] Ointment.

ungues (ŭng'gwēz). Plural of unguis.

Unguiculata (ŭng-gwik-yū-lā'tă) [L. *unguiculus,* nail or claw]. A division of Mammalia including all mammals having nails or claws, as distinguished from the Ungulata.

unguiculate (ŭng-gwik'yū-lāt). Having nails or claws, as distinguished from hooves.

unguiculus (ŭn-gwik'yū-lŭs) [L. dim. of *unguis,* nail]. A small nail or claw.

unguinal (ŭng'gwi-năl). Ungual.

unguis, pl. **ungues** (ŭng'gwis, -gwēz) [L.] [NA]. Onyx; nail plate; nail (1); one of the thin, horny, translucent plates covering the dorsal surface of the distal end of each terminal phalanx of fingers and toes. A nail consists of corpus or body, the visible part, and radix or root at the proximal end concealed under a fold of skin. The under part of the nail is formed from the stratum germinativum of the epidermis, the free surface from the stratum lucidum, the thin cuticular fold overlapping the lunula representing the stratum corneum.

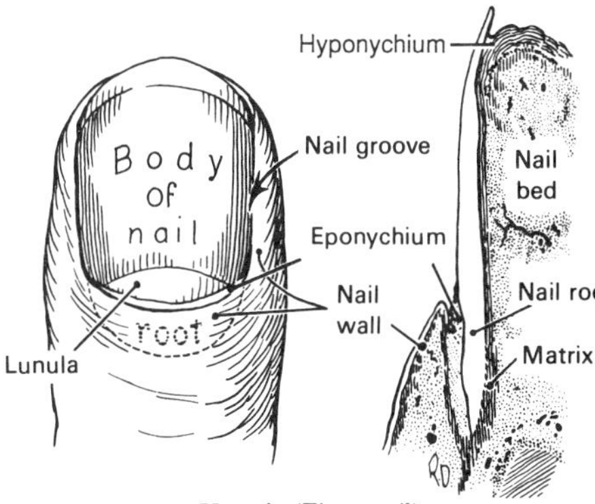

Unguis (Fingernail)

u. adun'cus, ingrown *nail.*
u. a'vis, *calcar* avis.
Haller's u., *calcar* avis.
u. incarna'tus, ingrown *nail.*

Ungulata (ŭng-gyū-lā'tă). A division of Mammalia containing the mammals with hooves, as distinguished from the Unguiculata.

ungulate (ŭng'gyū-lāt) [L. *ungulatus,* fr. *ungula,* hoof]. Having hooves.

unguligrade (ŭng'gyū-li-grād) [L. *ungula,* a hoof, + *gradus,* a step]. Walking on hooves, as by horses, pigs, and ruminants.

uni- [L. *unus,* one]. Prefix denoting one, single, not paired; corresponds to G. *mono-.*

uniarticular (yū-nē-ar-tik′yū-lăr). Monarticular.

uniaxial (yū-nēak′sē-ăl). Having but one axis; growing chiefly in one direction.

unibasal (yū-ni-bā′săl). Having but one base.

Uniblue A (yū′nē-blū) [C.I. 14553]. A protein stain used in electrophoresis.

unicameral, unicamerate (yū-nē-kam′ĕ-răl, -kam′ĕ-rāt). Monolocular.

unicellular (yū-ni-sel′yū-lăr). Composed of but one cell, as in the protozoons; for such u. organisms capable of undertaking life processes independently of other cells, the term acellular is also used.

unicentral (yū-ni-sen′trăl). Having a single center, as of growth or of ossification.

unicorn (yū′nē-kōrn). Unicornous.

unicornous (yū′ni-kōr′nŭs) [L. *unicornis,* fr. uni- + *cornu,* horn]. Unicorn; having but one horn, or cornu.

unicuspid, unicuspidate (yū-ni-kŭs′pid, -kŭs′pi-dāt). Having only one cusp, as a canine tooth.

unifamilial (yū′nē-fa-mil′ē-ăl). Relating to or occurring in a single family; denoting especially a nervous disease attacking several of the children in the same family in which no hereditary trait is apparent.

uniflagellate (yū-ni-flaj′ĕ-lāt). Monotrichous.

uniforate (yū-ni-fō′rāt). Having but one foramen, pore, or opening of any kind.

uniform (yū′ni-fōrm) [L. *uniformis,* fr. uni- + *forma,* form]. **1.** Having but one form; not variable in form. **2.** Of the same form or shape as another structure or object.

unigerminal (yū-ni-jer′mi-năl). Monogerminal; relating to a single germ or ovum.

uniglandular (yū-ni-glan′dū-lăr). Involving, relating to, or containing but one gland.

unilaminar, unilaminate (yū-ni-lam′i-năr, -lam′i-nāt). Having but one layer or lamina.

unilateral (yū-ni-lat′ĕ-răl). Confined to one side only.

unilobar (yū-ni-lō′băr). Having but one lobe.

unilocal (yū-ni-lō′kăl). Strictly, denoting a trait in which the genetic component is contributed exclusively by one locus; in practice, any trait in which the contribution from one locus is so large that the data are readily interpreted as mendelian.

unilocular (yū-ni-lok′yū-lăr) [uni- + L. *loculus,* compartment]. Having but one compartment or cavity, as in a fat cell.

unimolecular (yū′ni-mō-lek′yū-lăr). Monomolecular.

uninuclear, uninucleate (yū-ni-nū′klē-ăr, -nū′klē-āt). Having but one nucleus; *Cf.* mononuclear.

uniocular (yū-ni-ok′yū-lăr). **1.** Relating to one eye only. **2.** Having vision in only one eye.

union (yūn′yŭn) [L. *unus,* one]. **1.** The joining or amalgamation of two or more bodies. **2.** The structural adhesion or growing together of the edges of a wound.

autogenous u., in dentistry, the u. of two pieces of metal without solder.

faulty u., u. of fracture by fibrous tissue, without bone formation.

fibrous u., a persisting fibrous callus forming between fractured bone.

primary u., *healing* by first intention.

secondary u., *healing* by second intention.

vicious u., u. of the ends of a broken bone resulting in a deformity or a crooked limb; frequently used interchangeably with faulty u.

unioval, uniovular (yū-nē-ō′văl, -ov′yū-lăr). Relating to or formed from a single ovum.

unipennate (yū-ni-pen′āt) [uni- + L. *penna,* feather]. Demipenniform. **1.** Having a feather arrangement on one side; resembling one-half of a feather. **2.** Denoting certain muscles with fibers running at an acute angle from one side of a tendon.

unipolar (yū-ni-pō′lăr). **1.** Having but one pole; denoting a nerve cell from which the branches project from one side only. **2.** Situated at one extremity only of a cell.

uniport (yū′ni-pōrt) [uni- + L. *porto,* to carry]. Transport of a molecule or ion through a membrane by a carrier mechanism (uniporter), without known coupling to any other molecule or ion transport. *Cf.* antiport; symport.

uniporter (yū′ni-pōrt-er). A carrier mechanism that transports one molecule or ion through a membrane without known coupling to the transport of any other molecule or ion.

uniseptate (yū-ni-sep′tāt). Having but one septum or partition.

UNIT

unit (yū′nit) [L. *unus,* one]. **1.** One; a single person or thing. **2 (U).** A standard of measure, weight, or any other quality, by multiplications or fractions of which a scale or system is formed. **3.** A group of persons or things considered as a whole because of mutual activities or functions.

absolute u., a u. whose value is constant regardless of place or time.

alexin u., complement u.

Allen-Doisy u., mouse u.; the quantity of estrogen capable of producing in a spayed mouse a characteristic change in the vaginal epithelium, namely, disappearance of leukocytes and appearance of cornified cells, as determined by a vaginal smear; equal approximately to one-half of an estrone u.

alpha u.'s, cytoplasmic glycogen granules arranged in rosettes.

amboceptor u., hemolysin u.

androgen u. (international), the androgenic activity of 100 μg (0.1 mg) of crystalline androsterone as assayed by the comb growth response in capons.

Ångström u. (Å), see angstrom.

antigen u., the smallest amount of antigen that, in the presence of specific antiserum, will fix 1 complement u.

antitoxin u., standard antitoxin u.; a u. expressing the strength or activity of an antitoxin; in general, determined with reference to a preserved standard preparation of antitoxin. See also L *doses.*

antivenene u., the amount of antivenene which, injected in the ear vein, will protect 1 g weight of rabbit against a fatal dose of snake venom.

atomic mass u. (amu), a u. of mass by definition equal to $^{1}/_{12}$ of the mass of an atom of carbon-12, which equals $1.660{,}53 \times 10^{-27}$kg; in terms of energy, 1 amu equals 931 MeV.

base u.'s, the fundamental u.'s of length, mass, time, electric current, thermodynamic temperature, amount of substance, and luminous intensity in the International System of Units (SI); the names and symbols of the u.'s for these quantities are meter (m), kilogram (kg), second (s), ampere (A), kelvin (K), mole (mol), and candela (cd). See also International System of Units.

Bethesda u. [*Bethesda,* MD], a measure of inhibitor activity: the amount of inhibitor that will inactivate 50% or 0.5 unit of a coagulation factor during the incubation period.

biological standard u., a specific quantity of biologically active reference material (antibiotic, antitoxin, enzyme, hormone, vitamin, etc.) usually dried and stored in a central place in an atmo-

sphere of nitrogen, in the dark at −10°C.
bird u., a u. of prolactin activity: the minimal quantity of the hormone which will cause a certain increase in weight of the crop gland of pigeons.
Bodansky u., that amount of phosphatase that liberates 1 mg of phosphorus as inorganic phosphate during the first hour of incubation with a buffered substrate containing sodium β-glycerophosphate.
British thermal u. (BTU), the quantity of heat required to raise one pound of water from 3.9°C to 4.4°C; equal to 252 calories.
cat u., the dose of a drug (per kilogram of body weight of cat) which is just large enough to kill a cat when administered intravenously.
centimeter-gram-second (CGS, cgs) u., an absolute u. of the centimeter-gram-second system.
chlorophyll u., the number of chlorophyll molecules required to reduce one molecule of carbon dioxide by photosynthesis.
chorionic gonadotropin u. (international), the specific gonadotropic activity of 0.1 mg of the standard preparation of chorionic gonadotropin originating from the urine or placenta of pregnant women.
Clauberg u., see Clauberg *test*.
complement u., alexin u.; the smallest amount (highest dilution) of complement that will cause solution of the u. quantity of red blood cells in the presence of a hemolysin u.
Corner-Allen u., a u. of progestational activity, measured in rabbits; the minimum dose which, divided into five equal daily portions, produces on the sixth day the uterine changes characteristic of the eighth day of normal pregnancy; the u. has about the same potency as the international u.
coronary care u. (CCU), a group of beds within a hospital set aside for the care of patients having or suspected of having myocardial infarction.
corpus luteum hormone u., progesterone u. (international).
critical care u. (CCU), intensive care u.
CT u., an arbitrary index of x-ray attenuation in each pictured element of the CT image.
Dam u., a u. of activity of vitamin K; the smallest amount of vitamin K, per gram of chick per day, capable of producing normal coagulability in the blood of K-avitaminotic chicks after 3 days of oral administration.
digitalis u. (international), the activity of 0.1 g of the international standard powdered digitalis.
diphtheria antitoxin u., the antitoxin activity of 0.0628 mg standard diphtheria antitoxin.
dog u., the amount of adrenal cortical extract per kilogram of body weight which, given daily, will maintain an adrenalectomized dog in good condition for 7 to 10 days.
electromagnetic u. (emu), the u. in an absolute system (CGS) of u.'s utilizing the magnetic effects of current; *e.g.,* abampere, abfarad, abhenry, abohm, abvolt.
electrostatic u. (esu), the u. in an absolute system (CGS) of u.'s utilizing static electricity; *e.g.,* statampere, statcoulomb, statfarad, stathenry, statvolt.
u. of energy, **(1)** CGS system: erg, joule; **(2)** MKS system: newton-meter; **(3)** FPS system: foot-poundal; **(4)** gravitational u.: gram-centimeter, gram-meter, kilogram-meter, foot-pound; **(5)** SI: joule.
equine gonadotropin u. (international), the specific gonadotropic activity of 0.25 mg of standard preparation of the gonadotropic principle of pregnant mares' serum.
estradiol benzoate u. (international), the estrogenic activity of 0.1 μg of a standard preparation of estradiol benzoate.
estrone u. (international), the estrogenic activity of 0.1 μg (0.0001 mg) of a standard preparation of crystalline estrone.
Fishman-Lerner u., a u. of serum acid phosphatase activity based upon measurement of the amount of phenol released from a phenylphosphate substrate.
Florey u., Oxford u.
foot-pound-second (FPS, fps) u., an absolute u. of the foot-pound-second system.
u. of force, **(1)** CGS system: dyne; **(2)** FPS system: poundal; **(3)** MKS system: newton; **(4)** SI: newton.
G u. of streptomycin, see streptomycin u.'s.
gravitational u.'s (G), of energy: gram-centimeter, gram-meter, kilogram-meter, and foot-pound.
Hampson u., an obsolete u. of x-ray measurement, equal to $^1/_4$ erythema dose.
u. of heat, **(1)** calorie (gram calorie; kilocalorie); **(2)** British thermal u.; **(3)** joule.
hemolysin u., hemolytic u., amboceptor u.; the smallest quantity (highest dilution) of inactivated immune serum (hemolysin) that will sensitize the standard suspension of erythrocytes so that the standard complement will cause complete hemolysis.
heparin u., Howell u.; the quantity of heparin required to keep 1 ml of cat's blood fluid for 24 hr at 0°C; it is equivalent approximately to 0.002 mg of pure heparin.
Holzknecht u. (H), an obsolete u. of x-ray dosage equal to one-fifth of the erythema dose.
Hounsfield u., an arbitrary index of x-ray attenuation based on a scale of −1000 (air) to +1000 (bone), with water being 0; used in CT imaging.
Howell u., heparin u.
insulin u. (international), the activity contained in $^1/_{22}$ mg of the international standard of zinc-insulin crystals.
intensive care u. (ICU), critical care u.; a hospital facility for provision of intensive care of critically ill patients, characterized by high quality and quantity of continuous nursing and medical supervision and by use of sophisticated monitoring and resuscitative equipment; may be organized for the care of specific patient groups, *e.g.,* neonatal or, newborn ICU, neurological ICU.
u. of intermedin, a u. based upon the action of the hormone in causing the expansion of the melanophores in a hypophysectomized frog; equal to 1 μg of alkali-treated USP Posterior-pituitary Reference Standard.
international u. (IU), the amount of a substance, such as a drug, hormone, vitamin, etc., that produces a specific effect as defined by an international body and accepted internationally.
International System of Units (SI), see at International.
Jenner-Kay u., that amount of phosphatase that liberates 1 mg of phosphorus; approximately 2 Bodansky u.'s or 1 King u.
Karmen u., a formerly used enzyme u. for aminotransferase activity; a change of 0.001 in the absorbance of NADH/min.
Kienböck's u. (X), an obsolete u. of x-ray dosage equivalent to $^1/_{10}$ the erythema dose.
King u., King-Armstrong u.; the quantity of phosphatase that, acting upon disodium phenylphosphate in excess, at pH 9 for 30 min, liberates 1 mg of phenol.
King-Armstrong u., King u.
L u. of streptomycin, see streptomycin u.'s.
u. of length, **(1)** metric system and SI: meter; **(2)** CGS system: centimeter; **(3)** variable in the English system: inch for short distances, foot for moderate distances and for elevation, mile for long distances.
u. of light, see candela; footcandle; lumen; lux.
u. of luminous flux, see lumen.
u. of luminous intensity, see candela.
lung u., **(1)** a respiratory bronchiole together with the alveolar ducts and sacs and pulmonary alveoli into which the respiratory bronchiole leads; **(2)** considered by some to include the terminal bronchiole and its subdivisions, and called a pulmonary *acinus*.
u. of luteinizing activity (international), progesterone u. (international).
Mache u. (M.u.) in German, Mache Einheit (M.E.), obsolete u. of

measure of radium emanation.
u. of magnetic field intensity, see gauss; oersted; tesla.
u. of mass, **(1)** metric system: gram; **(2)** SI: kilogram; **(3)** English system: pound.
meter-kilogram-second (MKS, mks) u., an absolute u. of the meter-kilogram-second system.
motor u., a single somatic motor neuron and the group of muscle fibers innervated by it.
mouse u. (m.u.), Allen-Doisy u.
u. of ocular convergence, meter *angle.*
Oxford u., Florey u.; the minimum amount of penicillin which will prevent the growth of *Staphylococcus aureus* over an area 26 mm in diameter in a standard culture medium; 1 u. equals 0.6 μg of crystalline sodium salt of penicillin.
u. of oxytocin, the oxytocic activity of 0.5 mg of the USP Posterior-pituitary Reference Standard; 1 mg of synthetic oxytocin corresponds to 500 IU.
pantothenic acid u., filtrate factor u., measured in milligrams of the synthetic substance.
u. of penicillin, the penicillin activity of 0.6 μg of penicillin G.
phosphatase u., see Bodansky u.; Jenner-Kay u.; King u.
physiologic u., **(1)** the ultimate (hypothetical) vital u. of protoplasm, as conceived by Spencer; **(2)** the smallest division of an organ that will perform its function; *e.g.,* the renal nephron.
practical u.'s, u.'s of magnitudes convenient for use in the practical applications of electricity; as originally defined they were absolute u.'s (multiples of CGS electromagnetic u.'s); they include the ampere, coulomb, farad, henry, joule, ohm, volt, and watt.
u. of progestational activity (international), see progesterone u.
progesterone u. (international), corpus luteum hormone u.; u. of luteinizing activity (international); the progestational activity of 1 mg of u. of progestational activity (international); standard preparation of pure progesterone. See also Clauberg *test;* Corner-Allen u.
prolactin u. (international), the specific lactogenic activity contained in 0.1 mg of the standard preparation of the lactogenic substance of the anterior pituitary gland.
u. of radioactivity, see becquerel; curie; roentgen; Mache u.; uranium u.
riboflavin u., vitamin B_2 u.; potency usually expressed in terms of weight of pure riboflavin.
roentgen u., see roentgen.
S u. of streptomycin, see streptomycin u.'s.
Sherman u., u. of vitamin C, minimum protective dose; the minimum amount of vitamin C which, fed daily, will protect a 300-g guinea pig from scurvy for 90 days; equivalent to 0.5 to 0.6 mg of ascorbic acid.
Sherman-Bourquin u. of vitamin B_2, the amount of vitamin B_2 (G) required in the diet daily to sustain an average weekly gain of 3 g for 8 weeks in standard test rats; one u. is equivalent to 1 to 7 μg (0.001 to 0.007 mg) of riboflavin, depending on the deficiency diet used in the above assay.
Sherman-Munsell u., a rat growth u.; the daily amount of vitamin A which sustains a rate of gain amounting to 3 g a week in standard test rats.
SI u.'s, see base u.'s; International System of Units.
Somogyi u., a measure of the level of activity of amylase in blood serum, as analyzed by means of the Somogyi method (the most frequently used procedure); one u. is equivalent to 1 mg of reducing sugar liberated as glucose per 100 ml of serum, when an aliquot of the latter is mixed with a standard starch substrate (plus sodium chloride for maximal activation) and incubated for a standard time; normal range is 80 to 150 u.'s, but values are usually not regarded as clinically significant unless they are greater than 200 u.'s.
Steenbock u., a u. of vitamin D; the total amount of vitamin D which will produce within 10 days a narrow line of calcium deposit in the rachitic metaphyses of the distal ends of the radii and ulnae of standard rachitic rats.
streptomycin u.'s, **(1)** G u.: equals 1 g of the crystalline material or about 1,000,000 S u.'s; **(2)** L u.: equal to 1000 S u.'s; **(3)** S u.: the amount of streptomycin which will inhibit the growth of a standard strain of *Escherichia coli* in 1 ml of nutrient broth or other suitable medium.
Svedberg u. (S), a sedimentation constant of 1×10^{-13} seconds.
tetanus antitoxin u., the antitoxin activity of 0.3094 mg of standard tetanus antitoxin.
thiamin chloride u., thiamin hydrochloride u. (international).
thiamin hydrochloride u. (international), vitamin B_1 hydrochloride u.; thiamin chloride u.; the antineuritic activity of 0.003 mg of the standard crystalline vitamin B_1 hydrochloride.
u. of thyrotrophic activity, the activity of an amount of an extract of the anterior lobe of the hypophysis which, given daily for 5 days, will cause the thyroid of a guinea pig (weighing 200 g) to reach a weight of 600 mg.
toxic u., toxin u. (T.U.), a u. formerly synonymous with minimal lethal dose but which, because of the unstability of toxins, is now measured in terms of the quantity of standard antitoxin with which the toxin combines. See also L *doses,* minimal lethal *dose.*
uranium u., obsolete u. for the measurement of radioactivity, that of uranium being taken as 1.
USP u., a u. as defined and adopted by the *United States Pharmacopeia.*
u. of vasopressin, the pressor activity of 0.5 mg of the USP Posterior-pituitary Reference Standard; 1 mg of synthetic vasopressin corresponds to 600 IU.
vitamin A u. (international), the specific biologic activity of 0.3 μg of vitamin A (alcohol form). See also Sherman-Munsell u.
vitamin B_1 hydrochloride u., thiamin hydrochloride u.
vitamin B_2 u., riboflavin u. See also Sherman-Bourquin u. of vitamin B_2.
vitamin B_6 u., potency expressed in terms of weight of pure crystalline pyridoxine.
vitamin C u. (international), the vitamin C activity of 0.05 mg of the standard crystalline levoascorbic acid; 1 mg of crystalline vitamin C provides 20 USP u.'s. See also Sherman u.
vitamin D u. (international), the antirachitic activity contained in 0.025 μg of a preparation of crystalline vitamin D_3 (activated 7-dehydrocholesterol). See also Steenbock u.
vitamin E u., potency usually expressed in terms of weight of pure α-tocopherol.
vitamin K u., see Dam u.
volume u. (VU), a u. of a logarithmic scale for expressing the power level of a complex audio-frequency electrical signal, such as that transmitting music or speech; the power in volume u.'s equals the decibels of power above a reference level of one milliwatt, as measured with an appropriate meter.
u. of wavelength, see angstrom; nanometer.
u. of weight, see u. of mass.
u. of work, see u. of energy.

United States Adopted Names (USAN). Designation for nonproprietary names (for drugs) adopted by the USAN Council in cooperation with the manufacturers concerned; the designation USAN is applicable only to nonproprietary names coined since June 1961.

United States Pharmacopeia (USP). See Pharmacopeia.

United States Public Health Service (USPHS). A bureau of the U.S. Department of Health and Human Services, served by a corps of medical officers presided over by the Surgeon General, concerned with scientific research, domestic and insular quarantine, administration of government hospitals, publication of sanitary reports, and statistics; associated with it are the National Institutes of Health, Centers for Disease Control, and other units.

univalence, univalency (yū-ni-vā'lens, -vā'len-sē). Monovalence.

univalent (yū-ni-vā'lent). Monovalent (1).

unmedullated (ŭn-med'yū-lā-ted). Unmyelinated.

unmyelinated (ŭn-mī'ĕ-li-nā-ted). Amyelinated; amyelinic; nonmyelinated; unmedullated; nonmedullated; denoting nerve fibers (axons) lacking a myelin sheath.

Unna, Paul G., German dermatologist and staining expert, 1850–1929. See U.'s *disease, mark, stain;* U.-Pappenheim *stain;* U.-Taenzer *stain.*

unofficial (ŭn-ŏ-fish'ăl). Denoting a drug that is not listed in the *United States Pharmacopeia* or the *National Formulary.*

unphysiologic (ŭn-fis'ē-ō-loj'ik). Pertaining to conditions in the organism which are abnormal; can be used to refer to subjecting the body to abnormal amounts of substances normally present.

unsanitary (ŭn-san'i-tār-ē). Insanitary.

unsaturated (ŭn-sach'ŭr-āt-ed). **1.** Not saturated; denoting a solution in which the solvent is capable of dissolving more of the solute. **2.** Denoting a chemical compound in which all the affinities are not satisfied, so that still other atoms or radicals may be added to it. **3.** In organic chemistry, denoting compounds containing double and triple bonds.

unsex (ŭn'seks). To castrate; to deprive of the gonads.

unsoundness (ŭn-sownd'nes). In a horse, any deviation in form or function from the normal that interferes with the animal's usefulness.

unstriated (ŭn-strī'āt-ed). Without striations; not striped; denoting the structure of the smooth or involuntary muscles.

unthrifty (ŭn-thrif'tē). In animals, denoting a failure to grow or develop normally as a result of disease.

Unverricht, Heinrich, German physician, 1853–1912. See U.'s *disease.*

up-regulation. Opposite of down-regulation.

upsiloid (ŭp'si-loyd). Hypsiloid.

uptake (ŭp'tāk). The absorption by a tissue of some substance, food material, mineral, etc. and its permanent or temporary retention.

urachal (yūr'ă-kăl). Relating to the urachus.

urachus (yūr'ă-kŭs) [G. *ourachos,* the urinary canal of a fetus]. That portion of the reduced allantoic stalk between the apex of the bladder and the umbilicus; postnatally, the u. is normally merely a fibrous cord, but occasionally the old allantoic lumen may persist as a vesicoumbilical fistula.

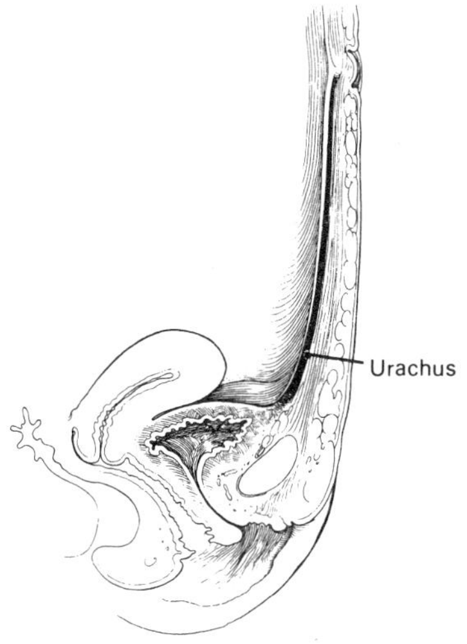

Urachus

uracil (yūr'ă-sil). 2,4-Dioxopyrimidine; 2,4-(1*H*,3*H*)-pyrimidinedione; a pyrimidine (base) present in ribonucleic acid.

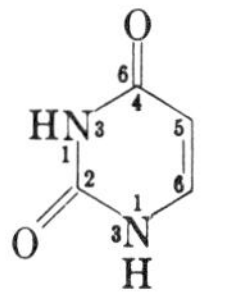

Uracil

Inner numbering, official international (IUPAC); *outer numbering,* original Fisher (abandoned).

u. dehydrogenase [EC 1.2.99.1], u. oxidase; an oxidoreductase catalyzing oxidation of uracil to barbituric acid; also oxidizes thymine.

u. mustard, uramustine; 5-[bis(2-chloroethyl)amino]uracil; an alkylating antineoplastic agent.

u. oxidase, u. dehydrogenase.

Uragoga (yūr'ă-gō-gă). *Cephaelis;* a genus of tropical plants (family Rubiaceae). *U. ipecacuanha (Cephaelis ipecacuanha)* is the source of Rio or Brazilian ipecac; *U. acuminata (C. acuminata)* is the source of Cartagena, Nicaragua, or Panama ipecac.

uragogue (yūr'ă-gog) [G. *ouron,* urine, + *agōgos,* drawing forth]. Obsolete term for diuretic (2).

uramustine (yūr-ă-mŭs'tēn). *Uracil* mustard.

uranin (yū'ră-nin). *Fluorescein* sodium.

uraninite (yū-ran'i-nīt). Pitchblende.

uranisco-. See urano-.

uraniscochasm (yū-ră-nis'kō-kazm) [uranisco- + G. *chasma,* cleft]. Uranoschisis.

uranisconitis (yū'ră-nis-kō-nī'tis). Palatitis.

uraniscoplasty (yū'ră-nis'kō-plas-tē) [uranisco- + G. *plassō,* to form]. Palatoplasty.

uraniscorrhaphy (yū'ră-nis-kōr'ă-fē) [uranisco- + G. *rhaphē,* suture]. Palatorrhaphy.

uraniscus (yū'ră-nis'kŭs) [G. *ouraniskos,* roof of the mouth, dim. of *ouranos,* sky]. Palatum.

uranium (yū-rā'nē-ŭm) [G. myth. character, *Uranus*]. A feebly radioactive metallic element, symbol U, atomic no. 92, atomic weight 238.03, occurring mainly in pitchblende and notable for its two isotopes: U-238 and U-235 (in 993:7 ratio), the latter of which was the first substance ever shown capable of supporting a self-sustaining chain reaction.

urano-, uranisco- [G. *ouranos,* sky vault, *ouraniskos,* roof of mouth (palate)]. Combining forms relating to the hard palate.

uranoplasty (yū'ră-nō-plas-tē). Palatoplasty.

uranorrhaphy (yū'ră-nōr'ă-fē) [urano- + G. *raphē,* suture]. Palatorrhaphy.

uranoschisis (yū'ră-nos'ki-sis) [urano- + G. *schisis,* fissure]. Uraniscochasm; cleft of the hard palate.

uranostaphyloplasty (yū'ră-nō-staf'i-lō-plas-tē)[urano- G. + *staphylē,* uvula, + *plassō,* to form]. Uranostaphylorrhaphy; repair of a cleft of both hard and soft palate.

uranostaphylorrhaphy (yū'ră-nō-staf-i-lōr'ă-fē). Uranostaphyloplasty.

uranostaphyloschisis (yū'ră-nō-staf'i-los'ki-sis) [urano- + G. *staphylē,* uvula, + *schisis,* fissure]. Uranoveloschisis; cleft of the soft and hard palates.

uranoveloschisis (yū'ră-nō-vē-los'ki-sis). Uranostaphyloschisis.

uranyl (yūr'ă-nil) The ion, UO_2^{2+} usually found in such salts as uranyl nitrate, $UO_2(NO_3)_2$.

urari (yū-rah'rē). Curare.

uraroma (yū'ră-rō'mă) [G. *ouron*, urine, + *arōma*, spice]. A spicy aromatic odor of the urine.

urarthritis (yū-rar-thrī'tis) [urate + arthritis]. Gouty inflammation of a joint.

urate (yūr'āt). A salt of uric acid.
u. oxidase [EC 1.7.3.3], uricase; an oxygen-requiring oxidoreductase that oxidizes uric acid.

uratemia (yū-rā-tē'mē-ă) [urate + G. *haima*, blood]. The presence of urates, especially sodium urate, in the blood.

urateribonucleotide phosphorylase (yūr'āt-rī-bō-nū'klē-ō-tīd) [EC 2.4.2.16]. A ribosyltransferase that phosphorylyzes urateribonucleotide to urate plus D-ribose 1-phosphate.

uratic (yū-rat'ik). Pertaining to a urate or to urates.

uratolysis (yū-rā-tol'i-sis) [urate + G. *lysis*, solution]. The decomposition or solution of urates.

uratolytic (yū'rā-tō-lit'ik). Causing the decomposition, or solution and removal of urates, from the tissues.

uratoma (yū-ră-tō'mă) [urate + G. *-oma*, tumor]. Gouty *tophus.*

uratosis (yū-rā-tō'sis). Any morbid condition due to the presence of urates in the blood or tissues.

uraturia (yū-rā-tū'rē-ă) [urate + G. *ouron*, urine]. The passage of an increased amount of urates in the urine.

Urbach, Erich, U.S. dermatologist, 1893-1946. See U.-Wiethe disease.

Urban, Jerome A., U.S. surgeon, *1914. See U.'s *operation.*

urceiform (yūr-sē'i-fōrm) [L. *urceus*, pitcher, + *forma*, form]. Urceolate; pitcher-shaped.

urceolate (yūr'sē-ō-lāt) [L. *urceolus*, dim. of *urceus*, pitcher]. Urceiform.

Urd Abbreviation for uridine.

ur-defenses (ūr'dē-fens-ez). Fundamental beliefs essential for man's psychological integrity; *e.g.*, religion, science.

ure-, urea-, ureo- [G. *ouron*, urine]. Combining forms denoting urea, urine. See also urin-, uro-.

urea (yū-rē'ă) [G. *ouron*, urine]. Carbamide; carbonyldiamide; NH_2–CO–NH_2; the chief end product of nitrogen metabolism in mammals, formed in the liver, by means of the Krebs-Henseleit cycle, and excreted in human urine in the amount of about 32 g a day (about $^6/_7$ of the nitrogen excreted from the body). It may be obtained artificially by heating a solution of ammonium cyanate. It occurs as colorless or white prismatic crystals, without odor but with a cooling saline taste, is soluble in water, and forms salts with acids; used as a diuretic in kidney function tests, and topically for various dermatitides.
u. peroxide, $CH_4N_2O{\cdot}H_2O_2$; a white crystalline compound used in an aqueous solution as an oxidizing mouthwash.
u. stibamine, a u. derivative of stibanilic acid, used in the treatment of kala azar and certain other tropical diseases.

ureagenesis (yū-rē-ă-jen'ĕ-sis) [urea + G. *genesis*, production]. Ureapoiesis; formation of urea, usually referring to the metabolism of amino acids to urea.

ureal (yū-rē'ăl). Ureic; relating to or containing urea.

Ureaplasma (yū-rē'ă-plaz'mă). *T-mycoplasma;* a genus of microaerophilic to anaerobic, nonmotile bacteria (family Mycoplasmataceae) containing Gram-negative, predominantly coccoidal to coccobacillary elements, approximately 0.3 μm in diameter, which frequently grow in short filaments; colonies are generally small, 20 to 30 μm in diameter, and are normally without zones of surface growth. These organisms hydrolyze urea with production of ammonia, and are found in the human genitourinary tract, occasionally in the pharynx and rectum. In males, they are associated with nongonococcal urethritis and prostatitis; in females, with genitourinary tract infections and reproductive failure. The type species is *U. urealyticum.*

ureapoiesis (yū-rē'ă-poy-ē'sis) [urea + G. *poiēsis*, a making]. Ureagenesis.

urease (yūr'ē-ās) [EC 3.5.1.5]. An amidohydrolase cleaving urea into CO_2 and NH_3.

urecchysis (yū-rek'i-sis) [G. *ouron*, urine, + *ekchysis*, a pouring out]. Extravasation of urine into the tissues.

uredema (yū-re-dē'mă) [G. *ouron*, urine, + *oidēma*, swelling]. Uroedema; edema due to infiltration of urine into the subcutaneous tissues.

uredo (yū-rē'dō) [L. a blight, a burning itch, fr. *uro*, pp. *ustus*, to burn]. **1.** Urticaria. **2.** A burning sensation in the skin.

ureic (yū-rē'ik). Ureal.

ureide (yūr'ē-īd). Any compound of urea in which one or more of its hydrogen atoms have been substituted by acid radicals.

3-ureidoisobutyric acid (yū-rē'i-dō-ī'sō-byū-tir'ik). H_2NCONH–$CH_2CH(CH_3)COOH$; an intermediate in thymine catabolism.

3-ureidopropionic acid (yū-rē'i-dō-prō-pi-on'ik). H_2NCONH–CH_2CH_2COOH; an intermediate in uracil catabolism.

ureidosuccinic acid (yū-rē'i-dō-sŭk-sin'ik). NH_2CONH-$CH(COOH)CH_2COOH$; *N*-carbamoylaspartic acid; a precursor of the pyrimidines.

urelcosis (yū-rel-kō'sis) [G. *ouron*, urine, + *helkōsis*, ulceration]. Ulceration of any part of the urinary tract.

uremia (yū-rē'mē-ă) [G. *ouron*, urine, + *haima*, blood]. Azotemia. **1.** An excess of urea and other nitrogenous waste in the blood. **2.** The complex of symptoms due to severe persisting renal failure that can be relieved by dialysis.
hypercalcemic u., u. due to renal failure caused by hypercalcemia with nephrocalcinosis.

uremic (yū-rē'mik). Relating to uremia.

uremigenic (yū-rē-mi-jen'ik). **1.** Of uremic origin or causation. **2.** Causing or resulting in uremia.

ureo-. See ure-.

ureotelic (yū'rē-ō-tel'ik) [ureo- + G. *telos*, end]. Excreting nitrogen in the form of urea.

urerythrin (yūr-er'i-thrin). Uroerythrin.

uresiesthesia (yū-rē'si-es-thē'zē-ă) [G. *ourēsis*, a urinating, + *aisthēsis*, sensation]. Uriesthesia; the desire to urinate.

uresis (yū-rē'sis) [G. *ourēsis*] Urination.

ureter (yū-rē'ter, yū'rē-ter) [G. *ourētēr*, urinary canal] [NA]. The thick-walled tube that conducts the urine from the renal pelvis of the kidney to the bladder; it consists of a pars abdominalis and a pars pelvina, is lined with transitional epithelium surrounded by smooth muscle, both circular and longitudinal, and is covered externally by a tunica adventitia.
curlicue u., term given to the twisted x-ray appearance of a u., herniated through the sciatic foramen; a very rare condition.

ureteral (yū-rē'tē-răl). Ureteric; relating to the ureter.

ureteralgia (yū-rē-ter-al'jē-ă) [ureter + G. *algos*, pain]. Pain in the ureter.

uretercystoscope (yū-rē'ter-sis'tō-skōp). Ureterocystoscope.

ureterectasia (yū-rē'ter-ek-tā'zē-ă) [ureter + G. *ektasis*, a stretching out]. Dilation of a ureter.

ureterectomy (yū-rē-ter-ek'tō-mē) [ureter + G. *ektomē*, excision].

Excision of a segment or all of a ureter.

ureteric (yū-rē-ter'ik). Ureteral.

ureteritis (yū-rē-ter-ī'tis). Inflammation of a ureter.

uretero- [G. *ourētēr,* urinary canal]. Combining form denoting the ureter.

ureterocele (yū-rē'ter-ō-sēl) [utero- + G. *kēlē,* hernia]. Saccular dilatation of the terminal portion of the ureter which protrudes into the lumen of the urinary bladder, probably due to a congenital stenosis of the ureteral meatus.

ureterocelorraphy (yū-rē'ter-ō-se-lōr'ă-fē) [ureterocele + G. *raphē,* suture]. Excision and suturing of a ureterocele performed through an open cystotomy incision.

ureterocervical (yū-rē'ter-ō-ser'vi-kal). Relating to a ureter and the cervix uteri.

ureterocolic (yū-rē'ter-ō-kol'ik). Relating to the ureter and the colon, especially to an anastomosis for lesions of the lower urinary tract.

ureterocolostomy (yū-rē'ter-ō-kō-los'tō-mē) [uretero- + G. *kolon,* colon, + *stoma,* mouth]. Implantation of the ureter into the colon.

ureterocystanastomosis (yū-rē'ter-ō-sist'ă-nas-tō-mō'sis). Ureteroneocystostomy.

ureterocystoscope (yū-rē'ter-ō-sis'tō-skōp). Uretercystoscope; a cystoscope with an attachment for catheterization of the ureters; the catheter is passed into the ureter when its orifice is brought into view with the cystoscope.

ureterocystostomy (yū-rē'ter-ō-sis-tos'tō-mē) [uretero- + G. *kystis,* bladder, + *stoma,* mouth]. Ureteroneocystostomy.

ureteroenteric (yū-rē'ter-ō-en-ter'ik). Relating to a ureter and the intestine.

ureteroenterostomy (yū-rē'ter-ō-en-ter-os'tō-mē) [uretero- + G. *enteron,* intestine, + *stoma,* mouth]. Formation of an opening between a ureter and the intestine.

ureterography (yū-rē'ter-og'ră-fē) [uretero- + G. *graphē,* a writing]. Radiography of the ureter after the injection of a contrast medium.

ureterohydronephrosis. (yū-rē'ter-ō-hī'drō-nef-rō'sis). Hydronephrosis involving also the ureters.

ureteroileoneocystostomy (yū-rē'ter-ō-il'ē-ō-nē'ō-sis-tos'tō-mē) [uretero- + ileum + G. *neos,* new, + *hystis,* bladder, + *stoma,* mouth]. Restoration of the continuity of the urinary tract by anastomosis of the upper segment of a partially destroyed ureter to a segment of ileum, the lower end of which is then implanted into the bladder.

ureteroileostomy (yū-rē'ter-ō-il-ē-os'tō-mē) [uretero- + ileum + G. *stoma,* mouth]. Implantation of a ureter into an isolated segment of ileum which drains through an abdominal stoma.

ureterolith (yū-rē'ter-ō-lith) [uretero- + G. *lithos,* stone]. A calculus in the ureter.

ureterolithiasis (yū-rē'ter-ō-li-thī'ă-sis) [ureterolith + G. *-iasis,* condition]. Lithureteria; the formation or presence of a calculus or calculi in one or both ureters.

ureterolithotomy (yū-rē'ter-ō-li-thot'ō-mē) [ureterolith + G. *tomē,* incision]. Surgical removal of a stone lodged in a ureter.

ureterolysis (yū'rē-ter-ol'i-sis) [uretero- + G. *lysis,* a loosening]. **1.** Ureterodialysis; rupture of a ureter. **2.** Paralysis of the ureter. **3.** Surgical freeing of the ureter from surrounding disease or adhesions.

ureteroneocystostomy (yū-rē'ter-ō-nē'ō-sis-tos'tō-mē) [uretero- + G. *neos,* new, + *kystis,* bladder, + *stoma,* mouth]. Ureterocystostomy; ureterocystanastomosis; an operation whereby the upper end of a transected ureter is implanted into the bladder.

ureteroneopyelostomy (yū-rē'ter-ō-nē'ō-pī-ĕ-los'tō-mē) [uretero- + G. *neos,* new, + *pyelos,* pelvis, + *stoma,* mouth]. Ureteropyeloneostomy; surgical reimplantation of the ureter into the pelvis of the opposite kidney.

ureteronephrectomy (yū-rē'ter-ō-nĕ-frek'tō-mē) [uretero- + G. *nephros,* kidney, + *ektomē,* excision]. Removal of a kidney with its ureter.

ureteropathy (yū-rē'ter-op'ă-thē) [uretero- + G. *pathos,* suffering]. Disease of the ureter.

ureteroplasty (yū-rē'ter-ō-plas-tē) [uretero- + G. *plastos,* formed]. Plastic surgery of the ureters.

ureteroproctostomy (yū-rē'ter-ō-prok-tos'tō-mē) [uretero- + G. *prōktos,* rectum, + *stoma,* mouth]. Ureterorectostomy; establishment of an opening between a ureter and the rectum.

ureteropyelitis (yū-rē'ter-ō-pī-ĕ-lī'tis) [uretero- + G. *pyelos,* pelvis, + *-itis,* inflammation]. Ureteropyelonephritis; inflammation of the pelvis of a kidney and its ureter.

ureteropyelography (yū-rē'ter-ō-pī'ĕ-log'ră-fē). Pyelography.

ureteropyeloneostomy (yū-rē'ter-ō-pī'ĕ-lō-nē-os'tō-mē). Ureteroneopyelostomy.

ureteropyelonephritis (yū-rē'ter-ō-pī'ĕ-lō-ne-frī'tis). Ureteropyelitis.

ureteropyelonephrostomy (yū-rē'ter-ō-pī'ĕ-lō-ne-fros'tō-mē) [uretero- + G. *pyelos,* pelvis, + *nephros,* kidney, + *stoma,* mouth]. Surgical formation of a new or more widely patent junction between the ureter and kidney pelvis.

ureteropyeloplasty (yū-rē'ter-ō-pī'ĕ-lō-plas-tē) [uretero- + G. *pyelos,* pelvis, + *plastos,* formed]. Plastic surgery of the ureter and of the pelvis of the kidney.

ureteropyelostomy (yū-rē'ter-ō-pī-ĕ-los'tō-mē) [uretero- + pelvis, + *stōma,* mouth]. Formation of a junction of the ureter and the renal pelvis.

ureteropyosis (yū-rē'ter-ō-pī-ō'sis) [uretero- + G. *pyōsis,* suppuration]. An accumulation of pus in the ureter.

ureterorectostomy (yū-rē'ter-ō-rek-tos'tō-mē). Ureteroproctostomy.

ureterorrhagia (yū-rē'ter-ō-rā'jē-ă) [uretero- + G. *rhēgnymi,* to burst forth]. Hemorrhage from a ureter.

ureterorrhaphy (yū-rē-ter-ōr'ă-fē) [uretero- + G. *rhaphē,* suture]. Suture of a ureter.

ureterosigmoid (yū-rē'ter-ō-sig'moyd). Relating to the ureter and the sigmoid colon, especially to an anastomosis between the two.

ureterosigmoidostomy (yū-rē'ter-ō-sig-moy-dos'tō-mē). Implantation of the ureters into the sigmoid colon.

ureterostegnosis (yū-rē'ter-ō-steg-nō'sis) [uretero- + G. *stegnōsis,* a making close]. Obsolete term for ureterostenosis.

ureterostenoma (yū-rē'ter-ō-sten-ō'mă) [uretero- + G. *stenōma,* a narrow place, fr. *stenos,* narrow]. The site of a stricture of a ureter.

ureterostenosis (yū-rē'ter-ō-ste-nō'sis) [uretero- + G. *stenōsis,* a narrowing]. Stricture of a ureter.

ureterostoma (yū-rē-ter-os'tō-mă) [uretero- + G. *stoma,* mouth]. A ureteral fistula.

ureterostomy (yū-rē-ter-os'tō-mē) [uretero- + G. *stoma,* mouth]. Establishment of an external opening into the ureter.

ureterotomy (yū-rē-ter-ot'ō-mē) [uretero- + G. *tomē,* incision]. Any surgical incision into a ureter.

ureterotrigonoenterostomy (yū-rē'ter-ō-tri-gō'nō-en-ter-os'tō-mē) [uretero-, + trigone (of bladder), + enterostomy]. Implantation of a ureter and its portion of the trigone of the bladder into the intestine.

ureteroureteral (yū-rē'ter-ō-yū-re'ter-ăl). Relating to two segments of the same ureter or to both ureters, especially an artificial anastomosis between them.

ureteroureterostomy (yū-rē'ter-ō-yū-rē'ter-os'tō-mē). Establishment of an anastomosis between the two ureters or between two segments of the same ureter.

ureterouterine (yū-rē'ter-ō-yū'ter-in). Relating to a ureter and the uterus, especially a fistula between the two.

ureterovaginal (yū-rē'ter-ō-vaj'i-năl). Relating to a ureter and the vagina; especially denoting a fistula, either surgical or pathologic, connecting the two.

ureterovesical (yū-rē'ter-ō-ves'i-kăl). Relating to the ureter and the bladder, specifically the junction of ureter with bladder.

ureterovesicostomy (yū-rē'ter-ō-ves-i-kos'tō-mē) [uretero- + L. *vesico,* bladder, + *stōma,* mouth]. Surgical joining of a ureter to the bladder.

urethan, urethane (yū'rĕ-than, -thān). Ethyl carbamate; $NH_2COOC_2H_5$; has antimitotic activity; formerly used medically as a hypnotic, but now more often used as an anesthetic for laboratory animals.

urethr-. See urethro-.

urethra (yū-rē'thră) [G. *ourēthra*]. Urogenital canal; a canal leading from the bladder, discharging the urine externally.
female u., u. feminina.
u. femini'na [NA], female u.; u. muliebris; a canal about 4 cm in length passing from the bladder, in close relation with the anterior wall of the vagina, opening in the vestibule behind the clitoris.
male u., u. masculina.
u. masculi'na [NA], male u.; u. virilis; a canal about 20 cm in length opening at the extremity of the glans penis; it gives passage to the spermatic fluid as well as the urine.
membranous u., *pars* membranacea urethrae masculinae.
u. mulie'bris, u. feminina.
penile u., *pars* spongiosa urethrae masculinae.
prostatic u., *pars* prostatica urethrae.
spongy u., *pars* spongiosa urethrae masculinae.
u. viri'lis, u. masculina.

urethral (yū-rē'thrăl). Relating to the urethra.

urethralgia (yū-rē-thral'jē-ă) [urethr- + G. *algos,* pain]. Urethrodynia; pain in the urethra.

urethrameter (yū-reth-ram'ĕ-ter). Urethrometer.

urethrascope (yū-rē'thră-skōp). Urethroscope.

urethratresia (yū-rē-thră-trē'zē-ă) [urethr- + G. *a-* priv. + *trēsis,* a boring]. Imperforation or occlusion of the urethra.

urethrectomy (yūr-ĕ-threk'tō-mē) [urethr- + G. *ektomē,* excision]. Excision of a segment or the entire urethra.

urethremorrhagia (yū-rē'threm-ō-rā'jē-ă) [urethr- + G. *haima,* blood, + *rhēgnymi,* to burst forth]. Urethrorrhagia; bleeding from the urethra.

urethremphraxis (yūr'ē-threm-frak'sis) [urethr- + G. *emphraxis,* a stoppage]. Urethrophraxis; obstruction of the free flow of urine through the urethra.

urethreurynter (yū-rē-thrū-rin'ter) [urethr- + G. *eurynō,* to dilate, fr. *eurys,* wide]. Obsolete instrument for dilating the urethra.

urethrism, urethrismus (yū'rē-thrizm, -thriz'mŭs). Urethrospasm; irritability or spasmodic stricture of the urethra.

urethritis (yū-rē-thrī'tis) [ureth- + G. *-itis,* inflammation]. Inflammation of the urethra.
anterior u., inflammation of the portion of the urethra anterior to the triangular ligament.
follicular u., granular u.; chronic u. with nodular lymphocytic infiltrations in the mucosa.
gonococcal u., gonorrhea in males.
granular u., follicular u.
nongonococcal u., u. not resulting from gonococcal infection; venereally transmitted *Chlamydia trachomatis* is the most common cause.
nonspecific u., simple u.; u. not resulting from gonococcal or other specific infectious agents.
u. petrif'icans, u., sometimes of gouty origin, in which there is a deposit of calcareous matter in the wall of the urethra.
posterior u., inflammation of the membranous and prostatic portions of the urethra.
simple u., nonspecific u.
specific u., gonorrhea.
u. vene'rea, gonorrhea.

urethro-, urethr- [G. *ourēthra,* urethra]. Combining forms denoting the urethra.

urethrobalanoplasty (yū-rē'thrō-bal'an-ō-plas-tē). Plastic repair of hypospadias and epispadias.

urethrobulbar (yū-rē'thrō-bŭl'băr). Bulbourethral.

urethrocele (yū-rē'thrō-sēl) [urethro- + G. *kēlē,* tumor, hernia]. Prolapse of the female urethra.

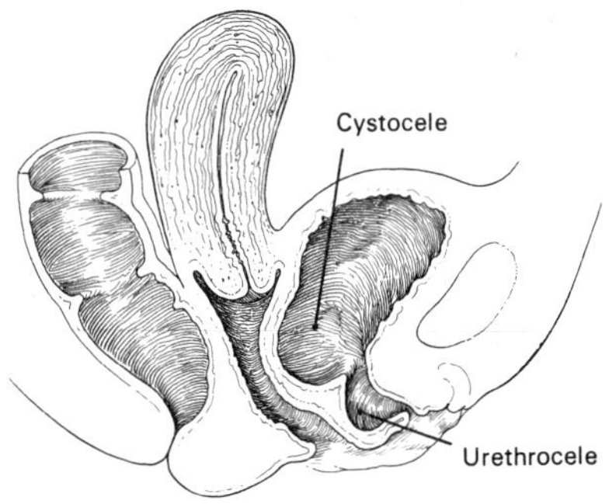

Urethrocele Accompanied by Cystocele

urethrocystitis (yū-rē'thrō-sis-tī'tis) [urethro- + G. *kystis,* bladder, + *-itis,* inflammation]. Inflammation of the urethra and bladder.

urethrocystometrography (yū-rē'thrō-sis'tō-me-trog'ră-fē) [urethro- + G. *kystis,* bladder, + *metron, measure,* + *skopeō,* to view]. Urethrocystometry.

urethrocystometry (yū-rē'thrō-sis-tom'ĕ-trē) [urethro- + G. *kystis,* bladder, + *metron,* measure]. Urethrocystometrography; a procedure that simultaneously measures pressures in urinary bladder and urethra.

urethrocystopexy (yū-rē'thrō-sis'tō-pek-sē) [urethro- + G. *kystis,* bladder, + *pēxis,* fixation]. Fixation of urethra and bladder for stress incontinence.

urethrodynia (yū-rē-thrō-din'ē-ă) [urethro- + G. *odynē,* pain]. Urethralgia.

urethrograph (yū-rē'thrō-graf) [urethro- + G. *graphō,* to write]. A recording urethrometer, indicating graphically the location and extent of urethral strictures.

urethrometer (yū-rē-throm'ĕ-ter) [urethro- + G. *metron,* measure]. Urethrameter; an instrument for measuring the caliber of the urethra.

urethropenile (yū-rē'thrō-pē'nīl). Relating to the urethra and the penis.

urethroperineal (yū-rē'thrō-pĕ-rī-nē'ăl). Relating to the urethra and the perineum.

urethroperineoscroal (yū-rē'thrō-pe-rī-nē-ō-skrō'tăl). Relating to the urethra, perineum, and scrotum.

urethropexy (yū-rē'thrō-pek-sē) [urethro- + G. *pēxis,* fixation]. Surgical suspension of the urethra from the posterior surface of the pubic symphysis for correction of urinary stress incontinence.

urethrophraxis (yū-rē'thrō-frak'sis). Urethremphraxis.

urethrophyma (yū-rē'thrō-fī'mă) [urethro- + G. *phyma,* a tumor]. Any tumor or circumscribed swelling of the urethra.

urethroplasty (yū-rē'thrō-plas-tē) [urethro- + G. *plastos,* formed]. Plastic surgery of the urethra.

urethroprostatic (yū-rē'thrō-pros-tat'ik). Relating to the urethra and the prostate.

urethrorectal (yū-rē'thrō-rek'tăl). Relating to the urethra and the rectum.

urethrorrhagia (yū-rē-thrō-rā'jē-ă). Urethremorrhagia.

urethrorrhaphy (yū-rē-thrōr'ă-fē) [urethro- + G. *rhaphē,* suture]. Suture of the urethra.

urethrorrhea (yū-rē-thrō-rē'ă) [urethro- + G. *rhoia,* a flow]. An abnormal discharge from the urethra.

urethroscope (yū-rē'thrō-skōp) [urethro- + G. *skopeō,* to view]. Urethrascope; an instrument for viewing the interior of the urethra.

urethroscopic (yū-rē-thrō-skop'ik) Relating to the urethroscope or to urethroscopy.

urethroscopy (yū-rē-thros'kŏ-pē). Inspection of the urethra with a urethroscope.

urethrospasm (yū-rē'thrō-spazm). Urethrism.

urethrostaxis (yū-rē'thrō-stak'sis) [urethro- + G. *staxis,* trickling]. Oozing of blood from the mucous membrane of the urethra.

urethrostenosis (yū-rē'thrō-ste-nō'sis) [urethro- + G. *stenōsis,* a narrowing]. Stricture of the urethra.

urethrostomy (yū-rē-thros'tō-mē) [urethro- + G. *stoma,* mouth]. Surgical formation of a permanent opening between the urethra and the skin.
perineal u., formation of a permanent opening into the bulbous portion of the urethra through a perineal skin incision.

urethrotome (yū-rē'thrō-tōm) [urethro- + G. *tomos,* cutting]. An instrument for dividing a stricture of the urethra.

urethrotomy (yū-rē-throt'ō-mē) [urethro- + G. *tomē,* incision]. Surgical incision of a stricture of the urethra.
external u., Wheelhouse's operation; perineal u.; u. via an external opening in the perineum or penile skin.
internal u., u. by means of an instrument passed through the urethra.
perineal u., external u.

urethrovaginal (yū-rē'thrō-vaj'i-năl). Relating to the urethra and the vagina.

urethrovesical (yū-rē'thrō-ves'i-kăl). Relating to the urethra and bladder.

urethrovesicopexy (yū-rē'thrō-ves'i-kŏ-pek-sē) [urethro- + L. *vesica,* bladder, + G. *pexis,* fixation]. Surgical suspension of the urethra and the base of the bladder from the posterior surface of the pubic symphysis for correction of urinary stress incontinence.

-uretic [G. *ourētikos,* relating to the urine]. Combining form denoting urine.

urgency (er'jen-sē). A strong desire to void accompanied by a fear of leakage.
motor u., u. from overactive detrusor function.
sensory u., u. due to vesicourethral hypersensitivity.

urginea (er-jin'ē-ă) [L. *urgeo,* to press, referring to the shape of the seeds]. The bulbs of *Urginea indica* (Indian squill) and *Urginea maritima* (white or Mediterranean squill); the source of squill.

urhidrosis (yūr-hi-drō'sis). Uridrosis.

uri-, uric-, urico- [G. *ouron,* urine]. Combining forms relating to uric acid.

urian (yūr'ē-ăn). Urochrome.

uric (yūr'ik). Relating to urine.

uric acid. Lithic acid; triketopurine; 2,6,8-trioxypurine; white crystals, poorly soluble, contained in solution in the urine of mammals and in solid form in the urine of birds and reptiles; sometimes solidified in small masses as stones or crystals or in larger concretions as calculi; with sodium and other bases it forms urates.
u. a. oxidase, see *urate* oxidase.

uricase (yūr'i-kās). *Urate* oxidase.

urico-. See uri-.

uricolysis (yūr-i-kol'i-sis) [urico- + G. *lysis,* a loosening]. Decomposition of uric acid.

uricolytic (yūr'i-kō-lit'ik). Relating to or effecting the hydrolysis of uric acid.

uricosuria (yū'ri-kō-sū'rē-ă) [urico- + G. *ouron,* urine]. Excessive amounts of uric acid in the urine.

uricosuric (yū'ri-kō-sū'rik). Tending to increase the excretion of uric acid.

uricotelic (yūr'i-kō-tel'ik) [urico- + G. *telos,* end]. Producing uric acid as the chief excretory product of nitrogen metabolism.

uridine (Urd) (yūr'i-dēn). 1-β-D-Ribofuranosyluracil; uracil ribonucleoside; one of the major nucleosides in RNA's; as the pyrophosphate (UDP, UDPG, etc.), u. is active in sugar metabolism.
u. diphosphate (UDP), uridine 5′-diphosphate; uridine 5′-pyrophosphate. See also entries under UDP.
u. phosphate (UMP), uridylic acid.
u. phosphorylase [EC 2.4.2.3], a ribosyltransferase that catalyzes the phosphorolysis of uridine to uracil plus ribose 1-phosphate.
u. triphosphate (UTP), uridine 5′-triphosphate; u. esterfied with triphosphoric acid at its 5′ position; the immediate precursor of uridylic acid residues in RNA.

uridinediphosphogalactose (UDPGal) (yūr'i-dēn-dī-fos'fō-gă-lak'tōs). UDPgalactose; a pyrophosphate group links the 5′ position of uridine and the 1 position of galactose.

uridinediphosphoglucose (UDPG, UDPGlc) (yūr'i-dēn-dī-fos'-fō-glū'kōs). UDPglucose; a pyrophosphate group links the 5′ position of uridine and the 1 position of glucose.

uridinediphosphoglucuronic acid (UDP-GlcUA) (yūr'i-dēn-dī-fos'fō-glū-kū-ron'ik). Uridine diphosphoglucose in which the 6 CH_2OH of the glucose has been oxidized to COOH (has become a glucuronyl residue).

uridrosis (yū-ri-drō'sis) [uri- + G. *hidrōs,* sweat]. Urhidrosis; sudor urinosus; the excretion of urea or uric acid in the sweat.
u. crystalli'na, urea *frost.*

uridylic acid (yūr-i-dil'ik). Uridine phosphate; uridine esterified by phosphoric acid on one or more sugar hydroxyl groups.

uridyltransferase (yūr'i-dil-trans'fer-ās). UDPglucose—hexose-1-phosphate.

uriesthesia (yūri-es-thē'zē-ă). Uresiesthesia.

urin-, urino- [G. *ouron,* urine]. Combining forms denoting urine. See also ure-, uro-.

urinal (yū'rin-ăl). A vessel into which urine is passed.

urinalysis (yū-ri-nal'i-sis). Analysis of the urine.

urinary (yūr'i-năr-ē). Relating to urine.

urinate (yūr'i-nāt). Micturate; to pass urine.

urination (yūr'i-nā'shŭn). Emiction; miction; micturition (1); uresis; the passing of urine. See Fig. on p. 1674.
stuttering u., the passage of urine in jets caused by intermittent spasmodic contraction of the bladder.

urine (yūr'in) [L. *urina;* G. *ouron*]. The fluid and dissolved substances excreted by the kidney.
ammoniacal u., ammoniuria.
black u., the dark u. of melanuria or hemoglobinuria.
chylous u., milky u.; u. of a milky appearance, containing chyle.

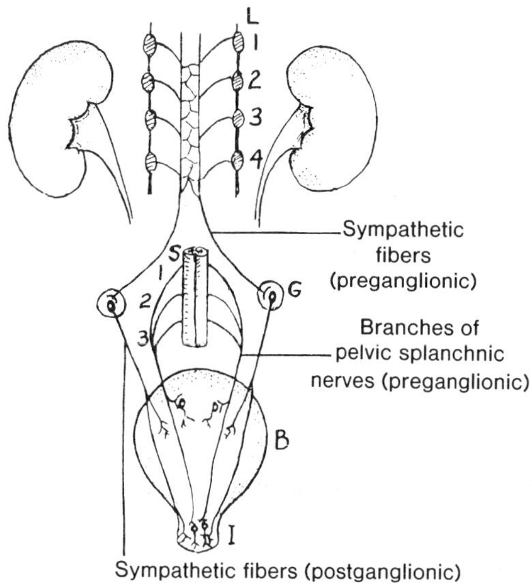

Innervation of Urination
B, urinary bladder; *G*, pelvic ganglion; *I*, internal sphincter; *L 1, 2, 3, 4*, ganglia of the lumbar sympathetic chain; *S 1, 2, 3*, sacral segments of the spinal cord.

cloudy u., nebulous u.; u. containing earthy phosphates in excess.
crude u., pale u. of low specific gravity, with very little sediment.
febrile u., feverish u., dark colored, concentrated u. of strong odor, passed by one suffering from fever.
gouty u., u. of a high color containing uric acid in excess.
honey u., old term for *diabetes* mellitus.
maple syrup u., see maple syrup urine *disease.*
milky u., chylous u.
nebulous u., cloudy u.
residual u., u. remaining in the bladder at the end of micturition in cases of prostatic obstruction, bladder atony, etc.

urinemia (yūr-i-nē'mē-ă). Obsolete term for uremia.

uriniferous (yūr-i-nif'ĕ-rŭs) [urine + L. *fero,* to carry]. Conveying urine; denoting the tubules of the kidney.

urinific (yūr-i-nif'ik) [urine + L. *facio,* to make]. Uriniparous.

uriniparous (yūr-i-nip'ă-rŭs) [urine + L. *pario,* to produce]. Urinific; producing or excreting urine; denoting the malpighian bodies and certain tubules in the renal cortex.

urino-. See urin-.

urinogenital (yūr'i-nō-jen'i-tăl). Genitourinary.

urinogenous (yūr-i-noj'ĕ-nŭs). Urogenous. **1.** Producing or excreting urine. **2.** Of urinary origin.

urinoma (yūr'i-nō'mă). A cystic collection of extravasated urine.

urinometer (yūr-i-nom'ĕ-ter) [urine + G. *metron,* measure]. Urometer; urogravimeter; a hydrometer for determining the specific gravity of the urine.

urinometry (yūr-i-nom'ĕ-trē). The determination of the specific gravity of the urine.

urinoscopy (yūr-i-nos'kŏ-pē). Uroscopy.

urinosexual (yūr-i-nō-sek'shū-ăl). Genitourinary.

urinous (yūr'i-nŭs). Relating to or of the nature of urine.

uriposia (yūr-i-pō'sē-ă) [urine + G. *posis,* drinking]. Urine-drinking.

uritis (yū-rī'tis) [L. *uro,* pp. *ustus,* to singe, burn, + G. *-itis,* inflammation]. Dermatitis *ambustionis.*

uro- [G. *ouron,* urine]. Combining form relating to urine. See also ure-, urin-.

uroammoniac (yū-rō-ă-mo'nē-ak). Relating to uric acid and ammonia; denoting a variety of urinary calculus.

uroanthelone (yūr-ō-an'thĕ-lōn). Urogastrone.

urobilin (yūr-ō-bī'lin, -bil'in). Urohematin; urohematoporphyrin; a uroporphyrin; an acyclic tetrapyrrole that is one of the natural breakdown products of hemoglobin via choleglobin, verdohemochrome, biliverdin, bilirubin, and *d*-urobilinogen; a urinary pigment that gives a varying orange-red coloration to urine according to its degree of oxidation.

urobilin IX-α. Mesobilene-b.

urobilinemia (yū'rō-bil-i-nē'mē-ă). The presence of urobilins in the blood.

urobilinogen (yūr-ō-bī-lin'ō-jen). Precursor of urobilin.

urobilinogen IXα. Mesobilane.

urobilinuria (yū'rō-bil-i-nū'rē-ă). The presence in the urine of urobilins in excessive amount, formed mainly from hemoglobin.

urocanase (yū'rō-kă-nās). Urocanate hydratase.

urocanate (yūr'ō-kă-nāt). A salt or ester of urocanic acid.
u. hydratase [EC 4.2.1.49], urocanase; an enzyme catalyzing the conversion of urocanic acid to an imidazolonepropionic acid, a step in histidine catabolism.

urocanic acid (yūr-ō-kan'ik). 4-Imidazoleacrylic acid; an acid derived from the oxidative deamination of histidine; present in dog's urine.

urocanicase (yūr-ō-kan'i-kās). One of a group of at least three enzymes that convert urocanic acid to glutamic acid.

urocele (yū'rō-sēl) [uro- + G. *kēlē,* hernia]. Uroscheocele; extravasation of urine into the scrotal sac.

urocheras (yū-rok'er-as) [uro- + G. *cheras,* gravel (an incorrect form of *cherados,* gravel)]. Uropsammus.

urochesia (yū-rō-kē'zē-ă) [uro- + G. *chezō,* to defecate]. Passage of urine from the anus.

urochrome (yūr'ō-krōm). Urian; the principal pigment of urine, a compound of urobilin and a peptide of unknown structure.

urochromogen (yūr-ō-krō'mō-jen). Originally, a body in the urine that, on taking up oxygen, formed urochrome; now, probably urobilinogen.

urocrisia (yū-rō-kris'ē-ă, -kriz'ē-ă) [uro- + G. *krinō,* to separate, judge]. **1.** Urocrisis. **2.** Obsolete term for diagnosis based upon the results of a urinary examination.

urocrisis (yū'rō-krī'sis) [uro- + G. *krisis,* crisis]. Urocrisia (1). **1.** Obsolete term for the critical stage of a disease accompanied by a copious discharge of urine. **2.** Severe pain in any of the urinary organs or passages occurring in tabes dorsalis.

urocyanin (yū'rō-sī'ă-nin) [uro- + G. *kyanos,* a blue substance]. Uroglaucin; an indigo blue pigment sometimes observed in the urine in certain diseases, especially scarlet fever.

urocyanogen (yū-rō-sī-an'ō-jen). A blue pigment sometimes observed in the urine in cases of cholera.

urocyanosis (yū'rō-sī-ă-nō'sis). A bluish discoloration of the urine in indicanuria.

urocyst (yū'rō-sist) [uro- + G. *kystis,* bladder]. *Vesica* urinaria.

urocystic (yū'rō-sis'tik). Relating to the urinary bladder.

urocystis (yū'rō-sis'tis). *Vesica* urinaria.

urocystitis (yūr'ō-sis-tī'tis) [uro- + G. *kystis,* bladder, + *-itis,* inflammation]. Inflammation of the urinary bladder. See also cystitis and subentries.

urodynamics (yū'rō-dī-nam'iks) [uro- + G. *dynamis,* force]. The study of the storage of urine within, and the flow of urine through and from, the urinary tract.

urodynia (yūr-ō-din′ē-ă) [uro- + G. *odynē*, pain]. Pain on urination.

urodysfunction (yūr′ō-dis-funk′shŭn). Urinary dysfunction.

uroedema (yūr′ō-e-dē′mă) [uro- + G. *oidēma*, swelling]. Uredema.

uroenterone (yūr-ō-en′ter-ōn). Urogastrone.

uroerythrin (yū-rō-er′i-thrin). Urerythrin; pupurin (1); a urinary pigment that gives a pink color to deposits of urates; presumably derived from melanin.

uroflavin (yūr-ō-flā′vin). A fluorescent product of riboflavin catabolism, or perhaps riboflavin itself, found in mammalian urine and feces.

urofollitropin (yūr-ō-fol′i-trō-pin). A preparation of gonadotropin extracted from the urine of postmenopausal women, used in conjunction with human chorionic gonadotropin to induce ovulation.

urofuscohematin (yū-rō-fŭs-kō-hē′mă-tin). A brownish red pigment found in the urine in a case of leprosy.

urogastrone (yūr-ō-gas′trōn). Anthelone; anthelone U; uroanthelone; uroenterone; a fluorescent pigment extracted from urine; an inhibitor of gastric secretion and motility. *Cf.* enterogastrone.

urogenital (yū′rō-jen′i-tăl). Genitourinary.

urogenous (yū-roj′ĕ-nŭs). Urinogenous.

uroglaucin (yū-rō-glaw′sin) [uro- + G. *glaukos*, bluish gray]. Urocyanin.

urogonadotropin (yūr′ō-gō-nad-ō-trō′pin). See human menopausal *gonadotropin.*

urogram (yūr′ō-gram). The roentgenographic record obtained by urography.

urography (yū-rog′ră-fē) [uro- + G. *graphō*, to write]. Roentgenography of any part (kidneys, ureters, or bladder) of the urinary tract.
antegrade u., x-ray examination of the urinary tract utilizing percutaneous injection of a contrast agent with a needle or catheter into the renal calices or pelvis (antegrade pyelography), or into the urinary bladder (antegrade cystography).
cystoscopic u., retrograde u.
intravenous u., exretory u., x-ray examination of kidneys, ureters, and bladder by means of a contrast agent injected into a vein.
retrograde u., cystoscopic u.; x-ray examination of the urinary tract by means of contrast fluid injected directly into the bladder, ureter, or renal pelvis.

urogravimeter (yū′rō-gră-vim′ĕ-ter) [uro- + L. *gravis*, heavy, + G. *metron*, measure]. Urinometer.

urohematin (yūr-ō-hēm′ă-tin). Urobilin.

urohematoporphyrin (yūr′ō-hēm′ă-tō-pōr′fi-rin). Urobilin.

uroheparin (yūr-ō-hep′ă-rin). An inactive form of heparin excreted in the urine.

urohypertensin (yūr′ō-hī-per-ten′sin). A pressor substance derived from the urine.

urokinase (yūr-ō-kī′nās). Plasminogen *activator.*

urolagnia (yūr-ō-lag′nē-ă) [uro- + G. *lagneia*, lust]. Sexual stimulation occasioned by the sight of a person urinating.

uroleucinic acid, uroleucic acid (yū′rō-lū-sin′ik, yū-rō-lū′sik). An aromatic compound, $C_9H_{10}O_5$, excreted in the urine of persons with alkaptonuria.

urolith (yū′rō-lith) [uro- + G. *lithos*, stone]. Urinary *calculus.*

urolithiasis (yū-rō-li-thī′ă-sis) Presence of calculi in the urinary system.

urolithic (yū-rō-lith′ik). Relating to urinary calculi.

urolithology (yū′rō-li-thol′ō-jē) [uro- + G. *lithos*, stone, + *logos*, study]. The branch of medicine concerned with the formation, composition, effects, and removal of urinary calculi.

urologic, urological (yū-rō-loj′ik, i-kăl). Relating to urology.

urologist (yū-rol′ō-jist). A specialist in urology.

urology (yū-rol′ō-jē) [uro- + G. *logos*, study]. The medical specialty concerned with the study, diagnosis, and treatment of diseases of the genitourinary tract, especially the urinary tract in both sexes and the genital organs in the male.

urolutein (yū-rō-lū′tē-in). Name given to yellow pigment in the urine. See urochrome; uroporphyrin (1).

uromelanin (yūr-ō-mel′ă-nin). A black pigment occasionally found in the urine, possibly a decomposition product of urochrome.

urometer (yū-rom′ĕ-ter). Urinometer.

uroncus (yū-rong′kŭs) [uro- + G. *onkos*, mass (tumor)]. A urinary cyst; a circumscribed area of extravasation of urine.

uronephrosis (yū′rō-ne-frō′sis). Hydronephrosis.

uronic acids (yū-ron′ik). Acids derived from monosaccharides by oxidation of the primary alcohol group ($-CH_2OH$) farthest removed from the carbonyl group to a carboxyl group ($-COOH$); *e.g.*, glucuronic acid.

uronoscopy (yū-rō-nos′kō-pē). Uroscopy.

uropathy (yū-rop′ă-thē) [uro- + G. *pathos*, suffering]. Any disorder involving the urinary tract.

urophanic (yūr-ō-fan′ik) [uro- + G. *phainō*, to appear]. Appearing in the urine; denoting any constituent, normal or pathologic, of the urine.

urophein (yū-rō-fē′in) [uro- + G. *phaios*, gray]. A grayish pigment occasionally found in the urine, possibly identical with urobilin.

uroplania (yū-rō-plā′nē-ă) [uro- + G. *planē*, a wandering]. Extravasation of urine.

uropoiesis (yū′rō-poy-ē′sis) [uro- + G. *poiēsis*, a making]. The production or secretion and excretion of urine.

uropoietic (yū′rō-poy-et′ik). Relating or pertaining to uropoiesis.

uroporphyrin (yūr-ō-pōr′fi-rin). **1.** Porphyrin excreted in the urine in porphyrinuria; *e.g.*, urobilin. **2.** Class name for all porphyrins containing 4 acetic acid groups and 4 propionic acid groups in positions 1 through 8. See also porphyrinogens.

uroporphyrinogen (yūr′ō-pōr-fi-rin′ō-jen). See porphyrinogens.

uropsammus (yū-rō-sam′ŭs) [uro- + G. *psammos*, sand]. Urocheras. **1.** Gravel. **2.** Any inorganic or uratic urinary sediment.

uropterin (yū-rop′ter-in). Urothion.

uropurpurin (yūr-ō-pŭr′pūr-in). A purple pigment in the urine.

uroradiology (yū′rō-rā-dē-ol′ō-jē). Examination of the urinary tract by one of the imaging methods of radiology.

urorectal (yū′rō-rek′tăl). Relating to the urinary tract and rectum.

urorosein (yūr-ō-rō′zē-in). A chromogen in the urine that forms a red color on the addition of nitric acid; normally exists in very minute quantity but is increased in tuberculosis and other wasting diseases, and is related to ingestion of indole compounds.

urorubin (yūr-ō-rū′bin). A red pigment in urine made more visible by treatment with hydrochloric acid.

urorubrohematin (yūr′ō-rū-brō-hē′mă-tin). A reddish pigment occasionally present in the urine in various chronic diseases.

uroscheocele (yū-ros′kē-ō-sēl) [uro- + G. *oscheon*, scrotum, + *kēlē*, tumor]. Urocele.

uroschesis (yū-ros′kē-sis) [uro- + G. *schesis*, a checking]. **1.** Retention of urine. **2.** Suppression of urine.

uroscopic (yūr-ō-skop′ik). Relating to uroscopy.

uroscopy (yū-ros′kō-pē) [uro- + G. *skopeō*, to view]. Uronoscopy; urinoscopy; examination of the urine, usually by means of a microscope.

urosemiology (yū′rō-sem-ē-ol′ō-jē) [uro- + G. *sēmeion*, a sign, +

logos, study]. The study of the urine as an aid to diagnosis.

urosepsin (yūr-ō-sep′sin). A substance formed by the decomposition of urine, supposed to be the cause of septic poisoning after urinary extravasation.

urosepsis (yūr-ō-sep′sis) [uro- + G. *sēpsis,* decomposition]. **1.** Sepsis resulting from the decomposition of extravasated urine. **2.** Sepsis from obstruction of infected urine.

uroseptic (yūr′ō-sep′tik). Relating to urosepsis.

urospectrin (yūr-ō-spek′trin). A pigment found in the urine, possibly the same as urobilin.

urothion (yūr-ō-thī′on). Uropterin; a sulfur-containing pteridine derivative isolated from urine.

urothorax (yūr-ō-thōr′aks). The presence of urine in the thoracic cavity, usually following complex multiple organ injuries.

uroureter (yūr-ō-yū-rē′ter). Hydroureter.

uroxanthin (yūr-ō-zan′thin). Indican (2).

uroxin (yū-rok′sin). Alloxantin.

urtica (er-tī′kă, er′ti-) [L. a nettle, fr. *uro,* pp. *ustus,* to burn]. Nettle; the herb, *Urtica dioica* (family Urticaceae); a weed, the leaves of which produce a stinging sensation when touching the skin. It has been used as a diuretic and hemostatic in metrorrhagia, epistaxis, and hematemesis.

urticant (er′ti-kant) [L. *urtica,* nettle; see urtica]. Producing a wheal or other similar itching agent.

urticaria (er′ti-kar′i-ă) [L. *urtica*]. Hives; nettle rash; cnidosis; uredo (1); urtication (3); an eruption of itching wheals, usually of systemic origin; it may be due to a state of hypersensitivity to foods or drugs, foci of infection, physical agents (heat, cold, light, friction), or psychic stimuli.

acute u., u. acu′ta, febrile u.

u. bullo′sa, u. vesiculosa; an eruption of wheals capped with subepidermal vesicles.

cholinergic u., heat u.; a form of physical or non-allergic u. initiated by heat (*e.g.,* hot baths, physical exercise, pyrexia, exposure to sun or to a warm room) or by excitement; the rather distinctive lesions consist of pruritic areas 1 to 2 mm in diameter surrounded by bright red macules.

chronic u., u. chron′ica, a form of u. in which the wheals recur frequently, or persist.

cold u., congelation u.; wheal formation that develops after exposure to lowered temperatures, with or without demonstrable passive-transfer antibodies.

u. confer′ta, a form of u. in which the wheals are aggregated in a group.

congelation u., cold u.

u. endem′ica, u. epidem′ica, u. caused by the nettling hairs of certain caterpillars.

factitious u., u. facti′tia, dermatographism.

febrile u., u. febri′lis, acute u.; u. accompanied by slight constitutional symptoms.

giant u., u. gi′gans, u. gigan′tea, angioneurotic *edema.*

heat u., cholinergic u.

u. hemorrhag′ica, u. bullosa in which the serous exudate contains blood.

u. maculo′sa, a chronic form of u. with lesions of a red color and little edema.

u. medicamento′sa, an urticarial form of drug eruption.

papular u., u. papulo′sa, *lichen* urticatus.

u. per′stans, a form of chronic u. in which the wheals persist unchanged for long periods.

u. pigmento′sa, cutaneous mastocytosis resulting from an excess of mast cells in the superficial dermis, producing a chronic eruption characterized by flat or slightly elevated brownish papules which urticate when stroked.

solar u., a form of u. resulting from exposure to specific light spectra; some patients have passive-transfer antibodies and others do not.

u. subcuta′nea, u. in which itching is present without the wheals.

u. tubero′sa, angioneurotic *edema.*

u. vesiculo′sa, u. bullosa.

vibratory u., a form of u. that occurs in response to vibratory stimuli.

urticarial, urticarious (er-ti-kar′ē-ăl, -kar′ē-ŭs). Relating to or marked by urticaria.

urticate (er′ti-kāt) [L. *urticatus*]. **1.** To perform urtication. **2.** Marked by the presence of wheals.

urtication (er-ti-kā′shŭn) [L. *urticatio*]. **1.** Whipping with nettles to induce counterirritation, formerly used in the treatment of peripheral paralysis. **2.** A burning sensation resembling that produced by urticaria or resulting from nettle poisoning. **3.** Urticaria.

urushiol (ū′rū-shē-ōl) [Jap. *urushi,* lac, + L. *oleum,* oil]. A mixture of nonvolatile hydrocarbons, derivatives of catechol with unsaturated C_{15}or C_{17}side chains, constituting the active allergen of the irritant oil of poison ivy, *Toxicodendron radicans,* poison oak, *T. diversilobum,* and the Asiatic laquer tree, *T. verniciferum.*

u. oxidase, laccase.

USAN Abbreviation for United States Adopted Names.

Usher, Barney, Canadian dermatologist, *1899. See Senear-U. *disease, syndrome.*

Usher, Charles Howard, British ophthalmologist, 1865–1942. See U.'s *syndrome.*

USP Abbreviation for *United States Pharmacopeia.* See Pharmacopeia.

USPHS Abbreviation for United States Public Health Service.

ustilaginism (ŭs-ti-laj′i-nizm). Poisoning by *Ustilago maydis* (corn smut) which produces burning, itching, hyperemia, acrocyanosis, and edema of the extremities; resembles ergotism, pellagra, or infantile acrocynia.

Ustilago (ŭs-ti-lā′gō) [L. a kind of thistle, fr. *ustio,* a burning]. A genus of smuts (order Ustilaginales).

U. may′dis, U. ze′ae, corn-smut; corn ergot; a species that resembles ergot of rye in its metabolic action; its black spores on the ears of corn are dispersed by wind and can cause contamination of laboratory cultures.

ustulation (ŭs-tyū-lā′shŭn) [L. *ustulo,* pp. *-atus,* to scorch]. **1.** Separation of compounds by heat, as in the process of freeing ores from sulfur by roasting. **2.** Drying of a drug by heat to prepare it for pulverization.

usurpation (yū′ser-pā′shŭn) [L. *usurpo,* pp. *-atus,* to seize]. Assumption of pacemaker function of the heart by a subsidiary focus as a result of its own increased automaticity; *e.g.,* accelerated A-V nodal pacemaker takes command when it exceeds the sinus rate.

uta (ū′tă) [Sp.]. A mild form of New World or American cutaneous leishmaniasis caused by *Leishmania peruana,* occurring in the high Andean valleys of Peru and Bolivia, and characterized by numerous small dermal lesions occurring almost exclusively on exposed skin surfaces; the dog is an important reservoir. Unlike all other forms of American cutaneous leishmaniasis, this disease is found at high elevations (2000 to 2500 m) in barren open country, rather than in lowland tropical forests.

uter-. See utero-.

uterectomy (yū-tĕ-rek′tō-mē). Hysterectomy.

uterine (yū′ter-in, yū′ter-īn). Relating to the uterus.

uterismus (yū-tĕ-riz′mŭs) [uter- + L. *-ismus,* action or condition, fr. G. *-ismos*]. Painful spasmodic contraction of the uterus.

uteritis (yū-tĕ-rī′tis). Metritis.

utero-, uter- [L. *uterus*]. Combining forms relating to the uterus. See also hystero- (1), metra-, metro-.

uteroabdominal (yū'ter-ō-ab-dom'i-năl). Uteroventral; relating to the uterus and the abdomen.

uterocervical (yū'ter-ō-ser'vi-kăl). Relating to the cervix uteri.

uterocystostomy (yū'ter-ō-sis-tos'tō-mē) [utero- + G. *kystis,* bladder, + *stoma,* mouth]. Formation of a communication between the uterus (cervix) and the bladder.

uterofixation (yū'ter-ō-fik-sā'shŭn). Hysteropexy.

uterolith (yū'ter-ō-lith) [utero- + G. *lithos,* stone]. Uterine *calculus.*

uterometer (yū-ter-om'ĕ-ter). Hysterometer.

utero-ovarian (yū'ter-ō-ō-vār'ē-an). Relating to the uterus and an ovary.

uteroparietal (yū'ter-ō-pa-rī'ĕ-tăl). Relating to the uterus and the abdominal wall.

uteropelvic (yū'ter-ō-pel'vik). Relating to the uterus and the pelvis.

uteropexy (yū'ter-ō-pek-sē). Hysteropexy.

uteroplacental (yū'ter-ō-pla-sen'tăl). Relating to the uterus and the placenta.

uteroplasty (yū'ter-ō-plas-tē) [utero- + G. *plastos,* formed]. Metroplasty; hysteroplasty; plastic surgery of the uterus.

uterosacral (yū'ter-ō-sā'krăl). Relating to the uterus and the sacrum.

uterosalpingography (yū'ter-ō-sal-pin-gog'ră-fē). Hysterosalpingography.

uteroscope (yū'ter-ō-skōp). Hysteroscope.

uteroscopy (yū-ter-os'kŏ-pē). Hysteroscopy.

uterotomy (yū-ter-ot'ō-mē). Hysterotomy.

uterotonic (yū'ter-ō-ton'ik) [utero- + G. *tonos,* tone, tension]. **1.** Giving tone to the uterine muscle. **2.** An agent that overcomes relaxation of the muscular wall of the uterus.

uterotubal (yū'ter-ō-tū'băl). Pertaining to the uterus and the uterine tubes.

uterotubography (yū'ter-ō-tū-bog'ră-fē). Hysterosalpingography.

uterovaginal (yū-ter-ō-vaj'i-năl). Relating to the uterus and the vagina.

uteroventral (yū'ter-ō-ven'trăl) [utero- + L. *venter,* belly]. Uteroabdominal.

uteroverdine (yū'ter-ō-ver'din). Biliverdin.

uterovesical (yū'ter-ō-ves'i-kăl). Relating to the uterus and the urinary bladder.

uterus, pl. uteri (yū'ter-ŭs, yū'ter-ī) [L.] [NA]. Womb; metra; the hollow muscular organ in which the impregnated ovum is developed into the child; it is about 7.5 cm in length in the nonpregnant woman, and consists of a main portion (corpus or body) with an elongated lower part (cervix or neck), at the extremity of which is the opening (os or mouth). The upper rounded portion of the u.,

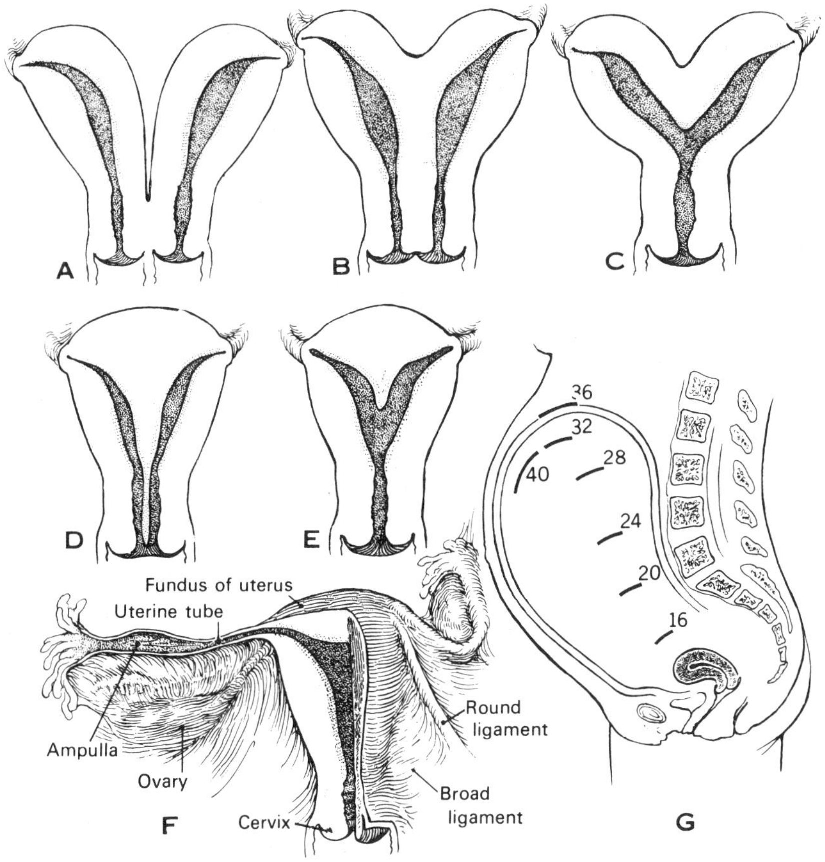

Uterus

A-E, types of abnormal uteri: *A*, uterus didelphys; *B*, uterus bicornis bicollis; *C*, uterus bicornis unicollis; *D*, uterus septus; *E*, uterus subseptus. *F*, normal uterus with adnexa. *G*, changes in size and position of the gravid uterus; numbers indicate weeks on the basis of "menstrual age."

opposite the os, is the fundus, at each extremity of which is the cornu or horn marking the part where the uterine (fallopian) tube joins the u. and through which the ovum reaches the uterine cavity after leaving the ovary. The organ is supported in the pelvic cavity by the broad ligaments, round ligaments, cardinal ligaments, and rectouterine and vesicouterine folds or ligaments.
u. acol'lis, a u. with atresia or absence of the cervix.
anomalous u., a malformed u. caused by abnormal development or fusion of the paramesonephric ducts.
arcuate u., u. arcua'tus, a u. with a depression at the fundus, an incomplete u. bicornis.
u. bicamera'tus vetula'rum a condition in which fluid accumulates in and distends the cervix and body of the u., the two ora being sealed by adhesions.
bicornate u., u. bicor'nis, bifid u.; u. bifidus; a u. that is more or less completely divided into two lateral horns, as a result of imperfect fusion of the paramesonephric ducts; it differs from septate u., in which there is no external mark of separation; in u. bicornis, the cervix may be single (**u. b. unicollis**) or double (**u. b. bicollis**).
bifid u., u. bi'fidus, bicornate u.
biforate u., u. bifor'is, double-mouthed u.; septate u. in which the cervix is divided into two by a septum.
u. bilocula'ris, septate u.
bipartite u., u. biparti'tus, septate u.
capped u., a condition of tonic contraction of the fundus musculature of the u.
cordiform u., u. cordiform'is, heart-shaped u.; an incomplete u. bicornis with a wedge-shaped depression at the fundus.
Couvelaire u., uteroplacental apoplexy; extravasation of blood into the uterine musculature and beneath the uterine peritoneum in association with severe forms of abruptio placentae.
u. didel'phys [G. *di-*, two, + *delphys,* womb], double u. with double cervix and double vagina; due to failure of the paramesonephric ducts to unite.
double-mouthed u., biforate u.
duplex u., u. du'plex, any u. with double lumen (u. didelphys, u. bicornis bicollis, or septate u.).
gravid u., the condition of the u. in pregnancy.
heart-shaped u., cordiform u.
incudiform u., u. incudiform'is, u. triangularis; u. bicornis in which the fundus between the two cornua is broad and flat.
masculine u., u. masculi'nus, *utriculus* prostaticus.
one-horned u., unicorn u.
u. parvicol'lis, a u. with an abnormal, disproportionately small cervix.
septate u., u. sep'tus, u. bilocularis or bipartitus; bipartite u.; a u. divided into two cavities by an anteroposterior septum.
subseptate u., u. subsep'tus, an incomplete u. septus.
triangular u., u. triangula'ris, incudiform u.
unicorn u., u. unicor'nis, one-horned u.; a u. in which only one lateral half exists, the other half being undeveloped or absent.

UTP Abbreviation for *uridine* triphosphate.

utricle (yū'tri-kl). Utriculus.
prostatic u., *utriculus* prostaticus.

utricular (yū-trik'yū-lăr). Relating to or resembling a utricle.

utriculi (yū-trik'yū-lī). Plural of utriculus.

utriculitis (yū-trik-yū-lī'tis) [utriculus + G. *-itis,* inflammation]. **1.** Inflammation of the internal ear. **2.** Inflammation of the utriculus prostaticus.

utriculosaccular (yū-trik'yū-lō-sak'yū-lăr). Relating to the utricle and the saccule of the labyrinth.

utriculus, pl. **utriculi** (yū'trik'yū-lŭs, -lī) [L. dim. of *uter,* leather bag] [NA]. Utricle; sacculus communis; the larger of the two membranous sacs in the vestibule of the labyrinth, lying in the elliptical recess; from it arise the semicircular ducts. See also vestibular *organ.*
u. prostat'icus [NA], prostatic utricle; alveus urogenitalis; sinus pocularis; uterus masculinus; vagina masculina; Weber's organ; Morgagni's sinus (2); a minute pouch in the prostate opening on the summit of the seminal colliculus, the analogue of the uterus and vagina in the female, being the remains of the fused caudal ends of the paramesonephric ducts.

utriform (yū'tri-fōrm) [L. *uter,* a skin bag, + *forma,* form]. Shaped like a leather bottle.

uvaeformis (yū-vē-fōr'mis) [L. *uva,* grape, + *forma,* form]. *Lamina* vasculosa choroideae.

uva ursi (ū'vă er'sī). The dried leaves of *Arctostaphylos uva-ursi* (family Ericaceae), bearberry, mountain box, a common plant of the North Temperate zone; contains antiseptic glycosides, arbutin, methylarbutin, and tannins; used in chronic inflammations of the urinary tract.

uvea (yū'vē-ă) [L. *uva,* grape]. *Tunica* vasculosa bulbi.

uveal (yū'vē-ăl). Relating to the uvea.

UVEB Abbreviation for unifocal ventricular ectopic beat.

uveitic (yū-vē-it'ik). Relating to the uvea.

uveitides (yū-vē-it'i-dēz). Plural of uveitis.

uveitis, pl. **uveitides** (yū-vē-ī'tis, -it'ī-dēz) [uvea + G. *-itis,* inflammation]. Inflammation of the uveal tract: iris, ciliary body, and choroid.
anterior u., inflammation involving the ciliary body and iris.
Förster's u., syphilitic inflammation, with diffuse nodules involving the choroid and retinal vasculitis.
Fuchs' u., heterochromic u.
heterochromic u., Fuch' u.; anterior uveitis and depigmentation of the iris.
lens-induced u., phacoanaphylactic u.
phacoanaphylactic u., lens-induced u.; intraocular inflammation occurring after extracapsular cataract extraction; probably an immune reaction to the patient's liberated lenticular proteins.
phacogenic u., u. secondary to hypermature cataract.
posterior u., choroiditis.
sympathetic u., a bilateral inflammation of the uveal tract caused by a perforating wound of one eye that injures the uvea.

uveoencephalitis (yū'vē-ō-en-sef-ă-lī'tis). Harada's *syndrome.*

uveoscleritis (yū'vē-ō-sklē-rī'tis). Inflammation of the sclera involved by extension from the uvea.

uviform (yū'vi-fōrm) [L. uva, grape, + *forma,* form]. Botryoid.

uviofast (yū'vē-ō-fast) [uviol (*u*ltra*viol*et), + fast]. Uvioresistant; not weakened or destroyed by subjection to ultraviolet radiation.

uviol (yū'vē-ol) [*u*ltra*viol*et]. A special kind of glass more than usually transparent to the ultraviolet or actinic rays.

uviometer (yū-vē-om'ĕ-ter) [uviol (*u*ltra*viol*et), + meter]. An instrument for measuring ultraviolet radiation.

uvioresistant (yū'vē-ō-rē-zis'tant). Uviofast.

uviosensitive (yū'vē-ō-sen'si-tiv) [uviol (*u*ltra*viol*et) + sensitive]. Sensitive to ultraviolet rays.

uvul-. See uvulo-.

uvula, pl. **uvuli** (yū'vyū-lă, -lī) [Mod. L. dim. of L. *uva,* a grape, the uvula] [NA]. An appendant fleshy mass; a structure bearing a fancied resemblance to the u. palatina.
bifid u., bifurcation of the u., constituting a partially cleft soft palate.
u. cerebel'li, u. vermis.
Lieutaud's u., u. vesicae.
u. palati'na [NA], pendulous palate; a conical projection from the

posterior edge of the middle of the soft palate, composed of connective tissue containing a number of racemose glands, and some muscular fibers (musculus uvulae).

u. ver'mis [NA], u. cerebelli; a triangular elevation on the vermis of the cerebellum, lying between the two tonsils anterior to the pyramis.

u. vesi'cae [NA], Lieutaud's u.; a slight projection into the cavity of the bladder, usually more prominent in old men, just behind the urethral opening, marking the location of the middle lobe of the prostate.

uvulaptosis (yū'vyū-lap-tō'sis). Uvuloptosis.

uvular (yū'vyū-lăr). Relating to the uvula.

uvularis (yū'vyū-lā'ris). *Musculus* uvulae.

uvulatome (yū'vyū-lă-tōm). Uvulotome.

uvulectomy (yū-vyū-lek'tō-mē) [uvula + G. *ektomē,* excision]. Staphylectomy; excision of the uvula.

uvulitis (yū-vyū-lī'tis). Inflammation of the uvula.

uvulo-, uvul- [L. *uvula*]. Combining forms denoting the uvula, usually the uvula palatina. See also staphylo-.

uvulopalatoplasty, uvulopalatopharyngoplasty (yū'vyū-lō-pal'ă-tō-plas-tē, -pal'ă-tō-fa-rin'gō-plas-tē). Palatopharyngoplasty.

uvuloptosis (yū'vyū-lop-tō'sis) [uvulo- + G. *ptōsis,* a falling]. Staphyloptosis; staphylodialysis; falling palate; uvulaptosis; relaxation or elongation of the uvula.

uvulotome (yū'vyū-lō-tōm). Staphylotome; uvulatome; an instrument for cutting the uvula.

uvulotomy (yū-vyū-lot'ō-mē) [uvulo- + G. *tomē,* a cutting]. Staphylotomy (1); any cutting operation on the uvula.

V

V **1.** Abbreviation for vision or visual acuity; volt; with subscript 1, 2, 3, etc., the abbreviation for unipolar chest electrocardiogram leads. **2.** Symbol for vanadium; volume, frequently with subscripts denoting location, chemical species, and conditions.

V_{max} Symbol for maximum *velocity.*

$\dot{V}$[volume + overdot denoting time derivative] **1.** Symbol for gas flow, frequently with subscripts indicating location and chemical species. See flow (3). **2.** Symbol for ventilation, frequently with a subscript; see subentries under ventilation.

$\dot{V}_{CO_2}$ Symbol for carbon dioxide *elimination.*

$\dot{V}_{O_2}$ Symbol for oxygen *consumption.*

v **1.** Abbreviation for volt. **2.** As a subscript, refers to venous *blood.*

$\bar{v}$ As a subscript, refers to mixed venous (pulmonary arterial) blood.

V-A Abbreviation for ventriculoatrial.

vaccenic acid (vak-sen'ik). 11-Octadecenoic acid; $CH_3(CH_2)_5CH{=}CH(CH_2)_9COOH$; an unsaturated fatty acid found in butter and other animal fats.

vaccina (vak-sin'ă). Vaccinia.

vaccinal (vak'si-năl). Relating to vaccine or vaccination.

vaccinate (vak'si-nāt). To administer a vaccine.

vaccination (vak'si-nā'shŭn). The act of administering a vaccine.

vaccinator (vak'si-nā-tŏr). **1.** Vaccinist; a person who vaccinates. **2.** A scarifier or other instrument used in vaccination.

VACCINE

vaccine (vak'sēn, vak-sēn') [L. *vaccinus,* relating to a cow]. Vaccinum; originally, the live v. (vaccinia, cowpox) virus inoculated in the skin as prophylaxis against smallpox and obtained from the skin of calves inoculated with seed virus. Usage has extended the meaning to include essentially any preparation intended for active immunological prophylaxis; *e.g.,* preparations of killed microbes of virulent strains or living microbes of attenuated (variant or mutant) strains; or microbial, fungal, plant, protozoal, or metazoan derivatives or products. Method of administration varies according to the v., inoculation being the most common, but ingestion is preferred in some instances and nasal spray is used occasionally.

adjuvant v., a v. that contains an adjuvant; most often the antigen (immunogen) is included in a water-in-oil emulsion (Freund incomplete type adjuvant), or is adsorbed onto an inorganic gel (alum, aluminum hydroxide or phosphate).

aqueous v., a v. having a liquid vehicle (*e.g.,* physiological salt solution) as distinguished from an emulsion.

autogenous v., a v. made from a culture of the patient's own bacteria.

bacillus Calmette-Guérin v., BCG v.

BCG v., bacillus Calmette-Guérin v.; Calmette-Guérin v.; tuberculosis v.; a suspension of an attenuated strain (bacillus Calmette-Guérin) of *Mycobacterium tuberculosis,* bovine type, which is inoculated into the skin for tuberculosis prophylaxis.

brucella strain 19 v., a live bacterial v. prepared from an attenuated variant strain of *Brucella abortus* (strain 19); used for vaccinating cattle against brucellosis.

Calmette-Guérin v., BCG v.

cholera v., an inactivated suspension of Inaba and Ogawa strains of *Vibrio cholerae* grown either on agar or in broth and preserved with phenol.

crystal violet v., see hog cholera v.'s.

Dakar v., yellow fever v. (2).

diphtheria, tetanus toxoids, and pertussis v., a v. available in three forms: 1) diphtheria and tetanus toxoids plus pertussis v. (DTP); 2) tetanus and diphtheria toxoids, adult type (Td); and 3) tetanus toxoid (T); used for active immunization against diphtheria, tetanus, and whooping cough.

duck embryo origin v. (DEV), see rabies v.

Flury strain v., see rabies v.'s, Flury strain egg-passage.

foot-and-mouth disease virus v.'s, v.'s either of inactivated virus from infected cattle tongue epithelium or, more recently, of live virus attenuated by embryonate egg or mouse passage and propagated in tissue culture.

Haffkine's v., (1) a killed culture of *Vibrio cholerae* in two strengths, a weaker one for the initial inoculation and a stronger one for the second inoculation 7 to 10 days after the first; **(2)** a killed plague bacillus (*Yersinia pestis*) v.

hepatitis B v., a formalin-inactivated v. prepared from the surface antigen (HBsAg) of the hepatitis B virus; the antigen can be obtained from the plasma of human carriers of the virus or by genetic engineering.

heterogenous v., v. that is not autogenous, but is prepared from the same species of bacterium.

high-egg-passage (HEP) v., see rabies v., Flury strain egg-passage.

hog cholera v.'s, v.'s either of virus from blood of infected swine, inactivated with crystal violet, or live virus attenuated in rabbits or tissue culture and frequently used in conjunction with hog cholera virus antiserum.

human diploid cell rabies v. (HDRV), in the U.S., rabies v. comprised of fixed virus grown on WI-38 cells and inactivated with tri-*n*-butyl phosphate.

inactivated poliovirus v. (IPV), see poliovirus v.'s (2).

influenza virus v.'s, influenza virus grown in embryonate eggs and inactivated, usually by the addition of formalin; because of the marked and progressive antigenic variation of the influenza viruses, the strains included are regularly changed following various outbreaks of influenza in order to include most recently isolated epidemic strains of both type A influenza and type B influenza.

live v., v. prepared from living, attenuated organisms.

live oral poliovirus v., see poliovirus v.'s (2).

low-egg-passage (LEP) v., see rabies v., Flury strain egg-passage.

measles virus v., v. containing live, attenuated strains of measles virus prepared in chick embryo cell culture.

measles, mumps, and rubella v. (MMR), a combination of live attenuated measles, mumps, and rubella viruses in an aqueous suspension; used for immunization against the respective diseases.

multivalent v., polyvalent v.

mumps virus v., v. containing live, attenuated mumps virus prepared in chick embryo cell cultures.

oil v., see adjuvant v.

oral poliovirus v. (OPV), see poliovirus v.'s (2).

Pasteur v., see rabies v.

pertussis v., see diphtheria, tetanus toxoids, and pertussis v.

plague v., v. (licensed for use in the U.S.) prepared from cultures of *Yersinia pestis,* inactivated with formaldehyde, and preserved with 0.5% phenol; injections are made intramuscularly, and booster inoculations are recommended every 6 to 12 months while individuals remain in an area of risk; live, attenuated bacterial and chemical fraction v.'s are also available.

pneumococcal v., v. comprised of purified capsular polysaccharide antigen from 23 types of *Streptococcus pneumoniae* (representing those types responsible for most of the reported pneumococcal diseases in the U.S.).

poliovirus v.'s, poliomyelitis v.'s, (1) inactivated poliovirus v. (IPV), an aqueous suspension of inactivated strains of poliomyelitis virus used by injection; has largely been replaced by the oral v.; **(2) oral poliovirus v. (OPV),** an aqueous suspension of live, attenuated strains of poliomyelitis virus given orally for active immunization against poliomyelitis.

polyvalent v., multivalent v.; a v. prepared from cultures of two or more strains of the same species or microorganism.

rabies v., a v. introduced by Pasteur as a method of treatment for the bite of a rabid animal: daily (14 to 21) injections of virus that increased serially from noninfective to fully infective "fixed" virus were given to render the central nervous system refractory to infection by virulent virus; this v., with but slight modification (*e.g.,* Semple v.), was used for many years but had the serious defect that the large quantity of heterologous nervous tissue inoculated along with the virus occasionally gave rise to an allergic (immunological) demyelinization. It has been largely replaced, in the case of man, by rabies v. of duck embryo origin (DEV), prepared from embryonate duck eggs infected with "fixed" virus and inactivated with β-propiolactone. Although still available, it is being replaced in turn by human diploid cell rabies v.

rabies v., Flury strain egg-passage, (1) high-egg-passage (HEP) v.: living Flury strain rabies virus at the 180th to 190th level egg passage (embryonate eggs), used for vaccination of cattle and cats; **(2)** low-egg-passage (LEP) v.: at the 40th to 50th passage level, containing 10^3 to 10^4 mouse LD_{50}; nonpathogenic in dogs but retains some pathogenicity for cattle and cats.

rickettsia v., attenuated, see typhus v.

Rocky Mountain spotted fever v., suspension of inactivated *Rickettsia rickettsii* prepared by growing the rickettsiae in the embryonate yolk sac of fowl eggs.

rubella virus v., live, a live virus v. prepared from duck embryo or human diploid cell culture infected with rubella virus; administered as a single subcutaneous injection.

Sabin v., an orally administered v. containing live, attenuated strains of poliovirus. See poliovirus v.'s.

Salk v., the original poliovirus v., composed of virus propagated in monkey kidney tissue culture and inactivated. See poliovirus v.'s.

Semple v., a modification of the original (Pasteur) rabies v., formerly widely used in the U.S., prepared from sheep brains, inactivated with formalin and administered in 14 to 21 daily injections; has variable potency and is associated with a high incidence of postvaccinal demyelination.

smallpox v., v. of vaccinia virus suspensions prepared from cutaneous vaccinial lesions of calves (calf lymph).

staphylococcus v., a suspension of organisms from cultures of one or more strains of *Staphylococcus;* used for furunculosis, acne, and other suppurative conditions.

stock v., a v. made from a stock microbial strain, in contradistinction to an autogenous v.

subunit v., a v. which, through chemical extraction, is free of viral nucleic acid and contains only minimal amounts of nonviral antigens (proteins derived from the culture medium); such v.'s are relatively free of the adverse reactions (*e.g.,* influenza virus) associated with v.'s containing the whole virion.

T.A.B. v., typhoid-paratyphoid A and B v.

tetanus v., see diphtheria, tetanus toxoids, and pertussis v.

tuberculosis v., BCG v.

typhoid v., a suspension of *Salmonella typhi* inactivated either by heat or by chemical (acetone) with an added preservative; in the U.S., the combined typhoid and paratyphoid A and B v.'s have been largely replaced by the monovalent typhoid v. because of the lack of evidence of effectiveness of paratyphoid A and paratyphoid B ingredients.

typhoid-paratyphoid A and B v., T.A.B. v.; a suspension of killed typhoid and paratyphoid A and B bacilli. See also typhoid v.

typhus v., a formaldehyde-inactivated suspension of *Rickettsia prowazekii* grown in embryonate eggs; effective against louse-borne (epidemic) typhus; primary immunization consists of two subcutaneous injections 4 or more weeks apart; booster doses are required every 6 to 12 months, as long as the possibility of exposure exists. A v. containing living rickettsiae of an attenuated strain of *R. prowazekii* has also been used.

whooping-cough v., see diphtheria, tetanus toxoids, and pertussis v. (3).

yellow fever v., (1) a living, attenuated strain (17D) of yellow fever virus propagated in embryonate fowl eggs; **(2)** Dakar v.; a suspension of dried mouse brain infected with French neurotropic (Dakar) strain of yellow fever virus, administered topically by the scratch method; not officially recommended in the United States because of meningoencephalitic reactions.

---

vaccinia (vak-sin'ē-ă) [L. *vaccinus,* relating to a cow, fr. *vacca,* a cow]. Vaccina; variola vaccine or vaccinia; primary reaction; an infection, primarily local and limited to the site of inoculation, induced in man by inoculation with the vaccinia virus in order to confer resistance to smallpox. On about the third day after this vaccination, papules form at the site of inoculation which become transformed into umbilicated vesicles and later pustules; they then dry up, and the scab falls off on about the 21st day, leaving a pitted scar; in some cases there are more or less marked constitutional disturbances.

v. gangreno'sa, progressive v.

generalized v., secondary lesions of the skin following vaccination which may occur in subjects with previously healthy skin but are more common in the case of traumatized skin, especially in the case of eczema (eczema vaccinatum). In the latter instance, generalized v. may result from mere contact with a vaccinated person. Secondary vaccinial lesions may also occur following transfer of virus from the vaccination to another site by means of the fingers.

progressive v., v. gangrenosa; a severe or even fatal form of v. occurring chiefly in subjects with an immunologic deficiency or dyscrasia and characterized by progressive enlargement of the initial and also of secondary lesions.

vaccinial (vak-sin'ē-ăl). Relating to vaccinia.

vacciniform (vak-sin'i-fōrm). Resembling vaccinia.

vaccinist (vak'si-nist). Vaccinator (1).

vaccinization (vak'sin-i-zā'shŭn). Vaccination repeated at short intervals until it will no longer take.

vaccinogen (vak-sin'-ō-jen). A source of vaccine, such as an inoculated heifer.

vaccinogenous (vak-si-noj'ĕ-nŭs). Producing vaccine, or relating to the production of vaccine.

vaccinoid (vak'si-noyd). Resembling vaccinia.

vaccinostyle (vak'si-nō-stīl). A pointed instrument used in vaccination.

vaccinum (vak'si-nŭm) [L.]. Vaccine.

vacuolar (vak-yū-ō'lăr). Relating to or resembling a vacuole.

vacuolate, vacuolated (vak'yū-ō-lāt, -lāt'ed). Having vacuoles.

vacuolation (vak'yū-ō-lā'shŭn). Vacuolization. **1.** Formation of vacuoles. **2.** The condition of having vacuoles.

vacuole (vak'yū-ōl) [Mod. L. *vacuolum,* dim. of L. *vacuum,* an empty space]. **1.** A minute space in any tissue. **2.** A clear space in the substance of a cell, sometimes degenerative in character, sometimes surrounding an englobed foreign body and serving as a temporary cell stomach for the digestion of the body.

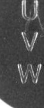

autophagic v., cytolysosome.

contractile v., a cavity formed by the accumulation of fluid in the ectoplasm of a protozoan; after increasing for a time it empties itself externally by a sudden contraction; it functions as an osmoregulatory mechanism for water balance, especially in freshwater protozoans.

parasitophorous v., a v. formed by layers of endoplasmic reticulum around an intracellular parasite which may serve to isolate the parasite and enclose it for lysozymal attack.

vacuolization (vak'yū-ō-li-zā'shŭn). Vacuolation.

vacuome (vak'yū-ōm) [vacuole + G. *-oma,* tumor]. A system of vacuoles which can be stained with neutral red in the living cell.

vacutome (vak'yū-tōm). Electrodermatome that applies suction to the skin to raise it before an advancing blade, usually for taking a split-thickness skin graft.

vacuum (vak'ūm) [L. ntr. of *vacuus,* empty]. An empty space, one practically exhausted of air or gas.

vadum (vā'dŭm) [L. a ford]. An occasional elevation from the bottom of a cerebral sulcus nearly obliterating it for a short distance.

vagal (vā'găl). Relating to the vagus nerve.

vagectomy (vā-jek'tō-mē). Surgical removal of a segment of a vagus nerve.

vagi (vā'gī, -jī). Plural of vagus.

vagin-. See vagino-.

vagina, gen. and pl. **vaginae** (vă-jī'nă, -nē) [L. sheath, the vagina] [NA]. **1.** Sheath (2); any sheathlike structure. **2.** The genital canal in the female, extending from the uterus to the vulva.

v. bul'bi [NA], sheath of eyeball; v. oculi; fascia bulbi; capsula bulbi; eye capsule; Tenon's capsule; a condensation of connective tissue on the outer aspect of the sclera from which it is separated by a narrow cleftlike space; the sheath is attached to the sclera near the sclerocorneal junction and blends with the fascia of the extraocular muscles.

v. carot'ica [NA], carotid sheath; the dense fibrous investment of the carotid artery, internal jugular vein, and vagus nerve on each side; the layers of cervical fascia blend with it.

v. cellulo'sa, the connective tissue sheath of a nerve or muscle (perineurium or perimysium, respectively).

v. commu'nis musculo'rum flexo'rum [NA], common flexor sheath; ulnar bursa; the synovial sheath that surrounds the tendons of the superficial and deep flexors of the digits as they pass through the carpal canal; it is commonly continuous with the digital sheath of the little finger.

v. exter'na ner'vi op'tici [NA], the outer sheath around the optic nerve, continuous with the pachymeninx (dura mater).

vagi'nae fibro'sae digito'rum ma'nus [NA], fibrous sheaths of the digits of the hand; the tubular fibrous layers that enclose the synovial sheaths and the superficial and deep flexor tendons and the tendon of the flexor pollicis longus in their passage along their respective digits; they are composed of annular and cruciform parts. See *pars* anularis vaginae fibrosae; *pars* cruciformis vaginae fibrosae.

vagi'nae fibro'sae digito'rum pe'dis [NA], fibrous sheaths of the toes; the tubular fibrous layer enclosing the synovial sheath and the tendons of the long and short flexors of the toes and the flexor hallucis longus in the digits; they are composed of annular and cruciform parts. See *pars* anularis vaginae fibrosae; *pars* cruciformis vaginae fibrosae.

v. fibro'sa ten'dinis [NA], fibrous sheath of a tendon.

v. inter'na ner'vi op'tici [NA], the innermost sheath around the optic nerve, continuous with the leptomeninges (pia-arachnoid).

v. intertubercula'ris [NA], intertubercular sheath; the extension of the synovial membrane of the shoulder joint downward in the intertubercular groove to surround the tendon of the long head of the biceps.

v. masculi'na, *utriculus* prostaticus.

v. muco'sa ten'dinis, v. synovialis tendinis.

v. mus'culi rec'ti abdo'minis [NA], sheath of the rectus abdominis, formed by the aponeuroses of the three anterolateral muscles of the abdominal wall that split to enclose the rectus and fuse medially to form the linea alba; it consists of a lamina anterior and a lamina posterior, the latter being absent below the linea arcuata (semicircular line).

v. musculo'rum obli'qui superio'ris [NA], sheath of superior oblique muscle; synovial trochlear or trochlear synovial bursa; v. synovialis trochleae; the synovial sheath enclosing the tendon of the superior oblique muscle as it passes through the trochlea.

v. musculo'rum perone'orum commu'nis [NA], the sheath that surrounds the tendons of the peroneus longus and brevis muscles in their passage across the ankle.

vagi'nae ner'vi op'tici, sheaths of the optic nerve, formed by extensions of the central meninges. See v. interna nervi optici; v. externa nervi optici.

v. oc'uli, v. bulbi.

v. proces'sus styloi'dei [NA], sheath of styloid process; vaginal process; a crest of bone (edge of the tympanic portion of the temporal bone) running from the front and medial side of the mastoid process to the spine of the sphenoid; it splits to ensheathe the base of the styloid process.

v. sep'tate, a bipartite v. caused by the presence of a more or less complete longitudinal septum.

vagi'nae synovia'les digito'rum ma'nus [NA], synovial sheaths of digits of hand; the synovial sheaths that enclose the flexor tendons of the fingers and line the inside of the fibrous tendon sheaths.

vagi'nae synovia'les digito'rum pe'dis [NA], synovial sheaths of digits of foot; similar in structure to the corresponding sheaths of the hand.

v. synovia'lis ten'dinis [NA], synovial or mucous sheath of a tendon; vaginal synovial membrane; theca tendinis; v. mucosa tendinis; a sheath of synovial membrane enveloping certain of the tendons; it contains a small amount of synovial fluid.

v. synovia'lis troch'leae, v. synovialis musculorum obliqui superioris.

v. ten'dinis mus'culi extenso'ris car'pi ulna'ris [NA], the synovial sheath surrounding the tendon of the extensor carpi ulnaris in its course deep to the extensor retinaculum.

v. ten'dinis mus'culi extenso'ris dig'iti min'imi [NA], the synovial sheath surrounding the tendon of the extensor digiti minimi in its passage deep to the extensor retinaculum.

v. ten'dinis mus'culi extenso'ris hallu'cis lon'gi [NA], the synovial sheath that surrounds the tendon of the extensor hallucis longus in its passage across the ankle.

v. ten'dinis mus'culi extenso'ris pol'licis lon'gi [NA], the synovial sheath surrounding the extensor pollicis longus tendon in its passage deep to the extensor retinaculum.

v. ten'dinis mus'culi flexo'ris car'pi radia'lis [NA], the synovial sheath enclosing the tendon of the flexor carpi radialis as it crosses the wrist.

v. ten'dinis mus'culi flexo'ris hallu'cis lon'gi [NA], the synovial sheath that envelops the tendon of the flexor hallucis longus as it passes into the foot deep to the flexor retinaculum.

v. ten'dinis mus'culi flexo'ris pol'licis lon'gi [NA], radial bursa; the synovial sheath that envelopes the tendon of the flexor pollicis longus in its course through the carpal canal; it is continuous with the digital sheath of the thumb, the two generally being considered as one sheath.

v. ten'dinis mus'culi perone'i lon'gi planta'ris [NA], the synovial sheath surrounding the tendon of the peroneus longus in its course across the sole of the foot.

v. ten'dinis mus'culi tibia'lis anterio'ris [NA], the synovial sheath, deep to the extensor retinaculum, that surrounds the tendon of the tibialis anterior as it crosses the ankle.

v. ten'dinis mus'culi tibia'lis posterio'ris [NA], the synovial sheath surrounding the tendon of the tibialis posterior as it passes into the foot deep to the flexor retinaculum.
v. ten'dinum mus'culi extenso'ris digito'rum pe'dis lon'gi [NA], the synovial sheath that surrounds the tendons of the long extensor and the peroneus tertius in their passage across the ankle.
v. ten'dinum mus'culi flexo'ris digito'rum pe'dis lon'gi [NA], the synovial sheath that envelopes the flexor digitorum longus tendons as they pass into the foot deep to the flexor retinaculum.
v. ten'dinum musculo'rum abducto'ris lon'gi et extenso'ris bre'vis pol'licis [NA], the synovial sheath lining the compartment of the extensor retinaculum that contains the abductor pollicis longus and extensor pollicis brevis tendons.
v. ten'dinum musculo'rum extenso'rum car'pi radia'lium [NA], the synovial sheath lining the compartment of the extensor retinaculum containing the tendons of the extensor carpi radialis longus and brevis muscles.
v. ten'dinum musculo'rum extenso'ris digitor'um et extenso'ris in'dicis [NA], the synovial sheath that surrounds the four tendons of the extensor digitorum muscle and the tendon of the extensor indicis deep to the extensor retinaculum.
vagi'nae vaso'rum, sheaths of vessels; fibrous envelopes ensheathing the arteries with their accompanying veins and sometimes nerves as well.

vaginal (vaj'i-năl) [Mod. L. *vaginalis*]. Relating to the vagina or to any sheath.

vaginalitis (vaj'i-nă-lī'tis). Inflammation of the tunica vaginalis testis.

vaginapexy (va-jī'nă-pek-sē). Vaginofixation.

vaginate (vaj'i-nāt). **1.** To ensheathe; to enclose in a sheath. **2.** Ensheathed; provided with a sheath.

vaginectomy (vaj-i-nek'tō-mē) [vagina + G. *ektomē*, excision]. Colpectomy; excision of the vagina or a segment thereof.

vaginism (vaj'i-nizm). Vaginismus.

vaginismus (vaj-i-niz'mŭs) [vagina + L. *-ismus*, action, condition]. Vaginism; vulvismus; painful involuntary spasm of the vagina preventing intercourse.
posterior v., spasmodic stenosis of the vagina caused by contraction of the levator ani muscle.

vaginitis, pl. **vaginitides** (vaj-i-nī'tis, -nī'ti-dēz) [vagina + G. *-itis*, inflammation]. Inflammation of the vagina.
adhesive v., v. adhesi'va, inflammation of vaginal mucosa with adhesions of the vaginal walls to each other.
amebic v., v. caused by *Entamoeba histolytica*.
atrophic v., thinning and atrophy of the vaginal epithelium usually resulting from diminished endocrine stimulation; a common occurrence in postmenopausal women.
v. cys'tica, v. emphysematosa.
desquamative inflammatory v., an acute inflammation of vagina of unknown cause, characterized by grayish pseudomembrane, free discharge, and easy bleeding on trauma; the discharge contains pus and immature epithelial cells, although estrogen levels are normal.
v. emphysemato'sa, v. or pachyvaginitis cystica; v. characterized by accumulation of gas in small connective tissue spaces lined by foreign-body giant cells.
granular v., a condition of cattle manifested by the appearance of small, spherical, transparent nodules in the mucosa of the vagina of cows and of the penis of bulls; the mucosa is reddened and a mucopurulent exudate appears on the affected surfaces; the precise cause is not known.
pinworm v., v. caused by *Enterobius vermicularis*.
senile v., v. seni'lis, v. occurring in old age, often assuming the form of adhesive v.; atrophic v. resulting from withdrawal of estrogen stimulation of mucosa.

vagino-, vagin- [L. *vagina, sheath*]. Combining forms denoting the vagina. See also colpo-.

vaginoabdominal (vaj'i-nō-ab-dom'i-năl). Relating to the vagina and the abdomen.

vaginocele (vaj'i-nō-sēl). Colpocele (1).

vaginodynia (vaj'i-nō-din'ē-ă). Colpodynia; colpalgia; vaginal pain.

vaginofixation (vaj'i-nō-fik-sā'shŭn). Colpopexy; vaginopexy; vaginapexy; suture of a relaxed and prolapsed vagina to the abdominal wall.

vaginohysterectomy (vaj'i-nō-his-ter-ek'tō-mē). Vaginal *hysterectomy.*

vaginolabial (vaj'i-nō-lā'bē-ăl). Relating to the vagina and the pudendal labia.

vaginomycosis (vaj'i-nō-mī-kō'sis). Colpomycosis; colpitis mycotica; vaginal infection due to a fungus.

vaginopathy (vaj-i-nop'ă-thē) [vagino- + G. *pathos*, suffering]. Colpopathy; any diseased condition of the vagina.

vaginoperineal (vaj'i-nō-per-i-nē'ăl). Relating to or involving the vagina and perineum.

vaginoperineoplasty (vaj'i-nō-per-i-nē'ō-plas-tē) [vagino- + perineum, + G. *plastos*, formed]. Colpoperineoplasty; plastic surgery of the perineum involving the vagina.

vaginoperineorrhaphy (vaj'i-nō-per-i-nē-ōr'ă-fē) [vagino- + perineum, + G. *raphē*, suture]. Colpoperineorrhaphy; repair of a lacerated vagina and perineum.

vaginoperineotomy (vaj'i-nō-per-i-nē-ot'ō-mē) [vagino- + perineum, + G. *tome*, incision]. Division of the outlet of the vagina and adjacent portion of the perineum to facilitate childbirth.

vaginoperitoneal (vaj'i-nō-per-i-tō-nē'ăl). Relating to the vagina and the peritoneum.

vaginopexy (vaj'i-nō-pek-sē). Vaginofixation.

vaginoplasty (vaj'i-nō-plas-tē). [vagino- + G. *plastos*, formed]. Colpoplasty; plastic surgery of the vagina.

vaginoscopy (vaj-i-nos'kō-pē). Inspection of the vagina, usually with an instrument.

vaginotomy (vaj-i-not'ō-mē). Colpotomy; coleotomy (2); a cutting operation in the vagina.

vaginovesical (vaj'i-nō-ves'i-kăl). Relating to the vagina and the urinary bladder.

vaginovulvar (vaj'i-nō-vŭl'văr). Relating to the vagina and the vulva.

Vaginulus plebeius (vaj-i-nū'lŭs plē'bē-ē-ŭs). The slug vector of *Angiostrongylus costaricensis*.

vagitus uterinus (va-jī'tŭs yū-ter-ī'nŭs) [L. fr. *vagio*, to squall; L. fr. *uterus*, womb]. Crying of the fetus while still within the uterus, possible when the membranes have been ruptured and air has entered the uterine cavity.

vago- [L. *vagus*]. Combining form denoting the vagus nerve.

vagoaccessorius (vā-gō-ak-ses-sō'rē-ŭs). The vagus and the accessory portion of the spinal accessory nerve, regarded as one nerve.

vagoglossopharyngeal (vā'gō-glos'ō-fă-rin'jē-ăl). Relating to the vagus and glossopharyngeal nerves; denoting their contiguous or common nuclei of origin and termination and regions innervated by both nerves such as the musculature of the pharynx.

vagolysis (vā-gol'i-sis) [vago- + G. *lysis*, a loosening]. Surgical destruction of the vagus nerve.

vagolytic (vā-gō-lit'ik) **1.** Pertaining to or causing vagolysis. **2.** A therapeutic or chemical agent that has inhibitory effects on the vagus nerve. **3.** Denoting an agent having such effects.

vagomimetic (vā'gō-mi-met'ik). Mimicking the action of the efferent fibers of the vagus nerve.

vagotomy (vā-got'ō-mē) [vago- + G. *tomē*, incision]. Division of the vagus nerve.

vagotonia (vā-gō-tō'nē-ă) [vago- + G. *tonos,* strain]. Sympathetic imbalance; parasympathotonia; irritability of the vagus nerve, often marked by excessive peristalsis and loss of the pharyngeal reflex; opposed to sympathicotonia.

vagotonic (vā-gō-ton'ik). Relating to or marked by vagotonia.

vagotropic (vā-gō-trop'ik) [vago- + G. *tropos,* turning]. Attracted by, hence acting upon, the vagus nerve.

vagovagal (vā'gō-vā'găl). Pertaining to a process that utilizes both afferent and efferent vagal fibers.

vagus, gen. and pl. **vagi** (vā'gŭs; vā'gī, -jī) [L. wandering, so-called because of the wide distribution of the nerve]. *Nervus* vagus.

Val Symbol for valine and its radicals.

valence, valency (vā'lens, -len-sē) [L. *valentia,* strength]. The combining power of one atom of an element (or a radical), that of the hydrogen atom being the unit of comparison, determined by the number of electrons in the outer shell of the atom (v. electrons); *e.g.,* in HCl, chlorine is monovalent; in H_2O, oxygen is bivalent; in NH_3, nitrogen is trivalent.
negative v., the number of v. electrons an atom can take up.
positive v., the number of v. electrons an atom can give up.

valent (vā'lent). Possessing valence.

Valentin, Gabriel G., German-Swiss physiologist, 1810–1883. See V.'s *corpuscles, ganglion, nerve.*

Valentine, Ferdinand C., U.S. surgeon, 1851–1909. See V.'s *position, test.*

valerate (val'ĕ-rāt). Valerianate; a salt of valeric acid; some are used in modern medicine.

valerian (vă-lēr'ē-an). Vandal root; garden heliotrope; the rhizome and roots of *Valeriana officinalis* (family Valerianaceae), a herb native in southern Europe and northern Asia, cultivated also in Great Britain and the U.S.; has been used as a sedative in hysteria and at the menopause.

valerianate (va-lē'rē-ă-nāt). Valerate.

valeric acid (vă-lēr'ik, vă-ler'ik). Pentanoic acid; normal aliphatic acid; C_4H_9COOH; distilled from valerian; some of its salts are used in medicine.

valethamate bromide (vă-leth'ă-māt). 2-Diethylaminoethyl 3-methyl-2-phenylvalerate methylbromide; an anticholinergic agent.

valetudinarian (val'ĕ-tū-di-nār'ē-ăn) [L. *valetudinarius,* sickly]. An invalid or person in chronically poor health.

valetudinarianism (val'ĕ-tū-di-nār'ē-ăn-izm). A weak or infirm state due to invalidism.

valgoid (val'goyd) [L. *valgus,* bowlegged, + G. *eidos,* resemblance]. Relating to valgus; knock-kneed; suffering from talipes valgus.

valgus (val'gŭs) [Mod. L. turned outward, fr. L. bowlegged]. Bent or twisted outward away from the midline or body; modern accepted usage, particularly in orthopedics, erroneously transposes the meaning of varus to v., as in *genu* valgum (knock-knee).

val'id [L. *valeo,* to be strong]. Effective; producing the desired result; verifiably correct.

validation (val-i-dā'shŭn). The act or process of making valid.
consensual v., the confirmation of the experience or judgment of one person by another.

validity (vă-lid'i-tē). An index of how well a test or procedure in fact measures what it purports to measure.
concurrent v., criterion-related v. used to predict performance in a real-life situation given at about the same time as the test or procedure.
construct v., the extent to which a test or procedure appears to measure a higher order, inferred theoretical construct, or trait in contrast to measuring a more limited, specific dimension.
content v., the extent to which the items of a test or procedure are in fact a representative sample of that which is to be measured.
criterion-related v., the degree of effectiveness with which performance on a test or procedure predicts performance in a real-life situation.
face v., the extent to which the items of a test or procedure appear superficially to sample that which is to be measured.
predictive v., criterion-related v. used to predict performance in a real-life task at a future time.

valine (Val) (val'in). 2-Amino-3-methylbutanoic acid; $(CH_3)_2CHCH(NH_2)COOH$; a constituent of most proteins.

valla (val'ă). Plural of vallum.

vallate (val'āt) [L. *vallo,* pp. *-atus,* to surround with, fr. *vallum,* a rampart]. Bordered with an elevation, as a cupped structure.

vallecula, pl. **valleculae** (vă-lek'yū-lă, -lē) [L. dim. of *vallis,* valley] [NA]. Valley; a crevice or depression on any surface.
v. cerebel'li [NA], vallis; a deep hollow on the inferior surface of the cerebellum, between the hemispheres, containing the medulla oblongata and the falx cerebelli.
v. epiglot'tica [NA], a depression between the median and lateral glossoepiglottic folds on either side.
v. syl'vii, *fossa* lateralis cerebri.
v. un'guis, *sulcus* matricis unguis.

Valleix, François L. I., French physician, 1807–1855. See V.'s *points.*

valley (val'ē). Vallecula.

vallis (val'is) [L. valley]. *Vallecula* cerebelli.

vallum, pl. **valla** (val'ŭm, -ă) [L. a rampart, fr. *vallus,* a stake]. **1** [NA]. Any raised, more or less circular ridge. **2.** The slightly raised outer wall of the circular depression, or fossa, surrounding a vallate papilla of the tongue.
v. un'guis [NA], wall of nail; nail fold; the fold of skin overlapping the lateral and proximal margins of the nail.

valmethamide (val-meth'ă-mīd). Valnoctamide.

valnoctamide (val-nok'tă-mīd). Valmethamide; 2-ethyl-3-methylvaleramide; an antianxiety agent.

valoid (val'oyd) [L. *valeo,* to be strong]. Equivalent *extract.*

valproic acid (val-prō'ik). 2-Propylvaleric acid; $C_8H_{16}O_2$; an anticonvulsant used to treat seizure disorders; also used as the sodium salt, valproate sodium.

Valsalva, Antonio M., Italian anatomist, 1666–1723. See V. *maneuver, test;* V.'s *antrum, ligaments, muscle, sinus; teniae* of V.

value (val'yū). A particular quantitative determination. For v.'s not given below, see the specific name. See also under index; number.
acetyl v., the milligrams of KOH required to neutralize the acetic acid produced by the hydrolysis of 1 g of acetylated fat; a measure of the hydroxy acids present in glycerides; notably high in castor oil.
buffer v., buffer index; the power of a substance in solution to absorb acid or alkali without change in pH; this is highest at a pH equal to the pK of the acid of the buffer pair. See also buffer *capacity.*
buffer v. of the blood, the ability of the blood to compensate for additions of acid or alkali without disturbance of the pH.
caloric v., the heat evolved by a food when burnt or metabolized.
globular v., color *index.*
homing v., in a cybernetic system such as homeostasis, that v. of a trait of interest which the restorative forces are directed to maintaining.
iodine v., iodine *number.*
maturation v., an indicator of the level of maturation attained by vaginal epithelium and used as a factor in cytohormonal evaluation from the maturation index by valuing the parabasal cells at 0.0, the intermediate cells at 0.5, and the superficial cells at 1.0; for special

investigations, subtypes of a major cell can be given different values.

normal v.'s, a set of laboratory test v.'s used to characterize apparently healthy individuals; now replaced by reference v.'s.

phenotypic v., in quantitative genetics, the metrical quantity of some trait associated with a particular phenotype.

predictive v., the proportion of individuals positive to a medical screening test which have the infection or disease under study.

reference v.'s, a set of laboratory test v.'s obtained from an individual or group in a defined state of health; this term replaces normal v.'s, since it is based on a defined state of health rather than on apparent health.

thiocyanogen v., thiocyanogen *number.*

threshold limit v. (TLV), the maximum concentration of a chemical recommended by the American Conference of Government Industrial Hygienists for repeated exposure without adverse health effects on workers.

valva, pl. valvae (val'vă, -vē) [L. one leaf of a double door] [NA]. Valve.

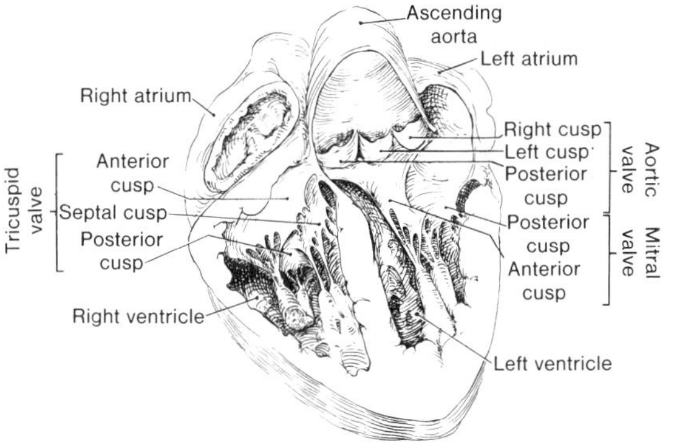

Valves of the Heart

v. aor'tae [NA], aortic valve; the valve between the left ventricle and the ascending aorta, consisting of three fibrous semilunar cusps (valvulae semilunares), located in the adult as anterior, right posterior, and left posterior; they are named in the NA, however, in accordance with the embryonic arrangement in which the cusps are posterior, left, and right.

v. atrioventricula'ris dex'tra [NA], right atrioventricular valve; tricuspid valve; v. tricuspidalis; valvula tricuspidalis; the valve closing the orifice between the right atrium and right ventricle of the heart; its three cusps are called anterior, posterior, and septal.

v. atrioventricula'ris sinis'tra [NA], left atrioventricular valve; mitral valve; v. mitralis; valvula bicuspidalis; bicuspid valve; the valve closing the orifice between the left atrium and left ventricle of the heart; its two cusps are called anterior and posterior.

v. ileoceca'lis [NA], ileocecal or ileocolic valve; Bauhin's or Tulp's (Tulpius') valve; valve of Varolius; ileocecal eminence; the bilabial prominence of the terminal ileum into the large intestine at the cecocolic junction as seen in cadavers; in the living individual it appears as a truncated cone with a star-shaped orifice.

v. mitra'lis, v. atrioventricularis sinistra.

v. tricuspida'lis, v. atrioventricularis dextra.

v. trun'ci pulmona'lis [NA], valve of pulmonary trunk; pulmonary valve; the valve at the entrance to the pulmonary trunk from the right ventricle; it consists of semilunar cusps (valvulae semilunares) which are usually arranged in the adult so that there is a right anterior, a left anterior, and a posterior cusp. The NA terminology names these cusps as right, left, and anterior, in conformity with their embryonic position.

valval, valvar (val'văl, val'văr). Relating to a valve.

valvate (val'vāt). Valvular; relating to or provided with a valve.

valve (valv) [L. *valva*]. Valva. **1.** A fold of the lining membrane of a canal or other hollow organ serving to retard or prevent a reflux of fluid. **2.** Any reduplication of tissue or flaplike structure resembling a valve. See also valva; valvula; plica.

Amussat's v., *plica* spiralis ductus cystici.

anal v.'s, *valvulae* anales.

anterior urethral v., a crescentic horizontal fold at the level of the penoscrotal junction.

aortic v., *valva* aortae.

atrioventricular v.'s, see *valva* atrioventricularis dextra and sinistra.

ball v., any of a variety of prosthetic cardiac v.'s comprised of a ball within a retaining cage affixed to the orifice; when appropriately sized, used in aortic, mitral, or tricuspid position.

Bauhin's v., *valva* ileocecalis.

Béraud's v., Krause's v.; a small fold in the interior of the lacrimal sac at its junction with the lacrimal duct.

Bianchi's v., *plica* lacrimalis.

bicuspid v., *valva* atrioventricularis sinistra.

Bochdalek's v., Foltz' valvule; a fold of mucous membrane in the lacrimal canaliculus at the punctum lacrimale.

Braune's v., a fold of mucous membrane at the junction of the esophagus with the stomach.

caval v., *valvula* venae cavae inferioris.

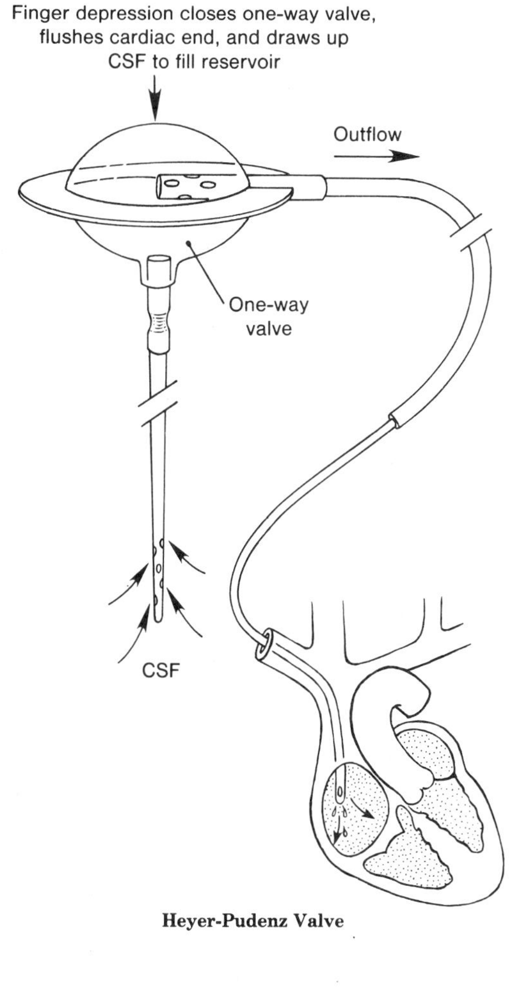

Heyer-Pudenz Valve

congenital v., an abnormal lining fold obstructing a passage; *e.g.*, of a mucous membrane in the urethra.
coronary v., *valvula* sinus coronarii.
v. of coronary sinus, *valvula* sinus coronarii.
eustachian v., *valvula* venae cavae inferioris.
Gerlach's v., valvula processus vermiformis; a fold of mucous membrane, simulating a v., sometimes found at the origin of the vermiform appendix.
Guérin's v., *valvula* fossae navicularis.
Hasner's v., *plica* lacrimalis.
Heister's v., *plica* spiralis ductus cystici.
Heyer-Pudenz v., a v. used in the shunting procedure for hydrocephaly; consisting of a catheter-valve system in which the ventricular catheter leads the cerebrospinal fluid into a one-way pump through which the cerebrospinal fluid passes down the distal catheter into the right atrium of the heart.
Hoboken's v.'s, the flangelike protrusions into the lumen of the umbilical arteries where they are twisted or kinked in their course through the umbilical cord.
Houston's v.'s, *plicae* transversales recti.
Huschke's v., *plica* lacrimalis.
ileocecal v., *valva* ileocecalis.
ileocolic v., *valva* ileocecalis.
v. of inferior vena cava, *valvula* venae cavae inferioris.
Kerckring's v.'s, *plicae* circulares.
Kohlrausch's v.'s, *plicae* transversales recti.
Krause's v., Béraud's v.
left atrioventricular v., *valva* atrioventricularis sinistra.
Mercier's v., an occasional fold of mucosa of the bladder partially occluding the ureteral orifice.
mitral v., *valva* atrioventricularis sinistra.
Morgagni's v.'s, *valvulae* anales.
nasal v., the variable aperture between the nasal septum and the moveable inferior margin of the lateral nasal cartilage.
nonrebreathing v., a type of v. that prevents mixture of inhaled and exhaled gases.
v. of oval foramen, *valvula* foraminis ovalis.
parachute mitral v., parachute deformity; congenital deformity of the mitral v. characterized by the presence of a single papillary muscle from which the chordae of both v. leaflets divide; thus the resemblance to a parachute; the condition often produces a stenosis as the combined result of the tugging action of the chordae on and the subsequent narrowing between the leaflets.
porcine v., a prosthetic cardiac v. derived from the pig heart, which is preserved and sterilized with glutaraldehyde, and permanently sutured to a shape-retaining artificial strut; in appropriate sizes, it can replace any natural heart v.
posterior urethral v.'s, Amussat's valvula; anomalous folds occurring at the level of the colliculus seminalis.
pulmonary v., *valva* trunci pulmonalis.
v. of pulmonary trunk, *valva* trunci pulmonalis.
pyloric v., *valvula* pylori.
rectal v.'s, *plicae* transversales recti.
reducing v., a v. designed to lower the pressure of a gas coming from a cylinder containing compressed gas under high pressure.
right atrioventricular v., *valva* atrioventricularis dextra.
Rosenmüller's v., *plica* lacrimalis.
semilunar v., *valvula* semilunaris.
spiral v., *plica* spiralis ductus cystici.
sylvian v., *valvula* venae cavae inferioris.
Tarin's v., *velum* medullare inferius.
Terrier's v., a valvelike fold between the gallbladder and the cystic duct.
thebesian v., *valvula* sinus coronarii.
toroidal v., a floating doughnut-shaped disc valve, retained by struts integral to the orifice ring, which seats or releases under the influence of intracardiac pressures, thus creating unidirectional blood flow in response to the cardiac beat.
tricuspid v., *valva* atrioventricularis dextra.
Tulp's v., Tulpius' v., *valva* ileocecalis.
urethral v.'s, folds in the urethral mucous membrane. See also anterior urethral v.; posterior urethral v.'s.
v. of Varolius, *valva* ileocecalis.
venous v., *valvula* venosa (2).
vesicoureteral v., a lock mechanism in the wall of the intravesical portion of the ureter that normally prevents urinary reflux.
Vieussens' v., *velum* medullare superius.

valveless (valv'les). Without valves; denoting certain veins, such as the portal, that are not provided with valves as are most of the veins.

valviform (val'vi-fōrm). Valve-shaped.

valvoplasty (val'vō-plas-tē) [valve + G. *plastos,* formed]. Valvuloplasty; surgical reconstruction of a deformed cardiac valve, for the relief of stenosis or incompetence.

valvotomy (val-vot'ō-mē) [valve + G. *tomē,* incision]. **1.** Valvulotomy; cutting through a stenosed cardiac valve to relieve the obstruction. **2.** Incision of a valvular structure.
rectal v., cutting through rectal folds that are too rigid or large.

valvula, pl. **valvulae** (val'vyū-lă, -lē) [Mod. L. dim. of *valva*] [NA]. Valvule; a valve, especially one of small size.
Amussat's v., posterior urethral *valves.*
val'vulae ana'les [NA], anal valves; Morgagni's valves; delicate crescent-shaped mucosal folds that pass between the lower ends of neighboring anal columns; the small pocket thus formed is an anal sinus.
v. bicuspida'lis, *valva* atrioventricularis sinistra.
val'vulae conniven'tes, *plicae* circulares.
v. fora'minis ova'lis [NA], valve of oval foramen; falx septi; a fold projecting into the left atrium from the margin of the foramen ovale in the fetus; when, with beginning inspiration, the blood pressure within the left atrium increases, the valve closes and its edges become adherent to the margin of the foramen ovale, occluding it.
v. fos'sae navicula'ris [NA], Guérin's valve or fold; a fold of mucous membrane sometimes found in the root of the fossa navicularis urethrae.
Gerlach's v., *reticulum* trabeculare.
v. lymphat'ica [NA], lymphatic valvule; one of the delicate semilunar valves found in lymphatic vessels; they are usually paired and similar in structure to venous valves and occur at close intervals along the vessel wall.
v. proces'sus vermifor'mis, Gerlach's *valve.*
v. pylor'i, pyloric valve; a prominent fold of mucous membrane at the gastroduodenal junction enclosing the gastroduodenal pylorus.
v. semiluna'ris [NA], semilunar valve; one of three semilunar segments serving as the three cusps of a valve preventing regurgitation at the beginning of the aorta; a similar valve guards the entrance of the pulmonary trunk; the segments are named, respectively, anterior, right, and left in the right ventricle, and posterior, right, and left in the left ventricle.
v. semiluna'ris tari'ni, *velum* medullare inferius.
v. si'nus corona'rii [NA], valve of coronary sinus; thebesian valve; coronary valve; a delicate fold of endocardium at the opening of the coronary sinus into the right atrium.
v. spiral'is, *plica* spiralis ductus cystici.
v. tricuspida'lis, *valva* atrioventricularis dextra.
v. ve'nae ca'vae inferio'ris [NA], valve of inferior vena cava; caval valve; eustachian or sylvian valve; an endocardial fold extending from the anterior inferior margin of the inferior vena cava to the anterior part of the limbus fossa ovalis.
v. veno'sa, (1) in the embryo, one of the pair of valves at the opening from the sinus venosus into the right atrium; **(2)** [NA] venous valve; a fold of the lining layer of a vein to prevent a reflux of blood.

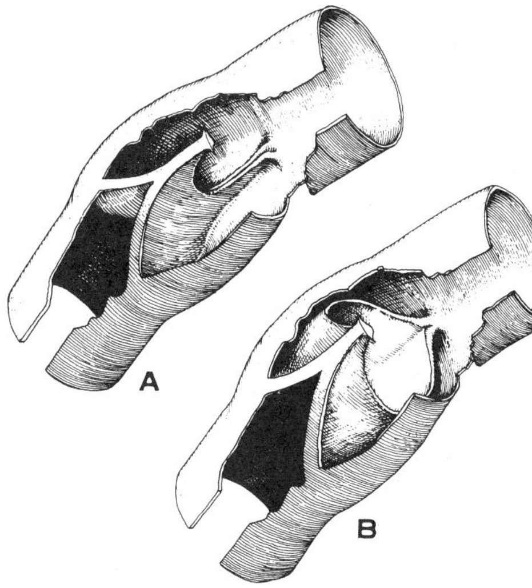

Venous Valves in Femoral Vein
A, closed; *B*, open.

v. vestib'uli, obsolete term for valvula venosa (1).

valvular (val'vyū-lăr). Valvate.

valvule (val'vūl) [L. *valvula*]. Valvula.
Foltz' v., Bochdalek's *valve.*
lymphatic v., *valvula* lymphatica.

valvulitis (val-vyū-lī'tis) [Mod. L. *valvula,* valve, + G. *-itis,* inflammation]. Inflammation of a valve, especially a heart valve.
rheumatic v., v. characterized in the acute stage by small fibrin vegetations along the lines of closure and by Aschoff bodies in the cusps; in the chronic stage, it is characterized by scarring, commissural adhesion, and stenosis or regurgitation.

valvuloplasty (val'vyū-lō-plas'tē). Valvoplasty.

valvulotome (val'vyū-lō-tōm). An instrument for sectioning a valve.

valvulotomy (val-vyū-lot'ō-mē). Valvotomy (1).

valyl (Val) (val'il). The radical of valine.

Van, van. For some names with this prefix not found below, see the principal part of the name.

vanadate (van'ă-dāt). A salt of vanadic acid.

vanadic acid (vă-nad'ik). An acid, H_3VO_4, derived from vanadium, forming salts with various bases.

vanadium (vă-nā'dē-ŭm) [*Vanadis,* Scand. myth.]. A metallic element, symbol V, atomic no. 23, atomic weight 50.95.

vanadium group. Those elements resembling vanadium in chemical and metallurgical properties; included with vanadium are niobium and tantalum.

van Bogaert, Ludo, Belgian neuropathologist, *1897. See v. B.'s *disease.*

Van Buchem, F.S. See V.B.'s *syndrome.*

van Buren, William H., U.S. surgeon, 1819–1883. See v. B. *sound;* v. B.'s *disease.*

vancomycin (van-kō-mī'sin). An antibiotic isolated from cultures of *Nocardia orientalis,* bactericidal and bacteriostatic against Gram-positive organisms; available as the hydrochloride.

van Creveld, S., Dutch physician, *1894. See Ellis-v. C. *syndrome.*

vandal root (van'dăl). Valerian.

van Deen, Izaak A., Dutch physiologist, 1804–1869. See v. D.'s *test.*

van den Bergh, A.A.H., Dutch physician, 1869–1943. See v. d. B.'s *test.*

van der Hoeve, J., Dutch ophthalmologist, 1878–1952. See v. d. H.'s *syndrome.*

van der Kolk, Jacobus L.C.S., Dutch physician, 1797–1862. See v. d. K.'s *law.*

van der Spieghel. See Spigelius.

van der Velden, Reinhardt, German physician, 1851–1903. See v. d. V.'s *test.*

van der Waals, Johannes D., Dutch physicist, 1837–1923. See v. d. W.'s *forces.*

van Ekenstein, W.A., 19th century scientist. See Lobry de Bruyn-v. E. *transformation.*

van Ermengen, Emile P., Belgian bacteriologist, 1851–1932. See v. E.'s *stain.*

van Gieson, Ira, U.S. histologist and bacteriologist, 1865–1913. See v. G.'s *stain.*

van Helmont, Jean B., French physician and chemist, 1577–1644. See v. H.'s *mirror.*

van Horne (Hoorn, Hoorne, Heurenius), Jan (Johannes), Dutch anatomist, 1621–1670. See v. H.'s *canal.*

vanilla (vă-nil'ă) [Sp. *vainilla,* little pod]. The cured, full-grown, unripe fruit of *Vanila planifolia* (Mexican or Bourbon v.) or of *V. tahitensis* (Tahiti v.), orchids (family Orchidaceae) native to Mexico and cultivated in other tropical countries; a flavoring agent.

vanillate (vă-nil'āt). A compound of vanillic acid; $C_8H_8O_4$.

vanillic acid (vă-nil'ik). Methylprotocatechuic acid; 4-hydroxy-3-methoxybenzoic acid; $CH_3O–C_6H_3(OH)COOH$; a flavoring agent.

vanillin (vă-nil'in). Methylprotocatechuic aldehyde; vanillic aldehyde; 4-hydroxy-3-methoxybenzaldehyde; obtained from vanilla and also prepared synthetically; a flavoring agent.

vanillism (vă-nil'izm). **1.** Symptoms of irritation of the skin, nasal mucous membrane, and conjunctiva from which workers with vanilla sometimes suffer. **2.** Infestation of the skin by sarcoptiform mites found in vanilla pods.

vanillylmandelic acid (VMA) (van'i-lil-man-del'ik, vă-nil'il-). Misnomer for 4-hydroxy-3-methoxymandelic acid (α,3-dihydroxy-2-methoxybenzeneacetic acid); the major urinary metabolite of adrenal and sympathetic catecholamines.

Van Slyke, Donald D., U.S. biochemist, 1883–1971, See *slyke;* V. S. *apparatus, formula.*

van't Hoff, Jacobus H., Dutch chemist, 1852–1911. See v. H.'s *law, theory;* Le Bel-v. H. *rule.*

vapor (vā'per) [L. steam]. **1.** Molecules in the gaseous phase of a solid or liquid substance exposed to a gas. **2.** A visible emanation of fine particles of a liquid. **3.** A medicinal preparation to be administered by inhalation.
anesthetic v., the gaseous phase of a liquid anesthetic with sufficient partial pressure at room temperature to produce general anesthesia when inhaled.

vaporization (vā-pōr-i-zā'shŭn). **1.** The change of a solid or liquid to a state of vapor. **2.** The therapeutic application of a vapor.

vaporize (vā'-per-īz). **1.** To convert a solid or liquid into a vapor. **2.** To apply a vapor therapeutically.

vaporizer (vā'per-īz-er). **1.** An apparatus for reducing medicated liquids to a state of vapor suitable for inhalation or application to accessible mucous membranes. See also nebulizer; atomizer. **2.** A device for volatizing liquid anesthetics.
Copper Kettle v., a high thermal capacity v. for volatile anesthetic agents; it uses copper as a conductor and reservoir of heat, and provides a large vaporizing interface by forcing the inflowing oxygen through a sintered bronze disk.

flow-over v., a device for vaporization of a liquid anesthetic by causing gases to pass over the anesthetic or over material saturated with the anesthetic.

temperature-compensated v., a v. of liquid anesthetics with graduated settings calibrated to deliver a known constant concentration of a specific anesthetic despite changes in inflow volume and despite cooling brought about by vaporization.

Vernitrol v., a high thermal capacity v. for volatile anesthetic agents, similar to the Copper Kettle v., that makes possible accurate calculation of the percentage of vapor delivered to the patient if the vapor pressure of the volatile liquid, the oxygen flow into the v., and the diluent flow are known.

vaporthorax (vāp-er-thō′raks). The existence of large water vapor bubbles in the pleural space between the lungs and the chest wall in an unprotected person exposed to altitudes above 63,000 ft., where the barometric pressure is less than 47 mm Hg and where water at body temperature vaporizes from the liquid state.

vapotherapy (vā′pō-ther′ă-pē). Treatment of disease by means of vapor or spray.

$\dot{V}$a/$\dot{Q}$ Abbreviation for ventilation/pefusion *ratio.*

Vaquez, Louis H., French physician, 1860–1936. See V.'s *disease.*

variability (vār′ē-ă-bil′i-tē). **1.** The capability of being variable. **2.** In genetics, the potential or actual differences, either quantitative or qualitative, in phenotype among individuals having the same genotype at a particular genetic locus.

baseline v. of fetal heart rate, the second-to-second changes in fetal heart rate as recorded on a graph.

variable (vār′ē-ă-bl) [L. *vario,* to vary, change, differ]. **1.** That which is inconstant, which can or does change, as contrasted with a constant. **2.** Deviating from the type in structure, form, physiology, or behavior.

dependent v., in experiments, a v. that is influenced by or dependent upon changes in the independent v.

independent v., in experiments, the v. controlled and manipulated by the experimenter.

intervening v., an event, such as an attitude or emotion, inferred to occur within an organism between the stimulation and response in such a way as to influence or determine the response.

variance (vār′ē-ans). The state of being variable, different, divergent, or deviate.

ball v., swelling and changes in shape and consistency of the ball in a ball-valve prosthesis, especially in one replacing the aortic valve.

variant (vār′ē-ant). **1.** That which, or one who, is variable. **2.** Having the tendency to alter or change, exhibit variety or diversity, not conform, or differ from the type.

inherited albumin v.'s, types of human serum albumin, distinguished by characteristic mobility patterns on electrophoresis, either faster or slower than those of normal albumin A; each type is due to a mutation of a gene controlling albumin synthesis; the mutant genes are codominant with the normal gene for albumin A, and the group forms a system of genetic polymorphism; types include: albumin b (slow), found occasionally in persons of European ancestry; albumin Ghent (fast), found first at Ghent, Belgium; albumin Mexico (slow), found in Indians of Mexico and the southwestern United States; albumin Naskapi (fast), found in the Naskapi and other Indians of northern North America; and albumin Reading (fast), found first at Reading, England.

L-phase v.'s, [L. fr. Lister Institute]. bacterial v.'s which do not have rigid cell walls but which may contain varying amounts of cell wall material; they are spherical to coccobacillary in shape and vary in size from small bodies that pass through filters which retain bacteria to bodies that are larger than the bacterial form; they are Gram-negative and resistant to penicillin; some revert to the bacterial phase upon removal of the inducing substance, whereas others do not; the v.'s differ greatly from the parent bacterial cells in mode of reproduction, physiology, growth requirements, and individual and colonial morphology; they are generally considered to be nonpathogenic, even if derived from a pathogenic bacterium.

variate (vār′ē-ăt). A measurable quantity capable of taking on a number of values; may be binary (*i.e.,* capable of taking on two values in a certain interval of values), continuous (*i.e.,* capable of taking on all values in a certain interval of real values), or discrete (*i.e.,* capable of taking on a limited number of values in a certain interval of real values).

variation (vār-ē-ā′shŭn) [L. *variatio,* fr. *vario,* to change, vary]. Deviation from the type, especially the parent type, in structure, form, physiology, or behavior.

beat-to-beat v. of fetal heart rate, variability of fetal heart rate from second to second.

continuous v., a series of very slight v.'s.

meristic v., in heredity, v. in characters that can be counted.

varication (vār-i-kā′shŭn). Formation or presence of varices.

variceal (vār-ĭ-sē′ăl, vă-ris′ē-ăl). Of or pertaining to a varix.

varicella (vār-i-sel′ă) [Mod. L. dim. of *variola*]. Chickenpox; waterpox; an acute contagious disease, usually occurring in children, caused by the varicella-zoster virus and marked by a sparse eruption of papules, which becoming vesicles and then pustules, like that of smallpox although less severe and varying in stages, usually with mild constitutional symptoms; incubation period is about 14 to 17 days.

v. gangreno′sa, gangrenous ulceration of varicella lesions with or without secondary infection, occurring mainly in children with severe underlying disease.

varicellation (vār-i-sē-lā′shŭn). Inoculation with the virus of chickenpox as a means of protection against that disease.

varicelliform (vār-ĭ-sel′ĭ-fōrm). Varicelloid; resembling varicella.

varicelloid (vār-ĭ-sel′oyd). Varicelliform.

varices (vār′i-sēz). Plural of varix.

variciform (vār′ĭ-si-fōrm, vă-ris′ĭ-fōrm). Varicoid; cirsoid; resembling a varix.

varico- [L. *varix,* a dilated vein]. Combining form denoting a varix or varicosity.

varicoblepharon (var′i-kō-blef′ă-ron) [varico- + G. *blepharon,* eyelid]. A varicosity of the eyelid.

varicocele (vār′i-kō-sēl) [varico- + G. *kēlē,* tumor, hernia]. Pampinocele; varicole; a condition manifested by abnormal dilation of the veins of the spermatic cord, caused by incompetency of valves in the internal spermatic vein and resulting in downward reflux of blood into the spermatic cord veins when the patient assumes the upright position.

ovarian v., tubo-ovarian or utero-ovarian v.; a varicose condition of the pampiniform plexus in the broad ligament of the uterus.

symptomatic v., a v. caused by obstruction of the internal spermatic vein, usually at the level of the renal vein and usually due to invasive renal cell carcinoma, characterized by failure of the dilated veins in the spermatic cord to empty when the patient assumes a recumbent position.

tubo-ovarian v., ovarian v.

utero-ovarian v., ovarian v.

varicocelectomy (vār′i-kō-sē-lek′tō-mē) [varicocele + G. *ektomē,* excision]. Operation for the relief of a varicocele by ligature and excision and by ligation of the dilated veins.

varicography (vār′ĭ-kog′ră-fē) [varico- + G. *graphō,* to write]. Roentgenography of the veins after injection of a radiopaque medium into varicose veins.

varicoid (vār′i-koyd). Variciform.

varicole (vār′i-kōl). Varicocele.

varicomphalus (văr-i-kom'fă-lŭs) [varico- + G. *omphalos,* navel]. A swelling formed by varicose veins at the umbilicus.

varicophlebitis (văr'i-kō-flĕ-bī'tis) [varico- + G. *phleps,* vein, + *-itis,* inflammation]. Inflammation of varicose veins.

varicose (văr'i-kōs). Relating to, affected with, or characterized by varices or varicosis.

varicosis, pl. **varicoses** (văr-i-kō'sis, -sēz) [varico- + G. *-osis,* condition]. A dilated or varicose state of a vein or veins.

varicosity (văr-i-kos'i-tē). A varix or varicose condition.

varicotomy (văr-i-kot'ō-mē) [varico- + G. *tomē,* a cutting]. An operation for varicose veins by subcutaneous incision.

varicula (vă-rik'yū-lă) [L. dim. of *varix*] Conjunctival varix; a varicose condition of the veins of the conjunctiva.

varicule (văr'i-kyūl) [L. *varicula,* dim. of *varix*]. A small varicose vein ordinarily seen in the skin; may be associated with venous stars, venous lakes, or larger varicose veins.

variola (vă-rī'ō-lă) [Med. L. dim of L. *varius,* spotted]. Smallpox.
v. benig'na, varioloid (2).
v. hemorrha'gica, hemorrhagic *smallpox.*
v. ma'jor, smallpox.
v. malig'na, malignant smallpox, usually of the hemorrhagic form.
v. milia'ris, a form of varioloid in which the eruption consists of miliary vesicles without the formation of pustules.
v. mi'nor, alastrim.
v. pemphigo'sa, a form of smallpox in which the eruption consists of pemphigus-like blebs.
v. si'ne eruptio'ne, an abortive form of smallpox in which the disease subsides without the appearance of any eruption, or at most a few papules that never go on to pustulation.
v. vaccine, v. vaccin'ia, vaccinia.
v. ve'ra, simple smallpox of ordinary severity in the unvaccinated.
v. verruco'sa, wartpox; a mild or abortive form of varioloid, the eruption of which consists mainly of papules, with occasionally minute vesicles at the apices, which persist for a time as wartlike lesions.

variolar (vă-rī'ō-lăr). Variolic; variolous; relating to smallpox.

variolate (văr'ē-ō-lāt). **1.** To inoculate with smallpox. **2.** Pitted or scarred, as if by smallpox.

variolation (văr'ē-ō-lā'shŭn). Variolization; the obsolete process of inoculating a susceptible person with material from a vesicle of a patient with smallpox.

variolic (văr-ē-ol'ik). Variolar.

varioliform (vă-rī'ō-li-fōrm, văr-ē-ō'li-fōrm) [variola + L. *forma,* form]. Varioloid (1).

variolization (văr'ē-ō-li-zā'shŭn). Variolation.

varioloid (văr'ē-ō-loyd) [variola + G. *eidos,* resemblance]. **1.** Varioliform; resembling smallpox. **2.** Modified or varicelloid smallpox; variola benigna; a mild form of smallpox occurring in persons who are relatively resistant, usually as a result of a previous vaccination; the course of the disease is significantly shorter and the different stages of the eruption follow each other rapidly, or the lesions may abort at any stage; may cause virulent smallpox in a nonimmune contact.

variolous (vă-rī'ō-lŭs). Variolar.

variolovaccine (vă-rī'ō-lō-vak'sēn). A vaccine obtained from the eruption following inoculation of a heifer with smallpox from the human.

varix, pl. **varices** (văr'iks, văr'i-sēz) [L. *varix* (*varic-*), a dilated vein]. **1.** A dilated vein. **2.** An enlarged and tortuous vein, artery, or lymphatic vessel.
v. anastomot'icus, aneurysmal v.
aneurysmal v., Pott's aneurysm; v. anastomoticus; dilation and tortuosity of a vein resulting from an acquired communication with an adjacent artery.
cirsoid v., cirsoid *aneurysm.*
conjunctival v., varicula.
esophageal varices, longitudinal venous varices at the lower end of the esophagus as a result of portal hypertension; they are superficial and liable to ulceration and massive bleeding.
gelatinous v., a lumpy or nodular condition of the umbilical cord.
lymph v., the formation of varices or cysts in the lymph nodes in consequence of obstruction in the efferent lymphatics.
turbinal v., a condition of permanent dilation of the veins of the turbinated bodies, especially of the inferior turbinate.

var'nish (dental). Cavity liner; solutions of natural resins and gums in a suitable solvent, of which a thin coating is applied over the surfaces of the cavity preparations before placement of restorations, used as a protective agent for the tooth against constituents of restorative materials.

Varolius (Varolio), Constantius (Costanzio), Italian anatomist and physician, 1543–1575. See V.'s *sphincter; valve* of V.; *pons* varolii.

varus (vā'rŭs) [Mod. L. bent inward, fr. L. knock-kneed]. Bent or twisted inward toward the midline of the limb or body; modern accepted usage, particularly in orthopedics, erroneously transposes the meaning of valgus to v., as in *genu* varum (bowleg).

vas- [L. *vas,* a vessel]. Combining form denoting a vas, blood vessel. See also vasculo-, vaso-.

vas, gen. **va'sis,** pl. **vasa,** gen. pl. **vasorum** (vas, vā'sis, vā'să, vā-sō'rŭm) [L. a vessel, dish] [NA]. A duct or canal conveying any liquid, such as blood, lymph, chyle, or semen. See also vessel.
v. aber'rans, *ductulus* aberrans.
v. aber'rans hep'atis, pl. **va'sa aberran'tia hep'atis,** one of numerous irregularly coursing arterial twigs found along with blind bile ducts in the fibrous appendix and in the capsule of the liver.
v. af'ferens, pl. **va'sa afferen'tia** [NA], afferent vessel; **(1)** any artery conveying blood to a part; **(2)** the arteriole that enters a renal glomerulus; **(3)** afferent lymphatic; a lymphatic vessel entering a lymph node.
v. anastomot'icum [NA], a vessel that establishes a connection between arteries, between veins, or between lymph vessels.
va'sa aur'is inter'nae [NA], vessels of the internal ear.
va'sa bre'via, *arteriae* gastricae breves.
v. capilla're [NA], capillary vessel. See blood *capillary;* lymph *capillary.*
va'sa chylif'era, chyle vessels. See lacteal (2).
v. collatera'le [NA], collateral vessel; a branch of an artery running parallel with the parent trunk.
v. def'erens, pl. **va'sa deferen'tia,** *ductus* deferens.
v. ef'ferens, pl. **va'sa efferen'tia** [NA], efferent vessel; **(1)** a vein carrying blood away from a part; **(2)** the arteriole that carries blood out of a renal glomerulus; it passes to the capillary bed surrounding the renal tubules; **(3)** efferent lymphatic; a lymphatic vessel leaving a lymph node.
Ferrein's vasa aberrantia, biliary canaliculi that are not connected with hepatic lobules.
Haller's v. aberrans, *ductulus* aberrans inferius.
va'sa lymphat'ica [NA], absorbant, lymphatic, or lymph vessels; the vessels that convey the lymph; they anastomose freely with each other.
v. lymphat'icum profun'dum [NA], deep lymphatic vessel; one of the vessels that drain lymph from the deep structures of the body; they tend to follow the courses of blood vessels to reach regional lymph nodes.
v. lymphat'icum superficia'le [NA], superficial lymphatic vessel; one of the lymphatic vessels that lie in the skin and subcutaneous tissues; they join the deep lymphatic vessels.
va'sa nervor'um [NA], vessels supplying a nerve trunk.
va'sa pre'via, umbilical vessels presenting in advance of the fetal

head, usually traversing the membranes and crossing the internal cervical os.
v. prom'inens [NA], a blood vessel in the substance of the prominentia spiralis of the cochlea.
va'sa rec'ta, **(1)** *arteriolae* rectae; **(2)** *tubuli* seminiferi recti.
Roth's v. aberrans, an occasional diverticulum of the rete testis.
va'sa sanguin'ea ret'inae [NA], blood vessels of the retina.
v. spira'le [NA], a blood vessel, larger than its fellows, in the basilar membrane just beneath the tunnel of Corti.
va'sa vaso'rum [NA], vessels of vessels; small arteries distributed to the outer and middle coats of the larger blood vessels, and their corresponding veins.
va'sa vortico'sa, *venae* vorticosae.

vasa (vā'să). Plural of vas.

vasal (vā'săl). Relating to a vas or to vasa.

vascular (vas'kyū-lăr) [L. *vasculum,* a small vessel, dim. of *vas*]. Relating to or containing blood vessels.

vascularity (vas-kyū-lar'i-tē). The condition of being vascular.

vascularization (vas'kyū-lăr-i-zā'shŭn). Arterialization (3); the formation of new blood vessels in a part.

vascularized (vas-kyū-lăr-īzd). Rendered vascular by the formation of new vessels.

vasculature (vas'kyū-lă-chūr). The vascular network of an organ.

vasculitis (vas-kyū-lī'tis). Angiitis.
cutaneous v., allergic, cutaneous systemic, or leukocytoclastic angiitis; Gougerot-Ruiter disease; trisymptome; a form of vasculitis which may affect the skin only, but also may involve other organs, with a polymorphonuclear infiltrate of the small (dermal) vessels.
leukocytoclastic v., cutaneous acute v. characterized clinically by palpable purpura, especially of the legs, and histologically by exudation of the neutrophils and sometimes fibrin around dermal venules, with nuclear dust and extravasation of red cells; may be limited to the skin or involve other tissues as in Henoch-Schönlein purpura.
livedo v., a hyalinizing segmented v. found in the cutaneous lesions of atrophie blanche, with occlusion of dermal blood vessels by fibrin.
nodular v., chronic or recurrent nodular lesions of subcutaneous tissue, especially of the legs of older women, with lobular panniculitis, focal necrosis, and obliterative inflammation of the arteries and veins, resembling erythema induratum but without evidence of associated tuberculosis.

vasculo- [L. *vasculum,* a small vessel, dim. of *vas*]. Combining form denoting a blood vessel. See also vas-, vaso-.

vasculocardiac (vas'kyū-lō-kar'dē-ak). Relating to the heart and blood vessels.

vasculogenesis (vas'kyū-lō-jen'ĕ-sis) [vasculo- + G. *genesis,* production]. Formation of the vascular system.

vasculomotor (vas'kū-lō-mō'ter). Vasomotor.

vasculomyelinopathy (vas'kyū-lō-mī-ĕ-li-nop'ă-thē). Small cerebral vessel vasculopathy with subsequent perivascular demyelination, presumably due to circulating immune complexes.

vasculopathy (vas-kyū-lop'ă-thē) [vasculo- + G. *pathos,* disease]. Any disease of the blood vessels.

vasculum, pl. vascula (vas'kyū-lŭm, -lă) [L. dim of *vas,* a vessel]. A small vessel.

vasectomy (va-sek'tō-mē) [vas- + G. *ektomē,* excision]. Deferentectomy; excision of a segment of the vas deferens, performed in association with prostatectomy, or to produce sterility.

vasifaction (vas-i-fak'shŭn). Angiopoiesis.

vasifactive (vas-i-fak'tiv). Angiopoietic.

vasiform (vas'i-fōrm). Having the shape of a vas or tubular structure.

vasitis (va-sī'tis). Deferentitis.

vaso- [L. *vas,* a vessel]. Combining form denoting a vas or blood vessel. See also vas-, vasculo-.

vasoactive (vā-sō-ak'tiv, vas-ō-). Influencing the tone and caliber of blood vessels.

vasoconstriction (vā'sō-kon-strik'shŭn, vas'ō-). Narrowing of the blood vessels.
active v., reduced caliber of a vessel caused by increased tonus in the smooth muscle in its walls.
passive v., reduced caliber of a vessel caused by decreased intraluminal pressure.

vasoconstrictive (vā'sō-kon-strik'tiv, vas'ō-). **1.** Causing narrowing of the blood vessels. **2.** Vasoconstrictor (1).

vasoconstrictor (vā'sō-kon-strik'ter, vas'ō-). **1.** Vasoconstrictive (2); an agent that causes narrowing of the blood vessels. **2.** A nerve, stimulation of which causes vascular constriction.

vasodentin (vā-sō-den'tin, vas-ō-). Vascular dentin; dentin in which the primitive capillaries have remained uncalcified and so are wide enough to give passage to the formed elements of the blood.

vasodepression (vā'sō-dē-presh'ŭn, vas'ō). Reduction of tone in blood vessels with vasodilation and resulting lowered blood pressure.

vasodepressor (vā'sō-dē-pres'er, vas'ō). **1.** Producing vasodepression. **2.** An agent that produces vasodepression.

vasodilatation (vā'sō-dil-ă-tā'shŭn, vas'ō-). Vasodilation.

vasodilation (vā'sō-dī-lā'shŭn, vas-ō-). Vasodilatation; phlebarteriectasia of the blood vessels.
active v., v. caused by decrease in tonus of smooth muscle in the wall of a vessel.
passive v., v. related to increased pressure in lumen of a vessel.

vasodilative (vā'sō-dī-lā'tiv, vas'ō-). **1.** Causing dilation of the blood vessels. **2.** Vasodilator (1).

vasodilator (vā'sō-dī-lā'ter, vas'ō-). **1.** Vasodilative (2); an agent that causes dilation of the blood vessels. **2.** A nerve, stimulation of which results in dilation of the blood vessels.

vasoepididymostomy (vā'sō-ep-i-did-i-mos'tō-mē, vas'ō-) [vaso- + epididymis + G. *stoma,* mouth]. Surgical anastomosis of the vasa deferentia to the epididymis, to bypass an obstruction at the level of the mid to distal epididymis or proximal vas.

vasofactive (vā-sō-fak'tiv, vas-ō-). Angiopoietic.

vasoformation (vā-sō-fōr-mā'shŭn, vas-ō-). Angiopoiesis.

vasoformative (vā-sō-fōr'mă-tiv, vas-ō-). Angiopoietic.

vasoganglion (vā-sō-gang'glē-on, vas-ō-). A mass of blood vessels.

vasography (vā-sog'ră-fē, vas-ō). **1.** Roentgenography of blood vessels. **2.** Roentgenographic study of the vas deferens, utilizing a contrast agent injected into the lumen, either transurethrally or by open vasotomy, *e.g.,* to determine its patency.

vasohypertonic (vā'sō-hī-per-ton'ik, vas'ō-) [vaso- + G. *hyper,* over, + *tonos,* tone]. Relating to increased arteriolar tension or vasoconstriction.

vasohypotonic (vā'sō-hī-po-ton'ik, vas'ō-) [vaso- + G. *hypo,* under, + *tonos,* tone]. Relating to reduced arteriolar tension or vasodilation.

vasoinhibitor (vā'sō-in-hib'i-ter, vas'ō-). An agent that restricts or prevents the functioning of the vasomotor nerves.

vasoinhibitory (vā'sō-in-hib'i-tōr-ē, vas'ō-). Restraining vasomotor action.

vasolabile (vā-sō-lā'bil, -bīl; vas-ō-). Characterizing the condition in which there is lability or active vasomotion of blood vessels.

vasoligation (vā'sō-li-gā'shŭn, vas'ō-). Ligation of the vas deferens, usually after its division.

vasomotion (vā-sō-mō'shŭn, vas-ō-). Angiokinesis; change in caliber of a blood vessel.

vasomotor (vā-sō-mō'ter, vas-ō-). Angiokinetic; vasculomotor. **1.** Causing dilation or constriction of the blood vessels. **2.** Denoting the nerves which have this action.

vasoneuropathy (vā'sō-nū-rop'ă-thē, vas'ō-). [vaso- + G. *neuron,* nerve, + *pathos,* suffering]. Any disease involving both the nerves and blood vessels.

vasoneurosis (vā'sō-nū-rō'sis, vas'ō-). Angioneurosis.

vaso-orchidostomy (vā'sō-ōr-ki-dos'tō-mē, vas'ō-) [vaso- + G. *orchis,* testis, + *stoma,* mouth]. Reestablishment of the interrupted seminiferous channels by uniting the tubules of the epididymis or of the rete testis to the divided end of the vas deferens.

vasoparalysis (vā'sō-pă-ral'i-sis, vas'ō-). Angioparalysis; angiohypotonia; paralysis, atonia, or hypotonia of blood vessels.

vasoparesis (vā'sō-pă-rē'sis, -par'ē-sis; vas'ō-) [vaso- + G. *paresis,* weakness]. Angioparesis; vasomotor paralysis; a mild degree of vasoparalysis.

vasopressin (VP) (vā-sō-pres'in, vas-ō-). Antidiuretic hormone; β-hypophamine; a nonapeptide hormone related to oxytocin and vasotocin; synthetically prepared or obtained from the neurohypophysis of healthy domestic animals used for food by man. In pharmacological doses v. causes contraction of smooth muscle, notably that of all blood vessels; large doses may produce cerebral or coronary arterial spasm.
arginine v., argipressin; [8-arginine]vasopressin; [Arg⁸]vasopressin; v. containing arginine in position 8 (as in most mammals and chickens).

Cys-Tyr-Phe-Gln-Asn-Cys-Pro-Arg-Gly-NH_2 (3 above Phe, 8 above Arg; Cys 1 and Cys 6 linked)

[8-Arginine] vasopressin

vasopressor (vā-sō-pres'er, vas-ō-). **1.** Producing vasoconstriction and a rise in blood pressure, usually understood to be systemic arterial pressure unless otherwise specified. **2.** An agent that has this effect.

vasopuncture (vā-sō-pŭnk'chūr, vas-ō-). The act of puncturing a vessel with a needle.

vasoreflex (vā-sō-rē'fleks, vas'ō-). A reflex that influences the caliber of blood vessels.

vasorelaxation (vā'sō-rē-lak-sā'shŭ, vas-ō), Reduction in tension of the walls of the blood vessels.

vasosection (vā-sō-sek'shŭn, vas-ō-). Vasotomy.

vasosensory (vā-sō-sen'ser-ē, vas-ō-). **1.** Relating to sensation in the blood vessels. **2.** Denoting sensory nerve fibers innervating blood vessels.

vasospasm (vā'sō-spazm, vas'ō-). Angiospasm; angiohypertonia; contraction or hypertonia of the muscular coats of the blood vessels.

vasospastic (vā-sō-spas'tik, vas-ō-). Angiospastic; relating to or characterized by vasospasm.

vasostimulant (va-sō-stim'yū-lant). **1.** Exciting vasomotor action. **2.** An agent that excites the vasomotor nerves to action. **3.** Vasotonic (2).

vasostomy (vă-sos'tō-mē) [vaso- + G. *stoma,* mouth]. Establishment of an artificial opening into the deferent duct.

vasothrombin (vā-sō-throm'bin, vas-ō-). Thrombin derived from the lining cells of the blood vessels.

vasotocin (vā-sō-tō'sin, vas-ō-). A nonapeptide hormone of the neurohypophysis of subvertebrates, with activities similar to that of vasopressin and oxytocin; chemically identical with human vasopressin except for isoleucine at position 3; thus [3-isoleucine]-vasopressin or [Ile³]vasopressin.
arginine v., v. with arginine at position 8 (identical with arginine oxytocin). See also arginine *vasopressin.*

vasotomy (vā-sot'ō-mē) [vaso- + G. *tomē,* incision]. Vasosection; incision into or division of the vas deferens.

vasotonia (vā-sō-tō'nē-ă, vas-ō-) [vaso- + G. *tonos,* tone]. Angiotonia; the tone of blood vessels, particularly the arterioles.

vasotonic (vā-sō-ton'ik, vas-ō-). **1.** Angiotonic; relating to vascular tone. **2.** Vasostimulant (3); an agent that increases vascular tension.

vasotribe (vā'sō-trīb, vas'ō-). Angiotribe.

vasotripsy (vā'sō-trip-sē, vas'ō-). Angiotripsy.

vasotrophic (vā-sō-trof'ik, vas-ō-) [vaso- + G. *trophē,* nourishment]. Relating to the nutrition of the blood vessels or the lymphatics.

vasotropic (vā-sō-trō'pik, vas-ō-) [vaso- + G. *tropē,* a turning]. Tending to act on the blood vessels.

vasovagal (vā-sō-vā'găl, vas-ō-). Relating to the action of the vagus nerve upon the blood vessels.

vasovasostomy (vā'sō-vă-sos'tō-mē, vas'ō-). [vaso- + vaso- + G. *stoma,* mouth]. Surgical anastomosis of vasa deferentia, to restore fertility in a previously vasectomized male.

vasovesiculectomy (vā'sō-vĕ-sik-yū-lek'tō-mē, vas'ō-) [vaso- + L. *vesicula,* vesicle, + G. *ektomē,* excision]. Excision of the vas deferens and seminal vesicles.

vastus (vas'tŭs) [L.]. Great. See under musculus.

VATER Acronym for *v*ertebral defects, *a*nal atresia, *t*racheoesophageal fistula with *e*sophageal atresia, and *r*adial and *r*enal anomalies. See VATER *complex.*

Vater, Abraham, German anatomist and botanist, 1684–1751. See V.'s *ampulla, fold;* V.-Pacini *corpuscles.*

vault (vawlt) [thr. O. Fr., fr. L. *volvo,* pp. *volutus,* to turn round]. A part resembling an arched roof or dome, *e.g.,* the v. of the pharynx, the upper part or roof of the rhinopharynx; the palatine v., palatum; v. of the vagina, fornix.

V-bends. V-shaped bends incorporated in an archwire, usually placed mesially or distally to the canines (cuspids) and used as a "dead" area of wire through which torquing bends may be placed.

VC Abbreviation for color *vision;* vital *capacity.*

VDRL Abbreviation for Venereal Disease Research Laboratories. See VDRL *test.*

vection (vek'shŭn) [L. *vectio,* conveyance]. Transference of the agents of disease from the sick to the well by a vector.

vectis (vek'tis) [L. a lever or bar]. Lever; an instrument resembling one of the blades of an obstetrical forceps, used as an aid in delivery by making traction on the presenting part of the fetus.

vector (vek'ter, tōr) [L. *vector,* a carrier]. **1.** An invertebrate animal (*e.g.,* tick, mite, mosquito, bloodsucking fly) capable of transmitting an infectious agent among vertebrates. **2.** Anything (*e.g.,* velocity, mechanical force, electromotive force) having magnitude, direction, and sense which can be represented by a straight line of appropriate length and direction. **3.** The electrical axis of the heart (represented by an arrow) whose length is proportional to the magnitude of the electrical force, whose direction gives the direction of the force, and whose tip represents the positive pole of the force. **4.** A DNA molecule that autonomously replicates in a cell to which another DNA segment may be artifically attached and be itself replicated.
biological v., a v., such as the *Anopheles* mosquito for malarial agents or the tsetse fly for agents of African sleeping sickness, that is essential in the life cycle of the pathogenic organism.

cloning v., an autonomously replicating plasmid with regions that are not essential for its propagation in bacteria and into which foreign DNA can be inserted; this foreign DNA is replicated and propagated as if it were a normal component of the v.
expression v., a v. (plasmid, yeast, or animal virus genome) used to introduce foreign genetic material into a propagatable host cell in order to replicate and amplify the foreign DNA sequences as a recombinant molecule (recombinant DNA cloning of sequences).
instantaneous v., the resultant v. of the heart's action currents at any given moment, usually represented as an arrow of appropriate direction and magnitude.
manifest v., projection of a spatial cardiac v. on a single plane.
mean v., a single cardiac v. representing the average of all v.'s present during a given time interval.
mechanical v., a v. that conveys pathogens to a susceptible individual without essential biological development of the pathogens in the v., as in the transfer of septic organisms on the feet or mouth parts of the housefly.
spatial v., a cardiac v. represented in more than one plane simultaneously; two- or three-dimensional orientation of a v.

vectorcardiogram (vek'tōr-kar'dē-ō-gram). A graphic representation of the magnitude and direction of the heart's action currents in the form of a vector loop.

vectorcardiography (vek'tōr-kar-dē-og'ră-fē). **1.** A variant of electrocardiography in which the heart's activation currents are represented by vector loops. **2.** The study and interpretation of vectorcardiograms.
spatial v., three-dimensional v. in which vector loops are inscribed in frontal, sagittal, and horizontal planes.

vectorial (vek-tōr'ē-ăl). Relating in any way to a vector.

vecuronium bromide (ve-kyū-rō'nē-ŭm). 1-[3,17-Bis(acetyloxy)-2-(1-piperidinyl)androstan-16-yl]-1-methylpiperidinium; a nondepolarizing neuromuscular relaxant with a relatively short duration of action; a monoquaternary homologue of pancuronium.

VEE Abbreviation for Venezuelan equine *encephalomyelitis.*

vegetable (vej'tă-bl, vej'ĕ-tă-bl) [M.E., fr. L. *vegetabilis* (see vegetation)]. **1.** A plant, specifically one used for food. **2.** Vegetal (1); relating to plants, as distinguished from animals or minerals.

vegetal (vej'ĕ-tăl). **1.** Vegetable (2). **2.** Denoting the vital functions common to plants and animals, such as respiration, metabolism, growth, generation, etc., distinguished from those peculiar to animals, such as conscious sensation and the mental faculties.

vegetality (vej-ĕ-tal'i-tē). The aggregate of the vital functions common to both plants and animals.

vegetarian (vej-ĕ-tār'ē-ăn). One whose diet is restricted to foods of vegetable origin, excluding primarily animal meats.

vegetarianism (vej-ĕ-tār'ē-ăn-izm). The practice as to diet of a vegetarian.

vegetation (vej-ĕ-tā'shŭn) [Mod. L. *vegetatio,* growth]. **1.** The process of growth in plants. **2.** A condition of sluggishness, comparable to the inactivity of plant life. **3.** A growth or excrescence of any sort. **4.** Specifically, a clot, composed largely of fused blood platelets, fibrin, and sometimes bacteria, adherent to a diseased heart valve.

vegetative (vej'ĕ-tā-tiv) [see vegetation]. **1.** Growing or functioning involuntarily or unconsciously, after the assumed manner of vegetable life; denoting especially a state of grossly impaired consciousness, as after severe head trauma or brain disease, in which an individual is incapable of voluntary or purposeful acts and only responds reflexively to painful stimuli. **2.** Resting; not active; denoting the stage of a cell or its nucleus in which the process of karyokinesis is quiescent.

vegetoanimal (vej'ĕ-tō-an'i-măl). Relating to both plants and animals.

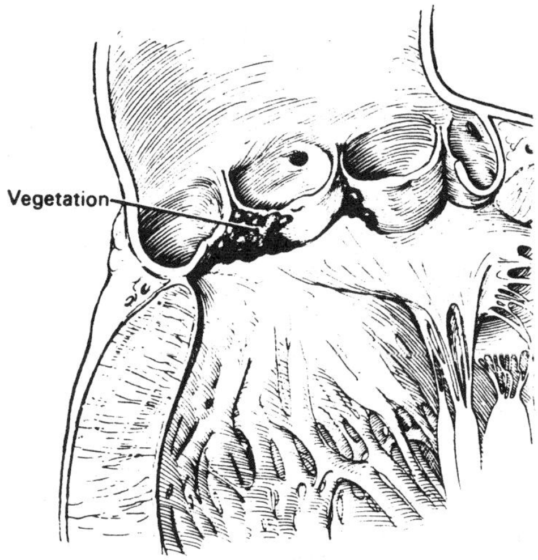

Vegetation on Aortic Valve

vehicle (vē'hi-kl) [L. *vehiculum,* a conveyance, fr. *veho,* to carry]. **1.** An excipient or a menstruum; a substance, usually without therapeutic action, used as a medium to give bulk for the administration of medicines. **2.** An inanimate substance (*e.g.,* food, milk, dust, clothing, instrument) by which or upon which an infectious agent passes from an infected to a susceptible host; v.'s consequently act as important sources of infection.

veil (vāl) [L. *velum*]. **1.** Velum (1). **2.** Caul (1).
aqueduct v., a membrane obstructing the sylvian aqueduct, causing a noncommunicating hydrocephalus.
Jackson's v., Jackson's *membrane.*
Sattler's v., a diffuse edema of the corneal epithelium that may develop after wearing contact lenses.

Veillonella (vā'yō-nel'ă) [Adrien *Veillon,* French bacteriologist, 1864–1931]. A genus of nonmotile, nonsporeforming, anaerobic bacteria (family Veillonellaceae) containing small (0.3 to 0.5 μm in diameter), Gram-negative cocci which occur as diplococci and in masses. Carbon dioxide is required for growth, and carbohydrates are not fermented. These organisms are parasitic in the mouth and the intestinal and respiratory tracts of humans and other animals. They produce serologically specific endotoxins (lipopolysaccharides) which induce pyrogenicity and the Schwarzman phenomenon in rabbits. The type species is *V. parvula.*
V. alcales'ens, a species found in the saliva of man and other animals.
V. alcales'cens subsp. **alcales'cens,** a subspecies found primarily in the mouth of humans but occasionally in the buccal cavity of rabbits and rats; it is the type subspecies of the species *V. alcalescens.*
V. alcales'cens subsp. **cri'ceti,** a subspecies found in the mouth of hamsters.
V. alcales'cens subsp. **dis'par,** a subspecies found in the mouth and respiratory tract of humans.
V. alcales'cens subsp. **rat'ti,** a subspecies found in the mouth and intestinal contents of rats.
V. par'vula, a species found normally as a harmless parasite in the natural cavities, especially the mouth and digestive tract, of man and other animals; it is the types species of the genus *V.*
V. par'vula subsp. **atyp'ica,** a subspecies found in the buccal cavity of rats and humans.
V. par'vula subsp. **par'vula,** a subspecies found in the mouth or the intestinal or respiratory tract of humans; it is the type subspe-

cies of the species *V. parvula*.

V. par'vula subsp. **roden'tium,** a subspecies found in the buccal cavity and intestinal tract of hamsters, rats, and rabbits.

Veillonellaceae (vā'yō-nĕ-lā'sē-ē). A family of nonmotile, nonsporeforming, anaerobic bacteria (order Eubacteriales) containing Gram-negative (with a tendency to resist decolorization) cocci which vary in diameter from small (0.3 to 0.5 μm) to large (2.5 μm). Characteristically, they occur in pairs; single cells, masses, or chains may also occur, but the chains may show gaps illustrating the basic diplococcal arrangement. These organisms are chemoorganotrophic; they may or may not ferment carbohydrates. They are parasites of homothermic animals such as humans, ruminants, rodents, and pigs, and are primarily found in the alimentary tract. The type genus is *Veillonella*.

VEIN

vein (vān) [L. *vena*] Vena.

accessory cephalic v., *vena* cephalica accessoria.
accessory hemiazygos v., *vena* hemiazygos accessoria.
accessory saphenous v., *vena* saphena accessoria.
accessory vertebral v., *vena* vertebralis accessoria.
accompanying v., vena comitans.
anastomotic v.'s, see *vena* anastomotica inferior; *vena* anastomotica superior.
angular v., *vena* angularis.
anonymous v.'s, *venae* brachiocephalicae.
anterior auricular v., *vena* auricularis anterior.
anterior cardiac v.'s, *venae* cordis anteriores.
anterior cardinal v.'s, see cardinal v.'s.
anterior cerebral v., *vena* cerebri anterior.
anterior facial v., *vena* facialis.
anterior intercostal v.'s, *venae* intercostales anteriores.
anterior jugular v., *vena* jugularis anterior.
anterior labial v.'s, *venae* labiales anteriores.
anterior pontomesencephalic v., *vena* pontomesencephalica anterior.
anterior scrotal v.'s, *venae* scrotales anteriores.
anterior v. of septum pellucidum, *vena* septi pellucidi anterior.
anterior tibial v.'s, *venae* tibiales anteriores.
anterior vertebral v., *vena* vertebralis anterior.
appendicular v., *vena* appendicularis.
aqueous v., a tributary of the anterior ciliary v. which receives aqueous humor from the venous sinus of the sclera.
arciform v.'s of kidney, *venae* arcuatae renis.
arcuate v.'s of kidney, *venae* arcuatae renis.
arterial v., vena arteriosa; so called because it ramifies like an artery (portal vein) or because, while proceeding from the heart like an artery, it contains unaerated blood, like a vein (pulmonary artery).
ascending lumbar v., *vena* lumbalis ascendens.
auricular v.'s, see *vena* auricularis anterior; *vena* auricularis posterior.
axillary v., *vena* axillaris.
azygos v., *vena* azygos.
basal v.'s, see entries under *vena* basalis.
basal v. of Rosenthal, *vena* basalis.
basilic v., *vena* basilica.
basivertebral v., *vena* basivertebralis.
Baumgarten's v.'s, nonobliterated remnants of the vena umbilicalis.
brachial v.'s, *venae* brachiales.
brachiocephalic v.'s, *venae* brachiocephalicae.
Breschet's v., *vena* diploica.
bronchial v.'s, *venae* bronchiales.
Browning's v., *vena* anastomotica inferior.
v. of bulb of penis, *vena* bulbi penis.
Burow's v., **(1)** an occasional v. passing from the inferior epigastric, sometimes receiving a tributary from the bladder, which empties into the portal v.; **(2)** one of the *venae* renis.
capillary v., venula.
cardiac v.'s, see entries under *vena* cordis.
cardinal v.'s, the major systemic venous channels in adult primitive vertebrates and in the embryos of higher vertebrates; the **anterior c. v.'s** are the major drainage channels from the cephalic part of the body, and the **posterior c. v.'s,** from the caudal part; the **common c. v.'s,** formed by the anastomosis of the anterior and posterior c. v.'s, are the main systemic return channels to the heart; in the older literature, sometimes called Cuvier's ducts.
v.'s of caudate nucleus, *venae* nuclei caudati.
central v.'s of liver, *venae* centrales hepatis.
central v. of retina, *vena* centralis retinae.
central v. of suprarenal gland, *vena* centralis glandulae suprarenalis.
cephalic v., *vena* cephalica.
v.'s of cerebellum, cerebellar v.'s, *venae* cerebelli.
cerebral v.'s, see entries under *vena* cerebri.
cervical v., see *vena* cervicalis profunda.
choroid v., see *vena* choroidea inferior; *vena* choroidea superior.
choroid v.'s of eye, *venae* vorticosae.
ciliary v.'s, *venae* ciliares.
circumflex v.'s, see entries under *vena* circumflexa.
v. of cochlear aqueduct, *vena* aqueductus cochleae.
v. of cochlear canaliculus, *vena* aqueductus cochleae.
colic v.'s, see *vena* colica dextra, media, sinistra.
common basal v., *vena* basalis communis.
common cardinal v.'s, see cardinal v.'s.
common facial v., vena facialis communis; a short vessel formed by the union of the facial v. and the retromandibular v., emptying into the jugular v.; considered to be a continuation of the facial v. in the NA.
common iliac v., *vena* iliaca communis.
companion v., *vena* comitans.
companion v.'s, *venae* comitantes.
condylar emissary v., *vena* emissaria condylaris.
conjunctival v.'s, *venae* conjunctivales.
coronary v., *vena* gastrica sinistra.
v. of corpus striatum, *vena* thalamostriata superior.
costoaxillary v., one of a number of anastomotic v.'s connecting the intercostal v.'s of the first to seventh intercostal spaces with the lateral thoracic or the thoracoepigastric v.
cutaneous v., *vena* cutanea.
Cuvier's v.'s, the common cardinal v.'s of the embryo. See cardinal v.'s.
cystic v., *vena* cystica.
deep cerebral v.'s, *venae* cerebri profundae.
deep cervical v., *vena* cervicalis profunda.
deep circumflex iliac v., *vena* circumflexa ilium profunda.
deep v.'s of clitoris, *venae* profundae clitoridis.
deep dorsal v. of clitoris, *vena* dorsalis clitoridis profunda.
deep dorsal v. of penis, *vena* dorsalis penis profunda.
deep epigastric v., *vena* epigastrica inferior.
deep facial v., *vena* faciei profunda.
deep femoral v., *vena* profunda femoris.
deep lingual v., *vena* profunda linguae.
deep middle cerebral v., *vena* cerebri media profunda.
deep v. of penis, *vena* profunda penis.
deep temporal v.'s, *venae* temporales profundae.
digital v.'s, see entries under *venae* digitales.
diploic v., *vena* diploica.

dorsal callosal v., *vena* corporis callosi dorsalis.
dorsal v.'s of clitoris, see *vena* dorsalis clitoridis profunda; *venae* dorsales clitoridis superficiales.
dorsal v. of corpus callosum, *vena* corporis callosi dorsalis.
dorsal digital v.'s of toes, *venae* digitales dorsales pedis.
dorsal lingual v., *vena* dorsalis linguae.
dorsal metacarpal v.'s, *venae* metacarpeae dorsales.
dorsal metatarsal v.'s, *venae* metatarseae dorsales.
dorsal v.'s of penis, see *vena* dorsalis penis profunda; *venae* dorsales penis superficiales.
dorsal scapular v., *vena* scapularis dorsalis.
dorsispinal v.'s, v.'s forming a plexus around the arches and processes of the vertebrae.
emissary v., *vena* emissaria. See also *vena* emissaria condylaris, mastoidea, occipitalis, parietalis.
epigastric v.'s, see *vena* epigastrica inferior and superficialis; *venae* epigastricae superiores.
episcleral v.'s, *venae* episclerales.
esophageal v.'s, *venae* esophageae.
ethmoidal v.'s, *venae* ethmoidales.
external iliac v., *vena* iliaca externa.
external jugular v., *vena* jugularis externa.
external nasal v.'s, *venae* nasales externae.
external pudendal v.'s, *venae* pudendae externae.
v.'s of eyelids, *venae* palpebrales.
facial v., *vena* facialis.
femoral v., *vena* femoralis.
fibular v.'s, *venae* peroneae.
frontal v.'s, **(1)** *venae* frontales; **(2)** *venae* supratrochleares.
v.'s of Galen, **(1)** see *vena* cerebri magna; **(2)** *venae* cerebri internae.
gastric v.'s, see *venae* gastricae breves; *vena* gastrica dextra and sinistra.
gastroepiploic v.'s, see *vena* gastro-omentalis dextra; *vena* gastro-omentalis sinistra.
gluteal v.'s, see *venae* gluteae inferiores; *venae* gluteae superiores.
great cardiac v., *vena* cordis magna.
great cerebral v., *vena* cerebri magna.
great v. of Galen, *vena* cerebri magna.
great saphenous v., *vena* saphena magna.
hemiazygos v., *vena* hemiazygos.
hemorrhoidal v.'s, see *venae* rectales inferiores and mediae; *vena* rectalis superior.
hepatic v.'s, *venae* hepaticae.
hepatic portal v., *vena* portae hepatis.
highest intercostal v., *vena* intercostalis suprema.
hypogastric v., *vena* iliaca interna.
ileal v.'s, see *venae* jejunales et ilei.
ileocolic v., *vena* ileocolica.
iliac v.'s, see entries under *vena* iliaca.
iliolumbar v., *vena* iliolumbalis.
inferior anastomotic v., *vena* anastomotica inferior.
inferior basal v., *vena* basalis inferior.
inferior cardiac v., *vena* cordis media.
inferior v.'s of cerebellar hemisphere, *venae* hemispherii cerebelli inferiores.
inferior cerebral v.'s, *venae* cerebri inferiores.
inferior choroid v., *vena* choroidea inferior.
inferior epigastric v., *vena* epigastrica inferior.
v.'s of inferior eyelid, *venae* palpebrales inferiores.
inferior gluteal v.'s, *venae* gluteae inferiores.
inferior hemorrhoidal v.'s, *venae* rectales inferiores.
inferior labial v., *vena* labialis inferior.
inferior laryngeal v., *vena* laryngea inferior.
inferior mesenteric v., *vena* mesenterica inferior.
inferior ophthalmic v., *vena* ophthalmica inferior.
inferior phrenic v., *vena* phrenica inferior.
inferior rectal v.'s, *venae* rectales inferiores.
inferior thalamostriate v.'s, *venae* thalamostriatae inferiores.
inferior thyroid v., *vena* thyroidea inferior.
inferior ventricular v., *vena* ventricularis inferior.
inferior v. of vermis, *vena* vermis inferior.
infrasegmental v.'s, see *pars* infrasegmentalis.
innominate v.'s, *venae* brachiocephalicae.
innominate cardiac v.'s, Vieussens' v.'s; the small superficial v.'s of the heart.
insular v.'s, *venae* insulares.
intercapitular v.'s, *venae* intercapitales.
intercostal v.'s, see entries under *venae* intercostales.
interlobar v.'s of kidney, *venae* interlobares renis.
interlobular v.'s of kidney, *venae* interlobulares renis.
interlobular v.'s of liver, *venae* interlobulares hepatis.
intermediate antebrachial v., *vena* intermedia antebrachii.
intermediate basilic v., *vena* intermedia basilica.
intermediate cephalic v., *vena* intermedia cephalica.
intermediate cubital v., *vena* intermedia cubiti.
intermediate v. of forearm, *vena* intermedia antebrachii.
internal auditory v.'s, *venae* labyrinthi.
internal cerebral v.'s, *venae* cerebri internae.
internal iliac v., *vena* iliaca interna.
internal jugular v., *vena* jugularis interna.
internal pudendal v., *vena* pudenda interna.
internal thoracic v., *vena* thoracica interna.
intersegmental v.'s, see *pars* infrasegmentalis.
intervertebral v., *vena* intervertebralis.
intrasegmental v.'s, see *pars* infrasegmentalis.
jejunal and ileal v.'s, *venae* jejunales et ilei.
jugular v.'s, see *vena* jugularis anterior, externa, and interna. See also posterior anterior jugular v.
key v., a deep-seated, dilated v. causing a "spider burst" on the surface.
v.'s of kidney, *venae* renis.
v.'s of knee, *venae* genus.
Krukenberg's v.'s, *venae* centrales hepatis.
Labbé's v., *vena* anastomotica inferior.
labial v.'s, see *venae* labiales anteriores and posteriores; *vena* labialis inferior and superior.
labyrinthine v.'s, *venae* labyrinthi.
lacrimal v., *vena* lacrimalis.
large v., a v., such as the inferior vena cava, characterized by having a reduced or absent tunica media and an adventitia with large bundles of longitudinally disposed smooth muscle.
large saphenous v., *vena* saphena magna.
laryngeal v.'s, see *vena* laryngea inferior and superior.
Latarget's v., *vena* prepylorica.
lateral atrial v., *vena* atrii lateralis.
lateral circumflex femoral v.'s, *venae* circumflexae femoris laterales.
lateral direct v.'s, *venae* directae laterales.
lateral v. of lateral ventricle, *vena* atrii lateralis.
v. of lateral recess of fourth ventricle, *vena* recessus lateralis ventriculi quarti.
lateral sacral v.'s, *venae* sacrales laterales.
lateral thoracic v., *vena* thoracica lateralis.
left colic v., *vena* colica sinistra.
left coronary v., *vena* cordis magna.
left gastric v., *vena* gastrica sinistra.
left gastroepiploic v., *vena* gastroomentalis sinistra.
left gastroomental v., *vena* gastroomentalis sinistra.
left hepatic v.'s, *venae* hepaticae sinistrae.
left inferior pulmonary v., *vena* pulmonalis inferior sinistra.
left ovarian v., *vena* ovarica sinistra.
left superior intercostal v., *vena* intercostalis superior sinistra.
left superior pulmonary v., *vena* pulmonalis superior sinistra.

left suprarenal v., *vena* suprarenalis sinistra.
left testicular v., *vena* testicularis sinistra.
left umbilical v., *vena* umbilicalis sinistra.
levoatrio-cardinal v., the communication of a systemic v. with the left atrium, other than a left superior vena cava or coronary sinus; may be the right superior vena cava.
lingual v., *vena* lingualis.
long saphenous v., *vena* saphena magna.
long thoracic v., *vena* thoracica lateralis.
lumbar v.'s, *venae* lumbales.
Marshall's oblique v., *vena* obliqua atrii sinistri.
masseteric v.'s, plexiform v.'s accompanying the masseteric artery that empty into the pterygoid venous plexus.
mastoid emissary v., *vena* emissaria mastoidea.
maxillary v., *vena* maxillaris.
Mayo's v., *vena* prepylorica.
medial atrial v., *vena* atrii medialis.
medial circumflex femoral v.'s, *venae* circumflexae femoris mediales.
medial v. of lateral ventricle, *vena* atrii medialis.
median antebrachial v., *vena* intermedia antebrachii.
median basilic v., *vena* intermedia basilica.
median cephalic v., *vena* intermedia cephalica.
median cubital v., *vena* intermedia cubiti.
median v. of forearm, *vena* intermedia antebrachii.
median v. of neck, a v. occasionally present due to fusion of the two anterior jugular v.'s.
median sacral v., *vena* sacralis mediana.
mediastinal v.'s, *venae* mediastinales.
medium v., a v. characterized by having a thinner wall and larger lumen than its corresponding artery, and a media with small bundles of circular muscle separated by considerable connective tissue; valves also occur.
v.'s of medulla oblongata, *venae* medullae oblongatae.
meningeal v.'s, *venae* meningeae.
mesencephalic v.'s, *venae* mesencephalicae.
mesenteric v.'s, see *vena* mesenterica inferior and superior.
metacarpal v.'s, see *venae* metacarpeae dorsales; *venae* metacarpeae palmares.
middle cardiac v., *vena* cordis media.
middle colic v., *vena* colica media.
middle hemorrhoidal v.'s, *venae* rectales mediae.
middle hepatic v.'s, *venae* hepaticae mediae.
middle meningeal v.'s, *venae* meningeae mediae.
middle rectal v.'s, *venae* rectales mediae.
middle temporal v., *vena* temporalis media.
middle thyroid v., *vena* thyroidea media.
musculophrenic v.'s, *venae* musculophrenicae.
nasofrontal v., *vena* nasofrontalis.
oblique v. of left atrium, *vena* obliqua atrii sinistri.
obturator v., *vena* obturatoria.
occipital v., *vena* occipitalis.
occipital v.'s, *venae* occipitales.
occipital emissary v., *vena* emissaria occipitalis.
v. of olfactory gyrus, *vena* gyri olfactorii.
ophthalmic v.'s, see *vena* ophthalmica inferior and superior.
ovarian v.'s, see *vena* ovarica dextra and sinistra.
palatine v., *vena* palatina.
palmar digital v.'s, *venae* digitales palmares.
palmar metacarpal v.'s, *venae* metacarpeae palmares.
pancreatic v.'s, *venae* pancreaticae.
pancreaticoduodenal v.'s, *venae* pancreaticoduodenales.
paraumbilical v.'s, *venae* paraumbilicales.
parietal v.'s, *venae* parietales.
parietal emissary v., *vena* emissaria parietalis.
parotid v.'s, *venae* parotideae.
pectoral v.'s, *venae* pectorales.
peduncular v.'s, *venae* pedunculares.
perforating v.'s, *venae* perforantes.
pericardiacophrenic v.'s, *venae* pericardiacophrenicae.
pericardial v.'s, *venae* pericardiacae.
peroneal v.'s, *venae* peroneae.
petrosal v., *vena* petrosa. See also *sinus* petrosus superior; *sinus* petrosus inferior.
pharyngeal v.'s, *venae* pharyngeae.
phrenic v.'s, see *vena* phrenica inferior; *venae* phrenicae superiores.
plantar digital v.'s, *venae* digitales plantares.
plantar metatarsal v.'s, *venae* metatarseae plantares.
v.'s of pons, *venae* pontis.
pontine v.'s, *venae* pontis.
popliteal v., *vena* poplitea.
portal v., *vena* portae hepatis.
posterior anterior jugular v., a variable tributary of the external jugular v. arising in the upper posterior part of the neck.
posterior auricular v., *vena* auricularis posterior.
posterior cardinal v.'s, see cardinal v.'s.
posterior facial v., *vena* retromandibularis.
v. of posterior horn, *vena* cornus posterioris.
posterior intercostal v.'s, *venae* intercostales posteriores.
posterior labial v.'s, *venae* labiales posteriores.
posterior v. of left ventricle, *vena* posterior ventriculi sinistri.
posterior marginal v., *vena* corporis callosi doralis.
posterior parotid v.'s, *venae* parotideae.
posterior pericallosal v., *vena* corporis callosi dorsalis.
posterior scrotal v.'s, *venae* scrotales posteriores.
posterior v. of septum pellucidum, *vena* septi pellucidi posterior.
posterior tibial v.'s, *venae* tibiales posteriores.
precentral cerebellar v., *vena* precentralis cerebelli.
prefrontal v.'s, *venae* prefrontales.
prepyloric v., *vena* prepylorica.
v. of pterygoid canal, *vena* canalis pterygoidei.
pudendal v.'s, see *venae* pudendae externae; *vena* pudenda interna.
pulmonary v.'s, *venae* pulmonales.
pyloric v., *vena* gastrica dextra.
radial v.'s, *venae* radiales.
renal v.'s, *venae* renales.
retromandibular v., *vena* retromandibularis.
Retzius' v.'s, Ruysch's v.'s; v.'s arising in the walls of the intestine and passing to the tributaries of the inferior vena cava instead of to those of the portal v.
right colic v., *vena* colica dextra.
right gastric v., *vena* gastrica dextra.
right gastroepiploic v., *vena* gastroomentalis dextra.
right gastroomental v., *vena* gastroomentalis dextra.
right hepatic v.'s, *venae* hepaticae dextrae.
right inferior pulmonary v., *vena* pulmonalis inferior dextra.
right ovarian v., *vena* ovarica dextra.
right superior intercostal v., *vena* intercostalis superior dextra.
right superior pulmonary v., *vena* pulmonalis superior dextra.
right suprarenal v., *vena* suprarenalis dextra.
right testicular v., *vena* testicularis dextra.
Rosenthal's v., *vena* basalis.
Ruysch's v.'s, Retzius' v.'s.
sacral v.'s, see *venae* sacrales laterales; *vena* sacralis mediana.
Santorini's v., *vena* emissaria parietalis.
saphenous v.'s, see *vena* saphena accessoria, magna, parva.
Sappey's v.'s, *venae* paraumbilicales.
scleral v.'s, *venae* sclerales.
scrotal v.'s, see *venae* scrotales anteriores; *venae* scrotales posteriores.
v. of septum pellucidum, see *vena* septi pellucidi anterior; *vena* septi pellucidi posterior.

short gastric v.'s, *venae* gastricae breves.
short saphenous v., *vena* saphena parva.
sigmoid v.'s, *venae* sigmoideae.
small v., a v. in which the three tunics are poorly defined and thin; longitudinal elastic networks occur and the smooth muscle of the media, which is circularly arranged, may be incomplete or in one or two layers.
small cardiac v., *vena* cordis parva.
small saphenous v., *vena* saphena parva.
smallest cardiac v.'s, *venae* cordis minimae.
spermatic v., see *vena* testicularis dextra and sinistra.
spinal v.'s, *venae* spinales.
spiral v. of modiolus, *vena* spiralis modioli.
splenic v., *vena* splenica.
stellate v.'s, *venulae* stellatae.
Stensen's v.'s, *venae* vorticosae.
sternocleidomastoid v., *vena* sternocleidomastoidea.
striate v.'s, *venae* thalamostriatae inferiores.
stylomastoid v., *vena* stylomastoidea.
subclavian v., *vena* subclavia.
subcutaneous v.'s of abdomen, *venae* subcutaneae abdominis.
sublingual v., *vena* sublingualis.
submental v., *vena* submentalis.
superficial v., *vena* cutanea.
superficial cerebral v.'s, *venae* cerebri superficiales.
superficial circumflex iliac v., *vena* circumflexa ilium superficialis.
superficial dorsal v.'s of clitoris, *venae* dorsales clitoridis superficiales.
superficial dorsal v.'s of penis, *venae* dorsales penis superficiales.
superficial epigastric v., *vena* epigastrica superficialis.
superficial middle cerebral v., *vena* cerebri media superficialis.
superficial temporal v.'s, *venae* temporales superficiales.
superior anastomotic v., *vena* anastomotica superior.
superior basal v., *vena* basalis superior.
superior v.'s of cerebellar hemisphere, *venae* hemispherii cerebelli superiores.
superior cerebral v.'s, *venae* cerebri superiores.
superior choroid v., *vena* choroidea superior.
superior epigastric v.'s, *venae* epigastricae superiores.
v.'s of superior eyelid, *venae* palpebrales superiores.
superior gluteal v.'s, *venae* gluteae superiores.
superior hemorrhoidal v., *vena* rectalis superior.
superior labial v., *vena* labialis superior.
superior laryngeal v., *vena* laryngea superior.
superior mesenteric v., *vena* mesenterica superior.
superior ophthalmic v., *vena* ophthalmica superior.
superior phrenic v.'s, *venae* phrenicae superiores.
superior rectal v., *vena* rectalis superior.
superior thalamostriate v., *vena* thalamostriata superior.
superior thyroid v., *vena* thyroidea superior.
superior v. of vermis, *vena* vermis superior.
supraorbital v., *vena* supraorbitalis.
suprarenal v.'s, see *vena* suprarenalis dextra and sinistra.
suprascapular v., *vena* suprascapularis.
supratrochlear v.'s, *venae* supratrochleares.
surface thalamic v.'s, *venae* directae laterales.
temporal v.'s, see *vena* temporalis media; *venae* temporales profundae and superficiales.
v.'s of temporomandibular joint, venae articulares temporomandibulares; several small tributaries to the retromandibular vein from the temporomandibular joint.
temporomaxillary v., *vena* retromandibularis.
terminal v., *vena* thalamostriata superior.
testicular v.'s, see *vena* testicularis dextra and sinistra.
thalamostriate v.'s, see *venae* thalamostriatae inferiores; vena thalamostriata superior.
thebesian v.'s, *venae* cordis minimae.
thoracic v.'s, see *vena* thoracica interna and lateralis.
thoracoacromial v., *vena* thoracoacromialis.
thoracoepigastric v., *vena* thoracoepigastrica.
thymic v.'s, *venae* thymicae.
thyroid v.'s, see *vena* thyroidea inferior, media, superior.
tracheal v.'s, *venae* tracheales.
transverse v. of face, *vena* transversa faciei.
transverse v.'s of neck, *venae* transversae colli.
transverse v. of scapula, *vena* suprascapularis.
Trolard's v., *vena* anastomotica superior.
tympanic v.'s, *venae* tympanicae.
ulnar v.'s, *venae* ulnares.
umbilical v., see *vena* umbilicalis sinistra.
v. of uncus, *vena* unci.
uterine v.'s, *venae* uterinae.
varicose v.'s, permanent dilation and tortuosity of v.'s, most commonly seen in the legs, probably as a result of congenitally incomplete valves; there is a predisposition to varicose v.'s among persons in occupations requiring long periods of standing, and in pregnant women.
vertebral v., *vena* vertebralis.
v.'s of vertebral column, *venae* columnae vertebralis.
Vesalius' v., the emissary v. passing through the foramen venosum.
vesical v.'s, *venae* vesicales.
vestibular v.'s, *venae* vestibulares.
v. of vestibular aqueduct, *vena* aqueductus vestibuli.
v. of vestibular bulb, *vena* bulbi vestibuli.
vidian v., *vena* canalis pterygoidei.
Vieussens' v.'s, innominate cardiac v.'s.
vitelline v., *vena* vitellina.
vortex v.'s, vorticose v.'s, *venae* vorticosae.

veined (vānd). Marked by veins or lines resembling veins on the surface.

veinlet (vān'let). Venula.

Vejovis (vē-jō'vis). A genus of scorpions (the so-called devil scorpions of North America), including *V. spinigerus,* the stripe-tailed devil scorpion; *V. carolinianus,* the southern devil scorpion; and *V. flavus,* the slender devil scorpion.

vela (vē'lă). Plural of velum.

velamen, pl. velamina (vĕ-lā'men, vĕ-lam'i-nă) [L. a veil]. Velum (1).
v. vul'vae, Hottentot apron; hypertrophy of the labia minora.

velamentous (vel-ă-men'tŭs). Veliform; expanded in the form of a sheet or veil.

velamentum, pl. **velamenta** (vel'ă-men'tŭm, -tă) [L. a cover]. Velum (1).

velamina (vĕ-lam'i-nă) Plural of velamen.

velar (vē'lăr). Relating to any velum, especially the velum palati.

veliform (vel'i-fōrm) [L. *velum,* veil, + *forma,* form]. Velamentous.

Vella, Luigi, Italian physiologist, 1825–1886. See V.'s *fistula;* Thiry-V. *fistula.*

vellicate (vel'i-kāt) [L. *vellico,* pp. *-atus,* to pluck, to twitch, fr. *vello,* to deprive of hair, pluck]. To twitch or contract spasmodically; said especially of fibrillary muscular spasms.

vellication (vel'i-kā'shŭn) A fibrillary muscular spasm.

vellus (vel'ŭs) [L. fleece]. **1.** Fine nonpigmented hair covering most of the body. **2.** A structure that is fleecy or soft and woolly in appearance.
v. oli'vae inferio'ris, a stratum of nerve fibers surrounding the inferior olive.

velocity (vĕ-los'i-tē) [L. *velocitas,* fr. *velox (veloc-),* quick, swift]. Rate of movement; specifically, distance traveled per unit time.
maximum v. (V_{max}), **(1)** the maximum rate of an enzymatic reaction that can be achieved by progressively increasing the substrate concentration, as in the Michaelis constant; **(2)** the maximum initial rate of shortening of a myocardial fiber that can be obtained under zero load; used to evaluate the contractility of the fiber.
nerve conduction v., the rate of impulse conductance in a peripheral nerve or its various component fibers, generally expressed in meters per second.

velogenic (vel-ō-jen'ik) [L. *velox,* rapid, + G. *-gen,* producing]. Denoting the virulence of a virus capable of inducing, after a brief incubation period, a fulminating and often lethal disease in embryonic, immature, and adult hosts; used in characterizing Newcastle disease virus.

velonoskiascopy (vē'lō-nō-ski-as'kŏ-pē) [G. *velonē (belonē),* needle, + skiascopy]. An obsolete subjective test for ametropia in which a thin rod is moved across the pupil while a distant light source is fixed; the shadow of the rod moves with the rod in myopia, and in the opposite direction in hyperopia.

velopharyngeal (vē'lō-fă-rin'jē-ăl). Pertaining to the soft palate (velum palatinum) and the posterior nasopharyngeal wall.

velosynthesis (vē'lō-sin'thĕ-sis). Palatorrhaphy.

Velpeau, Alfred A.L.M., French surgeon, 1795–1867. See V.'s *bandage, canal, fossa, hernia.*

velum, pl. **vela** (vē'lŭm, -lă) [L. veil, sail]. **1.** Velamen; velamentum; veil (1); any structure resembling a veil or curtain. **2.** Caul (1). **3.** *Omentum* majus. **4.** Any serous membrane or membranous envelope or covering.
anterior medullary v., v. medullaris superius.
inferior medullary v., v. medullare inferius.
v. interpos'itum, *tela* choroidea ventriculi tertii.
v. medulla're infe'rius [NA], inferior or posterior medullary v.; v. semilunare; v. tarini; Tarin's valve; valvula semilunaris tarini; a thin sheet of white matter, hidden by the tonsilla cerebelli, attached along the peduncle of the flocculus and, at and near the midline, to the nodulus of the vermis; it is continuous caudally with the lamina choroidea and plexus choroideus of the fourth ventricle.
v. medulla're supe'rius [NA], superior or anterior medullary v.; Vieussens' valve; the thin layer of white matter stretching between the two superior cerebellar peduncles, forming the roof of the superior recess of the fourth ventricle.
v. palati'num [NA], official alternate name for *palatum* molle.
v. pen'dulum pala'ti, *palatum* molle.
posterior medullary v., v. medullare inferius.
v. semiluna're, v. medullare inferius.
superior medullary v., v. medullaris superius.
v. tari'ni, v. medullare inferius.
v. termina'le, *lamina* terminalis cerebri.
v. transver'sum, a fold in the dorsal wall of the embryonic brain at the boundary between the telencephalon and diencephalon.
v. triangula're, *tela* choroidea ventriculi tertii.

VENA

vena, gen. and pl. **venae** (vē'nă, -nē) [L.] [NA]. Vein; a blood vessel carrying blood toward the heart; all the veins except the pulmonary carry dark or unaerated blood.
v. ad'vehens, pl. **ve'nae advehen'tes,** veins carrying blood to capillaries as in the portal circulation of the liver.
v. anastomot'ica infe'rior [NA], inferior anastomotic vein; Browning's or Labbé's vein; an inconstant vein that passes from the superficial middle cerebral vein posteriorly over the lateral aspect of the temporal lobe to enter the transverse sinus.
v. anastomot'ica supe'rior [NA], superior anastomotic vein; Trolard's vein; a large communicating vein between the superficial middle cerebral vein and the superior sagittal sinus; it passes upward from the lateral sulcus, often following the line of the sulcus centralis (Rolando's fissure).
v. angula'ris [NA], angular vein; a short vein at the anterior angle of the orbit, formed by the supraorbital and supratrochlear veins and continuing as the facial vein.
v. appendicula'ris [NA], appendicular vein; the tributary of the ileocolic vein that accompanies the appendicular artery.
v. aqueduc'tus coch'leae [NA], vein of cochlear aqueduct or canaliculus; v. canaliculi cochleae; it drains the cochlea and the sacculus, and empties into the superior bulb of the jugular vein by accompanying the cochlear aqueduct through the cochlear canal.
v. aqueduc'tus vestib'uli [NA], vein of vestibular aqueduct; a small vein accompanying the endolymphatic duct; it terminates in the inferior petrosal sinus.
ve'nae arcua'tae re'nis [NA], arcuate or arciform veins of kidney; veins that parallel the arcuate arteries, receive blood from interlobular veins and venulae rectae, and terminate in interlobar veins.
v. arterio'sa, arterial *vein.*
ve'nae articula'res temporomandibula'res, *veins* of temporomandibular joint.
v. a'trii latera'lis [NA], lateral atrial vein; lateral vein of lateral ventricle; v. ventriculi lateralis lateralis; a vein draining deep portions of the temporal and parietal lobes; it runs in the lateral wall of the lateral ventricle to terminate in the superior thalamostriate vein.
v. a'trii media'lis [NA], medial atrial vein; medial vein of lateral ventricle; v. ventriculi lateralis medialis; a vein that drains deep portions of the parietal and occipital lobes; it runs in the medial wall of the lateral ventricle to empty into the internal cerebral vein or the great cerebral vein.
v. auricula'ris ante'rior [NA], anterior auricular vein; v. preauricularis; one of several veins draining the auricle and acoustic meatus and emptying into the retromandibular vein.
v. auricula'ris poste'rior [NA], posterior auricular vein; a tributary to the external jugular vein, draining the region posterior to the ear.
v. axilla'ris [NA], axillary vein; a continuation of the basilic and brachial veins running from the lower border of the teres major muscle to the outer border of the first rib where it becomes the subclavian vein.
v. az'ygos [NA], azygos vein; v. azygos major; arises from the right ascending lumbar vein or the inferior v. cava, ascends through the aortic orifice of the diaphragm, lies in the posterior mediastinum, and terminates in the superior v. cava.
v. az'ygos ma'jor, v. azygos.
v. az'ygos mi'nor infe'rior, v. hemiazygos.
v. az'ygos mi'nor supe'rior, v. hemiazygos accessoria.
v. basa'lis [NA], basal vein of Rosenthal; Rosenthal's vein; a large vein passing caudally and dorsally along the medial surface of the temporal lobe from which it receives tributaries; it empties into the vena cerebri magna (of Galen) from the lateral side.
v. basa'lis commu'nis [NA], common basal vein; the tributary to the inferior pulmonary vein (right and left) that receives blood from the superior and inferior basal veins.
v. basa'lis infe'rior [NA], inferior basal vein; tributary to the common basal vein draining the medial and posterior part of the inferior lobe in each lung.
v. basa'lis supe'rior [NA], superior basal vein; tributary to the common basal vein draining the lateral and anterior part of the inferior lobe of each lung.
v. basil'ica [NA], basilic vein; arises on the back of the hand from

the ulnar side of the dorsal venous rete; it curves around the medial side of the forearm and passes up the medial side of the arm to join the axillary vein.
v. basivertebra'lis [NA], basivertebral vein; one of a number of veins in the spongy substance of the bodies of the vertebrae, emptying into the anterior internal vertebral venous plexus.
Billroth's venae cavernosae, *venae* cavernosae of spleen.
ve'nae brachia'les [NA], brachial veins; two veins in either arm accompanying the brachial artery and emptying into the axillary vein.
ve'nae brachiocephal'icae [NA], brachiocephalic veins; innominate or anonymous veins; formed by the union of the internal jugular and subclavian veins; tributaries are the right brachiocephalic vein, which receives the right vertebral and internal thoracic veins, and the right lymphatic duct, and the left brachiocephalic vein, which receives the left vertebral, internal thoracic, superior intercostal, thyroidea ima, and various anterior pericardial, bronchial, and mediastinal veins.
ve'nae bronchia'les [NA], bronchial veins; many veins running in front of and behind the bronchi and uniting into two main trunks which empty on the right side into the azygos vein, on the left into the accessory hemiazygos or the left superior intercostal vein.
v. bul'bi pe'nis [NA], vein of bulb of penis; a tributary of the internal pudendal vein that drains the bulb of the penis.
v. bul'bi vestib'uli [NA], vein of vestibular bulb; the vein draining the bulb of the vestibule; a tributary of the internal pudendal vein.
v. canalic'uli coch'leae, v. aqueductus cochleae.
v. cana'lis pterygoi'dei [NA], vein of pterygoid canal; vidian vein; a vein accompanying the nerve and artery through the pterygoid canal and emptying into the pharyngeal vein.
v. cardi'aca mag'na, v. cordis magna.
v. ca'va infe'rior [NA], inferior v. cava; postcava; receives the blood from the lower limbs and the greater part of the pelvic and abdominal organs; it begins at the level of the fifth lumbar vertebra on the right side, pierces the diaphragm at the level of the eighth thoracic vertebra, and empties into the back part of the right atrium of the heart.
v. ca'va supe'rior [NA], superior v. cava; precava; returns blood from the head and neck, upper limbs, and thorax; formed by union of the two brachiocephalic veins.
ve'nae caverno'sae pe'nis [NA], the cavernous venous spaces in the erectile tissue of the penis.
venae cavernosae of spleen, Billroth's venae cavernosae; small tributaries of the splenic vein in the pulp of the spleen.
v. centra'lis glan'dulae suprarena'lis [NA], central vein of suprarenal gland; the single draining vein of the gland; it receives a number of medullary veins; on the right side it empties directly into the inferior vena cava and on the left into the left renal vein.
ve'nae centra'les hep'atis [NA], central veins of the liver; Krukenberg's veins; the terminal branches of the hepatic veins that lie centrally in the hepatic lobules and receive blood from the liver sinusoids.
v. centra'lis ret'inae [NA], central vein of retina; formed by union of the retinal veins and accompanies the artery of the same name in the optic nerve.
v. cephal'ica [NA], cephalic vein; arises at the radial border of the dorsal venous rete of the hand, passes upward in front of the elbow and along the lateral side of the arm; it empties into the upper part of the axillary vein.
v. cephal'ica accesso'ria [NA], accessory cephalic vein; a variable vein that passes along the radial border of the forearm to join the cephalic vein near the elbow.
ve'nae cerebel'li [NA], veins of the cerebellum; cerebellar veins; the veins draining the cerebellum. See venae hemispherii cerebelli inferiores and superiores; v. petrosa; v. precentralis cerebelli; v. vermis inferior and superior.
ve'nae cerebel'li inferio'res, see venae hemispherii cerebelli inferiores.
ve'nae cerebel'li superio'res, see venae hemispherii cerebelli superiores.
v. cer'ebri ante'rior [NA], anterior cerebral vein; a small vein that parallels the anterior cerebral artery and drains into the basal vein.
ve'nae cer'ebri inferio'res [NA], inferior cerebral veins; numerous cerebral veins that drain the undersurface of the cerebral hemispheres and empty into the cavernous and transverse sinuses.
ve'nae cer'ebri inter'nae [NA], internal cerebral veins; veins of Galen (2); paired veins passing caudally near the midline in the tela choroidea of the third ventricle, formed by the union of the choroid vein, thalamostriate (terminal) vein, and v. septi pellucidi, and uniting caudally so as to form the v. cerebri magna.
v. cer'ebri mag'na [NA], great cerebral vein; great vein of Galen; a large, unpaired vein formed by the junction of the two internal cerebral veins in the caudal part of the tela choroidea of the third ventricle; it passes caudally between the splenium of the corpus callosum and the pineal gland, curving dorsally to continue into the sinus rectus.
v. cer'ebri me'dia profun'da [NA], deep middle cerebral vein; the vein that accompanies the middle cerebral artery in the depths of the lateral sulcus and empties into the basal vein of Rosenthal.
v. cer'ebri me'dia superficia'lis [NA], superficial middle cerebral vein; a large vein passing along the line of the sylvian fissure to join the cavernous sinus; it communicates with the superior sagittal sinus and transverse sinus via the superior and inferior anastomotic veins, respectively.
ve'nae cer'ebri profun'dae [NA], deep cerebral veins; the numerous veins draining the deep structures of the cerebral hemispheres; they empty into the tributaries of the great cerebral vein.
ve'nae cer'ebri superficia'les [NA], superficial cerebral veins; the veins on the superficial surface of the cerebral hemispheres; they comprise three groups: superior, middle, and inferior.
ve'nae cer'ebri superio'res [NA], superior cerebral veins; numerous (8 to 10) veins that drain the dorsal convexity of the cortical hemisphere and empty into the superior sagittal sinus, curving rostrally in passing through the subdural space so as to enter the sinus at an acute forward angle.
v. cervica'lis profun'da [NA], deep cervical vein; it runs with the artery of the same name between the semispinalis capitis and semispinalis cervicis and empties into the brachiocephalic or the vertebral vein.
v. choroi'dea infe'rior [NA], inferior choroid vein; a small vein draining the lower part of the choroid plexus of the lateral ventricle into the basal vein.
ve'nae choroi'deae oc'uli [NA], official alternate term for venae vorticosae.
v. choroi'dea supe'rior [NA], superior choroid vein; a tortuous vein that follows the choroid plexus of the lateral ventricle and unites with the superior thalamostriate vein and the anterior vein of the septum pellucidum to form the internal cerebral vein.
ve'nae cilia'res [NA], ciliary veins; several small veins, anterior and posterior, coming from the ciliary body.
ve'nae circumflex'ae fem'oris latera'les [NA], lateral circumflex femoral veins; the veins that accompany the lateral circumflex femoral artery.
ve'nae circumflex'ae fem'oris media'les [NA], medial circumflex femoral veins; the venae comitantes that parallel the medial circumflex femoral artery.
v. circumflex'a il'ium profun'da [NA], deep circumflex iliac vein; corresponds to the artery of the same name, and empties, near or in a common trunk with the inferior epigastric vein, into the external iliac vein.
v. circumflex'a il'ium superficia'lis [NA], superficial circumflex iliac vein; corresponding to the artery of the same name, emptying usually into the great saphenous vein, or sometimes into the femoral vein.

v. col'ica dex'tra [NA], right colic vein; the vein that parallels the right colic artery and drains blood from the ascending colon and right flexure.
v. col'ica me'dia [NA], middle colic vein; the tributary of the superior mesenteric vein that accompanies the middle colic artery.
v. col'ica sinis'tra [NA], left colic vein; a tributary of the inferior mesenteric vein that accompanies the left colic artery and drains the left flexure and descending colon.
ve'nae colum'nae vertebra'lis [NA], veins of vertebral column; includes the internal and external vertebral venous plexuses, the basivertebral veins, and the anterior and posterior spinal veins.
v. com'itans [NA], companion or accompanying vein; a vein accompanying another structure.
v. com'itans ner'vi hypoglos'si [NA], runs with the hypoglossal nerve below and lateral to the hyoglossus muscle, emptying usually into the lingual vein.
ve'nae comitan'tes [NA], companion veins; a pair of veins, occasionally more, that closely accompany an artery in such a manner that the pulsations of the artery aid venous return.
ve'nae conjunctiva'les [NA], conjunctival veins; the veins draining the conjunctiva.
ve'nae cor'dis anterio'res [NA], anterior cardiac veins; two or three small veins in the anterior wall of the right ventricle opening into the right atrium independently of the coronary sinus.
v. cor'dis mag'na [NA], great cardiac vein; v. cardiaca magna; left coronary vein; a tributary of the coronary sinus, beginning at the apex and running in the anterior interventricular sulcus.
v. cor'dis me'dia [NA], middle cardiac vein; inferior cardiac vein; begins at the apex of the heart and passes through the posterior interventricular sulcus to the coronary sinus.
ve'nae cor'dis min'imae [NA], smallest cardiac veins; thebesian veins; numerous small venous channels that open directly into the chambers of the heart from the capillary bed in the cardiac wall.
v. cor'dis par'va [NA], small cardiac vein; an inconstant vessel, accompanying the right coronary artery in the coronary sulcus, from the right margin of the right ventricle, and emptying into the coronary sinus or the middle cardiac vein.
v. cor'nus posterio'ris [NA], vein of posterior horn; a small vein draining the surface region of the posterior horn of the lateral ventricle; it is a tributary to the great cerebral vein.
v. corona'ria ventric'uli, v. gastrica sinistra.
v. cor'poris callo'si dorsa'lis [NA], dorsal vein of corpus callosum; posterior pericallosal vein; posterior marginal vein; dorsal callosal vein; it originates on the superior surface of the corpus callosum and runs posteriorly to terminate in the great cerebral vein.
v. cuta'nea [NA], cutaneous vein; superficial vein; one of a number of veins that course in the subcutaneous tissue and empty into deep veins; they form prominent systems of vessels in the limbs and are usually not accompanied by arteries.
v. cys'tica [NA], cystic vein; it drains the gallbladder, passing along the cystic duct to enter the right branch of the portal vein.
ve'nae digita'les dorsa'les pe'dis [NA], dorsal digital veins of toes; they receive intercapitular veins from the plantar venous arch, join to form four common dorsal digital veins, and terminate in the dorsal venous arch.
ve'nae digita'les palma'res [NA], palmar digital veins; they form paired venae comitantes along the proper and common digital arteries and empty into the superficial palmar venous arch.
ve'nae digita'les planta'res [NA], plantar digital veins; they arise in the toes and pass back to form four metatarsal veins that empty into the plantar venous arch.
v. diplo'ica [NA], diploic vein; Dupuytren's canal; Breschet's vein; one of the veins in the diploë of the cranial bones, connected with the cerebral sinuses by emissary veins; the main diploic veins are the frontal, anterior temporal, posterior temporal, and occipital.
ve'nae direc'tae latera'les [NA], lateral direct veins; surface thalamic veins; one or more veins running a subependymal course in a coronal plane over the thalamus, terminating in the internal cerebral vein.
v. dorsa'lis clitor'idis profun'da [NA], deep dorsal vein of clitoris; a tributary of the vesical venous plexus; it runs a course deep to the fascia on the dorsum of the clitoris.
ve'nae dorsa'les clitor'idis superficia'les [NA], superficial dorsal veins of clitoris; a pair of veins on the dorsum of the clitoris, tributary to the external pudendal vein on either side.
v. dorsa'lis lin'guae [NA], dorsal lingual vein; a tributary of the lingual.
v. dorsa'lis pe'nis profun'da [NA], deep dorsal vein of penis; a vein on the dorsum of the penis deep to the fascia penis; it is a tributary to the prostatic plexus.
ve'nae dorsa'les pe'nis superficia'les [NA], superficial dorsal veins of penis; a pair of veins on the dorsum of the penis superficial to the fascia penis; they are tributaries of the external pudendal veins on each side.
v. emissa'ria, pl. **ve'nae emissa'riae** [NA], emissary vein; emissary (2); emissarium; one of the channels of communication between the venous sinuses of the dura mater and the veins of the diploë and the scalp.
v. emissa'ria condyla'ris [NA], condylar emissary vein; emissarium condyloideum; a vein that connects the sigmoid sinus and the external vertebral venous plexuses through the condylar canal of the occipital bone.
v. emissa'ria mastoi'dea [NA], mastoid emissary vein; emissarium mastoideum; the vein that connects the sigmoid sinus with the occipital vein or one of the tributaries of the external jugular vein by way of the mastoid foramen.
v. emissa'ria occipita'lis [NA], occipital emissary vein; emissarium occipitale; an inconstant vessel connecting the occipital veins with the confluens sinuum.
v. emissa'ria parieta'lis [NA], parietal emissary vein; emissarium parietale; Santorini's vein; the vein that connects the superior sagittal sinus with the tributaries of the superficial temporal vein and other veins of the scalp.
v. epigas'trica infe'rior [NA], inferior epigastric vein; deep epigastric vein; corresponds to the artery of the same name and empties into the external iliac vein.
v. epigas'trica superficia'lis [NA], superficial epigastric vein; drains the lower and medial part of the anterior abdominal wall and empties into the great saphenous vein.
ve'nae epigas'tricae superio'res [NA], superior epigastric veins; the venae comitantes of the artery of the same name, tributaries of the internal thoracic vein.
ve'nae episclera'les [NA], episcleral veins; a series of small venules in the sclera close to the corneal margin that empty into the anterior ciliary veins.
ve'nae esopha'geae [NA], esophageal veins; several small venous trunks bringing blood from the esophagus and emptying into the brachiocephalic or the azygos veins.
ve'nae ethmoida'les [NA], ethmoidal veins; veins that accompany the anterior and posterior ethmoidal arteries and pass into the superior ophthalmic vein; they drain the ethmoidal sinuses.
v. facia'lis [NA], facial vein; anterior facial vein; v. facialis anterior; a continuation of the angular vein at the medial angle of the eye; it passes diagonally downward and outward, uniting with the retromandibular vein below the border of the lower jaw before emptying into the internal jugular vein
v. facia'lis ante'rior, v. facialis.
v. facia'lis commu'nis, common facial *vein.*
v. facia'lis poste'rior, v. retromandibularis.
v. facie'i profun'da [NA], deep facial vein; the communicating vein that passes from the facial vein to the pterygoid plexus in the infratemporal fossa; it is devoid of valves.
v. femora'lis [NA], femoral vein; it accompanies the femoral ar-

tery in the same sheath, being a continuation of the popliteal vein, and becomes the external iliac vein at the level of the inguinal (Poupart's) ligament.

ve'nae fibula'res [NA], official alternate term for venae peroneae.

ve'nae fronta'les, **(1)** [NA] frontal veins (1); the superficial veins draining the frontal cortex and emptying into the superior sagittal sinus; **(2)** venae supratrochleares.

ve'nae gas'tricae bre'ves [NA], short gastric veins; small vessels that drain the left portion of the wall of the stomach emptying into the splenic vein.

v. gas'trica dex'tra [NA], right gastric vein; pyloric vein; it receives veins from both surfaces of the upper portion of the stomach, runs to the right along the lesser curvature of the stomach, and empties into the portal vein.

v. gas'trica sinis'tra [NA], left gastric vein; coronary vein; v. coronaria ventriculi; arises from a union of veins from both surfaces of the cardia of the stomach; it runs in the lesser omentum and empties into the portal vein.

v. gastro-omenta'lis dex'tra [NA], right gastro-omental or gastroepiploic vein; a tributary of the superior mesenteric vein that parallels the right gastro-omental artery along the greater curvature of the stomach.

v. gastro-omenta'lis sinis'tra [NA], left gastro-omental or gastroepiploic vein; the vein that accompanies the left gastro-omental artery along the greater curvature of the stomach; it empties into the splenic vein.

ve'nae ge'nus [NA], veins of knee; the veins that accompany the genicular arteries; they drain blood from the structures around the knee, terminating in the popliteal vein.

ve'nae glu'teae inferio'res [NA], inferior gluteal veins; the venae comitantes of the inferior gluteal artery uniting at the sciatic foramen to form a common trunk which empties into the internal iliac vein.

ve'nae glu'teae superio'res [NA], superior gluteal veins; the veins that accompany the gluteal artery, entering the pelvis as two veins which unite into one and empty into the internal iliac vein.

v. gy'ri olfacto'rii [NA], vein of olfactory gyrus; a tributary of the basal vein which drains the medial olfactory stria.

v. hemiaz'ygos [NA], hemiazygos vein; v. azygos minor inferior; the continuation of the left ascending lumbar vein; it pierces the left crus of the diaphragm, ascends along the left side of the bodies of the lower thoracic vertebrae, opposite the eighth vertebra, crosses the midline behind the aorta, thoracic duct, and esophagus, and empties into the azygos vein.

v. hemiaz'ygos accesso'ria [NA], accessory hemiazygos vein; v. azygos minor superior; formed by the union of the fourth to seventh left posterior intercostal veins, passes along the side of the bodies of the fifth, sixth, and seventh thoracic vertebrae. then crosses the midline behind the aorta, esophagus, and thoracic duct, and empties into the azygos vein.

ve'nae hemisphe'rii cerebel'li inferio'res [NA], inferior veins of cerebellar hemisphere; several veins draining the inferior portion of the cerebellar hemispheres; they terminate in the petrosal vein.

ve'nae hemisphe'rii cerebel'li superio'res [NA], superior veins of cerebellar hemisphere; several veins draining the superior part of the cerebellar hemispheres; they terminate in the superior petrosal sinus or the petrosal vein.

ve'nae hemorrhoida'les inferio'res, venae rectales inferiores.

ve'nae hemorrhoida'les me'diae, venae rectales mediae.

v. hemorrhoida'lis supe'rior, v. rectalis superior.

ve'nae hepat'icae [NA], hepatic veins; the veins that drain the liver; they collect blood from the central veins and terminate in three large veins opening into the inferior vena cava below the diaphragm and several small inconstant veins entering the vena cava lower down.

ve'nae hepat'icae dex'trae [NA], right hepatic veins; veins draining the right lobe of the liver; they usually combine into one or two veins that empty into the inferior vena cava.

ve'nae hepat'icae me'diae [NA], middle hepatic veins; the veins draining the caudate lobe of the liver; they usually form one trunk before emptying into the inferior vena cava.

ve'nae hepat'icae sinis'trae [NA], left hepatic veins; the veins draining the left lobe of the liver; they usually form one or two veins that empty into the inferior vena cava.

v. hypogas'trica, v. iliaca interna.

v. ileocol'ica [NA], ileocolic vein; a large tributary of the superior mesenteric vein that runs parallel to the ileocolic artery and drains the terminal ileum, appendix, cecum, and the lower part of the ascending colon.

v. ili'aca commu'nis [NA], common iliac vein; formed by the union of the external and internal iliac veins at the brim of the pelvis and passes upward behind the internal iliac artery to the right side of the body of the fifth lumbar vertebra where it unites with its fellow of the opposite side to form the inferior v. cava; the left common iliac vein is submitted to a pulsating compression by the right common iliac artery against the vertebral column which may result in partial obstruction of the vein.

v. ili'aca exter'na [NA], external iliac vein; a direct continuation of the femoral vein above the inguinal ligament, uniting with the internal iliac vein to form the common iliac vein.

v. ili'aca inter'na [NA], internal iliac vein; hypogastric vein; v. hypogastrica; runs from the upper border of the greater sciatic notch to the brim of the pelvis where it joins the external iliac vein to form the common iliac vein; it drains most of the territory supplied by the internal iliac artery.

v. iliolumba'lis [NA], iliolumbar vein; accompanying the artery of the same name, anastomosing with the lumbar and deep circumflex iliac veins, and emptying into the internal iliac vein.

inferior v. cava, v. cava inferior.

v. innomina'ta, see venae brachiocephalicae.

ve'nae insula'res [NA], insular veins; veins draining the cortex of the insula, tributaries to the deep middle cerebral vein.

ve'nae intercapita'les [NA], intercapitular veins; the veins connecting the dorsal and palmar veins in the hand, or the dorsal and plantar veins in the foot.

ve'nae intercosta'les anterio'res [NA], anterior intercostal veins; tributaries to the musculophrenic or internal thoracic veins from the intercostal spaces.

ve'nae intercosta'les posterio'res [NA], posterior intercostal veins; veins draining the intercostal spaces posteriorly; from the fourth to the eleventh spaces on the right they are tributaries of the azygos vein; on the left they empty into either the hemiazygos or accessory hemiazygos veins.

v. intercosta'lis supe'rior dex'tra [NA], right superior intercostal vein; a tributary of the azygos vein formed by the union of the right second, third, and fourth posterior intercostal veins.

v. intercosta'lis supe'rior sinis'tra [NA], left superior intercostal vein; the vein formed by the union of the left second, third, and fourth intercostal veins; it passes forward across the arch of the aorta to empty into the left brachiocephalic vein and frequently communicates also with the accessory hemiazygos vein.

v. intercosta'lis supre'ma [NA], highest intercostal vein; the vein draining the first intercostal space into either the vertebral or the brachiocephalic vein.

ve'nae interloba'res re'nis [NA], interlobar veins of kidney; the veins in the kidney that parallel the interlobar arteries, receiving blood from arcuate veins, and terminate in the renal vein.

ve'nae interlobula'res hep'atis [NA], interlobular veins of liver; the terminal branches of the portal vein that course in the portal canals between liver lobules and empty into the liver sinusoids.

ve'nae interlobula'res re'nis [NA], interlobular veins of kidney; they parallel the interlobular arteries and drain the peritubular capillary plexus, emptying into the arcuate veins.

v. interme'dia antebra'chii [NA], intermediate or median antebrachial vein; intermediate or median vein of forearm; v. mediana antebrachii; it begins at the base of the dorsum of the thumb, curves around the radial side, ascends the middle of the forearm, and just below the bend of the elbow divides into the intermediate basilic and intermediate cephalic veins; sometimes it divides lower down, one branch going to the basilic vein, the other to the intermediate vein of the elbow.

v. interme'dia basil'ica [NA], intermediate or median basilic vein; v. mediana basilica; the medial branch of the intermediate antebrachial vein which joins the basilic vein.

v. interme'dia cephal'ica [NA], intermediate or median cephalic vein; v. mediana cephalica; the lateral branch of the intermediate antebrachial vein that joins the cephalic vein near the elbow.

v. interme'dia cu'biti [NA], intermediate or median cubital vein; v. mediana cubiti; a vein which passes across the bend of the elbow from the cephalic vein to the basilic vein; more commonly the vein in this location is called the intermediate basilic vein.

v. intervertebra'lis [NA], intervertebral vein; one of numerous veins accompanying the spinal nerves, emptying in the neck into the vertebral vein, in the thorax into the intercostal veins, in the lumbar and sacral regions into the lumbar and sacral veins.

ve'nae jejuna'les et il'ei [NA], jejunal and ileal veins; the veins that drain the jejunum and ileum; they terminate in the superior mesenteric vein.

v. jugula'ris ante'rior [NA], anterior jugular vein; it arises below the chin from veins draining the lower lip and mental region, descends the anterior portion of the neck superficially, and terminates in the external jugular vein at the lateral border of the scalenus anterior muscle.

v. jugula'ris exter'na [NA], external jugular vein; it is formed below the parotid gland by the junction of the posterior auricular vein and the retromandibular vein, and passes down the side of the neck superficial to the sternocleidomastoid muscle to empty into the subclavian vein.

v. jugula'ris inter'na [NA], internal jugular vein; a continuation of the sigmoid sinus of the dura mater, uniting, behind the cartilage of the first rib, with the subclavian vein to form the brachiocephalic vein.

ve'nae labia'les anterio'res [NA], anterior labial veins; they pass from the labia majora to the external pudendal veins.

v. labia'lis infe'rior [NA], inferior labial vein; a tributary of the facial vein draining the lower lip.

ve'nae labia'les posterio'res [NA], posterior labial veins; they pass posteriorly from the labia majora to the internal pudendal veins.

v. labia'lis supe'rior [NA], superior labial vein; veins taking blood from the upper lip and discharging into the facial vein.

ve'nae labyrin'thi [NA], labyrinthine veins; internal auditory veins; two veins accompanying each labyrinthine artery; they drain the internal ear, pass out through the internal acoustic meatus, and empty into the transverse sinus or the inferior petrosal sinus.

v. lacrima'lis [NA], lacrimal vein; it drains the lacrimal gland, passing posteriorly through the orbit with the lacrimal artery to empty into the superior ophthalmic vein.

v. laryn'gea infe'rior [NA], inferior laryngeal vein; the vein passing from the lower part of the larynx to the plexus thyroideus impar.

v. laryn'gea supe'rior [NA], superior laryngeal vein; it accompanies the superior laryngeal artery and empties into the superior thyroid vein.

v. liena'lis, v. splenica.

v. lingua'lis [NA], lingual vein; receives blood from the tongue, sublingual and submandibular glands, and muscles of the floor of the mouth; empties into the internal jugular or the facial vein.

ve'nae lumba'les [NA], lumbar veins; five in number, these veins accompany the lumbar arteries, drain the posterior body wall and the lumbar vertebral venous plexuses, and terminate anteriorly as follows: the first and second in the ascending lumbar vein, the third and fourth in the inferior vena cava, and the fifth in the iliolumbar vein.

v. lumba'lis ascen'dens [NA], ascending lumbar vein; it arises from the sacral and lumbar veins and at the diaphragm becomes the azygos vein on the right side, the hemiazygos vein on the left.

v. mamma'ria inter'na, v. thoracica interna.

v. maxilla'ris, pl. **ve'nae maxilla'res** [NA], maxillary vein; the posterior continuation of the pterygoid plexus; it joins the superficial temporal vein to form the retromandibular vein.

v. media'na antebra'chii, v. intermedia antebrachii.

v. media'na basil'ica, v. intermedia basilica.

v. media'na cephal'ica, v. intermedia cephalica.

v. media'na cu'biti, v. intermedia cubiti.

ve'nae mediastina'les [NA], mediastinal veins; several small veins from the mediastinum emptying into the brachiocephalic veins or the superior v. cava.

ve'nae medul'lae oblonga'tae [NA], veins of medulla oblongata; several veins draining the medulla oblongata; they are tributaries of the anterior spinal vein and the petrosal vein.

ve'nae menin'geae [NA], meningeal veins; veins that accompany the meningeal arteries; they communicate with venous sinuses and diploic veins and drain into regional veins outside the cranial vault.

ve'nae menin'geae me'diae [NA], middle meningeal veins; the venae comitantes of the middle meningeal artery that empty into the pterygoid plexus.

ve'nae mesencephal'icae [NA], mesencephalic veins; several veins draining the mesencephalon; the posterior ones are tributaries to the great cerebral vein; the lateral ones are tributaries to the basal vein.

v. mesenter'ica infe'rior [NA], inferior mesenteric vein; a continuation of the superior rectal vein at the brim of the pelvis, ascending to the left of the aorta behind the peritoneum and emptying into the splenic vein or into the superior mesenteric vein or rarely in the angle between these veins.

v. mesenter'ica supe'rior [NA], superior mesenteric vein; begins at the ileum in the right iliac fossa, ascends in the root of the mesentery, and unites behind the pancreas with the splenic vein to form the hepatic portal vein.

ve'nae metacar'peae dorsa'les [NA], dorsal metacarpal veins; three veins on the dorsum of the hand draining blood from the four medial digits into the dorsal venous network of the hand.

ve'nae metacar'peae palma'res [NA], palmar metacarpal veins; veins emptying into the deep venous arch from which the radial and ulnar veins arise.

ve'nae metatar'seae dorsa'les [NA], dorsal metatarsal veins; veins arising from the dorsal digital veins forming the dorsal venous arch of the foot.

ve'nae metatar'seae planta'res [NA], plantar metatarsal veins; veins formed from the plantar digital veins constituting the deep plantar venous arch, which empties into the medial and lateral plantar veins.

ve'nae mus'culophren'icae [NA], musculophrenic veins; the veins that accompany the musculophrenic artery and drain blood from the upper abdominal wall, lower intercostal spaces, and the diaphragm.

ve'nae nasa'les exter'nae [NA], external nasal veins; several vessels that drain the external nose, emptying into the angular or facial vein.

v. nasofronta'lis [NA], nasofrontal vein; the vein located in the anterior medial part of the orbit that connects the superior ophthalmic vein with the angular vein.

ve'nae nu'clei cauda'ti [NA], veins of caudate nucleus; small veins from the caudate nucleus draining into the superior thalamostriate vein.

v. obli'qua a'trii sinis'tri [NA], oblique vein of left atrium; Marshall's oblique vein; a small vein on the posterior wall of the left atrium, a tributary of the coronary sinus; it is developed from the left common cardinal vein.

v. obturato'ria, pl. **venae obturato'riae** [NA], obturator vein; formed by the union of tributaries draining the hip joint and the muscles of the upper and back part of the thigh; it enters the pelvis by the obturator canal and empties into the internal iliac vein.

ve'nae occipita'les [NA], occipital veins; the superficial veins draining the occipital cortex and emptying into the superior sagittal sinus and the transverse sinus.

v. occipita'lis [NA], occipital vein; drains the occipital region and empties into the internal jugular vein or the suboccipital plexus.

v. ophthal'mica infe'rior [NA], inferior ophthalmic vein; arises from the inferior palpebral and lacrimal and divides into two terminal branches, one of which runs to the pterygoid plexus while the other joins the superior ophthalmic vein or empties into the cavernous sinus.

v. ophthal'mica supe'rior [NA], superior ophthalmic vein; begins anteriorly from the nasofrontal vein, passes along the upper part of the medial wall of the orbit, passes through the superior orbital fissure, to empty into the cavernous sinus.

v. ova'rica dex'tra, [NA], right ovarian vein; begins at the pampiniform plexus at the hilum of the ovary and opens into the inferior v. cava.

v. ova'rica sinis'tra [NA], left ovarian vein; begins at the pampiniform plexus at the hilum of the ovary and empties into the left renal vein.

v. palati'na [NA], palatine vein; drains the palatine regions and empties into the facial vein.

ve'nae palpebra'les [NA], veins of eyelids; veins draining the superior eyelid, tributaries of the superior ophthalmic vein.

ve'nae palpebra'les inferio'res [NA], veins of inferior eyelid; veins originating in the inferior eyelid and emptying into the angular vein.

ve'nae palpebra'les superio'res [NA], veins of superior eyelid; veins draining the superior eyelid into the angular vein.

ve'nae pancreat'icae [NA], pancreatic veins; veins draining the pancreas, emptying into the splenic vein and the superior mesenteric vein.

ve'nae pancreat'icoduodena'les [NA], pancreaticoduodenal veins; veins that accompany the superior and inferior pancreaticoduodenal arteries, emptying into the superior mesenteric or portal vein.

ve'nae paraumbilica'les [NA], paraumbilical veins; Sappey's veins; several small veins arising from cutaneous veins about the umbilicus running along the ligamentum teres of the liver, and terminating as accessory portal veins in the substance of this organ.

ve'nae parieta'les [NA], parietal veins; the superficial veins draining the parietal cerebral cortex and emptying into the superior sagittal sinus.

ve'nae parotide'ae [NA], parotid veins; posterior parotid veins; parotid branches of the facial vein draining part of the parotid gland and emptying into the retromandibular vein.

ve'nae pectora'les [NA], pectoral veins; veins draining the pectoral muscles and emptying directly into the subclavian vein.

ve'nae peduncula'res [NA], peduncular veins; small tributaries of the basal vein from the cerebral peduncle.

ve'nae perforan'tes [NA], perforating veins; the veins that accompany the perforating arteries; they drain blood from the vastus lateralis and the hamstring muscles and terminate in the v. profunda femoris.

ve'nae pericardi'acae [NA], pericardial veins; several small veins from the pericardium emptying into the brachiocephalic veins or superior v. cava.

ve'nae pericardiacophren'icae [NA], pericardiacophrenic veins; the veins accompanying the pericardiacophrenic artery and emptying into the brachiocephalic veins or superior v. cava.

ve'nae perone'ae [NA], peroneal or fibular veins; venae fibulares; the veins that accompany the peroneal artery; they join the posterior tibial veins to enter the popliteal vein.

v. petro'sa [NA], petrosal vein; a short trunk formed by the union of four or five cerebellar and pontine veins opposite the brachium pontis; it terminates in the superior petrosal sinus.

ve'nae pharyn'geae [NA], pharyngeal veins; several veins from the pharyngeal plexus emptying into the internal jugular vein.

v. phren'ica infe'rior, pl. **ve'nae phren'icae inferio'res** [NA], inferior phrenic vein; the vein that drains the substance of the diaphragm and empties on the right side into the v. cava, on the left side into the left suprarenal vein; often a second vein on the left side passes transversely across the diaphragm anterior to the esophageal hiatus to enter the inferior v. cava.

ve'nae phren'icae superio'res [NA], superior phrenic veins; small veins that drain the upper surface of the diaphragm; they are tributaries of the azygos and hemiazygos veins.

ve'nae pon'tis [NA], veins of pons; pontine veins; several veins running transversely on the pons to join the petrosal vein.

v. pontomesencephal'ica ante'rior [NA], anterior pontomesencephalic vein; a vein in the midline of the interpeduncular fossa on the superior and anterior aspects of the pons; it communicates with the basal vein superiorly and the petrosal vein inferiorly.

v. poplite'a [NA], popliteal vein; arises at the lower border of the popliteus muscle by the union of the anterior and posterior tibial veins, ascends through the popliteal space, and pierces the adductor magnus muscle to become the femoral vein.

v. por'tae hep'atis [NA], hepatic portal vein; portal vein; v. portalis; a wide short vein formed by the superior mesenteric and splenic vein behind the pancreas, ascending in front of the inferior v. cava, and dividing at the right end of the transverse fissure of the liver into right and left branches, which ramify within the liver.

v. porta'lis, v. portae hepatis.

v. poste'rior ventric'uli sinis'tri [NA], posterior vein of left ventricle; arises on the diaphragmatic surface of the heart near the apex, runs to the left and parallel to the posterior interventricular sulcus, and empties in the coronary sinus.

v. preauricula'ris, v. auricularis anterior.

v. precentra'lis cerebel'li [NA], precentral cerebellar vein; an unpaired vein originating in the precentral cerebellar fissure passing anterior and superior to the culmen on its way to terminate in the great cerebral vein.

ve'nae prefronta'les [NA], prefrontal veins; the superficial veins draining the prefrontal cerebral cortex and emptying into the superior sagittal sinus.

v. prepylo'rica [NA], prepyloric vein; Latarjet's or Mayo's vein; a tributary of the right gastric vein that passes anterior to the pylorus at its junction with the duodenum.

ve'nae profun'dae clitor'idis [NA], deep veins of clitoris; the veins that pass from the dorsum of the clitoris to join the vesical plexus.

v. profun'da fem'oris [NA], deep femoral vein; the vein that accompanies the deep femoral artery, receiving perforating veins from the posterior aspect of the thigh. It joins the femoral vein in the femoral triangle, usually in common with the medial and lateral circumflex femoral veins.

v. profun'da lin'guae [NA], deep lingual vein; the vein that accompanies the deep lingual artery and joins the lingual vein. It drains the body and apex of the tongue.

v. profun'da pe'nis [NA], deep vein of penis; the vein deep to the deep fascia on the dorsum of the penis. It enters the prostatic plexus by passing through a gap between the arcuate pubic ligament and the transverse perineal ligament.

ve'nae puden'dae exter'nae [NA], external pudendal veins; these correspond to the arteries of the same name; they empty into the great saphenous vein or directly into the femoral vein, and receive the superficial dorsal vein of the penis (clitoris) and the anterior scrotal (or labial) veins.

v. puden'da inter'na [NA], internal pudendal vein; a tributary of

the internal iliac vein that accompanies the internal pudendal artery as a single or double vessel. It drains the perineum.
ve'nae pulmona'les [NA], pulmonary veins; four veins, two on each side, conveying blood from the lungs to the left atrium of the heart. The former veins are known as intersegmental or infrasegmental veins, whereas the latter veins, which emerge from the segments, are named intrasegmental.
v. pulmona'lis infe'rior dex'tra [NA], right inferior pulmonary vein; the vein returning blood from the inferior lobe of the right lung to the left atrium.
v. pulmona'lis infe'rior sinis'tra [NA], left inferior pulmonary vein; the vein returning blood from the inferior lobe of the left lung to the left atrium.
v. pulmona'lis supe'rior dex'tra [NA], right superior pulmonary vein; the vein returning blood from the superior and middle lobes of the right lung to the left atrium.
v. pulmona'lis supe'rior sinis'tra [NA], left superior pulmonary vein; the vein returning blood from the left superior lobe of the lung to the left atrium.
ve'nae radia'les [NA], radial veins; several veins continuing the deep palmar veins on the lateral side, and accompanying the radial artery.
v. reces'sus latera'lis ventric'uli quar'ti [NA], vein of lateral recess of fourth ventricle; a small vein originating in the cerebellar tonsil, coursing by the lateral recess of the fourth ventricle on its way to terminate in the petrosal vein.
ve'nae rec'tae, the ascending limbs of the vasa rectae in the renal medulla.
ve'nae recta'les inferio'res [NA], inferior rectal or hemorrhoidal veins; venae hemorrhoidales inferiores; veins that pass to the internal pudendal vein from the venous plexus around the anal canal.
ve'nae recta'les me'diae [NA], middle rectal or hemorrhoidal veins; venae hemorrhoidales mediae; several veins that pass from the rectal venous plexus to the internal iliac vein.
v. recta'lis supe'rior [NA], superior rectal or hemorrhoidal vein; v. hemorrhoidalis superior; it drains the greater part of the rectal venous plexus, and ascends between the layers of the mesorectum to the brim of the pelvis, where it becomes the inferior mesenteric vein.
ve'nae rena'les [NA], renal veins; they accompany the arteries of the same name, and open at right angles into the v. cava at the level of the second lumbar vertebra. The left renal vein receives the left suprarenal vein and the left gonadal vein.
ve'nae re'nis [NA], veins of kidney; the tributaries of the renal vein that drain the kidney; they parallel the arteries in the kidney and consist of interlobular, arcuate, and interlobar veins.
v. retromandibula'ris [NA], retromandibular vein; posterior facial vein; temporomaxillary vein; v. facialis posterior; it is formed by the union of the temporal veins in front of the ear, runs behind the ramus of the mandible through the parotid gland, and unites with the facial vein.
v. re'vehens, pl. **ve'nae revehen'tes,** veins in the embryo, passing from the sinusoid vessels in the liver to the inferior v. cava, that develop into the hepatic veins.
ve'nae sacra'les latera'les [NA], lateral sacral veins; several veins that accompany the corresponding artery and empty into the internal iliac vein on each side.
v. sacra'lis media'na [NA], median sacral vein; an unpaired vein accompanying the middle sacral artery emptying into the left common iliac vein.
v. saphe'na accesso'ria [NA], accessory saphenous vein; an occasional vein running in the thigh parallel to the great saphenous vein which it joins just before the latter empties into the femoral vein.
v. saphe'na mag'na [NA], great, large, or long saphenous vein; formed by the union of the dorsal vein of the great toe and the dorsal venous arch of the foot, ascends in front of the medial malleolus, behind the medial condyle of the femur, and empties into the femoral vein in the upper part of the femoral (Scarpa's) triangle.
v. saphe'na par'va [NA], small or short saphenous vein; arises on the lateral side of the foot from a union of the dorsal vein of the little toe with the dorsal venous arch, ascends behind the lateral malleolus, along the lateral border of the calcanean tendon and then through the middle of the calf to the lower portion of the popliteal space where it empties into the popliteal vein.
v. scapula'ris dorsa'lis [NA], dorsal scapular vein; the vein accompanying the descending scapular artery; it is a tributary to the subclavian or the external jugular vein.
ve'nae sclera'les [NA], scleral veins; small veins draining the sclera; they are tributaries to the anterior ciliary veins.
ve'nae scrota'les anterio'res [NA], anterior scrotal veins; veins passing from the scrotum to the external pudendal veins.
ve'nae scrota'les posterio'res [NA], posterior scrotal veins; veins passing posteriorly from the scrotum to the internal pudendal veins.
v. sep'ti pellu'cidi ante'rior [NA], anterior vein of septum pellucidum; vein draining the anterior part of the septum pellucidum; it empties into the superior thalamostriate vein.
v. sep'ti pellu'cidi poste'rior [NA], posterior vein of septum pellucidum; vein draining the posterior part of the septum pellucidum; it empties into the superior thalamostriate vein.
ve'nae sigmoi'deae [NA], sigmoid veins; the several tributaries of the inferior mesenteric vein that drain the sigmoid colon.
ve'nae spina'les [NA], spinal veins; the veins that drain the spinal cord; they form a plexus on the surface of the cord from which veins pass along the spinal roots to the internal vertebral venous plexus.
v. spira'lis modi'oli [NA], spiral vein of modiolus; the vein running a spiral course in the modiolus of the cochlea; it is tributary to both the labyrinthine vein and the vein of the cochlear aqueduct.
v. sple'nica [NA], splenic vein; v. lienalis; arises by the union of several small veins at the hilum on the anterior surface of the spleen, passes backward to the left kidney, then runs behind the upper border of the pancreas to the neck of the pancreas where it joins the superior mesenteric vein to form the portal vein.
ve'nae stella'tae, *venulae* stellatae.
v. sternocleidomastoi'dea [NA], sternocleidomastoid vein; it arises in the sternocleidomastoid muscle and drains into the internal jugular vein.
ve'nae stria'tae, venae thalamostriatae inferiores.
v. stylomastoi'dea [NA], stylomastoid vein; it drains the tympanic cavity and empties into the retromandibular vein.
v. subcla'via [NA], subclavian vein; the direct continuation of the axillary vein at the lateral border of the first rib; it passes medially to join the internal jugular vein and form the brachiocephalic vein on each side.
ve'nae subcuta'neae abdom'inis [NA], subcutaneous veins of abdomen; the network of superficial veins of the abdominal wall that empty into the thoracoepigastric, superficial epigastric, or superior epigastric veins.
v. sublingua'lis [NA], sublingual vein; a tributary of the lingualis.
v. submenta'lis [NA], submental vein; a vein situated below the chin, anastomosing with the sublingual vein, connecting with the anterior jugular vein, and emptying into the facial vein.
superior v. cava, v. cava superior.
v. supraorbita'lis [NA], supraorbital vein; drains the front of the scalp and unites with the supratrochlear veins to form the angular vein.
v. suprarena'lis dex'tra [NA], right suprarenal vein; the short vein that passes from the hilum of the right suprarenal to the inferior vena cava.
v. suprarena'lis sinis'tra [NA], left suprarenal vein; the vein from the hilum of the left suprarenal gland that passes downward to open into the left renal vein; it usually is joined by the left inferior phrenic vein.

v. suprascapula'ris [NA], suprascapular vein; transverse scapular vein; v. transversa scapulae; a vein that accompanies the suprascapular artery; it empties into the external jugular vein.
ve'nae supratrochlea'res [NA], supratrochlear veins; frontal veins (2); venae frontales (2); several veins that drain the front part of the scalp and unite with the supraorbital vein to form the angular vein.
v. tempora'lis me'dia [NA], middle temporal vein; it arises near the lateral angle of the eye and joins the superficial temporal veins to form the retromandibular vein.
ve'nae tempora'les profun'dae [NA], deep temporal veins; veins corresponding to the arteries of the same name; they empty into the pterygoid venous plexus.
ve'nae tempora'les superficia'les [NA], superficial temporal veins; veins that pass from the temporal region to join the retromandibular vein.
v. termina'lis [NA], v. thalamostriata superior.
v. testicula'ris dex'tra [NA], right testicular vein; it passes upward from the pampiniform plexus to join the inferior v. cava.
v. testicula'ris sinis'tra [NA], left testicular vein; originates from the pampiniform plexus and joins the left renal vein.
ve'nae thalamostria'tae inferio'res [NA], inferior thalamostriate veins; striate veins; venae striatae; veins draining the thalamus and corpus striatum exiting the anterior perforated substance; tributary to the basal vein.
v. thalamostria'ta supe'rior [NA], superior thalamostriate vein; terminal vein; v. terminalis; vein of corpus striatum; a long vein passing forward in the groove between the thalamus and caudate nucleus, covered by the lamina affixa, receiving the transverse caudate veins along its lateral side, and joining at the caudal wall of Monro's foramen with the v. choroidea and v. septi pellucidi to form the v. cerebri interna.
v. thora'cica inter'na, pl. **ve'nae thora'cicae inter'nae** [NA], internal thoracic vein; v. mammaria interna; usually two veins accompany each artery of the same name, fusing into one at the upper part of the thorax and emptying into the brachiocephalic vein of the same side.
v. thora'cica latera'lis [NA], lateral thoracic vein; long thoracic vein; a tributary of the axillary vein that drains the lateral thoracic wall and communicates with the thoracoepigastric and intercostal veins.
v. thoracoacromia'lis [NA], thoracoacromial vein; thoracic axis (2); corresponding to the artery of the same name, empties into the axillary vein, sometimes by a common trunk with the cephalic vein.
v. thoracoepigas'trica, pl. **ve'nae thoracoepigas'tricae** [NA], thoracoepigastric vein; one of two veins, sometimes a single vein, arising from the region of the superficial epigastric vein and opening into the axillary or the lateral thoracic vein.
ve'nae thy'micae [NA], thymic veins; a number of small veins from the thymus emptying into the left brachiocephalic vein.
v. thyroi'dea i'ma, v. thyroidea inferior.
v. thyroi'dea infe'rior [NA], inferior thyroid vein; v. thyroidea ima; formed by veins from the isthmus and lateral lobe of the thyroid gland and from the plexus thyroideus impar; it terminates in the left brachiocephalic vein.
v. thyroi'dea me'dia [NA], middle thyroid vein; it passes from the thyroid gland across the common carotid artery to empty into the internal jugular vein.
v. thyroi'dea supe'rior [NA], superior thyroid vein; receives blood from the upper part of the thyroid gland and larynx, accompanies the artery of the same name, and empties into the internal jugular vein.
ve'nae tibia'les anterio'res [NA], anterior tibial veins; the veins, usually two, that accompany the anterior tibial artery and empty into the popliteal vein.
ve'nae tibia'les posterio'res [NA], posterior tibial veins; the veins, usually two, that accompany the posterior tibial artery and terminate in the popliteal vein.
ve'nae trachea'les [NA], tracheal veins; several small venous trunks from the trachea, emptying into the brachiocephalic veins or the superior v. cava.
ve'nae transver'sae col'li [NA], transverse veins of the neck; they accompany the corresponding arteries, emptying into the external jugular vein or sometimes into the subclavian vein.
v. transver'sa facie'i [NA], transverse vein of the face; a tributary of the retromandibular vein, anastomosing with the facial vein.
v. transver'sa scap'ulae, v. suprascapularis.
ve'nae tympan'icae [NA], tympanic veins; veins exiting from the tympanic cavity through the petrotympanic fissure and emptying into the retromandibular vein.
ve'nae ulna'res [NA], ulnar veins; veins that accompany the ulnar artery.
v. umbilica'lis sinis'tra [NA], left umbilical vein; the vein that returns the blood from the placenta to the fetus; traversing the umbilical cord, it enters the fetal body at the umbilicus and passes thence into the liver, where it is joined by the portal vein; its blood then flows by way of the ductus venosus and the inferior v. cava to the right atrium.
v. un'ci [NA], vein of uncus; a vein draining the uncus into the inferior cerebral vein of the same side.
ve'nae uteri'nae [NA], uterine veins; two veins on each side which arise from the uterine plexus, pass through a part of the broad ligament and then through a peritoneal fold, and empty into the internal iliac vein.
v. ventricula'ris infe'rior [NA], inferior ventricular vein; vein draining the deep white matter of the superior and lateral portions of the temporal lobe; it begins in the body of the lateral ventricle and exits from the choroid fissure of the inferior horn where it joins the basal vein.
v. ventric'uli latera'lis latera'lis [NA], v. atrii lateralis.
v. ventric'uli latera'lis media'lis [NA], v. atrii medialis.
v. ver'mis infe'rior [NA], inferior vein of vermis; a vein draining part of the inferior part of the cerebellum; it courses on the inferior surface of the vermis and terminates in the straight sinus.
v. ver'mis supe'rior [NA], superior vein of the vermis; a vein draining part of the superior part of the cerebellum; it runs on the superior surface of the vermis to terminate in the internal cerebral vein.
v. vertebra'lis [NA], vertebral vein; a vein derived from tributaries which run through the foramina in the transverse processes of the first six cervical vertebrae and form a plexus around the vertebral artery; it empties as a single trunk into the brachiocephalic veins.
v. vertebra'lis accesso'ria [NA], accessory vertebral vein; a vein that accompanies the vertebral vein but passes through the foramen of the transverse process of the seventh cervical vertebra and opens independently into the brachiocephalic vein.
v. vertebra'lis ante'rior [NA], anterior vertebral vein; the small vein that accompanies the ascending cervical artery; it opens below into the vertebral vein.
ve'nae vesica'les [NA], vesical veins; veins that drain the vesical plexus; they join the internal iliac veins.
ve'nae vestibula'res [NA], vestibular veins; veins draining the saccule and utricle; they are tributaries of both the labyrinthine veins and the vein of the vestibular aqueduct.
v. vitelli'na, vitelline vein; a vein returning blood from the yolk sac to the embryo.
ve'nae vortico'sae [NA], vortex or vorticose veins; venae choroideae oculi; choroid veins of eye; Stensen's veins; vasa vorticosa; several veins in the tunica vasculosa formed of branches from the posterior surface of the eye and the ciliary body emptying into the superior or inferior ophthalmic vein.

venacavography (vē'nă-kā-vog'ră-fē). Cavography; angiography of a vena cava.

venation (vē-nā'shŭn) [L. *vena,* vein]. The arrangement and distribution of veins.

vene-. 1 [L. *vena,* vein]. Combining form denoting the veins. See also veno-. 2 [L. *venenum,* poison]. Combining form relating to venom.

venectasia (ve-nek-tā'sē-ă). Phlebectasia.

venectomy (ve-nek'tō-mē). Phlebectomy.

veneer (vĕ-nēr') [Fr. *fournir,* to furnish]. **1.** A thin surface layer laid over a base of common material. **2.** In dentistry, a layer of tooth-colored material, usually porcelain or acrylic resin, attached to and covering the surface of a metal crown or natural tooth structure.

venenation (ven-ĕ-nā'shŭn, vē-nĕ-) [L. *veneno,* pp. *-atus,* to poison, fr. *venenum,* poison]. Poisoning, as from a sting or bite.

veneniferous (ven-ĕ-nif'ĕ-rŭs) [L. *venenifer,* fr. *venenum,* poison, + *fero,* to carry]. Conveying poison, as through a sting or bite.

venenosalivary (ven'ĕ-nō-sal'i-văr-ē). Venomosalivary; secreting a poisonous saliva, said of venomous reptiles.

venenosity (ven-ĕ-nos'i-tē) [L. *venenosus,* poisonous]. The state of containing poison or being poisonous.

venenous (ven'ĕ-nŭs) [L. *venenosus*] Poisonous.

venereal (ve-nēr'ē-ăl) [L. *Venus* (*vener-*), goddess of love]. Relating to or resulting from sexual intercourse.

venereology (ve-nēr-ē-ol'ō-jē) [venereal (disease) + G. *logos,* study]. The study of venereal disease.

venereophobia (ve-nēr'ē-ō-fō'bē-ă) [venereal (disease) + G. *phobos,* fear]. Morbid fear of venereal disease.

venesection (ven-ē-sek'shŭn) [L. *vena,* vein, + *sectio,* a cutting]. Phlebotomy.

veni-. See veno-.

venin (ven'in) [see venom]. Any poisonous substance found in snake venom.

venipuncture (ven'i-pŭnk-chūr, vē'ni-) The puncture of a vein, usually to withdraw blood or inject a solution.

veno-, veni- [L. *vena,* vein]. Combining forms denoting the veins. See also vene- (1).

venoclysis (vē-nok'li-sis) [veno- + G. *klysis,* a washing out]. Phleboclysis.

venofibrosis (vē'nō-fī-brō'sis). Phlebosclerosis.

venogram (vē'nō-gram) [veno- + G. *gramma,* a writing]. **1.** X-ray demonstration of the veins. **2.** Phlebogram.

venography (vē-nog'ră-fē) [veno- + G. *grapho,* to write]. Phlebography (3); radiographic visualization of a vein, after the injection of a radiopaque substance.

splenic v., splenography; radiographic visualization of the spleen after injection of a contrast medium into it.

splenic portal v., visualization of the splenic and portal veins after the injection of radiopaque material into the spleen through a large needle; intra- or extrahepatic portal obstruction may be thus revealed.

transosseous v., radiographic visualization of veins along the drainage pathway of a bone's marrow by injection of a contrast medium into the marrow at an appropriate point, as in vertebral v.

vertebral v., radiographic visualization of epidural venous plexus by injection of contrast media into the spinous process.

venom (ven'ŏm) [M. Eng. and O. Fr. *venim,* fr. L. *venenum,* poison]. A poisonous fluid secreted by snakes, spiders, scorpions, etc.

kokoi v., a potent neurotoxin found in the frog *Phyllobates bicolor;* it is a nonprotein compound with a molecular weight of approximately 400, and is lethal in microgram quantities.

Russell's viper v., a v. used as a coagulant in the arrest of hemorrhage from accessible sites in hemophilia.

venomosalivary (ven'ō-mō-sal'i-var-ē). Venenosalivary.

venomotor (vē'nō-mō'ter) [veno- + L. *motor,* a move]. Causing change in the caliber of a vein.

venoperitoneostomy (vē'nō-per-i-tō-nē-os'tō-mē) [veno- + peritoneum + G. *stoma,* mouth]. Insertion of the cut end of the saphenous vein into the peritoneal cavity in cases of ascites; the vein is inverted so that the valves prevent regurgitation of blood into the cavity while the ascitic fluid flows into the vein.

venopressor (vē-nō-pres'er). Relating to the venous blood pressure and consequently the volume of venous supply to the right side of the heart.

venosclerosis (vē'nō-skle-rō'sis). Phlebosclerosis.

venose (vē'nōs) [L. *venosus*]. Having veins; veiny.

venosinal (vē'nō-sī'năl). Pertaining to the vena cava and the atrial sinus of the heart.

venosity (vē-nos'i-tē). **1.** A venous state; a condition in which the bulk of the blood is in the veins at the expense of the arteries. **2.** The unaerated condition of venous blood.

venostasis (vē-nō-stā'sis, vē-nos'tă-sis) [veno- + G. *stasis,* a standing]. Phlebostasis.

venostat (vē'nō-stat) [veno- + G. *statos,* standing, stationary]. Any instrument for arresting venous bleeding.

venostomy (vē-nos'tō-mē). Cutdown.

venotomy (vē-not'ō-mē). Phlebotomy.

venous (vē'nŭs) [L. *venosus*]. Phleboid (2); relating to a vein or to the veins.

venous return. The blood returning to the heart via the great veins and coronary sinus.

venovenostomy (vē'nō-vē-nos'tō-mē) [veno- + veno- + G. *stoma,* mouth]. Phlebophlebostomy; the formation of an anastomosis between two veins.

vent [O. Fr. *fente,* a chink, cleft]. An opening into a cavity or canal, especially one through which the contents of such a cavity are discharged, as the anus.

venter (ven'ter) [L. *venter* (*ventr-*), belly]. **1.** Abdomen. **2** [NA]. Belly (2); the wide swelling part of a muscle. **3.** One of the great cavities of the body. **4.** The uterus.

v. ante'rior mus'culi digas'trici [NA], the anterior belly of the digastric muscle, attached to the mandible.

v. fronta'lis [NA], frontal belly; the anterior belly of the occipitofrontalis muscle.

v. infe'rior mus'culi omohyoi'dei [NA], the inferior belly of the omohyoid muscle, attached to the superior border of the scapula.

v. occipita'lis [NA], occipital belly; the posterior belly of the occipitofrontalis muscle.

v. poste'rior mus'culi digas'trici [NA], the posterior belly of the digastric muscle, attached to the mastoid process.

v. propen'dens, **(1)** anteversion of the uterus; **(2)** a pendulous abdomen.

v. supe'rior mus'culi omohyoi'dei [NA], the superior belly of the omohyoid muscle, attached to the hyoid bone.

ventilate (ven'ti-lāt) [L. *ventilo,* pp. *-atus,* to fan, fr. *ventus,* the wind]. To aerate, or oxygenate, the blood in the pulmonary capillaries.

ventilation (ven-ti-lā'shŭn) [see ventilate]. **1.** Replacement of air or other gas in a space by fresh air or gas. **2.** Respiration (2); movement of gas(es) into and out of the lungs. **3 ($\dot{V}$).** In physiology, the tidal exchange of air between the lungs and the atmosphere that occurs in breathing. See also respiration.

alveolar v. ($\dot{V}_A$), the volume of gas expired from the alveoli to the outside of the body per minute; calculated as the respiratory frequency (f) multiplied by the difference between tidal volume and the dead space ($V_T - V_D$); units: ml/min BTPS.

artificial v., artificial respiration; application of mechanically or manually generated pressures, usually positive, to gas(es) in or about the airway as a means of producing gas exchange between the lungs and surrounding atmosphere.
assist-control v., artificial respiration in which inspiration is produced automatically after a set interval if the person has not already begun to inspire. *Cf.* assisted v.; controlled v.
assisted v., assisted respiration; application of mechanically or manually generated positive pressure to gas(es) in or about the airway during inhalation as a means of augmenting movement of gases into the lungs.
continuous positive pressure v. (CPPV), controlled mechanical v.
controlled v., controlled respiration; intermittent application of mechanically or manually generated positive pressure to gas(es) in or about the airway as a means of forcing gases into the lungs in the absence of spontaneous ventilatory efforts.
controlled mechanical v. (CMV), continuous or intermittent positive pressure breathing or v.; artificial v. in which all inspirations are provided by positive pressure applied to the airway.
intermittent mandatory v. (IMV), mechanical application of positive pressure at a predetermined frequency to the airway to increase tidal volume.
intermittent positive pressure v. (IPPV), controlled mechanical v.
manual v., use of the hands to generate, directly or indirectly, airway pressures; employed in assisted or controlled v.
maximum voluntary v. (MVV), maximum breathing capacity; the volume of air breathed when an individual breathes as deeply and as quickly as possible for a given time (*e.g.,* 15 sec.).
mechanical v., use of automatically cycling devices to generate airway pressures; employed in assisted or controlled v.
pulmonary v., respiratory minute volume, *i.e.,* the total volume of gas per minute inspired (V_I) or expired (V_E) expressed in liters per minute; differs from alveolar v. by including the exchange of dead space gas.
spontaneous intermittent mandatory v., synchronized intermittent mandatory v. (SIMV), intermittent mandatory v. spontaneously initiated by the patient, to increase tidal volume, and subsequently synchronized with his respiratory cycle.
wasted v., that part of the pulmonary v. which is ineffective in exchanging oxygen and carbon dioxide with pulmonary capillary blood; calculated as physiologic dead space multiplied by respiratory frequency.

vent'plant. An endo-osseous implant, usually made of titanium, utilized to provide support and fixation for a dental prosthesis by means of projections through the mucosa; also used to designate a family of implants.

ventrad (ven'trad) [L. *venter,* belly, + *ad,* to]. Toward the ventral aspect; opposed to dorsad.

ventral (ven'trăl) [L. *ventralis*]. **1.** Pertaining to the belly or to any venter. **2.** Anterior (2). **3.** In veterinary anatomy, the undersurface of an animal; often used to indicate the position of one structure relative to another, *i.e.,* situated nearer the undersurface of the body.

ventralis (ven-trā'lis) [L.] [NA]. Anterior (2).

ventricle (ven'tri-kl) [L. *ventriculus,* dim. of *venter,* belly]. Ventriculus.
Arantius' v., *calamus* scriptorius.
cerebral v.'s, see *ventriculus* lateralis, *ventriculus* quartus, *ventriculus* tertius, and *cavum* septi pellucidi.
v. of cerebral hemisphere, *ventriculus* lateralis.
v. of diencephalon, *ventriculus* tertius.
Duncan's v., *cavum* septi pellucidi.
fifth v., *cavum* septi pellucidi.
fourth v., *ventriculus* quartus.
v.'s of heart, see *ventriculus* cordis, dexter, sinister.
laryngeal v., *ventriculus* laryngis.
lateral v., *ventriculus* lateralis.
left v., *ventriculus* sinister.
Morgagni's v., *ventriculus* laryngis.
v. of rhombencephalon, *ventriculus* quartus.
right v., *ventriculus* dexter.
sixth v., Verga's v.
sylvian v., *cavum* septi pellucidi.
terminal v., *ventriculus* terminalis.
third v., *ventriculus* tertius.
Verga's v., cavum psalterii or vergae; sixth ventricle; an inconstant, horizontal, slitlike space between the posterior one-third of the corpus callosum and the underlying commissura fornicis (commissura hippocampi; psalterium) resulting from failure of these two commissural plates to fuse completely during fetal development; like the cavum septi pellucidi, the space is not a true v. in the sense that it did not develop from the central canal of the neural tube.
Vieussens' v., *cavum* septi pellucidi.
Wenzel's v., *cavum* septi pellucidi.

ventricose (ven'tri-kōs). Bulging or swollen on one side or unequally.

ventricular (ven-trik'yū-lăr) Relating to a ventricle, in any sense.

ventricularis (ven-trik'yū-lā'ris) [Mod. L. fr. L. *ventriculus*]. **1.** Ventricular. **2.** *Musculus* thyroepiglotticus.

ventricularization (ven-trik'yū-lar-i-zā'shŭn). Transformation of an atrial phenomenon to simulate a ventricular one, especially of the atrial (or venous) pulse tracing in tricuspid regurgitation.

ventriculitis (ven-trik-yū-lī'tis) [ventricle + G. *-itis,* inflammation]. Inflammation of the ventricles of the brain.

ventriculo- [L. *ventriculus,* ventricle]. Combining form denoting a ventricle.

ventriculoatrial (V-A) (ven-trik'yū-lō-ā'trē-ăl). Relating to both ventricles and atria, especially to the passage of conduction; *e.g.,* in the retrograde direction.

ventriculocisternostomy (ven-trik'yū-lō-sis'ter-nos'tō-mē) [ventriculo- + L. *cisterna,* cistern, + G. *stoma,* mouth]. An artificial opening between the ventricles of the brain and the cisterna magna. See also shunt (2).

ventriculography (ven-trik-yū-log'ră-fē) [ventriculo- + G. *graphē,* a writing]. **1.** Radiographic visualization of the cerebral ventricular system by injection of gaseous or radiopaque contrast material. **2.** Visualization of the ventricular activity of the heart by recording the distribution of radioactivity from an intravenously injected radionuclide.

ventriculomastoidostomy (ven-trik'yū-lō-mas'toy-dos'tō-mē) [ventriculo- + mastoid, + G. *stoma,* mouth]. Operation for the establishment of a communication between the lateral cerebral ventricle and the mastoid antrum by means of a polythene tube for the relief of hydrocephalus. See also shunt (2).

ventriculonector (ven-trik'yū-lō-nek'ter, -tōr) [ventriculo- + L. *necto,* to join]. *Truncus* atrioventricularis.

ventriculophasic (ven-trik'yū-lō-fā'zik). Influenced by ventricular contraction; applied to the atrial rhythm when this is modified by ventricular contraction; in v. sinus arrhythmia in complete A-V block the sinus impulse immediately following a ventricular contraction usually appears sooner than expected.

ventriculoplasty (ven-trik'yū-lō-plas-tē) [ventriculo- + G. *plastos,* formed]. Any surgical procedure to repair a defect of one of the ventricles of the heart.

ventriculopuncture (ven-trik'yū-lō-pŭnk'chūr). Insertion of a needle into a ventricle.

ventriculoscopy (ven-trik-yū-los'kŏ-pē) [ventriculo- + G. *skopeō,* to view]. Direct inspection of a ventricle with an endoscope.

ventriculostomy (ven-trik-yū-los'tō-mē) [ventriculo- + G. *stoma,* mouth]. Establishment of an opening in a ventricle, usually from the third ventricle to the subarachnoid space to relieve hydrocephalus. See also shunt (2).

third v., an operation to establish an opening from the third ventricle to the prechiasmal and interpeduncular cisterns (Stookey-Scarff operation) or from the third ventricle to the interpeduncular cistern (Dandy operation).

ventriculosubarachnoid (ven-trik'yū-lō-sŭb-ă-rak'noyd) [ventriculo- + subarachnoid]. Relating to the space occupied by the cerebrospinal fluid.

ventriculotomy (ven-trik-yū-lot'ō-mē) [ventriculo- + G. *tomē,* incision]. Incision into a ventricle; *e.g.,* into the third ventricle for the relief of hydrocephalus.

ventriculus, pl. **ventriculi** (ven-trik'yū-lŭs, -lī) [L. dim. of *venter,* belly]. Ventricle. **1** [NA]. Stomach. **2** [NA]. A normal cavity, as of the brain or heart. **3.** The enlarged posterior portion of the mesenteron of the insect alimentary canal, in which digestion occurs.

v. cor'dis [NA], ventricle of the heart; one of the two lower chambers of the heart.

v. dex'ter [NA], right ventricle; the cavity on the right side of the heart which receives the venous blood from the right atrium and drives it by the contraction of its walls into the pulmonary artery.

v. laryn'gis [NA], laryngeal ventricle or sinus; sinus laryngeus; Morgagni's ventricle; Morgagni's sinus (3); the recess in each lateral wall of the larynx between the vestibular and vocal folds.

v. latera'lis [NA], lateral ventricle; ventricle of cerebral hemisphere; a cavity shaped somewhat like a horseshoe in conformity with the general shape of the hemisphere; each lateral ventricle communicates with the third ventricle through the interventricular foramen of Monro, and expands from there forward into the frontal lobe as the cornu anterius as well as caudally over the thalamus as the pars centralis or cella media which, behind the thalamus, curves ventrally and laterally, then forward into the temporal lobe as the cornu inferius; from the apex of the curve a variably sized cornu posterius extends back into the white matter of the occipital lobe. The large choroid plexus of the lateral ventricle invades the cella media and the cornu inferius (but not the cornua anterius and posterius) from the medial side.

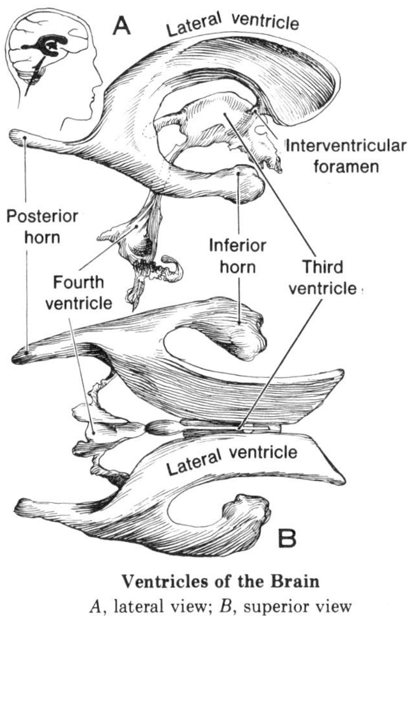

Ventricles of the Brain
A, lateral view; *B,* superior view

v. quar'tus [NA], fourth ventricle; ventricle of the rhombencephalon; a cavity of irregular tentlike shape extending from the obex rostralward to its communication with the sylvian aqueduct, enclosed between the cerebellum dorsally and the rhombencephalic tegmentum ventrally, having a rhomboid-shaped floor (fossa rhomboidea) and a tentlike roof which in its caudal part is formed by the tela choroidea and the velum medullare posterius, in its middle part by the white matter of the cerebellum, and in its narrowing rostral part (recessus superior) by the velum medullare anterius. The fourth ventricle reaches its greatest width at the pontomedullary transition, where it expands laterally behind the cerebellar peduncles into the spoutlike recessus lateralis, and its greatest height at the fastigial recess, which reaches up into the cerebellar white matter. Direct communication of the brain's ventricle system and the subarachnoid space is established at the level of the fourth ventricle by a median opening in the tela choroidea, the apertura mediana or foramen of Magendi, which opens into the cisterna magna, and on both sides by the apertura lateralis or foramen of Luschka, which connects the recessus lateralis with the cisterna basalis.

v. quin'tus, *cavum* septi pellucidi.

v. sinis'ter [NA], left ventricle; the cavity on the left side of the heart that receives the arterial blood from the left atrium and drives it by the contraction of its walls into the aorta.

v. termina'lis [NA], terminal ventricle; a dilation of the central canal of the spinal cord at the tip of the conus medullaris.

v. ter'tius [NA], third ventricle; diacele; ventricle of the diencephalon; a narrow, vertically oriented, irregularly quadrilateral cavity in the midplane, extending from the lamina terminalis to the rostral opening of the mesencephalic aqueduct. This ventricle communicates at its rostrodorsal corner with each of the two lateral ventricles through the left and right interventricular foramen of Monro. Its narrow roof is formed by the tela choroidea which is attached on either side to the tenia thalami; its lateral wall by the medial surface of the thalamus and, below the sulcus hypothalamicus, by the hypothalamus which also forms its floor. In lateral profile, the third ventricle exhibits a number of recesses: in its floor, from before backward, 1) the preoptic recess in the acute angle between the base of the lamina terminalis and the dorsum of the optic chiasm, 2) the infundibular recess extending ventrally into the infundibulum but (in man) not into the hypophysial stalk, and 3) the mamillary or inframamillary recess caused by the protrusion of the mamillary bodies into the ventricle. From its dorsocaudal corner, the pineal recess extends caudally into the pineal stalk.

ventriduct (ven'tri-dŭkt) [L. *venter,* belly, + *duco,* pp. *ductus,* to lead]. To draw toward the abdomen.

ventriduction (ven-tri-dŭk'shŭn). Drawing toward the abdomen or abdominal wall.

ventro- [L. *venter,* belly]. Combining form meaning ventral.

ventrocystorrhaphy (ven'trō-sis-tōr'ă-fē) [ventro- + G. *kystis,* cyst, + *rhaphē,* suture]. Cystopexy.

ventrodorsad (ven-trō-dōr'sad). In a direction from the venter to the dorsum.

ventroinguinal (ven'trō-ing'gwi-năl). Relating to the abdomen and the groin.

ventrolateral (ven-trō-lat'ĕ-răl). Both ventral and lateral.

ventromedian (ven-trō-mē'dē-an). Relating to the midline of the ventral surface.

ventroptosis, ventroptosia (ven-trō-tō'sis, -tō'sē-ă) [ventro- + G. *ptōsis,* a falling]. Gastroptosis.

ventroscopy (ven-tros'kŏ-pē) [ventro- + G. *skopeō,* to view]. Peritoneoscopy.

ventrotomy (ven-trot'ō-mē) [ventro- + G. *tomē,* incision]. Celiotomy.

Venturi, Giovanni B., Italian physicist, 1746–1822. See V. *effect, meter, tube.*

venula, pl. **venulae** (ven'yū-lă, -lē) [L. dim. of *vena,* vein] [NA]. Venule; veinlet; capillary vein; a minute vein; a venous radicle continuous with a capillary.

v. macula'ris infe'rior [NA], inferior macular venule; a small tributary of the central vein of the retina that drains the lower part of the macula.

v. macula'ris supe'rior [NA], superior macular venule; a small tributary of the central vein of the retina that drains the upper part of the macula.

v. media'lis ret'inae [NA], medial venule of retina; the small vein that passes from the part of the retina between the macula and the optic disk to join the central vein.

v. nasa'lis ret'inae infe'rior [NA], inferior nasal venule of retina; the small vein that passes from the inferior medial (nasal) part of the retina to join the central vein.

v. nasa'lis ret'inae supe'rior [NA], superior nasal venule of retina; the small vein that drains blood from the upper medial (nasal) part of the retina; it joins the central vein.

ven'ulae rec'tae re'nis [NA], straight venules of kidney; venules that drain the medullary pyramids of the kidney; they open into arcuate veins.

ven'ulae stella'tae [NA], stellate venules or veins; venae stellatae; Verheyen's stars; stellulae verheyenii; the star-shaped groups of venules in the renal cortex.

v. tempora'lis ret'inae infe'rior [NA], inferior temporal venule of retina; the small vein that passes from the lower lateral (temporal) part of the retina to enter the central vein.

v. tempora'lis ret'inae supe'rior [NA], superior temporal venule of retina; the venule that passes from the upper lateral (temporal) part of the retina to join the central vein.

venular (ven'yū-lăr). Venulous; pertaining to venules.

venule (ven'yūl, vē'nūl). Venula.

high endothelial postcapillary v.'s, v.'s in the lymph nodes, tonsils, and Peyer's patches that have a high-walled endothelium through which blood lymphocytes migrate into the lymphatic parenchyma.

inferior macular v., *venula* macularis inferior.

inferior nasal v. of retina, *venula* nasalis retinae inferior.

inferior temporal v. of retina, *venula* temporalis retinae inferior.

medial v. of retina, *venula* medialis retinae.

nasal v.'s of retina, see *venula* nasalis retinae inferior and superior.

pericytic v.'s, postcapillary v.'s.

postcapillary v.'s, pericytic v.'s; the microvasculature immediately following the capillaries, ranging in size from 10 to 50 μm, and characterized by investment of pericytes; they are the site of extravasation of blood cells, are particularly sensitive to histamine, and are believed to be important in blood-interstitial fluid exchanges.

stellate v.'s, *venulae* stellatae.

straight v.'s of kidney, *venulae* rectae renis.

superior macular v., *venula* macularis superior.

superior nasal v. of retina, *venula* nasalis retinae superior.

superior temporal v. of retina, *venula* temporalis retinae superior.

temporal v.'s of retina, see *venula* temporalis retinae inferior and superior.

venulous (ven'yū-lŭs). Venular.

VER Abbreviation for visual evoked response. See under evoked *response.*

verapamil (ver-ap'ă-mil). Iproveratril; 5-[(3,4-dimethoxyphenethyl)methylamino]-2-(3,4-dimethoxyphenyl)-2-isopropylvaleronitrile; a calcium channel blocking agent used to treat cardiac arrhythmias and angina pectoris.

veratric acid (vĕ-rat'ik). 3,4-Dimethoxybenzoic acid; $C_9H_{10}O_4$; obtained by methylation and subsequent oxidation of protocatechuic acid; present in the seeds of *Schoenocaulon officinale (Sabadilla officinarum).*

veratrine (ver'ă-trēn, -trin). A mixture of alkaloids from the seeds of *Schoenocaulon officinale (Sabadilla officinarum)* (family Liliaceae), including cevine, cevadine, cevadilline, sabadine, and veratridine; a powder of acrid taste, intensely irritating to the nasal mucous membrane, that has been used as an anodyne counterirritant in neuralgias and arthritis.

Veratrum (vĕ-rā'trŭm) [L. hellebore]. A genus of toxic liliaceous plants.

V. al'bum, white or European hellebore; the rhizome has emetic and cathartic actions.

V. vir'ide, American or green hellebore; the dried rhizome and roots contain therapeutically important alkaloids (cevadine, veratridine, jervine, pseudojervine, rubijervine, and several ester alkaloids of the base germine) used in the treatment of hypertensive disorders.

verbigeration (ver-bij-er-ā'shŭn) [L. *verbum,* word, + *gero,* to carry about]. Oral stereotypy; catalogia; constant repetition of meaningless words or phrases.

verbomania (ver-bō-mā'nē-ă) [L. *verbum,* word, + G. *mania,* frenzy]. An abnormal talkativeness; a psychotic flow of speech.

verdigris (ver'di-grēs, -gris, -grē) [O. Fr. *verd,* green, *de,* of, *Gris,* Greeks]. Cupric acetate (normal).

verdine (ver'din). Biliverdin.

verdoglobin (ver-dō-glō'bin). Choleglobin.

verdohemochrome (ver-dō-hē'mō-krōm). An intermediate stage in hemoglobin degradation to yield the bile pigments, *i.e.,* hemoglobin yields choleglobin (verdohemoglobin) and the loss of globin leaves v., the precursor of biliverdin.

verdohemoglobin (ver'dō-hē-mō-glō'bin). Choleglobin.

verdoperoxidase (ver'dō-per-oks'i-dās). A peroxidase, occurring in leukocytes, that contains a greenish ferriheme; responsible for the peroxidase activity of pus.

Verga, Andrea, Italian neurologist, 1811–1895. See V.'s *ventricle; cavum* vergae.

verge (verj). An edge or margin.

anal v., the transitional zone between the moist, hairless, modified skin of the anal canal and the perianal skin.

vergence (ver'jens) [L. *vergo,* to incline, to turn]. A disjunctive movement of the eyes in which the fixation axes are not parallel, as in convergence or divergence.

v. of lens, the reciprocal of the principal focal distance used as a measure of the divergence or convergence of parallel rays.

vergeture (ver'jĕ-chūr) [L. *virga,* a green twig, a stripe]. *Striae* cutis distensae.

Verheyen, Philippe, Flemish anatomist, 1648–1710. See V.'s *stars, stellulae* verheyenii.

Verhoeff, Frederick H., U.S. ophthalmologist, 1874–1968. See V.'s elastic tissue *stain;* Agnew-V. *incision.*

Vermes (ver'mēz) [L. *vermis,* worm]. Archaic term for a subkingdom of the animal kingdom containing worms and wormlike organisms; an unnatural division no longer in taxonomic use.

vermi- [L. *vermis,* worm]. Combining form denoting a worm, wormlike.

vermicidal (ver'mi-sī'dăl) [vermi- + L. *caedo,* to kill]. Destructive to worms; specifically, destructive to parasitic intestinal worms.

vermicide (ver'mi-sīd) [vermi- + L. *caedo,* to kill]. An agent that kills intestinal parasitic worms.

vermicular (ver-mik'yū-lăr) [L. *vermiculus,* dim. of *vermis,* worm]. Relating to, resembling, or moving like a worm.

vermiculation (ver-mik-yū-lā'shŭn). A wormlike movement, as in peristalsis.

vermicule (ver'mi-kūl) [L. *vermiculus,* a small worm]. Vermiculus. **1.** A small worm or wormlike organism or structure. **2.** Ookinete.

vermiculose, vermiculous (ver-mik'yū-lōs, -lŭs). **1.** Wormy; infected with worms or larvae. **2.** Wormlike. See also vermiform.

vermiculus (ver-mik'yū-lŭs) [L. dim. of *vermis,* worm]. Vermicule.

vermiform (ver'mi-fōrm) [vermi- + L. *forma,* form]. Worm-shaped; resembling a worm in form. See also lumbricoid; scolecoid (2).

vermifugal (ver-mif'yū-găl) [vermi- + L. *fugo,* to chase away]. Anthelmintic (2).

vermifuge (ver'mi-fūj) [vermi- + L. *fugo,* to chase away]. Anthelmintic (1).

vermilion (ver-mil'yon) [C.I. 77766]. A red pigment made from cinnabar or red mercuric sulfide.

vermilionectomy (ver-mil-yon-ek'tō-mē) [vermilion border + G. *ektomē,* cutting out]. Excision of the vermilion border.

vermin (ver'min) [L. *vermis,* a worm]. Parasitic insects, such as lice and bedbugs.

verminal (ver'mi-năl). Verminous.

vermination (ver-mi-nā'shŭn). **1.** The production or breeding of worms or larvae. **2.** Infestation with vermin.

verminous (ver'mi-nŭs) [L. *verminosus,* wormy]. Verminal; relating to, caused by, or infested with worms, larvae, or vermin.

vermis, pl. **vermes** (ver'mis, -mēz) [L. worm]. **1.** A worm; any structure or part resembling a worm in shape. **2** [NA]. V. cerebelli; the narrow middle zone between the two hemispheres of the cerebellum; the portion projecting above the level of the hemispheres on the upper surface is called the superior v.; the lower portion, sunken between the two hemispheres and forming the floor of the vallecula, is the inferior v.

vermix (ver'miks). *Appendix* vermiformis.

Verner, John V., U.S. internist, *1927. See V.-Morrison *syndrome.*

Vernet, Maurice, French neurologist, *1887. See V.'s *syndrome.*

Verneuil, Aristide A., French surgeon, 1823–1895. See V.'s *neuroma; hidradenitis* axillaris of V.

Vernier, Pierre, French mathematician, 1580–1637. See V. *acuity.*

vernix (ver'niks) [Mod. L.]. Varnish.

v. caseo'sa, the fatty substance, consisting of desquamated epithelial cells, lanugo hairs, and sebaceous matter, which covers the skin of the fetus.

Verocay, José, Czechoslovakian pathologist, 1876–1927. See V. *bodies.*

verruca, pl. **verrucae** (vĕ-rū'kă, -kē) [L.]. Verruga; wart; a flesh-colored growth characterized by circumscribed hypertrophy of the papillae of the corium, with thickening of the malpighian, granular, and keratin layers of the epidermis, and caused by human papilloma virus; also applied to epidermal verrucous tumors of nonviral etiology.

v. acumina'ta, *condyloma* acuminatum.

v. digita'ta, digitate wart; a wart in which the papillae project like fingers; they occur in groups, often on the scalp.

v. filifor'mis, filiform wart; a wart composed of greatly elongated papillae; appears more commonly on the face and neck.

v. gla'bra, a smooth wart.

v. mollusicfor'mis, condyloma.

v. necrogen'ica, postmortem *wart.*

v. perua'na, v. peruvia'na, *verruga* peruana.

v. pla'na, v. pla'na juveni'lis, flat or plane wart; a smooth, flat, flesh-colored wart of small size, occurring in groups, seen especially on the face of the young, and often associated with common warts of the hands.

v. pla'na seni'lis, solar *keratosis.*

v. planta'ris, plantar *wart.*

seborrheic v., seborrheic *keratosis.*

v. seni'lis, solar *keratosis.*

v. sim'plex, v. vulgaris.

v. vulga'ris, v. simplex; common, infectious, or viral wart; a keratotic papilloma of the epidermis caused by the human papilloma virus which occurs most frequently in young persons as a result of a localized infection and individual susceptibility or absence of immunity; the lesions are of variable duration, eventually undergoing spontaneous regression, and are superficial and vegetative, in contrast to those of the deep type of wart, myrmecia.

verruciform (vĕ-rū'si-fōrm) [L. *verruca,* wart, + *forma,* form]. Wart-shaped.

verrucose (vĕ-rū'kōs) [L. *verrucosus*] Verrucous; resembling a wart; denoting wartlike elevations.

verrucosis (ver-ū-kō'sis) [L. *verruca,* wart, + G. *-osis,* condition]. A condition marked by the appearance of multiple warts.

lymphostatic v., mossy *foot.*

verrucous (vĕ-rū'kŭs). Verrucose.

verruga (vĕ-rū'gă) [Sp.]. Verruca.

v. perua'na, v. peruvia'na, verruca peruana or peruviana; Peruvian wart; hemorrhagic pian; a stage or cutaneous form of Oroya fever (systemic form of bartonellosis), characterized by an eruption of soft conical or pedunculated papules the size of a pea and larger.

versicolor (ver-si-kŏl'ŏr) [L. particolored, fr. *verso,* to turn, twist, + *color,* color]. Variegated; marked by a variety of color.

version (ver'zhŭn, -shŭn) [L. *verto,* pp. *versus,* to turn]. **1.** Displacement of the uterus, with tilting of the entire organ without bending upon itself; such displacement may be anteversion, retroversion, or lateroversion. **2.** Change of position of the fetus in the uterus, occurring spontaneously or effected by manipulation. **3.** Inclination. **4.** Conjugate rotation of the eyes in the same direction; such rotation may be dextroversion, levoversion, supraversion, or infraversion.

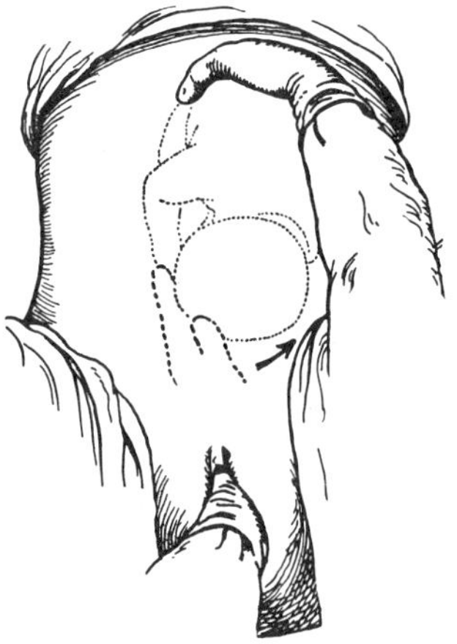

Version

bimanual v., bipolar v.; turning of the baby *in utero,* performed by the hands acting upon both extremities of the fetus; it may be external v. or combined v.

bipolar v., bimanual v.

Braxton Hicks v., internal v. of the fetus, substituting the breech for the head as the leading pole.

cephalic v., v. in which the fetus is turned so that the head presents.

combined v., bipolar v. by means of one hand in the vagina, the other on the abdominal wall.
external v., v. performed entirely by external manipulation.
internal v., v. performed by means of one hand within the vagina.
pelvic v., v. by means of which a transverse or oblique presentation is converted into a pelvic presentation by manipulating the buttocks of the fetus.
podalic v., a manual procedure that results in a podalic extraction.
postural v., nonmanual v. obtained by changing the position of the mother.
Potter's v., a v. in which both feet are brought down until the buttocks are delivered, the back is then rotated to an anterior position, the arms and shoulders are delivered by twisting and downward movements.
spontaneous v., turning of the fetus effected by the unaided contraction of the uterine muscle.
Wright's v., a cephalic v. employed in cases of shoulder presentation when the shoulders are pushed upward while the breech is moved toward the center of the uterus by the other hand; the head is then guided into the pelvis.

vertebra, gen. and pl. **vertebrae** (ver'tĕ-bră, -brē) [L. joint, fr. *verto,* to turn] [NA]. One of the segments of the spinal column; in man there are usually 33 vertebrae, 7 cervical, 12 thoracic, 5 lumbar, 5 sacral (fused into one bone, the sacrum), and 4 coccygeal (fused into one bone, the coccyx).
basilar v., the lowest lumbar v.
block vertebrae, fused vertebrae which, in radiographs, give the appearance of a more or less solid bony mass.
butterfly v., a hemivertebra or sagittally cleft v. that has a butterfly configuration in radiographs; congenital in origin.
caudal vertebrae, the vertebrae that form the skeleton of the tail.
cervical vertebrae, vertebrae cervicales.
ver'tebrae cervica'les [NA], cervical vertebrae; the seven segments of the vertebral column located in the neck.
ver'tebrae coccyg'eae [NA], coccygeal vertebrae; tail vertebrae; the four terminal segments of the vertebral column, usually fused to form the coccyx.
coccygeal vertebrae, vertebrae coccygeae.
codfish vertebrae, exaggeration of the concavity in the upper and lower surfaces of the vertebrae, as demonstrated radiographically in various types of osteopenia.
cranial v., a segment of the skull regarded as homologous with a segment of the vertebral column.
v. denta'ta, axis (5).
dorsal vertebrae, an old term for thoracic vertebrae.
false vertebrae, vertebrae spuriae; the fused vertebral segments of the sacrum and coccyx.
hourglass vertebrae, the radiographic appearance of some vertebrae in osteogenesis imperfecta tarda.
ver'tebrae lumba'les [NA], lumbar vertebrae; the vertebrae, usually five in number, located in the lumbar region of the back.
lumbar vertebrae, vertebrae lumbales.
v. mag'na, *os* sacrum.
odontoid v., axis (5).
v. pla'na, spondylitis with reduction of vertebral body to a thin disk.
v. prom'inens [NA], nuchal tubercle; the v. in the cervicothoracic region which has the most prominent spinous process (seventh cervical v. in 70% of the cases, sixth in 20%, and first thoracic v. in 10%).
sacral vertebrae, vertebrae sacrales.
ver'tebrae sacra'les [NA], sacral vertebrae; the segments of the vertebral column, usually five in number, that fuse to form the sacrum.
ver'tebrae spu'riae, false vertebrae.
tail vertebrae, vertebrae coccygeae.
thoracic vertebrae, vertebrae thoracicae.
ver'tebrae thora'cicae [NA], thoracic vertebrae; the segments of the vertebral column, usually twelve, which articulate with ribs to form part of the thoracic cage.
toothed v., axis (5).
true v., v. vera; any one of the cervical, thoracic, or lumbar vertebrae.
v. ve'ra, true v.

vertebral (ver'tĕ-brăl). Relating to a vertebra or the vertebrae.

vertebrarium (ver-tĕ-bră'rē-ŭm) [Mod. L.]. *Columna* vertebralis.

Vertebrata (ver-tĕ-brah'tă, -brā'tă) [L. *vertebratus,* jointed]. Craniata; the vertebrates, a major division of the phylum Chordata, consisting of those animals with a dorsal hollow nerve cord enclosed in a cartilaginous or bony spinal column; includes several classes of fishes, and the amphibians, reptiles, birds, and mammals.

vertebrate (ver'tĕ-brāt). **1.** Having a vertebral column. **2.** An animal having vertebrae.
notochordal v., a lower v. in which the notochord persists, unossified, in adult life.

vertebrated (ver'tĕ-brāt-ed). Jointed; composed of segments arranged longitudinally as in certain instruments.

vertebrectomy (ver'tĕ-brek'tō-mē) [vertebra + G. *ektomē,* excision]. Exsection of a vertebra.

vertebro- [L. *vertebra*]. Combining form denoting a vertebra, vertebral.

vertebroarterial (ver'tĕ-brō-ar-tēr'ē-ăl). Relating to a vertebra and an artery, or to the vertebral artery.

vertebrochondral (ver'tĕ-brō-kon'drăl) [vertebro- + G. *chondros,* cartilage]. Vertebrocostal (2); denoting the three false ribs (eighth, ninth, and tenth), which are connected with the vertebrae at one extremity and the costal cartilages at the other, these cartilages not articulating directly with the sternum.

vertebrocostal (ver'tĕ-brō-kos'tăl) [vertebro- + L. *costa,* rib]. **1.** Costovertebral. **2.** Vertebrochondral.

vertebrofemoral (ver-tĕ-brō-fem'ō-răl). Relating to the vertebrae and the femur.

vertebroiliac (ver'tĕ-brō-il'ē-ak). Relating to the vertebrae and the ilium.

vertebrosacral (ver-tĕ-brō-sā'krăl). Relating to the vertebrae and the sacrum.

vertebrosternal (ver'tĕ-brō-ster'năl). Sternovertebral.

vertex, pl. **vertices** (ver'teks, ver'ti-sēz) [L. whirl, whorl]. **1** [NA]. The topmost point of the vault of the skull, a landmark in craniometry. **2.** In obstetrics, the portion of the fetal head bounded by the planes of the trachelobregmatic and biparietal diameters, with the posterior fontanel at the apex.
v. cor'dis, *apex* cordis.
v. of cornea, v. corneae.
v. cor'neae [NA], vertex of cornea; the central part of the cornea, slightly thinner than the peripheral part.

vertical (ver'ti-kăl). **1.** Relating to the vertex, or crown of the head. **2.** Perpendicular. **3.** Verticalis.

verticalis (ver-ti-kā'lis) [L.] [NA]. Vertical (3); denoting any plane or line that passes longitudinally through the body in the anatomical position.

vertices (ver'ti-sēz). Plural of vertex.

verticil (ver'ti-sil) [L. *verticillus,* the whirl of a spindle, dim. of *vertex,* a whirl]. Whorl (4); vortex (1); a collection of similar parts radiating from a common axis.

verticillate (ver'ti-sil'āt). Disposed in the form of a verticil.

Verticillium (ver-ti-sil'ē-ŭm) [L. *verticillus,* the whirl of a spindle].

A genus of hyphomycetous fungi often found in clinical specimens as contaminants. They are occasionally found in the meatus in cases of otitis externa, but are of doubtful pathogenicity.

verticomental (ver-ti-kō-men′tăl). Relating to the crown of the head and the chin; denoting a diameter in craniometry.

vertiginous (ver-tij′i-nŭs). Relating to or suffering from vertigo.

vertigo (ver′ti-gō, ver-tī′gō) [L. *vertigo* (*vertigin-*), dizziness, fr. *verto,* to turn]. **1.** A sensation of irregular or whirling motion, either of oneself (**subjective v.**) or of external objects (**objective v**); v. implies a definite sensation of rotation of the subject or of objects about the subject in any plane. **2.** Imprecisely used as a general term to describe dizziness.
v. ab au′re lae′so, v. dependent upon chronic middle ear lesions.
auditory v., Ménière's *disease.*
aural v., v. caused by disease of the internal ear or pressure of cerumen on the drum membrane.
Charcot's v., laryngeal *syncope.*
chronic v., *status* vertigonosus.
endemic paralytic v., epidemic v.
epidemic v., Gerlier's disease; kubisagari; paralyzing v.; endemic paralytic v.; v. of sudden onset with headache, vomiting, paralyses, diplopia, pupillary disturbances, nystagmus, and sometimes tinnitus, that occurs in the same locality.
galvanic v., voltaic v.
gastric v., Trousseau's syndrome (1); v. symptomatic of disease of the stomach.
height v., vertical v.(1); dizziness experienced when looking down from a great height or in looking up at a high building or cliff.
horizontal v., dizziness experienced on lying down.
labyrinthine v., Ménière's *disease.*
laryngeal v., laryngeal *syncope.*
lateral v., dizziness caused by watching the telegraph poles and fences from the window of a fast-moving vehicle.
mechanical v., v. caused by continued rotation or vibration of the body.
nocturnal v., a feeling of falling when dropping off to sleep.
ocular v., dizziness attributed to refractive errors or imbalance of the extrinsic muscles.
organic v., v. due to brain damage.
paralyzing v., epidemic v.
postural v., v. which occurs particularly in elderly people with change of position, usually from lying or sitting to standing position.
rotary v., systematic v.; a form in which there is a sensation of rotation in a definite direction of the surrounding objects as well as oneself.
sham-movement v., gyrosa; dizziness accompanied by an impression that the body is rotating or that objects are rotating about the body.
systematic v., rotary v.
vertical v., **(1)** height v.; **(2)** dizziness experienced when standing upright.
voltaic v., galvanic v.; a lateral movement of the head upon galvanization of the vestibular nerve, the movement being in the direction opposed to the course of the current, *i.e.*, toward the positive pole.

vertometer (ver-tom′ĕ-ter) [vertex + G. *metron,* measure]. Lensometer.

verumontanitis (ver′ū-mon-tă-nī′tis) [see verumontanum]. Colliculitis.

verumontanum (ver-ū-mon-tā′nŭm) [L. *veru,* a spit, + *montanus,* mountainous]. *Colliculus* seminalis.

vesalianum (ve-sā′lē-ā′nŭm). *Os* vesalianum.

Vesalius (Vesal, Wesal), Andreas (Andre), Flemish anatomist, 1514–1564. See V.'s *bone, foramen, vein.*

vesic-. See vesico-.

vesica, gen. and pl. **vesicae** (ves′i-kă, -kē) [L.]. **1** [NA]. Bladder; a distensible musculomembranous organ serving as a receptacle for fluid, as the gallbladder. **2.** Any hollow structure or sac, normal or pathologic, containing a serous fluid.

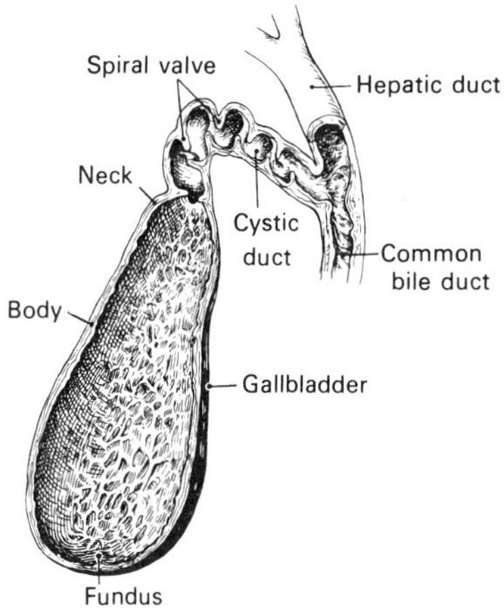

Vesica Biliaris (Gallbladder)

v. bilia′ris [NA], v. fellea; gallbladder; vesicula fellis; cystis fellea; cholecyst; cholecystis; bile cyst; a pear-shaped receptacle on the inferior surface of the liver, in a hollow between the right lobe and the quadrate lobe; it serves as a storage reservoir for bile.
v. fel′lea [NA], official alternate term for v. biliaris.
v. prostat′ica, *utriculus* prostaticus.
v. urina′ria [NA], urinary bladder; cystis urinaria; urocyst; urocystis; a musculomembranous elastic bag serving as a storage place for the urine.

vesical (ves′i-kăl). Relating to any bladder, but usually the urinary bladder.

vesicant (ves′i-kănt). Epispastic; vesicatory; an agent that produces a vesicle.

vesicate (ves′i-kāt). To form a vesicle.

vesication (ves-i-kā′shŭn). Vesiculation (1).

vesicatory (ves′i-kă-tōr-ē). Vesicant.

vesicle (ves′i-kl) [L. *vesicula,* a blister, dim. of *vesica,* bladder]. **1.** Vesicula. **2.** A small circumscribed elevation of the skin containing fluid. See also bleb; blister; bulla. **3.** A small sac containing liquid or gas.
acoustic v., auditory v.
acrosomal v., a v. derived from the Golgi apparatus during spermiogenesis whose limiting membrane adheres to the nuclear envelope; together with the acrosomal granule within, it spreads in a thin layer over the pole of the nucleus to form the acrosomal cap.
air v.'s, *alveoli* pulmonis.
allantoic v., the hollow portion of the allantois.
amniocardiac v., the rostral portion of the most primitive intraembryonic celom.
auditory v., acoustic or otic v.; one of the paired sacs of invaginated ectoderm that develop into the membranous labyrinth of the internal ear.
Baer's v., obsolete term for vesicular ovarian *follicle.*
blastodermic v., blastocyst.
cerebral v., encephalic or primary brain v.; each of the three divisions of the early embryonic brain (prosencephalon, mesencephalon, and rhombencephalon).
cervical v., an abnormally persisting vestige of the cervical sinus

or its associated branchial grooves.
encephalic v., cerebral v.
forebrain v., prosencephalon.
germinal v., archaic term for the nucleus of the ovum.
hindbrain v., rhombencephalon.
lens v., lenticular v.; in the embryo, the ectodermal invagination that forms opposite the optic cup; it is the primordium of the lens of the eye.
lenticular v., lens v.
malpighian v.'s, the minute air-filled v.'s on the surface of an expanded lung.
midbrain v., mesencephalon.
ocular v., *vesicula* ophthalmica.
optic v., *vesicula* ophthalmica.
otic v., auditory v.
pinocytotic v., a v., a fraction of a micrometer in diameter, containing fluid or solute being ingested into a cell by endocytosis. See also pinocytosis.
primary brain v., cerebral v.
seminal v., *vesicula* seminalis.
synaptic v.'s, the small (average diameter 30 nm), intracellular, membrane-bound v.'s near the presynaptic membrane of a synaptic junction, containing the transmitter substance which, in chemical synapses, mediates the passage of nerve impulses across the junction. See also synapse.
telencephalic v., paired diverticula arising from the prosencephalon, from which the forebrain develops.
umbilical v., yolk *sac.*

vesico-, vesic- [L. *vesica,* bladder]. Combining forms denoting a vesica, vesicle. See also vesiculo-.

vesicoabdominal (ves'i-kō-ab-dom'i-năl). Relating to the urinary bladder and the abdominal wall.

vesicobullous (ves'i-kō-bŭl'ŭs). Denoting an eruption of variously sized lesions containing fluid.

vesicocele (ves'i-kō-sēl). Cystocele.

vesicocervical (ves'i-kō-ser'vi-kăl). Relating to the urinary bladder and the cervix uteri.

vesicoclysis (ves'i-kok'li-sis) [vesico- + G. *klysis,* a washing out]. Washing out, or lavage, of the urinary bladder.

vesicofixation (ves'i-kō-fik-sā'shŭn). **1.** Cystopexy. **2.** Suture of the uterus to the bladder wall.

vesicointestinal (ves'i-kō-in-tes'ti-năl). Relating to the urinary bladder and the intestine.

vesicolithiasis (ves'i-kō-li-thī'ă-sis) [vesico- + G. *lithos,* stone, + *-iasis,* condition]. Cystolithiasis.

vesicoprostatic (ves'i-kō-pros-tat'ik). Relating to the bladder and the prostate gland.

vesicopubic (ves'i-kō-pyū'bik). Relating to the bladder and the os pubis.

vesicopustular (ves'i-kō-pŭs'tyū-lăr). Vesiculopustular (1); pertaining to a vesicopustule.

vesicopustule (ves'i-kō-pŭs'tyūl). A vesicle which is developing pus formation.

vesicorectal (ves'i-kō-rek'tăl). Relating to the bladder and the rectum.

vesicorectostomy (ves'i-kō-rek-tos'tō-mē) [vesico- + rectum + G. *stoma,* mouth]. Cystoproctostomy; cystorectostomy; surgical urinary tract diversion by anastomosis of the posterior bladder wall to the rectum.

vesicosigmoid (ves'i-kō-sig'moyd). Relating to the bladder and the sigmoid colon.

vesicosigmoidostomy (ves'ī-kō-sig-moy-dos'tō-mē) [vesico- + sigmoid + G. *stoma,* mouth]. Operative formation of a communication between the bladder and the sigmoid colon.

vesicospinal (ves'i-kō-spī'năl). Relating to the urinary bladder and the spinal cord; denoting the neural mechanisms that control retention and evacuation of urine by the bladder, located in the second lumbar and second sacral segment, respectively, of the spinal cord.

vesicostomy (ves'i-kos'tō-mē) [vesico- + G. *stoma,* mouth]. Cystostomy.

vesicotomy (ves'i-kot'ō-mē) Cystotomy.

vesicoumbilical (ves'i-kō-ŭm-bil'i-kăl). Omphalovesical; relating to the urinary bladder and the umbilicus.

vesicoureteral (ves'i-kō-yū-rē'ter-ăl). Relating to the bladder and the ureters.

vesicourethral (ves'i-kō-yū-rē'thrăl). Relating to the bladder and the urethra.

vesicouterine (ves'i-kō-yū'ter-in). Relating to the bladder and the uterus.

vesicouterovaginal (ves'i-kō-yū'ter-ō-vaj'i-năl). Relating to the bladder, uterus, and vagina.

vesicovaginal (ves-i-kō-vaj'i-năl). Relating to the bladder and vagina.

vesicovaginorectal (ves'i-kō-vaj'i-nō-rek'tăl). Relating to the bladder, vagina, and rectum.

vesicovisceral (ves'i-kō-vis'er-ăl). Relating to the urinary bladder and any other adjacent organ or viscus.

vesicula, gen. and pl. **vesiculae** (vĕ-sik'yū-lă, -lē) [L. blister, vesicle, dim. of *vesica,* bladder]. Vesicle (1); a small bladder or bladder-like structure.
v. fel'lis, *vesica* biliaris.
v. ophthal'mica [NA], optic or ocular vesicle; in the embryo, one of the paired evaginations from the ventrolateral walls of the forebrain from which sensory and pigment layers of the retina develop.
v. semina'lis [NA], seminal vesicle; seminal capsule or gland; glandula seminalis; gonecyst; gonecystis; one of two folded, sacculated, glandular structures which is a diverticulum of the ductus deferens; its secretion is one of the components of the semen; it normally does not store spermatozoa.

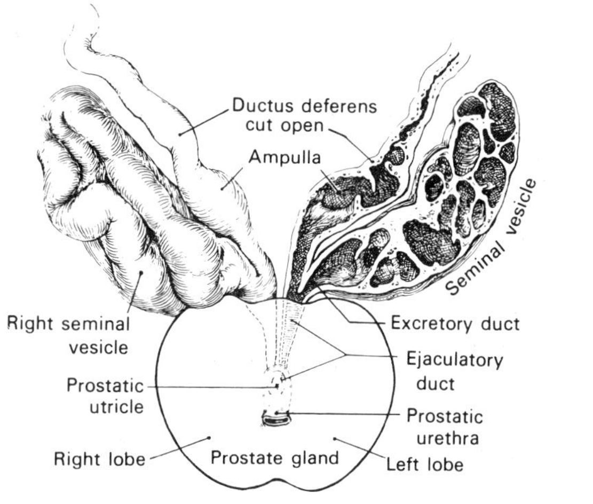

Seminal Vesicles

v. umbilica'lis, yolk *sac.*

vesicular (vĕ-sik'yū-lăr). **1.** Relating to a vesicle. **2.** Vesiculose; vesiculous; vesiculate (2); vesiculated; characterized by or containing vesicles.

vesiculate (vĕ-sik'yū-lāt). **1.** To become vesicular. **2.** Vesicular (2).

vesiculated (vĕ-sik'yū-lāt-ed). Vesicular (2).

vesiculation (vĕ-sik'yū-lā'shŭn). **1.** Blistering; vesication; the formation of vesicles. **2.** Inflation. **3.** Presence of a number of vesicles.

vesiculectomy (vĕ-sik'yū-lek'tō-mē) [L. *vesicula,* vesicle, + G. *ektomē,* excision]. Resection of a portion or all of each of the seminal vesicles.

vesiculiform (vĕ-sik'yū-li-fōrm). Resembling a vesicle.

vesiculitis (vĕ-sik-yū-lī'tis) [L. *vesicula,* vesicle, + G. *-itis,* inflammation]. Inflammation of any vesicle; especially of a seminal vesicle.

vesiculo- [L. *vesicula,* vesicle, dim. of *vesica,* bladder]. Combining form denoting a vesicle.

vesiculobronchial (vĕ-sik'yū-lō-brong'kē-ăl). Denoting an auscultatory sound having both a vesicular and a bronchial quality.

vesiculocavernous (vĕ-sik'yū-lō-kav'er-nŭs). Both vesicular and cavernous; denoting: **(1)** an auscultatory sound having both a vesicular and a cavernous quality; **(2)** the structure of certain neoplasms.

vesiculography (vĕ-sik-yū-log'ră-fī) [vesiculo- + G. *graphō,* to write]. X-ray examination of the seminal vesicles.

vesiculopapular (vĕ-sik'yū-lō-pap'yū-lăr). Pertaining to or consisting of a combination of vesicles and papules, or of papules becoming increasingly edematous with sufficient collection of fluid to form vesicles.

vesiculoprostatitis (vĕ-sik'yū-lō-pros'tă-tī'tis) [vesiculo- + prostate + G. *-itis,* inflammation]. Inflammation of the bladder and prostate.

vesiculopustular (vĕ-sik'yū-lō-pŭs'tyū-lăr). **1.** Vesicopustular. **2.** Pertaining to a mixed eruption of vesicles and pustules.

vesiculose (vĕ-sik'yū-lōs). Vesicular (2).

vesiculotomy (vĕ-sik-yū-lot'ō-mē) [vesiculo- + G. *tomē,* incision]. Surgical incision of the seminal vesicles.

vesiculotubular (vĕ-sik'yū-lō-tū'byū-ler). Denoting an auscultatory sound having both a vesicular and a tubular quality.

vesiculotympanic (vĕ-sik'yū-lō-tim-pan'ik). Denoting a percussion sound having both a vesicular and a tympanic quality.

vesiculous (vĕ-sik'yū-lŭs). Vesicular (2).

Vesiculovirus (vĕ-sik'yū-lō-vī'rŭs). A genus of viruses (family Rhabdoviridae) that includes the vesicular stomatitis virus (of cattle) and related viruses.

Veslingius (Vesling), Joannes, German anatomist, 1598–1649. See V.'s *line.*

vessel (ves'ĕl) [O. Fr. fr. L. *vascellum,* dim. of *vas*]. A structure conveying or containing a fluid, especially a liquid. See also vas.
absorbent v.'s, *vasa* lymphatica.
afferent v., *vas* afferens.
blood v., see *blood vessel.*
capillary v., vas capillare. See blood *capillary;* lymph *capillary.*
chyle v., lacteal (2).
collateral v., *vas* collaterale.
deep lymphatic v., *vas* lymphaticum profundum.
efferent v., *vas* efferens.
lacteal v., lacteal (2).
lymph v.'s, lymphatic v.'s, *vasa* lymphatica.
nutrient v., *arteria* nutricia.
superficial lymphatic v., *vas* lymphaticum superficiale.
v.'s of vessels, *vasa* vasorum.
vitelline v.'s, see *arteria* vitellina; *vena* vitellina.

vestibula (ves-tib'yū-lă). Plural of vestibulum.

vestibular (ves-tib'yū-lăr). Relating to a vestibule, especially the vestibule of the ear.

vestibularis (ves-tib-yū-lā'ris) [L.] [NA]. Vestibular.

vestibulate (ves-tib'yū-lăt). Possessing a vestibule.

vestibule (ves'ti-būl) [L. *vestibulum*]. Vestibulum.
aortic v., Sibson's aortic vestibule; *vestibulum* aortae; the portion of the left ventricle of the heart immediately below the aortic orifice, having fibrous walls and affording room for the segments of the closed aortic valve.
buccal v., that part of the vestibulum oris related to the cheek.
esophagogastric v., gastroesophageal v.
gastroesophageal v., esophagogastric v.; the dilated aboral portion of the esophagus, just above the esophagogastric orifice; usually it corresponds to the lumen of pars abdominalis of the esophagus although its relation to the diaphragm is variable.
labial v., that part of the vestibulum oris related to the lips.
v. of larynx, *vestibulum* laryngis.
v. of mouth, *vestibulum* oris.
v. of nose, *vestibulum* nasi.
v. of omental bursa, *vestibulum* bursae omentalis.
Sibson's aortic v., *vestibulum* aortae.
v. of vagina, *vestibulum* vaginae.

vestibulo- [L. *vestibulum,* vestibule]. Combining form denoting vestibule, vestibulum.

vestibulocerebellum (ves-tib'yū-lō-ser-ĕ-bel'ŭm) [vestibulo- + L. *cerebellum*]. Archicerebellum; those regions of the cerebellar cortex whose predominate afferent fibers arise from ganglion vestibulare and the nuclei vestibulares; structures included under this term are nodulus, flocculus, ventral parts of the uvula and small ventral parts of the lingula.

vestibulocochlear (ves-tib'yū-lō-kok'lē-ăr). **1.** Relating to the vestibulum and cochlea of the ear. **2.** Statoacoustic.

vestibuloplasty (ves-tib'yū-lō-plas-tē). [vestibulo- + G. *plassō,* to form]. Any of a series of surgical procedures designed to restore alveolar ridge height by lowering muscles attaching to the buccal, labial, and lingual aspects of the jaws.

vestibulospinal (ves-tib'yū-lō-spī'năl). See *tractus* vestibulospinalis.

vestibulotomy (ves-tib'yū-lot'ō-mē) [vestibulo- + G. *tomē,* incision]. Operation for an opening into the vestibule of the labyrinth.

vestibulourethral (ves-tib'yū-lō-ū-rē'thrăl). Relating to the vestibulum vaginae and urethra.

vestibulum, pl. **vestibula** (ves-tib'yū-lŭm, -lă) [L. antechamber, entrance court] [NA]. Vestibule. **1.** A small cavity or a space at the entrance of a canal. **2.** Specifically, the central, somewhat ovoid, cavity of the osseous labyrinth communicating with the semicircular canals posteriorly and the cochlea anteriorly.
v. aor'tae, aortic *vestibule.*
v. bur'sae omenta'lis [NA], vestibule of omental bursa; the upper part of the bursa omentalis, just within the epiploic foramen (of Winslow), behind the caudate lobe of the liver.
v. laryn'gis [NA], vestibule of larynx; atrium glottidis; the upper part of the laryngeal cavity from the superior aperture to the vestibular folds.
v. na'si [NA], vestibule of nose; the anterior part of the nasal cavity, especially that enclosed by cartilage.
v. o'ris [NA], vestibule of mouth; buccal cavity; that part of the mouth bounded laterally by the lips and the cheeks, medially by the teeth and/or gums, and above and below by the reflections of the mucosa from the lips and cheeks to the gums.
v. puden'di, v. vaginae.
v. vagi'nae [NA], vestibule of vagina; v. pudendi; the space behind the glans clitoridis between the labia minora, containing the openings of the vagina, urethra, and ducts of the greater vestibular glands.

vestige (ves'tij) [L. *vestigium*]. Vestigium.
v. of vaginal process, *vestigium* processus vaginalis.

vestigial (ves-tij'ē-ăl). Relating to a vestige.

vestigium, pl. **vestigia** (ves-tij'ē-ŭm, -ă) [L. footprint (trace), fr. *vestigo,* to track, trace]. Vestige; a trace or a rudimentary structure; the degenerated remains of any structure which occurs as an entity in the embryo or fetus.

v. proces'sus vagina'lis [NA], vestige of vaginal process; incompletely obliterated remnants of the vaginal process of the peritoneum remaining in the spermatic cord.

vesuvin (vĕ-sū'vin) [*Vesuvius,* volcano in Italy] [C.I. 21000]. Bismarck brown Y.

VESV Abbreviation for vesicular exanthema of swine *virus.*

veterinarian (vet'ĕ-rin-ār'ē-ăn) [see veterinary]. A person who holds an academic degree in veterinary medicine; a licensed practitioner of veterinary medicine.

Veterinarian's Oath. The official oath of the veterinary profession, adopted by the American Veterinary Medical Association in 1954: "Being admitted to the profession of veterinary medicine, I solemnly dedicate myself and the knowledge I possess to the benefit of society, to the conservation of our livestock resources and to the relief of suffering of animals. I will practice my profession conscientiously with dignity. The health of my patients, the best interest of their owners, and the welfare of my fellow man, will be my primary considerations. I will, at all times, be humane and temper pain with anesthesia where indicated. I will not use my knowledge contrary to the laws of humanity, nor in contravention to the ethical code of my profession. I will uphold and strive to advance the honor and noble traditions of the veterinary profession. These pledges I make freely in the eyes of God and upon my honor."

veterinary (vet'ĕ-rin-ār-ē) [L. *veterinarius,* fr. *veterina,* beast of burden]. Relating to the diseases of animals.

VHDL Abbreviation for very high density lipoprotein. See lipoprotein.

via, pl. **viae** (vī'ă, vē'ă, vī'ē) [L. way, road]. Any passage in the body, as the intestine, the vagina, etc.

viability (vī-ă-bil'i-tē) [Fr. *viabilité* fr. L. *vita,* life]. Capability of living; the state of being viable; usually connotes a fetus that has reached 500 g in weight and 20 gestational weeks.

viable (vī'ă-bl) [Fr. fr. *vie,* life, fr. L. *vita*]. Capable of living; denoting a fetus sufficiently developed to live outside of the uterus.

vial (vī'ăl) [G. *phialē,* a drinking cup]. Phial; a small bottle or receptacle for holding liquids, including medicines.

vibesate (vī'bĕ-sāt). A mixture of polvinate and malrosinol in organic solvent and a propellant; a modified polyvinyl plastic used as a topical spray for wounds.

vibration (vī-brā'shŭn) [L. *vibratio,* fr. *vibro,* pp. *-atus,* to quiver, shake]. **1.** A shaking. **2.** A to-and-fro movement, as in oscillation.

vibrative (vī'bră-tiv). Vibratory.

vibrator (vī'brā-ter, tōr). An instrument used for imparting vibrations.

vibratory (vī'bră-tōr-ē). Vibrative; marked by vibrations.

Vibrio (vib'rē-ō) [L. *vibro,* to vibrate]. A genus of motile (occasionally nonmotile), nonsporeforming, aerobic to facultatively anaerobic, Gram-negative bacteria (family Spirillaceae) containing short (0.5 to 3.0 μm), curved or straight rods which occur singly or which are occasionally united into S-shapes or spirals. Motile cells contain a single polar flagellum; in some species, two or more flagella occur in one polar tuft. Some of these organisms are saprophytes in salt and fresh water and in soil; others are parasites or pathogens. The type species is *V. cholerae.*

V. alginolyt'icus, a species associated with wound and ear infections, and with bacteremia in immunocompromised and in burn patients.

V. chol'erae, *V. comma;* cholera or comma bacillus; Koch's bacillus (2); a species that produces a soluble exotoxin (permeability factor) and is the cause of cholera in man; it is the type species of the genus *V.*

V. com'ma, *V. cholerae.*

V. fe'tus, *Campylobacter fetus.*

V. fluvia'lis, a species, similar to strains of *Aeromonas,* associated with diarrheal disease in humans.

V. furnis'sii, an aerogenic strain, similar to *V. fluvialis,* associated with diarrheal disease and outbreaks of gastroenteritis.

V. metschniko'vii, a species causing acute enteric disease in chickens and other avian species; also isolated from human stool.

V. mim'icus, a sucrose-negative strain, similar to *V. cholerae,* isolated from human stool in diarrheal disease and from human ear infections.

V. parahaemolyt'icus, a marine species which causes gastroenteritis, usually from eating contaminated shellfish.

V. sputo'rum, *Campylobacter sputorum.*

V. vulnif'icus, a species capable of causing septicemia in patients with an underlying chronic disease, especially hepatic disease; also a cause of wound infections, especially those associated with handling of shellfish.

vibrio (vib'rē-ō). A member of the genus *Vibrio.*

El Tor v., a bacterium regarded as a biovar of *V. cholerae.* It was originally isolated from six pilgrims who died of dysentery or gangrene of the colon at the Tor quarantine station on the Sinai Peninsula.

Nasik v., an organism differing from the cholera vibrio, being shorter and stouter and less comma-shaped; its cultures are very toxic to laboratory animals on intravenous injections.

vibrion septique (vē-brē-on' sep-tēk') [Fr. septic vibrio]. *Clostridium septicum.*

vibriosis, pl. **vibrioses** (vib-rē-ō'sis). Infection caused by species of *Vibrio.*

vibrissa, gen. and pl. **vibrissae** (vī-bris'ă, vī-bris'ē) [L. found only in pl. *vibrissae,* fr. *vibro,* to quiver] [NA]. One of the hairs growing at the anterior nares, or vestibulum nasi.

vibrissal (vib-ris'ăl). Relating to the vibrissae.

vibrocardiogram (vī'brō-kar'dē-ō-gram) [L. *vibro,* to shake, + G. *kardia,* heart, + *gramma,* a drawing]. A graphic record of chest vibrations produced by hemodynamic events of the cardiac cycle; the record provides an indirect, externally recorded measurement of isometric contraction and ejection times.

vibromasseur (vī'brō-ma-ser'). A type of vibrator for giving vibratory massage.

vibrotherapeutics (vī'brō-thār-ă-pyū'tiks). Vibratory *massage.*

vicarious (vī-ker'ē-ŭs) [L. *vicarius,* from *vicis,* supplying place of]. Acting as a substitute; occurring in an abnormal situation.

Vicat, L.J., French engineer, 1786–1861. See V. *needle.*

vicine (vī'sēn). 2,5-Diamino-4,6-diketopyrimidine-3-β-D-glucoside; a glucoside occurring in akta, a weed which contaminates *Lathyrus sativus* and is thought by some to be responsible for the symptoms of lathyrism.

Vicq d'Azyr, Félix, French anatomist, 1748–1794. See V. d'A.'s *bundle, centrum* semiovale *foramen.*

Victoria blue [Queen *Victoria*] Any of several blue diphenylnaphthylmethane derivatives; used as a stain in histology.

Victoria orange. An alkaline salt of dinitrocresol; a reddish yellow stain formerly used in histology.

Vidal, Jean Baptiste Emile, French dermatologist, 1825– 1893. See V.'s *disease.*

vidarabine (vī-der'ă-bēn). 9-β-D-Arabinofuranosyladenine monohydrate; a purine nucleoside obtained from fermentation cultures of *Streptomyces antibioticus* and used to treat herpes simplex infections.

vidian (vid'ē-an). Named after or described by Vidius.

Vidius (Vidus), Guidi (Guido), Italian anatomist and physician, 1500–1569. See vidian *artery, canal, nerve, vein.*

Vierordt, Karl, German physiologist, 1818–1884. See V.'s *hemotachometer.*

Vierra, J.P., 20th century Brazilian dermatologist. See V.'s *sign.*

Vieussens, Raymond de, French anatomist, 1641–1715. See V.'s *ansa, anulus, centrum foramina, ganglion, isthmus, limbus, loop, ring, valve, veins, ventricle.*

view (vyū). Projection (8).
axial v., axial *projection.*
base v., axial *projection.*
Caldwell v., Caldwell *projection.*
Stenvers v., Stenvers *projection.*
Towne v., Towne *projection.*
verticosubmental v., axial *projection.*

vigil (vij'il) [L. *vigilia,* wakefulness, alertness, fr. *vigeo,* to be active, to rouse]. A state of wakefulness or sleeplessness.
coma v., a state of muttering delirium in which the person is lethargic and partly conscious, yet never actually sleeping or completely comatose.

vigilambulism (vij-i-lam'byū-lizm) [L. *vigil,* awake, alert, + *ambulo,* to walk about]. A condition of unconsciousness regarding one's surroundings, with automatism, resembling somnambulism but occurring in the waking state.

vigilance (vij'i-lans) [L. *vigilantia,* wakefulness]. An attentiveness, alertness, or watchfulness for whatever may occur.

villi (vil'ī). Plural of villus.

villoma (vi-lō'mă). Papilloma.

villose (vil'ōs). Villous (2).

villositis (vil-ō-sī'tis) [villous + G. *-itis* inflammation]. Inflammation of the villous surface of the placenta.

villosity (vi-los'i-tē). Shagginess; an aggregation of villi.

villous (vil'ŭs). **1.** Relating to villi. **2.** Villose; shaggy; covered with villi.

villus, pl. villi (vil'ŭs, vil'ī) [L. shaggy hair (of beasts)]. **1.** A projection from the surface, especially of a mucous membrane. If the projection is minute, as from a cell surface, it is termed a microvillus. **2.** An elongated dermal papilla projecting into an intraepidermal vesicle or cleft.
anchoring v., a chorionic v. that is attached to the decidua basalis.
arachnoid villi, pacchionian corpuscles, glands; tufted prolongations of pia-arachnoid which protrude through the meningeal layer of the dura mater and have a thin limiting membrane; collections of a. v. form arachnoid granulations which lie in venous lacunae at the margin of the superior sagittal sinus; the spongy tissue of the a. v. contains tubules that serve as one-way valves for transfer of cerebrospinal fluid from the subarachnoid space to the venous system. Both a. v. and the granulations formed from them are major sites of fluid transfer. See also *granulationes* arachnoides.
chorionic villi, vascular processes of the chorion of the embryo entering into the formation of the placenta.
floating v., free v.
free v., floating v.; a chorionic v. that is not attached to the decidua basalis, but is "free" in the maternal blood of the intervillous spaces.
intestinal villi, villi intestinales.
vil'li intestina'les [NA], intestinal villi; projections (0.5 to 1.5 mm in length) of the mucous membrane of the intestine; they are leaf-shaped in the duodenum and become shorter, more finger-shaped, and sparser in the ileum.
vil'li pericardi'aci, pericardial villi; minute filiform projections from the surface of the serous pericardium.

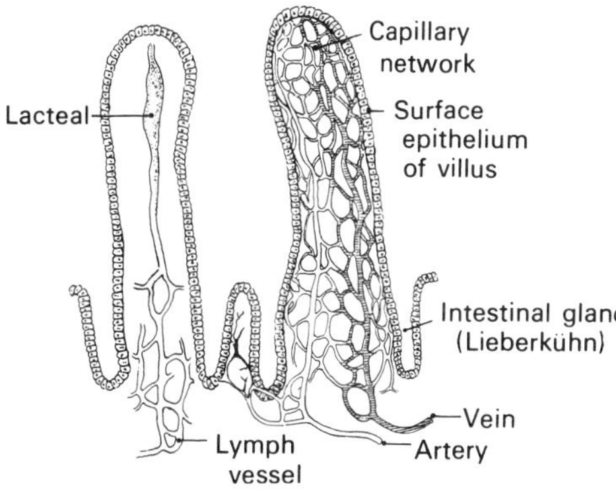

Intestinal Villus
Vertical section through intestinal mucosa (After Mall).

pericardial villi, villi pericardiaci.
peritoneal villi, villi peritoneales.
vil'li peritonea'les, peritoneal villi; villi on the surface of the peritoneum.
pleural villi, villi pleurales.
vil'li pleura'les, pleural villi; shaggy appendages on the pleura in the neighborhood of the costomediastinal sinus.
primary v., the first stage of chorionic v. development, with columns of cytotrophoblastic cells covered by syncytiotrophoblast.
secondary v., an intermediate stage of chorionic v. development following invasion by a connective tissue core.
synovial villi, villi synoviales.
vil'li synovia'les [NA], synovial villi; synovial tufts; synovial fringe; small vascular processes given off from a synovial membrane.
tertiary v., the definitive chorionic v. with a vascular core separated from maternal blood by connective tissue, cytotrophoblast, and syncytiotrophoblast.

villusectomy (vil-ŭs-ek'tō-mē) [villus + G. *ektomē,* excision]. Synovectomy.

vimentin (vī-men'tin). The major polypeptide which co-polymerizes with other subunits to form the intermediate filament cytoskeleton of mesenchymal cells. See also desmins.

vinbarbital (vin-bar'-bi-tahl). 5-Ethyl-5-(1-methyl-1-butenyl)barbituric acid; an intermediate-acting barbiturate used as a sedative and hypnotic.

vinblastine sulfate (vin-blas'tēn). Vincaleukoblastine; a dimeric alkaloid obtained from *Vinca rosea.* It arrests mitosis in metaphase (although vincristine is more active in this respect) and exhibits greater antimetabolic activity than does vincristine; used in the treatment of Hodgkin's disease, choriocarcinoma, acute and chronic leukemias, and other neoplastic diseases.

vincaleukoblastine (ving'kă-lū-kō-blas'tēn). Vinblastine sulfate.

Vinca rosea (ving'kă rō'zē-ă). Periwinkle; a species of myrtle (family Myrtaceae) used in various parts of the world as a home remedy; two active dimeric alkaloids obtained from this plant are vinblastine and vincristine.

Vincent, Henri, French physician, 1862–1950. See V.'s *angina, bacillus, disease, infection,* white *mycetoma, spirillum, tonsillitis.*

vincristine sulfate (vin-kris'tēn). A dimeric alkaloid obtained from *Vinca rosea;* its antineoplastic activity is similar to that of vinblastine, but no cross-resistance develops between these two agents, and it is more useful than vinblastine in lymphocytic lymphosarcoma and acute leukemia.

vinculum, pl. **vincula** (ving'kū-lŭm, -lă) [L. a fetter, fr. *vincio,* to bind] [NA]. A frenum, frenulum, or ligament.
v. bre've [NA], short v.; a triangular band that extends from the dorsal surface of each of the flexor tendons of a digit to the capsule of the nearby interphalangeal joint and to the phalanx proximal to the insertion of the tendon. See also vincula tendinum.
v. lin'guae, *frenulum* linguae.
vin'cula lin'gulae cerebell'i, alae lingulae cerebelli; small lateral prolongations of the lingula of the vermis of the cerebellum resting on the dorsal surface of the superior cerebellar peduncle.
long v., v. longum.
v. lon'gum [NA], long v.; a long, threadlike band that extends from the dorsal surface of each of the flexor tendons of a digit to the proximal phalanx. See also vincula tendinum.
v. prepu'tii, *frenulum* preputii.
short v., v. breve.
vin'cula ten'dinum [NA], vincula of tendons; synovial frenula or frena; tenacula tendinum; fibrous bands that extend from the flexor tendons of the fingers and toes to the capsules of the interphalangeal joints and to the phalanges; they convey small vessels to the tendons. See also v. breve; v. longum.
vincula of tendons, vincula tendinum.

Vineberg, Arthur M., Canadian thoracic surgeon, *1903. See V. *procedure.*

vinegar (vin'ē-găr) [Fr. *vinaigre,* fr. *vin,* wine, + *aigre,* sour]. Acetum; impure dilute acetic acid, made from wine, cider, malt, etc.
pyroligneous v., wood v.
wood v., pyroligneous v.; pyracetic acid; impure acetic acid produced by the destructive distillation of pine tar and wood.

vinic (vī'nik) [L. *vinum,* wine]. Relating to or derived from wine.

vinous (vī'nŭs). Relating to, containing, or of the nature of wine.

Vinson, Porter P., U.S. surgeon, 1890–1959. See Plummer-V. *syndrome.*

vinyl (vī'nil) Ethenyl; the hydrocarbon radical, $CH_2{=}CH{-}$.
v. carbinol, *allyl* alcohol.
v. chloride, chloroethylene; a substance used in the plastics industry and suspected of being a potent carcinogen in man.

vinylbenzene (vī'nil-ben'zēn). Styrene.

vinylene (vī'nil-ēn). Ethenylene; the bivalent radical, $-CH{=}CH-$.

vinyl ether. Divinyl ether.

vinylethyl ether (vī-nil-eth'il). Ethylvinyl ether.

vinylidene (vī-nil'i-dēn). The bivalent radical, $H_2C{=}C{=}$.

violaceous (vī-ō-lā'shŭs) [L. *viola,* violet]. Denoting a purple discoloration, usually of the skin.

violet (vī'ō-let) [L. *viola*]. The color evoked by wavelengths of the visible spectrum shorter than 450 nm. For individual violet dyes, see the specific name.
visual v., iodopsin.

viomycin (vī-ō-mī'sin). $C_{23}H_{36}N_{12}O_8$; an antibiotic agent obtained from *Streptomyces puniceus* var. *floridae;* active against acid-fast bacteria, including strains of tubercle bacilli resistant to streptomycin; may produce vestibular damage and deafness.

viosterol (vī-os'ter-ōl). Ergocalciferol.

VIP Abbreviation for vasoactive intestinal *polypeptide.*

viper vī'per) [L. *vipera,* serpent, snake]. A member of the snake family Viperidae.
Russell's v., daboia, daboya; *Vipera russelli,* the large, extremely deadly viper of the East Indies. The venom is coagulant in action and is used locally in a 1:10,000 solution for the arrest of hemorrhage in hemophilia.

Viperidae (vī-per'i-dē) [L. *vipera,* viper]. A family of poisonous Old World snakes, the true vipers, comprised of about 50 species and characterized by two relatively long caniculated fangs at the front of the upper jaw which are attached to movable bones, allowing them to be erect during the bite when the mouth is open, and folded into a palate skin fold when the jaws are shut.

vipoma (vi-pō'mă) [*v*asoactive *i*ntestinal *p*olypeptide + G. *-ōma,* tumor]. An endocrine tumor, usually originating in the pancreas, which produces a vasoactive intestinal polypeptide believed to cause profound cardiovascular and electrolyte changes with vasodilatory hypotension, watery diarrhea, hypokalemia, and dehydration.

Vipond, French physician. See V.'s *sign.*

viprynium embonate (vip-rin'ē-ŭm em'bō-nāt). Pyrvinium pamoate.

viraginity (vir'ă-jin'i-tē) [L. *virago* (*viragin-*), a female warrior]. Presence of pronounced masculine psychological qualities in a woman.

viral (vī'răl). Of, pertaining to, or caused by a virus.

Virchow, Rudolf, German pathologist and politician, 1821–1902. See V.'s *angle, cells, corpuscles, crystals, disease; law, node, psammoma;* V.-Holder angle; V.-Hassall bodies; V.-Robin *spaces.*

viremia (vī-rē'mē-ă) [virus + G. *haima,* blood]. The presence, as in smallpox, of a virus in the bloodstream.

vires (vī'rēz). Plural of vis.

virga (vir'gă) [L. a rod]. Penis.

virgin (ver'jin) [L. *virgo* (*virgin-*), maiden]. **1.** A person who has never had sexual intercourse. **2.** Virginal (2); fresh; unused; uncontaminated.

virginal (ver'ji-năl) [L. *virginalis*]. **1.** Relating to a virgin. **2.** Virgin (2).

virginity (ver-jin'i-tē) [L. *virginitas*] The virgin state.

virgophrenia (ver-gō-frē'nē-ă) [L. *virgo,* maiden, + G. *phrēn,* mind]. The receptive, capacious, and retentive mind of youth.

viricidal (vī-ri-sī'dă). Virucidal.

viricide (vī'ri-sīd). Virucide.

-viridae. Termination denoting a virus family.

virile (vir'il) [L. *virilis,* masculine, fr. *vir,* a man]. **1.** Relating to the male sex. **2.** Manly, strong, masculine. **3.** Possessing masculine traits.

virilescence (vir-i-les'ens). Assumption of male characteristics by the female.

virilia (vi-ril'ē-ă) [L. ntr. pl. of *virilis,* virile]. The male sexual organs.

virilism (vir'i-lizm) [L. *virilis,* masculine]. Possession of mature masculine somatic characteristics by a girl, woman, or prepubescent male; may be present at birth or may appear later, depending on its cause; may be relatively mild (e.g., hirsutism) or severe and is commonly the result of gonadal or adrenocortical dysfunction, or of androgenic therapy.
adrenal v., adrenal virilizing syndrome; v. produced by excessive or abnormal secretory patterns of adrenocortical steroids.

virility (vi-ril'i-tē) [L. *virilitas,* manhood, fr. *vir,* man]. The condition or quality of being virile.

virilization (vir'i-li-zā'shŭn). Production or acquisition of virilism.

virilizing (vir'i-līz-ing). Causing virilism.

-virinae. Termination denoting a subfamily of viruses.

virion (vī'rē-on, vir'ē-on). An elementary virus particle which, according to species, varies in size, from 15 to 300 nm, and in shape, being either spherical, polyhedral, rod-shaped, or tadpole-shaped. It is composed of a central core (nucleoid) containing either DNA or RNA, surrounded by a protein covering (capsid); this nucleic acid-protein complex (nucleocapsid) may be the complete v. (as in the case of the adenoviruses and the picornaviruses) or may be surrounded by an envelope (as in the herpetoviruses and the myxoviruses). Capsids may be icosahedral (cubic symmetry), helical, or complex; icosahedral capsids are composed of capsomeres, each of which consists either of five (pentamer, or pentagonal capsomere) or of six (hexamer, or hexagonal capsomere) protein units (monomers); helical capsids, not being in the form of icosahedrons, do not contain capsomeres, the protein monomers forming simpler, cylindrical structures around the nucleic acid core. The envelope is a membrane-like structure containing lipids, proteins, and carbohydrates, with structures that resemble spikes projecting from the surface; envelopes of some species of v.'s are disrupted by ether; those of other species are not.

viripotent (vir-i-pō'tent, vī-rip'ō-tent) [L. *viripotens,* fr. *vir,* man, + *potens,* having power]. Obsolete term denoting a sexually mature male.

viroid (vī'royd) [virus + G. *eidos,* resemblance]. An infectious pathogen of plants that is smaller than a virus (MW 75,000-100,000) and differs from one in that it consists only of single-stranded closed circular RNA, lacking a protein covering (capsid); replication does not depend on a helper virus, but is effected autonomously by the DNA-dependent polymerase of the infected host cell.

virologist (vī-rol'ō-jist). A specialist in virology.

virology (vī-rol'ō-jē, vi-) [virus + G. *logos,* study]. The study of viruses and of virus disease.

viropexis (vī-rō-pek'sis). Fixation of virus in tissue; specifically, the absorption (engulfment) of virus particles by a cell.

virucidal (vī-rū-sī'dăl). Viricidal; destructive to a virus.

virucide (vī-rŭ-sīd) [virus + L. *caedo,* to kill]. Viricide; an agent active against virus infections.

virucopria (vī-rŭ-kō'prē-ă). Presence of virus in feces.

virulence (vir'ū-lens) [L. *virulentia,* fr. *virulentus,* poisonous]. The quality of being toxic; the disease-evoking power of a microorganism in a given host.

virulent (vir'ū-lent) [L. *virulentus,* poisonous]. Extremely toxic, denoting a markedly pathogenic microorganism.

viruliferous (vī-rŭ-lif'er-ŭs). Conveying virus.

viruria (vī-rū'rē-ă) [virus + G. *ouron,* urine]. Presence of living viruses in the urine.

-virus. Termination denoting a genus of viruses.

VIRUS

virus, pl. viruses (vī'rŭs) [L. poison]. **1.** Formerly, the specific agent of an infectious disease. **2.** Filtrable v.; ultravirus; specifically, a term for a group of microbes which with few exceptions are capable of passing through fine filters that retain most bacteria, and are incapable of growth or reproduction apart from living cells. They have a procaryotic genetic apparatus but differ sharply from bacteria in other respects. During the early phase of replication the virion disintegrates, freeing elements that direct the host cell's metabolism in the process of producing v. Precise definition is difficult, and the criterion that a given v. contains only DNA or RNA, never both, may be subject to review, since v.'s included in the family Retroviridae seem to include not only RNA but also traces of DNA. Classification of v.'s depends upon characteristics of virions as well as upon mode of transmission, host range, symptomatology, and other factors. For v.'s not listed below, see the specific name. **3.** Relating to or caused by a v., as a virus disease.

v. III of rabbits [the third strain isolated, used for study], a herpetovirus causing latent infection of rabbits that can be activated by "blind" passage; may be carried in transplanted tumors.

2060 v., JH v.; a strain of common cold v. intermediate to *Enterovirus* and *Rhinovirus,* but usually grouped with the latter.

Abelson murine leukemia v., a retrovirus belonging to the Type C oncovirus group (family Oncovirinae) which is the only strain of murine leukemia v. associated with leukemia that produces *in vitro* transformation of mouse cells.

adeno-associated v. (AAV), *Dependovirus.*

adenoidal-pharyngeal-conjunctival (A-P-C) v., adenovirus.

adenosatellite v., *Dependovirus.*

African horse sickness v., a v. of the genus *Orbivirus;* the cause of African horse sickness.

African swine fever v., a DNA v. belonging to the family Iridoviridae and the etiologic agent of African swine fever.

AIDS-related v. (ARV), human immunodeficiency v.

Akabane v., a v. of the genus *Bunyavirus,* causing abortion in cattle and congenital arthrogryposis and hydrancephaly in bovine fetuses in Israel, Japan, and Australia; it is transmitted by mosquitoes.

Aleutian disease of mink v., an unclassified v., resistant to 0.3% formalin; the cause of Aleutian disease of mink.

amphotropic v., an oncornavirus that does not produce disease in its natural host but does replicate in tissue culture cells of the host species and also in cells from other species.

animal v.'s, v.'s occurring in man and other animals, causing inapparent infection or producing disease.

A-P-C v., adenovirus.

attenuated v., a variant strain of a pathogenic v., so modified as to excite the production of protective antibodies, yet not producing the specific disease.

Aujeszky's disease v., pseudorabies v.

Australian X disease v., Murray Valley encephalitis v.

avian encephalomyelitis v., a v. of the genus *Enterovirus* (family Picornaviridae) causing avian infectious encephalomyelitis in young chicks.

avian erythroblastosis v., avian leukosis-sarcoma *complex* (2).

avian infectious laryngotracheitis v., a herpesvirus causing avian infectious laryngotracheitis.

avian influenza v., fowl plague v.; a type A influenza v. (genus *Influenzavirus*) that causes fowl plague.

avian leukosis-sarcoma v., avian leukosis-sarcoma *complex* (2).

avian lymphomatosis v., **(1)** avian leukosis-sarcoma *complex* (2); **(2)** avian neurolymphomatosis v.

avian myeloblastosis v., avian leukosis-sarcoma *complex* (2).

avian neurolymphomatosis v., Marek's disease v.; fowl neurolymphomatosis v.; avian lymphomatosis v. (2); the herpetovirus that causes avian lymphomatosis (Marek's disease), but is believed to be distinct from those causing other forms of leukosis.

avian pneumoencephalitis v., Newcastle disease v.

avian sarcoma v., avian leukosis-sarcoma *complex* (2).

avian viral arthritis v., a v. of the genus *Reovirus* causing tenosynovitis and arthritis in chickens.

B v., monkey B v.; a herpetovirus, affecting Old World monkeys, that is very similar morphologically to herpes simplex v.; fatal infection may occur in humans following the bite of an infected monkey.

bacterial v., a v. which "infects" bacteria; a bacteriophage or a filamentous bacterial v.

BK v. [initials of patient from whom first isolated], a human polyomavirus of worldwide distribution which produces infections that are usually subclinical in immunocompetent individuals.

bluecomb v., transmissible turkey enteritis v.

bluetongue v., a v. of the genus *Orbivirus;* the agent of bluetongue in sheep.

Borna disease v., enzootic encephalomyelitis v.; an unclassified v. that is the cause of Borna disease.

Bornholm disease v., epidemic pleurodynia v.

bovine leukemia v. (BLV), bovine leukosis v.; a type C oncovirus commonly infecting cattle, especially dairy cows; in a small proportion of infected cattle, it will cause enzootic bovine leukosis.
bovine leukosis v., bovine leukemia v.
bovine papular stomatitis v., papular stomatitis v. of cattle; a poxvirus of the genus *Parapoxvirus,* reported from North America, Africa and Europe, causing bovine papular stomatitis.
bovine virus diarrhea v., mucosal disease v.; a v. of the genus *Pestivirus,* causing bovine virus diarrhea; New York, Oregon, and Indiana strains of the v. are recognized.
Bunyamwera v. [*Bunyamwera,* Uganda, where first isolated], a serologic group of the genus *Bunyavirus,* composed of 18 species, including Bunyamwera v. (the type species) and Guaroa v.
Bwamba v. [*Bwamba,* forest in Uganda where first isolated], a serologic group of the genus *Bunyavirus,* composed of two species, Bwamba v. (type species) and Pongola v.; associated with cases of Bwamba fever in Uganda.
CA v., croup-associated v. See parainfluenza v. type 2.
California v., a serologic group of the genus *Bunyavirus,* comprising 11 strains including La Crosse and Tahyna v., and the type strain, California v., which causes encephalitis, chiefly in the age group 4 to 14 years.
canarypox v., a poxvirus of the genus *Avipoxvirus* causing a fatal disease of canaries, and also infecting sparrows.
canine distemper v., dog distemper v.; an RNA v. of the genus *Morbillivirus* that causes canine distemper.
Capim v.'s, a serologic group of the genus *Bunyavirus,* the type species of which is Capim v.
Caraparu v., a species of C group *Bunyavirus* and an agent of bunyavirus encephalitis.
cat distemper v., feline panleukopenia v.
cattle plague v., rinderpest v.
Catu v., an arbovirus of the Guama subgroup of the genus *Bunyavirus;* an agent of bunyavirus encephalitis.
CELO v., chicken embryo lethal orphan v.; a v. with characteristics of adenovirus, and similar to quail bronchitis v.
Central European tick-borne encephalitis v., one of the v.'s of the tick-borne encephalitis complex of group B arboviruses (genus *Flavivirus*); the causative agent of tick-borne encephalitis (Central European subtype).
C group v.'s, a serologic group of the genus *Bunyavirus* (formerly called group C arboviruses), composed of 12 species including Caraparu, Murutucu, and Oriboca v.
Chagres v., a v., probably a bunyavirus, that is an agent of bunyavirus encephalitis.
chicken embryo lethal orphan v., CELO v.
chickenpox v., varicella-zoster v.
chikungunya v. [so named for the "bent up" position of persons so infected], a mosquito-transmitted arbovirus of the genus *Alphavirus* (family Togoviridae) found in parts of Africa and in India, Thailand, and Malaysia; causes a febrile illness with joint pains.
Coe v., a v. serologically identical with the A-21 strain of coxsackievirus; the cause of a common cold-like disease in military recruits.
cold v., common cold v.
Colorado tick fever v., a v. of the genus *Orbivirus,* found in the Rocky Mountain region of the United States and transmitted by the tick, *Dermacentor andersoni;* it causes Colorado tick fever.
Columbia S. K. v., a strain of encephalomyocarditis v.
common cold v., cold v.; any of the numerous strains of v. etiologically associated with the common cold, chiefly the rhinoviruses, but also strains of adenovirus, *Coxsackievirus,* ECHO v., and parainfluenza v.
contagious ecthyma (pustular dermatitis) v. of sheep, orf v.; soremouth v.; the poxvirus of the genus *Parapoxvirus* causing contagious ecthyma (pustular dermatitis) of sheep.
contagious pustular stomatitis v., horsepox v.
cowpox v., a v. of the genus *Orthopoxvirus* that causes cowpox.
Coxsackie v., see Coxsackievirus.
Crimean-Congo hemorrhagic fever v., a v. of the genus *Nairovirus* (family Bunyaviridae) from Africa and the southern USSR, carried by ticks (*Hyalomma* and *Amblyomma*) and found in human blood; the cause of Crimean-Congo hemorrhagic fever.
croup-associated v., parainfluenza v. type 2.
cytopathogenic v., a v. whose multiplication leads to degenerative changes in the host cell. See also cytopathic *effect.*
deer hemorrhagic fever v., a v. of the genus *Orbivirus* causing deer hemorrhagic fever.
defective v., a v. particle that contains insufficient nucleic acid to provide for production of all essential viral components; consequently, infectious v. is not produced except under certain conditions (*e.g.,* when the host cell is infected with a "helper" v. also).
delta v., hepatitis delta v.
dengue v., a v. of the genus *Flavivirus,* about 50 nm in diameter; the etiologic agent of dengue in man and also occurring in monkeys and chimpanzees, usually as inapparent infection; four serotypes are recognized; transmission is effected by mosquitoes of the genus *Aedes.*
distemper v., see canine distemper v.; feline panleukopenia v.
DNA v., deoxyvirus; a major group of animal v.'s in which the core consists of deoxyribonucleic acid (DNA); it includes adenoviruses, papovaviruses, herpesviruses, poxviruses, and other unclassified DNA v.'s.
dog distemper v., canine distemper v.
duck hepatitis v., a v. of the genus *Enterovirus* causing virus hepatitis of ducks.
duck influenza v., an influenza A v. distinct from human influenza A strains on bases of hemagglutination-inhibition.
duck plague v., a herpesvirus that causes duck plague.
eastern equine encephalomyelitis v., EEE v.; a v. of the genus *Alphavirus* (group A arbovirus) occurring in eastern United States; it is normally present in certain wild birds as an inapparent infection, but is capable of causing eastern equine encephalomyelitis in horses and man following transfer by the bites of culicine mosquitoes.
EB v., Epstein-Barr v.
Ebola v., viral hemorrhagic fever v.; a v. morphologically similar to but antigenically distinct from Marburg v. which causes viral hemorrhagic fever.
ECBO v., enteric cytopathogenic bovine orphan v.; former name for early isolates of enteroviruses.
ECHO v., echovirus; enteric cytopathogenic human orphan v.; an enterovirus belonging to the Picornaviridae, isolated from man; while there are many inapparent infections, certain of the several serotypes are associated with fever and aseptic meningitis, and some appear to cause mild respiratory disease.
ECMO v., enteric cytopathogenic monkey orphan v.; simian picornavirus recovered from monkey kidney cells and stools.
ecotropic v., an oncornavirus that does not produce disease in its natural host but does replicate in tissue culture cells derived from the host species.
ECSO v., enteric cytopathogenic swine orphan v.; a picornavirus isolated from outbreaks of enteritis in swine, but not known to be a natural pathogen.
ectromelia v., infectious ectromelia v.
EEE v., eastern equine encephalomyelitis v.
EMC v., encephalomyocarditis v.
encephalitis v., any one of a variety of v.'s that cause encephalitis.
encephalomyocarditis v., EMC v.; a picornavirus, probably of rodents, isolated from blood and stools of humans, other primates, pigs, and rabbits; occasionally causes febrile illness with central nervous system involvement in man, and an often fatal myocarditis in chimpanzees, monkeys and pigs; strains of this v. include Columbia S. K. v. and Mengo v.

enteric v.'s, v.'s of the genus Enterovirus.
enteric cytopathogenic bovine orphan v., ECBO v.
enteric cytopathogenic human orphan v., ECHO v.
enteric cytopathogenic monkey orphan v., ECMO v.
enteric cytopathogenic swine orphan v., ECSO v.
enteric orphan v.'s, enteroviruses isolated from man and other animals, "orphan"implying lack of known association with disease when isolated; many v.'s of the group are now known to be pathogenic; *e.g.,* include ECBO v.'s, ECHO v.'s, and ECSO v.'s.
enzootic encephalomyelitis v., Borna disease v.
ephemeral fever v., a rhabdovirus that causes ephemeral fever of cattle.
epidemic gastroenteritis v., gastroenteritis v. type A; an unclassified v., about 27 nm in diameter, which has not been cultured *in vitro;* it is the cause of epidemic nonbacterial gastroenteritis; at least three antigenically distinct serotypes have been recognized, including the Norwalk agent.
epidemic keratoconjunctivitis v., an adenovirus (type 8) causing epidemic keratoconjunctivitis, especially among shipyard workers, and also associated with outbreaks of swimming pool conjunctivitis.
epidemic myalgia v., epidemic pleurodynia v.
epidemic parotitis v., mumps v.
epidemic pleurodynia v., epidemic myalgia v.; Bornholm disease v.; a v. of *Enterovirus* coxsackievirus type B that causes epidemic pleurodynia.
Epstein-Barr v. (EBV), EB v.; a herpetovirus found in cell cultures of Burkitt's lymphoma; also, antibodies reactive with this v. have been reported in cases of infectious mononucleosis.
equine abortion v., equine rhinopneumonitis v.
equine arteritis v., infectious arteritis v. of horses; a v. of the genus *Pestivirus* that causes equine viral arteritis and, frequently, abortion; probably the most common cause of equine influenza.
equine coital exanthema v., a herpesvirus causing coital exanthema in male and female horses.
equine infectious anemia v., swamp fever v.; seemingly a non-type C retrovirus, unrelated to other members of the group, and the cause of equine infectious anemia.
equine influenza v.'s, strains of influenza v. type A which cause horse influenza; there are at least two subtypes.
equine rhinopneumonitis v., equine abortion v.; a herpesvirus reported in the U.S. Europe, and South Africa, causing equine rhinopneumonitis and equine virus abortion.
FA v., a strain of mouse encephalomyelitis v.
feline leukemia v. (FeLV), a v. causing many proliferative (neoplastic) and degenerative (blastopenic) diseases in domestic cats, including lymphosarcoma, thymic atrophy, immune complex glomerulonephritis, fetal abortions and resorptions, and several myeloproliferative and myelodegenerative conditions; it also causes immunosuppression in infected cats.
feline panleukopenia v., feline infectious agranulocytosis v.; cat distemper v.; panleukopenia v. of cats; a v. of the genus *Parvovirus* that causes panleukopenia; the v. infects all Felidae, raccoons and mink, but not dogs or other Canidae.
feline rhinotracheitis v., a herpesvirus that causes feline viral rhinotracheitis.
fibromatosis v. of rabbits, rabbit fibroma v.
fibrous bacterial v.'s, filamentous bacterial v.'s.
filamentous bacterial v.'s, fibrous bacterial v.'s; deoxyribonucleoproteins that "infect" and replicate in Gram- negative bacteria having sex pili and that, unlike bacteriophage, are released from infected bacteria without damage to the cell; they seem to be of two kinds, one of which has a specificity for F pili and the other for I pili.
filtrable v., virus (2).
fixed v., rabies v. of the utmost possible virulence for rabbits, obtained by numerous passages through this experimental host. See also street v.
Flury strain rabies v., see rabies v., Flury strain.
FMD v., foot-and-mouth disease v.
foamy v.'s, foamy agents; retroviruses of the subfamily Spumavirinae, found in primates and other mammals; so named because of lacelike changes produced in monkey kidney cells; syncytia are also produced.
foot-and-mouth disease v., FMD v.; a picornavirus of the genus *Rhinovirus* causing foot-and-mouth disease of cattle, swine, sheep, goats, and wild ruminants; it has wide distribution throughout Africa and Asia, causing serious economic losses; the v. is spread by contamination of the animal environment with infected saliva and excreta.
fowl erythroblastosis v., avian leukosis-sarcoma *complex* (2).
fowl lymphomatosis v., avian leukosis-sarcoma *complex* (2).
fowl myeloblastosis v., avian leukosis-sarcoma *complex* (2).
fowl neurolymphomatosis v., avian neurolymphomatosis v.
fowl plague v., avian influenza v.
fowlpox v., a v. of the genus *Avipoxvirus* causing fowlpox and avian diphtheria.
fox encephalitis v., infectious canine hepatitis v.
Friend v., Friend leukemia v., Swiss mouse leukemia v.; a strain of the splenic group of mouse leukemia v.'s, related to Moloney and Rauscher v.'s.
GAL v., gallus adeno-like v.; a v. with characteristics of adenovirus, not known to be associated with natural disease.
gallus adeno-like v., GAL v.
gastroenteritis v. type A, epidemic gastroenteritis v.
gastroenteritis v. type B, rotavirus.
German measles v., rubella v.
goatpox v., a v. of the genus *Capripoxvirus;* the cause of goatpox.
Graffi's v., a mouse myeloleukemia v. from filtrates of transplantable tumors; possibly related to Gross' v.
green monkey v., Marburg v.
Gross' v., Gross' leukemia v., a strain of mouse leukemia v.
Guama v., a serologic group of the genus *Bunyavirus,* composed of 6 species including Catu v., and the type strain, Guama v.
Guaroa v. a v. of the Bunyamwera group of the genus *Bunyavirus,* and an agent of bunyavirus encephalitis.
HA1 v., hemadsorption v. type 1. See parainfluenza v. type 3.
HA2 v., hemadsorption v. type 2. See parainfluenza v. type 1.
hand-foot-and-mouth disease v., the v. causing hand-foot-and-mouth disease; chiefly type A16 but also types A4, A5, A7, A9, or A10 *Entervirus* coxsackievirus.
Hantaan v., a v. of the family Bunyaviridae that causes Korean hemorrhagic fever.
hard pad v., the v. causing hard pad disease, probably canine distemper v., but sometimes not recovered.
helper v., a v. whose replication renders it possible for a defective v. or a virusoid (also present in the host cell) to develop into fully infectious agent.
hemadsorption v. type 1, parainfluenza v. type 3.
hemadsorption v. type 2, parainfluenza v. type 2.
hepatitis A v. (HAV), infectious hepatitis v.; the causative agent of viral hepatitis type A.
hepatitis B v. (HBV), serum hepatitis v.; the causative agent of viral hepatitis type B.
hepatitis delta v. (HDV), delta agent, antigen, or virus; a small "defective" v., similar to viroids and virusoids, that requires the presence of HBsAg provided by the hepatitis B v. for replication; it causes either acute or chronic delta hepatitis.
herpes v., see herpesvirus.
herpes simplex v. (HSV), herpesvirus.
herpes zoster v., varicella-zoster v.
hog cholera v., swine fever v.; an RNA virus of the genus *Pestivirus* that causes hog cholera.
horsepox v., contagious pustular stomatitis v.; the poxvirus causing horsepox.

human immunodeficiency v. (HIV), human T-cell lymphoma/-leukemia virus type III; human T-cell lymphotropic v. type III; lymphadenopathy-associated v.; AIDS-related v.; a cytopathic retrovirus (subfamily Oncovirinae, family Retroviridae) that is about 100 nm in diameter, has a lipid envelope, and has a characteristic dense cylindrical nucleoid containing core proteins and genomic RNA; it is the etiologic agent of acquired immunodeficiency syndrome (AIDS).

human papilloma v. (HPV), infectious papilloma v.; an icosahedral DNA v., 55 nm in diameter, of the genus *Papillomavirus;* certain types cause cutaneous and genital warts in man, including verruca vulgaris and condyloma acuminatum; other types are associated with severe cervical intraepithelial neoplasia and anogenital and laryngeal carcinomas.

human T-cell lymphoma/leukemia v., human T-cell lymphotropic v. (HTLV), a group of viruses (subfamily Lentivirinae, family Retroviridae) that are lymphotropic with a selective affinity for the helper/inducer cell subset of T lymphocytes and that are associated with adult T-cell leukemia and lymphoma. HTLV-III is the human immunodeficiency v. (HIV).

Ibaraki v., a v. of cattle in Japan, closely related to the bluetongue v.

IBR v., infectious bovine rhinotracheitis v.

Ilhéus v., a v. of the genus *Flavivirus* (group B arbovirus) first isolated in Brazil, later found in Colombia, Central America, and the Caribbean; the cause of Ilhéus encephalitis and Ilhéus fever.

inclusion conjunctivitis v.'s, former name for *Chlamydia trachomatis.*

infantile gastroenteritis v., rotavirus.

infectious arteritis v. of horses, equine arteritis v.

infectious bovine rhinotracheitis v., IBR v.; a herpesvirus causing infectious bovine rhinotracheitis.

infectious bronchitis v. (IBV), an RNA v. of the family Coronaviridae and the type species of the genus *Coronavirus,* causing infectious avian bronchitis, being most pathogenic in chicks up to about 4 weeks of age; not to be confused with avian infectious laryngotracheitis v.

infectious canine hepatitis v., fox encephalitis v.; Rubarth's disease v.; an adenovirus causing infectious canine hepatitis and fox encephalitis; coyotes, wolves, foxes, bears, and raccoons are also susceptible.

infectious ectromelia v., ectromelia v.; mousepox v.; pseudolymphocytic choriomeningitis v.; a poxvirus of the genus *Orthopoxvirus,* morphologically similar to vaccinia v., which occurs as a latent infection in laboratory mice, but which may be activated by stresses such as irradiation and transport to cause disease; inoculation into the footpad results in edema and necrosis.

infectious hepatitis v., hepatitis A v.

infectious papilloma v., human papilloma v.

infectious porcine encephalomyelitis v., Teschen disease v.

influenza v.'s, v.'s of the family Orthomyxoviridae which cause influenza and influenza-like infections of man and other animals; v.'s included are influenza v. types A and B of the genus *Influenzavirus,* causing, respectively, influenza A and B, and influenza v. type C, which probably belongs to a separate genus and causes influenza C.

insect v.'s, v.'s pathogenic for insects.

Jamestown Canyon v., a member of the California group of arboviruses (family Bunyaviridae) which has been associated with a mild febrile illness in man in North America.

Japanese B encephalitis v., Russian autumn encephalitis v.; a v. of the genus *Flavivirus* (group B arbovirus) occurring particularly in Japan but probably widespread throughout Southeast Asia; the v. is normally present in man, especially in children, as an inapparent infection, but may cause febrile response and sometimes encephalitis; it may cause encephalitis in horses and abortion in pigs; wild birds are probably the natural hosts and culicine mosquitoes the vectors.

JC v. [initials of patient from whom first isolated], a human polyomavirus of worldwide distribution which produces infections that are usually subclinical in immunocompetent individuals.

JH v. [*J* ohn *H* opkins University, where first isolated], 2060 v.

Junin v., a v. of the Tacaribe complex of arboviruses, genus *Arenavirus,* and the cause of Argentinian hemorrhagic fever; also isolated from mites and rodents.

K v., a papovavirus that causes pneumonia in young mice by various routes of inoculation.

Kelev strain rabies v., see rabies v., Kelev strain.

Kilham rat v., latent rat v.; a v. of the genus *Parvovirus* causing inapparent infection in rats; also recoverable from rat tumors.

Kisenyi sheep disease v., a v. that is probably the same as Nairobi sheep disease v.

Koongol v.'s, a serologic group of the genus *Bunyavirus,* comprising two species, Koongol (type species) and Wongal v.

Kyasanur Forest disease v., a group B arbovirus isolated from monkeys in India and capable of causing Kyasanur Forest disease in man; the v. is spread by monkeys and birds having mild infections; the vectors are probably species of the tick *Haemaphysalis.*

La Crosse v., a bunyavirus of the California group and an agent of bunyavirus encephalitis.

lactate dehydrogenase v., LDH agent; a togavirus present perhaps as a "passenger" in various transplantable mouse tumors.

Lassa v., an arenavirus that causes Lassa fever.

latent rat v., Kilham rat v.

LCM v., lymphocytic choriomeningitis v.

louping-ill v., a v. of the genus *Flavivirus* that causes louping ill and is transmitted by the hard tick *Ixodes ricinus.*

Lucké's v., a herpetovirus associated with Lucké's carcinoma.

lumpy skin disease v.'s, several poxviruses isolated from cattle with lumpy skin disease in South and East Africa; the Neethling v. has been most studied, and is serologically closely related to the v. of African sheep-pox.

Lunyo v., an atypical strain of Rift Valley fever v.

lymphadenopathy-associated v. (LAV), human immunodeficiency v.

lymphocytic choriomeningitis v., LCM v.; an RNA v. of the family Arenaviridae that infects mice, man, monkeys, dogs, and guinea pigs, and causes lymphocytic choriomeningitis; in man, infection may be inapparent, but sometimes the v. causes influenza-like disease, meningitis, or rarely meningoencephalomyelitis; *in utero* infections of mice establish a kind of immunological tolerance in which v. and antibody circulate together; the lesion responsible for the name of the v. is lymphocytic infiltration around blood vessels and choroid plexuses.

lymphogranuloma venereum v., former name for *Chlamydia trachomatis.*

Machupo v., a v. of the Tacaribe complex (genus *Arenavirus*); the cause of Bolivian hemorrhagic fever.

maedi v., medi or progressive pneumonia v.; a retrovirus (subfamily Lentivirinae) that is the cause of maedi; it is very similar to the visna v. and resembles C type RNA v. (Oncovirinae).

malignant catarrhal fever v., a herpesvirus of wide distribution causing malignant catarrhal fever of cattle; sheep and wildebeests harbor inapparent infections and may transmit the v. to cattle.

mammary cancer v. of mice, mammary tumor v. of mice.

mammary tumor v. of mice, mammary cancer v. of mice; mouse mammary tumor v.; Bittner's milk factor; milk factor; Bittner agent; an oncornavirus, antigenically distinct from the murine leukemia-sarcoma complex, that is associated with adenocarcinomatous tumors of the mammary gland, commonly latent in wild and laboratory mice and causing cancer only in genetically susceptible strains under certain hormonal influences.

Marburg v., green monkey v.; an unclassified, seemingly RNA-

containing v., first recognized at Marburg University (West Germany), where it was the cause of disease among handlers of green monkeys.
Marek's disease v., avian neurolymphomatosis v.
marmoset v., a herpetovirus obtained repeatedly from throat swabs and tissues of New World monkeys.
masked v., a v. ordinarily occurring in the host in a noninfective state, but which may be activated and demonstrated by special procedures such as blind passage in experimental animals.
Mayaro v., a v. of the genus *Alphavirus* causing epidemics of undifferentiated type fever in South America.
measles v., rubeola v.; an RNA v. of the genus *Morbillivirus* that causes measles in man and is transmitted via the respiratory tract; possesses hemagglutinating, hemadsorbing, and hemolyzing abilities.
medi v., maedi v.
Mengo v., a strain of encephalomyocarditis v.
mink enteritis v., a parvovirus that causes enteritis of mink.
MM v., a strain of encephalomyocarditis v.
Mokola v., a rabies related v. of the genus *Lyssavirus,* first isolated from shrews (*Crocidura* spp.) in Nigeria, which has caused fatal neurological disease in man and cats in Africa.
molluscum contagiosum v., the poxvirus causing molluscum contagiosum of man.
Moloney's v., a lymphoid leukemia v. of mice, isolated originally during propagation of S 37 mouse sarcoma.
monkey B v., B v.
monkeypox v., a v. of the genus *Orthopoxvirus* causing monkeypox.
mouse encephalomyelitis v., mouse poliomyelitis v.; Theiler's v.; Theiler's original v.; a v. of the genus *Enterovirus* normally associated with inapparent infections and found in the intestinal tracts of infected mice, occasionally causing mouse encephalomyelitis in experimentally inoculated susceptible mice.
mouse hepatitis v., a coronavirus that in the presence of *Eperythrozoon coccoides* causes fatal hepatitis in newly weaned mice; otherwise causes inapparent infection.
mouse leukemia v.'s, oncornaviruses of the murine leukemia-sarcoma complex that produce leukemia and sometimes lymphosarcomas in mice, including the Abelron, Gross, Moloney, Friend, and Rauscher strains of v.; they have been isolated from inbred mice having high incidence of spontaneous lymphoid leukemia.
mouse mammary tumor v., mammary tumor v. of mice.
mouse parotid tumor v., polyoma v.
mouse poliomyelitis v., mouse encephalomyelitis v.
mousepox v., infectious ectromelia v.
mouse thymic v., an unclassified ether-sensitive v., 75 to 100 nm in diameter, that causes necrosis of the thymus in young mice.
mucosal disease v., bovine virus diarrhea v.
mumps v., epidemic parotitis v.; a v. of the genus *Paramyxovirus* causing parotitis in man, sometimes with complications of orchitis, oophoritis, pancreatitis, meningoencephalitis and others, and transmitted by infected salivary secretions.
murine sarcoma v., a seemingly defective oncornavirus that produces sarcomas in mice when growing in the presence of a "helper" v.; *e.g.,* mouse leukemia v.
Murray Valley encephalitis v., MVE v.; Australian X disease v.; a group B arbovirus of the genus *Flavivirus* that causes Murray Valley encephalitis; it is transmitted by *Culex* mosquitoes, and also infects birds and horses.
Murutucu v., a C group mosquito-borne v. of the genus *Bunyavirus,* which has caused undifferentiated type fever in Brazil and French Guiana.
MVE v., Murray Valley encephalitis v.
myxomatosis v., rabbit myxoma v.
Nairobi sheep disease v., an unclassified arbovirus of the family Bunyaviridae causing Nairobi sheep disease, transmitted by the tick, *Rhipicephalus appendiculatus;* it is a serologic group of v.'s morphologically like *Bunyavirus* but antigenically unrelated to it.
naked v., a v. consisting only of a nucleocapsid; *i.e.,* one that does not possess an enclosing envelope.
ND v., Newcastle disease v.
Nebraska calf scours v., the bovine rotavirus. See rotavirus.
Neethling v., see lumpy skin disease v.'s.
negative strand v., a v. the genome of which is a strand of RNA that is complementary to messenger RNA; negative strand v.'s also carry RNA polymerases necessary for the synthesis of messenger RNA.
Negishi v., one of the group B arboviruses (genus *Flavivirus*) of the tick-borne encephalitis complex, isolated from fatal infections in Japan.
neonatal calf diarrhea v., one of two v.'s causing neonatal calf diarrhea; a reovirus-like v. is associated with disease in newborn calves, and a coronavirus is associated with disease in calves over 5 days of age.
neurotropic v., a v. that has an affinity for nervous tissue, *e.g.,* poliomyelitis v., neurotropic v. variant of yellow fever, and the "fixed" v. of rabies.
Newcastle disease v., ND v.; avian pneumoencephalitis v.; a v. of the genus *Paramyxovirus* causing Newcastle disease in chickens and, to a lesser extent, in turkeys and other birds; it may occasionally infect laboratory and poultry workers, causing conjunctivitis and lymphadenitis.
nonoccluded v., a v. not inclosed in an inclusion body, usually with reference to an insect v.
occluded v., a v. inclosed in an inclusion body, usually with reference to an insect v.
Omsk hemorrhagic fever v., a v. of the genus *Flavivirus* causing Omsk hemorrhagic fever.
oncogenic v., tumor v.; a v. of one of the two groups of tumor-evoking v.'s: the RNA tumor v.'s (*Oncovirinae*), which are well defined and rather homogeneous, or the DNA v.'s, which are more diverse.
O'nyong-nyong v., a v. of the genus *Alphavirus,* found in Uganda, Kenya, and Congo, which causes O'nyong-nyong fever.
orf v., contagious ecthyma v. of sheep.
Oriboca v., a C group v. of the genus *Bunyavirus,* and an agent of bunyavirus encephalitis.
ornithosis v., former name for *Chlamydia psittaci.*
orphan v.'s, v.'s, such as the enteric orphan v.'s, which when originally found were not specifically associated with disease; a number of these have since been shown to be pathogenic.
Pacheco's parrot disease v., parrot v. (2); probably a v. of the family Herpetoviridae, possibly related to the v. of infectious laryngotracheitis.
panleukopenia v. of cats, feline panleukopenia v.
pantropic v., the ordinary strain of yellow fever v., as distinguished from the neurotropic strain.
pappataci fever v.'s, phlebotomus fever v.'s.
papular stomatitis v. of cattle, bovine papular stomatitis v.
parainfluenza v.'s, v.'s of the genus *Paramyxovirus,* of five types: type 1 (hemadsorption v. type 2), which includes sendai v., causes acute laryngotracheitis in children and occasionally adults; type 2 (croup-associated v.) is associated especially with acute laryngotracheitis or croup in young children and minor upper respiratory infections in adults; type 3 (hemadsorption v. type 1; shipping fever v.) has been isolated from small children with pharyngitis, bronchiolitis, and pneumonia, and causes occasional respiratory infection in adults; bovine strains have been isolated from cattle with shipping fever, and the v. has also been isolated from sheep; type 4 has been isolated from a very few children with minor respiratory illness; type 5 has no known human pathogens but includes simian v's (*e.g.,* SV 5).
paravaccinia v., pseudocowpox v.

parrot v., **(1)** obsolete term for *Chlamydia psittaci;* **(2)** Pacheco's parrot disease v.
Patois v., a serologic group of the genus *Bunyavirus,* comprising 4 species.
pharyngoconjunctival fever v., one of several types of adenoviruses associated with outbreaks of fever and pharyngitis, sometimes with conjunctivitis, especially in service recruits and people in boarding schools.
phlebotomus fever v.'s, pappataci fever v.'s; sandfly fever v.'s; an unclassified serologic group of arboviruses morphologically like *Bunyavirus* but antigenically unrelated, transmitted by *Phlebotomus papatasi* (sandfly) and causing phlebotomus fever; there are 20 strains, including Icoarachi and Itaporanga.
plant v.'s, v.'s pathogenic to higher plants.
pneumonia v. of mice, PVM v.; an RNA v. of the genus *Pneumovirus,* occurring normally as latent infection in laboratory mice, but capable of activation by serial intranasal passage and causing pneumonia.
poliomyelitis v., poliovirus hominis; the picornavirus (genus *Enterovirus*) causing poliomyelitis in man; the route of infection is the alimentary tract, but the v. may enter the bloodstream and nervous system, sometimes causing paralysis of the limbs and, rarely, encephalitis; many infections are inapparent; serologic types 1, 2, and 3 are recognized, type 1 being responsible for most paralytic poliomyelitis and most epidemics.
polyoma v., mouse parotid tumor v.; a papovavirus (genus *Polyomavirus*) which normally occurs in inapparent infections in laboratory and wild mice, but after growth on tissue culture is capable of producing parotid tumors in mice and sarcomas in hamsters as well as tumors in other laboratory animals.
porcine hemagglutinating encephalitis v., swine encephalitis v.
Powassan v. [*Powassan,* Canada, where first isolated], a v. of the genus *Flavivirus,* (family Togaviridae), transmitted by ixodid ticks and causing Powassan encephalitis in children; also capable of producing meningoencephalomyelitis in rabbits and children.
progressive pneumonia v., maedi v.
pseudocowpox v., paravaccinia v.; a v. of the genus *Parapoxvirus* that causes pseudocowpox in humans and cattle; it is closely related to orf v. and papular stomatitis v.
pseudolymphocytic choriomeningitis v., infectious ectromelia v.
pseudorabies v., Aujesky's disease v.; a herpesvirus causing pseudorabies in swine.
psittacosis v., former name for *Chlamydia psittaci.*
PVM v., pneumonia v. of mice.
quail bronchitis v., a v., similiar to an adenovirus, closely related antigenically to CELO v.
Quaranfil v., an ungrouped arbovirus isolated from human blood and from herons.
rabbit fibroma v., fibromatosis v. of rabbits; Shope fibroma v.; a poxvirus of the genus *Leporipoxvirus,* closely related to vaccinia and myxoma v.'s, that causes Shope fibroma.
rabbit myxoma v., myxomatosis v.; the poxvirus of the genus *Leporipoxvirus* causing myxomatosis of rabbits.
rabbitpox v., an orthopoxvirus that causes epidemics of pox in laboratory rabbits; immunologically, it is closely related to vaccinia v. but is more virulent in rabbits.
rabies v., a rather large bullet-shaped v. of the genus *Lyssavirus* that is the causative agent of rabies.
rabies v., Flury strain, a v. isolated from human brain, attenuated (fixed) by serial propagation in nonmammalian hosts, and subsequently established in chick embryo culture.
rabies v., Kelev strain, an attenuated, embryonate fowl egg-passaged strain.
Rauscher's v., an RNA mouse leukemia v., similar to Friend v.
respiratory syncytial v., chimpanzee coryza agent; Rs v.; an RNA v. of the genus *Pneumovirus,* with a tendency to form syncytia in tissue culture, that causes minor respiratory infection with rhinitis and cough in adults, but is capable of causing bronchitis and bronchopneumonia in young children; first isolated from chimpanzees with respiratory disease; it resembles v.'s of the family Retroviridae in that it possesses an RNA genome, but it produces DNA intermediate forms which establish persistent infection of actively growing cells.
Rida v., a v. from chronic encephalopathy of sheep, resembling scrapie v.
Rift Valley fever v., a v. of the genus Phlebovirus (family Bunyaviridae) that occurs in central and southern Africa in sheep, goats, and cattle, causing abortions and severe febrile disease, especially in young lambs; humans, especially herdsmen and veterinarians, may become infected through close contact with infected animals, developing a dengue-like disease; the v. also infects buffaloes, camels and antelopes; it is mosquito-borne, but also probably infects by contact and respiratory tract.
rinderpest v., cattle plague v.; an RNA v. of the genus *Morbillivirus,* causing rinderpest; it is closely related to the measles and canine distemper v.'s.
RNA v., ribovirus; a group of v.'s in which the core consists of RNA; a major group of animal v.'s that includes the families Picornaviridae, Reoviridae, Togaviridae, Bunyaviridae, Arenaviridae, Paramyxoviridae, Retroviridae, Coronaviridae, Orthomyxoviridae, and Rhabdoviridae.
RNA tumor v.'s, v.'s of the subfamily Oncovirinae.
Ross River v., A mosquito-borne alphavirus that causes epidemic polyarthritis.
Rous-associated v. (RAV), a leukemia v. of the leukosis-sarcoma complex which by phenotypic mixing with a defective (noninfectious) strain of Rous sarcoma v. effects production of infectious sarcoma v. with envelope antigenicity of the RAV.
Rous sarcoma v. (RSV), a sarcoma-producing v. of the avian leukosis-sarcoma complex identified by Rous in 1911.
Rs v., respiratory syncytial v.
Rubarth's disease v., infectious canine hepatitis v.
rubella v., German measles v.; an RNA v. of the genus *Rubivirus;* the agent causing rubella (German measles) in man.
rubeola v., measles v.
Russian autumn encephalitis v., Japanese B encephalitis v.
Russian spring-summer encephalitis v., tick-borne encephalitis v.
Salisbury common cold v.'s, strains of rhinovirus of historical interest because of early studies that established the viral etiology of common colds.
salivary v., salivary gland v., a highly species-specific herpetovirus (cytomegalovirus) with particular affinity for the salivary gland tissue.
sandfly fever v.'s, phlebotomus fever v.'s.
San Miguel sea lion v., a calicivirus, first isolated from sea lions on San Miguel island off the California coast, which is indistinguishable from the vesicular exanthema of swine v. both biophysically and clinically in terms of the vesicular disease syndrome that it produces in swine.
Sendai v., a parainfluenza v. type 1 reported to cause pneumonia in pigs; also used extensively to effect fusion of tissue culture cells.
serum hepatitis v., hepatitis B v.
sheep-pox v., a poxvirus of the genus *Capripoxvirus* causing sheep-pox.
shipping fever v., parainfluenza v. type 3.
Shope fibroma v., rabbit fibroma v.
Simbu v., a serologic group of the genus *Bunyavirus,* comprising 16 species including the type strain, Simbu v.
simian v. (SV), any of a number of v.'s, belonging to various families, isolated from monkeys or from cultures of monkey cells.
simian v. 40 (SV40), vacuolating v.; simian vacuolating v; a small (40 to 45 nm) DNA v. of the genus *Polyomavirus;* the cause of seemingly inapparent infections in monkeys, especially rhesus, and a common contaminant of monkey cell cultures; the v. may cause

inapparent infection in man and may be excreted in stools of children for several weeks; it can produce fibrosarcoma in suckling hamsters, and transformation may occur in rhesus cell culture; it may also form "hybrid" v. in cells also infected with certain adenoviruses.
simian vacuolating v., simian v. 40.
Sindbis v. [village in Egypt where first isolated], the type species of the genus *Alphavirus* and causative agent of Sindbis fever.
slow v., a v., or a virus-like agent, etiologically associated with a slow v. disease.
smallpox v., variola v.
snowshoe hare v., a member of the California group of arboviruses (family Bunyaviridae) causing fever, severe headache, and nausea in man in North America.
soremouth v., contagious ecthyma v. of sheep.
Spondweni v., an arbovirus of the genus *Flavivirus* isolated from mosquitoes in Africa; may cause disease in humans.
St. Louis encephalitis v., a group B arbovirus occurring in the U.S., Trinidad, and Panama; normally present as inapparent infection in man, but sometimes a cause of encephalitis; the v. has been isolated from birds in Panama and from several mosquito species, especially *Psorophora.*
street v., an isolate of rabies v. from a naturally infected domestic animal.
swamp fever v., equine infectious anemia v.
swine encephalitis v., porcine hemagglutinating encephalitis v.; a coronavirus that causes swine encephalitis.
swine fever v., hog cholera v.
swine influenza v.'s, strains of influenza v. type A which cause influenza of swine and can infect man.
swinepox v., a poxvirus distinct from vaccinia v. and the cause of swinepox; the pig louse plays an important role in transmission.
Swiss mouse leukemia v., Friend v.
Tacaribe v., the type v. of the Tacaribe complex of v.'s (arenaviruses), isolated from bats and mosquitoes in Trinidad.
Tahyna v., a California group arbovirus from central Europe, known to infect man.
Teschen disease v., infectious porcine encephalomyelitis v.; a picornavirus causing Teschen disease of pigs; the v. is normally a harmless inhabitant of the intestinal tract, but virulent strains cause epizootics of the disease.
Tete v.'s, a serologic group of the genus *Bunyavirus,* comprising 4 species: Bahig, Matruh, Tete (the type species), and Tsuruse.
TGE v., transmissible gastroenteritis v. of swine.
Theiler's v., Theiler's original v., mouse encephalomyelitis v.
tick-borne encephalitis v., Russian spring-summer encephalitis v.; an arbovirus of the genus *Flavivirus* that occurs in Central Europe and the USSR in two subtypes, causing two forms of encephalitis in man: tick-borne encephalitis (Central European subtype) and tick-borne encephalitis (Eastern subtype); the vectors are ticks of the genus *Ixodes.*
TO v., Theiler's original v. See mouse encephalomyelitis v.
trachoma v., former name for *Chlamydia trachomatis.*
transmissible gastroenteritis v. of swine, TGE v.; a coronavirus that causes transmissible gastroenteritis of swine.
transmissible turkey enteritis v., bluecomb v.; a coronavirus causing bluecomb disease of turkeys.
tumor v., oncogenic v.
turkey meningoencephalitis v., a v. of the genus *Flavivirus* causing paralysis and enteritis in turkeys in Israel.
Turlock v., an unclassified serologic group of arboviruses morphologically like *Bunyavirus* but antigenically unrelated to it.
Umbre v., an arbovirus related serologically to the Turlock v.
vaccine v., see vaccine.
vaccinia v., poxvirus officinalis; the poxvirus (genus *Orthopoxvirus*) used in the immunization of people against variola (smallpox), usually causing a local reaction but sometimes generalized vaccinia, especially in children; the v. is closely related serologically to the v.'s of variola and cowpox, but certain differences have been demonstrated which indicate that they are perhaps distinct but closely related strains of a variola-vaccinia-cowpox complex; the lineage of vaccinia v. is uncertain, and it is very unlikely that it descended from Jenner's original v.
vacuolating v., simian v. 40.
varicella-zoster v., *Herpesvirus varicellae;* chickenpox or herpes zoster v.; a herpetovirus, morphologically identical to herpes simplex v., that causes varicella (chickenpox) and herpes zoster in man; varicella results from a primary infection with the v.; herpes zoster results from secondary invasion by the same v. or by reactivation of infection which in many instances has been latent for many years.
variola v., smallpox v.; a poxvirus of the genus *Orthopoxvirus,* the pathogen of smallpox in man.
VEE v., Venezuelan equine encephalomyelitis v.
Venezuelan equine encephalomyelitis v., VEE v.; a group A arbovirus of the genus *Alphavirus* occurring in Venezuela and several other South American countries, and in Panama and Trinidad, causing Venezuelan equine encephalomyelitis in horses and man; it seems to be more viscerotropic than neurotropic; the natural vector and reservoir host are unknown, but the v. can be transmitted experimentally by mosquitoes.
vesicular exanthema of swine v. (VESV), a calicivirus causing vesicular exanthema of swine. See also San Miguel sea lion v.
vesicular stomatitis v., VS v.; an RNA v. of the genus *Vesiculovirus,* causing vesicular stomatitis in horses, cattle, sheep, and pigs.
viral hemorrhagic fever v., Ebola v.
visceral disease v., cytomegalovirus.
visna v., an RNA v. (subfamily Lentivirinae) that causes visna; it is closely related antigenically to the similar maedi v.
VS v., vesicular stomatitis v.
WEE v., western equine encephalomyelitis v.
Wesselsbron disease v., a mosquito-borne group B arbovirus of the genus *Flavivirus* causing Wesselsbron fever.
West Nile v., an arbovirus of the genus *Flavivirus* reported in Egypt, Uganda, South Africa, Israel, and India, usually occurring as silent infection in humans, especially children, but capable of causing outbreaks of West Nile fever.
western equine encephalomyelitis v., WEE v.; a group A arbovirus of the genus *Alphavirus* occurring in the western United States and parts of South America; it occurs naturally, usually as a symptomless infection in birds, but causes western equine encephalomyelitis in horses and man following transfer by the bites of mosquitoes, chiefly *Culex tarsalis.*
xenotropic v., an oncornavirus that does not produce disease in its natural host and replicates only in tissue culture cells derived from a different species.
Yaba monkey v., a poxvirus, distinct from monkeypox v., that causes Yaba tumors in monkeys.
yellow fever v., an arbovirus, the type species of the genus *Flavivirus,* endemic in tropical Africa south of the Sahara and in tropical South America, occasionally spreading to countries outside these areas; it is the cause of yellow fever of man and other primates; the v. exists in wild primates, and probably also in edentates, marsupials, and rodents, and is transmitted to man by the *Aedes-Haemagogus* complex of tree-top mosquitoes which feed on arboreal mammals.
Zika v. [*Zika,* forest in Uganda, where first isolated]. a mosquito-borne virus of the genus *Flavivirus* (family Togoviridae), found in parts of Africa and in Malaysia, that causes Zika fever.

virusoid (vī′rŭs-oyd) [virus + G. *eidos,* resembling]. A plant pathogen resembling a viroid but having a much larger circular or linear RNA segment and a capsid; it is a satellite agent requiring RNA of an associated virus (helper virus) for replication.

virus shedding. Excretion of virus by any route from the infected host; route and duration of excretion vary according to the pathogenesis of the infection or disease.

vis, pl. **vires** (vis, vī'rēs) [L. force]. Force, energy, or power.
v. a fron'te, a force acting from in front; an obstructive, restraining, or impeding force.
v. a ter'go, a force acting from behind; a pushing or accelerating force.
v. conserva'trix, the inherent power in the organism resisting the effects of injury.
v. vi'tae, v. vita'lis, vitalism.

viscance (vis'kans). A measure of the energy dissipation due to a flow in a viscous system. In medicine and physiology, usually a measure of the energy dissipation in the flow of liquids, sols, or gels within cells and tissues, or of fluids (*e.g.*, blood, respiratory gases) in tubes. The v. is the pressure gradient from one end to the other of the flow path when unit flow occurs. The relationship between viscosity and v. is of the same nature as that between specific resistance, or resistivity, of a conductor material and the resistance of a particular conductor made from that material.

viscera (vis'er-ă). Plural of viscus.

viscerad (vis'er-ad) [viscera + L. *ad,* to]. In a direction toward the viscera.

visceral (vis'er-ăl). Splanchnic; relating to the viscera.

visceralgia (vis-er-al'jē-ă) [viscera + G. *algos,* pain]. Pain in any viscera.

viscerimotor (vis'er-i-mō'ter). Visceromotor.

viscero- [L. *viscus,* pl. *viscera,* the internal organs]. Combining form denoting the viscera. See also splanchno-.

viscerocranium (vis'er-ō-krā'nē-ŭm) [viscero- + cranium]. Splanchnocranium; jaw skeleton; that part of the skull derived from the embryonic pharyngeal arches; it comprises the bones of the facial skeleton.
cartilaginous v., those elements of the fetal skull derived from the second and succeeding pharyngeal arch cartilages.
membranous v., membranous bones, developed in the fetal skull, that overlie maxillary and mandibular components of the first pharyngeal arch cartilage.

viscerogenic (vis'er-ō-jen'ik) [viscero- + G. *-gen,* producing]. Of visceral origin; denoting a number of sensory and other reflexes.

viscerograph (vis'er-ō-graf) [viscero- + G. *graphō,* to write]. An instrument for recording the mechanical activity of the viscera.

visceroinhibitory (vis'er-ō-in-hib'i-tōr-ē). Restricting or arresting the functional activity of the viscera.

visceromegaly (vis'er-ō-meg'ă-lē) [viscero- + G. *megas,* large]. Splanchnomegaly; organomegaly; abnormal enlargement of the viscera, such as may be seen in acromegaly and other disorders.

visceromotor (vis'er-ō-mō'ter). Viscerimotor. **1.** Relating to or controlling movement in the viscera; denoting the autonomic nerves innervating the viscera, especially the intestines. **2.** Denoting a movement having a relation to the viscera; referring to reflex muscular contractions of the abdominal wall in cases of visceral disease.

visceroparietal (vis'er-ō-pă-rī'ĕ-tăl) [viscero- + L. *paries,* wall]. Relating to the viscera and the wall of the abdomen.

visceroperitoneal (vis'er-ō-per-i-tō-nē'ăl). Relating to the peritoneum and the abdominal viscera.

visceropleural (vis'er-ō-plū'răl). Pleurovisceral; relating to the pleural and the thoracic viscera.

visceroptosis, visceroptosia (vis'er-op-tō'sis, -tō'sē-ă) [viscero- + G. *ptōsis,* a falling]. Splanchnoptosis; splanchnoptosia; descent of the viscera from their normal positions.

viscerosensory (vis'er-ō-sen'sōr-ē). Relating to the sensory innervation of internal organs.

visceroskeletal (vis-er-ō-skel'ĕ-tăl). Splanchnoskeletal; relating to the visceroskeleton.

visceroskeleton (vis-er-ō-skel'ĕ-tŏn). **1.** Any bony formation in an organ, as in the heart, tongue, or penis of certain animals; the term also includes, according to some anatomists, the cartilaginous rings of the trachea and bronchi. **2.** Splanchnoskeleton, visceral skeleton; the bony framework protecting the viscera, such as the ribs and sternum, the pelvic bones, and the anterior portion of the skull.

viscerosomatic (vis'er-ō-sō-mat'ik) [viscero- + G. *sōma,* body]. Splanchnosomatic; relating to the viscera and the body.

viscerotome (vis'er-ō-tōm) [viscero- + G. *tomos,* cutting]. An instrument by means of which a section of an organ, *e.g.*, the liver, can be removed from a cadaver for examination without performing a general autopsy.

viscerotomy (vis-er-ot'ō-mē) [viscero- + G. *tomē,* incision]. Dissection of the viscera by incision, especially postmorten.

viscerotonia (vis'er-ō-tō'nē-ă) [viscero- + G. *tonos,* tone]. Personality traits of love of food, sociability, general relaxation, friendliness, and affection.

viscerotrophic (vis'er-ō-trof'ik) [viscero- + G. *trophē,* nourishment]. Relating to any trophic change determined by visceral conditions.

viscerotropic (vis'er-ō-trop'ik) [viscero- + G. *tropē,* a turning]. Affecting the viscera.

viscid (vis'id) [L. *viscidus,* stick, fr. *viscum,* birdlime]. Adhesive; sticky; glutinous.

viscidity (vi-sid'i-tē). Stickiness; adhesiveness.

viscidosis (vis-i-dō'sis). Cystic *fibrosis.*

viscoelasticity (vis'kō-ē-las-tis'i-tē). The property of a viscous material that also shows elasticity.

viscometer (vis-kom'ĕ-ter). Viscosimeter.

viscosimeter (vis-kō-sim'ĕ-ter). Viscometer; an apparatus for determining the viscosity of a fluid; in medicine, usually of the blood.

viscosimetry (vis-kō-sim'ĕ-trē) [viscosity + G. *metron,* measure]. Determination of the viscosity of a fluid, such as the blood.

viscosity (vis-kos'i-tē) [L. *viscositas,* fr. *viscosus,* viscous]. In general, the resistance to flow or alteration of shape, by any substance as a result of molecular cohesion; most frequently applied to liquids as the resistance of a fluid to flow because of a shearing force.
absolute v., force per unit area applied tangentially to a fluid, causing unit rate of displacement of parallel planes separated by a unit distance; units in CGS system: poise.
anomalous v., the viscous behavior of nonhomogenous fluids or suspensions, *e.g.*, blood, in which the apparent v. increases as flow or shear rate decreases toward zero.
apparent v., the v. calculated from Poiseuille's law at any particular flow and tube diameter; it is used for suspensions, such as blood, that exhibit anomalous v. and the Fåhraeus-Lindqvist effect.
dynamic v. (μ)**,** the internal or molecular frictional resistance of a fluid by Newton's law of v. as the ratio of the applied force per unit area to the relative velocity of adjacent fluid layers (produced by the force).
kinematic v. (υ)**,** a measure used in studies of fluid flow; the dynamic viscosity, μ, in poises divided by the density of the material; units: stokes.
newtonian v., the v. characteristics of a newtonian fluid.
relative v., the ratio of the v. of a solution or dispersion to the v. of the solvent or continuous phase.

viscous (vis'kŭs) [see viscid, viscosity]. Viscid; sticky; adhesive;

marked by high viscosity.

viscum (vis'kŭm). **1.** Mistletoe; the berries of *Viscum album* (family Loranthaceae), a parasitic plant growing on apple, pear, and other trees; has been used as an oxytocic. **2.** Herbage of *Phoradendron flavescens,* American mistletoe; has been used as an oxytocic and emmenagoque.

viscus, pl. **viscera** (vis'kŭs, vis'er-ă) [L. the soft parts, internal organs]. An organ of the digestive, respiratory, urogenital, and endocrine systems as well as the spleen, the heart, and great vessels; hollow and multilayered walled organs studied in splanchnology.

visile (viz'il). **1.** Denoting the type of mental imagery in which one recalls most readily that which has been seen. *Cf.* audile; motile. **2.** A person with such mental imagery. **3.** Visual.

vision (vizh'ŭn) [L. *visio,* fr. *video,* pp. *visus,* to see]. The act of seeing. See also sight.
achromatic v., achromatopsia.
binocular v., v. with a single image, by both eyes simultaneously.
blue v., cyanopsia.
central v., direct v.; v. stimulated by an object imaged on the fovea centralis.
chromatic v., chromatopsia.
color v. (VC), chromatopsia.
cone v., photopic v.
direct v., central v.
double v., diplopia.
facial v., sensing the proximity of objects by the nerves of the face, presumed in the case of the blind and also in sighted persons who are blindfolded or in darkness.
green v., chloropsia.
halo v., a condition in which colored or luminous rings are seen around lights.
haploscopic v., stereoscopic v. produced by the haploscope, or mirror-type stereoscope.
indirect v., peripheral v.
multiple v., polyopia.
night v., scotopic v.
oscillating v., oscillopsia.
peripheral v., indirect v.; v. resulting from retinal stimulation beyond the macula.
photopic v., photopia; cone v.; v. when the eye is light-adapted. See light *adaptation;* light-adapted *eye.*
red v., erythropsia.
rod v., scotopic v.
scotopic v., scotopia; rod, night, or twilight v.; v. when the eye is dark-adapted. See also dark *adaptation;* dark-adapted *eye.*
stereoscopic v., stereopsis; the single perception of a slightly different image from each eye.
subjective v., visual impressions that arise centrally and do not originate with ocular stimuli.
triple v., triplopia.
tubular v., tunnel v.; a constriction of the visual field, as though one were looking through a hollow cylinder or tube.
tunnel v., tubular v.
twilight v., scotopic v.
yellow v., xanthopsia.

visna (vis'nă). A chronic meningoencephalitis of sheep caused by a slow virus (subfamily Lentivirinae); it is now considered that visna and maedi are two histopathological and clinical manifestation of the same viral infection.

visual (vizh'ū-ăl) [Late L. *visualis,* fr. *visus,* vision]. Visile (2). **1.** Relating to vision. **2.** Denoting a person who learns and remembers more readily through sight than through hearing.

visualize (vizh'ū-ă-līz). To make visible.

visuoauditory (vizh'yū-ō-aw'di-tōr-ē). Relating to both vision and hearing; denoting nerves connecting the centers for these senses.

visuognosis (vizh'yū-og-nō'sis) [L. *visus,* vision, + G. *gnōsis,* knowledge]. Recognition and understanding of visual impressions.

visuomotor (viz'yū-ō-mō'ter). Denoting the ability to synchronize visual information with physical movement.

visuopsychic (vizh'yū-ō-sī'kik) [L. *visus,* vision, + G. *psychē,* mind]. Pertaining to the portion of the cerebral cortex concerned with the integration of visual impressions.

visuosensory (vizh'yū-ō-sen'sōr-ē). Pertaining to the perception of visual stimuli.

visuospatial (viz'yū-ō-spā'shăl). Denoting the ability to comprehend and conceptualize visual representations and spatial relationships in learning and performing a task.

visuscope (viz'yū-skōp). A modified ophthalmoscope that projects a black star on the patient's fundus.

vital (vīt-ăl) [L. *vitalis,* fr. *vita,* life]. Relating to life.

vitalism (vīt'ăl-izm) [L. *vitalis,* pertaining to life]. Vis vitae or vitalis; the theory that animal functions are dependent upon a special form of energy or force, the vital force, distinct from the physical forces.

vitalistic (vīt'ă-lis'tik). Pertaining to vitalism.

vitality (vīt-al'i-tē). Vital force or energy.

vitalize (vīt'ăl-īz). To endow with vital force.

vitalometer (vī-tă-lom'ĕ-ter). An electrical device for determining the vitality of the tooth pulp.

vital red [C.I. 23570]. Brilliant vital red; trisodium salt of a sulfonated diazo dye (a ditolyl group diazotized to sulfonated aminonaphthalene residues), used as a vital stain.

vitals (vīt'ălz). Viscera.

vitamer (vī'tă-mer). One of two or more similar compounds capable of fulfilling a specific vitamin function in the body; *e.g.,* niacin, niacinamide.

VITAMIN

vitamin (vīt'ă-min) [L. *vita,* life, + amine]. One of a group of organic substances, present in minute amount in natural foodstuffs, that are essential to normal metabolism; insufficient amounts in the diet may cause deficiency diseases.
v. A, (1) any β-ionone derivative, except provitamin A carotenoids, possessing qualitatively the biological activity of retinol; deficiency interferes with the production and resynthesis of rhodopsin, thereby causing night blindness, and produces a keratinizing metaplasia of epithelial cells that may result in xerophthalmia, keratosis, susceptibility to infections, and retarded growth; **(2)** the original v. A, now known as retinol.
v. A_1, retinol.
v. A_1 acid, retinoic acid.
v. A_1 alcohol, retinol.
v. A_1 aldehyde, retinaldehyde.
v. A_2, dehydroretinol.
v. A_2 aldehyde, dehydroretinaldehyde.
antiberiberi v., thiamin.
antihemorrhagic v., v. K.
antineuritic v., thiamin.
antirachitic v.'s, ergocalciferol (v. D_2) and cholecalciferol (v. D_3).
antiscorbutic v., ascorbic acid.
antisterility v., v. E(2).
v. B, a group of water-soluble substances originally considered as one v.
v. B_1, thiamin.

v. B_2, obsolete term for riboflavin.
v. B_3, obsolete term for nicotinamide.
v. B_4, once believed to be a factor necessary for nutrition of the chick, now identified simply as certain essential amino acids and/or adenine.
v. B_5, once used to describe biological activities now ascribed to pantothenic acid or nicotinic acid.
v. B_6, pyridoxine and related compounds (pyridoxal; pyridoxamine).
v. B_{12}, maturation, erythrocyte maturation, antipernicious anemia, or animal protein factor; generic descriptor for compounds exhibiting the biological activity of cyanocobalamin (cyanocob(III)alamin); the antianemia factor of liver extract that contains cobalt, a cyano group, and corrin in a cobamide structure. Several substances with similar formulas and with the characteristic hematinic action have been isolated and designated: B_{12a}, aquacobalamin; B_{12b}, hydroxocobalamin; B_{12c}, nitritocobalamin; B_{12r}, cob(II)alamin; B_{12s}, cob(I)alamin; B_{12III}, factors A and V_{1a} (cobyric acid), and pseudovitamin B_{12}. Vitamins B_{12a} and B_{12b} are known to be tautomeric compounds; B_{12b} has been obtained from cultures of *Streptomyces aureofaciens:* B_{12c} has been obtained from cultures of *Streptomyces griseus* and is distinguishable from B_{12} by differences in its absorption spectrum.
v. B_{12} with intrinsic factor concentrate, a combination of v. B_{12} with suitable preparations of the mucosa of the stomach or intestine of domestic animals used for food by man.
v. B_c conjugase, an enzyme catalyzing the hydrolysis of the pteroylpolyglutamic acids to pteroylmonoglutamic acid, with consequent increase in vitamin activity.
v. B_T, carnitine.
v. B_x, *p*-aminobenzoic acid.
v. B complex, a pharmaceutical term applied to drug products containing a mixture of the B v.'s, usually B_1, B_2, B_3, B_5, and B_6.
v. C, ascorbic acid.
v. D, generic descriptor for all steroids exhibiting the biological activity of ergocalciferol or cholecalciferol, the antirachitic v.'s popularly called the "sun-ray v.'s". They promote the proper utilization of calcium and phosphorus, thereby producing growth in young children, together with proper bone and tooth formation; the sulfate, a water-soluble conjugate, is found in the aqueous phase of human milk.
v. D_2, ergocalciferol.
v. D_3, cholecalciferol (1).
v. E, **(1)** α-tocopherol; **(2)** antisterility v. or factor; fertility v.; generic descriptor of tocol and tocotrienol derivatives possessing the biological activity of α-tocopherol; contained in various oils (wheat germ, cotton-seed, palm, rice) and whole grain cereals where it constitutes the nonsaponifiable fraction, also in animal tissue (liver, pancreas, heart) and lettuce; deficiency produces resorption or abortion in female rats and sterility in males.
v. F, term sometimes applied to the essential unsaturated fatty acids, linoleic, linolenic, and arachidonic acids.
fat-soluble v.'s, those v.'s, soluble in fat solvents (nonpolar solvents) and relatively insoluble in water, marked in chemical structure by the presence of large hydrocarbon moieties in the molecule; *e.g.*, v.'s A, D, E, K.
fertility v., v. E(2).
v. H, obsolete designation for biotin.
v. K, antihemorrhagic v. or factor; generic descriptor for compounds with the biological activity of phylloquinone; fat-soluble, thermostable compounds found in alfalfa, hog liver, fish meal, and vegetable oils, essential for the formation of normal amounts of prothrombin.
v. K_1, v. $K_1(20)$, phylloquinone.
v. K_2, v. $K_2(30)$, menaquinone-6.
v. $K_2(35)$, menaquinone-7.
v. K_4, menadiol diacetate.
v. K_5, 4-amino-2-methyl-1-naphthol; an antihemorrhagic v.
microbial v., a substance necessary for the growth of certain microorganisms, *e.g.*, biotin, *p*-aminobenzoic acid.
v. P, citrin; permeability v.; capillary permeability factor; a mixture of bioflavonoids extracted from plants (especially citrus fruits). It reduces the permeability and fragility of capillaries and is useful in the treatment of certain cases of purpura that are resistant to v. C therapy. See also hesperidin; quercetin; rutin.
permeability v., v. P.
v. U, term given to a factor in fresh cabbage juice that encourages the healing of peptic ulcer; thought to be a methionine derivative.

---

vitellarium (vit'ĕl-lar'ē-ŭm). Vitelline reservoir; in cestodes and trematodes, a common chamber receiving vitelline (yolk) material from the two vitelline ducts; the yolk material then passes into the ootype to surround the ovum with nutritive vitelline granules that are enclosed by a characteristically formed eggshell.
vitelliform (vī-tel'i-fōrm). Relating to or resembling the yolk of an egg.
vitellin (vī-tel'in). Lipovitellin; ovovitellin; a protein combined with lecithin in the yolk of egg.
vitelline (vī-tel'in, -ēn). Relating to the vitellus.
vitellogenesis (vī-tel'lō-jen'ĕ-sis, vī'tĕ-lō-) [L. *vitellus,* yolk, + G. *genesis,* production]. Formation of the yolk and its accumulation in the yolk-sac.
vitellolutein (vī-tel-ō-lū'tē-in). Lutein from the yolk of egg.
vitellorubin (vī-tel-ō-rū'bin). A reddish pigment from the yolk of egg.
vitellose (vī-tel'ōs). A protein fragment from vitellin.
vitellus (vī-tel'ŭs) [L.]. Yolk (1).
v. o'vi, yolk of egg; used in pharmacy for emulsifying oils and camphors.
vitiation (vish-ē-ā'shŭn) [L. *vitiatio* fr. *vitio,* pp. *vitiatus,* to corrupt, fr. *vitium,* vice]. A change that impairs utility or reduces efficiency.
vitiligines (vit-i-lij'i-nēz). Plural of vitiligo.
vitiliginous (vit-i-lij'i-nŭs). Relating to or characterized by vitiligo.
vitiligo, pl. vitiligines (vit-i-lī'gō, vit-i-lij'i-nēz) [L. a skin eruption, fr. *vitium,* blemish, vice]. Leukasmus; acquired leukoderma or leukopathia; piebald skin; the appearance on otherwise normal skin of nonpigmented white patches of varied sizes, often symmetrically distributed and usually bordered by hyperpigmented areas; hair in the affected areas is usually, but not always, white.
v. cap'itis, *alopecia* areata.
Cazenave's v., *alopecia* areata.
Celsus' v., *alopecia* areata.
circumnevic v., halo *nevus.*
v. i'ridis, small white patches in brown irides.
vitiligoidea (vit'i-lī-goy'dē-ă) [vitiligo + G. *eidos,* appearance]. Xanthoma.
vitrectomy (vi-trek'tō-mē) [vitreous + G. *ektomē,* excision]. Removal of the vitreous by means of an instrument which simultaneously removes vitreous by suction and cutting, and replaces it with saline or some other fluid.
anterior v., removal of the central vitreous gel.
posterior v., removal of the posterior cortical vitreous; sometimes the preretinal membranes are removed.
vitrein (vit'rē-in). Vitrosin; a collagen-like protein that, with hyaluronic acid, accounts for the gel state of the vitreous humor.
vitreitis (vit-rē-ī'tis) [L. *vitreus,* glassy, + G. *-itis,* inflammation]. Hyalitis; inflammation of the corpus vitreum.
vitreo- [L. *vitreus,* glassy]. Combining form denoting vitreous.
vitreodentin (vit'rē-ō-den'tin). Dentin of a particular brittle hardness.

vitreoretinal (vit'rē-ō-ret'i-năl). Pertaining to the retina and the corpus vitreum.

vitreoretinopathy (vit'rē-ō-ret'i-nop'ă-thē). Retinopathy with vitreous complications.
exudative v., a familial, slowly progressive ocular disease; characterized by posterior vitreous detachment, vitreous membranes, heterotopia of macula, retinal detachment, neovascularization, and recurrent hemorrhage.

vitreous (vit'rē-ŭs) [L. *vitreus,* glassy, fr. *vitrum,* glass]. **1.** Glassy; resembling glass. **2.** *Corpus* vitreum.
persistent anterior hyperplastic primary v., a unilateral congenital abnormality occurring in full-term infants; characterized by a retrolental fibrovascular membrane formed by persistent primary v. with remnants of the hyaloid artery and tunica vasculosa lentis; associated with leukokoria, microphthalmos, shallow anterior chamber, and elongated ciliary processes.
persistent posterior hyperplastic primary v., a unilateral congenital anomaly in full-term infants; associated with a congenital retinal fold and a v. membranous stalk containing remnants of the hyaloid artery.
primary v., the v. first formed in the embryo between the optic cup and the lens vesicle, and later vascularized by the hyaloid artery and its branches.
secondary v., avascular v. formed around the primary v.
tertiary v., v. fibrils derived from the neuroepithelium of the ciliary body and forming the zonula ciliaris.

vitreum (vit'rē-ŭm) [L. ntr. of *vitreus,* glassy]. *Corpus* vitreum.

vitrification (vit'ri-fi-kā'shŭn) [L. *vitrium,* glassy, + *facio,* to make]. Conversion of dental porcelain (frit) to a glassy substance by heat and fusion.

vitriol (vit'rē-ol) [L. *vitreolus,* glassy]. Any of the various salts of sulfuric acid, *e.g.,* blue v. (cupric sulfate), green v. (ferrous sulfate), white v. (zinc sulfate).

vitrosin (vit'rō-sin). Vitrein.

vivarium, pl. **vivaria** (vī-var'ē-ŭm, -ă) [L. *vivarius,* pertaining to living creatures]. Quarters in which animals are housed, particularly animals used in medical research.

vivi- [L. *vivus,* alive]. Combining form denoting living, alive.

vividialysis (viv'i-dī-al'i-sis). Removal by dialysis, as by lavage of peritoneal cavity.

vividiffusion (viv'i-di-fyū'zhŭn) [vivi- + diffusion]. A method by which circulating blood may be submitted to dialysis outside the body and returned to the circulation without exposure to the air or to any noxious influences; the principle used in the performance of renal dialysis with the artificial kidney.

vivification (viv'i-fi-kā'shŭn) [L. *vivifico,* pp. *-atus,* fr. *vivus,* alive, + *facio,* to make]. Revivification (2).

viviparity (viv'i-păr'i-tē). Zoogony; the quality or state of being viviparous, *i.e.,* producing offspring that are living at the time of birth.

viviparous (vī-vip'ă-rŭs) [vivi- + L. *pario,* to bear]. Zoogonous; giving birth to living young, in distinction to oviparous.

viviperception (viv'i-per-sep'shŭn) [vivi- + perception]. Observation of the vital processes in the organism without the aid of vivisection.

vivisect (viv-i-sekt'). To practice vivisection.

vivisection (viv-i-sek'shŭn) [vivi- + section]. Any cutting operation on a living animal for purposes of experimentation; often extended to denote any form of animal experimentation.

vivisectionist, vivisector (vi-vi-sek'shŭn-ist, vi-vi-sek'tŏr, -tōr). One who practices vivisection.

Vladimiroff, Vladimir D., Russian surgeon, 1837–1903. See Mikulicz-V. or V.-Mikulicz *amputation.*

VLDL Abbreviation for very low density lipoprotein. See lipoprotein.

VMA Abbreviation for vanillylmandelic acid.

VMC Abbreviation for void metal composite.

V.M.D. See D.V.M.

V-MI Abbreviation for Volpe-Manhold Index.

vocal (vō'kăl) [L. *vocalis*]. Pertaining to the voice or the organs of speech.

Vogel's law. See under law.

Voges, Otto, German physician, *1867. See V.-Proskauer *reaction.*

Vogt, Alfred, Swiss ophthalmologist, 1879–1943. See V.-Koyanagi *syndrome.*

Vogt, Cécile, German neurologist, 1875–1962. See V. *syndrome.*

Vogt, Heinrich, German neurologist, *1875. See Spielmeyer-V. *disease.*

Vogt, Karl, German physiologist, 1817–1895. See V.'s *angle.*

Vogt, Oskar, German neurologist, 1870–1959. See V. *syndrome.*

Vohwinkel syndrome. See under syndrome.

voice (voys) [L. *vox*]. The sound made by air passing out through the larynx and upper respiratory tract, the vocal cords being approximated and made tense.
amphoric v., amphorophony; a v. sound having a hollow, blowing character, heard over a pulmonary cavity when the patient speaks or whispers.
bronchial v., bronchophony.
cavernous v., the hollow or metallic v. sound heard over a pulmonary cavity.
epigastric v., the delusion of a v. proceeding from the epigastrium.
eunuchoid v., high pitched v. in the adult male resembling the v. of an immature boy; usually functional in origin.
myxedema v., the forced, rough, raucous v. of subjects of myxedema, probably due to myxedematous thickening of the vocal cords.

void (voyd). To evacuate urine or feces.

void metal composite (VMC). A porous metal structure that enables tissue growth within the openings to establish long-term attachment between prosthesis and tissue.

Voigt, Christian A., Austrian anatomist, 1809–1890. See V.'s *lines.*

vola (vō'lă) [L.]. Palm of the hand or sole of the foot.

volar vō'lăr). Referring to the vola; denoting either the palm of the hand or sole of the foot.

volaris (vō-lā'ris) [NA]. Volar.

volatile (vol'ă-til). **1.** Tending to evaporate rapidly. **2.** Tending toward violence, explosiveness, or rapid change.

volatilization (vol'ă-til-i-zā'shŭn) [fr. L. *volatilis,* volatile, fr. *volo,* pp. *volatus,* to fly]. Evaporation.

volatilize (vol'ă-til-īz). Evaporate.

Volhard, Franz, German physician, 1872–1950. See V.'s *test.*

volition (vō-lish'ŭn) [L. *volo,* fut. p. *voliturus,* to wish]. The conscious impulse to perform any act or to abstain from its performance; voluntary action.

volitional (vo-lish'ŭn-ăl). Done by an act of will; relating to volition.

Volkmann, Alfred W., German physiologist, 1800–1877. See V.'s *canals.*

Volkmann, Richard, German surgeon, 1830–1889. See V.'s *cheilitis, contracture, spoon.*

volley (vol'ē) [Fr. *volée,* fr. L. *volo,* to fly]. A synchronous group of impulses induced simultaneously by artificial stimulation of either nerve fibers or muscle fibers.

Vollmer, Herman, U.S. pediatrician, 1896–1959. See V. *test.*

Volpe-Manhold Index (V-MI). An index for comparing the amount of dental calculus in individuals.

volsella (vol-sel'ă) [see vulsella]. Vulsella *forceps.*

volt (V, v) vōlt) [Allesandro *Volta,* It. physicist, 1745–1827]. The unit of electromotive force; the electromotive force that will produce a current of 1 ampere in a circuit that has a resistance of 1 ohm.

voltage (vōl'tej). Electromotive force, pressure, or potential expressed in volts.

voltaic (vōl-tā'ik). Galvanic.

voltaism (vōl'tă-izm). Galvanism.

voltameter (vōl-tam'ĕ-ter) [volt + G. *metron,* measure]. An apparatus for measuring the strength of a galvanic current by its electrolytic action.

voltampere (vōlt'am-pēr). A unit of electrical power; the product of 1 volt by 1 ampere; equivalent to 1 watt or $^1/_{1000}$ kilowatt.

voltmeter (vōlt'mē-ter). An apparatus for measuring the electromotive force or difference of potential.

Voltolini, Friedrich E.R., German laryngologist, 1819–1889. See V.'s *disease.*

volume (V) (vol'yŭm) [L. *volumen,* something rolled up, scroll, fr. *volvo,* to roll]. Space occupied by matter, expressed usually in cubic millimeters, cubic centimeters, liters, etc. See also capacity.

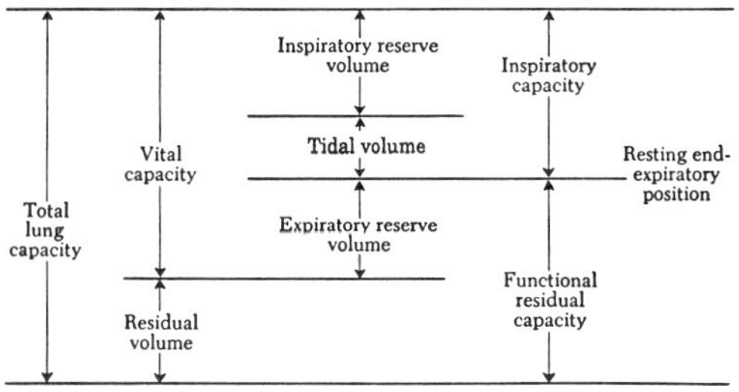

Nomenclature of Lung Volumes

atomic v., the atomic weight of an element divided by its density in the solid state; the v. of the gram-atomic weight of a solid element.

closing v. (CV), the lung v. at which the flow from the lower parts of the lungs becomes severely reduced or stops during expiration, presumably because of airway closure; measured by the sharp rise in expiratory concentration of a tracer gas that had been inspired at the beginning of a breath that started from residual volume.

distribution v., the v. throughout which an added tracer substance appears to have been evenly distributed, calculated by dividing the amount of tracer added by its concentration after equilibration.

end-diastolic v., the amount of blood in the ventricle immediately before a cardiac contraction begins; a measurement of cardiac filling between beats, *i.e.,* diastolic function.

end-systolic v., the amount of blood in the ventricle at the end of the cardiac ejection period and immediately preceding the beginning of ventricular relaxation; a measurement of the adequacy of cardiac emptying, *i.e.,* systolic function.

expiratory reserve v. (ERV), supplemental or reserve air; the maximal v. of air (about 1000 ml) that can be expelled from the lungs after a normal expiration.

forced expiratory v. (FEV, with subscript indicating time interval in seconds), the maximal v. that can be expired in a specific time interval when starting from maximal inspiration.

inspiratory reserve v. (IRV), complemental air; the maximal v. of air that can be inspired after a normal inspiration; the inspiratory capacity less the tidal v.

mean cell v. (MCV), the average v. of red cells, calculated from the hematocrit and the red cell count, in erythrocyte indices.

minute v., the v. of any fluid moved per minute; *e.g.,* the cardiac output or the respiratory minute v.

packed cell v., the v. of the blood cells in a sample of blood after it has been centrifuged in the hematocrit; normally, it amounts to 45% of the blood sample.

partial v., the actual v. occupied by one species of molecule or particle in a solution; the reciprocal of the density of the molecule.

residual v. (RV), residual air or capacity; the v. of air remaining in the lungs after a maximal expiratory effort.

respiratory minute v., the minute v. of breathing; the product of tidal v. times the respiratory frequency. See pulmonary *ventilation.*

resting tidal v., the tidal v. under normal conditions, *i.e.,* in the absence of exercise or other conditions that stimulate breathing.

standard v., the v. of a perfect gas at standard temperature and pressure, 22.414 liters.

stroke v., stroke output; the v. pumped out of one ventricle of the heart in a single beat.

tidal v. (V_T), tidal air; the v. of air that is inspired or expired in a single breath during regular breathing.

volumenometer (vol'yū-mĕ-nom'ĕ-ter) [volume + G. *metron,* measure]. Volumometer; a device for determining the volume of a solid by measuring the amount of liquid it displaces.

volumetric (vol-yū-met'rik). Relating to measurement by volume.

volumometer (vol-yū-mom'ĕ-ter). Volumenometer.

voluntary (vol'ŭn-tār-ē) [L. *voluntarius,* fr. *voluntas,* will, fr. *volo,* to wish]. Relating or acting in obedience to the will; not obligatory.

voluptuous (vō-lŭp'tyū-ŭs) [L. *voluptuosus,* fr. *voluptas,* pleasure]. Causing or caused by sensual pleasure; given to gratification of the senses.

volute (vō-lūt) [L. *voluta,* a scroll, fr. *volvo,* pp. *volutus,* to roll]. Rolled up; convoluted.

volutin (vol'ū-tin). Volutin granules; a nucleoprotein complex found as cytoplasmic granules in certain bacteria, yeasts, and protozoa (such as trypanosome flagellates) which serves as food reserves. Sometimes called metachromatic *granules* (2).

Volvox (vol'voks) [L. *volvo,* to roll]. A genus of highly organized colonial green flagellates of the class Phytomastigophorea.

volvulosis (vol-vū-lō'sis). Onchocerciasis.

volvulus (vol'vyū-lŭs) [L. *volvo,* to roll]. A twisting of the intestine causing obstruction.

gastric v., twisting of the stomach that may result in obstruction and impairment of the blood supply to the organ; it can occur in paraesophageal hernia and occasionally in eventration of the diaphragm.

vomer, gen. **vomeris** (vō'mer, vō'mer-is) [L. ploughshare] [NA]. A flat bone of trapezoidal shape forming the inferior and posterior portion of the nasal septum; it articulates with the sphenoid, ethmoid, two maxillae, and two palatine bones.

v. cartilagin'eus, *cartilago* vomeronasalis.

vomerine (vō'mer-ēn). Relating to the vomer.

vomerobasilar (vō'mer-ō-bas'i-lăr). Relating to the vomer and the base of the skull.

vomeronasal (vō'mer-ō-nā'săl). Relating to the vomer and the nasal bone.

vomica (vom'i-kă) [L. an ulcer, boil, fr. *vomo,* to vomit]. **1.** Vomicus; profuse expectoration of purulent matter. **2.** Obsolete term for a pulmonary cavity containing pus.

vomicose (vom'i-kōs) [L. *vomica,* an ulcer]. Profusely suppurating, as by many ulcers.

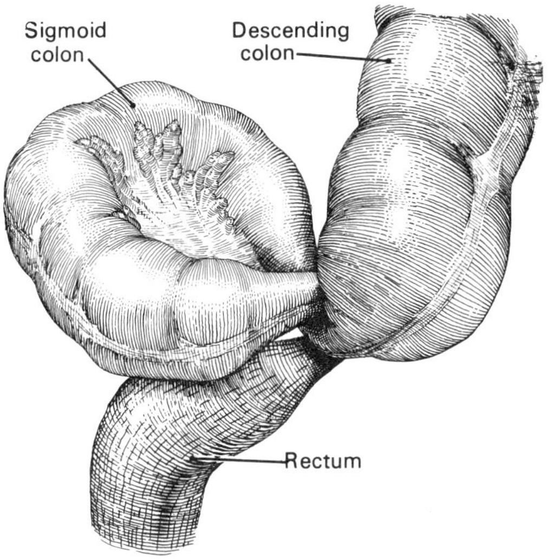

Volvulus

vomicus (vom'i-kŭs) [L.]. Vomica (1).

vom'it [L. *vomo,* pp. *vomitus,* to vomit]. **1.** To eject matter from the stomach through the mouth. **2.** Vomitis (2) the matter so ejected.
Barcoo v., attacks of nausea and vomiting accompanied by bulimia affecting those living in the interior of the southern part of Australia.
black v., coffee-ground v.; vomitus niger; the coffee-ground-colored material that is vomited, specifically, in severe yellow fever.
coffee-ground v., black v.

vomiting (vom'i-ting). Emesis; vomition; vomitus (1); the ejection of matter from the stomach through the esophagus and mouth.
dry v., retching.
epidemic v., epidemic nausea; nausea and v. that attacks a group of people (*e.g.,* in a school or small community) suddenly and without prodromal illness or malaise, is intense while it lasts, but ceases abruptly after a few hours or a day or so; symptoms are headache, abdominal pain, giddiness, and diarrhea in most of the cases, and extreme prostration in about 75%; probably one of several expressions of infection by gastroenteritis virus type A.
fecal v., stercoraceous v.; copremesis; ejection of fecal matter which has entered the stomach from the intestine, usually because of intestinal obstruction.
morning v., v. occurring on rising or immediately after breakfast in some women during early pregnancy.
pernicious v., uncontrollable v.
v. of pregnancy, v. occurring in the early months of pregnancy.
projectile v., expulsion of the contents of the stomach with great force.
psychogenic v., v. associated with emotional distress and anxiety, occurring usually during meals but without weight loss.
retention v., v. due to mechanical obstruction, usually hours after ingestion of a meal.
stercoraceous v., fecal v.

vomition (vō-mish'ŭn) [L. *vomitio,* fr. *vomo,* to vomit]. Vomiting.

vomitive (vom'i-tiv). Emetic.

vomitory (vom'i-tōr-ē). Emetic (2).

vomiturition (vom'i-tū-rish'ŭn). Retching.

vomitus (vom'i-tŭs) [L. a vomiting, vomit]. **1.** Vomiting. **2.** Vomit (2).
v. cruen'tes, hematemesis.
v. mari'nus, seasickness.
v. ni'ger, black *vomit.*

von. Often abbreviated to v. For names with this prefix not found here, see under the principal part of the name.

von Ebner, Victor, Austrian histologist, 1842–1925. See imbrication or incremental *lines* of v. E.; E.'s *glands, reticulum.*

von Economo, Constantin, Austrian neurologist, 1876–1931. See v. E.'s *disease.*

von Hippel, Eugen, German ophthalmologist, 1867–1939. See Hippel's *disease;* v. H.-Lindau *disease, syndrome.*

von Kossa, Julius, 19th century Austro-Hungarian pathologist. See v. K. *stain.*

von Schrötter, Leopold, Austrian laryngologist, 1837-1908. See Paget-von S. syndrome.

von Willebrand, E.A., Finnish physician, 1870–1949. See v. W.'s *disease, syndrome.*

Voorhees, James D., U.S. obstetrician, 1869–1929. See V. *bag.*

Voorhoeve, N., 20th century Dutch radiologist. See V.'s *disease.*

vortex, pl. **vortices** (vōr'teks, vōr'ti-sēz) [L. whirlpool, whorl, fr. *verto* or *vorto,* to turn around]. **1.** Verticil. **2.** Whorl (5). **3.** V. lentis.
v. coccyge'us, coccygeal whorl; a spiral arrangement of coarse hairs sometimes present over the region of the coccyx.
v. cor'dis [NA], whorl (2); a spiral arrangement of muscular fibers at the apex of the heart.
v. len'tis, vortex (3); one of the stellar figures on the surface of the lens of the eye.
vor'tices pilo'rum [NA], hair whorls; a spiral arrangement of the hairs, as at the crown of the head.

Vorticella (vōr-ti-sel'ă) [Mod. L. dim. of L. *vortex,* a whorl]. A genus of Ciliata of the order Peritrichida, of bell shape and with a spiral of cilia around the adoral zone; various free-living species have been found at times in the feces, urine, and mucous discharges.

vortices (vōr'ti-sēz). Plural of vortex.

vorticose (vōr'ti-kōs) [L. *vorticosus,* fr. *vortex,* a whorl]. Arranged in a whorl.

Vossius, Adolf, German pathologist, 1855–1925. See V.'s lenticular *ring.*

voussure (vū-sūr') [Fr.]. Prominence of the precordium due to enlargement of the heart during childhood.

vox (voks) [L.]. Voice.
v. cholera'ica, a peculiar, hoarse, almost inaudible, voice of a sufferer in the last stage of Asiatic cholera.

voxel (vok'sel). A contraction for volume element, which is the basic unit of CT reconstruction; represented as a pixel in the display of the CT image.

voyeur (vwah-yer'). One who practices voyeurism.

voyeurism (vwah-yer'izm) [Fr. *voir,* to see]. Scopophilia; the practice of obtaining sexual pleasure by looking, especially at the naked body or genitals of another or at erotic acts between others.

VP Abbreviation for vasopressin; variegate *porphyria.*

VR Abbreviation for vocal *resonance.*

VS Abbreviation for volumetric *solution.*

VU Abbreviation for volume *unit.*

vulgaris (vŭl-gā'ris) [L. fr. *vulgus,* a crowd]. Ordinary; of the usual type.

Vulpian, Edme F.A., French physician, 1826–1887. See V.'s *atrophy, effect.*

vulsella, vulsellum (vŭl-sel'ă, -lŭm) [L. pincers, fr. *vello,* pp. *vulsus,* to pluck]. Vulsella *forceps.*

vulva, pl. **vul'vae** (vŭ'vă) [L. a wrapper or covering, seed covering, womb, fr. *volvo,* to roll]. *Pudendum* femininum [NA]; pudendum muliebre; pudendum; cunnus; trema (2); the external genitalia of the female, comprised of the mons pubis, the labia majora and minora, the clitoris, the vestibule of the vagina and its glands, and the opening of the urethra and of the vagina.

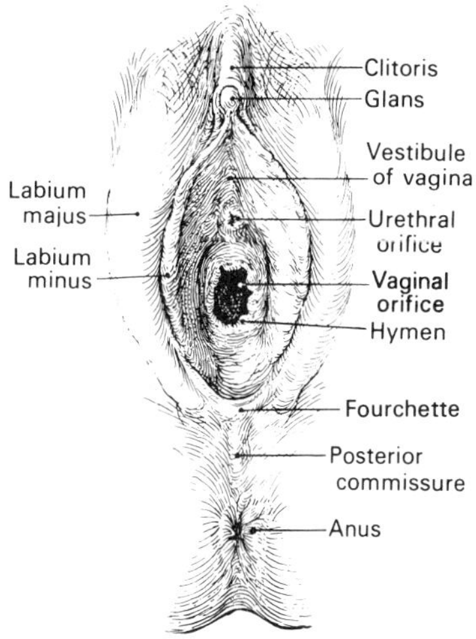

Vulva (Pudendum Femininum)

vulvar, vulval vŭl'văr, vŭl'văl). Relating to the vulva.

vulvectomy (vŭl-vek'tō-mē) [vulva + G. *ektomē,* excision]. Excision (either partial, complete, or radical) of the vulva.

vulvismus (vŭl-viz'mŭs). Vaginismus.

vulvitis (vŭl'vī'tis) [vulva + G. *-itis,* inflammation]. Inflammation of the vulva.

chronic atrophic v., an inflammation of atrophic vulvar skin, usually with severe pruritus.

chronic hypertrophic v., elephantiasis vulvae; swelling of the vulval tissues due to lymphatic obstruction; in some cases it may be caused by filariasis, with induration or ulceration of the skin.

follicular v., inflammation of the vulvar follicles.

leukoplakic v., *leukoplakia* vulvae.

vulvo- [L. *vulva*]. Combining form denoting the vulva.

vulvocrural (vŭl'vō-krū'răl). Relating to the vulva and the clitoris.

vulvouterine (vŭl-vō-yū'ter-in). Relating to the vulva and the uterus.

vulvovaginal (vŭl-vō-vaj'i-năl). Relating to the vulva and the vagina.

vulvovaginitis (vŭl'vō-vaj-i-nī'tis). Inflammation of both vulva and vagina, or of the vulvovaginal glands.

Vvedenskii. Alternate surname of *Wedensky,* Nikolai I.

V-Y-plasty. V-Y procedure; lengthening of tissues in one direction by incising in the lines of a V, sliding the two segments apart, and closing in the lines of a Y.

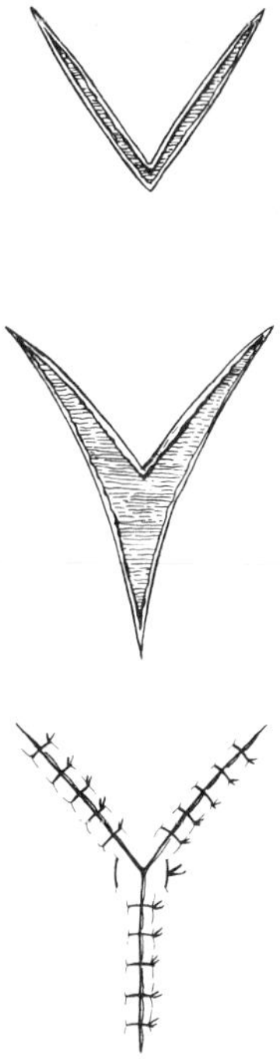

V-Y plasty

W

W Symbol for tungsten; watt.

Waage, P., Norwegian chemist, 1833–1900. See Guldberg-W. *law.*

Waaler, E., Norwegian pathologist. See Rose-W. *test.*

Waardenburg, Petrus Johannes, Dutch ophthalmologist, *1886. See W. *syndrome.*

Wachendorf, Eberhard J., German botanist and anatomist, 1702–1758. See W.'s *membrane.*

Wachstein, Max, U.S. histologist and pathologist, 1905–1965. See W.-Meissel *stain* for calcium-magnesium-ATPase.

Wachter, Herman J.G., German pathologist, *1878. See Bracht-W. *lesion.*

Wada, J.A., 20th century Japanese-Canadian neurologist. See W. *test.*

wadding (wahd'ing). Carded cotton or wool in sheets, used for surgical dressings.

waddle (wod'l). To walk with a side-to-side, swaying motion; occurring in pseudohypertrophic muscular dystrophy and certain other nervous conditions.

wafer (wā'fer). A thin sheet of dried flour paste, used to enclose a powder, the wafer being moistened and folded over the drug, so that it can be swallowed without taste.

Wagner, Hans, Swiss ophthalmologist, *1905. See W.'s *disease, syndrome.*

Wagstaffe, William W., English surgeon, 1843–1910. See W.'s *fracture.*

waist (wāst) [A.S. *waext*] The portion of the trunk between the ribs and the pelvis.

w. of the heart, in the chest x-ray, the middle segment of the cardiac silhouette, containing the pulmonary salient.

Walcher, Gustav A., German obstetrician, 1856–1935. See W. *position.*

Waldenström, Jan G., Swedish physician, *1906. See W.'s *macroglobulinemia, purpura, syndrome, test.*

Waldeyer (Waldeyer-Hartz), Heinrich W.G. von, German anatomist and pathologist, 1836–1921. See W.'s *fossae, glands,* zonal *layer,* throat *ring, sheath, space, tract.*

walk. 1. To move on foot. **2.** The characteristic manner in which one moves on foot. See also gait.

Walker, A. Earl, U.S. neurologist, *1907. See W. *tractotomy;* Dandy-W. *syndrome.*

Walker, J.T. Ainslie, British chemist, 1868–1930. See Rideal-W. *coefficient, method.*

Walker, James, British gynecologist, *1916. See W.'s *chart.*

Walker carcinoma, Walker carcinosarcoma. See under carcinosarcoma.

wall (wawl) [L. *vallum*]. An investing part enclosing a cavity such as the chest or abdomen, or covering a cell or any anatomical unit. See also paries.

anterior w. of middle ear, *paries* caroticus cavi tympani.

anterior w. of stomach, *paries* anterior ventriculi.

anterior w. of vagina, *paries* anterior vaginae.

axial w.'s of the pulp chambers, the w.'s parallel with the long axis of a tooth: the mesial, distal, buccal, and lingual w.'s.

carotid w. of middle ear, *paries* caroticus cavi tympani.

cavity w., one of the surfaces bounding a cavity.

cell w., the outer layer or membrane of some animal and plant cells; in the latter it is mainly cellulose.

chest w., thoracic w.; in respiratory physiology, the total system of structures outside the lungs that move as a part of breathing; it includes the rib cage, diaphragm, abdominal w., and abdominal contents.

enamel w., in dentistry, the part of the w. of a cavity consisting of enamel.

external w. of cochlear duct, *paries* externus ductus cochlearis.

inferior w. of orbit, *paries* inferior orbitae.

inferior w. of tympanic cavity, *paries* jugularis cavi tympani.

jugular w. of middle ear, *paries* jugularis cavi tympani.

labyrinthine w. of middle ear, *paries* labyrinthicus cavi tympani.

lateral w. of middle ear, *paries* membranaceus cavi tympani.

lateral w. of orbit, *paries* lateralis orbitae.

mastoid w. of middle ear, *paries* mastoideus cavi tympani.

medial w. of middle ear, *paries* labyrinthicus cavi tympani.

medial w. of orbit, *paries* medialis orbitae.

membranous w. of middle ear, *paries* membranaceus cavi tympani.

membranous w. of trachea, *paries* membranaceus tracheae.

w. of nail, *vallum* unguis.

parietal w., the body w. or the somatopleure from which it is formed.

posterior w. of middle ear, *paries* mastoideus cavi tympani.

posterior w. of stomach, *paries* posterior ventriculi.

posterior w. of vagina, *paries* posterior vaginae.

pulpal w., (1) one of the w.'s of the pulp cavity; **(2)** the w. of a cavity preparation adjacent to the pulp space; *e.g.,* mesial pulpal w.

splanchnic w., the w. of one of the viscera or the splanchnopleure from which it is formed.

superior w. of orbit, *paries* superior orbitae.

tegmental w. of middle ear, *paries* tegmentalis cavi tympani.

thoracic w., chest w.

tympanic w. of cochlear duct, *paries* tympanicus ductus cochlearis.

vestibular w. of cochlear duct, *paries* vestibularis ductus cochlearis.

Wallenberg, Adolf, German physician, 1862–1949. See W.'s *syndrome.*

Waller, Augustus V., British physiologist, 1816–1870. See wallerian *degeneration, law.*

wallerian (waw-ler'ē-an). Relating to or described by A.V. Waller.

wall-eye (wawl'ī). **1.** Exotropia. **2.** Absence of color in the iris, or leukoma of the cornea.

Walthard, Max, Swiss gynecologist, 1867–1933. See W.'s cell *rest.*

Walther, 19th century German surgeon and gynecologist. See W.'s *dilator.*

Walther, August F., German anatomist, 1688–1746. See W.'s *canals, ducts, ganglion, plexus.*

wandering (wahn'der-ing) [A.S. *wandrian,* to wander]. Moving about; not fixed; abnormally motile.

Wang, Chung T., Chinese pathologist, 1889–1931. See W.'s *test.*

Wangensteen, Owen H., U.S. surgeon, *1898. See W. *drainage, suction, tube.*

Wangiella (wang-gē-el'ă). A dematiaceous genus of fungi characterized by phialides without collarettes, a black yeastlike colony with yeast forms, and later hyphae; the fungi grow well at 40°C. *W. dermatitidis* is an etilogical agent of phaeohyphomycosis.

warble (war'bl) [M. Sw. *varbulde,* boil]. Small swelling in the skin on the back of cattle caused by the presence of larvae of *Hypoderma bovis* or *H. lineatum,* the so-called warble flies.

Warburg, Otto, German biochemist and Nobel laureate, 1883–

1970. See W.'s *apparatus*, old yellow *enzyme*, *theory;* W.-Lipmann-Dickens *shunt;* Barcroft-W. *apparatus, technique.*

Ward, Frederick O., British osteologist, 1818–1877. See W.'s *triangle.*

Ward, O.C., 20th century pediatrician. See Romano-W. *syndrome.*

ward (wōrd) [A.S. *weard*] A room or hall in a hospital containing a number of beds. See also unit.

Wardrop, James, British surgeon, 1782–1869. See W.'s *disease, method.*

warfarin sodium (war'fă-rin) [*W*isconsin *A*lumni *R*esearch *F*oundation + coum*arin*] [[3-(α-Acetonylbenzyl)-2-oxo-2*H*-1-benzopyran-4-yl]oxy]sodium; an anticoagulant with the same actions as dicumarol; also used as a rodenticide; also available as the potassium salt, with the same actions and uses.

warm-blooded (wărm'blŭd-ed). Homeothermic.

Warren, W. Dean, U.S. surgeon, *1924. See W. *shunt.*

wart (wōrt). Verruca.

anatomical w., postmortem w.
asbestos w., asbestos *corn.*
cattle w.'s, infectious *papilloma* of cattle.
common w., *verruca* vulgaris.
digitate w., *verruca* digitata.
fig w., *condyloma* acuminatum.
filiform w., *verruca* filiformis.
flat w., *verruca* plana.
fugitive w., a transitory w.; one that does not persist.
genital w., *condyloma* acuminatum.
Henle's w.'s, Hassall-Henle *bodies.*
infectious w.'s, *verruca* vulgaris.
moist w., *condyloma* acuminatum.
mosaic w., plantar growth of numerous closely aggregated w.'s forming a mosaic appearance.
necrogenic w., postmortem w.
Peruvian w., *verruga* peruana.
pitch w., a precancerous keratotic epidermal tumor, common among workers in pitch and coal tar derivatives. See pitch-worker's *cancer.*
plane w., *verruca* plana.
plantar w., verruca plantaris; a w. on the sole, often painful.
pointed w., *condyloma* acuminatum.
postmortem w., a tuberculous warty growth (tuberculosis cutis verrucosa) on the hand of one who performs postmorten examinations. Also called verruca necrogenica; anatomical, dissection, postmortem, or prosector's tubercle; anatomical, necrogenic, or prosector's w.
prosector's w., postmortem w.
seborrheic w., seborrheic *keratosis.*
senile w., solar *keratosis.*
soft w., skin *tag.*
soot w., the precancerous lesion of chimney sweep's cancer.
telangiectatic w., angiokeratoma.
tuberculous w., *tuberculosis* cutis verrucosa.
venereal w., *condyloma* acuminatum.
viral w., *verruca* vulgaris.

Wartenberg, Robert, German neurologist, 1887–1956. See W.'s *symptom.*

Warthin, Aldred S., U.S. pathologist, 1866–1931. See W.'s *tumor;* W.-Finkeldey *cells;* W.-Starry silver *stain.*

wartpox (wōrt'poks). *Variola* verrucosa.

warty (wōrt'ē). Relating to or covered with warts.

wash (wosh). A solution used to clean or bathe a part. For types of w.'s, see the specific term; *e.g.,* eyewash, mouthwash.

Wasmann, Adolphus, 19th century German anatomist. See W.'s *glands.*

Wassén, Erik, Swedish physician, *1901. See W. *test.*

Wassermann, August P. von, German bacteriologist, 1866–1925. See W. *antibody, reaction, test;* provocative W. *test.*

Wassermann-fast. A term used to designate a case in which the Wassermann reaction remains positive despite all treatment.

wasting (wāst'ing). **1.** Emaciation. **2.** Denoting a disease characterized by emaciation.

salt w., inappropriately large renal excretion of salt despite the apparent need of the body to retain it.

water (wah'ter) [A.S. *waeter*]. **1.** H_2O; a clear, odorless, tasteless liquid, solidifying at 32°F (0°C and R), and boiling at 212°F (100°C, 80°R), that is present in all animal and vegetable tissues and dissolves more substances than any other liquid. **2.** Euphemism for urine. **3.** Aromatic w.; a pharmacopeial preparation of a clear saturated aqueous solution (unless otherwise specified) of volatile oils, or other aromatic or volatile substances, prepared by processes involving distillation or solution (agitation followed by filtration).

w. of adhesion, w. held by molecular attraction in contact with solid surfaces, but not forming an essential part of their constitution.
alkaline w., a w. that contains appreciable amounts of the bicarbonates of calcium, lithium, potassium, or sodium.
aromatic w., w. (3).
baryta w., a saturated aqueous solution of barium hydroxide; used as an alkaline reagent.
bitter w., a natural mineral w. containing Epsom salt.
black w., *azoturia* of horses.
bound w., w. held to colloids and other substances and not removed by simple filtration.
bromine w., a w. containing the bromides of magnesium, potassium, or sodium in therapeutic amounts.
calcic w., a w. containing appreciable quantities of calcium salts in solution.
carbonated w., carbonic w., w. that contains a considerable amount of carbonic acid in solution.
carbon dioxide-free w., purified w. that has been boiled vigorously for 5 minutes or more.
chalybeate w., a w. that contains salts of iron in appreciable quantities.
chlorine w., a w. that contains the chlorides of sodium, potassium, calcium, and magnesium in varying amounts.
w. of combustion, w. of metabolism.
w. of constitution, w. held by a unit of structure as an essential part of its constitution, though not an ingredient of its molecules. See w. of crystallization.
w. of crystallization, w. of constitution that unites with certain salts and is essential to their arrangement in crystalline form; *e.g.,* $CuSO_4 \cdot 5H_2O$.
distilled w., w. purified by distillation.
earthy w., a w. containing a large amount of mineral matter, chiefly sulfate, in solution.
free w., w. in the body that can be removed by ultrafiltration and in which substances can be dissolved.
gentian aniline w., gentian violet with saturated aniline w., a more effective stain than simple gentian violet.
hard w., w. containing ions, such as Mg^{2+} and Ca^{2+}, that form insoluble salts with fatty acids so that ordinary soap will not lather in it.
heavy w., deuterium oxide; D_2O; w. in which most of the hydrogen atoms are deuterium, or heavy hydrogen (^2H), with properties that differ noticeably from those of ordinary w.
indifferent w., a mineral w. containing only a small quantity of saline matter.
w. for injection, w. purified by distillation for the preparation of products for parenteral use.
w. of metabolism, w. of combustion; the w. formed in the body by

oxidation of the hydrogen of the food, the greatest amount being produced in the metabolism of fat (about 117 g/100 g of fat).
mineral w., w. that contains appreciable amounts of certain salts, which give it therapeutic properties.
potable w., a w. fit for drinking, being free from contamination and not containing a sufficient quantity of saline material to be regarded as a mineral w.
purified w., w. obtained by distillation or deionization.
saline w., a w. that contains neutral salts (chlorides, bromides, iodides, sulfates) in appreciable amounts.
Selters w., Seltzer w. [Nieder *Selters,* a mineral spring in Prussia], a mineral w. containing carbonates of sodium, calcium, and magnesium, and chloride of sodium.
soft w., w. lacking those ions, such as Mg^{2+} and Ca^{2+}, that form insoluble salts with fatty acids, so that ordinary soap will lather easily in it.
sulfate w., a w. holding in solution appreciable quantities of the sulfates of calcium, magnesium, or sodium.
sulfur w., a w. containing hydrogen sulfide or the metallic sulfides.

waterfall (wah'ter-fawl). Sluice; a term used to describe flow in vascular beds where lateral pressure tending to collapse vessels greatly exceeds venous pressure. Flow is independent of venous pressure and occurs only when arterial pressure exceeds lateral pressure; likened to flow making a waterfall from a sluice or spillway over a dam, with arterial pressure being height of water behind the dam, lateral pressure being spillway height, and venous pressure being height of outflow stream below the dam.

Waterhouse, Rupert, British physician, 1873–1958. See W.-Friderichsen *syndrome.*

waterpox (wah'ter-poks). Varicella.

Waters, Charles Alexander, U.S. radiologist, 1888-1961. See W.'s view *roentgenogram.*

Waters, Edward G., U.S. obstetrician and gynecologist, *1898. See W.'s *operation.*

waters (wah'ters). Colloquialism for amniotic *fluid.*
bag of w., colloquialism for the amniotic sac and contained amniotic fluid.
false w., a leakage of fluid prior to or in beginning labor, before the rupture of the amnion.

watershed. 1. The area of marginal blood flow at the extreme periphery of a vascular bed. **2.** Slopes in the abdominal cavity formed by projections of the lumbar vertebrae and the pelvic brim which determine the direction in which a free effusion will gravitate when the body is in a supine position.

Waterston, David J., British thoracic and pediatric surgeon, *1910. See W. *shunt.*

Watson, James D., U.S. geneticist and Nobel laureate, 1928. See W.-Crick *helix.*

Watsonius watsoni (waht'sō'nē-ŭs waht-sō'nī). An amphistome intestinal fluke of primates in west Africa and east Asia (Singapore).

watt (waht) [James *Watt,* Scot. engineer, 1736–1819]. The SI unit of electrical power; the power available when the current is 1 ampere and the electromotive force is 1 volt; equal to 1 joule (10^7 ergs) per second or 1 voltampere.

wave (wāv) [A.S. *wafian,* to fluctuate]. **1.** A movement of particles in an elastic body, whether solid or fluid, whereby an advancing series of alternate elevations and depressions, or expansions and condensations, is produced. **2.** The elevation of the pulse, felt by the finger, or represented graphically in the curved line of the sphygmograph. **3.** The complete cycle of changes in the level of a source of energy that is repetitively varying with respect to time; in the electroencephalogram the w. is essentially a voltage-time graph. See also entries under rhythm.
A w., **(1)** the initial negative deflection in the electroretinogram, presumably reflecting retinal photoreceptor activity; **(2)** an atrial deflection in an electrocardiogram recorded from within the atrium of the heart.
acid w., acid *tide.*
alkaline w., alkaline *tide.*
alpha w., alpha *rhythm.*
arterial w., a w. in the jugular phlebogram due to transmission of carotid artery pulsation.
B w., the initial positive deflection in the electroretinogram, possibly arising from the inner nuclear layer of the retina.
beta w., beta *rhythm.*
brain w., colloquialism for electroencephalogram.
C w., a monophasic positive deflection in the electroretinogram arising in the pigment epithelium of the retina.
cannon w., an exaggerated A w. in the jugular pulse caused by right atrial contraction occurring after ventricular contraction has closed the tricuspid valve, as in ventricular premature beats and in complete heart block.
D w., a positive or negative deflection in the electroretinogram occurring when a light stimulus is removed (off-response).
delta w., **(1)** a slurring of the initial part of the upstroke of the R wave in the Wolff-Parkinson-White syndrome; **(2)** delta *rhythm.*
dicrotic w., recoil w.; the second rise in the tracing of a dicrotic pulse.
electrocardiographic w., a deflection of special shape and extent in the electrocardiogram representing the activity of a portion of the heart muscle.
excitation w., a w. of altered electrical conditions that is propagated along a muscle fiber preparatory to its contraction.
F w., FF w.'s, regular rapid atrial w.'s in the electrocardiogram characterizing atrial flutter.
f w., ff w.'s, fibrillary or flutter fibrillation w.'s; irregular undulations of the base line in the electrocardiogram, characterizing atrial fibrillation.
fibrillary w.'s, f w.'s.
flat top w.'s, activity in the electroencephalogram having a pattern suggesting a flat top; these w.'s are often found in temporal lobe discharges.
fluid w., a sign of free fluid in the abdominal cavity; percussion on one side of the abdomen transmits a w. that is felt on the opposite side.
flutter-fibrillation w.'s, ff w.'s.
microelectric w.'s, microwaves.
overflow w., the descending w. of the sphygmogram from the apex to the first anacrotic break.
P w., the first complex of the electrocardiogram, representing depolarization of the atria; if the P w. is retrograde or ectopic in form; it is labeled P′.
percussion w., the main positive w. of an arterial pulse tracing.
phrenic w., diaphragm *phenomenon.*
postextrasystolic T w., the T w. of the sinus beat immediately following an extrasystole.
pulse w., the progressive expansion of the arteries occurring with each contraction of the left ventricle of the heart.
Q w., the initial deflection of the QRS complex when such deflection is negative (downward).
R w., the first positive (upward) deflection of the QRS complex in the electrocardiogram; successive upward deflections within the same QRS complex are labeled R′, R″, etc.
random w.'s, w.'s in the electroencephalogram which occur paroxysmally and asynchronously.
recoil w., dicrotic w.
retrograde P w., the P w. pattern in the electrocardiogram representing retrograde depolarization of the atria, the impulse spreading from the A-V node upward.

S w., a negative (downward) deflection of the QRS complex following an R w; successive downward deflections within the same QRS complex are labeled S′, S″, etc.
sonic w.'s, audible sound w.'s, as distinguished from ultrasonic w.'s.
supersonic w.'s, see supersonic.
T w., the next deflection in the electrocardiogram following the QRS complex; represents ventricular repolarization.
theta w., theta *rhythm.*
tidal w., the w. between the percussion w. and the dicrotic w. in the downward limb of the arterial pulse tracing.
Traube-Hering w.'s, Traube-Hering *curves.*
U w., a positive w. following the T w. of the electrocardiogram.
ultrasonic w.'s, the periodic configuration of energy produced by sound having a frequency greater than 20,000 Hz.
V w., a large pressure w. visible in recordings from either the atrium or the incoming veins, normally produced by venous return but becoming very large when blood regurgitates through the A-V valve beyond the chamber from which the recording is made.

wavelength (wāv′length). The distance from one point on a wave (shaped like a sine curve) to the next point in the same phase; *i.e.,* from peak to peak or from trough to trough.

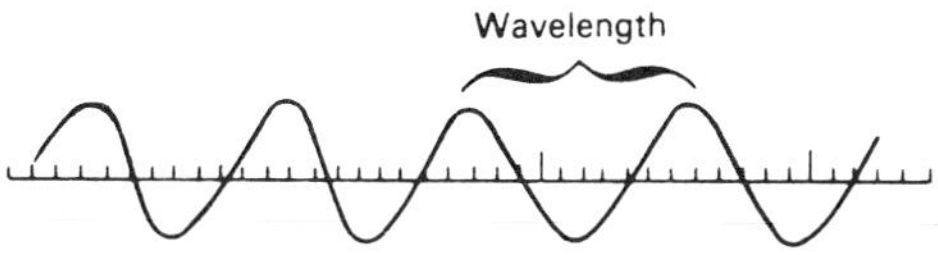

Wavelength

wavenumber (wāv′nŭm-ber). The number of waves per centimeter (cm^{-1}), used to simplify the large and unwieldy numbers heretofore used to designate frequency.

waveshape (wāv′shāp). Wave *form.*

wax (waks) [A.S. *weax*]. **1.** Cera; beeswax; a thick, tenacious substance, plastic at room temperature, secreted by bees for building the cells of their honeycomb. **2.** Any substance with physical properties similar to those of beeswax, of animal, vegetable, or mineral origin (oils, lipids, or fats that are solids at room temperature). **3.** Esters of high-molecular-weight fatty acids with monohydric or dihydric alcohols (aliphatic or cyclic), that are solid at room temperature.
animal w., beeswax, spermaceti, and any w. derived from the animal kingdom.
baseplate w., a hard pink w. used in dentistry for making occlusion rims.
bleached w., white w.
bone w., Horsley's bone w.; a mixture of antiseptic agents, oil, and w. used to stop bleeding by plugging bone cavities or haversian canals, especially of the skull.
boxing w., w. used for boxing impressions. See also boxing.
Brazil w., carnauba w.
carnauba w., Brazil or palm w.; a w. obtained from the Brazilian w. palm, *Copernica cerifera.*
casting w., inlay wax; any soft solid w. used in dentistry for patterns of all types and for many other purposes; most are basically paraffin but are modified by addition of gum dammar, carnauba w., or other ingredients, to meet various requirements.
Chinese w., **(1)** a vegetable w.; **(2)** a w. secreted by a scale insect, *Coccus ceriferus* or *C. pela,* and deposited in the twigs of a species of ash trees; used in China to make candles and also medicinally.
ear w., cerumen.
earth w., ceresin.
emulsifying w., a washable ointment base consisting of a mixture of cetostearyl alcohol, sodium lauryl sulfate, and water.
grave w., adipocere.
Horsley's bone w., bone w.
inlay w., casting w.
Japan w., a vegetable w. derived from *Rhus succedanea* and *Toxicodendron verniciferum.*
mineral w., **(1)** paraffin w.; **(2)** ceresin.
palm w., carnauba w.
paraffin w., mineral w. (1); a w. derived from petroleum.
vegetable w., palm w. or any w. derived from plants such as the bayberry.
white w., white beeswax; bleached w.; yellow w. bleached by being rolled very thin and exposed to the light and air, or bleached by chemical oxidants; same uses as yellow w.
yellow w., a yellowish, solid, brittle substance prepared from the honeycomb of the bee, *Apis mellifera;* the chief constituent is myricin (myricyl palmitate); others are cerotic acid (cerin), melissic acid, heptacosane, and hentriacontane; used in the preparation of ointments, cerates, plasters, and suppositories.

waxing, waxing-up (wak′sing). The contouring of a pattern in wax, generally applied to the shaping in wax of the contours of a trial denture or a crown prior to casting in metal.

Way, Stanley, British obstetrician-gynecologist. See Stanley Way *procedure.*

Wb Symbol for weber.

WBC Abbreviation for white blood *cell;* red *blood count.*

WDLL Abbreviation for well differentiated lymphocytic *lymphoma.*

wean (wēn) [A.S. *wenian*]. To implement weaning.

weaning (wēn′ing). **1.** Ablactation; permanent deprivation of breast milk and commencement of nourishment with other food. **2.** Gradual withdrawal of a patient from dependency on a life support system.

weanling (wēn′ling). A young animal that has become adjusted to food other than its mother's milk.

wear (wār). Wasting or deterioration caused by friction.
occlusal w., attritional loss of substance on opposing occlusal units or surfaces. See also abrasion (3).

web [A.S.]. A tissue or membrane bridging a space. See also tela.
esophageal w., a cribriform or w. formation in the esophagus caused by an irregular atrophy.
terminal w., a network of actin filaments in the apical end of columnar epithelial cells which anchor in the zonula adherans.

webbing (web′ing). Congenital condition apparent when adjacent structures are joined by a broad band of tissue not normally present to such a degree.

Weber, Ernst H., German physiologist and anatomist, 1795–1878. See W.'s *experiment, glands, law, paradox; test* for hearing; W.-Fechner *law.*

Weber, Frederick Parkes, British physician, 1863–1962. See W.-Christian *disease;* W.-Cockayne *syndrome;* Rendu-Osler-W. *disease, syndrome;* Sturge-Kalischer-W. *syndrome;* Sturge-W. *disease, syndrome;* Klippel-Trenaunay-W. *syndrome.*

Weber, Sir Hermann, English physician, 1823–1918. See W.'s *sign, syndrome.*

Weber, Moritz I., German anatomist, 1795–1875. See W.'s *organ.*

Weber, Wilhelm E., German physicist, 1804–1891. See W.'s *point, triangle.*

weber (Wb) (web′er). SI unit of magnetic flux, equal to volt-seconds (V·s).

Webster, John, British chemist, 1878–1927. See W.'s *test.*

Webster, John C., U.S. gynecologist, 1863–1950. See W.'s *operation.*

Wechsler, David, U.S. psychologist, *1896. See W. intelligence *scales;* W.-Bellevue *scale.*

Wedensky (Vvedenskii), Nikolai I., Russian neurophysiologist, 1852–1922. See W. *effect, facilitation, inhibition.*

wedge (wej) [A.S. *weeg*] A solid body having the shape of an acute-angled triangular prism.

dental w., a double inclined plane used for separating the teeth, maintaining the separation once obtained, or holding a matrix in place.

WEE Abbreviation for western equine *encephalomyelitis.*

Weeks, John E., U.S. ophthalmologist, 1853–1949. See W.'s *bacillus;* Koch-W. *bacillus, conjunctivitis.*

Wegener, F., 20th century German pathologist. See W.'s *granulomatosis.*

Wegner, Friedrich R.G., German pathologist, 1843–1917. See W.'s *disease, line.*

Weibel, Ewald R., 20th century Swiss physician. See W.-Pelade *bodies.*

Weichselbaum, Anthony, Austrian pathologist, 1845–1920. See W.'s *coccus;* Fraenkel-W. *pneumococcus.*

Weidel, Hugo, Austrian chemist, 1849–1899. See W.'s *reaction.*

Weigert, Carl, German pathologist, 1845–1904. See W.'s *law,* iodine *solution, stains;* W.-Gram *stain.*

weight (wāt) [A.S. *gewiht*] The product of the force of gravity, defined internationally as 980.665 cm/s^2, times the mass of the body.

atomic w. (AW, at wt), the mass in grams of 1 mole (6.02×10^{23}, atoms) of an atomic species; the mass of an atom of a chemical element in relation to the mass of an atom of carbon-12 (^{12}C), which is set equal to 12.000, thus a ratio and therefore dimensionless (although the actual mass, numerically the same, is sometimes expressed in daltons); not necessarily the w. of any individual atom of an element, since most elements are made up of several isotopes of different masses; *e.g.,* the atomic w. of chlorine is 35.457, because it is composed of ^{35}Cl and ^{37}Cl in proportions that give an average of 35.457. See also molecular w.

birth w., in humans, the first w. of an infant obtained within less than the first 60 completed minutes after birth; a full-size infant is one weighing 2500 g or more; a low birth w. is considered to be less than 2500 g.

combining w., gram *equivalent.*

equivalent w., gram *equivalent.*

gram-atomic w., atomic w. expressed in grams. *Cf.* mole.

gram-molecular w., molecular w. expressed in grams. *Cf.* mole.

molecular w. (MW, mol wt), molecular w. ratio; the sum of the atomic w.'s of all the atoms constituting a molecule; the mass of a molecule relative to the mass of a standard atom, now ^{12}C (taken as 12.000). See also atomic w.

weightlessness (wāt'les-nes). The psychophysiologic effect of zero-gravity, as experienced by someone falling freely in a vacuum (*e.g.,* astronauts in a stable orbit). A temporary state of simulated w. can be achieved during powered flight within the earth's atmosphere by traversing an inverted parabolic curve where gravitational pull and centrifugal force cancel each other out.

Weil, Adolf, German physician, 1848–1916. See W.'s *disease,* Larrey-W. *disease.*

Weil, Edmund, Austrian physician, 1880–1922. See W.-Felix *reaction, test.*

Weil, Ludwig A., German dentist, 1849–1895. See W.'s basal *layer, zone.*

Weill, G. See W.-Marchesani *syndrome.*

Weill, Jean, French physician. See Leri-W. *disease, syndrome.*

Weinberg, Michel, French pathologist, 1868– 1940. See W.'s *reaction.*

Weinberg, Wilhelm, German physician, 1862–1937. See Hardy-W. *equilibrium, law.*

Weingrow's reflex. See under reflex.

Weir, Robert F., U.S. surgeon, 1838–1927. See W.'s *operation.*

Weir Mitchell. See Mitchell, Silas Weir.

Weisbach, Albin, Austrian anthropologist, 1837–1914. See W.'s *angle.*

Weismann, August F.L., German biologist, 1834–1914. See weismannism; W.'s *theory.*

weismannism (vīs'man-izm). The concepts of heredity introduced by August Weismann. See Weismann's *theory.*

Weiss, Nathan, Austrian physician, 1851–1883. See W.'s *sign.*

Weiss, Soma, U.S. physician, 1898–1942. See Charcot-W.-Baker *syndrome;* Mallory-W. *lesion, syndrome, tear.*

Weitbrecht, Josias, German-Russian anatomist in St. Petersburg, 1702–1747. See W.'s *cartilage, cord, fibers, foramen, ligament.*

Welander, Lisa, Swedish neurologist, *1909. See Kugelberg-W. *disease;* Wohlfart-Kugelberg-W. *disease.*

Welch, William H., U.S. pathologist, 1850–1934. See W.'s *bacillus.*

Welcker, Hermann, German anthropologist and anatomist, 1822–1898. See W.'s *angle.*

Wells, G.C., 20th century British dermatologist. See W.'s *syndrome.*

Wells, M. See Muckle-W. *syndrome.*

welt [O.E. *waelt*]. Wheal.

wen [A.S.]. Old term for pilar *cyst.*

Wenckebach, Karel F., Dutch internist, 1864–1940. See W. *period, phenomenon.*

Wenzel, Joseph, German anatomist and physiologist, 1768–1808. See W.'s *ventricle.*

Wepfer, Johann J., 1620–1695. See W.'s *glands.*

Werdnig, Guido, Austrian neurologist, *1862. See W.-Hoffmann *disease.*

Werlhof, Paul G., German physician, 1699–1767. See W.'s *disease.*

Wermer, Paul, U.S. internist, 1898–1975. See W.'s *syndrome.*

Wernekinck (Werneking), Friedrich C.G., German anatomist and physician, 1798–1835. See W.'s *commissure, decussation.*

Werner, F.F., early 20th century German chemist. See W.'s *test.*

Werner, Otto, German physician, *1879. See W.'s *syndrome.*

Wernicke, Karl, German neurologist, 1848–1905. See W.'s *aphasia, area, center, disease, encephalopathy, field, radiation, reaction, region, sign, syndrome, zone;* W.-Korsakoff *encephalopathy, syndrome.*

Wertheim, Ernst, Austrian gynecologist, 1864–1920. See W.'s *operation.*

Werther, J. 20th century German physician. See W.'s *disease.*

West, Charles, British physician, 1816–1898. See W.'s *syndrome.*

Westberg, Friedrich, 19th century German physician. See W.'s *space.*

Westergren, Alf, Swedish physician, *1891. See W. *method.*

Westphal, Karl F.O., German neurologist, 1833–1890. See W.'s *disease, phenomenon, pseudosclerosis,* pupillary *reflex, sign;* W.-Erb *sign;* W.- Piltz *phenomenon;* W.-Strümpell *pseudosclerosis;* Edinger-W. *nucleus;* Strümpell-W. disease.

Wetzel, Norman C., U.S. pediatrician, *1897. See W. *grid.*

Wever, Ernest Glen, U.S. psychologist, *1902. See W.-Bray *phenomenon.*

Weyers, Helmut, 20th century German pediatrician. See W.-Thier *syndrome,* Meyer-Schwickerath and W. *syndrome.*

Wharton, Thomas, British anatomist and physician, 1614–1673. See W.'s *duct, jelly.*

whartonitis (hwar-tŏn-ī'tis). Inflammation of the submaxillary (Wharton's) duct.

wheal (hwēl) [A.S. *hwēle*]. Welt; a circumscribed, evanescent area of edema of the skin, appearing as an urticarial lesion, slightly reddened, often changing in size and shape and extending to adjacent areas, and usually accompanied by intense itching; produced by intradermal injection or test, or by exposure to allergenic substances in susceptible persons; also encountered in dermatitis herpetiformis (Darier's sign).

wheat germ oil (hwēt jerm). An oil obtained by expression from the germ of the wheat seed, *Triticum aestivum* (family Gramineae); one of the richest sources of natural vitamin E; used as a nutritional supplement.

Wheatstone, Charles, British physicist, 1802–1875. See W.'s *bridge.*

wheel (hwēl). A circular frame or disk designed to revolve around an axis.
Burlew w., Burlew *disk.*

Wheeler, Henry Lord, U.S. chemist, 1867–1914. See under W.-Johnson *test.*

Wheeler, John M., U.S. ophthalmologist, 1879–1938. See W. *method.*

Wheeler-Johnson test. See under test.

Wheelhouse, Claudius G., British surgeon, 1826–1909. See W.'s *operation.*

wheeze (hwēz) [A.S. *hwēsan*]. **1.** To breathe with difficulty and noisily. **2.** A whistling, squeaking, or puffing sound made by air passing through the fauces, glottis, or narrowed tracheobronchial airways in difficult breathing.
asthmatoid w., Jackson's sign; a puffing sound heard in front of the patient's open mouth in a case of foreign body in the trachea or a bronchus.

whelp (hwelp) [A.S.]. The act of a female dog (bitch) of giving birth to puppies.

whey (hwā) [A.S. *hwaeg*] Serum lactis; the watery part of milk remaining after the separation of the casein.
alum w., w. produced by curdling milk by means of powdered alum.
w. protein, see under protein.

whiplash (hwip'lash). See whiplash *injury.*

Whipple, Allen O., U.S. surgeon, 1881–1963. See W.'s *operation.*

Whipple, George H., U.S. pathologist and Nobel laureate, 1878–1976. See W's *disease.*

whipworm (hwip'werm). See *Trichuris trichiura.*

whisky, whiskey (hwis'kē) [Gael, *usquebaugh,* water of life]. Spiritus frumenti; an alcoholic liquid obtained by the distillation of the fermented mash of wholly or partly malted cereal grains, containing 47 to 53% by volume of C_2H_5OH, at 15.56°C; it must have been stored in charred wood containers for not less than 2 years. The various grains used in the manufacture of w. are barley, maize, rye, and wheat.

whisper (hwis'per) [A.S. *hwisprian*]. To speak without phonation.

whistle (hwis'l) [A.S. *hwistle*]. **1.** A sharp, shrill sound made by forcing air through a narrow opening. **2.** An instrument for producing a w.
Galton's w., a cylindrical w., attached to a compressible bulb, with a screw attachment that changes the note; used to test the hearing.

White, Paul Dudley, U.S. physician, 1886–1973. See Lee-W. *method,* Wolff-Parkinson-W. *syndrome.*

white (hwīt) [A.S. *hwīt*]. The color resulting from commingling of all the rays of the spectrum; the color of chalk or of snow.
w. of eye, the visible portion of the sclera.

Whitehead, Walter, British surgeon, 1840–1913. See W. *deformity;* W.'s *operation.*

whitehead (hwīt'hed). **1.** Milium. **2.** Closed *comedo.*

whitepox (hwīt'poks). Alastrim.

whites (hwīts). Colloquialism for leukorrhea or blennorrhea.

whiting (hwīt'ing). Chalk ($CaCO_3$) used for polishing metals or plastic appliances.

whitlow (hwit'lō) [M.E. *whitflawe*]. Felon.
herpetic w., painful herpes simplex virus infection of a finger, often accompanied by lymphangitis and regional adenopathy, lasting up to several weeks; most common in physicians, dentists, and nurses as a result of exposure to the virus in a patient's mouth.
melanotic w., subungual *melanoma.*
thecal w., suppurative lesion of distal phalanx; may involve tendon sheath and bone.

Whitman, Royal, U.S. surgeon, 1857–1946. See W.'s *frame.*

Whitmore, Alfred, British surgeon, 1876–1946. See W.'s *bacillus.*

Whitnall, Samuel E., British anatomist, 1876–1952. See W.'s *tubercle.*

whoop (hūp, hwūp). The sonorous inspiration in pertussis with which the paroxysm of coughing terminates, due to spasm of the larynx (glottis).
systolic w., systolic *honk.*

whooping cough (hūp'ing, hwūp'ing). Pertussis.

whorl (hwerl). **1.** A turn of the spiral cochlea of the ear. **2.** See *vortex* cordis. **3.** A turn of a concha nasalis. **4.** Verticil. **5.** Vortex (2); an area of hair growing in a radial manner suggesting whirling or twisting. See *vortices* pilorum. **6.** Digital w.; one of the distinguishing patterns comprising Galton's system of classification of fingerprints.
coccygeal w., *vortex* coccygeus.
digital w., whorl (6).
hair w.'s, *vortices* pilorum.

whorled (hwerld). Marked by or arranged in whorls. See also verticose; turbinate; convoluted; verticillate.

Wickham, Louis-Frédéric, French dermatologist, 1862–1929. See W.'s *striae.*

Widal, Georges F.I. French physician, 1862–1929. See W.'s *reaction, syndrome;* Gruber-W. *reaction;* Hayem-W. *anemia, syndrome.*

widow's peak. A sharp point of hair growth in the midline of the anterior scalp margin, usually resulting from recession of hair of the temple areas, or occurring as a congenital configuration of scalp hair.

width. Wideness; the distance from one side of an object or area to the other.
orbital w., the distance between the dacryon and the farthest point on the anterior edge of the outer border of the orbit (Broca), or between the latter point and the junction of the frontolacrimal suture and the posterior edge of the lacrimal groove.
window w., the amount of CT numbers encompassed by the range of the gray scale in the display of the CT image, ranging from 1 to 500 (or to 1000, depending on the type of machine).

Wiedemann, Hans R. See Beckwith-W. *syndrome.*

Wiener, H. See *tract* of Münzer and W.

Wiethe. See Urbach-Wiethe *disease.*

Wigand, J. Heinrich, German obstetrician and gynecologist, 1766–1817. See W. *maneuver.*

Wilde, Sir William R.W., Irish oculist and otologist, 1815–1876. See W.'s *cords, triangle.*

Wilder, Helenor C., 20th century U.S. scientist. See W.'s *stain* for reticulum.

Wilder, Joseph, U.S. neuropsychiatrist, *1895. See W.'s *law* of initial value.

Wilder, William H., U.S. ophthalmologst, 1860–1935. See W.'s *sign.*

Wildermuth, Hermann A., German psychiatrist, 1852–1907. See W.'s *ear.*

Wildervanck, L.S., 20th century Dutch geneticist. See W. *syndrome.*

wildfire (wīld'fīr). Fogo selvagem.

Wilhelmy, Ludwig F., German scientist, 1812–1864. See W. *balance.*

Wilkie, David P.D., Scottish surgeon, 1882–1938. See W.'s *artery, disease.*

Wilkinson, Daryl S., See Sneddon-W. *disease.*

Willebrand, E.A. von. See von Willebrand.

Willems, Charles, Belgian surgeon, 19th century. See W.'s *method.*

Willett, J. Abernethy, English obstetrician, †1932. See W.'s *clamp, forceps.*

Willi, H. See Prader-W. *syndrome.*

Williams, Anna W., U.S. bacteriologist, 1863–1955. See W.'s *stain;* Park-W. *bacillus, fixative.*

Williams, George A., U.S. obstetrician and gynecologist. See W.'s *operation.*

Williams, J.C.P., 20th century New Zealand cardiologist. See W. *syndrome.*

Williamson, Carl S., U.S. surgeon, 1896–1952. See Mann-W. *operation, ulcer.*

Willis, Thomas, British physician, 1621–1675. See W.'s *cords, pancreas, paracusis, pouch; circle* of W.; *centrum* nervosum.

Williston, Samuel Wendell, U.S. paleontologist, 1852–1918. See W.'s *law.*

willow (wil'ō) [A.S. *welig*] A tree of the genus *Salix;* the bark of several species, especially *S. fragilis,* is a source of salicin.

Wilms, Max, German surgeon, 1867–1918. See W.'s *tumor.*

Wilson, Clifford, British physician, *1906. See Kimmelstiel-W. *disease, syndrome.*

Wilson, Frank Norman, U.S. cardiologist, 1890–1952. See W. *block.*

Wilson, James, British anatomist, physilogist, and surgeon, 1765–1821. See W.'s *muscle.*

Wilson, Miriam G., U. S. pediatrician, *1922. See W.-Mikity *syndrome.*

Wilson, Samuel A. Kinnier, British neurologist, 1878–1937. See W.'s *disease, syndrome.*

Wilson, Sir William J. E., English dermatologist, 1809–1884. See W.'s *disease, lichen.*

Wilson's method. See under method.

windage (win'dej). Wind contusion; internal injury with no surface lesion, caused by collision with the pressure of compressed air or with an object propelled by compressed air.

wind-broken (wind'brō-ken) Heaving; asthmatic; said of a horse.

windburn (wind'bern). Erythema of the face due to exposure to wind.

windgall (wind'gawl). A soft, pulpy swelling in the neighborhood of the fetlock joint of the horse, varying in size from a pinhead to a large hen's egg.

window (win'dō). Fenestra.

aortic w., a radiolucent region below the aortic arch in the left anterior oblique view, formed by the bifurcation of the trachea and traversed by the left pulmonary artery.

cochlear w., *fenestra* cochleae.

oval w., *fenestra* vestibuli.

round w., *fenestra* cochleae.

tachycardia w., in paroxysmal tachycardia of the reentry type, the interval of time (the window) between the earliest and latest premature activation that can excite the paroxysm.

vestibular w., *fenestra* vestibuli.

windpipe (wind'pīp). Trachea.

windpuffs (wind'pŭfs). An affection of horses marked by a collection of synovial fluid between the tendons of the legs, particularly just above the fetlock joint, the prominence appearing on both sides of the tendon; most common in hard-worked animals and may end in lameness.

wine (wīn) [Fr. *vin;* L. *vinum*]. **1.** Vinous liquor; the fermented juice of the grape. **2.** A group of preparations consisting of a solution of one or more medicinal substances in w., usually white w. because of its comparative freedom from tannin. There are no official w.'s.

high w., the strong spirit obtained by rectification or redistillation of low w. in making whisky.

low w., the first weak distillate obtained from the mash in the process of making whisky.

red w., claret; an alcoholic liquor made by fermenting grapes, the fruit of *Vitis vinifera,* with their skins; has been used as a tonic.

sherry w., sherry; a w. of amber color, obtained originally from Jerez, Spain, containing about 20% alcohol; used in preparation of medicinal w.'s.

wing. 1. The anterior appendage of a bird. **2.** In anatomy, ala.

angel's w., a deformity in which both scapulae project conspicuously. See also winged *scapula.*

ashen w., *trigonum* nervi vagi.

w. of crista galli, *ala* cristae galli.

gray w., *trigonum* nervi vagi.

greater w. of sphenoid bone, *ala* major ossis sphenoidalis.

w. of ilium, *ala* ossis illi.

Ingrassia's w., *ala* minor ossis sphenoidalis.

lesser w. of sphenoid bone, *ala* minor ossis sphenoidalis.

w. of nose, *ala* nasi.

w. of sacrum, *ala* sacralis.

w. of vomer, *ala* vomeris.

Winiwarter, Felix von, German surgeon, 1852–1931. See W.-Buerger's *disease.*

wink [A.S. *wincian*]. To close and open the eyes rapidly; an involuntary act by which the tears are spread over the conjunctiva, keeping it moist.

Winkelman, Nathaniel W., U.S. neurologist, 1891–1956. See W.'s *disease.*

Winkler, Max, Swiss physician, 1875–1952. See W.'s *disease.*

Winslow, Jacob B., Danish anatomist, physicist, and surgeon in Paris, 1669–1760. See W.'s *foramen, ligament, pancreas, stars; stellulae* winslowii.

Winterbottom, Thomas M., British physician, 1765–1859. See W.'s *sign.*

wintergreen oil (win'ter-grēn). Gaultheria oil.

Winternitz, Wilhelm, Austrian physician, 1835–1917. See W.'s *sound.*

Wintersteiner, Hugo, Austrian ophthalmologist, 1865–1918. See W. *rosettes.*

Wintersteiner, Oskar, U.S. biochemist, 1898–1972. See W.'s *compounds.*

wire (wīr). Slender and pliable rod or thread of metal.

arch w., archwire.

Kirschner's w., Kirschner's apparatus; an apparatus for skeletal traction in long bone fracture.

ligature w., a soft thin w. of stainless steel used in dentistry to tie an archwire to band attachments or brackets.

separating w., a w. usually of soft brass used to gain separation between teeth. See also separation (2).

wrought w., a w. formed by drawing a cast structure through a die into a desired shape and size; used in dentistry for partial denture clasps and orthodontic appliances.

wiring (wīr'ing). Fastening together the ends of a broken bone by wire sutures.

circumferential w., fixation of mandibular fractures by passing wires around a section of bone with the ends exiting into the oral cavity; *i.e.,* circummandibular and circumzygomatic w.

continuous loop w., Stout's w.; the formation of wire loops on both maxillary and mandibular teeth, for the placement of intermaxillary elastics; used in reduction and fixation of fractures.

craniofacial suspension w., a method of w. using areas of bones not contiguous with the oral cavity for the support of fractured jaw segments (*e.g.,* pyriform aperture, zygomatic arch, zygomatic process of the frontal bone).

Gilmer w., a method of intermaxillary fixation in which single opposing teeth are wired circumferentially, and the wires are twisted together.

Ivy loop w., placement of a wire around two adjacent teeth to provide an attachment for intermaxillary elastics.

perialveolar w., fixing a splint to the maxillary arch by passing a wire through the alveolar process from the buccal plate to the palate.

pyriform aperture w., a method of w. using the nasal bones at the area of the pyriform aperture for the stabilization of fractures of the jaws.

Stout's w., continuous loop w.

Wirsung, Johann G., German anatomist in Padua, 1600–1643. See W.'s *canal, duct.*

wiry (wīr'ē). Resembling or having the feel of a wire; filiform and hard; denoting a variety of pulse.

Wiskott, Arthur, 20th century German pediatrician. See W.-Aldrich *syndrome.*

Wissler, Hans, Swiss pediatrician, *1906. See W.'s *syndrome.*

Wistar, Caspar, U.S. biologist, 1760–1818, after whom the Wistar Institute is named. See W. *rats.*

witch hazel (wich hāz'l). Hamamelis.

withdrawal (with-draw'ăl). **1.** The act of removal or retreating. **2.** A psychological and/or physical syndrome caused by the abrupt cessation of the use of a drug in an habituated individual. **3.** The therapeutic process of discontinuing a drug so as to avoid w. (2). **4.** A pattern of behavior, observed in schizophrenia and depression, characterized by a pathological retreat from interpersonal contact and social involvement, and leading to self-preoccupation.

withers (with'erz) [A.S. *wither,* against]. The region of the back of an animal, particularly of the horse, which lies between the shoulder blades.

fistulous w., a fistula, caused by bacterial infection, of the w.

wit'kop. A favoid condition of the scalp seen in South Africans.

witzelsucht (vit'sel-zŭkht) [Ger. *witzeln,* to affect wit, + *Sucht,* mania]. A morbid tendency to pun, make poor jokes, and tell pointless stories, while being oneself inordinately entertained thereby.

wobble (wah'bl). In molecular biology, unorthodox pairing between the base at the 5′ end of an anticodon and the base that pairs with it (in the 3′ position of the codon); thus, the anticodon 3′-UCU-5′ may pair with 5′AGA-3′ (normal or Watson-Crick pairing) or with 5′-AGG-3′ (wobble). Wobble pairings can occur between the unusual base hypoxanthine and adenine, uracil, or cytosine, between uracil and guanine, and between guanine and uracil, when in the 5′ position of an anticodon.

Wohlfahrtia (vōl-far'tē-ă) [P. *Wohlfahrt,* Ger. medical writer, †1726]. A genus of larviparous dipterous fleshflies (family Sarcophagidae), of which some species' larvae breed in ulcerated surfaces and flesh wounds of humans and animals. Important species include *W. magnifica,* a widely distributed obligatory fleshfly whose tissue-destroying maggots invade wounds or head cavities of domestic animals and humans; *W. nuba,* a facultative fleshfly of Old World distribution, also found in head wounds or head cavities but not in dermal sores; and *W. vigil* (*W. opaca*), which produces cutaneous myiasis in human infants in the northern U.S. and southern Canada by larvae that penetrate the skin and cause infected, boil-like, or furuncular lesions; mink and fox pups in fur farms, and probably rabbits and rodents, are attacked by this species.

wohlfahrtiosis (vōl-far-tē-ō'sis). Infection of animals and man with larvae of flies of the genus *Wohlfahrtia.*

Wohlfart, Gunnar, Swedish neurologist, 1910–1961. See W.-Kugelberg-Welander *disease.*

Wolf, A., 20th century U.S. pathologist. See W.-Orton *bodies.*

Wolfe, John R., Scottish ophthalmologist, 1824–1904. See W.'s *method;* W. *graft;* W.-Krause *graft.*

Wolff, Julius, German anatomist, 1836–1902. See W.'s *law.*

Wolff, Kaspar F., German embryologist in Russia, 1733–1794. See wolffian *body, cyst, duct, rest, ridge, tubules.*

Wolff, Louis, U.S. cardiologist, *1898. See W.-Chaikoff *block, effect;* W.-Parkinson-White *syndrome.*

wolffian (wulf'ē-an). Relating to or described by Kaspar Wolff.

Wölfler, Anton, Bohemian surgeon, 1850–1917. See W.'s *gland.*

wolfram, wolframium (wulf'ram, wulf-ram'ē-ŭm). Tungsten.

Wolfring, Emilj F. von, Polish ophthalmologist, 1832–1906. See W.'s *glands.*

wolfsbane (wulfs'bān). See aconite.

Wollaston, William H., British physician and physicist, 1766–1828. See W.'s *doublet, theory.*

Wolman, M., 20th century Israeli neuropathologist. See W.'s *disease.*

womb (wūm) [A.S. the belly]. Uterus.

falling of the w., *prolapse* of the uterus.

Wood, Robert W., U.S. physicist, 1868–1955. See W.'s *glass, lamp, light.*

wood alcohol (wud). *Methyl* alcohol.

wood wool. A specially prepared, not compressed, wood fiber used for surgical dressings.

wool (wul). Lana; the hair of the sheep; sometimes, when defatted, used as a surgical dressing.

wool alcohols. Wool wax alcohols; may be prepared by saponification of the grease of sheep wool and separation of the fraction that contains cholesterol (not less than 30%) and other alcohols; used to prepare w. a. ointment.

wool fat. Anhydrous lanolin; the purified, anhydrous, fatlike substance obtained from the wool of sheep. See also lanolin and subentries.

hydrous w. f., lanolin.

Woolner, Thomas, British sculptor, 1826–1892. See W.'s *tip.*

word salad (werd sal'ăd). A jumble of meaningless and unrelated words emitted by persons with certain kinds of schizophrenia.

Woringer, M.M.F., 20th century French dermatologist. See W.-Kolopp *disease.*

working out (werk'ing). In psychoanalysis, the state in the treatment process in which the patient's personal history and psychodynamics are uncovered.

working through. In psychoanalysis, the process of obtaining additional insight and personality changes in a patient through repeated and varied examination of a conflict or problem; the interactions between free association, resistance, interpretation, and working out constitute the fundamental facets of this process.

Worm, Ole, Danish anatomist, 1588–1654. See wormian *bones.*

worm (werm) [A.S. *wyrm*]. **1.** In anatomy, any structure resembling a w., *e.g.,* the midline part of the cerebellum. **2.** Lyssa (1). **3.** Term once used to designate any member of the invertebrate group or former subkingdom Vermes, a collective term no longer used taxonomically; now commonly used to designate any member of the separate phyla Annelida (the segmented or true w.'s), the Nematoda (roundworms), and the Platyhelminthes (flatworms). Important species include *Dracunculus medinensis* (dragon, guinea, Medina, or serpent w.), *Enterobius vermicularis* (seat w. or pinworm), *Haemonchus contortus* (stomach, barberpole, or twisted stomach w.), *Loa loa* (African eye w.), *Moniliformis* (phylum Acanthocephala, thorny-headed w.'s), *Oxyspirura mansoni* (Manson's eye w.), *Oxyuris* (animal pinworm), *Pentastomida* (tongue w.), *Stephanurus dentatus* (kidney or lard w. of swine), *Strongylus* (palisade w.), *Syngamus trachea* (gapeworm or forked w.), *Thelazia* (eye w.), *Trichinella spiralis* (pork or trichina w.), and *Trichostrongylus* (hairworm, or bankrupt or black scour w.). For some types of w.'s not listed as subentries here (because they are usually written as one word), see the full name.
caddis w., aquatic larva in the insect order Trichoptera.
fleece w., wool *maggot.*
Manson's eye w., *Oxyspirura mansoni.*
meal w., the larva of beetles of the genus *Tenebrio;* both larvae and adults are important pests, destroying flour, meal, and other cereal products; they are also intermediate hosts of the nematode parasite, *Gongylonema,* and of various tapeworms of the genus *Hymenolepis.*

worm bark. Andira.

wormian (werm'ē-an). Relating to or described by Ole Worm.

Wormley, Theodore G., U.S. chemist, 1826–1897. See W.'s *test.*

wormseed (werm'sēd). **1.** Santonica. **2.** Chenopodium.

wormwood (werm'wud). Absinthium.

wort (wōrt) [A.S. *wyrt,* a plant]. **1.** A suffix in the popular names of many plants, such as liverwort, lungwort, woundwort, etc. **2.** An infusion of malt.

Worth, Claud, British ophthalmologist, 1869–1936. See W.'s *amblyoscope.*

Woulfe, Peter, British chemist, 1727–1803. See W.'s *bottle.*

wound (wūnd). **1.** Trauma to any of the tissues of the body, especially that caused by physical means and with interruption of continuity. **2.** A surgical incision.
abraded w., abrasion (1).
avulsed w., a w. caused by or resulting from avulsion.
blowing w., open *pneumothorax.*
crease w., gutter w.
glancing w., gutter w.
gunshot w., a w. made with a bullet or other missile projected by a firearm.
gutter w., crease or glancing w.; a tangential w. that makes a furrow without perforating the skin.
incised w., a clean cut, as by a sharp instrument.
nonpenetrating w., injury, especially within the thorax or abdomen, produced without disruption of the surface of the body.
open w., a w. in which the tissues are exposed to the air.
penetrating w., a w. with disruption of the body surface that extends into underlying tissue or into a body cavity.
perforating w., a w. with an entrance and exit opening.
puncture w., a w. in which the opening is relatively small as compared to the depth, as produced by a narrow pointed object.
seton w., a tangential perforating w., the entrance and exit openings being on the same side of the body, head, or limb involved.
stab w., a puncture w. produced by the stabbing motion of a knife or similar object.
sucking w., open *pneumothorax.*
tangential w., a perforating w. or seton w. that involves only one side of the part.
traumatopneic w., open *pneumothorax.*

W-plasty. W procedure; surgery to prevent the contracture of a straight-line scar; the edges of the wound are trimmed in the shape of a W, or a series of W's, and closed in a zig-zag manner.

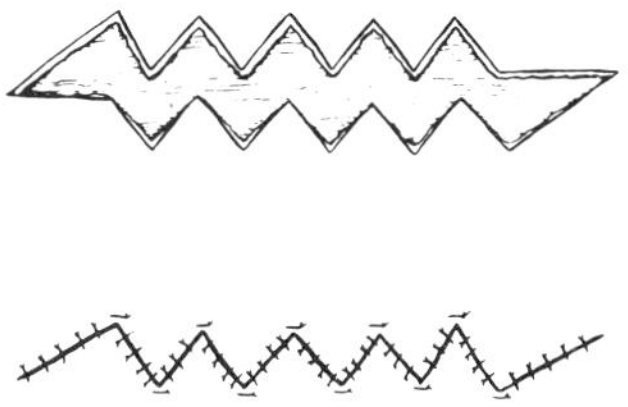

W-plasty

WR Abbreviation for Wassermann *reaction.*

Wr^{a} Abbreviation for Wright antigen. See low frequency blood groups, Blood Groups appendix.

wreath (rēth) [A.S. *wraeth,* a bandage]. A structure resembling a twisted or entwined band or a garland.
ciliary w., *corona* ciliaris.

Wright, Basil Martin, 20th century British physician. See W. *respirometer.*

Wright, James Homer, U.S. pathologist, 1871–1928. See W.'s *stain.*

Wright, Marmaduke Burr, U.S. obstetrician, 1803–1879. See W.'s *version.*

wrightine (rīt'ēn). Conessine.

wrinkle (ring'kl). A furrow, fold, or crease in the skin.

Wrisberg, Heinrich A., German anatomist and gynecologist, 1739–1808. See W.'s *cartilage, ganglia, ligament, nerve, tubercle.*

wrist (rist) [A.S. wrist joint, ankle joint]. Carpus.

wrist-drop. Carpoptosia; carpoptosis; drop hand; paralysis of the extensors of the wrist and fingers from a lesion of the radial nerve or from a polyneuropathy.

wryneck (rī'nek). Torticollis.

Wuchereria (vū-ker-er'ē-ă). A genus of filarial nematodes (family Onchocercidae, superfamily Filarioidea) characterized by adult forms that live chiefly in lymphatic vessels and produce large numbers of embryos or microfilariae that circulate in the bloodstream (microfilaremia), often appearing in the peripheral blood at regular intervals (see nocturnal *periodicity, W. bancrofti*). The extreme form of this infection (wuchereriasis or filariasis) is elephantiasis or pachydermia.

W. bancrof'ti, the bancroftian filaria, a species endemic in South Pacific islands, coastal China, India, and Burma, and throughout tropical Africa and northeastern South America (including certain Caribbean islands); transmitted to man (apparently the only definitive host) by mosquitoes, especially *Culex quinquefasciatus* and *Aedes pseudoscutellaris,* but also by several other species of *Culex, Aedes, Anopheles,* and *Mansonia,* depending on the specific geographic area; adults are white, 40-100 mm cylindroid, threadlike worms, and the microfilariae are ensheathed, with rounded anterior end and tapered, non-nucleated tail; the adult worms inhabit the larger lymphatic vessels (*e.g.,* in the extremities (especially lower), breasts, spermatic cord, and retroperitoneal tissues) and the sinuses of lymph nodes (*e.g.,* the popliteal, femoral, and inguinal groups, and also the epitrochlear and axillary nodes), where they sometimes cause temporary obstruction to the flow of lymph and slight or moderate degrees of inflammation.

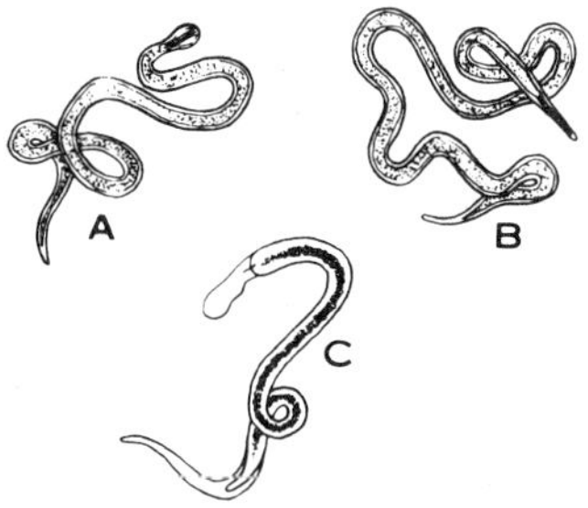

Wuchereria bancrofti
A, male, in man; *B*, female, in man; *C*, ensheathed microfilaria.

W. mala'yi, former name for *Brugia malayi.*

wuchereriasis (vū'ker-ē-rī'ă-sis). Infection with worms of the genus *Wuchereria.* See also filariasis.

Wurster, Casimir, German chemist, 1856–1913. See W.'s *reagent, test.*

Wyatt, W. See Brushfield-Wyatt *disease.*

Wyburn-Mason, R. See W.-M. *syndrome.*

X

X Symbol for Kienbock's *unit;* reactance; xanthosine.

xanchromatic (zan-krō-mat'ik). Xanthochromatic.

xanth-. See xantho-.

xanthelasma (zan-thĕ-laz'mă) [xanth- + G. *elasma,* a beaten metal plate]. Xanthoma.

generalized x., mormolipemic xanthoma planum; xanthoma planum of the neck, trunk, extremities, and eyelids in patients with normal plasma lipid levels.

x. palpebra'rum, *xanthoma* palpebrarum.

xanthelasmatosis (zan'thĕ-laz-mă-tō'sis). Obsolete term for xanthomatosis.

xanthelasmoidea (zan'thĕ-laz-moy'dē-ă) [xanthelasma + G. *eidos,* resemblance]. Obsolete term for *urticaria* pigmentosa.

xanthematin (zan-thēm'ă-tin). A yellow substance derived from hematin by treating with nitric acid.

xanthemia (zan-thē'mē-ă) [xanth- + G. *haima,* blood]. Carotenemia.

xanthene (zan'thēn). The basic structure of many natural products, drugs, dyes (*e.g.,* fluorescein, pyronin, eosins), indicators, pesticides, antibiotics, etc.

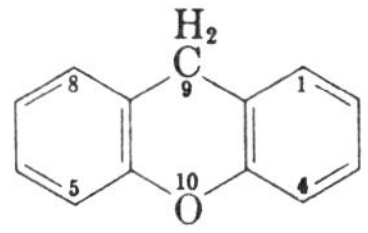

9*H*-Xanthene

xanthic (zan'thik). **1.** Yellow or yellowish in color. **2.** Relating to xanthine.

xanthine (zan'thin). 2,6-Dioxopurine; 2,6(1*H*,3*H*)-purinedione; oxidation product of guanine and hypoxanthine, precursor of uric acid; occurs in many organs and in the urine, occasionally forming urinary calculi.

x. dehydrogenase [EC 1.2.1.37], an oxidoreductase oxidizing x. to uric acid with NAD^+ as the oxidant.

x. nucleotide, *xanthosine* phosphate.

x. oxidase [EC 1.2.3.2], hypoxanthine oxidase; Schardinger enzyme; a flavoprotein containing molybdenum; an oxidoreductase catalyzing oxidation by O_2 of x. to uric acid, producing H_2O_2; also oxidizes hypoxanthine, some other purines and pterins, and aldehydes.

x. ribonucleoside, xanthosine.

xanthinol niacinate, xanthinol nicotinate (zan'thi-nōl). 7-[2-Hyroxy-3-[(2-hydroxyethyl)methylamino]propyl]theophylline compound with nicotinic acid; a peripheral vasodilator.

xanthinuria (zan-thi-nū'rē-ă) [xanthine + G. *ouron,* urine]. Xanthiuria; xanthuria. **1.** Excretion of abnormally large amounts of xanthine in the urine. **2.** A disorder resulting from defective synthesis of xanthine oxidase, characterized by urinary excretion of xanthine in place of uric acid, hypouricemia, and, in some cases, the formation of xanthine stones; autosomal recessive inheritance.

xanthism (zan'thizm) [G. *xanthos,* yellowish]. Rufous albinism; a pigmentary anomaly of blacks, characterized by red or yellow-red hair color, copper-red skin, and often by dilution of iris pigment.

xanthiuria (zan-thē-yū'rē-ă). Xanthinuria.

xantho-, xanth- [G. *xanthos,* yellow]. Combining forms denoting yellow, yellowish.

xanthochroia (zan-thō-kroy'ă). Xanthochromia.

xanthochromatic (zan'thō-krō-mat'ik). Xanthochromic; xanchromatic; yellow-colored.

xanthochromia (zan-thō-krō'mē-ă) [xantho- + G. *chrōma,* color]. The occurrence of patches of yellow color in the skin, resembling xanthoma, but without the nodules or plates. Also called xanthochroia; xanthopathy; xanthoderma (1); cholesteroderma; yellow disease.

xanthochromic (zan-thō-krō'mik). Xanthochromatic.

xanthochroous (zan-thok'rō-ŭs) [xantho- + G. *chroa,* complexion]. Having a fair yellowish complexion; light-skinned; blond.

xanthoderma (zan-thō-der'mă) [xantho- + G. *derma,* skin]. Yellow skin. **1.** Xanthochromia. **2.** Any yellow coloration of the skin.

xanthodont (zan'thō-dont) [xantho- + G. *odous,* tooth]. One who has yellow teeth.

xanthoerythrodermia perstans (zan'thō-ĕ-rith'rō-der'mē-ă per'-stanz). Parapsoriasis.

xanthogranuloma (zan'thō-gran'yū-lō'mă). A peculiar infiltration of retroperitoneal tissue by lipid macrophages, occurring most commonly in women.

juvenile x., nevoxanthoendothelioma; single or multiple reddish papules, usually found in young children, consisting of dermal infiltration by histiocytes and Touton giant cells.

necrobiotic x., a cutaneous and subcutaneous x. with focal necrosis, presenting as multiple large, sometimes ulcerated, nodules (especially around the eyes) associated with paraproteinemia.

xanthogranulomatous (zan'thō-gran'yū-lō'mă-tŭs). Relating to, of the nature of, or affected by xanthogranuloma.

xanthoma (zan-thō'mă) [xantho- + G. *-oma,* tumor]. Xanthelasma; vitiligoidea; a yellow nodule or plaque, especially of the skin, composed of lipid-laden histiocytes.

x. diabetico'rum, eruptive x. associated with severe diabetes.

x. dissemina'tum, a rare normolipemic disorder with coalescent cutaneous x.'s on flexural surfaces and mild diabetes insipidus.

eruptive x., x. diabeticorum; the sudden appearance of groups of waxy yellow or yellowish-brown lesions, especially over extensors of the elbows and knees, and on the back and buttocks of patients with severe hyperlipemia, or more rarely in severe diabetes.

fibrous x., see dermatofibroma.

x. mul'tiplex, xanthomatosis.

normolipemic x. pla'num, generalized *xanthelasma.*

x. palpebra'rum, xanthelasma palpebrarum; soft yellow-orange plaques found about the eyes; the most common type of x.

x. pla'num, a form marked by the occurrence of yellow bands or rectangular plates in the corium.

x. tubero'sum, x. tubero'sum sim'plex, xanthomatosis associated with familial type II, and occasionally type III, hyperlipoproteinemia.

verrucous x., histocytosis Y; a papilloma of the oral mucosa and skin in which squamous epithelium covers connective tissue papillae filled with large foamy histiocytes.

xanthomatosis (zan-thō-mă-tō'sis). Xanthoma multiplex; lipoid or lipid granulomatosis; cholesterosis cutis; widespread xanthomas, especially on the elbows and knees, that sometimes affect mucous membranes and are sometimes associated with metabolic disturbances.

biliary x., Rayer's disease; x. with hypercholesterolemia, resulting from biliary cirrhosis.

x. bul'bi, ulcerative fatty degeneration of the cornea after injury.

cerebrotendinous x., cerebrotendinous cholesterinosis; a disorder associated with deposition of cholestanol in the brain and other tissues and elevated levels in plasma but with normal cholesterol level; characterized by progressive cerebellar ataxia beginning after puberty, juvenile cataracts, spinal cord involvement, and tendinous or tuberous xanthomata; autosomal recessive inheritance.

familial hypercholesteremic x., type II familial *hyperlipoproteinemia.*

normal cholesteremic x., Hand-Schüller-Christian *disease.*

xanthomatous (zan-thō'mă-tŭs). Relating to xanthoma.

xanthopathy (zan-thop'ă-thē) [xantho- + G. *pathos,* suffering]. Xanthochromia.

xanthophyll (zan'thō-fil). Lutein (2); luteol; luteole; β,ε-carotene-3',3'-diol; oxygenated derivative of carotene; a yellow plant pigment, occurring also in egg yolk.

xanthoproteic (zan-thō-prō'tē-ik). Relating to xanthoprotein.

xanthoproteic acid. A noncrystallizable yellow substance derived from proteins upon treatment with nitric acid.

xanthoprotein (zan-thō-prō'tēn). The yellow product formed upon treating protein with hot nitric acid, probably from nitration of phenyl groups.

xanthopsia (zan-thop'sē-ă) [xantho- + G. *opsis,* vision]. Yellow vision; a condition in which objects appear yellow; may occur in picric acid and santonin poisoning, in jaundice, and in digitalis intoxication.

xanthopsin (zan-thop'sin). Obsolete term for all-*trans*-retinal.

xanthopsydracia (zan-thop-si-drā'sē-ă) [G. *xanthos,* yellow + *psydrax,* a blister on the tip of the tongue]. An eruption of small yellow pustules.

xanthopuccine (zan-thō-pŭk'sēn). Canadine.

xanthosine (X, Xao) (zan'thō-sēn, -sin). Xanthine ribonucleoside; 9-β-D-ribosylxanthine; the deamination product of guanosine (O replacing $-NH_2$).

x. phosphate, xanthine nucleotide; xanthylic acid; the phosphoric ester of x.

xanthosis (zan-thō'sis) [xantho- + G. *-osis,* condition]. A yellowish discoloration of degenerating tissues, especially seen in malignant neoplasms.

xanthous (zan'thŭs) [G. *xanthos,* yellow]. Yellow.

xanthurenic acid (zan-thū-rēn'ik). 4,8-Dihydroxyquinoline-2-carboxylic acid; 4,8-dihydroquinaldic acid; the sulfur-yellow crystals form a red compound with Millon reagent, or an intensely green one with ferrous sulfate; excreted in the urine of pyridoxine-deficient animals after the ingestion of tryptophan, and from rats fed almost exclusively with fibrin.

xanthuria (zan-thū'rē-ă). Xanthinuria.

xanthyl (zan'thil). A radical consisting of xanthine minus a hydrogen atom.

xanthylic (zan-thil'ik). Relating to xanthine.

xanthylic acid. *Xanthosine* phosphate.

Xao Symbol for xanthosine.

Xe Symbol for xenon.

xeno- [G. *xenos,* guest, host, stranger, foreign]. Combining form denoting strange or relationship to foreign material.

xenobiotic (zen'ō-bī-ot'ik). A pharmacologically, endocrinologically, or toxicologically active substance not endogenously produced and therefore foreign to an organism.

xenodiagno'sis (zen'ō-dī-ag-nō'sis). **1.** A method of diagnosing acute or early *Trypanosoma cruzi* infection (Chagas' disease) in man. Infection-free (laboratory-reared) triatomine bugs are fed on the suspected person and the trypanosome is identified by microscopic examination of the intestinal contents of the bug after a suitable incubation period. **2.** A similar method of biological diagnosis based upon experimental exposure of a parasite-free normal host capable of allowing the organism in question to multiply, enabling it to be more easily and reliably detected.

xenogeneic (zen'ō-jĕ-nē'ik) [xeno- + G. *-gen,* producing]. Xenogenic (2); heterologous, with respect to tissue grafts, especially when donor and recipient belong to widely separated species.

xenogenic (zen-ō-jen'ik) [xeno- + G. *-gen,* producing]. Xenogenous. **1.** Originating outside of the organism, or from a foreign substance that has been introduced into the organism. **2.** Xenogeneic.

xenogenous (zĕ-noj'ĕ-nŭs). Xenogenic.

xenograft (zen'ō-graft). Xenogeneic, heterologous, heteroplastic, heterospecific, or interspecific graft; heterograft; a graft transferred from an animal of one species to one of another species.

xenon (zen'on) [G. *xenos,* a stranger]. A gaseous element, symbol Xe, atomic no. 54, atomic weight 131.30; present in minute proportion in the atmosphere; produces general anesthesia in concentrations of 70 vol. percent.

xenon-133 (^{133}Xe). A radioisotope of xenon with a gamma emission and a physical half-life of 5.27 days; used in the study of pulmonary function and organ blood flow.

xenoparasite (zen-ō-par'ă-sīt). An ecoparasite that becomes pathogenic in consequence of weakened resistance on the part of its host.

xenophobia (zen-ō-fō'bē-ă) [xeno- + G. *phobos,* fear]. Morbid fear of strangers.

xenophonia (zen-ō-fō'nē-ă) [xeno- + G. *phōnē,* voice]. A speech defect marked by an alteration in accent and intonation.

xenophthalmia (zen'of-thal'mē-ă). Inflammation excited by the presence of a foreign body in the eye.

Xenopsylla (zen-op-sil'ă) [xeno- + G. *psylla,* flea]. The rat flea, a genus of fleas parasitic on the rat and involved in the transmission of bubonic plague. The species *X. cheopis* serves as a potent vector of *Yersinia pestis,* largely because its gut becomes "blocked" by a mass of *Y. pestis* cells which prevents the flea from feeding normally, so that it is inclined to attack man and other hosts; it is an important source of infection in traditional epidemic areas such as India. *X. astia* and *X. braziliensis* are also efficient vectors of plague.

xenyl (zen'il). A radical consisting of biphenyl minus a hydrogen atom.

xeransis (zē-ran'sis) [G. *xēransis,* fr. *xēros,* dry]. A gradual loss of moisture in the tissues.

xerantic (zē-ran'tik). Denoting xeransis.

xerasia (zē-rā'zē-ă) [G. *xērasia,* fr. *xēros,* dry]. A condition of the hair characterized by dryness and brittleness.

xero- [G. *xeros,* dry]. Combining form meaning dry.

xerochilia (zēr-ō-kī'lē-ă) [xero- + G. *cheilos,* lip]. Dryness of lips.

xeroderma (zēr'ō-der'mă) [xero- + G. *derma,* skin]. A mild form of ichthyosis characterized by excessive dryness of the skin due to a slight increase of the horny layer and diminished cutaneous secretion.

x. pigmento'sum, atrophoderma pigmentosum; an eruption of exposed skin occurring in childhood and characterized by numerous pigmented spots resembling freckles, larger atrophic lesions eventually resulting in glossy white thinning of the skin surrounded by telangiectases, and multiple solar keratoses which undergo malignant change at an early age; results from a single-gene autosomal recessive disorder in which DNA repair processes are defective, so that they are more liable to chromosome breaks and cancerous change when exposed to ultraviolet light.

xerogram (zē'rō-gram). Xeroradiograph.

xerography (zēr-og'ră-fē). Xeroradiography.

xeroma (zē-rō'mă). Xerophthalmia.

xeromammography (zēr'ō-mam-og'ră-fē). Radiographic examination of the breast with the image produced by dry powder toner on paper from an electrostatically charged plate (xeroradiography) rather than on radiographic film.

xeromenia (zēr-ō-mē'nē-ă) [xero- + G. *mēniaia,* menses]. Occurrence of the usual constitutional symptoms at the menstrual period without any show of blood.

xeromycteria (zēr'ō-mik-tēr'ē-ă) [xero- + G. *myktēr,* the nose]. Extreme dryness of the nasal mucous membrane.

xeronosus (zē-ron'ō-sŭs) [xero- + G. *nosos,* disease]. Xerosis.

xerophagia, xerophagy (zēr-ō-fā'jē-ă, zēr-of'ă-jē) [xero- + G. *phagein,* to eat]. The eating of dry foodstuffs; subsisting on a dry diet.

xerophthalmia (zēr-of-thal'mē-ă) [xero- + G. *ophthalmos,* eye]. Xerophthalmus; conjunctivitis arida; xeroma; excessive dryness of the conjunctiva and cornea, which lose their luster and become keratinized; may be due to local disease or to a systemic deficiency of vitamin A.

xerophthalmus (zēr'of-thal'mŭs). Xerophthalmia.

xeroradiograph (zē-rō-rā'dē-ō-graf). Xerogram; the permanent record made by xeroradiography.

xeroradiography (zēr'ō-rā'dē-og'ră-fē). Xerography; the making of a radiograph by means of a specially coated charged plate and developing with a dry powder rather than liquid chemicals.

xerosis (zē-rō'sis) [xero- + G. *-osis,* condition]. Xeronosus. **1.** Pathologic dryness of the skin (xeroderma), the conjunctiva (xerophthalmia), or mucous membranes. **2.** The normal evolutionary sclerosis of the tissues in old age.

x. parenchymato'sus, superficial drying of the conjunctiva due to diffuse scarring, with closure of the lacrimal gland openings.

xerostomia (zēr'ō-stō'mē-ă) [xero- + G. *stoma,* mouth]. A dryness of the mouth, having a varied etiology, resulting from diminished or arrested salivary secretion, or asialism.

xerotes (zē-rō'tēz) [G. *xērotēs*]. Dryness.

xerotic (zē-rot'ik). Dry; affected with xerosis.

xerotocia (zēr'ō-tō'sē-ă) [xero- + G. *tokos,* labor]. Dry *labor.*

xerotripsis (zēr-ō-trip'sis) [xero- + G. *tripsis,* a rubbing, fr. *tribō,* to rub]. Dry friction.

Xg blood group. See Blood Groups appendix.

X-inactivation. Lyonization.

xiph-, xiphi-. See xipho-.

xiphisternal (zif-i-ster'năl). Relating to the xiphisternum (xiphoid process).

xiphisternum (zif'i-ster'nŭm) [xiphoid + G. *sternon,* chest]. *Processus* xiphoideus.

xipho-, xiph-, xiphi- [G. *xiphos,* sword]. Combining forms denoting xiphoid, usually the processus xyphoideus.

xiphocostal (zif'ō-kos'tăl) [xipho- + L. *costa,* rib]. Relating to the xiphoid process and the ribs.

xiphodynia (zif-ō-din'ē-ă) [xipho- + G. *odynē,* pain]. Xyphoidalgia; pain of a neuralgic character, in the region of the xiphoid cartilage. See also hypersensitive xiphoid *syndrome.*

xiphoid (zif'oyd) [xipho- + G. *eidos,* appearance]. Ensiform; mucronate; gladiate; sword-shaped; applied especially to the processus xiphoideus.

xiphoidalgia (zif-oy-dal'jē-ă) [xiphoid + G. *algos,* pain]. Xiphodynia.

xiphoiditis (zif'oy-dī'tis) [xiphoid + G. *-itis,* inflammation]. Inflammation of the xiphoid process of the sternum.

xiphopagus (zi-fop'ă-gŭs) [xipho- + G. *pagos,* something fixed]. Conjoined twins united in the region of the xiphoid process of the sternum.

X-linked. Pertaining to genes situated on the X chromosome. Commonly but erroneously used synonymously with sex-linked, which would also comprise Y-linked traits.

x-radiation. Radiant energy from an x-ray tube. See also x-ray.

x-ray. Roentgen ray. **1.** The electromagnetic radiation emitted from a highly evacuated tube, excited by the bombardment of the target anode with a stream of electrons from a heated cathode. **2.** Electromagnetic radiation produced by the excitation of the inner orbital electrons of an atom.

xyl-, xylo- [G. *xylon,* wood]. Combining forms relating to wood or to xylose.

xylene (zī'lēn). Xylol.

x. cyanol FF [C.I. 43535], an acidic triphenylmethane dye used for histochemical staining of hemoglobin peroxidase and as a tracking dye for DNA sequencing in electrophoresis.

xylenol (zī'lĕ-nol). Dimethylphenol; $(CH_3)_2C_6H_3OH$, occurring in six isomeric forms; used in the manufacture of coal tar disinfectants and synthetic resins.

xylidine (zī'li-dēn). Aminoxylene; aminodimethylbenzene; $(CH_3)_2C_6H_3NH_2$; used as a reagent and in the manufacture of dyes.

xylo-. See xyl-.

xyloidin (zī-loy'din). Pyroxylin.

xyloketose (zī-lō-kē'tōs). Xylulose.

xylol (zī'lol). Xylene; dimethylbenzene; $C_6H_4(CH_3)_2$; a volatile liquid obtained from coal tar, having physical and chemical properties similar to those of benzene; it occurs as three isomers; *m-, o-,* and *p-* xylol; used as a solvent, in the manufacture of chemicals and synthetic fibers, and in histology as a clearing agent.

xylometazoline hydrochloride (zī'lō-mĕ-taz'ō-lēn). 2-(4'-*tert*-Butyl-2',6'-dimethylphenylmethyl)imidazoline hydrochloride; a sympathomimetic drug used as a nasal decongestant.

xylopyranose (zī-lō-pir'ă-nōs). Xylose in pyranose form.

xylose (zī'lōs). Wood or beechwood sugar; an aldopentose, isomeric with ribose, obtained by fermentation or hydrolysis of naturally occurring carbohydrate substances, *e.g.,* in wood fiber.

xylulose (zī'lū-lōs). Xyloketose; *threo*-pentulose; a 2-ketopentose. L-Xylulose appears in the urine in cases of essential pentosuria; D-xylulose 5-phosphate is an intermediate in pentose metabolism.

L-xylulosuria (zī'lū-lō-sū'rē-ă). Essential *pentosuria.*

xylyl (zī'lil). The radical consisting of xylene (xylol) minus a hydrogen atom.

x. bromide, $CH_3C_6H_4CH_2Br$; the *o-, m-,* and *p-* forms are powerful lacrimators.

xylylene (zī'li-lēn). The radical consisting of xylene (xylol) minus two hydrogen atoms.

xyrospasm (zī'rō-spazm) [G. *xyron,* razor, fr. *xyō,* to scrape]. Shaving *cramp.*

xysma (ziz'mă) [G. filings, shavings, fr. *xyō,* to scrape]. Membranous shreds in the feces.

Y

Y Symbol for yttrium.

yanggona (yang'gō-nă). Yaqona.

yaqona (yang'gō-nă) [Fijian name]. Kava (2); yanggona; a Fijian drink made from the powdered root of *Piper methysticum* (family Piperaceae); excessive drinking of it causes a state of hyperexcitability and a loss of power in the legs; chronic intoxication induces roughening of the skin and a state of debility. See also methysticum.

yaw. An individual lesion of the eruption of yaws.

mother y., buba madre; frambesioma; mamanpian; protopianoma; a large granulomatous lesion, considered to be the initial lesion in yaws, most commonly present on the hand, leg, or foot.

yawn [A.S. *gānian*]. **1.** To gape. **2.** An involuntary opening of the mouth, usually accompanied by a movement of respiration; it may be a sign of drowsiness or of vital depression, as after hemorrhage, but is often caused by suggestion.

yawn'ing. Oscitation; the act of producing a yawn.

yaws (yawz) [African, *yaw,* a raspberry]. An infectious tropical disease caused by *Treponema pertenue* and characterized by the development of crusted granulomatous ulcers on the extremities; may involve bone, but, unlike syphilis, does not produce central nervous system or cardiovascular pathology. Also called pian; rupia (2); boubas; bubas, Amboyna button; Charlouis' disease; mycosis framboesiodes; frambesia; polypapilloma (2); granuloma tropicum; zymotic papilloma.

bosch y., *pian* bois.

bush y., *pian* bois.

crab y., foot y.

foot y., crab u.; tubba; tubbae; dumas; y. of the feet with keratoderma of the palms and soles and ulcer formation.

forest y., *pian* bois.

guinea corn y., a form of y. in which the lesions resemble grains of Indian corn.

ringworm y., round, scaling, and crusted lesions that resemble ringworm.

Yb Symbol for ytterbium.

yearling (yēr'ling). An animal between one and two years of age; generally applied to horses and cattle.

yeast (yēst) [A.S. *gyst*]. A general term denoting true fungi of the family Saccharomycetaceae that are widely distributed in substrates that contain sugars (such as fruits), and in soil, animal excreta, the vegetative parts of plants, etc. Because of their ability to ferment carbohydrates, some y.'s are important to the brewing and baking industries.

brewers' y., y. produced by *Saccharomyces cerevisiae;* a by-product from the brewing of beer.

compressed y., the moist living cells of *Saccharomyces cerevisiae* combined with a starchy or absorbent base.

cultivated y., a form of y. propagated by culture and used in breadmaking, brewing, etc.

dried y., the dry cells of a suitable strain of *Saccharomyces cerevisiae;* brewers' dried y., debittered brewers' dried y., or primary dried y. are the sources of dried y.; it contains not less than 45% of protein, and in 1 g not less than 0.3 mg of nicotinic acid, 0.04 mg riboflavin, and 0.12 mg thiamin hydrochloride; used as a dietary supplement.

primary dried y., a source of dried y.; obtained from suitable strains of *Saccharomyces cerevisiae* grown in media other than those required for the production of beer.

wild y., any of the uncultivated forms of y.'s, useless as ferments and sometimes pathogenic.

yellow (yel'ō) [A.S. *geolu*]. A color occupying a position in the spectrum between green and orange. For individual yellow dyes see specific name.

indicator y., a compound formed in the bleaching of rhodopsin by light; it is chrome y. at pH 3.3-4.0 and pale y. at pH 9.0-10.0.

visual y., all-*trans*- retinal.

yellow root. Hydrastis.

yerba santa (yer'bă san'tă) [Sp. sacred herb]. Eriodictyon.

Yersinia (yer-sin'ē-ă) [A. J. E. *Yersin,* Swiss bacteriologist, 1862–1943]. A genus of motile and nonmotile, nonsporeforming bacteria (family Enterobacteriaceae) containing Gram-negative, unencapsulated, ovoid to rod-shaped cells. These organisms are nonmotile at 37°C, but some species are motile at temperatures below 30°C; motile cells are peritrichous. Citrate is not used as a sole source of carbon. These organisms are parasitic on humans and other animals. The type species is *Y. pestis.*

Y. enterocolit'ica, a species that causes yersiniosis in humans; it is found in the feces and lymph nodes of sick and healthy animals, including man, in material likely to be contaminated with feces, and in the cadavers of cattle, rabbits, hares, dogs, guinea pigs, horses, monkeys, pigs, and sheep.

Y. pes'tis, *Pasteurella pestis;* Kitasato's bacillus; plague bacillus; a species causing plague in man, rodents, and many other mammalian species, and transmitted from rat to rat and from rat to man by the rat flea, Xenopsylla; it is the type species of the genus *Y.*

Y. pseudotuberculo'sis, *Pasteurella pseudotuberculosis;* a species causing pseudotuberculosis in birds, rodents, and rarely in man.

yersiniosis (yer-sin-ē-ō'sis). A common human infectious disease caused by *Yersinia enterocolitica* and marked by diarrhea, enteritis, pseudoappendicitis, ileitis, erythema nodosum, and sometimes septicemia or acute arthritis.

pseudotubercular y., pseudotuberculosis.

yin-yang. In ancient Chinese thought, the concept of two complementary and opposing influences, Yin and Yang, underlying and controlling all nature, the aim of Chinese medicine being to produce proper balance between them. Used in modern terms to characterize any dualistic, reciprocal control system in which one influence tends to promote things that the opposing influence tends to inhibit, and vice versa; *e.g.,* the yin-yang hypothesis of biological control in which cyclic GMP and cyclic AMP are supposed to act in this dualistic, reciprocal way in controlling cellular functions.

-yl. Chemical suffix signifying that the substance is a radical by loss of an H atom (*e.g.,* alkyl, methyl, phenyl) or OH group (*e.g.,* acyl, acetyl, carbamoyl).

-ylene. Chemical suffix denoting a bivalent hydrocarbon radical (*e.g.,* methylene, $-CH_2-$) or possessing a double bond (*e.g.,* ethylene, $CH_2=CH_2$).

yogurt, yoghurt (yō'gert) [Bulg.]. Fermented, partially evaporated, whole milk prepared by maintaining it at 50°C for 12 hours after the addition of a mixed culture of *Lactobacillus bulgaricus, L. acidophilus,* and *Streptococcus lactis;* used as a food (a staple article of diet in Bulgaria).

yohimbine (yō-him'bēn). An alkaloid, the active principle of yohimbé, the bark of *Corynanthe yohimbi* (family Rubiaceae); it produces a competitive blockade, of limited duration, of adrenergic α-receptors; has also been used for its alleged aphrodisiac properties.

yoke (yōk) [A.S. *geoc*] Jugum (1).

alveolar y., *jugum* alveolare.

yolk (yōk, yōlk) [A.S. *geolca; geolu,* yellow]. **1.** Vitellus; one of the types of nutritive material stored in the ovum for the nutrition of the embryo; y. is particularly abundant and conspicuous in the eggs of birds. **2.** Fatty material found in the wool of sheep; when extracted and purified, it becomes lanolin.

white y., y. consisting of much finer particles those of yellow y.; thin layers of it lie between the zones of yellow y. and form the latebra.

yellow y., the chief constituent of the y. in a bird's egg; it consists of relatively coarse particles of stored food materials and is laid down in concentric zones with interposed thin layers of white y.

Yorke's autolytic reaction. See under reaction.

Young, Hugh H., U.S. urologist, 1870–1945. See Y. prostatic *tractor.*

Young, Thomas, British physician and physicist, 1773–1829. See Y.'s *modulus, rule;* Y.-Helmholtz *theory* of color vision.

Young, W.J. See Harden-Y. *ester.*

ypsiliform (ip'si-li-fōrm) [G. *ypsilon, upsilon,* the letter u or y, + L. *forma,* form]. Hypsiloid.

ytterbium (i-ter'bē-ŭm) [*Ytterby,* in Sweden]. A metallic element of the lanthanide group; symbol Yb; atomic no. 70, atomic weight 173.04.

yttrium (it'rē-ŭm) [*Ytterby,* in Sweden]. A metallic element, symbol Y, atomic no. 39, atomic weight 88.92.

yttrium-90. An artificially radioactive isotope with a physical half-life of 64 hours which decays with the emission of a 2.27 Mev β particle; used as an implant in pituitary ablation.

Yvon, Paul, French physician and chemist, 1848–1913. See Y.'s *test.*

Z

Z Abbreviation for benzyloxycarbonyl (carbobenzoxy); atomic *number.*

Zo_2 Symbol for microliters of oxygen taken up per hour by 10^8 spermatozoa; can vary as a function of temperature.

Zaglas, John, 19th century anatomist's assistant in Edinburgh. See Z.'s *ligament.*

Zahn, Friedrich W., German pathologist, 1845–1904. See Z.'s *infarct, lines, striae.*

Zambusch, Leo von, 20th century German physician. See generalized pustular *psoriasis* of Z.

Zappert, Julius, Austrian physician, 1867–1942. See Z. counting *chamber.*

Z-DNA A form of DNA, discovered by x-ray crystallography, that differs from the classical A and B forms.

zea (zē'ă) [Mod. L. maize]. Cornsilk; stigmata maydis; the styles and stigmas of *Zea mays* (family *Gramineae*), Indian corn; formerly used as a diuretic and antispasmodic.

zeatin (zē'ă-tin). 6-(*trans* -4-Hydroxy-3-methyl-2-butenylamino)purine; a cytokinin first isolated from kernels of sweet corn.

Zeeman, Pieter, Dutch physicist, 1865–1943. See Z. *effect.*

ZEEP Abbreviation for zero end-expiratory *pressure.*

zein (zē'in). A prolamine present in maize; it lacks chiefly the amino acids glycine and lysine, and is low in cystine content.

Zeis, Eduard, Dresden ophthalmologist, 1807–1868. See Z.'s *glands;* zeisian *sty.*

zeisian (zīs'ē-ăn). Relating to or described by Eduard Zeis.

Zeiss, Carl, German optician, 1816–1888. See Abbé-Z. *apparatus,* counting *chamber;* Thoma-Z. *hemocytometer.*

Zeitgeist (zīt'gīst) [Ger. *zeit,* time, + *geist,* spirit]. In psychology, the climate of opinion, conventions of thought, covert influences, and unquestioned assumptions that are implicit in a given culture, the arts, or science at any point in time, and in which the individual operates.

Zellweger, Hans U., U.S. pediatrician, *1909. See Z. *syndrome.*

zelophobia (zē-lō-fō'bē-ă) [G. *zēlos, zeal,* + *phobos,* fear]. Morbid fear of jealousy.

zelotypia (zē-lō-tip'ē-ă) [G. *zēlotypia;* rivalry, envy, fr. *zēlos,* zeal, + *typtō,* to strike]. Excessive zeal, carried to the point of morbidity, in the advocacy of any cause.

Zenker, Friedrich A., German pathologist, 1825–1898). See Z.'s *degeneration, diverticulum, fixative, necrosis, paralysis;* formol-Z. *fixative.*

zeolite (zē'ō-līt). A naturally occurring hydrated sodium aluminum silicate, $Na_2O{\cdot}Al_2O_3.(SiO_2)_x.(H_2O)_x$, used for softening of hard water by exchanging its Na^+ for the Ca^{2+} of the water; thus z. is an ion exchanger. Some synthetic ion exchangers are termed synthetic z.'s, although there is no chemical relationship.

zeoscope (zē'ō-skōp) [G. *zeō,* to boil, + *skopeō,* to examine]. A device for determining the alcoholic content of a liquid by ascertaining its exact boiling point.

zero (zē'rō) [Sp.; Ar. *sifr,* cipher]. **1.** The figure 0, indicating nothingness. **2.** In thermometry, the point from which the figures on the scale start in one or the other direction; in the Centigrade and Réaumur scales, z. indicates the freezing point for distilled water; in the Fahrenheit scale, it is 32° below the freezing point of water.

absolute z., the lowest possible temperature, that at which the form of motion constituting heat is assumed no longer to exist, determined as −273.2°C or 0 Kelvin.

zerogravity (zē-rō-grav'i-tē). A physical state existing in space or at a time in flight when the centrifugal thrust of a parabolic glide or turn exactly counteracts the force of gravity.

zetacrit (zā'tă-krit). The packed cell volume produced by vertical centrifugation of blood in capillary tubes, allowing controlled compaction and dispersion of red blood cells; read with a hematocrit to produce the zeta sedimentation ratio.

zeumatography (zū-mă-tog'ră-fē). A nuclear magnetic resonance technique that is sensitive to water in biologic systems and can give a three-dimensional picture of the interior of objects in a magnetic field.

zidovudine (zī-dō'vū-dēn). Azidothymidine, $C_{10}H_{13}N_5O_4$; a thymidine analogue that is an inhibitor of *in vitro* replication of HIV virus, the causative agent of AIDS and ARC, and is used in the management of these diseases.

Ziegler, S. Louis, U.S. ophthalmologist, 1861–1925. See Z.'s *operation.*

Ziehen, Georg T., German psychiatrist, 1862–1950. See Z.-Oppenheim *disease.*

Ziehl, Franz, German bacteriologist, 1857–1926. See Z.'s *stain,* Z.-Neelsen *stain.*

Ziemann, Hans R.P., German pathologist, *1865. See Z.'s *dots, stippling.*

Zieve, Leslie, U.S. physician, *1915. See Z.'s *syndrome.*

Zimmerlin, Franz, Swiss physician, 1858–1932. See Z.'s *atrophy.*

Zimmermann, Karl W., German histologist, 1861–1935. See Z.'s *corpuscle, granule,* elementary *particle, polkissen* of Z.

Zimmermann, Wilhelm, German physician, *1910. See Z. *reaction, test.*

zinc (zingk) [Ger. *Zink*]. A metallic element, symbol Zn, atomic no. 30, atomic weight 65.38; a number of salts of z. are used in medicine.

z. acetate, $Zn(C_2H_3O_2)2H_2O$; an emetic, styptic, and astringent.

z. caprylate, a topical antifungal compound.

z. chloride, butter of z.; $ZnCl_2$; formerly used as a caustic for the removal of cutaneous cancers, nevi, etc., and in weak solution in the treatment of gonorrhea and conjunctivitis.

z. gelatin, z. oxide, gelatin, glycerin, and purified water; used topically as a protectant.

z. iodide, ZnI_2; has been used as an antiseptic and astringent.

medicinal z. peroxide, a mixture of z. peroxide, z. carbonate, and z. hydroxide; a topical disinfectant, astringent, and deodorant.

z. oxide, ZnO; flowers of z.; z. white; used as a protective in ointment, as a dusting powder, and internally as an antispasmodic; also used in paint as a substitute for lead carbonate.

z. oxide and eugenol, used as a base material beneath metallic dental restorations and as a temporary filling material or impression material; setting and hardening result from complex reactions between the powder and the eugenol.

z. permanganate, action is similar to that of potassium permanganate, but more astringent; used in urethritis, by injection or douche in a 1:4000 solution.

z. peroxide, z. superoxide; ZnO_2; a yellowish white powder, insoluble in water and decomposed by acids; used in pharmaceutical preparations.

z. phenolsulfonate, z. sulfocarbolate; used as an intestinal antiseptic and locally as an astringent in chronic inflammation of the mucous membranes.

z. phosphide, Zn_3P_2; used as a bait poison for the extermination of rats and mice.

z. stearate, a z. compound with variable proportions of stearic and palmitic acids; a water-repellent, protective agent used in the treatment of eczema, acne, and other skin diseases.

z. sulfate, $ZnSo_4 \cdot 7H_2O$; used as a local astringent in the treatment of gonorrhea, indolent ulcers, conjunctivitis, and various skin diseases, and internally as an emetic.

z. sulfocarbolate, z. phenolsulfonate.

z. superoxide, z. peroxide.

z. undecylenate, z. undecenoate, $[CH_2{=}CH(CH_2)_8COO]_2Zn$; the z. salt of undecylenic acid; used in the treatment of fungal and other affections of the skin, including psoriasis.

z. white, z. oxide.

zinc-65 (^{65}Z). A radioactive zinc isotope that decays mainly by K-capture with a half-life of 245 days; used as tracer in studies of zinc metabolism.

zinciferous (zing-kif'er-ŭs). Containing zinc.

zincoid (zing'koyd) [G. *eidos,* resemblance]. Relating to or resembling zinc.

zingiber (zin'ji-ber). Ginger.

Zinn, Johann G., German anatomist, 1727–1759. See Z.'s *artery,* x-ray *cap,* vascular *circle, corona, ligament, membrane, ring, tendon, zonule.*

Zinsser, Hans, U.S. bacteriologist and immunologist, 1878–1940. See Brill-Z. *disease.*

zirconium (zir-kō'nē-ŭm) [*zircon,* a mineral, fr. Ar. *zarkūn,* cinnabar]. A metallic element, symbol Zr, atomic no. 40 atomic weight 91.22; widely distributed in nature, but never found in quantity in any one place.

Zn Symbol for zinc.

zo-. See zoo-.

zoacanthosis (zō'ă-kan-thō'sis) [G. *zōon,* animal, + acanthosis]. A cutaneous eruption due to introduction into the human skin of hair, bristles, stingers, etc., of lower animals.

zoamylin (zō-am'i-lin) [G. *zōē,* life, + *amylon,* starch]. Glycogen.

zoanthropic (zō-an-throp'ik). Relating to or marked by zoanthropy.

zoanthropy (zō-an'thrō-pē) [G. *zōon,* animal, + *anthrōpos,* man]. A delusion that one is an animal, such as a dog.

zoetic (zō-et'ik) [G. *zōē,* life]. Relating to life.

zoic (zō'ik) [G. *zōikos,* relating to an animal]. Relating to living things; having life.

zoite (zō'īt) [G. *zoōn,* animal]. Sporozoite.

Zollinger, Robert M., U.S. surgeon, *1903. See Z.-Ellison *syndrome, tumor.*

Zöllner, Johann F., German physicist, 1834–1882. See Z.'s *lines.*

zomepirac sodium (zō-mĕ-pir'ak). Sodium 5-(*p*-chlorodoenzoyl)-1,4-dimethylpyrrole-2-acetate dihydrate; an analgesic anti-inflammatory agent.

zona, pl. **zonae** (zō'nă, zō'nē) [L. fr. G. *zōnē,* a girdle, one of the zones of the sphere]. **1.** Zone; a segment; any encircling or beltlike structure, either external or internal, longitudinal or transverse. **2.** *Herpes* zoster.

z. arcua'ta, arcuate *zone.*

z. cilia'ris, ciliary *zone.*

z. coro'na, costal *fringe.*

z. dermat'ica, a ridge of thickened skin surrounding the protrusion in spina bifida.

z. epitheliosero'sa, the membranous ring, within the z. dermatica, surrounding the protrusion in spina bifida.

z. facia'lis, herpes zoster involving the face.

z. fascicula'ta, the layer of radially arranged cell cords in the cortical portion of the suprarenal gland, between the z. glomerulosa and z. reticularis; secretes cortisol and dehydroepiandrosterone.

z. glomerulo'sa, the outer layer of the cortex of the suprarenal gland just beneath the capsule; secretes aldosterone.

z. hemorrhoida'lis, annulus hemorrhoidalis; the part of the anal canal that contains the rectal venous plexus.

z. ig'nea, *herpes* zoster.

z. incer'ta [NA], a flat, obliquely disposed plate of gray matter in the subthalamic region situated between the thalamic fasciculus (tegmental field H_1 of Forel) and the lenticular fasciculus (tegmental field H_2). Medially, cells of this nucleus are adjacent to the prerubral area (tegmental field H) and, laterally, they are continuous with the reticular nucleus of the thalamus. Z. i. is a derivative of the ventral thalamus; it receives afferents from the precentral motor cortex and the cerebellum.

z. medullovasculo'sa, the fissured segment of the spinal cord that dorsally closes the sac in meningomyelocele.

z. ophthal'mica, herpes zoster in the distribution of the ophthalmic nerve.

z. orbicula'ris [NA], orbicular zone; zonular band; ring ligament; fibers of the articular capsule of the hip joint encircling the neck of the femur.

z. pectina'ta, pectinate *zone.*

z. pellu'cida, pellucid zone; a layer consisting of microvilli of the oocyte, cellular processes of follicular cells, and an intervening substance rich in glycoprotein; it appears homogeneous and translucent under the light microscope.

z. perfora'ta, *foramina* nervosa.

z. pupilla'ris, pupillary *zone.*

z. radia'ta, z. striata.

z. reticula'ris, the inner layer of the cortex of the adrenal gland, where the cell cords anastomose in a netlike fashion.

z. serpigino'sa, *herpes* zoster.

z. stria'ta, z. radiata; membrana striata; striated membrane; the thickened cell membrane of the ovum in forms, such as certain amphibia, in which it appears radially striated under the light microscope; with the electron microscope the striations can be seen to be microvilli.

z. tec'ta, arcuate *zone.*

z. vasculo'sa, vascular *zone.*

zonal (zō'năl). Relating to a zone.

zonary (zō'nar-ē). Relating to or having the form of a zone or belt.

zonate (zō'nāt). Zoned; ringed; having concentric layers of differing texture or pigmentation.

Zondek, Bernhardt, German obstetrician and gynecologist, 1891–1966. See Aschheim-Z. *test.*

ZONE

zone (zōn) [L. *zona*]. Zona (1). See also area; regio; region; space; spatium; spot.

abdominal z.'s, *regiones* abdominis.

androgenic z., **(1)** X z. (1); **(2)** fetal *cortex.* Named in the belief (as yet unsubstantiated) that the cells within this zone secrete androgens.

arcuate z., zona arcuata; zona tecta; the inner third of the lamina basilaris ductus cochlearis extending from the tympanic lip of the osseous spiral lamina to the outer pillar cell of the spiral organ (of Corti).

Barnes' z., cervical z.; the lower fourth of the pregnant uterus, attachment of the placenta to any part of which may cause dangerous hemorrhage.

cervical z., Barnes' z.

cervical z. of tooth, *cervix* dentis.

ciliary z., zona ciliaris; the outer, wider z. of the anterior surface of the iris, separated from the pupillary z. by the collarette.
comfort z., the temperature range between 28°C and 30°C at which the naked body is able to maintain the heat balance without either shivering or sweating; in the clothed body the range is from 13°C to 21°C.
z.'s of discontinuity, concentric z.'s of varying optical density in the lens of the eye, as seen in slitlamp biomicroscopy.
dolorogenic z., trigger *point.*
entry z., the area of the dorsal funiculus of the spinal cord, medial to the tip of the posterior horn, in which the entering fibers of the posterior nerve root divide into ascending and descending branches.
ependymal z., ependymal *layer.*
epileptogenic z., a cortical region which on stimulation reproduces the patient's spontaneous seizure or aura.
equivalence z., in a precipitin reaction, the z. in which neither antibody nor antigen is in excess. See also precipitation.
erogenous z., erotogenic z., a part of the body, stimulation of which excites sexual feelings.
fetal z., fetal *cortex.*
gingival z., that portion of the oral mucosa which surrounds the teeth and is firmly attached to the underlying alveolar bone.
Golgi z., **(1)** part of the cytoplasm occupied by the Golgi apparatus; **(2)** in secretory cells of exocrine glands, a z. between the nucleus and the luminal surface.
grenz z. (grents) [Ger. *Grenze,* borderline, boundary], in histopathology, a narrow layer beneath the epidermis which is not infiltrated or involved in the same way as are the lower layers of the dermis.
Head's z.'s, Head's *lines.*
interpalpebral z., the exposed area of the cornea and sclera between the lids of the open eye.
intertubular z., the dentinal matrix which lies between z.'s of peritubular dentin; it is less calcified and contains larger collagen fibers than does peritubular dentin.
isoelectric z., the range of H-ion concentration (pH) over which isoelectric precipitation occurs.
language z., a large area of the cerebral cortex on the left side (in right-handed persons) considered by some to embrace all the centers of memories and associations connected with language.
latent z., that portion of the cerebral cortex a lesion of which produces no symptoms.
Lissauer's marginal z., *fasciculus* dorsolateralis.
Looser's z.'s, incomplete fracture lines, resembling pseudofractures, usually seen in radiographs of persons with osteomalacia or ricketts.
mantle z., **(1)** mantle *layer;* **(2)** a layer of small B lymphocytes surrounding the paler-staining germinal centers of lymphoid follicles.
Marchant's z., the area on the sphenoid and occipital bones at the base of the skull from which the dura mater is readily detached.
marginal z., marginal *layer.*
motor z., that portion of the cerebral cortex which when stimulated produces a movement and when injured produces spasticity or paralysis.
neutral z., in dentistry, the potential space between the lips and cheeks on one side and the tongue on the other; natural or artificial teeth in this z. are subject to equal and opposite forces from the surrounding musculature.
nucleolar z., nucleolar *organizer.*
Obersteiner-Redlich z., Obersteiner-Redlich line; the narrow line along the course of a nerve (or nerve root) where the Schwann cells and connective tissue that support its axons are replaced by glia cells. The z. marks the true boundary between the central and the peripheral nervous system. Usually located at or near the surface of the spinal cord or brainstem, it can extend (*e.g.,* in the eighth nerve) several millimeters out along the nerve.
orbicular z., *zona* orbicularis.
pectinate z., zona pectinata; the outer two-thirds of the lamina basilaris ductus cochlearis.
pellucid z., *zona* pellucida.
peritubular z., the dentinal matrix surrounding the odontoblastic process; it is more highly calcified and contains finer collagen fibers than does the rest of the dentinal matrix.
polar z., the region in the vicinity of an electrode applied to the body. See also electrotonus.
protective z., the time in the cardiac cycle, immediately following the vulnerable period, during which a second stimulus will prevent the initiation of ventricular fibrillation by a previous stimulus applied during the vulnerable period, probably by blocking a reentrant pathway.
pupillary z., zona pupillaris; the central region of the anterior surface of the iris located between the collarette and the pupillary margin.
reflexogenic z., the area or z. where stimulation will elicit a given reflex.
secondary X z., an adrenocortical z., situated in the inner zona fasciculata, that appears upon postpubertal gonadectomy in some male rodents, most notably the mouse; the development of this z. is believed to be stimulated by pituitary gonadotropins.
segmental z., segmental plate; in a young embryo, the thickened dorsal portion of the mesoderm; either side of the midline that becomes metamerically divided to form the mesodermic somites.
Spitzka's marginal z., *fasciculus* dorsolateralis.
subplasmalemmal dense z., corneocyte *envelope.*
sudanophobic z., a z. of cells, at the periphery of the zona fasciculata in the adrenal cortex of the rat, that is not stained by Sudan dyes.
tender z.'s, Head's *lines.*
thymus-dependent z., paracortex.
trabecular z., *reticulum* trabeculare.
transitional z., **(1)** the equatorial region of the lens of the eye where the anterior epithelial cells become transformed into lens fibers; **(2)** that portion of a scleral contact lens between the corneal and scleral sections.
trigger z., trigger *point.*
trophotropic z. of Hess, an area in the hypothalamus concerned with positive rewarding bodily sensations.
vascular z., zona vasculosa; spongy spot; an area in the external acoustic meatus where a number of minute blood vessels enter from the mastoid bone.
vermilion z., vermilion transitional z., vermilion *border.*
Weil's basal z., Weil's basal *layer.*
Wernicke's z., Wernicke's *center.*
X z., **(1)** androgenic z. (1); a transient adrenocortical z. present in some rodents at birth, most notably in mice, situated between the zona reticularis and the adrenal medulla; it degenerates in males with the secretion at puberty and in females during their first pregnancy; it slowly enlarges in unmated females after puberty and does not degenerate until middle age; the X z. appears to secrete no hormone; **(2)** misnomer for the fetal *cortex* of primates.

zonesthesia (zōn-es-thē'zē-ă) [G. *zōnē,* girdle, + *aisthēsis,* sensation]. Girdle or cincture sensation; strangalesthesia; a sensation as if a cord were drawn around the body, constricting it.

zonifugal (zō-nif'yū-găl) [L. *zona,* zone, + *fugio,* to flee]. Passing from within any region outward; as in mapping out an area of disturbed sensation, when the stimulus is first applied to the affected region and is carried along into the part where sensation is normal.

zoning (zōn'ing). The occurrence of a stronger reaction in a lesser amount of suspected serum, observed sometimes in serologic tests used in the diagnosis of syphilis, and probably the result of high antibody titer.

zonipetal (zō-nip'ĕ-tăl) [L. *zona,* zone, + *peto,* to seek]. Passing from without toward and into any region; as in mapping out an area of disturbed sensation, when the stimulus begins in the normal part and is carried into the affected region.

zonoskeleton (zō'nō-skel'ĕ-tŏn) [L. *zona,* zone, + skeleton]. The proximal skeletal segments of the limbs, *i.e.,* scapula, clavicle, hip bone.

zonula, pl. **zonulae** (zō'nyū-lă, -lē; zon'yū-) [L. dim. of *zona,* zone] [NA]. Zonule; a small zone.

z. adhe'rens, intermediate junction; a belt-like desmosomal attachment between columnar epithelial cells, upon which filaments attach.

z. cilia'ris [NA], ciliary zonule; apparatus suspensorius lentis; Zinn's zonule; suspensory ligament of lens; a series of delicate meridional fibers arising from the inner surface of the orbiculus ciliaris and which run in bundles between, and in a very thin layer over, the ciliary processes; at the inner border of the corona, the fibers diverge into two groups that are attached to the capsule on the anterior and posterior surfaces of the lens close to the equator; the spaces between these two layers of fibers are filled with aqueous humor.

z. occlu'dens, tight junctions formed by the fusion of integral proteins of the lateral cell membranes of adjacent epithelial cells, limiting transepithelial permeability.

zonular (zō'nyū-lăr, zon'yū-). Relating to a zonula.

zonule (zō'nyūl, zon'yūl). Zonula.

ciliary z., *zonula* ciliaris.

Zinn's z., *zonula* ciliaris.

zonulitis (zō-nyū-lī'tis) [zonule + G. *-itis,* inflammation]. Assumed inflammation of the zonule of Zinn, or suspensory ligament of the lens of the eye.

zonulolysis, zonulysis (zō'nyū-lol'i-sis, -lī'sis) [zonule + G. *lysis,* dissolution]. Barraguer's method; dissolution of the zonula ciliaris by enzymes (α-chymotrypsin) to facilitate surgical removal of a cataract.

zoo-, zo- [G. *zōon,* animal]. Combining forms denoting an animal or animal life.

zooanthroponosis (zō'ō-an'thrō-pō-nō'sis). [zoo- + G. *anthrōpos,* man, + *nosos,* disease]. A zoonosis normally maintained by man but which can be transmitted to other vertebrates (*e.g.,* amebiasis to dogs, tuberculosis). *Cf.* anthropozoonosis; amphixenosis.

zooblast (zō'-ō-blast) [zoo- + G. *blastos,* germ]. An animal cell.

zoodermic (zō-ō-der'mik) [zoo- + G. *derma,* skin]. Relating to the skin of an animal.

zooerastia (zō'ō-ĕ-ras'tē-ă) [zoo- + G. *erastēs,* lover]. Bestiality.

zoofulvin (zō'ō-fŭl'vin). A yellow pigment obtained from the feathers of certain birds.

zoogenesis (zō-ō-jen'ĕ-sis) [zoo- + G. *genesis,* origin]. The doctrine of animal production or generation.

zoogeography (zō'ō-jē-og'ră-fē). The geography of animals; the study of the distribution of animals on the earth's surface.

zooglea (zō-og'lē-ă, zō'ō-glē'ă) [zoo- + G. *glia,* glue]. In bacteriology, an old term for a mass of bacteria held together by a clear gelatinous substance.

zoogonous (zō-oj'ō-nŭs). Viviparous.

zoogony (zō-oj'ō-nē). Viviparity.

zoograft (zō'ō-graft). Animal or zooplastic graft; a graft of tissue from an animal to a human.

zoografting (zō-ō-graft'ing). Zooplasty.

zooid (zō'oyd) [G. *zōodēs,* fr. *zōon,* animal, + *eidos,* resemblance]. **1.** Resembling an animal; an organism or object with an animal-like appearance. **2.** An animal cell capable of independent existence or movement, as the ovum or a spermatozoon, or the segment of a tapeworm. **3.** An individual of a colonial invertebrate, such as a coral.

zoolagnia (zō-ō-lag'nē-ă) [zoo- + G. *lagneia,* lust]. Sexual attraction toward animals.

zoolite, zoolith (zō'ō-līt, zō-ō-lith) [zoo- + G. *lithos,* stone]. A petrified animal.

zoologist (zō-ol'ō-jist). One who specializes in zoology.

zoology (zō-ol'ō-jē) [zoo- + G. *logos,* study]. The biology of animals.

zoom (zūm). The action of a varifocal lens system in a camera or microscope that maintains an object in focus while approaching it or receding from it; this effect may be obtained by moving two or more of the lens components at rates bearing a linear relation to one another.

zoomania (zō-ō-mā'nē-ă) [zoo- + G. *mania,* frenzy]. An excessive, abnormal love of animals.

Zoomastigina (zō'ō-mas-ti-jī'nă) [zoo- + G. *mastix,* whip]. Zoomastigophorea.

Zoomastigophorasida (zō'ō-mas-ti-gō-fō-ras'i-dă). Zoomastigophorea.

Zoomastigophorea (zō'ō-mas-ti-gō-fō'rē-ă) [zoo- + G. *mastix,* whip, + *phoros,* bearing]. Zoomastigina; Zoomastigophorasida; a class of flagellates (superclass Mastigophora) within the phylum Sarcomastigophora (flagellate and ameboid protozoans), of animal-like as opposed to plantlike characteristics. Chromatophores are absent; one to many flagella are found, although they may be absent in ameboid forms; sexuality is known in some groups. It includes many human parasites such as the trypanosomes and trichomonads, as well as a number of other parasitic and symbiotic forms.

zoomylus (zō-om'i-lŭs) [zoo- + G. *mylos,* stone]. Obsolete term for dermoid *cyst.*

Zoon, Jahannes Jacobus, Dutch dermatologist, *1902. See *balanitis* of Z.; Z.'s *erythroplasia.*

zoonosis (zō-ō-nō'sis) [zoo- + G. *nosos,* disease]. An infection or infestation shared in nature by man and other animals that are the normal or usual host; a disease of man acquired from an animal source. See also anthropozoonosis; cyclozoonosis; metazoonosis; saprozoonosis; zooanthroponosis.

direct z., a z. transmitted between animal and man from an infected to a susceptible host by contact, by a mechanical vector, or by some vehicle of transmission; the agent requires a single vertebrate host for completion of its life cycle and does not develop or show significant change during transmission; may include anthropozoonoses (rabies), zooanthroponoses (amebiasis), and amphixenoses (certain streptococcoses).

zoonotic (zō'ō-not'ik). Relating to a zoonosis.

zooparasite (zō-ō-par'ă-sīt). An animal parasite; an animal existing as a parasite.

zoopathology (zō-ō-pă-thol'ō-jē). The study or science of diseases of the lower animals.

zoophagous (zō-of'ă-gŭs) [G. *zōophagos,* fr. *zōon,* animal, + *phagein,* to eat]. Carnivorous.

zoophile (zō'ō-fīl) [zoo- + G. *philos,* fond]. **1.** A lover of animals; especially one more fond of animals than of people. **2.** One opposed to any animal experimentation; an antivivisectionist.

zoophilia (zō-ō-fil'ē-ă). Zoophilism.

zoophilic (zō-ō-fil'ik) [zoo- + G. *philos,* fond, loving]. **1.** Relating to or displaying zoophilism. **2.** Animal-seeking or animal-preferring; denoting preference of a parasite for an animal host over a human.

zoophilism (zō-of'i-lizm). Zoophilia; fondness for animals, espe-

cially an extravagant fondness for them.
erotic z., the deriving of sexual pleasure by patting or stroking animals.

zoophobia (zō-ō-fō'bē-ă) [zoo- + G. *phobos,* fear]. Morbid fear of animals.

zoophyte (zō'ō-fīt) [zoo- + G. *phyton,* plant]. An animal that resembles a plant, such as the sponges or sea anenomes.

zooplasty (zō'ō-plas-tē). Zoografting; grafting of tissue from an animal to a human.

zoosadism (zō-ō-sā'dizm). Sexual pleasure from cruelty to animals.

zoosmosis (zō-os-mō'sis) [G. *zōos,* living, + osmosis]. The process of osmosis in living tissues.

zootechnics (zō-ō-tek'niks) [zoo- + G. *technē,* art]. The art of managing domestic or captive animals, including handling, breeding, and keeping.

zootic (zō-ot'ik). Pertaining to animals other than man.

zootoxin (zō-ōtok'sin). Animal toxin; a substance, resembling the bacterial toxins in its antigenic properties, found in the fluids of certain animals; *e.g.,* in snake venom, the secretions of poisonous insects, eel-blood.

zootrophic (zō-ō-trof'ik) [zoo- + Gr. *trophē,* nourishment]. Relating to or serving for the nutrition of the lower animals.

zoster (zos'ter [G. *zōstēr,* a girdle]. *Herpes* zoster.

zosteriform (zos-ter'i-fōrm). Zosteroid.

zosteroid (zos'ter-oyd) [zoster + G. *eidos,* resemblance]. Zosteriform; resembling herpes zoster.

zoxazolamine (zok-să-zō'lă-mēn). 2-Amino-5-chlorobenzoxazole; a skeletal muscle relaxant that is no longer used because of its hepatic toxicity.

Z-plasty. Z procedure; surgery to elongate a contracted scar or to rotate tension 90°; the middle line of a Z-shaped incision is made along the line of greatest tension or contraction, and triangular flaps are raised on opposite sides of the two ends and transposed.

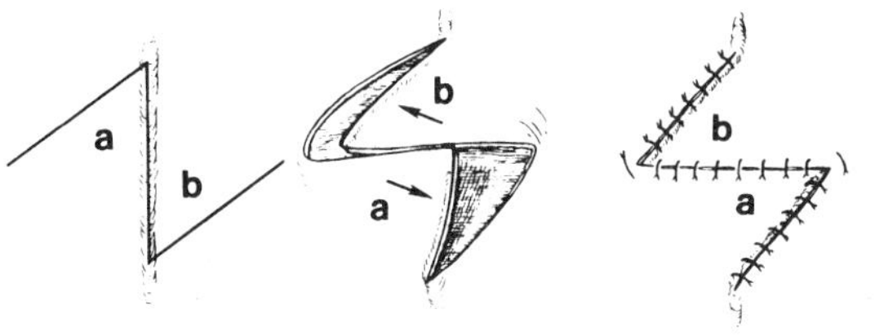

Z-plasty

Zr Symbol for zirconium.

Zsigmondy, Richard, German chemist, 1865–1929. See Z.'s *test;* brownian-Z. *movement.*

ZSR Abbreviation for zeta sedimentation *ratio.*

zuckergussleber (zuk'er-gus-lā-ber) [Ger. *Zuckerguss,* sugar frosting, + *Leber,* liver]. Frosted *liver.*

Zuckerkandl, Emil, Austrian anatomist, 1849–1910. See Z.'s *bodies, convolution, fascia, organs* of Z.

zwischenferment (tsvish'en-fer-ment'[Ger. *zwischen,* between, + *Ferment,* fermentation]. Glucose 6-phosphate dehydrogenase.

zwitterionic (tsvit'er-ī-on'ik). Denoting a substance with the properties of a zwitterion.

zwitterions (tsvit'er-ī-onz) [Ger. *Zwitter,* hermaphrodite, mongrel + ion]. Dipolar *ions.* See also zwitter *hypothesis.*

zyg-. See zygo-.

zygal (zī'găl). Relating to or shaped like a zygon or yoke; H-shaped.

zygapophysial, zygapophyseal (zī'gă-pō-fiz'ē-ăl, zī-gă-pof'i-se'ăl). Relating to a zygapophysis or articular process of a vertebra.

zygapophysis, pl. **zygapophyses** (zī'gă-pof'i-sis, -sēz) [G. *zygon,* yoke, + *apophysis,* offshoot] [NA]. Official alternate term for *processus* articularis.

zygion (zig'ē-on) [G. a later form of *zygon,* yoke]. In cephalometrics and craniometrics, the most lateral point of the zygomatic arch.

zygo-, zyg- [G. *zygon,* yoke, *zygōsis,* a joining]. Combining forms denoting yoke, a joining.

zygodactyly (zī-gō-dak'ti-lē). Syndactyly.

zygoma (zī-gō'mă) [G. a bar, bolt, the os jugale, fr. *zygon,* yoke]. **1.** *Os* zygomaticum. **2.** *Arcus* zygomaticus.

zygomatic (zī'gō-mat'ik). Rclating to the os zygomaticum.

zygomatico- [G. *zygoma*]. Combining form meaning zygomatic; relating usually to the zygomatic bone.

zygomaticoauricular (zī'gō-mat'i-kō-aw-rik'yū-lăr). Relating to the zygomatic bone and the auricle.

zygomaticoauricularis (zī'gō-mat'i-kō-aw-rik'yū-lăr'is). *Musculus* auricularis anterior.

zygomaticofacial (zī'gō-mat'i-kō-fā'shăl). Relating to the zygomatic bone and the face.

zygomaticofrontal (zī'gō-mat'i-kō-fron'tăl). Relating to the zygomatic and frontal bones.

zygomaticomaxillary (zī'gō-mat'i-kō-mak'si-lăr-ē). Relating to the zygomatic bone and the maxilla.

zygomatico-orbital (zī'gō-mat'i-kō-ōr'bi-tăl). Relating to the zygomatic bone and the orbit.

zygomaticosphenoid (zī'gō-mat'i-kō-sfē'noyd). Relating to the zygomatic and sphenoid bones.

zygomaticotemporal (zī'gō-mat'i-kō-tem'pŏ-răl). Relating to the zygomatic and temporal bones.

zygomaxillare (zī'gō-mak-si-lā'rē). Zygomaxillary point; key ridge; a craniometric point located externally at the lowest extent of the zygomaticomaxillary suture.

zygomaxillary (zī-gō-mak'si-lăr-ē). Relating to the zygomatic bone and the maxilla.

Zygomycetes (zī'gō-mī-sē'tēz) [zygo- + G. *mykēs* (*mykēt-*), fungus]. Phycomycetes; a class of fungi characterized by sexual reproduction resulting in the formation of a zygospore, and asexual reproduction by means of nonmotile spores called sporangiospores or conidia.

zygomycosis (zī'gō-mī-kō'sis). Phycomycosis; mucormycosis; a fungus infection associated with various genera of the class Zygomycetes, *e.g., Absidia, Mortierella, Mucor, Rhizopus.* The genera *Entomophthora, Conidiobolus,* and *Basidiobolus* are also causative agents.

zygon (zī'gon) [G. crossbar, yoke]. The short crossbar connecting the branches of a zygal fissure.

zygonema (zī-gōnē'mă) [zygo- + G. *nēma,* thread]. Zygotene.

zygopodium (zī-gō-pō'dē-ŭm) [zygo- + G. *podion,* small foot]. The distal intermediate segment of the limb skeleton, *i.e.,* radius and ulna, tibia and fibula.

zygosis (zī-gō'sis) [G. a joining]. True conjugation or sexual union of two unicellular organisms, consisting essentially in the fusion of the nuclei of the two cells.

zygosity (zī-gos'i-tē). The nature of the zygotes from which individuals are derived; *e.g.,* whether, with respect to a particular gene, they are homozygous or heterozygous or whether, in the case of twins, they are monozygotic or dizygotic.

zygosperm (zī'gō-sperm) [zygo- + G. *sperma,* seed]. Zygospore.

zygospore (zī'gō-spōr). Zygosperm; among the Phycomycetes, a thick-walled sexual spore arising from fusion of two morphologically identical structures, generally hyphal tips, bearing nuclei of opposite mating types (gametangia).

zygote (zī'gōt) [G. *zygōtos,* yoked]. **1.** The diploid cell resulting from union of a sperm and an ovum. **2.** The individual that develops from a fertilized ovum.

zygotene (zī'gō-tēn) [zygo- + G. *tainia* (L. *taenia*), band]. Zygonema; the stage of prophase in meiosis in which precise point for point pairing of homologous chromosomes begins.

zygotic (zī-got'ik). Pertaining to a zygote, or to zygosis.

zygotoblast (zī-gō'tō-blast) [G. *zygōtos,* yoked, + *blastos,* germ]. Sporozoite.

zygotomere (zī-gō'tō-mēr) [G. *zygōtos,* yoked, + *meros,* part]. Sporoblast.

zym-. See zymo-.

zymase (zī'mās). Obsolete term for enzyme; specifically, the intracellular enzyme of yeast that promotes alcoholic fermentation.

zymo-, zym- [G. *zymē,* leaven]. Combining forms denoting fermentation, enzymes.

zymodeme (zī'mō-dēm) [zymo- + G. *dēmos,* populace]. An isoenzyme pattern, as identified by isoenzyme electrophoresis.

zymogen (zī'mō-jen). Proenzyme.

zymogenesis (zī-mō-jen'ĕ-sis) [zymo- + G. *genesis,* production]. Transformation of a proenzyme (zymogen) into an active enzyme.

zymogenic (zī-mō-jen'ik). **1.** Zymogenous; relating to a zymogen or to zymogenesis. **2.** Causing fermentation.

zymogenous (zī-moj'ĕ-nŭs). Zymogenic (1).

zymogram (zī'mō-gram) [zymo- + G. *gramma,* something written]. Strips of paper, gels, etc. in which the locations of enzymes, separated electrophoretically or by other means, are demonstrated by histochemical methods.

zymohexase (zī-mō-heks'ās). Fructose-bisphosphate aldolase.

zymologist (zī-mol'ō-jist). Enzymologist.

zymology (zī-mol'ō-jē). Enzymology.

Zymonema (zī-mō-nē'mă) [zymo- + G. *nēma,* thread]. An obsolete generic designation formerly applied to certain dimorphic pathogenic fungi.

zymosan (zī'mō-san). Anticomplementary factor; a carbohydrate (glucose polymer) obtained from the walls of yeast cells; used in the assay of properdin.

zymoscope (zī'mō-skōp) [zymo- + G. *skopeō,* to view]. An instrument measuring CO_2 evolved and, therefore, the fermenting power of yeast.

zymose (zī'mōs). Obsolete term for β-fructofuranosidase.

zymosterol (zī-mos'ter-ol). 5α-Cholesta-8,24-dien-3β-ol; an intermediate in the biosynthesis of cholesterol from lanosterol.

APPENDICES

COMPARATIVE TEMPERATURE SCALES

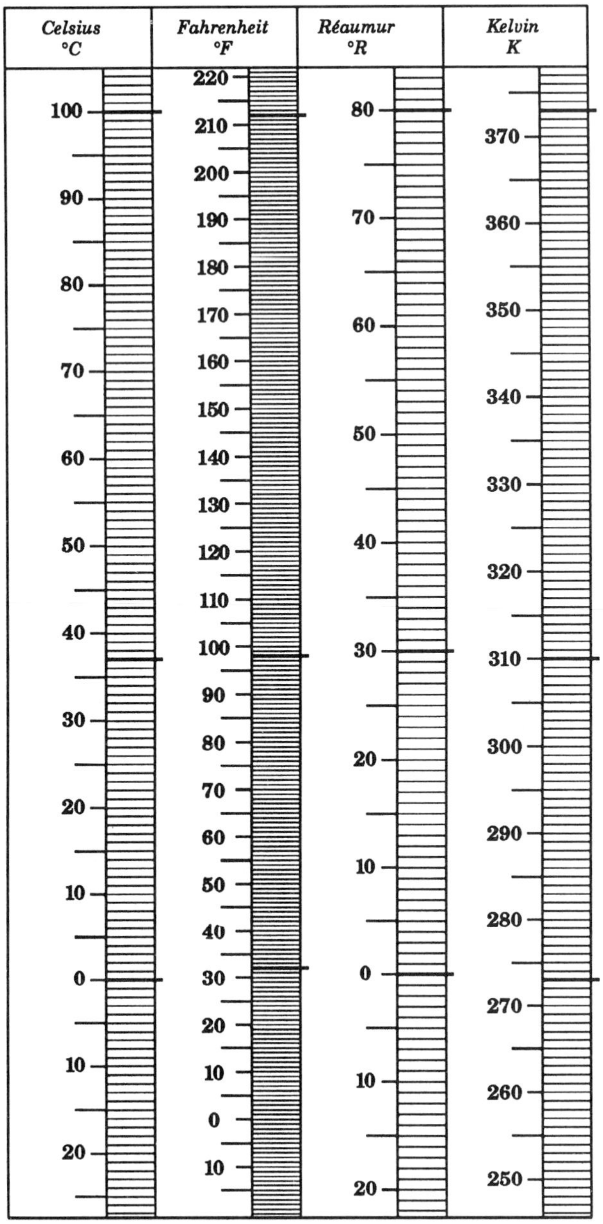

To convert Celsius, Fahrenheit, or Réaumur to Kelvin:

C to K: add 273.16
10°C to K: 10 + 273.16 = 283.16 K

F to K: convert to C, add 273.16
63°F = 17.2°C + 273.16 = 290.36 K

R to K: convert to C, add 273.16
34°R = 42.5°C + 273.16 = 315.66 K

To convert Fahrenheit to Celsius or Réaumur, Celsius to Fahrenheit or Réaumur, or Réaumur to Fahrenheit or Celsius:

Above 0°C and R, or 32°F

F to C: subtract 32, multiply by 5, divide by 9
63°F to C: 63 − 32 = 31 × 5 = 155 ÷ 9 = 17.2°C

F to R: subtract 32, multiply by 4, divide by 9
63°F to R: 63 − 32 = 31 × 4 = 124 ÷ 9 = 13.8°R

C to F: multiply by 9, divide by 5, add 32
37°C to F: 37 × 9 = 333 ÷ 5 = 66.6 + 32 = 98.6°F

C to R: multiply by 4, divide by 5
37°C to R: 37 × 4 = 148 ÷ 5 = 29.6°R

R to F: multiply by 9, divide by 4, add 32
34°R to F: 34 × 9 = 306 ÷ 4 = 76.5 + 32 = 108.5°F

R to C: multiply by 5, divide by 4
34°R to C: 34 × 5 = 170 ÷ 4 = 42.5°C

Between 0° and 32°F, −17.77° and 0°C, or −14.22° and 0°R

F to C: subtract from 32, multiply by 5, divide by 9
10°F to C: 32 − 10 = 22 × 5 = 110 ÷ 9 = −12.2°C

F to R: subtract from 32, multiply by 4, divide by 9
10°F to R: 32 − 10 = 22 × 4 = 88 ÷ 9 = −9.8°R

C to F: multiply by 9, divide by 5, subtract from 32
−12°C to F: 12 × 9 = 108 ÷ 5 = 21.6; 32 − 21.6 = 10.4°F

C to R: multiply by 4, divide by 5
−12°C to R: 12 × 4 = 48 ÷ 5 = 9.6°R

R to F: multiply by 9, divide by 4, subtract from 32
−12°R to F: 12 × 9 = 108 ÷ 4 = 27; 32 − 27 = 5°F

R to C: multiply by 5, divide by 4
−12°R to C: 12 × 5 = 60 ÷ 4 = 15°C

Below 0°F, −17.77°C, or −14.22°R

F to C: add 32, multiply by 5, divide by 9
−10°F to C: 10 + 32 = 42 × 5 = 210 ÷ 9 = −23.3°C

F to R: add 32, multiply by 4, divide by 9
−10°F to R: 10 + 32 = 42 × 4 = 168 ÷ 9 = −18.7°R

C to F: multiply by 9, divide by 5, subtract 32
−18°C to F: 18 × 9 = 162 ÷ 5 = 32.4 − 32 = 0.4°F

C to R: multiply by 4, divide by 5
−18°C to R: 18 × 4 = 72 ÷ 5 = 14.4°R

R to F: multiply by 9, divide by 4, subtract 32
−18°R to F: 18 × 9 = 162 ÷ 4 = 40.5 − 32 = −8.5°F

R to C: multiply by 5, divide by 4
−18°R to C: 18 × 5 = 90 ÷ 4 = 22.5°C

TEMPERATURE EQUIVALENTS

Celsius to Fahrenheit				Fahrenheit to Celsius					
°C	°F	°C	°F	°F	°C	°F	°C	°F	°C
−50	−58.0	49	120.2	−50	−46.7	99	37.2	157	69.4
−40	−40.0	50	122.0	−40	−40.0	100	37.7	158	70.0
−35	−31.0	51	123.8	−35	−37.2	101	38.3	159	70.5
−30	−22.0	52	125.6	−30	−34.4	102	38.8	160	71.1
−25	−13.0	53	127.4	−25	−31.7	103	39.4	161	71.6
−20	−4.0	54	129.2	−20	−28.9	104	40.0	162	72.2
−15	5.0	55	131.0	−15	−26.6	105	40.5	163	72.7
−10	14.0	56	132.8	−10	−23.3	106	41.1	164	73.3
−5	23.0	57	134.6	−5	−20.6	107	41.6	165	73.8
0	**32.0**	58	136.4	0	−17.7	108	42.2	166	74.4
1	33.8	59	138.2	1	−17.2	109	42.7	167	75.0
2	35.6	60	140.0	5	−15.0	110	43.3	168	75.5
3	37.4	61	141.8	10	−12.2	111	43.8	169	76.1
4	39.2	62	143.6	15	−9.4	112	44.4	170	76.6
5	41.0	63	145.4	20	−6.6	113	45.0	171	77.2
6	42.8	64	147.2	25	−3.8	114	45.5	172	77.7
7	44.6	65	149.0	30	−1.1	115	46.1	173	78.3
8	46.4	66	150.8	31	−0.5	116	46.6	174	78.8
9	48.2	67	152.6	**32**	**0**	117	47.2	175	79.4
10	50.0	68	154.4	33	0.5	118	47.7	176	80.0
11	51.8	69	156.2	34	1.1	119	48.3	177	80.5
12	53.6	70	158.0	35	1.6	120	48.8	178	81.1
13	55.4	71	159.8	36	2.2	121	49.4	179	81.6
14	57.2	72	161.6	37	2.7	122	50.0	180	82.2
15	59.0	73	163.4	38	3.3	123	50.5	181	82.7
16	60.8	74	165.2	39	3.8	124	51.1	182	83.3
17	62.6	75	167.0	40	4.4	125	51.6	183	83.8
18	64.4	76	168.8	41	5.0	126	52.2	184	84.4
19	66.2	77	170.6	42	5.5	127	52.7	185	85.0
20	68.0	78	172.4	43	6.1	128	53.3	186	85.5
21	69.8	79	174.2	44	6.6	129	53.8	187	86.1
22	71.6	80	176.0	45	7.2	130	54.4	188	86.6
23	73.4	81	177.8	46	7.7	131	55.0	189	87.2
24	75.2	82	179.6	47	8.3	132	55.5	190	87.7
25	77.0	83	181.4	48	8.8	133	56.1	191	88.3
26	78.8	84	183.2	49	9.4	134	56.6	192	88.8
27	80.6	85	185.0	50	10.0	135	57.2	193	89.4
28	82.4	86	186.8	55	12.7	136	57.7	194	90.0
29	84.2	87	188.6	60	15.5	137	58.3	195	90.5
30	86.0	88	190.4	65	18.3	138	58.8	196	91.1
31	87.8	89	192.2	70	21.1	139	59.4	197	91.6
32	89.6	90	194.0	75	23.8	140	60.0	198	92.2
33	91.4	91	195.8	80	26.6	141	60.5	199	92.7
34	93.2	92	197.6	85	29.4	142	61.1	200	93.3
35	95.0	93	199.4	86	30.0	143	61.6	201	93.8
36	96.8	94	201.2	87	30.5	144	62.2	202	94.4
37	**98.6**	95	203.0	88	31.0	145	62.7	203	95.0
38	100.4	96	204.8	89	31.6	146	63.3	204	95.5
39	102.2	97	206.6	90	32.2	147	63.8	205	96.1
40	104.0	98	208.4	91	32.7	148	64.4	206	96.6
41	105.8	99	210.2	92	33.3	149	65.0	207	97.2
42	107.6	**100**	**212.0**	93	33.8	150	65.5	208	97.7
43	109.4	101	213.8	94	34.4	151	66.1	209	98.3
44	111.2	102	215.6	95	35.0	152	66.6	210	98.8
45	113.0	103	217.4	96	35.5	153	67.2	211	99.4
46	114.8	104	219.2	97	36.1	154	67.7	**212**	**100.0**
47	116.6	105	221.0	98	36.6	155	68.3	213	100.5
48	118.4	106	222.8	**98.6**	**37.0**	156	68.8	214	101.1

WEIGHTS AND MEASURES

Scale of the Metric System and SI

Prefix	Symbol	Power	Multiple or Submultiple
exa-	E	10^{18}	1,000,000,000,000,000,000
peta-	P	10^{15}	1,000,000,000,000,000
tera-	T	10^{12}	1,000,000,000,000
giga-	G	10^{9}	1,000,000,000
mega-	M	10^{6}	1,000,000
kilo-	k	10^{3}	1,000
hecto-	h	10^{2}	100
deca-	da	10^{1}	10
UNIT			1
deci-	d	10^{-1}	0.1
centi-	c	10^{-2}	0.01
milli-	m	10^{-3}	0.001
micro-	μ	10^{-6}	0.000001
nano-	n	10^{-9}	0.000000001
pico-	p	10^{-12}	0.000000000001
femto-	f	10^{-15}	0.000000000000001
atto-	a	10^{-18}	0.000000000000000001

SI Base Units

Quantity	Name	Symbol
length	meter	m
mass*	kilogram†	kg
time	second	s
electric current	ampere	A
thermodynamic temperature	kelvin‡	K
luminous intensity	candela	cd
amount of substance	mole	mol

*In commercial and everyday use, "weight" usually means mass; *e.g.*, when speaking of a person's weight, the quantity referred to is mass.

†For historic reasons, kilogram is the only base unit with a prefix. Multiples and submultiples of the kilogram are formed by attaching the appropriate prefix to the stem word "gram" (*e.g.*, milligram) and the appropriate prefix symbol to the symbol "g" (*e.g.*, mg).

‡The degree Celsius (°C) is still widely accepted usage for expressing temperature and temperature intervals. Celsius (formerly centigrade) *temperature* is converted to kelvin (K) thermodynamic temperature by adding 273.16 to the Celsius scale. For *temperature interval,* 1°C equals 1 K.

Some SI Derived Units
Expressed in Terms of Base Units

Quantity	Name	Symbol
area	square meter	m^2
volume*	cubic meter	m^3
specific volume	cubic meter per kilogram	m^3/kg
speed, velocity	meter per second	m/s
acceleration	meter per second squared	m/s^2
mass density	kilogram per cubic meter	kg/m^3
concentration	mole per cubic meter	mol/m^3
luminance	candela per square meter	cd/m^2

*Liter (L, l), 10^{-3} m^3, is regarded as a special name for the cubic decimeter which is preferred for high accuracy measurement.

Some SI Derived Units with Special Names

Quantity	Name	Symbol	Expression
frequency	hertz	Hz	s^{-1}
force	newton	N	$m\ kg\ s^{-2}$
pressure, stress	pascal	Pa	$m^{-1}\ kg\ s^{-2}$
energy	joule	J	$m^2\ kg\ s^{-2}$
power	watt	W	$m^2\ kg\ s^{-3}$
quantity of electricity, electric charge	coulomb	C	s A
electric potential, electromotive force	volt	V	$m^2\ kg\ s^{-3}\ A^{-1}$
capacitance	farad	F	$m^{-2}\ kg^{-1}\ s^4\ A^2$
electric resistance	ohm	Ω	$m^2\ kg\ s^{-2}\ A^{-2}$
electric conductance	siemens	S	$m^{-2}\ kg^{-1}\ s^3\ A^2$
magnetic flux	weber	Wb	$m^2\ kg\ s^{-2}\ A^{-1}$
magnetic flux density	tesla	T	$kg\ s^{-2}\ A^{-1}$
activity of radionuclide	becquerel*	Bq	s^{-1}
absorbed dose of radiation	gray†	Gy	$m^2\ s^{-2}$
exposure (x and γ radiation)	coulomb per kilogram‡	C kg	$kg^{-1}\ s\ A$

*Replacing the curie (Ci), $3.7 \times 10^{10}\ s^{-1}$.

†Replacing the rad (rad), $10^{-2}\ J\ kg^{-1}$.

‡Replacing the roentgen (R), $2.58 \times 10^{-4}\ C\ kg^{-1}$.

Measures of Length

Micrometers	Millimeters	Centimeters	Meters	Kilometers	Miles	Yards	Feet	Inches
1	0.001	10^{-4}						0.000039
10^3	**1**	10^{-1}					0.00328	0.03937
10^4	10	**1**	0.01			0.0109	0.03281	0.3937
254,000	25.4	2.54	0.0254			0.0278	0.0833	**1**
	304.8	30.48	0.3048			0.333	**1**	12
10^6	10^3	10^2	**1**	0.001	0.0006213	1.0936	3.2808	39.37
914,400	914.40	91.44	0.9144	0.009	0.0005681	**1**	3	36
10^9	10^6	10^5	10^3	**1**	0.6215	1093.6121	3280.8	
			1609.0	1.609	**1**	1760.0	5280.0	

To convert:

Millimeters to inches: multiply by 10, divide by 254
Inches to millimeters: multiply by 254, divide by 10

Centimeters to feet: multiply by 10, divide by 307
Feet to centimeters: multiply by 307, divide by 10

Meters to yards: multiply by 70, divide by 64
Yards to meters: multiply by 64, divide by 70

Kilometers to miles: multiply by 5, divide by 8
Miles to kilometers: multiply by 8, divide by 5

Measures of Mass (Weight)

Avoirdupois Weights

				Metric Equivalents		
Grains	Drams	Ounces	Pounds	Milligrams	Grams	Kilograms
1	0.0366	0.0023	0.00014	64.8	0.0648	0.000065
27.34	**1**	0.0625	0.0039		1.772	0.001772
437.5	16	**1**	0.0625		28.350	0.028350
7,000	256	16	**1**		453.5924	0.453592
0.0154				**1**	0.001	
15.4324	0.5648	0.0353	0.002205	1000	**1**	0.001
15,432.358	564.32	35.27	2.2046		1000	**1**

To convert (approximately):

Kilograms to pounds: multiply by 1000, divide by 454
Pounds to kilograms: multiply by 454, divide by 1000

Grams to ounces: multiply by 20, divide by 567
Ounces to grams: multiply by 567, divide by 20

Apothecaries' Weights

Grains	Scruples	Drams	Ounces	Pounds	Metric Equivalents: Milligrams	Grams	Kilograms
1	0.05	0.0167	0.0021	0.00017	64.8	0.0648	0.000065
20	**1**	0.333	0.042	0.0035		1.296	0.001296
60	3	**1**	0.125	0.0104		3.888	0.000389
480	24	8	**1**	0.0833		31.103	0.031103
5,760	288	96	12	**1**		373.2418	0.373242
0.0154					**1**	0.001	
15.4324		0.2576	0.0322	0.0027	1000	**1**	0.001
15,432.358		257.2	32.15	2.6792		1000	**1**

Measures of Capacity

Apothecaries' Measures

Minims	Fluid Drams	Fluid Ounces	Pints	Quarts	Gallons	Metric Equivalents: Liters	Milliliters
1	0.0166	0.002	0.00013			0.0006	0.06161
60	**1**	0.125	0.0078	0.0039		0.0037	3.6967
480	8	**1**	0.0625	0.0312	0.0078	0.0296	29.5737
7,680	128	16	**1**	0.5	0.125	0.4732	473.166
15,360	256	32	2	**1**	0.25	0.9464	946.358
61,440	1024	128	8	4	**1**	3.7854	3785.434
16,230	270.52	33.8418	2.1134	1.0567	0.2642	**1**	1000
16.23	0.2705	0.0338	0.00212	0.00106	0.000265	0.001	**1**

To convert (approximately):

Liters to gallons: multiply by 264, divide by 1000
Gallons to liters: divide by 264, multiply by 1000

Liters to pints: multiply by 21, divide by 10
Pints to liters: multiply by 10, divide by 21

Approximate Household Measures and Weights*

Teaspoons	Tablespoons	Cups or Glasses	Drams	Fluid Ounces	Milliliters	Grams
1			1	0.125	5	5
3	**1**		4	0.50	15	15
48	16	**1**	64	8	237	240

*A drop is a measure of uncertain quantity, depending on the nature of the liquid as well as the shape of the container and of the opening from which the liquid falls. One drop of water is roughly equivalent to 1 minim.

LABORATORY REFERENCE RANGE VALUES

Thomas R. Koch, Ph.D., D.A.B.C.C., Department of Pathology, University of Maryland School of Medicine
Show-Hong Duh, Ph.D., Department of Pathology, University of Maryland School of Medicine

Reference range values are for apparently healthy individuals and often overlap significantly with values for persons who are sick. Actual values may vary significantly due to differences in assay methodologies and standardization. Institutions may also set up their own reference ranges based on the particular populations that they serve, thus there can be regional differences. Consequently, values reported by individual laboratories may differ from those listed in this appendix.

All values are given in conventional and SI units. However, where the SI units have not been widely accepted, conventional units are used. In case of the heterogenous nature of the materials measured or uncertainty of the exact molecular weight of the compounds, the SI system cannot be followed, and mass per volume is used as the unit of concentration.

Abbreviations:

ACD, acid-citrate-dextrose; **CHF**, congestive heart failure; **Cit**, citrate; **CNS**, central nervous system; **CSF**, cerebrospinal fluid; **cyclic AMP**, adenosine 3′:5′-cyclic phosphate; **EDTA**, ethylenediaminetetraacetic acid; **HDL**, high-density lipoprotein; **Hep**, heparin; **LDL-C**, low-density lipoprotein-cholesterol; **Ox**, oxalate; **RBC**, red blood cell(s); **RIA**, radioimmunoassay; **SD**, standard deviation

References:

Conn, R.B.: Laboratory values of clinical importance. In *Conn's Current Therapy 1988*. R.E. Rakel, Ed. Philadelphia, W.B. Saunders Co., 1988.

Tietz, N.W., and Logan, N.M. Reference ranges. In *Textbook of Clinical Chemistry*. N.W. Tietz, Ed. Philadelphia, W.B. Saunders Co., 1986.

National Cholesterol Education Program: Report of the expert panel on detection, evaluation, and treatment of high blood cholesterol in adults. *Arch. Intern. Med.* 1988;148:36–69.

Clinical Chemistry Laboratory: *Reference Range Values in Clinical Chemistry*. Professional services manual. Baltimore, Department of Pathology, University of Maryland Medical System, 1988.

Tests	Conventional Units	SI Units
Acetaminophen, serum or plasma (Hep or EDTA)		
Therapeutic	10–30 μg/mL	66–199 μmol/L
Toxic	>200 μg/mL	>1324 μmol/L
Acetoacetate plus acetone		
Serum		
Qualitative	Negative	Negative
Quantitative	0.3–2.0 mg/dL	3–20 mg/L
Urine		
Qualitative	Negative	Negative
Acid hemolysis test (Ham)	No hemolysis	No hemolysis
Adrenocorticotropin (ACTH), plasma		
6 AM	10–80 pg/mL	10–80 ng/L
6 PM	<50 pg/mL	<50 ng/L
Alanine aminotransferase (see Transaminase)		
Albumin		
Serum		
Adult	3.5–5.0 g/dL	35–50 g/L
>60 y	3.4–4.8 g/dL	34–48 g/L
	Avg. of 0.3 g/dL higher in upright individuals	Avg. of 3 g/L higher in upright individuals
Urine		
Qualitative	Negative	Negative
Quantitative	10–100 mg/24 h	10–100 mg/24 h
CSF	10–30 mg/dL	100–300 mg/L
*Aldolase, serum	0–11 mIU/mL (30°C)	0–11 U/L (30°C)
Aldosterone		
Serum		
Supine	3–10 ng/dL	0.08–0.3 nmol/L
Standing		
Male	6–22 ng/dL	0.17–0.61 nmol/L
Female	5–30 ng/dL	0.14–0.8 nmol/L
Urine	3–20 μg/24 h	8.3–55 nmol/24 h
Alpha amino nitrogen		
Serum	3.0–5.5 mg/dL	2.1–3.9 mmol/L
Urine	50–200 mg/24 h	3.6–14.3 nmol/24 h
Amikacin, serum or plasma (EDTA)		
Therapeutic		
Peak	25–35 μg/mL	43–60 μmol/L
Trough		
Less severe infection	1–4 μg/mL	1.7–6.8 μmol/L
Life-threatening infection	4–8 μg/mL	6.8–13.7 μmol/L
Toxic		
Peak	>35–40 μg/mL	>60–68 μmol/L
Trough	>10–15 μg/mL	>17–26 μmol/L
δ-Aminolevulinic acid, urine	1.3–7.0 mg/24 h	10–53 μmol/24 h

*Test values are method dependent.

Tests	Conventional Units		SI Units	
Amitriptyline, serum or plasma (Hep or EDTA); trough (≥12 h after dose)				
Therapeutic	120–250 ng/mL		433–903 nmol/L	
Toxic	>500 ng/mL		>1805 nmol/L	
Ammonia nitrogen				
Plasma	15–49 μg/dL		11–35 μmol/L	
Urine	20–70 mEq/24 h		20–70 nmol/24 h	
*Amylase				
Serum	25–125 mIU/mL		25–125 U/L	
Urine	1–17 U/h		1–17 U/h	
Amylase/creatinine clearance ratio	1–4%		0.01–0.04	
Anion gap	8–16 mEq/L		8–16 mmol/L	
Arsenic				
Whole blood (Hep)	0.2–6.2 μg/dL		0.03–0.83 μmol/L	
Chronic poisoning	10–50 μg/dL		1.33–6.65 μmol/L	
Acute poisoning	60–930 μg/dL		7.98–124 μmol/L	
Urine, 24 h	5–50 μg/d		0.07–0.67 μmol/d	
Ascorbic acid, blood	0.4–1.5 mg/dL		23–85 μmol/L	
Aspartate aminotransferase (see Transaminase)				
Base excess, blood	0 ± 2 mEq/L		0 ± 2 mmol/L	
Bicarbonate, serum	23–29 mEq/L		23–29 mmol/L	
Bile acids, serum	0.3–3.0 mg/dL		3.0–30.0 mg/L	
*Bilirubin				
Serum				
Adults				
Conjugated	0.0–0.3 mg/dL		0–5 μmol/L	
Unconjugated	0.01–1.1 mg/dL		0–19 μmol/L	
Delta	0–0.2 mg/dL		0–3 μmol/L	
Total	0.2–1.3 mg/L		3–22 μmol/L	
Neonates				
Conjugated	0–0.6 mg/dL		0–10 μmol/L	
Unconjugated	0.6–10.5 mg/dL		10–180 μmol/L	
Total	1.0–10.5 mg/dL		1.7–180 μmol/L	
Urine, qualitative	Negative		Negative	
Bone marrow, differential cell count	*Range (%)*	*Average (%)*	*Range*	*Average*
Myeloblasts	0.3–5.0	2.0	0.003–0.05	0.02
Promyelocytes	1.0–8.0	5.0	0.01–0.08	0.05
Myelocytes				
Neutrophilic	5.0–19.0	12.0	0.05–0.19	0.12
Eosinophilic	0.5–3.0	1.5	0.005–0.03	0.015
Basophilic	0.0–0.5	0.3	0.00–0.005	0.003
Metamyelocytes	13.0–32.0	22.0	0.13–0.32	0.22
Polymorphonuclear neutrophils	7.0–30.0	20.0	0.07–0.30	0.20
Polymorphonuclear eosinophils	0.5–4.0	2.0	0.005–0.04	0.02

*Test values are method dependent.

Tests	Conventional Units		SI Units	
Polymorphonuclear basophils	0.0–0.7	0.2	0.00–0.007	0.002
Lymphocytes	3.0–17.0	10.0	0.03–0.17	0.10
Plasma cells	0.0–2.0	0.4	0.00–0.02	0.004
Monocytes	0.5–5.0	2.0	0.005–0.05	0.02
Reticulum cells	0.1–2.0	0.2	0.001–0.02	0.002
Megakaryocytes	0.3–3.0	0.4	0.003–0.03	0.004
Pronormoblasts	1.0–8.0	4.0	0.01–0.08	0.04
Normoblasts	7.0–32.0	18.0	0.07–0.32	0.18
Cadmium, whole blood (Hep)	0.1–0.5 μg/dL		0.89–4.45 nmol/L	
Toxic	10–300 μg/dL		0.89–26.70 μmol/L	
Cadmium, urine, 24 h	<15 μg/d		<0.13 μmol/d	
Calcium, serum	4.5–5.5 mEq/L 9.0–11.0 mg/dL (Slightly higher in children) (Varies with protein concentration)		2.25–2.75 mmol/L (Slightly higher in children) (Varies with protein concentration)	
Calcium, ionized, serum	2.1–2.6 mEq/L 4.25–5.25 mg/dL		1.05–1.30 mmol/L	
Calcium, urine				
Low calcium diet	<150 mg/24 h		<3.8 nmol/24 h	
Usual diet (Hep or EDTA); trough	<250 mg/24 h		<6.3 nmol/24 h	
Therapeutic	8–12 μg/mL		34–51 μmol/L	
Toxic	>15 μg/mL		>63 μmol/L	
Carbon dioxide, total, serum/plasma (Hep)	22–29 mmol/L (lower in children)		Same	
Carbon dioxide tension (PCO_2), blood	35–45 mm Hg		35–45 mm Hg	
Carbon monoxide, as carboxyhemoglobin (HbCO), whole blood (EDTA)				
Nonsmokers	0.5–1.5% total Hb		0.005–0.015 HbCO fraction	
Smokers				
1–2 packs/d	4–5% total Hb		0.04–0.05 HbCO fraction	
>2 packs/d	8–9% total Hb		0.08–0.09 HbCO fraction	
Toxic	>20% total Hb		>0.20 HbCO fraction	
Lethal	>50% total Hb		>0.5 HbCO fraction	
Carotene, serum	40–200 μg/dL		0.74–3.72 μmol/L	
*Catecholamines, urine				
Epinephrine	<10 μg/24 h		<55 nmol/24 h	
Norepinephrine	<100 μg/24 h		< 590 nmol/24 h	
Total free catecholamines	4–126 μg/24 h		24–745 nmol/24 h (as norepinephrine)	
Total metanephrines	0.1–1.6 mg/24 h		0.5–8.1 μmol/24 h (as metanephrine)	
Cell counts				
Erythrocytes				
Males	4.6–6.2 million/mm^3		4.6–6.2 × 10^{12}/L	
Females	4.2–5.4 million/mm^3		4.2–5.4 × 10^{12}/L	
Children (varies with age)	4.5–5.1 million/mm^3		4.5–5.1 × 10^{12}/L	

*Test values are method dependent.

Tests	Conventional Units		SI Units
Leukocytes			
Total	4500–11,000/mm³		4.5–11.0 × 10^9/L
Differential	*Percentage*	*Absolute*	
Myelocytes	0	0/mm³	0/L
Band neutrophils	3–5	150–400/mm³	150–400 × 10^6/L
Segmented neutrophils	54–62	3000–5800/mm³	3000–5800 × 10^6/L
Lymphocytes	25–33	1500–3000/mm³	1500–3000 × 10^6/L
Monocytes	3–7	300–500/mm³	300–500 × 10^6/L
Eosinophils	1–3	50–250/mm³	50–250 × 10^6/L
Basophils	0–0.75	15–50/mm³	15–50 × 10^6/L
Platelets	150,000–350,000/mm³		150–350 × 10^9/L
Reticulocytes	25,000–75,000/mm³ 0.5–1.5% of erythrocytes		25–75 × 10^9/L
Cells, CSF	<5/mm³ (all mononucleocytes)		Same
Ceruloplasmin, serum	23–44 mg/dL		230–440 mg/L
Chloramphenicol, serum or plasma (Hep or EDTA); trough			
Therapeutic	10–25 μg/mL		31–77 μmol/L
Toxic	>25 μg/mL		>77 μmol/L
Chloride			
Serum	96–106 mEq/L		96–106 mmol/L
Sweat			
Normal	0–30 mmol/L		Same
Cystic fibrosis	60–200 mmol/L		Same
Urine, 24 h (vary greatly with Cl intake)			
Infant	2–10 mmol/d		Same
Child	14–50 mmol/d		Same
Adults	110–250 mmol/d		Same
CSF	120–130 mEq/L (20 mEq/L higher than serum)		120–130 mmol/L (20 mmol/L higher than serum)
Cholesterol, serum	Recommended desirable range: <200 mg/dL Borderline range: 200–230 mg/dL		Recommended desirable range: <5.2 mmol/L Borderline range: 5.2–6.0 mmol/L
Cholinesterase			
Serum	0.5–1.3 pH units		0.5–1.3 pH units
Erythrocytes	0.5–1.0 pH unit		0.5–1.0 pH unit
Chorionic gonadotropin, β-subunit (β-hCG)			
Serum or plasma (EDTA)			
Male and nonpregnant female	<3.0 mU/mL		<3.0 U/L
Female, post-conception			
7–10 d	>3.0 mU/mL		>3.0 U/L
30 d	100–5000 mU/mL		100–5000 U/L
40 d	>2000 mU/mL		>2000 U/L
10 wk	50,000–140,000 mU/mL		50,000–140,000 U/L
14 wk	10,000–50,000 mU/mL		10,000–50,000 U/L
Trophoblastic disease	>100,000 mU/mL		>100,000 U/L
Urine, 24 h			
Male and nonpregnant female	0 U/d		Same

Tests	Conventional Units	SI Units
Pregnancy (wk)		
6th	13,000 U/d (mean)	Same
8th	30,000 U/d (mean)	Same
12–14th	105,000 U/d (mean)	Same
16th	46,000 U/d (mean)	Same
Thereafter	5,000–20,000 U/d (mean)	Same
Clonazepam, serum or plasma (Hep or EDTA); trough		
Therapeutic	15–60 ng/mL	48–190 nmol/L
Toxic	>80 ng/mL	>254 nmol/L
Coagulation tests		
Antithrombin III (synthetic substrate)	80–120% of normal	0.8–1.2 of normal
Bleeding time (Duke)	1–5 min	1–5 min
Bleeding time (Ivy)	<5 min	<5 min
Bleeding time (template)	2.5–9.5 min	2.5–9.5 min
Clot retraction, qualitative	Begins in 30–60 min Complete in 24 h	Begins in 30–60 min Complete in 24 h
Coagulation time (Lee-White)	5–15 min (glass tubes) 19–60 min (siliconized tubes)	5–15 min (glass tubes) 19–60 min (siliconized tubes)
Cold hemolysin test (Donath-Landsteiner)	No hemolysis	No hemolysis
Complement components		
Total hemolytic complement activity, plasma (EDTA)	75–160 U/mL or >33% of plasma CH50	75–160 kU/L Fraction of CH50: >0.33
Total complement decay rate (functional), plasma (EDTA)	10–20% Deficiency: >50%	Fraction decay rate: 0.10–0.20 >0.50
$C1_q$, serum	6.5 ± 0.7 mg/dL (SD)	65 ± 7 mg/L (SD)
$C1_r$, serum	2.5–3.8 mg/dL	25–38 mg/L
$C1_s$ (C1 esterase), serum	2.5–3.8 mg/dL	25–38 mg/L
C2, serum	2.8 ± 0.6 mg/dL (SD)	28 ± 6 mg/L (SD)
C3, serum	80–155 mg/dL	800–1550 mg/L
C4, serum	13–37 mg/dL	130–370 mg/L
C5, serum	6.4 ± 1.3 mg/dL (SD)	64 ± 13 mg/L (SD)
C6, serum	5.6 ± 0.80 mg/dL (SD)	56 ± 8.0 mg/L (SD)
C7, serum	4.9–7.0 mg/dL	49–70 mg/L
C8, serum	4.3–6.3 mg/dL	43–63 mg/L
C9, serum	4.7–6.9 mg/dL	47–69 mg/L
Coombs' test		
Direct	Negative	Negative
Indirect	Negative	Negative
Copper		
Serum		
Males	70–140 μg/dL	11–22 μmol/L
Females	85–155 μg/dL	13–24 μmol/L
Urine	0–50 μg/24 h	0–0.80 μmol/24 h
Corpuscular values of erythrocytes (values are for adults; in children, values vary with age)		

Tests	Conventional Units	SI Units
Mean corpuscular hemoglobin (MCH)	27–31 pg	0.42–0.48 fmol
Mean corpuscular hemoglobin concentration (MCHC)	32–36%	0.32–0.36
Mean corpuscular volume (MCV)	80–96 μ^3	80–96 fL
Cortisol		
Plasma		
8 AM	6–23 μg/dL	170–635 nmol/L
4 PM	3–15 μg/dL	82–413 nmol/L
10 PM	<50% of 8 AM value	<0.5 of 8 AM value
Free, urine	10–100 μg/24 h	27.6–276 mmol/24 h
Creatine		
Serum	0.2–0.8 mg/dL	15–61 μmol/L
Urine		
Males	0–40 mg/24 h	0–0.30 mmol/24 h
Females	0–100 mg/24 h (Higher in children and pregnant women)	0–0.76 mmol/24 h (Higher in children and pregnant women)
*†Creatine kinase, serum (CK, CPK)		
White		
Male	60–320 mU/mL (37°C)	60–320 U/L (37°C)
Female	50–200 mU/mL (37°C)	50–200 U/L (37°C)
Black		
Male	130–450 mU/mL (37°C)	130–450 U/L (37°C)
Female	60–270 mU/mL (37°C)	60–270 U/L (37°C)
*Creatine kinase MB isoenzyme, serum	<15 U/L (37°C)	Same
Creatinine, enzymatic		
Serum or plasma, adult		
Male	0.8–1.5 mg/dL	71–133 μmol/L
Female	0.7–1.2 mg/dL	62–106 μmol/L
Urine	15–25 mg/kg body weight/24 h	0.13–0.22 mmol/kg body weight/24 h
*Creatinine clearance, enzymatic		
Males	110–150 mL/min	110–150 mL/min
Females	105–132 mL/min (1.73 m^2 surface area)	105–132 mL/min (1.73 m^2 surface area)
Cryoglobulins, serum	0	0
Cyanide		
Serum		
Nonsmokers	0.004 mg/L	0.15 μmol/L
Smokers	0.006 mg/L	0.23 μmol/L
Nitroprusside therapy	0.01–0.06 mg/L	0.38–2.30 μmol/L
Toxic	>0.1 mg/L	>3.84 μmol/L
Whole blood (Ox)		
Nonsmokers	0.016 mg/L	0.61 μmol/L
Smokers	0.041 mg/L	1.57 μmol/L
Nitroprusside therapy	0.05–0.5 mg/L	1.92–19.20 μmol/L
Toxic	>1 mg/L	>38.40 μmol/L

*Test values are method dependent.
†Test values are race dependent.

Tests	Conventional Units	SI Units
Cyclic AMP		
Plasma (EDTA)		
Males	5.6–10.9 ng/mL	17–33 nmol/L
Females	3.6–8.9 ng/mL	11–27 nmol/L
Urine, 24 h	<3.3 mg/d or <1.64 mg/g creatinine	<10 μmol/d or <565 μmol/mol creatinine
Cystine or cysteine, urine, qualitative	Negative	Negative
C-Peptide, serum		
Adult	4.0 ng/mL	4.0 μg/L
>60 y, male	1.5–5.0 ng/mL	1.5–5.0 μg/L
>60 y, female	1.4–5.5 ng/mL	1.4–5.5 μg/L
C-Reactive protein, serum		
Cord blood	1–35 μg/dL	10–350 μg/L
Adult	6.8–820 μg/dL	68–8200 μg/L
Dehydroepiandrosterone, urine	<15% of total 17-ketosteroids	<0.15 of total 17-ketosteroids
Males	0.2–2.0 mg/24 h	0.7–6.9 μm/24 h
Females	0.2–1.8 mg/24 h	0.7–6.2 μm/24 h
Desipramine, serum or plasma (Hep or EDTA); trough (12 h after dose)		
Therapeutic	75–160 ng/mL	281–600 nmol/L
Toxic	>1000 ng/mL	>3750 nmol/L
Diazepam, serum or plasma (Hep or EDTA); trough		
Therapeutic	100–1000 ng/mL	0.35–3.51 μmol/L
Toxic	>5000 ng/mL	>17.55 μmol/L
Digitoxin, serum or plasma (Hep or EDTA); 6 h after dose		
Therapeutic	20–35 ng/mL	26–46 nmol/L
Toxic	>45 ng/mL	>59 nmol/L
Digoxin, serum or plasma (Hep or EDTA); 12 h after dose		
Therapeutic		
CHF	0.8–1.5 ng/mL	1.0–1.9 nmol/L
Arrhythmias	1.5–2.0 ng/mL	1.9–2.6 nmol/L
Toxic		
Adult	>2.5 ng/mL	>3.2 nmol/L
Child	>3.0 ng/mL	>3.8 nmol/L
Disopyramide, serum or plasma (Hep or EDTA); trough		
Therapeutic arrhythmias		
Atrial	2.8–3.2 μg/mL	8.3–9.4 μmol/L
Ventricular	3.3–7.5 μg/mL	9.7–22 μmol/L
Toxic	>7 μg/mL	>20.7 μmol/L
Doxepin, serum or plasma (Hep or EDTA); trough (≥12 h after dose)		

Tests	Conventional Units	SI Units
Therapeutic	30–150 ng/mL	107–537 nmol/L
Toxic	>500 ng/mL	>1790 nmol/L
Electrophoresis, CSF	Predominantly albumin	Predominantly albumin
Estrogens, urine		
Males		
Estrone	3–8 μg/24 h	11–30 nmol/24 h
Estradiol	0–6 μg/24 h	0–22 nmol/24 h
Estriol	1–11 μg/24 h	3–38 nmol/24 h
‡Total	4–25 μg/24 h	14–90 nmol/24 h
Females		
Estrone	4–31 μg/24 h	15–115 nmol/24 h
Estradiol	0–14 μg/24 h	0–51 nmol/24 h
Estriol	0–72 μg/24 h	0–250 nmol/24 h
‡Total	5–100 μg/24 h (Markedly increased during pregnancy)	18–360 nmol/24 h (Markedly increased during pregnancy)
Ethanol, whole blood (Ox) or serum		
Depression of CNS	>100 mg/dL	>21.7 mmol/L
Fatalities reported	>400 mg/dL	>86.8 mmol/L
Ethosuximide, serum or plasma (Hep or EDTA); trough		
Therapeutic	40–100 μg/mL	283–708 μmol/L
Toxic	>150 μg/mL	>1062 μmol/L
Euglobulin lysis time	2–6 h at 37°C	2–6 h at 37°C
Factor VIII and other coagulation factors	50–150% of normal	0.50–1.5 or normal
Fibrin split products (Thrombo-Wellco test)	<10 μg/mL	<10 mg/L
Fibrinogen	200–400 mg/dL	5.9–11.7 μmol/L
Fibrinolysins	0	0
Partial thromboplastin time, activated (APTT)	20–35 sec	20–35 sec
Prothrombin consumption	Over 80% consumed in 1 h	Over 0.80 consumed in 1 h
Prothrombin content	100% (calculated from prothrombin time)	1.0 (calculated from prothrombin time)
Prothrombin time (one stage)	12.0–14.0 sec	12.0–14.0 sec
Tourniquet test	Ten or fewer petechiae in a 2.5 cm circle after 5 min	Ten or fewer petechiae in a 2.5 cm circle after 5 min
Fat, fecal, F, 72 h		
Infant, breast-fed	<1 g/d	Same
0–6 y	<2 g/d	Same
Adult	<7 g/d	Same
Adult (fat-free diet)	<4 g/d	Same
§Fatty acids, total, serum	190–420 mg/dL	7–15 mmol/L
Nonesterified, serum	8–25 mg/dL	0.30–0.90 mmol/L
Ferritin, serum		
Males	27–270 ng/mL	27–270 μg/L

‡Assuming a mixture of estrone, estradioles, and estriol in a molecular proportion of 2:1:2.

§"Fatty acids" include a mixture of different aliphatic acids of varying molecular weight; a mean molecular weight of 284 daltons has been assumed.

Tests	Conventional Units	SI Units
Females	9–180 ng/mL (higher if postmenopausal)	9–180 μg/L (higher if postmenopausal)
Ferritin values of <20 ng/mL (20 μg/L) have been reported to be generally associated with depleted iron stores		
Fibrinogen, plasma	200–400 mg/dL	5.9–11.7 μmol/L
Fluoride		
Plasma (Hep)	0.01–0.2 μg/mL	0.5–10.5 μmol/L
Urine	0.2–1.1 μg/mL	10.5–57.9 μmol/L
Urine, occupational exposure	4–5 μg/mL	210–263 μmol/L
Folate, serum	2.2–17.3 ng/mL	5.0–39.2 nmol/L
Erythrocytes	169–707 ng/mL	451–1602 nmol/L
Follicle-stimulating hormone (FSH), plasma		
Males	4–25 mU/mL	4–25 U/L
Females	4–30 mU/mL	4–30 U/L
Postmenopausal females	40–250 mU/mL	40–250 U/L
Gastrin, serum	0–200 pg/mL	0–200 ng/L
Gentamicin, serum or plasma (EDTA)		
Therapeutic		
Peak		
Less severe infection	5–8 μg/mL	10.4–16.7 μmol/L
Severe infection	8–10 μg/mL	16.7–20.9 μmol/L
Trough		
Less severe infection	<1 μg/mL	<2.1 μmol/L
Moderate infection	<2 μg/mL	<4.2 μmol/L
Severe infection	<2–4 μg/mL	<4.2–8.4 μmol/L
Toxic		
Peak	>10–12 μg/mL	>21–25 μmol/L
Trough	>2–4 μg/mL	>4.2–8.4 μmol/L
Glucose (fasting)		
Blood	60–100 mg/dL	3.33–5.55 mmol/L
Plasma or serum	70–115 mg/dL	3.89–6.38 mmol/L
Glucose, 2 h postprandial, serum	<120 mg/dL	<6.7 mmol/L
Glucose, urine		
Quantitative	<500 mg/24 h	<2.8 mmol/24 h
Qualitative	Negative	Negative
Glucose, CSF	50–75 mg/dL (20 mg/dL less than serum)	2.8–4.2 mmol/L (1.1 mmol/L less than serum)
*Glucose-6-phosphate dehydrogenase (G-6-PD) in erythrocytes, whole blood (ACD, EDTA, or Hep)	12.1 ± 2.9 U/g Hb (SD) 351 ± 60.6 U/10^{12} RBC 4.11 ± 0.71 U/mL RBC	0.78 ± 0.13 mU/mol Hb 0.35 ± 0.06 nU/RBC 4.11 ± 0.71 kU/L RBC
*γ-Glutamyltransferase		
Males	6–32 mU/mL (30°C)	6–32 U/L (30°C)
Females	4–18 mU/mL (30°C)	4–18 U/L (30°C)
Glutethimide, serum		
Therapeutic	2–6 μg/mL	9–28 μmol/L
Toxic	>5 μg/mL	>23 μmol/L

*Test values are method dependent.

Tests	Conventional Units	SI Units
Growth hormone, serum	0–10 ng/mL	0–10 μg/L
Haptoglobin, serum	100–200 mg/dL (As hemoglobin binding capacity)	16–31 μmol/L (As hemoglobin binding capacity)
Haptoglobin (as hemoglobin binding capacity)	100–200 mg/dL	16–31 μmol/L
HDL-cholesterol (HDL-C), serum or plasma (EDTA)	Recommended desirable range: >35 mg/dL	Recommended desirable range: >0.91 mmol/L
Hematocrit		
Males	40–54 mL/dL	0.40–0.54
Females	37–47 mL/dL	0.37–0.47
Newborn	49–54 mL/dL	0.49–0.54
Children (varies with age)	35–49 mL/dL	0.35–0.49
Hemoglobin (Hb)		
Males	14.0–18.0 g/dL	2.17–2.79 mmol/L
Females	12.0–16.0 g/dL	1.86–2.48 mmol/L
Newborn	16.5–19.5 g/dL	2.56–3.02 mmol/L
Children (varies with age)	11.2–16.5 g/dL	1.74–2.56 mmol/L
Hemoglobin, fetal	≥1 y old: <2% of total Hb	≥1 y old: <2% of total Hb
Hemoglobin, plasma	0–5.0 mg/dL	0–0.8 μmol/L
Hemoglobin and myoglobin, urine, qualitative	Negative	Negative
Hemoglobin electrophoresis, whole blood (EDTA, Cit, or Hep)		
HbA	>95%	>0.95 Hb fraction
HbA_{1c}	5.6–7.5%	0.056–0.075 Hb fraction
HbA_2	1.5–3.5%	0.015–0.035 Hb fraction
HbF	<2%	<0.02 Hb fraction
Homogentisic acid, urine, qualitative	Negative	Negative
*Hydroxybutyric dehydrogenase serum (HBD)	0–180 mU/mL (30°C)	0–180 U/L (30°C)
17-Hydroxycorticosteroids, urine		
Males	3–9 mg/24 h	8.3–25 μmol/24 h (as cortisol)
Females	2–8 mg/24 h	5.5–22 μmol/24 h (as cortisol)
5-Hydroxyindoleacetic acid, urine		
Qualitative	Negative	Negative
Quantitative	<9 mg/24 h	<47 μmol/24 h
Imipramine, serum or plasma (Hep or EDTA); trough (≥12 h after dose)		
Therapeutic	125–250 ng/mL	446–893 nmol/L
Toxic	>500 ng/mL	>1785 nmol/L

*Test values are method dependent.

Tests	Conventional Units	SI Units
Immunoglobulins, serum		
IgG	550–1900 mg/dL	5.5–19.0 g/L
IgA	60–333 mg/dL	0.60–3.3 g/L
IgM	45–145 mg/dL	0.45–1.5 g/L
IgD	0.5–3.0 mg/dL	5–30 mg/L
IgE	<500 ng/mL	<500 μg/L
	(Varies with age in children)	(Varies with age in children)
Immunoglobulin G (IgG), CSF		
Children under 14	<8% of total protein	<0.08 of total protein
Adults	<14% of total protein	<0.14 of total protein
Insulin, plasma (fasting)	5–25 μU/mL	36–179 pmol/L
Iron, serum	75–175 μg/dL	13–31 μmol/L
Iron binding capacity, serum		
Total	250–410 μg/dL	45–73 μmol/L
Saturation	20–55%	0.20–0.55
Ketosteroids, urine		
Males	6–18 mg/24 h	21–62 μmol/24 h
Females	4–13 mg/24 h (decrease with age)	14–45 μmol/24 h (decrease with age)
L-Lactate		
Plasma (NaF)		
Venous	4.5–19.8 mg/dL	0.5–2.2 mmol/L
Arterial	4.5–14.4 mg/dL	0.5–1.6 mmol/L
Whole blood (Hep), at bed rest		
Venous	8.1–15.3 mg/dL	0.9–1.7 mmol/L
Arterial	<11.3 mg/dL	<1.25 mmol/L
Urine, 24 h	496–1982 mg/d	5.5–22 mmol/d
CSF	<25.2 mg/dL	<2.8 mmol/L
*Lactate dehydrogenase (LDH)		
Total (L→P), 30°C, serum		
Newborn	160–450 U/L	Same
Neonate	300–1500 U/L	Same
Infant	100–250 U/L	Same
Child	60–170 U/L	Same
Adult	45–90 U/L	Same
>60 y	55–100 U/L	Same
*Isoenzymes, serum by agarose gel electrophoresis		
Fraction 1	14–26% of total	0.14–0.26 fraction of total
Fraction 2	29–39% of total	0.29–0.39 fraction of total
Fraction 3	20–26% of total	0.20–0.26 fraction of total
Fraction 4	8–16% of total	0.08–0.16 fraction of total
Fraction 5	6–16% of total	0.06–0.16 fraction of total
*Lactate dehydrogenase, CSF	10% of serum value	0.10 fraction of serum value
LDL-cholesterol (LDL-C), calculated, serum or plasma (EDTA)	Recommended desirable range for adults: <130 mg/dL	<3.37 mmol/L

*Test values are method dependent.

Tests	Conventional Units	SI Units
Lead		
Whole blood (Hep)		
Child	<25 μg/dL	<1.21 μmol/L
Adult	<25 μg/dL	<1.21 μmol/L
Toxic	≥60 μg/dL	≥2.90 μmol/L
Urine, 24 h	<80 μg/d	<0.39 μmol/d
Lecithin-sphingomyelin (L/S) ratio, amniotic fluid	2.0–5.0 indicates probable fetal lung maturity; >3.0 in diabetics	Same
*Leucine aminopeptidase, serum	14–40 mU/mL (30°C)	14–40 U/L (30°C)
Lidocaine, serum or plasma (Hep or EDTA); 45 min after bolus dose		
Therapeutic	1.5–6.0 μg/mL	6.4–26 μmol/L
Toxic		
CNS, cardiovascular depression	6–8 μg/mL	26–34.2 μmol/L
Seizures, obtundation, decreased cardiac output	>8 μg/mL	>34.2 μmol/L
*Lipase, serum	0–1.5 units (Cherry-Crandall)	0–1.5 units (Cherry-Crandall)
Lithium, serum or plasma (Hep or EDTA); 12 h after last dose		
Therapeutic	0.6–1.2 mEq/L	0.6–1.2 mmol/L
Toxic	>2 mEq/L	>2 mmol/L
Lorazepam, serum or plasma (Hep or EDTA), therapeutic	50–240 ng/mL	156–746 nmol/L
Luteinizing hormone (LH), serum		
Males	6–18 mU/mL	6–18 U/L
Females		
Premenopausal	5–22 mU/mL	5–22 U/L
Midcycle	3 times baseline	3 times baseline
Postmenopausal	>30 mU/mL	>30 U/L
Magnesium		
Serum	1.5–2.5 mEq/L 1.8–3.0 mg/dL	0.75–1.25 mmol/L
Urine	6.0–8.5 mEq/24 h	3.0–4.3 mmol/24 h
Mercury		
Whole blood (EDTA)	1–3 μg/dL	0.05–0.15 μmol/L
Urine, 24 h	<20 μg/d	<0.1 μmol/d
Toxic	>150 μg/d	>0.75 μmol/d
Metanephrines (see Catecholamines)		
Methemoglobin (MetHb, hemiglobin), whole blood (EDTA, Hep, or ACD)	0.06–0.24 g/dL or 0.78 ± 0.37% of total Hb (SD)	9.3–37.2 μmol/L or Mass fraction of total Hb: 0.008 ± 0.0037 (SD)

*Test values are method dependent.

Tests	Conventional Units	SI Units
Methotrexate, serum or plasma (Hep or EDTA)		
Therapeutic	Variable	Variable
Toxic		
1–2 wk after low-dose therapy	>9.1 ng/mL	>20 nmol/L
48 h after high-dose therapy	454 ng/mL	>1000 nmol/L
Myelin basic protein, CSF	<4 ng/mL	<4 μg/L
Nitroprusside, serum or plasma (EDTA), as thiocyanate, therapeutic	6–29 μg/mL	103–499 μmol/L
Nortriptyline, serum or plasma (Hep or EDTA); trough (≥12 h after dose)		
Therapeutic	50–150 ng/mL	190–570 nmol/L
Toxic	>500 ng/mL	>1900 nmol/L
*5′-Nucleotidase, serum	3.5–12.7 mU/mL (37°C)	3.5–12.5 U/L (37°C)
N-Acetylprocainamide, serum or plasma (Hep or EDTA); trough		
Therapeutic	5–30 μg/mL	18–108 μmol/L
Toxic	>40 μg/mL	>144 μmol/L
Occult blood, feces, random	Negative (<2 mL blood/150 g stool/d)	Negative (13.3 mL blood/kg stool/d)
Qualitative, urine, random	Negative	Negative
Osmolality		
Serum	285–295 mOsm/kg serum water	285–295 mmol/kg serum water
Urine	38–1400 mOsm/kg water	38–1400 mmol/kg water
Ratio, urine/serum	1.0–3.0 >3.0 after 12 h fluid restriction	Same
Osmotic fragility of erythrocytes	Begins in 0.45–0.39% NaCl Complete in 0.33–0.30% NaCl	Begins in 77–67 mmol/L NaCl Complete in 56–51 mmol/L NaCl
Oxazepam, serum or plasma (Hep or EDTA), therapeutic	0.2–1.4 μg/mL	0.70–4.9 μmol/L
Oxygen, blood		
Capacity	16–24 vol% (varies with hemoglobin)	7.14–10.7 mmol/L (varies with hemoglobin)
Content		
Arterial	15–23 vol%	6.69–10.3 mmol/L
Venous	10–16 vol%	4.46–7.14 mmol/L
Saturation		
Arterial	94–100% of capacity	0.94–1.00 of capacity
Venous	60–85% of capacity	0.60–0.85 of capacity
Tension, pO_2 arterial	75–100 mm Hg	75–100 mm Hg

*Test values are method dependent.

Tests	Conventional Units	SI Units
P50, blood	26–27 mm Hg	27–27 mm Hg
Pentobarbital, serum or plasma (Hep or EDTA); trough		
Therapeutic		
Hypnotic	1–5 μg/mL	4–22 μmol/L
Therapeutic coma	20–50 μg/mL	88–221 μmol/L
Toxic	>10 μg/mL	>44 μmol/L
pH		
Blood, arterial	7.35–7.45	7.35–7.45
Urine	4.6–8.0 (depends on diet)	Same
Phenacetin, plasma (EDTA)		
Therapeutic	1–20 μg/mL	6–112 μmol/L
Toxic	50–250 μg/mL	279–1395 μmol/L
Phenobarbital, serum or plasma (Hep or EDTA); trough		
Therapeutic	15–40 μg/mL	65–170 μmol/L
Toxic		
Slowness, ataxia, nystagmus	35–80 μg/mL	151–345 μmol/L
Coma with reflexes	65–117 μg/mL	280–504 μmol/L
Coma without reflexes	>100 μg/mL	>430 μmol/L
Phenolsulfonphthalein excretion (PSP), urine	25% or more in 15 min 40% or more in 30 min 55% or more in 2 h (After injection of 1 mL PSP intravenously)	0.25 or more in 15 min 0.40 or more in 30 min 0.55 or more in 2 h (After injection of 1 mL PSP intravenously)
Phenylalanine, serum	<3 mg/dL	<0.18 mmol/L
Phenylpyruvic acid, urine, qualitative	Negative	Negative
Phenytoin, serum or plasma (Hep or EDTA); trough		
Therapeutic	10–20 μg/mL	40–79 μmol/L
Toxic	>20 μg/mL	>79 μmol/L
*Phosphatase, acid, prostatic, serum		
RIA	<3.0 ng/mL	<3.0 μg/L
Enzymatic, 37°C	0.11–0.60 U/L (Roy, Brower, Hayden)	0.11–0.60 U/L
*Phosphatase, alkaline		
Leukocyte	Total score: 14–100	Total score: 14–100
Serum (ALP)	20–90 mU/mL (30°C) (Values are higher in children)	20–90 U/L (30°C) (Values are higher in children)
Phosphate, inorganic, serum		
Adults	3.0–4.5 mg/dL	1.0–1.5 mmol/L
Children	4.0–7.0 mg/dL	1.3–2.3 mmol/L
Phosphatidylglycerol (PG), amniotic fluid		
Absent	Fetal immaturity	Same
Present	Fetal maturity	Same

*Test values are method dependent.

Tests	Conventional Units	SI Units
Phospholipids, serum	6–12 mg/dL (As lipid phosphorus)	1.9–3.9 mmol/L (As lipid phosphorus)
Phosphorus, urine	0.4–1.3 g/24 h	12.9–42 mmol/24 h
Porphobilinogen, urine		
Qualitative	Negative	Negative
Quantitative	0–0.2 mg/dL <2.0 mg/24 h	0–0.9 μmol/L <9 μmol/24 h
Porphyrins, urine		
Coproporphyrin	50–250 μg/24 h	77–380 nmol/24 h
Uroporphyrin	10–30 μg/24 h	12–36 nmol/24 h
Potassium, plasma (Hep)		
Males	3.5–4.5 mEq/L	3.5–4.5 mmol/L
Females	3.4–4.4 mEq/L	3.4–4.4 mmol/L
Potassium		
Serum		
Premature		
Cord	5.0–10.2 mEq/L	5.0–10.2 mmol/L
48 h	3.0–6.0 mEq/L	3.0–6.0 mmol/L
Newborn, cord	5.6–12.0 mEq/L	5.6–12.0 mmol/L
Newborn	3.7–5.9 mEq/L	3.7–5.9 mmol/L
Infant	4.1–5.3 mEq/L	4.1–5.3 mmol/L
Child	3.4–4.7 mEq/L	3.4–4.7 mmol/L
Adult	3.5–5.1 mEq/L	3.5–5.1 mmol/L
Urine, 24 h	25–125 mEq/d, varies with diet	25–125 mmol/d; varies with diet
CSF	70% of plasma level or 2.5–3.2 mEq/L; rises with plasma hyperosmolality	0.70 of plasma level or 2.5–3.2 mmol/L; rises with plasma hyperosmolality
Pregnanediol, urine		
Males	0.4–1.4 mg/24 h	1.2–4.4 μmol/24 h
Females		
Proliferative phase	0.5–1.5 mg/24 h	1.6–4.7 μmol/24 h
Luteal phase	2.0–7.0 mg/24 h	6.2–22 μmol/24 h
Postmenopausal phase	0.2–1.0 mg/24 h	0.6–3.1 μmol/24 h
Pregnanetriol, urine	<2.5 mg/24 h in adults	<7.4 μmol/24 h in adults
Pressure, CSF	70–180 mm H_2O	Same
Primidone, serum or plasma (Hep or EDTA); trough		
Therapeutic	5–12 μg/mL	23–55 μmol/L
Toxic	>15 μg/mL	>69 μmol/L
Procainamide, serum or plasma (Hep or EDTA); trough		
Therapeutic	4–10 μg/mL	17–42 μmol/L
Toxic (also consider effect of metabolite (NAPA))	>10–12 μg/mL	>42–51 μmol/L
Prolactin, serum		
Males	1–20 ng/mL	1–20 μg/L
Females	1–25 ng/mL	1–25 μg/L
Propoxyphene, plasma (EDTA)		
Therapeutic	0.1–0.4 μg/mL	0.3–1.2 μmol/L
Toxic	>0.5 μg/mL	>1.5 μmol/L

Tests	Conventional Units	SI Units
Propranolol, serum or plasma (Hep or EDTA); trough		
Therapeutic	50–100 ng/mL	193–386 nmol/L
*Protein, serum		
Total	6.0–8.0 g/dL	60–80 g/L
Albumin	3.5–5.0 g/dL	35–50 g/L
	52–68% of total	0.52–0.68 of total
Globulin		
α_1	0.2–0.4 g/dL	2–4 g/L
	2–5% of total	0.02–0.05 of total
α_2	0.5–0.9 g/dL	5–9 g/L
	7–14% of total	0.07–0.14 of total
β	0.6–1.1 g/dL	6–11 g/L
	9–15% of total	0.09–0.15 of total
γ	0.7–1.7 g/dL	7–17 g/L
	11–21% of total	0.11–0.21 of total
Protein		
Urine		
Qualitative	Negative	Negative
Quantitative	10–150 mg/24 h	10–150 mg/24 h
CSF, total	15–45 mg/dL (higher, up to 70 mg/dL in the elderly and children)	0.150–0.450 g/L (higher, up to 0.70 g/L in the elderly and children)
Protoporphyrin, free, erythrocyte	27–61 μg/dL packed RBC	0.48–1.09 μmol/L packed RBC
Pyruvate, blood	0.3–0.9 mg/dL	0.03–0.10 mmol/L
Quinidine, serum or plasma (Hep or EDTA); trough		
Therapeutic	2–5 μg/mL	6–15 μmol/L
Toxic	>6 μg/mL	>18 μmol/L
Salicylates, serum or plasma (Hep or EDTA); trough		
Therapeutic	150–300 μg/mL	1086–2172 μmol/L
Toxic	>300 μg/mL	>2172 μmol/L
Sedimentation rate		
Wintrobe		
Males	0–5 mm in 1 h	0–5 mm/h
Females	0–15 mm in 1 h	0–15 mm/h
Westergren		
Males	0–15 mm in 1 h	0–15 mm/h
Females	0–20 mm in 1 h	0–20 mm/h
Sodium		
Serum or plasma (Hep)		
Premature		
Cord	116–140 mEq/L	116–140 mmol/L
48 h	128–148 mEq/L	128–148 mmol/L
Newborn, cord	126–166 mEq/L	126–166 mmol/L
Newborn	134–144 mEq/L	134–144 mmol/L
Infant	139–146 mEq/L	139–146 mmol/L

*Test values are method dependent.

Tests	Conventional Units	SI Units
Child	138–145 mEq/L	138–145 mmol/L
Adult	136–146 mEq/L	136–146 mmol/L
Urine, 24 h	40–220 mEq/d (diet dependent)	40–220 mmol/d (diet dependent)
Sweat		
Normal	10–40 mEq/L	10–40 mmol/L
Cystic fibrosis	>70 mEq/L	>70 mmol/L
Specific gravity	1.003–1.030	1.003–1.030
Sulfates, inorganic, serum	0.8–1.2 mg/dL	83–125 µmol/L
Testosterone, plasma		
Males	275–875 ng/dL	9.5–30 nmol/L
Females	23–75 ng/dL	0.8–2.6 nmol/L
Pregnant females	38–190 ng/dL	1.3–6.6 nmol/L
Theophylline, serum or plasma (Hep or EDTA)		
Therapeutic		
Bronchodilator	8–20 µg/mL	44–111 µmol/L
Prem. apnea	6–13 µg/mL	33–72 µmol/L
Toxic	>20 µg/mL	>110 µmol/L
Thiocyanate		
Serum or plasma (EDTA)		
Nonsmoker	1–4 µg/mL	17–69 µmol/L
Smoker	3–12 µg/mL	52–206 µmol/L
Therapeutic after nitroprusside infusion	6–29 µg/mL	103–499 µmol/L
Urine		
Nonsmoker	1–4 mg/d	17–69 µmol/d
Smoker	7–17 mg/d	120–292 µmol/d
Thiopental, serum or plasma (Hep or EDTA); trough		
Hypnotic	1.0–5.0 µg/mL	4.1–20.7 µmol/L
Coma	30–100 µg/mL	124–413 µmol/L
Anesthesia	7–130 µg/mL	29–536 µmol/L
Toxic concentration	>10 µg/mL	>41 µmol/L
Thyroid-stimulating hormone (TSH), serum	0.35–7 µU/mL	0.35–7 mU/L
Thyroxine (T_4) serum	5–12 µg/dL (varies with age, higher in children and pregnant women)	66–155 nmol/L (varies with age, higher in children and pregnant women)
Thyroxine, free, serum	1.0–2.1 ng/dL	13–27 pmol/L
Thyroxine binding globulin (TBG), serum (as thyroxine)	10–26 µg/dL	129–335 nmol/L
Titratable acidity, urine	20–40 mEq/24 h	20–40 mmol/24 h
Tobramycin, serum or plasma (Hep or EDTA)		
Therapeutic		
Peak		
Less severe infection	5–8 µg/mL	11–17 µmol/L
Severe infection	8–10 µg/mL	17–21 µmol/L
Trough		
Less severe infection	<1 µg/mL	<2 µmol/L
Moderate infection	<2 µg/mL	<4 µmol/L
Severe infection	<2–4 µg/mL	<4–9 µmol/L

Tests	Conventional Units	SI Units
Toxic		
Peak	>10–12 μg/mL	>21–26 μmol/L
Trough	>2–4 μg/mL	>4–9 μmol/L
*Transaminase, serum		
AST (asparate aminotransferase, SGOT)	7–40 mU/mL (37°C)	7–40 U/L (37°C)
ALT (alanine aminotransferase, SGPT)	5–35 mU/mL (37°C)	5–35 U/L (37°C)
Transferrin, serum		
Newborn	130–275 mg/dL	1.30–2.75 g/L
Adult	220–400 mg/dL	2.20–4.00 g/L
>60 y	180–380 mg/dL	1.80–3.80 g/L
Triglycerides, serum, fasting	40–150 mg/dl	0.4–1.5 g/L 0.45–1.71 mmol/L
Triiodothyronine (T_3), serum	150–250 ng/dL	2.3–3.9 nmol/L
*Triiodothyronine (T_3) uptake, resin (T3RU)	25–38% uptake	0.25–0.38 uptake
Uric acid		
Serum, enzymatic		
Male	3.5–7.2 mg/dL	0.21–0.42 mmol/L
Female	2.6–6.0 mg/dL	0.15–0.35 mmol/L
Child	2.0–5.5 mg/dL	0.12–0.32 mmol/L
*Urine	250–750 mg/24 h (with normal diet)	1.48–4.43 mmol/24 h (with normal diet)
Urea nitrogen, plasma or serum	11–23 mg/dL	7.9–16.4 mmol/L
Urea nitrogen/creatinine ratio, serum	12:1 to 20:1	12:1 to 20:1
Urobilinogen, urine	Up to 1.0 Ehrlich unit/2 h (1–3 PM) 0–4.0 mg/24 h	Up to 1.0 Ehrlich unit/2 h (1–3 PM) 0–6.8 μmol/24 h
Valproic acid, serum or plasma (Hep or EDTA); trough		
Therapeutic	50–100 μg/mL	347–693 μmol/L
Toxic	>100 μg/mL	>693 μmol/L
Vancomycin, serum or plasma (Hep or EDTA); trough		
Therapeutic	Not well established	
Toxic	>80–100 μg/mL	>80–100 mg/L
Vanillylmandelic acid (VMA), urine (4-hydroxy-3-methoxymandelic acid)	1–8 mg/24 h	5–40 μmol/24 h
Viscosity, serum	1.4–1.8 times water	1.4–1.8 times water
Vitamin A, serum	20–80 μg/dL	0.70–2.8 μmol/L
Vitamin B_{12}, serum	180–900 pg/mL	133–664 pmol/L
Vitamin E, serum		
Normal	7–20 μg/mL	16.2–46.4 μmol/L
Therapeutic	30–50 μg/mL	69.6–116 μmol/L
Zinc, serum	70–150 μg/dL	10.7–22.9 μmol/L

*Test values are method dependent.

BLOOD GROUPS

In this appendix, and in related terms defined in the dictionary proper, the term "blood group" is used to refer to an entire blood group system consisting of erythrocyte antigens whose specificity is controlled by a series of allelic genes or by a series of genes so closely linked on a single chromosome that they cannot be distinguished from alleles by available genetic methods. The terms "blood type" and "phenotype" are used to refer to a specific reaction pattern to testing antisera within a system. This usage is not universal. It should be noted that in current literature a single system may be referred to in the plural (*i.e.*, ABO blood groups) and the term "blood group" may be assigned to a single phenotype (*i.e.*, blood group A).

Each blood group is defined in terms of reaction to the original antiserum with which the system was discovered, with modification or extension as required by the discovery of additional antisera proved to be related to the same system. A "new" blood group antigen can be defined by showing that it is detected by an antiserum with reactions different from those of previously known antisera. If it can be shown that the "new" antigen is genetically independent of known blood group systems, it may qualify as the prototype antigen of a new blood group. If it can be shown that the "new" antigen is controlled by a gene allelic to one or more known blood group genes, it is assigned to the blood group of its alleles. Many known antigens have not been shown to be either genetically independent or related to certain other known antigens, and their status remains in doubt.

In the blood group definitions, emphasis has been placed on identification of symbols for genes, antigens, antisera, and phenotypes. These often appear in the literature without specification that they refer to a blood group. Attention is called to the general convention, followed here, that symbols for genes and genotypes are set in italics, whereas symbols for gene products or antigens, antisera, and phenotypes are set in Roman type. In the Rh-Hr terminology for tne Rh blood group, Roman type is used to designate antigenic substances, and boldface type is used to designate serologic factors and their corresponding antibodies. These conventions are in wide usage but are not consistently followed by all authors.

ABO blood group

This classical blood group system is defined by the agglutination reactions of erythrocytes to the natural isoantibodies anti-A and anti-B and related antisera (Landsteiner, 1900). In normal human blood there is a reciprocal relationship between the ABO antigens or agglutinogens on the surface of the erythrocyte and the natural antibodies or isoagglutinins found in serum. Individuals of type O do not have either A or B antigens on the erythrocytes, but their serum contains both anti-A and anti-B agglutinins. Individuals of type A have antigen A on the erythrocytes and anti-B in the serum. Individuals of type B have antigen B on the erythrocytes and anti-A in the serum. Individuals of type AB have both A and B antigens on the erythrocytes but no isoagglutinins in the serum. Types A and AB may be subdivided by anti-A_1 serum into types A_1 and A_2, and A_1B and A_2B. The A_2 antigen is weaker in reaction than the A_1, but their difference is also qualitative. Production of ABO antigens is controlled by a series of allelic genes A_1, A_2, B, and O (sometimes designated I^{A_1}, I^{A_2}, I^{B}, and i; i^{A_1}, i^{A_2}, i^{B}, and i; or A_1, A_2, a^B, and a). A_1 is dominant to A_2, and both are dominant to O; there is no dominance between A_1 and B or A_2 and B.

In the usual typing method a strong anti-A serum that agglutinates cells containing A_1 or A_2 antigen is used; cells agglutinated by this serum but not by anti-B are of type A but may be of genotype A_1A_1, A_1A_2, A_1O, A_2A_2, or

A_2O. Cells of persons of type A that are agglutinated by anti-A_1 are of type A_1 and may be of genotype A_1A_1, A_1A_2, or A_1O; type A cells not agglutinated by anti-A_1 are of type A_2 and may be of genotype A_2A_2 or A_2O. Cells agglutinated by anti-B but not anti-A are of type B and may be of genotype *BB* or *BO*. Cells agglutinated by both anti-A and anti-B are of type AB and can be divided into types A_1B (genotype A_1B) and A_2B (genotype A_2B) by anti-A_1. Cells not agglutinated by either anti-A or anti-B are of type O and genotype *OO*. Cells of type O do not simply lack antigenic substance; the vast majority possess an antigen called H that is chemically similar to antigens A and B and is probably the precursor antigen that is modified under the influence of genes A_1, A_2, and *B* into their corresponding antigens.

Rare individuals fail to form H antigen and, regardless of ABO genotype, do not produce A, B, or H antigens; such persons seem to be homozygous for a recessive gene called *h* or *x*. The postulated allele *H* or *X* is apparently necessary to convert a mucopolysaccharide precursor into H antigen. The term "Bombay" phenotype was assigned to such persons whose cells lack A, B, and H antigen and whose serum contains anti-A, anti-B,and anti-H; they are also referred to as the "Oh" phenotype. In addition, weak variants of antigen A have been described with phenotypes designated A_3, A_4, A_5, A_x, and A_z; more rarely, weak variants of B have been found. The ABO types are of prime importance with respect to blood transfusion, and maternal-fetal incompatibility is a frequent cause of fetal death and erythroblastosis fetalis.

Auberger blood group

This erythrocyte antigen is defined by reaction to an antibody designated anti-Au^a, originally found in the serum of a Madame Auberger who had received many transfusions (Salmon, Salmon, Liberge, Andre, Tippett, and Sanger, 1961). The Au^a antigen is inherited as a dominant trait and occurs in about 80 percent of whites and blacks.

Diego blood group

The erythrocyte antigen defined by anti-Di^a antibody was first found in Venezuela where it had been the cause of erythroblastosis fetalis (Layrisse, Arends, and Dominguez, 1955). An antibody with antithetical reactions, anti-Di^b, was discovered in 1967. The antigen system is controlled by two alleles, Di^a and Di^b. The Di^a antigen is common in American Indians and in Asiatics but is apparently absent in whites. This distribution is considered strong anthropological evidence to support the thesis that American Indians are derived from Mongolian or Asiatic ancestors.

Dombrock blood group

This erythrocyte antigen is defined by reaction to anti-Do^a antibody (Swanson, Polesky, Tippett, and Sanger, 1965). The Do^a antigen exhibits autosomal dominant inheritance and is found in about 65 to 66 percent of Northern Europeans, U.S. whites, and Israelis, in about 45 to 55 percent of U.S. blacks and American Indians, and in about 13 percent of Thais.

Duffy blood group

These erythrocyte antigens are defined by reactions to an immune serum called anti-Fy^a, first found in a hemophilic patient named Duffy who had received many transfusions (Cutbush, Mollison, and Parkin, 1950), and a serum with antithetical reactions, anti-Fy^b (Ikin, Mourant, Peffenkofer, and Blumenthal, 1951). The bloods of practically all whites are agglutinated by one, the other, or both of these antisera, but bloods of the majority of blacks and some Yemenite Jews give negative reactions to both antisera. It is therefore assumed that production of Duffy antigens is controlled by a series of at least three allelic genes, Fy^a, Fy^b, and *Fy*, with antibodies specific for only the first two of the series being now known. Persons with blood reacting positively to anti-Fy^a and negatively to anti-Fy^b are of phenotype Fy(a + b −), and their genotype may be either Fy^aFy^a or Fy^aFy. Persons of phenotype Fy(a + b +) are of genotype Fy^aFy^b. Those of phenotype Fy(a − b +) may be of genotype Fy^bFy^b or Fy^bFy. Those of phenotype Fy(a − b −) are of genotype *FyFy*. Duffy antibodies occasionally cause transfusion reactions or erythroblastosis fetalis.

High frequency blood groups

This group of antigens is found in almost all individuals but is absent in members of a very few families. Because of very high frequency they are often called "public" antigens. The antibodies usually have been found in the serum of a patient lacking the antigen who has become immunized by transfusion or pregnancy. Names or symbols applied to public antigens include: Vel, Yt^a, Ge, Lan, and Sm. See also low frequency blood groups.

I blood group

These erythrocyte antigens are defined by reactions to antibodies designated anti-I (Wiener, Unger, Cohen, and Feldman, 1956) and anti-i. Antigen I differs from other blood group antigens in the slowness of its development and in its wide range of strength in different individuals; the range approximates a normal distribution curve. Anti-I occurs in a wide range of strength and in two forms: autoanti-I is the antibody usually found in the serum of patients with acquired hemolytic anemia of the "cold agglutinin" type and in sera described as containing "nonspecific complete cold autoagglutinin"; natural anti-I or isoanti-I occurs regularly in the serum of persons of phenotype i. Phenotype i may be divided into types i_1 and i_2, both rare in adults.

Kell blood group

These erythrocyte antigens are defined by an immune antibody, anti-K, first found in the serum of a Mrs. Kell (Coombs, Mourant, and Race, 1946), and by anti-k (Levine, Backer, Wigod, and Ponder, 1949). Anti-k was known as anti-Cellano until its antithetical reactions to anti-K were established. An antiserum originally designated anti-Si was found to be identical to anti-K. The antigens K and k are controlled by a pair of allelic genes without dominance, hence three genotypes (*KK*, *Kk*, *kk*) may be recognized by agglutination of erythrocytes by anti-K alone, both anti-K and anti-k, or anti-k alone. Variant antigens of this system detected by human sera have been designated Kp^{a} and Kp^{b}. Very rare families have been found in which erythrocytes of certain persons give negative reactions with all antisera of the Kell group; this phenotype is designated K-k-Kp(a−b−). As a cause of transfusion reactions and erythroblastosis fetalis, the Kell blood group is next in clinical importance after the ABO and Rh blood groups.

Kidd blood group

These erythrocyte antigens are defined by reactions to an antibody designated anti-Jk^{a}, discovered in the serum of a Mrs. Kidd who had delivered an infant with erythroblastosis (Allen, Diamond, and Niedziela, 1951), and by reactions to its antithetical serum, anti-Jk^{b} (Plaut, Ikin, Mourant, Sanger, and Race, 1953). The antigens are controlled by a pair of genes without dominance, *Jk*^{a} and *Jk*^{b}, that are genetically independent of other blood group genes. Persons with erythrocytes that are agglutinated by anti-Jk^{a} but not by anti-Jk^{b} are of phenotype Jk(a+b−) and genotype *Jk*^{a}*Jk*^{a}; agglutination by both antisera indicates phenotype Jk(a+b+) and genotype *Jk*^{a}*Jk*^{b}; agglutination by only anti-Jk^{b} indicates phenotype Jk(a−b+) and genotype *Jk*^{b}*Jk*^{b}. The possibility that there may be a third allele at this locus or a modifier capable of suppressing the action of genes at this locus has been raised by the discovery of rare individuals (usually of Asiatic or South American Indian ancestry) whose erythrocytes give negative reactions to both antisera. Kidd antibodies occasionally cause transfusion reactions or erythroblastosis fetalis.

Lewis blood group

These antigens of erythrocytes, saliva, and certain other body fluids are defined by reactions to anti-Le^{a} antibody, first found in the serum of a Mrs. Lewis (Mourant, 1946), by reactions to related sera particularly anti-Le^{b}, and by interactions with the secretor factor. The Lewis antigens are formed in tissue under control of genes designated *Le* and *le* (*Le* dominant to *le*) and released into body fluids where they may be absorbed onto the surface of erythrocytes and determine the reactions of erythrocytes to antisera. The Lewis erythrocyte types of children may not develop fully until about age six years. The Lewis genes are genetically independent of those controlling the secretor factor (*Se* and *se*), but their products interact in certain phenotypic effects. Several theories have been proposed to account for the complex immunologic and genetic observations. The theory of Grubb and Ceppellini was summarized by Race and Sanger (1962) as shown in Table 1.

Variant antibodies of this system include: anti-Le^{X} (originally called anti-X), which seems to be anti-Le^{a} plus anti-Le^{b}; anti-Le^{c}, an immune rabbit serum that agglutinates Le(a−b−) cells; the Magard antiserum, obtained from a patient with carcinoma of the stomach, that agglutinates strongly the cells of A_1 Le(a−b−) secretors and less strongly those of A_2 Le(a−b−) secretors. Lewis antibodies have occasionally been implicated as a cause of transfusion reactions.

Low frequency blood groups

In this group of erythrocyte antigens, each is defined by a specific antiserum, and each is found only in members of a very few families. Because of their rarity they are often referred to as "private" antigens. The antibodies usually have been found in the sera of patients who have received transfusions or in mothers of erythroblastotic infants. They are often named for the family in which they were first discovered. The names or symbols assigned to some private

TABLE 1. *Secretor-Lewis Interactions**

Genotypes	Antigens				
	Of Saliva				Of Erythrocytes
	ABH	Le^{a}	Le^{bL}	Le^{bH}	
SeSe LeLe *SeSe Lele* *Sese LeLe* *Sese Lele*	+	+	+	+	Le(a−b+)
sese LeLe *sese Lele*	−	+	−	−	Le(a+b−)
SeSe lele *Sese lele*	+	−	−	+	Le(a−b−)
sese lele	−	−	−	−	Le(a−b−)

*From Race, R.R., and Sanger, R.: *Blood Groups in Man*, F
4. Oxford, England, Blackwell Scientific Publications,Ltd., 1

antigens are: Levay, Jobbins, Becker, Ven, Chr[a], Wright or Wr[a], Be[a], By, Swann or Sw[a], Good, Biles or Bi, Tr[a], Stobo, Ot, Ho, and Webb. See also high frequency blood groups.

Lutheran blood group

These blood group antigens are defined by reactions to an antibody designated anti-Lu[a], first found in serum of a patient who had received many transfusions (Callender, Race, and Paykoc, 1945), and its reciprocal, anti-Lu[b] (Cutbush and Chanarin, 1956). Production of the antigens is controlled by a pair of allelic genes, Lu^a and Lu^b, without dominance. The erythrocytes of persons with genotype Lu^aLu^a are agglutinated by anti-Lu[a] but not by anti-Lu[b], those of genotype Lu^aLu^b are agglutinated by both antisera, and those of genotype Lu^bLu^b are agglutinated by anti-Lu[b] but not by anti-Lu[a]. These antibodies are an uncommon cause of transfusion reactions.

MNSs blood group

This system of erythrocyte antigens was originally defined by reactions to immune rabbit sera designated anti-M and anti-N (Landsteiner and Levine, 1927) and has since been extended by reactions to sera anti-S, anti-s, and certain others. When tested with the readily available anti-M and anti-N sera only, the erythrocytes of all individuals may be assigned to one of three classes, M, N or MN, depending on whether they are agglutinated by one, the other, or both antisera. Production of M and N antigens is controlled by two allelic genes, *M* and *N*; persons of genotype *MM* are type M, those of genotype *NN* are type N, and those of the heterozygous genotype *MN* are type MN. As anti-M and anti-N sera are commercially available and the reactions are simple and reliable, they are widely used for medicolegal blood testing in disputed paternity actions and for genetic linkage and population studies. The *MN* locus is not genetically linked to loci of other major blood group systems. The MNSs antigens are only rarely the cause of hemolytic reactions to transfusion.

With the discovery of anti-S serum (1947) and its reciprocal anti-s (1951), it was shown that the MNS group is complex and that nine phenotypes representing ten genotypes may be defined by the four antisera (Table 2). In addition, nearly 1 percent of blood samples of blacks lack both S and s. An antibody designated as anti-U has been found that reacts with both S and s antigens. Weak variants of the M and N antigens that react with some anti-M or anti-N sera but not with others have been designated M_2 nd N_2. A qualitative variant of M has been designated . An antigen that gives intermediate reactions has been ignated M^c. An extremely rare variant of M detected a special serum has been designated M^g. Antigens

TABLE 2. *MNSs Phenotypes and Genotypes*

Antisera				Genotypes
M	N	S	s	
+	−	+	−	*MS/MS*
+	−	+	+	*MS/Ms*
+	−	−	+	*Ms/Ms*
+	+	+	−	*MS/Ns*
+	+	+	+	*MS/Ns* or *Ms/NS*
+	+	−	+	*Ms/Ns*
−	+	+	−	*NS/NS*
−	+	+	+	*NS/Ns*
−	+	−	+	*Ns/Ns*

designated Hu and He are detected by sera obtained from rabbits immunized with blood of certain blacks and are found almost entirely in persons of African ancestry; anti-Hu gives distinct reactions only with cells that also contain N, and most positives to anti-He possess both N and S. Other rare antigens that are associated with or are variants of the MNS group have been designated Mi^2, Vw (identical with Gr), and Mu.

P blood group

This system of erythrocyte antigens was originally defined by reaction to immune rabbit serum designated anti-P (Landsteiner and Levine, 1927) but has since been extended to include related antigens. An antibody previously known as anti-Tj[a] was shown to be related to anti-P in 1955, and the terminology presented in Table 3 was proposed by Sanger. In this terminology, P_1 is the phenotype previously called P+, P_2 is the phenotype previously called P−, and p is the phenotype previously called Tj(a−). A rare variant designated P^k has also been found.

TABLE 3. *P Blood Group**

Phenotypes		Phenotype Symbol	Genotypes
anti-P + P_1 (Tj[a])	anti-P_1 (P)		
+	+	P_1	P_1P_1; P_1P_2; P_1p
+	−	P_2	P_2P_2; P_2p
−	−	p	*pp*

*From Race, R.R., and Sanger, R.: *Blood Groups in Man*, Ed. 4. Oxford, England, Blackwell Scientific Publications, Ltd., 1962.

Rh blood group

This complex system of erythrocyte antigens was originally defined by reactions to serum from rabbits or guinea pigs immunized with blood of the rhesus monkey (Landsteiner and Wiener, 1940) but is now defined by reactions to a